GASTROENTEROLOGY AND HEPATOLOGY

HEMATOLOGY AND ONCOLOGY

INFECTIOUS DISEASES AND HIV/AIDS

NEPHROLOGY

NEUROLOGY AND PSYCHIATRY

PULMONARY

SYSTEMIC PRESENTATIONS

17th Edition

HARRISON'S
Principles of INTERNAL MEDICINE

EDITORS OF PREVIOUS EDITIONS

T. R. Harrison

Editor-in-Chief, Editions 1, 2, 3, 4, 5

W. R. Resnick

Editor, Editions 1, 2, 3, 4, 5

M. M. Wintrobe

Editor, Editions 1, 2, 3, 4, 5
Editor-in-Chief, Editions 6, 7

G. W. Thorn

Editor, Editions 1, 2, 3, 4, 5, 6, 7
Editor-in-Chief, Edition 8

R. D. Adams

Editor, Editions 2, 3, 4, 5, 6, 7, 8, 9, 10

P. B. Beeson

Editor, Editions 1, 2

I. L. Bennett, Jr.

Editor, Editions 3, 4, 5, 6

E. Braunwald

Editor, Editions 6, 7, 8, 9, 10, 12, 13, 14, 16
Editor-in-Chief, Editions 11, 15

K. J. Isselbacher

Editor, Editions 6, 7, 8, 10, 11, 12, 14
Editor-in-Chief, Editions 9, 13

R. G. Petersdorf

Editor, Editions 6, 7, 8, 9, 11, 12, 13
Editor-in-Chief, Edition 10

J. D. Wilson

Editor, Editions 9, 10, 11, 13, 14
Editor-in-Chief, Edition 12

J. B. Martin

Editor, Editions 10, 11, 12, 13, 14

A. S. Fauci

Editor, Editions 11, 12, 13, 15, 16
Editor-in-Chief, Edition 14

R. Root

Editor, Edition 12

D. L. Kasper

Editor, Editions 13, 14, 15
Editor-in-Chief, Edition 16

S. L. Hauser

Editor, Editions 14, 15, 16

D. L. Longo

Editor, Editions 14, 15, 16

J. L. Jameson

Editor, Editions 15, 16

17th Edition

HARRISON'S
Principles of
INTERNAL
MEDICINE

EDITORS

Anthony S. Fauci, MD
Chief, Laboratory of Immunoregulation; Director,
National Institute of Allergy and Infectious Diseases,
National Institutes of Health, Bethesda

Eugene Braunwald, MD
Distinguished Hersey Professor of Medicine,
Harvard Medical School; Chairman, TIMI Study Group,
Brigham and Women's Hospital, Boston

Dennis L. Kasper, MD
William Ellery Channing Professor of Medicine,
Professor of Microbiology and Molecular Genetics,
Harvard Medical School; Director, Channing Laboratory,
Department of Medicine, Brigham and Women's Hospital, Boston

Stephen L. Hauser, MD
Robert A. Fishman Distinguished Professor and Chairman,
Department of Neurology, University of California,
San Francisco, San Francisco

Dan L. Longo, MD
Scientific Director, National Institute on Aging,
National Institutes of Health, Bethesda and Baltimore

J. Larry Jameson, MD, PhD
Professor of Medicine;
Vice-President for Medical Affairs and Lewis Landsberg Dean,
Northwestern University Feinberg School of Medicine, Chicago

Joseph Loscalzo, MD, PhD
Hersey Professor of the Theory and Practice of Medicine,
Harvard Medical School; Chairman, Department of Medicine;
Physician-in-Chief, Brigham and Women's Hospital, Boston

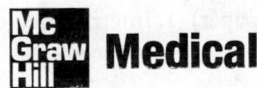

McGraw Hill Medical

New York   Chicago   San Francisco   Lisbon   London   Madrid   Mexico City
New Delhi   San Juan   Seoul   Singapore   Sydney   Toronto

Harrison's
PRINCIPLES OF INTERNAL MEDICINE
Seventeenth Edition

1234567890 DOWDOW 098

Single Edition Set ISBN 978-0-07-146633-2; MHID 0-07-146633-9
Single Edition Book ISBN 978-0-07-159991-7; MHID 0-07-159991-6

Two Volume Set ISBN 978-0-07-147691-1; MHID 0-07-147691-1
Volume 1 ISBN 978-0-07-147692-8; MHID 0-07-147692-X
Volume 2 ISBN 978-0-07-147693-5; MHID 0-07-147693-8

DVD ISBN 978-0-07-159990-0; MHID 0-07-159990-8

FOREIGN LANGUAGE EDITIONS
Arabic (13e): McGraw-Hill Libri Italia srl (1996)
Chinese Long Form (15e): McGraw-Hill International Enterprises, Inc., Taiwan
Chinese Short Form (15e): McGraw-Hill Education (Asia), Singapore
Croatian (16e): Placebo, Split, Croatia
French (16e): Medecine-Sciences Flammarion, Paris, France
German (16e): ABW Wissenschaftsverlagsgesellschaft mbH, Berlin, Germany
Greek (16e): Parissianos, S.A., Athens, Greece
Italian (16e): The McGraw-Hill Companies, Srl, Milan, Italy
Japanese (16e): MEDSI-Medical Sciences International Ltd, Tokyo, Japan

Korean (16e): McGraw-Hill Korea, Inc., Seoul, Korea
Polish (14e): Czelej Publishing Company, Lubin, Poland (2000)
Portuguese (16e): McGraw-Hill Interamericana do Brazil, Rio de Janeiro, Brazil
Romanian (14e): Teora Publishers, Bucharest, Romania (2000)
Serbian (15e): Publishing House Romanov, Bosnia & Herzegovina, Republic of Serbska
Spanish (16e): McGraw-Hill Interamericana de Espana S.A., Madrid, Spain
Turkish (15e): Nobel Tip Kitabevleri, Ltd., Istanbul, Turkey
Vietnamese (15e): McGraw-Hill Education (Asia), Singapore

This book was set in Minion, Myriad, and Dax by Silverchair Science + Communications, Inc. The editors were James Shanahan and Mariapaz Ramos Englis; editorial assistant was Jenna Esposito. The production director was Phil Galea and production manager was Catherine Saggese. The index was prepared by Barbara Littlewood. The text designer was Alan Barnett of alan barnett design; cover design was by David Dell'Accio. The medical illustrator was Daniel Knopsnyder.

R.R. Donnelley and Sons, Inc., was printer and binder.

Library of Congress Cataloging-in-Publication Data

Harrison's principles of internal medicine. -- 17th ed. / editors, Anthony S. Fauci ... [et al.].
    p. ; cm.
  Includes bibliographical references and index.
  ISBN-13: 978-0-07-146633-2 (hardcover : v. 2 : alk. paper)
  ISBN-10: 0-07-146633-9 (hardcover : v. 2 : alk. paper)
  ISBN-13: 978-0-07-147691-1 (hardcover : set : v. 2 : alk. paper)
  ISBN-10: 0-07-147691-1 (hardcover : set : v. 2 : alk. paper) 1. Internal medicine. I. Fauci, Anthony S.,
II. Title: Principles of internal medicine.
  [DNLM: 1. Internal Medicine. WB 115 H322 2008]
RC46.H333 2008
616--dc22

                                                                                2007012181

George W. Thorn
1906–2004

George W. Thorn was an editor of the first seven editions and Editor-in-Chief of the eighth edition. As a founding editor, he had an enormous impact on *Harrison's* and thereby on the education of countless thousands of physicians and medical students. His incisiveness, inventiveness, and originality, coupled with his broad knowledge of clinical medicine and medical science and his unswerving dedication to the application of techniques of contemporary science to the advancement of clinical medicine, played a vital role in the original organization of this textbook.

George Thorn began his remarkable career in endocrinologic research as a medical student at the University of Buffalo School of Medicine. Following a stint in general practice, which subsequently served him well as an educator, clinical investigator, and consultant, he obtained research training and held faculty positions at several institutions. In 1942, at the age of 36, he became Hersey Professor of the Theory and Practice of Physic (Medicine) at Harvard Medical School and Physician-in-Chief at Brigham and Women's. During the three decades in which he filled these positions with distinction, he created one of the first modern academic medical units where the education of physician-scientists, the highest standards of clinical care, and the conduct of exciting clinical research were inextricably intertwined and mutually reinforcing. Thorn's personal investigative interests focused on the adrenal cortex and the kidney. He developed techniques for the diagnosis of adrenal disease that are still in wide use. He characterized salt-losing nephritis and catalyzed the development of renal dialysis and the work that led to the development of renal transplantation.

George Thorn played many leadership roles in medicine and medical science. As a member of the governing board of the Massachusetts Institute of Technology (MIT) he was instrumental in the development of the Harvard-MIT program in Health Science and Technology. He was the founder, Director, and then President of the Howard Hughes Medical Institute, which became a major world force in the conduct of fundamental biomedical research under his leadership.

Thorn has influenced most profoundly a number of institutions: Harvard, the Brigham, MIT, and the Hughes Institute. To these and to *Harrison's*, he brought a unique blend of ebullience, imagination, curiosity, personal leadership, good humor, warmth, and compassion, which inspired generations of Harvard medical students, Brigham residents and research fellows, Hughes investigators, and editorial colleagues. The present Editors are pleased to express their admiration for this medical giant and beloved friend by dedicating this seventeenth edition of *Harrison's* to George W. Thorn, one of the founders of this book.

THE EDITORS

NOTICE

COVER ILLUSTRATIONS

(1) **Figure 222-10.** Three-dimensional reconstruction of a CT angiogram demonstrating a normal main left coronary artery arising from the aorta and its two branches, the left anterior descending artery (left) and the left circumflex artery (right).

(2) Computer rendition of chains of *Streptococcus pneumoniae* bacteria. This gram-positive oval-shaped bacterium is one of the causes of pneumonia. Although found living harmlessly in the body, *S. pneumoniae* can cause dangerous opportunistic infections of the lung. *(Credit: Hybrid Medical Animation/Photo Researchers, Inc.)*

(3) Three-dimensional representation of blood cells.

(4) Illustration of a myelinated axon with sodium channels clustered at the nodes of Ranvier where axonal depolarization occurs; this event results in saltatory conduction, with nerve impulse jumping from one node to the next.

(5) **Figure 364-15A.** A CT perfusion mean transit–time map showing delayed perfusion of the left middle cerebral artery distribution.

CONTENTS

PART 1 Introduction to Clinical Medicine

PART 2 Cardinal Manifestations and Presentation of Diseases

SECTION 1 PAIN

SECTION 2 ALTERATIONS IN BODY TEMPERATURE

SECTION 3 NERVOUS SYSTEM DYSFUNCTION

SECTION 4 DISORDERS OF EYES, EARS, NOSE, AND THROAT

SECTION 5 ALTERATIONS IN CIRCULATORY AND RESPIRATORY FUNCTIONS

CONTENTS

CONTENTS

PART 8 Bioterrorism and Clinical Medicine

PART 9 Disorders of the Cardiovascular System

CONTENTS

PART 15 Endocrinology and Metabolism

PART 16 Neurologic Disorders

For complete text for these chapters, see Harrison's, 17e, DVD

Chapter e1 ● The Safety and Quality of Health Care

A number of interventions that have been demonstrated to improve the safety and quality of care are available today and should be used more widely in clinical practice. Other interventions are undergoing evaluation, and still others are being developed in parallel with new technologies such as electronic health records systems. Many interventions will require changing the structure of care—for example, moving to a more team-oriented approach and ensuring that patients are more involved in their own care. Payers and the general public are now demanding better information about safety and quality as well as better performance in these areas. The clear implication is that these domains will need to be addressed directly by providers. Thus, physicians must learn about these two domains, how they can be improved, and the relative strengths and limitations of our current ability to measure them.

Chapter e2 ● Economic Considerations in the Practice of Medicine

Physicians need to develop and maintain an understanding of this topic and to reflect that understanding in their professional behavior. Covered in this chapter are the many causes of rising health care costs, with new technology being the main one; the ways in which insurance coverage (including Medicare and Medicaid) can drive demand for health care services; the influence of health professionals, hospitals, and the pharmaceutical and device industries on the supply of health care; and the different strategies available for cost control. With health care spending in the United States at >16% of the gross domestic product (as of 2005), this chapter should be of interest to all physicians.

Chapter e3 ● Racial and Ethnic Disparities in Health Care

This chapter illustrates how such disparities persist in spite of the great improvements in overall health and life expectancy. Many graphs and bar charts document the nature, extent, and root causes of differences in health care for minorities. These causes include social determinants, lack of access, complexity of the health care system, stereotyping, and patient-level factors such as mistrust. Key recommendations to bring about improvement are given, as is advice to the individual health care provider (e.g., being aware of disparities, practicing culturally competent care, avoiding stereotyping, and working to build trust).

Chapter e4 ● Ethical Issues in Clinical Medicine

This chapter discusses fundamental ethical guidelines, patients who lack decision-making capacity, decisions about life-sustaining interventions, conflicts of interest, and just allocation of resources. The chapter helps the physician to follow two fundamental but frequently conflicting ethical principles: respecting patient autonomy and acting in the patient's best interest. Also discussed are assessment of a patient's capacity to make medical decisions, choice of a surrogate, and standards for surrogate decision-making; care of dying patients, do-not-resuscitate orders, and decisions about when to withdraw or withhold life-sustaining interventions; and the risks of financial incentives, gifts from pharmaceutical companies, fear of treating HIV-infected patients, and reporting medical errors. The less-experienced physician will gain confidence in dealing with these perplexing and, at times, emotionally draining issues.

Chapter e5 ● Atlas of Rashes Associated with Fever

This chapter presents high-quality images of a variety of rashes that have an infectious etiology and are commonly associated with fever.

Even the most astute and experienced clinician is often diagnostically challenged by a patient with fever and rash, given the broad differential diagnosis. This atlas will help the physician to rapidly narrow the differential, promptly recognize key features, and administer appropriate and sometimes life-saving therapy.

Chapter e6 ● Memory Loss

This chapter discusses the formation of both long- and short-term memories. Long term memory is divided into declarative and non declarative memory; the former is further subdivided into semantic and episodic memories. Nondeclarative memory is subdivided into skills and habits (procedural memory), priming, conditioning, and nonassociative learning. Also covered are the associated anatomic substrates for each. Lesions in any of these associated areas cause deficits in storing, retaining, and retrieving information. Short-term, or working, memory relies on different regions of the brain, and lesions that disrupt their structure or function can be devastating. Testing of working memory can be effectively performed at the bedside. More detailed testing of memory should probably be done by a neuropsychologist, neuropsychiatrist, or behavioral neurologist.

Chapter e7 ● Atlas of Oral Manifestations of Disease

This atlas presents numerous outstanding photographs illustrating many oral conditions that indicate clinical disease either in the mouth or elsewhere. There is significant clinical value in examining the oral cavity for signs of disease, as the health status of the oral cavity is connected to cardiovascular disease and diabetes mellitus.

Chapter e8 ● Approach to the Patient with a Heart Murmur

This chapter provides comprehensive coverage of heart murmurs (systolic, diastolic, and continuous), their major attributes, and their response to bedside maneuvers, detected by auscultation. Together with the history, clinical context, and associated findings, this information allows the clinician to construct a differential diagnosis to guide the need for and urgency of further testing, such as echocardiography, transesophageal echocardiography, or cardiac CT or MRI.

Chapter e9 ● Atlas of Urinary Sediments and Renal Biopsies

This chapter illustrates key diagnostic features of selected kidney diseases, using light microscopy, immunofluorescence, and electron microscopy. Common urinalysis findings are also documented. The chapter amplifies the physician's knowledge of disorders of the kidney and urinary tract.

Chapter e10 ● Atlas of Skin Manifestations of Internal Disease

The atlas provides pictures of a selected group of inflammatory skin eruptions and neoplastic conditions, illustrating (1) common skin diseases and lesions, (2) nonmelanoma skin cancer, (3) melanoma and pigmented lesions, (4) infectious diseases and the skin, (5) immunologically mediated skin disease, and (6) skin manifestations of internal disease. Physicians frequently have to decide whether a cutaneous process is confined to the skin—a pure dermatologic event—or whether it is a manifestation of internal disease relating to the patient's overall medical condition, given the marked rise in both melanoma and nonmelanoma skin cancer.

Chapter e11 ⊘ Atlas of Hematology and Analysis of Peripheral Blood Smears

This atlas gives many examples of both normal and abnormal blood smears and a guide to blood smear interpretation. A normal peripheral blood smear is shown, as are normal granulocytes, monocytes, eosinophils, basophils, plasma cells, and bone marrow. Abnormal smears illustrate the defects found in conditions such as iron-deficiency anemia, sickle cell anemia, aplastic anemia, metastatic cancer, erythroid hyperplasia, acute myeloid and lymphoblastic leukemias, chronic myeloid and lymphoid leukemias, adult T cell leukemia, follicular lymphoma, and Burkitt's lymphoma, among others.

Chapter e12 ⊘ Thymoma

The chapter begins with a brief overview of the composition and function of the thymus and lists the various abnormalities that can occur. A thymoma develops when epithelial cells in the thymus become neoplastic. A link to myasthenia gravis (MG) is noted; about 30% of patients with a thymoma have MG, and MG patients have a high incidence of thymic abnormalities. Thymomas may be associated with other conditions (e.g., pure red cell aplasia) but to a lesser degree. Staging and histologic classification are presented. Early-stage disease is treated by surgical resection, with or without postoperative radiation. A multimodality approach is taken in late-stage disease: neoadjuvant chemotherapy followed by surgery, radiation therapy, and additional consolidation chemotherapy.

Chapter e13 ⊘ Late Consequences of Cancer and Its Treatment

This chapter discusses the long-term consequences of successful cancer treatment. Some problems may be related to the cancer itself or to the normal aging process, but many are caused by therapy, whether surgery, radiation, or chemotherapy. There may also be associated psychosocial problems. The consequences are covered in two ways—by organ system and by cancer type. It is now apparent that monitoring of cancer survivors is a critical component of their overall health care and that some aspects of primary treatment should be modified, where possible, to reduce later consequences.

Chapter e14 ⊘ Laboratory Diagnosis of Infectious Diseases

The chapter documents the evolution of methods used in the clinical microbiology laboratory to detect and identify viral, bacterial, fungal, and parasitic agents and to determine the antibiotic susceptibility of bacterial and fungal pathogens. Detection methods range from microscopic visualization, aided by a variety of stains, to systems that detect and amplify biologic signals. Identification methods include both classic biochemical phenotyping and more sophisticated methods such as gas chromatography and nucleic acid tests. Perhaps most useful to the nonspecialist is the large table giving clear and precise instructions for collection and transport of specimens to the laboratory for culture.

Chapter e15 ⊘ Infectious Complications of Burns and Bites

This chapter details the consequences of breaches in the skin from animal bites and scratches, which allow the inoculation of microorganisms into deeper, susceptible host tissues, and from burns, which may cause massive destruction of the integument and derangements in humoral and cellular immunity. The patient's own flora and organisms from the hospital environment can cause infections in burn injuries, and the frequency of infection parallels the extent and severity of the injury. Immunosuppression resulting from severe burns also puts patients at risk of infections, as do the necessary manipulations for clinical care. The risks of infection, both local and systemic, that can result from the variety of microorganisms involved in an animal or human bite are detailed. The treatment section covers wound management, antibiotic therapy for established infection and for prophylactic purposes, and rabies and tetanus prophylaxis.

Chapter e16 ⊘ Laboratory Diagnosis of Parasitic Infections

This chapter emphasizes the importance of the history and epidemiology of a patient's illness. Tables provide clear information on the geographic distribution, transmission, anatomic locations, and methods employed for the diagnosis of flatworm, roundworm, and protozoal infections. These tables should help the physician select the appropriate body fluid or biopsy site for microscopic examination. Other tables give information about the identification of parasites in samples from specific anatomic locations. Also listed are parasites frequently associated with eosinophilia and the serologic and molecular tests currently available for parasitic infections.

Chapter e17 ⊘ Pharmacology of Agents Used to Treat Parasitic Infections

This chapter deals exclusively with the pharmacologic properties of the agents used to treat infections due to parasites. Information on these agents' major toxicities, spectrum of activity, and safety for use during pregnancy and lactation is presented in Chap. 201.

Chapter e18 ⊘ Atlas of Blood Smears of Malaria and Babesiosis

This chapter provides both thin and thick blood films for *Plasmodium falciparum*, *P. vivax*, *P. ovale*, and *P. malariae*. The thick film allows detection of densities as low as 50 parasites per microliter, with great sensitivity; the thin film is better for speciation and provides useful prognostic information in severe falciparum malaria. One thin blood film showing trophozoites of *Babesia* is included.

Chapter e19 ⊘ Atlas of Electrocardiography

This chapter shows electrocardiograms to supplement those used in Chap. 221. The interpretations emphasize findings of specific teaching value.

Chapter e20 ⊘ Atlas of Noninvasive Cardiac Imaging

This chapter provides "real-time" image clips, as they are viewed in clinical practice, as well as additional static images. Noninvasive cardiac imaging is essential to the diagnosis and management of patients with known or suspected cardiovascular disease. This atlas supplements Chap. 222, which describes the principles and clinical applications of these important techniques.

Chapter e21 ⊘ Atlas of Cardiac Arrhythmias

This chapter shows electrocardiograms to supplement those used in Chaps. 225 and 226. The interpretations emphasize findings of specific teaching value.

Chapter e22 ⊘ Atlas of Atherosclerosis

The atlas consists of six videos that highlight some of the current understanding of atherosclerosis. Topics include pulse pressure, plaque instability, rudiments of the clinically important lipoproteins, formation and complications of atherosclerotic plaques, mechanisms of atherogenesis, and metabolic derangements that underlie the metabolic syndrome.

Chapter e23 ⊘ Atlas of Percutaneous Revascularization

The atlas presents seven case studies ranging from cardiogenic shock with left main coronary artery obstruction to percutaneous aortic valve replacement. The cases are illustrated by a selection of electrocardiograms, videos of angiograms, graphs, and CT scans, providing a good teaching tool.

Chapter e24 ⊘ Atlas of Chest Imaging

The atlas is a collection of chest x-rays and CT scans illustrative of specific major findings, which are categorized by those of volume loss, loss of parenchyma, interstitial processes, alveolar processes, bronchiectasis, pleural abnormalities, nodules and masses, and pulmonary vascular abnormalities.

Chapter e25 ⊘ Video Atlas of Gastrointestinal Endoscopy

This atlas demonstrates endoscopic findings in a variety of infectious, inflammatory, vascular, and neoplastic conditions. The premalignant conditions of Barrett's esophagus and colonic polyps are also illustrated. At the end of the chapter are several video clips demonstrating endoscopic treatment modalities for gastrointestinal bleeding, polyps, and biliary stones.

Chapter e26 ⊘ Atlas of Liver Biopsies

The atlas gives examples of common morphologic features of acute and chronic liver disorders—some involving the lobular areas and others the portal tracts. Liver biopsy is thought to represent the "gold standard" for assessing the degree of liver injury and fibrosis. Other important histologic features include those found in hepatic steatosis, injury of bile ducts in the portal tract, plasma cell infiltration, and portal inflammation affecting portal veins.

Chapter e27 ⊘ Primary Immunodeficiencies Associated with or Secondary to Other Diseases

The tables in this chapter add to the information given in Chap. 310 by listing (1) the primary immunodeficiencies associated with or secondary to other conditions, and (2) the genes or genetic loci associated with primary immunodeficiencies.

Chapter e28 ⊘ Atlas of Clinical Imaging in the Vasculitic Diseases

The atlas enhances the information given in Chap. 319 by images illustrating features associated with vasculitic syndromes such as Wegener's granulomatosis, Churg-Strauss syndrome, polyarteritis nodosa, and giant cell and Takayasu's arteritis. The images have been made using mainly CT scans and arteriograms.

Chapter e29 ⊘ Atlas of Clinical Manifestations of Metabolic Diseases

The atlas provides a visual survey of selected metabolic disorders, which can be used to facilitate learning and thereby enhance the recognition and care of patients with these disorders. The study of metabolic diseases has been invaluable for advancing understanding of human genetics, leading to novel approaches to therapy such as screening programs, blood and organ transplantation, gene therapy, and enzyme replacement.

Chapter e30 ⊘ Atlas of Neuroimaging

This atlas comprises 29 cases to assist the clinician caring for patients with neurologic symptoms. The majority of the images are MRIs; other techniques used are MR and conventional angiography and CT scans. Many neurologic diseases are illustrated, such as tuberculosis of the central nervous system (CNS), neurosyphilis, CNS aspergillosis, neurosarcoid, middle cerebral artery stenosis, CNS vasculitis, Huntington's disease, and acute transverse myelitis.

Chapter e31 ⊘ Electrodiagnostic Studies of Nervous System Disorders: EEG, Evoked Potentials, EMG

This chapter covers the two main techniques for electrodiagnosis of neurologic symptoms: the electroencephalogram (EEG) and the electromyogram (EMG). Evoked potentials (sensory, cognitive, and motor) are also covered. The EEG is most useful in evaluating patients with suspected epilepsy but is also helpful in assessing coma and as a noninvasive screening tool for focal structural abnormalities of the brain. EMG enables disorders of the motor units to be detected and characterized as neurogenic or myopathic, and the findings may provide a guide to the severity of an acute nerve disorder or, in chronic or degenerative disorders, whether the process is active or progressive—important for prognosis. Nerve conduction studies, which complement the EMG, are also covered.

Chapter e32 ⊘ Technique of Lumbar Puncture

This chapter covers the procedure of lumbar puncture (LP) in detail (with illustrations), from indications for imaging and laboratory studies prior to LP, analgesia, positioning, and the procedure itself (including dealing with complications that may arise during LP). Also included is a section on the main complication of LP—the post-LP headache—and its causes and therapy and strategies to avoid it.

Chapter e33 ⊘ Special Issues in Inpatient Neurologic Consultation

This chapter provides coverage of neurologic diseases and syndromes that are common reasons for inpatient consultation but that are not covered elsewhere in the text. Detailed here are central nervous system dysfunction (hyperperfusion states, post–cardiac bypass brain injury, and post–solid organ transplant injury); common neurologic complications of electrolyte disturbances (hyper- and hyponatremia, hyperosmolality, hypo- and hyperkalemia, and disturbances of calcium and magnesium); and peripheral nervous system dysfunction (including entrapment and obstetric neuropathies).

Chapter e34 ⊘ Heavy Metal Poisoning

This chapter provides specific information about the four main heavy metals that pose a significant threat to health via occupational and environmental exposures: lead, mercury, arsenic, and cadmium. A table clearly details the main sources, metabolism, toxic effects produced, diagnosis, and appropriate therapy for poisoning from these metals. Other metals covered, though not in the table, are copper, selenium, aluminum, chromium, manganese, and thallium.

Chapter e35 ⊘ Poisoning and Drug Overdosage

This chapter provides comprehensive coverage of the dose-related adverse effects following exposure to chemicals, drugs, or other xenobiotics. The section on diagnosis gives thorough coverage of the physical examination, laboratory assessment, electrocardiographic and radiologic studies, and toxicologic analysis. The treatment section gives detailed coverage of the general principles of care, supportive care, prevention of poison absorption, enhancement of poison elimination, administration of antidotes, and prevention of reexposure. Pathophysiologic features and treatment of specific toxic syndromes and poisonings are presented in tabular form.

Chapter e36 ⊘ Pulmonary Biomarkers in COPD

There has been increasing interest in using pulmonary biomarkers to understand and monitor the inflammation in the respiratory tracts of patients with COPD. A biomarker refers to any molecule or material (e.g., cells and tissue) that reflects the disease process. This chapter covers topics on bronchial biopsies, bronchoalveolar lavage, and sputum, among others.

Chapter e37 Chagas' Disease: Advances in Diagnosis and Management

Chagasic cardiomyopathy is the major complication resulting from infection by *Trypanosoma cruzi*. This infection is related to the close proximity between humans and triatomines carrying *T. cruzi*. This chapter discusses laboratory diagnosis and both etiologic and complementary treatments for the disease.

Chapter e38 The Polypill

Several risk factors contribute to causing atherosclerotic coronary artery disease, and some of these can be reduced by a variety of drugs. This chapter discusses the advantages and disadvantages of combining these drugs into one pill, the so-called polypill. The advantages include convenience of delivery, inclusion of all drugs thought to be essential for prevention, low cost, and possible enhanced compliance; disadvantages include possible overtreatment of low-risk patients, undertreatment of high-risk patients, and side effects from one or more components.

The authors emphasize that the role of a polypill in secondary and high-risk prevention is still speculative, and more trials need to be carried out. The polypill's greatest risk appears to be that both patients and physicians may give up on eliminating smoking and modifying sedentary lifestyles and unhealthy diets—tried and true risk-modification techniques.

Chapter e39 Mitochondrial DNA and Heritable Traits and Diseases

The structure and function of mitochondrial DNA (mtDNA) are discussed in depth in this chapter, which includes the proposition that the total cumulative burden of somatic mtDNA mutations acquired with age may contribute to aging and common age-related disturbances. Also included are an overview of the clinical and pathologic features of human mtDNA diseases and their presentations (enhanced by useful tables) and a discussion of the role of mtDNA mutations in the metabolic syndrome, type 2 diabetes mellitus, and neurodegenerative diseases in particular. Genetic counseling and treatment for mtDNA diseases round out the discussion.

INTERNATIONAL ADVISORY EDITORS

Oded Abramsky, MD, PhD
Professor and Head, Department of Neurology, Hebrew University Hadassah Medical School, Jerusalem, Israel

Peter J. Barnes, MA, DM, DSc
Professor and Head of Thoracic Medicine, National Heart & Lung Institute; Head of Respiratory Medicine, Imperial College London; Honorary Consultant Physician, Royal Brompton Hospital, London

Professor Dame Carol Black
Royal College of Physicians, Regents Park, London, United Kingdom

John Funder, MD
Professor, Prince Henry's Institute of Medical Research, Clayton, Victoria, Australia

Professor Donald Metcalf
Professor Emeritus, The Royal Melbourne Hospital, Victoria, Australia

Jose Antonio F. Ramires, MD, PhD
Heard Professor of Cardiology; General Director of the Heart Institute-INCOR, University of São Paulo Medical School, Brazil

Professor Philippe J. Sansonetti
Unité de Pathogénie Microbienne Moléculaire, INSERM U786 Institut Pasteur, Paris, France

Karl Skorecki, MD
Annie Chutick Professor and Chair in Medicine (Nephrology); Director, Rappaport Research Institute, Technion-Israel Institute of Technology; Director of Medicine and Research Development, Ramban Medical Center, Haifa, Israel

Professor K. Srinath Reddy
Professor and Head, Department of Cardiology, All India Institute of Medical Sciences, Ansari Nagar, New Delhi, India

George Stingl, MD
Department of Dermatology, Medical University of Vienna, Wahringer Gurtel 18-20, Vienna, Austria

Professor Nicholas J. White
Professor of Tropical Medicine, Oxford University, United Kingdom; Mahidol University, Bangkok, Thailand

---

Numbers in brackets refer to the chapters written or co-written by the contributor.

James L. Abbruzzese, MD
Chair and Professor, GI Medical Oncology; Associate Medical Director, GI and Endoscope Center, Ofc/EVP; University of Texas, MD Anderson Cancer Center, Houston [95]

Elias Abrutyn, MD†
Professor of Medicine and Public Health, Drexel University College of Medicine, Philadelphia [133, 134]

John C. Achermann, MD
Lecturer in Endocrinology, UCL Institute of Child Health, University College, London, United Kingdom [343]

John W. Adamson, MD
Clinical Professor of Medicine, UCSD Cancer Center, Hematology/Oncology, University of California at San Diego, La Jolla [58, 98]

Anthony A. Amato, MD
Associate Professor of Neurology, Harvard Medical School; Chief, Divison of Neuromuscular Diseases, Department of Neurology, Brigham and Women's Hospital, Boston [382]

Michael J. Aminoff, MD, DSc
Professor of Neurology, School of Medicine, University of California, San Francisco, San Francisco [23, 25, e31]

Neil M. Ampel, MD
Professor of Medicine, University of Arizona; Staff Physician, SAVAHCS, Tucson [193]

Jennifer Anderson, MD
Clinical Fellow, Department of Newborn Medicine, Children's Hospital of Boston, Boston [69]

Kenneth C. Anderson, MD
Kraft Family Professor of Medicine, Harvard Medical School; Chief, Division of Hematologic Neoplasia, Dana-Farber Cancer Institute, Boston [106, 107]

Elliott M. Antman, MD
Professor of Medicine, Harvard Medical School; Director, Samuel L. Levine Cardiac Unit, and Senior Investigator, TIMI Study Group, Brigham and Women's Hospital, Boston [237, 239]

Frederick R. Appelbaum, MD
Member and Director, Clinical Research Division, Fred Hutchinson Cancer Research Center; Professor and Head, Division of Medical Oncology, University of Washington School of Medicine, Seattle [108]

Gordon L. Archer, MD
Professor of Medicine and Microbiology/Immunology; Associate Dean for Research, School of Medicine, Virginia Commonwealth University, Richmond [127]

Valder Arruda, MD, PhD
Associate Professor of Pediatrics, University of Pennsylvania School of Medicine, Division of Hematology, The Children's Hospital of Philadelphia, Philadelphia [110]

Arthur K. Asbury, MD
Van Meter Professor of Neurology Emeritus, Philadelphia [25, 380]

John R. Asplin, MD
Clinical Associate, Department of Medicine, University of Chicago; Medical Director, Litholink Corporation, Chicago [281]

Kenneth H. Astrin, MD
Associate Professor, Department of Human Genetics, Mount Sinai School of Medicine of New York University, New York [352]

John C. Atherton, MD
Professor of Gastroenterology; Director, Wolfson Digestive Diseases Centre, University of Nottingham, United Kingdom [144]

Jane C. Atkinson, DDS
Program Director, Clinical Trials Program, Center for Clinical Research, National Institute of Dental and Craniofacial Research, National Institutes of Health, Bethesda [e7]

Paul S. Auerbach, MD, MS
Clinical Professor, Department of Surgery, Division of Emergency Medicine, Stanford University School of Medicine, Stanford [391]

K. Frank Austen, MD
AstraZeneca Professor of Respiratory and Inflammatory Diseases, Harvard Medical School; Director, Inflammation & Allergic Diseases Research Section, Division of Rheumatology, Immunology & Allergy, Brigham and Women's Hospital, Boston [311]

Eric H. Awtry, MD
Assistant Professor of Medicine, Boston University School of Medicine, Boston [233, 234]

Bruce R. Bacon, MD
James F. King Endowed Chair in Gastroenterology; Professor of Internal Medicine, Division of Gastroenterology & Hepatology, St. Louis [302, 303]

Lindsey R. Baden, MD
Assistant Professor of Medicine, Harvard Medical School, Boston [171]

†Deceased.

Kamal F. Badr, MD
Professor and Dean, School of Medicine, Lebanese American University, Byblos, Lebanon [280]

Donald S. Baim, MD
Professor of Medicine, Harvard Medical School; Executive Vice President, Chief Medical and Scientific Officer, Boston Scientific Corporation, Natick [223, 240, e23]

John R. Balmes, MD
Professor of Medicine, University of California, San Francisco; Chief, Division of Occupational and Environmental Medicine, San Francisco General Hospital; Professor of Environmental Health Sciences, School of Public Health, University of California, Berkeley [250]

Robert L. Barbieri, MD
Kate Macy Ladd Professor of Obstetrics, Gynecology and Reproductive Biology, Harvard Medical School, Boston [7]

Joanne M. Bargman, MD
Professor of Medicine, University of Toronto; Director, Peritoneal Dialysis Program, and Co-Director, Combined Renal-Rheumatology Lupus Clinic, University Health Network, Toronto [274]

Tamar F. Barlam, MD
Associate Professor of Medicine, Boston University School of Medicine, Boston [115, 140]

Peter J. Barnes, MA, DM, DSc
Professor and Head of Thoracic Medicine, National Heart & Lung Institute; Head of Respiratory Medicine, Imperial College London; Honorary Consultant Physician, Royal Brompton Hospital, London [248, e37]

Miriam J. Baron, MD
Instructor in Medicine, Harvard Medical School, Boston [121]

Kenneth J. Bart, MD, MPH, MSHPM
Professor Emeritus, Epidemiology and Biostatistics, San Diego State University, San Diego; Consultant, National Vaccine Program Office, Office of the Secretary, Department of Health and Human Services, Washington [116]

Shari S. Bassuk, ScD
Epidemiologist, Division of Preventive Medicine, Brigham and Women's Hospital, Boston [342]

David W. Bates, MD, MSc
Professor of Medicine, Harvard Medical School; Chief, General Medical Division, Brigham and Women's Hospital; Medical Director, Clinical and Qualitative Analysis Program, Partners Healthcare System, Boston [e1]

Robert P. Baughman, MD
Professor of Medicine, Cincinnati [322]

M. Flint Beal, MD
Anne Parrish Titzel Professor and Chair, Department of Neurology and Neuroscience, Weill Medical College of Cornell University; Neurologist-in-Chief, New York Presbyterian Hospital, New York [360, 371]

Nicholas J. Beeching, FFTM (RCPS Glas) DCH, DTM&H
Senior Lecturer in Infectious Diseases, Liverpool School of Tropical Medicine, University of Liverpool; Consultant and Clinical Lead, Tropical and Infectious Disease Unit, Royal Liverpool University Hospital, Liverpool, United Kingdom [150]

Robert S. Benjamin, MD
Professor of Medicine; Chairman, Department of Sarcoma Medical Oncology, The University of Texas MD Anderson Cancer Center, Houston [94]

Edward J. Benz, Jr., MD
Richard and Susan Smith Professor of Medicine; Professor of Pediatrics; Professor of Pathology, Harvard Medical School; President and CEO, Dana-Farber Cancer Institute; Director, Dana-Farber/Harvard Cancer Center, Boston [99]

Jean Bergounioux, MD
Medical Doctor of Pediatrics, Unité de Pathogénie Microbienne Moléculaire, Paris [147]

Joseph R. Betancourt, MD, MPH
Director, The Disparities Solutions Center, Massachusetts General Hospital; Assistant Professor of Medicine, Harvard Medical School [e3]

Shalender Bhasin, MD
Chief and Professor, Department of Endocrinology, Diabetes, & Nutrition, Boston University, Boston [340]

Atul K. Bhan, MBBS, MD
Professor of Pathology, Harvard Medical School; Director of the Immunopathology Unit, Department of Pathology, Massachusetts General Hospital, Boston [e26]

David R. Bickers, MD
Carl Truman Nelson Professor and Chair, Department of Dermatology, College of Physicians and Surgeons, Columbia University Medical Center, New York [57]

Henry J. Binder, MD
Professor of Medicine; Professor of Cellular & Molecular Physiology, Yale University, New Haven [288]

Thomas D. Bird, MD
Professor, Neurology and Medicine, University of Washington; Research Neurologist, Geriatric Research Education and Clinical Center, VA Puget Sound Health Care System, Seattle [365, e6]

William R. Bishai, MD, PhD
Professor of Medicine, The Johns Hopkins School of Medicine, Baltimore [131]

Bruce R. Bistrian, MD, PhD
Chief, Clinical Nutrition, Beth Israel Deaconess Medical Center; Professor of Medicine, Harvard Medical School, Boston [73]

Martin J. Blaser, MD
Frederick H. King Professor of Internal Medicine; Chair, Department of Medicine; Professor of Microbiology, New York University School of Medicine, New York [144, 148]

Clara D. Bloomfield, MD
Distinguished University Professor; William G. Pace III Professor of Cancer Research, Cancer Scholar and Senior Advisor, The Ohio State University Comprehensive Cancer Center and Arthur G. James Cancer Hospital and Richard J. Solove Research Institute, Columbus [104]

Richard S. Blumberg, MD
Professor of Medicine, Harvard Medical School; Chief, Division of Gastroenterology, Hepatology and Endoscopy, Brigham and Women's Hospital, Boston [289]

David Blumenthal, MD, MPP
Samuel O. Their Professor of Medicine; Professor of Health Care Policy, Harvard Medical School; Director, Institute for Health Policy, Massachusetts General Hospital/Partners HealthCare System, Boston [e3]

Jean L. Bolognia, MD
Professor of Dermatology, Yale Medical School [54]

George J. Bosl, MD
Chairman, Department of Medicine, Memorial Sloan-Kettering Cancer Center; Professor of Medicine, Joan and Sanford I Weill Medical College of Cornell University, New York [92]

Richard C. Boucher, Jr., MD
William Rand Kenan Professor of Medicine, University of North Carolina at Chapel Hill; Director, University of Carolina Cystic Fibrosis Center, Chapel Hill [253]

Eugene Braunwald, MD, MA (Hon), ScD (Hon)
Distinguished Hersey Professor of Medicine, Harvard Medical School; Chairman, TIMI Study Group, Brigham and Women's Hospital, Boston [1, 35, 36, 217, 219, 220, 230–232, 237–239, e8]

Irwin M. Braverman, MD
Professor of Dermatology, Yale University School of Medicine, New Haven [54]

Otis Webb Brawley, MD
Professor, Hematology, Oncology, Medicine & Epidemiology, Emory University; Chief Medical Officer, American Cancer Society, Atlanta [78]

Joel G. Breman, MD, DTPH
Senior Scientific Advisor, Fogarty International Center, National Institutes of Health, Bethesda [203, e18]

Barry M. Brenner, MD, AM, DSc (Hon), DMSc (Hon), Dipl (Hon)
Samuel A. Levine Professor of Medicine, Harvard Medical School; Director Emeritus, Renal Division, Brigham and Women's Hospital, Boston [45, 46, 279, 280, 283]

George J. Brewer, MD
Morton S. and Henrietta K. Sellner Active Emeritus Professor of Human Genetics; Active Emeritus Professor of Internal Medicine, University of Michigan Medical School, Ann Arbor [354]

F. Richard Bringhurst, MD
Senior Vice President for Medicine and Research Management , Massachusetts General Hospital; Associate Professor of Medicine, Harvard Medical School, Boston [346]

Kevin E. Brown, MD
Consultant Medical Virologist, Health Protection Agency, London [177]

Robert H. Brown, Jr., MD, DPhil
Neurologist, Massachusetts General Hospital; Professor of Neurology, Harvard Medical School, Boston [369, 382]

H. R. Büller, MD
Professor of Medicine; Chairman, Department of Vascular Medicine, Amsterdam [111]

David M. Burns, MD
Professor Emeritus, Department of Family and Preventive Medicine, University of California, San Diego School of Medicine, San Diego [390]

Michael J. Burns, MD
Assistant Professor of Medicine, Harvard Medical School, Boston [e35]

Joan R. Butterton, MD
Assistant Clinical Professor of Medicine, Harvard Medical School; Clinical Associate in Medicine, Massachusetts General Hospital, Boston [122]

John C. Byrd, MD
D. Warren Brown Professor of Leukemia Research Professor; Co-Director of Hematologic Malignancies, Division of Hematology and Oncology, Arthur G. James Cancer Hospital, Columbus [104]

Stephen B. Calderwood, MD
Morton N. Swartz, MD Academy Professor of Medicine (Microbiology and Molecular Genetics), Harvard Medical School; Chief, Division of Infectious Diseases, Massachusetts General Hospital, Boston [122]

Michael V. Callahan, MD, DTM&H (UK), MSPH
Clinical Associate Physician, Division of Infectious Diseases, Massachusetts General Hospital; Program Manager, Biodefense, Defense Advanced Research Project Agency (DARPA), United States Department of Defense, Washington [19]

Michael Camilleri, MD
Atherton and Winifred W. Bean Professor; Professor of Medicine and Physiology, Mayo Clinic College of Medicine, Rochester [40]

Grant L. Campbell, MD, PhD
Division of Vector-Borne Infectious Diseases, National Center for Infectious Diseases, Centers for Disease Control and Prevention, U.S. Public Health Service, Laporte [152]

Christopher P. Cannon, MD
Associate Professor of Medicine, Harvard Medical School; Associate Physician, Cardiovascular Division, Senior Investigator, TIMI Study Group, Brigham and Women's Hospital, Boston [238]

Jonathan R. Carapetis, MBBS, PhD
Director, Menzies School of Health Research; Professor, Charles Darwin University, Australia [315]

Mark Carlson, MD, MA
Chief Medical Officer and Senior Vice President, Clinical Affairs, St. Jude Medical, Sylmar; Adjunct Professor of Medicine, Case Western Reserve University, Cleveland[21]

Charles B. Carpenter, MD
Professor of Medicine, Harvard Medical School; Senior Physician, Brigham and Women's Hospital, Boston [276]

Brian I. Carr, MD, PhD
Professor of Medicine, Thomas Jefferson University; Director of the Liver Tumor Program, Kimmel Cancer Center, Philadelphia [88]

Lisa B. Caruso, MD, MPH
Assistant Professor of Medicine, Boston Medical Center, Boston [9]

Arturo Casadevall, MD, PhD
Professor of Microbiology and Immunology and of Medicine; Chair, Department of Microbiology and Immunology, Albert Einstein College of Medicine, New York [195]

Agustin Castellanos, MD
Professor of Medicine; Director, Clinical Electrophysiology, University of Miami Miller School of Medicine, Miami [267]

Stanley W. Chapman, MD
Professor of Medicine and Microbiology; Director, Division of Infectious Diseases; Vice-Chair for Academic Affairs, Department of Medicine, University of Mississippi School of Medicine, Jackson [194, 199]

Vinay Chaudhry, MD
Professor and Vice Chair, The Johns Hopkins University School of Medicine; Co-Director, EMG Laboratory, Johns Hopkins Hospital, Baltimore [379]

Lan X. Chen, MD
Clinical Assistant Professor of Medicine, University of Pennsylvania, Penn Presbyterian Medical Center & Philadelphia Veteran Affairs Medical Center, Philadelphia [327]

Yuan-Tsong Chen, MD
Distinguished Research Fellow and Director, Institute of Biomedical Sciences, Academia Sinica, Taiwan [356]

Glenn M. Chertow, MD
Professor of Medicine, Epidemiology and Biostatistics, University of California, San Francisco School of Medicine; Director, Clinical Services, Division of Nephrology, University of California, San Francisco Medical Center, San Francisco [273, 275]

John S. Child, MD
Director, Ahmanson-UCLA Adult Congenital Heart Disease Center; Streisand Professor of Medicine and Cardiology, David Geffen School of Medicine at UCLA, Los Angeles [229]

Yu Jo Chua, MBBS
Research Fellow (Medical Oncology), Royal Marsden Hospital, London [89]

Raymond T. Chung, MD
Associate Professor of Medicine, Harvard Medical School; Director of Hepatology, Massachusetts General Hospital; Medical Director, Liver Transplant Program, Massachusetts General Hospital, Boston [304]

Fredric L. Coe, MD
Professor of Medicine, University of Chicago, Chicago [281]

Jeffrey I. Cohen, MD
Chief, Medical Virology Section, Laboratory of Clinical Infectious Diseases, National Institute of Allergy and Infectious Diseases, National Institutes of Health, Bethesda [174, 184]

Ronit Cohen-Poradosu, MD
Channing Laboratory, Brigham and Women's Hospital, Boston [157]

Francis Collins, MD, PhD
Director, National Human Genome Research Institute, National Institutes of Health, Bethesda [79]

Wilson S. Colucci, MD
Thomas J. Ryan Professor of Medicine, Boston University School of Medicine; Chief, Cardiovascular Medicine, Boston University Medical Center, Boston [233, 234]

Max D. Cooper, MD
Professor of Medicine, Pediatrics, Microbiology, and Pathology, The University of Alabama at Birmingham, Birmingham [310, e27]

Michael J. Corbel, PhD, DSc(Med), FIBiol
Head, Division of Bacteriology, National Institute for Biological Standards and Control, Potters Bar, United Kingdom [150]

Lawrence Corey, MD
Professor of Medicine and Laboratory Medicine; Chair of Medical Virology, University of Washington; Head, Program in Infectious Diseases, Fred Hutchinson Cancer Research Center, Seattle [172]

Felicia Cosman, MD
Associate Professor of Clinical Medicine, Columbia University College of Physicians and Surgeons; Medical Director, Clinical Research Center, Helen Hayes Hospital, West Haverstraw, New York [348]

Mark A. Creager, MD
Professor of Medicine, Harvard Medical School; Simon C. Fireman Scholar in Cardiovascular Medicine; Director, Vascular Center, Brigham and Women's Hospital, Boston [242, 243]

Philip E. Cryer, MD
Irene E. and Michael M. Karl Professor of Endocrinology and Metabolism in Medicine, Washington University, St. Louis [339]

CONTRIBUTORS

David Cunningham, MD
Professor of Cancer Medicine, Institute of Cancer Research; Consultant Medical Oncologist, Head of Gastrointestinal Unit, Royal Marsden Hospital, London [89]

John J. Cush, MD
Director of Clinical Rheumatology, Baylor Research Institute; Professor of Medicine and Rheumatology, Baylor University Medical Center, Dallas [325]

Malwina Czarny-Ratajczak, PhD
Research Assistant Professor, Center for Gene Therapy, Tulane University Health Sciences Center, Tulane University, New Orleans [357]

Charles A. Czeisler, MD, PhD
Baldino Professor of Sleep Medicine, and Director, Division of Sleep Medicine, Harvard Medical School; Chief, Division of Sleep Medicine, Department of Medicine, Brigham and Women's Hospital, Boston [28]

Marinos C. Dalakas, MD
Professor of Neurology; Chief, Neuromuscular Diseases Section, NINDS, National Institute of Health, Bethesda [383]

Josep Dalmau, MD, PhD
Professor of Neurology, Division Neuro-Oncology, Department of Neurology, Philadelphia [97]

Daniel F. Danzl, MD
Professor and Chair, Department of Emergency Medicine, University of Louisville School of Medicine, Louisville [20]

Emily Darby, MD
Senior Fellow, Division of Infectious Diseases, University of Washington, Seattle [153]

Robert B. Daroff, MD
Gilbert W. Humphrey Professor of Neurology and Interim Chair, Department of Neurology, Case Western Reserve University School of Medicine and University Hospitals Case Medical Center, Cleveland [22]

Charles E. Davis, MD
Professor of Pathology and Medicine Emeritus, University of California San Diego School of Medicine; Director Emeritus, Microbiology Laboratory, University of California San Diego Medical Center, San Diego [e16]

Mahlon R. DeLong, MD
Timmie Professor of Neurology, Emory University School of Medicine, Atlanta [366]

John Del Valle, MD
Professor and Senior Associate Chair of Graduate Medical Education, Department of Internal Medicine, Division of Gastroenterology, University of Michigan Health System, Ann Arbor [287]

Marie B. Demay, MD
Associate Professor of Medicine, Harvard Medical School; Associate Physician, Massachusetts General Hospital, Boston [346]

Bradley M. Denker,
Associate Professor of Medicine, Harvard Medical School; Physician, Brigham and Women's Hospital; Chief of Nephrology, Harvard Vanguard Medical Associates, Boston [45]

David W. Denning, MBBS
Professor of Medicine and Medical Mycology, University of Manchester; Director, Regional Mycology Laboratory, Manchester Education and Research Centre, Wythenshawe Hospital, Manchester, United Kingdom [197]

David T. Dennis, MD, MPH
Faculty Affiliate, Department of Microbiology, Immunology and Pathology, Colorado State University; Medical Epidemiologist, Division of Influenza, Centers for Disease Control and Prevention, Atlanta [152, 165]

Robert J. Desnick, MD, PhD
Professor and Chair, Department of Genetics and Genomic Sciences, Mount Sinai School of Medicine of New York University, New York [352]

Betty Diamond, MD
Chief, Autoimmune Disease Center, The Feinstein Institute for Medical Research, New York [312]

Jules L. Dienstag, MD
Carl W. Walter Professor of Medicine and Dean for Medical Education, Harvard Medical School; Physician, Gastrointestinal Unit, Massachusetts General Hospital, Boston [298–300, 304, e26]

William P. Dillon, MD
Professor of Radiology, Neurology, and Neurosurgery; Vice-Chair, Department of Radiology; Chief, Neuroradiology, University of California, San Francisco [362, e30]

Charles A. Dinarello, MD
Professor of Medicine, University of Colorado Health Science Center, Denver [17]

Robert G. Dluhy, MD
Program Director, Fellowship in Endocrinology; Professor of Medicine, Brigham and Women's Hospital, Harvard Medical School; Associate Editor, New England Journal of Medicine, Boston [336]

Raphael Dolin, MD
Maxwell Finland Professor of Medicine (Microbiology and Molecular Genetics); Dean for Academic and Clinical Programs, Harvard Medical School, Boston [171, 179, 180]

Neil J. Douglas, MD
Professor of Respiratory and Sleep Medicine, University of Edinburgh; Honorary Consultant Physician, Royal Infirmary of Edinburgh, United Kingdom [259]

Daniel B. Drachman, MD
Professor of Neurology & Neuroscience; WW Smith Charitable Trust Professor of Neuroimmunology, The Johns Hopkins University School of Medicine, Baltimore [381]

David F. Driscoll, PhD
Assistant Professor of Medicine, Harvard Medical School, Boston [73]

Thomas D. DuBose, Jr., MD
Tinsley R. Harrison Professor and Chair of Internal Medicine; Professor of Physiology and Pharmacology, Wake Forest University School of Medicine, Winston-Salem [48]

J. Stephen Dumler, MD
Professor, Division of Medical Microbiology, Department of Pathology, The Johns Hopkins University School of Medicine and Immunology, The Johns Hopkins University Bloomberg School of Public Health, Baltimore [167]

Andrea E. Dunaif, MD
Charles F. Kettering Professor of Medicine and Chief, Division of Endocrinology, Metabolism, and Molecular Medicine, Northwestern University Feinberg School Medicine, Chicago [6]

Samuel C. Durso, MD, MBA
Associate Professor of Medicine, Clinical Director, Division of Geriatric Medicine and Gerontology, The Johns Hopkins University School of Medicine, Baltimore [32, e7]

Janice P. Dutcher, MD
Professor, New York Medical College; Associate Director, Our Lady of Mercy Cancer Center, Bronx [270]

Johanna Dwyer, DSc, RD
Professor of Medicine and Community Health, Tufts University School of Medicine and Friedman School of Nutrition Science and Policy; Senior Scientist Jean Mayer Human Nutrition Research Center on Aging at Tufts; Director of the Frances Stern Nutrition Center, Tufts-New England Medical Center Hospital, Boston [70]

Jeffery S. Dzieczkowski, MD
Physician, St. Alphonsus Regional Medical Center; Medical Director, Coagulation Clinic, Saint Alphonsus Medical Group/Internal Medicine, Boise [107]

Kim A. Eagle, MD
Albion Walter Hewlett Professor of Internal Medicine, Chief of Clinical Cardiology and Director, University of Michigan Cardiovascular Center, University of Michigan, Ann Arbor [8]

Robert H. Eckel, MD
Professor of Medicine, Division of Endocrinology, Metabolism and Diabetes, Division of Cardiology; Professor of Physiology and Biophysics; Charles A. Boettcher II Chair in Atherosclerosis; Program Director, Adult General Clinical Research Center, University of Colorado at Denver and Health Sciences Center; Director Lipid Clinic, University Hospital, Aurora [236]

John E. Edwards, Jr., MD
Chief, Division of Infectious Diseases, Harbor/University of California, Los Angeles Medical Center; Professor of Medicine, David Geffen School of Medicine at the University of California, Los Angeles, Torrance [191, 196]

David A. Ehrmann, MD
Professor of Medicine; Associate Director, University of Chicago General Clinical Research Center, Chicago [50]

Ezekiel J. Emanuel, MD, PhD
Chair, Department of Bioethics, The Warren G. Magnuson Clinical Center, National Institutes of Health, Bethesda [11]

Linda L. Emanuel, MD, PhD
Buehler Professor of Medicine; Director, Buehler Center on Aging, Health & Society, Northwestern University Feinberg School of Medicine, Chicago [11]

Joey English, MD, PhD
Assistant Professor of Neurology, University of California, San Francisco, San Francisco [364]

John W. Engstrom, MD
Professor of Neurology; Clinical Chief of Service; Neurology Residency Program Director, University of California, San Francisco, San Francisco [16, 370]

Paul Farmer, MD, PhD
Maude and Lillian Presley Professor of Medical Anthropology, Department of Social Medicine, Harvard Medical School; Associate Chief, Division of Social Medicine and Health Inequalities, Brigham and Women's Hospital; Co-Founder, Partners In Health, Boston [2]

Anthony S. Fauci, MD, DSc (Hon), DM&S (Hon), DHL (Hon), DPS (Hon), DLM (Hon), DMS (Hon)
Chief, Laboratory of Immunoregulation; Director, National Institute of Allergy and Infectious Diseases, National Institutes of Health, Bethesda [1, 181, 182, 214, 308, 319, e28]

Murray J. Favus, MD
Professor of Medicine, Interim Head, Endocrine Section; Director, Bone Section, University of Chicago Pritzker School of Medicine, Chicago [281, 349]

David T. Felson, MD, MPH
Professor of Medicine and Epidemiology; Chief, Clinical Epidemiology Unit, Boston University, Boston [326]

Robert G. Fenton, MD, PhD
Staff Clinician, National Institute on Aging, National Institutes of Health, Baltimore [80]

Howard L. Fields, MD, PhD
Professor of Neurology; Director, Wheeler Center for Neurobiology of Addiction, University of California, San Francisco, San Francisco [12]

Gregory A. Filice, MD
Professor of Medicine, University of Minnesota; Chief, Infectious Disease Section, Minneapolis Veterans Affairs Medical Center, Minneapolis [155]

Robert Finberg, MD
Professor and Chair, Department of Medicine, University of Massachusetts Medical School, Worcester [82, 126]

Joyce Fingeroth, MD
Associate Professor of Medicine, Harvard Medical School, Boston [126]

Daniel J. Fink, MD, MPH
Associate Professor of Clinical Pathology, College of Physicians and Surgeons, Columbia University, New York [Appendix]

Jeffrey S. Flier, MD
Caroline Shields Walker Professor of Medicine, Harvard Medical School; Dean of the Faculty of Medicine, Harvard School of Medicine, Boston [74]

Agnes B. Fogo, MD
Professor of Pathology, Medicine and Pediatrics; Director, Renal/EM Division, Department of Pathology, Vanderbilt University Medical Center, Nashville [e9]

Sonia Friedman, MD
Assistant Professor of Medicine, Harvard Medical School; Associate Physician, Brigham and Women's Hospital, Boston [289]

Andre D. Furtado, MD
Associate Specialist at the Department of Radiology, Neuroradiology Section, University of California, San Francisco, San Francisco [e30]

Robert F. Gagel, MD
Professor of Medicine and Head, Division of Internal Medicine, University of Texas MD Anderson Cancer Center, Houston [345]

John I. Gallin, MD
Director, The Warren G. Magnuson Clinical Center, National Institutes of Health, Bethesda [61]

J. Michael Gaziano, MD, MPH
Chief, Division of Aging, Brigham and Women's Hospital; Director, Massachusetts Veterans Epidemiology, Research and Information Center (MAVERIC) and Geriatric Research, Education and Clinical Center (GRECC), Boston VA Healthcare System; Associate Professor of Medicine, Harvard Medical School, Boston [218]

Thomas A. Gaziano, MD, MSc
Instructor in Medicine, Harvard Medical School; Associate Physician of Cardiovascular Medicine, Brigham and Women's Hospital, Boston [218]

Susan L. Gearhart, MD
Assistant Professor of Colorectal Surgery and Oncology, The Johns Hopkins University School of Medicine, Baltimore [291, 292, 293, 294]

Robert H. Gelber, MD
Scientific Director, Leonard Wood Memorial Leprosy Research Center, Cebu, Philippines; Clinical Professor of Medicine and Dermatology, University of California, San Francisco, San Francisco [159]

Jeffrey A. Gelfand, MD
Professor of Medicine, Harvard Medical School; Physician, Department of Medicine, Massachusetts General Hospital, Boston [19, 204]

Alfred L. George, MD
Grant W. Liddle Professor of Medicine and Pharmacology; Chief, Division of Genetic Medicine, Department of Medicine, Vanderbilt University, Nashville [271]

Dale N. Gerding, MD
Assistant Chief of Staff for Research, Hines VA Hospital, Hines; Professor, Stritch School of Medicine, Loyola University, Maywood [123]

Anne Gershon, MD
Professor of Pediatrics, Columbia University College of Physicians and Surgeons, New York [185–187]

Marc Ghany, MD
Staff Physician, Liver Diseases Branch, National Institute of Diabetes and Digestive and Kidney Diseases, National Institutes of Health, Bethesda [295]

Raymond J. Gibbons, MD
Arthur M. and Gladys D. Gray Professor of Medicine, Mayo Clinic College of Medicine; Consultant, Cardiovascular Diseases, Mayo Clinic, Rochester [222, e20]

Bruce C. Gilliland,† MD
Professor of Medicine and Laboratory Medicine, University of Washington School of Medicine, Seattle [321, 329–331]

Roger I. Glass, MD, PhD
Director, Fogarty International Center; Associate Director for International Research, National Institutes of Health, Bethesda [183]

Eli Glatstein, MD
Morton M. Kligerman Professor and Vice Chairman, Clinical Director, Department of Radiation Oncology, University of Pennsylvania Medical Center, Philadelphia [216]

Robert M. Glickman, MD
Professor of Medicine, New York University School of Medicine, New York [44]

James F. Glockner, MD
Assistant Professor of Radiology, Mayo Clinic College of Medicine, Rochester [222]

Peter J. Goadsby, MD, PhD, DSc
Professor of Clinical Neurology, Institute of Neurology, Queen Square London; Professor of Neurology, Department of Neurology, University of California, San Francisco, San Francisco [15]

Ary L. Goldberger, MD
Professor of Medicine, Harvard Medical School; Associate Director, Division of Interdisciplinary Medicine and Biotechnology, Beth Israel Deaconess Medical Center, Boston [221, e19, e21]

Samuel Z. Goldhaber, MD
Professor of Medicine, Harvard Medical School; Director, Venous Thromboembolism Research Group, Director, Anticoagulation Service, and Senior Staff Cardiologist, Department of Medicine, Brigham and Women's Hospital, Boston [256]

†Deceased.

Ralph Gonzales, MD, MSPH

Professor of Medicine, Epidemiology and Biostatistics, University of California, San Francisco, San Francisco [31]

Douglas S. Goodin, MD

Professor of Neurology, University of California, San Francisco, San Francisco [375]

Raj K. Goyal, MD

Mallinckrodt Professor of Medicine, Harvard Medical School, Boston; Physician, VA Boston Healthcare and Beth Israel Deaconess Medical Center, West Roxbury [38, 286]

Gregory A. Grabowski, MD

The A. Graeme Mitchell Chair of Human Genetics; Professor, University of Cincinnati College of Medicine, Department of Pediatrics; Director, Division of Human Genetics, Cincinnati Children's Hospital Medical Center, Cincinnati [355]

Norton J. Greenberger, MD

Clinical Professor of Medicine, Harvard Medical School; Senior Physician, Brigham and Women's Hospital, Boston [305–307]

David E. Griffith, MD

Professor of Medicine; William A. and Elizabeth B. Moncrief Distinguished Professor, University of Texas Health Center, Tyler [161]

Rasim Gucalp, MD

Professor of Clinical Medicine, Albert Einstein College of Medicine, Montefiore Medical Center, Bronx [270]

Chadi A. Hage, MD

Assistant Professor of Medicine, Indiana University School of Medicine, Roudebush VA Medical Center, Pulmonary-Critical Care and Infectious Diseases, Indianapolis [192]

Bevra Hannahs Hahn, MD

Professor of Medicine; Chief of Rheumatology; Vice Chair, Department of Medicine, David Geffen School of Medicine, University of California, Los Angeles, Los Angeles [313]

Janet E. Hall, MD

Associate Professor of Medicine, Harvard Medical School; Associate Physician, Massachusetts General Hospital, Boston [51, 341]

Jesse B. Hall, MD

Professor of Medicine, Anesthesia & Critical Care; Section Chief, Pulmonary and Critical Care Medicine, University of Chicago, Chicago [261]

Scott A. Halperin, MD

Professor of Pediatrics and of Microbiology and Immunology, Dalhousie University, Halifax, Nova Scotia [142]

Raymond C. Harris, Jr., MD

Ann and Roscoe R. Robinson Professor of Medicine; Chief, Division of Nephrology & Hypertension, Department of Medicine, Vanderbilt University, Nashville [272]

Gavin Hart, MD, MPH

Director, STD Services, Royal Adelaide Hospital; Clinical Associate Professor, School of Medicine, Flinders University, Adelaide, South Australia, Australia [154]

Rudy Hartskeerl, PhD

Head, FAO/OIE, World Health Organization and National Leptospirosis Reference Centre, KIT Biomedical Research, Royal Tropical Institute, Amsterdam, The Netherlands [164]

William L. Hasler, MD

Professor of Medicine, Division of Gastroenterology, University of Michigan Health System, Ann Arbor [39, 284]

Terry J. Hassold, PhD

Eastlick Distinguished Professor, Washington State University, Pullman [63]

Joshua Hauser, MD

Assistant Professor of Medicine and Palliative Care; Assistant Director of the Beuler Center on Aging, Northwestern University, Chicago [11]

Stephen L. Hauser, MD

Robert A. Fishman Distinguished Professor and Chairman, Department of Neurology, University of California, San Francisco, San Francisco [1, 360, 361, 371, 372, 375, 380, e32]

Barton F. Haynes, MD

Frederic M. Hanes Professor of Medicine and Immunology, Departments of Medicine and Immunology; Director, Duke Human Vaccine Institute, Duke University School of Medicine, Durham [308]

Douglas C. Heimburger, MD, MS

Professor of Nutrition Sciences; Professor of Medicine; Director, Clinical Nutrition Fellowship Program, University of Alabama at Birmingham, Birmingham [72]

J. Claude Hemphill III, MD, MAS

Associate Professor of Clinical Neurology and Neurological Surgery, University of California, San Francisco; Director, Neurocritical Care Program, San Francisco General Hospital, San Francisco [269]

Patrick H. Henry, MD

Adjunct Clinical Professor of Medicine, University of Iowa, Iowa City [60]

Barbara L. Herwaldt, MD, MPH

Medical Epidemiologist, Division of Parasitic Diseases, Centers for Disease Control and Prevention, Atlanta [205]

Katherine A. High, MD

William H. Bennett Professor of Pediatrics, University of Pennsylvania School of Medicine; Investigator, Howard Hughes Medical Institute, The Children's Hospital of Philadelphia, Philadelphia [65, 110]

Martin S. Hirsch, MD

Professor of Medicine, Harvard Medical School; Professor of Immunology and Infectious Diseases, Harvard School of Public Health; Physician, Massachusetts General Hospital, Boston [175]

Helen H. Hobbs, MD

Investigator, Howard Hughes Medical Institute; Professor of Internal Medicine and Molecular Genetics, University of Texas Southwestern Medical Center, Dallas [350]

Judith S. Hochman, MD

Harold Snyder Family Professor of Cardiology; Clinical Chief, the Leon H. Charney Division of Cardiology; New York University School of Medicine; Director, Cardiovascular Clinical Research, New York [226]

Elizabeth L. Hohmann, MD

Associate Professor of Medicine and Infectious Diseases, Harvard Medical School, Massachusetts General Hospital, Boston [132]

A. Victor Hoffbrand, DM

Emeritus Professor of Haematology, Royal Free and University College, London [100]

Steven M. Holland, MD

Senior Investigator and Head, Immunopathogenesis Unit, Clinical Pathophysiology Section, Laboratory of Host Defenses, National Institute of Allergy and Infectious Diseases, National Institutes of Health, Bethesda [61]

King K. Holmes, MD, PhD

William H. Foege Chair, Department of Global Health; Director, Center for AIDS and STD; Professor of Medicine and Global Health, University of Washington; Head, Infectious Diseases, Harborview Medical Center, Seattle [124]

Jay H. Hoofnagle, MD

Director, Liver Diseases Research Branch, Division of Digestive Diseases and Nutrition, National Institute of Diabetes and Digestive and Kidney Diseases, National Institutes of Health, Bethesda [295]

Robert J. Hopkin, MD

Assistant Professor of Clinical Pediatrics, The University of Cincinnati College of Medicine; Division and Program in Human Genetics, Cincinnati Children's Hospital Research Foundation, Cincinnati [355]

Jonathan C. Horton, MD, PhD

William F. Hoyt Professor of Neuro-Ophthalmology; Professor of Ophthalmology, Neurology, and Physiology, University of California, San Francisco, San Francisco [29]

Howard Hu, MD, MPH, ScD

NSF International Chair, Department of Environmental Health Sciences; Professor of Environmental Health, Epidemiology and Medicine, University of Michigan Schools of Public Health and Medicine, Ann Arbor [e34]

Gary W. Hunninghake, MD
Sterba Professor of Medicine; Director, Division of Pulmonary, Critical Care and Occupational Medicine; Director, Institute for Clinical and Translational Science; Director, Graduate Program in Translational Biomedicine; Senior Associate Dean for Clinical and Translational Science, Iowa City [249]

Sharon A. Hunt, MD
Professor, Cardiovascular Medicine, Stanford University, Palo Alto [228]

Charles G. Hurst, MD
Chief, Chemical Casualty Care Division, United States Medical Research Institute of Chemical Defense, Maryland [215]

Steven E. Hyman, MD
Provost, Harvard University; Professor of Neurobiology, Harvard Medical School, Boston [385]

David H. Ingbar, MD
Professor of Medicine, Physiology & Pediatrics; Director, Pulmonary, Allergy, Critical Care & Sleep Division; Executive Director, Center for Lung Science & Health, University of Minnesota School of Medicine; Co-Director, Medical ICU & Respiratory Care, University of Minnesota Medical Center, Fairview [266]

Edward P. Ingenito, MD, PhD
Assistant Professor, Harvard Medical School, Boston [263]

Mark A. Israel, MD
Professor of Pediatrics and Genetics, Dartmouth Medical School; Director, Norris Cotton Cancer Center, Dartmouth-Hitchcock Medical Center, Lebanon [374]

Alan C. Jackson, MD, FRCPC
Professor of Medicine (Neurology) and of Medical Microbiology, University of Manitoba; Section Head of Neurology, Winnipeg Regional Health Authority, Winnipeg, Manitoba, Canada [188]

Richard F. Jacobs, MD, FAAP
President, Arkansas Children's Hospital Research Institute; Horace C. Cabe Professor of Pediatrics, University of Arkansas for Medical Sciences, College of Medicine, Little Rock [151]

J. Larry Jameson, MD, PhD
Professor of Medicine; Vice President for Medical Affairs and Lewis Landsberg Dean, Northwestern University Feinberg School of Medicine, Chicago [1, 62, 64, 96, 332, 333, 335, 340, 343, e29]

Robert T. Jensen, MD
Chief, Digestive Diseases Branch, National Institute of Diabetes, Digestive and Kidney Diseases, National Institutes of Health, Bethesda [344]

Camilo Jimenez, MD
Assistant Professor, Department of Endocrine Neoplasia & Hormonal Disorders, The University of Texas, MD Cancer Center, Houston [345]

Eric C. Johannsen, MD
Assistant Professor, Department of Medicine, Harvard Medical School; Associate Physician, Division of Infectious Diseases, Brigham and Women's Hospital, Boston [188]

Bruce E. Johnson, MD
Director, Lowe Center for Thoracic Oncology, Department of Medical Oncology; Dana-Farber Cancer Institute, Department of Medicine, Brigham and Women's Hospital; Professor of Medicine, Harvard Medical School, Boston [96]

James R. Johnson, MD
Professor of Medicine, University of Minnesota, Minneapolis [143]

Stuart Johnson, MD
Associate Professor, Stritch School of Medicine, Loyola University, Maywood; Staff Physician, Hines VA Hospital, Hines [123]

S. Claiborne Johnston, MD, PhD
Professor, Neurology; Professor, Epidemiology and Biostatistics; Director, University of California, San Francisco Stroke Service, San Francisco [364]

S. Andrew Josephson, MD
Assistant Clinical Professor of Neurology, University of California, San Francisco, San Francisco [26, e33]

Jorge L. Juncos, MD
Associate Professor of Neurology, Emory University School of Medicine; Director of Neurology, Wesley Woods Hospital, Atlanta [366]

Eric Kandel, MD
University Professor; Fred Kavli Professor and Director, Kavli Institute for Brain Sciences; Senior Investigator, Howard Hughes Medical Institute, Columbia University, New York [385]

Marshall M. Kaplan, MD
Professor of Medicine, Tufts University School of Medicine; Chief Emeritus, Division of Gastroenterology, Tufts-New England Medical Center, Boston [43, 296]

Adolf W. Karchmer, MD
Professor of Medicine, Harvard Medical School, Boston [118]

Dennis L. Kasper, MD, MA (Hon)
William Ellery Channing Professor of Medicine, Professor of Microbiology and Molecular Genetics, Harvard Medical School; Director, Channing Laboratory, Department of Medicine, Brigham and Women's Hospital, Boston [1, 113, 115, 121, 135, 140, 157]

Lloyd H. Kasper, MD
Professor of Medicine and Microbiology/Immunology; Co-Director, Program in Immunotherapeutics, Dartmouth Medical School, Lebanon [207]

Daniel Kastner, MD, PhD
Chief, Genetics and Genomic Section, National Institute of Arthritis and Musculoskeletal and Skin Diseases, National Institutes of Health, Bethesda [323]

Elaine T. Kaye, MD
Clinical Assistant Professor of Dermatology, Harvard Medical School; Assistant in Medicine, Department of Medicine, Children's Hospital Medical Center, Boston [18, e5]

Kenneth M. Kaye, MD
Associate Professor of Medicine, Harvard Medical School; Associate Physician, Division of Infectious Diseases, Brigham and Women's Hospital, Boston [18, e5]

Jack A. Kessler, MD
Davis Professor of Stem Cell Biology; Chairman, Davis Department of Neurology, Northwestern University Feinberg School of Medicine, Chicago [67]

Gerald T. Keusch, MD
Associate Provost and Associate Dean for Global Health, Boston University School of Medicine, Boston [116, 149]

Jay S. Keystone, MD, FRCPC
Professor of Medicine, University of Toronto; Staff Physician, Centre for Travel and Tropical Medicine, Toronto General Hospital, Toronto [117]

Sundeep Khosla, MD
Professor of Medicine and Physiology, Mayo Clinic College of Medicine, Rochester [47]

Elliott Kieff, MD, PhD
Harriet Ryan Albee Professor of Medicine and Microbiology and Molecular Genetics, Harvard Medical School; Senior Physician, Brigham and Women's Hospital, Boston [170]

Jim Yong Kim, MD, PhD
Chief, Division of Social Medicine and Health Inequalities, Brigham and Women's Hospital; Director and Professor, François Xavier-Bagnoud Center for Health and Human Rights, Harvard School of Public Health; Professor of Social Medicine and Chair, Department of Social Medicine, Harvard Medical School, Boston [2]

Talmadge E. King, Jr., MD
Constance B. Wofsy Distinguished Professor and Interim Chair, Department of Medicine, University of California, San Francisco, San Francisco [255]

Louis V. Kirchhoff, MD, MPH
Professor, Departments of Internal Medicine and Epidemiology, University of Iowa; Staff Physician, Department of Veterans Affairs Medical Center, Iowa City [206]

Joel N. Kline, MD, MSc
Professor, Internal Medicine and Occupational & Environmental Health; Director, University of Iowa Asthma Center, Iowa City [249]

Minoru S. H. Ko, MD, PhD
Senior Investigator & Chief, Developmental Genomics & Aging Section, Laboratory of Genetics, National Institute on Aging, NIH, Baltimore [66]

Barbara A. Konkle, MD
Professor of Medicine and Hematology/Oncology, University of Pennsylvania; Director, Penn Comprehensive Hemophilia and Thrombosis Program, Philadelphia [59, 109]

Peter Kopp, MD
Associate Professor, Division of Endocrinology, Metabolism and Molecular Science, Northwestern University Feinberg School of Medicine, Chicago [62]

Walter J. Koroshetz, MD
Deputy Director, National Institute of Neurological Disorders and Stroke, National Institutes of Health, Bethesda [377]

Theodore A. Kotchen, MD
Associate Dean for Clinical Research; Director, General Clinical Research Center, Medical College of Wisconsin, Wisconsin [241]

Phyllis E. Kozarsky, MD
Professor of Medicine, Infectious Diseases; Co-Director, Travel and Tropical Medicine, Emory University School of Medicine, Atlanta [117]

Barnett S. Kramer, MD, MPH
Associate Director for Disease Prevention, Office of the Director, National Institutes of Health, Bethesda [78]

Stephen M. Krane, MD
Persis, Cyrus and Marlow B. Harrison Distinguished Professor of Medicine, Harvard Medical School, Massachusetts General Hospital, Boston [346]

Alexander Kratz, MD, PhD, MPH
Assistant Professor of Clinical Pathology, Columbia University College of Physicians and Surgeons; Associate Director, Core Laboratory, Columbia University Medical Center, New York-Presbyterian Hospital; Director, Allen Pavilion Laboratory, New York [Appendix]

John P. Kress, MD
Associate Professor of Medicine, Section of Pulmanary and Critical Care, University of Chicago, Chicago [261]

Patricia A. Kritek, MD, EdM
Instructor in Medicine, Harvard Medical School; Co-Director, Harvard Pulmonary and Critical Care Medicine Fellowship, Brigham and Women's Hospital, Boston [e24]

Henry M. Kronenberg, MD
Chief, Endocrine Unit, Massachusetts General Hospital; Professor of Medicine, Harvard Medical School, Boston [346]

Robert F. Kushner, MD
Professor of Medicine, Northwestern University Feinberg School of Medicine, Chicago [75]

Loren Laine, MD
Professor of Medicine, Keck School of Medicine, University of Southern California, Los Angeles [42]

Anil K. Lalwani, MD
Mendik Foundation Professor and Chairman, Department of Otolaryngology; Professor, Department of Pediatrics; Professor, Department of Physiology and Neuroscience, New York University School of Medicine, New York [30]

H. Clifford Lane, MD
Clinical Director; Director, Division of Clinical Research; Deputy Director, Clinical Research and Special Projects; Chief, Clinical and Molecular Retrovirology Section, Laboratory of Immunoregulation, National Institute of Allergy and Infectious Diseases, National Institutes of Health, Bethesda [182, 214]

Carol A. Langford, MD, MHS
Associate Professor of Medicine; Director, Center for Vasculitis Care and Research, Department of Rheumatic and Immunologic Diseases, Cleveland Clinic, Cleveland [319, 321, 329–331, e28]

Wei C. Lau, MD
Associate Professor; Medical Director, Cardiovascular Center Operating Rooms; Director, Adult Cardiovascular Anesthesiology, Ann Arbor [8]

Thomas J. Lawley, MD
William P. Timmie Professor of Dermatology; Dean, Emory University School of Medicine, Atlanta [52, 23, 55, e10]

Thomas H. Lee, MD
Professor of Medicine, Harvard Medical School; Chief Executive Officer, Partners Community Health Care, Inc; Network President, Partners Health Care, Boston [13]

Bruce D. Levy, MD
Associate Professor of Medicine, Harvard Medical School; Pulmonary and Critical Care Medicine, Brigham and Women's Hospital, Boston [262]

Julia B. Lewis, MD
Professor of Medicine, Division of Nephrology and Hypertension, Department of Medicine, Vanderbilt University School of Medicine, Nashville [277]

Peter Libby, MD
Mallinckrodt Professor of Medicine, Harvard Medical School; Chief, Cardiovascular Medicine, Brigham and Women's Hospital, Boston [217, 235, e22]

Richard W. Light, MD
Professor of Medicine, Vanderbilt University, Nashville [257]

Christopher H. Linden, MD
Professor, Department of Emergency Medicine, Division of Medical Toxicology, University of Massachusetts Medical School, Worcester [e35]

Robert Lindsay, MD, PhD
Professor of Clinical Medicine, Columbia University College of Physicians and Surgeons; Chief, Internal Medicine, Helen Hayes Hospital, West Havershaw, New York [348]

Marc E. Lippman, MD
Professor and Chair, Department of Medicine, University of Miami Leonard M. Miller School of Medicine, Miami [86]

Peter E. Lipsky, MD
Chief, Autoimmunity Branch, National Institute of Arthritis, Musculoskeletal, and Skin Diseases, National Institutes of Health, Department of Health and Human Services, Bethesda [312, 314, 325]

David A. Lipson, MD
Assistant Professor of Medicine, Pulmonary, Allergy & Critical Care Division, University of Pennsylvania Medical Center, King of Prussia [34, 345]

Kathleen D. Liu, MD, PhD, MCR
Assistant Professor, Division of Nephrology, San Francisco [273, 275]

Bernard Lo, MD
Professor of Medicine; Director, Program in Medical Ethics, University of California, San Francisco, San Francisco [e4]

Dan L. Longo, MD
Scientific Director, National Institute on Aging, National Institutes of Health, Bethesda and Baltimore [1, 58, 60, 68, 77, 80, 81, 105, 106, 181, e11–e13]

Nicola Longo, MD, PhD
Professor of Pediatrics; Chief, Division of Medical Genetics, Department of Pediatrics, University of Utah, Salt Lake City [358, 359]

Joseph Loscalzo, MD, PhD, MA (Hon)
Hersey Professor of the Theory and Practice of Medicine, Harvard Medical School; Chairman, Department of Medicine, Physician-in-Chief, Brigham and Women's Hospital, Boston [1, 36, 37, 217, 237, 242, 243]

Phillip A. Low, MD
Robert D and Patricia E Kern Professor of Neurology, Mayo Clinic College of Medicine, Rochester [370]

Daniel H. Lowenstein, MD
Professor of Neurology; Director, University of California, San Francisco Epilepsy Center; Associate Dean for Clinical/Translational Research, San Francisco [361, 363]

Elyse E. Lower, MD
Professor of Medicine, University of Cincinnati, Cincinnati [322]

Franklin D. Lowy, MD, PhD
Professor of Medicine and Pathology, Columbia University, College of Physicians & Surgeons, New York [129]

Sheila A. Lukehart, PhD
Professor of Medicine, University of Washington, Seattle [162, 163]

Lucio Luzzatto, MD, PhD
Professor of Hematology, University of Florence; Scientific Director, Instituto Toscano Tumori (ITT), Firenze, Italy [101]

Lawrence C. Madoff, MD
Associate Professor of Medicine, Harvard Medical School, Boston [113, 135, 328, e15]

James H. Maguire, MD, MPH
Professor and Director, International Health Division, Department of Epidemiology and Preventive Medicine, University of Maryland School of Medicine, Baltimore [392]

Adel A. F. Mahmoud, MD, PhD
Professor, Molecular Biology, Princeton University, Princeton [212]

Ronald V. Maier, MD
Jane and Donald D. Trunkey Professor and Vice Chair, Surgery, University of Washington; Surgeon-in-Chief, Harborview Medical Center, Seattle [264]

Mark E. Malliard, MD
Associate Professor and Chief, Division of Gastroenterology and Hepatology, Omaha [301]

Scott Manaker, MD, PhD
Associate Professor of Medicine and Pharmacology, Pulmonary and Critical Care Division, Department of Medicine, University of Pennsylvania, Philadelphia [247]

Hanna Mandel, MD
Director, Metabolic Disease Unit, Rambam Medical Health Care Campus, Haifa, Israel [e39]

Lionel A. Mandell, MD
Professor of Medicine, McMaster University, Hamilton, Ontario [251]

Douglas L. Mann, MD
Professor of Medicine, Molecular Physiology and Biophysics; Chief, Section of Cardiology, Baylor College of Medicine, St. Luke's Episcopal Hospital and Texas Heart Institute, Houston [227]

JoAnn E. Manson, MD, DrPH
Professor of Medicine and the Elizabeth Fay Brigham Professor of Women's Health, Harvard Medical School; Chief, Division of Preventive Medicine, Brigham and Women's Hospital, Boston [342]

Eleftheria Maratos-Flier, MD
Associate Professor of Medicine, Harvard Medical School; Chief, Obesity Section, Joslin Diabetes Center, Boston [74]

Francis Marchlinski, MD
Professor of Medicine; Director of Cardiac Electrophysiology, University of Pennsylvania Health System, University of Pennsylvania School of Medicine, Philadelphia [226]

Daniel B. Mark, MD, MPH
Professor of Medicine, Duke University Medical Center; Director, Outcomes Research, Duke Clinical Research Institute, Durham [3]

Thomas Marrie, MD
Professor, Department of Medicine; Dean, Faculty of Medicine and Dentistry, University of Alberta, Edmonton, Alberta [167]

Gary J. Martin, MD
Raymond J. Langenbach MD Professor of Medicine; Vice Chairman for Faculty Affairs and Education, Department of Medicine, Northwestern University Feinberg School of Medicine, Chicago [4]

Joseph B. Martin, MD, PhD, MA (Hon)
Dean Emeritus of the Faculty of Medicine, Edward R. and Anne G. Lefler Professor of Neurobiology, Harvard Medical School, Boston [12, 361]

Robert J. Mayer, MD
Stephen B. Kay Family Professor of Medicine, Harvard Medical School, Dana-Farber Cancer Institute, Boston [87]

Alexander J. McAdam, MD, PhD
Medical Director, Infectious Diseases Diagnostic Division, Children's Hospital, Boston; Assistant Professor, Department of Pathology, Harvard Medical School, Boston [e14]

Calvin O. McCall, MD
Associate Professor of Dermatology, Virginia Commonwealth University Medical Center, Richmond [53]

William M. McCormack, MD
Distinguished Teaching Professor of Medicine; Chief, Infectious Disease Division, SUNY Downstate Medical Center, Brooklyn [168]

Kevin T. McVary, MD
Associate Professor of Urology, Northwestern University Feinberg School of Medicine, Chicago [49]

Nancy K. Mello, PhD
Professor of Psychology (Neuroscience), Harvard Medical School, Boston [389]

Shlomo Melmed, MD
Senior Vice President, Academic Affairs; Associate Dean, Cedars Sinai Medical Center, David Geffen School of Medicine at UCLA, Los Angeles [333]

David Meltzer, MD, PhD
Associate Professor, Departments of Medicine and Economics, Harris School of Public Policy; Director of the Center for Health and the Social Sciences, The University of Chicago, Chicago [e2]

Jerry R. Mendell, MD
Professor of Pediatrics, Neurology and Pathology, The Ohio State University; Director, Center for Gene Therapy, The Research Institute at Nationwide Children's Hospital, Columbus [382]

Jack H. Mendelson, MD
Professor of Psychiatry (Neuroscience), Harvard Medical School, Belmont [389]

M.-Marsel Mesulam, MD
Director, Cognitive Neurology and Alzheimer's Disease Center; Dunbar Professor of Neurology and Psychiatry, Northwestern University Feinberg School of Medicine, Chicago [27]

Susan Miesfeldt, MD
Medical Oncology Medical Director, Cancer Risk and Prevention Clinic, Maine Medical Cancer and Maine Center for Cancer Medicine & Blood Disorders, Portland [64]

Edgar L. Milford, MD
Associate Professor of Medicine, Harvard Medical School; Director, Tissue Typing Laboratory, Brigham and Women's Hospital, Boston [276]

Bruce L. Miller, MD
AW and Mary Margaret Clausen Distinguished Professor of Neurology, University of California, San Francisco School of Medicine, San Francisco [26, 365, 378, e6]

Mark Miller, MD
Associate Director for Research, National Institutes of Health, Bethesda [116]

Samuel I. Miller, MD
Professor of Genome Sciences, Medicine, and Microbiology, University of Washington, Seattle [146]

John D. Minna, MD
Professor, Internal Medicine and Pharmacology; Director, Hamon Center for Therapeutic Oncology Research, University of Texas Southwestern Medical Center, Dallas [85]

Thomas A. Moore, MD
Clinical Professor and Associate Program Director, Department of Medicine, University of Kansas School of Medicine, Wichita [201, e17]

Pat J. Morin, PhD
Senior Investigator, Laboratory of Cellular and Molecular Biology, National Institute on Aging, National Institutes of Health, Bethesda [79]

Robert J. Motzer, MD
Attending Physician, Department of Medicine, Memorial Sloan-Kettering Cancer Center; Professor of Medicine, Weill Medical College of Cornell University, New York [90, 92]

Haralampos M. Moutsopoulos, MD
Professor and Chair, Department of Pathophysiology, School of Medicine, National University of Athens, Greece [317, 320]

Robert S. Munford, MD
Jan and Henri Bromberg Chair in Internal Medicine, University of Texas Southwestern Medical Center, Dallas [265]

Nikhil C. Munshi, MD
Associate Director, Jerome Lipper Multiple Myeloma Center, Dana-Farber Cancer Institute; Associate Professor, Harvard Medical School, Boston [106]

John R. Murphy, PhD
Professor of Medicine and Microbiology; Chief, Section of Molecular Medicine, Boston University School of Medicine, Boston [131]

Timothy F. Murphy, MD
UB Distinguished Professor, Department of Medicine and Microbiology; Chief, Infectious Diseases, State University of New York, Buffalo [139]

Joseph A. Murray, MD
Professor of Medicine, Division of Gastroenterology and Hepatology, The Mayo Clinic, Rochester [40]

Daniel M. Musher, MD

Chief, Infectious Disease Section, Michael E. DeBakey Veterans Affairs Medical Center; Professor of Medicine and Professor of Molecular Virology and Microbiology, Baylor College of Medicine, Houston [128, 138]

Mark B. Mycyk, MD

Assistant Professor of Emergency Medicine; Director of Clinical Toxicology and Toxicological Research, Northwestern University Feinberg School of Medicine, Chicago [e35]

Robert J. Myerberg, MD

Professor of Medicine and Physiology; AHA Chair in Cardiovascular Research, University of Miami Miller School of Medicine, Miami [267]

Nitish Naik, MD, DS

Department of Cardiology, All India Institute of Medical Sciences, Ansari Nagar, New Delhi, India [e38]

Eric G. Neilson, MD

Hugh J. Morgan Professor of Medicine and Cell Biology, Physician-in-Chief, Vanderbilt University Hospital; Chairman, Department of Medicine, Vanderbilt University School of Medicine, Nashville [271, 272, 277, e9]

Gerald T. Nepom, MD, PhD

Director, Benaroya Research Institute at Virginia Mason; Professor, University of Washington School of Medicine, Seattle [309]

Hartmut P. H. Neumann, MD

Head, Section Preventative Medicine, Department of Nephrology and General Medicine, Albert-Ludwigs-University of Freiburg, Germany [337]

Jonathan Newmark, MD, Colonel, Medical Corps, US Army

Deputy Joint Program Executive Officer, Medical Systems, Joint Program Executive Office for Chemical/Biological Defense, US Department of Defense Chemical Casualty Care; Consultant to the US Army Surgeon General; Adjunct Professor, Neurology, F. Edward Hébert School of Medicine, Uniformed Services University of the Health Sciences, Falls Church [215]

Rick A. Nishimura, MD

Judd and Mary Morris Leighton Professor of Cardiovascular Diseases; Professor of Medicine, Mayo Clinic College of Medicine, Rochester [222, e20]

Robert L. Norris, MD

Associate Professor, Department of Surgery, Division of Emergency Medicine, Stanford University School of Medicine, Stanford [391]

Thomas B. Nutman, MD

Head, Helminth Immunology Section; Head, Clinical Parasitology Unit; Laboratory of Parasitic Diseases, National Institute of Allergy and Infectious Diseases, National Insitutes of Health, Bethesda [210, 211]

Richard J. O'Brien, MD

Head of Scientific Evaluation, Foundation for Innovative New Diagnostics, Geneva, Switzerland [158]

Patrick O'Gara, MD

Associate Professor of Medicine, Harvard Medical School; Director, Clinical Cardiology, Brigham and Women's Hospital, Boston [230, e8]

Robert A. O'Rourke, MD

Distinguished Professor of Medicine Emeritus, University of Texas Health Science Center, San Antonio [220]

C. Warren Olanow, MD

Henry P. and Georgette Goldschmidt Professor and Chairman of the Department of Neurology, Professor of Neuroscience, The Mount Sinai School of Medicine, New York [367]

Andrew B. Onderdonk, PhD

Professor of Pathology, Harvard Medical School and Brigham and Women's Hospital, Boston [e14]

Chung Owyang, MD

Professor of Internal Medicine, H. Marvin Pollard Collegiate Professor; Chief, Division of Gastroenterology, University of Michigan Health System, Ann Arbor [284, 290]

Umesh D. Parashar, MBBS, MPH

Lead, Enteric and Respiratory Viruses Team, Epidemiology Branch, Division of Viral Diseases, National Center for Immunization and Respiratory Diseases, Centers for Disease Control and Prevention, Atlanta [183]

Jeffrey Parsonnet, MD

Associate Professor of Medicine and Microbiology, Dartmouth Medical School, Lebanon [120]

Parul S. Patel, MD

Transplant Neurologist, California Pacific Medical Center, San Francisco [278]

Shreyaskumar R. Patel, MD

Professor of Medicine, Deputy Chairman, Department of Sarcoma Medical Oncology, University of Texas, Houston [94]

Gustav Paumgartner, MD

Professor of Medicine, University of Munich, Munich, Germany [305]

David A. Pegues, MD

Professor of Medicine, Division of Infectious Diseases, David Geffen School of Medicine at UCLA, Los Angeles [146]

Florencia Pereyra, MD

Instructor in Medicine, Harvard Medical School; Division of Infectious Disease, Brigham and Women's Hospital, Boston [e15]

Michael C. Perry, MD, MS

Professor and Director, Division of Hematology/Medical Oncology, Department of Internal Medicine, Nellie B. Smith Chair of Oncology, Columbia [e13]

Michael A. Pesce, PhD

Clinical Professor of Pathology, Columbia University College of Physicians and Surgeons; Director of Specialty Laboratory, New York Presbyterian Hospital, Columbia University Medical Center, New York [Appendix]

Clarence J. Peters, MD

John Sealy Distinguished University Chair in Tropical and Emerging Virology, Director for Biodefense, Center for Biodefense and Emerging Infectious Diseases, University of Texas Medical Branch in Galveston, Galveston [189, 190]

Eliot A. Phillipson, MD

Professor, Department of Medicine, University of Toronto, Toronto [258]

Gerald B. Pier, PhD

Professor of Medicine (Microbiology and Molecular Genetics), Harvard Medical School; Microbiologist, Brigham and Women's Hospital, Boston [114]

Ronald E. Polk, PharmD

Chair, Department of Pharmacy, Professor of Pharmacy and Medicine, School of Pharmacy, Virginia Commonwealth University, Richmond [127]

Richard J. Pollack, MD

Research Associate in Immunology and Infectious Diseases, Harvard School of Public Health, Boston [392]

Reuven Porat, MD

Professor of Medicine; Director, Internal Medicine, Tel Aviv Sourasky Medical Center, Sackler Faculty of Medicine, Tel Aviv University, Tel Aviv [17]

Daniel A. Portnoy, PhD

Professor of Biochemistry and Molecular Biology, Department of Molecular and Cell Biology, University of California, Berkeley [132]

John T. Potts, Jr., MD

Jackson Distinguished Professor of Clinical Medicine, Harvard Medical School; Director of Research and Physician-in-Chief Emeritus, Massachusetts General Hospital, Charlestown [347]

Lawrie W. Powell, MD, PhD

Professor of Medicine, The University of Queensland and The Royal Brisbane and Women's Hospital, Brisbane, Queensland, Australia [351]

Alvin C. Powers, MD

Joe C. Davis Chair in Biomedical Science; Professor of Medicine, Molecular Physiology and Biophysics; Director, Vanderbilt Diabetes Research and Training Center; Director, Vanderbilt Diabetes Center, Nashville [338]

Daniel S. Pratt, MD

Assistant Professor of Medicine, Harvard Medical School; Director, Liver-Billary-Pancreas Center, Massachusetts General Hospital, Boston [43, 296]

Darwin J. Prockop, MD, PhD

Director of Center for Gene Therapy and Professor of Biochemistry, Tulane Health Sciences Center, New Orleans [357]

Stanley B. Prusiner, MD
Director, Institute for Neurodegenerative Diseases; Professor, Department of Neurology; Professor, Department of Biochemistry and Biophysics, University of California, San Francisco, San Francisco [378]

Daniel J. Rader, MD
Cooper-McClure Professor of Medicine, University of Pennsylvania School of Medicine, Philadelphia [350]

Roshini Rajapaksa, MD, BA
Assistant Professor, Department of Medicine, Gastroenterology, New York University Medical Center School of Medicine and Hospitals Center, New York [44]

Sanjay Ram, MD
Assistant Professor of Medicine, Division of Infectious Diseases and Immunology, University of Massachusetts Medical School, Worcester [137]

Jose A. F. Ramires
Head Professor of Cardiology; University of São Paulo Medical School and Heart Institute-INCOR, São Paulo, Brazil [e37]

Reuben Ramphal, MD
Professor, Division of Infectious Diseases, Department of Medicine, University of Florida College of Medicine, Gainesville [145]

Neil H. Raskin, MD
Professor of Neurology, University of California, San Francisco, San Francisco [15]

Mario C. Raviglione, MD
Director, StopTB Department, World Health Organization, Geneva [158]

K. Srinath Reddy, MD, DM, MSC
Department of Cardiology, All India Institute of Medical Sciences, Ansari Nagar, New Delhi, India [e38]

Sharon L. Reed, MD
Professor of Pathology and Medicine; Director, Microbiology and Virology Laboratories, University of California, San Diego Medical Center, San Diego [202, e16]

Richard C. Reichman, MD
Professor of Medicine and of Microbiology and Immunology; Director, Infectious Diseases Division, University of Rochester School of Medicine, Rochester [178]

Carol M. Reife, MD
Clinical Associate Professor of Medicine, Jefferson Medical College, Philadelphia [41]

John J. Reilly, Jr., MD
Associate Professor of Medicine, Harvard Medical School; Vice Chairman, Integrative Services, Department of Medicine, Brigham and Women's Hospital, Boston [254, e24]

John T. Repke, MD
University Professor and Chairman, Department of Obstetrics and Gynecology, Penn State University College of Medicine; Obstetrician-Gynecologist-In-Chief, The Milton S. Hershey Medical Center, Hershey [7]

Victor I. Reus, MD
Professor, Department of Psychiatry, University of California, San Francisco School of Medicine; Attending Physician, Langley Porter Hospital and Clinics, San Francisco [386]

Peter A. Rice, MD
Professor of Medicine, Division of Infectious Diseases and Immunology, University of Massachusetts Medical School, Worcester [137]

Stuart Rich, MD
Professor of Medicine, Section of Cardiology, University of Chicago, Chicago [244]

Gary S. Richardson, MD
Assistant Professor of Psychiatry, Case Western Reserve University, Cleveland; Senior Research Scientist, Sleep Disorders and Research Center, Henry Ford Hospital, Detroit [28]

Elizabeth Robbins, MD
Associate Clinical Professor, University of California, San Francisco, San Francisco [e32]

Gary L. Robertson, MD
Emeritus Professor of Medicine, Northwestern University Feinberg School of Medicine, Chicago [334]

Daniel M. Roden, MD
Professor of Medicine and Pharmacology, Assistant Vice-Chancellor for Personalized Medicine, Vanderbilt University, Nashville [5]

James A. Romano, Jr., PhD, DABT
Senior Principal Life Specialist, Science Applications International Corporation, Frederick [215]

Karen L. Roos, MD
John and Nancy Nelson Professor of Neurology, Indiana University School of Medicine, Indianapolis [376]

Allan H. Ropper, MD
Executive Vice-Chair, Department of Neurology, Brigham and Women's Hospital, Harvard Medical School, Boston [268, 372, 373]

Ilene M. Rosen, MD, MSc
Associate Director, Internal Medical Residency Program; Assistant Professor of Clinical Medicine, University of Pennsylvania School of Medicine, Philadelphia [246]

Roger N. Rosenberg, MD
Zale Distinguished Chair and Professor of Neurology, Department of Neurology, University of Texas Southwestern Medical Center, Dallas [368]

F. R. Rosendaal, MD
Professor of Clinical Epidemiology; Chairman, Department of Clinical Epidemiology, and Department of Thrombosis and Hemostasis, Leiden University Medical Center, The Netherlands [111]

Myrna R. Rosenfeld, MD, PhD
Associate Professor of Neurology, Division Neuro-Oncology, Department of Neurology, University of Pennsylvania, Philadelphia [97]

Jean-Claude Roujeau, MD
Professor of Dermatology, Hôpital Henri Mondor, Université Paris XII, Créteil, France [56]

Ambuj Roy, MD, DM
Department of Cardiology, All India Institute of Medical Sciences, Ansari Nagar, New Delhi, India [e38]

Michael A. Rubin, MD, PhD
Assistant Professor of Medicine, Division of Epidemiology and Infectious Diseases, Department of Internal Medicine, University of Utah School of Medicine, Salt Lake City [31]

Robert M. Russell, MD
Director, Jean Mayer USDA Human Nutrition Research Center on Aging at Tufts University; Professor of Medicine and Nutrition, Tufts University, Boston [71]

Thomas A. Russo, MD, CM
Professor of Medicine and Microbiology, State University of New York, Buffalo [143, 156]

Miguel Sabria, MD, PhD
Professor of Medicine, Autonomous University of Barcelona; Chief, Infectious Diseases Section, Germans Trias i Pujol Hospital, Barcelona, Spain [141]

Stephen M. Sagar, MD
Professor of Neurology, Case Western Reserve School of Medicine; Director of Neuro-Oncology, Ireland Cancer Center, University Hospitals of Cleveland, Cleveland [374]

David J. Salant, MD
Professor of Medicine, Pathology, and Laboratory Medicine, Boston University School of Medicine; Chief, Section of Nephrology, Boston Medical Center, Boston [278]

Martin A. Samuels, MD, DSc (Hon)
Chairman, Department of Neurology, Brigham and Women's Hospital; Professor of Neurology, Harvard Medical Center, Boston [e33]

Merle A. Sande,† MD
Professor of Medicine, University of Washington School of Medicine; President, Academic Alliance Foundation, Seattle [31]

Philippe Sansonetti
Professeur à l'Institut Pasteur, Paris, France [147]

Edward A. Sausville, MD, PhD
Professor of Medicine; Associate Director for Clinical Research, Marlene & Stewart Greenebaum Cancer Center, University of Maryland, Baltimore [81]

---

†Deceased.

xxxii

Mohamed H. Sayegh, MD
Director, Warren E. Grupe and John P. Morill Chair in Transplantation
Medicine; Professor of Medicine and Pediatrics, Harvard Medical School,
Boston [276]

David T. Scadden, MD
Gerald and Darlene Jordan Professor of Medicine, Harvard University;
Co-Chair, Department of Stem Cell and Regenerative Biology, Harvard
University, Boston [68]

Howard I. Scher, MD
Professor of Medicine, Weill Medical College of Cornell University; D. Wayne
Calloway Chair in Urologic Oncology; Chief, Genitourinary Oncology Service,
Memorial Sloan-Kettering Cancer Center, New York [90, 91]

Joan H. Schiller, MD
Professor of Medicine and Hematology/Oncology, University of Texas
Southwestern Medical School; Simmons Comprehensive Cancer Center,
Dallas [85]

Harry W. Schroeder, Jr., MD, PhD
Professor of Medicine, Microbiology, and Genetics, The University of Alabama,
Birmingham [310, e27]

Marc A. Schuckit, MD
Distinguished Professor of Psychiatry, School of Medicine, University of
California, San Diego; Director, Alcohol Research Center, VA San Diego
Healthcare System, San Diego [387, 388]

H. Ralph Schumacher, MD
Professor of Medicine, University of Pennsylvania School of Medicine,
Philadelphia [327]

Gordon E. Schutze, MD
Professor of Pediatrics and Pathology, University of Arkansas for Medical
Sciences, College of Medicine; Chief, Pediatric Infectious Diseases, Arkansas
Children's Hospital, Little Rock [151]

Stuart Schwartz, PhD
Professor of Human Genetics, Medicine and Pathology, University of Chicago,
Chicago [63]

Richard M. Schwartzstein, MD
Professor of Medicine, Harvard Medical School; Associate Chair, Pulmonary
and Critical Care Medicine; Vice-President for Education, Beth Israel
Deaconess Medical Center, Boston [33]

Julian L. Seifter, MD
Physician, Brigham and Women's Hospital; Associate Professor of Medicine,
Harvard Medical School, Boston [283]

David C. Seldin, MD, PhD
Professor of Medicine and Microbiology; Director, Amyloid Treatment and
Research Program Section of Hematology-Oncology, Department of Medicine,
Boston University School of Medicine and Boston Medical Center, Boston [324]

Andrew P. Selwyn, MA, MD
Professor of Medicine, Harvard Medical School, Boston [237]

Steven D. Shapiro, MD
Jack D. Myers Professor and Chair, University of Pittsburgh, Pittsburgh [254,
262]

William Silen, MD
Johnson and Johnson Distinguished Professor of Surgery, Emeritus, Harvard
Medical School, Boston [14, 293, 294]

Rebecca A. Silliman, MD, PhD
Professor of Medicine and Epidemiology, Boston University Schools of
Medicine and Public Health; Chief, Section of Geriatrics, Boston University
Medical Center, Boston [9]

Edwin K. Silverman, MD, PhD
Associate Professor of Medicine, Harvard Medical School, Brigham and
Women's Hospital, Boston [254]

Gary G. Singer, MD
Assistant Professor of Clinical Medicine, Washington University School of
Medicine, St. Louis [46]

Martha Skinner, MD
Professor of Medicine, Boston University School of Medicine; Director, Special
Projects, Amyloid Treatment and Research Program, Boston [324]

Karl Skorecki, MD
Annie Chutick Professor in Medicine (Nephrology); Director, Rappaport
Research Institute, Director of Medical and Research Development, Rambam
Medical Health Care Campus, Haifa, Israel [274, e39]

Wade S. Smith, MD, PhD
Professor of Neurology, Daryl R. Gress Endowed Chair of Neurocritical Care
and Stroke; Director, University of California, San Francisco Neurovascular
Service, San Francisco [269, 364]

A. George Smulian, MB, BCh
Associate Professor, University of Cincinnati College of Medicine; Chief,
Infectious Disease Section, Cincinnati VA Medical Center, Cincinnati [200]

Arthur J. Sober, MD
Professor, Department of Dermatology, Harvard Medical School; Associate
Chief, Department of Dermatology, Massachusetts General Hospital,
Boston [83]

Kelly A. Soderberg, PhD, MPH
Director, Program Management, Duke Human Vaccine Institute, Duke
University School of Medicine, Durham [308]

Michael F. Sorrell, MD
Robert L. Grissom Professor of Medicine, University of Nebraska Medical
Center, Omaha [301]

David H. Spach, MD
Professor of Medicine, Division of Infectious Diseases, University of
Washington, Seattle [153]

Peter Speelman, MD, PhD
Professor of Medicine and Infectious Diseases; Head, Division of Infectious
Diseases, Tropical Medicine and AIDS; Department of Internal Medicine,
Academic Medical Center, University of Amsterdam, The Netherlands [164]

Frank E. Speizer, MD
Edward H. Kass Professor of Medicine, Harvard Medical School, Channing
Laboratory, Department of Medicine, Brigham and Women's Hospital,
Boston [250]

Jerry L. Spivak, MD
Professor of Medicine, The Johns Hopkins University School of Medicine;
Attending Physician, Johns Hopkins Hospital, Baltimore [103]

Andrei C. Sposito
Professor of Medicine, University of Basilia Medical School, Basilia, Brazil [e37]

Walter E. Stamm, MD
Professor of Medicine; Head, Division of Allergy and Infectious Diseases,
University of Washington School of Medicine, Seattle [169, 282]

Allen C. Steere, MD
Professor of Medicine, Harvard Medical School, Boston [166]

Robert S. Stern, MD
Dermatologist-in-Chief; Carl J. Herzog Professor of Medicine, Harvard
Medical School, Boston [56]

Dennis L. Stevens, MD, PhD
Chief, Infectious Diseases Section, Veteran Affairs Medical Center, Boise; Professor
of Medicine, University of Washington School of Medicine, Seattle [119]

Stephen E. Straus,† MD
Senior Investigator, Laboratory of Clinical Investigation, National Institute of
Allergy and Infectious Diseases; Director, National Center for Complementary
and Alternative Medicine, National Institutes of Health, Bethesda [10, 384]

Lewis Sudarsky, MD
Associate Professor of Neurology, Harvard Medical School; Director of
Movement Disorders, Brigham and Women's Hospital, Boston [24]

Alan M. Sugar, MD
Professor of Medicine, Boston University School of Medicine; Medical
Director, Infectious Diseases Clinical Services, HIV/AIDS Program, and
Infection Control, Cape Cod Healthcare, Hyannis [198]

Donna C. Sullivan, PhD
Associate Professor of Medicine and Microbiology, Division of Infectious
Diseases, Department of Medicine, University of Mississippi School of
Medicine, Jackson [194, 199]

---

†Deceased.

Paolo M. Suter, MD, MS
Professor of Medicine, Medical Policlinic, Zurich, Switzerland [71]

Morton N. Swartz, MD
Professor of Medicine, Harvard Medical School; Chief, Jackson Firm Medical Service and Infectious Disease Unit, Massachusetts General Hospital, Boston [377]

A. Jamil Tajik, MD
Thomas J. Watson, Jr., Professor; Professor of Medicine and Pediatrics; Chairman (Emeritus), Zayed Cardiovascular Center, Mayo Clinic, Rochester, Minnesota; Consultant, Cardiovascular Division, Mayo Clinic, Scottsdale [222, e20]

Joel D. Taurog, MD
Professor of Internal Medicine, William M. and Gatha Burnett Professor for Arthritis Research, University of Texas Southwestern Medical Center, Dallas [318]

Stephen F. Templeton, MD
Clinical Assistant Professor of Dermatology, Emory University School of Medicine, Atlanta [e10]

Gregory Tino, MD
Associate Professor of Medicine, University of Pennsylvania School of Medicine; Chief, Pulmonary Clinical Service Hospital of the University of Pennsylvania, Philadelphia [252]

Zelig A. Tochner, MD
Associate Professor of Radiation Oncology; Clinical Director, Proton Therapy Project, University of Pennsylvania, Philadelphia [216]

Gordon F. Tomaselli, MD
David J. Carver Professor of Medicine, Vice Chairman, Department of Medicine for Research, The Johns Hopkins University, Baltimore [224, 225]

Mark Topazian, MD
Associate Professor of Medicine, Mayo College of Medicine, Rochester [285, e25]

Phillip P. Toskes, MD
Professor of Medicine, Division of Gastroenterology, Hepatology and Nutrition, University of Florida College of Medicine, Gainesville [306, 307]

Jeffrey M. Trent, PhD
President and Scientific Director, Translational Genomics Research Institute, Phoenix [79]

Elbert P. Trulock, MD
Professor of Medicine, Rosemary and I. Jerome Flance Professor of Pulmonary Medicine, Washington University School of Medicine, St. Louis [260]

Hensin Tsao, MD
Assistant Professor of Dermatology, Harvard Medical School; Clinical Director, Melanoma Genetics Program, Massachusetts General Hospital, Boston [83]

Kenneth L. Tyler, MD
Reuler-Lewin Family Professor of Neurology and Professor of Medicine and Microbiology, University of Colorado Health Sciences Center; Chief, Neurology Service, Denver Veterans Affairs Medical Center, Denver [376]

Joseph P. Vacanti, MD
John Homan Professor of Surgery, Harvard Medical School; Surgeon-in-Chief, Massachusetts General Hospital for Children, Boston [69]

Edouard Vannier, PhD
Assistant Professor, Department of Medicine, Division of Infectious Diseases, Tufts–New England Medical Center and Tufts University School of Medicine, Boston [204]

Gauri R. Varadhachary, MD
Associate Professor, Department of Gastrointestinal Medical Oncology, University of Texas MD Anderson Cancer Center, Houston [95]

John Varga, MD
Hughes Professor of Medicine, Northwestern University Feinberg School of Medicine, Chicago [316]

Bert Vogelstein, MD
Director, Ludwig Center for Cancer Genetics & Therapeutics; Investigator, Howard Hughes Medical Institute; Clayton Professor for Oncology & Pathology, Baltimore [79]

Everett E. Vokes, MD
Director, Section of Hematology/Oncology; Vice Chairman for Clinical Research, Department of Medicine; Deputy Director, Cancer Research Center; John E. Ultmann Professor of Medicine and Radiation and Cellular Oncology, Chicago [84]

Tamara J. Vokes, MD
Associate Professor, Section of Endocrinology, University of Chicago, Chicago [349]

C. Fordham von Reyn, MD
Professor of Medicine (Infectious Disease) and International Health; Director, DARDAR International Programs, Dartmouth Medical School, Lebanon [160]

Matthew K. Waldor, MD, PhD
Professor of Medicine (Microbiology and Molecular Genetics), Channing Laboratory, Brigham and Women's Hospital, Harvard Medical School, Boston [149]

David H. Walker, MD
The Carnage and Martha Walls Distinguished University Chair in Tropical Diseases; Professor and Chairman, Department of Pathology; Executive Director, Center for Biodefense and Emerging Infectious Disease, University of Texas Medical Branch, Galveston [167]

Richard J. Wallace, Jr., MD
Chairman, Department of Microbiology, University of Texas Health Center at Tyler, Tyler [161]

B. Timothy Walsh, MD
Professor of Psychiatry, College of Physicians & Surgeons, Columbia University; Director, Eating Disorders Research Unit, New York Psychiatric Institute, New York [76]

Peter D. Walzer, MD, MSc
Associate Chief of Staff for Research, Cincinnati VA Medical Center; Professor of Medicine, University of Cincinnati College of Medicine, Cincinnati [200]

Fred Wang, MD
Professor of Medicine, Harvard Medical School, Boston [170, 176]

Carl V. Washington, Jr., MD
Associate Professor of Dermatology, Emory University School of Medicine; Co-Director, Dermatologic Surgery Unit, The Emory Clinic, Atlanta [83]

Anthony P. Weetman, MD, DSc
Professor of Medicine and Dean of the School of Medicine and Biomedical Sciences, University of Sheffield, Sheffield, United Kingdom [335]

Steven E. Weinberger, MD
Senior Vice President for Medical Education Division, American College of Physicians; Senior Lecturer on Medicine, Harvard Medical School; Adjunct Professor of Medicine, University of Pennsylvania School of Medicine, Philadelphia [34, 245–247, 252]

Robert A. Weinstein, MD
Professor of Medicine, Rush University Medical Center; Chairman, Infectious Diseases, Cook County Hospital; Chief Operating Officer, CORE Center, Chicago [125]

Jeffrey I. Weitz, MD
Professor of Medicine and Biochemistry, McMaster University; Director, Henderson Research Centre, Heart and Stroke Foundation/J. Fraser Mustard Chair in Cardiovascular Research; Canada Research Chair (Tier1) in Thrombosis; Career Investigator, Heart and Stroke Foundation of Canada [112]

Peter F. Weller, MD
Professor of Medicine, Harvard Medical School; Co-Chief, Infectious Diseases Division; Chief, Allergy and Inflammation Division; Vice-Chair for Research, Department of Medicine, Beth Israel Deaconess Medical Center, Boston [208–211, 213]

Michael R. Wessels, MD
Professor of Pediatrics and Medicine (Microbiology and Molecular Genetics), Harvard Medical School; Chief, Division of Infectious Diseases, Children's Hospital, Boston [130]

Lee M. Wetzler, MD
Professor of Medicine, Associate Professor of Microbiology, Boston University School of Medicine, Boston [136]

Meir Wetzler, MD
Professor of Medicine, Roswell Park Cancer Institute, Buffalo [104]

L. Joseph Wheat, MD
President and Director, MiraVista Diagnostics and MiraBella Technology, Indianapolis [192]

xxxiv

A. Clinton White, Jr., MD
The Paul R. Stalnaker, MD, Distinguished Professor of Internal Medicine; Director, Infectious Disease Division, Department of Internal Medicine, University of Texas Medical Branch, Galveston [213]

Nicholas J. White, DSc
Professor of Tropical Medicine, Oxford University, United Kingdom; Mahidol University, Bangkok, Thailand [203, e18]

Richard J. Whitley, MD
Loeb Scholar in Pediatrics, Professor of Pediatrics, Microbiology, Medicine, and Neurosurgery, University of Alabama, Birmingham [173]

Gordon H. Williams, MD
Professor of Medicine, Harvard Medical School; Chief, Cardiovascular Endocrinology Section, Brigham and Women's Hospital, Boston [336]

John W. Winkleman, MD, PhD
Assistant Professor of Psychiatry, Harvard Medical School; Medical Director, Sleep Health Center, Brigham and Women's Hospital, Boston [28]

Bruce U. Wintroub, MD
Professor and Chair of Dermatology, Department of Dermatology; Vice Dean, School of Medicine Dean's Office, University of California, San Francisco, San Francisco [56]

Allan W. Wolkoff, MD
Professor of Medicine and Anatomy and Structural Biology; Director, Belfer Institute for Advanced Biomedical Studies; Associate Chair of Medicine for Research; Chief, Division of Hepatology, Albert Einstein College of Medicine, Bronx [297]

Louis Michel Wong-Kee-Song, MD
Assistant Professor of Medicine, Division of Gastroenterology and Hepatology, Mayo College of Medicine, Rochester [285, e25]

Robert L. Wortmann, MD
Dartmouth-Hitchcock Medical Center, Lebanon [353]

Richard Wunderink, MD
Professor, Division of Pulmonary and Critical Care, Department of Medicine, Northwestern University Feinberg School of Medicine; Director, Medical Intensive Care Unit, Northwestern Memorial Hospital, Chicago [251]

Joshua Wynne, MD, MBA, MPH
Executive Associate Dean, Professor of Medicine, University of North Dakota School of Medicine and Health Sciences, Grand Forks [231]

Kim B. Yancey, MD
Professor and Chair, Department of Dermatology, University of Texas, Southwestern, Dallas [52, 55]

Janet A. Yellowitz, DMD, MPH
Associate Professor; Director, Geriatric Dentistry, Baltimore [e7]

Neal S. Young, MD
Chief, Hematology Branch, National Heart, Lung, and Blood Institute, National Institutes of Health, Bethesda [102]

Robert C. Young, MD
Chancellor, Fox Chase Cancer Center, Philadelphia [93]

Alan S. L. Yu, MB, BChir
Associate Professor of Medicine, Physiology and Biophysics, University of Southern California Keck School of Medicine, Los Angeles [279]

Victor L. Yu, MD
Professor of Medicine, University of Pittsburgh, Pittsburgh [141]

The first edition of *Harrison's Principles of Internal Medicine* was published almost 60 years ago. Over the decades, the field of internal medicine has evolved greatly and has incorporated the spectacular advances that have occurred in the science of medicine into its armamentarium of diagnosis, prevention, and treatment. This textbook has evolved simultaneously to keep step with these advances while at the same time maintaining an appreciation of the art of medicine and the principles underlying the optimal care of the patient. In shaping and revising this latest edition, the Editors have committed themselves to making the textbook an invaluable resource for students and practitioners coping with the demands of modern medicine.

From the standpoint of physical appearance, one of the most striking elements of the textbook is the number of new and updated figures. The seventeenth edition features 300 additional illustrations (20% more than the previous edition); with the new illustrations included on the enclosed DVD, this edition has approximately 800 more images, a 60% increase in the course of just one edition. Many images have been redrawn by graphic artists working closely with the authors and editors to illustrate complex concepts, pathways, and algorithms in a clear and compelling manner. The seventeenth edition also features many additional plain film, CT, MRI, and ultrasound images, in recognition of the increased use of radiologic diagnosis in general medical practice. The notably increased use of pathologic and clinical photographs completes our concerted approach to a more robustly illustrated edition of *Harrison's*.

The seventeenth edition of *Harrison's* has a full-color format that draws from and extends the excellent appearance of the sixteenth edition to make the content more accessible and pleasant to read. The placement of color illustrations within the chapters rather than in the separate atlas was very favorably received by our sixteenth edition readers and has been continued in the current edition. Many changes to the design of this edition have been made in order to speed the reader's navigation through the textual and visual materials. For example, tables have been shaded for ease of reading, citations in tables and illustrations are now more instantly notable and in color, and our Treatment sections in each chapter have been redesigned to allow even faster access. The new global icons call greater attention to key epidemiologic and clinical differences in the practice of medicine throughout the world.

Evolving information technology enables us to broaden and deepen the nature, format, and medium of content included under the *Harrison's* name. Purchase of this textbook now includes a DVD, which has allowed the editors to expand the content in *Harrison's* by the use of "e-chapters," 39 in number. In addition to new chapters in traditional narrative format, the DVD includes a number of diagnostic and procedural atlases, which readers should find enormously helpful. The DVD also includes dozens of motion video clips of endoscopic and cardiac imaging. These diagnostic approaches have become central to the practice of medicine, and the video clips show crystal-clear depictions of abnormal anatomy, function, and results.

Globalization of economies and trade has had an enormous impact on nations throughout the world, both developing and developed. This phenomenon has underscored the reality of the globalization of medicine. In this regard, as this textbook is widely used by students and practitioners throughout the world and as we in the United States are more frequently confronted with issues related to global health, a special emphasis has been placed in this edition on global health in individual chapters together with an over-arching view presented by Dr. Kim and Dr. Farmer in a new chapter entitled "Global Issues in Medicine." We have highlighted, where appropriate, regional differences in the prevalence, approach, and treatment of diseases that need to be considered for delivery of the highest-quality medical care possible in various geographic settings. These are only highlights of the changes that the Editors hope will make the new *Harrison's* a helpful tool, not only for the student who needs an expert source of basic knowledge in internal medicine, but also for the pressured practitioner who needs a clear, concise, and balanced distillation of the best information on which to base daily clinical decisions.

The seventeenth edition has been enriched by the addition of a new editor, Joseph Loscalzo, MD, PhD, who joined with our most senior editor Eugene Braunwald, MD, in contributing to and/or editing of chapters in the Parts on Disorders of the Cardiovascular System, Disorders of the Respiratory System, and Disorders of the Kidney and Urinary Tract. The addition of Dr. Loscalzo provides a smooth editorial transition in preparation for the upcoming retirement from *Harrison's* of Dr. Braunwald who has served as an esteemed editor for 12 editions.

Part 1, "Introduction to Clinical Medicine," contains a new chapter that lays the framework for appreciating the global issues in medicine and the variations in disease incidence and patterns throughout the world. It sets the stage for the discussion in individual chapters of global issues related to specific diseases, a novel feature in this edition. In addition, there are e-chapters on quality and safety issues in patient care, economics of health care delivery, ethics in clinical medicine, and health care disparities. The last chapter addresses the evidence for racial and ethnic disparities in health care in the United States and globally and offers a variety of approaches for minimizing them.

Part 2, "Cardinal Manifestations and Presentation of Diseases," serves as a comprehensive introduction to clinical medicine as well as a practical guide to the care of patients with these manifestations. Each section focuses on a particular group of disorders, examining the concepts of pathophysiology and differential diagnosis that must be considered in caring for patients with these common clinical presentations. Major symptoms are reviewed and correlated with specific disease states, and clinical approaches to patients presenting with these symptoms are summarized. There are eleven new chapters in this Part. Every chapter that appeared in the sixteenth edition has been updated, and two chapters have new authors. Among the e-chapters are atlases of rashes associated with fever; oral manifestations of disease; renal biopsies and urinary sediments; skin manifestations of internal disease; and peripheral blood and bone marrow. A new chapter on Hypercalcemia and Hypocalcemia provides a succinct overview of the causes, clinical presentations, and management of these conditions as a complement to the more extensive discussion of these topics in Part 15, "Endocrinology and Metabolism." New chapters discuss common clinical presentations such as menstrual disorders and pelvic pain, the pathogenesis and treatment of headache, the clinical approach to imbalance, and the causes of confusion and delirium.

Part 3, "Genetics and Disease," has been extensively updated, reflecting the remarkable impact of the human genome project and its implications for clinical medicine. The material included in this edition is strongly geared toward clinical practice, in which genetic information increasingly comes into play. A new chapter on gene transfer in clinical medicine addresses the principles and strategies for this novel, but still experimental, therapeutic area.

Part 4, "Regenerative Medicine," is a new part initiated for this edition. It contains chapters on Stem Cell Biology, Applications of Stem Cell Biology in Clinical Medicine, Hematopoietic Stem Cells, and Tissue Engineering. These chapters summarize the state of the science in these emerging fields and outline the future directions for clinical applications of stem cell biology in regenerative medicine.

Part 5, "Nutrition," covers topics critical to clinical medicine, whether dealing with undernutrition in the context of chronic starvation or acute illness or the implications of overfeeding in industrialized nations. New authors with global expertise in nutrition have prepared the chapters on protein-energy malnutrition and enteral and parenteral nutrition therapy. A new chapter on the Management of Obesity and a complementary chapter on the Biology of Obesity address the explosion of new knowledge about pathways that regulate body weight and composition and the urgent need to provide effective means to prevent and treat the global epidemic of obesity and its complications.

The core of *Harrison's* continues to encompass the disorders of the organ systems and is contained in Parts 6 through 17. These sections include succinct accounts of the pathophysiology of diseases involving the major organ systems as well as infectious diseases, with an emphasis on clinical manifestations, diagnostic procedures, differential diagnosis, and treatment strategies and guidelines.

Part 6, "Oncology and Hematology," includes 11 chapters by new authors, including a completely revised section on Disorders of Hemostasis. A new e-chapter on Thymoma has also been added. As novel therapies are being added at a record pace to the armamentarium for oncologic and hematologic disorders, the mechanisms of action, pharmacology, clinical uses, and toxicities of these new agents have been included. Recent progress in the treatment of renal cell cancer, colorectal cancer, and breast cancer is highlighted. Revised chapters include the impact of genetic factors on cancer development and the use of gene expression data to define prognostic disease subsets.

Part 7, "Infectious Diseases," presents an overview of the latest information on disease epidemiology, pathogenesis, and genetics while focusing on the needs of clinicians who must accurately diagnose and treat infections under time pressure and cost constraints. Abundant illustrations offer key information in an easily accessible format to assist clinicians with these challenges. The expert authors of each chapter make specific recommendations regarding therapeutic regimens, including the drug(s) of choice, doses, durations, and alternatives. Current trends in antimicrobial resistance are discussed fully in light of their impact on therapeutic choices. In line with the international emphasis of this edition, the infectious diseases section includes expanded information on disease prevalences, distributions, features, and management in different regions of the world.

A total of 17 chapters have been completely rewritten by new authors, covering the latest advances in the management of important diseases such as pneumonia, shigellosis, and rabies and of infections due to *Pseudomonas*, *Bartonella*, *Listeria*, corynebacteria, and parvovirus. The section on fungal infections is entirely new and encompasses the expertise of current authorities on specific mycoses. Health care–associated infections, an area of enormous significance in terms of patient care in general and antimicrobial resistance in particular, are addressed by Robert Weinstein in a thorough, highly practical chapter. Another topic of ever-increasing importance—infections with gram-negative enteric bacilli, including *Escherichia coli*—is dealt with by Thomas Russo and James Johnson in a substantially reworked and updated chapter. The superb chapter on human papillomaviruses by Richard Reichman includes the latest information and recommendations regarding the recently licensed and widely publicized HPV vaccine. Finally, the chapter on HIV infection and AIDS by Anthony S. Fauci and H. Clifford Lane has once again been completely revised, with an emphasis on therapeutic strategies. This chapter is widely considered to be a classic in the field; its clinically pragmatic focus in combination with its comprehensive and analytical approach to the pathogenesis of HIV disease has led to its use as the sole complete reference on HIV/AIDS in medical schools.

New in this edition is a chapter on babesiosis, an important emerging infection that can cause severe disease in immunodeficient and elderly patients. Three additional new chapters of substantial clinical relevance appear in the electronic version of the textbook: an atlas of rashes associated with fever, an atlas of blood smears showing the various stages of the parasites causing malaria and babesiosis, and a chapter detailing the pharmacology of antiparasitic agents.

Terrorist attacks in various forms have become a frightening reality throughout the world. Important among these is the threat of bioterror attacks involving microbes or their toxins, chemicals, and radiation. This has become of particular concern in light of the anthrax attacks in the United States shortly after the September 11, 2001, airplane attacks on the World Trade Center in New York City and the Pentagon in Washington, DC. In the sixteenth edition, the editors developed a new Part on Bioterrorism and Clinical Medicine. Part 8 in the current edition has been updated with descriptions of the most recent countermeasures that have been developed as part of the United States

preparedness plan against bioterror attacks. Edited by *Harrison's* Anthony S. Fauci, these chapters are written succinctly and include easily readable charts, tables, and algorithms; their goal is to confer an understanding of the pathogenesis, diagnosis, treatment, and prognosis of the diseases in question.

Part 9, "Disorders of the Cardiovascular System," is now co-edited by two of the most preeminent experts in the field, Eugene Braunwald and Joseph Loscalzo, the newest addition to the team of *Harrison* editors. There are new chapters on the epidemiology of cardiovascular disease with an overview of the global nature of the growing pandemic, the basic biology of the cardiovascular system (written by Braunwald, Libby, and Loscalzo), and principles of electrophysiology. A new chapter on the metabolic syndrome summarizes the clinical features and complications of this disorder, which reflects the rapidly rising prevalence of obesity and insulin resistance. In addition, there are new e-chapters that provide atlases of basic electrocardiography, arrhythmias, noninvasive imaging, and percutaneous revascularization. Finally, every chapter has been revised to reflect the latest information on approaches to the diagnosis and treatment of specific cardiovascular diseases, and eight of these chapters have been written by new authors.

Part 10, "Disorders of the Respiratory System," includes a new e-chapter on chest imaging that provides an atlas of chest radiographs and computed tomographic studies of a wide range of chest diseases. In addition, three chapters have been written by new authors, including a superb chapter on asthma by Peter Barnes and an excellent chapter on pneumonia by Lionel Mandell.

With advances in health care delivery and pressures aimed at cost containment, critical care units account for a growing percentage of hospital beds. Part 11, "Critical Care Medicine," was first introduced as a separate Part for the sixteenth edition of *Harrison's*. It is devoted to the provision of optimal care in this medical setting of growing importance and deals with four main areas: respiratory critical care, shock and cardiac arrest, neurologic critical care, and a new section on oncologic emergencies.

Part 12, "Disorders of the Kidney and Urinary Tract," has undergone extensive revision and reorganization under the guidance of new editor Joseph Loscalzo. There is an outstanding new chapter on the cellular and molecular biology of the kidney by Eric Neilson, as well as a new e-chapter atlas of urinary sediments and renal pathology. In addition to a thorough updating of each revised chapter, five have new authors who bring a unique, contemporary perspective to their subject.

Part 13, "Disorders of the Gastrointestinal System," includes two new atlases of endoscopic findings, both static photographs and movies. New chapters have been added on mesenteric vascular insufficiency and common disorders of the colon and ano-rectum, and new authors have written two other chapters. The chapter on Cirrhosis and Its Complications has been completely rewritten by a new author, Bruce Bacon, who is also the new author for the chapter on Infiltrative, Genetic, and Metabolic Diseases Affecting the Liver. An Atlas of Liver Biopsies has been added as a new e-chapter.

Part 14, "Disorders of the Immune System, Connective Tissue, and Joints," has been extensively revised. The chapter on Introduction to the Immune System has been thoroughly updated. It has become a classic in its field and is often used as the textbook of immunology in postgraduate and medical school courses. This chapter combines an in-depth description and analysis of the principles of basic immunology with an easy flow into the application of these principles to clinical disease states. Its description of the relationship of innate to adaptive immunity is a model for understanding the intricacies of the human immune system. A new e-chapter written by Max Cooper on Primary Immunodeficiencies Associated with or Secondary to Other Diseases has been added to complement his printed book chapter on Primary Immunodeficiencies. The chapter on Systemic Sclerosis (Scleroderma) and Related Disorders has been rewritten by a new author. An Atlas of Clinical Imaging in the Vasculitis Syndromes has been added as a new e-chapter. The chapters on Sarcoidosis, Amyloidosis, Osteoarthritis, and Gout and Other Crystal Arthropathies have been rewritten by new authors. A highly skilled, academic, and clinical rheumatologist (Carol Langford) has joined the team as an author and has co-authored the chapters on the Vasculitis Syndromes, Relapsing Polychondritis, Fibromyalgia, and Arthritis Associated with Systemic Disease and Other Arthritides.

Part 15, "Endocrinology and Metabolism," includes several new authors, including those for the chapter on pheochromocytoma, which highlights recent advances in the genetic causes of these catecholamine-secreting tumors, as well as updated strategies for diagnosis and management. The chapter on the Ovary has a new author who integrates traditional hypothalamic-pituitary regulation of the menstrual cycle with the identification of multiple ovarian growth factors that regulate follicle development. Identification of these pathways has provided insight into the causes of premature ovarian failure and infertility. There have been rapid changes in the clinical management of many endocrine diseases, especially diabetes, lipoprotein disorders, and the menopause. These and other chapters have been updated extensively. A new Atlas of Metabolic Disorders has been added as an e-chapter.

Part 16, "Neurologic Disorders," has been extensively rewritten to highlight the many advances that have taken place in the understanding, diagnosis, treatment, and prevention of neurologic and psychiatric diseases. Notable are new chapters on essential tremor and movement disorders, peripheral neuropathy, and neurologic problems in hospitalized patients. Many illustrative neuroimaging figures appear throughout the section, and a new atlas of neuroimaging findings has been added. Knowledge of the dementias, Parkinson's disease, and related neurodegenerative disorders has been transformed by new findings from genetics, modular imaging, cell biology, and clinical research. The very latest information has been included, providing a practical guide to diagnosis and appropriate use of the latest treatments. New therapies are also revolutionizing the care of patients with stroke and multiple sclerosis, and these are also discussed in an evidence-based fashion that will be useful to all practitioners and not only to specialists. Another new chapter, authored by Stephen Hyman and Eric Kandel, reviews progress in deciphering the pathogenesis of common psychiatric disorders and discusses the remaining challenges to development of more effective treatments.

Part 17, "Poisoning, Drug Overdose, and Envenomation," focuses on topics most relevant to internal medicine.

Part 18 is a new feature to *Harrison's* and represents four brand new e-chapters from our International Advisory Editors. Dr. Peter Barnes addresses the emerging use of pulmonary biomarkers in COPD. This state of the art summary will be useful to clinicians and researchers alike. Chagas' disease continues to cause significant morbidity in Central and South America, and the long period between infection and cardiovascular complications can make the etiologic aspects of its diagnosis difficult. The cardiovascular pathologies and sequelae, as well as current approaches to diagnosis and treatment, are clearly described by Dr. Sposito and Dr. Ramires. Chapter e38 by Dr. Reddy, Dr. Naik, and Dr. Roy addresses the potential benefits and challenges of a polypill for multiple cardiovascular risk factors, an issue of global interest in light of increases in cardiovascular disease worldwide. Interest in the mitochondrial role in human health and disease has advanced considerably in recent years, and Chapter e39 by Dr. Skorecki and Dr. Mandel sets forth the current understanding of the role of the mitochondria in a large number of diseases and approaches to diagnosis and treatment.

Within the last 10 years, the *Harrison's* collection of publications has expanded as information delivery technology has evolved. *Harrison's Online (HOL)* is now one of the standard informational resources used in medical centers throughout the United States. In addition to the full content of the parent text, HOL offers frequent updates from and links to the emerging scientific and clinical literature; an expanded collection of reference citations; audio recordings and Podcasts of lectures by authorities in the various specialties of medicine; and other helpful supplementary materials such as a complete database of pharmacologic therapeutics, self-assessment questions for examination and board review; and an expanded collection of clinical photographs. The brand new "e-chapters" on the enclosed DVD, including the video clips of cardiac and endoscopic imaging, are also available on *HOL*. Future iterations of *HOL* will include expanded use of such supple-

mentary multimedia materials to illustrate further key concepts and clinical approaches discussed in the parent text.

In 2006, in recognition of the increasing time pressures placed on clinicians and the increasing use of electronic medical records systems, *Harrison's Practice of Medicine (HP)* made its debut. *HP* is a comprehensive database of specific clinical topics built from the ground up to provide authoritative guidance quickly at the point of care. *HP* is highly structured so that physicians and other health professionals can access the most salient features of any one of more than 700 diseases and clinical presentations within minutes. This innovative new application is updated regularly and includes fully integrated, detailed information on brand name and generic drugs. In addition, hyperlinks throughout *HP* enable quick access to the primary literature via PubMed. *HP* is available via the Internet and on PDA; samples of approximately 20 core topics from *HP* are included on the DVD packaged within this book.

The print publications within the *Harrison's* family are being revised for publication in new editions. The *Harrison's Manual of Medicine* is widely used by students and clinicians worldwide and, like the parent text, is available in print and digital formats. The PDA version of the *Harrison's Manual* provides full text coverage, the full complement of illustrations and tables from the print edition, and extensive cross-referencing between terms. In view of the requirements for continuing education for licensure and relicensure as well as emphasis on certification and recertification, a revision of the *Harrison's Self-Assessment and Board Review* will be published with this edition. This volume is again in the capable hands of Dr. Charles Wiener from Johns Hopkins. It consists of several hundred questions based on the seventeenth edition of *Harrison's*, along with answers and explanations for the answers.

Taken as a portfolio, *Harrison's* is now available in a wide variety of formats suitable for all levels of medical education and practice, and for all varieties of health care settings. It is gratifying that, whether in print or digital formats, the content within *Harrison's* remains so widely used and referenced by students and clinicians throughout medicine and health care across the globe.

We wish to express our appreciation to our many associates and colleagues, who, as experts in their fields, have offered us constructive criticisms and helpful suggestions. We acknowledge especially the contributions of the following individuals: Arv Vanagunas, Laura Kulik, Pat Lynch, Sundeep Khosla, Michael Bray, Mark D. Carlson, Daniel H. Lowenstein, Lawrence C. Madoff, Chung Owyang, Alice Pau, Mary Wright, and Gregory K. Folkers.

We thank in particular Kenneth and Elaine Kaye and Lindsey Baden, who gathered many high-quality illustrations of infectious disease manifestations. We also express our gratitude to Eileen J. Scott, who has applied her editorial expertise to the past six editions of *Harrison's*, and Alan Barnett, the text designer for this edition. This book could not have been edited without the dedicated help of our co-workers in the editorial offices of the individual editors. We are especially indebted to Patricia L. Duffey, Gregory K. Folkers, Sarah Matero, Julie B. McCoy, Elizabeth Robbins, Kathryn Saxon, Marie Scurti, Stephanie Tribuna, Karl Cremieux, and Kristina Shontz.

Finally, we continue to be highly indebted to the outstanding members of the McGraw-Hill organization: Mariapaz Ramos Englis, Senior Managing Editor, who will be retiring after serving the book and its Editors so well for four editions; Phil Galea and Catherine Saggese, Production Director and Manager, respectively; Jenna Esposito, the Editorial Assistant for this edition; James Halston, Digital Editing Manager; James F. Shanahan, Executive Editor; and Martin J. Wonsiewicz, Publisher, who recently left McGraw-Hill after serving as an extremely effective partner to the Editors for 10 years. They are an effective team who have given the Editors constant encouragement and sage advice. They have been instrumental in guiding the many changes instituted with this edition of *Harrison's* and in bringing this volume to fruition in a timely manner.

THE EDITORS

1 The Practice of Medicine
The Editors

THE MODERN-DAY PHYSICIAN

No greater opportunity, responsibility, or obligation can fall to the lot of a human being than to become a physician. In the care of the suffering, [the physician] needs technical skill, scientific knowledge, and human understanding.... Tact, sympathy, and understanding are expected of the physician, for the patient is no mere collection of symptoms, signs, disordered functions, damaged organs, and disturbed emotions. [The patient] is human, fearful, and hopeful, seeking relief, help, and reassurance.

—Harrison's Principles of Internal Medicine, 1950

The practice of medicine has changed in significant ways since the first edition of this book appeared in 1950. The advent of molecular biology with its enormous implications for the biological sciences (the sequencing of the human genome), sophisticated new imaging techniques, and advances in bioinformatics and information technology have contributed to an explosion of scientific information that has fundamentally changed the way we define, diagnose, treat, and prevent disease. This explosion of scientific knowledge is not at all static as it continues to intensify with time.

The widespread use of electronic medical records and the Internet have altered the way we practice medicine and exchange information. As today's physician struggles to integrate the copious amounts of scientific knowledge into everyday practice, it is important to remember that the ultimate goal of medicine is to treat the patient. Despite more than 50 years of scientific advances since the first edition of this text, it is critical to underscore that cultivating the intimate relationship that exists between physician and patient still lies at the heart of successful patient care.

The Science and Art of Medicine   Science-based technology and deductive reasoning form the foundation for the solution to many clinical problems. Spectacular advances in biochemistry, cell biology, and genomics, coupled with newly developed imaging techniques, allow access to the innermost parts of the cell and provide a window to the most remote recesses of the body. Revelations about the nature of genes and single cells have opened the portal for formulating a new molecular basis for the physiology of systems. Increasingly, we are understanding how subtle changes in many different genes can affect the function of cells and organisms. We are beginning to decipher the complex mechanisms by which genes are regulated. We have developed a new appreciation of the role of stem cells in normal tissue function and in the development of cancer, degenerative disease, and other disorders. The knowledge gleaned from the science of medicine has already improved and undoubtedly will further improve our understanding of complex disease processes and provide new approaches to disease treatment and prevention. Yet skill in the most sophisticated application of laboratory technology and in the use of the latest therapeutic modality alone does not make a good physician.

When a patient poses challenging clinical problems, an effective physician must be able to identify the crucial elements in a complex history and physical examination, to order the appropriate laboratory tests, and to extract the key results from the crowded computer printouts of data to determine whether to "treat" or to "watch." Deciding whether a clinical clue is worth pursuing or should be dismissed as a "red herring" and weighing whether a proposed treatment entails a greater risk than the disease itself are essential judgments that the skilled clinician must make many times each day. This combination of medical knowledge, intuition, experience, and judgment defines the *art of medicine*, which is as necessary to the practice of medicine as is a sound scientific base.

CLINICAL SKILLS
History-Taking   The written history of an illness should include all the facts of medical significance in the life of the patient. Recent events should be given the most attention. The patient should, at some early point, have the opportunity to tell his or her own story of the illness without frequent interruption and, when appropriate, receive expressions of interest, encouragement, and empathy from the physician. Any event related by the patient, however trivial or seemingly irrelevant, may provide the key to solving the medical problem. In general, only patients who feel comfortable will offer complete information, and thus putting the patient at ease to the greatest extent possible contributes substantially to obtaining an adequate history.

An informative history is more than an orderly listing of symptoms; by listening to patients and noting the way in which they describe their symptoms, physicians can gain valuable insight into the problem. Inflections of voice, facial expression, gestures, and attitude, i.e., "body language," may reveal important clues to the meaning of the symptoms to the patient. Because patients vary in their medical sophistication and ability to recall facts, the reported medical history should be corroborated whenever possible. The social history can also provide important insights into the types of diseases that should be considered. The family history not only identifies rare Mendelian disorders within a family but often reveals risk factors for common disorders such as coronary heart disease, hypertension, or asthma. A thorough family history may require input from multiple relatives to ensure completeness and accuracy. However, once recorded, it can be readily updated. The process of history-taking provides an opportunity to observe the patient's behavior and to watch for features to be pursued more thoroughly during the physical examination.

The very act of eliciting the history provides the physician with the opportunity to establish or enhance the unique bond that forms the basis for the ideal patient-physician relationship. This process helps the physician develop an appreciation of the patient's perception of the illness, the patient's expectations of the physician and the health care system, and the financial and social implications of the illness to the patient. Although current health care settings may impose time constraints on patient visits, it is important not to rush the history-taking since the patient may get the impression that what he or she is relating is not of importance to the physician and therefore may hold back relevant information. The confidentiality of the patient-physician relationship cannot be overemphasized.

Physical Examination   The purpose of the physical examination is to identify the physical signs of disease. The significance of these objective indications of disease is enhanced when they confirm a functional or structural change already suggested by the patient's history. At times, however, the physical signs may be the only evidence of disease.

The physical examination should be performed methodically and thoroughly, with consideration for the patient's comfort and modesty. Although attention is often directed by the history to the diseased organ or part of the body, the examination of a new patient must extend from head to toe in an objective search for abnormalities. Unless the physical examination is systematic and performed in a consistent manner from patient to patient, important segments may be inadvertently omitted. The results of the examination, like the details of the history, should be recorded at the time they are elicited, not hours later when they are subject to the distortions of memory. Skill in physical diagnosis is acquired with experience, but it is not merely technique that determines success in eliciting signs of disease. The detection of a few scattered petechiae, a faint diastolic murmur, or a small mass in the abdomen is not a question of keener eyes and ears or more sensitive fingers, but of a mind alert to these findings. Because physical findings can change with time, the physical examination should be repeated as frequently as the clinical situation warrants. Because a large number of highly sensitive diagnostic tests are available, particularly imaging techniques, it may be tempting to put less emphasis on the physical examination. Indeed, many patients are seen for the first time after a series of diagnostic tests have already been performed and the results known. This should not deter the physician from performing a thorough physical examination since clinical findings are often present that have "escaped" the barrage of preexamination diagnostic tests.

Diagnostic Studies We have become increasingly reliant on a wide array of laboratory tests to solve clinical problems. However, accumulated laboratory data do not relieve the physician from the responsibility of carefully observing, examining, and studying the patient. It is also essential to appreciate the limitations of diagnostic tests. By virtue of their impersonal quality, complexity, and apparent precision, they often gain an aura of authority regardless of the fallibility of the tests themselves, the instruments used in the tests, and the individuals performing or interpreting them. Physicians must weigh the expense involved in the laboratory procedures relative to the value of the information they are likely to provide.

Single laboratory tests are rarely ordered. Rather, physicians generally request "batteries" of multiple tests, which often prove useful. For example, abnormalities of hepatic function may provide the clue to such nonspecific symptoms as generalized weakness and increased fatigability, suggesting the diagnosis of chronic liver disease. Sometimes a single abnormality, such as an elevated serum calcium level, points to a particular disease, such as hyperparathyroidism or underlying malignancy.

The thoughtful use of screening tests, such as low-density lipoprotein cholesterol, may be quite useful. A group of laboratory determinations can be carried out conveniently on a single specimen at relatively low cost. Screening tests are most informative when directed toward common diseases or disorders and when their results indicate the need for other useful tests or interventions that may be costly to perform. On the one hand, biochemical measurements, together with simple laboratory examinations such as blood count, urinalysis, and sedimentation rate, often provide a major clue to the presence of a pathologic process. On the other hand, the physician must learn to evaluate occasional abnormalities among the screening tests that may not necessarily connote significant disease. An in-depth workup following a report of an isolated laboratory abnormality in a person who is otherwise well is almost invariably wasteful and unproductive. Among the more than 40 tests that are routinely performed as screening, it would not be unusual for one or two of them to be slightly abnormal. If there is no suspicion of an underlying illness, these tests are ordinarily repeated to ensure that the abnormality does not represent a laboratory error. If an abnormality is confirmed, it is important to consider its potential significance in the context of the patient's condition and other test results.

The development of technically improved imaging studies with greater sensitivity and specificity is one of the most rapidly advancing areas of medicine. These tests provide remarkably detailed anatomic information that can be a pivotal factor in medical decision-making. Ultrasonography, a variety of isotopic scans, CT, MRI, and positron emission tomography have benefited patients by supplanting older, more invasive approaches and opening new diagnostic vistas. Cognizant of their capabilities and the rapidity with which they can lead to a diagnosis, it is tempting to order a battery of imaging studies. All physicians have had experiences in which imaging studies turned up findings leading to an unexpected diagnosis. Nonetheless, patients must endure each of these tests, and the added cost of unnecessary testing is substantial. A skilled physician must learn to use these powerful diagnostic tools judiciously, always considering whether the results will alter management and benefit the patient.

PRINCIPLES OF PATIENT CARE
Evidence-Based Medicine Evidence-based medicine refers to the concept that clinical decisions are formally supported by data, preferably data that are derived from prospectively designed, randomized, controlled clinical trials. This is in sharp contrast to anecdotal experience, which may often be biased. Unless they are attuned to the importance of using larger, more objective studies for making decisions, even the most experienced physicians can be influenced by recent encounters with selected patients. Evidence-based medicine has become an increasingly important part of the routine practice of medicine and has led to the publication of a number of practice guidelines.

Practice Guidelines Professional organizations and government agencies are developing formal clinical-practice guidelines to aid physicians and other caregivers in making diagnostic and therapeutic decisions that are evidence-based, cost-effective, and most appropriate to a particular patient and clinical situation. As the evidence base of medicine increases, guidelines can provide a useful framework for managing patients with particular diagnoses or symptoms. They can protect patients—particularly those with inadequate health care benefits—from receiving substandard care. Guidelines can also protect conscientious caregivers from inappropriate charges of malpractice and society from the excessive costs associated with the overuse of medical resources. There are, however, caveats associated with clinical practice guidelines since they tend to oversimplify the complexities of medicine. Furthermore, groups with differing perspectives may develop divergent recommendations regarding issues as basic as the need for periodic sigmoidoscopy in middle-aged persons. Finally, guidelines do not—and cannot be expected to—account for the uniqueness of each individual and his or her illness. The physician's challenge is to integrate into clinical practice the useful recommendations offered by experts without accepting them blindly or being inappropriately constrained by them.

Medical Decision-Making Medical decision-making is an important responsibility of the physician and occurs at each stage of the diagnostic and treatment process. It involves the ordering of additional tests, requests for consults, and decisions regarding treatment and prognosis. This process requires an in-depth understanding of the pathophysiology and natural history of disease. As described above, medical decision-making should be evidence-based so that patients derive the full benefit of the scientific knowledge available to physicians. Formulating a differential diagnosis requires not only a broad knowledge base but also the ability to assess the relative probabilities of various diseases. Application of the scientific method, including hypothesis formation and data collection, is essential to the process of accepting or rejecting a particular diagnosis. Analysis of the differential diagnosis is an iterative process. As new information or test results are acquired, the group of disease processes being considered can be contracted or expanded appropriately.

Despite the importance of evidence-based medicine, much of medical decision-making relies on good clinical judgment—a process that is difficult to quantify or even to assess qualitatively. Physicians must use their knowledge and experience as a basis for weighing known factors along with the inevitable uncertainties and the need to use sound judgment; this is particularly important when a relevant evidence base is not available. Several quantitative tools may be invaluable in synthesizing the available information, including diagnostic tests, Bayes' theorem, and multivariate statistical models. *Diagnostic tests* serve to reduce uncertainty about a diagnosis or prognosis in a particular individual and to help the physician decide how best to manage that individual's condition. The battery of diagnostic tests complements the history and the physical examination. The accuracy of a given test is ascertained by determining its sensitivity (true positive rate) and specificity (true negative rate) as well as the predictive value of a positive and negative result. *Bayes' theorem* uses information on a test's sensitivity and specificity, in conjunction with the pretest probability of a diagnosis, to determine mathematically the posttest probability of the diagnosis. More complex clinical problems can be approached with *multivariate statistical models*, which generate highly accurate information even when multiple factors are acting individually or together to affect disease risk, progression, or response to treatment. Studies comparing the performance of statistical models with that of expert clinicians have documented equivalent accuracy, although the models tend to be more consistent. Thus, multivariate statistical models may be particularly helpful to less experienced clinicians. See Chap. 3 for a more thorough discussion of decision-making in clinical medicine.

Electronic Medical Records Our growing reliance on computers and the strength of information technology are playing an increasingly important role in medicine. Laboratory data are accessed almost universally through computers. Many medical centers now have electronic medical records, computerized order entry, and bar-coded tracking of medications. Some of these systems are interactive and provide reminders or warn of potential medical errors. In many ways, the health care system has lagged behind other industries in the adoption of information technology. Electronic medical records have extraordinary potential for providing rapid access to clinical information, imaging studies, laboratory results, and medications. This type of information is invaluable for ongoing efforts to enhance quality and improve patient safety. Ideally, patient records should be easily transferred across the health care system, providing reliable access to relevant data and historic information. However, technology limitations and concerns about privacy and cost continue to limit a broad-based utilization of electronic health records in most clinical settings. It should also be emphasized that information technology is merely a tool and can never replace the clinical decisions that are best made by the physician. In this regard, clinical knowledge and an understanding of the patient's needs, supplemented by quantitative tools, still seem to represent the best approach to decision-making in the practice of medicine.

Evaluation of Outcomes Clinicians generally use *objective* and readily measurable parameters to judge the outcome of a therapeutic intervention. For example, findings on physical or laboratory examination—such as the blood pressure level, the patency of a coronary artery on an angiogram, or the size of a mass on a radiologic examination—can provide critically important information. However, patients usually seek medical attention for *subjective* reasons; they wish to obtain relief from pain, to preserve or regain function, and to enjoy life. The components of a patient's health status or quality of life can include bodily comfort, capacity for physical activity, personal and professional function, sexual function, cognitive function, and overall perception of health. Each of these important areas can be assessed by means of structured interviews or specially designed questionnaires. Such assessments also provide useful parameters by which the physician can judge the patient's subjective view of his or her disability and the response to treatment, particularly in chronic illness. The practice of medicine requires consideration and integration of both objective and subjective outcomes.

Women's Health and Disease Although past epidemiologic studies and clinical trials have often focused predominantly on men, more recent studies have included more women, and some, like the Women's Health Initiative, have exclusively addressed women's health issues. Significant gender differences exist in diseases that afflict both men and women. Much is still to be learned in this arena, and ongoing studies should enhance our understanding of the mechanisms of gender differences in the course and outcome of certain diseases. For a more complete discussion of women's health, see Chap. 6.

Care of the Elderly The relative proportion of elderly individuals in the populations of developed nations has been growing considerably over the past few decades and will continue to grow. In this regard, the practice of medicine will continue to be greatly influenced by the health care needs of this growing elderly population. The physician must understand and appreciate the decline in physiologic reserve associated with aging; the diminished responses of the elderly to vaccinations such as those against influenza; the different responses of the

elderly to common diseases; and disorders that occur commonly with aging, such as depression, dementia, frailty, urinary incontinence, and fractures. For a more complete discussion of medical care for the elderly, see Chap. 9.

Errors in the Delivery of Health Care A report from the Institute of Medicine called for an ambitious agenda to reduce medical-error rates and improve patient safety by designing and implementing fundamental changes in health care systems. Adverse drug reactions occur in at least 5% of hospitalized patients, and the incidence increases with use of a large number of drugs. No matter what the clinical situation, it is the responsibility of the physician to use powerful therapeutic measures wisely, with due regard for their beneficial action, potential dangers, and cost. It is also the responsibility of hospitals and health care organizations to develop systems to reduce risk and ensure patient safety. Medication errors can be reduced through the use of ordering systems that eliminate misreading of handwriting. Implementation of infection-control systems, enforcement of hand-washing protocols, and careful oversight of antibiotic use can minimize complications of nosocomial infections.

The Role of the Physician in the Informed Consent of the Patient The fundamental principles of medical ethics require physicians to act in the patient's best interest and to respect the patient's autonomy. This is particularly relevant to the issue of informed consent. Most patients possess only limited medical knowledge and must rely on their physicians for advice. Physicians must respect their patients' autonomy, fully discussing the alternatives for care and the risks, benefits, and likely consequences of each alternative.

Patients are required to sign a consent form for essentially any diagnostic or therapeutic procedure. In such cases, it is particularly important for the patient to understand clearly the risks and benefits of these procedures; this is the definition of *informed consent*. It is incumbent on the physician to explain the procedures in a clear and understandable manner and to ascertain that the patient comprehends both the nature of the procedure and the attendant risks and benefits. The dread of the unknown, inherent in hospitalization, can be mitigated by such explanations.

The Approach to Grave Prognoses and Death No problem is more distressing than the diagnosis of an incurable disease, particularly when premature death is inevitable. What should the patient and family be told? What measures should be taken to maintain life? What can be done to maintain the quality of life?

Although some would argue otherwise, there is no ironclad rule that the patient must immediately be told "everything," even if the patient is an adult with substantial family responsibilities. How much is told at a given point in time should depend on the individual's ability to deal with the possibility of imminent death; often this capacity grows with time, and, whenever possible, gradual rather than abrupt disclosure is the best strategy. A wise and insightful physician is often guided by an understanding of what a patient wants to know and when he or she wants to know it. The patient's religious beliefs may also be taken into consideration. The patient must be given an opportunity to talk with the physician and ask questions. Patients may find it easier to share their feelings about death with their physician, who is likely to be more objective and less emotional, than with family members. As William Osler wrote, "One thing is certain; it is not for you to don the black cap and, assuming the judicial function, take hope away from any patient." Even when the patient directly inquires, "Am I dying?" the physician must attempt to determine whether this is a request for information or for reassurance. Only open communication between the patient and the physician can resolve this question and guide the physician in what to say and how to say it.

The physician should provide or arrange for emotional, physical, and spiritual support and must be compassionate, unhurried, and open. There is much to be gained by the laying on of hands. Pain should be adequately controlled, human dignity maintained, and isolation from family and close friends avoided. These aspects of care tend to be overlooked in hospitals, where the intrusion of life-sustaining apparati can so easily detract from attention to the whole person and encourage concentration instead on the life-threatening disease, against which the battle will ultimately be lost in any case. In the face of terminal illness, the goal of medicine must shift from *cure* to *care*, in the broadest sense of the term. In offering care to the dying patient, the physician must be prepared to provide information to family members and to deal with their grief and sometimes their feelings of guilt. It is important for the doctor to assure the family that everything possible has been done. For a more complete discussion of end-of-life care, see Chap. 11.

THE PATIENT-PHYSICIAN RELATIONSHIP

The significance of the intimate personal relationship between physician and patient cannot be too strongly emphasized, for in an extraordinarily large number of cases both the diagnosis and treatment are directly dependent on it. One of the essential qualities of the clinician is interest in humanity, **for the secret of the care of the patient is in caring for the patient.**

–Francis W. Peabody, 1881–1927

Physicians must never forget that patients are individual human beings with problems that all too often transcend their physical complaints. They are not "cases" or "admissions" or "diseases." This point is particularly important in this era of high technology in clinical medicine. Most patients are anxious and fearful. Physicians should instill confidence and should be reassuring but should never be arrogant. A professional attitude, coupled with warmth and openness, can do much to alleviate anxiety and to encourage patients to share all aspects of their medical history. Whatever the patient's attitude, the physician needs to consider the setting in which an illness occurs—in terms not only of the patients themselves but also of their familial, social, and cultural backgrounds. The ideal patient-physician relationship is based on thorough knowledge of the patient, on mutual trust, and on the ability to communicate.

The Dichotomy of Inpatient and Outpatient Internal Medicine
The hospital environment has transformed dramatically over the past few decades. In more recent times, emergency departments and critical care units have evolved to identify and manage critically ill patients, allowing them to survive formerly fatal diseases. There is increasing pressure to reduce the length of stay in the hospital and to manage complex disorders in the outpatient setting. This transition has been driven not only by efforts to reduce costs but also by the availability of new outpatient technologies, such as imaging and percutaneous infusion catheters for long-term antibiotics or nutrition, and by evidence that outcomes are often improved by minimizing inpatient hospitalization. Hospitals now consist of multiple distinct levels of care, such as the emergency department, procedure rooms, overnight observation units, critical care units, and palliative care units, in addition to traditional medical beds. A consequence of this differentiation has been the emergence of new specialties such as emergency medicine, intensivists, hospitalists, and end-of-life care. Moreover, these systems frequently involve "hand-offs" from the outpatient to the inpatient environment, from the critical care unit to a general medicine floor, and from the hospital to the outpatient environment. Clearly, one of the important challenges in internal medicine is to maintain continuity of care and information flow during these transitions, which threaten the traditional one-to-one relationship between patient and physician. In the current environment, teams of physicians, specialists, and other health care professionals have often replaced the personal interaction between doctor and patient. The patient can benefit greatly from effective collaboration among a number of health care professionals; however, *it is the duty of the patient's principal or primary physician to provide cohesive guidance through an illness.* In order to meet this challenge, the primary physician must be familiar with the techniques, skills, and objectives of specialist physicians and allied health professionals. The primary physician must ensure that the patient will benefit from scientific advances and from the expertise of specialists when they are needed, while still retaining responsibility for the major decisions concerning diagnosis and treatment.

Appreciation of the Patient's Hospital Experience
The hospital is an intimidating environment for most individuals. Hospitalized patients find themselves surrounded by air jets, buttons, and glaring lights; invaded by tubes and wires; and beset by the numerous members of the health care team—nurses, nurses' aides, physicians' assistants, social workers, technologists, physical therapists, medical students, house officers, attending and consulting physicians, and many others. They may be transported to special laboratories and imaging facilities replete with blinking lights, strange sounds, and unfamiliar personnel; they may be left unattended for periods of time; they may be obliged to share a room with other patients who have their own health problems. It is little wonder that patients may lose their sense of reality. Physicians who can appreciate the hospital experience from the patient's perspective and make an effort to develop a strong personal relationship with the patient whereby they may guide the patient through this experience can make a stressful situation more tolerable.

Trends in the Delivery of Health Care: A Challenge to the Humane Physician
Many trends in the delivery of health care tend to make medical care impersonal. These trends, some of which have been mentioned already, include (1) vigorous efforts to reduce the escalating costs of health care; (2) the growing number of managed-care programs, which are intended to reduce costs but in which the patient may have little choice in selecting a physician or in seeing that physician consistently; (3) increasing reliance on technological advances and computerization for many aspects of diagnosis and treatment; (4) the need for numerous physicians to be involved in the care of most patients who are seriously ill; and (5) an increased number of malpractice suits, some of which are justifiable because of medical errors, but others of which reflect an unrealistic expectation on the part of many patients that their disease will be cured or that complications will not occur during the course of complex illnesses or procedures.

Given these changes in the medical care system, it is a major challenge for physicians to maintain the *humane* aspects of medical care. The American Board of Internal Medicine, working together with the American College of Physicians–American Society of Internal Medicine and the European Federation of Internal Medicine, has published a *Charter on Medical Professionalism* that underscores three main principles in physicians' contract with society: (1) the primacy of patient welfare, (2) patient autonomy, and (3) social justice. Medical schools have also increased their emphasis on physician professionalism in recent years (Fig. 1-1). The humanistic qualities of a physician must encompass integrity, respect, and compassion. Availability, the expression of sincere concern, the willingness to take the time to explain all aspects of the illness, and a nonjudgmental attitude when dealing with patients whose cultures, lifestyles, attitudes, and values differ from those of the physician are just a few of the characteristics of the humane physician. Every physician will, at times, be challenged by patients who evoke strongly negative or positive emotional responses. Physicians should be alert to their own reactions to such patients and situations and should consciously monitor and control their behavior so that the patient's best interest remains the principal motivation for their actions at all times.

An important aspect of patient care involves an appreciation of the patient's "quality of life," a subjective assessment of what each patient values most. Such an assessment requires detailed, sometimes intimate knowledge of the patient, which can usually be obtained only through deliberate, unhurried, and often repeated conversations. Time pressures will always threaten these interactions, but they should not diminish the importance of understanding and seeking to fulfill the priorities of the patient.

FIGURE 1-1 A typical "white coat" ceremony in medical school where students are introduced to the responsibilities of patient care. *(Courtesy of The University of Texas Health Science Center at San Antonio; with permission.)*

THE TWENTY-FIRST CENTURY PHYSICIAN: EXPANDING FRONTIERS

The Era of Genomics In the spring of 2003, the complete sequencing of the human genome was announced, officially ushering in the genomic era. However, even before this landmark accomplishment, the practice of medicine had been evolving as a result of the insights gained from an understanding of the human genome as well as the genomes of a wide variety of microbes, whose genetic sequences were becoming widely available as a result of the breathtaking advances in sequencing techniques and informatics. Examples of the latter include the identification of a novel coronavirus as the etiologic agent of the severe acute respiratory syndrome (SARS) and the tracking of the evolution of a potentially pandemic influenza virus found in birds. Today, gene expression profiles are being used to guide therapy and inform prognosis for a number of diseases; the use of genotyping is providing a new means to assess the risk of certain diseases as well as variation in response to a number of drugs; we are understanding better the role of certain genes in the causality of certain common conditions such as obesity and allergies. Despite these advances, we are still in the infancy of understanding and utilizing the complexities of genomics in the diagnosis, prevention, and treatment of disease. Our task is complicated by the fact that phenotypes are generally determined not by genes alone but by the interplay of genetic and environmental factors. Indeed, we have just begun to scratch the surface of possibilities that the era of genomics will provide to the practice of medicine.

The rapidity of these advances may seem overwhelming to the practicing physician. However, he or she has an important role to play in ensuring that these powerful technologies and sources of new information are applied with sensitivity and intelligence to the patient. Since genomics is such a rapidly evolving field, physicians and other health care professionals must continue to educate themselves so that they can apply this new knowledge to the benefit of their patients' health and well-being. Genetic testing requires wise counsel based on an understanding of the value and limitations of the tests as well as the implications of their results for specific individuals. For a more complete discussion of genetic testing, see Chap. 64.

The Globalization of Medicine Physicians should be cognizant of diseases and health care services beyond local boundaries. Global travel has implications for disease spread, and it is not uncommon for diseases endemic to certain regions to be seen in other regions after a patient has traveled and returned from these regions. Patients have broader access to unique expertise or clinical trials at distant medical centers, and the cost of travel may be offset by the quality of care at these distant locations. As much as any other factor influencing global aspects of medicine, the Internet has transformed the transfer of medical information throughout the world. This change has been accompanied by the transfer of technological skills through telemedicine and international consultation for radiologic images and pathologic specimens. For a complete discussion of global issues, see Chap. 2.

Medicine on the Internet On the whole, the Internet has had a very positive effect on the practice of medicine; a wide range of information is available to physicians and patients through personal computers almost instantaneously at any time and from anywhere in the world. This medium holds enormous potential for delivering up-to-date information, practice guidelines, state-of-the-art conferences, journal contents, textbooks (including this text), and direct communications with other physicians and specialists, thereby expanding the depth and breadth of information available to the physician about the diagnosis and care of patients. Most medical journals are now accessible online, providing rapid and comprehensive sources of information. This medium also serves to lessen the information gap felt by physicians and health care providers in remote areas of the world by bringing them into direct and instant contact with the latest developments in medical care.

Patients, too, are turning to the Internet in increasing numbers to acquire information about their illnesses and therapies and to join Internet-based support groups. Physicians are increasingly faced with the prospect of dealing with patients who arrive with sophisticated information about their illness. In this regard, physicians are challenged in a positive way to keep themselves abreast of the latest relevant information while serving as an "editor" for the patients as they navigate through this seemingly endless source of information.

A critically important caveat is that virtually anything can be published on the Internet, with easy circumvention of the peer-review process that is an essential feature of quality publications. Physicians or patients who search the Internet for medical information must be aware of this danger. Notwithstanding this limitation, appropriate use of the Internet is revolutionizing information access for physicians and patients and in this regard is a great benefit that was not available to our predecessors.

Public Expectations and Accountability The level of knowledge and sophistication regarding health issues on the part of the general public has grown rapidly over the past few decades. As a result, expectations of the health care system in general and of physicians in particular have risen. Physicians are expected to master rapidly advancing fields (the *science* of medicine) while considering their patients' unique needs (the *art* of medicine). Thus, physicians are held accountable not only for the technical aspects of the care that they provide but also for their patients' satisfaction with the delivery and costs of care.

In many parts of the world, physicians are increasingly expected to account for the way in which they practice medicine by meeting certain standards prescribed by federal and local governments. The hospitalization of patients whose health care costs are reimbursed by the government and other third parties is subjected to utilization review. Thus, the physician must defend the cause for and duration of a patient's hospitalization if it falls outside certain "average" standards. Authorization for reimbursement is increasingly based on documentation of the nature and complexity of an illness, as reflected by recorded elements of the history and physical examination. There is a growing "pay for performance" movement, which seeks to link reimbursement to quality of care. The goal of this movement is to improve standards of health care and to contain spiraling health care costs. Physicians are also expected to give evidence of their continuing competence through mandatory continuing education, patient-record audits, maintenance of certification, or relicensing.

Medical Ethics and New Technologies The rapid pace of technological advances has profound implications for medical applications far beyond their traditional roles to prevent, treat, and cure disease. Cloning, genetic engineering, gene therapy, human-computer interfaces, nanotechnology, and designer drugs have the potential to modify inherited predispositions to disease, select desired characteristics in embryos, augment "normal" human performance, replace failing tissues, and substantially prolong life span. Because of their unique training, physicians have a responsibility to help shape the debate concerning the appropriate uses of, and limits that should be placed on, these new techniques.

The Physician as Perpetual Student It becomes all too apparent from the time we graduate from medical school that as physicians our lot is that of the "perpetual student" and the mosaic of our knowledge and experiences is eternally unfinished. This concept can be at the same time exhilarating and anxiety-provoking. It is exhilarating because we will continue to expand our knowledge that can be applied to our patients; it is anxiety-provoking because we realize that we will never know as much as we want or need to know. At best, we will translate this latter feeling into energy to continue to improve ourselves and realize our potential as physicians. In this regard, it is the responsibility of a physician to pursue new knowledge continually by reading, attending conferences and courses, and consulting colleagues and the Internet. This is often a difficult task for a busy practitioner; however, such a commitment to continued learning is an integral part of being a physician and must be given the highest priority.

Research, Teaching, and the Practice of Medicine The title *doctor* is derived from the Latin *docere*, "to teach," and physicians should share information and medical knowledge with colleagues, with students of medicine and related professions, and with their patients. The practice of medicine is dependent on the sum total of medical knowledge, which in turn is based on an unending chain of scientific discovery, clinical observation, analysis, and interpretation. Advances in medicine depend on the acquisition of new information through research,

and improved medical care requires the transmission of this information. As part of broader societal responsibilities, the physician should encourage patients to participate in ethical and properly approved clinical investigations if they do not impose undue hazard, discomfort, or inconvenience. On the other hand, physicians engaged in clinical research must be alert to potential conflicts of interest between their research goals and their obligations to individual patients; the best interests of the patient must always take priority.

To wrest from nature the secrets which have perplexed philosophers in all ages, to track to their sources the causes of disease, to correlate the vast stores of knowledge, that they may be quickly available for the prevention and cure of disease—these are our ambitions.

–William Osler, 1849–1919

FURTHER READINGS

BLANK L et al: Medical professionalism in the new millennium: A physician charter 15 months later. Ann Intern Med 138:839, 2003

COUNCIL ON GRADUATE MEDICAL EDUCATION: *Thirteenth Report: Physician Education for a Changing Health Care Environment.* US Department of Health and Human Services, March 1999

GUTTMACHER AE, COLLINS FS: Welcome to the genomic era. N Engl J Med 349:996, 2003

LUDMERER KM, JOHNS MME: Reforming graduate medical eduction. JAMA 294:1083, 2005

STRAUS SE et al: Teaching evidence-based medicine skills can change practice in a community hospital. J Gen Intern Med 20:340, 2005

2 Global Issues in Medicine
Jim Yong Kim, Paul Farmer

WHY GLOBAL HEALTH?

Global health, it has been noted, is not a discipline; it is, rather, a collection of problems. No single review can do much more than lay out the leading problems faced in applying evidence-based medicine in settings of great poverty or across national boundaries. In this chapter, we first introduce the major international bodies engaged in addressing these problems; identify the more significant barriers to improving the health of people who to date have not, by and large, had access to modern medicines; and summarize population-based data regarding the most common health problems faced by people living in poverty. Examining specific problems—notably AIDS (Chap. 182), but also tuberculosis (TB, Chap. 158), malaria (Chap. 203), severe acute respiratory syndrome (SARS; Chap. 179), and key noncommunicable diseases—helps to sharpen the discussion of barriers to prevention, diagnosis, and care as well as means of overcoming them. We next discuss global health equity, drawing on notions of social justice that once were central to international public health but have fallen out of favor over the past several decades. We close by acknowledging the importance of cost-effectiveness analysis linked to national economic data, while at the same time underlining the need to address disparities of disease risk and access to care.

HISTORY OF GLOBAL HEALTH INSTITUTIONS

Concern about health across national boundaries dates back many centuries, predating the Black Plague and other pandemics. Before the advent of germ theory, when epidemic disease began to be understood to be the result of microbes rather than of "miasmas" or the wrath of a divine being, the chief social responses to such epidemics often included accusations that this or that human group was responsible for propagat-

ing the affliction in question. Similarly inaccurate and ineffective beliefs abounded when the arrival of European colonists led to catastrophic outbreaks of communicable diseases among indigenous populations in the Americas, and these viewpoints continued to hold sway during subsequent pandemics of cholera. Many historians trace modern public health and epidemiology to the day in 1851 when Dr. John Snow, having discerned the link between cholera outbreaks in London and water sources used by the afflicted populace, removed the handle of the Broad Street water pump. Thus one cholera epidemic was stopped, but it would still be years before the etiology of cholera was discovered.

A proper understanding of etiology was necessary to the birth not only of epidemiology but also of efforts to apply public health measures across administrative boundaries; indeed, without agreement upon etiology and case definitions, there could be no sound metrics upon which to base either assessments of disease burden or effective interventions. The close of the nineteenth century marked the birth and rapid growth of microbiology and the development of some of the first effective vaccines, which, along with measures to promote sanitation, were for decades the mainstay of modern public health. Before the development of effective antibiotics in the mid-twentieth century, international health endeavors consisted largely of the transnational application of a small number of lessons learned from local or regional campaigns. Perhaps the first organization founded explicitly to tackle cross-border health issues was the Pan American Sanitary Bureau, which was formed by 11 countries in the Americas in 1902. The primary goal of what was later to become the Pan American Health Organization was the control of infectious diseases across the Americas. Of special concern was yellow fever, which had been running a deadly course through much of South and Central America and posed a threat to the construction of the Panama Canal. The identification of a mosquito vector in 1901 led public and private health authorities to focus on mosquito control; a vaccine was developed in the 1930s.

Even in the early heyday of vaccine development, no global institutions tackled the health problems of the world's poor. Colonial powers did address (with varying degrees of effectiveness and sources of motivation) the ranking infectious killers in regions now known as the developing world, but universal standards or even aspirations for international public health and medicine were still far in the future. Although the League of Nations concerned itself with health issues such as malaria in the early twentieth century, and although various organs of the nascent United Nations—including the United Nations Development Program and the United Nations Children's Fund (UNICEF)—also addressed health issues, the World Health Organization (WHO) was the first truly global health institution. Since its founding in 1948, the WHO has witnessed dramatic shifts in population health and in its own stature as the premier global health institution. In line with a long-standing focus on communicable diseases that readily cross administrative and political borders, leaders in global health, under the aegis of the WHO, initiated the effort that led to what some see as the greatest success in international health: the eradication of smallpox. Historians of the smallpox campaign note the preconditions that made eradication possible: international consensus regarding the potential for success, an effective vaccine, and the apparent lack of a nonhuman reservoir for the often-lethal and highly infectious etiologic agent. The primary obstacle was the lack of effective delivery mechanisms for the vaccine in settings of poverty, where health personnel were scarce and health systems weak. Close collaborations across administrative and political borders were clearly necessary. Naysayers were surprised when the smallpox eradication campaign, which engaged public health officials throughout the world, proved successful at the height of the Cold War.

The optimism born of the world's first successful disease-eradication campaign invigorated the international health community, if only briefly. Global consensus regarding the right to primary health care for all was reached at the International Conference on Primary Health Care in Alma-Ata (in what is now Kazakhstan) in 1978. However, the declaration of this collective vision was not followed by substantial funding, nor did the apparent consensus reflect universal commitment to the right to health care. Moreover, as is too often the case, success paradoxically weakened commitment. Basic-science research that might lead to effective vaccines and therapies for TB and malaria faltered in the latter decades of the twentieth century after these diseases were brought under control in the affluent countries where most such research is conducted. U.S. Surgeon General William H. Stewart declared in the late 1960s that it was time to "close the book on infectious diseases," and attention was turned to the main health problems of countries that had already undergone an "epidemiological transition"; that is, the focus shifted from premature deaths due to infectious diseases toward deaths from complications of chronic noncommunicable diseases, including malignancies and complications of heart disease.

In 1982, the visionary leader of UNICEF, James P. Grant, frustrated by the lack of action around the Health for All initiative announced in Alma-Ata, launched a "child survival revolution" focused on four inexpensive interventions collectively known by the acronym GOBI: growth monitoring; oral rehydration; breast-feeding; and immunizations for TB, diphtheria, whooping cough, tetanus, polio, and measles. GOBI, which was later expanded to GOBI-FFF (to include female education, food, and family planning), was controversial from the start, but Grant's advocacy led to enormous improvements in the health of poor children worldwide. The Expanded Programme on Immunization was especially successful and is thought to have raised the proportion of children worldwide who were receiving critical vaccines by more than threefold—i.e., from <20% to almost 80% (the target level).

For many reasons (including, perhaps, the success of the UNICEF-led campaign for child survival), the influence of the WHO waned during the 1980s. In the early 1990s, many observers argued that, with its vastly superior financial resources and close if unequal relationships with the governments of poor countries, the World Bank had eclipsed the WHO as the most important multilateral institution working in the area of health. One of the stated goals of the World Bank was to help poor countries identify "cost-effective" interventions worthy of international public support. At the same time, the World Bank encouraged many of these nations to reduce public expenditures in health and education as part of (later discredited) structural adjust-ment programs (SAPs), which were imposed as a condition for access to credit and assistance through international financial institutions such as the Bank and the International Monetary Fund (IMF). One trend related, at least in part, to these expenditure-reduction policies was the resurgence in Africa of many diseases that colonial regimes had brought under control, including malaria, trypanosomiasis, and schistosomiasis. Tuberculosis, an eminently curable disease, remained the world's leading infectious killer of adults. Half a million women per year died in childbirth during the last decade of the twentieth century, and few of the world's largest philanthropic or funding institutions focused on global health.

AIDS, first described in 1981, precipitated a change. In the United States, the advent of this newly described infectious killer marked the culmination of a series of events that discredited the grand talk of "closing the book" on infectious diseases. In Africa, which would emerge as the global epicenter of the pandemic, HIV disease further weakened TB control programs, while malaria continued to take as many lives as ever. At the dawn of the twenty-first century, these three diseases alone killed an estimated 6 million people each year. New research, new policies, and new funding mechanisms were called for. Some of the requisite innovations have emerged in the past few years. The leadership of the WHO has been challenged by the rise of institutions such as the Global Fund to Fight AIDS, Tuberculosis, and Malaria; the Joint United Nations Program on HIV/AIDS (UNAIDS); and the Bill & Melinda Gates Foundation and by bilateral efforts such as the U.S. President's Emergency Plan for AIDS Relief (PEPFAR). Yet with its 193 member states and 147 country offices, the WHO remains preeminent in matters relating to the cross-border spread of infectious and other health threats. In the aftermath of the SARS epidemic of 2003, the International Health Regulations—which provide a legal foundation for the WHO's direct investigation of a wide range of global health problems, including pandemic influenza, in any member state—were strengthened and brought into force in May 2007.

Even as attention to and resources for health problems in resource-poor settings grow, the lack of coherence in and among global health institutions may seriously undermine efforts to forge a more comprehensive and effective response. While UNICEF had great success in launching and sustaining the child survival revolution, the end of James Grant's term at UNICEF upon his death in 1995 was followed by a lamentable shift of focus away from immunizations; predictably, coverage dropped. The WHO has gone through two recent leadership transitions and is still woefully underfunded despite the ever-growing need to engage a wider and more complex range of health issues. In another instance of the paradoxical impact of success, the rapid growth of the Gates Foundation, while clearly one of the most important developments in the history of global health, has led other foundations to question the wisdom of continuing to invest their more modest resources in this field. We may indeed be living in what some have called "the golden age of global health," but leaders of major organizations such as the WHO, the Global Fund, UNICEF, UNAIDS, and the Gates Foundation must work together to design an effective architecture that will make the most of the extraordinary opportunities that now exist. To this end, new and old players in global health must invest heavily in *discovery* (relevant basic science); in the *development* of new tools (preventive, diagnostic, and therapeutic); and in a new science of implementation, or *delivery*.

THE ECONOMICS OF GLOBAL HEALTH

Political and economic concerns have often guided global health interventions. As mentioned previously, early efforts to control yellow fever were tied to the completion of the Panama Canal. However, the precise nature of the link between economics and health remains a matter for debate. Some economists and demographers argue that economic development is the key to improving the health status of populations, while others maintain that ill health is the chief barrier to development in poor countries. In either case, investment in health care, and especially in the control of communicable diseases, should lead to increased productivity. The question is where to find the necessary resources to start the predicted "virtuous cycle."

International financial institutions, including the World Bank and the IMF, have counseled limited investments and the capping of social expenditures in health and education. The socioeconomic argument was that a balanced budget and a "friendly investment climate"—that is, privatization, deregulation, decreased trade barriers, devalued currencies, and debt repayment—would favor development and thus improve health outcomes. The limitations on social-sector spending recommended for many poor countries by the World Bank and the IMF from the 1970s through the 1990s tended to confirm the opposite view. In the poorest countries, already-tiny health-sector budgets were further constricted. Moreover, health-sector spending in many poor countries channeled a majority of resources toward city hospitals that served mostly élites who were able to pay; consequently, in the past quarter-century, little spending went toward addressing the problems that most affected poor people in poor countries.

Since 1999, spurred by the leadership of the Gates Foundation and the growing interest in addressing novel and persistent challenges such as AIDS, spending on health in poor countries has increased, with $40 billion in new funds earmarked for the discovery and development of drugs and diagnostics targeting diseases of the poor; for comprehensive responses to the AIDS, TB, and malaria epidemics; for vaccine development and delivery; and even for improved methods of data collection in resource-poor settings. Nevertheless, in order to reach the United Nations' Millennium Development Goals, which include targets for poverty reduction, universal primary education, and gender equality, spending in the health sector will have to be further increased and sustained. To determine by how much and for how long, it is imperative that we improve our ability to assess the global burden of disease (GBD) and to plan interventions that more precisely match the need, which is glaring but often poorly understood. Refining metrics is an important task for global health: only recently have we had solid assessments of the GBD. Such assessments may serve as preliminaries or as correctives to effective interventions among the poor.

LIFE EXPECTANCY AND GLOBAL BURDEN OF DISEASE

Since the late 1980s, serious efforts have been made to calculate the GBD. The first GBD study, conducted in 1990, laid the foundation for the first report on *Disease Control Priorities in Developing Countries* (DCP1) and for the World Bank's 1993 World Development Report entitled *Investing in Health*. These efforts represented a major advance in our understanding of health status in developing countries. *Investing in Health* has been especially influential: it familiarized a broad audience with cost-effectiveness analysis for specific health interventions and with the notion of disability-adjusted life years (DALYs). The DALY, which has become a standard measure of the impact of a specific health condition on a population, combines in a single measure both absolute years of life lost and years lost due to disability for incident cases of a condition.

The second GBD analysis was carried out on health data from 2001. The latter report reflects growth in the available data on health in the poorest countries and in our capacity to measure the impact of specific conditions on a population. Yet, even in 2001, only 107 of 192 nations surveyed had reliable information on the causes of deaths within their own borders. It is essential to expand efforts to collect the most basic health data; this task falls to the WHO, national governments, and certain academic institutions. The lack of complete data has led to considerable uncertainty in estimates of overall mortality. The level of uncertainty ranges from as low as 1% for estimates of all-cause mortality in developed countries to well over 50% for disability resulting from diseases for which surveillance mechanisms are incomplete. As analytic methods and data quality have improved, however, important trends can be identified in a comparison of GBD estimates from 1990 and 2001.

Of the 56 million deaths worldwide in 2001, one-third were due to communicable diseases, maternal and perinatal conditions, and nutri-

tional deficiencies. While the proportion of all deaths attributable to these causes was unchanged from 1990, the share of all deaths due to the communicable disease HIV/AIDS grew from just 2% to an astonishing 14%. If these deaths were excluded, the fraction of all deaths related to communicable diseases, maternal and perinatal conditions, and nutritional deficiencies dropped from one-third to one-fifth. Of the deaths making up that one-fifth of the total figure, 97% occurred in middle- and low-income countries. The leading cause of death among adults in 2001 was ischemic heart disease, accounting for 17.3% of all deaths in high-income countries and for 11.8% in middle- and low-income countries. In second place was cerebrovascular disease, which accounted for 9.9% of deaths in high-income countries and for 9.5% of deaths in middle- and low-income countries. While the third leading cause of death in high-income countries was tracheal, bronchial, and lung cancers (which accounted for 5.8% of all deaths), these conditions do not even register in the top 10 places in middle- and low-income countries. Of the 10 leading causes of death in poorer countries, 5 were communicable diseases; in high-income countries, however, only 1 communicable disease—lower respiratory infection—was ranked among the top 10 causes of death.

Nearly 20% (10.6 million) of the 56 million dead in 2001 were children <5 years of age who died of acute respiratory infections, measles, diarrhea, malaria, and HIV/AIDS (Fig. 2-1). Of these deaths, 99% occurred in middle- and low-income countries, and fully 40% occurred in sub-Saharan Africa. If stillbirths are counted, the number of childhood deaths rises to 13.5 million worldwide (~25% of all deaths worldwide), of which more than half (i.e., one-eighth of all deaths) occurred before the first birthday. Between 1990 and 2001, under-five childhood mortality dropped by ≥30% in high-income countries, Latin America, the Caribbean, the Middle East, North Africa, and the middle- and low-income countries of Europe and Central Asia. Notably, the total number of deaths from diarrheal diseases dropped from 2.4 million in 1990 to 1.6 million in 2001, probably as a result of the increased use of oral rehydration therapy in poor countries. Malaria and HIV infection were the only two conditions for which childhood death rates increased between 1990 and 2001.

Among persons 15–59 years of age (Fig. 2-2), noncommunicable diseases accounted for more than half of all deaths in all regions except South Asia and sub-Saharan Africa, where communicable diseases, maternal and perinatal conditions, and nutritional deficiencies together accounted for one-third and two-thirds of all deaths, respectively. The 15- to 59-year-olds with noncommunicable conditions in low- and middle-income countries faced a 30% greater risk of death from their conditions than did their peers in high-income countries. In this age group, injuries accounted for 25% of all deaths; Europe and Central Asia registered even higher rates, with injuries accounting for one-third of all deaths. Overall, death rates in this age group declined between 1990 and 2001 in all regions except Europe and Central Asia, where cardiovascular diseases and injuries have caused increased mortality, and sub-Saharan Africa, where the impact of HIV/AIDS in this age cohort has been particularly devastating.

Noncommunicable diseases accounted for almost 60% of all deaths in 2001 but, because of the later onset of these diseases, accounted for only 40% of years of life lost. In contrast, because they occur more often in younger people, injuries accounted for 12% of years of life lost but for only 9% of deaths. Overall, males had an 11% higher death rate than females as well as a 15% higher rate of years of life lost; these figures reflect the earlier age of death of males worldwide. Notably, almost half of the disease burden in middle- and low-income countries in 2001 derived from noncommunicable disease—an increase of 10% since 1990.

Compared with years of life lost, there is greater uncertainty in calculating years of life lived with disability for specific conditions. Best estimates from 2001 reveal that, while the prevalence of diseases common in older populations (e.g., dementia and musculoskeletal disease) was higher in high-income countries, the disability experienced as a result of cardiovascular diseases, chronic respiratory diseases, and the long-term impact of communicable diseases was greater in low- and middle-income countries. Thus, predictably, in most low- and middle-income

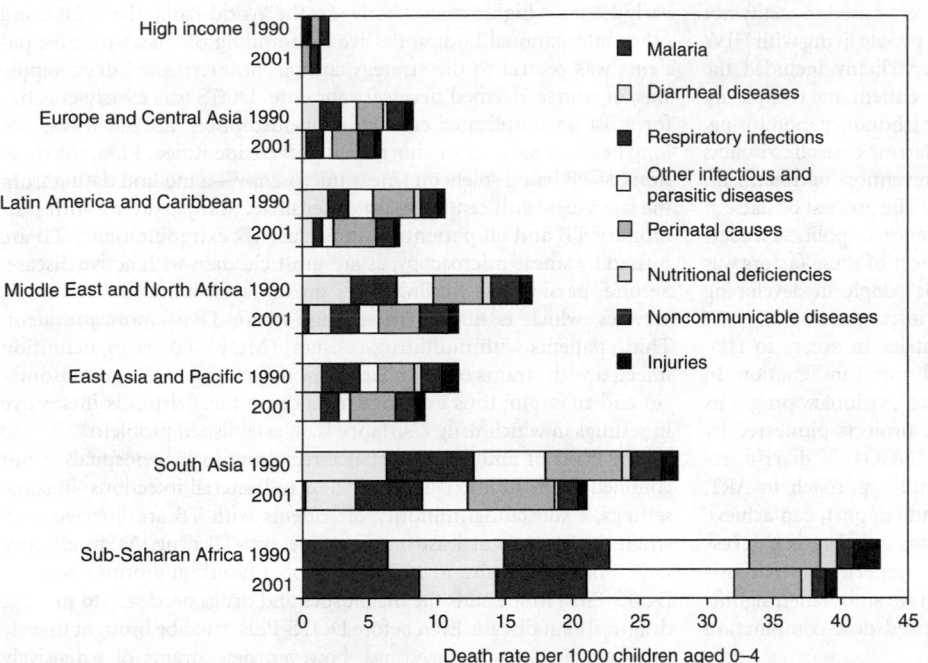

FIGURE 2-1 Death rates among children from birth through 4 years of age, by disease group and region, in 1990 and 2001. Cause-specific death rates for 1990, estimated from Murray and Lopez (1996), may not be completely comparable to those for 2001 because of changes in data availability and methods as well as some approximations in mapping 1990 estimates to the 2001 regions of East Asia and Pacific, South Asia, and Europe and Central Asia. For all geographic regions, high-income countries are excluded and are shown as a single group at the top of the graph. The geographic regions therefore refer to low- and middle-income countries only. *(Reprinted from Lopez et al, with permission from Elsevier.)*

and ambitions for global health grow, cost-effectiveness analyses (particularly those based on past conditions) must not hobble the increased worldwide commitment to provide resources and accessible services to all who need them. To illustrate this point, we turn in greater detail to AIDS, which has become, in the course of the last three decades, the world's leading infectious cause of death during adulthood.

AIDS

Chapter 182 provides an overview of the AIDS epidemic in the world today. Here we will limit ourselves to a discussion of AIDS in the developing world. Lessons learned in tackling AIDS in resource-constrained settings are highly relevant to discussions of other chronic diseases, including noncommunicable diseases, for which effective therapies have been developed. We highlight several of these lessons below.

In the United States, the availability of highly active antiretroviral therapy (ART) for AIDS has transformed this disease from an inescapably fatal destruction of cell-mediated immunity into a manageable chronic illness. In developing countries, treatment has been offered more broadly only since 2003, and only in the summer of 2006 did the number of patients receiving treatment exceed 25% of the number who currently need it. (It remains to be seen how many of

countries, people both lived shorter lives and experienced disability and poor health for a greater proportion of their lives. Indeed, 45% of the overall burden of disease occurred in South Asia and sub-Saharan Africa, which together comprise only one-third of the global population.

In its analysis of risk factors for ill health, the GBD project found that undernutrition was the leading cause of loss of DALYs in both 1990 and 2001. In an era that has seen obesity become a major health concern in so many developed countries, the persistence of undernutrition is surely cause for great consternation. Our inability to feed the hungry indicts many years of failed development projects and must be addressed as a problem of the highest priority. Indeed, no health care initiative, however generously funded and scientifically justified, will be effective without adequate nutrition.

The GBD analysis was used as the basis for the second edition of *Disease Control Priorities in Developing Countries* (DCP2). Published in 2006, DCP2 is a document of stunning breadth and ambition, providing cost-effectiveness analyses for >100 interventions and including 21 chapters focused on strategies for strengthening health systems. Cost-effectiveness analyses that compare two relatively equal interventions and facilitate the best choices under constraint are important; however, as both resources

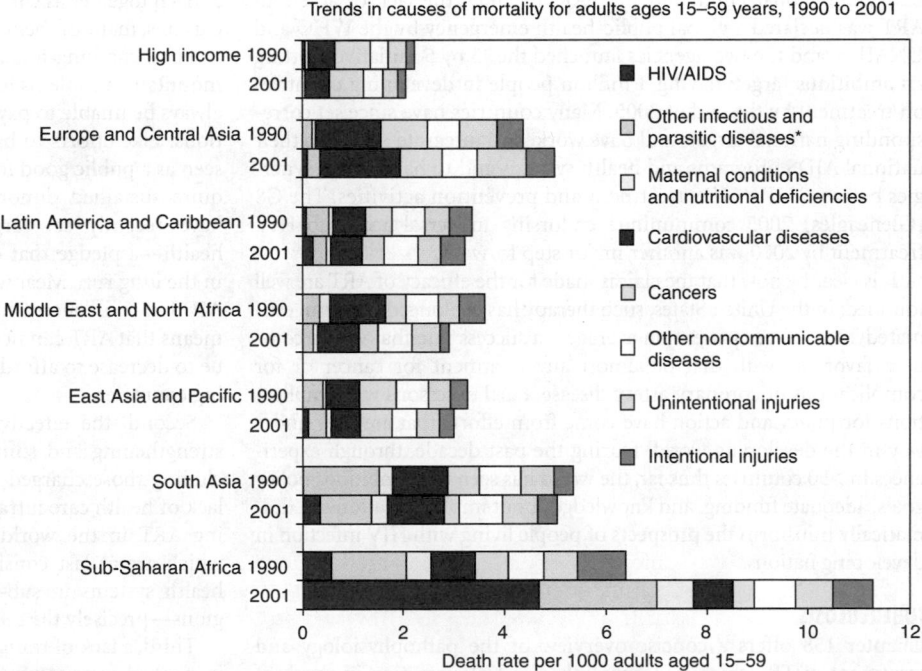

FIGURE 2-2 Death rates among persons 15–59 years old, by disease group and region, in 1990 and 2001. *Includes respiratory infections. Cause-specific death rates for 1990, estimated from Murray and Lopez (1996), may not be completely comparable to those for 2001 because of changes in data availability and methods as well as some approximations in mapping 1990 estimates to the 2001 regions of East Asia and Pacific, South Asia, and Europe and Central Asia. For all geographic regions, high-income countries are excluded and are shown as a single group at the top of the graph. The geographic regions therefore refer to low- and middle-income countries only. *(Reprinted from Lopez et al, with permission from Elsevier.)*

these fortunate few are receiving ART regularly and with the requisite social support.) Before 2003, many arguments were raised to justify not moving forward rapidly with ART programs for people living with HIV/AIDS in resource-limited settings. The standard litany included the price of therapy compared to the poverty of the patient, the complexity of the intervention, the lack of infrastructure for laboratory monitoring, and the lack of trained health care providers. Narrow cost-effectiveness arguments that created false dichotomies—prevention *or* treatment, rather than both—too often went unchallenged. The greatest obstacle at the time was the ambivalence, if not outright silence, of political leaders and experts in public health. The cumulative effect of these factors was to condemn to death tens of millions of poor people in developing countries who had become ill as a result of HIV infection.

The inequity between rich and poor countries in access to HIV treatment has rightly given rise to widespread moral indignation. In several middle-income countries, including Brazil, visionary programs have bridged the access gap. Other innovative projects pioneered by international nongovernmental organizations (NGOs) in diverse settings have clearly established that a very simple approach to ART, based on intensive community engagement and support, can achieve remarkable results. In 2000, the United Nations Accelerating Access Initiative finally brought the research-based and generic pharmaceutical industries into play, and AIDS drug prices have since fallen significantly. At the same time, easier-to-administer fixed-dose combination drugs have become more widely available.

Building on these lessons, the WHO advocated a public health approach to the treatment of people with AIDS in resource-limited settings. This approach, which was derived from models of care pioneered by the NGO Partners In Health and other groups, proposed standard first-line treatment regimens based on a simple five-drug formulary, with a more complex (and, up to now, more expensive) set of second-line options in reserve. Common clinical protocols were standardized, and intensive training packages for health and community workers were developed and implemented in many countries. These efforts were supported by unprecedented funding through the World Bank, the Global Fund, and PEPFAR. In 2003, the lack of access to ART was declared a global public-health emergency by the WHO and UNAIDS, and the two agencies launched the "3 by 5 initiative," setting an ambitious target: having 3 million people in developing countries on treatment by the end of 2005. Many countries have since set corresponding national targets and have worked to integrate ART into their national AIDS programs and health systems and to harness the synergies between HIV/AIDS treatment and prevention activities. The G8 (Gleneagles) 2005 communiqué endorsing universal access to HIV treatment by 2010 was another major step forward.

It is clear by now that the claims made for the efficacy of ART are well founded: in the United States, such therapy has prolonged life by an estimated 13 years per patient on average—a success rate that would compare favorably with that of almost any treatment for cancer or for complications of coronary artery disease. Further lessons with implications for policy and action have come from efforts that are now under way in the developing world. During the past decade, through experiences in >50 countries thus far, the world has seen that ambitious policy goals, adequate funding, and knowledge about implementation can dramatically transform the prospects of people living with HIV infection in developing nations.

TUBERCULOSIS

Chapter 158 offers a concise overview of the pathophysiology and treatment of TB, which is closely linked to HIV infection in much of the world. Indeed, a substantial proportion of the resurgence of TB registered in southern Africa may be attributed to HIV co-infection. Even before the advent of HIV, however, it was estimated that fewer than half of all cases of TB in developing countries were ever diagnosed, much less treated.

Primarily because of the common failure to diagnose and treat TB, international authorities devised a single strategy to reduce the burden of disease. The DOTS strategy (*d*irectly *o*bserved *t*herapy using short-

course isoniazid- and rifampin-based regimens) was promoted in the early 1990s as highly cost-effective by the World Bank, the WHO, and other international bodies. Passive case-finding of smear-positive patients was central to the strategy, and an uninterrupted drug supply was, of course, deemed necessary for cure. DOTS was clearly effective for most uncomplicated cases of drug-susceptible TB, but it was not long before a number of shortcomings were identified. First, the diagnosis of TB based solely on smear microscopy—a method dating from the late nineteenth century—is not sensitive. Many patients with pulmonary TB and all patients with exclusively extrapulmonary TB are missed by smear microscopy, as are most children with active disease. Second, passive case-finding relies on the availability of health care services, which is uneven in settings where TB is most prevalent. Third, patients with multidrug-resistant (MDR) TB are by definition infected with strains of *Mycobacterium tuberculosis* resistant to isoniazid and rifampin; thus exclusive reliance on these drugs is ineffective in settings in which drug resistance is an established problem.

The crisis of antibiotic resistance registered in U.S. hospitals is not confined to the industrialized world or to bacterial infections. In some settings, a substantial minority of patients with TB are infected with strains resistant to at least one first-line anti-TB drug. As an effective DOTS-based response to MDR TB, global health authorities adopted DOTS-Plus, which adds the diagnostics and drugs necessary to manage drug-resistant disease. Even before DOTS-Plus could be brought to scale in resource-constrained settings, however, new strains of extensively drug-resistant (XDR) *M. tuberculosis* began to threaten the success of TB control programs in already-beleaguered South Africa, for example, where high rates of HIV infection have led to a doubling of TB incidence over the past decade.

TUBERCULOSIS AND AIDS AS CHRONIC DISEASES: LESSONS LEARNED

Strategies effective against MDR TB have implications for the management of drug-resistant HIV infection and even drug-resistant malaria, which, through repeated infections and a lack of effective therapy, has become a chronic disease in parts of Africa. Indeed, examining AIDS and TB together as chronic diseases allows us to draw a number of conclusions, many of them pertinent to global health in general (Fig. 2-3).

First, charging fees for AIDS prevention and care will pose insurmountable problems for people living in poverty, many of whom will always be unable to pay even modest amounts for services or medications. Like efforts to battle airborne TB, such services might best be seen as a public good for public health. Initially, this approach will require sustained donor contributions, but many African countries have recently set targets for increased national investments in health—a pledge that could render ambitious programs sustainable in the long run. Meanwhile, as local investments increase, the price of AIDS care is decreasing. The development of generic medications means that ART can now cost <$0.50 (U.S.) per day, and costs continue to decrease to affordable levels for public health bodies in developing countries.

Second, the effective scale-up of pilot projects will require the strengthening and sometimes rebuilding of health care systems, including those charged with delivering primary care. In the past, the lack of health care infrastructure has been cited as a barrier to providing ART in the world's poorest regions; however, AIDS resources, which are at last considerable, may be marshaled to rebuild public health systems in sub-Saharan Africa and other HIV-burdened regions—precisely the settings in which TB is resurgent.

Third, a lack of trained health care personnel, most notably doctors, is invoked as a reason for the failure to treat AIDS in poor countries. The lack is real, and the "brain drain," which is discussed below, continues. However, one reason doctors leave Africa is that they lack the tools to practice their trade there. AIDS funding provides an opportunity not only to recruit physicians and nurses to underserved regions but also to train community health workers to supervise care for AIDS and many other diseases within their home villages and neighborhoods. Such training should be undertaken even in places where physicians are abundant, since community-based, closely supervised care

FIGURE 2-3 An HIV/TB co-infected patient in Rwanda, before (*left*) and after (*right*) 6 months of treatment.

represents the highest standard of care for chronic disease, whether in the First World or the Third.

Fourth, extreme poverty makes it difficult for many patients to comply with therapy for chronic diseases, whether communicable or not. Indeed, poverty in its many dimensions is far and away the greatest barrier to the scale-up of treatment and prevention programs. It is possible to remove many of the social and economic barriers to adherence, but only with what are sometimes termed "wrap-around services": food supplements for the hungry, help with transportation to clinics, child care, and housing. In many rural regions of Africa, hunger is the major coexisting condition in patients with AIDS or TB, and these consumptive diseases cannot be treated effectively without adequate caloric intake.

Finally, there is a need for a renewed basic-science commitment to the discovery and development of vaccines; of more reliable, less expensive diagnostic tools; and of new classes of therapeutic agents. This need applies not only to the three leading infectious killers—against none of which an effective vaccine exists—but also to many other neglected diseases of poverty.

MALARIA

We turn now to the world's third largest infectious killer, which has taken its greatest toll among children, especially African children, living in poverty.

The Cost of Malaria Malaria's human toll is enormous. An estimated 250 million people suffer from malarial disease each year, and the disease annually kills between 1 million and 2.5 million people, mostly pregnant women and children under the age of 5. The poor disproportionately suffer the consequences of malaria: 58% of malaria deaths occur in the poorest 20% of the world's population, and 90% are registered in sub-Saharan Africa. The differential magnitude of this mortality burden is greater than that associated with any other disease. Likewise, the morbidity differential is greater for malaria than for diseases caused by other pathogens, as documented in a study from Zambia that revealed a 40% greater prevalence of parasitemia among children under 5 in the poorest quintile than in the richest.

Despite suffering the greatest consequences of malaria, the poor are precisely those least able to access effective prevention and treatment tools. Economists describe the complex interactions between malaria and poverty from an opposite but complementary perspective: they de-

lineate ways in which malaria arrests economic development both for individuals and for whole nations. Microeconomic analyses focusing on direct and indirect costs estimate that malaria may consume up to 10% of a household's annual income. A Ghanaian study that categorized the population by income group highlighted the regressive nature of this cost: the burden of malaria represents only 1% of a wealthy family's income but 34% of a poor household's income.

At the national level, macroeconomic analyses estimate that malaria may reduce the per capita gross national product of a disease-endemic country by 50% relative to that of a non-malarial country. The causes of this drag include high fertility rates, impaired cognitive development of children, decreased schooling, decreased saving, decreased foreign investment, and restriction of worker mobility. Given this enormous cost, it is little wonder that an important review by the economists Sachs and Malaney concludes that "where malaria prospers most, human societies have prospered least."

Rolling Back Malaria In part because of differences in vector distribution and climate, resource-rich countries offer few blueprints for malaria control and treatment that are applicable in tropical (and resource-poor) settings. In 2001, African heads of state endorsed the WHO Roll Back Malaria (RBM) campaign, which prescribes strategies appropriate for sub-Saharan African countries. RBM recommends a three-pronged strategy to reduce malaria-related morbidity and mortality: the use of insecticide-treated bed nets (ITNs), combination antimalarial therapy, and indoor residual spraying.

ITNs are an efficacious and cost-effective public health intervention. A meta-analysis of controlled trials indicates that malaria incidence is reduced by 50% among persons who sleep under ITNs compared with that among those who do not use nets at all. Even untreated nets reduce malaria incidence by one-quarter. On an individual level, the utility of ITNs extends beyond protection from malaria. Several studies suggest that all-cause mortality is reduced among children under 5 to a greater degree than can be attributed to the reduction in malarial disease alone. Morbidity (specifically that due to anemia) predisposing children to diarrheal and respiratory illnesses and pregnant women to the delivery of low-birth-weight infants is also reduced in populations using ITNs. In some areas, ITNs offer a supplemental benefit by preventing transmission of lymphatic filariasis, cutaneous leishmaniasis, Chagas' disease, and tick-borne relapsing fever. At the community level, investigators suggest that the use of an ITN in just one household may reduce the number of mosquito bites in households up to several hundred meters away. The cost of ITNs per DALY saved is estimated at $10–$38 (U.S.), which qualifies ITNs as a "very efficient use of resources and [a] good candidate for public subsidy."[1]

Some RBM programs have had limited success, but overall the burden of malarial disease has continued to grow. In fact, annual malaria-attributable mortality increased between 1999 and 2003. While the RBM campaign's own report from that year is quick to note that morbidity and mortality data-collection methods in sub-Saharan Africa are inadequate and indicators may thus lag behind actual outcomes of ongoing campaigns, they nevertheless acknowledge that "RBM is acting against a background of increasing malaria burden."

Limited success in scaling-up ITN coverage reflects the inadequately acknowledged economic barriers that prevent the destitute sick from accessing critical preventive technologies. Despite proven efficacy and what are considered "reasonable costs," the 2003 RBM report reveals disappointing levels of ITN coverage. In 28 African countries surveyed, only 1.3% (range, 0.2–4.9%) of households owned at least one ITN, and <2% of children slept under an ITN. Why has the RBM campaign failed to achieve its goals? Do Africans not want to use bed nets? Do they not

[1]Nuwaha F: The challenge of chloroquine-resistant malaria in sub-Saharan Africa. Health Policy Plan 16:1, 2001.

recognize malaria as a health risk? Or have project managers and donors miscalculated most Africans' ability to obtain bed nets?

These are not rhetorical questions. The RBM strategy initially emphasized the importance of commercial markets as sources of ITNs for African populations. A precedent supporting this emphasis is the prior existence in countries such as Madagascar and Mali of local markets for untreated bed nets. Presumably, therefore, a demand for bed nets existed prior to the RBM campaign, as did a distribution system with points of sale. However, even with the application of subsidized social marketing strategies, this market approach has not resulted in large increases in coverage during the first years of the RBM campaign. Several studies have attempted to define willingness to pay (WTP) and actual payment for ITNs in African countries and thereby to determine why market-based strategies have been unsuccessful. Policy-makers often use WTP figures to determine appropriate pricing for social marketing projects and to project revenue and demand. A cross-sectional study in a rural Nigerian community administered two questionnaires, 1 month apart, to examine community members' WTP for ITNs, actual purchase of ITNs (with the second questionnaire accompanied by the opportunity to buy a subsidized ITN), and factors (such as socioeconomic status and recent history of malarial illness) contributing to hypothetical and actual ITN purchase. Among the 453 persons answering both surveys, the poorest quintile perceived a greater risk of malaria than the other quintiles (27.3% vs. 12.9–21.6%, $p < .05$). However, the poorest quintile was least likely to own a net, purchase a net, or express a hypothetical WTP. Even the most well-off quintile was willing to pay only 51% of the government-set price for an ITN. This finding suggests that even the relatively well-off may not be willing or able to pay for bed nets at set prices. The authors of this study concluded that reliance on the sale of nets alone may prove inadequate and that further studies are needed to define the degrees to which costs can be lowered and/or demand increased.

A 2002 study in highland Kenya compared the attitudes of people living in homesteads provided with heavily subsidized ITNs ($n = 190$) with those of residents of households that had no ITNs and had not been targeted by other health care initiatives ($n = 200$). Of all households, 97% expressed willingness to pay for ITNs. However, only 4% of those willing to pay offered spontaneously to meet the suggested price of 350 Kenyan shillings. After being prompted that "nets are expensive," 26% of respondents expressed willingness to pay the full price. This study did not offer nets for sale; therefore, the number of nets that would actually have been purchased is unknown. However, the study did contextualize the hypothetical WTP for ITNs by comparing their cost with other household costs: the price of one ITN is equal to the cost of sending three children to primary school for a year. By placing the nets' relative cost in context, the authors of this study call into question the likelihood that families in this district, over half of whom fall below the Kenyan poverty line, would actually be able to purchase ITNs.

Given the documented barriers to purchasing ITNs, especially among the poorest of the poor, many researchers and development professionals involved in malaria programs have called for the free distribution of ITNs, comparing their importance as a public health measure with that of childhood vaccination. The adoption of free ITN distribution strategies has been limited, however, by concerns about their feasibility and potential ITN misuse (for example, as nets for fishing). Evidence from a targeted free-distribution program discounts both concerns. In 2001, a Kenyan program sponsored by UNICEF sought to distribute 70,000 ITNs to pregnant women through antenatal clinics. Within 12 weeks, >50% of the ITNs had reached their intended recipients. A 1-year follow-up evaluation of 294 women who had received bed nets while pregnant—152 women from a high-transmission area and 142 from a low-transmission area—revealed that 84% of women in the high-transmission area used the ITNs throughout pregnancy. One year later, 77% continued to use the bed nets. In the low-transmission area, 57% of women used the ITNs during pregnancy, and 46% continued to use them a year later. These results contradict suppositions that free nets may not be used because recipients do not value them.

Given the scope and magnitude of the challenge posed by malaria, it is unlikely that any one strategy will work for every region or population

within a country or across the world. Encouraging results from an employer-based ITN distribution system in Kenya highlight the potential role of public-private partnerships. Potential synergies between antimalaria programs and measles vaccine campaigns or possibly lymphatic filariasis eradication campaigns have been reported or suggested. Concerns about discomfort associated with sleeping under ITNs or about insecticide toxicities must be addressed through educational campaigns.

Meeting the challenge of malaria control will continue to require careful study of appropriate preventive and therapeutic strategies in the context of our increasingly sophisticated molecular understanding of the pathogen, vector, and host. However, an appreciation for the economic and structural devastation wrought by malaria—like that inflicted by diarrhea, AIDS, and TB—on the most vulnerable populations should heighten our commitment to the critical analysis of ways to implement proven strategies for the prevention and treatment of these diseases.

CHRONIC NONCOMMUNICABLE DISEASES

While the burden of communicable diseases—especially HIV infection, tuberculosis, and malaria—still accounts for the majority of deaths in resource-poor regions such as sub-Saharan Africa, close to 60% of all deaths worldwide in 2005 were due to chronic noncommunicable diseases (NCDs). Moreover, 80% of deaths attributable to NCDs occurred in low- and middle-income countries, where 85% of the global population lives. In 2005, 8.5 million people in the world died of an NCD before their 60th birthday—a figure exceeding the total number of deaths due to AIDS, TB, and malaria combined. By 2020, NCDs will account for 80% of the GBD and for 7 of every 10 deaths in developing countries. The recent rise in resources for and attention to communicable diseases is both welcome and long overdue, but developing countries are already carrying a "double burden" of communicable and noncommunicable diseases.

Cardiovascular Disease Unlike TB, HIV infection, and malaria—diseases caused by single pathogens that damage multiple organs—cardiovascular diseases reflect injury to a single organ system downstream of a variety of insults. The burden of chronic cardiovascular disease in low-income countries represents one consequence of decades of health system neglect; furthermore, cardiovascular research and investment have long focused on the ischemic conditions that are increasingly common in high- and middle-income countries. Meanwhile, despite awareness of its health impact during the early twentieth century, cardiovascular damage in response to infection and malnutrition has fallen out of view until recently.

The perception of cardiovascular diseases as a problem of elderly populations in middle- and high-income countries has contributed to their neglect by global health institutions. Even in Eastern Europe and Central Asia, where the collapse of the Soviet Union was followed by a catastrophic surge in cardiovascular disease deaths (mortality rates from ischemic heart disease nearly doubled between 1991 and 1994 in Russia, for example), the modest flows of overseas development assistance to the health sector focused on the communicable causes that accounted for <1 in 20 excess deaths during this period.

Predictions of an imminent rise in the share of deaths and disabilities due to NCDs in developing countries have led to calls for preventive policies to restrict tobacco use, improve diet, and increase exercise alongside the prescription of multidrug regimens for persons with high levels of vascular risk. Although this agenda could do much to prevent pandemic NCD, it will do little to help those with established heart disease stemming from non-atherogenic pathologies.

The epidemiology of heart failure reflects inequalities in risk factor prevalence and treatment. Heart failure as a consequence of pericardial, myocardial, endocardial, or valvular injury accounts for as many as 1 in 10 admissions to hospitals around the world. Countries have reported a remarkably similar burden of this condition at the health system level since the 1950s, but the causes of heart failure and the age of the people affected vary with resources and ecology. In populations with a high human-development index, coronary artery disease and hypertension among the elderly account for most cases of heart failure. Among the world's poorest billion people, however, heart failure reflects poverty-driven exposure of children and young adults to rheumatogenic strains of streptococci and cardiotropic microorganisms (e.g., HIV, *Trypanosoma cruzi*, enteroviruses, *M. tuberculosis*), untreated high blood pressure, and nutrient deficiencies. The mechanisms of other causes of heart failure common in these populations—such as idiopathic dilated cardiomyopathy, peripartum cardiomyopathy, and endomyocardial fibrosis—remain unclear.

Of the 2.3 million annual cases of pediatric rheumatic heart disease, nearly half occur in sub-Saharan Africa. This disease leads to more than 33,000 cases of endocarditis, 252,000 strokes, and 680,000 deaths per year—almost all in developing countries. Researchers in Ethiopia have reported annual death rates as high as 12.5% in rural areas. In part because the prevention of rheumatic heart disease has not advanced since the disappearance of this disease in wealthy countries, no part of sub-Saharan Africa has yet eradicated rheumatic heart disease despite examples of success in Costa Rica, Cuba, and some Caribbean nations.

Strategies to eliminate rheumatic heart disease may depend on active case-finding confirmed by echocardiography among high-risk groups as well as efforts to extend access to surgical interventions among children with advanced valvular damage. Partnerships between established surgical programs and areas with limited or nonexistent facilities may help develop capacity and provide care to patients who would otherwise suffer an early and painful death. A long-term goal is the establishment of regional centers of excellence equipped to provide consistent, accessible, high-quality services.

In stark contrast to the extraordinary lengths to which patients in wealthy countries will go to treat ischemic cardiomyopathy, young patients with nonischemic cardiomyopathies in resource-poor settings have received little attention. These conditions account for as many as 25–30% of admissions for heart failure in sub-Saharan Africa and include poorly understood entities such as peripartum cardiomyopathy (which has an incidence in rural Haiti of 1 per 300 live births) and HIV cardiomyopathy. Multidrug regimens that include heart failure beta-blockers, ACE inhibitors, and other neurohormonal antagonists can dramatically reduce mortality risk and improve quality of life for these patients. Lessons learned in the scale-up of chronic care for HIV infection and TB may be illustrative as progress is made in establishing means to deliver cardiac therapies over a background of careful fluid management with diuretic drugs.

Because systemic investigation of the causes of stroke and heart failure in sub-Saharan Africa has begun only recently, little is known about the impact of elevated blood pressure in this portion of the continent. Modestly elevated blood pressure in the absence of tobacco use in populations with low rates of obesity may confer little risk of adverse events in the short run. In contrast, persistently elevated blood pressure above 180/110 goes largely undetected, untreated, and uncontrolled in this setting. In the Framingham cohort of men 45–74 years old, the prevalence of blood pressures above 210/120 declined from 1.8% in the 1950s to 0.1% in the 1990s with the introduction of effective antihypertensive agents. While debate continues about appropriate screening strategies and treatment thresholds, rural health centers staffed by nonphysicians must quickly gain access to essential antihypertensive medications.

In 1960, Paul Dudley White and colleagues reported on the prevalence of cardiovascular disease in the region near the Albert Schweitzer Hospital in Lambaréné, Gabon. Although the group found little evidence of myocardial infarction, they concluded that "*the high prevalence of mitral stenosis* [sic] *is astonishing.... We believe strongly that it is a duty to help bring to these sufferers the benefits of better penicillin prophylaxis and of cardiac surgery when indicated. The same responsibility exists for those with correctable congenital cardiovascular defects.*"[2] Leaders from tertiary centers in sub-Saharan Africa and elsewhere have continued to call for prevention and treatment of the cardiovascular conditions of the poor. The reconstruction of health services in response to pandemic infectious disease offers an opportunity to identify and treat patients with organ damage and to undertake the prevention of cardiovascular and other chronic conditions of poverty.

Cancer Low- and middle-income countries accounted for 53% and 56%, respectively, of the 10 million cases and 7 million deaths due to cancer in 2000. By 2020, the total number of new cancer cases will rise by 29% in developed countries and by 73% in developing countries. Also by 2020, overall mortality from cancer will increase by 104%, and the increase will be fivefold higher in developing than in developed countries. "Western" lifestyle changes will be responsible for the increased incidence of cancers of the breast, colon, and prostate, but historic realities, sociocultural and behavioral factors, genetics, and poverty itself will also have a profound impact on cancer-related mortality and morbidity. While infectious causes are responsible for <10% of cancers in developed countries, they account for 25% of all malignancies in low- and middle-income countries. Infectious causes of cancer such as human papillomavirus (cervical cancer), hepatitis B virus (liver cancer), and *Helicobacter pylori* (stomach cancer) will continue to have a much larger impact in developing countries. Environmental and dietary factors, such as indoor air pollution and high-salt diets, also help account for increased rates of certain cancers (e.g., lung and stomach cancers). Tobacco use (both smoking and chewing) is the most important source of increased mortality from lung and oral cancers. In contrast to decreasing tobacco use in many developed countries, the number of smokers is growing in developing countries, especially among women and young people.

For many reasons, outcomes of malignancies are far worse in developing countries than in developed nations. Overstretched health systems in poor countries simply are not capable of early detection; 80% of patients already have incurable malignancies at diagnosis. Treatment of cancers is available for only a very small number of mostly wealthy citizens in the majority of poor countries, and, even when treatment is available, the range and quality of services are often substandard.

Diabetes The International Diabetes Federation reports that the number of diabetics in the world is expected to increase from 194 million in 2003 to 330 million by 2030, when 3 of every 4 sufferers will live in developing countries. Because diabetics are far more frequently under the age of 65 in developing nations, the complications of micro- and macrovascular disease take a far greater toll. In 2005, an estimated 1.1 million people died of diabetes-related illnesses, and >80% of these deaths occurred in low- and middle-income countries.

Obesity and Tobacco Use In 2004, the WHO released its Global Strategy on Diet, Physical Activity and Health, which focused on the population-wide promotion of healthy diet and regular physical activity in an effort to reduce the growing global problem of overweight and obesity. Passing this strategy at the World Health Assembly proved difficult because of strong opposition from the food industry and from a number of WHO member states, including the United States. While globalization has had many positive effects, one negative aspect has been the growth in both developed and developing countries of well-financed lobbies that have aggressively promoted unhealthy dietary changes and increased consumption of alcohol and tobacco. Foreign direct investment in tobacco, beverage, and food products in developing countries reached $327 million in 2002—a figure nearly five times greater than the amount spent during that year to address NCDs by bilateral funding agencies, the WHO, and the World Bank combined.

The Three Pillars of Prevention The WHO estimates that 80% of all cases of cardiovascular disease and type 2 diabetes as well as 40% of all cancers can be prevented through the three pillars of healthy diet, physical activity, and avoidance of tobacco. While there is some evidence that population-based measures can have some impact on these behaviors, it is sobering to note that increasing obesity levels have not been successfully reversed in any population, including those of high-income countries with robust diet industries. Nonetheless, in Mauri-

---

[2]Miller DC et al: Survey of cardiovascular disease among Africans in the vicinity of the Albert Schweitzer Hospital in 1960. Am J Cardiol 19:432, 1962.

tius, for example, a single policy measure that changed the type of cooking oil available to the population led to a fall in mean serum cholesterol levels. Tobacco avoidance may be the most important and most difficult behavioral modification of all. In the twentieth century, 100 million people died worldwide of tobacco-related diseases; it is projected that >1 billion people will die of these diseases in the twenty-first century, with the vast majority of these deaths in developing countries. Today, 80% of the world's 1.2 billion smokers live in low- and middle-income countries, and, while tobacco consumption is falling in most developed countries, it continues to rise at a rate of ~3.4% per year in developing countries. The WHO's Framework Convention on Tobacco Control was a major advance, committing all of its signatories to a set of policy measures that have been shown to reduce tobacco consumption. However, most developing countries have continued to take a passive approach to the control of smoking.

ENVIRONMENTAL HEALTH

In a recent publication that examined how specific diseases and injuries are affected by environmental risk, the WHO determined that ~24% of the total GBD, one-third of the GBD among children, and 23% of all deaths are due to modifiable environmental factors. Many of these factors lead to deaths from infectious diseases; others lead to deaths from malignancies. Increasingly, etiology and nosology are difficult to parse. As much as 94% of diarrheal disease, which is linked to unsafe drinking water and poor sanitation, can be attributed to environmental factors. Risk factors such as indoor air pollution due to use of solid fuels, exposure to second-hand tobacco smoke, and outdoor air pollution account for 20% of lower respiratory infections in developed countries and for as many as 42% of such infections in developing countries. Various forms of unintentional injury and malaria top the list of health problems to which environmental factors contribute. Some 4 million children die every year from causes related to unhealthy environments, and the number of infant deaths due to environmental factors in developing countries is 12 times that in developed countries.

MENTAL HEALTH

The WHO reports that some 450 million people worldwide are affected by mental, neurologic, or behavioral problems at any given time and that ~873,000 people die by suicide every year. Major depression is the leading cause of lost DALYs in the world today. One in four patients visiting a health service has at least one mental, neurologic, or behavioral disorder, but most of these disorders are neither diagnosed nor treated. Most low- and middle-income countries devote <1% of their already-paltry health expenditures to mental health.

Increasingly effective therapies exist for many of the major causes of mental disorder. Effective treatments for many neurologic diseases, including seizure disorders, have long been available. One of the greatest barriers to delivery of such therapies is the paucity of skilled personnel. Most sub-Saharan African countries have only a handful of psychiatrists, for example; most of them practice in cities and are unavailable within the public sector or to patients living in poverty. Of the few patients who are fortunate enough to see a psychiatrist or neurologist, fewer still are able to adhere to treatment regimens: several surveys of already-diagnosed patients ostensibly receiving daily therapy have revealed that, among the poor, few can take their medications as prescribed. The same barriers that prevent the poor from having reliable access to insulin or ART also prevent them from benefiting from antidepressant, antipsychotic, and antiepileptic agents. To alleviate this problem, some authorities are proposing the training of health workers to provide community-based adherence support, counseling services, and referrals for patients in need of mental health services.

World Mental Health: Problems and Priorities in Low-Income Countries offers a comprehensive analysis of the burden of mental, behavioral, and social problems in low-income countries and relates the mental health consequences of social forces such as violence, dislocation, poverty, and the disenfranchisement of women to current economic, political, and environmental concerns.

HEALTH SYSTEMS AND THE "BRAIN DRAIN"

A significant and oft-invoked barrier to effective health care in resource-poor settings is the lack of medical personnel. In what is termed the *brain drain*, many physicians and nurses emigrate from their home countries to pursue opportunities abroad, leaving behind health systems that are understaffed and ill-equipped to deal with the epidemic diseases that ravage local populations. The WHO recommends a minimum of 20 physicians and 100 nurses per 100,000 persons, but recent reports from that organization and others confirm that many countries, especially in sub-Saharan Africa, fall far short of those target numbers. More than half of these countries register fewer than 10 physicians per 100,000 population. In contrast, the United States and Cuba register 279 and 596 doctors per 100,000 population, respectively. Similarly, the majority of sub-Saharan African countries do not have even half of the WHO-recommended minimum number of nurses. In addition to these appalling national aggregates, further inequalities in health care staffing exist *within* countries. Rural-urban disparities in health care personnel mirror disparities of both wealth and health. In 1992, the poorest districts in southern Africa reported 5.5 doctors, 188.1 nurses, and 0.5 pharmacists per 100,000 population. The same survey found, in the richest districts, 35.6 doctors, 375.3 nurses, and 5.4 pharmacists per 100,000 population. Nearly 90% of Malawi's population is rural, but >95% of clinical officers were at urban facilities, and 47% of nurses were at tertiary care facilities. Even community health workers, trained to provide first-line services to rural populations, often transfer to urban districts. In 1989 in Kenya, for example, there were only 138 health workers per 100,000 persons in the rural North Eastern Province, whereas there were 688 per 100,000 in Nairobi.

In addition to inter- and intranational transfer of personnel, the AIDS epidemic contributes to personnel shortages across Africa. Although data on the prevalence of HIV infection among health professionals are scarce, the available numbers suggest substantial and adverse impacts on an already-overburdened health sector. In 1999, it was estimated that 17–32% of health care workers in Botswana had HIV disease, and this number is expected to increase in the coming years. A recent study that examined the fates of a small cohort of Ugandan physicians found that at least 22 of the 77 doctors who graduated from Makerere University Medical School in 1984 had died by 2004—most, presumably, of AIDS. Similar numbers have been registered in South Africa, where a small study by the Human Sciences Research Council found an HIV seroprevalence among health professionals similar to that among the general population—in this case, 15.7% of all health care workers surveyed. The shortage of medical personnel in the areas hardest hit by HIV has profound implications for prevention and treatment efforts in these regions. The cycle of health-sector impoverishment, brain drain, and lack of personnel to fill positions when they are available conspires against ambitious programs to bring ART to persons living with both AIDS and poverty. The president of Botswana recently declared that one of his country's main obstacles to rapid expansion of HIV/AIDS treatment is "a dearth of doctors, nurses, pharmacists, and other health workers."[3] In South Africa, the departure of nearly 600 pharmacists in 2001, coupled with standing vacancies for 32,000 nurses, has put continued strain on that relatively affluent country's ability to respond to calls for expanded treatment programs. In Malawi, only 28% of established nursing posts are filled. Furthermore, the education of medical trainees is jeopardized as the ranks of the health and academic communities continue to shrink as a result of migration or disease. The long-term implications are sobering.

A proper biosocial analysis of the brain drain reminds us that the flight of health personnel—almost always, as most reviews suggest, from poor to less-poor regions—is not simply a question of desire for more equitable remuneration. Epidemiologic trends and access to the tools of the trade are also relevant, as are working conditions in general. In many settings now losing skilled health personnel, the advent of HIV has led to a sharp rise in TB incidence; in the eyes of health care providers, other

---

[3]Dugger C: Botswana's brain drain cripples war on AIDS. *New York Times* A10 (13 November 2003).

opportunistic infections have also become insuperable challenges. Together, these forces have conspired to render the provision of proper care impossible, as the comments of a Kenyan medical resident suggest: "Regarding HIV/AIDS, it is impossible to go home and forget about it. Even the simplest opportunistic infections we have no drugs for. Even if we do, there is only enough for a short course. It is impossible to forget about it. . . . Just because of the numbers, I am afraid of going to the floors. It is a nightmare thinking of going to see the patients. You are afraid of the risk of infection, diarrhea, urine, vomit, blood. . . . It is frightening to think about returning."[4] Another resident noted, "Before training we thought of doctors as supermen. . . . [Now] we are only mortuary attendants."[5] Nurses and other providers are, of course, similarly affected.

Given the difficult conditions under which these health care personnel work, is it any surprise when the U.S. government's appointed Global AIDS Coordinator notes that there are more Ethiopian physicians practicing in Chicago than in all of Ethiopia? In Zambia, only 50 of the 600 doctors trained since the country's independence in 1964 remain in their home country. Nor is it surprising that a 1999 survey of medical students in Ghana in their final year of training revealed that 40 of 43 students planned to leave the country upon graduation. When providing care for the sick becomes a nightmare for those at the beginning of clinical training, physician burn-out soon follows among those who carry on in settings of impoverishment. In the public-sector institutions put in place to care for the poorest people, the confluence of epidemic disease, lack of resources with which to respond, and unrealistically high user fees has led to widespread burn-out among health workers. Patients and their families are those who pay most dearly for provider burn-out, just as they bear the burden of disease and—with the introduction of user fees—much of the cost of responding, however inadequately, to new epidemics and persistent plagues.

CONCLUSION: TOWARD A SCIENCE OF IMPLEMENTATION

Public-health strategies draw largely on quantitative methods—from epidemiology and biostatistics, but also from economics. Clinical practice, including internal medicine, draws on a rapidly expanding knowledge base but remains focused on individual patient care; clinical interventions are rarely population-based. In fact, neither public-health nor clinical approaches alone will prove adequate in addressing the problems of global health. There is a long way to go before evidence-based internal medicine is applied effectively among the world's poor. Complex infectious diseases such as AIDS and TB have proven difficult but not impossible to manage; drug resistance and a lack of effective health systems have further complicated such work. Beyond communicable disease, in the arena of chronic diseases (e.g., cardiovascular disease), global health is a nascent endeavor. Efforts to address any one of these problems in settings of great scarcity need to be integrated into broader efforts to strengthen failing health systems and to alleviate the growing personnel crisis within these systems.

For these reasons, scholarly work and practice in the field once known as international health and now often designated *global health equity* are changing rapidly. Such work is still informed by the tension between clinical practice and population-based interventions, between analysis and action. Once metrics are refined, how might they inform efforts to lessen the premature morbidity and mortality registered among the world's poor? As in the nineteenth century, human rights perspectives have proven helpful in turning attention to the problems of the destitute sick; such perspectives may also inform strategies of delivering care equitably. A number of university hospitals are developing training programs for physicians with interests in global health. In medical schools across the United States and in other wealthy countries, interest in global health has been exploding. An informal survey at Harvard Medical School in 2006 revealed that nearly one-quarter of the 160 entering students either had significant global health experience or were planning a career in global health. A similar sea-change among trainees has been reported at other medical schools. Half a century or even a decade ago, such high levels of interest would have been unimaginable.

Persistent epidemics, improved metrics, and growing interest have only recently been matched by an unprecedented investment in addressing the health problems of poor people in the developing world. Ours is a moment of opportunity. To ensure that the opportunity is not wasted, the basic facts need to be laid out for specialists and laypeople alike. More than 12 million people die each year simply because they live in poverty. An absolute majority of these premature deaths occur in Africa, with the poorer regions of Asia not far behind. Most of these deaths occur because the world's poorest do not have access to the fruits of science. They include deaths from vaccine-preventable illness; deaths during childbirth; deaths from infectious diseases that might be cured with access to antibiotics and other essential medicines; deaths from malaria that would have been prevented by bed nets and access to therapy; and deaths from water-borne illnesses. Other excess mortality is attributable to the inadequacy of efforts to develop new tools. Those funding the discovery and development of new tools typically neglect the concurrent need for strategies to make them available to the poor. Indeed, some would argue that the biggest challenge facing those who seek to address this outcome gap is the lack of practical means of distribution in the regions most heavily affected.

The development of tools must be followed in short order by their equitable distribution. When new preventive and therapeutic tools are developed without concurrent attention to delivery or implementation, we face what are sometimes termed *perverse effects:* even as new tools are developed, inequalities of outcome—less morbidity and mortality among those who can afford access, with sustained high morbidity and mortality among those who cannot—will grow in the absence of an equity plan to deliver the tools to those most at risk. Preventing such a future is the most important goal of global health.

FURTHER READINGS

COHEN J: The new world of global health. Science 311:162, 2006

DESJARLAIS R et al (eds): *World Mental Health: Problems and Priorities in Low-Income Countries.* New York, Oxford University Press, 1995

FARMER PE: *Infections and Inequalities: The Modern Plagues*, 2d ed. Berkeley, University of California Press, 2001

———: From "marvelous momentum" to healthcare for all. Response to Garrett L: The challenge of global health. Foreign Affairs 86:155, 2007

FAUCI AS et al: Emerging infectious diseases: A 10-year perspective from the National Institute of Allergy and Infectious Diseases. Emerg Infect Dis 11:519, 2005

GARRETT L: The challenge of global health. Foreign Affairs 86:14, 2007

HOTEZ PJ et al: Neglected tropical diseases and HIV/AIDS. Lancet 368:1865, 2006

JAMISON DT et al (eds): *Disease Control Priorities in Developing Countries*, 2d ed. Washington, DC, Oxford University Press and The World Bank, 2006

KIM JY et al (eds): *Dying for Growth: Global Inequality and the Health of the Poor.* Monroe, ME, Common Courage Press, 2000

LOPEZ AD et al: Global and regional burden of disease and risk factors, 2001: Systematic analysis of population health data. Lancet 367:1747, 2006

MURRAY CJL, LOPEZ AD (eds): The global burden of disease: A comprehensive assessment of mortality and disability from diseases, injuries, and risk factors in 1990 and projected to 2020. Cambridge, MA, Harvard University Press, 1996

SACHS J, MALANEY O: The economic and social burden of malaria. Nature 415:680, 2002

WORLD BANK: *World Development Report 1993: Investing in Health.* New York, Oxford University Press, 1993

WORLD HEALTH ORGANIZATION: *Macroeconomics and Health: Investing in Health for Economic Development.* Geneva, Commission on Macroeconomics and Health, 2001

———: *World Health Report 2006: Working Together for Health.* Geneva, World Health Organization, 2006

---

[4]Raviola G et al: HIV, disease plague, demoralization, and "burnout": Resident experience of the medical profession in Nairobi, Kenya. Cult Med Psychiatry 26:55, 2002.
[5]Ibid.

3 Decision-Making in Clinical Medicine
Daniel B. Mark

To the medical student who requires 2 h to collect a patient's history and perform a physical examination, and several additional hours to organize them into a coherent presentation, the experienced clinician's ability to reach a diagnosis and decide on a management plan in a fraction of the time seems extraordinary. While medical knowledge and experience play a significant role in the senior clinician's ability to arrive at a differential diagnosis and plan quickly, much of the process involves skill in clinical decision-making. The first goal of this chapter is to provide an introduction to the study of clinical reasoning.

Equally bewildering to the student are the proper use of diagnostic tests and the integration of the results into the clinical assessment. The novice medical practitioner typically uses a "shotgun" approach to testing, hoping to hit a target without knowing exactly what that target is. The expert, on the other hand, usually has a specific target in mind and efficiently adjusts the testing strategy to it. The second goal of this chapter is to review briefly some of the crucial basic statistical concepts that govern the proper interpretation and use of diagnostic tests. Quantitative tools available to assist in clinical decision-making will also be discussed.

Evidence-based medicine is the term used to describe the integration of the best available research evidence with clinical judgment and experience in the care of patients. The third goal of this chapter is to provide a brief overview of some of the tools of evidence-based medicine.

CLINICAL DECISION-MAKING

CLINICAL REASONING

The most important clinical actions are not procedures or prescriptions but the judgments from which all other aspects of clinical medicine flow. In the modern era of large randomized trials and evidence-based medicine, it is easy to overlook the importance of this elusive mental activity and focus instead on the algorithmic practice guidelines constructed to improve care. One reason for this apparent neglect is that much more research has been done on how doctors *should* make decisions (e.g., using a Bayesian model, discussed below) than on how they actually *do*. Thus, much of what we know about clinical reasoning comes from empirical studies of nonmedical problem-solving behavior.

Despite the great technological advances of medicine over the last century, uncertainty still plays a pivotal role in all aspects of medical decision-making. We may know that a patient does not have long to live, but we cannot be certain how long. We may prescribe a potent new receptor blocker to reverse the course of a patient's illness, but we cannot be certain that the therapy will achieve the desired result and that result alone. Uncertainty in medical outcomes creates the need for probabilities and other mathematical/statistical tools to help guide decision-making. (These tools are reviewed later in the chapter.)

Uncertainty is compounded by the information overload that characterizes modern medicine. Today's experienced clinician needs close to 2 million pieces of information to practice medicine. Doctors subscribe to an average of seven journals, representing over 2500 new articles each year. Computers offer the obvious solution both for management of information and for better quantitation and management of the daily uncertainties of medical care. While the technology to computerize medical practice is available, many practical problems remain to be solved before patient information can be standardized and integrated with medical evidence on a single electronic platform.

The following three examples introduce the subject of clinical reasoning:

- A 46-year-old man presents to his internist with a chief complaint of hemoptysis. The physician knows that the differential diagnosis of hemoptysis includes over 100 different conditions, including cancer and tuberculosis. The examination begins with some general background questions, and the patient is asked to describe his symptoms and their chronology. By the time the examination is completed, and even before any tests are run, the physician has formulated a working diagnostic hypothesis and planned a series of steps to test it. In an otherwise healthy and nonsmoking patient recovering from a viral bronchitis, the doctor's hypothesis would be that the acute bronchitis is responsible for the small amount of blood-streaked sputum the patient observed. In this case, a chest x-ray may provide sufficient reassurance that a more serious disorder is not present.

- A second 46-year-old patient with the same chief complaint who has a 100-pack-year smoking history, a productive morning cough, and episodes of blood-streaked sputum may generate the principal diagnostic hypothesis of carcinoma of the lung. Consequently, along with the chest x-ray, the physician obtains a sputum cytology examination and refers this patient for fiberoptic bronchoscopy.

- A third 46-year-old patient with hemoptysis who is from a developing country is evaluated with an echocardiogram as well, because the physician thinks she hears a soft diastolic rumbling murmur at the apex on cardiac auscultation, suggesting rheumatic mitral stenosis.

These three simple vignettes illustrate two aspects of expert clinical reasoning: (1) the use of cognitive shortcuts as a way to organize the complex unstructured material that is collected in the clinical evaluation, and (2) the use of diagnostic hypotheses to consolidate the information and indicate appropriate management steps.

THE USE OF COGNITIVE SHORTCUTS

Cognitive shortcuts or rules of thumb, sometimes referred to as *heuristics*, can help solve complex problems, of the sort encountered daily in clinical medicine, with great efficiency. Clinicians rely on three basic types of heuristics. When assessing a particular patient, clinicians often weigh the probability that this patient's clinical features match those of the class of patients with the leading diagnostic hypotheses being considered. In other words, the clinician is searching for the diagnosis for which the patient appears to be a representative example; this cognitive shortcut is called the *representativeness heuristic*.

It may take only a few characteristics from the history for an expert clinician using the representativeness heuristic to arrive at a sound diagnostic hypothesis. For example, an elderly patient with new-onset fever, cough productive of copious sputum, unilateral pleuritic chest pain, and dyspnea is readily identified as fitting the pattern for acute pneumonia, probably of bacterial origin. Evidence of focal pulmonary consolidation on the physical examination will increase the clinician's confidence in the diagnosis because it fits the expected pattern of acute bacterial pneumonia. Knowing this allows the experienced clinician to conduct an efficient, directed, and therapeutically productive patient evaluation since there may be little else in the history or physical examination of direct relevance. The inexperienced medical student or resident, who has not yet learned the patterns most prevalent in clinical medicine, must work much harder to achieve the same result and is often at risk of missing the important clinical problem in a sea of compulsively collected but unhelpful data.

However, physicians using the representativeness heuristic can reach erroneous conclusions if they fail to consider the underlying prevalence of two competing diagnoses (i.e., the prior, or pretest, probabilities). Consider a patient with pleuritic chest pain, dyspnea, and a low-grade fever. A clinician might consider acute pneumonia and acute pulmonary embolism to be the two leading diagnostic alternatives. Using the representativeness heuristic, the clinician might judge both diagnostic candidates to be equally likely, although to do so would be wrong if pneumonia was much more prevalent in the underlying population. Mistakes may also result from a failure to consider that a pattern based on a small number of prior observations will likely be less reliable than one based on larger samples.

A second commonly used cognitive shortcut, the *availability heuristic*, involves judgments made on the basis of how easily prior similar cases or outcomes can be brought to mind. For example, the experienced clinician may recall 20 elderly patients seen over the past few years who presented with painless dyspnea of acute onset and were found to have acute myocardial infarction. The novice clinician may spend valuable time seeking a pulmonary cause for the symptoms before considering and then confirming the cardiac diagnosis. In this situation, the patient's clinical pattern does not fit the expected pattern of acute myocardial infarction, but experience with this atypical presentation, and the ability to recall it, can help direct the physician to the diagnosis.

Errors with the availability heuristic can come from several sources of recall bias. For example, rare catastrophes are likely to be remembered with a clarity and force out of proportion to their value, and recent experience is, of course, easier to recall and therefore more influential on clinical judgments.

The third commonly used cognitive shortcut, the *anchoring heuristic*, involves estimating a probability by starting from a familiar point (the anchor) and adjusting to the new case from there. Anchoring can be a powerful tool for diagnosis but is often used incorrectly. For example, a clinician may judge the probability of coronary artery disease (CAD) to be very high after a positive exercise thallium test, because the prediction has been anchored to the test result ("positive test = high probability of CAD"). Yet, as discussed below, this prediction would be inaccurate if the clinical (pretest) picture of the patient being tested indicates a low probability of disease (e.g., a 30-year-old woman with no risk factors). As illustrated in this example, anchors are not necessarily the same as the pretest probability (see "Measures of Disease Probability and Bayes' Theorem," below).

DIAGNOSTIC HYPOTHESIS GENERATION

Cognitive scientists studying the thought processes of expert clinicians have observed that clinicians group data into packets, or "chunks," which are stored in their memories and manipulated to generate diagnostic hypotheses. Because short-term memory can typically hold only 7–10 items at a time, the number of packets that can be actively integrated into hypothesis-generating activities is similarly limited. The cognitive shortcuts discussed above play a key role in the generation of diagnostic hypotheses, many of which are discarded as rapidly as they are formed.

A diagnostic hypothesis sets a context for diagnostic steps to follow and provides testable predictions. For example, if the enlarged and quite tender liver felt on physical examination is due to acute hepatitis (the hypothesis), certain specific liver function tests should be markedly elevated (the prediction). If the tests come back normal, the hypothesis may need to be discarded or substantially modified.

One of the factors that make teaching diagnostic reasoning difficult is that expert clinicians do not follow a fixed pattern in patient examinations. From the outset, they are generating, refining, and discarding diagnostic hypotheses. The questions they ask in the history are driven by the hypotheses they are working with at the moment. Even the physical examination is driven by specific questions rather than a pre-ordained checklist. While the student is palpating the abdomen of the alcoholic patient, waiting for a finding to strike him, the expert clinician is on a focused search mission. Is the spleen enlarged? How big is the liver? Is it tender? Are there any palpable masses or nodules? Each question focuses the attention of the examiner to the exclusion of all other inputs until answered, allowing the examiner to move on to the next specific question.

Negative findings are often as important as positive ones in establishing and refining diagnostic hypotheses. Chest discomfort that is not provoked or worsened by exertion in an active patient reduces the likelihood that chronic ischemic heart disease is the underlying cause. The absence of a resting tachycardia and thyroid gland enlargement reduces the likelihood of hyperthyroidism in a patient with paroxysmal atrial fibrillation.

The acuity of a patient's illness can play an important role in overriding considerations of prevalence and other issues described above. For example, clinicians are taught to consider aortic dissection routinely as a possible cause of acute severe chest discomfort along with myocardial infarction, even though the typical history of dissection is different from myocardial infarction and dissection is far less prevalent (Chap. 242). This recommendation is based on the recognition that a relatively rare but catastrophic diagnosis like aortic dissection is very difficult to make unless it is explicitly considered. If the clinician fails to elicit any of the characteristic features of dissection by history and finds equivalent blood pressures in both arms and no pulse deficits, he or she may feel comfortable in discarding the aortic dissection hypothesis. If, however, the chest x-ray shows a widened mediastinum, the hypothesis may be reinstated and a diagnostic test ordered [e.g., thoracic computed tomography (CT) scan, transesophageal echocardiogram] to evaluate it more fully. In nonacute situations, the prevalence of potential alternative diagnoses should play a much more prominent role in diagnostic hypothesis generation.

Generation of Diagnostic Hypotheses   Because the generation and evaluation of appropriate diagnostic hypotheses is a skill that not all clinicians possess to an equal degree, errors in this process can occur; in the patient with serious acute illness, these may lead to tragic consequences. Consider the following hypothetical example. A 45-year-old male patient with a 3-week history of a "flulike" upper respiratory infection (URI) presented to his physician with symptoms of dyspnea and a productive cough. Based on the presenting complaint, the clinician pulled out a "URI Assessment Form" to improve quality and efficiency of care. The physician quickly completed the examination components outlined on this structured form, noting in particular the absence of fever and a clear chest examination. He then prescribed an antibiotic for presumed bronchitis, showed the patient how to breathe into a paper bag to relieve his "hyperventilation," and sent him home with the reassurance that his illness was not serious. After a sleepless night with significant dyspnea unrelieved by breathing into a bag, the patient developed nausea and vomiting and collapsed. He was brought into the Emergency Department in cardiac arrest and could not be resuscitated. Autopsy showed a posterior wall myocardial infarction and a fresh thrombus in an atherosclerotic right coronary artery. What went wrong? The clinician decided, even before starting the history, that the patient's complaints were not serious. He therefore felt confident that he could perform an abbreviated and focused examination using the URI assessment protocol rather than considering the full range of possibilities and performing appropriate tests to confirm or refute his initial hypotheses. In particular, by concentrating on the "URI," the clinician failed to elicit the full dyspnea history, which would have suggested a far more serious disorder, and neglected to search for other symptoms that could have directed him to the correct diagnosis.

This example illustrates how patients can diverge from textbook symptoms and the potential consequences of being unable to adapt the diagnostic process to real-world challenges. The expert, while recognizing that common things occur commonly, approaches each evaluation on high alert for clues that the initial diagnosis may be wrong. Patients often provide information that "does not fit" with any of the leading diagnostic hypotheses being considered. Distinguishing real clues from false trails can only be achieved by practice and experience. A less-experienced clinician who tries to be too efficient (as in the above example) can make serious errors. Use of a rapid systematic clinical survey of symptoms and organ systems can help prevent the clinician from overlooking important but inapparent clues.

MAJOR INFLUENCES ON CLINICAL DECISION-MAKING

More than a decade of research on variations in clinician practice patterns has shed much light on forces that shape clinical decisions. The use of heuristic "shortcuts," as detailed above, provides a partial explanation, but several other key factors play an important role in shaping diagnostic hypotheses and management decisions. These factors can be grouped conceptually into three overlapping categories: (1) factors related to physicians' personal characteristics and practice style, (2) factors related to the practice setting, and (3) factors related to economic incentives.

Factors Related to Practice Style One of the key roles of the physician in medical care is to serve as the patient's agent to ensure that necessary care is provided at a high level of quality. Factors that influence this role include the physician's knowledge, training, and experience. It is obvious that physicians cannot practice evidence-based medicine (EBM; described later in the chapter) if they are unfamiliar with the evidence. As would be expected, specialists generally know the evidence in their field better than do generalists. Surgeons may be more enthusiastic about recommending surgery than medical doctors because their belief in the beneficial effects of surgery is stronger. For the same reason, invasive cardiologists are much more likely to refer chest pain patients for diagnostic catheterization than are noninvasive cardiologists or generalists. The physician beliefs that drive these different practice styles are based on personal experience, recollection, and interpretation of the available medical evidence. For example, heart failure specialists are much more likely than generalists to achieve target angiotensin-converting enzyme (ACE) inhibitor therapy in their heart failure patients because they are more familiar with what the targets are (as defined by large clinical trials), have more familiarity with the specific drugs (including dosages and side effects), and are less likely to overreact to foreseeable problems in therapy such as a rise in creatinine levels or symptomatic hypotension. Other intriguing research has shown a wide distribution of acceptance times of antibiotic therapy for peptic ulcer disease following widespread dissemination of the "evidence" in the medical literature. Some gastroenterologists accepted this new therapy before the evidence was clear (reflecting, perhaps, an aggressive practice style), and some gastroenterologists lagged behind (a conservative practice style, associated in this case with older physicians). As a group, internists lagged several years behind gastroenterologists.

The opinion of influential leaders can also have an important effect on practice patterns. Such influence can occur at both the national level (e.g., expert physicians teaching at national meetings) and the local level (e.g., local educational programs, "curbside consultations"). Opinion leaders do not have to be physicians. When conducting rounds with clinical pharmacists, physicians are less likely to make medication errors and more likely to use target levels of evidence-based therapies.

The patient's welfare is not the only concern that drives clinical decisions. The physician's perception about the risk of a malpractice suit resulting from either an erroneous decision or a bad outcome creates a style of practice referred to as *defensive medicine*. This practice involves using tests and therapies with very small marginal returns to preclude future criticism in the event of an adverse outcome. For example, a 40-year-old woman who presents with a long-standing history of intermittent headache and a new severe headache along with a normal neurologic examination has a very low likelihood of structural intracranial pathology. Performance of a head CT or magnetic resonance imaging (MRI) scan in this situation would constitute defensive medicine. On the other hand, the results of the test could provide reassurance to an anxious patient.

Practice Setting Factors Factors in this category relate to the physical resources available to the physician's practice and the practice environment. *Physician-induced demand* is a term that refers to the repeated observation that physicians have a remarkable ability to accommodate to and employ the medical facilities available to them. One of the foundational studies in outcomes research showed that physicians in Boston had an almost 50% higher hospital admission rate than did physicians in New Haven, despite there being no obvious differences in the health of the cities' inhabitants. The physicians in New Haven were not aware of using fewer hospital beds for their patients, nor were the Boston physicians aware of using less stringent criteria to admit patients. In both cities, physicians unconsciously adopted their practice styles to the available level of hospital beds.

Other environmental factors that can influence decision-making include the local availability of specialists for consultations and procedures, "high tech" facilities such as angiography suites, a heart surgery program, and MRI machines.

Economic Incentives Economic incentives are closely related to the other two categories of practice-modifying factors. Financial issues can exert both stimulatory and inhibitory influences on clinical practice. In general, physicians are paid on a fee-for-service, capitation, or salary basis. In fee-for-service, the more the physician does, the more the physician gets paid. The economic incentive in this case is to do more. When fees are reduced (discounted fee-for-service), doctors tend to increase the number of services billed for. Capitation, in contrast, provides a fixed payment per patient per year, encouraging physicians to take on more patients but to provide each patient with fewer services. Expensive services are more likely to be affected by this type of incentive than inexpensive preventive services. Salary compensation plans pay physicians the same regardless of the amount of clinical work performed. The incentive here is to see fewer patients.

In summary, expert clinical decision-making can be appreciated as a complex interplay between cognitive devices used to simplify large amounts of complex information interacting with physician biases reflecting education, training, and experience, all of which are shaped by powerful, sometimes perverse, external forces. In the next section, a set of statistical tools and concepts that can assist in making clinical decisions in the presence of uncertainty are reviewed.

QUANTITATIVE METHODS TO AID CLINICAL DECISION-MAKING

The process of medical decision-making can be divided into two parts: (1) defining the available courses of action and estimating the likely outcomes with each, and (2) assessing the desirability of the outcomes. The former task involves integrating key information about the patient along with relevant evidence from the medical literature to create the structure of a decision. The remainder of this chapter will review some quantitative tools available to assist the clinician in these activities.

QUANTITATIVE MEDICAL PREDICTIONS

Diagnostic Testing: Measures of Test Accuracy The purpose of performing a test on a patient is to reduce uncertainty about the patient's diagnosis or prognosis and to aid the clinician in making management decisions. Although diagnostic tests are commonly thought of as laboratory tests (e.g., measurement of serum amylase level) or procedures (e.g., colonoscopy or bronchoscopy), any technology that changes our understanding of the patient's problem qualifies as a diagnostic test. Thus, even the history and physical examination can be considered a form of diagnostic test. In clinical medicine, it is common to reduce the results of a test to a dichotomous outcome, such as positive or negative, normal or abnormal. In many cases, this simplification results in the waste of useful information. However, such simplification makes it easier to demonstrate some of the quantitative ways in which test data can be used.

The accuracy of diagnostic tests is defined in relation to an accepted "gold standard," which is presumed to reflect the true state of the patient (Table 3-1). To define the diagnostic performance of a new test, an appropriate population must be identified (ideally patients in whom the new test would be used) and both the new and the gold standard tests are applied to all subjects. The results of the two tests are then compared. The *sensitivity* or *true-positive rate* of the new test is the proportion of patients with disease (defined by the gold standard) who have a positive (new) test. This measure reflects how well the test identifies patients with disease. The proportion of patients with disease who have a negative test is the *false-negative rate* and is calculated as 1 − sensitivity. The proportion of patients without disease who have a negative test is the *specificity* or *true-negative rate*. This measure reflects how well the test correctly identifies patients without disease. The proportion of patients without disease who have a positive test is the *false-positive rate*, calculated as 1 − specificity. A perfect test would have a sensitivity of 100% and a specificity of 100% and would completely separate patients with disease from those without it.

Calculating sensitivity and specificity requires selection of a decision value for the test to define the threshold value at or above which the test is considered "positive." For any given test, as this cut point is moved to

| TABLE 3-1 | MEASURES OF DIAGNOSTIC TEST ACCURACY |

	Disease Status	
Test Result	**Present**	**Absent**
Positive	True-positive (*TP*)	False-positive (*FP*)
Negative	False-negative (*FN*)	True-negative (*TN*)

Identification of Patients with Disease

True-positive rate (sensitivity) = *TP*/(*TP*+*FN*)
False-negative rate = *FN*/(*TP*+*FN*)
True-positive rate = 1 − false-negative rate

Identification of Patients without Disease

True-negative rate (specificity) = *TN*/(*TN*+*FP*)
False-positive rate = *FP*/(*TN*+*FP*)
True-negative rate = 1 − false-positive rate

| TABLE 3-2 | MEASURES OF DISEASE PROBABILITY |

Pretest probability of disease = probability of disease before test is done. May use population prevalence of disease or more patient-specific data to generate this probability estimate.

Posttest probability of disease = probability of disease accounting for both pretest probability and test results. Also called predictive value of the test.

Bayes' theorem: Computational version:

$$\text{Posttest probability} = \frac{\text{Pretest probability} \times \text{test sensitivity}}{\begin{array}{c}\text{Pretest probability} \times \text{test sensitivity} + \\ (1 - \text{pretest probability}) \times \text{test false-positive rate}\end{array}}$$

Example [with a pretest probability of 0.50 and a "positive" diagnostic test result (test sensitivity = 0.90, test specificity = 0.90)]:

$$\text{Posttest probability} = \frac{(0.50)(0.90)}{(0.50)(0.90) + (0.50)(0.10)}$$
$$= 0.90$$

improve sensitivity, specificity typically falls and vice versa. This dynamic tradeoff between more accurate identification of subjects with disease versus those without disease is often displayed graphically as a receiver operating characteristic (ROC) curve (Fig. 3-1). An ROC curve plots sensitivity (*y*-axis) versus 1 − specificity (*x*-axis). Each point on the curve represents a potential cut point with an associated sensitivity and specificity value. The area under the ROC curve is often used as a quantitative measure of the information content of a test. Values range from 0.5 (no diagnostic information at all, test is equivalent to flipping a coin) to 1.0 (perfect test).

In the testing literature, ROC areas are often used to compare alternative tests that can be used for a particular diagnostic problem (Fig. 3-1). The test with the highest area (i.e., closest to 1.0) is presumed to be the most accurate. However, ROC curves are not a panacea for evaluation of diagnostic test utility. Like Bayes' theorem (discussed below), they are typically focused on only one possible test parameter (e.g., ST-segment response in a treadmill exercise test) to the exclusion of

FIGURE 3-1 The receiver operating characteristic (ROC) curves for three diagnostic exercise tests for detection of CAD: exercise ECG, exercise SPECT, and exercise echo. Each ROC curve illustrates the trade-off that occurs between improved test sensitivity (accurate detection of patients with disease) and improved test specificity (accurate detection of patients without disease), as the test value defining when the test turns from "negative" to "positive" is varied. A 45° line would indicate a test with no information (sensitivity = specificity at every test value). The area under each ROC curve is a measure of the information content of the test. Moving to a test with a larger ROC area (e.g., from exercise ECG to exercise echo) improves diagnostic accuracy. However, these curves are not measured in the same populations and the effect of referral biases on the results cannot easily be discerned. *(From KE Fleischmann et al: JAMA 280:913, 1998, with permission.)*

other potentially relevant data. In addition, ROC area comparisons do not simulate the way test information is actually used in clinical practice. Finally, biases in the underlying population used to generate the ROC curves (e.g., related to an unrepresentative test sample) can bias the ROC area and the validity of a comparison among tests.

Measures of Disease Probability and Bayes' Theorem Unfortunately, there are no perfect tests; after every test is completed, the true disease state of the patient remains uncertain. Quantitating this residual uncertainty can be done with Bayes' theorem. This theorem provides a simple mathematical way to calculate the posttest probability of disease from three parameters: the pretest probability of disease, the test sensitivity, and the test specificity (Table 3-2). The pretest probability is a quantitative expression of the confidence in a diagnosis before the test is performed. In the absence of more relevant information, it is usually estimated from the prevalence of the disease in the underlying population. For some common conditions, such as coronary artery disease (CAD), nomograms and statistical models have been created to generate better estimates of pretest probability from elements of the history and physical examination. The posttest probability, then, is a revised statement of the confidence in the diagnosis, taking into account what was known both before and after the test.

The term *predictive value* is often used as a synonym for the posttest probability. Unfortunately, clinicians commonly misinterpret reported predictive values as intrinsic measures of test accuracy. Studies of diagnostic tests compound the confusion by calculating predictive values on the same sample used to measure sensitivity and specificity. Since all posttest probabilities are a function of the prevalence of disease in the tested population, such calculations are clinically irrelevant unless the test is subsequently applied to populations with the same disease prevalence. For these reasons, the term *predictive value* is best avoided in favor of the more informative *posttest probability*.

To understand conceptually how Bayes' theorem estimates the posttest probability of disease, it is useful to examine a nomogram version of Bayes' theorem (Fig. 3-2). In this nomogram, the accuracy of the diagnostic test in question is summarized by the *likelihood ratio*, which is defined as the ratio of the probability of a given test result (e.g., "positive" or "negative") in a patient with disease to the probability of that result in a patient without disease.

For a positive test, the likelihood ratio is calculated as the ratio of the true-positive rate to the false-positive rate [or sensitivity/(1 − specificity)]. For example, a test with a sensitivity of 0.90 and a specificity of 0.90 has a likelihood ratio of 0.90/(1 − 0.90), or 9. Thus, for this hypothetical test, a "positive" result is 9 times more likely in a patient with the disease than in a patient without it. Most tests in medicine have likelihood ratios for a positive result between 1.5 and 20. Higher values are associated with tests that are more accurate at identifying patients with disease, with values of 10 or greater of particular note. If sensitivity is excellent but specificity is less so, the likelihood ratio will be substantially reduced (e.g., with a 90% sensitivity but a 60% specificity, the likelihood ratio is 2.25).

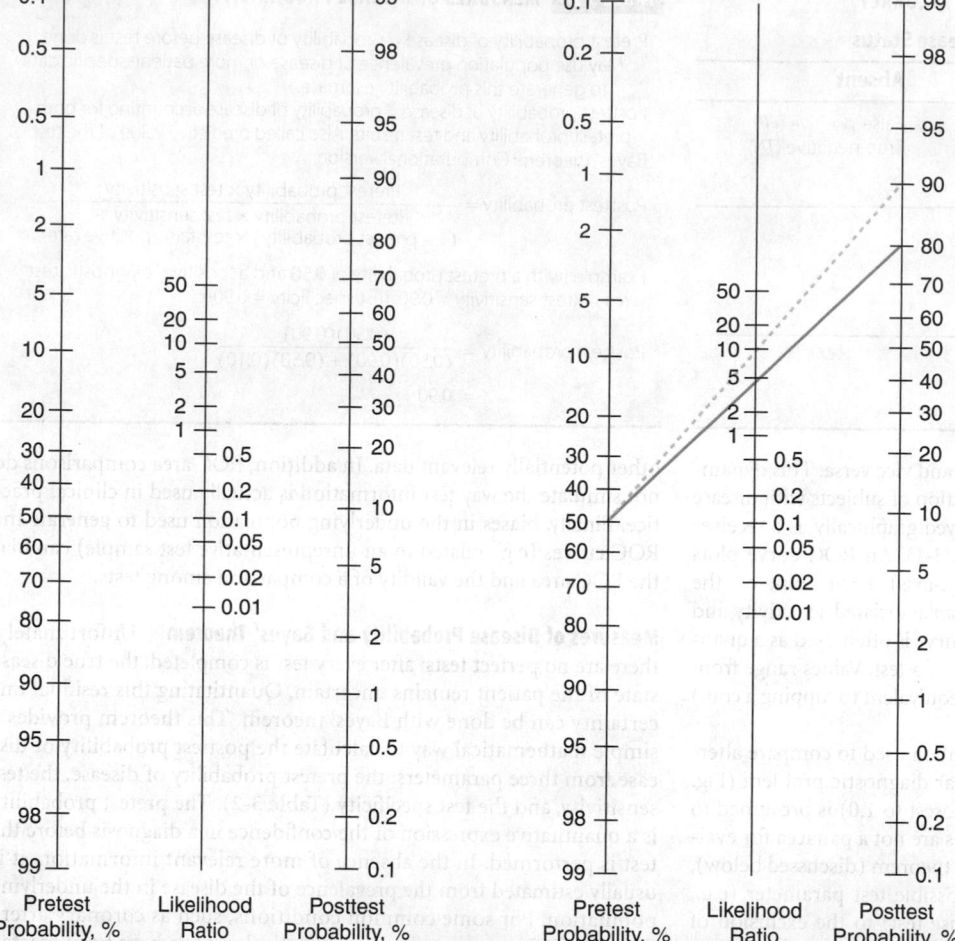

| Pretest Probability, % | Likelihood Ratio | Posttest Probability, % | | Pretest Probability, % | Likelihood Ratio | Posttest Probability, % |

FIGURE 3-2 Nomogram version of Bayes' Theorem used to predict the posttest probability of disease (right-hand scale) using the pretest probability of disease (left-hand scale) and the likelihood ratio for a positive test (middle scale). See text for information on calculation of likelihood ratios. To use, place a straightedge connecting the pretest probability and the likelihood ratio and read off the posttest probability. The right-hand part of the figure illustrates the value of a positive exercise treadmill test (likelihood ratio 4, green line) and a positive exercise thallium SPECT perfusion study (likelihood ratio 9, broken yellow line) in the patient with a pretest probability of coronary artery disease of 50%. Treadmill results shown in solid line; thallium perfusion results in dashed line. *(From DB Mark: Screening Tests, in Atlas of Cardiovascular Risk Factors. Philadelphia, Current Medicine, LLC, 2006, with permission.)*

For a negative test, the corresponding likelihood ratio is the ratio of the false negative rate to the true negative rate [or (1 − sensitivity)/specificity]. The smaller the likelihood ratio (i.e., closer to 0) the better the test performs at ruling out disease. The hypothetical test we considered above with a sensitivity of 0.9 and a specificity of 0.9 would have a likelihood ratio for a negative test result of (1 − 0.9)/0.9 of 0.11, meaning that a negative result is almost 10 times more likely if the patient is disease-free than if he has disease.

Applications to Diagnostic Testing in CAD

Consider two tests commonly used in the diagnosis of CAD, an exercise treadmill and an exercise single photon emission CT (SPECT) myocardial perfusion imaging test (Chap. 222). Meta-analysis has shown a positive treadmill ST-segment response to have an average sensitivity of 66% and an average specificity of 84%, yielding a likelihood ratio of 4.1 [0.66/(1 − 0.84)]. If we use this test on a patient with a pretest probability of CAD of 10%, the posttest probability of disease following a positive result rises to only about 30%. If a patient with a pretest probability of CAD of 80% has a positive test result, the posttest probability of disease is about 95%.

The exercise SPECT myocardial perfusion test is a more accurate test for the diagnosis of CAD. For our purposes, assume that the finding of a reversible exercise-induced perfusion defect has both a sensi-

tivity and specificity of 90%, yielding a likelihood ratio for a positive test of 9.0 [0.90/(1 − 0.90)]. If we again test our low pretest probability patient and he has a positive test, using Fig. 3-2 we can demonstrate that the posttest probability of CAD rises from 10 to 50%. However, from a decision-making point of view, the more accurate test has not been able to improve diagnostic confidence enough to change management. In fact, the test has moved us from being fairly certain that the patient did not have CAD to being completely undecided (a 50:50 chance of disease). In a patient with a pretest probability of 80%, using the more accurate exercise SPECT test raises the posttest probability to 97% (compared with 95% for the exercise treadmill). Again, the more accurate test does not provide enough improvement in posttest confidence to alter management, and neither test has improved much upon what was known from clinical data alone.

If the pretest probability is low (e.g., 20%), even a positive result on a very accurate test will not move the posttest probability to a range high enough to rule in disease (e.g., 80%). Conversely, with a high pretest probability, a negative test will not adequately rule out disease. Thus, the largest gain in diagnostic confidence from a test occurs when the clinician is most uncertain before performing it (e.g., pretest probability between 30 and 70%). For example, if a patient has a pretest probability for CAD of 50%, a positive exercise treadmill test will move the posttest probability to 80% and a positive exercise SPECT perfusion test will move it to 90% (Fig. 3-2).

Bayes' theorem, as presented above, employs a number of important simplifications that should be considered. First, few tests have only two useful outcomes, positive or negative, and many tests provide numerous pieces of data about the patient. Even if these can be integrated into a summary result, multiple levels of useful information may be present (e.g., strongly positive, positive, indeterminate, negative, strongly negative). While Bayes' theorem can be adapted to this more detailed test result format, it is computationally complex to do so.

Finally, it has long been asserted that sensitivity and specificity are prevalence-independent parameters of test accuracy, and many texts still make this statement. This statistically useful assumption, however, is clinically simplistic. A treadmill exercise test, for example, has a sensitivity in a population of patients with one-vessel CAD of around 30%, whereas its sensitivity in severe three-vessel CAD approaches 80%. Thus, the best estimate of sensitivity to use in a particular decision will often vary, depending on the distribution of disease stages present in the tested population. A hospitalized population typically has a higher prevalence of disease and in particular a higher prevalence of more advanced disease than an outpatient population. As a consequence, test sensitivity will tend to be higher in hospitalized patients, whereas test specificity will be higher in outpatients.

Statistical Prediction Models Bayes' theorem, as presented above, deals with a clinical prediction problem that is unrealistically simple relative to most problems a clinician faces. Prediction models, based on multivariable statistical models, can handle much more complex problems and substantially enhance predictive accuracy for specific situations. Their particular advantage is the ability to take into account many overlapping pieces of information and assign a relative weight to each based on its unique contribution to the prediction in question. For example, a logistic regression model to predict the probability of CAD takes into account all of the relevant independent factors from the clinical examination and diagnostic testing instead of the small handful of data that clinicians can manage in their heads or with Bayes' theorem. However, despite this strength, the models are too complex computationally to use without a calculator or computer (although this limit may be overcome once medicine is practiced from a fully computerized platform).

To date, only a handful of prediction models have been properly validated. The importance of independent validation in a population separate from the one used to develop the model cannot be overstated. An unvalidated prediction model should be viewed with the same skepticism appropriate for a new drug or medical device that has not been through rigorous clinical trial testing.

When statistical models have been compared directly with expert clinicians, they have been found to be more consistent, as would be expected, but not significantly more accurate. Their biggest promise, then, would seem to be to make less-experienced clinicians more accurate predictors of outcome.

DECISION SUPPORT TOOLS

DECISION SUPPORT SYSTEMS

Over the past 35 years, many attempts have been made to develop computer systems to help clinicians make decisions and manage patients. Conceptually, computers offer a very attractive way to handle the vast information load that today's physicians face. The computer can help by making accurate predictions of outcome, simulating the whole decision process, or providing algorithmic guidance. Computer-based predictions using Bayesian or statistical regression models inform a clinical decision but do not actually reach a "conclusion" or "recommendation." Artificial intelligence systems attempt to simulate or replace human reasoning with a computer-based analogue. To date, such approaches have achieved only limited success. Reminder or protocol-directed systems do not make predictions but use existing algorithms, such as practice guidelines, to guide clinical practice. In general, however, decision support systems have shown little impact on practice. Reminder systems, although not yet in widespread use, have shown the most promise, particularly in correcting drug dosing and in promoting adherence to guidelines. The full impact of these approaches will only be evaluable when computers are fully integrated into medical practice.

DECISION ANALYSIS

Compared with the methods discussed above, decision analysis represents a completely different approach to decision support. Its principal application is in decision problems that are complex and involve a substantial risk, a high degree of uncertainty in some key area, or an idiosyncratic feature that does not "fit" the available evidence. Five general steps are involved. First, the decision problem must be clearly defined. Second, the elements of the decision must be made explicit. This involves specifying the alternatives being considered, their relevant outcomes, the probabilities attached to each outcome, and the relative desirability (called "utility") of each outcome. Cost can also be assigned to each branch of the decision tree, allowing calculation of cost effectiveness. Typically, the data to populate a decision model are derived from the literature, from unpublished sources, from expert opinion and from other secondary sources. Third, the decision model must be "evaluated" to determine the net long-term health benefits and costs of each strategy being considered. Fourth, the incremental health benefits and costs of the more effective strategies must be calculated. Finally, extensive sensitivity analyses must be used to examine the effects on the results of varying the starting assumptions through plausible alternative values.

An example decision tree created to evaluate strategies for screening for human immunodeficiency virus (HIV) infection is shown in **Fig. 3-3**. Up to 20,000 new cases of HIV infection are believed to be caused each year in the United States by infected individuals who are unaware of their illness. In addition, about 40% of HIV-positive patients progress to AIDS within a year of their diagnosis. Early identification offers the opportunity both to prevent progression to AIDS through use of serial CD4 counts and measurements of viral load linked to selective use of combination antiretroviral therapy and to encourage reduction of risky sexual behavior.

The Centers for Disease Control and Prevention (CDC) proposed in 2003 that routine HIV testing should be a part of standard medical care. In a decision-model exploration of this proposed strategy compared with usual care, assuming a 1% prevalence of unidentified HIV infection in the population, routine screening of a cohort of 43-year-old men and women increased life expectancy by 5.5 days and cost $194 per subject screened. The cost-effectiveness ratio for screening relative to usual care was $15,078 per quality-adjusted life year. Results were sensitive to assumptions about the effectiveness of behavior modification on subsequent sexual behavior, the benefits of early therapy of HIV infection and the prevalence and incidence of HIV infection in the population targeted. This model, which required over 75 separate data points, provides novel insights into a clinical management problem that has not been subjected to a randomized clinical trial.

The process of building and evaluating decision models is generally too complex for use in real-time clinical management. The potential for this tool therefore lies in the development of a set of published models addressing a particular decision or policy area that can serve to highlight key pressure points in the problem. Although many published models tend to focus excessively on providing an "answer," their better role is to enhance understanding of the most important questions that deserve particular attention in clinical decision-making.

EVIDENCE-BASED MEDICINE

The "art of medicine" is traditionally defined as a practice combining medical knowledge (including scientific evidence), intuition, and judgment in the care of patients (Chap. 1). Evidence-based medicine (EBM) updates this construct by placing a much-greater emphasis on the processes by which the clinician gains knowledge of the most up-to-date and relevant clinical research. The key processes of EBM can be summarized in four steps:

1. Formulating the management question to be answered
2. Searching the literature and on-line databases for applicable research data

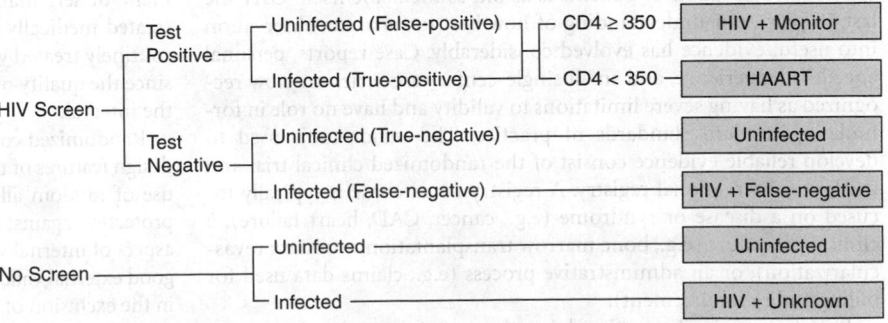

FIGURE 3-3 Basic structure of decision model used to evaluate strategies for screening for HIV in the general population. HIV, human immunodeficiency virus; HAART, highly active antiretroviral therapy. *(Figure provided courtesy of G. Sanders; with permission.)*

TABLE 3-3 **SELECTED TOOLS FOR FINDING THE EVIDENCE IN EVIDENCE-BASED MEDICINE**

Name	Description	Web Address	Availability
Evidence-Based Medicine Reviews	Comprehensive electronic database that combines and integrates: 1. The Cochrane Database of Systematic Reviews 2. ACP Journal Club 3. The Database of Abstracts of Reviews of Effectiveness	*http://www.ovid.com*	Subscription required; available through medical center libraries and other institutions
Cochrane Library	Collection of EBM databases including The Cochrane Database of Systematic Reviews—full text articles reviewing specific health care topics	*http://www.cochrane.org*	Subscription required; abstracts of systematic reviews available free online; some countries have funding to provide free access to all residents
ACP Journal Club	Collection of summaries of original studies and systematic reviews; published bimonthly; all data since 1991 available on Web site, updated yearly	*http://www.acpjc.org*	Subscription required
Clinical Evidence	Monthly updated directory of concise overviews of common clinical interventions	*http://www.clinicalevidence.com*	Subscription required; free access for UK and for developing countries
MEDLINE	National Library of Medicine database with citations back to 1966	*http://www.nlm.nih.gov*	Free via Internet

Note: ACP, American College of Physicians; EBM, evidence-based medicine.

3. Appraising the evidence gathered with regard to its validity and relevance
4. Integrating this appraisal with knowledge about the unique aspects of the patient (including preferences)

Steps 2 and 3 are the heart of EBM as it is currently used in practice. The process of searching the world's research literature and appraising the quality and relevance of studies thus identified can be quite time-consuming and requires skills and training that most clinicians do not possess. Thus, the best starting point for most EBM searches is the identification of recent systematic overviews of the problem in question (Table 3-3).

Generally, the EBM tools listed in Table 3-3 provide access to research information in one of two forms. The first, primary research reports, is the original peer-reviewed research work that is published in medical journals. Initial access to this information in an EBM search may be gained through MEDLINE, which provides access to a huge amount of data in abstract form. However, it is often difficult, using MEDLINE, to locate reports that are on point in a sea of irrelevant or unhelpful information and being reasonably certain that important reports have not been overlooked. The second form, systematic reviews, comprehensively summarizes the available evidence on a particular topic up to a certain date and provides the interpretation of the reviewer. Explicit criteria are used to find all the relevant scientific research and grade its quality. The prototype for this kind of resource is the Cochrane Database of Systematic Reviews. One of the key components of a systematic review is a meta-analysis. In the next two sections, we will review some of the major types of clinical research reports available in the literature and the process of aggregating those data into meta-analyses.

Sources of Evidence: Clinical Trials and Registries The notion of learning from observation of patients is as old as medicine itself. Over the last 50 years, our understanding of how best to turn raw observation into useful evidence has evolved considerably. Case reports, personal anecdotal experience, and small single-center case series are now recognized as having severe limitations to validity and have no role in formulating modern standards of practice. The major tools used to develop reliable evidence consist of the randomized clinical trial and the large observational registry. A registry or database is typically focused on a disease or syndrome (e.g., cancer, CAD, heart failure), a clinical procedure (e.g., bone marrow transplantation, coronary revascularization), or an administrative process (e.g., claims data used for billing and reimbursement).

By definition, in observational data the care of the patient is not controlled by the investigator. Carefully collected *prospective* observational data can achieve a level of quality approaching that of major clinical trial data. At the other end of the spectrum, data collected retrospectively

(e.g., chart review) are limited in form and content to what previous observers thought was important to record, which may not serve the research question under study particularly well. Data not specifically collected for research (e.g., claims data) will often have important limitations that cannot be overcome in the analysis phase of the research. Advantages to observational data include the ability to capture a broader population than is typically represented in clinical trials. In addition, observational data are the primary source of evidence for questions where a randomized trial cannot or will not be performed. For example, it may be difficult to randomize patients to test diagnostic or therapeutic strategies that are unproven but widely accepted in practice. In addition, we cannot randomize patients to a gender, racial/ethnic group, socioeconomic status, or country of residence. We are also not willing to randomize patients to a potentially harmful intervention, such as smoking or overeating to develop obesity.

The major difference between a well-done clinical trial and a well-done prospective observational study of a particular management strategy is the lack of protection from treatment selection bias in the latter. The underlying concept in the use of observational data to compare diagnostic or therapeutic strategies is that there is enough uncertainty in practice that similar patients will be managed differently by different physicians. In short, the assumption is that there is an element of randomness (in the sense of disorder rather than in the formal statistical sense) to clinical management. In such cases, statistical models can be used to adjust for important imbalances and "level the playing field" so that a fair comparison among treatment options can be made. When management is clearly not random (e.g., all eligible left main coronary artery disease patients are referred for coronary bypass surgery), the problem may be too confounded for statistical correction, and observational data may not provide reliable evidence.

In general, use of concurrent controls is vastly preferable to historical controls. For example, comparison of current surgical management of left main coronary artery disease with left main patients treated medically during the 1970s (the last time these patients were routinely treated with medicine alone) would be extremely misleading since the quality of "medical therapy" has made huge improvements in the interval.

Randomized controlled clinical trials include the careful prospective design features of the best observational data studies but also include the use of random allocation of treatment. This design provides the best protection against confounding due to treatment selection bias (a major aspect of internal validity). However, the randomized trial may not have good external validity if the process of recruitment into the trial resulted in the exclusion of many potentially eligible subjects.

Consumers of medical evidence need to be aware that randomized trials vary widely in their quality and applicability to practice. The process of designing such a trial often involves a great many compromises. For example, trials designed to gain FDA approval for an investigational drug or device will need to address certain regulatory requirements that may result in a different trial design from what practicing clinicians would find useful.

Meta-Analysis The Greek prefix *meta* signifies something at a later or higher stage of development. Meta-analysis is research done on research data for the purpose of combining and summarizing the available evidence quantitatively. Although it can be used to combine nonrandomized studies, meta-analysis is most valuable when used to summarize all of the randomized trials on a particular therapeutic problem. Ideally, unpublished trials should be identified and included to avoid publication bias (i.e., "positive" trials are more likely to be published). Furthermore, some of the best meta-analyses obtain and analyze the raw patient-level data from the individual trials rather than working only with what is available in the published reports of each trial. Not all published meta-analyses are reliable sources of evidence on a particular problem. Their methodology must be carefully scrutinized to ensure proper study design and analysis. The results of a well-done meta-analysis are likely to be most persuasive if it includes at least several large-scale, properly performed randomized trials. In cases where the available trials are small or poorly done, meta-analysis should not be viewed as a remedy for the deficiency in primary trial data.

Meta-analyses typically focus on summary measures of relative treatment benefit, such as odds ratios or relative risks. Clinicians should also examine what absolute risk reduction (ARR) can be expected from the therapy. A useful summary metric of absolute treatment benefit is the number needed to treat (NNT) to prevent one adverse outcome event (e.g., death, stroke). NNT is simply 1/ARR. For example, if a hypothetical therapy reduced mortality over a 5-year follow-up by 33% (the relative treatment benefit) from 12% (control arm) to 8% (treatment arm), the absolute risk reduction would be 12% − 8% = 4% and the NNT = $1/4$ or 25. Thus, we would need to treat 25 patients for 5 years to prevent 1 death. If we applied our hypothetical treatment to a lower-risk population, say with a 6% 5-year mortality, the 33% relative treatment benefit would reduce absolute mortality by 2% (from 6 to 4%) and the NNT for the same therapy in this different group of patients would be 50. Although not always made explicit, comparisons of NNT estimates from different studies need to take account of the duration of follow-up used to create each estimate.

Clinical Practice Guidelines According to the 1990 Institute of Medicine definition, clinical practice guidelines are "systematically developed statements to assist practitioner and patient decisions about appropriate health care for specific clinical circumstances." This definition provides emphasis to several crucial features of modern guideline development. First, guidelines are created using the tools of EBM. In particular, the core of the development process is a systematic literature search followed by a review of the relevant peer-reviewed literature. Second, guidelines are usually focused around a clinical disorder (e.g., adult diabetes, stable angina pectoris) or a health care intervention (e.g., cancer screening). Third, guidelines are intended to "assist" decision-making, not to define explicitly what decisions should be made in a particular situation. The primary objective is to improve the quality of medical care by identifying areas where care should be standardized, based on compelling evidence.

Guidelines are narrative documents constructed by an expert panel whose composition is often chosen by interested professional organizations. These panels vary in the degree to which they represent all relevant stakeholders. The guideline documents consist of a series of specific management recommendations, a summary indication of the quantity and quality of evidence supporting each recommendation, and a narrative discussion of the recommendations. Many recommendations have little or no supporting evidence and, thus, reflect the expert consensus of the guideline panel. In part to protect against errors by individual panels, the final step in guideline construction is peer review, followed by a final revision in response to the critiques provided.

Guidelines are closely tied to the process of quality improvement in medicine through their identification of evidence-based best practices. Such practices can be used as quality indicators. Examples include the proportion of acute MI patients who receive aspirin upon admission to a hospital and the proportion of heart-failure patients with depressed ejection fraction who are on an ACE inhibitor. Routine measurement and reporting of such quality indicators can produce selective improvements in quality, since many physicians prefer not to be outliers.

CONCLUSIONS

In this era of EBM, it is tempting to think that all the difficult decisions practitioners face have been or soon will be solved and digested into practice guidelines and computerized reminders. However, EBM provides practitioners with an ideal rather than a finished set of tools with which to manage patients. The significant contribution of EBM has been to promote the development of more powerful and user-friendly EBM tools that can be accessed by the busy practitioners. This is an enormously important contribution that is slowly changing the way medicine is practiced. One of the repeated admonitions of EBM pioneers has been to replace reliance on the local "gray-haired expert" (who may be often wrong but is rarely in doubt) with a systematic search for and evaluation of the evidence. But EBM has not eliminated the need for subjective judgments. Each systematic review or clinical practice guideline presents the interpretation of "experts" whose biases remain largely invisible to the review's consumers. In addition, meta-analyses cannot generate evidence where there are no adequate randomized trials, and most of what clinicians confront in practice will never be thoroughly tested in a randomized trial. For the foreseeable future, excellent clinical reasoning skills and experience supplemented by well-designed quantitative tools and a keen appreciation for individual patient preferences will continue to be of paramount importance in the professional life of medical practitioners.

FURTHER READINGS

BALK EM et al: Correlation of quality measures with estimates of treatment effect in meta-analyses of randomized controlled trials. JAMA 287:2973, 2002

DEL MAR C et al: *Clinical Thinking: Evidence, Communication and Decision Making.* Malden, Mass., Blackwell, 2006

GRIMES DA et al: Refining clinical diagnosis with likelihood ratios. Lancet 365:1500, 2005

HAYNES RB et al: *Clinical Epidemiology: How to Do Clinical Practice Research.* Philadelphia, Lippincott Williams & Wilkins, 2006

PETERSON ED et al: Association between hospital process performance and outcomes among patients with acute coronary syndromes JAMA 295:1912, 2006

REILLY BM et al: Translating clinical research into clinical practice: Impact of using prediction rules to make decisions. Ann Intern Med 144:201, 2006

SANDERS GD et al: Cost-effectiveness of screening for HIV in the era of highly active antiretroviral therapy. N Engl J Med 352:570, 2005

4 Screening and Prevention of Disease

Gary J. Martin

A primary goal of health care is to prevent disease or to detect it early enough that intervention will be more effective. Strategies for disease screening and prevention are driven by evidence that testing and intervention are practical and effective. Currently most screening tests are readily available and inexpensive. Examples include tests that are biochemical (e.g., cholesterol, glucose), physiologic (e.g., blood pressure, growth curves), radiologic (e.g., mammogram, bone densitometry), or tissue specimens (e.g., Pap smear, fine-needle aspirations). In the future, it is anticipated that genetic testing will play an increasingly important role for predicting disease risk (Chap. 64). However, such tests are not widely used except for individuals at risk for high-penetrance genes based on family or ethnic history (e.g., *BRCA1, BRCA2*). The identification of low-penetrance but high-frequency genes that cause common disorders such as diabetes, hypertension, or macular degeneration offers the possibility of new genetic tests. However, any new screening test, whether based on genetic or other methods, must be subjected to rigorous evaluation of its sensitivity, specificity, impact on disease, and cost-effectiveness. Physicians and patients are continuously introduced to new screening tests, often in advance of complete evaluation. For example, the use of whole-body CT imaging has been advocated as a means to screen for a variety of disorders. Though appealing in concept, there is currently no evidence to justify this approach, which is associated with high cost and a substantial risk of false-positive results.

This chapter will review the basic principles of screening and prevention in the primary care setting. Recommendations for specific disorders, such as cardiovascular disease, diabetes, or cancer, are provided in the chapters dedicated to these topics.

BASIC PRINCIPLES OF SCREENING

In general, screening is most effective when applied to relatively common disorders that carry a large disease burden (Table 4-1). The five leading causes of mortality in the United States are heart diseases, malignant neoplasms, accidents, cerebrovascular diseases, and chronic obstructive pulmonary disease. Thus, many prevention strategies are targeted at these conditions. From a global health perspective, these same conditions are priorities, but malaria, malnutrition, AIDS, tuberculosis, and violence carry a heavy disease burden (Chap. 2).

A primary goal of screening is the early detection of a risk factor or disease at a stage when it can be corrected or cured. For example, most cancers have a better prognosis when identified as premalignant lesions or when they are still resectable. Similarly, early identification of hypertension or hyperlipidemia allows therapeutic interventions that reduce the long-term risk of cardiovascular or cerebrovascular events. However, early detection does not necessarily influence survival. For example, in some studies of lung cancer screening, tumors are identified at an earlier stage, but overall mortality does not differ between screened and unscreened populations. The apparent improvement in 5-year survival rates can be attributed to the detection of smaller tumors rather than a real change in clinical course after diagnosis. Similarly, the detection of prostate cancer may not lead to a mortality difference because the disease is often indolent and competing morbidities, such as coronary artery disease, may ultimately cause mortality (Chap. 78).

Disorders with a long latency period increase the potential gains associated with detection. For example, cancer of the cervix has a long latency between dysplasia and invasive carcinoma, providing an opportunity for detection by routine screening. It is hoped that the introduction of new papilloma virus vaccines will provide additional disease prevention, ultimately reducing the reliance on screening for cervical cancer. For colon cancer, an adenomatous polyp progresses to invasive cancer over 4–12 years, providing an opportunity to detect early lesions by fecal occult blood testing (FOBT) or endoscopy. On the other hand, breast cancer screening in premenopausal women is more challenging because of the relatively short interval between development of a localized breast cancer and metastasis to regional nodes (estimated to be ~12 months).

METHODS OF MEASURING HEALTH BENEFITS

It is not practical to perform all possible screening procedures. For example, screening for laryngeal cancer in smokers is not currently recommended. It is necessary to examine the strength of evidence in favor of screening measures relative to the cost and risk of false-positive tests. For example, should ultrasound be used to screen for ovarian cancer in average-risk women? It is currently estimated that the unnecessary laparotomies triggered by finding benign ovarian masses would actually cause more harm than the benefit derived from detecting the occasional curable ovarian cancer.

A variety of endpoints are used to assess the potential gain from screening and prevention interventions:

1. *The number of subjects screened to alter the outcome in one individual.* It is estimated, for example, that 731 women ages 65–69 would need to be screened by dual-energy x-ray absorptiometry (DEXA) and then treated appropriately to prevent one hip fracture from osteoporosis.
2. *The absolute and relative impact of screening on disease outcome.* A meta-analysis of Swedish mammography trials (ages 40–70) found that ~1.2 fewer women per thousand would die from breast cancer if they were screened over a 12-year period. By comparison, ~3 lives per 1000 might be saved from colon cancer in a population (ages 50–75) screened with annual FOBT over a 13-year period. Based on this analysis, colon cancer screening may actually save more women's lives than mammography. The impact of FOBT (8.8/1000 versus 5.9/1000) might be stated either as 3 lives per 1000 or as a 30% reduction in colon cancer death; thus, it is important to consider both the relative and absolute impact on numbers of lives saved.
3. *The cost per year of life saved* is used to assess the effectiveness of many screening and prevention strategies. Typically, strategies that cost <$30,000–50,000 per year of life saved are considered "cost-effective" (Chap. 3). For example, using alendronate to treat 65-year-old women with osteoporosis approaches this threshold of approximately $30,000 per year of life saved.
4. *Increase in average life expectancy for a population.* Predicted increases in life expectancy for various screening procedures are listed in Table 4-2. It should be noted, however, that the life-expectancy increase is an average that applies to a population and not to an individual. In reality, the vast majority of the screened population does not derive any benefit and possibly incurs a slight risk from false-positive results. A small subset of patients, however, will benefit greatly from being screened. For example, Pap smears do not benefit the 98% of women who never develop cancer of the cervix. However, for the 2% who would develop localized cervical cancer, Pap smears may add as much as 25 years to their lives. Some studies suggest that a 1-month gain of life expectancy is a reasonable goal for a population-based preventive strategy.

The U.S. Preventive Services Task Force (USPSTF) provides recommendations for evidence-based screening (Table 4-3). In addition to these population-based guidelines, it is reasonable to consider family and social history to identify individuals with special risk (*www.ahrq.gov/clinic/uspstfix.htm*). For example, when there is a significant family history of breast, colon, or prostate cancer, it is prudent to initiate screening about 10 years before the age when the youngest

TABLE 4-1 LIFETIME CUMULATIVE RISK	
Breast cancer for women	10%
Colon cancer	6%
Cancer of the cervix for women[a]	2%
Domestic violence for women	Up to 15%
Hip fracture for Caucasian women	16%

[a]Assuming an unscreened population.

TABLE 4-2 ESTIMATED AVERAGE INCREASE IN LIFE EXPECTANCY FOR A POPULATION

Screening Procedure	Average Increase
Mammography:	
Women, 40–50 years	0–5 days
Women, 50–70 years	1 month
Pap smears, age 18–65	2–3 months
Screening treadmill for a 50-year-old (asymptomatic) man	8 days
PSA and digital rectal exam for a man >50 years	Up to 2 weeks
Getting a 35-year-old smoker to quit	3–5 years
Beginning regular exercise for a 40-year-old man (30 min 3 times a week)	9 months to 2 years

Note: PSA, prostate-specific antigen.

family member developed cancer. Screening should also be considered for many other common disorders pending the development of further evidence. Three examples are screening for diabetes (using fasting blood glucose), domestic violence, and coronary artery disease in intermediate-risk asymptomatic individuals.

Cost-Effectiveness Screening techniques must be cost-effective if they are to be applied to large populations. Costs include not only the expense of testing but also time away from work and potential risks. When the risk-to-benefit ratio is less favorable, it is useful to provide information to patients and factor their perspectives into the decision-making process. For example, many expert groups, including the USPSTF, recommend an individualized discussion about prostate cancer screening, as the decision-making process is complex and relies heavily on personal

TABLE 4-3 CLINICAL PREVENTIVE SERVICES FOR NORMAL-RISK ADULTS RECOMMENDED BY THE U.S. PREVENTIVE SERVICES TASK FORCE

Test or Disorder	Population,[a] Years	Frequency	Chapter Reference
Blood pressure, height and weight	>18	Periodically	64
Cholesterol	Men > 35	Every 5 years	225
	Women > 45	Every 5 years	
Diabetes	>45 or earlier, if there are additional risk factors	Every 3 years	323
Pap smear[b]	Within 3 years of onset of sexual activity or 21–65	Every 1–3 years	67
Chlamydia	Women 18–25	Every 1–2 years	160
Mammography[a]	Women > 40	Every 1–2 years	67, 76
Colorectal cancer[a]	>50		67, 77
fecal occult blood and/or		Every year	
sigmoidoscopy or		Every 5 years	
colonoscopy		Every 10 years	
Osteoporosis	Women > 65; >60 at risk	Periodically	333
Abdominal aortic aneurysm (ultrasound)	Men 65–75 who have ever smoked	Once	
Alcohol use	>18	Periodically	372
Vision, hearing	>65	Periodically	25, 26
Adult immunization			107, 108
Tetanus-diptheria (Td)	>18	Every 10 years	
Varicella (VZV)	Susceptibles only, >18	Two doses	
Measles, mumps, rubella (MMR)	Women, childbearing age	One dose	
Pneumococcal	>65	One dose	
Influenza	>50	Yearly	
Human papillomavirus (HPV)	Up to age 26	If not done prior	

[a]Screening is performed earlier and more frequently when there is a strong family history. Randomized, controlled trials have documented that fecal occult blood testing (FOBT) confers a 15 to 30% reduction in colon cancer mortality. Although randomized trials have not been performed for sigmoidoscopy or colonoscopy, well-designed case-control studies suggest similar or greater efficacy relative to FOBT.
[b]In the future, Pap smear frequency may be influenced by HPV testing and the HPV vaccine.
Note: Prostate-specific antigen (PSA) testing is capable of enhancing the detection of early-stage prostate cancer, but evidence is inconclusive that it improves health outcomes. PSA testing is recommended by several professional organizations and is widely used in clinical practice, but it is not currently recommended by the U.S. Preventive Services Task Force (Chap. 81).
Source: Adapted from the U.S. Preventive Services Task Force, 2005. *Guide to Clinical Prevention Services*, 3d ed. http://www.ahrq.gov/clinic/uspstfix.htm

TABLE 4-4 COUNSELING TO PREVENT DISEASE

Topic	Chapter Reference
Tobacco cessation	375
Drug and alcohol use	372, 373
Nutrition to maintain caloric balance and vitamin intake	60
Calcium intake in women >18 years	333
Folic acid: Women of childbearing age	61
Oral health	28
Aspirin use to prevent cardiovascular disease in selected men >40 years and women >50 years	225
Chemoprevention of breast cancer in women at high risk	76
STDs and HIV prevention	115, 173
Physical activity	
Sun exposure	51
Injury prevention (loaded handgun, seat belts, bicycle helmet)	
Issues in the elderly	8
Polypharmacy	
Fall prevention	
Hot water heater <120°	
Vision, hearing, dental evaluations	
Immunizations (pneumococcal, influenza)	

Note: STDs, sexually transmitted diseases.

issues. Although the early detection of prostate cancer may intuitively seem desirable, risks include false-positive results that can lead to anxiety and unnecessary surgery. Potential complications from surgery and radiation treatment include erectile dysfunction, urinary incontinence, and bowel dysfunction. Some men may decline screening, while others may be more willing to accept the risks of an early-detection strategy.

Another example of shared decision-making is the choice of colon cancer screening techniques (Chap. 78). In controlled studies, the use of annual FOBT reduces colon cancer deaths by 15–30%. Flexible sigmoidoscopy reduces colon cancer deaths by ~60%. Colonoscopy offers the same, or greater, benefit than flexible sigmoidoscopy, but its use incurs additional costs and risks. These screening procedures have not been directly compared in the same population, but the estimated cost to society is similar: $10,000–25,000 per year of life saved. Thus, while one patient may prefer the ease of preparation, less time disruption, and the lower risk of flexible sigmoidoscopy, others may prefer the sedation and thoroughness of colonoscopy.

When considering the impact of screening tests, it is important to recognize that tobacco and alcohol use, diet, and exercise comprise the vast majority of factors that influence preventable deaths in developed countries. Perhaps the single greatest preventive health care measure is to help patients quit smoking (Chap. 390).

COMMONLY ENCOUNTERED ISSUES
Despite compelling evidence that prevention strategies can have major health care benefits, implementation of these services is challenging because of competing demands on physician and patient time and because of gaps in health care reimbursement. Moreover, efforts to reduce disease risk frequently involve behavior changes (e.g., weight loss, exercise, seatbelts) or managing addictive conditions (e.g., tobacco and alcohol use) that are often recalcitrant to intervention. Public education and economic incentives are often useful, in addition to counseling by health care providers (Table 4-4).

A number of techniques can assist the physician with the growing number of recommended screening tests. An appropriately configured electronic health record can provide reminder systems that make it easier for physicians to track and meet guidelines. Some systems provide patients with secure access to their medical records, providing an additional means to enhance adherence to routine screening. Systems that provide nurses and other staff with standing orders are effective for smoking prevention and immunizations. The Agency for Healthcare Research and Quality and the Centers for Disease Control and Prevention have developed flow sheets as part of their "Put Prevention into Practice" program (*http://www.ahcpr.gov/clinic/ppipix.htm*). Age-specific recommendations for screening and counseling are summarized in Table 4-5.

A routine health care examination should be performed every 1–3 years before age 50 and every year thereafter. History should include medication use (prescription and non-prescription), allergies, dietary history, use of alcohol and tobacco, sexual practices, and a thorough family history, if not obtained previously. Routine measurements should include assessments of height, weight (body mass index), and blood pressure, in addition to the relevant physical examination. The increasing incidence of skin cancer underscores the importance of screening for suspicious skin lesions. Hearing and vision should be tested after age 65, or earlier if the patient describes difficulties. Other gender- and age-specific examinations are listed in Table 4-3. Counseling and instruction about self-examination (e.g., skin, breast) can be provided during the routine examination.

Many patients see a physician for ongoing care of chronic illnesses, and this visit provides an opportunity to include a "measure of prevention" for other health problems. For example, the patient seen for management of hypertension or diabetes can have breast cancer screening incorporated into one visit and a discussion about colon cancer screening at the next visit. Other patients may respond more favorably to a clearly defined visit that addresses all relevant screening and prevention interventions. Because of age or comorbidities, it may be appropriate in some patients to abandon certain screening and prevention activities, although there are fewer data about when to "sunset" these services. The risk of certain cancers, like cancer of the cervix, ultimately declines, and it is reasonable to cease Pap smears after about age 65 if previous recent Pap smears have been negative. For breast, colon, and prostate cancer, it is reasonable to reevaluate the need for screening after about age 75. For some older patients with advanced diseases such as severe chronic obstructive pulmonary disease or congestive heart failure or who are immobile, the benefit of some screening procedures is low, and other priorities emerge when life expectancy is <10 years. This shift in focus needs to be done tactfully and allows greater focus on the conditions likely to impact quality and length of life.

TABLE 4-5 AGE-SPECIFIC CAUSES OF MORTALITY AND CORRESPONDING PREVENTATIVE OPTIONS

Age Group	Leading Causes of Age-Specific Mortality	Screening Prevention Interventions to Consider for Each Specific Population
15–24	1. Accident 2. Homicide 3. Suicide 4. Malignancy 5. Heart disease	• Counseling on routine seat belt use, bicycle/motorcycle/ATV helmets (1) • Counseling on diet and exercise (5) • Discuss dangers of alcohol use while driving, swimming, boating (1) • Ask about vaccination status (tetanus, diphtheria, hepatitis B, MMR, rubella, varicella, meningitis, HPV) • Ask about gun use and/or gun possession (2,3) • Assess for substance abuse history including alcohol (2,3) • Screen for domestic violence (2,3) • Screen for depression and/or suicidal/homicidal ideation (2,3) • Pap smear for cervical cancer screening, discuss STD prevention (4) • Recommend skin, breast, and testicular self-exams (4) • Recommend UV light avoidance and regular sun screen use (4) • Measurement of blood pressure, height, weight and body mass index (5) • Discuss health risks of tobacco use, consider emphasis of cosmetic and economic issues to improve quit rates for younger smokers (4,5) • *Chlamydia* screening and contraceptive counseling for sexually active females • HIV, hepatitis B, and syphilis testing if there is high-risk sexual behavior(s) or any prior history of sexually transmitted disease
25–44	1. Accident 2. Malignancy 3. Heart disease 4. Suicide 5. Homicide 6. HIV	*As above plus consider the following:* • Readdress smoking status, encourage cessation at every visit (2,3) • Obtain detailed family history of malignancies and begin early screening/prevention program if patient is at significant increased risk (2) • Assess all cardiac risk factors (including screening for diabetes and hyperlipidemia) and consider primary prevention with aspirin for patients at >3% 5-year risk of a vascular event (3) • Assess for chronic alcohol abuse, risk factors for viral hepatitis, or other risks for development of chronic liver disease • Begin breast cancer screening with mammography at age 40 (2)
45–64	1. Malignancy 2. Heart disease 3. Accident 4. Diabetes mellitus 5. Cerebrovascular disease 6. Chronic lower respiratory disease 7. Chronic liver disease and cirrhosis 8. Suicide	• Consider prostate cancer screen with annual PSA and digital rectal exam at age 50 (or possibly earlier in African Americans or patients with family history) (1) • Begin colorectal cancer screening at age 50 with either fecal occult blood testing, flexible sigmoidoscopy, or colonoscopy (1) • Reassess vaccination status at age 50 and give special consideration to vaccines against *Streptococcus pneumoniae*, influenza, tetanus, and viral hepatitis • Consider screening for coronary disease in higher risk patients (2,5)
≥65	1. Heart disease 2. Malignancy 3. Cerebrovascular disease 4. Chronic lower respiratory disease 5. Alzheimer's disease 6. Influenza and pneumonia 7. Diabetes mellitus 8. Kidney disease 9. Accidents 10. Septicemia	*As above plus consider the following:* • Readdress smoking status, encourage cessation at every visit (1,2,3) • One-time ultrasound for AAA in men 65–75 who have ever smoked • Consider pulmonary function testing for all long-term smokers to assess for development of chronic obstructive pulmonary disease (3,7) • Vaccinate all smokers against influenza and *S. pneumoniae* at age 50 (6) • Screen all postmenopausal women (and all men with risk factors) for osteoporosis • Reassess vaccination status at age 65, emphasis on influenza and *S. pneumoniae* (3,7) • Screen for dementia and depression (5) • Screen for visual and hearing problems, home safety issues, and elder abuse (9)

Note: The numbers in parentheses refer to areas of risk in the mortality column affected by the specified intervention.
Abbreviations: MMR, measles-mumps-rubella; HPV, human papilloma virus; STD, sexually transmitted disease; UV, ultraviolet; PSA, prostate-specific antigen; AAA, abdominal aortic aneurysm.

ACKNOWLEDGMENTS

The author is grateful to Dan Evans, MD, for contributions to this topic in Harrison's Manual of Medicine.

FURTHER READINGS

BARRETT-CONNOR E et al: The rise and fall of menopausal hormone therapy. Annu Rev Public Health 26:115, 2005

FENTON JJ et al: Delivery of cancer screening: How important is the preventive health examination? Arch Intern Med 167(6):580, 2007

GREENLAND P et al: Coronary artery calcium score combined with Framingham score for risk prediction in asymptomatic individuals. JAMA 291:210, 2004

RANSOHOFF DF, SANDLER RS: Clinical practice: Screening for colorectal cancer. N Engl J Med 346:40, 2002

U.S. PREVENTIVE SERVICES TASK FORCE: Clinical preventive services for normal-risk adults. Put prevention into practice. Agency for Healthcare Research and Quality, Rockville, MD, January 2003. Available at *www.ahrq.gov/ppip/adulttm.htm*

WRIGHT JC, WEINSTEIN MC: Gains in life expectancy from medical interventions—standardizing data on outcomes. N Engl J Med 339:380, 1998

5 Principles of Clinical Pharmacology
Dan M. Roden

Drugs are the cornerstone of modern therapeutics. Nevertheless, it is well recognized among physicians and among the lay community that the outcome of drug therapy varies widely among individuals. While this variability has been perceived as an unpredictable, and therefore inevitable, accompaniment of drug therapy, this is not the case. The goal of this chapter is to describe the principles of clinical pharmacology that can be used for the safe and optimal use of available and new drugs.

Drugs interact with specific target molecules to produce their beneficial and adverse effects. The chain of events between administration of a drug and production of these effects in the body can be divided into two components, both of which contribute to variability in drug actions. The first component comprises the processes that determine drug delivery to, and removal from, molecular targets. The resultant description of the relationship between drug concentration and time is termed *pharmacokinetics*. The second component of variability in drug action comprises the processes that determine variability in drug actions despite equivalent drug delivery to effector drug sites. This description of the relationship between drug concentration and effect is termed *pharmacodynamics*. As discussed further below, pharmacodynamic variability can arise as a result of variability in function of the target molecule itself or of variability in the broad biologic context in which the drug-target interaction occurs to achieve drug effects.

Two important goals of the discipline of clinical pharmacology are (1) to provide a description of conditions under which drug actions vary among human subjects; and (2) to determine mechanisms underlying this variability, with the goal of improving therapy with available drugs as well as pointing to new drug mechanisms that may be effective in the treatment of human disease. The first steps in the discipline were empirical descriptions of the influence of disease X on drug action Y or of individuals or families with unusual sensitivities to adverse drug effects. These important descriptive findings are now being replaced by an understanding of the molecular mechanisms underlying variability in drug actions. Thus, the effects of disease, drug coadministration, or familial factors in modulating drug action can now be reinterpreted as variability in expression or function of specific genes whose products determine pharmacokinetics and pharmacodynamics. Nevertheless, it is the personal interaction of the patient with the physician or other health care provider that first identifies unusual variability in drug actions; maintained alertness to unusual drug responses continues to be a key component of improving drug safety.

Unusual drug responses, segregating in families, have been recognized for decades and initially defined the field of *pharmacogenetics*. Now, with an increasing appreciation of common polymorphisms across the human genome, comes the opportunity to reinterpret descriptive mechanisms of variability in drug action as a consequence of specific DNA polymorphisms, or sets of DNA polymorphisms, among individuals. This approach defines the nascent field of *pharmacogenomics*, which may hold the opportunity of allowing practitioners to integrate a molecular understanding of the basis of disease with an individual's genomic make-up to prescribe personalized, highly effective, and safe therapies.

INDICATIONS FOR DRUG THERAPY

It is self-evident that the benefits of drug therapy should outweigh the risks. Benefits fall into two broad categories: those designed to alleviate a symptom and those designed to prolong useful life. An increasing emphasis on the principles of evidence-based medicine and techniques such as large clinical trials and meta-analyses have defined benefits of drug therapy in specific patient subgroups. Establishing the balance between risk and benefit is not always simple: for example, therapies that provide symptomatic benefits but shorten life may be entertained in patients with serious and highly symptomatic diseases such as heart failure or cancer. These decisions illustrate the continuing highly personal nature of the relationship between the prescriber and the patient.

Some adverse effects are so common and so readily associated with drug therapy that they are identified very early during clinical use of a drug. On the other hand, serious adverse effects may be sufficiently uncommon that they escape detection for many years after a drug begins to be widely used. The issue of how to identify rare but serious adverse effects (that can profoundly affect the benefit-risk perception in an individual patient) has not been satisfactorily resolved. Potential approaches range from an increased understanding of the molecular and genetic basis of variability in drug actions to expanded postmarketing surveillance mechanisms. None of these have been completely effective, so practitioners must be continuously vigilant to the possibility that unusual symptoms may be related to specific drugs, or combinations of drugs, that their patients receive.

Beneficial and adverse reactions to drug therapy can be described by a series of dose-response relations (Fig. 5-1). Well-tolerated drugs

FIGURE 5-1 The concept of a therapeutic ratio. Each panel illustrates the relationship between increasing dose and cumulative probability of a desired or adverse drug effect. **Top.** A drug with a wide therapeutic ratio, i.e., a wide separation of the two curves. **Bottom.** A drug with a narrow therapeutic ratio; here, the likelihood of adverse effects at therapeutic doses is increased because the curves are not well separated. Further, a steep dose-response curve for adverse effects is especially undesirable, as it implies that even small dosage increments may sharply increase the likelihood of toxicity. When there is a definable relationship between drug concentration (usually measured in plasma) and desirable and adverse effect curves, concentration may be substituted on the abscissa. Note that not all patients necessarily demonstrate a therapeutic response (or adverse effect) at any dose, and that some effects (notably some adverse effects) may occur in a dose-independent fashion.

FIGURE 5-2 Idealized time-plasma concentration curves after a single dose of drug. A. The time course of drug concentration after an instantaneous IV bolus or an oral dose in the one-compartment model shown. The area under the time-concentration curve is clearly less with the oral drug than the IV, indicating incomplete bioavailability. Note that despite this incomplete bioavailability, concentration after the oral dose can be higher than after the IV dose at some time points. The inset shows that the decline of concentrations over time is linear on a log-linear plot, characteristic of first-order elimination, and that oral and IV drug have the same elimination (parallel) time course. **B.** The decline of central compartment concentration when drug is distributed both to and from a peripheral compartment and eliminated from the central compartment. The rapid initial decline of concentration reflects not drug elimination but distribution.

demonstrate a wide margin, termed the *therapeutic ratio, therapeutic index*, or *therapeutic window*, between the doses required to produce a therapeutic effect and those producing toxicity. In cases where there is a similar relationship between plasma drug concentration and effects, monitoring plasma concentrations can be a highly effective aid in managing drug therapy by enabling concentrations to be maintained above the minimum required to produce an effect and below the concentration range likely to produce toxicity. Such monitoring has been widely used to guide therapy with specific agents, such as certain antiarrhythmics, anticonvulsants, and antibiotics. Many of the principles in clinical pharmacology and examples outlined below, which can be applied broadly to therapeutics, have been developed in these arenas.

PRINCIPLES OF PHARMACOKINETICS

The processes of absorption, distribution, metabolism, and excretion—collectively termed *drug disposition*—determine the concentration of drug delivered to target effector molecules.

ABSORPTION

Bioavailability   When a drug is administered orally, subcutaneously, intramuscularly, rectally, sublingually, or directly into desired sites of action, the amount of drug actually entering the systemic circulation may be less than with the intravenous route (Fig. 5-2A). The fraction of drug available to the systemic circulation by other routes is termed *bioavailability*. Bioavailability may be <100% for two reasons: (1) absorption is reduced, or (2) the drug undergoes metabolism or elimination prior to entering the systemic circulation.

When a drug is administered by a nonintravenous route, the peak concentration occurs later and is lower than after the same dose given by rapid intravenous injection, reflecting absorption from the site of administration (Fig. 5-2). The extent of absorption may be reduced because a drug is incompletely released from

its dosage form, undergoes destruction at its site of administration, or has physicochemical properties such as insolubility that prevent complete absorption from its site of administration. Slow absorption is deliberately designed into "slow-release" or "sustained-release" drug formulations in order to minimize variation in plasma concentrations during the interval between doses.

"First-Pass" Effect   When a drug is administered orally, it must transverse the intestinal epithelium, the portal venous system, and the liver prior to entering the systemic circulation (Fig. 5-3). Once a drug enters the enterocyte, it may undergo metabolism, be transported into the portal vein, or undergo excretion back into the intestinal lumen. Both excretion into the intestinal lumen and metabolism decrease systemic bioavailability. Once a drug passes this enterocyte barrier, it may also be taken up into the hepatocyte, where bioavailability can be further limited by metabolism or excretion into the bile. This elimination in intestine and liver, which reduces the amount of drug delivered to the systemic circulation, is termed *presystemic elimination*, or *first-pass elimination*.

Drug movement across the membrane of any cell, including enterocytes and hepatocytes, is a combination of passive diffusion and active transport, mediated by specific drug uptake and efflux molecules. The drug transport molecule that has been most widely studied is P-glycoprotein, the product of the normal expression of the *MDR1* gene. P-glycoprotein is expressed on the apical aspect of the enterocyte and on the canalicular aspect of the hepatocyte (Fig. 5-3); in both locations, it serves as an efflux pump, thus limiting availability of drug to the systemic circulation. P-glycoprotein is also an important component of the blood-brain barrier, discussed further below.

Drug metabolism generates compounds that are usually more polar and hence more readily excreted than parent drug. Metabolism takes place predominantly in the liver but can occur at other sites such as kidney, intestinal epithelium, lung, and plasma. "Phase I" metabolism involves chemical modification, most often oxidation accomplished by members of the cytochrome P450 (CYP) monooxygenase superfamily. CYPs that are especially important for drug metabolism (Table 5-1)

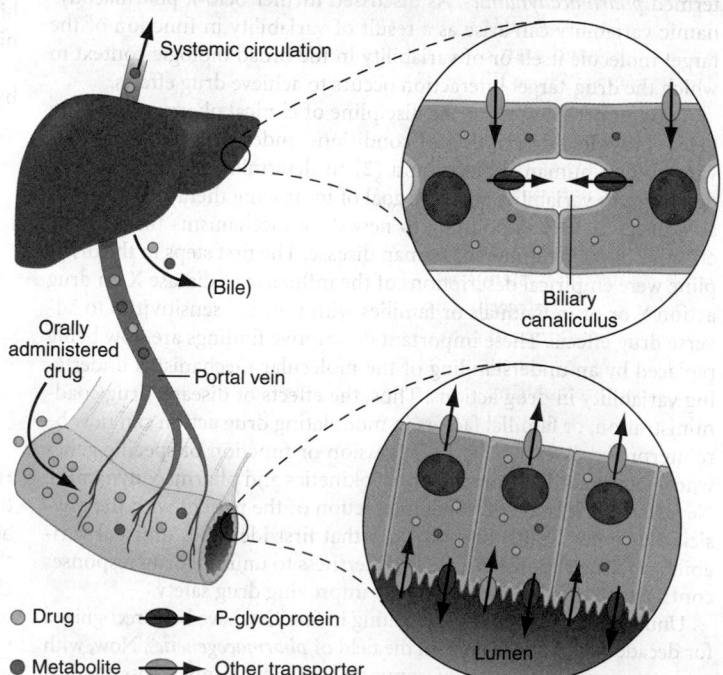

FIGURE 5-3 Mechanism of presystemic clearance. After drug enters the enterocyte, it can undergo metabolism, excretion into the intestinal lumen, or transport into the portal vein. Similarly, the hepatocyte may accomplish metabolism and biliary excretion prior to the entry of drug and metabolites to the systemic circulation. [*Adapted by permission from DM Roden, in DP Zipes, J Jalife (eds): Cardiac Electrophysiology: From Cell to Bedside, 4th ed. Philadelphia, Saunders, 2003. Copyright 2003 with permission from Elsevier.*]

TABLE 5-1 MOLECULAR PATHWAYS MEDIATING DRUG DISPOSITION

Molecule	Substrates[a]	Inhibitors[a]
CYP3A	Calcium channel blockers	Amiodarone
	Antiarrhythmics (lidocaine, quinidine, mexiletine)	Ketoconazole, itraconazole
	HMG-CoA reductase inhibitors ("statins"; see text)	Erythromycin, clarithromycin
	Cyclosporine, tacrolimus	Ritonavir
	Indinavir, saquinavir, ritonavir	
CYP2D6[b]	Timolol, metoprolol, carvedilol	Quinidine (even at ultra-low doses)
	Phenformin	Tricyclic antidepressants
	Codeine	Fluoxetine, paroxetine
	Propafenone, flecainide	
	Tricyclic antidepressants	
	Fluoxetine, paroxetine	
CYP2C9[b]	Warfarin	Amiodarone
	Phenytoin	Fluconazole
	Glipizide	Phenytoin
	Losartan	
CYP2C19[b]	Omeprazole	
	Mephenytoin	
Thiopurine S-methyltransferase[b]	6-Mercaptopurine, azathioprine	
N-acetyltransferase[b]	Isoniazid	
	Procainamide	
	Hydralazine	
	Some sulfonamides	
UGT1A1[b]	Irinotecan	
Pseudocholinesterase[b]	Succinylcholine	
P-glycoprotein	Digoxin	Quinidine
	HIV protease inhibitors	Amiodarone
	Many CYP3A substrates	Verapamil
		Cyclosporine
		Itraconazole
		Erythromycin

[a]Inhibitors affect the molecular pathway, and thus may affect substrate.
[b]Clinically important genetics variants described.
A listing of CYP substrates, inhibitors, and inducers is maintained at *http://medicine.iupui.edu/flockhart/table.htm*.

include CYP3A4, CYP3A5, CYP2D6, CYP2C9, CYP2C19, CYP1A2, and CYP2E1, and each drug may be a substrate for one or more of these enzymes. "Phase II" metabolism involves conjugation of specific endogenous compounds to drugs or their metabolites. The enzymes that accomplish phase II reactions include glucuronyl-, acetyl-, sulfo- and methyltransferases. Drug metabolites may exert important pharmacologic activity, as discussed further below.

Clinical Implications of Altered Bioavailability

Some drugs undergo near-complete presystemic metabolism and thus cannot be administered orally. Nitroglycerin cannot be used orally because it is completely extracted prior to reaching the systemic circulation. The drug is therefore used by the sublingual or transdermal routes, which bypass presystemic metabolism.

Some drugs with very extensive presystemic metabolism can still be administered by the oral route, using much higher doses than those required intravenously. Thus, a typical intravenous dose of verapamil is 1–5 mg, compared to the usual single oral dose of 40–120 mg. Administration of low-dose aspirin can result in exposure of cyclooxygenase in platelets in the portal vein to the drug, but systemic sparing because of first-pass aspirin deacylation in the liver. This is an example of presystemic metabolism being exploited to therapeutic advantage.

DISTRIBUTION AND ELIMINATION

Most pharmacokinetic processes are first-order; i.e., the rate of the process depends on the amount of drug present. Clinically important exceptions are discussed below (see "Principles of Dose Selection"). In the simplest pharmacokinetic model (Fig. 5-2A), a drug bolus is administered instantaneously to a central compartment, from which drug elimination occurs as a first-order process. The first-order nature of drug elimination leads directly to the relationship describing drug concentration (C) at any time (t) following the bolus:

$$C = (dose/V_c) \cdot e^{(-0.69t/t_{1/2})}$$

where V_c is the volume of the compartment into which drug is delivered and $t_{1/2}$ is elimination half-life. As a consequence of this relationship, a plot of the logarithm of concentration vs time is a straight line (Fig. 5-2A, inset). *Half-life* is the time required for 50% of a first-order process to be complete. Thus, 50% of drug elimination is accomplished after one drug-elimination half-life, 75% after two, 87.5% after three, etc. In practice, first-order processes such as elimination are near-complete after four–five half-lives.

In some cases, drug is removed from the central compartment not only by elimination but also by distribution into peripheral compartments. In this case, the plot of plasma concentration vs time after a bolus may demonstrate two (or more) exponential components (Fig. 5-2B). In general, the initial rapid drop in drug concentration represents not elimination but drug distribution into and out of peripheral tissues (also first-order processes), while the slower component represents drug elimination; the initial precipitous decline is usually evident with administration by intravenous but not other routes. Drug concentrations at peripheral sites are determined by a balance between drug distribution to and redistribution from peripheral sites, as well as by elimination. Once the distribution process is near-complete (four to five distribution half-lives), plasma and tissue concentrations decline in parallel.

Clinical Implications of Half-Life Measurements The elimination half-life not only determines the time required for drug concentrations to fall to near-immeasurable levels after a single bolus; it is also the key determinant of the time required for steady-state plasma concentrations to be achieved after any change in drug dosing (Fig. 5-4). This applies to the initiation of chronic drug therapy (whether by multiple oral doses or by continuous intravenous infusion), a change in chronic drug dose or dosing interval, or discontinuation of drug.

Steady state describes the situation during chronic drug administration when the amount of drug administered per unit time equals drug eliminated per unit time. With a continuous intravenous infusion, plasma concentrations at steady state are stable, while with chronic oral drug administration, plasma concentrations vary during the dosing interval but the time-concentration profile between dosing intervals is stable (Fig. 5-4).

DRUG DISTRIBUTION

In a typical 70-kg human, plasma volume is ~3 L, blood volume is ~5.5 L, and extracellular water outside the vasculature is ~42 L. The volume of distribution of drugs extensively bound to plasma proteins but not to tissue components approaches plasma volume; warfarin is an example. By contrast, for drugs highly bound to tissues, the volume of distribution can be far greater than any physiologic space. For example, the volume of distribution of digoxin and tricyclic antidepressants is hundreds of liters, obviously exceeding total-body volume. Such drugs are not readily removed by dialysis, an important consideration in overdose.

Clinical Implications of Drug Distribution Digoxin accesses its cardiac site of action slowly, over a distribution phase of several hours. Thus,

FIGURE 5-4 Drug accumulation to steady state. In this simulation, drug was administered (arrows) at intervals = 50% of the elimination half-life. Steady state is achieved during initiation of therapy after ~5 elimination half-lives, or 10 doses. A loading dose did not alter the eventual steady state achieved. A doubling of the dose resulted in a doubling of the steady state but the same time course of accumulation. Once steady state is achieved, a change in dose (increase, decrease, or drug discontinuation) results in a new steady state in ~5 elimination half-lives. *[Adapted by permission from DM Roden, in DP Zipes, J Jalife (eds): Cardiac Electrophysiology: From Cell to Bedside, 4th ed. Philadelphia, Saunders, 2003. Copyright 2003 with permission from Elsevier.]*

after an intravenous dose, plasma levels fall, but those at the site of action increase over hours. Only when distribution is near-complete does the concentration of digoxin in plasma reflect pharmacologic effect. For this reason, there should be a 6–8 h wait after administration before plasma levels of digoxin are measured as a guide to therapy.

Animal models have suggested, and clinical studies are confirming, that limited drug penetration into the brain, the "blood-brain barrier," often represents a robust P-glycoprotein–mediated efflux process from capillary endothelial cells in the cerebral circulation. Thus, drug distribution into the brain may be modulated by changes in P-glycoprotein function.

LOADING DOSES For some drugs, the indication may be so urgent that the time required to achieve steady-state concentrations may be too long. Under these conditions, administration of "loading" dosages may result in more rapid elevations of drug concentration to achieve therapeutic effects earlier than with chronic maintenance therapy (Fig. 5-4). Nevertheless, the time required for true steady state to be achieved is still determined only by elimination half-life. This strategy is only appropriate for drugs exhibiting a defined relationship between drug dose and effect.

Disease can alter loading requirements: in congestive heart failure, the central volume of distribution of lidocaine is reduced. Therefore, lower-than-normal loading regimens are required to achieve equivalent plasma drug concentrations and to avoid toxicity.

RATE OF INTRAVENOUS ADMINISTRATION Although the simulations in Fig. 5-2 use a single intravenous bolus, this is very rarely appropriate in practice because side effects related to transiently very high concentrations can result. Rather, drugs are more usually administered orally or as a slower intravenous infusion. Some drugs are so predictably lethal when infused too rapidly that special precautions should be taken to prevent accidental boluses. For example, solutions of potassium for intravenous administration >20 meq/L should be avoided in all but the most exceptional and carefully monitored circumstances. This minimizes the possibility of cardiac arrest due to accidental increases in infusion rates of more concentrated solutions.

While excessively rapid intravenous drug administration can lead to catastrophic consequences, transiently high drug concentrations after

intravenous administration can occasionally be used to advantage. The use of midazolam for intravenous sedation, for example, depends upon its rapid uptake by the brain during the distribution phase to produce sedation quickly, with subsequent egress from the brain during the redistribution of the drug as equilibrium is achieved.

Similarly, adenosine must be administered as a rapid bolus in the treatment of reentrant supraventricular tachycardias (Chap. 226) to prevent elimination by very rapid ($t_{1/2}$ of seconds) uptake into erythrocytes and endothelial cells before the drug can reach its clinical site of action, the atrioventricular node.

PLASMA PROTEIN BINDING

Many drugs circulate in the plasma partly bound to plasma proteins. Since only unbound (free) drug can distribute to sites of pharmacologic action, drug response is related to the free rather than the total circulating plasma drug concentration.

Clinical Implications of Altered Protein Binding For drugs that are normally highly bound to plasma proteins (>90%), small changes in the extent of binding (e.g., due to disease) produce a large change in the amount of unbound drug, and hence drug effect. The acute-phase reactant α_1-acid glycoprotein binds to basic drugs, such as lidocaine or quinidine, and is increased in a range of common conditions, including myocardial infarction, surgery, neoplastic disease, rheumatoid arthritis, and burns. This increased binding can lead to reduced pharmacologic effects at therapeutic concentrations of total drug. Conversely, conditions such as hypoalbuminemia, liver disease, and renal disease can decrease the extent of drug binding, particularly of acidic and neutral drugs, such as phenytoin. Here, plasma concentration of free drug is increased, so drug efficacy and toxicity are enhanced if total (free + bound) drug concentration is used to monitor therapy.

CLEARANCE

When drug is eliminated from the body, the amount of drug in the body declines over time. An important approach to quantifying this reduction is to consider that drug concentration at the beginning and end of a time period are unchanged, and that a specific volume of the body has been "cleared" of the drug during that time period. This defines clearance as volume/time. Clearance includes both drug metabolism and excretion.

Clinical Implications of Altered Clearance • *ADJUSTING DRUG DOSAGES* While elimination half-life determines the time required to achieve steady-state plasma concentrations (C_{ss}), the *magnitude* of that steady state is determined by clearance (Cl) and dose alone. For a drug administered as an intravenous infusion, this relationship is

$$Css = \text{dosing rate}/Cl \qquad \text{or} \qquad \text{dosing rate} = Cl \times Css$$

When drug is administered orally, the average plasma concentration within a dosing interval ($C_{avg,ss}$) replaces C_{ss}, and bioavailability (F) must be included:

$$F \times \text{dosing rate} = Cl \times C_{avg,ss}$$

Genetic variants, drug interactions, or diseases that reduce the activity of drug-metabolizing enzymes or excretory mechanisms may lead to decreased clearance and hence a requirement for downward dose adjustment to avoid toxicity. Conversely, some drug interactions and genetic variants increase CYP expression, and hence increased drug dosage may be necessary to maintain a therapeutic effect.

THE CONCEPT OF HIGH-RISK PHARMACOKINETICS When drugs utilize a single pathway exclusively for elimination, any condition that inhibits that pathway (be it disease-related, genetic, or due to a drug interaction) can lead to dramatic changes in drug concentrations and thus increase the risk of concentration-related drug toxicity. For example, administration of drugs that inhibit P-glycoprotein reduces digoxin clearance, since P-glycoprotein is the major mediator of digoxin elimination; the risk of digoxin toxicity is high with this drug interaction unless digoxin dosages are reduced. Conversely, when drugs undergo elimination by multiple drug metabolizing or excretory pathways, absence of one pathway (due to a genetic variant or drug interaction) is much less likely to have a large impact on drug concentrations or drug actions.

ACTIVE DRUG METABOLITES

From an evolutionary point of view, drug metabolism probably developed as a defense against noxious xenobiotics (foreign substances, e.g., from plants) to which our ancestors inadvertently exposed themselves. The organization of the drug uptake and efflux pumps and the location of drug metabolism in the intestine and liver prior to drug entry to the systemic circulation (Fig. 5-3) support this idea of a primitive protective function.

However, drug metabolites are not necessarily pharmacologically inactive. Metabolites may produce effects similar to, overlapping with, or distinct from those of the parent drug. For example, N-acetyl-procainamide (NAPA) is a major metabolite of the antiarrhythmic procainamide. While it exerts antiarrhythmic effects, its electrophysiologic properties differ from those of the parent drug. Indeed, NAPA accumulation is the usual explanation for marked QT prolongation and torsades des pointes ventricular tachycardia (Chap. 226) during therapy with procainamide. Thus, the common laboratory practice of adding procainamide to NAPA concentrations to estimate a total therapeutic effect is inappropriate.

Prodrugs are inactive compounds that require metabolism to generate active metabolites that mediate the drug effects. Examples include many angiotensin-converting enzyme (ACE) inhibitors, the angiotensin receptor blocker losartan, the antineoplastic irinotecan, and the analgesic codeine (whose active metabolite morphine probably underlies the opioid effect during codeine administration). Drug metabolism has also been implicated in bioactivation of procarcinogens and in generation of reactive metabolites that mediate certain adverse drug effects (e.g., acetaminophen hepatotoxicity, discussed below).

PRINCIPLES OF PHARMACODYNAMICS

Once a drug accesses a molecular site of action, it alters the function of that molecular target, with the ultimate result of a drug effect that the patient or physician can perceive. For drugs used in the urgent treatment of acute symptoms, little or no delay is anticipated (or desired) between the drug-target interaction and the development of a clinical effect. Examples of such acute situations include vascular thrombosis, shock, malignant hypertension, or status epilepticus.

For many conditions, however, the indication for therapy is less urgent, and a delay between the interaction of a drug with its pharmacologic target(s) and a clinical effect is common. Pharmacokinetic mechanisms that can contribute to such a delay include uptake into peripheral compartments or accumulation of active metabolites. Commonly, the clinical effect develops as a downstream consequence of the initial molecular effect the drug produces. Thus, administration of a proton-pump inhibitor or an H_2-receptor blocker produces an immediate increase in gastric pH but ulcer healing that is delayed. Cancer chemotherapy inevitably produces delayed therapeutic effects, often long after drug is undetectable in plasma and tissue. Translation of a molecular drug action to a clinical effect can thus be highly complex and dependent on the details of the pathologic state being treated. These complexities have made pharmacodynamics and its variability less amenable than pharmacokinetics to rigorous mathematical analysis. Nevertheless, some clinically important principles can be elucidated.

A drug effect often depends on the presence of underlying pathophysiology. Thus, a drug may produce no action or a different spectrum of actions in unaffected individuals compared to patients. Further, concomitant disease can complicate interpretation of response to drug therapy, especially adverse effects. For example, high doses of anticonvulsants such as phenytoin may cause neurologic symptoms, which may be confused with the underlying neurologic disease. Similarly, increasing dyspnea in a patient with chronic lung disease receiving amiodarone therapy could be due to drug, underly-

ing disease, or an intercurrent cardiopulmonary problem. Thus the presence of chronic lung disease may alter the risk-benefit ratio in a specific patient to argue against the use of amiodarone.

The concept that a drug interacts with a specific molecular receptor does not imply that the drug effect will be constant over time, even if stable drug and metabolite concentrations are maintained. The drug-receptor interaction occurs in a complex biologic milieu that it can vary to modulate the drug effect. For example, ion channel blockade by drugs, an important anticonvulsant and antiarrhythmic effect, is often modulated by membrane potential, itself a function of factors such as extracellular potassium or local ischemia. Thus, the effects of these drugs may vary depending on the external milieu. Receptors may be up- or down-regulated by disease or by the drug itself. For example, β-adrenergic blockers upregulate β-receptor density during chronic therapy. While this effect does not usually result in resistance to the therapeutic effect of the drugs, it may produce severe agonist–mediated effects (such as hypertension or tachycardia) if the blocking drug is abruptly withdrawn.

PRINCIPLES OF DOSE SELECTION

The desired goal of therapy with any drug is to maximize the likelihood of a beneficial effect while minimizing the risk of adverse effects. Previous experience with the drug, in controlled clinical trials or in postmarketing use, defines the relationships between dose (or plasma concentration) and these dual effects and provides a starting point for initiation of drug therapy.

Figure 5-1 illustrates the relationships among dose, plasma concentrations, efficacy, and adverse effects and carries with it several important implications:

1. *The target drug effect should be defined when drug treatment is started.* With some drugs, the desired effect may be difficult to measure objectively, or the onset of efficacy can be delayed for weeks or months; drugs used in the treatment of cancer and psychiatric disease are examples. Sometimes a drug is used to treat a symptom, such as pain or palpitations, and here it is the patient who will report whether the selected dose is effective. In yet other settings, such as anticoagulation or hypertension, the desired response is more readily measurable.

2. *The nature of anticipated toxicity often dictates the starting dose.* If side effects are minor, it may be acceptable to start at a dose highly likely to achieve efficacy and downtitrate if side effects occur. However, this approach is rarely if ever justified if the anticipated toxicity is serious or life-threatening; in this circumstance, it is more appropriate to initiate therapy with the lowest dose that may produce a desired effect.

3. *The above considerations do not apply if these relationships between dose and effects cannot be defined.* This is especially relevant to some adverse drug effects (discussed in further detail below) whose development is not readily related to drug dose.

4. *If a drug dose does not achieve its desired effect, a dosage increase is justified only if toxicity is absent and the likelihood of serious toxicity is small.* For example, a small percentage of patients with strong seizure foci require plasma levels of phenytoin >20 μg/mL to control seizures. Dosages to achieve this effect may be appropriate, if tolerated. Conversely, clinical experience with flecainide suggests that levels >1000 ng/mL, or dosages >400 mg/d, may be associated with an increased risk of sudden death; thus dosage increases beyond these limits are ordinarily not appropriate, even if the higher dosage appears tolerated.

Other mechanisms that can lead to failure of drug effect should also be considered; drug interactions and noncompliance are common examples. This is one situation in which measurement of plasma drug concentrations, if available, can be especially useful. Noncompliance is an especially frequent problem in the long-term treatment of diseases such as hypertension and epilepsy, occurring in ≥25% of patients in therapeutic environments in which no special effort is made to involve patients in the responsibility for their own health. Multidrug regimens with multiple doses per day are especially prone to noncompliance.

Monitoring response to therapy, by physiologic measures or by plasma concentration measurements, requires an understanding of the relationships between plasma concentration and anticipated effects. For example, measurement of QT interval is used during treatment with sotalol or dofetilide to avoid marked QT prolongation that can herald serious arrhythmias. In this setting, evaluating the electrocardiogram at the time of anticipated peak plasma concentration and effect (e.g., 1–2 h postdose at steady state) is most appropriate. Maintained high aminoglycoside levels carry a risk of nephrotoxicity, so dosages should be adjusted on the basis of plasma concentrations measured at trough (predose). On the other hand, ensuring aminoglycoside efficacy is accomplished by adjusting dosage so that peak drug concentrations are above a minimal antibacterial concentration. For dose adjustment of other drugs (e.g., anticonvulsants), concentration should be measured at its lowest during the dosing interval, just prior to a dose at steady state (Fig. 5-4), to ensure a maintained therapeutic effect.

CONCENTRATION OF DRUGS IN PLASMA AS A GUIDE TO THERAPY

Factors such as interactions with other drugs, disease-induced alterations in elimination and distribution, and genetic variation in drug disposition combine to yield a wide range of plasma levels in patients given the same dose. Hence, if a predictable relationship can be established between plasma drug concentration and beneficial or adverse drug effect, measurement of plasma levels can provide a valuable tool to guide selection of an optimal dose. This is particularly true when there is a narrow range between the plasma levels yielding therapeutic and adverse effects, as with digoxin, theophylline, some antiarrhythmics, aminoglycosides, cyclosporine, and anticonvulsants. On the other hand, if drug access to important sites of action outside plasma is highly variable, monitoring plasma concentration may not provide an accurate guide to therapy (Fig. 5-5A).

The common situation of first-order elimination implies that average, maximum, and minimum steady-state concentrations are related linearly to the dosing rate. Accordingly, the maintenance dose may be adjusted on the basis of the ratio between the desired and measured concentrations *at steady state*; for example, if a doubling of the steady-state plasma concentration is desired, the dose should be doubled. In some cases, elimination becomes saturated at high doses, and the process then occurs at a fixed amount per unit time (zero order). For drugs with this property (e.g., phenytoin and theophylline), plasma concentrations change disproportionately more than the alteration in the dosing rate. In this situation, changes in dose should be small to minimize the degree of unpredictability, and plasma concentration monitoring should be used to ensure that dose modification achieves the desired level.

DETERMINATION OF MAINTENANCE DOSE

An increase in dosage is usually best achieved by changing the drug dose but not the dosing interval, e.g., by giving 200 mg every 8 h instead of 100 mg every 8 h. However, this approach is acceptable only if the resulting maximum concentration is not toxic and the trough value does not fall

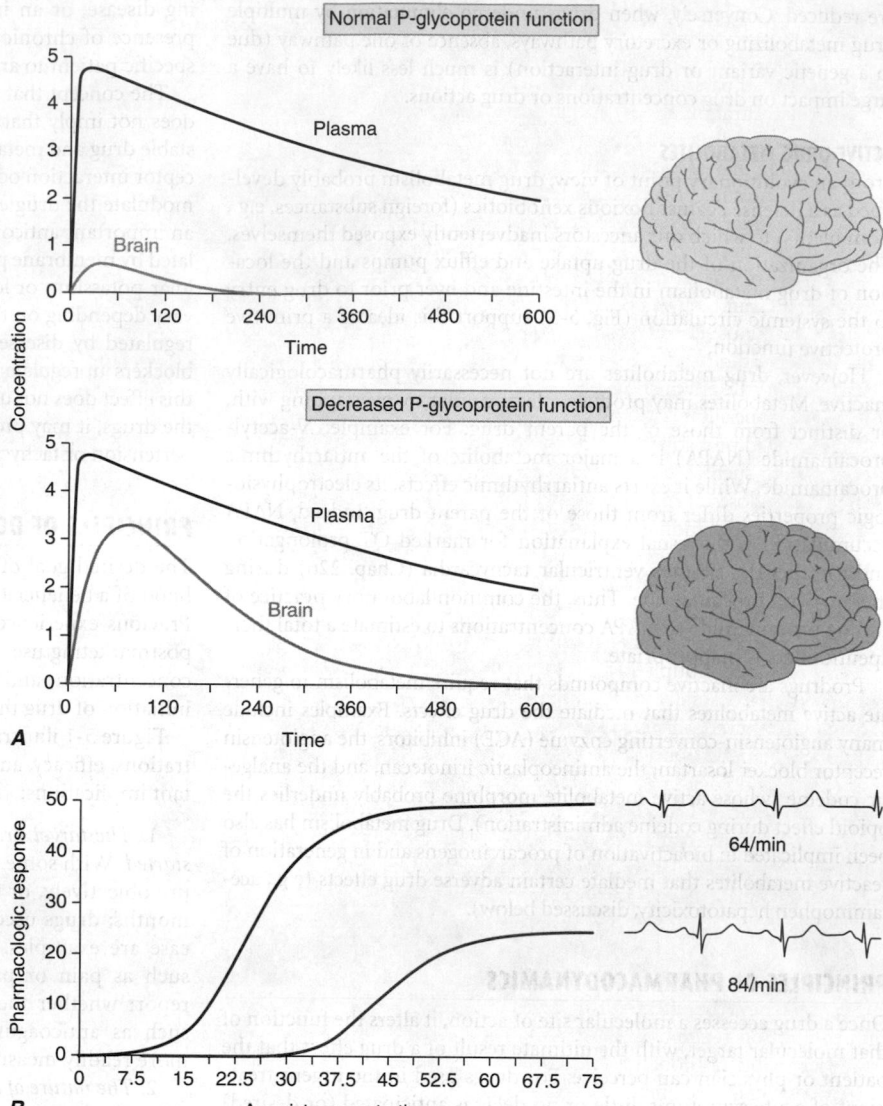

FIGURE 5-5 A. The efflux pump P-glycoprotein excludes drugs from the endothelium of capillaries in the brain, and so constitutes a key element of the blood-brain barrier. Thus, reduced P-glycoprotein function (e.g., due to drug interactions or genetically determined variability in gene transcription) increases penetration of substrate drugs into the brain, even when plasma concentrations are unchanged. **B.** The graph shows an effect of a β₁-receptor polymorphism on receptor function in vitro. Patients with the hypofunctional variant may display greater heart-rate slowing or blood pressure lowering on exposure to receptor blocking agents.

below the minimum effective concentration for an undesirable period of time. Alternatively, the steady state may be changed by altering the frequency of intermittent dosing but not the size of each dose. In this case, the magnitude of the fluctuations around the average steady-state level will change—the shorter the dosing interval, the smaller the difference between peak and trough levels.

Fluctuation within a dosing interval is determined by the relationship between the dosing interval and the drug's half-life. If the dosing interval is equal to the drug's half-life, fluctuation is about twofold, which is usually acceptable. With drugs that have a low therapeutic ratio, dosage changes should be conservative (<50% dose change) and not more frequent than every three–four half-lives. Other drugs, such as many antihypertensives, have little dose-related toxicity, so the therapeutic ratio is large. Even if drug is eliminated rapidly, it can be given infrequently. Thus, 75 mg of captopril will result in reduced blood pressure for up to 12 h, even though captopril elimination half-life is about 2 h; this is because the dose raises the concentration of drug in plasma many times higher than the threshold for its pharmacologic effect.

EFFECTS OF DISEASE ON DRUG CONCENTRATION AND RESPONSE

RENAL DISEASE

Renal excretion of parent drug and metabolites is generally accomplished by glomerular filtration and by specific drug transporters, only now being identified. If a drug or its metabolites are primarily excreted through the kidneys and increased drug levels are associated with adverse effects, drug dosages must be reduced in patients with renal dysfunction to avoid toxicity. The antiarrhythmics dofetilide and sotalol undergo predominant renal excretion and carry a risk of QT prolongation and arrhythmias if doses are not reduced in renal disease. Thus, in end-stage renal disease, sotalol can be given as 40 mg after dialysis (every second day), compared to the usual daily dose, 80–120 mg every 12 h. The narcotic analgesic meperidine undergoes extensive hepatic metabolism, so that renal failure has little effect on its plasma concentration. However, its metabolite, normeperidine, does undergo renal excretion, accumulates in renal failure, and probably accounts for the signs of central nervous system excitation, such as irritability, twitching, and seizures, that appear when multiple doses of meperidine are administered to patients with renal disease. Protein binding of some drugs (e.g., phenytoin) may be altered in uremia, so measuring free drug concentration may be desirable.

In non-end-stage renal disease, changes in renal drug clearance are generally proportional to those in creatinine clearance, which may be measured directly or estimated from the serum creatinine (Chap. 272). This estimate, coupled with the knowledge of how much drug is normally excreted renally vs nonrenally, allows an estimate of the dose adjustment required. In practice, most decisions involving dosing adjustment in patients with renal failure use published recommended adjustments in dosage or dosing interval based on the severity of renal dysfunction indicated by creatinine clearance. Any such modification of dose is a first approximation and should be followed by plasma concentration data (if available) and clinical observation to further optimize therapy for the individual patient.

LIVER DISEASE

In contrast to the predictable decline in renal clearance of drugs in renal insufficiency, the effects of diseases like hepatitis or cirrhosis on drug disposition range from impaired to increased drug clearance, in an unpredictable fashion. Standard tests of liver function are not useful in adjusting doses. First-pass metabolism may decrease—and thus oral bioavailability increases—as a consequence of disrupted hepatocyte function, altered liver architecture, and portacaval shunts. The oral availability for high-first-pass drugs such as morphine, meperidine, midazolam, and nifedipine is almost doubled in patients with cirrhosis, compared to those with normal liver function. Therefore the size of the oral dose of such drugs should be reduced in this setting.

HEART FAILURE AND SHOCK

Under conditions of decreased tissue perfusion, the cardiac output is redistributed to preserve blood flow to the heart and brain at the expense of other tissues (Chap. 227). As a result, drugs may be distributed into a smaller volume of distribution, higher drug concentrations will be present in the plasma, and the tissues that are best perfused (the brain and heart) will be exposed to these higher concentrations. If either the brain or heart is sensitive to the drug, an alteration in response will occur. As well, decreased perfusion of the kidney and liver may impair drug clearance. Thus, in severe congestive heart failure, in hemorrhagic shock, and in cardiogenic shock, response to usual drug doses may be excessive, and dosage reduction may be necessary. For example, the clearance of lidocaine is reduced by about 50% in heart failure, and therapeutic plasma levels are achieved at infusion rates of 50% or less than those usually required. The volume of distribution of lidocaine is also reduced, so loading regimens should be reduced.

DRUG USE IN THE ELDERLY

In the elderly, multiple pathologies and medications used to treat them result in more drug interactions and adverse effects. Aging also results in changes in organ function, especially of the organs involved in drug disposition. Initial doses should be less than the usual adult dosage and should be increased slowly. The number of medications, and doses per day, should be kept as low as possible.

Even in the absence of kidney disease, renal clearance may be reduced by 35–50% in elderly patients. Dosage adjustments are therefore necessary for drugs that are eliminated mainly by the kidneys. Because muscle mass and therefore creatinine production are reduced in older individuals, a normal serum creatinine concentration can be present even though creatinine clearance is impaired; dosages should be adjusted on the basis of creatinine clearance, as discussed above. Aging also results in a decrease in the size of, and blood flow to, the liver and possibly in the activity of hepatic drug-metabolizing enzymes; accordingly, the hepatic clearance of some drugs is impaired in the elderly. As with liver disease, these changes are not readily predicted.

Elderly patients may display altered drug sensitivity. Examples include increased analgesic effects of opioids, increased sedation from benzodiazepines and other CNS depressants, and increased risk of bleeding while receiving anticoagulant therapy, even when clotting parameters are well controlled. Exaggerated responses to cardiovascular drugs are also common because of the impaired responsiveness of normal homeostatic mechanisms. Conversely, the elderly display decreased sensitivity to β-adrenergic receptor blockers.

Adverse drug reactions are especially common in the elderly because of altered pharmacokinetics and pharmacodynamics, the frequent use of multidrug regimens, and concomitant disease. For example, use of long half-life benzodiazepines is linked to the occurrence of hip fractures in elderly patients, perhaps reflecting both a risk of falls from these drugs (due to increased sedation) and the increased incidence of osteoporosis in elderly patients. In population surveys of the noninstitutionalized elderly, as many as 10% had at least one adverse drug reaction in the previous year.

GENETIC DETERMINANTS OF THE RESPONSE TO DRUGS

PRINCIPLES OF GENETIC VARIATION AND HUMAN TRAITS

(See also Chaps. 62 and 64) Variants in the human genome resulting in variation in level of expression or function of molecules important for pharmacokinetics and pharmacodynamics are increasingly recognized. These may be mutations (very rare variants, often associated with disease) or polymorphisms, variants that are much more common in a population. Variants may occur at a single nucleotide [known as single nucleotide polymorphism (SNP)] or involve insertion or deletion of one or more nucleotides. They may be in the exons (coding regions) or introns (noncoding intervening sequences). Exonic polymorphisms may or may not alter the encoded protein, and variant proteins may or may not display altered function. Similarly, polymorphisms in intronic regions may or may not alter gene expression and protein level.

As variation in the human genome is increasingly well documented, associations are being described between polymorphisms and various traits (including response to drug therapy). Some of these rely on well-developed chains of evidence, including in vitro studies demonstrating variant protein function, familial aggregation of the variant allele with the trait, and association studies in large populations. In other cases, the associations are less compelling. Identifying "real" associations is one challenge that must be overcome before the concept of genotyping to identify optimal drugs (or dosages) in individual patients prior to prescribing can be considered for widespread clinical practice. Nevertheless, the appeal of using genomic information to guide therapy is considerable.

Rates of drug efficacy and adverse effects often vary among ethnic groups. Many explanations for such differences are plausible; genomic approaches have now established that functionally important variants determining differences in drug response often display differing distributions among ethnic groups. This finding may have importance for drug use among ethnic groups, as well as in drug development.

GENETICALLY DETERMINED DRUG DISPOSITION AND VARIABLE EFFECTS

The concept that genetically determined variations in drug metabolism might be associated with variable drug levels, and hence effect, was advanced at the end of the nineteenth century, and the first exam-

FIGURE 5-6 A. CYP2D6 metabolic activity was assessed in 290 subjects by administration of a test dose of a probe substrate and measurement of urinary formation of the CYP2D6-generated metabolite. The heavy arrow indicates a clear antimode, separating poor metabolizer subjects (PMs, green), with two loss-of-function CYP2D6 alleles, indicated by the intron-exon structures below the bar chart. Individuals with one or two functional alleles are grouped together as extensive metabolizers (EMs, blue). Also shown are ultrarapid metabolizers (UMs), with 2–12 functional copies of the gene (red), displaying the greatest enzyme activity. *(Adapted by permission from M-L Dahl et al: J Pharmacol Exp Ther 274:516, 1995.)* **B.** These simulations show the predicted effects of CYP2D6 genotype on disposition of a substrate drug. With a single dose (*left*), there is an inverse "gene-dose" relationship between the number of active alleles and the areas under the time-concentration curves (smallest in UM subjects; highest in PM subjects); this indicates that clearance is greatest in UM subjects. In addition, elimination half-life is longest in PM subjects. The right panel shows that these single dose differences are exaggerated during chronic therapy: steady-state concentration is much higher in PM subjects (decreased clearance), as is the time required to achieve steady state (longer elimination half-life).

ples of familial clustering of unusual drug responses due to this mechanism were noted in the mid-twentieth century. Clinically important genetic variants have been described in multiple molecular pathways of drug disposition (Table 5-1). A distinct multimodal distribution of drug disposition (as shown in **Fig. 5-6**) argues for a predominant effect of variants in a single gene in the metabolism of that substrate. Individuals with two alleles (variants) encoding for nonfunctional protein make up one group, often termed *poor metabolizers* (PM phenotype); many variants can produce such a loss of function, complicating the use of genotyping in clinical practice. Individuals with one functional allele make up a second (*intermediate metabolizers*) and may or may not be distinguishable from those with two functional alleles (*extensive metabolizers*, EMs). *Ultra-rapid metabolizers* with especially high enzymatic activity (occasionally due to gene duplication; Fig. 5-6) have also been described for some traits. Many drugs in widespread use can inhibit specific drug disposition pathways (Table 5-1), and so EM individuals receiving such agents can respond like PM patients (*phenocopying*). Polymorphisms in genes encoding drug uptake or drug efflux transporters may be another contributor to variability

in drug delivery to target sites and, hence, drug effects. However, loss-of-function alleles in these genes have not yet been described.

CYP Variants CYP3A4 is the most abundant hepatic and intestinal CYP and is also the enzyme responsible for metabolism of the greatest number of drugs in therapeutic use. CYP3A4 activity is highly variable (up to an order of magnitude) among individuals, but the underlying mechanisms are not yet well understood. A closely related gene, encoding CYP3A5 (which shares substrates with CYP3A4), does display loss-of-function variants, especially in African-derived populations. CYP3A refers to both enzymes.

CYP2D6 is second to CYP3A4 in the number of commonly used drugs that it metabolizes. CYP2D6 is polymorphically distributed, with about 7% of European- and African-derived populations (but very few Asians) displaying the PM phenotype (Fig. 5-6). Dozens of loss-of-function variants in the CYP2D6 gene have been described; the PM phenotype arises in individuals with two such alleles. In addition, ultrarapid metabolizers with multiple functional copies of the CYP2D6 gene have been identified, particularly among northern Africans.

CYP2D6 represents the main metabolic pathway for a number of drugs (Table 5-1). Codeine is biotransformed by CYP2D6 to the potent active metabolite morphine, so its effects are blunted in PMs and exaggerated in ultrarapid metabolizers. In the case of drugs with beta-blocking properties metabolized by CYP2D6, including ophthalmic timolol and the sodium channel–blocking antiarrhythmic propafenone, PM subjects display greater signs of beta blockade (including bradycardia and bronchospasm) than EMs. Further, in EM subjects, propafenone elimination becomes zero-order at higher doses; so, for example, a tripling of the dose may lead to a tenfold increase in drug concentration. The oral hypoglycemic agent phenformin was withdrawn because it occasionally caused profound lactic acidosis; this likely arose as a result of high concentrations in CYP2D6 PMs. Ultrarapid metabolizers may require very high dosages of tricyclic antidepressants to achieve a therapeutic effect and, with codeine, may display transient euphoria and nausea due to very rapid generation of morphine. Tamoxifen undergoes CYP2D6-mediated biotransformation to an active metabolite, so its efficacy may be in part related to this polymorphism. In addition, the widespread use of selective serotonin reuptake inhibitors (SSRIs) to treat tamoxifen-related hot flashes may also alter the drug's effects since many SSRIs (fluoxetine, paroxetine) are also CYP2D6 inhibitors.

The PM phenotype for CYP2C19 is common (20%) among Asians and rarer (3–5%) in European-derived populations. The impact of polymorphic CYP2C19-mediated metabolism has been demonstrated with the proton pump inhibitor omeprazole, where ulcer cure rates with "standard" dosages were markedly lower in EM patients (29%) than in PMs (100%). Thus, understanding the importance of this polymorphism would have been important in developing the drug, and knowing a patient's CYP2C19 genotype should improve therapy.

There are common allelic variants of *CYP2C9* that encode proteins with loss of catalytic function. These variant alleles are associated increased rates of neurologic complications with phenytoin and of hypoglycemia with glipizide. The angiotensin-receptor blocker losartan is a prodrug that is bioactivated by CYP2C9; as a result, PMs and those receiving inhibitor drugs may display little response to therapy.

Transferase Variants One of the most extensively studied phase II polymorphisms is the PM trait for thiopurine S-methyltransferase (TPMT). TPMT bioinactivates the antileukemic drug 6-mercaptopurine. Further, 6-mercaptopurine is itself an active metabolite of the immunosuppressive azathioprine. Homozygotes for alleles encoding the inactive TPMT (1 in 300 individuals) predictably exhibit severe and potentially fatal pancytopenia on standard doses of azathioprine or 6-mercaptopurine. On the other hand, homozygotes for fully functional alleles may display less anti-inflammatory or antileukemic effect with the drugs.

N-acetylation is catalyzed by hepatic *N*-acetyl transferase (NAT), which represents the activity of two genes, *NAT-1* and *NAT-2*. Both enzymes transfer an acetyl group from acetyl coenzyme A to the drug; NAT-1 activity is generally constant, while polymorphisms in *NAT-2* result in individual differences in the rate at which drugs are acetylated and thus define "rapid acetylators" and "slow acetylators." Slow acetylators make up ~50% of European- and African-derived populations but are less common among Asians.

Slow acetylators have an increased incidence of the drug-induced lupus syndrome during procainamide and hydralazine therapy and of hepatitis with isoniazid. Induction of CYPs (e.g., by rifampin) also increases the risk of isoniazid-related hepatitis, likely reflecting generation of reactive metabolites of acetylhydrazine, itself an isoniazid metabolite.

Individuals homozygous for a common promoter polymorphism that reduces transcription of uridine diphosphate glucuronosyltransferase (*UGT1A1*) have benign hyperbilirubinemia (Gilbert's syndrome; Chap. 297). This variant has also been associated with diarrhea and increased bone marrow depression with the antineoplastic prodrug irinotecan, whose active metabolite is normally detoxified by this UGT1A1-mediated glucuronidation.

VARIABILITY IN THE MOLECULAR TARGETS WITH WHICH DRUGS INTERACT

As molecular approaches identify specific gene products as targets of drug action, polymorphisms that alter the expression or function of these drug targets—and thus modulate their actions in patients—are also being recognized. Multiple polymorphisms identified in the β_2-adrenergic receptor appear to be linked to specific phenotypes in asthma and congestive heart failure, diseases in which β_2-receptor function might be expected to determine prognosis. Polymorphisms in the β_2-receptor gene have also been associated with response to inhaled β_2-receptor agonists, while those in the β_1-adrenergic receptor gene have been associated with variability in heart rate slowing and blood pressure lowering (Fig. 5-5B). In addition, in heart failure, a common polymorphism in the β_1-adrenergic receptor gene has been implicated in variable clinical outcome during therapy with the beta blocker bucindolol. Response to the 5-lipoxygenase inhibitor zileuton in asthma has been linked to polymorphisms that determine the expression level of the 5-lipoxygenase gene. Herceptin, which potentiates anthracycline-related cardiotoxicity, is ineffective in breast cancers that do not express the herceptin receptor; thus, "genotyping" the tumor is a mechanism to avoid potentially toxic therapy in patients who would derive no benefit.

Drugs may also interact with genetic pathways of disease, to elicit or exacerbate symptoms of the underlying conditions. In the porphyrias, CYP inducers are thought to increase the activity of enzymes proximal to the deficient enzyme, exacerbating or triggering attacks (Chap. 352). Deficiency of glucose-6-phosphate dehydrogenase (G6PD), most often in individuals of African or Mediterranean descent, increases

risk of hemolytic anemia in response to primaquine and a number of other drugs that do not cause hemolysis in patients with normal amounts of the enzyme (Chap. 101). Patients with mutations in the ryanodine receptor, which controls intracellular calcium in skeletal muscle and other tissues, may be asymptomatic until exposed to certain general anesthetics, which trigger the syndrome of malignant hyperthermia. Certain antiarrhythmics and other drugs can produce marked QT prolongation and torsades des pointes (Chap. 226), and in some patients this adverse effect represents unmasking of previously subclinical congenital long QT syndrome.

POLYMORPHISMS THAT MODULATE THE BIOLOGIC CONTEXT WITHIN WHICH THE DRUG-TARGET INTERACTIONS OCCUR

The interaction of a drug with its molecular target is translated into a clinical action in a complex biologic milieu that is itself often perturbed by disease. Thus, polymorphisms that determine variability in this biology may profoundly influence drug response, although the genes involved are not themselves directly targets of drug action. Polymorphisms in genes important for lipid homeostasis (such as the ABCA1 transporter and the cholesterol ester transport protein) modulate response to 3-hydroxymethylglutaryl-CoA (HMG-CoA) reductase inhibitors, "statins." In one large study, the combination of diuretic use combined with a variant in the adducin gene (encoding a cytoskeletal protein important for renal tubular sodium absorption) decreased stroke or myocardial infarction risk, while neither factor alone had an effect. Common polymorphisms in ion channel genes that are not themselves the target of QT-prolonging drugs may nevertheless influence the extent to which those drugs affect the electrocardiogram and produce arrhythmias. These findings not only point to new mechanisms for understanding drug action, but also can be used for drug development. For example, a set of polymorphisms in the gene encoding 5-lipoxygenase activating protein (FLAP) has been identified as a risk factor for myocardial infarction in an Icelandic population, and an initial clinical trial of a FLAP inhibitor was conducted only in subjects with the high risk allele.

MULTIPLE VARIANTS MODULATING DRUG EFFECTS

As this discussion makes clear, for each drug with a defined mechanism of action and disposition pathways, a set of "candidate genes," in which polymorphisms may mediate variable clinical responses, can be identified. Indeed, polymorphisms in multiple genes have been associated with variability in the effect of a single drug. CYP2C9 loss-of-function variants are associated with a requirement for lower maintenance doses of the vitamin K antagonist anticoagulant warfarin. In rarer (<2%) individuals homozygous for these variant alleles, maintenance warfarin dosages may be difficult to establish, and the risk of bleeding complications appears increased. In addition to *CYP2C9*, variants in the promoter region of *VKORC1*, encoding a vitamin K epoxide reductase, predict warfarin dosages; these promoter variants are in tight *linkage disequilibrium*, i.e. genotyping at one polymorphic site within this *haplotype block* provides reliable information on the identity of genotypes at other linked sites (Chap. 62). Thus, variability in response to warfarin can be linked to both coding region polymorphisms in CYP2C9 and promoter haplotypes in the warfarin target *VKORC1*.

As genotyping technologies improve and data sets of patients with well-documented drug responses are accumulated, it is becoming possible to interrogate hundreds of polymorphisms in dozens of candidate genes. This approach has been applied to implicate linked noncoding polymorphisms in the HMG-CoA reductase gene as predicting efficacy of HMG-CoA reductase inhibitors, and in variants in the gene-encoding corticotrophin-releasing hormone receptor 1 as predicting efficacy of inhaled steroids in asthma.

Technologies are now evolving to interrogate hundreds of thousands of SNPs across the genome, or to rapidly resequence each patient's genome. These approaches, which have been applied to identify new genes modulating disease susceptibility (Chap. 62), may be applicable to the problem of identifying genomic predictors of variable drug effects.

PROSPECTS FOR INCORPORATING GENETIC INFORMATION INTO CLINICAL PRACTICE

The examples of associations between specific genotypes and drug responses raise the tantalizing prospect that patients will undergo routine genotyping for loci known to modulate drug levels or response prior to receiving a prescription. Indeed, clinical tests for some of the polymorphisms described above, including those in *TPMT*, *UGT1A1*, *CYP2D6*, and *CYP2C19*, have been approved by the U.S. Food and Drug Administration (FDA). The twin goals are to identify patients likely to exhibit adverse effects and those most likely to respond well. Obstacles that must be overcome before this vision becomes a reality include replication of even the most compelling associations, demonstrations of cost-effectiveness, development of readily useable genotyping technologies, and ethical issues involved in genotyping. While these barriers seem daunting, the field is very young and evolving rapidly. Indeed, one major result of understanding of the role of genetics in drug action has been improved screening of drugs during the development process to reduce the likelihood of highly variable metabolism or unanticipated toxicity (such as torsades des pointes).

INTERACTIONS BETWEEN DRUGS

Drug interactions can complicate therapy by increasing or decreasing the action of a drug; interactions may be based on changes in drug disposition or in drug response in the absence of changes in drug levels. *Interactions must be considered in the differential diagnosis of any unusual response occurring during drug therapy.* Prescribers should recognize that patients often come to them with a legacy of drugs acquired during previous medical experiences, often with multiple physicians who may not be aware of all the patient's medications. A meticulous drug history should include examination of the patient's medications and, if necessary, calls to the pharmacist to identify prescriptions. It should also address the use of agents not often volunteered during questioning, such as over-the-counter (OTC) drugs, health food supplements, and topical agents such as eye drops. Lists of interactions are available from a number of electronic sources. While it is unrealistic to expect the practicing physician to memorize these, certain drugs consistently run the risk of generating interactions, often by inhibiting or inducing specific drug elimination pathways. Examples are presented below and in Table 5-2. Accordingly, when these drugs are started or stopped, prescribers must be especially alert to the possibility of interactions.

PHARMACOKINETIC INTERACTIONS CAUSING DECREASED DRUG EFFECTS

Gastrointestinal absorption can be reduced if a drug interaction results in drug binding in the gut, as with aluminum-containing antacids, kaolin-pectin suspensions, or bile acid sequestrants. Drugs such as histamine H_2 receptor antagonists or proton pump inhibitors that alter gastric pH may decrease the solubility and hence absorption of weak bases such as ketoconazole.

Expression of some genes responsible for drug elimination, notably *CYP3A* and *MDR1*, can be markedly increased by "inducing" drugs, such as rifampin, carbamazepine, phenytoin, St. John's wort, and glutethimide and by smoking, exposure to chlorinated insecticides such as DDT (CYP1A2), and chronic alcohol ingestion. Administration of

Drug	**Mechanism**	**Examples**
Antacids Bile acid sequestrants	Reduced absorption	Antacids/tetracyclines Cholestryamine/digoxin
Proton pump inhibitors H₂-receptor blockers	Altered gastric pH	Ketoconazole absorption decreased

Rifampin
Carbamazepine
Barbiturates
Phenytoin
St. John's wort
Glutethimide
	Induction of hepatic metabolism	Decreased concentration and effects of
		    warfarin
		    quinidine
		    cyclosporine
		    losartan
		    oral contraceptives
		    methadone

Tricyclic antidepressants Fluoxetine Quinidine	Inhibitors of CYP2D6	Increased β-blockade Decreased codeine effect

Cimetidine	Inhibitor of multiple CYPs	Increased concentration and effects of
		    warfarin
		    theophylline
		    phenytoin

Ketoconazole, itraconazole
Erythromycin, clarithromycin
Calcium channel blockers
Ritonavir
	Inhibitor of CYP3A	Increased concentration and toxicity of
		    some HMG-CoA reductase inhibitors
		    cyclosporine
		    cisapride, terfenadine (now withdrawn)
		Increased concentration and effects of
		    indinavir (with ritonavir)
		Decreased clearance and dose requirement for cyclosporine (with calcium channel blockers)

Allopurinol	Xanthine oxidase inhibitor	Azathioprine and 6-mercaptopurine toxicity

Amiodarone	Inhibitor of many CYPs and of P-glycoprotein	Decreased clearance (risk of toxicity) for
		    warfarin
		    digoxin
		    quinidine

Gemfibrazol (and other fibrates)	CYP3A inhibition	Rhabdomyolysis when co-prescribed with some HMG-CoA reductase inhibitors
Quinidine Amiodarone Verapamil Cyclosporine Itraconazole Erythromycin	P-glycoprotein inhibition	Risk of digoxin toxicity
Phenylbutazone Probenecid Salicylates	Inhibition of renal tubular transport	Salicylates → increased risk of methotrexate toxicity

TABLE 5-2 DRUGS WITH A HIGH RISK OF GENERATING PHARMACOKINETIC INTERACTIONS

inducing agents lowers plasma levels over 2–3 weeks as gene expression is increased. If a drug dose is stabilized in the presence of an inducer that is subsequently stopped, major toxicity can occur as clearance returns to preinduction levels and drug concentrations rise. Individuals vary in the extent to which drug metabolism can be induced, likely through genetic mechanisms.

Interactions that inhibit the bioactivation of prodrugs will similarly decrease drug effects. The analgesic effect of codeine depends on its metabolism to morphine via CYP2D6. Thus, the CYP2D6 inhibitor quinidine reduces the analgesic efficacy of codeine in EMs.

Interactions that decrease drug delivery to intracellular sites of action can decrease drug effects: tricyclic antidepressants can blunt the antihypertensive effect of clonidine by decreasing its uptake into adrenergic neurons. Reduced CNS penetration of multiple HIV protease inhibitors (with the attendant risk of facilitating viral replication in a sanctuary site) appears attributable to P-glycoprotein-mediated exclusion of the drug from the CNS; indeed, inhibition of P-glycoprotein has been proposed as a therapeutic approach to enhance drug entry to the CNS (Fig. 5-5A).

PHARMACOKINETIC INTERACTIONS CAUSING INCREASED DRUG EFFECTS

The most common mechanism here is inhibition of drug elimination. In contrast to induction, new protein synthesis is not involved, and the effect develops as drug and any inhibitor metabolites accumulate (a function of their elimination half-lives). Since shared substrates of a single enzyme can compete for access to the active site of the protein, many CYP substrates can also be considered inhibitors. However, some drugs are especially potent as inhibitors (and occasionally may not even be substrates) of specific drug-elimination pathways, and so it is in the use of these agents that clinicians must be most alert to the potential for interactions (Table 5-2). Commonly implicated interacting drugs of this type include cimetidine, erythromycin and some other macrolide antibiotics (clarithromycin but not azithromycin), ketoconazole and other azole antifungals, the antiretroviral agent ritonavir, and high concentrations of grapefruit juice (Table 5-2). The consequences of such interactions will depend on the drug whose elimination is being inhibited; high-risk drugs are those for which alternate pathways of elimination are not available and for which drug accumulation increases the risk of serious toxicity (see "The Concept of High-Risk Pharmacokinetics," above). Examples include CYP3A inhibitors increasing the risk of cyclosporine toxicity or of rhabdomyolysis with some HMG-CoA reductase inhibitors (lovastatin, simvastatin, atorvastatin), and P-glycoprotein inhibitors increasing risk of digoxin toxicity.

Phenytoin, an inducer of many systems, including CYP3A, inhibits CYP2C9. CYP2C9 metabolism of losartan to its active metabolite is inhibited by phenytoin, with potential loss of antihypertensive effect.

The antiviral ritonavir is a very potent CYP3A4 inhibitor that has been added to anti-HIV regimens, not because of its antiviral effects but because it decreases clearance, and hence increases efficacy, of other anti-HIV agents. Grapefruit (but not orange) juice inhibits CYP3A, especially at high doses; patients receiving drugs where even modest CYP3A inhibition may increase the risk of adverse effects (e.g., cyclosporine, some HMG-CoA reductase inhibitors) should therefore avoid grapefruit juice.

CYP2D6 is markedly inhibited by quinidine, a number of neuroleptic drugs (chlorpromazine and haloperidol), and the SSRIs fluoxetine and paroxetine. Clinical consequences of fluoxetine's interaction with CYP2D6 substrates may not be apparent for weeks after the drug is started, because of its very long half-life and slow generation of a CYP2D6-inhibiting metabolite.

6-Mercaptopurine, the active metabolite of azathioprine, is metabolized not only by TPMT but also by xanthine oxidase. When allopurinol, a potent inhibitor of xanthine oxidase, is administered with standard doses of azathioprine or 6-mercaptopurine, life-threatening toxicity (bone marrow suppression) can result.

A number of drugs are secreted by the renal tubular transport systems for organic anions. Inhibition of these systems can cause excessive drug accumulation. Salicylate, for example, reduces the renal clearance of methotrexate, an interaction that may lead to methotrexate toxicity. Renal tubular secretion contributes substantially to the elimination of penicillin, which can be inhibited (to increase its therapeutic effect) by probenecid. Similarly, inhibition of the tubular cation transport system by cimetidine decreases the renal clearance of dofetilide and of procainamide and its active metabolite NAPA.

DRUG INTERACTIONS NOT MEDIATED BY CHANGES IN DRUG DISPOSITION

Drugs may act on separate components of a common process to generate effects greater than either has alone. Antithrombotic therapy with combinations of antiplatelet agents (glycoprotein IIb/IIIa inhibitors, aspirin, clopidogrel) and anticoagulants (warfarin, heparins) are often used in the treatment of vascular disease, although such combinations carry an increased risk of bleeding.

Nonsteroidal anti-inflammatory drugs (NSAIDs) cause gastric ulcers, and in patients treated with warfarin, the risk of bleeding from a peptic ulcer is increased almost threefold by concomitant use of an NSAID.

Indomethacin, piroxicam, and probably other NSAIDs antagonize the antihypertensive effects of β-adrenergic receptor blockers, diuretics, ACE inhibitors, and other drugs. The resulting elevation in blood pressure ranges from trivial to severe. This effect is not seen with aspirin and sulindac but has been found with the cyclooxygenase 2 (COX-2) inhibitor celecoxib.

Torsades des pointes during administration of QT-prolonging antiarrhythmics (quinidine, sotalol, dofetilide) occur much more frequently in patients receiving diuretics, probably reflecting hypokalemia. In vitro, hypokalemia not only prolongs the QT interval in the absence of drug but also potentiates drug block of ion channels that results in QT prolongation. Also, some diuretics have direct electrophysiologic actions that prolong QT.

The administration of supplemental potassium leads to more frequent and more severe hyperkalemia when potassium elimination is reduced by concurrent treatment with ACE inhibitors, spironolactone, amiloride, or triamterene.

The pharmacologic effects of sildenafil result from inhibition of the phosphodiesterase type 5 isoform that inactivates cyclic GMP in the vasculature. Nitroglycerin and related nitrates used to treat angina produce vasodilation by elevating cyclic GMP. Thus, coadministration of these nitrates with sildenafil can cause profound hypotension, which can be catastrophic in patients with coronary disease.

Sometimes, combining drugs can increase overall efficacy and/or reduce drug-specific toxicity. Such therapeutically useful interactions are described in chapters dealing with specific disease entities, elsewhere in this text.

ADVERSE REACTIONS TO DRUGS

The beneficial effects of drugs are coupled with the inescapable risk of untoward effects. The morbidity and mortality from these untoward effects often present diagnostic problems because they can involve every organ and system of the body; these may be mistaken for signs of underlying disease.

Adverse reactions can be classified in two broad groups. One type results from exaggeration of an intended pharmacologic action of the drug, such as increased bleeding with anticoagulants or bone marrow suppression with antineoplastics. The other type of adverse reactions ensues from toxic effects unrelated to the intended pharmacologic actions. The latter effects are often unanticipated (especially with new drugs) and frequently severe and result from recognized as well as undiscovered mechanisms.

Drugs may increase the frequency of an event that is common in a general population, and this may be especially difficult to recognize; the increase in myocardial infarctions with the COX-2 inhibitor rofecoxib is an excellent example. Drugs can also cause rare and serious adverse effects, such as hematologic abnormalities, arrhythmias, or hepatic or renal dysfunction. Prior to regulatory approval and marketing, new drugs are tested in relatively few patients who tend to be less sick and to have fewer concomitant diseases than those patients who subsequently receive the drug therapeutically. Because of the relatively small number of patients studied in clinical trials and the selected nature of these patients, rare adverse effects are generally not detected prior to a drug's approval, and physicians therefore need to be cautious in the prescription of new drugs and alert for the appearance of previously unrecognized adverse events.

Elucidating mechanisms underlying adverse drug effects can assist development of safer compounds or allow a patient subset at especially high risk to be excluded from drug exposure. National adverse reaction reporting systems, such as those operated by the FDA (suspected adverse reactions can be reported online at *http://www.fda.gov/medwatch/report/hcp.htm*) and the Committee on Safety of Medicines in Great Britain, can prove useful. The publication or reporting of a newly recognized adverse reaction can in a short time stimulate many similar such reports of reactions that previously had gone unrecognized.

Occasionally, "adverse" effects may be exploited to develop an entirely new indication for a drug. Unwanted hair growth during minoxidil treatment of severely hypertensive patients led to development of the drug for hair growth. Sildenafil was initially developed as an antianginal, but its effects to alleviate erectile dysfunction not only led to a new drug indication but also to increased understanding of the role of type 5 phosphodiesterase in erectile tissue. These examples further reinforce the concept that prescribers must remain vigilant to the possibility that unusual symptoms may reflect unappreciated drug effects.

Some 25–50% of patients make errors in self-administration of prescribed medicines, and these errors can be responsible for adverse drug effects. Similarly, patients commit errors in taking OTC drugs by not reading or following the directions on the containers. Physicians must recognize that providing directions with prescriptions does not always guarantee compliance.

In hospital, drugs are administered in a controlled setting, and patient compliance is, in general, ensured. Errors may occur nevertheless—the wrong drug or dose may be given or the drug may be given to the wrong patient—and improved drug distribution and administration systems are addressing this problem.

EPIDEMIOLOGY

Patients receive, on average, 10 different drugs during each hospitalization. The sicker the patient, the more drugs are given, and there is a corresponding increase in the likelihood of adverse drug reactions. When <6 different drugs are given to hospitalized patients, the probability of an adverse reaction is ~5%, but if >15 drugs are given, the probability is >40%. Retrospective analyses of ambulatory patients have revealed adverse drug effects in 20%. Serious adverse reactions are also well recognized with "herbal" remedies and OTC compounds: examples include kava-associated hepatotoxicity, L-tryptophan–associated eosinophilia-myalgia, and phenylpropanolamine-associated stroke, each of which has caused fatalities.

A small group of widely used drugs accounts for a disproportionate number of reactions. Aspirin and other NSAIDs, analgesics, digoxin, anticoagulants, diuretics, antimicrobials, glucocorticoids, antineoplastics, and hypoglycemic agents account for 90% of reactions, although the drugs involved differ between ambulatory and hospitalized patients.

TOXICITY UNRELATED TO A DRUG'S PRIMARY PHARMACOLOGIC ACTIVITY

Cytotoxic Reactions Drugs or more commonly reactive metabolites generated by CYPs can covalently bind to tissue macromolecules (such as proteins or DNA) to cause tissue toxicity. Because of the reactive nature of these metabolites, covalent binding often occurs close to the site of production, typically the liver.

The most common cause of drug-induced hepatotoxicity is acetaminophen overdosage. Normally, reactive metabolites are detoxified by combining with hepatic glutathione. When glutathione becomes exhausted, the metabolites bind instead to hepatic protein, with resultant hepatocyte damage. The hepatic necrosis produced by the ingestion of acetaminophen can be prevented or attenuated by the administration of substances such as N-acetylcysteine that reduce the binding of electrophilic metabolites to hepatic proteins. The risk of acetaminophen-related hepatic necrosis is increased in patients receiving drugs such as phenobarbital or phenytoin that increase the rate of drug metabolism or ethanol that exhaust glutathione stores. Such toxicity has even occurred with therapeutic dosages, so patients at risk through these mechanisms should be warned.

Immunologic Mechanisms Most pharmacologic agents are small molecules with low molecular weights (<2000) and thus are poor immunogens. Generation of an immune response to a drug therefore usually requires in vivo activation and covalent linkage to protein, carbohydrate, or nucleic acid.

Drug stimulation of antibody production may mediate tissue injury by several mechanisms. The antibody may attack the drug when the drug is covalently attached to a cell and thereby destroy the cell. This occurs in penicillin-induced hemolytic anemia. Antibody-drug-antigen complexes may be passively adsorbed by a bystander cell, which is then destroyed by activation of complement; this occurs in quinine- and quinidine-induced thrombocytopenia. Heparin-induced thrombocytopenia arises when antibodies against complexes of platelet factor 4 peptide and heparin generate immune complexes that activate platelets; thus, the thrombocytopenia is accompanied by "paradoxical" thrombosis and is treated with thrombin inhibitors. Drugs or their reactive metabolites may alter a host tissue, rendering it antigenic and eliciting autoantibodies. For example, hydralazine and procainamide (or their reactive metabolites) can chemically alter nuclear material, stimulating the formation of antinuclear antibodies and occasionally causing lupus erythematosus. Drug-induced pure red cell aplasia (Chap. 102) is due to an immune-based drug reaction. Red cell formation in bone marrow cultures can be inhibited by phenytoin and purified IgG obtained from a patient with pure red cell aplasia associated with phenytoin.

Serum sickness (Chap. 311) results from the deposition of circulating drug-antibody complexes on endothelial surfaces. Complement activation occurs, chemotactic factors are generated locally, and an inflammatory response develops at the site of complex entrapment. Arthralgias, urticaria, lymphadenopathy, glomerulonephritis, or cerebritis may result. Foreign proteins (vaccines, streptokinase, therapeutic antibodies) and antibiotics are common causes. Many drugs, particularly antimicrobial agents, ACE inhibitors, and aspirin, can elicit anaphylaxis with production of IgE, which binds to mast cell membranes. Contact with a drug antigen initiates a series of biochemical events in the mast cell and results in the release of mediators that can produce the characteristic urticaria, wheezing, flushing, rhinorrhea, and (occasionally) hypotension.

Drugs may also elicit cell-mediated immune responses. Topically administered substances may interact with sulfhydryl or amino groups in the skin and react with sensitized lymphocytes to produce the rash characteristic of contact dermatitis. Other types of rashes may also result from the interaction of serum factors, drugs, and sensitized lymphocytes.

DIAGNOSIS AND TREATMENT OF ADVERSE DRUG REACTIONS

The manifestations of drug-induced diseases frequently resemble those of other diseases, and a given set of manifestations may be produced by different and dissimilar drugs. Recognition of the role of a drug or drugs in an illness depends on appreciation of the possible adverse reactions to drugs in any disease, on identification of the temporal relationship between drug administration and development of the illness, and on familiarity with the common manifestations of the drugs. Many associations between particular drugs and specific reactions have been described, but there is always a "first time" for a novel association, and any drug should be suspected of causing an adverse effect if the clinical setting is appropriate.

Illness related to a drug's intended pharmacologic action is often more easily recognized than illness attributable to immune or other mechanisms. For example, side effects such as cardiac arrhythmias in patients receiving digitalis, hypoglycemia in patients given insulin, and bleeding in patients receiving anticoagulants are more readily related to a specific drug than are symptoms such as fever or rash, which may be caused by many drugs or by other factors.

Electronic sources of adverse drug reactions can be useful. However, exhaustive compilations often provide little sense of perspective in terms of frequency and seriousness, which can vary considerably among patients.

Eliciting a drug history from patients is important for diagnosis. Attention must be directed to OTC drugs and herbal preparations as well as to prescription drugs. Each type can be responsible for adverse drug effects, and adverse interactions may occur between OTC drugs and prescribed drugs. Loss of efficacy of oral contraceptives or cyclosporine by concurrent use of St. John's wort are examples. In addition, it is common for patients to be cared for by several physicians, and duplicative, additive, counteractive, or synergistic drug combinations may therefore be administered if the physicians are not aware of the patients' drug histories. Every physician should determine what drugs a patient has been taking, for the previous month or two ideally, before prescribing any medications. Medications stopped for inefficacy or adverse effects should be documented to avoid pointless and potentially dangerous reexposure. A frequently overlooked source of additional drug exposure is topical therapy; for example, a patient complaining of bronchospasm may not mention that an ophthalmic beta blocker is being used unless specifically asked. A history of previous adverse drug effects in patients is common. Since these patients have shown a predisposition to drug-induced illnesses, such a history should dictate added caution in prescribing drugs.

Laboratory studies may include demonstration of serum antibody in some persons with drug allergies involving cellular blood elements, as in agranulocytosis, hemolytic anemia, and thrombocytopenia. For example, both quinine and quinidine can produce platelet agglutination in vitro in the presence of complement and the serum from a patient who has developed thrombocytopenia following use of this drug. Biochemical abnormalities such as G6PD deficiency, serum pseudocholinesterase level, or genotyping may also be useful in diagnosis, often after an adverse effect has occurred in the patient or a family member.

Once an adverse reaction is suspected, discontinuation of the suspected drug followed by disappearance of the reaction is presumptive evidence of a drug-induced illness. Confirming evidence may be sought by cautiously reintroducing the drug and seeing if the reaction reappears. However, that should be done only if confirmation would be useful in the future management of the patient and if the attempt would not entail undue risk. With concentration-dependent adverse reactions, lowering the dosage may cause the reaction to disappear, and raising it may cause the reaction to reappear. When the reaction is thought to be allergic, however, readministration of the drug may be hazardous, since anaphylaxis may develop. Readministration is unwise under these conditions unless no alternative drugs are available and treatment is necessary.

If the patient is receiving many drugs when an adverse reaction is suspected, the drugs likeliest to be responsible can usually be identified; this should include both potential culprit agents as well as drugs that alter their elimination. All drugs may be discontinued at once or, if this is not practical, discontinued one at a time, starting with the ones most suspect, and the patient observed for signs of improvement. The time needed for a concentration-dependent adverse effect to disappear depends on the time required for the concentration to fall below the range associated with the adverse effect; that, in turn, depends on the initial blood level and on the rate of elimination or metabolism of the drug. Adverse effects of drugs with long half-lives or those not directly related to serum concentration may take a considerable time to disappear.

SUMMARY

Modern clinical pharmacology aims to replace empiricism in the use of drugs with therapy based on in-depth understanding of factors that determine an individual's response to drug treatment. Molecular pharmacology, pharmacokinetics, genetics, clinical trials, and the educated prescriber all contribute to this process. No drug response should ever be termed *idiosyncratic*; all responses have a mechanism whose understanding will help guide further therapy with that drug or successors. This rapidly expanding understanding of variability in drug actions makes the process of prescribing drugs increasingly daunting for the practitioner. However, fundamental principles should guide this process:

- The benefits of drug therapy, however defined, should always outweigh the risk.

- The smallest dosage necessary to produce the desired effect should be used.
- The number of medications and doses per day should be minimized.
- Although the literature is rapidly expanding, accessing it is becoming easier; tools such as computers and hand-held devices to search databases of literature and unbiased opinion will become increasingly commonplace.
- Genetics play a role in determining variability in drug response and may become a part of clinical practice.
- Prescribers should be particularly wary when adding or stopping specific drugs that are especially liable to provoke interactions and adverse reactions.
- Prescribers should use only a limited number of drugs, with which they are thoroughly familiar.

FURTHER READINGS

BAILEY DG, DRESSER GK: Interactions between grapefruit juice and cardiovascular drugs. Am J Cardiovasc Drugs 4:281, 2004

CHASMAN DI et al: Pharmacogenetic study of statin therapy and cholesterol reduction. JAMA 291:2821, 2004

EICHELBAUM M et al: Pharmacogenomics and individualized drug therapy. Annu Rev Med 57:119, 2006

GURWITZ JH: Serious adverse drug effects—Seeing the trees through the forest. N Engl J Med 354:1413, 2006

HAKONARSON H et al: Effects of a 5-lipoxygenase-activating protein inhibitor on biomarkers associated with risk of myocardial infarction: a randomized trial. JAMA 293:2245, 2005

JOHNSON JA, TURNER ST: Hypertension pharmacogenomics: Current status and future directions. Curr Opin Mol Ther 7:218, 2005

KIM RB: Transporters and drug discovery: Why, when, and how. Mol Pharm 3:26, 2006

LIGGETT SB et al: A polymorphism within a conserved β_1-adrenergic receptor motif alters cardiac function and β-blocker response in human heart failure. Proc Natl Acad Sci USA 103:11288–11293, 2006

NAVARRO VJ, SENIOR JR: Drug-related hepatotoxicity. N Engl J Med 354:731, 2006

PIRMOHAMED M et al: Adverse drug reactions as cause of admission to hospital: Prospective analysis of 18,820 patients. Br Med J 329:15, 2004

RIEDER MJ et al: Effect of VKORC1 haplotypes on transcriptional regulation and warfarin dose. N Engl J Med 352:2285, 2005

RODEN DM: Drug-induced prolongation of the QT Interval. N Engl J Med 350:1013, 2004

———— et al: Pharmacogenomics: challenges and opportunities. Ann Intern Med, 145:745, 2006

SHU Y et al: Evolutionary conservation predicts function of variants of the human organic cation transporter, OCT1. Proc Natl Acad Sci USA 100:5902, 2003

WEISS ST et al: Asthma steroid pharmacogenetics: A study strategy to identify replicated treatment responses. Proc Am Thorac Soc 1:364, 2004

6 Women's Health
Andrea Dunaif

The study of biologic differences between sexes has emerged as a distinct scientific discipline. A report from the Institute of Medicine (IOM) found that sex has a broad impact on biologic and disease processes and succinctly concluded: sex matters. The National Institutes of Health established the Office of Research on Women's Health in 1990 to develop an agenda for future research in the field. In parallel, women's health has become a distinct clinical discipline with a focus on disorders that are disproportionately represented in women. The

integration of women's health into internal medicine and other specialties has been accompanied by novel approaches to health care delivery, including greater attention to patient education and involvement in disease prevention and medical decision-making.

The IOM report recommended the term *sex difference* to describe biologic processes that differ between males and females and *gender difference* for features related to social influences. Disorders highlighted here are reviewed in detail in other chapters.

DISEASE RISK: REALITY AND PERCEPTION

The leading causes of death are the same in women and men: (1) heart disease, (2) cancer, and (3) cerebrovascular disease (Table 6-1; Fig.

TABLE 6-1 **DEATHS AND PERCENT OF TOTAL DEATHS FOR THE 15 LEADING CAUSES OF DEATH BY SEX IN THE UNITED STATES, 2003**

Cause of Death	Women Rank	Women Deaths	Women Total Deaths, %	Men Rank	Men Deaths	Men Total Deaths, %
Diseases of heart	1	348,994	28.0	1	336,095	28.0
Malignant neoplasms	2	268,912	21.6	2	287,990	24.0
Cerebrovascular diseases	3	96,263	7.7	4	61,426	5.1
Chronic lower respiratory diseases	4	65,668	5.3	5	60,714	5.1
Alzheimer's disease	5	45,122	3.6	10	18,335	1.5
Diabetes mellitus	6	38,781	3.1	6	35,438	2.9
Accidents	7	38,745	3.1	3	70,532	5.9
Influenza, pneumonia	8	36,385	2.9	7	28,778	2.4
Nephritis, nephrotic syndrome, nephrosis	9	21,972	1.8	9	20,481	1.7
Septicemia	10	19,082	1.5	12	14,987	1.2
Essential (primary) hypertension, hypertensive renal disease	11	13,727	1.1	15	8,213	0.7
Chronic liver disease, cirrhosis	12	9,591	0.8	11	17,912	1.5
Parkinson's disease	13	7,817	0.6	14	10,180	0.8
Intentional self-harm (suicide)	14	6,281	0.5	8	25,203	2.1
Assault (homicide)	15	3,850	0.3	13	13,882	1.2

Source: Data from Centers for Disease Control and Prevention: National Vital Statistics Reports, Vol. 54, No. 13, April 19, 2006, Table 12, http://www.cdc.gov/nchs/data/nvsr/nvsr54/nvsr54_13.pdf.

6-1). The leading cause of cancer death, lung cancer, is the same in both sexes, with higher mortality rates than breast, colon, and prostate cancer combined. Breast cancer is the second leading cause of cancer death in women, but it causes about 60% fewer deaths than lung cancer. Men are substantially more likely to die from suicide, homicide, and accidents than women.

Women's risk for many diseases increases at menopause, which occurs at a median age of 51.4 years. In the industrialized world, women spend one-third of their lives in the postmenopausal period. Estrogen levels fall abruptly at menopause, inducing a variety of physiologic and metabolic responses. Rates of cardiovascular disease increase and bone density begins to decrease rapidly after menopause. In the United States, women live on average about 5 years longer than men, with a life expectancy at birth in 2004 of 80.4 years, compared to 75.2 years in men. Elderly women outnumber elderly men, so that age-related conditions, such as hypertension, have a female preponderance. However, the difference in life expectancy between men and women has decreased an average of 0.1 year every year since 1980, and, if this convergence in mortality figures continues, it is projected that mortality rates will be similar by 2054.

Women's perception of disease risk is often inaccurate. Public awareness campaigns have resulted in almost 50% of U.S. women knowing that cardiovascular disease is the leading cause of death in women. Nevertheless, the condition they fear most is breast cancer, despite the fact that death rates from breast cancer have been falling since the 1990s. In any given decade of life, a woman's risk for breast cancer never exceeds 1 in 34. Although a woman's lifetime risk of developing breast cancer if she lives past 85 years is about 1 in 9, it is much more likely that she will die from cardiovascular disease than from breast cancer. In other words, many elderly women have breast cancer but die from other causes. Similarly, a minority of women are aware that lung cancer is the leading cause of cancer death in women. These misconceptions are unfortunate as they perpetuate inadequate attention to modifiable risk factors, such as dyslipidemia, hypertension, and cigarette smoking.

Physicians are also less likely to recognize women's risk for cardiovascular disease. A survey of physicians in 2004 found that women with intermediate risk for cardiovascular disease, according to Framingham risk score, were significantly more likely to be assigned to a lower risk category than men with similar risk profiles. Moreover, when presented with actors portraying patients with chest pain, physicians' estimates

for probability of coronary heart disease (CHD) were significantly lower for women than for men and lower for black women than for white women. These perceptions on the part of both the patient and her physician lead to important differences in cardiac care.

SEX DIFFERENCES IN HEALTH AND DISEASE

ALZHEIMER'S DISEASE

(See also Chap. 365) Alzheimer's disease (AD) affects approximately twice as many women as men. Because the risk for AD increases with age, part of this sex difference is accounted for by the fact that women live longer than men. However, additional factors likely contribute to the increased risk for AD in women, including sex differences in brain size, structure, and functional organization. There is emerging evidence for sex-specific differences in gene expression, not only for genes on the X and Y chromosomes but also for some autosomal genes. Estrogens have pleiotropic genomic and nongenomic effects on the central nervous system, including neurotrophic actions in key areas involved in cognition and memory. Women with AD have lower endogenous estrogen levels compared to women without AD. These observations have led to the hypothesis that estrogen is neuroprotective.

Some studies have suggested that estrogen administration improves cognitive function in nondemented postmenopausal women as well as in women with AD, and several observational studies have suggested that postmenopausal hormone therapy (PHT) may decrease the risk of AD. However, recent placebo-controlled trials have found no improvement in disease progression or cognitive function after up to 15 months of PHT in women with AD. Further, the Women's Health Initiative Memory Study (WHIMS), an ancillary study in the Women's Health Initiative (WHI), found no benefit compared to placebo of estrogen alone [combined continuous equine estrogen (CEE), 0.625 mg qd] or estrogen with progestin [CEE, 0.625 mg qd, and medroxyprogesterone acetate (MPA), 2.5 mg qd] on cognitive function or the development of dementia in women 65 years and older. Indeed, there was a significantly increased risk for both dementia and mild cognitive impairment in women receiving hormone therapy. The possible explanations for the discrepant results between the observational studies and the randomized clinical trials remain unclear (Chap. 342).

CORONARY HEART DISEASE

(See also Chap. 237) There are major sex differences in CHD, the leading cause of death in men and women in developed countries. CHD death rates have been falling in men over the past 30 years, but they have been increasing in women. Since 1984, more women than men have died of cardiovascular disease. Gonadal steroids have major effects on the cardiovascular system and lipid metabolism. Estrogen increases high-density lipoprotein (HDL) and lowers low-density lipoprotein (LDL), whereas androgens have the opposite effect. Estrogen has direct vasodilatory effects on the vascular endothelium, enhances insulin sensitivity, and has antioxidant properties. There is a striking increase in CHD after both natural and surgical menopause suggesting that endogenous estrogens are cardioprotective. Women also have longer QT intervals on electrocardiograms, which increases their susceptibility to certain arrhythmias. Animal studies suggest that the sex difference in QT interval duration is caused by sex steroid effects on cardiac repolarization, in part related to their effects on cardiac voltage-gated potassium channels; there is a lower density of the

FIGURE 6-1 Death rates per 100,000 population for 2003 by 5-year age groups in U.S. women. Note that the scale of the y-axis is increased by tenfold in the graph on the right compared to that on the left. Accidents and HIV/AIDS are the leading causes of death in young women 20–34 years of age. Accidents, breast cancer, and ischemic heart disease (IHD) are the leading causes of death in women 35–44 years of age. Breast cancer is the leading cause of death in women 45–49 years of age, and IHD

becomes the leading cause of death in women beginning at 50 years of age. In older women, IHD remains the leading cause of death, cerebrovascular disease becomes the second leading cause of death, and lung cancer is the leading cause of cancer-related deaths. AD, Alzheimer's disease; Ca, cancer; CLRD, chronic lower respiratory disease; DM, diabetes mellitus. *(Data adapted from Centers for Disease Control and Prevention, www.cdc.gov/nchs/data/statab/Mortfinal2003_worktable210r.pdf.)*

rapid component (I_{Kr}) of the delayed rectifier potassium current (I_K) in females.

CHD presents differently in women, who are usually 10–15 years older than their male counterparts and are more likely to have comorbidities such as hypertension, congestive heart failure, and diabetes mellitus (DM). In the Framingham study, angina was the most frequent initial symptom of CHD in women, whereas myocardial infarction was the most frequent initial presentation in men. Women more often have atypical symptoms, such as nausea, vomiting, indigestion, and upper back pain.

Women with myocardial infarction are more likely to present with cardiac arrest or cardiogenic shock, whereas men are more likely to present with ventricular tachycardia. Further, younger women with myocardial infarction are more likely to die than men of similar age, with women under 50 experiencing twice the mortality rate of men, even after adjustment for differences in disease severity and management. Indeed, the younger the woman, the greater the risk of death from myocardial infarction compared to men (Fig. 6-2).

Physicians are less likely to suspect heart disease in women with chest pain and less likely to perform diagnostic and therapeutic cardiac procedures in women. In addition, there are sex differences in the accuracy of certain diagnostic procedures. The exercise electrocardiogram has substantial false-positive as well as false-negative rates in women compared to men. Women are less likely to receive therapies such as angioplasty, thrombolytic therapy, coronary artery bypass grafts (CABGs), beta blockers, or aspirin. There are also sex differences in outcomes when women with CHD do receive therapeutic interventions. Women undergoing CABG surgery have more advanced disease, a higher perioperative mortality rate, less relief of angina, and less graft patency; however, 5- and 10-year survival rates are similar. Women undergoing percutaneous transluminal coronary angioplasty have lower rates of initial angiographic and clinical success than men, but they also have a lower rate of restenosis and a better long-term outcome. Women may benefit less and have more frequent serious bleeding complications from thrombolytic therapy than do men. Factors such as older age, more comorbid conditions, and more severe CHD in women at the time of events or procedures appear to account in part for the observed sex differences.

Elevated cholesterol levels, hypertension, smoking, obesity, low HDL cholesterol levels, DM, and lack of physical activity are important risk factors for CHD in both men and women. Total triglyceride levels are an independent risk factor for CHD in women but not in men. Low HDL cholesterol and DM are more important risk factors for CHD in women than in men. Smoking is an important risk factor for CHD in women—it accelerates atherosclerosis, exerts direct negative effects on cardiac function, and is associated with an earlier age of menopause. Cholesterol-lowering drugs are equally effective in men and women for primary and secondary prevention of CHD. However, because of perceptions that women are at lower risk for CHD, they receive fewer interventions for modifiable risk factors than do men. In contrast to men, randomized

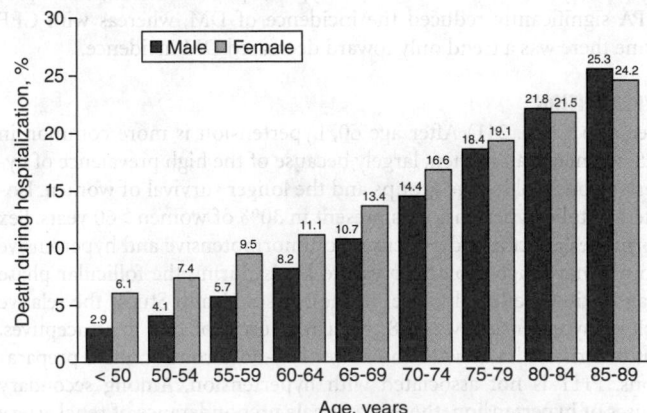

FIGURE 6-2 Rates of death during hospitalization for myocardial infarction among women and men according to age. The overall mortality rate during hospitalization was 16.7% among women and 11.5% among men but was twice the rate in women <50 years compared to men in the same age range. The interaction between sex and age was significant ($p <.001$). *(From V Vaccarino et al: N Engl J Med 341:217, 1999; with permission.)*

trials have shown that aspirin was not effective in the primary prevention of CHD in women; it did significantly reduce the risk of ischemic stroke. Secondary prevention in women with known CHD is also suboptimal. At baseline, only about 30% of women enrolled in the Heart and Estrogen/progestin Replacement Study (HERS), a secondary prevention trial in women with established CHD, were taking beta blockers, and only 45% received lipid-lowering medications.

The sex differences in CHD prevalence, beneficial biologic effects of estradiol on the cardiovascular system, and reduced risk for CHD in observational studies of women receiving PHT led to the widespread use of PHT for the prevention of CHD. However, the WHI, which studied more than 16,000 women on CEE plus MPA or placebo and more than 10,000 women with hysterectomy on CEE alone or placebo, did not demonstrate a benefit of PHT for the primary or secondary prevention of CHD. In addition, CEE plus MPA was associated with an increased risk for CHD, particularly in the first year of therapy, whereas CEE alone neither increased nor decreased CHD risk. There was no evidence for cardioprotective effects of estrogens in smaller randomized trials that used either oral or transdermal estradiol, arguing against the hypothesis that the type of estrogen or its route of administration accounted for the lack of CHD risk reduction. In the WHI, there was a suggestion of a reduction in CHD risk in women ages 50–59 at baseline who received CEE alone. This finding suggests that the time at which PHT is initiated is critical for cardioprotection and is consistent with the "timing hypothesis." According to this hypothesis, PHT has differential effects depending on the stage of atherosclerosis; adverse effects are seen with advanced, unstable lesions. This hypothesis is currently under investigation in randomized clinical trials. **PHT is discussed further in Chap. 342.**

DIABETES MELLITUS

(See also Chap. 338) Women are more sensitive to insulin than men. Despite this, the prevalence of type 2 DM is similar in men and women. There is a sex difference in the relationship between endogenous androgen levels and DM risk: higher bioavailable testosterone levels are associated with increased risk in women, whereas lower bioavailable testosterone levels are associated with increased risk in men. Polycystic ovary syndrome and gestational DM—common conditions in premenopausal women—are associated with a significantly increased risk for type 2 DM. Premenopausal women with DM lose the cardioprotective effect of female sex and have identical rates of CHD to those in males. These women have impaired endothelial function and reduced coronary vasodilatory responses, which may predispose to cardiovascular complications. In individuals with DM, women have a greater risk for myocardial infarction than men. Women with DM are more likely to have left ventricular hypertrophy. In the WHI, CEE plus MPA significantly reduced the incidence of DM, whereas with CEE alone there was a trend only toward decreased DM incidence.

HYPERTENSION

(See also Chap. 241) After age 60, hypertension is more common in U.S. women than in men, largely because of the high prevalence of hypertension in older age groups and the longer survival of women. Isolated systolic hypertension is present in 30% of women >60 years. Sex hormones affect blood pressure. Both normotensive and hypertensive women have higher blood pressure levels during the follicular phase than during the luteal phase. In the Nurses Health Study, the relative risk of hypertension was 1.8 in current users of oral contraceptives, but this risk is lower with the newer low-dose contraceptive preparations. PHT is not associated with hypertension. Among secondary causes of hypertension, there is a female preponderance of renal artery fibromuscular dysplasia.

The benefits of treatment for hypertension have been dramatic in both women and men. In a meta-analysis of the effects of hypertension treatment, the Individual Data Analysis of Antihypertensive Intervention Trial found a reduction of risk for stroke and for major cardiovascular events in women. The effectiveness of various antihypertensive drugs appears to be comparable in women and men; however, women

may experience more side effects. For example, women are more likely to develop cough with angiotensin-converting enzyme inhibitors.

AUTOIMMUNE DISORDERS

(See also Chap. 312) Most autoimmune disorders occur more commonly in women than in men; these include autoimmune thyroid and liver diseases, lupus, rheumatoid arthritis (RA), scleroderma, multiple sclerosis (MS), and idiopathic thrombocytopenic purpura. However, there is no sex difference in the incidence of type 1 DM, and ankylosing spondylitis occurs more commonly in men. There are relatively few differences in bacterial disease infection rates in men and women. In general, sex differences in viral diseases can be accounted for by differences in behaviors, such as exposures or rates of immunization. Sex differences in both immune responses and adverse reactions to vaccines have been reported. For example, there is a female preponderance of postvaccination arthritis.

The mechanisms for these sex differences remain obscure. Adaptive immune responses are more robust in women than in men, which may be explained by the stimulatory actions of estrogens and the inhibitory actions of androgens on the cellular mediators of immunity. Consistent with an important role for gonadal hormones, there is variation in immune responses during the menstrual cycle, and the activity of certain autoimmune disorders is altered by castration or pregnancy (e.g., RA and MS may remit during pregnancy). Nevertheless, the majority of studies show that exogenous estrogens and progestins in the form of PHT or oral contraceptives do not alter autoimmune disease incidence or activity. Exposure to fetal antigens, including circulating fetal cells that persist in certain tissues, has been speculated to increase the risk of autoimmune responses. There is clearly an important genetic component to autoimmunity, as indicated by the familial clustering and HLA association of many such disorders. However, HLA types are not sexually dimorphic.

HIV INFECTION

(See also Chap. 182) Women account for almost 50% of the 40 million persons infected with HIV-1 worldwide. AIDS is an important cause of death in younger women (Fig. 6-1). Heterosexual contact with an at-risk partner is the fastest-growing transmission category, and women are more susceptible to HIV infection than men. This increased susceptibility is in part accounted for by an increased prevalence of sexually transmitted diseases in women. Some studies have suggested that hormonal contraceptives may increase the risk of HIV transmission. Progesterone has been shown to increase susceptibility to infection in nonhuman primate models of HIV. Women are also more likely to be infected by multiple variants of the virus than men. Women with HIV have more rapid decreases in their CD4 cell counts than men. Compared with men, HIV-infected women more frequently develop candidiasis, but Kaposi's sarcoma is less common than in men.

Other sexually transmitted diseases, such as chlamydial infection and gonorrhea, are important causes of infertility in women, and papilloma virus infection predisposes to cervical cancer.

OBESITY

(See also Chap. 75) The prevalence of obesity is higher in women than in men. However, according to a recent study by the Agency for Healthcare Research and Quality, >80% of patients undergoing bariatric surgery are women. Pregnancy and menopause are risk factors for obesity. There are major sex differences in body fat distribution. Women characteristically have gluteal and femoral or gynoid pattern of fat distribution, whereas men typically have a central or android pattern. Gonadal steroids appear to be the major regulators of fat distribution through a number of direct effects on adipose tissue. Studies in humans also suggest that gonadal steroids play a role in modulating food intake and energy expenditure.

In men and women, upper-body obesity characterized by increased visceral fat is associated with an increased risk for cardiovascular disease and DM. In women, endogenous androgen levels are positively associated with upper-body obesity, and androgen administration increases visceral fat. In contrast, there is an inverse relationship between endogenous androgen levels and central obesity in men. Further, androgen administration decreases visceral fat in centrally obese men. The reasons for these sex differences in the relationship between visceral fat and androgens are unknown. Obesity increases a woman's risk for certain cancers, in particular postmenopausal breast and endometrial cancer, in part because adipose tissue provides an extragonadal source of estrogen through aromatization of circulating adrenal and ovarian androgens, especially the conversion of androstenedione to estrone. Obesity increases the risk of infertility, miscarriage, and complications of pregnancy.

OSTEOPOROSIS

(See also Chap. 348) Osteoporosis is about five times more common in postmenopausal women than in age-matched men, and osteoporotic hip fractures are a major cause of morbidity in elderly women. Men accumulate more bone mass and lose bone more slowly than women. Sex differences in bone mass are found as early as infancy. Calcium intake, vitamin D, and estrogen all play important roles in bone formation and bone loss. Particularly during adolescence, calcium intake is an important determinant of peak bone mass. Vitamin D deficiency is surprisingly common in elderly women, occurring in >40% of women living in northern latitudes. Receptors for estrogens and androgens have been identified in bone. Estrogen deficiency is associated with increased osteoclast activity and a decreased number of bone-forming units, leading to net bone loss. The aromatase enzyme, which converts androgens to estrogens, is also present in bone. Recent studies show that estrogen is an important determinant of bone mass in men (derived from the aromatization of androgens) as well as in women.

PHARMACOLOGY

On average, women have lower body weights, smaller organs, higher percent body fat, and lower total-body water than men. There are also important sex differences in drug action and metabolism that are not accounted for by these differences in body size and composition. Gonadal steroids alter the binding and metabolism of a number of drugs. Further, menstrual cycle phase and pregnancy can alter drug action. Two-thirds of cases of drug-induced torsades des pointes, a rare, life-threatening ventricular arrhythmia, occur in women because they have a longer, more vulnerable QT interval. These drugs, which include certain antihistamines, antibiotics, antiarrhythmics, and antipsychotics, can prolong cardiac repolarization by blocking cardiac voltage-gated potassium channels, particularly I_{Kr}. Women require lower doses of neuroleptics to control schizophrenia. Women awaken from anesthesia faster than men given the same doses of anesthetics. Women also take more medications than men, including over-the-counter formulations and supplements. The greater use of medications combined with these biologic differences may account for the reported higher frequency of adverse drug reactions in women than in men.

PSYCHOLOGICAL DISORDERS

(See also Chap. 386) Depression, anxiety, and affective and eating disorders (bulimia and anorexia nervosa) are more common in women than in men. Epidemiologic studies from both developed and developing nations consistently find major depression to be twice as common in women as in men, with the sex difference becoming evident in early adolescence. Depression occurs in 10% of women during pregnancy and in 10–15% of women during the postpartum period. There is a high likelihood of recurrence of postpartum depression with subsequent pregnancies. The incidence of major depression diminishes after age 45 years and does not increase with the onset of menopause. Depression in women appears to have a worse prognosis than in men; episodes last longer, and there is a lower rate of spontaneous remission. Schizophrenia and bipolar disorders occur at equal rates in men and women, although there may be sex differences in symptoms.

Both biologic and social factors account for the greater prevalence of depressive disorders in women. Men have higher levels of the neurotransmitter serotonin. Gonadal steroids also affect mood, and fluctuations during the menstrual cycle have been linked to symptoms of premenstrual syndrome. Sex hormones differentially affect the hypothalamic-pituitary-adrenal responses to stress. Testosterone appears to blunt cortisol responses to corticotropin-releasing hormone. Both low and high levels of estrogen can activate the hypothalamic-pituitary-adrenal axis.

SLEEP DISORDERS

(See also Chap. 28) There are striking sex differences in sleep and its disorders. During sleep, women have an increased amount of slow-wave activity, differences in timing of delta activity, and an increase in the number of sleep spindles. Testosterone modulates neural control of breathing and upper airway mechanics. Men have a higher prevalence of sleep apnea. Testosterone administration to hypogonadal men as well as to women increases apneic episodes during sleep. Women with the hyperandrogenic disorder polycystic ovary syndrome have an increased prevalence of obstructive sleep apnea, and apneic episodes are positively correlated with their circulating testosterone levels. In contrast, progesterone accelerates breathing, and, in the past, progestins were used for treatment of sleep apnea.

SUBSTANCE ABUSE AND TOBACCO

(See also Chaps. 387 and 390) Substance abuse is more common in men than in women. However, one-third of Americans who suffer from alcoholism are women. Women alcoholics are less likely to be diagnosed than men. A greater proportion of men than women seek help for alcohol and drug abuse. Men are more likely to go to an alcohol or drug treatment facility, while women tend to approach a primary care physician or mental health professional for help under the guise of a psychosocial problem. Late-life alcoholism is more common in women than men. On average, alcoholic women drink less than alcoholic men but exhibit the same degree of impairment. Blood alcohol levels are higher in women than in men after drinking equivalent amounts of alcohol, adjusted for body weight. This greater bioavailability of alcohol in women is due to both the smaller volume of distribution and the slower gastric metabolism of alcohol secondary to lower activity of gastric alcohol dehydrogenase than is the case in men. In addition, alcoholic women are more likely to abuse tranquilizers, sedatives, and amphetamines. Women alcoholics have a higher mortality rate than do nonalcoholic women and alcoholic men. Women also appear to develop alcoholic liver disease and other alcohol-related diseases with shorter drinking histories and lower levels of alcohol consumption. Alcohol abuse also poses special risks to a woman, adversely affecting fertility and the health of the baby (fetal alcohol syndrome). Even moderate alcohol use increases the risk of breast cancer, hypertension, and stroke in women.

More men than women smoke tobacco, but the prevalence of smoking is declining faster in men than in women. Smoking markedly increases the risk of cardiovascular disease in premenopausal women and is also associated with a decrease in the age of menopause. Women who smoke are more likely to develop chronic obstructive pulmonary disease and lung cancer than men and at lower levels of tobacco exposure.

VIOLENCE AGAINST WOMEN

Domestic violence is the most common cause of physical injury in women, exceeding the combined incidence of all other types of injury (such as from rape, mugging, and auto accidents). Sexual assault is one of the most common crimes against women. One in five adult women in the United States reports having experienced sexual assault during her lifetime. Adult women are much more likely to be raped by a spouse, ex-spouse, or acquaintance than by a stranger. Domestic violence may be an unrecognized feature of certain clinical presentations such as chronic abdominal pain, headaches, substance abuse, and eating disorders, in addition to more obvious manifestations such as trauma.

SUMMARY

Women's health is now a mature discipline, and the importance of sex differences in biologic processes is well-recognized. It is clear that understanding the mechanisms of these differences will have an impact on both women's and men's health. For example, estrogen is now recognized as an important regulator of bone density in men as well as in women. Elucidating the biology of sex hormone action has resulted in the design of drugs with tissue-specific hormone agonist and antagonist effects. These discoveries will make it feasible to selectively modulate the actions of sex hormones in both women and men to prevent and treat disease.

FURTHER READINGS

Hsia J et al: Conjugated equine estrogens and coronary heart disease: The Women's Health Initiative. Arch Intern Med 166:357, 2006

Mendelsohn ME, Karas RH: Molecular and cellular basis of cardiovascular gender differences. Science 308:1583, 2005

Mosca L et al: National Study of Physician Awareness and Adherence to Cardiovascular Disease Prevention Guidelines. Circulation 111:499, 2005

Ridker PM et al: A randomized trial of low-dose aspirin in the primary prevention of cardiovascular disease in women. N Engl J Med 352:1293, 2005

Special Section Women's Health. Science 308:1569, 2005

Turgeon JL et al: Hormone therapy: Physiological complexity belies therapeutic simplicity. Science 304:1269, 2004

Wizemann TM, Pardue M-L (eds): *Exploring the Biological Contributions to Human Health: Does Sex Matter?* Washington, DC, National Academy of Sciences, 2001

7 Medical Disorders during Pregnancy
Robert L. Barbieri, John T. Repke

Approximately 4 million births occur in the United States each year. A significant proportion of these are complicated by one or more medical disorders. Three decades ago, many medical disorders were contraindications to pregnancy. Advances in obstetrics, neonatology, obstetric anesthesiology, and medicine have increased the expectation that pregnancy will result in an excellent outcome for both mother and fetus despite most of these conditions. Successful pregnancy requires important physiologic adaptations, such as a marked increase in cardiac output. Medical problems that interfere with the physiologic adaptations of pregnancy increase the risk for poor pregnancy outcome; conversely, in some instances pregnancy may adversely impact an underlying medical disorder.

HYPERTENSION (See also Chap. 241)

In pregnancy, cardiac output increases by 40%, most of which is due to an increase in stroke volume. Heart rate increases by ~10 beats/min during the third trimester. In the second trimester of pregnancy, systemic vascular resistance decreases and this is associated with a fall in blood pressure. During pregnancy, a blood pressure of 140/90 mmHg is considered to be abnormally elevated and is associated with an increase in perinatal morbidity and mortality. In all pregnant women, the measurement of blood pressure should be performed in the sitting position, because for many the lateral recumbent position is associated with a blood pressure lower than that recorded in the sitting position. The diagnosis of hypertension requires the measurement of two elevated blood pressures, at least 6 h apart. Hypertension during pregnancy is usually caused by preeclampsia, chronic hypertension, gestational hypertension, or renal disease.

PREECLAMPSIA

Approximately 5–7% of all pregnant women develop *preeclampsia*, the new onset of hypertension (blood pressure >140/90 mmHg) and proteinuria (>300 mg/24 h) after 20 weeks of gestation. Although the precise placental factors that cause preeclampsia are unknown, the end result is vasospasm and endothelial injury in multiple organs. Excessive placental secretion of a soluble fms-like tyrosine kinase 1, a naturally occurring vascular endothelial growth factor antagonist, and decreased secretion of placental growth factor may contribute to the endothelial dysfunction, hypertension, and proteinuria observed in preeclampsia. Glomerular endothelial cells demonstrate swelling and encroach on the vascular lumen. Preeclampsia is associated with abnormalities of cerebral circulatory autoregulation, which increase the risk of stroke at near-normal blood pressures. Risk factors for the development of preeclampsia include nulliparity, diabetes mellitus, a history of renal disease or chronic hypertension, a prior history of preeclampsia, extremes of maternal age (>35 years or <15 years), obesity, factor V Leiden mutation, angiotensinogen gene T235, G20210A prothrombin gene mutation, antiphospholipid antibody syndrome, and multiple gestation.

Severe preeclampsia is the presence of new-onset hypertension and proteinuria accompanied by central nervous system (CNS) dysfunction (headaches, blurred vision, seizures, coma), marked elevations of blood pressure (>160/110 mmHg), severe proteinuria (>5 g/24 h), oliguria or renal failure, pulmonary edema, hepatocellular injury (ALT > 2 × the upper limits of normal), thrombocytopenia (platelet count < 100,000/L), or disseminated intravascular coagulation. Women with *mild preeclampsia* are those with the diagnosis of new-onset hypertension, proteinuria, and edema without evidence of severe preeclampsia. The HELLP (hemolysis, elevated liver enzymes, low platelets) syndrome is a special subgroup of severe preeclampsia and is a major cause of morbidity and mortality in this disease. The presence of platelet dysfunction and coagulation disorders further increases the risk of stroke.

℞ PREECLAMPSIA

Preeclampsia resolves within a few weeks after delivery. For pregnant women with preeclampsia prior to 37 weeks' gestation, delivery reduces the mother's morbidity but exposes the fetus to the risk of premature delivery. The management of preeclampsia is challenging because it requires the clinician to balance the health of both mother and fetus simultaneously and to make management decisions that afford both the best opportunities for infant survival. In general, prior to term, women with *mild* preeclampsia can be managed conservatively with bed rest, close monitoring of blood pressure and renal function, and careful fetal surveillance. For women with *severe* preeclampsia, delivery is recommended unless the patient is eligible for expectant management in a tertiary hospital setting. Expectant management of severe preeclampsia remote from term affords some benefits for the fetus with significant risks for the mother.

The definitive treatment of preeclampsia is delivery of the fetus and placenta. For women with severe preeclampsia, aggressive management of blood pressures > 160/110 mmHg reduces the risk of cerebrovascular accidents. Intravenous labetalol or hydralazine are the drugs most commonly used to manage preeclampsia. Intravenous hydralazine may be associated with more episodes of maternal hypotension than labetalol. Alternative agents such as calcium channel blockers may be used. Elevated arterial pressure should be reduced slowly to avoid hypotension and a decrease in blood flow to the fetus. *Angiotensin-converting enzyme (ACE) inhibitors as well as angiotensin-receptor blockers should be avoided in the second and third trimesters of pregnancy because of their adverse effects on fetal development.* Pregnant women treated with ACE inhibitors often develop oligohydramnios, which may be caused by decreased fetal renal function.

Magnesium sulfate is the treatment of choice for the prevention and treatment of eclamptic seizures. Two large randomized clinical trials have demonstrated the superiority of magnesium sulfate over phenytoin and diazepam, and a recent large randomized clinical trial has demonstrated the efficacy of magnesium sulfate in reducing the risk of seizure and possibly reducing the risk of maternal death. Magnesium may prevent seizures by interacting with N-methyl-D-aspartate (NMDA) receptors in the CNS. Given the difficulty of predicting eclamptic seizures on the basis of disease severity, it is recommended that once the decision to proceed with delivery is made, all patients carrying a diagnosis of preeclampsia be treated with magnesium sulfate (see **Regimens**, below).

REGIMENS FOR THE ADMINISTRATION OF MAGNESIUM SULFATE FOR SEIZURE PROPHYLAXIS IN WOMEN IN LABOR WITH PREECLAMPSIA

Intramuscular	Intravenous
10 g (5 g IM deep in each buttock)[a]	6-g bolus over 15 min
5 g IM deep q4h, alternating sides	1–3 g/h by continuous infusion pump
	May be mixed in 100 mL crystalloid; if given by intravenous push, make up as 20% solution; push at maximum rate of 1 g/min
	40-g MgSO₄·7H₂O in 1000 mL Ringers lactate; run at 25–75 mL/h (1–3 g/h)[a]

[a]Made up as 50% solution

CHRONIC ESSENTIAL HYPERTENSION

Pregnancy complicated by chronic essential hypertension is associated with intrauterine growth restriction and increased perinatal mortality. Pregnant women with chronic hypertension are at increased risk for superimposed preeclampsia and abruptio placenta. Women with chronic hypertension should have a thorough prepregnancy evaluation, both to identify remediable causes of hypertension and to ensure that the prescribed antihypertensive agents are not associated with an adverse outcome of pregnancy (e.g., ACE inhibitors, angiotensin-receptor blockers). α-Methyldopa, labetalol, and nifedipine are the most commonly used medications for the treatment of chronic hypertension in pregnancy. Baseline evaluation of renal function is necessary to help differentiate the effects of chronic hypertension versus superimposed preeclampsia should the hypertension worsen during pregnancy. There are no convincing data that demonstrate that treatment of mild chronic hypertension improves perinatal outcome.

GESTATIONAL HYPERTENSION

This is the development of elevated blood pressure during pregnancy or in the first 24 h post partum in the absence of preexisting chronic hypertension and other signs of preeclampsia. Uncomplicated gestational hypertension that does not progress to preeclampsia has not been associated with adverse pregnancy outcome or adverse long-term prognosis.

RENAL DISEASE (See also Chaps. 272 and 280)

Normal pregnancy is characterized by an increase in glomerular filtration rate and creatinine clearance. This occurs secondary to a rise in renal plasma flow and increased glomerular filtration pressures. Patients with underlying renal disease and hypertension may expect a worsening of hypertension during pregnancy. If superimposed preeclampsia develops, the additional endothelial injury results in a capillary leak syndrome that may make the management of these patients challenging. In general, patients with underlying renal disease and hypertension benefit from aggressive management of blood pressure. Preconception counseling is also essential for these patients so that accurate risk assessment can occur prior to the establishment of pregnancy and important medication changes and adjustments can be made. In general, a prepregnancy serum creatinine level <133 μmol/L (<1.5 mg/dL) is associated with a favorable prognosis. When renal disease worsens during pregnancy, close collaboration between the nephrologist and the maternal-fetal medicine specialist is essential so that decisions regarding delivery can be weighed in the context of sequelae of prematurity for the neonate versus long-term sequelae for the mother with respect to future renal function.

CARDIAC DISEASE

VALVULAR HEART DISEASE

(See also Chap. 230) This is the most common cardiac problem complicating pregnancy.

Mitral Stenosis This is the valvular disease most likely to cause death during pregnancy. The pregnancy-induced increase in blood volume, cardiac output, and tachycardia can increase the transmitral pressure gradient and cause pulmonary edema in women with mitral stenosis. Pregnancy associated with long-standing mitral stenosis may result in pulmonary hypertension. Sudden death has been reported when hypovolemia has been allowed to occur in this condition. Careful control of heart rate, especially during labor and delivery, minimizes the impact of tachycardia and reduced ventricular filling times on cardiac function. Pregnant women with mitral stenosis are at increased risk for the development of atrial fibrillation and other tachyarrhythmias. Medical management of severe mitral stenosis and atrial fibrillation with digoxin and beta blockers is recommended. Balloon valvulotomy can be carried out during pregnancy.

Mitral Regurgitation and Aortic Regurgitation and Stenosis These are generally well tolerated during pregnancy. The pregnancy-induced decrease in systemic vascular resistance reduces the risk of cardiac failure with these conditions. As a rule, mitral valve prolapse does not present problems for the pregnant patient, and aortic stenosis, unless very severe, is well tolerated. In the most severe cases of aortic stenosis, limitation of activity or balloon valvuloplasty may be indicated.

CONGENITAL HEART DISEASE

(See also Chap. 229) The presence of a congenital cardiac lesion in the mother increases the risk of congenital cardiac disease in the newborn. Prenatal screening of the fetus for congenital cardiac disease with ultrasound is recommended. Atrial or ventricular septal defect is usually well tolerated during pregnancy in the absence of pulmonary hypertension, provided that the woman's prepregnancy cardiac status is favorable. Use of air filters on IV sets during labor and delivery in patients with intracardiac shunts is generally recommended.

OTHER CARDIAC DISORDERS

Supraventricular tachycardia (Chap. 226) is a common cardiac complication of pregnancy. Treatment is the same as in the nonpregnant patient, and fetal tolerance of medications such as adenosine and calcium channel blockers is acceptable. When necessary, electrocardioversion may be performed and is generally well tolerated by mother and fetus.

Peripartum cardiomyopathy (Chap. 231) is an uncommon disorder of pregnancy associated with myocarditis, and its etiology remains unknown. Treatment is directed toward symptomatic relief and improvement of cardiac function. Many patients recover completely; others are left with a progressive dilated cardiomyopathy. Recurrence in a subsequent pregnancy has been reported, and women should be counseled to avoid pregnancy after a diagnosis of peripartum cardiomyopathy.

SPECIFIC HIGH-RISK CARDIAC LESIONS

Marfan Syndrome (See also Chap. 357) This is an autosomal dominant disease, associated with a high risk of maternal morbidity. Approximately 15% of pregnant women with Marfan syndrome develop a major cardiovascular manifestation during pregnancy, with almost all women surviving. An aortic root diameter <40 mm is considered to be associated with a favorable outcome of pregnancy. Prophylactic therapy with beta blockers has been advocated, although large-scale clinical trials in pregnancy have not been performed.

Pulmonary Hypertension (See also Chap. 244) Maternal mortality in the setting of severe pulmonary hypertension is high, and primary pulmonary hypertension is a contraindication to pregnancy. Termination of pregnancy may be advisable in these circumstances to preserve the life of the mother. In the Eisenmenger syndrome, i.e., the combination of pulmonary hypertension with right-to-left shunting due to congenital abnormalities (Chap. 229), maternal and fetal death occur frequently. Systemic hypotension may occur after blood loss, prolonged Valsalva maneuver, or regional anesthesia; sudden death secondary to hypotension is a dreaded complication. Management of these patients is challenging, and invasive hemodynamic monitoring during labor and delivery is generally recommended.

In patients with pulmonary hypertension, vaginal delivery is less stressful hemodynamically than cesarean section, which should be reserved for accepted obstetric indications.

DEEP VENOUS THROMBOSIS AND PULMONARY EMBOLISM (See also Chap. 256)

A hypercoagulable state is characteristic of pregnancy, and deep venous thrombosis (DVT) occurs in about 1 in 2000 pregnancies. Pulmonary embolism is one of the most common causes of maternal death in the United States. In pregnant women, DVT occurs much more commonly in the left leg than in the right leg, due to the compression of the left iliac vein by the iliac artery and the uterus. Activated protein C resistance caused by the factor V Leiden mutation increases the risk for DVT and pulmonary embolism during pregnancy. Approximately 25% of women with DVT during pregnancy carry the factor V Leiden allele. The presence of the factor V Leiden mutation also increases the risk for severe preeclampsia. Additional genetic mutations associated with DVT during pregnancy include the prothrombin G20210A mutation (heterozygotes and homozygotes) and the methylenetetrahydrofolate reductase C677T mutation (homozygotes).

℞ DEEP VENOUS THROMBOSIS

Aggressive diagnosis and management of DVT and suspected pulmonary embolism optimize the outcome for mother and fetus. In general, all diagnostic and therapeutic modalities afforded the nonpregnant patient should be utilized in pregnancy. Anticoagulant therapy with low-molecular-weight heparin (LMWH) or unfractionated heparin is indicated in pregnant women with DVT. LMWH may be associated with an increased risk of epidural hematoma in women receiving an epidural anesthetic in labor. One approach to this problem is to switch from LMWH to unfractionated heparin before the anticipated delivery date. Warfarin therapy is contraindicated in the first trimester due to its association with fetal chondrodysplasia punctata. In the second and third trimesters, warfarin may cause fetal optic atrophy and mental retardation. When DVT occurs in the postpartum period, LMWH therapy for 7–10 days may be followed by warfarin therapy for 3–6 months. Warfarin is not contraindicated in breast-feeding women.

ENDOCRINE DISORDERS

DIABETES MELLITUS

(See also Chap. 338) In pregnancy, the fetoplacental unit induces major metabolic changes, the purpose of which is to shunt glucose and amino acids to the fetus while the mother uses ketones and triglycerides to fuel her metabolic needs. These metabolic changes are accompanied by maternal insulin resistance, caused in part by placental production of steroids, a growth hormone variant, and placental lactogen. Although pregnancy has been referred to as a state of "accelerated starvation," it is better characterized as "accelerated ketosis." In pregnancy, after an overnight fast, plasma glucose is lower by 0.8–1.1 mmol/L (15–20 mg/dL) than in the nonpregnant state. This is due to the use of glucose by the fetus. In early pregnancy, fasting may result in circulating glucose concentrations in the range of 2.2 mmol/L (40 mg/dL) and may be associated with symptoms of hypoglycemia. In contrast to the decrease in maternal glucose concentration, plasma hydroxybutyrate and acetoacetate levels rise to two to four times normal after a fast.

℞ DIABETES MELLITUS IN PREGNANCY

Pregnancy complicated by diabetes mellitus is associated with higher maternal and perinatal morbidity and mortality rates. Preconception counseling and treatment are important for the diabetic patient contemplating pregnancy and can reduce the risk of congenital malformations and improve pregnancy outcome. Folate supplementation reduces the incidence of fetal neural tube defects, which occur with greater frequency in fetuses of diabetic mothers. In addition, optimizing glucose control during key pe-

riods of organogenesis reduces other congenital anomalies including sacral agenesis, caudal dysplasia, renal agenesis, and ventricular septal defect.

Once pregnancy is established, glucose control should be managed more aggressively than in the nonpregnant state. In addition to dietary changes, this requires more frequent blood glucose monitoring and often involves additional injections of insulin or conversion to an insulin pump. Fasting blood glucose levels should be maintained at <5.8 mmol/L (<105 mg/dL) with no values >7.8 mmol/L (140 mg/dL). Commencing in the third trimester, regular surveillance of maternal glucose control as well as assessment of fetal growth (obstetric sonography) and fetoplacental oxygenation (fetal heart rate monitoring or biophysical profile) optimizes pregnancy outcome. Pregnant diabetic patients without vascular disease are at greater risk for delivering a macrosomic fetus, and attention to fetal growth via clinical and ultrasound examinations is important. Fetal macrosomia is associated with an increased risk of maternal and fetal birth trauma. Pregnant women with diabetes have an increased risk of developing preeclampsia, and those with vascular disease are at greater risk for developing intrauterine growth restriction, which is associated with an increased risk of fetal and neonatal death. Excellent pregnancy outcomes in patients with diabetic nephropathy and proliferative retinopathy have been reported with aggressive glucose control and intensive maternal and fetal surveillance.

Glycemic control may become more difficult to achieve as pregnancy progresses due to an increase in insulin resistance. Because of delayed pulmonary maturation of the fetuses of diabetic mothers, early delivery should be avoided unless there is biochemical evidence of fetal lung maturity. In general, efforts to control glucose and maintain the pregnancy until the estimated date of delivery result in the best overall outcome for both mother and newborn.

GESTATIONAL DIABETES

All pregnant women should be screened for gestational diabetes unless they are in a low-risk group. Women at low risk for gestational diabetes are those <25 years of age; those with a body mass index < 25 kg/m^2, no maternal history of macrosomia or gestational diabetes, and no diabetes in a first-degree relative; and those not members of a high-risk ethnic group (African American, Hispanic, Native American). A typical two-step strategy for establishing the diagnosis of gestational diabetes involves administration of a 50-g oral glucose challenge with a single serum glucose measurement at 60 min. If the plasma glucose is <7.8 mmol/L (<140 mg/dL), the test is considered normal. Serum glucose > 7.8 mmol/L (>140 mg/dL) warrants administration of a 100-g oral glucose challenge with serum glucose measurements obtained in the fasting state, and at 1, 2, and 3 h. Normal values are plasma glucose concentrations <5.8 mmol/L (<105 mg/dL), 10.5 mmol/L (190 mg/dL), 9.1 mmol/L (165 mg/dL), and 8.0 mmol/L (145 mg/dL), respectively. Some centers have adopted more conservative criteria, using <7.5 mmol/L (<135 mg/dL) as the screening threshold, and values of <5.3 mmol/L (<95 mg/dL), <10 mmol/L (<180 mg/dL), <8.6 mmol/L (<155 mg/dL), and <7.8 mmol/L (<140 mg/dL) as the upper norms for a 3-h glucose tolerance test.

Pregnant women with gestational diabetes are at increased risk of preeclampsia, delivering infants who are large for their gestational age, and birth lacerations. Their fetuses are at risk of hypoglycemia and birth trauma (brachial plexus) injury.

℞ GESTATIONAL DIABETES

Treatment of gestational diabetes with a two-step strategy of dietary intervention followed by insulin injections if diet alone does not adequately control blood sugar [fasting glucose < 5.6 mmol/L (<100 mg/dL) and 2-h post-prandial <7.0 mmol/L (<126 mg/dL)] is associated with a decreased risk of birth trauma for the fetus. More recently the use of the oral hypoglycemic agent glyburide has become popular for managing gestational diabetes refractory to nutritional management. More data on the safety and efficacy of glyburide for the management of gestational diabetes are needed before it supplants insulin as the treatment agent of choice. For women with gestational diabetes, within the 10 years after the index pregnancy there is a 40% risk of being diagnosed with diabetes. All women with a history of gestational diabetes should be counseled about prevention strategies and evaluated regularly for diabetes.

THYROID DISEASE

(See also Chap. 335) In pregnancy, the estrogen-induced increase in thyroxine-binding globulin causes an increase in circulating levels of total T_3 and total T_4. The normal range of circulating levels of free T_4, free T_3, and thyroid-stimulating hormone (TSH) remain unaltered by pregnancy.

The thyroid gland normally enlarges during pregnancy. Maternal hyperthyroidism occurs at a rate of ~2 per 1000 pregnancies and is generally well tolerated by pregnant women. Clinical signs and symptoms should alert the physician to the occurrence of this disease. Many of the physiologic adaptations to pregnancy may mimic subtle signs of hyperthyroidism. Although pregnant women are able to tolerate mild hyperthyroidism without adverse sequelae, more severe hyperthyroidism can cause spontaneous abortion or premature labor, and thyroid storm is associated with a significant risk of maternal mortality.

℞ HYPERTHYROIDISM IN PREGNANCY

Hyperthyroidism in pregnancy should be aggressively evaluated and treated. The treatment of choice is propylthiouracil. Because it crosses the placenta, the minimum effective dose should be used to maintain free T_4 in the upper normal range. Methimazole crosses the placenta to a greater degree than propylthiouracil and has been associated with fetal aplasia cutis. Radioiodine should not be used during pregnancy, either for scanning or treatment, because of effects on the fetal thyroid. In emergent circumstances, additional treatment with beta blockers and a saturated solution of potassium iodide may be necessary. Hyperthyroidism is most difficult to control in the first trimester of pregnancy and easiest to control in the third trimester.

The goal of therapy for *hypothyroidism* is to maintain the serum TSH in the normal range, and thyroxine is the drug of choice. Children born to women with an elevated serum TSH (and a normal total thyroxine) during pregnancy have impaired performance on neuropsychologic tests. During pregnancy, the dose of thyroxine required to keep the TSH in the normal range rises. In one study, the mean replacement dose of thyroxine required to maintain the TSH in the normal range was 0.1 mg daily before pregnancy, and it increased to 0.15 mg daily during pregnancy. Since the increased thyroxine requirement occurs as early as the fifth week of pregnancy, one approach is to increase the thyroxine dose by 30% as soon as pregnancy is diagnosed and then adjust the dose by serial measurement of TSH.

HEMATOLOGIC DISORDERS

Pregnancy has been described as a state of physiologic anemia. Part of the reduction in hemoglobin concentration is dilutional, but iron and folate deficiencies are the major causes of correctable anemia during pregnancy.

In populations at high risk for hemoglobinopathies (Chap. 99), hemoglobin electrophoresis should be performed as part of the prenatal screen. Hemoglobinopathies can be associated with increased maternal and fetal morbidity and mortality. Management is tailored to the specific hemoglobinopathy and is generally the same for both pregnant and nonpregnant women. Prenatal diagnosis of hemoglobinopathies in the fetus is readily available and should be discussed with prospective parents either prior to or early in pregnancy.

Thrombocytopenia occurs commonly during pregnancy. The majority of cases are benign gestational thrombocytopenias, but the differential diagnosis should include immune thrombocytopenia (Chap. 109) and preeclampsia. Maternal thrombocytopenia may also be caused by catastrophic obstetric events such as retention of a dead fetus, sepsis, abruptio placenta, and amniotic fluid embolism.

NEUROLOGIC DISORDERS

Headache appearing during pregnancy is usually due to migraine (Chap. 15), a condition that may worsen, improve, or be unaffected by pregnancy. A new or worsening headache, particularly if associated with visual blurring, may signal eclampsia (above) or pseudotumor cerebri (benign intracranial hypertension; Chap. 29); diplopia due to a sixth nerve palsy suggests pseudotumor cerebri. The risk of seizures in patients with epilepsy increases in the postpartum period but not consistently during pregnancy; management is discussed in Chap. 363. The risk of stroke is generally thought to increase during pregnancy because of a hypercoagulable state; however, studies suggest that the period of risk occurs primarily in the postpartum period and that both ischemic and hemorrhagic strokes may occur at this time. Guidelines for use of heparin therapy are summarized above (see "Deep Venous Thrombosis and Pulmonary Embolism"); warfarin is teratogenic and should be avoided.

The onset of a new movement disorder during pregnancy suggests chorea gravidarum, a variant of Sydenham's chorea associated with rheumatic fever and streptococcal infection (Chap. 315); the chorea may recur with subsequent pregnancies. Patients with preexisting multiple sclerosis (Chap. 375) experience a gradual decrease in the risk of relapses as pregnancy progresses and, conversely, an increase in attack risk during the postpartum period. Beta interferons should *not* be administered to pregnant MS patients, but moderate or severe relapses can be safely treated with pulse glucocorticoid therapy. Finally, certain tumors, particularly pituitary adenoma and meningioma (Chap. 374), may manifest during pregnancy because of accelerated growth, possibly driven by hormonal factors.

Peripheral nerve disorders associated with pregnancy include Bell's palsy (idiopathic facial paralysis, Chap. 379), which is approximately threefold more likely to occur during the third trimester and immediate postpartum period than in the general population. Therapy with glucocorticoids should follow the guidelines established for nonpregnant patients. Entrapment neuropathies are common in the later stages of pregnancy, presumably as a result of fluid retention. Carpal tunnel syndrome (median nerve) presents as pain and paresthesia in the hand, often worse at night, and later with weakness in the thenar muscles. Treatment is generally conservative; wrist splints may be helpful, and glucocorticoid injections or surgical section of the carpal tunnel can usually be postponed. Meralgia paresthetica (lateral femoral cutaneous nerve) consists of pain and numbness in the lateral aspect of the thigh without weakness. Patients are usually reassured to learn that these symptoms are benign and can be expected to remit spontaneously after the pregnancy has been completed.

Judicious use of neuroimaging procedures is reasonable during pregnancy. Some centers require that formal consent be obtained from pregnant patients before MRI scans are administered. Experimental data indicate that high-field-strength MRI may be teratogenic to rodents; however, studies in pregnant MRI technicians have failed to show any risk to the fetus, even with chronic exposure. The paramagnetic MRI contrast agent gadolinium is usually not administered, particularly during the first trimester, because it crosses the blood-brain barrier. CT scanning of the brain is also considered safe, particularly as the procedure is fast, little radioactive scatter is produced, and pelvic contents are easily shielded; iodinated contrast media should be avoided whenever possible.

GASTROINTESTINAL AND LIVER DISEASE

Up to 90% of pregnant women experience nausea and vomiting during the first trimester of pregnancy. Occasionally, hyperemesis gravidarum requires hospitalization to prevent dehydration, and sometimes parenteral nutrition is required.

Crohn's disease may be associated with exacerbations in the second and third trimesters. Ulcerative colitis is associated with disease exacerbations in the first trimester and during the early postpartum period. Medical management of these diseases during pregnancy is identical to the management in the nonpregnant state (Chap. 289).

Exacerbation of gall bladder disease is commonly observed during pregnancy. In part this may be due to pregnancy-induced alteration in the metabolism of bile and fatty acids. Intrahepatic cholestasis of pregnancy is generally a third-trimester event. Profound pruritus may accompany this condition, and it may be associated with increased fetal mortality. It has been suggested that placental bile salt deposition may contribute to progressive uteroplacental insufficiency. Therefore, regular fetal surveillance should be undertaken once the diagnosis of intrahepatic cholestasis is made. Favorable results with ursodiol have been reported.

Acute fatty liver is a rare complication of pregnancy. Frequently confused with the HELLP syndrome (see "Preeclampsia," above) and severe preeclampsia, the diagnosis of acute fatty liver of pregnancy may be facilitated by imaging studies and laboratory evaluation. Acute fatty liver of pregnancy is generally characterized by markedly increased levels of bilirubin and ammonia and by hypoglycemia. Management of acute fatty liver of pregnancy is supportive; recurrence in subsequent pregnancies has been reported.

All pregnant women should be screened for hepatitis B. This information is important for pediatricians after delivery of the infant. All infants receive hepatitis B vaccine. Infants born to mothers who are carriers of hepatitis B surface antigen should also receive hepatitis B immune globulin as soon after birth as possible and preferably within the first 72 h. Screening for hepatitis C is recommended for individuals at high risk for exposure.

INFECTIONS

BACTERIAL INFECTIONS

Other than bacterial vaginosis, the most common bacterial infections during pregnancy involve the urinary tract (Chap. 282). Many pregnant women have asymptomatic bacteriuria, most likely due to stasis caused by progestational effects on ureteral and bladder smooth muscle and later in pregnancy due to compression effects of the enlarging uterus. In itself, this condition is not associated with an adverse outcome of pregnancy. However, if asymptomatic bacteriuria is left untreated, symptomatic pyelonephritis may occur. Indeed, ~75% of cases of pregnancy-associated pyelonephritis are the result of untreated asymptomatic bacteriuria. All pregnant women should be screened with a urine culture for asymptomatic bacteriuria at the first prenatal visit. Subsequent screening with nitrite/leukocyte esterase strips is indicated for high-risk women, such as those with sickle cell trait or a history of urinary tract infections. All women with positive screens should be treated.

Abdominal pain and fever during pregnancy create a clinical dilemma. The diagnosis of greatest concern is intrauterine amniotic infection. While amniotic infection most commonly follows rupture of the membranes, this is not always the case. In general, antibiotic therapy is not recommended as a temporizing measure in these circumstances. If intrauterine infection is suspected, induced delivery with concomitant antibiotic therapy is generally indicated. Intrauterine amniotic infection is most often caused by pathogens such as *Escherichia coli* and group B streptococcus. In high-risk patients at term or in preterm patients, routine intrapartum prophylaxis of group B streptococcal (GBS) disease is recommended. Penicillin G and ampicillin are the drugs of choice. In penicillin-allergic patients, clindamycin is recommended. For the reduction of neonatal morbidity due to GBS, universal screening of pregnant women for GBS between 35 and 37 weeks gestation with intrapartum antibiotic treatment of infected women is recommended.

Postpartum infection is a significant cause of maternal morbidity and mortality. While rare after vaginal delivery, postpartum endomyometritis develops in 5% of patients having elective repeat cesarean section and in 25% of patients after emergency cesarean section following prolonged labor. Prophylactic antibiotics should be given to all patients undergoing cesarean section. As most cases of postpartum endomyometritis are polymicrobial, broad-spectrum antibiotic coverage with a penicillin, aminoglycoside, and metronidazole is recommended (Chap. 157). Most cases resolve within 72 h. Women who do not respond to antibiotic treatment for postpartum endomyometritis should be evaluated for septic pelvic thrombophlebitis. Imaging studies may be helpful in establishing the diagnosis, which is primarily a clinical diagnosis of exclusion. Patients with septic pelvic thrombophlebitis generally have tachycardia out of proportion to their fever and respond rapidly to intravenous administration of heparin.

All patients are screened prenatally for gonorrhea and chlamydial infections, and the detection of either should result in prompt treatment. Ceftriaxone and azithromycin are the agents of choice (Chaps. 137 and 169).

VIRAL INFECTIONS

Cytomegalovirus Infection   Viral infection in pregnancy presents a significant challenge. The most common cause of congenital viral infection in the United States is cytomegalovirus (CMV) (Chap. 175). As many as 50–90% of women of childbearing age have antibodies to CMV, but only rarely does CMV reactivation result in neonatal infection. More commonly, primary CMV infection during pregnancy creates a risk of congenital CMV. No currently accepted treatment of CMV during pregnancy has been demonstrated to protect the fetus effectively. Moreover, it is impossible to predict which fetus will sustain life-threatening CMV infection. Severe CMV disease in the newborn is characterized most often by petechiae, hepatosplenomegaly, and jaundice. Chorioretinitis, microcephaly, intracranial calcifications, hepatitis, hemolytic anemia, and purpura may also develop. CNS involvement, resulting in the development of psychomotor, ocular, auditory, and dental abnormalities over time, has been described.

Rubella   (See also Chap. 186) Rubella virus is a known teratogen; first-trimester rubella carries a high risk of fetal anomalies, though the risk decreases significantly later in pregnancy. Congenital rubella may be diagnosed by percutaneous umbilical blood sampling with the detection of IgM antibodies in fetal blood. All pregnant women should be screened for their immune status to rubella. Indeed, all women of childbearing age, regardless of pregnancy status, should have their immune status for rubella verified and be immunized if necessary. The incidence of congenital rubella in the United States is extremely low.

Herpesvirus   (See also Chap. 172) The acquisition of genital herpes during pregnancy is associated with spontaneous abortion, prematurity, and congenital and neonatal herpes. A recent cohort study of pregnant women without evidence of previous herpes infection demonstrated that ~2% of the women acquired a new herpes infection during the pregnancy. Approximately 60% of the newly infected women had no clinical symptoms. Infection occurred equally in all three trimesters. If herpes seroconversion occurred early in pregnancy, the risk of transmission to the newborn was very low. In women who acquired genital herpes shortly before delivery, the risk of transmission was high. The risk of active genital herpes lesions at term can be reduced by prescribing acyclovir for the last 4 weeks of pregnancy to women who have had their first episode of genital herpes during the pregnancy.

Herpesvirus infection in the newborn can be devastating. Disseminated neonatal herpes carries with it high mortality and morbidity rates from CNS involvement. It is recommended that pregnant women with active genital herpes lesions at the time of presentation in labor be delivered by cesarean section.

Parvovirus   (See also Chap. 177) Parvovirus infection (human parvovirus B19) may occur during pregnancy. It rarely causes sequelae, but susceptible women infected during pregnancy may be at risk for fetal hydrops secondary to erythroid aplasia and profound anemia.

HIV Infection   (See also Chap. 182) The predominant cause of HIV infection in children is transmission of the virus from the mother to the newborn during the perinatal period. Exposures, which increase the risk of mother-to-child transmission, include vaginal delivery, preterm delivery, trauma to the fetal skin, and maternal bleeding. Additionally, recent infection with high maternal viral load, low maternal CD4+ T cell count, prolonged labor, prolonged length of membrane rupture, and the presence of other genital tract infections, such as syphilis or herpes, increase the risk of transmission. Breast-feeding may also transmit HIV to the newborn and is therefore contraindicated in most developed countries for HIV-infected mothers. There is no clear evidence to suggest that the course of HIV disease is altered by pregnancy. There is also no clear evidence to suggest that uncomplicated HIV disease adversely impacts pregnancy other than by its inherent infection risk.

Rx HIV INFECTION IN PREGNANCY

The majority of cases of mother-to-child (vertical) transmission of HIV-1 occur during the intrapartum period. Mechanisms of vertical transmission include infection after rupture of the membranes and direct contact of the fetus with infected secretions or blood from the maternal genital tract. Zidovudine (ZDV) administered during pregnancy and labor and to the newborn reduces the risk of vertical transmission by 70%. Cesarean section is associated with additional risk reduction compared to vaginal delivery, especially in women with a viral load >1000 copies/mL. Regardless of the mode of delivery, intrapartum ZDV should be provided.

SUMMARY

Maternal mortality has decreased steadily during the past 70 years. The maternal death rate has decreased from nearly 600/100,000 live births in 1935 to 8/100,00 live births in 2002. The most common causes of maternal death in the United States today are, in decreasing order of frequency, pulmonary embolism, obstetric hemorrhage, hypertension, sepsis, cardiovascular conditions including peripartum cardiomyopathy, and ectopic pregnancy. With improved diagnostic and therapeutic modalities as well as with advances in the treatment of infertility, more patients with medical complications will be seeking, and be in need of, complex obstetric care. Improving outcome of pregnancy in these women will be best obtained by assembling a team of internists, specialists in maternal-fetal medicine (high-risk obstetrics), and anesthesiologists to counsel these patients about the risks of pregnancy and to plan their treatment prior to conception. The importance of preconception counseling cannot be overstated. It is the responsibility of all physicians caring for women in the reproductive age group to assess their patient's reproductive plans as part of their overall health evaluation.

FURTHER READINGS

ALEXANDER EK et al: Timing and magnitude of increases in levothyroxine requirements during pregnancy in women with hypothyroidism. N Engl J Med 351:292, 2005

BATES SM et al: Use of antithrombotic agents during pregnancy: The Seventh ACCP Conference on antithrombotic and thrombolytic therapy. Chest 126:627S, 2004

BUCHANAN TA, XIANG AH: Gestational diabetes mellitus. J Clin Invest 115:485, 2005

CROWTHER CA et al: Effect of treatment of gestational diabetes mellitus on pregnancy outcomes. N Engl J Med 352:2477, 2005

DENEUX-THARAUX C et al: Underreporting of pregnancy-related mortality in the United States and Europe. Obstet Gynecol 106:684, 2005

KAAJA RJ, GREER IA: Manifestations of chronic disease during pregnancy. JAMA 294:2751, 2005

LEVINE RJ: Circulating angiogenic factors and the risk of preeclampsia. N Engl J Med 350:672, 2004

MAGEE LA et al: Hydralazine for treatment of severe hypertension in pregnancy: Meta-analysis. BMJ 327:955, 2003

SIBAI BM: Chronic hypertension in pregnancy. Obstet Gynecol 100:369, 2002

THE MAGPIE TRIAL COLLABORATIVE GROUP: Do women with preeclampsia, and their babies, benefit from magnesium sulfate? The Magpie Trial: A randomised placebo-controlled trial. Lancet 359:1877, 2002

8 Medical Evaluation of the Surgical Patient
Wei C. Lau, Kim A. Eagle

Over 40 million persons undergo noncardiac surgical procedures in the United States annually. Cardiovascular and pulmonary complications continue to account for major morbidity and mortality in such patients. Emerging evidence-based practices dictate that the internist should perform an individualized evaluation of the surgical patient to provide an accurate preoperative risk assessment and stratification in order to guide optimum perioperative risk-reduction strategies. This chapter reviews cardiovascular and pulmonary preoperative risk assessment, targeting intermediate- and high-risk patients to strategically guide perioperative therapies in order to improve outcome. It also reviews perioperative management and prophylaxis of diabetes mellitus, endocarditis, and venous thromboembolism.

ANESTHETICS

Mortality is extremely low with safe delivery of modern anesthesia, especially in low-risk patients undergoing low-risk surgery (Table 8-1). Inhaled anesthetics have predictable circulatory and respiratory effects; all decrease arterial pressure in a dose-dependent manner by reducing sympathetic tone, causing systemic vasodilation, myocardial depression, and decreased cardiac output. Inhaled anesthetics also cause respiratory depression with diminished responses to both hypercapnia and hypoxemia in a dose-dependent manner, and they have a variable effect on heart rate. In combination with neuromuscular blockade, inhaled anesthetic agents also cause reduction in functional residual lung capacity due to loss of diaphragmatic and intercostal muscle function. This decreases lung volume, which may lead to atelectasis in the dependent lung regions and, in turn, may result in arterial hypoxemia from ventilation-perfusion mismatch as well as an increased risk of postoperative pulmonary complications.

Several meta-analyses have examined the safety of general (inhaled) and neuroaxial (epidural or spinal) anesthesia and found that overall mortality was lower in patients receiving neuroaxial anesthesia. Lower rates of venous thrombosis, pulmonary embolism, pneumonia, and respiratory depression were also observed in patients who were provided neuroaxial anesthesia. However, there were no significant differences in cardiac events between the two approaches. A combination of neuroaxial blockade and general anesthesia is useful when it is desired to reduce general anesthesia requirements. Evidence from a meta-analysis of randomized controlled trials also supports postoperative epidural analgesia for the purpose of pain relief for more than 24 h.

EVALUATION OF INTERMEDIATE- TO HIGH-RISK PATIENTS

Simple, standardized preoperative screening questionnaires, such as the one shown in Table 8-2, have been developed for the purpose of identifying patients at intermediate or high risk who would benefit from a more detailed clinical evaluation. Evaluation of such patients for operation should always begin with a thorough history and physical examination and with a 12-lead resting ECG, in accordance with the American College of Cardiology/American Heart Association (ACC/AHA) guideline recommendations. The history should focus on symptoms of occult cardiac or pulmonary disease. The urgency of the surgery should be determined, as true emergent procedures are associ-

TABLE 8-1 SURGERY: GRADATION OF RISK OF COMMON NONCARDIAC SURGICAL PROCEDURES

Higher	• Emergent major operations, especially elderly • Aortic and other noncarotid major vascular surgery (endovascular and nonendovascular) • Prolonged surgery associated with large fluid shift and/or blood loss
Intermediate	• Major thoracic surgery • Major abdominal surgery • Carotid endarterectomy surgery • Head/neck surgery • Orthopedic surgery • Prostate surgery
Lower	• Eye, skin, and superficial surgery • Endoscopic procedures

Source: From KA Eagle et al.

ated with an unavoidably higher morbidity and mortality. Preoperative laboratory testing should be carried out only for specific clinical conditions based on the clinical examination. Thus, healthy patients of any age undergoing elective surgical procedures without coexisting medical conditions should not require any testing unless the degree of surgical stress may result in unusual changes from the baseline state.

PREOPERATIVE CARDIAC RISK ASSESSMENT

Assessment of exercise tolerance in the prediction of in-hospital perioperative risk is most helpful in patients who self-report worsening exercise-induced cardiopulmonary symptoms, those who may benefit from noninvasive or invasive cardiac testing regardless of scheduled surgical procedure, and those with known coronary artery disease (CAD) or with multiple risk factors who are able to exercise. For predicting perioperative events, poor exercise tolerance has been defined as the inability to walk four blocks or climb two flights of stairs at a normal pace or to meet a metabolic equivalent (MET) level of four (e.g., carrying objects of 15–20 lb, playing golf or doubles tennis) because of the development of dyspnea, angina, or excessive fatigue (Table 8-3).

TABLE 8-2 STANDARDIZED PREOPERATIVE QUESTIONNAIRES[a]

1. Age, weight, height
2. Are you:
   Female and 55 years of age or older or male and 45 years of age of older?
   If yes, are you also 70 years of age or older?
3. Do you take anticoagulant ("blood thinners") medications?
4. Do you have or have you had any of the following heart related conditions?
   Heart disease
   Heart attack within the last 6 months
   Angina (chest pain)
   Irregular heartbeat
   Heart failure
5. Do you have or have you ever had any of the following?
   Rheumatoid arthritis
   Kidney disease
   Liver disease
   Diabetes
6. Do you get short of breath when you lie flat?
7. Are you currently on oxygen treatment?
8. Do you have a chronic cough that produces any discharge or fluid?
9. Do you have lung problems or diseases?
10. Have you or any blood member of your family ever had a problem with any anesthesia other than nausea?
    If yes, describe:
11. If female, is it possible that you could be pregnant?
    Pregnancy test:
    Please list date of last menstrual period:

[a]University of Michigan Health System patient information report. Patients who answer yes to any of questions 2–9 should receive a more detailed clinical evaluation.
Source: Adapted from KK Tremper, P Benedict: Anesthesiology 92:1212, 2000; with permission.

TABLE 8-3 FUNCTIONAL STATUS

Higher ↕ Risk ↕ Lower	• Difficulty with adult activities of daily living • Cannot walk four blocks or up two flights of stairs or unable to meet a MET level of 4 • Inactive but no limitation • Active: easily does vigorous tasks • Performs regular vigorous exercises

Source: From KA Eagle et al.

Previous studies have prospectively compared several cardiac risk indices. Given its accuracy and simplicity, the revised cardiac risk index (RCRI) (Table 8-4) is favored. The RCRI relies on the presence or absence of six identifiable predictive factors, which include high-risk surgery, ischemic heart disease, congestive heart failure, cerebrovascular disease, diabetes mellitus, and renal dysfunction. Each of these predictors is assigned one point. The risk of major cardiac events—defined as myocardial infarction, pulmonary edema, ventricular fibrillation or primary cardiac arrest, and complete heart block—can then be predicted. Based on the presence of none, one, two, three, or more of these clinical predictors, the rate of development of one of these major cardiac events is estimated to be 0.5, 1, 5, and 10%, respectively (Fig. 8-1). RCRI 0 has 0.4–0.5% risk of cardiac events; RCRI 1 has 0.9–1.3%; RCRI 2 has 4–6.6%; and RCRI ≥3 has 9–11% risk of cardiac events. The clinical utility of the RCRI is to identify patients with three or more predictors who are at higher risk (≥10%) for cardiac complications, and who may benefit from further risk stratification with noninvasive cardiac testing or initiation of preoperative preventive medical management.

PREOPERATIVE NONINVASIVE CARDIAC TESTING FOR RISK STRATIFICATION

There is little evidence to support widespread application of preoperative noninvasive cardiac testing for all patients undergoing major surgery. Rather, a selective approach based on clinical risk categorization appears to be both useful clinically and cost-effective. There is potential benefit in identifying asymptomatic but high-risk patients, such as those with left main or left main–equivalent CAD, or those with three-vessel CAD with poor left ventricular function who may benefit from coronary revascularization (Chap. 237). However, evidence does not support aggressive attempts to identify patients at intermediate risk with asymp-

TABLE 8-4 REVISED CARDIAC RISK INDEX CLINICAL MARKERS

High-risk surgical procedures
   Vascular surgery
   Major intraperitoneal or intrathoracic procedures
Ischemic heart disease
   History of myocardial infarction
   Current angina considered to be ischemic
   Requiring sublingual nitroglycerin
   Positive exercise test
   Pathological Q-waves on ECG
   History of PTCA and/or CABG with current angina considered to be ischemic
Congestive heart failure
   Left ventricular failure by physical examination
   History of paroxysmal nocturnal dyspnea
   History of pulmonary edema
   S3 gallop on cardiac auscultation
   Bilateral rales on pulmonary auscultation
   Pulmonary edema on chest x-ray
Cerebrovascular disease
   History of transient ischemic attack
   History of cerebrovascular accident
Diabetes mellitus
   Treatment with insulin
Chronic renal insufficiency
   Serum creatinine >2 mg/dL

Note: ECG, electrocardiogram; PTCA, percutaneous transluminal coronary angioplasty; CABG, coronary artery bypass grafting.
Source: Adapted from TH Lee et al, with permission.

FIGURE 8-1 Risk stratification based on the Revised Cardiac Risk Index. Derivation and prospective validation of a simple index for prediction of cardiac risk of major noncardiac surgery. Cardiac events include myocardial infarction, pulmonary edema, ventricular fibrillation, cardiac asystole, and complete heart block. *(Adapted from TH Lee et al, with permission.)*

tomatic but advanced coronary artery disease, since coronary revascularization appears to offer little advantage over medical therapy.

An RCRI score ≥3 in patients with severe myocardial ischemia on stress testing should lead to consideration of coronary revascularization prior to noncardiac surgery. Noninvasive cardiac testing is most appropriate if it is anticipated that in the event of a strongly positive test a patient will meet guidelines for coronary angiography and coronary revascularization. Pharmacologic stress tests are more useful than exercise testing in patients with functional limitations. Dobutamine echocardiography and persantine, adenosine or dobutamine nuclear perfusion testing (Chap. 222) have excellent negative predictive values (near 100%) but poor positive predictive values (< 20%) for identification of patients at risk for perioperative myocardial infarction or death. Thus, a negative study is reassuring, but a positive study is a relatively weak predictor of a "hard" perioperative cardiac event. A stepwise approach is illustrated in **Fig. 8-2.**

RISK MODIFICATION USING PREVENTIVE STRATEGIES TO REDUCE CARDIAC RISK
Perioperative Coronary Revascularization Currently, potential options for reducing perioperative cardiovascular risk include coronary artery revascularization and/or perioperative medical preventive therapies

ALGORITHM FOR CARDIAC RISK ASSESSMENT

[algorithm flowchart]

FIGURE 8-2 Composite algorithm for cardiac risk assessment and stratification in patients undergoing noncardiac surgery. Stepwise clinical evaluation: [1] Emergency surgery; [2] Prior coronary revascularization; [3] Prior coronary evaluation; [4] Clinical assessment; [5] Revised cardiac risk index; [6] Risk modification strategies. Preventative medical therapy = beta blocker and statin therapy. RCRI, revised cardiac risk index. *(Adapted from KA Eagle et al and TH Lee et al.)*

(Chap. 237). *Prophylactic* coronary revascularization with either coronary artery bypass grafting (CABG) or percutaneous coronary intervention (PCI) provides no short- or midterm survival benefit for patients *without* left main CAD or three-vessel CAD in the presence of poor left ventricular systolic function. Although PCI is associated with lower procedural risk than is CABG in the perioperative setting, the placement of a coronary artery stent in a short period of time prior to noncardiac surgery may increase the risk of bleeding during surgery if dual antiplatelet therapy (aspirin and clopidogrel) is administered, or it increases the perioperative risk of myocardial infarction and cardiac death due to stent thrombosis if such therapy is withdrawn prematurely (Chap. 240). It is recommended that, if possible, noncardiac surgery be delayed 4–6 weeks after placement of a bare metal coronary stent and 3–6 months after a drug-eluting stent. For patients who *must* undergo noncardiac surgery early (first few days to 4 weeks) after PCI, simple balloon angioplasty without stent placement appears to be a reasonable alternative, since dual antiplatelet therapy is not necessary in such patients.

PERIOPERATIVE MEDICAL PREVENTIVE THERAPIES

Perioperative preventive medical therapy with β-adrenergic antagonists, HMG-CoA reductase inhibitors (statins), and aspirin has the goal of reducing perioperative adrenergic stimulation, ischemia, and inflammation, which are triggered during the perioperative period.

β-ADRENERGIC ANTAGONISTS

A recent expedited update of the ACC/AHA guideline focusing on recommendations for perioperative beta blocker therapy recommended the following: (1) Beta blockers *should be continued* in high-risk patients previously receiving these drugs who undergo vascular surgery, and they *should be administered* to high-risk patients identified by myocardial ischemia on preoperative assessment who are scheduled to undergo vascular surgery (Class I indications). (2) Beta blockers are *probably recommended* (Class IIa indication) for high-risk patients defined by multiple clinical predictors who undergo intermediate- or high-risk procedures. They *may be considered* (Class IIb indication) for intermediate-risk patients who undergo intermediate- or high-risk procedures and for low-risk patients who undergo vascular surgery.

HMG-COA REDUCTASE INHIBITORS (STATINS)

A number of prospective and retrospective studies support the perioperative prophylactic use of statins for reduction of cardiac complications in patients with established atherosclerosis. Although the future role of statin prophylaxis in the reduction of perioperative cardiac risk awaits definitive clarification by an ongoing trial, perioperative statin therapy to reduce perioperative cardiac risk may now be considered in intermediate- or high-risk patients with atherosclerotic cardiovascular disease undergoing major noncardiac surgery.

ANGIOTENSIN-CONVERTING ENZYME (ACE) INHIBITORS

Evidence supports the discontinuation of ACE inhibitors and angiotensin receptor blockers for 24 hours prior to noncardiac surgery due to adverse circulatory effects after induction of anesthesia.

ORAL ANTIPLATELET AGENTS

Evidence-based recommendations regarding perioperative use of aspirin and/or clopidogrel to reduce cardiac risk currently lack clarity. A substantial increase in perioperative bleeding and transfusion requirement in patients receiving dual antiplatelet therapy has been observed. The discontinuation of clopidogrel and aspirin for 5–7 days prior to major surgery to minimize the risk of perioperative bleeding and transfusion must be balanced with the potential increased risk of an acute coronary syndrome and of subacute stent thrombosis in patients with recent coronary stent implantation. If clinicians elect to withhold antiplatelet agents prior to surgery, they should be restarted as soon as possible postoperatively.

CALCIUM CHANNEL BLOCKERS

Evidence is lacking to support the use of calcium channel blockers as a prophylactic strategy to decrease perioperative risk in major noncardiac surgery.

TABLE 8-5	PREDISPOSING RISK FACTORS FOR PULMONARY COMPLICATIONS

1. Upper respiratory tract infection: cough, dyspnea
2. Age >60 years
3. COPD
4. American Society of Anesthesiologists Class ≥2
5. Functionally dependent
6. Congestive heart failure
7. Serum albumin <3.5 g/dL
8. FEV_1 <2 L
9. MVV <50% of predicted
10. PEF <100 L or 50% predicted value
11. P_{CO_2} ≥45 mmHg
12. P_{O_2} ≤50 mmHg

Note: COPD, chronic obstructive pulmonary disease; FEV_1, forced expiratory volume in one second; MVV, maximum voluntary ventilation; PEF, peak expiratory flow rate; P_{CO_2}, partial pressure of carbon dioxide; P_{O_2}, partial pressure of oxygen.
Source: Modified from GW Smetana et al and from DN Mohr et al: Postgrad Med 100:247, 1996, with permission.

PREOPERATIVE PULMONARY ASSESSMENT

Perioperative pulmonary complications occur frequently and lead to significant morbidity and mortality. The guidelines from the American College of Physicians recommend the following:

(1) All patients undergoing noncardiac surgery should be assessed for risk of pulmonary complications (Table 8-5).

(2) Patients undergoing emergency or prolonged (>3 h) surgery; aortic aneurysm repair; vascular surgery; major abdominal, thoracic, neuro, head, and neck surgery; and general anesthesia should be considered to be at higher risk for postoperative pulmonary complications.

(3) Patients at higher risk of pulmonary complications should receive deep breathing exercises and/or incentive spirometry, as well as selective use of a nasogastric tube for postoperative nausea, vomiting, or symptomatic abdominal distention to reduce postoperative risk (Table 8-6).

(4) Routine preoperative spirometry and chest radiography are less helpful for predicting risk of postoperative pulmonary complications, but may be appropriate for patients with chronic obstructive pulmonary disease (COPD) or asthma.

(5) Pulmonary artery catheterization, total parenteral nutrition, and total enteral nutrition are not encouraged for postoperative pulmonary risk reduction.

Other Preoperative Pulmonary Risk-Modification Strategies Risk-modification strategies to reduce postoperative pulmonary complications should be implemented, particularly in higher-risk patients. Patients with cough or dyspnea preoperatively should be evaluated to

TABLE 8-6	RISK MODIFICATION TO REDUCE PERIOPERATIVE PULMONARY COMPLICATIONS

Preoperatively
- Cessation of smoking
- Training in proper breathing (incentive spirometry)
- Inhalation bronchodilator therapy
- Control of infection and secretion, when indicated
- Weight reduction, when appropriate

Intraoperatively
- Limited duration of anesthesia
- Select shorter acting neuromuscular blocking drugs when indicated
- Prevention of aspiration
- Maintenance of optimal bronchodilation

Postoperatively
- Continuation of preoperative measures, with particular attention to
  inspiratory capacity maneuvers
  mobilization of secretions
  early ambulation
  encouragement of coughing
  selective use of a nasogastric tube
  adequate pain control without excessive narcotics

Source: From VA Lawrence et al and from WF Dunn, PD Scanlon, Mayo Clin Proc 68:371, 1993, with permission.

determine the underlying cause of these symptoms. Patients who smoke should be counseled to quit for at least 8 weeks prior to elective surgery. Patients with asthma or COPD can be given steroids and bronchodilators pre- and postoperatively to optimize pulmonary function. Bacterial pulmonary infection should be treated preoperatively.

DIABETES MELLITUS

(See also Chap. 338) Many patients with diabetes mellitus have significant symptomatic or asymptomatic CAD and may have silent myocardial ischemia due to autonomic dysfunction. Evidence supports intensive perioperative glycemic control to achieve near-normal glucose levels (90–110 mg/dL) versus moderate glycemic control (120–200 mg/dL), using insulin infusion. This practice must be balanced against the risk of hypoglycemic complications. Oral hypoglycemic agonists should be held on the morning of operation. Perioperative hyperglycemia should be treated with intravenous infusion of short-acting insulin or subcutaneous sliding-scale insulin. Patients who are diet-controlled may proceed to surgery with close postoperative monitoring.

PROPHYLAXIS FOR INFECTIVE ENDOCARDITIS

(See also Chap. 118) Perioperative prophylactic antibiotics should be administered to patients with congenital or valvular heart disease, prosthetic valves, mitral valve prolapse, or other cardiac abnormalities in accordance with ACC/AHA practice guidelines.

PROPHYLAXIS OF VENOUS THROMBOEMBOLISM

(See also Chap. 256) Perioperative prophylaxis of venous thromboembolism should follow established guidelines of the American College of Chest Physicians. Aspirin is not supported as a single agent for thromboprophylaxis. Low-dose unfractionated heparin (≤5000 units subcutaneous bid), low-molecular-weight heparin (e.g., enoxaparin 30 mg bid or 40 mg od) or a pentasaccharide (fondaparinux 2.5 mg od) for patients at moderate risk, and unfractionated heparin (5000 units subcutaneous tid) for patients at high risk. Graduated compression stockings and pneumatic compression devices are useful supplements to anticoagulant therapy.

EAGLE KA et al: ACC/AHA guideline update for perioperative cardiovascular evaluation for noncardiac surgery—executive summary: A report of the American College of Cardiology/American Heart Association Task Force on Practice Guidelines (Committee to Update the 1996 Guidelines on Perioperative Cardiovascular Evaluation for Noncardiac Surgery). J Am Coll Cardiol 39:542, 2002

FLEISHER LA et al: ACC/AHA 2006 guideline update for perioperative cardiovascular evaluation for noncardiac surgery: Focused update on perioperative beta-blocker therapy. A report of the American College of Cardiology/American Heart Association Task Force on Practice Guidelines (writing committee to update the 2002 guidelines on perioperative cardiovascular evaluation for noncardiac surgery). J Am Coll Cardiol 47:2343, 2006

GEERTS WH et al: Prevention of venous thromboembolism: The Seventh ACCP Conference on Antithrombotic and Thrombolytic Therapy. Chest 126(Suppl 3):338S, 2004

LAWRENCE VA et al: Strategies to reduce postoperative pulmonary complications after noncardiothoracic surgery: Systematic review for the American College of Physicians. Ann Intern Med 144:596, 2006

LEE TH et al: Derivation and prospective validation of a simple index for prediction of cardiac risk of major noncardiac surgery. Circulation 100:1043, 1999

LINDENAUER PK et al: Perioperative beta-blocker therapy and mortality after major noncardiac surgery. N Engl J Med 353:349, 2005

McFALLS EO et al: Coronary-artery revascularization before elective major vascular surgery. N Engl J Med 351:2795, 2004

QASEEM A et al: Risk assessment for and strategies to reduce perioperative pulmonary complications for patients undergoing noncardiothoracic surgery: A guideline from the American College of Physicians. Ann Intern Med 144:575, 2006

SMETANA GW et al: Preoperative pulmonary risk stratification for noncardiothoracic surgery: Systematic review for the American College of Physicians. Ann Intern Med 144:581, 2006

9 Geriatric Medicine
Lisa B. Caruso, Rebecca A. Silliman

AGING

Aging is the progressive, universal decline first in functional reserve and then in function that occurs in organisms over time. Aging is heterogeneous. It varies widely in different individuals and in different organs within a particular individual. Aging is not a disease; however, the risk of developing disease is increased, often dramatically, as a function of age. The biochemical composition of tissues changes with age; physiologic capacity decreases, the ability to maintain homeostasis in adapting to stressors declines, and vulnerability to disease processes increases with age. After maturation, mortality rate increases exponentially with age.

DEMOGRAPHY OF AGING

Populations worldwide are aging. Improvements in environmental (e.g., clean water and improved sanitation) and behavioral (nutrition, reduced risk exposures) factors and the treatment and prevention of infectious diseases are largely responsible for the 30-year increase in life expectancy since 1900. In the United States, by 2030, 1 person in 5 will be >65 years. Old people are not evenly distributed geographically. Half of older people in the United States live in nine states, led by California, Florida, New York, and Texas.

🌐 GLOBAL AGING

Between 2000 and 2030, the number of older adults worldwide is expected to increase from 420 to 974 million. At present 59% of older adults live in the developing countries of Africa, Asia, Latin America, the Caribbean, and Oceania. The developing world has the largest absolute number of older adults and is experiencing the largest percentage increase.

Only 13% of those ≥80 years live in the United States; over 40% of those ≥80 years live in Asia. Embedded within these figures are additional critically important factors. Women outlive men; only 15% of centenarians are men. Men also remarry more frequently than do women; consequently, older women are frequently single and live alone. Women are more likely to have inadequate financial resources. Women also spend a greater portion of their surviving years being disabled than do men. In the United States, rates of disability decreased during the 1980s and 1990s, but the epidemics of obesity and physical inactivity may reverse these trends. A further concern for countries that already have high proportions of older adults (e.g., Japan, Sweden, Greece, and Italy, whose citizens >65 are 17–18% of their population) is the ratio of the >65 age group to the 15- to 64-year age group—the so-called dependency ratio. This ratio currently ranges from 22% in Europe to 6% in Africa but is expected to rise to >50% in Europe by 2050, with all other areas of the world exceeding 25% by 2050, except Africa.

LIFE EXPECTANCY

Often life-extending therapies are not offered to older patients because of an underestimate of life expectancy. Figure 9-1 shows average life expectancy as a function of age together with values for the lowest and highest quartiles of the population. White women currently have the highest life expectancy. Black women and white men have nearly identical life expectancies, and black men have the poorest life expectancy. At age 85 years, racial differences in life expectancy largely disappear. The average 75-year-

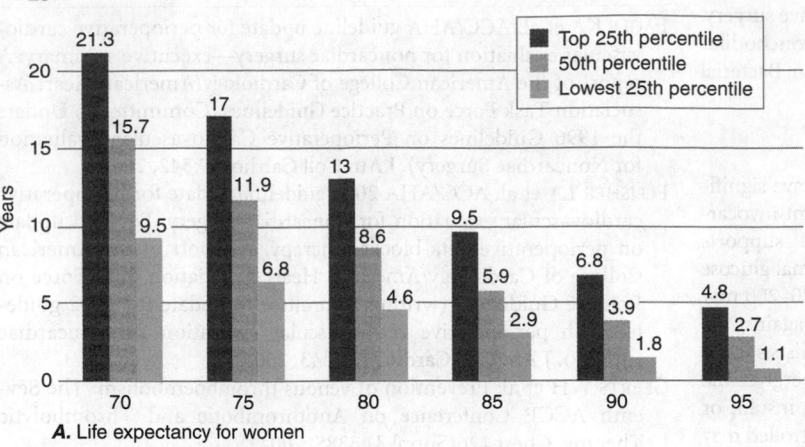

A. Life expectancy for women

B. Life expectancy for men

FIGURE 9-1 Upper, middle, and lower quartiles of life expectancy for women and men at selected ages. *(From LC Walter, KE Covinsky, JAMA 285:2751, 2001.)*

old is expected to live to age 86 and the average 85-year-old to age 91. Furthermore, where the issue has been examined, age is not a factor in determining the efficacy of a particular intervention. Thus, age alone generally should not be used to withhold life-extending interventions.

BIOLOGY OF AGING

As we age, we become increasingly unlike one another. For any variable one can measure, the variation in the distribution of values in a population increases with age. While the mean value may trend up or down, the age-related increase in the range of values is striking testimony to the diverse manifestations of the aging process. In addition, homeostatic mechanisms are slower to respond to stressors and take longer to restore normal function as we age. The ability to maintain stable function in the face of a change in the environment is called *allostasis* and it declines with age.

One problem as we age is nosologic; when is a particular change considered a normal age-related alteration and when does it become a disease? Ideas about the range of normal for a particular age continue to evolve. At one time, a 75-year-old with a blood pressure of 170/90 mmHg might have been considered to have an age-related increase in systolic blood pressure that did not require intervention. However, we now know that such a reading is a reflection of increased vascular stiffness, one of the most important risk factors for cardiovascular morbidity and mortality. Similarly, follow-up of individuals with fasting serum glucose levels of 6.1–6.7 mmol/L (110–120 mg/dL) have shown them to be at increased risk of diabetes complications. Accordingly impaired glucose metabolism is now defined as a fasting glucose level > 6.1 mmol/L (>110 mg/dL). Thus, the indications for interventions to alter natural history have changed and will continue to change as we learn more about aging.

Whether age-related changes that produce an aging phenotype have a common origin in a global process that alters cell or organ function or have heterogeneous contributions in different systems or different

individuals is unclear. Studies of aging (*gerontology*) are aimed at understanding the cellular and molecular basis of age-related changes and have two ultimate therapeutic goals: preserving function as long as possible and extending life span. These two goals may not be linked.

The lack of model systems for studying aging has hampered progress. For many years, researchers have studied replicative senescence of normal cells in culture. Why do normal cells have a finite replicative potential in vitro and why do cells from older individuals undergo fewer divisions than cells from younger individuals? Many have hoped that insights from such studies would reveal information about the aging process. However, the link between the failure of cells to divide in a synthetic culture medium and the aging phenotype of a whole organism is tenuous, at best. The body tissues with the greatest replicative potential should identify the organs most susceptible to age-related defective replication. In humans, these organs are the lining of the small intestine and the hematopoietic system. In the absence of disease, no age-related problem is caused by the inability of cells to replicate. Old people do not run out of absorptive surface in the small intestine or fail to make blood cells. Better in vitro models of aging are needed.

Experimental aging studies rely heavily on manipulation of life span in intact organisms such as worms, flies, and rodents. Such studies have revealed important insights. Alteration of genes involved in DNA repair often leads to premature aging. Alteration of genes involved in insulin signaling often leads to life extension. In the worm, life extension can be accomplished by alteration of gene expression in a single tissue, neurons. Calorie restriction (at least 30% lower than an ad lib diet) increases both average and maximal life span in a wide range of species. In several species, interventions associated with increased life span activate the expression of one or more of a family of genes, called *sirtuins*, that function by silencing the expression of certain other genes. However, these and other important observations have not yet led to a complete picture of the molecular basis of aging. Some ideas are summarized in Table 9-1.

Additional insights about aging may be derived by understanding the clinical syndromes that produce a premature aging phenotype, the so-called segmental progerias. These syndromes are rare inherited disorders that mimic normal aging imperfectly. They include Werner

TABLE 9-1	SOME THEORIES OF AGING
Hypothesis	**How It May Work**
Genetic	Aging is a genetic program activated in post-reproductive life when an individual's evolutionary mission is accomplished
Oxidative stress	Accumulation of oxidative damage to DNA, proteins, and lipids interferes with normal function and produces a decrease in stress responses
Mitochondrial dysfunction	A common deletion in mitochondrial DNA with age compromises function and alters cell metabolic processes and adaptability to environmental change
Hormonal changes	The decline and loss of circadian rhythm in secretion of some hormones produces a functional hormone deficiency state
Telomere shortening	Aging is related to a decline in the ability of cells to replicate
Defective host defenses	The failure of the immune system to respond to infectious agents and the overactivity of natural immunity create vulnerability to environmental stresses
Accumulation of senescent cells	Renewing tissues become dysfunctional through loss of ability to renew

syndrome, Bloom syndrome, Cockayne syndrome, Hutchinson-Gilford progeria, and Rothmund-Thomson syndrome. Hutchinson-Gilford progeria involves a mutation in lamin A, a component of the nuclear envelope. The symptoms have an onset in early childhood, and median survival is only about 13 years. All the other well-studied progeria syndromes involve mutations in DNA helicases, which are involved in DNA repair and recombination. The syndromes have features of accelerated aging and are associated with an increased risk of cancers. Werner syndrome has accelerated atherosclerosis as a prominent feature. Whether these conditions can reveal secrets of normal aging is not yet clear. However, they suggest that the maintenance of the integrity of the genome is a vulnerable function that can lead to premature aging if it is performed suboptimally.

Genetics and Exceptional Longevity Just as genetics is revealing information about premature aging, family studies may also identify features of delayed or successful aging. Twin studies suggest that ~30% of the variation in longevity can be attributed to genetic factors, with the remainder being attributable to environmental and behavioral factors. Long life span runs in families, and studies of centenarians and their offspring may define particularly adaptive phenotypes. For example, centenarians are less likely to be carriers of the apolipoprotein E ε4 allele, which is associated both with risk for heart disease and Alzheimer's disease. Ashkenazi Jewish centenarians and their offspring have been found to have larger high-density lipoprotein (HDL) and low-density lipoprotein (LDL) particle sizes; a lower prevalence of hypertension, cardiovascular disease, and the metabolic syndrome; and a greater likelihood of carrying an atheroprotective variant of the cholesteryl ester transfer protein gene. As studies of genetically more homogeneous populations such as those in Iceland and Sardinia progress, additional genetic contributions to healthy aging may be identified.

Frailty, Disabilty, and Comorbid Illness Frailty is defined as a clinical syndrome in which three or more of the following are present: unintentional weight loss of ≥4.5 kg (≥10 lb) in the past year (reflecting poor nutrition, catabolic metabolism, and sarcopenia), feeling exhausted (poor endurance), poor grip strength (weakness), slow walking speed, and low physical activity. Frailty overlaps with disability and comorbid illness but is not synonymous with them. Frailty is associated with a high risk of falls, disability, and death. It is unknown whether frailty is a single clinical syndrome or multiple syndromes and whether it has a central cause or multiple causes. Frail patients often share many physical and biochemical characteristics, and studies are underway to assess whether the syndrome or parts of it are responsive to interventions.

CHRONIC DISEASES AND THEIR IMPLICATIONS
The incidence, prevalence, and burden of chronic diseases increase with age, and this increased burden of disease is also associated with an increased risk of disability and decreased ability to recover from disability once it occurs.

The Global Perspective In 2005, chronic diseases accounted for 20 million deaths worldwide among those ≥70 years. The major disease contributors were cardiovascular disease (30%), cancer (13%), chronic respiratory disease (7%), and diabetes mellitus (2%). These diseases, driven to a large extent by tobacco use and obesity, are not concentrated in the developed world; rather, they are a large and growing problem in developing/low-income countries that lack the resources to prevent and manage chronic diseases and their consequences.

General Considerations Hypertension and diabetes mellitus are two common chronic conditions whose prevalence increases with age. In the United States, the National Health and Nutrition Examination Survey estimates that the prevalence of hypertension is between 60 and 84% and the prevalence of diabetes mellitus is between 18 and 21% in adults >65 years. The prevalence of both hypertension and di-

abetes is projected to increase substantially based on the demographics of aging and obesity. Moreover, rates of uncontrolled blood pressure in older adults are increasing, not decreasing. Both hypertension and diabetes accelerate functional decline in older adults, with hypertension accelerating cognitive decline and diabetes accelerating physical decline. Diabetes is also associated with a greater risk and severity of urinary incontinence (UI) and of falls in older women. Moreover, diabetes and stroke are the conditions most consistently associated with a diminished capacity for functional recovery in the aged.

The incidence of most cancers and cancer-specific mortality both increase with age. The age-adjusted incidence of cancer is ten times higher in the 65+ population than in those <65, and the age-adjusted cancer mortality is 15-fold higher. As a result, the incidence of cancer is expected to increase disproportionately in relation to overall population growth, and this trend is observed in countries throughout the world. Moreover, the majority of cancer survivors (>60%) are 65+ years of age.

In 2000, the leading causes of death among older Americans were heart disease (33%), cancer (22%), and cerebrovascular disease (8%). The death rate from heart disease has continued to decline; in 2006, cancer was the leading cause of death in persons <85 years. The management of chronic disease in older adults is particularly challenging. As examples, both hypertension and diabetes are established risk factors for micro- and macrovascular disease. Randomized clinical trials have demonstrated treatment efficacy, and guidelines for therapy are well established. Yet substantial evidence indicates that both conditions are inadequately treated, particularly in older adults with comorbidity. A portion of the problem is related to the fact that most clinical trials omit patients with comorbidities, making their results difficult to extrapolate to older patients with comorbid illness who are taking several other medications. The risks of drug-drug or drug-food interactions increase as a function of the number of medications used and patient age. In addition, the physician must take into account the impact of the disease and its treatment on the quality of life. Here, current functional status and rate of previous decline are helpful factors in estimating the level of functioning to which the patient may return. In concert with patient preferences and life goals, this information can help physicians and patients make decisions that are optimal at the individual patient level.

One attempt to develop an evidence-based quality of care framework for older adults cared for in ambulatory settings has been the Assessing Care of Vulnerable Elders (ACOVE) project. Designed to inform the care of persons >65 years who are at high risk for death or functional decline over a 2-year period, based on age, self-rated health, self-report of physical capability, and functional limitations, the ACOVE indicators cover 22 topics, including diseases, syndromes, impairments, and clinical situations that are prevalent, have strong influence on health/quality of life, and are amenable to available interventions. The tool has drawbacks. The indicators are generally focused on the care of one disease or condition at a time, and the total number of indicators is overwhelmingly large (236). However, it appears that better quality of care is associated with improved survival. Better strategies to target clusters of interventions to those who will benefit most are needed.

APPROACH TO:
The Geriatric Patient

FUNCTIONAL ASSESSMENT While the geriatric patient may have multiple chronic illnesses, functional status is the best indicator of prognosis and longevity. Functional status is defined as how well a person is able to provide for his or her own daily needs. Changes in function may signal a medical illness, advancing cognitive impairment, changes in social support, depression, substance abuse, or a combination of these. These changes should not be accepted as "just part of getting old." Documentation of a patient's baseline functional status is essential so that changes can be identified and addressed.

TABLE 9-2 SUGGESTED BRIEF GERIATRIC ASSESSMENT INSTRUMENTS

Domain	Instrument	Sensitivity	Specificity	Time (min)	Cutpoint	Comments
Cognition						
Dementia	MMSE	79–100%[a]	46–100%	9	<24[b]	Widely studied and accepted
	Timed time and change test	94–100%	37–46%	<2	<3 s for time and <10 s for change	Sensitive and quick
Delirium	CAM	94–100%	90–95%	<5		Sensitive and easy to apply
Affective disorders	GDS 5-question form	97%	85%	1	2	Rapid screen
Visual impairment	Snellen chart	"Gold standard"	"Gold standard"	2	Inability to read at 20/40 line	Universally used
Hearing impairment	Whispered voice	80–90%	70–89%	0.5	50% correct	No special equipment needed
	Pure tone audiometry	94–100%	70–94%	<5	Inability to hear >2 of 4 40-db tones (0.5, 1, 2, and 3 kHz)	Can be performed by trained office staff
Dental health	DENTAL[c]	82%	90%	<2 (estimated)	Score >2	
Nutritional status	Weight loss of >4.5 kg (>10 lb) in 6 months or weight <45 kg (<100 lb)	65–70%	87–88%		Yes to either	
Gait and balance	"Timed Get Up and Go" test	88%	94%	<1	>20s	Requires no special equipment

[a]Some studies have found lower sensitivities, but most studies of dementia subjects fall in this range.

[b]Cutoff is dependent on a number of variables including age, education, and racial or ethnic background.

[c]KA Atchinson, TA Dolan. Development of the geriatric oral health assessment index. J Dent Educ 11:680, 1990; with permission.

Note: MMSE, Mini-Mental Status Examination; CAM, confusion assessment method; GDS, geriatric depression scale.

Source: From CK Cassel et al. *Geriatric Medicine: An Evidence-Based Approach,* 4th ed. New York, Springer-Verlag, 2003; with permission.

Table 9-2 lists some suggested brief screening strategies for assessing functional status.

The first opportunity to assess the functional status of an older adult is when the patient is greeted and taken for a short walk into an examination room. In what way is the greeting received? Does the patient need assistance in getting out of a chair? Does he or she use an assistive device, such as a cane or walker? What is the patient's gait speed? How stable is the patient's gait? Is the patient fatigued after a short walk? These observations provide important initial information about how chronic illnesses affect the life of an older adult.

The basic activities of daily living (ADLs), which comprise activities essential for physical independence, and the instrumental activities of daily living (IADLs), which are necessary for independence in the community, are the most commonly used tools to assess functional status. The ADLs are dressing, bathing, feeding, toileting, transferring, and ambulating. The IADLs are money management, medication administration, using transportation, using the telephone, shopping, housekeeping, and meal preparation. These activities should be reviewed with the patient at the initial encounter and at periodic intervals. Cognitive deficits and psychosocial factors, however, may invalidate a patient's self-report, requiring the assistance of a third party for an accurate assessment. When functional deficits are identified, services provided by community (formal) or familial (informal) supports can be implemented to help the older adult continue to live in the least restrictive setting possible.

Other dimensions of the geriatric functional assessment include assessments of gait and balance, cognition, vision and hearing, dental and nutritional health, and driving ability. The Timed Get Up and Go Test is a valid clinical measure of balance in older adults. The patient is observed and timed as he or she rises from a chair, walks 3 m, turns around, and returns to sit down in the chair. A healthy older adult should be able to complete the test in <10 s. Difficulty performing this test is associated with increased fall risk and warrants further evaluation of mobility.

The screening tools to assess cognition in the older adult assist in identifying dementia and delirium, two common geriatric syndromes, both of which have a major effect on the functional status of the older adult. In addition, history-taking can be inaccurate and misleading if cognitive impairment is not recognized before a medical evaluation. The Mini-Mental State Examination (MMSE) is the most commonly used test to assess cognitive function (Chap. 26). The Mini-Cog assessment instrument is an alternative to the MMSE and may be superior in assessing culturally diverse populations. The Mini-Cog consists of repeating three unrelated words, followed by a clock-drawing test (CDT) showing a specific time. The times 11:10 or 8:20 are often used. The patient is then asked to recall the three words. The patient receives one point for each recalled word after the CDT and two points for a normal clock. A score of 0–2 is a positive screen for dementia.

Delirium can cause loss of independence, prolonged hospitalizations, and increased health care costs and can be life threatening. It is often undiagnosed by health care providers and not recognized as a symptom of other medical illnesses. The Confusion Assessment Method (CAM) is highly sensitive and specific for identifying delirium. Delirium is diagnosed when the confusional state is both (1) acute in onset with a fluctuating course and (2) associated with inattention, and either (3) manifested by disorganized thinking or (4) an altered level of consciousness. Simple tests of attention include having the patient repeat a series of numbers or stating the months of the year backwards.

While specialists perform full vision and hearing assessments, any provider caring for an older adult should be able to screen for deficits in these areas because they commonly present in older patients, they can lead to loss of patient independence, and they often result from treatable conditions. Basic tests for visual acuity such as the handheld Jaeger card for testing near vision and the wall-mounted Snellen chart for testing far vision are the tests most commonly used in office-based practices. Visual impairment is defined as being unable to read the 20/40 line or worse. Visual acuity itself has not been associated with increased fall risk in most studies; however, binocular vision, depth perception, and contrast sensitivity contribute to postural stability and object recognition. Hearing impairment can lead to decreased physical function, depression, and social isolation. The whisper test and testing with a handheld audioscope are used frequently as screening tests. To perform the whisper test, the examiner covers the opposite ear of the patient being tested, exhales completely, and then whispers an easily answered question from a distance of 60 cm (2 ft) from the ear being tested. Treatment of hearing loss with amplification by a hearing aid has been shown to improve quality of life. Patients demonstrating vision or hearing impairment should be referred for full ophthalmologic and audiologic evaluation. Hearing and vision impairment together are associated with lower functional status than either impairment alone.

Malnutrition is not uncommon in older adults and is associated with increased mortality, morbidity, and admission to nursing homes. In community-dwelling adults, the following definitions of malnutrition may be used: (1) involuntary weight loss [e.g., ≥4.5 kg (≥10 lb) over 6 months, ≥4% over 1 year], (2) abnormal body mass index [BMI: weight/height^2 (in kg/m^2) (e.g., BMI < 22 or BMI > 27], (3) hypoalbuminemia [e.g., ≤38 g/L (≤3.8 g/dL)], (4) hypocholesterolemia [e.g., <4.1 mmol/L (<160 mg/dL)], or (5) specific vitamin or micronutrient deficiency (e.g., vitamin B$_{12}$). When any one of these is present, a multidimensional assessment should be undertaken. The clinician should review the patient's access to food. Are there economic or other barriers to receiving high-quality food? Are there dental problems that might interfere with eating such as loose dentures, missing teeth, or other oral pathology? Many medical illnesses interfere with digestion or absorption of food, increase nutritional requirements, or require dietary restrictions. Is the patient unable to shop, prepare meals, or feed him- or herself? Does the patient have cultural habits or food preferences that could affect his or her nutritional status? Poor appetite may be related to medications, medical illnesses, or depression.

For many older adults, being independent depends on driving an automobile. However, the traffic violation rate per driver is increased in both teenagers and older drivers. One study has identified poor design copying on the MMSE, fewer blocks walked, and more foot abnormalities as the best predictors of adverse driving events. While a patient can undergo a formal driving assessment, often done by rehabilitation experts, the clinician can also indirectly assess a patient's driving skills by performing vision, cognition, and motor assessments in the office. Making the decision that an older adult is no longer able to drive is often done by the patient, but when the patient has limited insight into his or her physical and/or cognitive impairments, family, friends, health care providers, and sometimes government employees are responsible for keeping the older patient, as well as other drivers, safe.

GERIATRIC SYNDROMES

Geriatric syndrome refers to a symptom presentation that is common in older adults; most are multifactorial in origin. Several of these topics are covered in more detail elsewhere in the text.

Dementia and Delirium   Dementia is a syndrome of progressive decline in which multiple intellectual abilities deteriorate, causing both cognitive and functional impairment. While dementia is a state of chronic confusion, delirium is an acute state of confusion. It is important to differentiate delirium from dementia. Early identification and treatment of the underlying causes of delirium can improve outcomes. Delirium may be the only manifestation of a life-threatening illness in the older adult. Both dementia and delirium are characterized by disorientation, memory impairment, paranoia, hallucinations, emotional lability, and sleep-wake cycle reversal. Key features of delirium are acute onset, impaired attention, and an altered level of consciousness. Dementia and delirium are described more fully in Chaps. 365 and 26, respectively.

The main goals of care of a patient with dementia are to maintain an optimal quality of life and to maximize cognitive and physical functioning. Therefore, when an older patient presents with cognitive impairment, a key goal is to identify and treat reversible causes of cognitive impairment, such as infections, electrolyte abnormalities, vitamin deficiencies, thyroid disease, substance abuse, medication, and psychiatric illnesses. The clinician must then ask key questions: (1) Is the patient safe in the community? (2) Is the patient able to perform his or her own ADLs and IADLs? (3) What assistance is needed to maximize the patient's functioning in his or her living situation? The

patient may not be able to answer these questions accurately, so an objective, cognitively intact informant will be helpful.

If the patient has dangerous behaviors, such as leaving the stove on or getting lost, a plan of care involving increased patient supervision should be put in place. As dementia progresses, more caregiving services, both formal and informal, will need to be added to support the patient in the community. *Formal caregivers* are paid care providers. Examples are visiting nurses, home health aides who assist with personal hygiene, homemakers who assist with housework and meal preparation, Meals-on-Wheels, adult day programs, state aging services, and hospice services. *Informal caregivers* are persons who provide an older adult with unpaid care. Examples are family members, friends, neighbors, or church members.

The primary caregiver of a patient with dementia may need more physician support than the patient. Caring for a disabled spouse or parent is associated with an increased risk of depression or anxiety. Caregivers experiencing mental or emotional strain have an increased risk of dying compared to non-caregivers. Predictors of nursing home admission for patients with Alzheimer's disease include aggression, assault, paranoia, nighttime wandering, and loss of capacity to recognize the caregiver. Adult day care and respite programs may help to alleviate some caregiver burden. Support groups, through organizations such as the Alzheimer's Association, can also help to educate caregivers and decrease stress.

When patients with dementia exhibit agitated behaviors, medical illnesses, such as infections, pain syndromes, and drug side effects, must be ruled out as causes. These behaviors are, however, often part of a dementing illness. If the agitated behavior is harmful to the patient or others and does not respond to non-pharmacologic therapies, such as redirecting the patient, providing a calm environment, or familiar surroundings, then low doses of psychotropic medication may be helpful. Antipsychotics, anxiolytics, or antidepressants can be used, depending on the type of symptoms. Low-dose risperidone (0.25–1.5 mg/d) or olanzapine (2.5–10 mg/d) can be used if a patient has upsetting delusions or hallucinations. Antidepressants such as citalopram (10–30 mg/d) can be used for depressive symptoms. Patients on antipsychotics should be monitored closely for the development of extrapyramidal side effects, such as tremor, rigidity, and bradykinesia. The lowest dose possible should be used; dosage reductions should be attempted, if possible, at 6-month intervals. Sometimes, as cognitive functioning worsens, patients will no longer have the psychoses or the depression causing the agitated behaviors.

Falls   This discussion of falls excludes falls occurring from seizure, stroke, syncope, or an insurmountable environmental hazard (Chap. 24). Fall rates and risk of injury from falls increase with age. Annually, ~30% of community dwelling adults >65 years fall, while 50% of individuals >80 years fall. Injuries in 20–30% of fallers reduce subsequent mobility and independence, with 3–5% of falls resulting in fracture. Falling is an independent risk factor for nursing home placement. Often the occurrence of a fall does not come to the attention of the health care provider. Given fall frequency and resulting morbidity and mortality from falling in older adults, all older patients should have a fall risk assessment and be asked about falls in the past year.

While most falls are multifactorial, falling is sometimes a symptom of another disease, such as an infection or neurologic disorder, or a medication side effect. In addition, age-related physiologic changes contribute to fall risk. These include decreased proprioception, increased postural sway, and declines in baroreflex sensitivity resulting in orthostatic hypotension. The evaluation of a fall should begin with a history, including the circumstances at the time of the fall, any associated symptoms, and a thorough medication review of both prescription and over-the-counter medications. The physical examination should include postural vital signs, vision evaluation, gait and balance testing, and a musculoskeletal evaluation of joint stability and range of motion. An environmental assessment of the patient's home by a visiting nurse or other health care provider can reveal additional hazards that can increase fall risk, such as clutter, loose carpets, and poor lighting.

58 Interventions designed to reduce fall rates must also preserve mobility and independence. Physical restraint use has been found to be strongly associated with increased fall risk and increased risk for serious injury from a fall in nursing home residents. The major risk factors for falls are shown in Table 9-3. Several factors associated with increased risk for falling include low creatinine clearance [<1.1 mL/s (< 65 mL/min)], low serum 25-hydroxyvitamin D levels (< 39 nmol/L) and high serum parathyroid hormone levels, insomnia, and fear of falling. Table 9-3 also outlines suggested interventions targeted at common fall risk factors. General exercise and balance training; t'ai chi; psychotropic medication elimination; and multidisciplinary, multifactorial, risk factor screening and intervention have been shown to reduce fall risk.

Urinary Incontinence UI is a major problem for older adults, afflicting up to 30% of community-dwelling elders and 50% of nursing home residents. Up to age 80 years, UI affects women twice as commonly as men; after age 80, the sexes are equally affected. In addition to the great impact of UI on a patient's well-being, including embarrassment, social isolation, and depression, UI is also a risk factor for nursing home placement. While certainly not a normal part of aging, advanced age, functional impairment, dementia, obesity, smoking, affective disorder, constipation, certain medical illnesses (such as chronic obstructive pulmonary disease and heart failure), and a history of pelvic surgery are associated with UI. UI is often due to a combination of these risk factors.

Older patients must be asked directly whether they have symptoms of UI, since only half of community-dwelling women with incontinence will discuss their incontinence with a health care provider. UI can then be determined to be either *transient* or *established*, although "transient" UI may be misdiagnosed as "established" if left untreated. The "DRIIIPP" mnemonic (Table 9-4) is very useful when evaluating a patient for reversible conditions that may cause or contribute to UI. If these conditions are identified and treated, the older adult benefits from relief of UI and symptoms of other comorbidities.

Leaking of urine occurs in four ways. The bladder can be limited in its ability to empty *or* in its ability to store urine; or one or both of the urethral sphincters may be unable to allow storage of urine *or* to allow passage of urine. Impairments can exist in one or in several of the urine storage mechanisms of the lower urinary tract. Four classifications of established UI have been proposed based on this understanding of the lower urinary tract: stress incontinence, urge incontinence, mixed stress and urge incontinence, and overflow incontinence.

Stress incontinence, which is rare in men, results when the urethral sphincter mechanisms are inadequate to hold urine during bladder filling. Patients describe symptoms of leaking small amounts of urine during activities that increase intraabdominal pressure, such as coughing, laughing, sneezing, lifting, or standing up. Patient history is very sensitive (0.906) but not very specific (0.511) in diagnosing stress incontinence. A stress test in the office can be performed by having the patient stand with a full bladder and cough. The test is positive if urine leakage coincides with the cough. An involuntary bladder contraction induced by the cough may cause leakage several seconds after the cough. The most common causes of stress incontinence in women are insufficient pelvic support due to childbearing, gynecologic surgery, and the decreased effects of estrogen on tissues of the lower urinary tract. Surgical interventions are the most effective treatments; pelvic muscle exercises can be helpful, although treatment failure is higher in patients who have two or more leakages per day.

Urge incontinence, also known as detrusor overactivity (DO), is characterized by uninhibited bladder contractions and is the most common form of UI in older adults. Patients often describe symptoms of an uncontrollable need to void. Urinary frequency and nocturnal incontinence are common, particularly accompanied by loss of larger urine

TABLE 9-3 **RECOMMENDED COMPONENTS OF CLINICAL ASSESSMENT AND MANAGEMENT FOR OLDER PERSONS LIVING IN THE COMMUNITY WHO ARE AT RISK FOR FALLING**

Assessment and Risk Factor	Management
Circumstances of previous falls[a]	Changes in environment and activity to reduce the likelihood of recurrent falls
Medication use High-risk medications (e.g., benzodiazepines, other sleeping medications, neuroleptics, antidepressants, anticonvulsants, or class IA antiarrhythmics)[a,b,c] Four or more medications[c]	Review and reduction of medications
Vision[a] Acuity <20/60 Decreased depth perception Decreased contrast sensitivity Cataracts	Ample lighting without glare; avoidance of multifocal glasses while walking; referral to an ophthalmologist
Postural blood pressure (after ≥5 min in a supine position, immediately after standing, and 2 min after standing)[c] ≥20 mmHg (or ≥20%) drop in systolic pressure, with or without symptoms, either immediately or after 2 min of standing	Diagnosis and treatment of underlying cause, if possible; review and reduction of medications; modification of salt restriction; adequate hydration; compensatory strategies (e.g., elevation of head of bed, rising slowly, or dorsiflexion exercises); pressure stockings; pharmacologic therapy if the above strategies fail
Balance and gait[b,c] Patient's report or observation of unsteadiness Impairment on brief assessment (e.g., the Get-Up and Go test or performance-oriented assessment of mobility)	Diagnosis and treatment of underlying cause, if possible; reduction of medications that impair balance; environmental interventions; referral to physical therapist for assistive devices and for gait and progressive balance training
Targeted neurologic examination Impaired proprioception[a] Impaired cognition[a] Decreased muscle strength[b,c]	Diagnosis and treatment of underlying cause, if possible; increase in proprioceptive input (with an assistive device or appropriate footwear that encases the foot and has a low heel and thin sole); reduction of medications that impede cognition; awareness on the part of caregivers of cognitive deficits; reduction of environmental risk factors; referral to physical therapist for gait, balance, and strength training
Targeted musculoskeletal examination: examination of legs (joints and range of motion) and examination of feet[a]	Diagnosis and treatment of the underlying cause, if possible; referral to physical therapist for strength, range-of-motion, and gait and balance training and for assistive devices; use of appropriate footwear; referral to podiatrist
Targeted cardiovascular examination[b] Syncope Arrhythmia (if there is known cardiac disease, an abnormal electrocardiogram, and syncope)	Referral to cardiologist; carotid-sinus massage (in the case of syncope)
Home-hazard evaluation after hospital discharge[b,c]	Removal of loose rugs and use of nightlights; nonslip bath-mats, and stair rails; other interventions as necessary

[a]Recommendation of this assessment is based on observational data that the finding is associated with an increased risk of falling.
[b]Recommendation of this assessment is based on one or more randomized controlled trials of a single intervention.
[c]Recommendation of this assessment is based on one or more randomized controlled trials of a multifactorial intervention strategy that included this component.
Source: ME Tinetti: N Engl J Med 348:45, 2003; with permission.

<table>
<tr><td colspan="2">

TABLE 9-4 REVERSIBLE CONDITIONS ASSOCIATED WITH URINARY INCONTINENCE

</td></tr>
</table>

Delirium
Restricted mobility—illness, injury, gait disorder, restraint
Infection—acute, symptomatic urinary tract infection
Inflammation—atrophic vaginitis
Impaction—of feces
Polyuria—diabetes, caffeine intake, volume overload
Pharmaceuticals—diuretics, α-adrenergic agonists or antagonists, anticholinergic agents (psychotropics, antidepressants, anti-Parkinsonians)

Source: After DB Reuben et al.

volumes (>100 mL). Urge incontinence may be idiopathic, associated with lesions of the central nervous system, such as a stroke, or be due to bladder irritation from infection, stones, or tumors. The term *detrusor hyperactivity with impaired contractility* (DHIC) is a type of urge incontinence characterized by involuntary bladder contractions with a weak detrusor muscle leading to incomplete emptying of the bladder. The diagnosis is primarily based on a patient's symptoms in the absence of urinary retention and the leakage of urine with stress maneuvers.

Measurement of postvoid residual (PVR) should be part of an incontinence evaluation in all patients. Under sterile conditions, the patient's bladder is catheterized 5–10 min after the patient has voided. Generally, a PVR > 200 mL suggests detrusor underactivity or obstruction. The patient should be referred for further urologic evaluation.

Initial treatment of urge incontinence should be bladder retraining by encouraging the patient to void every 2 h or based on the patient's symptom frequency. The patient can also try urgency control by sitting or standing quietly while focusing on allowing the urgency to pass before slowly walking to the bathroom to void. If the patient has no incontinence for 2 days, the voiding interval can be increased by 30–60 minutes until the patient is only voiding every 3–4 h. The anticholinergic drugs, oxybutinin and tolterodine, which cause bladder relaxation, can be added to this therapy. Their use in older adults may be limited by anticholinergic symptoms such as urinary retention, confusion, constipation, and dry mouth. Patients using tolterodine have a reduced risk of dry mouth and fewer withdrawals due to side effects, but the efficacy of oxybutinin and tolterodine is similar.

Mixed incontinence refers to UI where symptoms of both stress and urge incontinence are present. A simple, quick questionnaire consisting of three incontinence questions (3IQ) may help to classify urge and stress incontinence in women in the primary care setting. Question one asks if the patient has leaked urine in the past 3 months. Question two familiarizes patients with types of incontinence: stress, urge, or other. Question three asks the patient for the category of incontinence based on her symptoms during the past 3 months: stress, urge, mixed, or other. The 3IQ improved the likelihood of a positive diagnosis of urge incontinence (+likelihood ratio of 3.29) and of stress incontinence (+likelihood ratio of 2.13).

Overflow incontinence is due to either bladder outlet obstruction or an atonic bladder. Male patients, but rarely females, may complain of dribbling after voiding, an incessant urge to urinate, or straining to urinate. On physical examination, patients may have a palpable distended bladder. Prostatic hypertrophy, prostate cancer, and urethral strictures are the most common causes of overflow incontinence in men, while a cystocele can cause this problem in women. Detrusor atonicity or underactivity can be caused by spinal cord disease, autonomic neuropathy of diabetes, alcoholism, vitamin B_{12} deficiency, Parkinson's disease, tabes dorsalis, or chronic outlet obstruction. Urodynamic testing is helpful in distinguishing urethral obstruction from detrusor underactivity. The most effective treatment for bladder outlet obstruction is surgical removal of the obstruction. Intermittent or indwelling catheterization may be required for nonoperative candidates with obstruction or for patients with detrusor underactivity. For men who have benign prostatic hypertrophy (BPH) and are not in retention, α-adrenergic blockers such as terazosin, doxazosin, or tamulosin can decrease symptoms of urinary frequency and nocturia. Finasteride, a 5α-reductase inhibitor, may be useful in combination with doxazosin for decreasing lower urinary tract symptoms due to BPH in men with a total prostate volume of ≥25 mL.

The diagnosis of *functional incontinence* describes individuals who have UI and have either cognitive or functional impairments which limit their ability to toilet themselves. However, other treatable causes of UI may be missed if one assumes dementia or immobility is the cause of UI in these patients.

Pressure Ulcers Pressure ulcers, also known as pressure sores, bedsores, or decubitus ulcers, occur in older patients with reduced mobility. A pressure ulcer occurs when increased pressure between skin and a bony prominence produces tissue necrosis. While pressure ulcers can occur anywhere, 80% of pressure ulcers occur over the heels, lateral malleoli, sacrum, ischia, and greater trochanters. Shear forces, causing stretching and angulation of blood vessels, and frictional forces, causing separation of the epidermal or dermal layers, can also lead to tissue necrosis and open ulceration. Moisture can increase friction leading to maceration and superficial skin erosions.

Reported incidence data for the United States vary widely by site of care: general acute care, 0.4–38%; long-term care, 2.2–23.9%; and home care, 0–17%. Prevalence rates range from 10–18% in general acute care, 2.3–28% in long-term care, and 0–29% in home care. In older adults and nursing home residents, the development of a pressure ulcer increases mortality by fourfold. Osteomyelitis and sepsis are important, morbid complications of pressure ulcers.

The notion that all pressure ulcers are preventable is controversial. While repositioning patients at risk for developing pressure ulcers every 2 h and providing bedbound patients mattresses with pressure-relieving capabilities are standard interventions to prevent pressure ulcers, other immutable risk factors may ultimately contribute to skin breakdown in certain patients. Major risk factors associated with the development of pressure ulcers are listed in Table 9-5.

When an ulcer is identified, one must try to identify its etiology. Pressure ulcers lie at sites of pressure. Diabetic ulcers can also be caused by pressure in extremities compromised by neuropathy and vascular disease, including both large and small blood vessels. Venous stasis ulcers develop on the lower extremities with or without edema due to incompetent valves of the veins. Arterial ischemic ulcers develop at sites of decreased blood flow. Since adequate blood supply is necessary for tissue to heal, assessment of pulses and ankle-brachial indices (ABI) for ulcers of the lower extremities can provide prognostic information. An ABI of <0.4 is associated with a low likelihood of wound healing. If the patient is not a surgical candidate for revascularization, the goal of care must be to keep the wound free of infection and to alleviate any related patient discomfort.

When an ulcer is identified as a pressure ulcer, the ulcer should be staged so that the appropriate therapy may be instituted. The staging in

<table>
<tr><td colspan="2">

TABLE 9-5 MAJOR RISK FACTORS ASSOCIATED WITH THE DEVELOPMENT OF PRESSURE ULCERS IN THE OLDER ADULT

</td></tr>
</table>

Alterations in sensation or response to discomfort
Degenerative neurologic disease
Cerebrovascular disease
Central nervous system (CNS) injury
Depression
Drugs that adversely affect alertness

Alterations in mobility
Neurologic disease/injury
Fractures
Pain
Restraints

Significant changes in weight (≥5% in 30 days or ≥10% in the previous 180 days)
Protein-calorie undernutrition
Edema

Incontinence
Bowel and bladder

Source: From American Medical Directors Association (AMDA): *Pressure Ulcers.* Columbia, MD, American Medical Directors Association, 1996.

TABLE 9-6 STAGING SYSTEM FOR PRESSURE ULCERS

Stage 1
Nonblanchable erythema of intact skin, or dislocation, edema, induration, and warmth over a bony prominence among patients with darker skin; the heralding lesion of skin ulceration.

Stage 2
Partial thickness skin loss involving epidermis, dermis, or both. The ulcer is superficial and presents clinically as an abrasion, blister, or shallow crater.

Stage 3
Full thickness skin loss involving damage to, or necrosis of, subcutaneous tissue that may extend down to, but not through, fascia. The ulcer presents clinically as a deep crater with or without undermining adjacent tissue.

Stage 4
Full thickness skin loss with extensive destruction, tissue necrosis or damage to muscle, bone, or supporting structures (e.g., tendon, joint capsule). Undermining and sinus tracts also may be associated with Stage 4 pressure ulcers.

Source: From American Medical Directors Association (AMDA): *Pressure Ulcers.* Columbia, MD, American Medical Directors Association, 1996.

Table 9-6 is based on a system developed in 1989 by the National Pressure Ulcer Advisory Panel. Nonblanching erythema constitutes vascular damage and hemorrhage. Stage 1 ulcers can progress to stage 4 ulcers in as little as a day or two, depending on how deeply the necrosis extends. Once a hard, dark eschar develops, the ulcer cannot be staged until the necrotic tissue is removed. Three major steps in pressure ulcer management lead to wound healing: debridement, cleansing, and dressing. *Debridement*, either surgical or chemical, is necessary to remove necrotic tissue to allow new granulation tissue to grow. Necrotic tissue can also contain bacteria that impede wound healing. *Cleansing* the wound helps to lower bacteria counts. Normal saline is best, as its use protects new granulation tissue. In foul-smelling, infected wounds, bacteriocidal agents such as 1% povidine-iodine, 0.25% acetic acid, or 0.5% sodium hypochlorite (Dakin's solution) can be used as disinfectants, but not for more than a week at a time as they are cytotoxic to fibroblasts and delay wound healing. A discussion of which *dressing* to use is beyond the scope of this chapter, but the choice of a dressing should be based on the ulcer stage, whether or not local infection is present, whether or not excessive exudate is present, and whether continued debridement is necessary. Management of pressure ulcers should be interdisciplinary involving physicians, nurses, wound care specialists, occupational or physical therapists, and nutritionists. Usually, stage 1 and 2 pressure ulcers heal in days to weeks, whereas healing of stage 3 and 4 ulcers may be seen at 2–4 weeks, but they often take many months to heal.

PREVENTION AND HEALTHY AGING

Central to the care of older adults is the prevention of functional decline, accidents, and the development of new diseases or worsening of prevalent ones. When asked, most older adults identify maintenance of independence as their top priority. Thus, although the U.S. Preventive Services Task Force (USPSTF) has 30 recommendations for primary and secondary disease prevention in older adults, those most likely to help elders achieve their goal of maintaining independence are emphasized here. Specific discussions of vision and hearing, safe driving, and falls risk are discussed elsewhere in this chapter.

Nutrition Adequate nutrition is fundamental to healthy aging. In general, energy requirements decrease with age due to a decline in lean body mass and decreased physical activity. Despite this decrease, older adults may be at risk of undernutrition due to medication side effects; functional, visual, or cognitive impairment; oral disease, swallowing disorders, or loss of smell/taste; depression and social isolation; and chronic illnesses.

Although the proportional requirements of protein, fat, and carbohydrates do not change with age, calories from carbohydrate sources gradually substitute for those from fat. To maintain adequate caloric intake and also promote cardiovascular health, substitution of mononounsaturated (olive oil, canola oil, peanuts, avocados, nuts, seeds),

omega-3 (sardines, mackerel, salmon, tuna, flounder, haddock), and omega-6 (liquid vegetable oils) fatty acids (the so-called "Mediterranean Diet") for *trans* fatty acids may be beneficial. As older adults tend to have lower intakes of both dietary fiber and fluids, increased intake of both should be encouraged, particularly as antidotes for age-related constipation. Although vitamin requirements do not change with age, older adults are particularly prone to inadequate intake of vitamins D and B_{12} and calcium, and supplementation should be considered.

Functional Decline There are 14 million noninstitutionalized older adults with functional disabilities, with a greater proportion of women being disabled (43%) than men (40%). Exercise improves body composition, psychological well-being, and disease outcomes, and reduces risk of injurious falls. Physical and cognitive exercise may also reduce the risk of dementia. Even the most sedentary of individuals appear to benefit from increasing physical activity. All patients should be asked about their level of physical activity, e.g., the number of days during an average week that they spend at least 15 min walking, bicycling, swimming, weight training, etc. An exercise prescription may be beneficial. It should consider flexibility, endurance, strength, and balance but should be preceded by attention to musculoskeletal problems, footwear, and risk factors for cardiovascular disease. Guidelines for such a prescription are shown in Table 9-7.

An exercise program should be initiated gradually. Increasingly, community organizations provide supervised group programs. The National Institute on Aging also has a range of on-line and video resources for older adults.

Accident Prevention In addition to exercise, attention to accident prevention is critical. Falls risk assessment is addressed above. In addition, exercise, particularly directed at balance, resistance, and aerobic training, decreases risk. Seatbelt use should be encouraged. Per mile driven, older adults are at highest risk of serious injury or death as a result of motor vehicle accidents. Assessment of the ability to drive safely is critical to motor vehicle safety (see above). With many older adults riding bicycles, motorcycles, and mopeds, patients should be encouraged to use helmets. Head injuries are common among riders and are particularly devastating to older adults; helmets mitigate this risk.

Although moderate alcohol consumption has been associated with many salutary effects, it is not without consequences for older adults who, because of age-related changes in alcohol distribution, increased brain sensitivity to its effects, and the potential for medication-alcohol interactions, are at risk for alcohol side effects at lower levels of consumption than their younger counterparts. When the definition of at least 12 drinks per year is used, 29% of older adults are classified as regular consumers: 40% of men and 21% of women. The National Institute on Alcohol Abuse and Alcoholism recommends that both men and women aged ≥65 consume no more than three drinks in a day and no more than seven drinks in a week, while the American Geriatrics Society recommends no more than two drinks on any single drinking occasion. Lower drinking limits or abstinence is recommended for those who take medications that interact with alcohol or who have a health condition exacerbated by alcohol. An approach to screening for heavy drinking is first to ask about heavy drinking days in the past year. If a man reports that he consumed five or more drinks in a day, or a woman reports that she consumed four or more drinks in a day, further questioning is warranted. The 10-item AUDIT (Alcohol Use Disorders Identification Test) is a validated strategy for identifying unhealthy drinking.

DISEASE PREVENTION AND EARLY DETECTION

Immunizations Although vaccine efficacy declines with age, the risks of no vaccination far outweigh the consequences of less than complete protection. Influenza vaccination is thus recommended annually, and all adults ≥65 should receive the pneumococcal vaccine at least once. In addition, a one-time revaccination should be given if the original vaccination was ≥5 years earlier and persons were ≤65 years at the time of primary vaccination. Tetanus vaccinations should be administered every 10 years.

TABLE 9-7 RECOMMENDATIONS FOR OPTIMAL AGING AND PREVENTION AND TREATMENT OF DISEASE IN OLDER ADULTS

Modality	Resistance Training	Cardiovascular Endurance Training	Flexibility Training	Balance Training
Dose				
Frequency	2–3 days/week	3–7 days/week	1–7 days/week	3–7 days/week
Volume	1–3 sets of 8–12 repetitions, 8–10 major muscle groups	20–60 min per session	Major muscle groups 1 sustained stretch (20 s) of each	1–2 sets of 4–10 different exercises emphasizing dynamic postures[a]
Intensity	15–18 on Perceived Exertion Scale (70–80% 1 RM), 6 s/repetition, 1–2 min rest between sets	12–14 on Perceived Exertion Scale (50–60% heart rate reserve or maximal exercise capacity)	Progressive neuromuscular facilitation technique[b]	Progressive difficulty as tolerated, at the level that is not yet mastered[c]
Requirements for safety and maximal efficacy	Slow speed, no ballistic movements, day of rest between sessions Good form, no substitution of muscles No breath holding, Valsalva maneuver Increase weight progressively to maintain relative intensity at high load If possible, power training (high-velocity, high-loading) provides benefits of increased strength, power, endurance, balance, and bone density	Low-impact activity if arthritis present; high impact more potent for bone remodeling Weight-bearing, best include hills/stairs if possible Increase workload progressively to maintain relative intensity Perceived exertion better than monitoring pulse to gauge intensity May accumulate short bouts (10 min) of exercise to reach volume goal One hour/week high-intensity endurance exercise equivalent to 3–4 hours/week moderate-intensity endurance exercise for cardiovascular/metabolic benefits	Static rather than ballistic stretching Stretch warmed muscles after other exercises are complete, as part of cooldown	Safe environment or monitoring Dynamic as well as static modes of training Gradual increase in difficulty as competence is demonstrated

[a]Examples of balance enhancing activities include t'ai chi movements, standing yoga or ballet movements, tandem walking, standing on one leg, stepping over objects, climbing up and down steps slowly, turning, standing on heels and toes, walking on compliant surface such as foam mattresses, maintaining balance on moving vehicle such as bus or train, and dual tasking (addition of a cognitive distractor such as naming animals while balancing), etc.
[b]Proprioceptive neuromuscular facilitation involves stretching as far as possible, then relaxing the involved muscles, then attempting to stretch further, and finally holding the maximal stretch position for at least 20 s.
[c]Intensity is increased by decreasing the base of support (e.g., progressing from standing on two feet while holding onto the back of a chair to standing on one foot with no hand support); by decreasing other sensory input (e.g., closing eyes or standing on a foam pillow); or by perturbing the center of mass (e.g., holding a heavy object out to one side while maintaining balance, standing on one leg while lifting other leg out behind body, or leaning forward as far as possible without falling or moving feet).
Note: 1 RM, one repetition maximum that is a measure of maximal dynamic strength: the maximal weight one can lift with a particular muscle group one time in good form; the Perceived Exertion Scale of is a self-rating of how hard one's body is working.
Source: From MAF Singh: J Gerontol: Med Sci 57A:M274, 2002; with permission.

Bone Health Some 70% of women ≥80 years have osteoporosis. Given this substantial risk, the significant morbidity and mortality associated with osteoporotic fractures, and the proven efficacy of bisphosphonates in increasing bone mineral density and preventing fractures, all women >65 years should receive dual-energy x-ray absorptiometry (DEXA) screening at least once. The most appropriate interval between screening tests has not been determined, although a minimum of 2 years is recommended to reliably measure a change in bone density. Although routine measurement of vitamin D levels is not recommended, women who are at high risk for deficiency by virtue of dietary insufficiency and/or lack of sun exposure should be considered for screening.

Cancer Screening The effect of cancer screening is not evident for at least 3–5 years; thus, screening is not likely to be of benefit in persons with a limited life expectancy. Individual values and preferences are clearly also important considerations.

BREAST CANCER The incidence of breast cancer increases with age and peaks in the eighth decade. The sensitivity and specificity of mammography reaches its maximum in the ninth decade. Over 25% of breast cancer deaths occur in women ≥80 years. These facts suggest that mammographic screening would be of benefit in older women; however, only two clinical trials have examined the efficacy of mammographic screening in women ≥70 years, and both were inconclusive. The best supporting observational evidence comes from two Surveillance, Epidemiology, and End Results Medicare studies that found an association between screening mammography and decreased breast cancer mortality. Mammography screening in the 2 years preceding a diagnosis of breast cancer eliminated the age-related disparities in size and stage of the breast tumor at diagnosis.

Annual clinical breast examination (CBE) is a potentially attractive screening alternative to mammography, since the postmenopausal atrophy of breast tissue improves CBE sensitivity in older women compared to younger women. It is also less uncomfortable and cheaper than a mammogram. However, it should be used to complement mammographic screening and reserved as a stand alone strategy only for women who refuse or cannot undergo mammography.

PROSTATE CANCER Prostate cancer screening in older men is a particularly challenging topic as many more older men die with prostate cancer than from it. Nonetheless, 92% of prostate cancer deaths occur in men who are >65 years. Although prostate cancer can be detected earlier via prostate-specific antigen testing, mortality from prostate cancer has not been reduced as a result of screening. The U.S. Preventive Services Task Force has concluded that evidence to recommend for or against screening is lacking. Other organizations such as the American Cancer Society and American Urological Society recommend screening among those with at least a 10-year life expectancy. The matter is complicated by the fact that techniques to treat prostate cancer often greatly affect quality of life. Furthermore, we are not able to reliably predict whether a particular prostate cancer is life-threatening. Given the uncertainties, PSA screening should be reserved for the most robust of older men and only after a thorough discussion of the arguments for and against screening.

COLORECTAL CANCER Annual or biennial fecal occult blood testing (FOBT) reduces mortality in those up to age 80. Other screening options include sigmoidoscopy (every 5 years), FOBT and sigmoidoscopy (every 5 years), double-contrast barium enema (every 5–10 years), and colonoscopy (every 10 years). No one method has been shown to be superior, and all methods are cost effective. Digital rectal examination (DRE) alone or with a FOBT is not recommended (though DRE is used to screen for prostate cancer). The choice of a colorectal cancer screening strategy is based on many considerations, including procedure risk. Colonoscopy might seem the most attractive option; the colon can be completely visualized and biopsies taken if the examination is positive. If the examination is negative, it does not need to be repeated for 10 years. However, adequate preparation requires lower extremity strength and mobility, and the ability to tolerate substantial fluid losses. Furthermore, the procedure has a small risk of bowel perforation or bleeding. Yet about half of colon cancers occur beyond the reach of a sigmoidoscope.

LUNG CANCER   Although lung cancer is also a leading killer, no screening interventions have been shown to be effective.

Disease Risk Modification   Longitudinal studies are providing evidence that risk factor modification, especially smoking cessation and blood pressure reduction, particularly in mid-life but also up to age 75, results in greater gains in life-years than do medical and surgical therapies, especially in men. In addition, lower levels of risk factors in mid-life are associated with survival free of major morbidity to age 85. Although lifestyle modifications in mid-life are important, modifications even late in life may make a difference. A person is never too old to benefit from smoking cessation.

Older adults are also at risk for obesity, which is becoming more common among successive birth cohorts. Among men, 33.4% of those 65–74 years are obese compared to 20.4% among those >75 years. For women, the comparable figures are 38.8% and 25.1%. Weight loss in obese older adults has the potential advantage of improving mobility and decreasing the severity of comorbidities. Nonetheless, it should be pursued cautiously and be coupled with aerobic and resistance training, since many obese persons are relatively sarcopenic. No data confirm the efficacy and safety of pharmacotherapies for obesity in older persons. Although bariatric surgery has higher perioperative morbidity/mortality in older adults, if successful it can also result in improvements in the severity of comorbidities.

FURTHER READINGS

BROWN JS et al: The sensitivity and specificity of a simple test to distinguish between urge and stress urinary incontinence. Ann Intern Med 144:715, 2006

CASSEL CK et al (eds): *Geriatric Medicine: An Evidence-Based Approach*, 4th ed. New York, Springer-Verlag, 2003

KIRKLAND JL et al: Adipogenesis and aging: Does aging make fat go MAD? Exp Gerontol 37:757, 2002

PERLS T, TERRY D: Understanding the determinants of exceptional longevity. Ann Intern Med 139:445, 2003

REUBEN DB et al: *Geriatrics At Your Fingertips: 2006–2007*, 8th ed. New York: The American Geriatrics Society, 2006

TINETTI ME et al: Potential pitfalls of disease-specific guidelines for patients with multiple conditions. N Engl J Med 351:2870, 2004

WALTER LC et al: Screening for colorectal, breast, and cervical cancer in the elderly: A review of the evidence. Am J Med 118:1078, 2005

10 Complementary and Alternative Medicine

Stephen E. Straus[†]

BACKGROUND

Medicine, not long ago the domain of solitary generalists and their nurse assistants, now engages scores of specialists and allied professionals—radiation physicists, cytologists, nurse practitioners, psychiatric social workers, dental hygienists, and many more—who wield tools of unprecedented ability to extend life and sustain its quality. This evolution of the health care system has been achieved, in part, by a formidable enterprise of critical observation and formal investigation that disproves some once-accepted practices and stimulates emergence of new approaches that compete for acceptance. One need only peruse the serial editions of this textbook to comprehend the scope of these changes.

Other factors have also affected evolutionary changes in medicine. Immigration and related demographic changes yield increasingly diverse populations who value their own health traditions. The public's expectations of health and the nature of the health care system itself have been altered by unprecedented access to sources of information, goods, and services; the disposable income to afford them; and a patchwork quilt of regulations and laws that constrain medical practice on the one hand and facilitate increased choice in health care on the other. The emergence of complementary and alternative medicine is one manifestation of these changes in health care.

DEFINITIONS

In every generation, medical practices exist that are not accepted by the mainstream: they are viewed with suspicion and dismissed as implausible or irrational. For a time, approaches that evoked some appeal, but which had not been thoroughly tested, were deemed *unconventional*. Over the past decade or so, they have been called *complementary and alternative medicine* (CAM), to reflect their use as adjuncts to or as substitutes for more generally accepted practices, respectively. CAM does not encompass practices that have yet to be translated fully from the laboratory into the clinic or practices that were well studied and disproved, but which manage to sustain some public appeal. Rather, CAM entails approaches with surprising pervasiveness, many of which can claim at least some evidentiary support. Until recently, CAM could also be defined as practices that are neither widely taught in medical schools nor reimbursed. However, medical students increasingly seek and receive some instruction about CAM, while third-party payers have identified in CAM a marketing tool to attract new, well-heeled clients. In the past few years, another term has been coined—*integrative medicine*—to suggest encouragingly that some CAM approaches, and the practitioners who deliver them, will be shown worthy of being added to the health care repertoire.

SCOPE

The myriad practices and products that encompass CAM (Table 10-1) can be organized into five somewhat overlapping domains. Special diets, high doses of vitamins and minerals, and extracts of animal or botanical products are grouped together as *biologically based* CAM approaches. Massage, osteopathic and chiropractic manipulation, and cranial-sacral therapies are grouped as *manipulative and body-based* CAM approaches. Diverse forms of meditation, spirituality, and various uses of hypnosis are CAM approaches that attempt to harness brain pathways to affect health and behavior. All three of these CAM domains have well-accepted analogues in conventional medicine—low-fat, low-cholesterol diets; physical therapy; and psychotherapy, to name but a few.

A fourth CAM domain is known as *energy medicine*, to reflect its exploitation of veritable or putative energy fields. Today, magnets are increasingly popular health products. Over 2000 years ago, however, while Greek physicians believed that health requires a balance of vital humors, Asian practitioners postulated the flow and balance of vital energies and described tools to restore them. Acupuncture aims to correct energies that flow through special meridians, or channels. Reiki, a Japanese approach, and healing touch, a modern variant, purport to diagnose and correct one's energy by passing the hands of an adept therapist over the patient.

[†]Deceased. Dr. Straus was a contributor to *Harrison's* since the 13th edition. He died on May 14, 2007.

TABLE 10-1 SOME COMPLEMENTARY AND ALTERNATIVE MEDICAL PRACTICES

Type	Description
Acupuncture	A Chinese medical practice that involves the insertion of hair-thin needles into nonanatomic energy channels, called meridians
Alexander technique	A movement therapy that emphasizes efficient use of muscles to relieve pain, decrease skeletal strain, and improve posture
Anthroposophic medicine	A spiritually based system of medicine that incorporates herbs, homeopathy, diet, and a movement therapy called eurythmy
Aromatherapy	The use of essential plant oils (distilled concentrates) in massage, baths, or inhalation
Ayurvedic medicine	The major East Indian traditional medicine system, utilizing pulse and tongue diagnosis; treatment includes diet, exercise, herbs, oil massages, and elimination regimens (utilizing emetics, diarrheals, etc.)
Bach flower remedies	Dilute flower infusions used to treat emotional conditions
Biofeedback	The use of machinery that translates physiologic processes into audio or visual signals
Chiropractic	Adjustments of spinal vertebrae in an effort to affect neuromuscular function
Cranial-sacral therapy	Gentle manipulation of the cranium and spine
Curanderismo	A spiritual healing tradition common in Mexican-American communities that utilizes ritual cleansing, herbs and incantations
Dance therapy	Therapeutic method that uses movement to facilitate emotional expression and release
Feldenkrais bodywork	Highly structured movement sequences that emphasize proper head positioning
Guided imagery	The use of imagination to invoke specific images that are hoped to affect physiologic function
Hydropathy	Treatment utilizing water at various temperatures, sometimes aerated or under pressure, sometimes with added salts or other substances
Hypnosis	The induction of an altered state of mind within which a subject becomes receptive to specific suggestions
Massage	The use of specific gliding and kneading strokes and friction to achieve muscle relaxation
Meditation	A process by which one tries to achieve awareness without thought
Music therapy	Singing, playing instruments, or listening to music
Naturopathy	A mixture of modalities that may include herbs, homeopathy, acupuncture, hydropathy, diet, and exercise
Native American medicine	Diverse systems, many of which incorporate prayer, chant, music, healing ceremonies, counseling, herbs, laying on of hands, and smudging (ritual cleansing with smoke from sacred plants)
Osteopathy	A medical field incorporating manipulative techniques for correcting abnormalities of the musculoskeletal system
Reflexology/zone therapy	Manual stimulation of points on the hands or feet, believed to affect distant organs
Rolfing/structural integration	A manual therapy that attempts to realign the body by deep tissue manipulation of fasciae
Shiatsu/acupressure	Finger pressure at points along nonanatomic meridians
Siddha medicine	An East Indian medical system (prevalent among Tamil-speaking people) utilizing breathing techniques, incantations, herbs, and muppu (a tri-salt preparation)
T'ai chi ch'aun	Chinese dancelike exercises described as a "moving meditation"
Therapeutic touch	Secular version of the laying on of hands, described as a "healing meditation"
Tibetan medicine	A medical system that utilizes diagnosis by pulse and urine examination; therapies include herbs, diet, and massage
Traditional Chinese medicine	A medical system that utilizes examination of the tongue and pulses for diagnosis and acupuncture, herbal mixtures, massage, exercise, and diet
Trager bodywork	Light massage combined with gentle passive movements to help patients maximize freedom of movement
Unani medicine	An East Indian medical system, derived from Persian medicine, practiced primarily in the Muslim community; also called "hikmat"
Yoga	An Indian practice that includes postures (asanas), breathing exercises (pranayama), and cleansing practices (kriyas)

The fifth domain, termed *alternative systems of medicine*, combines elements of the four other domains and aims to provide primary approaches to all health needs, rather than just adjunctive solutions to them. Western variants include practices developed by Native Americans, homeopathy, and naturopathic medicine. Eastern variants such as Ayurvedic medicine of India, traditional Chinese medicine, and Tibetan medicine are rich in their use of meditative exercises and herbal products.

PATTERNS OF USE

Despite its enormous success in prolonging life and sustaining its quality, contemporary western biomedicine has features that discourage some patients: many diseases, especially chronic ones, are neither curable nor well palliated; existing treatments can impose serious adverse reactions; and provision of care is fragmented and impersonal. CAM, despite lack of proof of efficacy, appeals to many because its practitioners are optimistic, and they invest the time to speak with and touch their patients. CAM empowers patients to make their own health choices, its natural products are believed to be inherently healthier and safer than synthetic ones, and care is provided in a "holistic" fashion, meaning that the broader medical, social, and emotional contexts of illness are considered in designing the treatment plan.

The first large survey by Eisenberg in 1993 surprised the medical community by showing that >30% of Americans use CAM approaches. Many studies since then have extended these conclusions by surveying specific demographic groups and patient populations. The Centers for Disease Control and Prevention (CDC) study of nearly 31,000 American adults revealed that in 2002 36% had used one or

more modalities, with spiritual approaches, herbal medicine, chiropractic, and massage being the most prevalent. Over 1% underwent acupuncture treatment that year. Surveys among patients with cancer showed that 30 to 86% used CAM, with highest rates in those with more advanced disease and undergoing aggressive treatments. Similarly, among AIDS patients, 36 to 91% are reported to use CAM. In devastating chronic illnesses like these, CAM is called upon to provide hope of cures when conventional medicine cannot, to extend life, to ameliorate treatment side effects, and to provide emotional and physical comfort. While somewhat subject to vagaries of definition as to what counts as a CAM treatment, surveys have shown that Americans are willing to pay for these services out of pocket, with an estimated $7 billion each year on vitamins and mineral supplements, $4 billion on herbals and other natural products, and nearly $4 billion more on sports supplements. Eisenberg reported that total CAM expenditures in 1997 approached $30 billion, with more visits to practitioners for CAM services than to physicians in general.

FIELDS OF PRACTICE

Osteopathic Medicine Founded in 1892 in the American heartland by the physician Andrew Taylor Still, osteopathic medicine was based originally on the belief that manipulation of soft tissue and bone can correct a wide range of diseases of the musculoskeletal and other organ systems. Over the ensuing century, osteopathy evolved progressively towards conventional (allopathic) medicine. Today, the training, practice, credentialing, licensure, and reimbursement of osteopathic physicians is virtually indistinguishable from those of allopathic physicians, with 4 years of osteopathic medical school followed by specialty and subspecialty training and certification by organizations such as the American Board of Internal Medicine. Some osteopathic physicians continue to practice spinal manipulation, primarily as a tool to address specific musculoskeletal complaints.

Chiropractic Medicine In 1895, Daniel David Palmer founded in Missouri the first school of chiropractic medicine to teach manipulation of the spine. Palmer believed that subluxations, or partial dislocations of vertebrae, cause disease by impinging on key nerve roots. Today, chiropractors undertake 5 years of training in basic and relevant clinical sciences. Increasingly, they complete additional postgraduate training in radiology and outpatient therapeutics, primarily of musculoskeletal conditions, although within the discipline there are factions that continue to perform manipulation for many other pathologic entities. Chiropractors also advise on nutrition, exercise, and other health maintenance approaches. Over 70,000 doctors of chiropractic medicine are licensed to practice in the United States.

Acupuncture A venerable component of traditional Chinese medicine, acupuncture emerged in recent decades as a free-standing clinical discipline. Over 3000 American physicians have acquired targeted postgraduate training that permits them to practice acupuncture in over 40 states and the District of Columbia. Over 4000 non-MDs have taken far more extended training, leading to licensure to practice independently or under the supervision of a physician.

Massage Therapy Drawing upon millennia of empirical knowledge, some 80 American schools instruct students in an array of the soft tissue manipulative approaches that constitute massage. Thirty-one states and the District of Columbia license trainees to perform therapeutic massage.

Naturopathic Medicine Twelve states license practitioners of naturopathy, a discipline that emerged in central Europe in the late eighteenth century. That conventional treatments of the day were usually ineffective, if not overtly harmful, stimulated the search for safer and more "natural" approaches—naturopathy is one of them. The concept underlying this discipline is that the body possesses powerful mechanisms for self-healing that a properly instructed practitioner could harness. About 1400 naturopathic physicians have completed 4 years of education in basic and clinical sciences and are licensed to manage a predominantly outpatient population. Conventional and unconventional diagnostic tests and medications are prescribed with an emphasis on relatively low doses of drugs, herbal medicines, special diets, and exercises.

Homeopathic Medicine The late eighteenth century also witnessed the emergence of homeopathy, another discipline that arose at least in part as a reaction to the toxicity inherent to many of the allopathic approaches of the day. Homeopathy was developed by Samuel Hahnemann, a German physician, who postulated that substances that cause particular side effects in a well person may be used to treat or prevent such symptoms in an ill person if administered in miniscule amounts—what is known as "the doctrine of similars." For example, contact with poison ivy (*Rhus toxicodendron*) causes susceptible persons to experience an itchy, blistering rash. Homeopathy espouses administration of highly diluted extracts of poison ivy to treat other blistering, pruritic eruptions such as varicella. During the early nineteenth century, the then-nascent field of homeopathy used blinded tests on volunteers, presaging wider use of placebo-controlled trials, to "prove" which materials were the most able to induce or relieve symptoms. By the mid-nineteenth century homeopathy had gained considerable presence in the American medical establishment and may, in fact, have facilitated the development of immunization and allergen desensitization, both of which utilize very small quantities of materials to elicit measurable biologic outcomes. Today, however, homeopathy is accepted less fully in the United States than in some other countries: it is the largest of all CAM practices in the United Kingdom, Germany, and France and is widely used in India. In America, only three states currently license the practice of homeopathy. The relative decline of homeopathy relates, at least in part, to the field's inability to articulate a rational mechanism as to why products that are diluted more than 10^{60}-fold, greater than Avogadro's number, could incite biologic effects. Nonetheless, homeopathic remedies are readily available and commonly recommended by naturopathic physicians and other licensed and unlicensed practitioners.

Other Disciplines There are numerous other CAM practices, among which some involve formal training, such as that leading to a Doctorate of Oriental Medicine, or extended apprenticeships, as in learning herbal medicine. Unfortunately, most of the other fields have not agreed upon practice standards, credentialing processes, requirements for continuing education, or external accountability.

REGULATION

As indicated above, some CAM disciplines are carefully regulated. CAM products, however, are not strongly regulated. Herbal medicines, and dietary supplements more generally, occupy a unique regulatory status that affords the public remarkable freedom of choice but also many undesired challenges, summarized below.

Elements of virtually all traditional healing approaches, herbal medicines were presumed safe long before the implementation of stringent drug regulations by the U.S. Food and Drug Administration (FDA). In 1994, the United States Congress passed the Dietary Supplements Health and Education Act (DSHEA) that permits sale of dietary supplements "over-the-counter," as it were, but without the requirement imposed on manufacturers of prescription or conventional over-the-counter drugs to prove their products to be safe and effective before marketing. Supplements can be removed by the FDA from the market only if they are proven to be hazardous. Purveyors of dietary supplements cannot claim them to prevent or treat any disease. They can, however, claim that they maintain "normal structure and function" of body systems. For example, a product cannot claim to treat arthritis, but it can claim to maintain "normal joint health."

Homeopathic products predate FDA drug regulations and are sold with no requirement that they be proven effective. It would be reasonable to assume, however, given the extent to which homeopathic products are diluted, that most of them are safe.

SAFETY

Despite their lack of apparent toxicities, homeopathic products, like all other CAM products and practices, do convey one type of risk, namely, that individuals will pursue them in lieu of more conventional modalities that are proven to be beneficial. Members of the public have considerable freedom to determine what is in their own best interest, even if those decisions deny them effective treatment, although the courts have found the rights of parents to withhold treatment of their children to be limited in instances of life-threatening illnesses. Investigators have a broad ethical obligation to not withhold proven treatments for serious illnesses for the sake of testing unproven ones.

Additional risks are imposed by the use of other CAM approaches: injuries inflicted by a practice, inherent toxicities of the modality, and interference by the modality with more conventional treatments.

Injury Physical and manipulative interventions can harm patients. In past decades, reused acupuncture needles transmitted hepatitis B virus infection; today, the standard of care requires disposable needles. Aggressive massage can cause soft tissue injuries. Spinal manipulation of patients with unrecognized vertebral lesions has been associated with cord injuries, and cervical manipulation has been associated with stroke. These appear to be rare events.

Inherent Toxicity While the public may believe that "natural" equates with "safe," it is abundantly clear that natural products can be toxic.

Misidentification of medicinal mushrooms has led to liver failure. Contamination of tryptophan supplements caused the eosinophilia-myalgia syndrome. Herbal products containing particular species of *Aristolochia* were associated with genitourinary malignancies. In 2001, extracts of kava, long used by Pacific Islanders for its mild anxiolytic and sedative properties, were associated with fulminant liver failure. A number of products, including the popular *Ginkgo biloba*, are known to prolong bleeding times and have been associated with postoperative hemorrhage. Among the most controversial of dietary supplements is *Ephedra sinica*, or ma huang, a product used in traditional Chinese medicine for short-term treatment of asthma and bronchial congestion. The scientific basis for these indications was revealed when ephedra was shown to contain the ephedrine alkaloids, especially ephedrine and pseudoephedrine. With the promulgation of the DSHEA regulations, supplements containing ephedra and herbs rich in caffeine sold widely in the U.S. marketplace, because of their claims to promote weight loss and to enhance athletic performance. Reports of severe and fatal adverse events associated with use of ephedra-containing products led to an evidence-based review of the data surrounding them, and finally, in 2004, the FDA banned their sale in the United States.

Herbal-Drug Interactions   The constituents of a few natural products are toxic; others are known to interfere with the metabolism of life-saving drugs. This effect was illustrated most compellingly with the demonstration in 2000 that consumption of St.-John's-wort interferes with the bioavailability of the HIV protease inhibitor indinavir. Later studies showed its similar interference with metabolism of topoisomerase inhibitors such as irinotecan, with cyclosporine, and with many other drugs. The breadth of interference stems from the ability of hyperforin in St.-John's-wort to upregulate expression of the pregnane X receptor, a promiscuous nuclear regulatory factor that promotes the expression of many hepatic oxidative, conjugative, and efflux enzymes engaged in drug and food metabolism.

ACQUIRING EVIDENCE

CAM evolved through an entirely different epistemologic framework than contemporary biomedicine. Empirical observations of individual patients constitute the primary evidentiary base on which CAM practices are guided and taught. Nonetheless, over the past few decades, thousands of studies have been performed of various CAM approaches, including hundreds of trials involving herbals, acupuncture, or homeopathy. To date, very few CAM approaches have been proved effective. Several factors contribute to this lack of convincing evidence. The vast majority of CAM studies have been seriously flawed by lack of appropriate controls, bias on the part of the investigators, small sample sizes, reliance on highly subjective and nonvalidated measures of benefit, and by inappropriate statistical tests.

In addition, a series of methodologic issues challenge even the better-designed CAM studies. No uniform practice guidelines exist, and the herbal products marketed in the United States are highly variable in quality and composition. Some CAM practices are not amenable to blinding. For example, both the patient and the practitioner would know if spinal manipulation had been performed. These problems are not unique to CAM, as they also complicate attempts to study conventional practices such as psychotherapy or surgery. Efforts are now being made to randomize patients to other equally demanding control interventions, and acupuncture at traditional needling points is being compared to needling at what are arguably irrelevant points.

Even with ongoing improvements in study design and conduct, issues of belief stand in the way of comprehending and accepting the results of some CAM studies. Many physicians are reluctant to believe positive outcomes of clinical approaches that have not emerged through the classic experimental paradigm by which drugs and biologic agents are developed, namely, the orderly progression from preclinical testing through serial phases of clinical trials. More importantly, it is difficult to accept results that are counterintuitive or whose underlying mechanism still defies rational explanation. As suggested above, an example of this

dilemma involves studies of homeopathy. Some clinical trials of homeopathy for asthma, infantile diarrhea, and other common conditions reported positive results. Two systematic reviews of homeopathy trials gleaned an overall favorable impression of the clinical trials data, concluding that the treatments were more beneficial than placebo. Even the best trials and these reviews have been criticized on methodologic grounds. It remains unclear what evidence could compel a change in belief about the benefits of homeopathy when there remain no cogent explanations for how substances diluted beyond the point at which only solute remains could exert physiologic effects.

By contrast, while methodologic problems continue to plague acupuncture trials, belief has been growing even in academic centers that acupuncture may be effective. The emerging acceptance of acupuncture results, in part, from its widespread availability and use in the United States today, even within the walls of major medical centers where it is used as an ancillary approach to pain management. Yet, its acceptance appears to stem from more than just its communal appeal. Since the mid-1970s, biochemical and imaging studies began to yield evidence that needling can trigger release of endogenous opioids that bind to specific receptors in the very brain regions that mediate the beneficial effects of narcotic analgesics.

EXISTING EVIDENCE

While it is difficult to conclude decisively that a particular CAM approach lacks any merit, it is quite feasible to discern that its effect size, or degree of benefit, is too small or inconsistent to be worth pursuing further. Over the past century, many once unconventional medical approaches failed—one need only think back to the exotic electrical devices, procedures, and tonics that fell out of fashion. Two questions are often asked: (1) Whether any of the more contemporary CAM modalities deserve to be rejected? (2) Whether data showing them to be ineffective would change anyone's mind about using them?

The case of laetrile is instructive. This extract of apricot seeds was touted in the 1970s as a cure for solid tumors. Thousands crossed the Mexican border to secure laetrile for their own use. The lack of any positive preclinical data discouraged oncologists from agreeing at first to study laetrile, until public pressure required that an answer be obtained. Two studies in the 1980s showed no benefit of laetrile treatment. Today, some continue to seek the product, but the numbers are vastly smaller than before meaningful data were obtained. A similar fate befell a cocktail of drugs used for cancer patients through the 1970s and 1980s by Dr. Luigi DiBella in Italy, once large studies revealed it to have no detectable impact on the course of a variety of advanced cancers.

In contrast, modalities that have been well tested and found ineffective are still in fairly common practice. For example, the renowned biochemist Linus Pauling proclaimed vitamin C able to effectively treat and even prevent the common cold. Several high-quality studies failed to demonstrate clinically important effects of vitamin C in preventing or treating viral colds. The early studies were criticized for using too little of the vitamin, yet doses that well exceeded its bioavailability also proved negative. Nonetheless, ingestion of extra vitamin C remains a common habit of individuals who perceive the onset of cold symptoms. For most people, this practice is wasteful but not harmful; however, people with iron overload (either hemochromatosis or chronic transfusion requirement) can be damaged by vitamin C, which generates free radicals in the setting of iron excess.

Despite the failure of some CAM approaches, early studies have yielded positive or at least encouraging data for a number of them. Good sources of information include the Natural Medicines Comprehensive Database (*www.NaturalDatabase.com*) and National Institutes of Health (NIH) websites such as *http://ods.od.nih.gov*; *http://nccam.nih.gov/health/* and *http://www3.cancer.gov/occam/information.html*.

Vitamins/Minerals

- *Vitamin A:* Large studies in a number of developing nations proved that vitamin A deficiency is prevalent and associated with increased risks of mortality in young children. Prospective trials showed that ingestion of 100,000 to 200,000 IU of vitamin A twice a year reduces the overall death rate in early childhood and possibly also the progression of HIV/AIDS significantly.

- *Folic acid:* Rates of neural tube defects in newborns are significantly diminished by folate food supplementation.
- *Folic acid, vitamin B_6, and vitamin B_{12}:* Some high-quality randomized, double-blind, controlled trials suggested that this vitamin combination lowers serum homocysteine levels, but this has not lowered the risk of cardiovascular end points.
- *Vitamins C and E, β-carotene, and zinc:* A large randomized controlled trial showed that these supplements combined reduce the progression of age-related macular degeneration.

Even vitamins and minerals, which are presumed safe in moderate doses, can have unexpected adverse effects. Two large controlled trials of β-carotene for prevention of cancer or retinal diseases found increased rates of lung cancer in those randomized to the supplement. Ongoing large prospective trials are seeking benefits from ingestion of supplements on rates of prostate cancer (vitamin E and selenium) and Alzheimer's disease (vitamin E).

Herbals and Other Natural Products

- *Glucosamine and/or chondroitin sulfate:* Systematic surveys of smaller controlled trials led to a large multicenter trial that concluded that these products are superior to placebo in improving performance and slowing the narrowing of the joint space in patients with moderate to severely painful and disabling osteoarthritis of the knee. It remains uncertain whether their use also slows degradation of joint cartilage.
- *Ginkgo biloba:* Americans spent nearly $250 million on this herbal product in 2000. The literature shows no evidence that it improves cognition, but over 3000 older Americans currently participate in a randomized blinded trial to ascertain whether its use can reduce the rate of onset and progression of dementia.
- *Saw palmetto (Serenoa repens) and African plum (Pygeum africanum):* Each of these botanicals has been advocated for aging men to obtain symptomatic relief treatment of benign prostatic hyperplasia. Sales of saw palmetto are growing, with an estimated $131 million spent on the product consumed by Americans in 2000. However, clinical trials have shown that saw palmetto is ineffective in this setting.
- *St.-John's-wort (Hypericum perforatum):* Among the most popular herbal products worldwide, numerous small studies and systematic reviews suggested it to benefit patients with a wide range of depressive syndromes. High-quality, randomized, placebo-controlled trials found St.-John's-wort to not be superior to placebo for treatment of major depression of moderate severity, a spectrum of illness that clearly warrants professional evaluation and treatment.
- *Echinacea species:* Echinacea roots are widely used to treat or prevent respiratory infections, with over $200 million in sales in 2000. Although in vitro studies have shown that *Echinacea* constituents stimulate humoral and cellular immune responses, systematic reviews of the clinical trials have not concluded that they are beneficial.

Other Modalities

- *Acupuncture:* A frequently cited NIH-led consensus development conference in 1997 concluded that acupuncture relieves nausea from chemotherapy and pain following extraction of molars. Some subsequent studies confirmed these earlier impressions regarding acute nausea and vomiting, but the data regarding pain management have been mixed, with little evidence that it benefits neuropathic pain. A well-conducted study reported in 2004, however, concluded that acupuncture provides significant adjunctive relief for patients with osteoarthritis of the knee.
- *Mind-body medicine:* Clinical trials support the use of biofeedback for incontinence, headache, and stroke rehabilitation. Hypnosis may be beneficial in relieving pain due to minor surgical interventions, chemotherapy-associated nausea, and irritable bowel syndrome.
- *Spinal manipulation:* Systematic reviews of some well-designed trials concluded that chiropractic or osteopathic manipulation provides significant improvement for patients with uncomplicated acute back pain. No proof exists that they are superior to, or more cost-effective than, other conventional approaches, nor do they alter the long-term outcome.

SUMMARY

An array of unproven modalities will always be used by the patients under our care. Physicians must approach each encounter as an opportunity to better understand their patient's beliefs and expectations and use those insights to help guide their personal health care practices in a constructive way. Many of these choices are entirely innocuous and can be accommodated in the context of the established diagnostic and therapeutic interventions. Some of these choices should be actively discouraged. Along the way, scientific evidence will drive many CAM approaches out of favor. Some modalities will garner sufficient support to become part of mainstream care: the next generation of physicians will never know they were once controversial.

FURTHER READINGS

ADAMS M, JEWELL AP: The use of complementary and alternative medicine by cancer patients. Int Semin Surg Oncol 4:10, 2007

BARNES PM et al: Complementary and alternative medicine use among adults: United States, 2002. Adv Data 27:1, 2004

BENT S et al: Saw palmetto for benign prostatic hyperplasia. N Engl J Med 354: 557, 2006

BERMAN B et al: Effectiveness of acupuncture as adjunctive therapy in osteoarthritis of the knee: A randomized, controlled trial. Ann Intern Med 141: 120, 2004

DE SMET PA: Herbal remedies. N Engl J Med 347:2046, 2002

EISENBERG DM et al: Trends in alternative medicine use in the United States, 1990–1997: Results of a follow-up national survey. JAMA 280:1569, 1998

KAPTCHUK TJ: Acupuncture: Theory, efficacy and practice. Ann Intern Med 136:374, 2002

KINSEL JF, STRAUS SE: Complementary and alternative therapeutics: Rigorous research is needed to support claims. Annu Rev Pharmacol Toxicol 43:463, 2003

11 Palliative and End-of-Life Care
Ezekiel J. Emanuel, Joshua Hauser, Linda L. Emanuel

EPIDEMIOLOGY

In 2003, 2,448,288 individuals died in the United States (Table 11-1). Over 70% of all deaths occur in those >65 years of age. The epidemiology of mortality is similar in most developed countries; cardiovascular diseases and cancer are the predominant causes of death, a marked change since 1900, when heart disease caused ~8% of all deaths and cancer accounted for <4% of all deaths. In 2003, AIDS accounted for <1% of all deaths, although among those age 35–44, it remains a leading cause of death.

It is estimated that in developed countries ~70% of all deaths are preceded by a disease or condition such that it is reasonable to plan for dying in the foreseeable future. Cancer has served as the paradigm for terminal care, but it is not the only type of illness with a recognizable and predictable terminal phase. Since heart failure, chronic obstructive pulmonary disease (COPD), chronic liver failure, dementia, and many

TABLE 11-1 TEN LEADING CAUSES OF DEATH IN THE UNITED STATES AND BRITAIN

	United States			Britain	
Cause of Death	Number of Deaths	Percent of Total	Number of Deaths Among People ≥65 Years of Age	Number of Deaths	Percent of Total
All deaths	2,448,288	100	1,804,373	538,254	100
Heart disease	685,089	28	563,390	129,009	24
Cancer	556,902	22.7	388,390	135,955	25.3
Stroke	157,689	6.4	138,134	57,808	10.7
Chronic obstructive pulmonary disease	126,382	5.2	109,139	27,905	5.2
Accidents	109,277	4.5	34,335	10,979	2
Diabetes	74,219	3	54,919	6316	1.2
Pneumonia/influenza	65,163	2.7	57,670	34,477	6.4
Alzheimer's disease	63,457	2.6	62,814	5055	0.9
Nephritis, nephritic syndrome, nephrosis	42,453	1.7	35,254	3287	0.6
Septicemia	34,069	1.3	26,445	2206	0.4

Source: National Center for Health Statistics (2003) *http://www.cdc.gov/nchs*; National Statistics (Great Britain, 2003) *http://www.statistics.gov.uk.*

other conditions have recognizable terminal phases, a systematic approach to end-of-life care should be part of all medical specialties. Many patients with illness-related suffering can also benefit from palliative care, regardless of prognosis. Ideally, palliative care should be considered as a part of comprehensive care for all patients.

Over the past few decades in the United States, a significant change in the site of death has occurred that coincides with patient and family preferences. Nearly 60% of Americans died as inpatients in hospitals in 1980. By 2000, the trend was reversing, with ~40% of Americans dying as hospital inpatients (Fig. 11-1). This shift has been most dramatic for those dying from cancer and COPD and for younger and very old individuals. In the past decade, it is associated with the increased use of hospice care; in 2005, ~33% of all decedents in the United States received such care. Cancer patients currently constitute ~50% of hospice users, with ~60% of all terminal cancer patients receiving hospice care. About 70% of patients receiving hospice care die out of the hospital. In addition, with shortening of hospital stays, many serious conditions are being treated at home or on an outpatient basis. Consequently, providing optimal palliative and end-of-life care requires ensuring that appropriate services are available in a variety of settings, including noninstitutional settings.

HOSPICE AND THE PALLIATIVE CARE FRAMEWORK

Central to this type of care is an interdisciplinary team approach that typically encompasses pain and symptom management, spiritual and psychological care for the patient, and support for family caregivers during the patient's illness and the bereavement period.

Terminally ill patients have a wide variety of advanced diseases, often with multiple symptoms demanding relief, and require noninvasive therapeutic regimens to be delivered in flexible care settings. Fundamental to ensuring quality palliative and end-of-life care is a focus on four broad domains: (1) physical symptoms; (2) psychological symptoms; (3) social needs that include interpersonal relationships, caregiving, and economic concerns; and (4) existential or spiritual needs.

A comprehensive assessment screens for and evaluates needs in each of these four domains. Goals for care are established in discussion with the patient and/or family based on the assessment in each of these domains. Interventions are then aimed at improving or managing symptoms and needs. While physicians are responsible for certain especially technical interventions, and for coordinating the interventions, they cannot be responsible for providing all of them. Since failing to address any one of the domains is likely to preclude a good death, a well coordinated, effectively communicating interdisciplinary team takes on special importance in end-of-life care. Depending on the setting, critical members of the interdisciplinary team will include physicians, nurses, social workers, chaplains, nurse's aides, physical therapists, bereavement counselors, and volunteers.

ASSESSMENT AND CARE PLANNING
Comprehensive Assessment Standardized methods for conducting a comprehensive assessment focus on evaluating the patient's condition in all four domains affected by illness: physical, psychological, social, and spiritual. The assessment of physical and mental symptoms should follow a modified version of the traditional medical history and physical examination that emphasizes symptoms. Questions should aim at elucidating symptoms and discerning sources of suffering and gauging how much these symptoms interfere with the patient's quality of life. Standardized assessment is critical. Currently, there are 21 symptom assessment instruments for cancer alone. Instruments with good psychometric properties that assess a wide range of symptoms include the Memorial Symptom Assessment Scale (MSAS), the Rotterdam Symptom Checklist, the Worthing Chemotherapy Questionnaire, and the Computerized Symptom Assessment Instrument. These are long and may be useful for initial clinical or for research assessments. Shorter instruments are useful for patients whose performance status does not permit comprehensive assessments. Suitable shorter instruments include the Condensed Memorial Symptom Assessment Scale, the Edmonton Symptom Assessment System, the M.D. Anderson Symptom Assessment Inventory, and the Symptom Distress Scale. Using such instruments ensures that the assessment is comprehensive and does not just focus on pain and a few other physical symptoms. Invasive tests are best avoided in end-of-life care, and even minimally invasive tests should be carefully evaluated for their benefit-to-burden ratio for the patient. Aspects of the physical examination that are uncomfortable and unlikely to yield useful information can also be omitted.

Regarding social needs, health care providers should assess the status of important relationships, financial burdens, care-giving needs, and access to medical care. Relevant questions will include: *How often is there someone to feel close to? How has this illness been for your family? How has it affected your relationships? How much help do you need with things like getting meals or getting around? How much trouble do you have getting the medical care you need?* In the area of existential needs,

FIGURE 11-1 Graph showing trends in the site of death in the past two decades. ◆, percentage of hospital inpatient deaths; ■, percentage of decedents enrolled in a hospice.

providers should assess distress and the patient's sense of being emotionally and existentially settled and of finding purpose or meaning. Helpful assessment questions can include: *How much are you able to find meaning since your illness began? What things are most important to you at this stage?* In addition, it can be helpful to ask about how well the patient perceives his or her care to be: *How much do you feel your doctors and nurses respect you? How clear is the information from us about what to expect regarding your illness? How much do you feel that the medical care you are getting fits with your goals?* If concern is detected in any of these areas, deeper evaluative questions are warranted.

Communication Especially when an illness is life-threatening, there are many emotionally charged and potentially conflict-creating moments, collectively called "bad news" situations, in which empathic and effective communication skills are essential. These moments include communicating to the patient and/or family about a terminal diagnosis, the patient's prognosis, any treatment failures, deemphasizing efforts to cure and prolong life while focusing more on symptom management and palliation, advance care planning, and the patient's death.

Just as surgeons plan and prepare for major operations or investigators rehearse a presentation of research results, physicians and health care providers caring for patients with significant or advanced illness can develop a practiced approach to sharing important information and planning interventions. In addition, families identify as important both how well the physician was prepared to deliver bad news and the setting in which it was delivered. For instance, 27% of families making critical decisions for patients in an intensive care unit (ICU) desired better and more private physical space to communicate with physicians, and 48% found having clergy present reassuring.

An organized and effective procedure for communicating bad news with seven steps goes by the acronym P-SPIKES: (1) *p*repare for the discussion, (2) *s*et up a suitable environment, (3) begin the discussion by finding out what the *pa*tient and/or family understand, (4) determine how they will comprehend new *i*nformation best and how much they want to know, (5) provide needed new *k*nowledge accordingly, (6) allow for *e*motional responses, and (7) *s*hare plans for the next steps in care. Table 11-2 provides a summary of these steps along with suggested phrases and underlying rationales for each.

Continuous Goal Assessment Major barriers to ensuring quality palliative and end-of-life care include difficulty in providing an accurate prognosis and emotional resistance of patients and their families to accepting the implications of a poor prognosis. A practical solution to these barriers is to integrate palliative care with curative care regardless of prognosis. With this approach, palliative care no longer conveys the message of

failure, having no more treatments, or "giving up hope." Fundamental to integrating palliative care with curative therapy is to include continuous goal assessment as part of the routine patient reassessment that occurs at most patient-physician encounters.

Goals for care are numerous, ranging from cure of a specific disease, to prolonging life, to relief of a symptom, to delaying the course of an incurable disease, to adapting to progressive disability without disrupting the family, to finding peace of mind or personal meaning, to dying in a manner that leaves loved ones with positive memories. Discernment of goals for care can be approached through a seven-step protocol: (1) ensure that medical and other information is as complete as reasonably possible and understood by all relevant parties (see above); (2) explore what the patient and/or family are hoping for while identifying relevant and realistic goals; (3) share all the options with the patient and family; (4) respond with empathy as they adjust to changing expectations; (5) make a plan, emphasizing what can be done toward the realistic

TABLE 11-2 ELEMENTS OF COMMUNICATING BAD NEWS—THE P-SPIKES APPROACH

Acronym	Steps	Aim of the Interaction	Preparations, Questions, or Phrases
P	Preparation	Mentally prepare for the interaction with the patient and/or family.	Review what information needs to be communicated. Plan how you will provide emotional support. Rehearse key steps and phrases in the interaction.
S	Setting of the interaction	Ensure the appropriate setting for a serious and potentially emotionally charged discussion.	Ensure patient, family, and appropriate social supports are present. Devote sufficient time. Ensure privacy and prevent interruptions by people or beeper. Bring a box of tissues.
P	Patient's perception and preparation	Begin the discussion by establishing the baseline and whether the patient and family can grasp the information. Ease tension by having the patient and family contribute.	Start with open-ended questions to encourage participation. Possible phrases to use: *What do you understand about your illness? When you first had symptom X, what did you think it might be? What did Dr. X tell you when he sent you here? What do you think is going to happen?*
I	Invitation and information needs	Discover what information needs the patient and/or family have and what limits they want regarding the bad information.	Possible phrases to use: *If this condition turns out to be something serious, do you want to know? Would you like me to tell you all the details of your condition? If not, then who would you like me to talk to?*
K	Knowledge of the condition	Provide the bad news or other information to the patient and/or family sensitively.	Do not just dump the information on the patient and family. Check for patient and family understanding. Possible phrases to use: *I feel badly to have to tell you this, but… Unfortunately, the tests showed… I'm afraid the news is not good…*
E	Empathy and exploration	Identify the cause of the emotions—e.g., poor prognosis. Empathize with the patient and/or family's feeling. Explore by asking open-ended questions.	Strong feelings in reaction to bad news are normal. Acknowledge what the patient and family are feeling. Remind them such feelings are normal, even if frightening. Give them time to respond. Remind patient and family you won't abandon them. Possible phrases to use: *I imagine this is very hard for you to hear. You look very upset. Tell me how you are feeling. I wish the news were different. We'll do whatever we can to help you.*
S	Summary and planning	Delineate for the patient and the family the next steps, including additional tests or interventions.	It is the unknown and uncertain that can increase anxiety. Recommend a schedule with goals and landmarks. Provide your rationale for the patient and/or family to accept (or reject). If the patient and/or family are not ready to discuss the next steps, schedule a follow-up visit.

Source: Adapted from Buckman.

goals; (6) follow through with the plan; and (7) review and revise this plan periodically, considering at every encounter whether the goals of care should be reviewed with the patient and/or family. Each of these steps need not be followed in rote order, but together they provide a helpful framework for interactions with patients and their families about goals for care. It can be especially challenging if a patient or family member has difficulty letting go of an unrealistic goal. One strategy is to help them refocus on more realistic goals, and also suggest that, while hoping for the best, it is still prudent to plan for other outcomes as well.

Advance Care Planning · PRACTICES

Advance care planning is a process of planning for future medical care in case the patient becomes incapable of making medical decisions. Ideally, such planning would occur before a health care crisis or the terminal phase of an illness. Unfortunately, diverse barriers prevent this. While 80% of Americans endorse advance care planning and completing living wills, only 29% have actually done so. Most patients expect physicians to initiate advance care planning and will wait for physicians to broach the subject. Patients also wish to discuss advance care planning with their families. Yet patients with unrealistic expectations are significantly more likely to prefer aggressive treatments. Fewer than one-third of health care providers have completed advance care planning for themselves. Hence, a good first step is for health care providers to complete advance care planning for themselves. This makes providers aware of the critical choices in the process and the issues that are especially charged and allows them to tell their patients truthfully that they have done advance planning themselves.

Steps in effective advance care planning center on (1) introducing the topic, (2) structuring a discussion, (3) reviewing plans that have been discussed by the patient and family, (4) documenting the plans, (5) updating them periodically, and (6) implementing the advance care directives (Table 11-3). Two of the main barriers to advance care planning are problems in raising the topic and structuring a succinct discussion. Raising the topic can be done efficiently as a routine matter, noting that it is recommended for all patients, analogous to purchasing insurance or estate planning. Almost all of the most difficult cases have involved unexpected, acute episodes of brain damage in young individuals.

Structuring a focused discussion is a central communication skill. Identify the health care proxy and recommend his or her involvement in the advance care planning process. Select a worksheet, preferably one that has been evaluated and demonstrated to produce reliable and valid expressions of patient preferences, and orient the patient and proxy to it. Such worksheets exist for both general and disease-specific situations. Discuss with the patient and proxy one scenario as an example to demonstrate how to think about the issues. It is often helpful to begin with a scenario in which

the patient is likely to have settled preferences for care, such as being in a persistent vegetative state. Once the patient's preferences for interventions in this scenario are determined, suggest that the patient and proxy discuss and complete the worksheet for the others. If appropriate, suggest they involve other family members in the discussion. On a return visit, go over the patient's preferences, checking and resolving any inconsistencies. After having the patient and proxy sign the document, place it in the medical chart and be sure that copies are provided to relevant family members and care sites. Since patients' preferences can change, these documents need to be reviewed periodically.

TYPES OF DOCUMENTS Advance care planning documents are of two broad types. The first includes living wills or instructional directives; these are advisory documents that describe the types of decisions that should direct care. Some are more specific, delineating different scenarios and interventions for the patient to choose from. Among these, some are for general use and others are designed for use by

---

TABLE 11-3 STEPS IN ADVANCE CARE PLANNING

Step	Goals to be Achieved and Measures to Cover	Useful Phrases or Points to Make
Introducing advance care planning	Ask the patient what he or she knows about advance care planning and if he or she has already completed an advanced care directive. Indicate that you as a physician have completed advance care planning. Indicate that you try to perform advance care planning with all patients regardless of prognosis. Explain the goals of the process as empowering the patient and ensuring you and the proxy understand the patient's preferences. Provide the patient relevant literature including the advance care directive that you prefer to use. Recommend the patient identify a proxy decision-maker who should attend the next meeting.	*I'd like to talk with you about something I try to discuss with all my patients. It's called advance care planning. In fact, I feel that this is such an important topic that I have done this myself. Are you familiar with advance care planning or living wills?* *Have you thought about the type of care you would want if you ever became too sick to speak for yourself? That is the purpose of advance care planning.* *There is no change in health that we have not discussed. I am bringing this up now because it is sensible for everyone, no matter how well or ill, old or young.* Have many copies of advance care directives available, including in the waiting room, for patients and families. Know resources for state-specific forms (available at *www.nhpco.org*).
Structured discussion of scenarios and patient	Affirm that the goal of the process is to follow the patient's wishes if the patient loses decision-making capacity. Elicit the patient's overall goals related to health care. Elicit the patient's preferences for specific interventions in a few salient and common scenarios. Help the patient define the threshold for withdrawing and withholding interventions. Define the patient's preference for the role of the proxy.	Use a structured worksheet with typical scenarios. Begin the discussion with persistent vegetative state and consider other scenarios, such as recovery from an acute event with serious disability, asking the patient about his or her preferences regarding specific interventions, such as ventilators, artificial nutrition, and CPR, and then proceeding to less-invasive interventions, such as blood transfusions and antibiotics.
Review the patient's preferences	After the patient has made choices of interventions, review them to ensure they are consistent and the proxy is aware of them.	
Document the patient's preferences	Formally complete the advance care directive and have witness sign it. Provide a copy for the patient and the proxy. Insert a copy into the patient's medical record and summarize in a progress note.	
Update the directive	Periodically, and with major changes in health status, review the directive with the patient and make any modifications.	
Apply the directive	The directive goes into effect only when the patient becomes unable to make medical decisions for him- or herself. Re-read the directive to be sure about its content. Discuss your proposed actions based on the directive with the proxy.	

Note: CPR, cardiopulmonary resuscitation.

patients with a specific type of disease, such as cancer or HIV. Less specific directives can be general statements of not wanting life-sustaining interventions or forms that describe the values that should guide specific terminal care decisions. The second type of advance directive allows the designation of a health care proxy (sometimes also referred to as a durable attorney for health care) who is an individual selected by the patient to make decisions. The choice is not either/or; a combined directive that includes a living will and designates a proxy is often used, and the directive should clearly indicate whether the specified patient preferences or the proxy's choice takes precedence if they conflict.

A potentially misleading distinction relates to statutory as opposed to advisory documents. Statutory documents are drafted to fulfill relevant state laws. Advisory documents are drafted to reflect the patient's wishes. Both are legal, the first under state law, and the latter under common or constitutional law.

LEGAL ASPECTS   As of 2006, 48 states and the District of Columbia had enacted living will legislation. Many states have their own statutory forms. Massachusetts and Michigan do not have living will laws, although both have health care proxy laws. In 25 states, the laws state that the living will is not valid if a woman is pregnant. However, like all other states except Alaska, these states have enacted durable power of attorney for health care laws that permit patients to designate a proxy decision-maker with authority to terminate life-sustaining treatments. Only in Alaska does the law prohibit proxies from terminating life-sustaining treatments.

The U.S. Supreme Court has ruled that patients have a constitutional right to decide about refusing and terminating medical interventions, including life-sustaining interventions, and that mentally incompetent patients can exercise this right by providing "clear and convincing evidence" of their preferences. Since advance care directives permit patients to provide such evidence, commentators agree that they are constitutionally protected. Most commentators believe that a state is required to honor any clear advance care directive, whether or not it is written on an "official" form. Many states have enacted laws to explicitly honor out-of-state directives. If a patient is not using a statutory form, then it might be advisable to attach a statutory form to the advance care directive being used. State-specific forms are readily available free of charge for health care providers and patients and families through the website of the National Hospice and Palliative Care Organization (*http://www.nhpco.org*).

INTERVENTIONS

PHYSICAL SYMPTOMS AND THEIR MANAGEMENT

Great emphasis has been placed on addressing dying patients' pain. Some institutions have made pain assessment a fifth vital sign to emphasize its importance. This has also been advocated by large health care systems, such as the Veterans' Administration and accrediting bodies such as the Joint Commission on the Accreditation of Health Care Organizations (JCAHO). Although this embrace of pain as the fifth vital sign has been symbolically important, no data document that it has changed pain management practices. While good palliative care requires good pain management, it also requires more. The frequency of symptoms varies by disease and other factors. The most common physical and psychological symptoms among all terminally ill patients include pain, fatigue, insomnia, anorexia, dyspnea, depression, anxiety, and nausea and vomiting. In the last days of life, terminal delirium is also common. Assessments of patients with advanced cancer have shown that patients experienced an average of 11.5 different physical and psychological symptoms (Table 11-4).

Evaluations to determine the etiology of these symptoms can usually be limited to the history and physical examination. In some cases, radiologic or other diagnostic examinations will provide sufficient benefit in directing optimal palliative care to warrant the risks, potential discomfort, and inconvenience especially to the seriously ill pa-

TABLE 11-4 COMMON PHYSICAL AND PSYCHOLOGICAL SYMPTOMS OF TERMINALLY ILL PATIENTS

Physical Symptoms	Psychological Symptoms
Pain	Anxiety
Fatigue and weakness	Depression
Dyspnea	Hopelessness
Insomnia	Meaninglessness
Dry mouth	Irritability
Anorexia	Impaired concentration
Nausea and vomiting	Confusion
Constipation	Delirium
Cough	Loss of libido
Swelling of arms or legs	
Itching	
Diarrhea	
Dysphagia	
Dizziness	
Fecal and urinary incontinence	
Numbness/tingling in hands/feet	

tient. Only a few of the common symptoms presenting difficult management issues will be addressed in this chapter. Additional information on the management of other symptoms, such as nausea and vomiting, insomnia, and diarrhea can be found in Chaps. 39 and 77, Chap. 28, and Chap. 40, respectively.

Pain • *FREQUENCY*   The frequency of pain among terminally ill patients varies widely. Substantial pain occurs in 36–90% of patients with advanced cancer. In the SUPPORT study of hospitalized patients with diverse conditions and an estimated survival of ≤6 months, 22% reported moderate to severe pain, and caregivers of these patients noted that 50% had similar levels of pain during the last few days of life.

ETIOLOGY   *Nociceptive pain* is the result of direct mechanical or chemical stimulation of nociceptors and normal neural signaling to the brain. It tends to be localized, aching, throbbing, and cramping. The classic example is bone metastases. *Visceral pain* is caused by nociceptors in gastrointestinal, respiratory, and other organ systems. It is a deep or colicky type of pain classically associated with pancreatitis, myocardial infarction, or tumor invasion of viscera. *Neuropathic pain* arises from disordered nerve signals. It is described by patients as burning, electrical, or shocklike pain. Classic examples are post-stroke pain, tumor invasion of the brachial plexus, and herpetic neuralgia.

ASSESSMENT   Pain is a subjective experience. Depending upon the patient's circumstances, perspective, and physiologic condition, the same physical lesion or disease state can produce different levels of reported pain and need for pain relief. Systematic assessment includes eliciting the following: (1) type: throbbing, cramping, burning, etc. (2) periodicity: continuous, with or without exacerbations, or incident; (3) location; (4) intensity; (5) modifying factors; (6) effects of treatments; (7) functional impact; and (8) impact on patient. Several validated pain assessment measures may be used, such as the Visual Analogue Scale, the Brief Pain Inventory, and the pain component of one of the more comprehensive symptom assessment instruments. Frequent reassessments are essential to assess the effects of interventions.

INTERVENTIONS   Interventions for pain must be tailored to each individual with the goal of preempting chronic pain and relieving breakthrough pain. At the end of life, there is rarely reason to doubt the patient's report of pain. Pain medications are the cornerstone of management. If these are failing and nonpharmacologic interventions—including radiotherapy, anesthetic or neurosurgical procedures, such as peripheral nerve blocks or epidural medications—are required, a pain consultation is appropriate.

Pharmacologic interventions follow the World Health Organization three-step approach involving nonopioid analgesics, mild opioids, and strong opioids, with or without adjuvants (Chap. 12). Nonopioid analgesics, especially nonsteroidal anti-inflammatory drugs (NSAIDs), are the initial treatments for mild pain. They work primarily by inhibiting peripheral prostaglandins, reducing inflammation, but may also have central nervous system (CNS) effects. They have a ceiling effect. Ibuprofen, up to 1600 mg/d qid, has a minimal risk of bleeding and renal impairment and is a good initial choice. In patients with a history of severe gastrointestinal (GI) or other bleeding, it should be avoided. In patients with a history of mild gastritis or gastroesophageal reflux disease (GERD), acid-lowering therapy, such as a proton-pump inhibitor, should be used. Acetaminophen is an alternative in patients with a history of GI bleeding and can be used safely at up to 4 g/d, qid. In patients with liver dysfunction due to metastases or other causes or in patients with heavy alcohol use, doses should be reduced.

If nonopioid analgesics are insufficient, then opioids should be introduced. They work by interacting with mu opioid receptors in the CNS to activate pain-inhibitory neurons; most are receptor antagonists. The mixed agonist/antagonist opioids useful for post-acute pain should not be used for the chronic pain in end-of-life care. Weak opioids, such as codeine, can be used initially. However, if these are escalated and fail to relieve pain, then strong opioids, such as morphine 5–10 mg every 4 h, should be used. Nonopioid analgesics should be combined with opioids because they potentiate the effect of opioids.

For continuous pain, opioids should be administered on a regular, around-the-clock basis consistent with their duration of analgesia. They should not be provided only when the patient experiences pain; the goal is to prevent patients from experiencing pain. Patients should also be provided rescue medication, such as liquid morphine, for breakthrough pain that should generally be 20% of the baseline dose. Patients should be informed that using the rescue medication does not obviate their taking the next standard dose of pain medication. If after 24 h the patient's pain remains uncontrolled and recurs before the next dose, requiring the patient to utilize the rescue medication, the daily opioid dose can be increased by the total dose of rescue medications used by the patient, or by 50% for moderate pain and 100% for severe pain of the standing opioid daily dose.

It is inappropriate to start with extended-release preparations. Instead, an initial focus on using short-acting preparations in order to determine how much is required in the first 24–48 h will allow clinicians to determine opioid needs. Once pain relief is obtained with short-acting preparations, then switch to extended-release preparations. Even with a stable extended-release preparation regimen, the patient may have incident pain, such as during movement or dressing changes. Short-acting preparations should be taken before such predictable episodes. Although less common, patients may have "end-of-dose failure" with long-acting opioids, meaning that they develop pain after 8 h in the case of an every 12-h medication. In these cases, a trial of giving an every 12-h medication every 8 h is appropriate.

Because of differences in opioid receptors, cross-tolerance among opioids is incomplete and patients may experience different side effects with different opioids. Therefore, if a patient is not experiencing pain relief or is experiencing too many side effects, change to another opioid preparation is appropriate. When switching, begin with 50–75% of the published equianalgesic dose of the new opioid.

Unlike NSAIDs, opioids have no ceiling effect; therefore, there is no maximum dose no matter how many milligrams the patient is receiving. The appropriate dose is the dose needed to achieve pain relief. This is an important point for clinicians to explain to patients and families. Addiction or excessive respiratory depression is extremely unlikely in the terminally ill; fear of these side effects should neither prevent escalating opioid medications when the patient is experiencing insufficient pain relief nor justify using opioid antagonists.

Opioid side effects should be anticipated and treated preemptively. Nearly all patients experience constipation that can be debilitating (see below). Failure to prevent constipation often results in noncompliance with opioid therapy. Methylnaltrexone is a drug that targets opioid-induced constipation by blocking peripheral opioid receptors but not central receptors for analgesia. In placebo-controlled trials, it has been shown to cause laxation within 24 h of administration. As with the use

of opioids, about a third of patients using methylnaltrexone experience nausea and vomiting, but unlike constipation, tolerance develops, usually within a week. Therefore, when beginning opioids, an antiemetic, such as metoclopramide or a serotonin antagonist, is often prescribed prophylactically and stopped after 1 week. Olanzapine has also been shown to have anti-nausea properties and can also be effective in countering delirium or anxiety, with the advantage of some weight gain.

Drowsiness, a common side effect of opioids, also usually abates within a week. During this period, drowsiness can be treated with psychostimulants, such as dextroamphetamine, methylphenidate, or modafinil. Modafinil has the advantage of every day dosing. Pilot reports suggest that donepezil may also be helpful for opiate-induced drowsiness, as well as relieving fatigue and anxiety. Metabolites of morphine and most opioids are cleared renally; doses may need to be adjusted for patients with renal failure.

Seriously ill patients with chronic pain relief rarely if ever become addicted. Suspicion of addiction should not be a reason to withhold pain medications from terminally ill patients. Patients and families may withhold prescribed opioids for fear of addiction or dependence. Physicians and health care providers should reassure patients and families that the patient will not become addicted to opioids if used as prescribed for pain relief; this fear should not prevent the patient from taking the medications around the clock. However, diversion of drugs for use by other family members or illicit sale may occur. It may be necessary to advise the patient and caregiver about secure storage of opioids. Contract writing with the patient and family can help. If that fails, transfer to a safe facility may be necessary.

Tolerance is the need for increasing medication dosage for the same pain relief without a change in disease. In the case of patients with advanced disease, the need for increasing opioid dosage for pain relief is usually caused by disease progression rather than tolerance. Physical dependence is indicated by symptoms from the abrupt withdrawal of opioids and should not be confused with addiction.

Adjuvant analgesic medications are nonopioids that potentiate the analgesic effects of opioids. They are especially important in the management of neuropathic pain. Gabapentin, an anticonvulsant initially studied in the setting of herpetic neuralgia, is now the first-line treatment for neuropathic pain from a variety of causes. It is begun at 100–300 mg bid or tid, with 50–100% dose increments every 3 days. Usually 900–3600 mg/d in two or three doses is effective. One potential side effect to be aware of is confusion and drowsiness, especially in the elderly. Other effective adjuvant medications include pregabalin, which has the same mechanism of action as gabapentin but is more efficiently absorbed from the GI tract. Lamotrigine is a novel agent whose mechanism of action is unknown, but it has shown effectiveness. It is recommended to begin at 25–50 mg/d increasing to 100 mg/d. Carbamazepine, a first-generation agent, has been proven effective in randomized trials for neuropathic pain. Other potentially effective anticonvulsant adjuvants include topiramate (25–50 mg qd or bid rising to 100–300 mg/d) and oxcarbazepine (75–300 mg bid, rising to 1200 mg bid). Glucocorticoids, preferably dexamethasone given once a day, can be useful in reducing inflammation that causes pain while elevating mood, energy, and appetite. Its main side effects include confusion, sleep difficulties, and fluid retention. Glucocorticoids are especially effective for bone pain and abdominal pain from distention of the GI tract or liver. Other drugs, including clonidine and baclofen, can be effective in pain relief. These drugs are adjuvants and should generally be used in conjunction with—not instead of—opioids. Methadone, carefully dosed because of unpredictable half-life in many patients, has activity at the N-methyl D-aspartamate (NMDA) receptor and is useful for complex pain syndromes and neuropathic pain. It is generally reserved for cases when first-line opioids (morphine, oxycodone, hydromorphone) are either ineffective or unavailable.

Radiation therapy can treat bone pain from single metastatic lesions. Bone pain from multiple metastases can be amenable to radiopharmaceuticals, such as strontium 89 and samarium 153. Bisphosphonates [such as pamidronate (90 mg every 4 weeks)] and calcitonin (200 IU intranasally once or twice a day) also provide relief from bone pain but have onset of action of days.

Constipation • *FREQUENCY* Constipation is reported in up to 90% of terminally ill patients.

ETIOLOGY While hypercalcemia and other factors can cause constipation, it is most frequently a predictable consequence of the use of opioids for the relief of pain and dyspnea and of tricyclic antidepressants, from their anticholinergic effects, as well as of the inactivity and poor diet that are common among seriously ill patients. If untreated, constipation can cause substantial pain and vomiting and is also associated with confusion and delirium. Whenever opioids and other medications known to cause constipation are used, preemptive treatment for constipation should be instituted.

ASSESSMENT Establish the patient's previous bowel habits, including the frequency, consistency, and volume. Abdominal and rectal examinations should be performed to exclude impaction or acute abdomen. Radiographic assessments beyond a simple flat plate of the abdomen in cases where obstruction is suspected are rarely necessary.

INTERVENTION While physical activity, adequate hydration, and dietary treatments with fiber can be helpful, each is limited in its effectiveness for most seriously ill patients, and fiber may exacerbate problems in the setting of dehydration and if impaired motility is the etiology. Fiber is contraindicated in the presence of opioid use. Stimulant and osmotic laxatives, stool softeners, fluids, and enemas are the mainstays of therapy (Table 11-5). When preventing constipation from opioids and other medications, a combination of a laxative and stool softener (such as senna and docusate) should be used. If after several days of treatment a bowel movement has not occurred, a rectal examination to remove impacted stool and to place a suppository is necessary. For patients with impending bowel obstruction or gastric stasis, octreotide to reduce secretions can be helpful. For patients in whom the suspected mechanism is dysmotility, metoclopramide can be helpful.

Nausea • *FREQUENCY* Up to 70% of patients with advanced cancer have nausea, defined as the subjective sensation of wanting to vomit.

ETIOLOGY Nausea and vomiting are both caused by stimulation at one of four sites: the GI tract, the vestibular system, the chemoreceptor trigger zone (CTZ), and the cerebral cortex. Medical treatments of nausea are aimed at receptors at each of these sites: The GI tract contains mechanoreceptors, chemoreceptors, and 5-hydroxytryptamine type 3 (5-HT3) receptors; the vestibular system likely contains histamine and acetylcholine receptors; and the CTZ contains chemoreceptors, dopamine type 2 receptors, and 5-HT3 receptors. An example of nausea that is most likely mediated by the cortex is anticipatory nausea before a dose of chemotherapy or other noxious stimuli.

Specific causes of nausea include metabolic changes (liver failure, uremia from renal failure, hypercalcemia), bowel obstruction, constipation, infection, GERD, vestibular disease, brain metastases, medications (including antibiotics, NSAIDs, proton-pump inhibitors, opioids, chemotherapy), and radiation therapy. Anxiety can also contribute to nausea.

INTERVENTION Medical treatment of nausea is directed at the anatomic and receptor-mediated cause that a careful history and physical examination reveals. When a single specific cause is not found, many advocate beginning treatment with dopamine antagonists such as haloperidol or prochlorperazine. Prochlorperazine is usually more sedating than haloperidol. When decreased motility is suspected, metoclopramide can be an effective treatment. When inflammation of the GI tract is suspected, glucocorticoids such as dexamethasone are

an appropriate treatment. For post-chemotherapy and -radiation therapy nausea, one of the 5-HT3 receptor antagonists (ondansetron, granisetron, dolasetron) is recommended. When a vestibular cause (such as "motion sickness" or labyrinthitis) is suspected, antihistamines such as meclizine (whose primary side effect is drowsiness) or anticholinergics such as scopolamine can be effective. In anticipatory nausea, a benzodiazepine such as lorazepam is indicated. As with antihistamines, drowsiness and confusion are the main side effects.

Dyspnea • *FREQUENCY* Dyspnea is a subjective experience of being short of breath. Nearly 75% of dying patients experience dyspnea at some point in their illness. Dyspnea is among the most distressing of physical symptoms and can be even more distressing than pain.

ASSESSMENT As with pain, dyspnea is a subjective experience that may not correlate with objective measures of P_{O_2}, P_{CO_2}, or respiratory rate. Consequently, measurements of oxygen saturation through pulse oximetry or blood gases are rarely helpful in guiding therapy. Potentially reversible or treatable causes of dyspnea include infection, pleural effusions, pulmonary emboli, pulmonary edema, asthma, or tumor encroachment on the airway. However, the risk-benefit ratio of the diagnostic and therapeutic interventions for patients with little time left to live must be carefully considered before undertaking diagnostic steps. Frequently, the specific etiology cannot be identified, and dyspnea is the consequence of progression of the underlying disease that cannot be treated. The anxiety caused by dyspnea and the choking sensation can significantly exacerbate the underlying dyspnea in a negatively reinforcing cycle.

INTERVENTIONS When reversible or treatable etiologies are diagnosed, they should be treated as long as the side effects of treatment, such as repeated drainage of effusions or anticoagulants, are less burdensome than the dyspnea itself. More aggressive treatments, such as stenting a bronchial lesion may be warranted if it is clear that the dyspnea is due to tumor invasion at that site and if the patient and family understand the risks of such a procedure. Usually, treatment will be symptomatic (Table 11-6). Low-dose opioids reduce the sensitivity of the central respiratory center and the sensation of dyspnea. If patients are not receiving opioids, weak opioids can be initiated; if patients are already receiving opioids, then morphine or other strong opioids should be used. Controlled trials do not support the use of nebulized opioids for dyspnea at the end of life. Phenothiazines and chlorpromazine may be helpful when combined with opioids. Benzodiazepines can be helpful if anxiety is present but should be neither first-line therapy nor used alone in the treatment of dyspnea. If the patient has a history of COPD or asthma, inhaled bronchodilators and glucocorticoids may also be helpful. If the patient has pulmonary edema due to heart failure, di-

TABLE 11-5 **MEDICATIONS FOR THE MANAGEMENT OF CONSTIPATION**

Intervention	Dose	Comment
Stimulant laxatives		These agents directly stimulate peristalsis and may reduce colonic absorption of water.
Prune juice	120–240 mL/d	
Senna (Senokot)	2–8 tablets PO bid	
Bisacodyl	5–15 mg/d PO, PR	Work in 6–12 h.
Osmotic laxatives		These agents are not absorbed. They attract and retain water in the gastrointestinal tract.
Lactulose	15–30 mL PO q4–8h	
Magnesium hydroxide (Milk of Magnesia)	15–30 mL/d PO	Lactulose may cause flatulence and bloating.
Magnesium citrate	125–250 mL/d PO	Lactulose works in 1 day; magnesium products in 6 h.
Stool softeners		These agents work by increasing water secretion and as detergents increasing water penetration into the stool.
Sodium docusate (Colace)	300–600 mg/d PO	
Calcium docusate	300–600 mg/d PO	Work in 1–3 days.
Suppositories and enemas		
Bisacodyl	10–15 PR qd	
Sodium phosphate enema	PR qd	Fixed dose, 4.5 oz, Fleet's.

TABLE 11-6 MEDICATIONS FOR THE MANAGEMENT OF DYSPNEA

Intervention	Dose	Comments
Weak opioids		For patients with mild dyspnea
Codeine (or codeine with 325 mg acetaminophen)	30 mg PO q4h	For opioid-naïve patient
Hydrocodone	5 mg PO q4h	
Strong opioids		For opioid-naïve patients with moderate to severe dyspnea
Morphine	5–10 mg PO q4h	
	30–50% of baseline opioid dose q4h	For patients already taking opioids for pain or other symptoms
Oxycodone	5–10 mg PO q4h	
Hydromorphone	1–2 mg PO q4h	
Anxiolytics		Give a dose every hour until the patient is relaxed, then provide a dose for maintenance
Lorazepam	0.5–2.0 mg PO/SL/IV qh then q4–6h	
Clonazepam	0.25–2.0 mg PO q12h	
Midazolam	0.5 mg IV q15min	

uresis with a medication such as furosemide is indicated. Excess secretions can be dried with scopolamine, transdermally or intravenously. Oxygen can be used, although it may only be an expensive placebo. For some families and patients, oxygen is distressing; for some it is reassuring. More general interventions that medical staff can do include: sitting the patient upright, removing smoke or other irritants such as perfume, ensuring a supply of fresh air with sufficient humidity, and minimizing other factors that can increase anxiety.

Fatigue · *FREQUENCY* More than 90% of terminally ill patients experience fatigue and/or weakness. Fatigue is frequently cited as among the most distressing of symptoms.

ETIOLOGY The multiple causes of fatigue in the terminally ill can be categorized as resulting from the underlying disease; from disease-induced factors, such as tumor necrosis factor and other cytokines; and from secondary factors such as dehydration, anemia, infection, hypothyroidism, and drug side effects. Apart from low caloric intake, loss of muscle mass and changes in muscle enzymes may play an important role in fatigue of terminal illness. The importance of changes in the CNS, especially the reticular activating system, have been hypothesized based on reports of fatigue in patients receiving cranial radiation, experiencing depression, or with chronic pain in the absence of cachexia or other physiologic changes. Finally, depression and other causes of psychological distress can contribute to fatigue.

ASSESSMENT Fatigue is subjective; objective changes, even in body mass, may be absent. Consequently, assessment must rely on patient self-reporting. Scales used to measure fatigue, such as the Edmonton Functional Assessment Tool, the Fatigue Self-Report scales, or the Rhoten Fatigue scale, are usually appropriate for research rather than clinical purposes. In clinical practice, a simple performance assessment such as the Karnofsky Performance Status or the Eastern Cooperative Oncology Group's question "How much of the day does the patient spend in bed?" may be the best measure. In this 0–4 performance status assessment, a 0 = normal activity; 1 = symptomatic without being bedridden; 2 = requiring some, but <50%, bed time; 3 = bedbound more than half the day; and 4 = bedbound all the time. Such a scale allows for assessment over time and correlates with overall disease severity and prognosis.

INTERVENTIONS At the end of life, fatigue will not be "cured." The goal is to ameliorate it and help patients and families to adjust expectations. Behavioral interventions should be utilized to avoid blaming the patient for inactivity and to educate both the family and patient that the underlying disease causes physiologic changes producing low energy levels. Understanding that the problem is physiologic not psychological can help to alter expectations regarding the patient's level of physical activity. Practically, this may mean reducing routine activities, such as housework and cooking, or social events outside the house,

and making it acceptable to receive guests lying on a couch. At the same time, institution of exercise regimens and physical therapy can raise endorphins, reduce muscle wasting, and reduce the risk of depression. In addition, ensuring good hydration without worsening edema may help reduce fatigue. Discontinuing medications that worsen fatigue may help, including cardiac medications, benzodiazepines, certain antidepressants or opioids, if pain is well-controlled.

Only a few pharmacologic interventions target fatigue and weakness. Glucocorticoids can increase energy and enhance mood. Dexamethasone is preferred for its once-a-day dosing and minimal mineralocorticoid activity. Benefit, if any, will usually be seen within the first month. Psychostimulants, such as dextroamphetamine (5–10 mg PO) and methylphenidate (2.5–5 mg PO), may also enhance energy levels, although a randomized trial did not show methylphenidate beneficial compared to placebo in cancer fatigue. Dosages should be given in the morning and at noon to minimize the risk of counterproductive insomnia. Modafinil, developed for narcolepsy, has shown some promise in the treatment of fatigue and has the advantage of once-daily dosing. Its precise role in the fatigue at the end of life is yet to be determined. Anecdotal evidence suggests that L-carnitine might improve fatigue, depression, and sleep disruption.

PSYCHOLOGICAL SYMPTOMS AND THEIR MANAGEMENT

Depression · *FREQUENCY* Depression at the end of life presents an apparently paradoxical situation. Many people believe that depression is normal among seriously ill patients because they are dying. People frequently say "wouldn't you be depressed?" However, depression is not a necessary part of terminal illness and can contribute to needless suffering. While sadness, anxiety, anger, and irritability are normal responses to a serious condition, they are typically of modest intensity and transient. Persistent sadness and anxiety and the physically disabling symptoms that these can lead to are abnormal and suggestive of major depression. While as many as 75% of terminally ill patients experience depressive symptoms, <25% of terminally ill patients have major depression.

ETIOLOGY Previous history of depression, family history of depression or bipolar disorder, and prior suicide attempts are associated with increased risk for depression among terminally ill patients. Other symptoms, such as pain and fatigue, are associated with higher rates of depression; uncontrolled pain can exacerbate depression, and depression can cause patients to be more distressed by pain. Many medications used in the terminal stages, including glucocorticoids, and some anticancer agents, such as tamoxifen, interleukin 2, interferon α, and vincristine, are also associated with depression. Some terminal conditions, such as pancreatic cancer, certain strokes, and heart failure have been reported to be associated with higher rates of depression, although this is controversial. Finally, depression may be attributable to grief over the loss of a role or function, social isolation, or loneliness.

ASSESSMENT Diagnosing depression among seriously ill patients is complicated because many of the vegetative symptoms in the DSM-IV criteria for clinical depression—insomnia, anorexia and weight loss, fatigue, decreased libido, and difficulty concentrating—are associated with the dying process itself. The assessment of depression in seriously ill patients should therefore focus on the dysphoric mood, helplessness, hopelessness, and lack of interest and enjoyment and concentration in normal activities. The single questions "how often do you feel downhearted and blue?" (more than a good bit of the time or similar responses) or "do you feel depressed most of the time?" are appropriate for screening.

Certain conditions may be confused with depression. Endocrinopathies, such as hypothyroidism or Cushing's syndrome, electrolyte abnormalities such as hypercalcemia, and akathisia, especially from dopamine-blocking antiemetics such as metoclopramide and prochlorperazine, can mimic depression and should be excluded.

INTERVENTIONS Physicians must treat any physical symptom, such as pain, that may be causing or exacerbating depression. Fostering adaptation to the many losses that the patient is experiencing can also be helpful. Nonpharmacologic interventions, including group or individual psychological counseling, and behavioral therapies, such as relaxation or imagery, can be helpful, especially in combination with drug therapy.

Pharmacologic interventions remain the core of therapy. The same medications are used to treat depression in terminally ill as in non-terminally ill patients. Psychostimulants may be preferred for patients with a poor prognosis or for those with fatigue or opioid-induced somnolence. Psychostimulants are comparatively fast acting, working within a few days, instead of the weeks required for selective serotonin reuptake inhibitors (SSRIs). Dextroamphetamine or methylphenidate should be started at 2.5–5.0 mg in the morning and at noon, the same starting dosages used for treating fatigue. The dose can be escalated up to 15 mg bid. Modafinil is started at 100 mg qd and can be increased to 200 mg if there is no effect at the lower dose. Pemoline is a nonamphetamine psychostimulant with minimal abuse potential. It is also effective as an antidepressant beginning at 18.75 mg in the morning and at noon. Because it can be absorbed through the buccal mucosa, it is preferred for patients with intestinal obstruction or dysphagia. If used for prolonged periods, liver function must be monitored. The psychostimulants can also be combined with more traditional antidepressants, while waiting for the latter to become effective, and then tapered after a few weeks if necessary. Psychostimulants have side effects, particularly initial anxiety, insomnia, and rarely paranoia, which may necessitate lowering the dose or discontinuing treatment.

Mirtazapine, an antagonist at the postsynaptic serotonin receptors, is a promising psychostimulant. It should be started at 7.5 mg before bed. It has sedating, antiemetic and anxiolytic properties with few drug interactions. Its side effect of weight gain may also be beneficial for seriously ill patients; it is available in orally disintegrating tablets.

For patients with a prognosis of several months or longer, SSRIs, including fluoxetine, sertraline, paroxetine and citalopram, and serotonin-noradrenaline reuptake inhibitors, such as venlafaxine, are the preferred treatment because of their efficacy and comparatively few side effects. Because low doses of these medications may be effective for seriously ill patients, use half the usual starting dose for healthy adults. The starting dose for fluoxetine is 10 mg once a day. In most cases, once-a-day dosing is possible. The choice of which SSRI to use should be driven by (1) the patient's past success or failure with the specific medication, and (2) the most favorable side effect profile for that specific agent. For instance, for a patient in whom fatigue is a major symptom, a more activating SSRI (fluoxetine) would be appropriate. For a patient in whom anxiety and sleeplessness are major symptoms, a more sedating SSRI (paroxetine) would be appropriate.

Atypical antidepressants are recommended only in selected circumstances, usually with the assistance of a specialty consultation. Trazodone can be an effective antidepressant but is sedating and can cause orthostatic hypotension and, rarely, priapism. Therefore, it should be used only when a sedating effect is desired and is often used for patients with insomnia, at a dose starting at 25 mg. In addition to its antidepressant effects, bupropion is energizing, making it useful for depressed patients suffering from fatigue. However, it can cause seizures, preventing its use for patients with a risk of CNS neoplasms or terminal delirium. Finally, alprazolam, a benzodiazepine, starting at 0.25–1.0 mg tid, can be effective in seriously ill patients suffering from a combination of anxiety and depression. While it is potent and works quickly, it has many drug interactions and may cause delirium, especially among very ill patients, because of its strong binding to the benzodiazepine–GABA receptor complex.

Unless used as adjuvants for the treatment of pain, tricyclic antidepressants are not recommended. Similarly, the monoamine oxidase (MAO) inhibitors are not recommended because of their side effects and dangerous drug interactions.

Delirium • FREQUENCY In the weeks or months before death, delirium is uncommon, although it may be significantly underdiagnosed. However, delirium becomes relatively common in the hours and days immediately before death. Up to 85% of patients dying from cancer may experience terminal delirium.

ETIOLOGY Delirium is a global cerebral dysfunction characterized by alterations in cognition and consciousness. It is frequently preceded by anxiety, changes in sleep patterns (especially reversal of day and night), and decreased attention. In contrast to dementia, delirium has an acute onset, fluctuating consciousness and inattention, and is reversible, although reversibility may be more theoretical than real for patients near death. Delirium may occur in a patient with dementia; indeed, patients with dementia are more vulnerable to delirium.

Causes of delirium include metabolic encephalopathy arising from liver or renal failure, hypoxemia, or infection; electrolyte imbalances such as hypercalcemia; paraneoplastic syndromes; dehydration; and primary brain tumors, brain metastases, or leptomeningeal spread of tumor. Commonly, among dying patients, delirium can be caused by side effects of treatments, including radiation for brain metastases, and medications, including opioids, glucocorticoids, anticholinergic drugs, antihistamines, antiemetics, benzodiazepines, and chemotherapeutic agents. The etiology may be multifactorial; e.g., dehydration may exacerbate opioid-induced delirium.

ASSESSMENT Delirium should be recognized in any terminally ill patient with new onset of disorientation, impaired cognition, somnolence, fluctuating levels of consciousness, or delusions with or without agitation. Delirium must be distinguished from acute anxiety and depression, as well as dementia. The central distinguishing feature is altered consciousness, which is not usually noted in anxiety, depression, and dementia. Although "hyperactive" delirium characterized by overt confusion and agitation is likely more common, patients should also be assessed for "hypoactive" delirium characterized by sleep-wake reversal and decreased alertness.

In some cases, use of formal assessment tools such as the Mini-Mental Status Examination (which does not distinguish delirium from dementia) or the Delirium Rating Scale (which does distinguish delirium from dementia) may be helpful in distinguishing delirium from other processes. The patient's list of medications must be carefully evaluated. Nonetheless, a reversible etiologic factor for delirium is found in fewer than half of terminally ill patients. Because most terminally ill patients experiencing delirium will be very close to death and may be at home, extensive diagnostic evaluations, such as lumbar punctures or neuroradiologic examinations, are usually inappropriate.

INTERVENTIONS One of the most important objectives of terminal care is to provide terminally ill patients the lucidity to say goodbye to the people they love. Delirium, especially with agitation during the final days, is distressing to family and caregivers. A strong determinant of bereavement difficulties is witnessing a difficult death. Thus, terminal delirium should be treated aggressively.

At the first sign of delirium, such as day-night reversal with slight changes in mentation, let the family know that it is time to be sure that everything they want to have said has been said. The family should be informed that delirium is common just before death.

If medications are suspected of being a cause of the delirium, then unnecessary agents should be discontinued. Other potentially reversible causes such as constipation, urinary retention, and metabolic abnormalities should be treated. Supportive measures aimed at providing a familiar environment should be instituted, including restricting visits only to individuals with whom the patient is familiar and eliminating new experiences; orienting the patient, if possible, by providing a clock and calendar; and gently correcting the patient's hallucinations or cognitive mistakes.

Pharmacologic management focuses on the use of neuroleptics and, in the extreme, anesthetics (Table 11-7). Haloperidol remains first-line therapy. Usually, patients can be controlled with a low dose (1–3 mg/d),

TABLE 11-7 MEDICATIONS FOR THE MANAGEMENT OF DELIRIUM	
Interventions	**Dose**
Neuroleptics	
Haloperidol	0.5–5 mg q2–12h, PO/IV/SC/IM
Thioridazine	10–75 mg q4–8h, PO
Chlorpromazine	12.5–50 mg q4–12h, PO/IV/IM
Atypical neuroleptics	
Olanzapine	2.5–5 mg qd or bid, PO
Risperidone	1–3 mg q12h, PO
Anxiolytics	
Lorazepam	0.5–2 mg q1–4h, PO/IV/IM
Midazolam	1–5 mg/h continuous infusion, IV/SC
Anesthetics	
Propofol	0.3–2.0 mg/h continuous infusion, IV

usually given every 6 h, although some may require as much as 20 mg/d. It can be administered PO, SC, or IV. IM injections should not be used, except when it is the only way to get a patient under control. Olanzapine, an atypical neuroleptic, has shown significant effectiveness in completely resolving delirium in cancer patients. It has other beneficial effects for terminally ill patients, including antinausea, antianxiety, and weight gain. It is useful for patients with longer anticipated life expectancy because it is less likely to cause dysphoria and has a lower risk of dystonic reactions. Also, because it is metabolized through multiple pathways, it can be used in patients with hepatic and renal dysfunction. Olanzapine has the disadvantage that it is only available orally and that it takes a week to reach steady state. The usual dose is 2.5–5 mg PO bid. Chlorpromazine (10–25 mg every 4–6 h) can be useful if sedation is desired and can be administered IV or PR in addition to PO. Dystonic reactions resulting from dopamine blockade are a side effect of neuroleptics, although they are reported to be rare when used to treat terminal delirium. If patients develop dystonic reactions, benztropine should be administered. Neuroleptics may be combined with lorazepam to reduce agitation when the delirium is the result of alcohol or sedative withdrawal.

If no response to first-line therapy is seen, a specialty consultation should be obtained with a change to a different medication. If patients fail to improve after a second neuroleptic, then sedation with an anesthetic such as propofol or continuous-infusion midazolam may be necessary. By some estimates, at the very end of life as many as 25% of patients experiencing delirium, especially restless delirium with myoclonus or convulsions, may require sedation.

Physical restraints should be used with great reluctance only when the patient's violence is threatening to self or others. If used, their appropriateness should be reevaluated frequently.

Insomnia • *FREQUENCY* Sleep disorders, defined as either difficulty initiating sleep or maintaining sleep, sleep difficulty at least 3 nights a week or sleep difficulty that causes impairment of daytime functioning, occurs in between 19 and 63% of patients with advanced cancer.

ETIOLOGY Patients with cancer may have changes in sleep efficiency such as an increase in stage I sleep. Other etiologies of insomnia are coexisting physical illness, such as thyroid disease, or coexisting psychological illnesses, such as depression and anxiety. Medications, including antidepressants, psychostimulants, steroids, and β agonists, are significant contributors to sleep disorders, as are caffeine and alcohol. Multiple over-the-counter medications contain caffeine and antihistamines, which can contribute to sleep disorders.

ASSESSMENT Assessment should include specific questions concerning sleep onset, sleep maintenance, and early morning wakening as these will provide clues to the causative agents and to management. Patients should be asked about previous sleep problems, screened for depression and anxiety, and asked about symptoms of thyroid disease. Caffeine and alcohol are prominent causes of sleep problems, and a careful history of these substances should be obtained. Both excessive use and withdrawal from alcohol can be causes of sleep problems.

INTERVENTIONS The mainstays of intervention include improvement of sleep hygiene (encouraging regular time for sleep, decreased nighttime distractions, elimination of caffeine and other stimulants and alcohol), intervention to treat anxiety and depression, and finally treatment for the insomnia itself. For patients with depression who have insomnia and anxiety, a sedating antidepressant such as mirtazapine can be helpful. In the elderly, trazodone, beginning at 25 mg at nighttime, is an effective sleep aid at doses lower than its antidepressant effect. Zolpidem may have a decreased incidence of delirium in patients compared with traditional benzodiazepines, but this has not been clearly established. When benzodiazepines are prescribed, short-acting ones (such as lorazepam) are favored over longer-acting (such as diazepam). Patients who receive these medications should be observed for signs of increased confusion and delirium.

SOCIAL NEEDS AND THEIR MANAGEMENT
Financial Burdens • *FREQUENCY* Dying can impose substantial economic strains on patients and families, causing distress. In the United States, with one of the least comprehensive health insurance systems among the developed countries, ~20% of terminally ill patients and their families spend >10% of family income on health care costs over and above health insurance premiums. Between 10 and 30% of families sell assets, use savings, or take out a mortgage to pay for the patient's health care costs. Nearly 40% of terminally ill patients in the United States report that the cost of their illness is a moderate or great economic hardship for their family.

The patient is likely to reduce and stop working. In 20% of cases, a family member of the terminally ill patient also stops working to provide care. The major underlying causes of economic burden are related to poor physical functioning and care needs, such as the need for housekeeping, nursing, and personal care. More debilitated patients and poor patients experience greater economic burdens.

INTERVENTION This economic burden should not be ignored as a private matter. It has been associated with a number of adverse health outcomes, including preferring comfort care over life-prolonging care as well as consideration of euthanasia or physician-assisted suicide. Economic burdens increase the psychological distress of families and caregivers of terminally ill patients, and poverty is associated with many adverse health outcomes. Assistance from a social worker, early on if possible, to ensure access to all available benefits may be helpful. Many patients, families, and health care providers are unaware of options for long-term care insurance, respite care, the Family Medical Leave Act (FMLA), and other sources of assistance. Some of these options (such as respite care) may be part of a formal hospice program but others (such as the FMLA) do not require enrollment in a hospice program.

Relationships • *FREQUENCY* Settling personal issues and closing the narrative of lived relationships are universal needs. When asked if sudden death or death after an illness is preferable, respondents often initially select the former but soon change to the latter as they reflect on the importance of saying goodbye. Bereaved family members who have not had the chance to say goodbye often have a more difficult grief process.

INTERVENTIONS Care of seriously ill patients requires efforts to facilitate the types of encounters and time spent with family and friends that are necessary to meet these needs. Family and close friends may need to be accommodated with unrestricted visiting hours, which may include sleeping near the patient even in otherwise regimented institutional settings. Physicians and other health care providers may be able to facilitate and resolve strained interactions between the patient and other family members. Assistance for patients and family members who are unsure about how to create or help preserve memories, whether by providing materials such as a scrap book or memory box or by offering them suggestions and informational resources, can be deeply appreciated. Taking photographs and creating videos can be especially helpful to terminally ill patients who have younger children or grandchildren.

FREQUENCY Caring for seriously ill patients places a heavy burden on families. Families are frequently required to provide transportation and homemaking as well as other services. Typically, paid professionals such as home health nurses and hospice workers supplement family care; only about a quarter of all care giving is exclusively paid professional assistance. The trend toward more out-of-hospital deaths will increase reliance on families for end-of-life care. Increasingly, family members are being called upon to provide physical care (such as moving and bathing patients) and medical care (such as assessing symptoms and giving medications) in addition to emotional care and support.

Three-quarters of family caregivers of terminally ill patients are women—wives, daughters, and even sisters. Since many are widowed, women themselves tend to be able to rely less on family for caregiving assistance and may need more paid assistance. About 20% of terminally ill patients report substantial unmet needs for nursing and personal care. The impact of caregiving on family caregivers is substantial: both bereaved and current caregivers have a higher mortality compared to non-caregiving controls.

INTERVENTIONS It is imperative to inquire about unmet needs and to try to ensure those needs are met either through the family or paid professional services when possible. Community assistance through houses of worship or other community groups can often be mobilized by one or two phone calls from the medical team to someone the patient or family identifies. Sources of support specifically for family caregivers should be identified through local sources or nationally through groups such as the National Family Caregivers Association (*www.nfcacares.org*), the American Cancer Society (*www.cancer.org*), and the Alzheimer's Association (*www.alz.org*).

EXISTENTIAL NEEDS AND THEIR MANAGEMENT

FREQUENCY Religion and spirituality are often important to dying patients. Nearly 70% of patients report becoming more religious or spiritual when they became terminally ill, and many find comfort in various religious or spiritual practices such as prayer. However, ~20% of terminally ill patients become less religious, frequently feeling cheated or betrayed by becoming terminally ill. For other patients, the need is for existential meaning and purpose that is distinct from and may even be antithetical to religion or spirituality. When asked, patients and family caregivers frequently report wanting their professional caregivers to be more attentive to religion and spirituality.

ASSESSMENT Health care providers are often hesitant about involving themselves in the religious, spiritual, and existential experiences of their patients, because it may seem private or not relevant to the current illness. But physicians and other members of the care team should be able to at least detect spiritual and existential needs. Screening questions have been developed for a physician's spiritual history taking. Spiritual distress can amplify other types of suffering and even masquerade as intractable physical pain, anxiety, or depression. The screening questions in the comprehensive assessment are usually sufficient. Deeper evaluation and intervention are rarely appropriate for the physician unless no other member of a care team is available or suitable. Pastoral care providers may be helpful, whether from the medical institution or the patient's own community.

INTERVENTIONS Precisely how religious practices, spirituality, and existential explorations can be facilitated and improve end-of-life care is not well established. What is clear is that for physicians, one main intervention is to inquire about the role and importance of spirituality and religion in a patient's life. This will help a patient feel heard and help physicians to identify specific needs. In one study, only 36% of respondents indicated that a clergy member would be comforting. Nevertheless, the increase in religious and spiritual interest among a substantial fraction of dying patients suggests inquiring of individual patients how this need can be addressed.

MANAGING THE LAST STAGES

WITHDRAWING AND WITHHOLDING LIFE-SUSTAINING TREATMENT

LEGAL ASPECTS For centuries, it has been deemed ethical to withhold or withdraw life-sustaining interventions. The current legal consensus is that patients have a constitutional and common law right to refuse medical interventions. Courts have also held that incompetent patients have a right to refuse medical interventions. For patients who are incompetent and terminally ill and who have not completed an advance care directive, next of kin can exercise this right, although this may be restricted in some states depending how clear and convincing the evidence is of the patient's preferences. Courts have limited families' ability to terminate life-sustaining treatments from patients who are conscious, incompetent, but not terminally ill. In theory, patients' right to refuse medical therapy can be limited by four countervailing interests: (1) preservation of life, (2) prevention of suicide, (3) protection of third parties such as children, and (4) preserving the integrity of the medical profession. In practice, these interests almost never override the right of competent patients and incompetent patients who have left explicit and advance care directives.

Regarding incompetent patients who either appointed a proxy without specific indications of their wishes or who never completed an advance care directive, three criteria have been suggested to guide the decision to terminate medical interventions. First, some commentators suggest that ordinary care should be administered but extraordinary care could be terminated. Because the ordinary/extraordinary distinction is too vague, courts and commentators widely agree that it should not be used to justify decisions about stopping treatment. Second, many courts have advocated use of the substituted-judgment criterion, which holds that the proxy decision-makers should try to imagine what the incompetent patient would do if he or she were competent. However, multiple studies indicate that many proxies, even close family members, cannot accurately predict what the patient would have wanted. Therefore, substituted judgment becomes more of a guessing game than a way of fulfilling the patient's wishes. Finally, the best-interests criterion holds that proxies should evaluate treatments by balancing their benefits and risks and select those treatments in which the benefits maximally outweigh the burdens of treatment. Clinicians have a clear and crucial role in this by carefully and dispassionately explaining the known benefits and burdens of specific treatments. Yet, even when information is as clear as possible, different individuals can have very different views of what is in the patient's best interests, and families may have disagreements or even overt conflicts. This criterion has been criticized because no single way exists of determining the balance between benefits and burdens; it depends on a patient's personal values. As a matter of practice, physicians rely on family members to make decisions that they feel are best and object only if these decisions seem to demand treatments that the physicians consider not beneficial.

PRACTICES Withholding and withdrawing acutely life-sustaining medical interventions from terminally ill patients are now standard practice. More than 90% of American patients die without cardiopulmonary resuscitation (CPR), and just as many forgo other potentially life-sustaining interventions. For instance, during 1987–1988 in ICUs, CPR was performed 49% of the time, but only 10% of the time in 1992–1993. On average, 3.8 interventions, such as vasopressors and transfusions, were stopped for each dying ICU patient. However, practices vary widely among hospitals and ICUs, suggesting an important element of physician preferences rather than objective data.

Mechanical ventilation may be the most challenging intervention to withdraw. The two approaches are *terminal extubation*, which is the removal of the endotracheal tube, and *terminal weaning*, which is the gradual reduction of the FI_{O_2} or ventilator rate. One-third of ICU physicians prefer to use the terminal wean technique, while 13% extubate; the majority of physicians utilize both techniques. Some recommend terminal weaning because patients do not develop upper airway obstruction and the distress caused by secretions or stridor; however, terminal weaning can also prolong the dying process and not allow a patient's family to be with him or her unencumbered by an endotracheal tube. To ensure comfort for conscious or semiconscious patients before withdrawal of the ventilator, neuromuscular blocking agents should be terminated and sedatives and analgesics administered. Removing the neuromuscular blocking agents permits patients to show discomfort, facilitating the titration of sedatives and analgesics; it also permits interactions between patients and their families. A common practice is to inject a bolus of midazolam (2–4 mg) or lorazepam (2–4 mg) before withdrawal, followed by 5–10 mg of morphine and continuous infusion of morphine (50% of the bolus dose per hour) during weaning. In patients who have significant upper airway secretions, IV scopolamine at a rate of 100 μg/h can be administered. Additional boluses of morphine or increases in the infusion rate should be administered for respiratory distress or signs of pain. Higher doses will be needed for patients already receiving sedatives and opioids. Families need to be reassured about treatments for common symptoms after withdrawal of ventilatory support such as dyspnea or agitation and warned about the uncertainty of length of survival after withdrawal of ventilatory support: up to 10% of patients unexpectedly survive for 1 day or more after mechanical ventilation is stopped.

FUTILE CARE

Beginning in the late 1980s, some commentators argued that physicians could terminate futile treatments demanded by families of terminally ill patients. Although no objective definition or standard of futility exists, several categories have been proposed. Physiologic futility means that an intervention will have no physiologic effect. Some have defined qualitative futility as those that "fail to end a patient's total dependence on intensive medical care." Quantitative futility occurs "when physicians conclude (either through personal experience, experiences shared with colleagues, or consideration of reported empiric data) that in the last 100 cases, a medical treatment has been useless." The term conceals subjective value judgments about when a treatment is "not beneficial." Deciding whether a treatment that obtains an additional 6 weeks of life or a 1% survival advantage confers benefit depends upon patients' preferences and goals. Furthermore, physicians' predictions of when treatments were futile deviated markedly from the quantitative definition. When residents thought CPR was quantitatively futile, more than one in five patients had a >10% chance of survival to hospital discharge. Quantitative futility rarely applies in ICU settings. Many commentators reject using futility as a criterion of withdrawing care, preferring instead to consider futility situations as ones that represent conflict that can benefit from careful negotiation between families and health care providers.

Some hospitals have enacted "unilateral DNR" policies to allow clinicians to provide a do-not-resuscitate order in cases where consensus cannot be reached with families and medical opinion is that resuscitation would be futile if attempted. This type of a policy is not a replacement for careful and patient communication and negotiation, but recognizes that agreement cannot always be reached. Texas, Virginia, Maryland, and California and have enacted so-called medical futility laws that provide physicians a "safe harbor" from liability if they terminate life-sustaining treatments over the wishes of the patient's family. For instance, in Texas when a disagreement about terminating interventions between the medical team and family has not been resolved by an ethics consultation, then the hospital is supposed to try to facilitate transfer of the patient to another institution willing to provide treatment. If this fails after 10 days, then the hospital and physician may unilaterally withdraw treatments determined to be futile. The family may appeal to a state court. Early data suggest the law increases futility consultations for the ethics committee and that while most families concur with withdrawal, about 10–15% of families refuse to withdraw treatment. Approximately 12 cases have gone to court in Texas in 7 years after adoption of the law.

EUTHANASIA AND PHYSICIAN-ASSISTED SUICIDE

Euthanasia and physician-assisted suicide are defined in Table 11-8. Terminating life-sustaining care and providing opioid medications to manage symptoms have long been considered ethical by the medical profession and legal by courts and should not be confused with euthanasia or physician-assisted suicide.

LEGAL ASPECTS Euthanasia is legal in the Netherlands and Belgium. Euthanasia was legalized in the Northern Territory of Australia but then repealed. Euthanasia is not legal in any state in the United States. Physician-assisted suicide is legal in Oregon but only if multiple criteria are met and then only after a process that includes a 15-day waiting period. In Switzerland, a layperson can legally assist suicide. In all other countries and all other states in the United States, physician-assisted suicide and euthanasia are illegal explicitly or by common law.

PRACTICES Fewer than 10–20% of terminally ill patients actually consider euthanasia and/or physician-assisted suicide for themselves. In the Netherlands and Oregon, >70% of patients utilizing these interventions are dying of cancer; <5% of deaths by euthanasia or physician-assisted suicide involve patients with AIDS or amyotrophic lateral sclerosis. In the Netherlands, if all legal and illegal acts are grouped, euthanasia and physician-assisted suicide account for 3.5% of all deaths. In Oregon, ~0.1% of patients die by physician-assisted suicide, although this may be an underestimate.

Pain is not a primary motivator for patients' requests for or interest in euthanasia and/or physician-assisted suicide. Among the first patients to receive physician-assisted suicide in Oregon, only 1 patient of 15 had inadequate pain control compared to 15 of 43 patients in a control group experiencing inadequate pain relief. Depression, hopelessness, and, more profoundly, concerns about loss of dignity or autonomy or being a burden on family members, appear to be primary factors motivating a desire for euthanasia or physician-assisted suicide. A study from the Netherlands showed that depressed terminally ill cancer patients were four times more likely to request euthanasia, and confirmed that uncontrolled pain was not associated with greater interest in euthanasia.

Euthanasia and physician-assisted suicide are no guarantee of a painless, quick death. Data from the Netherlands indicate that in as many as 20% of cases technical and other problems arose, including patients waking from coma, not becoming comatose, regurgitating medications, and a prolonged time to death. Problems were significantly more common in physician-assisted suicide, sometimes requiring the physician to intervene and provide euthanasia.

Whether practicing in a setting where euthanasia is legal or not, over a career, between 12 and 54% of physicians will receive a request for euthanasia or physician-assisted suicide from a patient. Competency in dealing with such a request is crucial. While challenging, such a request can also be a chance to address intense suffering. After receiving a request for euthanasia and/or physician-assisted suicide, health care providers should carefully clarify the request with empathic, open-ended questions to help elucidate the underlying cause for the request such as: "What makes you

TABLE 11-8 DEFINITIONS OF ASSISTED SUICIDE AND EUTHANASIA

Term	Definition	Legal Status
Voluntary active euthanasia	Intentionally administering medications or other interventions to cause the patient's death with the patient's informed consent	Netherlands Belgium
Involuntary active euthanasia	Intentionally administering medications or other interventions to cause the patient's death when the patient was competent to consent but did not—e.g., the patient may not have been asked	Nowhere
Passive euthanasia	Withholding or withdrawing life-sustaining medical treatments from a patient to let him or her die (terminating life-sustaining treatments)	Everywhere
Physician-assisted suicide	A physician provides medications or other interventions to a patient with the understanding that the patient can use them to commit suicide	Oregon Netherlands Belgium Switzerland

want to consider this option?" Endorsing either moral opposition or moral support for the act tends to be counterproductive, either lending an impression of being judgmental or of endorsing the idea that the patient's life is worthless. Health care providers must reassure the patient of continued care and commitment. The patient should be educated about alternative, less controversial options, such as symptom management and withdrawing any unwanted treatments; the reality of euthanasia and/or physician-assisted suicide, since the patient may have misconceptions about their effectiveness; and also the legal implications of the choice. Depression, hopelessness, and other symptoms of psychological distress as well as physical suffering and economic burdens are likely factors motivating the request, and such factors should be assessed and treated aggressively. After these interventions and clarification of options, most patients proceed with another approach, declining life-sustaining interventions, possibly including refusal of nutrition and hydration.

CARE DURING THE LAST HOURS

Most laypersons have limited experiences with the actual dying process and death. They frequently do not know what to expect of the final hours, and afterwards. The family and other caregivers must be prepared, especially if the plan is for the patient to die at home.

Patients in the last days of life typically experience extreme weakness and fatigue and become bedbound; this can lead to pressure sores. The issue of turning patients who are near the end of life, however, must be balanced against the potential discomfort that movement may cause. Patients stop eating and drinking with drying of mucosal membranes and dysphagia. Careful attention to oral swabbing, lubricants for lips, and use of artificial tears can provide a form of care to substitute for attempts at feeding the patient. With loss of the gag reflex and dysphagia, patients may also experience accumulation of oral secretions, producing noises during respiration sometimes called "the death rattle." Scopolamine can reduce the secretions. Patients also experience changes in respiration with periods of apnea or Cheyne-Stokes breathing. Decreased intravascular volume and cardiac output cause tachycardia, hypotension, peripheral coolness, and livedo reticularis (skin mottling). Patients can have urinary and, less frequently, fecal incontinence. Changes in consciousness and neurologic function generally lead to two different paths to death (Fig. 11-2).

Each of these terminal changes can cause patients and families distress, requiring reassurance and targeted interventions (Table 11-9). Informing families that these changes might occur, and even providing them an information sheet, can help to preempt problems and minimize distress. Understanding that patients stop eating because they are dying, not dying because they have stopped eating, can reduce family and caregiver anxiety. Similarly, informing the family and caregivers that the "death rattle" may occur and that it is not indicative of suffocation or choking can reduce their worry from the breathing sounds.

Families and caregivers may also feel guilty about stopping treatments, fearing that they are "killing" the patient. This may lead to demands for interventions that may be ineffective. In such cases, the physician should remind the family and caregivers about the inevitability of events and the palliative goals. Interventions may prolong the dying process and cause discomfort. Physicians should also emphasize that withholding treatments is both legal and ethical, and that the family members are not the cause of the patient's death. This reassurance may need to be provided multiple times.

Hearing and touch are said to be the last senses to stop functioning. Whether this is the case or not, families and caregivers can be encouraged to communicate with the dying patient. Encouraging them to talk directly to the patient, even if he or she is unconscious, and hold the patient's hand or demonstrate affection in other ways can be an effective way to channel their urge "to do something" for the patient.

When the plan is for the patient to die at home, the physician must inform the family and caregivers how to determine that the patient has died. The cardinal signs are cessation of cardiac function and respiration; the pupils become fixed; the body becomes cool; muscles relax; and incontinence may occur. Remind the family and caregivers that the eyes may remain open even when the patient has died because the

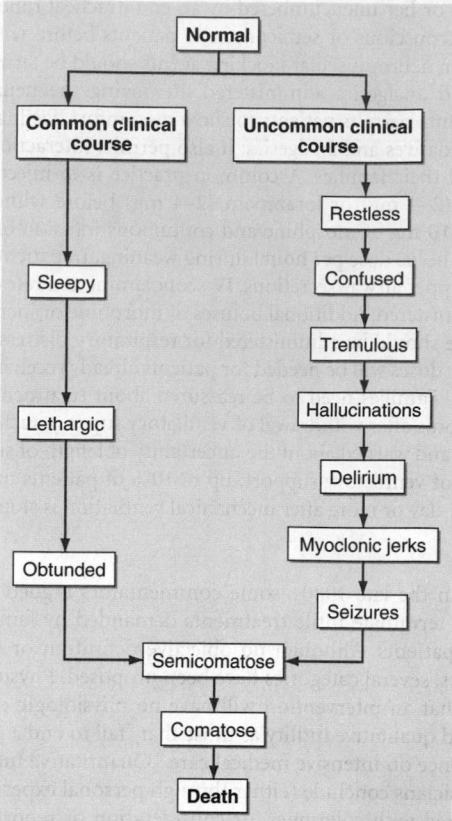

FIGURE 11-2 Common and uncommon clinical courses in the last days of terminally ill patients. (*Adapted from FD Ferris et al: Module 4: Palliative care, in Comprehensive Guide for the Care of Persons with HIV Disease. Toronto: Mt. Sinai Hospital and Casey Hospice, 1995, at www.cpsonline.info/content/resources/hivmodule4.html.*)

retroorbital fat pad may be depleted, permitting the orbit to fall posteriorly, which makes it difficult for the eyelids to cover the eyeball.

The physician should establish a plan for who the family or caregivers will contact when the patient is dying or has died. Without a plan, they may panic and call 911, unleashing a cascade of unwanted events from arrival of emergency personnel and resuscitation to hospital admission. The family and caregivers should be instructed to contact the hospice (if one is involved), the covering physician, or the on-call member of the palliative care team. They should also be told that the medical examiner need not be called, unless the state requires it for all deaths. Unless foul play is suspected, the health care team need not contact the medical examiner either.

Just after the patient dies, even the best-prepared family may experience shock and loss and be emotionally distraught. They need time to assimilate the event and be comforted. Health care providers may find it meaningful to write a bereavement card or letter to the family. The purpose is to communicate about the patient, perhaps emphasizing the patient's virtues, the honor it was to care for the patient, and express concern for the family's hardship. Some physicians attend the funerals of their patients. While this is beyond any medical obligation, the presence of the physician can be a source of support to the grieving family and provides an opportunity for closure for the physician.

Death of a spouse is a strong predictor of poor health, and even mortality, for the surviving spouse. It may be important to alert the spouse's physician about the death to be aware of symptoms that might require professional attention.

PALLIATIVE CARE SERVICES: HOW AND WHERE

Determining the best approach to providing palliative care to patients will depend upon patient preferences, the availability of caregivers and specialized services in close proximity, institutional resources, and re-

TABLE 11-9 **MANAGING CHANGES IN THE PATIENT'S CONDITION DURING THE FINAL DAYS AND HOURS**

Changes in the Patient's Condition	Potential Complication	Family's Possible Reaction and Concern	Advice and Intervention
Profound fatigue	Bedbound with development of pressure ulcers that are prone to infection, malodor, and pain, and joint pain	Patient is lazy and giving up.	Reassure family and caregivers that terminal fatigue will not respond to interventions and should not be resisted. Use an air mattress if necessary.
Anorexia	None	Patient is giving up; patient will suffer from hunger and will starve to death.	Reassure family and caregivers that the patient is not eating because he or she is dying; not eating at the end of life does not cause suffering or death. Forced feeding, whether oral, parenteral, or enteral, does not reduce symptoms or prolong life.
Dehydration	Dry mucosal membranes (see below)	Patient will suffer from thirst and die of dehydration.	Reassure family and caregivers that dehydration at the end of life does not cause suffering because patients lose consciousness before any symptom distress. Intravenous hydration can worsen symptoms of dyspnea by pulmonary edema and peripheral edema as well as prolong dying process.
Dysphagia	Inability to swallow oral medications needed for palliative care		Do not force oral intake. Discontinue unnecessary medications that may have been continued including antibiotics, diuretics, anti-depressants, and laxatives. If swallowing pills is difficult, convert essential medications (analgesics, antiemetics, anxiolytics, and psychotropics) to oral solutions, buccal, sublingual, or rectal administration.
"Death rattle"—noisy breathing		Patient is choking and suffocating.	Reassure the family and caregivers that this is caused by secretions in the oropharynx and the patient is not choking. Reduce secretions with scopolamine (0.2–0.4 mg SC q4h or 1–3 patches q3d) Reposition patient to permit drainage of secretions. Do not suction. Suction can cause patient and family discomfort, and is usually ineffective.
Apnea, Cheyne-Stokes respirations, dyspnea		Patient is suffocating.	Reassure family and caregivers that unconscious patients do not experience suffocation or air hunger. Apneic episodes are frequently a premorbid change. Opioids or anxiolytics may be used for dyspnea. Oxygen is unlikely to relieve dyspneic symptoms and may prolong the dying process.
Urinary or fecal incontinence	Skin breakdown if days until death Potential transmission of infectious agents to caregivers	Patient is dirty, malodorous, and physically repellent.	Remind family and caregivers to use universal precautions. Frequent changes of bedclothes and bedding. Use diapers, urinary catheter, or rectal tube if diarrhea or high urine output.
Agitation or delirium	Day/night reversal Hurt self or caregivers	Patient is in horrible pain and going to have a horrible death.	Reassure family and caregivers that agitation and delirium do not necessarily connote physical pain. Depending upon the prognosis and goals of treatment, consider evaluating for causes of delirium and modify medications. Manage symptoms with haloperidol, chlorpromazine, diazepam, or midazolam.
Dry mucosal membranes	Cracked lips, mouth sores, and candidiasis can also cause pain. Odor	Patient may be malodorous, physically repellent.	Use baking soda mouthwash or saliva preparation q15–30min. Use topical nystatin for candidiasis. Coat lips and nasal mucosa with petroleum jelly q60–90min. Use ophthalmic lubricants q4h or artificial tears q30min.

imbursement. Hospice is a leading, but not the only, model of palliative care services. In the United States, the vast majority of hospice care is provided in residential homes. By 2002, just over 20% of hospice was provided in nursing homes. In the United States, Medicare pays for hospice services under Part A, the hospital insurance part of reimbursement. Two physicians must certify that the patient has a prognosis of ≤6 months, if the disease runs its usual course. Prognoses are probabilistic by their nature; patients are not required to die within 6 months but rather to have a condition from which half the individuals with it would not be alive within 6 months. Patients sign a hospice enrollment form that states their intent to forgo curative services related to their terminal illness, but they can still receive medical services for other comorbid conditions. Patients can also withdraw enrollment and re-enroll later; the hospice Medicare benefit can be revoked later to secure traditional Medicare benefits. Payments to the hospice are per diem (or capitated), not fee-for-service. Payments are intended to cover physician services for the medical direction of the care team; regular home care visits by registered nurses and licensed practical nurses; home health aid and homemaker services; chaplain services; social work services; bereavement counseling; and medical equipment, supplies, and medications. No specific therapy is excluded and the goal is for each therapy to be considered for its symptomatic (as opposed to disease-modifying) effect. Additional clinical care, including services of the primary physician, is covered by Medicare Part B, even while the hospice Medicare benefit is in place.

By 2005, the mean length of enrollment in a hospice was 59 days, with the median being 26 days. Such short stays create barriers to establishing high-quality palliative services in patients' homes and also place financial strains on hospice providers since the initial assessments are resource intensive. Physicians should initiate early referrals to the hospice to allow more time for patients to receive palliative care.

Hospice care has been the main way of securing palliative services for terminally ill patients. However, efforts are now being made to ensure continuity of palliative care across settings and through time. Palliative care services are becoming available as consultative services and more rarely as palliative care units in hospitals, in day care and other outpatient settings, and in nursing homes. Palliative care consultations for non-hospice patients can be billed as for other consultations under Medicare

Part B, the physician reimbursement part. Many believe palliative care should be offered to patients regardless of their prognosis. A patient, his or her family, and physicians should not have to make a "curative vs. palliative care" decision because it is rarely possible to make such a decisive switch to embracing mortality.

FUTURE DIRECTIONS

OUTCOME MEASURES

Care near the end of life cannot be measured by most of the available validated outcome measures since palliative care does not consider death a bad outcome. Similarly, the family and patients receiving end-of-life care may not desire the elements elicited in current quality-of-life measurements. Symptom control, enhanced family relationships, and quality of bereavement are difficult to measure and are rarely the primary focus of carefully developed or widely used outcome measures. Nevertheless, outcomes are as important in end-of-life care as in any other field of medical care. Specific end-of-life care instruments are being developed both for assessment, such as The Brief Hospice Inventory and NEST (*needs near the end of life screening tool*), and for outcome measures, such as the Palliative Care Outcomes Scale, and for prognosis, such as the Palliative Prognostic Index. The field of end-of-life care is entering an era of evidence-based practice and continuous improvement through clinical trials.

FURTHER READINGS

Web Sites

Education in Palliative and End of Life Care (EPEC): *http://www.epec.net*

End of Life—Palliative Education Resource Center: *http://www.eperc.mcw.edu*

National Hospice and Palliative Care Organization (including state-specific advance directives): *http://www.nhpco.org*

NCCN: The National Comprehensive Cancer Network palliative care guidelines: *http://www.nccn.org*

Center to Advance Palliative Care: *http://www.capc.org*

Family Caregiver Alliance: *http://www.caregiver.org*

National Family Caregivers Association: *http://www.nfcacares.org/*

The Medical Directive: *http://www.medicaldirective.org*

American Academy of Hospice and Palliative Medicine: *www.aahpm.org*

Books

AMERICAN SOCIETY OF CLINICAL ONCOLOGY: *Optimizing Cancer Care—The Importance of Symptom Management.* vols 1 and 2. Alexandria, VA, ASCO, 2001

BUCKMAN R: *How to Break Bad News: A Guide for Health Care Professionals.* Baltimore, Johns Hopkins University Press, 1992

Articles

CHRISTAKIS NA, ALLISON PD: Mortality after the hospitalization of a spouse. N Engl J Med 354:719, 2006.

EMANUEL L et al, for the Palliative Care Guidelines Group of the American Hospice Foundation: Integrating palliative care into disease management guidelines. Journal of Palliative Medicine 7:774, 2004

KAPO J et al: Palliative care for the older adult. J Palliat Med 10:185, 2007

LYNN J: Serving patients who may die soon and their families: The role of hospice and other services. JAMA 285:925, 2001

MEISEL A et al, for the American College of Physicians–American Society of Internal Medicine End-of-Life Care Consensus Panel: Seven legal barriers to end-of-life care: Myths, realities, and grains of truth. JAMA 284:2495, 2000

MURRAY SA et al: Illness trajectories and palliative care. BMJ 330:1007, 2005

PART 2: Cardinal Manifestations and Presentation of Diseases

SECTION 1   PAIN

12 Pain: Pathophysiology and Management

Howard L. Fields, Joseph B. Martin

The task of medicine is to preserve and restore health and to relieve suffering. Understanding pain is essential to both these goals. Because pain is universally understood as a signal of disease, it is the most common symptom that brings a patient to a physician's attention. The function of the pain sensory system is to protect the body and maintain homeostasis. It does this by detecting, localizing, and identifying tissue-damaging processes. Since different diseases produce characteristic patterns of tissue damage, the quality, time course, and location of a patient's pain complaint and the location of tenderness provide important diagnostic clues and are used to evaluate the response to treatment. Once this information is obtained, it is the obligation of the physician to provide rapid and effective pain relief.

THE PAIN SENSORY SYSTEM

Pain is an unpleasant sensation localized to a part of the body. It is often described in terms of a penetrating or tissue-destructive process (e.g., stabbing, burning, twisting, tearing, squeezing) and/or of a bodily or emotional reaction (e.g., terrifying, nauseating, sickening). Furthermore, any pain of moderate or higher intensity is accompanied by anxiety and the urge to escape or terminate the feeling. These properties illustrate the duality of pain: it is both sensation and emotion. When acute, pain is characteristically associated with behavioral arousal and a stress response consisting of increased blood pressure, heart rate, pupil diameter, and plasma cortisol levels. In addition, local muscle contraction (e.g., limb flexion, abdominal wall rigidity) is often present.

PERIPHERAL MECHANISMS

The Primary Afferent Nociceptor
A peripheral nerve consists of the axons of three different types of neurons: primary sensory afferents, motor neurons, and sympathetic postganglionic neurons (Fig. 12-1). The cell bodies of primary sensory afferents are located in the dorsal root ganglia in the vertebral foramina. The primary afferent axon bifurcates to send one process into the spinal cord and the other to innervate tissues. Primary afferents are classified by their diameter, degree of myelination, and conduction velocity. The largest-diameter fibers, A-beta (Aβ), respond maximally to light touch and/or moving stimuli; they are present primarily in nerves that innervate the skin. In normal individuals, the activity of these fibers does not produce pain. There are two other classes of primary afferents: the small-diameter myelinated A-delta (Aδ) and the unmyelinated (C fiber) axons (Fig. 12-1). These fibers are present in nerves to the skin and to deep somatic and visceral structures. Some tissues, such as the cornea, are innervated only by Aδ and C af-

ferents. Most Aδ and C afferents respond maximally only to intense (painful) stimuli and produce the subjective experience of pain when they are electrically stimulated; this defines them as *primary afferent nociceptors* (*pain receptors*). The ability to detect painful stimuli is completely abolished when Aδ and C axons are blocked.

Individual primary afferent nociceptors can respond to several different types of noxious stimuli. For example, most nociceptors respond to heating, intense cold, intense mechanical stimuli such as a pinch, and application of irritating chemicals including ATP, serotonin, bradykinin and histamine.

Sensitization   When intense, repeated, or prolonged stimuli are applied to damaged or inflamed tissues, the threshold for activating primary afferent nociceptors is lowered and the frequency of firing is higher for all stimulus intensities. Inflammatory mediators such as bradykinin, nerve growth factor, some prostaglandins, and leukotrienes contribute to this process, which is called *sensitization*. In sensitized tissues, normally innocuous stimuli can produce pain. Sensitization is a clinically important process that contributes to tenderness, soreness, and hyperalgesia. A striking example of sensitization is sunburned skin, in which severe pain can be produced by a gentle slap on the back or a warm shower.

Sensitization is of particular importance for pain and tenderness in deep tissues. Viscera are normally relatively insensitive to noxious mechanical and thermal stimuli, although hollow viscera do generate significant discomfort when distended. In contrast, when affected by a disease process with an inflammatory component, deep structures such as joints or hollow viscera characteristically become exquisitely sensitive to mechanical stimulation.

A large proportion of Aδ and C afferents innervating viscera are completely insensitive in normal noninjured, noninflamed tissue. That is, they cannot be activated by known mechanical or thermal stimuli and are not spontaneously active. However, in the presence of inflammatory mediators, these afferents become sensitive to mechanical stimuli. Such afferents have been termed *silent nociceptors*, and

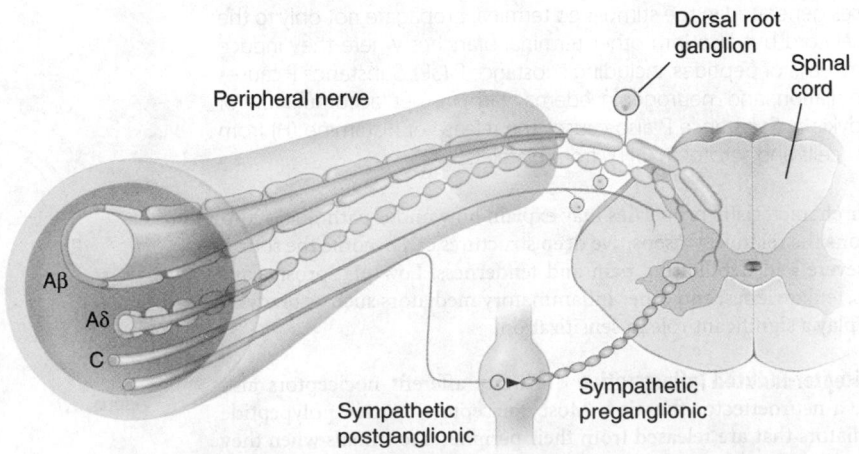

FIGURE 12-1 Components of a typical cutaneous nerve. There are two distinct functional categories of axons: primary afferents with cell bodies in the dorsal root ganglion, and sympathetic postganglionic fibers with cell bodies in the sympathetic ganglion. Primary afferents include those with large-diameter myelinated (Aβ), small-diameter myelinated (Aδ), and unmyelinated (C) axons. All sympathetic postganglionic fibers are unmyelinated.

A

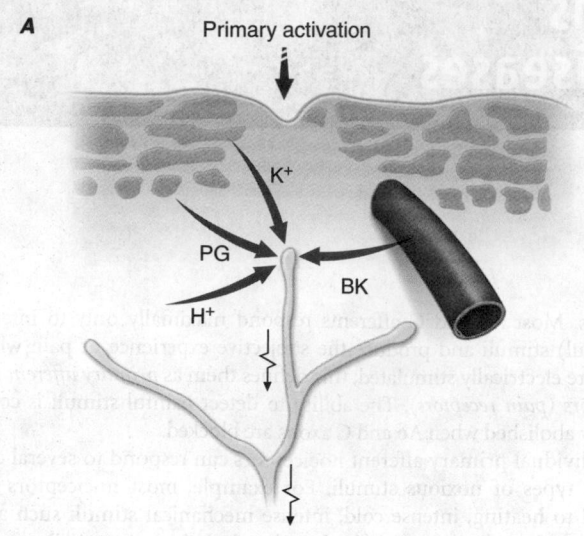

Primary activation

B

Secondary activation

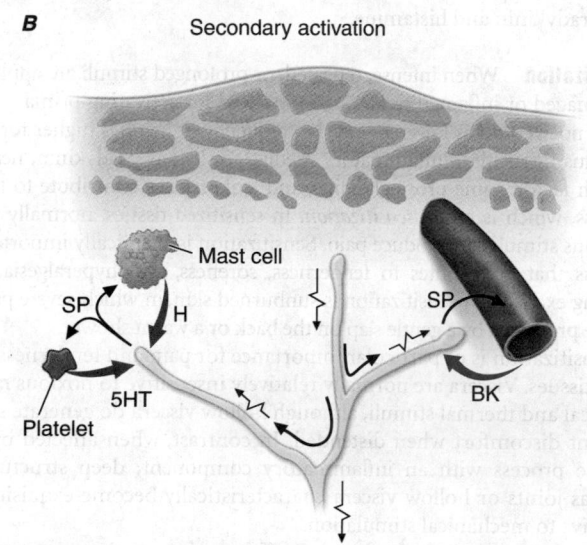

FIGURE 12-2 Events leading to activation, sensitization, and spread of sensitization of primary afferent nociceptor terminals. A. Direct activation by intense pressure and consequent cell damage. Cell damage induces lower pH (H^+) and leads to release of potassium (K^+) and to synthesis of prostaglandins (PG) and bradykinin (BK). Prostaglandins increase the sensitivity of the terminal to bradykinin and other pain-producing substances. **B.** Secondary activation. Impulses generated in the stimulated terminal propagate not only to the spinal cord but also into other terminal branches where they induce the release of peptides, including substance P (SP). Substance P causes vasodilation and neurogenic edema with further accumulation of bradykinin. Substance P also causes the release of histamine (H) from mast cells and serotonin (5HT) from platelets.

their characteristic properties may explain how under pathologic conditions the relatively insensitive deep structures can become the source of severe and debilitating pain and tenderness. Low pH, prostaglandins, leukotrienes, and other inflammatory mediators such as bradykinin play a significant role in sensitization.

Nociceptor-Induced Inflammation Primary afferent nociceptors also have a neuroeffector function. Most nociceptors contain polypeptide mediators that are released from their peripheral terminals when they are activated (Fig. 12-2). An example is substance P, an 11-amino-acid peptide. Substance P is released from primary afferent nociceptors and has multiple biologic activities. It is a potent vasodilator, degranulates mast cells, is a chemoattractant for leukocytes, and increases the production and release of inflammatory mediators. Interestingly, depletion of substance P from joints reduces the severity of experimental

arthritis. Primary afferent nociceptors are not simply passive messengers of threats to tissue injury but also play an active role in tissue protection through these neuroeffector functions.

CENTRAL MECHANISMS

The Spinal Cord and Referred Pain The axons of primary afferent nociceptors enter the spinal cord via the dorsal root. They terminate in the dorsal horn of the spinal gray matter (Fig. 12-3). The terminals of primary afferent axons contact spinal neurons that transmit the pain signal to brain sites involved in pain perception. When primary afferents are activated by noxious stimuli, they release neurotransmitters from their terminals that excite the spinal cord neurons. The major neurotransmitter they release is glutamate, which rapidly excites dorsal horn neurons. Primary afferent nociceptor terminals also release peptides, including substance P and calcitonin gene-related peptide, which produce a slower and longer-lasting excitation of the dorsal horn neurons. The axon of each primary afferent contacts many spinal neurons, and each spinal neuron receives convergent inputs from many primary afferents.

The convergence of sensory inputs to a single spinal pain-transmission neuron is of great importance because it underlies the phenomenon of referred pain. All spinal neurons that receive input from the viscera and deep musculoskeletal structures also receive input from the skin. The convergence patterns are determined by the spinal segment of the dorsal root ganglion that supplies the afferent innervation of a structure. For example, the afferents that supply the central diaphragm are derived from the third and fourth cervical dorsal root ganglia. Primary afferents with cell bodies in these same ganglia supply the skin of the shoulder and lower neck. Thus, sensory inputs from both the shoulder skin and the central diaphragm converge on pain-transmission neurons in the third and fourth cervical spinal segments. *Because of this convergence and the fact that the spinal neurons are most often activated by inputs from the skin, activity evoked in spinal neurons by input from deep structures is mislocalized by the patient to a place that is roughly coextensive with the region of skin innervated by the same spinal segment.* Thus, inflammation near the central diaphragm is usually reported as discomfort near the shoulder. This spatial displacement of pain sensation from the site of the injury that produces it is known as *referred pain*.

Ascending Pathways for Pain A majority of spinal neurons contacted by primary afferent nociceptors send their axons to the contralateral thalamus. These axons form the contralateral spinothalamic tract, which lies in the anterolateral white matter of the spinal cord, the lateral edge of the medulla, and the lateral pons and midbrain. The spinothalamic pathway is crucial for pain sensation in humans. Interruption of this pathway produces permanent deficits in pain and temperature discrimination.

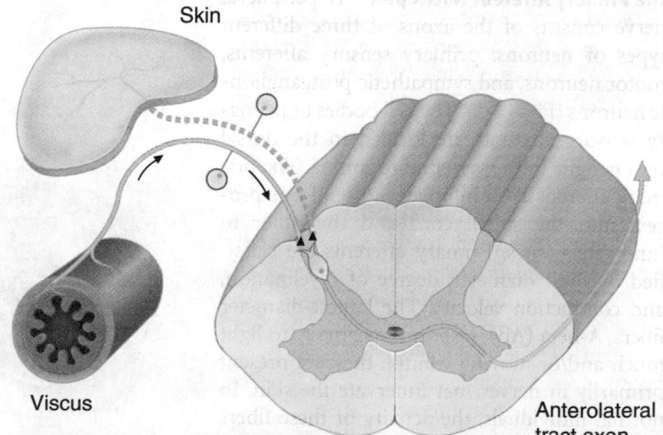

FIGURE 12-3 The convergence-projection hypothesis of referred pain. According to this hypothesis, visceral afferent nociceptors converge on the same pain-projection neurons as the afferents from the somatic structures in which the pain is perceived. The brain has no way of knowing the actual source of input and mistakenly "projects" the sensation to the somatic structure.

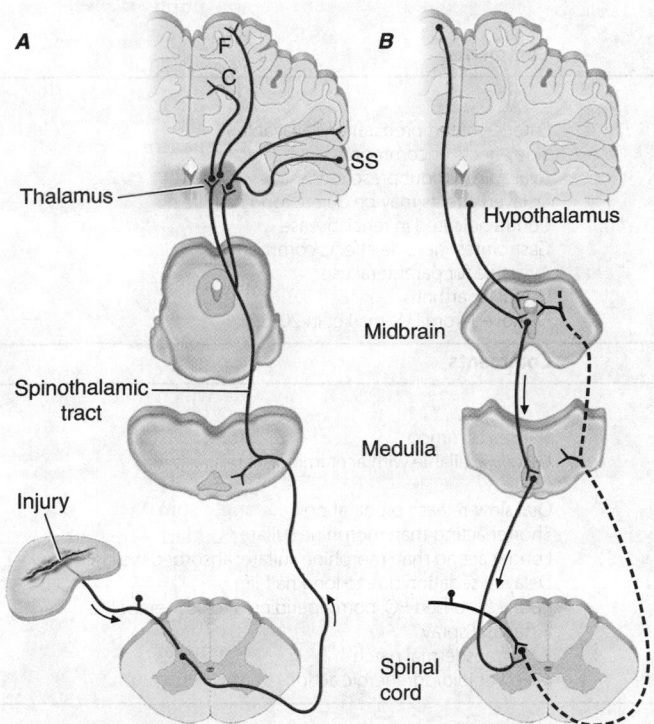

FIGURE 12-4 Pain transmission and modulatory pathways. A. Transmission system for nociceptive messages. Noxious stimuli activate the sensitive peripheral ending of the primary afferent nociceptor by the process of transduction. The message is then transmitted over the peripheral nerve to the spinal cord, where it synapses with cells of origin of the major ascending pain pathway, the spinothalamic tract. The message is relayed in the thalamus to the anterior cingulate (C), frontal insular (F), and somatosensory cortex (SS). **B.** Pain-modulation network. Inputs from frontal cortex and hypothalamus activate cells in the midbrain that control spinal pain-transmission cells via cells in the medulla.

Spinothalamic tract axons ascend to several regions of the thalamus. There is tremendous divergence of the pain signal from these thalamic sites to broad areas of the cerebral cortex that subserve different aspects of the pain experience (Fig. 12-4). One of the thalamic projections is to the somatosensory cortex. This projection mediates the purely sensory aspects of pain, i.e., its location, intensity, and quality. Other thalamic neurons project to cortical regions that are linked to emotional responses, such as the cingulate gyrus and other areas of the frontal lobes, including the insular cortex. These pathways to the frontal cortex subserve the affective or unpleasant emotional dimension of pain. This affective dimension of pain produces suffering and exerts potent control of behavior. Because of this dimension, fear is a constant companion of pain.

PAIN MODULATION

The pain produced by injuries of similar magnitude is remarkably variable in different situations and in different individuals. For example, athletes have been known to sustain serious fractures with only minor pain, and Beecher's classic World War II survey revealed that many soldiers in battle were unbothered by injuries that would have produced agonizing pain in civilian patients. Furthermore, even the suggestion of relief can have a significant analgesic effect (placebo). On the other hand, many patients find even minor injuries (such as venipuncture) frightening and unbearable, and the expectation of pain has been demonstrated to induce pain without a noxious stimulus.

The powerful effect of expectation and other psychological variables on the perceived intensity of pain implies the existence of brain circuits that can modulate the activity of the pain-transmission pathways. One of these circuits has links in the hypothalamus, midbrain, and medulla, and it selectively controls spinal pain-transmission neurons through a descending pathway (Fig. 12-4).

Human brain imaging studies have implicated this pain-modulating circuit in the pain-relieving effect of attention, suggestion, and opioid analgesic medications. Furthermore, each of the component structures of the pathway contains opioid receptors and is sensitive to the direct application of opioid drugs. In animals, lesions of the system reduce the analgesic effect of systemically administered opioids such as morphine. Along with the opioid receptor, the component nuclei of this pain-modulating circuit contain endogenous opioid peptides such as the enkephalins and β-endorphin.

The most reliable way to activate this endogenous opioid-mediated modulating system is by prolonged pain and/or fear. There is evidence that pain-relieving endogenous opioids are released following surgical procedures and in patients given a placebo for pain relief.

Pain-modulating circuits can enhance as well as suppress pain. Both pain-inhibiting and pain-facilitating neurons in the medulla project to and control spinal pain-transmission neurons. Since pain-transmission neurons can be activated by modulatory neurons, it is theoretically possible to generate a pain signal with no peripheral noxious stimulus. In fact, human functional imaging studies have demonstrated increased activity in this circuit during migraine headache. A central circuit that facilitates pain could account for the finding that pain can be induced by suggestion or enhanced by expectation, and it could provide a framework for understanding how psychological factors can contribute to chronic pain.

NEUROPATHIC PAIN

Lesions of the peripheral or central nervous pathways for pain typically result in a loss or impairment of pain sensation. Paradoxically, damage to or dysfunction of these pathways can produce pain. For example, damage to peripheral nerves, as occurs in diabetic neuropathy, or to primary afferents, as in herpes zoster, can result in pain that is referred to the body region innervated by the damaged nerves. Though rare, pain may also be produced by damage to the central nervous system, particularly the spinothalamic pathway or thalamus. Such neuropathic pains are often severe and are notoriously intractable to standard treatments for pain.

Neuropathic pains typically have an unusual burning, tingling, or electric shock–like quality and may be triggered by very light touch. These features are rare in other types of pain. On examination, a sensory deficit is characteristically present in the area of the patient's pain. Hyperpathia is also characteristic of neuropathic pain; patients often complain that the very lightest moving stimuli evoke exquisite pain (allodynia). In this regard it is of clinical interest that a topical preparation of 5% lidocaine in patch form is effective for patients with postherpetic neuralgia who have prominent allodynia.

A variety of mechanisms contribute to neuropathic pain. As with sensitized primary afferent nociceptors, damaged primary afferents, including nociceptors, become highly sensitive to mechanical stimulation and begin to generate impulses in the absence of stimulation. There is evidence that this increased sensitivity and spontaneous activity is due to an increased concentration of sodium channels. Damaged primary afferents may also develop sensitivity to norepinephrine. Interestingly, spinal cord pain-transmission neurons cut off from their normal input may also become spontaneously active. Thus, both central and peripheral nervous system hyperactivity contribute to neuropathic pain.

Sympathetically Maintained Pain Patients with peripheral nerve injury can develop a severe burning pain (causalgia) in the region innervated by the nerve. The pain typically begins after a delay of hours to days or even weeks. The pain is accompanied by swelling of the extremity, periarticular osteoporosis, and arthritic changes in the distal joints. The pain is dramatically and immediately relieved by blocking the sympathetic innervation of the affected extremity. Damaged primary afferent nociceptors acquire adrenergic sensitivity and can be activated by stimulation of the sympathetic outflow. A similar syndrome called *reflex sympathetic dystrophy* can be produced without obvious nerve damage by a variety of injuries, including fractures of bone, soft tissue trauma, myocardial infarction, and stroke (Chap. 370). Although the pathophysiology of this condition is poorly understood, the pain and the signs of inflammation are rapidly relieved by blocking the sympathetic nervous

TABLE 12-1 DRUGS FOR RELIEF OF PAIN

Generic Name	Dose, mg	Interval	Comments
Nonnarcotic Analgesics: Usual Doses and Intervals			
Acetylsalicylic acid	650 PO	q 4 h	Enteric-coated preparations available
Acetaminophen	650 PO	q 4 h	Side effects uncommon
Ibuprofen	400 PO	q 4–6 h	Available without prescription
Naproxen	250–500 PO	q 12 h	Delayed effects may be due to long half-life
Fenoprofen	200 PO	q 4–6 h	Contraindicated in renal disease
Indomethacin	25–50 PO	q 8 h	Gastrointestinal side effects common
Ketorolac	15–60 IM/IV	q 4–6 h	Available for parenteral use
Celecoxib	100–200 PO	q 12–24 h	Useful for arthritis
Valdecoxib	10–20 PO	q12–24 h	Removed from U.S. market in 2005

Generic Name	Parenteral Dose, mg	PO Dose, mg	Comments
Narcotic Analgesics: Usual Doses and Intervals			
Codeine	30–60 q 4 h	30–60 q 4 h	Nausea common
Oxycodone	—	5–10 q 4–6 h	Usually available with acetaminophen or aspirin
Morphine	10 q 4 h	60 q 4 h	
Morphine sustained release	—	30–200 bid to tid	Oral slow-release preparation
Hydromorphone	1–2 q 4 h	2–4 q 4 h	Shorter acting than morphine sulfate
Levorphanol	2 q 6–8 h	4 q 6–8 h	Longer acting than morphine sulfate; absorbed well PO
Methadone	10 q 6–8 h	20 q 6–8 h	Delayed sedation due to long half-life
Meperidine	75–100 q 3–4 h	300 q 4 h	Poorly absorbed PO; normeperidine a toxic metabolite
Butorphanol	—	1–2 q 4 h	Intranasal spray
Fentanyl	25–100 µg/h	—	72 h Transdermal patch
Tramadol	—	50–100 q 4–6 h	Mixed opioid/adrenergic action

Generic Name	Uptake Blockade 5-HT	Uptake Blockade NE	Sedative Potency	Anticholinergic Potency	Orthostatic Hypotension	Cardiac Arrhythmia	Ave. Dose, mg/d	Range, mg/d
Antidepressants[a]								
Doxepin	++	+	High	Moderate	Moderate	Less	200	75–400
Amitriptyline	++++	++	High	Highest	Moderate	Yes	150	25–300
Imipramine	++++	++	Moderate	Moderate	High	Yes	200	75–400
Nortriptyline	+++	++	Moderate	Moderate	Low	Yes	100	40–150
Desipramine	+++	++++	Low	Low	Low	Yes	150	50–300
Venlafaxine	+++	++	Low	None	None	No	150	75–400
Duloxetine	+++	+++	Low	None	None	No	40	30–60

Generic Name	PO Dose, mg	Interval	Generic Name	PO Dose, mg	Interval
Anticonvulsants and Antiarrhythmics[a]					
Phenytoin	300	daily/qhs	Clonazepam	1	q 6 h
Carbamazepine	200–300	q 6 h	Gabapentin[b]	600–1200	q 8 h
Oxcarbazine	300	bid	Pregabalin	150–600	bid

[a]Antidepressants, anticonvulsants, and antiarrhythmics have not been approved by the U.S. Food and Drug Administration (FDA) for the treatment of pain.

[b]Gabapentin in doses up to 1800 mg/d is FDA approved for postherpetic neuralgia.
Note: 5-HT, serotonin; NE, norepinephrine.

system. This implies that sympathetic activity can activate undamaged nociceptors when inflammation is present. Signs of sympathetic hyperactivity should be sought in patients with posttraumatic pain and inflammation and no other obvious explanation.

℞ ACUTE PAIN

The ideal treatment for any pain is to remove the cause; thus, diagnosis should always precede treatment planning. Sometimes treating the underlying condition does not immediately relieve pain. Furthermore, some conditions are so painful that rapid and effective analgesia is essential (e.g., the postoperative state, burns, trauma, cancer, sickle cell crisis). Analgesic medications are a first line of treatment in these cases, and all practitioners should be familiar with their use.

ASPIRIN, ACETAMINOPHEN, AND NONSTEROIDAL ANTI-INFLAMMATORY AGENTS (NSAIDS) These drugs are considered together because they are used for similar problems and may have a similar mechanism of action (Table 12-1). All these compounds inhibit cyclooxygenase (COX), and, except for acetaminophen, all have anti-inflammatory actions, especially at higher dosages. They are particularly effective for mild to moderate headache and for pain of musculoskeletal origin.

Since they are effective for these common types of pain and are available without prescription, COX inhibitors are by far the most commonly used anal-

gesics. They are absorbed well from the gastrointestinal tract and, with occasional use, have only minimal side effects. With chronic use, gastric irritation is a common side effect of aspirin and NSAIDs and is the problem that most frequently limits the dose that can be given. Gastric irritation is most severe with aspirin, which may cause erosion and ulceration of the gastric mucosa leading to bleeding or perforation. Because aspirin irreversibly acetylates platelets and thereby interferes with coagulation of the blood, gastrointestinal bleeding is a particular risk. Increased age and history of gastrointestinal disease increase the risks of aspirin and NSAIDs. In addition to NSAIDs' well-known gastrointestinal toxicity, nephrotoxicity is a significant problem for patients using them on a chronic basis, and patients at risk for renal insufficiency should be monitored closely. NSAIDs also cause an increase in blood pressure in a significant number of individuals. Long-term treatment with NSAIDs requires regular blood pressure monitoring and treatment if necessary. Although toxic to the liver when taken in a high dose, acetaminophen rarely produces gastric irritation and does not interfere with platelet function.

The introduction of a parenteral form of NSAID, ketorolac, extends the usefulness of this class of compounds in the management of acute severe pain. Ketorolac is sufficiently potent and rapid in onset to supplant opioids for many patients with acute severe headache and musculoskeletal pain.

There are two major classes of COX: COX-1 is constitutively expressed, and COX-2 is induced in the inflammatory state. COX-2–selective drugs have moderate analgesic potency and produce less gastric irritation than the nonselective COX inhibitors. It is not yet clear whether the use of COX-2–selective drugs is associated with a lower risk of nephrotoxicity compared to nonselective NSAIDs. On the other hand, COX-2–selective drugs offer a significant benefit in the management of acute postoperative pain because they do not affect blood coagulation. This is a situation in which the nonselective COX inhibitors would be contraindicated because they impair platelet-mediated blood clotting and are thus associated with increased bleeding at the operative site. COX-2 inhibitors, including celecoxib (Celebrex), and valdecoxib (Bextra), are associated with increased cardiovascular risk. It is possible that this is a class effect of NSAIDs, excluding aspirin. These drugs are contraindicated in patients in the immediate period after coronary artery bypass surgery and should be used with caution in patients having a history of or significant risk factors for cardiovascular disease.

OPIOID ANALGESICS   Opioids are the most potent pain-relieving drugs currently available. Furthermore, of all analgesics, they have the broadest range of efficacy, providing the most reliable and effective method for rapid pain relief. Although side effects are common, they are usually not serious except for respiratory depression and can be reversed rapidly with the narcotic antagonist naloxone. The physician should not hesitate to use opioid analgesics in patients with acute severe pain. **Table 12-1** lists the most commonly used opioid analgesics.

Opioids produce analgesia by actions in the central nervous system. They activate pain-inhibitory neurons and directly inhibit pain-transmission neurons. Most of the commercially available opioid analgesics act at the same opioid receptor (μ-receptor), differing mainly in potency, speed of onset, duration of action, and optimal route of administration. Although the dose-related side effects (sedation, respiratory depression, pruritus, constipation) are similar among the different opioids, some side effects are due to accumulation of nonopioid metabolites that are unique to individual drugs. One striking example of this is normeperidine, a metabolite of meperidine. Normeperidine produces hyperexcitability and seizures that are not reversible with naloxone. Normeperidine accumulation is increased in patients with renal failure.

The most rapid relief with opioids is obtained by intravenous administration; relief with oral administration is significantly slower. Common side effects include nausea, vomiting, constipation, and sedation. The most serious side effect is respiratory depression. Patients with any form of respiratory compromise must be kept under close observation following opioid administration; an oxygen saturation monitor may be useful. The opioid antagonist naloxone should be readily available. Opioid effects are dose-related, and there is great variability among patients in the doses that relieve pain and produce side effects. Because of this, initiation of therapy requires titration to optimal dose and interval. The most important principle is to provide adequate pain relief. This requires determining whether the drug has adequately relieved the pain and the duration of the relief. *The most common error made by physicians in managing severe pain with opioids is to prescribe an inadequate dose. Since many patients are reluctant to complain, this practice leads to needless suffering.* In the absence of sedation at the expected time of peak effect, a physician should not hesitate to repeat the initial dose to achieve satisfactory pain relief.

An innovative approach to the problem of achieving adequate pain relief is the use of patient-controlled analgesia (PCA). PCA requires a device that can deliver a baseline continuous dose of an opioid drug, as well as preprogrammed additional doses whenever the patient pushes a button. The patient can then titrate the dose to the optimal level. This approach is used most extensively for the management of postoperative pain, but there is no reason why it should not be used for any hospitalized patient with persistent severe pain. PCA is also used for short-term home care of patients with intractable pain, such as that caused by metastatic cancer.

Because of patient variability in analgesia requirement, intravenous PCA is generally begun after the patient's pain has been controlled. The bolus dose of the drug (typically 1 mg morphine or 40 μg fentanyl) can then be delivered repeatedly as needed. To prevent overdosing, PCA devices are programmed with a lockout period after each demand dose is delivered (5–10 min) and a limit on the total dose delivered per hour. While some have advocated the use of a simultaneous background infusion of the PCA drug, this increases the risk of respiratory depression and has not been shown to increase the overall efficacy of the technique.

Many physicians, nurses, and patients have a certain trepidation about using opioids that is based on an exaggerated fear of addiction. In fact, there is a vanishingly small chance of patients becoming addicted to narcotics as a result of their appropriate medical use.

The availability of new routes of administration has extended the usefulness of opioid analgesics. Most important is the availability of spinal ad-

ministration. Opioids can be infused through a spinal catheter placed either intrathecally or epidurally. By applying opioids directly to the spinal cord, regional analgesia can be obtained using a relatively low total dose. In this way, such side effects as sedation, nausea, and respiratory depression can be minimized. This approach has been used extensively in obstetric procedures and for lower-body postoperative pain. Opioids can also be given intranasally (butorphanol), rectally, and transdermally (fentanyl), thus avoiding the discomfort of frequent injections in patients who cannot be given oral medication. The fentanyl transdermal patch has the advantage of providing fairly steady plasma levels, which maximizes patient comfort.

Opioid and COX Inhibitor Combinations   When used in combination, opioids and COX inhibitors have additive effects. Because a lower dose of each can be used to achieve the same degree of pain relief, and their side effects are nonadditive, such combinations can be used to lower the severity of dose-related side effects. Fixed-ratio combinations of an opioid with acetaminophen carry a special risk. Dose escalation as a result of increased severity of pain or decreased opioid effect as a result of tolerance may lead to levels of acetaminophen that are toxic to the liver.

CHRONIC PAIN

Managing patients with chronic pain is intellectually and emotionally challenging. The patient's problem is often difficult to diagnose; such patients are demanding of the physician's time and often appear emotionally distraught. The traditional medical approach of seeking an obscure organic pathology is usually unhelpful. On the other hand, psychological evaluation and behaviorally based treatment paradigms are frequently helpful, particularly in the setting of a multidisciplinary pain-management center.

There are several factors that can cause, perpetuate, or exacerbate chronic pain. First, of course, the patient may simply have a disease that is characteristically painful for which there is presently no cure. Arthritis, cancer, migraine headaches, fibromyalgia, and diabetic neuropathy are examples of this. Second, there may be secondary perpetuating factors that are initiated by disease and persist after that disease has resolved. Examples include damaged sensory nerves, sympathetic efferent activity, and painful reflex muscle contraction. Finally, a variety of psychological conditions can exacerbate or even cause pain.

There are certain areas to which special attention should be paid in the medical history. Because depression is the most common emotional disturbance in patients with chronic pain, patients should be questioned about their mood, appetite, sleep patterns, and daily activity. A simple standardized questionnaire, such as the Beck Depression Inventory, can be a useful screening device. It is important to remember that major depression is a common, treatable, and potentially fatal illness.

Other clues that a significant emotional disturbance is contributing to a patient's chronic pain complaint include: pain that occurs in multiple unrelated sites; a pattern of recurrent, but separate, pain problems beginning in childhood or adolescence; pain beginning at a time of emotional trauma, such as the loss of a parent or spouse; a history of physical or sexual abuse; and past or present substance abuse.

On examination, special attention should be paid to whether the patient guards the painful area and whether certain movements or postures are avoided because of pain. Discovering a mechanical component to the pain can be useful both diagnostically and therapeutically. Painful areas should be examined for deep tenderness, noting whether this is localized to muscle, ligamentous structures, or joints. Chronic myofascial pain is very common, and in these patients deep palpation may reveal highly localized trigger points that are firm bands or knots in muscle. Relief of the pain following injection of local anesthetic into these trigger points supports the diagnosis. A neuropathic component to the pain is indicated by evidence of nerve damage, such as sensory impairment, exquisitely sensitive skin, weakness and muscle atrophy, or loss of deep tendon reflexes. Evidence suggesting sympathetic nervous system involvement includes the presence of diffuse swelling, changes in skin color and temperature, and hypersensitive skin and joint tenderness compared with the normal side. Relief of the pain with a sympathetic block is diagnostic.

A guiding principle in evaluating patients with chronic pain is to assess both emotional and organic factors before initiating therapy. Addressing these issues together, rather than waiting to address emotional issues after organic causes of pain have been ruled out, improves compliance in part because it assures patients that a psychological evaluation does not mean that the physician is questioning the validity of their complaint. Even when an organic cause for a patient's pain can be found, it is still wise to look for other factors. For example, a cancer patient with painful bony metastases may have additional pain due to nerve damage and may also be depressed. Optimal therapy requires that each of these factors be looked for and treated.

℞ CHRONIC PAIN

Once the evaluation process has been completed and the likely causative and exacerbating factors identified, an explicit treatment plan should be developed. An important part of this process is to identify specific and realistic functional goals for therapy, such as getting a good night's sleep, being able to go shopping, or returning to work. A multidisciplinary approach that utilizes medications, counseling, physical therapy, nerve blocks, and even surgery may be required to improve the patient's quality of life. There are also some newer, relatively invasive procedures that can be helpful for some patients with intractable pain. These procedures include implanting intraspinal cannulae to deliver morphine or intraspinal electrodes for spinal stimulation. There are no set criteria for predicting which patients will respond to these procedures. They are generally reserved for patients who have not responded to conventional pharmacologic approaches. Referral to a multidisciplinary pain clinic for a full evaluation should precede any invasive procedures. Such referrals are clearly not necessary for all chronic pain patients. For some, pharmacologic management alone can provide adequate relief.

ANTIDEPRESSANT MEDICATIONS   The tricyclic antidepressants [amitriptyline, imipramine, nortriptyline, desipramine (TCAs; Table 12-1)] are extremely useful for the management of patients with chronic pain. Although developed for the treatment of depression, the tricyclics have a spectrum of dose-related biologic activities that include the production of analgesia in a variety of clinical conditions. Although the mechanism is unknown, the analgesic effect of TCAs has a more rapid onset and occurs at a lower dose than is typically required for the treatment of depression. Furthermore, patients with chronic pain who are not depressed obtain pain relief with antidepressants. There is evidence that tricyclic drugs potentiate opioid analgesia, so they may be useful adjuncts for the treatment of severe persistent pain such as occurs with malignant tumors. **Table 12-2** lists some of the painful conditions that respond to tricyclics. TCAs are of particular value in the management of neuropathic pain such as occurs in diabetic neuropathy and postherpetic neuralgia, for which there are few other therapeutic options.

The TCAs that have been shown to relieve pain have significant side effects (Table 12-1; Chap. 386). Some of these side effects, such as orthostatic hypotension, drowsiness, cardiac conduction delay, memory impairment, constipation, and urinary retention, are particularly problematic in elderly patients, and several are additive to the side effects of opioid analgesics. The serotonin-selective reuptake inhibitors such as fluoxetine (Prozac) have fewer and less serious side effects than TCAs, but they are much less effective for relieving pain. It is of interest that venlafaxine (Effexor) and duloxetine (Cymbalta), which are nontricyclic antidepressants that block both serotonin and norepinephrine reuptake, appear to retain most of the pain-relieving effect of TCAs with a side-effect profile more like that of the serotonin-selective reuptake inhibitors. These drugs may be particularly useful in patients who cannot tolerate the side effects of tricyclics.

ANTICONVULSANTS AND ANTIARRHYTHMICS   These drugs are useful primarily for patients with neuropathic pain. Phenytoin (Dilantin) and carbamazepine (Tegretol) were first shown to relieve the pain of trigeminal neuralgia. This pain has a characteristic brief, shooting, electric shock–like quality. In fact, anticonvulsants seem to be helpful largely for pains that have such a lancinating quality. Newer anticonvulsants, gabapentin (Neurontin) and pregabalin (Lyrica), are effective for a broad range of neuropathic pains.

Antiarrhythmic drugs such as low-dose lidocaine and mexiletine (Mexitil) can also be effective for neuropathic pain. These drugs block the spontaneous activity of damaged primary afferent nociceptors.

CHRONIC OPIOID MEDICATION   The long-term use of opioids is accepted for patients with pain due to malignant disease. Although opioid use for chronic pain of nonmalignant origin is controversial, it is clear that for many such patients opioid analgesics are the best available option. This is understandable since opioids are the most potent and have the broadest range of efficacy of any analgesic medications. Although addiction is rare in patients who first use opioids for pain relief, some degree of tolerance and physical dependence are likely with long-term use. Therefore, before embarking on opioid therapy, other options should be explored, and the limitations and risks of opioids should be explained to the patient. It is also important to point out that some opioid analgesic medications have mixed agonist-antagonist properties (e.g., pentazocine and butorphanol). From a practical standpoint, this means that they may worsen pain by inducing an abstinence syndrome in patients who are physically dependent on other opioid analgesics.

With long-term outpatient use of orally administered opioids, it is desirable to use long-acting compounds such as levorphanol, methadone, or sustained-release morphine (Table 12-1). Transdermal fentanyl is another excellent option. The pharmacokinetic profile of these drug preparations enables prolonged pain relief, minimizes side effects such as sedation that are associated with high peak plasma levels, and reduces the likelihood of rebound pain associated with a rapid fall in plasma opioid concentration. Constipation is a virtually universal side effect of opioid use and should be treated expectantly.

TREATMENT OF NEUROPATHIC PAIN   It is important to individualize treatment for patients with neuropathic pain. Several general principles should guide therapy: the first is to move quickly to provide relief; a second is to minimize drug side effects. For example, in patients with postherpetic neuralgia and significant cutaneous hypersensitivity, topical lidocaine (Lidoderm patches) can provide immediate relief without side effects. Anticonvulsants (gabapentin or pregabalin, see above) or antidepressants can be used as first-line drugs for patients with neuropathic pain. Antiarrhythmic drugs such as lidocaine and mexiletene can be effective (see above). There is no consensus on which class of drug should be used as a first-line treatment for any chronically painful condition. However, because relatively high doses of anticonvulsants are required for pain relief, sedation is very common. Sedation is also a problem with the tricyclic antidepressants but is much less of a problem with serotonin/norepinephrine reuptake inhibitors (SNRIs, e.g., venlafaxine and duloxetine). Thus, in the elderly or in those patients whose daily activities require high-level mental activity, these drugs should be considered as the first line. In contrast, opioid medications should be used as a second- or third-line drug class. While highly effective for many painful conditions, opioids are sedating, and their effect tends to lessen over time, leading to dose escalation and, occasionally, a worsening of pain due to physical dependence. Drugs of different classes can be used in combination to optimize pain control.

It is worth emphasizing that many patients, especially those with chronic pain, seek medical attention primarily because they are suffering and because only physicians can provide the medications required for pain relief. A primary responsibility of all physicians is to minimize the physical and emotional discomfort of their patients. Familiarity with pain mechanisms and analgesic medications is an important step toward accomplishing this aim.

TABLE 12-2	PAINFUL CONDITIONS THAT RESPOND TO TRICYCLIC ANTIDEPRESSANTS

Postherpetic neuralgia[a]
Diabetic neuropathy[a]
Tension headache[a]
Migraine headache[a]
Rheumatoid arthritis[a,b]
Chronic low back pain[b]
Cancer
Central post-stroke pain

[a]Controlled trials demonstrate analgesia.
[b]Controlled studies indicate benefit but not analgesia.

FURTHER READINGS

CRAIG AD: How do you feel? Interoception: The sense of the physiological condition of the body. Nat Rev Neurosci 8:655, 2002

FIELDS HL: Should we be reluctant to prescribe opioids for chronic nonmalignant pain? Pain 129:233, 2007

KELTNER JR et al: Isolating the modulatory effect of expectation on pain transmission: A functional magnetic resonance imaging study. J Neurosci 26:4437, 2006

MACINTYRE PE: Safety and efficacy of patient-controlled analgesia. Br J Anaesth 87:36, 2001

WAGER TD et al: Placebo-induced changes in FMRI in the anticipation and experience of pain. Science 303:1162, 2004

13 Chest Discomfort

Thomas H. Lee

Chest discomfort is one of the most common challenges for clinicians in the office or emergency department. The differential diagnosis includes conditions affecting organs throughout the thorax and abdomen, with prognostic implications that vary from benign to life-threatening (Table 13-1). Failure to recognize potentially serious conditions such as acute ischemic heart disease, aortic dissection, tension pneumothorax, or pulmonary embolism can lead to serious complications, including death. Conversely, overly conservative management of low-risk patients leads to unnecessary hospital admissions, tests, procedures, and anxiety.

CAUSES OF CHEST DISCOMFORT

Myocardial Ischemia and Injury   Myocardial ischemia occurs when the oxygen supply to the heart is not sufficient to meet metabolic needs. This mismatch can result from a decrease in oxygen supply, a rise in demand, or both. The most common underlying cause of myocardial ischemia is obstruction of coronary arteries by atherosclerosis; in the presence of such obstruction, transient ischemic episodes are usually precipitated by an increase in oxygen demand as a result of physical exertion. However, ischemia can also result from psychological stress, fever, or large meals or from compromised oxygen delivery due to anemia, hypoxia, or hypotension. Ventricular hypertrophy due to valvular heart disease, hypertrophic cardiomyopathy, or hypertension can predispose the myocardium to ischemia because of impaired penetration of blood flow from epicardial coronary arteries to the endocardium.

ANGINA PECTORIS   (See also Chap. 237) The chest discomfort of myocardial ischemia is a visceral discomfort that is usually described as a heaviness, pressure, or squeezing (Table 13-2). Other common adjectives for anginal pain are burning and aching. Some patients deny any "pain" but may admit to dyspnea or a vague sense of anxiety. The word "sharp" is sometimes used by patients to describe intensity rather than quality.

The location of angina pectoris is usually retrosternal; most patients do not localize the pain to any small area. The discomfort may radiate to the neck, jaw, teeth, arms, or shoulders, reflecting the common origin in the posterior horn of the spinal cord of sensory neurons supplying the heart and these areas. Some patients present with aching in sites of radiated pain as their only symptoms of ischemia. Occasional patients report epigastric distress with ischemic episodes. Less common is radiation to below the umbilicus or to the back.

Stable angina pectoris usually develops gradually with exertion, emotional excitement, or after heavy meals. Rest or treatment with sublingual nitroglycerin typically leads to relief within several minutes. In contrast, pain that is fleeting (lasting only a few seconds) is rarely ischemic in origin. Similarly, pain that lasts for several hours is unlikely to represent angina, particularly if the patient's electrocardiogram (ECG) does not show evidence of ischemia.

Anginal episodes can be precipitated by any physiologic or psychological stress that induces tachycardia. Most myocardial perfusion occurs during diastole, when there is minimal pressure opposing coronary artery flow from within the left ventricle. Since tachycardia decreases the percentage of the time in which the heart is in diastole, it decreases myocardial perfusion.

UNSTABLE ANGINA AND MYOCARDIAL INFARCTION   (See also Chaps. 238 and 239) Patients with these acute ischemic syndromes usually complain of symptoms similar in quality to angina pectoris, but more prolonged and severe. The onset of these syndromes may occur with the patient at rest, or awakened from sleep, and sublingual nitroglycerin may lead to transient or no relief. Accompanying symptoms may include diaphoresis, dyspnea, nausea, and light-headedness.

The physical examination may be completely normal in patients with chest discomfort due to ischemic heart disease. Careful auscultation during ischemic episodes may reveal a third or fourth heart sound, reflecting myocardial systolic or diastolic dysfunction. A transient murmur of mitral regurgitation suggests ischemic papillary muscle dysfunction. Severe episodes of ischemia can lead to pulmonary congestion and even pulmonary edema.

OTHER CARDIAC CAUSES   Myocardial ischemia caused by hypertrophic cardiomyopathy or aortic stenosis leads to angina pectoris similar to that caused by coronary atherosclerosis. In such cases, a loud systolic murmur or other findings usually suggest that abnormalities other than coronary atherosclerosis may be contributing to the patient's symptoms. Some patients with chest pain and normal coronary angiograms have functional abnormalities of the coronary circulation, ranging from coronary spasm visible on coronary angiography to abnormal vasodilator responses and heightened vasoconstrictor responses. The term "cardiac syndrome X" is used to describe patients with angina-like chest pain and ischemic-appearing ST-segment depression during stress despite normal coronary arteriograms. Some data indicate that many such patients have limited changes in coronary flow in response to pacing stress or coronary vasodilators. Despite the possibility that chest pain may be due to myocardial ischemia in such patients, their prognosis is excellent.

Pericarditis   (See also Chap. 232) The pain in pericarditis is believed to be due to inflammation of the adjacent parietal pleura, since most of the pericardium is believed to be insensitive to pain. Thus, infectious pericarditis, which usually involves adjoining pleural surfaces, tends to be associated with pain, while conditions that cause only local inflammation (e.g., myocardial infarction or uremia) and cardiac tamponade tend to result in mild or no chest pain.

TABLE 13-1 DIFFERENTIAL DIAGNOSES OF PATIENTS ADMITTED TO HOSPITAL WITH ACUTE CHEST DISCOMFORT RULED NOT MYOCARDIAL INFARCTION

Diagnosis	Percent
Gastroesophageal disease[a]	42
Gastroesophageal reflux	
Esophageal motility disorders	
Peptic ulcer	
Gallstones	
Ischemic heart disease	31
Chest wall syndromes	28
Pericarditis	4
Pleuritis/pneumonia	2
Pulmonary embolism	2
Lung cancer	1.5
Aortic aneurysm	1
Aortic stenosis	1
Herpes zoster	1

[a]In order of frequency.

Source: P Fruergaard et al: Eur Heart J 17:1028, 1996.

TABLE 13-2 TYPICAL CLINICAL FEATURES OF MAJOR CAUSES OF ACUTE CHEST DISCOMFORT

Condition	Duration	Quality	Location	Associated Features
Angina	More than 2 and less than 10 min	Pressure, tightness, squeezing, heaviness, burning	Retrosternal, often with radiation to or isolated discomfort in neck, jaw, shoulders, or arms—frequently on left	Precipitated by exertion, exposure to cold, psychologic stress S_4 gallop or mitral regurgitation murmur during pain
Unstable angina	10–20 min	Similar to angina but often more severe	Similar to angina	Similar to angina, but occurs with low levels of exertion or even at rest
Acute myocardial infarction	Variable; often more than 30 min	Similar to angina but often more severe	Similar to angina	Unrelieved by nitroglycerin May be associated with evidence of heart failure or arrhythmia
Aortic stenosis	Recurrent episodes as described for angina	As described for angina	As described for angina	Late-peaking systolic murmur radiating to carotid arteries
Pericarditis	Hours to days; may be episodic	Sharp	Retrosternal or toward cardiac apex; may radiate to left shoulder	May be relieved by sitting up and leaning forward Pericardial friction rub
Aortic dissection	Abrupt onset of unrelenting pain	Tearing or ripping sensation; knifelike	Anterior chest, often radiating to back, between shoulder blades	Associated with hypertension and/or underlying connective tissue disorder, e.g., Marfan syndrome Murmur of aortic insufficiency, pericardial rub, pericardial tamponade, or loss of peripheral pulses
Pulmonary embolism	Abrupt onset; several minutes to a few hours	Pleuritic	Often lateral, on the side of the embolism	Dyspnea, tachypnea, tachycardia, and hypotension
Pulmonary hypertension	Variable	Pressure	Substernal	Dyspnea, signs of increased venous pressure including edema and jugular venous distention
Pneumonia or pleuritis	Variable	Pleuritic	Unilateral, often localized	Dyspnea, cough, fever, rales, occasional rub
Spontaneous pneumothorax	Sudden onset; several hours	Pleuritic	Lateral to side of pneumothorax	Dyspnea, decreased breath sounds on side of pneumothorax
Esophageal reflux	10–60 min	Burning	Substernal, epigastric	Worsened by postprandial recumbency Relieved by antacids
Esophageal spasm	2–30 min	Pressure, tightness, burning	Retrosternal	Can closely mimic angina
Peptic ulcer	Prolonged	Burning	Epigastric, substernal	Relieved with food or antacids
Gallbladder disease	Prolonged	Burning, pressure	Epigastric, right upper quadrant, substernal	May follow meal
Musculoskeletal disease	Variable	Aching	Variable	Aggravated by movement May be reproduced by localized pressure on examination
Herpes zoster	Variable	Sharp or burning	Dermatomal distribution	Vesicular rash in area of discomfort
Emotional and psychiatric conditions	Variable; may be fleeting	Variable	Variable; may be retrosternal	Situational factors may precipitate symptoms Anxiety or depression often detectable with careful history

The adjacent parietal pleura receives its sensory supply from several sources, so the pain of pericarditis can be experienced in areas ranging from the shoulder and neck to the abdomen and back. Most typically, the pain is retrosternal and is aggravated by coughing, deep breaths, or changes in position—all of which lead to movements of pleural surfaces. The pain is often worse in the supine position and relieved by sitting upright and leaning forward. Less common is a steady aching discomfort that mimics acute myocardial infarction.

Diseases of the Aorta   (See also Chap. 242) *Aortic dissection* is a potentially catastrophic condition that is due to spread of a subintimal hematoma within the wall of the aorta. The hematoma may begin with a tear in the intima of the aorta or with rupture of the vasa vasorum within the aortic media. This syndrome can occur with trauma to the aorta, including motor vehicle accidents or medical procedures in which catheters or intraaortic balloon pumps damage the intima of the aorta. Nontraumatic aortic dissections are rare in the absence of hypertension and/or conditions associated with deterioration of the elastic or muscular components of the media within the aorta's wall. Cystic medial degeneration is a feature of several inherited connective tissue diseases, including Marfan and Ehlers-Danlos syndromes. About half of all aortic dissections in women under 40 years of age occur during pregnancy.

Almost all patients with acute dissections present with severe chest pain, although some patients with chronic dissections are identified without associated symptoms. Unlike the pain of ischemic heart disease, symptoms of aortic dissection tend to reach peak severity immediately, often causing the patient to collapse from its intensity. The classic teaching is that the adjectives used to describe the pain reflect the process oc-

curring within the wall of the aorta—"ripping" and "tearing"—but more recent data suggest that the most common presenting complaint is sudden onset of severe, sharp pain. The location often correlates with the site and extent of the dissection. Thus, dissections that begin in the ascending aorta and extend to the descending aorta tend to cause pain in the front of the chest that extends into the back, between the shoulder blades.

Physical findings may also reflect extension of the aortic dissection that compromises flow into arteries branching off the aorta. Thus, loss of a pulse in one or both arms, cerebrovascular accident, or paraplegia can all be catastrophic consequences of aortic dissection. Hematomas that extend proximally and undermine the coronary arteries or aortic valve apparatus may lead to acute myocardial infarction or acute aortic insufficiency. Rupture of the hematoma into the pericardial space leads to pericardial tamponade.

Another abnormality of the aorta that can cause chest pain is a *thoracic aortic aneurysm*. Aortic aneurysms are frequently asymptomatic but can cause chest pain and other symptoms by compressing adjacent structures. This pain tends to be steady, deep, and sometimes severe.

Pulmonary Embolism   (See also Chap. 256) Chest pain due to pulmonary embolism is believed to be due to distention of the pulmonary artery or infarction of a segment of the lung adjacent to the pleura. Massive pulmonary emboli may lead to substernal pain that is suggestive of acute myocardial infarction. More commonly, smaller emboli lead to focal pulmonary infarctions that cause pain that is lateral and pleuritic. Associated symptoms include dyspnea and, occasionally, hemoptysis. Tachycardia is usually present. Although not always present, certain characteristic ECG changes can support the diagnosis.

Pneumothorax (See also Chap. 257) Sudden onset of pleuritic chest pain and respiratory distress should lead to consideration of spontaneous pneumothorax, as well as pulmonary embolism. Such events may occur without a precipitating event in persons without lung disease, or as a consequence of underlying lung disorders.

Pneumonia or Pleuritis (See also Chaps. 251 and 257) Lung diseases that damage and cause inflammation of the pleura of the lung usually cause a sharp, knifelike pain that is aggravated by inspiration or coughing.

Gastrointestinal Conditions (See also Chap. 286) Esophageal pain from acid reflux from the stomach, spasm, obstruction, or injury can be difficult to discern from myocardial syndromes. Acid reflux typically causes a deep burning discomfort that may be exacerbated by alcohol, aspirin, or some foods; this discomfort is often relieved by antacid or other acid-reducing therapies. Acid reflux tends to be exacerbated by lying down and may be worse in early morning when the stomach is empty of food that might otherwise absorb gastric acid.

Esophageal spasm may occur in the presence or absence of acid reflux and leads to a squeezing pain indistinguishable from angina. Prompt relief of esophageal spasm is often provided by antianginal therapies such as sublingual nifedipine, further promoting confusion between these syndromes. Chest pain can also result from injury to the esophagus, such as a Mallory-Weiss tear caused by severe vomiting.

Chest pain can result from diseases of the gastrointestinal tract below the diaphragm, including *peptic ulcer disease, biliary disease,* and *pancreatitis.* These conditions usually cause abdominal pain as well as chest discomfort; symptoms are not likely to be associated with exertion. The pain of ulcer disease typically occurs 60 to 90 min after meals, when postprandial acid production is no longer neutralized by food in the stomach. Cholecystitis usually causes a pain that is described as aching, occurring an hour or more after meals.

Neuromusculoskeletal Conditions *Cervical disk disease* can cause chest pain by compression of nerve roots. Pain in a dermatomal distribution can also be caused by *intercostal muscle cramps* or by *herpes zoster.* Chest pain symptoms due to herpes zoster may occur before skin lesions are apparent.

Costochondral and *chondrosternal syndromes* are the most common causes of anterior chest musculoskeletal pain. Only occasionally are physical signs of costochondritis such as swelling, redness, and warmth (Tietze's syndrome) present. The pain of such syndromes is usually fleeting and sharp, but some patients experience a dull ache that lasts for hours. Direct pressure on the chondrosternal and costochondral junctions may reproduce the pain from these and other musculoskeletal syndromes. Arthritis of the shoulder and spine and bursitis may also cause chest pain. Some patients who have these conditions and myocardial ischemia blur and confuse symptoms of these syndromes.

Emotional and Psychiatric Conditions As many as 10% of patients who present to emergency departments with acute chest discomfort have panic disorder or other emotional conditions. The symptoms in these populations are highly variable, but frequently the discomfort is described as visceral tightness or aching that lasts more than 30 min. Some patients offer other atypical descriptions, such as pain that is fleeting, sharp, and/or localized to a small region. The ECG in patients with emotional conditions may be difficult to interpret if hyperventilation causes ST-T-wave abnormalities. A careful history may elicit clues of depression, prior panic attacks, somatization, agoraphobia, or other phobias.

APPROACH TO THE PATIENT:
Chest Discomfort

The evaluation of the patient with chest discomfort must accommodate two goals—determining the diagnosis and assessing the safety of the immediate management plan. The latter issue is often dominant when the patient has acute chest discomfort, such as patients

TABLE 13-3 CONSIDERATIONS IN THE ASSESSMENT OF THE PATIENT WITH CHEST DISCOMFORT

1. Could the chest discomfort be due to an acute, potentially life-threatening condition that warrants immediate hospitalization and aggressive evaluation?

Acute ischemic heart disease	Pulmonary embolism
Aortic dissection	Spontaneous pneumothorax

2. If not, could the discomfort be due to a chronic condition likely to lead to serious complications?
   Stable angina
   Aortic stenosis
   Pulmonary hypertension
3. If not, could the discomfort be due to an acute condition that warrants specific treatment?
   Pericarditis
   Pneumonia/pleuritis
   Herpes zoster
4. If not, could the discomfort be due to another treatable chronic condition?

Esophageal reflux	Cervical disk disease
Esophageal spasm	Arthritis of the shoulder or spine
Peptic ulcer disease	Costochondritis
Gallbladder disease	Other musculoskeletal disorders
Other gastrointestinal conditions	Anxiety state

seen in the emergency department. In such settings, the clinician must focus first on identifying patients who require aggressive interventions to diagnose or manage potentially life-threatening conditions, including acute ischemic heart disease, acute aortic dissection, pulmonary embolism, and tension pneumothorax. If such conditions are unlikely, the clinician must address questions such as the safety of discharge to home, admission to a non-coronary care unit facility, or immediate exercise testing. Table 13-3 displays a sequence of questions that can be used in the evaluation of the patient with chest discomfort, with the diagnostic entities that are most important for consideration at each stage of the evaluation.

ACUTE CHEST DISCOMFORT In patients with acute chest discomfort, the clinician must first assess the patient's respiratory and hemodynamic status. If either is compromised, initial management should focus on stabilizing the patient before the diagnostic evaluation is pursued. If, however, the patient does not require emergent interventions, then a focused history, physical examination, and laboratory evaluation should be performed to assess the patient's risk of life-threatening conditions.

Clinicians who are seeing patients in the office setting should not assume that they do not have acute ischemic heart disease, even if the prevalence may be lower. Malpractice litigation related to myocardial infarctions that were missed during office evaluations is becoming increasingly common, and ECGs were not performed in many such cases. The prevalence of high-risk patients seen in office settings may be increasing due to congestion in emergency departments.

In either setting, the *history* should include questions about the quality and location of the chest discomfort (Table 13-2). The patient should also be asked about the nature of onset of the pain and its duration. Myocardial ischemia is usually associated with a gradual intensification of symptoms over a period of minutes. Pain that is fleeting or that lasts hours without being associated with electrocardiographic changes is not likely to be ischemic in origin. Although the presence of risk factors for coronary artery disease may heighten concern for this diagnosis, the absence of such risk factors does not lower the risk for myocardial ischemia enough to be used to justify a decision to discharge a patient.

Wide radiation of chest pain increases probability that pain is due to myocardial infarction. Radiation of chest pain to the left arm is common with acute ischemic heart disease, but radiation to the right arm is also highly consistent with this diagnosis. Figure 13-1 shows estimates derived from several studies of the impact of various clinical features from the history on the probability that a patient has an acute myocardial infarction.

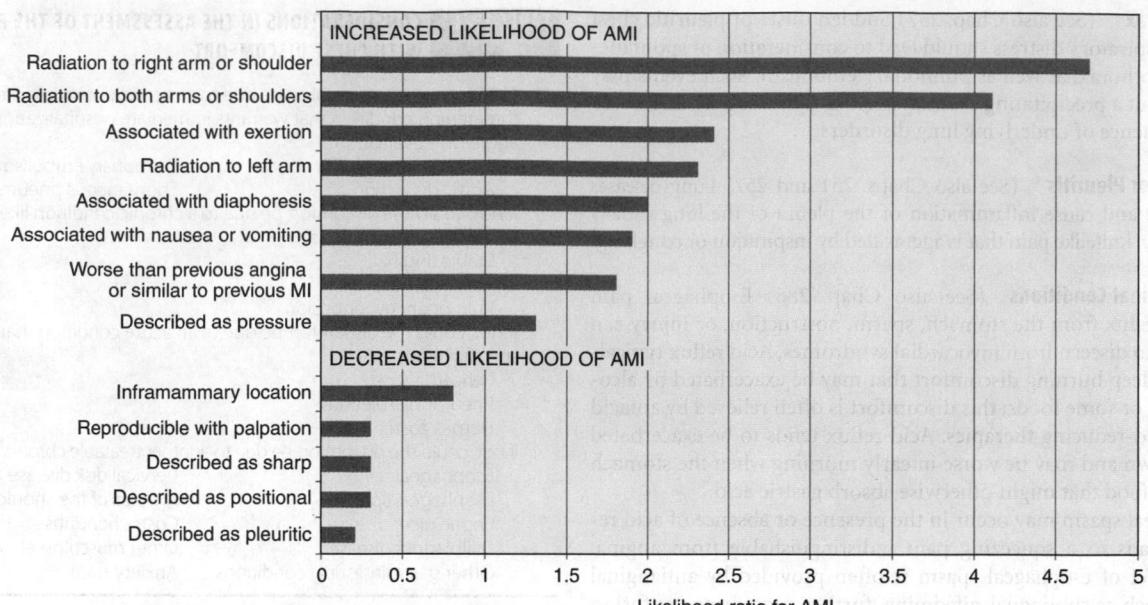

FIGURE 13-1 Impact of chest pain characteristics on odds of acute myocardial infarction (AMI). *(Figure prepared from data in Swap and Nagurney.)*

Right shoulder pain is also common with acute cholecystitis, but this syndrome is usually accompanied by pain that is located in the abdomen rather than chest. Chest pain that radiates between the scapulae raises the question of aortic dissection.

The *physical examination* should include evaluation of blood pressure in both arms and of pulses in both legs. Poor perfusion of a limb may be due to an aortic dissection that has compromised flow to an artery branching from the aorta. Chest auscultation may reveal diminished breath sounds; a pleural rub; or evidence of pneumothorax, pulmonary embolism, pneumonia, or pleurisy. Tension pneumothorax may lead to a shift in the trachea from the midline, away from the side of the pneumothorax. The cardiac examination should seek pericardial rubs, systolic and diastolic murmurs, and third or fourth heart sounds. Pressure on the chest wall may reproduce symptoms in patients with musculoskeletal causes of chest pain; it is important that the clinician ask the patient if the chest pain syndrome is being completely reproduced before drawing too much reassurance that more serious underlying conditions are not present.

An *ECG* is an essential test for adults with chest discomfort that is not due to an obvious traumatic cause. In such patients, the presence of electrocardiographic changes consistent with ischemia or infarction (Chap. 221) is associated with high risks of acute myocardial infarction or unstable angina (Table 13-4); such patients should be admitted to a unit with electrocardiographic monitoring and the capacity to respond to a cardiac arrest. The absence of such changes does not exclude acute ischemic heart disease, but the risk of life-threatening complications is low for patients with normal electrocardiograms or only nonspecific ST-T-wave changes. If these patients are not considered appropriate for immediate discharge, they are often candidates for early or immediate exercise testing.

Markers of myocardial injury are often obtained in the emergency department evaluation of acute chest discomfort. The most commonly used markers are creatine kinase (CK), CK-MB, and the cardiac troponins (I and T). Rapid bedside assays of the cardiac troponins have been developed and shown to be sufficiently accurate to predict prognosis and guide management. Some data support the use of other markers, such as serum myoglobin, C-reactive protein (CRP), placental growth factor, myeloperoxidase, and B-type natriuretic peptide (BNP); their roles are the subject of ongoing research. Single values of any of these markers do not have high sensitivity for acute myocardial infarction or for prediction of

complications. Hence, decisions to discharge patients home should not be made on the basis of single negative values of these tests.

Provocative tests for coronary artery disease are not appropriate for patients with ongoing chest pain. In such patients, rest myocardial perfusion scans can be considered; a normal scan reduces the likelihood of coronary artery disease and can help avoid admission of low-risk patients to the hospital. Promising early results suggest that 64-slice CT and cardiac MRI may be of sufficient accuracy for diagnosis of coronary disease that these technologies may become widely used for patients with acute chest pain in whom the diagnosis is not clear.

Clinicians frequently employ therapeutic trials with sublingual nitroglycerin or antacids or, in the stable patient seen in the office setting, a proton pump inhibitor. A common error is to assume that a response to any of these interventions clarifies the diagnosis. While such information is often helpful, the patient's response may be due to the placebo effect. Hence, myocardial ischemia should never be considered excluded solely because of a response to antacid therapy. Similarly, failure of nitroglycerin to relieve pain does not exclude the diagnosis of coronary disease.

TABLE 13-4 PREVALENCE OF MYOCARDIAL INFARCTION AND UNSTABLE ANGINA AMONG SUBSETS OF PATIENTS WITH ACUTE CHEST DISCOMFORT IN THE EMERGENCY DEPARTMENT

Finding	Prevalence	
	Myocardial Infarction, %	Unstable Angina, %
ST elevation (≥1 mm) or Q waves on ECG not known to be old	79	12
Ischemia or strain on ECG not known to be old (ST depression ≥1 mm or ischemic T waves)	20	41
None of the preceding ECG changes but a prior history of angina or myocardial infarction (history of heart attack or nitroglycerin use)	4	51
None of the preceding ECG changes and no prior history of angina or myocardial infarction (history of heart attack or nitroglycerin use)	2	14

Note: ECG, electrocardiogram.
Unpublished data from Brigham and Women's Hospital Chest Pain Study, 1997–1999.

If the patient's history or examination is consistent with aortic dissection, imaging studies to evaluate the aorta must be pursued promptly because of the high risk of catastrophic complications with this condition. Appropriate tests include a chest CT scan with contrast, MRI, or transesophageal echocardiography.

Acute pulmonary embolism should be considered in patients with respiratory symptoms, pleuritic chest pain, hemoptysis, or a history of venous thromboembolism or coagulation abnormalities. Initial tests usually include CT angiography or a lung scan, which are sometimes combined with lower extremity venous ultrasound or D-dimer testing.

If patients with acute chest discomfort show no evidence of life-threatening conditions, the clinician should then focus on serious chronic conditions with the potential to cause major complications, the most common of which is stable angina. Early use of exercise electrocardiography, stress echocardiography, or stress perfusion imaging for such patients, whether in the office or the emergency department, is now an accepted management strategy for low-risk patients. Exercise testing is not appropriate, however, for patients who (1) report pain that is believed to be ischemic occurring at rest or (2) have electrocardiographic changes not known to be old that are consistent with ischemia.

Patients with sustained chest discomfort who do not have evidence for life-threatening conditions should be evaluated for evidence of conditions likely to benefit from acute treatment (Table 13-3). Pericarditis may be suggested by the history, physical examination, and ECG (Table 13-2). Clinicians should carefully assess blood pressure patterns and consider echocardiography in such patients to detect evidence of impending pericardial tamponade. Chest x-rays can be used to evaluate the possibility of pulmonary disease.

GUIDELINES AND CRITICAL PATHWAYS FOR ACUTE CHEST DISCOMFORT

Guidelines for the initial evaluation for patients with acute chest pain have been developed by the American College of Cardiology, American Heart Association, and other organizations. These guidelines recommend performance of an ECG for virtually all patients with chest pain who do not have an obvious noncardiac cause of their pain, and performance of a chest x-ray for patients with signs or symptoms consistent with congestive heart failure, valvular heart disease, pericardial disease, or aortic dissection or aneurysm.

The American College of Cardiology/American Heart Association guidelines on exercise testing support its use in low-risk patients presenting to the emergency department, as well as in selected intermediate-risk patients. However, these guidelines emphasize that exercise tests should be performed only after patients have been screened for high-risk features or other indicators for hospital admission.

Many medical centers have adopted critical pathways and other forms of guidelines to increase efficiency and to expedite the treatment of patients with high-risk acute ischemic heart disease syndromes. These guidelines emphasize the following strategies:

- Rapid identification and treatment of patients for whom emergent reperfusion therapy, either via percutaneous coronary interventions or thrombolytic agents, is likely to lead to improved outcomes.

- Triage to non-coronary care unit monitored facilities such as intermediate-care units or chest pain units of patients with a low risk for complications, such as patients without new ischemic changes on their ECGs and without ongoing chest pain. Such patients can usually be safely observed in non-coronary care unit settings, undergo early exercise testing, or be discharged home. Risk stratification can be assisted through use of prospectively validated multivariate algorithms that have been published for acute ischemic heart disease and its complications.
- Shortening lengths of stay in the coronary care unit and hospital. Recommendations regarding the minimum length of stay in a monitored bed for a patient who has no further symptoms have decreased in recent years to 12 h or less if exercise testing or other risk stratification technologies are available.

NONACUTE CHEST DISCOMFORT

The management of patients who do not require admission to the hospital or who no longer require inpatient observation should seek to identify the cause of the symptoms and the likelihood of major complications. Noninvasive tests for coronary disease serve both to diagnose this condition and to identify patients with high-risk forms of coronary disease who may benefit from revascularization. Gastrointestinal causes of chest pain can be evaluated via endoscopy or radiology studies, or with trials of medical therapy. Emotional and psychiatric conditions warrant appropriate evaluation and treatment; randomized trial data indicate that cognitive therapy and group interventions lead to decreases in symptoms for such patients.

FURTHER READINGS

BRENNAN M-L et al: Prognostic value of myeloperoxidase in patients with chest pain. N Engl J Med 349:1595, 2003

GIBBONS RJ et al: ACC/AHA 2002 guideline update for exercise testing. A report of the American College of Cardiology/American Heart Association Task Force on Practice Guidelines (Committee on Exercise Testing). Available at *www.acc.org/qualityandscience/clinical/guidelines/exercise/dirindex.htm*. Accessed on January 22, 2006

GIBSON PB et al: Low event rate for stress-only perfusion imaging in patients evaluated for chest pain. J Am Coll Cardiol 39:999, 2002

HEESCHEM C et al: Prognostic value of placental growth factor in patients with chest pain. JAMA 291:435, 2004

KWONG RY et al: Detecting acute coronary syndrome in the emergency department with cardiac magnetic resonance imaging. Circulation 197:531, 2003

LEBER AW et al: Quantification of obstructive and nonobstructive coronary lesions of 64-slice computed tomography. J Am Coll Cardiol 46:147, 2005

SWAP CJ, NAGURNEY JT: Value and limitations of chest pain history in the evaluation of patients with suspected acute coronary syndromes. JAMA 294:2623, 2005

TONG KL et al: Myocardial contrast echocardiography versus Thrombolysis in Myocardial Infarction score in patients presenting to the emergency department with chest pain and a nondiagnostic electrocardiogram. J Am Coll Cardiol 46:928, 2005

TSAI TT et al: Acute aortic syndromes. Circulation 205:3802, 2005

14 Abdominal Pain
William Silen

The correct interpretation of acute abdominal pain is challenging. Since proper therapy may require urgent action, the unhurried approach suitable for the study of other conditions is sometimes denied. Few other clinical situations demand greater judgment, because the most catastrophic of events may be forecast by the subtlest of symptoms and signs. A meticulously executed, detailed history and physical examination are of great importance. The etiologic classification in Table 14-1, although not complete, forms a useful basis for the evaluation of patients with abdominal pain.

The diagnosis of "acute or surgical abdomen" is not an acceptable one because of its often misleading and erroneous connotation. The most obvious of "acute abdomens" may not require operative intervention, and the mildest of abdominal pains may herald an urgently correctable lesion. Any patient with abdominal pain of recent onset requires early and thorough evaluation and accurate diagnosis.

Inflammation of the Parietal Peritoneum   The pain of parietal peritoneal inflammation is steady and aching in character and is located directly over the inflamed area, its exact reference being possible because it is transmitted by somatic nerves supplying the parietal peritoneum. The intensity of the pain is dependent on the type and amount of material to which the peritoneal surfaces are exposed in a given time period. For example, the sudden release into the peritoneal cavity of a small quantity of *sterile* acid gastric juice causes much more pain than the same amount of grossly contaminated neutral feces. Enzymatically active pancreatic juice incites more pain and inflammation than does the same amount of sterile bile containing no potent enzymes. Blood and urine are often so bland as to go undetected if their contact with the peritoneum has not been sudden and massive. In the case of bacterial contamination, such as in pelvic inflammatory disease, the pain is frequently of low intensity early in the illness until bacterial multiplication has caused the elaboration of irritating substances.

The rate at which the irritating material is applied to the peritoneum is important. Perforated peptic ulcer may be associated with entirely different clinical pictures dependent only on the rapidity with which the gastric juice enters the peritoneal cavity.

The pain of peritoneal inflammation is invariably accentuated by pressure or changes in tension of the peritoneum, whether produced by palpation or by movement, as in coughing or sneezing. The patient with peritonitis lies quietly in bed, preferring to avoid motion, in contrast to the patient with colic, who may writhe incessantly.

Another characteristic feature of peritoneal irritation is tonic reflex spasm of the abdominal musculature, localized to the involved body segment. The intensity of the tonic muscle spasm accompanying peritoneal inflammation is dependent on the location of the inflammatory process, the rate at which it develops, and the integrity of the nervous system. Spasm over a perforated retrocecal appendix or perforated ulcer into the lesser peritoneal sac may be minimal or absent because of the protective effect of overlying viscera. A slowly developing process often greatly attenuates the degree of muscle spasm. Catastrophic abdominal emergencies such as a perforated ulcer may be associated with minimal or no detectable pain or muscle spasm in obtunded, seriously ill, debilitated elderly patients or in psychotic patients.

Obstruction of Hollow Viscera   The pain of obstruction of hollow abdominal viscera is classically described as intermittent, or colicky. Yet the lack of a truly cramping character should not be misleading, because distention of a hollow viscus may produce steady pain with only very occasional exacerbations. It is not nearly as well localized as the pain of parietal peritoneal inflammation.

The colicky pain of obstruction of the small intestine is usually periumbilical or supraumbilical and is poorly localized. As the intestine becomes progressively dilated with loss of muscular tone, the colicky nature of the pain may diminish. With superimposed strangulating obstruction, pain may spread to the lower lumbar region if there is traction on the root of the mesentery. The colicky pain of colonic obstruction is of lesser intensity than that of the small intestine and is often located in the infraumbilical area. Lumbar radiation of pain is common in colonic obstruction.

Sudden distention of the biliary tree produces a steady rather than colicky type of pain; hence the term *biliary colic* is misleading. Acute distention of the gallbladder usually causes pain in the right upper quadrant with radiation to the right posterior region of the thorax or to the tip of the right scapula, and distention of the common bile duct is often associated with pain in the epigastrium radiating to the upper part of the lumbar region. Considerable variation is common, however, so that differentiation between these may be impossible. The typical subscapular pain or lumbar radiation is frequently absent. Gradual dilatation of the biliary tree, as in carcinoma of the head of the pancreas, may cause no pain or only a mild aching sensation in the epigastrium or right upper quadrant. The pain of distention of the pancreatic ducts is similar to that described for abstention of the common bile duct but, in addition, is very frequently accentuated by recumbency and relieved by the upright position.

TABLE 14-1   **SOME IMPORTANT CAUSES OF ABDOMINAL PAIN**

Pain Originating in the Abdomen

Parietal peritoneal inflammation
  Bacterial contamination
    Perforated appendix or other perforated viscus
    Pelvic inflammatory disease
  Chemical irritation
    Perforated ulcer
    Pancreatitis
    Mittelschmerz
Mechanical obstruction of hollow viscera
  Obstruction of the small or large intestine
  Obstruction of the biliary tree
  Obstruction of the ureter
Vascular disturbances
  Embolism or thrombosis
  Vascular rupture
  Pressure or torsional occlusion
  Sickle cell anemia
Abdominal wall
  Distortion or traction of mesentery
  Trauma or infection of muscles
Distension of visceral surfaces, e.g. by hemorrhage
  Hepatic or renal capsules
Inflammation of a viscus
  Appendicitis
  Typhoid fever
  Typhlitis

Pain Referred from Extraabdominal Source

Cardiothoracic
  Acute myocardial infarction
  Myocarditis, endocarditis, pericarditis
  Congestive heart failure
  Pneumonia
  Pulmonary embolus
  Pleurodynia
  Pneumothorax
  Empyema
  Esophageal disease, spasm, rupture, inflammation
Genitalia
  Torsion of the testis

Metabolic Causes

Diabetes
Uremia
Hyperlipidemia
Hyperparathyroidism
Acute adrenal insufficiency
Familial Mediterranean fever
Porphyria
C'1 esterase inhibitor deficiency (angioneurotic edema)

Neurologic/Psychiatric Causes

Herpes zoster
Tabes dorsalis
Causalgia
Radiculitis from infection or arthritis
Spinal cord or nerve root compression
Functional disorders
Psychiatric disorders

Toxic Causes

Lead poisoning
Insect or animal envenomations
  Black widow spiders
  Snake bites

Uncertain Mechanisms

Narcotic withdrawal
Heat stroke

Obstruction of the urinary bladder results in dull suprapubic pain, usually low in intensity. Restlessness without specific complaint of pain may be the only sign of a distended bladder in an obtunded patient. In contrast, acute obstruction of the intravesicular portion of the ureter is characterized by severe suprapubic and flank pain that radiates to the penis, scrotum, or inner aspect of the upper thigh. Obstruction of the ureteropelvic junction is felt as pain in the costovertebral angle, whereas obstruction of the remainder of the ureter is associated with flank pain that often extends into the same side of the abdomen.

Vascular Disturbances A frequent misconception, despite abundant experience to the contrary, is that pain associated with intraabdominal vascular disturbances is sudden and catastrophic in nature. The pain of embolism or thrombosis of the superior mesenteric artery or that of impending rupture of an abdominal aortic aneurysm certainly may be severe and diffuse. Yet, just as frequently, the patient with occlusion of the superior mesenteric artery has only mild continuous diffuse pain for 2 or 3 days before vascular collapse or findings of peritoneal inflammation appear. The early, seemingly insignificant discomfort is caused by hyperperistalsis rather than peritoneal inflammation. Indeed, absence of tenderness and rigidity in the presence of continuous, diffuse pain in a patient likely to have vascular disease is quite characteristic of occlusion of the superior mesenteric artery. Abdominal pain with radiation to the sacral region, flank, or genitalia should always signal the possible presence of a rupturing abdominal aortic aneurysm. This pain may persist over a period of several days before rupture and collapse occur.

Abdominal Wall Pain arising from the abdominal wall is usually constant and aching. Movement, prolonged standing, and pressure accentuate the discomfort and muscle spasm. In the case of hematoma of the rectus sheath, now most frequently encountered in association with anticoagulant therapy, a mass may be present in the lower quadrants of the abdomen. Simultaneous involvement of muscles in other parts of the body usually serves to differentiate myositis of the abdominal wall from an intraabdominal process that might cause pain in the same region.

REFERRED PAIN IN ABDOMINAL DISEASES

Pain referred to the abdomen from the thorax, spine, or genitalia may prove a vexing diagnostic problem, because diseases of the upper part of the abdominal cavity such as acute cholecystitis or perforated ulcer are frequently associated with intrathoracic complications. A most important, yet often forgotten, dictum is that the possibility of intrathoracic disease must be considered in every patient with abdominal pain, especially if the pain is in the upper part of the abdomen. Systematic questioning and examination directed toward detecting myocardial or pulmonary infarction, pneumonia, pericarditis, or esophageal disease (the intrathoracic diseases that most often masquerade as abdominal emergencies) will often provide sufficient clues to establish the proper diagnosis. Diaphragmatic pleuritis resulting from pneumonia or pulmonary infarction may cause pain in the right upper quadrant and pain in the supraclavicular area, the latter radiation to be distinguished from the referred subscapular pain caused by acute distention of the extrahepatic biliary tree. The ultimate decision as to the origin of abdominal pain may require deliberate and planned observation over a period of several hours, during which repeated questioning and examination will provide the diagnosis or suggest the appropriate studies.

Referred pain of thoracic origin is often accompanied by splinting of the involved hemithorax with respiratory lag and decrease in excursion more marked than that seen in the presence of intraabdominal disease. In addition, apparent abdominal muscle spasm caused by referred pain will diminish during the inspiratory phase of respiration, whereas it is persistent throughout both respiratory phases if it is of abdominal origin. Palpation over the area of referred pain in the abdomen also does not usually accentuate the pain and in many instances actually seems to relieve it. Thoracic disease and abdominal disease frequently coexist and may be difficult or impossible to differentiate. For example, the patient with known biliary tract disease often has epigastric pain during myocardial infarction, or biliary colic may be referred to the precordium or left shoulder in a patient who has suffered previously from angina pectoris. For an explanation of the radiation of pain to a previously diseased area, see Chap. 12.

Referred pain from the spine, which usually involves compression or irritation of nerve roots, is characteristically intensified by certain motions such as cough, sneeze, or strain and is associated with hyperesthesia over the involved dermatomes. Pain referred to the abdomen from the testes or seminal vesicles is generally accentuated by the slightest pressure on either of these organs. The abdominal discomfort is of dull aching character and is poorly localized.

METABOLIC ABDOMINAL CRISES

Pain of metabolic origin may simulate almost any other type of intraabdominal disease. Several mechanisms may be at work. In certain instances, such as hyperlipidemia, the metabolic disease itself may be accompanied by an intraabdominal process such as pancreatitis, which can lead to unnecessary laparotomy unless recognized. C1 esterase deficiency associated with angioneurotic edema is often associated with episodes of severe abdominal pain. Whenever the cause of abdominal pain is obscure, a metabolic origin always must be considered. Abdominal pain is also the hallmark of familial Mediterranean fever (Chap. 323).

The problem of differential diagnosis is often not readily resolved. The pain of porphyria and of lead colic is usually difficult to distinguish from that of intestinal obstruction, because severe hyperperistalsis is a prominent feature of both. The pain of uremia or diabetes is nonspecific, and the pain and tenderness frequently shift in location and intensity. Diabetic acidosis may be precipitated by acute appendicitis or intestinal obstruction, so if prompt resolution of the abdominal pain does not result from correction of the metabolic abnormalities, an underlying organic problem should be suspected. Black widow spider bites produce intense pain and rigidity of the abdominal muscles and back, an area infrequently involved in intraabdominal disease.

NEUROGENIC CAUSES

Causalgic pain may occur in diseases that injure sensory nerves. It has a burning character and is usually limited to the distribution of a given peripheral nerve. Normal stimuli such as touch or change in temperature may be transformed into this type of pain, which is frequently present in a patient at rest. The demonstration of irregularly spaced cutaneous pain spots may be the only indication of an old nerve lesion underlying causalgic pain. Even though the pain may be precipitated by gentle palpation, rigidity of the abdominal muscles is absent, and the respirations are not disturbed. Distention of the abdomen is uncommon, and the pain has no relationship to the intake of food.

Pain arising from spinal nerves or roots comes and goes suddenly and is of a lancinating type (Chap. 16). It may be caused by herpes zoster, impingement by arthritis, tumors, herniated nucleus pulposus, diabetes, or syphilis. It is not associated with food intake, abdominal distention, or changes in respiration. Severe muscle spasm, as in the gastric crises of tabes dorsalis, is common but is either relieved or is not accentuated by abdominal palpation. The pain is made worse by movement of the spine and is usually confined to a few dermatomes. Hyperesthesia is very common.

Pain due to functional causes conforms to none of the aforementioned patterns. Mechanism is hard to define. Irritable bowel syndrome (IBS) is a functional gastrointestinal disorder characterized by abdominal pain and altered bowel habits. The diagnosis is made on the basis of clinical criteria (Chap. 290) and after exclusion of demonstrable structural abnormalities. The episodes of abdominal pain are often brought on by stress, and the pain varies considerably in type and location. Nausea and vomiting are rare. Localized tenderness and muscle spasm are inconsistent or absent. The causes of IBS or related functional disorders are not known.

APPROACH TO THE PATIENT:
Abdominal Pain

Few abdominal conditions require such urgent operative intervention that an orderly approach need be abandoned, no matter how ill the patient. Only those patients with exsanguinating intraabdominal hemorrhage (e.g., ruptured aneurysm) must be rushed to the operating room immediately, but in such instances only a few minutes are required to assess the critical nature of the problem. Under these circumstances, all obstacles must be swept aside, adequate venous access for fluid replacement obtained, and the operation begun. Many patients of this type have died in the radiology department or the emergency room while awaiting such unnecessary examinations as electrocardiograms or abdominal films. *There are no contraindications to operation when massive intraabdominal hemorrhage is present.* Fortunately, this situation is relatively rare. These comments do not pertain to gastrointestinal hemorrhage, which can often be managed by other means (Chap. 42).

Nothing will supplant an orderly, painstakingly *detailed history*, which is far more valuable than any laboratory or radiographic examination. This kind of history is laborious and time-consuming, making it not especially popular, even though a reasonably accurate diagnosis can be made on the basis of the history alone in the majority of cases. Computer-aided diagnosis of abdominal pain provides no advantage over clinical assessment alone. In cases of *acute* abdominal pain, a diagnosis is readily established in most instances, whereas success is not so frequent in patients with *chronic* pain. IBS is one of the most common causes of abdominal pain and must always be kept in mind (Chap. 290). The location of the pain can assist in narrowing the differential diagnosis (see Table 14-2); however, the *chronological sequence of events* in the patient's history is often more important than emphasis on the location of pain. If the examiner is sufficiently open-minded and unhurried, asks the proper questions, and listens, the patient will usually provide the diagnosis. Careful attention should be paid to the extraabdominal regions that may be responsible for abdominal pain. An accurate menstrual history in a female patient is essential. Narcotics or analgesics should *not* be withheld until a definitive diagnosis or a definitive plan has been formulated; obfuscation of the diagnosis by adequate analgesia is unlikely.

In the examination, simple critical inspection of the patient, e.g., of facies, position in bed, and respiratory activity, may provide valuable clues. The amount of information to be gleaned is directly proportional to the *gentleness* and thoroughness of the examiner. Once a patient with peritoneal inflammation has been examined brusquely, accurate assessment by the next examiner becomes almost impossible. Eliciting rebound tenderness by sudden release of a deeply palpating hand in a patient with suspected peritonitis is cruel and unnecessary. The same information can be obtained by gentle percussion of the abdomen (rebound tenderness on a miniature scale), a maneuver that can be far more precise and localizing. Asking the patient to cough will elicit true rebound tenderness without the need for placing a hand on the abdomen. Furthermore, the forceful demonstration of rebound tenderness will startle and induce protective spasm in a nervous or worried patient in whom true rebound tenderness is not present. A palpable gallbladder will be missed if palpation is so brusque that voluntary muscle spasm becomes superimposed on involuntary muscular rigidity.

As in history taking, sufficient time should be spent in the examination. Abdominal signs may be minimal but nevertheless, if accompanied by consistent symptoms, may be exceptionally meaningful. Abdominal signs may be virtually or totally absent in cases of pelvic peritonitis, so careful *pelvic and rectal examinations are mandatory in every patient with abdominal pain.* Tenderness on pelvic or rectal examination in the absence of other abdominal signs can be caused by operative indications such as perforated appendicitis, diverticulitis, twisted ovarian cyst, and many others.

Much attention has been paid to the presence or absence of peristaltic sounds, their quality, and their frequency. Auscultation of the abdomen is one of the least revealing aspects of the physical examination of a patient with abdominal pain. Catastrophes such as strangulating small intestinal obstruction or perforated appendicitis may occur in the presence of normal peristaltic sounds. Conversely, when the proximal part of the intestine above an obstruction becomes markedly distended and edematous, peristaltic sounds may lose the characteristics of borborygmi and become weak or absent, even when peritonitis is not present. It is usually the severe chemical peritonitis of sudden onset that is associated with the truly silent abdomen. Assessment of the patient's state of hydration is important.

Laboratory examinations may be of great value in assessment of the patient with abdominal pain, yet with few exceptions they rarely establish a diagnosis. Leukocytosis should never be the single deciding factor as to whether or not operation is indicated. A white blood cell count >20,000/μL may be observed with perforation of a viscus, but pancreatitis, acute cholecystitis, pelvic inflammatory disease, and intestinal infarction may be associated with marked leukocytosis. A normal white blood cell count is not rare in cases of perforation of abdominal viscera. The diagnosis of anemia may be more helpful than the white blood cell count, especially when combined with the history.

The urinalysis may reveal the state of hydration or rule out severe renal disease, diabetes, or urinary infection. Blood urea nitrogen, glucose, and serum bilirubin levels may be helpful. Serum amylase levels may be increased by many diseases other than pancreatitis, e.g., perforated ulcer, strangulating intestinal obstruction, and acute cholecystitis; thus, elevations of serum amylase do not rule out the need for an operation. The determination of the serum lipase may have greater accuracy than that of the serum amylase.

Plain and upright or lateral decubitus radiographs of the abdomen may be of value in cases of intestinal obstruction, perforated ulcer, and a variety of other conditions. They are usually unnecessary in patients with acute appendicitis or strangulated external hernias. In rare instances, barium or water-soluble contrast study of the upper part of the gastrointestinal tract may demonstrate partial intestinal obstruction that may elude diagnosis by other means. If there is any question of obstruction of the colon, oral administration of barium sulfate should be avoided. On the other hand, in cases of suspected colonic obstruction (without perforation), contrast enema may be diagnostic.

In the absence of trauma, peritoneal lavage has been replaced as a diagnostic tool by ultrasound, CT, and laparoscopy. Ultrasonog-

TABLE 14-2	DIFFERENTIAL DIAGNOSES OF ABDOMINAL PAIN BY LOCATION	
Right Upper Quadrant	**Epigastric**	**Left Upper Quadrant**
Cholecystitis	Peptic ulcer disease	Splenic infarct
Cholangitis	Gastritis	Splenic rupture
Pancreatitis	GERD	Splenic abscess
Pneumonia/empyema	Pancreatitis	Gastritis
Pleurisy/pleurodynia	Myocardial infarction	Gastric ulcer
Subdiaphragmatic abscess	Pericarditis	Pancreatitis
Hepatitis	Ruptured aortic aneurysm	Subdiaphragmatic abscess
Budd-Chiari syndrome	Esophagitis	
Right Lower Quadrant	**Periumbilical**	**Left Lower Quadrant**
Appendicitis	Early appendicitis	Diverticulitis
Salpingitis	Gastroenteritis	Salpingitis
Inguinal hernia	Bowel obstruction	Inguinal hernia
Ectopic pregnancy	Ruptured aortic aneurysm	Ectopic pregnancy
Nephrolithiasis		Nephrolithiasis
Inflammatory bowel disease		Irritable bowel syndrome
Mesenteric lymphadenitis		Inflammatory bowel disease
Typhlitis		

Diffuse Nonlocalized Pain	
Gastroenteritis	Diabetes
Mesenteric ischemia	Malaria
Bowel obstruction	Familial Mediterranean fever
Irritable bowel syndrome	Metabolic diseases
Peritonitis	Psychiatric disease

raphy has proved to be useful in detecting an enlarged gallbladder or pancreas, the presence of gallstones, an enlarged ovary, or a tubal pregnancy. Laparoscopy is especially helpful in diagnosing pelvic conditions, such as ovarian cysts, tubal pregnancies, salpingitis, and acute appendicitis. Radioisotopic scans (HIDA) may help differentiate acute cholecystitis from acute pancreatitis. A CT scan may demonstrate an enlarged pancreas, ruptured spleen, or thickened colonic or appendiceal wall and streaking of the mesocolon or mesoappendix characteristic of diverticulitis or appendicitis.

Sometimes, even under the best circumstances with all available aids and with the greatest of clinical skill, a definitive diagnosis cannot be established at the time of the initial examination. Nevertheless, despite lack of a clear anatomic diagnosis, it may be abundantly clear to an experienced and thoughtful physician and surgeon that on clinical grounds alone operation is indicated.

15 Headache
Peter J. Goadsby, Neil H. Raskin

Headache is among the most common reasons that patients seek medical attention. Diagnosis and management is based on a careful clinical approach that is augmented by an understanding of the anatomy, physiology, and pharmacology of the nervous system pathways that mediate the various headache syndromes.

GENERAL PRINCIPLES

A classification system developed by the International Headache Society characterizes headache as primary or secondary (Table 15-1). *Primary headaches* are those in which headache and its associated features are the disorder in itself, whereas *secondary headaches* are those caused by exogenous disorders. Primary headache often results in considerable disability and a decrease in the patient's quality of life. Mild secondary headache, such as that seen in association with upper respiratory tract infections, is common but rarely worrisome. Life-threatening headache is relatively uncommon, but vigilance is required in order to recognize and appropriately treat patients with this category of head pain.

ANATOMY AND PHYSIOLOGY OF HEADACHE

Pain usually occurs when peripheral nociceptors are stimulated in response to tissue injury, visceral distension, or other factors (Chap. 12). In such situations, pain perception is a normal physiologic response mediated by a healthy nervous system. Pain can also result when pain-producing pathways of the peripheral or central nervous system (CNS) are damaged or activated inappropriately. Headache may originate from either or both mechanisms. Relatively few cranial structures are pain-producing; these include the scalp, middle meningeal artery, dural sinuses, falx cerebri, and proximal segments of the large pial arteries. The ventricular ependyma, choroid plexus, pial veins, and much of the brain parenchyma are not pain-producing.

TABLE 15-1 COMMON CAUSES OF HEADACHE

Primary Headache		Secondary Headache	
Type	%	Type	%
Migraine	16	Systemic infection	63
Tension-type	69	Head injury	4
Cluster	0.1	Vascular disorders	1
Idiopathic stabbing	2	Subarachnoid hemorrhage	<1
Exertional	1	Brain tumor	0.1

Source: After J Olesen et al: *The Headaches*. Philadelphia, Lippincott, Williams & Wilkins, 2005.

Should that decision be questionable, watchful waiting with repeated questioning and examination will often elucidate the true nature of the illness and indicate the proper course of action.

FURTHER READINGS

CERVERO F, LAIRD JM: Visceral pain. Lancet 353:2145, 1999

JONES PF: Suspected acute appendicitis: Trends in management over 30 years. Br J Surg 88:1570, 2001

LYON C, CLARK DC: Diagnosis of acute abdominal pain in older patients. Am Fam Physician 74:1537, 2006

SILEN W: Cope's Early Diagnosis of the Acute Abdomen, 21st ed, New York and Oxford: Oxford University Press, 2005

TAIT IS et al: Do patients with abdominal pain wait unduly long for analgesia? J R Coll Surg Edinb 44:181, 1999

The key structures involved in primary headache appear to be

- the large intracranial vessels and dura mater
- the peripheral terminals of the trigeminal nerve that innervate these structures
- the caudal portion of the trigeminal nucleus, which extends into the dorsal horns of the upper cervical spinal cord and receives input from the first and second cervical nerve roots (the trigeminocervical complex)
- the pain modulatory systems in the brain that receive input from trigeminal nociceptors

The innervation of the large intracranial vessels and dura mater by the trigeminal nerve is known as the *trigeminovascular system*. Autonomic symptoms, such as *lacrimation* and *nasal congestion*, are prominent in the trigeminal autonomic cephalalgias, including cluster headache and paroxysmal hemicrania, and may also be seen in migraine. These autonomic symptoms reflect activation of cranial parasympathetic pathways, and functional imaging studies indicate that vascular changes in migraine and cluster headache, when present, are similarly driven by these cranial autonomic systems. Migraine and other primary headache types are not "vascular headaches"; these disorders do not reliably manifest vascular changes, and treatment outcomes cannot be predicted by vascular effects.

CLINICAL EVALUATION OF ACUTE, NEW-ONSET HEADACHE

The patient who presents with a new, severe headache has a differential diagnosis that is quite different from the patient with recurrent headaches over many years. In new-onset and severe headache, the probability of finding a potentially serious cause is considerably greater than in recurrent headache. Patients with recent onset of pain require prompt evaluation and often treatment. Serious causes to be considered include meningitis, subarachnoid hemorrhage, epidural or subdural hematoma, glaucoma, and purulent sinusitis. When worrisome symptoms and signs are present (Table 15-2), rapid diagnosis and management is critical.

TABLE 15-2 HEADACHE SYMPTOMS THAT SUGGEST A SERIOUS UNDERLYING DISORDER

"Worst" headache ever
First severe headache
Subacute worsening over days or weeks
Abnormal neurologic examination
Fever or unexplained systemic signs
Vomiting that precedes headache
Pain induced by bending, lifting, cough
Pain that disturbs sleep or presents immediately upon awakening
Known systemic illness
Onset after age 55
Pain associated with local tenderness, e.g., region of temporal artery

A complete neurologic examination is an essential first step in the evaluation. In most cases, patients with an abnormal examination or a history of recent-onset headache should be evaluated by a CT or MRI study. As an initial screening procedure for intracranial pathology in this setting, CT and MRI methods appear to be equally sensitive. In some circumstances a lumbar puncture (LP) is also required, unless a benign etiology can be otherwise established. A general evaluation of acute headache might include the investigation of cardiovascular and renal status by blood pressure monitoring and urine examination; eyes by fundoscopy, intraocular pressure measurement, and refraction; cranial arteries by palpation; and cervical spine by the effect of passive movement of the head and by imaging.

The psychological state of the patient should also be evaluated since a relationship exists between head pain and depression. Many patients in chronic daily pain cycles become depressed, although depression itself is rarely a cause of headache. Drugs with antidepressant actions are also effective in the prophylactic treatment of both tension-type headache and migraine.

Underlying recurrent headache disorders may be activated by pain that follows otologic or endodontic surgical procedures. Thus, pain about the head as the result of diseased tissue or trauma may reawaken an otherwise quiescent migrainous syndrome. Treatment of the headache is largely ineffective until the cause of the primary problem is addressed.

Serious underlying conditions that are associated with headache are described below. Brain tumor is a rare cause of headache and even less commonly a cause of severe pain. The vast majority of patients presenting with severe headache have a benign cause.

SECONDARY HEADACHE

The management of secondary headache focuses on diagnosis and treatment of the underlying condition.

MENINGITIS

Acute, severe headache with stiff neck and fever suggests meningitis. LP is mandatory. Often there is striking accentuation of pain with eye movement. Meningitis can be easily mistaken for migraine in that the cardinal symptoms of pounding headache, photophobia, nausea, and vomiting are present. Meningitis is discussed in Chaps. 376 and 377.

INTRACRANIAL HEMORRHAGE

Acute, severe headache with stiff neck but without fever suggests subarachnoid hemorrhage. A ruptured aneurysm, arteriovenous malformation, or intraparenchymal hemorrhage may also present with headache alone. Rarely, if the hemorrhage is small or below the foramen magnum, the head CT scan can be normal. Therefore, LP may be required to definitively diagnose subarachnoid hemorrhage. Intracranial hemorrhage is discussed in Chap. 269.

BRAIN TUMOR

Approximately 30% of patients with brain tumors consider headache to be their chief complaint. The head pain is usually nondescript—an intermittent deep, dull aching of moderate intensity, which may worsen with exertion or change in position and may be associated with nausea and vomiting. This pattern of symptoms results from migraine far more often than from brain tumor. The headache of brain tumor disturbs sleep in about 10% of patients. Vomiting that precedes the appearance of headache by weeks is highly characteristic of posterior fossa brain tumors. A history of amenorrhea or galactorrhea should lead one to question whether a prolactin-secreting pituitary adenoma (or the polycystic ovary syndrome) is the source of headache. Headache arising de novo in a patient with known malignancy suggests either cerebral metastases or carcinomatous meningitis, or both. Head pain appearing abruptly after bending, lifting, or coughing can be due to a posterior fossa mass (or a Chiari malformation). Brain tumors are discussed in Chap. 374.

TEMPORAL ARTERITIS

(See also Chaps. 29 and 319) Temporal (giant cell) arteritis is an inflammatory disorder of arteries that frequently involves the extracranial carotid circulation. It is a common disorder of the elderly; its annual incidence is 77 per 100,000 individuals ages 50 and older. The average age of onset is 70 years, and women account for 65% of cases. About half of patients with untreated temporal arteritis develop blindness due to involvement of the ophthalmic artery and its branches; indeed, the ischemic optic neuropathy induced by giant cell arteritis is the major cause of rapidly developing bilateral blindness in patients >60 years. Because treatment with glucocorticoids is effective in preventing this complication, prompt recognition of the disorder is important.

Typical presenting symptoms include headache, polymyalgia rheumatica (Chap. 319), jaw claudication, fever, and weight loss. Headache is the dominant symptom and often appears in association with malaise and muscle aches. Head pain may be unilateral or bilateral and is located temporally in 50% of patients but may involve any and all aspects of the cranium. Pain usually appears gradually over a few hours before peak intensity is reached; occasionally, it is explosive in onset. The quality of pain is only seldom throbbing; it is almost invariably described as dull and boring, with superimposed episodic stabbing pains similar to the sharp pains that appear in migraine. Most patients can recognize that the origin of their head pain is superficial, external to the skull, rather than originating deep within the cranium (the pain site for migraineurs). Scalp tenderness is present, often to a marked degree; brushing the hair or resting the head on a pillow may be impossible because of pain. Headache is usually worse at night and often aggravated by exposure to cold. Additional findings may include reddened, tender nodules or red streaking of the skin overlying the temporal arteries, and tenderness of the temporal or, less commonly, the occipital arteries.

The erythrocyte sedimentation rate (ESR) is often, though not always, elevated; a normal ESR does not exclude giant cell arteritis. A temporal artery biopsy followed by treatment with prednisone 80 mg daily for the first 4–6 weeks should be initiated when clinical suspicion is high. The prevalence of migraine among the elderly is substantial, considerably higher than that of giant cell arteritis. Migraineurs often report amelioration of their headaches with prednisone; thus, caution must be used when interpreting the therapeutic response.

GLAUCOMA

Glaucoma may present with a prostrating headache associated with nausea and vomiting. The headache often starts with severe eye pain. On physical examination, the eye is often red with a fixed, moderately dilated pupil. Glaucoma is discussed in Chap. 29.

PRIMARY HEADACHE SYNDROMES

Primary headaches are disorders in which headache and associated features occur in the absence of any exogenous cause (Table 15-1). The most common are migraine, tension-type headache, and cluster headache.

MIGRAINE HEADACHE

Migraine, the second most common cause of headache, afflicts approximately 15% of women and 6% of men. It is usually an episodic headache that is associated with certain features such as sensitivity to light, sound, or movement; nausea and vomiting often accompany the headache. A useful description of migraine is a benign and recurring syndrome of headache associated with other symptoms of neurologic dysfunction in varying admixtures (Table 15-3). Migraine can often be recognized by its activators, referred to as *triggers*.

The brain of the migraineur is particularly sensitive to environmental and sensory stimuli; migraine-prone patients do not habituate easily to sensory stimuli. This sensitivity is amplified in females during the menstrual cycle. Headache can be initiated or amplified by various triggers, including glare, bright lights, sounds, or other afferent stimulation; hunger; excess stress; physical exertion; stormy weather or barometric pressure changes; hormonal fluctuations during menses; lack of or excess sleep; and alcohol or other chemical stimulation. Knowledge of a patient's susceptibility to specific triggers can be useful in management strategies involving lifestyle adjustments.

TABLE 15-3	SYMPTOMS ACCOMPANYING SEVERE MIGRAINE ATTACKS IN 500 PATIENTS

Symptom	Patients Affected, %
Nausea	87
Photophobia	82
Lightheadedness	72
Scalp tenderness	65
Vomiting	56
Visual disturbances	36
Photopsia	26
Fortification spectra	10
Paresthesias	33
Vertigo	33
Alteration of consciousness	18
Syncope	10
Seizure	4
Confusional state	4
Diarrhea	16

Source: From NH Raskin, *Headache*, 2d ed. New York, Churchill Livingston, 1988; with permission.

Pathogenesis The sensory sensitivity that is characteristic of migraine is probably due to dysfunction of monoaminergic sensory control systems located in the brainstem and thalamus (Fig. 15-1).

Activation of cells in the trigeminal nucleus results in the release of vasoactive neuropeptides, particularly calcitonin gene-related peptide (CGRP), at vascular terminations of the trigeminal nerve. Recently, antagonists of CGRP have shown some early promise in the therapy of migraine. Centrally, the second-order trigeminal neurons cross the midline and project to ventrobasal and posterior nuclei of the thalamus for further processing. Additionally, there are projections to the periaqueductal gray and hypothalamus, from which reciprocal descending systems have established anti-nociceptive effects. Other brainstem regions likely to be involved in descending modulation of trigeminal pain include the nucleus locus coeruleus in the pons and the rostroventromedial medulla.

Pharmacologic and other data point to the involvement of the neurotransmitter 5-hydroxytryptamine (5-HT; also known as serotonin) in migraine. Approximately 50 years ago, methysergide was found to antagonize certain peripheral actions of 5-HT and was introduced as the first drug capable of preventing migraine attacks. The triptans are designed to selectively stimulate subpopulations of 5-HT receptors; at least 14 different 5-HT receptors exist in humans. The triptans are potent agonists of 5-HT$_{1B}$, 5-HT$_{1D}$, and 5-HT$_{1F}$ receptors and are less potent at the 5-HT$_{1A}$ receptor. A growing body of data indicates that the antimigraine efficacy of the triptans relates to their ability to stimulate 5-HT$_{1B/1D}$ receptors, which are located on both blood vessels and nerve terminals.

Data also support a role for dopamine in the pathophysiology of certain subtypes of migraine. Most migraine symptoms can be induced by dopaminergic stimulation. Moreover, there is dopamine receptor hypersensitivity in migraineurs, as demonstrated by the induction of yawning, nausea, vomiting, hypotension, and other symptoms of a migraine attack by dopaminergic agonists at doses that do not affect nonmigraineurs. Dopamine receptor antagonists are effective therapeutic agents in migraine, especially when given parenterally or concurrently with other antimigraine agents.

Migraine genes identified by studying families with familial hemiplegic migraine (FHM) reveal involvement of ion channels, suggesting that alterations in membrane excitability can predispose to migraine. Mutations involving the Ca$_v$2.1 (P/Q) type voltage-gated calcium channel *CACNA1A* gene are now known to cause FHM 1; this mutation is responsible for about 50% of FHM. Mutations in the Na$^+$-K$^+$ATPase *ATP1A2* gene, designated FHM 2, are responsible for about 20% of FHM. Mutations in the neuronal voltage-gated sodium channel *SCN1A* cause FHM 3. Functional neuroimaging has suggested that brainstem regions in migraine (Fig. 15-2) and the posterior hypothalamic gray matter region close to the human circadian pacemaker cells of the suprachiasmatic nucleus in cluster headache (Fig. 15-3) are good candidates for specific involvement in primary headache.

Diagnosis and Clinical Features Diagnostic criteria for migraine headache are listed in Table 15-4. A high index of suspicion is required to diagnose migraine: the migraine aura, consisting of visual disturbances with flashing lights or zigzag lines moving across the visual field or of other neurologic symptoms, is reported in only 20–25% of patients. A headache diary can often be helpful in making the diagnosis; this is also helpful in assessing disability and the frequency of treatment for acute attacks. Patients with episodes of migraine that occur daily or near-daily are considered to have chronic migraine (see "Chronic Daily Headache," below). Migraine must be differentiated from tension-type headache (discussed below), the most common primary headache syndrome seen in clinical practice. *Migraine at its most basic level is headache with associated features, and tension-type headache is headache that is featureless. Most patients with disabling headache probably have migraine.*

Patients with acephalgic migraine experience recurrent neurologic symptoms, often with nausea or vomiting, but with little or no headache. Vertigo can be prominent; it has been estimated that one-third of patients referred for vertigo or dizziness have a primary diagnosis of migraine.

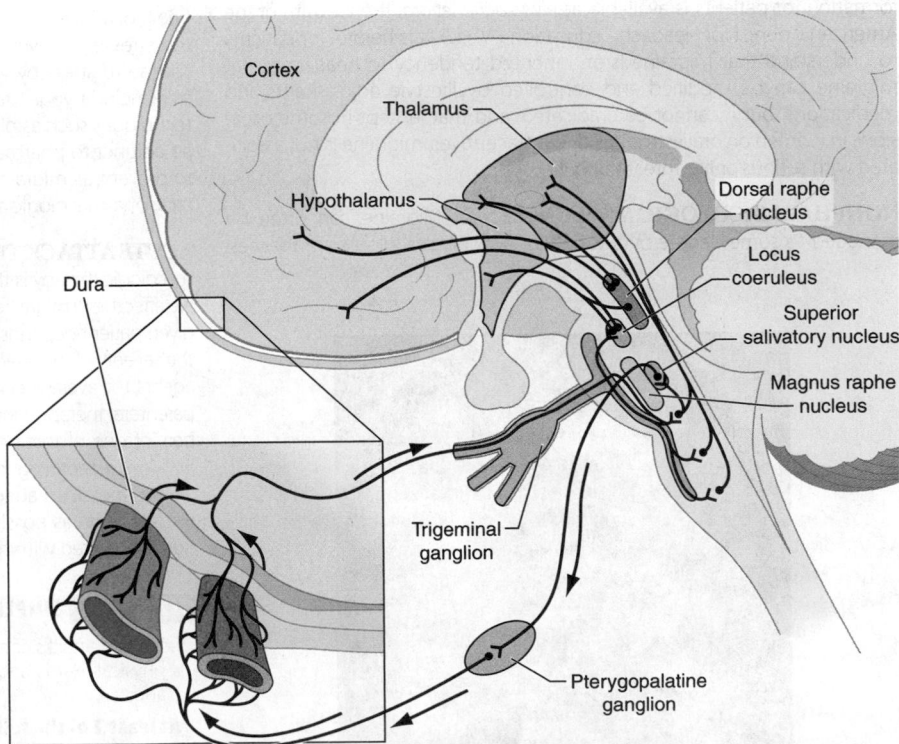

FIGURE 15-1 Brainstem pathways that modulate sensory input. The key pathway for pain in migraine is the trigeminovascular input from the meningeal vessels, which passes through the trigeminal ganglion and synapses on second-order neurons in the trigeminocervical complex. These neurons in turn project in the quintothalamic tract and, after decussating in the brainstem, synapse on neurons in the thalamus. Important modulation of the trigeminovascular nociceptive input comes from the dorsal raphe nucleus, locus coeruleus, and nucleus raphe magnus.

A   **B**   **C**

FIGURE 15-2 Positron emission tomography (PET) activation in migraine. In spontaneous attacks of episodic migraine (**A**) there is activation of the region of the dorsolateral pons (intersection of dark blue lines); an identical pattern is found in chronic migraine (not shown). This area, which includes the noradrenergic locus coeruleus, is fundamental to the expression of migraine. Moreover, lateralization of changes in this region of the brainstem correlates with lateralization of the head pain in hemicranial migraine; the scans shown in panels **B** and **C** are of patients with acute migraine headache on the right and left side, respectively. *(From S Afridi et al: Arch Neurol 62:1270, 2005; Brain 128:932, 2005.)*

℞ MIGRAINE HEADACHES

Once a diagnosis of migraine has been established, it is important to assess the extent of a patient's disease and disability. The Migraine Disability Assessment Score (MIDAS) is a well-validated, easy-to-use tool (**Fig. 15-4**).

Patient education is an important aspect of migraine management. Information for patients is available at *www.achenet.org*, the website of the American Council for Headache Education (ACHE). It is helpful for patients to understand that migraine is an inherited tendency to headache; that migraine can be modified and controlled by lifestyle adjustments and medications, but it cannot be eradicated; and that, except in some occasions in women on oral estrogens or contraceptives, migraine is not associated with serious or life-threatening illnesses.

NONPHARMACOLOGIC MANAGEMENT   Migraine can often be managed to some degree by a variety of nonpharmacologic approaches.

Most patients benefit by the identification and avoidance of specific headache triggers. A regulated lifestyle is helpful, including a healthful diet, regular exercise, regular sleep patterns, avoidance of excess caffeine and alcohol, and avoidance of acute changes in stress levels.

The measures that benefit a given individual should be used routinely since they provide a simple, cost-effective approach to migraine management. Patients with migraine do not encounter more stress than headache-free individuals; overresponsiveness to stress appears to be the issue. Since the stresses of everyday living cannot be eliminated, lessening one's response to stress by various techniques is helpful for many patients. These may include yoga, transcendental meditation, hypnosis, and conditioning techniques such as biofeedback. For most patients, this approach is, at best, an adjunct to pharmacotherapy. Nonpharmacologic measures are unlikely to prevent all migraine attacks. When these measures fail to prevent an attack, pharmacologic approaches are then needed to abort an attack.

ACUTE ATTACK THERAPIES FOR MIGRAINE   The mainstay of pharmacologic therapy is the judicious use of one or more of the many drugs that are effective in migraine (**Table 15-5**). The selection of the optimal regimen for a given patient depends on a number of factors, the most important of which is the severity of the attack. Mild migraine attacks can usually be managed by oral agents; the average efficacy rate is 50–70%. Severe migraine attacks may require parenteral therapy. Most drugs effective in the treatment of migraine are members of one of three major pharmacologic classes: anti-inflammatory agents, $5HT_{1B/1D}$ receptor agonists, and dopamine receptor antagonists.

In general, an adequate dose of whichever agent is chosen should be used as soon as possible after the onset of an attack. If additional medication is required within 60 min because symptoms return or have not abat-

FIGURE 15-3 Posterior hypothalamic gray matter activation on positron emission tomography (PET) in a patient with acute cluster headache. Posterior hypothalamic gray matter activation on positron emission tomography (PET) in a patient with acute cluster headache. *(From A May et al: Lancet 352:275, 1998.)*

TABLE 15-4	SIMPLIFIED DIAGNOSTIC CRITERIA FOR MIGRAINE
Repeated attacks of headache lasting 4–72 h in patients with a normal physical examination, no other reasonable cause for the headache, and:	
At least 2 of the following features:	**Plus at least 1 of the following features:**
Unilateral pain	Nausea/vomiting
Throbbing pain	Photophobia and phonophobia
Aggravation by movement	
Moderate or severe intensity	

Source: Adapted from the International Headache Society Classification (Headache Classification Committee of the International Headache Society, 2004).

*MIDAS Questionnaire

INSTRUCTIONS: Please answer the following questions about ALL headaches you have had over the last 3 months. Write zero if you did not do the activity in the last 3 months.

1. On how many days in the last 3 months did you miss work or school because of your headaches? .... _____ days

2. How many days in the last 3 months was your productivity at work or school reduced by half or more because of your headaches *(do not include days you counted in question 1 where you missed work or school)*? .... _____ days

3. On how many days in the last 3 months did you **not** do household work because of your headaches? .... _____ days

4. How many days in the last 3 months was your productivity in household work reduced by half or more because of your headaches *(do not include days you counted in question 3 where you did not do household work)*? .... _____ days

5. On how many days in the last 3 months did you miss family, social, or leisure activities because of your headaches? .... _____ days

A. On how many days in the last 3 months did you have a headache? *(If a headache lasted more than one day, count each day.)* .... _____ days

B. On a scale of 0–10, on average how painful were these headaches? *(Where 0 = no pain at all, and 10 = pain as bad as it can be.)* .... _____

*Migraine Disability Assessment Score
(Questions 1–5 are used to calculate the MIDAS score.)
Grade I—Minimal or Infrequent Disability: 0–5
Grade II—Mild or Infrequent Disability: 6–10
Grade III—Moderate Disability: 11–20
Grade IV—Severe Disability: > 20

© Innovative Medical Research 1997

FIGURE 15-4 MIDAS Questionnaire.

ed, the initial dose should be increased for subsequent attacks. Migraine therapy must be individualized; a standard approach for all patients is not possible. A therapeutic regimen may need to be constantly refined until one is identified that provides the patient with rapid, complete, and consistent relief with minimal side effects **(Table 15-6)**.

Nonsteroidal Anti-Inflammatory Drugs (NSAIDs) Both the severity and duration of a migraine attack can be reduced significantly by anti-inflammatory agents (Table 15-5). Indeed, many undiagnosed migraineurs are self-treated with nonprescription NSAIDs. A general consensus is that NSAIDs are most effective when taken early in the migraine attack. However, the effectiveness of anti-inflammatory agents in migraine is usually less than optimal in moderate or severe migraine attacks. The combination of acetaminophen, aspirin, and caffeine has been approved for use by the U.S. Food and Drug Administration (FDA) for the treatment of mild to moderate migraine. The combination of aspirin and metoclopramide has been shown to be equivalent to a single dose of sumatriptan. Important side effects of NSAIDs include dyspepsia and gastrointestinal irritation.

5-HT$_1$ AGONISTS **Oral** Stimulation of 5-HT$_{1B/1D}$ receptors can stop an acute migraine attack. Ergotamine and dihydroergotamine are nonselective receptor agonists, while the triptans are selective 5-HT$_{1B/1D}$ receptor agonists. A variety of triptans (e.g., naratriptan, rizatriptan, eletriptan, sumatriptan, zolmitriptan, almotriptan, frovatriptan) are now available for the treatment of migraine.

Each drug in the triptan class has similar pharmacologic properties but varies slightly in terms of clinical efficacy. Rizatriptan and eletriptan are the most efficacious of the triptans currently available in the United States. Sumatriptan and zolmitriptan have similar rates of efficacy as well as time to onset, whereas naratriptan and frovatriptan are the slowest-acting and least efficacious. Clinical efficacy appears to be related more to the t_{max} (time to peak plasma level) than to the potency, half-life, or bioavailability. This observation is consistent with a large body of data indicating that faster-acting analgesics are more effective than slower-acting agents.

Unfortunately, monotherapy with a selective oral 5-HT$_{1B/1D}$ agonist does not result in rapid, consistent, and complete relief of migraine in all patients. Triptans are not effective in migraine with aura unless given after the aura is completed and the headache initiated. Side effects are common though often mild and transient. Moreover, 5-HT$_{1B/1D}$ agonists are contraindicated in individuals with a history of cardiovascular and cere-

brovascular disease. Recurrence of headache is another important limitation of triptan use and occurs at least occasionally in most patients.

Ergotamine preparations offer a nonselective means of stimulating 5-HT$_1$ receptors. A nonnauseating dose of ergotamine should be sought since a dose that provokes nausea is too high and may intensify head pain. Except for a sublingual formulation of ergotamine, oral formulations of ergotamine also contain 100 mg caffeine (theoretically to enhance ergotamine absorption and possibly to add additional analgesic activity). The average oral ergotamine dose for a migraine attack is 2 mg. Since the clinical studies demonstrating the efficacy of ergotamine in migraine predated the clinical trial methodologies used with the triptans, it is difficult to assess the clinical efficacy of ergotamine versus the triptans. In general, ergotamine appears to have a much higher incidence of nausea than triptans, but less headache recurrence.

Nasal The fastest-acting nonparenteral antimigraine therapies that can be self-administered include nasal formulations of dihydroergotamine (Migranal), zolmitriptan (Zomig nasal), or sumatriptan. The nasal sprays result in substantial blood levels within 30–60 min. Although in theory nasal sprays might provide faster and more effective relief of a migraine attack than oral formulations, their reported efficacy is only approximately 50–60%.

Parenteral Parenteral administration of drugs such as dihydroergotamine and sumatriptan is approved by the FDA for the rapid relief of a migraine attack. Peak plasma levels of dihydroergotamine are achieved 3 min after intravenous dosing, 30 min after intramuscular dosing, and 45 min after subcutaneous dosing. If an attack has not already peaked, subcutaneous or intramuscular administration of 1 mg dihydroergotamine suffices for about 80–90% of patients. Sumatriptan, 6 mg subcutaneously, is effective in ~70–80% of patients.

DOPAMINE ANTAGONISTS **Oral** Oral dopamine antagonists should be considered as adjunctive therapy in migraine. Drug absorption is impaired during migraine because of reduced gastrointestinal motility. Delayed absorption occurs even in the absence of nausea and is related to the severity of the attack and not its duration. Therefore, when oral NSAIDs and/or triptan agents fail, the addition of a dopamine antagonist such as metoclopramide, 10 mg, should be considered to enhance gastric absorption. In addition, dopamine antagonists decrease nausea/vomiting and restore normal gastric motility.

Parenteral Parenteral dopamine antagonists (e.g., chlorpromazine, prochlorperazine, metoclopramide) can also provide significant acute relief of migraine; they can be used in combination with parenteral 5-HT$_{1B/1D}$ agonists. A common intravenous protocol used for the treatment of severe migraine is the administration over 2 min of a mixture of 5 mg of prochlorperazine and 0.5 mg of dihydroergotamine.

OTHER MEDICATIONS FOR ACUTE MIGRAINE **Oral** The combination of acetaminophen, dichloralphenazone, and isometheptene, one to two capsules, has been classified by the FDA as "possibly" effective in the treatment of migraine. Since the clinical studies demonstrating the efficacy of this combination analgesic in migraine predated the clinical trial methodologies used with the triptans, it is difficult to compare the efficacy of this sympathomimetic compound to other agents.

Nasal A nasal preparation of butorphanol is available for the treatment of acute pain. As with all narcotics, the use of nasal butorphanol should be limited to a select group of migraineurs, as described below.

Parenteral Narcotics are effective in the acute treatment of migraine. For example, intravenous meperidine (50–100 mg) is given frequently in the emergency room. This regimen "works" in the sense that the pain of migraine is eliminated. However, this regimen is clearly suboptimal for patients with recurrent headache. Narcotics do not treat the underlying headache mechanism; rather, they act to alter the pain sensation. Moreover, in patients taking oral narcotics such as oxycodone or hydrocodone, narcotic addiction can greatly con-

TABLE 15-5   TREATMENT OF ACUTE MIGRAINE

Drug	Trade Name	Dosage
Simple Analgesics		
Acetaminophen, aspirin, caffeine	Excedrin Migraine	Two tablets or caplets q6h (max 8 per day)
NSAIDs		
Naproxen	Aleve, Anaprox, generic	220–550 mg PO bid
Ibuprofen	Advil, Motrin, Nuprin, generic	400 mg PO q3–4h
Tolfenamic acid	Clotam Rapid	200 mg PO. May repeat x 1 after 1–2 h
5-HT$_1$ Agonists		
Oral		
Ergotamine	Ergomar	One 2 mg sublingual tablet at onset and q$^1/_2$h (max 3 per day, 5 per week)
Ergotamine 1 mg, caffeine 100 mg	Ercaf, Wigraine	One or two tablets at onset, then one tablet q$^1/_2$h (max 6 per day, 10 per week)
Naratriptan	Amerge	2.5 mg tablet at onset; may repeat once after 4 h
Rizatriptan	Maxalt Maxalt-MLT	5–10 mg tablet at onset; may repeat after 2 h (max 30 mg/d)
Sumatriptan	Imitrex	50–100 mg tablet at onset; may repeat after 2 h (max 200 mg/d)
Frovatriptan	Frova	2.5 mg tablet at onset, may repeat after 2 h (max 5 mg/d)
Almotriptan	Axert	12.5 mg tablet at onset, may repeat after 2 h (max 25 mg/d)
Eletriptan	Relpax	40 or 80 mg
Zolmitriptan	Zomig Zomig Rapimelt	2.5 mg tablet at onset; may repeat after 2 h (max 10 mg/d)
Nasal		
Dihydroergotamine	Migranal Nasal Spray	Prior to nasal spray, the pump must be primed 4 times; 1 spray (0.5 mg) is administered, followed in 15 min by a second spray
Sumatriptan	Imitrex Nasal Spray	5–20 mg intranasal spray as 4 sprays of 5 mg or a single 20 mg spray (may repeat once after 2 h, not to exceed a dose of 40 mg/d)
Zolmitriptan	Zomig	5 mg intranasal spray as one spray (may repeat once after 2 h, not to exceed a dose of 10 mg/d)
Parenteral		
Dihydroergotamine	DHE-45	1 mg IV, IM, or SC at onset and q1h (max 3 mg/d, 6 mg per week)
Sumatriptan	Imitrex Injection	6 mg SC at onset (may repeat once after 1 h for max of 2 doses in 24 h)
Dopamine Antagonists		
Oral		
Metoclopramide	Reglan,^{a} generic^a	5–10 mg/d
Prochlorperazine	Compazine,^{a} generic^a	1–25 mg/d
Parenteral		
Chlorpromazine	Generic^a	0.1 mg/kg IV at 2 mg/min; max 35 mg/d
Metoclopramide	Reglan,^{a} generic	10 mg IV
Prochlorperazine	Compazine,^{a} generic^a	10 mg IV
Other		
Oral		
Acetaminophen, 325 mg, *plus* dichloralphenazone, 100 mg, *plus* isometheptene, 65 mg	Midrin, Duradrin, generic	Two capsules at onset followed by 1 capsule q1h (max 5 capsules)
Nasal		
Butorphanol	Stadol^a	1 mg (1 spray in 1 nostril), may repeat if necessary in 1–2 h
Parenteral		
Narcotics	Generic^a	Multiple preparations and dosages; see Table 12-1

^{a}Not all drugs are specifically indicated by the FDA for migraine. Local regulations and guidelines should be consulted.

Note: Antiemetics (e.g., domperidone 10 mg or ondansetron) or prokinetics (e.g., metoclopramide 10 mg) are sometimes useful adjuncts.

Abbreviations: NSAIDs, nonsteroidal anti-inflammatory drugs; 5-HT, 5-hydroxytryptamine.

fuse the treatment of migraine. Narcotic craving and/or withdrawal can aggravate and accentuate migraine. Therefore, it is recommended that narcotic use in migraine be limited to patients with severe, but infrequent, headaches that are unresponsive to other pharmacologic approaches.

MEDICATION-OVERUSE HEADACHE

Acute attack medications, particularly codeine or barbiturate-containing compound analgesics, have a propensity to aggravate headache frequency and induce a state of refractory daily or near-daily headache called *medication-overuse headache*. This condition is likely not a separate headache entity but a reaction of the migraine patient to a particular medicine. Migraine patients who have two or more headache days a week should be cautioned about frequent analgesic use (see "Chronic Daily Headache," below).

PREVENTIVE TREATMENTS FOR MIGRAINE

Patients with an increasing frequency of migraine attacks, or with attacks that are either unresponsive or poorly responsive to abortive treatments, are good candidates for preventive agents. In general, a preventive medication should be considered in the subset of patients with five or more attacks a month. Significant side effects are associated with the use of many of these agents; furthermore, determination of dose can be difficult since the recommended doses have been derived for conditions other than migraine. The mechanism of action of these drugs is unclear; it seems likely that the brain sensitivity that underlies migraine is modified. Patients are usually started on a low dose of a chosen treatment; the dose is then gradually increased, up to a reasonable maximum to achieve clinical benefit.

Drugs that have the capacity to stabilize migraine are listed in **Table 15-7**. Drugs must be taken daily, and there is usually a lag of at least 2–12 weeks before an effect is seen. The drugs that have been approved by the FDA for the prophylactic treatment of migraine include propranolol, timolol, sodium valproate, topiramate, and methysergide (not available in the United States). In addition, a number of other drugs appear to display prophylactic efficacy. This group includes amitriptyline, nortriptyline, flunarizine, phenelzine, gabapentin, topiramate, and cyproheptadine. Phenelzine and methysergide are usually reserved for recalcitrant cases because of their serious potential side effects. Phenelzine is a monoamine oxidase inhibitor (MAOI); therefore, tyramine-containing foods, decongestants, and meperidine are contraindicated. Methysergide may cause retroperitoneal or cardiac valvular fibrosis when it is used for >6 months, and thus monitoring is required for patients using this drug; the risk of fibrosis is about 1:1500 and is likely to reverse after the drug is stopped.

The probability of success with any one of the antimigraine drugs is 50–75%. Many patients are managed adequately with low-dose amitriptyline, propranolol, topiramate, gabapentin, or valproate. If these agents fail or lead to unacceptable side effects, second-line agents such as methysergide or phenelzine can be used. Once effective stabilization is achieved, the drug is continued for 5–6 months and then slowly tapered to assess the continued need. Many patients are able to discontinue medication and experience fewer and milder attacks for long periods, suggesting that these drugs may alter the natural history of migraine.

TENSION-TYPE HEADACHE
Clinical Features The term *tension-type headache* (TTH) is commonly used to describe a chronic head-pain syndrome characterized by bilateral tight, bandlike discomfort. The pain typically builds slowly,

TABLE 15-6   CLINICAL STRATIFICATION OF ACUTE SPECIFIC MIGRAINE TREATMENTS

Clinical Situation	Treatment Options
Failed NSAIDS/analgesics	**First tier**
	Sumatriptan 50 mg or 100 mg PO
	Almotriptan 12.5 mg PO
	Rizatriptan 10 mg PO
	Eletriptan 40 mg PO
	Zolmitriptan 2.5 mg PO
	Slower effect/better tolerability
	Naratriptan 2.5 mg PO
	Frovatriptan 2.5 mg PO
	Infrequent headache
	Ergotamine 1–2 mg PO
	Dihydroergotamine nasal spray 2 mg
Early nausea or difficulties taking tablets	Zolmitriptan 5 mg nasal spray
	Sumatriptan 20 mg nasal spray
	Rizatriptan 10 mg MLT wafer
Headache recurrence	Ergotamine 2 mg (most effective PR/usually with caffeine)
	Naratriptan 2.5 mg PO
	Almotriptan 12.5 mg PO
	Eletriptan 40 mg
Tolerating acute treatments poorly	Naratriptan 2.5 mg
	Almotriptan 12.5 mg
Early vomiting	Zolmitriptan 5 mg nasal spray
	Sumatriptan 25 mg PR
	Sumatriptan 6 mg SC
Menses-related headache	**Prevention**
	Ergotamine PO at night
	Estrogen patches
	Treatment
	Triptans
	Dihydroergotamine nasal spray
Very rapidly developing symptoms	Zolmitriptan 5 mg nasal spray
	Sumatriptan 6 mg SC
	Dihydroergotamine 1 mg IM

fluctuates in severity, and may persist more or less continuously for many days. The headache may be episodic or chronic (present >15 days per month).

A useful clinical approach is to diagnose TTH in patients whose headaches are completely without accompanying features such as nausea, vomiting, photophobia, phonophobia, osmophobia, throbbing, and aggravation with movement. Such an approach neatly separates migraine, which has one or more of these features and is the main differential diagnosis, from TTH. However, the International Headache Society's definition of TTH allows an admixture of nausea, photophobia, or phonophobia in various combinations, illustrating the difficulties in distinguishing these two clinical entities. Patients whose headaches fit the TTH phenotype and who have migraine at other times, along with a family history of migraine, migrainous illnesses of childhood, or typical migraine triggers to their migraine attacks, may be biologically different from those who have TTH headache with none of the features.

Pathophysiology   The pathophysiology of TTH is incompletely understood. It seems likely that TTH is due to a primary disorder of CNS pain modulation alone, unlike migraine, which involves a more generalized disturbance of sensory modulation. Data suggest a genetic contribution to TTH, but this may not be a valid finding: given the current diagnostic criteria, the studies undoubtedly included many migraine patients. The name *tension-type headache* implies that pain is a product of *nervous tension*, but there is no clear evidence for tension as an etiology. Muscle contraction has been considered to be a feature that distinguishes TTH from migraine, but there appear to be no differences in contraction between the two headache types.

℞ TENSION-TYPE HEADACHE

The pain of TTH can generally be managed with simple analgesics such as acetaminophen, aspirin, or NSAIDs. Behavioral approaches including relaxation can also be effective. Clinical studies have demonstrated that triptans in pure TTH are not helpful, although triptans are effective in TTH when the patient also has migraine. For chronic TTH, amitriptyline is the only proven treatment (Table 15-7); other tricyclics, selective serotonin reuptake inhibitors, and the benzodiazepines have not been shown to be effective. There is no evidence for the efficacy of acupuncture. Placebo controlled trials of botulinum toxin type A in chronic TTH have not shown benefit.

TRIGEMINAL AUTONOMIC CEPHALALGIAS, INCLUDING CLUSTER HEADACHE

The trigeminal autonomic cephalalgias (TACs) are a group of primary headaches that includes cluster headache, paroxysmal hemicrania, and SUNCT (short-lasting unilateral neuralgiform headache attacks with conjunctival injection and tearing). TACs are characterized by relatively short-lasting attacks of head pain associated with cranial autonomic symptoms, such as lacrimation, conjunctival injection, or nasal congestion (Table 15-8). Pain is usually severe and may occur more than once a day. Because of the associated nasal congestion or rhinorrhea, patients are often misdiagnosed with "sinus headache" and treated with decongestants, which are ineffective.

TACs must be differentiated from short-lasting headaches that do not have prominent cranial autonomic syndromes, notably trigeminal neuralgia, primary stabbing headache, and hypnic headache. The cycling pattern and length, frequency, and timing of attacks are useful in classifying patients. Patients with TACs should undergo pituitary imaging and pituitary function tests as there is an excess of TAC presentations in patients with pituitary tumor–related headache.

Cluster Headache   Cluster headache is a rare form of primary headache with a population frequency of 0.1%. The pain is deep, usually retroorbital, often excruciating in intensity, nonfluctuating, and explosive in quality. A core feature of cluster headache is periodicity. At least one of the daily attacks of pain recurs at about the same hour each day for the duration of a cluster bout. The typical cluster headache patient has daily bouts of one to two attacks of relatively short-duration unilateral pain for 8–10 weeks a year; this is usually followed by a pain-free interval that averages 1 year. Cluster headache is characterized as chronic when there is no period of sustained remission. Patients are generally perfectly well between episodes. Onset is nocturnal in about 50% of patients, and men are affected three times more often than women. Patients with cluster headache tend to move about during attacks, pacing, rocking, or rubbing their head for relief; some may even become aggressive during attacks. This is in sharp contrast to patients with migraine, who prefer to remain motionless during attacks.

Cluster headache is associated with ipsilateral symptoms of cranial parasympathetic autonomic activation: conjunctival injection or lacrimation, rhinorrhea or nasal congestion, or cranial sympathetic dysfunction such as ptosis. The sympathetic deficit is peripheral and likely to be due to parasympathetic activation with injury to ascending sympathetic fibers surrounding a dilated carotid artery as it passes into the cranial cavity. When present, photophobia and phonophobia are far more likely to be unilateral and on the same side of the pain, rather than bilateral, as is seen in migraine. This phenomenon of unilateral photophobia/phonophobia is characteristic of TACs. Cluster headache is likely to be a disorder involving central pacemaker neurons in the region of the posterior hypothalamus (Fig. 15-2).

℞ CLUSTER HEADACHE

The most satisfactory treatment is the administration of drugs to prevent cluster attacks until the bout is over. However, treatment of acute attacks is required for all cluster headache patients at some time.

ACUTE ATTACK TREATMENT   Cluster headache attacks peak rapidly, and thus a treatment with quick onset is required. Many patients with acute cluster headache respond very well to oxygen inhalation. This should be given as 100% oxygen at 10–12 L/min for 15–20 min. It appears that high flow and high oxygen content are important. Sumatriptan 6 mg subcutaneously is rapid in onset and will usually shorten an attack to 10–15 min; there is no evidence of tachyphylaxis. Sumatriptan (20 mg) and zolmitriptan (5 mg) nasal sprays are both effective in acute cluster head-

TABLE 15-7 PREVENTIVE TREATMENTS IN MIGRAINE[a]

Drug	Dose	Selected Side Effects
Pizotifen[b]	0.5–2 mg qd	Weight gain Drowsiness
Beta blocker		
Propranolol	40–120 mg bid	Reduced energy Tiredness Postural symptoms *Contraindicated in asthma*
Tricyclics		
Amitriptyline	10–75 mg at night	Drowsiness
Dothiepin	25–75 mg at night	
Nortriptyline	25–75 mg at night	**Note:** Some patients may only need a total dose of 10 mg, although generally 1–1.5 mg/kg body weight is required
Anticonvulsants		
Topiramate	25–200 mg/d	Paresthesias Cognitive symptoms Weight loss Glaucoma Caution with nephrolithiasis
Valproate	400–600 mg bid	Drowsiness Weight gain Tremor Hair loss Fetal abnormalities Hematologic or liver abnormalities
Gabapentin	900–3600 mg qd	Dizziness Sedation
Serotonergic drugs		
Methysergide	1–4 mg qd	Drowsiness Leg cramps Hair loss Retroperitoneal fibrosis (1-month drug holiday is required every 6 months)
Flunarizine[b]	5–15 mg qd	Drowsiness Weight gain Depression Parkinsonism
No convincing evidence from controlled trials		
Verapamil		
Controlled trials demonstrate *no effect*		
Nimodipine		
Clonidine		
SSRIs: fluoxetine		

[a]Commonly used preventives are listed with reasonable doses and common side effects. Not all listed medicines are approved by the FDA; local regulations and guidelines should be consulted.
[b]Not available in the United States.

---

ache, offering a useful option for patients who may not wish to self-inject daily. Oral sumatriptan is not effective for prevention or for acute treatment of cluster headache.

PREVENTIVE TREATMENTS (Table 15-9) The choice of a preventive treatment in cluster headache depends in part on the length of the bout. Patients with long bouts or those with chronic cluster headache require medicines that are safe when taken for long periods. For patients with relatively short bouts, limited courses of oral glucocorticoids or methysergide (not available in the United States) can be very useful. A 10-day course of prednisone, beginning at 60 mg daily for 7 days and followed by a rapid taper, may interrupt the pain bout for many patients. When ergotamine (1–2 mg) is used, it is most effective when given 1–2 h before an expected attack. Patients who use ergotamine daily must be educated regarding the early symptoms of ergotism, which may include vomiting, numbness, tingling, pain, and cyanosis of the limbs; a weekly limit of 14 mg should be adhered to. Lithi-

um (600–900 mg qd) appears to be particularly useful for the chronic form of the disorder.

Many experts favor verapamil as the first-line preventive treatment for patients with chronic cluster headache or prolonged bouts. While verapamil compares favorably with lithium in practice, some patients require verapamil doses far in excess of those administered for cardiac disorders. The initial dose range is 40–80 mg twice daily; effective doses may be as high as 960 mg/d. Side effects such as constipation and leg swelling can be problematic. Of paramount concern, however, is the cardiovascular safety of verapamil, particularly at high doses. Verapamil can cause heart block by slowing conduction in the atrioventricular node, a condition that can be monitored by following the PR interval on a standard EKG. Approximately 20% of patients treated with verapamil develop EKG abnormalities, which can be observed with doses as low as 240 mg/d; these abnormalities can worsen over time in patients on stable doses. A baseline EKG is recommended for all patients. The EKG is repeated 10 days after a dose change in those patients whose dose is being increased above 240 mg daily. Dose increases are usually made in 80-mg increments. For patients on long-term verapamil, EKG monitoring every 6 months is advised.

NEUROSTIMULATION THERAPY When medical therapies fail in chronic cluster headache, neurostimulation therapy strategies can be employed. Deep-brain stimulation of the region of the posterior hypothalamic gray matter has proven successful in a substantial proportion of patients. Favorable results have also been reported with the less-invasive approach of occipital nerve stimulation.

Paroxysmal Hemicrania Paroxysmal hemicrania (PH) is characterized by frequent unilateral, severe, short-lasting episodes of headache. Like cluster headache, the pain tends to be retroorbital but may be experienced all over the head and is associated with autonomic phe-

---

TABLE 15-8 CLINICAL FEATURES OF THE TRIGEMINAL AUTONOMIC CEPHALALGIAS

	Cluster Headache	Paroxysmal Hemicrania	SUNCT
Gender	M>F	F=M	F~M
Pain			
Type	Stabbing, boring	Throbbing, boring, stabbing	Burning, stabbing, sharp
Severity	Excruciating	Excruciating	Severe to excruciating
Site	Orbit, temple	Orbit, temple	Periorbital
Attack frequency	1/alternate day–8/d	1–40/d (>5/d for more than half the time)	3–200/d
Duration of attack	15–180 min	2–30 min	5–240 s
Autonomic features	Yes	Yes	Yes (prominent conjunctival injection and lacrimation)[a]
Migrainous features[b]	Yes	Yes	Yes
Alcohol trigger	Yes	No	No
Cutaneous triggers	No	No	Yes
Indomethacin effect	—	Yes[c]	—
Abortive treatment	Sumatriptan injection or nasal spray Oxygen	No effective treatment	Lidocaine (IV)
Prophylactic treatment	Verapamil Methysergide Lithium	Indomethacin	Lamotrigine Topiramate Gabapentin

[a]If conjunctival injection and tearing not present, consider SUNA.
[b]Nausea, photophobia, or phonophobia; photophobia and phonophobia are typically unilateral on the side of the pain.
[c]Indicates complete response to indomethacin.
Note: SUNCT, short-lasting unilateral neuralgiform headache attacks with conjunctival injection and tearing.

TABLE 15-9	PREVENTIVE MANAGEMENT OF CLUSTER HEADACHE
Short-Term Prevention	**Long-Term Prevention**
Episodic Cluster Headache	**Episodic Cluster Headache & Prolonged Chronic Cluster Headache**
Prednisone 1 mg/kg up to 60 mg qd, tapering over 21 days Methysergide 3–12 mg/d Verapamil 160–960 mg/d Greater occipital nerve injection	Verapamil 160–960 mg/d Lithium 400–800 mg/d Methysergide 3–12 mg/d Topiramate[a] 100–400 mg/d Gabapentin[a] 1200–3600 mg/d Melatonin[a] 9–12 mg/d

[a]Unproven but of potential benefit.

nomena such as lacrimation and nasal congestion. Patients with re-missions are said to have episodic PH, while those with the nonremitting form are said to have chronic PH. The essential features of PH are: unilateral, very severe pain; short-lasting attacks (2–45 min); very frequent attacks (usually more than five a day); marked autonomic features ipsilateral to the pain; rapid course (<72 h); and excellent response to indomethacin. In contrast to cluster headache, which predominantly affects males, the male:female ratio in PH is close to 1:1.

Indomethacin (25–75 mg tid), which can completely suppress attacks of PH, is the treatment of choice. Although therapy may be complicated by indomethacin-induced gastrointestinal side effects, currently there are no consistently effective alternatives. Topiramate is helpful in some cases. Piroxicam has been used, although it is not as effective as indomethacin. Verapamil, an effective treatment for cluster headache, does not appear to be useful for PH. In occasional patients, PH can coexist with trigeminal neuralgia (PH-tic syndrome); similar to cluster-tic syndrome, each component may require separate treatment.

Secondary PH has been reported with lesions in the region of the sella turcica, including arteriovenous malformation, cavernous sinus meningioma, and epidermoid tumors. Secondary PH is more likely if the patient requires high doses (>200 mg/d) of indomethacin. In patients with apparent bilateral PH, raised CSF pressure should be suspected. It is important to note that indomethacin reduces CSF pressure. When a diagnosis of PH is considered, MRI is indicated to exclude a pituitary lesion.

SUNCT/SUNA SUNCT is a rare primary headache syndrome characterized by severe, unilateral orbital or temporal pain that is stabbing or throbbing in quality. Diagnosis requires at least 20 attacks, lasting for 5–240 s; ipsilateral conjunctival injection and lacrimation should be present. In some patients conjunctival injection or lacrimation are missing, and the diagnosis of SUNA (short-lasting *u*nilateral *n*euralgiform headache attacks with cranial *a*utonomic symptoms) has been suggested.

DIAGNOSIS The pain of SUNCT/SUNA is unilateral and may be located anywhere in the head. Three basic patterns can be seen: single stabs, which are usually short-lived; groups of stabs; or a longer attack comprising many stabs between which the pain does not completely resolve, thus giving a "saw-tooth" phenomenon with attacks lasting many minutes. Each pattern may be seen in the context of an underlying continuous head pain. Characteristics that lead to a suspected diagnosis of SUNCT are the cutaneous (or other) triggerability of attacks, a lack of refractory period to triggering between attacks, and the lack of a response to indomethacin. Apart from trigeminal sensory disturbance, the neurologic examination is normal in primary SUNCT.

The diagnosis of SUNCT is often confused with trigeminal neuralgia (TN) particularly in first-division TN (Chap. 371). Minimal or no cranial autonomic symptoms and a clear refractory period to triggering indicate a diagnosis of TN.

SECONDARY (SYMPTOMATIC) SUNCT SUNCT can be seen with posterior fossa or pituitary lesions. All patients with SUNCT/SUNA should be evaluated with pituitary function tests and a brain MRI with pituitary views.

TABLE 15-10	CLASSIFICATION OF CHRONIC DAILY HEADACHE		
	Primary		
	>4 h Daily	**<4 h Daily**	**Secondary**
	Chronic migraine[a]	Chronic cluster headache[b]	Posttraumatic Head injury Iatrogenic Postinfectious
	Chronic tension-type headache[a]	Chronic paroxysmal hemicrania	Inflammatory, such as Giant cell arteritis Sarcoidosis Behçet's syndrome
	Hemicrania continua[a] New daily persistent headache[a]	SUNCT/SUNA Hypnic headache	Chronic CNS infection Medication-overuse headache[a]

[a]May be complicated by analgesic overuse.
[b]Some patients may have headache > 4 h per day.
Note: SUNCT, short-lasting *u*nilateral *n*euralgiform headache attacks with conjunctival injection and tearing; SUNA, short-lasting *u*nilateral *n*euralgiform headache attacks with cranial *a*utonomic symptoms.

℞ SUNCT/SUNA

ABORTIVE THERAPY Therapy of acute attacks is not a useful concept in SUNCT/SUNA since the attacks are of such short duration. However, intravenous lidocaine, which arrests the symptoms, can be used in hospitalized patients.

PREVENTIVE THERAPY Long-term prevention to minimize disability and hospitalization is the goal of treatment. The most effective treatment for prevention is lamotrigine, 200–400 mg/d. Topiramate and gabapentin may also be effective. Carbamazepine, 400–500 mg/d, has been reported by patients to offer modest benefit.

Surgical approaches such as microvascular decompression or destructive trigeminal procedures are seldom useful and often produce long-term complications. Greater occipital nerve injection has produced limited benefit in some patients. Mixed success with occipital nerve stimulation has been observed. Complete control with deep-brain stimulation of the posterior hypothalamic region was reported in a single patient. For intractable cases, short-term prevention with intravenous lidocaine can be effective.

CHRONIC DAILY HEADACHE

The broad diagnosis of chronic daily headache (CDH) can be applied when a patient experiences headache on 15 days or more per month. CDH is not a single entity; it encompasses a number of different headache syndromes, including chronic TTH as well as headache secondary to trauma, inflammation, infection, medication overuse, and other causes (Table 15-10). Population-based estimates suggest that about 4% of adults have daily or near-daily headache. Daily headache may be primary or secondary, an important consideration in guiding management of this complaint.

APPROACH TO THE PATIENT:
Chronic Daily Headache

The first step in the management of patients with CDH is to diagnose any underlying condition (Table 15-10). For patients with primary headaches, diagnosis of the headache type will guide therapy. Preventive treatments such as tricyclics, either amitriptyline or doxepin at doses up to 1 mg/kg, are very useful in patients with CDH. Tricyclics are started in low doses (10–25 mg) daily and may be given 12 h before the expected time of awakening in order to avoid excess morning sleepiness. Anticonvulsants, such as topiramate, valproate, and gabapentin, are also useful in migraineurs. Flunarizine can also be very effective for some patients, as can methysergide or phenelzine.

MANAGEMENT OF MEDICALLY INTRACTABLE DISABLING CHRONIC DAILY HEADACHE The management of medically intractable headache is difficult. At this time, the only promising approach is occipital nerve stimulation, which appears to modulate thalamic processing in migraine and has shown promise in both chronic cluster headache and hemicrania continua (see below). Clinical trials using botulinum toxin in chronic migraine have failed to show any objective benefit.

MEDICATION-OVERUSE HEADACHE Overuse of analgesic medication for headache can aggravate headache frequency and induce a state of refractory daily or near-daily headache called *medication-overuse headache*. A proportion of patients who stop taking analgesics will experience substantial improvement in the severity and frequency of their headache. However, even after cessation of analgesic use, many patients continue to have headache, although they may feel clinically improved in some way, especially if they have been using codeine or barbiturates regularly. The residual symptoms probably represent the underlying headache disorder.

Management of Medication Overuse: Outpatients For patients who overuse medications, it is essential that analgesic use be reduced and eliminated. One approach is to reduce the medication dose by 10% every 1–2 weeks. Immediate cessation of analgesic use is possible for some patients, provided there is no contraindication. Both approaches are facilitated by the use of a medication diary maintained during the month or two before cessation; this helps to identify the scope of the problem. A small dose of an NSAID such as naproxen, 500 mg bid if tolerated, will help relieve residual pain as analgesic use is reduced. NSAID overuse is not usually a problem for patients with daily headache when the dose is taken once or twice daily; however, overuse problems may develop with more frequent dosing schedules. Once the patient has substantially reduced analgesic use, a preventive medication should be introduced. It must be emphasized that *preventives generally do not work in the presence of analgesic overuse*. The most common cause of unresponsiveness to treatment is the use of a preventive when analgesics continue to be used regularly. For some patients, discontinuing analgesics is very difficult; often the best approach is to directly inform the patient that some degree of pain is inevitable during this initial period.

Management of Medication Overuse: Inpatients Some patients will require hospitalization for detoxification. Such patients have typically failed efforts at outpatient withdrawal or have a significant medical condition, such as diabetes mellitus, which would complicate withdrawal as an outpatient. Following admission to the hospital, acute medications are withdrawn completely on the first day, in the absence of a contraindication. Antiemetics and fluids are administered as required; clonidine is used for opiate withdrawal symptoms. For acute intolerable pain during the waking hours aspirin, 1 g (not approved in United States) intravenously, is useful. Intramuscular chlorpromazine can be helpful at night; patients must be adequately hydrated. If the patient does not improve within 3–5 days, a course of intravenous dihydroergotamine (DHE) can be employed. DHE, administered every 8 h for 3 consecutive days, can induce a significant remission that allows a preventive treatment to be established. 5-HT$_3$ antagonists, such as ondansetron or granisetron, are often required with DHE to prevent significant nausea.

NEW DAILY PERSISTENT HEADACHE New daily persistent headache (NDPH) is a clinically distinct syndrome; its causes are listed in Table 15-11.

TABLE 15-11 DIFFERENTIAL DIAGNOSIS OF NEW DAILY PERSISTENT HEADACHE

Primary	Secondary
Migrainous-type	Subarachnoid hemorrhage
Featureless (tension-type)	Low CSF volume headache
	Raised CSF pressure headache
	Posttraumatic headache[a]
	Chronic meningitis

[a]Includes postinfectious forms.

Clinical Presentation The patient with NDPH presents with headache on most if not all days; the onset is recent and clearly recalled by the patient. The headache usually begins abruptly, but onset may be more gradual; evolution over 3 days has been proposed as the upper limit for this syndrome. Patients typically recall the exact day and circumstances of the onset of headache; the new, persistent head pain does not remit. The first priority is to distinguish between a primary and a secondary cause of this syndrome. Subarachnoid hemorrhage is the most serious of the secondary causes and must be excluded either by history or appropriate investigation (Chap. 269).

Secondary NDPH *Low CSF Volume Headache* In these syndromes, head pain is positional: it begins when the patient sits or stands upright and resolves upon reclining. The pain, which is occipitofrontal, is usually a dull ache but may be throbbing. Patients with chronic low CSF volume headache typically present with a history of headache from one day to the next that is generally not present on waking but worsens during the day. Recumbency usually improves the headache within minutes, but it takes only minutes to an hour for the pain to return when the patient resumes an upright position.

The most common cause of headache due to persistent low CSF volume is CSF leak following lumbar puncture (LP). Post-LP headache usually begins within 48 h but may be delayed for up to 12 days. Its incidence is between 10 and 30%. Beverages with caffeine may provide temporary relief. Besides LP, index events may include epidural injection or a vigorous Valsalva maneuver, such as from lifting, straining, coughing, clearing the eustachian tubes in an airplane, or multiple orgasms. Spontaneous CSF leaks are well recognized, and the diagnosis should be considered whenever the headache history is typical, even when there is no obvious index event. As time passes from the index event, the postural nature may become less apparent; cases in which the index event occurred several years before the eventual diagnosis have been recognized. Symptoms appear to result from low volume rather than low pressure: although low CSF pressures, typically 0–50 mmH$_2$O, are usually identified, a pressure as high as 140 mmH$_2$O has been noted with a documented leak. Postural orthostatic tachycardia syndrome [POTS (Chap. 370)] can present with orthostatic headache similar to low CSF volume headache and is a diagnosis that needs consideration here.

When imaging is indicated to identify the source of a presumed leak, an MRI with gadolinium is the initial study of choice (Fig. 15-5). A striking pattern of diffuse meningeal enhancement is so typical that in the appropriate clinical context the diagnosis is established. Chiari malformations may sometimes be noted on MRI; in such cases surgery to decompress the posterior fossa usually worsens the headache. The source of CSF leakage may be identified by spinal MRI, by CT myelogram, or with ^{111}In-DTPA CSF studies; in the absence of a directly identified site of leakage, early emptying of ^{111}In-DTPA tracer into the bladder or slow progress of tracer across the brain suggests a CSF leak.

Initial treatment for low CSF volume headache is bed rest. For patients with persistent pain, intravenous caffeine (500 mg in 500 mL saline administered over 2 h) is often very effective. An EKG to screen for arrhythmia should be performed before administration. It is reasonable to administer at least two infusions of caffeine before embarking on additional tests to identify the source of the CSF leak. Since intravenous caffeine is safe and can be curative, it spares many patients the need for further investigations. If unsuccessful, an abdominal binder may be helpful. If a leak can be identified, an autologous blood patch is usually curative. A blood patch is also effective for post-LP headache; in this setting the location is empirically determined to be the site of the LP. In patients with intractable pain, oral theophylline is a useful alternative; however, its effect is less rapid than caffeine.

Raised CSF Pressure Headache Raised CSF pressure is well recognized as a cause of headache. Brain imaging can often reveal the

FIGURE 15-5 Magnetic resonance image showing diffuse meningeal enhancement after gadolinium administration in a patient with low CSF volume headache.

cause, such as a space-occupying lesion. NDPH due to raised CSF pressure can be the presenting symptom for patients with idiopathic intracranial hypertension (pseudotumor cerebri) without visual problems, particularly when the fundi are normal. Persistently raised intracranial pressure can trigger chronic migraine. These patients typically present with a history of generalized headache that is present on waking and improves as the day goes on. It is generally worse with recumbency. Visual obscurations are frequent. The diagnosis is relatively straightforward when papilledema is present, but the possibility must be considered even in patients without fundoscopic changes. Formal visual-field testing should be performed even in the absence of overt ophthalmic involvement. Headache on rising in the morning or nocturnal headache is also characteristic of obstructive sleep apnea or poorly controlled hypertension.

Evaluation of patients suspected to have raised CSF pressure requires brain imaging. It is most efficient to obtain an MRI, including an MR venogram as the initial study. If there are no contraindications, the CSF pressure should be measured by LP; this should be done when the patient is symptomatic so that both the pressure and the response to removal of 20–30 mL of CSF can be determined. An elevated opening pressure and improvement in headache following removal of CSF is diagnostic.

Initial treatment is with acetazolamide (250–500 mg bid); the headache may improve within weeks. If ineffective, topiramate is the next treatment of choice; it has many actions that may be useful in this setting, including carbonic anhydrase inhibition, weight loss, and neuronal membrane stabilization, likely mediated via effects on phosphorylation pathways. Severely disabled patients who do not respond to medical treatment require intracranial pressure monitoring and may require shunting.

Post-Traumatic Headache A traumatic event can trigger a headache process that lasts for many months or years after the event. The term *trauma* is used in a very broad sense: headache can develop following an injury to the head, but it can also develop after an infectious episode, typically viral meningitis, a flulike illness, or a parasitic infection. Complaints of dizziness, vertigo, and impaired memory can accompany the headache. Symptoms may remit after several weeks or persist for months and even years after the injury. Typically the neurologic examination is normal and CT or MRI studies are unrevealing. Chronic subdural hematoma may on occasion mimic this disorder. In one series, one-third of patients with NDPH reported headache beginning after a transient flulike illness characterized

by fever, neck stiffness, photophobia, and marked malaise. Evaluation reveals no apparent cause for the headache. There is no convincing evidence that persistent Epstein-Barr infection plays a role in this syndrome. A complicating factor is that many patients undergo LP during the acute illness; iatrogenic low CSF volume headache must be considered in these cases. Post-traumatic headache may also be seen after carotid dissection and subarachnoid hemorrhage, and following intracranial surgery. The underlying theme appears to be that a traumatic event involving the pain-producing meninges can trigger a headache process that lasts for many years.

Treatment is largely empirical. Tricyclic antidepressants, notably amitriptyline, and anticonvulsants such as topiramate, valproate, and gabapentin, have been used with reported benefit. The MAOI phenelzine may also be useful in carefully selected patients. The headache usually resolves within 3–5 years, but it can be quite disabling.

Primary NDPH Primary NDPH occurs in both males and females. It can be of the migrainous type, with features of migraine, or it can be featureless, appearing as new-onset TTH (Table 15-11). Migrainous features are common and include unilateral headache and throbbing pain; each feature is present in about one-third of patients. Nausea, photophobia, and/or phonophobia occur in about half of patients. Some patients have a previous history of migraine; however, the proportion of NDPH sufferers with preexisting migraine is no greater than the frequency of migraine in the general population. At 24 months, ~86% of patients are headache-free. Treatment of migrainous-type primary NDPH consists of using the preventive therapies effective in migraine (Table 15-7). Featureless NDPH is one of the primary headache forms most refractory to treatment. Standard preventive therapies can be offered but are often ineffective.

OTHER PRIMARY HEADACHES

Hemicrania Continua The essential features of hemicrania continua are moderate and continuous unilateral pain associated with fluctuations of severe pain; complete resolution of pain with indomethacin; and exacerbations that may be associated with autonomic features, including conjunctival injection, lacrimation, and photophobia on the affected side. The age of onset ranges from 11 to 58 years; women are affected twice as often as men. The cause is unknown.

℞ HEMICRANIA CONTINUA

Treatment consists of indomethacin; other NSAIDs appear to be of little or no benefit. The intramuscular injection of 100 mg indomethacin has been proposed as a diagnostic tool; administration with a placebo injection has been recommended. Alternatively, a trial of oral indomethacin, starting with 25 mg tid, then 50 mg tid, and then 75 mg tid, can be given. Up to 2 weeks may be necessary to assess whether a dose has a useful effect. Topiramate can be helpful in some patients. Occipital nerve stimulation may have a role in patients with hemicrania continua who are unable to tolerate indomethacin.

Primary Stabbing Headache The essential features of primary stabbing headache are stabbing pain confined to the head or, rarely, the face, lasting from 1 to many seconds or minutes and occurring as a single stab or a series of stabs; absence of associated cranial autonomic features; absence of cutaneous triggering of attacks; and a pattern of recurrence at irregular intervals (hours to days). The pains have been variously described as "ice-pick pains" or "jabs and jolts." They are more common in patients with other primary headaches, such as migraine, the TACs, and hemicrania continua.

℞ PRIMARY STABBING HEADACHE

The response of primary stabbing headache to indomethacin (25–50 mg two to three times daily) is usually excellent. As a general rule the symptoms wax and wane, and after a period of control on indomethacin, it is appropriate to withdraw treatment and observe the outcome.

Primary Cough Headache Primary cough headache is a generalized headache that begins suddenly, lasts for several minutes, and is precipitated by coughing; it is preventable by avoiding coughing or other precipitating events, which can include sneezing, straining, laughing, or stooping. In all patients with this syndrome serious etiologies must be excluded before a diagnosis of "benign" primary cough headache can be established. A Chiari malformation or any lesion causing obstruction of CSF pathways or displacing cerebral structures can be the cause of the head pain. Other conditions that can present with cough or exertional headache as the initial symptom include cerebral aneurysm, carotid stenosis, and vertebrobasilar disease. Benign cough headache can resemble benign exertional headache (below), but patients with the former condition are typically older.

Rx PRIMARY COUGH HEADACHE

Indomethacin 25–50 mg two to three times daily is the treatment of choice. Some patients with cough headache obtain pain relief with LP; this is a simple option when compared to prolonged use of indomethacin, and it is effective in about one-third of patients. The mechanism of this response is unclear.

Primary Exertional Headache Primary exertional headache has features resembling both cough headache and migraine. It may be precipitated by any form of exercise; it often has the pulsatile quality of migraine. The pain, which can last from 5 min to 24 h, is bilateral and throbbing at onset; migrainous features may develop in patients susceptible to migraine. Primary exertional headache can be prevented by avoiding excessive exertion, particularly in hot weather or at high altitude.

The mechanism of primary exertional headache is unclear. Acute venous distension likely explains one syndrome, the acute onset of headache with straining and breath holding, as in weightlifter's headache. As exertion can result in headache in a number of serious underlying conditions, these must be considered in patients with exertional headache. Pain from angina may be referred to the head, probably by central connections of vagal afferents, and may present as exertional headache (cardiac cephalgia). The link to exercise is the main clinical clue that headache is of cardiac origin. Pheochromocytoma may occasionally cause exertional headache. Intracranial lesions and stenosis of the carotid arteries are other possible etiologies.

Rx PRIMARY EXERTIONAL HEADACHE

Exercise regimens should begin modestly and progress gradually to higher levels of intensity. Indomethacin at daily doses from 25 to 150 mg is generally effective in benign exertional headache. Indomethacin (50 mg), ergotamine (1 mg orally), dihydroergotamine (2 mg by nasal spray), or methysergide (1–2 mg orally given 30–45 min before exercise) are useful prophylactic measures.

Primary Sex Headache Sex headache is precipitated by sexual excitement. The pain usually begins as a dull bilateral headache which suddenly becomes intense at orgasm. The headache can be prevented or eased by ceasing sexual activity before orgasm. Three types of sex headache are reported: a dull ache in the head and neck that intensifies as sexual excitement increases; a sudden, severe, explosive headache occurring at orgasm; and a postural headache developing after coitus that resembles the headache of low CSF pressure. The latter arises from vigorous sexual activity and is a form of low CSF pressure headache. Headaches developing at the time of orgasm are not always benign; 5–12% of cases of subarachnoid hemorrhage are precipitated by sexual intercourse. Sex headache is reported by men more often than women and may occur at any time during the years of sexual activity.

It may develop on several occasions in succession and then not trouble the patient again, even without an obvious change in sexual activity. In patients who stop sexual activity when headache is first noticed, the pain may subside within a period of 5 min to 2 h. In about half of patients, sex headache will subside within 6 months. About half of patients with sex headache have a history of exertional headaches, but there is no excess of cough headache. Migraine is probably more common in patients with sex headache.

Rx PRIMARY SEX HEADACHE

Benign sex headaches recur irregularly and infrequently. Management can often be limited to reassurance and advice about ceasing sexual activity if a mild, warning headache develops. Propranolol can be used to prevent headache that recurs regularly or frequently, but the dosage required varies from 40 to 200 mg/d. An alternative is the calcium channel-blocking agent diltiazem, 60 mg tid. Ergotamine (1 mg) or indomethacin (25–50 mg) taken about 30–45 min prior to sexual activity can also be helpful.

Primary Thunderclap Headache Sudden onset of severe headache may occur in the absence of any known provocation. The differential diagnosis includes the sentinel bleed of an intracranial aneurysm, cervicocephalic arterial dissection, and cerebral venous thrombosis. Headaches of explosive onset may also be caused by the ingestion of sympathomimetic drugs or of tyramine-containing foods in a patient who is taking MAOIs, or they may be a symptom of pheochromocytoma. Whether thunderclap headache can be the presentation of an unruptured cerebral aneurysm is uncertain. When neuroimaging studies and LP exclude subarachnoid hemorrhage, patients with thunderclap headache usually do very well over the long term. In one study of patients whose CT scans and CSF findings were negative, ~15% had recurrent episodes of thunderclap headache, and nearly half subsequently developed migraine or tension-type headache.

The first presentation of any sudden-onset severe headache should be vigorously investigated with neuroimaging (CT or, when possible, MRI with MR angiography) and CSF examination. Formal cerebral angiography should be reserved for those cases in which no primary diagnosis is forthcoming and for clinical situations that are particularly suggestive of intracranial aneurysm. Reversible segmental cerebral vasoconstriction may be seen in primary thunderclap headache without an intracranial aneurysm. In the presence of posterior leukoencephalopathy, the differential diagnosis includes cerebral angiitis, drug toxicity (cyclosporine, intrathecal methotrexate/cytarabine, pseudoephedrine, or cocaine), posttransfusion effects, and postpartum angiopathy. Treatment with nimodipine may be helpful, although by definition the vasoconstriction of primary thunderclap headache resolves spontaneously.

Hypnic Headache This headache syndrome typically begins a few hours after sleep onset. The headaches last from 15 to 30 min and are typically moderately severe and generalized, although they may be unilateral and can be throbbing. Patients may report falling back to sleep only to be awakened by a further attack a few hours later; up to three repetitions of this pattern occur through the night. Daytime naps can also precipitate head pain. Most patients are female, and the onset is usually after age 60. Headaches are bilateral in most, but may be unilateral. Photophobia or phonophobia and nausea are usually absent. The major secondary consideration in this headache type is poorly controlled hypertension; 24-h blood pressure monitoring is recommended to detect this treatable condition.

Rx HYPNIC HEADACHE

Patients with hypnic headache generally respond to a bedtime dose of lithium carbonate (200–600 mg). For those intolerant of lithium, verapamil (160 mg) or methysergide (1–4 mg at bedtime) may be alternative strategies. One to two cups of coffee or caffeine, 60 mg orally, at bedtime may be effective in approximately one-third of patients. Case reports suggest that flunarizine, 5 mg nightly, can be effective.

FURTHER READINGS

COHEN AS et al: Trigeminal autonomic cephalalgias: Current and future treatments. Headache 47:969, 2007

GOADSBY PJ: Is medication-overuse headache a distinct biological entity? Nat Clin Pract Neurol 2:401, 2006

HEADACHE CLASSIFICATION COMMITTEE OF THE INTERNATIONAL HEADACHE SOCIETY: The international classification of headache disorders (second edition). Cephalalgia 24:1, 2004

LANCE JW, GOADSBY PJ: *Mechanism and Management of Headache.* New York, Elsevier, 2005

LEVY M et al: The clinical characteristics of headache in patients with pituitary tumours. Brain 128:1921, 2005

OLESEN J et al: *The Headaches.* Philadelphia, Lippincott, Williams & Wilkins, 2005

16 Back and Neck Pain
John W. Engstrom

The importance of back and neck pain in our society is underscored by the following: (1) the cost of back pain in the United States is ~$100 billion annually, including direct health care expenses plus costs due to loss of productivity; (2) back symptoms are the most common cause of disability in those <45 years; (3) low back pain is the second most common reason for visiting a physician in the United States; and (4) ~1% of the U.S. population is chronically disabled because of back pain.

ANATOMY OF THE SPINE

The anterior portion of the spine consists of cylindrical vertebral bodies separated by intervertebral disks and held together by the anterior and posterior longitudinal ligaments. The intervertebral disks are composed of a central gelatinous nucleus pulposus surrounded by a tough cartilaginous ring, the annulus fibrosis; disks are responsible for 25% of spinal column length (Figs. 16-1 and 16-2). The disks are largest in the cervical and lumbar regions where movements of the spine are greatest. The disks are elastic in youth and allow the bony vertebrae to move easily upon each other. Elasticity is lost with age. The function of the anterior spine is to absorb the shock of body movements such as walking and running.

The posterior portion of the spine consists of the vertebral arches and seven processes. Each arch consists of paired cylindrical pedicles anteriorly and paired laminae posteriorly. The vertebral arch gives rise to two transverse processes laterally, one spinous process posteriorly, plus two superior and two inferior articular facets. The apposition of a superior and inferior facet constitutes a *facet joint.* The functions of the posterior spine are to protect the spinal cord and nerves within the spinal canal and to stabilize the spine by providing sites for the attachment of muscles and ligaments. The contraction of muscles attached to the spinous and transverse processes produces a system of pulleys and levers that results in flexion, extension, and lateral bending movements of the spine.

Nerve root injury (*radiculopathy*) is a common cause of neck, arm, low back, and leg pain (Figs. 25-2 and 25-3). The nerve roots exit at a level above their respective vertebral bodies in the cervical region (the C7 nerve root exits at the C6-C7 level) and below their respective vertebral bodies in the thoracic and lumbar regions (the T1 nerve root exits at the T1-T2 level). The cervical nerve roots follow a short intraspinal course before exiting. By contrast, because the spinal cord ends at the vertebral L1 or L2 level, the lumbar nerve roots follow a long intraspinal course and can be injured anywhere from the upper lumbar spine to their exit at the intervertebral foramen. For example, disk herniation at the L4-L5 level commonly produces compression of the traversing S1 nerve root (Fig. 16-3).

Pain-sensitive structures in the spine include the periosteum of the vertebrae, dura, facet joints, annulus fibrosus of the intervertebral disk, epidural veins, and the posterior longitudinal ligament. Disease of these diverse structures may explain many cases of back pain without nerve root compression. The nucleus pulposus of the intervertebral disk is not pain-sensitive under normal circumstances. Pain sensation is conveyed partially by the sinuvertebral nerve that arises from the spinal nerve at each spine segment and reenters the spinal canal through the intervertebral foramen at the same level. The lumbar and cervical spine possess the greatest potential for movement and injury.

APPROACH TO THE PATIENT:
Back Pain

TYPES OF BACK PAIN   Understanding the type of pain experienced by the patient is the essential first step. Attention is also focused on identification of risk factors for serious underlying diseases; the majority of these are due to radiculopathy, fracture, tumor, infection, or referred pain from visceral structures (Table 16-1).

Local pain is caused by stretching of pain-sensitive structures that compress or irritate sensory nerve endings. The site of the pain is near the affected part of the back.

Pain referred to the back may arise from abdominal or pelvic viscera. The pain is usually described as primarily abdominal or pelvic but is accompanied by back pain and usually unaffected by posture. The patient may occasionally complain of back pain only.

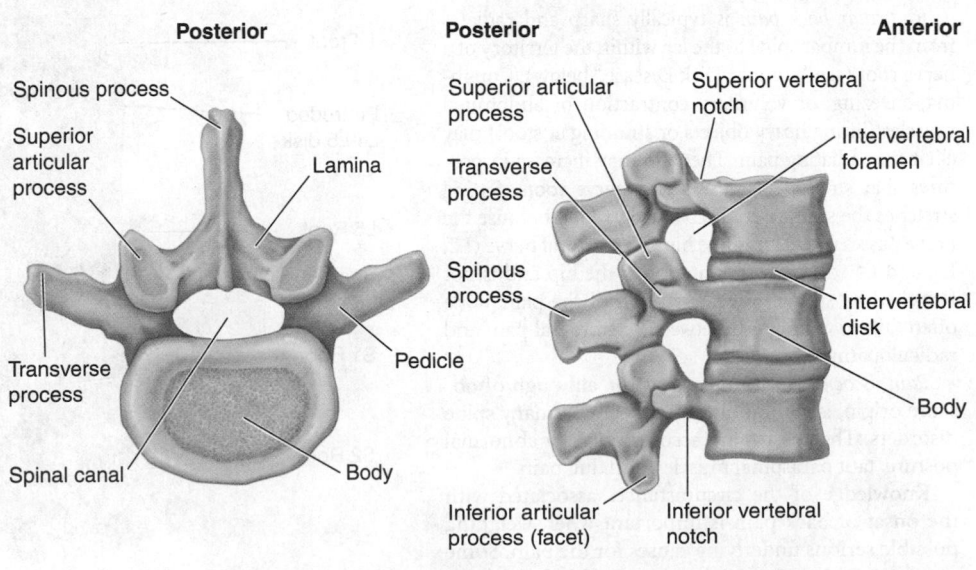

FIGURE 16-1 Vertebral anatomy. (*From A Gauthier Cornuelle, DH Gronefeld: Radiographic Anatomy Positioning. New York, McGraw-Hill, 1998; with permission.*)

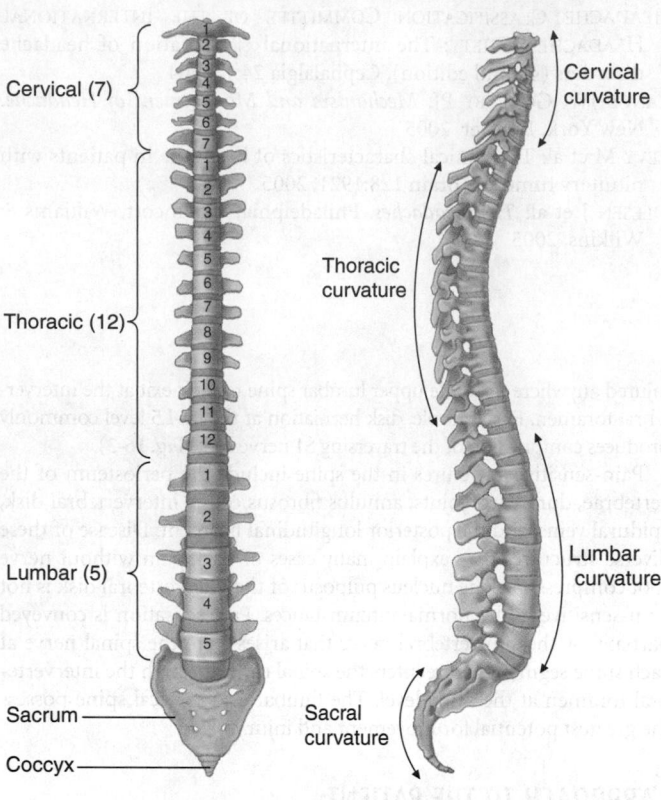

FIGURE 16-2 Spinal column. (*From: A Gauthier Cornuelle, DH Gronefeld: Radiographic Anatomy Positioning. New York, McGraw-Hill, 1998; with permission.*)

Pain of spine origin may be located in the back or referred to the buttocks or legs. Diseases affecting the upper lumbar spine tend to refer pain to the lumbar region, groin, or anterior thighs. Diseases affecting the lower lumbar spine tend to produce pain referred to the buttocks, posterior thighs, or rarely the calves or feet. Provocative injections into pain-sensitive structures of the lumbar spine may produce leg pain that does not follow a dermatomal distribution. This "sclerotomal" pain may explain some cases of back and leg pain without evidence of nerve root compression.

Radicular back pain is typically sharp and radiates from the lumbar spine to the leg within the territory of a nerve root (see "Lumbar Disk Disease," below). Coughing, sneezing, or voluntary contraction of abdominal muscles (lifting heavy objects or straining at stool) may elicit the radiating pain. The pain may increase in postures that stretch the nerves and nerve roots. Sitting stretches the sciatic nerve (L5 and S1 roots) because the nerve passes posterior to the hip. The femoral nerve (L2, L3, and L4 roots) passes anterior to the hip and is not stretched by sitting. The description of the pain alone often fails to distinguish between sclerotomal pain and radiculopathy.

Pain associated with muscle spasm, although of obscure origin, is commonly associated with many spine disorders. The spasms are accompanied by abnormal posture, taut paraspinal muscles, and dull pain.

Knowledge of the circumstances associated with the onset of back pain is important when weighing possible serious underlying causes for the pain. Some patients involved in accidents or work-related injuries may exaggerate their pain for the purpose of compensation or for psychological reasons.

EXAMINATION OF THE BACK A physical examination that includes the abdomen and rectum is advisable. Back pain referred from visceral organs may be reproduced during palpation of the abdomen [pancreatitis, abdominal aortic aneurysm (AAA)] or percussion over the costovertebral angles (pyelonephritis).

The normal spine has cervical and lumbar lordosis, and a thoracic kyphosis. Exaggeration of these normal alignments may result in hyperkyphosis of the thoracic spine or hyperlordosis of the lumbar spine. Inspection may reveal a lateral curvature of the spine (scoliosis) or an asymmetry in the paraspinal muscles, suggesting muscle spasm. Back pain of bony spine origin is often reproduced by palpation or percussion over the spinous process of the affected vertebrae.

Forward bending is often limited by paraspinal muscle spasm; the latter may flatten the usual lumbar lordosis. Flexion of the hips is normal in patients with lumbar spine disease, but flexion of the lumbar spine is limited and sometimes painful. Lateral bending to the side opposite the injured spinal element may stretch the damaged tissues, worsen pain, and limit motion. Hyperextension of the spine (with the patient prone or standing) is limited when nerve root compression, facet joint pathology, or other bony spine disease is present.

Pain from hip disease may mimic pain of lumbar spine disease. Hip pain can be reproduced by internal and external rotation at the hip with the knee and hip in flexion (Patrick sign) and by tapping the heel with the examiner's palm while the leg is extended.

With the patient lying flat, passive flexion of the extended leg at the hip stretches the L5 and S1 nerve roots and the sciatic nerve. Passive dorsiflexion of the foot during the maneuver adds to the stretch. While flexion to at least 80° is normally possible without causing pain, tight hamstring muscles are a source of pain in some patients. The *straight leg–raising (SLR)* test is positive if the maneuver reproduces the patient's usual back or limb pain. Eliciting the SLR sign in the sitting position may help determine if the finding is reproducible. The patient may describe pain in the low back, buttocks, posterior thigh, or lower leg, but the key feature is reproduction of the patient's usual pain. The *crossed*

FIGURE 16-3 Compression of L5 and S1 roots by herniated disks. (*From: RD Adams et al: Principles of Neurology, 8th ed. New York, McGraw-Hill, 2005; with permission.*)

TABLE 16-1 ACUTE LOW BACK PAIN: RISK FACTORS FOR AN IMPORTANT STRUCTURAL CAUSE

History
  Pain worse at rest or at night
  Prior history of cancer
  History of chronic infection (esp. lung, urinary tract, skin)
  History of trauma
  Incontinence
  Age > 50 years
  Intravenous drug use
  Glucocorticoid use
  History of a rapidly progressive neurologic deficit

Examination
  Unexplained fever
  Unexplained weight loss
  Percussion tenderness over the spine
  Abdominal, rectal, or pelvic mass
  Patrick's sign or heel percussion sign
  Straight leg or reverse straight-leg raising signs
  Progressive focal neurologic deficit

SLR sign is positive when flexion of one leg reproduces the pain in the opposite leg or buttocks. The crossed SLR sign is less sensitive but more specific for disk herniation than the SLR sign. The nerve or nerve root lesion is always on the side of the pain. The *reverse SLR sign* is elicited by standing the patient next to the examination table and passively extending each leg with the knee fully extended. This maneuver, which stretches the L2-L4 nerve roots and the femoral nerve, is considered positive if the patient's usual back or limb pain is reproduced.

The neurologic examination includes a search for focal weakness or muscle atrophy, focal reflex changes, diminished sensation in the legs, and signs of spinal cord injury. The examiner should be alert to the possibility of breakaway weakness, defined as fluctuating strength during muscle testing. Breakaway weakness may be due to pain or a combination of pain and underlying true weakness. Breakaway weakness without pain is due to lack of effort. In uncertain cases, electromyography (EMG) can determine whether or not true weakness is present. Findings with specific nerve root lesions are shown in Table 16-2 and are discussed below.

LABORATORY, IMAGING, AND EMG STUDIES   Routine laboratory studies are rarely needed for the initial evaluation of nonspecific acute (<3 months duration) low back pain (ALBP). If risk factors for a serious underlying cause are present, then laboratory studies [complete blood count (CBC), erythrocyte sedimentation rate (ESR), urinalysis] are indicated.

CT scanning is superior to routine x-rays for the detection of fractures involving posterior spine structures, craniocervical and craniothoracic junctions, C1 and C2 vertebrae, bone fragments within the spinal canal, or malalignment; CT scans are increasingly used as a primary screening modality for moderate to severe trauma. In the absence of risk factors, these imaging studies are rarely helpful in nonspecific ALBP. MRI and CT-myelography are the radiologic tests of choice for evaluation of most serious diseases involving the spine. MRI is superior for the definition of soft tissue structures, whereas CT-myelography provides optimal imaging of the lateral recess of the spinal canal and bony lesions and is tolerated by claustrophobic patients. While the added diagnostic value of modern neuroimaging is significant, there is concern that these studies may be overutilized in patients with ALBP.

Electrodiagnostic studies can be used to assess the functional integrity of the peripheral nervous system (**Chap. e30**). Sensory nerve conduction studies are normal when focal sensory loss is due to nerve root damage because the nerve roots are proximal to the nerve cell bodies in the dorsal root ganglia. The diagnostic yield of needle EMG is higher than that of nerve conduction studies for radiculopathy. Denervation changes in a myotomal (segmental) distribution are detected by sampling multiple muscles supplied by different nerve roots and nerves; the pattern of muscle involvement indicates the nerve root(s) responsible for the injury. Needle EMG provides objective information about motor nerve fiber injury when the clinical evaluation of weakness is limited by pain or poor effort. EMG and nerve conduction studies will be normal when only limb pain or sensory nerve root injury or irritation is present.

CAUSES OF BACK PAIN   (Table 16-3)

CONGENITAL ANOMALIES OF THE LUMBAR SPINE

Spondylolysis is a bony defect in the pars interarticularis (a segment near the junction of the pedicle with the lamina) of the vertebra; the etiology may be a stress fracture in a congenitally abnormal segment. The defect (usually bilateral) is best visualized on oblique projections in plain x-rays, CT scan, or single photon emission CT (SPECT) bone scan and occurs in the setting of a single injury, repeated minor injuries, or growth. Although frequently asymptomatic, it is the most common cause of persistent low back pain in adolescents and is often activity-related.

Spondylolisthesis is the anterior slippage of the vertebral body, pedicles, and superior articular facets, leaving the posterior elements behind. Spondylolisthesis can be associated with spondylolysis, congenital anomalies of the lumbosacral junction, infection, osteoporosis, tumor, trauma, prior surgery, or degenerative spine disease. It occurs more frequently in women. The slippage may be asymptomatic or may cause low back pain and hamstring tightness, nerve root injury (the L5 root most frequently), or symptomatic spinal stenosis. Tenderness may be elicited near the segment that has "slipped" forward (most often L4 on L5 or occasionally L5 on S1). A "step" may be present on deep palpation of the posterior elements of the segment above the spondylolisthetic joint. The trunk may be shortened and the abdomen protu-

TABLE 16-2 LUMBOSACRAL RADICULOPATHY—NEUROLOGIC FEATURES

Lumbosacral Nerve Roots	Examination Findings			Pain Distribution
	Reflex	**Sensory**	**Motor**	
L2[a]	—	Upper anterior thigh	Psoas (hip flexion)	Anterior thigh
L3[a]	—	Lower anterior thigh Anterior knee	Psoas (hip flexion) Quadriceps (knee extension) Thigh adduction	Anterior thigh, knee
L4[a]	Quadriceps (knee)	Medial calf	Quadriceps (knee extension)[b] Thigh adduction Tibialis anterior (foot dorsiflexion)	Knee, medial calf Anterolateral thigh
L5[c]	—	Dorsal surface—foot Lateral calf	Peroneii (foot eversion)[b] Tibialis anterior (foot dorsiflexion) Gluteus medius (hip abduction) Toe dorsiflexors	Lateral calf, dorsal foot, posterolateral thigh, buttocks
S1[c]	Gastrocnemius/ soleus (ankle)	Plantar surface—foot Lateral aspect—foot	Gastrocnemius/soleus (foot plantar flexion)[b] Abductor hallucis (toe flexors)[b] Gluteus maximus (hip extension)	Bottom foot, posterior calf, posterior thigh, buttocks

[a]Reverse straight leg–raising sign present—see "Examination of the Back."
[b]These muscles receive the majority of innervation from this root.
[c]Straight leg–raising sign present—see "Examination of the Back."

TABLE 16-3   CAUSES OF BACK AND NECK PAIN

Congenital/developmental
  Spondylolysis and spondylolisthesis[a]
  Kyphoscoliosis[a]
  Spina bifida occulta[a]
  Tethered spinal cord[a]
Minor trauma
  Strain or sprain
  Whiplash injury[b]
Fractures
  Traumatic—falls, motor vehicle accidents
  Atraumatic—osteoporosis, neoplastic infiltration, exogenous steroids
Intervertebral disk herniation
Degenerative
  Disk-osteophyte complex
  Internal disk disruption
  Spinal stenosis with neurogenic claudication[a]
  Uncovertebral joint disease[b]
  Atlantoaxial joint disease (e.g., rheumatoid arthritis)[a]
Arthritis
  Spondylosis
  Facet or sacroiliac arthropathy
  Autoimmune (e.g., anklyosing spondylitis, Reiter's syndrome)
Neoplasms—metastatic, hematologic, primary bone tumors
Infection/inflammation
  Vertebral osteomyelitis
  Spinal epidural abscess
  Septic disk
  Meningitis
  Lumbar arachnoiditis[a]
Metabolic
  Osteoporosis—hyperparathyroidism, immobility
  Osteosclerosis (e.g., Paget's disease)
Vascular
  Abdominal aortic aneurysm
  Vertebral artery dissection[b]
Other
  Referred pain from visceral disease
  Postural
  Psychiatric, malingering, chronic pain syndromes

[a]Low back pain only.
[b]Neck pain only.

berant as a result of extreme forward displacement of L4 on L5; in severe cases cauda equina syndrome (CES) may occur (see below). Surgery is considered for symptoms persisting for >1 year that do not respond to conservative measures (e.g., rest, physical therapy). Surgery is usually indicated for cases with progressive neurologic deficit, abnormal gait or postural deformity, slippage > 50%, or scoliosis.

Spina bifida occulta is a failure of closure of one or several vertebral arches posteriorly; the meninges and spinal cord are normal. A dimple or small lipoma may overlie the defect. Most cases are asymptomatic and discovered incidentally during evaluation for back pain.

Tethered cord syndrome usually presents as a progressive cauda equina disorder (see below), although myelopathy may also be the initial manifestation. The patient is often a young adult who complains of perineal or perianal pain, sometimes following minor trauma. Neuroimaging studies reveal a low-lying conus (below L1-L2) and a short and thickened filum terminale.

TRAUMA

A patient complaining of back pain and inability to move the legs may have a spinal fracture or dislocation, and, with fractures above L1, spinal cord compression. Care must be taken to avoid further damage to the spinal cord or nerve roots by immobilizing the back pending results of x-rays.

Sprains and Strains   The terms *low back sprain*, *strain*, or *mechanically induced muscle spasm* refer to minor, self-limited injuries associated with lifting a heavy object, a fall, or a sudden deceleration such as in an automobile accident. These terms are used loosely and do not clearly describe a specific anatomic lesion. The pain is usually confined to the

lower back, and there is no radiation to the buttocks or legs. Patients with paraspinal muscle spasm often assume unusual postures.

Traumatic Vertebral Fractures   Most traumatic fractures of the lumbar vertebral bodies result from injuries producing anterior wedging or compression. With severe trauma, the patient may sustain a fracture-dislocation or a "burst" fracture involving the vertebral body and posterior elements. Traumatic vertebral fractures are caused by falls from a height (a pars interarticularis fracture of the L5 vertebra is common), sudden deceleration in an automobile accident, or direct injury. Neurologic impairment is common, and early surgical treatment is indicated. In victims of blunt trauma, CT scans of the chest, abdomen, or pelvis can be reformatted to detect associated vertebral fractures.

LUMBAR DISK DISEASE

This is a common cause of chronic or recurrent low back and leg pain (Figs. 16-3 and 16-4). Disk disease is most likely to occur at the L4-L5 and L5-S1 levels, but upper lumbar levels are involved occasionally. The cause is often unknown; the risk is increased in overweight individuals. Disk herniation is unusual prior to age 20 and is rare in the fibrotic disks of the elderly. Degeneration of the nucleus pulposus and the annulus fibrosus increases with age and may be asymptomatic or painful. Genetic factors may play a role in predisposing some patients to disk degeneration. The pain may be located in the low back only or referred to the leg, buttock, or hip. A sneeze, cough, or trivial movement may cause the nucleus pulposus to prolapse, pushing the frayed and weakened annulus posteriorly. With severe disk disease, the nucleus may protrude through the annulus (herniation) or become extruded to lie as a free fragment in the spinal canal.

The mechanism by which intervertebral disk injury causes back pain is controversial. The inner annulus fibrosus and nucleus pulposus are normally devoid of innervation. Inflammation and production of proinflammatory cytokines within the protruding or ruptured disk may trigger or perpetuate back pain. Ingrowth of nociceptive (pain) nerve fibers into inner portions of a diseased disk may be responsible for chronic "diskogenic" pain. Nerve root injury (radiculopathy) from disk herniation may be due to compression, inflammation, or both; pathologically, demyelination and axonal loss are usually present.

Symptoms of a ruptured disk include back pain, abnormal posture, limitation of spine motion (particularly flexion), or radicular pain. A dermatomal pattern of sensory loss or a reduced or absent deep ten-

FIGURE 16-4 MRI of lumbar herniated disk; left S1 radiculopathy. Sagittal T1-weighted image on the left with arrows outlining disk margins. Sagittal T2 image on the right reveals a protruding disk at the L5-S1 level (*arrows*), which displaces the central thecal sac.

don reflex is more suggestive of a specific root lesion than is the pattern of pain. Motor findings (focal weakness, muscle atrophy, or fasciculations) occur less frequently than focal sensory or reflex changes. Symptoms and signs are usually unilateral, but bilateral involvement does occur with large central disk herniations that compress multiple descending nerve roots within the spinal canal. Clinical manifestations of specific nerve root lesions are summarized in Table 16-2. There is suggestive evidence that lumbar disk herniation with a nonprogressive nerve root deficit can be managed nonsurgically. The size of the disk protrusion may naturally decrease over time.

The differential diagnosis covers a variety of serious and treatable conditions, including epidural abscess, hematoma, or tumor. Fever, constant pain uninfluenced by position, sphincter abnormalities, or signs of spinal cord disease suggest an etiology other than lumbar disk disease. Bilateral absence of ankle reflexes can be a normal finding in old age or a sign of bilateral S1 radiculopathy. An absent deep tendon reflex or focal sensory loss may indicate injury to a nerve root, but other sites of injury along the nerve must also be considered. For example, an absent knee reflex may be due to a femoral neuropathy or an L4 nerve root injury. A loss of sensation over the foot and lateral lower calf may result from a peroneal or lateral sciatic neuropathy or an L5 nerve root injury. Focal muscle atrophy may reflect a nerve root or peripheral nerve injury, an anterior horn cell disease, or disuse.

An MRI scan or CT-myelogram is necessary to establish the location and type of pathology. Spinal MRI yields exquisite views of intraspinal and adjacent soft tissue anatomy. Bony lesions of the lateral recess or intervertebral foramen are optimally visualized by CT-myelography. The correlation of neuroradiologic findings to symptoms, particularly pain, is not simple. Contrast-enhancing tears in the annulus fibrosus or disk protrusions are widely accepted as common sources of back pain; however, many studies have found that most asymptomatic adults have similar findings. Asymptomatic disk protrusions are also common and may enhance with contrast. Furthermore, in patients with known disk herniation treated either medically or surgically, persistence of the herniation 10 years later had no relationship to the clinical outcome. In summary, MRI findings of disk protrusion, tears in the annulus fibrosus, or contrast enhancement are common incidental findings that, by themselves, should not dictate management decisions for patients with back pain.

There are four indications for intervertebral disk surgery: (1) progressive motor weakness from nerve root injury demonstrated on clinical examination or EMG, (2) bowel or bladder disturbance or other signs of spinal cord compression, (3) incapacitating nerve root pain despite conservative treatment for 4 weeks at a minimum, and (4) recurrent incapacitating pain despite conservative treatment. The latter two criteria are more subjective and less well established than the others. Surgical treatment should also be considered if steady pain and/or neurologic findings do not substantially improve over 4–12 weeks.

The usual surgical procedure is a partial hemilaminectomy with excision of the prolapsed disk. Fusion of the involved lumbar segments should be considered only if significant spinal instability is present (i.e., degenerative spondylolisthesis or isthmic spondylolysis). Over a recent 5-year period, the number of lumbar fusion procedures performed in the United States more than doubled, for uncertain reasons. There are no large prospective, randomized trials comparing fusion to other types of surgical intervention. In one study, patients with persistent low back pain despite an initial diskectomy fared no better with spine fusion than with a conservative regimen of cognitive intervention and exercise.

Cauda equina syndrome (CES) signifies an injury of multiple lumbosacral nerve roots within the spinal canal. Low back pain, weakness and areflexia in the legs, saddle anesthesia, and loss of bladder function may occur. The problem must be distinguished from disorders of the lower spinal cord (conus medullaris syndrome), acute transverse myelitis (Chap. 372), and Guillain-Barré syndrome (Chap. 380). Combined involvement of the conus medullaris and cauda equina can occur. CES is commonly due to a ruptured lumbosacral intervertebral disk, lumbosacral spine fracture, hematoma within the spinal canal (e.g., following lumbar puncture in patients with coagulopathy), compressive tumor, or

other mass lesion. Treatment options include surgical decompression, sometimes urgently in an attempt to restore or preserve motor or sphincter function, or radiotherapy for metastatic tumors (Chap. 374).

DEGENERATIVE CONDITIONS

Lumbar spinal stenosis describes a narrowed lumbar spinal canal. *Neurogenic claudication* is the usual symptom, consisting of back and buttock or leg pain induced by walking or standing and relieved by sitting. Symptoms in the legs are usually bilateral. Lumbar stenosis, by itself, is frequently asymptomatic, and the correlation between the severity of symptoms and degree of stenosis of the spinal canal is poor. Unlike vascular claudication, symptoms are often provoked by standing without walking. Unlike lumbar disk disease, symptoms are usually relieved by sitting. Focal weakness, sensory loss, or reflex changes may occur when spinal stenosis is associated with radiculopathy. Severe neurologic deficits, including paralysis and urinary incontinence, occur rarely. Spinal stenosis can be acquired (75%), congenital, or due to a combination of these factors. Congenital forms (achondroplasia, idiopathic) are characterized by short, thick pedicles that produce both spinal canal and lateral recess stenosis. Acquired factors that contribute to spinal stenosis include degenerative diseases (spondylosis, spondylolisthesis, scoliosis), trauma, spine surgery, metabolic or endocrine disorders (epidural lipomatosis, osteoporosis, acromegaly, renal osteodystrophy, hypoparathyroidism), and Paget's disease. MRI provides the best definition of the abnormal anatomy (Fig. 16-5).

Conservative treatment of symptomatic spinal stenosis includes nonsteroidal anti-inflammatory drugs (NSAIDs), exercise programs, and symptomatic treatment of acute pain episodes. Surgical therapy is considered when medical therapy does not relieve symptoms sufficiently to allow for activities of daily living or when significant focal neurologic signs are present. Most patients with neurogenic claudication treated surgically experience at least 75% relief of back and leg pain. Up to 25% develop recurrent stenosis at the same spinal level or an adjacent level 5 years after the initial surgery; recurrent symptoms usually respond to a second surgical decompression.

Facet joint hypertrophy can produce unilateral radicular symptoms or signs due to bony compression; symptoms are often indistinguishable from disk-related radiculopathy. Stretch signs, focal motor weakness, hyporeflexia, or dermatomal sensory loss may be present. Hypertrophic superior or inferior facets can be visualized by x-rays, CT, or MRI. Surgical foraminotomy results in long-term relief of leg and back pain in 80–90% of these patients. The usefulness of therapeutic facet joint blocks for pain has not been rigorously studied.

ARTHRITIS

Spondylosis, or osteoarthritic spine disease, typically occurs in later life and primarily involves the cervical and lumbosacral spine. Patients of-

FIGURE 16-5 Spinal stenosis. Sagittal T2 fast spin echo magnetic resonance imaging of a normal (*left*) and stenotic (*right*) lumbar spine, revealing multifocal narrowing (*arrows*) of the cerebrospinal fluid spaces surrounding the nerve roots within the thecal sac.

ten complain of back pain that is increased with movement and associated with stiffness. The relationship between clinical symptoms and radiologic findings is usually not straightforward. Pain may be prominent when x-ray, CT, or MRI findings are minimal, and large osteophytes can be seen in asymptomatic patients. Radiculopathy occurs when hypertrophied facets and osteophytes compress nerve roots in the lateral recess or intervertebral foramen. Osteophytes arising from the vertebral body may cause or contribute to central spinal canal stenosis. Disc degeneration may also play a role in reducing the cross-sectional area of the intervertebral foramen; the descending pedicle may compress the exiting nerve root. Rarely, osteoarthritic changes in the lumbar spine are sufficient to compress the cauda equina.

Ankylosing Spondylitis (See also Chap. 318) This distinctive arthritic spine disease typically presents with the insidious onset of low back and buttock pain. Patients are often males below age 40. Associated features include morning back stiffness, nocturnal pain, pain unrelieved by rest, an elevated ESR, and the histocompatibility antigen HLA-B27. Onset at a young age and back pain improving with exercise are characteristic. Loss of the normal lumbar lordosis and exaggeration of thoracic kyphosis develop as the disease progresses. Inflammation and erosion of the outer fibers of the annulus fibrosus at the point of contact with the vertebral body are followed by ossification and bony growth that bridges adjacent vertebral bodies and reduces spine mobility in all planes. Radiologic hallmarks are periarticular destructive changes, sclerosis of the sacroiliac joints, and bridging of vertebral bodies to produce the fused "bamboo spine."

Stress fractures through the spontaneously ankylosed posterior bony elements of the rigid, osteoporotic spine may produce focal pain, spinal instability, spinal cord compression, or CES. Atlantoaxial subluxation with spinal cord compression occasionally occurs. Ankylosis of the ribs to the spine and a decrease in the height of the thoracic spine may compromise respiratory function. For many patients, therapy with anti-tumor necrosis factor agents is effective in reducing disease activity. Similar to ankylosing spondylitis, restricted movements may accompany Reiter's syndrome, psoriatic arthritis, and chronic inflammatory bowel disease.

NEOPLASMS
(See also Chap. 374) Back pain is the most common neurologic symptom in patients with systemic cancer and may be the presenting symptom. The cause is usually vertebral metastases. Metastatic carcinoma (breast, lung, prostate, thyroid, kidney, gastrointestinal tract), multiple myeloma, and non-Hodgkin's and Hodgkin's lymphomas frequently involve the spine. Cancer-related back pain tends to be constant, dull, unrelieved by rest, and worse at night. By contrast, mechanical low back pain usually improves with rest. Plain x-rays may or may not show destructive lesions in one or several vertebral bodies without disk space involvement. MRI, CT, and CT-myelography are the studies of choice when spinal metastasis is suspected. MRI is preferred, but the most rapidly available procedure is best because the patient's condition may worsen quickly. Fewer than 5% of patients who are nonambulatory at the time of diagnosis ever regain the ability to walk, thus early diagnosis is crucial.

INFECTIONS/INFLAMMATION
Vertebral osteomyelitis is usually caused by staphylococci, but other bacteria or tuberculosis (Pott's disease) may be responsible. The primary source of infection is usually the urinary tract, skin, or lungs. Intravenous drug use is a well-recognized risk factor. Whenever pyogenic osteomyelitis is found, the possibility of bacterial endocarditis should be considered. Back pain exacerbated by motion and unrelieved by rest, spine tenderness over the involved spine segment, and an elevated ESR are the most common findings in vertebral osteomyelitis. Fever or an elevated white blood cell count is found in a minority of patients. Plain radiographs may show a narrowed disk space with erosion of adjacent vertebrae; however, these diagnostic changes may take weeks or months to appear. MRI and CT are sensitive and specific for osteomyelitis; CT may be more readily available in emergency settings and better tolerated by some patients with severe back pain.

Spinal epidural abscess (Chap. 372) presents with back pain (aggravated by movement or palpation) and fever. Signs of nerve root injury or spinal cord compression may be present. The abscess may track over multiple spinal levels and is best delineated by spine MRI.

Lumbar adhesive arachnoiditis with radiculopathy is due to fibrosis following inflammation within the subarachnoid space. The fibrosis results in nerve root adhesions, and presents as back and leg pain associated with motor, sensory, or reflex changes. Causes of arachnoiditis include multiple lumbar operations, chronic spinal infections, spinal cord injury, intrathecal hemorrhage, myelography (rare), intrathecal injection of glucocorticoids or anesthetics, and foreign bodies. The MRI shows clumped nerve roots located centrally or adherent to the dura peripherally, or loculations of cerebrospinal fluid within the thecal sac. Clumped nerve roots may also occur with demyelinating polyneuropathy or neoplastic infiltration. Treatment is usually unsatisfactory. Microsurgical lysis of adhesions, dorsal rhizotomy, and dorsal root ganglionectomy have been tried, but outcomes have been poor. Dorsal column stimulation for pain relief has produced varying results. Epidural injections of glucocorticoids have been of limited value.

METABOLIC CAUSES
Osteoporosis and Osteosclerosis Immobilization or underlying conditions such as osteomalacia, hyperparathyroidism, hyperthyroidism, multiple myeloma, metastatic carcinoma, or glucocorticoid use may accelerate osteoporosis and weaken the vertebral body, leading to compression fractures and pain. The most common causes of nontraumatic vertebral body fractures are postmenopausal (type 1) or senile (type 2) osteoporosis (Chap. 348). Compression fractures occur in up to half of patients with severe osteoporosis, and those who sustain a fracture have a 4.5-fold increased risk for recurrence. The sole manifestation of a compression fracture may be localized back pain or radicular pain exacerbated by movement and often reproduced by palpation over the spinous process of the affected vertebra. The clinical context, neurologic signs, and x-ray appearance of the spine establish the diagnosis. Antiresorptive drugs including bisphosphonates (e.g., alendronate), transdermal estrogen, and tamoxifen have been shown to reduce the risk of osteoporotic fractures. Fewer than one-third of patients with prior compression fractures are adequately treated for osteoporosis despite the increased risk for future fractures; rates of primary prevention among individuals at risk, but without a history of fracture, are even less. Compression fractures above the midthoracic region suggest malignancy; if tumor is suspected, a bone biopsy or diagnostic search for a primary tumor is indicated. For a complete discussion of diagnosis and management of osteoporosis, see Chap. 348.

Interventions [percutaneous vertebroplasty (PVP), kyphoplasty] exist for osteoporotic compression fractures associated with debilitating pain. Candidates for PVP have midline back pain, palpation tenderness over the spinous process of the affected vertebral body, <80% loss of vertebral body height, and onset of symptoms within the prior 4 months. The PVP technique consists of injection of polymethylmethacrylate, under fluoroscopic guidance, into the affected vertebral body. Kyphoplasty adds the inflation of a balloon in the vertebral body prior to the injection of cement. Rare complications can include extravasation of cement into the epidural space (resulting in myelopathy) or fatal pulmonary embolism from migration of cement into paraspinal veins. Approximately three-quarters of patients who meet selection criteria have reported enhanced quality of life. Relief of pain following PVP has also been reported in patients with vertebral metastases, myeloma, or hemangiomas.

Osteosclerosis, an abnormally increased bone density often due to Paget's disease, is readily identifiable on routine x-ray studies and may or may not produce back pain. Spinal cord or nerve root compression may result from bony encroachment. For further discussion of these bone disorders, see Chaps. 347–349.

REFERRED PAIN FROM VISCERAL DISEASE
Diseases of the thorax, abdomen, or pelvis may refer pain to the posterior portion of the spinal segment that innervates the diseased organ. Oc-

casionally, back pain may be the first and only manifestation. Upper abdominal diseases generally refer pain to the lower thoracic or upper lumbar region (eighth thoracic to the first and second lumbar vertebrae), lower abdominal diseases to the mid-lumbar region (second to fourth lumbar vertebrae), and pelvic diseases to the sacral region. Local signs (pain with spine palpation, paraspinal muscle spasm) are absent, and little or no pain accompanies routine movements of the spine.

Low Thoracic or Lumbar Pain with Abdominal Disease Peptic ulcers or tumors of the posterior wall of the stomach or duodenum typically produce epigastric pain (Chaps. 87 and 287), but midline back or paraspinal pain may occur if retroperitoneal extension is present. Fatty foods are more likely to induce back pain associated with biliary disease. Diseases of the pancreas produce back pain to the right of the spine (head of the pancreas involved) or to the left (body or tail involved). Pathology in retroperitoneal structures (hemorrhage, tumors, pyelonephritis) produces paraspinal pain that radiates to the lower abdomen, groin, or anterior thighs. A mass in the iliopsoas region often produces unilateral lumbar pain with radiation toward the groin, labia, or testicles. The sudden appearance of lumbar pain in a patient receiving anticoagulants suggests retroperitoneal hemorrhage.

Isolated low back pain occurs in 15–20% of patients with a contained rupture of an abdominal aortic aneurysm (AAA). The classic clinical triad of abdominal pain, shock, and back pain occurs in <20% of patients. Two of these three features are present in two-thirds of patients, and hypotension is present in half. The typical patient is an elderly male smoker with back pain. Frequently, the diagnosis is initially missed because the symptoms and signs can be nonspecific. Common misdiagnoses include nonspecific back pain, diverticulitis, renal colic, sepsis, and myocardial infarction. A careful abdominal examination revealing a pulsatile mass (present in 50–75% of patients) is an important physical finding. Patients with suspected AAA should be evaluated with abdominal ultrasound, CT, or MRI (Chap. 242).

Inflammatory bowel disorders (colitis, diverticulitis) or cancers of the colon may produce lower abdominal pain, midlumbar back pain, or both. The pain may have a beltline distribution around the body. A lesion in the transverse or proximal descending colon may refer pain to the mid or left back at the L2-L3 level. Lesions of the sigmoid colon may refer pain to the upper sacral or midline suprapubic regions or left lower quadrant of the abdomen.

Sacral Pain with Gynecologic and Urologic Disease Pelvic organs rarely cause low back pain, except for gynecologic disorders involving the uterosacral ligaments. The pain is referred to the sacral region. Endometriosis or uterine cancers may invade the uterosacral ligaments. Pain associated with endometriosis is typically premenstrual and often continues until it merges with menstrual pain. Uterine malposition may cause uterosacral ligament traction (retroversion, descensus, and prolapse) or produce sacral pain after prolonged standing.

Menstrual pain may be felt in the sacral region. The poorly localized, cramping pain can radiate down the legs. Pain due to neoplastic infiltration of nerves is typically continuous, progressive in severity, and unrelieved by rest at night. Less commonly, radiation therapy of pelvic tumors may produce sacral pain from late radiation necrosis of tissue or nerves. Low back pain that radiates into one or both thighs is common in the last weeks of pregnancy.

Urologic sources of lumbosacral back pain include chronic prostatitis, prostate cancer with spinal metastasis (Chap. 91), and diseases of the kidney and ureter. Lesions of the bladder and testes do not usually produce back pain. Infectious, inflammatory, or neoplastic renal diseases may produce ipsilateral lumbosacral pain, as can renal artery or vein thrombosis. Paraspinal lumbar pain may be a symptom of ureteral obstruction due to nephrolithiasis.

OTHER CAUSES OF BACK PAIN

Postural Back Pain There is a group of patients with nonspecific chronic low back pain (CLBP) in whom no anatomic lesion can be found despite exhaustive investigation. These individuals complain of vague, diffuse back pain with prolonged sitting or standing that is relieved by rest. The physical examination is unrevealing except for "poor posture." Imaging studies and laboratory evaluations do not identify a specific cause. Exercises to strengthen the paraspinal and abdominal muscles are sometimes helpful.

Psychiatric Disease CLBP may be encountered in patients who seek financial compensation; in malingerers; or in those with concurrent substance abuse, chronic anxiety states, or depression. Many patients with CLBP have a history of psychiatric illness (depression, anxiety, substance abuse) or childhood trauma (physical or sexual abuse) that antedates the onset of back pain. Preoperative psychological assessment has been used to exclude patients with marked psychological impairments that predict a poor surgical outcome.

Unidentified The cause of low back pain occasionally remains unclear. Some patients have had multiple operations for disk disease but have persistent pain and disability. The original indications for surgery may have been questionable, with back pain only, no definite neurologic signs, or a minor disk bulge noted on CT or MRI. Scoring systems based upon neurologic signs, psychological factors, physiologic studies, and imaging studies have been devised to minimize the likelihood of unsuccessful surgery.

℞ BACK PAIN

ACUTE LOW BACK PAIN (ALBP) ALBP is defined as pain of <3 months' duration. Full recovery can be expected in 85% of adults with ALBP without leg pain. Most have purely "mechanical" symptoms (i.e., pain that is aggravated by motion and relieved by rest).

Observational studies have been used to justify a minimalist approach to this problem. These studies share a number of limitations: (1) a true placebo control group is often lacking; (2) patients who consult different provider groups (generalists, orthopedists, neurologists) are assumed to have similar etiologies for their back pain; (3) no information is provided about the details of treatment; and (4) no attempt to tabulate structural causes of ALBP is made.

The algorithms for the treatment of back pain (**Fig. 16-6**) draw from published clinical practice guidelines (CPGs). However, since CPGs are based on incomplete evidence, guidelines should not substitute for clinical judgment.

The initial assessment excludes serious causes of spine pathology that require urgent intervention, including infection, cancer, and trauma. Risk factors for a serious cause of ALBP are shown in Table 16-1. Laboratory studies are unnecessary if risk factors are absent. Plain spine films or CT are rarely indicated in the first month of symptoms unless a spine fracture is suspected.

Clinical trials have shown no benefit of >2 days of bed rest for uncomplicated ALBP. There is evidence that bed rest is also ineffective for patients with sciatica or for acute back pain with signs of nerve root injury. Similarly, traction is not effective for ALBP. Possible advantages of early ambulation for ALBP include maintenance of cardiovascular conditioning, improved disk and cartilage nutrition, improved bone and muscle strength, and increased endorphin levels. One trial of early vigorous exercise was negative, but the value of less vigorous exercise or other exercise programs are unknown. Early resumption of normal physical activity (without heavy manual labor) is likely to be beneficial.

Proof is lacking to support the treatment of acute back and neck pain with acupuncture, transcutaneous electrical nerve stimulation, massage, ultrasound, diathermy, magnets, or electrical stimulation. Cervical collars can be modestly helpful by limiting spontaneous and reflex neck movements that exacerbate pain. Evidence regarding the efficacy of ice is lacking; heat may provide a short-term reduction in pain and disability. These interventions are optional given the lack of negative evidence, low cost, and low risk. Biofeedback has not been studied rigorously. Facet joint, trigger point, and ligament injections are not recommended for acute treatment.

A role for modification of posture has not been validated by rigorous clinical studies. As a practical matter, temporary suspension of activity known to increase mechanical stress on the spine (heavy lifting, prolonged sitting, bending or twisting, straining at stool) may be helpful.

Education is an important part of treatment. Satisfaction and the likelihood of follow-up increase when patients are educated about prognosis,

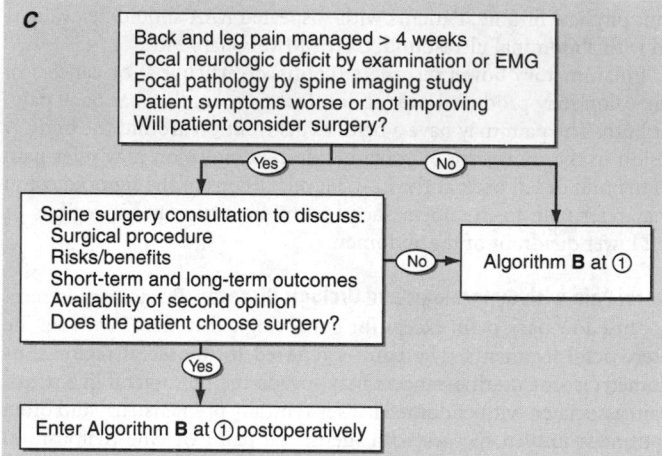

FIGURE 16-6 Algorithms for management of acute low back pain, age ≥ 18 years. A. Symptoms <3 months, first 4 weeks. **B.** Management weeks 4–12. ①, entry point from Algorithm *C* postoperatively or if patient declines surgery. **C.** Surgical options. (NSAIDs, nonsteroidal anti-inflammatory drugs; CBC, complete blood count; ESR, erythrocyte sedimentation rate; UA, urinalysis; EMG, electromyography; NCV, nerve conduction velocity studies; MRI, magnetic resonance imaging; CT, computed tomography; CNS, central nervous system.)

treatment methods, activity modifications, and strategies to prevent future exacerbations. In one study, patients who felt they did not receive an adequate explanation for their symptoms wanted further diagnostic tests. Evidence for the efficacy of structured education programs ("back school") is inconclusive; there is modest evidence for a short-term benefit, but evidence for a long-term benefit is lacking. Randomized studies of back school for primary prevention of low back injury and pain have failed to demonstrate any benefit.

NSAIDs and acetaminophen (see Table 12-1) are effective over-the-counter agents for ALBP. Muscle relaxants (cyclobenzaprine, 10 mg PO qhs as initial dose, up to 10 mg PO tid) provide short-term (4–7 days) benefit, particularly at night if sleep is affected, but drowsiness limits daytime use. Opioid analgesics are no more effective than NSAIDs or acetaminophen for initial treatment of ALBP, nor do they increase the likelihood of return to work. Short-term use of opioids may be necessary in patients unresponsive

to or intolerant of acetaminophen or NSAIDs. There is no evidence to support the use of oral glucocorticoids or tricyclic antidepressants for ALBP.

Epidural glucocorticoids may occasionally produce short-term pain relief in ALBP with radiculopathy, but proof is lacking for pain relief beyond 1 month. Epidural glucocorticoids, anesthetics, or opioids are not indicated in the initial treatment of ALBP without radiculopathy. Diagnostic nerve root blocks have been advocated to determine if pain originates from a specific nerve root. However, improvement may result even when the nerve root is not responsible for the pain; this may occur as a placebo effect, from a pain-generating lesion located distally along the peripheral nerve, or from anesthesia of the sinuvertebral nerve. Therapeutic nerve root blocks with injection of glucocorticoids and a local anesthetic should be considered only after conservative measures fail, particularly when temporary relief of pain is necessary.

A short course of lumbar spinal manipulation or physical therapy (PT) for symptomatic relief of uncomplicated ALBP is a reasonable option. Prospective,

TABLE 16-4 CERVICAL RADICULOPATHY—NEUROLOGIC FEATURES

Cervical Nerve Roots	Examination Findings			Pain Distribution
	Reflex	Sensory	Motor	
C5	Biceps	Over lateral deltoid	Supraspinatus[a] (initial arm abduction) Infraspinatus[a] (arm external rotation) Deltoid[a] (arm abduction) Biceps (arm flexion)	Lateral arm, medial scapula
C6	Biceps	Thumb, index fingers Radial hand/ forearm	Biceps (arm flexion) Pronator teres (internal forearm rotation)	Lateral forearm, thumb, index finger
C7	Triceps	Middle fingers Dorsum forearm	Triceps[a] (arm extension) Wrist extensors[a] Extensor digitorum[a] (finger extension)	Posterior arm, dorsal forearm, lateral hand
C8	Finger flexors	Little finger Medial hand and forearm	Abductor pollicis brevis (abduction D1) First dorsal interosseous (abduction D2) Abductor digiti minimi (abduction D5)	4th and 5th fingers, medial forearm
T1	Finger flexors	Axilla and medial arm	Abductor pollicis brevis (abduction D1) First dorsal interosseous (abduction D2) Abductor digiti minimi (abduction D5)	Medial arm, axilla

[a]These muscles receive the majority of innervation from this root.

randomized studies are difficult to perform in part because there is no consensus about what constitutes an adequate placebo control. Specific PT or chiropractic protocols that may provide benefit have not been fully defined.

CHRONIC LOW BACK PAIN CLBP, defined as pain lasting >12 weeks, accounts for 50% of total back pain costs. Risk factors include obesity, female gender, older age, prior history of back pain, restricted spinal mobility, pain radiating into a leg, high levels of psychological distress, poor self-rated health, minimal physical activity, smoking, job dissatisfaction, and widespread pain. Combinations of these premorbid factors have been used to predict which individuals with ALBP are likely to develop CLBP. The initial approach to these patients is similar to that for ALBP. Treatment of this heterogeneous group of patients is directed toward the underlying cause when known; the ultimate goal is to restore function to the maximum extent possible.

Many conditions that produce CLBP can be identified by a combination of neuroimaging and electrophysiologic studies. Spine MRI and CT-myelography are almost always the imaging techniques of choice. Imaging studies should be performed only in circumstances when the results are likely to influence management.

Injection studies can be used diagnostically to help determine the anatomic source of back pain. Reproduction of the patient's typical pain with diskography has been used as evidence that a specific disk is the pain generator. Pain relief following a foraminal nerve root block or glucocorticoid injection into a facet has been similarly used as evidence that the facet joint or nerve root is the source. However, the possibility that the injection response was a placebo effect or due to systemic absorption of the glucocorticoids is usually not considered. The value of these procedures in the treatment of CLBP or in the selection of candidates for surgery is largely unknown despite their widespread use. The value of thermography in the assessment of radiculopathy also has not been rigorously studied.

The diagnosis of nerve root injury is most secure when the history, examination, results of imaging studies, and the EMG are concordant. The correlation between CT and EMG for localization of nerve root injury is between 65 and 73%. Up to one-third of asymptomatic adults have a disk protrusion detected by CT or MRI scans. Thus, surgical intervention based solely upon radiologic findings increases the likelihood of an unsuccessful outcome.

An unblinded study in patients with chronic sciatica found that surgery could hasten relief of symptoms by ~2 months; however, at 1 year there was no advantage of surgery over conservative medical therapy, and nearly all patients (95%) in both groups made a full recovery regardless of the treatment approach.

CLBP can be treated with a variety of conservative measures. Acute and subacute exacerbations are managed with NSAIDs and comfort measures. There is no good evidence to suggest that one NSAID is more effective than another. Bed rest should not exceed 2 days. Activity tolerance is the primary goal, while pain relief is secondary. Exercise programs can reverse atrophy in paraspinal muscles and strengthen extensors of the trunk. Intensive physical exercise or "work hardening" regimens (under the guidance of a physical therapist) have been effective in returning some patients to work, improving walking distances, and diminishing pain. The benefit can be sustained with home exercise regimens. It is difficult to endorse one specific exercise or PT regimen given the heterogeneous nature of this patient group. The role of manipulation, back school, or epidural steroid injections in the treatment of CLBP is unproven. There is no strong evidence to support the use of acupuncture or traction. A reduction in sick leave days, long-term health care utilization, and pension expenditures may offset the initial expense of multidisciplinary treatment programs. Studies of hydrotherapy for CLBP have yielded mixed results; however, given its low risk and cost, hydrotherapy can be considered as a treatment option. Transcutaneous electrical nerve stimulation (TENS) has not been adequately studied in CLBP.

PAIN IN THE NECK AND SHOULDER (Table 16-4)

Neck pain, which usually arises from diseases of the cervical spine and soft tissues of the neck, is common (4.6% of adults in one study). Neck pain arising from the cervical spine is typically precipitated by movement and may be accompanied by focal tenderness and limitation of motion. Pain arising from the brachial plexus, shoulder, or peripheral nerves can be confused with cervical spine disease, but the history and examination usually identify a more distal origin for the pain. Cervical spine trauma, disk disease, or spondylosis may be asymptomatic or painful and can produce a myelopathy, radiculopathy, or both. The nerve roots most commonly affected are C7 and C6.

TRAUMA TO THE CERVICAL SPINE

Trauma to the cervical spine (fractures, subluxation) places the spinal cord at risk for compression. Motor vehicle accidents, violent crimes, or falls account for 87% of spinal cord injuries (Chap. 372). Immediate immobilization of the neck is essential to minimize further spinal cord injury from movement of unstable cervical spine segments. A CT scan is the diagnostic procedure of choice for detection of acute fractures. Following major trauma to the cervical spine, injury to the vertebral arteries is common; most lesions are asymptomatic and can be visualized by MRI and angiography.

Whiplash injury is due to trauma (usually automobile accidents) causing cervical musculoligamental sprain or strain due to hyperflexion or hyperextension. This diagnosis should not be applied to patients with fractures, disk herniation, head injury, focal neurologic findings, or altered consciousness. Imaging of the cervical spine is not cost-effective acutely but is useful to detect disk herniations when symptoms persist for >6 weeks following the injury. Severe initial symptoms have been associated with a poor long-term outcome.

CERVICAL DISK DISEASE

Herniation of a lower cervical disk is a common cause of neck, shoulder, arm, or hand pain or tingling. Neck pain, stiffness, and a range of motion limited by pain are the usual manifestations. A herniated cervical disk is responsible for ~25% of cervical radiculopathies. Extension and lateral rotation of the neck narrows the ipsilateral intervertebral foramen and may reproduce radicular symptoms (Spurling's sign). In young persons, acute nerve root compression from a ruptured cervical disk is often due to trauma. Cervical disk herniations are usually posterolateral near the lateral recess and intervertebral foramen. Typical patterns of reflex, sensory, and motor changes that accompany specific cervical nerve root lesions are summarized in Table 16-4; however, (1) overlap in function between adjacent nerve roots is common, (2) symptoms and signs may be evident in only part of the injured nerve root territory, and (3) the location of pain is the most variable of the clinical features.

CERVICAL SPONDYLOSIS

Osteoarthritis of the cervical spine may produce neck pain that radiates into the back of the head, shoulders, or arms, or may be the source of headaches in the posterior occipital region (supplied by the C2-C4 nerve roots). Osteophytes, disk protrusions, and hypertrophic facet or uncovertebral joints may compress one or several nerve roots at the intervertebral foramina (**Fig. 16-7**); this compression accounts for 75% of cervical radiculopathies. The roots most commonly affected are C7 and C6. Narrowing of the spinal canal by osteophytes, ossification of the posterior longitudinal ligament (OPLL), or a large central disk may compress the cervical spinal cord. Combinations of radiculopathy and myelopathy may also be present. Spinal cord involvement is suggested by Lhermitt's symptom, an electrical sensation elicited by neck flexion and radiating down the spine from the neck. When little or no neck pain accompanies cord compression, the diagnosis may be confused with amyotrophic lateral sclerosis (Chap. 369), multiple sclerosis (Chap. 375), spinal cord tumors, or syringomyelia (Chap. 372). The possibility of cervical spondylosis should be considered even when the patient presents with symptoms or signs in the legs only. MRI is the study of choice to define the anatomic abnormalities, but plain CT is adequate to assess bony spurs, foraminal narrowing, or OPLL. EMG and nerve conduction studies can localize and assess the severity of the nerve root injury.

OTHER CAUSES OF NECK PAIN

Rheumatoid arthritis (RA) (Chap. 314) of the cervical apophyseal joints produces neck pain, stiffness, and limitation of motion. In advanced RA, synovitis of the atlantoaxial joint (C1-C2; Fig. 16-2) may damage the transverse ligament of the atlas, producing forward displacement of the atlas on the axis (atlantoaxial subluxation). Radiologic evidence of atlantoaxial subluxation occurs in 30% of patients with RA. Not surprisingly, the degree of subluxation correlates with the severity of erosive disease. When subluxation is present, careful assessment is important to identify early signs of myelopathy. Occasional patients develop high spinal cord compression leading to quadriparesis, respiratory insufficiency, and death. Surgery should be considered when myelopathy or spinal instability is present.

Ankylosing spondylitis can cause neck pain and less commonly atlantoaxial subluxation; surgery may be required to prevent spinal cord compression. Acute *herpes zoster* presents as acute posterior occipital or neck pain prior to the outbreak of vesicles. *Neoplasms* metastatic to the cervical spine, *infections* (osteomyelitis and epidural abscess), and *metabolic bone diseases* may be the cause of neck pain. Neck pain may also be referred from the heart with coronary artery ischemia (cervical angina syndrome).

THORACIC OUTLET

The thoracic outlet contains the first rib, the subclavian artery and vein, the brachial plexus, the clavicle, and the lung apex. Injury to these structures may result in postural or movement-induced pain around the shoulder and supraclavicular region. *True neurogenic thoracic outlet syndrome* (TOS) results from compression of the lower trunk of the brachial plexus or ventral rami of the C8 or T1 nerve roots by an anomalous band of tissue connecting an elongate transverse process at C7 with the first rib. Signs include weakness of intrinsic muscles of the hand and diminished sensation on the palmar aspect of the fourth and fifth digits. EMG and nerve conduction studies confirm the diag-

nosis. Treatment consists of surgical resection of the anomalous band. The weakness and wasting of intrinsic hand muscles typically does not improve, but surgery halts the insidious progression of weakness. *Arterial TOS* results from compression of the subclavian artery by a cervical rib; the compression results in poststenotic dilatation of the artery and thrombus formation. Blood pressure is reduced in the affected limb, and signs of emboli may be present in the hand. Neurologic signs are absent. Ultrasound can confirm the diagnosis noninvasively. Treatment is with thrombolysis or anticoagulation (with or without embolectomy) and surgical excision of the cervical rib compressing the subclavian artery or vein. *Disputed TOS* includes a large number of patients with chronic arm and shoulder pain of unclear cause. The lack of sensitive and specific findings on physical examination or laboratory markers for this condition frequently results in diagnostic uncertainty. The role of surgery in disputed TOS is controversial. Multidisciplinary pain management is a conservative approach, although treatment is often unsuccessful.

BRACHIAL PLEXUS AND NERVES

Pain from injury to the brachial plexus or peripheral nerves of the arm can occasionally mimic pain of cervical spine origin. Neoplastic infiltration of the lower trunk of the brachial plexus may produce shoulder pain radiating down the arm, numbness of the fourth and fifth fingers, and weakness of intrinsic hand muscles innervated by the ulnar and median nerves. Postradiation fibrosis (most commonly from treatment of breast cancer) may produce similar findings, although pain is less often present. A Pancoast tumor of the lung (Chap. 85) is another cause and should be considered, especially when a Horner's syndrome is present. *Suprascapular neuropathy* may produce severe shoulder pain, weakness, and wasting of the supraspinatus and infraspinatus muscles. *Acute brachial neuritis* is often confused with radiculopathy; the acute onset of severe shoulder or scapular pain is followed over days to weeks by weakness of the proximal arm and shoulder girdle muscles innervated by the upper brachial plexus. The onset is often preceded by an infection. The suprascapular and long thoracic nerves are most often affected; the latter results in a winged scapula. Brachial neuritis may also present as an isolated paralysis of the diaphragm. Complete recovery occurs in 75% of patients after 2 years and in 89% after 3 years.

Occasional cases of carpal tunnel syndrome produce pain and paresthesias extending into the forearm, arm, and shoulder resembling a

FIGURE 16-7 Cervical spondylosis; left C6 radiculopathy. **A.** Sagittal T2 fast spin echo magnetic resonance imaging reveals a hypointense osteophyte that protrudes from the C5-C6 level into the thecal sac, displacing the spinal cord posteriorly (*white arrow*). **B.** Axial 2-mm section from a 3-D volume gradient echo sequence of the cervical spine. The high signal of the right C5-C6 intervertebral foramen contrasts with the narrow high signal of the left C5-C6 intervertebral foramen produced by osteophytic spurring (*arrows*).

C5 or C6 root lesion. Lesions of the radial or ulnar nerve can mimic a radiculopathy at C7 or C8, respectively. EMG and nerve conduction studies can accurately localize lesions to the nerve roots, brachial plexus, or peripheral nerves. For further discussion of peripheral nerve disorders, see Chap. 379.

SHOULDER

Pain arising from the shoulder can on occasion mimic pain from the spine. If symptoms and signs of radiculopathy are absent, then the differential diagnosis includes mechanical shoulder pain (tendonitis, bursitis, rotator cuff tear, dislocation, adhesive capsulitis, and cuff impingement under the acromion) and referred pain (subdiaphragmatic irritation, angina, Pancoast tumor). Mechanical pain is often worse at night, associated with local shoulder tenderness and aggravated by abduction, internal rotation, or extension of the arm. Pain from shoulder disease may radiate into the arm or hand, but sensory, motor, and reflex changes are absent.

℞ NECK PAIN

There are few well-designed clinical trials that address optimal treatment of neck pain or cervical radiculopathy. Relief of pain, prevention of recurrence, and improved neurologic function are reasonable goals. Symptomatic treatment includes the use of analgesic medications and/or a soft cervical collar. Most treatment recommendations reflect anecdotal experience, case series, or conclusions derived from studies of the lumbar spine. Controlled studies of oral prednisone or transforaminal glucocorticoid injections have not been performed. Reasonable indications for cervical disk surgery include a progressive radicular motor deficit, pain that fails to respond to conservative management and limits activities of daily living, or cervical spinal cord compression. Surgical management of herniated cervical disks usually consists of an anterior approach with diskectomy followed by anterior interbody fusion. A simple posterior partial laminectomy with diskectomy is an acceptable alternative approach. Another surgical approach involves implantation of an artificial disk; in one prospective trial, outcomes after 2 years favored the implant over a traditional anterior cervical discectomy with fusion. The artificial disk is not yet approved for general use in the United States. The risk of subsequent radiculopathy or myelopathy at cervical segments adjacent to the fusion is ~3% per year and 26% per decade. Although this risk is sometimes portrayed as a late complication of surgery, it may also reflect the natural history of degenerative cervical disk disease.

Nonprogressive cervical radiculopathy due to a herniated cervical disk may be treated conservatively, even if a focal neurologic deficit is present, with a high rate of success. However, if the cervical radiculopathy is due to bony compression from cervical spondylosis, then surgical decompression is generally indicated to forestall the progression of neurologic signs.

Cervical spondylotic myelopathy is typically managed with either anterior decompression and fusion or laminectomy in order to forestall progression of the myelopathy known to occur in 20–30% of untreated patients. However, one prospective study comparing surgery vs. conservative treatment for mild cervical spondylotic myelopathy showed no difference in outcome after 2 years of follow-up.

FURTHER READINGS

ATLAS SJ, NARDIN RA: Evaluation and treatment of low back pain: An evidence-based approach to clinical care. Muscle Nerve 27:265, 2003

BAGLEY LJ: Imaging of spinal trauma. Radiol Clin North Am 44:1, 2006

CASSIDY JD et al: Effect of eliminating compensation for pain and suffering on the outcome of insurance claims for whiplash injury. N Engl J Med 342:1179, 2000

CAVALIER R et al: Spondylolysis and spondylolisthesis in children and adolescents: Diagnosis, natural history, and non-surgical management. J Am Acad Orthop Surg 14:417, 2006

COWAN JA JR et al: Changes in the utilization of spinal fusion in the United States. Neurosurgery 59:1, 2006

GORBACH C et al: Therapeutic efficacy of facet joint blocks. AJR Am J Roentgenol 186:5, 2006

MUMMANENI PV et al: Clinical and radiographic analysis of cervical disk arthroplasty compared with allograft fusion: A randomized controlled clinical trial. J Neurosurg Spine 6:198, 2007

PEUL WC et al: Surgery versus prolonged conservative treatment for sciatica. N Engl J Med 356:2245, 2007

VAN ALFEN N, VAN ENGELEN BG: The clinical spectrum of neuralgic amyotrophy in 246 cases. Brain 129:438, 2006

WEINSTEIN JN et al: Surgical versus nonsurgical treatment for lumbar degenerative spondylolisthesis. N Engl J Med 356:2257, 2007

——— et al: Surgical vs nonoperative treatment for lumbar disc herniation. The spine patient outcomes research trial (SPORT): A randomized trial. JAMA 296:2441, 2006

SECTION 2 ALTERATIONS IN BODY TEMPERATURE

17 Fever and Hyperthermia
Charles A. Dinarello, Reuven Porat

Body temperature is controlled by the hypothalamus. Neurons in both the preoptic anterior hypothalamus and the posterior hypothalamus receive two kinds of signals: one from peripheral nerves that transmit information from warmth/cold receptors in the skin and the other from the temperature of the blood bathing the region. These two types of signals are integrated by the thermoregulatory center of the hypothalamus to maintain normal temperature. In a neutral temperature environment, the metabolic rate of humans produces more heat than is necessary to maintain the core body temperature at 37°C.

A normal body temperature is ordinarily maintained, despite environmental variations, because the hypothalamic thermoregulatory center balances the excess heat production derived from metabolic activity in muscle and the liver with heat dissipation from the skin and lungs. According to studies of healthy individuals 18–40 years of age, the mean oral temperature is 36.8° ± 0.4°C (98.2° ± 0.7°F), with low levels at 6 A.M. and higher levels at 4–6 P.M. The maximum normal oral temperature is 37.2°C (98.9°F) at 6 A.M. and 37.7°C (99.9°F) at 4 P.M.; these values define the 99th percentile for healthy individuals. In light of these studies, an A.M. temperature of >37.2°C (>98.9°F) or a P.M. temperature of >37.7°C (>99.9°F) would define a fever. The normal daily temperature variation is typically 0.5°C (0.9°F). However, in some individuals recovering from a febrile illness, this daily variation can be as great as 1.0°C. During a febrile illness, the diurnal variation is usually maintained but at higher, febrile levels. The daily temperature variation appears to be fixed in early childhood; in contrast, elderly individuals can exhibit a reduced ability to develop fever, with only a modest fever even in severe infections.

Rectal temperatures are generally 0.4°C (0.7°F) higher than oral readings. The lower oral readings are probably attributable to mouth breathing, which is a factor in patients with respiratory infections and rapid breathing. Lower-esophageal temperatures closely reflect core temperature. Tympanic membrane (TM) thermometers measure radiant heat from the tympanic membrane and nearby ear canal and display that absolute value (unadjusted mode) or a value automatically calculated from the absolute reading on the basis of nomograms relating the radiant temperature measured to actual core temperatures obtained in clinical studies (adjusted mode). These measurements, although convenient, may be more variable than directly determined oral or rectal values. Studies in adults show that readings are lower with unadjusted-mode than with adjusted-mode TM thermometers and that unadjusted-mode TM values are 0.8°C (1.6°F) lower than rectal temperatures.

In women who menstruate, the A.M. temperature is generally lower in the 2 weeks before ovulation; it then rises by ~0.6°C (1°F) with ovulation and remains at that level until menses occur. Body temperature can be elevated in the postprandial state. Pregnancy and endocrinologic dysfunction also affect body temperature.

FEVER VERSUS HYPERTHERMIA

FEVER

Fever is an elevation of body temperature that exceeds the normal daily variation and occurs *in conjunction with an increase in the hypothalamic set point* (e.g., from 37°C to 39°C). This shift of the set point from "normothermic" to febrile levels very much resembles the resetting of the home thermostat to a higher level in order to raise the ambient temperature in a room. Once the hypothalamic set point is raised, neurons in the vasomotor center are activated and vasoconstriction commences. The individual first notices vasoconstriction in the hands and feet. Shunting of blood away from the periphery to the internal organs essentially decreases heat loss from the skin, and the person feels cold. For most fevers, body temperature increases by 1°–2°C. Shivering, which increases heat production from the muscles, may begin at this time; however, shivering is not required if heat conservation mechanisms raise blood temperature sufficiently. Nonshivering heat production from the liver also contributes to increasing core temperature. In humans, behavioral adjustments (e.g., putting on more clothing or bedding) help raise body temperature by decreasing heat loss.

The processes of heat conservation (vasoconstriction) and heat production (shivering and increased nonshivering thermogenesis) continue until the temperature of the blood bathing the hypothalamic neurons matches the new thermostat setting. Once that point is reached, the hypothalamus maintains the temperature at the febrile level by the same mechanisms of heat balance that function in the afebrile state. When the hypothalamic set point is again reset downward (in response to either a reduction in the concentration of pyrogens or the use of antipyretics), the processes of heat loss through vasodilation and sweating are initiated. Loss of heat by sweating and vasodilation continues until the blood temperature at the hypothalamic level matches the lower setting. Behavioral changes (e.g., removal of clothing) facilitate heat loss.

A fever of >41.5°C (>106.7°F) is called *hyperpyrexia*. This extraordinarily high fever can develop in patients with severe infections but most commonly occurs in patients with central nervous system (CNS) hemorrhages. In the preantibiotic era, fever due to a variety of infectious diseases rarely exceeded 106°F, and there has been speculation that this natural "thermal ceiling" is mediated by neuropeptides functioning as central antipyretics.

In rare cases, the hypothalamic set point is elevated as a result of local trauma, hemorrhage, tumor, or intrinsic hypothalamic malfunction. The term *hypothalamic fever* is sometimes used to describe elevated temperature caused by abnormal hypothalamic function. However, most patients with hypothalamic damage have *sub*normal, not *supra*normal, body temperatures.

HYPERTHERMIA

Although most patients with elevated body temperature have fever, there are circumstances in which elevated temperature represents not fever but hyperthermia (Table 17-1). Hyperthermia is characterized by an uncontrolled increase in body temperature that exceeds the body's ability to lose heat. The setting of the hypothalamic thermoregulatory center is unchanged. In contrast to fever in infections, hyperthermia does not involve pyrogenic molecules (see "Pyrogens," below). Exogenous heat exposure and endogenous heat production are two mechanisms by which hyperthermia can result in dangerously high internal temperatures. Excessive heat production can easily cause hyperthermia despite physiologic and behavioral control of body temperature.

TABLE 17-1 CAUSES OF HYPERTHERMIA SYNDROMES

Heat Stroke

Exertional: Exercise in higher-than-normal heat and/or humidity
Nonexertional: Anticholinergics, including antihistamines; antiparkinsonian drugs; diuretics; phenothiazines

Drug-Induced Hyperthermia

Amphetamines, cocaine, phencyclidine (PCP), methylenedioxymethamphetamine (MDMA; "ecstasy"), lysergic acid diethylamide (LSD), salicylates, lithium, anticholinergics, sympathomimetics

Neuroleptic Malignant Syndrome

Phenothiazines; butyrophenones, including haloperidol and bromperidol; fluoxetine; loxapine; tricyclic dibenzodiazepines; metoclopramide; domperidone; thiothixene; molindone; withdrawal of dopaminergic agents

Serotonin Syndrome

Selective serotonin reuptake inhibitors (SSRIs), monoamine oxidase inhibitors (MAOIs), tricyclic antidepressants

Malignant Hyperthermia

Inhalational anesthetics, succinylcholine

Endocrinopathy

Thyrotoxicosis, pheochromocytoma

Central Nervous System Damage

Cerebral hemorrhage, status epilepticus, hypothalamic injury

Source: After FJ Curley, RS Irwin, JM Rippe et al (eds): *Intensive Care Medicine*, 3d ed. Boston, Little, Brown, 1996.

For example, work or exercise in hot environments can produce heat faster than peripheral mechanisms can lose it.

Heat stroke in association with a warm environment may be categorized as exertional or nonexertional. *Exertional heat stroke* typically occurs in individuals exercising at elevated ambient temperatures and/or humidities. In a dry environment and at maximal efficiency, sweating can dissipate ~600 kcal/h, requiring the production of >1 L of sweat. Even in healthy individuals, dehydration or the use of common medications (e.g., over-the-counter antihistamines with anticholinergic side effects) may precipitate exertional heat stroke. *Nonexertional heat stroke* typically occurs in either very young or elderly individuals, particularly during heat waves. According to the Centers for Disease Control and Prevention, there were 7000 deaths attributed to heat injury in the United States from 1979 to 1997. The elderly, the bedridden, persons taking anticholinergic or antiparkinsonian drugs or diuretics, and individuals confined to poorly ventilated and non-air-conditioned environments are most susceptible.

Drug-induced hyperthermia has become increasingly common as a result of the increased use of prescription psychotropic drugs and illicit drugs. Drug-induced hyperthermia may be caused by monoamine oxidase inhibitors (MAOIs), tricyclic antidepressants, and amphetamines and by the illicit use of phencyclidine (PCP), lysergic acid diethylamide (LSD), methylenedioxymethamphetamine (MDMA, "ecstasy"), or cocaine.

Malignant hyperthermia occurs in individuals with an inherited abnormality of skeletal-muscle sarcoplasmic reticulum that causes a rapid increase in intracellular calcium levels in response to halothane and other inhalational anesthetics or to succinylcholine. Elevated temperature, increased muscle metabolism, muscle rigidity, rhabdomyolysis, acidosis, and cardiovascular instability develop within minutes. This rare condition is often fatal. The *neuroleptic malignant syndrome* occurs in the setting of neuroleptic agent use (antipsychotic phenothiazines, haloperidol, prochlorperazine, metoclopramide) or the withdrawal of dopaminergic drugs and is characterized by "lead-pipe" muscle rigidity, extrapyramidal side effects, autonomic dysregulation, and hyperthermia. This disorder appears to be caused by the inhibition of central dopamine receptors in the hypothalamus, which results in increased heat generation and decreased heat dissipation. The *serotonin syndrome*, seen with selective serotonin uptake inhibitors (SSRIs), MAOIs, and other serotonergic medications, has many overlapping features, including hyperthermia, but may be distinguished by the presence of diarrhea, tremor, and myoclonus rather than the lead-pipe rigidity of the neuroleptic malignant syndrome. Thyrotoxicosis and pheochromocytoma can also cause increased thermogenesis.

It is important to distinguish between fever and hyperthermia since hyperthermia can be rapidly fatal and characteristically does not respond to antipyretics. In an emergency situation, however, making this distinction can be difficult. For example, in systemic sepsis, fever (hyperpyrexia) can be rapid in onset, and temperatures can exceed 40.5°C. Hyperthermia is often diagnosed on the basis of the events immediately preceding the elevation of core temperature—e.g., heat exposure or treatment with drugs that interfere with thermoregulation. In patients with heat stroke syndromes and in those taking drugs that block sweating, the skin is hot but dry, whereas in fever the skin can be cold as a consequence of vasoconstriction. Antipyretics do not reduce the elevated temperature in hyperthermia, whereas in fever—and even in hyperpyrexia—adequate doses of either aspirin or acetaminophen usually result in some decrease in body temperature.

PATHOGENESIS OF FEVER

PYROGENS

The term *pyrogen* is used to describe any substance that causes fever. *Exogenous* pyrogens are derived from outside the patient; most are microbial products, microbial toxins, or whole microorganisms. The classic example of an exogenous pyrogen is the lipopolysaccharide (endotoxin) produced by all gram-negative bacteria. Pyrogenic products of gram-positive organisms include the enterotoxins of *Staphylococcus aureus* and the group A and B streptococcal toxins, also called *superantigens*. One staphylococcal toxin of clinical importance is that associated with isolates of *S. aureus* from patients with toxic shock syndrome. These products of staphylococci and streptococci cause fever in experimental animals when injected intravenously at concentrations of 1–10 μg/kg. Endotoxin is a highly pyrogenic molecule in humans: when injected intravenously into volunteers, a dose of 2–3 ng/kg produces fever, leukocytosis, acute-phase proteins, and generalized symptoms of malaise.

PYROGENIC CYTOKINES

Cytokines are small proteins (molecular mass, 10,000–20,000 Da) that regulate immune, inflammatory, and hematopoietic processes. For example, the elevated leukocytosis seen in several infections with an absolute neutrophilia is the result of the cytokines interleukin (IL) 1 and IL-6. Some cytokines also cause fever; formerly referred to as *endogenous pyrogens*, they are now called *pyrogenic cytokines*. The pyrogenic cytokines include IL-1, IL-6, tumor necrosis factor (TNF), ciliary neurotropic factor (CNTF), and interferon (IFN) α. (IL-18, a member of the IL-1 family, does not appear to be a pyrogenic cytokine.) Other pyrogenic cytokines probably exist. Each cytokine is encoded by a separate gene, and each pyrogenic cytokine has been shown to cause fever in laboratory animals and in humans. When injected into humans, IL-1 and TNF produce fever at low doses (10–100 ng/kg); in contrast, for IL-6, a dose of 1–10 μg/kg is required for fever production.

A wide spectrum of bacterial and fungal products induce the synthesis and release of pyrogenic cytokines, as do viruses. However, fever can be a manifestation of disease in the absence of microbial infection. For example, inflammatory processes, trauma, tissue necrosis, or antigen-antibody complexes can induce the production of IL-1, TNF, and/or IL-6, which—individually or in combination—trigger the hypothalamus to raise the set point to febrile levels.

ELEVATION OF THE HYPOTHALAMIC SET POINT BY CYTOKINES

During fever, levels of prostaglandin E$_2$ (PGE$_2$) are elevated in hypothalamic tissue and the third cerebral ventricle. The concentrations of PGE$_2$ are highest near the circumventricular vascular organs (organum vasculosum of lamina terminalis)—networks of enlarged cap-

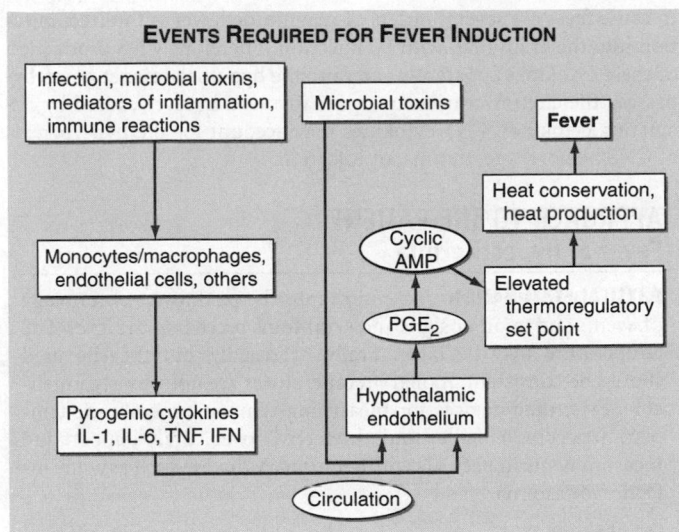

EVENTS REQUIRED FOR FEVER INDUCTION

FIGURE 17-1 Chronology of events required for the induction of fever. AMP, adenosine 5′-monophosphate; IFN, interferon; IL, interleukin; PGE$_2$, prostaglandin E$_2$; TNF, tumor necrosis factor.

illaries surrounding the hypothalamic regulatory centers. Destruction of these organs reduces the ability of pyrogens to produce fever. Most studies in animals have failed to show, however, that pyrogenic cytokines pass from the circulation into the brain itself. Thus, it appears that both exogenous and endogenous pyrogens interact with the endothelium of these capillaries and that this interaction is the first step in initiating fever—i.e., in raising the set point to febrile levels.

The key events in the production of fever are illustrated in Fig. 17-1. As has been mentioned, several cell types can produce pyrogenic cytokines. Pyrogenic cytokines such as IL-1, IL-6, and TNF are released from the cells and enter the systemic circulation. Although the systemic effects of these circulating cytokines lead to fever by inducing the synthesis of PGE$_2$, they also induce PGE$_2$ in peripheral tissues. The increase in PGE$_2$ in the periphery accounts for the nonspecific myalgias and arthralgias that often accompany fever. It is thought that some systemic PGE$_2$ escapes destruction by the lung and gains access to the hypothalamus via the internal carotid. However, it is the elevation of PGE$_2$ in the brain that starts the process of raising the hypothalamic set point for core temperature.

There are four receptors for PGE$_2$, and each signals the cell in different ways. Of the four receptors, the third (EP-3) is essential for fever: when the gene for this receptor is deleted in mice, no fever follows the injection of IL-1 or endotoxin. Deletion of the other PGE$_2$ receptor genes leaves the fever mechanism intact. Although PGE$_2$ is essential for fever, it is not a neurotransmitter. Rather, the release of PGE$_2$ from the brain side of the hypothalamic endothelium triggers the PGE$_2$ receptor on glial cells, and this stimulation results in the rapid release of cyclic adenosine 5′-monophosphate (cyclic AMP), which is a neurotransmitter. As shown in Fig. 17-1, the release of cyclic AMP from the glial cells activates neuronal endings from the thermoregulatory center that extend into the area. The elevation of cyclic AMP is thought to account for changes in the hypothalamic set point either directly or indirectly (by inducing the release of neurotransmitters). Distinct receptors for microbial products are located on the hypothalamic endothelium. These receptors are called *Toll-like receptors* and are similar in many ways to IL-1 receptors. The direct activation of Toll-like receptors also results in PGE$_2$ production and fever.

PRODUCTION OF CYTOKINES IN THE CNS

Several viral diseases produce active infection in the brain. Glial and possibly neuronal cells synthesize IL-1, TNF, and IL-6. CNTF is also synthesized by neural as well as neuronal cells. What role in the production of fever is played by these cytokines produced in the brain itself? In experimental animals, the concentrations of cytokine required to cause fever are several orders of magnitude lower with direct injection into the brain than with IV injection. Therefore, CNS production of these cytokines apparently can raise the hypothalamic set point, bypassing the circumventricular organs involved in fever caused by circulating cytokines. CNS cytokines may account for the hyperpyrexia of CNS hemorrhage, trauma, or infection.

APPROACH TO THE PATIENT:
Fever or Hyperthermia

PHYSICAL EXAMINATION Attention must be paid to the chronology of events and to other signs and symptoms preceding the fever. The temperature may be taken orally or rectally, but the site used should be consistent. Axillary temperatures are notoriously unreliable. Electronic devices for measuring tympanic membrane temperatures are reliable and preferred over oral temperature measurements in patients with pulmonary disease such as acute infection or asthma.

LABORATORY TESTS The workup should include a complete blood count; a differential count should be performed manually or with an instrument sensitive to the identification of eosinophils, juvenile or band forms, toxic granulations, and Döhle bodies, the last three of which are suggestive of bacterial infection. Neutropenia may be present with some viral infections.

Measurement of circulating cytokines in patients with fever is of little use since levels of pyrogenic cytokines in the circulation often are below the detection limit of the assay or do not coincide with the fever. Although some studies have shown correlations between circulating IL-6 levels and peak febrile elevations, the most valuable measurements in patients with fever are C-reactive protein level and erythrocyte sedimentation rate. These markers of pathologic processes are particularly helpful in identifying disease in patients with small elevations in body temperature.

FEVER IN RECIPIENTS OF ANTICYTOKINE THERAPY As of this writing, more than 750,000 patients in the United States are receiving chronic anticytokine therapy for Crohn's disease, rheumatoid arthritis, or psoriasis. Does such therapy mask infection by preventing fever? With the increasing use of anticytokines to reduce the activity of IL-1, IL-6, IL-12, and TNF, the effect of these agents on the febrile response must be considered.

The blocking of cytokine activity has the distinct clinical drawback of lowering the level of host defenses against both routine bacterial and opportunistic infections. The opportunistic infections reported in patients given neutralizing antibodies to TNF-α (infliximab or adalimumab) are similar to those reported in the HIV-1-infected population (e.g., new infection with or reactivation of *Mycobacterium tuberculosis*, with dissemination). A soluble receptor for TNF, etanercept, is also associated with opportunistic infections but less so than the neutralizing antibodies.

In nearly all reported cases of infection associated with anticytokine therapy, fever is among the presenting signs. However, the extent to which the febrile response is reduced in these patients remains unknown. Fever in a patient who develops an infection during anticytokine treatment is likely to be due to the direct action of microbial products on the hypothalamic thermoregulatory center, with induction of PGE$_2$. For example, blocking the activity of IL-1 or TNF during experimental endotoxin-induced fever in volunteers does not affect the febrile response.

℞ FEVER AND HYPERTHERMIA

THE DECISION TO TREAT FEVER Most fevers are associated with self-limited infections, such as common viral diseases. The use of antipyretics is not contraindicated in these infections: there is no significant clinical evidence that antipyretics delay the resolution of viral or bacterial infections, nor is there evidence that fever facilitates recovery from infection or acts as an adjuvant to the immune system. In fact, peripheral PGE$_2$ production is a potent immunosuppressant. In short, treatment of fever and its symptoms does no harm and does not slow the resolution of common viral and bacterial infections.

However, in bacterial infections, withholding antipyretic therapy can be helpful in evaluating the effectiveness of a particular antibiotic therapy, particularly in the absence of cultural identification of the infecting organism. The routine use of antipyretics can mask an inadequately treated bacterial infection. Withholding antipyretics in some cases may facilitate the diagnosis of an unusual febrile disease. For example, the usual times of peak and trough temperatures may be reversed in typhoid fever and disseminated tuberculosis. Temperature-pulse dissociation (relative bradycardia) occurs in typhoid fever, brucellosis, leptospirosis, some drug-induced fevers, and factitious fever. In newborns, the elderly, patients with chronic renal failure, and patients taking glucocorticoids, fever may not be present despite infection, or core temperature may be hypothermic. Hypothermia is often observed in patients with septic shock.

Some infections have characteristic patterns in which febrile episodes are separated by intervals of normal temperature. For example, *Plasmodium vivax* causes fever every third day, whereas fever occurs every fourth day with *P. malariae*. Other relapsing fevers are related to *Borrelia* infections, with days of fever followed by a several-day afebrile period and then a relapse of days of fever. In the Pel-Ebstein pattern, fever lasting 3–10 days is followed by afebrile periods of 3–10 days; this pattern can be classic for Hodgkin's disease and other lymphomas. In cyclic neutropenia, fevers occur every 21 days and accompany the neutropenia. There is no periodicity of fever in patients with familial Mediterranean fever.

Recurrent fever is documented at some point in most autoimmune diseases and all autoinflammatory diseases. The autoinflammatory diseases include adult and juvenile Still's disease, familial Mediterranean fever, hyper-IgD syndrome, familial cold-induced autoinflammatory syndrome, neonatal-onset multisystem autoinflammatory disease, Blau syndrome, Schnitzler syndrome, Muckle-Wells syndrome, and TNF receptor–associated periodic syndrome. Besides recurrent fevers, neutrophilia and serosal inflammation characterize these diseases. The fevers associated with these illnesses are dramatically reduced by blocking of IL-1β activity. Anticytokines therefore reduce fever in autoimmune and autoinflammatory diseases. Although fevers in autoinflammatory diseases are mediated by IL-1β, patients also respond to antipyretics.

MECHANISMS OF ANTIPYRETIC AGENTS The reduction of fever by lowering of the elevated hypothalamic set point is a direct function of reducing the level of PGE$_2$ in the thermoregulatory center. The synthesis of PGE$_2$ depends on the constitutively expressed enzyme cyclooxygenase. The substrate for cyclooxygenase is arachidonic acid released from the cell membrane, and this release is the rate-limiting step in the synthesis of PGE$_2$. Therefore, inhibitors of cyclooxygenase are potent antipyretics. The antipyretic potency of various drugs is directly correlated with the inhibition of brain cyclooxygenase. Acetaminophen is a poor cyclooxygenase inhibitor in peripheral tissue and lacks noteworthy anti-inflammatory activity; in the brain, however, acetaminophen is oxidized by the p450 cytochrome system, and the oxidized form inhibits cyclooxygenase activity. Moreover, in the brain, the inhibition of another enzyme, COX-3, by acetaminophen may account for the antipyretic effect of this agent. However, COX-3 is not found outside the CNS.

Oral aspirin and acetaminophen are equally effective in reducing fever in humans. Nonsteroidal anti-inflammatory drugs (NSAIDs) such as ibuprofen and specific inhibitors of COX-2 are also excellent antipyretics. Chronic, high-dose therapy with antipyretics such as aspirin or any NSAID does not reduce normal core body temperature. Thus, PGE$_2$ appears to play no role in normal thermoregulation.

As effective antipyretics, glucocorticoids act at two levels. First, similar to the cyclooxygenase inhibitors, glucocorticoids reduce PGE$_2$ synthesis by inhibiting the activity of phospholipase A$_2$, which is needed to release arachidonic acid from the cell membrane. Second, glucocorticoids block the transcription of the mRNA for the pyrogenic cytokines. Limited experimental evidence indicates that ibuprofen and COX-2 inhibitors reduce IL-1-induced IL-6 production and may contribute to the antipyretic activity of NSAIDs.

REGIMENS FOR THE TREATMENT OF FEVER The objectives in treating fever are first to reduce the elevated hypothalamic set point and second to facilitate heat loss. Reducing fever with antipyretics also reduces systemic symptoms of headache, myalgias, and arthralgias.

Oral aspirin and NSAIDs effectively reduce fever but can adversely affect platelets and the gastrointestinal tract. Therefore, acetaminophen is preferred to all of these agents as an antipyretic. In children, acetaminophen must be used because aspirin increases the risk of Reye's syndrome. If the patient cannot take oral antipyretics, parenteral preparations of NSAIDs and rectal suppository preparations of various antipyretics can be used.

Treatment of fever in some patients is highly recommended. Fever increases the demand for oxygen (i.e., for every increase of 1°C over 37°C, there is a 13% increase in oxygen consumption) and can aggravate preexisting cardiac, cerebrovascular, or pulmonary insufficiency. Elevated temperature can induce mental changes in patients with organic brain disease. Children with a history of febrile or nonfebrile seizure should be aggressively treated to reduce fever, although it is unclear what triggers the febrile seizure and there is no correlation between absolute temperature elevation and onset of a febrile seizure in susceptible children.

In hyperpyrexia, the use of cooling blankets facilitates the reduction of temperature; however, cooling blankets should not be used without oral antipyretics. In hyperpyretic patients with CNS disease or trauma, reducing core temperature mitigates the ill effects of high temperature on the brain.

TREATING HYPERTHERMIA A high core temperature in a patient with an appropriate history (e.g., environmental heat exposure or treatment with anticholinergic or neuroleptic drugs, tricyclic antidepressants, succinylcholine, or halothane) along with appropriate clinical findings (dry skin, hallucinations, delirium, pupil dilation, muscle rigidity, and/or elevated levels of creatine phosphokinase) suggests hyperthermia. Attempts to lower the already normal hypothalamic set point are of little use. Physical cooling with sponging, fans, cooling blankets, and even ice baths should be initiated immediately in conjunction with the administration of IV fluids and appropriate pharmacologic agents (see below). If insufficient cooling is achieved by external means, internal cooling can be achieved by gastric or peritoneal lavage with iced saline. In extreme circumstances, hemodialysis or even cardiopulmonary bypass with cooling of blood may be performed.

Malignant hyperthermia should be treated immediately with cessation of anesthesia and IV administration of dantrolene sodium. The recommended dose of dantrolene is 1–2.5 mg/kg given intravenously every 6 h for at least 24–48 h—until oral dantrolene can be administered, if needed. Procainamide should also be administered to patients with malignant hyperthermia because of the likelihood of ventricular fibrillation in this syndrome. Dantrolene at similar doses is indicated in the neuroleptic malignant syndrome and in drug-induced hyperthermia and may even be useful in the hyperthermia of the serotonin syndrome and thyrotoxicosis. The neuroleptic malignant syndrome may also be treated with bromocriptine, levodopa, amantadine, or nifedipine or by induction of muscle paralysis with curare and pancuronium. Tricyclic antidepressant overdose may be treated with physostigmine.

ACKNOWLEDGMENT
The substantial contributions of Jeffrey A. Gelfand to this chapter in previous editions are gratefully acknowledged.

FURTHER READINGS

De Koning HD et al: Beneficial response to anakinra and thalidomide in Schnitzler's syndrome. Ann Rheum Dis 65:542, 2006

Dinarello CA: Infection, fever, and exogenous and endogenous pyrogens: Some concepts have changed. J Endotoxin Res 10:202, 2004

Hawkins PN et al: Spectrum of clinical features in Muckle-Wells syndrome and response to anakinra. Arthritis Rheum 50:607, 2004

Hoffman HM et al: Prevention of cold-associated acute inflammation in familial cold autoinflammatory syndrome by interleukin-1 receptor antagonist. Lancet 364:1779, 2004

Keane J et al: Tuberculosis associated with infliximab, a tumor necrosis factor-α-neutralizing agent. N Engl J Med 345:1098, 2001

Pascual V et al: Role of interleukin-1 (IL-1) in the pathogenesis of systemic onset juvenile idiopathic arthritis and clinical response to IL-1 blockade. J Exp Med 201:1479, 2005

Simon A, van der Meer JW: Pathogenesis of familial periodic fever syndromes or hereditary autoinflammatory syndromes. Am J Physiol Regul Integr Comp Physiol 292:R86, 2007

——— et al: Beneficial response to interleukin-1 receptor antagonist in TRAPS. Am J Med 117:208, 2004

Wallis RS et al: Differential effects of TNF blockers on TB immunity. Ann Rheum Dis 64(Suppl3):132, 2005

——— et al: Granulomatous infectious diseases associated with tumor necrosis factor antagonists. Clin Infect Dis 38:1261, 2004

18 Fever and Rash
Elaine T. Kaye, Kenneth M. Kaye

The acutely ill patient with fever and rash often presents a diagnostic challenge for physicians. The distinctive appearance of an eruption in concert with a clinical syndrome may facilitate a prompt diagnosis and the institution of life-saving therapy or critical infection-control interventions. Representative images of many of the rashes discussed in this chapter are included in Chap. e5.

APPROACH TO THE PATIENT:
Fever and Rash

A thorough history of patients with fever and rash includes the following relevant information: immune status, medications taken within the previous month, specific travel history, immunization status, exposure to domestic pets and other animals, history of animal (including arthropod) bites, existence of cardiac abnormalities, presence of prosthetic material, recent exposure to ill individuals, and exposure to sexually transmitted diseases. The history should also include the site of onset of the rash and its direction and rate of spread.

A thorough physical examination entails close attention to the rash, with an assessment and precise definition of its salient features. First, it is critical to determine the *type* of lesions that make up the eruption. *Macules* are flat lesions defined by an area of changed color (i.e., a blanchable erythema). *Papules* are raised, solid lesions <5 mm in diameter; *plaques* are lesions >5 mm in diameter with a flat, plateau-like surface; and *nodules* are lesions >5 mm in diameter with a more rounded configuration. *Wheals* (urticaria, hives) are papules or plaques that are pale pink and may appear annular (ringlike) as they enlarge; classic (nonvasculitic) wheals are transient, lasting only 24–48 h in any defined area. *Vesicles* (<5 mm) and *bullae* (>5 mm) are circumscribed, elevated lesions containing fluid. *Pustules* are raised lesions containing purulent exudate; vesicular processes such as varicella or herpes simplex may evolve to pustules. *Nonpalpable purpura* is a flat lesion that is due to bleeding into the skin; if <3 mm in diameter, the purpuric lesions are termed *petechiae*; if >3 mm, they are termed *ecchymoses*. *Palpable purpura* is a raised lesion that is due to inflammation of the vessel wall (vasculitis) with subsequent hemorrhage. An *ulcer* is a defect in the skin extending at least into the upper layer of the dermis, and an *eschar* (tâche noire) is a necrotic lesion covered with a black crust.

Other pertinent features of rashes include their *configuration* (i.e., annular or target), the *arrangement* of their lesions, and their *distribution* (i.e., central or peripheral). For further discussion, see Chaps. 52, 54, and 115.

CLASSIFICATION OF RASH

This chapter reviews rashes that reflect systemic disease, but it does not include localized skin eruptions (i.e., cellulitis, impetigo) that may also be associated with fever (Chap. 119). Rashes are classified herein on the basis of the morphology and distribution of lesions. For practical purposes, this classification system is based on the most typical disease presentations. However, morphology may vary as rashes evolve, and the presentation of diseases with rashes is subject to many variations (Chap. 54). For instance, the classic petechial rash of Rocky Mountain spotted fever (RMSF; Chap. 167) may initially consist of blanchable erythematous macules distributed peripherally; at times, the rash associated with RMSF may not be predominantly acral, or a rash may not develop at all.

Diseases with fever and rash may be classified by type of eruption: centrally distributed maculopapular, peripheral, confluent desquamative erythematous, vesiculobullous, urticarial, nodular, purpuric, ulcerated, or eschar (Table 18-1). For a more detailed discussion of each disease associated with a rash, the reader is referred to the chapter dealing with that specific disease. (Reference chapters are cited in the text and listed in Table 18-1.)

TABLE 18-1 DISEASES ASSOCIATED WITH FEVER AND RASH

Disease	Etiology	Description	Group Affected/ Epidemiologic Factors	Clinical Syndrome	Chapter
Centrally Distributed Maculopapular Eruptions					
Acute meningococcemia[a]	—	—	—	—	136
Rubeola (measles, first disease)	Paramyxovirus	Discrete lesions that become confluent as rash spreads from hairline downward, sparing palms and soles; lasts ≥3 days; Koplik's spots	Nonimmune individuals	Cough, conjunctivitis, coryza, severe prostration	185
Rubella (German measles, third disease)	Togavirus	Spreads from hairline downward, clearing as it spreads; Forschheimer spots	Nonimmune individuals	Adenopathy, arthritis	186
Erythema infectiosum (fifth disease)	Human parvovirus B19	Bright-red "slapped-cheek" appearance followed by lacy reticular rash that waxes and wanes over 3 weeks; rarely, papular-purpuric "gloves-and-socks" syndrome on hands and feet	Most common in children aged 3–12 years; occurs in winter and spring	Mild fever; arthritis in adults; rash following resolution of fever	177
Exanthem subitum (roseola, sixth disease)	Human herpesvirus 6	Diffuse maculopapular eruption (sparing face); resolves within 2 days	Usually affects children <3 years old	Rash following resolution of fever; similar to Boston exanthem (echovirus 16)	175
Primary HIV infection	HIV	Nonspecific diffuse macules and papules; may be urticarial; oral or genital ulcers in some cases	Individuals recently infected with HIV	Pharyngitis, adenopathy, arthralgias	182
Infectious mononucleosis	Epstein-Barr virus	Diffuse maculopapular eruption (10–15% of cases; 90% if ampicillin is given); urticaria in some cases; periorbital edema (50%); palatal petechiae (25%)	Adolescents, young adults	Hepatosplenomegaly, pharyngitis, cervical lymphadenopathy, atypical lymphocytosis, heterophile antibody	174
Other viral exanthems	Echoviruses 2, 4, 9, 11, 16, 19, and 25; coxsackieviruses A9, B1, and B5; etc.	Skin findings mimicking rubella or measles	Affect children more commonly than adults	Nonspecific viral syndromes	184
Exanthematous drug-induced eruption	Drugs (antibiotics, anticonvulsants, diuretics, etc.)	Intensely pruritic, bright-red macules and papules, symmetric on trunk and extremities; may become confluent	Occurs 2–3 d after exposure in previously sensitized individuals; otherwise, after 2–3 weeks (but can occur anytime, even shortly after drug is discontinued)	Variable findings: fever and eosinophilia	56
Epidemic typhus	Rickettsia prowazekii	Maculopapular eruption appearing in axillae, spreading to trunk and later to extremities; usually spares face, palms, soles; evolves from blanchable macules to confluent eruption with petechiae; rash evanescent in recrudescent typhus (Brill-Zinsser disease)	Exposure to body lice; occurrence of recrudescent typhus as relapse after 30–50 years	Headache, myalgias; 10–40% mortality if untreated; milder clinical presentation in recrudescent form	167
Endemic (murine) typhus	Rickettsia typhi	Maculopapular eruption, usually sparing palms, soles	Exposure to rat or cat fleas	Headache, myalgias	167
Scrub typhus	Orientia tsutsugamushi	Diffuse macular rash starting on trunk; eschar at site of mite bite	Endemic in South Pacific, Australia, Asia; transmitted by mites	Headache, myalgias, regional adenopathy; mortality up to 30% if untreated	167
Rickettsial spotted fevers	Rickettsia conorii (boutonneuse fever), Rickettsia australis (North Queensland tick typhus), Rickettsia sibirica (Siberian tick typhus), and others	Eschar common at bite site; maculopapular (rarely, vesicular and petechial) eruption on proximal extremities, spreading to trunk and face	Exposure to ticks; R. conorii in Mediterranean region, India, Africa; R. australis in Australia; R. sibirica in Siberia, Mongolia	Headache, myalgias, regional adenopathy	167

(continued)

TABLE 18-1 DISEASES ASSOCIATED WITH FEVER AND RASH (CONTINUED)

Disease	Etiology	Description	Group Affected/ Epidemiologic Factors	Clinical Syndrome	Chapter
Human monocytotropic ehrlichiosis[b]	*Ehrlichia chaffeensis*	Maculopapular eruption (40% of cases), involves trunk and extremities; may be petechial	Tick-borne; most common in U.S. Southeast, southern Midwest, and mid-Atlantic regions	Headache, myalgias, leukopenia	167
Leptospirosis	*Leptospira interrogans*	Maculopapular eruption; conjunctivitis; scleral hemorrhage in some cases	Exposure to water contaminated with animal urine	Myalgias; aseptic meningitis; *fulminant form*: icterohemorrhagic fever (Weil's disease)	164
Lyme disease	*Borrelia burgdorferi*	Papule expanding to erythematous annular lesion with central clearing (erythema chronicum migrans or ECM; average diameter, 15 cm), sometimes with concentric rings, sometimes with indurated or vesicular center; multiple secondary ECM lesions in some cases	Bite of tick vector	Headache, myalgias, chills, photophobia occurring acutely; CNS disease, myocardial disease, arthritis weeks to months later in some cases	166
Typhoid fever	*Salmonella typhi*	Transient, blanchable erythematous macules and papules, 2–4 mm, usually on trunk (rose spots)	Ingestion of contaminated food or water (rare in U.S.)	Variable abdominal pain and diarrhea; headache, myalgias, hepatosplenomegaly	146
Dengue fever[c]	Dengue virus (4 serotypes; flaviviruses)	Rash in 50% of cases; initially diffuse flushing; midway through illness, onset of maculopapular rash, which begins on trunk and spreads centrifugally to extremities and face; pruritus, hyperesthesia in some cases; after defervescence, petechiae on extremities in some cases	Occurs in tropics and subtropics; transmitted by mosquito	Headache, musculoskeletal pain ("breakbone fever"); leukopenia; occasionally biphasic ("saddleback") fever	189
Rat-bite fever (sodoku)	*Spirillum minus*	Eschar at bite site; then blotchy violaceous or red-brown rash involving trunk and extremities	Rat bite; primarily found in Asia; rare in U.S.	Regional adenopathy, recurrent fevers if untreated	...
Relapsing fever	*Borrelia* species	Central rash at end of febrile episode; petechiae in some cases	Exposure to ticks or body lice	Recurrent fever, headache, myalgias, hepatosplenomegaly	165
Erythema marginatum (rheumatic fever)	Group A *Streptococcus*	Erythematous annular papules and plaques occurring as polycyclic lesions in waves over trunk, proximal extremities; evolving and resolving within hours	Patients with rheumatic fever	Pharyngitis preceding polyarthritis, carditis, subcutaneous nodules, chorea	315
Systemic lupus erythematosus	Autoimmune disease	Macular and papular erythema, often in sun-exposed areas; discoid lupus lesions (local atrophy, scale, pigmentary changes); periungual telangiectasis; malar rash; vasculitis sometimes causing urticaria, palpable purpura; oral erosions in some cases	Most common in young to middle-aged women; flares precipitated by sun exposure	Arthritis; cardiac, pulmonary, renal, hematologic, and vasculitic disease	313
Still's disease	Autoimmune disease	Transient 2- to 5-mm erythematous papules appearing at height of fever on trunk, proximal extremities; lesions evanescent	Children and young adults	High spiking fever, polyarthritis, splenomegaly; erythrocyte sedimentation rate, >100 mm/h	331
Arcanobacterial pharyngitis	*Arcanobacterium (Corynebacterium) haemolyticum*	Diffuse, erythematous, maculopapular eruption involving trunk and proximal extremities; may desquamate	Children and young adults	Exudative pharyngitis, lymphadenopathy	131
Peripheral Eruptions					
Chronic meningococcemia, disseminated gonococcal infection[a], human parvovirus B19 infection[g]	—	—	—	—	136, 137, 177
Rocky Mountain spotted fever	*Rickettsia rickettsii*	Rash beginning on wrists and ankles and spreading centripetally; appears on palms and soles later in disease; lesion evolution from blanchable macules to petechiae	Tick vector; widespread but more common in southeastern and southwest-central U.S.	Headache, myalgias, abdominal pain; mortality up to 40% if untreated	167

(continued)

TABLE 18-1   DISEASES ASSOCIATED WITH FEVER AND RASH (CONTINUED)

Disease	Etiology	Description	Group Affected/ Epidemiologic Factors	Clinical Syndrome	Chapter
Secondary syphilis	*Treponema pallidum*	Coincident primary chancre in 10% of cases; copper-colored, scaly papular eruption, diffuse but prominent on palms and soles; rash never vesicular in adults; condyloma latum, mucous patches, and alopecia in some cases	Sexually transmitted	Fever, constitutional symptoms	162
Atypical measles	Paramyxovirus	Maculopapular eruption beginning on distal extremities and spreading centripetally; may evolve into vesicles or petechiae; edema of extremities; Koplik's spots absent	Individuals contracting measles who received killed measles vaccine in 1963–1967 in U.S. without subsequent live vaccine	Headache, nodular pneumonia	185
Hand-foot-and-mouth disease	Coxsackievirus A16 most common cause	Tender vesicles, erosions in mouth; 0.25-cm papules on hands and feet with rim of erythema evolving into tender vesicles	Summer and fall; primarily children <10 years old; multiple family members	Transient fever	184
Erythema multiforme	Drugs, infection, idiopathic causes	Target lesions (central erythema surrounded by area of clearing and another rim of erythema) up to 2 cm; symmetric on knees, elbows, palms, soles; may become diffuse; may involve mucosal surfaces; life-threatening in maximal form (Stevens-Johnson syndrome)	Drug intake (i.e., sulfa, phenytoin, penicillin); herpes simplex virus or *Mycoplasma pneumoniae* infection	Varies with predisposing factor	—[d]
Rat-bite fever (Haverhill fever)	*Streptobacillus moniliformis*	Maculopapular eruption over palms, soles, and extremities; tends to be more severe at joints; eruption sometimes becoming generalized; may be purpuric; may desquamate	Rat bite, ingestion of contaminated food	Myalgias; arthritis (50%); fever recurrence in some cases	…
Bacterial endocarditis	*Streptococcus, Staphylococcus*, etc.	*Subacute course*: Osler's nodes (tender pink nodules on finger or toe pads); petechiae on skin and mucosa; splinter hemorrhages. *Acute course (Staphylococcus aureus)*: Janeway lesions (painless erythematous or hemorrhagic macules, usually on palms and soles)	Abnormal heart valve, intravenous drug use	New heart murmur	118

Confluent Desquamative Erythemas

Disease	Etiology	Description	Group Affected/ Epidemiologic Factors	Clinical Syndrome	Chapter
Scarlet fever (second disease)	Group A *Streptococcus* (pyrogenic exotoxins A, B, C)	Diffuse blanchable erythema beginning on face and spreading to trunk and extremities; circumoral pallor; "sandpaper" texture to skin; accentuation of linear erythema in skin folds (Pastia's lines); enanthem of white evolving into red "strawberry" tongue; desquamation in second week	Most common in children aged 2–10 years; usually follows group A streptococcal pharyngitis	Fever, pharyngitis, headache	130
Kawasaki disease	Idiopathic causes	Rash similar to scarlet fever (scarlatiniform) or erythema multiforme; fissuring of lips, strawberry tongue; conjunctivitis; edema of hands, feet; desquamation later in disease	Children <8 years	Cervical adenopathy, pharyngitis, coronary artery vasculitis	54, 319
Streptococcal toxic shock syndrome	Group A *Streptococcus* (associated with pyrogenic exotoxin A and/ or B or certain M types)	When present, rash often scarlatiniform	May occur in setting of severe group A streptococcal infections, such as necrotizing fasciitis, bacteremia, pneumonia	Multiorgan failure, hypotension; 30% mortality rate	130
Staphylococcal toxic shock syndrome	*S. aureus* (toxic shock syndrome toxin 1, enterotoxin B or C)	Diffuse erythema involving palms; pronounced erythema of mucosal surfaces; conjunctivitis; desquamation 7–10 days into illness	Colonization with toxin-producing *S. aureus*	Fever >39°C (102°F), hypotension, multiorgan dysfunction	129
Staphylococcal scalded-skin syndrome	*S. aureus*, phage group II	Diffuse tender erythema, often with bullae and desquamation; Nikolsky's sign	Colonization with toxin-producing *S. aureus*; occurs in children <10 years old (termed "Ritter's disease" in neonates) or adults with renal dysfunction	Irritability; nasal or conjunctival secretions	129

(continued)

TABLE 18-1 DISEASES ASSOCIATED WITH FEVER AND RASH (CONTINUED)

Disease	Etiology	Description	Group Affected/ Epidemiologic Factors	Clinical Syndrome	Chapter
Exfoliative erythroderma syndrome	Underlying psoriasis, eczema, drug eruption, mycosis fungoides	Diffuse erythema (often scaling) interspersed with lesions of underlying condition	Usually occurs in adults over age 50; more common in men	Fever, chills (i.e., difficulty with thermoregulation); lymphadenopathy	53, 56
Stevens-Johnson syndrome (SJS), toxic epidermal necrolysis (TEN)	Drugs, other causes (infection, neoplasm, graft-vs.-host disease)	Diffuse erythema or target-like lesions progressing to bullae, with sloughing and necrosis of entire epidermis; Nikolsky's sign. *TEN:* maximal form of SJS. *SJS:* maximal form of erythema multiforme	Uncommon in children; more common in patients with HIV infection or graft-vs.-host disease	Dehydration, sepsis sometimes resulting from lack of normal skin integrity; 25% mortality	56
Vesiculobullous Eruptions					
Hand-foot-and-mouth syndrome[e]; staphylococcal scalded-skin syndrome; toxic epidermal necrolysis[f]	—	—	—	—	—[d]
Varicella (chickenpox)	Varicella-zoster virus	Macules (2–3 mm) evolving into papules, then vesicles (sometimes umbilicated), on an erythematous base ("dewdrops on a rose petal"); pustules then forming and crusting; lesions appearing in crops; may involve scalp, mouth; intensely pruritic	Usually affects children; 10% of adults susceptible; most common in late winter and spring	Malaise; generally mild disease in healthy children; more severe disease with complications in adults and immunocompromised children	173
Pseudomonas "hot-tub" folliculitis	*Pseudomonas aeruginosa*	Pruritic, erythematous follicular, papular, vesicular, or pustular lesions that may involve axillae, buttocks, abdomen, and especially areas occluded by bathing suits; can manifest as tender isolated nodules on palmar or plantar surfaces (the latter designated "*Pseudomonas* hot-foot syndrome")	Bathers in hot tubs or swimming pools; occurs in outbreaks	Earache, sore eyes and/or throat; generally self-limited	145
Variola (smallpox)	Variola major virus	Red macules on tongue, palate evolving to papules and vesicles; skin macules evolving to papules, then vesicles, then pustules over 1 week, with subsequent lesion crusting; lesions initially appearing on face and spreading centrifugally from trunk to extremities; differs from varicella in that (1) skin lesions in any given area are at same stage of development and (2) there is a prominent distribution of lesions on face and extremities (including palms, soles) as opposed to prominent rash on trunk	Nonimmune individuals exposed to smallpox	Prodrome of fever, headache, backache, myalgias; vomiting in 50% of cases	214
Primary herpes simplex virus (HSV) infection	HSV	Erythema rapidly followed by hallmark *grouped vesicles* that may evolve into pustules; painful lesions that may ulcerate, especially on mucosal surfaces; lesions at site of inoculation: commonly gingivostomatitis for HSV-1 and genital lesions for HSV-2; recurrent disease milder (e.g., herpes labialis does not involve oral mucosa)	Primary infection most common in children and young adults for HSV-1 and in sexually active young adults for HSV-2; no fever in recurrent infection	Regional lymphadenopathy	172

(continued)

TABLE 18-1   DISEASES ASSOCIATED WITH FEVER AND RASH (CONTINUED)

Disease	Etiology	Description	Group Affected/ Epidemiologic Factors	Clinical Syndrome	Chapter
Disseminated her-pesvirus infection	Varicella-zoster virus or HSV	Generalized vesicles that can evolve to pustules and ulcerations; individual lesions similar for varicella-zoster and HSV. *Zoster cutaneous dissemination*: >25 lesions extending outside involved dermatome. *HSV*: extensive, progressive mucocutaneous lesions in some cases; HSV lesions sometimes disseminate in eczematous skin (eczema herpeticum); HSV visceral dissemination may occur with only limited skin lesions	Immunosuppressed individuals, eczema	Visceral organ involvement (especially liver) in some cases	172, 173, 376
Rickettsialpox	*Rickettsia akari*	Eschar found at site of mite bite; generalized rash involving face, trunk, extremities; may involve palms and soles; <100 papules and plaques (2–10 mm); tops of lesions develop vesicles that may evolve into pustules	Seen in urban settings; transmitted by mouse mites	Headache, myalgias, regional adenopathy; mild disease	167
Disseminated *Vibrio vulnificus* infection	*V. vulnificus*	Erythematous lesions evolving into hemorrhagic bullae and then into necrotic ulcers	Patients with cirrhosis, diabetes, renal failure; exposure by ingestion of contaminated saltwater seafood	Hypotension; 50% mortality	149
Ecthyma gangrenosum	*P. aeruginosa*, other gram-negative rods, fungi	Indurated plaque evolving into hemorrhagic bulla or pustule that sloughs, resulting in eschar formation; erythematous halo; most common in axillary, groin, perianal regions	Usually affects neutropenic patients; occurs in up to 28% of individuals with *Pseudomonas* bacteremia	Clinical signs of sepsis	145
Urticarial Eruptions					
Urticarial vasculitis	Serum sickness, often due to infection (including hepatitis B viral, enteroviral, parasitic), drugs (including penicillins, sulfonamides, salicylates, barbiturates); connective tissue disease; idiopathic causes	Erythematous, circumscribed areas of edema; occasionally indurated; pruritic or burning; lesions sometimes purpuric; individual lesions lasting up to 5 days	In serum sickness, occurs 8–14 days after antigen exposure in nonsensitized individuals; may occur within 36 h in sensitized individuals	Malaise, lymphadenopathy, myalgias, arthralgias	319[d]
Nodular Eruptions					
Disseminated infection	Fungi (e.g., candidiasis, histoplasmosis, cryptococcosis, sporotrichosis, coccidioidomycosis); mycobacteria	Subcutaneous nodules (up to 3 cm); fluctuance, draining common with mycobacteria; necrotic nodules (extremities, periorbital or nasal regions) common with *Aspergillus*, *Mucor*	Immunocompromised hosts (i.e., bone marrow transplant recipients, patients undergoing chemotherapy, HIV-infected patients, alcoholics)	Features vary with organism	—[d]
Erythema nodosum (septal panniculitis)	Infections (e.g., streptococcal, fungal, mycobacterial, yersinial); drugs (e.g., sulfas, penicillins, oral contraceptives); sarcoidosis; idiopathic causes	Large, violaceous, nonulcerative, subcutaneous nodules; exquisitely tender; usually on lower legs but also on upper extremities	More common in females 15–30 years old	Arthralgias (50%); features vary with associated condition	—[d]
Sweet's syndrome (acute febrile neutrophilic dermatosis)	Yersinial infection; lymphoproliferative disorders; idiopathic causes	Tender red or blue edematous nodules giving impression of vesiculation; usually on face, neck, upper extremities; when on lower extremities, may mimic erythema nodosum	More common in women and in persons 30–60 years old; 20% of cases associated with malignancy (men and women equally affected in this group)	Headache, arthralgias, leukocytosis	54
Bacillary angiomatosis	*Bartonella henselae* or *Bartonella quintana*	Many forms, including erythematous, smooth vascular nodules; friable, exophytic lesions; erythematous plaques (may be dry, scaly); subcutaneous nodules (may be erythematous)	Usually in HIV infection	Peliosis of liver and spleen in some cases; lesions may involve multiple organs; bacteremia	153

(continued)

TABLE 18-1 **DISEASES ASSOCIATED WITH FEVER AND RASH (CONTINUED)** 127

Disease	Etiology	Description	Group Affected/ Epidemiologic Factors	Clinical Syndrome	Chapter
Purpuric Eruptions					
Rocky Mountain spotted fever, rat-bite fever, endocarditis[e]; epidemic typhus[g]; dengue fever[c]; human parvovirus B19 infection[g]	—	—	—	—	—[d]
Acute meningococcemia	*Neisseria meningitidis*	Initially pink maculopapular lesions evolving into petechiae; petechiae rapidly becoming numerous, sometimes enlarging and becoming vesicular; trunk, extremities most commonly involved; may appear on face, hands, feet; may include purpura fulminans reflecting disseminated intravascular coagulation (see below)	Most common in children, individuals with asplenia or terminal complement component deficiency (C5-C8)	Hypotension, meningitis (sometimes preceded by upper respiratory infection)	136
Purpura fulminans	Severe disseminated intravascular coagulation	Large ecchymoses with sharply irregular shapes evolving into hemorrhagic bullae and then into black necrotic lesions	Individuals with sepsis (e.g., involving *N. meningitidis*), malignancy, or massive trauma; asplenic patients at high risk for sepsis	Hypotension	136, 265
Chronic meningococcemia	*N. meningitidis*	Variety of recurrent eruptions, including pink maculopapular; nodular (usually on lower extremities); petechial (sometimes developing vesicular centers); purpuric areas with pale blue-gray centers	Individuals with complement deficiencies	Fevers, sometimes intermittent; arthritis, myalgias, headache	136
Disseminated gonococcal infection	*Neisseria gonorrhoeae*	Papules (1–5 mm) evolving over 1–2 days into hemorrhagic pustules with gray necrotic centers; hemorrhagic bullae occurring rarely; lesions (usually fewer than 40) distributed peripherally near joints (more commonly on upper extremities)	Sexually active individuals (more often females), some with complement deficiency	Low-grade fever, tenosynovitis, arthritis	137
Enteroviral petechial rash	Usually echovirus 9 or coxsackievirus A9	Disseminated petechial lesions (may also be maculopapular, vesicular, or urticarial)	Often occurs in outbreaks	Pharyngitis, headache; aseptic meningitis with echovirus 9	184
Viral hemorrhagic fever	Arboviruses and arenaviruses	Petechial rash	Residence in or travel to endemic areas or other virus exposure	Triad of fever, shock, hemorrhage from mucosa or gastrointestinal tract	189, 190
Thrombotic thrombocytopenic purpura/hemolytic-uremic syndrome	Idiopathic, *Escherichia coli* O157:H7 (Shiga toxin), drugs	Petechiae	Individuals with *E. coli* O157:H7 gastroenteritis (especially children), cancer chemotherapy, HIV infection, autoimmune diseases; pregnant/postpartum women	Fever (not always present), hemolytic anemia, thrombocytopenia, renal dysfunction, neurologic dysfunction; coagulation studies normal	54, 101, 109, 143, 147
Cutaneous small-vessel vasculitis (leukocytoclastic vasculitis)	Infections (including group A *Streptococcus*, viral hepatitis), drugs, chemicals, food allergens, idiopathic causes	Palpable purpuric lesions appearing in crops on legs or other dependent areas; may become vesicular or ulcerative; usually resolve over 3–4 weeks	Occurs in a wide spectrum of diseases, including connective tissue disease, cryoglobulinemia, malignancy, Henoch-Schönlein purpura (HSP); more common in children	Fever, malaise, arthralgias, myalgias; systemic vasculitis in some cases; renal, joint, and gastrointestinal involvement commonly seen in HSP	54

(continued)

TABLE 18-1 **DISEASES ASSOCIATED WITH FEVER AND RASH (CONTINUED)**

Disease	Etiology	Description	Group Affected/ Epidemiologic Factors	Clinical Syndrome	Chapter
Eruptions with Ulcers and/or Eschars					
Scrub typhus, rickettsial spotted fevers, rat-bite fever[g]; rickettsialpox, ecthyma gangrenosum[h]	—	—	—	—	—[d]
Tularemia	*Francisella tularensis*	Ulceroglandular form: erythematous, tender papule evolves into necrotic, tender ulcer with raised borders; in 35% of cases, eruptions (maculopapular, vesiculopapular, acneiform, urticarial, erythema nodosum, or erythema multiforme) may occur	Exposure to ticks, biting flies, infected animals	Fever, headache, lymphadenopathy	151
Anthrax	*Bacillus anthracis*	Pruritic papule enlarging and evolving into a 1- by 3-cm painless ulcer surrounded by vesicles and then developing a central eschar with edema; residual scar	Exposure to infected animals or animal products or other exposure to anthrax spores	Lymphadenopathy, headache	214

[a]See "Purpuric eruptions."
[b]In human granulocytotropic ehrlichiosis, or anaplasmosis (caused by *Anaplasma phagocytophila*; most common in the upper midwestern and northeastern regions of the United States), rash is rare.
[c]See "Viral hemorrhagic fever" under "Purpuric eruptions" for dengue hemorrhagic fever/ dengue shock syndrome.

[d]See etiology-specific chapters.
[e]See "Peripheral eruptions."
[f]See "Confluent desquamative erythemas."
[g]See "Centrally distributed maculopapular eruptions."
[h]See "Vesiculobullous eruptions."

CENTRALLY DISTRIBUTED MACULOPAPULAR ERUPTIONS

Centrally distributed rashes, in which lesions are primarily truncal, are the most common type of eruption. The rash of *rubeola* (measles) starts at the hairline 2–3 days into the illness and moves down the body, sparing the palms and soles (Chap. 185). It begins as discrete erythematous lesions, which become confluent as the rash spreads. Koplik's spots (1- to 2-mm white or bluish lesions with an erythematous halo on the buccal mucosa) are pathognomonic for measles and are generally seen during the first 2 days of symptoms. They should not be confused with Fordyce's spots (ectopic sebaceous glands), which have no erythematous halos and are found in the mouth of healthy individuals. Koplik's spots may briefly overlap with the measles exanthem.

Rubella (German measles) also spreads from the hairline downward; unlike that of measles, however, the rash of rubella tends to clear from originally affected areas as it migrates, and it may be pruritic (Chap. 186). Forchheimer spots (palatal petechiae) may develop but are nonspecific since they also develop in mononucleosis (Chap. 174) and scarlet fever (Chap. 130). Postauricular and suboccipital adenopathy and arthritis are common among adults with German measles. Exposure of pregnant women to ill individuals should be avoided, as rubella causes severe congenital abnormalities. Numerous strains of enteroviruses (Chap. 184), primarily echoviruses and coxsackieviruses, cause nonspecific syndromes of fever and eruptions that may mimic rubella or measles. Patients with infectious mononucleosis caused by Epstein-Barr virus (Chap. 174) or with primary infection caused by HIV (Chap. 182) may exhibit pharyngitis, lymphadenopathy, and a nonspecific maculopapular exanthem.

The rash of *erythema infectiosum* (fifth disease), which is caused by human parvovirus B19, primarily affects children 3–12 years old; it develops after fever has resolved as a bright blanchable erythema on the cheeks ("slapped cheeks") with perioral pallor (Chap. 177). A more diffuse rash (often pruritic) appears the next day on the trunk and extremities and then rapidly develops into a lacy reticular eruption that may wax and wane (especially with temperature change) over 3 weeks. Adults with fifth disease often have arthritis, and fetal hydrops can develop in association with this condition in pregnant women.

Exanthem subitum (roseola) is caused by human herpesvirus 6 and is most common among children <3 years of age (Chap. 175). As in erythema infectiosum, the rash usually appears after fever has subsided. It consists of 2- to 3-mm rose-pink macules and papules that rarely coalesce, occur initially on the trunk and sometimes on the extremities (sparing the face), and fade within 2 days.

Although drug reactions have many manifestations, including urticaria, exanthematous *drug-induced eruptions* (Chap. 56) are most common and are often difficult to distinguish from viral exanthems. Eruptions elicited by drugs are usually more intensely erythematous and pruritic than viral exanthems, but this distinction is not reliable. A history of new medications and an absence of prostration may help to distinguish a drug-related rash from an eruption of another etiology. Rashes may persist for up to 2 weeks after administration of the offending agent is discontinued. Certain populations are more prone than others to drug rashes. Of HIV-infected patients, 50–60% develop a rash in response to sulfa drugs; 90% of patients with mononucleosis due to Epstein-Barr virus develop a rash when given ampicillin.

Rickettsial illnesses (Chap. 167) should be considered in the evaluation of individuals with centrally distributed maculopapular eruptions. The usual setting for *epidemic typhus* is a site of war or natural disaster in which people are exposed to body lice. A diagnosis of recrudescent typhus should be considered in European immigrants to the United States. However, an indigenous form of typhus, presumably transmitted by flying squirrels, has been reported in the southeastern United States. *Endemic typhus* or *leptospirosis* (the latter caused by a spirochete; Chap. 164) may be seen in urban environments where rodents proliferate. Outside the United States, other rickettsial diseases cause a spotted-fever syndrome and should be considered in residents of or travelers to endemic areas. Similarly, *typhoid fever*, a nonrickettsial disease caused by *Salmonella typhi* (Chap. 146), is usually acquired during travel outside the United States. Dengue fever, caused by a mosquito-transmitted flavivirus, occurs in tropical and subtropical regions of the world (Chap. 189).

Some centrally distributed maculopapular eruptions have distinctive features. Erythema chronicum migrans (ECM), the rash of Lyme disease (Chap. 166), typically manifests as singular or multiple annular plaques. Untreated ECM lesions usually fade within a month but may persist for more than a year. *Erythema marginatum*, the rash of acute rheumatic fever (Chap. 315), has a distinctive pattern of enlarging and shifting transient annular lesions.

Collage vascular diseases may cause fever and rash. Patients with *systemic lupus erythematosus* (Chap. 313) typically develop a sharply defined, erythematous eruption in a butterfly distribution on the cheeks (malar rash) as well as many other skin manifestations. *Still's disease* (Chap. 331) manifests as an evanescent salmon-colored rash on the trunk and proximal extremities that coincides with fever spikes.

PERIPHERAL ERUPTIONS

These rashes are alike in that they are most prominent peripherally or begin in peripheral (acral) areas before spreading centripetally. Early diagnosis and therapy are critical in RMSF (Chap. 167) because of its grave prognosis if untreated. Lesions evolve from macular to petechial, start on the wrists and ankles, spread centripetally, and appear on the palms and soles only later in the disease. The rash of *secondary syphilis* (Chap. 162), which may be generalized but is prominent on the palms and soles, should be considered in the differential diagnosis of pityriasis rosea, especially in sexually active patients. *Atypical measles* (Chap. 185) is seen in individuals contracting measles who received the killed measles vaccine between 1963 and 1967 in the United States and who were not subsequently protected with the live vaccine. *Hand-foot-and-mouth disease* (Chap. 184), most commonly caused by coxsackievirus A16, is distinguished by tender vesicles distributed peripherally and in the mouth; outbreaks commonly occur within families. The classic target lesions of *erythema multiforme* (EM) appear symmetrically on the elbows, knees, palms, soles, and face. In severe cases, these lesions spread diffusely and involve mucosal surfaces. Stevens-Johnson syndrome is considered a maximal form of erythema multiforme and is life-threatening. Lesions may develop on the hands and feet in *endocarditis* (Chap. 118).

CONFLUENT DESQUAMATIVE ERYTHEMAS

These eruptions consist of diffuse erythema frequently followed by desquamation. The eruptions caused by group A *Streptococcus* or *Staphylococcus aureus* are toxin mediated. *Scarlet fever* (Chap. 130) usually follows pharyngitis; patients have a facial flush, a "strawberry" tongue, and accentuated petechiae in body folds (Pastia's lines). *Kawasaki disease* (Chaps. 54 and 319) presents in the pediatric population as fissuring of the lips, a strawberry tongue, conjunctivitis, adenopathy, and sometimes cardiac abnormalities. *Streptococcal toxic shock syndrome* (Chap. 130) manifests with hypotension, multiorgan failure, and often a severe group A streptococcal infection (e.g., necrotizing fasciitis). *Staphylococcal toxic shock syndrome* (Chap. 129) also presents with hypotension and multiorgan failure, but usually only *S. aureus* colonization—not a severe *S. aureus* infection—is documented. *Staphylococcal scalded-skin syndrome* (Chap. 129) is seen primarily in children and in immunocompromised adults. Generalized erythema is often evident during the prodrome of fever and malaise; profound tenderness of the skin is distinctive. In the exfoliative stage, the skin can be induced to form bullae with light lateral pressure (Nikolsky's sign). In a mild form, a scarlatiniform eruption mimics scarlet fever, but the patient does not exhibit a strawberry tongue or circumoral pallor. In contrast to the staphylococcal scalded-skin syndrome, in which the cleavage plane is superficial in the epidermis, *toxic epidermal necrolysis* (Chap. 56), a maximal variant of Stevens-Johnson syndrome, involves sloughing of the entire epidermis, resulting in severe disease. *Exfoliative erythroderma syndrome* (Chaps. 53 and 56) is a serious reaction associated with systemic toxicity that is often due to eczema, psoriasis, mycosis fungoides, or a severe drug reaction.

VESICULOBULLOUS ERUPTIONS

Varicella (Chap. 173) is highly contagious, often occurring in winter or spring. At any point in time, within a given region of the body, varicella lesions are in different stages of development. In immunocompromised hosts, varicella vesicles may lack the characteristic erythematous base or may appear hemorrhagic. Lesions of *Pseudomonas* "hot-tub" folliculitis (Chap. 145) are also pruritic and may appear similar to those of varicella. However, hot-tub folliculitis generally occurs in outbreaks after bathing in hot tubs or swimming pools, and lesions occur in regions occluded by bathing suits. Lesions of *variola* (smallpox; Chap. 214) also appear similar to those of varicella but are all at the same stage of development in a given region of the body. Variola lesions are most prominent on the face and extremities, while varicella lesions are most prominent on the trunk. Herpes simplex virus infection (Chap. 172) is characterized by hallmark grouped vesicles on an erythematous base. Primary herpes infection is accompanied by fever and toxicity, while recurrent disease is milder. *Rickettsialpox* (Chap. 167) is often documented in urban settings and is characterized by vesicles. It can be distinguished from varicella by an eschar at the site of the mouse-mite bite and the papule/plaque base of each vesicle. Disseminated *Vibrio vulnificus* infection (Chap. 149) or *ecthyma gangrenosum* due to *Pseudomonas aeruginosa* (Chap. 145) should be considered in immunosuppressed individuals with sepsis and hemorrhagic bullae.

URTICARIAL ERUPTIONS

Individuals with classic urticaria ("hives") usually have a hypersensitivity reaction without associated fever. In the presence of fever, urticarial eruptions are usually due to *urticarial vasculitis* (Chap. 319). Unlike individual lesions of classic urticaria, which last up to 48 h, these lesions may last up to 5 days. Etiologies include serum sickness (often induced by drugs such as penicillins, sulfas, salicylates, or barbiturates), connective-tissue disease (e.g., systemic lupus erythematosus or Sjögren's syndrome), and infection (e.g., with hepatitis B virus, enteroviruses, or parasites). Malignancy may be associated with fever and chronic urticaria (Chap. 54).

NODULAR ERUPTIONS

In immunocompromised hosts, nodular lesions often represent disseminated infection. Patients with disseminated *candidiasis* (often due to *Candida tropicalis*) may have a triad of fever, myalgias, and eruptive nodules (Chap. 196). Disseminated *cryptococcosis* lesions (Chap. 195) may resemble molluscum contagiosum (Chap. 176). Necrosis of nodules should raise the suspicion of *aspergillosis* (Chap. 197) or *mucormycosis* (Chap. 198). *Erythema nodosum* presents with exquisitely tender nodules on the lower extremities. *Sweet's syndrome* (Chap. 54) should be considered in individuals with multiple nodules and plaques, often so edematous that they give the appearance of vesicles or bullae. Sweet's syndrome may affect either healthy individuals or persons with lymphoproliferative disease.

PURPURIC ERUPTIONS

Acute meningococcemia (Chap. 136) classically presents in children as a petechial eruption, but initial lesions may appear as blanchable macules or urticaria. RMSF should be considered in the differential diagnosis of acute meningococcemia. *Echovirus 9 infection* (Chap. 184) may mimic acute meningococcemia; patients should be treated as if they have bacterial sepsis since prompt differentiation of these conditions may be impossible. Large ecchymotic areas of *purpura fulminans* (Chaps. 136 and 265) reflect severe underlying disseminated intravascular coagulation, which may be due to infectious or noninfectious causes. The lesions of *chronic meningococcemia* (Chap. 136) may have a variety of morphologies, including petechial. Purpuric nodules may develop on the legs and resemble erythema nodosum but lack its exquisite tenderness. Lesions of *disseminated gonococcemia* (Chap. 137) are distinctive, sparse, countable hemorrhagic pustules, usually located near joints. The lesions of chronic meningococcemia and those of gonococcemia may be indistinguishable in terms of appearance and distribution. *Viral hemorrhagic fever* (Chaps. 189 and 190) should be considered in patients with an appropriate travel history and a petechial rash. *Thrombotic thrombocytopenic purpura* (Chaps. 54, 101, and 109) and *hemolytic-uremic syndrome* (Chaps. 109, 143, and 147) are closely related and are noninfectious causes of fever and petechiae. *Cutaneous small-vessel vasculitis* (leukocytoclastic vasculitis) typically manifests as palpable purpura and has a wide variety of causes (Chap. 54).

ERUPTIONS WITH ULCERS OR ESCHARS

The presence of an ulcer or eschar in the setting of a more widespread eruption can provide an important diagnostic clue. For example, the presence of an eschar may suggest the diagnosis of scrub typhus or rickettsialpox (Chap. 167) in the appropriate setting. In other illnesses (e.g., anthrax; Chap. 214), an ulcer or eschar may be the only skin manifestation.

FURTHER READINGS

CHERRY JD: Contemporary infectious exanthems. Clin Infect Dis 16:199, 1993

———: Cutaneous manifestations of systemic infections, in *Textbook of Pediatric Infectious Diseases*, vol. 1, 4th ed, RD Feigin, JD Cherry (eds). Philadelphia, Saunders, 1998, pp 713–737

EICHENFIELD LF et al (eds): *Textbook of Neonatal Dermatology*. Philadelphia, Saunders, 2001

FREEDBERG IM et al (eds): *Fitzpatrick's Dermatology in General Medicine*, 6th ed. New York, McGraw-Hill, 2003

LEVIN S, GOODMAN LJ: An approach to acute fever and rash (AFR) in the adult. Curr Clin Top Infect Dis 15:19, 1995

PALLER AS, MANCINI AJ (eds): *Hurwitz Clinical Pediatric Dermatology*, 3d ed. Philadelphia, Elsevier Saunders, 2006

SCHLOSSBERG D: Fever and rash. Infect Dis Clin North Am 10:101, 1996

WEBER DJ et al: The acutely ill patient with fever and rash, in *Principles and Practice of Infectious Diseases*, vol 1, 6th ed, GL Mandell et al (eds). Philadelphia, Elsevier Churchill Livingstone, 2005, pp 729–746

WENNER HA: Virus diseases associated with cutaneous eruptions. Prog Med Virol 16:269, 1973

WOLFF K, JOHNSON RAJ: *Fitzpatrick's Color Atlas and Synopsis of Clinical Dermatology*, 5th ed. New York, McGraw-Hill, 2005

19 Fever of Unknown Origin
Jeffrey A. Gelfand, Michael V. Callahan

DEFINITION AND CLASSIFICATION

Fever of unknown origin (FUO) was defined by Petersdorf and Beeson in 1961 as (1) temperatures of >38.3°C (>101°F) on several occasions; (2) a duration of fever of >3 weeks; and (3) failure to reach a diagnosis despite 1 week of inpatient investigation. While this classification has stood for more than 30 years, Durack and Street have proposed a new system for classification of FUO: (1) classic FUO; (2) nosocomial FUO; (3) neutropenic FUO; and (4) FUO associated with HIV infection.

Classic FUO corresponds closely to the earlier definition of FUO, differing only with regard to the prior requirement for 1 week's study in the hospital. The newer definition is broader, stipulating three outpatient visits or 3 days in the hospital without elucidation of a cause or 1 week of "intelligent and invasive" ambulatory investigation. In *nosocomial FUO*, a temperature of ≥38.3°C (≥101°F) develops on several occasions in a hospitalized patient who is receiving acute care and in whom infection was not manifest or incubating on admission. Three days of investigation, including at least 2 days' incubation of cultures, is the minimum requirement for this diagnosis. *Neutropenic FUO* is defined as a temperature of ≥38.3°C (≥101°F) on several occasions in a patient whose neutrophil count is <500/μL or is expected to fall to that level in 1–2 days. The diagnosis of neutropenic FUO is invoked if a specific cause is not identified after 3 days of investigation, including at least 2 days' incubation of cultures. *HIV-associated FUO* is defined by a temperature of ≥38.3°C (≥101°F) on several occasions over a period of >4 weeks for outpatients or >3 days for hospitalized patients with HIV infection. This diagnosis is invoked if appropriate investigation over 3 days, including 2 days' incubation of cultures, reveals no source.

Adoption of these categories of FUO in the literature has allowed a more rational compilation of data regarding these disparate groups. In the remainder of this chapter, the discussion will focus on classic FUO in the adult unless otherwise specified.

CAUSES OF CLASSIC FUO

Table 19-1 summarizes the findings of several large studies of FUO carried out since the advent of the antibiotic era, including a prospective study of 167 adult patients with FUO encompassing all eight university hospitals in the Netherlands and using a standardized protocol in which the first author reviewed every patient. Coincident with the widespread use of antibiotics, increasingly useful diagnostic technologies—both noninvasive and invasive—have been developed. Newer studies reflect not only changing patterns of disease but also the impact of diagnostic techniques that make it possible to eliminate many patients with specific illness from the FUO category. The ubiquitous use of potent broad-spectrum antibiotics may have decreased the number of infections causing FUO. The wide availability of ultrasonography, CT, MRI, radionuclide scanning, and positron emission tomography (PET) scanning has enhanced the detection of localized infections and of occult neoplasms and lymphomas in patients previously thought to have FUO. Likewise, the widespread availability of highly specific and sensitive immunologic testing has reduced the number of undetected cases of systemic lupus erythematosus and other autoimmune diseases.

Infections, especially extrapulmonary tuberculosis, remain the leading diagnosable cause of FUO. Prolonged mononucleosis syndromes caused by Epstein-Barr virus, cytomegalovirus (CMV), or HIV are conditions whose consideration as a cause of FUO is sometimes confounded by delayed antibody responses. Intraabdominal abscesses (sometimes poorly localized) and renal, retroperitoneal, and paraspinal abscesses continue to be difficult to diagnose. Renal malacoplakia, with submucosal plaques or nodules involving the urinary tract, may cause FUO and is often fatal if untreated. It is associated with intracellular bacterial infection, is seen most often in patients with defects of intracellular bacterial killing, and is treated with fluoroquinolones or trimethoprim-sulfamethoxazole. Occasionally, other organs may be involved. Osteomyelitis, especially where prosthetic devices have been implanted, and infective endocarditis must be considered. Although true culture-negative infective endocarditis is rare, one may be misled by slow-growing organisms of the HACEK group (*Haemophilus aphrophilus, Actinobacillus actinomycetemcomitans, Cardiobacterium hominis, Eikenella corrodens,* and *Kingella kingae*; Chap. 140), *Bartonella* spp. (previously *Rochalimaea*), *Legionella* spp., *Coxiella burnetii, Chlamydophila psittaci,* and fungi. Prostatitis, dental abscesses, sinusitis, and cholangitis continue to be sources of occult fever.

Fungal disease, most notably histoplasmosis involving the reticuloendothelial system, may cause FUO. FUO with headache should

TABLE 19-1	CLASSIC FUO IN ADULTS						
Authors (Year of Publication)	Years of Study	No. of Cases	Infections (%)	Neoplasms (%)	Noninfectious Inflammatory Diseases (%)	Miscellaneous Causes (%)	Undiagnosed Causes (%)
Petersdorf and Beeson (1961)	1952–1957	100	36	19	19[a]	19[a]	7
Larson and Featherstone (1982)	1970–1980	105	30	31	16[a]	11[a]	12
Knockaert and Vanneste (1992)	1980–1989	199	22.5	7	23[a]	21.5[a]	25.5
de Kleijn et al. (1997, Part I)	1992–1994	167	26	12.5	24	8	30

[a]Authors' raw data retabulated to conform to altered diagnostic categories.
Source: Modified from de Kleijn et al., 1997 (Part I).

prompt examination of spinal fluid for *Cryptococcus neoformans.* Malaria (which may result from transfusion, the failure to take a prescribed prophylactic agent, or infection with a drug-resistant strain) continues to be a cause, particularly of asynchronous FUO. A related protozoan infection, babesiosis, may cause FUO and is increasing in geographic distribution and in incidence, especially among the elderly and immunosuppressed.

In most earlier series, neoplasms were the next most common cause of FUO after infections (Table 19-1). In more recent series, a decrease in the percentage of FUO cases due to malignancy was attributed to improvement in diagnostic technologies—in particular, high-resolution tomography, MRI, PET scanning, and tumor antigen assays. This observation does not diminish the importance of considering neoplasia in the initial diagnostic evaluation of a patient with fever. A number of patients in these series had temporal arteritis, adult Still's disease, drug-related fever, and factitious fever. In recent series, ~25–30% of cases of FUO have remained undiagnosed. The general term *noninfectious inflammatory diseases* applies to systemic rheumatologic or vasculitic diseases such as polymyalgia rheumatica, lupus, and adult Still's disease as well as to granulomatous diseases such as sarcoidosis and Crohn's and granulomatous hepatitis.

In the elderly, multisystem disease is the most frequent cause of FUO, giant-cell arteritis being the leading etiologic entity in this category. In patients >50 years of age, this disease accounts for 15–20% of FUO cases. Tuberculosis is the most common infection causing FUO in the elderly, and colon cancer is an important cause of FUO with malignancy in this age group.

Many diseases have been grouped in the various studies as "miscellaneous." On this list are drug fever, pulmonary embolism, factitious fever, the hereditary periodic fever syndromes (familial Mediterranean fever, hyper-IgD syndrome, tumor necrosis factor receptor–associated periodic syndrome, familial cold urticaria, and the Muckle-Wells syndrome), and Fabry disease.

A drug-related etiology must be considered in any case of prolonged fever. Any febrile pattern may be elicited by a drug. Virtually all classes of drugs cause fever, but antimicrobial agents (especially β-lactam antibiotics), cardiovascular drugs (e.g., quinidine), antineoplastic drugs, and drugs acting on the central nervous system (e.g., phenytoin) are particularly common causes.

It is axiomatic that, as the duration of fever increases, the likelihood of an infectious cause decreases, even for the more indolent infectious etiologies (e.g., brucellosis, paracoccidioidomycosis, malaria due to *Plasmodium malariae*). In a series of 347 patients referred to the National Institutes of Health from 1961 to 1977, only 6% had an infection (Table 19-2). A significant proportion (9%) had factitious fevers—i.e., fevers due either to false elevations of temperature or to self-induced disease. A substantial number of these factitious cases were in young women in the health professions. It is worth noting that 8% of the patients with prolonged fevers (some of whom had completely normal liver function studies) had granulomatous hepatitis, and 6% had adult Still's disease. After prolonged investigation, 19% of cases still had no specific diagnosis. A total of 27% of patients had no actual fever during inpatient observation or had an exaggerated circadian temperature rhythm without chills, elevated pulse, or other abnormalities.

More than 200 conditions may be considered in the differential diagnosis of classic FUO in adults; the most common of these are listed in Table 19-3. This list applies strictly to the United States. Geographic considerations are paramount. For example, in Japan, human T cell lymphotropic virus type I is a consideration; in China, infection plays a greater role and tuberculosis is prominent; and in Spain, visceral leishmaniasis may be a more common cause of FUO. The frequency of global travel underscores the need for a detailed travel history, and the continuing emergence of new infectious diseases makes this listing potentially incomplete. The possibility of international and domestic terrorist activity involving the intentional release of infectious agents, many of which cause illnesses presenting with prolonged fever, underscores the need for obtaining an insightful environmental, occupational, and professional

TABLE 19-2 CAUSES OF FUO LASTING >6 MONTHS

Cause	Cases, %
None identified	19
Miscellaneous causes	13
Factitious causes	9
Granulomatous hepatitis	8
Neoplasm	7
Still's disease	6
Infection	6
Collagen vascular disease	4
Familial Mediterranean fever	3
No fever[a]	27

[a]No actual fever observed during 2–3 weeks of inpatient observation. Includes patients with exaggerated circadian rhythm.

Source: From a study of 347 patients referred to the National Institutes of Health from 1961 to 1977 with a presumptive diagnosis of FUO of >6 months' duration (R Aduan et al. Prolonged fever of unknown origin. Clin Res 26:558A, 1978).

history, with early notification of public health authorities in cases of suspicious etiology (Chap. 214).

SPECIALIZED DIAGNOSTIC STUDIES

Classic FUO A stepwise flow chart depicting the diagnostic workup and therapeutic management of FUO is provided in Fig. 19-1. In this flow chart, reference is made to "potentially diagnostic clues," as outlined by de Kleijn and colleagues; these clues may be key findings in the history (e.g., travel), localizing signs, or key symptoms. Certain specific diagnostic maneuvers become critical in dealing with prolonged fevers. If factitious fever is suspected, electronic thermometers should be used, temperature-taking should be supervised, and simultaneous urine and body temperatures should be measured. Thick blood smears should be examined for *Plasmodium*; thin blood smears, prepared with proper technique and quality stains and subjected to expert microscopy, should be used to speciate *Plasmodium* and to identify *Babesia, Trypanosoma, Leishmania, Rickettsia,* and *Borrelia.* Any tissue removed during prior relevant surgery should be reexamined; slides should be requested, and, if need be, paraffin blocks of fixed pathologic material should be reexamined and additional special studies performed. Relevant x-rays should be reexamined; reviewing of prior radiologic reports may be insufficient. Serum should be set aside in the laboratory as soon as possible and retained for future examination for rising antibody titers.

Febrile agglutinins is a vague term that in most laboratories refers to serologic studies for salmonellosis, brucellosis, and rickettsial diseases. These studies are seldom useful, having low sensitivity and variable specificity. Multiple blood samples (no fewer than three and rarely more than six, including samples for anaerobic culture) should be cultured in the laboratory for at least 2 weeks to ensure that any HACEK group organisms that may be present have ample time to grow (Chap. 140). Lysis-centrifugation blood culture techniques should be employed in cases where prior antimicrobial therapy or fungal or atypical mycobacterial infection is suspected. Blood culture media should be supplemented with L-cysteine or pyridoxal to assist in the isolation of nutritionally variant streptococci. It should be noted that sequential cultures positive for multiple organisms may reflect self-injection of contaminated substances. Urine cultures, including cultures for mycobacteria, fungi, and CMV, are indicated. In the setting of recurrent fevers with lymphocytic meningitis (Mollaret's meningitis), cerebrospinal fluid can be tested for herpesvirus, with use of the polymerase chain reaction (PCR) to amplify and detect viral nucleic acid (Chap. 172). A recent report described a highly multiplexed oligonucleotide microarray using PCR amplification and containing probes for all recognized vertebrate virus species and for 135 bacterial, 73 fungal, and 63 parasitic genera and species. The eventual clinical validation of such microarrays will further diminish rates of undiagnosed FUO of infectious etiology.

In any FUO workup, the erythrocyte sedimentation rate (ESR) should be determined. Striking elevation of the ESR and anemia of chronic disease are frequently seen in association with giant-cell arteritis

Infections

Localized pyogenic infections
  Appendicitis
  Cat-scratch disease
  Cholangitis
  Cholecystitis
  Dental abscess
  Diverticulitis/abscess
  Lesser sac abscess
  Liver abscess
  Mesenteric lymphadenitis
  Osteomyelitis
  Pancreatic abscess
  Pelvic inflammatory disease
  Perinephric/intrarenal abscess
  Prostatic abscess
  Renal malacoplakia
  Sinusitis
  Subphrenic abscess
  Suppurative thrombophlebitis
  Tuboovarian abscess
Intravascular infections
  Bacterial aortitis
  Bacterial endocarditis
  Vascular catheter infection
Systemic bacterial infections
  Bartonellosis
  Brucellosis
  Campylobacter infection
  Cat-scratch disease/bacillary angiomatosis
    (*B. henselae*)
  Gonococcemia
  Legionnaires' disease
  Leptospirosis
  Listeriosis
  Lyme disease
  Melioidosis
  Meningococcemia
  Rat-bite fever
  Relapsing fever
  Salmonellosis
  Syphilis
  Tularemia
  Typhoid fever
  Vibriosis
  Yersinia infection
Mycobacterial infections
  M. avium/M. intracellulare infections
  Other atypical mycobacterial infections
  Tuberculosis
Other bacterial infections
  Actinomycosis
  Bacillary angiomatosis
  Nocardiosis
  Whipple's disease
Rickettsial infections
  Anaplasmosis
  Ehrlichiosis
  Murine typhus
  Q fever
  Rickettsialpox
  Rocky Mountain spotted fever

Mycoplasmal infections
Chlamydial infections
  Lymphogranuloma venereum
  Psittacosis
  TWAR (*C. pneumoniae*) infection
Viral infections
  Colorado tick fever
  Coxsackievirus group B infection
  Cytomegalovirus infection
  Dengue
  Epstein-Barr virus infection
  Hepatitis A, B, C, D, and E
  Human herpesvirus 6 infection
  Human immunodeficiency virus
    infection
  Lymphocytic choriomeningitis
  Parvovirus B19 infection
Fungal infections
  Aspergillosis
  Blastomycosis
  Candidiasis
  Coccidioidomycosis
  Cryptococcosis
  Histoplasmosis
  Mucormycosis
  Paracoccidioidomycosis
  Pneumocystis infection
  Sporotrichosis
Parasitic infections
  Amebiasis
  Babesiosis
  Chagas' disease
  Leishmaniasis
  Malaria
  Strongyloidiasis
  Toxocariasis
  Toxoplasmosis
  Trichinosis
Presumed infections, agent undetermined
  Kawasaki's disease (mucocutaneous lymph
    node syndrome)
  Kikuchi's necrotizing lymphadenitis

Neoplasms

Malignant
  Colon cancer
  Gall bladder carcinoma
  Hepatoma
  Hodgkin's lymphoma
  Immunoblastic T-cell lymphoma
  Leukemia
  Lymphomatoid granulomatosis
  Malignant histiocytosis
  Non-Hodgkin's lymphoma
  Pancreatic cancer
  Renal cell carcinoma
  Sarcoma
Benign
  Atrial myxoma
  Castleman's disease
  Renal angiomyolipoma

Habitual Hyperthermia

(Exaggerated circadian rhythm)

Collagen Vascular/Hypersensitivity Diseases

Adult Still's disease
Behçet's disease
Erythema multiforme
Erythema nodosum
Giant-cell arteritis/polymyalgia rheumatica
Hypersensitivity pneumonitis
Hypersensitivity vasculitis
Mixed connective-tissue disease
Polyarteritis nodosa
Relapsing polychondritis
Rheumatic fever
Rheumatoid arthritis
Schnitzler's syndrome
Systemic lupus erythematosus
Takayasu's aortitis
Weber-Christian disease
Wegener's granulomatosis

Granulomatous Diseases

Crohn's disease
Granulomatous hepatitis
Midline granuloma
Sarcoidosis

Miscellaneous Conditions

Aortic dissection
Drug fever
Gout
Hematomas
Hemoglobinopathies
Laennec's cirrhosis
PFPA syndrome: periodic fever, adenitis,
  pharyngitis, aphthae
Postmyocardial infarction syndrome
Recurrent pulmonary emboli
Subacute thyroiditis (de Quervain's)
Tissue infarction/necrosis

Inherited and Metabolic Diseases

Adrenal insufficiency
Cyclic neutropenia
Deafness, urticaria, and amyloidosis
Fabry disease
Familial cold urticaria
Familial Mediterranean fever
Hyperimmunoglobulinemia D and periodic
  fever
Muckle-Wells syndrome
Tumor necrosis factor receptor–associated
  periodic syndrome
Type V hypertriglyceridemia

Thermoregulatory Disorders

Central
  Brain tumor
  Cerebrovascular accident
  Encephalitis
  Hypothalamic dysfunction
Peripheral
  Hyperthyroidism
  Pheochromocytoma

Factitious Fevers

"Afebrile" FUO (<38.3°C)

Source: Modified from RK Root, RG Petersdorf, in JD Wilson et al (eds): *Harrison's Principles of Internal Medicine,* 12th ed. New York, McGraw-Hill, 1991.

or polymyalgia rheumatica—common causes of FUO in patients >50 years of age. Still's disease is suggested by elevations of ESR, leukocytosis, and anemia and is often accompanied by arthralgias, polyserositis (pleuritis, pericarditis), lymphadenopathy, splenomegaly, and rash. The C-reactive protein level may be a useful cross-reference for the ESR and is a more sensitive and specific indicator of an "acute-phase" inflammatory metabolic response. Antinuclear antibody, antineutrophil cytoplasmic antibody, rheumatoid factor, and serum cryoglobulins should be measured to rule out other collagen vascular diseases and vasculitis. Elevated levels of angiotensin-converting enzyme in serum may point to sarcoi-

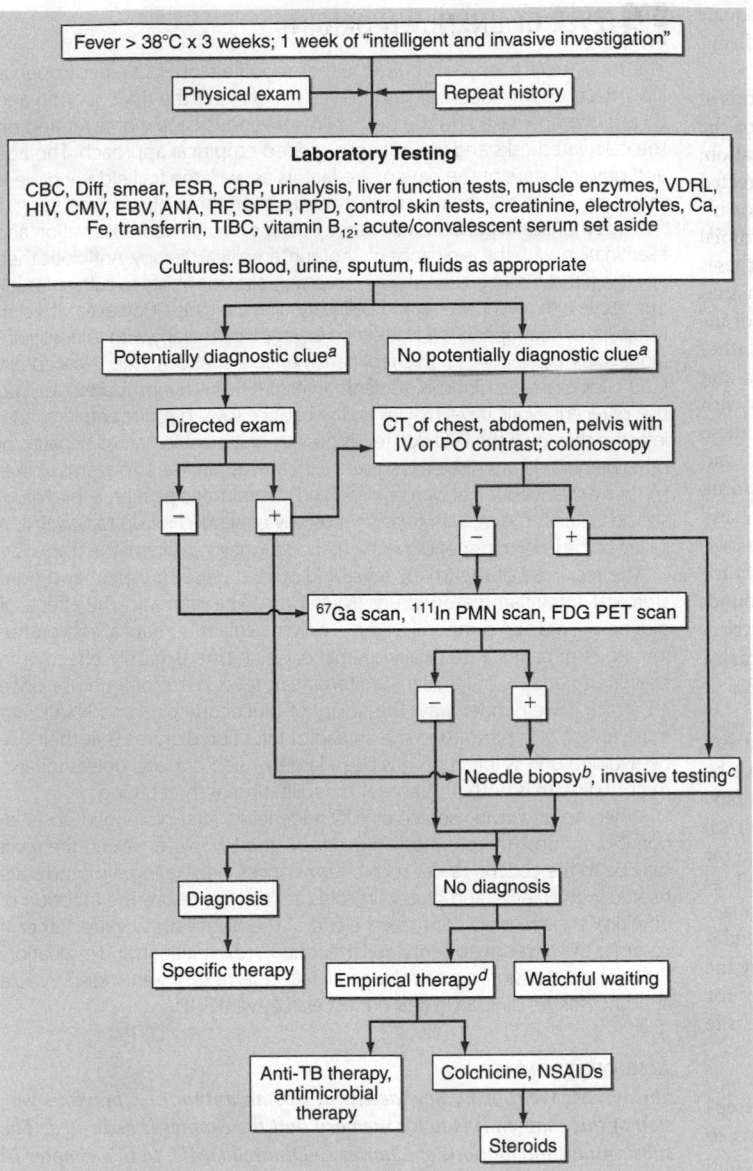

FIGURE 19-1 Approach to the patient with classic FUO. [a]"Potentially diagnostic clues," as outlined by de Kleijn and colleagues (1997, Part II), may be key findings in the history, localizing signs, or key symptoms. ANA, antinuclear antibody; CBC, complete blood count; CMV, cytomegalovirus; CRP, C-reactive protein; CT, computed tomography; Diff, differential; EBV, Epstein-Barr virus; ESR, erythrocyte sedimentation rate; FDG, fluorodeoxyglucose F18; NSAIDs, nonsteroidal anti-inflammatory drugs; PET, positron emission tomography; PMN, polymorphonuclear leukocyte; PPD, purified protein derivative; RF, rheumatoid factor; SPEP, serum protein electrophoresis; TB, tuberculosis; TIBC, total iron-binding capacity; VDRL, Venereal Disease Research Laboratory test. [b]Needle biopsy of liver as well as any other tissue indicated by "potentially diagnostic clues." [c]Invasive testing could involve laparoscopy. [d]Empirical therapy is a last resort, given the good prognosis of most patients with FUO persisting without a diagnosis.

dosis. With rare exceptions, the intermediate-strength purified protein derivative (PPD) skin test should be used to screen for tuberculosis in patients with classic FUO. Concurrent control tests, such as the mumps skin test antigen (Aventis-Pasteur, Swiftwater, PA), should be employed. It should be kept in mind that both the PPD skin test and control tests may yield negative results in miliary tuberculosis, sarcoidosis, Hodgkin's disease, malnutrition, or AIDS.

Noninvasive procedures should include an upper gastrointestinal contrast study with small-bowel follow-through and colonoscopy to examine the terminal ileum and cecum. Colonoscopy is especially strongly indicated in the elderly. Chest x-rays should be repeated if new symp-

toms arise. Sputum should be induced with an ultrasonic nebulizer for cultures and cytology. If there are pulmonary signs or symptoms, bronchoscopy with bronchoalveolar lavage for cultures and cytology should be considered. High-resolution spiral CT of the chest and abdomen should be performed with both IV and oral contrast. If a spinal or paraspinal lesion is suspected, however, MRI is preferred. MRI may be superior to CT in demonstrating intraabdominal abscesses and aortic dissection, but the relative utility of MRI and CT in the diagnosis of FUO is unknown. At present, abdominal CT with contrast should be used unless MRI is specifically indicated. Arteriography may be useful for patients in whom systemic necrotizing vasculitis is suspected. Saccular aneurysms may be seen, most commonly in renal or hepatic vessels, and may permit diagnosis of arteritis when biopsy is difficult. Ultrasonography of the abdomen is useful for investigation of the hepatobiliary tract, kidneys, spleen, and pelvis. Echocardiography may be helpful in an evaluation for bacterial endocarditis, pericarditis, nonbacterial thrombotic endocarditis, and atrial myxomas. Transesophageal echocardiography is especially sensitive for these lesions.

Radionuclide scanning procedures using technetium (Tc) 99m sulfur colloid, gallium (Ga) 67 citrate, or indium (In) 111–labeled leukocytes may be useful in identifying and/or localizing inflammatory processes. In one study, Ga scintigraphy yielded useful diagnostic information in almost one-third of cases, and it was suggested that this procedure might actually be used before other imaging techniques if no specific organ is suspected of being abnormal. It is likely that PET scanning, which provides quicker results (hours vs days), will prove even more sensitive and specific than ^{67}Ga scanning in FUO. ^{99m}Tc bone scan should be undertaken to look for osteomyelitis or bony metastases; ^{67}Ga scan may be used to identify sarcoidosis (Chap. 322) or *Pneumocystis* infection (Chap. 200) in the lungs or Crohn's disease (Chap. 289) in the abdomen. ^{111}In-labeled white blood cell (WBC) scan may be used to locate abscesses. With these scans, false-positive and false-negative findings are common. Fluorodeoxyglucose F18 (FDG) PET scanning appears to be superior to other forms of nuclear imaging. The FDG used in PET scans accumulates in tumors and at sites of inflammation and has even been shown to accumulate reliably at sites of vasculitis. Where available, FDG PET scanning should therefore be chosen over ^{67}Ga scanning in the diagnosis of FUO.

Biopsy of the liver and bone marrow should be considered in the workup of FUO if the studies mentioned above are unrevealing and if fever is prolonged. Granulomatous hepatitis has been diagnosed by liver biopsy, even when liver enzymes are normal and no other diagnostic clues point to liver disease. All biopsy specimens should be cultured for bacteria, mycobacteria, and fungi. Likewise, in the absence of clues pointing to the bone marrow, bone marrow biopsy (not simple aspiration) for histology and culture has yielded diagnoses late in the workup. When possible, a section of the tissue block should be retained for further sections or stains. PCR technology makes it possible in some cases to identify and speciate mycobacterial DNA in paraffin-embedded, fixed tissues at some research centers. Thus, in some cases, a retrospective diagnosis can be made on the basis of studies of long-fixed pathologic tissues. In a patient over age 50 (or occasionally in a younger patient) with the appropriate symptoms and laboratory findings, "blind biopsy" of one or both temporal arteries may yield a diagnosis of arteritis. Tenderness or decreased pulsation, if noted, should guide the selection of a site for biopsy. Lymph node biopsy may be helpful if nodes are enlarged, but inguinal nodes are often palpable and are seldom diagnostically useful.

Exploratory laparotomy has been performed when all other diagnostic procedures fail but has largely been replaced by imaging and guided-biopsy techniques. Laparoscopic biopsy may provide more adequate guided sampling of lymph nodes or liver, with less invasive morbidity.

Nosocomial FUO (See also Chap. 125) The primary considerations in diagnosing nosocomial FUO are the underlying susceptibility of the patient coupled with the potential complications of hospitalization. The original surgical or procedural field is the place to begin a directed physical and laboratory examination for abscesses, hematomas, or infected foreign bodies. More than 50% of patients with nosocomial FUO are infected. Intravascular lines, septic phlebitis, and prostheses are all suspect. In this setting, the best approach is to focus on sites where occult infections may be sequestered, such as the sinuses of intubated patients or a prostatic abscess in a man with a urinary catheter. *Clostridium difficile* colitis may be associated with fever and leukocytosis before the onset of diarrhea. In ~25% of patients with nosocomial FUO, the fever has a noninfectious cause. Among these causes are acalculous cholecystitis, deep-vein thrombophlebitis, and pulmonary embolism. Drug fever, transfusion reactions, alcohol/drug withdrawal, adrenal insufficiency, thyroiditis, pancreatitis, gout, and pseudogout are among the many possible causes to consider. As in classic FUO, repeated meticulous physical examinations, coupled with focused diagnostic techniques, are imperative. Multiple blood, wound, and fluid cultures are mandatory. The pace of diagnostic tests is accelerated, and the threshold for procedures—CT scans, ultrasonography, ^{111}In WBC scans, noninvasive venous studies—is low. Even so, 20% of cases of nosocomial FUO may go undiagnosed.

Like diagnostic measures, therapeutic maneuvers must be swift and decisive, as many patients are already critically ill. IV lines must be changed (and cultured), drugs stopped for 72 h, and empirical therapy started if bacteremia is a threat. In many hospital settings, empirical antibiotic coverage for nosocomial FUO now includes vancomycin for coverage of methicillin-resistant *Staphylococcus aureus* as well as broad-spectrum gram-negative coverage with piperacillin/tazobactam, ticarcillin/clavulanate, imipenem, or meropenem. Practice guidelines covering many of these issues have been published jointly by the Infectious Diseases Society of America (IDSA) and the Society for Critical Care Medicine and can be accessed on the IDSA website (*www.journals.uchicago.edu/IDSA/guidelines*).

Neutropenic FUO (See also Chap. 82) Neutropenic patients are susceptible to focal bacterial and fungal infections, to bacteremic infections, to infections involving catheters (including septic thrombophlebitis), and to perianal infections. *Candida* and *Aspergillus* infections are common. Infections due to herpes simplex virus or CMV are sometimes causes of FUO in this group. While the duration of illness may be short in these patients, the consequences of untreated infection may be catastrophic; 50–60% of febrile neutropenic patients are infected, and 20% are bacteremic. The IDSA has published extensive practice guidelines covering these critically ill neutropenic patients; these guidelines appear on the website cited in the previous section. In these patients, severe mucositis, quinolone prophylaxis, colonization with methicillin-resistant *S. aureus*, obvious catheter-related infection, or hypotension dictates the use of vancomycin plus ceftazidime, cefepime, or a carbapenem with or without an aminoglycoside to provide empirical coverage for bacterial sepsis.

HIV-Associated FUO HIV infection alone may be a cause of fever. Infection due to *Mycobacterium avium* or *Mycobacterium intracellulare*, tuberculosis, toxoplasmosis, CMV infection, *Pneumocystis* infection, salmonellosis, cryptococcosis, histoplasmosis, non-Hodgkin's lymphoma, and (of particular importance) drug fever are all possible causes of FUO. Mycobacterial infection can be diagnosed by blood cultures and by liver, bone marrow, and lymph node biopsies. Chest CT should be performed to identify enlarged mediastinal nodes. Serologic studies may reveal cryptococcal antigen, and ^{67}Ga scan may help identify *Pneumocystis* pulmonary infection. FUO has an infectious etiology in >80% of HIV-infected patients, but drug fever and lymphoma remain important considerations. Treatment of HIV-associated FUO depends on many factors and is discussed in Chap. 182.

℞ FEVER OF UNKNOWN ORIGIN

The focus here is on classic FUO. Other modifiers of FUO—neutropenia, HIV infection, a nosocomial setting—all vastly affect the risk equation and dictate therapy based on the probability of various causes of fever and on the calculated risks and benefits of a guided empirical approach. The age and physical state of the patient are factors as well: the frail elderly patient may merit a trial of empirical therapy earlier than the robust young adult.

The emphasis in patients with classic FUO is on continued observation and examination, with the avoidance of "shotgun" empirical therapy. Antibiotic therapy (even that for tuberculosis) may irrevocably alter the ability to culture fastidious bacteria or mycobacteria and delineate ultimate cause. However, vital-sign instability or neutropenia is an indication for empirical therapy with a fluoroquinolone plus piperacillin or the regimen mentioned above (see "Nosocomial FUO"), for example. Cirrhosis, asplenia, intercurrent immunosuppressive drug use, or recent exotic travel may all tip the balance toward earlier empirical anti-infective therapy. If the PPD skin test is positive or if granulomatous hepatitis or other granulomatous disease is present with anergy (and sarcoid seems unlikely), then a therapeutic trial with isoniazid and rifampin (and possibly a third drug) should be undertaken, with treatment usually continued for up to 6 weeks. A failure of the fever to respond over this period suggests an alternative diagnosis.

The response of rheumatic fever and Still's disease to aspirin and non-steroidal anti-inflammatory drugs (NSAIDs) may be dramatic. The effects of glucocorticoids on temporal arteritis, polymyalgia rheumatica, and granulomatous hepatitis are equally dramatic. Colchicine is highly effective in preventing attacks of familial Mediterranean fever but is of little use once an attack is well under way. The ability of glucocorticoids and NSAIDs to mask fever while permitting the spread of infection dictates that their use be avoided unless infection has been largely ruled out and unless inflammatory disease is both probable and debilitating or threatening.

When no underlying source of FUO is identified after prolonged observation (>6 months), the prognosis is generally good, however vexing the fever may be to the patient. Under such circumstances, debilitating symptoms are treated with NSAIDs, and glucocorticoids are the last resort. The initiation of empirical therapy does not mark the end of the diagnostic workup; rather, it commits the physician to continued thoughtful reexamination and evaluation. Patience, compassion, equanimity, and intellectual flexibility are indispensable attributes for the clinician in dealing successfully with FUO.

ACKNOWLEDGMENTS
Sheldon M. Wolff, MD, now deceased, was an author of a previous version of this chapter. It is to his memory that the chapter is dedicated. The substantial contributions of Charles A. Dinarello, MD, to this chapter in previous editions are gratefully acknowledged.

FURTHER READINGS

BLEEKER-ROVERS CP et al: A prospective multicenter study on fever of unknown origin: The yield of a structured diagnostic protocol. Medicine 86:26, 2007

DE KLEIJN EM et al: Fever of unknown origin (FUO): I. A prospective multicenter study of 167 patients with FUO, using fixed epidemiologic entry criteria. Medicine 76:392, 1997

——— et al: Fever of unknown origin (FUO): II. Diagnostic procedures in a prospective multicenter study of 167 patients. Medicine 76:401, 1997

GOTO M et al: A retrospective review of 226 hospitalized patients with fever. Intern Med 46:17, 2007

HIRSCHMANN JV: Fever of unknown origin in adults. Clin Infect Dis 24:291, 1997

HUGHES WT et al: 2002 guidelines for the use of antimicrobial agents in neutropenic patients with cancer. Clin Infect Dis 34:730, 2002

KNOCKAERT DC et al: Fever of unknown origin in adults: 40 years on. J Intern Med 253:263, 2003

MOURAD O et al: A comprehensive evidence-based approach to fever of unknown origin. Arch Intern Med 163:545, 2003

O'GRADY NP et al: Practice guidelines for evaluating new fever in critically ill adult patients. Clin Infect Dis 26:1042, 1998

ZENONE T: Fever of unknown origin in adults: Evaluation of 144 cases in a non-university hospital. Scand J Infect Dis 38:632, 2006

20 Hypothermia and Frostbite
Daniel F. Danzl

HYPOTHERMIA

Accidental hypothermia occurs when there is an unintentional drop in the body's core temperature below 35°C (95°F). At this temperature, many of the compensatory physiologic mechanisms to conserve heat begin to fail. *Primary accidental hypothermia* is a result of the direct exposure of a previously healthy individual to the cold. The mortality rate is much higher for those patients who develop *secondary hypothermia* as a complication of a serious systemic disorder.

CAUSES

Primary accidental hypothermia is geographically and seasonally pervasive. Although most cases occur in the winter months and in colder climates, it is surprisingly common in warmer regions as well. Multiple variables make individuals at the extremes of age, the elderly and neonates, particularly vulnerable to hypothermia (Table 20-1). The elderly have diminished thermal perception and are more susceptible to immobility, malnutrition, and systemic illnesses that interfere with heat generation or conservation. Dementia, psychiatric illness, and socioeconomic factors often compound these problems by impeding adequate measures to prevent hypothermia. Neonates have high rates of heat loss because of their increased surface-to-mass ratio and their lack of effective shivering and adaptive behavioral responses. In addition, malnutrition can contribute to heat loss because of diminished subcutaneous fat and because of depleted energy stores used for thermogenesis.

Individuals whose occupations or hobbies entail extensive exposure to cold weather are at increased risk for hypothermia. Military history is replete with hypothermic tragedies. Hunters, sailors, skiers, and climbers also are at great risk of exposure, whether it involves injury, changes in weather, or lack of preparedness.

Ethanol causes vasodilatation (which increases heat loss), reduces thermogenesis and gluconeogenesis, and may impair judgment or lead to obtundation. Phenothiazines, barbiturates, benzodiazepines, cyclic antidepressants, and many other medications reduce centrally mediated vasoconstriction. Up to 25% of patients admitted to an intensive care unit because of drug overdose are hypothermic. Anesthetics can block the shivering responses; their effects are compounded when patients are not covered adequately in the operating or recovery rooms.

Several types of endocrine dysfunction can lead to hypothermia. Hypothyroidism—particularly when extreme, as in myxedema coma—reduces the metabolic rate and impairs thermogenesis and be-

havioral responses. Adrenal insufficiency and hypopituitarism also increase susceptibility to hypothermia. Hypoglycemia, most commonly caused by insulin or oral hypoglycemic drugs, is associated with hypothermia, in part the result of neuroglycopenic effects on hypothalamic function. Increased osmolality and metabolic derangements associated with uremia, diabetic ketoacidosis, and lactic acidosis can lead to altered hypothalamic thermoregulation.

Neurologic injury from trauma, cerebrovascular accident, subarachnoid hemorrhage, or hypothalamic lesions increases susceptibility to hypothermia. Agenesis of the corpus callosum, or Shapiro syndrome, is one cause of episodic hypothermia, characterized by profuse perspiration followed by a rapid fall in temperature. Acute spinal cord injury disrupts the autonomic pathways that lead to shivering and prevents cold-induced reflex vasoconstrictive responses.

Hypothermia associated with sepsis is a poor prognostic sign. Hepatic failure causes decreased glycogen stores and gluconeogenesis, as well as a diminished shivering response. In acute myocardial infarction associated with low cardiac output, hypothermia may be reversed after adequate resuscitation. With extensive burns, psoriasis, erythrodermas, and other skin diseases, increased peripheral blood flow leads to excessive heat loss.

THERMOREGULATION

Heat loss occurs through five mechanisms: radiation (55–65% of heat loss), conduction (10–15% of heat loss, but much greater in cold water), convection (increased in the wind), respiration, and evaporation (which are affected by the ambient temperature and the relative humidity).

The preoptic anterior hypothalamus normally orchestrates thermoregulation (Chap. 17). The immediate defense of thermoneutrality is via the autonomic nervous system, whereas delayed control is mediated by the endocrine system. Autonomic nervous system responses include the release of norepinephrine, increased muscle tone, and shivering, leading to thermogenesis and an increase in the basal metabolic rate. Cutaneous cold thermoreception causes direct reflex vasoconstriction to conserve heat. Prolonged exposure to cold also stimulates the thyroid axis, leading to an increased metabolic rate.

CLINICAL PRESENTATION

In most cases of hypothermia, the history of exposure to environmental factors, such as prolonged exposure to the outdoors without adequate clothing, makes the diagnosis straightforward. In urban settings, however, the presentation is often more subtle and other disease processes, toxin exposures, or psychiatric diagnoses should be considered.

After initial stimulation by hypothermia, there is progressive depression of all organ systems. The timing of the appearance of these clinical manifestations varies widely (Table 20-2). Without knowing the core temperature, it can be difficult to interpret other vital signs. For example, a tachycardia disproportionate to the core temperature suggests secondary hypothermia resulting from hypoglycemia, hypovolemia, or a toxin overdose. Because carbon dioxide production declines progressively, the respiratory rate should be low; persistent hyperventilation suggests a central nervous system (CNS) lesion or one of the organic acidoses. A markedly depressed level of consciousness in a patient with mild hypothermia should raise suspicion of an overdose or CNS dysfunction due to infection or trauma.

Physical examination findings can also be altered by hypothermia. For instance, the assumption that areflexia is solely attributable to hypothermia can obscure and delay the diagnosis of a spinal cord lesion. Patients with hypothermia may be confused or combative; these symptoms abate more rapidly with rewarming than with the use of restraints. A classic example of maladaptive behavior in patients with hypothermia is paradoxical undressing, which involves the inappropriate removal of clothing in response to a cold stress. The cold-induced ileus and abdominal rectus spasm can mimic, or mask, the presentation of an acute abdomen (Chap. 14).

When a patient in hypothermic cardiac arrest is first discovered, cardiopulmonary resuscitation is indicated, unless (1) a do-not-resuscitate status is verified, (2) obviously lethal injuries are identified, or

TABLE 20-1	RISK FACTORS FOR HYPOTHERMIA
Age extremes	Endocrine-related
Elderly	Diabetes mellitus
Neonates	Hypoglycemia
Environmental exposure	Hypothyroidism
Occupational	Adrenal insufficiency
Sports-related	Hypopituitarism
Inadequate clothing	Neurologic-related
Immersion	Cerebrovascular accident
Toxicologic & pharmacologic	Hypothalamic disorders
Ethanol	Parkinson's disease
Phenothiazines	Spinal cord injury
Barbiturates	Multisystem
Carcinomatosis	Trauma
Anesthetics	Sepsis
Neuromuscular blockers	Shock
Antidepressants	Hepatic or renal failure
Insufficient fuel	Burns and exfoliative dermatologic
Malnutrition	disorders
Marasmus	Immobility or debilitation
Kwashiorkor	

TABLE 20-2 PHYSIOLOGIC CHANGES ASSOCIATED WITH ACCIDENTAL HYPOTHERMIA

Severity	Body Temperature	Central Nervous System	Cardiovascular	Respiratory	Renal and Endocrine	Neuromuscular
Mild	35°C (95°F)–32.2°C (90°F)	Linear depression of cerebral metabolism; amnesia; apathy; dysarthria; impaired judgment; maladaptive behavior	Tachycardia, then progressive bradycardia; cardiaccycle prolongation; vasoconstriction; increase in cardiac output and blood pressure	Tachypnea, then progressive decrease in respiratory minute volume; declining oxygen consumption; bronchorrhea; bronchospasm	Diuresis; increase in catecholamines, adrenal steroids, triiodothyronine and thyroxine; increase in metabolism with shivering	Increased preshivering muscle tone, then fatiguing
Moderate	<32.2°C (90°F)–28°C (82.4°F)	EEG abnormalities; progressive depression of level of consciousness; pupillary dilatation; paradoxical undressing; hallucinations	Progressive decrease in pulse and cardiac output; increased atrial and ventricular arrhythmias; suggestive (J-wave) ECG changes	Hypoventilation; 50% decrease in carbon dioxide production per 8°C drop in temperature; absence of protective airway reflexes	50% increase in renal blood flow; renal autoregulation intact; impaired insulin action	Hyporeflexia; diminishing shivering-induced thermogenesis; rigidity
Severe	<28°C (82.4°F)	Loss of cerebrovascular autoregulation; decline in cerebral blood flow; coma; loss of ocular reflexes; progressive decrease in EEG	Progressive decrease in blood pressure, heart rate, and cardiac output; re-entrant dysrhythmias; maximum risk of ventricular fibrillation; asystole	Pulmonic congestion and edema; 75% decrease in oxygen consumption; apnea	Decrease in renal blood flow parallels decrease in cardiac output; extreme oliguria; poikilothermia; 80% decrease in basal metabolism	No motion; decreased nerve-conduction velocity; peripheral areflexia; no corneal or oculocephalic reflexes

Source: Modified from RR Kempainen, DD Brunette: Resp. Care 49:192, 2004.

(3) the depression of a frozen chest wall is not possible. As the resuscitation proceeds, the prognosis is grave if there is evidence of widespread cell lysis, as reflected by potassium levels > 10 mmol/L (10 meq/L). Other findings that may preclude continuing resuscitation include a core temperature < 10–12°C, a pH < 6.5, or evidence of intravascular thrombosis with a fibrinogen value < 0.5 g/L (<50 mg/dL). The decision to terminate resuscitation before rewarming the patient past 33°C should be predicated on the type and severity of the precipitants of hypothermia. There are no validated prognostic indicators for recovery from hypothermia. A history of asphyxia with secondary cooling is the most important negative predictor of survival.

DIAGNOSIS AND STABILIZATION

Hypothermia is confirmed by measuring the core temperature, preferably at two sites. Rectal probes should be placed to a depth of 15 cm and not adjacent to cold feces. A simultaneous esophageal probe should be placed 24 cm below the larynx; it may read falsely high during heated inhalation therapy. Relying solely on infrared tympanic thermography is not advisable.

After a diagnosis of hypothermia is established, cardiac monitoring should be instituted, along with attempts to limit further heat loss. If the patient is in ventricular fibrillation, one defibrillation attempt (2 J/kg) should be administered. If the rhythm does not convert, rewarm the patient to 30–32°C before repeating defibrillation attempts. Supplemental oxygenation is always warranted, since tissue oxygenation is adversely affected by the leftward shift of the oxyhemoglobin dissociation curve. Pulse oximetry may be unreliable in patients with vasoconstriction. If protective airway reflexes are absent, gentle endotracheal intubation should be performed. Adequate pre-oxygenation will prevent ventricular arrhythmias. Although cardiac pacing for hypothermic bradydysrhythmias is rarely indicated, the transthoracic technique is preferable.

Insertion of a gastric tube prevents dilatation secondary to decreased bowel motility. Indwelling bladder catheters facilitate monitoring of cold-induced diuresis. Dehydration is commonly encountered with chronic hypothermia, and most patients benefit from a bolus of crystalloid. Normal saline is preferable to lactated Ringer's solution, as the liver in hypothermic patients inefficiently metabolizes lactate. The placement of a pulmonary artery catheter risks perforation of the less compliant pulmonary artery. Insertion of a central venous catheter into the cold right atrium should be avoided, since this can precipitate arrhythmias.

Arterial blood gases should not be corrected for temperature (Chap. 48). An uncorrected pH of 7.42 and a P_{CO_2} of 40 mmHg reflects appropriate alveolar ventilation and acid-base balance at any core temperature. Acid-base imbalances should be corrected gradually, since the bicarbonate buffering system is inefficient. A common error is overzealous hyperventilation in the setting of depressed CO_2 production. When the P_{CO_2} decreases 10 mmHg at 28°C, it doubles the pH increase of 0.08 that occurs at 37°C.

The severity of anemia may be underestimated because the hematocrit increases 2% for each 1°C drop in temperature. White blood cell sequestration and bone marrow suppression are common, potentially masking an infection. Although hypokalemia is more common in chronic hypothermia, hyperkalemia also occurs; the expected electrocardiographic changes can be obscured by hypothermia. Patients with renal insufficiency, metabolic acidoses, or rhabdomyolysis are at greatest risk for electrolyte disturbances.

Coagulopathies are common because cold inhibits the enzymatic reactions required for activation of the intrinsic cascade. In addition, thromboxane B_2 production by platelets is temperature-dependent, and platelet function is impaired. The administration of platelets and fresh frozen plasma is, therefore, not effective. The prothrombin or partial thromboplastin times or INR (international normalized ratio) reported by the laboratory appear deceptively normal and contrast with the observed in vivo coagulopathy. This contradiction occurs because all coagulation tests are routinely performed at 37°C, and the enzymes are thus rewarmed.

REWARMING STRATEGIES

The key initial decision is whether to rewarm the patient passively or actively. *Passive external rewarming* simply involves covering and insulating the patient in a warm environment. With the head also covered, the rate of rewarming is usually 0.5° to 2.0°C per hour. This technique is ideal for previously healthy patients who develop acute, mild primary accidental hypothermia. The patient must have sufficient glycogen to support endogenous thermogenesis.

The application of heat directly to the extremities of patients with chronic severe hypothermia should be avoided because it can induce peripheral vasodilatation and precipitate core temperature "afterdrop"—a response characterized by a continual decline in the core temperature after removal of the patient from the cold. Truncal heat application reduces the risk of afterdrop.

Active rewarming is necessary under the following circumstances: core temperature < 32°C (poikilothermia), cardiovascular instability, age extremes, CNS dysfunction, hormone insufficiency, or suspicion of secondary hypothermia. *Active external rewarming* is best accomplished with forced-air heating blankets. Other options include radiant heat sources and hot packs. Monitoring a patient with hypothermia in a heated tub is extremely difficult. Electric blankets should be avoided because vasoconstricted skin is easily burned.

There are numerous widely available *active core rewarming* options. Airway rewarming with heated humidified oxygen (40°–45°C) is a convenient option via mask or endotracheal tube. Although airway rewarming provides less heat than some other forms of active core rewarming, it eliminates respiratory heat loss and adds 1°–2°C to the overall rewarming rate. Crystalloids should be heated to 40°–42°C, but the quantity of heat provided is significant only during massive volume resuscitation. The most efficient method for heating and delivering fluid or blood is with a countercurrent in-line heat exchanger. Heated irrigation of the gastrointestinal tract or bladder transfers minimal heat because of the limited available surface area. These methods should be reserved for patients in cardiac arrest and then used in combination with all available active rewarming techniques. Closed thoracic lavage is far more efficient in severely hypothermic patients with cardiac arrest. The hemithoraces are irrigated through two large-bore thoracostomy tubes that are inserted into the hemithoraces. Thoracostomy tubes should not be placed in the left chest of a spontaneously perfusing patient for purposes of rewarming. Peritoneal lavage with the dialysate at 40°–45°C efficiently transfers heat when delivered through two catheters with outflow suction. Like peritoneal dialysis, standard hemodialysis is especially useful for patients with electrolyte abnormalities, rhabdomyolysis, or toxin ingestions.

Extracorporeal blood rewarming options (Table 20-3) should be considered in severely hypothermic patients, especially those with *primary accidental hypothermia.* Cardiopulmonary bypass should be considered in nonperfusing patients without documented contraindications to resuscitation. Circulatory support may be the only effective option in patients with completely frozen extremities, or those with significant tissue destruction coupled with rhabdomyolysis. There is no evidence that extremely rapid rewarming improves survival in perfusing patients. The best strategy is usually a combination of passive, truncal active, and active core rewarming techniques.

℞ HYPOTHERMIA

When a patient is hypothermic, target organs and the cardiovascular system respond minimally to most medications. Moreover, cumulative doses can cause toxicity during rewarming because of increased binding of drugs to proteins, and impaired metabolism and excretion. As an example, the administration of repeated doses of digoxin or insulin would be ineffective while the patient is hypothermic, and the residual drugs are potentially toxic during rewarming.

Achieving a mean arterial pressure of at least 60 mmHg should be an early objective. If the hypotension does not respond to crystalloid/colloid infusion and rewarming, low-dose dopamine (2–5 μg/kg per min) support should be considered. Perfusion of the vasoconstricted cardiovascular system may also be improved with low-dose IV nitroglycerin.

Atrial arrhythmias should initially be monitored without intervention, as the ventricular response will be slow, and unless preexistent, most will convert spontaneously during rewarming. The role of prophylaxis and treatment of ventricular arrhythmias is problematic. Preexisting ventricular ectopy may be suppressed by hypothermia and reappear during rewarming. None of the class I agents has proved to be safe and efficacious. When available, bretylium tosylate was the class III ventricular antiarrhythmic of choice. There is no evidence that amiodarone is safe.

Initiating empirical therapy for adrenal insufficiency is usually not warranted unless there is a history suggesting steroid dependence, hypoadrenalism, or a failure to rewarm with standard therapy. The administration of parenteral levothyroxine to euthyroid patients with hypothermia, however, is potentially hazardous. Because laboratory results can be delayed and confounded by the presence of the sick euthyroid syndrome (Chap. 335), historic clues or physical findings suggestive of hypothyroidism should be sought. When myxedema is the cause of hypothermia, the relaxation phase of the Achilles reflex is prolonged more than the contraction phase.

Hypothermia obscures most of the symptoms and signs of infection, notably fever and leukocytosis. Shaking rigors from infection may be mistaken for shivering. Except in mild cases, extensive cultures and repeated physical examinations are essential. Unless an infectious source is identified, empirical antibiotic prophylaxis is most warranted in the elderly, neonates, and immunocompromised patients.

Preventive measures should be discussed with high-risk individuals, such as the elderly or people whose work frequently exposes them to extreme cold. The importance of layered clothing and headgear, adequate shelter, increased caloric intake, and the avoidance of ethanol should be emphasized, along with access to rescue services.

TABLE 20-3 OPTIONS FOR EXTRACORPOREAL BLOOD REWARMING

Extracorporeal Rewarming (ECR) Technique	Considerations
Venovenous (VV)	Circuit—CV catheter to CV or peripheral catheter No oxygenator/circulatory support Flow rates 150–400 mL/min ROR 2°–3°C/h
Hemodialysis (HD)	Circuit—single or dual vessel cannulation Stabilizes electrolyte or toxicologic abnormalities Exchange cycle volumes 200–500 mL/min ROR 2°–3°C/h
Continuous arteriovenous rewarming (CAVR)	Circuit—percutaneous 8.5 Fr femoral catheters Requires BP 60 mmHg systolic No perfusionist/pump/anticoagulation Flow rates 225–375 mL/min ROR 3°–4°C/h
Cardiopulmonary bypass (CPB)	Circuit—full circulatory support with pump and oxygenator Perfusate-temperature gradient (5°–10°C) Flow rates 2–7 L/min (ave. 3–4) ROR up to 9.5°C/h

Note: BP, blood pressure; CV, central venous; ROR, rate of rewarming.

FROSTBITE

Peripheral cold injuries include both freezing and nonfreezing injuries to tissue. Tissue freezes quickly when in contact with thermal conductors such as metal or volatile solutions. Other predisposing factors include constrictive clothing or boots, immobility, or vasoconstrictive medications. Frostbite occurs when the tissue temperature drops below 0°C. Ice crystal formation subsequently distorts and destroys the cellular architecture. Once the vascular endothelium is damaged, stasis progresses rapidly to microvascular thrombosis. After the tissue thaws, there is progressive dermal ischemia. The microvasculature begins to collapse, arteriovenous shunting increases tissue pressures, and edema forms. Finally, thrombosis, ischemia, and superficial necrosis appear. The development of mummification and demarcation may take weeks to months.

CLINICAL PRESENTATION

The initial presentation of frostbite can be deceptively benign. The symptoms always include a sensory deficiency affecting light touch, pain, and temperature perception. The acral areas and distal extremities are the most common insensate areas. Some patients complain of a clumsy or "chunk of wood" sensation in the extremity.

FIGURE 20-1 Frostbite with vesiculation, surrounded by edema and erythema.

Deep frostbitten tissue can appear waxy, mottled, yellow, or violaceous-white. Favorable presenting signs include some warmth or sensation with normal color. The injury is often superficial if the subcutaneous tissue is pliable or if the dermis can be rolled over boney prominences.

Clinically, it is most practical to classify frostbite as superficial or deep. Superficial does not entail tissue loss. Classically, frostbite is retrospectively graded like a burn. First-degree frostbite causes only anesthesia and erythema. The appearance of superficial vesiculation surrounded by edema and erythema is considered second degree (**Fig.**

20-1). Hemorrhagic vesicles reflect a serious injury to the microvasculature and indicate third-degree frostbite. Fourth-degree injuries damage subcuticular, muscular, and osseous tissues.

The two most common nonfreezing peripheral cold injuries are *chilblain (pernio)* and *immersion (trench) foot*. Chilblain results from neuronal and endothelial damage induced by repetitive exposure to dry cold. Young females, particularly those with a history of Raynaud's phenomenon, are at greatest risk. Persistent vasospasticity and vasculitis can cause erythema, mild edema, and pruritus. Eventually plaques, blue nodules, and ulcerations develop. These lesions typically involve the dorsa of the hands and feet. In contrast, immersion (trench) foot results from repetitive exposure to wet cold above the freezing point. The feet initially appear cyanotic, cold, and edematous. The subsequent development of bullae is often indistinguishable from frostbite. This vesiculation rapidly progresses to ulceration and liquefaction gangrene. Patients with milder cases complain of hyperhidrosis, cold sensitivity, and painful ambulation for many years.

℞ FROSTBITE

Frozen tissue should be rapidly and completely thawed by immersion in circulating water at 37°–40°C. Rapid rewarming often produces an initial hyperemia. The early formation of large clear distal blebs is more favorable than smaller proximal dark hemorrhagic blebs. A common error is the premature termination of thawing, since the reestablishment of perfusion is intensely painful. Parenteral narcotics will be necessary with deep frostbite. If cyanosis persists after rewarming, the tissue compartment pressures should be monitored carefully.

Numerous experimental antithrombotic and vasodilatory treatment regimens have been evaluated. There is no conclusive evidence that dextran, heparin, steroids, calcium channel blockers, hyperbaric oxygen, or prostaglandin inhibitors salvage tissue. A treatment protocol for frostbite is summarized in **Table 20-4**.

Unless infection develops, any decision regarding debridement or amputation should be deferred until there is clear evidence of demarcation, mummification, and sloughing. Magnetic resonance angiography may demonstrate the line of demarcation earlier than clinical demarcation. The most common symptomatic sequelae reflect neuronal injury and the persistently abnormal sympathetic tone, including paresthesias, thermal misperception, and hyperhidrosis. Delayed findings include nail deformities, cutaneous carcinomas, and epiphyseal damage in children.

Management of the chilblain syndrome is usually supportive. With refractory perniosis, alternatives include nifedipine, steroids, or limaprost, a prostaglandin E_1 analogue.

FURTHER READINGS

BRIEVA J et al: Severe hypothermia: Challenging normal physiology. Anesth Intensive Care 33:662, 2005

DANZL DF: Accidental hypothermia, in *Rosen's Emergency Medicine: Concepts and Clinical Practice*, 6th ed, J Marx et al (eds). St. Louis, Mosby, 2006, p 2236

ERVASTI O et al: The occurrence of frostbite and its risk factors in young men. Int J Circumpolar Health 63:71, 2004

GIESBRECHT GG: Cold stress, near drowning and accidental hypothermia: A review. Aviat Space Environ Med 71:733, 2000

JURKOVICH GJ: Environmental cold-induced injury. Surg Clin North Am 87(1):247, viii, 2007

KEMPAINEN RR, BRUNETTE DD: The evaluation and management of accidental hypothermia. Respir Care 49:192, 2004

VASSAL T et al: Severe accidental hypothermia treated in an ICU: Prognosis and outcome. Chest 120:1998, 2001

TABLE 20-4	TREATMENT FOR FROSTBITE	
Before Thawing	**During Thawing**	**After Thawing**
Remove from environment	Consider parenteral analgesia and ketorolac	Gently dry and protect part; elevate; pledgets between toes, if macerated
Prevent partial thawing and refreezing	Administer ibuprofen, 400 mg PO	If clear vesicles are intact, aspirate sterilely; if broken, debride and dress with antibiotic or sterile aloe vera ointment
Stabilize core temperature and treat hypothermia	Immerse part in 37°–40°C (thermometer-monitored) circulating water containing an antiseptic soap until distal flush (10–45 min)	Leave hemorrhagic vesicles intact to prevent dessication and infection
Protect frozen part—no friction or massage	Encourage patient to gently move part	Continue ibuprofen 400 mg PO (12 mg/kg per day) q8–12h
Address medical or surgical conditions	If pain is refractory, reduce water temperature to 35°–37°C and administer parenteral narcotics	Consider tetanus and streptococcal prophylaxis; elevate part
Hydrotherapy at 37°C
Consider phenoxybenzamine in severe cases

SECTION 3 NERVOUS SYSTEM DYSFUNCTION

21 Syncope
Mark D. Carlson

Syncope, a transient loss of consciousness and postural tone due to reduced cerebral blood flow, is associated with spontaneous recovery. It may occur suddenly, without warning, or may be preceded by symptoms of faintness ("presyncope"). These symptoms include lightheadedness, dizziness, a feeling of warmth, diaphoresis, nausea, and visual blurring occasionally proceeding to transient blindness. Presyncopal symptoms vary in duration and may increase in severity until loss of consciousness occurs, or they may resolve prior to loss of consciousness if the cerebral ischemia is corrected. The differentiation of syncope from seizure is an important, sometimes difficult, diagnostic problem.

Syncope may be benign when it occurs as a result of normal cardiovascular reflex effects on heart rate and vascular tone, or serious when due to a life-threatening cardiac arrhythmia. Syncope may occur as a single event or may be recurrent. Recurrent, unexplained syncope, particularly in an individual with structural heart disease, is associated with a high risk of death (40% mortality within 2 years).

PATHOPHYSIOLOGY

Under normal circumstances systemic blood pressure is regulated by a complex process that includes the musculature, venous valves, autonomic nervous system, and renin-aldosterone-angiotensin system. Knowledge of these processes is important to understanding the pathophysiology of syncope. Approximately three-fourths of the systemic blood volume is contained in the venous bed, and any interference in venous return may lead to a reduction in cardiac output. Cerebral blood flow can be maintained if cardiac output and systemic arterial vasoconstriction compensate, but when these adjustments fail, hypotension with resultant cerebral underperfusion to less than half of normal results in syncope. Normally, the pooling of blood in the lower parts of the body is prevented by (1) pressor reflexes that induce constriction of peripheral arterioles and venules, (2) reflex acceleration of the heart by means of aortic and carotid reflexes, and (3) improvement of venous return to the heart by activity of the muscles of the limbs. Tilting a normal person upright on a tilt table causes some blood to accumulate in the lower limbs and diminishes cardiac output slightly; this may be followed by a slight transitory fall in systolic blood pressure. However, in a patient with defective vasomotor reflexes, upright tilt may produce an abrupt and sustained fall in blood pressure, precipitating a faint.

CAUSES OF SYNCOPE

Transiently decreased cerebral blood flow is usually due to one of three general mechanisms: disorders of vascular tone or blood volume, cardiovascular disorders including obstructive lesions and cardiac arrhythmias, or cerebrovascular disease (Table 21-1). Not infrequently, however, the cause of syncope is multifactorial.

DISORDERS OF VASCULAR TONE OR BLOOD VOLUME

Disorders of vascular tone or blood volume that can cause syncope include the reflex syncopes and a number of conditions resulting in orthostatic intolerance. The reflex syncopes—including neurocardiogenic syncope, situational syncope, and carotid sinus hypersensitivity—share common autonomic nervous system pathophysiologic mechanisms: a cardioinhibitory component (e.g., bradycardia due to increased vagal activity), a vasodepressor component (e.g., inappropriate vasodilatation due to sympathetic withdrawal), or both.

Neurocardiogenic (Vasovagal and Vasodepressor) Syncope   The term *neurocardiogenic* is generally used to encompass both vasovagal and vasodepressor syncope. Strictly speaking, vasovagal syncope is associated with both sympathetic withdrawal (vasodilatation) and increased parasympathetic activity (bradycardia), whereas vasodepressor syncope is associated with sympathetic withdrawal alone.

These forms of syncope are the common faint that may be experienced by normal persons; they account for approximately half of all episodes of syncope. Neurocardiogenic syncope is frequently recurrent and commonly precipitated by a hot or crowded environment, alcohol, extreme fatigue, severe pain, hunger, prolonged standing, and emotional or stressful situations. Episodes are often preceded by a presyncopal prodrome lasting seconds to minutes, and rarely occur in the supine position. The individual is usually sitting or standing and experiences

TABLE 21-1	CAUSES OF SYNCOPE

I. Disorders of Vascular Tone or Blood Volume
  A. Reflex syncopes
    1. Neurocardiogenic
    2. Situational
      Cough
      Micturition
      Defecation
      Valsalva
      Deglutition
    3. Carotid sinus hypersensitivity
  B. Orthostatic hypotension
    1. Drug-induced (antihypertensive or vasodilator drugs)
    2. Pure autonomic failure (idiopathic orthostatic hypotension)
    3. Multisystem atrophies
    4. Peripheral neuropathy (diabetic, alcoholic, nutritional, amyloid)
    5. Physical deconditioning
    6. Sympathectomy
    7. Decreased blood volume
II. Cardiovascular Disorders
  A. Structural and obstructive causes
    1. Pulmonary embolism
    2. Pulmonary hypertension
    3. Atrial myxoma
    4. Mitral valvular stenosis
    5. Myocardial disease (massive acute myocardial infarction)
    6. Left ventricular myocardial restriction or constriction
    7. Pericardial constriction or tamponade
    8. Aortic outflow tract obstruction
    9. Aortic valvular stenosis
    10. Hypertrophic obstructive cardiomyopathy
  B. Cardiac arrhythmias
    1. Bradyarrhythmias
      a. Sinus bradycardia, sinoatrial block, sinus arrest, sick-sinus syndrome
      b. Atrioventricular block
    2. Tachyarrhythmias
      a. Supraventricular tachycardia with structural cardiovascular disease
      b. Atrial fibrillation with the Wolff-Parkinson-White syndrome
      c. Atrial flutter with 1:1 atrioventricular conduction
      d. Ventricular tachycardia
III. Cerebrovascular Disease
  A. Vertebrobasilar insufficiency
  B. Basilar artery migraine
IV. Other Disorders that May Resemble Syncope
  A. Metabolic
    1. Hypoxia
    2. Anemia
    3. Diminished carbon dioxide due to hyperventilation
    4. Hypoglycemia
  B. Psychogenic
    1. Anxiety attacks
    2. Hysterical fainting
  C. Seizures

weakness, nausea, diaphoresis, lightheadedness, blurred vision, and often a forceful heartbeat with tachycardia followed by cardiac slowing and decreasing blood pressure prior to loss of consciousness. The individual appears pale or ashen; in dark-skinned individuals, the pallor may only be notable in the conjunctivae and lips. Patients with a gradual onset of presyncopal symptoms have time to protect themselves against injury; in others, syncope occurs suddenly, without warning.

The depth and duration of unconsciousness vary. Sometimes the patient remains partly aware of the surroundings, or there may be complete unresponsiveness. The unconscious patient usually lies motionless, with skeletal muscles relaxed, but a few clonic jerks of the limbs and face may occur. Sphincter control is usually maintained, in contrast to a seizure. The pulse may be feeble or apparently absent, the blood pressure low or undetectable, and breathing may be almost imperceptible. The duration of unconsciousness is rarely longer than a few minutes if the conditions that provoke the episode are reversed. Once the patient is placed in a horizontal position, the strength of the pulse improves, color begins to return to the face, breathing becomes quicker and deeper, and consciousness is restored. Some patients may experience a sense of residual weakness after regaining consciousness, and rising too soon may precipitate another faint. Unconsciousness may be prolonged if an individual remains upright; thus, it is essential that individuals with vasovagal syncope assume a recumbent position as soon as possible. Although usually benign, neurocardiogenic syncope can be associated with prolonged asystole and hypotension, resulting in hypoxic-ischemic injury.

Neurocardiogenic syncope often occurs in the setting of increased peripheral sympathetic activity and venous pooling. Under these conditions, vigorous myocardial contraction of a relatively empty left ventricle is thought to activate myocardial mechanoreceptors and vagal afferent nerve fibers that inhibit sympathetic activity and increase parasympathetic activity. The resultant vasodilatation and bradycardia induce hypotension and syncope. Although the reflex involving myocardial mechanoreceptors is the mechanism usually accepted as responsible for neurocardiogenic syncope, other reflexes may also be operative. Patients with transplanted (denervated) hearts have experienced cardiovascular responses identical to those present during neurocardiogenic syncope. This should not be possible if the response depends solely on the reflex mechanisms described above, unless the transplanted heart has become reinnervated. Moreover, neurocardiogenic syncope often occurs in response to stimuli (fear, emotional stress, or pain) that may not be associated with venous pooling in the lower extremities, which suggests a cerebral component to the reflex.

As distinct from the peripheral mechanisms, the central nervous system (CNS) mechanisms responsible for neurocardiogenic syncope are uncertain, but a sudden surge in central serotonin levels may contribute to the sympathetic withdrawal. Endogenous opiates (endorphins) and adenosine are also putative participants in the pathogenesis.

Situational Syncope A variety of activities, including cough, deglutition, micturition, and defecation, are associated with syncope in susceptible individuals. Like neurocardiogenic syncope, these syndromes may involve a cardioinhibitory response, a vasodepressor response, or both. Cough, micturition, and defecation are associated with maneuvers (such as Valsalva's, straining, and coughing) that may contribute to hypotension and syncope by decreasing venous return. Increased intracranial pressure secondary to the increased intrathoracic pressure may also contribute by decreasing cerebral blood flow.

Cough syncope typically occurs in men with chronic bronchitis or chronic obstructive lung disease during or after prolonged coughing fits. Micturition syncope occurs predominantly in middle-aged and older men, particularly those with prostatic hypertrophy and obstruction of the bladder neck; loss of consciousness usually occurs at night during or immediately after voiding. Deglutition syncope and defecation syncope occur in men and women. Deglutition syncope may be associated with esophageal disorders, particularly esophageal spasm. In some individuals, particular foods and carbonated or cold beverages initiate episodes by activating esophageal sensory receptors that trigger reflex sinus bradycardia or atrioventricular (AV) block. Defecation syncope is probably secondary to Valsalva's maneuver in older individuals with constipation.

Carotid Sinus Hypersensitivity Syncope due to carotid sinus hypersensitivity is precipitated by pressure on the carotid sinus baroreceptors, which are located just cephalad to the bifurcation of the common carotid artery. This typically occurs in the setting of shaving, a tight collar, or turning the head to one side. Carotid sinus hypersensitivity occurs predominantly in men ≥50 years old. Activation of carotid sinus baroreceptors gives rise to impulses carried via the nerve of Hering, a branch of the glossopharyngeal nerve, to the medulla in the brainstem. These afferent impulses activate efferent sympathetic nerve fibers to the heart and blood vessels, cardiac vagal efferent nerve fibers, or both. In patients with carotid sinus hypersensitivity, these responses may cause sinus arrest or AV block (a cardioinhibitory response), vasodilatation (a vasodepressor response), or both (a mixed response). The underlying mechanisms responsible for the carotid sinus hypersensitivity are not clear, and validated diagnostic criteria do not exist.

Postural (Orthostatic) Hypotension Orthostatic intolerance can result from hypovolemia or from disturbances in vascular control. The latter may occur due to agents that affect the vasculature or due to primary or secondary abnormalities of autonomic control. Sudden rising from a recumbent position or standing quietly are precipitating circumstances. *Orthostatic hypotension may be the cause of syncope in up to 30% of the elderly; polypharmacy with antihypertensive or antidepressant drugs is often a contributor in these patients.*

Postural syncope may occur in otherwise normal persons with defective postural reflexes. Pure autonomic failure (formerly called *idiopathic postural hypotension*) is characterized by orthostatic hypotension, syncope and near syncope, neurocardiogenic bladder, constipation, heat intolerance, inability to sweat, and erectile dysfunction (Chap. 370). The disorder is more common in men than women and typically begins between the ages of 50 and 75 years.

Orthostatic hypotension, often accompanied by disturbances in sweating, impotence, and sphincter difficulties, is also a primary feature of a variety or other autonomic nervous system disorders (Chap. 370). Among the most common causes of neurogenic orthostatic hypotension are chronic diseases of the peripheral nervous system that involve postganglionic unmyelinated fibers (e.g., diabetic, nutritional, and amyloid polyneuropathy). Much less common are the multiple system atrophies; these are CNS disorders in which orthostatic hypotension is associated with (1) parkinsonism (Shy-Drager syndrome), (2) progressive cerebellar degeneration, or (3) a more variable parkinsonian and cerebellar syndrome (Chap. 366). A rare, acute postganglionic dysautonomia may represent a variant of Guillain-Barré syndrome (Chap. 380); a related disorder, autoimmune autonomic neuropathy, is associated with autoantibodies to the ganglionic acetylcholine receptor.

There are several additional causes of postural syncope: (1) after physical deconditioning (such as after prolonged illness with recumbency, especially in elderly individuals with reduced muscle tone) or after prolonged weightlessness, as in space flight; (2) after sympathectomy that has abolished vasopressor reflexes; and (3) in patients receiving antihypertensive or vasodilator drugs and those who are hypovolemic because of diuretics, excessive sweating, diarrhea, vomiting, hemorrhage, or adrenal insufficiency.

Glossopharyngeal Neuralgia Syncope due to glossopharyngeal neuralgia (Chap. 371) is preceded by pain in the oropharynx, tonsillar fossa, or tongue. Loss of consciousness is usually associated with asystole rather than vasodilatation. The mechanism is thought to involve activation of afferent impulses in the glossopharyngeal nerve that terminate in the nucleus solitarius of the medulla and, via collaterals, activate the dorsal motor nucleus of the vagus nerve.

CARDIOVASCULAR DISORDERS

Cardiac syncope results from a sudden reduction in cardiac output, caused most commonly by a cardiac arrhythmia. In normal individuals, heart rates between 30 and 180 beats/min do not reduce cerebral blood flow, especially if the person is in the supine position. As the heart rate decreases, ventricular filling time and stroke volume increase to maintain normal cardiac output. At rates <30 beats/min, stroke volume can no longer increase to compensate adequately for the decreased heart rate. At rates greater than ~180 beats/min, ventricular filling time is inadequate to maintain adequate stroke volume. In either case, cerebral hypoperfusion and syncope may occur. Upright posture; cerebrovascular disease; anemia; loss of atrioventricular synchrony; and coronary, myocardial, or valvular disease all reduce the tolerance to alterations in rate.

Bradyarrhythmias (Chap. 225) may occur as a result of an abnormality of impulse generation (e.g., sinoatrial arrest) or impulse conduction (e.g., AV block). Either may cause syncope if the escape pacemaker rate is insufficient to maintain cardiac output. Syncope due to bradyarrhythmias may occur abruptly, without presyncopal symptoms, and recur several times daily. Patients with *sick sinus syndrome* may have sinus pauses (>3 s), and those with syncope due to high-degree AV block (*Stokes-Adams-Morgagni syndrome*) may have evidence of conduction system disease (e.g., prolonged PR interval, bundle branch block). However, the arrhythmia is often transitory, and the surface electrocardiogram or continuous electrocardiographic monitor (Holter monitor) taken later may not reveal the abnormality. The *bradycardia-tachycardia syndrome* is a common form of sinus node dysfunction in which syncope generally occurs as a result of marked sinus pauses, some following termination of paroxysms of atrial tachyarrhythmias. Drugs are a common cause for bradyarrhythmias, particularly in patients with underlying structural heart disease. Digoxin, β-adrenergic receptor antagonists, calcium channel blockers, and many antiarrhythmic drugs may suppress sinoatrial node impulse generation or slow AV nodal conduction.

Syncope due to a *tachyarrhythmia* (Chap. 226) is usually preceded by palpitation or lightheadedness but may occur abruptly with no warning symptoms. *Supraventricular tachyarrhythmias* are unlikely to cause syncope in individuals with structurally normal hearts but may do so if they occur in patients with (1) heart disease that also compromises cardiac output, (2) cerebrovascular disease, (3) a disorder of vascular tone or blood volume, or (4) a rapid ventricular rate. These tachycardias result most commonly from paroxysmal atrial flutter, atrial fibrillation, or reentry involving the AV node or accessory pathways that bypass part or all of the AV conduction system. Patients with *Wolff-Parkinson-White syndrome* may experience syncope when a very rapid ventricular rate occurs due to reentry across an accessory AV connection.

In patients with structural heart disease, ventricular tachycardia is a common cause of syncope, particularly in those with a prior myocardial infarction. Patients with aortic valvular stenosis and hypertrophic obstructive cardiomyopathy are also at risk for ventricular tachycardia. Individuals with abnormalities of ventricular repolarization (prolongation of the QT interval) are at risk to develop polymorphic ventricular tachycardia (torsades des pointes). Those with the inherited form of this syndrome often have a family history of sudden death in young individuals. Genetic markers can identify some patients with familial long-QT syndrome, but the clinical utility of these markers remains unproven. Drugs (i.e., certain antiarrhythmics and erythromycin) and electrolyte disorders (i.e., hypokalemia, hypocalcemia, hypomagnesemia) can prolong the QT interval and predispose to torsades des pointes. Antiarrhythmic medications may precipitate ventricular tachycardia, particularly in patients with structural heart disease.

In addition to arrhythmias, syncope may also occur with a variety of structural cardiovascular disorders. Episodes are usually precipitated when the cardiac output cannot increase to compensate adequately for peripheral vasodilatation. Peripheral vasodilatation may be appropriate, such as following exercise, or may occur due to inappropriate activation of left ventricular mechanoreceptor reflexes, as occurs in aortic outflow tract obstruction (aortic valvular stenosis or hypertrophic obstructive cardiomyopathy). Obstruction to forward flow is the most common reason that cardiac output cannot increase. Pericardial tamponade is a rare cause of syncope. Syncope occurs in up to 10% of patients with massive pulmonary embolism and may occur with exertion in patients with severe primary pulmonary hypertension. The cause is an inability of the right ventricle to provide appropriate cardiac output in the presence of obstruction or increased pulmonary vascular resistance. Loss of consciousness is usually accompanied by other symptoms such as chest pain and dyspnea. Atrial myxoma, a prosthetic valve thrombus, and, rarely, mitral stenosis may impair left ventricular filling, decrease cardiac output, and cause syncope.

CEREBROVASCULAR DISEASE

Cerebrovascular disease alone rarely causes syncope but may lower the threshold for syncope in patients with other causes. The vertebrobasilar arteries, which supply brainstem structures responsible for maintaining consciousness, are usually involved when cerebrovascular disease causes or contributes to syncope. An exception is the rare patient with tight bilateral carotid stenosis and recurrent syncope, often precipitated by standing or walking. Most patients who experience lightheadedness or syncope due to cerebrovascular disease also have symptoms of focal neurologic ischemia, such as arm or leg weakness, diplopia, ataxia, dysarthria, or sensory disturbances. Basilar artery migraine is a rare disorder that causes syncope in adolescents.

DIFFERENTIAL DIAGNOSIS

ANXIETY ATTACKS AND HYPERVENTILATION SYNDROME

Anxiety, such as occurs in panic attacks, is frequently interpreted as a feeling of faintness or dizziness resembling presyncope. However, the symptoms are not accompanied by facial pallor and are not relieved by recumbency. The diagnosis is made on the basis of the associated symptoms such as a feeling of impending doom, air hunger, palpitations, and tingling of the fingers and perioral region. Attacks can often be reproduced by hyperventilation, resulting in hypocapnia, alkalosis, increased cerebrovascular resistance, and decreased cerebral blood flow. The release of epinephrine also contributes to the symptoms.

SEIZURES

A seizure may be heralded by an aura, which is caused by a focal seizure discharge and hence has localizing significance (Chap. 363). The aura is usually followed by a rapid return to normal or by a loss of consciousness. Injury from falling is frequent in a seizure and rare in syncope, since only in generalized seizures are protective reflexes abolished instantaneously. Sustained tonic-clonic movements are characteristic of convulsive seizures, but brief clonic, or tonic-clonic, seizure-like activity can accompany fainting episodes. The period of unconsciousness in seizures tends to be longer than in syncope. Urinary incontinence is frequent in seizures and rare in syncope. The return of consciousness is prompt in syncope and slow after a seizure. Mental confusion, headache, and drowsiness are common sequelae of seizures, whereas physical weakness with a clear sensorium characterizes the postsyncopal state. Repeated spells of unconsciousness in a young person at a rate of several per day or month are more suggestive of epilepsy than syncope. See Table 363-7 for a comparison of seizures and syncope.

HYPOGLYCEMIA

Severe hypoglycemia is usually due to a serious disease such as a tumor of the islets of Langerhans or advanced adrenal, pituitary, or hepatic disease; or to excessive administration of insulin.

HYSTERICAL FAINTING

The attack is usually unattended by an outward display of anxiety. Lack of change in pulse and blood pressure or color of the skin and mucous membranes distinguish it from the vasodepressor faint.

APPROACH TO THE PATIENT:
Syncope

The diagnosis of syncope is often challenging. The cause may only be apparent at the time of the event, leaving few, if any, clues when the patient is seen later by the physician. The physician should think first of those causes that constitute a therapeutic emergency, including massive internal hemorrhage or myocardial infarction, which may be painless, and cardiac arrhythmias. In elderly persons, a sudden faint, without obvious cause, should arouse the sus-

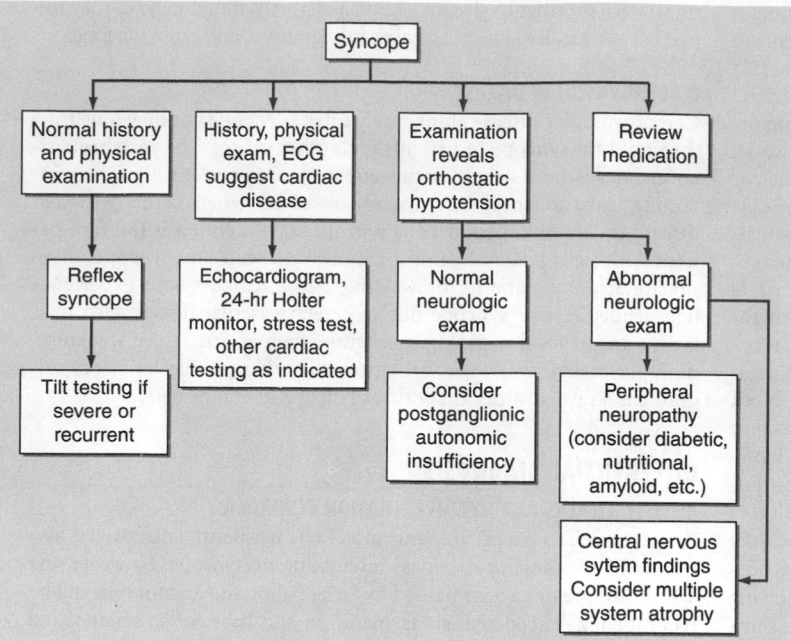

FIGURE 21-1 Approach to the patient with syncope.

picion of complete heart block or a tachyarrhythmia, even though all findings are negative when the patient is seen.

Figure 21-1 depicts an algorithmic approach to syncope. A careful history is the most important diagnostic tool, both to suggest the correct cause and to exclude important potential causes (Table 21-1). The nature of the events and their time course immediately prior to, during, and after an episode of syncope often provide valuable etiologic clues. Loss of consciousness in particular situations, such as during venipuncture or micturition or with volume depletion, suggests an abnormality of vascular tone. The position of the patient at the time of the syncopal episode is important; syncope in the supine position is unlikely to be vasovagal and suggests an arrhythmia or a seizure. Syncope due to carotid sinus syndrome may occur when the individual is wearing a shirt with a tight collar, turning the head (turning to look while driving in reverse), or manipulating the neck (as in shaving). The patient's medications must be noted, including nonprescription drugs or health store supplements, with particular attention to recent changes.

The physical examination should include evaluation of heart rate and blood pressure in the supine, sitting, and standing positions. In patients with unexplained recurrent syncope, an attempt to reproduce an attack may assist in diagnosis. Anxiety attacks induced by hyperventilation can be reproduced readily by having the patient breathe rapidly and deeply for 2–3 min. Cough syncope may be reproduced by inducing the Valsalva's maneuver. Carotid sinus massage should generally be avoided, unless carotid ultrasound is negative for atheroma, because its diagnostic specificity is unknown and it may provoke a transient ischemic attack (TIA) or stroke in individuals with carotid atheromas.

DIAGNOSTIC TESTS The choice of diagnostic tests should be guided by the history and the physical examination. Measurements of serum electrolytes, glucose, and the hematocrit are usually indicated. Cardiac enzymes should be evaluated if myocardial ischemia is suspected. Blood and urine toxicology screens may reveal the presence of alcohol or other drugs. In patients with possible adrenocortical insufficiency, plasma aldosterone and mineralocorticoid levels should be obtained.

Although the surface electrocardiogram is unlikely to provide a definitive diagnosis, it may provide clues to the cause of syncope *and should be performed in almost all patients*. The presence of conduction

abnormalities (PR prolongation and bundle branch block) suggests a bradyarrhythmia, whereas pathologic Q waves or prolongation of the QT interval suggests a ventricular tachyarrhythmia. Inpatients should undergo continuous electrocardiographic monitoring; outpatients should wear a Holter monitor for 24–48 h. Whenever possible, symptoms should be correlated with the occurrence of arrhythmias. Continuous electrocardiographic monitoring may establish the cause of syncope in as many as 15% of patients. Cardiac event monitors may be useful in patients with infrequent symptoms, particularly in patients with presyncope. An implantable event monitor may be necessary for patients with extremely infrequent episodes. The presence of a late potential on a signal-averaged electrocardiogram is associated with increased risk for ventricular tachyarrhythmias in patients with a prior myocardial infarction. Low-voltage (visually inapparent) T wave alternans is also associated with development of sustained ventricular arrhythmias.

Invasive cardiac electrophysiologic testing provides diagnostic and prognostic information regarding sinus node function, AV conduction, and supraventricular and ventricular arrhythmias (Chaps. 225 and 226). Prolongation of the sinus node recovery time (>1500 ms) is a specific finding (85–100%) for diagnosis of sinus node dysfunction but has a low sensitivity; continuous electrocardiographic monitoring is usually more effective for diagnosing this abnormality. Prolongation of the HV interval and conduction block below the His bundle indicate that His-Purkinje disease may be responsible for syncope. Programmed stimulation for ventricular arrhythmias is most useful in patients who have experienced a myocardial infarction; the sensitivity and specificity of this technique is lower in patients with normal hearts or those with heart disease other than coronary artery disease.

Upright tilt table testing is indicated for recurrent syncope, a single syncopal episode that caused injury, or a single syncopal event in a "high-risk" setting (pilot, commercial vehicle driver, etc.), whether or not there is a history of preexisting heart disease or prior vasovagal episodes. In susceptible patients, upright tilt at an angle between 60° and 80° for 30–60 min induces a vasovagal episode. The protocol can be shortened if upright tilt is combined with administration of drugs that cause venous pooling or increase adrenergic stimulation (isoproterenol, nitroglycerin, edrophonium, or adenosine). The sensitivity and specificity of tilt-table testing is difficult to ascertain because of the lack of validated criteria. Moreover, the reflexes responsible for vasovagal syncope can be elicited in most, if not all, individuals given the appropriate stimulus. The specificity of tilt-table testing has been reported to be near 90%, but it is lower when pharmacologic provocation is employed. The reported sensitivity of the test ranges between 20 and 74%, the variability due to differences in populations studied, techniques used, and the absence of a true "gold standard" against which to compare test results. The reproducibility (in a time ranging from several hours to weeks) is 80–90% for an initially positive response, but may be less for an initially negative response (ranging from 30 to 90%).

A variety of other tests may be useful to determine the presence of structural heart disease that may cause syncope. The echocardiogram with Doppler examination detects valvular, myocardial, and pericardial abnormalities. The echocardiogram is the "gold standard" for the diagnosis of hypertrophic cardiomyopathy and atrial myxoma. Cardiac cine MRI provides an alternative noninvasive modality that may be useful for patients in whom diagnostic-quality echocardiographic images cannot be obtained. This test is also indicated for patients suspected of having arrhythmogenic right ventricular dysplasia or right ventricular outflow tract ventricular tachycardia. Both are associated with right ventricular structural abnormalities that are better visualized on MR imaging than by echocardiogram. Exercise testing may detect ischemia or exercise-induced arrhythmias. In some patients, cardiac catheterization may be necessary to diagnose the presence or severity of coronary artery disease or valvular abnormalities. Ultrafast CT scan, ventilation-perfusion scan, or pulmonary angiography is indicated in patients in whom syncope may be due to pulmonary embolus.

In cases of possible cerebrovascular syncope, neuroimaging tests may be indicated, including Doppler ultrasound studies of the carotid and vertebrobasilar systems, MRI, magnetic resonance angiography, and x-ray angiography of the cerebral vasculature (Chap. 364). Electroencephalography is indicated if seizures are suspected.

Rx SYNCOPE

The treatment of syncope is directed at the underlying cause. This discussion will focus on disorders of autonomic control. **Arrhythmias are discussed in Chaps. 225 and 226, valvular heart diseases in Chap. 230, and cerebrovascular disorders in Chap. 364.**

Certain precautions should be taken regardless of the cause of syncope. At the first sign of symptoms, patients should make every effort to avoid injury should they lose consciousness. Patients with frequent episodes, or those who have experienced syncope without warning symptoms, should avoid situations in which sudden loss of consciousness might result in injury (e.g., climbing ladders, swimming alone, operating heavy machinery, driving). Patients should lower their head to the extent possible and preferably should lie down. Lowering the head by bending at the waist should be avoided because it may further compromise venous return to the heart. When appropriate, family members or other close contacts should be educated as to the problem. This will ensure appropriate therapy and may prevent delivery of inappropriate therapy (chest compressions associated with cardiopulmonary resuscitation) that may inflict trauma.

Patients who have lost consciousness should be placed in a position that maximizes cerebral blood flow, offers protection from trauma, and secures the airway. Whenever possible, the patient should be placed supine with the head turned to the side to prevent aspiration and the tongue from blocking the airway. Assessment of the pulse and direct cardiac auscultation may assist in determining if the episode is associated with a bradyarrhythmia or a tachyarrhythmia. Clothing that fits tightly around the neck or waist should be loosened. Peripheral stimulation, such as sprinkling cold water on the face, may be helpful. Patients should not be given anything by mouth or be permitted to rise until the sense of physical weakness has passed.

Patients with vasovagal syncope should be instructed to avoid situations or stimuli that have caused them to lose consciousness and to assume a recumbent position when premonitory symptoms occur. These behavioral modifications alone may be sufficient for patients with infrequent and relatively benign episodes of vasovagal syncope, particularly when loss of consciousness occurs in response to a specific stimulus. Tilt training (standing and leaning against a wall for progressively longer periods each day) has been used with limited success, particularly for patients with orthostatic intolerance. Episodes associated with intravascular volume depletion may be prevented by salt and fluid loading prior to provocative events.

Drug therapy may be necessary when vasovagal syncope is resistant to the above measures, when episodes occur frequently, or when syncope is associated with a significant risk for injury. β-Adrenergic receptor antagonists (metoprolol, 25–50 mg bid; atenolol, 25–50 mg qd; or nadolol, 10–20 mg bid; all starting doses), the most widely used agents, mitigate the increase in myocardial contractility that stimulates left ventricular mechanoreceptors and also block central serotonin receptors. Serotonin reuptake inhibitors (paroxetine, 20–40 mg qd; or sertraline, 25–50 mg qd), appear to be effective for some patients. Bupropion SR (150 mg qd), another antidepressant, has also been used with success. β-Adrenergic receptor antagonists and serotonin reuptake inhibitors are well tolerated and are often used as first-line agents for younger patients. Hydrofludrocortisone (0.1–0.2 mg qd), a mineralocorticoid, promotes sodium retention, volume expansion, and peripheral vasoconstriction by increasing β-receptor sensitivity to endogenous catecholamines. Hydrofludrocortisone is useful for patients with intravascular volume depletion and for those who also have postural hypotension. Proamatine (2.5–10 mg bid or tid), an α-agonist, has been used as a first-line agent for some patients. In a randomized controlled trial, proamatine was more effective than placebo in preventing

syncope during an upright tilt-test. However, in some patients, proamatine and hydrofludrocortisone may increase resting supine systemic blood pressure, which may be problematic for those with hypertension.

Disopyramide (150 mg bid), a vagolytic antiarrhythmic drug with negative inotropic properties, and transdermal scopolamine, another vagolytic, have been used to treat vasovagal syncope, as have theophylline and ephedrine. Side effects associated with these drugs have limited their use for this indication. Disopyramide is a type 1A antiarrhythmic drug and should be used with great caution, if at all, in patients who are at risk for ventricular arrhythmias.

Although several clinical trials have suggested that pharmacologic therapy for neurocardiogenic syncope is effective, the few long-term prospective randomized controlled trials have yielded mixed results. In the Prevention of Syncope Trial (POST), metoprolol was ineffective in patients <42 years of age but decreased the incidence of syncope in patients >42, raising the possibility that there may be significant age-related differences in response to pharmacologic therapy.

Studies of permanent pacing for neurocardiogenic syncope have also yielded mixed results. Dual-chamber cardiac pacing may be effective for patients with frequent episodes of vasovagal syncope, particularly for those with prolonged asystole associated with vasovagal episodes. Pacemakers that can be programmed to transiently pace at a high rate (90–100 beats/min) after a profound drop in the patient's intrinsic heart rate are most effective.

Patients with orthostatic hypotension should be instructed to rise slowly and systematically (supine to seated, seated to standing) from the bed or a chair. Movement of the legs prior to rising facilitates venous return from the lower extremities. Whenever possible, medications that aggravate the problem (vasodilators, diuretics, etc.) should be discontinued. Elevation of the head of the bed [20–30 cm (8–12 in.)] and use of compression stockings may help.

Additional therapeutic modalities include salt loading and a variety of pharmacologic agents including sympathomimetic amines, monoamine oxidase inhibitors, beta blockers, and levodopa. The treatment of orthostatic hypotension secondary to central or peripheral disorders of the autonomic nervous system is discussed in Chap. 370.

Glossopharyngeal neuralgia is treated with carbamazepine, which is effective for syncope as well as for pain. Patients with carotid sinus hypersensitivity should be instructed to avoid clothing and situations that stimulate carotid sinus baroreceptors. They should turn their entire body, rather than just their head, when looking to the side. Those with intractable syncope due to the cardioinhibitory response to carotid sinus stimulation should undergo permanent pacemaker implantation.

Patients with syncope should be hospitalized when there is a possibility that the episode may have resulted from a life-threatening abnormality or if recurrence with significant injury seems likely. These individuals should be admitted to a bed with continuous electrocardiographic monitoring. Patients who are known to have a normal heart and for whom the history strongly suggests vasovagal or situational syncope may be treated as outpatients if the episodes are neither frequent nor severe.

FURTHER READINGS

GRUBB BP: Neurocardiogenic syncope and related disorders of orthostatic intolerance. Circulation 111:2997, 2005

———, OLSHANSKY B (eds): *Syncope: Mechanisms and Management,* 2d ed. Malden, Mass., Blackwell Futura, 2005

KAPOOR WN: Current evaluation in management of syncope. Circulation 106:1606, 2002

KAUFMAN H et al: Midodrine in neurally mediated syncope: A double-blind, randomized, crossover study. Ann Neurol 52:342, 2002

KAUFMANN H, BHATTACHARYA K: Diagnosis and treatment of neurally mediated syncope. Neurologist 8:175, 2002

KERR SRJ et al: Carotid sinus hypersensitivity in asymptomatic older persons: Implications for diagnosis of syncope and falls. Arch Intern Med 166:515, 2006

MAISEL W, STEBENSON W: Syncope—getting to the heart of the matter. N Engl J Med 347:931, 2002

SOTERIADES E et al: Incidence and prognosis of syncope. N Engl J Med 347:878, 2002

144 STRICKBERGER SA et al: AHA/ACCF scientific statement on the evaluation of syncope: From the American Heart Association Councils on Clinical Cardiology, Cardiovascular Nursing, Cardiovascular Disease in the Young, and Stroke, and the Quality of Care and Outcomes Research Interdisciplinary Working Group; and the American College of Cardiology Foundation: In collaboration with the Heart Rhythm Society: Endorsed by the American Autonomic Society. Circulation 113(2):316, 2006

VAN DIJK N et al: Quality of life within one year following presentation after transient loss of consciousness. Am J Cardio 100:672, 2007

22 Dizziness and Vertigo
Robert B. Daroff

Dizziness is a common and often vexing symptom. Patients use the term to encompass a variety of sensations, including those that seem semantically appropriate (e.g., lightheadedness, faintness, spinning, giddiness) and those that are misleadingly inappropriate, such as mental confusion, blurred vision, headache, or tingling. Moreover, some individuals with gait disorders caused by peripheral neuropathy, myelopathy, spasticity, parkinsonism, or cerebellar ataxia complain of "dizziness" despite the absence of vertigo or other abnormal cephalic sensations. In this context, the term *dizziness* is being used to describe disturbed ambulation. There may be mild associated lightheadedness, particularly with impaired sensation from the feet or poor vision; this is known as *multiple-sensory-defect dizziness* and occurs in elderly individuals who complain of dizziness only when walking. Decreased position sense (secondary to neuropathy or myelopathy) and poor vision (from cataracts or retinal degeneration) create an overreliance on the aging vestibular apparatus. A less precise but sometimes comforting designation to patients is *benign dysequilibrium of aging*. Thus, a careful history is necessary to determine exactly what a patient who states, "Doctor, I'm dizzy," is experiencing. After eliminating the misleading symptoms or gait disturbance, "dizziness" usually means either *faintness* (presyncope) or *vertigo* (an illusory or hallucinatory sense of movement of the body or environment, most often a feeling of spinning). Operationally, after obtaining the history, dizziness may be classified into three categories: (1) faintness, (2) vertigo, and (3) miscellaneous head sensations.

FAINTNESS

Prior to an actual faint (syncope), there are often prodromal presyncopal symptoms (faintness) reflecting ischemia to a degree insufficient to impair consciousness. These include lightheadedness, "dizziness" without true vertigo, a feeling of warmth, diaphoresis, nausea, and visual blurring occasionally proceeding to blindness. Presyncopal symptoms vary in duration and may increase in severity until loss of consciousness occurs or may resolve prior to loss of consciousness if the cerebral ischemia is corrected. Faintness and syncope are discussed in detail in Chap. 21.

VERTIGO

Vertigo is usually due to a disturbance in the vestibular system. The end organs of this system, situated in the bony labyrinths of the inner ears, consist of the three semicircular canals and the otolithic apparatus (utricle and saccule) on each side. The canals transduce angular acceleration, while the otoliths transduce linear acceleration and the static gravitational forces that provide a sense of head position in space. The neural output of the end organs is conveyed to the vestibular nuclei in the brainstem via the eighth cranial nerves. The principal projections from the vestibular nuclei are to the nuclei of cranial nerves III, IV, and VI; spinal cord; cerebral cortex; and cerebellum. The vestibuloocular reflex (VOR) serves to maintain visual stability during head movement and depends on direct projections from the vestibular nuclei to the sixth cranial nerve (abducens) nuclei in the pons and, via the medial longitudinal fasciculus, to the third (oculomotor) and fourth (trochlear) cranial nerve nuclei in the midbrain. These connections account for the nystagmus (to-and-fro oscillation of the eyes) that is an almost invariable accompaniment of vestibular dysfunction. The vestibular nerves and nuclei project to areas of the cerebellum (primarily the flocculus and nodulus) that modulate the VOR. The vestibulospinal pathways assist in the maintenance of postural stability. Projections to the cerebral cortex, via the thalamus, provide conscious awareness of head position and movement.

The vestibular system is one of three sensory systems subserving spatial orientation and posture; the other two are the visual system (retina to occipital cortex) and the somatosensory system that conveys peripheral information from skin, joint, and muscle receptors. The three stabilizing systems overlap sufficiently to compensate (partially or completely) for each other's deficiencies. Vertigo may represent either physiologic stimulation or pathologic dysfunction in any of the three sensory systems.

Physiologic Vertigo This occurs in normal individuals when (1) the brain is confronted with an intersensory mismatch among the three stabilizing sensory systems; (2) the vestibular system is subjected to unfamiliar head movements to which it is unadapted, such as in seasickness; (3) unusual head/neck positions, such as the extreme extension when painting a ceiling; or (4) following a spin. Intersensory mismatch explains carsickness, height vertigo, and the visual vertigo most commonly experienced during motion picture chase scenes; in the latter, the visual sensation of environmental movement is unaccompanied by concomitant vestibular and somatosensory movement cues. *Space sickness*, a frequent transient effect of active head movement in the weightless zero-gravity environment, is another example of physiologic vertigo.

Pathologic Vertigo This results from lesions of the visual, somatosensory, or vestibular systems. Visual vertigo is caused by new or incorrect eyeglasses or by the sudden onset of an extraocular muscle paresis with diplopia; in either instance, central nervous system (CNS) compensation rapidly counteracts the vertigo. Somatosensory vertigo, rare in isolation, is usually due to a peripheral neuropathy or myelopathy that reduces the sensory input necessary for central compensation when there is dysfunction of the vestibular or visual systems.

The most common cause of pathologic vertigo is vestibular dysfunction involving either its end organ (labyrinth), nerve, or central connections. The vertigo is associated with jerk nystagmus and is frequently accompanied by nausea, postural unsteadiness, and gait ataxia. Since vertigo increases with rapid head movements, patients tend to hold their heads still.

LABYRINTHINE DYSFUNCTION This causes severe rotational or linear vertigo. When rotational, the hallucination of movement, whether of environment or self, is directed away from the side of the lesion. The fast phases of nystagmus beat away from the lesion side, and the tendency to fall is toward the side of the lesion, particularly in darkness or with the eyes closed.

Under normal circumstances, when the head is straight and immobile, the vestibular end organs generate a tonic resting firing frequency that is equal from the two sides. With any rotational acceleration, the anatomic positions of the semicircular canals on each side necessitate an increased firing rate from one and a commensurate decrease from the other. This change in neural activity is ultimately projected to the cerebral cortex, where it is summed with inputs from the visual and somatosensory systems to produce the appropriate conscious sense of rotational movement. After cessation of prolonged rotation, the firing frequencies of the two end organs reverse; the side with the initially increased rate decreases, and the other side increases. A sense of rotation in the opposite direction is experienced; since there is no actual head movement, this hallucinatory sensation is *physiologic postrotational vertigo*.

Any disease state that changes the firing frequency of an end organ, producing unequal neural input to the brainstem and ultimately the cerebral cortex, causes vertigo. The symptom can be conceptualized as the cortex inappropriately interpreting the abnormal neural input as indicating actual head rotation. Transient abnormalities produce short-lived symptoms. With a fixed unilateral deficit, central compensatory mechanisms ultimately diminish the vertigo. Since compensation depends on the plasticity of connections between the vestibular nuclei and the cerebellum, patients with brainstem or cerebellar disease have diminished adaptive capacity, and symptoms may persist indefinitely. Compensation is always inadequate for severe fixed bilateral lesions despite normal cerebellar connections; these patients are permanently symptomatic when they move their heads.

Acute unilateral labyrinthine dysfunction is caused by infection, trauma, and ischemia. Often, no specific etiology is uncovered, and the nonspecific terms *acute labyrinthitis*, *acute peripheral vestibulopathy*, or *vestibular neuritis* are used to describe the event. The vertiginous attacks are brief and leave the patient with mild vertigo for several days. Infection with herpes simplex virus type 1 has been implicated. It is impossible to predict whether a patient recovering from the first bout of vertigo will have recurrent episodes.

Labyrinthine ischemia, presumably due to occlusion of the labyrinthine branch of the internal auditory artery, may be the sole manifestation of vertebrobasilar insufficiency (Chap. 364); patients with this syndrome present with the abrupt onset of severe vertigo, nausea, and vomiting, but without tinnitus or hearing loss.

Acute bilateral labyrinthine dysfunction is usually the result of toxins such as drugs or alcohol. The most common offending drugs are the aminoglycoside antibiotics that damage the hair cells of the vestibular end organs and may cause a permanent disorder of equilibrium.

Recurrent unilateral labyrinthine dysfunction, in association with signs and symptoms of cochlear disease (progressive hearing loss and tinnitus), is usually due to Ménière's disease (Chap. 30). When auditory manifestations are absent, the term *vestibular neuronitis* denotes recurrent monosymptomatic vertigo. Transient ischemic attacks of the posterior cerebral circulation (vertebrobasilar insufficiency) only infrequently cause recurrent vertigo without concomitant motor, sensory, visual, cranial nerve, or cerebellar signs (Chap. 364).

Positional vertigo is precipitated by a recumbent head position, either to the right or to the left. Benign paroxysmal positional (or positioning) vertigo (BPPV) of the posterior semicircular canal is particularly common. Although the condition may be due to head trauma, usually no precipitating factors are identified. It generally abates spontaneously after weeks or months. The vertigo and accompanying nystagmus have a distinct pattern of latency, fatigability, and habituation that differs from the less common central positional vertigo (Table 22-1) due to lesions in and around the fourth ventricle. Moreover, the pattern of nystagmus in posterior canal BPPV is distinctive. When supine, with the head turned to the side of the offending ear (bad ear down), the lower eye displays a large-amplitude torsional nystagmus, and the upper eye has a lesser degree of torsion combined with upbeating nystagmus. If the eyes are directed to the upper ear, the vertical nystagmus in the upper eye increases in amplitude. Mild dysequilibrium when upright may also be present.

A *perilymphatic fistula* should be suspected when episodic vertigo is precipitated by Valsalva or exertion, particularly upon a background of a

TABLE 22-1 BENIGN PAROXYSMAL POSITIONAL VERTIGO AND CENTRAL POSITIONAL VERTIGO

Features	BPPV	Central
Latency[a]	3–40 s	None: immediate vertigo and nystagmus
Fatigability[b]	Yes	No
Habituation[c]	Yes	No
Intensity of vertigo	Severe	Mild
Reproducibility[d]	Variable	Good

[a]Time between attaining head position and onset of symptoms.
[b]Disappearance of symptoms with maintenance of offending position.
[c]Lessening of symptoms with repeated trials.
[d]Likelihood of symptom production during any examination session.

TABLE 22-2 FEATURES OF PERIPHERAL AND CENTRAL VERTIGO

Sign or Symptom	Peripheral (Labyrinth)	Central (Brainstem or Cerebellum)
Direction of associated nystagmus	Unidirectional; fast phase opposite lesion[a]	Bidirectional or unidirectional
Purely horizontal nystagmus without torsional component	Uncommon	Common
Vertical or purely torsional nystagmus	Never present	May be present
Visual fixation	Inhibits nystagmus and vertigo	No inhibition
Severity of vertigo	Marked	Often mild
Direction of spin	Toward fast phase	Variable
Direction of fall	Toward slow phase	Variable
Duration of symptoms	Finite (minutes, days, weeks) but recurrent	May be chronic
Tinnitus and/or deafness	Often present	Usually absent
Associated CNS abnormalities	None	Extremely common (e.g., diplopia, hiccups, cranial neuropathies, dysarthria)
Common causes	BPPV, infection (labyrinthitis), Ménière's, neuronitis, ischemia, trauma, toxin	Vascular, demyelinating, neoplasm

[a]In Ménière's disease, the direction of the fast phase is variable.

stepwise progressive sensory-neural hearing loss. The condition is usually caused by head trauma or barotrauma or occurs after middle ear surgery.

VERTIGO OF VESTIBULAR NERVE ORIGIN This occurs with diseases that involve the nerve in the petrous bone or the cerebellopontine angle. Although less severe and less frequently paroxysmal, it has many of the characteristics of labyrinthine vertigo. The adjacent auditory division of the eighth cranial nerve is usually affected, which explains the frequent association of vertigo with unilateral tinnitus and hearing loss. The most common cause of eighth cranial nerve dysfunction is a tumor, usually a schwannoma (*acoustic neuroma*) or a meningioma. These tumors grow slowly and produce such a gradual reduction of labyrinthine output that central compensatory mechanisms can prevent or minimize the vertigo; auditory symptoms are the most common manifestations.

CENTRAL VERTIGO Lesions of the brainstem or cerebellum can cause acute vertigo, but associated signs and symptoms usually permit distinction from a labyrinthine etiology (Table 22-2). Occasionally, an acute lesion of the vestibulocerebellum may present with monosymptomatic vertigo indistinguishable from a labyrinthopathy.

Vertigo may be a manifestation of a migraine aura (Chap. 15), but some patients with migraine have episodes of vertigo unassociated with their headaches. Antimigrainous treatment should be considered in such patients with otherwise enigmatic vertiginous episodes.

Vestibular epilepsy, vertigo secondary to temporal lobe epileptic activity, is rare and almost always intermixed with other epileptic manifestations.

PSYCHOGENIC VERTIGO This is sometimes called phobic postural vertigo and is usually a concomitant of panic attacks (Chap. 386) or agoraphobia (fear of large open spaces, crowds, or leaving the safety of home). It should be suspected in patients so "incapacitated" by their symptoms that they adopt a prolonged housebound status. Most patients with organic vertigo attempt to function despite their discomfort. Organic vertigo is accompanied by nystagmus; a psychogenic etiology is almost certain when nystagmus is absent during a vertiginous episode. The symptoms often develop after an episode of acute labyrinthine dysfunction.

MISCELLANEOUS HEAD SENSATIONS

This designation is used, primarily for purposes of initial classification, to describe dizziness that is neither faintness nor vertigo. Cephalic ischemia or vestibular dysfunction may be of such low intensity that the usual symptomatology is not clearly identified. For example, a small decrease in blood pressure or a slight vestibular imbalance may cause sensations different from distinct faintness or vertigo but that may be identified properly by provocative testing techniques (see below). Other causes of dizziness in this category are hyperventilation syndrome, hypoglycemia, and the somatic symptoms of a clinical depression; these patients should all have normal neurologic examinations and vestibular function tests. Depressed patients often insist that the depression is "secondary" to the dizziness.

APPROACH TO THE PATIENT:
Dizziness and Vertigo

The most important diagnostic tool is a detailed history focused on the meaning of "dizziness" to the patient. Is it faintness (presyncope)? Is there a sensation of spinning? If either of these is affirmed and the neurologic examination is normal, appropriate investigations for the multiple causes of cephalic ischemia, presyncope (Chap. 21), or vestibular dysfunction are undertaken.

When the meaning of "dizziness" is uncertain, provocative tests may be helpful. These office procedures simulate either cephalic ischemia or vestibular dysfunction. Cephalic ischemia is obvious if the dizziness is duplicated during maneuvers that produce orthostatic hypotension. Further provocation involves the Valsalva maneuver, which decreases cerebral blood flow and should reproduce ischemic symptoms.

Hyperventilation is the cause of dizziness in many anxious individuals; tingling of the hands and face may be absent. Forced hyperventilation for 1 min is indicated for patients with enigmatic dizziness and normal neurologic examinations.

The simplest provocative test for vestibular dysfunction is rapid rotation and abrupt cessation of movement in a swivel chair. This always induces vertigo that the patients can compare with their symptomatic dizziness. The intense induced vertigo may be unlike the spontaneous symptoms, but shortly thereafter, when the vertigo has all but subsided, a lightheadedness supervenes that may be identified as "my dizziness." When this occurs, the dizzy patient, originally classified as suffering from "miscellaneous head sensations," is now properly diagnosed as having mild vertigo secondary to a vestibulopathy.

Patients with symptoms of positional vertigo should be appropriately tested (Table 22-1). A final provocative and diagnostic vestibular test, requiring the use of Frenzel eyeglasses (self-illuminated goggles with convex lenses that blur out the patient's vision, but allow the examiner to see the eyes greatly magnified), is vigorous head shaking in the horizontal plane for about 10 s. If nystagmus develops after the shaking stops, even in the absence of vertigo, vestibular dysfunction is demonstrated. The maneuver can then be repeated in the vertical plane. If the provocative tests establish the dizziness as a vestibular symptom, an evaluation of vestibular vertigo is undertaken.

EVALUATION OF PATIENTS WITH PATHOLOGIC VESTIBULAR VERTIGO
The evaluation depends on whether a central etiology is suspected (Table 22-2). If so, MRI of the head is mandatory. Such an examination is rarely helpful in cases of recurrent monosymptomatic vertigo with a normal neurologic examination. Typical BPPV requires no investigation after the diagnosis is made (Table 22-1).

Vestibular function tests serve to (1) demonstrate an abnormality when the distinction between organic and psychogenic is uncertain, (2) establish the side of the abnormality, and (3) distinguish between peripheral and central etiologies. The standard test is electronystagmography (calorics), where warm and cold water (or air) are applied, in a prescribed fashion, to the tympanic membranes, and the slow-phase velocities of the resultant nystagmus from the two are compared. A velocity decrease from one side indicates hypofunction ("canal paresis"). An inability to induce nystagmus with ice water denotes a "dead labyrinth." Some institutions have the capability of quantitatively determining various aspects of the VOR using computer-driven rotational chairs and precise oculographic recording of the eye movements.

TABLE 22-3 TREATMENT OF VERTIGO

Agent[a]	Dose[b]
Antihistamines	
Meclizine	25–50 mg 3 times/day
Dimenhydrinate	50 mg 1–2 times/day
Promethazine[c]	25–50-mg suppository or IM
Benzodiazepines	
Diazepam	2.5 mg 1–3 times/day
Clonazepam	0.25 mg 1–3 times/day
Phenothiazines	
Prochlorperazine[c]	5 mg IM or 25 mg suppository
Anticholinergic[d]	
Scopolamine transdermal	Patch
Sympathomimetics[d]	
Ephedrine	25 mg/d
Combination preparations[d]	
Ephedrine and promethazine	25 mg/d of each
Exercise therapy	
Repositioning maneuvers[e]	
Vestibular rehabilitation[f]	
Other	
Diuretics or low-salt (1 g/d) diet[g]	
Antimigrainous drugs[h]	
Inner ear surgery[i]	
Glucocorticoids[c]	100 mg/d for 3 days, tapered by 20 mg every 3 days

[a]All listed drugs are U.S. Food and Drug Administration approved, but most are not approved for the treatment of vertigo.
[b]Usual oral (unless otherwise stated) starting dose in adults; maintenance dose can be reached by a gradual increase.
[c]For acute vertigo only.
[d]For motion sickness only.
[e]For benign paroxysmal positional vertigo.
[f]For vertigo other than Ménière's and positional.
[g]For Ménière's disease.
[h]For migraine-associated vertigo (see Chap. 15 for a listing of prophylactic antimigrainous drugs).
[i]For perilymphatic fistula and refractory cases of Ménière's disease.

CNS disease can produce dizzy sensations of all types. Consequently, a neurologic examination is always required even if the history or provocative tests suggest a cardiac, peripheral vestibular, or psychogenic etiology. Any abnormality on the neurologic examination should prompt appropriate neurodiagnostic studies.

Rx VERTIGO

Treatment of acute vertigo consists of bed rest (1–2 days maximum) and vestibular suppressant drugs such as antihistaminics (meclizine, dimenhydrinate, promethazine), tranquilizers with GABA-ergic effects (diazepam, clonazepam), phenothiazines (prochlorperazine), or glucocorticoids (Table 22-3). If the vertigo persists beyond a few days, most authorities advise ambulation in an attempt to induce central compensatory mechanisms, despite the short-term discomfort to the patient. Chronic vertigo of labyrinthine origin may be treated with a systematized vestibular rehabilitation program to facilitate central compensation.

Posterior semicircular canal BPPV, the most common type, is often self-limited but, when persistent, may respond dramatically to specific repositioning exercise programs designed to empty particulate debris from the canal. One of these exercises, the Epley procedure, is graphically demonstrated, in four languages, on a website for use in both physicians' offices and self-treatment (www.charite.de/ch/neuro/vertigo.html).

Prophylactic measures to prevent recurrent vertigo are variably effective. Antihistamines are commonly utilized but are of limited value. Ménière's disease may respond to a diuretic or, more effectively, to a very low salt diet (1 g/d). Recurrent episodes of migraine-associated vertigo should be treated with antimigrainous therapy (Chap. 15). There are a variety of inner ear surgical procedures for refractory Ménière's disease, but these are only rarely necessary.

Psychogenic ("phobic postural") vertigo is best treated with cognitive-behavioral therapy.

Global Considerations There are no epidemiologic studies indicating an increased frequency of specific types of vertigo in different geographical areas. However, whereas BPPV of the posterior semicircular canal is overwhelmingly the most common form of positional vertigo in most countries, there seems to be an unusually large number of reports of horizontal (lateral) BPPV from Italy and Korea.

FURTHER READINGS

DIETERICH M: Dizziness. The Neurologist 10:154, 2004

HALMAGI GM: Diagnosis and management of vertigo. Clin Med 5:159, 2005

LEIGH RJ, ZEE DS: *Neurology of Eye Movement*, 4th ed. New York, Oxford, 2006, pp 76–79; 559–597

STRUPP M et al: Methylprednisolone, valacyclovir, or the combination for vestibular neuritis. N Engl J Med 351:354, 2004

———, BRANDT T: Pharmacological advances in the treatment of neuro-otological and eye movement disorders. Curr Opin Neurol 19:33, 2006

WHITE J et al: Canalith repositioning for benign paroxysmal positional vertigo. Otol Neurotol 26:704, 2005

ZINGLER VC et al: Causative factors and epidemiology of bilateral vestibulopathy in 255 patients. Ann Neurol 61:524, 2007

23 Weakness and Paralysis
Michael J. Aminoff

Normal motor function involves integrated muscle activity that is modulated by the activity of the cerebral cortex, basal ganglia, cerebellum, and spinal cord. Motor system dysfunction leads to weakness or paralysis, which is discussed in this chapter, or to ataxia (Chap. 368) or abnormal movements (Chap. 367). The mode of onset, distribution, and accompaniments of weakness help to suggest its cause.

Weakness is a reduction in the power that can be exerted by one or more muscles. Increased fatigability or limitation in function due to pain or articular stiffness is often confused with weakness by patients. *Increased fatigability* is the inability to sustain the performance of an activity that should be normal for a person of the same age, gender, and size. Increased time is sometimes required for full power to be exerted, and this *bradykinesia* may be misinterpreted as weakness. Severe proprioceptive sensory loss may also lead to complaints of weakness because adequate feedback information about the direction and power of movements is lacking. Finally, *apraxia*, a disorder of planning and initiating a skilled or learned movement unrelated to a significant motor or sensory deficit (Chap. 27), is sometimes mistaken for weakness by inexperienced medical staff.

Paralysis indicates weakness that is so severe that the muscle cannot be contracted at all, whereas *paresis* refers to weakness that is mild or moderate. The prefix "hemi-" refers to one half of the body, "para-" to both legs, and "quadri-" to all four limbs. The suffix "-plegia" signifies severe weakness or paralysis.

Weakness or paralysis is typically accompanied by other neurologic abnormalities that help to indicate the site of the responsible lesion. These include changes in tone, muscle bulk, muscle stretch reflexes, and cutaneous reflexes (Table 23-1).

Tone is the resistance of a muscle to passive stretch. Central nervous system (CNS) abnormalities that cause weakness generally produce *spasticity*, an increase in tone associated with disease of upper motor neurons. Spasticity is velocity-dependent, has a sudden release after reaching a maximum (the "clasp-knife" phenomenon), and predominantly affects the antigravity muscles (i.e., upper-limb flexors and lower-limb extensors). Spasticity is distinct from rigidity and paratonia, two other types of hypertonia. *Rigidity* is increased tone that is present throughout the range of motion (a "lead pipe" or "plastic" stiffness) and affects flexors and extensors equally; it sometimes has a cogwheel quality that is enhanced by voluntary movement of the contralateral limb (reinforcement). Rigidity occurs with certain extrapyramidal disorders such as Parkinson's disease. *Paratonia* (or *gegenhalten*) is increased tone that varies irregularly in a manner that may seem related to the degree of relaxation, is present throughout the range of motion, and affects flexors and extensors equally; it usually results from disease of the frontal lobes. Weakness with *decreased tone* (*flaccidity*) or normal tone occurs with disorders of *motor units*. A motor unit consists of a single lower motor neuron and all of the muscle fibers that it innervates.

Muscle bulk is generally unaffected in patients with upper motor neuron lesions, although mild disuse atrophy may eventually occur. By contrast, atrophy is often conspicuous when a lower motor neuron lesion is responsible for weakness and may also occur with advanced muscle disease.

Muscle stretch (tendon) reflexes are usually increased with upper motor neuron lesions, although they may be decreased or absent for a variable period immediately after onset of an acute lesion. This is usually—but not invariably—accompanied by abnormalities of *cutaneous reflexes* (such as superficial abdominals; Chap. 361) and, in particular, by an extensor plantar (Babinski) response. The muscle stretch reflexes are depressed in patients with lower motor neuron lesions when there is direct involvement of specific reflex arcs. The stretch reflexes are generally preserved in patients with myopathic weakness except in advanced stages, when they are sometimes attenuated. In disorders of the neuromuscular junction, the intensity of the reflexes may be affected by preceding voluntary activity of affected muscles—such activity may lead to enhancement of initially depressed reflexes in Lambert-Eaton myasthenic syndrome and, conversely, to depression of initially normal reflexes in myasthenia gravis (Chap. 381).

The distinction of *neuropathic* (lower motor neuron) from *myopathic* weakness is sometimes difficult clinically, although distal weakness is likely to be neuropathic and symmetric proximal weakness myopathic. *Fasciculations* (visible or palpable twitch within a muscle due to the spontaneous discharge of a motor unit) and early atrophy indicate that weakness is neuropathic.

PATHOGENESIS

Upper Motor Neuron Weakness This pattern of weakness results from disorders that affect the upper motor neurons or their axons in the cerebral cortex, subcortical white matter, internal capsule, brainstem, or spinal cord (Fig. 23-1). Such lesions produce weakness through decreased activation of the lower motor neurons. In general, distal muscle groups are affected more severely than proximal ones, and axial movements are spared unless the lesion is severe and bilateral. With corticobulbar involvement, weakness is usually observed only in the lower face and tongue; extraocular, upper facial, pharyngeal, and jaw muscles are almost always spared. With bilateral corticobulbar lesions, *pseudobulbar palsy* often develops: dysarthria, dysphagia, dysphonia, and emotional

TABLE 23-1	SIGNS THAT DISTINGUISH ORIGIN OF WEAKNESS		
Sign	**Upper Motor Neuron**	**Lower Motor Neuron**	**Myopathic**
Atrophy	None	Severe	Mild
Fasciculations	None	Common	None
Tone	Spastic	Decreased	Normal/decreased
Distribution of weakness	Pyramidal/regional	Distal/segmental	Proximal
Tendon reflexes	Hyperactive	Hypoactive/absent	Normal/hypoactive
Babinski's sign	Present	Absent	Absent

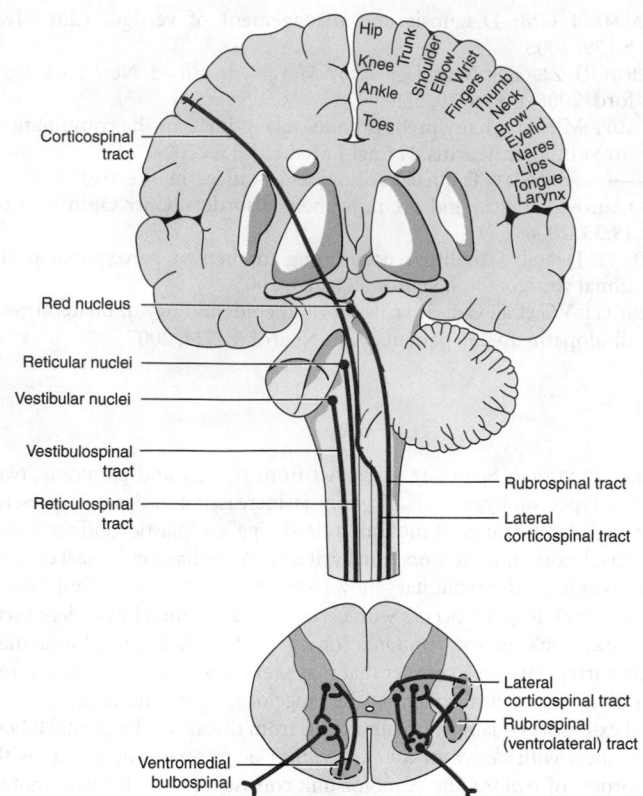

FIGURE 23-1 The corticospinal and bulbospinal upper motor neuron pathways. Upper motor neurons have their cell bodies in layer V of the primary motor cortex (the precentral gyrus, or Brodmann's area 4) and in the premotor and supplemental motor cortex (area 6). The upper motor neurons in the primary motor cortex are somatotopically organized as illustrated on the right side of the figure.

Axons of the upper motor neurons descend through the subcortical white matter and the posterior limb of the internal capsule. Axons of the *pyramidal* or *corticospinal system* descend through the brainstem in the cerebral peduncle of the midbrain, the basis pontis, and the medullary pyramids. At the cervicomedullary junction, most pyramidal axons decussate into the contralateral corticospinal tract of the lateral spinal cord, but 10–30% remain ipsilateral in the anterior spinal cord. Pyramidal neurons make direct monosynaptic connections with lower motor neurons. They innervate most densely the lower motor neurons of hand muscles and are involved in the execution of learned, fine movements. Corticobulbar neurons are similar to corticospinal neurons but innervate brainstem motor nuclei.

Bulbospinal upper motor neurons influence strength and tone but are not part of the pyramidal system. The descending *ventromedial bulbospinal pathways* originate in the tectum of the midbrain (tectospinal pathway), the vestibular nuclei (vestibulospinal pathway), and the reticular formation (reticulospinal pathway). These pathways influence axial and proximal muscles and are involved in the maintenance of posture and integrated movements of the limbs and trunk. The descending *ventrolateral bulbospinal pathways*, which originate predominantly in the red nucleus (rubrospinal pathway), facilitate distal limb muscles. The bulbospinal system is sometimes referred to as the *extrapyramidal upper motor neuron system*. In all figures, nerve cell bodies and axon terminals are shown, respectively, as closed circles and forks.

lability accompany bilateral facial weakness and a brisk jaw jerk. Spasticity accompanies upper motor neuron weakness but may not be present in the acute phase. Upper motor neuron lesions also affect the ability to perform rapid repetitive movements. Such movements are slow and coarse, but normal rhythmicity is maintained. Finger-nose-finger and heel-knee-shin maneuvers are performed slowly but adequately.

Lower Motor Neuron Weakness This pattern results from disorders of cell bodies of lower motor neurons in the brainstem motor nuclei and

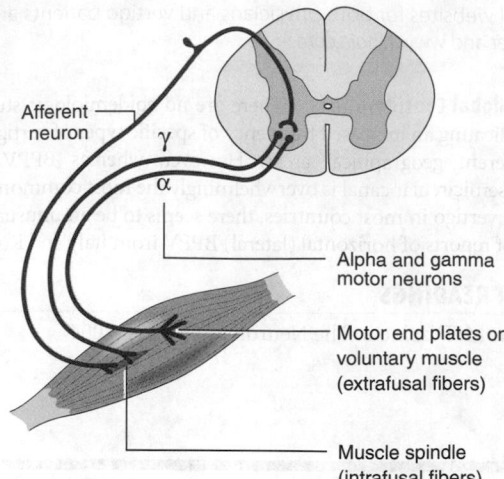

FIGURE 23-2 Lower motor neurons are divided into α and γ types. The larger α motor neurons are more numerous and innervate the extrafusal muscle fibers of the motor unit. Loss of α motor neurons or disruption of their axons produces lower motor neuron weakness. The smaller, less numerous γ motor neurons innervate the intrafusal muscle fibers of the muscle spindle and contribute to normal tone and stretch reflexes. The α motor neuron receives direct excitatory input from corticomotoneurons and primary muscle spindle afferents. The α and γ motor neurons also receive excitatory input from other descending upper motor neuron pathways, segmental sensory inputs, and interneurons. The α motor neurons receive direct inhibition from Renshaw cell interneurons, and other interneurons indirectly inhibit the α and γ motor neurons.

A tendon reflex requires the function of all illustrated structures. A tap on a tendon stretches muscle spindles (which are tonically activated by γ motor neurons) and activates the primary spindle afferent neurons. These stimulate the α motor neurons in the spinal cord, producing a brief muscle contraction, which is the familiar tendon reflex.

the anterior horn of the spinal cord, or from dysfunction of the axons of these neurons as they pass to skeletal muscle (**Fig. 23-2**). Weakness is due to a decrease in the number of muscle fibers that can be activated, through a loss of α motor neurons or disruption of their connections to muscle. Loss of γ motor neurons does not cause weakness but decreases tension on the muscle spindles, which decreases muscle tone and attenuates the stretch reflexes elicited on examination. An absent stretch reflex suggests involvement of spindle afferent fibers.

When a motor unit becomes diseased, especially in anterior horn cell diseases, it may spontaneously discharge, producing *fasciculations* that may be seen or felt clinically or recorded by electromyography (EMG). When α motor neurons or their axons degenerate, the denervated muscle fibers may also discharge spontaneously. These single muscle fiber discharges, or *fibrillation potentials*, cannot be seen or felt but can be recorded with EMG. If lower motor neuron weakness is present, recruitment of motor units is delayed or reduced, with fewer than normal activated at a given discharge frequency. This contrasts with weakness of upper motor neuron type, in which a normal number of motor units is activated at a given frequency but with a diminished maximal discharge frequency.

Myopathic Weakness Myopathic weakness is produced by disorders of the muscle fibers. Disorders of the neuromuscular junctions also produce weakness, but this is variable in degree and distribution and is influenced by preceding activity of the affected muscle. At a muscle fiber, if the nerve terminal releases a normal number of acetylcholine molecules presynaptically and a sufficient number of postsynaptic acetylcholine receptors are opened, the end plate reaches threshold and thereby generates an action potential that spreads across the muscle fiber membrane and into the transverse tubular system. This electrical excitation activates intracellular events that produce an energy-dependent contraction of the muscle fiber (excitation-contraction coupling).

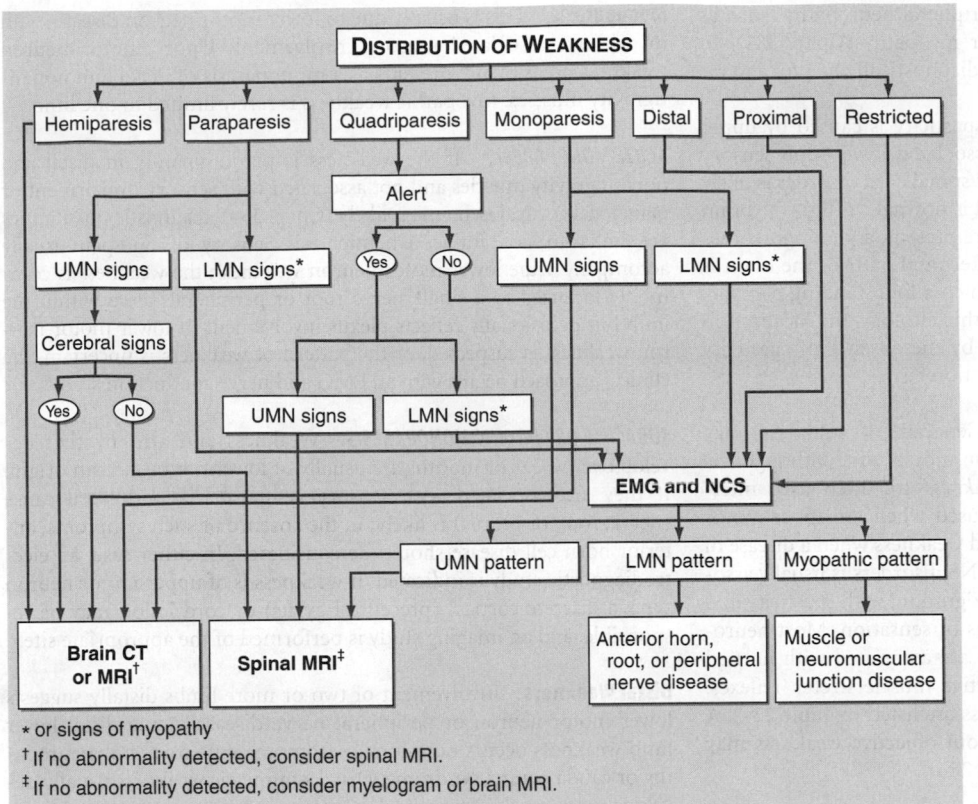

FIGURE 23-3 An algorithm for the initial workup of a patient with weakness. EMG, electromyography; LMN, lower motor neuron; NCS, nerve conduction studies; UMN, upper motor neuron.

In the figure:

DISTRIBUTION OF WEAKNESS

Hemiparesis | Paraparesis | Quadriparesis | Monoparesis | Distal | Proximal | Restricted

Alert — Yes / No

UMN signs | LMN signs*

Cerebral signs — Yes / No

UMN signs | LMN signs*

UMN signs | LMN signs*

EMG and NCS

UMN pattern | LMN pattern | Myopathic pattern

Brain CT or MRI† | Spinal MRI‡

Anterior horn, root, or peripheral nerve disease | Muscle or neuromuscular junction disease

* or signs of myopathy
† If no abnormality detected, consider spinal MRI.
‡ If no abnormality detected, consider myelogram or brain MRI.

Myopathic weakness is produced by a decrease in the number or contractile force of muscle fibers activated within motor units. With muscular dystrophies, inflammatory myopathies, or myopathies with muscle fiber necrosis, the number of muscle fibers is reduced within many motor units. On EMG, the size of each motor unit action potential is decreased, and motor units must be recruited more rapidly than normal to produce the desired power. Some myopathies produce weakness through loss of contractile force of muscle fibers or through relatively selective involvement of the type II (fast) fibers. These may not affect the size of individual motor unit action potentials and are detected by a discrepancy between the electrical activity and force of a muscle.

Diseases of the neuromuscular junction, such as myasthenia gravis, produce weakness in a similar manner, but the loss of muscle fibers is functional (due to inability to activate them) rather than related to muscle fiber loss. The number of muscle fibers that are activated varies over time, depending on the state of rest of the neuromuscular junctions. Thus, fatigable weakness is suggestive of myasthenia gravis or other disorders of the neuromuscular junction.

Hemiparesis Hemiparesis results from an upper motor neuron lesion above the midcervical spinal cord; most such lesions are above the foramen magnum. The presence of other neurologic deficits helps to localize the lesion. Thus, language disorders, cortical sensory disturbances, cognitive abnormalities, disorders of visual-spatial integration, apraxia, or seizures point to a cortical lesion. Homonymous visual field defects reflect either a cortical or a subcortical hemispheric lesion. A "pure motor" hemiparesis of the face, arm, or leg is often due to a small, discrete lesion in the posterior limb of the internal capsule, cerebral peduncle, or upper pons. Some brainstem lesions produce "crossed paralyses," consisting of ipsilateral cranial nerve signs and contralateral hemiparesis (Chap. 364). The absence of cranial nerve signs or facial weakness suggests that a hemiparesis is due to a lesion in the high cervical spinal cord, especially if associated with ipsilateral loss of proprioception and contralateral loss of pain and temperature sense (the Brown-Séquard syndrome).

Acute or episodic hemiparesis usually results from ischemic or hemorrhagic stroke, but may also relate to hemorrhage occurring into brain tumors or as a result of trauma; other causes include a focal structural lesion or inflammatory process as in multiple sclerosis, abscess, or sarcoidosis. Evaluation begins immediately with a CT scan of the brain (Fig. 23-3) and laboratory studies. If the CT is normal and an ischemic stroke is unlikely, MRI of the brain or cervical spine is performed.

Subacute hemiparesis that evolves over days or weeks has an extensive differential diagnosis. A common cause is subdural hematoma, especially in elderly or anticoagulated patients, even when there is no history of trauma. Infectious possibilities include cerebral abscess, fungal granuloma or meningitis, and parasitic infection. Weakness from primary and metastatic neoplasms may evolve over days to weeks. AIDS may present with subacute hemiparesis due to toxoplasmosis or primary CNS lymphoma. Noninfectious inflammatory processes, such as multiple sclerosis or, less commonly, sarcoidosis, merit consideration. If the brain MRI is normal and there are no cortical and hemispheric signs, MRI of the cervical spine should be undertaken.

Chronic hemiparesis that evolves over months is usually due to a neoplasm or vascular malformation, a chronic subdural hematoma, or a degenerative disease. If an MRI of the brain is normal, the possibility of a foramen magnum or high cervical spinal cord lesion should be considered.

Paraparesis An intraspinal lesion at or below the upper thoracic spinal cord level is most commonly responsible, but a paraparesis may also result from lesions at other locations that disturb upper motor neurons (especially parasagittal intracranial lesions) and lower motor neurons [anterior horn cell disorders, cauda equina syndromes due to involvement of nerve roots derived from the lower spinal cord (Chap. 372), and peripheral neuropathies].

Acute paraparesis may not be recognized as due to spinal cord disease at an early stage if the legs are flaccid and areflexic. Usually, however, there is sensory loss in the legs with an upper level on the trunk; a dissociated sensory loss suggestive of a central cord syndrome; or exaggerated stretch reflexes in the legs with normal reflexes in the arms. It is important to image the spinal cord (Fig. 23-3). Compressive lesions (particularly epidural tumor, abscess, or hematoma, but also a prolapsed intervertebral disk and vertebral involvement by malignancy or infection), spinal cord infarction (proprioception is usually spared), an arteriovenous fistula or other vascular anomaly, and transverse myelitis, are among the possible causes (Chap. 372).

Diseases of the cerebral hemispheres that produce acute paraparesis include anterior cerebral artery ischemia (shoulder shrug is also affected), superior sagittal sinus or cortical venous thrombosis, and acute hydrocephalus. If upper motor neuron signs are associated with drowsiness, confusion, seizures, or other hemispheric signs, MRI of the brain should be undertaken.

Paraparesis may result from a cauda equina syndrome, for example, following trauma to the low back, a midline disk herniation, or an intraspinal tumor; although sphincters are affected, hip flexion is often spared, as is sensation over the anterolateral thighs. Rarely, paraparesis is caused by a rapidly evolving anterior horn cell disease (such as poliovirus or West Nile virus infection), peripheral neuropathy (such as Guillain-Barré syndrome; Chap. 380) or myopathy (Chap. 382). In such cases, electrophysiologic studies are diagnostically helpful and refocus the subsequent evaluation.

Subacute or chronic paraparesis with spasticity is caused by upper motor neuron disease. When there is associated lower-limb sensory loss and sphincter involvement, a chronic spinal cord disorder is likely (Chap. 372). If an MRI of the spinal cord is normal, MRI of the brain may be indicated. If hemispheric signs are present, a parasagittal meningioma or chronic hydrocephalus is likely and MRI of the brain is the initial test. In the rare situation in which a longstanding paraparesis has a lower motor neuron or myopathic etiology, the localization is usually suspected on clinical grounds by the absence of spasticity and confirmed by EMG and nerve conduction tests.

Quadriparesis or Generalized Weakness Generalized weakness may be due to disorders of the CNS or of the motor unit. Although the terms *quadriparesis* and *generalized weakness* are often used interchangeably, quadriparesis is commonly used when an upper motor neuron cause is suspected, and generalized weakness when a disease of the motor unit is likely. Weakness from CNS disorders is usually associated with changes in consciousness or cognition, with spasticity and brisk stretch reflexes, and with alterations of sensation. Most neuromuscular causes of generalized weakness are associated with normal mental function, hypotonia, and hypoactive muscle stretch reflexes. The major causes of intermittent weakness are listed in Table 23-2. A patient with generalized fatigability without objective weakness may have the chronic fatigue syndrome (Chap. 384).

ACUTE QUADRIPARESIS Acute quadriparesis with onset over minutes may result from disorders of upper motor neurons (e.g., anoxia, hypotension, brainstem or cervical cord ischemia, trauma, and systemic metabolic abnormalities) or muscle (electrolyte disturbances, certain inborn errors of muscle energy metabolism, toxins, or periodic paralyses). Onset over hours to weeks may, in addition to the above, be due to lower motor neuron disorders. Guillain-Barré syndrome (Chap. 380) is the most common lower motor neuron weakness that progresses over days to 4 weeks; the finding of an elevated protein level in the cerebrospinal fluid is helpful but may be absent early in the course.

In obtunded patients, evaluation begins with a CT scan of the brain. If upper motor neuron signs are present but the patient is alert, the initial test is usually an MRI of the cervical cord. If weakness is lower motor neuron, myopathic, or uncertain in origin, the clinical approach begins with blood studies to determine the level of muscle enzymes and electrolytes and an EMG and nerve conduction study.

SUBACUTE OR CHRONIC QUADRIPARESIS When quadriparesis due to upper motor neuron disease develops over weeks, months, or years, the distinction between disorders of the cerebral hemispheres, brainstem, and cervical spinal cord is usually possible clinically. An MRI is obtained of the clinically suspected site of pathology. EMG and nerve conduction studies help to distinguish lower motor neuron disease (which usually presents with weakness that is most profound distally) from myopathic weakness, which is typically proximal.

TABLE 23-2 CAUSES OF EPISODIC GENERALIZED WEAKNESS

1. Electrolyte disturbances, e.g., hypokalemia, hyperkalemia, hypercalcemia, hypernatremia, hyponatremia, hypophosphatemia, hypermagnesemia
2. Muscle disorders
   a. Channelopathies (periodic paralyses)
   b. Metabolic defects of muscle (impaired carbohydrate or fatty acid utilization; abnormal mitochondrial function)
3. Neuromuscular junction disorders
   a. Myasthenia gravis
   b. Lambert-Eaton myasthenic syndrome
4. Central nervous system disorders
   a. Transient ischemic attacks of the brainstem
   b. Transient global cerebral ischemia
   c. Multiple sclerosis

Monoparesis This is usually due to lower motor neuron disease, with or without associated sensory involvement. Upper motor neuron weakness occasionally presents as a monoparesis of distal and nonantigravity muscles. Myopathic weakness is rarely limited to one limb.

ACUTE MONOPARESIS If the weakness is predominantly in distal and nonantigravity muscles and not associated with sensory impairment or pain, focal cortical ischemia is likely (Chap. 364); diagnostic possibilities are similar to those for acute hemiparesis. Sensory loss and pain usually accompany acute lower motor neuron weakness; the weakness is commonly localized to a single nerve root or peripheral nerve within the limb but occasionally reflects plexus involvement. If lower motor neuron weakness is suspected, or the pattern of weakness is uncertain, the clinical approach begins with an EMG and nerve conduction study.

SUBACUTE OR CHRONIC MONOPARESIS Weakness and atrophy that develop over weeks or months are usually of lower motor neuron origin. If they are associated with sensory symptoms, a peripheral cause (nerve, root, or plexus) is likely; in the absence of such symptoms, anterior horn cell disease should be considered. In either case, an electrodiagnostic study is indicated. If weakness is of upper motor neuron type, a discrete cortical (precentral gyrus) or cord lesion may be responsible, and an imaging study is performed of the appropriate site.

Distal Weakness Involvement of two or more limbs distally suggests lower motor neuron or peripheral nerve disease. Acute distal lower limb weakness occurs occasionally from an acute toxic polyneuropathy or cauda equina syndrome. Distal symmetric weakness usually develops over weeks, months, or years and, when associated with numbness, is due to metabolic, toxic, hereditary, degenerative, or inflammatory diseases of peripheral nerves (Chap. 379). Anterior horn cell disease may begin distally but is typically asymmetric and without accompanying numbness (Chap. 369). Rarely, myopathies present with distal weakness (Chap. 382). Electrodiagnostic studies help to localize the disorder (Fig. 23-3).

Proximal Weakness Myopathy often produces symmetric weakness of the pelvic or shoulder girdle muscles (Chap. 382). Diseases of the neuromuscular junction [such as myasthenia gravis (Chap. 381)], may present with symmetric proximal weakness often associated with ptosis, diplopia, or bulbar weakness and fluctuating in severity during the day. Extreme fatigability present in some cases of myasthenia gravis may even suggest episodic weakness, but strength rarely returns fully to normal. In anterior horn cell disease proximal weakness is usually asymmetric, but may be symmetric if familial. Numbness does not occur with any of these diseases. The evaluation usually begins with determination of the serum creatine kinase level and electrophysiologic studies.

Weakness in a Restricted Distribution Weakness may not fit any of the above patterns, being limited, for example, to the extraocular, hemifacial, bulbar, or respiratory muscles. If unilateral, restricted weakness is usually due to lower motor neuron or peripheral nerve disease, such as in a facial palsy (Chap. 379) or an isolated superior oblique muscle paresis (Chap. 382). Weakness of part of a limb is usually due to a peripheral nerve lesion such as carpal tunnel syndrome or another entrapment neuropathy. Relatively symmetric weakness of extraocular or bulbar muscles is usually due to a myopathy (Chap. 382) or neuromuscular junction disorder (Chap. 381). Bilateral facial palsy with areflexia suggests Guillain-Barré syndrome (Chap. 380). Worsening of relatively symmetric weakness with fatigue is characteristic of neuromuscular junction disorders. Asymmetric bulbar weakness is usually due to motor neuron disease. Weakness limited to respiratory muscles is uncommon and is usually due to motor neuron disease, myasthenia gravis, or polymyositis/dermatomyositis (Chap. 383).

ACKNOWLEDGMENT
Richard K. Olney, MD, was the author of this chapter in previous editions, and his contributions in the last three editions of Harrison's are appreciated.

24 Gait and Balance Disorders
Lewis Sudarsky

PREVALENCE, MORBIDITY, AND MORTALITY

Gait and balance problems are common in the elderly and contribute to the risk of falls and injury. Gait disorders have been described in 15% of individuals over the age of 65. By age 80, one person in four will use a mechanical aid to assist ambulation. Among those 85 and older, the prevalence of gait abnormality approaches 40%. In epidemiologic studies, gait disorders are consistently identified as a major risk factor for falls and injury.

A substantial number of older persons report insecure balance and experience falls and fear of falling. Prospective studies indicate that 20–30% of those over age 65 fall each year, and the proportion is even higher in hospitalized elderly and nursing home patients. Each year 8% of individuals >75 suffer a serious fall-related injury. Hip fractures often result in hospitalization and nursing home admission. For each person who is physically disabled, there are others whose functional independence is constrained by anxiety and fear of falling. Nearly one in five of elderly individuals voluntarily limit their activity because of fear of falling. With loss of ambulation, there is a diminished quality of life and increased morbidity and mortality.

ANATOMY AND PHYSIOLOGY

Upright bipedal gait depends on the successful integration of postural control and locomotion. These functions are widely distributed in the central nervous system. The biomechanics of bipedal walking are complex, and the performance is easily compromised by injury at any level. Command and control centers in the brainstem, cerebellum, and forebrain modify the action of spinal pattern generators to promote stepping. While a form of "fictive locomotion" can be elicited from quadrupedal animals after spinal transection, this capacity is limited in primates. Step generation in primates is dependent on locomotor centers in the pontine tegmentum, midbrain, and subthalamic region. Locomotor synergies are executed through the reticular formation and descending pathways in the ventromedial spinal cord. Cerebral control provides a goal and purpose for walking and is involved in avoidance of obstacles and adaptation of locomotor programs to context and terrain.

Postural control requires the maintenance of the center of mass over the base of support through the gait cycle. Unconscious postural adjustments maintain standing balance: long latency responses are measurable in the leg muscles, beginning 110 ms after a perturbation. Forward motion of the center of mass provides propulsive force for stepping, but failure to maintain the center of mass within stability limits results in falls. The anatomic substrate for dynamic balance has not been well defined, but the vestibular nucleus and midline cerebellum contribute to balance control in animals. Human patients with damage to these structures have impaired balance with standing and walking.

Standing balance depends on good quality sensory information about the position of the body center with respect to the environment, support surface, and gravitational forces. Sensory information for postural control is primarily generated by the visual system, the vestibular system, and by proprioceptive receptors in the muscle spindles and joints. A healthy redundancy of sensory afferent information is generally available, but loss of two of the three pathways is sufficient to compromise standing balance. Balance disorders in older individuals sometimes result from multiple insults in the peripheral sensory systems (e.g., visual loss, vestibular deficit, peripheral neuropathy), critically degrading the quality of afferent information needed for balance stability.

Older patients with mental status abnormalities and dementia from neurodegenerative diseases appear to be particularly prone to falls and injury. Frailty, muscle weakness, and deconditioning undoubtedly contribute to the risk. There is a growing literature on the use of attentional resources to manage locomotion. The ability to walk while attending to a cognitive task (dual tasking) may be particularly compromised in older adults with a history of falls. Walking is generally considered to be unconscious and automatic, but older patients with deficits in executive function may be unable to manage the attention needed for dynamic balance when distracted.

DISORDERS OF GAIT

The heterogeneity of gait disorders observed in clinical practice reflects the large network of neural systems involved in the task. There is the potential for abnormalities to develop, and walking is vulnerable to neurologic disease at every level. Gait disorders have been classified descriptively, based on the abnormal physiology and biomechanics. One problem with this approach is that many failing gaits look fundamentally similar. This overlap reflects common patterns of adaptation to threatened balance stability and declining performance. *The gait disorder observed clinically must be viewed as the product of a neurologic deficit and a functional adaptation.* Unique features of the failing gait are often overwhelmed by the adaptive response. Some of the common patterns of abnormal gait are summarized below. Gait disorders can also be classified by etiology, as listed in Table 24-1.

Cautious Gait The term *cautious gait* is used to describe the patient who walks with an abbreviated stride and lowered center of mass, as if walking on a slippery surface. This disorder is both common and nonspecific. It is, in essence, an adaptation to a perceived postural threat. A fear of falling may be associated. In one study, this disorder was observed in more than one-third of older patients with a higher level gait disturbance. Physical therapy often improves walking to the degree that follow-up observation may reveal a more specific underlying disorder.

Stiff-Legged Gait Spastic gait is characterized by stiffness in the legs, an imbalance of muscle tone, and a tendency to circumduct and scuff the feet. The disorder reflects compromise of corticospinal command and overactivity of spinal reflexes. The patient may walk on his or her toes. In extreme instances, the legs cross due to increased tone in the adductors. Upper motor neuron signs are present on physical examination. Shoes often reflect an uneven pattern of wear across the outside. The disorder may be cerebral or spinal in origin.

Myelopathy from cervical spondylosis is a common cause of spastic or spastic-ataxic gait. Demyelinating disease and trauma are the leading causes of myelopathy in younger patients. In a chronic progressive myelopathy of unknown cause, workup with laboratory and imaging tests may establish a diagnosis of multiple sclerosis. A family history should suggest hereditary spastic paraplegia (HSP). Genetic testing is now available for some of the common HSP mutations. Tropical spastic paraparesis related to the retrovirus HTLV-I is endemic in parts of the Caribbean and South America. A structural lesion, such as tumor or spinal vascular malformation, should be excluded with appropriate testing. Spinal cord disorders are discussed in detail in Chap. 372.

With cerebral spasticity asymmetry is common, involvement of the upper extremities is usually observed, and dysarthria is often an associated feature. Common causes include vascular disease (stroke), multiple sclerosis, and perinatal injury to the nervous system (cerebral palsy).

Other stiff-legged gaits include dystonia (Chap. 382) and stiff-person syndrome. Dystonia is a disorder characterized by sustained muscle con-

TABLE 24-1 ETIOLOGY OF GAIT DISORDER		
	Cases	**Percent**
Sensory deficits	22	18.3
Myelopathy	20	16.7
Multiple infarcts	18	15.0
Parkinsonism	14	11.7
Cerebellar degeneration	8	6.7
Hydrocephalus	8	6.7
Toxic/metabolic	3	2.5
Psychogenic	4	3.3
Other	6	5.0
Unknown cause	17	14.2
Total	120	100%

Source: Reproduced with permission from Masdeu et al.

tractions, resulting in repetitive twisting movements and abnormal posture. It often has a genetic basis. Dystonic spasms produce plantar flexion and inversion of the feet, sometimes with torsion of the trunk. In autoimmune stiff-person syndrome, there is exaggerated lordosis of the lumbar spine and overactivation of antagonist muscles, which restricts trunk and lower limb movement and results in a wooden or fixed posture.

Parkinsonism and Freezing Gait Parkinson's disease (Chap. 366) is common, affecting 1% of the population >55. The stooped posture and shuffling gait are characteristic and distinctive features. Patients sometimes accelerate (festinate) with walking or display retropulsion. There may be difficulty with gait initiation (freezing) and a tendency to turn en bloc. Imbalance and falls may develop as the disease progresses over years. Other progressive neurodegenerative disorders may also involve a freezing gait; these include progressive supranuclear palsy, multiple system atrophy, corticobasal degeneration, and primary pallidal degeneration. Such patients with atypical parkinsonian syndromes frequently present with axial stiffness, postural instability, and a shuffling gait but tend to lack the characteristic pill-rolling tremor of Parkinson's disease. Falls within the first year suggest the possibility of progressive supranuclear palsy.

Hyperkinetic movement disorders also produce characteristic and recognizable disturbances in gait. In Huntington's disease (Chap. 367), the unpredictable occurrence of choreic movements gives the gait a dancing quality. Tardive dyskinesia is the cause of many odd, stereotypic gait disorders seen in chronic psychiatric patients.

Frontal Gait Disorder Frontal gait disorder, sometimes known as "gait apraxia," is common in the elderly and has a variety of causes. Typical features include a wide base of support, short stride, shuffling along the floor, and difficulty with starts and turns. Many patients exhibit difficulty with gait initiation, descriptively characterized as the "slipping clutch" syndrome or "gait ignition failure." The term *lower body parkinsonism* is also used to describe such patients. Strength is generally preserved, and patients are able to make stepping movements when not standing and maintaining balance at the same time. This disorder is a higher level motor control disorder, as opposed to an apraxia.

The most common cause of frontal gait disorder is vascular disease, particularly subcortical small-vessel disease. Lesions are frequently found in the deep frontal white matter and centrum ovale. Gait disorder may be the salient feature in hypertensive patients with ischemic lesions of the deep hemisphere white matter (Binswanger's disease). The clinical syndrome includes mental change (variable in degree), dysarthria, pseudobulbar affect (emotional disinhibition), increased tone, and hyperreflexia in the lower limbs.

Communicating hydrocephalus in the adult also presents with a gait disorder of this type. Other features of the diagnostic triad (mental change, incontinence) may be absent in the initial stages. MRI demonstrates ventricular enlargement, an enlarged flow void about the aqueduct, and a variable degree of periventricular white matter change. A lumbar puncture or dynamic test is necessary to confirm the presence of hydrocephalus.

Cerebellar Gait Ataxia Disorders of the cerebellum have a dramatic impact on gait and balance. Cerebellar gait ataxia is characterized by a wide base of support, lateral instability of the trunk, erratic foot placement, and decompensation of balance when attempting to walk tandem. Difficulty maintaining balance when turning is often an early feature. Patients are unable to walk tandem heel to toe, and display truncal sway in narrow-based or tandem stance. They show considerable variation in their tendency to fall in daily life.

Causes of cerebellar ataxia in older patients include stroke, trauma, tumor, and neurodegenerative disease, including multiple system atrophy (Chaps. 366 and 370) and various forms of hereditary cerebellar degeneration (Chap. 368). MRI demonstrates the extent and topography of cerebellar atrophy. A short expansion at the site of the fragile X mutation (fragile X pre-mutation) has been associated with gait ataxia in older men. Alcoholic cerebellar degeneration can be screened by history and often confirmed by MRI.

Sensory Ataxia As reviewed above, balance depends on high-quality afferent information from the visual and the vestibular systems and proprioception. When this information is lost or degraded, balance during locomotion is impaired and instability results. The sensory ataxia of tabetic neurosyphilis is a classic example. The contemporary equivalent is the patient with neuropathy affecting large fibers. Vitamin B_{12} deficiency is a treatable cause of large-fiber sensory loss in the spinal cord and peripheral nervous system. Joint position and vibration sense are diminished in the lower limbs. The stance in such patients is destabilized by eye closure; they often look down at their feet when walking and do poorly in the dark. Patients have been described with imbalance from bilateral vestibular loss, caused by disease or by exposure to ototoxic drugs. Table 24-2 compares sensory ataxia with cerebellar ataxia and frontal gait disorder. Some patients exhibit a syndrome of imbalance from the combined effect of multiple sensory deficits. Such patients, often elderly and diabetic, have disturbances in proprioception, vision, and vestibular sense that impair postural support.

Neuromuscular Disease Patients with neuromuscular disease often have an abnormal gait, occasionally as a presenting feature. With distal weakness (peripheral neuropathy) the step height is increased to compensate for foot drop, and the sole of the foot may slap on the floor during weight acceptance. Neuropathy may be associated with a degree of sensory imbalance, as described above. Patients with myopathy or muscular dystrophy more typically exhibit proximal weakness. Weakness of the hip girdle may result in a degree of excess pelvic sway during locomotion.

Toxic and Metabolic Disorders Alcohol intoxication is the most common cause of acute walking difficulty. Chronic toxicity from medications and metabolic disturbances can impair motor function and gait. Mental status changes may be present, and examination may reveal asterixis or myoclonus. Static equilibrium is disturbed, and such patients are easily thrown off balance. Disequilibrium is particularly evident in patients with chronic renal disease and those with hepatic failure, in whom asterixis may impair postural support. Sedative drugs, especially neuroleptics and long-acting benzodiazepines, affect postural control and increase the risk for falls. These disorders are important to recognize because they are often treatable.

Psychogenic Gait Disorder Psychogenic disorders are common in outpatient practice, and the presentation often involves gait. Some patients with extreme anxiety or phobia walk with exaggerated caution with abduction of the arms, as if walking on ice. This inappropriately overcautious gait differs in degree from the gait of the patient who is insecure and making adjustments for imbalance. Depressed patients exhibit primarily slowness, a manifestation of psychomotor retardation, and lack of purpose in their stride. Hysterical gait disorders are among the most spectacular encountered. Odd gyrations of posture with wastage of muscular energy (astasia-abasia), extreme slow mo-

TABLE 24-2 FEATURES OF CEREBELLAR ATAXIA, SENSORY ATAXIA, AND FRONTAL GAIT DISORDERS

	Cerebellar Ataxia	Sensory Ataxia	Frontal Gait
Base of support	Wide-based	Narrow base, looks down	Wide-based
Velocity	Variable	Slow	Very slow
Stride	Irregular, lurching	Regular with path deviation	Short, shuffling
Romberg	+/−	Unsteady, falls	+/−
Heel→ shin	Abnormal	+/−	Normal
Initiation	Normal	Normal	Hesitant
Turns	Unsteady	+/−	Hesitant, multistep
Postural instability	+	+++	++++
			Poor postural synergies getting up from a chair
Falls	Late event	Frequent	Frequent

tion, and dramatic fluctuations over time may be observed in patients with somatoform disorders and conversion reaction.

APPROACH TO THE PATIENT:
Slowly Progressive Disorder of Gait

When reviewing the history it is helpful to inquire about the onset and progression of disability. Initial awareness of an unsteady gait often follows a fall. Stepwise evolution or sudden progression suggest vascular disease. Gait disorder may be associated with urinary urgency and incontinence, particularly in patients with cervical spine disease or hydrocephalus. It is always important to review the use of alcohol and medications that affect gait and balance. Information on localization derived from the neurologic examination can be helpful to narrow the list of possible diagnoses.

Gait observation provides an immediate sense of the patient's degree of disability. Characteristic patterns of abnormality are sometimes observed, though failing gaits often look fundamentally similar. Cadence (steps/min), velocity, and stride length can be recorded by timing a patient over a fixed distance. Watching the patient get out of a chair provides a good functional assessment of balance.

Brain imaging studies may be informative in patients with an undiagnosed disorder of gait. MRI is sensitive for cerebral lesions of vascular or demyelinating disease and is a good screening test for occult hydrocephalus. Patients with recurrent falls are at risk for subdural hematoma. Many elderly patients with gait and balance difficulty have white matter abnormalities in the periventricular region and centrum semiovale. While these lesions may be an incidental finding, a substantial burden of white matter disease will ultimately impact cerebral control of locomotion.

DISORDERS OF BALANCE

Balance is the ability to maintain equilibrium: a state in which opposing physical forces cancel. In physiology, this is taken to mean the ability of the organism to control the center of mass with respect to gravity and the support surface. In reality, no one is aware of what or where the center of mass is, but everyone, including gymnasts, figure skaters, and platform divers, move so as to manage it. Imbalance implies a disturbance of equilibrium. Disorders of balance present with difficulty maintaining posture standing and walking and with a subjective sense of disequilibrium, a form of dizziness.

The cerebellum and vestibular system organize antigravity responses needed to maintain the upright posture. As reviewed above, these responses are physiologically complex, and the anatomic representation is not well understood. Failure, resulting in disequilibrium, can occur at several levels: cerebellar, vestibular, somatosensory, and higher level disequilibrium. Patients with hereditary ataxia or alcoholic cerebellar degeneration do not generally complain of dizziness, but balance is visibly impaired. Neurologic examination will reveal a variety of cerebellar signs. Postural compensation may prevent falls early on, but falls inevitably occur with disease progression. The progression of a neurodegenerative ataxia is often measured by the number of years to loss of stable ambulation. Vestibular disorders have symptoms and signs in three categories: vertigo, the subjective appreciation or illusion of movement; nystagmus, a vestibulo-oculomotor sign; and poor balance, an impairment of vestibulo-spinal function. Not every patient has all manifestations. Patients with vestibular deficits related to ototoxic drugs may lack vertigo or obvious nystagmus, but balance is impaired on standing and walking, and the patient cannot navigate in the dark. Laboratory testing is available to explore vestibulo-oculomotor and vestibulo-spinal deficits.

Somatosensory deficits also produce imbalance and falls. There is often a subjective sense of insecure balance and fear of falling. Postural control is compromised by eye closure (Romberg's sign); these patients also have difficulty navigating in the dark. A dramatic example is the patient with autoimmune subacute sensory neuropathy, sometimes a paraneoplastic disorder (Chap. 97). Compensatory strategies enable such patients to walk in the virtual absence of proprioception, but the task requires active visual monitoring. Patients with higher level disorders of equilibrium

TABLE 24-3	RISK FACTORS FOR FALLS, A META-ANALYSIS: SUMMARY OF SIXTEEN CONTROLLED STUDIES	
Risk Factor	**Mean RR (OR)**	**Range**
Weakness	4.9	1.9–10.3
Balance deficit	3.2	1.6–5.4
Gait disorder	3.0	1.7–4.8
Visual deficit	2.8	1.1–7.4
Mobility limitation	2.5	1.0–5.3
Cognitive impairment	2.4	2.0–4.7
Impaired functional status	2.0	1.0–3.1
Postural hypotension	1.9	1.0–3.4

Note: RR, relative risks from prospective studies; OR, odds ratios from retrospective studies.

Source: Reprinted from Masdeu et al, with permission.

have difficulty maintaining balance in daily life and may present with falls. There may be reduced awareness of balance impairment. Classic examples include patients with progressive supranuclear palsy and normal pressure hydrocephalus. Patients on sedating medications are also in this category. In prospective studies, cognitive impairment and the use of sedative medications substantially increase the risk for falls.

FALLS

Falls are a common event, particularly among the elderly. Modest changes in balance function have been described in fit older subjects as a result of normal aging. Subtle deficits in sensory systems, attention, and motor reaction time contribute to the risk, and environmental hazards abound. Epidemiologic studies have identified a number of risk factors for falls, summarized in Table 24-3. A fall is not a neurologic problem, nor reason for referral to a specialist, but there are circumstances in which neurologic evaluation is appropriate. In a classic study, 90% of fall events occurred among 10% of individuals, a group known as *recurrent fallers*. Some of these are frail older persons with chronic diseases. Recurrent falls sometimes indicate the presence of serious balance impairment. Syncope, seizure, or falls related to loss of consciousness require appropriate evaluation and treatment (Chaps. 21 and 363).

The descriptive classification of falls is as difficult as the classification of gait disorders, for many of the same reasons. Postural control systems are widely distributed, and a number of disease-related abnormalities occur. Unlike gait problems that are apparent on observation, falls are rarely observed in the office. The patient and family may have limited information about what triggered the fall. Injuries can complicate the physical examination. While there is no standard nosology of falls, common patterns can be identified.

Slipping, Tripping, and "Mechanical Falls" Slipping on icy pavement, tripping on obstacles, and falls related to obvious environmental factors are often termed *mechanical falls*. They occasionally occur in healthy individuals with good balance compensation. Frequent tripping falls raise suspicion about an underlying neurologic deficit. Patients with spasticity, leg weakness, or foot drop experience tripping falls.

Weakness and Frailty Patients who lack strength in antigravity muscles have difficulty rising from a chair, fatigue easily when walking, and have difficulty maintaining their balance after a perturbation. These patients are often unable to get up after a fall and may be on the floor for an hour or more before help arrives. Deconditioning of this sort is often treatable. Resistance strength training can increase muscle mass and leg strength in people in their 80s and 90s.

Drop Attacks and Collapsing Falls Drop attacks are sudden collapsing falls without loss of consciousness. Patients who collapse from lack of postural tone present a diagnostic challenge. The patient may report that his or her legs just gave out underneath; the family may describe the patient as "collapsing in a heap." Orthostatic hypotension may be a factor in some such falls. Asterixis or epilepsy may impair postural support. A colloid cyst of the third ventricle can present with intermittent obstruction of the foramen of Monroe, resulting in a drop attack. While collapsing falls are more common in older patients with vascular risk factors, they should not be confused with vertebrobasilar ischemic attacks.

Toppling Falls Some patients maintain tone in antigravity muscles but fall over like a tree trunk, as if postural defenses had disengaged. There may be a consistent direction to such falls. The patient with cerebellar pathology may lean and topple over toward the side of the lesion. Patients with lesions of the vestibular system or its central pathways may experience lateral pulsion and toppling falls. Patients with progressive supranuclear palsy often fall over backwards. Falls of this nature occur in patients with advanced Parkinson's disease once postural instability has developed.

Gait Freezing Another fall pattern in Parkinson's disease and related disorders is the fall due to freezing of gait. The feet stick to the floor and the center of mass keeps moving, resulting in a disequilibrium from which the patient cannot recover. This can result in a forward fall. Gait freezing can also occur as the patient attempts to turn and change direction. Similarly, the patient with Parkinson's disease and festinating gait may find his feet unable to keep up, resulting in a forward fall.

Falls Related to Sensory Deficit Patients with somatosensory, visual, or vestibular deficits are prone to falls. These patients have particular difficulty dealing with poor illumination or walking on uneven ground. These patients often express subjective imbalance, apprehension, and fear of falling. Deficits in joint position and vibration sense are apparent on physical examination.

℞ INTERVENTIONS TO REDUCE THE RISK OF FALLS AND INJURY

Efforts should be made to define the etiology of the gait disorder and mechanism of the falls. Standing blood pressure should be recorded. Specific treatment may be possible, once a diagnosis is established. Therapeutic intervention is often recommended for older patients at substantial risk for falls, even if no neurologic disease is identified. A home visit to look for environmental hazards can be helpful. A variety of modifications may be recommended to improve safety, including improved lighting and the installation of grab bars and nonslip surfaces.

Rehabilitation interventions attempt to improve muscle strength and balance stability and to make the patient more resistant to injury. High-intensity resistance strength training with weights and machines is useful to improve muscle mass, even in frail older patients. Improvements are realized in posture and gait, which should translate to reduced risk of falls and injury. The goal of sensory balance training is to improve balance stability. Measurable gains can be achieved in a few weeks of training, and benefits can be maintained over 6 months by a 10- to 20-min home exercise program. This strategy is particularly successful in patients with vestibular and somatosensory balance disorders. The Yale Health and Aging study used a strategy of targeted, multiple risk factor abatement to reduce falls in the elderly. Prescription medications were adjusted, and home-based exercise programs were tailored to the patient's need, based on an initial geriatric assessment. The program realized a 44% reduction in falls, compared with a control group of patients who had periodic social visits.

FURTHER READINGS

BRONSTEIN A et al: *Clinical Disorders of Balance, Posture and Gait.* London, Arnold Press, 2003

GANZ DA et al: Will my patient fall? JAMA 297:77, 2007

MASDEU J et al: *Gait Disorders of Aging: With Special Reference to Falls.* Boston, Little Brown, 1995

SNIJDERS AH et al: Neurological gait disorders in elderly people: Clinical approach and classification. Lancet Neurol 6:63, 2007

SPRINGER S et al: Dual-tasking effects on gait variability: The role of aging, falls, and executive function. Mov Disord 21:950, 2006

SUDARSKY L: Gait disorders in the elderly. N Engl J Med 322:1441, 1990

TINETTI ME: Preventing falls in elderly persons. N Engl J Med 348:42, 2003

25 Numbness, Tingling, and Sensory Loss
Michael J. Aminoff, Arthur K. Asbury

Normal somatic sensation reflects a continuous monitoring process, little of which reaches consciousness under ordinary conditions. By contrast, disordered sensation, particularly when experienced as painful, is alarming and dominates the sufferer's attention. Physicians should be able to recognize abnormal sensations by how they are described, know their type and likely site of origin, and understand their implications.

POSITIVE AND NEGATIVE SYMPTOMS

Abnormal sensory symptoms may be divided into two categories, positive and negative. The prototypical positive symptom is tingling (pins-and-needles); other positive sensory phenomena include altered sensations that are described as pricking, bandlike, lightning-like shooting feelings (lancinations), aching, knifelike, twisting, drawing, pulling, tightening, burning, searing, electrical, or raw feelings. Such symptoms are often painful.

Positive phenomena usually result from trains of impulses generated at sites of lowered threshold or heightened excitability along a peripheral or central sensory pathway. The nature and severity of the abnormal sensation depend on the number, rate, timing, and distribution of ectopic impulses and the type and function of nervous tissue in which they arise. Because positive phenomena represent excessive activity in sensory pathways, they are not necessarily associated with a sensory deficit (loss) on examination.

Negative phenomena represent loss of sensory function and are characterized by diminished or absent feeling, often experienced as numbness, and by abnormal findings on sensory examination. In disorders affecting peripheral sensation, it is estimated that at least half the afferent axons innervating a given site are lost or functionless before a sensory deficit can be demonstrated by clinical examination. This threshold varies according to how rapidly function is lost in sensory nerve fibers. If the rate of loss is slow, lack of cutaneous feeling may be unnoticed by the patient and difficult to demonstrate on examination, even though few sensory fibers are functioning; if rapid, both positive and negative phenomena are usually conspicuous. Subclinical degrees of sensory dysfunction may be revealed by sensory nerve conduction studies or somatosensory evoked potentials (**Chap. e31**).

Whereas sensory symptoms may be either positive or negative, sensory signs on examination are always a measure of negative phenomena.

TERMINOLOGY

Words used to characterize sensory disturbance are descriptive and based on convention. Paresthesias and dysesthesias are general terms used to denote positive sensory symptoms. The term *paresthesias* typically refers to tingling or pins-and-needles sensations but may include a wide variety of other abnormal sensations, except pain; it sometimes implies that the abnormal sensations are perceived spontaneously. The more general term *dysesthesias* denotes all types of abnormal sensations, including painful ones, regardless of whether a stimulus is evident.

Another set of terms refers to sensory abnormalities found on examination. *Hypesthesia* or *hypoesthesia* refers to a reduction of cutaneous sensation to a specific type of testing such as pressure, light touch, and warm or cold stimuli; *anesthesia,* to a complete absence of skin sensation to the same stimuli plus pinprick; and *hypalgesia* or *analgesia* to reduced or absent pain perception (nociception), such as perception of the pricking quality elicited by a pin. *Hyperesthesia* means pain or increased sensitivity in response to touch. Similarly, *allodynia* describes the situation in which a nonpainful stimulus, once perceived, is experienced as painful, even excruciating. An example is elicitation of a painful sensation by application of a vibrating tuning fork. *Hyperalgesia* denotes severe pain in response to a mildly noxious stimulus, and *hyperpathia*, a broad term, encompasses all the phenomena described by hyperesthesia, allodynia, and hyperalgesia. With hyperpathia, the threshold for a sensory stimulus is increased and perception is delayed, but once felt, is unduly painful.

Disorders of deep sensation, arising from muscle spindles, tendons, and joints, affect proprioception (position sense). Manifestations include imbalance (particularly with eyes closed or in the dark), clumsiness of precision movements, and unsteadiness of gait, which are referred to collectively as *sensory ataxia*. Other findings on examination usually, but not invariably, include reduced or absent joint position and vibratory sensibility and absent deep tendon reflexes in the affected limbs. Romberg's sign is positive, which means that the patient sways markedly or topples when asked to stand with feet close together and eyes closed. In severe states of deafferentation involving deep sensation, the patient cannot walk or stand unaided or even sit unsupported. Continuous involuntary movements (*pseudoathetosis*) of the outstretched hands and fingers occur, particularly with eyes closed.

ANATOMY OF SENSATION

Cutaneous afferent innervation is conveyed by a rich variety of receptors, both naked nerve endings (nociceptors and thermoreceptors) and encapsulated terminals (mechanoreceptors). Each type of receptor has its own set of sensitivities to specific stimuli, size and distinctness of receptive fields, and adaptational qualities. Much of the knowledge about these receptors has come from the development of techniques to study single intact nerve fibers intraneurally in awake, unanesthetized human subjects. It is possible not only to record from but also to stimulate single fibers in isolation. A single impulse, whether elicited by a natural stimulus or evoked by electrical microstimulation in a large myelinated afferent fiber may be both perceived and localized.

Afferent fibers of all sizes in peripheral nerve trunks traverse the dorsal roots and enter the dorsal horn of the spinal cord (Fig. 25-1). From there the smaller fibers take a different route to the parietal cortex than the larger fibers. The polysynaptic projections of the smaller fibers (unmyelinated and small myelinated), which subserve mainly nociception, temperature sensibility, and touch, cross and ascend in the opposite anterior and lateral columns of the spinal cord, through the brainstem, to the ventral posterolateral (VPL) nucleus of the thalamus, and ultimately project to the postcentral gyrus of the parietal cortex (Chap. 12). This is the *spinothalamic pathway* or *anterolateral system*. The larger fibers, which subserve tactile and position sense and kinesthesia, project rostrally in the posterior column on the same side of the spinal cord and make their first synapse in the gracile or cuneate nucleus of the lower medulla. Axons of the second-order neuron decussate and ascend in the medial lemniscus located medially in the medulla and in the tegmentum of the pons and midbrain and synapse in the VPL nucleus; the third-order neurons project to parietal cortex. This large-fiber system is referred to as the *posterior column–medial lemniscal pathway* (lemniscal, for short). Note that although the lemniscal and the anterolateral pathways both project up the spinal cord to the thalamus, it is the (crossed) anterolateral pathway that is referred to as the *spinothalamic tract*, by convention.

Although the fiber types and functions that make up the spinothalamic and lemniscal systems are relatively well known, many other fibers, particularly those associated with touch, pressure, and position sense, ascend in a diffusely distributed pattern both ipsilaterally and contralaterally in the anterolateral quadrants of the spinal cord. This explains why a complete lesion of the posterior columns of the spinal cord may be associated with little sensory deficit on examination.

EXAMINATION OF SENSATION

The main components of the sensory examination are tests of primary sensation (pain, touch, vibration, joint position, and thermal sensation; Table 25-1).

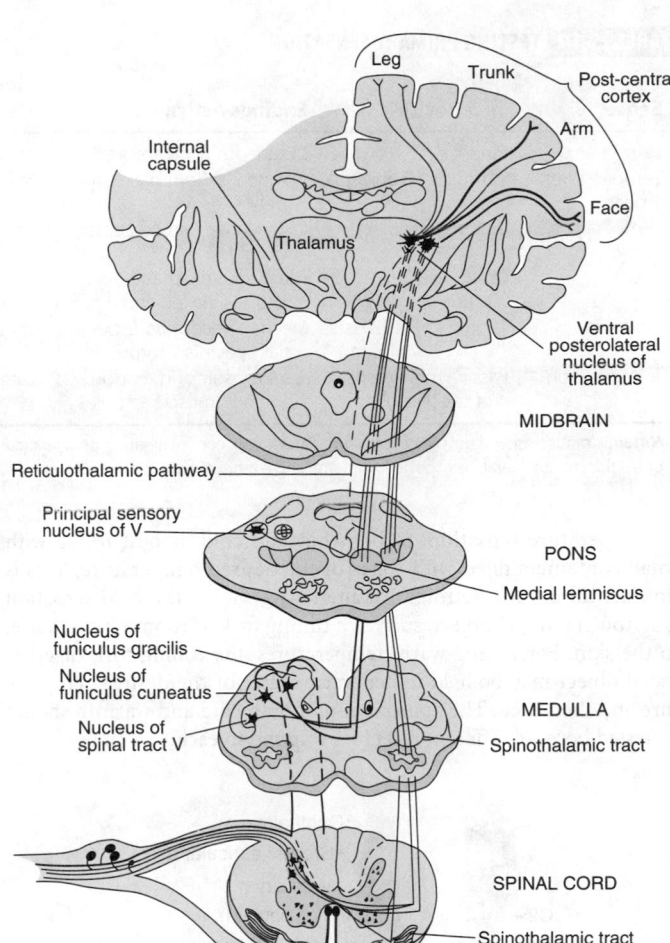

FIGURE 25-1 The main somatosensory pathways. The spinothalamic tract (pain, thermal sense) and the posterior column–lemniscal system (touch, pressure, joint position) are shown. Offshoots from the ascending anterolateral fasciculus (spinothalamic tract) to nuclei in the medulla, pons, and mesencephalon and nuclear terminations of the tract are indicated. *(From AH Ropper, RH Brown, in Adams and Victor's Principles of Neurology, 8th ed. New York, McGraw-Hill, 2007.)*

Some general principles pertain. The examiner must depend on patient responses, particularly when testing cutaneous sensation (pin, touch, warm, or cold), which complicates interpretation. Further, examination may be limited in some patients. In a stuporous patient, for example, sensory examination is reduced to observing the briskness of withdrawal in response to a pinch or other noxious stimulus. Comparison of response on one side of the body to the other is essential. In the alert but uncooperative patient, it may not be possible to examine cutaneous sensation, but some idea of proprioceptive function may be gained by noting the patient's best performance of movements requiring balance and precision. Frequently, patients present with sensory symptoms that do not fit an anatomic localization and that are accompanied by either no abnormalities or gross inconsistencies on examination. The examiner should then consider whether the sensory symptoms are a disguised request for help with psychological or situational problems. Discretion must be used in pursuing this possibility. Finally, sensory examination of a patient who has no neurologic complaints can be brief and consist of pinprick, touch, and vibration testing in the hands and feet plus evaluation of stance and gait, including the Romberg maneuver. Evaluation of stance and gait also tests the integrity of motor and cerebellar systems.

Primary Sensation (See Table 25-1) The sense of pain is usually tested with a clean pin, asking the patient to focus on the pricking or unpleasant quality of the stimulus and not just the pressure or touch sensation elicited. Areas of hypalgesia should be mapped by proceeding radially from the most hypalgesic site (Figs. 25-2 and 25-3).

TABLE 25-1 | TESTING PRIMARY SENSATION

Sense	Test Device	Endings Activated	Fiber Size Mediating	Central Pathway
Pain	Pinprick	Cutaneous nociceptors	Small	SpTh, also D
Temperature, heat	Warm metal object	Cutaneous thermoreceptors for hot	Small	SpTh
Temperature, cold	Cold metal object	Cutaneous thermoreceptors for cold	Small	SpTh
Touch	Cotton wisp, fine brush	Cutaneous mechanoreceptors, also naked endings	Large and small	Lem, also D and SpTh
Vibration	Tuning fork, 128 Hz	Mechanoreceptors, especially pacinian corpuscles	Large	Lem, also D
Joint position	Passive movement of specific joints	Joint capsule and tendon endings, muscle spindles	Large	Lem, also D

Note: D, diffuse ascending projections in ipsilateral and contralateral anterolateral columns; SpTh, spinothalamic projection, contralateral; Lem, posterior column and lemniscal projection, ipsilateral.

Touch is usually tested with a wisp of cotton or a fine camelhair brush. In general, it is better to avoid testing touch on hairy skin because of the profusion of sensory endings that surround each hair follicle.

Joint position testing is a measure of proprioception, one of the most important functions of the sensory system. With the patient's eyes closed, joint position is tested in the distal interphalangeal joint of the great toe and fingers. If errors are made in recognizing the direction of passive movements, more proximal joints are tested. A test of proximal joint position sense, primarily at the shoulder, is performed by asking the patient to bring the two index fingers together with arms extended and eyes closed. Normal individuals can do this accurately, with errors of 1 cm or less.

Temperature sensation, to both hot and cold, is best tested with small containers filled with water of the desired temperature. This is impractical in most settings. An alternative way to test cold sensation is to touch a metal object, such as a tuning fork at room temperature, to the skin. For testing warm temperatures, the tuning fork or other metal object may be held under warm water of the desired temperature and then used. The appreciation of both cold and warmth should be tested because different receptors respond to each.

The sense of vibration is tested with a tuning fork that vibrates at 128 Hz. Vibration is usually tested over bony points, beginning distally; in the feet, it is tested over the dorsal surface of the distal phalanx of the big toes and at the malleoli of the ankles, and in the hands dorsally at the distal phalanx of the fingers. If abnormalities are found, more proximal sites can be examined. Vibratory thresholds at the same site in the patient and the examiner may be compared for control purposes.

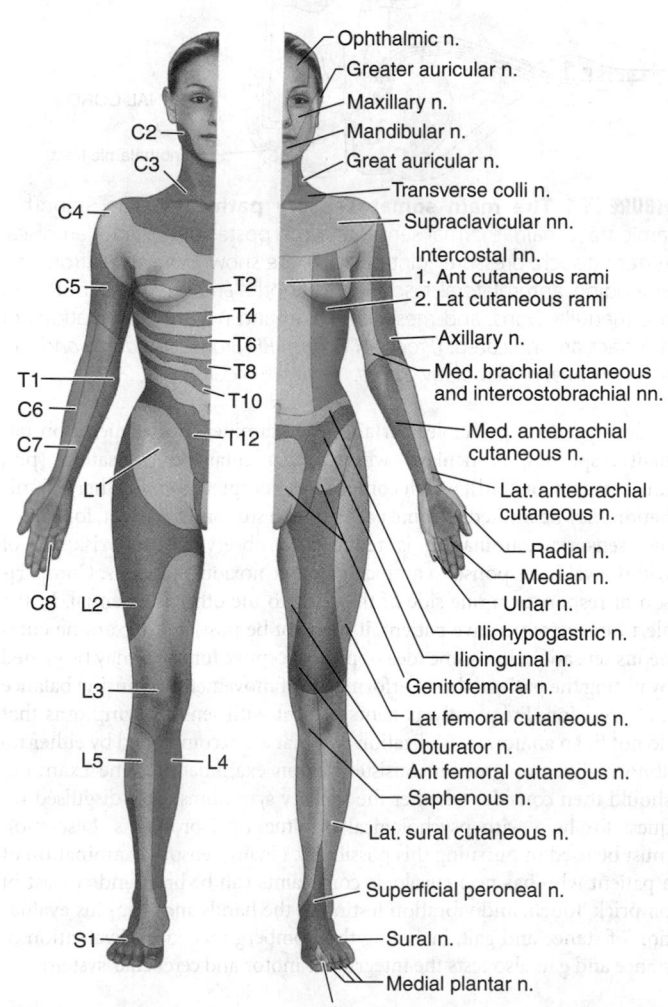

FIGURE 25-2 Anterior view of dermatomes (*left*) and cutaneous areas (*right*) supplied by individual peripheral nerves. (*Modified from MB Carpenter and J Sutin, in Human Neuroanatomy, 8th ed, Baltimore, Williams & Wilkins, 1983.*)

FIGURE 25-3 Posterior view of dermatomes (*left*) and cutaneous areas (*right*) supplied by individual peripheral nerves. (*Modified from MB Carpenter and J Sutin, in Human Neuroanatomy, 8th ed, Baltimore, Williams & Wilkins, 1983.*)

Quantitative Sensory Testing Effective sensory testing devices are now available commercially. Quantitative sensory testing is particularly useful for serial evaluation of cutaneous sensation in clinical trials. Threshold testing for touch and vibratory and thermal sensation is the most widely used application.

Cortical Sensation The most commonly used tests of cortical function are two-point discrimination, touch localization, and bilateral simultaneous stimulation and tests for graphesthesia and stereognosis. Abnormalities of these sensory tests, in the presence of normal primary sensation in an alert cooperative patient, signify a lesion of the parietal cortex or thalamocortical projections to the parietal lobe. If primary sensation is altered, these cortical discriminative functions will usually be abnormal also. Comparisons should always be made between analogous sites on the two sides of the body because the deficit with a specific parietal lesion is likely to be unilateral. Interside comparisons are important for all cortical sensory testing.

Two-point discrimination is tested by special calipers, the points of which may be set from 2 mm to several centimeters apart and then applied simultaneously to the site to be tested. The pulp of the fingertips is a common site to test; a normal individual can distinguish about 3-mm separation of points there.

Touch localization is performed by light pressure for an instant with the examiner's fingertip or a wisp of cottonwool; the patient, whose eyes are closed, is required to identify the site of touch with the fingertip. *Bilateral simultaneous stimulation* at analogous sites (e.g., the dorsum of both hands) can be carried out to determine whether the perception of touch is extinguished consistently on one side or the other. The phenomenon is referred to as *extinction*. *Graphesthesia* means the capacity to recognize with eyes closed letters or numbers drawn by the examiner's fingertip on the palm of the hand. Once again, interside comparison is of prime importance. Inability to recognize numbers or letters is termed *agraphesthesia*.

Stereognosis refers to the ability to identify common objects by palpation, recognizing their shape, texture, and size. Common standard objects, such as a key, paper clip, or coins, are best used. Patients with normal stereognosis should be able to distinguish a dime from a penny and a nickel from a quarter without looking. Patients should only be allowed to feel the object with one hand at a time. If they are unable to identify it in one hand, it should be placed in the other for comparison. Individuals unable to identify common objects and coins in one hand and who can do so in the other are said to have *astereognosis* of the abnormal hand.

LOCALIZATION OF SENSORY ABNORMALITIES

Sensory symptoms and signs can result from lesions at almost any level of the nervous system from parietal cortex to the peripheral sensory receptor. Noting the distribution and nature of sensory symptoms and signs is the most important way to localize their source. Their extent, configuration, symmetry, quality, and severity are the key observations.

Dysesthesias without sensory findings by examination may be difficult to interpret. To illustrate, tingling dysesthesias in an acral distribution (hands and feet) can be systemic in origin, e.g., secondary to hyperventilation, or induced by a medication such as acetazolamide. Distal dysesthesias can also be an early event in an evolving polyneuropathy or may herald a myelopathy, such as from vitamin B_{12} deficiency. Sometimes distal dysesthesias have no definable basis. In contrast, dysesthesias that correspond to a particular peripheral nerve territory denote a lesion of that nerve trunk. For instance, dysesthesias restricted to the fifth digit and the adjacent one-half of the fourth finger on one hand reliably point to disorder of the ulnar nerve, most commonly at the elbow.

Nerve and Root In focal nerve trunk lesions severe enough to cause a deficit, sensory abnormalities are readily mapped and generally have discrete boundaries (Figs. 25-2 and 25-3). Root ("radicular") lesions are frequently accompanied by deep, aching pain along the course of the related nerve trunk. With compression of a fifth lumbar (L5) or first sacral (S1) root, as from a ruptured intervertebral disc, sciatica (radicular pain relating to the sciatic nerve trunk) is a frequent manifestation

(Chap. 16). With a lesion affecting a single root, sensory deficits may be minimal or absent because adjacent root territories overlap extensively.

With polyneuropathies, sensory deficits are generally graded, distal, and symmetric in distribution (Chap. 379). Dysesthesias, followed by numbness, begin in the toes and ascend symmetrically. When dysesthesias reach the knees, they have usually also appeared in the fingertips. The process appears to be nerve length–dependent, and the deficit is often described as "stocking-glove" in type. Involvement of both hands and feet also occurs with lesions of the upper cervical cord or the brainstem, but an upper level of the sensory disturbance may then be found on the trunk and other evidence of a central lesion may be present, such as sphincter involvement or signs of an upper motor neuron lesion (Chap. 23). Although most polyneuropathies are pansensory and affect all modalities of sensation, selective sensory dysfunction according to nerve fiber size may occur. Small-fiber polyneuropathies are characterized by burning, painful dysesthesias with reduced pinprick and thermal sensation but sparing of proprioception, motor function, and deep tendon reflexes. Touch is involved variably; when spared, the sensory pattern is referred to as exhibiting *sensory dissociation*. Sensory dissociation may occur with spinal cord lesions as well as small-fiber neuropathies. Large-fiber polyneuropathies are characterized by vibration and position sense deficits, imbalance, absent tendon reflexes, and variable motor dysfunction but preservation of most cutaneous sensation. Dysesthesias, if present at all, tend to be tingling or bandlike in quality.

Spinal Cord (See also Chap. 372) If the spinal cord is transected, all sensation is lost below the level of transection. Bladder and bowel function are also lost, as is motor function. Hemisection of the spinal cord produces the Brown-Séquard syndrome, with absent pain and temperature sensation contralaterally and loss of proprioceptive sensation and power ipsilaterally below the lesion (see Figs. 25-1 and 372-1).

Numbness or paresthesias in both feet may arise from a spinal cord lesion; this is especially likely when the upper level of the sensory loss extends to the trunk. When all extremities are affected, the lesion is probably in the cervical region or brainstem unless a peripheral neuropathy is responsible. The presence of upper motor neuron signs (Chap. 23) supports a central lesion; a hyperesthetic band on the trunk may suggest the level of involvement.

A dissociated sensory loss can reflect spinothalamic tract involvement in the spinal cord, especially if the deficit is unilateral and has an upper level on the torso. Bilateral spinothalamic tract involvement occurs with lesions affecting the center of the spinal cord, such as in syringomyelia. There is a dissociated sensory loss with impairment of pinprick and temperature appreciation but relative preservation of light touch, position sense, and vibration appreciation.

Dysfunction of the posterior columns in the spinal cord or of the posterior root entry zone may lead to a bandlike sensation around the trunk or a feeling of tight pressure in one or more limbs. Flexion of the neck sometimes leads to an electric shock–like sensation that radiates down the back and into the legs (Lhermitte's sign) in patients with a cervical lesion affecting the posterior columns, such as from multiple sclerosis, cervical spondylosis, or recent irradiation to the cervical region.

Brainstem Crossed patterns of sensory disturbance, in which one side of the face and the opposite side of the body are affected, localize to the lateral medulla. Here a small lesion may damage both the ipsilateral descending trigeminal tract and ascending spinothalamic fibers subserving the opposite arm, leg, and hemitorso (see "Lateral medullary syndrome" in Fig. 364-10). A lesion in the tegmentum of the pons and midbrain, where the lemniscal and spinothalamic tracts merge, causes pansensory loss contralaterally.

Thalamus Hemisensory disturbance with tingling numbness from head to foot is often thalamic in origin but can also arise from the anterior parietal region. If abrupt in onset, the lesion is likely to be due to a small stroke (lacunar infarction), particularly if localized to the thalamus. Occasionally, with lesions affecting the VPL nucleus or adjacent white matter, a syndrome of thalamic pain, also called *Déjerine-Roussy* *syndrome*, may ensue. The persistent, unrelenting unilateral pain is often described in dramatic terms.

Cortex With lesions of the parietal lobe involving either the cortex or subjacent white matter, the most prominent symptoms are contralateral hemineglect, hemi-inattention, and a tendency not to use the affected hand and arm. On cortical sensory testing (e.g., two-point discrimination, graphesthesia), abnormalities are often found but primary sensation is usually intact. Anterior parietal infarction may present as a pseudothalamic syndrome with contralateral loss of primary sensation from head to toe. Dysesthesias or a sense of numbness may also occur, and rarely, a painful state.

26 Confusion and Delirium
S. Andrew Josephson, Bruce L. Miller

Confusion, a mental and behavioral state of reduced comprehension, coherence, and capacity to reason, is one of the most common problems encountered in medicine, accounting for a large number of emergency department visits, hospital admissions, and inpatient consultations. *Delirium*, a term used to describe an acute confusional state, remains a major cause of morbidity and mortality, contributing billions of dollars yearly to health care costs in the United States alone. Delirium often goes unrecognized despite clear evidence that it is usually the cognitive manifestation of serious underlying medical or neurologic illness.

CLINICAL FEATURES OF DELIRIUM

A multitude of terms are used to describe delirium, including encephalopathy, acute brain failure, acute confusional state, and postoperative or intensive care unit (ICU) psychosis. Delirium has many clinical manifestations, but essentially it is defined as a relatively acute decline in cognition that fluctuates over hours or days. The hallmark of delirium is a deficit of attention, although all cognitive domains—including memory, executive function, visuospatial tasks, and language—are variably involved. Associated symptoms may include altered sleep-wake cycles, perceptual disturbances such as hallucinations or delusions, affect changes, and autonomic findings including heart rate and blood pressure instability.

Delirium is a clinical diagnosis that can only be made at the bedside. Two broad clinical categories of delirium have been described, hyperactive and hypoactive subtypes, based on differential psychomotor features. The cognitive syndrome associated with severe alcohol withdrawal remains the classic example of the hyperactive subtype, featuring prominent hallucinations, agitation, and hyperarousal, often accompanied by life-threatening autonomic instability. In striking contrast is the hypoactive subtype of delirium, exemplified by opiate intoxication, in which patients are withdrawn and quiet, with prominent apathy and psychomotor slowing.

This dichotomy between subtypes of delirium is a useful construct, but patients often fall somewhere along a spectrum between the hyperactive and hypoactive extremes, sometimes fluctuating from one to the other within minutes. Therefore, clinicians must recognize the broad range of presentations of delirium in order to identify all patients with this potentially reversible cognitive disturbance. Hyperactive patients, such as those with delirium tremens, are easily recognized by their characteristic severe agitation, tremor, hallucinations, and autonomic instability. Patients who are quietly disturbed are more often overlooked on the medical wards and in the ICU, yet multiple studies suggest that this under-recognized hypoactive subtype is associated with worse outcomes.

The reversibility of delirium is emphasized because many etiologies, such as systemic infection and medication effects, can be easily treated. However, the long-term cognitive effects of delirium remain largely unknown and understudied. Some episodes of delirium continue for weeks, months, or even years. The persistence of delirium in some patients and its high recurrence rate may be due to inadequate treatment of the underlying etiology for the syndrome. In some instances, deliri-

Focal Sensory Seizures These are generally due to lesions in the area of the postcentral or precentral gyrus. The principal symptom of focal sensory seizures is tingling, but additional, more complex sensations may occur, such as a rushing feeling, a sense of warmth, or a sense of movement without detectable motion. Symptoms typically are unilateral; commonly begin in the arm or hand, face, or foot; and often spread in a manner that reflects the cortical representation of different bodily parts, as in a Jacksonian march. Duration of seizures is variable; they may be transient, lasting only for seconds, or persist for an hour or more. Focal motor features may supervene, often becoming generalized with loss of consciousness and tonic-clonic jerking.

um does not disappear because there is underlying permanent neuronal damage. Even after an episode of delirium resolves, there may still be lingering effects of the disorder. A patient's recall of events after delirium varies widely, ranging from complete amnesia to repeated reexperiencing of the frightening period of confusion in a disturbing manner, similar to what is seen in patients with posttraumatic stress disorder.

RISK FACTORS

An effective primary prevention strategy for delirium begins with identification of patients at highest risk, including those preparing for elective surgery or being admitted to the hospital. Although no single validated scoring system has been widely accepted as a screen for asymptomatic patients, there are multiple well-established risk factors for delirium.

The two most consistently identified risks are older age and baseline cognitive dysfunction. Individuals who are over age 65 or exhibit low scores on standardized tests of cognition develop delirium upon hospitalization at a rate approaching 50%. Whether age and baseline cognitive dysfunction are truly independent risk factors is uncertain. Other predisposing factors include sensory deprivation, such as preexisting hearing and visual impairment, as well as indices for poor overall health, including baseline immobility, malnutrition, and underlying medical or neurologic illness.

In-hospital risks for delirium include the use of bladder catheterization, physical restraints, sleep and sensory deprivation, and the addition of three or more new medications. Avoiding such risks remains a key component of delirium prevention as well as treatment. Surgical and anesthetic risk factors for the development of postoperative delirium include specific procedures such as those involving cardiopulmonary bypass and inadequate or excessive treatment of pain in the immediate postoperative period.

The relationship between delirium and dementia (Chap. 365) is complicated by significant overlap between these two conditions, and it is not always simple to distinguish between the two. Dementia and preexisting cognitive dysfunction serve as major risk factors for delirium, and at least two-thirds of cases of delirium occur in patients with coexisting underlying dementia. A form of dementia with parkinsonism, termed *dementia with Lewy bodies*, is characterized by a fluctuating course, prominent visual hallucinations, parkinsonism, and an attentional deficit that clinically resembles hyperactive delirium. Delirium in the elderly often reflects an insult to the brain that is vulnerable due to an underlying neurodegenerative condition. Therefore, the development of delirium sometimes heralds the onset of a previously unrecognized brain disorder.

EPIDEMIOLOGY

Delirium is a common disease, but its reported incidence has varied widely based on the criteria used to define the disorder. Estimates of delirium in hospitalized patients range from 14 to 56%, with higher rates reported for elderly patients and patients undergoing hip surgery. Older patients in the ICU have especially high rates of delirium ranging from 70 to 87%. The condition is not recognized in up to one-third of delirious inpatients, and the diagnosis is especially problematic in the ICU environment where cognitive dysfunction is often difficult to appreciate in the setting of serious systemic illness and sedation. Delirium in the ICU should be viewed as an important manifestation of organ dysfunction not unlike liver, kidney, or heart failure.

Outside of the acute hospital setting, delirium occurs in nearly two-thirds of patients in nursing homes and in over 80% of those at the end of life. These estimates emphasize the remarkably high frequency of this cognitive syndrome in older patients, a population expected to grow in the upcoming decade with the aging of the "baby boom" generation.

In previous decades an episode of delirium was viewed as a transient condition that carried a benign prognosis. Delirium has now been clearly associated with substantial morbidity and increased mortality, and is increasingly recognized as a sign of serious underlying illness. Recent estimates of in-hospital mortality among delirious patients have ranged from 25 to 33%, a rate that is similar to patients with sepsis. Patients with an in-hospital episode of delirium have a higher mortality in the months and years following their illness compared with age-matched nondelirious hospitalized patients. Delirious hospitalized patients have a longer length of stay, are more likely to be discharged to a nursing home, and are more likely to experience subsequent episodes of delirium; as a result, this condition has enormous economic implications.

PATHOGENESIS

The pathogenesis and anatomy of delirium are incompletely understood. The attentional deficit that serves as the neuropsychological hallmark of delirium appears to have a diffuse localization with the brainstem, thalamus, prefrontal cortex, thalamus, and parietal lobes. Rarely, focal lesions such as ischemic strokes have led to delirium in otherwise healthy persons; right parietal and medial dorsal thalamic lesions have been reported most commonly, stressing the relevance of these areas to delirium pathogenesis. In most cases, delirium results from widespread disturbances in cortical and subcortical regions, rather than a focal neuroanatomic cause. Electroencephalogram (EEG) data in persons with delirium usually show symmetric slowing, a nonspecific finding supporting diffuse cerebral dysfunction.

Deficiency of acetylcholine often plays a key role in delirium pathogenesis. Medications with anticholinergic properties can precipitate delirium in susceptible individuals, and therapies designed to boost cholinergic tone such as cholinesterase inhibitors have, in small trials, been shown to relieve symptoms of delirium. Dementia patients are susceptible to episodes of delirium, and those with Alzheimer's pathology are known to have a chronic cholinergic deficiency state due to degeneration of acetylcholine-producing neurons in the basal forebrain. Another common dementia associated with decreased acetylcholine levels, dementia with Lewy bodies, clinically mimics delirium in some patients. Other neurotransmitters are also likely involved in this diffuse cerebral disorder. For example, increases in dopamine can also lead to delirium. Patients with Parkinson's disease treated with dopaminergic medications can develop a delirious-like state that features visual hallucinations, fluctuations, and confusion. In contrast, reducing dopaminergic tone with dopamine antagonists such as typical and atypical antipsychotic medications has long been recognized as effective symptomatic treatment in patients with delirium.

Not all individuals exposed to the same insult will develop signs of delirium. A low dose of an anticholinergic medication may have no cognitive effects on a healthy young adult but may produce a florid delirium in an elderly person with known underlying dementia. However, an extremely high dose of the same anticholinergic medication may lead to delirium even in healthy young persons. This concept of delirium developing as the result of an insult in predisposed individuals is currently the most widely accepted pathogenic construct. Therefore, if a previously healthy individual with no known history of cognitive illness develops delirium in the setting of a relatively minor insult such as elective surgery or hospitalization, then an unrecognized underlying neurologic illness such as a neurodegenerative disease, multiple previous strokes, or another diffuse cerebral cause should be considered. In this context, delirium can be viewed as the symptom resulting from a "stress test for the brain" induced by the insult. Exposure to known inciting factors such as systemic infection or offending drugs can unmask a decreased cerebral reserve and herald a serious underlying and potentially treatable illness.

TABLE 26-1	THE CONFUSION ASSESSMENT METHOD (CAM) DIAGNOSTIC ALGORITHM

The diagnosis of delirium requires the presence of features 1 and 2 and of *either* 3 or 4.[a]

Feature 1: Acute onset and fluctuating course
This feature is satisfied by positive responses to these questions: Is there evidence of an acute change in mental status from the patient's baseline? Did the (abnormal) behavior fluctuate during the day—that is, tend to come and go—or did it increase and decrease in severity?

Feature 2: Inattention
This feature is satisfied by a positive response to this question: Did the patient have difficulty focusing attention—for example, was easily distractible—or have difficulty keeping track of what was being said?

Feature 3: Disorganized thinking
This feature is satisfied by a positive response to this question: Was the patient's thinking disorganized or incoherent, such as rambling or irrelevant conversation, unclear or illogical flow of ideas, or unpredictable switching from subject to subject?

Feature 4: Altered level of consciousness
This feature is satisfied by any answer other than "alert" to this question: Overall, how would you rate this patient's level of consciousness: alert (normal), vigilant (hyperalert), lethargic (drowsy, easily aroused), stupor (difficult to arouse), or coma (unarousable)?

[a]Information is usually obtained from a reliable reporter, such as a family member, caregiver, or nurse.
Source: Modified from Inouye SK et al: Ann Intern Med 113:941, 1990.

APPROACH TO THE PATIENT:
Delirium

As the diagnosis of delirium is clinical and made at the bedside, a careful history and physical examination is necessary when evaluating patients with possible confusional states. Screening tools can aid physicians and nurses in identifying patients with delirium, including the Confusion Assessment Method (CAM) (Table 26-1); the Organic Brain Syndrome Scale; the Delirium Rating Scale; and, in the ICU, the Delirium Detection Score and the ICU version of the CAM. These scales are based on criteria from the American Psychiatric Association's *Diagnostic and Statistical Manual of Mental Disorders* (DSM) or the World Health Organization's International Classification of Diseases (ICD). Unfortunately, these scales themselves do not identify the full spectrum of patients with delirium. All patients who are acutely confused should be presumed delirious regardless of their presentation due to the wide variety of possible clinical features. A course that fluctuates over hours or days and may worsen at night (termed *sundowning*) is typical but not essential for the diagnosis. Observation of the patient will usually reveal an altered level of consciousness or a deficit of attention. Other hallmark features that may be present in the delirious patient include alteration of sleep-wake cycles, thought disturbances such as hallucinations or delusions, autonomic instability, and changes in affect.

HISTORY It may be difficult to elicit an accurate history in delirious patients who have altered levels of consciousness or impaired attention. Information from a collateral source such as a spouse or other family member is therefore invaluable. The three most important pieces of history include the patient's baseline cognitive function, the time course of the present illness, and current medications.

Premorbid cognitive function can be assessed through the collateral source or, if needed, via a review of outpatient records. Delirium by definition represents a change that is relatively acute, usually over hours to days, from a cognitive baseline. As a result, an acute confusional state is nearly impossible to diagnose without some knowledge of baseline cognitive function. Without this information, many patients with dementia or depression may be mistaken as delirious during a single initial evaluation. Patients with a more hypoactive, apathetic presentation with psychomotor slowing may only be identified as being different from baseline through conversations with family members. A number of validated instruments have been shown to accurately diagnose cognitive dysfunction using a collateral source including the modified Blessed Dementia Rating Scale and Clinical Dementia Rating (CDR). Baseline cognitive impairment is common in patients with delirium. Even when no such history of cognitive impairment is elicited, there should still be a high suspicion for previously unrecognized underlying neurologic disorder.

Establishing the time course of cognitive change is important not only to make a diagnosis of delirium but also to correlate the onset of the illness with potentially treatable etiologies such as recent medication changes or symptoms of systemic infection.

Medications remain a common cause of delirium, especially those compounds with anticholinergic or sedative properties. It is estimated that nearly one-third of all cases of delirium are secondary to medications, especially in the elderly. Medication histories should include all prescription as well as over-the-counter and herbal substances taken by the patient and any recent changes in dosing or formulation, including substitution of generics for brand-name medications.

Other important elements of the history include screening for symptoms of organ failure or systemic infection, which often contributes to delirium in the elderly. A history of illicit drug use, alcoholism, or toxin exposure is common in younger delirious patients. Finally, asking the patient and collateral source about other symptoms that may accompany delirium, such as depression or hallucinations, may help identify potential therapeutic targets.

PHYSICAL EXAMINATION The general physical examination in a delirious patient should include a careful screening for signs of infection such as fever, tachypnea, pulmonary consolidation, heart murmur, or stiff neck. The patient's fluid status should be assessed; both dehydration and fluid overload with resultant hypoxia have been associated with delirium, and each is usually easily rectified. The appearance of the skin can be helpful, showing jaundice in hepatic encephalopathy, cyanosis in hypoxia, or needle tracks in patients using intravenous drugs.

The neurologic examination requires a careful assessment of mental status. Patients with delirium often present with a fluctuating course; therefore the diagnosis can be missed when relying on a single time point of evaluation. Some but not all patients exhibit the characteristic pattern of sundowning, a worsening of their condition in the evening. In these cases, assessment only during morning rounds may be falsely reassuring.

An altered level of consciousness ranging from hyperarousal to lethargy to coma is present in most patients with delirium and can be easily assessed at the bedside. In the patient with a relatively normal level of consciousness, a screen for an attentional deficit is in order, as this deficit is the classic neuropsychological hallmark of delirium. Attention can be assessed while taking a history from the patient. Tangential speech, a fragmentary flow of ideas, or inability to follow complex commands often signifies an attentional problem. Formal neuropsychological tests to assess attention exist, but a simple bedside test of digit span forward is quick and fairly sensitive. In this task, patients are asked to repeat successively longer random strings of digits beginning with two digits in a row. Average adults can repeat a string of between five to seven digits before faltering; a digit span of four or less usually indicates an attentional deficit unless hearing or language barriers are present.

More formal neuropsychological testing can be extraordinarily helpful in assessing the delirious patient, but it is usually too cumbersome and time-consuming in the inpatient setting. A simple Mini Mental Status Examination (MMSE) (see Table 365-5) can provide some information regarding orientation, language, and visuospatial skills; however, performance of some tasks on the MMSE such as spelling "world" backwards or serial subtraction of digits will be impaired by delirious patients' attentional deficits alone and are therefore unreliable.

The remainder of the screening neurologic examination should focus on identifying new focal neurologic deficits. Focal strokes or

mass lesions in isolation are rarely the cause of delirium, but patients with underlying extensive cerebrovascular disease or neurodegenerative conditions may not be able to cognitively tolerate even relatively small new insults. Patients should also be screened for additional signs of neurodegenerative conditions such as parkinsonism, which is seen not only in idiopathic Parkinson's disease but also in other dementing conditions such as Alzheimer's disease, dementia with Lewy bodies, and progressive supranuclear palsy. The presence of multifocal myoclonus or asterixis on the motor examination is nonspecific but usually indicates a metabolic or toxic etiology of the delirium.

ETIOLOGY   Some etiologies can be easily discerned through a careful history and physical examination, while others require confirmation with laboratory studies, imaging, or other ancillary tests. A large, diverse group of insults can lead to delirium, and the cause in many patients is often multifactorial. Common etiologies are listed in Table 26-2.

Prescribed, over-the-counter, and herbal medications are common precipitants of delirium. Drugs with anticholinergic properties, narcotics, and benzodiazepines are especially frequent offenders, but nearly any compound can lead to cognitive dysfunction in a predisposed patient. While an elderly patient with baseline dementia may become delirious upon exposure to a relatively low dose of a medication, other less-susceptible individuals may only become delirious with very high doses of the same medication. This observation emphasizes the importance of correlating the timing of recent medication changes, including dose and formulation, with the onset of cognitive dysfunction.

TABLE 26-2   COMMON ETIOLOGIES OF DELIRIUM

Toxins
   Prescription medications: especially those with anticholinergic properties, narcotics and benzodiazepines
   Drugs of abuse: alcohol intoxication and alcohol withdrawal, opiates, ecstasy, LSD, GHB, PCP, ketamine, cocaine
   Poisons: inhalants, carbon monoxide, ethylene glycol, pesticides
Metabolic conditions
   Electrolyte disturbances: hypoglycemia, hyperglycemia, hyponatremia, hypernatremia, hypercalcemia, hypocalcemia, hypomagnesemia
   Hypothermia and hyperthermia
   Pulmonary failure: hypoxemia and hypercarbia
   Liver failure/hepatic encephalopathy
   Renal failure/uremia
   Cardiac failure
   Vitamin deficiencies: B_{12}, thiamine, folate, niacin
   Dehydration and malnutrition
   Anemia
Infections
   Systemic infections: urinary tract infections, pneumonia, skin and soft tissue infections, sepsis
   CNS infections: meningitis, encephalitis, brain abscess
Endocrinologic conditions
   Hyperthyroidism, hypothyroidism
   Hyperparathyroidism
   Adrenal insufficiency
Cerebrovascular disorders
   Global hypoperfusion states
   Hypertensive encephalopathy
   Focal ischemic strokes and hemorrhages: especially nondominant parietal and thalamic lesions
Autoimmune disorders
   CNS vasculitis
   Cerebral lupus
Seizure-related disorders
   Nonconvulsive status epilepticus
   Intermittent seizures with prolonged post-ictal states
Neoplastic disorders
   Diffuse metastases to the brain
   Gliomatosis cerebri
   Carcinomatous meningitis
Hospitalization
Terminal end of life delirium

Abbreviations: LSD, lysergic acid diethylamide; GHB, γ-hydroxybutyrate; PCP, phencyclidine; CNS, central nervous system.

In younger patients especially, illicit drugs and toxins are common causes of delirium. In addition to more classic drugs of abuse, the recent rise in availability of so-called club drugs, such as methylene-dioxymethamphetamine (MDMA, ecstasy), γ-hydroxybutyrate (GHB), and the PCP-like agent ketamine, has led to an increase in delirious young persons presenting to acute care settings. Many common prescription drugs such as oral narcotics and benzodiazepines are now often abused and readily available on the street. Alcohol intoxication with high serum levels can cause confusion, but more commonly it is withdrawal from alcohol that leads to a classic hyperactive delirium. Alcohol and benzodiazepine withdrawal should be considered in all cases of delirium as even patients who drink only a few servings of alcohol every day can experience relatively severe withdrawal symptoms upon hospitalization.

Metabolic abnormalities such as electrolyte disturbances of sodium, calcium, magnesium, or glucose can cause delirium, and mild derangements can lead to substantial cognitive disturbances in susceptible individuals. Other common metabolic etiologies include liver and renal failure, hypercarbia and hypoxia, vitamin deficiencies of thiamine and B_{12}, autoimmune disorders including CNS vasculitis, and endocrinopathies such as thyroid and adrenal disorders.

Systemic infections often cause delirium, especially in the elderly. A common scenario involves the development of an acute cognitive decline in the setting of a urinary tract infection in a patient with baseline dementia. Pneumonia, skin infections such as cellulitis, and frank sepsis can also lead to delirium. This so-called septic encephalopathy, often seen in the ICU, is likely due to the release of proinflammatory cytokines and their diffuse cerebral effects. CNS infections such as meningitis, encephalitis, and abscess are less-common etiologies of delirium; however, given the high mortality associated with these conditions when not treated quickly, clinicians must always maintain a high index of suspicion.

In some susceptible individuals, exposure to the unfamiliar environment of a hospital can lead to delirium. This etiology usually occurs as part of a multifactorial delirium and should be considered a diagnosis of exclusion after all other causes have been thoroughly investigated. Many primary prevention and treatment strategies for delirium involve relatively simple methods to address those aspects of the inpatient setting that are most confusing.

Cerebrovascular etiologies are usually due to global hypoperfusion in the setting of systemic hypotension from heart failure, septic shock, dehydration, or anemia. Focal strokes in the right parietal lobe and medial dorsal thalamus can rarely lead to a delirious state. A more common scenario involves a new focal stroke or hemorrhage causing confusion in a patient who has decreased cerebral reserve. In these individuals, it is sometimes difficult to distinguish between cognitive dysfunction resulting from the new neurovascular insult itself and delirium due to the infectious, metabolic, and pharmacologic complications that can accompany hospitalization after stroke.

Because a fluctuating course is often seen in delirium, intermittent seizures may be overlooked when considering potential etiologies. Both nonconvulsive status epilepticus as well as recurrent focal or generalized seizures followed by post-ictal confusion can cause delirium; EEG remains essential for this diagnosis. Seizure activity spreading from an electrical focus in a mass or infarct can explain global cognitive dysfunction caused by relatively small lesions.

It is very common for patients to experience delirium at the end of life in palliative care settings. This condition, sometimes described as *terminal restlessness*, must be identified and treated aggressively as it is an important cause of patient and family discomfort at the end of life. It should be remembered that these patients may also be suffering from more common etiologies of delirium such as systemic infection.

LABORATORY AND DIAGNOSTIC EVALUATION A cost-effective approach to the diagnostic evaluation of delirium allows the history and physical examination to guide tests. No established algorithm for workup will fit all delirious patients due to the staggering number

TABLE 26-3 STEP-WISE EVALUATION OF A PATIENT WITH DELIRIUM 161

Initial evaluation
  History with special attention to medications (including over-the-counter and herbals)
  General physical examination and neurologic examination
  Complete blood count
  Electrolyte panel including calcium, magnesium, phosphorus
  Liver function tests including albumin
  Renal function tests
First-tier further evaluation guided by initial evaluation
  Systemic infection screen
    Urinalysis and culture
    Chest radiograph
    Blood cultures
  Electrocardiogram
  Arterial blood gas
  Serum and/or urine toxicology screen (perform earlier in young persons)
  Brain imaging with MRI with diffusion and gadolinium (preferred) or CT
  Suspected CNS infection: lumbar puncture following brain imaging
  Suspected seizure-related etiology: electroencephalogram (EEG) (if high suspicion should be performed immediately)
Second-tier further evaluation
  Vitamin levels: B_{12}, folate, thiamine
  Endocrinologic laboratories: thyroid-stimulating hormone (TSH) and free T4; cortisol
  Serum ammonia
  Sedimentation rate
  Autoimmune serologies: antinuclear antibodies (ANA), complement levels; p-ANCA, c-ANCA
  Infectious serologies: rapid plasmin reagin (RPR); fungal and viral serologies if high suspicion; HIV antibody
  Lumbar puncture (if not already performed)
  Brain MRI with and without gadolinium (if not already performed)

Note: p-ANCA, perinuclear antineutrophil cytoplasmic antibody; c-ANCA, cytoplasmic antineutrophil cytoplasmic antibody.

of potential etiologies, but one step-wise approach is detailed in Table 26-3. If a clear precipitant is identified early, such as an offending medication, then little further workup is required. If, however, no likely etiology is uncovered with initial evaluation, an aggressive search for an underlying cause should be initiated.

Basic screening labs, including a complete blood count, electrolyte panel, and tests of liver and renal function, should be obtained in all patients with delirium. In elderly patients, screening for systemic infection, including chest radiography, urinalysis and culture, and possibly blood cultures, is important. In younger individuals, serum and urine drug and toxicology screening may be appropriate early in the workup. Additional laboratory tests addressing other autoimmune, endocrinologic, metabolic, and infectious etiologies should be reserved for patients in whom the diagnosis remains unclear after initial testing.

Multiple studies have demonstrated that brain imaging in patients with delirium is often unhelpful. However, if the initial workup is unrevealing, most clinicians quickly move toward imaging of the brain in order to exclude structural causes. A noncontrast CT scan can identify large masses and hemorrhages but is otherwise relatively insensitive for discovering an etiology of delirium. The ability of MRI to identify most acute ischemic strokes as well as to provide neuroanatomic detail that gives clues to possible infectious, inflammatory, neurodegenerative, and neoplastic conditions makes it the test of choice. Since MRI techniques are limited by availability, speed of imaging, patient cooperation, and contraindications to magnetic exposure, many clinicians begin with CT scanning and proceed to MRI if the etiology of delirium remains elusive.

Lumbar puncture (LP) must be obtained immediately, after appropriate neuroimaging, in all patients in whom CNS infection is suspected. Spinal fluid examination can also be useful in identifying inflammatory and neoplastic conditions as well as in the diagnosis of hepatic encephalopathy through elevated CSF glutamine levels. As a result, LP should be considered in any delirious patient with a negative workup. EEG does not have a routine role in the workup of delirium, but it remains invaluable if seizure-related etiologies are considered.

℞ DELIRIUM

Management of delirium begins with treatment of the underlying inciting factor (e.g., patients with systemic infections should be given appropriate antibiotics and underlying electrolyte disturbances judiciously corrected). These treatments often lead to prompt resolution of delirium. Blindly targeting the symptoms of delirium pharmacologically only serves to prolong the time patients remain in the confused state and may mask important diagnostic information.

Relatively simple methods of supportive care can be highly effective in treating patients with delirium. Reorientation by the nursing staff and family combined with visible clocks, calendars, and outside-facing windows can reduce confusion. Sensory isolation should be prevented by providing glasses and hearing aids to those patients who need them. Sundowning can be addressed to a large extent through vigilance to appropriate sleep-wake cycles. During the day, a well-lit room should be accompanied by activities or exercises to prevent napping. At night, a quiet, dark environment with limited interruptions by staff can assure proper rest. These sleep-wake cycle interventions are especially important in the ICU setting as the usual constant 24-h activity commonly provokes delirium. Attempting to mimic the home environment as much as possible has also been shown to help treat and even prevent delirium. Visits from friends and family throughout the day minimize the anxiety associated with the constant flow of new faces of staff and physicians. Allowing hospitalized patients to have access to home bedding, clothing, and nightstand objects makes the hospital environment less foreign and therefore less confusing. Simple standard nursing practices such as maintaining proper nutrition and volume status as well as managing incontinence and skin breakdown also help to alleviate discomfort and resulting confusion.

In some instances, patients pose a threat to their own safety or to the safety of staff members, and acute management is required. Bed alarms and personal sitters are more effective and much less disorienting than physical restraints. Chemical restraints should be avoided, but, when necessary, very-low-dose typical or atypical antipsychotic medications administered on an as-needed basis are effective. The recent association of atypical antipsychotic use in the elderly with increased mortality underscores the importance of using these medications judiciously and only as a last resort. Benzodiazepines are not as effective as antipsychotics and often worsen confusion via their sedative properties. Although many clinicians still use benzodiazepines to treat acute confusion, their use should be limited only to cases in which delirium is caused by alcohol or benzodiazepine withdrawal.

PREVENTION

Given the high morbidity associated with delirium and the tremendously increased health care costs that accompany it, development of an effective strategy to prevent delirium in hospitalized patients is extremely important. Successful identification of high-risk patients is the first step, followed by initiation of appropriate interventions. One trial randomized more than 850 elderly inpatients to simple standardized protocols used to manage risk factors for delirium, including cognitive impairment, immobility, visual impairment, hearing impairment, sleep deprivation, and dehydration. Significant reductions in the number and duration of episodes of delirium were observed in the treatment group, but unfortunately delirium recurrence rates were unchanged. All hospitals and health care systems should work toward developing standardized protocols to address common risk factors with the goal of decreasing the incidence of delirium.

ACKNOWLEDGMENT

In the previous edition, Allan H. Ropper contributed to a section on acute confusional states that was incorporated into this current chapter.

FURTHER READINGS

ELY EW et al: Delirium as a predictor of mortality in mechanically ventilated patients in the intensive care unit. JAMA 291:1753, 2004

INOUYE SK: Delirium in older persons. N Engl J Med 354:1157, 2006

——— et al: A multicomponent intervention to prevent delirium in hospitalized older patients. N Engl J Med 340:669, 1999

KALISVAART KJ et al: Risk factors and prediction of postoperative delirium in elderly hip-surgery patients: Implementation and validation of a medical risk factor model. J Am Geriatr Soc 54:817, 2006

YOUNG J, INOUYE SK: Delirium in older people. BMJ 334:842, 2007

27 Aphasia, Memory Loss, and Other Focal Cerebral Disorders
M.-Marsel Mesulam

The cerebral cortex of the human brain contains ~20 billion neurons spread over an area of 2.5 m^2. The *primary sensory* areas provide an obligatory portal for the entry of sensory information into cortical circuitry, whereas the *primary motor* areas provide final common pathways for coordinating complex motor acts. The primary sensory and motor areas constitute 10% of the cerebral cortex. The rest is subsumed by unimodal, heteromodal, paralimbic, and limbic areas, collectively known as the *association cortex* (Fig. 27-1). The association cortex mediates the integrative processes that subserve cognition, emotion, and behavior. A systematic testing of these mental functions is necessary for the effective clinical assessment of the association cortex and its diseases.

According to current thinking, there are no centers for "hearing words," "perceiving space," or "storing memories." Cognitive and behavioral functions (domains) are coordinated by intersecting *large-scale neural networks* that contain interconnected cortical and subcortical components. The network approach to higher cerebral function has at least four implications of clinical relevance: (1) a single domain such as language or memory can be disrupted by damage to any one of several areas, as long as these areas belong to the same network; (2) damage confined to a single area can give rise to multiple deficits, involving the functions of all networks that intersect in that region; (3) damage to a network component may give rise to minimal or transient deficits if other parts of the network undergo compensatory reorganization; and (4) individual anatomic sites within a network display a relative (but not absolute) specialization for different behavioral aspects of the relevant function. Five anatomically defined large-scale networks are most relevant to clinical practice: a perisylvian network for language; a parietofrontal network for spatial cognition; an occipitotemporal network for face and object recognition; a limbic network for retentive memory; and a prefrontal network for attention and behavior.

THE LEFT PERISYLVIAN NETWORK FOR LANGUAGE: APHASIAS AND RELATED CONDITIONS

Language allows the communication and elaboration of thoughts and experiences by linking them to arbitrary symbols known as words. The neural substrate of language is composed of a distributed network centered in the perisylvian region of the *left* hemisphere. The posterior pole of this network is located at the temporoparietal junction and includes a region known as *Wernicke's area*. An essential function of Wernicke's area is to transform sensory inputs into their lexical representations so that these can establish the distributed associations that give the word its meaning. The anterior pole of the language network is located in the inferior frontal gyrus and includes a region known as *Broca's area*. An essential function of this area is to transform lexical representations into their articulatory sequences so that the words can be uttered in the form of spoken language. The sequencing function of Broca's area also appears to involve the ordering of words into sentences that contain a meaning-appropriate *syntax* (grammar). Wernicke's and Broca's areas are interconnected with each other and with additional perisylvian, temporal, prefrontal, and posterior parietal regions, making up a neural network subserving the various aspects of lan-

FIGURE 27-1 Lateral (*top*) and medial (*bottom*) views of the cerebral hemispheres. The numbers refer to the Brodmann cytoarchitectonic designations. Area 17 corresponds to the primary visual cortex, 41–42 to the primary auditory cortex, 1–3 to the primary somatosensory cortex, and 4 to the primary motor cortex. The rest of the cerebral cortex contains association areas. AG, angular gyrus; B, Broca's area; CC, corpus callosum; CG, cingulate gyrus; DLPFC, dorsolateral prefrontal cortex; FEF, frontal eye fields (premotor cortex); FG, fusiform gyrus; IPL, inferior parietal lobule; ITG, inferior temporal gyrus; LG, lingual gyrus; MPFC, medial prefrontal cortex; MTG, middle temporal gyrus; OFC, orbitofrontal cortex; PHG, parahippocampal gyrus; PPC, posterior parietal cortex; PSC, peristriate cortex; SC, striate cortex; SMG, supramarginal gyrus; SPL, superior parietal lobule; STG, superior temporal gyrus; STS, superior temporal sulcus; TP, temporopolar cortex; W, Wernicke's area.

guage function. Damage to any one of these components or to their interconnections can give rise to language disturbances (*aphasia*). Aphasia should be diagnosed only when there are deficits in the formal aspects of language such as naming, word choice, comprehension, spelling, and syntax. Dysarthria and mutism do not, by themselves, lead to a diagnosis of aphasia. The language network shows a left hemisphere dominance pattern in the vast majority of the population. In ~90% of right handers and 60% of left handers, aphasia occurs only after lesions of the left hemisphere. In some individuals no hemispheric dominance for language can be discerned, and in some others (including a small minority of right handers) there is a right hemisphere dominance for language. A language disturbance occurring after a right hemisphere lesion in a right hander is called *crossed aphasia*.

CLINICAL EXAMINATION

The clinical examination of language should include the assessment of naming, spontaneous speech, comprehension, repetition, reading, and writing. A deficit of naming (*anomia*) is the single most common finding

in aphasic patients. When asked to name common objects (pencil or wristwatch), the patient may fail to come up with the appropriate word, may provide a circumlocutious description of the object ("the thing for writing"), or may come up with the wrong word (*paraphasia*). If the patient offers an incorrect but legitimate word ("pen" for "pencil"), the naming error is known as a *semantic paraphasia*; if the word approximates the correct answer but is phonetically inaccurate ("plentil" for "pencil"), it is known as a *phonemic paraphasia*. Asking the patient to name body parts, geometric shapes, and component parts of objects (lapel of coat, cap of pen) can elicit mild forms of anomia in patients who can otherwise name common objects. In most anomias, the patient cannot retrieve the appropriate name when shown an object but can point to the appropriate object when the name is provided by the examiner. This is known as a one-way (or retrieval-based) naming deficit. A two-way naming deficit exists if the patient can neither provide nor recognize the correct name, indicating the presence of a language comprehension impairment. *Spontaneous speech* is described as "fluent" if it maintains appropriate output volume, phrase length, and melody or as "nonfluent" if it is sparse, halting, and average utterance length is below four words. The examiner should also note if the speech is paraphasic or circumlocutious; if it shows a relative paucity of substantive nouns and action verbs versus function words (prepositions, conjunctions); and if word order, tenses, suffixes, prefixes, plurals, and possessives are appropriate. *Comprehension* can be tested by assessing the patient's ability to follow conversation, by asking yes-no questions ("Can a dog fly?", "Does it snow in summer?") or asking the patient to point to appropriate objects ("Where is the source of illumination in this room?"). Statements with embedded clauses or passive voice construction ("If a tiger is eaten by a lion, which animal stays alive?") help to assess the ability to comprehend complex syntactic structure. Commands to close or open the eyes, stand up, sit down, or roll over should not be used to assess overall comprehension since appropriate responses aimed at such axial movements can be preserved in patients who otherwise have profound comprehension deficits.

Repetition is assessed by asking the patient to repeat single words, short sentences, or strings of words such as "No ifs, ands, or buts." The testing of repetition with tongue-twisters such as "hippopotamus" or "Irish constabulary" provides a better assessment of dysarthria and palilalia than aphasia. Aphasic patients may have little difficulty with tongue-twisters but have a particularly hard time repeating a string of function words. It is important to make sure that the number of words does not exceed the patient's attention span. Otherwise, the failure of repetition becomes a reflection of the narrowed attention span rather than an indication of an aphasic deficit. *Reading* should be assessed for deficits in reading aloud as well as comprehension. *Writing* is assessed for spelling errors, word order, and grammar. *Alexia* describes an inability to either read aloud or comprehend single words and simple sentences; *agraphia* (or *dysgraphia*) is used to describe an acquired deficit in the spelling or grammar of written language.

The correspondence between individual deficits of language function and lesion location does not display a rigid one-to-one relationship and should be conceptualized within the context of the distributed network model. Nonetheless, the classification of aphasias of acute onset into specific clinical syndromes helps to determine the most likely anatomic distribution of the underlying neurologic disease and has implications for etiology and prognosis (Table 27-1). The syndromes listed in Table 27-1 are most applicable to aphasias caused by cerebrovascular accidents (CVA). They can be divided into "central" syndromes, which result from damage to the two epicenters of the language network (Broca's and Wernicke's areas), and "disconnection" syndromes, which arise from lesions that interrupt the functional connectivity of these centers with each other and with the other components of the language network. The syndromes outlined below are idealizations; pure syndromes occur rarely.

Wernicke's Aphasia
Comprehension is impaired for spoken and written language. Language output is fluent but is highly paraphasic and circumlocutious. The tendency for paraphasic errors may be so pronounced that it leads to strings of neologisms, which form the basis of what is known as "jargon aphasia." Speech contains large

numbers of function words (e.g., prepositions, conjunctions) but few substantive nouns or verbs that refer to specific actions. The output is therefore voluminous but uninformative. For example, a patient attempts to describe how his wife accidentally threw away something important, perhaps his dentures: "We don't need it anymore, she says. And with it when that was downstairs was my teeth-tick . . . a . . . den . . . dentith . . . my dentist. And they happened to be in that bag . . . see? How could this have happened? How could a thing like this happen...So she says we won't need it anymore...I didn't think we'd use it. And now if I have any problems anybody coming a month from now, 4 months from now, or 6 months from now, I have a new dentist. Where my two . . . two little pieces of dentist that I use . . . that I . . . all gone. If she throws the whole thing away . . . visit some friends of hers and she can't throw them away."

Gestures and pantomime do not improve communication. The patient does not seem to realize that his or her language is incomprehensible and may appear angry and impatient when the examiner fails to decipher the meaning of a severely paraphasic statement. In some patients this type of aphasia can be associated with severe agitation and paranoid behaviors. One area of comprehension that may be preserved is the ability to follow commands aimed at axial musculature. The dissociation between the failure to understand simple questions ("What is your name?") in a patient who rapidly closes his or her eyes, sits up, or rolls over when asked to do so is characteristic of Wernicke's aphasia and helps to differentiate it from deafness, psychiatric disease, or malingering. Patients with Wernicke's aphasia cannot express their thoughts in meaning-appropriate words and cannot decode the meaning of words in any modality of input. This aphasia therefore has expressive as well as receptive components. Repetition, naming, reading, and writing are also impaired.

The lesion site most commonly associated with Wernicke's aphasia is the posterior portion of the language network and tends to involve at least parts of Wernicke's area. An embolus to the inferior division of the middle cerebral artery, and to the posterior temporal or angular branches in particular, is the most common etiology (Chap. 364). Intracerebral hemorrhage, severe head trauma, or neoplasm are other causes. A coexisting right hemi- or superior quadrantanopia is common, and mild right nasolabial flattening may be found, but otherwise the examination is often unrevealing. The paraphasic, neologistic speech in an agitated patient with an otherwise unremarkable neurologic examination may lead to the suspicion of a primary psychiatric disorder such as schizophrenia or mania, but the other components characteristic of acquired aphasia and the absence of prior psychiatric disease usually settle the issue. Some patients with Wernicke's aphasia due to intracerebral hemorrhage or head trauma may improve as the hemorrhage or the injury heals. In most other patients, prognosis for recovery is guarded.

Broca's Aphasia Speech is nonfluent, labored, interrupted by many word-finding pauses, and usually dysarthric. It is impoverished in function words but enriched in meaning-appropriate nouns and verbs. Abnormal word order and the inappropriate deployment of *bound morphemes* (word endings used to denote tenses, possessives, or plurals) lead to a characteristic agrammatism. Speech is telegraphic and pithy but quite informative. In the following passage, a patient with Broca's aphasia describes his medical history: "I see . . . the dotor, dotor sent me . . . Bosson. Go to hospital. Dotor . . . kept me beside. Two, tee days, doctor send me home."

Output may be reduced to a grunt or single word ("yes" or "no"), which is emitted with different intonations in an attempt to express approval or disapproval. In addition to fluency, naming and repetition are

TABLE 27-1 CLINICAL FEATURES OF APHASIAS AND RELATED CONDITIONS

	Comprehension	Repetition of Spoken Language	Naming	Fluency
Wernicke's	Impaired	Impaired	Impaired	Preserved or increased
Broca's	Preserved (except grammar)	Impaired	Impaired	Decreased
Global	Impaired	Impaired	Impaired	Decreased
Conduction	Preserved	Impaired	Impaired	Preserved
Nonfluent (motor) transcortical	Preserved	Preserved	Impaired	Impaired
Fluent (sensory) transcortical	Impaired	Preserved	Impaired	Preserved
Isolation	Impaired	Echolalia	Impaired	No purposeful speech
Anomic	Preserved	Preserved	Impaired	Preserved except for word-finding pauses
Pure word deafness	Impaired only for spoken language	Impaired	Preserved	Preserved
Pure alexia	Impaired only for reading	Preserved	Preserved	Preserved

also impaired. Comprehension of spoken language is intact, except for syntactically difficult sentences with passive voice structure or embedded clauses. Reading comprehension is also preserved, with the occasional exception of a specific inability to read small grammatical words such as conjunctions and pronouns. The last two features indicate that Broca's aphasia is not just an "expressive" or "motor" disorder and that it may also involve a comprehension deficit for function words and syntax. Patients with Broca's aphasia can be tearful, easily frustrated, and profoundly depressed. Insight into their condition is preserved, in contrast to Wernicke's aphasia. Even when spontaneous speech is severely dysarthric, the patient may be able to display a relatively normal articulation of words when singing. This dissociation has been used to develop specific therapeutic approaches (melodic intonation therapy) for Broca's aphasia. Additional neurologic deficits usually include right facial weakness, hemiparesis or hemiplegia, and a buccofacial apraxia characterized by an inability to carry out motor commands involving oropharyngeal and facial musculature (e.g., patients are unable to demonstrate how to blow out a match or suck through a straw). Visual fields are intact. The cause is most often infarction of Broca's area (the inferior frontal convolution; "B" in Fig. 27-1) and surrounding anterior perisylvian and insular cortex, due to occlusion of the superior division of the middle cerebral artery (Chap. 364). Mass lesions including tumor, intracerebral hemorrhage, or abscess may also be responsible. Small lesions confined to the posterior part of Broca's area may lead to a nonaphasic and often reversible deficit of speech articulation, usually accompanied by mild right facial weakness. When the cause of Broca's aphasia is stroke, recovery of language function generally peaks within 2–6 months, after which time further progress is limited.

Global Aphasia Speech output is nonfluent, and comprehension of spoken language is severely impaired. Naming, repetition, reading, and writing are also impaired. This syndrome represents the combined dysfunction of Broca's and Wernicke's areas and usually results from strokes that involve the entire middle cerebral artery distribution in the left hemisphere. Most patients are initially mute or say a few words, such as "hi" or "yes." Related signs include right hemiplegia, hemisensory loss, and homonymous hemianopia. Occasionally, a patient with a lesion in Wernicke's area will present with a global aphasia that soon resolves into Wernicke's aphasia.

Conduction Aphasia Speech output is fluent but paraphasic, comprehension of spoken language is intact, and repetition is severely impaired. Naming and writing are also impaired. Reading aloud is impaired, but reading comprehension is preserved. The lesion sites spare Broca's and Wernicke's areas but may induce a functional disconnection between the two so that lexical representations formed in Wernicke's area and adjacent regions cannot be conveyed to Broca's area for assembly into corresponding articulatory patterns. Occasionally, a Wernicke's area lesion gives rise to a transient Wernicke's aphasia that rapidly resolves into a conduction aphasia. The paraphasic output in conduction aphasia interferes with the ability to express meaning, but this deficit is not nearly as severe as the one displayed by patients with Wernicke's aphasia. Associated neurologic signs in conduction aphasia vary according to the primary lesion site.

Nonfluent Transcortical Aphasia (Transcortical Motor Aphasia) The features are similar to Broca's aphasia, but repetition is intact and agrammatism may be less pronounced. The neurologic examination may be otherwise intact, but a right hemiparesis can also exist. The lesion site disconnects the intact language network from prefrontal areas of the brain and usually involves the anterior watershed zone between anterior and middle cerebral artery territories or the supplementary motor cortex in the territory of the anterior cerebral artery.

Fluent Transcortical Aphasia (Transcortical Sensory Aphasia) Clinical features are similar to those of Wernicke's aphasia, but repetition is intact. The lesion site disconnects the intact core of the language network from other temporoparietal association areas. Associated neurologic findings may include hemianopia. Cerebrovascular lesions (e.g., infarctions in the posterior watershed zone) or neoplasms that involve the temporoparietal cortex posterior to Wernicke's area are the most common causes.

Isolation Aphasia This rare syndrome represents a combination of the two transcortical aphasias. Comprehension is severely impaired, and there is no purposeful speech output. The patient may parrot fragments of heard conversations (*echolalia*), indicating that the neural mechanisms for repetition are at least partially intact. This condition represents the pathologic function of the language network when it is isolated from other regions of the brain. Broca's and Wernicke's areas tend to be spared, but there is damage to the surrounding frontal, parietal, and temporal cortex. Lesions are patchy and can be associated with anoxia, carbon monoxide poisoning, or complete watershed zone infarctions.

Anomic Aphasia This form of aphasia may be considered the "minimal dysfunction" syndrome of the language network. Articulation, comprehension, and repetition are intact, but confrontation naming, word finding, and spelling are impaired. Speech is enriched in function words but impoverished in substantive nouns and verbs denoting specific actions. Language output is fluent but paraphasic, circumlocutious, and uninformative. The lesion sites can be anywhere within the left hemisphere language network, including the middle and inferior temporal gyri. *Anomic aphasia is the single most common language disturbance seen in head trauma, metabolic encephalopathy, and Alzheimer's disease.*

Pure Word Deafness The most common causes are either bilateral or left-sided middle cerebral artery strokes affecting the superior temporal gyrus. The net effect of the underlying lesion is to interrupt the flow of information from the unimodal auditory association cortex to Wernicke's area. Patients have no difficulty understanding written language and can express themselves well in spoken or written language. They have no difficulty interpreting and reacting to environmental sounds since primary auditory cortex and subcortical auditory relays are intact. Since auditory information cannot be conveyed to the language network, however, it cannot be decoded into lexical representations and the patient reacts to speech as if it were in an alien tongue that cannot be deciphered. Patients cannot repeat spoken language but have no difficulty naming objects. In time, patients with pure word deafness teach themselves lip reading and may appear to have improved. There may be no additional neurologic findings, but agitated paranoid reactions are frequent in the acute stages. Cerebrovascular lesions are the most frequent cause.

Pure Alexia without Agraphia This is the visual equivalent of pure word deafness. The lesions (usually a combination of damage to the left occipital cortex and to a posterior sector of the corpus callosum—the splenium) interrupt the flow of visual input into the language network.

There is usually a right hemianopia, but the core language network remains unaffected. The patient can understand and produce spoken language, name objects in the left visual hemifield, repeat, and write. However, the patient acts as if illiterate when asked to read even the simplest sentence because the visual information from the written words (presented to the intact left visual hemifield) cannot reach the language network. Objects in the left hemifield may be named accurately because they activate nonvisual associations in the right hemisphere, which, in turn, can access the language network through transcallosal pathways anterior to the splenium. Patients with this syndrome may also lose the ability to name colors, although they can match colors. This is known as a *color anomia*. The most common etiology of pure alexia is a vascular lesion in the territory of the posterior cerebral artery or an infiltrating neoplasm in the left occipital cortex that involves the optic radiations as well as the crossing fibers of the splenium. Since the posterior cerebral artery also supplies medial temporal components of the limbic system, the patient with pure alexia may also experience an amnesia, but this is usually transient because the limbic lesion is unilateral.

Aphemia There is an acute onset of severely impaired fluency (often mutism), which cannot be accounted for by corticobulbar, cerebellar, or extrapyramidal dysfunction. Recovery is the rule and involves an intermediate stage of hoarse whispering. Writing, reading, and comprehension are intact, so this is not a true aphasic syndrome. Partial lesions of Broca's area or subcortical lesions that undercut its connections with other parts of the brain may be present. Occasionally, the lesion site is on the medial aspects of the frontal lobes and may involve the supplementary motor cortex of the left hemisphere.

Apraxia This generic term designates a complex motor deficit that cannot be attributed to pyramidal, extrapyramidal, cerebellar, or sensory dysfunction and that does not arise from the patient's failure to understand the nature of the task. The form that is most frequently encountered in clinical practice is known as *ideomotor apraxia*. Commands to perform a specific motor act ("cough," "blow out a match") or to pantomime the use of a common tool (a comb, hammer, straw, or toothbrush) in the absence of the real object cannot be followed. The patient's ability to comprehend the command is ascertained by demonstrating multiple movements and establishing that the correct one can be recognized. Some patients with this type of apraxia can imitate the appropriate movement (when it is demonstrated by the examiner) and show no impairment when handed the real object, indicating that the sensorimotor mechanisms necessary for the movement are intact. Some forms of ideomotor apraxia represent a disconnection of the language network from pyramidal motor systems: commands to execute complex movements are understood but cannot be conveyed to the appropriate motor areas, even though the relevant motor mechanisms are intact. *Buccofacial apraxia* involves apraxic deficits in movements of the face and mouth. *Limb apraxia* encompasses apraxic deficits in movements of the arms and legs. Ideomotor apraxia is almost always caused by lesions in the left hemisphere and is commonly associated with aphasic syndromes, especially Broca's aphasia and conduction aphasia. Its presence cannot be ascertained in patients with language comprehension deficits. The ability to follow commands aimed at axial musculature ("close the eyes," "stand up") is subserved by different pathways and may be intact in otherwise severely aphasic and apraxic patients. Patients with lesions of the anterior corpus callosum can display a special type of ideomotor apraxia confined to the left side of the body. Since the handling of real objects is not impaired, ideomotor apraxia, by itself, causes no major limitation of daily living activities.

Ideational apraxia refers to a deficit in the execution of a goal-directed sequence of movements in patients who have no difficulty executing the individual components of the sequence. For example, when asked to pick up a pen and write, the sequence of uncapping the pen, placing the cap at the opposite end, turning the point toward the writing surface, and writing may be disrupted, and the patient may be seen trying to write with the wrong end of the pen or even with the removed cap. These motor sequencing problems are usually seen in the context of confusional states and dementias rather than focal lesions associated with aphasic conditions. *Limb-kinetic apraxia* involves a clumsiness in the actual use of tools that cannot be attributed to sensory, pyramidal, extrapyramidal, or cerebellar dysfunction. This condition can emerge in the context of focal premotor cortex lesions or *corticobasal ganglionic degeneration*.

Gerstmann's Syndrome The combination of *acalculia* (impairment of simple arithmetic), *dysgraphia* (impaired writing), *finger anomia* (an inability to name individual fingers such as the index or thumb), and *right-left confusion* (an inability to tell whether a hand, foot, or arm of the patient or examiner is on the right or left side of the body) is known as Gerstmann's syndrome. In making this diagnosis it is important to establish that the finger and left-right naming deficits are not part of a more generalized anomia and that the patient is not otherwise aphasic. When Gerstmann's syndrome is seen in isolation, it is commonly associated with damage to the inferior parietal lobule (especially the angular gyrus) in the left hemisphere.

Aprosodia Variations of melodic stress and intonation influence the meaning and impact of spoken language. For example, the two statements "He *is* clever." and "He is *clever?*" contain an identical word choice and syntax but convey vastly different messages because of differences in the intonation and stress with which the statements are uttered. This aspect of language is known as *prosody*. Damage to perisylvian areas in the right hemisphere can interfere with speech prosody and can lead to syndromes of aprosodia. Damage to right hemisphere regions corresponding to Wernicke's area can selectively impair decoding of speech prosody, whereas damage to right hemisphere regions corresponding to Broca's area yields a greater impairment in the ability to introduce meaning-appropriate prosody into spoken language. The latter deficit is the most common type of aprosodia identified in clinical practice—the patient produces grammatically correct language with accurate word choice but the statements are uttered in a monotone that interferes with the ability to convey the intended stress and affect. Patients with this type of aprosodia give the mistaken impression of being depressed or indifferent.

Subcortical Aphasia Damage to subcortical components of the language network (e.g., the striatum and thalamus of the left hemisphere) can also lead to aphasia. The resulting syndromes contain combinations of deficits in the various aspects of language but rarely fit the specific patterns described in Table 27-1. In a patient with a CVA, an anomic aphasia accompanied by dysarthria or a fluent aphasia with hemiparesis should raise the suspicion of a subcortical lesion site.

Progressive Aphasias In clinical practice, acquired aphasias are most commonly encountered in one of two contexts: CVAs and degenerative diseases. Aphasias caused by CVAs start suddenly and display maximal deficits at the onset. The underlying lesion is relatively circumscribed and associated with a total loss of neural function at the lesion site. These are the "classic" aphasias described above where relatively reproducible relationships between lesion site and aphasia pattern can be discerned. Aphasias caused by neurodegenerative diseases have an insidious onset and relentless progression so that the symptomatology changes over time. Since the neuronal loss within the areas encompassed by the neurodegeneration is partial and since it tends to include multiple components of the language network, distinctive clinical patterns and clinico-anatomic correlations are less obvious.

Dementia is a generic term used to designate a neurodegenerative disease that impairs intellect and behavior to the point where customary daily living activities become compromised (Chap. 365). Alzheimer's disease is the single most common cause of dementia. The neuropathology of Alzheimer's disease causes the earliest and most profound neuronal loss in memory-related parts of the brain such as the entorhinal cortex and the hippocampus. This is why progressive forgetfulness for recent events and experiences is the cardinal feature of Alzheimer's disease. In time, the neuronal pathology in Alzheimer's disease spreads to the language network and a progressive aphasia, usually of the anomic

type, becomes added to the progressive amnesia. There are other patterns of dementia, however, where neurodegeneration initially targets the language rather than memory network of the brain, leading to the emergence of a progressive aphasia that becomes the most prominent aspect of the clinical picture during the initial phases of the disease. Primary progressive aphasia (PPA) is the most widely recognized syndrome with this pattern of selective language impairment.

CLINICAL PRESENTATION AND DIAGNOSIS OF PPA The patient with PPA comes to medical attention because of word-finding difficulties, abnormal speech patterns, and spelling errors of recent onset. PPA is diagnosed when other mental faculties such as memory for daily events, visuospatial skills (assessed by tests of drawing and face recognition), and comportment (assessed by history obtained from a third party) remain relatively intact; when language is the major area of dysfunction for the first few years of the disease; and when structural brain imaging does not reveal a specific lesion, other than atrophy, to account for the language deficit. Impairments in other cognitive functions may also emerge, but the language dysfunction remains the most salient feature and deteriorates most rapidly throughout the illness.

LANGUAGE IN PPA The language impairment in PPA varies from patient to patient. Some patients cannot find the right words to express thoughts; others cannot understand the meaning of heard or seen words; still others cannot name objects in the environment. The language impairment can be fluent (that is, with normal articulation, flow, and number of words per utterance) or nonfluent. The single most common sign of primary progressive aphasia is anomia, manifested by an inability to come up with the right word during conversation and/or an inability to name objects shown by the examiner. Many patients remain in an anomic phase through most of the disease and experience a gradual intensification of word-finding deficits to the point of near-mutism. Others, however, proceed to develop distinct forms of agrammatism and/or word comprehension deficits. The agrammatism consists of inappropriate word order and misuse of small grammatical words. One patient, for example, sent the following e-mail to her daughter: "I will come my house in your car and drive my car into chicago. . . . You will back get your car and my car park in my driveway. Love, Mom." Comprehension deficits, if present, start with an occasional inability to understand single low-frequency words and gradually progress to encompass the comprehension of conversational speech.

The impairments of syntax, comprehension, naming, or writing in PPA are no different from those seen in aphasias of cerebrovascular causes. However, they form slightly different patterns. According to a classification proposed by Gorno-Tempini and colleagues, three variants of PPA can be recognized: an agrammatical variant characterized by poor fluency and impaired syntax, a semantic variant characterized by preserved fluency and syntax but poor single word comprehension, and a logopenic variant characterized by preserved syntax and comprehension but frequent word-finding pauses during spontaneous speech. The agrammatical variant is also known as *progressive nonfluent aphasia* and displays similarities to Broca's aphasia. However, dysarthria is usually absent. The semantic variant of PPA is also known as *semantic dementia* and displays similarities to Wernicke's aphasia, but the comprehension difficulty tends to be milder. The most obvious difference between aphasias caused by CVA and those caused by neurodegenerative disease is the post-stroke improvement in CVA-related aphasias, leading to a progressive crystallization of the subtypes listed in Table 27-1, versus the gradual deterioration that leads to a loss of syndromic specificity as the disease progresses.

PATHOPHYSIOLOGY Patients with PPA display progressive atrophy (indicative of neuronal loss), electroencephalographic slowing, decreased blood flow (measured by single photon emission CT) and decreased glucose utilization (measured by positron emission tomography) that are most pronounced within the language network of the brain. The abnormalities may remain confined to left hemisphere perisylvian and anterior temporal cortices for many years. The clinical focality of primary progressive aphasia is thus matched by the anatomic selectivity of the underlying pathologic process.

The three variants display overlapping distributions of neuronal loss but the agrammatical variant is most closely associated with atrophy in the anterior parts of the language network (where Broca's area is located), the semantic variant with atrophy in the temporal components of the language network, and the logopenic variant with atrophy in the temporoparietal component of the language network. The relationship between poor language comprehension and damage to Wernicke's area, which is a feature of CVA-related aphasias, is not present in PPA. Instead, poor comprehension is most closely associated with neuronal loss in the lateral and anterior temporal cortex.

NEUROPATHOLOGY Approximately 30% of patients have shown the microscopic pathology of Alzheimer's disease, presumably with an atypical distribution of lesions. In the majority of cases, the neuropathology falls within the family of frontotemporal lobar degenerations (FTLD) and displays various combinations of focal neuronal loss, gliosis, tau-positive inclusions, Pick bodies, and tau-negative ubiquitin inclusions (Chap. 365). Familial forms of PPA with tau-negative ubiquinated inclusions have recently been linked to mutations of the progranulin gene on chromosome 17. Apolipoprotein E and prion protein genotyping has shown differences between patients with typical clinical patterns of Alzheimer's disease and those with a diagnosis of PPA. The intriguing possibility has been raised that a personal or family history of dyslexia may be a risk factor for primary progressive aphasia, at least in some patients, suggesting that this disease may arise on a background of genetic or developmental vulnerability affecting language-related areas of the brain.

THE PARIETOFRONTAL NETWORK FOR SPATIAL ORIENTATION: NEGLECT AND RELATED CONDITIONS

HEMISPATIAL NEGLECT

Adaptive orientation to significant events within the extrapersonal space is subserved by a large-scale network containing three major cortical components. The *cingulate cortex* provides access to a limbic-motivational mapping of the extrapersonal space, the *posterior parietal cortex* to a sensorimotor representation of salient extrapersonal events, and the *frontal eye fields* to motor strategies for attentional behaviors (Fig. 27-2). Subcortical components of this network include the striatum and the thalamus. Contralesional hemispatial neglect represents one outcome of damage to any of the cortical or subcortical components of this network. *The traditional view that hemispatial neglect always denotes a parietal lobe lesion is inaccurate.* In keeping with this anatomic organization, the clinical manifestations of neglect display three behavioral components: sensory events (or their mental representations) within the neglected hemispace have a lesser impact on overall awareness; there is a paucity of exploratory and orienting acts directed toward the neglected hemispace; and the patient behaves as if the neglected hemispace was motivationally devalued.

According to one model of spatial cognition, the right hemisphere directs attention within the *entire* extrapersonal space, whereas the left hemisphere directs attention mostly within the contralateral right hemispace. Consequently, unilateral left hemisphere lesions do not give rise to much contralesional neglect since the global attentional mechanisms of the right hemisphere can compensate for the loss of the *contralaterally* directed attentional functions of the left hemisphere. Unilateral right hemisphere lesions, however, give rise to severe contralesional left hemispatial neglect because the unaffected left hemisphere does not contain ipsilateral attentional mechanisms. This model is consistent with clinical experience, which shows that contralesional neglect is more common, severe, and lasting after damage to the right hemisphere than after damage to the left hemisphere. Severe neglect for the right hemispace is rare, even in left handers with left hemisphere lesions.

Patients with severe neglect may fail to dress, shave, or groom the left side of the body; may fail to eat food placed on the left side of the tray; and may fail to read the left half of sentences. When the examiner

FIGURE 27-2 Functional magnetic resonance imaging of language and spatial attention in neurologically intact subjects. The dark areas show regions of task-related significant activation. (*Top*) The subjects were asked to determine if two words were synonymous. This language task led to the simultaneous activation of the two epicenters of the language network, Broca's area (B) and Wernicke's area (W). The activations are exclusively in the left hemisphere. (*Bottom*) The subjects were asked to shift spatial attention to a peripheral target. This task led to the simultaneous activation of the three epicenters of the attentional network, the posterior parietal cortex (P), the frontal eye fields (F), and the cingulate gyrus (CG). The activations are predominantly in the right hemisphere. (*Courtesy of Darren Gitelman, MD; with permission.*)

draws a large circle [12–15 cm (5–6 in.) in diameter] and asks the patient to place the numbers 1–12 as if the circle represented the face of a clock, there is a tendency to crowd the numbers on the right side and leave the left side empty. When asked to copy a simple line drawing, the patient fails to copy detail on the left; and when asked to write, there is a tendency to leave an unusually wide margin on the left.

Two bedside tests that are useful in assessing neglect are *simultaneous bilateral stimulation* and *visual target cancellation*. In the former, the examiner provides either unilateral or simultaneous bilateral stimulation in the visual, auditory, and tactile modalities. Following right hemisphere injury, patients who have no difficulty detecting unilateral stimuli on either side experience the bilaterally presented stimulus as coming only from the right. This phenomenon is known as *extinction* and is a manifestation of the sensory-representational aspect of hemispatial neglect. In the target detection task, targets (e.g., As) are interspersed with foils (e.g., other letters of the alphabet) on a 21.5 × 28.0 cm (8.5 × 11 in.) sheet of paper and the patient is asked to circle all the targets. A failure to detect targets on the left is a manifestation of the exploratory deficit in hemispatial neglect (Fig. 27-3A). Hemianopia, by itself, does not interfere with performance in this task since the patient is free to turn the head and eyes to the left. The normal tendency in target detection tasks is to start from the left upper quadrant and move systematically in horizontal or vertical sweeps. Some patients show a tendency to start the process from the right and proceed in a haphazard fashion. This represents a subtle manifestation of left neglect, even if the patient eventually manages to detect all the appropriate targets. Some patients with neglect may also deny the existence of hemiparesis and may even deny ownership of the paralyzed limb, a condition known as *anosognosia*.

Cerebrovascular lesions and neoplasms in the right hemisphere are the most common causes of hemispatial neglect. Depending on the

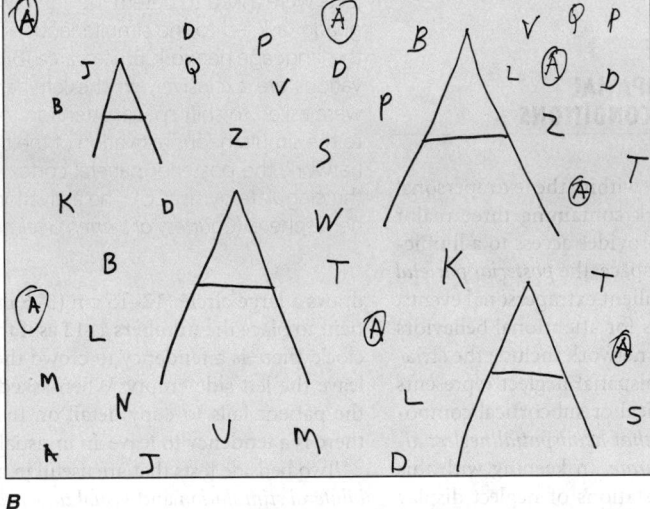

FIGURE 27-3 Evidence of left hemispatial neglect and simultanagnosia. **A.** A 47-year-old man with a large frontoparietal lesion in the right hemisphere was asked to circle all the As. Only targets on the right are circled. This is a manifestation of left hemispatial neglect. **B.** A 70-year-old woman with a 2-year history of degenerative dementia was able to circle most of the small targets but ignored the larger ones. This is a manifestation of simultanagnosia.

site of the lesion, the patient with neglect may also have hemiparesis, hemihypesthesia, and hemianopia on the left, but these are not invariant findings. The majority of patients display considerable improvement of hemispatial neglect, usually within the first several weeks.

BÁLINT'S SYNDROME, SIMULTANAGNOSIA, DRESSING APRAXIA, AND CONSTRUCTION APRAXIA

Bilateral involvement of the network for spatial attention, especially its parietal components, leads to a state of severe spatial disorientation known as *Bálint's syndrome*. Bálint's syndrome involves deficits in the orderly visuomotor scanning of the environment (*oculomotor apraxia*) and in accurate manual reaching toward visual targets (*optic ataxia*). The third and most dramatic component of Bálint's syndrome is known as *simultanagnosia* and reflects an inability to integrate visual information in the center of gaze with more peripheral information. The patient gets stuck on the detail that falls in the center of gaze without attempting to scan the visual environment for additional information. The patient with simultanagnosia "misses the forest for the trees." Complex visual scenes cannot be grasped in their entirety, leading to severe limitations in the visual identification of objects and scenes. For example, a patient who is

shown a table lamp and asked to name the object may look at its circular base and call it an ash tray. Some patients with simultanagnosia report that objects they look at may suddenly vanish, probably indicating an inability to look back at the original point of gaze after brief saccadic displacements. Movement and distracting stimuli greatly exacerbate the difficulties of visual perception. Simultanagnosia can sometimes occur without the other two components of Bálint's syndrome.

A modification of the letter cancellation task described above can be used for the bedside diagnosis of simultanagnosia. In this modification, some of the targets (e.g., As) are made to be much larger than the others [7.5–10 cm vs 2.5 cm (3–4 in. vs 1 in.) in height], and all targets are embedded among foils. Patients with simultanagnosia display a counterintuitive but characteristic tendency to miss the larger targets (Fig. 27-3*B*). This occurs because the information needed for the identification of the larger targets cannot be confined to the immediate line of gaze and requires the integration of visual information across a more extensive field of view. The greater difficulty in the detection of the larger targets also indicates that poor acuity is not responsible for the impairment of visual function and that the problem is central rather than peripheral. Bálint's syndrome results from bilateral dorsal parietal lesions; common settings include watershed infarction between the middle and posterior cerebral artery territories, hypoglycemia, sagittal sinus thrombosis, or atypical forms of Alzheimer's disease. In patients with Bálint's syndrome due to stroke, bilateral visual field defects (usually inferior quadrantanopias) are common.

Another manifestation of bilateral (or right-sided) dorsal parietal lobe lesions is *dressing apraxia*. The patient with this condition is unable to align the body axis with the axis of the garment and can be seen struggling as he or she holds a coat from its bottom or extends his or her arm into a fold of the garment rather than into its sleeve. Lesions that involve the posterior parietal cortex also lead to severe difficulties in copying simple line drawings. This is known as a *construction apraxia* and is much more severe if the lesion is in the right hemisphere. In some patients with right hemisphere lesions, the drawing difficulties are confined to the left side of the figure and represent a manifestation of hemispatial neglect; in others, there is a more universal deficit in reproducing contours and three-dimensional perspective. Dressing apraxia and construction apraxia represent special instances of a more general disturbance in spatial orientation.

THE OCCIPITOTEMPORAL NETWORK FOR FACE AND OBJECT RECOGNITION: PROSOPAGNOSIA AND OBJECT AGNOSIA

Perceptual information about faces and objects is initially encoded in primary (striate) visual cortex and adjacent (upstream) peristriate visual association areas. This information is subsequently relayed first to the downstream visual association areas of occipitotemporal cortex and then to other heteromodal and paralimbic areas of the cerebral cortex. Bilateral lesions in the fusiform and lingual gyri of the occipitotemporal cortex disrupt this process and interfere with the ability of otherwise intact perceptual information to activate the distributed multimodal associations that lead to the recognition of faces and objects. The resultant face and object recognition deficits are known as *prosopagnosia* and *visual object agnosia*.

The patient with prosopagnosia cannot recognize familiar faces, including, sometimes, the reflection of his or her own face in the mirror. This is not a perceptual deficit since prosopagnosic patients can easily tell if two faces are identical or not. Furthermore, a prosopagnosic patient who cannot recognize a familiar face by visual inspection alone can use auditory cues to reach appropriate recognition if allowed to listen to the person's voice. The deficit in prosopagnosia is therefore modality-specific and reflects the existence of a lesion that prevents the activation of otherwise intact multimodal templates by relevant visual input. Damasio has pointed out that the deficit in prosopagnosia is not limited to the recognition of faces but that it can also extend to the recognition of individual members of larger generic object groups. For example, prosopagnosic patients characteristically have no difficulty with the generic identification of a face as a face or of a car as a car, but they cannot recognize the identity of an individual face or the make of an individual car. This reflects a visual recognition deficit for proprietary features that characterize individual members of an object class. When recognition problems become more generalized and extend to the generic identification of common objects, the condition is known as visual object agnosia. In contrast to prosopagnosic patients, those with object agnosia cannot recognize a face as a face or a car as a car.

It is important to distinguish visual object agnosia from anomia. The patient with anomia cannot name the object but can describe its use. In contrast, the patient with visual agnosia is unable either to name a visually presented object or to describe its use. The characteristic lesions in prosopagnosia and visual object agnosia consist of bilateral infarctions in the territory of the posterior cerebral arteries. Associated deficits can include visual field defects (especially superior quadrantanopias) or a centrally based color blindness known as *achromatopsia*. Rarely, the responsible lesion is unilateral. In such cases, prosopagnosia is associated with lesions in the right hemisphere and object agnosia with lesions in the left.

THE LIMBIC NETWORK FOR MEMORY: AMNESIAS

Limbic and paralimbic areas (such as the hippocampus, amygdala, and entorhinal cortex), the anterior and medial nuclei of the thalamus, the medial and basal parts of the striatum, and the hypothalamus collectively constitute a distributed network known as the *limbic system*. The behavioral affiliations of this network include the coordination of emotion, motivation, autonomic tone, and endocrine function. An additional area of specialization for the limbic network, and the one which is of most relevance to clinical practice, is that of declarative (conscious) memory for recent episodes and experiences. A disturbance in this function is known as an *amnestic state*. In the absence of deficits in motivation, attention, language, or visuospatial function, the clinical diagnosis of a persistent global amnestic state is always associated with bilateral damage to the limbic network, usually within the hippocampo-entorhinal complex or the thalamus.

Although the limbic network is the site of damage for amnestic states, it is almost certainly not the storage site for memories. Memories are stored in widely distributed form throughout the cerebral cortex. The role attributed to the limbic network is to bind these distributed fragments into coherent events and experiences that can sustain conscious recall. Damage to the limbic network does not necessarily destroy memories but interferes with their conscious (declarative) recall in coherent form. The individual fragments of information remain preserved despite the limbic lesions and can sustain what is known as *implicit memory*. For example, patients with amnestic states can acquire new motor or perceptual skills, even though they may have no conscious knowledge of the experiences that led to the acquisition of these skills.

The memory disturbance in the amnestic state is multimodal and includes retrograde and anterograde components. The *retrograde amnesia* involves an inability to recall experiences that occurred before the onset of the amnestic state. Relatively recent events are more vulnerable to retrograde amnesia than more remote and more extensively consolidated events. A patient who comes to the emergency room complaining that he cannot remember his identity but who can remember the events of the previous day is almost certainly not suffering from a neurologic cause of memory disturbance. The second and most important component of the amnestic state is the *anterograde amnesia*, which indicates an inability to store, retain, and recall new knowledge. Patients with amnestic states cannot remember what they ate a few minutes ago or the details of an important event they may have experienced a few hours ago. In the acute stages, there may also be a tendency to fill in memory gaps with inaccurate, fabricated, and often implausible information. This is known as *confabulation*. Patients with the amnestic syndrome forget that they forget and tend to deny the existence of a memory problem when questioned.

The patient with an amnestic state is almost always disoriented, especially to time. Accurate temporal orientation and accurate knowledge of current news rule out a major amnestic state. The anterograde component of an amnestic state can be tested with a list of four to five words read aloud by the examiner up to five times or until the patient can immediately repeat the entire list without intervening delay. In the next phase of testing, the patient is allowed to concentrate on the words and to rehearse them internally for 1 min before being asked to recall them. Accurate performance in this phase indicates that the patient is motivated and sufficiently attentive to hold the words online for at least 1 min. The final phase of the testing involves a retention period of 5–10 min, during which the patient is engaged in other tasks. Adequate recall at the end of this interval requires offline storage, retention, and retrieval. Amnestic patients fail this phase of the task and may even forget that they were given a list of words to remember. Accurate recognition of the words by multiple choice in a patient who cannot recall them indicates a less severe memory disturbance that affects mostly the retrieval stage of memory. The retrograde component of an amnesia can be assessed with questions related to autobiographical or historic events. The anterograde component of amnestic states is usually much more prominent than the retrograde component. In rare instances, usually associated with temporal lobe epilepsy or benzodiazepine intake, the retrograde component may dominate.

The assessment of memory can be quite challenging. Bedside evaluations may only detect the most severe impairments. Less severe memory impairments, as in the case of patients with temporal lobe epilepsy, mild head injury, or early dementia, require quantitative evaluations by neuropsychologists. Confusional states caused by toxic-metabolic encephalopathies and some types of frontal lobe damage interfere with attentional capacity and lead to secondary memory impairments, even in the absence of any limbic lesions. This sort of memory impairment can be differentiated from the amnestic state by the presence of additional impairments in the attention-related tasks described below in the section on the frontal lobes.

Many neurologic diseases can give rise to an amnestic state. These include tumors (of the sphenoid wing, posterior corpus callosum, thalamus, or medial temporal lobe), infarctions (in the territories of the anterior or posterior cerebral arteries), head trauma, herpes simplex encephalitis, Wernicke-Korsakoff encephalopathy, paraneoplastic limbic encephalitis, and degenerative dementias such as Alzheimer's or Pick's disease. The one common denominator of all these diseases is that they lead to the bilateral lesions within one or more components in the limbic network, most commonly the hippocampus, entorhinal cortex, the mammillary bodies of the hypothalamus, and the limbic thalamus. Occasionally, unilateral left-sided lesions can give rise to an amnestic state, but the memory disorder tends to be transient. Depending on the nature and distribution of the underlying neurologic disease, the patient may also have visual field deficits, eye movement limitations, or cerebellar findings.

Transient global amnesia is a distinctive syndrome usually seen in late middle age. Patients become acutely disoriented and repeatedly ask who they are, where they are, what they are doing. The spell is characterized by anterograde amnesia (inability to retain new information) and a retrograde amnesia for relatively recent events that occurred before the onset. The syndrome usually resolves within 24–48 h and is followed by the filling-in of the period affected by the retrograde amnesia, although there is persistent loss of memory for the events that occurred during the ictus. Recurrences are noted in ~20% of patients. Migraine, temporal lobe seizures, and transient ischemic events in the posterior cerebral territory have been postulated as causes of transient global amnesia. The absence of associated neurologic findings may occasionally lead to the incorrect diagnosis of a psychiatric disorder.

THE PREFRONTAL NETWORK FOR ATTENTION AND BEHAVIOR

Approximately one-third of all the cerebral cortex in the human brain is located in the frontal lobes. The frontal lobes can be subdivided into motor-premotor, dorsolateral prefrontal, medial prefrontal, and orbitofrontal components. The terms *frontal lobe syndrome* and *prefrontal cortex* refer only to the last three of these four components. These are the parts of the cerebral cortex that show the greatest phylogenetic expansion in primates and especially in humans. The dorsolateral prefrontal, medial prefrontal, and orbitofrontal areas, and the subcortical structures with which they are interconnected (i.e., the head of the caudate and the dorsomedial nucleus of the thalamus), collectively make up a large-scale network that coordinates exceedingly complex aspects of human cognition and behavior.

The prefrontal network plays an important role in behaviors that require an integration of thought with emotion and motivation. There is no simple formula for summarizing the diverse functional affiliations of the prefrontal network. Its integrity appears important for the simultaneous awareness of context, options, consequences, relevance, and emotional impact so as to allow the formulation of adaptive inferences, decisions, and actions. Damage to this part of the brain impairs mental flexibility, reasoning, hypothesis formation, abstract thinking, foresight, judgment, the online (attentive) holding of information, and the ability to inhibit inappropriate responses. Behaviors impaired by prefrontal cortex lesions, especially those related to the manipulation of mental content, are often referred to as "executive functions."

Even very large bilateral prefrontal lesions may leave all sensory, motor, and basic cognitive functions intact while leading to isolated but dramatic alterations of personality and behavior. The most common clinical manifestations of damage to the prefrontal network take the form of two relatively distinct syndromes. In the *frontal abulic syndrome*, the patient shows a loss of initiative, creativity, and curiosity and displays a pervasive emotional blandness and apathy. In the *frontal disinhibition syndrome*, the patient becomes socially disinhibited and shows severe impairments of judgment, insight, and foresight. The dissociation between intact cognitive function and a total lack of even rudimentary common sense is striking. Despite the preservation of all essential memory functions, the patient cannot learn from experience and continues to display inappropriate behaviors without appearing to feel emotional pain, guilt, or regret when such behaviors repeatedly lead to disastrous consequences. The impairments may emerge only in real-life situations when behavior is under minimal external control and may not be apparent within the structured environment of the medical office. Testing judgment by asking patients what they would do if they detected a fire in a theater or found a stamped and addressed envelope on the road is not very informative since patients who answer these questions wisely in the office may still act very foolishly in the more complex real-life setting. The physician must therefore be prepared to make a diagnosis of frontal lobe disease on the basis of historic information alone even when the office examination of mental state may be quite intact.

The abulic syndrome tends to be associated with damage to the dorsolateral prefrontal cortex, and the disinhibition syndrome with the medial prefrontal or orbitofrontal cortex. These syndromes tend to arise almost exclusively after bilateral lesions, most frequently in the setting of head trauma, stroke, ruptured aneurysms, hydrocephalus, tumors (including metastases, glioblastoma, and falx or olfactory groove meningiomas), or focal degenerative diseases. Unilateral lesions confined to the prefrontal cortex may remain silent until the pathology spreads to the other side. The emergence of developmentally primitive reflexes, also known as frontal release signs, such as grasping (elicited by stroking the palm) and sucking (elicited by stroking the lips) are seen primarily in patients with large structural lesions that extend into the premotor components of the frontal lobes or in the context of metabolic encephalopathies. The vast majority of patients with prefrontal lesions and frontal lobe behavioral syndromes do not display these reflexes.

Damage to the frontal lobe disrupts a variety of attention-related functions including working memory (the transient online holding of information), concentration span, the scanning and retrieval of stored information, the inhibition of immediate but inappropriate responses, and mental flexibility. The capacity for focusing on a trend of thought and the ability to voluntarily shift the focus of attention from one thought or stimulus to another can become impaired. Digit span (which should be seven forward and five reverse) is decreased; the recitation of the months of the year in reverse order (which should take less than 15 s) is slowed; and the fluency in producing words starting with a, f, or s that can be generated in 1 min (normally ≥12 per letter) is diminished even in nonaphasic patients. Characteristically, there is a progressive slowing of performance as the task proceeds; e.g., the patient asked to count backwards by 3s may say "100, 97, 94, . . . 91, . . . 88," etc., and may not complete the task. In "go–no-go" tasks (where the instruction is to raise the finger upon hearing one tap but to keep it still upon hearing two taps), the patient shows a characteristic inability to keep still in response to the "no-go" stimulus; mental flexibility (tested by the ability to shift from one criterion to another in sorting or matching tasks) is impoverished; distractibility by irrelevant stimuli is increased; and there is a pronounced tendency for impersistence and perseveration.

These attentional deficits disrupt the orderly registration and retrieval of new information and lead to *secondary* memory deficits. Such memory deficits can be differentiated from the *primary* memory impairments of the amnestic state by showing that they improve when the attentional load of the task is decreased. Working memory (also known as immediate memory) is an attentional function based on the temporary online holding of information. It is closely associated with the integrity of the prefrontal network and the ascending reticular activating system. Retentive memory, on the other hand, depends on the stable (offline) storage of information and is associated with the integrity of the limbic network. The distinction of the underlying neural mechanisms is illustrated by the observation that severely amnestic patients who cannot remember events that occurred a few minutes ago may have intact if not superior working memory capacity as shown in tests of digit span.

Lesions in the caudate nucleus or in the dorsomedial nucleus of the thalamus (subcortical components of the prefrontal network) can also produce a frontal lobe syndrome. This is one reason why the mental state changes associated with degenerative basal ganglia diseases, such as Parkinson's or Huntington's disease, may take the form of a frontal lobe syndrome. Because of its widespread connections with other regions of association cortex, one essential computational role of the prefrontal network is to function as an integrator, or "orchestrator," for other networks. Bilateral multifocal lesions of the cerebral hemispheres, none of which are individually large enough to cause specific cognitive deficits such as aphasia or neglect, can collectively interfere with the connectivity and integrating function of the prefrontal cortex. A frontal lobe syndrome is the single most common behavioral profile associated with a variety of bilateral multifocal brain diseases including metabolic encephalopathy, multiple sclerosis, vitamin B_{12} deficiency, and others. In fact, the vast majority of patients with the clinical diagnosis of a frontal lobe syndrome tend to have lesions that do not involve prefrontal cortex but involve either the subcortical components of the prefrontal network or its connections with other parts of the brain. In order to avoid making a diagnosis of "frontal lobe syndrome" in a patient with no evidence of frontal cortex disease, it is advisable to use the diagnostic term *frontal network syndrome*, with the understanding that the responsible lesions can lie anywhere within this distributed network.

The patient with frontal lobe disease raises potential dilemmas in differential diagnosis: the abulia and blandness may be misinterpreted as depression, and the disinhibition as idiopathic mania or acting-out. Appropriate intervention may be delayed while a treatable tumor keeps expanding. An informed approach to frontal lobe disease and its behavioral manifestations may help to avoid such errors.

CARING FOR THE PATIENT WITH DEFICITS OF HIGHER CEREBRAL FUNCTION

Some of the deficits described in this chapter are so complex that they may bewilder not only the patient and family but also the physician. It is imperative to carry out a systematic clinical evaluation in order to characterize the nature of the deficits and explain them in lay terms to the patient and family. Such an explanation can allay at least some of the anxieties, address the mistaken impression that the deficit (e.g., social disinhibition or inability to recognize family members) is psychologically motivated, and lead to practical suggestions for daily living activities. The consultation of a skilled neuropsychologist may aid in the formulation of diagnosis and management. Patients with simultanagnosia, for example, may benefit from the counterintuitive instruction to stand back when they cannot find an item so that a greater search area falls within the immediate field of gaze. Some patients with frontal lobe disease can be extremely irritable and abusive to spouses and yet display all the appropriate social graces during the visit to the medical office. In such cases, the history may be more important than the bedside examination in charting a course of treatment.

Reactive depression is common in patients with higher cerebral dysfunction and should be treated. These patients may be sensitive to the usual doses of antidepressants or anxiolytics and deserve a careful titration of dosage. Brain damage may cause a dissociation between feeling states and their expression, so that a patient who may superficially appear jocular could still be suffering from an underlying depression that deserves to be treated. In many cases, agitation may be controlled with reassurance. In other cases, treatment with sedating antidepressants may become necessary. The use of neuroleptics for the control of agitation should be reserved for refractory cases since extrapyramidal side effects are frequent in patients with coexisting brain damage.

Spontaneous improvement of cognitive deficits due to acute neurologic lesions is common. It is most rapid in the first few weeks but may continue for up to 2 years, especially in young individuals with single brain lesions. The mechanisms for this recovery are incompletely understood. Some of the initial deficits appear to arise from remote dysfunction (diaschisis) in parts of the brain that are interconnected with the site of initial injury. Improvement in these patients may reflect, at least in part, a normalization of the remote dysfunction. Other mechanisms may involve functional reorganization in surviving neurons adjacent to the injury or the compensatory use of homologous structures, e.g., the right superior temporal gyrus with recovery from Wernicke's aphasia. In some patients with large lesions involving Broca's and Wernicke's areas, only Wernicke's area may show contralateral compensatory reorganization (or bilateral functionality), giving rise to a situation where a lesion that should have caused a global aphasia becomes associated with a residual Broca's aphasia. Prognosis for recovery from aphasia is best when Wernicke's area is spared. Cognitive rehabilitation procedures have been used in the treatment of higher cortical deficits. There are few controlled studies, but some do show a benefit of rehabilitation in the recovery from hemispatial neglect and aphasia. Some types of deficits may be more prone to recovery than others. For example, patients with nonfluent aphasias are more likely to benefit from speech therapy than patients with fluent aphasias and comprehension deficits. In general, lesions that lead to a denial of illness (e.g., anosognosia) are associated with cognitive deficits that are more resistant to rehabilitation. The recovery from higher cortical dysfunction is rarely complete. Periodic neuropsychological assessment is necessary for quantifying the pace of the improvement and for generating specific recommendations for cognitive rehabilitation, modifications in the home environment, and the timetable for returning to school or work.

In general medical practice, most patients with deficits in higher cognitive functions will be suffering from dementia. There is a mistaken belief that dementias are anatomically diffuse and that they cause global cognitive impairments. This is only true at the terminal stages. During most of the clinical course, dementias are exquisitely selective with respect to anatomy and cognitive pattern. Alzheimer's disease, for example, causes the greatest destruction in medial temporal areas belonging to the memory network and is clinically characterized by a correspondingly severe amnesia. There are other dementias where memory is intact. Frontal lobe dementia results from a selective degeneration of the frontal lobe and leads to a gradual dissolution of behavior and complex attention. Primary progressive aphasia is characterized by a gradual atrophy of the left perisylvian language network and leads to a progressive dissolution of language that can remain isolated for up to 10 years. An enlightened approach to the differential diagnosis and treatment of these patients requires an understanding of the principles that link neural networks to higher cerebral functions.

FURTHER READINGS

CATANI M, FFYCHTE H: The rises and falls of disconnection syndromes. Brain 128:2224, 2005

CRUTS M et al: Null mutations in progranulin cause ubiquitin-positive frontotemporal dementia linked to chromosome 17q21. Nature 442:916, 2006

GITELMAN DR et al: A large-scale distributed network for covert spatial attention. Further anatomical delineation based on stringent behavioral and cognitive controls. Brain 122:1093, 1999

HEISS W-D et al: Differential capacity of left and right hemispheric areas for compensation of poststroke aphasia. Ann Neurol 45:430, 1999

HILLIS AE: Aphasia: Progress in the last quarter of a century. Neurology 69:200, 2007

KNIBB JA et al: Clinical and pathological characterization of progressive aphasia. Ann Neurol 59:156, 2006

LEIGUARDA RC, MARSDEN CD: Limb apraxias: Higher-order disorders of sensorimotor integration. Brain 123:860, 2000

LI X et al: Prion protein codon 129 genotype is altered in primary progressive aphasia. Ann Neurol 58:858, 2005

MESULAM M-M: Behavioral neuroanatomy: Large-scale networks, association cortex, frontal syndromes, the limbic system and hemispheric specializations, in *Principles of Behavioral and Cognitive Neurology*, 2d ed, M-M Mesulam (ed). New York, Oxford University Press, 2000, pp 1–120

———: Current concepts: Primary progressive aphasia—a language-based dementia. New Engl J Med 348:1535, 2003

———: The human frontal lobes: Transcending the default mode through contingent encoding, in *Principles of Frontal Lobe Function*, DT Stuss, RT Knight (eds). New York, Oxford University Press, 2002, pp 8–30

SUMMERFIELD JJ et al: Orienting attention based on long-term memory experience. Neuron 49:905, 2006

28 Sleep Disorders
Charles A. Czeisler, John W. Winkelman, Gary S. Richardson

Disturbed sleep is among the most frequent health complaints physicians encounter. More than one-half of adults in the United States experience at least intermittent sleep disturbances. For most, it is an occasional night of poor sleep or daytime sleepiness. However, the Institute of Medicine estimates that 50–70 million Americans suffer from a chronic disorder of sleep and wakefulness, which can lead to serious impairment of daytime functioning. In addition, such problems may contribute to or exacerbate medical or psychiatric conditions. Thirty years ago, many such complaints were treated with hypnotic medications without further diagnostic evaluation. Since then, a distinct class of sleep and arousal disorders has been identified.

PHYSIOLOGY OF SLEEP AND WAKEFULNESS

Most adults sleep 7–8 h per night, although the timing, duration, and internal structure of sleep vary among healthy individuals and as a

FIGURE 28-1 Stages of REM sleep (solid bars), the four stages of NREM sleep, and wakefulness over the course of the entire night for representative young and older adult men. Characteristic features of sleep in older people include reduction of slow-wave sleep, frequent spontaneous awakenings, early sleep onset, and early morning awakening. *(From the Division of Sleep Medicine, Brigham and Women's Hospital.)*

function of age. At the extremes, infants and the elderly have frequent interruptions of sleep. In the United States, adults of intermediate age tend to have one consolidated sleep episode per day, although in some cultures sleep may be divided into a mid-afternoon nap and a shortened night sleep. Two principal systems govern the sleep-wake cycle: one actively generates sleep and sleep-related processes and another times sleep within the 24-h day. Either intrinsic abnormalities in these systems or extrinsic disturbances (environmental, drug- or illness-related) can lead to sleep or circadian rhythm disorders.

STATES AND STAGES OF SLEEP

States and stages of human sleep are defined on the basis of characteristic patterns in the electroencephalogram (EEG), the electrooculogram (EOG—a measure of eye-movement activity), and the surface electromyogram (EMG) measured on the chin and neck. The continuous recording of this array of electrophysiologic parameters to define sleep and wakefulness is termed *polysomnography*.

Polysomnographic profiles define two states of sleep: (1) rapid-eye-movement (REM) sleep, and (2) non-rapid-eye-movement (NREM) sleep. NREM sleep is further subdivided into four stages, characterized by increasing arousal threshold and slowing of the cortical EEG. REM sleep is characterized by a low-amplitude, mixed-frequency EEG similar to that of NREM stage 1 sleep. The EOG shows bursts of REM similar to those seen during eyes-open wakefulness. Chin EMG activity is absent, reflecting the brainstem-mediated muscle atonia that is characteristic of that state.

ORGANIZATION OF HUMAN SLEEP

Normal nocturnal sleep in adults displays a consistent organization from night to night (Fig. 28-1). After sleep onset, sleep usually progresses through NREM stages 1–4 within 45–60 min. Slow-wave sleep (NREM stages 3 and 4) predominates in the first third of the night and comprises 15–25% of total nocturnal sleep time in young adults. The percentage of slow-wave sleep is influenced by several factors, most notably age (see below). Prior sleep deprivation increases the rapidity of sleep onset and both the intensity and amount of slow-wave sleep.

The first REM sleep episode usually occurs in the second hour of sleep. More rapid onset of REM sleep in a young adult (particularly if <30 min) may suggest pathology such as endogenous depression, narcolepsy, circadian rhythm disorders, or drug withdrawal. NREM and REM alternate through the night with an average period of 90–110 min (the "ultradian" sleep cycle). Overall, REM sleep constitutes 20–25% of total sleep, and NREM stages 1 and 2 are 50–60%.

Age has a profound impact on sleep state organization (Fig. 28-1). Slow-wave sleep is most intense and prominent during childhood, decreasing sharply at puberty and across the second and third decades of

life. After age 30, there is a progressive decline in the amount of slow-wave sleep, and the amplitude of delta EEG activity comprising slow-wave sleep is profoundly reduced. The depth of slow-wave sleep, as measured by the arousal threshold to auditory stimulation, also decreases with age. In the otherwise healthy older person, slow-wave sleep may be completely absent, particularly in males.

A different age profile exists for REM sleep than for slow-wave sleep. In infancy, REM sleep may comprise 50% of total sleep time, and the percentage is inversely proportional to developmental age. The amount of REM sleep falls off sharply over the first postnatal year as a mature REM-NREM cycle develops; thereafter, REM sleep occupies a relatively constant percentage of total sleep time.

NEUROANATOMY OF SLEEP

Experimental studies in animals have variously implicated the medullary reticular formation, the thalamus, and the basal forebrain in the generation of sleep, while the brainstem reticular formation, the midbrain, the subthalamus, the thalamus, and the basal forebrain have all been suggested to play a role in the generation of wakefulness or EEG arousal.

Current models suggest that the capacity for sleep and wakefulness generation is distributed along an axial "core" of neurons extending from the brainstem rostrally to the basal forebrain. A cluster of γ-aminobutyric acid (GABA) and galaninergic neurons in the ventrolateral preoptic (VLPO) hypothalamus is selectively activated coincident with sleep onset. These neurons project to and inhibit multiple distinct wakefulness centers including the tuberomammillary (histaminergic) nucleus that are important to the ascending arousal system, indicating that the hypothalamic VLPO neurons play a key executive role in sleep regulation.

Specific regions in the pons are associated with the neurophysiologic correlates of REM sleep. Small lesions in the dorsal pons result in the loss of the descending muscle inhibition normally associated with REM sleep; microinjections of the cholinergic agonist carbachol into the pontine reticular formation appear to produce a state with all of the features of REM sleep. These experimental manipulations are mimicked by pathologic conditions in humans and animals. In narcolepsy, for example, abrupt, complete, or partial paralysis (cataplexy) occurs in response to a variety of stimuli. In dogs with this condition, physostigmine, a central cholinesterase inhibitor, increases the frequency of cataplectic attacks, while atropine decreases their frequency. Conversely, in REM sleep behavior disorder (see below), patients suffer from incomplete motor inhibition during REM sleep, resulting in involuntary, occasionally violent movement during REM sleep.

NEUROCHEMISTRY OF SLEEP

Early experimental studies that focused on the raphe nuclei of the brainstem appeared to implicate serotonin as the primary sleep-promoting neurotransmitter, while catecholamines were considered to be responsible for wakefulness. Simple neurochemical models have given way to more complex formulations involving multiple parallel waking systems. Pharmacologic studies suggest that histamine, acetylcholine, dopamine, serotonin, and noradrenaline are all involved in wake promotion. In addition, pontine cholinergic neurotransmission is known to play a role in REM sleep generation. The alerting influence of caffeine implicates adenosine, whereas the hypnotic effect of benzodiazepines and barbiturates suggests a role for endogenous ligands of the GABA$_A$ receptor complex. A newly characterized neuropeptide, hypocretin (orexin), has recently been implicated in the pathophysiology of narcolepsy (see below), but its role in normal sleep regulation remains to be defined.

A variety of sleep-promoting substances have been identified, although it is not known whether they are involved in the endogenous sleep-wake regulatory process. These include prostaglandin D$_2$, delta

E-Box   Per1 gene

FIGURE 28-2 Model of the molecular feedback loop at the core of the mammalian circadian clock. The positive element of the feedback loop (+) is the transcriptional activation of the *Per1* gene (and probably other clock genes) by a heterodimer of the transcription factors CLOCK and BMAL1 (also called MOP3) bound to an E-box DNA regulatory element. The *Per1* transcript and its product, the clock component PER1 protein, accumulate in the cell cytoplasm. As it accumulates, the PER1 protein is recruited into a multiprotein complex thought to contain other circadian clock component proteins such as cryptochromes (CRYs), Period proteins (PERs), and others. This complex is then transported into the cell nucleus (across the dotted line), where it functions as the negative element in the feedback loop (–) by inhibiting the activity of the CLOCK-BMAL1 transcription factor heterodimer. As a consequence of this action, the concentration of PER1 and other clock proteins in the inhibitory complex falls, allowing CLOCK-BMAL1 to activate transcription of *Per1* and other genes and begin another cycle. The dynamics of the 24-h molecular cycle are controlled at several levels, including regulation of the rate of PER protein degradation by casein kinase-1 epsilon (CK1E). Additional limbs of this genetic regulatory network, omitted for the sake of clarity, are thought to contribute stability. Question marks denote putative clock proteins, such as Timeless (TIM), as yet lacking genetic proof of a role in the mammalian clock mechanism. (*Copyright Charles J. Weitz, Ph.D., Department of Neurobiology, Harvard Medical School.*)

sleep–inducing peptide, muramyl dipeptide, interleukin 1, fatty acid primary amides, and melatonin. The hypnotic effect of these substances is commonly limited to NREM or slow-wave sleep, although peptides that increase REM sleep have also been reported. Many putative "sleep factors," including interleukin 1 and prostaglandin D_2, are immunologically active as well, suggesting a link between immune function and sleep-wake states.

PHYSIOLOGY OF CIRCADIAN RHYTHMICITY

The sleep-wake cycle is the most evident of the many 24-h rhythms in humans. Prominent daily variations also occur in endocrine, thermoregulatory, cardiac, pulmonary, renal, gastrointestinal, and neurobehavioral functions. At the molecular level, endogenous circadian rhythmicity is driven by self-sustaining transcriptional/translational feedback loops (**Fig. 28-2**). In evaluating a daily variation in humans, it is important to distinguish between those rhythmic components passively evoked by periodic environmental or behavioral changes (e.g., the increase in blood pressure and heart rate upon assumption of the upright posture) and those actively driven by an endogenous oscillatory process (e.g., the circadian variation in plasma cortisol that persists under a variety of environmental and behavioral conditions).

While it is now recognized that many peripheral tissues in mammals have circadian clocks that regulate diverse physiologic processes, these independent tissue-specific oscillations are coordinated by a central neural pacemaker located in the suprachiasmatic nuclei (SCN) of the hypothalamus. Bilateral destruction of these nuclei results in a loss of the endogenous circadian rhythm of locomotor activity, which can be restored only by transplantation of the same structure from a donor animal. The genetically determined period of this endogenous neural oscillator, which averages ~24.2 h in humans, is normally synchro-

nized to the 24-h period of the environmental light-dark cycle. Small differences in circadian period underlie variations in diurnal preference, with the circadian period shorter in individuals who typically rise early compared to those who typically go to bed late. Entrainment of mammalian circadian rhythms by the light-dark cycle is mediated via the retinohypothalamic tract, a monosynaptic pathway that links specialized, photoreceptive retinal ganglion cells directly to the SCN. Humans are exquisitely sensitive to the resetting effects of light, particularly at the blue end (~460–480 nm) of the visible spectrum.

The timing and internal architecture of sleep are directly coupled to the output of the endogenous circadian pacemaker. Paradoxically, the endogenous circadian rhythms of sleep tendency, sleepiness, and REM sleep propensity all peak near the habitual wake time, just after the nadir of the endogenous circadian temperature cycle, whereas the circadian wake propensity rhythm peaks 1–3 h before the habitual bedtime. These rhythms are thus timed to oppose the homeostatic decline of sleep tendency during the habitual sleep episode and the rise of sleep tendency throughout the usual waking day, respectively. Misalignment of the output of the endogenous circadian pacemaker with the desired sleep-wake cycle can, therefore, induce insomnia, decreased alertness, and impaired performance evident in night-shift workers and airline travelers.

BEHAVIORAL CORRELATES OF SLEEP STATES AND STAGES

Polysomnographic staging of sleep correlates with behavioral changes during specific states and stages. During the transitional state between wakefulness and sleep (stage 1 sleep), subjects may respond to faint auditory or visual signals without "awakening." Memory incorporation is inhibited at the onset of NREM stage 1 sleep, which may explain why individuals aroused from that transitional sleep stage frequently deny having been asleep. Such transitions may intrude upon behavioral wakefulness after sleep deprivation, notwithstanding attempts to remain continuously awake (see "Shift-Work Disorder," below).

Awakenings from REM sleep are associated with recall of vivid dream imagery >80% of the time. The reliability of dream recall increases with REM sleep episodes occurring later in the night. Imagery may also be reported after NREM sleep interruptions, though these typically lack the detail and vividness of REM sleep dreams. The incidence of NREM sleep dream recall can be increased by selective REM sleep deprivation, suggesting that REM sleep and dreaming per se are not inexorably linked.

PHYSIOLOGIC CORRELATES OF SLEEP STATES AND STAGES

All major physiologic systems are influenced by sleep. Changes in cardiovascular function include a decrease in blood pressure and heart rate during NREM and particularly during slow-wave sleep. During REM sleep, phasic activity (bursts of eye movements) is associated with variability in both blood pressure and heart rate mediated principally by the vagus. Cardiac dysrhythmias may occur selectively during REM sleep. Respiratory function also changes. In comparison to relaxed wakefulness, respiratory rate becomes more regular during NREM sleep (especially slow-wave sleep) and tonic REM sleep and becomes very irregular during phasic REM sleep. Minute ventilation decreases in NREM sleep out of proportion to the decrease in metabolic rate at sleep onset, resulting in a higher P_{CO_2}.

Endocrine function also varies with sleep. Slow-wave sleep is associated with secretion of growth hormone, while sleep in general is associated with augmented secretion of prolactin. Sleep has a complex effect on the secretion of luteinizing hormone (LH): during puberty, sleep is associated with increased LH secretion, whereas sleep in the postpubertal female inhibits LH secretion in the early follicular phase of the menstrual cycle. Sleep onset (and probably slow-wave sleep) is associated with inhibition of thyroid-stimulating hormone and of the adrenocorticotropic hormone–cortisol axis, an effect that is superimposed on the prominent circadian rhythms in the two systems.

The pineal hormone melatonin is secreted predominantly at night in both day- and night-active species, reflecting the direct modulation of pineal activity by the circadian pacemaker through a circuitous neural pathway from the SCN to the pineal gland. Melatonin secretion is not dependent upon the occurrence of sleep, persisting in individuals kept awake at night. In addition, exogenous melatonin increases sleepiness and increases sleep duration when administered to healthy adults attempting to sleep during daylight hours, at a time when endogenous melatonin levels are low. The efficacy of melatonin as a sleep-promoting therapy for patients with insomnia is currently not known.

Sleep is also accompanied by alterations of thermoregulatory function. NREM sleep is associated with an attenuation of thermoregulatory responses to either heat or cold stress, and animal studies of thermosensitive neurons in the hypothalamus document an NREM-sleep-dependent reduction of the thermoregulatory set-point. REM sleep is associated with complete absence of thermoregulatory responsiveness, effectively resulting in functional poikilothermy. However, the potential adverse impact of this failure of thermoregulation is blunted by inhibition of REM sleep by extreme ambient temperatures.

TABLE 28-1 EVALUATION OF THE PATIENT WITH THE COMPLAINT OF EXCESSIVE DAYTIME SOMNOLENCE

Findings on History and Physical Examination	Diagnostic Evaluation	Diagnosis	Therapy
Obesity, snoring, hypertension	Polysomnography with respiratory monitoring	Obstructive sleep apnea	Continuous positive airway pressure; ENT surgery (e.g., uvulopalatopharyngoplasty); dental appliance; pharmacologic therapy (e.g., protriptyline); weight loss
Cataplexy, hypnogogic hallucinations, sleep paralysis, family history	Polysomnography with multiple sleep latency testing	Narcolepsy-cataplexy syndrome	Stimulants (e.g., modafinil, methylphenidate); REM-suppressant antidepressants (e.g., protriptyline); genetic counseling
Restless legs, disturbed sleep, predisposing medical condition (e.g., iron deficiency or renal failure)	Assessment for predisposing medical conditions	Restless legs syndrome	Treatment of predisposing condition, if possible; dopamine agonists (e.g., pramipexole, ropinirole)
Disturbed sleep, predisposing medical conditions (e.g., asthma) and/or predisposing medical therapies (e.g., theophylline)	Sleep-wake diary recording	Insomnias (see text)	Treatment of predisposing condition and/or change in therapy, if possible; behavioral therapy; short-acting benzodiazepine receptor agonist (e.g., zolpidem)

Note: ENT, ears, nose, throat; REM, rapid eye movement; EMG, electromyogram.

DISORDERS OF SLEEP AND WAKEFULNESS

APPROACH TO THE PATIENT:
Sleep Disorders

Patients may seek help from a physician because of one of several symptoms: (1) an acute or chronic inability to initiate or maintain sleep adequately at night (insomnia); (2) chronic fatigue, sleepiness, or tiredness during the day; or (3) a behavioral manifestation associated with sleep itself. Complaints of insomnia or excessive daytime sleepiness should be approached as symptoms (much like fever or pain) of underlying disorders. Knowledge of the differential diagnosis of these presenting complaints is essential to identify any underlying medical disorder. Only then can appropriate treatment, rather than nonspecific approaches (e.g., over-the-counter sleeping aids), be applied. Diagnoses of exclusion, such as primary insomnia, should be made only after other diagnoses have been ruled out. Table 28-1 outlines the diagnostic and therapeutic approach to the patient with a complaint of excessive daytime sleepiness.

A careful history is essential. In particular, the duration, severity, and consistency of the symptoms are important, along with the patient's estimate of the consequences of the sleep disorder on waking function. Information from a friend or family member can be invaluable; some patients may be unaware of, or will underreport, such potentially embarrassing symptoms as heavy snoring or falling asleep while driving. Patients with excessive sleepiness should be advised to avoid all driving until effective therapy has been achieved.

Completion by the patient of a day-by-day sleep-work-drug log for at least 2 weeks can help the physician better understand the nature of the complaint. Work times and sleep times (including daytime naps and nocturnal awakenings) as well as drug and alcohol use, including caffeine and hypnotics, should be noted each day.

Polysomnography is necessary for the diagnosis of specific disorders such as narcolepsy and sleep apnea and may be of utility in other settings as well. In addition to the three electrophysiologic variables used to define sleep states and stages, the standard clinical polysomnogram includes measures of respiration (respiratory effort, air flow, and oxygen saturation), anterior tibialis EMG, and electrocardiogram.

EVALUATION OF INSOMNIA

Insomnia is the complaint of inadequate sleep; it can be classified according to the nature of sleep disruption and the duration of the complaint.

Insomnia is subdivided into difficulty falling asleep (*sleep onset insomnia*), frequent or sustained awakenings (*sleep maintenance insomnia*), early morning awakenings (*sleep offset insomnia*), or persistent sleepiness/fatigue despite sleep of adequate duration (*nonrestorative sleep*). Similarly, the duration of the symptom influences diagnostic and therapeutic considerations. An insomnia complaint lasting one to several nights (within a single episode) is termed *transient insomnia* and is typically the result of situational stress or a change in sleep schedule or environment (e.g., jet lag disorder). *Short-term insomnia* lasts from a few days to 3 weeks. Disruption of this duration is usually associated with more protracted stress, such as recovery from surgery or short-term illness. *Long-term insomnia*, or *chronic insomnia*, lasts for months or years and, in contrast with short-term insomnia, requires a thorough evaluation of underlying causes (see below). Chronic insomnia is often a waxing and waning disorder, with spontaneous or stressor-induced exacerbations.

An occasional night of poor sleep, typically in the setting of stress or excitement about external events, is both common and without lasting consequences. However, persistent insomnia can lead to impaired daytime function, injury due to accidents, and the development of major depression. In addition, there is emerging evidence that individuals with chronic insomnia have increased utilization of health care resources, even after controlling for co-morbid medical and psychiatric disorders.

All insomnias can be exacerbated and perpetuated by behaviors that are not conducive to initiating or maintaining sleep. *Inadequate sleep hygiene* is characterized by a behavior pattern prior to sleep or a bedroom environment that is not conducive to sleep. Noise or light in the bedroom can interfere with sleep, as can a bed partner with periodic limb movements during sleep or one who snores loudly. Clocks can heighten the anxiety about the time it has taken to fall asleep. Drugs that act on the central nervous system, large meals, vigorous exercise, or hot showers just before sleep may all interfere with sleep onset. Many individuals participate in stressful work-related activities in the evening, producing a state incompatible with sleep onset. In preference to hypnotic medications, patients should be counseled to avoid stressful activities before bed, develop a soporific bedtime ritual, and to prepare and reserve the bedroom environment for sleeping. Consistent, regular rising times should be maintained daily, including weekends.

PRIMARY INSOMNIA

Many patients with chronic insomnia have no clear, single identifiable underlying cause for their difficulties with sleep. Rather, such patients often have multiple etiologies for their insomnia, which may evolve over the years. In addition, the chief sleep complaint may change over time, with initial insomnia predominating at one point, and multiple awakenings or nonrestorative sleep occurring at other times. Subsyndromal psychiatric disorders (e.g., anxiety and mood complaints), negative conditioning to the sleep environment (psychophysiologic insomnia, see below), amplification of the time spent awake (paradoxical insomnia), physiologic hyperarousal, and poor sleep hygiene (see above) may all be present. As these processes may be both causes and consequences of chronic insomnia, many individuals will have a progressive course to their symptoms in which the severity is proportional to the chronicity, and much of the complaint may persist even after effective treatment of the initial inciting etiology. Treatment of insomnia is often directed to each of the putative contributing factors: behavior therapies for anxiety and negative conditioning (see below), pharmacotherapy and/or psychotherapy for mood/anxiety disorders, and an emphasis on maintenance of good sleep hygiene.

If insomnia persists after treatment of these contributing factors, empirical pharmacotherapy is often used on a nightly or intermittent basis. A variety of sedative compounds are used for this purpose. Alcohol and antihistamines are the most commonly used nonprescription sleep aids. The former may help with sleep onset but is associated with sleep disruption during the night and can escalate into abuse, dependence, and withdrawal in the predisposed individual. Antihistamines may be of benefit when used intermittently but often produce rapid tolerance and may have multiple side effects (especially anticholinergic), which limit their use, particularly in the elderly. Benzodiazepine-receptor agonists are the most effective and well-tolerated class of medications for insomnia. The broad range of half-lives allows flexibility in the duration of sedative action. The most commonly prescribed agents in this family are zaleplon (5–20 mg), with a half-life of 1–2 h; zolpidem (5–10 mg) and triazolam (0.125–0.25 mg), with half-lives of 2–3 h; eszopiclone (1–3 mg), with a half-life of 5.5–8 h; and temazepam (15–30 mg) and lorazepam (0.5–2 mg), with half-lives of 6–12 h. Generally, side effects are minimal when the dose is kept low and the serum concentration is minimized during the waking hours (by using the shortest-acting, effective agent). Recent data suggest that at least one benzodiazepine receptor agonist (eszopiclone) continues to be effective for 6 months of nightly use. However, longer durations of use have not been evaluated, and it is unclear whether this is true of other agents in this class. Moreover, with even brief continuous use of benzodiazepine-receptor agonists, rebound insomnia can occur upon discontinuation. The likelihood of rebound insomnia and tolerance can be minimized by short durations of treatment, intermittent use, or gradual tapering of the dose. For acute insomnia, nightly use of a benzodiazepine receptor agonist for a maximum of 2–4 weeks is advisable. For chronic insomnia, intermittent use is recommended, unless the consequences of untreated insomnia outweigh concerns regarding chronic use. Benzodiazepine receptor agonists should be avoided, or used very judiciously, in patients with a history of substance or alcohol abuse. The heterocyclic antidepressants (trazodone, amitriptyline, and doxepin) are the most commonly prescribed alternatives to benzodiazepine receptor agonists due to their lack of abuse potential and lower cost. Trazodone (25–100 mg) is used more commonly than the tricyclic antidepressants as it has a much shorter half-life (5–9 h), has much less anticholinergic activity (sparing patients, particularly the elderly, constipation, urinary retention, and tachycardia), is associated with less weight gain, and is much safer in overdose. The risk of priapism is small (~1 in 10,000).

Psychophysiologic Insomnia Persistent *psychophysiologic insomnia* is a behavioral disorder in which patients are preoccupied with a perceived inability to sleep adequately at night. This sleep disorder begins like any other acute insomnia; however, the poor sleep habits and sleep-related anxiety ("insomnia phobia") persist long after the initial incident. Such patients become hyperaroused by their own efforts to sleep or by the sleep environment, and the insomnia becomes a conditioned or learned response. Patients may be able to fall asleep more easily at unscheduled times (when not trying) or outside the home environment. Polysomnographic recording in patients with psychophysiologic insomnia reveals an objective sleep disturbance, often with an abnormally long sleep latency; frequent nocturnal awakenings; and an increased amount of stage 1 transitional sleep. Rigorous attention should be paid to improving sleep hygiene, correction of counterproductive, arousing behaviors before bedtime, and minimizing

exaggerated beliefs regarding the negative consequences of insomnia. Behavioral therapies are the treatment modality of choice, with intermittent use of medications. When patients are awake for >20 min, they should read or perform other relaxing activities to distract themselves from insomnia-related anxiety. In addition, bedtime and wake time should be scheduled to restrict time in bed to be equal to their perceived total sleep time. This will generally produce sleep deprivation, greater sleep drive, and, eventually, better sleep. Time in bed can then be gradually expanded. In addition, methods directed towards producing relaxation in the sleep setting (e.g., meditation, muscle relaxation) are encouraged.

Adjustment Insomnia (Acute Insomnia) This typically develops after a change in the sleeping environment (e.g., in an unfamiliar hotel or hospital bed) or before or after a significant life event, such as a change of occupation, loss of a loved one, illness, or anxiety over a deadline or examination. Increased sleep latency, frequent awakenings from sleep, and early morning awakening can all occur. Recovery is generally rapid, usually within a few weeks. Treatment is symptomatic, with intermittent use of hypnotics and resolution of the underlying stress. *Altitude insomnia* describes a sleep disturbance that is a common consequence of exposure to high altitude. Periodic breathing of the Cheyne-Stokes type occurs during NREM sleep about half the time at high altitude, with restoration of a regular breathing pattern during REM sleep. Both hypoxia and hypocapnia are thought to be involved in the development of periodic breathing. Frequent awakenings and poor quality sleep characterize altitude insomnia, which is generally worse on the first few nights at high altitude but may persist. Treatment with acetazolamide can decrease time spent in periodic breathing and substantially reduce hypoxia during sleep.

COMORBID INSOMNIA

Insomnia Associated with Mental Disorders Approximately 80% of patients with psychiatric disorders describe sleep complaints. There is considerable heterogeneity, however, in the nature of the sleep disturbance both between conditions and among patients with the same condition. *Depression* can be associated with sleep onset insomnia, sleep maintenance insomnia, or early morning wakefulness. However, hypersomnia occurs in some depressed patients, especially adolescents and those with either bipolar or seasonal (fall/winter) depression (Chap. 386). Indeed, sleep disturbance is an important vegetative sign of depression and may commence before any mood changes are perceived by the patient. Consistent polysomnographic findings in depression include decreased REM sleep latency, lengthened first REM sleep episode, and shortened first NREM sleep episode; however, these findings are not specific for depression, and the extent of these changes varies with age and symptomatology. Depressed patients also show decreased slow-wave sleep and reduced sleep continuity.

In *mania* and *hypomania*, sleep latency is increased and total sleep time can be reduced. Patients with *anxiety disorders* tend not to show the changes in REM sleep and slow-wave sleep seen in endogenously depressed patients. *Chronic alcoholics* lack slow-wave sleep, have decreased amounts of REM sleep (as an acute response to alcohol), and have frequent arousals throughout the night. This is associated with impaired daytime alertness. The sleep of chronic alcoholics may remain disturbed for years after discontinuance of alcohol usage. Sleep architecture and physiology are disturbed in *schizophrenia* (with a decreased amount of stage 4 sleep and a lack of augmentation of REM sleep following REM sleep deprivation); chronic schizophrenics often show day-night reversal, sleep fragmentation, and insomnia.

Insomnia Associated with Neurologic Disorders A variety of neurologic diseases result in sleep disruption through both indirect, nonspecific mechanisms (e.g., pain in cervical spondylosis or low back pain) or by impairment of central neural structures involved in the generation and control of sleep itself. For example, *dementia* from any cause has long been associated with disturbances in the timing of the sleep-wake cycle, often characterized by nocturnal wandering and an exacerbation of symptomatology at night (so-called sundowning).

Epilepsy may rarely present as a sleep complaint (Chap. 363). Often the history is of abnormal behavior, at times with convulsive movements during sleep. The differential diagnosis includes REM sleep behavior disorder, sleep apnea syndrome, and periodic movements of sleep (see above). Diagnosis requires nocturnal polysomnography with a full EEG montage. Other neurologic diseases associated with abnormal movements, such as *Parkinson's disease, hemiballismus, Huntington's chorea,* and *Tourette syndrome* (Chap. 366), are also associated with disrupted sleep, presumably through secondary mechanisms. However, the abnormal movements themselves are greatly reduced during sleep. Headache syndromes (*migraine* or *cluster headache*) may show sleep-associated exacerbations (Chap. 15) by unknown mechanisms.

Fatal familial insomnia is a rare hereditary disorder caused by degeneration of anterior and dorsomedial nuclei of the thalamus. Insomnia is a prominent early symptom. Patients develop progressive autonomic dysfunction, followed by dysarthria, myoclonus, coma, and death. The pathogenesis is a mutation in the prion gene (Chap. 378).

Insomnia Associated with Other Medical Disorders   A number of medical conditions are associated with disruptions of sleep. The association is frequently nonspecific, e.g., sleep disruption due to chronic pain from rheumatologic disorders. Attention to this association is important in that sleep-associated symptoms are often the presenting or most bothersome complaint. Treatment of the underlying medical problem is the most useful approach. Sleep disruption can also result from the use of medications such as glucocorticoids (see below).

One prominent association is between sleep disruption and *asthma*. In many asthmatics there is a prominent daily variation in airway resistance that results in marked increases in asthmatic symptoms at night, especially during sleep. In addition, treatment of asthma with theophylline-based compounds, adrenergic agonists, or glucocorticoids can independently disrupt sleep. When sleep disruption is a side effect of asthma treatment, inhaled glucocorticoids (e.g., beclomethasone) that do not disrupt sleep may provide a useful alternative.

Cardiac ischemia may also be associated with sleep disruption. The ischemia itself may result from increases in sympathetic tone as a result of sleep apnea. Patients may present with complaints of nightmares or vivid, disturbing dreams, with or without awareness of the more classic symptoms of angina or of the sleep disordered breathing. Treatment of the sleep apnea may substantially improve the angina and the nocturnal sleep quality. *Paroxysmal nocturnal dyspnea* can also occur as a consequence of sleep-associated cardiac ischemia that causes pulmonary congestion exacerbated by the recumbent posture.

Chronic obstructive pulmonary disease is also associated with sleep disruption, as is *cystic fibrosis, menopause, hyperthyroidism, gastroesophageal reflux, chronic renal failure,* and *liver failure.*

Medication-, Drug-, or Alcohol-Dependent Insomnia   Disturbed sleep can result from ingestion of a wide variety of agents. Caffeine is perhaps the most common pharmacologic cause of insomnia. It produces increased latency to sleep onset, more frequent arousals during sleep, and a reduction in total sleep time for up to 8–14 h after ingestion. Even small amounts of coffee can significantly disturb sleep in some patients; therefore, a 1- to 2-month trial without caffeine should be attempted in patients with these symptoms. Similarly, alcohol and nicotine can interfere with sleep, despite the fact that many patients use them to relax and promote sleep. Although alcohol can increase drowsiness and shorten sleep latency, even moderate amounts of alcohol increase awakenings in the second half of the night. In addition, alcohol ingestion prior to sleep is contraindicated in patients with sleep apnea because of the inhibitory effects of alcohol on upper airway muscle tone. Acutely, amphetamines and cocaine suppress both REM sleep and total sleep time, which return to normal with chronic use. Withdrawal leads to a REM sleep rebound. A number of prescribed medications can produce insomnia. Antidepressants, sympathomimetics, and glucocorticoids are common causes. In addition, severe rebound insomnia can result from the acute withdrawal of hypnotics, especially following the use of high doses of benzodiazepines with a short half-life. For this reason, hypnotic doses should be low to moderate and prolonged drug tapering is encouraged.

RESTLESS LEGS SYNDROME (RLS)

Patients with this sensory-motor disorder report an irresistible urge to move the legs, or sometimes the upper extremities, that is often associated with a creepy-crawling or aching dysesthesias deep within the affected limbs. For most patients with RLS, the dysesthesias and restlessness are much worse in the evening or night compared to the daytime and frequently interfere with the ability to fall asleep. The symptoms appear with inactivity and are temporarily relieved by movement. In contrast, paresthesias secondary to peripheral neuropathy persist with activity. The severity of this chronic disorder may wax and wane over time and can be exacerbated by sleep deprivation, caffeine, alcohol, serotonergic antidepressants, and pregnancy. The prevalence is 1–5% of young to middle-age adults and 10–20% of those >60 years. There appear to be important differences in RLS prevalence among racial groups, with higher prevalence in those of Northern European ancestry. Roughly one-third of patients (particularly those with an early age of onset) will have multiple affected family members. At least three separate chromosomal loci have been identified in familial RLS, though no gene has been identified to date. Iron deficiency and renal failure may cause RLS, which is then considered secondary RLS. The symptoms of RLS are exquisitely sensitive to dopaminergic drugs (e.g., pramipexole 0.25–0.5 mg q8PM or ropinirole 0.5–4.0 mg q8PM), which are the treatments of choice. Opioids, benzodiazepines, and gabapentin may also be of therapeutic value. Most patients with restless legs also experience periodic limb movements of sleep, although the reverse is not the case.

PERIODIC LIMB MOVEMENT DISORDER (PLMD)

Periodic limb movements of sleep (PLMS), previously known as *nocturnal myoclonus*, consists of stereotyped, 0.5- to 5.0-s extensions of the great toe and dorsiflexion of the foot, which recur every 20–40 s during NREM sleep, in episodes lasting from minutes to hours, as documented by bilateral surface EMG recordings of the anterior tibialis on polysomnography. PLMS is the principal objective polysomnographic finding in 17% of patients with insomnia and 11% of those with excessive daytime somnolence (Fig. 28-3). It is often unclear whether it is an incidental finding or the cause of disturbed sleep. When deemed to be the latter, PLMS is called PLMD. PLMS occurs in a wide variety of sleep disorders (including narcolepsy, sleep apnea, REM sleep behavior disorder, and various forms of insomnia) and may be associated with frequent arousals and an increased number of sleep-stage transitions. The pathophysiology is not well understood, though individuals with high spinal transections can exhibit periodic leg movements during sleep, suggesting the existence of a spinal generator. Treatment options include dopaminergic medications or benzodiazepines.

EVALUATION OF DAYTIME SLEEPINESS

Daytime impairment due to sleep loss may be difficult to quantify for several reasons. First, sleepiness is not necessarily proportional to subjectively assessed sleep deprivation. In obstructive sleep apnea, for example, the repeated brief interruptions of sleep associated with resumption of respiration at the end of apneic episodes result in daytime sleepiness, despite the fact that the patient may be unaware of the sleep fragmentation. Second, subjective descriptions of waking impairment vary from patient to patient. Patients may describe themselves as "sleepy," "fatigued," or "tired" and may have a clear sense of the meaning of those terms, while others may use the same terms to describe a completely different condition. Third, sleepiness, particularly when profound, may affect judgment in a manner analogous to ethanol, such that subjective awareness of the condition and the consequent cognitive and motor impairment is reduced. Finally, patients may be reluctant to admit that sleepiness is a problem, both because they are generally unaware of what constitutes normal alertness and because sleepiness is generally viewed pejoratively, ascribed more often to a deficit in motivation than to an inadequately addressed physiologic sleep need.

Specific questioning about the occurrence of sleep episodes during normal waking hours, both intentional and unintentional, is necessary to determine the extent of the adverse effects of sleepiness on a patient's day-

A

B

FIGURE 28-3 Polysomnographic recordings of (A) obstructive sleep apnea and (B) periodic limb movement of sleep. Note the snoring and reduction in air flow in the presence of continued respiratory effort, associated with the subsequent oxygen desaturation (upper panel). Periodic limb movements occur with a relatively constant intermovement interval and are associated with changes in the EEG and heart rate acceleration (lower panel). Abbreviations: R.A.T., right anterior tibialis; L.A.T., left anterior tibialis. *(From the Division of Sleep Medicine, Brigham and Women's Hospital.)*

time function. Specific areas to be addressed include the occurrence of inadvertent sleep episodes while driving or in other safety-related settings, sleepiness while at work or school (and the relationship of sleepiness to work and school performance), and the effect of sleepiness on social and family life. Driving is particularly hazardous for patients with increased sleepiness. Reaction time is equally impaired by 24 h of sleep loss as by a blood alcohol level of 0.10 g/dL. More than half of Americans admit to driving when drowsy. An estimated 250,000 motor vehicle crashes per year are due to drowsy drivers, thus causing 20% of all serious crash injuries. Drowsy driving legislation, aimed at improving education of all drivers about the hazards of driving drowsy and establishing sanctions comparable to those for drunk driving, is pending in several states. Screening for sleep disorders, provision of an adequate number of safe highway rest areas, maintenance of unobstructed shoulder rumble strips, and strict enforcement and compliance monitoring of hours-of-service policies are needed to reduce the risk of sleep-related transportation crashes. Evidence for significant daytime impairment [in association either with the diagnosis of a primary sleep disorder, such as narcolepsy or sleep apnea, or with imposed or self-selected sleep-wake schedules (see "Shift-Work Disorder," below)] raises the issue of the physician's responsibility to notify motor vehicle licensing authorities of the increased risk of sleepiness-related vehicle accidents. As with epilepsy, legal requirements vary from state to state, and existing legal precedents do not provide a consistent interpretation of the balance between the physician's responsibility and the patient's right to privacy. At a minimum, physicians should document discussions with the patient regarding the increased risk of operating a vehicle, as well as a recommendation that driving be suspended until successful treatment or a schedule modification can be instituted.

The distinction between fatigue and sleepiness can be useful in the differentiation of patients with complaints of fatigue or tiredness in the setting of disorders such as fibromyalgia (Chap. 329), chronic fatigue syndrome (Chap. 384), or endocrine deficiencies such as hypothyroidism (Chap. 335) or Addison's disease (Chap. 336). While patients with these disorders can typically distinguish their daytime symptoms from the sleepiness that occurs with sleep deprivation, substantial overlap can occur. This is particularly true when the primary disorder also results in chronic sleep disruption (e.g., sleep apnea in hypothyroidism) or in abnormal sleep (e.g., fibromyalgia).

While clinical evaluation of the complaint of excessive sleepiness is usually adequate, objective quantification is sometimes necessary. Assessment of daytime functioning as an index of the adequacy of sleep can be made with the multiple sleep latency test (MSLT), which involves repeated measurement of sleep latency (time to onset of sleep) under standardized conditions during a day following quantified nocturnal sleep. The average latency across four to six tests (administered every 2 h across the waking day) provides an objective measure of daytime sleep tendency. Disorders of sleep that result in pathologic daytime somnolence can be reliably distinguished with the MSLT. In addition, the multiple measurements of sleep onset may identify direct transitions from wakefulness to REM sleep that are suggestive of specific pathologic conditions (e.g., narcolepsy).

NARCOLEPSY

Narcolepsy is both a disorder of the ability to sustain wakefulness voluntarily and a disorder of REM sleep regulation (Table 28-2). The classic "narcolepsy tetrad" consists of excessive daytime somnolence plus three specific symptoms related to an intrusion of REM sleep characteristics (e.g., muscle atonia, vivid dream imagery) into the transition between wakefulness and sleep: (1) sudden weakness or loss of muscle tone without loss of consciousness, often elicited by emotion (cataplexy); (2) hallucinations at sleep onset (hypnogogic hallucinations) or upon awakening (hypnopompic hallucinations); and (3) muscle paralysis upon awakening (sleep paralysis). The severity of cataplexy varies, as patients may have two to three attacks per day or per decade. Some patients with objectively confirmed narcolepsy (see below) may show no evidence of cataplexy. In those with cataplexy, the extent and duration of an attack may also vary, from a transient sagging of the jaw lasting a few seconds to rare cases of flaccid paralysis of the entire voluntary musculature for up to 20–30 min. Symptoms of narcolepsy typically begin in the second decade, although the onset ranges from ages 5–50. Once established, the disease is chronic without remissions. Secondary forms of narcolepsy have been described (e.g., after head trauma).

Narcolepsy affects about 1 in 4000 people in the United States and appears to have a genetic basis. Recently, several convergent lines of evidence suggest that the hypothalamic neuropeptide hypocretin (orexin) is involved in the pathogenesis of narcolepsy: (1) a mutation in the hypocretin receptor 2 gene has been associated with canine narcolepsy; (2) hypocretin "knockout" mice that are genetically unable to produce this neuropeptide exhibit behavioral and electrophysiologic features resembling human narcolepsy; and (3) cerebrospinal fluid levels of hypocretin are reduced in most patients who have narcolepsy

TABLE 28-2	PREVALENCE OF SYMPTOMS IN NARCOLEPSY
Symptom	**Prevalence, %**
Excessive daytime somnolence	100
Disturbed sleep	87
Cataplexy	76
Hypnagogic hallucinations	68
Sleep paralysis	64
Memory problems	50

Source: Modified from TA Roth, L Merlotti in SA Burton et al (eds), *Narcolepsy 3rd International Symposium: Selected Symposium Proceedings*, Chicago, Matrix Communications, 1989.

with cataplexy. The inheritance pattern of narcolepsy in humans is more complex than in the canine model. However, almost all narcoleptics with cataplexy are positive for HLA DQB1*0602 (Chap. 309), suggesting that an autoimmune process may be responsible.

Diagnosis　The diagnostic criteria continue to be a matter of debate. Certainly, objective verification of excessive daytime somnolence, typically with MSLT mean sleep latencies <8 min, is an essential if nonspecific diagnostic feature. Other conditions that cause excessive sleepiness, such as sleep apnea or chronic sleep deprivation, must be rigorously excluded. The other objective diagnostic feature of narcolepsy is the presence of REM sleep in at least two of the naps during the MSLT. Abnormal regulation of REM sleep is also manifested by the appearance of REM sleep immediately or within minutes after sleep onset in 50% of narcoleptic patients, a rarity in unaffected individuals maintaining a conventional sleep-wake schedule. The REM-related symptoms of the classic narcolepsy tetrad are variably present. There is increasing evidence that narcoleptics with cataplexy (one-half to two-thirds of patients) may represent a more homogeneous group than those without this symptom. However, a history of cataplexy can be difficult to establish reliably. Hypnogogic and hypnopompic hallucinations and sleep paralysis are often found in non-narcoleptic individuals and may be present in only one-half of narcoleptics. Nocturnal sleep disruption is commonly observed in narcolepsy but is also a nonspecific symptom. Similarly, a history of "automatic behavior" during wakefulness (a trancelike state during which simple motor behaviors persist) is not specific for narcolepsy and serves principally to corroborate the presence of daytime somnolence.

℞ NARCOLEPSY

The treatment of narcolepsy is symptomatic. Somnolence is treated with wake-promoting therapeutics. Modafinil is now the drug of choice, principally because it is associated with fewer side effects than older stimulants and has a long half-life; 200–400 mg is given as a single daily dose. Older drugs such as methylphenidate (10 mg bid to 20 mg qid) or dextroamphetamine (10 mg bid) are still used as alternatives, particularly in refractory patients. These latter medications are now available in slow-release formulations, extending their duration of action and allowing once daily dosing.

Treatment of the REM-related phenomena cataplexy, hypnogogic hallucinations, and sleep paralysis requires the potent REM sleep suppression produced by antidepressant medications. The tricyclic antidepressants [e.g., protriptyline (10–40 mg/d) and clomipramine (25–50 mg/d)] and the selective serotonin reuptake inhibitors (SSRIs) [e.g., fluoxetine (10–20 mg/d)] are commonly used for this purpose. Efficacy of the antidepressants is limited largely by anticholinergic side effects (tricyclics) and by sleep disturbance and sexual dysfunction (SSRIs). Alternately, gamma hydroxybutyrate (GHB), given at bed time, and 4 h later, is effective in reducing daytime cataplectic episodes. Adequate nocturnal sleep time and planned daytime naps (when possible) are important preventative measures.

SLEEP APNEA SYNDROMES

Respiratory dysfunction during sleep is a common, serious cause of excessive daytime somnolence as well as of disturbed nocturnal sleep. An estimated 2–5 million individuals in the United States have a reduction or cessation of breathing for 10–150 s, from thirty to several hundred times every night during sleep. These episodes may be due to either an occlusion of the airway (*obstructive sleep apnea*), absence of respiratory effort (*central sleep apnea*), or a combination of these factors (*mixed sleep apnea*) (Fig. 28-3). Failure to recognize and treat these conditions appropriately may lead to impairment of daytime alertness, increased risk of sleep-related motor vehicle accidents, hypertension and other serious cardiovascular complications, and increased mortality. Sleep apnea is particularly prevalent in overweight men and in the elderly, yet it is estimated to remain undiagnosed in 80–90% of affected individuals. This is unfortunate since effective treatments are available. Readers are referred to Chap. 259 for a comprehensive review of the diagnosis and treatment of patients with these conditions.

PARASOMNIAS

The term *parasomnia* refers to abnormal behaviors or experiences that arise from or occur during sleep. A continuum of parasomnias arise from NREM sleep, from brief confusional arousals to sleepwalking and night terrors. The presenting complaint is usually related to the behavior itself, but the parasomnias can disturb sleep continuity or lead to mild impairments in daytime alertness. Two main parasomnias occur in REM sleep: REM sleep behavior disorder (RBD), which will be described below, and nightmare disorder.

Sleepwalking (Somnambulism)　Patients affected by this disorder carry out automatic motor activities that range from simple to complex. Individuals may walk, urinate inappropriately, eat, or exit from the house while remaining only partially aware. Full arousal may be difficult, and individuals may rarely respond to attempted awakening with agitation or even violence. Sleepwalking arises from stage 3 or 4 NREM sleep, usually in the first 2 hours of the night, and is most common in children and adolescents, when these sleep stages are most robust. Episodes are usually isolated but may be recurrent in 1–6% of patients. The cause is unknown, though it has a familial basis in roughly one-third of cases.

Sleep Terrors　This disorder, also called *pavor nocturnus*, occurs primarily in young children during the first several hours after sleep onset, in stages 3 and 4 of NREM sleep. The child suddenly screams, exhibiting autonomic arousal with sweating, tachycardia, and hyperventilation. The individual may be difficult to arouse and rarely recalls the episode on awakening in the morning. Parents are usually reassured to learn that the condition is self-limited and benign and that no specific therapy is indicated. Both sleep terrors and sleepwalking represent abnormalities of arousal. In contrast, *nightmares* occur during REM sleep and cause full arousal, with intact memory for the unpleasant episode.

Sleep Bruxism　Bruxism is an involuntary, forceful grinding of teeth during sleep that affects 10–20% of the population. The patient is usually unaware of the problem. The typical age of onset is 17–20 years, and spontaneous remission usually occurs by age 40. Sex distribution appears to be equal. In many cases, the diagnosis is made during dental examination, damage is minor, and no treatment is indicated. In more severe cases, treatment with a rubber tooth guard is necessary to prevent disfiguring tooth injury. Stress management or, in some cases, biofeedback can be useful when bruxism is a manifestation of psychological stress. There are anecdotal reports of benefit using benzodiazepines.

Sleep Enuresis　Bedwetting, like sleepwalking and night terrors, is another parasomnia that occurs during sleep in the young. Before age 5 or 6, nocturnal enuresis should probably be considered a normal feature of development. The condition usually improves spontaneously by puberty, has a prevalence in late adolescence of 1–3%, and is rare in adulthood. In older patients with enuresis a distinction must be made between primary and secondary enuresis, the latter being defined as bedwetting in patients who have previously been fully continent for 6–12 months. Treatment of primary enuresis is reserved for patients of appropriate age (>5 or 6 years) and consists of bladder training exercises and behavioral therapy. Urologic abnormalities are more common in primary enuresis and must be assessed by urologic examination. Important causes of secondary enuresis include emotional disturbances, urinary tract infections or malformations, cauda equina lesions, epilepsy, sleep apnea, and certain medications. Symptomatic pharmacotherapy is usually accomplished with desmopressin (0.2 mg qhs), oxybutynin chloride (5–10 mg qhs) or imipramine (10–50 mg qhs).

Miscellaneous Parasomnias　Other clinical entities may be characterized as a parasomnia or a sleep-related movement disorder in that they occur selectively during sleep and are associated with some degree of sleep disruption. Examples include *jactatio capitis nocturna* (nocturnal headbanging, rhythmic movement disorder), confusional arousals, sleep-related eating disorder, and nocturnal leg cramps.

REM Sleep Behavior Disorder (RBD) RBD is a rare condition that is distinct from other parasomnias in that it occurs during REM sleep. It primarily afflicts men of middle age or older, many of whom have an existing, or developing, neurologic disease. Approximately one-half of patients with RBD will develop Parkinson's disease (Chap. 366) within 10–20 years. Presenting symptoms consist of agitated or violent behavior during sleep, as reported by a bed partner. In contrast to typical somnambulism, injury to the patient or bed partner is not uncommon, and, upon awakening, the patient reports vivid, often unpleasant, dream imagery. The principal differential diagnosis is nocturnal seizures, which can be excluded with polysomnography. In RBD, seizure activity is absent on the EEG, and disinhibition of the usual motor atonia is observed in the EMG during REM sleep, at times associated with complex motor behaviors. The pathogenesis is unclear, but damage to brainstem areas mediating descending motor inhibition during REM sleep may be responsible. In support of this hypothesis are the remarkable similarities between RBD and the sleep of animals with bilateral lesions of the pontine tegmentum in areas controlling REM sleep motor inhibition. Treatment with clonazepam (0.5–1.0 mg qhs) provides sustained improvement in almost all reported cases.

CIRCADIAN RHYTHM SLEEP DISORDERS

A subset of patients presenting with either insomnia or hypersomnia may have a disorder of sleep *timing* rather than sleep *generation*. Disorders of sleep timing can be either organic (i.e., due to an intrinsic defect in the circadian pacemaker or its input from entraining stimuli) or environmental (i.e., due to a disruption of exposure to entraining stimuli from the environment). Regardless of etiology, the symptoms reflect the influence of the underlying circadian pacemaker on sleep-wake function. Thus, effective therapeutic approaches should aim to entrain the oscillator at an appropriate phase.

Jet Lag Disorder More than 60 million persons experience transmeridian air travel annually, which is often associated with excessive daytime sleepiness, sleep onset insomnia, and frequent arousals from sleep, particularly in the latter half of the night. Gastrointestinal discomfort is common. The syndrome is transient, typically lasting 2–14 d depending on the number of time zones crossed, the direction of travel, and the traveler's age and phase-shifting capacity. Travelers who spend more time outdoors reportedly adapt more quickly than those who remain in hotel rooms, presumably due to bright (outdoor) light exposure. Avoidance of antecedent sleep loss and obtaining nap sleep on the afternoon prior to overnight travel greatly reduces the difficulty of extended wakefulness. Laboratory studies suggest that sub-milligram doses of the pineal hormone melatonin can enhance sleep efficiency, but only if taken when endogenous melatonin concentrations are low (i.e., during biologic daytime), and that melatonin may induce phase shifts in human rhythms. A large-scale clinical trial evaluating the safety and efficacy of melatonin as a treatment for jet lag disorder and other circadian sleep disorders is needed.

Shift-Work Disorder More than 7 million workers in the United States regularly work at night, either on a permanent or rotating schedule. In addition, each week millions more elect to remain awake at night to meet deadlines, drive long distances, or participate in recreational activities. This results in both sleep loss and misalignment of the circadian rhythm with respect to the sleep-wake cycle.

Studies of regular night-shift workers indicate that the circadian timing system usually fails to adapt successfully to such inverted schedules. This leads to a misalignment between the desired work-rest schedule and the output of the pacemaker and in disturbed daytime sleep in most individuals. Sleep deprivation, increased length of time awake prior to work, and misalignment of circadian phase produce decreased alertness and performance, increased reaction time, and increased risk of performance lapses, thereby resulting in greater safety hazards among night workers and other sleep-deprived individuals. Sleep disturbance nearly doubles the risk of a fatal work accident. Additional problems include higher rates of cancer and of cardiac, gastrointestinal, and reproductive disorders in chronic night-shift workers.

Sleep onset is associated with marked attenuation in perception of both auditory and visual stimuli and lapses of consciousness. The sleepy individual may thus attempt to perform routine and familiar motor tasks during the transition state between wakefulness and sleep (stage 1 sleep) in the absence of adequate processing of sensory input from the environment. Motor vehicle operators are especially vulnerable to sleep-related accidents since the sleep-deprived driver or operator often fails to heed the warning signs of fatigue. Such attempts to override the powerful biologic drive for sleep by the sheer force of will can yield a catastrophic outcome when sleep processes intrude involuntarily upon the waking brain. Such sleep-related attentional failures typically last only seconds but are known on occasion to persist for longer durations. These frequent brief intrusions of stage 1 sleep into behavioral wakefulness are a major component of the impaired psychomotor performance seen with sleepiness. There is a significant increase in the risk of sleep-related, fatal-to-the-driver highway crashes in the early morning and late afternoon hours, coincident with bimodal peaks in the daily rhythm of sleep tendency.

Medical housestaff constitute another group of workers at risk for accidents and other adverse consequences of lack of sleep and misalignment of the circadian rhythm. Recent research has demonstrated that the practice of scheduling interns and residents to work shifts of 30 consecutive hours both doubles the risk of attentional failures among intensive care unit interns working at night and significantly increases the risk of serious medical errors in intensive care units. Moreover, working for >24 h consecutively increases the risk of needlestick injuries and more than doubles the risk of motor vehicle crashes on the commute home. Some 20% of hospital interns report making a fatigue-related mistake that injured a patient, and 5% admit making a mistake that results in the death of a patient.

From 5–10% of individuals scheduled to work at night or in the early morning hours have much greater than average difficulties remaining awake during night work and sleeping during the day; these individuals are diagnosed with chronic and severe shift-work disorder (SWD). Patients with this disorder have a level of excessive sleepiness during night work and insomnia during day sleep that the physician judges to be clinically significant; the condition is associated with an increased risk of sleep-related accidents and with some of the illnesses associated with night-shift work. Patients with chronic and severe SWD are profoundly sleepy at night. In fact, their sleep latencies during night work average just 2 min, comparable to mean sleep latency durations of patients with narcolepsy or severe daytime sleep apnea.

℞ SHIFT-WORK DISORDER

Caffeine is frequently used to promote wakefulness. However, it cannot forestall sleep indefinitely, and it does not shield users from sleep-related performance lapses. Postural changes, exercise, and strategic placement of nap opportunities can sometimes temporarily reduce the risk of fatigue-related performance lapses. Properly timed exposure to bright light can facilitate rapid adaptation to night-shift work.

While many techniques (e.g., light treatment) used to facilitate adaptation to night shift work may help patients with this disorder, modafinil is the only therapeutic intervention that has ever been evaluated as a treatment for this specific patient population. Modafinil (200 mg, taken 30–60 min before the start of each night shift) is approved by the U.S. Food and Drug Administration as a treatment for the excessive sleepiness during night work in patients with SWD. Although treatment with modafinil significantly increases sleep latency and reduces the risk of lapses of attention during night work, SWD patients remain excessively sleepy at night, even while being treated with modafinil.

Safety programs should promote education about sleep and increase awareness of the hazards associated with night work. The goal should be to minimize both sleep deprivation and circadian disruption. Work schedules should be designed to minimize: (1) exposure to night work, (2) the frequency of shift rotation so that shifts do not rotate more than once every 2–3 weeks, (3) the number of consecutive night shifts, and (4) the duration of night shifts. Shift durations of >16 h should be universally recognized as increasing the risk of sleep-related errors and performance lapses to a level that is unacceptable in nonemergency circumstances.

Delayed Sleep Phase Disorder Delayed sleep phase disorder is characterized by: (1) reported sleep onset and wake times intractably later than desired, (2) actual sleep times at nearly the same clock hours daily, and (3) essentially normal all-night polysomnography except for delayed sleep onset. Patients exhibit an abnormally delayed endogenous circadian phase, with the temperature minimum during the constant routine occurring later than normal. This delayed phase could be due to: (1) an abnormally long, genetically determined intrinsic period of the endogenous circadian pacemaker; (2) an abnormally reduced phase-advancing capacity of the pacemaker; or (3) an irregular prior sleep-wake schedule, characterized by frequent nights when the patient chooses to remain awake well past midnight (for social, school, or work reasons). In most cases, it is difficult to distinguish among these factors, since patients with an abnormally long intrinsic period are more likely to "choose" such late-night activities because they are unable to sleep at that time. Patients tend to be young adults. This self-perpetuating condition can persist for years and does not usually respond to attempts to reestablish normal bedtime hours. Treatment methods involving bright-light phototherapy during the morning hours or melatonin administration in the evening hours show promise in these patients, although the relapse rate is high.

Advanced Sleep Phase Disorder Advanced sleep phase disorder (ASPD) is the converse of the delayed sleep phase syndrome. Most commonly, this syndrome occurs in older people, 15% of whom report that they cannot sleep past 5 A.M., with twice that number complaining that they wake up too early at least several times per week. Patients with ASPD experience excessive daytime sleepiness during the evening hours, when they have great difficulty remaining awake, even in social settings. Typically, patients awaken from 3–5 A.M. each day, often several hours before their desired wake times. In addition to age-related ASPD, an early-onset familial variant of this condition has also been reported. In one such family, autosomal dominant ASPD was due to a missense mutation in a circadian clock component (PER2, as shown in Fig. 28-2) that altered the circadian period. Patients with ASPD may benefit from bright-light phototherapy during the evening hours, designed to reset the circadian pacemaker to a later hour.

Non-24-Hour Sleep-Wake Disorder This condition can occur when the maximal phase-advancing capacity of the circadian pacemaker is not adequate to accommodate the difference between the 24-h geophysical day and the intrinsic period of the pacemaker in the patient. Alternatively, patients' self-selected exposure to artificial light may drive the circadian pacemaker to a >24-h schedule. Affected patients are not able to maintain a stable phase relationship between the output of the pacemaker and the 24-h day. Such patients typically present with an incremental pattern of successive delays in sleep onsets and wake times,

progressing in and out of phase with local time. When the patient's endogenous rhythms are out of phase with the local environment, insomnia coexists with excessive daytime sleepiness. Conversely, when the endogenous rhythms are in phase with the local environment, symptoms remit. The intervals between symptomatic periods may last several weeks to several months. Blind individuals unable to perceive light are particularly susceptible to this disorder. Nightly low-dose (0.5 mg) melatonin administration has been reported to improve sleep and, in some cases, to induce synchronization of the circadian pacemaker.

MEDICAL IMPLICATIONS OF CIRCADIAN RHYTHMICITY

Prominent circadian variations have been reported in the incidence of acute myocardial infarction, sudden cardiac death, and stroke, the leading causes of death in the United States. Platelet aggregability is increased after arising in the early morning hours, coincident with the peak incidence of these cardiovascular events. A better understanding of the possible role of circadian rhythmicity in the acute destabilization of a chronic condition such as atherosclerotic disease could improve the understanding of the pathophysiology.

Diagnostic and therapeutic procedures may also be affected by the time of day at which data are collected. Examples include blood pressure, body temperature, the dexamethasone suppression test, and plasma cortisol levels. The timing of chemotherapy administration has been reported to have an effect on the outcome of treatment. Few physicians realize the extent to which routine measures are affected by the time (or sleep/wake state) when the measurement is made.

In addition, both the toxicity and effectiveness of drugs can vary during the day. For example, more than a fivefold difference has been observed in mortality rates following administration of toxic agents to experimental animals at different times of day. Anesthetic agents are particularly sensitive to time-of-day effects. Finally, the physician must be increasingly aware of the public health risks associated with the ever-increasing demands made by the duty-rest-recreation schedules in our round-the-clock society.

FURTHER READINGS

FLEMONS WW: Clinical practice. Obstructive sleep apnea. N Engl J Med 347:498, 2002

PACK AI et al: Risk factors for excessive sleepiness in older adults. Ann Neurol 59:893, 2006

SCAMMELL TE: The neurobiology, diagnosis, and treatment of narcolepsy. Ann Neurol 53:154, 2003

SILBER MH: Clinical practice. Chronic insomnia. N Engl J Med 353:803, 2005

SECTION 4 | DISORDERS OF EYES, EARS, NOSE, AND THROAT

29 Disorders of the Eye
Jonathan C. Horton

THE HUMAN VISUAL SYSTEM

The visual system provides a supremely efficient means for the rapid assimilation of information from the environment to aid in the guidance of behavior. The act of seeing begins with the capture of images focused by the cornea and lens upon a light-sensitive membrane in the back of the eye, called the *retina*. The retina is actually part of the brain, banished to the periphery to serve as a transducer for the conversion of patterns of light energy into neuronal signals. Light is absorbed by photopigment in two types of receptors: rods and cones.

In the human retina there are 100 million rods and 5 million cones. The rods operate in dim (scotopic) illumination. The cones function under daylight (photopic) conditions. The cone system is specialized for color perception and high spatial resolution. The majority of cones are located within the macula, the portion of the retina serving the central 10° of vision. In the middle of the macula a small pit termed the *fovea*, packed exclusively with cones, provides best visual acuity.

Photoreceptors hyperpolarize in response to light, activating bipolar, amacrine, and horizontal cells in the inner nuclear layer. After processing of photoreceptor responses by this complex retinal circuit, the flow of sensory information ultimately converges upon a final common pathway: the ganglion cells. These cells translate the visual image impinging upon the retina into a continuously varying barrage of action potentials that propagates along the primary optic pathway to visual centers within the brain. There are a million ganglion cells in each retina, and hence a million fibers in each optic nerve.

Ganglion cell axons sweep along the inner surface of the retina in the nerve fiber layer, exit the eye at the optic disc, and travel through the optic nerve, optic chiasm, and optic tract to reach targets in the brain. The majority of fibers synapse upon cells in the lateral geniculate body, a thalamic relay station. Cells in the lateral geniculate body project in turn to the primary visual cortex. This massive afferent retinogeniculocortical sensory pathway provides the neural substrate for visual perception. Although the lateral geniculate body is the main target of the retina, separate classes of ganglion cells project to other subcortical visual nuclei involved in different functions. Ganglion cells that mediate pupillary constriction and circadian rhythms are light sensitive, owing to a novel visual pigment, melanopsin. Pupil responses are mediated by input to the pretectal olivary nuclei in the midbrain. The pretectal nuclei send their output to the Edinger-Westphal nuclei, which in turn provide parasympathetic innervation to the iris sphincter via an interneuron in the ciliary ganglion. Circadian rhythms are timed by a retinal projection to the suprachiasmatic nucleus. Visual orientation and eye movements are served by retinal input to the superior colliculus. Gaze stabilization and optokinetic reflexes are governed by a group of small retinal targets known collectively as the *brainstem accessory optic system*.

The eyes must be rotated constantly within their orbits to place and maintain targets of visual interest upon the fovea. This activity, called *foveation*, or looking, is governed by an elaborate efferent motor system. Each eye is moved by six extraocular muscles, supplied by cranial nerves from the oculomotor (III), trochlear (IV), and abducens (VI) nuclei. Activity in these ocular motor nuclei is coordinated by pontine and midbrain mechanisms for smooth pursuit, saccades, and gaze stabilization during head and body movements. Large regions of the frontal and parietooccipital cortex control these brainstem eye movement centers by providing descending supranuclear input.

CLINICAL ASSESSMENT OF VISUAL FUNCTION

REFRACTIVE STATE

In approaching the patient with reduced vision, the first step is to decide whether refractive error is responsible. In *emmetropia*, parallel rays from infinity are focused perfectly upon the retina. Sadly, this condition is enjoyed by only a minority of the population. In *myopia*, the globe is too long, and light rays come to a focal point in front of the retina. Near objects can be seen clearly, but distant objects require a diverging lens in front of the eye. In *hyperopia*, the globe is too short, and hence a converging lens is used to supplement the refractive power of the eye. In *astigmatism*, the corneal surface is not perfectly spherical, necessitating a cylindrical corrective lens. In recent years it has become possible to correct refractive error with the excimer laser by performing LASIK (laser in situ keratomileusis) to alter the curvature of the cornea.

With the onset of middle age, *presbyopia* develops as the lens within the eye becomes unable to increase its refractive power to accommodate upon near objects. To compensate for presbyopia, the emmetropic patient must use reading glasses. The patient already wearing glasses for distance correction usually switches to bifocals. The only exception is the myopic patient, who may achieve clear vision at near simply by removing glasses containing the distance prescription.

Refractive errors usually develop slowly and remain stable after adolescence, except in unusual circumstances. For example, the acute onset of diabetes mellitus can produce sudden myopia because of lens edema induced by hyperglycemia. Testing vision through a pinhole aperture is a useful way to screen quickly for refractive error. If the visual acuity is better through a pinhole than with the unaided eye, the patient needs a refraction to obtain best corrected visual acuity.

VISUAL ACUITY

The Snellen chart is used to test acuity at a distance of 6 m (20 ft). For convenience, a scale version of the Snellen chart, called the Rosenbaum card, is held at 36 cm (14 in) from the patient (Fig. 29-1). All subjects should be able to read the 6/6 m (20/20 ft) line with each eye

FIGURE 29-1 The Rosenbaum card is a miniature, scale version of the Snellen chart for testing visual acuity at near. When the visual acuity is recorded, the Snellen distance equivalent should bear a notation indicating that vision was tested at near, not at 6 m (20 ft), or else the Jaeger number system should be used to report the acuity.

using their refractive correction, if any. Patients who need reading glasses because of presbyopia must wear them for accurate testing with the Rosenbaum card. If 6/6 (20/20) acuity is not present in each eye, the deficiency in vision must be explained. If worse than 6/240 (20/800), acuity should be recorded in terms of counting fingers, hand motions, light perception, or no light perception. Legal blindness is defined by the Internal Revenue Service as a best corrected acuity of 6/60 (20/200) or less in the better eye, or a binocular visual field subtending 20° or less. For driving the laws vary by state, but most require a corrected acuity of 6/12 (20/40) in at least one eye for unrestricted privileges. Patients with a homonymous hemianopia should not drive.

PUPILS

The pupils should be tested individually in dim light with the patient fixating on a distant target. If they respond briskly to light, there is no need to check the near response, because isolated loss of constriction (miosis) to accommodation does not occur. For this reason, the ubiquitous abbreviation PERRLA (pupils equal, round, and reactive to light and accommodation) implies a wasted effort with the last step.

FIGURE 29-2 Demonstration of a relative afferent pupil defect (Marcus Gunn pupil) in the left eye, done with the patient fixating upon a distant target. **A.** With dim background lighting, the pupils are equal and relatively large. **B.** Shining a flashlight into the right eye evokes equal, strong constriction of both pupils. **C.** Swinging the flashlight over to the damaged left eye causes dilation of both pupils, although they remain smaller than in **A.** Swinging the flashlight back over to the healthy right eye would result in symmetric constriction back to the appearance shown in **B.** Note that the pupils always remain equal; the damage to the left retina/optic nerve is revealed by weaker bilateral pupil constriction to a flashlight in the left eye compared with the right eye. *(From P Levatin, Arch Ophthalmol 62:768, 1959.)*

However, it is important to test the near response if the light response is poor or absent. Light-near dissociation occurs with neurosyphilis (Argyll Robertson pupil), lesions of the dorsal midbrain (obstructive hydrocephalus, pineal region tumors), and after aberrant regeneration (oculomotor nerve palsy, Adie's tonic pupil).

An eye with no light perception has no pupillary response to direct light stimulation. If the retina or optic nerve is only partially injured, the direct pupillary response will be weaker than the consensual pupillary response evoked by shining a light into the other eye. This *relative afferent pupillary defect* (Marcus Gunn pupil) can be elicited with the swinging flashlight test (**Fig. 29-2**). It is an extremely useful sign in retrobulbar optic neuritis and other optic nerve diseases, where it may be the sole objective evidence for disease.

Subtle inequality in pupil size, up to 0.5 mm, is a fairly common finding in normal persons. The diagnosis of essential or physiologic anisocoria is secure as long as the relative pupil asymmetry remains constant as ambient lighting varies. Anisocoria that increases in dim light indicates a sympathetic paresis of the iris dilator muscle. The triad of miosis with ipsilateral ptosis and anhidrosis constitutes *Horner's*

syndrome, although anhidrosis is an inconstant feature. Brainstem stroke, carotid dissection, or neoplasm impinging upon the sympathetic chain are occasionally identified as the cause of Horner's syndrome, but most cases are idiopathic.

Anisocoria that increases in bright light suggests a parasympathetic palsy. The first concern is an oculomotor nerve paresis. This possibility is excluded if the eye movements are full and the patient has no ptosis or diplopia. Acute pupillary dilation (mydriasis) can occur from damage to the ciliary ganglion in the orbit. Common mechanisms are infection (herpes zoster, influenza), trauma (blunt, penetrating, surgical), or ischemia (diabetes, temporal arteritis). After denervation of the iris sphincter the pupil does not respond well to light, but the response to near is often relatively intact. When the near stimulus is removed, the pupil redilates very slowly compared with the normal pupil, hence the term *tonic pupil*. In *Adie's syndrome*, a tonic pupil occurs in conjunction with weak or absent tendon reflexes in the lower extremities. This benign disorder, which occurs predominantly in healthy young women, is assumed to represent a mild dysautonomia. Tonic pupils are also associated with Shy-Drager syndrome, segmental hypohidrosis, diabetes, and amyloidosis. Occasionally, a tonic pupil is discovered incidentally in an otherwise completely normal, asymptomatic individual. The diagnosis is confirmed by placing a drop of dilute (0.125%) pilocarpine into each eye. Denervation hypersensitivity produces pupillary constriction in a tonic pupil, whereas the normal pupil shows no response. Pharmacologic dilation from accidental or deliberate instillation of anticholinergic agents (atropine, scopolamine drops) into the eye can also produce pupillary mydriasis. In this situation, normal strength (1%) pilocarpine causes no constriction.

Both pupils are affected equally by systemic medications. They are small with narcotic use (morphine, heroin) and large with anticholinergics (scopolamine). Parasympathetic agents (pilocarpine, demecarium bromide) used to treat glaucoma produce miosis. In any patient with an unexplained pupillary abnormality, a slit-lamp examination is helpful to exclude surgical trauma to the iris, an occult foreign body, perforating injury, intraocular inflammation, adhesions (synechia), angle-closure glaucoma, and iris sphincter rupture from blunt trauma.

EYE MOVEMENTS AND ALIGNMENT

Eye movements are tested by asking the patient with both eyes open to pursue a small target such as a penlight into the cardinal fields of gaze. Normal ocular versions are smooth, symmetric, full, and maintained in all directions without nystagmus. Saccades, or quick refixation eye movements, are assessed by having the patient look back and forth between two stationary targets. The eyes should move rapidly and accurately in a single jump to their target. Ocular alignment can be judged by holding a penlight directly in front of the patient at about 1 m. If the eyes are straight, the corneal light reflex will be centered in the middle of each pupil. To test eye alignment more precisely, the cover test is useful. The patient is instructed to gaze upon a small fixation target in the distance. One eye is covered suddenly while observing the second eye. If the second eye shifts to fixate upon the target, it was misaligned. If it does not move, the first eye is uncovered and the test is repeated on the second eye. If neither eye moves, the eyes are aligned orthotropically. If the eyes are orthotropic in primary gaze but the patient complains of diplopia, the cover test should be performed with the head tilted or turned in whatever direction elicits diplopia. With practice the examiner can detect an ocular deviation (heterotropia) as small as 1–2° with the cover test. Deviations can be measured by placing prisms in front of the misaligned eye to determine the power required to neutralize the fixation shift evoked by covering the other eye.

STEREOPSIS

Stereoacuity is determined by presenting targets with retinal disparity separately to each eye using polarized images. The most popular office tests measure a range of thresholds from 800–40 seconds of arc. Normal stereoacuity is 40 seconds of arc. If a patient achieves this level of stereoacuity, one is assured that the eyes are aligned orthotropically and that vision is intact in each eye. Random dot stereograms have no monocular depth cues and provide an excellent screening test for strabismus and amblyopia in children.

COLOR VISION

The retina contains three classes of cones, with visual pigments of differing peak spectral sensitivity: red (560 nm), green (530 nm), and blue (430 nm). The red and green cone pigments are encoded on the X chromosome; the blue cone pigment on chromosome 7. Mutations of the blue cone pigment are exceedingly rare. Mutations of the red and green pigments cause congenital X-linked color blindness in 8% of males. Affected individuals are not truly color blind; rather, they differ from normal subjects in how they perceive color and how they combine primary monochromatic lights to match a given color. Anomalous trichromats have three cone types, but a mutation in one cone pigment (usually red or green) causes a shift in peak spectral sensitivity, altering the proportion of primary colors required to achieve a color match. Dichromats have only two cone types and will therefore accept a color match based upon only two primary colors. Anomalous trichromats and dichromats have 6/6 (20/20) visual acuity, but their hue discrimination is impaired. Ishihara color plates can be used to detect red-green color blindness. The test plates contain a hidden number, visible only to subjects with color confusion from red-green color blindness. Because color blindness is almost exclusively X-linked, it is worth screening only male children.

The Ishihara plates are often used to detect acquired defects in color vision, although they are intended as a screening test for congenital color blindness. Acquired defects in color vision frequently result from disease of the macula or optic nerve. For example, patients with a history of optic neuritis often complain of color desaturation long after their visual acuity has returned to normal. Color blindness can also occur from bilateral strokes involving the ventral portion of the occipital lobe (cerebral achromatopsia). Such patients can perceive only shades of gray and may also have difficulty recognizing faces (prosopagnosia). Infarcts of the dominant occipital lobe sometimes give rise to color anomia. Affected patients can discriminate colors, but they cannot name them.

VISUAL FIELDS

Vision can be impaired by damage to the visual system anywhere from the eyes to the occipital lobes. One can localize the site of the lesion with considerable accuracy by mapping the visual field deficit by finger confrontation and then correlating it with the topographic anatomy of the visual pathway (Fig. 29-3). Quantitative visual field mapping is performed by computer-driven perimeters (Humphrey, Octopus) that present a target of variable intensity at fixed positions in the visual field (Fig. 29-3A). By generating an automated printout of light thresholds, these static perimeters provide a sensitive means of detecting scotomas in the visual field. They are exceedingly useful for serial assessment of visual function in chronic diseases such as glaucoma or pseudotumor cerebri.

The crux of visual field analysis is to decide whether a lesion is before, at, or behind the optic chiasm. If a scotoma is confined to one eye, it must be due to a lesion anterior to the chiasm, involving either the optic nerve or retina. Retinal lesions produce scotomas that correspond optically to their location in the fundus. For example, a superior-nasal retinal detachment results in an inferior-temporal field cut. Damage to the macula causes a central scotoma (Fig. 29-3B).

Optic nerve disease produces characteristic patterns of visual field loss. Glaucoma selectively destroys axons that enter the superotemporal or inferotemporal poles of the optic disc, resulting in arcuate scotomas shaped like a Turkish scimitar, which emanate from the blind spot and curve around fixation to end flat against the horizontal meridian (Fig. 29-3C). This type of field defect mirrors the arrangement of the nerve fiber layer in the temporal retina. Arcuate or nerve fiber layer scotomas also occur from optic neuritis, ischemic optic neuropathy, optic disc drusen, and branch retinal artery or vein occlusion.

Damage to the entire upper or lower pole of the optic disc causes an altitudinal field cut that follows the horizontal meridian (Fig. 29-3D). This pattern of visual field loss is typical of ischemic optic neuropathy

but also occurs from retinal vascular occlusion, advanced glaucoma, and optic neuritis.

About half the fibers in the optic nerve originate from ganglion cells serving the macula. Damage to papillomacular fibers causes a cecocentral scotoma encompassing the blind spot and macula (Fig. 29-3E). If the damage is irreversible, pallor eventually appears in the temporal portion of the optic disc. Temporal pallor from a cecocentral scotoma may develop in optic neuritis, nutritional optic neuropathy, toxic optic neuropathy, Leber's hereditary optic neuropathy, and compressive optic neuropathy. It is worth mentioning that the temporal side of the optic disc is slightly more pale than the nasal side in most normal individuals. Therefore, it can sometimes be difficult to decide whether the temporal pallor visible on fundus examination represents a pathologic change. Pallor of the nasal rim of the optic disc is a less equivocal sign of optic atrophy.

At the optic chiasm, fibers from nasal ganglion cells decussate into the contralateral optic tract. Crossed fibers are damaged more by compression than uncrossed fibers. As a result, mass lesions of the sellar region cause a temporal hemianopia in each eye. Tumors anterior to the optic chiasm, such as meningiomas of the tuberculum sella, produce a junctional scotoma characterized by an optic neuropathy in one eye and a superior-temporal field cut in the other eye (Fig. 29-3G). More symmetric compression of the optic chiasm by a pituitary adenoma (Fig. 333-4), meningioma, craniopharyngioma, glioma, or aneurysm results in a bitemporal hemianopia (Fig. 29-3H). The insidious development of a bitemporal hemianopia often goes unnoticed by the patient and will escape detection by the physician unless each eye is tested separately.

It is difficult to localize a postchiasmal lesion accurately, because injury anywhere in the optic tract, lateral geniculate body, optic radiations, or visual cortex can produce a homonymous hemianopia, i.e., a temporal hemifield defect in the contralateral eye and a matching nasal hemifield defect in the ipsilateral eye (Fig. 29-3I). A unilateral postchiasmal lesion leaves the visual acuity in each eye unaffected, although the patient may read the letters on only the left or right half of the eye chart. Lesions of the optic radiations tend to cause poorly matched or incongruous field defects in each eye. Damage to the optic radiations in the temporal lobe (Meyer's loop) produces a superior quadrantic homonymous hemianopia (Fig. 29-3J), whereas injury to the optic radiations in the parietal lobe results in an inferior quadrantic homonymous hemianopia (Fig. 29-3K). Lesions of the primary visual cortex give rise to dense, congruous hemianopic field defects. Occlusion of the posterior cerebral artery supplying the occipital lobe is a frequent cause of total homonymous hemianopia. Some patients with hemianopia after occipital stroke have macular sparing, because the macular representation at the tip of the occipital lobe is supplied by collaterals from the middle cerebral artery (Fig. 29-3L). Destruction of both occipital lobes produces cortical blindness. This condition can be distinguished from bilateral prechiasmal visual loss by noting that the pupil responses and optic fundi remain normal.

DISORDERS

RED OR PAINFUL EYE

Corneal Abrasions These are seen best by placing a drop of fluorescein in the eye and looking with the slit lamp using a cobalt-blue light. A penlight with a blue filter will suffice if no slit lamp is available. Damage to the corneal epithelium is revealed by yellow fluorescence of the exposed basement membrane underlying the epithelium. It is important to check for foreign bodies. To search the conjunctival fornices, the lower lid should be pulled down and the upper lid everted. A foreign body can be removed with a moistened cotton-tipped applicator after placing a drop of topical anesthetic, such as proparacaine, in the eye. Alternatively, it may be possible to flush the foreign body from the eye by irrigating copiously with saline or artificial tears. If the corneal epithelium has been abraded, antibiotic ointment and a patch should be applied to the eye. A drop of an intermediate-acting cycloplegic, such as cyclopentolate hydrochloride 1%, helps to reduce pain by relaxing the ciliary body. The eye should be reexamined the next day. Minor abrasions may not require patching and cycloplegia.

Subconjunctival Hemorrhage This results from rupture of small vessels bridging the potential space between the episclera and conjunctiva. Blood dissecting into this space can produce a spectacular red eye, but vision is not affected and the hemorrhage resolves without treatment. Subconjunctival hemorrhage is usually spontaneous but can occur from blunt trauma, eye rubbing, or vigorous coughing. Occasionally it is a clue to an underlying bleeding disorder.

Pinguecula This is a small, raised conjunctival nodule at the temporal or nasal limbus. In adults such lesions are extremely common and have little significance, unless they become inflamed (pingueculitis). A *pterygium* resembles a pinguecula but has crossed the limbus to encroach upon the corneal surface. Removal is justified when symptoms of irritation or blurring develop, but recurrence is a common problem.

Blepharitis This refers to inflammation of the eyelids. The most common form occurs in association with acne rosacea or seborrheic dermatitis. The eyelid margins are usually colonized heavily by staphylococci. Upon close inspection, they appear greasy, ulcerated, and crusted with scaling debris that clings to the lashes. Treatment consists of warm compresses, strict eyelid hygiene, and topical antibiotics such as *erythromycin*. An external *hordeolum* (sty) is caused by staphylococcal infection of the superficial accessory glands of Zeis or Moll located in the eyelid margins. An internal hordeolum occurs after suppurative infection of the oil-secreting meibomian glands within the tarsal plate of the eyelid. Systemic antibiotics, usually tetracyclines, are sometimes necessary for treatment of meibomian gland inflammation (meibomitis) or chronic, severe blepharitis. A *chalazion* is a painless, granulomatous inflammation of a meibomian gland that produces a pealike nodule within the eyelid. It can be incised and drained, or injected with glucocorticoids. Basal cell, squamous cell, or meibomian gland carcinoma should be suspected for any nonhealing, ulcerative lesion of the eyelids.

Dacrocystitis An inflammation of the lacrimal drainage system, this can produce epiphora (tearing) and ocular injection. Gentle pressure over the lacrimal sac evokes pain and reflux of mucus or pus from the tear puncta. Dacrocystitis usually occurs after obstruction of the lacrimal system. It is treated with topical and systemic antibiotics, followed by probing or surgery to reestablish patency. *Entropion* (inversion of the eyelid) or *ectropion* (sagging or eversion of the eyelid) can also lead to epiphora and ocular irritation.

Monocular Prechiasmal Field Defects:

A — Normal Field Right Eye (30°) — blind spot
B — Central Scotoma (30°)
C — Nerve-Fiber Bundle (Arcuate) Scotoma (30°)
D — Altitudinal Scotoma (30°)
E — Ceco-central Scotoma (30°)
F — Enlarged Blind-Spot with Peripheral Constriction (30°)

Binocular Chiasmal or Postchiasmal Field Defects:

(Left eye) (Right eye)

G — Junctional Scotoma (30°)
H — Bitemporal Hemianopia (30°)
I — Homonymous Hemianopia (30°)
J — Superior Quadrantanopia (30°)
K — Inferior Quadrantanopia (30°)
L — Homonymous Hemianopia with Macular Sparing (30°)

Right — 100° 60° — Left

Optic Nerve
Optic Chiasm — G
H
Optic Tract
Lateral Geniculate Body — J
Optic Radiations — L
Primary Visual Cortex
K — I

FIGURE 29-3 Ventral view of the brain, correlating patterns of visual field loss with the sites of lesions in the visual pathway. The visual fields overlap partially, creating 120° of central binocular field flanked by a 40° monocular crescent on either side. The visual field maps in this figure were done with a computer-driven perimeter (Humphrey Instruments, Carl Zeiss, Inc.). It plots the retinal sensitivity to light in the central 30° using a gray scale format. Areas of visual field loss are shown in black. The examples of common monocular, prechiasmal field defects are all shown for the right eye. By convention, the visual fields are always recorded with the left eye's field on the left, and the right eye's field on the right, just as the patient sees the world.

Conjunctivitis This is the most common cause of a red, irritated eye. Pain is minimal, and the visual acuity is reduced only slightly. The most common viral etiology is adenovirus infection. It causes a watery discharge, mild foreign-body sensation, and photophobia. Bacterial infection tends to produce a more mucopurulent exudate. Mild cases of infectious conjunctivitis are usually treated empirically with broad-spectrum topical ocular antibiotics, such as sulfacetamide 10%, polymixin-bacitracin-neomycin, or trimethoprim-polymixin combination. Smears and cultures are usually reserved for severe, resistant, or recurrent cases of conjunctivitis. To prevent contagion, patients should be admonished to wash their hands frequently, not to touch their eyes, and to avoid direct contact with others.

Allergic Conjunctivitis This condition is extremely common and often mistaken for infectious conjunctivitis. Itching, redness, and epiphora are typical. The palpebral conjunctiva may become hypertropic with giant excrescences called cobblestone papillae. Irritation from contact lenses or any chronic foreign body can also induce formation of cobblestone papillae. *Atopic conjunctivitis* occurs in subjects with atopic dermatitis or asthma. Symptoms caused by allergic conjunctivitis can be alleviated with cold compresses, topical vasoconstrictors, antihistamines, and mast cell stabilizers such as cromolyn sodium. Topical glucocorticoid solutions provide dramatic relief of immune-mediated forms of conjunctivitis, but their long-term use is ill-advised because of the complications of glaucoma, cataract, and secondary infection. Topical nonsteroidal anti-inflammatory agents (NSAIDs) such as ketorolac tromethamine are a better alternative.

Keratoconjunctivitis Sicca   Also known as dry eye, it produces a burning, foreign-body sensation, injection, and photophobia. In mild cases the eye appears surprisingly normal, but tear production measured by wetting of a filter paper (Schirmer strip) is deficient. A variety of systemic drugs, including antihistaminic, anticholinergic, and psychotropic medications, result in dry eye by reducing lacrimal secretion. Disorders that involve the lacrimal gland directly, such as sarcoidosis or Sjögren's syndrome, also cause dry eye. Patients may develop dry eye after radiation therapy if the treatment field includes the orbits. Problems with ocular drying are also common after lesions affecting cranial nerves V or VII. Corneal anesthesia is particularly dangerous, because the absence of a normal blink reflex exposes the cornea to injury without pain to warn the patient. Dry eye is managed by frequent and liberal application of artificial tears and ocular lubricants. In severe cases the tear puncta can be plugged or cauterized to reduce lacrimal outflow.

Keratitis   This is a threat to vision because of the risk of corneal clouding, scarring, and perforation. Worldwide, the two leading causes of blindness from keratitis are trachoma from chlamydial infection and vitamin A deficiency related to malnutrition. In the United States, contact lenses play a major role in corneal infection and ulceration. They should not be worn by anyone with an active eye infection. In evaluating the cornea, it is important to differentiate between a superficial infection (*keratoconjunctivitis*) and a deeper, more serious ulcerative process. The latter is accompanied by greater visual loss, pain, photophobia, redness, and discharge. Slit-lamp examination shows disruption of the corneal epithelium, a cloudy infiltrate or abscess in the stroma, and an inflammatory cellular reaction in the anterior chamber. In severe cases, pus settles at the bottom of the anterior chamber, giving rise to a hypopyon. Immediate empirical antibiotic therapy should be initiated after corneal scrapings are obtained for Gram's stain, Giemsa stain, and cultures. Fortified topical antibiotics are most effective, supplemented with subconjunctival antibiotics as required. A fungal etiology should always be considered in the patient with keratitis. Fungal infection is common in warm humid climates, especially after penetration of the cornea by plant or vegetable material.

Herpes Simplex   The *herpes viruses* are a major cause of blindness from keratitis. Most adults in the United States have serum antibodies to herpes simplex, indicating prior viral infection (Chap. 172). Primary ocular infection is generally caused by herpes simplex type 1, rather than type 2. It manifests as a unilateral follicular blepharoconjunctivitis, easily confused with adenoviral conjunctivitis unless telltale vesicles appear on the periocular skin or conjunctiva. A dendritic pattern of corneal epithelial ulceration revealed by fluorescein staining is pathognomonic for herpes infection but is seen in only a minority of primary infections. Recurrent ocular infection arises from reactivation of the latent herpes virus. Viral eruption in the corneal epithelium may result in the characteristic herpes dendrite. Involvement of the corneal stroma produces edema, vascularization, and iridocyclitis. Herpes keratitis is treated with topical antiviral agents, cycloplegics, and oral acyclovir. Topical glucocorticoids are effective in mitigating corneal scarring but must be used with extreme caution because of the danger of corneal melting and perforation. Topical glucocorticoids also carry the risk of prolonging infection and inducing glaucoma.

Herpes Zoster   Herpes zoster from reactivation of latent varicella (chickenpox) virus causes a dermatomal pattern of painful vesicular dermatitis. Ocular symptoms can occur after zoster eruption in any branch of the trigeminal nerve but are particularly common when vesicles form on the nose, reflecting nasociliary (V1) nerve involvement (Hutchinson's sign). Herpes zoster ophthalmicus produces corneal dendrites, which can be difficult to distinguish from those seen in herpes simplex. Stromal keratitis, anterior uveitis, raised intraocular pressure, ocular motor nerve palsies, acute retinal necrosis, and postherpetic scarring and neuralgia are other common sequelae. Herpes zoster ophthalmicus is treated with antiviral agents and cycloplegics. In severe cases, glucocorticoids may be added to prevent permanent visual loss from corneal scarring.

Episcleritis   This is an inflammation of the episclera, a thin layer of connective tissue between the conjunctiva and sclera. Episcleritis resembles conjunctivitis but is a more localized process and discharge is absent. Most cases of episcleritis are idiopathic, but some occur in the setting of an autoimmune disease. *Scleritis* refers to a deeper, more severe inflammatory process, frequently associated with a connective tissue disease such as rheumatoid arthritis, lupus erythematosus, polyarteritis nodosa, Wegener's granulomatosis, or relapsing polychondritis. The inflammation and thickening of the sclera can be diffuse or nodular. In anterior forms of scleritis, the globe assumes a violet hue and the patient complains of severe ocular tenderness and pain. With posterior scleritis the pain and redness may be less marked, but there is often proptosis, choroidal effusion, reduced motility, and visual loss. Episcleritis and scleritis should be treated with NSAIDs. If these agents fail, topical or even systemic glucocorticoid therapy may be necessary, especially if an underlying autoimmune process is active.

Uveitis   Involving the anterior structures of the eye, this is also called *iritis* or *iridocyclitis*. The diagnosis requires slit-lamp examination to identify inflammatory cells floating in the aqueous humor or deposited upon the corneal endothelium (keratic precipitates). Anterior uveitis develops in sarcoidosis, ankylosing spondylitis, juvenile rheumatoid arthritis, inflammatory bowel disease, psoriasis, Reiter's syndrome, and Behçet's disease. It is also associated with herpes infections, syphilis, Lyme disease, onchocerciasis, tuberculosis, and leprosy. Although anterior uveitis can occur in conjunction with many diseases, no cause is found to explain the majority of cases. For this reason, laboratory evaluation is usually reserved for patients with recurrent or severe anterior uveitis. Treatment is aimed at reducing inflammation and scarring by judicious use of topical glucocorticoids. Dilation of the pupil reduces pain and prevents the formation of synechiae.

Posterior Uveitis   This is diagnosed by observing inflammation of the vitreous, retina, or choroid on fundus examination. It is more likely than anterior uveitis to be associated with an identifiable systemic disease. Some patients have panuveitis, or inflammation of both the anterior and posterior segments of the eye. Posterior uveitis is a manifestation of autoimmune diseases such as sarcoidosis, Behçet's disease, Vogt-Koyanagi-Harada syndrome, and inflammatory bowel disease (Fig. 29-4). It also accompanies diseases such as toxoplasmosis, onchocerciasis, cysticercosis, coccidioidomycosis, toxocariasis, and histoplasmosis; infections caused by organisms such as *Candida*, *Pneumocystis carinii*, *Cryptococcus*, *Aspergillus*, herpes, and cytomegalovirus (see Fig. 175-1); and other diseases such as syphilis, Lyme disease, tuberculosis, cat-scratch disease, Whipple's disease, and brucellosis. In multiple sclerosis, chronic inflammatory changes can develop in the extreme periphery of the retina (pars planitis or intermediate uveitis).

Acute Angle-Closure Glaucoma   This is a rare and frequently misdiagnosed cause of a red, painful eye. Susceptible eyes have a shallow anterior chamber, either because the eye has a short axial length (hyperopia) or a lens enlarged by the gradual development of cataract. When the pupil becomes mid-dilated, the peripheral iris blocks aqueous outflow via the anterior chamber angle and the intraocular pressure rises

FIGURE 29-4 Retinal vasculitis, uveitis, and hemorrhage in a 32-year-old woman with Crohn's disease. Note that the veins are frosted with a white exudate. Visual acuity improved from 20/400 to 20/20 following treatment with intravenous methylprednisolone.

FIGURE 29-5 Hollenhorst plaque lodged at the bifurcation of a retinal arteriole proves that a patient is shedding emboli from either the carotid artery, great vessels, or heart.

abruptly, producing pain, injection, corneal edema, obscurations, and blurred vision. In some patients, ocular symptoms are overshadowed by nausea, vomiting, or headache, prompting a fruitless workup for abdominal or neurologic disease. The diagnosis is made by measuring the intraocular pressure during an acute attack or by observing a narrow chamber angle by means of a specially mirrored contact lens. Acute angle closure is treated with acetazolamide (PO or IV), topical beta blockers, prostaglandin analogues, α_2-adrenergic agonists, and pilocarpine to induce miosis. If these measures fail, a laser can be used to create a hole in the peripheral iris to relieve pupillary block. Many physicians are reluctant to dilate patients routinely for fundus examination because they fear precipitating an angle-closure glaucoma. The risk is actually remote and more than outweighed by the potential benefit to patients of discovering a hidden fundus lesion visible only through a fully dilated pupil. Moreover, a single attack of angle closure after pharmacologic dilation rarely causes any permanent damage to the eye and serves as an inadvertent provocative test to identify patients with narrow angles who would benefit from prophylactic laser iridectomy.

Endophthalmitis This occurs from bacterial, viral, fungal, or parasitic infection of the internal structures of the eye. It is usually acquired by hematogenous seeding from a remote site. Chronically ill, diabetic, or immunosuppressed patients, especially those with a history of indwelling IV catheters or positive blood cultures, are at greatest risk for endogenous endophthalmitis. Although most patients have ocular pain and injection, visual loss is sometimes the only symptom. Septic emboli, from a diseased heart valve or a dental abscess, that lodge in the retinal circulation can give rise to endophthalmitis. White-centered retinal hemorrhages (Roth's spots) are considered pathognomonic for subacute bacterial endocarditis, but they also appear in leukemia, diabetes, and many other conditions. Endophthalmitis also occurs as a complication of ocular surgery, occasionally months or even years after the operation. An occult penetrating foreign body or unrecognized trauma to the globe should be considered in any patient with unexplained intraocular infection or inflammation.

TRANSIENT OR SUDDEN VISUAL LOSS

Amaurosis Fugax This term refers to a transient ischemic attack of the retina (Chap. 364). Because neural tissue has a high rate of metabolism, interruption of blood flow to the retina for more than a few seconds results in *transient monocular blindness*, a term used interchangeably with amaurosis fugax. Patients describe a rapid fading of vision like a curtain descending, sometimes affecting only a portion of the visual field. Amaurosis fugax usually occurs from an embolus that becomes stuck within a retinal arteriole (Fig. 29-5). If the embolus breaks up or passes, flow is restored and vision returns quickly to normal without per-

manent damage. With prolonged interruption of blood flow, the inner retina suffers infarction. Ophthalmoscopy reveals zones of whitened, edematous retina following the distribution of branch retinal arterioles. Complete occlusion of the central retinal artery produces arrest of blood flow and a milky retina with a cherry-red fovea (Fig. 29-6). Emboli are composed of either cholesterol (Hollenhorst plaque), calcium, or platelet-fibrin debris. The most common source is an atherosclerotic plaque in the carotid artery or aorta, although emboli can also arise from the heart, especially in patients with diseased valves, atrial fibrillation, or wall motion abnormalities.

In rare instances, amaurosis fugax occurs from low central retinal artery perfusion pressure in a patient with a critical stenosis of the ipsilateral carotid artery and poor collateral flow via the circle of Willis. In this situation, amaurosis fugax develops when there is a dip in systemic blood pressure or a slight worsening of the carotid stenosis. Sometimes there is contralateral motor or sensory loss, indicating concomitant hemispheric cerebral ischemia.

Retinal arterial occlusion also occurs rarely in association with retinal migraine, lupus erythematosus, anticardiolipin antibodies (Fig. 29-6), anticoagulant deficiency states (protein S, protein C, and antithrombin III deficiency), pregnancy, IV drug abuse, blood dyscrasias, dysproteinemias, and temporal arteritis.

Marked *systemic hypertension* causes sclerosis of retinal arterioles, splinter hemorrhages, focal infarcts of the nerve fiber layer (cotton-wool spots), and leakage of lipid and fluid (hard exudate) into the macula (Fig. 29-7). In hypertensive crisis, sudden visual loss can result

FIGURE 29-6 Central retinal artery occlusion combined with ischemic optic neuropathy in a 19-year-old woman with an elevated titer of anticardiolipin antibodies. Note the orange dot (rather than cherry red) corresponding to the fovea and the spared patch of retina just temporal to the optic disc.

FIGURE 29-7 Hypertensive retinopathy with scattered flame (splinter) hemorrhages and cotton-wool spots (nerve fiber layer infarcts) in a patient with headache and a blood pressure of 234/120.

FIGURE 29-9 Anterior ischemic optic neuropathy from temporal arteritis in a 78-year-old woman with pallid disc swelling, hemorrhage, visual loss, myalgia, and an erythrocyte sedimentation rate of 86 mm/h.

from vasospasm of retinal arterioles and retinal ischemia. In addition, acute hypertension may produce visual loss from ischemic swelling of the optic disc. Patients with acute hypertensive retinopathy should be treated by lowering the blood pressure. However, the blood pressure should not be reduced precipitously, because there is a danger of optic disc infarction from sudden hypoperfusion.

Impending *branch* or *central retinal vein occlusion* can produce prolonged visual obscurations that resemble those described by patients with amaurosis fugax. The veins appear engorged and phlebitic, with numerous retinal hemorrhages (Fig. 29-8). In some patients, venous blood flow recovers spontaneously, while others evolve a frank obstruction with extensive retinal bleeding ("blood and thunder" appearance), infarction, and visual loss. Venous occlusion of the retina is often idiopathic, but hypertension, diabetes, and glaucoma are prominent risk factors. Polycythemia, thrombocythemia, or other factors leading to an underlying hypercoagulable state should be corrected; aspirin treatment may be beneficial.

Anterior Ischemic Optic Neuropathy (AION) This is caused by insufficient blood flow through the posterior ciliary arteries supplying the optic disc. It produces painless, monocular visual loss that is usually sudden, although some patients have progressive worsening. The optic disc appears swollen and surrounded by nerve fiber layer splinter hemorrhages (Fig. 29-9). AION is divided into two forms: arteritic and nonarteritic. The nonarteritic form of AION is most common. No specific cause can be identified, although diabetes and hypertension are frequent risk factors. No treatment is available. About 5% of patients, especially those over age 60, develop the arteritic form of AION in conjunction with giant cell (temporal) arteritis (Chap. 319). It is urgent to recognize arteritic AION so that high doses of glucocorticoids

can be instituted immediately to prevent blindness in the second eye. Symptoms of polymyalgia rheumatica may be present; the sedimentation rate and C-reactive protein level are usually elevated. In a patient with visual loss from suspected arteritic AION, temporal artery biopsy is mandatory to confirm the diagnosis. Glucocorticoids should be started immediately, without waiting for the biopsy to be completed. The diagnosis of arteritic AION is difficult to sustain in the face of a negative temporal artery biopsy, but such cases do occur rarely.

Posterior Ischemic Optic Neuropathy This is an infrequent cause of acute visual loss, induced by the combination of severe anemia and hypotension. Cases have been reported after major blood loss during surgery, exsanguinating trauma, gastrointestinal bleeding, and renal dialysis. The fundus usually appears normal, although optic disc swelling develops if the process extends far enough anteriorly. Vision can be salvaged in some patients by prompt blood transfusion and reversal of hypotension.

Optic Neuritis This is a common inflammatory disease of the optic nerve. In the Optic Neuritis Treatment Trial (ONTT), the mean age of patients was 32 years, 77% were female, 92% had ocular pain (especially with eye movements), and 35% had optic disc swelling. In most patients, the demyelinating event was retrobulbar and the ocular fundus appeared normal on initial examination (Fig. 29-10), although optic disc pallor slowly developed over subsequent months.

Virtually all patients experience a gradual recovery of vision after a single episode of optic neuritis, even without treatment. This rule is so reliable that failure of vision to improve after a first attack of optic

FIGURE 29-8 Central retinal vein occlusion can produce massive retinal hemorrhage ("blood and thunder"), ischemia, and vision loss.

FIGURE 29-10 Retrobulbar optic neuritis is characterized by a normal fundus examination initially, hence the rubric, "the doctor sees nothing, and the patient sees nothing." Optic atrophy develops after severe or repeated attacks.

neuritis casts doubt upon the original diagnosis. Treatment with high-dose IV methylprednisolone (250 mg every 6 h for 3 days) followed by oral prednisone (1 mg/kg per day for 11 days) makes no difference in final acuity (measured 6 months after the attack), but the recovery of visual function occurs more rapidly.

For some patients, optic neuritis remains an isolated event. However, the ONTT showed that the 10-year cumulative probability of developing clinically definite multiple sclerosis following optic neuritis is 38%. In patients with two or more demyelinating plaques on brain magnetic resonance (MR) imaging, treatment with interferon beta-1a can retard the development of more lesions. In summary, an MR scan is recommended in every patient with a first attack of optic neuritis. When visual loss is severe (worse than 20/100), treatment with intravenous followed by oral glucocorticoids hastens recovery. If multiple lesions are present on the MR scan, treatment with interferon β-1a should be considered.

Leber's Hereditary Optic Neuropathy

This disease usually affects young men, causing gradual, painless, severe, central visual loss in one eye, followed weeks or months later by the same process in the other eye. Acutely, the optic disc appears mildly plethoric with surface capillary telangiectases, but no vascular leakage on fluorescein angiography. Eventually optic atrophy ensues. Leber's optic neuropathy is caused by a point mutation at codon 11778 in the mitochondrial gene encoding nicotinamide adenine dinucleotide dehydrogenase (NADH) subunit 4. Additional mutations responsible for the disease have been identified, most in mitochondrial genes encoding proteins involved in electron transport. Mitochondrial mutations causing Leber's neuropathy are inherited from the mother by all her children, but usually only sons develop symptoms. There is no treatment.

Toxic Optic Neuropathy

This can result in acute visual loss with bilateral optic disc swelling and central or cecocentral scotomas. Such cases have been reported to result from exposure to ethambutol, methyl alcohol (moonshine), ethylene glycol (antifreeze), or carbon monoxide. In toxic optic neuropathy, visual loss can also develop gradually and produce optic atrophy (Fig. 29-11) without a phase of acute optic disc edema. Many agents have been implicated as a cause of toxic optic neuropathy, but the evidence supporting the association for many is weak. The following is a partial list of potential offending drugs or toxins: disulfiram, ethchlorvynol, chloramphenicol, amiodarone, monoclonal anti-CD3 antibody, ciprofloxacin, digitalis, streptomycin, lead, arsenic, thallium, D-penicillamine, isoniazid, emetine, and sulfonamides. Deficiency states, induced either by starvation, malabsorption, or alcoholism, can lead to insidious visual loss. Thiamine, vitamin B_{12}, and folate levels should be checked in any patient with unexplained, bilateral central scotomas and optic pallor.

FIGURE 29-11 Optic atrophy is not a specific diagnosis, but refers to the combination of optic disc pallor, arteriolar narrowing, and nerve fiber layer destruction produced by a host of eye diseases, especially optic neuropathies.

FIGURE 29-12 Papilledema means optic disc edema from raised intracranial pressure. This obese young woman with pseudotumor cerebri was misdiagnosed as a migraineur until fundus examination was performed, showing optic disc elevation, hemorrhages, and cotton-wool spots.

Papilledema

This connotes bilateral optic disc swelling from raised intracranial pressure (Fig. 29-12). Headache is a frequent, but not invariable, accompaniment. All other forms of optic disc swelling, e.g., from optic neuritis or ischemic optic neuropathy, should be called "optic disc edema." This convention is arbitrary but serves to avoid confusion. Often it is difficult to differentiate papilledema from other forms of optic disc edema by fundus examination alone. Transient visual obscurations are a classic symptom of papilledema. They can occur in only one eye or simultaneously in both eyes. They usually last seconds but can persist longer. Obscurations follow abrupt shifts in posture or happen spontaneously. When obscurations are prolonged or spontaneous, the papilledema is more threatening. Visual acuity is not affected by papilledema unless the papilledema is severe, long-standing, or accompanied by macular edema and hemorrhage. Visual field testing shows enlarged blind spots and peripheral constriction (Fig. 29-3F). With unremitting papilledema, peripheral visual field loss progresses in an insidious fashion while the optic nerve develops atrophy. In this setting, reduction of optic disc swelling is an ominous sign of a dying nerve rather than an encouraging indication of resolving papilledema.

Evaluation of papilledema requires neuroimaging to exclude an intracranial lesion. MR angiography is appropriate in selected cases to search for a dural venous sinus occlusion or an arteriovenous shunt. If neuroradiologic studies are negative, the subarachnoid opening pressure should be measured by lumbar puncture. An elevated pressure, with normal cerebrospinal fluid, points by exclusion to the diagnosis of *pseudotumor cerebri* (idiopathic intracranial hypertension). The majority of patients are young, female, and obese. Treatment with a carbonic anhydrase inhibitor such as acetazolamide lowers intracranial pressure by reducing the production of cerebrospinal fluid. Weight reduction is vital but often unsuccessful. If acetazolamide and weight loss fail, and visual field loss is progressive, a shunt should be performed without delay to prevent blindness. Occasionally, emergency surgery is required for sudden blindness caused by fulminant papilledema.

Optic Disc Drusen

These are refractile deposits within the substance of the optic nerve head (Fig. 29-13). They are unrelated to drusen of the retina, which occur in age-related macular degeneration. Optic disc drusen are most common in people of northern European descent. Their diagnosis is obvious when they are visible as glittering particles upon the surface of the optic disc. However, in many patients they are hidden beneath the surface, producing pseudo-papilledema. It is important to recognize optic disc drusen to avoid an unnecessary evaluation for papilledema. Ultrasound or CT scanning is sensitive for detection of buried optic disc drusen because they contain calcium. In most patients, optic disc drusen are an incidental, innocuous finding, but they can produce visual obscurations. On perimetry they give rise

FIGURE 29-13 Optic disc drusen are calcified deposits of unknown etiology within the optic disc. They are sometimes confused with papilledema.

FIGURE 29-14 Retinal detachment appears as an elevated sheet of retinal tissue with folds. In this patient the fovea was spared, so acuity was normal, but a superior detachment produced an inferior scotoma.

to enlarged blind spots and arcuate scotomas from damage to the optic disc. With increasing age, drusen tend to become more exposed on the disc surface as optic atrophy develops. Hemorrhage, choroidal neovascular membrane, and AION are more likely to occur in patients with optic disc drusen. No treatment is available.

Vitreous Degeneration This occurs in all individuals with advancing age, leading to visual symptoms. Opacities develop in the vitreous, casting annoying shadows upon the retina. As the eye moves, these distracting "floaters" move synchronously, with a slight lag caused by inertia of the vitreous gel. Vitreous traction upon the retina causes mechanical stimulation, resulting in perception of flashing lights. This photopsia is brief and confined to one eye, in contrast to the bilateral, prolonged scintillations of cortical migraine. Contraction of the vitreous can result in sudden separation from the retina, heralded by an alarming shower of floaters and photopsia. This process, known as *vitreous detachment*, is a frequent involutional event in the elderly. It is not harmful unless it damages the retina. A careful examination of the dilated fundus is important in any patient complaining of floaters or photopsia to search for peripheral tears or holes. If such a lesion is found, laser application can forestall a retinal detachment. Occasionally a tear ruptures a retinal blood vessel, causing vitreous hemorrhage and sudden loss of vision. On attempted ophthalmoscopy the fundus is hidden by a dark red haze of blood. Ultrasound is required to examine the interior of the eye for a retinal tear or detachment. If the hemorrhage does not resolve spontaneously, the vitreous can be removed surgically. Vitreous hemorrhage also occurs from the fragile neovascular vessels that proliferate on the surface of the retina in diabetes, sickle cell anemia, and other ischemic ocular diseases.

Retinal Detachment This produces symptoms of floaters, flashing lights, and a scotoma in the peripheral visual field corresponding to the detachment (Fig. 29-14). If the detachment includes the fovea, there is an afferent pupil defect and the visual acuity is reduced. In most eyes, retinal detachment starts with a hole, flap, or tear in the peripheral retina (rhegmatogenous retinal detachment). Patients with peripheral retinal thinning (lattice degeneration) are particularly vulnerable to this process. Once a break has developed in the retina, liquified vitreous is free to enter the subretinal space, separating the retina from the pigment epithelium. The combination of vitreous traction upon the retinal surface and passage of fluid behind the retina leads inexorably to detachment. Patients with a history of myopia, trauma, or prior cataract extraction are at greatest risk for retinal detachment. The diagnosis is confirmed by ophthalmoscopic examination of the dilated eye.

Classic Migraine (See also Chap. 15) This usually occurs with a visual aura lasting about 20 min. In a typical attack, a small central disturbance in the field of vision marches toward the periphery, leaving a transient scotoma in its wake. The expanding border of migraine sco-

toma has a scintillating, dancing, or zig-zag edge, resembling the bastions of a fortified city, hence the term *fortification spectra*. Patients' descriptions of fortification spectra vary widely and can be confused with amaurosis fugax. Migraine patterns usually last longer and are perceived in both eyes, whereas amaurosis fugax is briefer and occurs in only one eye. Migraine phenomena also remain visible in the dark or with the eyes closed. Generally they are confined to either the right or left visual hemifield, but sometimes both fields are involved simultaneously. Patients often have a long history of stereotypic attacks. After the visual symptoms recede, headache develops in most patients.

Transient Ischemic Attacks Vertebrobasilar insufficiency may result in acute homonymous visual symptoms. Many patients mistakenly describe symptoms in their left or right eye, when in fact they are occurring in the left or right hemifield of both eyes. Interruption of blood supply to the visual cortex causes a sudden fogging or graying of vision, occasionally with flashing lights or other positive phenomena that mimic migraine. Cortical ischemic attacks are briefer in duration than migraine, occur in older patients, and are not followed by headache. There may be associated signs of brainstem ischemia, such as diplopia, vertigo, numbness, weakness, or dysarthria.

Stroke This occurs when interruption of blood supply from the posterior cerebral artery to the visual cortex is prolonged. The only finding on examination is a homonymous visual field defect that stops abruptly at the vertical meridian. Occipital lobe stroke is usually due to thrombotic occlusion of the vertebrobasilar system, embolus, or dissection. Lobar hemorrhage, tumor, abscess, and arteriovenous malformation are other common causes of hemianopic cortical visual loss.

Factitious (Functional, Nonorganic) Visual Loss This is claimed by hysterics or malingerers. The latter comprise the vast majority, seeking sympathy, special treatment, or financial gain by feigning loss of sight. The diagnosis is suspected when the history is atypical, physical findings are lacking or contradictory, inconsistencies emerge on testing, and a secondary motive can be identified. In our litigious society, the fraudulent pursuit of recompense has spawned an epidemic of factitious visual loss.

CHRONIC VISUAL LOSS

Cataract This is a clouding of the lens sufficient to reduce vision. Most cataracts develop slowly as a result of aging, leading to gradual impairment of vision. The formation of cataract occurs more rapidly in patients with a history of ocular trauma, uveitis, or diabetes mellitus. Cataracts are acquired in a variety of genetic diseases, such as myotonic dystrophy, neurofibromatosis type 2, and galactosemia. Radiation therapy and glucocorticoid treatment can induce cataract as a side effect. The cataracts associated with radiation or glucocorticoids have a typical posterior subcapsular location. Cataract can be detected by noting an impaired red reflex when viewing light reflected from the fundus with an ophthalmoscope or by examining the dilated eye using the slit lamp.

The only treatment for cataract is surgical extraction of the opacified lens. Over a million cataract operations are performed each year in the United States. The operation is generally done under local anesthesia on an outpatient basis. A plastic or silicone intraocular lens is placed within the empty lens capsule in the posterior chamber, substituting for the natural lens and leading to rapid recovery of sight. More than 95% of patients who undergo cataract extraction can expect an improvement in vision. In some patients, the lens capsule remaining in the eye after cataract extraction eventually turns cloudy, causing secondary loss of vision. A small opening is made in the lens capsule with a laser to restore clarity.

Glaucoma   This is a slowly progressive, insidious optic neuropathy, usually associated with chronic elevation of intraocular pressure. In Americans of African descent it is the leading cause of blindness. The mechanism whereby raised intraocular pressure injures the optic nerve is not understood. Axons entering the inferotemporal and superotemporal aspects of the optic disc are damaged first, producing typical nerve fiber bundle or arcuate scotomas on perimetric testing. As fibers are destroyed, the neural rim of the optic disc shrinks and the physiologic cup within the optic disc enlarges (Fig. 29-15). This process is referred to as pathologic "cupping." The cup-to-disc diameter is expressed as a ratio, e.g., 0.2/1. The cup-to-disc ratio ranges widely in normal individuals, making it difficult to diagnose glaucoma reliably simply by observing an unusually large or deep optic cup. Careful documentation of serial examinations is helpful. In the patient with physiologic cupping, the large cup remains stable, whereas in the patient with glaucoma it expands relentlessly over the years. Detection of visual field loss by computerized perimetry also contributes to the diagnosis. Finally, most patients with glaucoma have raised intraocular pressure. However, many patients with typical glaucomatous cupping and visual field loss have intraocular pressures that apparently never exceed the normal limit of 20 mmHg (so-called low-tension glaucoma).

In acute angle-closure glaucoma, the eye is red and painful due to abrupt, severe elevation of intraocular pressure. Such cases account for only a minority of glaucoma cases: most patients have open, anterior chamber angles. The cause of raised intraocular pressure in open angle glaucoma is unknown, but it is associated with gene mutations in the heritable forms.

Glaucoma is usually painless (except in angle-closure glaucoma). Foveal acuity is spared until end-stage disease is reached. For these reasons, severe and irreversible damage can occur before either the patient or physician recognizes the diagnosis. Screening of patients for glaucoma by noting the cup-to-disc ratio on ophthalmoscopy and by measuring intraocular pressure is vital. Glaucoma is treated with topical adrenergic agonists, cholinergic agonists, beta blockers, and prostaglandin analogues. Occasionally, systemic absorption of beta blocker from

FIGURE 29-15 Glaucoma results in "cupping" as the neural rim is destroyed and the central cup becomes enlarged and excavated. The cup-to-disc ratio is about 0.7/1.0 in this patient.

FIGURE 29-16 Age-related macular degeneration begins with the accumulation of drusen within the macula. They appear as scattered yellow subretinal deposits.

eye drops can be sufficient to cause side effects of bradycardia, hypotension, heart block, bronchospasm, or depression. Topical or oral carbonic anhydrase inhibitors are used to lower intraocular pressure by reducing aqueous production. Laser treatment of the trabecular meshwork in the anterior chamber angle improves aqueous outflow from the eye. If medical or laser treatments fail to halt optic nerve damage from glaucoma, a filter must be constructed surgically (trabeculectomy) or a valve placed to release aqueous from the eye in a controlled fashion.

Macular Degeneration   This is a major cause of gradual, painless, bilateral central visual loss in the elderly. The old term, "senile macular degeneration," misinterpreted by many patients as an unflattering reference, has been replaced with "age-related macular degeneration." It occurs in a nonexudative (dry) form and an exudative (wet) form. Inflammation may be important in both forms of macular degeneration; recent genetic data indicates that susceptibility is associated with variants in the gene for complement factor H, an inhibitor of the alternative complement pathway. The nonexudative process begins with the accumulation of extracellular deposits, called drusen, underneath the retinal pigment epithelium. On ophthalmoscopy, they are pleomorphic but generally appear as small discrete yellow lesions clustered in the macula (Fig. 29-16). With time they become larger, more numerous, and confluent. The retinal pigment epithelium becomes focally detached and atrophic, causing visual loss by interfering with photoreceptor function. Treatment with vitamins C and E, beta carotene, and zinc may retard dry macular degeneration.

Exudative macular degeneration, which develops in only a minority of patients, occurs when neovascular vessels from the choroid grow through defects in Bruch's membrane into the potential space beneath the retinal pigment epithelium. Leakage from these vessels produces elevation of the retina and pigment epithelium, with distortion (metamorphopsia) and blurring of vision. Although onset of these symptoms is usually gradual, bleeding from subretinal choroidal neovascular membranes sometimes causes acute visual loss. The neovascular membranes can be difficult to see on fundus examination because they are beneath the retina. Fluorescein or indocyanine green angiography is extremely useful for their detection. Neovascular membranes are treated with either photodynamic therapy or intraocular injection of vascular endothelial growth factor antagonists. Surgical attempts to remove subretinal membranes in age-related macular degeneration have not improved vision in most patients. However, outcomes have been more encouraging for patients with choroidal neovascular membranes from ocular histoplasmosis syndrome.

Major or repeated hemorrhage under the retina from neovascular membranes results in fibrosis, development of a round (disciform) macular scar, and permanent loss of central vision.

Central Serous Chorioretinopathy   This primarily affects males between the ages of 20 and 50. Leakage of serous fluid from the choroid causes small, localized detachment of the retinal pigment epithelium and the neurosensory retina. These detachments produce acute or chronic symptoms of metamorphopsia and blurred vision when the macula is involved. They are difficult to visualize with a direct ophthalmoscope because the detached retina is transparent and only slightly elevated. Diagnosis of central serous chorioretinopathy is made easily by fluorescein angiography, which shows dye streaming into the subretinal space. The cause of central serous chorioretinopathy is unknown. Symptoms may resolve spontaneously if the retina reattaches, but recurrent detachment is common. Laser photocoagulation has benefited some patients with this condition.

Diabetic Retinopathy A rare disease until 1921, when the discovery of insulin resulted in a dramatic improvement in life expectancy for patients with diabetes mellitus, it is now a leading cause of blindness in the United States. The retinopathy of diabetes takes years to develop but eventually appears in nearly all cases. Regular surveillance of the dilated fundus is crucial for any patient with diabetes. In advanced diabetic retinopathy, the proliferation of neovascular vessels leads to blindness from vitreous hemorrhage, retinal detachment, and glaucoma (see Fig. 338-9). These complications can be avoided in most patients by administration of panretinal laser photocoagulation at the appropriate point in the evolution of the disease. For further discussion of the manifestations and management of diabetic retinopathy, see Chap. 338.

Retinitis Pigmentosa This is a general term for a disparate group of rod and cone dystrophies characterized by progressive night blindness, visual field constriction with a ring scotoma, loss of acuity, and an abnormal electroretinogram (ERG). It occurs sporadically or in an autosomal recessive, dominant, or X-linked pattern. Irregular black deposits of clumped pigment in the peripheral retina, called *bone spicules* because of their vague resemblance to the spicules of cancellous bone, give the disease its name (Fig. 29-17). The name is actually a misnomer because retinitis pigmentosa is not an inflammatory process. Most cases are due to a mutation in the gene for rhodopsin, the rod photopigment, or in the gene for peripherin, a glycoprotein located in photoreceptor outer segments. Vitamin A (15,000 IU/day) slightly retards the deterioration of the ERG in patients with retinitis pigmentosa but has no beneficial effect on visual acuity or fields. Some forms of retinitis pigmentosa occur in association with rare, hereditary systemic diseases (olivopontocerebellar degeneration, Bassen-Kornzweig disease, Kearns-Sayre syndrome, Refsum's disease). Chronic treatment with chloroquine, hydroxychloroquine, and phenothiazines (especially thioridazine) can produce visual loss from a toxic retinopathy that resembles retinitis pigmentosa.

Epiretinal Membrane This is a fibrocellular tissue that grows across the inner surface of the retina, causing metamorphopsia and reduced visual

FIGURE 29-17 Retinitis pigmentosa with black clumps of pigment in the retinal periphery known as "bone spicules." There is also atrophy of the retinal pigment epithelium, making the vasculature of the choroid easily visible.

FIGURE 29-18 Melanoma of the choroid, appearing as an elevated dark mass in the inferior temporal fundus, just encroaching upon the fovea.

acuity from distortion of the macula. A crinkled, cellophane-like membrane is visible on the retinal examination. Epiretinal membrane is most common in patients over 50 years of age and is usually unilateral. Most cases are idiopathic, but some occur as a result of hypertensive retinopathy, diabetes, retinal detachment, or trauma. When visual acuity is reduced to the level of about 6/24 (20/80), vitrectomy and surgical peeling of the membrane to relieve macular puckering are recommended. Contraction of an epiretinal membrane sometimes gives rise to a *macular hole*. Most macular holes, however, are caused by local vitreous traction within the fovea. Vitrectomy can improve acuity in selected cases.

Melanoma and Other Tumors Melanoma is the most common primary tumor of the eye (Fig. 29-18). It causes photopsia, an enlarging scotoma, and loss of vision. A small melanoma is often difficult to differentiate from a benign choroidal nevus. Serial examinations are required to document a malignant pattern of growth. Treatment of melanoma is controversial. Options include enucleation, local resection, and irradiation. *Metastatic tumors* to the eye outnumber primary tumors. Breast and lung carcinoma have a special propensity to spread to the choroid or iris. Leukemia and lymphoma also commonly invade ocular tissues. Sometimes their only sign on eye examination is cellular debris in the vitreous, which can masquerade as a chronic posterior uveitis. *Retrobulbar tumor* of the optic nerve (meningioma, glioma) or *chiasmal tumor* (pituitary adenoma, meningioma) produces gradual visual loss with few objective findings, except for optic disc pallor. Rarely, sudden expansion of a pituitary adenoma from infarction and bleeding (*pituitary apoplexy*) causes acute retrobulbar visual loss, with headache, nausea, and ocular motor nerve palsies. In any patient with visual field loss or optic atrophy, CT or MR scanning should be considered if the cause remains unknown after careful review of the history and thorough examination of the eye.

PROPTOSIS

When the globes appear asymmetric, the clinician must first decide which eye is abnormal. Is one eye recessed within the orbit (*enophthalmos*) or is the other eye protuberant (*exophthalmos*, or *proptosis*)? A small globe or a Horner's syndrome can give the appearance of enophthalmos. True enophthalmos occurs commonly after trauma, from atrophy of retrobulbar fat, or fracture of the orbital floor. The position of the eyes within the orbits is measured using a Hertel exophthalmometer, a hand-held instrument that records the position of the anterior corneal surface relative to the lateral orbital rim. If this instrument is not available, relative eye position can be judged by bending the patient's head forward and looking down upon the orbits. A proptosis of only 2 mm in one eye is detectable from this perspective. The development of proptosis implies a space-occupying lesion in the orbit, and usually warrants CT or MR imaging.

Graves' Ophthalmopathy This is the leading cause of proptosis in adults (Chap. 335). The proptosis is often asymmetric and can even appear to be unilateral. Orbital inflammation and engorgement of the extraocular muscles, particularly the medial rectus and the inferior rectus, account for the protrusion of the globe. Corneal exposure, lid retraction, conjunctival injection, restriction of gaze, diplopia, and visual loss from optic nerve compression are cardinal symptoms. Graves' ophthalmopathy is treated with oral prednisone (60 mg/d) for 1 month, followed by a taper over several months, topical lubricants, eyelid surgery, eye muscle surgery, or orbital decompression. Radiation therapy is not effective.

Orbital Pseudotumor   This is an idiopathic, inflammatory orbital syndrome, frequently confused with Graves' ophthalmopathy. Symptoms are pain, limited eye movements, proptosis, and congestion. Evaluation for sarcoidosis, Wegener's granulomatosis, and other types of orbital vasculitis or collagen-vascular disease is negative. Imaging often shows swollen eye muscles (orbital myositis) with enlarged tendons. By contrast, in Graves' ophthalmopathy the tendons of the eye muscles are usually spared. The Tolosa-Hunt syndrome may be regarded as an extension of orbital pseudotumor through the superior orbital fissure into the cavernous sinus. The diagnosis of orbital pseudotumor is difficult. Biopsy of the orbit frequently yields nonspecific evidence of fat infiltration by lymphocytes, plasma cells, and eosinophils. A dramatic response to a therapeutic trial of systemic glucocorticoids indirectly provides the best confirmation of the diagnosis.

Orbital Cellulitis   This causes pain, lid erythema, proptosis, conjunctival chemosis, restricted motility, decreased acuity, afferent pupillary defect, fever, and leukocytosis. It often arises from the paranasal sinuses, especially by contiguous spread of infection from the ethmoid sinus through the lamina papyracea of the medial orbit. A history of recent upper respiratory tract infection, chronic sinusitis, thick mucous secretions, or dental disease is significant in any patient with suspected orbital cellulitis. Blood cultures should be obtained, but they are usually negative. Most patients respond to empirical therapy with broad-spectrum IV antibiotics. Occasionally, orbital cellulitis follows an overwhelming course, with massive proptosis, blindness, septic cavernous sinus thrombosis, and meningitis. To avert this disaster, orbital cellulitis should be managed aggressively in the early stages, with immediate imaging of the orbits and antibiotic therapy that includes coverage of methicillin-resistant *Staphylococcus aureus*. Prompt surgical drainage of an orbital abscess or paranasal sinusitis is indicated if optic nerve function deteriorates despite antibiotics.

Tumors   Tumors of the orbit cause painless, progressive proptosis. The most common primary tumors are hemangioma, lymphangioma, neurofibroma, dermoid cyst, adenoid cystic carcinoma, optic nerve glioma, optic nerve meningioma, and benign mixed tumor of the lacrimal gland. Metastatic tumor to the orbit occurs frequently in breast carcinoma, lung carcinoma, and lymphoma. Diagnosis by fine-needle aspiration followed by urgent radiation therapy can sometimes preserve vision.

Carotid Cavernous Fistulas   With anterior drainage through the orbit these produce proptosis, diplopia, glaucoma, and corkscrew, arterialized conjunctival vessels. Direct fistulas usually result from trauma. They are easily diagnosed because of the prominent signs produced by high-flow, high-pressure shunting. Indirect fistulas, or dural arteriovenous malformations, are more likely to occur spontaneously, especially in older women. The signs are more subtle and the diagnosis is frequently missed. The combination of slight proptosis, diplopia, enlarged muscles, and an injected eye is often mistaken for thyroid ophthalmopathy. A bruit heard upon auscultation of the head, or reported by the patient, is a valuable diagnostic clue. Imaging shows an enlarged superior ophthalmic vein in the orbits. Carotid cavernous shunts can be eliminated by intravascular embolization.

PTOSIS
Blepharoptosis   This is an abnormal drooping of the eyelid. Unilateral or bilateral ptosis can be congenital, from dysgenesis of the levator palpebrae superioris, or from abnormal insertion of its aponeurosis into the eyelid. Acquired ptosis can develop so gradually that the patient is unaware of the problem. Inspection of old photographs is helpful in dating the onset. A history of prior trauma, eye surgery, contact lens use, diplopia, systemic symptoms (e.g., dysphagia or peripheral muscle weakness), or a family history of ptosis should be sought. Fluctuating ptosis that worsens late in the day is typical of myasthenia gravis. Examination should focus upon evidence for proptosis, eyelid masses or deformities, inflammation, pupil inequality, or limitation of motility. The width of the palpebral fissures is measured in primary gaze to quantitate the degree of ptosis. The ptosis will be underestimated if the patient compensates by lifting the brow with the frontalis muscle.

Mechanical Ptosis   This occurs in many elderly patients from stretching and redundancy of eyelid skin and subcutaneous fat (dermatochalasis). The extra weight of these sagging tissues causes the lid to droop. Enlargement or deformation of the eyelid from infection, tumor, trauma, or inflammation also results in ptosis on a purely mechanical basis.

Aponeurotic Ptosis   This is an acquired dehiscence or stretching of the aponeurotic tendon, which connects the levator muscle to the tarsal plate of the eyelid. It occurs commonly in older patients, presumably from loss of connective tissue elasticity. Aponeurotic ptosis is also a frequent sequela of eyelid swelling from infection or blunt trauma to the orbit, cataract surgery, or hard contact lens usage.

Myogenic Ptosis   The causes of *myogenic ptosis* include myasthenia gravis (Chap. 381) and a number of rare myopathies that manifest with ptosis. The term *chronic progressive external ophthalmoplegia* refers to a spectrum of systemic diseases caused by mutations of mitochondrial DNA. As the name implies, the most prominent findings are symmetric, slowly progressive ptosis and limitation of eye movements. In general, diplopia is a late symptom because all eye movements are reduced equally. In the *Kearns-Sayre* variant, retinal pigmentary changes and abnormalities of cardiac conduction develop. Peripheral muscle biopsy shows characteristic "ragged-red fibers." *Oculopharyngeal dystrophy* is a distinct autosomal dominant disease with onset in middle age, characterized by ptosis, limited eye movements, and trouble swallowing. *Myotonic dystrophy*, another autosomal dominant disorder, causes ptosis, ophthalmoparesis, cataract, and pigmentary retinopathy. Patients have muscle wasting, myotonia, frontal balding, and cardiac abnormalities.

Neurogenic Ptosis   This results from a lesion affecting the innervation to either of the two muscles that open the eyelid: Müller's muscle or the levator palpebrae superioris. Examination of the pupil helps to distinguish between these two possibilities. In Horner's syndrome, the eye with ptosis has a smaller pupil and the eye movements are full. In an oculomotor nerve palsy, the eye with the ptosis has a larger, or a normal, pupil. If the pupil is normal but there is limitation of adduction, elevation, and depression, a pupil-sparing oculomotor nerve palsy is likely (see next section). Rarely, a lesion affecting the small, central subnucleus of the oculomotor complex will cause bilateral ptosis with normal eye movements and pupils.

DOUBLE VISION (DIPLOPIA)
The first point to clarify is whether diplopia persists in either eye after covering the opposite eye. If it does, the diagnosis is monocular diplopia. The cause is usually intrinsic to the eye and therefore has no dire implications for the patient. Corneal aberrations (e.g., keratoconus, pterygium), uncorrected refractive error, cataract, or foveal traction may give rise to monocular diplopia. Occasionally it is a symptom of malingering or psychiatric disease. Diplopia alleviated by covering one eye is binocular diplopia and is caused by disruption of ocular alignment. Inquiry should be made into the nature of the double vision (purely side-by-side versus partial vertical displacement of images), mode of onset, duration, intermittency, diurnal variation, and associ-

ated neurologic or systemic symptoms. If the patient has diplopia while being examined, motility testing should reveal a deficiency corresponding to the patient's symptoms. However, subtle limitation of ocular excursions is often difficult to detect. For example, a patient with a slight left abducens nerve paresis may appear to have full eye movements, despite a complaint of horizontal diplopia upon looking to the left. In this situation, the cover test provides a more sensitive method for demonstrating the ocular misalignment. It should be conducted in primary gaze, and then with the head turned and tilted in each direction. In the above example, a cover test with the head turned to the right will maximize the fixation shift evoked by the cover test.

Occasionally, a cover test performed in an asymptomatic patient during a routine examination will reveal an ocular deviation. If the eye movements are full and the ocular misalignment is equal in all directions of gaze (concomitant deviation), the diagnosis is strabismus. In this condition, which affects about 1% of the population, fusion is disrupted in infancy or early childhood. To avoid diplopia, vision is suppressed from the nonfixating eye. In some children, this leads to impaired vision (amblyopia, or "lazy" eye) in the deviated eye.

Binocular diplopia occurs from a wide range of processes: infectious, neoplastic, metabolic, degenerative, inflammatory, and vascular. One must decide if the diplopia is neurogenic in origin or due to restriction of globe rotation by local disease in the orbit. Orbital pseudotumor, myositis, infection, tumor, thyroid disease, and muscle entrapment (e.g., from a blowout fracture) cause restrictive diplopia. The diagnosis of restriction is usually made by recognizing other associated signs and symptoms of local orbital disease in conjunction with imaging.

Myasthenia Gravis (See also Chap. 381) This is a major cause of diplopia. The diplopia is often intermittent, variable, and not confined to any single ocular motor nerve distribution. The pupils are always normal. Fluctuating ptosis may be present. Many patients have a purely ocular form of the disease, with no evidence of systemic muscular weakness. The diagnosis can be confirmed by an IV edrophonium injection or by an assay for antiacetylcholine receptor antibodies. Negative results from these tests do not exclude the diagnosis. *Botulism* from food or wound poisoning can mimic ocular myasthenia.

After restrictive orbital disease and myasthenia gravis are excluded, a lesion of a cranial nerve supplying innervation to the extraocular muscles is the most likely cause of binocular diplopia.

Oculomotor Nerve The third cranial nerve innervates the medial, inferior, and superior recti; inferior oblique; levator palpebrae superioris; and the iris sphincter. Total palsy of the oculomotor nerve causes ptosis, a dilated pupil, and leaves the eye "down and out" because of the unopposed action of the lateral rectus and superior oblique. This combination of findings is obvious. More challenging is the diagnosis of early or partial oculomotor nerve palsy. In this setting, any combination of ptosis, pupil dilation, and weakness of the eye muscles supplied by the oculomotor nerve may be encountered. Frequent serial examinations during the evolving phase of the palsy help ensure that the diagnosis is not missed. The advent of an oculomotor nerve palsy with a pupil involvement, especially when accompanied by pain, suggests a compressive lesion, such as a tumor or circle of Willis aneurysm. Neuroimaging should be obtained, along with a CT or MR angiogram. Occasionally, a catheter arteriogram must be done to exclude an aneurysm.

A lesion of the oculomotor nucleus in the rostral midbrain produces signs that differ from those caused by a lesion of the nerve itself. There is bilateral ptosis because the levator muscle is innervated by a single central subnucleus. There is also weakness of the contralateral superior rectus, because it is supplied by the oculomotor nucleus on the other side. Occasionally both superior recti are weak. Isolated nuclear oculomotor palsy is rare. Usually neurologic examination reveals additional signs to suggest brainstem damage from infarction, hemorrhage, tumor, or infection.

Injury to structures surrounding fascicles of the oculomotor nerve descending through the midbrain has given rise to a number of classic eponymic designations. In *Nothnagel's syndrome*, injury to the superior cerebellar peduncle causes ipsilateral oculomotor palsy and contralateral cerebellar ataxia. In *Benedikt's syndrome*, injury to the red nucleus results in ipsilateral oculomotor palsy and contralateral tremor, chorea, and athetosis. *Claude's syndrome* incorporates features of both the aforementioned syndromes, by injury to both the red nucleus and the superior cerebellar peduncle. Finally, in *Weber's syndrome*, injury to the cerebral peduncle causes ipsilateral oculomotor palsy with contralateral hemiparesis.

In the subarachnoid space the oculomotor nerve is vulnerable to aneurysm, meningitis, tumor, infarction, and compression. In cerebral herniation the nerve becomes trapped between the edge of the tentorium and the uncus of the temporal lobe. Oculomotor palsy can also occur from midbrain torsion and hemorrhages during herniation. In the cavernous sinus, oculomotor palsy arises from carotid aneurysm, carotid cavernous fistula, cavernous sinus thrombosis, tumor (pituitary adenoma, meningioma, metastasis), herpes zoster infection, and the Tolosa-Hunt syndrome.

The etiology of an isolated, pupil-sparing oculomotor palsy often remains an enigma, even after neuroimaging and extensive laboratory testing. Most cases are thought to result from microvascular infarction of the nerve, somewhere along its course from the brainstem to the orbit. Usually the patient complains of pain. Diabetes, hypertension, and vascular disease are major risk factors. Spontaneous recovery over a period of months is the rule. If this fails to occur, or if new findings develop, the diagnosis of microvascular oculomotor nerve palsy should be reconsidered. Aberrant regeneration is common when the oculomotor nerve is injured by trauma or compression (tumor, aneurysm). Miswiring of sprouting fibers to the levator muscle and the rectus muscles results in elevation of the eyelid upon downgaze or adduction. The pupil also constricts upon attempted adduction, elevation, or depression of the globe. Aberrant regeneration is not seen after oculomotor palsy from microvascular infarct and hence vitiates that diagnosis.

Trochlear Nerve The fourth cranial nerve originates in the midbrain, just caudal to the oculomotor nerve complex. Fibers exit the brainstem dorsally and cross to innervate the contralateral superior oblique. The principal actions of this muscle are to depress and to intort the globe. A palsy therefore results in hypertropia and excyclotorsion. The cyclotorsion is seldom noticed by patients. Instead, they complain of vertical diplopia, especially upon reading or looking down. The vertical diplopia is also exacerbated by tilting the head toward the side with the muscle palsy, and alleviated by tilting it away. This "head tilt test" is a cardinal diagnostic feature.

Isolated trochlear nerve palsy occurs from all the causes listed above for the oculomotor nerve, except aneurysm. The trochlear nerve is particularly apt to suffer injury after closed head trauma. The free edge of the tentorium is thought to impinge upon the nerve during a concussive blow. Most isolated trochlear nerve palsies are idiopathic and hence diagnosed by exclusion as "microvascular." Spontaneous improvement occurs over a period of months in most patients. A base-down prism (conveniently applied to the patient's glasses as a stick-on Fresnel lens) may serve as a temporary measure to alleviate diplopia. If the palsy does not resolve, the eyes can be realigned by weakening the inferior oblique muscle.

Abducens Nerve The sixth cranial nerve innervates the lateral rectus muscle. A palsy produces horizontal diplopia, worse on gaze to the side of the lesion. A nuclear lesion has different consequences, because the abducens nucleus contains interneurons that project via the medial longitudinal fasciculus to the medial rectus subnucleus of the contralateral oculomotor complex. Therefore, an abducens nuclear lesion produces a complete lateral gaze palsy, from weakness of both the ipsilateral lateral rectus and the contralateral medial rectus. *Foville's syndrome* following dorsal pontine injury includes lateral gaze palsy, ipsilateral facial palsy, and contralateral hemiparesis incurred by damage to descending corticospinal fibers. *Millard-*

Gubler syndrome from ventral pontine injury is similar, except for the eye findings. There is lateral rectus weakness only, instead of gaze palsy, because the abducens fascicle is injured rather than the nucleus. Infarct, tumor, hemorrhage, vascular malformation, and multiple sclerosis are the most common etiologies of brainstem abducens palsy.

After leaving the ventral pons, the abducens nerve runs forward along the clivus to pierce the dura at the petrous apex, where it enters the cavernous sinus. Along its subarachnoid course it is susceptible to meningitis, tumor (meningioma, chordoma, carcinomatous meningitis), subarachnoid hemorrhage, trauma, and compression by aneurysm or dolichoectatic vessels. At the petrous apex, mastoiditis can produce deafness, pain, and ipsilateral abducens palsy (*Gradenigo's syndrome*). In the cavernous sinus, the nerve can be affected by carotid aneurysm, carotid cavernous fistula, tumor (pituitary adenoma, meningioma, nasopharyngeal carcinoma), herpes infection, and Tolosa-Hunt syndrome.

Unilateral or bilateral abducens palsy is a classic sign of raised intracranial pressure. The diagnosis can be confirmed if papilledema is observed on fundus examination. The mechanism is still debated but is probably related to rostral-caudal displacement of the brainstem. The same phenomenon accounts for abducens palsy from low intracranial pressure (e.g., after lumbar puncture, spinal anesthesia, or spontaneous dural cerebrospinal fluid leak).

Treatment of abducens palsy is aimed at prompt correction of the underlying cause. However, the cause remains obscure in many instances, despite diligent evaluation. As mentioned above for isolated trochlear or oculomotor palsy, most cases are assumed to represent microvascular infarcts because they often occur in the setting of diabetes or other vascular risk factors. Some cases may develop as a postinfectious mononeuritis (e.g., following a viral flu). Patching one eye or applying a temporary prism will provide relief of diplopia until the palsy resolves. If recovery is incomplete, eye muscle surgery can nearly always realign the eyes, at least in primary position. A patient with an abducens palsy that fails to improve should be reevaluated for an occult etiology (e.g., chordoma, carcinomatous meningitis, carotid cavernous fistula, myasthenia gravis).

Multiple Ocular Motor Nerve Palsies   These should not be attributed to spontaneous microvascular events affecting more than one cranial nerve at a time. This remarkable coincidence does occur, especially in diabetic patients, but the diagnosis is made only in retrospect after exhausting all other diagnostic alternatives. Neuroimaging should focus on the cavernous sinus, superior orbital fissure, and orbital apex, where all three ocular motor nerves are in close proximity. In the diabetic or compromised host, fungal infection (*Aspergillus*, Mucorales, *Cryptococcus*) is a frequent cause of multiple nerve palsies. In the patient with systemic malignancy, carcinomatous meningitis is a likely diagnosis. Cytologic examination may be negative despite repeated sampling of the cerebrospinal fluid. The cancer-associated Lambert-Eaton myasthenic syndrome can also produce ophthalmoplegia. Giant cell (temporal) arteritis occasionally manifests as diplopia from ischemic palsies of extraocular muscles. Fisher syndrome, an ocular variant of Guillain-Barré, produces ophthalmoplegia with areflexia and ataxia. Often the ataxia is mild, and the reflexes are normal. Antiganglioside antibodies (GQ1b) can be detected in about 50% of cases.

Supranuclear Disorders of Gaze   These are often mistaken for multiple ocular motor nerve palsies. For example, Wernicke's encephalopathy can produce nystagmus and a partial deficit of horizontal and vertical gaze that mimics a combined abducens and oculomotor nerve palsy. The disorder occurs in malnourished or alcoholic patients and can be reversed by thiamine. Infarct, hemorrhage, tumor, multiple sclerosis, encephalitis, vasculitis, and Whipple's disease are other important causes of supranuclear gaze palsy. Disorders of vertical gaze, especially downwards saccades, are an early feature of progressive supranuclear palsy. Smooth pursuit is affected later in the course of the disease. Par-

kinson's disease, Huntington's chorea, and olivopontocerebellar degeneration can also affect vertical gaze.

The *frontal eye field* of the cerebral cortex is involved in generation of saccades to the contralateral side. After hemispheric stroke, the eyes usually deviate towards the lesioned side because of the unopposed action of the frontal eye field in the normal hemisphere. With time, this deficit resolves. Seizures generally have the opposite effect: the eyes deviate conjugately away from the irritative focus. *Parietal lesions* disrupt smooth pursuit of targets moving toward the side of the lesion. Bilateral parietal lesions produce *Balint's syndrome*, characterized by impaired eye-hand coordination (optic ataxia), difficulty initiating voluntary eye movements (ocular apraxia), and visuospatial disorientation (simultanagnosia).

Horizontal Gaze   Descending cortical inputs mediating horizontal gaze ultimately converge at the level of the pons. Neurons in the paramedian pontine reticular formation are responsible for controlling conjugate gaze toward the same side. They project directly to the ipsilateral abducens nucleus. A lesion of either the paramedian pontine reticular formation or the abducens nucleus causes an ipsilateral conjugate gaze palsy. Lesions at either locus produce nearly identical clinical syndromes, with the following exception: vestibular stimulation (oculocephalic maneuver or caloric irrigation) will succeed in driving the eyes conjugately to the side in a patient with a lesion of the paramedian pontine reticular formation, but not in a patient with a lesion of the abducens nucleus.

INTERNUCLEAR OPHTHALMOPLEGIA   This results from damage to the medial longitudinal fasciculus ascending from the abducens nucleus in the pons to the oculomotor nucleus in the midbrain (hence, "internuclear"). Damage to fibers carrying the conjugate signal from abducens interneurons to the contralateral medial rectus motoneurons results in a failure of adduction on attempted lateral gaze. For example, a patient with a left internuclear ophthalmoplegia will have slowed or absent adducting movements of the left eye (Fig. 29-19). A patient with bilateral injury to the medial longitudinal fasciculus will have bilateral internuclear ophthalmoplegia. Multiple sclerosis is the most common cause, although tumor, stroke, trauma, or any brainstem process may be responsible. *One-and-a-half syndrome* is due to a combined lesion of the medial longitudinal fasciculus and the abducens nucleus on the same side. The patient's only horizontal eye movement is abduction of the eye on the other side.

Vertical Gaze   This is controlled at the level of the midbrain. The neuronal circuits affected in disorders of vertical gaze are not fully elucidated, but lesions of the rostral interstitial nucleus of the medial longitudinal fasciculus and the interstitial nucleus of Cajal cause supranuclear paresis of upgaze, downgaze, or all vertical eye movements. Distal basilar artery ischemia is the most common etiology. *Skew deviation* refers to a vertical misalignment of the eyes, usually constant in all positions of gaze. The finding has poor localizing value because skew deviation has been reported after lesions in widespread regions of the brainstem and cerebellum.

PARINAUD'S SYNDROME   Also known as dorsal midbrain syndrome, this is a distinct supranuclear vertical gaze disorder from damage to the posterior commissure. It is a classic sign of hydrocephalus from aqueductal stenosis. Pineal region tumors, cysticercosis, and stroke also cause Parinaud's syndrome. Features include loss of upgaze (and sometimes downgaze), convergence-retraction nystagmus on attempted upgaze, downwards ocular deviation ("setting sun" sign), lid retraction (Collier's sign), skew deviation, pseudoabducens palsy, and light-near dissociation of the pupils.

Nystagmus   This is a rhythmical oscillation of the eyes, occurring physiologically from vestibular and optokinetic stimulation or pathologically in a wide variety of diseases (Chap. 22). Abnormalities of the eyes or optic nerves, present at birth or acquired in childhood, can

FIGURE 29-19 Left internuclear ophthalmoplegia (INO). *A.* In primary position of gaze the eyes appear normal. ***B.*** Horizontal gaze to the left is intact. ***C.*** On attempted horizontal gaze to the right, the left eye fails to adduct. In mildly affected patients the eye may adduct partially, or more slowly than normal. Nystagmus is usually present in the abducted eye. ***D.*** T2-weighted axial MRI image through the pons showing a demyelinating plaque in the left medial longitudinal fasciculus (*arrow*).

produce a complex, searching nystagmus with irregular pendular (sinusoidal) and jerk features. This nystagmus is commonly referred to as *congenital sensory nystagmus.* It is a poor term, because even in children with congenital lesions, the nystagmus does not appear until several months of age. *Congenital motor nystagmus,* which looks similar to congenital sensory nystagmus, develops in the absence of any abnormality of the sensory visual system. Visual acuity is also reduced in congenital motor nystagmus, probably by the nystagmus itself, but seldom below a level of 20/200.

JERK NYSTAGMUS This is characterized by a slow drift off the target, followed by a fast corrective saccade. By convention, the nystagmus is named after the quick phase. Jerk nystagmus can be downbeat, upbeat, horizontal (left or right), and torsional. The pattern of nystagmus may vary with gaze position. Some patients will be oblivious to their nystagmus. Others will complain of blurred vision, or a subjective, to-and-fro movement of the environment (oscillopsia) corresponding to their nystagmus. Fine nystagmus may be difficult to see upon gross examination of the eyes. Observation of nystagmoid movements of the optic disc on ophthalmoscopy is a sensitive way to detect subtle nystagmus.

GAZE-EVOKED NYSTAGMUS This is the most common form of jerk nystagmus. When the eyes are held eccentrically in the orbits, they have a natural tendency to drift back to primary position. The subject compensates by making a corrective saccade to maintain the deviated eye position. Many normal patients have mild gaze-evoked nystagmus. Exaggerated gaze-evoked nystagmus can be induced by drugs (sedatives, anticonvulsants, alcohol); muscle paresis; myasthenia gravis; demyelinating disease; and cerebellopontine angle, brainstem, and cerebellar lesions.

VESTIBULAR NYSTAGMUS *Vestibular nystagmus* results from dysfunction of the labyrinth (Ménière's disease), vestibular nerve, or vestibular nucleus in the brainstem. Peripheral vestibular nystagmus often occurs in discrete attacks, with symptoms of nausea and vertigo. There may be associated tinnitus and hearing loss. Sudden shifts in head position may provoke or exacerbate symptoms.

DOWNBEAT NYSTAGMUS *Downbeat nystagmus* occurs from lesions near the craniocervical junction (Chiari malformation, basilar invagination). It has also been reported in brainstem or cerebellar stroke, lithium or anticonvulsant intoxication, alcoholism, and multiple sclerosis. *Upbeat nystagmus* is associated with damage to the pontine tegmentum, from stroke, demyelination, or tumor.

Opsoclonus This rare, dramatic disorder of eye movements consists of bursts of consecutive saccades (saccadomania). When the saccades are confined to the horizontal plane, the term *ocular flutter* is preferred. It can occur from viral encephalitis, trauma, or a paraneoplastic effect of neuroblastoma, breast carcinoma, and other malignancies. It has also been reported as a benign, transient phenomenon in otherwise healthy patients.

FURTHER READINGS

ALBERT DM et al (eds): *Albert and Jakobiec's Principles and Practice of Ophthalmology,* 3d ed. Philadelphia, Saunders, 2007

BALCER LJ et al: Natalizumab reduces visual loss in patients with relapsing multiple sclerosis. Neurology 68:1299, 2007

GARIANO RF, GARDNER TW: Retinal angiogenesis in development and disease. Nature 438:960, 2005

ROSENFELD PJ et al: Ranibizumab for neovascular age-related macular degeneration. N Engl J Med 355:1419, 2006

RUTAR T et al: Ophthalmic manifestations of infections caused by the USA300 clone of community-associated methicillin-resistant *Staphylococcus aureus.* Ophthalmology 113:1455, 2006

30 Disorders of Smell, Taste, and Hearing

Anil K. Lalwani

SMELL

The sense of smell determines the flavor and palatability of food and drink and serves, along with the trigeminal system, as a monitor of inhaled chemicals, including dangerous substances such as natural gas, smoke, and air pollutants. Olfactory dysfunction affects ~1% of people under age 60 and more than half of the population beyond this age.

DEFINITIONS

Smell is the perception of odor by the nose. *Taste* is the perception of salty, sweet, sour, or bitter by the tongue. Related sensations during eating such as somatic sensations of coolness, warmth, and irritation are mediated through the trigeminal, glossopharyngeal, and vagal afferents in the nose, oral cavity, tongue, pharynx, and larynx. *Flavor* is the complex interaction of taste, smell, and somatic sensation. Terms relating to disorders of smell include *anosmia*, an absence of the ability to smell; *hyposmia*, a decreased ability to smell; *hyperosmia*, an increased sensitivity to an odorant; *dysosmia*, distortion in the perception of an odor; *phantosmia*, perception of an odorant where none is present; and *agnosia*, inability to classify, contrast, or identify odor sensations verbally, even though the ability to distinguish between odorants or to recognize them may be normal. An odor stimulus is referred to as an *odorant*. Each category of smell dysfunction can be further subclassified as total (applying to all odorants) or partial (dysfunction of only select odorants).

PHYSIOLOGY OF SMELL

The *olfactory epithelium* is located in the superior part of the nasal cavities and is highly variable in its distribution between individuals. Over time the olfactory epithelium loses its homogeneity, as small areas undergo metaplasia producing islands of respiratory-like epithelium. This process is thought to be secondary to insults from environmental toxins, bacteria, and viruses. The primary sensory neuron in the olfactory epithelium is the bipolar cell. The dendritic process of the bipolar cell has a bulb-shaped vesicle that projects into the mucous layer and bears six to eight cilia containing odorant receptors. On average, each bipolar cell elaborates 56 cm^2 (9 in.^{2}) of surface area to receive olfactory stimuli. These primary sensory neurons are unique among sensory systems in that they are short-lived, regularly replaced, and regenerate and establish new central connections after injury. Basal stem cells, located on the basal surface of the olfactory epithelium, are the progenitors that differentiate into new bipolar cells (Fig. 30-1).

Between 50 and 200 unmyelinated axons of receptor cells form the fila of the olfactory nerve; they pass through the cribriform plate to terminate within spherical masses of neuropil, termed *glomeruli*, in the olfactory bulb. Olfactory ensheathing cells, which have features resembling glia of both the central and peripheral nervous systems, surround the axons along their course. The glomeruli are the focus of a high degree of convergence of information, since many more fibers enter than leave them. The main second-order neurons are mitral cells. The primary dendrite of each mitral cell extends into a single glomerulus. Axons of the mitral cells project along with the axons of adjacent tufted cells to the limbic system, including the anterior olfactory nucleus and the amygdala. Cognitive awareness of smell requires stimulation of the prepiriform cortex or amygdaloid nuclei.

A secondary site of olfactory chemosensation is located in the epithelium of the vomeronasal organ, a tubular structure that opens on the ventral aspect of the nasal septum. In humans, this structure is rudimentary and nonfunctional, without central projections. Sensory neurons located in the vomeronasal organ detect pheromones, nonvolatile chemical signals that in lower mammals trigger innate and stereotyped reproductive and social behaviors, as well as neuroendocrine changes.

The sensation of smell begins with introduction of an odorant to the cilia of the bipolar neuron. Most odorants are hydrophobic; as they move from the air phase of the nasal cavity to the aqueous phase of the olfactory mucous, they are transported toward the cilia by small water-soluble proteins called *odorant-binding proteins* and reversibly bind to receptors on the cilia surface. Binding leads to conformational changes in the receptor protein, activation of G protein–coupled second messengers, and generation of action potentials in the primary neurons. Intensity appears to be coded by the amount of firing in the afferent neurons.

Olfactory receptor proteins belong to the large family of G protein–coupled receptors that also includes rhodopsins; α- and β-adrenergic receptors; muscarinic acetylcholine receptors; and neurotransmitter receptors for dopamine, serotonin, and substance P. In humans, there are 300–1000 olfactory receptor genes belonging to 20 different families located in clusters at >25 different chromosomal locations. Each olfactory neuron expresses only one or, at most, a few receptor genes, thus providing the molecular basis of odor discrimination. Bipolar cells that express similar receptors appear to be scattered across discrete spatial zones. These similar cells converge on a select few glomeruli in the olfactory bulb. The result is a potential spatial map of how we receive odor stimuli, much like the tonotopic organization of how we perceive sound.

DISORDERS OF THE SENSE OF SMELL

These are caused by conditions that interfere with the access of the odorant to the olfactory neuroepithelium (transport loss), injure the receptor region (sensory loss), or damage central olfactory pathways (neural loss). Currently no clinical tests exist to differentiate these different types of olfactory losses. Fortunately, the history of the disease provides important clues to the cause. The leading causes of olfactory disorders are summarized in Table 30-1; the most common etiologies are head trauma in children and young adults, and viral infections in older adults.

Head trauma is followed by unilateral or bilateral impairment of smell in up to 15% of cases; anosmia is more common than hyposmia. Olfactory dysfunction is more common when trauma is associated with loss of consciousness, moderately severe head injury (grades II–

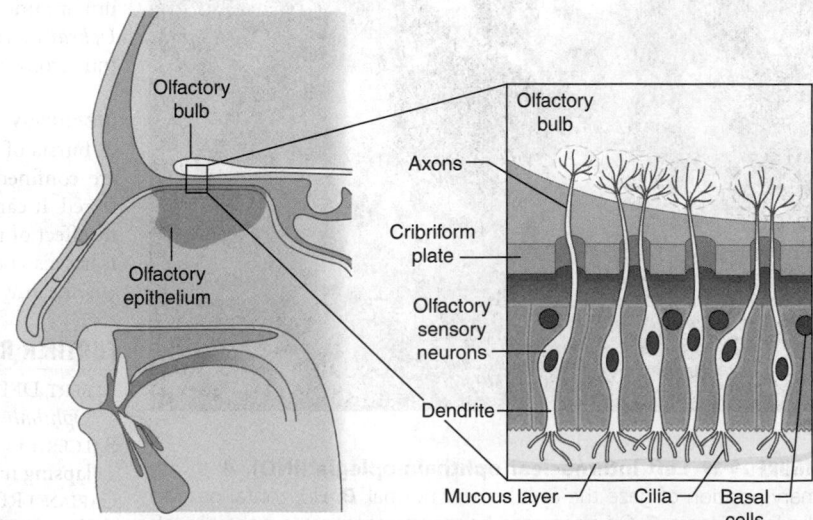

FIGURE 30-1 Olfaction. Olfactory sensory neurons (bipolar cells) are embedded in a small area of specialized epithelium in the dorsal posterior recess of the nasal cavity. These neurons project axons to the olfactory bulb of the brain, a small ovoid structure that rests on the cribriform plate of the ethmoid bone. Odorants bind to specific receptors on olfactory cilia and initiate a cascade of action potential events that lead to the production of action potentials in the sensory axons.

TABLE 30-1   CAUSES OF OLFACTORY DYSFUNCTION

Transport Losses	Neural Losses
Allergic rhinitis	AIDS
Bacterial rhinitis and sinusitis	Alcoholism
Congenital abnormalities	Alzheimer's disease
Nasal neoplasms	Cigarette smoke
Nasal polyps	Depression
Nasal septal deviation	Diabetes mellitus
Nasal surgery	Drugs/toxins
Viral infections	Huntington's chorea
Sensory Losses	Hypothyroidism
Drugs	Kallmann syndrome
Neoplasms	Malnutrition
Radiation therapy	Neoplasms
Toxin exposure	Neurosurgery
Viral infections	Parkinson's disease
	Trauma
	Vitamin B_{12} deficiency
	Zinc deficiency

V), and skull fracture. Frontal injuries and fractures disrupt the cribriform plate and olfactory axons that perforate it. Sometimes there is an associated cerebrospinal fluid (CSF) rhinorrhea resulting from a tearing of the dura overlying the cribriform plate and paranasal sinuses. Anosmia may also follow blows to the occiput. Once traumatic anosmia develops, it is usually permanent; only 10% of patients ever improve or recover. Perversion of the sense of smell may occur as a transient phase in the recovery process.

Viral infections can destroy the olfactory neuroepithelium, which is then replaced by respiratory epithelium. Parainfluenza virus type 3 appears to be especially detrimental to human olfaction. HIV infection is associated with subjective distortion of taste and smell, which may become more severe as the disease progresses. The loss of taste and smell may play an important role in the development and progression of HIV-associated wasting. Congenital anosmias are rare but important. Kallmann syndrome is an X-linked disorder characterized by congenital anosmia and hypogonadotropic hypogonadism resulting from a failure of migration from the olfactory placode of olfactory receptor neurons and neurons synthesizing gonadotropin-releasing hormone (Chap. 340). Anosmia can also occur in albinos. The receptor cells are present but are hypoplastic, lack cilia, and do not project above the surrounding supporting cells.

Meningiomas of the inferior frontal region are the most frequent neoplastic cause of anosmia; loss of smell may be the only neurologic abnormality. Rarely, anosmia can occur with gliomas of the frontal lobe. Occasionally, pituitary adenomas, craniopharyngiomas, suprasellar meningiomas, and aneurysms of the anterior part of the circle of Willis extend forward and damage olfactory structures. These tumors and hamartomas may also induce seizures with olfactory hallucinations, indicating involvement of the uncus of the temporal lobe.

Olfactory dysfunction is common in a variety of neurologic diseases, including Alzheimer's disease, Parkinson's disease, amyotrophic lateral sclerosis, and multiple sclerosis. In Alzheimer's and Parkinson's, olfactory loss may be the first clinical sign of the disease. In Parkinson's disease, bilateral olfactory deficits occur more commonly than the cardinal signs of the disorder such as tremor. In multiple sclerosis, olfactory loss is related to lesions visible by MRI, in olfactory processing areas in the temporal and frontal lobes.

Dysosmia, subjective distortions of olfactory perception, may occur with intranasal diseases that partially impair smell or during recovery from a neurogenic anosmia. Most dysosmic disorders consist of disagreeable odors, sometimes accompanied by distortions of taste. Dysosmia also can occur with depression.

APPROACH TO THE PATIENT:
Disorders of the Sense of Smell

Unilateral anosmia is rarely a complaint and is only recognized by testing of smell in each nasal cavity separately. Bilateral anosmia, on the other hand, brings patients to medical attention. Anosmic patients usually complain of a loss of the sense of taste even though their taste thresholds may be within normal limits. In actuality, they are complaining of a loss of flavor detection, which is mainly an olfactory function. The physical examination should include a thorough inspection of the ears, upper respiratory tract, and head and neck. A neurologic examination emphasizing the cranial nerves and cerebellar and sensorimotor function is essential. Any signs of depression should be noted.

Sensory olfactory function can be assessed by several methods. The Odor Stix test uses a commercially available odor-producing magic marker–like pen held approximately 8–15 cm (3–6 in.) from the patient's nose. The 30-cm alcohol test uses a freshly opened isopropyl alcohol packet held ~30 cm (12 in.) from the patient's nose. There is a commercially available scratch-and-sniff card containing three odors available for gross testing of olfaction. A superior test is the University of Pennsylvania Smell Identification Test (UPSIT). This consists of a 40-item, forced choice, scratch-and-sniff paradigm. For example, one of the items reads, "This odor smells most like (a) chocolate, (b) banana, (c) onion, or (d) fruit punch." The test is highly reliable, is sensitive to age and sex differences, and provides an accurate quantitative determination of the olfactory deficit. The UPSIT, which is a forced-choice test, can also be used to identify malingerers who typically report fewer correct responses than would be expected by chance. The average score for total anosmics is slightly higher than that expected on the basis of chance because of the inclusion of some odorants that act by trigeminal stimulation.

Olfactory threshold testing is another method of assessing olfactory function. Following assessment of sensory olfactory function, the detection threshold for an odorant such as methyl ethyl carbinol is established using graduated concentrations for each side of the nose. Nasal resistance can also be measured with anterior rhinomanometry for each side of the nose.

CT or MRI of the head is required to rule out paranasal sinusitis; neoplasms of the anterior cranial fossa, nasal cavity, or paranasal sinuses; or unsuspected fractures of the anterior cranial fossa. Bone abnormalities are best seen with CT. MRI is the most sensitive method to visualize olfactory bulbs, ventricles, and other soft tissue of the brain. Coronal CT is optimal for assessing cribriform plate, anterior cranial fossa, and sinus anatomy.

Biopsy of the olfactory epithelium is possible. However, given the widespread degeneration of the olfactory epithelium and intercalation of respiratory epithelium in the olfactory area of adults with no apparent olfactory dysfunction, biopsy results must be interpreted with caution.

℞ DISORDERS OF THE SENSE OF SMELL

Therapy for patients with transport olfactory losses due to allergic rhinitis, bacterial rhinitis and sinusitis, polyps, neoplasms, and structural abnormalities of the nasal cavities can be undertaken with a high likelihood for improvement. Allergy management; antibiotic therapy; topical and systemic glucocorticoid therapy; and surgery for nasal polyps, deviation of the nasal septum, and chronic hyperplastic sinusitis are frequently effective in restoring the sense of smell.

There is no proven treatment for sensorineural olfactory losses. Fortunately, spontaneous recovery often occurs. Zinc and vitamin therapy (especially with vitamin A) are advocated by some. Profound zinc deficiency can produce loss and distortion of the sense of smell but is not a clinically important problem except in very limited geographic areas (Chap. 71). The epithelial degeneration associated with vitamin A deficiency can cause anosmia, but in western societies the prevalence of vitamin A deficiency is low. Exposure to cigarette smoke and other airborne toxic chemicals can cause metaplasia of the olfactory epithelium, and spontaneous recovery can occur if the insult is removed. Counseling of patients is therefore helpful in such cases.

More than half of people over age 60 suffer from olfactory dysfunction. No effective treatment exists for presbyosmia, but patients are often reassured to learn that this problem is common in their age group. In addition, early recognition and counseling can help patients to compensate for the loss of smell. The incidence of natural gas–related accidents is disproportionately high in the elderly, perhaps due in part to the gradual loss of smell. Mercaptan, the pungent odor in natural gas, is an olfactory stimulant that does not activate taste receptors. Many elderly with olfactory dysfunction experience a decrease in flavor sensation and find it necessary to hyperflavor food, usually by increasing the amount of salt in their diet.

TASTE

Compared with disorders of smell, gustatory disorders are uncommon. Loss of olfactory sensitivity is often accompanied by complaints of loss of the sense of taste, usually with normal detection thresholds for taste.

DEFINITIONS

Disturbances of the sense of taste may be categorized as *total ageusia*, total absence of gustatory function or inability to detect the qualities of sweet, salt, bitter, or sour; *partial ageusia*, ability to detect some but not all of the qualitative gustatory sensations; *specific ageusia*, inability to detect the taste quality of certain substances; *total hypogeusia*, decreased sensitivity to all tastants; *partial hypogeusia*, decreased sensitivity to some tastants; and *dysgeusia* or *phantogeusia*, distortion in the perception of a tastant, i.e., the perception of the wrong quality when a tastant is presented or the perception of a taste when there has been no tastant ingested. Confusion between sour and bitter, and less commonly between salty and bitter, may represent a semantic misunderstanding or have a true pathophysiologic basis. It may be possible to differentiate between the loss of flavor recognition in patients with olfactory losses who complain of a loss of taste as well as smell by asking if they are able to taste sweetness in sodas, saltiness in potato chips, etc.

PHYSIOLOGY OF TASTE

The taste receptor cells are located in the taste buds, spherical groups of cells arranged in a pattern resembling the segments of a citrus fruit (**Fig. 30-2**). At the surface, the taste bud has a pore into which microvilli of the receptor cells project. Unlike the olfactory system, the receptor cell is not the primary neuron. Instead, gustatory afferent nerve fibers contact individual taste receptor cells. The papillae lie along the lateral margin and dorsum of the tongue; at the junction of the dorsum and the base of the tongue; and in the palate, epiglottis, larynx, and esophagus.

Tastants gain access to the receptor cells through the taste pore. Four classes of taste have been traditionally recognized: sweet, salt, sour, and bitter, and more recently "umami" (monosodium glutamate, disodium gluanylate, disodium inosinate). Tastants enter the taste pore in a solution and initiate transduction by either activating receptors coupled to G-proteins or by directly activating ion channels on the microvillae within the taste bud. Individual gustatory afferent fibers almost always respond to a number of different chemicals. As with olfaction and other sensory systems, intensity appears to be encoded by the quantity of neural activity.

The sense of taste is mediated through the facial, glossopharyngeal, and vagal nerves. The chorda tympani branch of the facial nerve subserves taste from the anterior two-thirds of the tongue. The posterior third of the tongue is supplied by the lingual branch of the glossopharyngeal nerve. Afferents from the palate travel with the greater superficial petrosal nerve to the geniculate ganglion and then via the facial nerve to the brainstem. The internal branch of the superior laryngeal nerve of the vagus nerve contains the taste afferents from the larynx, including the epiglottis and esophagus.

The central connections of the nerves terminate in the brainstem in the nucleus of the tractus solitarius. The central pathway from the nucleus of the tractus solitarius projects to the ipsilateral parabrachial nuclei of the pons. Two divergent pathways project from the parabrachial nuclei. One ascends to the gustatory relay in the dorsal thalamus, synapses, and continues to the cortex of the insula. There is also evidence for a direct pathway from the parabrachial nuclei to the cortex. (Olfaction and gustation appear to be unique among sensory systems in that at least some fibers bypass the thalamus.) The other pathway from the parabrachial nuclei goes to the ventral forebrain, including the lateral hypothalamus, substantia innominata, central nucleus of the amygdala, and the stria terminalis.

FIGURE 30-2 Taste. A. The taste buds of the anterior two-thirds of the tongue are innervated by the gustatory fibers that travel in a branch of the facial nerve (VII) called the chorda tympani. The taste buds of the posterior third of the tongue are innervated by gustatory fibers that travel in the lingual branch of the glossopharyngeal nerve (IX). [*Adapted from ER Kandel et al (eds): Principles of Neural Science, 4th ed, New York, McGraw-Hill, 2000; with permission.*] **B.** The main types of taste papillae are shown in schematic cross sections. Each type predominates in specific areas of the tongue, as indicated by the arrows from **A. C.** Each taste bud contains 50–150 taste cells that extend from the base of the taste bud to the taste pore, where the apical microvilli of taste cells have contact with tastants dissolved in saliva and taste pore mucus. Access of tastants to the basolateral regions of these cells is generally prevented by tight junctions between taste cells. Taste cells are short-lived cells that are replaced from stem cells at the base of the taste bud. Three types of taste cells in each taste bud (light cells, dark cells, and intermediate cells) may represent different stages of differentiation or different cell lineages. Taste stimuli, detected at the apical end of the taste cell, induce action potentials that cause the release of neurotransmitter at synapses formed at the base of the taste cell with gustatory fibers that transmit signals to the brain.

DISORDERS OF THE SENSE OF TASTE

Disorders of the sense of taste are caused by conditions that interfere with the access of the tastant to the receptor cells in the taste bud (transport loss), injure receptor cells (sensory loss), or damage gustatory afferent nerves and central gustatory pathways (neural loss) (**Table 30-2**). *Transport gustatory losses* result from xerostomia due to many causes, including Sjögren's syndrome, radiation therapy, heavy-metal intoxication, and bacterial colonization of the taste pore. *Sensory gustatory losses* are caused by inflammatory and degenerative diseases in the oral cavity; a vast number of drugs, particularly those that interfere with cell turnover such as antithyroid and antineoplastic agents;

TABLE 30-2   CAUSES OF GUSTATORY DYSFUNCTION

Transport Gustatory Losses	Neural Gustatory Losses
Drugs	Diabetes mellitus
Heavy-metal intoxication	Hypothyroidism
Radiation therapy	Oral neoplasms
Sjögren's syndrome	Oral surgery
Xerostomia	Radiation therapy
Sensory Gustatory Losses	Renal disease
Aging	Stroke and other CNS disorders
Candidiasis	Trauma
Drugs (antithyroid and	Upper respiratory tract infections
antineoplastic)	
Endocrine disorders	
Oral neoplasms	
Pemphigus	
Radiation therapy	
Viral infections (especially with	
herpes viruses)	

radiation therapy to the oral cavity and pharynx; viral infections; endocrine disorders; neoplasms; and aging. *Neural gustatory losses* occur with neoplasms, trauma, and surgical procedures in which the gustatory afferents are injured. Taste buds degenerate when their gustatory afferents are transected but remain when their somatosensory afferents are severed. Patients with renal disease have increased thresholds for sweet and sour tastes, which resolves with dialysis.

A side effect of medication is the single most common cause of taste dysfunction in clinical practice. Xerostomia, regardless of the etiology, can be associated with taste dysfunction. It is associated with poor oral clearance and poor dental hygiene and can adversely affect the oral mucosa, all leading to dysgeusia. However, severe salivary gland failure does not necessarily lead to taste complaints. Xerostomia, the use of antibiotics or glucocorticoids, or immunodeficiency can lead to overgrowth of *Candida*; overgrowth alone, without thrush or overt signs of infection, can be associated with bad taste or hypogeusia. When taste dysfunction occurs in a patient at risk for fungal overgrowth, a trial of nystatin or other antifungal medication is warranted.

Upper respiratory infections and head trauma can lead to both smell and taste dysfunction; taste is more likely to improve than smell. The mechanism of taste disturbance in these situations is not well understood. Trauma to the chorda tympani branch of the facial nerve during middle ear surgery or third molar extractions is relatively common and can cause dysgeusia. Bilateral chorda tympani injuries are usually associated with hypogeusia, whereas unilateral lesions produce only limited symptoms.

As noted above, aging itself may be associated with reduced taste sensitivity. The taste dysfunction may be limited to a single compound and may be mild.

APPROACH TO THE PATIENT:
Disorders of the Sense of Taste

Patients who complain of loss of taste should be evaluated for both gustatory and olfactory function. Clinical assessment of taste is not as well developed or standardized as that of smell. The first step is to perform suprathreshold whole-mouth taste testing for quality, intensity, and pleasantness perception of four taste qualities: sweet, salty, sour, and bitter. Most commonly used reagents for taste testing are sucrose, citric acid or hydrochloric acid, caffeine or quinine (sulfate or hydrochloride), and sodium chloride. The taste stimuli should be freshly prepared and have similar viscosity. For quantification, detection thresholds are obtained by applying graduated dilutions to the tongue quadrants or by whole-mouth sips. Electric taste testing (*electrogustometry*) is used clinically to identify taste deficits in specific quadrants of the tongue. Regional gustatory testing may also be performed to assess for the possibility of loss localized to one or several receptor fields as a result of a peripheral or central lesion. The history of the disease and localization studies provide important clues to the causes of the taste disturbance. For example, absence of taste on the anterior two-thirds of the tongue associated with a facial paralysis indicates that the lesion is proximal to the juncture of the chorda tympani branch with the facial nerve in the mastoid.

Rx DISORDERS OF THE SENSE OF TASTE

Treatment of gustatory disorders is limited. No effective therapies exist for the sensorineural disorders of taste. Altered taste due to surgical stretch injury of the chorda tympani nerve usually improves within 3–4 months, while dysfunction is usually permanent with transection of the nerve. Taste dysfunction following trauma may resolve spontaneously without intervention and is more likely to do so than posttraumatic smell dysfunction. Idiopathic alterations of taste sensitivity usually remain stable or worsen; zinc and vitamin therapy are of unproven value. Directed therapy to address factors that affect taste perception can be of value. Xerostomia can be treated with artificial saliva, providing some benefit to patients with a disturbed salivary milieu. Oral pilocarpine may be beneficial for a variety of forms of xerostomia. Appropriate treatment of bacterial and fungal infections of the oral cavity can be of great help in improving taste function. Taste disturbance related to drugs can often be resolved by changing the prescribed medication.

HEARING

Hearing loss is one of the most common sensory disorders in humans and can present at any age. Nearly 10% of the adult population has some hearing loss, and one-third of individuals >65 years have a hearing loss of sufficient magnitude to require a hearing aid.

PHYSIOLOGY OF HEARING

(**Fig. 30-3**) The function of the external and middle ear is to amplify sound to facilitate mechanotransduction by hair cells in the inner ear. Sound waves enter the external auditory canal and set the tympanic membrane in motion, which in turn moves the malleus, incus, and stapes of the middle ear. Movement of the footplate of the stapes causes pressure changes in the fluid-filled inner ear eliciting a traveling wave in the basilar membrane of the cochlea. The tympanic membrane and the ossicular chain in the middle ear serve as an impedance-matching mechanism, improving the efficiency of energy transfer from air to the fluid-filled inner ear.

Stereocilia of the hair cells of the organ of Corti, which rests on the basilar membrane, are in contact with the tectorial membrane and are deformed by the traveling wave. A point of maximal displacement of the basilar membrane is determined by the frequency of the stimulating tone. High-frequency tones cause maximal displacement of the basilar membrane near the base of the cochlea. As the frequency of the stimulating tone decreases, the point of maximal displacement moves toward the apex of the cochlea.

The inner and outer hair cells of the organ of Corti have different innervation patterns, but both are mechanoreceptors. The afferent innervation relates principally to the inner hair cells, and the efferent innervation relates principally to outer hair cells. The motility of the outer hair cells alters the micromechanics of the inner hair cells, creating a cochlear amplifier, which explains the exquisite sensitivity and frequency selectivity of the cochlea.

Beginning in the cochlea, the frequency specificity is maintained at each point of the central auditory pathway: dorsal and ventral cochlear nuclei, trapezoid body, superior olivary complex, lateral lemniscus, inferior colliculus, medial geniculate body, and auditory cortex. At low frequencies, individual auditory nerve fibers can respond more or less synchronously with the stimulating tone. At higher frequencies, phase-locking occurs so that neurons alternate in response to particular phases of the cycle of the sound wave. Intensity is encoded by the amount of neural activity in individual neurons, the number of neurons that are active, and the specific neurons that are activated.

GENETIC CAUSES OF HEARING LOSS

More than half of childhood hearing impairment is thought to be hereditary; hereditary hearing impairment (HHI) can also manifest later in life. HHI may be classified as either nonsyndromic, when hearing loss is the only clinical abnormality, or syndromic, when hearing loss is associated with anomalies in other organ systems. Near-

FIGURE 30-3 Ear anatomy. A. Drawing of modified coronal section through external ear and temporal bone, with structures of the middle and inner ear demonstrated. **B.** High-resolution view of inner ear.

ly two-thirds of HHIs are nonsyndromic, and the remaining one-third are syndromic. Between 70 and 80% of nonsyndromic HHI is inherited in an autosomal recessive manner and designated DFNB; another 15–20% is autosomal dominant (DFNA). Less than 5% is X-linked or maternally inherited via the mitochondria.

Nearly 100 loci harboring genes for nonsyndromic HHI have been mapped, with equal numbers of dominant and recessive modes of inheritance; numerous genes have now been cloned (Table 30-3). The hearing genes fall into the categories of structural proteins (MYH9, MYO7A, MYO15, TECTA, DIAPH1), transcription factors (POU3F4, POU4F3), ion channels (KCNQ4, SLC26A4), and gap junction proteins (GJB2, GJB3, GJB6). Several of these genes, including connexin 26 (GJB2), TECTA, and TMC1, cause both autosomal dominant and recessive forms of nonsyndromic HHI. In general, the hearing loss associated with dominant genes has its onset in adolescence or adulthood and varies in severity, whereas the hearing loss associated with recessive inheritance is congenital and profound. Connexin 26 is particularly important because it is associated with nearly 20% of cases of childhood deafness. Two frame-shift mutations, 35delG and 167delT, account for >50% of the cases; however, screening for these two mutations alone is insufficient to diagnose GJB2-related recessive deafness. The 167delT mutation is highly prevalent in Ashkenazi Jews; ~1 in 1765 individuals in this population are homozygous and affected. The hearing loss can also vary among the members of the same family, suggesting that other genes or factors influence the auditory phenotype.

The contribution of genetics to presbycusis (see below) is also becoming better understood. In addition to GJB2, several other nonsyndromic genes are associated with hearing loss that progresses with age. Sensitivity to aminoglycoside ototoxicity can be maternally transmitted through a mitochondrial mutation. Susceptibility to noise-induced hearing loss may also be genetically determined.

There are >400 syndromic forms of hearing loss. These include Usher syndrome (retinitis pigmentosa and hearing loss), Waardenburg syndrome (pigmentary abnormality and hearing loss), Pendred syndrome (thyroid organification defect and hearing loss), Alport syndrome (renal disease and hearing loss), Jervell and Lange-Nielsen syndrome (prolonged QT interval and hearing loss), neurofibromatosis type 2 (bilateral acoustic schwannoma), and mitochondrial disorders [mitochondrial encephalopathy, lactic acidosis, and stroke-like episodes (MELAS); myoclonic epilepsy and ragged red fibers (MERRF); progressive external ophthalmoplegia (PEO)] (Table 30-4).

DISORDERS OF THE SENSE OF HEARING

Hearing loss can result from disorders of the auricle, external auditory canal, middle ear, inner ear, or central auditory pathways (Fig. 30-4). *In general, lesions in the auricle, external auditory canal, or middle ear*

TABLE 30-3   HEREDITARY HEARING IMPAIRMENT GENES

Designation	Gene	Function
Autosomal Dominant		
	CRYM	Thyroid hormone binding protein
DFNA1	DIAPH1	Cytoskeletal protein
DFNA2	GJB3 (Cx31)	Gap junctions
DFNA2	KCNQ4	Potassium channel
DFNA3	GJB2 (Cx26)	Gap junctions
DFNA3	GJB6 (Cx30)	Gap junctions
DFNA4	MYH14	Class II nonmuscle myosin
DFNA5	DFNA5	Unknown
DFNA6/14/38	WFS	Transmembrane protein
DFNA8/12	TECTA	Tectorial membrane protein
DFNA9	COCH	Unknown
DFNA10	EYA4	Developmental gene
DFNA11	MYO7A	Cytoskeletal protein
DFNA13	COL11A2	Cytoskeletal protein
DFNA15	POU4F3	Transcription factor
DFNA17	MYH9	Cytoskeletal protein
DFNA20/26	ACTG1	Cytoskeletal protein
DFNA22	MYO6	Unconventional myosin
DFNA28	TFCP2L3	Transcription factor
DFNA36	TMC1	Transmembrane protein
DFNA48	MYO1A	Unconventional myosin
Autosomal Recessive		
	SLC26A5 (Prestin)	Motor protein
DFNB1	GJB2 (CX26)	Gap junction
	GJB6 (CX30)	Gap junction
DFNB2	MYO7A	Cytoskeletal protein
DFNB3	MYO15	Cytoskeletal protein
DFNB4	PDS (SLC26A4)	Chloride/iodide transporter
DFNB6	TMIE	Transmembrane protein
DFNB7/B11	TMC1	Transmembrane protein
DFNB9	OTOF	Trafficking of membrane vesicles
DFNB8/10	TMPRSS3	Transmembrane serine protease
DFNB12	CDH23	Intercellular adherence protein
DFNB16	STRC	Stereocilia protein
DFNB18	USH1C	Unknown
DFNB21	TECTA	Tectorial membrane protein
DFNB22	OTOA	Gel attachement to nonsensory cell
DFNB23	PCDH15	Morphogenesis and cohesion
DFNB28	TRIOBP	Cytoskeletal-organizing protein
DFNB29	CLDN14	Tight junctions
DFNB30	MYO3A	Hybrid motor-signaling myosin
DFNB31	WHRN	PDZ domain–containing protein
DFNB36	ESPN	Ca-insensitive actin-bundling protein
DFNB37	MYO6	Unconventional myosin
DFNB67	TMHS	Unknown function; tetraspan protein

TABLE 30-4 SYNDROMIC HEREDITARY HEARING IMPAIRMENT GENES

Syndrome	Gene	Function
Alport syndrome	COL4A3-5	Cytoskeletal protein
BOR syndrome	EYA1	Developmental gene
	SIX1	Developmental gene
Jervell and Lange-Nielsen syndrome	KVLQT1	Delayed rectifier K+ channel
	KCNE1	Delayed rectifier K+ channel
Norrie disease	Norrin	Cell-cell interactions
Pendred syndrome	SLC26A4	Chloride/iodide transporter
Treacher Collins	TCOF1	Nucleolar-cytoplasmic transport
Usher syndrome	MYO7A	Cytoskeletal protein
	USH1C	Unknown
	CDH23	Intercellular adherence protein
	PCDH15	Cell adhesion molecule
	SANS	Harmonin associated protein
	USH2A	Cell adhesion molecule
	VLGR1	G protein–coupled receptor
	USH3	Unknown
WS type I, III	PAX3	Transcription factor
WS type II	MITF	Transcription factor
	SLUG	Transcription factor
WS type IV	EDNRB	Endothelin-B receptor
	EDN3	Endothelin-B receptor ligand
	SOX10	Transcription factor

Note: BOR, branchio-oto-renal syndrome; WS, Waardenburg syndrome.

cause conductive hearing losses, whereas lesions in the inner ear or eighth nerve cause sensorineural hearing losses.

Conductive Hearing Loss This results from obstruction of the external auditory canal by cerumen, debris, and foreign bodies; swelling of the lin-

ing of the canal; atresia or neoplasms of the canal; perforations of the tympanic membrane; disruption of the ossicular chain, as occurs with necrosis of the long process of the incus in trauma or infection; otosclerosis; or fluid, scarring, or neoplasms in the middle ear. Rarely, inner-ear malformations may present as conductive hearing loss beginning in adulthood.

Cholesteatoma, stratified squamous epithelium in the middle ear or mastoid, occurs frequently in adults. This is a benign, slowly growing lesion that destroys bone and normal ear tissue. Theories of pathogenesis include traumatic implantation and invasion, immigration and invasion through a perforation, and metaplasia following chronic infection and irritation. On examination, there is often a perforation of the tympanic membrane filled with cheesy white squamous debris. A chronically draining ear that fails to respond to appropriate antibiotic therapy should raise suspicion of a cholesteatoma. Conductive hearing loss secondary to ossicular erosion is common. Surgery is required to remove this destructive process.

Conductive hearing loss with a normal ear canal and intact tympanic membrane suggests ossicular pathology. Fixation of the stapes from *otosclerosis* is a common cause of low-frequency conductive hearing loss. It occurs equally in men and women and is inherited as an autosomal dominant trait with incomplete penetrance. Hearing impairment usually presents between the late teens to the forties. In women, the otosclerotic process is accelerated during pregnancy, and the hearing loss is often first noticeable at this time. A hearing aid or a simple outpatient surgical procedure (stapedectomy) can provide adequate auditory rehabilitation. Extension of otosclerosis beyond the stapes footplate to involve the cochlea (cochlear otosclerosis) can lead to mixed or sensorineural hearing loss. Fluoride therapy to prevent hearing loss from cochlear otosclerosis is of uncertain value.

Eustachian tube dysfunction is extremely common in adults and may predispose to acute otitis media (AOM) or serous otitis media (SOM). Trauma, AOM, or chronic otitis media are the usual factors

CHAPTER 30 Disorders of Smell, Taste, and Hearing

FIGURE 30-4 An algorithm for the approach to hearing loss. HL, hearing loss; SNHL, sensorineural hearing loss; TM, tympanic membrane; SOM, serous otitis media; AOM, acute otitis media; *, CT scan of temporal bone; †, MRI scan.

responsible for tympanic membrane perforation. While small perforations often heal spontaneously, larger defects usually require surgical intervention. Tympanoplasty is highly effective (>90%) in the repair of tympanic membrane perforations. Otoscopy is usually sufficient to diagnose AOM, SOM, chronic otitis media, cerumen impaction, tympanic membrane perforation, and eustachian tube dysfunction.

Sensorineural Hearing Loss Damage to the hair cells of the organ of Corti may be caused by intense noise, viral infections, ototoxic drugs (e.g., salicylates, quinine and its synthetic analogues, aminoglycoside antibiotics, loop diuretics such as furosemide and ethacrynic acid, and cancer chemotherapeutic agents such as cisplatin), fractures of the temporal bone, meningitis, cochlear otosclerosis (see above), Ménière's disease, and aging. Congenital malformations of the inner ear may be the cause of hearing loss in some adults. Genetic predisposition alone or in concert with environmental exposures may also be responsible.

Presbycusis (age-associated hearing loss) is the most common cause of sensorineural hearing loss in adults. In the early stages, it is characterized by symmetric, gentle to sharply sloping high-frequency hearing loss. With progression, the hearing loss involves all frequencies. More importantly, the hearing impairment is associated with significant loss in clarity. There is a loss of discrimination for phonemes, recruitment (abnormal growth of loudness), and particular difficulty in understanding speech in noisy environments. Hearing aids may provide limited rehabilitation once the word recognition score deteriorates below 50%. Cochlear implants are the treatment of choice when hearing aids prove inadequate, even when hearing loss is incomplete.

Ménière's disease is characterized by episodic vertigo, fluctuating sensorineural hearing loss, tinnitus, and aural fullness. Tinnitus and/or deafness may be absent during the initial attacks of vertigo, but invariably appear as the disease progresses and increase in severity during acute attacks. The annual incidence of Ménière's disease is 0.5–7.5 per 1000; onset is most frequently in the fifth decade of life but may also occur in young adults or the elderly. Histologically, there is distention of the endolymphatic system (endolymphatic hydrops) leading to degeneration of vestibular and cochlear hair cells. This may result from endolymphatic sac dysfunction secondary to infection, trauma, autoimmune disease, inflammatory causes, or tumor; an idiopathic etiology constitutes the largest category and is most accurately referred to as Ménière's disease. Although any pattern of hearing loss can be observed, typically, low-frequency, unilateral sensorineural hearing impairment is present. MRI should be obtained to exclude retrocochlear pathology such as a cerebellopontine angle tumor or demyelinating disorder. Therapy is directed towards the control of vertigo. A low-salt diet is the mainstay of treatment for control of rotatory vertigo. Diuretics, a short course of glucocorticoids, and intratympanic gentamicin may also be useful adjuncts in recalcitrant cases. Surgical therapy of vertigo is reserved for unresponsive cases and includes endolymphatic sac decompression, labyrinthectomy, and vestibular nerve section. Both labyrinthectomy and vestibular nerve section abolish rotatory vertigo in >90% of cases. Unfortunately, there is no effective therapy for hearing loss, tinnitus, or aural fullness from Ménière's disease.

Sensorineural hearing loss may also result from any neoplastic, vascular, demyelinating, infectious, or degenerative disease or trauma affecting the central auditory pathways. HIV leads to both peripheral and central auditory system pathology and is associated with sensorineural hearing impairment.

A finding of conductive and sensory hearing loss in combination is termed *mixed hearing loss*. Mixed hearing losses are due to pathology of both the middle and inner ear, as can occur in otosclerosis involving the ossicles and the cochlea, head trauma, chronic otitis media, cholesteatoma, middle ear tumors, and some inner ear malformations.

Trauma resulting in temporal bone fractures may be associated with conductive, sensorineural, or mixed hearing loss. If the fracture spares the inner ear, there may simply be conductive hearing loss due to rupture of the tympanic membrane or disruption of the ossicular chain. These abnormalities can be surgically corrected. Profound hearing loss and severe vertigo are associated with temporal bone fractures involving the inner ear. A perilymphatic fistula associated with leakage of inner-ear fluid into the middle ear can occur and may require surgical repair. An associated facial nerve injury is not uncommon. CT is best suited to assess fracture of the traumatized temporal bone, evaluate the ear canal, and determine the integrity of the ossicular chain and the involvement of the inner ear. CSF leaks that accompany temporal bone fractures are usually self-limited; the value of prophylactic antibiotics is uncertain.

Tinnitus is defined as the perception of a sound when there is no sound in the environment. It may have a buzzing, roaring, or ringing quality and may be pulsatile (synchronous with the heartbeat). Tinnitus is often associated with either a conductive or sensorineural hearing loss. The pathophysiology of tinnitus is not well understood. The cause of the tinnitus can usually be determined by finding the cause of the associated hearing loss. Tinnitus may be the first symptom of a serious condition such as a vestibular schwannoma. Pulsatile tinnitus requires evaluation of the vascular system of the head to exclude vascular tumors such as glomus jugulare tumors, aneurysms, and stenotic arterial lesions; it may also occur with SOM.

APPROACH TO THE PATIENT:
Disorders of the Sense of Hearing

The goal in the evaluation of a patient with auditory complaints is to determine (1) the nature of the hearing impairment (conductive vs. sensorineural vs. mixed), (2) the severity of the impairment (mild, moderate, severe, profound), (3) the anatomy of the impairment (external ear, middle ear, inner ear, or central auditory pathway), and (4) the etiology. The history should elicit characteristics of the hearing loss, including the duration of deafness, unilateral vs. bilateral involvement, nature of onset (sudden vs. insidious), and rate of progression (rapid vs. slow). Symptoms of tinnitus, vertigo, imbalance, aural fullness, otorrhea, headache, facial nerve dysfunction, and head and neck paresthesias should be noted. Information regarding head trauma, exposure to ototoxins, occupational or recreational noise exposure, and family history of hearing impairment may also be important. A sudden onset of unilateral hearing loss, with or without tinnitus, may represent a viral infection of the inner ear or a stroke. Patients with unilateral hearing loss (sensory or conductive) usually complain of reduced hearing, poor sound localization, and difficulty hearing clearly with background noise. Gradual progression of a hearing deficit is common with otosclerosis, noise-induced hearing loss, vestibular schwannoma, or Ménière's disease. Small vestibular schwannomas typically present with asymmetric hearing impairment, tinnitus, and imbalance (rarely vertigo); cranial neuropathy, in particular of the trigeminal or facial nerve, may accompany larger tumors. In addition to hearing loss, Ménière's disease may be associated with episodic vertigo, tinnitus, and aural fullness. Hearing loss with otorrhea is most likely due to chronic otitis media or cholesteatoma.

Examination should include the auricle, external ear canal, and tympanic membrane. The external ear canal of the elderly is often dry and fragile; it is preferable to clean cerumen with wall-mounted suction and cerumen loops and to avoid irrigation. In examining the eardrum, the topography of the tympanic membrane is more important than the presence or absence of the light reflex. In addition to the pars tensa (the lower two-thirds of the eardrum), the pars flaccida above the short process of the malleus should also be examined for retraction pockets that may be evidence of chronic eustachian tube dysfunction or cholesteatoma. Insufflation of the ear canal is necessary to assess tympanic membrane mobility and compliance. Careful inspection of the nose, nasopharynx, and upper respiratory tract is indicated. Unilateral serous effusion should prompt a fiberoptic examination of the nasopharynx to exclude neoplasms. Cranial nerves should be evaluated with special attention to facial and trigeminal nerves, which are commonly affected with tumors involving the cerebellopontine angle.

The Rinne and Weber tuning fork tests, with a 512-Hz tuning fork, are used to screen for hearing loss, differentiate conductive from sensorineural hearing losses, and to confirm the findings of audiologic evaluation. Rinne's test compares the ability to hear by air conduction with the ability to hear by bone conduction. The tines of a vibrating tuning fork are held near the opening of the external auditory canal, and then the stem is placed on the mastoid process; for direct contact, it may be placed on teeth or dentures. The patient is asked to indicate whether the tone is louder by air conduction or bone conduction. Normally, and in the presence of sensorineural hearing loss, a tone is heard louder by air conduction than by bone conduction; however, with conductive hearing loss of ≥30 dB (see "Audiologic Assessment," below), the bone-conduction stimulus is perceived as louder than the air-conduction stimulus. For the Weber test, the stem of a vibrating tuning fork is placed on the head in the midline and the patient asked whether the tone is heard in both ears or better in one ear than in the other. With a unilateral conductive hearing loss, the tone is perceived in the affected ear. With a unilateral sensorineural hearing loss, the tone is perceived in the unaffected ear. A 5-dB difference in hearing between the two ears is required for lateralization.

LABORATORY ASSESSMENT OF HEARING
Audiologic Assessment The minimum audiologic assessment for hearing loss should include the measurement of pure tone air-conduction and bone-conduction thresholds, speech reception threshold, discrimination score, tympanometry, acoustic reflexes, and acoustic-reflex decay. This test battery provides a screening evaluation of the entire auditory system and allows one to determine whether further differentiation of a sensory (cochlear) from a neural (retrocochlear) hearing loss is indicated.

Pure tone audiometry assesses hearing acuity for pure tones. The test is administered by an audiologist and is performed in a sound-attenuated chamber. The pure tone stimulus is delivered with an audiometer, an electronic device that allows the presentation of specific frequencies (generally between 250 and 8000 Hz) at specific intensities. Air and bone conduction thresholds are established for each ear. Air conduction thresholds are determined by presenting the stimulus in air with the use of headphones. Bone conduction thresholds are determined by placing the stem of a vibrating tuning fork or an oscillator of an audiometer in contact with the head. In the presence of a hearing loss, broad-spectrum noise is presented to the nontest ear for *masking* purposes so that responses are based on perception from the ear under test.

The responses are measured in decibels. An *audiogram* is a plot of intensity in decibels of hearing threshold versus frequency. A decibel (dB) is equal to 20 times the logarithm of the ratio of the sound pressure required to achieve threshold in the patient to the sound pressure required to achieve threshold in a normal hearing person. Therefore, a change of 6 dB represents doubling of sound pressure, and a change of 20 dB represents a tenfold change in sound pressure. Loudness, which depends on the frequency, intensity, and duration of a sound, doubles with approximately each 10-dB increase in sound pressure level. Pitch, on the other hand, does not directly correlate with frequency. The perception of pitch changes slowly in the low and high frequencies. In the middle tones, which are important for human speech, pitch varies more rapidly with changes in frequency.

Pure tone audiometry establishes the presence and severity of hearing impairment, unilateral vs. bilateral involvement, and the type of hearing loss. Conductive hearing losses with a large mass component, as is often seen in middle-ear effusions, produce elevation of thresholds that predominate in the higher frequencies. Conductive hearing losses with a large stiffness component, as in fixation of the footplate of the stapes in early otosclerosis, produce threshold elevations in the lower frequencies. Often, the conductive hearing loss involves all frequencies, suggesting involvement of both stiffness and mass. In general, sensorineural hearing losses such as presbycusis affect higher frequencies more than lower frequencies. An exception is Ménière's disease, which is characteristically associated with low-frequency sensorineural hearing loss. Noise-induced hearing loss has an unusual pattern of hearing impairment in which the loss at 4000 Hz is greater than at higher frequencies. Vestibular schwannomas characteristically affect the higher frequencies, but any pattern of hearing loss can be observed.

Speech recognition requires greater synchronous neural firing than is necessary for appreciation of pure tones. *Speech audiometry* tests the clarity with which one hears. The *speech reception threshold* (SRT) is defined as the intensity at which speech is recognized as a meaningful symbol and is obtained by presenting two-syllable words with an equal accent on each syllable. The intensity at which the patient can repeat 50% of the words correctly is the SRT. Once the SRT is determined, discrimination or word recognition ability is tested by presenting one-syllable words at 25–40 dB above the SRT. The words are phonetically balanced in that the phonemes (speech sounds) occur in the list of words at the same frequency that they occur in ordinary conversational English. An individual with normal hearing or conductive hearing loss can repeat 88–100% of the phonetically balanced words correctly. Patients with a sensorineural hearing loss have variable loss of discrimination. As a general rule, neural lesions produce greater deficits in discrimination than do lesions in the inner ear. For example, in a patient with mild asymmetric sensorineural hearing loss, a clue to the diagnosis of vestibular schwannoma is the presence of a substantial deterioration in discrimination ability. Deterioration in discrimination ability at higher intensities above the SRT also suggests a lesion in the eighth nerve or central auditory pathways.

Tympanometry measures the impedance of the middle ear to sound and is useful in diagnosis of middle-ear effusions. A *tympanogram* is the graphic representation of change in impedance or compliance as the pressure in the ear canal is changed. Normally, the middle ear is most compliant at atmospheric pressure, and the compliance decreases as the pressure is increased or decreased; this pattern is seen with normal hearing or in the presence of sensorineural hearing loss. Compliance that does not change with change in pressure suggests middle-ear effusion. With a negative pressure in the middle ear, as with eustachian tube obstruction, the point of maximal compliance occurs with negative pressure in the ear canal. A tympanogram in which no point of maximal compliance can be obtained is most commonly seen with discontinuity of the ossicular chain. A reduction in the maximal compliance peak can be seen in otosclerosis.

During tympanometry, an intense tone elicits contraction of the stapedius muscle. The change in compliance of the middle ear with contraction of the stapedius muscle can be detected. The presence or absence of this *acoustic reflex* is important in the anatomic localization of facial nerve paralysis as well as hearing loss. Normal or elevated acoustic reflex thresholds in an individual with sensorineural hearing impairment suggests a cochlear hearing loss. Assessment of *acoustic reflex decay* helps differentiate sensory from neural hearing losses. In neural hearing loss, the reflex adapts or decays with time.

Otoacoustic emissions (OAE) can be measured with microphones inserted into the external auditory canal. The emissions may be spontaneous or evoked with sound stimulation. The presence of OAEs indicates that the outer hair cells of the organ of Corti are intact and can be used to assess auditory thresholds and to distinguish sensory from neural hearing losses.

Evoked Responses *Electrocochleography* measures the earliest evoked potentials generated in the cochlea and the auditory nerve. Receptor potentials recorded include the cochlear microphonic, generated by the outer hair cells of the organ of Corti, and the summating potential, generated by the inner hair cells in response to sound. The whole nerve action potential representing the composite firing of the first-order neurons can also be recorded during electrocochleography. Clinically, the test is useful in the diagnosis of Ménière's disease, where an elevation of the ratio of summating potential to action potential is seen.

Brainstem auditory evoked responses (BAERs) are useful in differentiating the site of sensorineural hearing loss. In response to sound, five distinct electrical potentials arising from different stations along the peripheral and central auditory pathway can be identified using computer averaging from scalp surface electrodes. BAERs are valuable in situations in which patients cannot or will not give reliable voluntary thresholds. They are also used to assess the integrity of the auditory nerve and brainstem in various clinical situations, including intraoperative monitoring and in determination of brain death.

The *vestibular-evoked myogenic potential (VEMP) test* elicits a vestibulocollic reflex whose afferent limb arises from acoustically sensitive cells in the saccule, with signals conducted via the inferior vestibular nerve. VEMP is a biphasic, short-latency response recorded from the tonically contracted sternocleidomastoid muscle in response to loud auditory clicks or tones. VEMPs may be diminished or absent in patients with early and late Ménière's disease, vestibular neuritis, benign paroxysmal positional vertigo, and vestibular schwannoma. On the other hand, the threshold for VEMPs may be lower in cases of superior canal dehiscence and perilymphatic fistula.

Imaging Studies   The choice of radiologic tests is largely determined by whether the goal is to evaluate the bony anatomy of the external, middle, and inner ear or to image the auditory nerve and brain. Axial and coronal CT of the temporal bone with fine 1-mm cuts is ideal for determining the caliber of the external auditory canal, integrity of the ossicular chain, and presence of middle-ear or mastoid disease; it can also detect inner-ear malformations. CT is also ideal for the detection of bone erosion with chronic otitis media and cholesteatoma. MRI is superior to CT for imaging of retrocochlear pathology such as vestibular schwannoma, meningioma, other lesions of the cerebellopontine angle, demyelinating lesions of the brainstem, and brain tumors. Both CT and MRI are equally capable of identifying inner-ear malformations and assessing cochlear patency for preoperative evaluation of patients for cochlear implantation.

℞ DISORDERS OF THE SENSE OF HEARING

In general, conductive hearing losses are amenable to surgical correction, while sensorineural hearing losses are more difficult to manage. Atresia of the ear canal can be surgically repaired, often with significant improvement in hearing. Tympanic membrane perforations due to chronic otitis media or trauma can be repaired with an outpatient tympanoplasty. Likewise, conductive hearing loss associated with otosclerosis can be treated by stapedectomy, which is successful in 90–95% of cases. Tympanostomy tubes allow the prompt return of normal hearing in individuals with middle-ear effusions. Hearing aids are effective and well-tolerated in patients with conductive hearing losses.

Patients with mild, moderate, and severe sensorineural hearing losses are regularly rehabilitated with hearing aids of varying configuration and strength. Hearing aids have been improved to provide greater fidelity and have been miniaturized. The current generation of hearing aids can be placed entirely within the ear canal, thus reducing any stigma associated with their use. In general, the more severe the hearing impairment, the larger the hearing aid required for auditory rehabilitation. Digital hearing aids lend themselves to individual programming, and multiple and directional microphones at the ear level may be helpful in noisy surroundings. Since all hearing aids amplify noise as well as speech, the only absolute solution to the problem of noise is to place the microphone closer to the speaker than the noise source. This arrangement is not possible with a self-contained, cosmetically acceptable device.

In many situations, including lectures and the theater, hearing-impaired persons benefit from assistive devices that are based on the principle of having the speaker closer to the microphone than any source of noise. Assistive devices include infrared and frequency-modulated (FM) transmission as well as an electromagnetic loop around the room for transmission to the individual's hearing aid. Hearing aids with telecoils can also be used with properly equipped telephones in the same way.

In the event that the hearing aid provides inadequate rehabilitation, cochlear implants may be appropriate. Criteria for implantation include severe to profound hearing loss with word recognition score ≤30% under best aided conditions. Worldwide, >20,000 deaf individuals (including 4000 children) have received cochlear implants. Cochlear implants are neural prostheses that convert sound energy to electrical energy and can be used to stimulate the auditory division of the eighth nerve directly. In most cases of profound hearing impairment, the auditory hair cells are lost but the ganglionic cells of the auditory division of the eighth nerve are preserved. Cochlear implants consist of electrodes that are inserted into the cochlea through the round window, speech processors that extract acoustical elements of speech for conversion to electrical currents, and a means of transmitting the electrical energy through the skin. Patients with implants experience sound that helps with speech reading, allows open-set word recognition, and helps in modulating the person's own voice. Usually, within 3 months after implantation, adult patients can understand speech without visual cues. With the current generation of multichannel cochlear implants, nearly 75% of patients are able to converse on the telephone. For individuals who have had both eighth nerves destroyed by trauma or bilateral vestibular schwannomas (e.g., neurofibromatosis type 2), brainstem auditory implants placed near the cochlear nucleus may provide auditory rehabilitation.

Tinnitus often accompanies hearing loss. As for background noise, tinnitus can degrade speech comprehension in individuals with hearing impairment. Therapy for tinnitus is usually directed towards minimizing the appreciation of tinnitus. Relief of the tinnitus may be obtained by masking it with background music. Hearing aids are also helpful in tinnitus suppression, as are tinnitus maskers, devices that present a sound to the affected ear that is more pleasant to listen to than the tinnitus. The use of a tinnitus masker is often followed by several hours of inhibition of the tinnitus. Antidepressants have been shown to be beneficial in helping patients cope with tinnitus.

Hard-of-hearing individuals often benefit from a reduction in unnecessary noise (e.g., radio or television) to enhance the signal-to-noise ratio. Speech comprehension is aided by lip reading; therefore the impaired listener should be seated so that the face of the speaker is well-illuminated and easily seen. Although speech should be in a loud, clear voice, one should be aware that in sensorineural hearing losses in general and in hard-of-hearing elderly in particular, recruitment (abnormal perception of loud sounds) may be troublesome. Above all, optimal communication cannot take place without both parties giving it their full and undivided attention.

PREVENTION

Conductive hearing losses may be prevented by prompt antibiotic therapy of adequate duration for AOM and by ventilation of the middle ear with tympanostomy tubes in middle-ear effusions lasting ≥12 weeks. Loss of vestibular function and deafness due to aminoglycoside antibiotics can largely be prevented by careful monitoring of serum peak and trough levels.

Some 10 million Americans have noise-induced hearing loss, and 20 million are exposed to hazardous noise in their employment. Noise-induced hearing loss can be prevented by avoidance of exposure to loud noise or by regular use of ear plugs or fluid-filled ear muffs to attenuate intense sound. High-risk activities for noise-induced hearing loss include wood and metal working with electrical equipment and target practice and hunting with small firearms. All internal-combustion and electric engines, including snow and leaf blowers, snowmobiles, outboard motors, and chain saws, require protection of the user with hearing protectors. Virtually all noise-induced hearing loss is preventable through education, which should begin before the teenage years. Programs of industrial conservation of hearing are required when the exposure over an 8-h period averages 85 dB. Workers in such noisy environments can be protected with preemployment audiologic assessment, the mandatory use of hearing protectors, and annual audiologic assessments.

ACKNOWLEDGMENT
The author acknowledges the contributions of Dr. James B. Snow, Jr., to this chapter.

FURTHER READINGS

Benton R: On the origin of smell: Odorant receptors in insects. Cell Mol Life Sci 63:1579, 2006

Breer H et al: The sense of smell: Multiple olfactory subsystems. Cell Mol Life Sci 63:1465, 2004

Breslin PA, Huang L: Human taste: Peripheral anatomy, taste transduction, and coding. Adv Otorhinolaryngol 63:152, 2006

Dulac C: Sparse encoding of natural scents. Neuron 50:816, 2006

Gates GA, Mills JH: Presbycusis. Lancet 366:1111, 2005

Gudziol V et al: Clinical significance of results from olfactory testing. Laryngoscope 116:1858, 2006

Heckmann JG, Lang CJ: Neurological causes of taste disorders. Adv Otorhinolaryngol 63:255, 2006

Lalwani AK (ed): *Current Diagnosis and Treatment in Otolaryngology—Head & Neck Surgery*, 2d ed. New York, McGraw-Hill, 2007

Rennels M, Pickering LK: Sensorineural hearing loss in children. Lancet 365:2085, 2005

31 Pharyngitis, Sinusitis, Otitis, and Other Upper Respiratory Tract Infections

Michael A. Rubin, Ralph Gonzales, Merle A. Sande

Infections of the upper respiratory tract (URIs) have a tremendous impact on public health. They are among the most common reasons for visits to primary care providers, and, although the illnesses are typically mild, their high incidence and transmission rates place them among the leading causes of time lost from work or school. Even though the minority (~25%) of cases are caused by bacteria, URIs are the leading diagnoses for which antibiotics are prescribed on an outpatient basis in the United States. The enormous consumption of antibiotics for these illnesses has contributed to the rise in antibiotic resistance among common community-acquired pathogens such as *Streptococcus pneumoniae*—a trend that in itself has had an enormous influence on public health.

Although most URIs are caused by viruses, distinguishing patients with primary viral infection from those with primary bacterial infection is difficult. Signs and symptoms of bacterial and viral URIs are, in fact, indistinguishable. Because routine, rapid testing is neither available nor practical for most syndromes, acute infections are diagnosed largely on clinical grounds. Thus the judicious use of antibiotics in this setting is challenging.

NONSPECIFIC INFECTIONS OF THE UPPER RESPIRATORY TRACT

Nonspecific URIs are a broadly defined group of disorders that collectively constitute the leading cause of ambulatory care visits in the United States. By definition, nonspecific URIs have no prominent localizing features. They are identified by a variety of descriptive names, including *acute infective rhinitis*, *acute rhinopharyngitis/nasopharyngitis*, *acute coryza*, and *acute nasal catarrh*, as well as by the inclusive label *common cold*.

Etiology The large assortment of URI classifications reflects the wide variety of causative infectious agents and the varied manifestations of common pathogens. Nearly all nonspecific URIs are caused by viruses spanning multiple virus families and many antigenic types. For instance, there are at least 100 immunotypes of rhinovirus (Chap. 179), the most common cause of URI (~30–40% of cases); other causes include influenza virus (three immunotypes; Chap. 180) as well as parainfluenza virus (four immunotypes), coronavirus (at least three immunotypes), and adenovirus (47 immunotypes) (Chap. 179). Respiratory syncytial virus (RSV) also accounts for a small percentage of cases each year, as do some viruses not typically associated with URIs (e.g., enteroviruses, rubella virus, and varicella-zoster virus). Even with sophisticated diagnostic and culture techniques, a substantial proportion (25–30%) of cases have no assigned pathogen.

Clinical Manifestations The signs and symptoms of nonspecific URI are similar to those of other URIs but lack a pronounced localization to one particular anatomic location, such as the sinuses, pharynx, or lower airway. Nonspecific URI is commonly described as an acute, mild, and self-limited catarrhal syndrome, with a median duration of ~1 week. Signs and symptoms are diverse and frequently variable across patients. The principal signs and symptoms of nonspecific URI include rhinorrhea (with or without purulence), nasal congestion, cough, and sore throat. Other manifestations, such as fever, malaise, sneezing, and hoarseness, are more variable, with fever more common among infants and young children. Occasionally, clinical features reflect the underlying viral pathogen; myalgias and fatigue, for example, are sometimes seen with influenza and parainfluenza infections, while conjunctivitis may suggest infection with adenovirus or enterovirus. Findings on physical examination are frequently nonspecific and unimpressive. Between 0.5 and 2% of colds are complicated by secondary bacterial infections (e.g., rhinosinusitis, otitis media, and pneumonia), particularly in high-risk

Secondary bacterial infections are usually associated with a prolonged course of illness, increased severity of illness, and localization of signs and symptoms. Purulent secretions from the nares or throat have often been used as an indication of sinusitis or pharyngitis. However, these secretions are also seen in nonspecific URI and, in the absence of other clinical features, are poor predictors of bacterial infection.

℞ UPPER RESPIRATORY INFECTIONS

Antibiotics have no role in the treatment of uncomplicated nonspecific URI. In the absence of clinical evidence of bacterial infection, treatment remains entirely symptom-based, with use of decongestants and nonsteroidal anti-inflammatory drugs. Other therapies directed at specific symptoms are often useful, including dextromethorphan for cough and lozenges with topical anesthetic for sore throat. Clinical trials of zinc, vitamin C, echinacea, and other alternative remedies have revealed no consistent benefit for the treatment of nonspecific URI.

INFECTIONS OF THE SINUS

Sinusitis refers to an inflammatory condition involving the four paired structures surrounding the nasal cavities. Although most cases of sinusitis involve more than one sinus, the maxillary sinus is most commonly involved; next in frequency are the ethmoid, frontal, and sphenoid sinuses. Each sinus is lined with a respiratory epithelium that produces mucus, which is transported out by ciliary action through the sinus ostium and into the nasal cavity. Normally, mucus does not accumulate in the sinuses, which remain sterile despite their adjacency to the bacterium-filled nasal passages. When the sinus ostia are obstructed, however, or when ciliary clearance is impaired or absent, the secretions can be retained, producing the typical signs and symptoms of sinusitis. The retained secretions may become infected with a variety of pathogens, including viruses, bacteria, and fungi. Sinusitis affects a tremendous proportion of the population, accounts for millions of visits to primary care physicians each year, and is the fifth leading diagnosis for which antibiotics are prescribed. It is typically classified by duration of illness (acute vs. chronic); by etiology (infectious vs. noninfectious); and, when infectious, by the offending pathogen type (viral, bacterial, or fungal).

ACUTE SINUSITIS

Acute sinusitis—defined as sinusitis of <4 weeks' duration—constitutes the vast majority of sinusitis cases. Most cases are diagnosed in the ambulatory care setting and occur primarily as a consequence of a preceding viral URI. Differentiating acute bacterial and viral sinusitis on clinical grounds is difficult. Therefore, it is perhaps unsurprising that antibiotics are prescribed frequently (in 85–98% of all cases) for this condition.

Etiology A number of infectious and noninfectious factors can contribute to acute obstruction of the sinus ostia or impairment of ciliary clearance, with consequent sinusitis. Noninfectious causes include allergic rhinitis (with either mucosal edema or polyp obstruction), barotrauma (e.g., from deep-sea diving or air travel), or chemical irritants. Illnesses such as nasal and sinus tumors (e.g., squamous cell carcinoma) or granulomatous diseases (e.g., Wegener's granulomatosis or rhinoscleroma) can also produce obstruction of the sinus ostia, while conditions leading to altered mucus content (e.g., cystic fibrosis) can cause sinusitis through impaired mucus clearance. In the hospital setting, nasotracheal intubation is a major risk factor for nosocomial sinusitis in intensive care units.

Acute infectious sinusitis can be caused by a variety of organisms, including viruses, bacteria, and fungi. Viral rhinosinusitis is far more common than bacterial sinusitis, although relatively few studies have sampled sinus aspirates for the presence of different viruses. In those studies that have done so, the viruses most commonly isolated—both alone and with bacteria—have been rhinovirus, parainfluenza virus, and influenza virus. Bacterial causes of sinusitis have been better described. Among community-acquired cases, *S. pneumoniae* and nontypable *Haemophilus influenzae* are the most common pathogens, accounting for 50–60% of cases.

Moraxella catarrhalis causes disease in a significant percentage (20%) of children but less often in adults. Other streptococcal species and *Staphylococcus aureus* cause only a small percentage of cases, although there is increasing concern about community strains of methicillin-resistant *S. aureus* (MRSA) as an emerging cause. Anaerobes are occasionally found in association with infections of the roots of premolar teeth that spread into the adjacent maxillary sinuses. The role of *Chlamydophila pneumoniae* and *Mycoplasma pneumoniae* in the pathogenesis of acute sinusitis is still unclear. Nosocomial cases are commonly associated with bacteria found in the hospital environment, including *S. aureus, Pseudomonas aeruginosa, Serratia marcescens, Klebsiella pneumoniae,* and *Enterobacter* species. Often, these infections are polymicrobial and involve organisms that are highly resistant to numerous antibiotics. Fungi are also established causes of sinusitis, although most acute cases are in immunocompromised patients and represent invasive, life-threatening infections. The best-known example is rhinocerebral mucormycosis caused by fungi of the order Mucorales, which includes *Rhizopus, Rhizomucor, Mucor, Absidia,* and *Cunninghamella*. These infections usually occur in diabetic patients with ketoacidosis but also develop in transplant recipients, patients with hematologic malignancies, and patients receiving chronic glucocorticoid or deferoxamine therapy. Other hyaline molds, such as *Aspergillus* and *Fusarium* species, are also occasional causes of this disease.

Clinical Manifestations   Most cases of acute sinusitis present after or in conjunction with a viral URI, and it can be difficult to discriminate the clinical features of one from the other. A large proportion of patients with colds have sinus inflammation, although bacterial sinusitis complicates only 0.2–2% of these viral infections. Common presenting symptoms of sinusitis include nasal drainage and congestion, facial pain or pressure, and headache. Thick, purulent or discolored nasal discharge is often thought to indicate bacterial sinusitis but also occurs early in viral infections such as the common cold and is not specific to bacterial infection. Other nonspecific manifestations include cough, sneezing, and fever. Tooth pain, most often involving the upper molars, is associated with bacterial sinusitis, as is halitosis.

In acute sinusitis, sinus pain or pressure often localizes to the involved sinus (particularly the maxillary sinus) and can be worse when the patient bends over or is supine. Although rare, manifestations of advanced sphenoid or ethmoid sinus infection can be profound, including severe frontal or retroorbital pain radiating to the occiput, thrombosis of the cavernous sinus, and signs of orbital cellulitis. Acute focal sinusitis is uncommon but should be considered in the patient with severe symptoms over the maxillary sinus and fever, regardless of illness duration. Similarly, advanced frontal sinusitis can present with a condition known as *Pott's puffy tumor*, with soft tissue swelling and pitting edema over the frontal bone from a communicating subperiosteal abscess. Life-threatening complications include meningitis, epidural abscess, and cerebral abscess.

Patients with acute fungal sinusitis (such as mucormycosis) often present with symptoms related to pressure effects, particularly when the infection has spread to the orbits and cavernous sinus. Signs such as orbital swelling and cellulitis, proptosis, ptosis, and decreased extraocular movement are common, as is retroorbital or periorbital pain. Nasopharyngeal ulcerations, epistaxis, and headaches are also frequent, and involvement of cranial nerves V and VII has been described in more advanced cases. Bony erosion may be evident on examination. Oftentimes, the patient does not appear seriously ill despite the rapidly progressive nature of these infections.

Patients with acute nosocomial sinusitis are often critically ill and thus do not manifest the typical clinical features of sinus disease. This diagnosis should be suspected, however, when hospitalized patients who have appropriate risk factors (e.g., nasotracheal intubation) develop fever of unknown origin.

Diagnosis   Distinguishing viral from bacterial sinusitis in the ambulatory setting is usually difficult, given the relatively low sensitivity and specificity of the common clinical features. One clinical feature that has been used to help guide diagnostic and therapeutic decision-making is illness duration. Because acute bacterial sinusitis is uncommon in patients whose symptoms have lasted <7 days, several authorities now recommend reserving this diagnosis for patients with "persistent" symptoms (i.e., symptoms lasting >7 days in adults or >10–14 days in children) accompanied by purulent nasal discharge (Table 31-1). Even among the patients who meet these criteria, only 40–50% have true bacterial sinusitis. The use of CT or sinus radiography is not recommended for routine cases, particularly early in the course of illness (i.e., at <7 days), given the high prevalence of similar abnormalities among cases of acute viral rhinosinusitis. In the evaluation of persistent, recurrent, or chronic sinusitis, CT of the sinuses is the radiographic study of choice.

The clinical history and/or setting can often identify cases of acute anaerobic bacterial sinusitis, acute fungal sinusitis, or sinusitis from noninfectious causes (e.g., allergic rhinosinusitis). In the case of an immunocompromised patient with acute fungal sinus infection, immediate examination by an otolaryngologist is required. Biopsy specimens from involved areas should be examined by a pathologist for evidence of fungal hyphal elements and tissue invasion. Cases of suspected acute nosocomial sinusitis should be confirmed by sinus CT. Because therapy should target the offending organism, a sinus aspirate should be obtained, if possible, for culture and susceptibility testing.

℞ ACUTE SINUSITIS

Most patients with a diagnosis of acute rhinosinusitis based on clinical grounds improve without antibiotic therapy. The preferred initial approach in patients with mild to moderate symptoms of short duration is therapy aimed at facilitating sinus drainage, such as oral and topical decongestants, nasal saline lavage, and—in patients with a history of chronic sinusitis or allergies—nasal glucocorticoids. Adult patients who do not improve after 7 days, children who do not improve after 10–14 days, and patients with more severe symptoms (regardless of duration) should be treated with antibiotics (Table 31-1). Empirical therapy should consist of the narrowest-spectrum agent active against the most common bacterial pathogens, including *S. pneumoniae* and *H. influenzae*—e.g., amoxicillin. No clinical trials support the use of broad-spectrum agents for routine cases of bacterial sinusitis, even in the current era of drug-resistant *S. pneumoniae*. Up to 10% of patients do not respond to initial antimicrobial therapy; sinus aspiration and/or lavage by an otolaryngologist should be considered in these cases. Antibiotic prophylaxis to prevent episodes of recurrent acute bacterial sinusitis is not recommended.

Surgical intervention and IV antibiotic administration are usually reserved for patients with severe disease or those with intracranial complications, such as abscess or orbital involvement. Immunocompromised patients with acute invasive fungal sinusitis usually require extensive surgical debridement and treatment with IV antifungal agents active against fungal hyphal forms, such as amphotericin B. Specific therapy should be individualized according to the fungal species and the individual patient's characteristics.

Treatment of nosocomial sinusitis should begin with broad-spectrum antibiotics to cover common pathogens such as *S. aureus* and gram-negative bacilli. Therapy should then be tailored to the results of culture and susceptibility testing of sinus aspirates.

CHRONIC SINUSITIS

Chronic sinusitis is characterized by symptoms of sinus inflammation lasting >12 weeks. This illness is most commonly associated with either bacteria or fungi, and clinical cure in most cases is very difficult. Many patients have undergone treatment with repeated courses of antibacterial agents and multiple sinus surgeries, increasing their risk of colonization with antibiotic-resistant pathogens and of surgical complications. Patients often suffer significant morbidity, sometimes over many years.

In *chronic bacterial sinusitis*, infection is thought to be due to the impairment of mucociliary clearance from repeated infections rather than to persistent bacterial infection. However, the pathogenesis of this condition is poorly understood. Although certain conditions (e.g., cystic fibrosis) can predispose patients to chronic bacterial sinusitis, most patients with this infection do not have obvious underlying conditions that result in the obstruction of sinus drainage, the impairment of ciliary action, or immune dysfunction. Patients experience constant nasal congestion and sinus pressure, with intermittent periods of greater severity,

TABLE 31-1   GUIDELINES FOR THE DIAGNOSIS AND TREATMENT OF ACUTE SINUSITIS

Age Group	Diagnostic Criteria	Treatment Recommendations[a]
Adults	Moderate symptoms (e.g., nasal purulence/ congestion or cough) for >7 d *or* Severe symptoms of any duration, including unilateral/focal facial swelling or tooth pain	*Initial therapy* Amoxicillin, 500 mg PO tid or 875 mg PO bid, *or* TMP-SMX, 1 DS tablet PO bid for 10–14 d *Exposure to antibiotics within 30 d or >30% prevalence of penicillin-resistant S. pneumoniae* Amoxicillin, 1000 mg PO tid, *or* Amoxicillin/clavulanate (extended release), 2000 mg PO bid, *or* Antipneumococcal fluoroquinolone (e.g., levofloxacin, 500 mg PO qd) *Recent treatment failure* Amoxicillin/clavulanate (extended release), 2000 mg PO bid, *or* Amoxicillin, 1500 mg bid, plus clindamycin, 300 mg PO qid, *or* Antipneumococcal fluoroquinolone (e.g., levofloxacin, 500 mg PO qd)
Children	Moderate symptoms (e.g., nasal purulence/congestion or cough) for >10–14 d *or* Severe symptoms of any duration, including fever (>102°F), unilateral/focal facial swelling or pain	*Initial therapy* Amoxicillin, 45–90 mg/kg qd (up to 2 g) PO in divided doses (bid or tid), *or* Cefuroxime axetil, 30 mg/kg qd PO in divided doses (bid), *or* Cefdinir, 14 mg/kg PO qd *Exposure to antibiotics within 30 d, recent treatment failure, or >30% prevalence of penicillin-resistant S. pneumoniae* Amoxicillin, 90 mg/kg qd (up to 2 g) PO in divided doses (bid), plus clavulanate, 6.4 mg/kg qd PO in divided doses (bid) (extra-strength suspension), *or* Cefuroxime axetil, 30 mg/kg qd PO in divided doses (bid), *or* Cefdinir, 14 mg/kg PO qd

[a]Unless otherwise specified, the duration of therapy is generally 10 d, with appropriate follow-up.

Note: DS, double-strength; TMP-SMX, trimethoprim-sulfamethoxazole.

Sources: American Academy of Pediatrics Subcommittee on Management of Sinusitis and Committee on Quality Improvement, 2001; Hickner et al, 2001; Piccirillo, 2004; and Sinus and Allergy Health Partnership, 2004.

which may persist for years. CT can be helpful in determining the extent of disease and the response to therapy. The management team should include an otolaryngologist to conduct endoscopic examinations and obtain tissue samples for histologic examination and culture.

Chronic fungal sinusitis is a disease of immunocompetent hosts and is usually noninvasive, although slowly progressive invasive disease is sometimes seen. Noninvasive disease, which is typically associated with hyaline molds such as *Aspergillus* species and dematiaceous molds such as *Curvularia* or *Bipolaris* species, can present as a number of different scenarios. In mild, indolent disease, which usually occurs in the setting of repeated failures of antibacterial therapy, only nonspecific mucosal changes may be seen on sinus CT. Endoscopic surgery is usually curative in these patients, with no need for antifungal therapy. Another form of disease presents with long-standing, often unilateral symptoms and opacification of a single sinus on imaging studies as a result of a mycetoma (fungus ball) within the sinus. Treatment for this condition is also surgical, although systemic antifungal therapy may be warranted in the rare case where bony erosion occurs. A third form of disease, known as *allergic fungal sinusitis*, is seen in patients with a history of nasal polyposis and asthma, who often have had multiple sinus surgeries. Patients with this condition produce a thick, eosinophilic mucus with the consistency of peanut butter that contains sparse fungal hyphae on histologic examination. Patients often present with pansinusitis.

℞ CHRONIC SINUSITIS

Treatment of chronic bacterial sinusitis can be challenging and consists primarily of repeated culture-guided courses of antibiotics, sometimes for 3–4 weeks at a time; administration of intranasal glucocorticoids; and me-chanical irrigation of the sinus with sterile saline solution. When this management approach fails, sinus surgery may be indicated and sometimes provides significant, albeit short-term, alleviation. Treatment of chronic fungal sinusitis consists of surgical removal of impacted mucus. Recurrence, unfortunately, is common.

INFECTIONS OF THE EAR AND MASTOID

Infections of the ear and associated structures can involve both the middle and external ear, including the skin, cartilage, periosteum, ear canal, and tympanic and mastoid cavities. Both viruses and bacteria are known causes of these infections, some of which result in significant morbidity if not treated appropriately.

INFECTIONS OF THE EXTERNAL EAR STRUCTURES

Infections involving the structures of the external ear are often difficult to differentiate from noninfectious inflammatory conditions with similar clinical manifestations. Clinicians should consider inflammatory disorders as a possible cause of external ear irritation, particularly in the absence of local or regional adenopathy. Aside from the more salient causes of inflammation such as trauma, insect bite, and overexposure to sunlight or extreme cold, the differential diagnosis should include less common conditions such as autoimmune disorders (e.g., lupus or relapsing polychondritis) and vasculitides (e.g., Wegener's granulomatosis).

Auricular Cellulitis   Auricular cellulitis is an infection of the skin overlying the external ear and typically follows minor local trauma. It presents with the typical signs and symptoms of a skin/soft tissue infection, with tenderness, erythema, swelling, and warmth of the external ear (particularly the lobule) but without apparent involvement of the ear canal or inner structures. Treatment consists of warm compresses and oral antibiotics such as dicloxacillin that are active against typical skin and soft tissue pathogens (specifically, *S. aureus* and streptococci). IV antibiotics, such as a first-generation cephalosporin (e.g., cefazolin) or a penicillinase-resistant penicillin (e.g., nafcillin), are occasionally needed for more severe cases.

Perichondritis   Perichondritis, an infection of the perichondrium of the auricular cartilage, typically follows local trauma (e.g., ear piercing, burns, or lacerations). Occasionally, when the infection spreads down to the cartilage of the pinna itself, patients may also have chondritis. The infection may closely resemble auricular cellulitis, with erythema, swelling, and extreme tenderness of the pinna, although the lobule is less often involved in perichondritis. The most common pathogens are *P. aeruginosa* and *S. aureus*, although other gram-negative and gram-positive organisms are occasionally involved. Treatment consists of systemic antibiotics active against both *P. aeruginosa* and *S. aureus*. An antipseudomonal penicillin (e.g., piperacillin) or a combination of a penicillinase-resistant penicillin plus an antipseudomonal quinolone (e.g., nafcillin plus ciprofloxacin) is typically used. Incision and drainage may be helpful for culture and for resolution of infection, which often takes weeks. When perichondritis fails to respond to adequate antimicrobial therapy, clinicians should consider a noninfectious inflammatory etiology; for example, relapsing polychondritis is often mistaken for infectious perichondritis.

Otitis Externa   The term *otitis externa* refers to a collection of diseases involving primarily the auditory meatus. Otitis externa usually results from a combination of heat, retained moisture, and desquamation and maceration of the epithelium of the outer ear canal. The disease exists in several forms: localized, diffuse, chronic, and invasive. All forms are predominantly bacterial in origin, with *P. aeruginosa* and *S. aureus* the most common pathogens.

Acute localized otitis externa (*furunculosis*) can develop in the outer third of the ear canal, where skin overlies cartilage and hair follicles are numerous. As in furunculosis elsewhere on the body, *S. aureus* is the usual pathogen, and treatment typically consists of an oral antistaphylococcal penicillin (e.g., dicloxacillin), with incision and drainage in cases of abscess formation.

Acute diffuse otitis externa is also known as *swimmer's ear*, although it can develop in patients who have not recently been swimming. Heat, humidity, and the loss of protective cerumen lead to excessive moisture and elevation of the pH in the ear canal, which in turn lead to skin maceration and irritation. Infection may then occur; the predominant pathogen is *P. aeruginosa*, although other gram-negative and gram-positive organisms have been recovered from patients with this condition. The illness often starts with itching and progresses to severe pain, which is usually triggered by manipulation of the pinna or tragus. The onset of pain is generally accompanied by the development of an erythematous, swollen ear canal, often with scant white, clumpy discharge. Treatment consists of cleansing the canal to remove debris and to enhance the activity of topical therapeutic agents—usually hypertonic saline or mixtures of alcohol and acetic acid. Inflammation can also be decreased by adding glucocorticoids to the treatment regimen or by using Burow's solution (aluminum acetate in water). Antibiotics are most effective when given topically. Otic mixtures provide adequate pathogen coverage; these preparations usually combine neomycin with polymyxin, with or without glucocorticoids.

Chronic otitis externa is caused primarily by repeated local irritation, most commonly arising from persistent drainage from a chronic middle-ear infection. Other causes of repeated irritation, such as insertion of cotton swabs or other foreign objects into the ear canal, can lead to this condition, as can rare chronic infections such as syphilis, tuberculosis, or leprosy. Chronic otitis externa typically presents as erythematous, scaling dermatitis in which the predominant symptom is pruritus rather than pain; this condition must be differentiated from several others that produce a similar clinical picture, such as atopic dermatitis, seborrheic dermatitis, psoriasis, and dermatomycosis. Therapy consists of identifying and treating or removing the offending process, although successful resolution is frequently difficult.

Invasive otitis externa, also known as *malignant* or *necrotizing* otitis externa, is an aggressive and potentially life-threatening disease that occurs predominantly in elderly diabetic patients and other immunocompromised patients. The disease begins in the external canal, progresses slowly over weeks to months, and often is difficult to distinguish from a severe case of chronic otitis externa because of the presence of purulent otorrhea and an erythematous swollen ear and external canal. Severe, deep-seated otalgia is often noted and can help differentiate invasive from chronic otitis externa. The characteristic finding on examination is granulation tissue in the posteroinferior wall of the external canal, near the junction of bone and cartilage. If left unchecked, the infection can migrate to the base of the skull (resulting in skull-base osteomyelitis) and on to the meninges and brain, with a high associated mortality rate. Cranial nerve involvement is occasionally seen, with the facial nerve usually affected first and most often. Thrombosis of the sigmoid sinus can occur if the infection extends to that area. CT, which can reveal osseous erosion of the temporal bone and skull base, can be used to help determine the extent of disease, as can gallium and technetium-99 scintigraphy studies. *P. aeruginosa* is by far the most common pathogen, although *S. aureus*, *Staphylococcus epidermidis*, *Aspergillus*, *Actinomyces*, and some gram-negative bacteria have also been associated with this disease. In all cases, the external ear canal should be cleansed and a biopsy specimen of the granulation tissue within the canal (or of deeper tissues) should be obtained for culture of the offending organism. IV antibiotic therapy is directed specifically toward the recovered pathogen. For *P. aeruginosa*, the regimen typically includes an antipseudomonal penicillin or cephalosporin (e.g., piperacillin or ceftazidime) with an aminoglycoside. A fluoroquin-

olone antibiotic is frequently used in place of the aminoglycoside and can even be administered orally, given the excellent bioavailability of this drug class. In addition, antibiotic drops containing an agent active against *Pseudomonas* (e.g., ciprofloxacin) are usually prescribed and are combined with glucocorticoids to reduce inflammation. Cases of invasive *Pseudomonas* otitis externa recognized in the early stages can sometimes be treated with oral and otic fluoroquinolones alone, albeit with close follow-up. Extensive surgical debridement, once an important component of the treatment approach, is now rarely indicated.

INFECTIONS OF MIDDLE-EAR STRUCTURES

Otitis media is an inflammatory condition of the middle ear that results from dysfunction of the eustachian tube in association with a number of illnesses, including URIs and chronic rhinosinusitis. The inflammatory response to these conditions leads to the development of a sterile transudate within the middle-ear and mastoid cavities. Infection may occur if bacteria or viruses from the nasopharynx contaminate this fluid, producing an acute (or sometimes chronic) illness.

Acute Otitis Media Acute otitis media results when pathogens from the nasopharynx are introduced into the inflammatory fluid collected in the middle ear (e.g., by nose blowing during a URI). The proliferation of these pathogens in this space leads to the development of the typical signs and symptoms of acute middle-ear infection. The diagnosis of acute otitis media requires the demonstration of fluid in the middle ear (with tympanic membrane immobility) and the accompanying signs or symptoms of local or systemic illness (Table 31-2).

ETIOLOGY Acute otitis media typically follows a viral URI. The causative viruses (most commonly RSV, influenza virus, rhinovirus, and enterovirus) can themselves cause subsequent acute otitis media; more often, they predispose the patient to bacterial otitis media. Studies using tympanocentesis have consistently found *S. pneumoniae* to be the most common bacterial cause, isolated in up to 35% of cases. *H. influenzae* (nontypable strains) and *M. catarrhalis* are also common bacterial causes of acute otitis media, and concern is increasing about community strains of MRSA as an emerging etiologic agent. Viruses, such as those mentioned above, have been recovered either alone or with bacteria in 17–40% of cases.

CLINICAL MANIFESTATIONS Fluid in the middle ear is typically demonstrated or confirmed with pneumatic otoscopy. In the absence of fluid, the tympanic membrane moves visibly with the application of positive and negative pressure, but this movement is dampened when fluid is present. With bacterial infection, the tympanic membrane can also be erythematous, bulging, or retracted and occasionally can spontaneously perforate. The signs and symptoms accompanying infection can be local or systemic, including otalgia, otorrhea, diminished hearing, fever, or irritability. Erythema of the tympanic membrane is often evident but is nonspecific as it is frequently seen in association with inflammation of the upper respiratory mucosa (e.g., during examination of young children). Other signs and symptoms that are occasionally reported include vertigo, nystagmus, and tinnitus.

℞ ACUTE OTITIS MEDIA

There has been considerable debate on the usefulness of antibiotics for the treatment of acute otitis media. Although most cases resolve clinically 1 week after the onset of illness, antibiotics appear to be of some benefit. A higher proportion of treated than of untreated patients are free of illness 3–5 days after diagnosis. The difficulty of predicting which patients will benefit from antibiotic therapy has led to different approaches. In the Netherlands, for instance, physicians typically manage acute otitis media with initial observation, administering anti-inflammatory agents for aggressive pain management and reserving antibiotics for high-risk patients, patients with complicated disease, or patients who do not improve after 48–72 h. In contrast, many experts in the United States continue to recommend antibiotic therapy for children <6 months old in light of the higher

TABLE 31-2 GUIDELINES FOR THE DIAGNOSIS AND TREATMENT OF ACUTE OTITIS MEDIA

Illness Severity	Diagnostic Criteria	Treatment Recommendations
Mild to moderate	Fluid in the middle ear, evidenced by decreased tympanic membrane mobility, air/fluid level behind tympanic membrane, bulging tympanic membrane, purulent otorrhea *and* Acute onset of signs and symptoms of middle-ear inflammation, including fever, otalgia, decreased hearing, tinnitus, vertigo, erythematous tympanic membrane	*Initial therapy* [a] Observation alone (symptom relief only)[b] *or* Amoxicillin, 80–90 mg/kg qd (up to 2 g) PO in divided doses (bid or tid), *or* Cefdinir, 14 mg/kg qd PO in 1 dose or divided doses (bid), *or* Cefuroxime, 30 mg/kg qd PO in divided doses (bid), *or* Azithromycin, 10 mg/kg qd PO on day 1 followed by 5 mg/kg qd PO for 4 d *Exposure to antibiotics within 30 d or recent treatment failure*[a,c] Amoxicillin, 90 mg/kg qd (up to 2 g) PO in divided doses (bid), plus clavulanate, 6.4 mg/kg qd PO in divided doses (bid), *or* Ceftriaxone, 50 mg/kg IV/IM qd for 3 d, *or* Clindamycin, 30–40 mg/kg qd PO in divided doses (tid)
Severe	As above, with temperature ≥39.0°C *or* Moderate to severe otalgia	*Initial therapy* [a] Amoxicillin, 90 mg/kg qd (up to 2 g) PO in divided doses (bid), plus clavulanate, 6.4 mg/kg qd PO in divided doses (bid), *or* Ceftriaxone, 50 mg/kg IV/IM qd for 3 d *Exposure to antibiotics within 30 d or recent treatment failure*[a,c] Ceftriaxone, 50 mg/kg IV/IM qd for 3 d, *or* Clindamycin, 30–40 mg/kg qd PO in divided doses (tid), *or* Consider tympanocentesis with culture

[a]Duration (unless otherwise specified): 10 d for patients <6 years old and patients with severe disease; 5–7 d (with consideration of observation only in previously healthy individuals with mild disease) for patients ≥6 years old.
[b]Observation (deferring antibacterial treatment for 48–72 h and limiting management to symptom relief) is an option for mild to moderate disease in children 6 months to 2 years of age with an uncertain diagnosis and for children ≥2 years of age.
[c]Failure to improve and/or clinical worsening after 48–72 h of observation or treatment.
Sources: American Academy of Pediatrics Subcommittee on Management of Acute Otitis Media, 2004; Dowell et al, 1998.

frequency of secondary complications in this young and functionally immunocompromised population. However, observation without antimicrobial therapy is now generally considered a reasonable option in the United States for mild to moderate disease in children 6 months to 2 years of age with an uncertain diagnosis and for children ≥2 years of age (Table 31-2).

Given that most studies of the etiologic agents of acute otitis media consistently document similar pathogen profiles, therapy is generally empirical except in those few cases where tympanocentesis is warranted—e.g., cases in newborns, cases refractory to therapy, and cases in patients who are severely ill or immunodeficient. Despite resistance to penicillin and amoxicillin in roughly one-quarter of *S. pneumoniae* isolates, one-third of *H. influenzae* isolates, and nearly all *M. catarrhalis* isolates, outcome studies continue to find that amoxicillin is as successful as any other agent, and it remains the drug of first choice in recommendations from multiple sources (Table 31-2). Therapy for uncomplicated acute otitis media is typically administered for 5–7 days to patients ≥6 years old; longer courses (e.g., 10 days) should be reserved for children <6 years old and patients with severe disease, in whom short-course therapy may be inadequate.

A switch in regimen is recommended if there is no clinical improvement by the third day of therapy, given the possibility of infection with a β-lactamase-producing strain of *H. influenzae* or *M. catarrhalis* or with a strain of penicillin-resistant *S. pneumoniae*. Decongestants and antihistamines are frequently used as adjunctive agents to reduce congestion and relieve obstruction of the eustachian tube, but clinical trials have yielded no significant evidence of benefit with either class of agents.

Recurrent Acute Otitis Media Recurrent acute otitis media (more than three episodes within 6 months or four episodes within 12 months) is generally due to relapse or reinfection, although data indicate that the majority of early recurrences are new infections. In general, the same pathogens responsible for acute otitis media cause recurrent disease; even so, the recommended treatment consists of antibiotics active against β-lactamase-producing organisms. Antibiotic prophylaxis [e.g., with trimethoprim-sulfamethoxazole (TMP-SMX) or amoxicillin] can reduce recurrences in patients with recurrent acute otitis media by an average of one episode per year, but this benefit is small compared with the cost of the drug and the high likelihood of colonization with antibiotic-resistant pathogens. Other approaches, including placement of tympanostomy tubes, adenoidectomy, and tonsillectomy plus adenoidectomy, are of questionable overall value, given the relatively small benefit compared with the potential for complications.

Serous Otitis Media In serous otitis media (otitis media with effusion), fluid is present in the middle ear for an extended period and in the absence of signs and symptoms of infection. In general, acute effusions are self-limited; most resolve in 2–4 weeks. In some cases, however (in particular after an episode of acute otitis media), effusions can persist for months. These chronic effusions are often associated with a significant hearing loss in the affected ear. In younger children, persistent effusions and decreased hearing can be associated with impairment of language acquisition skills. The great majority of cases of otitis media with effusion resolve spontaneously within 3 months without antibiotic therapy. Antibiotic therapy or myringotomy with insertion of tympanostomy tubes is typically reserved for patients in whom bilateral effusion (1) has persisted for at least 3 months and (2) is associated with significant bilateral hearing loss. With this conservative approach and the application of strict diagnostic criteria for acute otitis media and otitis media with effusion, it is estimated that 6–8 million courses of antibiotics could be avoided each year in the United States.

Chronic Otitis Media Chronic suppurative otitis media is characterized by persistent or recurrent purulent otorrhea in the setting of tympanic membrane perforation. Usually, there is also some degree of conductive hearing loss. This condition can be categorized as active or inactive. Inactive disease is characterized by a central perforation of the tympanic membrane, which allows drainage of purulent fluid from the middle ear. When the perforation is more peripheral, squamous epithelium from the auditory canal may invade the middle ear through the perforation, forming a mass of keratinaceous debris (*cholesteatoma*) at the site of invasion. This mass can enlarge and has the potential to erode bone and promote further infection, which can lead to meningitis, brain abscess, or paralysis of cranial nerve VII. Treatment of chronic active otitis media is surgical; mastoidectomy, myringoplasty, and tympanoplasty can be performed as outpatient surgical procedures, with an overall success rate of ~80%. Chronic inactive otitis media is more difficult to cure, usually requiring repeated courses of topical antibiotic drops during periods of drainage. Systemic antibiotics may offer better cure rates, but their role in the treatment of this condition remains unclear.

Mastoiditis Acute mastoiditis was relatively common among children before the introduction of antibiotics. Because the mastoid air cells connect with the middle ear, the process of fluid collection and infection is usually the same in the mastoid as in the middle ear. Early and frequent treatment of acute otitis media is most likely the reason that

FIGURE 31-1 Acute mastoiditis. Axial CT image shows an acute fluid collection within the mastoid air cells on the left.

the incidence of acute mastoiditis has declined to only 1.2–2.0 cases per 100,000 person-years in countries with high prescribing rates for acute otitis media. In countries like the Netherlands, where antibiotics are used sparingly for acute otitis media, the incidence rate of acute mastoiditis is roughly twice that in countries like the United States. However, neighboring Denmark has a rate of acute mastoiditis similar to that in the Netherlands but an antibiotic-prescribing rate for acute otitis media more similar to that in the United States.

In typical acute mastoiditis, purulent exudate collects in the mastoid air cells (Fig. 31-1), producing pressure that may result in erosion of the surrounding bone and the formation of abscess-like cavities that are usually evident on CT. Patients typically present with pain, erythema, and swelling of the mastoid process along with displacement of the pinna, usually in conjunction with the typical signs and symptoms of acute middle-ear infection. Rarely, patients can develop severe complications if the infection tracks under the periosteum of the temporal bone to cause a subperiosteal abscess, erodes through the mastoid tip to cause a deep neck abscess, or extends posteriorly to cause septic thrombosis of the lateral sinus.

Purulent fluid should be cultured whenever possible to help guide antimicrobial therapy. Initial empirical therapy is usually directed against the typical organisms associated with acute otitis media, such as *S. pneumoniae*, *H. influenzae*, and *M. catarrhalis*. Some patients with more severe or prolonged courses of illness should be treated for infection with *S. aureus* and gram-negative bacilli (including *Pseudomonas*). Broad empirical therapy is usually narrowed once culture results become available. Most patients can be treated conservatively with IV antibiotics; surgery (cortical mastoidectomy) can be reserved for complicated cases and those in which conservative treatment has failed.

INFECTIONS OF THE PHARYNX AND ORAL CAVITY

Oropharyngeal infections range from mild, self-limited viral illnesses to serious, life-threatening bacterial infections. The most common presenting symptom is sore throat—one of the most frequent reasons for ambulatory care visits by both adults and children. Although sore throat is a symptom in many noninfectious illnesses as well, the overwhelming majority of patients with a new sore throat have acute pharyngitis of viral or bacterial etiology.

ACUTE PHARYNGITIS

Millions of visits to primary care providers each year are for sore throat; the majority of cases of acute pharyngitis are caused by typical respiratory viruses. The most important source of concern is infection with group A β-hemolytic *Streptococcus* (*S. pyogenes*), which is associated with acute glomerulonephritis and acute rheumatic fever. The risk of rheumatic fever can be reduced by timely penicillin therapy.

Etiology A wide variety of organisms cause acute pharyngitis. The relative importance of the different pathogens can only be estimated, since a significant proportion of cases (~30%) have no identified cause. Together, respiratory viruses are the most common identifiable cause of acute pharyngitis, with rhinoviruses and coronaviruses accounting for large proportions of cases (~20% and at least 5%, respectively). Influenza virus, parainfluenza virus, and adenovirus also account for a measurable share of cases, the latter as part of the more clinically severe syndrome of pharyngoconjunctival fever. Other important but less common viral causes include herpes simplex virus (HSV) types 1 and 2, coxsackievirus A, cytomegalovirus (CMV), and Epstein-Barr virus (EBV). Acute HIV infection can present as acute pharyngitis and should be considered in high-risk populations.

Acute bacterial pharyngitis is typically caused by *S. pyogenes*, which accounts for ~5–15% of all cases of acute pharyngitis in adults; rates vary with the season and with utilization of the health care system. Group A streptococcal pharyngitis is primarily a disease of children 5–15 years of age; it is uncommon among children <3 years old, as is rheumatic fever. Streptococci of groups C and G account for a minority of cases, although these serogroups are nonrheumatogenic. The remaining bacterial causes of acute pharyngitis are seen infrequently (<1% each) but should be considered in appropriate exposure groups because of the severity of illness if left untreated; these etiologic agents include *Neisseria gonorrhoeae*, *Corynebacterium diphtheriae*, *Corynebacterium ulcerans*, *Yersinia enterocolitica*, and *Treponema pallidum* (in secondary syphilis). Anaerobic bacteria can also cause acute pharyngitis (*Vincent's angina*) and can contribute to more serious polymicrobial infections, such as peritonsillar or retropharyngeal abscess (see below). Atypical organisms such as *M. pneumoniae* and *C. pneumoniae* have been recovered from patients with acute pharyngitis; whether these agents are commensals or causes of acute infection is debatable.

Clinical Manifestations Although the signs and symptoms accompanying acute pharyngitis are not reliable predictors of the etiologic agent, the clinical presentation occasionally suggests that one etiology is more likely than another. Acute pharyngitis due to respiratory viruses such as rhinovirus or coronavirus is usually not severe and is typically associated with a constellation of coryzal symptoms better characterized as nonspecific URI. Findings on physical examination are uncommon; fever is rare, and tender cervical adenopathy and pharyngeal exudates are not seen. In contrast, acute pharyngitis from influenza virus can be severe and is much more likely to be associated with fever as well as with myalgias, headache, and cough. The presentation of pharyngoconjunctival fever due to adenovirus infection is similar. Since pharyngeal exudate may be present on examination, this condition can be difficult to differentiate from streptococcal pharyngitis. However, adenoviral pharyngitis is distinguished by the presence of conjunctivitis in one-third to one-half of patients. Acute pharyngitis from primary HSV infection can also mimic streptococcal pharyngitis in some cases, with pharyngeal inflammation and exudate, but the presence of vesicles and shallow ulcers on the palate can help differentiate the two diseases. This HSV syndrome is distinct from pharyngitis caused by coxsackievirus (*herpangina*), which is associated with small vesicles that develop on the soft palate and uvula and then rupture to form shallow white ulcers. Acute exudative pharyngitis coupled with fever, fatigue, generalized lymphadenopathy, and (on occasion) splenomegaly is characteristic of infectious mononucleosis due to EBV or CMV. Acute primary infection with HIV is frequently associated with fever and acute pharyngitis as well as with myalgias, arthralgias, malaise, and occasionally a nonpruritic maculopapular rash, which later may be followed by lymphadenopathy and mucosal ulcerations without exudate.

The clinical features of acute pharyngitis caused by streptococci of groups A, C, and G are all similar, ranging from a relatively mild illness without many accompanying symptoms to clinically severe cases with profound pharyngeal pain, fever, chills, and abdominal pain. A hyperemic pharyngeal membrane with tonsillar hypertrophy and exudate is usually seen, along with tender anterior cervical adenopathy. Coryzal manifestations, including cough, are typically absent; when present, they suggest a viral etiology. Strains of *S. pyogenes* that generate erythrogenic toxin can also produce scarlet fever characterized by an erythematous rash and strawberry tongue. The other types of acute bacterial pharyngitis (e.g., gonococcal, diphtherial, and yersinial) often present as exudative pharyngitis with or without other clinical features. Their etiologies are often suggested only by the clinical history.

Diagnosis The primary goal of diagnostic testing is to separate acute streptococcal pharyngitis from pharyngitis of other etiologies (particularly viral) so that antibiotics can be prescribed more efficiently for patients to whom they may be beneficial. The most appropriate standard for the diagnosis of streptococcal pharyngitis, however, has not been definitively established. Throat swab culture is generally regarded as such. However, this method cannot distinguish between infection and colonization, and it takes 24–48 h to yield results that vary according to technique and culture conditions. Rapid antigen-detection tests offer good specificity (>90%) but lower sensitivity when implemented in routine practice. The sensitivity has also been shown to vary across the clinical spectrum of disease (65–90%). Several clinical prediction systems (Table 31-3) can increase the sensitivity of rapid antigen-detection tests to >90% in controlled settings. Since the sensitivities achieved in routine clinical practice are often lower, several medical and professional societies continue to recommend that all negative rapid antigen-detection tests in children be confirmed by a throat culture to limit transmission and complications of illness caused by group A streptococci. The Centers for Disease Control and Prevention, the Infectious Diseases Society of America, the American College of Physicians, and the American Academy of Family Physicians do not recommend backup culture when adults have negative results in a high-sensitivity, rapid antigen-detection test, however, given the lower prevalence and smaller benefit in this age group.

Cultures and rapid diagnostic tests for other causes of acute pharyngitis, such as influenza virus, adenovirus, HSV, EBV, CMV, and *M. pneumoniae*, are available in some locations and can be used when these infections are suspected. The diagnosis of acute EBV infection depends primarily on the detection of antibodies to the virus with a heterophile agglutination assay (monospot slide test) or enzyme-linked immunosorbent assay. Testing for HIV RNA or antigen (p24) should be performed when acute primary HIV infection is suspected. If other bacterial causes are suspected (particularly *N. gonorrhoeae*, *C. diphtheriae*, or *Y. enterocolitica*), specific cultures should be requested since these organisms may be missed on routine throat swab culture.

℞ PHARYNGITIS

Antibiotic treatment of pharyngitis due to *S. pyogenes* confers numerous benefits, including a decrease in the risk of rheumatic fever. The magnitude of this benefit is fairly small, however, since rheumatic fever is now a rare disease, even among untreated patients. When therapy is started within 48 h of illness onset, however, symptom duration is also decreased. An additional benefit of therapy is the potential to reduce the spread of streptococcal pharyngitis, particularly in areas of overcrowding or close contact. Antibiotic therapy for acute pharyngitis is therefore recommended in cases where *S. pyogenes* is confirmed as the etiologic agent by rapid antigen-detection test or throat swab culture. Otherwise, antibiotics should be given in routine cases only when another bacterial cause has been identified. Effective therapy for streptococcal pharyngitis consists of either a single dose of IM benzathine penicillin or a full 10-day course of oral penicillin

TABLE 31-3   GUIDELINES FOR THE DIAGNOSIS AND TREATMENT OF ACUTE PHARYNGITIS

Age Group	Diagnostic Criteria	Treatment Recommendations[a]
Adults	*Clinical suspicion of streptococcal pharyngitis* (e.g., fever, tonsillar swelling, exudate, enlarged/tender anterior cervical lymph nodes, absence of cough or coryza)[b] *with:* History of rheumatic fever *or* Documented household exposure *or* Positive rapid strep screen	Penicillin V, 500 mg PO tid, *or* Amoxicillin, 500 mg PO bid, *or* Erythromycin, 250 mg PO qid, *or* Benzathine penicillin G, single dose of 1.2 million units IM
Children	*Clinical suspicion of streptococcal pharyngitis* (e.g., tonsillar swelling, exudate, enlarged/tender anterior cervical lymph nodes, absence of coryza) *with:* History of rheumatic fever *or* Documented household exposure *or* Positive rapid strep screen *or* Positive throat culture (for patients with negative rapid strep screen)	Amoxicillin, 45 mg/kg qd PO in divided doses (bid or tid), *or* Penicillin VK, 50 mg/kg qd PO in divided doses (bid), *or* Cephalexin, 50 mg/kg qd PO in divided doses (qid), *or* Benzathine penicillin G, single dose of 25,000 units/kg IM

[a]Unless otherwise specified, the duration of therapy is generally 10 d, with appropriate follow-up.
[b]Some organizations support treating adults who have these symptoms and signs without administering a rapid streptococcal antigen test.
Sources: Cooper et al, 2001; Schwartz et al, 1998.

(Table 31-3). Erythromycin can be used in place of penicillin, although resistance to erythromycin among *S. pyogenes* strains in some parts of the world (particularly Europe) can prohibit the use of this drug. Newer (and more expensive) antibiotics are also active against streptococci but offer no greater efficacy than the above agents. Testing for cure is unnecessary and may reveal only chronic colonization. There is no evidence to support antibiotic treatment of group C or G streptococcal pharyngitis or of pharyngitis in which *Mycoplasma* or *Chlamydophila* has been recovered. Penicillin prophylaxis (benzathine penicillin G, 1.2 million units IM every 3–4 weeks) is indicated for patients at risk of recurrent rheumatic fever.

Treatment of viral pharyngitis is entirely symptom-based except in infection with influenza virus or HSV. For influenza, a number of therapeutic agents exist, including amantadine, rimantadine, and the two newer agents oseltamivir and zanamivir. All of these agents need to be started within 36–48 h of symptom onset to reduce illness duration meaningfully. Of these agents, only oseltamivir and zanamivir are active against both influenza A and influenza B and therefore can be used when local infection patterns are unknown. Oropharyngeal HSV infection sometimes responds to treatment with antiviral agents such as acyclovir, although these drugs are often reserved for immunosuppressed patients.

Complications Although rheumatic fever is the best-known complication of acute streptococcal pharyngitis, the risk of its following acute infection remains quite low. Other complications include acute glomerulonephritis and numerous suppurative conditions, such as peritonsillar abscess (*quinsy*), otitis media, mastoiditis, sinusitis, bacteremia, and pneumonia—all of which occur at low rates. Although antibiotic treatment of acute streptococcal pharyngitis can prevent the development of rheumatic fever, there is no evidence that it can prevent acute glomerulonephritis. Some evidence supports antibiotic use to prevent the suppurative complications of streptococcal pharyngitis, particularly peritonsillar abscess, which can also involve oral anaerobes such as *Fusobacterium*. Abscesses are usually accompanied by severe pharyngeal pain, dysphagia, fever, and dehydration; in addition, medial displacement of the tonsil and lateral displacement of the uvula are often evident on examination. Although early use of IV antibiotics (e.g., clindamycin; penicillin G with metronidazole) may obviate the need for surgical drainage in some cases, treatment typically involves needle aspiration or incision and drainage.

ORAL INFECTIONS

Aside from periodontal disease such as gingivitis, infections of the oral cavity most commonly involve HSV or *Candida* species. In addition to causing painful cold sores on the lips, HSV can infect the tongue and buccal mucosa, causing the formation of irritating vesicles. Although topical antiviral agents (e.g., acyclovir and penciclovir) can be used externally for cold sores, oral or IV acyclovir is often needed for primary infections, extensive oral infections, and infections in immunocompromised patients. Oropharyngeal candidiasis (*thrush*) is caused by a variety of *Candida* species, most often *C. albicans*. Thrush occurs predominantly in neonates, immunocompromised patients (especially those with AIDS), and recipients of prolonged antibiotic or glucocorticoid therapy. In addition to sore throat, patients often report a burning tongue, and physical examination reveals friable white or gray plaques on the gingiva, tongue, and oral mucosa. Treatment, which usually consists of an oral antifungal suspension (nystatin or clotrimazole) or oral fluconazole, is frequently successful. In the uncommon cases of fluconazole-refractory thrush that are seen in some patients with AIDS, other therapeutic options include oral formulations of itraconazole, amphotericin B, or voriconazole as well as the IV echinocandins (caspofungin, micafungin, and anidulafungin).

Vincent's angina, also known as *acute necrotizing ulcerative gingivitis* or *trench mouth*, is a unique and dramatic form of gingivitis characterized by painful, inflamed gingiva with ulcerations of the interdental papillae that bleed easily. Since oral anaerobes are the cause, patients typically have halitosis and frequently present with fever, malaise, and lymphadenopathy. Treatment consists of debridement and oral administration of penicillin plus metronidazole, with clindamycin alone as an alternative.

Ludwig's angina is a rapidly progressive, potentially fulminant cellulitis that involves the sublingual and submandibular spaces and that typically originates from an infected or recently extracted tooth, most commonly the lower second and third molars. Improved dental care has substantially reduced the incidence of this disorder. Infection in these areas leads to dysphagia, odynophagia, and "woody" edema in the sublingual region, forcing the tongue up and back with the potential for airway obstruction. Fever, dysarthria, and drooling may also be noted, and patients may speak in a "hot potato" voice. Intubation or tracheostomy may be necessary to secure the airway, as asphyxiation is the most common cause of death. Patients should be monitored closely and treated promptly with IV antibiotics directed against streptococci and oral anaerobes. Recommended agents include ampicillin/sulbactam and high-dose penicillin plus metronidazole.

Postanginal septicemia (*Lemierre's disease*) is a rare anaerobic oropharyngeal infection caused predominantly by *Fusobacterium necrophorum*. The illness typically starts as a sore throat (most commonly in adolescents and young adults), which may present as exudative tonsillitis or peritonsillar abscess. Infection of the deep pharyngeal tissue allows organisms to drain into the lateral pharyngeal space, which contains the carotid artery and internal jugular vein. Septic thrombophlebitis of the internal jugular vein can result, with associated pain, dysphagia, and neck swelling and stiffness. Sepsis usually occurs 3–10 days after the onset of sore throat and is often coupled with metastatic infection to the lung and other distant sites. Occasionally, the infection can extend along the carotid sheath and into the posterior mediastinum, resulting in mediastinitis, or it can erode into the carotid artery, with the early sign of repeated small bleeds into the mouth. The mortality rate from these invasive infections can be as high as 50%. Treatment consists of IV antibiotics (penicillin G or clindamycin) and surgical drainage of any purulent collections. The concomitant use of anticoagulants to prevent embolization remains controversial but is often advised.

INFECTIONS OF THE LARYNX AND EPIGLOTTIS

LARYNGITIS

Laryngitis is defined as any inflammatory process involving the larynx and can be caused by a variety of infectious and noninfectious processes. The vast majority of laryngitis cases seen in clinical practice in developed countries are acute. Acute laryngitis is a common syndrome caused predominantly by the same viruses responsible for many other URIs. In fact, most cases of acute laryngitis occur in the setting of a viral URI.

Etiology   Nearly all major respiratory viruses have been implicated in acute viral laryngitis, including rhinovirus, influenza virus, parainflu-

enza virus, adenovirus, coxsackievirus, coronavirus, and RSV. Acute laryngitis can also be associated with acute bacterial respiratory infections, such as those caused by group A *Streptococcus* or *C. diphtheriae* (although diphtheria has been all but eliminated in the United States). Another bacterial pathogen thought to play a role (albeit unclear) in the pathogenesis of acute laryngitis is *M. catarrhalis*, which has been recovered on nasopharyngeal culture from a significant percentage of people with acute laryngitis. Chronic laryngitis of infectious etiology is much less common in developed than in developing countries. Laryngitis due to *Mycobacterium tuberculosis* is often difficult to distinguish from laryngeal cancer, in part because of the frequent absence of signs, symptoms, and radiographic findings typical of pulmonary disease. *Histoplasma* and *Blastomyces* may cause laryngitis, often as a complication of systemic infection. *Candida* species can cause laryngitis as well, often in association with thrush or esophagitis and particularly in immunosuppressed patients. Rare cases of chronic laryngitis are due to *Coccidioides* and *Cryptococcus*.

Clinical Manifestations   Laryngitis is characterized by hoarseness and can also be associated with reduced vocal pitch or aphonia. As acute laryngitis is caused predominantly by respiratory viruses, these symptoms usually occur in association with other symptoms and signs of URI, including rhinorrhea, nasal congestion, cough, and sore throat. Direct laryngoscopy often reveals diffuse laryngeal erythema and edema, along with vascular engorgement of the vocal folds. In addition, chronic disease (e.g., tuberculous laryngitis) often includes mucosal nodules and ulcerations visible on laryngoscopy; these lesions are sometimes mistaken for laryngeal cancer.

℞ LARYNGITIS

Acute laryngitis is usually treated with humidification and voice rest alone. Antibiotics are not recommended except when group A *Streptococcus* is cultured, in which case penicillin is the drug of choice. The choice of therapy for chronic laryngitis depends on the pathogen, whose identification usually requires biopsy with culture. Patients with laryngeal tuberculosis are highly contagious because of the large number of organisms that are easily aerosolized. These patients should be managed in the same way as patients with active pulmonary disease.

CROUP

The term *croup* actually denotes a group of diseases collectively referred to as "croup syndrome," all of which are acute and predominantly viral respiratory illnesses characterized by marked swelling of the subglottic region of the larynx. Croup primarily affects children <6 years old. For a detailed discussion of this entity, the reader is referred to a text of pediatric medicine.

EPIGLOTTITIS

Acute epiglottitis (supraglottitis) is an acute, rapidly progressive cellulitis of the epiglottis and adjacent structures that can result in complete—and potentially fatal—airway obstruction in both children and adults. Before the widespread use of *H. influenzae* type b (Hib) vaccine, this entity was much more common among children, with a peak incidence at ~3.5 years of age. In some countries, mass vaccination against Hib has reduced the annual incidence of acute epiglottitis in children by >90%; in contrast, the annual incidence in adults has changed little since the introduction of Hib vaccine. Because of the danger of airway obstruction, acute epiglottitis constitutes a medical emergency, particularly in children, and prompt diagnosis and airway protection are of utmost importance.

Etiology   After the introduction of the Hib vaccine in the mid-1980s, disease incidence among children in the United States declined dramatically. Nevertheless, lack of vaccination or vaccine failure has meant that many pediatric cases seen today are still due to Hib. In adults and (more recently) in children, a variety of other bacterial pathogens have been associated with epiglottitis, the most common

FIGURE 31-2 Acute epiglottitis. In this lateral soft tissue radiograph of the neck, the arrow indicates the enlarged edematous epiglottis (the "thumbprint sign").

being group A *Streptococcus*. Other pathogens seen less frequently include *S. pneumoniae*, *Haemophilus parainfluenzae*, and *S. aureus*. Viruses have not yet been established as causes of acute epiglottitis.

Clinical Manifestations and Diagnosis Epiglottitis typically presents more acutely in young children than in adolescents or adults. On presentation, most children have had symptoms for <24 h, including high fever, severe sore throat, tachycardia, systemic toxicity, and (in many cases) drooling while sitting forward. Symptoms and signs of respiratory obstruction may also be present and may progress rapidly. The somewhat milder illness in adolescents and adults often follows 1–2 days of severe sore throat and is commonly accompanied by dyspnea, drooling, and stridor. Physical examination of patients with acute epiglottitis may reveal moderate or severe respiratory distress, with inspiratory stridor and retractions of the chest wall. These findings *diminish* as the disease progresses and the patient tires. Conversely, oropharyngeal examination reveals injection that is much less severe than would be predicted from the symptoms—a finding that should alert the clinician to a cause of symptoms and obstruction that lies beyond the tonsils. The diagnosis is often made on clinical grounds, although direct fiberoptic laryngoscopy is frequently performed in a controlled environment (e.g., an operating room) in order to visualize and culture the typical edematous "cherry-red" epiglottis and to facilitate placement of an endotracheal tube. Direct visualization in an examination room (e.g., with a tongue blade and indirect laryngoscopy) is not recommended because of the risk of immediate laryngospasm and complete airway obstruction. Lateral neck radiographs and laboratory tests can assist in the diagnosis but may delay the critical securing of the airway and cause the patient to be moved or repositioned more than is necessary, thereby increasing the risk of further airway compromise. Neck radiographs typically reveal an enlarged edematous epiglottis (the "thumbprint sign," Fig. 31-2), usually with a dilated hypopharynx and normal subglottic structures. Laboratory tests characteristically document mild to moderate leukocytosis with a predominance of neutrophils. Blood cultures are positive in a significant proportion of cases.

℞ EPIGLOTTITIS

Security of the airway is always of primary concern in acute epiglottitis, even if the diagnosis is only suspected. Mere observation for signs of impending airway obstruction is not routinely recommended, particularly in children. Many adults have been managed with observation only since the

illness is perceived to be milder in this age group, but some data suggest that this approach may be risky and probably should be reserved only for adult patients who have yet to develop dyspnea or stridor. Once the airway has been secured and specimens of blood and epiglottis tissue have been obtained for culture, treatment with IV antibiotics should be given to cover the most likely organisms, particularly *H. influenzae*. Because rates of ampicillin resistance in this organism have risen significantly in recent years, therapy with a β-lactam/β-lactamase inhibitor combination or a second- or third-generation cephalosporin is recommended. Typically, ampicillin/sulbactam, cefuroxime, cefotaxime, or ceftriaxone is given, with clindamycin and TMP-SMX reserved for patients allergic to β-lactams. Antibiotic therapy should be continued for 7–10 days and should be tailored, if necessary, to the organism recovered in culture. If the household contacts of a patient with *H. influenzae* epiglottitis include an unvaccinated child under the age of 4, all members of the household (including the patient) should receive prophylactic rifampin for 4 days to eradicate carriage of *H. influenzae*.

INFECTIONS OF THE DEEP NECK STRUCTURES

Deep neck infections are usually extensions of infection from other primary sites, most often within the pharynx or oral cavity. Many of these infections are life-threatening but are difficult to detect at early stages when they may be more easily managed. Three of the most clinically relevant spaces in the neck are the submandibular (and sublingual) space, the lateral pharyngeal (or parapharyngeal) space, and the retropharyngeal space. These spaces communicate with one another and with other important structures in the head, neck, and thorax, providing pathogens with easy access to areas including the mediastinum, carotid sheath, skull base, and meninges. Once infection reaches these sensitive areas, mortality rates can be as high as 20–50%.

Infection of the submandibular and/or sublingual space typically originates from an infected or recently extracted lower tooth. The result is the severe, life-threatening infection referred to as Ludwig's angina (see "Oral Infections," above). Infection of the lateral pharyngeal (or parapharyngeal) space is most often a complication of common infections of the oral cavity and upper respiratory tract, including tonsillitis, peritonsillar abscess, pharyngitis, mastoiditis, or periodontal infection. This space, located deep to the lateral wall of the pharynx, contains a number of sensitive structures, including the carotid artery, internal jugular vein, cervical sympathetic chain, and portions of cranial nerves IX through XII; at its distal end, it opens into the posterior mediastinum. Involvement of this space with infection can therefore be rapidly fatal. Examination may reveal some tonsillar displacement, trismus, and neck rigidity, but swelling of the lateral pharyngeal wall can easily be missed. The diagnosis can be confirmed by CT. Treatment consists of airway management, operative drainage of fluid collections, and at least 10 days of IV therapy with an antibiotic active against streptococci and oral anaerobes (e.g., ampicillin/sulbactam). A particularly severe form of this infection involving the components of the carotid sheath (postanginal septicemia, Lemierre's disease) is described above (see "Oral Infections"). Infection of the retropharyngeal space can also be extremely dangerous, as this space runs posterior to the pharynx from the skull base to the superior mediastinum. Infections in this space are more common among children <5 years old because of the presence of several small retropharyngeal lymph nodes that typically atrophy by the age of 4 years. Infection is usually a consequence of extension from another site of infection, most commonly acute pharyngitis. Other sources include otitis media, tonsillitis, dental infections, Ludwig's angina, and anterior extension of vertebral osteomyelitis. Retropharyngeal space infection can also follow penetrating trauma to the posterior pharynx (e.g., from an endoscopic procedure). Infections are commonly polymicrobial, involving a mixture of aerobes and anaerobes; group A β-hemolytic streptococci and *S. aureus* are the most common pathogens. *M. tuberculosis* was a frequent cause in the past but now is rarely involved in the United States.

Patients with retropharyngeal abscess typically present with sore throat, fever, dysphagia, and neck pain and are often drooling because of difficulty and pain with swallowing. Examination may reveal tender cervical adenopathy, neck swelling, and diffuse erythema and edema of the posterior pharynx as well as a bulge in the posterior pharyngeal wall that may not be obvious on routine inspection. A soft tissue mass is usually demonstrable by lateral neck radiography or CT. Because of the risk of airway obstruction, treatment begins with securing of the airway, which is followed by a combination of surgical drainage and IV antibiotic administration. Initial empirical therapy should cover streptococci, oral anaerobes, and *S. aureus*; ampicillin/sulbactam, clindamycin alone, or clindamycin plus ceftriaxone is usually effective. Complications result primarily from extension to other areas; for example, rupture into the posterior pharynx may lead to aspiration pneumonia and empyema. Extension may also occur to the lateral pharyngeal space and mediastinum, resulting in mediastinitis and pericarditis, or into nearby major blood vessels. All these events are associated with a high mortality rate.

FURTHER READINGS

AMERICAN ACADEMY OF PEDIATRICS SUBCOMMITTEE ON MANAGEMENT OF ACUTE OTITIS MEDIA: Diagnosis and management of acute otitis media. Pediatrics 113:1451, 2004

AMERICAN ACADEMY OF PEDIATRICS SUBCOMMITTEE ON MANAGEMENT OF SINUSITIS AND COMMITTEE ON QUALITY IMPROVEMENT: Clinical practice guideline: Management of sinusitis. Pediatrics 108:798, 2001

COOPER RJ et al: Principles of appropriate antibiotic use for acute pharyngitis in adults: Background. Ann Intern Med 134:509, 2001

DOWELL SF et al: Otitis media—principles of judicious use of antimicrobial agents. Pediatrics 101:165, 1998

GONZALES R et al: Principles of appropriate antibiotic use for treatment of nonspecific upper respiratory tract infections in adults: Background. Ann Intern Med 134:490, 2001

HICKNER JM et al: Principles of appropriate antibiotic use for acute rhinosinusitis in adults: Background. Ann Intern Med 134:498, 2001

PICCIRILLO JF: Acute bacterial sinusitis. N Engl J Med 351:902, 2004

RAFEI K et al: Airway infectious disease emergencies. Pediatr Clin North Am 53:215, 2006

SCHWARTZ B et al: Pharyngitis—principles of judicious use of antimicrobial agents. Pediatrics 101:171, 1998

SINUS AND ALLERGY HEALTH PARTNERSHIP: Antimicrobial treatment guidelines for acute bacterial rhinosinusitis. Otolaryngol Head Neck Surg 130:1, 2004

VAN ZUIJLEN DA et al: National differences in incidence of acute mastoiditis: Relationship to prescribing patterns of antibiotics for acute otitis media? Pediatr Infect Dis J 20:140, 2001

WENZEL RP et al: Acute bronchitis. N Engl J Med 355:2125, 2006

32 Oral Manifestations of Disease
Samuel C. Durso

As primary care physicians and consultants, internists are often asked to evaluate patients with disease of the oral soft tissues, teeth, and pharynx. Knowledge of the oral milieu and its unique structures is necessary to guide preventive services and recognize oral manifestations of local or systemic disease (**Chap. e7**). Furthermore, internists frequently collaborate with dentists in the care of patients who have a variety of medical conditions that affect oral health or who undergo dental procedures that increase their risk of medical complications.

DISEASES OF THE TEETH AND PERIODONTAL STRUCTURES

TOOTH AND PERIODONTAL STRUCTURE

Tooth formation begins during the sixth week of embryonic life and continues through the first 17 years of age. Tooth development begins in utero and continues until after the tooth erupts. Normally all 20 deciduous teeth have erupted by age 3 and have been shed by age 13. Permanent teeth, eventually totaling 32, begin to erupt by age 6 and have completely erupted by age 14, though third molars (wisdom teeth) may erupt later.

The erupted tooth consists of the visible crown covered with enamel and the root submerged below the gum line and covered with bonelike cementum. *Dentin*, a material that is denser than bone and exquisitely sensitive to pain, forms the majority of the tooth substance. Dentin surrounds a core of myxomatous *pulp* containing the vascular and nerve supply. The tooth is held firmly in the alveolar socket by the *periodontium*, supporting structures that consist of the gingivae, alveolar bone, cementum, and periodontal ligament. The periodontal ligament tenaciously binds the tooth's cementum to the alveolar bone. Above this ligament is a collar of attached gingiva just below the crown. A few millimeters of unattached or free gingiva (1–3 mm) overlap the base of the crown, forming a shallow sulcus along the gum-tooth margin.

Dental Caries, Pulpal and Periapical Disease, and Complications Dental caries begin asymptomatically as a destructive process of the hard surface of the tooth. *Streptococcus mutans*, principally, along with other bacteria colonize the organic buffering film on the tooth surface to produce *plaque*. If not removed by brushing or the natural cleaning action of saliva and oral soft tissues, bacterial acids demineralize the enamel. Fissures and pits on the occlusion surfaces are the most frequent sites of decay. Surfaces adjacent to tooth restorations and exposed roots are also vulnerable, particularly as teeth are retained in an aging population. Over time, dental caries extend to the underlying dentin, leading to cavitation of the enamel and ultimately penetration to the tooth pulp, producing *acute pulpitis*. At this early stage, when the pulp infection is limited, the tooth becomes sensitive to percussion and hot or cold, and pain resolves immediately when the irritating stimulus is removed. Should the infection spread throughout the pulp, *irreversible pulpitis* occurs, leading to pulp necrosis. At this late stage pain is severe and has a sharp or throbbing visceral quality that may be worse when the patient lies down. Once pulp necrosis is complete, pain may be constant or intermittent, but cold sensitivity is lost.

Treatment of caries involves removal of the softened and infected hard tissue; sealing the exposed dentin; and restoration of the tooth structure with silver amalgam, composite plastic, gold, or porcelain. Once irreversible pulpitis occurs, root canal therapy is necessary, and the contents of the pulp chamber and root canals are removed, followed by thorough cleaning, antisepsis, and filling with an inert material. Alternatively, the tooth may be extracted.

Pulpal infection, if it does not egress through the decayed enamel, leads to *periapical abscess* formation, which produces pain on chewing. If the infection is mild and chronic, a *periapical granuloma* or eventually a *periapical cyst* forms, either of which produces radiolucency at the root apex. When unchecked, a periapical abscess can erode into the alveolar bone producing osteomyelitis, penetrate and drain through the gingivae (parulis or gumboil), or track along deep fascial planes, producing a virulent cellulitis (Ludwig's angina) involving the submandibular space and floor of the mouth (Chap. 157). Elderly patients, those with diabetes mellitus, and patients taking glucocorticoids may experience little or no pain and fever as these complications develop.

Periodontal Disease Periodontal disease accounts for more tooth loss than caries, particularly in the elderly. Like dental caries, chronic infection of the gingiva and anchoring structures of the tooth begins with formation of bacterial plaque. The process begins invisibly above the gum line and in the gingival sulcus. Plaque, including mineralized plaque (calculus), is preventable by appropriate dental hygiene, including periodic professional cleaning. Left undisturbed, chronic inflammation ensues and produces a painless hyperemia of the free and attached gingivae (*gingivitis*) that typically bleeds with brushing. If ignored, severe *periodontitis* occurs, leading to deepening of the physiologic sulcus and destruction of the periodontal ligament. Pockets develop around the teeth and become filled with pus and debris. As the periodontium is destroyed, teeth loosen and exfoliate. Eventually there is resorption of the alveolar bone. A role for the chronic inflammation resulting from chronic periodontal disease in promoting coronary heart disease and stroke has been proposed. Epidemiologic studies demonstrate a moderate but significant association between chronic periodontal inflammation and atherogenesis, though a causal role remains unproven.

Acute and aggressive forms of periodontal disease are less common than the chronic forms described above. However, if the host is stressed or exposed to a new pathogen, rapidly progressive and destructive disease of the periodontal tissue can occur. A virulent example is *acute necrotizing ulcerative gingivitis* (ANUG), or *Vincent's infection*, characterized as "trench mouth" during World War I. Stress, poor oral hygiene, and tobacco and alcohol use are risk factors. The presentation includes sudden gingival inflammation, ulceration, bleeding, interdental gingival necrosis, and fetid halitosis. *Localized juvenile periodontitis*, seen in adolescents, is particularly destructive and appears to be associated with impaired neutrophil chemotaxis. *AIDS-related periodontitis* resembles ANUG in some patients or a more destructive form of adult chronic periodontitis in others. It may also produce a gangrene-like destructive process of the oral soft tissues and bone that resembles *noma*, seen in severely malnourished children in developing nations.

Prevention of Tooth Decay and Periodontal Infection Despite the reduced prevalence of dental caries and periodontal disease in the United States due in large part to water fluoridation and improved dental care, respectively, both diseases constitute a major public health problem worldwide and for certain groups. The internist should promote preventive dental care and hygiene as part of health maintenance. Special populations at high risk for dental caries and periodontal disease include those with xerostomia, diabetics, alcoholics, tobacco users, those with Down's syndrome, and those with gingival hyperplasia. Furthermore, patients lacking dental care access (low socioeconomic status) and those with reduced ability to provide self-care (e.g., nursing home residents, those with dementia or upper extremity disability) suffer at a disproportionate rate. It is important to provide counseling regarding regular dental hygiene and professional cleaning, use of fluoride-containing toothpaste, professional fluoride treatments, and use of electric toothbrushes for patients with limited dexterity and to give instruction to caregivers for those unable to perform self-care. Internists caring for international students studying in the United States should be aware of the high prevalence of dental decay in this population. Cost, fear of dental care, and language and cultural differences may create barriers that prevent some from seeking preventive dental services.

Developmental and Systemic Disease Affecting the Teeth and Periodontium Malocclusion is the most common developmental problem, which, in addition to a problem with cosmesis, can interfere with mastication unless corrected through orthodontic techniques. Impacted third molars are common and occasionally become infected. Acquired prognathism due to *acromegaly* may also lead to malocclusion, as may deformity of the maxilla and mandible due to *Paget's disease* of the bone. Delayed tooth eruption, receding chin, and a protruding tongue are occasional features of *cretinism* and *hypopituitarism*. Congenital syphilis produces tapering, notched (Hutchinson's) incisors and finely nodular (mulberry) molar crowns.

Enamel hypoplasia results in crown defects ranging from pits to deep fissures of primary or permanent teeth. Intrauterine infection (syphilis, rubella), vitamin deficiency (A, C, or D), disorders of calcium metabolism (malabsorption, vitamin D–resistant rickets, hypoparathyroidism), prematurity, high fever, or rare inherited defects (*amelogenesis imperfecta*) are all causes. Tetracycline, given in sufficiently high doses during the first 8 years, may produce enamel hypoplasia and discoloration. Exposure to endogenous pigments can discolor developing teeth: *erythroblastosis fetalis* (green or bluish-black), congenital liver disease (green or yellow-brown), and porphyria (red or brown that fluoresces with ultraviolet light). *Mottled enamel* occurs if excessive fluoride is ingested during development. Worn enamel is seen with age, bruxism, or excessive acid exposure (e.g., chronic gastric reflux or bulimia).

Premature tooth loss resulting from periodontitis is seen with cyclic neutropenia, Papillon-Lefèvre syndrome, Chédiak-Higashi syndrome, and leukemia. Rapid focal tooth loosening is most often due to infection, but rarer causes include histiocytosis X, Ewing's sarcoma, osteosarcoma, or Burkitt's lymphoma. Early loss of primary teeth is a feature of *hypophosphatasia*, a rare inborn error of metabolism.

Pregnancy may produce severe gingivitis and localized *pyogenic granulomas*. Severe periodontal disease occurs with Down's syndrome and diabetes mellitus. *Gingival hyperplasia* may be caused by phenytoin, calcium channel blockers (e.g., nifedipine), and cyclosporine. *Idiopathic familial gingival fibromatosis* and several syndrome-related disorders appear similar. Removal of the medication often reverses the drug-induced form, though surgery may be needed to control both. *Linear gingival erythema* is variably seen in patients with advanced HIV infection and probably represents immune deficiency and decreased neutrophil activity. Diffuse or focal gingival swelling may be a feature of early or late acute myelomonocytic leukemia (AML) as well as of other lymphoproliferative disorders. A rare, but pathognomonic, sign of Wegener's granulomatosis is a red-purplish, granular gingivitis (strawberry gums).

DISEASES OF THE ORAL MUCOSA

Infection Most oral mucosal diseases involve microorganisms (Table 32-1).

Pigmented Lesions See Table 32-2.

Dermatologic Diseases See Tables 32-1, 32-2, and 32-3 and Chaps. 52–56.

Diseases of the Tongue See Table 32-4.

HIV Disease and AIDS See Tables 32-1, 32-2, 32-3, and 32-5; Chap. 182; and Figs. 174-1 and 196-1.

Ulcers Ulceration is the most common oral mucosal lesion. Although there are many causes, the host and pattern of lesions, including the presence of systemic features, narrow the differential diagnosis (Table 32-1). Most acute ulcers are painful and self-limited. Recurrent aphthous ulcers and herpes simplex infection constitute the majority. Persistent and deep aphthous ulcers can be idiopathic or seen with HIV/AIDS. Aphthous lesions are often the presenting symptom in *Behçet's syndrome* (Chap. 320). Similar-appearing, though less painful, lesions may occur with Reiter's syndrome, and aphthous ulcers are occasionally present during phases of discoid or *systemic lupus erythematosus* (Chap. 316). Aphthous-like ulcers are seen in Crohn's disease (Chap. 289), but unlike the common aphthous variety, they may exhibit granulomatous inflammation histologically. Recurrent aphthae in some patients with *celiac disease* have been reported to remit with elimination of gluten.

Of major concern are chronic, relatively painless ulcers and mixed red/white patches (erythroplakia and leukoplakia) of more than 2 weeks' duration. Squamous cell carcinoma and premalignant dysplasia should be considered early and a diagnostic biopsy obtained. The importance is underscored because early-stage malignancy is vastly more treatable than late-stage disease. High-risk sites include the lower lip, floor of the mouth, ventral and lateral tongue, and soft palate–tonsillar pillar complex. Significant risk factors for oral cancer in Western countries include sun exposure (lower lip) and tobacco and alcohol use. In India and some other Asian countries, smokeless tobacco mixed with betel nut, slaked lime, and spices is a common cause of oral cancer. Less common etiologies include syphilis and Plummer-Vinson syndrome (iron deficiency).

Rarer causes of chronic oral ulcer such as tuberculosis, fungal infection, Wegener's granulomatosis, and midline granuloma may look identical to carcinoma. Making the correct diagnosis depends on recognizing other clinical features and biopsy of the lesion. The syphilitic chancre is typically painless and therefore easily missed. Regional lymphadenopathy is invariably present. Confirmation is achieved using appropriate bacterial and serologic tests.

TABLE 32-1   VESICULAR, BULLOUS, OR ULCERATIVE LESIONS OF THE ORAL MUCOSA

Condition	Usual Location	Clinical Features	Course
Viral Diseases			
Primary acute herpetic gingivo-stomatitis [herpes simplex virus (HSV) type 1, rarely type 2]	Lip and oral mucosa (buccal, gingival, lingual mucosa)	Labial vesicles that rupture and crust, and intraoral vesicles that quickly ulcerate; extremely painful; acute gingivitis, fever, malaise, foul odor, and cervical lymphadenopathy; occurs primarily in infants, children, and young adults	Heals spontaneously in 10–14 days. Unless secondarily infected, lesions lasting >3 weeks are not due to primary HSV infection.
Recurrent herpes labialis	Mucocutaneous junction of lip, perioral skin	Eruption of groups of vesicles that may coalesce, then rupture and crust; painful to pressure or spicy foods	Lasts about 1 week, but condition may be prolonged if secondarily infected. If severe, topical or oral antiviral may reduce healing time.
Recurrent intraoral herpes simplex	Palate and gingiva	Small vesicles on keratinized epithelium that rupture and coalesce; painful	Heals spontaneously in about 1 week. If severe, topical or oral antiviral may reduce healing time.
Chickenpox (varicella-zoster virus)	Gingiva and oral mucosa	Skin lesions may be accompanied by small vesicles on oral mucosa that rupture to form shallow ulcers; may coalesce to form large bullous lesions that ulcerate; mucosa may have generalized erythema	Lesions heal spontaneously within 2 weeks.
Herpes zoster (reactivation of varicella-zoster virus)	Cheek, tongue, gingiva, or palate	Unilateral vesicular eruptions and ulceration in linear pattern following sensory distribution of trigeminal nerve or one of its branches	Gradual healing without scarring unless secondarily infected; post-herpetic neuralgia is common. Oral acyclovir, famcyclovir, or val-acyclovir reduce healing time and postherpetic neuralgia
Infectious mononucleosis (Epstein-Barr virus)	Oral mucosa	Fatigue, sore throat, malaise, fever, and cervical lymphadenopathy; numerous small ulcers usually appear several days before lymphadenopathy; gingival bleeding and multiple petechiae at junction of hard and soft palates	Oral lesions disappear during convalescence; no treatment though glucocorticoids indicated if tonsillar swelling compromises airway
Herpangina (coxsackievirus A; also possibly coxsackie B and echovirus)	Oral mucosa, pharynx, tongue	Sudden onset of fever, sore throat, and oropharyngeal vesicles, usually in children under 4 years, during summer months; diffuse pharyngeal congestion and vesicles (1–2 mm), grayish-white surrounded by red areola; vesicles enlarge and ulcerate	Incubation period 2–9 days; fever for 1–4 days; recovery uneventful
Hand, foot, and mouth disease (coxsackievirus A16 most common)	Oral mucosa, pharynx, palms, and soles	Fever, malaise, headache with oropharyngeal vesicles that become painful, shallow ulcers; highly infectious; usually affects children under age 10	Incubation period 2–18 days; lesions heal spontaneously in 2–4 weeks
Primary HIV infection	Gingiva, palate, and pharynx	Acute gingivitis and oropharyngeal ulceration, associated with febrile illness resembling mononucleosis and including lymphadenopathy	Followed by HIV seroconversion, asymptomatic HIV infection, and usually ultimately by HIV disease
Bacterial or Fungal Diseases			
Acute necrotizing ulcerative gingivitis ("trench mouth," Vincent's infection)	Gingiva	Painful, bleeding gingiva characterized by necrosis and ulceration of gingival papillae and margins plus lymphadenopathy and foul odor	Debridement and diluted (1:3) peroxide lavage provide relief within 24 h; antibiotics in acutely ill patients; relapse may occur
Prenatal (congenital) syphilis	Palate, jaws, tongue, and teeth	Gummatous involvement of palate, jaws, and facial bones; Hutchinson's incisors, mulberry molars, glossitis, mucous patches, and fissures on corner of mouth	Tooth deformities in permanent dentition irreversible
Primary syphilis (chancre)	Lesion appears where organism enters body; may occur on lips, tongue, or tonsillar area	Small papule developing rapidly into a large, painless ulcer with indurated border; unilateral lymphadenopathy; chancre and lymph nodes containing spirochetes; serologic tests positive by third to fourth weeks	Healing of chancre in 1–2 months, followed by secondary syphilis in 6–8 weeks
Secondary syphilis	Oral mucosa frequently involved with mucous patches, primarily on palate, also at commissures of mouth	Maculopapular lesions of oral mucosa, 5–10 mm in diameter with central ulceration covered by grayish membrane; eruptions occurring on various mucosal surfaces and skin accompanied by fever, malaise, and sore throat	Lesions may persist from several weeks to a year
Tertiary syphilis	Palate and tongue	Gummatous infiltration of palate or tongue followed by ulceration and fibrosis; atrophy of tongue papillae produces characteristic bald tongue and glossitis	Gumma may destroy palate, causing complete perforation
Gonorrhea	Lesions may occur in mouth at site of inoculation or secondarily by hematogenous spread from a primary focus elsewhere	Most pharyngeal infection is asymptomatic; may produce burning or itching sensation; oropharynx and tonsils may be ulcerated and erythematous; saliva viscous and fetid	More difficult to eradicate than urogenital infection, though pharyngitis usually resolves with appropriate antimicrobial treatment

(continued)

TABLE 32-1   VESICULAR, BULLOUS, OR ULCERATIVE LESIONS OF THE ORAL MUCOSA (CONTINUED)

Condition	Usual Location	Clinical Features	Course
Tuberculosis	Tongue, tonsillar area, soft palate	A painless, solitary, 1–5 cm, irregular ulcer covered with a persistent exudate; ulcer has a firm undermined border	Autoinnoculation from pulmonary infection usual; lesions resolve with appropriate antimicrobial therapy
Cervicofacial actinomycosis	Swellings in region of face, neck, and floor of mouth	Infection may be associated with an extraction, jaw fracture, or eruption of molar tooth; in acute form resembles an acute pyogenic abscess, but contains yellow "sulfur granules" (gram-positive mycelia and their hyphae)	Typically swelling is hard and grows painlessly; multiple abscesses with draining tracks develop; penicillin first choice; surgery usually necessary
Histoplasmosis	Any area of the mouth, particularly tongue, gingiva, or palate	Nodular, verrucous, or granulomatous lesions; ulcers are indurated and painful; usual source hematogenous or pulmonary, but may be primary	Systemic antifungal therapy necessary to treat
Candidiasis (Table 32-3)			
Dermatologic Diseases			
Mucous membrane pemphigoid	Typically produces marked gingival erythema and ulceration; other areas of oral cavity, esophagus, and vagina may be affected	Painful, grayish-white collapsed vesicles or bullae of full-thickness epithelium with peripheral erythematous zone; gingival lesions desquamate, leaving ulcerated area	Protracted course with remissions and exacerbations; involvement of different sites occurs slowly; glucocorticoids may temporarily reduce symptoms but do not control the disease
Erythema multiforme minor and major (Stevens-Johnson syndrome)	Primarily the oral mucosa and the skin of hands and feet	Intraoral ruptured bullae surrounded by an inflammatory area; lips may show hemorrhagic crusts; the "iris," or "target," lesion on the skin is pathognomonic; patient may have severe signs of toxicity	Onset very rapid; usually idiopathic, but may be associated with trigger such as drug reaction; condition may last 3–6 weeks; mortality with EM major 5–15% if untreated
Pemphigus vulgaris	Oral mucosa and skin; sites of mechanical trauma (soft/hard palate, frenulum, lips, buccal mucosa)	Usually (>70%) presents with oral lesions; fragile, ruptured bullae and ulcerated oral areas; mostly in older adults	With repeated occurrence of bullae, toxicity may lead to cachexia, infection, and death within 2 years; often controllable with oral glucocorticoids
Lichen planus	Oral mucosa and skin	White striae in mouth; purplish nodules on skin at sites of friction; occasionally causes oral mucosal ulcers and erosive gingivitis	White striae alone usually asymptomatic; erosive lesions often difficult to treat, but may respond to glucocorticoids
Other Conditions			
Recurrent aphthous ulcers	Usually on nonkeratinized oral mucosa (buccal and labial mucosa, floor of mouth, soft palate, lateral and ventral tongue)	Single or clusters of painful ulcers with surrounding erythematous border; lesions may be 1–2 mm in diameter in crops (herpetiform), 1–5 mm (minor), or 5–15 mm (major)	Lesions heal in 1–2 weeks but may recur monthly or several times a year; protective barrier with orabase and topical steroids give symptomatic relief; systemic glucocorticoids may be needed in severe cases
Behçet's syndrome	Oral mucosa, eyes, genitalia, gut, and CNS	Multiple aphthous ulcers in mouth; inflammatory ocular changes, ulcerative lesions on genitalia; inflammatory bowel disease and CNS disease	Oral lesions often first manifestation; persist several weeks and heal without scarring
Traumatic ulcers	Anywhere on oral mucosa; dentures frequently responsible for ulcers in vestibule	Localized, discrete ulcerated lesions with red border; produced by accidental biting of mucosa, penetration by a foreign object, or chronic irritation by a denture	Lesions usually heal in 7–10 days when irritant is removed, unless secondarily infected
Squamous cell carcinoma	Any area in the mouth, most commonly on lower lip, tongue, and floor of mouth	Ulcer with elevated, indurated border; failure to heal, pain not prominent; lesions tend to arise in areas of erythro/leukoplakia or in smooth atrophic tongue	Invades and destroys underlying tissues; frequently metastasizes to regional lymph nodes
Acute myeloid leukemia (usually monocytic)	Gingiva	Gingival swelling and superficial ulceration followed by hyperplasia of gingiva with extensive necrosis and hemorrhage; deep ulcers may occur elsewhere on the mucosa complicated by secondary infection	Usually responds to systemic treatment of leukemia; occasionally requires local radiation therapy
Lymphoma	Gingiva, tongue, palate and tonsillar area	Elevated, ulcerated area that may proliferate rapidly, giving the appearance of traumatic inflammation	Fatal if untreated; may indicate underlying HIV infection
Chemical or thermal burns	Any area in mouth	White slough due to contact with corrosive agents (e.g., aspirin, hot cheese) applied locally; removal of slough leaves raw, painful surface	Lesion heals in several weeks if not secondarily infected

Note: CNS, central nervous system.

TABLE 32-2 PIGMENTED LESIONS OF THE ORAL MUCOSA

Condition	Usual Location	Clinical Features	Course
Oral melanotic macule	Any area of the mouth	Discrete or diffuse localized, brown to black macule	Remains indefinitely; no growth
Diffuse melanin pigmentation	Any area of the mouth	Diffuse pale to dark-brown pigmentation; may be physiologic ("racial") or due to smoking	Remains indefinitely
Nevi	Any area of the mouth	Discrete, localized, brown to black pigmentation	Remains indefinitely
Malignant melanoma	Any area of the mouth	Can be flat and diffuse, painless, brown to black, or can be raised and nodular	Expands and invades early; metastasis leads to death
Addison's disease	Any area of the mouth, but mostly buccal mucosa	Blotches or spots of bluish-black to dark-brown pigmentation occurring early in the disease, accompanied by diffuse pigmentation of skin; other symptoms of adrenal insufficiency	Condition controlled by adrenal steroid replacement
Peutz-Jeghers syndrome	Any area of the mouth	Dark-brown spots on lips, buccal mucosa, with characteristic distribution of pigment around lips, nose, eyes, and on hands; concomitant intestinal polyposis	Oral pigmented lesions remain indefinitely; gastrointestinal polyps may become malignant
Drug ingestion (neuroleptics, oral contraceptives, minocycline, zidovudine, quinine derivatives)	Any area of the mouth	Brown, black, or gray areas of pigmentation	Gradually disappears following cessation of drug
Amalgam tattoo	Gingiva and alveolar mucosa	Small blue-black pigmented areas associated with embedded amalgam particles in soft tissues; these may show up on radiographs as radiopaque particles in some cases	Remains indefinitely
Heavy metal pigmentation (bismuth, mercury, lead)	Gingival margin	Thin blue-black pigmented line along gingival margin; rarely seen except for children exposed to lead-based paint	Indicative of systemic absorption; no significance for oral health
Black hairy tongue	Dorsum of tongue	Elongation of filiform papillae of tongue, which become stained by coffee, tea, tobacco, or pigmented bacteria	Improves within 1–2 weeks with gentle brushing of tongue or discontinuation of antibiotic if due to bacterial overgrowth
Fordyce "spots"	Buccal and labial mucosa	Numerous small yellowish spots just beneath mucosal surface; no symptoms; due to hyperplasia of sebaceous glands	Benign; remains without apparent change
Kaposi's sarcoma	Palate most common, but may occur in any other site	Red or blue plaques of variable size and shape; often enlarge, become nodular and may ulcerate	Usually indicative of HIV infection or non-Hodgkin's lymphoma; rarely fatal, but may require treatment for comfort or cosmesis
Mucous retention cysts	Buccal and labial mucosa	Bluish-clear fluid-filled cyst due to extravasated mucous from injured minor salivary gland	Benign; painless unless traumatized; may be removed surgically

TABLE 32-3 WHITE LESIONS OF ORAL MUCOSA

Condition	Usual Location	Clinical Features	Course
Lichen planus	Buccal mucosa, tongue, gingiva, and lips; skin	Striae, white plaques, red areas, ulcers in mouth; purplish papules on skin; may be asymptomatic, sore, or painful; lichenoid drug reactions may look similar	Protracted; responds to topical glucocorticoids
White sponge nevus	Oral mucosa, vagina, anal mucosa	Painless white thickening of epithelium; adolescent/early adult onset; familial	Benign and permanent
Smoker's leukoplakia and smokeless tobacco lesions	Any area of oral mucosa, sometimes related to location of habit	White patch that may become firm, rough, or red-fissured and ulcerated; may become sore and painful but usually painless	May or may not resolve with cessation of habit; 2% develop squamous cell carcinoma; early biopsy essential
Erythroplakia with or without white patches	Floor of mouth common in men; tongue and buccal mucosa in women	Velvety, reddish plaque; occasionally mixed with white patches or smooth red areas	High risk of squamous cell cancer; early biopsy essential
Candidiasis	Any area in mouth	*Pseudomembranous type* ("thrush"): creamy white curdlike patches that reveal a raw, bleeding surface when scraped; found in sick infants, debilitated elderly patients receiving high doses of glucocorticoids or broad-spectrum antibiotics, or in patients with AIDS	Responds favorably to antifungal therapy and correction of predisposing causes where possible
		Erythematous type: flat, red, sometimes sore areas in same groups of patients	Course same as for pseudomembranous type
		Candidal leukoplakia: nonremovable white thickening of epithelium due to *Candida*	Responds to prolonged antifungal therapy
		Angular cheilitis: sore fissures at corner of mouth	Responds to topical antifungal therapy
Hairy leukoplakia	Usually lateral tongue, rarely elsewhere on oral mucosa	White areas ranging from small and flat to extensive accentuation of vertical folds; found in HIV carriers in all risk groups for AIDS	Due to EBV; responds to high dose acyclovir but recurs; rarely causes discomfort unless secondarily infected with *Candida*
Warts (papillomavirus)	Anywhere on skin and oral mucosa	Single or multiple papillary lesions, with thick, white keratinized surfaces containing many pointed projections; cauliflower lesions covered with normal-colored mucosa or multiple pink or pale bumps (focal epithelial hyperplasia)	Lesions grow rapidly and spread; consider squamous cell carcinoma and rule out with biopsy; excision or laser therapy; may regress in HIV infected patients on antiretroviral therapy

Note: EBV, Epstein-Barr virus.

TABLE 32-4 ALTERATIONS OF THE TONGUE

Type of Change	Clinical Features
Size or Morphology Changes	
Macroglossia	Enlarged tongue that may be part of a syndrome found in developmental conditions such as Down syndrome, Simpson-Golabi-Behmel syndrome, or Beckwith-Wiedemann syndrome may be due to tumor (hemangioma or lymphangioma), metabolic disease (such as primary amyloidosis), or endocrine disturbance (such as acromegaly or cretinism)
Fissured ("scrotal") tongue	Dorsal surface and sides of tongue covered by painless shallow or deep fissures that may collect debris and become irritated
Median rhomboid glossitis	Congenital abnormality of tongue with ovoid, denuded area in median posterior portion of the tongue; may be associated with candidiasis and may respond to antifungals
Color Changes	
"Geographic" tongue (benign migratory glossitis)	Asymptomatic inflammatory condition of the tongue, with rapid loss and regrowth of filiform papillae, leading to appearance of denuded red patches "wandering" across the surface of the tongue
Hairy tongue	Elongation of filiform papillae of the medial dorsal surface area due to failure of keratin layer of the papillae to desquamate normally; brownish-black coloration may be due to staining by tobacco, food, or chromogenic organisms
"Strawberry" and "raspberry" tongue	Appearance of tongue during scarlet fever due to the hypertrophy of fungiform papillae plus changes in the filiform papillae
"Bald" tongue	Atrophy may be associated with xerostomia, pernicious anemia, iron-deficiency anemia, pellagra, or syphilis; may be accompanied by painful burning sensation; may be an expression of erythmematous candidiasis and respond to antifungals

Disorders of mucosal fragility often produce painful oral ulcers that fail to heal within 2 weeks. *Mucous membrane pemphigoid* and *pemphigus vulgaris* are the major acquired disorders. While clinical features are often distinctive, immunohistochemical examination should be performed for diagnosis and to distinguish these entities from *lichen planus* and drug reactions.

Hematologic and Nutritional Disease Internists are more likely to encounter patients with acquired, rather than congenital, bleeding disorders. Bleeding after minor trauma should stop after 15 min and within an hour of tooth extraction if local pressure is applied. More prolonged bleeding, if not due to continued injury or rupture of a large vessel, should lead to investigation for a clotting abnormality. In addition to bleeding, petechiae and ecchymoses are prone to occur at the line of vibration between the soft and hard palates in patients with platelet dysfunction or thrombocytopenia.

All forms of leukemia, but particularly acute myelomonocytic leukemia, can produce gingival bleeding, ulcers, and gingival enlargement. Oral ulcers are a feature of agranulocytosis, and ulcers and mucositis are often severe complications of chemotherapy and radiation therapy for hematologic and other malignancies. Plummer-Vinson syndrome (iron deficiency, angular stomatitis, glossitis, and dysphagia) raises the risk of oral squamous cell cancer and esophageal cancer at the postcricoidal tissue web. Atrophic papillae and a red, burning tongue may occur with pernicious anemia. B group vitamin deficiencies produce many of these same symptoms as well as oral ulceration and cheilosis. Cheilosis may also be seen in iron deficiency. Swollen, bleeding gums, ulcers, and loosening of the teeth are a consequence of scurvy.

NONDENTAL CAUSES OF ORAL PAIN

Most but not all oral pain emanates from inflamed or injured tooth pulp or periodontal tissues. Nonodontogenic causes may be overlooked. In most instances toothache is predictable and proportional to the stimulus applied, and an identifiable condition (e.g., caries, abscess) is found. Local anesthesia eliminates pain originating from dental or periodontal structures, but not referred pains. The most common nondental origin is myofascial pain referred from muscles of mastication, which become tender and ache with increased use. Many sufferers exhibit bruxism (the grinding of teeth, often during sleep) that is secondary to stress and anxiety. *Temporomandibular disorder* is closely related. It predominantly affects females ages 15–45. Features include pain, limited mandibular movement, and temporomandibular joint sounds. The etiologies are complex, and malocclusion does not play the primary role once attributed to it. *Osteoarthritis* is a common cause of masticatory pain. Anti-inflammatory medication, jaw rest, soft foods, and heat provide relief. The temporomandibular joint is involved in 50% of patients with *rheumatoid arthritis* and is usually a late feature of severe disease. Bilateral preauricular pain, particularly in the morning, limits range of motion.

Migrainous neuralgia may be localized to the mouth. Episodes of pain and remission without identifiable cause and absence of relief with local anesthesia are important clues. *Trigeminal neuralgia* (*tic douloureaux*) may involve the entire branch or part of the mandibular or maxillary branches of the fifth cranial nerve and produce pain in one or a few teeth. Pain may occur spontaneously or may be triggered by touching the lip or gingiva, brushing the teeth, or chewing. *Glossopharyngeal neuralgia* produces similar acute neuropathic symptoms in the distribution of the ninth cranial nerve. Swallowing, sneezing, coughing, or pressure on the tragus of the ear triggers pain that is felt in the base of the tongue, pharynx, and soft palate and may be referred to the temporomandibular joint. *Neuritis* involving the maxillary and mandibular divisions of the trigeminal nerve (e.g., maxillary sinusitis, neuroma, and leukemic infiltrate) is distinguished from ordinary toothache by the neuropathic quality of the pain. Occasionally *phantom pain* follows tooth extraction.

TABLE 32-5 ORAL LESIONS ASSOCIATED WITH HIV INFECTION

Lesion Morphology	Etiologies
Papules, nodules, plaques	Candidiasis (hyperplastic and pseudomembranous)[a] Condyloma acuminatum (human papillomavirus infection) Squamous cell carcinoma (preinvasive and invasive) Non-Hodgkin's lymphoma[a] Hairy leukoplakia[a]
Ulcers	Recurrent aphthous ulcers[a] Angular cheilitis Squamous cell carcinoma Acute necrotizing ulcerative gingivitis[a] Necrotizing ulcerative periodontitis[a] Necrotizing ulcerative stomatitis Non-Hodgkin's lymphoma[a] Viral infection (herpes simplex, herpes zoster, cytomegalovirus) *Mycobacterium tuberculosis, Mycobacterium avium-intracellulare* Fungal infection (histoplasmosis, cryptococcosis, candidiasis, geotrichosis, aspergillosis) Bacterial infection (*Escherichia coli, Enterobacter cloacae, Klebsiella pneumoniae, Pseudomonas aeruginosa*) Drug reactions (single or multiple ulcers)
Pigmented lesions	Kaposi's sarcoma[a] Bacillary angiomatosis (skin and visceral lesions more common than oral) Zidovudine pigmentation (skin, nails, and occasionally oral mucosa) Addison's disease
Miscellaneous	Linear gingival erythema[a]

[a]Strongly associated with HIV infection.

Often the earliest symptom of Bell's palsy in the day or so before facial weakness develops is pain and hyperalgesia behind the ear and side of the face. Likewise, similar symptoms may precede visible lesions of herpes zoster infecting the seventh nerve (Ramsey-Hunt syndrome) or trigeminal nerve. *Postherpetic neuralgia* may follow either condition. *Coronary ischemia* may produce pain exclusively in the face and jaw and, like typical angina pectoris, is usually reproducible with increased myocardial demand. Aching in several upper molar or premolar teeth that is unrelieved by anesthetizing the teeth may point to *maxillary sinusitis*.

Giant cell arteritis is notorious for producing headache, but it may also produce facial pain or sore throat without headache. Jaw and tongue claudication with chewing or talking is relatively common. Tongue infarction is rare. Patients with subacute thyroiditis often experience pain referred to the face or jaw before the tender thyroid gland and transient hyperthyroidism are appreciated.

Burning mouth syndrome (glossodynia) is present in the absence of an identifiable cause (e.g., vitamin B_{12} deficiency, iron deficiency, Plummer-Vinson syndrome, diabetes mellitus, low-grade *Candida* infection, food sensitivity, or subtle xerostomia) and predominantly affects postmenopausal women. The etiology may be neuropathic. Clonazepam, alpha-lipoic acid and cognitive behavioral therapy have benefited some.

DISEASES OF THE SALIVARY GLANDS

Saliva is essential to oral health. Its major components, water and mucin, serve as a cleansing solvent and lubricating fluid. In addition, it contains antimicrobial factors (e.g., lysozyme, lactoperoxidase, secretory IgA), epidermal growth factor, minerals, and buffering systems. The major salivary glands secrete intermittently in response to autonomic stimulation, which is high during a meal but low otherwise. Hundreds of minor glands in the lips and cheeks secrete mucus continuously. Consequently, oral function becomes impaired when salivary function is reduced. Dry mouth (*xerostomia*) is perceived when salivary flow is reduced by 50%. The most common etiology is medication, especially drugs with anticholinergic properties, but also alpha and beta blockers, calcium channel blockers, and diuretics. Other causes include Sjögren's syndrome, chronic parotitis, salivary duct obstruction, diabetes mellitus, HIV/AIDS, and irradiation for head and neck cancer. Management involves eliminating or limiting drying medications, preventive dental care, and supplementing oral liquid. Sugarless mints or chewing gum may stimulate salivary secretion if dysfunction is mild. When sufficient exocrine tissue remains, pilocarpine or cevimeline has been shown to increase secretions. Commercial saliva substitutes or gels relieve dryness but must be supplemented with fluoride applications to prevent caries.

Sialolithiasis presents most often as painful swelling but in some instances as just swelling or pain. The obstructing stone produces spasm upon eating. Conservative therapy consists of local heat, massage, and hydration. Promotion of salivary secretion with mints or lemon drops may flush out small stones. Antibiotic treatment is necessary when bacterial infection in suspected. In adults, *acute bacterial parotitis* is typically unilateral and most commonly affects postoperative patients within the first 2 weeks of surgery. *Staphylococcus aureus* is the most common bacterial agent. Dehydration, advanced age, and chronic debilitating disease are major risks. Chronic bacterial sialadenitis results from lowered salivary secretion and recurrent bacterial infection. When suspected bacterial infection is not responsive to therapy, the differential diagnosis should be expanded to include benign and malignant neoplasms, lymphoproliferative disorders, Sjögren's syndrome, sarcoidosis, tuberculosis, lymphadenitis, actinomycosis, and Wegener's granulomatosis. Bilateral nontender parotid enlargement occurs with diabetes mellitus, cirrhosis, bulimia, HIV/AIDS, and drugs (e.g., iodide, propylthiouracil).

Pleomorphic adenoma comprises two-thirds of all salivary neoplasms. The parotid is the principal salivary gland affected, and the tumor presents as a firm, slow-growing mass. Though benign, recurrence is common if resection is incomplete. Malignant tumors such as mucoepidermoid carcinoma, adenoid cystic carcinoma, and adenocarcinoma tend to grow relatively fast, depending upon grade. They may ulcerate and invade nerves, producing numbness and facial paralysis.

Neutron-beam radiation therapy is an effective treatment; 5-year survival is about 68% for malignant salivary gland tumors.

DENTAL CARE OF MEDICALLY COMPLEX PATIENTS

Routine dental care (e.g., extraction, scaling and cleaning, tooth restoration, and root canal) is remarkably safe. The most common concerns regarding care of dental patients with medical disease are fear of excessive bleeding for patients on anticoagulants, infection of the heart valves and prosthetic devices from hematogenous seeding of oral flora, and cardiovascular complications resulting from vasopressors used with local anesthetics during dental treatment. Experience confirms that the risks of any of these complications are very low.

Patients undergoing tooth extraction or alveolar and gingival surgery rarely experience uncontrolled bleeding when warfarin anticoagulation is maintained within the therapeutic range currently recommended for prevention of venous thrombosis, atrial fibrillation, or mechanical heart valve. Embolic complications and death, however, have been reported during subtherapeutic anticoagulation. Therapeutic anticoagulation should be confirmed before and continued through the procedure. Likewise, low-dose aspirin (e.g., 81–325 mg) can be safely continued.

Patients at high or moderate risk for bacterial endocarditis (Chap. 118) should maintain optimal oral hygiene, including flossing, and have regular professional cleaning. Prophylactic antibiotics are recommended for all at-risk patients who undergo dental and oral procedures likely to cause significant bleeding and bacteremia. Should unexpected bleeding occur, antibiotics given within 2 h following the procedure provide effective prophylaxis.

Hematogenous bacterial seeding from oral infection can undoubtedly produce late prosthetic joint infection and therefore requires removal of the infected tissue (e.g., drainage, extraction, root canal) and appropriate antibiotic therapy. However, evidence that late prosthetic joint infection occurs following routine dental procedures is lacking. For this reason, antibiotic prophylaxis is not recommended before dental surgery in patients with orthopedic pins, screws, and plates. It is, however, advised within the first 2 years after joint replacement for patients who have inflammatory arthropathies, immunosuppression, type 1 diabetes mellitus, previous prosthetic joint infection, hemophilia, or malnourishment.

Concern often arises regarding the use of vasoconstrictors in patients with hypertension and heart disease. Vasoconstrictors enhance the depth and duration of local anesthesia, thus reducing the anesthetic dose and potential toxicity. If intravascular injection is avoided, 2% lidocaine with 1:100,000 epinephrine (limited to a total of 0.036 mg epinephrine) can be used safely in those with controlled hypertension and stable coronary heart disease, arrhythmia, or congestive heart failure. Precaution should be taken with patients taking tricyclic antidepressants and nonselective beta blockers as these drugs may potentiate the effect of epinephrine.

Elective dental treatments should be postponed for at least 1 month after myocardial infarction, after which the risk of reinfarction is low provided the patient is medically stable (e.g., stable rhythm, stable angina, and free of heart failure). Patients who have suffered a stroke should have elective dental care deferred for 6 months. In both situations, effective stress reduction requires good pain control, including the use of the minimal amount of vasoconstrictor necessary to provide good hemostasis and local anesthesia.

Bisphosphonate therapy can be associated with *osteonecrosis* of the jaw. Most patients affected have received high dose aminobisphosphonate therapy for multiple myeloma or metastatic breast cancer and have undergone tooth extraction or dental surgery. Intra-oral lesions appear as exposed yellow-white hard bone involving the mandible or maxilla. Two-thirds are painful. Patients about to receive aminobisphosphonate therapy should receive preventive dental care that reduces the risk of infection and need for future dentoalveolar surgery.

HALITOSIS

Halitosis typically emanates from the oral cavity or nasal passages. Volatile sulfur compounds resulting from bacterial decay of food and cellular debris account for the malodor. Periodontal disease, caries, acute forms of gingivitis, poorly fitting dentures, oral abscess, and tongue coating are usual causes. Treatment includes correcting poor hygiene, treating infection, and tongue brushing. Xerostomia can produce and exacerbate halitosis. Pockets of decay in the tonsillar crypts, esophageal diverticulum, esophageal stasis (e.g., achalasia, stricture), sinusitis, and lung abscess account for some instances. A few systemic diseases produce distinctive odors: renal failure (ammoniacal), hepatic (fishy), and ketoacidosis (fruity). *Helicobacter pylori* gastritis can also produce ammoniac breath. If no odor is detectable, then pseudohalitosis or even halitophobia must be considered. These conditions represent varying degrees of psychiatric illness.

AGING AND ORAL HEALTH

While tooth loss and dental disease are not normal consequences of aging, a complex array of structural and functional changes occurs with age that can affect oral health. Subtle changes in tooth structure (e.g., diminished pulp space and volume, sclerosis of dentinal tubules, altered proportions of nerve and vascular pulp content) result in diminished or altered pain sensitivity, reduced reparative capacity, and increased tooth brittleness. In addition, age-associated fatty replacement of salivary acini may reduce physiologic reserve, thus increasing the risk of xerostomia.

Poor oral hygiene often results when vision fails or when patients lose manual dexterity and upper extremity flexibility. This is particularly common for nursing home residents and must be emphasized since regular oral cleaning and dental care has been shown to reduce the incidence of pneumonia. Other risks for dental decay include limited lifetime fluoride exposure and preference by some older adults for intensely sweet foods when taste and olfaction wane. These factors occur in an increasing proportion of persons over age 75 who retain teeth that have extensive restorations and exposed roots. Without assiduous care, decay can become quite advanced yet remain asymptomatic. Consequently, much or all of the tooth can be destroyed before the process is detected.

Periodontal disease, a leading cause of tooth loss, is indicated by loss of alveolar bone height. Over 90% of Americans have some degree of periodontal disease by age 50. Healthy adults who have not experienced significant alveolar bone loss by the sixth decade do not typically develop significant worsening with advancing age.

Complete edentulousness with advanced age, though less common than in previous decades, is still present in approximately 50% of Americans age ≥85. Speech, mastication, and facial contours are dramatically affected. Edentulousness may also worsen obstructive sleep apnea, particularly in those without symptoms while wearing dentures. Dentures can improve speech articulation and restore diminished facial contours. Mastication is restored less predictably, and those expecting dentures to improve oral intake are often disappointed. Dentures require periodic adjustment to accommodate inevitable remodeling that leads to a diminished volume of the alveolar ridge. Pain can result from friction or traumatic lesions produced by loose dentures. Poor fit and poor oral hygiene may permit candidiasis to develop. This may be asymptomatic or painful and is indicated by erythematous smooth or granular tissue conforming to an area covered by the appliance.

ACKNOWLEDGMENT
The author acknowledges the contribution to this chapter by the previous author, Dr. John S. Greenspan.

FURTHER READINGS

DURSO SC: Interaction with other health team members in caring for elderly patients. Dent Clin N Am 49:377, 2005

LITTLE JW et al (eds): *Dental Management of the Medically Compromised Patient*, 6th ed. St. Louis, Mosby, 2002

REGEZI JA, SCIUBBA JJ: *Oral Pathology: Clinical Pathologic Correlations*, 4th ed. Philadelphia, Saunders, 2002

SPAHR A et al: Periodontal infection and coronary heart disease. Role of periodontal bacteria and importance of total pathogen burden in the coronary event and periodontal disease (CORODONT) study. Arch Intern Med 166:554, 2006

WOO SB et al: Systematic Review: Bisphosphonates and osteonecrosis of the jaws. Ann Intern Med 144:753, 2006

SECTION 5 · ALTERATIONS IN CIRCULATORY AND RESPIRATORY FUNCTIONS

33 Dyspnea and Pulmonary Edema
Richard M. Schwartzstein

DYSPNEA

The American Thoracic Society defines *dyspnea* as a "subjective experience of breathing discomfort that consists of qualitatively distinct sensations that vary in intensity. The experience derives from interactions among multiple physiological, psychological, social, and environmental factors, and may induce secondary physiological and behavioral responses." Dyspnea, a symptom, must be distinguished from the signs of increased work of breathing.

MECHANISMS OF DYSPNEA

Respiratory sensations are the consequence of interactions between the *efferent*, or outgoing, motor output from the brain to the ventilatory muscles (feed-forward) and the *afferent*, or incoming, sensory input from receptors throughout the body (feedback), as well as the integrative processing of this information that we infer must be occurring in the brain (Fig. 33-1). A given disease state may lead to dyspnea by one or more mechanisms, some of which may be operative under some circumstances but not others.

Motor Efferents Disorders of the ventilatory pump are associated with increased work of breathing or a sense of an increased effort to breathe. When the muscles are weak or fatigued, greater effort is required, even though the mechanics of the system are normal. The increased neural output from the motor cortex is thought to be sensed due to a corollary discharge that is sent to the sensory cortex at the same time that signals are sent to the ventilatory muscles.

Sensory Afferents Chemoreceptors in the carotid bodies and medulla are activated by hypoxemia, acute hypercapnia, and acidemia. Stimulation of these receptors, as well as others that lead to an increase in ventilation, produce a sensation of air hunger. Mechanoreceptors in the lungs, when stimulated by bronchospasm, lead to a sensation of chest tightness. J-receptors, sensitive to interstitial edema, and pulmonary vascular receptors, activated by acute changes in pulmonary artery pressure, appear to contribute to air hunger. Hyperinflation is associated with the sensation of an inability to get a deep breath or of an unsatisfying breath. It is not clear if this sensation arises from receptors in the lungs or chest wall, or if it is a variant of the sensation of air hunger. Metaboreceptors, located in skeletal muscle, are believed to be activated by changes in the local biochemical milieu of the tissue active during exercise and, when stimulated, contribute to the breathing discomfort.

ALGORITHM FOR THE INPUTS IN DYSPNEA PRODUCTION

FIGURE 33-1 Hypothetical model for integration of sensory inputs in the production of dyspnea. Afferent information from the receptors throughout the respiratory system projects directly to the sensory cortex to contribute to primary qualitative sensory experiences and provide feedback on the action of the ventilatory pump. Afferents also project to the areas of the brain responsible for control of ventilation. The motor cortex, responding to input from the control centers, sends neural messages to the ventilatory muscles and a corollary discharge to the sensory cortex (feed-forward with respect to the instructions sent to the muscles). If the feed-forward and feedback messages do not match, an error signal is generated and the intensity of dyspnea increases. *(Adapted from Gillette and Schwartzstein.)*

Integration: Efferent-Reafferent Mismatch   A discrepancy or mismatch between the feed-forward message to the ventilatory muscles and the feedback from receptors that monitor the response of the ventilatory pump increases the intensity of dyspnea. This is particularly important when there is a mechanical derangement of the ventilatory pump, such as in asthma or chronic obstructive pulmonary disease (COPD).

Anxiety   Acute anxiety may increase the severity of dyspnea either by altering the interpretation of sensory data or by leading to patterns of breathing that heighten physiologic abnormalities in the respiratory system. In patients with expiratory flow limitation, for example, the increased respiratory rate that accompanies acute anxiety leads to hyperinflation, increased work of breathing, a sense of an increased effort to breathe, and a sense of an unsatisfying breath.

ASSESSING DYSPNEA
Quality of Sensation
As with pain, dyspnea assessment begins with a determination of the quality of the discomfort (Table 33-1). Dyspnea questionnaires, or lists of phrases commonly used by patients, assist those who have difficulty describing their breathing sensations.

Sensory Intensity   A modified Borg scale or visual analogue scale can be utilized to measure dyspnea at rest, immediately following exercise, or on recall of a reproducible physical task, e.g., climbing the stairs at home. An alternative approach is to inquire about the activities a pa-

TABLE 33-1	ASSOCIATION OF QUALITATIVE DESCRIPTORS AND PATHOPHYSIOLOGIC MECHANISMS OF SHORTNESS OF BREATH
Descriptor	**Pathophysiology**
Chest tightness or constriction	Bronchoconstriction, interstitial edema (asthma, myocardial ischemia)
Increased work or effort of breathing	Airway obstruction, neuromuscular disease (COPD, moderate to severe asthma, myopathy, kyphoscoliosis)
Air hunger, need to breathe, urge to breathe	Increased drive to breathe (CHF, pulmonary embolism, moderate to severe airflow obstruction)
Cannot get a deep breath, unsatisfying breath	Hyperinflation (asthma, COPD) and restricted tidal volume (pulmonary fibrosis, chest wall restriction)
Heavy breathing, rapid breathing, breathing more	Deconditioning

Note: CHF, congestive heart failure; COPD, chronic obstructive pulmonary disease.
Source: From Schwartzstein and Feller-Kopman.

tient can do, i.e., to gain a sense of the patient's disability. The Baseline Dyspnea Index and the Chronic Respiratory Disease Questionnaire are commonly used tools for this purpose.

Affective Dimension   For a sensation to be reported as a symptom, it must be perceived as unpleasant and interpreted as abnormal. We are still in the early stages of learning the best ways to assess the affective dimension of dyspnea. Some therapies for dyspnea, such as pulmonary rehabilitation, may reduce breathing discomfort, in part, by altering this dimension.

DIFFERENTIAL DIAGNOSIS
Dyspnea is the consequence of deviations from normal function in the cardiopulmonary systems. Alterations in the respiratory system can be considered in the context of the controller (stimulation of breathing); the ventilatory pump (the bones and muscles that form the chest wall, the airways, and the pleura); and the gas exchanger (the alveoli, pulmonary vasculature, and surrounding lung parenchyma). Similarly, alterations in the cardiovascular system can be grouped into three categories: conditions associated with high, normal, and low cardiac output (Fig. 33-2).

Respiratory System Dyspnea · *CONTROLLER*   Acute hypoxemia and hypercapnia are associated with increased activity in the controller. Stimulation of pulmonary receptors, as occurs in acute bronchospasm, interstitial edema, and pulmonary embolism, also leads to hyperventilation and air hunger, as well as a sense of chest tightness in the case of asthma. High altitude, high progesterone states such as pregnancy, and drugs such as aspirin stimulate the controller and can cause dyspnea even when the respiratory system is normal.

VENTILATORY PUMP   Disorders of the airways (e.g., asthma, emphysema, chronic bronchitis, bronchiectasis) lead to increased airway resis-

ALGORITHM FOR DYSPNEA PATHOPHYSIOLOGY

FIGURE 33-2 Pathophysiology of dyspnea. When confronted with a patient with shortness of breath of unclear cause, it is useful to begin the analysis with a consideration of the broad pathophysiologic categories that explain the vast majority of cases. COPD, chronic obstructive pulmonary disease. *(Adapted from Schwartzstein and Feller-Kopman.)*

tance and work of breathing. Hyperinflation further increases the work of breathing and can produce a sense of an inability to get a deep breath. Conditions that stiffen the chest wall, such as kyphoscoliosis, or that weaken ventilatory muscles, such as myasthenia gravis or the Guillain-Barré syndrome, are also associated with an increased effort to breathe. Large pleural effusions may contribute to dyspnea, both by increasing the work of breathing and by stimulating pulmonary receptors if there is associated atelectasis.

GAS EXCHANGER Pneumonia, pulmonary edema, and aspiration all interfere with gas exchange. Pulmonary vascular and interstitial lung disease and pulmonary vascular congestion may produce dyspnea by direct stimulation of pulmonary receptors. In these cases, relief of hypoxemia typically has only a small impact on the intensity of dyspnea.

Cardiovascular System Dyspnea • *HIGH CARDIAC OUTPUT* Mild to moderate anemia is associated with breathing discomfort during exercise. Left-to-right intracardiac shunts may lead to high cardiac output and dyspnea, although in their later stages these conditions may be complicated by the development of pulmonary hypertension, which contributes to dyspnea. The breathlessness associated with obesity is probably due to multiple mechanisms, including high cardiac output and impaired ventilatory pump function.

NORMAL CARDIAC OUTPUT Cardiovascular deconditioning is characterized by early development of anaerobic metabolism and stimulation of chemoreceptors and metaboreceptors. Diastolic dysfunction—due to hypertension, aortic stenosis, or hypertrophic cardiomyopathy—is an increasingly frequent recognized cause of exercise-induced breathlessness. Pericardial disease, e.g., constrictive pericarditis, is a relatively rare cause of chronic dyspnea.

LOW CARDIAC OUTPUT Diseases of the myocardium resulting from coronary artery disease and nonischemic cardiomyopathies result in a greater left ventricular end-diastolic volume and an elevation of the left ventricular end-diastolic as well as pulmonary capillary pressures. Pulmonary receptors are stimulated by the elevated vascular pressures and resultant interstitial edema, causing dyspnea.

APPROACH TO THE PATIENT:
Dyspnea

(Fig. 33-3) In obtaining a *history*, the patient should be asked to describe in his/her own words what the discomfort feels like, as well as the effect of position, infections, and environmental stimuli on the dyspnea. Orthopnea is a common indicator of congestive heart failure, mechanical impairment of the diaphragm associated with obesity, or asthma triggered by esophageal reflux. Nocturnal dyspnea suggests congestive heart failure or asthma. Acute, intermittent episodes of dyspnea are more likely to reflect episodes of myocardial ischemia, bronchospasm, or pulmonary embolism, while chronic persistent dyspnea is typical of COPD and interstitial lung disease. Risk factors for occupational lung disease and for coronary artery disease should be solicited. Left atrial myxoma or hepatopulmonary syndrome should be considered when the patient complains of *platypnea*, defined as dyspnea in the upright position with relief in the supine position.

The *physical examination* should begin during the interview of the patient. Inability of the patient to speak in full sentences before stopping to get a deep breath suggests a condition that leads to stimulation of the controller or an impairment of the ventilatory pump with reduced vital capacity. Evidence for increased work of breathing (supraclavicular retractions, use of accessory muscles of ventilation, and the tripod position, characterized by sitting with one's hands braced on the knees) is indicative of disorders of the ventilatory pump, most commonly increased airway resistance or stiff lungs and chest wall. When measuring the vital signs, an accurate assessment of the respiratory rate should be obtained and examination for a pulsus paradox-

us carried out (Chap. 232); if it is >10 mm Hg, consider the presence of COPD. During the general examination, signs of anemia (pale conjunctivae), cyanosis, and cirrhosis (spider angiomata, gynecomastia) should be sought. Examination of the chest should focus on symmetry of movement; percussion (dullness indicative of pleural effusion, hyper-resonance a sign of emphysema); and auscultation (wheezes, rales, rhonchi, prolonged expiratory phase, diminished breath sounds, which are clues to disorders of the airways, and interstitial edema or fibrosis). The cardiac examination should focus on signs of elevated right heart pressures (jugular venous distention, edema, accentuated pulmonic component to the second heart sound); left ventricular dysfunction (S3 and S4 gallops); and valvular disease (murmurs). When examining the abdomen with the patient in the supine position, it should be noted whether there is paradoxical movement of the abdomen (inward motion during inspiration), a sign of diaphragmatic weakness. Clubbing of the digits may be an indication of interstitial pulmonary fibrosis, and the presence of joint swelling or deformation as well as changes consistent with Raynaud's disease may be indicative of a collagen-vascular process that can be associated with pulmonary disease.

Patients with exertional dyspnea should be asked to walk under observation in order to reproduce the symptoms. The patient should be examined for new findings that were not present at rest and for oxygen saturation. A "picture" of the patient while symptomatic may be worth thousands of dollars in laboratory tests.

Following the history and physical examination, a *chest radiograph* should be obtained. The lung volumes should be assessed (hyperinflation indicates obstructive lung disease, low lung volumes suggest interstitial edema or fibrosis, diaphragmatic dysfunction, or impaired chest wall motion). The pulmonary parenchyma should be examined for evidence of interstitial disease and emphysema. Prominent pulmonary vasculature in the upper zones indicates pulmonary venous hypertension, while enlarged central pulmonary arteries suggest pulmonary artery hypertension. An enlarged cardiac silhouette suggests a dilated cardiomyopathy or valvular disease. Bilateral pleural effusions are typical of congestive heart failure and some forms of collagen vascular disease. Unilateral effusions raise the specter of carcinoma and pulmonary embolism but may also occur in heart failure. *Computed tomography* (CT) *of the chest* is generally reserved for further evaluation of the lung parenchyma (interstitial lung disease) and possible pulmonary embolism.

Laboratory studies should include an electrocardiogram to look for evidence of ventricular hypertrophy and prior myocardial infarction. Echocardiography is indicated in patients in whom systolic dysfunction, pulmonary hypertension, or valvular heart disease is suspected.

Distinguishing Cardiovascular from Respiratory System Dyspnea If a patient has evidence of both pulmonary and cardiac disease, a cardiopulmonary exercise test should be carried out to determine which system is responsible for the exercise limitation. If, at peak exercise, the patient achieves predicted maximal ventilation, demonstrates an increase in dead space or hypoxemia (oxygen saturation below 90%), or develops bronchospasm, the respiratory system is probably the cause of the problem. Alternatively, if the heart rate is >85% of the predicted maximum, if anaerobic threshold occurs early, if the blood pressure becomes excessively high or drops during exercise, if the O_2 pulse (O_2 consumption/heart rate, an indicator of stroke volume) falls, or if there are ischemic changes on the electrocardiogram, an abnormality of the cardiovascular system is likely the explanation for the breathing discomfort.

℞ DYSPNEA

The first goal is to correct the underlying problem responsible for the symptom. If this is not possible, one attempts to lessen the intensity of the symptom and its effect on the patient's quality of life. Supplemental O_2 should be administered if the resting O_2 saturation is ≤90% or if the pa-

ALGORITHM FOR THE EVALUATION OF THE PATIENT WITH DYSPNEA

History

↓

Quality of sensation, timing, positional disposition
Persistent vs. intermittent

↓

Physical Exam

↓

General appearance: Speak in full sentences? Accessory muscles? Color?
Vital Signs: Tachypnea? Pulsus paradoxus? Oximetry-evidence of desaturation?
Chest: Wheezes, rales, rhonchi, diminished breath sounds? Hyperinflated?
Cardiac exam: JVP elevated? Precordial impulse? Gallop? Murmur?
Extremities: Edema? Cyanosis?

↓

At this point, diagnosis may be evident—if not, proceed to further evaluation

↓

Chest radiograph
Assess cardiac size, evidence of CHF
Assess for hyperinflation
Assess for pneumonia, interstitial lung disease, pleural effusions

↓

Suspect low cardiac output, myocardial ischemia, or pulmonary vascular disease

Suspect respiratory pump or gas exchange abnormality

Suspect high cardiac output

↓

ECG and echocardiogram to assess left ventricular function and pulmonary artery pressure

Pulmonary function testing—if diffusing capacity reduced, consider CT angiogram to assess for interstitial lung disease and pulmonary embolism

Hematocrit, thyroid function tests

↓

If diagnosis still uncertain, obtain cardiopulmonary exercise test

FIGURE 33-3 An algorithm for the evaluation of the patient with dyspnea. JVP, jugular venous pulse; CHF, congestive heart failure; ECG, electrocardiogram; CT, computed tomography. *(Adapted from Schwartzstein and Feller-Kopman.)*

tient's saturation drops to these levels with activity. For patients with COPD, pulmonary rehabilitation programs have demonstrated positive effects on dyspnea, exercise capacity, and rates of hospitalization. Studies of anxiolytics and antidepressants have not demonstrated consistent benefit. Experimental interventions—e.g., cold air on the face, chest wall vibration, and inhaled furosemide—to modulate the afferent information from receptors throughout the respiratory system are being studied.

PULMONARY EDEMA

MECHANISMS OF FLUID ACCUMULATION

The extent to which fluid accumulates in the interstitium of the lung depends on the balance of hydrostatic and oncotic forces within the pulmonary capillaries and in the surrounding tissue. Hydrostatic pressure favors movement of fluid from the capillary into the interstitium. The oncotic pressure, which is determined by the protein concentration in the blood, favors movement of fluid into the vessel. Albumin, the primary protein in the plasma, may be low in conditions such as cirrhosis and nephrotic syndrome. While hypoalbuminemia favors movement of fluid into the tissue for any given hydrostatic pressure in the capillary, it is usually not sufficient by itself to cause interstitial edema. In a healthy individual, the tight junctions of the capillary endothelium are impermeable to proteins, and the lymphatics in the tissue carry away the small amounts of protein that may leak out; together these factors result in an oncotic force that maintains fluid in the capillary. Disruption of the endothelial barrier, however, allows protein to escape the capillary bed and enhances the movement of fluid into the tissue of the lung.

Cardiogenic Pulmonary Edema (See also Chap. 266) Cardiac abnormalities that lead to an increase in pulmonary venous pressure shift the balance of forces between the capillary and the interstitium. Hydrostatic pressure is increased and fluid exits the capillary at an increased rate, resulting in interstitial and, in more severe cases, alveolar edema. The development of pleural effusions may further compromise respiratory system function and contribute to breathing discomfort.

Early signs of pulmonary edema include exertional dyspnea and orthopnea. Chest radiographs show peribronchial thickening, prominent vascular markings in the upper lung zones, and Kerley B lines. As the pulmonary edema worsens, alveoli fill with fluid; the chest radiograph shows patchy alveolar filling, typically in a perihilar distribution, which then progresses to diffuse alveolar infiltrates. Increasing airway edema is associated with rhonchi and wheezes.

Noncardiogenic Pulmonary Edema By definition, hydrostatic pressures are normal in noncardiogenic pulmonary edema. Lung water increases due to damage of the pulmonary capillary lining with leakage of proteins and other macromolecules into the tissue; fluid follows the protein as oncotic forces are shifted from the vessel to the surrounding lung tissue. This process is associated with dysfunction of the surfactant lining the alveoli, increased surface forces, and a propensity for the alveoli to collapse at low lung volumes. Physiologically, noncardiogenic pulmonary edema is characterized by intrapulmonary shunt with hypoxemia and decreased pulmonary compliance. Pathologically, hyaline membranes are evident in the alveoli, and inflammation leading to pulmonary fibrosis may be seen. Clinically, the picture ranges from mild dyspnea to respiratory failure. Auscultation of the lungs may be relatively normal despite chest radiographs that show diffuse alveolar infiltrates. CT scans demonstrate that the distribution of alveolar edema is more heterogeneous than was once thought.

It is useful to categorize the causes of noncardiogenic pulmonary edema in terms of whether the injury to the lung is likely to result from direct, indirect, or pulmonary vascular causes (Table 33-2). Direct inju-

TABLE 33-2 COMMON CAUSES OF NONCARDIOGENIC PULMONARY EDEMA

| **Direct Injury to Lung** |
| Chest trauma, pulmonary contusion |
| Aspiration |
| Smoke inhalation |
| Pneumonia |
| Oxygen toxicity |
| Pulmonary embolism, reperfusion |

| **Hematogenous Injury to Lung** |
| Sepsis |
| Pancreatitis |
| Nonthoracic trauma |
| Leukoagglutination reactions |
| Multiple transfusions |
| Intravenous drug use, e.g., heroin |
| Cardiopulmonary bypass |

| **Possible Lung Injury Plus Elevated Hydrostatic Pressures** |
| High altitude pulmonary edema |
| Neurogenic pulmonary edema |
| Reexpansion pulmonary edema |

ries are mediated via the airways (e.g. aspiration) or as the consequence of blunt chest trauma. Indirect injury is the consequence of mediators that reach the lung via the blood stream. The third category includes conditions that may be the consequence of acute changes in pulmonary vascular pressures, possibly the result of sudden autonomic discharge in the case of neurogenic and high-altitude pulmonary edema, or sudden swings of pleural pressure, as well as transient damage to the pulmonary capillaries in the case of reexpansion pulmonary edema.

Distinguishing Cardiogenic from Noncardiogenic Pulmonary Edema The *history* is essential for assessing the likelihood of underlying cardiac disease as well as for identification of one of the conditions associated with noncardiogenic pulmonary edema. The *physical examination* in cardiogenic pulmonary edema is notable for evidence of increased intracardiac pressures (S3 gallop, elevated jugular venous pulse, peripheral edema), and rales and/or wheezes on auscultation of the chest. In contrast, the physical examination in noncardiogenic pulmonary edema is dominated by the findings of the precipitating condition; pulmonary findings may be relatively normal in the early stages. The *chest radiograph* in cardiogenic pulmonary edema typically shows an enlarged cardiac silhouette, vascular redistribution, interstitial thickening, and perihilar alveolar infiltrates; pleural effusions are common. In noncardiogenic pulmonary edema, heart size is normal, alveolar infiltrates are distributed more uniformly throughout the lungs, and pleural effusions are uncommon. Finally, the *hypoxemia* of cardiogenic

pulmonary edema is due largely to ventilation-perfusion mismatch and responds to the administration of supplemental oxygen. In contrast, hypoxemia in noncardiogenic pulmonary edema is due primarily to intrapulmonary shunting and typically persists despite high concentrations of inhaled O_2.

FURTHER READINGS

ABIDOV A et al: Prognostic significance of dyspnea in patients referred for cardiac stress testing. N Engl J Med 353:1889, 2005

Dyspnea mechanisms, assessment, and management: A consensus statement. Am Rev Resp Crit Care Med 159:321, 1999

GILLETTE MA, SCHWARTZSTEIN RM: Mechanisms of dyspnea, in *Supportive Care in Respiratory Disease*, SH Ahmedzai and MF Muer (eds). Oxford, U.K., Oxford University Press, 2005

MAHLER DA et al. Descriptors of breathlessness in cardiorespiratory diseases. Am J Respir Crit Care Med 154:1357, 1996

———, O'DONNELL DE (eds): *Dyspnea: Mechanisms, Measurement, and Management*. New York, Marcel Dekker, 2005

SCHWARTZSTEIN RM. The language of dyspnea, in *Dyspnea: Mechanisms, Measurement, and Management*, DA Mahler and DE O'Donnell (eds). New York, Marcel Dekker, 2005

———, FELLER-KOPMAN D. Shortness of breath, in *Primary Care Cardiology*, 2d ed, E Braunwald and L Goldman (eds). Philadelphia: WB Saunders, 2003

34 Cough and Hemoptysis
Steven E. Weinberger, David A. Lipson

COUGH

Cough is an explosive expiration that provides a normal protective mechanism for clearing the tracheobronchial tree of secretions and foreign material. When excessive or bothersome, it is also one of the most common symptoms for which patients seek medical attention. Reasons for this include discomfort from the cough itself, interference with normal lifestyle, and concern for the cause of the cough, especially fear of cancer.

MECHANISM

Coughing may be initiated either voluntarily or reflexively. As a defensive reflex it has both afferent and efferent pathways. The *afferent limb* includes receptors within the sensory distribution of the trigeminal, glossopharyngeal, superior laryngeal, and vagus nerves. The *efferent limb* includes the recurrent laryngeal nerve and the spinal nerves. The cough starts with a deep inspiration followed by glottic closure, relaxation of the diaphragm, and muscle contraction against a closed glottis. The resulting markedly positive intrathoracic pressure causes narrowing of the trachea. Once the glottis opens, the large pressure differential between the airways and the atmosphere coupled with tracheal narrowing produces rapid flow rates through the trachea. The shearing forces that develop aid in the elimination of mucus and foreign materials.

ETIOLOGY

Cough can be initiated by a variety of irritant triggers either from an exogenous source (smoke, dust, fumes, foreign bodies) or from an endogenous origin (upper airway secretions, gastric contents). These stimuli may affect receptors in the upper airway (especially the pharynx and larynx) or in the lower respiratory tract, following access to the tracheobronchial tree by inhalation or aspiration. When cough is triggered by upper airway secretions (as with postnasal drip) or gastric contents (as with gastroesophageal reflux), the initiating factor can go unrecognized and the cough may persist. Additionally, prolonged exposure to such irritants may initiate airway inflammation, which can

itself precipitate cough and sensitize the airway to other irritants. Cough associated with gastroesophageal reflux is due only in part to irritation of upper airway receptors or to aspiration of gastric contents, as a vagally mediated reflex mechanism secondary to acid in the distal esophagus may also contribute.

Any disorder resulting in inflammation, constriction, infiltration, or compression of airways can be associated with cough. Inflammation commonly results from airway infections, ranging from viral or bacterial bronchitis to bronchiectasis. In viral bronchitis, airway inflammation sometimes persists long after resolution of the typical acute symptoms, thereby producing a prolonged cough that may last for weeks. Pertussis infection is also a possible cause of persistent cough in adults; however, diagnosis is generally made on clinical grounds (Chap. 142). Asthma is a common cause of cough. Although the clinical setting commonly suggests when a cough is secondary to asthma, some patients present with cough in the absence of wheezing or dyspnea, thus making the diagnosis more subtle ("cough variant asthma"). A neoplasm infiltrating the airway wall, such as bronchogenic carcinoma or a carcinoid tumor, is commonly associated with cough. Airway infiltration with granulomas may also trigger a cough, as seen with endobronchial sarcoidosis or tuberculosis. Compression of airways results from extrinsic masses such as lymph nodes or mediastinal tumors, or rarely from an aortic aneurysm.

Examples of parenchymal lung disease potentially producing cough include interstitial lung disease, pneumonia, and lung abscess. Congestive heart failure may be associated with cough, probably as a consequence of interstitial as well as peribronchial edema. A nonproductive cough complicates the use of angiotensin-converting enzyme (ACE) inhibitors in 5–20% of patients taking these agents. Onset is usually within 1 week of starting the drug but can be delayed up to 6 months. Although the mechanism is not known with certainty, it may relate to accumulation of bradykinin or substance P, both of which are degraded by ACE. In contrast, angiotensin II receptor antagonists do not seem to increase cough, likely because these drugs do not significantly increase bradykinin levels.

The most common causes of cough can be categorized according to the duration of the cough. Acute cough (<3 weeks) is most often due to upper respiratory infection (especially the common cold, acute bacterial sinusitis, and pertussis), but more serious disorders, such as pneumonia, pulmonary embolus, and congestive heart failure, can also present in this fashion. Subacute cough (between 3 and 8 weeks) is commonly post-infectious, resulting from persistent airway inflammation and/or postnasal drip following viral infection, pertussis, or infection with *Mycoplasma* or *Chlamydia*. In the patient with subacute cough that is not clearly post-infectious, the varied causes of chronic cough should be considered. Chronic cough (>8 weeks) in a smoker raises the possibilities of chronic obstructive lung disease or bronchogenic carcinoma. In a nonsmoker who has a normal chest radiograph and is not taking an ACE inhibitor, the most common causes of chronic cough are postnasal drip (sometimes termed the *upper airway cough syndrome*), asthma, and gastroesophageal reflux. Eosinophilic bronchitis in the absence of asthma has also been recognized as a potential cause of chronic cough.

APPROACH TO THE PATIENT:
Cough

A detailed *history* frequently provides the most valuable clues for the etiology of the cough. Particularly important questions include:

1. Is the cough acute, subacute, or chronic?
2. At its onset, were there associated symptoms suggestive of a respiratory infection?
3. Is it seasonal or associated with wheezing?
4. Is it associated with symptoms suggestive of postnasal drip (nasal discharge, frequent throat clearing, a "tickle in the throat") or gastroesophageal reflux (heartburn or sensation of regurgitation)? However, the absence of such suggestive symptoms does not exclude either of these diagnoses.
5. Is it associated with fever or sputum? If sputum is present, what is its character?
6. Does the patient have any associated diseases or risk factors for disease (e.g., cigarette smoking, risk factors for infection with HIV, environmental exposures)?
7. Is the patient taking an ACE inhibitor?

The general *physical examination* may point to a systemic or nonpulmonary cause of cough, such as heart failure or primary nonpulmonary neoplasm. Examination of the oropharynx may provide suggestive evidence for postnasal drip, including oropharyngeal mucus or erythema, or a "cobblestone" appearance to the mucosa. Auscultation of the chest may demonstrate inspiratory stridor (indicative of upper airway disease), rhonchi or expiratory wheezing (indicative of lower airway disease), or inspiratory crackles (suggestive of a process involving the pulmonary parenchyma, such as interstitial lung disease, pneumonia, or pulmonary edema).

Chest radiography may be particularly helpful in suggesting or confirming the cause of the cough. Important potential findings include the presence of an intrathoracic mass lesion, localized pulmonary parenchymal opacification, or diffuse interstitial or alveolar disease. An area of honeycombing or cyst formation may suggest bronchiectasis, while symmetric bilateral hilar adenopathy may suggest sarcoidosis.

Pulmonary function testing (Chap. 246) is useful for assessing the functional abnormalities that accompany certain disorders producing cough. Measurement of forced expiratory flow rates can demonstrate reversible airflow obstruction characteristic of asthma. When asthma is considered but flow rates are normal, bronchoprovocation testing with methacholine or cold-air inhalation can demonstrate hyperreactivity of the airways to a bronchoconstrictive stimulus. Measurement of lung volumes and diffusing capacity is useful primarily for demonstration of a restrictive pattern, often seen with any of the diffuse interstitial lung diseases.

If *sputum* is produced, gross and microscopic examination may provide useful information. Purulent sputum suggests chronic bronchitis, bronchiectasis, pneumonia, or lung abscess. Blood in the sputum may be seen in the same disorders, but its presence also raises the question of an endobronchial tumor. Greater than 3% eosinophils seen on staining of induced sputum in a patient with-

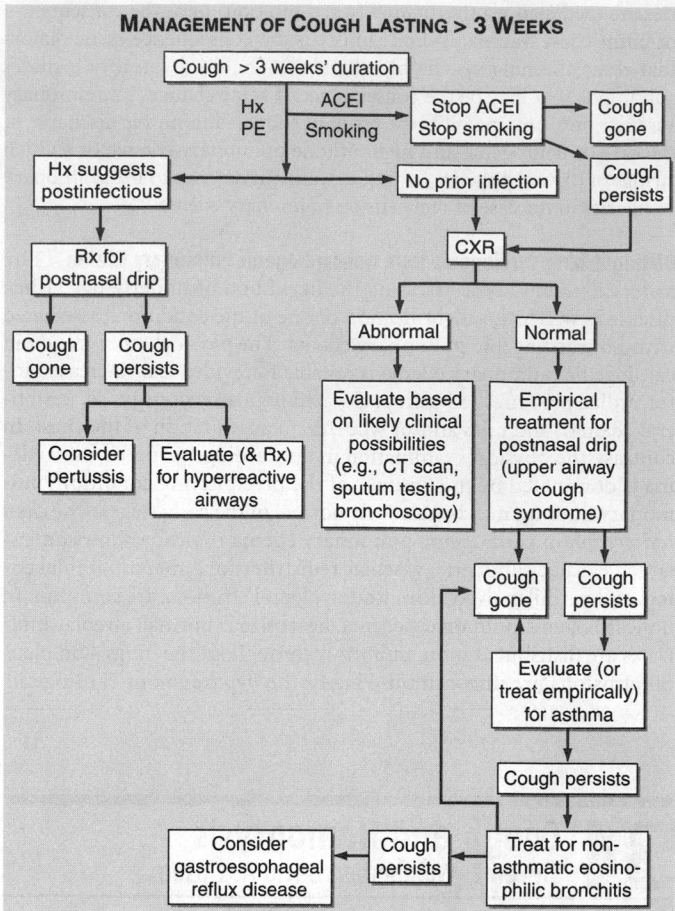

FIGURE 34-1 Algorithm for management of cough lasting >3 weeks. Cough between 3 and 8 weeks is considered subacute; cough >8 weeks is considered chronic. Hx, history; PE, physical examination; ACEI, angiotensin-converting enzyme inhibitor; Rx, treat; CXR, chest x-ray.

out asthma suggests the possibility of eosinophilic bronchitis. Gram and acid-fast stains and cultures may demonstrate a particular infectious pathogen, while sputum cytology may provide a diagnosis of a pulmonary malignancy.

More specialized studies are helpful in specific circumstances. *Fiberoptic bronchoscopy* is the procedure of choice for visualizing an endobronchial tumor and collecting cytologic and histologic specimens. Inspection of the tracheobronchial mucosa can demonstrate endobronchial granulomas often seen in sarcoidosis, and endobronchial biopsy of such lesions or transbronchial biopsy of the lung interstitium can confirm the diagnosis. Inspection of the airway mucosa by bronchoscopy may also demonstrate the characteristic appearance of endobronchial Kaposi's sarcoma in patients with AIDS. *High-resolution computed tomography* (HRCT) can confirm the presence of interstitial lung disease and frequently suggests a diagnosis based on the specific abnormal pattern. It is the procedure of choice for demonstrating dilated airways and confirming the diagnosis of bronchiectasis.

A diagnostic algorithm for evaluation of subacute and chronic cough is presented in **Fig. 34-1.**

COMPLICATIONS

Common complications of coughing include chest and abdominal wall soreness, urinary incontinence, and exhaustion. On occasion, paroxysms of coughing may precipitate syncope (cough syncope; Chap. 21), consequent to markedly positive intrathoracic and alveolar pressures, diminished venous return, and decreased cardiac output. Although cough fractures of the ribs may occur in otherwise normal patients, their occurrence should at least raise the possibility of pathologic fractures, which are seen with multiple myeloma, osteoporosis, and osteolytic metastases.

℞ COUGH

Definitive treatment of cough depends on determining the underlying cause and then initiating specific therapy. Elimination of an exogenous inciting agent (cigarette smoke, ACE inhibitors) or an endogenous trigger (postnasal drip, gastroesophageal reflux) is usually effective when such a precipitant can be identified. Other important management considerations are treatment of specific respiratory tract infections, bronchodilators for potentially reversible airflow obstruction, inhaled glucocorticoids for eosinophilic bronchitis, chest physiotherapy and other methods to enhance clearance of secretions in patients with bronchiectasis, and treatment of endobronchial tumors or interstitial lung disease when such therapy is available and appropriate. In patients with chronic, unexplained cough, an empirical approach to treatment is often used for both diagnostic and therapeutic purposes, starting with an antihistamine-decongestant combination, nasal glucocorticoids, or nasal ipratropium spray to treat unrecognized postnasal drip. If ineffective, this may be followed sequentially by empirical treatment for asthma, nonasthmatic eosinophilic bronchitis, and gastroesophageal reflux.

Symptomatic or nonspecific therapy of cough should be considered when: (1) the cause of the cough is not known or specific treatment is not possible, and (2) the cough performs no useful function or causes marked discomfort or sleep disturbance. An irritative, nonproductive cough may be suppressed by an antitussive agent, which increases the latency or threshold of the cough center. Such agents include codeine (15 mg qid) or nonnarcotics such as dextromethorphan (15 mg qid). These drugs provide symptomatic relief by interrupting prolonged, self-perpetuating paroxysms. However, a cough productive of significant quantities of sputum should usually not be suppressed, since retention of sputum in the tracheobronchial tree may interfere with the distribution of alveolar ventilation and the ability of the lung to resist infection.

HEMOPTYSIS

Hemoptysis is defined as the expectoration of blood from the respiratory tract, a spectrum that varies from blood-streaking of sputum to coughing up large amounts of pure blood. *Massive hemoptysis* is variably defined as the expectoration of >100–600 mL over a 24-h period, although the patient's estimation of the amount of blood is notoriously unreliable. Expectoration of even relatively small amounts of blood is a frightening symptom and may be a marker for potentially serious disease, such as bronchogenic carcinoma. Massive hemoptysis, on the other hand, can represent an acutely life-threatening problem. Blood can fill the airways and the alveolar spaces, not only seriously disturbing gas exchange but potentially causing asphyxiation.

ETIOLOGY

Because blood originating from the nasopharynx or the gastrointestinal tract can mimic blood coming from the lower respiratory tract, it is important to determine initially that the blood is not coming from one of these alternative sites. Clues that the blood is originating from the gastrointestinal tract include a dark red appearance and an acidic pH, in contrast to the typical bright red appearance and alkaline pH of true hemoptysis.

An etiologic classification of hemoptysis can be based on the site of origin within the lungs (Table 34-1). The most common site of bleeding is the tracheobronchial tree, which can be affected by inflammation (acute or chronic bronchitis, bronchiectasis) or by neoplasm (bronchogenic carcinoma, endobronchial metastatic carcinoma, or bronchial carcinoid tumor). The bronchial arteries, which originate either from the aorta or from intercostal arteries and are therefore part of the high-pressure systemic circulation, are the source of bleeding in bronchitis or bronchiectasis or with endobronchial tumors. Blood originating from the pulmonary parenchyma can be either from a localized source, such as an infection (pneumonia, lung abscess, tuberculosis), or from a process diffusely affecting the parenchyma (as with a coagulopathy or with an autoimmune process such as Goodpasture's

TABLE 34-1	DIFFERENTIAL DIAGNOSIS OF HEMOPTYSIS

Source other than the lower respiratory tract
  Upper airway (nasopharyngeal) bleeding
  Gastrointestinal bleeding
Tracheobronchial source
  Neoplasm (bronchogenic carcinoma, endobronchial metastatic tumor, Kaposi's sarcoma, bronchial carcinoid)
  Bronchitis (acute or chronic)
  Bronchiectasis
  Broncholithiasis
  Airway trauma
  Foreign body
Pulmonary parenchymal source
  Lung abscess
  Pneumonia
  Tuberculosis
  Mycetoma ("fungus ball")
  Goodpasture's syndrome
  Idiopathic pulmonary hemosiderosis
  Wegener's granulomatosis
  Lupus pneumonitis
  Lung contusion
Primary vascular source
  Arteriovenous malformation
  Pulmonary embolism
  Elevated pulmonary venous pressure (esp. mitral stenosis)
  Pulmonary artery rupture secondary to balloon-tip pulmonary artery catheter manipulation
Miscellaneous/rare causes
  Pulmonary endometriosis (catamenial hemoptysis)
  Systemic coagulopathy or use of anticoagulants or thrombolytic agents

Adapted from SE Weinberger: *Principles of Pulmonary Medicine*, 4th ed. Philadelphia, Saunders, 2004, with permission.

syndrome). Disorders primarily affecting the pulmonary vasculature include pulmonary embolic disease and those conditions associated with elevated pulmonary venous and capillary pressures, such as mitral stenosis or left ventricular failure.

Although the relative frequency of the different etiologies of hemoptysis varies from series to series, most recent studies indicate that bronchitis and bronchogenic carcinoma are the two most common causes in the United States. Despite the lower frequency of tuberculosis and bronchiectasis seen in recent compared to older series, these two disorders still represent the most common causes of massive hemoptysis in several series, especially worldwide. Even after extensive evaluation, a sizable proportion of patients (up to 30% in some series) have no identifiable etiology for their hemoptysis. These patients are classified as having idiopathic or cryptogenic hemoptysis, and subtle airway or parenchymal disease is presumably responsible for the bleeding.

APPROACH TO THE PATIENT:
Hemoptysis

The *history* is extremely valuable. Hemoptysis that is described as blood-streaking of mucopurulent or purulent sputum often suggests bronchitis. Chronic production of sputum with a recent change in quantity or appearance favors an acute exacerbation of chronic bronchitis. Fever or chills accompanying blood-streaked purulent sputum suggests pneumonia, whereas a putrid smell to the sputum raises the possibility of lung abscess. When sputum production has been chronic and copious, the diagnosis of bronchiectasis should be considered. Hemoptysis following the acute onset of pleuritic chest pain and dyspnea is suggestive of pulmonary embolism.

A history of previous or coexisting disorders should be sought, such as renal disease (seen with Goodpasture's syndrome or Wegener's granulomatosis), lupus erythematosus (with associated pulmonary hemorrhage from lupus pneumonitis), or a previous malignancy (either recurrent lung cancer or endobronchial metastasis from a nonpulmonary primary tumor) or treatment for malignancy (with recent chemotherapy or a bone marrow transplant). In a patient with AIDS, endobronchial or pulmonary parenchymal Kaposi's sarcoma should be considered. Risk factors for bronchogenic carcinoma, particularly smoking and asbestos exposure, should be sought. Patients should be questioned about previous bleeding disorders, treatment with anticoagulants, or use of drugs that can be associated with thrombocytopenia.

The *physical examination* may also provide helpful clues to the diagnosis. For example, examination of the lungs may demonstrate a pleural friction rub (pulmonary embolism), localized or diffuse crackles (parenchymal bleeding or an underlying parenchymal process associated with bleeding), evidence of airflow obstruction (chronic bronchitis), or prominent rhonchi, with or without wheezing or crackles (bronchiectasis). Cardiac examination may demonstrate findings of pulmonary arterial hypertension, mitral stenosis, or heart failure. Skin and mucosal examination may reveal Kaposi's sarcoma, arteriovenous malformations of Osler-Rendu-Weber disease, or lesions suggestive of systemic lupus erythematosus.

Diagnostic evaluation of hemoptysis starts with a chest radiograph (often followed by a CT scan) to look for a mass lesion, findings suggestive of bronchiectasis (Chap. 252), or focal or diffuse parenchymal disease (representing either focal or diffuse bleeding or a focal area of pneumonitis). Additional initial screening evaluation often includes a complete blood count, a coagulation profile, and assessment for renal disease with a urinalysis and measurement of blood urea nitrogen and creatinine levels. When sputum is present, examination by Gram and acid-fast stains (along with the corresponding cultures) is indicated.

Fiberoptic bronchoscopy is particularly useful for localizing the site of bleeding and for visualization of endobronchial lesions. When bleeding is massive, rigid bronchoscopy is often preferable to fiberoptic bronchoscopy because of better airway control and greater suction capability. In patients with suspected bronchiectasis, HRCT is the diagnostic procedure of choice.

A diagnostic algorithm for evaluation of nonmassive hemoptysis is presented in Fig. 34-2.

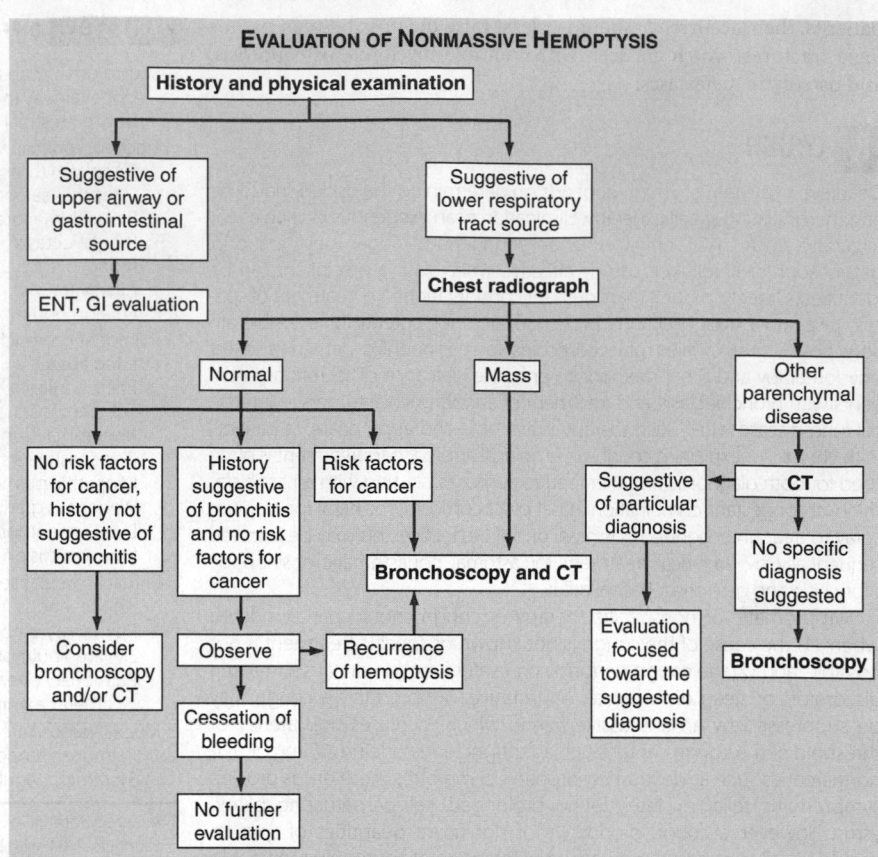

FIGURE 34-2 An algorithm for the evaluation of nonmassive hemoptysis. ENT, ear, nose, and throat; GI, gastrointestinal; CT, computed tomography.

℞ HEMOPTYSIS

The rapidity of bleeding and its effect on gas exchange determine the urgency of management. When the bleeding is confined to either blood-streaking of sputum or production of small amounts of pure blood, gas exchange is usually preserved; establishing a diagnosis is the first priority. When hemoptysis is massive, maintaining adequate gas exchange, preventing blood from spilling into unaffected areas of lung, and avoiding asphyxiation are the highest priorities. Keeping the patient at rest and partially suppressing cough may help the bleeding to subside. If the origin of the blood is known and is limited to one lung, the bleeding lung should be placed in the dependent position, so that blood is not aspirated into the unaffected lung.

With massive bleeding, the need to control the airway and maintain adequate gas exchange may necessitate endotracheal intubation and mechanical ventilation. In patients in danger of flooding the lung contralateral to the side of hemorrhage despite proper positioning, isolation of the right and left mainstem bronchi from each other can be achieved by selectively intubating the nonbleeding lung (often with bronchoscopic guidance) or by using specially designed double-lumen endotracheal tubes. Another option involves inserting a balloon catheter through a bronchoscope by direct visualization and inflating the balloon to occlude the bronchus leading to the bleeding site. This technique not only prevents aspiration of blood into unaffected areas but also may promote tamponade of the bleeding site and cessation of bleeding.

Other available techniques for control of significant bleeding include laser phototherapy, electrocautery, bronchial artery embolization, and surgical resection of the involved area of lung. With bleeding from an endobronchial tumor, argon plasma coagulation or the neodymium:yttrium-aluminum-garnet (Nd:YAG) laser can often achieve at least temporary hemostasis by coagulating the bleeding site. Electrocautery, which uses an electric current for thermal destruction of tissue, can be used similarly for management of bleeding from an endobronchial tumor. Bronchial artery embolization involves an arteriographic procedure in which a vessel proximal to the bleeding site is cannulated, and a material such as Gelfoam is injected to occlude the bleeding vessel. Surgical resection is a therapeutic option either for the emergent therapy of life-threatening hemoptysis that fails to respond to other measures or for the elective but definitive management of localized disease subject to recurrent bleeding.

FURTHER READINGS

AMERICAN COLLEGE OF CHEST PHYSICIANS: Diagnosis and management of cough: ACCP evidence-based clinical practice guidelines. Chest 129:1S, 2006

GIBSON PG et al: Eosinophilic bronchitis: Clinical manifestations and implications for treatment. Thorax 57:178, 2002

HAQUE RA et al: Chronic idiopathic cough. A discrete clinical entity? Chest 127:1710, 2005

IRWIN RS, MADISON JM: The diagnosis and treatment of cough. N Engl J Med 343:1715, 2000

————, ————: The persistently troublesome cough. Am J Respir Crit Care Med 165:1469, 2002

JEAN-BAPTISTE E: Clinical assessment and management of massive hemoptysis. Crit Care Med 28:1642, 2000

KHALIL A et al: Role of MDCT in identification of the bleeding site and the vessels causing hemoptysis. AJR Am J Roentgenol 188:W117, 2007

35 Hypoxia and Cyanosis
Eugene Braunwald

HYPOXIA

The fundamental task of the cardiorespiratory system is to deliver O_2 (and substrates) to the cells and to remove CO_2 (and other metabolic products) from them. Proper maintenance of this function depends on intact cardiovascular and respiratory systems, an adequate number of red blood cells and hemoglobin, and a supply of inspired gas containing adequate O_2.

EFFECTS

Decreased O_2 availability to cells results in an inhibition of the respiratory chain and increased anaerobic glycolysis. This switch from aerobic to anaerobic metabolism, Pasteur's effect, maintains some, albeit markedly reduced, adenosine triphosphate (ATP) production. In severe hypoxia, when ATP production is inadequate to meet the energy requirements of ionic and osmotic equilibrium, cell membrane depolarization leads to uncontrolled Ca^{2+} influx and activation of Ca^{2+}-dependent phospholipases and proteases. These events, in turn, cause cell swelling and ultimately cell necrosis.

The adaptations to hypoxia are mediated, in part, by the upregulation of genes encoding a variety of proteins, including glycolytic enzymes such as phosphoglycerate kinase and phosphofructokinase, as well as the glucose transporters Glut-1 and Glut-2; and by growth factors, such as vascular endothelial growth factor (VEGF) and erythropoietin, which enhance erythrocyte production.

During hypoxia systemic arterioles dilate, at least in part, by opening of K_{ATP} channels in vascular smooth-muscle cells due to the hypoxia-induced reduction in ATP concentration. By contrast, in pulmonary vascular smooth-muscle cells, inhibition of K^+ channels causes depolarization which, in turn, activates voltage-gated Ca^{2+} channels raising the cytosolic $[Ca^{2+}]$ and causing smooth-muscle cell contraction. Hypoxia-induced pulmonary arterial constriction shunts blood away from poorly ventilated toward better-ventilated portions of the lung; however, it also increases pulmonary vascular resistance and right ventricular afterload.

Effects on the Central Nervous System

Changes in the central nervous system, particularly the higher centers, are especially important consequences of hypoxia. Acute hypoxia causes impaired judgment, motor incoordination, and a clinical picture resembling acute alcoholism. High-altitude illness is characterized by headache secondary to cerebral vasodilatation, and by gastrointestinal symptoms, dizziness, insomnia, and fatigue, or somnolence. Pulmonary arterial and sometimes venous constriction cause capillary leakage and high-altitude pulmonary edema (HAPE) (Chap. 33), which intensifies hypoxia and can initiate a vicious circle. Rarely, high-altitude cerebral edema (HACE) develops. This is manifest by severe headache and papilledema and can cause coma. As hypoxia becomes more severe, the centers of the brainstem are affected, and death usually results from respiratory failure.

CAUSES OF HYPOXIA

Respiratory Hypoxia When hypoxia occurs consequent to respiratory failure, Pa_{O_2} declines, and when respiratory failure is persistent, the hemoglobin-oxygen (Hb-O_2) dissociation curve (see Fig. 99-2) is displaced to the right, with greater quantities of O_2 released at any level of tissue P_{O_2}. Arterial hypoxemia, i.e., a reduction of O_2 saturation of arterial blood (Sa_{O_2}), and consequent cyanosis are likely to be more marked when such depression of Pa_{O_2} results from pulmonary disease than when the depression occurs as the result of a decline in the fraction of oxygen in inspired air (Fi_{O_2}). In this latter situation, Pa_{CO_2} falls secondary to anoxia-induced hyperventilation and the Hb-O_2 dissociation curve is displaced to the left, limiting the decline in Sa_{O_2} at any level of Pa_{O_2}.

The most common cause of respiratory hypoxia is *ventilation-perfusion mismatch* resulting from perfusion of poorly ventilated alveoli. Respiratory hypoxemia may also be caused by *hypoventilation*, and it is then associated with an elevation of Pa_{CO_2} (Chap. 246). These two forms of respiratory hypoxia are usually correctable by inspiring 100% O_2 for several minutes. A third cause is shunting of blood across the lung from the pulmonary arterial to the venous bed (*intrapulmonary right-to-left shunting*) by perfusion of nonventilated portions of the lung, as in pulmonary atelectasis or through pulmonary arteriovenous connections. The low Pa_{O_2} in this situation is correctable only in part by an Fi_{O_2} of 100%.

Hypoxia Secondary to High Altitude As one ascends rapidly to 3000 m (~10,000 ft), the reduction of the O_2 content of inspired air (Fi_{O_2}) leads to a decrease in alveolar P_{O_2} to about 60 mmHg, and a condition termed *high-altitude illness* develops (see above). At higher altitudes, arterial saturation declines rapidly and symptoms become more serious; and at 5000 m, unacclimatized individuals usually cease to be able to function normally.

Hypoxia Secondary to Right-to-Left Extrapulmonary Shunting From a physiologic viewpoint, this cause of hypoxia resembles intrapulmonary right-to-left shunting but is caused by congenital cardiac malformations such as tetralogy of Fallot, transposition of the great arteries, and Eisenmenger's syndrome (Chap. 229). As in pulmonary right-to-left shunting, the Pa_{O_2} cannot be restored to normal with inspiration of 100% O_2.

Anemic Hypoxia A reduction in hemoglobin concentration of the blood is attended by a corresponding decline in the O_2-carrying capacity of the blood. Although the Pa_{O_2} is normal in anemic hypoxia, the absolute quantity of O_2 transported per unit volume of blood is diminished. As the anemic blood passes through the capillaries and the usual quantity of O_2 is removed from it, the P_{O_2} and saturation in the venous blood decline to a greater degree than normal.

Carbon Monoxide (CO) Intoxication (See also **Chap. e34**) Hemoglobin that is combined with CO (carboxyhemoglobin, COHb) is unavailable for O_2 transport. In addition, the presence of COHb shifts the Hb-O_2 dissociation curve to the left (see Fig. 99-2) so that O_2 is unloaded only at lower tensions, contributing further to tissue hypoxia.

Circulatory Hypoxia As in anemic hypoxia, the Pa_{O_2} is usually normal, but venous and tissue P_{O_2} values are reduced as a consequence of reduced tissue perfusion and greater tissue O_2 extraction. This pathophysiology leads to an increased arterial–mixed venous O_2 difference, or $(a - \bar{v})$ gradient. Generalized circulatory hypoxia occurs in heart failure (Chap. 227) and in most forms of shock (Chap. 264).

Specific Organ Hypoxia Localized circulatory hypoxia may occur consequent to decreased perfusion secondary to organic arterial obstruction, as in localized atherosclerosis in any vascular bed, or as a consequence of vasoconstriction, as observed in Raynaud's phenomenon (Chap. 243). Localized hypoxia may also result from venous obstruction and the resultant expansion of interstitial fluid causing arterial compression and, thereby, reduction of arterial inflow. Edema, which increases the distance through which O_2 must diffuse before it reaches cells, can also cause localized hypoxia. In an attempt to maintain adequate perfusion to more vital organs in patients with reduced cardiac output secondary to heart failure or hypovolemic shock, vasoconstriction may reduce perfusion in the limbs and skin, causing hypoxia of these regions.

Increased O_2 Requirements If the O_2 consumption of tissues is elevated without a corresponding increase in perfusion, tissue hypoxia ensues and the P_{O_2} in venous blood declines. Ordinarily, the clinical picture of patients with hypoxia due to an elevated metabolic rate, as in fever or thyrotoxicosis, is quite different from that in other types of hypoxia; the skin is warm and flushed owing to increased cutaneous blood flow that dissipates the excessive heat produced, and cyanosis is usually absent.

Exercise is a classic example of increased tissue O_2 requirements. These increased demands are normally met by several mechanisms operating simultaneously: (1) increasing the cardiac output and ventilation and, thus, O_2 delivery to the tissues; (2) preferentially directing the blood to the exercising muscles by changing vascular resistances in the circulatory beds of exercising tissues, directly and/or reflexly; (3) increasing O_2 extraction from the delivered blood and widening the arteriovenous O_2 difference; and (4) reducing the pH of the tissues and capillary blood, shifting the Hb-O_2 curve to the right (see Fig. 99-2) and unloading more O_2 from hemoglobin. If the capacity of these mechanisms is exceeded, then hypoxia, especially of the exercising muscles, will result.

Improper Oxygen Utilization Cyanide (**Chap. e35**) and several other similarly acting poisons cause cellular hypoxia. The tissues are unable to utilize O_2, and as a consequence, the venous blood tends to have a high O_2 tension. This condition has been termed *histotoxic hypoxia.*

ADAPTATION TO HYPOXIA
An important component of the respiratory response to hypoxia originates in special chemosensitive cells in the carotid and aortic bodies and in the respiratory center in the brainstem. The stimulation of these cells by hypoxia increases ventilation, with a loss of CO_2, and can lead to respiratory alkalosis. When combined with the metabolic acidosis resulting from the production of lactic acid, the serum bicarbonate level declines (Chap. 48).

With the reduction of Pa_{O_2}, cerebrovascular resistance decreases and cerebral blood flow increases in an attempt to maintain O_2 delivery to the brain. However, when the reduction of Pa_{O_2} is accompanied by hyperventilation and a reduction of Pa_{CO_2}, cerebrovascular resistance rises, cerebral blood flow falls, and hypoxia is intensified.

The diffuse, systemic vasodilation that occurs in generalized hypoxia raises the cardiac output. In patients with underlying heart disease, the requirements of peripheral tissues for an increase of cardiac output with hypoxia may precipitate congestive heart failure. In patients with ischemic heart disease, a reduced Pa_{O_2} may intensify myocardial ischemia and further impair left ventricular function.

One of the important mechanisms of compensation for chronic hypoxia is an increase in the hemoglobin concentration and in the number of red blood cells in the circulating blood, i.e., the development of polycythemia secondary to erythropoietin production (Chap. 103). In persons with chronic hypoxemia secondary to prolonged residence at a high altitude (>13,000 ft, 4200 m), a condition termed *chronic mountain sickness* develops. It is characterized by a blunted respiratory drive, reduced ventilation, erythrocytosis, cyanosis, weakness, right ventricular enlargement secondary to pulmonary hypertension, and even stupor.

CYANOSIS

Cyanosis refers to a bluish color of the skin and mucous membranes resulting from an increased quantity of reduced hemoglobin, or of hemoglobin derivatives, in the small blood vessels of those areas. It is usually most marked in the lips, nail beds, ears, and malar eminences. Cyanosis, especially if developed recently, is more commonly detected by a family member than the patient. The florid skin characteristic of polycythemia vera (Chap. 103) must be distinguished from the true cyanosis discussed here. A cherry-colored flush, rather than cyanosis, is caused by COHb (**Chap. e35**).

The degree of cyanosis is modified by the color of the cutaneous pigment and the thickness of the skin, as well as by the state of the cutaneous capillaries. The accurate clinical detection of the presence and degree of cyanosis is difficult, as proved by oximetric studies. In some instances, central cyanosis can be detected reliably when the Sa_{O_2} has fallen to 85%; in others, particularly in dark-skinned persons, it may not be detected until it has declined to 75%. In the latter case, examination of the mucous membranes in the oral cavity and the conjunctivae rather than examination of the skin is more helpful in the detection of cyanosis.

The increase in the quantity of reduced hemoglobin in the mucocutaneous vessels that produces cyanosis may be brought about either by an increase in the quantity of venous blood as a result of dilation of the venules and venous ends of the capillaries or by a reduction in the Sa_{O_2} in the capillary blood. In general, cyanosis becomes apparent when the concentration of reduced hemoglobin in capillary blood exceeds 40 g/L (4 g/dL).

It is the *absolute*, rather than the *relative*, quantity of reduced hemoglobin that is important in producing cyanosis. Thus, in a patient with severe anemia, the *relative* quantity of reduced hemoglobin in the venous blood may be very large when considered in relation to the total quantity of hemoglobin in the blood. However, since the concentration of the latter is markedly reduced, the *absolute* quantity of reduced hemoglobin may still be small, and, therefore, patients with severe anemia and even *marked* arterial desaturation may not display cyanosis. Conversely, the higher the total hemoglobin content, the greater is the tendency toward cyanosis; thus, patients with marked polycythemia tend to be cyanotic at higher levels of Sa_{O_2} than patients with normal hematocrit values. Likewise, local passive congestion, which causes an increase in the total quantity of reduced hemoglobin in the vessels in a given area, may cause cyanosis. Cyanosis is also observed when nonfunctional hemoglobin, such as methemoglobin or sulfhemoglobin (Chap. 99), is present in blood.

Cyanosis may be subdivided into central and peripheral types. In the *central* type, the Sa_{O_2} is reduced or an abnormal hemoglobin derivative is present, and the mucous membranes and skin are both affected. *Peripheral* cyanosis is due to a slowing of blood flow and abnormally great extraction of O_2 from normally saturated arterial blood. It results from vasoconstriction and diminished peripheral blood flow, such as occurs in cold exposure, shock, congestive failure, and peripheral vascular disease. Often in these conditions, the mucous membranes of the oral cavity or those beneath the tongue may be spared. Clinical differentiation between central and peripheral cyanosis may not always be simple, and in conditions such as cardiogenic shock with pulmonary edema there may be a mixture of both types.

DIFFERENTIAL DIAGNOSIS
Central Cyanosis (Table 35-1) Decreased Sa_{O_2} results from a marked reduction in the Pa_{O_2}. This reduction may be brought about by a decline in the Fi_{O_2} without sufficient compensatory alveolar hyperventilation to maintain alveolar P_{O_2}. Cyanosis usually becomes manifest in an ascent to an altitude of 4000 m (13,000 ft).

Seriously *impaired pulmonary function,* through perfusion of unventilated or poorly ventilated areas of the lung or alveolar hypoventilation, is a common cause of central cyanosis (Chap. 246). This condition may occur acutely, as in extensive pneumonia or pulmonary edema, or chronically with chronic pulmonary diseases (e.g., emphysema). In the latter situation, secondary polycythemia is generally present and clubbing of the fingers (see below) may occur. Another cause of reduced

TABLE 35-1	CAUSES OF CYANOSIS

Central Cyanosis

Decreased arterial oxygen saturation
  Decreased atmospheric pressure—high altitude
  Impaired pulmonary function
    Alveolar hypoventilation
    Uneven relationships between pulmonary ventilation and perfusion
    (perfusion of hypoventilated alveoli)
    Impaired oxygen diffusion
  Anatomic shunts
    Certain types of congenital heart disease
    Pulmonary arteriovenous fistulas
    Multiple small intrapulmonary shunts
  Hemoglobin with low affinity for oxygen
Hemoglobin abnormalities
  Methemoglobinemia—hereditary, acquired
  Sulfhemoglobinemia—acquired
  Carboxyhemoglobinemia (not true cyanosis)

Peripheral Cyanosis

Reduced cardiac output
Cold exposure
Redistribution of blood flow from extremities
Arterial obstruction
Venous obstruction

Sa_{O_2} is *shunting of systemic venous blood into the arterial circuit.* Certain forms of congenital heart disease are associated with cyanosis on this basis (see above and Chap. 229).

Pulmonary arteriovenous fistulae may be congenital or acquired, solitary or multiple, microscopic or massive. The severity of cyanosis produced by these fistulae depends on their size and number. They occur with some frequency in hereditary hemorrhagic telangiectasia. Sa_{O_2} reduction and cyanosis may also occur in some patients with cirrhosis, presumably as a consequence of pulmonary arteriovenous fistulae or portal vein–pulmonary vein anastomoses.

In patients with cardiac or pulmonary right-to-left shunts, the presence and severity of cyanosis depend on the size of the shunt relative to the systemic flow as well as on the $Hb-O_2$ saturation of the venous blood. With increased extraction of O_2 from the blood by the exercising muscles, the venous blood returning to the right side of the heart is more unsaturated than at rest, and shunting of this blood intensifies the cyanosis. Secondary polycythemia occurs frequently in patients with arterial O_2 unsaturation and contributes to the cyanosis.

Cyanosis can be caused by small quantities of circulating methemoglobin and by even smaller quantities of sulfhemoglobin (Chap. 99). Although they are uncommon causes of cyanosis, these abnormal oxyhemoglobin derivatives should be sought by spectroscopy when cyanosis is not readily explained by malfunction of the circulatory or respiratory systems. Generally, digital clubbing does not occur with them.

Peripheral Cyanosis Probably the most common cause of peripheral cyanosis is the normal vasoconstriction resulting from exposure to cold air or water. When cardiac output is reduced, cutaneous vasoconstriction occurs as a compensatory mechanism so that blood is diverted from the skin to more vital areas such as the central nervous system and heart, and cyanosis of the extremities may result even though the arterial blood is normally saturated.

Arterial obstruction to an extremity, as with an embolus, or arteriolar constriction, as in cold-induced vasospasm (Raynaud's phenomenon, Chap. 243), generally results in pallor and coldness, and there may be associated cyanosis. Venous obstruction, as in thrombophlebitis, dilates the subpapillary venous plexuses and thereby intensifies cyanosis.

APPROACH TO THE PATIENT:
Cyanosis

Certain features are important in arriving at the cause of cyanosis:

1. It is important to ascertain the time of onset of cyanosis. Cyanosis present since birth or infancy is usually due to congenital heart disease.
2. Central and peripheral cyanosis must be differentiated. Evidence of disorders of the respiratory or cardiovascular systems are helpful. Massage or gentle warming of a cyanotic extremity will increase peripheral blood flow and abolish peripheral, but not central, cyanosis.
3. The presence or absence of clubbing of the digits (see below) should be ascertained. The combination of cyanosis and clubbing is frequent in patients with congenital heart disease and right-to-left shunting, and is seen occasionally in patients with pulmonary disease such as lung abscess or pulmonary arteriovenous fistulae. In contrast, peripheral cyanosis or acutely developing central cyanosis is *not* associated with clubbed digits.
4. Pa_{O_2} and Sa_{O_2} should be determined, and in patients with cyanosis in whom the mechanism is obscure, spectroscopic examination of the blood performed to look for abnormal types of hemoglobin (critical in the differential diagnosis of cyanosis).

CLUBBING

The selective bullous enlargement of the distal segments of the fingers and toes due to proliferation of connective tissue, particularly on the dorsal surface, is termed *clubbing*; there is also increased sponginess of the soft tissue at the base of the nail. Clubbing may be hereditary, idiopathic, or acquired and associated with a variety of disorders, including cyanotic congenital heart disease (see above), infective endocarditis, and a variety of pulmonary conditions (among them primary and metastatic lung cancer, bronchiectasis, lung abscess, cystic fibrosis, and mesothelioma), as well as with some gastrointestinal diseases (including inflammatory bowel disease and hepatic cirrhosis). In some instances it is occupational, e.g., in jackhammer operators.

Clubbing in patients with primary and metastatic lung cancer, mesothelioma, bronchiectasis, and hepatic cirrhosis may be associated with *hypertrophic osteoarthropathy.* In this condition, the subperiosteal formation of new bone in the distal diaphyses of the long bones of the extremities causes pain and symmetric arthritis-like changes in the shoulders, knees, ankles, wrists, and elbows. The diagnosis of hypertrophic osteoarthropathy may be confirmed by bone radiographs. Although the mechanism of clubbing is unclear, it appears to be secondary to a humoral substance that causes dilation of the vessels of the fingertip.

FURTHER READINGS

Fawcett RS et al: Nail abnormalities: Clues to systemic disease. Am Fam Physician 69:1417, 2004

Giordano FJ: Oxygen, oxidative stress, hypoxia, and heart failure. J Clin Invest 115:500, 2005

Griffey RT et al: Cyanosis. J Emerg Med 18:369, 2000

Hackett PH, Roach RC: Current concepts: High altitude illness. N Engl J Med 345:107, 2001

Levy MM: Pathophysiology of oxygen delivery in respiratory failure. Chest 128(Suppl 2):547S, 2005

Michiels C: Physiological and pathological responses to hypoxia. Am J Pathol 164:1875, 2004

Tsai BM et al: Hypoxic pulmonary vasoconstriction in cardiothoracic surgery: Basic mechanisms to potential therapies. Ann Thorac Surg 78:360, 2004

36 Edema
Eugene Braunwald, Joseph Loscalzo

Edema is defined as a clinically apparent increase in the interstitial fluid volume, which may expand by several liters before the abnormality is evident. Therefore, a weight gain of several kilograms usually precedes overt manifestations of edema, and a similar weight loss from diuresis can be induced in a slightly edematous patient before "dry weight" is achieved. *Anasarca* refers to gross, generalized edema. *Ascites* (Chap. 44) and *hydrothorax* refer to accumulation of excess fluid in the peritoneal and pleural cavities, respectively, and are considered to be special forms of edema.

Depending on its cause and mechanism, edema may be localized or have a generalized distribution; it is recognized in its generalized form by puffiness of the face, which is most readily apparent in the periorbital areas, and by the persistence of an indentation of the skin following pressure; this is known as "pitting" edema. In its more subtle form, edema may be detected by noting that after the stethoscope is removed from the chest wall, the rim of the bell leaves an indentation on the skin of the chest for a few minutes. When the ring on a finger fits more snugly than in the past or when a patient complains of difficulty in putting on shoes, particularly in the evening, edema may be present.

About one-third of total-body water is confined to the extracellular space. Approximately 75% of the latter, in turn, is interstitial fluid and the remainder is the plasma.

Starling Forces The forces that regulate the disposition of fluid between these two components of the extracellular compartment are frequently referred to as the *Starling forces*. The hydrostatic pressure within the vascular system and the colloid oncotic pressure in the interstitial fluid tend to promote movement of fluid from the vascular to the extravascular space. On the other hand, the colloid oncotic pressure contributed by plasma proteins and the hydrostatic pressure within the interstitial fluid, referred to as the *tissue tension*, promote the movement of fluid into the vascular compartment.

As a consequence of these forces, there is a movement of water and diffusible solutes from the vascular space at the arteriolar end of the capillaries. Fluid is returned from the interstitial space into the vascular system at the venous end of the capillaries and by way of the lymphatics. Unless these channels are obstructed, lymph flow rises with increases in net movement of fluid from the vascular compartment to the interstitium. These flows are usually balanced so that a steady state exists in the sizes of the intravascular and interstitial compartments, and, yet, a large exchange between them occurs. However, should either the hydrostatic or oncotic pressure gradient be altered significantly, a further net movement of fluid between the two components of the extracellular space will take place. The development of edema, then, depends on one or more alterations in the Starling forces so that there is increased flow of fluid from the vascular system into the interstitium or into a body cavity.

Edema due to an increase in capillary pressure may result from an elevation of venous pressure due to obstruction to venous and/or lymphatic drainage. An increase in capillary pressure may be generalized, as occurs in congestive heart failure (see below). The Starling forces may also be imbalanced when the colloid oncotic pressure of the plasma is reduced, owing to any factor that may induce hypoalbuminemia, such as severe malnutrition, liver disease, loss of protein into the urine or into the gastrointestinal tract, or a severe catabolic state. Edema may be localized to one extremity when venous pressure is elevated due to unilateral thrombophlebitis (see below).

Capillary Damage Edema may also result from damage to the capillary endothelium, which increases its permeability and permits the transfer of protein into the interstitial compartment. Injury to the capillary wall can result from drugs, viral or bacterial agents, and thermal or mechanical trauma. Increased capillary permeability may also be a consequence of a hypersensitivity reaction and is characteristic of immune injury. Damage to the capillary endothelium is presumably responsible for inflammatory edema, which is usually nonpitting, localized, and accompanied by other signs of inflammation—redness, heat, and tenderness.

Reduction of Effective Arterial Volume In many forms of edema, the effective arterial blood volume, a parameter that represents the filling of the arterial tree, is reduced. Underfilling of the arterial tree may be caused by a reduction of cardiac output and/or systemic vascular resistance. As a consequence of underfilling, a series of physiologic responses designed to restore the effective arterial volume to normal are set into motion. A key element of these responses is the retention of salt and, therefore, of water, ultimately leading to edema.

Renal Factors and the Renin-Angiotensin-Aldosterone (RAA) System (See also Chap. 336) In the final analysis, renal retention of Na^+ is central to the development of generalized edema. The diminished renal blood flow characteristic of states in which the effective arterial blood volume is reduced is translated by the renal juxtaglomerular cells (specialized myoepithelial cells surrounding the afferent arteriole) into a signal for increased renin release (Chap. 336). Renin is an enzyme with a molecular mass of about 40,000 Da that acts on its substrate, angiotensinogen, an α_2-globulin synthesized by the liver, to release angiotensin I,

a decapeptide, which is broken down to angiotensin II (AII), an octapeptide. AII has generalized vasoconstrictor properties; it is especially active on the efferent arterioles. This efferent arteriolar constriction reduces the hydrostatic pressure in the peritubular capillaries, while the increased filtration fraction raises the colloid osmotic pressure in these vessels, thereby enhancing salt and water reabsorption in the proximal tubule as well as in the ascending limb of the loop of Henle.

The RAA system has long been recognized as a hormonal system; however, it also operates locally. Intrarenally produced AII contributes to glomerular efferent arteriolar constriction, and this "tubuloglomerular feedback" causes salt and water retention. These renal effects of AII are mediated by activation of AII type 1 receptors, which can be blocked by specific antagonists [angiotensin receptor blockers (ARBs)].

The mechanisms responsible for the increased release of renin when renal blood flow is reduced include: (1) a baroreceptor response in which reduced renal perfusion results in incomplete filling of the renal arterioles and diminished stretch of the juxtaglomerular cells, a signal that increases the elaboration and/or release of renin; (2) reduced glomerular filtration, which lowers the NaCl load reaching the distal renal tubules and the macula densa, cells in the distal convoluted tubules that act as chemoreceptors and that signal the neighboring juxtaglomerular cells to secrete renin; and (3) activation of the β-adrenergic receptors in the juxtaglomerular cells by the sympathetic nervous system and by circulating catecholamines, which also stimulates renin release. These three mechanisms generally act in concert to enhance Na^+ retention and, thereby, contribute to the formation of edema.

AII that enters the systemic circulation stimulates the production of aldosterone by the zona glomerulosa of the adrenal cortex. Aldosterone, in turn, enhances Na^+ reabsorption (and K^+ excretion) by the collecting tubule. In patients with heart failure, not only is aldosterone secretion elevated but the biologic half-life of aldosterone is prolonged, which increases further the plasma level of the hormone. A depression of hepatic blood flow, especially during exercise, is responsible for reduced hepatic catabolism of aldosterone. The activation of the RAA system is most striking in the early phase of acute, severe heart failure and is less intense in patients with chronic, stable, compensated heart failure.

Increased quantities of aldosterone are secreted in heart failure and in other edematous states, and blockade of the action of aldosterone by spironolactone (an aldosterone antagonist) or amiloride (a blocker of epithelial Na^+ channels) often induces a moderate diuresis in edematous states. Yet, persistently augmented levels of aldosterone (or other mineralocorticoids) alone do not always promote accumulation of edema, as witnessed by the lack of striking fluid retention in most instances of primary aldosteronism (Chap. 336). Furthermore, although normal individuals retain some NaCl and water with the administration of potent mineralocorticoids, such as deoxycorticosterone acetate or fludrocortisone, this accumulation is self-limiting, despite continued exposure to the steroid, a phenomenon known as *mineralocorticoid escape*. The failure of normal individuals who receive large doses of mineralocorticoids to accumulate large quantities of extracellular fluid and to develop edema is probably a consequence of an increase in glomerular filtration rate (pressure natriuresis) and the action of natriuretic substance(s) (see below). The continued secretion of aldosterone may be more important in the accumulation of fluid in edematous states because patients with edema secondary to heart failure, nephrotic syndrome, and hepatic cirrhosis are generally unable to repair the deficit in effective arterial blood volume. As a consequence, they do not develop pressure natriuresis.

Arginine Vasopressin (AVP) (See also Chap. 334) The secretion of AVP occurs in response to increased intracellular osmolar concentration, and by stimulating V_2 receptors, AVP increases the reabsorption of free water in the renal distal tubule and collecting duct, thereby increasing total-body water. Circulating AVP is elevated in many patients with heart failure secondary to a nonosmotic stimulus associated with decreased effective arterial volume. Such patients fail to show the normal reduction of AVP with a reduction of osmolality, contributing to edema formation and hyponatremia.

Endothelin This potent peptide vasoconstrictor is released by endothelial cells; its concentration is elevated in heart failure and contributes to renal vasoconstriction, Na⁺ retention, and edema in heart failure.

Natriuretic Peptides Atrial distention and/or a Na⁺ load cause release into the circulation of atrial natriuretic peptide (ANP), a polypeptide; a high-molecular-weight precursor of ANP is stored in secretory granules within atrial myocytes. Release of ANP causes (1) excretion of sodium and water by augmenting glomerular filtration rate, inhibiting sodium reabsorption in the proximal tubule, and inhibiting release of renin and aldosterone; and (2) arteriolar and venous dilation by antagonizing the vasoconstrictor actions of AII, AVP, and sympathetic stimulation. Thus, ANP has the capacity to oppose Na⁺ retention and arterial pressure elevation in hypervolemic states.

The closely related brain natriuretic peptide (BNP) is stored primarily in ventricular myocardium and is released when ventricular diastolic pressure rises. Its actions are similar to those of ANP. Circulating levels of ANP and BNP are elevated in congestive heart failure and in cirrhosis with ascites, but obviously not sufficiently to prevent edema formation. In addition, in edematous states there is abnormal resistance to the actions of natriuretic peptides.

CLINICAL CAUSES OF EDEMA
Obstruction of Venous (and Lymphatic) Drainage of a Limb
In this condition the hydrostatic pressure in the capillary bed upstream (proximal) to the obstruction increases so that an abnormal quantity of fluid is transferred from the vascular to the interstitial space. Since the alternative route (i.e., the lymphatic channels) may also be obstructed or maximally filled, an increased volume of interstitial fluid in the limb develops, i.e., there is trapping of fluid in the extremity. Tissue tension rises in the affected limb until it counterbalances the primary alterations in the Starling forces, at which time no further fluid accumulates. The net effect is a local increase in the volume of interstitial fluid, causing local edema. The displacement of fluid into a limb may occur at the expense of the blood volume in the remainder of the body, thereby reducing effective arterial blood volume and leading to the retention of NaCl and H₂O until the deficit in plasma volume has been corrected. This same sequence occurs in ascites and hydrothorax, in which fluid is trapped or accumulates in the cavitary space, depleting the intravascular volume and leading to secondary salt and fluid retention.

Congestive Heart Failure
(See also Chap. 227) In this disorder the impaired systolic emptying of the ventricle(s) and/or the impairment of ventricular relaxation promotes an accumulation of blood in the venous circulation at the expense of the effective arterial volume, and the aforementioned sequence of events (Fig. 36-1) is initiated. In mild heart failure, a small increment of total blood volume may repair the deficit of arterial volume and establish a new steady state. Through the operation

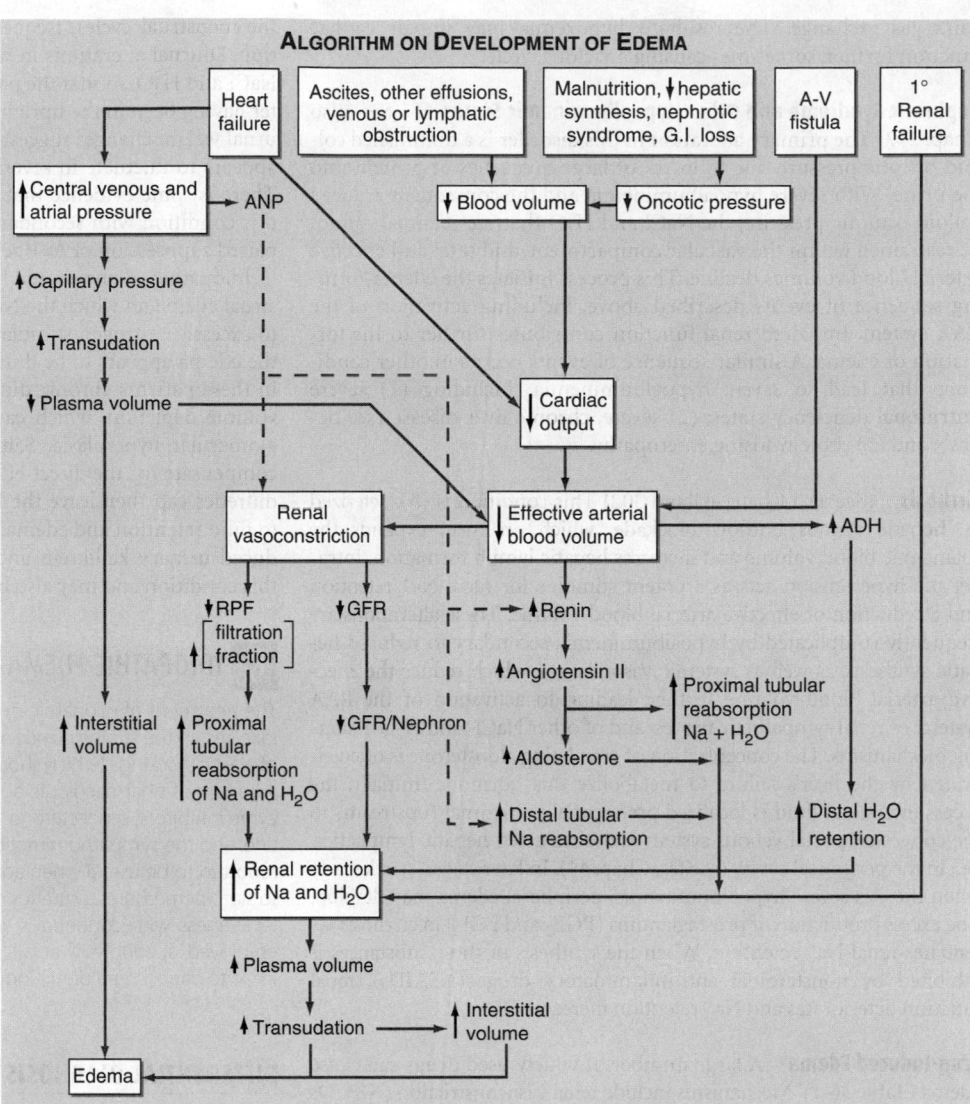

ALGORITHM ON DEVELOPMENT OF EDEMA

FIGURE 36-1 Sequence of events leading to the formation and retention of salt and water and the development of edema. ANP, atrial natriuretic peptide; RPF, renal plasma flow; GFR, glomerular filtration rate; ADH, antidiuretic hormone. Inhibitory influences are shown by broken lines.

of Starling's law of the heart, an increase in ventricular diastolic volume promotes a more forceful contraction and may thereby restore the cardiac output. However, if the cardiac disorder is more severe, fluid retention continues, and the increment in blood volume accumulates in the venous circulation. With reduction in cardiac output, a decrease in baroreflex-mediated inhibition of the vasomotor center activates renal vasoconstrictor nerves and the RAA system, causing Na⁺ and H₂O retention.

Incomplete ventricular emptying (systolic heart failure) and/or inadequate ventricular relaxation (diastolic heart failure) both lead to an elevation of ventricular diastolic pressure. If the impairment of cardiac function primarily involves the right ventricle, pressures in the systemic veins and capillaries rise, augmenting the transudation of fluid into the interstitial space and enhancing the likelihood of peripheral edema. The elevated systemic venous pressure is transmitted to the thoracic duct with consequent reduction of lymph drainage, further increasing the accumulation of edema.

If the impairment of cardiac function (incomplete ventricular emptying and/or inadequate relaxation) involves the left ventricle primarily, then pulmonary venous and capillary pressures rise. Pulmonary artery pressure rises and this, in turn, interferes with the emptying of the right ventricle, leading to an elevation of right ventricular diastolic and of central and systemic venous pressures, thereby enhancing the likelihood of the formation of peripheral edema. The elevation of pulmonary capillary pressure may cause pulmonary edema, which impairs gas exchange. The resultant hypoxemia may impair cardiac function further, sometimes causing a vicious circle.

Nephrotic Syndrome and Other Hypoalbuminemic States
(See also Chap. 277) The primary alteration in this disorder is a diminished colloid oncotic pressure due to losses of large quantities of protein into the urine. With severe hypoalbuminemia and the consequent reduced colloid osmotic pressure, the NaCl and H_2O that are retained cannot be restrained within the vascular compartment, and total and effective arterial blood volumes decline. This process initiates the edema-forming sequence of events described above, including activation of the RAA system. Impaired renal function contributes further to the formation of edema. A similar sequence of events occurs in other conditions that lead to *severe* hypoalbuminemia, including (1) severe nutritional deficiency states; (2) severe, chronic liver disease (see below); and (3) protein-losing enteropathy.

Cirrhosis
(See also Chaps. 44 and 302) This condition is characterized by hepatic venous outflow blockade, which, in turn, expands the splanchnic blood volume and increases hepatic lymph formation. Intrahepatic hypertension acts as a potent stimulus for renal Na^+ retention and a reduction of effective arterial blood volume. These alterations are frequently complicated by hypoalbuminemia secondary to reduced hepatic synthesis, as well as systemic vasodilation, which reduce the effective arterial blood volume further, leading to activation of the RAA system, of renal sympathetic nerves, and of other NaCl- and H_2O-retaining mechanisms. The concentration of circulating aldosterone is often elevated by the liver's failure to metabolize this hormone. Initially, the excess interstitial fluid is localized preferentially proximal (upstream) to the congested portal venous system and obstructed hepatic lymphatics, i.e., in the peritoneal cavity (ascites, Chap. 44). In later stages, particularly when there is severe hypoalbuminemia, peripheral edema may develop. The excess production of prostaglandins (PGE_2 and PGI_2) in cirrhosis attenuates renal Na^+ retention. When the synthesis of these substances is inhibited by nonsteroidal anti-inflammatory drugs (NSAIDs), renal function deteriorates and Na^+ retention increases.

Drug-Induced Edema
A large number of widely used drugs can cause edema (Table 36-1). Mechanisms include renal vasoconstriction (NSAIDs and cyclosporine), arteriolar dilatation (vasodilators), augmented renal Na^+ reabsorption (steroid hormones), and capillary damage (interleukin 2).

Idiopathic Edema
This syndrome, which occurs almost exclusively in women, is characterized by periodic episodes of edema (unrelated to the menstrual cycle), frequently accompanied by abdominal distention. Diurnal alterations in weight occur with orthostatic retention of NaCl and H_2O, so that the patient may weigh several pounds more after having been in the upright posture for several hours. Such large diurnal weight changes suggest an increase in capillary permeability that appears to fluctuate in severity and to be aggravated by hot weather. There is some evidence that a reduction in plasma volume occurs in this condition with secondary activation of the RAA system and impaired suppression of AVP release.

Idiopathic edema should be distinguished from cyclical or premenstrual edema, in which the NaCl and H_2O retention may be secondary to excessive estrogen stimulation. There are also some cases in which the edema appears to be diuretic-induced. It has been postulated that in these patients chronic diuretic administration leads to mild blood volume depletion, which causes chronic hyperreninemia and juxtaglomerular hyperplasia. Salt-retaining mechanisms appear to overcompensate for the direct effects of the diuretics. *Acute* withdrawal of diuretics can then leave the Na^+-retaining forces unopposed, leading to fluid retention and edema. Decreased dopaminergic activity and reduced urinary kallikrein and kinin excretion have been reported in this condition and may also be of pathogenetic importance.

Rx IDIOPATHIC EDEMA

The treatment of idiopathic cyclic edema includes a reduction in NaCl intake, rest in the supine position for several hours each day, and the wearing of elastic stockings (which should be put on before arising in the morning). A variety of pharmacologic agents, including angiotensin-converting enzyme inhibitors, progesterone, the dopamine receptor agonist bromocriptine, and the sympathomimetic amine dextroamphetamine, have all been reported to be useful when administered to patients who do not respond to simpler measures. Diuretics may be helpful initially but may lose their effectiveness with continuous administration; accordingly, they should be employed sparingly, if at all. Discontinuation of diuretics paradoxically leads to diuresis in diuretic-induced edema, described above.

DIFFERENTIAL DIAGNOSIS

LOCALIZED EDEMA
(See also Chap. 243) Edema originating from inflammation or hypersensitivity is usually readily identified. Localized edema due to venous or lymphatic obstruction may be caused by thrombophlebitis, chronic lymphangitis, resection of regional lymph nodes, filariasis, etc. Lymphedema is particularly intractable because restriction of lymphatic flow results in increased protein concentration in the interstitial fluid, a circumstance that aggravates retention of fluid.

GENERALIZED EDEMA
The differences among the three major causes of generalized edema are shown in Table 36-2.

The great majority of patients with generalized edema suffer from advanced cardiac, renal, hepatic, or nutritional disorders. Consequently, the differential diagnosis of generalized edema should be directed toward identifying or excluding these several conditions.

Edema of Heart Failure
(See also Chap. 227) The presence of heart disease, as manifested by cardiac enlargement and a gallop rhythm, together with evidence of cardiac failure, such as dyspnea, basilar rales, venous distention, and hepatomegaly, usually indicate that edema results from heart failure. Noninvasive tests, such as echocardiography, may be helpful in establishing the diagnosis of heart disease. The edema of heart failure typically occurs in the dependent portions of the body.

Edema of the Nephrotic Syndrome
(See also Chap. 277) Marked proteinuria (>3.5 g/d), hypoalbuminemia (<35 g/L), and, in some instances, hypercholesterolemia are present. This syndrome may occur during the course of a variety of kidney diseases, which include glo-

TABLE 36-1	DRUGS ASSOCIATED WITH EDEMA FORMATION

Nonsteroidal anti-inflammatory drugs
Antihypertensive agents
    Direct arterial/arteriolar vasodilators
        Hydralazine
        Clonidine
        Methyldopa
        Guanethidine
        Minoxidil
    Calcium channel antagonists
    α-Adrenergic antagonists
    Thiazolidinediones
Steroid hormones
    Glucocorticoids
    Anabolic steroids
    Estrogens
    Progestins
Cyclosporine
Growth hormone
Immunotherapies
    Interleukin 2
    OKT3 monoclonal antibody

Source: From Chertow.

TABLE 36-2 PRINCIPAL CAUSES OF GENERALIZED EDEMA: HISTORY, PHYSICAL EXAMINATION, AND LABORATORY FINDINGS

Organ System	History	Physical Examination	Laboratory Findings
Cardiac	Dyspnea with exertion prominent—often associated with orthopnea—or paroxysmal nocturnal dyspnea	Elevated jugular venous pressure, ventricular (S_3) gallop; occasionally with displaced or dyskinetic apical pulse; peripheral cyanosis, cool extremities, small pulse pressure when severe	Elevated urea nitrogen-to-creatinine ratio common; elevated uric acid; serum sodium often diminished; liver enzymes occasionally elevated with hepatic congestion
Hepatic	Dyspnea infrequent, except if associated with significant degree of ascites; most often a history of ethanol abuse	Frequently associated with ascites; jugular venous pressure normal or low; blood pressure lower than in renal or cardiac disease; one or more additional signs of chronic liver disease (jaundice, palmar erythema, Dupuytren's contracture, spider angiomata, male gynecomastia; asterixis and other signs of encephalopathy) may be present	If severe, reductions in serum albumin, cholesterol, other hepatic proteins (transferrin, fibrinogen); liver enzymes elevated, depending on the cause and acuity of liver injury; tendency toward hypokalemia, respiratory alkalosis; macrocytosis from folate deficiency
Renal	Usually chronic: may be associated with uremic signs and symptoms, including decreased appetite, altered (metallic or fishy) taste, altered sleep pattern, difficulty concentrating, restless legs or myoclonus; dyspnea can be present, but generally less prominent than in heart failure	Blood pressure may be elevated; hypertensive or diabetic retinopathy in selected cases; nitrogenous fetor; periorbital edema may predominate; pericardial friction rub in advanced cases with uremia	Albuminuria, hypoalbuminemia; sometimes, elevation of serum creatinine and urea nitrogen; hyperkalemia, metabolic acidosis, hyperphosphatemia, hypocalcemia, anemia (usually normocytic)

Source: From Chertow.

merulonephritis, diabetic glomerulosclerosis, and hypersensitivity reactions. A history of previous renal disease may or may not be elicited.

Edema of Acute Glomerulonephritis and Other Forms of Renal Failure

(See also Chap. 277) The edema occurring during the acute phases of glomerulonephritis is characteristically associated with hematuria, proteinuria, and hypertension. Although some evidence supports the view that the fluid retention is due to increased capillary permeability, in most instances the edema results from primary retention of NaCl and H_2O by the kidneys owing to renal insufficiency. This state differs from congestive heart failure in that it is characterized by a normal (or sometimes even increased) cardiac output and a normal arterial–mixed venous oxygen difference. Patients with edema due to renal failure commonly have evidence of arterial hypertension as well as pulmonary congestion on chest roentgenograms even without cardiac enlargement, but they may not develop orthopnea. Patients with *chronic* renal failure may also develop edema due to primary renal retention of NaCl and H_2O.

Edema of Cirrhosis

(See also Chap. 302) Ascites and biochemical and clinical evidence of hepatic disease (collateral venous channels, jaundice, and spider angiomas) characterize edema of hepatic origin. The ascites (Chap. 44) is frequently refractory to treatment because it collects as a result of a combination of obstruction of hepatic lymphatic drainage, portal hypertension, and hypoalbuminemia. A sizable accumulation of ascitic fluid may increase intraabdominal pressure and impede venous return from the lower extremities; hence, it tends to promote accumulation of edema in this region as well.

Edema of Nutritional Origin

A diet grossly deficient in protein over a prolonged period may produce hypoproteinemia and edema. The latter may be intensified by the development of beriberi heart disease, also of nutritional origin, in which multiple peripheral arteriovenous fistulae result in reduced effective systemic perfusion and effective arterial blood volume, thereby enhancing edema formation (Chap. 71). Edema may actually become intensified when famished subjects are first provided with an adequate diet. The ingestion of more food may increase the quantity of NaCl ingested, which is then retained along with H_2O. So-called refeeding edema may also be linked to increased release of insulin, which directly increases tubular Na^+ reabsorption. In addition to hypoalbuminemia, hypokalemia and caloric deficits may be involved in the edema of starvation.

Other Causes of Edema

These include hypothyroidism, in which the edema (myxedema) is located typically in the pretibial region and which may also be associated with periorbital puffiness; exogenous hyperadrenocortism; pregnancy; and administration of estrogens and vasodilators, particularly dihydropyridines such as nifedipine.

DISTRIBUTION OF EDEMA

The distribution of edema is an important guide to its cause. Thus, edema limited to one leg or to one or both arms is usually the result of venous and/or lymphatic obstruction. Edema resulting from hypoproteinemia characteristically is generalized, but it is especially evident in the very soft tissues of the eyelids and face and tends to be most pronounced in the morning because of the recumbent posture assumed during the night. Less common causes of facial edema include trichinosis, allergic reactions, and myxedema. Edema associated with heart failure, by contrast, tends to be more extensive in the legs and to be accentuated in the evening, a feature also determined largely by posture. When patients with heart failure have been confined to bed, edema may be most prominent in the presacral region. Paralysis reduces lymphatic and venous drainage on the affected side and may be responsible for unilateral edema.

ADDITIONAL FACTORS IN DIAGNOSIS

The color, thickness, and sensitivity of the skin are significant. Local tenderness and warmth suggest inflammation. Local cyanosis may signify venous obstruction. In individuals who have had repeated episodes of prolonged edema, the skin over the involved areas may be thickened, indurated, and often red.

Estimation of the venous pressure is of importance in evaluating edema. Ordinarily, a significant generalized increase in venous pressure can be recognized by the level at which cervical veins collapse (Chap. 220). In patients with obstruction of the superior vena cava, edema is confined to the face, neck, and upper extremities, in which the venous pressure is elevated compared with that in the lower extremities. Severe heart failure may cause ascites that may be distinguished from the ascites caused by hepatic cirrhosis by the jugular venous pressure, which is usually elevated in heart failure and normal in cirrhosis.

Determination of the concentration of serum albumin aids importantly in identifying those patients in whom edema is due, at least in part, to diminished intravascular colloid oncotic pressure. The presence of proteinuria also affords useful clues. The absence of proteinuria excludes nephrotic syndrome but cannot exclude nonproteinuric causes of renal failure. Slight to moderate proteinuria is the rule in patients with heart failure.

APPROACH TO THE PATIENT:
Edema

An important first question is whether the edema is localized or generalized. If it is localized, those local phenomena that may be responsible should be considered. If the edema is generalized, it should be determined, first, if there is serious hypoalbuminemia, e.g., serum albumin <25 g/L. If so, the history, physical examination, urinalysis, and other laboratory data will help evaluate the question of cirrhosis, severe malnutrition, or the nephrotic syndrome as the underlying disorder. If hypoalbuminemia is not present, it should be determined if there is evidence of congestive heart failure of a severity to promote generalized edema. Finally, it should be determined whether the patient has an adequate urine output, or if there is significant oliguria or anuria. These abnormalities are discussed in Chaps. 45, 273, and 274.

FURTHER READINGS

ABASSI ZA et al: Control of extracellular fluid volume and the pathophysiology of edema formation, in *The Kidney*, 7th ed, BM Brenner (ed). Philadelphia, Saunders, 2004, pp 777–856

CHERTOW GM: Approach to the patient with edema, in *Cardiology for the Primary Care Physician*, 2d ed, E Braunwald, L Goldman (eds). Philadelphia, Saunders, 2003, pp 117–128

DISKIN CJ et al: Edema, oncotic pressure, and free entropy: Novel considerations for treatment of edema through attention to thermodynamics. Nephron 78:131, 1998

MCCULLOUGH JC: Renal disorders and heart disease, in *Braunwald's Heart Disease*, 7th ed, D Zipes et al (eds). Philadelphia, Saunders, 2005

O'BRIEN JG et al: Treatment of edema. Am Fam Physician 71:2111, 2005

STREETEN DH: Idiopathic edema. Pathogenesis, clinical features, and treatment. Endocrinol Metab Clin North Am 24:531, 1995

37 Palpitations
Joseph Loscalzo

Palpitations are extremely common among patients who present to their caregiver and can best be defined as an intermittent "thumping," "pounding," or "fluttering" sensation in the chest. This sensation can be either intermittent or sustained, and either regular or irregular. Most patients interpret palpitations as an unusual awareness of the heart beat and become especially concerned when they sense that they have had "skipped" or "missing" heart beats. Palpitations are often noted when the patient is quietly resting, during which time other stimuli are minimal. Palpitations that are positional may reflect a structural process within (e.g., atrial myxoma) or adjacent to (e.g., mediastinal mass) the heart.

Palpitations are brought about by cardiac (43%), psychiatric (31%), miscellaneous (10%), and unknown (16%) causes, according to one large series. Cardiac causes include premature atrial and ventricular contractions, supraventricular and ventricular arrhythmias, mitral valve prolapse, aortic regurgitation, and atrial myxoma. Intermittent palpitations are commonly caused by premature atrial or ventricular contractions: the postextrasystolic beat is sensed by the patient owing to the increase in ventricular end-diastolic dimension following the pause in the cardiac cycle and the increased strength of contraction (*postextrasystolic potentiation*) of that beat. Regular, sustained palpitations can be caused by regular supraventricular and ventricular tachycardias (Chap. 226). Irregular, sustained palpitations can be caused by atrial fibrillation.

It is important to note that most arrhythmias are not associated with palpitations. In those that are, it is often useful either to ask the patient to "tap out" the rhythm of the palpitations or to take his or her pulse while palpitations are occurring. In general, hyperdynamic cardiovascular states caused by catecholaminergic stimulation from exercise, stress, or pheochromocytoma can lead to palpitations. In addition, the enlarged ventricle of aortic regurgitation and accompanying hyperdynamic precordium frequently lead to the sensation of palpitations. Other factors that enhance the strength of myocardial contraction, including tobacco, caffeine, aminophylline, atropine, thyroxine, cocaine, and amphetamines, can cause palpitations.

Psychiatric causes of palpitations include panic attack or disorder, anxiety states, and somatization, alone or in combination. Patients with psychiatric causes for palpitations more commonly report a longer duration of the sensation (>15 min) and other accompanying symptoms than do patients with other causes. Among the miscellaneous causes of palpitations are included thyrotoxicosis, drugs (see above) and ethanol, spontaneous skeletal muscle contractions of the chest wall, pheochromocytoma, and systemic mastocytosis.

APPROACH TO THE PATIENT:
Palpitations

The principal goal in assessing patients with palpitations is to determine if the symptom is caused by a life-threatening arrhythmia. Patients with preexisting coronary artery disease (CAD) or risk factors for CAD are at greatest risk for ventricular arrhythmias as a cause for palpitations. In addition, the association of palpitations with other symptoms suggesting hemodynamic compromise, including syncope or lightheadedness, supports this diagnosis. Palpitations caused by sustained tachyarrhythmias in patients with CAD can be accompanied by angina pectoris or dyspnea. In patients with ventricular dysfunction (systolic or diastolic), aortic stenosis, hypertrophic cardiomyopathy, or mitral stenosis, with or without CAD, palpitations can be accompanied by dyspnea from increased left atrial and pulmonary capillary wedge pressure.

Key features of the physical examination that will help confirm or refute the presence of an arrhythmia as a cause for the palpitations and its adverse hemodynamic consequences include measurement of the vital signs, assessment of the jugular venous pressure and pulse, and auscultation of the chest and precordium. A resting electrocardiogram can be used to document the arrhythmia. If exertion is known to induce the arrhythmia and accompanying palpitations, exercise electrocardiography can be used to make the diagnosis. If the arrhythmia is sufficiently infrequent, other methods must be used, including continuous electrocardiographic (Holter) monitoring; telephonic monitoring, through which the patient can transmit an electrocardiographic tracing during a sensed episode; and loop recordings (external or implantable), which can capture the electrocardiographic event for later review.

Most patients with palpitations do not have serious arrhythmias or underlying structural heart disease. Occasional benign atrial or ventricular premature contractions can often be managed with beta blocker therapy if sufficiently troubling to the patient. Palpitations incited by alcohol, tobacco, or illicit drugs need to be managed by abstention, while those caused by pharmacologic agents should be addressed by considering alternative therapies. Psychiatric causes of palpitations may benefit from cognitive or pharmacotherapies. The physician should note that palpitations are at the very least bothersome and, on occasion, frightening to the patient. Once serious causes for the symptom have been excluded, the patient should be reassured the palpitations will not adversely affect his or her prognosis.

ACKNOWLEDGMENT

Dr. Thomas Lee authored this chapter in previous editions. Some of the material from the 16th edition have been carried forward.

FURTHER READINGS

ABBOTT AV: Diagnostic approach to palpitations. Am Fam Physician 71:743, 2005

PICKETT CC, ZIMETBAUM PJ: Palpitations: A proper evaluation and approach to effective medical therapy. Curr Cardiol Rep 7:362, 2005

WEBER BE, KAPOOR WN: Evaluation and outcomes of patients with palpitations. Am J Med 100:138, 1996

SECTION 6 ALTERATIONS IN GASTROINTESTINAL FUNCTION

38 Dysphagia
Raj K. Goyal

Dysphagia is defined as a sensation of "sticking" or obstruction of the passage of food through the mouth, pharynx, or esophagus. However, it is often used as an umbrella term to include other symptoms related to swallowing difficulty. *Aphagia* signifies complete esophageal obstruction, which is usually due to bolus impaction and represents a medical emergency. *Difficulty in initiating a swallow* occurs in disorders of the voluntary phase of swallowing. However, once initiated, swallowing is completed normally. *Odynophagia* means painful swallowing. Frequently, odynophagia and dysphagia occur together. *Globus pharyngeus* is the sensation of a lump lodged in the throat. However, no difficulty is encountered when swallowing is performed. *Misdirection of food*, resulting in nasal regurgitation and laryngeal and pulmonary aspiration during swallowing, is characteristic of oropharyngeal dysphagia. *Phagophobia*, meaning fear of swallowing, and *refusal to swallow* may occur in hysteria, rabies, tetanus, and pharyngeal paralysis due to fear of aspiration. Painful inflammatory lesions that cause odynophagia may also cause refusal to swallow. Some patients may feel the food as it goes down the esophagus. This esophageal sensitivity is not associated with either food sticking or obstruction.

PHYSIOLOGY OF SWALLOWING

The process of swallowing begins with a voluntary (oral) phase that includes a preparatory phase during which a food bolus suitable for swallowing is prepared and a transfer phase during which the bolus is pushed into the pharynx by contraction of the tongue. The bolus then activates oropharyngeal sensory receptors that initiate the deglutition reflex. The deglutition reflex is centrally mediated and involves a complex series of events. It serves both to propel food through the pharynx and the esophagus and to prevent its entry into the airway. When the bolus is propelled backward by the tongue, the larynx moves forward and the upper esophageal sphincter (UES) opens. As the bolus moves into the pharynx, contraction of the superior pharyngeal constrictor against the contracted soft palate initiates a peristaltic contraction that proceeds rapidly downward to move the bolus through the pharynx and the esophagus. The lower esophageal sphincter (LES) opens as the food enters the esophagus and remains open until the peristaltic contraction has swept the bolus into the stomach. Peristaltic contraction in response to a swallow is called *primary peristalsis*. It involves inhibition followed by sequential contraction of muscles along the entire swallowing passage. The inhibition that precedes the peristaltic contraction is called *deglutitive inhibition*. Local distention of the esophagus from residual food activates *secondary peristalsis*.

Muscles of the oral cavity, pharynx, UES, and cervical esophagus are striated and are directly innervated by the lower motor neurons carried in the cranial nerves. Oral cavity muscles are innervated by the Vth and the VIIth cranial nerves and the tongue muscles by the XIIth cranial nerve. Pharyngeal muscles are innervated by the IXth and the Xth cranial nerves.

The UES consists of constrictor and dilator muscles. The constrictor muscles include the cricopharyngeus and inferior pharyngeal constrictor muscles. The dilator muscles include a number of suprahyoid muscles including the geniohyoid muscle. The constrictor muscles are innervated by the Xth cranial nerves and the dilator muscles are innervated by the XIIth and also the Vth and the VIIth cranial nerves. The UES remains closed owing to the elastic properties of its wall and to neurogenic tonic contraction of the cricopharyngeus muscle. Inhibition of the vagal excitatory activity in the central nervous system relaxes the cricopharyngeus, and contraction of the dilator muscles opens the UES by causing upward and forward displacement of the larynx.

The neuromuscular apparatus for peristalsis is different in cervical and thoracic parts of the esophagus. The cervical esophagus, like the pharyngeal muscles, is composed of striated muscles and is innervated by lower motor neurons in the vagus (Xth cranial) nerve. Peristalsis in the cervical esophagus is due to sequential activation of the vagal motor neurons in the nucleus ambiguus.

In contrast, the thoracic esophagus and LES are composed of smooth-muscle fibers and are innervated by excitatory and inhibitory neurons within the esophageal myenteric plexus. Neurotransmitters of the excitatory nerves are acetylcholine and substance P, and of the inhibitory nerves are vasoactive intestinal peptide (VIP) and nitric oxide. Separate groups of parasympathetic preganglionic nerve fibers in the Xth cranial nerve arising from its dorsal motor nucleus project onto the inhibitory and excitatory postganglionic myenteric neurons. Patterned activation of inhibitory followed by excitatory vagal pathways is responsible for peristalsis, which consists of a sequence of inhibition (deglutitive inhibition) followed by contraction. The LES relaxes, with deglutitive inhibition, at the onset of esophageal peristalsis.

The LES is closed at rest because of its intrinsic myogenic tone, influenced by excitatory and inhibitory nerves. The function of the LES is supplemented by the striated muscle of the diaphragmatic crura, which surrounds the LES and acts as an external LES.

PATHOPHYSIOLOGY OF DYSPHAGIA

Based on anatomic site of involvement, dysphagia may be divided into oral, pharyngeal, and esophageal dysphagia. Normal transport of an ingested bolus through the swallowing passage depends on the size of the ingested bolus and size of the lumen, the force of peristaltic contraction, and deglutitive inhibition, including normal relaxation of UES and LES during swallowing. Dysphagia caused by a large bolus or a narrow lumen is called *mechanical dysphagia*, whereas dysphagia due to weakness of peristaltic contractions or to impaired deglutitive inhibition causing nonperistaltic contractions and impaired sphincter relaxation is called *motor dysphagia*.

Oral and Pharyngeal (Oropharyngeal) Dysphagia Oral-phase dysphagia is associated with poor bolus formation and control, so that food may either drool out of the mouth or overstay in the mouth or the patient may experience difficulty in initiating the swallowing reflex. Poor bolus control may also lead to premature spillage of food into the pharynx and aspiration into the unguarded larynx and/or nasal cavity. Pharyngeal-phase dysphagia is associated with stasis of food in the pharynx due to poor pharyngeal propulsion and obstruction at the UES. Pharyngeal stasis leads to nasal regurgitation and laryngeal aspiration during or after a swallow. Nasal regurgitation and laryngeal aspiration during the process of swallowing are hallmarks of oropharyngeal dysphagia.

Oropharyngeal dysphagia may be due to mechanical causes, including a variety of developmental abnormalities, head and neck tumors, radiation therapy, and inflammatory processes (Table 38-1).

TABLE 38-1 OROPHARYNGEAL DYSPHAGIA

Oropharyngeal Mechanical Dysphagia

I. Wall defects
  A. Congenital
    1. Cleft lip, cleft palate
    2. Laryngeal clefts
  B. Post surgical
II. Intrinsic narrowing
  A. Inflammatory
    1. Viral (herpes simplex, varicella-zoster, cytomegalovirus)
    2. Bacterial (peritonsillar abscess)
    3. Fungal (Candida)
    4. Mucocutaneous bullous diseases
    5. Caustic, chemical, thermal injury
  B. Web
    1. Plummer-Vinson syndrome
  C. Strictures
    1. Congenital microganthia
    2. Caustic ingestion
    3. Post-radiation
  D. Tumors
    1. Benign
    2. Malignant
III. Extrinsic compression
  A. Retropharyngeal abscess, mass
  B. Zenker's diverticulum
  C. Thyroid disorders
  D. Vertebral osteophytes

Oropharyngeal Motor Dysphagia

I. Diseases of cerebral cortex and brainstem
  A. With altered consciousness or dementia
    1. Dementias including Alzheimer's disease
    2. Altered consciousness, metabolic encephalopathy, encephalitis, meningitis, cerebrovascular accident, brain injury
  B. With normal cognitive functions
    1. Brain injury
    2. Cerebral palsy
    3. Rabies, tetanus, neurosyphilis
    4. Cerebrovascular disease
    5. Parkinson's disease and other extrapyramidal lesions
    6. Multiple sclerosis (bulbar and pseudobulbar palsy)
    7. Amyotrophic lateral sclerosis (motor neuron disease)
    8. Poliomyelitis and post-poliomyelitis syndrome
II. Diseases of cranial nerves (V, VII, IX, X, XII)
  A. Basilar meningitis (chronic inflammatory, neoplastic)
  B. Nerve injury
  C. Neuropathy (Guillain-Barré syndrome, familial dysautonomia, sarcoid, diabetic and other causes)
III. Neuromuscular
  A. Myasthenia gravis
  B. Eaton-Lambert syndrome
  C. Botulinum toxin
  D. Aminoglycoside and other drugs
IV. Muscle disorders
  A. Myositis (polymyositis, dermatomyositis, sarcoidosis)
  B. Metabolic myopathy (mitochondrial myopathy, thyroid myopathy)
  C. Primary myopathies (myotonic dystrophy, oculopharyngeal myopathy)

Oropharyngeal motor dysphagia results from impairment of the voluntary effort required in bolus preparation or neuromuscular disorders affecting bolus preparation, initiation of the swallowing reflex, timely passage of food through the pharynx, and prevention of entry of food into the nasal and the laryngeal opening. Paralysis of the suprahyoid muscles leads to loss of opening of the UES and severe dysphagia. Because each side of the pharynx is innervated by ipsilateral nerves, a unilateral lesion of motor neurons leads to unilateral pharyngeal paralysis.

Neuromuscular disorders causing dysphagia are listed in Table 38-1. They include a variety of cortical and suprabulbar disorders, lesions of the cranial nerves in their nuclei in the brain stem or their course to the muscles, defects of neurotransmission at the motor end plates, and muscular diseases. Some of these disorders also involve laryngeal muscles and vocal cords, causing hoarseness.

Since the oropharyngeal phase of swallowing lasts no more than a second, rapid-sequence videofluoroscopy is necessary to permit detection and analysis of abnormalities of oral and pharyngeal function. However, such studies can only be performed in a fully conscious and cooperative patient. A videofluoroscopic swallowing study (VFSS) using barium of different consistencies may reveal difficulties in the oral phase of swallowing. The pharynx is examined to detect stasis of barium in the valleculae and pyriform sinuses and regurgitation of barium into the nose and tracheobronchial tree. Pharyngeal contraction waves and opening of UES with a swallow are carefully monitored. Manometric studies may demonstrate reduced amplitude of pharyngeal contractions and reduced UES pressure without further fall in pressure on swallowing (see Fig. 286-3). General treatment consists of maneuvers to reduce pharyngeal stasis and to enhance airway protection under the direction of a trained swallow therapist. Feeding by a naso-gastric tube or an endoscopically placed gastrostomy tube may be necessary for nutritional support; however, these maneuvers do not provide protection against aspiration of salivary secretions. Gastrostomy tube feeding may actually increase gastroesophageal reflux and lead to more aspiration. Jejunostomy tube feeding may lessen reflux.

Dysphagia resulting from a cerebrovascular accident usually improves with time, although often not completely. Patients with myasthenia gravis (Chap. 381) and polymyositis (Chap. 383) may respond to treatment of the primary disease. Cricopharyngeal myotomy is usually not helpful. Extensive operative procedures to prevent aspiration are rarely needed. Death is often due to pulmonary complications.

A cricopharyngeal bar results from failure of the cricopharyngeus to relax but with normal activity of the suprahyoid muscles on swallowing. Barium swallow shows a prominent projection on the posterior wall of the pharynx at the level of the lower part of the cricoid cartilage (see Fig. 286-1). A transient cricopharyngeal bar is seen in up to 5% of individuals without dysphagia undergoing upper gastrointestinal studies; it can be produced in normal individuals during a Valsalva maneuver. A persistent cricopharyngeal bar may be caused by fibrosis in the cricopharyngeus. Cricopharyngeal myotomy may be helpful in severely symptomatic case with functional evidence of obstruction by the cricopharyngeus muscle, but is contraindicated in the presence of gastroesophageal reflux because it may lead to pharyngeal and pulmonary aspiration. Globus pharyngeus mainly occurs in individuals with emotional disorders, particularly in women. Results of barium studies and manometry are normal. Treatment consists primarily of reassurance. Some patients with globus pharyngeus have associated reflux esophagitis, and they may respond to treatment of the esophagitis.

Esophageal Dysphagia In an adult, the esophageal lumen can distend up to 4 cm in diameter. When the esophagus cannot dilate beyond 2.5 cm in diameter, dysphagia to normal solid food can occur. Dysphagia is always present when the esophagus cannot distend beyond 1.3 cm. Circumferential lesions produce dysphagia more consistently than do lesions that involve only a portion of circumferences of the esophageal wall, as uninvolved segments retain their distensibility. The esophageal causes of mechanical dysphagia are listed in Table 38-2. Common causes include carcinoma, peptic and other benign strictures, and lower esophageal ring. Esophageal motor dysphagia may result from abnormalities in peristalsis and deglutitive inhibition due to diseases of the esophageal striated or smooth muscle.

Diseases of the striated muscle often also involve the cervical part of the esophagus, in addition to affecting the oropharyngeal muscles. Clinical manifestations of the cervical esophageal involvement are usually overshadowed by those of the oropharyngeal dysphagia.

Diseases of the smooth-muscle segment involve the thoracic part of the esophagus and the LES. Dysphagia occurs when the peristaltic contractions are weak or absent or when the contractions are nonperistaltic. Loss of peristalsis may be associated with failure of LES relaxation. Weakness of contractile power occurs due to muscle weakness, as in scleroderma or impaired cholinergic effect. Nonperistaltic contractions and failure of LES relaxation occur due to impaired inhibitory innervation. In diffuse esophageal spasm (DES), inhibitory innervation only to the esophageal body is impaired, whereas in achalasia inhibitory innervation to both the esophageal body and LES is impaired. Dysphagia due to esophageal muscle

TABLE 38-2 **ESOPHAGEAL DYSPHAGIA**

Esophageal Mechanical Dysphagia

I. Wall defects
   A. Congenital
   B. Tracheoesophageal fistula
II. Intrinsic narrowing
   A. Inflammatory esophagitis
      1. Viral (herpes simplex, varicella-zoster, cytomegalovirus)
      2. Bacterial
      3. Fungal (*Candida*)
      4. Mucocutaneous bullous diseases
      5. Caustic, chemical, thermal injury
      6. Eosinophilic esophagitis
   B. Webs and rings
      1. Esophageal (congenital, inflammatory)
      2. Lower esophageal mucosal ring (Schatzki's ring)
      3. Eosinophilic esophagitis
      4. Host-versus-graft disease, mucocutaneous disorders
   C. Benign strictures
      1. Peptic
      2. Caustic
      3. Pill-induced
      4. Inflammatory (Crohn's disease, *Candida*, mucocutaneous lesions)
      5. Ischemic
      6. Postoperative
      7. Post-radiation
      8. Congenital
   D. Tumors
      1. Benign
      2. Malignant
III. Extrinsic compression
   A. Vascular compression (dysphagia lusoria, aberrant right subclavian artery, right-sided aorta, left atrial enlargement, aortic aneurysm)
   B. Posterior mediastinal mass
   C. Postvagotomy hematoma and fibrosis

Esophageal Motor Dysphagia

I. Disorders of cervical esophagus
   (see oropharyngeal motor disorders, Table 38-1)
II. Disorders of thoracic esophagus
   A. Diseases of smooth muscle or excitatory nerves
      1. Weak muscle contraction or LES tone
         a. Idiopathic
         b. Scleroderma and related collagen vascular diseases
         c. Hollow visceral myopathy
         d. Myotonic dystrophy
         e. Metabolic neuromyopathy (amyloid, alcohol?, diabetes?)
         f. Drugs: anticholinergics, smooth muscle relaxants
      2. Enhanced muscle contraction
         a. Hypertensive peristalsis (nutcracker esophagus)
         b. Hypertensive LES, hypercontracting LES
   B. Disorders of inhibitory innervation
      1. Diffuse esophageal spasm
      2. Achalasia
         a. Primary
         b. Secondary (Chagas' disease, carcinoma, lymphoma, neuropathic intestinal pseudo-obstruction syndrome)
      3. Contractile (muscular) lower esophageal ring

Note: LES, lower esophageal sphincter.

weakness is often associated with symptoms of gastroesophageal reflux disease (GERD). Dysphagia due to loss of the inhibitory innervation is typically not associated with GERD but may be associated with chest pain.

The causes of esophageal motor dysphagia are also listed in Table 38-2; they include scleroderma of the esophagus, achalasia, DES, and other motor disorders.

APPROACH TO THE PATIENT:
Dysphagia

Figure 38-1 shows an algorithm of approach to a patient with dysphagia.

HISTORY The history can provide a presumptive diagnosis in >80% of patients. The site of dysphagia described by the patient helps to determine the site of esophageal obstruction; the lesion is at or below the perceived location of dysphagia.

Associated symptoms provide important diagnostic clues. Nasal regurgitation and tracheobronchial aspiration with swallowing are hallmarks of pharyngeal paralysis or a tracheoesophageal fistula. Tracheobronchial aspiration unrelated to swallowing may be due to achalasia, Zenker's diverticulum, or gastroesophageal reflux.

Association of laryngeal symptoms and dysphagia occurs in various neuromuscular disorders. The presence of hoarseness may be an important diagnostic clue. When hoarseness precedes dysphagia, the primary lesion is usually in the larynx; hoarseness following dysphagia may suggest involvement of the recurrent laryngeal nerve by extension of esophageal carcinoma. Sometimes hoarseness may be due to laryngitis secondary to gastroesophageal reflux. Hiccups may rarely occur with a lesion in the distal portion of the esophagus. Unilateral wheezing with dysphagia may indicate a mediastinal mass involving the esophagus and a large bronchus.

The type of food causing dysphagia provides useful information. Difficulty only with solids implies mechanical dysphagia with a lumen that is not severely narrowed. In advanced obstruction, dysphagia occurs with liquids as well as solids. In contrast, motor dysphagia due to achalasia and DES is equally affected by solids and liquids from the very onset. Patients with scleroderma have dysphagia to solids that is unrelated to posture and to liquids while recumbent but not upright. When peptic stricture develops in patients with scleroderma, dysphagia becomes more persistent.

The duration and course of dysphagia are helpful in diagnosis. Transient dysphagia may be due to an inflammatory process. Progressive dysphagia lasting a few weeks to a few months is suggestive of carcinoma of the esophagus. Episodic dysphagia to solids lasting several years indicates a benign disease characteristic of a lower esophageal ring.

Severe weight loss that is out of proportion to the degree of dysphagia is highly suggestive of carcinoma.

Chest pain with dysphagia occurs in DES and related motor disorders. Chest pain resembling DES may occur in esophageal obstruction due to a large bolus. A prolonged history of heartburn and reflux preceding dysphagia indicates peptic stricture. A history of prolonged nasogastric intubation, ingestion of caustic agents, ingestion of pills without water, previous radiation therapy, or associated mucocutaneous diseases may provide the cause of esophageal stricture. If odynophagia is present, candidal, herpes, or pill-induced esophagitis should be suspected.

In patients with AIDS or other immunocompromised states, esophagitis due to opportunistic infections such as *Candida*, herpes simplex virus, or cytomegalovirus and to tumors such as Kaposi's sarcoma and lymphoma should be considered.

PHYSICAL EXAMINATION Physical examination is important in oral and pharyngeal motor dysphagia. Signs of bulbar or pseudobulbar palsy, including dysarthria, dysphonia, ptosis, tongue atrophy, and hyperactive jaw jerk, in addition to evidence of generalized neuromuscular disease, should be sought. The neck should be examined for thyromegaly or a spinal abnormality. A careful inspection of the mouth and pharynx should disclose lesions that may interfere with passage of food. Pulmonary complications such as acute or chronic aspiration pneumonia may be present.

Physical examination is often unrevealing in esophageal dysphagia. Changes in the skin and extremities may suggest a diagnosis of scleroderma and other collagen vascular diseases or mucocutaneous diseases such as pemphigoid or epidermolysis bullosa, which may involve the esophagus. Cancer spread to lymph nodes and liver may be evident.

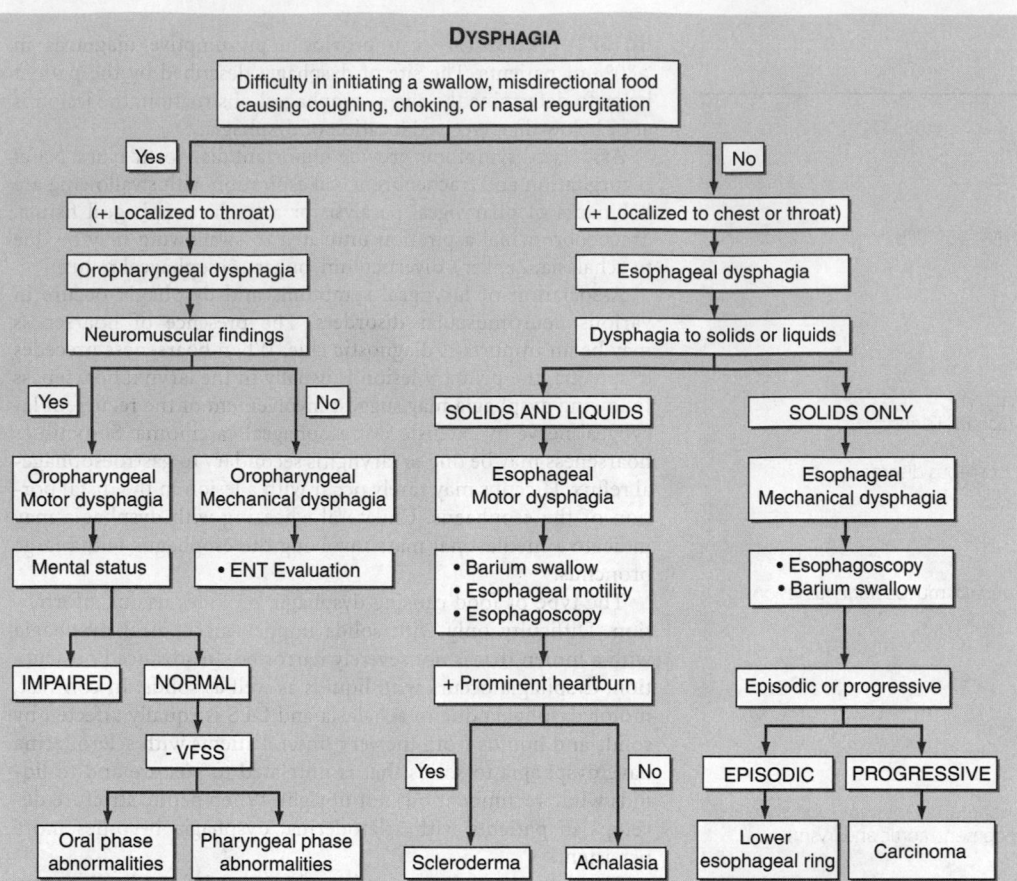

FIGURE 38-1 Approach to the patient with dysphagia. ENT, ear, nose, and throat; VFSS, videofluoroscopic swallowing study.

DIAGNOSTIC PROCEDURES Dysphagia is usually a symptom of organic disease rather than a functional complaint. If oral or pharyngeal dysphagia is suspected, VFSS by both a radiologist and a swallow therapist is the procedure of choice. Videoendoscopy is currently performed only in specialized centers. Otolaryngoscopic and neurologic evaluation are also usually required.

If esophageal mechanical dysphagia is suspected on clinical history, barium swallow and esophagogastroscopy with or without mucosal biopsies are the diagnostic procedures of choice. In some cases, CT examination and endoscopic ultrasound may be useful. For motor esophageal dysphagia, barium swallow, esophageal manometry, esophageal pH, and impedance testing are useful diagnostic tests. Esophagogastroscopy is also often performed in patients with motor dysphagia to exclude an associated structural abnormality (Chap. 286).

FURTHER READINGS

MASSEY B, SHAKER R: Oral pharyngeal and upper esophageal sphincter motility disorders. *www.GImotilityonline.com; doi:10.1038/gimo19*, 2006

MCCULLOUGH TM, JAFFE D: Head and neck disorders causing dysphagia. *www.GI motilityonline.com; doi:10.1038/gimo36*, 2006

PATERSON WG et al: Esophageal motility disorders. *www.GImotility online.com; doi:10.1038/gimo20*, 2006

39 Nausea, Vomiting, and Indigestion
William L. Hasler

Nausea is the subjective feeling of a need to vomit. *Vomiting* (emesis) is the oral expulsion of gastrointestinal contents resulting from contractions of gut and thoracoabdominal wall musculature. Vomiting is contrasted with *regurgitation*, the effortless passage of gastric contents into the mouth. *Rumination* is the repeated regurgitation of stomach contents, which may be rechewed and reswallowed. In contrast to vomiting, these phenomena often exhibit volitional control. *Indigestion* is a nonspecific term that encompasses a variety of upper abdominal complaints including nausea, vomiting, heartburn, regurgitation, and dyspepsia (the presence of symptoms thought to originate in the gastroduodenal region). Some individuals with dyspepsia report predominantly epigastric burning, gnawing discomfort, or pain. Others with dyspepsia experience a constellation of symptoms including postprandial fullness, early satiety (an inability to complete a meal due to premature fullness), bloating, eructation (belching), and anorexia.

NAUSEA AND VOMITING

MECHANISMS
Vomiting is coordinated by the brain stem and is effected by neuromuscular responses in the gut, pharynx, and thoracoabdominal wall.

The mechanisms underlying nausea are poorly understood but likely involve the cerebral cortex, as nausea requires conscious perception. This is supported by electroencephalographic studies showing activation of temporofrontal cortical regions during nausea.

Coordination of Emesis Several brain stem nuclei—including the nucleus tractus solitarius, dorsal vagal and phrenic nuclei, medullary nuclei that regulate respiration, and nuclei that control pharyngeal, facial, and tongue movements—coordinate the initiation of emesis. Neurotransmitters involved in this coordination are uncertain; however, roles for neurokinin NK_1, serotonin 5-HT_3, and vasopressin pathways are postulated.

Somatic and visceral muscles exhibit stereotypic responses during emesis. Inspiratory thoracic and abdominal wall muscles contract, producing high intrathoracic and intraabdominal pressures that facilitate expulsion of gastric contents. The gastric cardia herniates across the diaphragm and the larynx moves upward to promote oral propulsion of the vomitus. Under normal conditions, distally migrating gut contractions are regulated by an electrical phenomenon, the slow wave, which cycles at 3 cycles/min in the stomach and 11 cycles/min in the duodenum. With emesis, there is slow-wave abolition and initiation of orally propagating spike activity, which evokes retrograde contractions that assist in oral expulsion of intestinal contents.

Activators of Emesis Emetic stimuli act at several sites. Emesis provoked by unpleasant thoughts or smells originates in the cerebral cortex, whereas cranial nerves mediate vomiting after gag reflex activation. Motion sickness and inner ear disorders act on the labyrinthine apparatus, whereas gastric irritants and cytotoxic agents such as cisplatin stimulate gastroduodenal vagal afferent nerves. Nongastric visceral afferents are activated by intestinal and colonic obstruction and mesenteric ischemia. The area postrema, a medullary nucleus, responds to bloodborne emetic stimuli and is termed the *chemoreceptor trigger zone.* Many emetogenic drugs act on the area postrema, as do bacterial toxins and metabolic factors produced during uremia, hypoxia, and ketoacidosis.

Neurotransmitters that mediate induction of vomiting are selective for these anatomic sites. Labyrinthine disorders stimulate vestibular cholinergic muscarinic M_1 and histaminergic H_1 receptors, whereas gastroduodenal vagal afferent stimuli activate serotonin 5-HT_3 receptors. The area postrema is richly served by nerve fibers acting on 5-HT_3, M_1, H_1, and dopamine D_2 receptor subtypes. Transmitter mediators in the cerebral cortex are poorly understood, although cortical cannabinoid CB_1 pathways have been characterized. Optimal pharmacologic management of vomiting requires understanding of these pathways.

DIFFERENTIAL DIAGNOSIS

Nausea and vomiting are caused by conditions within and outside the gut as well as by drugs and circulating toxins (**Table 39-1**).

Intraperitoneal Disorders Visceral obstruction and inflammation of hollow and solid viscera may produce vomiting as the main symptom. Gastric obstruction results from ulcer disease and malignancy, while small-bowel and colonic obstruction occur because of adhesions, benign or malignant tumors, volvulus, intussusception, or inflammatory diseases such as Crohn's disease. The superior mesenteric artery syndrome, occurring after weight loss or prolonged bed rest, results when the duodenum is compressed by the overlying superior mesenteric artery. Abdominal irradiation impairs intestinal contractile function and induces strictures. Biliary colic causes nausea via action on visceral afferent nerves. Vomiting with pancreatitis, cholecystitis, and appendicitis is due to localized visceral irritation and induction of ileus. Enteric infections with viruses or bacteria such as *Staphylococcus aureus* and *Bacillus cereus* are common causes of acute vomiting, especially in children. Opportunistic infections such as cytomegalovirus or herpes simplex virus induce emesis in immunocompromised individuals.

Disordered gut sensorimotor function also commonly causes nausea and vomiting. *Gastroparesis* is defined as a delay in emptying of food from the stomach and occurs after vagotomy, with pancreatic adenocarcinoma, with mesenteric vascular insufficiency, or in systemic diseases such as diabetes, scleroderma, and amyloidosis. Idiopathic gastroparesis occurring in the absence of systemic illness may follow a viral prodrome, suggesting an infectious etiology. Intestinal pseudoobstruction is characterized by disrupted intestinal and colonic motor activity and leads to retention of food residue and secretions, bacterial overgrowth, nutrient malabsorption, and symptoms of nausea, vomiting, bloating, pain, and altered defecation. *Intestinal pseudoobstruction* may be idiopathic or inherited as a familial visceral myopathy or neuropathy, or it may result from systemic disease or as a paraneoplastic complication of a malignancy such as small cell lung carcinoma. Patients with gastroesophageal reflux may report nausea and vomiting, as do some individuals with functional dyspepsia and irritable bowel syndrome.

Three other functional disorders without organic abnormalities have been characterized in adults. *Chronic idiopathic nausea* is defined as nausea without vomiting occurring several times weekly, whereas *functional vomiting* is defined as one or more vomiting episodes weekly in

TABLE 39-1 CAUSES OF NAUSEA AND VOMITING		
Intraperitoneal	**Extraperitoneal**	**Medications/Metabolic Disorders**
Obstructing disorders	Cardiopulmonary disease	Drugs
Pyloric obstruction	Cardiomyopathy	Cancer chemotherapy
Small bowel obstruction	Myocardial infarction	Antibiotics
Colonic obstruction	Labyrinthine disease	Cardiac antiarrhythmics
Superior mesenteric artery syndrome	Motion sickness	Digoxin
Enteric infections	Labyrinthitis	Oral hypoglycemics
Viral	Malignancy	Oral contraceptives
Bacterial	Intracerebral disorders	Endocrine/metabolic disease
Inflammatory diseases	Malignancy	Pregnancy
Cholecystitis	Hemorrhage	Uremia
Pancreatitis	Abscess	Ketoacidosis
Appendicitis	Hydrocephalus	Thyroid and parathyroid disease
Hepatitis	Psychiatric illness	Adrenal insufficiency
Altered sensorimotor function	Anorexia and bulimia nervosa	Toxins
Gastroparesis	Depression	Liver failure
Intestinal pseudoobstruction	Postoperative vomiting	Ethanol
Functional dyspepsia		
Gastroesophageal reflux		
Chronic idiopathic nausea		
Functional vomiting		
Cyclic vomiting syndrome		
Biliary colic		
Abdominal irradiation		

the absence of an eating disorder or psychiatric disease. *Cyclic vomiting syndrome* is a rare disorder of unknown etiology that produces periodic discrete episodes of relentless nausea and vomiting. The syndrome shows a strong association with migraine headaches, suggesting that some cases may be migraine variants. Cyclic vomiting is most common in children, although adult cases have been described in association with rapid gastric emptying and with chronic cannabis use.

Extraperitoneal Disorders Myocardial infarction and congestive heart failure are cardiac causes of nausea and vomiting. Postoperative emesis occurs after 25% of surgeries, most commonly laparotomy and orthopedic surgery, and is more prevalent in women. Increased intracranial pressure from tumors, bleeding, abscess, or obstruction to cerebrospinal fluid outflow produces prominent vomiting with or without nausea. Motion sickness, labyrinthitis, and Ménière's disease evoke symptoms via labyrinthine pathways. Patients with psychiatric illnesses including anorexia nervosa, bulimia nervosa, anxiety, and depression may report significant nausea that may be associated with delayed gastric emptying.

Medications and Metabolic Disorders Drugs evoke vomiting by action on the stomach (analgesics, erythromycin) or area postrema (digoxin, opiates, anti-Parkinsonian drugs). Emetogenic agents include antibiotics, cardiac antiarrhythmics, antihypertensives, oral hypoglycemics, and contraceptives. Cancer chemotherapy causes vomiting that is acute (within hours of administration), delayed (after 1 or more days), or anticipatory. Acute emesis resulting from highly emetogenic agents such as cisplatin is mediated by 5-HT_3 pathways, whereas delayed emesis is 5-HT_3-independent. Anticipatory nausea often responds better to anxiolytic therapy than to antiemetics.

Several metabolic disorders elicit nausea and vomiting. Pregnancy is the most prevalent endocrinologic cause of nausea, occurring in 70% of women in the first trimester. Hyperemesis gravidarum is a severe form of nausea of pregnancy which can produce significant fluid loss and electrolyte disturbances. Uremia, ketoacidosis, and adrenal insufficiency, as well as parathyroid and thyroid disease, are other metabolic causes of emesis.

Circulating toxins evoke symptoms via effects on the area postrema. Endogenous toxins are generated in fulminant liver failure, whereas exogenous enterotoxins may be produced by enteric bacterial infection. Ethanol intoxication is a common toxic etiology of nausea and vomiting.

APPROACH TO THE PATIENT:
Nausea and Vomiting

HISTORY AND PHYSICAL EXAMINATION The history helps define the etiology of unexplained nausea and vomiting. Drugs, toxins, and gastrointestinal infections commonly cause acute symptoms, whereas established illnesses evoke chronic complaints. Pyloric obstruction and gastroparesis produce vomiting within 1 h of eating, whereas emesis from intestinal obstruction occurs later. In severe cases of gastroparesis, the vomitus may contain food residue ingested hours or days previously. Hematemesis raises suspicion of an ulcer, malignancy, or Mallory-Weiss tear, whereas feculent emesis is noted with distal intestinal or colonic obstruction. Bilious vomiting excludes gastric obstruction, while emesis of undigested food is consistent with a Zenker's diverticulum or achalasia. Relief of abdominal pain by emesis characterizes small-bowel obstruction, whereas vomiting has no effect on pancreatitis or cholecystitis pain. Pronounced weight loss raises concern about malignancy or obstruction. Fevers suggest inflammation; an intracranial source is considered if there are headaches or visual field changes. Vertigo or tinnitus indicates labyrinthine disease.

The physical examination complements information obtained in the history. Demonstration of orthostatic hypotension and reduced skin turgor indicate intravascular fluid loss. Pulmonary abnormalities raise concern for aspiration of vomitus. Abdominal auscultation may reveal absent bowel sounds with ileus. High-pitched rushes suggest bowel obstruction, while a succussion splash upon abrupt lateral movement of the patient is found with gastroparesis or pyloric obstruction. Tenderness or involuntary guarding raises suspicion of inflammation, whereas fecal blood suggests mucosal injury from ulcer, ischemia, or tumor. Neurologic etiologies present with papilledema, visual field loss, or focal neural abnormalities. Neoplasm is suggested by palpation of masses or adenopathy.

DIAGNOSTIC TESTING For intractable symptoms or an elusive diagnosis, selected diagnostic tests can direct clinical management. Electrolyte replenishment is indicated for hypokalemia or metabolic alkalosis. Detection of iron-deficiency anemia mandates a search for mucosal injury. Pancreaticobiliary disease is indicated by abnormal pancreatic enzymes or liver biochemistries, whereas endocrinologic, rheumatologic, or paraneoplastic etiologies are suggested by specific hormone or serologic testing. If luminal obstruction is suspected, supine and upright abdominal radiographs may show intestinal air-fluid levels with reduced colonic air. Ileus is characterized by diffusely dilated air-filled bowel loops.

Anatomic studies may be indicated if initial testing is nondiagnostic. Upper endoscopy detects ulcers or malignancy, while small-bowel barium radiography diagnoses partial small-bowel obstruction. Colonoscopy or contrast enema radiography can detect colonic obstruction. Abdominal ultrasound or computed tomography (CT) defines intraperitoneal inflammatory processes, while CT or magnetic resonance imaging (MRI) of the head can delineate intracranial disease. Mesenteric angiography or MRI is useful when ischemia is considered.

Gastrointestinal motility testing may detect a motor disorder that contributes to symptoms when anatomic abnormalities are absent. Gastroparesis commonly is diagnosed using gastric scintigraphy, by which emptying of a radiolabeled meal is measured. Isotopic breath tests and telemetry capsule methods also have been validated. Electrogastrography, a noninvasive test of gastric slow-wave activity using cutaneous electrodes placed over the stomach, has been proposed as an alternate means of diagnosing gastroparesis. The diagnosis of intestinal pseudoobstruction often is suggested by abnormal barium transit and luminal dilation on small-bowel contrast radiography. Small-intestinal manometry can confirm the diagnosis and further characterize the motor abnormality as neuropathic or myopathic based on contractile patterns. Such investigation can obviate the need for open intestinal biopsy to evaluate for smooth muscle or neuronal degeneration.

R_x NAUSEA AND VOMITING

GENERAL PRINCIPLES Therapy of vomiting is tailored to correction of medically or surgically remediable abnormalities if possible. Hospitalization is considered for severe dehydration especially if oral fluid replenishment cannot be sustained. Once oral intake is tolerated, nutrients are restarted with liquids that are low in fat, as lipids delay gastric emptying. Foods high in indigestible residues are avoided as these also prolong gastric retention.

ANTIEMETIC MEDICATIONS The most commonly used antiemetic agents act on sites within the central nervous system **(Table 39-2)**. Antihistamines such as meclizine and dimenhydrinate and anticholinergic drugs like scopolamine act on labyrinthine-activated pathways and are useful in motion sickness and inner ear disorders. Dopamine D_2 antagonists treat emesis evoked by area postrema stimuli and are useful for medication, toxic, and metabolic etiologies. Dopamine antagonists freely cross the blood-brain barrier and cause anxiety, dystonic reactions, hyperprolactinemic effects (galactorrhea and sexual dysfunction), and irreversible tardive dyskinesia.

Other drug classes exhibit antiemetic properties. Serotonin 5-HT$_3$ antagonists such as ondansetron and granisetron exhibit utility in postoperative vomiting, after radiation therapy, and in the prevention of cancer chemotherapy–induced emesis. The usefulness of 5-HT$_3$ antagonists for other causes of emesis is less well established. Low-dose tricyclic antidepressant agents provide symptomatic benefit in patients with chronic idiopathic nausea and functional vomiting as well as in diabetic patients with nausea and vomiting whose disease is of long standing.

GASTROINTESTINAL MOTOR STIMULANTS Drugs that stimulate gastric emptying are indicated for gastroparesis (Table 39-2). Metoclopramide, a combined 5-HT$_4$ agonist and D_2 antagonist, exhibits efficacy in gastroparesis, but antidopaminergic side effects limit its use in 25% of patients. Erythromycin, a macrolide antibiotic, increases gastroduodenal motility by action on receptors for motilin, an endogenous stimulant of fasting motor activity. Intravenous erythromycin is useful for inpatients with refractory gastroparesis; however, oral forms also have some utility. Domperidone, a D_2 antagonist not available in the United States, exhibits prokinetic and antiemetic effects but does not cross into most other brain regions; thus, anxiety and dystonic reactions are rare. The main side effects of domperidone relate to induction of hyperprolactinemia via effects on pituitary regions served by a porous blood-brain barrier. The 5-HT$_4$ agonist tegaserod potently stimulates gastric emptying in patients with gastroparesis; however, its effects on symptoms of gastric retention are unproven.

Patients with refractory upper gut motility disorders pose significant challenges. Liquid suspensions of prokinetic drugs may be beneficial, as liquids empty from the stomach more rapidly than pills. Metoclopramide can be administered subcutaneously in patients unresponsive to oral drugs. Intestinal pseudoobstruction may respond to the somatostatin analogue octreotide, which induces propagative small intestinal motor complexes. Pyloric injections of botulinum toxin are reported in uncontrolled studies to benefit patients with gastroparesis. Placement of a feeding jejunostomy reduces hospitalizations and improves overall health in some patients with gastroparesis who do not respond to drug therapy. Surgical options are limited for refractory cases, but postvagotomy gastroparesis may improve with near-total resection of the stomach. Implanted gastric electrical stimulators may reduce symptoms, enhance nutrition, improve quality of life, and decrease health care expenditures in patients with medication-refractory gastroparesis.

SELECTED CLINICAL SETTINGS Cancer chemotherapeutic agents such as cisplatin are intensely emetogenic (Chap. 77). Given prophylactically, 5-HT$_3$ antagonists prevent chemotherapy-induced acute vomiting in most cases (Table 39-2). Optimal antiemetic effects often are obtained with a 5-HT$_3$ antagonist combined with a glucocorticoid. High-dose metoclopramide also exhibits efficacy in chemotherapy-evoked emesis, while benzodiazepines such as lorazepam are useful in reducing anticipatory nausea and vomiting. Therapy of delayed emesis 1–5 days after chemotherapy is less successful. Neurokinin NK$_1$ antagonists (e.g., aprepitant) exhibit antiemetic and antinausea effects during both the acute and delayed periods after chemotherapy. Cannabinoids such as tetrahydrocannabinol, long advocated for cancer-associated emesis, produce significant side effects and exhibit no

TABLE 39-2   TREATMENT OF NAUSEA AND VOMITING

Treatment	Mechanism	Examples	Clinical Indications
Antiemetic agents	Antihistaminergic	Dimenhydrinate, meclizine	Motion sickness, inner ear disease
	Anticholinergic	Scopolamine	Motion sickness, inner ear disease
	Antidopaminergic	Prochlorperazine, thiethylperazine	Medication-, toxin-, or metabolic-induced emesis
	5-HT$_3$ antagonist	Ondansetron, granisetron	Chemotherapy- and radiation-induced emesis, postoperative emesis
	NK$_1$ antagonist	Aprepitant	Chemotherapy-induced nausea and vomiting
	Tricyclic antidepressant	Amitriptyline, nortriptyline	Chronic idiopathic nausea, functional vomiting, cyclic vomiting syndrome
Prokinetic agents	5-HT$_4$ agonist and antidopaminergic	Metoclopramide	Gastroparesis
	Motilin agonist	Erythromycin	Gastroparesis, ?intestinal pseudoobstruction
	Peripheral antidopaminergic	Domperidone	Gastroparesis
	5-HT$_4$ agonist	Tegaserod	?Gastroparesis, ?intestinal pseudoobstruction
	Somatostatin analogue	Octreotide	Intestinal pseudoobstruction
Special settings	Benzodiazepines	Lorazepam	Anticipatory nausea and vomiting with chemotherapy
	Glucocorticoids	Methylprednisolone, dexamethasone	Chemotherapy-induced emesis
	Cannabinoids	Tetrahydrocannabinol	?Chemotherapy-induced emesis

CHAPTER 39

Nausea, Vomiting, and Indigestion

more efficacy than antidopaminergic agents. Most current drug regimens produce greater reductions in vomiting than in nausea.

The clinician should exercise caution in managing the pregnant patient with nausea. Studies of the teratogenic effects of available antiemetic agents provide conflicting results. Few controlled trials have been performed in nausea of pregnancy, although antihistamines such as meclizine and antidopaminergics such as prochlorperazine demonstrate efficacy greater than placebo. Some obstetricians offer alternative therapies such as pyridoxine, acupressure, or ginger.

Controlling emesis in cyclic vomiting syndrome is a challenge. In many individuals, prophylactic treatment with tricyclic antidepressants, cyproheptadine, or β-adrenoceptor antagonists can reduce the frequency of attacks. Intravenous 5-HT$_3$ antagonists combined with the sedating effects of a benzodiazepine such as lorazepam are a mainstay of treatment of acute symptom flares. Small studies report benefits with antimigraine therapies, including the serotonin 5-HT$_1$ agonist sumatriptan as well as certain newer anticonvulsant drugs.

INDIGESTION

MECHANISMS
The most common causes of indigestion are gastroesophageal acid reflux and functional dyspepsia. Other cases are a consequence of a more serious organic illness.

Gastroesophageal Acid Reflux   Acid reflux can result from a variety of physiologic defects. Reduced lower esophageal sphincter (LES) tone is an important cause of reflux in scleroderma and pregnancy; it may also be a factor in patients without other systemic conditions. Many individuals exhibit frequent transient LES relaxations during which acid bathes the esophagus. Overeating and aerophagia can transiently override the barrier function of the LES, whereas impaired esophageal body motility and reduced salivary secretion prolong acid exposure. The role of hiatal hernias is controversial—although most reflux patients exhibit hiatal hernias, most individuals with hiatal hernias do not have excess heartburn.

Gastric Motor Dysfunction   Disturbed gastric motility is purported to cause acid reflux in some cases of indigestion. Delayed gastric emptying is also found in 25–50% of functional dyspeptics. The relation of these defects to symptom induction is uncertain; many studies show poor correlation between symptom severity and the degree of motor dysfunction. Impaired gastric fundus relaxation after eating may underlie selected dyspeptic symptoms like bloating, nausea, and early satiety.

Visceral Afferent Hypersensitivity   Disturbed gastric sensory function is proposed as a pathogenic factor in functional dyspepsia. Visceral afferent hypersensitivity was first demonstrated in patients with irritable bowel syndrome who had heightened perception of rectal balloon inflation without changes in rectal compliance. Similarly, dyspeptic patients experience discomfort with fundic distention to lower pressures

than healthy controls. Some patients with heartburn exhibit normal esophageal acid exposure. These individuals with functional heartburn are believed to have heightened perception of normal esophageal pH.

Other Factors   *Helicobacter pylori* has a clear etiologic role in peptic ulcer disease, but ulcers cause a minority of cases of dyspepsia. Infection with *H. pylori* is considered to be a minor factor in the genesis of functional dyspepsia. In contrast, functional dyspepsia is associated with a reduced sense of physical and mental well-being and is exacerbated by stress, suggesting an important role for psychological factors. Analgesics cause dyspepsia, while nitrates, calcium channel blockers, theophylline, and progesterone promote acid reflux. Other exogenous stimuli that induce acid reflux include ethanol, tobacco, and caffeine via LES relaxation. Genetic factors may contribute to development of acid reflux.

DIFFERENTIAL DIAGNOSIS
Gastroesophageal Reflux Disease   Gastroesophageal reflux disease (GERD) is prevalent in Western society. Heartburn is reported once monthly by 40% of Americans and daily by 7–10%. Most cases of heartburn occur because of excess acid reflux; however, approximately 10% of patients with functional heartburn exhibit normal degrees of esophageal acid exposure.

Functional Dyspepsia   Nearly 25% of the populace has dyspeptic symptoms at least six times yearly, but only 10–20% of these individuals present to physicians. Functional dyspepsia, the cause of symptoms in 60% of dyspeptic patients, is defined as ≥3 months of bothersome postprandial fullness, early satiety, epigastric pain, or epigastric burning with symptom onset at least 6 months before diagnosis in the absence of organic cause. Most patients follow a benign course, but a small number with *H. pylori* infection or on nonsteroidal anti-inflammatory drugs (NSAIDs) progress to ulcer formation. As with idiopathic gastroparesis, some cases of functional dyspepsia result from prior gastrointestinal infection.

Ulcer Disease   In most cases of GERD, there is no destruction of the esophagus. However, 5% of patients develop esophageal ulcers, and some form strictures. Symptoms do not reliably distinguish nonerosive from erosive or ulcerative esophagitis. Some 15–25% of cases of dyspepsia stem from ulcers of the stomach or duodenum. The most common causes of ulcer disease are gastric infection with *H. pylori* and use of NSAIDs. Other rare causes of gastroduodenal ulcer include Crohn's disease (Chap. 289) and Zollinger-Ellison syndrome (Chap. 287), a condition resulting from gastrin overproduction by an endocrine tumor.

Malignancy   Dyspeptic patients often seek care because of fear of cancer. However, <2% of cases result from gastroesophageal malignancy. Esophageal squamous cell carcinoma occurs most often in those with histories of tobacco or ethanol intake. Other risk factors include prior caustic ingestion, achalasia, and the hereditary disorder tylosis. Esophageal adenocarcinoma usually complicates long-standing acid reflux. Between 8 and 20% of GERD patients exhibit intestinal metaplasia of the esophagus, termed *Barrett's metaplasia*. This condition predisposes to esophageal adenocarcinoma (Chap. 87). Gastric malignancies include adenocarcinoma, which is prevalent in certain Asian societies, and lymphoma.

Other Causes Alkaline reflux esophagitis produces GERD-like symptoms in patients who have had surgery for peptic ulcer disease. Opportunistic fungal or viral esophageal infections may produce heartburn or chest discomfort but more often cause odynophagia. Other causes of esophageal inflammation include eosinophilic esophagitis and pill esophagitis. Biliary colic is in the differential diagnosis of dyspepsia, but most patients with true biliary colic report discrete episodes of right upper quadrant or epigastric pain rather than chronic burning discomfort, nausea, and bloating. Intestinal lactase deficiency produces gas, bloating, discomfort, and diarrhea after lactose ingestion. Lactase deficiency occurs in 15–25% of Caucasians of northern European descent but is more common in African Americans and Asians. Intolerance of other carbohydrates (e.g., fructose, sorbitol) produces similar symptoms. Small-intestinal bacterial overgrowth may produce dyspepsia, often with bowel dysfunction, distention, and malabsorption. Pancreatic disease (chronic pancreatitis and malignancy), hepatocellular carcinoma, celiac disease, Ménétrier's disease, infiltrative diseases (sarcoidosis and eosinophilic gastroenteritis), mesenteric ischemia, thyroid and parathyroid disease, and abdominal wall strain cause dyspepsia. Extraperitoneal etiologies of indigestion include congestive heart failure and tuberculosis.

APPROACH TO THE PATIENT:
Indigestion

HISTORY AND PHYSICAL EXAMINATION Care of the patient with indigestion requires a thorough interview. GERD classically produces heartburn, a substernal warmth in the epigastrium that moves toward the neck. Heartburn often is exacerbated by meals and may awaken the patient. Associated symptoms include regurgitation of acid and water brash, the reflex release of salty salivary secretions into the mouth. Atypical symptoms include pharyngitis, asthma, cough, bronchitis, hoarseness, and chest pain that mimics angina. Some patients with acid reflux on esophageal pH testing do not report heartburn and note abdominal pain or other symptoms.

Some individuals with dyspepsia report a predominance of epigastric pain or burning that is intermittent and not generalized or localized to other regions. Others experience a postprandial distress syndrome characterized by fullness occurring after normal-sized meals and early satiety that prevents completion of regular meals several times weekly, with associated bloating, belching, or nausea. Functional dyspepsia overlaps with other functional bowel disorders such as irritable bowel syndrome.

The physical exam with GERD and functional dyspepsia usually is normal. In atypical GERD, pharyngeal erythema and wheezing may be noted. Poor dentition may be seen with prolonged acid regurgitation. Functional dyspeptics may exhibit epigastric tenderness or abdominal distention.

Discrimination between functional and organic causes of indigestion mandates exclusion of selected historic and examination features. Odynophagia suggests esophageal infection, while dysphagia is worrisome for a benign or malignant esophageal blockage. Other alarming features include unexplained weight loss, recurrent vomiting, occult or gross gastrointestinal bleeding, jaundice, a palpable mass or adenopathy, and a family history of gastrointestinal malignancy.

DIAGNOSTIC TESTING As indigestion is prevalent and because most cases result from GERD or functional dyspepsia, a general principle is to perform only limited and directed diagnostic testing of selected individuals.

TABLE 39-3	ALARM SYMPTOMS IN GERD

Odynophagia
Unexplained weight loss
Recurrent vomiting
Occult or gross gastrointestinal bleeding
Jaundice
Palpable mass or adenopathy
Family history of gastrointestinal malignancy

Once alarm factors are excluded (Table 39-3), patients with typical GERD do not need further evaluation and are treated empirically. Upper endoscopy is indicated to exclude mucosal injury in cases with atypical symptoms, symptoms unresponsive to acid suppressing drugs, or alarm factors. For heartburn >5 years in duration, especially in patients >50 years old, endoscopy is recommended to screen for Barrett's metaplasia. However, the clinical benefits and cost-effectiveness of this approach have not been validated in controlled studies. Ambulatory esophageal pH testing using a catheter method or an implanted esophageal capsule device is considered for drug-refractory symptoms and atypical symptoms like unexplained chest pain. Esophageal manometry most commonly is ordered when surgical treatment of GERD is considered. A low LES pressure may predict failure of drug therapy and helps select patients who may require surgery. Demonstration of disordered esophageal body peristalsis may affect the decision to operate or modify the type of operation chosen. Manometry with provocative testing may clarify the diagnosis in patients with atypical symptoms. Blind perfusion of saline and then acid into the esophagus, known as the *Bernstein test*, can delineate whether unexplained chest discomfort results from acid reflux.

Upper endoscopy is performed as the initial diagnostic test in patients with unexplained dyspepsia who are >55 years old or have alarm factors because of the elevated risks of malignancy and ulcer in these groups. The management approach to patients <55 years old without alarm factors is dependent on the prevalence of *H. pylori* infection in the local population. For individuals who reside in regions with low *H. pylori* prevalence (<10%), a 4-week trial of a potent acid-suppressing medication such as a proton pump inhibitor is recommended. If this fails, a "test and treat" approach is most commonly applied. *H. pylori* status is determined with urea breath testing, stool antigen measurement, or blood serology testing. Those who are *H. pylori* positive are given therapy to eradicate the infection. If symptoms resolve on either of these regimens, no further intervention is required. For patients in areas with high *H. pylori* prevalence (>10%), an initial test and treat approach is advocated, with a subsequent trial of an acid-suppressing regimen offered for those who fail *H. pylori* treatment or for those who are negative for the infection. In each of these patient subsets, upper endoscopy is reserved for those who fail to respond to therapy.

Further testing is indicated if other factors are present. If bleeding is reported, a blood count is obtained to exclude anemia. Thyroid chemistries or calcium levels screen for metabolic disease, whereas specific serologies may suggest celiac disease. For suspected pancreaticobiliary causes, pancreatic and liver chemistries are obtained. If abnormalities are found, abdominal ultrasound or CT may give important information. Gastric emptying scintigraphy is considered to exclude gastroparesis in patients whose dyspeptic symptoms resemble postprandial distress when drug treatment fails. Gastric scintigraphy also assesses for gastroparesis in patients with GERD, especially if surgical intervention is being considered. Breath testing after carbohydrate ingestion may detect lactase deficiency, intolerance to other dietary carbohydrates, or small-intestinal bacterial overgrowth.

℞ INDIGESTION

GENERAL PRINCIPLES For mild indigestion, reassurance that a careful evaluation revealed no serious organic disease may be the only intervention needed. Drugs that cause acid reflux or dyspepsia should be stopped if possible. Patients with GERD should limit ethanol, caffeine, chocolate, and tobacco use because of their effects on the LES. Other measures in GERD include ingesting a low-fat diet, avoiding snacks before bedtime, and elevating the head of the bed.

Specific therapies for organic disease should be offered when possible. Surgery is appropriate in disorders like biliary colic, while diet changes are indicated for lactase deficiency or celiac disease. Some illnesses such as peptic ulcer disease may be cured by specific medical regimens. However, as most indigestion is caused by GERD or functional dyspepsia, medications that reduce gastric acid, stimulate motility, or blunt gastric sensitivity are indicated.

ACID-SUPPRESSING OR NEUTRALIZING MEDICATIONS Drugs that reduce or neutralize gastric acid are most often prescribed for GERD. Histamine H_2 antagonists such as cimetidine, ranitidine, famotidine, and nizatidine are useful in mild to moderate GERD. For severe symptoms or many cases of erosive or ulcerative esophagitis, proton pump inhibitors such as omeprazole, lansoprazole, rabeprazole, pantoprazole, or esomeprazole are needed. These drugs, which inhibit gastric H^+, K^+-ATPase activity, are more potent than H_2 antagonists. Acid suppressants may be taken continuously or on demand depending on symptom severity. Many patients initially started on a proton pump inhibitor can be stepped down to an H_2 antagonist. Combination therapy with a proton pump inhibitor and an H_2 antagonist has been proposed for some refractory cases.

Acid-suppressing drugs are also effective in appropriately selected patients with functional dyspepsia. Meta-analysis of eight controlled trials calculated a risk ratio of 0.86, with a 95% confidence interval of 0.78–0.95, favoring proton pump inhibitor therapy over placebo. The benefits of less potent acid reducing therapies such as H_2 antagonists are unproven.

Liquid antacids are useful for short-term control of mild GERD but are less effective for severe disease unless given at high doses that elicit side effects (diarrhea and constipation with magnesium- and aluminum-containing agents, respectively). Alginic acid in combination with antacids may form a floating barrier to acid reflux in individuals with upright symptoms. Sucralfate is a salt of aluminum hydroxide and sucrose octasulfate that buffers acid and binds pepsin and bile salts. Its efficacy in GERD is felt to be comparable to that of H_2 antagonists.

***HELICOBACTER PYLORI* ERADICATION** *H. pylori* eradication is clearly indicated only for peptic ulcer and mucosa-associated lymphoid tissue gastric lymphoma. The utility of eradication therapy in functional dyspepsia is less well established, but <15% of cases relate to this infection. Meta-analysis of 13 controlled trials calculated a risk ratio of 0.91, with a 95% confidence interval of 0.87–0.96, favoring *H. pylori* eradication therapy over placebo. Several drug combinations show efficacy in eliminating the infection (Chap. 287); most include 10–14 days of a proton pump inhibitor or bismuth subsalicylate in concert with two antibiotics. *H. pylori* infection is associated with reduced prevalence of GERD, especially in the elderly. However, eradication of the infection does not worsen GERD symptoms. To date, no consensus recommendations regarding *H. pylori* eradication in GERD patients have been offered.

GASTROINTESTINAL MOTOR STIMULANTS Motor stimulants (also known as prokinetics) such as metoclopramide, erythromycin, domperidone, and tegaserod have limited utility in GERD. The γ-aminobutyric acid B (GABA-B) agonist baclofen reduces esophageal acid exposure by inhibiting transient LES relaxations; the clinical benefits of this drug are yet to be defined in large trials. Several studies have evaluated the effectiveness of motor-stimulating drugs in functional dyspepsia; however, convincing evidence of their benefits has not been found. Some clinicians suggest that patients with symptoms resembling postprandial distress may respond preferentially to prokinetic drugs.

OTHER OPTIONS Antireflux surgery (fundoplication) is offered to GERD patients who are young and may require lifelong therapy, have typical heartburn and regurgitation, and are responsive to proton pump inhibitors. Individuals who may respond less well to operative therapy include those with atypical symptoms, those with poor response to proton pump inhibitors, and those who have esophageal motor disturbances. Fundoplications are performed laparoscopically when possible and include the Nissen and Toupet procedures in which the proximal stomach is partly or completely wrapped around the distal esophagus to increase LES pressure. Dysphagia, gas-bloat syndrome, and gastroparesis may be long-term complications of these procedures. Endoscopic therapies for increasing the barrier function of the gastroesophageal junction, including radiofrequency energy delivery, suturing, biopolymer implantation, and gastroplication, have been investigated in patients with refractory GERD with variable results and some adverse consequences.

Some patients with functional heartburn and functional dyspepsia refractory to standard therapies may respond to low-dose tricyclic antidepressants. Their mechanism of action is unknown but may involve blunting of visceral pain processing in the brain. Gas and bloating are among the most troubling symptoms in some patients with indigestion and can be difficult to treat. Dietary exclusion of gas-producing foods such as legumes and use of simethicone or activated charcoal provide symptom benefits in some patients. Therapies that modify gut flora, including antibiotics and probiotic preparations containing active bacterial cultures, are useful for cases of bacterial overgrowth and functional lower gastrointestinal disorders, but their utility in functional dyspepsia is unproven. Psychological treatments may be offered for refractory functional dyspepsia, but no convincing data suggest their efficacy.

FURTHER READINGS

ABELL TL et al: Treatment of gastroparesis: A multidisciplinary clinical review. Neurogastroenterol Motil 18:263, 2006

DeVAULT KR, CASTELL DO: American College of Gastroenterology. Updated guidelines for the diagnosis and treatment of gastroesophageal reflux disease. Am J Gastroenterol 100:190, 2005

GALMICHE JP et al: Functional esophageal disorders. Gastroenterology 130:1459, 2006

HASLER WL, CHEY WD: Nausea and vomiting. Gastroenterology 125:1860, 2003

KAHRILAS PJ, LEE TJ: Pathophysiology of gastroesophageal reflux disease. Thor Surg Clin 15:323, 2005

PARKMAN HP et al: American Gastroenterological Association technical review on the diagnosis and treatment of gastroparesis. Gastroenterology 127:1592, 2004

SCHWARTZBERG LS: Chemotherapy-induced nausea and vomiting: Clinician and patient perspectives. J Support Oncol 5(suppl 1):5, 2007

TACK J et al: Functional gastroduodenal disorders. Gastroenterology 130:1466, 2006

TALLEY NJ et al: American Gastroenterological Association technical review on the evaluation of dyspepsia. Gastroenterology 129:1756, 2005

TALLEY NJ et al: Guidelines for the management of dyspepsia. Am J Gastroenterol 100:2324, 2005

40 Diarrhea and Constipation
Michael Camilleri, Joseph A. Murray

Diarrhea and constipation are exceedingly common and together exact an enormous toll in terms of mortality, morbidity, social inconvenience, loss of work productivity, and consumption of medical resources. Worldwide, >1 billion individuals suffer one or more episodes of acute diarrhea each year. Among the 100 million persons affected annually by acute diarrhea in the United States, nearly half must restrict activities, 10% consult physicians, ~250,000 require hospitalization, and ~5000 die (primarily the elderly). The annual economic burden to society may exceed $20 billion. Acute infectious diarrhea remains one of the most common causes of mortality in developing countries, particularly among children, accounting for 2–3 million deaths per year. Constipation, by contrast, is rarely associated with mortality and is exceedingly common in developed countries, leading to frequent self-medication and, in a third of those, to medical consultation. Population statistics on chronic diarrhea and constipation are more uncertain, perhaps due to variable definitions and reporting, but the frequency of these conditions is also high. United States population surveys put prevalence rates for chronic diarrhea at 2–7% and for chronic constipation at 12–19%, with women being affected twice as often as men. Diarrhea and constipation are among the most common patient complaints faced by internists and primary care physicians, and they account for nearly 50% of referrals to gastroenterologists.

Although diarrhea and constipation may present as mere nuisance symptoms at one extreme, they can be severe or life-threatening at the other. Even mild symptoms may signal a serious underlying gastrointestinal lesion, such as colorectal cancer, or systemic disorder, such as thyroid disease. Given the heterogeneous causes and potential severity of these common complaints, it is imperative for clinicians to appreciate the pathophysiology, etiologic classification, diagnostic strategies, and principles of management of diarrhea and constipation, so that rational and cost-effective care can be delivered.

NORMAL PHYSIOLOGY

While the primary function of the small intestine is the digestion and assimilation of nutrients from food, the small intestine and colon together perform important functions that regulate the secretion and absorption of water and electrolytes, the storage and subsequent transport of intraluminal contents aborally, and the salvage of some nutrients after bacterial metabolism of carbohydrate that are not absorbed in the small intestine. The main motor functions are summarized in Table 40-1. Alterations in fluid and electrolyte handling contribute significantly to diarrhea. Alterations in motor and sensory functions of the colon result in highly prevalent syndromes such as irritable bowel syndrome (IBS), chronic diarrhea, and chronic constipation.

NEURAL CONTROL

The small intestine and colon have intrinsic and extrinsic innervation. The *intrinsic innervation*, also called the enteric nervous system, comprises myenteric, submucosal, and mucosal neuronal layers. The function of these layers is modulated by interneurons through the actions of neurotransmitter amines or peptides, including acetylcholine, vasoactive intestinal peptide (VIP), opioids, norepinephrine, serotonin, ATP, and nitric oxide. The myenteric plexus regulates smooth-muscle function, and the submucosal plexus affects secretion, absorption, and mucosal blood flow.

The *extrinsic innervations* of the small intestine and colon are part of the autonomic nervous system and also modulate motor and secretory functions. The parasympathetic nerves convey visceral sensory and excitatory pathways to the colon. Parasympathetic fibers via the vagus nerve reach the small intestine and proximal colon along the branches of the superior mesenteric artery. The distal colon is supplied by sacral parasympathetic nerves (S_{2-4}) via the pelvic plexus; these fibers course through the wall of the colon as ascending intracolonic fibers as far as, and in some instances including, the proximal colon. The chief excitatory neurotransmitters controlling motor function are acetylcholine and the tachykinins, such as substance P. The sympathetic nerve supply modulates motor functions and reaches the small intestine and colon alongside their arterial vessels. Sympathetic input to the gut is generally excitatory to sphincters and inhibitory to non-sphincteric muscle. Visceral afferents convey sensation from the gut to the central nervous system; initially, they course along sympathetic fibers; but as they approach the spinal cord they separate, have cell bodies in the dorsal root ganglion, and enter the dorsal horn of the spinal cord. Afferent signals are conveyed to the brain along the lateral spinothalamic tract and the nociceptive dorsal column pathway and are then projected beyond the thalamus and brainstem to the insula and cerebral cortex to be perceived. Other afferent fibers synapse in the prevertebral ganglia and reflexly modulate intestinal motility.

INTESTINAL FLUID ABSORPTION AND SECRETION

On an average day, 9 L of fluid enter the gastrointestinal (GI) tract; ~1 L of residual fluid reaches the colon; the stool excretion of fluid constitutes about 0.2 L/d. The colon has a large capacitance and functional reserve and may recover up to four times its usual volume of 0.8 L/d, provided the rate of flow permits reabsorption to occur. Thus, the colon can partially compensate for excess fluid delivery to the colon because of intestinal absorptive or secretory disorders.

In the colon, sodium absorption is predominantly electrogenic, and uptake takes place at the apical membrane; it is compensated for by the export functions of the basolateral sodium pump. A variety of neural and non-neural mediators regulate colonic fluid and electrolyte balance, including cholinergic, adrenergic, and serotonergic mediators. Angiotensin and aldosterone also influence colonic absorption, reflecting the common embryologic development of the distal colonic epithelium and the renal tubules.

SMALL-INTESTINAL MOTILITY

During fasting, the motility of the small intestine is characterized by a cyclical event called the migrating motor complex (MMC), which serves to clear nondigestible residue from the small intestine (the intestinal "housekeeper"). This organized, propagated series of contractions lasts on average 4 min, occurs every 60–90 min, and usually involves the entire small intestine. After food ingestion, the small intestine produces irregular, mixing contractions of relatively low amplitude, except in the distal ileum where more powerful contractions occur intermittently and empty the ileum by bolus transfers.

ILEOCOLONIC STORAGE AND SALVAGE

The distal ileum acts as a reservoir, emptying intermittently by bolus movements. This action allows time for salvage of fluids, electrolytes, and nutrients. Segmentation by haustra compartmentalizes the colon and facilitates mixing, retention of residue, and formation of solid stools. There is increased appreciation of the intimate interaction between the colonic function and the luminal ecology. The resident bacteria in the colon are necessary for the digestion of unabsorbed carbohydrates that reach the colon even in health, thereby providing a vital source of nutrients to the mucosa. Normal colonic flora also keeps pathogens at bay by a variety of mechanisms. In health, the ascending and transverse regions of colon function as reservoirs (average transit, 15 h), and the descending colon acts as a conduit (average transit, 3 h). The colon is efficient at conserving sodium and water, a function that is particularly important in sodium-depleted patients in whom the small intestine alone is unable to maintain sodium balance. Diarrhea or constipation may result from alteration in the reservoir function of the proximal colon or the propulsive function of the left colon. Constipation may also result from disturbances of the rectal or sigmoid reservoir, typically as a result of dysfunction of the pelvic floor or the coordination of defecation.

COLONIC MOTILITY AND TONE

The small intestinal MMC only rarely continues into the colon. However, short duration or phasic contractions mix colonic contents, and high-amplitude (>75 mmHg) propagated contractions (HAPCs) are sometimes associated with mass movements through the colon and normally occur approximately five times per day, usually on awakening in the morning and postprandially. Increased frequency of HAPCs may result in diarrhea or urgency. The predominant phasic contractions in the colon are irregular and nonpropagated and serve a "mixing" function.

TABLE 40-1	NORMAL GASTROINTESTINAL MOTILITY: FUNCTIONS AT DIFFERENT ANATOMIC LEVELS

Stomach and small bowel
  Synchronized MMCs in fasting
  Accommodation, trituration, mixing, transit
    Stomach ~3 h
    Small bowel ~3 h
  Ileal reservoir empties boluses
Colon: irregular mixing, fermentation, absorption, transit
  Ascending, transverse: reservoirs
  Descending: conduit
  Sigmoid/rectum: volitional reservoir

Note: MMC, migrating motor complex.

Colonic tone refers to the background contractility upon which phasic contractile activity (typically contractions lasting <15 s) is superimposed. It is an important cofactor in the colon's capacitance (volume accommodation) and sensation.

COLONIC MOTILITY AFTER MEAL INGESTION

After meal ingestion, colonic phasic and tonic contractility increase for a period of ~2 h. The initial phase (~10 min) is mediated by the vagus nerve in response to mechanical distention of the stomach. The subsequent response of the colon requires caloric stimulation and is mediated at least in part by hormones, e.g., gastrin and serotonin.

DEFECATION

Tonic contraction of the puborectalis muscle, which forms a sling around the rectoanal junction, is important to maintain continence; during defecation, sacral parasympathetic nerves relax this muscle, facilitating the straightening of the rectoanal angle (Fig. 40-1). Distention of the rectum results in transient relaxation of the internal anal sphincter via intrinsic and reflex sympathetic innervation. As sigmoid and rectal contractions increase the pressure within the rectum, the rectosigmoid angle opens by >15°. Voluntary relaxation of the external anal sphincter (striated muscle innervated by the pudendal nerve) in response to the sensation produced by distention permits the evacuation of feces; this evacuation process can be augmented by an increase in intraabdominal pressure created by the Valsalva maneuver. Defecation can also be delayed voluntarily by contraction of the external anal sphincter.

DIARRHEA

DEFINITION

Diarrhea is loosely defined as passage of abnormally liquid or unformed stools at an increased frequency. For adults on a typical Western diet, stool weight >200 g/d can generally be considered diarrheal. Diarrhea may be further defined as *acute* if <2 weeks, *persistent* if 2–4 weeks, and *chronic* if >4 weeks in duration.

Two common conditions, usually associated with the passage of stool totaling <200 g/d, must be distinguished from diarrhea, as diagnostic and therapeutic algorithms differ. *Pseudodiarrhea*, or the frequent passage of small volumes of stool, is often associated with rectal urgency and accompanies IBS or proctitis. *Fecal incontinence* is the involuntary discharge of rectal contents and is most often caused by neuromuscular disorders or structural anorectal problems. Diarrhea and urgency, especially if severe, may aggravate or cause incontinence. Pseudodiarrhea and fecal incontinence occur at prevalence rates comparable to or higher than that of chronic diarrhea and should always be considered in patients complaining of "diarrhea." Overflow diarrhea may occur in nursing home patients due to fecal impaction that is readily detectable by rectal examination. A careful history and physical examination generally allow these conditions to be discriminated from true diarrhea.

ACUTE DIARRHEA

More than 90% of cases of acute diarrhea are caused by infectious agents; these cases are often accompanied by vomiting, fever, and abdominal pain. The remaining 10% or so are caused by medications, toxic ingestions, ischemia, and other conditions.

Infectious Agents Most infectious diarrheas are acquired by fecal-oral transmission or, more commonly, via ingestion of food or water contaminated with pathogens from human or animal feces. In the immunocompetent person, the resident fecal microflora, containing >500 taxonomically distinct species, are rarely the source of diarrhea and may actually play a role in suppressing the growth of ingested pathogens. Disturbances of flora by antibiotics can lead to diarrhea by reducing the digestive function or by allowing the overgrowth of pathogens, such as *Clostridium difficile* (Chap. 123). Acute infection or injury occurs when

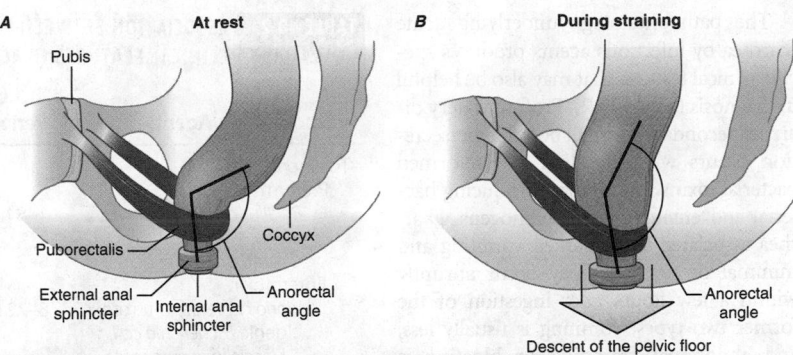

FIGURE 40-1 Sagittal view of the anorectum (*A*) at rest and (*B*) during straining to defecate. Continence is maintained by normal rectal sensation and tonic contraction of the internal anal sphincter and the puborectalis muscle, which wraps around the anorectum, maintaining an anorectal angle between 80° and 110°. During defecation, the pelvic floor muscles (including the puborectalis) relax, allowing the anorectal angle to straighten by at least 15°, and the perineum descends by 1.0–3.5 cm. The external anal sphincter also relaxes and reduces pressure on the anal canal. *(Reproduced with permission from Lembo and Camilleri.)*

the ingested agent overwhelms the host's mucosal immune and nonimmune (gastric acid, digestive enzymes, mucus secretion, peristalsis, and suppressive resident flora) defenses. Established clinical associations with specific enteropathogens may offer diagnostic clues.

In the United States, five high-risk groups are recognized:

1. *Travelers.* Nearly 40% of tourists to endemic regions of Latin America, Africa, and Asia develop so-called traveler's diarrhea, most commonly due to enterotoxigenic or enteroaggregative *Escherichia coli* as well as to *Campylobacter, Shigella, Aeromonas,* norovirus, *Coronavirus* and *Salmonella*. Visitors to Russia (especially St. Petersburg) may have increased risk of *Giardia*-associated diarrhea; visitors to Nepal may acquire *Cyclospora*. Campers, backpackers, and swimmers in wilderness areas may become infected with *Giardia*. Cruise ships may be affected by outbreaks of gastroenteritis caused by agents such as Norwalk virus.

2. *Consumers of certain foods.* Diarrhea closely following food consumption at a picnic, banquet, or restaurant may suggest infection with *Salmonella, Campylobacter,* or *Shigella* from chicken; enterohemorrhagic *E. coli* (O157:H7) from undercooked hamburger; *Bacillus cereus* from fried rice; *Staphylococcus aureus* or *Salmonella* from mayonnaise or creams; *Salmonella* from eggs; and *Vibrio* species, *Salmonella,* or acute hepatitis A from seafood, especially if raw.

3. *Immunodeficient persons.* Individuals at risk for diarrhea include those with either primary immunodeficiency (e.g., IgA deficiency, common variable hypogammaglobulinemia, chronic granulomatous disease) or the much more common secondary immunodeficiency states (e.g., AIDS, senescence, pharmacologic suppression). Common enteric pathogens often cause a more severe and protracted diarrheal illness, and, particularly in persons with AIDS, opportunistic infections, such as by *Mycobacterium* species, certain viruses (cytomegalovirus, adenovirus, and herpes simplex), and protozoa (*Cryptosporidium, Isospora belli,* Microsporida, and *Blastocystis hominis*) may also play a role (Chap. 182). In patients with AIDS, agents transmitted venereally per rectum (e.g., *Neisseria gonorrhoeae, Treponema pallidum, Chlamydia*) may contribute to proctocolitis. Persons with hemochromatosis are especially prone to invasive, even fatal, enteric infections with *Vibrio* species and *Yersinia* infections and should avoid raw fish.

4. *Daycare attendees and their family members.* Infections with *Shigella, Giardia, Cryptosporidium,* rotavirus, and other agents are very common and should be considered.

5. *Institutionalized persons.* Infectious diarrhea is one of the most frequent categories of nosocomial infections in many hospitals and long-term care facilities; the causes are a variety of microorganisms but most commonly *C. difficile*.

The pathophysiology underlying acute diarrhea by infectious agents produces specific clinical features that may also be helpful in diagnosis (Table 40-2). Profuse watery diarrhea secondary to small bowel hypersecretion occurs with ingestion of preformed bacterial toxins, enterotoxin-producing bacteria, and enteroadherent pathogens. Diarrhea associated with marked vomiting and minimal or no fever may occur abruptly within a few hours after ingestion of the former two types; vomiting is usually less, and abdominal cramping or bloating is greater; fever is higher with the latter. Cytotoxin-producing and invasive microorganisms all cause high fever and abdominal pain. Invasive bacteria and *Entamoeba histolytica* often cause bloody diarrhea (referred to as *dysentery*). *Yersinia* invades the terminal ileal and proximal colon mucosa and may cause especially severe abdominal pain with tenderness mimicking acute appendicitis.

Finally, infectious diarrhea may be associated with systemic manifestations. Reiter's syndrome (arthritis, urethritis, and conjunctivitis) may accompany or follow infections by *Salmonella, Campylobacter, Shigella,* and *Yersinia*. Yersiniosis may also lead to an autoimmune-type thyroiditis, pericarditis, and glomerulonephritis. Both enterohemorrhagic *E. coli* (O157:H7) and *Shigella* can lead to the *hemolytic-uremic syndrome* with an attendant high mortality rate. The syndrome of postinfectious IBS has now been recognized as a complication of infectious diarrhea. Acute diarrhea can also be a major symptom of several systemic infections including *viral hepatitis, listeriosis, legionellosis,* and *toxic shock syndrome.*

Other Causes Side effects from medications are probably the most common noninfectious cause of acute diarrhea, and etiology may be suggested by a temporal association between use and symptom onset. Although innumerable medications may produce diarrhea, some of the more frequently incriminated include antibiotics, cardiac antidysrhythmics, antihypertensives, nonsteroidal anti-inflammatory drugs (NSAIDs), certain antidepressants, chemotherapeutic agents, bronchodilators, antacids, and laxatives. Occlusive or nonocclusive *ischemic colitis* typically occurs in persons >50 years; often presents as acute lower abdominal pain preceding watery, then bloody diarrhea; and generally results in acute inflammatory changes in the sigmoid or left colon while sparing the rectum. Acute diarrhea may accompany colonic *diverticulitis* and *graft-versus-host disease.* Acute diarrhea, often associated with systemic compromise, can follow ingestion of toxins including organophosphate insecticides, amanita and other mushrooms, arsenic, and preformed environmental toxins in seafood, such as ciguatera and scombroid. Conditions causing chronic diarrhea can also be confused with acute diarrhea early in their course. This confusion may occur with inflammatory bowel disease (IBD) and some of the other inflammatory chronic diarrheas that may have an abrupt rather than insidious onset and exhibit features that mimic infection.

APPROACH TO THE PATIENT:
Acute Diarrhea

The decision to evaluate acute diarrhea depends on its severity and duration and on various host factors (Fig. 40-2). Most episodes of

	TABLE 40-2	**ASSOCIATION BETWEEN PATHOBIOLOGY OF CAUSATIVE AGENTS AND CLINICAL FEATURES IN ACUTE INFECTIOUS DIARRHEA**				
Pathobiology/Agents	**Incubation Period**	**Vomiting**	**Abdominal Pain**	**Fever**	**Diarrhea**
Toxin producers					
Preformed toxin					
Bacillus cereus, Staphylococcus aureus,	1–8 h	3–4+	1–2+	0–1+	3–4+, watery
Clostridium perfringens	8–24 h				
Enterotoxin					
Vibrio cholerae, enterotoxigenic *Escherichia coli, Klebsiella pneumoniae, Aeromonas* species	8–72 h	2–4+	1–2+	0–1+	3–4+, watery
Enteroadherent					
Enteropathogenic and enteroadherent *E. coli, Giardia* organisms, cryptosporidiosis, helminths	1–8 d	0–1+	1–3+	0–2+	1–2+, watery, mushy
Cytotoxin-producers					
Clostridium difficile	1–3 d	0–1+	3–4+	1–2+	1–3+, usually watery, occasionally bloody
Hemorrhagic *E. coli*	12–72 h	0–1+	3–4+	1–2+	1–3+, initially watery, quickly bloody
Invasive organisms					
Minimal inflammation					
Rotavirus and Norwalk agent	1–3 d	1–3+	2–3+	3–4+	1–3+, watery
Variable inflammation					
Salmonella, Campylobacter, and *Aeromonas* species, *Vibrio parahaemolyticus, Yersinia*	12 h–11 d	0–3+	2–4+	3–4+	1–4+, watery or bloody
Severe inflammation					
Shigella species, enteroinvasive *E. coli, Entamoeba histolytica*	12 h–8 d	0–1+	3–4+	3–4+	1–2+, bloody

Source: Adapted from DW Powell, in T Yamada (ed): *Textbook of Gastroenterology and Hepatology,* 4th ed. Philadelphia, Lippincott Williams & Wilkins, 2003; and DR Syndman, in SL Gorbach (ed): *Infectious Diarrhea.* London, Blackwell, 1986.

acute diarrhea are mild and self-limited and do not justify the cost and potential morbidity of diagnostic or pharmacologic interventions. Indications for evaluation include profuse diarrhea with dehydration, grossly bloody stools, fever ≥ 38.5° C, duration > 48 h without improvement, recent antibiotic use, new community outbreaks, associated severe abdominal pain in patients >50 years, and elderly (≥70 years) or immunocompromised patients. In some cases of moderately severe febrile diarrhea associated with fecal leukocytes (or increased fecal levels of the leukocyte proteins) or with gross blood, a diagnostic evaluation might be avoided in favor of an empirical antibiotic trial (see below).

The cornerstone of diagnosis in those suspected of severe acute infectious diarrhea is microbiologic analysis of the stool. Workup includes cultures for bacterial and viral pathogens, direct inspection for ova and parasites, and immunoassays for certain bacterial toxins (*C. difficile*), viral antigens (rotavirus), and protozoal antigens (*Giardia, E. histolytica*). The aforementioned clinical and epidemiologic associations may assist in focusing the evaluation. If a particular pathogen or set of possible pathogens is so implicated, then either the whole panel of routine studies may not be necessary or, in some instances, special cultures may be appropriate as for enterohemorrhagic and other types of *E. coli, Vibrio* species, and *Yersinia*. Molecular diagnosis of pathogens in stool can be made by identification of unique DNA sequences; and evolving microarray technologies could lead to a more rapid, sensitive, specific, and cost-effective diagnostic approach in the future.

Persistent diarrhea is commonly due to *Giardia* (Chap. 202), but additional causative organisms that should be considered include *C. difficile* (especially if antibiotics had been administered), *E. his-*

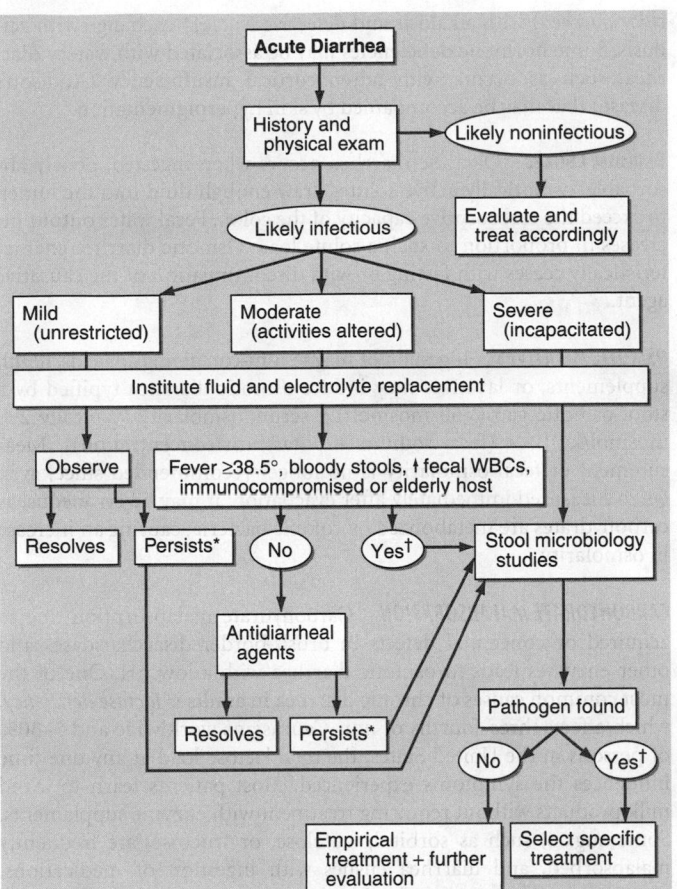

FIGURE 40-2 Algorithm for the management of acute diarrhea.
Consider empirical Rx before evaluation with (*) metronidazole and with (†) quinolone. WBCs, white blood cells.

tolytica, Cryptosporidium, Campylobacter, and others. If stool studies are unrevealing, then flexible sigmoidoscopy with biopsies and upper endoscopy with duodenal aspirates and biopsies may be indicated. Brainerd diarrhea is an increasingly recognized entity characterized by an abrupt-onset diarrhea that persists for at least 4 weeks, but may last 1–3 years, and is thought to be of infectious origin. It may be associated with subtle inflammation of the distal small intestine or proximal colon.

Structural examination by sigmoidoscopy, colonoscopy, or abdominal CT scanning (or other imaging approaches) may be appropriate in patients with uncharacterized persistent diarrhea to exclude IBD, or as an initial approach in patients with suspected noninfectious acute diarrhea such as might be caused by ischemic colitis, diverticulitis, or partial bowel obstruction.

℞ ACUTE DIARRHEA

Fluid and electrolyte replacement are of central importance to all forms of acute diarrhea. Fluid replacement alone may suffice for mild cases. Oral sugar-electrolyte solutions (sport drinks or designed formulations) should be instituted promptly with severe diarrhea to limit dehydration, which is the major cause of death. Profoundly dehydrated patients, especially infants and the elderly, require IV rehydration.

In moderately severe nonfebrile and nonbloody diarrhea, antimotility and antisecretory agents such as loperamide can be useful adjuncts to control symptoms. Such agents should be avoided with febrile dysentery, which may be exacerbated or prolonged by them. Bismuth subsalicylate may reduce symptoms of vomiting and diarrhea but should not be used to treat immunocompromised patients or those with renal impairment because of the risk of bismuth encephalopathy.

Judicious use of antibiotics is appropriate in selected instances of acute diarrhea and may reduce its severity and duration (Fig. 40-2). Many phy-

sicians treat moderately to severely ill patients with febrile dysentery empirically without diagnostic evaluation using a quinolone, such as ciprofloxacin (500 mg bid for 3–5 d). Empirical treatment can also be considered for suspected giardiasis with metronidazole (250 mg qid for 7 d). Selection of antibiotics and dosage regimens are otherwise dictated by specific pathogens, geographic patterns of resistance, and conditions found (Chaps. 122, 143, and 146–152). Antibiotic coverage is indicated whether or not a causative organism is discovered in patients who are immunocompromised, have mechanical heart valves or recent vascular grafts, or are elderly. Antibiotic prophylaxis is indicated for certain patients traveling to high-risk countries in whom the likelihood or seriousness of acquired diarrhea would be especially high, including those with immunocompromise, IBD, hemochromatosis, or gastric achlorhydria. Use of trimethoprim/sulfamethoxazole, ciprofloxacin, or rifaximin may reduce bacterial diarrhea in such travelers by 90%, though rifaximin may not be suitable for invasive disease. Finally, physicians should be vigilant to identify if an outbreak of diarrheal illness is occurring and to alert the public health authorities promptly. This may reduce the ultimate size of the affected population.

CHRONIC DIARRHEA

Diarrhea lasting >4 weeks warrants evaluation to exclude serious underlying pathology. In contrast to acute diarrhea, most of the causes of chronic diarrhea are noninfectious. The classification of chronic diarrhea by pathophysiologic mechanism facilitates a rational approach to management, though many diseases cause diarrhea by more than one mechanism (Table 40-3).

Secretory Causes Secretory diarrheas are due to derangements in fluid and electrolyte transport across the enterocolonic mucosa. They are characterized clinically by watery, large-volume fecal outputs that are typically painless and persist with fasting. Because there is no malab-

TABLE 40-3	MAJOR CAUSES OF CHRONIC DIARRHEA ACCORDING TO PREDOMINANT PATHOPHYSIOLOGIC MECHANISM
Secretory causes	**Inflammatory causes**
Exogenous stimulant laxatives	Idiopathic inflammatory bowel
Chronic ethanol ingestion	disease (Crohn's, chronic
Other drugs and toxins	ulcerative colitis)
Endogenous laxatives (dihydroxy bile acids)	Lymphocytic and collagenous colitis
Idiopathic secretory diarrhea	Immune-related mucosal
Certain bacterial infections	disease (1° or 2° immuno-
Bowel resection, disease, or fistula (↓ absorption)	deficiencies, food allergy, eosinophilic gastroenteritis,
Partial bowel obstruction or fecal impaction	graft-vs-host disease) Infections (invasive bacteria,
Hormone-producing tumors (carcinoid, VIPoma, medullary cancer of thyroid, mastocytosis, gastrinoma, colorectal villous adenoma)	viruses, and parasites, Brainerd diarrhea) Radiation injury Gastrointestinal malignancies
Addison's disease	**Dysmotile causes**
Congenital electrolyte absorption defects	Irritable bowel syndrome (including post-infectious IBS)
Osmotic causes	Visceral neuromyopathies
Osmotic laxatives (Mg^{2+}, PO_4^{-3}, SO_4^{-2})	Hyperthyroidism Drugs (prokinetic agents)
Lactase and other disaccharide deficiencies	Postvagotomy **Factitial causes**
Nonabsorbable carbohydrates (sorbitol, lactulose, polyethylene glycol)	Munchausen Eating disorders **Iatrogenic causes**
Steatorrheal causes	Cholecystectomy
Intraluminal maldigestion (pancreatic exocrine insufficiency, bacterial overgrowth, bariatric surgery, liver disease)	Ileal resection Bariatric surgery Vagotomy, fundoplication
Mucosal malabsorption (celiac sprue, Whipple's disease, infections, abetalipoproteinemia, ischemia)	
Post-mucosal obstruction (1° or 2° lymphatic obstruction)	

sorbed solute, stool osmolality is accounted for by normal endogenous electrolytes with no fecal osmotic gap.

MEDICATIONS Side effects from regular ingestion of drugs and toxins are the most common secretory causes of chronic diarrhea. Hundreds of prescription and over-the-counter medications (see "Other Causes of Acute Diarrhea," above) may produce unwanted diarrhea. Surreptitious or habitual use of stimulant laxatives [e.g., senna, cascara, bisacodyl, ricinoleic acid (castor oil)] must also be considered. Chronic ethanol consumption may cause a secretory-type diarrhea due to enterocyte injury with impaired sodium and water absorption as well as rapid transit and other alterations. Inadvertent ingestion of certain environmental toxins (e.g., arsenic) may lead to chronic rather than acute forms of diarrhea. Certain bacterial infections may occasionally persist and be associated with a secretory-type diarrhea.

BOWEL RESECTION, MUCOSAL DISEASE, OR ENTEROCOLIC FISTULA These conditions may result in a secretory-type diarrhea because of inadequate surface for reabsorption of secreted fluids and electrolytes. Unlike other secretory diarrheas, this subset of conditions tends to worsen with eating. With disease (e.g., Crohn's ileitis) or resection of <100 cm of terminal ileum, dihydroxy bile acids may escape absorption and stimulate colonic secretion (cholorrheic diarrhea). This mechanism may contribute to so-called *idiopathic secretory diarrhea*, in which bile acids are functionally malabsorbed from a normal-appearing terminal ileum. Partial bowel obstruction, ostomy stricture, or fecal impaction may paradoxically lead to increased fecal output due to fluid hypersecretion.

HORMONES Although uncommon, the classic examples of secretory diarrhea are those mediated by hormones. *Metastatic gastrointestinal carcinoid tumors* or, rarely, *primary bronchial carcinoids* may produce watery diarrhea alone or as part of the carcinoid syndrome that comprises episodic flushing, wheezing, dyspnea, and right-sided valvular heart disease. Diarrhea is due to the release into the circulation of potent intestinal secretagogues including serotonin, histamine, prostaglandins, and various kinins. Pellagra-like skin lesions may rarely occur as the result of serotonin overproduction with niacin depletion. *Gastrinoma*, one of the most common neuroendocrine tumors, most typically presents with refractory peptic ulcers, but diarrhea occurs in up to one-third of cases and may be the only clinical manifestation in 10%. While other secretagogues released with gastrin may play a role, the diarrhea most often results from fat maldigestion owing to pancreatic enzyme inactivation by low intraduodenal pH. The watery diarrhea hypokalemia achlorhydria syndrome, also called *pancreatic cholera*, is due to a non-β cell pancreatic adenoma, referred to as a *VIPoma*, that secretes VIP and a host of other peptide hormones including pancreatic polypeptide, secretin, gastrin, gastrin-inhibitory polypeptide (also called glucose-dependent insulinotropic peptide), neurotensin, calcitonin, and prostaglandins. The secretory diarrhea is often massive with stool volumes >3 L/d; daily volumes as high as 20 L have been reported. Life-threatening dehydration; neuromuscular dysfunction from associated hypokalemia, hypomagnesemia, or hypercalcemia; flushing; and hyperglycemia may accompany a VIPoma. *Medullary carcinoma of the thyroid* may present with watery diarrhea caused by calcitonin, other secretory peptides, or prostaglandins. This tumor occurs sporadically or, in 25–50% of cases, as a feature of multiple endocrine neoplasia type 2a with pheochromocytomas and hyperparathyroidism. Prominent diarrhea is often associated with metastatic disease and poor prognosis. *Systemic mastocytosis*, which may be associated with the skin lesion urticaria pigmentosa, may cause diarrhea that is either secretory, and mediated by histamine, or inflammatory due to intestinal infiltration by mast cells. Large *colorectal villous adenomas* may rarely be associated with a secretory diarrhea that may cause hypokalemia, can be inhibited by NSAIDs, and is apparently mediated by prostaglandins.

CONGENITAL DEFECTS IN ION ABSORPTION Rarely, defects in specific carriers associated with ion absorption cause watery diarrhea from birth, and these disorders include defective Cl⁻/HCO₃⁻ exchange (*congenital chloridorrhea*) with alkalosis and defective Na⁺/H⁺ exchange with acidosis. Some hormone deficiencies may be associated with watery diarrhea, such as occurs with adrenocortical insufficiency (Addison's disease) that may be accompanied by skin hyperpigmentation.

Osmotic Causes Osmotic diarrhea occurs when ingested, poorly absorbable, osmotically active solutes draw enough fluid into the lumen to exceed the reabsorptive capacity of the colon. Fecal water output increases in proportion to such a solute load. Osmotic diarrhea characteristically ceases with fasting or with discontinuation of the causative agent.

OSMOTIC LAXATIVES Ingestion of magnesium-containing antacids, health supplements, or laxatives may induce osmotic diarrhea typified by a stool osmotic gap (>50 mosmol/L): serum osmolarity (typically 290 mosmol/kg)[2 × (fecal sodium + potassium concentration)]. Measurement of fecal osmolarity is no longer recommended since, even when measured immediately after evacuation, it may be erroneous, as carbohydrates are metabolized by colonic bacteria, causing an increase in osmolarity.

CARBOHYDRATE MALABSORPTION Carbohydrate malabsorption due to acquired or congenital defects in brush-border disaccharidases and other enzymes leads to osmotic diarrhea with a low pH. One of the most common causes of chronic diarrhea in adults is *lactase deficiency*, which affects three-fourths of non-Caucasians worldwide and 5–30% of persons in the United States; the total lactose load at any one time influences the symptoms experienced. Most patients learn to avoid milk products without requiring treatment with enzyme supplements. Some sugars, such as sorbitol, lactulose, or fructose, are frequently malabsorbed, and diarrhea ensues with ingestion of medications, gum, or candies sweetened with these poorly or incompletely absorbed sugars.

Steatorrheal Causes Fat malabsorption may lead to greasy, foul-smelling, difficult-to-flush diarrhea often associated with weight loss and nutritional deficiencies due to concomitant malabsorption of amino acids and vitamins. Increased fecal output is caused by the osmotic effects of fatty acids, especially after bacterial hydroxylation, and, to a lesser extent, by the neutral fat. Quantitatively, steatorrhea is defined as stool fat exceeding the normal 7 g/d; rapid-transit diarrhea may result in fecal fat up to 14 g/d; daily fecal fat averages 15–25 g with small intestinal diseases and is often >32 g with pancreatic exocrine insufficiency. Intraluminal maldigestion, mucosal malabsorption, or lymphatic obstruction may produce steatorrhea.

INTRALUMINAL MALDIGESTION This condition most commonly results from pancreatic exocrine insufficiency, which occurs when >90% of pancreatic secretory function is lost. *Chronic pancreatitis*, usually a sequel of ethanol abuse, most frequently causes pancreatic insufficiency. Other causes include *cystic fibrosis*, *pancreatic duct obstruction*, and rarely, *somatostatinoma*. Bacterial overgrowth in the small intestine may deconjugate bile acids and alter micelle formation, impairing fat digestion; it occurs with stasis from a blind-loop, small bowel diverticulum or dysmotility and is especially likely in the elderly. Finally, cirrhosis or biliary obstruction may lead to mild steatorrhea due to deficient intraluminal bile acid concentration.

MUCOSAL MALABSORPTION Mucosal malabsorption occurs from a variety of enteropathies, but most commonly from *celiac disease*. This gluten-sensitive enteropathy affects all ages and is characterized by villous atrophy and crypt hyperplasia in the proximal small bowel and can present with fatty diarrhea associated with multiple nutritional deficiencies of varying severity. Celiac disease is much more frequent than previously thought; it affects ~1% of the population, frequently presents without steatorrhea, can mimic IBS, and has many other GI and extraintestinal manifestations. *Tropical sprue* may produce a similar histologic and clinical syndrome but occurs in residents of or travelers to tropical climates; abrupt onset and response to antibiotics suggest an infectious etiology. *Whipple's disease*, due to the bacillus *Tropheryma whipplei* and histiocytic infiltration of the small-bowel mucosa, is a less common cause of steatorrhea that most typically occurs in young or middle-aged men; it is frequently associated with arthralgias, fever, lymphadenopathy, and extreme fatigue and may affect the central nervous system and endocardium. A similar clinical and histologic picture results from *Mycobacterium avium-intracellulare* infection in patients with AIDS. *Abetalipoproteinemia* is a rare defect of chylomicron formation and fat malabsorption in children, associated with acanthocytic erythrocytes, ataxia, and retinitis pigmentosa. Several other conditions may cause mucosal malabsorption including infections, especially with protozoa such as *Giardia*, numerous medications (e.g., colchicine, cholestyramine, neomycin), and chronic ischemia.

POSTMUCOSAL LYMPHATIC OBSTRUCTION The pathophysiology of this condition, which is due to the rare *congenital intestinal lymphangiectasia* or to *acquired lymphatic obstruction* secondary to trauma, tumor, or infection, leads to the unique constellation of fat malabsorption with enteric losses of protein (often causing edema) and lymphocytopenia. Carbohydrate and amino acid absorption are preserved.

Inflammatory Causes Inflammatory diarrheas are generally accompanied by pain, fever, bleeding, or other manifestations of inflammation. The mechanism of diarrhea may not only be exudation but, depending on lesion site, may include fat malabsorption, disrupted fluid/electrolyte absorption, and hypersecretion or hypermotility from release of cytokines and other inflammatory mediators. The unifying feature on stool analysis is the presence of leukocytes or leukocyte-derived proteins such as calprotectin. With severe inflammation, exudative protein loss can lead to anasarca (generalized edema). Any middle-aged or older person with chronic inflammatory-type diarrhea, especially with blood, should be carefully evaluated to exclude a colorectal tumor.

IDIOPATHIC INFLAMMATORY BOWEL DISEASE The illnesses in this category, which include *Crohn's disease* and *chronic ulcerative colitis*, are among the most common organic causes of chronic diarrhea in adults and range in severity from mild to fulminant and life-threatening. They may be associated with uveitis, polyarthralgias, cholestatic liver disease (primary sclerosing cholangitis), and skin lesions (erythema nodosum, pyoderma gangrenosum). *Microscopic colitis*, including both lymphocytic and *collagenous colitis*, is an increasingly recognized cause of chronic watery diarrhea, especially in middle-aged women and those on NSAIDS; biopsy of a normal-appearing colon is required for histologic diagnosis. It may coexist with symptoms suggesting IBS or with celiac sprue. It typically responds well to anti-inflammatory drugs (e.g., bismuth), to the opioid agonist loperamide, or to budesonide.

PRIMARY OR SECONDARY FORMS OF IMMUNODEFICIENCY Immunodeficiency may lead to prolonged infectious diarrhea. With common variable *hypogammaglobulinemia*, diarrhea is particularly prevalent and often the result of giardiasis.

EOSINOPHILIC GASTROENTERITIS Eosinophil infiltration of the mucosa, muscularis, or serosa at any level of the GI tract may cause diarrhea, pain, vomiting, or ascites. Affected patients often have an atopic history, Charcot-Leyden crystals due to extruded eosinophil contents may be seen on microscopic inspection of stool, and peripheral eosinophilia is present in 50–75% of patients. While hypersensitivity to certain foods occurs in adults, true food allergy causing chronic diarrhea is rare.

OTHER CAUSES Chronic inflammatory diarrhea may be caused by *radiation enterocolitis, chronic graft-versus-host disease, Behçet's syndrome*, and *Cronkite-Canada syndrome*, among others.

Dysmotility Causes Rapid transit may accompany many diarrheas as a secondary or contributing phenomenon, but primary dysmotility is an unusual etiology of true diarrhea. Stool features often suggest a secretory diarrhea, but mild steatorrhea of up to 14 g of fat per day can be produced by maldigestion from rapid transit alone. *Hyperthyroidism, carcinoid syndrome*, and certain drugs (e.g., prostaglandins, prokinetic agents) may produce hypermotility with resultant diarrhea. Primary visceral neuromyopathies or idiopathic acquired intestinal pseudoobstruction may lead to stasis with secondary bacterial overgrowth causing diarrhea. *Diabetic diarrhea*, often accompanied by peripheral and generalized autonomic neuropathies, may occur in part because of intestinal dysmotility.

The exceedingly common *irritable bowel syndrome* (10% point prevalence, 1–2% per year incidence) is characterized by disturbed intestinal and colonic motor and sensory responses to various stimuli. Symptoms of stool frequency typically cease at night, alternate with periods of constipation, are accompanied by abdominal pain relieved with defecation, and rarely result in weight loss or true diarrhea.

Factitial Causes Factitial diarrhea accounts for up to 15% of unexplained diarrheas referred to tertiary care centers. Either as a form of *Munchausen syndrome* (deception or self-injury for secondary gain) or *eating disorders*, some patients covertly self-administer laxatives alone or in combination with other medications (e.g., diuretics) or surreptitiously add water or urine to stool sent for analysis. Such patients are typically women, often with histories of psychiatric illness and disproportionately from careers in health care. Hypotension and hypokalemia are common co-presenting features. The evaluation of such patients may be difficult: contamination of the stool with water or urine is suggested by very low or high stool osmolarity, respectively. Such patients often deny this possibility when confronted, but they do benefit from psychiatric counseling when they acknowledge their behavior.

APPROACH TO THE PATIENT:
Chronic Diarrhea

The laboratory tools available to evaluate the very common problem of chronic diarrhea are extensive, and many are costly and invasive. As such, the diagnostic evaluation must be rationally directed by a careful history and physical examination (**Fig. 40-3A**). When this strategy is unrevealing, simple triage tests are often warranted to direct the choice of more complex investigations (**Fig. 40-3B**). The history, physical examination (**Table 40-4**), and routine blood studies should attempt to characterize the mechanism of diarrhea, identify diagnostically helpful associations, and assess the patient's fluid/electrolyte and nutritional status. Patients should be questioned about the onset, duration, pattern, aggravating (especially diet) and relieving factors, and stool characteristics of their diarrhea. The presence or absence of fecal incontinence, fever, weight loss, pain, certain exposures (travel, medications, contacts with diarrhea), and common extraintestinal manifestations (skin changes, arthralgias, oral aphthous ulcers) should be noted. A family history of IBD or sprue may indicate those possibilities. Physical findings may offer clues such as a thyroid mass, wheezing, heart murmurs, edema, hepatomegaly, abdominal masses, lymphadenopathy, mucocutaneous abnormalities, perianal fistulae, or anal sphincter laxity. Peripheral blood leukocytosis, elevated sedimentation rate, or C-reactive protein suggests inflammation; anemia reflects blood loss or nutritional deficiencies; or eosinophilia may occur with parasitoses, neoplasia, collagen-vascular disease, allergy, or eosinophilic gastroenteritis. Blood chemistries may demonstrate electrolyte, hepatic, or other metabolic disturbances. Measuring tissue transglutaminase antibodies may help detect celiac disease.

A therapeutic trial is often appropriate, definitive, and highly cost effective when a specific diagnosis is suggested on the initial physician encounter. For example, chronic watery diarrhea, which ceases with fasting in an otherwise healthy young adult, may justify a trial of a lactose-restricted diet; bloating and diarrhea persisting since a mountain backpacking trip may warrant a trial of metronidazole for likely giardiasis; and postprandial diarrhea persisting

A

B

FIGURE 40-3 Chronic diarrhea. A. Initial management based on accompanying symptoms or features. **B.** Evaluation based on findings from a limited age appropriate screen for organic disease. p.r., per rectum; bm, bowel movement; IBS, irritable bowel syndrome; Hb, hemoglobin; Alb, albumin; MCV, mean corpuscular volume; MCH, mean corpuscular hemoglobin; OSM, osmolality. *(Reprinted from M Camilleri: Clin Gastroenterol Hepatol. 2:198, 2004.)*

since an ileal resection might be due to bile acid malabsorption and be treated with cholestyramine before further evaluation. Persistent symptoms require additional investigation.

Certain diagnoses may be suggested on the initial encounter, e.g., idiopathic IBD; however, additional focused evaluations may be necessary to confirm the diagnosis and characterize the severity or extent of disease so that treatment can be best guided. Patients suspected of having IBS should be initially evaluated with flexible sigmoidoscopy with colorectal biopsies; those with normal findings might be reassured and, as indicated, treated empirically with antispasmodics, antidiarrheals, bulk agents, anxiolytics, or antidepressants. Any patient who presents with chronic diarrhea and hematochezia should be evaluated with stool microbiologic studies and colonoscopy.

In an estimated two-thirds of cases, the cause for chronic diarrhea remains unclear after the initial encounter, and further testing is required. Quantitative stool collection and analyses can yield important objective data that may establish a diagnosis or characterize the type of diarrhea as a triage for focused additional studies (Fig. 40-3*B*). If stool weight is >200 g/d, additional stool analyses should be performed that might include electrolyte concentration,

pH, occult blood testing, leukocyte inspection (or leukocyte protein assay), fat quantitation, and laxative screens.

For secretory diarrheas (watery, normal osmotic gap), possible medication-related side effects or surreptitious laxative use should be reconsidered. Microbiologic studies should be done including fecal bacterial cultures (including media for *Aeromonas* and *Pleisiomonas*), inspection for ova and parasites, and *Giardia* antigen assay (the most sensitive test for giardiasis). Small-bowel bacterial overgrowth can be excluded by intestinal aspirates with quantitative cultures or with glucose or lactulose breath tests involving measurement of breath hydrogen, methane, or other metabolite (e.g., $^{14}CO_2$). However, interpretation of these breath tests may be confounded by disturbances of intestinal transit. When suggested by history or other findings, screens for peptide hormones should be pursued (e.g., serum gastrin, VIP, calcitonin, and thyroid hormone/thyroid-stimulating hormone, or urinary 5-hydroxyindolacetic acid and histamine). Upper endoscopy and colonoscopy with biopsies and small-bowel barium x-rays are helpful to rule out structural or occult inflammatory disease.

Further evaluation of osmotic diarrhea should include tests for lactose intolerance and magnesium ingestion, the two most common causes. Low fecal pH suggests carbohydrate malabsorption; lactose malabsorption can be confirmed by lactose breath testing or by a therapeutic trial with lactose exclusion and observation of the effect of lactose challenge (e.g., a liter of milk). Lactase determination on small-bowel biopsy is generally not available. If fecal magnesium or laxative levels are elevated, then inadvertent or surreptitious ingestion should be considered and psychiatric help should be sought.

For those with proven fatty diarrhea, endoscopy with small-bowel biopsy (including aspiration for *Giardia* and quantitative cultures) should be performed; if this procedure is unrevealing, a small-bowel radiograph is often an appropriate next step. If small-bowel studies are negative or if pancreatic disease is suspected, pancreatic exocrine insufficiency should be excluded with direct tests, such as the secretin-cholecystokinin stimulation test or a variation that could be performed endoscopically. In general, indirect tests such as assay of fecal chymotrypsin activity or a bentiromide test have fallen out of favor because of low sensitivity and specificity.

TABLE 40-4	**PHYSICAL EXAMINATION IN PATIENTS WITH CHRONIC DIARRHEA**

1. Are there general features to suggest malabsorption or inflammatory bowel disease (IBD) such as anemia, dermatitis herpetiformis, edema, or clubbing?
2. Are there features to suggest underlying autonomic neuropathy or collagen-vascular disease in the pupils, orthostasis, skin, hands, or joints?
3. Is there an abdominal mass or tenderness?
4. Are there any abnormalities of rectal mucosa, rectal defects, or altered anal sphincter functions?
5. Are there any mucocutaneous manifestations of systemic disease such as dermatitis herpetiformis (celiac disease), erythema nodosum (ulcerative colitis), flushing (carcinoid), or oral ulcers for IBD or celiac disease?

Chronic inflammatory-type diarrheas should be suspected by the presence of blood or leukocytes in the stool. Such findings warrant stool cultures, inspection for ova and parasites, *C. difficile* toxin assay, colonoscopy with biopsies, and, if indicated, small-bowel contrast studies.

Rx CHRONIC DIARRHEA

Treatment of chronic diarrhea depends on the specific etiology and may be curative, suppressive, or empirical. If the cause can be eradicated, treatment is curative as with resection of a colorectal cancer, antibiotic administration for Whipple's disease, or discontinuation of a drug. For many chronic conditions, diarrhea can be controlled by suppression of the underlying mechanism. Examples include elimination of dietary lactose for lactase deficiency or gluten for celiac sprue, use of glucocorticoids or other anti-inflammatory agents for idiopathic IBDs, adsorptive agents such as cholestyramine for ileal bile acid malabsorption, proton pump inhibitors such as omeprazole for the gastric hypersecretion of gastrinomas, somatostatin analogues such as octreotide for malignant carcinoid syndrome, prostaglandin inhibitors such as indomethacin for medullary carcinoma of the thyroid, and pancreatic enzyme replacement for pancreatic insufficiency. When the specific cause or mechanism of chronic diarrhea evades diagnosis, empirical therapy may be beneficial. Mild opiates, such as diphenoxylate or loperamide, are often helpful in mild or moderate watery diarrhea. For those with more severe diarrhea, codeine or tincture of opium may be beneficial. Such antimotility agents should be avoided with IBD, as toxic megacolon may be precipitated. Clonidine, an α_2-adrenergic agonist, may allow control of diabetic diarrhea. For all patients with chronic diarrhea, fluid and electrolyte repletion is an important component of management (see "Acute Diarrhea," above). Replacement of fat-soluble vitamins may also be necessary in patients with chronic steatorrhea.

CONSTIPATION

DEFINITION

Constipation is a common complaint in clinical practice and usually refers to persistent, difficult, infrequent, or seemingly incomplete defecation. Because of the wide range of normal bowel habits, constipation is difficult to define precisely. Most persons have at least three bowel movements per week; however, low stool frequency alone is not the sole criterion for the diagnosis of constipation. Many constipated patients have a normal frequency of defecation but complain of excessive straining, hard stools, lower abdominal fullness, or a sense of incomplete evacuation. The individual patient's symptoms must be analyzed in detail to ascertain what is meant by "constipation" or "difficulty" with defecation.

Stool form and consistency are well correlated with the time elapsed from the preceding defecation. Hard, pellety stools occur with slow transit, while loose watery stools are associated with rapid transit. Both small pellety or very large stools are more difficult to expel than normal stools.

The perception of hard stools or excessive straining is more difficult to assess objectively, and the need for enemas or digital disimpaction is a clinically useful way to corroborate the patient's perceptions of difficult defecation.

Psychosocial or cultural factors may also be important. A person whose parents attached great importance to daily defecation will become greatly concerned when he or she misses a daily bowel movement; some children withhold stool to gain attention or because of fear of pain from anal irritation; and some adults habitually ignore or delay the call to have a bowel movement.

CAUSES

Pathophysiologically, chronic constipation generally results from inadequate fiber or fluid intake or from disordered colonic transit or anorectal function. These result from neurogastroenterologic disturbance, certain drugs, advancing age, or in association with a large number of systemic diseases that affect the gastrointestinal tract (**Table 40-5**). Constipation of recent onset may be a symptom of significant

TABLE 40-5 CAUSES OF CONSTIPATION IN ADULTS

Types of Constipation and Causes	Examples
Recent onset	
Colonic obstruction	Neoplasm; stricture: ischemic, diverticular, inflammatory
Anal sphincter spasm	Anal fissure, painful hemorrhoids
Medications	
Chronic	
Irritable bowel syndrome	Constipation-predominant, alternating
Medications	Ca²⁺ blockers, antidepressants
Colonic pseudo-obstruction	Slow-transit constipation, megacolon (rare Hirschprung's, Chagas)
Disorders of rectal evacuation	Pelvic floor dysfunction; anismus; descending perineum syndrome; rectal mucosal prolapse; rectocele
Endocrinopathies	Hypothyroidism, hypercalcemia, pregnancy
Psychiatric disorders	Depression, eating disorders, drugs
Neurologic disease	Parkinsonism, multiple sclerosis, spinal cord injury
Generalized muscle disease	Progressive systemic sclerosis

organic disease such as tumor or stricture. In *idiopathic constipation*, a subset of patients exhibit delayed emptying of the ascending and transverse colon with prolongation of transit (often in the proximal colon) and a reduced frequency of propulsive HAPCs. *Outlet obstruction to defecation* (also called *evacuation disorders*) may cause delayed colonic transit, which is usually corrected by biofeedback retraining of the disordered defecation. Constipation of any cause may be exacerbated by hospitalization or chronic illnesses that lead to physical or mental impairment and result in inactivity or physical immobility.

APPROACH TO THE PATIENT:
Constipation

A careful history should explore the patient's symptoms and confirm whether he or she is indeed constipated based on frequency (e.g., fewer than three bowel movements per week), consistency (lumpy/hard), excessive straining, prolonged defecation time, or need to support the perineum or digitate the anorectum. In the vast majority of cases (probably >90%), there is no underlying cause (e.g., cancer, depression, or hypothyroidism), and constipation responds to ample hydration, exercise, and supplementation of dietary fiber (15–25 g/d). A good diet and medication history and attention to psychosocial issues are key. Physical examination and, particularly, a rectal examination should exclude fecal impaction and most of the important diseases that present with constipation and possibly indicate features suggesting an evacuation disorder (e.g., high anal sphincter tone).

The presence of weight loss, rectal bleeding, or anemia with constipation mandates either flexible sigmoidoscopy plus barium enema or colonoscopy alone, particularly in patients >40 years, to exclude structural diseases such as cancer or strictures. Colonoscopy alone is most cost effective in this setting since it provides an opportunity to biopsy mucosal lesions, perform polypectomy, or dilate strictures. Barium enema has advantages over colonoscopy in the patient with isolated constipation, since it is less costly and identifies colonic dilatation and all significant mucosal lesions or strictures that are likely to present with constipation. Melanosis coli, or pigmentation of the colon mucosa, indicates the use of anthraquinone laxatives such as cascara or senna; however, this is usually apparent from a careful history. An unexpected disorder such as megacolon or cathartic colon may also be detected by colonic radiographs. Measurement of serum calcium, potassium, and thyroid-stimulating hormone levels will identify rare patients with metabolic disorders.

Patients with more troublesome constipation may not respond to fiber alone and may be helped by a bowel training regimen: tak-

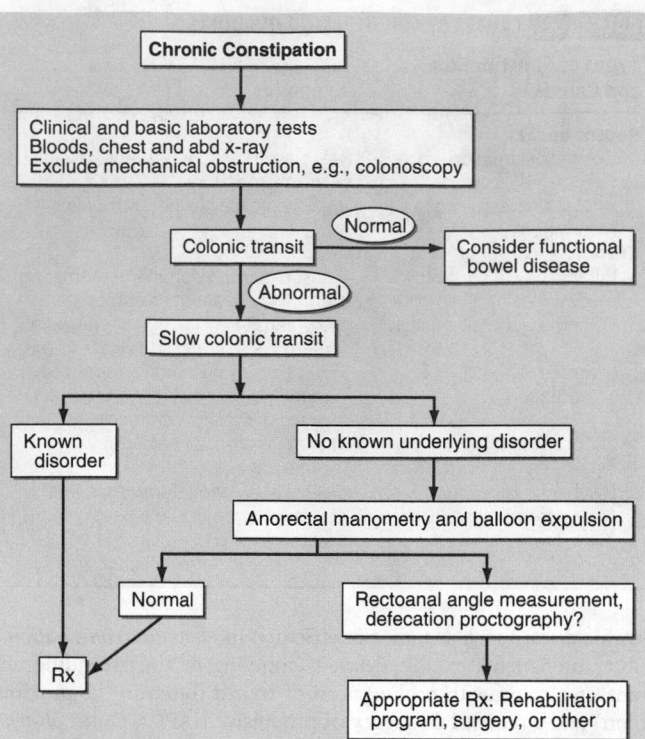

FIGURE 40-4 Algorithm for the management of constipation.

ing an osmotic laxative (lactulose, sorbitol, polyethylene glycol) and evacuating with enema or glycerine suppository as needed. After breakfast, a distraction-free 15–20 min on the toilet without straining is encouraged. Excessive straining may lead to development of hemorrhoids, and, if there is weakness of the pelvic floor or injury to the pudendal nerve, may result in obstructed defecation from descending perineum syndrome several years later. Those few who do not benefit from the simple measures delineated above or require long-term treatment with potent laxatives with the attendant risk of developing laxative abuse syndrome are assumed to have severe or intractable constipation and should have further investigation (Fig. 40-4). Novel agents that induce secretion (e.g., lubiprostone, a chloride channel activator) are also available.

INVESTIGATION OF SEVERE CONSTIPATION

A small minority (probably <5%) of patients have severe or "intractable" constipation. These are the patients most likely to be seen by gastroenterologists or in referral centers. Further observation of the patient may occasionally reveal a previously unrecognized cause, such as an evacuation disorder, laxative abuse, malingering, or psychological disorder. In these patients, evaluations of the physiologic function of the colon and pelvic floor and of psychological status aid in the rational choice of treatment. Even among these highly selected patients with severe constipation, a cause can be identified in only about two-thirds of tertiary referral patients (see below).

Measurement of Colonic Transit Radiopaque marker transit tests are easy, repeatable, generally safe, inexpensive, reliable, and highly applicable in evaluating constipated patients in clinical practice. Several validated methods are very simple. For example, radiopaque markers are ingested; an abdominal flat film taken 5 days later should indicate passage of 80% of the markers out of the colon without the use of laxatives or enemas. This test does not provide useful information about the transit profile of the stomach and small bowel.

Radioscintigraphy with a delayed-release capsule containing radiolabeled particles has been used to noninvasively characterize normal, accelerated, or delayed colonic function over 24–48 h with low radiation exposure. This approach simultaneously assesses gastric, small bowel

(which may be important in ~20% of patients with delayed colonic transit since they reflect a more generalized GI motility disorder), and colonic transit. The disadvantages are the greater cost and the need for specific materials prepared in a nuclear medicine laboratory.

Anorectal and Pelvic Floor Tests Pelvic floor dysfunction is suggested by the inability to evacuate the rectum, a feeling of persistent rectal fullness, rectal pain, the need to extract stool from the rectum digitally, application of pressure on the posterior wall of the vagina, support of the perineum during straining, and excessive straining. These significant symptoms should be contrasted with the sense of incomplete rectal evacuation, which is common in IBS.

Formal psychological evaluation may identify eating disorders, "control issues," depression, or post-trauma stress disorders that may respond to cognitive or other intervention and may be important in restoring quality of life to patients who might present with chronic constipation.

A simple clinical test in the office to document a nonrelaxing puborectalis muscle is to have the patient strain to expel the index finger during a digital rectal examination. Motion of the puborectalis posteriorly during straining indicates proper coordination of the pelvic floor muscles.

Measurement of perineal descent is relatively easy to gauge clinically by placing the patient in the left decubitus position and watching the perineum to detect inadequate descent (<1.5 cm, a sign of pelvic floor dysfunction) or perineal ballooning during straining relative to bony landmarks (>4 cm, suggesting excessive perineal descent).

A useful overall test of evacuation is the balloon expulsion test. A balloon-tipped urinary catheter is placed and inflated with 50 mL of water. Normally, a patient can expel it while seated on a toilet or in the left lateral decubitus position. In the lateral position, the weight needed to facilitate expulsion of the balloon is determined; normally expulsion occurs with <200 g added.

Anorectal manometry when used in the evaluation of patients with severe constipation may find an excessively high resting (>80 mmHg) or squeeze anal sphincter tone, suggesting anismus (anal sphincter spasm). This test also identifies rare syndromes, such as adult Hirschsprung's disease, by the absence of the rectoanal inhibitory reflex.

Defecography (a dynamic barium enema including lateral views obtained during barium expulsion) reveals "soft abnormalities" in many patients; the most relevant findings are the measured changes in rectoanal angle, anatomic defects of the rectum such as internal mucosal prolapse, and enteroceles or rectoceles. Surgically remediable conditions are identified in only a few patients. These include severe, whole-thickness intussusception with complete outlet obstruction due to funnel-shaped plugging at the anal canal or an extremely large rectocele that fills preferentially during attempts at defecation instead of expulsion of the barium through the anus. In summary, defecography requires an interested and experienced radiologist, and abnormalities are not pathognomonic for pelvic floor dysfunction. The most common cause of outlet obstruction is failure of the puborectalis muscle to relax; this is not identified by defecography but requires a dynamic study such as proctography. MRI is being developed as an alternative and provides more information about the structure and function of the pelvic floor, distal colorectum, and anal sphincters.

Dynamic imaging studies such as proctography during defecation or scintigraphic expulsion of artificial stool help measure perineal descent and the rectoanal angle during rest, squeezing, and straining, and scintigraphic expulsion quantitates the amount of "artificial stool" emptied. Lack of straightening of the rectoanal angle by at least 15° during defecation confirms pelvic floor dysfunction.

Neurologic testing (electromyography) is more helpful in the evaluation of patients with incontinence than of those with symptoms suggesting obstructed defecation. The absence of neurologic signs in the lower extremities suggests that any documented denervation of the puborectalis results from pelvic (e.g., obstetric) injury or from stretching of the pudendal nerve by chronic, long-standing straining. Constipation is common among patients with spinal cord injuries, neurologic diseases such as Parkinson's disease, multiple sclerosis, and diabetic neuropathy.

Spinal-evoked responses during electrical rectal stimulation or stimulation of external anal sphincter contraction by applying magnetic stimulation over the lumbosacral cord identify patients with limited sacral neuropathies with sufficient residual nerve conduction to attempt biofeedback training.

In summary, a balloon expulsion test is an important screening test for anorectal dysfunction. If positive, an anatomic evaluation of the rectum or anal sphincters and an assessment of pelvic floor relaxation are the tools for evaluating patients in whom obstructed defecation is suspected.

℞ CONSTIPATION

After the cause of constipation is characterized, a treatment decision can be made. Slow-transit constipation requires aggressive medical or surgical treatment; anismus or pelvic floor dysfunction usually responds to biofeedback management (Fig. 40-4). However, only ~60% of patients with severe constipation are found to have such a physiologic disorder (half with colonic transit delay and half with evacuation disorder). Patients with spinal cord injuries or other neurologic disorders require a dedicated bowel regime that often includes rectal stimulation, enema therapy, and carefully timed laxative therapy.

Patients with slow-transit constipation are treated with bulk, osmotic, prokinetic, secretory, and stimulant laxatives including fiber, psyllium, milk of magnesia, lactulose, polyethylene glycol (colonic lavage solution), lubiprostone, and bisacodyl. Newer treatment aimed at enhancing motility and secretion may have application in circumstances such as constipation-predominant IBS in females or severe constipation. If a 3- to 6-month trial of medical therapy fails and patients continue to have documented slow-transit constipation unassociated with obstructed defecation, the patients should be considered for laparoscopic colectomy with ileorectostomy; however, this should not be undertaken if there is continued evidence of an evacuation disorder or a generalized GI dysmotility. Referral to a specialized center for further tests of colonic motor function is warranted. The decision to resort to surgery is facilitated in the presence of megacolon and megarectum. The complications after surgery include small-bowel obstruction (11%) and fecal soiling, particularly at night during the first postoperative year. Frequency of defecation is 3–8 per day during the first year, dropping to 1–3 per day from the second year after surgery.

Patients who have a combined (evacuation and transit/motility) disorder should pursue pelvic floor retraining (biofeedback and muscle relaxation), psychological counseling, and dietetic advice first, followed by colectomy and ileorectosomy if colonic transit studies do not normalize and symptoms are intractable despite biofeedback and optimized medical therapy. In patients with pelvic floor dysfunction alone, biofeedback training has a 70–80% success rate, measured by the acquisition of comfortable stool habits. Attempts to manage pelvic floor dysfunction with operations (internal anal sphincter or puborectalis muscle division) have achieved only mediocre success and have been largely abandoned.

FURTHER READINGS

BARTLETT JG: Narrative review: The new epidemic of *Clostridium difficile*-associated enteric disease. Ann Intern Med 145:758, 2006

CAMILLERI M: Chronic diarrhea: A review on pathophysiology and management for the clinical gastroenterologist. Clin Gastroenterol Hepatol 2:198, 2004

FARRELL RJ, KELLY CP: Celiac sprue. N Engl J Med 346:180, 2002

GADEWAR S, FASANO A: Current concepts in the evaluation, diagnosis and management of acute infectious diarrhea. Curr Opin Pharmacol 5:559, 2005

LEMBO A, CAMILLERI M: Chronic constipation. N Engl J Med 349:1360, 2003

MUSHER DM, MUSHER BL: Contagious acute gastrointestinal infections. N Engl J Med 351:2417, 2004

WALD A: Constipation in the primary care setting: Current concepts and misconceptions. Am J Med 119:736, 2006

WALD A: Clinical practice. Fecal incontinence in adults. N Engl J Med 356:1648, 2007

41 Weight Loss
Carol M. Reife

Significant unintentional weight loss in a previously healthy individual is often a harbinger of underlying systemic disease. During the routine medical examination, changes in weight should always be assessed; loss of 5% of body weight over 6–12 months should prompt further evaluation.

PHYSIOLOGY OF WEIGHT REGULATION

The normal individual maintains body weight at a remarkably stable "set point," given the wide variation in daily caloric intake and level of activity. Because of the physiologic importance of maintaining energy stores, voluntary weight loss is difficult to achieve and sustain.

Appetite and metabolism are regulated by an intricate network of neural and hormonal factors. The hypothalamic feeding and satiety centers play a central role in these processes (Chap. 74). Neuropeptides such as corticotropin-releasing hormone (CRH), α-melanocyte-stimulating hormone (α-MSH), and cocaine- and amphetamine-related transcript (CART) induce anorexia by acting centrally on satiety centers. The gastrointestinal peptides ghrelin, glucagon, somatostatin, and cholecystokinin signal satiety and thus decrease food intake. Hypoglycemia suppresses insulin, reducing glucose utilization and inhibiting the satiety center.

Leptin is produced by adipose tissue, and it plays a central role in the long-term maintenance of weight homeostasis by acting on the hypothalamus to decrease food intake and increase energy expenditure (Chap. 74). Leptin suppresses expression of hypothalamic neuropeptide Y, a potent appetite stimulatory peptide, and it increases the expression of α-MSH, which acts through the MC4R melanocortin receptor to decrease appetite. Thus, leptin activates a series of downstream neural pathways that alter food-seeking behavior and metabolism. Leptin deficiency, which occurs in conjunction with the loss of adipose tissue, stimulates appetite and induces adaptive responses including inhibition of hypothalamic thyrotropin-releasing hormone (TRH) and gonadotropin-releasing hormone (GnRH).

A variety of cytokines, including tumor necrosis factor α (TNF-α), interleukin (IL) 6 (IL-6), IL-1, interferon γ (IFN-γ), ciliary neurotrophic factor (CNTF), and leukemia inhibitory factor (LIF), can induce cachexia (Chap. 17). In addition to causing anorexia, these factors may stimulate fever, depress myocardial function, modulate immune and inflammatory responses, and induce a variety of specific metabolic alterations. TNF-α, for example, preferentially mobilizes fat but spares skeletal muscle. Levels of these cytokines may be increased in patients with cancer, sepsis, chronic inflammatory conditions, AIDS, or congestive heart failure.

Weight loss occurs when energy expenditure exceeds calories available for energy utilization (Chap. 72). In most individuals, approximately half of food energy is utilized for basal processes such as maintenance of body temperature. In a 70-kg person, basal activity consumes ~1800 kcal/d. About 40% of caloric intake is used for physical activity, although athletes may use >50% during vigorous exercise. About 10% of caloric intake is used for dietary thermogenesis, the energy expended for digestion, absorption, and metabolism of food.

Mechanisms of weight loss include decreased food intake, malabsorption, loss of calories, and increased energy requirements (Fig. 41-1). Changes in weight may involve loss of tissue mass or body fluid content. A deficit of 3500 kcal generally correlates with the loss of 0.45 kg (1 lb) of body fat, but one must also consider water weight [1 kg/L (2.2 lb/L)] gained or lost. Weight loss that persists over weeks to months reflects the loss of tissue mass.

Food intake may be influenced by a wide variety of visual, olfactory, and gustatory stimuli as well as by genetic, psychological, and social fac-

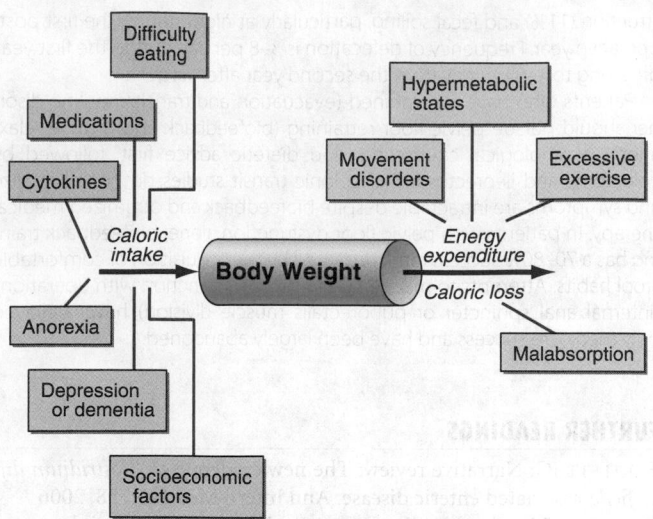

FIGURE 41-1 Energy balance and pathophysiology of weight loss.

TABLE 41-1	CAUSES OF WEIGHT LOSS
Cancer	Medications
Endocrine and metabolic	Antibiotics
Hyperthyroidism	Nonsteroidal anti-inflammatory
Diabetes mellitus	drugs
Pheochromocytoma	Serotonin reuptake inhibitors
Adrenal insufficiency	Metformin
Gastrointestinal disorders	Levodopa
Malabsorption	ACE inhibitors
Obstruction	Other drugs
Pernicious anemia	Disorders of the mouth and teeth
Cardiac disorders	Age-related factors
Chronic ischemia	Physiologic changes
Chronic congestive heart failure	Decreased taste and smell
Respiratory disorders	Functional disabilities
Emphysema	Neurologic
Chronic obstructive pulmonary	Stroke
disease	Parkinson's disease
Renal insufficiency	Neuromuscular disorders
Rheumatologic disease	Dementia
Infections	Social
HIV	Isolation
Tuberculosis	Economic hardship
Parasitic infection	Psychiatric and behavioral
Subacute bacterial endocarditis	Depression
	Anxiety
	Bereavement
	Alcoholism
	Eating disorders
	Increased activity or exercise
	Idiopathic

tors. Absorption may be impaired because of pancreatic insufficiency, cholestasis, celiac sprue, intestinal tumors, radiation injury, inflammatory bowel disease, infection, or medication effect. These disease processes may be manifest as changes in stool frequency and consistency. Calories may also be lost due to vomiting or diarrhea, glucosuria in diabetes mellitus, or fistulous drainage. Resting energy expenditure decreases with age and can be affected by thyroid status. Beginning at about age 60, body weight declines by an average of 0.5% per year. Body composition is also affected by aging; adipose tissue increases and lean muscle mass decreases with age.

SIGNIFICANCE OF WEIGHT LOSS

Unintentional weight loss, especially in the elderly, is relatively common and is associated with increased morbidity and mortality rates, even after comorbid conditions have been taken into account. Prospective studies indicate that significant involuntary weight loss is associated with a mortality rate of 25% over the next 18 months. Retrospective studies of significant weight loss in the elderly document mortality rates of 9–38% over a 2- to 3-year period.

Cancer patients with weight loss have decreased performance status, impaired responses to chemotherapy, and reduced median survival (Chap. 77). Marked weight loss also predisposes to infection. Patients undergoing elective surgery, who have lost >4.5 kg (>10 lb) in 6 months, have higher surgical mortality rates. Vitamin and nutrient deficiencies may also accompany significant weight loss (Chap. 71).

CAUSES OF WEIGHT LOSS

The list of possible causes of weight loss is extensive (Table 41-1). In the elderly, the most common causes of weight loss are depression, cancer, and benign gastrointestinal disease. Lung and gastrointestinal cancer are the most common malignancies in patients presenting with weight loss. In younger individuals, diabetes mellitus, hyperthyroidism, psychiatric disturbances including eating disorders, and infection, especially with HIV, should be considered.

The cause of involuntary weight loss is rarely occult. Careful history and physical examination, in association with directed diagnostic testing, will identify the cause of weight loss in 75% of patients. The etiology of weight loss may not be found in the remaining patients, despite extensive testing. Patients with negative evaluations tend to have lower mortality rates than those found to have organic disease.

Patients with medical causes of weight loss usually have signs or symptoms that suggest involvement of a particular organ system. Gastrointestinal tumors, including those of the pancreas and liver, may affect food intake early in the course of illness, causing weight loss before other symptoms are apparent. Lung cancer may present with post-obstructive pneumonia, dyspnea, or cough and hemoptysis; however, it may be silent and should be considered even in those without a history of cigarette smoking. Depression and isolation can cause profound weight loss, especially in the

elderly. Chronic pulmonary disease and congestive heart failure can produce anorexia, and they also increase resting energy expenditure. Weight loss may be the presenting sign of infectious diseases such as HIV infection, tuberculosis, endocarditis, and fungal or parasitic infections. Hyperthyroidism or pheochromocytoma increases metabolism. Elderly patients with apathetic hyperthyroidism may present with weight loss and weakness, with few other manifestations of thyrotoxicosis. New-onset diabetes mellitus is often accompanied by weight loss, reflecting glucosuria and loss of the anabolic actions of insulin. Adrenal insufficiency may be suggested by increased pigmentation, hyponatremia, and hyperkalemia.

APPROACH TO THE PATIENT:
Weight Loss

Before extensive evaluation is undertaken, it is important to confirm weight loss and to determine the time interval over which it has occurred. Almost half of patients who claim significant weight loss have no actual change when body weight is measured objectively. In the absence of documentation, changes in belt notch position or the fit of clothing may be confirmatory. Not infrequently, patients who have actually sustained significant weight loss are unaware that it has occurred. Routine documentation of weight during office visits is therefore important.

The review of systems should focus on signs or symptoms that are associated with disorders that commonly cause weight loss. These include fever, pain, shortness of breath or cough, palpitations, and evidence of neurologic disease. Gastrointestinal isturbances, including difficulty eating, dysphagia, anorexia, nausea, and change in bowel habits, should be sought. Travel history, use of cigarettes and alcohol, and all medications should be reviewed, and patients should be questioned about previous illness or surgery as well as diseases in family members. Risk factors for HIV infection should be assessed. Signs of depression, evidence of dementia, and social factors, including financial issues that might affect food intake, should be considered.

Physical examination should begin with weight determination and documentation of vital signs. The skin should be examined for pallor, jaundice, turgor, scars from prior surgery, and stigmata of systemic disease. The search for oral thrush or dental disease, thyroid gland enlargement, adenopathy, and respiratory or cardiac abnormalities and a detailed examination of the abdomen often lead to clues for further evaluation. Rectal examination, including prostate examination, should be performed in men; and all women should have a pelvic examination, even if they have had a hysterectomy. Neurologic examination should include mental status assessment and screening for depression.

Laboratory testing should confirm or exclude possible diagnoses elicited from the history and physical examination (Table 41-2). An initial phase of testing should include a complete blood count with differential, serum chemistry tests including glucose, electrolytes, renal and liver tests, calcium, thyroid-stimulating hormone (TSH), urinalysis, and chest x-ray. Patients at risk for HIV infection should have HIV antibody testing. In all cases, recommended cancer screening tests appropriate for the gender and age group, such as mammograms and colonoscopies, should be updated (Chap. 78).

TABLE 41-2	SCREENING TESTS FOR EVALUATION OF INVOLUNTARY WEIGHT LOSS
Initial testing	Additional testing
CBC	HIV test
Electrolytes, calcium, glucose	Upper and/or lower
Renal and liver function tests	gastrointestinal endoscopy
Urinalysis	Abdominal CT scan or MRI
TSH	Chest CT scan
Chest x-ray	
Recommended cancer screening	

42 Gastrointestinal Bleeding
Loren Laine

Bleeding from the gastrointestinal (GI) tract may present in five ways. *Hematemesis* is vomitus of red blood or "coffee-grounds" material. *Melena* is black, tarry, foul-smelling stool. *Hematochezia* is the passage of bright red or maroon blood from the rectum. *Occult GI bleeding* (GIB) may be identified in the absence of overt bleeding by a fecal occult blood test or the presence of iron deficiency. Finally, patients may present only with *symptoms of blood loss or anemia* such as lightheadedness, syncope, angina, or dyspnea.

SOURCES OF GASTROINTESTINAL BLEEDING
Upper Gastrointestinal Sources of Bleeding (Table 42-1) The annual incidence of hospital admissions for upper GIB (UGIB) in the United States and Europe is ~0.1%, with a mortality rate of ~5–10%. Patients rarely die from exsanguination; rather, they die due to decompensation from other underlying illnesses. The mortality rate for patients <60 years in the absence of major concurrent illness is <1%. Independent predictors of rebleeding and death in patients hospitalized with UGIB include increasing age, comorbidities, and hemodynamic compromise (tachycardia or hypotension).

Peptic ulcers are the most common cause of UGIB, accounting for up to ~50% of cases; an increasing proportion is due to nonsteroidal anti-inflammatory drugs (NSAIDs), with the prevalence of *Helicobacter pylori* decreasing. Mallory-Weiss tears account for ~5–10 or 15% of cases. The proportion of patients bleeding from varices varies widely from ~5 to 30%, depending on the population. Hemorrhagic or erosive gastropathy (e.g., due to NSAIDs or alcohol) and erosive esophagitis often cause mild UGIB, but major bleeding is rare.

PEPTIC ULCERS In addition to clinical features, characteristics of an ulcer at endoscopy provide important prognostic information. One-third of patients with active bleeding or a nonbleeding visible vessel have further bleeding that requires urgent surgery if they are treated conservatively. These patients clearly benefit from endoscopic therapy

If gastrointestinal signs or symptoms are present, upper and/or lower endoscopy and abdominal imaging with either CT or MRI have a relatively high yield, consistent with the high prevalence of gastrointestinal disorders in patients with weight loss. If an etiology of weight loss is not found, careful clinical follow-up, rather than persistent undirected testing, is reasonable.

FURTHER READINGS
ALIBHAI S: An approach to the management of unintentional weight loss in elderly people. CMAJ 172:773, 2005

BOURAS EP, LANGE SM: Rational approach to patients with unintentional weight loss. Mayo Clinic Proc 76:923, 2001

HERNANDEZ JL, MATORRAS JA: Involuntary weight loss without specific symptoms: A clinical prediction score for malignant neoplasm. Q J Med 96: 649, 2003

INUI A: Cancer anorexia-cachexia syndrome: Current issues in research and management. Cancer J Clinicians 52:72, 2002

NORA E, RAMAN A: Hypermetabolism, cachexia and wasting. Curr Opin Endocrinol Diabetes 12: 326, 2005

SCHWARTZ MW: Brain pathways controlling food intake and body weight. Exp Biol Med 226:978, 2001

STRASSER F, BRUERA ED: Update on anorexia and cachexia. Hematol Oncol Clin North Am 16:589, 2002

WALLACE JI: Involuntary weight loss in elderly outpatients: Recognition, etiologies, and treatment. Clin Geriatr Med 13:717, 1997

with bipolar electrocoagulation, heater probe, injection therapy (e.g., absolute alcohol, 1:10,000 epinephrine), and/or clips with reductions in bleeding, hospital stay, mortality rate, and costs. In contrast, patients with clean-based ulcers have rates of recurrent bleeding approaching zero. If there is no other reason for hospitalization, such patients may be discharged on the first hospital day, following stabilization. Patients without clean-based ulcers should usually remain in the hospital for 3 days, as most episodes of recurrent bleeding occur within 3 days.

Randomized controlled trials document that a high-dose constant-infusion IV proton pump inhibitor (PPI) (e.g., omeprazole 80-mg bolus and 8-mg/h infusion), designed to sustain intragastric pH > 6 and enhance clot stability, decreases further bleeding (but not mortality), in patients with high-risk ulcers (active bleeding, nonbleeding visible vessel, adherent clot), even after appropriate endoscopic therapy. Institution of therapy at presentation in all patients with UGIB does not significantly improve outcomes such as further bleeding, transfusions, or mortality as compared to initiating therapy only when high-risk ulcers are identified at the time of endoscopy.

One-third of patients with a bleeding ulcer will rebleed within the next 1–2 years. Prevention of recurrent bleeding focuses on the three main factors in ulcer pathogenesis, *H. pylori*, NSAIDs, and acid. Eradi-

TABLE 42-1	SOURCES OF BLEEDING IN PATIENTS HOSPITALIZED FOR UPPER GI BLEEDING IN YEARS 2000–2002
Sources of Bleeding	**Proportion of Patients, %**
Ulcers	31–59
Varices	7–20
Mallory-Weiss tears	4–8
Gastroduodenal erosions	2–7
Erosive esophagitis	1–13
Neoplasm	2–7
Vascular ectasias	0–6
No source identified	8–14

Source: Data from M Van Leerdam et al: Am J Gastroenterol 98:1494, 2003; DM Jensen et al: Gastrointest Endosc 57:AB147, 2003; KC Thomopoulos et al: Eur J Gastroenterol Hepatol 16:177, 2004; F Di Fiore et al: Eur J Gastroenterol Hepatol 17:641, 2005.

cation of *H. pylori* in patients with bleeding ulcers decreases rates of rebleeding to <5%. If a bleeding ulcer develops in a patient taking NSAIDs, the NSAIDs should be discontinued, if possible. If NSAIDs must be continued, initial treatment should be with a PPI. Long-term preventive strategies to decrease NSAID-associated ulcers include use of a cyclooxygenase 2 (COX-2) selective inhibitor (coxib) or addition of GI co-therapy to a traditional NSAID. PPIs and misoprostol are effective co-therapies, but PPIs are more commonly used due to less frequent dosing (once daily) and fewer side effects (e.g., diarrhea). However, either PPI co-therapy alone or use of a coxib alone is associated with an annual rebleeding rate of ~10% in high-risk patients (i.e., a recent bleeding ulcer). Combination of a coxib and PPI provides a further significant decrease in ulcers and recurrent bleeding and should be employed in very high-risk patients. Patients with bleeding ulcers unrelated to *H. pylori* or NSAIDs should remain on full-dose antisecretory therapy indefinitely. **Peptic ulcers are discussed in Chap. 287.**

MALLORY-WEISS TEARS   The classic history is vomiting, retching, or coughing preceding hematemesis, especially in an alcoholic patient. Bleeding from these tears, which are usually on the gastric side of the gastroesophageal junction, stops spontaneously in 80–90% of patients and recurs in only 0–7%. Endoscopic therapy is indicated for actively bleeding Mallory-Weiss tears. Angiographic therapy with embolization and operative therapy with oversewing of the tear are rarely required. **Mallory-Weiss tears are discussed in Chap. 286.**

ESOPHAGEAL VARICES   Patients with variceal hemorrhage have poorer outcomes than patients with other sources of UGIB. Endoscopic therapy for acute bleeding and repeated sessions of endoscopic therapy to eradicate esophageal varices significantly reduce rebleeding and mortality. Ligation is the endoscopic therapy of choice for esophageal varices because it has less rebleeding, a lower mortality rate, fewer local complications, and requires fewer treatment sessions to achieve variceal eradication than sclerotherapy.

Octreotide (50-μg bolus and 50-μg/h IV infusion for 2–5 days) further helps in the control of acute bleeding when used in combination with endoscopic therapy. Other vasoactive agents such as somatostatin and terlipressin, available outside the United States, are also effective. Antibiotic therapy (e.g., quinolones) is also recommended for patients with cirrhosis presenting with UGIB, as antibiotics decrease bacterial infections and mortality in this population. Over the long term, treatment with nonselective beta blockers decreases recurrent bleeding from esophageal varices. Chronic therapy with beta blockers plus endoscopic ligation is recommended for prevention of recurrent esophageal variceal bleeding.

In patients who have persistent or recurrent bleeding despite endoscopic and medical therapy, more invasive therapy is warranted. Transjugular intrahepatic portosystemic shunt (TIPS) decreases rebleeding more effectively than endoscopic therapy, although hepatic encephalopathy is more common and the mortality rates are comparable. Most patients with TIPS have shunt stenosis within 1–2 years and require reintervention to maintain shunt patency, although the use of coated stents appears to markedly decrease shunt dysfunction, at least in the first year. A randomized comparison of TIPS and distal splenorenal shunt in Child-Pugh class A or B cirrhotic patients with refractory variceal bleeding revealed no significant difference in rebleeding, encephalopathy, or survival, but a much higher rate of reintervention with TIPS (82% vs. 11%). Therefore, TIPS is most appropriate in patients with more severe liver disease and those in whom transplant is anticipated. Patients with milder, well-compensated cirrhosis should require fewer re-interventions with decompressive surgery, although the higher initial risks of surgery must also be considered.

Portal hypertension is also responsible for bleeding from gastric varices, varices in the small and large intestine, and portal hypertensive gastropathy and enterocolopathy.

HEMORRHAGIC AND EROSIVE GASTROPATHY ("GASTRITIS")   Hemorrhagic and erosive gastropathy, often labeled gastritis, refers to endoscopically visualized subepithelial hemorrhages and erosions. These are mucosal lesions and thus do not cause major bleeding. They develop in various clinical settings, the most important of which are NSAID use, alcohol intake, and stress. Half of patients who chronically ingest NSAIDs have erosions (15–30% have ulcers), while up to 20% of actively drinking alcoholic patients with symptoms of UGIB have evidence of subepithelial hemorrhages or erosions.

Stress-related gastric mucosal injury occurs only in extremely sick patients: those who have experienced serious trauma, major surgery, burns covering more than one-third of the body surface area, major intracranial disease, and severe medical illness (i.e., ventilator dependence, coagulopathy). Significant bleeding probably does not develop unless ulceration occurs. The mortality rate in these patients is quite high because of their serious underlying illnesses.

The incidence of bleeding from stress-related gastric mucosal injury or ulceration has decreased dramatically in recent years, most likely due to better care of critically ill patients. Pharmacologic prophylaxis for bleeding may be considered in the high-risk patients mentioned above. Multiple trials document the efficacy of intravenous H_2-receptor antagonist therapy, which is more effective than sucralfate but not superior to a PPI immediate-release suspension given via nasogastric tube. Prophylactic therapy decreases bleeding but does not lower the mortality rate.

OTHER CAUSES   Other, less frequent causes of UGIB include erosive duodenitis, neoplasms, aortoenteric fistulas, vascular lesions [including hereditary hemorrhagic telangiectasias (Osler-Weber-Rendu) and gastric antral vascular ectasia ("watermelon stomach")], Dieulafoy's lesion (in which an aberrant vessel in the mucosa bleeds from a pinpoint mucosal defect), prolapse gastropathy (prolapse of proximal stomach into esophagus with retching, especially in alcoholics), and hemobilia and hemosuccus pancreaticus (bleeding from the bile duct or pancreatic duct).

Small-Intestinal Sources of Bleeding   Small-intestinal sources of bleeding (bleeding from sites beyond the reach of the standard upper endoscope) are difficult to diagnose and are responsible for the majority of cases of obscure GIB. Fortunately, small-intestinal bleeding is uncommon. The most common causes are vascular ectasias and tumors (e.g., adenocarcinoma, leiomyoma, lymphoma, benign polyps, carcinoid, metastases, and lipoma). Other less common causes include Crohn's disease, infection, ischemia, vasculitis, small-bowel varices, diverticula, Meckel's diverticulum, duplication cysts, and intussusception. NSAIDs induce small-intestinal erosions and ulcers and may be a relatively common cause of chronic, obscure GIB; coxibs induce less small-intestinal injury than traditional NSAIDs.

Meckel's diverticulum is the most common cause of significant lower GIB (LGIB) in children, decreasing in frequency as a cause of bleeding with age. In adults <40–50 years, small-bowel tumors often account for obscure GIB; in patients >50–60 years, vascular ectasias are usually responsible.

Vascular ectasias should be treated with endoscopic therapy if possible. Surgical therapy can be used for vascular ectasias isolated to a segment of the small intestine when endoscopic therapy is unsuccessful. Although estrogen/progesterone compounds have been used for vascular ectasias, a double-blind trial found no benefit in prevention of recurrent bleeding. Isolated lesions, such as tumors, diverticula, or duplications, are generally treated with surgical resection.

Colonic Sources of Bleeding   The incidence of hospitalizations for LGIB is about one-fifth that for UGIB. Hemorrhoids are probably the most common cause of LGIB; anal fissures also cause minor bleeding and pain. If these local anal processes, which rarely require hospitalization, are excluded, the most common causes of LGIB in adults are diverticula, vascular ectasias (especially in the proximal colon of patients >70 years), neoplasms (primarily adenocarcinoma), and colitis—most commonly infectious or idiopathic inflammatory bowel disease, but occasionally ischemic or radiation-induced. Uncommon causes include post-polypectomy bleeding, solitary rectal ulcer

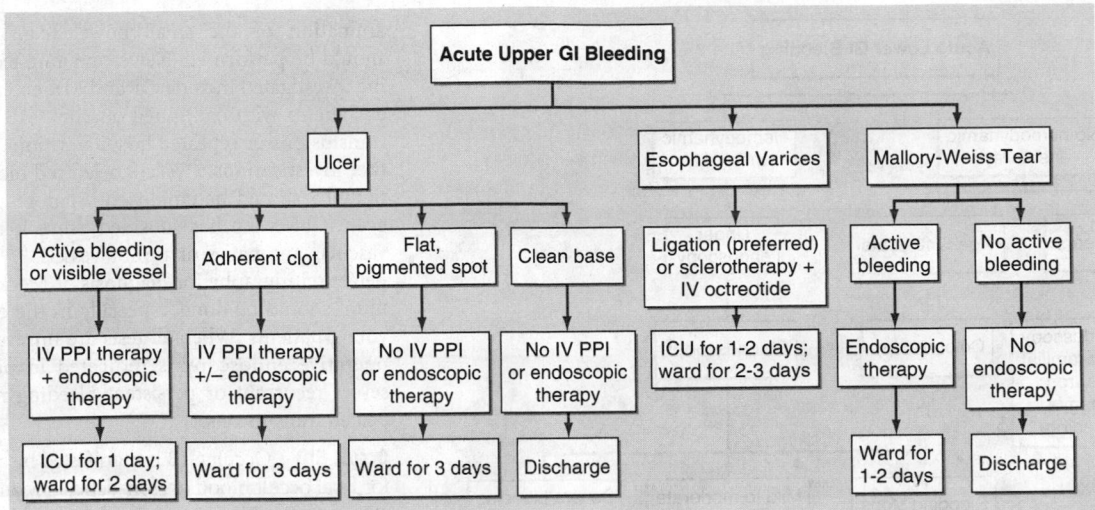

FIGURE 42-1 Suggested algorithm for patients with acute upper gastrointestinal bleeding. Recommendations on level of care and time of discharge assume patient is stabilized without further bleed-ing or other concomitant medical problems. PPI, proton pump inhibitor; ICU, intensive care unit.

syndrome, NSAID-induced ulcers or colitis, trauma, varices (most commonly rectal), lymphoid nodular hyperplasia, vasculitis, and aortocolic fistulas. In children and adolescents, the most common colonic causes of significant GIB are inflammatory bowel disease and juvenile polyps.

Diverticular bleeding is abrupt in onset, usually painless, sometimes massive, and often from the right colon; minor and occult bleeding is not characteristic. Clinical reports suggest that bleeding colonic diverticula stop bleeding spontaneously in ~80% of patients and rebleed in about 20–25% of patients. Intraarterial vasopressin or embolization by superselective technique should stop bleeding in a majority of patients. If bleeding persists or recurs, segmental surgical resection is indicated.

Bleeding from right colonic vascular ectasias in the elderly may be overt or occult; it tends to be chronic and only occasionally is hemodynamically significant. Endoscopic hemostatic therapy may be useful in the treatment of vascular ectasias, as well as discrete bleeding ulcers and post-polypectomy bleeding, while endoscopic polypectomy, if possible, is used for bleeding colonic polyps. Surgical therapy is generally required for major, persistent, or recurrent bleeding from the wide variety of colonic sources of GIB that cannot be treated medically, angiographically, or endoscopically.

APPROACH TO THE PATIENT:
Gastrointestinal Bleeding

Measurement of the heart rate and blood pressure is the best way to assess a patient with GIB. Clinically significant bleeding leads to postural changes in heart rate or blood pressure, tachycardia, and, finally, recumbent hypotension. In contrast, the hemoglobin does not fall immediately with acute GIB, due to proportionate reductions in plasma and red cell volumes (i.e., "people bleed whole blood"). Thus, hemoglobin may be normal or only minimally decreased at the initial presentation of a severe bleeding episode. As extravascular fluid enters the vascular space to restore volume, the hemoglobin falls, but this process may take up to 72 h. Patients with slow, chronic GIB may have very low hemoglobin values despite normal blood pressure and heart rate. With the development of iron-deficiency anemia, the mean corpuscular volume will be low and red blood cell distribution width will be increased.

DIFFERENTIATION OF UPPER FROM LOWER GIB Hematemesis indicates an upper GI source of bleeding (above the ligament of Treitz). Melena indicates that blood has been present in the GI tract for at least 14 h. Thus, the more proximal the bleeding site, the more likely melena will occur. Hematochezia usually represents a lower GI source of bleeding, although an upper GI lesion may bleed so briskly that blood does not remain in the bowel long enough for melena to develop. When hematochezia is the presenting symptom of UGIB, it is associated with hemodynamic instability and dropping hemoglobin. Bleeding lesions of the small bowel may present as melena or hematochezia. Other clues to UGIB include hyperactive bowel sounds and an elevated blood urea nitrogen level (due to volume depletion and blood proteins absorbed in the small intestine).

A nonbloody nasogastric aspirate may be seen in up to 18% of patients with UGIB—usually from a duodenal source. Even a bile-stained appearance does not exclude a bleeding postpyloric lesion since reports of bile in the aspirate are incorrect in ~50% of cases. Testing of aspirates that are not grossly bloody for occult blood is not useful.

DIAGNOSTIC EVALUATION OF THE PATIENT WITH GIB Upper GIB (Fig. 42-1) History and physical examination are not usually diagnostic of the source of GIB. Upper endoscopy is the test of choice in patients with UGIB and should be performed urgently in patients with hemodynamic instability (hypotension, tachycardia, or postural changes in heart rate or blood pressure). Early endoscopy is also beneficial in cases of milder bleeding for management decisions. Patients with major bleeding and high-risk endoscopic findings (e.g., varices, ulcers with active bleeding or a visible vessel) benefit from endoscopic hemostatic therapy, while patients with low-risk lesions (e.g., clean-based ulcers, nonbleeding Mallory-Weiss tears, erosive or hemorrhagic gastropathy) who have stable vital signs and hemoglobin, and no other medical problems, can be discharged home.

Lower GIB (Fig. 42-2) Patients with hematochezia and hemodynamic instability should have upper endoscopy to rule out an upper GI source before evaluation of the lower GI tract. Patients with presumed LGIB may undergo early sigmoidoscopy for the detection of obvious, low-lying lesions. However, the procedure is difficult with brisk bleeding, and it is usually not possible to identify the area of bleeding. Sigmoidoscopy is useful primarily in patients <40 years with minor bleeding.

Colonoscopy after an oral lavage solution is the procedure of choice in patients admitted with LGIB unless bleeding is too massive or unless sigmoidoscopy has disclosed an obvious actively bleeding lesion. ^{99m}Tc-labeled red cell scan allows repeated imaging for up to 24 h and may identify the general location of bleeding. However, radionuclide scans should be interpreted with caution

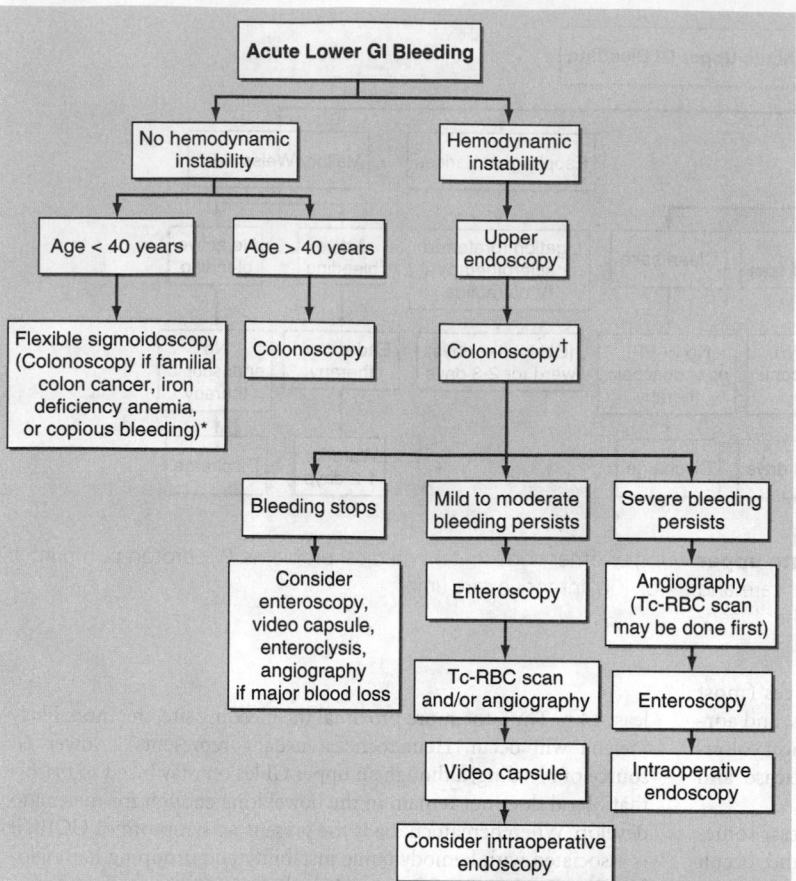

FIGURE 42-2 Suggested algorithm for patients with acute lower gastrointestinal bleeding. Sequential recommendations under "Hemodynamic instability" assume a test is found to be nondiagnostic before next test is performed. *Some suggest colonoscopy for any degree of rectal bleeding in patients <40 years as well. †If massive bleeding does not allow time for colonic lavage, proceed to angiography. Tc-RBC, [99m]technetium-labeled red blood cell.

because results, especially from later images, are highly variable. In active LGIB, angiography can detect the site of bleeding (extravasation of contrast into the gut) and permits treatment with intraarterial infusion of vasopressin or embolization. Even after bleeding has stopped, angiography may identify lesions with abnormal vasculature, such as vascular ectasias or tumors.

GIB of Obscure Origin Obscure GIB is defined as persistent or recurrent bleeding for which no source has been identified by routine endoscopic and contrast x-ray studies; it may be overt (e.g., melena, hematochezia) or occult. Push enteroscopy, with a specially designed enteroscope or a pediatric colonoscope to inspect the entire duodenum and part of the jejunum, is generally the next step. Push enteroscopy may identify probable bleeding sites in 20–40% of patients with obscure GIB. Video capsule endoscopy, which allows endoscopic examination of the entire small intestine, increases diagnostic yield in obscure GIB: a systematic review of 14 trials comparing push enteroscopy to capsule revealed "clinically significant findings" in 26% and 56% of patients, respectively. However, lack of control of the capsule prevents its manipulation and full visualization of the intestine; in addition, tissue cannot be sampled and therapy cannot be applied. A new endoscopic technique, double-balloon enteroscopy, allows the endoscopist to potentially examine and provide therapy to much or all of the small intestine. If enteroscopy and video capsule endoscopy are negative or unavailable, a specialized radiographic ex-

amination of the small bowel (e.g., enteroclysis) should be performed. Newer imaging techniques being investigated include CT and MR enterography.

Patients with continued obscure GIB who require transfusions or repeated hospitalizations warrant further investigations. ^{99m}Tc-labeled red blood cell scintigraphy should be employed. Angiography is useful even if bleeding has subsided, since it may disclose vascular anomalies or tumor vessels. ^{99m}Tc-pertechnetate scintigraphy for diagnosis of Meckel's diverticulum should be done, especially in the evaluation of young patients. When all tests are unrevealing, intraoperative endoscopy is indicated in patients with severe recurrent or persistent bleeding requiring repeated transfusions.

Occult GIB Occult GIB is manifested by a positive test for fecal occult blood or iron-deficiency anemia. Evaluation of a positive test for fecal occult blood generally should begin with colonoscopy, particularly in patients >40 years. If evaluation of the colon is negative, many perform upper endoscopy only if iron-deficiency anemia or upper GI symptoms are present, while others recommend upper endoscopy in all patients since up to 25–40% of these patients may have some abnormality noted on upper endoscopy. If standard endoscopic tests are unrevealing, enteroscopy, video capsule endoscopy, and/or enteroclysis may be considered in patients with iron-deficiency anemia.

FURTHER READINGS

CHAN FK et al: Proton pump inhibitor plus a COX-2 inhibitor for the prevention of recurrent ulcer bleeding in patients with arthritis: A double blinded, randomized trial. Gastroenterology 130:A-105, 2006

CIPOLLETTA L et al: Outpatient management for low-risk nonvariceal upper GI bleeding: A randomized controlled trial. Gastrointest Endosc 55:1, 2002

CONRAD SA et al: Randomized, double-blind comparison of immediate-release omeprazole oral suspension versus intravenous cimetidine for the prevention of upper gastrointestinal bleeding in critically ill patients. Crit Care Med 33:760, 2005

D'AMICO G et al: Pharmacological treatment of portal hypertension: An evidence-based approach. Semin Liver Dis 19:475, 1999

HENDERSON JM et al: Distal splenorenal shunt versus transjugular intrahepatic portal systematic shunt for variceal bleeding: A randomized trial. Gastroenterology 130:1643, 2006

LAINE L, COOK D: Endoscopic ligation compared with sclerotherapy for treatment of esophageal variceal bleeding: A meta-analysis. Ann Intern Med 123:280, 1995

LAU JYW et al: Effect of intravenous omeprazole on recurrent bleeding after endoscopic treatment of bleeding peptic ulcers. N Engl J Med 343:310, 2000

MARMO R et al: Dual therapy versus monotherapy in endoscopic treatment of high-risk bleeding ulcers: A meta-analysis of controlled trials. Am J Gastroenterol 102:279, 2007

ROCKALL TA et al: Risk assessment after acute upper gastrointestinal haemorrhage. Gut 38:316, 1996

TRIESTER SL et al. A meta-analysis of the yield of capsule endoscopy compared to other diagnostic modalities in patients with obscure gastrointestinal bleeding. Am J Gastroenterol 100:2407, 2005

43 Jaundice
Daniel S. Pratt, Marshall M. Kaplan

Jaundice, or icterus, is a yellowish discoloration of tissue resulting from the deposition of bilirubin. Tissue deposition of bilirubin occurs only in the presence of serum hyperbilirubinemia and is a sign of either liver disease or, less often, a hemolytic disorder. The degree of serum bilirubin elevation can be estimated by physical examination. Slight increases in serum bilirubin are best detected by examining the sclerae, which have a particular affinity for bilirubin due to their high elastin content. The presence of scleral icterus indicates a serum bilirubin of at least 51 μmol/L (3.0 mg/dL). The ability to detect scleral icterus is made more difficult if the examining room has fluorescent lighting. If the examiner suspects scleral icterus, a second place to examine is underneath the tongue. As serum bilirubin levels rise, the skin will eventually become yellow in light-skinned patients and even green if the process is long-standing; the green color is produced by oxidation of bilirubin to biliverdin.

The differential diagnosis for yellowing of the skin is limited. In addition to jaundice, it includes carotenoderma, the use of the drug quinacrine, and excessive exposure to phenols. Carotenoderma is the yellow color imparted to the skin by the presence of carotene; it occurs in healthy individuals who ingest excessive amounts of vegetables and fruits that contain carotene, such as carrots, leafy vegetables, squash, peaches, and oranges. Unlike jaundice, where the yellow coloration of the skin is uniformly distributed over the body, in carotenoderma the pigment is concentrated on the palms, soles, forehead, and nasolabial folds. Carotenoderma can be distinguished from jaundice by the sparing of the sclerae. Quinacrine causes a yellow discoloration of the skin in 4–37% of patients treated with it. Unlike carotene, quinacrine can cause discoloration of the sclerae.

Another sensitive indicator of increased serum bilirubin is darkening of the urine, which is due to the renal excretion of conjugated bilirubin. Patients often describe their urine as tea or cola colored. Bilirubinuria indicates an elevation of the direct serum bilirubin fraction and therefore the presence of liver disease.

Increased serum bilirubin levels occur when an imbalance exists between bilirubin production and clearance. A logical evaluation of the patient who is jaundiced requires an understanding of bilirubin production and metabolism.

PRODUCTION AND METABOLISM OF BILIRUBIN

(See also Chap. 297) Bilirubin, a tetrapyrrole pigment, is a breakdown product of heme (ferroprotoporphyrin IX). About 70–80% of the 250–300 mg of bilirubin produced each day is derived from the breakdown of hemoglobin in senescent red blood cells. The remainder comes from prematurely destroyed erythroid cells in bone marrow and from the turnover of hemoproteins such as myoglobin and cytochromes found in tissues throughout the body.

The formation of bilirubin occurs in reticuloendothelial cells, primarily in the spleen and liver. The first reaction, catalyzed by the microsomal enzyme heme oxygenase, oxidatively cleaves the α bridge of the porphyrin group and opens the heme ring. The end products of this reaction are biliverdin, carbon monoxide, and iron. The second reaction, catalyzed by the cytosolic enzyme biliverdin reductase, reduces the central methylene bridge of biliverdin and converts it to bilirubin. Bilirubin formed in the reticuloendothelial cells is virtually insoluble in water. This is due to tight internal hydrogen bonding between the water-soluble moieties of bilirubin, proprionic acid carboxyl groups of one dipyrrolic half of the molecule with the imino and lactam groups of the opposite half. This configuration blocks solvent access to the polar residues of bilirubin and places the hydrophobic residues on the outside. To be transported in blood, bilirubin must be solubilized. This is accomplished by its reversible, noncovalent binding to albumin. Unconjugated bilirubin bound to albumin is transported to the liver, where it, but not the albumin, is taken up by hepatocytes via a process that at least partly involves carrier-mediated membrane transport. No specific bilirubin transporter has yet been identified (Chap. 297, Fig. 297-1).

After entering the hepatocyte, unconjugated bilirubin is bound to the cytosolic protein ligandin, or glutathione S-transferase B. Whereas ligandin was initially thought to be a transport protein, responsible for delivering unconjugated bilirubin from the plasma membrane to the endoplasmic reticulum, it now appears that its role may in fact be to reduce bilirubin efflux back into the plasma. Studies suggest that unconjugated bilirubin may well rapidly diffuse unaided through the aqueous cytosol between membranes. In the endoplasmic reticulum, bilirubin is solubilized by conjugation to glucuronic acid, a process that disrupts the internal hydrogen bonds and yields bilirubin monoglucuronide and diglucuronide. The conjugation of glucuronic acid to bilirubin is catalyzed by bilirubin uridine diphosphate-glucuronosyl transferase (UDPGT). The now hydrophilic bilirubin conjugates diffuse from the endoplasmic reticulum to the canalicular membrane, where bilirubin monoglucuronide and diglucuronide are actively transported into canalicular bile by an energy-dependent mechanism involving the multiple drug resistance protein 2.

The conjugated bilirubin excreted into bile drains into the duodenum and passes unchanged through the proximal small bowel. Conjugated bilirubin is not taken up by the intestinal mucosa. When the conjugated bilirubin reaches the distal ileum and colon, it is hydrolyzed to unconjugated bilirubin by bacterial β-glucuronidases. The unconjugated bilirubin is reduced by normal gut bacteria to form a group of colorless tetrapyrroles called urobilinogens. About 80–90% of these products are excreted in feces, either unchanged or oxidized to orange derivatives called urobilins. The remaining 10–20% of the urobilinogens are passively absorbed, enter the portal venous blood, and are reexcreted by the liver. A small fraction (usually <3 mg/dL) escapes hepatic uptake, filters across the renal glomerulus, and is excreted in urine.

MEASUREMENT OF SERUM BILIRUBIN

The terms direct- and indirect-reacting bilirubin are based on the original van den Bergh reaction. This assay, or a variation of it, is still used in most clinical chemistry laboratories to determine the serum bilirubin level. In this assay, bilirubin is exposed to diazotized sulfanilic acid, splitting into two relatively stable dipyrrylmethene azopigments that absorb maximally at 540 nm, allowing for photometric analysis. The direct fraction is that which reacts with diazotized sulfanilic acid in the absence of an accelerator substance such as alcohol. The direct fraction provides an approximate determination of the conjugated bilirubin in serum. The total serum bilirubin is the amount that reacts after the addition of alcohol. The indirect fraction is the difference between the total and the direct bilirubin and provides an estimate of the unconjugated bilirubin in serum.

With the van den Bergh method, the normal serum bilirubin concentration usually is 17 μmol/L (<1 mg/dL). Up to 30%, or 5.1 μmol/L (0.3 mg/dL), of the total may be direct-reacting (conjugated) bilirubin. Total serum bilirubin concentrations are between 3.4 and 15.4 μmol/L (0.2 and 0.9 mg/dL) in 95% of a normal population.

Several new techniques, although less convenient to perform, have added considerably to our understanding of bilirubin metabolism. First, they demonstrate that in normal persons or those with Gilbert's syndrome, almost 100% of the serum bilirubin is unconjugated; <3% is monoconjugated bilirubin. Second, in jaundiced patients with hepatobiliary disease, the total serum bilirubin concentration measured by these new, more accurate methods is lower than the values found with diazo methods. This suggests that there are diazo-positive compounds distinct from bilirubin in the serum of patients with hepatobiliary disease. Third, these studies indicate that in jaundiced patients with hepatobiliary disease, monoglucuronides of bilirubin predominate over the diglucuronides. Fourth, part of the direct-reacting bilirubin fraction includes conjugated bilirubin that is covalently linked to albumin. This albumin-linked bilirubin fraction (*delta fraction*, or *biliprotein*) represents an important fraction of total serum bilirubin in patients with cholestasis and hepatobiliary disorders. Albumin-bound conjugated bilirubin is formed in serum when hepatic excretion of bilirubin glucuronides is impaired and the glucuronides are present in serum in increasing amounts. By virtue of its tight binding to albumin, the clearance rate of albumin-bound bilirubin from serum approximates the half-life of albumin, 12–14 days, rather than the short half-life of bilirubin, about 4 h.

The prolonged half-life of albumin-bound conjugated bilirubin explains two previously unexplained enigmas in jaundiced patients with liver disease: (1) that some patients with conjugated hyperbilirubinemia do not exhibit bilirubinuria during the recovery phase of their disease because the bilirubin is covalently bound to albumin and therefore not filtered by the renal glomeruli, and (2) that the elevated serum bilirubin level declines more slowly than expected in some patients who otherwise appear to be recovering satisfactorily. Late in the recovery phase of hepatobiliary disorders, all the conjugated bilirubin may be in the albumin-linked form. Its value in serum falls slowly because of the long half-life of albumin.

MEASUREMENT OF URINE BILIRUBIN

Unconjugated bilirubin is always bound to albumin in the serum, is not filtered by the kidney, and is not found in the urine. Conjugated bilirubin is filtered at the glomerulus and the majority is reabsorbed by the proximal tubules; a small fraction is excreted in the urine. Any bilirubin found in the urine is conjugated bilirubin. The presence of bilirubinuria implies the presence of liver disease. A urine dipstick test (Ictotest) gives the same information as fractionation of the serum bilirubin. This test is very accurate. A false-negative test is possible in patients with prolonged cholestasis due to the predominance of conjugated bilirubin covalently bound to albumin.

APPROACH TO THE PATIENT:
Bilirubin

The bilirubin present in serum represents a balance between input from production of bilirubin and hepatic/biliary removal of the pigment. Hyperbilirubinemia may result from (1) overproduction of bilirubin; (2) impaired uptake, conjugation, or excretion of bilirubin; or (3) regurgitation of unconjugated or conjugated bilirubin from damaged hepatocytes or bile ducts. An increase in unconjugated bilirubin in serum results from either overproduction, impairment of uptake, or conjugation of bilirubin. An increase in conjugated bilirubin is due to decreased excretion into the bile ductules or backward leakage of the pigment. The initial steps in evaluating the patient with jaundice are to determine (1) whether the hyperbilirubinemia is predominantly conjugated or unconjugated in nature, and (2) whether other biochemical liver tests are abnormal. The thoughtful interpretation of limited data will allow for a rational evaluation of the patient (Fig. 43-1). This discussion will focus solely on the evaluation of the adult patient with jaundice.

ISOLATED ELEVATION OF SERUM BILIRUBIN Unconjugated Hyperbilirubinemia
The differential diagnosis of an isolated unconjugated hyperbilirubinemia is limited (Table 43-1). The critical determination is whether the patient is suffering from a hemolytic process resulting in an overproduction of bilirubin (hemolytic disorders and ineffective erythropoiesis) or from impaired hepatic uptake/conjugation of bilirubin (drug effect or genetic disorders).

ALGORITHM FOR PATIENT WITH JAUNDICE

History (focus on medication/drug exposure)
Physical examination
Lab tests: Bilirubin with fractionation, ALT, AST, alkaline phosphatase, prothrombin time, and albumin

Isolated elevation of the bilirubin

Direct hyperbilirubinemia (direct > 15%) See Table 43-1
→ Inherited disorders Dubin-Johnson syndrome Rotor's syndrome

Indirect hyperbilirubinemia (direct < 15%) See Table 43-1
→ Drugs Rifampicin Probenecid
→ Inherited disorders Gilbert's syndrome Crigler-Najjar syndromes
→ Hemolytic disorders Ineffective erythropoiesis

Bilirubin and other liver tests elevated

Hepatocellular pattern: ALT/AST elevated out of proportion to alkaline phosphatase See Table 43-2
1. Viral serologies
   Hepatitis A IgM
   Hepatitis B surface antigen and core antibody (IgM)
   Hepatitis C RNA
2. Toxicology screen
   Acetaminophen level
3. Ceruloplasmin (if patient less than 40 years of age)
4. ANA, SMA, LKM, SPEP

Results negative
Additional virologic testing CMV DNA, EBV capsid antigen Hepatitis D antibody (if indicated) Hepatitis E IgM (if indicated)
Results negative
Liver biopsy

Cholestatic pattern: Alkaline phosphatase out of proportion ALT/AST See Table 43-3
→ Ultrasound
Dilated ducts Extrahepatic cholestasis → CT/ERCP
Ducts not dilated Intrahepatic cholestasis
Serologic testing AMA Hepatitis serologies Hepatitis A, CMV, EBV Review drugs (see Table 43-3)
Results negative → MRCP/Liver biopsy
AMA positive → Liver biopsy

FIGURE 43-1 Evaluation of the patient with jaundice. MRCP, magnetic resonance cholangiopancreatography; ALT, alanine aminotransferase; AST, aspartate aminotransferase; SMA, smooth-muscle antibody; AMA, antimitochondrial antibody; LKM, liver-kidney microsomal antibody; SPEP, serum protein electrophoresis; CMV, cytomegalovirus; EBV, Epstein-Barr virus.

Hemolytic disorders that cause excessive heme production may be either inherited or acquired. Inherited disorders include spherocytosis, sickle cell anemia, thalassemia, and deficiency of red cell enzymes such as pyruvate kinase and glucose-6-phosphate dehydrogenase. In these conditions, the serum bilirubin rarely exceeds 86 μmol/L (5 mg/dL). Higher levels may occur when there is coexistent renal or hepatocellular dysfunction or in acute hemolysis such as a sickle cell crisis. In evaluating jaundice in patients with chronic hemolysis, it is important to remember the high incidence of pigmented (calcium bilirubinate) gallstones found in these patients, which increases the likelihood of choledocholithiasis as an alternative explanation for hyperbilirubinemia.

Acquired hemolytic disorders include microangiopathic hemolytic anemia (e.g., hemolytic-uremic syndrome), paroxysmal nocturnal hemoglobinuria, spur cell anemia, and immune hemolysis. Ineffective erythropoiesis occurs in cobalamin, folate, and iron deficiencies.

In the absence of hemolysis, the physician should consider a problem with the hepatic uptake or conjugation of bilirubin. Certain drugs, including rifampicin and probenecid, may cause unconjugated hyperbilirubinemia by diminishing hepatic uptake of

TABLE 43-1   CAUSES OF ISOLATED HYPERBILIRUBINEMIA

I. Indirect hyperbilirubinemia
  A. Hemolytic disorders
    1. Inherited
      a. Spherocytosis, elliptocytosis
        Glucose-6-phosphate dehydrogenase and pyruvate kinase
        deficiencies
      b. Sickle cell anemia
    2. Acquired
      a. Microangiopathic hemolytic anemias
      b. Paroxysmal nocturnal hemoglobinuria
      c. Spur cell anemia
      d. Immune hemolysis
  B. Ineffective erythropoiesis
    1. Cobalamin, folate, thalassemia, and severe iron deficiencies
  C. Drugs
    1. Rifampicin, probenecid, ribavirin
  D. Inherited conditions
    1. Crigler-Najjar types I and II
    2. Gilbert's syndrome
II. Direct hyperbilirubinemia
  A. Inherited conditions
    1. Dubin-Johnson syndrome
    2. Rotor's syndrome

bilirubin. Impaired bilirubin conjugation occurs in three genetic conditions: Crigler-Najjar syndrome, types I and II, and Gilbert's syndrome. *Crigler-Najjar type I* is an exceptionally rare condition found in neonates and characterized by severe jaundice [bilirubin > 342 μmol/L (>20 mg/dL)] and neurologic impairment due to kernicterus, frequently leading to death in infancy or childhood. These patients have a complete absence of bilirubin UDPGT activity, usually due to mutations in the critical 3′ domain of the *UDPGT* gene, and are totally unable to conjugate, hence cannot excrete bilirubin. The only effective treatment is orthotopic liver transplantation. Use of gene therapy and allogeneic hepatocyte infusion are experimental approaches of future promise for this devastating disease.

Crigler-Najjar type II is somewhat more common than type I. Patients live into adulthood with serum bilirubin levels that range from 103–428 μmol/L (6–25 mg/dL). In these patients, mutations in the bilirubin *UDPGT* gene cause reduced but not completely absent activity of the enzyme. Bilirubin *UDPGT* activity can be induced by the administration of phenobarbital, which can reduce serum bilirubin levels in these patients. Despite marked jaundice, these patients usually survive into adulthood, although they may be susceptible to kernicterus under the stress of intercurrent illness or surgery.

Gilbert's syndrome is also marked by the impaired conjugation of bilirubin due to reduced bilirubin UDPGT activity. Patients with Gilbert's syndrome have a mild unconjugated hyperbilirubinemia with serum levels almost always <103 μmol/L (6 mg/dL). The serum levels may fluctuate, and jaundice is often identified only during periods of fasting. One molecular defect that has been identified in patients with Gilbert's syndrome is in the TATAA element in the 5′ promoter region of the bilirubin *UDPGT* gene upstream of exon 1. This defect alone is not necessarily sufficient for producing the clinical syndrome of Gilbert's as there are patients who are homozygous for this defect yet do not have the levels of hyperbilirubinemia typically seen in Gilbert's syndrome. An enhancer polymorphism that lowers transcriptional activity has recently been identified. The decrease in transcription caused by both mutations together may be critical for producing the syndrome. Unlike both Crigler-Najjar syndromes, Gilbert's syndrome is very common. The reported incidence is 3–7% of the population with males predominating over females by a ratio of 2–7:1.

Conjugated Hyperbilirubinemia   Elevated conjugated hyperbilirubinemia is found in two rare inherited conditions: *Dubin-Johnson syndrome* and *Rotor's syndrome* (Table 43-1). Patients with both conditions present with asymptomatic jaundice, typically in the second generation of life. The defect in Dubin-Johnson syndrome is mutations in the gene for multiple drug resistance protein 2.

These patients have altered excretion of bilirubin into the bile ducts. Rotor's syndrome seems to be a problem with the hepatic storage of bilirubin. Differentiating between these syndromes is possible, but clinically unnecessary, due to their benign nature.

ELEVATION OF SERUM BILIRUBIN WITH OTHER LIVER TEST ABNORMALITIES   The remainder of this chapter will focus on the evaluation of the patient with a conjugated hyperbilirubinemia in the setting of other liver test abnormalities. This group of patients can be divided into those with a primary hepatocellular process and those with intra- or extrahepatic cholestasis. Being able to make this differentiation will guide the physician's evaluation (Fig. 43-1). This differentiation is made on the basis of the history and physical examination as well as the pattern of liver test abnormalities.

History   A complete medical history is perhaps the single most important part of the evaluation of the patient with unexplained jaundice. Important considerations include the use of or exposure to any chemical or medication, either physician-prescribed, over-the-counter, complementary or alternative medicines such as herbal and vitamin preparations, or other drugs such as anabolic steroids. The patient should be carefully questioned about possible parenteral exposures, including transfusions, IV and intranasal drug use, tattoos, and sexual activity. Other important questions include recent travel history, exposure to people with jaundice, exposure to possibly contaminated foods, occupational exposure to hepatotoxins, alcohol consumption, the duration of jaundice, and the presence of any accompanying symptoms such as arthralgias, myalgias, rash, anorexia, weight loss, abdominal pain, fever, pruritus, and changes in the urine and stool. While none of these latter symptoms are specific for any one condition, they can suggest a particular diagnosis. A history of arthralgias and myalgias predating jaundice suggests hepatitis, either viral or drug-related. Jaundice associated with the sudden onset of severe right upper quadrant pain and shaking chills suggests choledocholithiasis and ascending cholangitis.

Physical Examination   The general assessment should include assessment of the patient's nutritional status. Temporal and proximal muscle wasting suggests long-standing diseases such as pancreatic cancer or cirrhosis. Stigmata of chronic liver disease, including spider nevi, palmar erythema, gynecomastia, caput medusae, Dupuytren's contractures, parotid gland enlargement, and testicular atrophy are commonly seen in advanced alcoholic (Laennec's) cirrhosis and occasionally in other types of cirrhosis. An enlarged left supraclavicular node (Virchow's node) or periumbilical nodule (Sister Mary Joseph's nodule) suggests an abdominal malignancy. Jugular venous distention, a sign of right-sided heart failure, suggests hepatic congestion. Right pleural effusion, in the absence of clinically apparent ascites, may be seen in advanced cirrhosis.

The abdominal examination should focus on the size and consistency of the liver, whether the spleen is palpable and hence enlarged, and whether there is ascites present. Patients with cirrhosis may have an enlarged left lobe of the liver, which is felt below the xiphoid, and an enlarged spleen. A grossly enlarged nodular liver or an obvious abdominal mass suggests malignancy. An enlarged tender liver could be viral or alcoholic hepatitis, an infiltrative process such as amyloid, or, less often, an acutely congested liver secondary to right-sided heart failure. Severe right upper quadrant tenderness with respiratory arrest on inspiration (Murphy's sign) suggests cholecystitis or, occasionally, ascending cholangitis. Ascites in the presence of jaundice suggests either cirrhosis or malignancy with peritoneal spread.

Laboratory Tests   When the physician encounters a patient with unexplained jaundice, there is a battery of tests that are helpful in the initial evaluation. These include total and direct serum bilirubin with fractionation, aminotransferases, alkaline phosphatase, albumin, and prothrombin time tests. Enzyme tests [alanine aminotransferase (ALT), aspartate aminotransferase (AST), and alkaline phosphatase] are helpful in differentiating between a hepatocellular process and a cholestatic process (Table 296-1; Fig. 43-1), a critical step in determining what additional workup is indicated. Patients with a hepatocellular process generally have a disproportionate rise in the aminotransferases compared to the alkaline phosphatase. Patients with a cholestatic process have a disproportionate rise in the alkaline phosphatase compared to the aminotransferases. The bilirubin can be prominently elevated in both hepatocellular and cholestatic conditions and therefore is not necessarily helpful in differentiating between the two.

In addition to the enzyme tests, all jaundiced patients should have additional blood tests, specifically an albumin level and a prothrombin time, to assess liver function. A low albumin suggests a chronic process such as cirrhosis or cancer. A normal albumin is suggestive of a more acute process such as viral hepatitis or choledocholithiasis. An elevated prothrombin time indicates either vitamin K deficiency due to prolonged jaundice and malabsorption of vitamin K or significant hepatocellular dysfunction. The failure of the prothrombin time to correct with parenteral administration of vitamin K indicates severe hepatocellular injury.

The results of the bilirubin, enzyme tests, albumin, and prothrombin time tests will usually indicate whether a jaundiced patient has a hepatocellular or a cholestatic disease, as well as some indication of the duration and severity of the disease. The causes and evaluation of hepatocellular and cholestatic diseases are quite different.

Hepatocellular Conditions

Hepatocellular diseases that can cause jaundice include viral hepatitis, drug or environmental toxicity, alcohol, and end-stage cirrhosis from any cause (Table 43-2). Wilson's disease, once believed to occur primarily in young adults, should be considered in all adults if no other cause of jaundice is found. Autoimmune hepatitis is typically seen in young to middle-aged women but may affect men and women of any age. Alcoholic hepatitis can be differentiated from viral and toxin-related hepatitis by the pattern of the aminotransferases. Patients with alcoholic hepatitis typically have an AST:ALT ratio of at least 2:1. The AST rarely exceeds 300 U/L. Patients with acute viral hepatitis and toxin-related injury severe enough to produce jaundice typically have aminotransferases > 500 U/L, with the ALT greater than or equal to the AST. The degree of aminotransferase elevation can occasionally help in differentiating between hepatocellular and cholestatic processes. While ALT and AST values less than 8 times normal may be seen in either hepatocellular or cholestatic liver disease, values 25 times normal or higher are seen primarily in acute hepatocellular diseases. Patients with jaundice from cirrhosis can have normal or only slight elevations of the aminotransferases.

When the physician determines that the patient has a hepatocellular disease, appropriate testing for acute viral hepatitis includes a hepatitis A IgM antibody, a hepatitis B surface antigen and core IgM antibody, and a hepatitis C viral RNA test. It can take many weeks for the hepatitis C antibody to become detectable, making it an unreliable test if acute hepatitis C is suspected. Depending on circumstances, studies for hepatitis D, E, Epstein-Barr virus (EBV), and cytomegalovirus (CMV) may be indicated. Ceruloplasmin is the initial screening test for Wilson's disease. Testing for autoimmune hepatitis usually includes an antinuclear antibody and measurement of specific immunoglobulins.

Drug-induced hepatocellular injury can be classified either as predictable or unpredictable. Predictable drug reactions are dose-dependent and affect all patients who ingest a toxic dose of the drug in question. The classic example is acetaminophen hepatotoxicity. Unpredictable or idiosyncratic drug reactions are not dose-dependent and occur in a minority of patients. A great number of drugs can cause idiosyncratic hepatic injury. Environmental toxins are also an important cause of hepatocellular injury. Examples include industrial chemicals such as vinyl chloride, herbal preparations containing pyrrolizidine alkaloids (Jamaica bush tea) and Kava Kava, and the mushrooms *Amanita phalloides* or *A. verna* that contain highly hepatotoxic amatoxins.

Cholestatic Conditions

When the pattern of the liver tests suggests a cholestatic disorder, the next step is to determine whether it is intra- or extrahepatic cholestasis (Fig. 43-1). Distinguishing intrahepatic

TABLE 43-2	HEPATOCELLULAR CONDITIONS THAT MAY PRODUCE JAUNDICE

Viral hepatitis
    Hepatitis A, B, C, D, and E
    Epstein-Barr virus
    Cytomegalovirus
    Herpes simplex
Alcohol
Drug toxicity
    Predictable, dose-dependent, e.g., acetaminophen
    Unpredictable, idosyncratic, e.g., isoniazid
Environmental toxins
    Vinyl chloride
    Jamaica bush tea—pyrrolizidine alkaloids
    Kava Kava
    Wild mushrooms—*Amanita phalloides* or *A. verna*
Wilson's disease
Autoimmune hepatitis

from extrahepatic cholestasis may be difficult. History, physical examination, and laboratory tests are often not helpful. The next appropriate test is an ultrasound. The ultrasound is inexpensive, does not expose the patient to ionizing radiation, and can detect dilation of the intra- and extrahepatic biliary tree with a high degree of sensitivity and specificity. The absence of biliary dilatation suggests intrahepatic cholestasis, while the presence of biliary dilatation indicates extrahepatic cholestasis. False-negative results occur in patients with partial obstruction of the common bile duct or in patients with cirrhosis or primary sclerosing cholangitis (PSC) where scarring prevents the intrahepatic ducts from dilating.

Although ultrasonography may indicate extrahepatic cholestasis, it rarely identifies the site or cause of obstruction. The distal common bile duct is a particularly difficult area to visualize by ultrasound because of overlying bowel gas. Appropriate next tests include CT, magnetic resonance cholangiography (MRCP), and endoscopic retrograde cholangiopancreatography (ERCP). CT scanning and MRCP are better than ultrasonography for assessing the head of the pancreas and for identifying choledocholithiasis in the distal common bile duct, particularly when the ducts are not dilated. ERCP is the "gold standard" for identifying choledocholithiasis. It is performed by introducing a side-viewing endoscope perorally into the duodenum. The ampulla of Vater is visualized and a catheter is advanced through the ampulla. Injection of dye allows for the visualization of the common bile duct and the pancreatic duct. The success rate for cannulation of the common bile duct ranges from 80–95%, depending on the operator's experience. Beyond its diagnostic capabilities, ERCP allows for therapeutic interventions, including the removal of common bile duct stones and the placement of stents. In patients in whom ERCP is unsuccessful and there is a high likelihood of the need for a therapeutic intervention, transhepatic cholangiography can provide the same information and allow for intervention. MRCP is a now widely available, noninvasive technique for imaging the bile and pancreatic ducts; it has replaced ERCP as the initial diagnostic test in cases where the need for intervention is felt to be small.

In patients with apparent *intrahepatic cholestasis*, the diagnosis is often made by serologic testing in combination with percutaneous liver biopsy. The list of possible causes of intrahepatic cholestasis is long and varied (Table 43-3). A number of conditions that typically cause a hepatocellular pattern of injury can also present as a cholestatic variant. Both hepatitis B and C can cause a cholestatic hepatitis (fibrosing cholestatic hepatitis). This disease variant has been reported in patients who have undergone solid organ transplantation. Hepatitis A, alcoholic hepatitis, EBV, and CMV may also present as cholestatic liver disease.

Drugs may cause intrahepatic cholestasis, a variant of drug-induced hepatitis. Drug-induced cholestasis is usually reversible after eliminating the offending drug, although it may take many

TABLE 43-3   CHOLESTATIC CONDITIONS THAT MAY PRODUCE JAUNDICE

I. Intrahepatic
  A. Viral hepatitis
    1. Fibrosing cholestatic hepatitis—hepatitis B and C
    2. Hepatitis A, Epstein-Barr virus, cytomegalovirus
  B. Alcoholic hepatitis
  C. Drug toxicity
    1. Pure cholestasis—anabolic and contraceptive steroids
    2. Cholestatic hepatitis—chlorpromazine, erythromycin estolate
    3. Chronic cholestasis—chlorpromazine and prochlorperazine
  D. Primary biliary cirrhosis
  E. Primary sclerosing cholangitis
  F. Vanishing bile duct syndrome
    1. Chronic rejection of liver transplants
    2. Sarcoidosis
    3. Drugs
  G. Inherited
    1. Progressive familial intrahepatic cholestasis
    2. Benign recurrent cholestasis
  H. Cholestasis of pregnancy
  I. Total parenteral nutrition
  J. Nonhepatobiliary sepsis
  K. Benign postoperative cholestasis
  L. Paraneoplastic syndrome
  M. Venooclusive disease
  N. Graft-versus-host disease
  O. Infiltrative disease
    1. TB
    2. Lymphoma
    3. Amyloid
II. Extrahepatic
  A. Malignant
    1. Cholangiocarcinoma
    2. Pancreatic cancer
    3. Gallbladder cancer
    4. Ampullary cancer
    5. Malignant involvement of the porta hepatis lymph nodes
  B. Benign
    1. Choledocholithiasis
    2. Postoperative biliary structures
    3. Primary sclerosing cholangitis
    4. Chronic pancreatitis
    5. AIDS cholangiopathy
    6. Mirizzi syndrome
    7. Parasitic disease (ascariasis)

months for cholestasis to resolve. Drugs most commonly associated with cholestasis are the anabolic and contraceptive steroids. Cholestatic hepatitis has been reported with chlorpromazine, imipramine, tolbutamide, sulindac, cimetidine, and erythromycin estolate. It also occurs in patients taking trimethoprim, sulfamethoxazole, and penicillin-based antibiotics such as ampicillin, dicloxacillin, and clavulinic acid. Rarely, cholestasis may be chronic and associated with progressive fibrosis despite early discontinuation of the drug. Chronic cholestasis has been associated with chlorpromazine and prochlorperazine.

Primary biliary cirrhosis is an autoimmune disease predominantly of middle-aged women in which there is a progressive destruction of interlobular bile ducts. The diagnosis is made by the presence of the antimitochondrial antibody that is found in 95% of patients. *Primary sclerosing cholangitis* is characterized by the destruction and fibrosis of larger bile ducts. The disease may involve only the intrahepatic ducts and present as intrahepatic cholestasis. However, in 95% of patients with PSC, both intra- and extrahepatic ducts are involved. The diagnosis of PSC is made by imaging the biliary tree. The pathognomonic findings are multiple strictures of bile ducts with dilatations proximal to the strictures. Approximately 75% of patients with PSC have inflammatory bowel disease.

The *vanishing bile duct syndrome* and *adult bile ductopenia* are rare conditions in which there are a decreased number of bile ducts seen in liver biopsy specimens. The histologic picture is similar to that found in primary biliary cirrhosis. This picture is seen in pa-

tients who develop chronic rejection after liver transplantation and in those who develop graft-versus-host disease after bone marrow transplantation. Vanishing bile duct syndrome also occurs in rare cases of sarcoidosis, in patients taking certain drugs including chlorpromazine, and idiopathically.

There are also familial forms of intrahepatic cholestasis. The familial intrahepatic cholestatic syndromes include *progressive familial intrahepatic cholestasis* (PFIC) *types 1–3*, and *benign recurrent cholestasis* (BRC). PFIC1 and BRC are autosomal recessive diseases that result from mutations in the *ATP8B1* gene that encodes a protein belonging to the subfamily of P-type ATPases; the exact function of this protein remains poorly defined. While PFIC1 is a progressive condition that manifests in childhood, BRC presents later than PFIC1 and is marked by recurrent episodes of jaundice and pruritus; the episodes are self-limited but can be debilitating. PFIC2 is caused by mutations in the *ABCB11* gene, which encodes the bile salt export pump, and PFIC3 is caused by mutations in the multidrug-resistant P-glycoprotein 3. *Cholestasis of pregnancy* occurs in the second and third trimesters and resolves after delivery. Its cause is unknown, but the condition is probably inherited and cholestasis can be triggered by estrogen administration.

Other causes of intrahepatic cholestasis include total parenteral nutrition (TPN), nonhepatobiliary sepsis, benign postoperative cholestasis, and a paraneoplastic syndrome associated with a number of different malignancies, including Hodgkin's disease, medullary thyroid cancer, renal cell cancer, renal sarcoma, T cell lymphoma, prostate cancer, and several gastrointestinal malignancies. The term *Stauffer's syndrome* has been used for intrahepatic cholestasis specifically associated with renal cell cancer. In patients developing cholestasis in the intensive care unit, the major considerations should be sepsis, shock liver, and TPN jaundice. Jaundice occurring after bone marrow transplantation is most likely due to venooclusive disease or graft-versus-host disease.

Causes of *extrahepatic cholestasis* can be split into malignant and benign (Table 43-3). Malignant causes include pancreatic, gallbladder, ampullary, and cholangiocarcinoma. The latter is most commonly associated with PSC and is exceptionally difficult to diagnose because its appearance is often identical to that of PSC. Pancreatic and gallbladder tumors, as well as cholangiocarcinoma, are rarely resectable and have poor prognoses. Ampullary carcinoma has the highest surgical cure rate of all the tumors that present as painless jaundice. Hilar lymphadenopathy due to metastases from other cancers may cause obstruction of the extrahepatic biliary tree.

Choledocholithiasis is the most common cause of extrahepatic cholestasis. The clinical presentation can range from mild right upper quadrant discomfort with only minimal elevations of the enzyme tests to ascending cholangitis with jaundice, sepsis, and circulatory collapse. PSC may occur with clinically important strictures limited to the extrahepatic biliary tree. In cases where there is a dominant stricture, patients can be effectively managed with serial endoscopic dilatations. Chronic pancreatitis rarely causes strictures of the distal common bile duct, where it passes through the head of the pancreas. AIDS cholangiopathy is a condition, usually due to infection of the bile duct epithelium with CMV or cryptosporidia, which has a cholangiographic appearance similar to that of PSC. These patients usually present with greatly elevated serum alkaline phosphatase levels (mean, 800 IU/L), but the bilirubin is often near normal. These patients do not typically present with jaundice.

SUMMARY

The goal of this chapter is not to provide an encyclopedic review of all of the conditions that can cause jaundice. Rather, it is intended to provide a framework that helps a physician to evaluate the patient with jaundice in a logical way (Fig. 43-1).

Simply stated, the initial step is to obtain appropriate blood tests to determine if the patient has an isolated elevation of serum bilirubin. If so, is the bilirubin elevation due to an increased unconjugated or conjugated fraction? If the hyperbilirubinemia is accompanied by other liver test abnormalities, is the disorder hepatocellular or cholestatic? If cholestatic, is it intra- or extrahepatic? All of these questions can be answered with a thoughtful history, physical examination, and interpretation of laboratory and radiologic tests and procedures.

FURTHER READINGS

BOSMA PJ: Inherited disorders of bilirubin metabolism. J Hepatol 38:107, 2003

FERENCI P: Wilson's disease. Clin Gastroenterol Hepatol 3:726, 2005

FOX IJ et al: Treatment of the Crigler-Najjar syndrome type I with hepatocyte transplantation. N Engl J Med 338:1422, 1998

GLASOVA H, BEUERS U: Extrahepatic manifestations of cholestasis. J Gastroenterol Hepatol 9:938, 2002

PRATT DS, KAPLAN MM: Laboratory tests, in Schiff's Diseases of the Liver, 9th ed, ER Schiff et al (eds). Philadelphia, Lippincott Williams & Wilkins, 2003

TRAUNER M et al: Molecular pathogenesis of cholestasis. N Engl J Med 339:1217, 1998

44 Abdominal Swelling and Ascites
Robert M. Glickman, Roshini Rajapaksa

ABDOMINAL SWELLING

Abdominal swelling or distention is a common problem in clinical medicine and may be the initial manifestation of a systemic disease or of otherwise unsuspected abdominal disease. *Subjective* abdominal enlargement, often described as a sensation of fullness or bloating, is usually transient and is often related to a functional gastrointestinal disorder when it is not accompanied by objective physical findings of increased abdominal girth or local swelling. *Obesity* and lumbar lordosis, which may be associated with prominence of the abdomen, may usually be distinguished from true increases in the volume of the peritoneal cavity by history and careful physical examination.

CLINICAL HISTORY

Abdominal swelling may first be noticed by the patient because of a progressive increase in belt or clothing size, the appearance of abdominal or inguinal hernias, or the development of a localized swelling. Often, considerable abdominal enlargement has gone unnoticed for weeks or months, either because of coexistent obesity or because the ascites formation has been insidious, without pain or localizing symptoms. Progressive abdominal distention may be associated with a sensation of "pulling" or "stretching" of the flanks or groins and vague low back pain. Localized pain usually results from involvement of an abdominal organ (e.g., a passively congested liver, large spleen, or colonic tumor). Pain is uncommon in cirrhosis with ascites, and when it is present, pancreatitis, hepatocellular carcinoma, or peritonitis should be considered. Tense ascites or abdominal tumors may produce increased intraabdominal pressure, resulting in indigestion and heartburn due to gastroesophageal reflux or dyspnea, abdominal wall hernias (inguinal and umbilical), orthopnea, and tachypnea from elevation of the diaphragm. A coexistent pleural effusion, more commonly on the right, presumably due to leakage of ascitic fluid through lymphatic channels in the diaphragm, may also contribute to respiratory embarrassment. A large pleural effusion, obscuring most of the lung, is known as a *hepatic hydrothorax.* The patient with diffuse abdominal swelling should be questioned about increased alcohol intake, a prior episode of jaundice or hematuria, or a change in bowel habits. Such historic information may provide the clues that will lead one to suspect an occult cirrhosis, a colonic tumor with peritoneal seeding, congestive heart failure, or nephrosis.

PHYSICAL EXAMINATION

A carefully executed general physical examination can yield valuable clues concerning the etiology of abdominal swelling. Thus palmar erythema and spider angiomas suggest an underlying cirrhosis, while supraclavicular adenopathy (Virchow's node) should raise the question of an underlying gastrointestinal malignancy.

Inspection of the abdomen is important. By noting the abdominal contour, one may be able to distinguish localized from generalized swelling. The tensely distended abdomen with tightly stretched skin, bulging flanks, and everted umbilicus is characteristic of ascites. A prominent abdominal venous pattern with the direction of flow away from the umbilicus is often a reflection of portal hypertension; venous collaterals with flow from the lower part of the abdomen toward the umbilicus suggest obstruction of the inferior vena cava; flow downward toward the umbilicus suggests superior vena cava obstruction. "Doming" of the abdomen with visible ridges from underlying intestinal loops is usually due to intestinal obstruction or distention. An epigastric mass, with evident peristalsis proceeding from left to right, usually indicates underlying pyloric obstruction. A liver with metastatic deposits may be visible as a nodular right upper quadrant mass moving with respiration.

Auscultation may reveal the high-pitched, rushing sounds of early intestinal obstruction or a succussion sound due to increased fluid and gas in a dilated hollow viscus. Careful auscultation over an enlarged liver occasionally reveals a harsh bruit signifying a vascular tumor (especially a hepatocellular carcinoma) or alcoholic hepatitis, or the leathery friction rub of a surface nodule. A venous hum at the umbilicus may signify portal hypertension and an increased collateral blood flow around the liver. A fluid wave and flank dullness that shifts with change in position of the patient are important signs that indicate the presence of peritoneal fluid, although a minimum of 1500 mL of fluid is usually required to produce these findings. In obese patients, small amounts of fluid may be difficult to demonstrate and often can only be detected by ultrasound examination of the abdomen, which can detect as little as 100 mL of fluid. Careful percussion should serve to distinguish generalized abdominal enlargement from localized swelling due to an enlarged uterus, ovarian cyst, or distended bladder. Percussion can also outline an abnormally small or large liver. Loss of normal liver dullness may result from massive hepatic necrosis; it also may be a clue to free gas in the peritoneal cavity, as from perforation of a hollow viscus.

Palpation is often difficult with massive ascites, and ballottement of overlying fluid may be the only method of palpating the liver or spleen. A slightly enlarged spleen in association with ascites may be the only evidence of an occult cirrhosis. When there is evidence of portal hypertension, a soft liver suggests that obstruction to portal flow is extrahepatic; a firm liver suggests cirrhosis as the likely cause of the portal hypertension. A very hard or nodular liver is a clue that the liver is infiltrated with tumor, and when accompanied by ascites, it suggests that the latter is due to peritoneal seeding. The presence of a hard periumbilical nodule (Sister Mary Joseph's nodule) suggests metastatic disease from a pelvic or gastrointestinal primary tumor. A pulsatile liver and ascites may be found in tricuspid insufficiency.

An attempt should be made to determine whether a mass is solid or cystic, smooth or irregular, and whether it moves with respiration. The liver, spleen, and gallbladder should descend with respiration unless they are fixed by adhesions or extension of tumor beyond the organ. A fixed mass not descending with respiration may indicate that it is retroperitoneal. Tenderness, especially if localized, may indicate an inflammatory process such as an abscess; it also may be due to stretching of the visceral peritoneum or tumor necrosis. Rectal and pelvic examinations are mandatory; they may reveal otherwise undetected masses due to tumor or infection.

Radiographic and laboratory examinations are essential for confirming or extending the impressions gained on physical examination. Upright and recumbent films of the abdomen may demonstrate the dilated loops of intestine with fluid levels characteristic of intestinal obstruction or the diffuse abdominal haziness and loss of psoas margins suggestive of ascites. Ultrasonography is often of value in detecting ascites, determining the presence of a mass, or evaluating the size of the liver and

Condition	Gross Appearance	Protein, g/L	Serum-Ascites Albumin Gradient, g/dL	Cell Count Red Blood Cells, >10,000/μL	Cell Count White Blood Cells, per μL	Other Tests
Cirrhosis	Straw-colored or bile-stained	<25 (95%)	>1.1	1%	<250 (90%)[a]; predominantly mesothelial	
Neoplasm	Straw-colored, hemorrhagic, mucinous, or chylous	>25 (75%)	<1.1	20%	>1000 (50%); variable cell types	Cytology, cell block, peritoneal biopsy
Tuberculous peritonitis	Clear, turbid, hemorrhagic, chylous	>25 (50%)	<1.1	7%	>1000 (70%); usually >70% lymphocytes	Peritoneal biopsy, stain and culture for acid-fast bacilli
Pyogenic peritonitis	Turbid or purulent	If purulent, >25	<1.1	Unusual	Predominantly polymorphonuclear leukocytes	Positive Gram's stain, culture
Congestive heart failure	Straw-colored	Variable, 15–53	>1.1	10%	<1000 (90%); usually mesothelial, mononuclear	
Nephrosis	Straw-colored or chylous	<25 (100%)	<1.1	Unusual	<250; mesothelial, mononuclear	If chylous, ether extraction, Sudan staining
Pancreatic ascites (pancreatitis, pseudocyst)	Turbid, hemorrhagic, or chylous	Variable, often >25	<1.1	Variable, may be blood-stained	Variable	Increased amylase in ascitic fluid and serum

[a]Because the conditions of examining fluid and selecting patients were not identical in each series, the percentage figures (in parentheses) should be taken as an indication of the order of magnitude rather than as the precise incidence of any abnormal finding.

spleen. CT scanning provides similar information and is often necessary to visualize the retroperitoneum, pancreas, and lymph nodes. A plain film of the abdomen may reveal the distended colon of otherwise unsuspected ulcerative colitis and give valuable information as to the size of the liver and spleen. An irregular and elevated right side of the diaphragm may be a clue to a liver abscess or hepatocellular carcinoma. Studies of the gastrointestinal tract with barium or other contrast media are usually necessary in the search for a primary tumor.

Laboratory abnormalities that are highly suggestive of cirrhosis as the cause of ascites include unexplained thrombocytopenia, decreased albumin, and a prolonged prothrombin time.

ASCITES

The evaluation of a patient with ascites requires that the cause of the ascites be established. In most cases ascites appears as part of a well-recognized illness, i.e., cirrhosis, congestive heart failure, nephrosis, or disseminated carcinomatosis. In these situations, the physician should determine that the development of ascites is indeed a consequence of the basic underlying disease and not due to the presence of a separate or related disease process. This distinction is necessary even when the cause of ascites seems obvious. For example, when the patient with compensated cirrhosis and minimal ascites develops progressive ascites that is increasingly difficult to control with sodium restriction or diuretics, the temptation is to attribute the worsening of the clinical picture to progressive liver disease. However, an occult hepatocellular carcinoma, portal vein thrombosis, spontaneous bacterial peritonitis, alcoholic hepatitis, viral infection, or even tuberculosis may be responsible for the decompensation. The disappointingly low success in diagnosing tuberculous peritonitis or hepatocellular carcinoma in the patient with cirrhosis and ascites reflects the too-low index of suspicion for the development of such superimposed conditions. Similarly, the patient with congestive heart failure may develop ascites from a disseminated carcinoma with peritoneal seeding. It is important to note, however, that while there are many different causes of ascites, in the United States >80% of cases are due to cirrhosis. Risk factors for the development of cirrhosis include alcoholism, viral hepatitis, nonalcoholic steatohepatitis, and a family history of liver disease.

Diagnostic paracentesis (50–100 mL) should be part of the routine evaluation of the patient with ascites, and does not routinely require the prior administration of platelets or fresh-frozen plasma unless disseminated intravascular coagulation is suspected. The fluid should be examined for its gross appearance; protein content, albumin level, cell count, and differential cell count should be determined; and Gram's and acid-fast stains and culture should be performed. Cytologic and cell-block examination may disclose an otherwise unsuspected carcinoma. A serum ascites–albumin gradient (SAAG) should be calculated to determine if the fluid has the features of a transudate or an exudate. The gradient correlates directly with portal pressure. A gradient >1.1 g/dL (high gradient) is characteristic of uncomplicated cirrhotic ascites and differentiates ascites due to portal hypertension from ascites not due to portal hypertension >97% of the time. Other etiologies of high-gradient ascites include alcoholic hepatitis, congestive heart failure, hepatic metastases, constrictive pericarditis, and Budd-Chiari syndrome. A gradient <1.1 g/dL (low gradient) suggests that the ascites is not due to portal hypertension with >97% accuracy and mandates a search for other causes such as peritoneal carcinomatosis, tuberculous peritonitis, pancreatitis, serositis, pyogenic peritonitis, and nephrotic syndrome (Table 44-1). Table 44-1 presents some of the disease states that produce high-SAAG and low-SAAG ascites. Although there is variability of the ascitic fluid in any given disease state, some features are sufficiently characteristic to suggest certain diagnostic possibilities. For example, blood-stained fluid with >25 g/L protein is unusual in uncomplicated cirrhosis but is consistent with tuberculous peritonitis or neoplasm. Cloudy fluid with a predominance of polymorphonuclear cells (>250/μL) and a positive Gram's stain are characteristic of bacterial peritonitis, which requires antibiotic therapy; if most cells are lymphocytes, tuberculosis should be suspected. The complete examination of each fluid is most important, for occasionally only one finding may be abnormal. For example, if the fluid is a typical transudate but contains >250 white blood cells per microliter, the finding should be recognized as atypical for cirrhosis and should warrant a search for tumor or infection. This is especially true in the evaluation of cirrhotic ascites where occult peritoneal infection may be present with only minor elevations in the white blood cell count of the peritoneal fluid (300–500/μL). Since Gram's stain of the fluid may be negative in a high proportion of such cases, careful culture of the peritoneal fluid is mandatory. Bedside inoculation of blood culture flasks with ascitic fluid results in a dramatically increased incidence of positive cultures when bacterial infection is present (90 vs. 40% positivity with conventional cultures done by the laboratory). Direct visualization of the peritoneum (laparoscopy) may disclose peritoneal deposits of tumor, tuberculosis, or metastatic disease of the liver. Biopsies are taken under direct vision, often adding to the diagnostic accuracy of the procedure.

Chylous ascites refers to a turbid, milky, or creamy peritoneal fluid due to the presence of thoracic or intestinal lymph. Such a fluid shows Sudan-staining fat globules microscopically and an increased triglyceride content by chemical examination. Opaque milky fluid usually has a triglyceride concentration of >11.3 mmol/L (>1000 mg/dL), but a triglyceride concentration of >2.3 mmol/L (>200 mg/dL) is sufficient for the diagnosis. A turbid fluid due to leukocytes or tumor cells may be confused with chylous fluid (pseudochylous), and it is often helpful to carry out alkalinization and ether extraction of the specimen. Alkali tend to dissolve cellular proteins and thereby reduce turbidity; ether extraction leads to clearing if the turbidity of the fluid is due to lipid. Chylous ascites is most often the result of lymphatic disruption or obstruction from cirrhosis, tumor, trauma, tuberculosis, filariasis (Chap. 211), or congenital abnormalities. It may also be seen in the nephrotic syndrome.

Rarely, ascitic fluid may be *mucinous* in character, suggesting either pseudomyxoma peritonei (Chap. 291) or rarely a colloid carcinoma of the stomach or colon with peritoneal implants.

On occasion, ascites may develop as a seemingly isolated finding in the absence of a clinically evident underlying disease. Then, a careful analysis of ascitic fluid may indicate the direction the evaluation should take. A useful framework for the workup starts with an analysis of whether the fluid is classified as a high (transudate) or low (exudate) gradient fluid. *High-gradient (transudative) ascites* of unclear etiology is most often due to occult cirrhosis, right-sided venous hypertension raising hepatic sinusoidal pressure, Budd-Chiari syndrome, or massive hepatic metastases. Cirrhosis with well-preserved liver function (normal albumin) resulting in ascites is invariably associated with significant portal hypertension (Chap. 301). Evaluation should include liver function tests and a hepatic imaging procedure (i.e., CT or ultrasound) to detect nodular changes in the liver suggesting portal hypertension. On occasion, a wedged hepatic venous pressure can be useful to document portal hypertension. Finally, if clinically indicated, a liver biopsy will confirm the diagnosis of cirrhosis and perhaps suggest its etiology. Other etiologies may result in hepatic venous congestion and resultant ascites. Right-sided cardiac valvular disease and particularly constrictive pericarditis should raise a high index of suspicion and may require cardiac imaging and cardiac catheterization for definitive diagnosis. Hepatic vein thrombosis is evaluated by visualizing the hepatic veins with imaging techniques (Doppler ultrasound, angiography, CT scans, MRI) to demonstrate obliteration, thrombosis, or obstruction by tumor. Uncommonly, transudative ascites may be associated with benign tumors of the ovary, particularly fibroma (Meigs' syndrome) with ascites and hydrothorax.

Low-gradient (exudative) ascites should initiate an evaluation for primary peritoneal processes, most importantly infection and tumor. Tuberculous peritonitis (Table 44-1) is best diagnosed by peritoneal biopsy, either percutaneously or via laparoscopy. Histologic examination invariably shows granulomata that may contain acid-fast bacilli. Since cultures of peritoneal fluid and biopsies for tuberculosis may require 6 weeks, characteristic histology with appropriate stains allows antituberculosis therapy to be started promptly. Similarly, the diagnosis of peritoneal seeding by tumor can usually be made by cytologic analysis of peritoneal fluid or by peritoneal biopsy if cytology is negative. Appropriate diagnostic studies can then be undertaken to determine the nature and site of the primary tumor. Pancreatic ascites (Table 44-1) is invariably associated with an extravasation of pancreatic fluid from the pancreatic ductal system, most commonly from a leaking pseudocyst. Ultrasound or CT examination of the pancreas followed by visualization of the pancreatic duct by direct cannulation [viz., endoscopic retrograde cholangiopancreatography (ERCP)] usually discloses the site of leakage and permits resective surgery to be carried out.

An analysis of the physiologic and metabolic factors involved in the production of ascites (detailed in Chap. 301), coupled with a complete evaluation of the nature of the ascitic fluid, invariably discloses the etiology of the ascites and permits appropriate therapy to be instituted.

ACKNOWLEDGMENT

Dr. Kurt J. Isselbacher was the co-author of this chapter in previous editions.

FURTHER READINGS

LIPSKY MS, STERNBACH MR: Evaluation and initial management of patients with ascites. Am Fam Physician 54:1327, 1996

MCHUTCHISON JG: Differential diagnosis of ascites. Semin Liver Dis 17:191, 1997

PARSONS SL et al: Malignant ascites. Br J Surg 83:6, 1996

PINTO PC et al: Large volume paracentesis in nonedematous patients with tense ascites: Its effect on intravascular volume. Hepatology 8:207, 1988

RUNYON BA: Management of adult patients with ascites due to cirrhosis. Hepatology 39:841, 2004

SECTION 7 — ALTERATIONS IN RENAL AND URINARY TRACT FUNCTION

45 Azotemia and Urinary Abnormalities

Bradley M. Denker, Barry M. Brenner

Normal kidney functions occur through numerous cellular processes to maintain body homeostasis. Disturbances in any of these functions can lead to a constellation of abnormalities that may be detrimental to survival. The clinical manifestations of these disorders will depend upon the pathophysiology of the renal injury and will often be initially identified as a complex of symptoms, abnormal physical findings, and laboratory changes that together make possible the identification of specific syndromes. These renal syndromes (Table 45-1) may arise as the consequence of a systemic illness or can occur as a primary renal disease. Nephrologic syndromes usually consist of several elements that reflect the underlying pathologic processes. The duration and severity of the disease will affect these findings and typically include one or more of the following: (1) disturbances in urine volume (oliguria, anuria, polyuria); (2) abnormalities of urine sediment [red blood cells (RBC); white blood cells, casts, and crystals]; (3) abnormal excretion of serum proteins (proteinuria); (4) reduction in glomerular filtration rate (GFR) (azotemia); (5) presence of hypertension and/or expanded total body fluid volume (edema); (6) electrolyte abnormalities; or (7) in some syndromes, fever/pain. The combination of these findings should permit identification of one of the major nephrologic syndromes (Table 45-1) and will allow differential diagnoses to be narrowed and the appropriate diagnostic evaluation and therapeutic course to be determined. Each of these syndromes and their associated diseases are discussed in more detail in subsequent chapters. This chapter will focus on several aspects of renal abnormalities that are critically important to distinguishing among these processes: (1) reduction in GFR leading to azotemia, (2) alterations of the urinary sediment and/or protein excretion, and (3) abnormalities of urinary volume.

TABLE 45-1   INITIAL CLINICAL AND LABORATORY DATA BASE FOR DEFINING MAJOR SYNDROMES IN NEPHROLOGY

Syndromes	Important Clues to Diagnosis	Findings That Are Common	Location of Discussion of Disease-Causing Syndrome
Acute or rapidly progressive renal failure	Anuria Oliguria Documented recent decline in GFR	Hypertension, hematuria Proteinuria, pyuria Casts, edema	Chaps. 273, 277, 279, 283
Acute nephritis	Hematuria, RBC casts Azotemia, oliguria Edema, hypertension	Proteinuria Pyuria Circulatory congestion	Chap. 277
Chronic renal failure	Azotemia for >3 months Prolonged symptoms or signs of uremia Symptoms or signs of renal osteodystrophy Kidneys reduced in size bilaterally Broad casts in urinary sediment	Proteinuria Casts Polyuria, nocturia Edema, hypertension Electrolyte disorders	Chaps. 272, 274
Nephrotic syndrome	Proteinuria >3.5 g per 1.73 m^2 per 24 h Hypoalbuminemia Edema Hyperlipidemia	Casts Lipiduria	Chap. 277
Asymptomatic urinary abnormalities	Hematuria Proteinuria (below nephrotic range) Sterile pyuria, casts		Chap. 277
Urinary tract infection/pyelonephritis	Bacteriuria >10^5 colonies per milliliter Other infectious agent documented in urine Pyuria, leukocyte casts Frequency, urgency Bladder tenderness, flank tenderness	Hematuria Mild azotemia Mild proteinuria Fever	Chap. 282
Renal tubule defects	Electrolyte disorders Polyuria, nocturia Renal calcification Large kidneys Renal transport defects	Hematuria "Tubular" proteinuria (<1 g/24 h) Enuresis	Chaps. 278, 279
Hypertension	Systolic/diastolic hypertension	Proteinuria Casts Azotemia	Chaps. 241, 280
Nephrolithiasis	Previous history of stone passage or removal Previous history of stone seen by x-ray Renal colic	Hematuria Pyuria Frequency, urgency	Chap. 281
Urinary tract obstruction	Azotemia, oliguria, anuria Polyuria, nocturia, urinary retention Slowing of urinary stream Large prostate, large kidneys Flank tenderness, full bladder after voiding	Hematuria Pyuria Enuresis, dysuria	Chap. 283

Note: GFR; glomerular filtration rate; RBC, red blood cell.

AZOTEMIA

ASSESSMENT OF GLOMERULAR FILTRATION RATE

Monitoring the GFR is important in both the hospital and outpatient settings, and several different methodologies are available (discussed below). In most acute clinical circumstances a measured GFR is not available, and the serum creatinine level is used to estimate the GFR in order to supply appropriate doses of renally excreted drugs and to follow short-term changes in GFR. Serum creatinine is the most widely used marker for GFR, and the GFR is related directly to the urine creatinine excretion and inversely to the serum creatinine (U_{Cr}/P_{Cr}). The creatinine clearance is calculated from these measurements for a defined time period (usually 24 h) and is expressed in mL/min. Based upon this relationship and some important caveats (discussed below), the GFR will fall in roughly inverse proportion to the rise in P_{Cr}. Failure to account for GFR reductions in drug dosing can lead to significant morbidity and mortality from drug toxicities (e.g., digoxin, aminoglycosides). In the outpatient setting, the serum creatinine is often used as a surrogate for GFR (although much less accurate; see below). In patients with chronic progressive renal disease there is an approximately linear relationship between $1/P_{Cr}$ and time. The slope of this line will remain constant for an individual patient, and when values are obtained that do not fall on this line, an investigation for a superimposed acute process (e.g., volume depletion, drug reaction) should be initiated. It should be emphasized that the signs and symptoms of uremia will develop at significantly different levels of serum creatinine depending upon the patient (size, age, and sex), the underlying renal disease, existence of concurrent diseases, and true GFR. In general, patients do not develop symptomatic uremia until renal insufficiency is usually quite severe (GFR < 15 mL/min).

A reduced GFR leads to retention of nitrogenous waste products (azotemia) such as urea and creatinine. Azotemia may result from reduced renal perfusion, intrinsic renal disease, or postrenal processes (ureteral obstruction; see below and **Fig. 45-1**). Precise determination of GFR is problematic as both commonly measured indices (urea and creatinine) have characteristics that affect their accuracy as markers of clearance. Urea clearance may significantly underestimate GFR because of tubule urea reabsorption. Creatinine is derived from muscle metabolism of creatine, and its generation varies little from day to day. Creatinine is useful for estimating GFR because it is a small, freely filtered solute. However, serum creatinine levels can increase acutely from dietary ingestion of cooked meat, and creatinine can be secreted into the proximal tubule through an organic cation pathway, leading to overestimation of the GFR. There are many clinical settings where a creatinine clearance is not available, and decisions concerning drug dosing must be made based on the serum creatinine. Two formulas are widely used to estimate GFR: (1) Cockcroft-Gault, which accounts for age and muscle mass (this value should be multiplied by 0.85 for women, since a lower fraction of the body weight is composed of muscle):

$$\frac{\text{Creatinine}}{\text{clearance (mL/min)}} = \frac{(140 - \text{age}) \times \text{lean body weight (kg)}}{\text{plasma creatinine (mg/dL)} \times 72}$$

and (2) MDRD (modification of diet in renal disease):

$$\text{GFR (mL/min per 1.73 m}^2) = 186.3 \times P_{Cr} \, (e^{-1.154}) \times \text{age} \, (e^{-0.203})$$
$$\times (0.742 \text{ if female}) \times (1.21 \text{ if black}).$$

FIGURE 45-1 Approach to the patient with azotemia. WBC, white blood cell; RBC, red blood cell; GBM, glomerular basement membrane.

Although more cumbersome than Cockcroft-Gault, the MDRD equation is felt to be more accurate, and numerous websites are available for making the calculation (*www.kidney.org/professionals/kdoqi/ gfr_calculator.cfm*).

The gradual loss of muscle from chronic illness, chronic use of glucocorticoids, or malnutrition can mask significant changes in GFR with small or imperceptible changes in serum creatinine concentration. More accurate determinations of GFR are available using inulin clearance or radionuclide-labeled markers such as ^{125}I-iothalamate or EDTA. These methods are highly accurate due to precise quantitation and the absence of any renal reabsorption/secretion and should be used to follow GFR in patients in whom creatinine is not likely to be a reliable indicator (patients with decreased muscle mass secondary to age, malnutrition, concurrent illnesses). (See also Table 274-2.) Cystatin C is a member of the cystatin superfamily of cysteine protease inhibitors and is produced at a relatively constant rate from all nucleated cells. Cystatin C production is not affected by diet or nutritional status and may provide a more sensitive indicator of GFR than the plasma creatinine concentration. However, it remains to be validated in many clinical settings.

APPROACH TO THE PATIENT:
Azotemia

Once it has been established that GFR is reduced, the physician must decide if this represents acute or chronic renal injury. The clinical situa-

tion, history, and laboratory data often make this an easy distinction. However, the laboratory abnormalities characteristic of chronic renal failure, including anemia, hypocalcemia, and hyperphosphatemia, are often also present in patients presenting with acute renal failure. Radiographic evidence of renal osteodystrophy (Chap. 274) would be seen only in chronic renal failure but is a very late finding, and these patients are usually on dialysis. The urinalysis and renal ultrasound can occasionally facilitate distinguishing acute from chronic renal failure. An approach to the evaluation of azotemic patients is shown in Fig. 45-1. Patients with advanced chronic renal insufficiency often have some proteinuria, nonconcentrated urine (isosthenuria; isoosmotic with plasma), and small kidneys on ultrasound, characterized by increased echogenicity and cortical thinning. Treatment should be directed toward slowing the progression of renal disease and providing symptomatic relief for edema, acidosis, anemia, and hyperphosphatemia, as discussed in Chap. 274. Acute renal failure (Chap. 273) can result from processes affecting renal blood flow (prerenal azotemia), intrinsic renal diseases (affecting small vessels, glomeruli, or tubules), or postrenal processes (obstruction to urine flow in ureters, bladder, or urethra) (Chap. 283).

Prerenal Failure Decreased renal perfusion accounts for 40–80% of acute renal failure and, if appropriately treated, is readily reversible. The etiologies of prerenal azotemia include any cause of decreased circulating blood volume (gastrointestinal hemorrhage, burns, diarrhea, diuretics), volume sequestration (pancreatitis, peritonitis, rhabdomyolysis), or decreased effective arterial volume (cardiogenic shock, sepsis). Renal perfusion can also be affected by reductions in cardiac output from peripheral vasodilatation (sepsis, drugs) or profound renal vasoconstriction [severe heart failure, hepatorenal syndrome, drugs such as nonsteroidal anti-inflammatory drugs (NSAIDs)]. True, or "effective," arterial hypovolemia leads to a fall in mean arterial pressure, which in turn triggers a series of neural and humoral responses that include activation of the sympathetic nervous and renin-angiotensin-aldosterone systems and ADH release. GFR is maintained by prostaglandin-mediated relaxation of afferent arterioles and angiotensin II–mediated constriction of efferent arterioles. Once the mean arterial pressure falls below 80 mmHg, there is a steep decline in GFR.

Blockade of prostaglandin production by NSAIDs can result in severe vasoconstriction and acute renal failure. Angiotensin-converting enzyme (ACE) inhibitors decrease efferent arteriolar tone and in turn decrease glomerular capillary perfusion pressure. Patients on NSAIDs and/or ACE inhibitors are most susceptible to hemodynamically mediated acute renal failure when blood volume is reduced for any reason. Patients with bilateral renal artery stenosis (or stenosis in a solitary kidney) are dependent upon efferent arteriolar vasoconstriction for maintenance of glomerular filtration pressure and are particularly susceptible to precipitous decline in GFR when given ACE inhibitors.

Prolonged renal hypoperfusion can lead to acute tubular necrosis (ATN; an intrinsic renal disease discussed below). The urinalysis and urinary electrolytes can be useful in distinguishing prerenal azotemia from ATN (Table 45-2). The urine of patients with prerenal azotemia can be predicted from the stimulatory actions of norepinephrine, angiotensin II, ADH, and low tubule fluid flow rate on salt and water reabsorption. In prerenal conditions, the tubules are intact leading to a concentrated urine (>500 mosm), avid Na retention (urine Na concentration < 20 mM/L; fractional excretion of Na < 1%), and $U_{Cr}/P_{Cr} > 40$ (Table 45-2). The prerenal urine sediment is usually normal or has occasional hyaline and granular casts, while the sediment of ATN is usually filled with cellular debris and dark (muddy brown) granular casts.

Postrenal Azotemia Urinary tract obstruction accounts for <5% of cases of acute renal failure, but it is usually reversible and must be ruled out early in the evaluation (Fig. 45-1). Since a single kidney is capable of adequate clearance, acute renal failure from obstruction requires obstruction at the urethra or bladder outlet, bilateral ureteral obstruction, or unilateral obstruction in a patient with a single functioning kidney. Obstruction is usually diagnosed by the presence of ureteral and renal pelvic dilatation on renal ultrasound. However, early in the course of obstruction or if the ureters are unable to dilate (such as encasement by pelvic tumors or periureteral), the ultrasound examination may be negative. The specific urologic conditions that cause obstruction are discussed in Chap. 283.

Intrinsic Renal Disease When prerenal and postrenal azotemia have been excluded as etiologies of renal failure, an intrinsic parenchymal renal disease is present. Intrinsic renal disease can arise from processes involving large renal vessels, intrarenal microvasculature and glomeruli, or tubulointerstitium. Ischemic and toxic ATN account for ~90% of acute intrinsic renal failure. As outlined in Fig. 45-1, the clinical setting and urinalysis are helpful in separating the possible etiologies of acute intrinsic renal failure. Prerenal azotemia and ATN are part of a spectrum of renal hypoperfusion; evidence of structural tubule injury is present in ATN, whereas prompt reversibility occurs with prerenal azotemia upon restoration of adequate renal perfusion. Thus, ATN can often be distinguished from prerenal azotemia by urinalysis and urine electrolyte composition (Table 45-2 and Fig. 45-1). Ischemic ATN is observed most frequently in patients who have undergone major surgery, trauma, severe hypovolemia, overwhelming sepsis, or extensive burns. Nephrotoxic ATN complicates the administration of many common medications, usually by inducing a combination of intrarenal vasoconstriction, direct tubule toxicity, and/or tubule obstruction. The kidney is vulnerable to toxic injury by virtue of its rich blood supply (25% of cardiac output) and its ability to concentrate and metabolize toxins. A diligent search for hypotension and nephrotoxins will usually uncover the specific etiology of ATN.

Discontinuation of nephrotoxins and stabilizing blood pressure will often suffice without the need for dialysis while the tubules recover. An extensive list of potential drugs and toxins implicated in ATN can be found in Chap. 273.

Processes that involve the tubules and interstitium can lead to acute renal failure. These include drug-induced interstitial nephritis (especially antibiotics, NSAIDs, and diuretics), severe infections (both bacterial and viral), systemic diseases (e.g., systemic lupus erythematosus), or infiltrative disorders (e.g., sarcoid, lymphoma, or leukemia). A list of drugs associated with allergic interstitial nephritis can be found in Chap. 279. The urinalysis usually shows mild to moderate proteinuria, hematuria, and pyuria (~75% of cases) and occasionally white blood cell casts. The finding of RBC casts in interstitial nephritis has been reported but should prompt a search for glomerular diseases (Fig. 45-1). Occasionally renal biopsy will be needed to distinguish among these possibilities. The finding of eosinophils in the urine is suggestive of allergic interstitial nephritis or atheroembolic renal disease and is optimally observed by using a Hansel stain. The absence of eosinophiluria, however, does not exclude these possible etiologies.

Occlusion of large renal vessels including arteries and veins is an uncommon cause of acute renal failure. A significant reduction in GFR by this mechanism suggests bilateral processes or a unilateral process in a patient with a single functioning kidney. Renal arteries can be occluded with atheroemboli, thromboemboli, in situ thrombosis, aortic dissection, or vasculitis. Atheroembolic renal failure can occur spontaneously but is most often associated with recent aortic instrumentation. The emboli are cholesterol-rich and lodge in medium and small renal arteries, leading to an eosinophil-rich inflammatory reaction. Patients with atheroembolic acute renal failure often have a normal urinalysis, but the urine may contain eosinophils and casts. The diagnosis can be confirmed by renal biopsy, but this is often unnecessary when other stigmata of atheroemboli are present (livedo reticularis, distal peripheral infarcts, eosinophilia). Renal artery thrombosis may lead to mild proteinuria and hematuria, whereas renal vein thrombosis typically induces heavy proteinuria and hematuria. These vascular complications often require angiography for confirmation and are discussed in Chap. 280.

Diseases of glomeruli (glomerulonephritis or vasculitis) and the renal microvasculature (hemolytic uremic syndromes, thrombotic thrombocytopenic purpura, or malignant hypertension) usually present with various combinations of glomerular injury: proteinuria, hematuria, reduced GFR, and alterations of Na excretion leading to hypertension, edema, and circulatory congestion (acute nephritic syndrome). These findings may occur as primary renal diseases or as renal manifestations of systemic diseases. The clinical setting and other laboratory data will help distinguish primary renal from systemic diseases. The finding of RBC casts in the urine is an indication for early renal biopsy (Fig. 45-1) as the pathologic pattern has important implications for diagnosis, prognosis, and treatment. Hematuria without RBC casts can also be an indication of glomerular disease, and this evaluation is summarized in Fig. 45-2. A detailed discussion of glomerulonephritis and diseases of the microvasculature can be found in Chap. 277.

Oliguria and Anuria Oliguria refers to a 24-h urine output of <500 mL, and anuria is the complete absence of urine formation (<50 mL). Anuria can be caused by total urinary tract obstruction, total renal artery or vein occlusion, and shock (manifested by severe hypotension and intense renal vasoconstriction). Cortical necrosis, ATN, and rapidly progressive glomerulonephritis can occasionally cause anuria. Oliguria can accompany any cause of acute renal failure and carries a more serious prognosis for renal recovery in all conditions except prerenal azotemia. Nonoliguria refers to urine output >500 mL/d in patients with acute or chronic azotemia. With nonoliguric ATN, disturbances of potassium and hydrogen balance are less severe than in oliguric patients, and recovery to normal renal function is usually more rapid.

TABLE 45-2 LABORATORY FINDINGS IN ACUTE RENAL FAILURE

Index	Prerenal Azotemia	Oliguric Acute Renal Failure
BUN/P_{Cr} Ratio	>20:1	10–15:1
Urine sodium (U_{Na}), meq/L	<20	>40
Urine osmolality, mosmol/L H_2O	>500	<350
Fractional excretion of sodium	<1%	>2%
$FE_{Na} = \dfrac{U_{Na} \times P_{Cr} \times 100}{P_{Na} \times U_{Cr}}$		
Urine/plasma creatinine (U_{Cr}/P_{Cr})	>40	<20

Note: BUN, Blood urea nitrogen; P_{Cr}, plasma creatinine; U_{Na}, urine sodium concentration; P_{Na}, plasma sodium concentration; U_{Cr}, urine creatinine concentration.

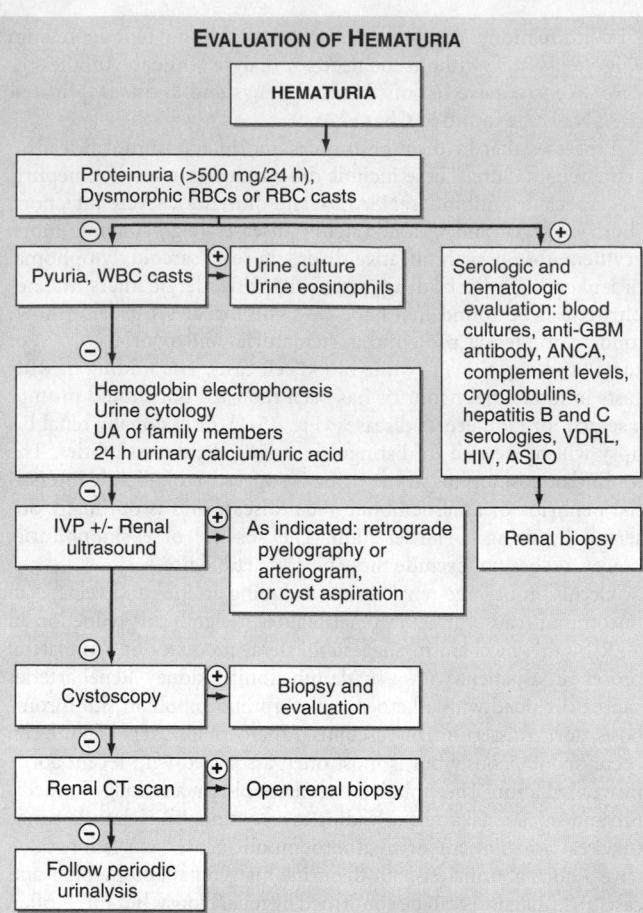

EVALUATION OF HEMATURIA

```
                    HEMATURIA
                        │
                        ▼
            Proteinuria (>500 mg/24 h),
            Dysmorphic RBCs or RBC casts
              │ (−)                │ (+)
              ▼                    ▼
    Pyuria, WBC casts  (+)   Serologic and
              │────────►  Urine culture   hematologic
              │           Urine eosinophils   evaluation: blood
              │ (−)                        cultures, anti-GBM
              ▼                            antibody, ANCA,
    Hemoglobin electrophoresis            complement levels,
    Urine cytology                        cryoglobulins,
    UA of family members                  hepatitis B and C
    24 h urinary calcium/uric acid        serologies, VDRL,
              │                           HIV, ASLO
              │ (−)                        │
              ▼                            ▼
    IVP +/- Renal   (+)   As indicated: retrograde    Renal biopsy
    ultrasound  ────►  pyelography or
              │           arteriogram,
              │           or cyst aspiration
              │ (−)
              ▼
    Cystoscopy   (+)   Biopsy and
              │────►   evaluation
              │ (−)
              ▼
    Renal CT scan  (+)   Open renal biopsy
              │──────►
              │ (−)
              ▼
    Follow periodic
    urinalysis
```

FIGURE 45-2 Approach to the patient with hematuria. RBC, red blood cell; WBC, white blood cell; GBM, glomerular basement membrane; ANCA, antineutrophil cytoplasmic antibody; VDRL, venereal disease research laboratory; ASLO, antistreptolysin O; UA, urinalysis; IVP, intravenous pyelography; CT, computed tomography.

ABNORMALITIES OF THE URINE

PROTEINURIA

The evaluation of proteinuria is shown schematically in **Fig. 45-3** and is typically initiated after detection of proteinuria by dipstick examination. The dipstick measurement detects mostly albumin and gives false-positive results when pH > 7.0 and the urine is very concentrated or contaminated with blood. A very dilute urine may obscure significant proteinuria on dipstick examination, and proteinuria that is not predominantly albumin will be missed. This is particularly important for the detection of Bence-Jones proteins in the urine of patients with multiple myeloma. Tests to measure total urine concentration accurately rely on precipitation with sulfosalicylic or trichloracetic acids. Currently, ultrasensitive dipsticks are available to measure microalbuminuria (30–300 mg/d), an early marker of glomerular disease that has been shown to predict glomerular injury in early diabetic nephropathy (Fig. 45-3).

The magnitude of proteinuria and the protein composition of the urine depend upon the mechanism of renal injury leading to protein losses. Both charge and size selectivity normally prevent virtually all plasma albumin, globulins, and other large-molecular-weight proteins from crossing the glomerular wall. However, if this barrier is disrupted, there can be leakage of plasma proteins into the urine (glomerular proteinuria; Fig. 45-3). Smaller proteins (<20 kDa) are freely filtered but are readily reabsorbed by the proximal tubule. Normal individuals excrete <150 mg/d of total protein and <30 mg/d of albumin. The remainder of the protein in the urine is secreted by the tubules (Tamm-Horsfall, IgA, and urokinase) or represents small amounts of filtered β_2-microglobulin, apoproteins, enzymes, and peptide hormones. Another mechanism of proteinuria occurs when there is excessive production of an abnormal protein that exceeds the capacity of the tubule for reabsorption. This most commonly occurs with plasma cell dyscrasias such as multiple myeloma, amyloidosis, and lymphomas that are associated with monoclonal production of immunoglobulin light chains.

The normal glomerular endothelial cell forms a barrier composed of pores of ~100 nm that hold back blood cells but offer little impediment to passage of most proteins. The glomerular basement membrane traps most large proteins (>100 kDa), while the foot processes of epithelial cells (podocytes) cover the urinary side of the glomerular basement membrane and produce a series of narrow channels (slit diaphragms) to normally allow molecular passage of small solutes and water but not proteins. Some glomerular diseases, such as minimal change disease, cause fusion of glomerular epithelial cell foot processes, resulting in predominantly "selective" (Fig. 45-3) loss of albumin. Other glomerular diseases can present with disruption of the basement membrane and slit diaphragms (e.g., by immune complex deposition), resulting in losses of albumin and other plasma proteins. The fusion of foot processes causes increased pressure across the capillary basement membrane, resulting in areas with larger pore sizes. The combination of increased pressure and larger pores results in significant proteinuria ("nonselective"; Fig. 45-3).

When the total daily excretion of protein is >3.5 g, there is often associated hypoalbuminemia, hyperlipidemia, and edema (nephrotic syndrome; Fig. 45-3). However, total daily urinary protein excretion >3.5 g can occur without the other features of the nephrotic syndrome in a variety of other renal diseases (Fig. 45-3). Plasma cell dyscrasias (multiple myeloma) can be associated with large amounts of excreted light chains in the urine, which may not be detected by dipstick (which detects mostly albumin). The light chains produced from these disorders are filtered by the glomerulus and overwhelm the reabsorptive capacity of the proximal tubule. A sulfosalicylic acid precipitate that is out of proportion to the dipstick estimate is suggestive of light chains (Bence Jones protein), and light chains typically redissolve upon warming of the precipitate. Renal failure from these disorders occurs through a variety of mechanisms including tubule obstruction (cast nephropathy) and light chain deposition.

Hypoalbuminemia in nephrotic syndrome occurs through excessive urinary losses and increased proximal tubule catabolism of filtered albumin. Hepatic rates of albumin synthesis are increased although not to levels sufficient to prevent hypoalbuminemia. Edema forms from renal sodium retention and from reduced plasma oncotic pressure, which favors fluid movement from capillaries to interstitium. The mechanisms designed to correct the decrease in effective intravascular volume contribute to edema formation in some patients. These mechanisms include activation of the renin-angiotensin system, antidiuretic hormone, and the sympathetic nervous system, all of which promote excessive renal salt and water reabsorption.

The severity of edema correlates with the degree of hypoalbuminemia and is modified by other factors such as heart disease or peripheral vascular disease. The diminished plasma oncotic pressure and urinary losses of regulatory proteins appear to stimulate hepatic lipoprotein synthesis. The resulting hyperlipidemia results in lipid bodies (fatty casts, oval fat bodies) in the urine. Other proteins are lost in the urine, leading to a variety of metabolic disturbances. These include thyroxine-binding globulin, cholecalciferol-binding protein, transferrin, and metal-binding proteins. A hypercoagulable state frequently accompanies severe nephrotic syndrome due to urinary losses of antithrombin III, reduced serum levels of proteins S and C, hyperfibrinogenemia, and enhanced platelet aggregation. Some patients develop severe IgG deficiency with resulting defects in immunity. Many diseases (some listed in Fig. 45-3) and drugs can cause the nephrotic syndrome, and a complete list can be found in Chap. 277.

HEMATURIA, PYURIA, AND CASTS

Isolated hematuria without proteinuria, other cells, or casts is often indicative of bleeding from the urinary tract. Normal red blood cell excretion is up to 2 million RBCs per day. Hematuria is defined as two to five RBCs per high-power field (HPF) and can be detected by dipstick. Common causes of isolated hematuria include stones, neoplasms, tuberculosis, trauma, and prostatitis. Gross hematuria with blood clots is

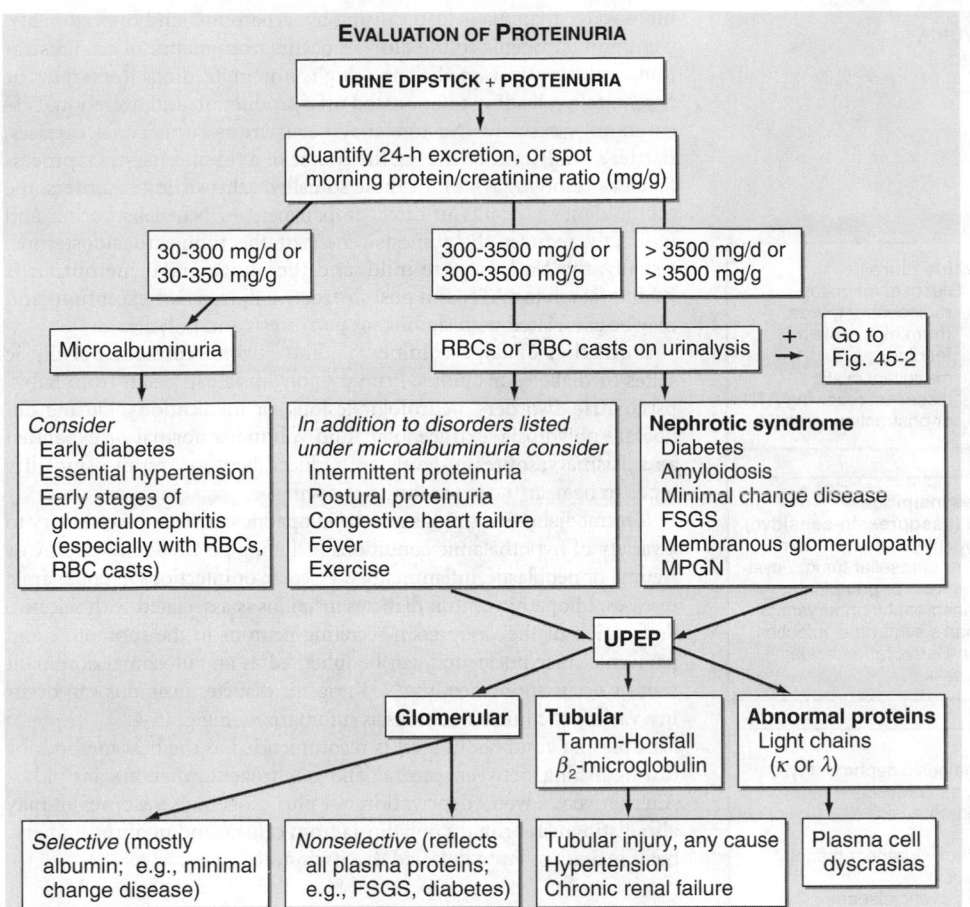

FIGURE 45-3 Approach to the patient with proteinuria. Investigation of proteinuria is often initiated by a positive dipstick on routine urinalysis. Conventional dipsticks detect predominantly albumin and cannot detect urinary albumin levels of 30–300 mg/d. However, more exact determination of proteinuria should employ a 24-h urine collection or a spot morning protein/creatinine ratio (mg/g). The pattern of proteinuria on UPEP (urine protein electrophoresis) can be classified as "glomerular," "tubular," or "abnormal" depending upon the origin of the urine proteins. Glomerular proteinuria is due to abnormal glomerular permeability. "Tubular proteins" such as Tamm-Horsfall are normally produced by the renal tubule and shed into the urine. Abnormal circulating proteins such as kappa or lambda light chains are readily filtered because of their small size. RBC, red blood cell; FSGS, focal segmental glomerulosclerosis; MPGN, membranoproliferative glomerulonephritis.

almost never indicative of glomerular bleeding; rather, it suggests a posttrenal source in the urinary collecting system. Evaluation of patients presenting with microscopic hematuria is outlined in Fig. 45-2. A single urinalysis with hematuria is common and can result from menstruation, viral illness, allergy, exercise, or mild trauma. Annual urinalysis of servicemen over a 10-year period showed an incidence of 38%. However, persistent or significant hematuria (>three RBCs/HPF on three urinalyses, or a single urinalysis with >100 RBCs, or gross hematuria) identified significant renal or urologic lesions in 9.1%. Even patients who are chronically anticoagulated should be investigated as outlined in Fig. 45-2. The suspicion for urogenital neoplasms in patients with isolated painless hematuria (nondysmorphic RBCs) increases with age. Neoplasms are rare in the pediatric population, and isolated hematuria is more likely to be "idiopathic" or associated with a congenital anomaly. Hematuria with pyuria and bacteriuria is typical of infection and should be treated with antibiotics after appropriate cultures. Acute cystitis or urethritis in women can cause gross hematuria. Hypercalciuria and hyperuricosuria are also risk factors for unexplained isolated hematuria in both children and adults. In some of these patients (50–60%), reducing calcium and uric acid excretion through dietary interventions can eliminate the microscopic hematuria.

Isolated microscopic hematuria can be a manifestation of glomerular diseases. The RBCs of glomerular origin are often dysmorphic when ex-amined by phase-contrast microscopy. Irregular shapes of RBCs may also occur due to pH and osmolarity changes produced along the distal nephron. There is, however, significant observer variability in detecting dysmorphic RBCs. The most common etiologies of isolated glomerular hematuria are IgA nephropathy, hereditary nephritis, and thin basement membrane disease. IgA nephropathy and hereditary nephritis can lead to episodic gross hematuria. A family history of renal failure is often present in patients with hereditary nephritis, and patients with thin basement membrane disease often have other family members with microscopic hematuria. A renal biopsy is needed for the definitive diagnosis of these disorders, which are discussed in more detail in Chap. 277. Hematuria with dysmorphic RBCs, RBC casts, and protein excretion >500 mg/d is virtually diagnostic of glomerulonephritis. RBC casts form as RBCs that enter the tubule fluid become trapped in a cylindrical mold of gelled Tamm-Horsfall protein. Even in the absence of azotemia, these patients should undergo serologic evaluation and renal biopsy as outlined in Fig. 45-2.

Isolated pyuria is unusual since inflammatory reactions in the kidney or collecting system are also associated with hematuria. The presence of bacteria suggests infection, and white blood cell casts with bacteria are indicative of pyelonephritis. White blood cells and/or white blood cell casts may also be seen in tubulointerstitial processes such as interstitial nephritis, systemic lupus erythematosus, and transplant rejection. In chronic renal diseases, degenerated cellular casts called *waxy casts* can be seen in the urine. *Broad casts* are thought to arise in the dilated tubules of enlarged nephrons that have undergone compensatory hypertrophy in response to reduced renal mass (i.e., chronic renal failure). A mixture of broad casts typically seen with chronic renal failure together with cellular casts and RBCs may be seen in smoldering processes such as chronic glomerulonephritis.

ABNORMALITIES OF URINE VOLUME

The volume of urine produced varies depending upon the fluid intake, renal function, and physiologic demands of the individual. See "Azotemia," above, for discussion of decreased (oliguria) or absent urine production (anuria). The physiology of water formation and renal water conservation are discussed in Chap. 272.

POLYURIA

By history, it is often difficult for patients to distinguish urinary frequency (often of small volumes) from polyuria (>3 L/d), and a 24-h urine collection is needed for evaluation (Fig. 45-4). Polyuria results from two potential mechanisms: (1) excretion of nonabsorbable solutes (such as glucose) or (2) excretion of water (usually from a defect in ADH production or renal responsiveness). To distinguish a solute diuresis from a water diuresis and to determine if the diuresis is appropriate for the clinical circumstances, a urine osmolality is measured.

EVALUATION OF POLYURIA

POLYURIA (>3 L/24 h)

Urine osmolality

< 250 mosmol   > 300 mosmol

Solute diuresis
Glucose, mannitol, radiocontrast, urea (from high protein feeding), medullary cystic diseases, resolving ATN, or obstruction, diuretics

History, low serum sodium

Water deprivation test or ADH level

Primary polydipsia
Psychogenic
Hypothalamic disease
Drugs (thioridazine, chlorpromazine, anticholinergic agents)

Diabetes insipidus
Central (vasopressin-sensitive)
posthypophysectomy, trauma, supra- or intrasellar tumor / cyst histiocystosis or granuloma, encroachment by aneurysm, Sheehan's syndrome, infection, Guillain-Barré, fat embolus, empty sella

Nephrogenic (vasopressin-insensitive)
Acquired tubular diseases: pyelonephritis, analgesic nephropathy, multiple myeloma, amyloidosis, obstruction, sarcoidosis, hypercalcemia, hypokalemia, Sjögren's syndrome, sickle cell anemia
Drugs or toxins: lithium, demeclocycline, methoxyflurane, ethanol, diphenylhydantoin, propoxyphene, amphotericin
Congenital: hereditary, polycystic or medullary cystic disease

FIGURE 45-4 Approach to the patient with polyuria. ATN, acute tubular necrosis; ADH, antidiuretic hormone.

The average person excretes between 600 and 800 mosmol of solutes per day, primarily as urea and electrolytes. If the urine output is >3 L/d and the urine is dilute (<250 mosmol/L), then total mosmol excretion is normal and a water diuresis is present. This circumstance could arise from polydipsia, inadequate secretion of vasopressin (central diabetes insipidus), or failure of renal tubules to respond to vasopressin (nephrogenic diabetes insipidus). If the urine volume is >3 L/d and urine osmolality is >300 mosmol/L, then a solute diuresis is clearly present and a search for the responsible solute(s) is mandatory.

Excessive filtration of a poorly reabsorbed solute such as glucose, mannitol, or urea can depress reabsorption of NaCl and water in the proximal tubule and lead to enhanced excretion in the urine. Poorly controlled diabetes mellitus with glucosuria is the most common cause of a solute diuresis, leading to volume depletion and serum hypertonicity. Since the urine Na concentration is less than that of blood,

more water than Na is lost, causing hypernatremia and hypertonicity. Common iatrogenic solute diuresis occurs from mannitol administration, radiocontrast media, and high-protein feedings (enterally or parenterally), leading to increased urea production and excretion. Less commonly, excessive Na loss may occur from cystic renal diseases, Bartter's syndrome, or during the course of a tubulointerstitial process (such as resolving ATN). In these so-called salt-wasting disorders, the tubule damage results in direct impairment of Na reabsorption and indirectly reduces the responsiveness of the tubule to aldosterone. Usually, the Na losses are mild, and the obligatory urine output is <2 L/d (resolving ATN and postobstructive diuresis are exceptions and may be associated with significant natriuresis and polyuria).

Formation of large volumes of dilute urine represent polydipsic states or diabetes insipidus. Primary polydipsia can result from habit, psychiatric disorders, neurologic lesions, or medications. During deliberate polydipsia, extracellular fluid volume is normal or expanded and plasma vasopressin levels are reduced because serum osmolality tends to be near the lower limits of normal.

Central diabetes insipidus may be idiopathic in origin or secondary to a variety of hypothalamic conditions including posthypophysectomy or trauma or neoplastic, inflammatory, vascular, or infectious hypothalamic diseases. Idiopathic central diabetes insipidus is associated with selective destruction of the vasopressin-secreting neurons in the supraoptic and paraventricular nuclei and can be inherited as an autosomal dominant trait or occur spontaneously. Nephrogenic diabetes insipidus can occur in a variety of clinical situations as summarized in Fig. 45-4.

A plasma vasopressin level is recommended as the best method for distinguishing between central and nephrogenic diabetes insipidus. Alternatively, a water deprivation test plus exogenous vasopressin may also distinguish primary polydipsia from central and nephrogenic diabetes insipidus. **For a detailed discussion, see Chap. 334.**

FURTHER READINGS

ANDERSON S et al: Renal and systemic manifestations of glomerular disease, in *Brenner & Rector's The Kidney*, 7th ed, BM Brenner (ed). Philadelphia, Saunders, 2004, pp 1927–1954

BERL T, VERBALIS J: Pathophysiology of water metabolism, in *Brenner & Rector's The Kidney*, 7th ed, BM Brenner (ed). Philadelphia, Saunders, 2004, pp 857–920

KASISKE BL, KEANE WF: Laboratory assessment of renal disease: Clearance, urinalysis and renal biopsy, in *Brenner & Rector's The Kidney*, 7th ed, BM Brenner (ed). Philadelphia, Saunders, 2004, pp 1107–1150

KHADRA MH et al: A prospective analysis of 1,930 patients with hematuria to evaluate current diagnostic practice. J Urol 163:524, 2000

RODRIGO E et al: Measurement of renal function in pre-ESRD patients. Kidney Int Suppl 80:11, 2002

SASAKI S: Nephrogenic diabetes insipidus: Update of genetic and clinical aspects. Nephrol Dial Transplant 19:1351, 2004

SHRIER RW et al: Acute renal failure: Definitions, diagnosis, pathogenesis and therapy. J Clin Invest 114:5, 2004

46 Fluid and Electrolyte Disturbances
Gary G. Singer, Barry M. Brenner

SODIUM AND WATER

Composition of Body Fluids   Water is the most abundant constituent in the body, comprising approximately 50% of body weight in women and 60% in men. This difference is attributable to differences in the relative proportions of adipose tissue in men and women. Total body water is distributed in two major compartments: 55–75% is intracellular [intracellular fluid (ICF)], and 25–45% is extracellular [extracellular fluid (ECF)]. The ECF is further subdivided into intravascular (plasma water) and extravascular (interstitial) spaces in a ratio of 1:3.

The solute or particle concentration of a fluid is known as its *osmolality* and is expressed as milliosmoles per kilogram of water (mosmol/kg). Water crosses cell membranes to achieve osmotic equilibrium (ECF osmolality = ICF osmolality). The extracellular and intracellular solutes or osmoles are markedly different due to disparities in permeability and the presence of transporters and active pumps. The major ECF particles are Na^+ and its accompanying anions Cl^- and HCO_3^-, whereas K^+ and organic phosphate esters (ATP, creatine phosphate, and phospholipids) are the predominant ICF osmoles. Solutes that are restricted to the ECF or the ICF determine the *effective osmolality* (or *tonicity*) of that compartment. Since Na$^+$ is largely restricted to the extracellular compartment, total body Na$^+$ content is a reflection of ECF volume. Likewise, K$^+$ and its attendant anions are predominantly limited to the ICF and are necessary for normal cell function. Therefore, the number of intracellular particles is relatively constant, and a change in ICF osmolality is usually due to a change in ICF water content. However, in certain situations, brain cells can vary the number of intracellular solutes in order to defend against large water shifts. This process of *osmotic adaptation* is important in the defense of cell volume and occurs in chronic hyponatremia and hypernatremia. This response is mediated initially by transcellular shifts of K$^+$ and Na$^+$, followed by synthesis, import, or export of organic solutes (so-called osmolytes) such as inositol, betaine, and glutamine. During chronic hyponatremia, brain cells lose solutes, thereby defending cell volume and diminishing neurologic symptoms. The converse occurs during chronic hypernatremia. Certain solutes, such as urea, do not contribute to water shift across cell membranes and are known as *ineffective osmoles*.

Fluid movement between the intravascular and interstitial spaces occurs across the capillary wall and is determined by the Starling forces—capillary hydraulic pressure and colloid osmotic pressure. The transcapillary hydraulic pressure gradient exceeds the corresponding oncotic pressure gradient, thereby favoring the movement of plasma ultrafiltrate into the extravascular space. The return of fluid into the intravascular compartment occurs via lymphatic flow.

Water Balance   (See also Chap. 272) The normal plasma osmolality is 275–290 mosmol/kg and is kept within a narrow range by mechanisms capable of sensing a 1–2% change in tonicity. To maintain a steady state, water intake must equal water excretion. Disorders of water homeostasis result in hypo- or hypernatremia. Normal individuals have an obligate water loss consisting of urine, stool, and evaporation from the skin and respiratory tract. Gastrointestinal excretion is usually a minor component of total water output, except in patients with vomiting, diarrhea, or high enterostomy output states. Evaporative or insensitive water losses are important in the regulation of core body temperature. Obligatory renal water loss is mandated by the minimum solute excretion required to maintain a steady state. Normally, about 600 mosmols must be excreted per day, and since the maximal urine osmolality is 1200 mosmol/kg, a minimum urine output of 500 mL/d is required for neutral solute balance.

WATER INTAKE   The primary stimulus for water ingestion is *thirst*, mediated either by an increase in effective osmolality or a decrease in ECF volume or blood pressure. *Osmoreceptors*, located in the anterolateral hypothalamus, are stimulated by a rise in tonicity. Ineffective osmoles, such as urea and glucose, do not play a role in stimulating thirst. The average osmotic threshold for thirst is approximately 295 mosmol/kg and varies among individuals. Under normal circumstances, daily water intake exceeds physiologic requirements.

WATER EXCRETION   In contrast to the ingestion of water, its excretion is tightly regulated by physiologic factors. The principal determinant of renal water excretion is *arginine vasopressin* (AVP; formerly antidiuretic hormone), a polypeptide synthesized in the supraoptic and paraventricular nuclei of the hypothalamus and secreted by the posterior pituitary gland. The binding of AVP to V$_2$ receptors on the basolateral membrane of principal cells in the collecting duct activates adenylyl cyclase and initiates a sequence of events that leads to the insertion of water channels into the luminal membrane. These water channels that are specifically activated by AVP are encoded by the *aquaporin-2* gene (Chap. 334). The net effect is passive water reabsorption along an osmotic gradient from the lumen of the collecting duct to the hypertonic medullary interstitium. The major stimulus for AVP secretion is hypertonicity. Since the major ECF solutes are Na$^+$ salts, effective osmolality is primarily determined by the plasma Na$^+$ concentration. An increase or decrease in tonicity is sensed by hypothalamic osmoreceptors as a decrease or increase in cell volume, respectively, leading to enhancement or suppression of AVP secretion. The osmotic threshold for AVP release is 280–290 mos-

mol/kg, and the system is sufficiently sensitive that plasma osmolality varies by no more than 1–2%.

Nonosmotic factors that regulate AVP secretion include *effective circulating (arterial) volume*, nausea, pain, stress, hypoglycemia, pregnancy, and numerous drugs. The hemodynamic response is mediated by baroreceptors in the carotid sinus. The sensitivity of these receptors is significantly lower than that of the osmoreceptors. In fact, depletion of blood volume sufficient to result in a decreased mean arterial pressure is necessary to stimulate AVP release, whereas small changes in effective circulating volume have little effect.

To maintain homeostasis and a normal plasma Na$^+$ concentration, the ingestion of solute-free water must eventually lead to the loss of the same volume of electrolyte-free water. Three steps are required for the kidney to excrete a water load: (1) filtration and delivery of water (and electrolytes) to the diluting sites of the nephron; (2) active reabsorption of Na$^+$ and Cl$^-$ without water in the thick ascending limb of the loop of Henle (TALH) and, to a lesser extent, in the distal nephron; and (3) maintenance of a dilute urine due to impermeability of the collecting duct to water in the absence of AVP. Abnormalities of any of these steps can result in impaired free water excretion, and eventual hyponatremia.

Sodium Balance   Sodium is actively pumped out of cells by the Na$^+$, K$^+$-ATPase pump. As a result, 85–90% of all Na$^+$ is extracellular, and the ECF volume is a reflection of total body Na$^+$ content. Normal volume regulatory mechanisms ensure that Na$^+$ loss balances Na$^+$ gain. If this does not occur, conditions of Na$^+$ excess or deficit ensue and are manifest as edematous or hypovolemic states, respectively. It is important to distinguish between disorders of osmoregulation and disorders of volume regulation since water and Na$^+$ balance are regulated independently. Changes in Na$^+$ concentration generally reflect disturbed water homeostasis, whereas alterations in Na$^+$ content are manifest as ECF volume contraction or expansion and imply abnormal Na$^+$ balance.

SODIUM INTAKE   Individuals eating a typical western diet consume approximately 150 mmol of NaCl daily. This normally exceeds basal requirements. As noted above, sodium is the principal extracellular cation. Therefore, dietary intake of Na$^+$ results in ECF volume expansion, which in turn promotes enhanced renal Na$^+$ excretion to maintain steady state Na$^+$ balance.

SODIUM EXCRETION   (See also Chap. 272) The regulation of Na$^+$ excretion is multifactorial and is the major determinant of Na$^+$ balance. A Na$^+$ deficit or excess is manifest as a decreased or increased effective circulating volume, respectively. Changes in effective circulating volume tend to lead to parallel changes in glomerular filtration rate (GFR). However, tubule Na$^+$ reabsorption, and not GFR, is the major regulatory mechanism controlling Na$^+$ excretion. Almost two-thirds of filtered Na$^+$ is reabsorbed in the proximal convoluted tubule; this process is electroneutral and isoosmotic. Further reabsorption (25–30%) occurs in the TALH via the apical *Na$^+$-K$^+$-2Cl$^-$ co-transporter;* this is an active process and is also electroneutral. Distal convoluted tubule reabsorption of Na$^+$ (5%) is mediated by the *thiazide-sensitive Na$^+$-Cl$^-$ co-transporter.* Final Na$^+$ reabsorption occurs in the cortical and medullary collecting ducts, the amount excreted being reasonably equivalent to the amount ingested per day.

HYPOVOLEMIA

Etiology   True volume depletion, or hypovolemia, generally refers to a state of combined salt and water loss exceeding intake, leading to ECF volume contraction. The loss of Na$^+$ may be renal or extrarenal (Table 46-1).

RENAL   Many conditions are associated with excessive urinary NaCl and water losses, including diuretics. Pharmacologic diuretics inhibit specific pathways of Na$^+$ reabsorption along the nephron with a consequent increase in urinary Na$^+$ excretion. Enhanced filtration of nonreabsorbed solutes, such as glucose or urea, can also impair tubular reabsorption of Na$^+$ and water, leading to an osmotic or solute diuresis. This often occurs in poorly controlled diabetes mellitus and in patients receiving high-protein hyperalimentation. Mannitol is a diuretic

TABLE 46-1 CAUSES OF HYPOVOLEMIA

I. ECF volume contracted
  A. Extrarenal Na⁺ loss
    1. Gastrointestinal (vomiting, nasogastric suction, drainage, fistula, diarrhea)
    2. Skin/respiratory (insensible losses, sweat, burns)
    3. Hemorrhage
  B. Renal Na⁺ and water loss
    1. Diuretics
    2. Osmotic diuresis
    3. Hypoaldosteronism
    4. Salt-wasting nephropathies
  C. Renal water loss
    1. Diabetes insipidus (central or nephrogenic)
II. ECF volume normal or expanded
  A. Decreased cardiac output
    1. Myocardial, valvular, or pericardial disease
  B. Redistribution
    1. Hypoalbuminemia (hepatic cirrhosis, nephrotic syndrome)
    2. Capillary leak (acute pancreatitis, ischemic bowel, rhabdomyolysis)
  C. Increased venous capacitance
    1. Sepsis

Note: ECF, extracellular fluid.

that produces an osmotic diuresis because the renal tubule is impermeable to mannitol. Many tubule and interstitial renal disorders are associated with Na⁺ wasting. Excessive renal losses of Na⁺ and water may also occur during the diuretic phase of acute tubular necrosis (Chap. 273) and following the relief of bilateral urinary tract obstruction. Finally, mineralocorticoid deficiency (hypoaldosteronism) causes salt wasting in the presence of normal intrinsic renal function.

Massive renal water excretion can also lead to hypovolemia. The ECF volume contraction is usually less severe since two-thirds of the volume lost is intracellular. Conditions associated with excessive urinary water loss include *central diabetes insipidus* (CDI) and *nephrogenic diabetes insipidus* (NDI). These two disorders are due to impaired secretion of and renal unresponsiveness to AVP, respectively, and are discussed below.

EXTRARENAL Nonrenal causes of hypovolemia include fluid loss from the gastrointestinal tract, skin, and respiratory system and third-space accumulations (burns, pancreatitis, peritonitis). Approximately 9 L of fluid enters the gastrointestinal tract daily, 2 L by ingestion and 7 L by secretion. Almost 98% of this volume is reabsorbed so that fecal fluid loss is only 100–200 mL/d. Impaired gastrointestinal reabsorption or enhanced secretion leads to volume depletion. Since gastric secretions have a low pH (high H⁺ concentration) and biliary, pancreatic, and intestinal secretions are alkaline (high HCO_3^- concentration), vomiting and diarrhea are often accompanied by metabolic alkalosis and acidosis, respectively.

Water evaporation from the skin and respiratory tract contributes to thermoregulation. These *insensible losses* amount to 500 mL/d. During febrile illnesses, prolonged heat exposure, exercise, or increased salt and water loss from skin, in the form of sweat, can be significant and lead to volume depletion. The Na⁺ concentration of sweat is normally 20–50 mmol/L and decreases with profuse sweating due to the action of aldosterone. Since sweat is hypotonic, the loss of water exceeds that of Na⁺. The water deficit is minimized by enhanced thirst. Nevertheless, ongoing Na⁺ loss is manifest as hypovolemia. Enhanced evaporative water loss from the respiratory tract may be associated with hyperventilation, especially in mechanically ventilated febrile patients.

Certain conditions lead to fluid sequestration in a *third space*. This compartment is extracellular but is not in equilibrium with either the ECF or the ICF. The fluid is effectively lost from the ECF and can result in hypovolemia. Examples include the bowel lumen in gastrointestinal obstruction, subcutaneous tissues in severe burns, retroperitoneal space in acute pancreatitis, and peritoneal cavity in peritonitis. Finally, severe hemorrhage from any source can result in volume depletion.

Pathophysiology ECF volume contraction is manifest as a decreased plasma volume and hypotension. Hypotension is due to decreased venous return (preload) and diminished cardiac output; it triggers baroreceptors in the carotid sinus and aortic arch and leads to activation of the sympathetic nervous system and the renin-angiotensin system. The net effect is to maintain mean arterial pressure and cerebral and coronary perfusion. In contrast to the cardiovascular response, the renal response is aimed at restoring the ECF volume by decreasing the GFR and filtered load of Na⁺ and, most importantly, by promoting tubular reabsorption of Na⁺. Increased sympathetic tone increases proximal tubular Na⁺ reabsorption and decreases GFR by causing preferential afferent arteriolar vasoconstriction. Sodium is also reabsorbed in the proximal convoluted tubule in response to increased angiotensin II and altered peritubular capillary hemodynamics (decreased hydraulic and increased oncotic pressure). Enhanced reabsorption of Na⁺ by the collecting duct is an important component of the renal adaptation to ECF volume contraction. This occurs in response to increased *aldosterone* and AVP secretion and suppressed *atrial natriuretic peptide* secretion.

Clinical Features A careful history is often helpful in determining the etiology of ECF volume contraction (e.g., vomiting, diarrhea, polyuria, diaphoresis). Most symptoms are nonspecific and secondary to electrolyte imbalances and tissue hypoperfusion and include fatigue, weakness, muscle cramps, thirst, and postural dizziness. More severe degrees of volume contraction can lead to end-organ ischemia manifest as oliguria, cyanosis, abdominal and chest pain, and confusion or obtundation. Diminished skin turgor and dry oral mucous membranes are poor markers of decreased interstitial fluid. Signs of intravascular volume contraction include decreased jugular venous pressure, postural hypotension, and postural tachycardia. Larger and more acute fluid losses lead to hypovolemic shock, manifest as hypotension, tachycardia, peripheral vasoconstriction, and hypoperfusion—cyanosis, cold and clammy extremities, oliguria, and altered mental status.

Diagnosis A thorough history and physical examination are generally sufficient to diagnose the etiology of hypovolemia. Laboratory data usually confirm and support the clinical diagnosis. The blood urea nitrogen (BUN) and plasma creatinine concentrations tend to be elevated, reflecting a decreased GFR. Normally, the BUN:creatinine ratio is about 10:1. However, in *prerenal azotemia*, hypovolemia leads to increased urea reabsorption, a proportionately greater elevation in BUN than plasma creatinine, and a BUN:creatinine ratio of 20:1 or higher. An increased BUN (relative to creatinine) may also be due to increased urea production that occurs with hyperalimentation (high-protein), glucocorticoid therapy, and gastrointestinal bleeding.

The appropriate response to hypovolemia is enhanced renal Na⁺ and water reabsorption, which is reflected in the urine composition. Therefore, the urine Na⁺ concentration should usually be <20 mmol/L except in conditions associated with impaired Na⁺ reabsorption, as in acute tubular necrosis (Chap. 273). Another exception is hypovolemia due to vomiting, since the associated metabolic alkalosis and increased filtered HCO_3^- impair proximal Na⁺ reabsorption. In this case, the urine Cl⁻ is low (<20 mmol/L). The urine osmolality and specific gravity in hypovolemic subjects are generally >450 mosmol/kg and 1.015, respectively, reflecting the presence of enhanced AVP secretion. However, in hypovolemia due to diabetes insipidus, urine osmolality and specific gravity are indicative of inappropriately dilute urine.

℞ HYPOVOLEMIA

The therapeutic goals are to restore normovolemia with fluid similar in composition to that lost and to replace ongoing losses. Symptoms and signs, including weight loss, can help estimate the degree of volume contraction and should also be monitored to assess response to treatment. Mild volume contraction can usually be corrected via the oral route. More severe hypovolemia requires intravenous therapy. Isotonic or normal saline (0.9% NaCl or 154 mmol/L Na⁺) is the solution of choice in normonatremic and most hyponatremic individuals and should be administered initially in patients with hypotension or shock. Hypernatremia reflects a proportionately greater deficit of water than Na⁺, and its correction will therefore require a hypotonic solution such as half-normal saline (0.45% NaCl or 77 mmol/L Na⁺) or 5% dextrose in water. Patients with significant hemorrhage, anemia, or intravascular volume depletion may require blood transfusion or colloid-containing solutions (albumin, dextran). Hypokalemia may be present initially or may ensue as a result of increased urinary K$^+$ excretion; it should be corrected by adding appropriate amounts of KCl to replacement solutions.

HYPONATREMIA

Etiology A plasma Na$^+$ concentration <135 mmol/L usually reflects a hypotonic state. However, plasma osmolality may be normal or increased in some cases of hyponatremia. Isotonic or slightly hypotonic hyponatremia may complicate transurethral resection of the prostate or bladder because large volumes of isoosmotic (mannitol) or hypoosmotic (sorbitol or glycine) bladder irrigation solution can be absorbed and result in a dilutional hyponatremia. The metabolism of sorbitol and glycine to CO_2 and water may lead to hypotonicity if the accumulated fluid and solutes are not rapidly excreted. Hypertonic hyponatremia is usually due to hyperglycemia or, occasionally, intravenous administration of mannitol. Relative insulin deficiency causes myocytes to become impermeable to glucose. Therefore, during poorly controlled diabetes mellitus, glucose is an effective osmole and draws water from muscle cells, resulting in hyponatremia. Plasma Na$^+$ concentration falls by 1.4 mmol/L for every 100 mg/dL rise in the plasma glucose concentration.

Most causes of hyponatremia are associated with a low plasma osmolality (Table 46-2). In general, hypotonic hyponatremia is due either to a primary water gain (and secondary Na$^+$ loss) or a primary Na$^+$ loss (and secondary water gain). In the absence of water intake or hypotonic fluid replacement, hyponatremia is usually associated with hypovolemic shock due to a profound sodium deficit and transcellular water shift. Contraction of the ECF volume stimulates thirst and AVP secretion. The increased water ingestion and impaired renal excretion result in hyponatremia. It is important to note that *diuretic-induced hyponatremia* is almost always due to thiazide diuretics. Loop diuretics decrease the tonicity of the medullary interstitium and impair maximal urinary concentrating capacity. This limits the ability of AVP to promote water retention. In contrast, thiazide diuretics lead to Na$^+$ and K$^+$ depletion and AVP-mediated water retention. Hyponatremia can also occur by a process of *desalination*. This occurs when the urine tonicity (the sum of the concentrations of Na$^+$ and K$^+$) exceeds that of administered intravenous fluids (including isotonic saline). This accounts for some cases of acute postoperative hyponatremia and cerebral salt wasting after neurosurgery.

Hyponatremia in the setting of ECF volume expansion is usually associated with edematous states, such as congestive heart failure, hepat-

TABLE 46-2 CAUSES OF HYPONATREMIA

I. Pseudohyponatremia
  A. Normal plasma osmolality
    1. Hyperlipidemia
    2. Hyperproteinemia
    3. Posttransurethral resection of prostate/bladder tumor
  B. Increased plasma osmolality
    1. Hyperglycemia
    2. Mannitol
II. Hypoosmolal hyponatremia
  A. Primary Na$^+$ loss (secondary water gain)
    1. Integumentary loss: sweating, burns
    2. Gastrointestinal loss: vomiting, tube drainage, fistula, obstruction, diarrhea
    3. Renal loss: diuretics, osmotic diuresis, hypoaldosteronism, salt-wasting nephropathy, postobstructive diuresis, nonoliguric acute tubular necrosis
  B. Primary water gain (secondary Na$^+$ loss)
    1. Primary polydipsia
    2. Decreased solute intake (e.g., beer potomania)
    3. AVP release due to pain, nausea, drugs
    4. Syndrome of inappropriate AVP secretion
    5. Glucocorticoid deficiency
    6. Hypothyroidism
    7. Chronic renal insufficiency
  C. Primary Na$^+$ gain (exceeded by secondary water gain)
    1. Heart failure
    2. Hepatic cirrhosis
    3. Nephrotic syndrome

ic cirrhosis, and the nephrotic syndrome. These disorders all have in common a decreased effective circulating arterial volume, leading to increased thirst and increased AVP levels. Additional factors impairing the excretion of solute-free water include a reduced GFR, decreased delivery of ultrafiltrate to the diluting site (due to increased proximal fractional reabsorption of Na$^+$ and water), and diuretic therapy. The degree of hyponatremia often correlates with the severity of the underlying condition and is an important prognostic factor. Oliguric acute and chronic renal failure may be associated with hyponatremia if water intake exceeds the ability to excrete equivalent volumes.

Hyponatremia in the absence of ECF volume contraction, decreased effective circulating arterial volume, or renal insufficiency is usually due to increased AVP secretion resulting in impaired water excretion. Ingestion or administration of water is also required since high levels of AVP alone are usually insufficient to produce hyponatremia. This disorder, commonly termed the *syndrome of inappropriate antidiuretic hormone secretion* (SIADH), is the most common cause of normovolemic hyponatremia and is due to the nonphysiologic release of AVP from the posterior pituitary or an ectopic source (Chap. 334). Renal free-water excretion is impaired while the regulation of Na$^+$ balance is unaffected. The most common causes of SIADH include neuropsychiatric and pulmonary diseases, malignant tumors, major surgery (postoperative pain), and pharmacologic agents. Severe pain and nausea are physiologic stimuli of AVP secretion; these stimuli are inappropriate in the absence of hypovolemia or hyperosmolality. The pattern of AVP secretion can be used to classify SIADH into four subtypes: (1) erratic autonomous AVP secretion (ectopic production); (2) normal regulation of AVP release around a lower osmolality set point or *reset osmostat* (cachexia, malnutrition); (3) normal AVP response to hypertonicity with failure to suppress completely at low osmolality (incomplete pituitary stalk section); and (4) normal AVP secretion with increased sensitivity to its actions or secretion of some other antidiuretic factor (rare). Patients with the nephrogenic syndrome of inappropriate antidiuresis have clinical and laboratory features consistent with SIADH but undetectable levels of AVP. It is hypothesized that this disorder is due to gain of function mutations in the V2 receptor.

Hormonal excess or deficiency may cause hyponatremia. Adrenal insufficiency (Chap. 336) and hypothyroidism (Chap. 335) may present with hyponatremia and should not be confused with SIADH. Although decreased mineralocorticoids may contribute to the hyponatremia of adrenal insufficiency, it is the cortisol deficiency that leads to hypersecretion of AVP both indirectly (secondary to volume depletion) and directly (cosecreted with corticotropin-releasing factor). The mechanisms by which hypothyroidism leads to hyponatremia include decreased cardiac output and GFR and increased AVP secretion in response to hemodynamic stimuli.

Finally, hyponatremia may occur in the absence of AVP or renal failure if the kidney is unable to excrete the dietary water load. In psychogenic or primary polydipsia, compulsive water consumption may overwhelm the normally large renal excretory capacity of 12 L/d (Chap. 334). These patients often have psychiatric illnesses and may be taking medications, such as phenothiazines, that enhance the sensation of thirst by causing a dry mouth. The maximal urine output is a function of the minimum urine osmolality achievable and the mandatory solute excretion. Metabolism of a normal diet generates about 600 mosmol/d, and the minimum urine osmolality in humans is 50 mosmol/kg. Therefore, the maximum daily urine output will be about 12 L (600 ÷ 50 = 12). A solute excretion rate of greater than ~750 mosmol/d is, by definition, an *osmotic diuresis*. A low-protein diet may yield as few as 250 mosmol/d, which translates into a maximal urine output of 5 L/d at a minimum urine tonicity of 50 mosmol/kg. Beer drinkers typically have a poor dietary intake of protein and electrolytes and consume large volumes (of beer), which may exceed the renal excretory capacity and result in hyponatremia. This phenomenon is referred to as *beer potomania*.

Clinical Features The clinical manifestations of hyponatremia are related to osmotic water shift leading to increased ICF volume, specifically brain cell swelling or cerebral edema. Therefore the symptoms are primarily neurologic, and their severity is dependent on the rapidity of on-

CLINICAL APPROACH TO HYPONATREMIA

Plasma Osmolality

High → Hyperglycemia, Mannitol

Normal → Hyperproteinemia, Hyperlipidemia, Bladder irrigation

Low → Maximal volume of maximally dilute urine (<100 mosmol/kg)

ECF volume (No) / Primary polydipsia, Reset osmostat (Yes)

Increased → Heart failure, Hepatic cirrhosis, Nephrotic syndrome, Renal insufficiency

Normal → SIADH, Exclude hypothyroidism, Exclude adrenal insufficiency

Decreased → Urine Na+ concentration

<10 mmol/L → Extrarenal Na+ loss, Remote diuretic use, Remote vomiting

>20 mmol/L → Na+-wasting nephropathy, Hypoaldosteronism, Diuretic, Vomiting

FIGURE 46-1 Algorithm depicting clinical approach to hyponatremia. ECF, extracellular fluid; SIADH, syndrome of inappropriate antidiuretic hormone secretion.

set and absolute decrease in plasma Na+ concentration. Patients may be asymptomatic or complain of nausea and malaise. As the plasma Na+ concentration falls, the symptoms progress to include headache, lethargy, confusion, and obtundation. Stupor, seizures, and coma do not usually occur unless the plasma Na+ concentration falls acutely below 120 mmol/L or decreases rapidly. As described above, adaptive mechanisms designed to protect cell volume occur in chronic hyponatremia. Loss of Na+ and K+, followed by organic osmolytes, from brain cells decreases brain swelling due to secondary transcellular water shifts (from ICF to ECF). The net effect is to minimize cerebral edema and its symptoms.

Diagnosis (Fig. 46-1) Hyponatremia is not a disease but a manifestation of a variety of disorders. The underlying cause can often be ascertained from an accurate history and physical examination, including an assessment of ECF volume status and effective circulating arterial volume. The differential diagnosis of hyponatremia, an expanded ECF volume, and decreased effective circulating volume includes congestive heart failure, hepatic cirrhosis, and the nephrotic syndrome. Hypothyroidism and adrenal insufficiency tend to present with a near-normal ECF volume and decreased effective circulating arterial volume. All of these diseases have characteristic signs and symptoms. Patients with SIADH are usually euvolemic.

Four laboratory findings often provide useful information and can narrow the differential diagnosis of hyponatremia: (1) the plasma osmolality, (2) the urine osmolality, (3) the urine Na+ concentration, and (4) the urine K+ concentration. Since ECF tonicity is determined primarily by the Na+ concentration, most patients with hyponatremia have a decreased plasma osmolality. The appropriate renal response to hypoosmolality is to excrete the maximum volume of dilute urine, i.e., urine osmolality and specific gravity of <100 mosmol/kg and 1.003, respectively. This occurs in patients with primary polydipsia. If this is not present, it suggests impaired free-water excretion due to the action of AVP on the kidney. The

secretion of AVP may be a physiologic response to hemodynamic stimuli or it may be inappropriate in the presence of hyponatremia and euvolemia. Since Na+ is the major ECF cation and is largely restricted to this compartment, ECF volume contraction represents a deficit in total body Na+ content. Therefore, volume depletion in patients with normal underlying renal function results in enhanced tubule Na+ reabsorption and a urine Na+ concentration <20 mmol/L. The finding of a urine Na+ concentration >20 mmol/L in hypovolemic hyponatremia implies a salt-wasting nephropathy, diuretic therapy, hypoaldosteronism, or occasionally vomiting. Both the urine osmolality and the urine Na+ concentration can be followed serially when assessing response to therapy.

SIADH is characterized by hypoosmotic hyponatremia in the setting of an inappropriately concentrated urine (urine osmolality >100 mosmol/kg). Patients are typically normovolemic and have normal Na+ balance. They tend to be mildly volume-expanded secondary to water retention and have a urine Na+ excretion rate equal to intake (urine Na+ concentration usually >40 mmol/L). By definition, they have normal renal, adrenal, and thyroid function and usually have normal K+ and acid-base balance. SIADH is often associated with hypouricemia due to the uricosuric state induced by volume expansion. In contrast, hypovolemic patients tend to be hyperuricemic secondary to increased proximal urate reabsorption.

℞ HYPONATREMIA

The goals of therapy are twofold: (1) to raise the plasma Na+ concentration by restricting water intake and promoting water loss and (2) to correct the underlying disorder. Mild asymptomatic hyponatremia is generally of little clinical significance and requires no treatment. The management of asymptomatic hyponatremia associated with ECF volume contraction should include Na+ repletion, generally in the form of isotonic saline. The direct effect of the administered NaCl on the plasma Na+ concentration is trivial. However, restoration of euvolemia removes the hemodynamic stimulus for AVP release, allowing the excess free water to be excreted. The hyponatremia associated with edematous states tends to reflect the severity of the underlying disease and is usually asymptomatic. These patients have increased total body water that exceeds the increase in total body Na+ content. Treatment should include restriction of Na+ and water intake, correction of hypokalemia, and promotion of water loss in excess of Na+. The latter may require the use of loop diuretics with replacement of a proportion of the urinary Na+ loss to ensure net free-water excretion. Dietary water restriction should be less than the urine output. Correction of the K+ deficit may raise the plasma Na+ concentration by favoring a shift of Na+ out of cells as K+ moves in. Water restriction is also a component of the therapeutic approach to hyponatremia associated with primary polydipsia, renal failure, and SIADH (Chap. 334). The recent development of nonpeptide vasopressin antagonists has introduced a new selective treatment for euvolemic and hypervolemic hyponatremia.

The rate of correction of hyponatremia depends on the absence or presence of neurologic dysfunction. This, in turn, is related to the rapidity of onset and magnitude of the fall in plasma Na+ concentration. In asymptomatic patients, the plasma Na+ concentration should be raised by no more than 0.5–1.0 mmol/L per h and by less than 10–12 mmol/L over the first 24 h. Acute or severe hyponatremia (plasma Na+ concentration <110–115 mmol/L) tends to present with altered mental status and/or seizures and requires more rapid correction. Severe symptomatic hyponatremia should be treated with hypertonic saline, and the plasma Na+ concentration should be raised by 1–2 mmol/L per hour for the first 3–4 h or until the seizures subside. Once again, the plasma Na+ concentration should probably be raised by no more than 12 mmol/L during the first 24 h. The quantity of Na+ required to increase the plasma Na+ concentration by a given amount can be estimated by multiplying the deficit in plasma Na+ concentration by the total body water.

Under normal conditions, total body water is 50 or 60% of lean body weight in women or men, respectively. Therefore, to raise the plasma Na+ concentration from 105 to 115 mmol/L in a 70-kg man requires 420 mmol [(115 − 105) × 70 × 0.6] of Na+. The risk of correcting hyponatremia too rapidly is the development of the *osmotic demyelination syndrome* (ODS). This is a neurologic disorder characterized by flaccid paralysis, dysarthria, and dysphagia. The diagnosis is usually suspected clinically and can be confirmed by appropriate neuroimaging studies. There is no specific treatment for the disorder, which is associated with significant morbidity and mortality. Patients with chronic hyponatremia are most susceptible to the development of

ODS, since their brain cell volume has returned to near normal as a result of the osmotic adaptive mechanisms described above. Therefore, administration of hypertonic saline to these individuals can cause sudden osmotic shrinkage of brain cells. In addition to rapid or overcorrection of hyponatremia, risk factors for ODS include prior cerebral anoxic injury, hypokalemia, and malnutrition, especially secondary to alcoholism. Water restriction in primary polydipsia and intravenous saline therapy in ECF volume–contracted patients may also lead to overly rapid correction of hyponatremia as a result of AVP suppression and a brisk water diuresis. This can be prevented by administration of water or use of an AVP analogue to slow down the rate of free water excretion. **For further discussion, see Chap. 334.**

HYPERNATREMIA

Etiology Hypernatremia is defined as a plasma Na^+ concentration >145 mmol/L. Since Na^+ and its accompanying anions are the major effective ECF osmoles, hypernatremia is a state of hyperosmolality. As a result of the fixed number of ICF particles, maintenance of osmotic equilibrium in hypernatremia results in ICF volume contraction. Hypernatremia may be due to primary Na^+ gain or water deficit. The two components of an appropriate response to hypernatremia are increased water intake stimulated by thirst and the excretion of the minimum volume of maximally concentrated urine reflecting AVP secretion in response to an osmotic stimulus.

In practice, the majority of cases of hypernatremia result from the loss of water. Since water is distributed between the ICF and the ECF in a 2:1 ratio, a given amount of solute-free water loss will result in a twofold greater reduction in the ICF compartment than the ECF compartment. For example, consider three scenarios: the loss of 1 L of water, isotonic NaCl, or half-isotonic NaCl. If 1 L of water is lost, the ICF volume will decrease by 667 mL, whereas the ECF volume will fall by only 333 mL. Due to the fact that Na^+ is largely restricted to the ECF, this compartment will decrease by 1 L if the fluid lost is isoosmotic. One liter of half-isotonic NaCl is equivalent to 500 mL of water (one-third ECF, two-thirds ICF) plus 500 mL of isotonic saline (all ECF). Therefore, the loss of 1 L of half-isotonic saline decreases the ECF and ICF volumes by 667 mL and 333 mL, respectively.

The degree of hyperosmolality is typically mild unless the thirst mechanism is abnormal or access to water is limited. The latter occurs in infants, the physically handicapped, and patients with impaired mental status; in the postoperative state; and in intubated patients in the intensive care unit. On rare occasions, impaired thirst may be due to *primary hypodipsia*. This usually occurs as a result of damage to the hypothalamic osmoreceptors that control thirst and tends to be associated with abnormal osmotic regulation of AVP secretion. Primary hypodipsia may be due to a variety of pathologic changes, including granulomatous disease, vascular occlusion, and tumors. A subset of hypodipsic hypernatremia, referred to as *essential hypernatremia*, does not respond to forced water intake. This appears to be due to a specific osmoreceptor defect resulting in nonosmotic regulation of AVP release. Thus, the hemodynamic effects of water loading lead to AVP suppression and excretion of dilute urine.

The source of free water loss is either renal or extrarenal. Nonrenal loss of water may be due to evaporation from the skin and respiratory tract (insensible losses) or loss from the gastrointestinal tract. Insensible losses are increased with fever, exercise, heat exposure, and severe burns and in mechanically ventilated patients. Furthermore, the Na^+ concentration of sweat decreases with profuse perspiration, thereby increasing solute-free water loss. Diarrhea is the most common gastrointestinal cause of hypernatremia. Specifically, osmotic diarrheas (induced by lactulose, sorbitol, or malabsorption of carbohydrate) and viral gastroenteritides result in water loss exceeding that of Na^+ and K^+. In contrast, secretory diarrheas (e.g., cholera, carcinoid, VIPoma) have a fecal osmolality (twice the sum of the concentrations of Na^+ and K^+) similar to that of plasma and present with ECF volume contraction and a normal plasma Na^+ concentration or hyponatremia.

Renal water loss is the most common cause of hypernatremia and is due to drug-induced or osmotic diuresis or diabetes insipidus (Chap. 334). Loop diuretics interfere with the countercurrent mechanism and produce an isoosmotic solute diuresis. This results in a decreased med-

ullary interstitial tonicity and impaired renal concentrating ability. The presence of non-reabsorbed organic solutes in the tubule lumen impairs the osmotic reabsorption of water. This leads to water loss in excess of Na^+ and K^+, known as an osmotic diuresis. The most frequent cause of an osmotic diuresis is hyperglycemia and glucosuria in poorly controlled diabetes mellitus. Intravenous administration of mannitol and increased endogenous production of urea (high-protein diet) can also result in an osmotic diuresis.

Hypernatremia secondary to nonosmotic urinary water loss is usually due to: (1) Central diabetes insipidus (CDI) characterized by impaired AVP secretion, or (2) NDI resulting from end-organ (renal) resistance to the actions of AVP. The most common cause of CDI is destruction of the neurohypophysis. This may occur as a result of trauma, neurosurgery, granulomatous disease, neoplasms, vascular accidents, or infection. In many cases, CDI is idiopathic and may occasionally be hereditary. The familial form of the disease is inherited in an autosomal dominant fashion and has been attributed to mutations in the propressophysin (AVP precursor) gene. Nephrogenic diabetes insipidus (NDI) may be either inherited or acquired. Congenital NDI is an X-linked recessive trait due to mutations in the V_2 receptor gene. Mutations in the autosomal *aquaporin-2* gene may also result in NDI. The *aquaporin-2* gene encodes the water channel protein whose membrane insertion is stimulated by AVP. The causes of sporadic NDI are numerous and include drugs (especially lithium), hypercalcemia, hypokalemia, and conditions that impair medullary hypertonicity (e.g., papillary necrosis or osmotic diuresis). Pregnant women, in the second or third trimester, may develop NDI as a result of excessive elaboration of vasopressinase by the placenta.

Finally, although infrequent, a primary Na^+ gain may cause hypernatremia. For example, inadvertent administration of hypertonic NaCl or $NaHCO_3$ or replacing sugar with salt in infant formula can produce this complication.

Clinical Features As a consequence of hypertonicity, water shifts out of cells, leading to a contracted ICF volume. A decreased brain cell volume is associated with an increased risk of subarachnoid or intracerebral hemorrhage. Hence, the major symptoms of hypernatremia are neurologic and include altered mental status, weakness, neuromuscular irritability, focal neurologic deficits, and occasionally coma or seizures. Patients may also complain of polyuria or thirst. For unknown reasons, patients with polydipsia from CDI tend to prefer ice-cold water. The signs and symptoms of volume depletion are often present in patients with a history of excessive sweating, diarrhea, or an osmotic diuresis. As with hyponatremia, the severity of the clinical manifestations is related to the acuity and magnitude of the rise in plasma Na^+ concentration. Chronic hypernatremia is generally less symptomatic as a result of adaptive mechanisms designed to defend cell volume. Brain cells initially take up Na^+ and K^+ salts, later followed by accumulation of organic osmolytes such as inositol. This serves to restore the brain ICF volume toward normal.

Diagnosis (Fig. 46-2) A complete history and physical examination will often provide clues as to the underlying cause of hypernatremia. Relevant symptoms and signs include the absence or presence of thirst, diaphoresis, diarrhea, polyuria, and the features of ECF volume contraction. The history should include a list of current and recent medications, and the physical examination is incomplete without a thorough mental status and neurologic assessment. Measurement of urine volume and osmolality are essential in the evaluation of hyperosmolality. The appropriate renal response to hypernatremia is the excretion of the minimum volume (500 mL/d) of maximally concentrated urine (urine osmolality >800 mosmol/kg). These findings suggest extrarenal or remote renal water loss or administration of hypertonic Na^+ salt solutions. The presence of a primary Na^+ excess can be confirmed by the presence of ECF volume expansion and natriuresis (urine Na^+ concentration usually >100 mmol/L).

Many causes of hypernatremia are associated with polyuria and a submaximal urine osmolality. The product of the urine volume and osmolality, i.e., the solute excretion rate, is helpful in determining the

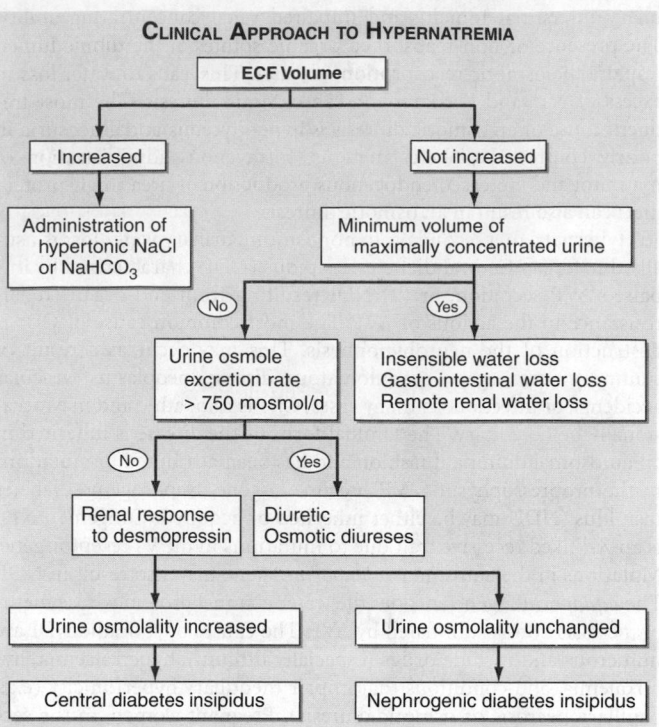

CLINICAL APPROACH TO HYPERNATREMIA

FIGURE 46-2 Algorithm depicting clinical approach to hypernatremia.

basis of the polyuria (see above). To maintain a steady state, total solute excretion must equal solute production. As stated above, individuals eating a normal diet generate ~600 mosmol/d. Therefore, daily solute excretion in excess of 750 mosmol defines an osmotic diuresis. This can be confirmed by measuring the urine glucose and urea. In general, both CDI and NDI present with polyuria and hypotonic urine (urine osmolality <250 mosmol/kg). The degree of hypernatremia is usually mild unless there is an associated thirst abnormality. The clinical history, physical examination, and pertinent laboratory data can often rule out causes of acquired NDI. CDI and NDI can generally be distinguished by administering the AVP analogue desmopressin (10 μg intranasally) after careful water restriction. The urine osmolality should increase by at least 50% in CDI and will not change in NDI. Unfortunately, the diagnosis may sometimes be difficult due to partial defects in AVP secretion and action.

℞ HYPERNATREMIA

The therapeutic goals are to stop ongoing water loss by treating the underlying cause and to correct the water deficit. The ECF volume should be restored in hypovolemic patients. The quantity of water required to correct the deficit can be calculated from the following equation:

$$\text{Water deficit} = \frac{\text{Plasma Na}^+ \text{ concentration} - 140}{140} \times \text{Total body water}$$

In hypernatremia due to water loss, total body water is approximately 50 and 40% of lean body weight in men and women, respectively. For example, a 50-kg woman with a plasma Na$^+$ concentration of 160 mmol/L has an estimated free-water deficit of 2.9 L {[(160 − 140) ÷ 140] × (0.4 × 50)}. As in hyponatremia, rapid correction of hypernatremia is potentially dangerous. In this case, a sudden decrease in osmolality could potentially cause a rapid shift of water into cells that have undergone osmotic adaptation. This would result in swollen brain cells and increase the risk of seizures or permanent neurologic damage. Therefore, the water deficit should be corrected slowly over at least 48–72 h. When calculating the rate of water replacement, ongoing losses should be taken into account, and the plasma Na$^+$ concentration should be lowered by 0.5 mmol/L per h and by no more than 12 mmol/L over the first 24 h.

The safest route of administration of water is by mouth or via a nasogastric tube (or other feeding tube). Alternatively, 5% dextrose in water or half-isotonic saline can be given intravenously. The appropriate treatment of CDI consists of administering desmopressin intranasally (Chap. 334). Other options for decreasing urine output include a low-salt diet in combination with low-dose thiazide diuretic therapy. In some patients with partial CDI, drugs that either stimulate AVP secretion or enhance its action on the kidney have been useful. These include chlorpropamide, clofibrate, carbamazepine, and nonsteroidal anti-inflammatory drugs (NSAIDs). The concentrating defect in NDI may be reversible by treating the underlying disorder or eliminating the offending drug. Symptomatic polyuria due to NDI can be treated with a low-Na$^+$ diet and thiazide diuretics, as described above. This induces mild volume depletion, which leads to enhanced proximal reabsorption of salt and water and decreased delivery to the site of action of AVP, the collecting duct. By impairing renal prostaglandin synthesis, NSAIDs potentiate AVP action and thereby increase urine osmolality and decrease urine volume. Amiloride may be useful in patients with NDI who need to be on lithium. The nephrotoxicity of lithium requires the drug to be taken up into collecting duct cells via the amiloride-sensitive Na$^+$ channel.

POTASSIUM

Potassium Balance   Potassium is the major intracellular cation. The normal plasma K$^+$ concentration is 3.5–5.0 mmol/L, whereas that inside cells is about 150 mmol/L. Therefore, the amount of K$^+$ in the ECF (30–70 mmol) constitutes <2% of the total body K$^+$ content (2500–4500 mmol). The ratio of ICF to ECF K$^+$ concentration (normally 38:1) is the principal result of the resting membrane potential and is crucial for normal neuromuscular function. The basolateral Na$^+$, K$^+$-ATPase pump actively transports K$^+$ in and Na$^+$ out of the cell in a 2:3 ratio, and the passive outward diffusion of K$^+$ is quantitatively the most important factor that generates the resting membrane potential. The activity of the electrogenic Na$^+$, K$^+$-ATPase pump may be stimulated as a result of an increased intracellular Na$^+$ concentration and inhibited in the setting of digoxin toxicity or chronic illness such as heart failure or renal failure.

The K$^+$ intake of individuals on an average western diet is 40–120 mmol/d, or approximately 1 mmol/kg per day, 90% of which is absorbed by the gastrointestinal tract. Maintenance of the steady state necessitates matching K$^+$ ingestion with excretion. Initially, extrarenal adaptive mechanisms, followed later by urinary excretion, prevent a doubling of the plasma K$^+$ concentration that would occur if the dietary K$^+$ load remained in the ECF compartment. Immediately following a meal, most of the absorbed K$^+$ enters cells as a result of the initial elevation in the plasma K$^+$ concentration and facilitated by insulin release and basal catecholamine levels. Eventually, however, the excess K$^+$ is excreted in the urine (see below). The regulation of gastrointestinal K$^+$ handling is not well understood. The amount of K$^+$ lost in the stool can increase from 10 to 50% or 60% (of dietary intake) in chronic renal insufficiency. In addition, colonic secretion of K$^+$ is stimulated in patients with large volumes of diarrhea, resulting in potentially severe K$^+$ depletion.

Potassium Excretion   (See also Chap. 272) Renal excretion is the major route of elimination of dietary and other sources of excess K$^+$. The filtered load of K$^+$ (GFR × plasma K$^+$ concentration = 180 L/d × 4 mmol/L = 720 mmol/d) is ten- to twentyfold greater than the ECF K$^+$ content. Some 90% of filtered K$^+$ is reabsorbed by the proximal convoluted tubule and loop of Henle. Proximally, K$^+$ is reabsorbed passively with Na$^+$ and water, whereas the luminal Na$^+$-K$^+$-2Cl$^-$ co-transporter mediates K$^+$ uptake in the thick ascending limb of the loop of Henle. Therefore, K$^+$ delivery to the distal nephron [distal convoluted tubule and cortical collecting duct (CCD)] approximates dietary intake. Net distal K$^+$ secretion or reabsorption occurs in the setting of K$^+$ excess or depletion, respectively. The cell responsible for K$^+$ secretion in the late distal convoluted tubule (or connecting tubule) and CCD is the principal cell. Virtually all regulation of renal K$^+$ excretion and total body K$^+$ balance occurs in the distal nephron. Potassium secretion is regulated by two physiologic stimuli—aldosterone and hyperkalemia. Aldosterone is secreted by the zona glomerulosa cells of the adrenal cortex in response to high renin and angiotensin II or hyperkalemia. The plasma K$^+$ concentration, independent of

TABLE 46-3 CAUSES OF HYPOKALEMIA

I. Decreased intake
   A. Starvation
   B. Clay ingestion
II. Redistribution into cells
   A. Acid-base
      1. Metabolic alkalosis
   B. Hormonal
      1. Insulin
      2. β_2-Adrenergic agonists (endogenous or exogenous)
      3. α-Adrenergic antagonists
   C. Anabolic state
      1. Vitamin B_{12} or folic acid (red blood cell production)
      2. Granulocyte-macrophage colony stimulating factor (white blood cell production)
      3. Total parenteral nutrition
   D. Other
      1. Pseudohypokalemia
      2. Hypothermia
      3. Hypokalemic periodic paralysis
      4. Barium toxicity
III. Increased loss
   A. Nonrenal
      1. Gastrointestinal loss (diarrhea)
      2. Integumentary loss (sweat)
   B. Renal
      1. Increased distal flow: diuretics, osmotic diuresis, salt-wasting nephropathies
      2. Increased secretion of potassium
         a. Mineralocorticoid excess: primary hyperaldosteronism, secondary hyperaldosteronism (malignant hypertension, renin-secreting tumors, renal artery stenosis, hypovolemia), apparent mineralocorticoid excess (licorice, chewing tobacco, carbenoxolone), congenital adrenal hyperplasia, Cushing's syndrome, Bartter's syndrome
         b. Distal delivery of non-reabsorbed anions: vomiting, nasogastric suction, proximal (type 2) renal tubular acidosis, diabetic ketoacidosis, glue-sniffing (toluene abuse), penicillin derivatives
         c. Other: amphotericin B, Liddle's syndrome, hypomagnesemia

aldosterone, can directly affect K^+ secretion. In addition to the K^+ concentration in the lumen of the CCD, renal K^+ loss depends on the urine flow rate, a function of daily solute excretion (see above). Since excretion is equal to the product of concentration and volume, increased distal flow rate can significantly enhance urinary K^+ output. Finally, in severe K^+ depletion, secretion of K^+ is reduced and reabsorption in the cortical and medullary collecting ducts is upregulated.

HYPOKALEMIA

Etiology (Table 46-3) Hypokalemia, defined as a plasma K^+ concentration <3.5 mmol/L, may result from one (or more) of the following: decreased net intake, shift into cells, increased net loss. Diminished intake is seldom the sole cause of K^+ depletion since urinary excretion can be effectively decreased to <15 mmol/d as a result of net K^+ reabsorption in the distal nephron. With the exception of the urban poor and certain cultural groups, the amount of K^+ in the diet almost always exceeds that excreted in the urine. However, dietary K^+ restriction may exacerbate the hypokalemia secondary to increased gastrointestinal or renal loss. An unusual cause of decreased K^+ intake is ingestion of clay (geophagia), which binds dietary K^+ and iron. This custom was previously common among African Americans in the American South.

REDISTRIBUTION INTO CELLS Movement of K^+ into cells may transiently decrease the plasma K^+ concentration without altering total body K^+ content. For any given cause, the magnitude of the change is relatively small, often <1 mmol/L. However, a combination of factors may lead to a significant fall in the plasma K^+ concentration and may amplify the hypokalemia due to K^+ wasting. Metabolic alkalosis is often associated with hypokalemia. This occurs as a result of K^+ redistribution as well as excessive renal K^+ loss. Treatment of diabetic ketoacidosis with insulin may lead to hypokalemia due to stimulation of the Na^+-H^+ antiporter and (secondarily) the Na^+, K^+-ATPase pump. Furthermore, uncontrolled hy-

perglycemia often leads to K^+ depletion from an osmotic diuresis (see below). Stress-induced catecholamine release and administration of β_2-adrenergic agonists directly induce cellular uptake of K^+ and promote insulin secretion by pancreatic islet β cells. *Hypokalemic periodic paralysis* is a rare condition characterized by recurrent episodic weakness or paralysis (Chap. 382). Since K^+ is the major ICF cation, anabolic states can potentially result in hypokalemia due to a K^+ shift into cells. This may occur following rapid cell growth seen in patients with pernicious anemia treated with vitamin B_{12} or with neutropenia after treatment with granulocyte-macrophage colony stimulating factor. Massive transfusion with thawed washed red blood cells (RBCs) could cause hypokalemia since frozen RBCs lose up to half of their K^+ during storage.

NONRENAL LOSS OF POTASSIUM Excessive sweating may result in K^+ depletion from increased integumentary and renal K^+ loss. Hyperaldosteronism, secondary to ECF volume contraction, enhances K^+ excretion in the urine (Chap. 336). Normally, K^+ lost in the stool amounts to 5–10 mmol/d in a volume of 100–200 mL. Hypokalemia subsequent to increased gastrointestinal loss can occur in patients with profuse diarrhea (usually secretory), villous adenomas, VIPomas, or laxative abuse. However, the loss of gastric secretions does not account for the moderate to severe K^+ depletion often associated with vomiting or nasogastric suction. Since the K^+ concentration of gastric fluid is 5–10 mmol/L, it would take 30–80 L of vomitus to achieve a K^+ deficit of 300–400 mmol typically seen in these patients. In fact, the hypokalemia is primarily due to increased renal K^+ excretion. Loss of gastric contents results in volume depletion and metabolic alkalosis, both of which promote kaliuresis. Hypovolemia stimulates aldosterone release, which augments K^+ secretion by the principal cells. In addition, the filtered load of HCO_3^- exceeds the reabsorptive capacity of the proximal convoluted tubule, thereby increasing distal delivery of $NaHCO_3$, which enhances the electrochemical gradient favoring K^+ loss in the urine.

RENAL LOSS OF POTASSIUM (See also Chap. 336) In general, most cases of chronic hypokalemia are due to renal K^+ wasting. This may be due to factors that increase the K^+ concentration in the lumen of the CCD or augment distal flow rate. Mineralocorticoid excess commonly results in hypokalemia. *Primary hyperaldosteronism* is due to dysregulated aldosterone secretion by an adrenal adenoma (Conn's syndrome) or carcinoma or to adrenocortical hyperplasia. In a rare subset of patients, the disorder is familial (autosomal dominant) and aldosterone levels can be suppressed by administering low doses of exogenous glucocorticoid. The molecular defect responsible for *glucocorticoid-remediable hyperaldosteronism* is a rearranged gene (due to a chromosomal crossover), containing the 5′-regulatory region of the 11β-hydroxylase gene and the coding sequence of the aldosterone synthase gene. Consequently, mineralocorticoid is synthesized in the zona fasciculata and regulated by corticotropin. A number of conditions associated with hyperreninemia result in secondary hyperaldosteronism and renal K^+ wasting. High renin levels are commonly seen in both renovascular and malignant hypertension. Renin-secreting tumors of the juxtaglomerular apparatus are a rare cause of hypokalemia. Other tumors that have been reported to produce renin include renal cell carcinoma, ovarian carcinoma, and Wilms' tumor. Hyperreninemia may also occur secondary to decreased effective circulating arterial volume.

In the absence of elevated renin or aldosterone levels, enhanced distal nephron secretion of K^+ may result from increased production of non-aldosterone mineralocorticoids in *congenital adrenal hyperplasia*. Glucocorticoid-stimulated kaliuresis does not normally occur due to the conversion of cortisol to cortisone by 11β-hydroxysteroid dehydrogenase (11β-HSDH). Therefore, 11β-HSDH deficiency or suppression allows cortisol to bind to the aldosterone receptor and leads to the *syndrome of apparent mineralocorticoid excess*. Drugs that inhibit the activity of 11β-HSDH include glycyrrhetinic acid, present in licorice, chewing tobacco, and carbenoxolone. The presentation of Cushing's syndrome may include hypokalemia if the capacity of 11β-HSDH to inactivate cortisol is overwhelmed by persistently elevated glucocorticoid levels.

Liddle's syndrome is a rare familial (autosomal dominant) disease characterized by hypertension, hypokalemic metabolic alkalosis, renal

K$^+$ wasting, and suppressed renin and aldosterone secretion. Increased distal delivery of Na$^+$ with a nonreabsorbable anion (not Cl$^-$) enhances K$^+$ secretion. Classically, this is seen with *proximal (type 2) renal tubular acidosis* (RTA) and vomiting, associated with bicarbonaturia. Diabetic ketoacidosis and toluene abuse (glue sniffing) can lead to increased delivery of β-hydroxybutyrate and hippurate, respectively, to the CCD and to renal K$^+$ loss. High doses of penicillin derivatives administered to volume-depleted patients may likewise promote renal K$^+$ secretion as well as an osmotic diuresis. *Classic distal (type 1) RTA* is associated with hypokalemia due to increased renal K$^+$ loss, the mechanism of which is uncertain. Amphotericin B causes hypokalemia due to increased distal nephron permeability to Na$^+$ and K$^+$ and to renal K$^+$ wasting.

Bartter's syndrome is a disorder characterized by hypokalemia, metabolic alkalosis, hyperreninemic hyperaldosteronism secondary to ECF volume contraction, and juxtaglomerular apparatus hyperplasia. Finally, diuretic use and abuse are common causes of K$^+$ depletion. Carbonic anhydrase inhibitors, loop diuretics, and thiazides are all kaliuretic. The degree of hypokalemia tends to be greater with long-acting agents and is dose-dependent. Increased renal K$^+$ excretion is due primarily to increased distal solute delivery and secondary hyperaldosteronism (due to volume depletion). See also Chap. 278.

Clinical Features The clinical manifestations of K$^+$ depletion vary greatly between individual patients, and their severity depends on the degree of hypokalemia. Symptoms seldom occur unless the plasma K$^+$ concentration is <3 mmol/L. Fatigue, myalgia, and muscular weakness of the lower extremities are common complaints and are due to a lower (more negative) resting membrane potential. More severe hypokalemia may lead to progressive weakness, hypoventilation (due to respiratory muscle involvement), and eventually complete paralysis. Impaired muscle metabolism and the blunted hyperemic response to exercise associated with profound K$^+$ depletion increase the risk of rhabdomyolysis. Smooth-muscle function may also be affected and manifest as paralytic ileus.

The electrocardiographic changes of hypokalemia (Fig. 221-16) are due to delayed ventricular repolarization and do not correlate well with the plasma K$^+$ concentration. Early changes include flattening or inversion of the T wave, a prominent U wave, ST-segment depression, and a prolonged QU interval. Severe K$^+$ depletion may result in a prolonged PR interval, decreased voltage and widening of the QRS complex, and an increased risk of ventricular arrhythmias, especially in patients with myocardial ischemia or left ventricular hypertrophy. Hypokalemia may also predispose to digitalis toxicity. Hypokalemia is often associated with acid-base disturbances related to the underlying disorder. In addition, K$^+$ depletion results in intracellular acidification and an increase in net acid excretion or new HCO$_3^-$ production. This is a consequence of enhanced proximal HCO$_3^-$ reabsorption, increased renal ammoniagenesis, and increased distal H$^+$ secretion. This contributes to the generation of metabolic alkalosis frequently present in hypokalemic patients. NDI (see above) is not uncommonly seen in K$^+$ depletion and is manifest as polydipsia and polyuria. Glucose intolerance may also occur with hypokalemia and has been attributed to either impaired insulin secretion or peripheral insulin resistance.

Diagnosis (Fig. 46-3) In most cases, the etiology of K$^+$ depletion can be determined by a careful history. Diuretic and laxative abuse as well as surreptitious vomiting may be difficult to identify but should be excluded. Rarely, patients with a marked leukocytosis (e.g., acute myeloid leukemia) and normokalemia may have a low measured plasma K$^+$ concentration due to white blood cell uptake of K$^+$ at room temperature. This *pseudohypokalemia* can be avoided by storing the blood sample on ice or rapidly separating the plasma (or serum) from the cells.

After eliminating decreased intake and intracellular shift as potential causes of hypokalemia, examination of the renal response can help to clarify the source of K$^+$ loss. The appropriate response to K$^+$ depletion is to excrete <15 mmol/d of K$^+$ in the urine, due to increased reabsorption and decreased distal secretion. Hypokalemia with minimal renal K$^+$ excretion suggests that K$^+$ was lost via the skin or gastrointestinal tract or that there is a remote history of vomiting or diuretic use. As described

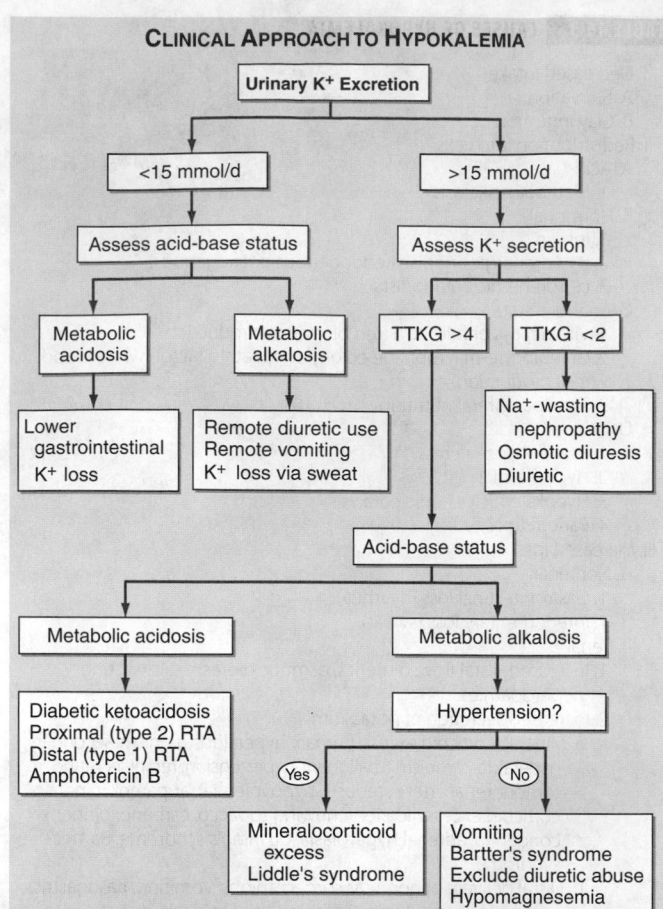

FIGURE 46-3 Algorithm depicting clinical approach to hypokalemia. TTKG, transtubular K$^+$ concentration gradient; RTA, renal tubular acidosis.

above, renal K$^+$ wasting may be due to factors that either increase the K$^+$ concentration in the CCD or increase the distal flow rate (or both). The ECF volume status, blood pressure, and associated acid-base disorder may help to differentiate the causes of excessive renal K$^+$ loss. A rapid and simple test designed to evaluate the driving force for net K$^+$ secretion is the *transtubular K$^+$ concentration gradient* (TTKG). The TTKG is the ratio of the K$^+$ concentration in the lumen of the CCD ([K$^+$]$_{CCD}$) to that in peritubular capillaries or plasma ([K$^+$]$_P$). The validity of this measurement depends on three assumptions: (1) few solutes are reabsorbed in the medullary collecting duct (MCD), (2) K$^+$ is neither secreted nor reabsorbed in the MCD, and (3) the osmolality of the fluid in the terminal CCD is known. Significant reabsorption or secretion of K$^+$ in the MCD seldom occurs, except in profound K$^+$ depletion or excess, respectively. When AVP is acting (OSM$_U$ ≥ OSM$_P$), the osmolality in the terminal CCD is the same as that of plasma, and the K$^+$ concentration in the lumen of the distal nephron can be estimated by dividing the urine K$^+$ concentration ([K$^+$]$_U$) by the ratio of the urine to plasma osmolality (OSM$_U$/OSM$_P$):

$$[K^+]_{CCD} = [K^+]_U \div (OSM_U/OSM_P)TTKG$$
$$= [K^+]_{CCD}/[K^+]_P = [K^+]_U \div (OSM_U/OSM_P)/[K^+]_P$$

Hypokalemia with a TTKG greater than 4 suggests renal K$^+$ loss due to increased distal K$^+$ secretion. Plasma renin and aldosterone levels are often helpful in differentiating the various causes of hyperaldosteronism. Bicarbonaturia and the presence of other non-reabsorbed anions also increase the TTKG and lead to renal K$^+$-wasting.

℞ HYPOKALEMIA

The therapeutic goals are to correct the K$^+$ deficit and to minimize ongoing losses. With the exception of periodic paralysis, hypokalemia resulting from transcellular shifts rarely requires intravenous K⁺ supplementation, which can lead to rebound hyperkalemia. It is generally safer to correct hypokalemia via the oral route. The degree of K⁺ depletion does not correlate well with the plasma K⁺ concentration. A decrement of 1 mmol/L in the plasma K⁺ concentration (from 4.0 to 3.0 mmol/L) may represent a total body K⁺ deficit of 200–400 mmol, and patients with plasma levels under 3.0 mmol/L often require in excess of 600 mmol of K⁺ to correct the deficit. Furthermore, factors promoting K⁺ shift out of cells (e.g., insulin deficiency in diabetic ketoacidosis) may result in underestimation of the K⁺ deficit. Therefore, the plasma K⁺ concentration should be monitored frequently when assessing the response to treatment. Potassium chloride is usually the preparation of choice and will promote more rapid correction of hypokalemia and metabolic alkalosis. Potassium bicarbonate and citrate (metabolized to HCO_3^-) tend to alkalinize the patient and would be more appropriate for hypokalemia associated with chronic diarrhea or RTA.

Patients with severe hypokalemia or those unable to take anything by mouth require intravenous replacement therapy with KCl. The maximum concentration of administered K⁺ should be no more than 40 mmol/L via a peripheral vein or 60 mmol/L via a central vein. The rate of infusion should not exceed 20 mmol/h unless paralysis or malignant ventricular arrhythmias are present. Ideally, KCl should be mixed in normal saline since dextrose solutions may initially exacerbate hypokalemia due to insulin-mediated movement of K⁺ into cells. Rapid intravenous administration of K⁺ should be used judiciously and requires close observation of the clinical manifestations of hypokalemia (electrocardiogram and neuromuscular examination).

HYPERKALEMIA

Etiology Hyperkalemia, defined as a plasma K⁺ concentration >5.0 mmol/L, occurs as a result of either K⁺ release from cells or decreased renal loss. Increased K⁺ intake is rarely the sole cause of hyperkalemia since the phenomenon of *potassium adaptation* ensures rapid K⁺ excretion in response to increases in dietary consumption. Iatrogenic hyperkalemia may result from overzealous parenteral K⁺ replacement or in patients with renal insufficiency. *Pseudohyperkalemia* represents an artificially elevated plasma K⁺ concentration due to K⁺ movement out of cells immediately prior to or following venipuncture. Contributing factors include prolonged use of a tourniquet with or without repeated fist clenching, hemolysis, and marked leukocytosis or thrombocytosis. The latter two result in an elevated serum K⁺ concentration due to release of intracellular K⁺ following clot formation. Pseudohyperkalemia should be suspected in an otherwise asymptomatic patient with no obvious underlying cause. If proper venipuncture technique is used and a plasma (not serum) K⁺ concentration is measured, it should be normal. Intravascular hemolysis, tumor lysis syndrome, and rhabdomyolysis all lead to K⁺ release from cells as a result of tissue breakdown.

Metabolic acidoses, with the exception of those due to the accumulation of organic anions, can be associated with mild hyperkalemia resulting from intracellular buffering of H⁺ (see above). Insulin deficiency and hypertonicity (e.g., hyperglycemia) promote K⁺ shift from the ICF to the ECF. The severity of exercise-induced hyperkalemia is related to the degree of exertion. It is due to release of K⁺ from muscles and is usually rapidly reversible, often associated with rebound hypokalemia. Treatment with beta blockers rarely causes hyperkalemia but may contribute to the elevation in plasma K⁺ concentration seen with other conditions. *Hyperkalemic periodic paralysis* (Chap. 382) is a rare autosomal dominant disorder characterized by episodic weakness or paralysis, precipitated by stimuli that normally lead to mild hyperkalemia (e.g., exercise). The genetic defect appears to be a single amino acid substitution due to a mutation in the gene for the skeletal muscle Na⁺ channel. Hyperkalemia may occur with severe digitalis toxicity due to inhibition of the Na⁺,K⁺-ATPase pump. Depolarizing muscle relaxants such as succinylcholine can increase the plasma K⁺ concentration, especially in patients with massive trauma, burns, or neuromuscular disease.

Chronic hyperkalemia is virtually always associated with decreased renal K⁺ excretion due to either impaired secretion or diminished distal solute delivery (Table 46-4). The latter is seldom the only cause of impaired K⁺ excretion but may significantly contribute to hyperkalemia in protein-malnourished (low urea excretion) and ECF volume–contracted (decreased distal NaCl delivery) patients. Decreased K⁺ se-

TABLE 46-4 **CAUSES OF HYPERKALEMIA**

I. Renal failure
II. Decreased distal flow (i.e., decreased effective circulating arterial volume)
III. Decreased K⁺ secretion
  A. Impaired Na⁺ reabsorption
    1. Primary hypoaldosteronism: adrenal insufficiency, adrenal enzyme deficiency (21-hydroxylase, 3β-hydroxysteroid dehydrogenase, corticosterone methyl oxidase)
    2. Secondary hypoaldosteronism: hyporeninemia, drugs (ACE inhibitors, NSAIDs, heparin)
    3. Resistance to aldosterone: pseudohypoaldosteronism, tubulointerstitial disease, drugs (K⁺-sparing diuretics, trimethoprim, pentamidine)
  B. Enhanced Cl⁻ reabsorption (chloride shunt)
    1. Gordon's syndrome
    2. Cyclosporine

Note: ACE, angiotensin-converting enzyme; NSAIDs, nonsteroidal anti-inflammatory drugs.

cretion by the principal cells results from either impaired Na⁺ reabsorption or increased Cl⁻ reabsorption.

Hyporeninemic hypoaldosteronism is a syndrome characterized by euvolemia or ECF volume expansion and suppressed renin and aldosterone levels (Chaps. 336 and 338). This disorder is commonly seen in mild renal insufficiency, diabetic nephropathy, or chronic tubulointerstitial disease. Patients frequently have an impaired kaliuretic response to exogenous mineralocorticoid administration, suggesting that enhanced distal Cl⁻ reabsorption (electroneutral Na⁺ reabsorption) may account for many of the findings of hyporeninemic hypoaldosteronism. NSAIDs inhibit renin secretion and the synthesis of vasodilatory renal prostaglandins. The resultant decrease in GFR and K⁺ secretion is often manifest as hyperkalemia. As a rule, the degree of hyperkalemia due to hypoaldosteronism is mild in the absence of increased K⁺ intake or renal dysfunction.

Angiotensin-converting enzyme (ACE) inhibitors block the conversion of angiotensin I to angiotensin II. Angiotensin receptor antagonists directly inhibit the actions of angiotensin II on AT1 angiotensin II receptors. The actions of both of these classes of drugs result in impaired aldosterone release. Patients at increased risk of ACE inhibitor or angiotensin receptor antagonist–induced hyperkalemia include those with diabetes mellitus, renal insufficiency, decreased effective circulating arterial volume, bilateral renal artery stenosis, or concurrent use of K⁺-sparing diuretics or NSAIDs.

Decreased aldosterone synthesis may be due to *primary adrenal insufficiency* (Addison's disease) or congenital adrenal enzyme deficiency (Chap. 336). Heparin (including low-molecular-weight heparin) inhibits production of aldosterone by the cells of the zona glomerulosa and can lead to severe hyperkalemia in a subset of patients with underlying renal disease, diabetes mellitus, or those receiving K⁺-sparing diuretics, ACE inhibitors, or NSAIDs. *Pseudohypoaldosteronism* is a rare familial disorder characterized by hyperkalemia, metabolic acidosis, renal Na⁺ wasting, hypotension, high renin and aldosterone levels, and end-organ resistance to aldosterone. The gene encoding the mineralocorticoid receptor is normal in these patients, and the electrolyte abnormalities can be reversed with suprapharmacologic doses of an exogenous mineralocorticoid (e.g., 9α-fludrocortisone) or an inhibitor of 11β-HSDH (e.g., carbenoxolone). The kaliuretic response to aldosterone is impaired by K⁺-sparing diuretics. Spironolactone is a competitive mineralocorticoid antagonist, whereas amiloride and triamterene block the apical Na⁺ channel of the principal cell. Two other drugs that impair K⁺ secretion by blocking distal nephron Na⁺ reabsorption are trimethoprim and pentamidine. These antimicrobial agents may contribute to the hyperkalemia often seen in patients infected with HIV who are being treated for *Pneumocystis carinii* pneumonia.

Hyperkalemia frequently complicates acute oliguric renal failure due to increased K⁺ release from cells (acidosis, catabolism) and decreased excretion. Increased distal flow rate and K⁺ secretion per nephron compensate for decreased renal mass in chronic renal insufficiency. However, these adaptive mechanisms eventually fail to maintain K⁺ balance when the GFR falls below 10–15 mL/min or oliguria ensues. Otherwise asymptomatic urinary tract obstruction is an often overlooked cause of hyperkalemia. Other nephropathies associated with impaired K⁺ excretion include drug-induced interstitial nephritis, lupus nephritis, sickle cell disease, and diabetic nephropathy.

Gordon's syndrome is a rare condition characterized by hyperkalemia, metabolic acidosis, and a normal GFR. These patients are usually volume-expanded with suppressed renin and aldosterone levels as well as refractory to the kaliuretic effect of exogenous mineralocorticoids. It has been suggested that these findings could all be accounted for by increased distal Cl⁻ reabsorption (electroneutral Na⁺ reabsorption), also referred to as a *Cl⁻ shunt*. A similar mechanism may be partially responsible for the hyperkalemia associated with cyclosporine nephrotoxicity. *Hyperkalemic distal (type 4) RTA* may be due to either hypoaldosteronism or a Cl⁻ shunt (aldosterone-resistant).

Clinical Features Since the resting membrane potential is related to the ratio of the ICF to ECF K⁺ concentration, hyperkalemia partially depolarizes the cell membrane. Prolonged depolarization impairs membrane excitability and is manifest as weakness, which may progress to flaccid paralysis and hypoventilation if the respiratory muscles are involved. Hyperkalemia also inhibits renal ammoniagenesis and reabsorption of NH₄⁺ in the TALH. Thus, net acid excretion is impaired and results in metabolic acidosis, which may further exacerbate the hyperkalemia due to K⁺ movement out of cells.

The most serious effect of hyperkalemia is cardiac toxicity, which does not correlate well with the plasma K⁺ concentration. The earliest electrocardiographic changes include increased T-wave amplitude, or peaked T waves. More severe degrees of hyperkalemia result in a prolonged PR interval and QRS duration, atrioventricular conduction delay, and loss of P waves. Progressive widening of the QRS complex and merging with the T wave produces a sine wave pattern. The terminal event is usually ventricular fibrillation or asystole.

Diagnosis (Fig. 46-4) With rare exceptions, chronic hyperkalemia is always due to impaired K⁺ excretion. If the etiology is not readily apparent and the patient is asymptomatic, pseudohyperkalemia should be excluded, as described above. Oliguric acute renal failure and severe chronic renal insufficiency should also be ruled out. The history should focus on medications that impair K⁺ handling and potential sources of K⁺ intake. Evaluation of the ECF compartment, effective circulating volume, and urine output are essential components of the physical examination. The severity of hyperkalemia is determined by the symptoms, plasma K⁺ concentration, and electrocardiographic abnormalities.

The appropriate renal response to hyperkalemia is to excrete at least 200 mmol of K⁺ daily. In most cases, diminished renal K⁺ loss is due to impaired K⁺ secretion, which can be assessed by measuring the transtubular K⁺ concentration gradient (TTKG). A TTKG <10 implies a decreased driving force for K⁺ secretion due to either hypoaldosteronism or resistance to the renal effects of mineralocorticoid. This can be determined by evaluating the kaliuretic response to administration of mineralocorticoid (e.g., 9α-fludrocortisone). Primary adrenal insufficiency can be differentiated from hyporeninemic hypoaldosteronism by examining the renin-aldosterone axis. Renin and aldosterone levels should be measured in the supine and upright positions following 3 days of Na⁺ restriction (Na⁺ intake <10 mmol/d) in combination with a loop diuretic to induce mild volume contraction. Aldosterone-resistant hyperkalemia can result from the various causes of impaired distal Na⁺ reabsorption or from a Cl⁻ shunt. The former leads to salt wasting, ECF volume contraction, and high renin and aldosterone levels. In contrast, enhanced distal Cl⁻ reabsorption is associated with volume expansion and suppressed renin and aldosterone secretion. As mentioned above, hypoaldosteronism seldom causes severe hyperkalemia in the absence of increased dietary K⁺ intake, renal insufficiency, transcellular K⁺ shifts, or antikaliuretic drugs.

℞ HYPERKALEMIA

The approach to therapy depends on the degree of hyperkalemia as determined by the plasma K⁺ concentration, associated muscular weakness, and changes on the electrocardiogram. Potentially fatal hyperkalemia rarely occurs unless the plasma K⁺ concentration exceeds 7.5 mmol/L and is usually

CLINICAL APPROACH TO HYPERKALEMIA

FIGURE 46-4 Algorithm depicting clinical approach to hyperkalemia. NSAID, nonsteroidal anti-inflammatory drug; ACE, angiotensin-converting enzyme; RTA, renal tubular acidosis; TTKG, transtubular K⁺ concentration gradient.

associated with profound weakness and absent P waves, QRS widening, or ventricular arrhythmias on the electrocardiogram.

Severe hyperkalemia requires emergent treatment directed at minimizing membrane depolarization, shifting K⁺ into cells, and promoting K⁺ loss. In addition, exogenous K⁺ intake and antikaliuretic drugs should be discontinued. Administration of calcium gluconate decreases membrane excitability. The usual dose is 10 mL of a 10% solution infused over 2–3 min. The effect begins within minutes but is short-lived (30–60 min), and the dose can be repeated if no change in the electrocardiogram is seen after 5–10 min. Insulin causes K⁺ to shift into cells by mechanisms described previously and will temporarily lower the plasma K⁺ concentration. Although glucose alone will stimulate insulin release from normal pancreatic β cells, a more rapid response generally occurs when exogenous insulin is administered (with glucose to prevent hypoglycemia). A commonly recommended combination is 10–20 units of regular insulin and 25–50 g of glucose. Obviously, hyperglycemic patients should not be given glucose. If effective, the plasma K⁺ concentration will fall by 0.5–1.5 mmol/L in 15–30 min, and the effect will last for several hours. Alkali therapy with intravenous NaHCO₃ can also shift K⁺ into cells. This is safest when administered as an isotonic solution of 3 ampules per liter (134 mmol/L NaHCO₃) and ideally should be reserved for severe hyperkalemia associated with metabolic acidosis. Patients with end-stage renal disease seldom respond to this intervention and may not tolerate the Na⁺ load and resultant volume expansion. When administered parenterally or in nebulized form, β₂-adrenergic agonists promote cellular uptake of K⁺ (see above). The onset of action is 30 min, lowering the plasma K⁺ concentration by 0.5 to 1.5 mmol/L, and the effect lasts 2–4 h.

Removal of K⁺ can be achieved using diuretics, cation-exchange resin, or dialysis. Loop and thiazide diuretics, often in combination, may enhance K⁺ excretion if renal function is adequate. Sodium polystyrene sulfonate is a cation-exchange resin that promotes the exchange of Na⁺ for K⁺ in the gastrointestinal tract. Each gram binds 1 mmol of K⁺ and releases 2–3 mmol of Na⁺. When given by mouth, the usual dose is 25–50 g mixed with 100 mL of 20% sorbitol to prevent constipation. This will generally lower the plasma K⁺ concentration by 0.5–1.0 mmol/L within 1–2 h and last for 4–6 h. Sodium polystyrene sulfonate can also be administered as a retention enema consisting of 50 g of resin and 50 mL of 70% sorbitol mixed in 150 mL of tap water. The sorbitol should be omitted from the enema in postoperative patients due to the increased incidence of sorbitol-induced colonic necrosis, especially following renal transplantation. The most rapid and effective way of lowering the plasma K$^+$ concentration is hemodialysis. This should be reserved for patients with renal failure and those with severe life-threatening hyperkalemia unresponsive to more conservative measures. Peritoneal dialysis also removes K$^+$ but is only 15–20% as effective as hemodialysis. Finally, the underlying cause of the hyperkalemia should be treated. This may involve dietary modification, correction of metabolic acidosis, cautious volume expansion, and administration of exogenous mineralocorticoid.

FURTHER READINGS

ADROGUE HJ, MADIAS NE: Hypernatremia. N Engl J Med 342:1493, 2000

———: Hyponatremia. N Engl J Med 342:1581, 2000

BERL T, VERBALIS J: Pathophysiology of water metabolism, in *Brenner & Rector's The Kidney*, 7th ed, BM Brenner (ed). Philadelphia, Saunders, 2004

COHN JN et al: New guidelines for potassium replacement in clinical practice: A contemporary review by the National Council on Potassium in Clinical Practice. Arch Intern Med 160:2429, 2000

GOLDSZMIDT MA, ILIESCU EA: DDAVP to prevent rapid correction in hyponatremia. Clin Nephrol 53:226, 2000

GREENBERG A, VERBALIS JG: Vasopressin receptor antagonists. Kidney Int 69:2124, 2006

GROSS P: Treatment of severe hyponatremia. Kidney Int 60:2417, 2001

HARRIGAN MR: Cerebral salt wasting syndrome. Crit Care Clin 17:125, 2001

MOUNT DB: Disorders of potassium balance, in *Brenner & Rector's The Kidney*, 7th ed, BM Brenner (ed). Philadelphia, Saunders, 2004

NIELSEN S et al: Aquaporins in the kidney: From molecules to medicine. Physiol Rev 82:205, 2002

WARNOCK DG: Genetic forms of renal potassium and magnesium wasting. Am J Med 112:235, 2002

47 Hypercalcemia and Hypocalcemia
Sundeep Khosla

The calcium ion plays a critical role in normal cellular function and signaling, regulating diverse physiologic processes such as neuromuscular signaling, cardiac contractility, hormone secretion, and blood coagulation. Thus, extracellular calcium concentrations are maintained within an exquisitely narrow range through a series of feedback mechanisms that involve parathyroid hormone (PTH) and the active vitamin D metabolite 1,25-dihydroxyvitmin D [1,25(OH)$_2$D]. These feedback mechanisms are orchestrated by integrating signals between the parathyroid glands, kidney, intestine, and bone (Fig. 47-1) (Chap. 346).

Disorders of serum calcium concentration are relatively common and often serve as a harbinger of underlying disease. This chapter provides a brief summary of the approach to patients with altered serum calcium levels. See Chap. 347 for a detailed discussion of this topic.

HYPERCALCEMIA

ETIOLOGY

The causes of hypercalcemia can be understood and classified based on derangements in the normal feedback mechanisms that regulate serum calcium (Table 47-1). Excess PTH production, which is not appropriately suppressed by increased serum calcium concentrations, occurs in primary neoplastic disorders of the parathyroid glands (parathyroid adenomas, hyperplasia, or, rarely, carcinoma) that are associated with increased parathyroid cell mass and impaired feedback inhibition by calcium. Inappropriate PTH secretion for the ambient level of serum calcium also occurs with heterozygous inactivating calcium sensor receptor (CaSR) mutations, which impair extracellular calcium sensing by the parathyroid glands and the kidneys, resulting in familial hypocalciuric hypercalcemia (FHH). Although PTH secretion by tumors is extremely rare, many solid tumors produce PTH-related peptide (PTHrP), which shares homology with PTH in the first 13 amino acids and binds the PTH receptor, thus mimicking effects of PTH on bone and the kidney. In PTHrP-mediated hypercalcemia of malignancy, PTH levels are suppressed by the high serum calcium levels. Hypercalcemia associated with granulomatous disease (e.g., sarcoidosis) or lymphomas is caused by enhanced conversion of 25(OH)D to the potent 1,25(OH)$_2$D. In these disorders, 1,25(OH)$_2$D enhances intestinal calcium absorption, resulting in hypercalcemia and suppressed PTH. Disorders that directly increase calcium mobilization from bone, such as hyperthyroidism or osteolytic metastases,

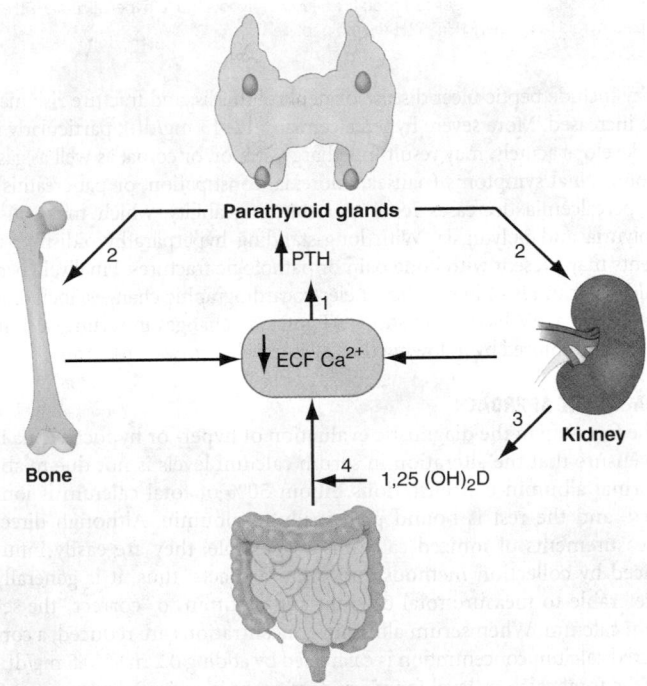

FIGURE 47-1 Feedback mechanisms maintaining extracellular calcium concentrations within a narrow, physiologic range [8.9–10.1 mg/dL (2.2–2.5 mM)]. A decrease in extracellular (ECF) calcium (Ca^{2+}) triggers an increase in parathyroid hormone (PTH) secretion (1) via activation of the calcium sensor receptor on parathyroid cells. PTH, in turn, results in increased tubular reabsorption of calcium by the kidney (2) and resorption of calcium from bone (2) and also stimulates renal 1,25(OH)$_2$D production (3). 1,25(OH)$_2$D, in turn, acts principally on the intestine to increase calcium absorption (4). Collectively, these homeostatic mechanisms serve to restore serum calcium levels to normal.

also lead to hypercalcemia with suppressed PTH secretion, as does exogenous calcium overload, as in milk-alkali syndrome, or total parenteral nutrition with excessive calcium supplementation.

CLINICAL MANIFESTATIONS

Mild hypercalcemia (up to 11–11.5 mg/dL) is usually asymptomatic and recognized only on routine calcium measurements. Some patients may complain of vague neuropsychiatric symptoms, including trouble concentrating, personality changes, or depression. Other presenting symptoms

TABLE 47-1 CAUSES OF HYPERCALCEMIA

Excessive PTH production
    Primary hyperparathyroidism (adenoma, hyperplasia, rarely carcinoma)
    Tertiary hyperparathyroidism (long-term stimulation of PTH secretion in renal insufficiency)
    Ectopic PTH secretion (very rare)
    Inactivating mutations in the CaSR (FHH)
    Alterations in CaSR function (lithium therapy)
Hypercalcemia of malignancy
    Overproduction of PTHrP (many solid tumors)
    Lytic skeletal metastases (breast, myeloma)
Excessive 1,25(OH)$_2$D production
    Granulomatous diseases (sarcoidosis, tuberculosis, silicosis)
    Lymphomas
    Vitamin D intoxication
Primary increase in bone resorption
    Hyperthyroidism
    Immobilization
Excessive calcium intake
    Milk-alkali syndrome
    Total parenteral nutrition
Other causes
    Endocrine disorders (adrenal insufficiency, pheochromocytoma, VIPoma)
    Medications (thiazides, vitamin A, antiestrogens)

Note: CaSR, calcium sensor receptor; FHH, familial hypocalciuric hypercalcemia; PTH, parathyroid hormone; PTHrP, PTH-related peptide.

may include peptic ulcer disease or nephrolithiasis, and fracture risk may be increased. More severe hypercalcemia (>12–13 mg/dL), particularly if it develops acutely, may result in lethargy, stupor, or coma, as well as gastrointestinal symptoms (nausea, anorexia, constipation, or pancreatitis). Hypercalcemia decreases renal concentrating ability, which may cause polyuria and polydipsia. With long-standing hyperparathyroidism, patients may present with bone pain or pathologic fractures. Finally, hypercalcemia can result in significant electrocardiographic changes, including bradycardia, AV block, and short QT interval; changes in serum calcium can be monitored by following the QT interval (Fig. 221-16).

DIAGNOSTIC APPROACH

The first step in the diagnostic evaluation of hyper- or hypocalcemia is to ensure that the alteration in serum calcium levels is not due to abnormal albumin concentrations. About 50% of total calcium is ionized, and the rest is bound principally to albumin. Although direct measurements of ionized calcium are possible, they are easily influenced by collection methods and other artifacts; thus, it is generally preferable to measure total calcium and albumin to "correct" the serum calcium. When serum albumin concentrations are reduced, a corrected calcium concentration is calculated by adding 0.2 mM (0.8 mg/dL) to the total calcium level for every decrement in serum albumin of 1.0 g/dL below the reference value of 4.1 g/dL for albumin, and conversely for elevations in serum albumin.

A detailed history may provide important clues regarding the etiology of the hypercalcemia (Table 47-1). Chronic hypercalcemia is most commonly caused by primary hyperparathyroidism, as opposed to the second most common etiology of hypercalcemia, an underlying malignancy. The history should include medication use, previous neck surgery, and systemic symptoms suggestive of sarcoidosis or lymphoma.

Once true hypercalcemia is established, the second most important laboratory test in the diagnostic evaluation is a PTH level using a two-site assay for the intact hormone. Increases in PTH are often accompanied by hypophosphatemia. In addition, serum creatinine should be measured to assess renal function; hypercalcemia may impair renal function, and renal clearance of PTH may be altered depending on the fragments detected by the assay. If the PTH level is increased (or "inappropriately normal") in the setting of an elevated calcium and low phosphorus, the diagnosis is almost always primary hyperparathyroidism. Since individuals with familial hypocalciuric hypercalcemia (FHH) may also present with mildly elevated PTH levels and hypercalcemia, this diagnosis should be considered and excluded because parathyroid surgery is ineffective in this condition. A calcium/creatinine clearance ratio (calculated as urine calcium/serum cal-

cium divided by urine creatinine/serum creatinine) of <0.01 is suggestive of FHH, particularly when there is a family history of mild, asymptomatic hypercalcemia. Ectopic PTH secretion is extremely rare.

A suppressed PTH level in the face of hypercalcemia is consistent with non-parathyroid-mediated hypercalcemia, most often due to underlying malignancy. Although a tumor that causes hypercalcemia is generally overt, a PTHrP level may be needed to establish the diagnosis of hypercalcemia of malignancy. Serum 1,25(OH)$_2$D levels are increased in granulomatous disorders, and clinical evaluation in combination with laboratory testing will generally provide a diagnosis for the various disorders listed in Table 47-1.

℞ HYPERCALCEMIA

Mild, asymptomatic hypercalcemia does not require immediate therapy, and management should be dictated by the underlying diagnosis. By contrast, significant, symptomatic hypercalcemia usually requires therapeutic intervention independent of the etiology of hypercalcemia. Initial therapy of significant hypercalcemia begins with volume expansion since hypercalcemia invariably leads to dehydration; 4–6 L of intravenous saline may be required over the first 24 h, keeping in mind that underlying comorbidities (e.g., congestive heart failure) may require the use of loop diuretics to enhance sodium and calcium excretion. However, loop diuretics should not be initiated until the volume status has been restored to normal. If there is increased calcium mobilization from bone (as in malignancy or severe hyperparathyroidism), drugs that inhibit bone resorption should be considered. Zoledronic acid (e.g., 4 mg intravenously over ~30 min), pamidronate (e.g., 60–90 mg intravenously over 2–4 h), and etidronate (e.g., 7.5 mg/kg per day for 3–7 consecutive days) are approved by the U.S. Food and Drug Administration for the treatment of hypercalcemia of malignancy in adults. Onset of action is within 1–3 days, with normalization of serum calcium levels occurring in 60–90% of patients. Bisphosphonate infusions may need to be repeated if hypercalcemia relapses. Because of their effectiveness, bisphosphonates have replaced calcitonin or plicamycin, which are rarely used in current practice for the management of hypercalcemia. In rare instances, dialysis may be necessary. Finally, while intravenous phosphate chelates calcium and decreases serum calcium levels, this therapy can be toxic because calcium-phosphate complexes may deposit in tissues and cause extensive organ damage.

In patients with 1,25(OH)$_2$D-mediated hypercalcemia, glucocorticoids are the preferred therapy, as they decrease 1,25(OH)$_2$D production. Intravenous hydrocortisone (100–300 mg daily) or oral prednisone (40–60 mg daily) for 3–7 days are used most often. Other drugs, such as ketoconazole, chloroquine, and hydroxychloroquine, may also decrease 1,25(OH)$_2$D production and are used occasionally.

HYPOCALCEMIA

ETIOLOGY

The causes of hypocalcemia can be differentiated according to whether serum PTH levels are low (hypoparathyroidism) or high (secondary hyperparathyroidism). Although there are many potential causes of hypocalcemia, impaired PTH or vitamin D production are the most common etiologies (Table 47-2) (Chap. 347). Because PTH is the main defense against hypocalcemia, disorders associated with deficient PTH production or secretion may be associated with profound, life-threatening hypocalcemia. In adults, hypoparathyroidism most commonly results from inadvertent damage to all four glands during thyroid or parathyroid gland surgery. Hypoparathyroidism is a cardinal feature of autoimmune endocrinopathies (Chap. 345); rarely, it may be associated with infiltrative diseases such as sarcoidosis. Impaired PTH secretion may be secondary to magnesium deficiency or to activating mutations in the CaSR, which suppress PTH, leading to effects that are opposite to those that occur in FHH.

Vitamin D deficiency, impaired 1,25(OH)$_2$D production (primarily secondary to renal insufficiency), or, rarely, vitamin D resistance also cause hypocalcemia. However, the degree of hypocalcemia in these disorders is generally not as severe as that seen with hypoparathyroidism because the parathyroids are capable of mounting a compensatory increase in PTH secretion. Hypocalcemia may also occur in conditions associated with severe tissue injury such as burns, rhabdomyolysis, tumor lysis, or pancreatitis. The cause of hypocalcemia in these settings

TABLE 47-2 CAUSES OF HYPOCALCEMIA

Low Parathyroid Hormone Levels (Hypoparathyroidism)

Parathyroid agenesis
  Isolated
  DiGeorge syndrome
Parathyroid destruction
  Surgical
  Radiation
  Infiltration by metastases or systemic diseases
  Autoimmune
Reduced parathyroid function
  Hypomagnesemia
  Activating CaSR mutations

High Parathyroid Hormone Levels (Secondary Hyperparathyroidism)

Vitamin D deficiency or impaired $1,25(OH)_2D$ production/action
  Nutritional vitamin D deficiency (poor intake or absorption)
  Renal insufficiency with impaired $1,25(OH)_2D$ production
  Vitamin D resistance, including receptor defects
Parathyroid hormone resistance syndromes
  PTH receptor mutations
  Pseudohypoparathyroidism (G protein mutations)
Drugs
  Calcium chelators
  Inhibitors of bone resorption (bisphosphonates, plicamycin)
  Altered vitamin D metabolism (phenytoin, ketoconazole)
Miscellaneous causes
  Acute pancreatitis
  Acute rhabdomyolysis
  Hungry bone syndrome after parathyroidectomy
  Osteoblastic metastases with marked stimulation of bone formation
    (prostate cancer)

Note: CaSR, calcium sensor receptor; PTH, parathyroid hormone.

may include a combination of low albumin, hyperphosphatemia, tissue deposition of calcium, and impaired PTH secretion.

CLINICAL MANIFESTATIONS

Patients with hypocalcemia may be asymptomatic if the decreases in serum calcium are relatively mild and chronic, or they may present with life-threatening complications. Moderate to severe hypocalcemia is associated with paresthesias, usually of the fingers, toes, and circumoral regions, and is caused by increased neuromuscular irritability. On physical examination, a Chvostek's sign (twitching of the circumoral muscles in response to gentle tapping of the facial nerve just anterior to the ear) may be elicited, although it is also present in ~10% of normal individuals. Carpal spasm may be induced by inflation of a blood pressure cuff to 20 mmHg above the patient's systolic blood pressure for 3 min (Trousseau's sign). Severe hypocalcemia can induce seizures, carpopedal spasm, bronchospasm, laryngospasm, and prolongation of the QT interval.

DIAGNOSTIC APPROACH

In addition to measuring serum calcium, it is useful to determine albumin, phosphorus, and magnesium levels. As for the evaluation of hypercalcemia, determining the PTH level is central to the evaluation

of hypocalcemia. A suppressed (or "inappropriately low") PTH level in the setting of hypocalcemia establishes absent or reduced PTH secretion (hypoparathyroidism) as the cause of the hypocalcemia. Further history will often elicit the underlying cause (i.e., parathyroid agenesis vs. destruction). By contrast, an elevated PTH level (secondary hyperparathyroidism) should direct attention to the vitamin D axis as the cause of the hypocalcemia. Nutritional vitamin D deficiency is best assessed by obtaining serum 25-hydroxyvitamin D levels, which reflect vitamin D stores. In the setting of renal insufficiency or suspected vitamin D resistance, serum $1,25(OH)_2D$ levels are informative.

R_x HYPOCALCEMIA

The approach to treatment depends on the severity of the hypocalcemia, the rapidity with which it develops, and the accompanying complications (e.g., seizures, laryngospasm). Acute, symptomatic hypocalcemia is initially managed with calcium gluconate, 10 mL 10% wt/vol (90 mg or 2.2 mmol) intravenously, diluted in 50 mL of 5% dextrose or 0.9% sodium chloride, given intravenously over 5 min. Continuing hypocalcemia often requires a constant intravenous infusion (typically 10 ampuls of calcium gluconate or 900 mg of calcium in 1 L of 5% dextrose or 0.9% sodium chloride administered over 24 h). Accompanying hypomagnesemia, if present, should be treated with appropriate magnesium supplementation.

Chronic hypocalcemia due to hypoparathyroidism is treated with calcium supplements (1000–1500 mg/d elemental calcium in divided doses) and either vitamin D_2 or D_3 (25,000–100,000 U daily) or calcitriol [$1,25(OH)_2D$, 0.25–2 μg/d]. Other vitamin D metabolites (dihydrotachysterol, alfacalcidiol) are now used less frequently. Vitamin D deficiency, however, is best treated using vitamin D supplementation, with the dose depending on the severity of the deficit and the underlying cause. Thus, nutritional vitamin D deficiency generally responds to relatively low doses of vitamin D (50,000 U, 2–3 times per week for several months), while vitamin D deficiency due to malabsorption may require much higher doses (100,000 U/d or more). The treatment goal is to bring serum calcium into the low normal range and to avoid hypercalciuria, which may lead to nephrolithiasis.

FURTHER READINGS

BILEZIKIAN JP, SILVERBERG SJ: Asymptomatic primary hyperparathyroidism. N Engl J Med 350:1746, 2004

FARFORD B et al: Nonsurgical management of primary hyperparathyroidism. Mayo Clin Proc 82(3):351, 2007

FINKELSTEIN JS, POTTS JT JR: Medical management of hypercalcemia, in *Endocrinology*, 5th ed, LJ DeGroot, JL Jameson (eds). Philadelphia, Elsevier, 2006

KIFOR O et al: Activating antibodies to the calcium-sensing receptor in two patients with autoimmune hypoparathyroidism. J Clin Endocrinol Metab 89:548, 2004

MARX SJ: Hyperparathyroid and hypoparathyroid disorders. N Engl J Med 343:1863, 2000

STEWART AF: Hypercalcemia associated with cancer. N Engl J Med 352:373, 2005

THAKKER RV: Genetics of endocrine and metabolic disorders: parathyroid. Rev Endocr Metab Disord 5:37, 2004

48 Acidosis and Alkalosis
Thomas D. DuBose, Jr.

NORMAL ACID-BASE HOMEOSTASIS

Systemic arterial pH is maintained between 7.35 and 7.45 by extracellular and intracellular chemical buffering together with respiratory and renal regulatory mechanisms. The control of arterial CO_2 tension (Pa_{CO_2}) by the central nervous system and respiratory systems and the

control of the plasma bicarbonate by the kidneys stabilize the arterial pH by excretion or retention of acid or alkali. The metabolic and respiratory components that regulate systemic pH are described by the Henderson-Hasselbalch equation:

$$pH = 6.1 + \log \frac{HCO_3^-}{Pa_{CO_2} \times 0.0301}$$

Under most circumstances, CO_2 production and excretion are matched, and the usual steady-state Pa_{CO_2} is maintained at 40 mmHg.

Underexcretion of CO_2 produces hypercapnia, and overexcretion causes hypocapnia. Nevertheless, production and excretion are again matched at a new steady-state Pa_{CO_2}. Therefore, the Pa_{CO_2} is regulated primarily by neural respiratory factors (Chap. 258) and is not subject to regulation by the rate of CO_2 production. Hypercapnia is usually the result of hypoventilation rather than of increased CO_2 production. Increases or decreases in Pa_{CO_2} represent derangements of neural respiratory control or are due to compensatory changes in response to a primary alteration in the plasma $[HCO_3^-]$.

The kidneys regulate plasma $[HCO_3^-]$ through three main processes: (1) "reabsorption" of filtered HCO_3^-, (2) formation of titratable acid, and (3) excretion of NH_4^+ in the urine. The kidney filters ~4000 mmol of HCO_3^- per day. To reabsorb the filtered load of HCO_3^-, the renal tubules must therefore secrete 4000 mmol of hydrogen ions. Between 80 and 90% of HCO_3^- is reabsorbed in the proximal tubule. The distal nephron reabsorbs the remainder and secretes protons, as generated from metabolism, to defend systemic pH. While this quantity of protons, 40–60 mmol/d, is small, it must be secreted to prevent chronic positive H^+ balance and metabolic acidosis. This quantity of secreted protons is represented in the urine as titratable acid and NH_4^+. Metabolic acidosis in the face of normal renal function increases NH_4^+ production and excretion. NH_4^+ production and excretion are impaired in chronic renal failure, hyperkalemia, and renal tubular acidosis.

In sum, these regulatory responses, including chemical buffering, the regulation of Pa_{CO_2} by the respiratory system, and the regulation of $[HCO_3^-]$ by the kidneys, act in concert to maintain a systemic arterial pH between 7.35 and 7.45.

DIAGNOSIS OF GENERAL TYPES OF DISTURBANCES

The most common clinical disturbances are simple acid-base disorders, i.e., metabolic acidosis or alkalosis or respiratory acidosis or alkalosis. Since compensation is not complete, the pH is abnormal in simple disturbances. More complicated clinical situations can give rise to mixed acid-base disturbances.

SIMPLE ACID-BASE DISORDERS

Primary respiratory disturbances (primary changes in Pa_{CO_2}) invoke compensatory metabolic responses (secondary changes in $[HCO_3^-]$), and primary metabolic disturbances elicit predictable compensatory respiratory responses. Physiologic compensation can be predicted from the relationships displayed in Table 48-1. Metabolic acidosis due to an increase in endogenous acids (e.g., ketoacidosis) lowers extracellular fluid $[HCO_3^-]$ and decreases extracellular pH. This stimulates the medullary chemoreceptors to increase ventilation and to return the ratio of $[HCO_3^-]$ to Pa_{CO_2}, and thus pH, toward normal, although not to normal. The degree of respiratory compensation expected in a simple form of metabolic acidosis can be predicted from the relationship: $Pa_{CO_2} = (1.5 \times [HCO_3^-]) + 8 \pm 2$, i.e., the Pa_{CO_2} is expected to decrease 1.25 mmHg for each mmol per liter decrease in $[HCO_3^-]$. Thus, a patient with metabolic acidosis and $[HCO_3^-]$ of 12 mmol/L would be expected to have a Pa_{CO_2} between 24 and 28 mmHg. Values for Pa_{CO_2} <24 or >28 mmHg define a mixed disturbance (metabolic acidosis and respiratory alkalosis or metabolic alkalosis and respiratory acidosis, respectively). Another way to judge the appropriateness of the response in $[HCO_3^-]$ or Pa_{CO_2} is to use an acid-base nomogram (Fig. 48-1). While the shaded areas of the nomogram show the 95% confidence limits for normal compensation in simple disturbances, finding acid-base values within the shaded area does not necessarily rule out a mixed disturbance. Imposition of one disorder over another may result in values lying within the area of a third. Thus, the nomogram, while convenient, is not a substitute for the equations in Table 48-1.

MIXED ACID-BASE DISORDERS

Mixed acid-base disorders—defined as independently coexisting disorders, not merely compensatory responses—are often seen in patients in critical care units and can lead to dangerous extremes of pH (Table 48-2). A patient with diabetic ketoacidosis (metabolic acidosis) may devel-

TABLE 48-1	PREDICTION OF COMPENSATORY RESPONSES ON SIMPLE ACID-BASE DISTURBANCES AND PATTERN OF CHANGES			
Disorder	**Prediction of Compensation**	**Range of Values**		
		pH	**HCO_3^-**	**Pa_{CO_2}**
Metabolic acidosis	$Pa_{CO_2} = (1.5 \times HCO_3^-) + 8 \pm 2$ *or* Pa_{CO_2} will ↓ 1.25 mmHg per mmol/L ↓ in $[HCO_3^-]$ *or* $Pa_{CO_2} = [HCO_3^-] + 15$	Low	Low	Low
Metabolic alkalosis	Pa_{CO_2} will ↑ 0.75 mmHg per mmol/L ↑ in $[HCO_3^-]$ *or* Pa_{CO_2} will ↑ 6 mmHg per 10 mmol/L ↑ in $[HCO_3^-]$ *or* $Pa_{CO_2} = [HCO_3^-] + 15$	High	High	High
Respiratory alkalosis		High	Low	Low
Acute	$[HCO_3^-]$ will ↓ 0.2 mmol/L per mmHg ↓ in Pa_{CO_2}			
Chronic	$[HCO_3^-]$ will ↓ 0.4 mmol/L per mmHg ↓ in Pa_{CO_2}			
Respiratory acidosis		Low	High	High
Acute	$[HCO_3^-]$ will ↑ 0.1 mmol/L per mmHg ↑ in Pa_{CO_2}			
Chronic	$[HCO_3^-]$ will ↑ 0.4 mmol/L per mmHg ↑ in Pa_{CO_2}			

op an independent respiratory problem leading to respiratory acidosis or alkalosis. Patients with underlying pulmonary disease may not respond to metabolic acidosis with an appropriate ventilatory response because of insufficient respiratory reserve. Such imposition of respiratory acidosis on metabolic acidosis can lead to severe acidemia and a poor outcome. When metabolic acidosis and metabolic alkalosis coexist in the same patient, the pH may be normal or near normal. When the pH is normal, an elevated anion gap (AG; see below) denotes the presence of a metabolic acidosis. A discrepancy in the ΔAG (prevailing minus nor-

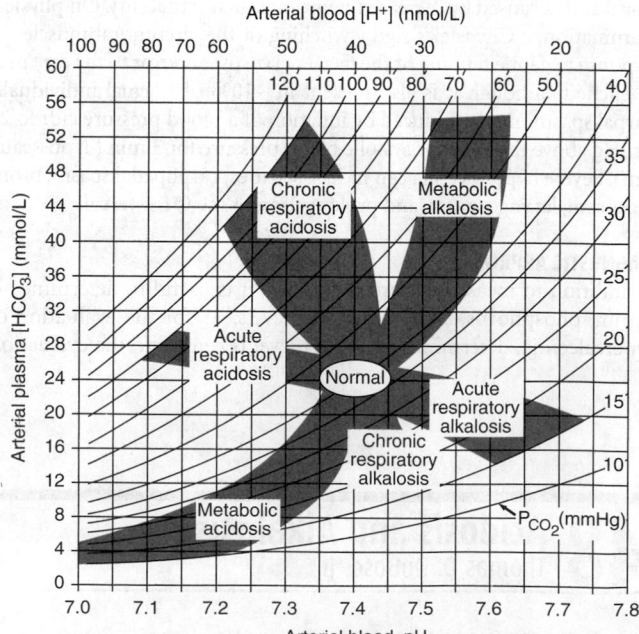

FIGURE 48-1 Acid-base nomogram. Shown are the 90% confidence limits (range of values) of the normal respiratory and metabolic compensations for primary acid-base disturbances. *(From DuBose, used with permission.)*

PART 2

Cardinal Manifestations and Presentation of Diseases

TABLE 48-2 EXAMPLES OF MIXED ACID-BASE DISORDERS

Mixed Metabolic and Respiratory

Metabolic acidosis – respiratory alkalosis
  Key: High- or normal-AG metabolic acidosis; prevailing Pa_{CO_2} *below* predicted value (Table 48-1)
  Example: Na^+, 140; K^+, 4.0; Cl^-, 106; HCO_3^-, 14; AG, 20; Pa_{CO_2}, 24; pH, 7.39 (lactic acidosis, sepsis in ICU)

Metabolic acidosis – respiratory acidosis
  Key: High- or normal-AG metabolic acidosis; prevailing Pa_{CO_2} *above* predicted value (Table 48-1)
  Example: Na^+, 140; K^+, 4.0; Cl^-, 102; HCO_3^-, 18; AG, 20; Pa_{CO_2}, 38; pH, 7.30 (severe pneumonia, pulmonary edema)

Metabolic alkalosis – respiratory alkalosis
  Key: Pa_{CO_2} does not increase as predicted; pH higher than expected
  Example: Na^+, 140; K^+, 4.0; Cl^-, 91; HCO_3^-, 33; AG, 16; Pa_{CO_2}, 38; pH, 7.55 (liver disease and diuretics)

Metabolic alkalosis – respiratory acidosis
  Key: Pa_{CO_2} higher than predicted; pH normal
  Example: Na^+, 140; K^+, 3.5; Cl^-, 88; HCO_3^-, 42; AG, 10; Pa_{CO_2}, 67; pH, 7.42 (COPD on diuretics)

Mixed Metabolic Disorders

Metabolic acidosis – metabolic alkalosis
  Key: Only detectable with high-AG acidosis; $\Delta AG \gg \Delta HCO_3^-$
  Example: Na^+, 140; K^+, 3.0; Cl^-, 95; HCO_3^-, 25; AG, 20; Pa_{CO_2}, 40; pH, 7.42 (uremia with vomiting)

Metabolic acidosis – metabolic acidosis
  Key: Mixed high-AG – normal-AG acidosis; ΔHCO_3^- accounted for by combined change in ΔAG and ΔCl^-
  Example: Na^+, 135; K^+, 3.0; Cl^-, 110; HCO_3^-, 10; AG, 15; Pa_{CO_2}, 25; pH, 7.20 (diarrhea and lactic acidosis, toluene toxicity, treatment of diabetic ketoacidosis)

Note: AG, anion gap; ICU, intensive care unit; COPD, chronic obstructive pulmonary disease.

mal AG) and the ΔHCO_3^- (normal minus prevailing HCO_3^-) indicates the presence of a mixed high-gap acidosis—metabolic alkalosis (see example below). A diabetic patient with ketoacidosis may have renal dysfunction resulting in simultaneous metabolic acidosis. Patients who have ingested an overdose of drug combinations such as sedatives and salicylates may have mixed disturbances as a result of the acid-base response to the individual drugs (metabolic acidosis mixed with respiratory acidosis or respiratory alkalosis, respectively). Even more complex are triple acid-base disturbances. For example, patients with metabolic acidosis due to alcoholic ketoacidosis may develop metabolic alkalosis due to vomiting and superimposed respiratory alkalosis due to the hyperventilation of hepatic dysfunction or alcohol withdrawal.

APPROACH TO THE PATIENT:
Acid-Base Disorders

A stepwise approach to the diagnosis of acid-base disorders follows (Table 48-3). Care should be taken when measuring blood gases to obtain the arterial blood sample without using excessive heparin. Blood for electrolytes and arterial blood gases should be drawn simultaneously prior to therapy, since an increase in $[HCO_3^-]$ occurs

TABLE 48-3 STEPS IN ACID-BASE DIAGNOSIS

1. Obtain arterial blood gas (ABG) and electrolytes simultaneously.
2. Compare $[HCO_3^-]$ on ABG and electrolytes to verify accuracy.
3. Calculate anion gap (AG).
4. Know four causes of high-AG acidosis (ketoacidosis, lactic acid acidosis, renal failure, and toxins).
5. Know two causes of hyperchloremic or nongap acidosis (bicarbonate loss from GI tract, renal tubular acidosis).
6. Estimate compensatory response (Table 48-1).
7. Compare ΔAG and ΔHCO_3^-.
8. Compare change in $[Cl^-]$ with change in $[Na^+]$.

with metabolic alkalosis and respiratory acidosis. Conversely, a decrease in $[HCO_3^-]$ occurs in metabolic acidosis and respiratory alkalosis. In the determination of arterial blood gases by the clinical laboratory, both pH and Pa_{CO_2} are measured, and the $[HCO_3^-]$ is calculated from the Henderson-Hasselbalch equation. This calculated value should be compared with the measured $[HCO_3^-]$ (total CO_2) on the electrolyte panel. These two values should agree within 2 mmol/L. If they do not, the values may not have been drawn simultaneously, a laboratory error may be present, or an error could have been made in calculating the $[HCO_3^-]$. After verifying the blood acid-base values, one can then identify the precise acid-base disorder.

CALCULATE THE ANION GAP All evaluations of acid-base disorders should include a simple calculation of the AG; it represents those unmeasured anions in plasma (normally 10 to 12 mmol/L) and is calculated as follows: $AG = Na^+ - (Cl^- + HCO_3^-)$. The unmeasured anions include anionic proteins, phosphate, sulfate, and organic anions. When acid anions, such as acetoacetate and lactate, accumulate in extracellular fluid, the AG increases, causing a high-AG acidosis. An increase in the AG is most often due to an increase in unmeasured anions and less commonly is due to a decrease in unmeasured cations (calcium, magnesium, potassium). In addition, the AG may increase with an increase in anionic albumin, because of either increased albumin concentration or alkalosis, which alters albumin charge. A decrease in the AG can be due to (1) an increase in unmeasured cations; (2) the addition to the blood of abnormal cations, such as lithium (lithium intoxication) or cationic immunoglobulins (plasma cell dyscrasias); (3) a reduction in the major plasma anion albumin concentration (nephrotic syndrome); (4) a decrease in the effective anionic charge on albumin by acidosis; or (5) hyperviscosity and severe hyperlipidemia, which can lead to an underestimation of sodium and chloride concentrations. A fall in serum albumin by 1 g/dL from the normal value (4.5 g/dL) decreases the anion gap by 2.5 meq/L. Know the common causes of a high-AG acidosis (Table 48-3).

In the face of a normal serum albumin, a high AG is usually due to non-chloride-containing acids that contain inorganic (phosphate, sulfate), organic (ketoacids, lactate, uremic organic anions), exogenous (salicylate or ingested toxins with organic acid production), or unidentified anions. The high AG is significant even if an additional acid-base disorder is superimposed to modify the $[HCO_3^-]$ independently. Simultaneous metabolic acidosis of the high-AG variety plus either chronic respiratory acidosis or metabolic alkalosis represents such a situation in which $[HCO_3^-]$ may be normal or even high (Table 48-2). Compare the change in $[HCO_3^-]$ (ΔHCO_3^-) and the change in the AG (ΔAG).

Similarly, normal values for $[HCO_3^-]$, Pa_{CO_2}, and pH do not ensure the absence of an acid-base disturbance. For instance, an alcoholic who has been vomiting may develop a metabolic alkalosis with a pH of 7.55, Pa_{CO_2} of 48 mmHg, $[HCO_3^-]$ of 40 mmol/L, $[Na^+]$ of 135, $[Cl^-]$ of 80, and $[K^+]$ of 2.8. If such a patient were then to develop a superimposed alcoholic ketoacidosis with a β-hydroxybutyrate concentration of 15 mM, arterial pH would fall to 7.40, $[HCO_3^-]$ to 25 mmol/L, and the Pa_{CO_2} to 40 mmHg. Although these blood gases are normal, the AG is elevated at 30 mmol/L, indicating a mixed metabolic alkalosis and metabolic acidosis. A mixture of high-gap acidosis and metabolic alkalosis is recognized easily by comparing the differences (Δ values) in the normal to prevailing patient values. In this example, the ΔHCO_3^- is 0 (25 – 25 mmol/L) but the ΔAG is 20 (30 – 10 mmol/L). Therefore, 20 mmol/L is unaccounted for in the Δ/Δ value (ΔAG to ΔHCO_3^-).

METABOLIC ACIDOSIS

Metabolic acidosis can occur because of an increase in endogenous acid production (such as lactate and ketoacids), loss of bicarbonate (as in diarrhea), or accumulation of endogenous acids (as in renal failure). Metabolic acidosis has profound effects on the respiratory, cardiac, and

TABLE 48-4 CAUSES OF HIGH-ANION-GAP METABOLIC ACIDOSIS

Lactic acidosis	Toxins
Ketoacidosis	Ethylene glycol
Diabetic	Methanol
Alcoholic	Salicylates
Starvation	Propylene glycol
	Pyroglutamic acid
	Renal failure (acute and chronic)

nervous systems. The fall in blood pH is accompanied by a characteristic increase in ventilation, especially the tidal volume (Kussmaul respiration). Intrinsic cardiac contractility may be depressed, but inotropic function can be normal because of catecholamine release. Both peripheral arterial vasodilation and central venoconstriction can be present; the decrease in central and pulmonary vascular compliance predisposes to pulmonary edema with even minimal volume overload. Central nervous system function is depressed, with headache, lethargy, stupor, and, in some cases, even coma. Glucose intolerance may also occur.

There are two major categories of clinical metabolic acidosis: high-AG and normal-AG, or hyperchloremic acidosis (Table 48-3 and Table 48-4).

Rx METABOLIC ACIDOSIS

Treatment of metabolic acidosis with alkali should be reserved for severe acidemia except when the patient has no "potential HCO_3^-" in plasma. Potential $[HCO_3^-]$ can be estimated from the increment (Δ) in the AG (ΔAG = patient's AG − 10). It must be determined if the acid anion in plasma is metabolizable (i.e., β-hydroxybutyrate, acetoacetate, and lactate) or nonmetabolizable (anions that accumulate in chronic renal failure and after toxin ingestion). The latter requires return of renal function to replenish the $[HCO_3^-]$ deficit, a slow and often unpredictable process. Consequently, patients with a normal AG acidosis (hyperchloremic acidosis), a slightly elevated AG (mixed hyperchloremic and AG acidosis), or an AG attributable to a nonmetabolizable anion in the face of renal failure should receive alkali therapy, either PO (NaHCO₃ or Shohl's solution) or IV (NaHCO₃), in an amount necessary to slowly increase the plasma $[HCO_3^-]$ into the 20–22 mmol/L range.

Controversy exists, however, in regard to the use of alkali in patients with a pure AG acidosis owing to accumulation of a metabolizable organic acid anion (ketoacidosis or lactic acidosis). In general, severe acidosis (pH < 7.20) warrants the IV administration of 50–100 meq of NaHCO₃, over 30–45 min, during the initial 1–2 h of therapy. Provision of such modest quantities of alkali in this situation seems to provide an added measure of safety, but it is essential to monitor plasma electrolytes during the course of therapy, since the [K⁺] may decline as pH rises. The goal is to increase the $[HCO_3^-]$ to 10 meq/L and the pH to 7.15, not to increase these values to normal.

HIGH-ANION-GAP ACIDOSES

APPROACH TO THE PATIENT:
High-Anion-Gap Acidoses

There are four principal causes of a high-AG acidosis: (1) lactic acidosis, (2) ketoacidosis, (3) ingested toxins, and (4) acute and chronic renal failure (Table 48-4). Initial screening to differentiate the high-AG acidoses should include (1) a probe of the history for evidence of drug and toxin ingestion and measurement of arterial blood gas to detect coexistent respiratory alkalosis (salicylates); (2) determination of whether diabetes mellitus is present (diabetic ketoacidosis); (3) a search for evidence of alcoholism or increased levels of β-hydroxybutyrate (alcoholic ketoacidosis); (4) observation for clinical signs of uremia and determination of the blood urea nitrogen (BUN) and creatinine (uremic acidosis); (5) inspection of the urine for oxalate crystals (ethylene glycol); and (6) recognition of the numerous clinical settings in which lactate levels may be increased (hypotension, shock, cardiac failure, leukemia, cancer, and drug or toxin ingestion).

Lactic Acidosis An increase in plasma L-lactate may be secondary to poor tissue perfusion (type A)—circulatory insufficiency (shock, car-

diac failure), severe anemia, mitochondrial enzyme defects, and inhibitors (carbon monoxide, cyanide)—or to aerobic disorders (type B)—malignancies, nucleoside analogue reverse transcriptase inhibitors in HIV, diabetes mellitus, renal or hepatic failure, thiamine deficiency, severe infections (cholera, malaria), seizures, or drugs/toxins (biguanides, ethanol, methanol, propylene glycol, isoniazid, and fructose). Propylene glycol may be used as a vehicle for IV medications including lorazepam, and toxicity has been reported in several settings. Unrecognized bowel ischemia or infarction in a patient with severe atherosclerosis or cardiac decompensation receiving vasopressors is a common cause of lactic acidosis. Pyroglutamic acidemia has been reported in critically ill patients receiving acetaminophen, which is associated with depletion of glutathione. D-Lactic acid acidosis, which may be associated with jejunoileal bypass, short bowel syndrome, or intestinal obstruction, is due to formation of D-lactate by gut bacteria.

APPROACH TO THE PATIENT:
Lactic Acid Acidosis

The underlying condition that disrupts lactate metabolism must first be corrected; tissue perfusion must be restored when inadequate. Vasoconstrictors should be avoided, if possible, since they may worsen tissue perfusion. Alkali therapy is generally advocated for acute, severe acidemia (pH < 7.15) to improve cardiac function and lactate utilization. However, NaHCO₃ therapy may paradoxically depress cardiac performance and exacerbate acidosis by enhancing lactate production (HCO₃⁻ stimulates phosphofructokinase). While the use of alkali in moderate lactic acidosis is controversial, it is generally agreed that attempts to return the pH or $[HCO_3^-]$ to normal by administration of exogenous NaHCO₃ are deleterious. A reasonable approach is to infuse sufficient NaHCO₃ to raise the arterial pH to no more than 7.2 over 30–40 min.

NaHCO₃ therapy can cause fluid overload and hypertension because the amount required can be massive when accumulation of lactic acid is relentless. Fluid administration is poorly tolerated because of central venoconstriction, especially in the oliguric patient. When the underlying cause of the lactic acidosis can be remedied, blood lactate will be converted to HCO₃⁻ and may result in an overshoot alkalosis.

Ketoacidosis • DIABETIC KETOACIDOSIS (DKA) This condition is caused by increased fatty acid metabolism and the accumulation of ketoacids (acetoacetate and β-hydroxybutyrate). DKA usually occurs in insulin-dependent diabetes mellitus in association with cessation of insulin or an intercurrent illness, such as an infection, gastroenteritis, pancreatitis, or myocardial infarction, which increases insulin requirements temporarily and acutely. The accumulation of ketoacids accounts for the increment in the AG and is accompanied most often by hyperglycemia [glucose > 17 mmol/L (300 mg/dL)]. The relationship between the ΔAG and ΔHCO₃⁻ is ~1:1 in DKA but may decrease in the well-hydrated patient with preservation of renal function. Ketoacid excretion in the urine reduces the anion gap in this situation. It should be noted that since insulin prevents production of ketones, bicarbonate therapy is rarely needed except with extreme acidemia (pH < 7.1), and then in only limited amounts. Patients with DKA are typically volume depleted and require fluid resuscitation with isotonic saline. Volume overexpansion is not uncommon, however, after IV fluid administration, and contributes to the development of a hyperchloremic acidosis during treatment of DKA because volume expansion increases urinary ketoacid anion excretion (loss of potential bicarbonate). The mainstay for treatment of this condition is IV regular insulin and is described in Chap. 338 in more detail.

ALCOHOLIC KETOACIDOSIS (AKA) Chronic alcoholics can develop ketoacidosis when alcohol consumption is abruptly curtailed and nutrition is poor. AKA is usually associated with binge drinking, vomiting, abdominal pain, starvation, and volume depletion. The glucose concentration is variable, and acidosis may be severe because of elevated ketones, predominantly β-hydroxybutyrate. Hypoperfusion may enhance lactic acid production, chronic respiratory alkalosis may accompany liver disease, and metabolic alkalosis can result from vomiting (refer to the relationship between ΔAG and ΔHCO_3^-). Thus, mixed acid-base disorders are common in AKA. As the circulation is restored by administration of isotonic saline, the preferential accumulation of β-hydroxybutyrate is then shifted to acetoacetate. This explains the common clinical observation of an increasingly positive nitroprusside reaction as the patient improves. The nitroprusside ketone reaction (Acetest) can detect acetoacetic acid but not β-hydroxybutyrate, so that the degree of ketosis and ketonuria can not only change with therapy, but can be underestimated initially. Patients with AKA usually present with relatively normal renal function, as opposed to DKA where renal function is often compromised because of volume depletion (osmotic diuresis) or diabetic nephropathy. The AKA patient with normal renal function may excrete relatively large quantities of ketoacids in the urine, therefore, and may have a relatively normal AG and a discrepancy in the $\Delta AG/\Delta HCO_3^-$ relationship. Typically, insulin levels are low, and concentrations of triglyceride, cortisol, glucagon, and growth hormone are increased.

℞ ALCOHOLIC KETOACIDOSIS

Extracellular fluid deficits almost always accompany AKA and should be repleted by IV administration of saline and glucose (5% dextrose in 0.9% NaCl). Hypophosphatemia, hypokalemia, and hypomagnesemia may coexist and should be corrected. Hypophosphatemia usually emerges 12–24 h after admission, may be exacerbated by glucose infusion, and, if severe, may induce rhabdomyolysis. Upper gastrointestinal hemorrhage, pancreatitis, and pneumonia may accompany this disorder.

Drug- and Toxin-Induced Acidosis • *SALICYLATES* (See also **Chap. e34**) Salicylate intoxication in adults usually causes respiratory alkalosis or a mixture of high-AG metabolic acidosis and respiratory alkalosis. Only a portion of the AG is due to salicylates. Lactic acid production is also often increased.

℞ SALICYLATE-INDUCED ACIDOSIS

Vigorous gastric lavage with isotonic saline (not $NaHCO_3$) should be initiated immediately followed by administration of activated charcoal per NG tube. In the acidotic patient, to facilitate removal of salicylate, intravenous $NaHCO_3$ is administered in amounts adequate to alkalinize the urine and to maintain urine output (urine pH > 7.5). While this form of therapy is straightforward in acidotic patients, a coexisting respiratory alkalosis may make this approach hazardous. Alkalemic patients should not receive $NaHCO_3^-$. Acetazolamide may be administered in the face of alkalemia, when an alkaline diuresis cannot be achieved, or to ameliorate volume overload associated with $NaHCO_3^-$ administration, but this drug can cause systemic metabolic acidosis if HCO_3^- is not replaced. Hypokalemia should be anticipated with an alkaline diuresis and should be treated promptly and aggressively. Glucose-containing fluids should be administered because of the danger of hypoglycemia. Excessive insensible fluid losses may cause severe volume depletion and hypernatremia. If renal failure prevents rapid clearance of salicylate, hemodialysis can be performed against a bicarbonate dialysate.

ALCOHOLS Under most physiologic conditions, sodium, urea, and glucose generate the osmotic pressure of blood. Plasma osmolality is calculated according to the following expression: $P_{osm} = 2Na^+ + Glu + BUN$ (all in mmol/L), or, using conventional laboratory values in which glucose and BUN are expressed in milligrams per deciliter: $P_{osm} = 2Na^+ + Glu/18 + BUN/2.8$. The calculated and determined osmolality should agree within 10–15 mmol/kg H_2O. When the measured osmolality exceeds the calculated osmolality by >15–20 mmol/kg H_2O, one of two circumstances prevails. Either the serum sodium is spuriously low, as with hyperlipidemia or hyperproteinemia (pseudohyponatremia), or osmolytes other than sodium salts, glucose, or urea have accumulated in plasma. Examples include mannitol, radiocontrast media, isopropyl alcohol, ethylene glycol, propylene glycol, ethanol, methanol, and acetone. In this situation, the difference between the calculated osmolality and the measured osmolality (*osmolar gap*) is proportional to the concentration of the unmeasured solute. With an appropriate clinical history and index of suspicion, identification of an osmolar gap is helpful in identifying the presence of poison-associated AG acidosis. Three alcohols may cause fatal intoxications: ethylene glycol, methanol, and isopropyl alcohol. All cause an elevated osmolal gap, but only the first two cause a high-AG acidosis.

ETHYLENE GLYCOL (See also **Chap. e34**) Ingestion of ethylene glycol (commonly used in antifreeze) leads to a metabolic acidosis and severe damage to the central nervous system, heart, lungs, and kidneys. The increased AG and osmolar gap are attributable to ethylene glycol and its metabolites, oxalic acid, glycolic acid, and other organic acids. Lactic acid production increases secondary to inhibition of the tricarboxylic acid cycle and altered intracellular redox state. Diagnosis is facilitated by recognizing oxalate crystals in the urine, the presence of an osmolar gap in serum, and a high-AG acidosis. If antifreeze containing a fluorescent dye is ingested, a Wood's lamp applied to the urine may be revealing. Treatment should not be delayed while awaiting measurement of ethylene glycol levels in this setting.

℞ ETHYLENE GLYCOL–INDUCED ACIDOSIS

This includes the prompt institution of a saline or osmotic diuresis, thiamine and pyridoxine supplements, fomepizole or ethanol, and hemodialysis. The IV administration of the alcohol dehydrogenase inhibitor fomepizole (4-methylpyrazole; 7 mg/kg as a loading dose) or ethanol IV to achieve a level of 22 mmol/L (100 mg/dL) serves to lessen toxicity because they compete with ethylene glycol for metabolism by alcohol dehydrogenase. Fomepizole, although expensive, offers the advantages of a predictable decline in ethylene glycol levels without excessive obtundation during ethyl alcohol infusion.

METHANOL (See also **Chap. e34**) The ingestion of methanol (wood alcohol) causes metabolic acidosis, and its metabolites formaldehyde and formic acid cause severe optic nerve and central nervous system damage. Lactic acid, ketoacids, and other unidentified organic acids may contribute to the acidosis. Due to its low molecular weight (32 Da), an osmolar gap is usually present.

℞ METHANOL-INDUCED ACIDOSIS

This is similar to that for ethylene glycol intoxication, including general supportive measures, fomepizole or ethanol administration, and hemodialysis.

ISOPROPYL ALCOHOL Ingested isopropanol is absorbed rapidly and may be fatal when as little as 150 mL of rubbing alcohol, solvent, or de-icer is consumed. A plasma level >400 mg/dL is life threatening. Isopropyl alcohol differs from ethylene glycol and methanol in that the parent compound, not the metabolites, causes toxicity, and acidosis is not present because acetone is rapidly excreted.

℞ ISOPROPYL ALCOHOL TOXICITY

Isopropanol alcohol toxicity is treated by watchful waiting and supportive therapy; IV fluids, pressors, ventilatory support if needed, and occasionally hemodialysis for prolonged coma or levels >400 mg/dL.

Renal Failure (See also Chaps. 273 and 274) The hyperchloremic acidosis of moderate renal insufficiency is eventually converted to the high-AG acidosis of advanced renal failure. Poor filtration and reabsorption of organic anions contribute to the pathogenesis. As renal disease progresses, the number of functioning nephrons eventually becomes insufficient to keep pace with net acid production. Uremic acidosis is characterized, therefore, by a reduced rate of NH_4^+ production and excretion, primarily due to decreased renal mass. [HCO_3^-] rarely falls to <15 mmol/L, and the AG is rarely >20 mmol/L. The acid retained in chronic renal disease is buffered by alkaline salts from bone. Despite significant retention of acid (up to 20 mmol/d), the serum [HCO_3^-] does not decrease further, indicating participation of buffers

TABLE 48-5 CAUSES OF NON-ANION-GAP ACIDOSIS

I. Gastrointestinal bicarbonate loss
  A. Diarrhea
  B. External pancreatic or small-bowel drainage
  C. Ureterosigmoidostomy, jejunal loop, ileal loop
  D. Drugs
    1. Calcium chloride (acidifying agent)
    2. Magnesium sulfate (diarrhea)
    3. Cholestyramine (bile acid diarrhea)
II. Renal acidosis
  A. Hypokalemia
    1. Proximal RTA (type 2)
    2. Distal (classic) RTA (type 1)
  B. Hyperkalemia
    1. Generalized distal nephron dysfunction (type 4 RTA)
      a. Mineralocorticoid deficiency
      b. Mineralocorticoid resistance (autosomal dominant PHA I)
      c. Voltage defect (autosomal dominant PHA I and PHA II)
      d. Tubulointerstitial disease
III. Drug-induced hyperkalemia (with renal insufficiency)
  A. Potassium-sparing diuretics (amiloride, triamterene, spironolactone)
  B. Trimethoprim
  C. Pentamidine
  D. ACE-Is and ARBs
  E. Nonsteroidal anti-inflammatory drugs
  F. Cyclosporine and tacrolimus
IV. Other
  A. Acid loads (ammonium chloride, hyperalimentation)
  B. Loss of potential bicarbonate: ketosis with ketone excretion
  C. Expansion acidosis (rapid saline administration)
  D. Hippurate
  E. Cation exchange resins

Note: RTA, renal tubular acidosis; ACE-I, angiotensin-converting enzyme inhibitors; ARB, angiotensin receptor blocker; PHA, pseudohypoaldosteronism.

outside the extracellular compartment. Chronic metabolic acidosis results in significant loss of bone mass due to reduction in bone calcium carbonate. Chronic acidosis also increases urinary calcium excretion, proportional to cumulative acid retention.

 RENAL FAILURE

Because of the association of renal failure acidosis with muscle catabolism and bone disease, both uremic acidosis and the hyperchloremic acidosis of renal failure require oral alkali replacement to maintain the [HCO$_3^-$] between 20 and 24 mmol/L. This can be accomplished with relatively modest amounts of alkali (1.0–1.5 mmol/kg body weight per day). Sodium citrate (Shohl's solution) or NaHCO$_3$ tablets (650-mg tablets contain 7.8 meq) are equally effective alkalinizing salts. Citrate enhances the absorption of aluminum from the gastrointestinal tract and should never be given together with aluminum-containing antacids because of the risk of aluminum intoxication. When hyperkalemia is present, furosemide (60–80 mg/d) should be added.

HYPERCHLOREMIC (NONGAP) METABOLIC ACIDOSES

Alkali can be lost from the gastrointestinal tract in diarrhea or from the kidneys (renal tubular acidosis, RTA). In these disorders (Table 48-5), reciprocal changes in [Cl$^-$] and [HCO$_3^-$] result in a normal AG. In pure hyperchloremic acidosis, therefore, the increase in [Cl$^-$] above the normal value approximates the decrease in [HCO$_3^-$]. The absence of such a relationship suggests a mixed disturbance.

APPROACH TO THE PATIENT:
Hyperchloremic Metabolic Acidoses

In diarrhea, stools contain a higher [HCO$_3^-$] and decomposed HCO$_3^-$ than plasma so that metabolic acidosis develops along with volume depletion. Instead of an acid urine pH (as anticipated with systemic acidosis), urine pH is usually around 6 because metabolic acidosis and hypokalemia increase renal synthesis and excretion of NH$_4^+$, thus providing a urinary buffer that increases urine pH. Meta-

bolic acidosis due to gastrointestinal losses with a high urine pH can be differentiated from RTA (Chap. 278) because urinary NH$_4^+$ excretion is typically low in RTA and high with diarrhea. Urinary NH$_4^+$ levels can be estimated by calculating the urine anion gap (UAG): UAG = [Na$^+$ + K$^+$]$_u$ − [Cl$^-$]$_u$. When [Cl$^-$]$_u$ > [Na$^+$ + K$^+$], the urine gap is negative by definition. This indicates that the urine ammonium level is appropriately increased, suggesting an extrarenal cause of the acidosis. Conversely, when the urine anion gap is positive, the urine ammonium level is low, suggesting a renal cause of the acidosis.

Loss of functioning renal parenchyma by progressive renal disease leads to hyperchloremic acidosis when the glomerular filtration rate (GFR) is between 20 and 50 mL/min and to uremic acidosis with a high AG when the GFR falls to <20 mL/min. Such a progression occurs commonly with tubulointerstitial forms of renal disease, but hyperchloremic metabolic acidosis can persist with advanced glomerular disease. In advanced renal failure, ammoniagenesis is reduced in proportion to the loss of functional renal mass, and ammonium accumulation and trapping in the outer medullary collecting tubule may also be impaired. Because of adaptive increases in K$^+$ secretion by the collecting duct and colon, the acidosis of chronic renal insufficiency is typically normokalemic.

Proximal RTA (type 2 RTA) (Chap. 278) is most often due to generalized proximal tubular dysfunction manifested by glycosuria, generalized aminoaciduria, and phosphaturia (Fanconi syndrome). With a low plasma [HCO$_3^-$], the urine pH is acid (pH < 5.5). The fractional excretion of [HCO$_3^-$] may exceed 10–15% when the serum HCO$_3^-$ > 20 mmol/L. Since HCO$_3^-$ is not reabsorbed normally in the proximal tubule, therapy with NaHCO$_3$ will enhance renal potassium wasting and hypokalemia.

The typical findings in acquired or inherited forms of classic distal RTA (type 1 RTA) include hypokalemia, hyperchloremic acidosis, low urinary NH$_4^+$ excretion (positive UAG, low urine [NH$_4^+$]), and inappropriately high urine pH (pH > 5.5). Such patients are unable to acidify the urine below a pH of 5.5. Most patients have hypocitraturia and hypercalciuria, so nephrolithiasis, nephrocalcinosis, and bone disease are common. In generalized distal nephron dysfunction (type 4 RTA), hyperkalemia is disproportionate to the reduction in GFR because of coexisting dysfunction of potassium and acid secretion. Urinary ammonium excretion is invariably depressed, and renal function may be compromised, for example, due to diabetic nephropathy, amyloidosis, or tubulointerstitial disease.

Hyporeninemic hypoaldosteronism typically causes hyperchloremic metabolic acidosis, most commonly in older adults with diabetes mellitus or tubulointerstitial disease and renal insufficiency. Patients usually have mild to moderate renal insufficiency (GRF, 20–50 mL/min) and acidosis, with elevation in serum [K$^+$] (5.2–6.0 mmol/L), concurrent hypertension, and congestive heart failure. Both the metabolic acidosis and the hyperkalemia are out of proportion to impairment in GFR. Nonsteroidal anti-inflammatory drugs, trimethoprim, pentamidine, and angiotensin-converting enzyme (ACE) inhibitors can also cause hyperkalemia with hyperchloremic metabolic acidosis in patients with renal insufficiency (Table 48-5). See Chap. 278 for the pathophysiology, diagnosis, and treatment of RTA.

METABOLIC ALKALOSIS

Metabolic alkalosis is manifested by an elevated arterial pH, an increase in the serum [HCO$_3^-$], and an increase in Pa$_{CO_2}$ as a result of compensatory alveolar hypoventilation (Table 48-1). It is often accompanied by hypochloremia and hypokalemia. The arterial pH establishes the diagnosis, since it is increased in metabolic alkalosis and decreased or normal in respiratory acidosis. Metabolic alkalosis frequently occurs in association with other disorders such as respiratory acidosis or alkalosis or metabolic acidosis.

PATHOGENESIS

Metabolic alkalosis occurs as a result of net gain of [HCO$_3^-$] or loss of nonvolatile acid (usually HCl by vomiting) from the extracellular fluid. Since it is unusual for alkali to be added to the body, the disorder involves a generative stage, in which the loss of acid usually causes alkalosis, and a maintenance stage, in which the kidneys fail to compensate by excreting HCO_3^-.

Under normal circumstances, the kidneys have an impressive capacity to excrete HCO_3^-. Continuation of metabolic alkalosis represents a failure of the kidneys to eliminate HCO_3^- in the usual manner. For HCO_3^- to be added to the extracellular fluid, it must be administered exogenously or synthesized endogenously, in part or entirely by the kidneys. The kidneys will retain, rather than excrete, the excess alkali and maintain the alkalosis if (1) volume deficiency, chloride deficiency, and K^+ deficiency exist in combination with a reduced GFR, which augments distal tubule H^+ secretion; or (2) hypokalemia exists because of autonomous hyperaldosteronism. In the first example, alkalosis is corrected by administration of NaCl and KCl, whereas in the latter it is necessary to repair the alkalosis by pharmacologic or surgical intervention, not with saline administration.

DIFFERENTIAL DIAGNOSIS

To establish the cause of metabolic alkalosis (Table 48-6), it is necessary to assess the status of the extracellular fluid volume (ECFV), the recumbent and upright blood pressure, the serum $[K^+]$, and the renin-aldosterone system. For example, the presence of chronic hypertension and chronic hypokalemia in an alkalotic patient suggests either mineralocorticoid excess or that the hypertensive patient is receiving diuretics. Low plasma renin activity and normal urine $[Na^+]$ and $[Cl^-]$ in a patient who is not taking diuretics indicate a primary mineralocorticoid excess syn-drome. The combination of hypokalemia and alkalosis in a normotensive, nonedematous patient can be due to Bartter's or Gitelman's syndrome, magnesium deficiency, vomiting, exogenous alkali, or diuretic ingestion. Determination of urine electrolytes (especially the urine $[Cl^-]$) and screening of the urine for diuretics may be helpful. If the urine is alkaline, with an elevated $[Na^+]$ and $[K^+]$ but low $[Cl^-]$, the diagnosis is usually either vomiting (overt or surreptitious) or alkali ingestion. If the urine is relatively acid and has low concentrations of Na^+, K^+, and Cl^-, the most likely possibilities are prior vomiting, the posthypercapnic state, or prior diuretic ingestion. If, on the other hand, neither the urine sodium, potassium, nor chloride concentrations are depressed, magnesium deficiency, Bartter's or Gitelman's syndrome, or current diuretic ingestion should be considered. Bartter's syndrome is distinguished from Gitelman's syndrome because of hypocalciuria and hypomagnesemia in the latter disorder. The genetic and molecular basis of these two disorders has been elucidated recently (Chap. 278).

Alkali Administration   Chronic administration of alkali to individuals with normal renal function rarely, if ever, causes alkalosis. However, in patients with coexistent hemodynamic disturbances, alkalosis can develop because the normal capacity to excrete HCO_3^- may be exceeded or there may be enhanced reabsorption of HCO_3^-. Such patients include those who receive HCO_3^- (PO or IV), acetate loads (parenteral hyperalimentation solutions), citrate loads (transfusions), or antacids plus cation-exchange resins (aluminum hydroxide and sodium polystyrene sulfonate).

METABOLIC ALKALOSIS ASSOCIATED WITH ECFV CONTRACTION, K^+ DEPLETION, AND SECONDARY HYPERRENINEMIC HYPERALDOSTERONISM

Gastrointestinal Origin   Gastrointestinal loss of H^+ from vomiting or gastric aspiration results in retention of HCO_3^-. The loss of fluid and NaCl in vomitus or nasogastric suction results in contraction of the ECFV and an increase in the secretion of renin and aldosterone. Volume contraction through a reduction in GFR results in an enhanced capacity of the renal tubule to reabsorb HCO_3^-. During active vomiting, however, the filtered load of bicarbonate is acutely increased to the point that the reabsorptive capacity of the proximal tubule for HCO_3^- is exceeded. The excess $NaHCO_3$ issuing out of the proximal tubule reaches the distal tubule, where H^+ secretion is enhanced by an aldosterone and the delivery of the poorly reabsorbed anion, HCO_3^-. Correction of the contracted ECFV with NaCl and repair of K^+ deficits corrects the acid-base disorder, and chloride deficiency.

Renal Origin · DIURETICS   (See also Chap. 227) Drugs that induce chloruresis, such as thiazides and loop diuretics (furosemide, bumetanide, torsemide, and ethacrynic acid), acutely diminish the ECFV without altering the total body bicarbonate content. The serum $[HCO_3^-]$ increases because the reduced ECFV "contracts" the $[HCO_3^-]$ in the plasma (contraction alkalosis). The chronic administration of diuretics tends to generate an alkalosis by increasing distal salt delivery, so that K^+ and H^+ secretion are stimulated. The alkalosis is maintained by persistence of the contraction of the ECFV, secondary hyperaldosteronism, K^+ deficiency, and the direct effect of the diuretic (as long as diuretic administration continues). Repair of the alkalosis is achieved by providing isotonic saline to correct the ECFV deficit.

SOLUTE LOSING DISORDERS: BARTTER'S SYNDROME AND GITELMAN'S SYNDROME   See Chap. 278.

NONREABSORBABLE ANIONS AND MAGNESIUM DEFICIENCY   Administration of large quantities of nonreabsorbable anions, such as penicillin or carbenicillin, can enhance distal acidification and K^+ secretion by increasing the transepithelial potential difference (lumen negative). Mg^{2+} deficiency results in hypokalemic alkalosis by enhancing distal acidification through stimulation of renin and hence aldosterone secretion.

POTASSIUM DEPLETION   Chronic K^+ depletion may cause metabolic alkalosis by increasing urinary acid excretion. Both NH_4^+ production and absorption are enhanced and HCO_3^- reabsorption is stimulated.

TABLE 48-6   CAUSES OF METABOLIC ALKALOSIS

I. Exogenous HCO_3^- loads
   A. Acute alkali administration
   B. Milk-alkali syndrome
II. Effective ECFV contraction, normotension, K^+ deficiency, and secondary hyperreninemic hyperaldosteronism
   A. Gastrointestinal origin
      1. Vomiting
      2. Gastric aspiration
      3. Congenital chloridorrhea
      4. Villous adenoma
   B. Renal origin
      1. Diuretics
      2. Posthypercapnic state
      3. Hypercalcemia/hypoparathyroidism
      4. Recovery from lactic acidosis or ketoacidosis
      5. Nonreabsorbable anions including penicillin, carbenicillin
      6. Mg^{2+} deficiency
      7. K^+ depletion
      8. Bartter's syndrome (loss of function mutations in TALH)
      9. Gitelman's syndrome (loss of function mutation in Na^+-Cl^- cotransporter in DCT)
III. ECFV expansion, hypertension, K^+ deficiency, and mineralocorticoid excess
   A. High renin
      1. Renal artery stenosis
      2. Accelerated hypertension
      3. Renin-secreting tumor
      4. Estrogen therapy
   B. Low renin
      1. Primary aldosteronism
         a. Adenoma
         b. Hyperplasia
         c. Carcinoma
      2. Adrenal enzyme defects
         a. 11 β-Hydroxylase deficiency
         b. 17 α-Hydroxylase deficiency
      3. Cushing's syndrome or disease
      4. Other
         a. Licorice
         b. Carbenoxolone
         c. Chewer's tobacco
IV. Gain-of-function mutation of renal sodium channel with ECFV expansion, hypertension, K^+ deficiency, and hyporeninemic-hypoaldosteronism
   A. Liddle's syndrome

Note: ECFV, extracellular fluid volume; TALH, thick ascending limb of Henle's loop; DCT, distal convoluted tubule.

Chronic K⁺ deficiency upregulates the renal H⁺, K⁺-ATPase to increase K⁺ absorption at the expense of enhanced H⁺ secretion. Alkalosis associated with severe K⁺ depletion is resistant to salt administration, but repair of the K⁺ deficiency corrects the alkalosis.

AFTER TREATMENT OF LACTIC ACIDOSIS OR KETOACIDOSIS When an underlying stimulus for the generation of lactic acid or ketoacid is removed rapidly, as with repair of circulatory insufficiency or with insulin therapy, the lactate or ketones are metabolized to yield an equivalent amount of HCO_3^-. Other sources of new HCO_3^- are additive with the original amount generated by organic anion metabolism to create a surfeit of HCO_3^-. Such sources include (1) new HCO_3^- added to the blood by the kidneys as a result of enhanced acid excretion during the preexisting period of acidosis, and (2) alkali therapy during the treatment phase of the acidosis. Acidosis-induced contraction of the ECFV and K⁺ deficiency act to sustain the alkalosis.

POSTHYPERCAPNIA Prolonged CO_2 retention with chronic respiratory acidosis enhances renal HCO_3^- absorption and the generation of new HCO_3^- (increased net acid excretion). If the Pa_{CO_2} is returned to normal, metabolic alkalosis results from the persistently elevated $[HCO_3^-]$. Alkalosis develops if the elevated Pa_{CO_2} is abruptly returned toward normal by a change in mechanically controlled ventilation. Associated ECFV contraction does not allow complete repair of the alkalosis by correction of the Pa_{CO_2} alone, and alkalosis persists until Cl⁻ supplementation is provided.

METABOLIC ALKALOSIS ASSOCIATED WITH ECFV EXPANSION, HYPERTENSION, AND HYPERALDOSTERONISM

Increased aldosterone levels may be the result of autonomous primary adrenal overproduction or of secondary aldosterone release due to renal overproduction of renin. Mineralocorticoid excess increases net acid excretion and may result in metabolic alkalosis, which may be worsened by associated K⁺ deficiency. ECFV expansion from salt retention causes hypertension. The kaliuresis persists because of mineralocorticoid excess and distal Na⁺ absorption causing enhanced K⁺ excretion, continued K⁺ depletion with polydipsia, inability to concentrate the urine, and polyuria.

Liddle's syndrome (Chap. 278) results from increased activity of the collecting duct Na⁺ channel (ENaC) and is a rare inherited disorder associated with hypertension due to volume expansion manifested as hypokalemic alkalosis and normal aldosterone levels.

Symptoms With metabolic alkalosis, changes in central and peripheral nervous system function are similar to those of hypocalcemia (Chap. 346); symptoms include mental confusion, obtundation, and a predisposition to seizures, paresthesia, muscular cramping, tetany, aggravation of arrhythmias, and hypoxemia in chronic obstructive pulmonary disease. Related electrolyte abnormalities include hypokalemia and hypophosphatemia.

℞ METABOLIC ALKALOSIS

This is primarily directed at correcting the underlying stimulus for HCO_3^- generation. If primary aldosteronism, renal artery stenosis, or Cushing's syndrome is present, correction of the underlying cause will reverse the alkalosis. $[H^+]$ loss by the stomach or kidneys can be mitigated by the use of proton pump inhibitors or the discontinuation of diuretics. The second aspect of treatment is to remove the factors that sustain the inappropriate increase in HCO_3^- reabsorption, such as ECFV contraction or K⁺ deficiency. Although K⁺ deficits should be repaired, NaCl therapy is usually sufficient to reverse the alkalosis if ECFV contraction is present, as indicated by a low urine $[Cl^-]$.

If associated conditions preclude infusion of saline, renal HCO_3^- loss can be accelerated by administration of acetazolamide, a carbonic anhydrase inhibitor, which is usually effective in patients with adequate renal function but can worsen K⁺ losses. Dilute hydrochloric acid (0.1 N HCl) is also effective but can cause hemolysis, and must be delivered centrally and slowly. Hemodialysis against a dialysate low in $[HCO_3^-]$ and high in $[Cl^-]$ can be effective when renal function is impaired.

TABLE 48-7 RESPIRATORY ACID-BASE DISORDERS

I. Alkalosis
  A. Central nervous system stimulation
    1. Pain
    2. Anxiety, psychosis
    3. Fever
    4. Cerebrovascular accident
    5. Meningitis, encephalitis
    6. Tumor
    7. Trauma
  B. Hypoxemia or tissue hypoxia
    1. High altitude, ↓Pa_{CO_2}
    2. Pneumonia, pulmonary edema
    3. Aspiration
    4. Severe anemia
  C. Drugs or hormones
    1. Pregnancy, progesterone
    2. Salicylates
    3. Cardiac failure
  D. Stimulation of chest receptors
    1. Hemothorax
    2. Flail chest
    3. Cardiac failure
    4. Pulmonary embolism
  E. Miscellaneous
    1. Septicemia
    2. Hepatic failure
    3. Mechanical hyperventilation
    4. Heat exposure
    5. Recovery from metabolic acidosis

II. Acidosis
  A. Central
    1. Drugs (anesthetics, morphine, sedatives)
    2. Stroke
    3. Infection
  B. Airway
    1. Obstruction
    2. Asthma
  C. Parenchyma
    1. Emphysema
    2. Pneumoconiosis
    3. Bronchitis
    4. Adult respiratory distress syndrome
    5. Barotrauma
  D. Neuromuscular
    1. Poliomyelitis
    2. Kyphoscoliosis
    3. Myasthenia
    4. Muscular dystrophies
  E. Miscellaneous
    1. Obesity
    2. Hypoventilation
    3. Permissive hypercapnia

RESPIRATORY ACIDOSIS

Respiratory acidosis can be due to severe pulmonary disease, respiratory muscle fatigue, or abnormalities in ventilatory control and is recognized by an increase in Pa_{CO_2} and decrease in pH (Table 48-7). In acute respiratory acidosis, there is an immediate compensatory elevation (due to cellular buffering mechanisms) in HCO_3^-, which increases 1 mmol/L for every 10-mmHg increase in Pa_{CO_2}. In chronic respiratory acidosis (>24 h), renal adaptation increases the $[HCO_3^-]$ by 4 mmol/L for every 10-mmHg increase in Pa_{CO_2}. The serum HCO_3^- usually does not increase above 38 mmol/L.

The clinical features vary according to the severity and duration of the respiratory acidosis, the underlying disease, and whether there is accompanying hypoxemia. A rapid increase in Pa_{CO_2} may cause anxiety, dyspnea, confusion, psychosis, and hallucinations and may progress to coma. Lesser degrees of dysfunction in chronic hypercapnia include sleep disturbances, loss of memory, daytime somnolence, personality changes, impairment of coordination, and motor disturbances such as tremor, myoclonic jerks, and asterixis. Headaches and other signs that mimic raised intracranial pressure, such as papilledema, abnormal reflexes, and focal muscle weakness, are due to vasoconstriction secondary to loss of the vasodilator effects of CO_2.

Depression of the respiratory center by a variety of drugs, injury, or disease can produce respiratory acidosis. This may occur acutely with general anesthetics, sedatives, and head trauma or chronically with sedatives, alcohol, intracranial tumors, and the syndromes of sleep-disordered breathing, including the primary alveolar and obesity-hypoventilation syndromes (Chaps. 258 and 259). Abnormalities or disease in the motor neurons, neuromuscular junction, and skeletal muscle can cause hypoventilation via respiratory muscle fatigue. Mechanical ventilation, when not properly adjusted and supervised, may result in respiratory acidosis, particularly if CO_2 production suddenly rises (because of fever, agitation, sepsis, or overfeeding) or alveolar ventilation falls because of worsening pulmonary function. High levels of positive end-expiratory pressure in the presence of reduced cardiac output may cause hypercapnia as a result of large increases in alveolar dead space (Chap. 246). Permissive hypercapnia is being used with increasing frequency because of studies suggesting lower mortality rates than with conventional mechanical ventilation, especially with severe central nervous system or heart disease. The potential beneficial effects of permissive hypercapnia may be mitigated by correction of the acidemia by administration of $NaHCO_3$.

Acute hypercapnia follows sudden occlusion of the upper airway or generalized bronchospasm as in severe asthma, anaphylaxis, inhalational burn, or toxin injury. Chronic hypercapnia and respiratory acidosis occur in end-stage obstructive lung disease. Restrictive disorders involving both the chest wall and the lungs can cause respiratory acidosis because the high metabolic cost of respiration causes ventilatory muscle fatigue. Advanced stages of intrapulmonary and extrapulmonary restrictive defects present as chronic respiratory acidosis.

The diagnosis of respiratory acidosis requires, by definition, the measurement of Pa_{CO_2} and arterial pH. A detailed history and physical examination often indicate the cause. Pulmonary function studies (Chap. 246), including spirometry, diffusion capacity for carbon monoxide, lung volumes, and arterial Pa_{CO_2} and O_2 saturation, usually make it possible to determine if respiratory acidosis is secondary to lung disease. The workup for nonpulmonary causes should include a detailed drug history, measurement of hematocrit, and assessment of upper airway, chest wall, pleura, and neuromuscular function.

Rx RESPIRATORY ACIDOSIS

The management of respiratory acidosis depends on its severity and rate of onset. Acute respiratory acidosis can be life threatening, and measures to reverse the underlying cause should be undertaken simultaneously with restoration of adequate alveolar ventilation. This may necessitate tracheal intubation and assisted mechanical ventilation. Oxygen administration should be titrated carefully in patients with severe obstructive pulmonary disease and chronic CO_2 retention who are breathing spontaneously (Chap. 254). When oxygen is used injudiciously, these patients may experience progression of the respiratory acidosis. Aggressive and rapid correction of hypercapnia should be avoided, because the falling Pa_{CO_2} may provoke the same complications noted with acute respiratory alkalosis (i.e., cardiac arrhythmias, reduced cerebral perfusion, and seizures). The Pa_{CO_2} should be lowered gradually in chronic respiratory acidosis, aiming to restore the Pa_{CO_2} to baseline levels and to provide sufficient Cl^- and K^+ to enhance the renal excretion of HCO_3^-.

Chronic respiratory acidosis is frequently difficult to correct, but measures aimed at improving lung function (Chap. 254) can help some patients and forestall further deterioration in most.

RESPIRATORY ALKALOSIS

Alveolar hyperventilation decreases Pa_{CO_2} and increases the HCO_3^-/Pa_{CO_2} ratio, thus increasing pH (Table 48-7). Nonbicarbonate cellular buffers respond by consuming HCO_3^-. Hypocapnia develops when a sufficiently strong ventilatory stimulus causes CO_2 output in the lungs to exceed its metabolic production by tissues. Plasma pH and $[HCO_3^-]$ appear to vary proportionally with Pa_{CO_2} over a range from 40–15 mmHg. The relationship between arterial $[H^+]$ concentration and Pa_{CO_2} is ~0.7 mmol/L per mmHg (or 0.01 pH unit/mmHg), and that for plasma $[HCO_3^-]$ is 0.2 mmol/L per mmHg. Hypocapnia sustained for >2–6 h is further compensated by a decrease in renal ammonium and titratable acid excretion and a reduction in filtered HCO_3^- reabsorption. Full renal adaptation to respiratory alkalosis may take several days and requires normal volume status and renal function. The kidneys appear to respond directly to the lowered Pa_{CO_2} rather than to alkalosis per se. In chronic respiratory alkalosis a 1-mmHg fall in Pa_{CO_2} causes a 0.4- to 0.5-mmol/L drop in $[HCO_3^-]$ and a 0.3-mmol/L fall (or 0.003 rise in pH) in $[H^+]$.

The effects of respiratory alkalosis vary according to duration and severity but are primarily those of the underlying disease. Reduced cerebral blood flow as a consequence of a rapid decline in Pa_{CO_2} may cause dizziness, mental confusion, and seizures, even in the absence of hypoxemia. The cardiovascular effects of acute hypocapnia in the conscious human are generally minimal, but in the anesthetized or mechanically ventilated patient, cardiac output and blood pressure may fall because of the depressant effects of anesthesia and positive-pressure ventilation on heart rate, systemic resistance, and venous return. Cardiac arrhythmias may occur in patients with heart disease as a result of changes in oxygen unloading by blood from a left shift in the hemoglobin-oxygen dissociation curve (Bohr

effect). Acute respiratory alkalosis causes intracellular shifts of Na^+, K^+, and PO_4^- and reduces free $[Ca^{2+}]$ by increasing the protein-bound fraction. Hypocapnia-induced hypokalemia is usually minor.

Chronic respiratory alkalosis is the most common acid-base disturbance in critically ill patients and, when severe, portends a poor prognosis. Many cardiopulmonary disorders manifest respiratory alkalosis in their early to intermediate stages, and the finding of normocapnia and hypoxemia in a patient with hyperventilation may herald the onset of rapid respiratory failure and should prompt an assessment to determine if the patient is becoming fatigued. Respiratory alkalosis is common during mechanical ventilation.

The hyperventilation syndrome may be disabling. Paresthesia, circumoral numbness, chest wall tightness or pain, dizziness, inability to take an adequate breath, and, rarely, tetany may themselves be sufficiently stressful to perpetuate the disorder. Arterial blood-gas analysis demonstrates an acute or chronic respiratory alkalosis, often with hypocapnia in the range of 15–30 mmHg and no hypoxemia. Central nervous system diseases or injury can produce several patterns of hyperventilation and sustained Pa_{CO_2} levels of 20–30 mmHg. Hyperthyroidism, high caloric loads, and exercise raise the basal metabolic rate, but ventilation usually rises in proportion so that arterial blood gases are unchanged and respiratory alkalosis does not develop. Salicylates are the most common cause of drug-induced respiratory alkalosis as a result of direct stimulation of the medullary chemoreceptor (**Chap. e34**). The methylxanthines, theophylline, and aminophylline stimulate ventilation and increase the ventilatory response to CO_2. Progesterone increases ventilation and lowers arterial Pa_{CO_2} by as much as 5–10 mmHg. Therefore, chronic respiratory alkalosis is a common feature of pregnancy. Respiratory alkalosis is also prominent in liver failure, and the severity correlates with the degree of hepatic insufficiency. Respiratory alkalosis is often an early finding in gram-negative septicemia, before fever, hypoxemia, or hypotension develops.

The diagnosis of respiratory alkalosis depends on measurement of arterial pH and Pa_{CO_2}. The plasma $[K^+]$ is often reduced and the $[Cl^-]$ increased. In the acute phase, respiratory alkalosis is not associated with increased renal HCO_3^- excretion, but within hours net acid excretion is reduced. In general, the HCO_3^- concentration falls by 2.0 mmol/L for each 10-mmHg decrease in Pa_{CO_2}. Chronic hypocapnia reduces the serum $[HCO_3^-]$ by 4.0 mmol/L for each 10-mmHg decrease in Pa_{CO_2}. It is unusual to observe a plasma $HCO_3^- < 12$ mmol/L as a result of a pure respiratory alkalosis.

When a diagnosis of respiratory alkalosis is made, its cause should be investigated. The diagnosis of hyperventilation syndrome is made by exclusion. In difficult cases, it may be important to rule out other conditions such as pulmonary embolism, coronary artery disease, and hyperthyroidism.

Rx RESPIRATORY ALKALOSIS

The management of respiratory alkalosis is directed toward alleviation of the underlying disorder. If respiratory alkalosis complicates ventilator management, changes in dead space, tidal volume, and frequency can minimize the hypocapnia. Patients with the hyperventilation syndrome may benefit from reassurance, rebreathing from a paper bag during symptomatic attacks, and attention to underlying psychological stress. Antidepressants and sedatives are not recommended. β-Adrenergic blockers may ameliorate peripheral manifestations of the hyperadrenergic state.

FURTHER READINGS

DuBose TD Jr: Acid-base disorders, in *Brenner and Rector's The Kidney*, 8th ed, BM Brenner (ed). Philadelphia, Saunders, 2007, in press

———, Alpern RJ: Renal tubular acidosis, in *The Metabolic and Molecular Bases of Inherited Disease*, 8th ed, CR Scriver et al (eds). New York, McGraw-Hill, 2001

Galla JH: Metabolic alkalosis, in *Acid-Base and Electrolyte Disorders—A Companion to Brenner and Rector's The Kidney*, TD DuBose, LL Hamm (eds). Philadelphia, Saunders, 2002, pp 109–128

296 LASKI ME, WESSON DE: Lactic acidosis, in *Acid-Base and Electrolyte Disorders—A Companion to Brenner and Rector's The Kidney*, TD DuBose, LL Hamm (eds). Philadelphia, Saunders, 2002, pp 83–107

MADIAS NE: Respiratory alkalosis, in *Acid-Base and Electrolyte Disorders—A Companion to Brenner and Rector's The Kidney*, TD DuBose, LL Hamm (eds). Philadelphia, Saunders, 2002, pp 147–164

WESSON DE et al: Clinical syndromes of metabolic alkalosis, in *The Kidney: Physiology and Pathophysiology*, 3d ed, DW Seldin, G Giebisch (eds). Philadelphia, Lippincott Williams and Wilkins, 2000, pp 2055–2072

SECTION 8 · ALTERATIONS IN SEXUAL FUNCTION AND REPRODUCTION

49 Sexual Dysfunction
Kevin T. McVary

Male sexual dysfunction affects 10–25% of middle-aged and elderly men. Female sexual dysfunction occurs with a similar frequency. Demographic changes, the popularity of newer treatments, and greater awareness of sexual dysfunction by patients and society have led to increased diagnosis and associated health care expenditures for the management of this common disorder. Because many patients are reluctant to initiate discussion of their sex lives, the physician should address this topic directly to elicit a history of sexual dysfunction.

MALE SEXUAL DYSFUNCTION

PHYSIOLOGY OF MALE SEXUAL RESPONSE
Normal male sexual function requires (1) an intact libido, (2) the ability to achieve and maintain penile erection, (3) ejaculation, and (4) detumescence. *Libido* refers to sexual desire and is influenced by a variety of visual, olfactory, tactile, auditory, imaginative, and hormonal stimuli. Sex steroids, particularly testosterone, act to increase libido. Libido can be diminished by hormonal or psychiatric disorders or by medications.

Penile tumescence leading to erection depends on the increased flow of blood into the lacunar network accompanied by the complete relaxation of the arteries and corporal smooth muscle. The microarchitecture of the corpora is composed of a mass of smooth muscle (trabecula) which contains a network of endothelial-lined vessels (lacunar spaces). Subsequent compression of the trabecular smooth muscle against the fibroelastic tunica albuginea causes a passive closure of the emissary veins and accumulation of blood in the corpora. In the presence of a full erection and a competent valve mechanism, the corpora become noncompressible cylinders from which blood does not escape.

The central nervous system (CNS) exerts an important influence by either stimulating or antagonizing spinal pathways that mediate erectile function and ejaculation. The erectile response is mediated by a combination of central (psychogenic) and peripheral (reflexogenic) innervation. Sensory nerves that originate from receptors in the penile skin and glans converge to form the dorsal nerve of the penis, which travels to the S2-S4 dorsal root ganglia via the pudendal nerve. Parasympathetic nerve fibers to the penis arise from neurons in the intermediolateral columns of S2-S4 sacral spinal segments. Sympathetic innervation originates from the T-11 to the L-2 spinal segments and descends through the hypogastric plexus.

Neural input to smooth-muscle tone is crucial to the initiation and maintenance of an erection. There is also an intricate interaction between the corporal smooth muscle cell and its overlying endothelial cell lining (Fig. 49-1A). Nitric oxide, which induces vascular relaxation, promotes erection and is opposed by endothelin-1 (ET-1) and Rho kinase, which mediate vascular contraction. Nitric oxide is synthesized from L-arginine by nitric oxide synthase and is released from the nonadrenergic, noncholinergic (NANC) autonomic nerve supply to act postjunctionally on smooth-muscle cells. Nitric oxide increases the production of cyclic 3′,5′-guanosine monophosphate (cyclic

GMP), which induces relaxation of the smooth muscle (Fig. 49-1B). Cyclic GMP is gradually broken down by phosphodiesterase type 5 (PDE-5). Inhibitors of PDE-5, such as the oral medications sildenafil, vardenifil, and tadalafil maintain erections by reducing the breakdown of cyclic GMP. However, if nitric oxide is not produced at some level, PDE-5 inhibitors are ineffective, as these drugs facilitate, but do not initiate, the initial enzyme cascade. In addition to nitric oxide, vasoactive prostaglandins (PGE_1, $PGF_{2\alpha}$) are synthesized within the cavernosal tissue and increase cyclic AMP levels, also leading to relaxation of cavernosal smooth-muscle cells.

Ejaculation is stimulated by the sympathetic nervous system, which results in contraction of the epididymis, vas deferens, seminal vesicles,

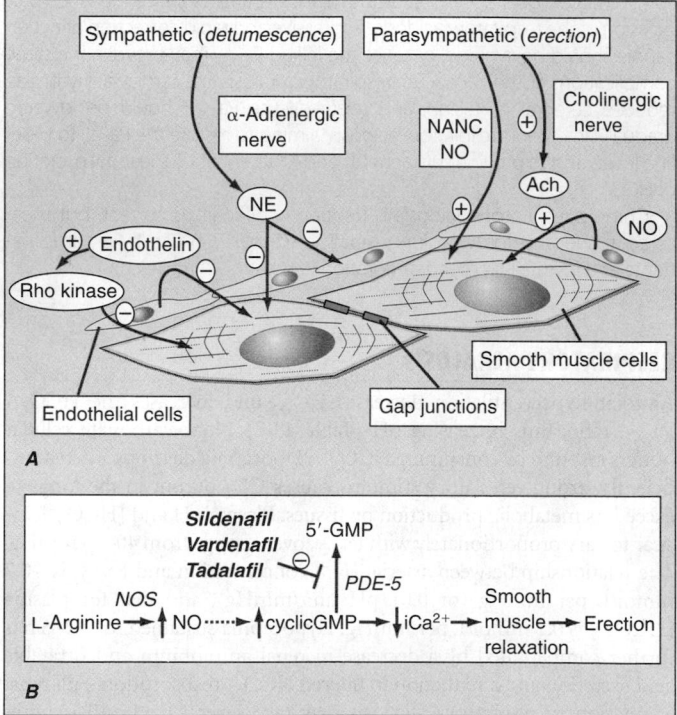

FIGURE 49-1 Pathways that control erection and detumescence. **A.** Erection is mediated by cholinergic parasympathetic pathways, and nonadrenergic, noncholinergic (NANC) pathways, which release nitric oxide (NO). Endothelial cells also release NO, which induces vascular smooth-muscle cell relaxation, allowing enhanced blood flow, and leading to erection. Detumescence is mediated by sympathetic pathways that release norepinephrine and stimulate α-adrenergic pathways, leading to contraction of vascular smooth-muscle cells. Endothelin, released from endothelial cells, also induces contraction. Rho kinase activation via endothelin activity (among others) also contributes to detumescence by alteration of calcium signaling. **B.** Biochemical pathways of NO synthesis and action. Sildenafil, vardenafil, and tadalafil enhance erectile function by inhibiting phosphodiesterase type 5 (PDE-5), thereby maintaining high levels of cyclic 3′,5′-guanosine monophosphate (cyclic GMP). NOS, nitric oxide synthase; iCa^{2+}, intracellular calcium.

and prostate, causing seminal fluid to enter the urethra. Seminal fluid emission is followed by rhythmic contractions of the bulbocavernosus and ischiocavernosus muscles, leading to ejaculation. *Premature ejaculation* is usually related to anxiety or a learned behavior and is amenable to behavioral therapy or treatment with medications such as selective serotonin reuptake inhibitors (SSRIs). *Retrograde ejaculation* results when the internal urethral sphincter does not close; it may occur in men with diabetes or after surgery involving the bladder neck.

Detumescence is mediated by norepinephrine from the sympathetic nerves, endothelin from the vascular surface, and smooth-muscle contraction induced by postsynaptic α-adrenergic receptors and activation of Rho kinase. These events increase venous outflow and restore the flaccid state. Venous leak can cause premature detumescence and is caused by insufficient relaxation of the corporal smooth muscle rather than a specific anatomic defect. *Priapism* refers to a persistent and painful erection and may be associated with sickle cell anemia, hypercoagulable states, spinal cord injury, or injection of vasodilator agents into the penis.

ERECTILE DYSFUNCTION

Epidemiology Erectile dysfunction (ED) is not considered a normal part of the aging process. Nonetheless, it is associated with certain physiologic and psychological changes related to age. In the Massachusetts Male Aging Study (MMAS), a community-based survey of men between the ages of 40 and 70, 52% of responders reported some degree of ED. Complete ED occurred in 10% of respondents, moderate ED occurred in 25%, and minimal ED in 17%. The incidence of moderate or severe ED more than doubled between the ages of 40 and 70. In the National Health and Social Life Survey (NHSLS), which was a nationally representative sample of men and women ages 18–59, 10% of men reported being unable to maintain an erection (corresponding to the proportion of men in the MMAS reporting severe ED). Incidence was highest among men in the 50–59 age group (21%) and among men who were poor (14%), divorced (14%), and less educated (13%).

The incidence of ED is also higher among men with certain medical disorders such as diabetes mellitus, obesity, lower urinary tract symptoms secondary to benign prostatic hyperplasia (BPH), heart disease, hypertension, and decreased HDL levels. Smoking is a significant risk factor in the development of ED. Medications used to treat diabetes or cardiovascular disease are additional risk factors (see below). There is a higher incidence of ED among men who have undergone radiation or surgery for prostate cancer and in those with a lower spinal cord injury. Psychological causes of ED include depression, anger, or stress from unemployment or other causes.

Pathophysiology ED may result from three basic mechanisms: (1) failure to initiate (psychogenic, endocrinologic, or neurogenic); (2) failure to fill (arteriogenic); or (3) failure to store adequate blood volume within the lacunar network (venoocclusive dysfunction). These categories are not mutually exclusive, and multiple factors contribute to ED in many patients. For example, diminished filling pressure can lead secondarily to venous leak. Psychogenic factor frequently coexist with other etiologic factors and should be considered in all cases. Diabetic, atherosclerotic, and drug-related causes account for >80% of cases of ED in older men.

VASCULOGENIC The most frequent organic cause of ED is a disturbance of blood flow to and from the penis. Atherosclerotic or traumatic arterial disease can decrease flow to the lacunar spaces, resulting in decreased rigidity and an increased time to full erection. Excessive outflow through the veins, despite adequate inflow, may also contribute to ED. Structural alterations to the fibroelastic components of the corpora may cause a loss of compliance and an inability to compress the tunical veins. This condition may result from aging, increased cross-linking of collagen fibers induced by nonenzymatic glycosylation, hypoxia, or altered synthesis of collagen associated with hypercholesterolemia.

NEUROGENIC Disorders that affect the sacral spinal cord or the autonomic fibers to the penis preclude nervous system relaxation of penile smooth muscle, thus leading to ED. In patients with spinal cord injury,

the degree of ED depends on the completeness and level of the lesion. Patients with incomplete lesions or injuries to the upper part of the spinal cord are more likely to retain erectile capabilities than those with complete lesions or injuries to the lower part. Although 75% of patients with spinal cord injuries have some erectile capability, only 25% have erections sufficient for penetration. Other neurologic disorders commonly associated with ED include multiple sclerosis and peripheral neuropathy. The latter is often due to either diabetes or alcoholism. Pelvic surgery may cause ED through disruption of the autonomic nerve supply.

ENDOCRINOLOGIC Androgens increase libido, but their exact role in erectile function remains unclear. Individuals with castrate levels of testosterone can achieve erections from visual or sexual stimuli. Nonetheless, normal levels of testosterone appear to be important for erectile function, particularly in older males. Androgen replacement therapy can improve depressed erectile function when it is secondary to hypogonadism; however, it is not useful for ED when endogenous testosterone levels are normal. Increased prolactin may decrease libido by suppressing gonadotropin-releasing hormone (GnRH), and it also leads to decreased testosterone levels. Treatment of hyperprolactinemia with dopamine agonists can restore libido and testosterone.

DIABETIC ED occurs in 35–75% of men with diabetes mellitus. Pathologic mechanisms are primarily related to diabetes-associated vascular and neurologic complications. Diabetic macrovascular complications are mainly related to age, whereas microvascular complications correlate with the duration of diabetes and the degree of glycemic control (Chap. 338). Individuals with diabetes also have reduced amounts of nitric oxide synthase in both endothelial and neural tissues.

PSYCHOGENIC Two mechanisms contribute to the inhibition of erections in psychogenic ED. First, psychogenic stimuli to the sacral cord may inhibit reflexogenic responses, thereby blocking activation of vasodilator outflow to the penis. Second, excess sympathetic stimulation in an anxious man may increase penile smooth-muscle tone. The most common causes of psychogenic ED are performance anxiety, depression, relationship conflict, loss of attraction, sexual inhibition, conflicts over sexual preference, sexual abuse in childhood, and fear of pregnancy or sexually transmitted disease. Almost all patients with ED, even when it has a clear-cut organic basis, develop a psychogenic component as a reaction to ED.

MEDICATION-RELATED Medication-induced ED (Table 49-1) is estimated to occur in 25% of men seen in general medical outpatient clinics. Among the antihypertensive agents, the thiazide diuretics and beta blockers have been implicated most frequently. Calcium channel blockers and angiotensin-converting enzyme inhibitors are less frequently cited. These drugs may act directly at the corporal level (e.g., calcium channel blockers) or indirectly by reducing pelvic blood pressure, which is important in the development of penile rigidity. α Adrenergic blockers are less likely to cause ED. Estrogens, GnRH agonists, H_2 antagonists, and spironolactone cause ED by suppressing gonadotropin production or by blocking androgen action. Antidepressant and antipsychotic agents—particularly neuroleptics, tricyclics, and SSRIs—are associated with erectile, ejaculatory, orgasmic, and sexual desire difficulties.

Although many medications can cause ED, patients frequently have concomitant risk factors that confound the clinical picture. If there is a strong association between the institution of a drug and the onset of ED, alternative medications should be considered. Otherwise, it is often practical to treat the ED without attempting multiple changes in medications, as it may be difficult to establish a causal role for the drug.

APPROACH TO THE PATIENT:
Erectile Dysfunction

A good physician-patient relationship helps to unravel the possible causes of ED, many of which require discussion of personal and some-

TABLE 49-1 DRUGS ASSOCIATED WITH ERECTILE DYSFUNCTION

Classification	Drugs
Diuretics	Thiazides
	Spironolactone
Antihypertensives	Calcium channel blockers
	Methyldopa
	Clonidine
	Reserpine
	β-Blockers
	Guanethidine
Cardiac/anti-hyperlipidemics	Digoxin
	Gemfibrozil
	Clofibrate
Antidepressants	Selective serotonin reuptake inhibitors
	Tricyclic antidepressants
	Lithium
	Monoamine oxidase inhibitors
Tranquilizers	Butyrophenones
	Phenothiazines
H_2 antagonists	Ranitidine
	Cimetidine
Hormones	Progesterone
	Estrogens
	Corticosteroids
	GnRH agonists
	5α-Reductase inhibitors
	Cyproterone acetate
Cytotoxic agents	Cyclophosphamide
	Methotrexate
	Roferon-A
Anticholinergics	Disopyramide
	Anticonvulsants
Recreational	Ethanol
	Cocaine
	Marijuana

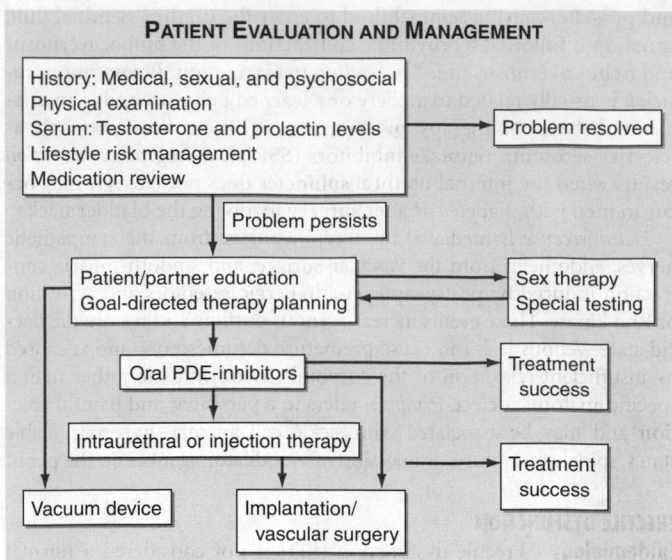

FIGURE 49-2 Algorithm for the evaluation and management of patients with ED.

times embarrassing topics. For this reason, a primary care provider is often ideally suited to initiate the evaluation. A complete medical and sexual history should be taken in an effort to assess whether the cause of ED is organic, psychogenic, or multifactorial (Fig. 49-2). Initial questions should focus on the onset of symptoms, the presence and duration of partial erections, and the progression of ED. A history of nocturnal or early morning erections is useful for distinguishing physiologic from psychogenic ED. Nocturnal erections occur during rapid eye movement (REM) sleep and require intact neurologic and circulatory systems. Organic causes of ED are generally characterized by a gradual and persistent change in rigidity or the inability to sustain nocturnal, coital, or self-stimulated erections. The patient should be questioned about the presence of penile curvature or pain with coitus. It is also important to address libido, as decreased sexual drive and ED are sometimes the earliest signs of endocrine abnormalities (e.g., increased prolactin, decreased testosterone levels). It is useful to ask whether the problem is confined to coitus with one or other partners; ED arises not uncommonly in association with new or extramarital sexual relationships. Situational ED, as opposed to consistent ED, suggests psychogenic causes. Ejaculation is much less commonly affected than erection, but questions should be asked about whether ejaculation is normal, premature, delayed, or absent. Relevant risk factors should be identified, such as diabetes mellitus, coronary artery disease (CAD), or neurologic disorders. The patient's surgical history should be explored with an emphasis on bowel, bladder, prostate, or vascular procedures. A complete drug history is also important. Social changes that may precipitate ED are also crucial to the evaluation, including health worries, spousal death, divorce, relationship difficulties, and financial concerns.

Because ED commonly involves a host of endothelial cell risk factors, men with ED report higher rates of overt and silent myocardial infarction. As such, ED in an otherwise asymptomatic male warrants consideration of other vascular disorders including CAD.

The physical examination is an essential element in the assessment of ED. Signs of hypertension as well as evidence of thyroid,

hepatic, hematologic, cardiovascular, or renal diseases should be sought. An assessment should be made of the endocrine and vascular systems, the external genitalia, and the prostate gland. The penis should be carefully palpated along the corpora to detect fibrotic plaques. Reduced testicular size and loss of secondary sexual characteristics are suggestive of hypogonadism. Neurologic examination should include assessment of anal sphincter tone, the bulbocavernosus reflex, and testing for peripheral neuropathy.

Although hyperprolactinemia is uncommon, a serum prolactin level should be measured, as decreased libido and/or erectile dysfunction may be the presenting symptoms of a prolactinoma or other mass lesions of the sella (Chap. 333). The serum testosterone level should be measured and, if low, gonadotropins should be measured to determine whether hypogonadism is primary (testicular) or secondary (hypothalamic-pituitary) in origin (Chap. 340). If not performed recently, serum chemistries, CBC, and lipid profiles may be of value, as they can yield evidence of anemia, diabetes, hyperlipidemia, or other systemic diseases associated with ED. Determination of serum prostate specific antigen (PSA) should be conducted according to recommended clinical guidelines (Chap. 91).

Additional diagnostic testing is rarely necessary in the evaluation of ED. However, in selected patients, specialized testing may provide insight into pathologic mechanisms of ED and aid in the selection of treatment options. Optional specialized testing includes: (1) studies of nocturnal penile tumescence and rigidity; (2) vascular testing (in-office injection of vasoactive substances, penile Doppler ultrasound, penile angiography, dynamic infusion cavernosography/cavernosometry); (3) neurologic testing (biothesiometry-graded vibratory perception; somatosensory evoked potentials); and (4) psychological diagnostic tests. The information potentially gained from these procedures must be balanced against their invasiveness and cost.

℞ MALE SEXUAL DYSFUNCTION

PATIENT EDUCATION Patient and partner education is essential in the treatment of ED. In goal-directed therapy, education facilitates understanding of the disease, results of the tests, and selection of treatment. Discussion of treatment options helps to clarify how treatment is best offered and stratify first- and second-line therapies. Patients with high-risk lifestyle issues, such as smoking, alcohol abuse, or recreational drug use, should be counseled on the role these factors play in the development of ED.

ORAL AGENTS Sildenafil, tadalafil, and vardenifil are the only approved and effective oral agents for the treatment of ED. These three medications have markedly improved the management of ED because they are effective for the treatment of a broad range of causes, including psychogenic, diabetic, vasculogenic, postradical prostatectomy (nerve-sparing procedures), and spinal cord injury. They belong to a class of medications that are selective and potent inhibitors of PDE-5, the predominant phosphodiesterase isoform found in the penis. They are administered in graduated doses and enhance erections after sexual stimulation. The onset of action is approximately 60–120 min, depending on the medication used and other factors such as recent food intake. Reduced initial doses should be considered for patients who are elderly, taking concomitant alpha blockers, have renal insufficiency, or are taking medications that inhibit the CYP3A4 metabolic pathway in the liver (e.g., erythromycin, cimetidine, ketoconazole, and, possibly, itraconazole and mibefradil), as they may increase the serum concentration of the PDE-5 inhibitors or promote hypotension. Testosterone supplementation combined with a PDE-5 inhibitor may be beneficial in improving erectile function in hypogonadal men with erectile dysfunction who are unresponsive to PDE-5 inhibitors alone. These drugs do not affect ejaculation, orgasm, or sexual drive. Side effects associated with PDE-5 inhibitors include headaches (19%), facial flushing (9%), dyspepsia (6%), and nasal congestion (4%). Approximately 7% of men using sildenafil may experience transient altered color vision (blue halo effect), while 6% of men taking tadalafil may experience loin pain. PDE-5 inhibitors are contraindicated in men receiving nitrate therapy for cardiovascular disease, including agents delivered by oral, sublingual, transnasal, or topical routes. These agents can potentiate its hypotensive effect and may result in profound shock. Likewise, amyl/butyl nitrate "poppers" may have a fatal synergistic effect on blood pressure. PDE-5 inhibitors should also be avoided in patients with congestive heart failure and cardiomyopathy because of the risk of vascular collapse. Because sexual activity leads to an increase in physiologic expenditure [5–6 metabolic equivalents (METS)], physicians have been advised to exercise caution in prescribing any drug for sexual activity to those with active coronary disease, heart failure, borderline hypotension, or hypovolemia, and to those on complex antihypertensive regimens.

Although the PDE-5 inhibitors share a common mechanism of action, there are a few differences among the three agents. Having been on the market the longest, sildenafil has the most robust data confirming its activity, safety, and tolerability. It has recently been released for use in pulmonary hypertension as well as ED. Tadalafil is unique in its longer half-life. All three drugs are effective for patients with ED of all ages, severities, and etiologies. While there are pharmacokinetic and pharmacodynamic differences among these agents, clinically relevant differences are not clear.

ANDROGEN THERAPY   Testosterone replacement is used to treat both primary and secondary causes of hypogonadism (Chap. 340). Androgen supplementation in the setting of normal testosterone is rarely efficacious and is discouraged. Methods of androgen replacement include transdermal patches and gels, parenteral administration of long-acting testosterone esters (enanthate and cypionate), and oral preparations (17 α-alkylated derivatives) (Chap. 340). Transdermal delivery of testosterone using patches or gels (50–100 mg/d) more closely mimics physiologic testosterone levels, but it is unclear whether this translates into improved sexual function. The administration of 200–300 mg intramuscularly every 2–3 weeks provides another option but is far from an ideal physiologic replacement. Oral androgen preparations have the potential for hepatotoxicity and should be avoided. Testosterone therapy is contraindicated in men with androgen-sensitive cancers (e.g., prostate) and may be inappropriate for men with bladder neck obstruction. It is generally advisable to measure PSA before giving androgen. Hepatic function should be tested before and during testosterone therapy.

VACUUM CONSTRICTION DEVICES   Vacuum constriction devices (VCD) are a well-established, noninvasive therapy. They are a reasonable treatment alternative for select patients who cannot take sildenafil or do not desire other interventions. VCD draw venous blood into the penis and use a constriction ring to restrict venous return and maintain tumescence. Adverse events with VCD include pain, numbness, bruising, and altered ejaculation. Additionally, many patients complain that the devices are cumbersome and that the induced erections have a nonphysiologic appearance and feel.

INTRAURETHRAL ALPROSTADIL   If a patient fails to respond to oral agents, a reasonable next choice is intraurethral or self-injection of vasoactive substances. Intraurethral prostaglandin E_1 (alprostadil), in the form of a semisolid pellet (doses of 125–1000 μg), is delivered with an applicator. Approximately 65% of men receiving intraurethral alprostadil respond with an erection when tested in the office, but only 50% of those achieve successful

coitus at home. Intraurethral insertion is associated with a markedly reduced incidence of priapism in comparison to intracavernosal injection.

INTRACAVERNOSAL SELF-INJECTION   Injection of synthetic formulations of alprostadil is effective in 70–80% of patients with ED, but discontinuation rates are high because of the invasive nature of administration. Doses range between 1 and 40 μg. Injection therapy is contraindicated in men with a history of hypersensitivity to the drug and in men at risk for priapism (hypercoaguable states, sickle cell disease). Side effects include local adverse events, prolonged erections, pain, and fibrosis with chronic use. Various combinations of alprostadil, phentolamine, and/or papaverine are sometimes used.

SURGERY   A less frequently used form of therapy for ED involves the surgical implantation of a semirigid or inflatable penile prosthesis. These surgical treatments are invasive, associated with potential complications, and generally reserved for treatment of refractory ED. Despite their high cost and invasiveness, penile prostheses are associated with high rates of patient and partner satisfaction.

SEX THERAPY   A course of sex therapy may be useful for addressing specific interpersonal factors that may affect sexual functioning. Sex therapy generally consists of in-session discussion and at-home exercises specific to the person and the relationship. It is preferable if therapy includes both partners, provided the patient is involved in an ongoing relationship.

FEMALE SEXUAL DYSFUNCTION

Female sexual dysfunction (FSD) has traditionally included disorders of desire, arousal, pain, and muted orgasm. The associated risk factors for FSD are similar to those in males: cardiovascular disease, endocrine disorders, hypertension, neurologic disorders, and smoking (Table 49-2).

EPIDEMIOLOGY

Epidemiologic data are limited, but the available estimates suggest that as many as 43% of women complain of at least one sexual problem. Despite the recent interest in organic causes of FSD, desire and arousal phase disorders (including lubrication complaints) remain the most common presenting problems when surveyed in a community-based population.

PHYSIOLOGY OF THE FEMALE SEXUAL RESPONSE

The female sexual response requires the presence of estrogens. A role for androgens is also likely but less well-established. In the CNS, estrogens and androgens work synergistically to enhance sexual arousal and response. A number of studies report enhanced libido in women during preovulatory phases of the menstrual cycle, suggesting that hormones involved in the ovulatory surge (e.g., estrogens) increase desire.

Sexual motivation is heavily influenced by context, including the environment and partner factors. Once sufficient sexual desire is reached, sexual arousal is mediated by the central and autonomic nervous systems. Cerebral sympathetic outflow is thought to increase desire, while peripheral parasympathetic activity results in clitoral vasocongestion and vaginal secretion (lubrication).

The neurotransmitters for clitoral corporal engorgement are similar to those in the male, with a prominent role for neural, smooth muscle,

TABLE 49-2	RISK FACTORS FOR FEMALE SEXUAL DYSFUNCTION

Neurologic disease: stroke, spinal cord injury, Parkinsonism
Trauma, genital surgery, radiation
Endocrinopathies: diabetes, hyperprolactinemia
Liver and/or renal failure
Cardiovascular disease
Psychological factors and interpersonal relationship disorders: sexual abuse, life stressors
Medications
   Antiandrogens: cimetidine, spironolactone
   Antidepressants, alcohol, hypnotics, sedatives
   Antiestrogens or GnRH antagonists
   Antihistamines, sympathomimetic amines
   Antihypertensives: diuretics, calcium channel blockers
   Alkylating agents
   Anticholinergics

and endothelial released nitric oxide (NO). A fine network of vaginal nerves and arterioles promote a vaginal transudate. The major transmitters of this complex vaginal response are not certain, but roles for NO and vasointestinal polypeptide (VIP) are suspected. Investigators studying the normal female sexual response have challenged the long-held construct of a linear and unmitigated relationship between initial desire, arousal, vasocongestion, lubrication, and eventual orgasm. Caregivers should consider a paradigm of a positive emotional and physical outcome with one, many, or no orgasmic peak and release.

Although there are the obvious anatomic differences as well as variation in the density of vascular and neural beds in males and females, the primary effectors of sexual response are strikingly similar. Intact sensation is important for arousal. Thus, reduced levels of sexual functioning are more common in women with peripheral neuropathies (e.g., diabetes). Vaginal lubrication is a transudate of serum that results from the increased pelvic blood flow associated with arousal. Vascular insufficiency from a variety of causes may compromise adequate lubrication and result in dyspareunia. Cavernosal and arteriole smooth-muscle relaxation occurs via increased nitric oxide synthase (NOS) activity and produces engorgement in the clitoris and surrounding vestibule. Orgasm requires an intact sympathetic outflow tract; hence, orgasmic disorders are common in female patients with spinal cord injuries.

APPROACH TO THE PATIENT:
Female Sexual Dysfunction

Many women do not volunteer information concerning their sexual response. Open-ended questions in a supportive atmosphere are helpful for initiating a discussion of sexual fitness in women who are reluctant to discuss such issues. Once a complaint has been voiced, a comprehensive evaluation should be performed, including a medical history, psychosocial history, physical examination, and limited laboratory testing.

The history should include the usual medical, surgical, obstetric, psychological, gynecologic, sexual, and social information. Past experiences, intimacy, knowledge, and partner availability should also be ascertained. Medical disorders that may impact sexual health should be delineated. These include diabetes, cardiovascular disease, gynecologic conditions, obstetric history, depression, anxiety disorders, and neurologic disease. Medications should be reviewed as they may impact arousal, libido, and orgasm. The need for counseling and life stresses should be identified. The physical examination should assess the genitalia, including clitoris. Pelvic floor examination may identify prolapse or other disorders. Laboratory studies are needed, especially if menopausal status is uncertain. Estradiol, FSH, and LH are usually obtained, and dehydroepiandrosterone (DHEA) should be considered as it reflects adrenal androgen secretion. A complete blood count, liver function assessment, and lipid studies may be useful, if not otherwise obtained. Complicated diagnostic evaluation, such as clitoral Doppler ultrasonography and biothesiometry, require expensive equipment and are of uncertain utility. It is important for the patient to identify which symptoms are most distressing.

The evaluation of FSD previously occurred mainly in a psychosocial context. However, inconsistencies between diagnostic categories based on only psychosocial considerations, and the emerging recognition of organic etiologies, has led to a new classification of FSD. This diagnostic scheme is based on four components that are not mutually exclusive: (1) *Hypoactive sexual desire*—the persistent or recurrent lack of sexual thoughts and/or receptivity to sexual activity, which causes personal distress. Hypoactive sexual desire may result from endocrine failure or may be associated with psychological or emotional disorders, (2) *Sexual arousal disorder*—the persistent or recurrent inability to attain or maintain sexual excitement, which causes personal distress, (3) *Orgasmic disorder*—the persistent or recurrent loss of orgasmic potential after sufficient sexual stimulation and arousal, which causes personal distress, (4) *Sexual pain disorder*—persistent or recurrent genital pain associated with noncoital sexual stimulation, which causes personal distress. This newer classification emphasizes "personal distress" as a requirement for dysfunction and provides clinicians with an organized framework for evaluation prior to or in conjunction with more traditional counseling methods.

℞ FEMALE SEXUAL DYSFUNCTION

GENERAL An open discussion with the patient is important as couples may need to be educated about normal anatomy and physiologic responses, including role of orgasm in sexual encounters. Physiologic changes associated with aging and/or disease should be explained. Couples may need to be reminded that clitoral stimulation rather than coital intromission may be more beneficial.

Behavioral modification and nonpharmacologic therapies should be a first step. Patient and partner counseling may improve communication and relationship strains. Lifestyle changes involving known risk factors can be an important part of the treatment process. Emphasis on maximizing physical health and avoiding lifestyles (e.g., smoking, alcohol abuse) and medications likely to produce FSD is important (Table 49-2). The use of topical lubricants may address complaints of dyspareunia and dryness. Contributing medications, such as antidepressants, may need to be altered, including the use of medications with less impact on sexual function, dose reduction, medication switching, or drug holidays.

HORMONAL THERAPY In postmenopausal women, estrogen replacement therapy may be helpful in treating vaginal atrophy, decreasing coital pain, and improving clitoral sensitivity (Chap. 342). Estrogen replacement in the form of local cream is the preferred method, as it avoids systemic side effects. Androgen levels in women decline substantially before menopause. However, low levels of testosterone or DHEA are not effective predictors of a positive therapeutic outcome with androgen therapy. The widespread use of exogenous androgens is not supported by the literature except in select circumstances (premature ovarian failure or menopausal states) and in secondary arousal disorders.

ORAL AGENTS The efficacy of PDE-5 inhibitors in FDS has been a marked disappointment given the proposed role of nitric oxide-dependent physiology in the normal female sexual response. The use of PDE-5 inhibitors for FSD should be discouraged pending proof that it is effective.

CLITORAL VACUUM DEVICE In patients with arousal and orgasmic difficulties, the option of using a clitoral vacuum device may be explored. This handheld battery-operated device has a small soft plastic cup that applies a vacuum over the stimulated clitoris. This causes increased cavernosal blood flow, engorgement, and vaginal lubrication.

FURTHER READINGS

ARAUJO AB et al: Changes in sexual function in middle-aged and older men: Longitudinal data from the Massachusetts male aging study. J Am Geriatr Soc 52:1502, 2004

BASSON R: Recent advances in women's sexual function and dysfunction. Menopause 11:714, 2004

BHASIN S et al: Sexual dysfunction in men and women with endocrine disorders. Lancet 369(9561):597, 2007

BURNETT AL: Erectile dysfunction. J Urol 175:S25, 2006

DAVIS SR et al: Endocrine aspects of female sexual dysfunction. J Sex Med 1:82, 2004

DOGGRELL SA: Comparison of clinical trials with sildenafil, vardenafil, and tadalafil in erectile dysfunction. Expert Opin Pharmacother 6:75, 2005

PAULS RN et al: Female sexual dysfunction: principles of diagnosis and therapy. Obstet Gynecol Surv 60:196, 2005

REES PM et al: Sexual function in men and women with neurological disorders. Lancet 369(9560):512, 2007

50 Hirsutism and Virilization
David A. Ehrmann

Hirsutism, defined as excessive male-pattern hair growth, affects approximately 10% of women. It usually represents a variation of normal hair growth, but rarely it is a harbinger of a serious underlying condition. Hirsutism is often idiopathic but may be caused by conditions associated with androgen excess, such as polycystic ovarian syndrome (PCOS) or congenital adrenal hyperplasia (CAH) (Table 50-1). Cutaneous manifestations commonly associated with hirsutism include acne and male-pattern balding (androgenic alopecia). *Virilization* refers to a condition in which androgen levels are sufficiently high to cause additional signs and symptoms such as deepening of the voice, breast atrophy, increased muscle bulk, clitoromegaly, and increased libido; virilization is an ominous sign that suggests the possibility of an ovarian or adrenal neoplasm.

HAIR FOLLICLE GROWTH AND DIFFERENTIATION

Hair can be categorized as either *vellus* (fine, soft, and not pigmented) or *terminal* (long, coarse, and pigmented). The number of hair follicles does not change over an individual's lifetime, but the follicle size and type of hair can change in response to numerous factors, particularly androgens. Androgens are necessary for terminal hair and sebaceous gland development and mediate differentiation of pilosebaceous units (PSUs) into either a terminal hair follicle or a sebaceous gland. In the former case, androgens transform the vellus hair into a terminal hair; in the latter, the sebaceous component proliferates and the hair remains vellus.

There are three phases in the cycle of hair growth: (1) *anagen* (growth phase), (2) *catagen* (involution phase), and (3) *telogen* (rest phase). Depending on the body site, hormonal regulation may play an important role in the hair growth cycle. For example, the eyebrows, eyelashes, and vellus hairs are androgen-insensitive, whereas the axillary and pubic areas are sensitive to low levels of androgens. Hair growth on the face, chest, upper abdomen, and back requires greater levels of androgens and is therefore more characteristic of the pattern typically seen in men. Androgen excess in women leads to increased hair growth in most androgen-

sensitive sites except in the scalp region, where hair loss occurs because androgens cause scalp hairs to spend less time in the anagen phase.

Although androgen excess underlies most cases of hirsutism, there is only a modest correlation between androgen levels and the quantity of hair growth. This is due to the fact that hair growth from the follicle also depends on local growth factors, and there is variability in end-organ sensitivity. Genetic factors and ethnic background also influence hair growth. In general, dark-haired individuals tend to be more hirsute than blonde or fair individuals. Asians and Native Americans have relatively sparse hair in regions sensitive to high androgen levels, whereas people of Mediterranean descent are more hirsute.

CLINICAL ASSESSMENT

Historic elements relevant to the assessment of hirsutism include the age of onset and rate of progression of hair growth and associated symptoms or signs (e.g., acne). Depending on the cause, excess hair growth is typically first noted during the second and third decades. The growth is usually slow but progressive. Sudden development and rapid progression of hirsutism suggest the possibility of an androgen-secreting neoplasm, in which case virilization also may be present.

The age of onset of menstrual cycles (menarche) and the pattern of the menstrual cycle should be ascertained; irregular cycles from the time of menarche onward are more likely to result from ovarian rather than adrenal androgen excess. Associated symptoms such as galactorrhea should prompt evaluation for hyperprolactinemia (Chap. 333) and possibly hypothyroidism (Chap. 335). Hypertension, striae, easy bruising, centripetal weight gain, and weakness suggest hypercortisolism (Cushing's syndrome; Chap. 336). Rarely, patients with growth hormone excess (i.e., acromegaly) will present with hirsutism. Use of medications such as phenytoin, minoxidil, or cyclosporine may be associated with androgen-independent excess hair growth (i.e., hypertrichosis). A family history of infertility and/or hirsutism may indicate disorders such as nonclassic CAH (Chap. 336).

Physical examination should include measurement of height, weight, and calculation of body mass index (BMI). A BMI >25 kg/m^2 is indicative of excess weight for height, and values >30 kg/m^2 are often seen in association with hirsutism. Notation should be made of blood pressure, as adrenal causes may be associated with hypertension. Cutaneous signs sometimes associated with androgen excess and insulin resistance include acanthosis nigricans and skin tags.

An objective clinical assessment of hair distribution and quantity is central to the evaluation in any woman presenting with hirsutism. This assessment permits the distinction between hirsutism and hypertrichosis and provides a baseline reference point to gauge the response to treatment. A simple and commonly used method to grade hair growth is the modified scale of Ferriman and Gallwey (Fig. 50-1), where each of nine androgen-sensitive sites is graded from 0 to 4. Approximately 95% of Caucasian women have a score below 8 on this scale; thus, it is normal for most women to have some hair growth in androgen-sensitive sites. Scores above 8 suggest excess androgen-mediated hair growth, a finding that should be assessed further by hormonal evaluation (see below). In racial/ethnic groups that are less likely to manifest hirsutism (e.g., Asian women), additional cutaneous evidence of androgen excess should be sought, including pustular acne or thinning hair.

HORMONAL EVALUATION

Androgens are secreted by the ovaries and adrenal glands in response to their respective tropic hormones, luteinizing hormone (LH) and adrenocorticotropic hormone (ACTH). The principal circulating steroids involved in the etiology of hirsutism are testosterone, androstenedione, and dehydroepiandrosterone (DHEA) and its sulfated form (DHEAS). The ovaries and adrenal glands normally contribute about equally to testosterone production. Approximately half of the total testosterone originates from direct glandular secretion, and the remainder is derived from peripheral conversion of androstenedione and DHEA (Chap. 340).

Although it is the most important circulating androgen, testosterone is, in effect, the penultimate androgen in mediating hirsutism;

TABLE 50-1	CAUSES OF HIRSUTISM

Gonadal hyperandrogenism
  Ovarian hyperandrogenism
  Polycystic ovary syndrome/functional ovarian hyperandrogenism
  Ovarian steroidogenic blocks
  Syndromes of extreme insulin resistance
  Ovarian neoplasms
Adrenal hyperandrogenism
  Premature adrenarche
  Functional adrenal hyperandrogenism
  Congenital adrenal hyperplasia (nonclassic and classic)
  Abnormal cortisol action/metabolism
  Adrenal neoplasms
Other endocrine disorders
  Cushing's syndrome
  Hyperprolactinemia
  Acromegaly
Peripheral androgen overproduction
  Obesity
  Idiopathic
Pregnancy-related hyperandrogenism
  Hyperreactio luteinalis
  Thecoma of pregnancy
Drugs
  Androgens
  Oral contraceptives containing androgenic progestins
  Minoxidil
  Phenytoin
  Diazoxide
  Cyclosporine
  True hermaphroditism

FIGURE 50-1 Hirsutism scoring scale of Ferriman and Gallwey.
The nine body areas possessing androgen-sensitive areas are graded
from 0 (no terminal hair) to 4 (frankly virile) to obtain a total score. A
normal hirsutism score is less than 8. [*Modified from DA Ehrmann et al:*

*Hyperandrogenism, hirsutism, and polycystic ovary syndrome, in LJ De-
Groot and JL Jameson (eds), Endocrinology, 5th ed. Philadelphia, Saunders, 2006; with permission.*]

it is converted to the more potent dihydrotestosterone (DHT) by the
enzyme 5α-reductase, which is located in the PSU. DHT has a higher
affinity for, and slower dissociation from, the androgen receptor. The
local production of DHT allows it to serve as the primary mediator

of androgen action at the level of the pilosebaceous unit. There are
two isoenzymes of 5α-reductase: type 2 is found in the prostate
gland and in hair follicles, whereas type 1 is found primarily in sebaceous glands.

CLINICAL EVALUATION OF HIRSUTISM

FIGURE 50-2 Algorithm for the evaluation and differential diagnosis of hirsutism. ACTH, adrenocorticotropic hormone; CAH, congenital adrenal hyperplasia; DHEAS, sulfated form of dehydroepiandrosterone; PCOS, polycystic ovarian syndrome.

One approach to testing for hyperandrogenemia is depicted in **Fig. 50-2**. In addition to measuring blood levels of testosterone and DHEAS, it is also important to measure the level of free (or unbound) testosterone. The fraction of testosterone that is not bound to its carrier protein, sex-hormone binding globulin (SHBG), is biologically available for conversion to DHT and for binding to androgen receptors. Hyperinsulinemia and/or androgen excess decrease hepatic production of SHBG, resulting in levels of total testosterone within the high-normal range, whereas the unbound hormone is more substantially elevated. Although there is a decline in ovarian testosterone production after menopause, ovarian estrogen production decreases to an even greater extent, and the concentration of SHBG is reduced. Consequently, there is an increase in the relative proportion of unbound testosterone, and it may exacerbate hirsutism after menopause.

A baseline plasma total testosterone level >12 nmol/L (>3.5 ng/mL) usually indicates a virilizing tumor, whereas a level >7 nmol/L (>2 ng/mL) is suggestive. A basal DHEAS level >18.5 μmol/L (>7000 μg/L) suggests an adrenal tumor. Although DHEAS has been proposed as a "marker" of predominant adrenal androgen excess, it is not unusual to find modest elevations in DHEAS among women with PCOS. Computed tomography (CT) or magnetic resonance imaging (MRI) should be used to localize an adrenal mass, and ultrasound will usually suffice to identify an ovarian mass if clinical evaluation and hormonal levels suggest these possibilities.

PCOS is the most common cause of ovarian androgen excess (Chap. 341). However, the increased ratio of LH to follicle-stimulating hormone that is characteristic of carefully studied patients with PCOS is not seen in up to half of these women due to the pulsatility of gonadotropins. If performed, ultrasound shows enlarged ovaries and increased stroma in many women with PCOS. However, polycystic ovaries may also be found in women without clinical or laboratory features of PCOS. Therefore, polycystic ovaries are a relatively insensitive and nonspecific finding for the diagnosis of ovarian hyperandrogenism. Although not usually necessary, gonadotropin-releasing hormone agonist testing can be used to make a specific

diagnosis of ovarian hyperandrogenism. A peak 17-hydroxyprogesterone level ≥7.8 nmol/L (≥2.6 μg/L), after the administration of 100 μg nafarelin (or 10 μg/kg leuprolide) subcutaneously, is virtually diagnostic of ovarian hyperandrogenism.

Because adrenal androgens are readily suppressed by low doses of glucocorticoids, the dexamethasone androgen-suppression test may broadly distinguish ovarian from adrenal androgen overproduction. A blood sample is obtained before and after administering dexamethasone (0.5 mg orally every 6 h for 4 days). An adrenal source is suggested by suppression of unbound testosterone into the normal range; incomplete suppression suggests ovarian androgen excess. An overnight 1-mg dexamethasone suppression test, with measurement of 8:00 A.M. serum cortisol, is useful when there is clinical suspicion of Cushing's syndrome (Chap. 336).

Nonclassic CAH is most commonly due to 21-hydroxylase deficiency but can also be caused by autosomal recessive defects in other steroidogenic enzymes necessary for adrenal corticosteroid synthesis (Chap. 336). Because of the enzyme defect, the adrenal gland cannot secrete glucocorticoids efficiently (especially cortisol). This results in diminished negative feedback inhibition of ACTH, leading to compensatory adrenal hyperplasia and the accumulation of steroid precursors that are subsequently converted to androgen. Deficiency of 21-hydroxylase can be reliably excluded by determining a morning 17-hydroxyprogesterone level <6 nmol/L (<2 μg/L) (drawn in the follicular phase). Alternatively, 21-hydroxylase deficiency can be diagnosed by measurement of 17-hydroxyprogesterone 1 h after administration of 250 μg of synthetic ACTH (cosyntropin) intravenously.

Rx HIRSUTISM

Treatment of hirsutism may be accomplished pharmacologically or by mechanical means of hair removal. Nonpharmacologic treatments should be considered in all patients, either as the only treatment or as an adjunct to drug therapy.

Nonpharmacologic treatments include (1) bleaching; (2) depilatory (removal from the skin surface) such as shaving and chemical treatments; or (3) epilatory (removal of the hair including the root) such as plucking, waxing, electrolysis, and laser therapy. Despite perceptions to the contrary, shaving does not increase the rate or density of hair growth. Chemical depilatory treatments may be useful for mild hirsutism that affects only limited skin areas, though they can cause skin irritation. Wax treatment removes hair temporarily but is uncomfortable. Electrolysis is effective for more permanent hair removal, particularly in the hands of a skilled electrologist. Laser phototherapy appears to be efficacious for hair removal. It delays hair regrowth and causes permanent hair removal in most patients. The long-term effects and complications associated with laser treatment are still being evaluated.

Pharmacologic therapy is directed at interrupting one or more of the steps in the pathway of androgen synthesis and action: (1) suppression of adrenal and/or ovarian androgen production; (2) enhancement of androgen-binding to plasma-binding proteins, particularly SHBG; (3) impairment of the peripheral conversion of androgen precursors to active androgen; and (4) inhibition of androgen action at the target tissue level. Attenuation of hair growth is typically not evident until 4–6 months after initiation of medical treatment and, in most cases, leads to only a modest reduction in hair growth.

Combination estrogen-progestin therapy, in the form of an oral contraceptive, is usually the first-line endocrine treatment for hirsutism and acne, after cosmetic and dermatologic management. The estrogenic component of most oral contraceptives currently in use is either ethinyl estradiol or mestranol. The suppression of LH leads to reduced production of ovarian androgens. The reduced androgen levels also result in a dose-related increase in SHBG, thereby lowering the fraction of unbound plasma testosterone. Combination therapy has also been demonstrated to decrease DHEAS, perhaps by reducing ACTH levels. Estrogens also have a direct, dose-dependent suppressive effect on sebaceous cell function.

The choice of a specific oral contraceptive should be predicated on the progestational component, as progestins vary in their suppressive effect on SHBG levels and in their androgenic potential. Ethynodiol diacetate has relatively low androgenic potential, whereas progestins such as norgestrel and levonorgestrel are particularly androgenic, as judged from their attenuation of the estrogen-induced increase in SHBG. Norgestimate exemplifies the newer generation of progestins that are virtually nonandrogenic. Drospirenone, an analogue of spironolactone that has both antimineralocorticoid and antiandrogenic activities, has been approved for use as a progestational agent in combination with ethinyl estradiol. Its properties suggest that it should be the preferred choice for the treatment of hirsutism.

Oral contraceptives are contraindicated in women with a history of thromboembolic disease or in women with increased risk of breast or other estrogen-dependent cancers (Chap. 342). There is a relative contraindication to the use of oral contraceptives in smokers or in those with hypertension or a history of migraine headaches. In most trials, estrogen-progestin therapy alone improves the extent of acne by a maximum of 50–70%. The effect on hair growth may not be evident for 6 months, and the maximum effect may require 9–12 months owing to the length of the hair growth cycle. Improvements in hirsutism are typically in the range of 20%, but there may be an arrest of further progression of hair growth.

Adrenal androgens are more sensitive than cortisol to the suppressive effects of glucocorticoids. Therefore, glucocorticoids are the mainstay of treatment in patients with CAH. Although glucocorticoids have been reported to restore ovulatory function in some women with PCOS, this effect is highly variable. Because of side effects from excessive glucocorticoids, low doses should be used. Dexamethasone (0.2–0.5 mg) or prednisone (5–10 mg) should be taken at bedtime to achieve maximal suppression by inhibiting the nocturnal surge of ACTH.

Cyproterone acetate is the prototypic antiandrogen. It acts mainly by competitive inhibition of the binding of testosterone and DHT to the androgen receptor. In addition, it may enhance the metabolic clearance of testosterone by inducing hepatic enzymes. Although not available for use in the United States, cyproterone acetate is widely used in Canada, Mexico, and Europe. Cyproterone (50–100 mg) is given on days 1–15 and ethinyl estradiol (50 μg) is given on days 5–26 of the menstrual cycle. Side effects include irregular uterine bleeding, nausea, headache, fatigue, weight gain, and decreased libido.

Spironolactone, usually used as a mineralocorticoid antagonist, is also a weak antiandrogen. It is almost as effective as cyproterone acetate when used at high enough doses (100–200 mg daily). Patients should be monitored intermittently for hyperkalemia or hypotension, though these side effects are uncommon. Pregnancy should be avoided because of the risk of feminization of a male fetus. Spironolactone can also cause menstrual irregularity. It is often used in combination with an oral contraceptive, which suppresses ovarian androgen production and helps prevent pregnancy.

Flutamide is a potent nonsteroidal antiandrogen that is effective in treating hirsutism, but concerns about the induction of hepatocellular dysfunction have limited its use. Finasteride is a competitive inhibitor of 5α-reductase type 2. Beneficial effects on hirsutism have been reported, but the predominance of 5α-reductase type 1 in the PSU appears to account for its limited efficacy. Finasteride would also be expected to impair sexual differentiation in a male fetus, and it should not be used in women who may become pregnant.

Eflornithine cream (Vaniqa) has been approved as a novel treatment for unwanted facial hair in women, but long-term efficacy remains to be established. It can cause skin irritation under exaggerated conditions of use. Ultimately, the choice of any specific agent(s) must be tailored to the unique needs of the patient being treated. As noted previously, pharmacologic treatments for hirsutism should be used in conjunction with nonpharmacologic approaches. It is also helpful to review the pattern of female hair distribution in the normal population to dispel unrealistic expectations.

FURTHER READINGS

CARMINA E: Antiandrogens for the treatment of hirsutism. Expert Opin Investig Drugs 11:357, 2002

EHRMANN DA: Polycystic ovary syndrome. N Engl J Med 352:1223, 2005

HORDINSKY M et al: Hair loss and hirsutism in the elderly. Clin Geriatr Med 18:121, 2002

LANIGAN SW: Management of unwanted hair in females. Clin Exp Dermatol 26:644, 2001

ROSENFIELD RL: Clinical practice. Hirsutism. N Engl J Med 353:2578, 2005

SANCHEZ LA et al: Laser hair reduction in the hirsute patient: A critical assessment. Hum Reprod Update 8:169, 2002

51 Menstrual Disorders and Pelvic Pain
Janet E. Hall

Menstrual dysfunction can signal an underlying abnormality that may have long-term health consequences. Although frequent or prolonged bleeding usually prompts a woman to seek medical attention, infrequent or absent bleeding may seem less troubling, and the patient may not bring it to the attention of the physician. Thus, a focused menstrual history is a critical part of every female patient encounter. Pelvic pain is a common complaint that may relate to an abnormality of the reproductive organs but may also be of gastrointestinal, urinary tract, or musculoskeletal origin. Depending on its cause, pelvic pain may require urgent surgical attention.

MENSTRUAL DISORDERS

DEFINITION AND PREVALENCE

Amenorrhea refers to the absence of menstrual periods. Amenorrhea is classified as *primary* if menstrual bleeding has never occurred in the absence of hormonal treatment or *secondary* if menstrual periods are absent for 3–6 months. *Oligoamenorrhea* is defined as a cycle length >35 days or <10 menses per year. Both the frequency and amount of vaginal bleeding are irregular in oligoamenorrhea. It is often associated with anovulation, which can also occur with intermenstrual intervals of <24 days or vaginal bleeding for >7 days. Frequent or heavy

irregular bleeding is termed *dysfunctional uterine bleeding* if anatomic uterine lesions or a bleeding diathesis have been excluded.

Primary Amenorrhea This is a rare disorder occurring in <1% of the female population. However, between 3 and 5% of women experience at least 3 months of secondary amenorrhea in a given year. There is no evidence that race or ethnicity influence the prevalence of amenorrhea. However, because of the importance of adequate nutrition for normal reproductive function, both the age at menarche and the prevalence of secondary amenorrhea vary significantly in different parts of the world.

The absence of menses by age 16 has been used traditionally to define primary amenorrhea. However, other factors such as growth, secondary sexual characteristics, the presence of cyclic pelvic pain, and the secular trend to an earlier age of menarche, particularly in African-American girls, also influence the age at which primary amenorrhea should be investigated. Thus, an evaluation for amenorrhea should be initiated by age 15 or 16 in the presence of normal growth and secondary sexual characteristics; age 13 in the absence of secondary sexual characteristics or if height is less than the third percentile; age 12 or 13 in the presence of breast development and cyclic pelvic pain; or within 2 years of breast development if menarche has not occurred.

Secondary Amenorrhea or Oligoamenorrhea Anovulation and irregular cycles are relatively common for 2–4 years after menarche and for 1–2 years before the final menstrual period. In the intervening years, menstrual cycle length is ~28 days, with an intermenstrual interval normally ranging between 25 and 35 days. Cycle-to-cycle variability in an individual woman who is consistently ovulating is generally +/– 2 days. Pregnancy is the most common cause of amenorrhea and should be excluded early in any evaluation of menstrual irregularity. However, many women will occasionally miss a single period. Three or more months of secondary amenorrhea should prompt an evaluation, as should a history of intermenstrual intervals of >35 or <21 days, or bleeding that persists for >7 days.

DIAGNOSIS

Evaluation of menstrual dysfunction depends on understanding the interrelationships between the four critical components of the reproductive tract: (1) the hypothalamus, (2) the pituitary, (3) the ovaries, and (4) the uterus and outflow tract (Fig. 51-1; Chap. 341). This system is maintained by complex negative and positive feedback loops involving the ovarian steroids (estradiol and progesterone) and peptides (inhibin B and inhibin A) and the hypothalamic [gonadotropin-releasing hormone (GnRH)] and pituitary [follicle-stimulating hormone (FSH) and luteinizing hormone (LH)] components of this system (Fig. 51-1).

Disorders of menstrual function can be thought of in two main categories: disorders of the uterus and outflow tract and disorders of ovulation. Many of the conditions that cause primary amenorrhea are congenital but go unrecognized until the time of normal puberty (e.g., genetic, chromosomal, and anatomic abnormalities). All causes of secondary amenorrhea can also cause primary amenorrhea.

Disorders of the Uterus or Outflow Tract Abnormalities of the uterus and outflow tract typically present as primary amenorrhea. In patients with normal pubertal development and a blind vagina, the differential diagnosis includes *obstruction* by a transverse vaginal septum or imperforate hymen; *müllerian agenesis* (Mayer-Rokitansky-Kuster-Hauser syndrome), which has been associated with mutations in the *WNT4* gene; and *androgen insensitivity syndrome* (AIS), which is an X-linked recessive disorder that accounts for ~10% of all cases of primary amenorrhea (Chap. 340). Patients with AIS have a 46, XY karyotype, but because of the lack of androgen receptor responsiveness, they have severe underandrogenization and female external genitalia. The absence of pubic and axillary hair distinguishes them clinically from patients with müllerian agenesis. *Asherman syndrome* presents as secondary amenorrhea or hypomenorrhea and results from partial or complete obliteration of the uterine cavity by adhesions that prevent normal growth and shedding of the endometrium. Curettage performed for pregnancy complications accounts for >90% of cases; genital tuberculosis is an important cause in endemic regions.

℞ DISORDERS OF UTERUS OR OUTFLOW TRACT

Obstruction of the outflow tract requires surgical correction. The risk of endometriosis is increased with this condition, perhaps because of retrograde menstrual flow. *Müllerian agenesis* may also require surgical intervention, although vaginal dilatation is adequate in some patients. Because ovarian function is normal, assisted reproductive techniques can be used with a surrogate carrier. *Androgen resistance syndrome* requires gonadectomy because there is risk of gonadoblastoma in the dysgenetic gonads. Whether this should be performed in early childhood or after completion of breast development is controversial. Estrogen replacement is indicated after gonadectomy, and vaginal dilatation may be required to allow sexual intercourse.

Disorders of Ovulation Once uterus and outflow tract abnormalities have been excluded, all other causes of amenorrhea involve disorders of ovulation. The differential diagnosis is based on the results of initial

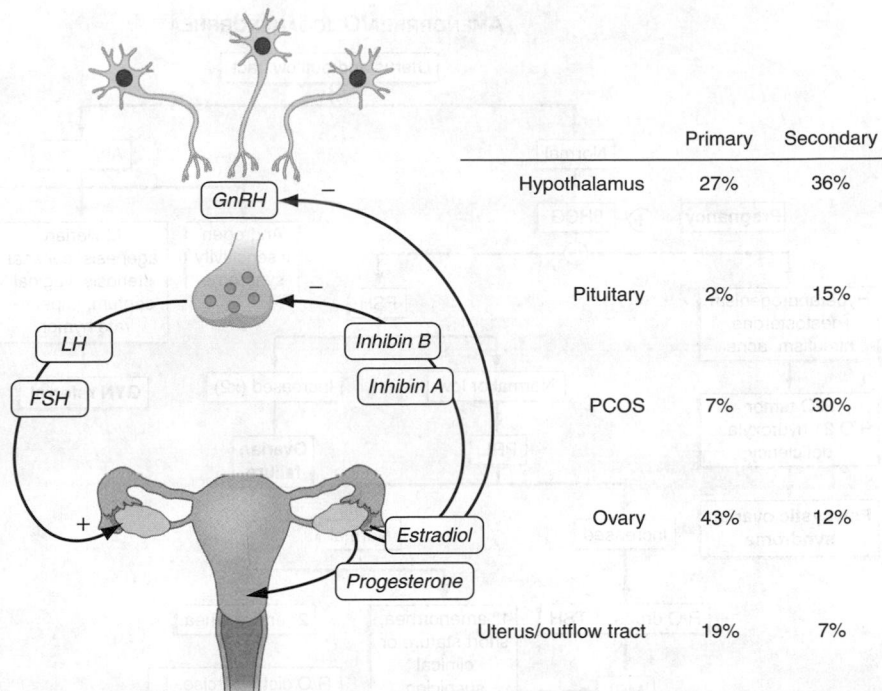

	Primary	Secondary
Hypothalamus	27%	36%
Pituitary	2%	15%
PCOS	7%	30%
Ovary	43%	12%
Uterus/outflow tract	19%	7%

FIGURE 51-1 Role of the hypothalamic-pituitary-gonadal axis in the etiology of amenorrhea. Gonadotropin-releasing hormone (GnRH) secretion from the hypothalamus stimulates follicle-stimulating hormone (FSH) and luteinizing hormone (LH) secretion from the pituitary to induce ovarian folliculogenesis and steroidogenesis. Ovarian secretion of estradiol and progesterone controls the shedding of the endometrium, resulting in menses and, in combination with the inhibins, provides feedback regulation of the hypothalamus and pituitary to control secretion of FSH and LH. The prevalence of amenorrhea resulting from abnormalities at each level of the reproductive system (hypothalamus, pituitary, ovary, uterus, and outflow tract) varies depending on whether amenorrhea is primary or secondary. PCOS, polycystic ovarian syndrome.

tests including a pregnancy test, gonadotropins, and assessment of hyperandrogenism (Fig. 51-2).

HYPOGONADOTROPIC HYPOGONADISM Low estrogen levels in combination with normal or low levels of LH and FSH are seen with anatomic, genetic, or functional abnormalities that interfere with hypothalamic GnRH secretion or normal pituitary responsiveness to GnRH. Although relatively uncommon, tumors and infiltrative diseases should be considered in the differential diagnosis of hypogonadotropic hypogonadism (Chap. 333). These disorders may present with primary or secondary amenorrhea. They may occur in association with other features suggestive of hypothalamic or pituitary dysfunction such as short stature, diabetes insipidus, galactorrhea, or headache. Hypogonadotropic hypogonadism may also be seen following cranial irradiation. In the postpartum period, it may be due to pituitary necrosis (Sheehan syndrome) or lymphocytic hypophysitis. Because reproductive dysfunction is commonly associated with hyperprolactinemia, either from neuroanatomic lesions or medications, prolactin should be measured in all patients with hypogonadotropic hypogonadism (Chap. 333).

Isolated hypogonadotropic hypogonadism (IHH) is more common in men than women and is often associated with anosmia. IHH generally presents with primary amenorrhea. A number of genetic causes of IHH have been identified (Chaps. 340 and 341).

Functional hypothalamic amenorrhea (HA) is caused by a mismatch between energy expenditure and energy intake. Leptin secretion may play a key role in transducing the signals from the periphery to the hypothalamus in HA. The hypothalamic-pituitary-adrenal axis may also play a role. The diagnosis of HA can generally be made on the basis of a careful history, physical examination, and the demonstration of low levels of gonadotropins and normal prolactin levels. Eating disorders and chronic disease must be specifically excluded (Chap. 76). An atypical history, headache, signs of other hypothalamic dysfunction, or hyper-

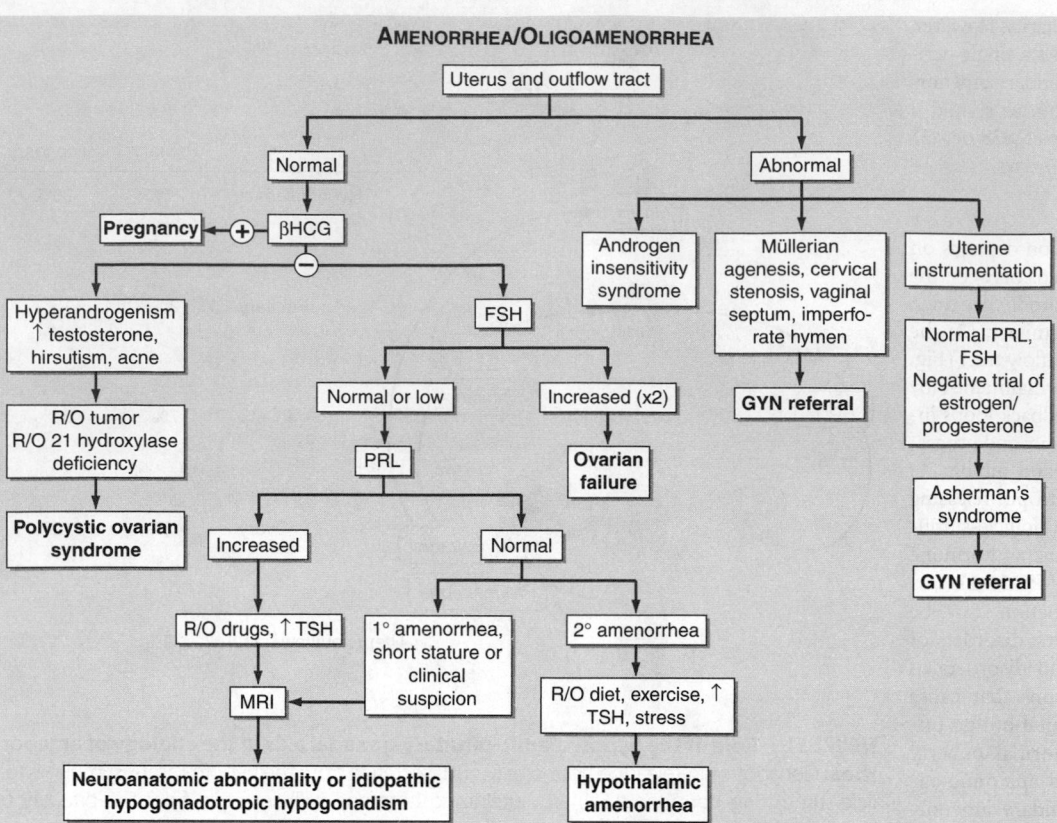

FIGURE 51-2 Algorithm for evaluation of amenorrhea. β-hCG, human chorionic gonadotropin; PRL, prolactin; FSH, follicle-stimulating hormone; TSH, thyroid-stimulating hormone.

prolactinemia, even if mild, necessitates cranial imaging with CT or MRI to exclude a neuroanatomic cause.

HYPERGONADOTROPIC HYPOGONADISM   Ovarian failure is considered premature when it occurs in women younger than age 40. Ovarian failure is associated with the loss of negative-feedback restraint on the hypothalamus and pituitary, resulting in increased FSH and LH levels. FSH is a better marker of ovarian failure as its levels are less variable than LH. As with natural menopause, premature ovarian failure (POF) may wax and wane, and serial measurements may be necessary to establish the diagnosis.

Once the diagnosis of POF has been established, further evaluation is indicated because of other health problems that may be associated with POF. For example, POF is seen in association with a variety of chromosomal abnormalities including Turner syndrome, autoimmune polyglandular failure syndromes, radio- and chemotherapy, and galactosemia. In the majority of cases, however, a cause is not determined. The recognition that early ovarian failure occurs in premutation carriers of the fragile X syndrome is important because of increased risk of severe mental retardation in male children with *FMR1* mutations.

Hypergonadotropic hypogonadism occurs rarely in other disorders, such as mutations in the FSH or LH receptors. Aromatase deficiency and 17α-hydroxylase deficiency are associated with elevated gonadotropins with hyperandrogenism and hypertension, respectively. Gonadotropin-secreting tumors in women of reproductive age generally present with high, rather than low, estrogen levels and cause ovarian hyperstimulation or dysfunctional bleeding.

℞ AMENORRHEA CAUSED BY OVULATORY DISORDERS

Amenorrhea is almost always associated with chronically low levels of estrogen, whether it is caused by hypogonadotropic hypogonadism or ovarian failure. Development of secondary sexual characteristics requires gradual titration of estradiol replacement with eventual addition of a progestin. Symptoms of hypoestrogenism can be treated with hormone replacement therapy or oral contraceptive pills. Patients with hypogonadotropic hypogonadism who are interested in fertility require treatment with pulsatile GnRH or exogenous FSH and LH, whereas patients with

ovarian failure can consider oocyte donation, which has a high chance of success in this population.

POLYCYSTIC OVARIAN SYNDROME (PCOS)   This is diagnosed based on the presence of clinical or biochemical evidence of hyperandrogenism in association with amenorrhea or oligomenorrhea. Symptoms generally begin shortly after menarche and are slowly progressive. Lean patients with PCOS generally have high LH levels in the presence of normal to low levels of FSH and estradiol. The LH/FSH abnormality is less pronounced in obese patients in whom insulin resistance is a more prominent feature. Most patients also have a polycystic ovarian morphology on ultrasound, although there is controversy as to whether this morphology in combination with hyperandrogenism is sufficient for the diagnosis of PCOS.

℞ POLYCYSTIC OVARIAN SYNDROME

The major abnormality in patients with PCOS is the failure of regular, predictable ovulation. Thus, these patients are at risk for the development of dysfunctional bleeding and endometrial hyperplasia associated with unopposed estrogen exposure. Endometrial protection can be achieved with the use of oral contraceptives or progestins (medroxyprogesterone acetate, 5–10 mg, or prometrium, 200 mg daily for 10–14 days of each month). Oral contraceptives are also useful for management of hyperandrogenic symptoms, as is spironolactone, which functions as a weak androgen receptor antagonist. Management of the associated metabolic syndrome may be appropriate for some patients (Chap. 236). For patients interested in fertility, weight control is a critical first step. Clomiphene citrate is highly effective as first-line treatment, with or without the addition of metformin. Exogenous gonadotropins can be used by experienced practitioners.

PELVIC PAIN

The mechanisms causing pelvic pain are similar to those causing abdominal pain (Chap. 14) and include inflammation of the parietal peritoneum, obstruction of hollow viscera, vascular disturbances, and pain originating in the abdominal wall. Pelvic pain may reflect pelvic disease per se but may also reflect extrapelvic disorders that refer pain to the pel-

TABLE 51-1 CAUSES OF PELVIC PAIN

	Acute	Chronic
Cyclic pelvic pain		Premenstrual symptoms Mittelschmerz Dysmenorrhea Endometriosis
Noncyclic pelvic pain	Pelvic inflammatory disease Ruptured or hemorrhagic ovarian cyst or ovarian torsion Ectopic pregnancy Endometritis Acute growth or degeneration of uterine myoma	Pelvic congestion syndrome Adhesions and retroversion of the uterus Pelvic malignancy Vulvodynia History of sexual abuse

vis. In up to 60% of cases, pelvic pain can be attributed to gastrointestinal problems including appendicitis, cholecystitis, infections, intestinal obstruction, diverticulitis, or inflammatory bowel disease. Urinary tract and musculoskeletal disorders are also common causes of pelvic pain.

APPROACH TO THE PATIENT:
Pelvic Pain

A thorough history including the type, location, radiation, and status with respect to increasing or decreasing severity can help to identify the cause of acute pelvic pain. Specific associations with vaginal bleeding, sexual activity, defecation, urination, movement, or eating should be specifically sought. A careful menstrual history is essential to assess the possibility of pregnancy. Determination of whether the pain is acute versus chronic and cyclic versus noncyclic will direct further investigation (Table 51-1). However, disorders that cause cyclic pain may occasionally cause noncyclic pain, and the converse is also true.

ACUTE PELVIC PAIN

Pelvic inflammatory disease most commonly presents with bilateral lower abdominal pain. It is generally of recent onset and is exacerbated by intercourse or jarring movements. Fever is present in about half of patients; abnormal uterine bleeding occurs in about one-third. New vaginal discharge, urethritis, and chills may be present but are less specific signs. *Adnexal pathology* can present acutely and may be due to rupture, bleeding or torsion of cysts, or, much less commonly, neoplasms of the ovary, fallopian tubes, or paraovarian areas. Fever may be present with ovarian torsion. *Ectopic pregnancy* is associated with right or left sided lower abdominal pain, vaginal bleeding and menstrual cycle abnormalities, with clinical signs generally appearing 6–8 weeks after the last normal menstrual period. Orthostatic signs and fever may be present. Risk factors include the presence of known tubal disease, previous ectopic pregnancies, or a history of infertility, DES exposure of the mother in utero, or a history of pelvic infections. *Uterine pathology* includes endometritis and, less frequently, degenerating leiomyomas (fibroids). Endometritis is often associated with vaginal bleeding and systemic signs of infection. It occurs in the setting of sexually transmitted infections, uterine instrumentation, or postpartum infection.

A sensitive pregnancy test, complete blood count with differential, urinalysis, tests for chlamydial and gonococcal infections, and abdominal ultrasound aid in making the diagnosis and directing further management.

℞ ACUTE PELVIC PAIN

Treatment of acute pelvic pain depends on the suspected etiology but may require surgical or gynecologic intervention. Conservative management is an important consideration for ovarian cysts, if torsion is not suspected, to avoid unnecessary pelvic surgery and the subsequent risk of infertility due to adhesions. The majority of unruptured ectopic pregnan-

cies are now treated with methotrexate, which is effective in 84–96% of cases. However, surgical treatment may be required.

CHRONIC PELVIC PAIN

Some women experience discomfort at the time of ovulation (*mittelschmerz*). Pain can be quite intense but is generally of short duration. The mechanism is thought to involve rapid expansion of the dominant follicle, although it may also be caused by peritoneal irritation by follicular fluid released at the time of ovulation. Many women experience premenstrual symptoms such as breast discomfort, food cravings, and abdominal bloating or discomfort. These moliminal symptoms are a good predictor of ovulation, although their absence is less helpful.

Dysmenorrhea *Dysmenorrhea* refers to the crampy lower abdominal discomfort that begins with the onset of menstrual bleeding and gradually decreases over the next 12–72 h. It may be associated with nausea, diarrhea, fatigue, and headache and occurs in 60–93% of adolescents, beginning with the establishment of regular ovulatory cycles. Its prevalence decreases after pregnancy and with the use of oral contraceptives.

Primary dysmenorrhea results from increased stores of prostaglandin precursors, which are generated by sequential stimulation of the uterus by estrogen and progesterone. During menstruation these precursors are converted to prostaglandins, which cause intense uterine contractions, decreased blood flow, and increased peripheral nerve hypersensitivity, resulting in pain.

Secondary dysmenorrhea is caused by underlying pelvic pathology. *Endometriosis* results from the presence of endometrial glands and stroma outside of the uterus. These deposits of ectopic endometrium respond to hormonal stimulation and cause dysmenorrhea, which generally precedes menstruation by several days. Endometriosis may also be associated with painful intercourse, painful bowel movements, and tender nodules in the uterosacral ligament. Fibrosis and adhesions can produce lateral displacement of the cervix. The CA125 level may be increased, but it has low negative predictive value. Definitive diagnosis requires laparoscopy. Symptomatology does not always predict the extent of endometriosis. Other secondary causes of dysmenorrhea include adenomyosis, a condition caused by the presence of ectopic endometrial glands and stroma within the myometrium. Cervical stenosis may result from trauma, infection, or surgery.

℞ DYSMENORRHEA

Local application of heat; use of vitamins B_1, B_6, and E and magnesium; acupuncture; yoga; and exercise are of some benefit for the treatment of dysmenorrhea. However, nonsteroidal anti-inflammatory drugs (NSAIDs) are the most effective treatment and provide >80% sustained response rates. Ibuprofen, naproxen, ketoprofen, mefanamic acid, and nimesulide are all superior to placebo. Treatment should be started a day before expected menses and is generally continued for 2–3 days. Oral contraceptives also reduce symptoms of dysmenorrhea. Failure of response to NSAIDs and oral contraceptives is suggestive of a pelvic disorder, such as endometriosis, and diagnostic laparoscopy should be considered to guide further treatment.

FURTHER READINGS

DAWOOD MY: Primary dysmenorrhea: Advances in pathogenesis and management. Obstet Gynecol 108:428, 2006

GENAZZANI AD et al: Diagnostic and therapeutic approach to hypothalamic amenorrhea. Ann NY Acad Sci 1092:103, 2006

HALL JE: Neuroendocrine control of the menstrual cycle, in *Yen and Jaffe's Reproductive Endocrinology*, 5th ed. JF Strauss, RL Barbieri (eds). Philadelphia, Elsevier, 2004, pp 195–211

LATTHE P et al: Factors predisposing women to chronic pelvic pain: Systematic review. BMJ 332(7544):749, 2006

PITTOCK ST et al: Mayer-Rokitansky-Kuster-Hauser anomaly and its associated malformations. Am J Med Genet A 135:314, 2005

WITTENBERGER MD et al: The FMR1 premutation and reproduction. Fertil Steril 87:456, 2007

52 Approach to the Patient with a Skin Disorder

Thomas J. Lawley, Kim B. Yancey

The challenge of examining the skin lies in distinguishing normal from abnormal, significant findings from trivial ones, and in integrating pertinent signs and symptoms into an appropriate differential diagnosis. The fact that the largest organ in the body is visible is both an advantage and a disadvantage to those who examine it. It is advantageous because no special instrumentation is necessary and because the skin can be biopsied with little morbidity. However, the casual observer can be misled by a variety of stimuli and overlook important, subtle signs of skin or systemic disease. For instance, the sometimes minor differences in color and shape that distinguish a melanoma (Fig. 52-1) from a benign nevomelanocytic nevus (Fig. 52-2) can be difficult to recognize. To aid in the interpretation of skin lesions, a variety of descriptive terms have been developed to characterize cutaneous lesions (Tables 52-1, 52-2, and 52-3 as well as Fig. 52-3) and to formulate a differential diagnosis (Table 52-4). For instance, the finding of scaling papules (present in patients with psoriasis or atopic dermatitis) places the patient in a different diagnostic category than would hemorrhagic papules, which may indicate vasculitis or sepsis (Figs. 52-4 and 52-5, respectively). It is also important to differentiate primary from secondary skin lesions. If the examiner focuses on linear erosions overlying an area of erythema and scaling, he or she may incorrectly assume that the erosion is the primary lesion and the redness and scale are secondary, while the correct interpretation would be that the patient has a pruritic eczematous dermatitis with erosions caused by scratching.

APPROACH TO THE PATIENT:
Skin Disorder

In examining the skin it is usually advisable to assess the patient before taking an extensive history. This way, the entire cutaneous surface is sure to be evaluated, and objective findings can be integrated

FIGURE 52-1 Superficial spreading melanoma. This is the most common type of melanoma. Such lesions usually demonstrate asymmetry, border irregularity, color variegation (black, blue, brown, pink, and white), a diameter >6 mm, and a history of change (e.g., an increase in size or development of associated symptoms such as pruritus or pain).

FIGURE 52-2 Nevomelanocytic nevus. Nevi are benign proliferations of nevomelanocytes characterized by regularly shaped hyperpigmented macules or papules of a uniform color.

with relevant historic data. Four basic features of a skin lesion must be noted and considered during a physical examination: the distribution of the eruption, the types of primary and secondary lesions, the shape of individual lesions, and the arrangement of the lesions. An ideal skin examination includes evaluation of the skin, hair, and

---

TABLE 52-1 DESCRIPTION OF PRIMARY SKIN LESIONS

Macule: A flat, colored lesion, <2 cm in diameter, not raised above the surface of the surrounding skin. A "freckle," or ephelid, is a prototype pigmented macule.

Patch: A large (>2 cm) flat lesion with a color different from the surrounding skin. This differs from a macule only in size.

Papule: A small, solid lesion, <0.5 cm in diameter, raised above the surface of the surrounding skin and hence palpable (e.g., a closed comedone, or whitehead, in acne).

Nodule: A larger (0.5–5.0 cm), firm lesion raised above the surface of the surrounding skin. This differs from a papule only in size (e.g., a dermal nevomelanocytic nevus).

Tumor: A solid, raised growth >5 cm in diameter.

Plaque: A large (>1 cm), flat-topped, raised lesion; edges may either be distinct (e.g., in psoriasis) or gradually blend with surrounding skin (e.g., in eczematous dermatitis).

Vesicle: A small, fluid-filled lesion, <0.5 cm in diameter, raised above the plane of surrounding skin. Fluid is often visible, and the lesions are translucent [e.g., vesicles in allergic contact dermatitis caused by *Toxicodendron* (poison ivy)].

Pustule: A vesicle filled with leukocytes. Note: The presence of pustules does not necessarily signify the existence of an infection.

Bulla: A fluid-filled, raised, often translucent lesion >0.5 cm in diameter.

Wheal: A raised, erythematous, edematous papule or plaque, usually representing short-lived vasodilatation and vasopermeability.

Telangiectasia: A dilated, superficial blood vessel.

TABLE 52-2 DESCRIPTION OF SECONDARY SKIN LESIONS

Lichenification: A distinctive thickening of the skin that is characterized by accentuated skin-fold markings.

Scale: Excessive accumulation of stratum corneum.

Crust: Dried exudate of body fluids that may be either yellow (i.e., serous crust) or red (i.e., hemorrhagic crust).

Erosion: Loss of epidermis without an associated loss of dermis.

Ulcer: Loss of epidermis and at least a portion of the underlying dermis.

Excoriation: Linear, angular erosions that may be covered by crust and are caused by scratching.

Atrophy: An acquired loss of substance. In the skin, this may appear as a depression with intact epidermis (i.e., loss of dermal or subcutaneous tissue) or as sites of shiny, delicate, wrinkled lesions (i.e., epidermal atrophy).

Scar: A change in the skin secondary to trauma or inflammation. Sites may be erythematous, hypopigmented, or hyperpigmented depending on their age or character. Sites on hair-bearing areas may be characterized by destruction of hair follicles.

TABLE 52-3 · COMMON DERMATOLOGIC TERMS

Alopecia: Hair loss; it may be partial or complete.

Annular: Ring-shaped lesions.

Cyst: A soft, raised, encapsulated lesion filled with semisolid or liquid contents.

Herpetiform: Grouped lesions.

Lichenoid: Violaceous to purple, polygonal lesions that resemble those seen in lichen planus.

Milia: Small, firm, white papules filled with keratin.

Morbilliform: Generalized, small erythematous macules and/or papules that resemble lesions seen in measles.

Nummular: Coin-shaped lesions.

Poikiloderma: Skin that displays variegated pigmentation, atrophy, and telangiectases.

Polycyclic: A configuration of skin lesions formed from coalescing rings or incomplete rings.

Pruritus: A sensation that elicits the desire to scratch. Pruritus is often the predominant symptom of inflammatory skin diseases (e.g., atopic dermatitis, allergic contact dermatitis); it is also commonly associated with xerosis and aged skin. Systemic conditions that can be associated with pruritus include chronic renal disease, cholestasis, pregnancy, malignancy, thyroid disease, polycythemia vera, and delusions of parasitosis.

FIGURE 52-3 A schematic representation of several common primary skin lesions (see Table 52-1).

nails as well as the mucous membranes of the mouth, eyes, nose, nasopharynx, and anogenital region. In the initial examination it is important that the patient be disrobed as completely as possible. This will minimize chances of missing important individual skin

TABLE 52-4 · SELECTED COMMON DERMATOLOGIC CONDITIONS

Diagnosis	Common Distribution	Usual Morphology	Diagnosis	Common Distribution	Usual Morphology
Acne vulgaris	Face, upper back	Open and closed comedones, erythematous papules, pustules, cysts	Seborrheic keratosis	Trunk, face	Brown plaques with adherent, greasy scale; "stuck on" appearance
Rosacea	Blush area of cheeks, nose, forehead, chin	Erythema, telangiectases, papules, pustules	Folliculitis	Any hair-bearing area	Follicular pustules
			Impetigo	Anywhere	Papules, vesicles, pustules, often with honey-colored crusts
Seborrheic dermatitis	Scalp, eyebrows, perinasal areas	Erythema with greasy yellow-brown scale	Herpes simplex	Lips, genitalia	Grouped vesicles progressing to crusted erosions
Atopic dermatitis	Antecubital and popliteal fossae; may be widespread	Patches and plaques of erythema, scaling, and lichenification; pruritus	Herpes zoster	Dermatomal, usually trunk but may be anywhere	Vesicles limited to a dermatome (often painful)
Stasis dermatitis	Ankles, lower legs	Patches of erythema and scaling on background of hyperpigmentation associated with signs of venous insufficiency	Varicella	Face, trunk, relative sparing of extremities	Lesions arise in crops and quickly progress from erythematous macules to papules to vesicles to pustules to crusted sites
Dyshidrotic eczema	Palms, soles, sides of fingers and toes	Deep vesicles	Pityriasis rosea	Trunk (Christmas tree pattern); herald patch followed by multiple smaller lesions	Symmetric erythematous patches with a collarette of scale
Allergic contact dermatitis	Anywhere	Localized erythema, vesicles, scale, and pruritus (e.g., fingers, earlobes—nickel; dorsal aspect of foot—shoe; exposed surfaces—poison ivy)	Tinea versicolor	Chest, back, abdomen, proximal extremities	Scaly hyper- or hypopigmented macules
Psoriasis	Elbows, knees, scalp, lower back, fingernails (may be generalized)	Papules and plaques covered with silvery scale; nails have pits	Candidiasis	Groin, beneath breasts, vagina, oral cavity	Erythematous macerated areas with satellite pustules; white, friable patches on mucous membranes
Lichen planus	Wrists, ankles, mouth (may be widespread)	Violaceous flat-topped papules and plaques	Dermatophytosis	Feet, groin, beard, or scalp	Varies with site, (e.g., tinea corporis—scaly annular patch)
Keratosis pilaris	Extensor surfaces of arms and thighs, buttocks	Keratotic follicular papules with surrounding erythema	Scabies	Groin, axillae, between fingers and toes, beneath breasts	Excoriated papules, burrows, pruritus
Melasma	Forehead, cheeks, temples, upper lip	Tan to brown patches	Insect bites	Anywhere	Erythematous papules with central puncta
Vitiligo	Periorificial, trunk, extensor surfaces of extremities, flexor wrists, axillae	Chalk-white macules	Cherry angioma	Trunk	Red, blood-filled papules
			Keloid	Anywhere (site of previous injury)	Firm tumor, pink, purple, or brown
			Dermatofibroma	Anywhere	Firm red to brown nodule that shows dimpling of overlying skin with lateral compression
Actinic keratosis	Sun-exposed areas	Skin-colored or red-brown macule or papule with dry, rough, adherent scale	Acrochordons (skin tags)	Groin, axilla, neck	Fleshy papules
Basal cell carcinoma	Face	Papule with pearly, telangiectatic border on sun-damaged skin	Urticaria	Anywhere	Wheals, sometimes with surrounding flare; pruritus
Squamous cell carcinoma	Face, especially lower lip, ears	Indurated and possibly hyperkeratotic lesions often showing ulceration and/or crusting	Transient acantholytic dermatosis	Trunk, especially anterior chest	Erythematous papules
			Xerosis	Extensor extremities, especially legs	Dry, erythematous, scaling patches; pruritus

FIGURE 52-4 Necrotizing vasculitis. Palpable purpuric papules on the lower legs are seen in this patient with cutaneous small vessel vasculitis. *(Courtesy of Robert Swerlick, MD; with permission.)*

FIGURE 52-5 Meningococcemia. An example of fulminant meningococcemia with extensive angular purpuric patches. *(Courtesy of Stephen E. Gellis, MD; with permission.)*

lesions and make it possible to assess the distribution of the eruption accurately. The patient should first be viewed from a distance of about 1.5–2 m (4–6 ft) so that the general character of the skin and the distribution of lesions can be evaluated. Indeed, distribution of lesions often correlates highly with diagnosis (Fig. 52-6). For example, a hospitalized patient with a generalized erythematous exanthem is more likely to have a drug eruption than is a patient with a similar rash limited to the sun-exposed portions of the face. Once the distribution of the lesions has been established, the nature of the primary lesion must be determined. Thus, when lesions are distributed on elbows, knees, and scalp, the most likely possibility based solely on distribution is psoriasis or dermatitis herpetiformis (Figs. 52-7 and 52-8, respectively). The primary lesion in psoriasis is a scaly papule that soon forms erythematous plaques covered with a white scale, whereas that of dermatitis herpetiformis is an urticarial papule that quickly becomes a small vesicle. In this manner, identification of the primary lesion directs the examiner toward the proper diagnosis. Secondary changes in skin can also be quite helpful. For example, scale represents excessive epidermis, while crust is the result of a discontinuous epithelial cell layer. Palpation of skin lesions can also yield insight into the character of an eruption. Thus, red papules on the lower extremities that blanch with pressure can be a manifestation of many different diseases, but hemorrhagic red papules that do not blanch with pressure indicate palpable purpura characteristic of necrotizing vasculitis (Fig. 52-4).

The shape of lesions is also an important feature. Flat, round, erythematous papules and plaques are common in many cutaneous diseases. However, target-shaped lesions that consist in part of erythematous plaques are spe-

cific for erythema multiforme (Fig. 52-9). In the same way, the arrangement of individual lesions is important. Erythematous papules and vesicles can occur in many conditions, but their arrangement in a specific linear array suggests an external etiology such as allergic contact (Fig. 52-10) or primary irritant dermatitis. In contrast, lesions with a generalized arrangement are common and suggest a systemic etiology.

As in other branches of medicine, a complete history should be obtained to emphasize the following features:

1. Evolution of lesions
   a. Site of onset
   b. Manner in which the eruption progressed or spread

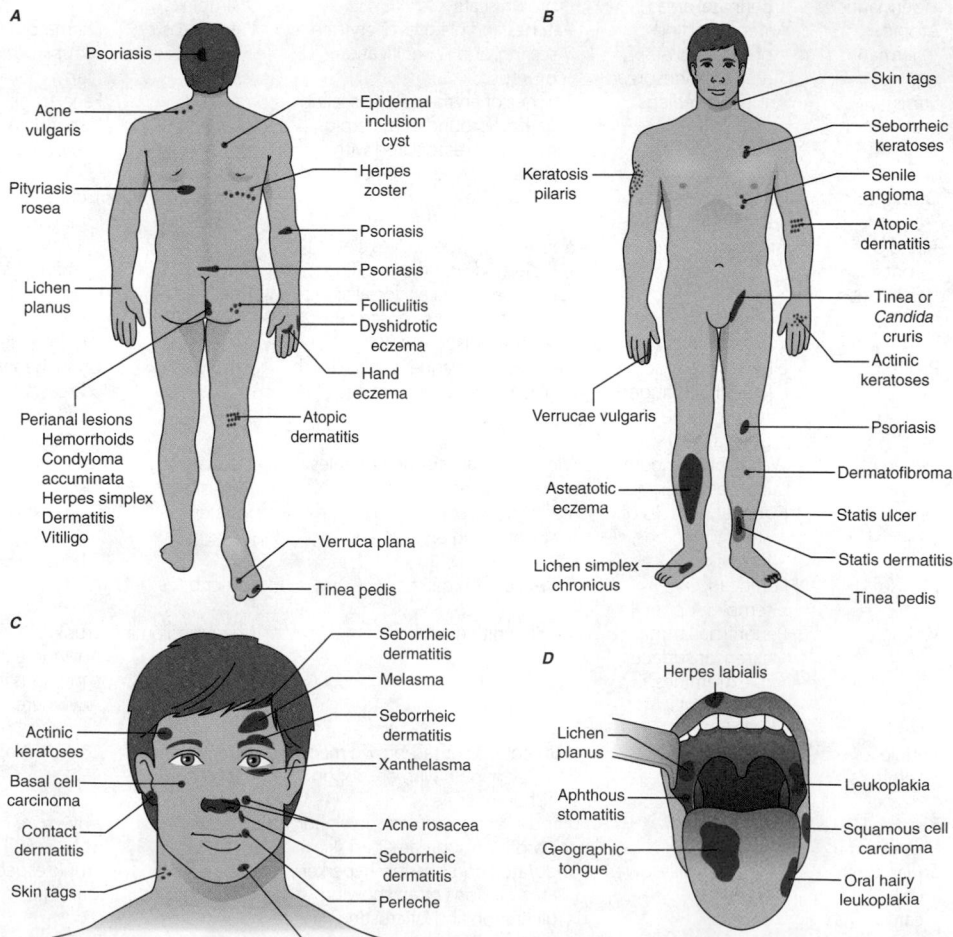

FIGURE 52-6 A–D. The distribution of some common dermatologic diseases and lesions.

FIGURE 52-7 Psoriasis. This papulosquamous skin disease is characterized by small and large erythematous papules and plaques with overlying adherent silvery scale.

c. Duration
d. Periods of resolution or improvement in chronic eruptions
2. Symptoms associated with the eruption
a. Itching, burning, pain, numbness
b. What, if anything, has relieved symptoms
c. Time of day when symptoms are most severe
3. Current or recent medications (prescribed as well as over-the-counter)
4. Associated systemic symptoms (e.g., malaise, fever, arthralgias)
5. Ongoing or previous illnesses
6. History of allergies
7. Presence of photosensitivity
8. Review of systems
9. Family history (particularly relevant for patients with melanoma, atopy, psoriasis, or acne)
10. Social, sexual, or travel history as relevant to the patient

DIAGNOSTIC TECHNIQUES

Many skin diseases can be diagnosed on gross clinical appearance, but sometimes relatively simple diagnostic procedures can yield valuable information. In most instances, they can be performed at the bedside with a minimum of equipment.

Skin Biopsy A skin biopsy is a straightforward minor surgical procedure; however, it is important to biopsy a lesion that is most likely to yield diagnostic findings. This decision may require expertise in skin diseases and knowledge of superficial anatomic structures in selected areas of the body. In this procedure, a small area of skin is anesthetized

FIGURE 52-8 Dermatitis herpetiformis. This disorder typically displays pruritic, grouped papulovesicles on elbows, knees, buttocks, and posterior scalp. Vesicles are often excoriated due to associated pruritus.

FIGURE 52-9 Erythema multiforme. This eruption is characterized by multiple erythematous plaques with a target or iris morphology. It usually represents a hypersensitivity reaction to drugs (e.g., sulfonylamides) or infections (e.g., HSV). *(Courtesy of the Yale Resident's Slide Collection; with permission.)*

with 1% lidocaine with or without epinephrine. The skin lesion in question can be excised or saucerized with a scalpel or removed by punch biopsy. In the latter technique, a punch is pressed against the surface of the skin and rotated with downward pressure until it penetrates to the subcutaneous tissue. The circular biopsy is then lifted with forceps, and the bottom is cut with iris scissors. Biopsy sites may or may not need suture closure, depending on size and location.

A

B

FIGURE 52-10 Allergic contact dermatitis (ACD). A. An example of ACD in its acute phase, with sharply demarcated, weeping, eczematous plaques in a perioral distribution. **B.** ACD in its chronic phase demonstrating an erythematous, lichenified, weeping plaque on skin chronically exposed to nickel in a metal snap. *(B, Courtesy of Robert Swerlick, MD; with permission.)*

CHAPTER 52 Approach to the Patient with a Skin Disorder

FIGURE 52-11 Urticaria. Discrete and confluent, edematous, erythematous papules and plaques are characteristic of this whealing eruption.

FIGURE 52-12 Vitiligo. Characteristic lesions display an acral distribution and striking depigmentation as a result of loss of melanocytes.

KOH Preparation A potassium hydroxide (KOH) preparation is performed on scaling skin lesions where a fungal infection is suspected. The edge of such a lesion is scraped gently with a no. 15 scalpel blade, and the removed scale is collected on a glass microscope slide then treated with 1 to 2 drops of a solution of 10–20% KOH. KOH dissolves keratin and allows easier visualization of fungal elements. Brief heating of the slide accelerates dissolution of keratin. When the preparation is viewed under the microscope, the refractile hyphae will be seen more easily when the light intensity is reduced and the condenser is lowered. This technique can be utilized to identify hyphae in dermatophyte infections, pseudohyphae and budding yeast in *Candida* infections (see Fig. 196-1), and "spaghetti and meatballs" yeast forms in tinea versicolor. The same sampling technique can be used to obtain scale for culture of selected pathogenic organisms.

Tzanck Smear A Tzanck smear is a cytologic technique most often used in the diagnosis of herpesvirus infections [herpes simplex virus (HSV) or varicella zoster virus (VZV)] (see Figs. 173-1 and 173-3). An early vesicle, not a pustule or crusted lesion, is unroofed, and the base of the lesion is scraped gently with a scalpel blade. The material is placed on a glass slide, air-dried, and stained with Giemsa or Wright's stain. Multinucleated epithelial giant cells suggest the presence of HSV or VZV; culture or immunofluorescence testing must be performed to identify the specific virus.

Diascopy Diascopy is designed to assess whether a skin lesion will blanch with pressure as, for example, in determining whether a red lesion is hemorrhagic or simply blood-filled. Urticaria (Fig. 52-11) will blanch with pressure, whereas a purpuric lesion caused by necrotizing vasculitis (Fig. 52-4) will not. Diascopy is performed by pressing a microscope slide or magnifying lens against a lesion and noting the

amount of blanching that occurs. Granulomas often have an opaque to transparent, brown-pink "apple jelly" appearance on diascopy.

Wood's Light A Wood's lamp generates 360-nm ultraviolet (or "black") light that can be used to aid the evaluation of certain skin disorders. For example, a Wood's lamp will cause erythrasma (a superficial, intertriginous infection caused by *Corynebacterium minutissimum*) to show a characteristic coral pink color, and wounds colonized by *Pseudomonas* to appear pale blue. Tinea capitis caused by certain dermatophytes such as *Microsporum canis* or *M. audouini* exhibits a yellow fluorescence. Pigmented lesions of the epidermis such as freckles are accentuated, while dermal pigment such as postinflammatory hyperpigmentation fades under a Wood's light. Vitiligo (Fig. 52-12) appears totally white under a Wood's lamp, and previously unsuspected areas of involvement often become apparent. A Wood's lamp may also aid in the demonstration of tinea versicolor and in recognition of ash leaf spots in patients with tuberous sclerosis.

Patch Tests Patch testing is designed to document sensitivity to a specific antigen. In this procedure, a battery of suspected allergens is applied to the patient's back under occlusive dressings and allowed to remain in contact with the skin for 48 h. The dressings are removed, and the area is examined for evidence of delayed hypersensitivity reactions (e.g., erythema, edema, or papulovesicles). This test is best performed by physicians with special expertise in patch testing and is often helpful in the evaluation of patients with chronic dermatitis.

FURTHER READINGS

DERMATOLOGY LEXICON PROJECT: *www.futurehealth.rochester.edu/dlp2/*
JAMES WD et al: *Andrews' Diseases of the Skin: Clinical Dermatology*, 10th ed. Philadelphia, Elsevier, 2006
WOLFF K et al (eds): *Fitzpatrick's Dermatology in General Medicine*, 7th ed. New York, McGraw-Hill, 2008

53 Eczema, Psoriasis, Cutaneous Infections, Acne, and Other Common Skin Disorders
Calvin O. McCall, Thomas J. Lawley

ECZEMA AND DERMATITIS

Eczema is a type of dermatitis and these terms are often used synonymously (atopic eczema or atopic dermatitis). Eczema is a reaction pattern that presents with variable clinical findings and the common

histologic finding of spongiosis (intercellular edema of the epidermis). Eczema is the final common expression for a number of disorders, including those discussed in the following sections. Primary lesions may include erythematous macules, papules, and vesicles, which can coalesce to form patches and plaques. In severe eczema, secondary lesions from infection or excoriation, marked by weeping and crusting, may predominate. In chronic eczematous conditions, lichenification (cutaneous hypertrophy and accentuation of normal skin markings) may alter the characteristic appearance of eczema.

ATOPIC DERMATITIS

Atopic dermatitis (AD) is the cutaneous expression of the atopic state, characterized by a family history of asthma, allergic rhinitis, or ecze-

TABLE 53-1 CLINICAL FEATURES OF ATOPIC DERMATITIS

1. Pruritus and scratching
2. Course marked by exacerbations and remissions
3. Lesions typical of eczematous dermatitis
4. Personal or family history of atopy (asthma, allergic rhinitis, food allergies, or eczema)
5. Clinical course lasting longer than 6 weeks
6. Lichenification of skin

ma. The prevalence of AD is increasing worldwide. Some of its features are shown in Table 53-1.

The etiology of AD is only partially defined, but there is a clear genetic predisposition. When both parents are affected by AD, >80% of their children manifest the disease. When only one parent is affected, the prevalence drops to slightly over 50%. Patients with AD may display a variety of immunoregulatory abnormalities including increased IgE synthesis, increased serum IgE, and impaired delayed-type hypersensitivity reactions.

The clinical presentation often varies with age. Half of patients with AD present within the first year of life, and 80% present by 5 years of age. About 80% ultimately coexpress allergic rhinitis or asthma. The infantile pattern is characterized by weeping inflammatory patches and crusted plaques on the face, neck, and extensor surfaces. The childhood and adolescent pattern is marked by dermatitis of flexural skin, particularly in the antecubital and popliteal fossae (Fig. 53-1). AD may resolve spontaneously, but over half of all individuals affected as children will have dermatitis in adult life. The distribution of lesions may be similar to those seen in childhood; however, adults frequently have localized disease, manifesting as lichen simplex chronicus or hand eczema (see below). In patients with localized disease, AD may be suspected because of a typical personal history, family history, or the presence of cutaneous stigmata of AD such as perioral pallor, an extra fold of skin beneath the lower eyelid (Dennie's line), increased palmar skin markings, and an increased incidence of cutaneous infections, particularly with *Staphylococcus aureus*. Regardless of other manifestations, pruritus is a prominent characteristic of AD in all age groups and is exacerbated by dry skin. Many of the cutaneous findings in affected patients, such as lichenification, are secondary to rubbing and scratching.

℞ ATOPIC DERMATITIS

Therapy of AD should include avoidance of cutaneous irritants, adequate moisturizing through the application of emollients, judicious use of topical anti-inflammatory agents, and prompt treatment of secondary infection. Patients should be instructed to bathe no more often than daily using warm or cool water, and to use only mild bath soap. Immediately after bathing while the skin is still moist, a topical anti-inflammatory agent in a cream or ointment base should be applied to areas of dermatitis, and all other skin areas should be lubricated with a moisturizer. Approximately 30 g of a topical agent is required to cover the entire body surface of an average adult.

Low- to midpotency topical glucocorticoids are employed in most treatment regimens for AD. Skin atrophy and the potential for systemic absorption are constant concerns, especially with more potent agents. Low-potency topical glucocorticoids or non-glucocorticoid anti-inflammatory agents should be selected for use on the face and intertriginous areas to minimize the risk of skin atrophy. Two non-glucocorticoid anti-inflammatory agents are now available, tacrolimus ointment and pimecrolimus cream. These agents are macrolide immunosuppressants that are approved by the U.S. Food and Drug Administration (FDA) for topical use in AD. Reports of broader effectiveness appear in the literature. These agents do not cause skin atrophy, nor do they suppress the hypothalamic-pituitary-adrenal axis. Recently, however, concerns have emerged regarding the potential for lymphomas in patients treated with these agents. Thus, caution should be exercised when considering these agents. Currently, they are also more costly than topical glucocorticoids.

Secondary infection of eczematous skin may lead to exacerbation of AD. Crusted and weeping skin lesions may be infected with *S. aureus*. When secondary infection is suspected, eczematous lesions should be cultured and patients treated with systemic antibiotics active against *S. aureus*. The initial use of penicillinase-resistant penicillins or cephalosporins is preferable. Dicloxacillin or cephalexin (250 mg qid for 7–10 days) is generally adequate; however, antibiotic selection must be directed by culture results and clinical response. More than 50% of *S. aureus* (SA) isolates are now methacillin resistant (MR) in some communities—community acquired MRSA (CA-MRSA). Current recommendations for the treatment of CA-MRSA infection in adults include trimethoprim/sulfamethoxazole (1–2 double strength bid), minocycline (100 mg bid), doxycycline (100 mg bid), or clindamycin (300–450 mg qid). Duration of therapy should be 7–10 days. Inducible resistance may limit clindamycin's usefulness. The latter can be detected by the double-disc diffusion test, which should be ordered if the isolate is erythromycin-resistant and clindamycin-sensitive. As an adjunct, the use of triclosan-containing antibacterial washes and intermittent nasal mupirocin may be useful.

Control of pruritus is essential for treatment, since AD often represents "an itch that rashes." Antihistamines are most often used to control pruritus, and mild sedation may be responsible for their antipruritic action. Sedation may also limit their usefulness; however, when used at bedtime, sedating antihistamines may improve the patient's sleep. Unlike their effects in urticaria, nonsedating antihistamines and selective H_2 blockers are of little use in controlling the pruritus of AD.

Treatment with systemic glucocorticoids should be limited to severe exacerbations unresponsive to topical therapy. In the patient with chronic AD, therapy with systemic glucocorticoids will generally clear the skin only briefly, and cessation of the systemic therapy will invariably be accompanied by return, if not worsening, of the dermatitis. Patients who do not respond to conventional therapies should be considered for patch testing to rule out allergic contact dermatitis. The role of dietary allergens in atopic dermatitis is controversial, and there is little evidence they play any role outside of infancy. Immunotherapy with aeroallergens has not proven useful in AD.

LICHEN SIMPLEX CHRONICUS

Lichen simplex chronicus may represent the end stage of a variety of pruritic and eczematous disorders, including atopic dermatitis. It consists of a circumscribed plaque or plaques of lichenified skin (thickening of the skin and accentuation of normal skin markings) due to chronic scratching or rubbing. Common areas involved include the posterior nuchal region, dorsum of the feet, and ankles. Treatment of lichen simplex chronicus centers on breaking the cycle of chronic itching and scratching. High-potency topical glucocorticoids are helpful in most cases, but in recalcitrant cases, application of topical glucocorticoids under occlusion, or intralesional injection of glucocorticoids may be required. Oral antihistamines such as hydroxyzine (10–25 mg every 6 h) or tricyclic antidepressants with antihistaminic activity, such as doxepin (10–25 mg at bedtime), are useful primarily due to their sedating action. Higher doses of these agents may be required, but sedation can become bothersome. Patients need to be counseled regarding driving or operating heavy equipment after taking these medications.

CONTACT DERMATITIS

Contact dermatitis is an inflammatory process in skin caused by an exogenous agent or agents that directly or indirectly injure the skin. This

FIGURE 53-1 Atopic dermatitis. Hyperpigmentation, lichenification, and scaling in the antecubital fossae are seen in this patient with atopic dermatitis. (*Courtesy of Robert Swerlick, MD; with permission.*)

injury may be caused by an inherent characteristic of a compound—irritant contact dermatitis (ICD). An example of ICD would be dermatitis induced by a concentrated acid or base. Agents that cause allergic contact dermatitis (ACD) induce an antigen-specific immune response (poison ivy dermatitis). The clinical lesions of contact dermatitis may be acute (wet and edematous) or chronic (dry, thickened, and scaly), depending on the persistence of the insult (see Fig. 52-10).

Irritant Contact Dermatitis ICD is generally well demarcated and often localized to areas of thin skin (eyelids, intertriginous areas) or to areas where the irritant was occluded. Lesions may range from minimal skin erythema to areas of marked edema, vesicles, and ulcers. Chronic low-grade irritant dermatitis is the most common type of ICD, and the most common area of involvement is the hands (see below). The most common irritants encountered are chronic wet work, soaps, and detergents. Treatment should be directed to avoidance of irritants and use of protective gloves or clothing.

Allergic Contact Dermatitis ACD is a manifestation of delayed-type hypersensitivity mediated by memory T lymphocytes in the skin. The most common cause of ACD is exposure to plants, especially to members of the family Anacardiaceae, including the genus *Toxicodendron*. Poison ivy, poison oak, and poison sumac are members of this genus and cause an allergic reaction marked by erythema, vesiculation, and severe pruritus. The eruption is often linear or angular, corresponding to areas where plants have touched the skin. The sensitizing antigen common to these plants is urushiol, an oleoresin containing the active ingredient pentadecylcatechol. The oleoresin may adhere to skin, clothing, tools, and pets, and contaminated articles may cause dermatitis even after prolonged storage. Blister fluid does not contain urushiol and is not capable of inducing skin eruption in exposed subjects.

℞ CONTACT DERMATITIS

If contact dermatitis is suspected and an offending agent is identified and removed, the eruption will resolve. Usually, treatment with high-potency topical glucocorticoids is enough to relieve symptoms while the dermatitis runs its course. For those patients who require systemic therapy, daily oral prednisone beginning at 1 mg/kg, but usually ≤60 mg/d, is sufficient. It should be tapered over 2–3 weeks, and each daily dose given in the morning with food.

Identification of a contact allergen can be a difficult and time-consuming task. Patients with dermatitis unresponsive to conventional therapy or with an unusual and patterned distribution should be suspected of having ACD. They should be questioned carefully regarding occupational exposures and topical medications. Common sensitizers include preservatives in topical preparations, nickel sulfate, potassium dichromate, thimerosal, neomycin sulfate, fragrances, formaldehyde, and rubber-curing agents. Patch testing is helpful in identifying these agents but should not be attempted on patients with widespread active dermatitis or on those taking systemic glucocorticoids.

HAND ECZEMA

Hand eczema is a very common, chronic skin disorder in which both exogenous and endogenous factors play important roles. It may be associated with other cutaneous disorders such as atopic dermatitis, and contact with various agents may be involved. It represents a large proportion of occupation-associated skin disease. Chronic, excessive exposure to water and detergents, harsh chemicals, or allergens may initiate or aggravate this disorder. It may present with dryness and cracking of the skin of the hands as well as with variable amounts of erythema and edema. Often, the dermatitis will begin under rings where water and irritants are trapped. Dyshidrotic eczema, a variant of hand eczema, presents with multiple, intensely pruritic, small papules and vesicles occurring on the thenar and hypothenar eminences and the sides of the fingers (**Fig. 53-2**). Lesions tend to occur in crops that slowly form crusts and heal.

The evaluation of a patient with hand eczema should include an assessment of potential occupation-associated exposures. The history should be directed to identifying possible irritant or allergen exposures.

FIGURE 53-2 Dyshidrotic eczema. This example is characterized by deep-seated vesicles and scaling on palms and lateral fingers, and the disease is often associated with an atopic diathesis.

℞ HAND ECZEMA

Therapy of hand dermatitis is directed toward avoidance of irritants, identification of possible contact allergens, treatment of coexistent infection, and application of topical glucocorticoids. Whenever possible, the hands should be protected by gloves, preferably vinyl. The use of rubber gloves (latex) to protect dermatitic skin is sometimes associated with the development of hypersensitivity reactions to components of the gloves. Patients can be treated with cool moist compresses, followed by application of a mid- to high-potency topical glucocorticoid in a cream or ointment base. As with atopic dermatitis, treatment of secondary infection is essential for good control. Additionally, patients with hand dermatitis should be examined for dermatophyte infection by KOH preparation and culture (see below).

NUMMULAR ECZEMA

Nummular eczema is characterized by circular or oval "coinlike" lesions, beginning as small edematous papules that become crusted and scaly. The etiology of nummular eczema is unknown, but dry skin is a contributing factor. Common locations are the trunk or the extensor surfaces of the extremities, particularly on the pretibial areas or dorsum of the hands. It occurs more frequently in men and is most commonly seen in middle age. The treatment of nummular eczema is similar to that for atopic dermatitis.

ASTEATOTIC ECZEMA

Asteatotic eczema, also known as *xerotic eczema* or "*winter itch,*" is a mildly inflammatory dermatitis that develops in areas of extremely dry skin, especially during the dry winter months. Clinically, there may be considerable overlap with nummular eczema. This form of eczema accounts for a large number of physician visits because of the associated pruritus. Fine cracks and scale, with or without erythema, characteristically develop in areas of dry skin, especially on the anterior surfaces of the lower extremities in elderly patients. Asteatotic eczema responds well to topical moisturizers and the avoidance of cutaneous irritants. Overbathing and the use of harsh soaps exacerbate asteatotic eczema.

STASIS DERMATITIS AND STASIS ULCERATION

Stasis dermatitis develops on the lower extremities secondary to venous incompetence and chronic edema. Patients may give a history of deep venous thrombosis, have evidence of vein removal, or varicose veins. Early findings in stasis dermatitis consist of mild erythema and scaling associated with pruritus. The typical initial site of involvement is the medial aspect of the ankle, often over a distended vein (**Fig. 53-3**). Stasis dermatitis may become acutely inflamed, with crusting and exudate. In this state, it is easily confused with cellulitis. Chronic stasis dermatitis is often associated with dermal fibrosis that is recognized clinically as

FIGURE 53-3 Stasis dermatitis. An example of stasis dermatitis showing erythematous, scaly, and oozing patches over the lower leg. Several stasis ulcers are also seen in this patient.

brawny edema of the skin. As the disorder progresses, the dermatitis becomes progressively pigmented, due to chronic erythrocyte extravasation leading to cutaneous hemosiderin deposition. Stasis dermatitis may be complicated by secondary infection and contact dermatitis. Severe stasis dermatitis may precede the development of stasis ulcers.

℞ STASIS DERMATITIS AND STASIS ULCERATION

Patients with stasis dermatitis and stasis ulceration benefit greatly from leg elevation and the routine use of compression stockings with a gradient of at least 30–40 mmHg. Stockings providing less compression, such as anti-embolism hose, are poor substitutes. Use of emollients and/or midpotency topical glucocorticoids and avoidance of irritants are also helpful in treating stasis dermatitis. Protecting the legs from injury, including scratching, and control of chronic edema are essential to prevent ulcers. Diuretics may be required to adequately control chronic edema.

Stasis ulcers are difficult to treat, and resolution is slow. It is extremely important to elevate the affected limb as much as possible. The ulcer should be kept clear of necrotic material by gentle debridement and covered with a semipermeable dressing and a compression dressing or compression stocking. Glucocorticoids should not be applied to ulcers, since they may retard healing; however, they may be applied to the surrounding skin to control itching, scratching, and additional trauma. Secondarily infected lesions should be treated with appropriate oral antibiotics, but it should be noted that all ulcers will become colonized with bacteria, and the purpose of antibiotic therapy should not be to clear all bacterial growth. Care must be taken to exclude treatable causes of leg ulcers (hypercoagulation, vasculitis) before beginning the chronic management outlined above.

SEBORRHEIC DERMATITIS

Seborrheic dermatitis is a common, chronic disorder, characterized by greasy scales overlying erythematous patches or plaques. Induration and scale are generally less prominent than in psoriasis, but clinical overlap exists between these diseases—"sebopsoriasis." The most common location is in the scalp where it may be recognized as severe dandruff. On the face, seborrheic dermatitis affects the eyebrows, eyelids, glabella, and nasolabial

FIGURE 53-4 Seborrheic dermatitis. Central facial erythema with overlying greasy, yellowish scale is seen in this patient. (*Courtesy of Jean Bolognia, MD; with permission.*)

folds (**Fig. 53-4**). Scaling of the external auditory canal is common in seborrheic dermatitis. Additionally, the postauricular areas often become macerated and tender. Seborrheic dermatitis may also develop in the central chest, axilla, groin, submammary folds, and gluteal cleft. Rarely, it may cause a widespread generalized dermatitis. Pruritus is variable.

Seborrheic dermatitis may be evident within the first few weeks of life, and within this context it occurs in the scalp ("cradle cap"), face, or groin. It is rarely seen in children beyond infancy but becomes evident again during adult life. Although it is frequently seen in patients with Parkinson's disease, in those who have had cerebrovascular accidents, and in those with HIV infection, the overwhelming majority of individuals with seborrheic dermatitis have no underlying disorder.

℞ SEBORRHEIC DERMATITIS

Treatment with low-potency topical glucocorticoids in conjunction with a topical antifungal agent, such as ketoconazole cream or ciclopirox cream, is often effective. The scalp and beard areas may benefit from anti-dandruff shampoos, which should be left in place 3–5 min before rinsing. High-potency topical glucocorticoid solutions (betamethasone or clobetasol) are effective for control of severe scalp involvement. High potency glucocorticoids should not be used on the face since this is often associated with steroid-induced rosacea or atrophy. Tacrolimus and pimecrolimus are alternatives to topical glucocorticoids, especially when seborrheic dermatitis involves eyelids, although they are not FDA-approved for these indications.

PAPULOSQUAMOUS DISORDERS (Table 53-2)

PSORIASIS

Psoriasis is one of the most common dermatologic diseases, affecting up to 1% of the world's population. It is a chronic inflammatory skin disor-

	Clinical Features	Other Notable Features	Histologic Features
Psoriasis	Sharply demarcated, erythematous plaques with mica-like scale; predominantly elbows, knees, and scalp; atypical forms may localize to intertriginous areas; eruptive forms may be associated with infection	May be aggravated by certain drugs, infection; severe forms seen associated with HIV	Acanthosis, vascular proliferation
Lichen planus	Purple polygonal papules marked by severe pruritus; lacy white markings, especially associated with mucous membrane lesions	Certain drugs may induce: thiazides, antimalarial drugs	Interface dermatitis
Pityriasis rosea	Rash often preceded by herald patch; oval to round plaques with trailing scale; most often affects the trunk, and eruption lines up in skin folds giving a "fir tree"-like appearance; generally spares palms and soles	Variable pruritus; self-limited resolving in 2–8 weeks; may be imitated by secondary syphilis	Pathologic features often nonspecific
Dermatophytosis	Polymorphous appearance depending on dermatophyte, body site, and host response; sharply defined to ill-demarcated scaly plaques with or without inflammation; may be associated with hair loss	KOH preparation may show branching hyphae; culture helpful	Hyphae and neutrophils in stratum corneum

TABLE 53-2 PAPULOSQUAMOUS DISORDERS

der clinically characterized by erythematous, sharply demarcated papules and rounded plaques, covered by silvery micaceous scale. The skin lesions of psoriasis are variably pruritic. Traumatized areas often develop lesions of psoriasis (Koebner or isomorphic phenomenon). Additionally, other external factors may exacerbate psoriasis including infections, stress, and medications (lithium, beta blockers, and antimalarials).

The most common variety of psoriasis is called *plaque-type*. Patients with plaque-type psoriasis will have stable, slowly enlarging plaques, which remain basically unchanged for long periods of time. The most commonly involved areas are the elbows, knees, gluteal cleft, and the scalp. Involvement tends to be symmetric. Plaque psoriasis generally develops slowly and runs an indolent course. It rarely remits spontaneously. *Inverse psoriasis* affects the intertriginous regions including the axilla, groin, submammary region, and navel; it also tends to affect the scalp, palms, and soles. The individual lesions are sharply demarcated plaques (see Fig. 52-7), but they may be moist and without scale due to their location.

Guttate psoriasis (eruptive psoriasis) is most common in children and young adults. It develops acutely in individuals without psoriasis or in those with chronic plaque psoriasis. Patients present with many small erythematous, scaling papules, frequently after upper respiratory tract infection with β-hemolytic streptococci. The differential diagnosis should include pityriasis rosea and secondary syphilis.

Pustular psoriasis is another variant. Patients may have disease localized to the palms and soles, or the disease may be generalized. Regardless of the extent of disease, the skin is erythematous with pustules and variable scale. Localized to the palms and soles, it is easily confused with eczema. When generalized, episodes are characterized by fever (39°–40°C) lasting several days, an accompanying generalized eruption of sterile pustules, and a background of intense erythema; patients may become erythrodermic. Episodes of fever and pustules are recurrent. Local irritants, pregnancy, medications, infections, and systemic glucocorticoid withdrawal can precipitate this form of psoriasis. Oral retinoids are the treatment of choice in nonpregnant patients.

About half of all patients with psoriasis have fingernail involvement, appearing as punctate pitting, onycholysis, nail thickening, or subungual hyperkeratosis. About 5–10% of patients with psoriasis have associated arthralgias, and these are most often found in patients with fingernail involvement. Although some have the coincident occurrence of classic rheumatoid arthritis (Chap. 314), many have psoriatic arthritis that falls into one of three types: (1) asymmetric inflammatory arthritis most commonly involving the distal and proximal interphalangeal joints and less commonly the knees, hips, ankles, and wrists; (2) a seronegative rheumatoid arthritis–like disease; a significant portion of these patients go on to develop a severe destructive arthritis; or (3) disease limited to the spine (psoriatic spondylitis).

The etiology of psoriasis is still poorly understood, but there is clearly a genetic component to the disease. Over 50% of patients with psoriasis report a positive family history. Psoriatic lesions demonstrate infiltrates of activated T cells that are thought to elaborate cytokines responsible for keratinocyte hyperproliferation, which results in the characteristic clinical findings. Agents inhibiting T cell activation, clonal expansion, or release of proinflammatory cytokines are often effective for the treatment of severe psoriasis (see below).

Rx PSORIASIS

Treatment of psoriasis depends on the type, location, and extent of disease. All patients should be instructed to avoid excess drying or irritation of their skin and to maintain adequate cutaneous hydration. Most patients with localized, plaque-type psoriasis can be managed with midpotency topical glucocorticoids, although their long-term use is often accompanied by loss of effectiveness (tachyphylaxis) and atrophy of the skin. A topi-

TABLE 53-3 FDA-APPROVED SYSTEMIC THERAPY FOR PSORIASIS

Agent	Medication Class	Administration		Adverse Events (Selected)
		Route	Frequency	
Methotrexate	Antimetabolite	Oral	Weekly	Hepatotoxicity, pulmonary toxicity, pancytopenia, potential for increased malignancies, ulcerative stomatitis, nausea, diarrhea, teratogenicity
Acitretin	Retinoid	Oral	Daily	Teratogenicity, osteophyte formation, hyperlipidemia, flare of inflammatory bowel disease, hepatoxicity, depression
Cyclosporine	Calcineurin inhibitor	Oral	Twice daily	Renal dysfunction, hypertension, hyperkalemia, hyperuricemia, hypomagnesemia, hyperlipidemia, increased risk of malignancies

cal vitamin D analogue (calcipotriene) and a retinoid (tazarotene) are also efficacious in the treatment of limited psoriasis and have largely replaced other topical agents such as coal tar, salicylic acid, and anthralin.

Ultraviolet light, natural or artificial, is an effective therapy for many patients with widespread psoriasis. Ultraviolet B (UV-B) light, narrowband UV-B, and ultraviolet A (UV-A) spectrum with either oral or topical psoralens (PUVA) are also extremely effective. The long-term use of UV light may be associated with an increased incidence of non-melanoma and melanoma skin cancer. UV light therapy is contraindicated in patients receiving cyclosporine and should be used with great care in all immunocompromised patients due to an increased risk of developing skin cancers.

Various systemic agents can be used for severe, widespread psoriatic disease (Table 53-3). Oral glucocorticoids should not be used for the treatment of psoriasis due to the potential for developing life-threatening pustular psoriasis when therapy is discontinued. Methotrexate is an effective agent, especially in patients with psoriatic arthritis. The synthetic retinoid, acitretin, is useful, especially when immunosuppression must be avoided; however, teratogenicity limits its use.

The evidence implicating psoriasis as a T cell–mediated disorder has directed therapeutic efforts to immunoregulation. Cyclosporine and other immunosuppressive agents can be very effective in the treatment of psoriasis, and much attention is currently directed toward the development of biologic agents with more selective immunosuppressive properties and better safety profiles (Table 53-4). Experience with these agents is limited and information regarding combination therapy and adverse events continues to emerge. Use of TNF-α inhibitors may worsen congestive heart failure (CHF), and they should be used with caution in those at risk of or known to have CHF. Further, none of the immunosuppressive agents used in the treatment of psoriasis should be initiated if the patient has a severe infection; patients on such therapy should be routinely screened for tuberculosis. Malignancies, including a risk or history of certain malignancies, may limit the use of these systemic agents.

LICHEN PLANUS

Lichen planus (LP) is a papulosquamous disorder that may affect the skin, scalp, nails, and mucous membranes. The primary cutaneous lesions are pruritic, polygonal, flat-topped, violaceous papules. Close examination of the surface of these papules often reveals a network of gray lines (Wickham's striae). The skin lesions may occur anywhere but have a predilection for the wrists, shins, lower back, and genitalia (Fig. 53-5). Involvement of the scalp, lichen planopilaris, may lead to scarring alopecia, and nail involvement may lead to permanent deformity or loss of fingernails and toenails. LP commonly involves mucous membranes, particularly the buccal mucosa, where it can present a spectrum of disease from a mild, white, reticulate eruption of the mucosa, to a severe, erosive stomatitis. Erosive stomatitis may persist for years and may be linked to an increased risk of oral squamous cell carcinoma. Cutaneous eruptions clinically resembling LP have been observed after administration of numerous drugs, including thiazide diuretics, gold, antimalarials, penicillamine, and phenothiazines, and in patients with skin lesions of chronic graft-versus-host disease. Additionally, LP may be associated with hepatitis C infection. The course of LP is variable, but most patients have spontaneous remissions 6 months to 2 years after the onset of disease. Topical glucocorticoids are the mainstay of therapy.

TABLE 53-4 BIOLOGICS APPROVED FOR PSORIASIS OR PSORIATIC ARTHRITIS

Agent	Mechanism of Action	Indication	Administration		Warnings
			Route	Frequency	
Alefacept	Anti-CD-2	Ps	IM	Once weekly × 12 weeks; may repeat	Lymphopenia, potential for increased malignancies, serious infections
Etanercept	Anti TNF-α	Ps, PsA	SC	Once or twice weekly	Serious infections, neurologic events, hematologic events, potential for increased malignancies
Efalizumab	Anti CD-11a	Ps	SC	Once weekly	Serious infections, potential for increased malignancies, thrombocytopenia, hemolytic anemia, psoriasis worsening
Adalimumab	Anti TNF-α	PsA	SC	Every other week	Serious infections, neurologic events, potential for increased malignancies, hypersensitivity reactions, hematologic events
Infliximab	Anti TNF-α	PsA	IV	Initial infusion followed by infusions at week 2, 6, then every 8 weeks	Serious infections, hepatotoxicity, hematologic events, hypersensitivity reactions, neurologic events, potential for increased malignancies

Ps, psoriasis; PsA, psoriatic arthritis; IM, intramuscular; SC, subcutaneous; TNF, tumor necrosis factor.

PITYRIASIS ROSEA

Pityriasis rosea (PR) is a papulosquamous eruption of unknown etiology occurring more commonly in the spring and fall. Its first manifestation is the development of a 2- to 6-cm annular lesion (the herald patch). This is followed in a few days to a few weeks by the appearance of many smaller annular or papular lesions with a predilection to occur on the trunk (Fig. 53-6). The lesions are generally oval, with their long axis parallel to the skin-fold lines. Individual lesions may range in color from red to brown and have a trailing scale. PR shares many clinical features with the eruption of secondary syphilis, but palm and sole lesions are extremely rare in PR and common in secondary syphilis. The eruption tends to be moderately pruritic and lasts 3–8 weeks. Treatment is directed at alleviating pruritus and consists of oral antihistamines, midpotency topical glucocorticoids, and, in some cases, the use of UV-B phototherapy.

CUTANEOUS INFECTIONS (Table 53-5)

IMPETIGO, ECTHYMA, AND FURUNCULOSIS

Impetigo is a common superficial bacterial infection of skin caused most often by *S. aureus* (Chap. 129), and in some cases by group A β-hemolytic streptococci (Chap. 130). The primary lesion is a superficial pustule that ruptures and forms a characteristic yellow-brown honey-colored crust (Chap. 130). Lesions may occur on normal skin—primary infection—or in areas already affected by another skin disease—secondary infection. Lesions caused by staphylococci may be tense, clear bullae, and this less common form of the disease is called *bullous impetigo*. Blisters are caused by the production of exfoliative toxin by

S. aureus phage type II. This is the same toxin responsible for staphylococcal scalded-skin syndrome (SSSS), often resulting in dramatic loss of the superficial epidermis due to blistering. SSSS is much more common in children than in adults; however, it should be considered along with toxic epidermal necrolysis and severe drug eruptions in patients with widespread blistering of the skin. *Ecthyma* is a variant of impetigo that causes punched-out ulcerative lesions. It may result from neglected or inadequately treated impetigo. Treatment of both ecthyma and impetigo involves gentle debridement of adherent crusts, which is facilitated by the use of soaks and topical antibiotics, in conjunction with appropriate oral antibiotics. *Furunculosis* is also caused by *S. aureus*, and this disorder has gained prominence in the last decade because of CA-MRSA. A furuncle, or boil, is a painful, erythematous, nodule that can occur on any cutaneous surface. The lesions may be solitary but are most often multiple. Patients frequently believe they have been bitten by spiders or insects. Family members or close contacts may also be affected. Furuncles can rupture and drain spontaneously or may need incision and drainage, which may be adequate therapy for small solitary furuncles without cellulitis or systemic symptoms. Whenever possible, lesional material should be sent for culture. Current recommendations for methicillin-sensitive infections are β-lactam antibiotics. Therapy for CA-MRSA was discussed previously (see "Atopic Dermatitis"). Warm compresses and nasal mupirocin are helpful therapeutic additions. Severe infections may require IV antibiotics.

ERYSIPELAS AND CELLULITIS

See Chap. 119

FIGURE 53-5 Lichen planus. An example of lichen planus showing multiple flat-topped, violaceous papules and plaques. Nail dystrophy as seen in this patient's thumbnail may also be a feature. (*Courtesy of Robert Swerlick, MD; with permission.*)

FIGURE 53-6 Pityriasis rosea. In this patient with pityriasis rosea, multiple round to oval erythematous patches with fine central scale are distributed along the skin tension lines on the trunk.

TABLE 53-5 COMMON SKIN INFECTIONS

	Clinical Features	Etiologic Agent	Treatment
Impetigo	Honey-colored crusted papules, plaques, or bullae	Group A Streptococcus and *Staphylococcus aureus*	Systemic or topical antistaphylococcal antibiotics
Dermatophytosis	Inflammatory or noninflammatory annular scaly plaques; may have hair loss; groin involvement spares scrotum; hyphae on KOH preparation	*Trichophyton*, *Epidermophyton*, or *Microsporum* sp.	Topical azoles, systemic griseofulvin, terbinafine, or azoles
Candidiasis	Inflammatory papules and plaques with satellite pustules, frequently in intertriginous areas; may involve scrotum; pseudohyphae on KOH preparation	*Candida albicans* and other *Candida* species	Topical nystatin or azoles; systemic azoles for resistant disease
Tinea versicolor	Hyperpigmented or hypopigmented scaly patches on the trunk; characteristic mixture of hyphae and spores on KOH preparation ("spaghetti and meatballs")	*Malassezia furfur*	Topical selenium sulfide lotion or azoles

DERMATOPHYTOSIS

Dermatophytes are fungi that infect skin, hair, and nails and include members of the genera *Trichophyton*, *Microsporum*, and *Epidermophyton*. Tinea corporis, or infection of the relatively hairless skin of the body (glabrous skin), may have a variable appearance depending on the extent of the associated inflammatory reaction (see Fig. 52-11). Typical infections have an annular appearance that patients refer to as "ringworm." Deep inflammatory nodules or granulomas occur in some infections—especially in those infections inappropriately treated with mid- to high-potency topical glucocorticoids. Involvement of the groin (tinea cruris) is more common in males than females. It presents as a scaling, erythematous eruption sparing the scrotum. Infection of the foot (tinea pedis) is the most common dermatophyte infection and is often chronic; it is characterized by variable erythema, edema, scaling, pruritus, and occasionally vesiculation. Involvement may be widespread or localized but generally involves the web space between the fourth and fifth toes. Infection of the nails (tinea unguium or onychomycosis) occurs in many patients with tinea pedis and is characterized by opacified, thickened nails and subungual debris. The distal-lateral variant is most common. Proximal subungual onychomycosis may be a marker for HIV infection or other immunocompromised states. Dermatophyte infection of the scalp (tinea capitis) has returned in epidemic proportions, particularly affecting inner-city children, but it also affects adults. The predominant organism is *T. tonsurans*, which can produce a relatively noninflammatory infection with mild scale and hair loss that is diffuse or localized. *T. tonsurans* can also cause a markedly inflammatory dermatosis with edema and nodules. This latter presentation is a kerion.

The diagnosis of tinea can be made from skin scrapings, nail scrapings, or hair by culture or direct microscopic examination with potassium hydroxide (KOH). Nail clippings may be sent for histologic examination with periodic acid Schiff (PAS) stain.

℞ DERMATOPHYTOSIS

Both topical and systemic therapies may be used to treat dermatophyte infections. Treatment depends on the site involved and the type of infection. Topical therapy is generally effective for uncomplicated tinea corporis, tinea cruris, and limited tinea pedis. It is not effective as a monotherapy for tinea capitis or onychomycosis. Topical imidazoles, triazoles, and allylamines may be effective therapies for dermatophyte infections, but nystatin is not active against dermatophytes. Topicals are generally applied twice daily, and treatment should continue 1 week beyond clinical resolution of the infection. Tinea pedis often requires longer treatment courses and frequently relapses. Oral antifungal agents may be required for recalcitrant tinea pedis or tinea corporis.

Oral antifungal agents are required for dermatophyte infections involving the hair and nails and for other infections unresponsive to topical therapy. A fungal etiology should be confirmed by direct microscopic examination or by culture prior to prescribing oral antifungal agents. All of the oral agents may cause hepatotoxicity and should not be used in women who are pregnant or breast-feeding.

Griseofulvin is the only oral agent approved in the United States for dermatophyte infections involving the skin, hair, or nails. When griseofulvin is used, a daily dose of 500 mg microsized or 375 mg ultramicrosized griseofulvin administered with a fatty meal is an adequate dose for most dermatophyte infections. Higher doses are required for some cases of tinea pedis and tinea capitis. The usual adult dose of griseofulvin for tinea capitis is 1 g microsized or 0.5 g ultramicrosized given daily. Markedly inflammatory tinea capitis may result in scarring and hair loss, and systemic or topical glucocorticoids may be helpful in preventing these sequelae. The duration of therapy may be 2 weeks for uncomplicated tinea corporis, 8–12 weeks for tinea capitis, or as long as 6–18 months for nail infections. Due to high relapse rates, griseofulvin is seldom used for nail infections. Common side effects of griseofulvin include gastrointestinal distress, headache, and urticaria.

Oral itraconazole and terbinafine are approved for onychomycosis. Itraconazole is given as either continuous daily therapy (200 mg/d) or pulses (200 mg bid for 1 week per month) administered with food. Fingernails require 2 months of continuous therapy or two pulses. Toenails require 3 months of continuous therapy or three pulses. Itraconazole has the potential for serious interactions with other drugs requiring the P450 enzyme system for metabolism. Terbinafine (250 mg/d) is also effective for onychomycosis. Therapy with terbinafine is continued for 6 weeks for fingernail infections and 12 weeks for toenail infections. Terbinafine has fewer drug-drug interactions, but caution should be used when patients are on multiple medications.

TINEA VERSICOLOR

Tinea versicolor is caused by a non-dermatophyte, dimorphic fungus, *Malassezia furfur*, a normal inhabitant of the skin. The expression of infection is promoted by heat and humidity. The typical lesions consist of oval scaly macules, papules, and patches concentrated on the chest, shoulders, and back but only rarely on the face or distal extremities. On dark skin, they often appear as hypopigmented areas, while on light skin, they are slightly erythematous or hyperpigmented. A KOH preparation from scaling lesions will demonstrate a confluence of short hyphae and round spores ("spaghetti and meatballs"). Lotions or shampoos containing sulfur, salicylic acid, or selenium sulfide will clear the infection if used daily for 1–2 weeks and then weekly thereafter. These preparations are irritating if left on the skin for more than 10 min; thus, they should be washed off completely. Treatment with some oral antifungal agents is also effective, but they do not provide lasting results, and they are not FDA-approved for this indication. Ketoconazole has been used as a single 400-mg dose; the patient waits 1 h, exercises to the point of sweating, then lets the skin dry. Itraconazole and fluconazole have also been used at various doses and frequencies. Griseofulvin is not effective, and terbenifine is not reliably effective for tinea versicolor.

CANDIDIASIS

Candidiasis is a fungal infection caused by a related group of yeasts, whose manifestations may be localized to the skin, or rarely, may be systemic and life-threatening. The causative organism is usually *Candida albicans*, but may also be *C. tropicalis*, *C. parapsilosis*, or *C. krusei*. These organisms are normal saprophytic inhabitants of the gastrointestinal tract but may overgrow (usually due to broad-spectrum antibiotic therapy) and cause disease at a number of cutaneous sites. Other predisposing factors include diabetes mellitus, chronic intertrigo, oral contraceptive use, and cellular immune deficiency. Candidiasis is a very common infection in HIV-infected individuals (Chap. 182). The oral cavity is commonly involved. Lesions may occur on the tongue or buccal mucosa (thrush) and appear as white plaques (see Fig. 52-12). Microscopic examination of scrapings demonstrate both pseudohyphae and yeast forms. Fissured, macerated lesions at the corners of the mouth (perlèche) are often seen in individuals with poorly fitting dentures and may also be associated with candidal infection. Additionally, candidal infections have an affinity for sites that are chronically wet and macerated, including the skin around nails (onycholysis and paronychia) and in intertriginous areas. Intertriginous lesions are characteristically edematous, erythematous, and scaly, with scattered "satellite pustules." In males, there is often involvement of the penis and scrotum as well as the inner aspect of the thighs. In contrast to dermatophyte infections, candidal infections are frequently painful and accompanied by a marked inflammatory response. Diagnosis of candidal infection is based upon the clinical pattern and demonstration of yeast on KOH preparation or culture.

℞ CANDIDIASIS

Treatment involves removing any predisposing factors such as antibiotic therapy or chronic wetness and the use of appropriate topical or systemic antifungal agents. Effective topicals include nystatin or azoles (miconazole, clotrimazole, econazole, or ketoconazole). The associated inflammatory response accompanying candidal infection on glabrous skin can be treated with a mild glucocorticoid lotion or cream (2.5% hydrocortisone). Systemic therapy is usually reserved for immunosuppressed patients or individuals with chronic or recurrent disease who fail to respond to appropriate topical therapy. Oral agents approved for the treatment of candidiasis include itraconazole and fluconazole. Oral nystatin is only effective for candidiasis of the gastrointestinal tract. Griseofulvin and terbenifine are not effective.

WARTS

Warts are cutaneous neoplasms caused by papilloma viruses. More than 100 different human papilloma viruses (HPV) have been described. A typical wart, verruca vulgaris, is sessile, dome-shaped, and usually about a centimeter in diameter. Its surface is hyperkeratotic consisting of many small filamentous projections. The HPV that cause typical verruca vulgaris also cause typical plantar warts, flat warts (or verruca plana), and filiform warts. Plantar warts are endophytic and are covered by thick keratin. Paring of the wart will generally demonstrate a central core of keratinized debris and punctate bleeding points. Filiform warts are most commonly seen on the face, neck, and skin folds and present as papillomatous lesions on a narrow base. Flat warts are only slightly elevated and have a velvety, nonverrucous surface. They have a propensity for the face, arms, and legs and are often spread by shaving.

Genital warts begin as small papillomas that may grow to form large fungating lesions. In women, they may involve either the labia, perineum, or perianal skin. Additionally, the mucosa of the vagina, urethra, and anus can be involved, as well as the cervical epithelium. In men, the lesions often occur initially in the coronal sulcus but may be seen on the shaft of the penis, the scrotum, perianal skin, or in the urethra.

Appreciable evidence has accumulated that suggests HPV plays a role in the development of neoplasia of the uterine cervix and anogenital skin (Chap. 93). HPV types 16 and 18 have been most intensely studied and are the major risk factors for intraepithelial neoplasia and squamous cell carcinoma of the cervix, anus, vulva, and penis. The risk is higher in patients immunosuppressed after solid organ transplantation and in those infected with HIV. Recent evidence also implicates other types. Histologic examination of biopsies from affected sites may reveal changes associated with typical warts and/or features typical of intraepidermal carcinoma (Bowen's disease). Squamous cell carcinomas associated with HPV infections have also been observed in extragenital skin (Chap. 83). This is most commonly seen in patients immunosuppressed after organ transplantation. Patients on long-term immunosuppression should be monitored for the development of squamous cell carcinoma and other cutaneous malignancies.

℞ WARTS

Treatment of warts, other than anogenital warts, should be tempered by the observation that a majority of warts in normal individuals resolve spontaneously within 1–2 years. There are many modalities available to treat warts, but no single therapy is universally effective. Factors that influence the choice of therapy include the location of the wart, extent of disease, the age and immunologic status of the patient, and the patient's desire for therapy. Perhaps the most useful and convenient method for treating warts in almost any location is cryotherapy with liquid nitrogen. Equally effective for non-genital warts, but requiring much more patient compliance, is the use of keratolytic agents such as salicylic acid plasters or solutions. For genital warts, in-office application of a podophyllin solution is moderately effective but may be associated with marked local reactions. Prescription preparations of dilute, purified podophyllin are available for home use. Topical imiquimod, a potent inducer of local cytokine release, has also been approved for use in genital warts. Conventional and laser surgical procedures may be required for recalcitrant warts. Recurrence of warts appears to be common to all these modalities. A highly effective vaccine for selected types of HPV has been recently approved by the FDA, and its use will likely reduce the incidence of anogenital and cervical carcinoma.

HERPES SIMPLEX
See Chap. 172

HERPES ZOSTER
See Chap. 173

ACNE

ACNE VULGARIS
Acne vulgaris is a self-limited disorder primarily of teenagers and young adults, although perhaps 10–20% of adults may continue to experience some form of the disorder. The permissive factor for the expression of the disease in adolescence is the increase in sebum production by sebaceous glands after puberty. Small cysts, called *comedones*, form in hair follicles due to blockage of the follicular orifice by retention of keratinous material and sebum. The activity of bacteria (*Proprionobacterium acnes*) within the comedones releases free fatty acids from sebum, causes inflammation within the cyst, and results in rupture of the cyst wall. An inflammatory foreign-body reaction develops as result of extrusion of oily and keratinous debris from the cyst.

The clinical hallmark of acne vulgaris is the comedone, which may be closed (whitehead) or open (blackhead). Closed comedones appear as 1- to 2-mm pebbly white papules, which are accentuated when the skin is stretched. They are the precursors of inflammatory lesions of acne vulgaris. The contents of closed comedones are not easily expressed. Open comedones, which rarely result in inflammatory acne lesions, have a large dilated follicular orifice and are filled with easily expressible oxidized, darkened, oily debris. Comedones are usually accompanied by inflammatory lesions: papules, pustules, or nodules.

The earliest lesions seen in adolescence are generally mildly inflamed or noninflammatory comedones on the forehead. Subsequently, more typical inflammatory lesions develop on the cheeks, nose, and chin (Fig. 53-7). The most common location for acne is the face, but involvement of the chest and back is common. Most disease remains mild and does not lead to scarring. A small number of patients develop large inflam-

FIGURE 53-7 Acne vulgaris. An example of acne vulgaris with inflammatory papules, pustules, and comedones. (*Courtesy of Kalman Watsky, MD; with permission.*)

CHAPTER 53

Eczema, Psoriasis, Cutaneous Infections, Acne, and Other Common Skin Disorders matory cysts and nodules, which may drain and result in significant scarring. Regardless of the severity, acne may affect a patient's quality of life. If adequately treated, this may be a transient effect. In the case of severe, scarring acne, the effects can be permanent and profound. Early therapeutic intervention in severe acne is essential.

Exogenous and endogenous factors can alter the expression of acne vulgaris. Friction and trauma (from headbands or chin straps of athletic helmets), application of comedogenic topical agents (cosmetics or hair preparations), or chronic topical exposure to certain industrial compounds may elicit or aggravate acne. Glucocorticoids, topical or systemic, may also elicit acne. Other systemic medications such as oral contraceptive pills, lithium, isoniazid, androgenic steroids, halogens, phenytoin, and phenobarbital may produce acneiform eruptions or aggravate preexisting acne. Genetic factors and polycystic ovary disease may also play a role.

℞ ACNE VULGARIS

Treatment of acne vulgaris is directed toward elimination of comedones by normalization of follicular keratinization, decreasing sebaceous gland activity, decreasing the population of *P. acnes*, and decreasing inflammation. Minimal to moderate, pauci-inflammatory disease may respond adequately to local therapy alone. Although areas affected with acne should be kept clean, overly vigorous scrubbing may aggravate acne due to mechanical rupture of comedones. Topical agents such as retinoic acid, benzoyl peroxide, or salicylic acid may alter the pattern of epidermal desquamation, preventing the formation of comedones and aiding in the resolution of preexisting cysts. Topical antibacterial agents such as azelaic acid, topical erythromycin (with or without zinc), or clindamycin are also useful adjuncts to therapy.

Patients with moderate to severe acne with a prominent inflammatory component will benefit from the addition of systemic therapy, such as tetracycline in doses of 250–500 mg bid, or doxycycline, 100 mg bid. Minocycline may also be useful. Such antibiotics appear to have an anti-inflammatory effect independent of their antibacterial effect. Female patients who do not respond to oral antibiotics may benefit from hormonal therapy. Women placed on oral contraceptives containing ethinyl estradiol and norgestimate have demonstrated improvement in their acne when compared to a placebo control.

Patients with severe nodulocystic acne unresponsive to the therapies discussed above may benefit from treatment with the synthetic retinoid, isotretinoin. Its dose is based on the patient's weight, and it is given once daily for 5 months. Results are excellent in appropriately selected patients. Its use is highly regulated due to its potential for severe adverse events, primarily teratogenicity. Additionally, patients receiving this medication develop extremely dry skin, cheilitis, and must be followed for development of hypertriglyceridemia. Recently there have also been concerns that it is associated with severe depression in some patients. The latter has not been proved. At present, prescribers must enroll in a program designed to prevent pregnancy and adverse events while patients are taking isotretinoin. These measures are imposed to ensure that all prescribers are familiar with the risks of isotretinoin; that all female patients have two negative pregnancy tests prior to initiating therapy and a negative pregnancy test prior to each refill; and that all patients have been warned about the risks associated with isotretinoin.

ACNE ROSACEA

Acne rosacea, commonly referred to as rosacea, is an inflammatory disorder predominantly affecting the central face. Those most often affected are Caucasians of northern European background, but it is seen in patients with dark skin also. It is seen almost exclusively in adults, only rarely affecting patients <30 years. Rosacea is more common in women, but those most severely affected are men. It is characterized by the presence of erythema, telangiectases, and superficial pustules (Fig. 53-8), but is not associated with the presence of comedones. Rosacea only rarely involves the chest or back.

FIGURE 53-8 Acne rosacea. Prominent facial erythema, telangiectasia, scattered papules, and small pustules are seen in this patient with acne rosacea. (*Courtesy of Robert Swerlick, MD; with permission.*)

There is a relationship between the tendency for facial flushing and the subsequent development of acne rosacea. Often, individuals with rosacea initially demonstrate a pronounced flushing reaction. This may be in response to heat, emotional stimuli, alcohol, hot drinks, or spicy foods. As the disease progresses, the flush persists longer and longer and may eventually become permanent. Papules, pustules, and telangiectases can become superimposed on the persistent flush. Rosacea of very long standing may lead to connective tissue overgrowth, particularly of the nose (rhinophyma). Rosacea may also be complicated by various inflammatory disorders of the eye, including keratitis, blepharitis, iritis, and recurrent chalazion. These ocular problems are potentially sight-threatening and warrant ophthalmologic evaluation.

℞ ACNE ROSACEA

Acne rosacea can be treated topically or systemically. Mild disease often responds to topical metronidazole or sodium sulfacetamide. More severe disease requires oral tetracyclines: tetracycline 250–500 mg bid, doxycycline 100 mg bid, or minocycline 50–100 mg bid. Residual telangiectasia may respond to laser therapy. Topical glucocorticoids, especially potent agents, should be avoided since chronic use of these preparations may elicit rosacea. Topical therapy of the skin is not effective treatment for ocular disease.

SKIN DISEASES AND SMALLPOX VACCINATION

Given the potential threat of a bioterrorism attack with smallpox, vaccinations against smallpox are available to the general public, although they are not recommended. Because of a higher incidence of adverse events associated with smallpox vaccination in patients with a history of certain skin diseases, including atopic dermatitis, eczema, and psoriasis, such vaccination is contraindicated in patients with these conditions in the absence of a bioterrorism attack and a real or potential exposure to smallpox. In the case of such exposure, the risk of smallpox infection outweighs the risk of adverse events from the vaccine (Chap. 214).

FURTHER READINGS

JAMES WD et al: *Andrews' Diseases of the Skin Clinical Dermatology,* 10th ed. Philadelphia, Saunders-Elsevier, 2006

WOLFF K, JOHNSON RA: *Fitzpatrick's Color Atlas and Synopsis of Clinical Dermatology,* 5th ed. New York, McGraw-Hill, 2005

WOLFF K et al (eds): *Fitzpatrick's Dermatology in General Medicine,* 7th ed. New York, McGraw-Hill, 2008

WOLVERTON SE (ed): *Comprehensive Dermatologic Drug Therapy.* Philadelphia, Saunders, 2001

54 Skin Manifestations of Internal Disease

Jean L. Bolognia, Irwin M. Braverman

It is now a generally accepted concept in medicine that the skin can show signs of internal disease. Therefore, in textbooks of medicine one finds a chapter describing in detail the major systemic disorders that can be identified by cutaneous signs. The underlying assumption of such a chapter is that the clinician has been able to identify the disorder in the patient and needs only to read about it in the textbook. In reality, concise differential diagnoses and the identification of these disorders are actually difficult for the nondermatologist because he or she is not well versed in the recognition of cutaneous lesions or their spectrum of presentations. Therefore, the authors of this chapter have decided to cover this particular topic of cutaneous medicine not by discussing individual disorders but by describing and discussing the various presenting clinical signs and symptoms that indicate the presence of these disorders. Concise differential diagnoses will be generated in which the significant diseases will be briefly discussed and distinguished from the more common disorders that have no significance for internal diseases. The latter disorders are reviewed in table form and always need to be excluded when considering the former. For a detailed description of individual diseases, the reader should consult a dermatologic text.

PAPULOSQUAMOUS SKIN LESIONS

(Table 54-1) When an eruption is characterized by elevated lesions, papules (<1 cm), or plaques (>1 cm), in association with scale, it is referred to as a *papulosquamous lesion*. The most common papulosquamous diseases—*psoriasis, tinea, pityriasis rosea,* and *lichen planus*—are primary cutaneous disorders (Chap. 53). When psoriatic lesions are accompanied by arthritis, the possibility of psoriatic arthritis or *Reiter's disease* should be considered. A history of oral ulcers, conjunctivitis, uveitis, and/or urethritis points to the latter diagnosis. Lithium, beta blockers, HIV or streptococcal infections, and a rapid taper of systemic glucocorticoids are known to exacerbate psoriasis.

Whenever the diagnosis of pityriasis rosea or lichen planus is made, it is important to review the patient's medications because the eruption can be treated by simply discontinuing the offending agent. Pityriasis rosea–like drug eruptions are seen most commonly with beta blockers, angiotensin-converting enzyme (ACE) inhibitors, gold, and metronidazole, while the drugs that can produce a lichenoid eruption include thiazides, antimalarials, gold, quinidine, phenothiazines, sulfonylureas, and ACE inhibitors. In some populations, there is a higher prevalence of hepatitis C viral infection in patients with lichen planus. Lichen planus–like lesions are also observed in chronic graft-versus-host disease.

In its early stages, *cutaneous T cell lymphoma* (CTCL) may be confused with eczema or psoriasis, but it often fails to respond to the appropriate therapy for those inflammatory diseases. CTCL can develop within lesions of large-plaque parapsoriasis and is suggested by an increase in the thickness of the lesions. The diagnosis of CTCL is established by skin biopsy in which collections of atypical T lymphocytes are found in the epidermis and dermis. As the disease progresses, cutaneous tumors and lymph node involvement may appear.

In *secondary syphilis* there are scattered red-brown papules with thin scale. The eruption often involves the palms and soles and can resemble pityriasis rosea. Associated findings are helpful in making the diagnosis and include annular plaques on the face, nonscarring alopecia, condyloma lata (broad-based and moist), and mucous patches as well as lymphadenopathy, malaise, fever, headache, and myalgias. The interval between the primary chancre and the secondary stage is usually 4–8 weeks, and spontaneous resolution without appropriate therapy is seen.

ERYTHRODERMA

(Table 54-2) *Erythroderma* is the term used when the majority of the skin surface is erythematous (red in color). There may be associated scale, erosions, or pustules as well as shedding of the hair and nails. Potential systemic manifestations include fever, chills, hypothermia, reactive lymphadenopathy, peripheral edema, hypoalbuminemia, and high-output cardiac failure. The major etiologies of erythroderma are (1) cutaneous diseases such as psoriasis and dermatitis (Table 54-3); (2) drugs; (3) systemic diseases, most commonly CTCL; and (4) idiopathic. In the first three groups, the location and description of the initial lesions, prior to the development of the erythroderma, aid in the diagnosis. For example, a history of red scaly plaques on the elbows and knees would point to psoriasis. It is also important to examine the skin carefully for a migration of the erythema and associated secondary changes such as pustules or erosions. Migratory waves of erythema studded with superficial pustules are seen in *pustular psoriasis*.

Drug-induced erythroderma (exfoliative dermatitis) may begin as an exanthematous (morbilliform) eruption (Chap. 56) or may arise as diffuse erythema. A number of drugs can produce an erythroderma, including penicillins, sulfonamides, carbamazepine, phenytoin, gold, allopurinol, and zalcitabine. Fever and peripheral eosinophilia often accompany the eruption, and there may also be facial swelling, hepatitis, and allergic interstitial nephritis; this constellation is frequently referred to as *drug reaction with eosinophilia and systemic symptoms* (DRESS). In addition, reactions to anticonvulsants can lead to a pseudolymphoma syndrome (with adenopathy and circulating atypical lymphocytes), while reactions to allopurinol may be accompanied by gastrointestinal bleeding.

The most common malignancy that is associated with erythroderma is CTCL; in some series, up to 25% of the cases of erythroderma were due to CTCL. The patient may progress from isolated plaques and tumors, but more commonly the erythroderma is present throughout the course of the disease (Sézary syndrome). In the Sézary syndrome, there are circulating atypical T lymphocytes, pruritus, and lymphadenopathy. In cases of erythroderma where there is no apparent cause (idiopathic), longitudinal follow-up is mandatory to monitor for the possible development of CTCL. There have been isolated case reports of erythroderma secondary to some solid tumors—lung, liver, prostate, thyroid, and colon—but it is usually in a late stage of the disease.

TABLE 54-1 SELECTED CAUSES OF PAPULOSQUAMOUS SKIN LESIONS

1. Primary cutaneous disorders
   a. Psoriasis[a]
   b. Tinea[a]
   c. Pityriasis rosea[a]
   d. Lichen planus[a]
   e. Parapsoriasis
   f. Bowen's disease (squamous cell carcinoma in situ)[b]
2. Drugs
3. Systemic diseases
   a. Lupus erythematosus[c]
   b. Cutaneous T cell lymphoma
   c. Secondary syphilis
   d. Reiter's disease
   e. Sarcoidosis[d]

[a]Discussed in detail in Chap. 53.
[b]Associated with chronic sun exposure and exposure to arsenic.
[c]See also Red Lesions in "Papulonodular Skin Lesions."
[d]See also Red-Brown Lesions in "Papulonodular Skin Lesions."

TABLE 54-2 CAUSES OF ERYTHRODERMA

1. Primary cutaneous disorders
   a. Psoriasis[a]
   b. Dermatitis [atopic, contact >> seborrheic or stasis (with autosensitization)][a]
   c. Pityriasis rubra pilaris
2. Drugs
3. Systemic diseases
   a. Cutaneous T cell lymphoma
   b. Lymphoma
4. Idiopathic

[a]Discussed in detail in Chap. 53.

TABLE 54-3 ERYTHRODERMA (PRIMARY CUTANEOUS DISORDERS)

	Initial Lesions	Location of Initial Lesions	Other Findings	Diagnostic Aids	Treatment
Psoriasis[a]	Pink-red, silvery scale, sharply demarcated	Elbows, knees, scalp, presacral area	Nail dystrophy, arthritis, pustules	Skin biopsy	Topical glucocorticoids, vitamin D; UV-B (narrowband); oral retinoid and/or PUVA; MTX, cyclosporine, anti-TNF agents
Dermatitis[a] Atopic	Acute: Erythema, fine scale, crust, indistinct borders Chronic: Lichenification (increased skin markings)	Antecubital and popliteal fossae, neck, hands	Pruritus Family history of atopy, including asthma, allergic rhinitis or conjunctivitis, and atopic dermatitis Exclude secondary infection with *S. aureus* Exclude superimposed irritant or allergic contact dermatitis	Skin biopsy	Topical glucocorticoids, tacrolimus, pimecrolimus, tar, and antipruritics; oral antihistamines; open wet dressings; UV-B ± UV-A; PUVA; oral/IM glucocorticoids; MTX; cyclosporine Topical or oral antibiotics
Contact	Local: Erythema, crusting, vesicles, and bullae	Depends on offending agent	Irritant—onset often within hours Allergic—delayed-type hypersensitivity; lag time of 48 h	Patch testing	Remove irritant or allergen; topical glucocorticoids; oral antihistamines; oral/IM glucocorticoids
	Systemic: Erythema, fine scale, crust	Generalized	Patient has history of allergic contact dermatitis to topical agent and then receives systemic medication that is structurally related, e.g., ethylenediamine (topical), aminophylline (IV)	Patch testing	Same as local
Seborrheic (rare)	Pink-red, greasy scale	Scalp, nasolabial folds, eyebrows, intertriginous zones	Flares with stress, HIV infection Associated with Parkinson's disease	Skin biopsy	Topical glucocorticoids and imidazoles
Stasis (with autosensitization)	Erythema, crusting, excoriations	Lower extremities	Pruritus, lower extremity edema History of venous ulcers, thrombophlebitis, and/or cellulitis Exclude cellulitis Exclude superimposed contact dermatitis, e.g., topical neomycin	Skin biopsy	Topical glucocorticoids; open wet dressings; leg elevation; pressure stockings
Pityriasis rubra pilaris	Orange-red, perifollicular papules	Generalized, but characteristic "skip" areas of normal skin	Wax-like keratoderma Exclude cutaneous T cell lymphoma	Skin biopsy	Isotretinoin or acitretin; methotrexate

[a]Discussed in detail in Chap. 53.

Note: PUVA, psoralens + ultraviolet A irradiation; UV-B, ultraviolet B; UV-A, ultraviolet A; MTX, methotrexate; TNF, tumor necrosis factor.

ALOPECIA

(Table 54-4) The two major forms of alopecia are scarring and nonscarring. In *scarring alopecia* there are associated fibrosis, inflammation, and loss of hair follicles. A smooth scalp with a decreased number of follicular openings is usually observed clinically, but in some cases the changes are seen only in biopsy specimens from the affected areas. In *nonscarring alopecia* the hair shafts are gone, but the hair follicles are preserved, explaining the reversible nature of nonscarring alopecia.

The most common causes of nonscarring alopecia include *telogen effluvium, androgenetic alopecia, alopecia areata, tinea capitis,* and some cases of *traumatic alopecia* (Table 54-5). In women with androgenetic alopecia, an elevation in circulating levels of androgens may be seen as a result of ovarian or adrenal gland dysfunction. When there are signs of virilization, such as a deepened voice and enlarged clitoris, the possibility of an ovarian or adrenal gland tumor should be considered.

Exposure to various drugs can also cause diffuse hair loss, usually by inducing a telogen effluvium. An exception is the anagen effluvium observed with antimitotic agents such as daunorubicin. Alopecia is a side effect of the following drugs: warfarin, heparin, propylthiouracil, carbimazole, vitamin A, isotretinoin, acitretin, lithium, beta blockers, colchicine, and amphetamines. Fortunately, spontaneous regrowth usually follows discontinuation of the offending agent.

Less commonly, nonscarring alopecia is associated with *lupus erythematosus* and *secondary syphilis*. In systemic lupus there are two forms of alopecia—one is scarring secondary to discoid lesions (see below) and the other is nonscarring. The latter form may be diffuse and involve the entire

TABLE 54-4 CAUSES OF ALOPECIA

I. Nonscarring alopecia
  A. Primary cutaneous disorders
    1. Telogen effluvium
    2. Androgenetic alopecia
    3. Alopecia areata
    4. Tinea capitis
    5. Traumatic alopecia[a]
  B. Drugs
  C. Systemic diseases
    1. Lupus erythematosus
    2. Secondary syphilis
    3. Hypothyroidism
    4. Hyperthyroidism
    5. Hypopituitarism
    6. Deficiencies of protein, iron, biotin, and zinc
II. Scarring alopecia
  A. Primary cutaneous disorders
    1. Cutaneous lupus (chronic discoid)
    2. Lichen planus
    3. Folliculitis decalvans
    4. Linear scleroderma (morphea)
    5. Central centrifugal cicatricial alopecia
  B. Systemic diseases
    1. Lupus erythematosus
    2. Sarcoidosis
    3. Cutaneous metastases

[a]Most patients with trichotillomania, pressure-induced alopecia.

TABLE 54-5 NONSCARRING ALOPECIA (PRIMARY CUTANEOUS DISORDERS)

	Clinical Characteristics	Pathogenesis	Treatment
Telogen effluvium	Diffuse shedding of normal hairs Follows either major stress (high fever, severe infection) or change in hormones (post partum) Reversible without treatment	Stress causes the normally asynchronous growth cycles of individual hairs to become synchronous; therefore, large numbers of growing (anagen) hairs simultaneously enter the dying (telogen) phase	Observation; discontinue any drugs that have alopecia as a side effect; must exclude underlying metabolic causes, e.g., hypothyroidism, hyperthyroidism
Androgenetic alopecia (male pattern; female pattern)	Miniaturization of hairs along the midline of the scalp Recession of the anterior scalp line in men and some women	Increased sensitivity of affected hairs to the effects of testosterone Increased levels of circulating androgens (ovarian or adrenal source in women)	If no evidence of hyperandrogen state, then topical minoxidil; finasteride[a]; hair transplant
Alopecia areata	Well-circumscribed, circular areas of hair loss, 2–5 cm in diameter In extensive cases, coalescence of lesions and/or involvement of other hair-bearing surfaces of the body Pitting of the nails	The germinative zones of the hair follicles are surrounded by T lymphocytes Occasional associated diseases: hyperthyroidism, hypothyroidism, vitiligo, Down syndrome	Topical anthralin; intralesional glucocorticoids; topical contact sensitizers
Tinea	Varies from scaling with minimal hair loss to discrete patches with "black dots" (broken hairs) to boggy plaque with pustules (kerion)	Invasion of hairs by dermatophytes, most commonly *Trichophyton tonsurans*	Oral griseofulvin or terbinafine plus 2.5% selenium sulfide or ketoconazole shampoo; examine family members
Traumatic alopecia[b]	Broken hairs Irregular outline	Traction with curlers, rubber bands, braiding Exposure to heat or chemicals (e.g., hair straighteners) Mechanical pulling (trichotillomania)	Discontinuation of offending hair style or chemical treatments; trichotillomania may require hair clipping and observation of shaved hairs or biopsy for diagnosis, possibly followed by psychotherapy

[a]To date, FDA-approved for men. [b]May also be scarring.

scalp, or it may be localized to the frontal scalp, eventually resulting in multiple short hairs ("lupus hairs"). Scattered, poorly circumscribed patches of alopecia with a "moth-eaten" appearance are a manifestation of the secondary stage of syphilis. Diffuse thinning of the hair is also associated with hypothyroidism and hyperthyroidism (Table 54-4).

Scarring alopecia is more frequently the result of a primary cutaneous disorder such as *lichen planus, folliculitis decalvans, chronic cutaneous (discoid) lupus,* or *linear scleroderma (morphea)* than it is a sign of systemic disease. Although the scarring lesions of *discoid lupus* can be seen in patients with systemic lupus, in the majority of cases the disease process is limited to the skin. Less common causes of scarring alopecia include *sarcoidosis* (see "Papulonodular Skin Lesions," below) and *cutaneous metastases.*

In the early phases of discoid lupus, lichen planus, and folliculitis decalvans, there are circumscribed areas of alopecia. Fibrosis and subsequent loss of follicles are observed primarily in the center of the individual lesions, while the inflammatory process is most prominent at the periphery. The areas of active inflammation in discoid lupus are erythematous with scale, whereas the areas of previous inflammation are often hypopigmented with a rim of hyperpigmentation. In lichen planus the peripheral perifollicular macules are usually violet-colored. Complete examination of the skin and oral mucosa combined with a biopsy and direct immunofluorescence microscopy will aid in distinguishing these two entities. The peripheral active lesions in folliculitis decalvans are follicular pustules; these patients can develop a reactive arthritis.

FIGURATE SKIN LESIONS

(Table 54-6) In *figurate eruptions*, the lesions form rings and arcs that are usually erythematous but can be skin-colored to brown. Most commonly, they are due to primary cutaneous diseases such as *tinea, urticaria, erythema annulare centrifugum,* and *granuloma annulare* (Chaps. 53 and 55). An underlying systemic illness is found in a second, less common group of migratory annular erythemas. It includes *erythema gyratum repens, erythema migrans, erythema marginatum,* and *necrolytic migratory erythema.*

In erythema gyratum repens, one sees numerous mobile concentric arcs and wavefronts that resemble the grain in wood. A search for an underlying malignancy is mandatory in a patient with this eruption. Erythema migrans is the cutaneous manifestation of Lyme disease, which is

caused by the spirochete *Borrelia burgdorferi.* In the initial stage (3–30 days after tick bite), a single annular lesion is usually seen, which can expand to ≥10 cm in diameter. Within several days, approximately half the patients develop multiple smaller erythematous lesions at sites distant from the bite. Associated symptoms include fever, headache, photophobia, myalgias, arthralgias, and malar rash. Erythema marginatum is seen in patients with rheumatic fever, primarily on the trunk. Lesions are pink-red in color, flat to mildly elevated, and transient.

There are additional cutaneous diseases that present as annular eruptions but lack an obvious migratory component. Examples include *CTCL, subacute cutaneous lupus, secondary syphilis,* and *sarcoidosis* (see "Papulonodular Skin Lesions," below).

ACNE

(Table 54-7) In addition to *acne vulgaris* and *acne rosacea,* the two major forms of acne (Chap. 53), there are drugs and systemic diseases that can lead to acneiform eruptions (Table 54-7).

TABLE 54-6 CAUSES OF FIGURATE SKIN LESIONS

I. Primary cutaneous disorders
  A. Tinea
  B. Urticaria (≥90% of cases)
  C. Erythema annulare centrifugum
  D. Granuloma annulare
  E. Psoriasis
II. Systemic diseases
  A. Migratory
    1. Erythema migrans
    2. Urticaria (≤10% of cases)
    3. Erythema gyratum repens
    4. Erythema marginatum
    5. Pustular psoriasis
    6. Necrolytic migratory erythema (glucagonoma syndrome)[a]
  B. Nonmigratory
    1. Sarcoidosis
    2. Subacute lupus erythematosus
    3. Secondary syphilis
    4. Cutaneous T cell lymphoma (e.g., mycosis fungoides)

[a]Migratory erythema with erosions; favors lower extremities and girdle area.

PART 2 | Cardinal Manifestations and Presentation of Diseases

TABLE 54-7	CAUSES OF ACNEIFORM ERUPTIONS

I. Primary cutaneous disorders
   A. Acne vulgaris
   B. Acne rosacea
II. Drugs, e.g., anabolic steroids, glucocorticoids, lithium, iodides, EGFR[a] inhibitors
III. Systemic diseases
   A. Increased androgen production
      1. Adrenal origin, e.g., Cushing's disease, 21-hydroxylase deficiency
      2. Ovarian origin, e.g., polycystic ovary syndrome
   B. Cryptococcosis, disseminated
   C. Dimorphic fungi
   D. Behçet's disease

[a]EGFR, epidermal growth factor receptor.

Patients with the *carcinoid syndrome* have episodes of flushing of the head, neck, and sometimes the trunk. Resultant skin changes of the face, in particular telangiectasias, may mimic the clinical appearance of acne rosacea.

PUSTULAR LESIONS

Acneiform eruptions (see "Acne," above) and *folliculitis* represent the most common pustular dermatoses. An important consideration in the evaluation of follicular pustules is a determination of the associated pathogen, e.g., normal flora, *Staphylococcus aureus*, *Pseudomonas aeruginosa* ("hot tub" folliculitis), *Malassezia*, dermatophytes (Majocchi's granuloma). Noninfectious forms of folliculitis include HIV-associated eosinophilic folliculitis and folliculitis secondary to drugs such as glucocorticoids and lithium. Administration of high-dose systemic glucocorticoids can result in a widespread eruption of follicular pustules on the trunk, characterized by lesions in the same stage of development. With regard to underlying systemic diseases, nonfollicular-based pustules are a characteristic component of pustular psoriasis and can be seen in septic emboli of bacterial or fungal origin (see "Purpura," below).

TELANGIECTASIAS

(Table 54-8) In order to distinguish the various types of telangiectasias, it is important to examine the shape and configuration of the dilated blood vessels. *Linear telangiectasias* are seen on the face of patients with *actinically damaged skin* and *acne rosacea*, and they are found on the legs of patients with *venous hypertension* and *essential telangiectasia*. Patients with an unusual form of *mastocytosis* (telangiectasia macularis eruptiva perstans) and the *carcinoid syndrome* (see "Acne," above) also have linear telangiectasias. Lastly, linear telangiectasias are found in areas of cutaneous inflammation. For example, lesions of discoid lupus frequently have telangiectasias within them.

TABLE 54-8	CAUSES OF TELANGIECTASIAS

I. Primary cutaneous disorders
  A. Linear
    1. Acne rosacea
    2. Actinically damaged skin
    3. Venous hypertension
    4. Essential telangiectasia
    5. Within basal cell carcinomas
  B. Poikiloderma
    1. Ionizing radiation[a]
    2. Poikiloderma vasculare atrophicans
  C. Spider angioma
    1. Idiopathic
    2. Pregnancy
II. Systemic diseases
  A. Linear
    1. Carcinoid
    2. Ataxia-telangiectasia
    3. Mastocytosis
  B. Poikiloderma
    1. Dermatomyositis
    2. Cutaneous T cell lymphoma
    3. Xeroderma pigmentosum
  C. Mat
    1. Scleroderma
  D. Periungual
    1. Lupus erythematosus
    2. Scleroderma
    3. Dermatomyositis
    4. Hereditary hemorrhagic telangiectasia
  E. Papular
    1. Hereditary hemorrhagic telangiectasia
  F. Spider angioma
    1. Cirrhosis

[a]Becoming less common.

Poikiloderma is a term used to describe a patch of skin with (1) reticulated hypo- and hyperpigmentation, (2) wrinkling secondary to epidermal atrophy, and (3) telangiectasias. Poikiloderma does not imply a single disease entity—although becoming less common, it is seen in skin damaged by *ionizing radiation* as well as in patients with autoimmune connective tissue diseases, primarily *dermatomyositis* (DM), and rare genodermatoses (e.g., Kindler syndrome).

In *scleroderma*, the dilated blood vessels have a unique configuration and are known as *mat telangiectasias*. The lesions are broad macules that usually measure 2–7 mm in diameter but occasionally are larger. Mats have a polygonal or oval shape, and their erythematous color may be uniform or the result of delicate telangiectasias. The most common locations for mat telangiectasias are the face, oral mucosa, and hands—peripheral sites that are prone to intermittent ischemia. The CREST (calcinosis cutis, Raynaud's phenomenon, esophageal dysmotility, sclerodactyly, and telangiectasia) variant of scleroderma (Chap. 316) is associated with a chronic course and anticentromere antibodies. Mat telangiectasias are an important clue to the diagnosis of the CREST syndrome as well as systemic scleroderma, for they may be the only cutaneous finding.

Periungual telangiectasias are pathognomonic signs of the three major autoimmune connective tissue diseases—lupus erythematosus, scleroderma, and DM. They are easily visualized by the naked eye and occur in at least two-thirds of these patients. In both DM and lupus there is associated nailfold erythema, and in DM the erythema is often accompanied by "ragged" cuticles and fingertip tenderness. Under 10× magnification, the blood vessels in the nailfolds of lupus patients are tortuous and resemble "glomeruli," whereas in scleroderma and DM there is a loss of capillary loops and those that remain are markedly dilated.

In *hereditary hemorrhagic telangiectasia* (Osler-Rendu-Weber disease), the lesions usually appear during adulthood and are most commonly seen on the mucous membranes, face, and distal extremities, including under the nails. They represent arteriovenous (AV) malformations of the dermal microvasculature, are dark red in color, and are usually slightly elevated. When the skin is stretched over an individual lesion, an eccentric punctum with radiating legs is seen. Although the degree of systemic involvement varies in this autosomal dominant disease (due to mutations in either the endoglin or activin receptor–like kinase gene), the major symptoms are recurrent epistaxis and gastrointestinal bleeding. The fact that these mucosal telangiectasias are actually AV communications helps to explain their tendency to bleed.

HYPOPIGMENTATION

(Table 54-9) Disorders of hypopigmentation are often classified as either diffuse or localized. The classic example of *diffuse hypopigmentation* is *oculocutaneous albinism* (OCA). The most common forms are due to mutations in the tyrosinase gene (type I) or the *P* gene (type II); patients with type IA OCA have a total lack of enzyme activity. At birth, different forms of OCA can appear similar—white hair, gray-blue eyes, and pink-white skin. However, the patients with no tyrosinase activity maintain this phenotype, whereas those with decreased activity will acquire some pigmentation of the eyes, hair, and skin as they age. The degree of pigment formation is also a function of racial background, and the pigmentary dilution is readily apparent when patients are compared to their first-degree relatives. The ocular findings in OCA correlate with the degree of hypopigmentation and include decreased visual acuity, nystagmus, photophobia, and a lack of normal binocular vision.

The differential diagnosis of *localized hypomelanosis* includes the following primary cutaneous disorders: *idiopathic guttate hypomelanosis, postinflammatory hypopigmentation, tinea (pityriasis) versicolor, vitiligo, chemical leukoderma, nevus depigmentosus* (see below), and *piebaldism* (Table 54-9). In this group of diseases, the areas of involvement are macules or patches with a decrease or absence of pigmentation. Patients with vitiligo also have an increased incidence of several autoimmune disorders, including hypothyroidism, Graves' disease, pernicious anemia, Addison's disease, uveitis, alopecia areata, chronic mucocutaneous candidiasis, and the polyglandular autoimmune syndromes (types I and II). Diseases of the thyroid gland are the most frequently associated disorders, occurring in up to 30% of patients with

TABLE 54-9 CAUSES OF HYPOPIGMENTATION

I. Primary cutaneous disorders
   A. Diffuse
     1. Generalized vitiligo^a
   B. Localized
     1. Idiopathic guttate hypomelanosis
     2. Postinflammatory
     3. Tinea (pityriasis) versicolor
     4. Vitiligo
     5. Chemical leukoderma
     6. Nevus depigmentosus
     7. Piebaldism
II. Systemic diseases
   A. Diffuse
     1. Oculocutaneous albinism^b
       a. Hermansky-Pudlak syndrome^c
       b. Chédiak-Higashi syndrome^d
     2. Phenylketonuria
     3. Homocystinuria
   B. Localized
     1. Vogt-Koyanagi-Harada
     2. Scleroderma
     3. Melanoma-associated leukoderma
     4. Tuberous sclerosis
     5. Hypomelanosis of Ito/mosaicism
     6. Incontinentia pigmenti (stage IV)
     7. Sarcoidosis
     8. Tuberculoid and indeterminate leprosy
     9. Cutaneous T cell lymphoma
     10. Onchocerciasis

^aAbsence of melanocytes.
^bNormal number of melanocytes.
^cPlatelet storage defect and restrictive lung disease secondary to deposits of ceroid-like material; one form due to mutations in β subunit of adaptor protein.
^dGiant lysosomal granules and recurrent infections.

vitiligo. Circulating autoantibodies are often found, and the most common ones are antithyroglobulin, antimicrosomal, and antithyroid-stimulating hormone receptor antibodies.

There are four systemic diseases that should be considered in a patient with skin findings suggestive of vitiligo—*Vogt-Koyanagi-Harada syndrome, scleroderma, onchocerciasis,* and *melanoma-associated leukoderma.* A history of aseptic meningitis, nontraumatic uveitis, tinnitus, hearing loss, and/or dysacusis points to the diagnosis of the Vogt-Koyanagi-Harada syndrome. In these patients, the face and scalp are the most common locations of pigment loss. The vitiligo-like leukoderma seen in patients with scleroderma has a clinical resemblance to idiopathic vitiligo that has begun to repigment as a result of treatment; that is, perifollicular macules of normal pigmentation are seen within areas of depigmentation. The basis of this leukoderma is unknown; there is no evidence of inflammation in areas of involvement, but it can resolve if the underlying connective tissue disease becomes inactive. In contrast to idiopathic vitiligo, melanoma-associated leukoderma often begins on the trunk, and its appearance should prompt a search for metastatic disease. It is also seen in patients undergoing immunotherapy for melanoma, with cytotoxic T lymphocytes presumably recognizing cell surface antigens common to melanoma cells and melanocytes.

There are two systemic disorders (neurocristopathies) that may have the cutaneous findings of piebaldism (Table 54-10). They are *Shah-Waardenburg syndrome* and *Waardenburg syndrome.* A possible explanation for both disorders is an abnormal embryonic migration or survival of two neural crest–derived elements, one of them being melanocytes and the other myenteric ganglion cells (leading to Hirschsprung disease in Shah-Waardenburg syndrome) or auditory nerve cells (Waardenburg syndrome). The latter syndrome is characterized by congenital sensorineural hearing loss, dystopia canthorum (lateral displacement of the inner canthi but normal interpupillary distance), heterochromic irises, and a broad nasal root, in addition to the piebaldism. Patients with Waardenburg syndrome have been shown to have mutations in three genes including two (*PAX-3* and *MITF*) that encode DNA-binding proteins, while patients with Hirschsprung disease plus white spotting have mutations in one of three genes—endothelin 3, endothelin B receptor, and *SOX-10.*

In *tuberous sclerosis,* the earliest cutaneous sign is an ash leaf spot. These lesions are often present at birth and are usually multiple; however, detection may require Wood's lamp examination, especially in fair-skinned individuals. The pigment within them is reduced but not absent. The average size is 1–3 cm, and the common shapes are polygonal and lance-ovate. Examination of the patient for additional cutaneous signs such as multiple angiofibromas of the face (adenoma sebaceum), ungual and gingival fibromas, fibrous plaques of the forehead, and connective tissue nevi (shagreen patches) is recommended. It is important to remember that an ash leaf spot on the scalp will result in *poliosis,* which is a circumscribed patch of gray-white hair. Internal manifestations include seizures, mental retardation, central nervous system (CNS) and retinal hamartomas, renal angiomyolipomas, and cardiac rhabdomyomas. The latter can be detected in up to 60% of children (<18 years) with tuberous sclerosis by echocardiography.

Nevus depigmentosus is a stable, well-circumscribed hypomelanosis that is present at birth. There is usually a single oval or rectangular lesion, but occasionally the nevus has a segmental or whorled pattern (also referred to as *linear nevoid hypopigmentation*). It is important to distinguish this more common entity from ash leaf spots of tuberous sclerosis, especially when there are multiple lesions. In *hypomelanosis of Ito,* swirls and streaks of hypopigmentation run parallel to one another in a pattern that resembles a marble cake. Lesions may progress or regress with time, and in up to a third of patients, associated abnormalities are found involving the musculoskeletal system (asymmetry), the CNS (seizures and mental retardation), and the eyes (strabismus and hypertelorism). Chromosomal mosaicism has been detected in these patients, lending support to the hypothesis that the pattern is the result of the migration of two clones of primordial melanocytes, each with a different pigment potential.

Localized areas of decreased pigmentation are commonly seen as a result of cutaneous inflammation (Table 54-10) and have been observed in the skin overlying active lesions of sarcoidosis (see "Papulonodular Skin Lesions," below) as well as in CTCL. Cutaneous infections also present as disorders of hypopigmentation, and in *tuberculoid leprosy* there are a few asymmetric patches of hypomelanosis that have associated anesthesia, anhidrosis, and alopecia. Biopsy specimens of the palpable border show dermal granulomas that contain rare, if any, *Mycobacterium leprae* organisms.

HYPERPIGMENTATION

(Table 54-11) Disorders of hyperpigmentation are also divided into two groups—localized and diffuse. The localized forms are due to an epidermal alteration, a proliferation of melanocytes, or an increase in pigment production. Both seborrheic keratoses and acanthosis nigricans belong to the first group. *Seborrheic keratoses* are common lesions, but in one rare clinical setting they are a sign of systemic disease, and that setting is the sudden appearance of multiple lesions, often with an inflammatory base and in association with acrochordons (skin tags) and acanthosis nigricans. This is termed the *sign of Leser-Trélat* and alerts the clinician to search for an internal malignancy. *Acanthosis nigricans* can also be a reflection of an internal malignancy, most commonly of the gastrointestinal tract, and it appears as velvety hyperpigmentation, primarily in flexural areas. In the majority of patients, acanthosis nigricans is associated with obesity and insulin resistance, but it may be a reflection of an endocrinopathy such as acromegaly, Cushing's syndrome, polycystic ovary syndrome, or insulin-resistant diabetes mellitus (type A, type B, and lipoatrophic forms).

A proliferation of melanocytes results in the following pigmented lesions: *lentigo, melanocytic nevus,* and *melanoma* (Chap. 83). In an adult, the majority of lentigines are related to sun exposure, which explains their distribution. However, in the Peutz-Jeghers and LEOPARD [*l*entigines; *E*CG abnormalities, primarily conduction defects; *o*cular hypertelorism; *p*ulmonary stenosis and subaortic valvular stenosis; *a*bnormal genitalia (cryptorchidism, hypospadias); *r*etardation of growth; and *d*eafness (sensorineural)] syndromes, lentigines do serve

TABLE 54-10 HYPOPIGMENTATION (PRIMARY CUTANEOUS DISORDERS, LOCALIZED)

	Clinical Characteristics	Wood's Lamp Examination (UV-A; Peak = 365 nm)	Skin Biopsy Specimen	Pathogenesis	Treatment
Idiopathic guttate hypomelanosis	Common; acquired; 1–4 mm in diameter Shins and extensor forearms	Less enhancement than vitiligo	Abrupt decrease in epidermal melanin content	Possible somatic mutations as a reflection of aging; UV exposure	None
Postinflammatory hypopigmentation	Can develop within active lesions, as in subacute lupus, or after the lesion fades, as in dermatitis	Depends on particular disease Usually less enhancement than in vitiligo	Type of inflammatory infiltrate depends on specific disease	Block in transfer of melanin from melanocytes to keratinocytes could be secondary to edema or decrease in contact time Destruction of melanocytes if inflammatory cells attack basal layer	Treat underlying inflammatory disease
Tinea (pityriasis) versicolor	Common disorder Upper trunk and neck Shawl-like distribution Young adults Macules have fine white scale when scratched	Golden fluorescence	Hyphae and budding yeast in stratum corneum	Invasion of stratum corneum by the yeast *Malassezia* Yeast is lipophilic and produces C_9 and C_{11} dicarboxylic acids, which in vitro inhibit tyrosinase	Selenium sulfide 2.5%; topical imidazoles; oral imidazoles or triazoles
Vitiligo	Acquired; progressive Symmetric areas of complete pigment loss Periorificial—around mouth, nose, eyes, nipples, umbilicus, anus Other areas—flexor wrists, extensor distal extremities Segmental form is less common—unilateral, dermatomal-like	More apparent Chalk-white	Absence of melanocytes Mild inflammation	Possible autoimmune phenomenon that results in destruction of melanocytes—cellular and/or humoral Alternative hypothesis is self-destruction of melanocytes and circulating antibodies or cytotoxic T cells as a secondary phenomenon	Topical glucocorticoids; topical calcineurin inhibitors; UV-B; PUVA; transplants; depigmentation if widespread
Chemical leukoderma	Similar appearance to vitiligo Often begins on hands Satellite lesions in areas not exposed to chemicals	More apparent Chalk-white	Decreased number or absence of melanocytes	Exposure to chemicals that selectively destroy melanocytes, in particular phenols and catechols (germicides; adhesives) Release of cellular antigens and activation of circulating lymphocytes may explain satellite phenomenon	Avoid exposure to offending agent, then treat as vitiligo
Piebaldism	Autosomal dominant Congenital, stable White forelock Areas of hypomelanosis contain normally pigmented and hyperpigmented macules of various sizes Symmetric involvement of central forehead, ventral trunk, and mid regions of upper and lower extremities	Enhancement of leukoderma and hyperpigmented macules	Hypomelanotic areas—few to no melanocytes	Defect in migration of melanoblasts from neural crest to ventral skin or failure of melanoblasts to survive or differentiate in these areas Mutations within the c-*kit* proto-oncogene that encodes the tyrosine kinase receptor for stem cell growth factor	None; occasionally transplants

Note: PUVA, psoralens +ultraviolet A irradiation; UV-B, ultraviolet B.

as a clue to systemic disease. In *LEOPARD syndrome*, hundreds of lentigines develop during childhood and are scattered over the entire surface of the body. The lentigines in patients with *Peutz-Jeghers syndrome* are located primarily around the nose and mouth, on the hands and feet, and within the oral cavity. While the pigmented macules on the face may fade with age, the oral lesions persist. However, similar intraoral lesions are also seen in Addison's disease and as a normal finding in darkly pigmented individuals. Patients with this autosomal dominant syndrome (due to mutations in a novel serine threonine kinase gene) have multiple benign polyps of the gastrointestinal tract, testicular tumors, and an increased risk of developing gastrointestinal (primarily colon), pancreatic, and gynecologic cancers.

In the Carney complex, numerous lentigines are also seen, but in association with cardiac myxomas. This autosomal dominant disorder is also known as the *LAMB* (lentigines, atrial myxomas, mucocutaneous myxomas, and blue nevi) *syndrome* or *NAME* [nevi, atrial myxoma, myxoid neurofibroma, and ephelides (freckles)] *syndrome*. These patients can also have evidence of endocrine overactivity in the form of Cushing's syndrome, acromegaly, or sexual precocity.

The third type of localized hyperpigmentation is due to a local increase in pigment production, and it includes *ephelides* and café au lait macules (CALM). The latter are most commonly associated with two disorders—neurofibromatosis (NF) and McCune-Albright syndrome. *CALM* are flat, uniformly brown in color (usually two shades darker than uninvolved skin), and can vary in size from 0.5–12 cm. Approximately 80–90% of adult patients with *type I NF* will have six or more CALM measuring ≥1.5 cm in diameter. Additional findings are discussed in the section on neurofibromas (see "Papulonodular Skin Le-

TABLE 54-11 CAUSES OF HYPERPIGMENTATION

I. Primary cutaneous disorders
  A. Localized
    1. Epidermal alteration
      a. Seborrheic keratosis
      b. Acanthosis nigricans (obesity)
      c. Pigmented actinic keratosis
    2. Proliferation of melanocytes
      a. Lentigo
      b. Nevus
      c. Melanoma
    3. Increased pigment production
      a. Ephelides (freckles)
      b. Café au lait macule
      c. Postinflammatory hyperpigmentation
  B. Localized and diffuse
    1. Drugs
II. Systemic diseases
  A. Localized
    1. Epidermal alteration
      a. Seborrheic keratoses (sign of Leser-Trélat)
      b. Acanthosis nigricans (endocrine disorders, paraneoplastic)
    2. Proliferation of melanocytes
      a. Lentigines (Peutz-Jeghers and LEOPARD syndromes; xeroderma pigmentosum)
      b. Nevi [Carney complex (LAMB and NAME syndromes)][a]
    3. Increased pigment production
      a. Café au lait macules (neurofibromatosis, McCune-Albright syndrome[b])
      b. Urticaria pigmentosa[c]
    4. Dermal pigmentation
      a. Incontinentia pigmenti (stage III)
      b. Dyskeratosis congenita
  B. Diffuse
    1. Endocrinopathies
      a. Addison's disease
      b. Nelson syndrome
      c. Ectopic ACTH syndrome
    2. Metabolic
      a. Porphyria cutanea tarda
      b. Hemochromatosis
      c. Vitamin B_{12}, folate deficiency
      d. Pellagra
      e. Malabsorption, Whipple's disease
    3. Melanosis secondary to metastatic melanoma
    4. Autoimmune
      a. Biliary cirrhosis
      b. Scleroderma
      c. POEMS syndrome
      d. Eosinophilia-myalgia syndrome[d]
    5. Drugs and metals

[a]Also lentigines.
[b]Polyostotic fibrous dysplasia.
[c]See also "Papulonodular Skin Lesions."
[d]Late 1980s.

Localized hyperpigmentation is seen as a side effect of several other *systemic medications*, including those that produce fixed drug reactions [nonsteroidal anti-inflammatory drugs (NSAIDs), sulfonamides, barbiturates, and tetracyclines] and those that can complex with melanin (antimalarials) or iron (minocycline). Fixed drug eruptions recur in the exact same location as circular areas of erythema that can become bullous and then resolve as brown macules. The eruption usually appears within hours of administration of the offending agent, and common locations include the genitalia, extremities, and perioral region. Chloroquine and hydroxychloroquine produce gray-brown to blue-black discoloration of the shins, hard palate, and face, while blue macules (often misdiagnosed as bruises) can be seen on the lower extremities and in sites of inflammation with prolonged minocycline administration. Estrogen in oral contraceptives can induce melasma—symmetric brown patches on the face, especially the cheeks, upper lip, and forehead. Similar changes are seen in pregnancy and in patients receiving phenytoin.

In the diffuse forms of hyperpigmentation, the darkening of the skin may be of equal intensity over the entire body or may be accentuated in sun-exposed areas. The causes of diffuse hyperpigmentation can be divided into four major groups—endocrine, metabolic, autoimmune, and drugs. The endocrinopathies that frequently have associated hyperpigmentation include *Addison's disease, Nelson syndrome*, and *ectopic ACTH syndrome*. In these diseases, the increased pigmentation is diffuse but is accentuated in the palmar creases, sites of friction, scars, and the oral mucosa. An overproduction of the pituitary hormones α-MSH (melanocyte-stimulating hormone) and ACTH can lead to an increase in melanocyte activity. These peptides are products of the proopiomelanocortin gene and exhibit homology; e.g., α-MSH and ACTH share 13 amino acids. A minority of the patients with Cushing's disease or hyperthyroidism have generalized hyperpigmentation.

The metabolic causes of hyperpigmentation include *porphyria cutanea tarda* (PCT), *hemochromatosis, vitamin B_{12} deficiency, folic acid deficiency, pellagra, malabsorption*, and *Whipple's disease*. In patients with PCT (see "Vesicles/Bullae," below), the skin darkening is seen in sun-exposed areas and is a reflection of the photoreactive properties of porphyrins. The increased level of iron in the skin of patients with hemochromatosis stimulates melanin pigment production and leads to the classic bronze color. Patients with pellagra have a brown discoloration of the skin, especially in sun-exposed areas, as a result of nicotinic acid (niacin) deficiency. In the areas of increased pigmentation, there is a thin varnish-like scale. These changes are also seen in patients who are vitamin B_6 deficient, have functioning carcinoid tumors (increased consumption of niacin), or take isoniazid. Approximately 50% of the patients with Whipple's disease have an associated generalized hyperpigmentation in association with diarrhea, weight loss, arthritis, and lymphadenopathy. A diffuse slate-blue color is seen in patients with melanosis secondary to metastatic melanoma. Although there is a debate as to whether the color is due to single-cell metastases in the dermis or to a widespread deposition of melanin resulting from the high concentration of circulating melanin precursors, there is more evidence to support the latter.

Of the autoimmune diseases associated with diffuse hyperpigmentation, *biliary cirrhosis* and *scleroderma* are the most common, and occasionally both disorders are seen in the same patient. The skin is dark brown in color, especially in sun-exposed areas. In biliary cirrhosis the hyperpigmentation is accompanied by pruritus, jaundice, and xanthomas, whereas in scleroderma it is accompanied by sclerosis of the extremities, face, and, less commonly, the trunk. Additional clues to the diagnosis of scleroderma are telangiectasias, calcinosis cutis, Raynaud's phenomenon, and distal ulcerations (see "Telangiectasias," above). The differential diagnosis of cutaneous sclerosis with hyperpigmentation includes the POEMS [*p*olyneuropathy; *o*rganomegaly (liver, spleen, lymph nodes); *e*ndocrinopathies (impotence, gynecomastia); *M*-protein; and *s*kin changes] syndrome. The skin changes include hyperpigmentation, skin thickening, hypertrichosis, and angiomas.

Diffuse hyperpigmentation that is due to drugs or metals can result from one of several mechanisms—induction of melanin pigment formation, complexing of the drug or its metabolites to melanin, and deposits of the drug in the dermis. Busulfan, cyclophosphamide, 5-fluorouracil,

sions," below). In comparison with NF, the CALM in patients with *McCune-Albright syndrome* [polyostotic fibrous dysplasia with precocious puberty in females due to mosaicism for an activating mutation in a G protein ($G_s\alpha$) gene] are usually larger, more irregular in outline, and tend to respect the midline. CALM have also been associated with pulmonary stenosis (Watson syndrome), tuberous sclerosis, the LEOPARD syndrome, and multiple endocrine neoplasia (MEN), but a few such lesions can be found in normal individuals.

In incontinentia pigmenti, dyskeratosis congenita, and bleomycin pigmentation, the areas of localized hyperpigmentation form a pattern—swirled in the first, reticulated in the second, and flagellate in the third. In *dyskeratosis congenita*, atrophic reticulated hyperpigmentation is seen on the neck, trunk, and thighs and is accompanied by nail dystrophy, pancytopenia, and leukoplakia of the oral and anal mucosae. The latter often develops into squamous cell carcinoma. In addition to the flagellate pigmentation (linear streaks) on the trunk, patients receiving bleomycin often have hyperpigmentation overlying the elbows, knees, and small joints of the hand.

and inorganic arsenic induce pigment production. Complexes containing melanin or hemosiderin plus the drug or its metabolites are seen in patients receiving chlorpromazine and minocycline. The sun-exposed skin as well as the conjunctivae of patients on long-term, high-dose chlorpromazine can become blue-gray in color. Patients taking minocycline may develop a diffuse blue-gray, muddy appearance in sun-exposed areas in addition to pigmentation of the mucous membranes, teeth, nails, bones, and thyroid. Administration of amiodarone can result in both a phototoxic eruption (exaggerated sunburn) and/or a brown or blue-gray discoloration of sun-exposed skin. Biopsy specimens of the latter show yellow-brown granules in dermal macrophages, which represent intralysosomal accumulations of lipids, amiodarone, and its metabolites. Actual deposits of a particular drug or metal in the skin are seen with silver (argyria), where the skin appears blue-gray in color; gold (chrysiasis), where the skin has a brown to blue-gray color; and clofazimine, where the skin appears reddish brown. The associated hyperpigmentation is accentuated in sun-exposed areas, and discoloration of the eye is seen with gold (sclerae) and clofazimine (conjunctivae).

VESICLES/BULLAE

(Table 54-12) Depending on their size, cutaneous blisters are referred to as *vesicles* (<0.5 cm) or *bullae* (>0.5 cm). The primary blistering disorders include *pemphigus vulgaris, pemphigus foliaceus, pemphigus erythematosus, paraneoplastic pemphigus, bullous pemphigoid, gestational pemphigoid, cicatricial pemphigoid, epidermolysis bullosa acquisita, linear IgA bullous dermatosis,* and *dermatitis herpetiformis* (Chap. 55).

Vesicles and bullae are also seen in *contact dermatitis,* both allergic and irritant forms (Chap. 53). When there is a linear arrangement of vesicular lesions, an exogenous cause should be suspected. Bullous dis-

TABLE 54-12   CAUSES OF VESICLES/BULLAE

I. Primary cutaneous diseases
  A. Primary blistering diseases (autoimmune)
    1. Pemphigus[a]
    2. Bullous pemphigoid[b]
    3. Gestational pemphigoid[b]
    4. Cicatricial pemphigoid[b]
    5. Dermatitis herpetiformis[b,c]
    6. Linear IgA bullous dermatosis[b]
    7. Epidermolysis bullosa acquisita[b,d]
  B. Secondary blistering diseases
    1. Contact dermatitis[a]
    2. Erythema multiforme[a,b]
    3. Stevens-Johnson syndrome
    4. Toxic epidermal necrolysis[b]
  C. Infections
    1. Varicella/zoster virus[a,e]
    2. Herpes simplex virus[a,e]
    3. Enteroviruses, e.g., hand-foot-and-mouth disease
    4. Staphylococcal scalded-skin syndrome[a,f]
    5. Bullous impetigo[a]
II. Systemic diseases
  A. Autoimmune
    1. Paraneoplastic pemphigus[a]
  B. Infections
    1. Cutaneous emboli[b]
  C. Metabolic
    1. Diabetic bullae[a,b]
    2. Porphyria cutanea tarda[b]
    3. Porphyria variegata[b]
    4. Pseudoporphyria[b]
    5. Bullous dermatosis of hemodialysis[b]
  D. Ischemia
    1. Coma bullae

[a]Intraepidermal.
[b]Subepidermal.
[c]Associated with gluten enteropathy.
[d]Associated with inflammatory bowel disease.
[e]Also systemic.
[f]In adults, associated with renal failure and immunocompromised state.

ease secondary to the ingestion of drugs can take one of several forms, including phototoxic eruptions, isolated bullae, Stevens-Johnson syndrome (SJS), and toxic epidermal necrolysis (TEN) (Chap. 56). Clinically, phototoxic eruptions resemble an exaggerated sunburn with diffuse erythema and bullae in sun-exposed areas. The most commonly associated drugs are doxycycline, sulfonamides, thiazides, NSAIDs, and psoralens. The development of a phototoxic eruption is dependent on the doses of both the drug and ultraviolet (UV)-A irradiation.

Toxic epidermal necrolysis is characterized by bullae that arise on widespread areas of erythema and then slough. This results in large areas of denuded skin. The associated morbidity, such as sepsis, and mortality are relatively high and are a function of the extent of epidermal necrosis. In addition, these patients may also have involvement of the mucous membranes and intestinal tract. Drugs are the primary cause of TEN, and the most common offenders are phenytoin, barbiturates, carbamazepine, sulfonamides, penicillins, and NSAIDs. Severe acute graft-versus-host disease (grade 4) can also resemble TEN.

In *erythema multiforme* (EM), the primary lesions are pink-red macules and edematous papules, the centers of which may become vesicular. The clue to the diagnosis of EM, as opposed to a morbilliform exanthem, is the development of a "dusky" violet color or petechiae in the center of the lesions. Target or iris lesions are also characteristic of EM and arise as a result of active centers and borders in combination with centrifugal spread. However, iris lesions need not be present to make the diagnosis of EM.

EM has been subdivided into two major groups: (1) EM minor due to herpes simplex virus (HSV); and (2) EM major due to HSV, *Mycoplasma pneumoniae,* or rarely drugs. Involvement of the mucous membranes (oral, nasal, ocular, and genital) is seen more commonly in the latter form. Hemorrhagic crusts of the lips are characteristic of EM major and SJS as well as herpes simplex, pemphigus vulgaris, and paraneoplastic pemphigus. Fever, malaise, myalgias, sore throat, and cough may precede or accompany the eruption. The lesions of EM usually resolve over 3–6 weeks but may be recurrent, especially when due to HSV. In addition to HSV (in which lesions appear 7–12 days after the viral eruption), EM can also follow vaccinations, radiation therapy, and exposure to environmental toxins.

Induction of SJS is most often due to drugs, especially sulfonamides, phenytoin, barbiturates, penicillins, and carbamazepine. Widespread dusky macules and significant mucosal involvement are characteristic of SJS, and the cutaneous lesions may or may not develop epidermal detachment. If the latter occurs, by definition, it is limited to <10% of the body surface area (BSA). Greater involvement leads to the diagnosis of SJS/TEN overlap (10–30% BSA) or TEN (>30% BSA).

In addition to primary blistering disorders and hypersensitivity reactions, bacterial and viral infections can lead to vesicles and bullae. The most common infectious agents are HSV (Chap. 172), varicella-zoster virus (Chap. 173), and *S. aureus* (Chap. 129).

Staphylococcal scalded-skin syndrome (SSSS) and *bullous impetigo* are two blistering disorders associated with staphylococcal (phage group II) infection. In SSSS, the initial findings are redness and tenderness of the central face, neck, trunk, and intertriginous zones. This is followed by short-lived flaccid bullae and a slough or exfoliation of the superficial epidermis. Crusted areas then develop, characteristically around the mouth. SSSS is distinguished from TEN by the following features: younger age group (primarily infants), more superficial site of blister formation, no oral lesions, shorter course, less morbidity and mortality, and an association with staphylococcal exfoliative toxin ("exfoliatin"), not drugs. A rapid diagnosis of SSSS versus TEN can be made by a frozen section of the blister roof or exfoliative cytology of the blister contents. In SSSS the site of staphylococcal infection is usually extracutaneous (conjunctivitis, rhinorrhea, otitis media, pharyngitis, tonsillitis), and the cutaneous lesions are sterile, whereas in bullous impetigo the skin lesions are the site of infection. Impetigo is more localized than SSSS and usually presents with honey-colored crusts. Occasionally, superficial purulent blisters also form. *Cutaneous emboli* from gram-negative infections may present as isolated bullae, but the base of the lesion is purpuric or necrotic, and it may develop into an ulcer (see "Purpura," below).

Several metabolic disorders are associated with blister formation, including diabetes mellitus, renal failure, and porphyria. Local hypoxia secondary to decreased cutaneous blood flow can also produce blisters, which explains the presence of bullae over pressure points in comatose patients (coma bullae). In *diabetes mellitus*, tense bullae with clear viscous fluid arise on normal skin. The lesions can be as large as 6 cm in diameter and are located on the distal extremities. There are several types of porphyria, but the most common form with cutaneous findings is *PCT*. In sun-exposed areas (primarily the face and hands), the skin is very fragile, and trauma leads to erosions and tense vesicles. These lesions then heal with scarring and formation of milia; the latter are firm, 1- to 2-mm white or yellow papules that represent epidermoid inclusion cysts. Associated findings can include hypertrichosis of the lateral malar region (men) or face (women) and, in sun-exposed areas, hyperpigmentation and firm sclerotic plaques. An elevated level of urinary uroporphyrins confirms the diagnosis and is due to a decrease in uroporphyrinogen decarboxylase activity. Precipitating agents include alcohol, iron, chlorinated hydrocarbons, hepatitis C infection, and hepatomas.

The differential diagnosis of PCT includes (1) *porphyria variegata*—the skin signs of PCT plus the systemic findings of acute intermittent porphyria; it has a diagnostic plasma porphyrin fluorescence emission at 626 nm; (2) *drug-induced* pseudoporphyria—the clinical and histologic findings are similar to PCT, but porphyrins are normal; etiologic agents include naproxen, furosemide, tetracycline, and nalidixic acid; (3) *bullous dermatosis of hemodialysis*—the same appearance as PCT, but porphyrins are usually normal or occasionally borderline elevated; patients have chronic renal failure and are on hemodialysis; (4) PCT associated with hepatomas, hepatic carcinomas, and hemodialysis; and (5) *epidermolysis bullosa acquisita* (Chap. 55).

EXANTHEMS

(Table 54-13) Exanthems are characterized by an acute generalized eruption. The two most common presentations are erythematous macules and papules (morbilliform) and confluent blanching erythema (scarlatiniform). *Morbilliform* eruptions are usually due to either drugs or viral infections. For example, up to 5% of the patients receiving penicillins, sulfonamides, phenytoin, or gold will develop a maculopapular eruption. Accompanying signs may include pruritus, fever, eosinophilia, and transient lymphadenopathy. Similar maculopapular eruptions are seen in the classic childhood viral exanthems, including (1) *rubeola* (measles)—a prodrome of coryza, cough, and conjunctivitis followed by Koplik's spots on the buccal mucosa; the eruption begins behind the ears, at the hairline, and on the forehead and then spreads down the body, often becoming confluent; (2) *rubella*—the eruption begins on the forehead and face and then spreads down the body; it resolves in the same order and is associated with retroauricular and suboccipital lymphadenopathy; and (3) *erythema infectiosum* (fifth disease)—erythema of the cheeks is followed by a reticulated pattern on extremities; it is secondary to a parvovirus B19 infection, and an associated arthritis is seen in adults.

Both measles and rubella are seen in unvaccinated young adults, and an atypical form of measles is seen in adults immunized with either killed measles vaccine or killed vaccine followed in time by live vaccine. In contrast to classic measles, the eruption of atypical measles begins on the palms, soles, wrists, and knuckles, and the lesions may become purpuric. The patient with atypical measles can have pulmonary involvement and be quite ill. Rubelliform and roseoliform eruptions are also associated with *Epstein-Barr virus* (5–15% of patients), *echovirus*, *coxsackievirus*, *cytomegalovirus*, and *adenovirus* infections. Detection of specific IgM antibodies or fourfold elevations in IgG antibodies allows the proper diagnosis. Occasionally, a maculopapular drug eruption is a reflection of an underlying viral infection. For example, about 95% of the patients with infectious mononucleosis who are given ampicillin will develop a rash.

Of note, early in the course of infections with *Rickettsia* and meningococcus, prior to the development of purpura, the lesions may be erythematous macules and papules. This is also the case in chickenpox prior to the development of vesicles. Maculopapular eruptions are associated with early *HIV infection*, early secondary *syphilis*, *typhoid fever*, and *acute graft-versus-host disease*. In the last, lesions frequently begin on the palms and soles; the macular rose spots of typhoid fever involve primarily the anterior trunk.

The prototypic *scarlatiniform* eruption is seen in *scarlet fever* and is due to an erythrotoxin produced by group A β-hemolytic streptococcal infections, most commonly pharyngitis. This eruption is characterized by diffuse erythema, which begins on the neck and upper trunk, and red follicular puncta. Additional findings include a white strawberry tongue (white coating with red papillae) followed by a red strawberry tongue (red tongue with red papillae); petechiae of the palate; a facial flush with circumoral pallor; linear petechiae in the antecubital fossae; and desquamation of the involved skin, palms, and soles 5–20 days after onset of the eruption. A similar desquamation of the palms and soles is seen in toxic shock syndrome (TSS), Kawasaki's disease, and after severe febrile illnesses. Certain strains of staphylococci also produce an erythrotoxin that leads to the same clinical findings as in streptococcal scarlet fever, except that the anti-streptolysin O or -DNase B titers are not elevated.

In *toxic shock syndrome*, staphylococcal (phage group I) infections produce an exotoxin (TSST-1) that causes the fever and rash, as well as enterotoxins. Initially, the majority of cases were reported in menstruating women who were using tampons. However, other sites of infection, including wounds and vaginitis, can lead to TSS. The diagnosis of TSS is based on clinical criteria (Chap. 129), and three of these involve mucocutaneous sites (diffuse erythema of the skin, desquamation of the palms and soles 1–2 weeks after onset of illness, and involvement of the mucous membranes). The latter is characterized as hyperemia of the vagina, oropharynx, or conjunctivae. Similar systemic findings have been described in *streptococcal toxic shock–like syndrome* (Chap. 130), and although an exanthem is seen less often than in TSS due to a staphylococcal infection, the underlying infection is often in the soft tissue.

The cutaneous eruption in *Kawasaki's disease* (mucocutaneous lymph node syndrome) (Chap. 319) is polymorphous, but the two most common forms are morbilliform and scarlatiniform. Additional mucocutaneous findings include bilateral conjunctival injection; erythema and edema of the hands and feet followed by desquamation; and diffuse erythema of the oropharynx, red strawberry tongue, and erosions with crusting on the lips. This clinical picture can resemble TSS and scarlet fever, but clues to the diagnosis of Kawasaki's disease are cervical lymphadenopathy, lip erosions, and thrombocytosis. The most serious associated systemic finding in this disease is coronary aneurysm secondary to arteritis. Aneurysms may lead to sudden death, primarily within the first 30 days of the illness. Scarlatiniform eruptions are also seen in the early phase of SSSS (see "Vesicles/Bullae," above) and as reactions to drugs.

TABLE 54-13	CAUSES OF EXANTHEMS

I. Morbilliform
  A. Drugs
  B. Viral
    1. Rubeola (measles)
    2. Rubella
    3. Erythema infectiosum
    4. Epstein-Barr virus, echovirus, coxsackievirus, CMV,[a] and adenovirus
    5. Early HIV (plus mucosal ulcerations)
  C. Bacterial
    1. Typhoid fever
    2. Early secondary syphilis
    3. Early *Rickettsia*
    4. Early meningococcemia
  D. Acute graft-versus-host disease
  E. Kawasaki disease
II. Scarlatiniform
  A. Scarlet fever
  B. Toxic shock syndrome
  C. Kawasaki disease
  D. Early staphylococcal scalded-skin syndrome

[a]CMV, cytomegalovirus.

URTICARIA

(Table 54-14) *Urticaria* (hives) are transient lesions that are composed of a central wheal surrounded by an erythematous halo. Individual lesions are round, oval, or figurate and are often pruritic. Acute and chronic urticaria has a wide variety of allergic etiologies and reflect edema in the dermis. Urticarial lesions can also be seen in patients with mastocytosis (urticaria pigmentosa), hyperthyroidism, and systemic-onset juvenile idiopathic arthritis (Still's disease). In both juvenile- and adult-onset Still's disease, the lesions coincide with the fever spike, are transient, and are due to dermal infiltrates of neutrophils.

The common *physical urticarias* include dermographism, solar urticaria, cold urticaria, and cholinergic urticaria. Patients with *dermographism* exhibit linear wheals following minor pressure or scratching of the skin. It is a common disorder, affecting ~5% of the population. *Solar urticaria* characteristically occurs within minutes of sun exposure and is a skin sign of one systemic disease—erythropoietic protoporphyria. In addition to the urticaria, these patients have subtle pitted scarring of the nose and hands. *Cold urticaria* is precipitated by exposure to the cold, and therefore exposed areas are usually affected. In some patients, the disease is associated with abnormal circulating proteins—more commonly cryoglobulins and less commonly cryofibrinogens or cold agglutinins. Additional systemic symptoms include wheezing and syncope, thus explaining the need for these patients to avoid swimming in cold water. *Cholinergic urticaria* is precipitated by heat, exercise, or emotion and is characterized by small wheals with relatively large flares. It is occasionally associated with wheezing.

Whereas urticarias are the result of dermal edema, subcutaneous edema leads to the clinical picture of *angioedema*. Sites of involvement include the eyelids, lips, tongue, larynx, and gastrointestinal tract as well as the subcutaneous tissue. Angioedema occurs alone or in combination with urticaria, including urticarial vasculitis and the physical urticarias. Both acquired and hereditary (autosomal dominant) forms of angioedema occur (Chap. 311), and in the latter, urticaria is rarely, if ever, seen.

Urticarial vasculitis is an immune complex disease that may be confused with simple urticaria. In contrast to simple urticaria, individual lesions tend to last longer than 24 h and usually develop central petechiae that can be observed even after the urticarial phase has resolved. The patient may also complain of burning rather than pruritus. On biopsy, there is a leukocytoclastic vasculitis of the small blood vessels. Although many cases of urticarial vasculitis are idiopathic in origin, it can be a reflection of an underlying systemic illness such as lupus erythematosus, Sjögren's syndrome, or hereditary complement deficiency. There is a spectrum of urticarial vasculitis that ranges from purely cutaneous to multisystem involvement. The most common systemic signs and symptoms are arthralgias and/or arthritis, nephritis, and crampy abdominal pain, with asthma and chronic obstructive lung disease seen less often. Hypocomplementemia occurs in one- to two-thirds of patients, even in the idiopathic cases. Urticarial vasculitis can also be seen in patients with *hepatitis B* and *hepatitis C* infections, *serum sickness*, and *serum sickness–like illnesses*.

TABLE 54-14 CAUSES OF URTICARIA AND ANGIOEDEMA

I. Primary cutaneous disorders
  A. Acute and chronic urticaria[a]
  B. Physical urticaria
    1. Dermatographism
    2. Solar urticaria[b]
    3. Cold urticaria[b]
    4. Cholinergic urticaria[b]
  C. Angioedema (hereditary and acquired)[b]
II. Systemic diseases
  A. Urticarial vasculitis
  B. Hepatitis B or C infection
  C. Serum sickness
  D. Angioedema (hereditary and acquired)

[a]A small minority develop anaphylaxis.
[b]Also systemic.

PAPULONODULAR SKIN LESIONS

(Table 54-15) In the *papulonodular diseases*, the lesions are elevated above the surface of the skin and may coalesce to form plaques. The location, consistency, and color of the lesions are the keys to their diagnosis; this section is organized on the basis of color.

WHITE LESIONS

In *calcinosis cutis* there are firm white to white-yellow papules with an irregular surface. When the contents are expressed, a chalky white material is seen. *Dystrophic calcification* is seen at sites of previous inflammation or damage to the skin. It develops in acne scars as well as on the distal extremities of patients with scleroderma and in the subcutaneous tissue and intermuscular fascial planes in DM. The latter is more extensive and is more commonly seen in children. An elevated calcium phosphate product, most commonly due to secondary hyperparathyroidism in the setting of renal failure, can lead to nodules of *metastatic calcinosis cutis*, which tend to be subcutaneous and periarticular. These patients can also develop calcification of muscular arteries and subsequent ischemic necrosis (calciphylaxis).

SKIN-COLORED LESIONS

There are several types of skin-colored lesions, including epidermoid inclusion cysts, lipomas, rheumatoid nodules, neurofibromas, angiofibromas, neuromas, and adnexal tumors such as tricholemmomas. Both *epidermoid inclusion cysts* and *lipomas* are very common mobile subcutaneous nodules—the former are rubbery and drain cheeselike material (sebum and keratin) if incised. Lipomas are firm and somewhat lobulated on palpation. When extensive facial epidermoid inclusion cysts develop during childhood or there is a family history of such lesions, the patient should be examined for other signs of Gardner syndrome, including osteomas and desmoid tumors. *Rheumatoid nodules* are firm, 0.5- to 4-cm nodules that tend to localize around pressure points, especially the elbows. They are seen in ~20% of patients with rheumatoid arthritis and 6% of patients with Still's disease. Biopsies of the nodules show palisading granulomas. Similar lesions that are smaller and shorter-lived are seen in rheumatic fever.

Neurofibromas (benign Schwann cell tumors) are soft papules or nodules that exhibit the "button-hole" sign, that is, they invaginate into the skin with pressure in a manner similar to a hernia. Single lesions are seen in normal individuals, but multiple neurofibromas, usually in combination with six or more CALM measuring >1.5 cm (see "Hyperpigmentation," above), axillary freckling, and multiple Lisch nodules, are seen in von Recklinghausen's disease (NF type I; Chap. 375). In some patients the neurofibromas are localized and unilateral due to somatic mosaicism.

Angiofibromas are firm, pink to skin-colored papules that measure from 3 mm to a few centimeters in diameter. When multiple lesions are located on the central cheeks (adenoma sebaceum), the patient has tuberous sclerosis or MEN syndrome, type 1. The former is an autosomal disorder due to mutations in two different genes, and the associated findings are discussed in the section on ash leaf spots as well as in Chap. 375.

Neuromas (benign proliferations of nerve fibers) are also firm, skin-colored papules. They are more commonly found at sites of amputation and as rudimentary supernumerary digits. However, when there are multiple neuromas on the eyelids, lips, distal tongue, and/or oral mucosa, the patient should be investigated for other signs of the MEN syndrome, type 2b. Associated findings include marfanoid habitus, protuberant lips, intestinal ganglioneuromas, and medullary thyroid carcinoma (>75% of patients; Chap. 345).

Adnexal tumors are derived from pluripotent cells of the epidermis that can differentiate toward hair, sebaceous, apocrine, or eccrine glands or remain undifferentiated. *Basal cell carcinomas* (BCCs) are examples of adnexal tumors that have little or no evidence of differentiation. Clinically, they are translucent papules with rolled borders, telangiectasias, and central erosion. BCCs commonly arise in sun-damaged skin of the head and neck as well as the upper trunk. When a patient has multiple BCCs, especially prior to age 30, the possibility of the nevoid basal cell carcinoma syndrome should be raised. It is inherited as an autosomal

TABLE 54-15	PAPULONODULAR SKIN LESIONS ACCORDING TO COLOR GROUPS

I. White
   A. Calcinosis cutis
II. Skin-colored
   A. Rheumatoid nodules
   B. Neurofibromas (von Recklinghausen's disease)
   C. Angiofibromas (tuberous sclerosis, MEN syndrome, type 1)
   D. Neuromas (MEN syndrome, type 2b)
   E. Adnexal tumors
      1. Basal cell carcinomas (nevoid basal cell carcinoma syndrome)
      2. Tricholemmomas (Cowden disease)
   F. Osteomas (Gardner syndrome)
   G. Primary cutaneous disorders
      1. Epidermal inclusion cysts
      2. Lipomas
III. Pink/translucent[a]
   A. Amyloidosis
   B. Papular mucinosis
IV. Yellow
   A. Xanthomas
   B. Tophi
   C. Necrobiosis lipoidica
   D. Pseudoxanthoma elasticum
   E. Sebaceous adenomas (Torre syndrome)
V. Red[a]
   A. Papules
      1. Angiokeratomas (Fabry disease)
      2. Bacillary angiomatosis (primarily in AIDS)
   B. Papules/plaques
      1. Cutaneous lupus
      2. Lymphoma cutis
      3. Leukemia cutis
   C. Nodules
      1. Panniculitis
      2. Cutaneous polyarteritis nodosa
      3. Systemic vasculitis
   D. Primary cutaneous disorders
      1. Arthropod bites
      2. Cherry hemangiomas
      3. Infections, e.g., erysipelas, sporotrichosis
      4. Polymorphous light eruption
      5. Lymphocytoma cutis (pseudolymphoma)
VI. Red-brown[a]
   A. Sarcoidosis
   B. Sweet's syndrome
   C. Urticaria pigmentosa
   D. Erythema elevatum diutinum (chronic leukocytoclastic vasculitis)
   E. Lupus vulgaris
VII. Blue[a]
   A. Venous malformations (blue rubber bleb syndrome)
   B. Primary cutaneous disorders
      1. Venous lake
      2. Blue nevus
VIII. Violaceous
   A. Lupus pernio (sarcoidosis)
   B. Lymphoma cutis
   C. Cutaneous lupus
IX. Purple
   A. Kaposi's sarcoma
   B. Angiosarcoma
   C. Palpable purpura
X. Brown-black[b]
XI. Any color
   A. Metastases

[a]May have darker hue in more darkly pigmented individuals.
[b]See also "Hyperpigmentation."
Note: MEN, multiple endocrine neoplasia.

dominant trait and is associated with jaw cysts, palmar and plantar pits, frontal bossing, medulloblastomas, and calcification of the falx cerebri and diaphragma sellae. *Tricholemmomas* are also skin-colored adnexal tumors but differentiate toward hair follicles and can have a wartlike appearance. The presence of multiple tricholemmomas on the face and cobblestoning of the oral mucosa points to the diagnosis of Cowden dis-

ease (multiple hamartoma syndrome) due to mutations in the *PTEN* gene. Internal organ involvement (in decreasing order of frequency) includes fibrocystic disease and carcinoma of the breast, adenomas and carcinomas of the thyroid, and gastrointestinal polyposis. Keratoses of the palms, soles, and dorsal aspect of the hands are also seen.

PINK LESIONS

The cutaneous lesions associated with primary systemic *amyloidosis* are often pink in color and translucent. Common locations are the face, especially the periorbital and perioral regions, and flexural areas. On biopsy, homogeneous deposits of amyloid are seen in the dermis and in the walls of blood vessels; the latter lead to an increase in vessel wall fragility. As a result, petechiae and purpura develop in clinically normal skin as well as in lesional skin following minor trauma, hence the term *pinch purpura*. Amyloid deposits are also seen in the striated muscle of the tongue and result in macroglossia.

Even though specific mucocutaneous lesions are rarely seen in secondary amyloidosis and are present in only ~30% of the patients with primary amyloidosis, a rapid diagnosis of systemic amyloidosis can be made by an examination of abdominal subcutaneous fat. By special staining, deposits are seen around blood vessels or individual fat cells in 40–50% of patients. There are also three forms of amyloidosis that are limited to the skin and that should not be construed as cutaneous lesions of systemic amyloidosis. They are macular amyloidosis (upper back), lichenoid amyloidosis (usually lower extremities), and nodular amyloidosis. In macular and lichenoid amyloidosis, the deposits are composed of altered epidermal keratin. Recently, macular and lichenoid amyloidosis have been associated with MEN syndrome, type 2a.

Patients with *multicentric reticulohistiocytosis* also have pink-colored papules and nodules on the face and mucous membranes as well as on the extensor surface of the hands and forearms. They have a polyarthritis that can mimic rheumatoid arthritis clinically. On histologic examination, the papules have characteristic giant cells that are not seen in biopsies of rheumatoid nodules. Pink to skin-colored papules that are firm, 2–5 mm in diameter, and often in a linear arrangement are seen in patients with *papular mucinosis*. This disease is also referred to as *generalized lichen myxedematosus* or *scleromyxedema*. The latter name comes from the brawny induration of the face and extremities that may accompany the papular eruption. Biopsy specimens of the papules show localized mucin deposition, and serum protein electrophoresis and/or immunofixation electrophoresis demonstrates a monoclonal spike of IgG, usually with a λ light chain.

YELLOW LESIONS

Several systemic disorders are characterized by yellow-colored cutaneous papules or plaques—hyperlipidemia (xanthomas), gout (tophi), diabetes (necrobiosis lipoidica), pseudoxanthoma elasticum, and Torre syndrome (sebaceous tumors). Eruptive xanthomas are the most common form of *xanthomas* and are associated with hypertriglyceridemia (types I, III, IV, and V). Crops of yellow papules with erythematous halos occur primarily on the extensor surfaces of the extremities and the buttocks, and they spontaneously involute with a fall in serum triglycerides. Increased β-lipoproteins (primarily types II and III) result in one or more of the following types of xanthoma: xanthelasma, tendon xanthomas, and plane xanthomas. Xanthelasma are found on the eyelids, whereas tendon xanthomas are frequently associated with the Achilles and extensor finger tendons; plane xanthomas are flat and favor the palmar creases, face, upper trunk, and scars. Tuberous xanthomas are frequently associated with hypertriglyceridemia, but they are also seen in patients with hypercholesterolemia (type II) and are found most frequently over the large joints or hand. Biopsy specimens of xanthomas show collections of lipid-containing macrophages (foam cells).

Patients with several disorders, including biliary cirrhosis, can have a secondary form of hyperlipidemia with associated tuberous and planar xanthomas. However, patients with myeloma have *normolipemic flat xanthomas*. This latter form of xanthoma may be ≥12 cm in diameter and is most frequently seen on the upper trunk or side of the neck. It is important to note that the most common setting for eruptive xanthomas is uncontrolled diabetes mellitus. The least specific sign for hyperlipidemia is xanthelasma, because at least 50% of the patients with this finding have normal lipid profiles.

In *tophaceous gout* there are deposits of monosodium urate in the skin around the joints, particularly those of the hands and feet. Additional sites of *tophi* formation include the helix of the ear and the olecranon and prepatellar bursae. The lesions are firm, yellow in color, and occasionally discharge a chalky material. Their size varies from 1 mm to 7 cm, and the diagnosis can be established by polarization of the aspirated contents of a lesion. Lesions of *necrobiosis lipoidica* are found primarily on the shins (90%), and patients can have diabetes mellitus or develop it subsequently. Characteristic findings include a central yellow color, atrophy (transparency), telangiectasias, and an erythematous border. Ulcerations can also develop within the plaques. Biopsy specimens show necrobiosis of collagen, granulomatous inflammation, and obliterative endarteritis.

In *pseudoxanthoma elasticum* (PXE) there is an abnormal deposition of calcium on the elastic fibers of the skin, eye, and blood vessels. In the skin, the flexural areas such as the neck, axillae, antecubital fossae, and inguinal area are the primary sites of involvement. Yellow papules coalesce to form reticulated plaques that have an appearance similar to that of plucked chicken skin. In severely affected skin, hanging, redundant folds develop. Biopsy specimens of involved skin show swollen and irregularly clumped elastic fibers with deposits of calcium. In the eye, the calcium deposits in Bruch's membrane lead to angioid streaks and choroiditis; in the arteries of the heart, kidney, gastrointestinal tract, and extremities, the deposits lead to angina, hypertension, gastrointestinal bleeding, and claudication, respectively. Long-term administration of D-penicillamine can lead to PXE-like skin changes as well as elastic fiber alterations in internal organs.

Adnexal tumors that have differentiated toward sebaceous glands include sebaceous adenoma, sebaceous carcinoma, and sebaceous hyperplasia. Except for sebaceous hyperplasia, which is commonly seen on the face, these tumors are fairly rare. Patients with Torre syndrome have one or more *sebaceous adenoma(s)*, and they can also have sebaceous carcinomas and sebaceous hyperplasia as well as keratoacanthomas. The internal manifestations of Torre syndrome include *multiple carcinomas* of the gastrointestinal tract (primarily colon) as well as cancers of the larynx, genitourinary tract, and endometrium.

RED LESIONS

Cutaneous lesions that are red in color have a wide variety of etiologies; in an attempt to simplify their identification, they will be subdivided into papules, papules/plaques, and subcutaneous nodules. Common red papules include *arthropod bites* and *cherry hemangiomas*; the latter are small, bright-red, dome-shaped papules that represent benign proliferation of capillaries. In patients with AIDS, the development of multiple red hemangioma-like lesions points to bacillary angiomatosis, and biopsy specimens show clusters of bacilli that stain positive with the Warthin-Starry stain; the pathogens have been identified as *Bartonella henselae* and *B. quintana*. Disseminated visceral disease is seen primarily in immunocompromised hosts but can occur in immunocompetent individuals.

Multiple *angiokeratomas* are seen in Fabry disease, an X-linked recessive lysosomal storage disease that is due to a deficiency of α-galactosidase A. The lesions are red to red-blue in color and can be quite small in size (1–3 mm), with the most common location being the lower trunk. Associated findings include chronic renal failure, peripheral neuropathy, and corneal opacities (cornea verticillata). Electron photomicrographs of angiokeratomas and clinically normal skin demonstrate lamellar lipid deposits in fibroblasts, pericytes, and endothelial cells that are diagnostic of this disease. Widespread acute eruptions of erythematous papules are discussed in the section on exanthems.

There are several infectious diseases that present as erythematous papules or nodules in a lymphocutaneous or sporotrichoid pattern, i.e., in a linear arrangement along the lymphatic channels. The two most common etiologies are *Sporothrix schenckii* (sporotrichosis) and *M. marinum* (mycobacteria other than tuberculosis; atypical mycobacteria). The organisms are introduced as a result of trauma, and a primary inoculation site is often seen in addition to the lymphatic nodules. Additional causes include *Nocardia*, *Leishmania*, and other dimorphic fungi; culture of lesional tissue will aid in the diagnosis.

The diseases that are characterized by erythematous plaques with scale are reviewed in the papulosquamous section, and the various forms of dermatitis are discussed in the section on erythroderma. Additional disorders in the differential diagnosis of red papules/plaques include *erysipelas*, *polymorphous light eruption* (PMLE), *cutaneous lymphoid hyperplasia* (lymphocytoma cutis), *cutaneous lupus*, *lymphoma cutis*, and *leukemia cutis*. The first three diseases represent primary cutaneous disorders. PMLE is characterized by erythematous papules and plaques in a primarily sun-exposed distribution—dorsum of the hand, extensor forearm, and upper trunk. Lesions follow exposure to UV-B and/or UV-A, and in northern latitudes PMLE is most severe in the late spring and early summer. A process referred to as "hardening" occurs with continued UV exposure, and the eruption fades, but in temperate climates it will recur in the spring. PMLE must be differentiated from cutaneous lupus, and this is accomplished by histologic examination and direct immunofluorescence of the lesions. Cutaneous lymphoid hyperplasia (pseudolymphoma) is a *benign* polyclonal proliferation of lymphocytes in the skin that presents as infiltrated pink-red to red-purple papules and plaques; it must be distinguished from lymphoma cutis.

Several types of red plaques are seen in patients with systemic *lupus*, including (1) erythematous urticarial plaques across the cheeks and nose in the classic butterfly rash; (2) erythematous discoid lesions with fine or "carpet-tack" scale, telangiectasias, central hypopigmentation, peripheral hyperpigmentation, follicular plugging, and atrophy located on the face, scalp, external ears, arms, and upper trunk; and (3) psoriasiform or annular lesions of subacute lupus with hypopigmented centers located primarily on the extensor arms and upper trunk. Additional cutaneous findings include (1) a violaceous flush on the face and V of the neck; (2) urticarial vasculitis (see "Urticaria," above); (3) lupus panniculitis (see below); (4) diffuse alopecia; (5) alopecia secondary to discoid lesions; (6) periungual telangiectasias and erythema; (7) EM-like lesions that may become bullous; and (8) distal ulcerations secondary to Raynaud's phenomenon, vasculitis, or livedoid vasculopathy. Patients with only discoid lesions usually have the form of lupus that is limited to the skin. However, 2–10% of these patients eventually develop systemic lupus. Direct immunofluorescence of involved skin shows deposits of IgG or IgM and C3 in a granular distribution along the dermal-epidermal junction.

In *lymphoma cutis* there is a proliferation of malignant lymphocytes or histiocytes in the skin, and the clinical appearance resembles that of cutaneous lymphoid hyperplasia—infiltrated pink-red to red-purple papules and plaques. Lymphoma cutis can occur anywhere on the surface of the skin, whereas the sites of predilection for lymphocytomas include the malar ridge, tip of the nose, and earlobes. Patients with non-Hodgkin lymphomas have specific cutaneous lesions more often than those with Hodgkin disease, and occasionally, the skin nodules precede the development of extracutaneous non-Hodgkin lymphoma or represent the only site of involvement (e.g., primary cutaneous B cell lymphoma). Arcuate lesions are sometimes seen in lymphoma and lymphocytoma cutis as well as in CTCL. *Adult T cell leukemia/lymphoma* that develops in association with HTLV-1 infection is characterized by cutaneous plaques, hypercalcemia, and circulating CD25+ lymphocytes. *Leukemia cutis* has the same appearance as lymphoma cutis, and specific lesions are seen more commonly in monocytic leukemias than in lymphocytic or granulocytic leukemias. Cutaneous chloromas (granulocytic sarcomas) may precede the appearance of circulating blasts in acute myelogeneous leukemia and, as such, represent a form of aleukemic leukemia cutis.

Common causes of erythematous subcutaneous nodules include inflamed epidermoid inclusion cysts, acne cysts, and furuncles. *Panniculitis*, an inflammation of the fat, also presents as subcutaneous nodules and is frequently a sign of systemic disease. There are several forms of panniculitis, including erythema nodosum, erythema induratum/nodular vasculitis, lupus profundus, lipodermatosclerosis, α1-antitrypsin deficiency, factitial, and fat necrosis secondary to pancreatic disease. Except for erythema nodosum, these lesions may break down and ulcerate or heal with a scar. The shin is the most common location for the nodules of erythema nodosum, whereas the calf is the most common location for lesions of erythema induratum. In erythema nodosum the nodules are initially red but then develop a blue color as they resolve. Patients with erythema nodosum but no underlying systemic illness can still have fever, malaise, leukocytosis, arthralgias, and/or arthritis. However, the possibility of an underlying illness should be excluded, and the most common associations are streptococcal infections, upper respiratory viral infections, sarcoidosis, and inflammatory bowel disease in addition to drugs (oral contraceptives, sulfonamides, penicillins, bromides, iodides). Less common associations include bacterial gastroenteritis (*Yersinia, Salmonella*) and coccidioidomycosis followed by tuberculosis, histoplasmosis, brucellosis, and infections with *Chlamydophila pneumoniae* or *Chlamydia trachomatis, M. pneumoniae*, or hepatitis B virus.

Erythema induratum and nodular vasculitis share a similar histology and were thought to represent the clinical spectrum of a single entity; subsequently they have been separated, with the latter usually idiopathic and the former associated with the presence of *M. tuberculosis* DNA by polymerase chain reaction (PCR) within skin lesions. The lesions of lupus profundus are found primarily on the upper arms and buttocks (sites of abundant fat) and are seen in both the cutaneous and systemic forms of lupus. The overlying skin may be normal, erythematous, or have the changes of discoid lupus. The subcutaneous fat necrosis that is associated with pancreatic disease is presumably secondary to circulating lipases and is seen in patients with pancreatic carcinoma as well as in patients with acute and chronic pancreatitis. In this disorder there may be an associated arthritis, fever, and inflammation of visceral fat. Histologic examination of deep incisional biopsy specimens will aid in the diagnosis of the particular type of panniculitis.

Subcutaneous erythematous nodules are also seen in *cutaneous polyarteritis nodosa* (PAN) and as a manifestation of *systemic vasculitis*, e.g., systemic PAN, allergic granulomatosis, or Wegener's granulomatosis (Chap. 319). Cutaneous PAN presents with painful subcutaneous nodules and ulcers within a red-purple, netlike pattern of livedo reticularis. The latter is due to slowed blood flow through the superficial horizontal venous plexus. The majority of lesions are found on the lower extremity, and while arthralgias and myalgias may accompany cutaneous PAN, there is no evidence of systemic involvement. In both the cutaneous and systemic forms of vasculitis, skin biopsy specimens of the associated nodules will show the changes characteristic of a vasculitis; the size of the vessel involved will depend on the particular disease.

RED-BROWN LESIONS

The cutaneous lesions in *sarcoidosis* (Chap. 322) are classically red to red-brown in color, and with diascopy (pressure with a glass slide) a yellow-brown residual color is observed that is secondary to the granulomatous infiltrate. The waxy papules and plaques may be found anywhere on the skin, but the face is the most common location. Usually there are no surface changes, but occasionally the lesions will have scale. Biopsy specimens of the papules show "naked" granulomas in the dermis, i.e., granulomas surrounded by a minimal number of lymphocytes. Other cutaneous findings in sarcoidosis include annular lesions with an atrophic or scaly center, papules within scars, hypopigmented macules and papules, alopecia, acquired ichthyosis, erythema nodosum, and lupus pernio (see below).

The differential diagnosis of sarcoidosis includes foreign-body granulomas produced by chemicals such as beryllium and zirconium, late secondary syphilis, and *lupus vulgaris*. Lupus vulgaris is a form of cutaneous tuberculosis that is seen in previously infected and sensitized individuals. There is often underlying active tuberculosis elsewhere, usually in the lungs or lymph nodes. At least 90% of the lesions occur in the head and neck area and are red-brown plaques with a yellow-brown color on diascopy. Secondary scarring and squamous cell carcinomas can develop within the plaques. Cultures or PCR analysis of the lesions should be done because it is rare for the acid-fast stain to show bacilli within the dermal granulomas.

Sweet's syndrome is characterized by red to red-brown plaques and nodules that are frequently painful and occur primarily on the head, neck, and upper extremities. The patients also have fever, neutrophilia, and a dense dermal infiltrate of neutrophils in the lesions. In ~10% of the patients there

is an associated malignancy, most commonly acute myelogenous leukemia. Sweet's syndrome has also been reported with lymphoma, myeloma, myelodysplastic syndromes, and solid tumors (primarily of the genitourinary tract) as well as drugs (e.g., *all-trans*-retinoic acid). The differential diagnosis includes neutrophilic eccrine hidradenitis and atypical forms of pyoderma gangrenosum. Extracutaneous sites of involvement include joints, muscles, eye, kidney (proteinuria, occasionally glomerulonephritis), and lung (neutrophilic infiltrates). The idiopathic form of Sweet's syndrome is seen more often in women, following a respiratory tract infection.

A generalized distribution of red-brown macules and papules is seen in the form of mastocytosis known as *urticaria pigmentosa* (Chap. 311). Each lesion represents a collection of mast cells in the dermis, with hyperpigmentation of the overlying epidermis. Stimuli such as rubbing cause these mast cells to degranulate, and this leads to the formation of localized urticaria (Darier's sign). Additional symptoms can result from mast cell degranulation and include headache, flushing, diarrhea, and pruritus. Mast cells also infiltrate various organs such as the liver, spleen, and gastrointestinal tract, and accumulations of mast cells in the bones may produce either osteosclerotic or osteolytic lesions on radiographs. In the majority of these patients, however, the internal involvement remains indolent. A subtype of chronic cutaneous small-vessel vasculitis, *erythema elevatum diutinum* (EED), also presents with papules that are red-brown in color. The papules coalesce into plaques on the extensor surfaces of knees, elbows, and the small joints of the hand. Flares of EED have been associated with streptococcal infections.

BLUE LESIONS

Lesions that are blue in color are the result of either vascular ectasias and tumors or melanin pigment in the dermis. *Venous lakes* (ectasias) are compressible dark-blue lesions that are found commonly in the head and neck region. *Venous malformations* are also compressible blue papulonodules and plaques that can occur anywhere on the body, including the oral mucosa. When there are multiple rather than single congenital lesions, the patient may have the blue rubber bleb syndrome or Mafucci's syndrome. Patients with the blue rubber bleb syndrome also have vascular anomalies of the gastrointestinal tract that may bleed, whereas patients with Mafucci's syndrome have associated dyschondroplasia and osteochondromas. *Blue nevi* (moles) are seen when there are collections of pigment-producing nevus cells in the dermis. These benign papular lesions are dome-shaped and occur most commonly on the dorsum of the hand or foot or in the head and neck region.

VIOLACEOUS LESIONS

Violaceous papules and plaques are seen in *lupus pernio, lymphoma cutis*, and *cutaneous lupus*. Lupus pernio is a particular type of sarcoidosis that involves the tip and alar rim of the nose as well as the earlobes, with lesions that are violaceous in color rather than red-brown. This form of sarcoidosis is associated with involvement of the upper respiratory tract. The plaques of lymphoma cutis and cutaneous lupus may be red or violaceous in color and were discussed above.

PURPLE LESIONS

Purple-colored papules and plaques are seen in vascular tumors, such as *Kaposi's sarcoma* (Chap. 182) and *angiosarcoma*, and when there is extravasation of red blood cells into the skin in association with inflammation, as in *palpable purpura* (see "Purpura," below). Patients with congenital or acquired AV fistulas and venous hypertension can develop purple papules on the lower extremities that can resemble Kaposi's sarcoma clinically and histologically; this condition is referred to as pseudo-Kaposi sarcoma (acral angiodermatitis). Angiosarcoma is found most commonly on the scalp and face of elderly patients or within areas of chronic lymphedema and presents as purple papules and plaques. In the head and neck region the tumor often extends beyond the clinically defined borders and may be accompanied by facial edema.

BROWN AND BLACK LESIONS

Brown- and black-colored papules are reviewed in "Hyperpigmentation," above.

These are discussed last because they can have a wide range of colors. Most commonly they present as either firm, skin-colored subcutaneous nodules or firm, red to red-brown papulonodules. The lesions of lymphoma cutis range from pink-red to plum in color, whereas metastatic melanoma can be pink, blue, or black in color. Cutaneous metastases develop from hematogenous or lymphatic spread and are most often due to the following primary carcinomas: in men, lung, colon, melanoma, and oral cavity; and in women, breast, melanoma, and lung. These metastatic lesions may be the initial presentation of the carcinoma, especially when the primary site is the lung, kidney, or ovary.

PURPURA

(Table 54-16) *Purpura* are seen when there is an extravasation of red blood cells into the dermis and, as a result, the lesions do not blanch with pressure. This is in contrast to those erythematous or violet-colored lesions that are due to localized vasodilatation—they do blanch with pressure. Purpura (≥3 mm) and petechiae (≤2 mm) are divided into two major groups, palpable and nonpalpable. The most frequent causes of *nonpalpable* petechiae and purpura are primary cutaneous disorders such as *trauma, solar (actinic) purpura,* and *capillaritis.* Less common causes are *steroid purpura* and *livedoid vasculopathy* (see "Ulcers," below). Solar purpura are seen primarily on the extensor forearms, while steroid purpura secondary topotent topical glucocorticoids or endogenous or exogenous Cushing's syndrome can be more widespread. In both cases there is alteration of the supporting connective tissue that surrounds the dermal blood vessels. In contrast, the petechiae that result from capillaritis are found primarily on the lower extremities. In capillaritis there is an

TABLE 54-16 CAUSES OF PURPURA

I. Primary cutaneous disorders
  A. Nonpalpable
    1. Trauma
    2. Solar purpura
    3. Steroid purpura
    4. Capillaritis
    5. Livedoid vasculopathy[a]
II. Systemic diseases
  A. Nonpalpable
    1. Clotting disturbances
      a. Thrombocytopenia (including ITP)
      b. Abnormal platelet function
      c. Clotting factor defects
    2. Vascular fragility
      a. Amyloidosis
      b. Ehlers-Danlos syndrome
      c. Scurvy
    3. Thrombi
      a. Disseminated intravascular coagulation
      b. Monoclonal cryoglobulinemia
      c. Heparin-induced thrombocytopenia and thrombosis
      d. Thrombotic thrombocytopenic purpura
      e. Warfarin reaction
    4. Emboli
      a. Cholesterol
      b. Fat
    5. Possible immune complex
      a. Gardner-Diamond syndrome (autoerythrocyte sensitivity)
      b. Waldenström's hypergammaglobulinemic purpura
  B. Palpable
    1. Vasculitis
      a. Cutaneous small-vessel vasculitis
      b. Polyarteritis nodosa
    2. Emboli[b]
      a. Acute meningococcemia
      b. Disseminated gonococcal infection
      c. Rocky Mountain spotted fever
      d. Ecthyma gangrenosum

[a]Also associated with systemic diseases.
[b]Bacterial, fungal, or parasitic.
Note: ITP, idiopathic thrombocytopenic purpura.

extravasation of erythrocytes as a result of perivascular lymphocytic inflammation. The petechiae are bright red, 1–2 mm in size, and scattered within annular or coin-shaped yellow-brown macules. The yellow-brown color is caused by hemosiderin deposits within the dermis.

Systemic causes of nonpalpable purpura fall into several categories, and those secondary to clotting disturbances and vascular fragility will be discussed first. The former group includes *thrombocytopenia* (Chap. 109), *abnormal platelet function* as is seen in uremia, and *clotting factor defects.* The initial site of presentation for thrombocytopenia-induced petechiae is the distal lower extremity. Capillary fragility leads to nonpalpable purpura in patients with systemic *amyloidosis* (see "Papulonodular Skin Lesions," above), disorders of collagen production such as *Ehlers-Danlos syndrome,* and *scurvy.* In scurvy there are flattened corkscrew hairs with surrounding hemorrhage on the lower extremities, in addition to gingivitis. Vitamin C is a cofactor for lysyl hydroxylase, an enzyme involved in the posttranslational modification of procollagen that is necessary for cross-link formation.

In contrast to the previous group of disorders, the purpura seen in the following group of diseases are associated with thrombi formation within vessels. It is important to note that these thrombi are demonstrable in skin biopsy specimens. This group of disorders includes disseminated intravascular coagulation (DIC), monoclonal cryoglobulinemia, thrombotic thrombocytopenic purpura, and reactions to warfarin and heparin (heparin-induced thrombocytopenia and thrombosis). DIC is triggered by several types of infection (gram-negative, gram-positive, viral, and rickettsial) as well as by tissue injury and neoplasms. Widespread purpura and hemorrhagic infarcts of the distal extremities are seen. Similar lesions are found in purpura fulminans, which is a form of DIC associated with fever and hypotension that occurs more commonly in children following an infectious illness such as varicella, scarlet fever, or an upper respiratory tract infection. In both disorders, hemorrhagic bullae can develop in involved skin.

Monoclonal cryoglobulinemia is associated with multiple myeloma, Waldenström's macroglobulinemia, lymphocytic leukemia, and lymphoma. Purpura, primarily of the lower extremities, and hemorrhagic infarcts of the fingers and toes are seen in these patients. Exacerbations of disease activity can follow cold exposure or an increase in serum viscosity. Biopsy specimens show precipitates of the cryoglobulin within dermal vessels. Similar deposits have been found in the lung, brain, and renal glomeruli. Patients with *thrombotic thrombocytopenic purpura* can also have hemorrhagic infarcts as a result of intravascular thromboses. Additional signs include thrombocytopenic purpura, fever, and microangiopathic hemolytic anemia (Chap. 101).

Administration of *warfarin* can result in painful areas of erythema that become purpuric and then necrotic with an adherent black eschar; the condition is referred to as warfarin-induced necrosis. This reaction is seen more often in women and in areas with abundant subcutaneous fat—breasts, abdomen, buttocks, thighs, and calves. The erythema and purpura develop between the third and tenth day of therapy, most likely as a result of a transient imbalance in the levels of anticoagulant and procoagulant vitamin K–dependent factors. Continued therapy does not exacerbate preexisting lesions, and patients with an inherited or acquired deficiency of protein C are at increased risk for this particular reaction as well as for purpura fulminans.

Purpura secondary to *cholesterol emboli* are usually seen on the lower extremities of patients with atherosclerotic vascular disease. They often follow anticoagulant therapy or an invasive vascular procedure such as an arteriogram but also occur spontaneously from disintegration of atheromatous plaques. Associated findings include livedo reticularis, gangrene, cyanosis, and ischemic ulcerations. Multiple step sections of the biopsy specimen may be necessary to demonstrate the cholesterol clefts within the vessels. Petechiae are also an important sign of *fat embolism* and occur primarily on the upper body 2–3 days after a major injury. By using special fixatives, the emboli can be demonstrated in biopsy specimens of the petechiae. Emboli of tumor or thrombus are seen in patients with atrial myxomas and marantic endocarditis.

In the *Gardner-Diamond syndrome* (autoerythrocyte sensitivity), female patients develop large ecchymoses within areas of painful, warm erythema. Intradermal injections of autologous erythrocytes or phosphatidyl serine derived from the red cell membrane can reproduce the lesions in some patients; however, there are instances where a reaction is seen at an injection site of the forearm but not in the midback region. The latter has led some observers to view Gardner-Diamond syndrome as a cutaneous manifestation of severe emotional stress. More recently, the possibility of platelet dysfunction (as assessed via aggregation studies) has been raised. *Waldenström's hypergammaglobulinemic purpura* is a chronic disorder characterized by petechiae on the lower extremities. There are circulating complexes of IgG–anti-IgG molecules, and exacerbations are associated with prolonged standing or walking.

Palpable purpura are further subdivided into vasculitic and embolic. In the group of vasculitic disorders, cutaneous small-vessel vasculitis, also known as *leukocytoclastic vasculitis* (LCV), is the one most commonly associated with palpable purpura (Chap. 319). Underlying etiologies include drugs (e.g., antibiotics), infections (e.g., hepatitis C virus), and autoimmune connective tissue diseases. *Henoch-Schönlein purpura* is a subtype of acute LCV that is seen primarily in children and adolescents following an upper respiratory infection. The majority of lesions are found on the lower extremities and buttocks. Systemic manifestations include fever, arthralgias (primarily of the knees and ankles), abdominal pain, gastrointestinal bleeding, and nephritis. Direct immunofluorescence examination shows deposits of IgA within dermal blood vessel walls. In *polyarteritis nodosa*, specific cutaneous lesions result from a vasculitis of arterial vessels or there may be an associated LCV. The arteritis leads to ischemia of the skin, and this explains the irregular outline of the purpura (see below).

Several types of infectious emboli can give rise to palpable purpura. These embolic lesions are usually *irregular* in outline as opposed to the lesions of LCV, which are *circular* in outline. The irregular outline is indicative of a cutaneous infarct, and the size corresponds to the area of skin that received its blood supply from that particular arteriole or artery. The palpable purpura in LCV are circular because the erythrocytes simply diffuse out evenly from the postcapillary venules as a result of inflammation. Infectious emboli are most commonly due to gram-negative cocci (meningococcus, gonococcus), gram-negative rods (Enterobacteriaceae), and gram-positive cocci (*Staphylococcus*). Additional causes include *Rickettsia* and, in immunocompromised patients, *Candida* and opportunistic fungi.

The embolic lesions in *acute meningococcemia* are found primarily on the trunk, lower extremities, and sites of pressure, and a gunmetal-gray color often develops within them. Their size varies from 1 mm to several centimeters, and the organisms can be cultured from the lesions. Associated findings include a preceding upper respiratory tract infection, fever, meningitis, DIC, and, in some patients, a deficiency of the terminal components of complement. In *disseminated gonococcal infection* (arthritis-dermatitis syndrome), a small number of papules and vesicopustules with central purpura or hemorrhagic necrosis are found on the distal extremities. Additional symptoms include arthralgias, tenosynovitis, and fever. To establish the diagnosis, a Gram stain of these lesions should be performed. *Rocky Mountain spotted fever* is a tick-borne disease that is caused by *R. rickettsii*. A several-day history of fever, chills, severe headache, and photophobia precedes the onset of the cutaneous eruption. The initial lesions are erythematous macules and papules on the wrists, ankles, palms, and soles. With time, the lesions spread centripetally and become purpuric.

Lesions of *ecthyma gangrenosum* begin as edematous, erythematous papules or plaques and then develop central purpura and necrosis. Bullae formation also occurs in these lesions, and they are frequently found in the girdle region. The organism that is classically associated with ecthyma gangrenosum is *Pseudomonas aeruginosa*, but other gram-negative rods such as *Klebsiella*, *Escherichia coli*, and *Serratia* can produce similar lesions. In immunocompromised hosts, the list of potential pathogens is expanded to include *Candida* and opportunistic fungi.

ULCERS

The approach to the patient with a cutaneous ulcer is outlined in Table 54-17. Peripheral vascular diseases of the extremities are reviewed in Chap. 243, as is Raynaud's phenomenon.

TABLE 54-17 CAUSES OF CUTANEOUS ULCERS

I. Primary cutaneous disorders
  A. Peripheral vascular disease (Chap. 243)
    1. Venous
    2. Arterial
  B. Livedoid vasculopathy[a]
  C. Squamous cell carcinoma, e.g., within scars
  D. Infections, e.g., ecthyma caused by *Streptococcus* (Chap. 130)
II. Systemic diseases
  A. Lower legs
    1. Cutaneous small-vessel vasculitis[b]
    2. Hemoglobinopathies (Chap. 99)
    3. Cryoglobulinemia,[b] cryofibrinogenemia
    4. Cholesterol emboli[b]
    5. Necrobiosis lipoidica[c]
    6. Antiphospholipid syndrome (Chap. 110)
    7. Neuropathic[d] (Chap. 338)
    8. Panniculitis
  B. Hands and feet
    1. Raynaud's phenomenon (Chap. 243)
  C. Generalized
    1. Pyoderma gangrenosum
    2. Calciphylaxis (Chap. 347)
    3. Infections, e.g., dimorphic fungi, chronic herpes simplex
    4. Lymphoma
  D. Mucosal
    1. Behçet's syndrome (Chap. 320)
    2. Erythema multiforme major, Stevens-Johnson syndrome, TEN
    3. Primary blistering disorders (Chap. 55)
    4. Lupus erythematosus
    5. Inflammatory bowel disease

[a]Also associated with systemic diseases.
[b]Reviewed in section on Purpura.
[c]Reviewed in section on Papulonodular Skin Lesions.
[d]Favors plantar surface of the foot.
Note: TEN, toxic epidermal necrolysis.

Livedoid vasculopathy (livedoid vasculitis; atrophie blanche) represents a combination of a vasculopathy plus intravascular thrombosis. Purpuric lesions and livedo reticularis are found in association with *painful* ulcerations of the lower extremities. These ulcers are often slow to heal, but when they do, irregularly shaped white scars are formed. The majority of cases are secondary to venous hypertension, but possible underlying illnesses include cryofibrinogenemia and disorders of hypercoagulability, e.g., the antiphospholipid syndrome (Chaps. 111 and 313).

In *pyoderma gangrenosum*, the border of the ulcers has a characteristic appearance of an undermined necrotic violaceous edge and a peripheral erythematous halo. The ulcers often begin as pustules that then expand rather rapidly to a size as large as 20 cm. Although these lesions are most commonly found on the lower extremities, they can arise anywhere on the surface of the body, including sites of trauma (pathergy). An estimated 30–50% of cases are idiopathic, and the most common associated disorders are ulcerative colitis and Crohn's disease. Less commonly, pyoderma gangrenosum is associated with seropositive rheumatoid arthritis, acute and chronic myelogenous leukemia, hairy cell leukemia, and myelofibrosis. Additional findings in these patients, even those with idiopathic disease, are cutaneous anergy and a monoclonal gammopathy, usually IgA. Because the histology of pyoderma gangrenosum may be nonspecific (dermal infiltrate of neutrophils when in untreated state), the diagnosis is usually made clinically and includes excluding less common causes of similar-appearing ulcers such as necrotizing vasculitis, Meleney's ulcer (synergistic infection at a site of trauma or surgery), dimorphic fungi, cutaneous amebiasis, spider bites, and factitial. In the myeloproliferative disorders, the ulcers may be more superficial with a pustulobullous border, and these lesions provide a connection between classic pyoderma gangrenosum and acute febrile neutrophilic dermatosis (Sweet's syndrome).

FEVER AND RASH

The major considerations in a patient with a fever and a rash are inflammatory diseases versus infectious diseases. In the hospital setting, the most common scenario is a patient who has a drug rash plus a fever secondary to an underlying infection. However, it should be emphasized that a drug reaction can lead to both a cutaneous eruption and a fever ("drug fever"), especially in the setting of DRESS. Additional inflammatory diseases that are often associated with a fever include pustular psoriasis, erythroderma, and Sweet's syndrome. Lyme disease, secondary syphilis, and viral and bacterial exanthems (see "Exanthems," above) are examples of infectious diseases that produce a rash and a fever. Lastly, it is important to determine whether or not the cutaneous lesions represent septic emboli (see "Purpura," above). Such lesions usually have evidence of ischemia in the form of purpura, necrosis, or impending necrosis (gunmetal-gray color). In the patient with thrombocytopenia, however, purpura can be seen in inflammatory reactions such as morbilliform drug eruptions and infectious lesions.

FURTHER READINGS

BOLOGNIA JL et al: *Dermatology*, 2d ed. Philadelphia, Mosby, 2007
BRAVERMAN IM: *Skin Signs of Systemic Disease*, 3d ed. Philadelphia, Saunders, 1998
CALLEN JP et al: *Dermatological Signs of Internal Disease*, 3d ed. Philadelphia, Saunders, 2003
MCKEE PH et al: *Pathology of the Skin*, 3d ed. London, Elsevier, 2005
SPITZ JL: *Genodermatoses: A Clinical Guide to Genetic Skin Disorders*, 2d ed. Lippincott Williams & Wilkins, 2004

55 Immunologically Mediated Skin Diseases

Kim B. Yancey, Thomas J. Lawley

A number of immunologically mediated skin diseases and immunologically mediated systemic disorders with cutaneous manifestations are now recognized as distinct entities with consistent clinical, histologic, and immunopathologic findings. Many of these disorders are due to autoimmune mechanisms. Clinically, they are characterized by morbidity (pain, pruritus, disfigurement) and in some instances by mortality (largely due to loss of epidermal barrier function and/or secondary infection). The major features of the more common immunologically mediated skin diseases are summarized in this chapter (Table 55-1), as are the systemic disorders with cutaneous manifestations.

AUTOIMMUNE CUTANEOUS DISEASES

PEMPHIGUS VULGARIS

Pemphigus refers to a group of autoantibody-mediated intraepidermal blistering diseases characterized by loss of cohesion between epidermal cells (a process termed *acantholysis*). Manual pressure to the skin of these patients may elicit the separation of the epidermis (Nikolsky's sign). This finding, while characteristic of pemphigus, is not specific to this group of disorders and is also seen in toxic epidermal necrolysis, Stevens-Johnson syndrome, and a few other skin diseases.

Pemphigus vulgaris (PV) is a mucocutaneous blistering disease that predominates in patients >40 years. PV typically begins on mucosal surfaces; it often progresses to a mucocutaneous disease in which fragile, flaccid blisters rupture to produce extensive denudation of the skin (Fig. 55-1). PV typically involves the mouth, scalp, face, neck, axilla, groin, and trunk. PV may be associated with severe skin pain; some patients experience pruritus as well. Lesions usually heal without scarring, except at sites complicated by secondary infection or mechanically induced dermal wounds. Postinflammatory

TABLE 55-1	IMMUNOLOGICALLY MEDIATED BLISTERING DISEASES			
Disease	**Clinical**	**Histology**	**Immunopathology**	**Autoantigens**[a]
Pemphigus foliaceus	Crusts and shallow erosions on scalp, central face, upper chest, and back	Acantholytic blister formed in superficial layer of epidermis	Cell surface deposits of IgG on keratinocytes	Dsg1
Pemphigus vulgaris	Flaccid blisters, denuded skin, oromucosal lesions	Acantholytic blister formed in suprabasal layer of epidermis	Cell surface deposits of IgG on keratinocytes	Dsg3 (plus Dsg1 in patients with skin involvement)
Paraneoplastic pemphigus	Painful stomatitis with papulosquamous or lichenoid eruptions that progress to blisters	Acantholysis, keratinocyte necrosis and vacuolar interface dermatitis	Cell surface deposits of IgG and C3 on keratinocytes and (variably) similar immunoreactants in epidermal BMZ	Plakin protein family members and desmosomal cadherins (see text for details)
Bullous pemphigoid	Large tense blisters on flexor surfaces and trunk	Subepidermal blister with eosinophil-rich infiltrate	Linear band of IgG and/or C3 in epidermal BMZ	BPAG1, BPAG2
Pemphigoid gestationis	Pruritic, urticarial plaques, rimmed by vesicles and bullae on the trunk and extremities	Teardrop-shaped, subepidermal blisters in dermal papillae; eosinophil-rich infiltrate	Linear band of C3 in epidermal BMZ	BPAG2 (plus BPAG1 in some patients)
Linear IgA disease	Pruritic small papules on extensor surfaces; occasionally larger, arciform blisters	Subepidermal blister with neutrophil-rich infiltrate	Linear band of IgA in epidermal BMZ	BPAG2 (see text for specific details)
Cicatricial pemphigoid	Erosive and/or blistering lesions of mucous membranes and possibly the skin; scarring of some sites	Subepidermal blister that may or may not include a leukocytic infiltrate	Linear band of IgG, IgA, and/or C3 in epidermal BMZ	BPAG2, laminin 5, or others
Epidermolysis bullosa acquisita	Blisters, erosions, scars, and milia on sites exposed to trauma; widespread, inflammatory, tense blisters may be seen initially	Subepidermal blister that may or may not include a leukocytic infiltrate	Linear band of IgG and/or C3 in epidermal BMZ	Type VII collagen
Dermatitis herpetiformis	Extremely pruritic small papules and vesicles on elbows, knees, buttocks, and posterior neck	Subepidermal blister with neutrophils in dermal papillae	Granular deposits of IgA in dermal papillae	Epidermal transglutaminase

[a]Autoantigens bound by these patients' autoantibodies are defined as follows: Dsg1, desmoglein 1; Dsg3, desmoglein 3; BPAG1, bullous pemphigoid antigen 1; BPAG2, bullous pemphigoid antigen 2.
Note: BMZ, basement membrane zone.

A

B

FIGURE 55-1 Pemphigus vulgaris. A. Pemphigus vulgaris demonstrating flaccid bullae that are easily ruptured, resulting in multiple erosions and crusted plaques. **B.** Pemphigus vulgaris almost invariably involves the oral mucosa and may present with erosions involving the gingiva, buccal mucosa, palate, posterior pharynx, or the tongue. (**B**, *Courtesy of Robert Swerlick, MD; with permission.*)

hyperpigmentation is usually present at sites of healed lesions for some time.

Biopsies of early lesions demonstrate intraepidermal vesicle formation secondary to loss of cohesion between epidermal cells (i.e., acantholytic blisters). Blister cavities contain acantholytic epidermal cells, which appear as round homogeneous cells containing hyperchromatic nuclei. Basal keratinocytes remain attached to the epidermal basement membrane, hence blister formation is within the suprabasal portion of the epidermis. Lesional skin may contain focal collections of intraepidermal eosinophils within blister cavities; dermal alterations are slight, often limited to an eosinophil-predominant leukocytic infiltrate. Direct immunofluorescence microscopy of lesional or intact patient skin shows deposits of IgG on the surface of keratinocytes; deposits of complement components are typically found in lesional but not uninvolved skin. Deposits of IgG on keratinocytes are derived from circulating autoantibodies directed against cell-surface autoantigens. Such circulating autoantibodies can be demonstrated in 80–90% of PV patients by indirect immunofluorescence microscopy; monkey esophagus is the optimal substrate for these

to the cadherin family of calcium-dependent adhesion molecules. Such autoantibodies can be precisely quantitated by enzyme-linked immunosorbent assay (ELISA). Patients with early PV (i.e., mucosal disease) have only IgG autoantibodies directed against Dsg3; patients with advanced PV (i.e., mucocutaneous disease) have IgG autoantibodies directed against both Dsg3 and Dsg1. Experimental studies have shown that autoantibodies from patients with PV are pathogenic (i.e., responsible for blister formation) and that their titer correlates with disease activity. Recent studies have shown that the anti-Dsg autoantibody profile in these patients' sera as well as the tissue distribution of Dsg3 and Dsg1 determine the site of blister formation in patients with pemphigus. Coexpression of Dsg3 and Dsg1 by epidermal cells protects against pathogenic IgG directed against either cadherin but not pathogenic autoantibodies directed against both.

PV can be life-threatening. Prior to the availability of glucocorticoids, the mortality ranged from 60–90%; the current mortality is ~5%. Common causes of morbidity and mortality are infection and complications of treatment with glucocorticoids. Bad prognostic factors include advanced age, widespread involvement, and the requirement for high doses of glucocorticoids (with or without other immunosuppressive agents) for control of disease. The course of PV in individual patients is variable and difficult to predict. Some patients achieve remission, while others may require long-term treatment or succumb to complications of their disease or its treatment. The mainstay of treatment is systemic glucocorticoids. Patients with moderate to severe PV are usually started on prednisone, 1 mg/kg per day. If new lesions continue to appear after 1–2 weeks of treatment, the dose may need to be increased. Many regimens combine an immunosuppressive agent with systemic glucocorticoids for control of PV. The most frequently used are azathioprine (2–2.5 mg/kg per day), mycophenolate mofetil (20–35 mg/kg per day), or cyclophosphamide (1–2 mg/kg per day). Patients with severe, treatment-resistant disease may derive benefit from plasmapheresis [six high-volume exchanges (i.e., 2–3 liters per exchange) over ~2 weeks], IV immunoglobulin (2 g/kg over 3–5 days every 6–8 weeks), or rituximab (375 mg/m^2 per week × 4). It is important to bring severe or progressive disease under control quickly to lessen the severity and/or duration of this disorder.

PEMPHIGUS FOLIACEUS

Pemphigus foliaceus (PF) is distinguished from PV by several features. In PF, acantholytic blisters are located high within the epidermis, usually just beneath the stratum corneum. Hence PF is a more superficial blistering disease than PV. The distribution of lesions in the two disorders is much the same, except that in PF mucous membranes are almost always spared. Patients with PF rarely demonstrate intact blisters but rather exhibit shallow erosions associated with erythema, scale, and crust formation. Mild cases of PF resemble severe seborrheic dermatitis; severe PF may cause extensive exfoliation. Sun exposure (ultraviolet irradiation) may be an aggravating factor. *Fogo selvagem* (FS), an endemic form of PF thought to develop as a consequence of environmental stimuli (e.g., insect bites), is found in south central rural Brazil as well as selected sites in Latin America and Tunisia.

Patients with PF have immunopathologic features in common with PV. Specifically, direct immunofluorescence microscopy of perilesional skin demonstrates IgG on the surface of keratinocytes. Similarly, patients with PF have circulating IgG autoantibodies directed against the surface of keratinocytes. Guinea pig esophagus is the optimal substrate for indirect immunofluorescence microscopy studies of sera from patients with PF. In PF, autoantibodies are directed against Dsg1, a 160-kDa desmosomal cadherin. As noted for PV, the autoantibody profile in patients with PF (i.e., anti-Dsg1 IgG) and the tissue distribution of this autoantigen (i.e., expression in oral mucosa that is compensated by coexpression of Dsg3) is thought to account for the distribution of lesions in this disease.

Although pemphigus has been associated with several autoimmune diseases, its association with thymoma and/or myasthenia gravis is particularly notable. To date, >30 cases of thymoma and/or myasthenia gravis have been reported in association with pemphigus, usually with PF. Patients may also develop pemphigus as a consequence of drug exposure; drug-induced pemphigus usually resembles PF rather than PV. Drugs containing a thiol group in their chemical structure (e.g., penicillamine, captopril, enalapril) are most commonly associated with drug-induced pemphigus. Nonthiol drugs linked to pemphigus include penicillins, cephalosporins, and piroxicam. It has been suggested that thiol- and nonthiol-containing drugs induce pemphigus via biochemical and immunologic mechanisms, respectively. Hence, the better prognosis upon drug withdrawal in cases of pemphigus induced by thiol-containing medications. Some cases of drug-induced pemphigus are durable and require treatment with systemic glucocorticoids and/or immunosuppressive agents.

PF is generally a less severe disease than PV and carries a better prognosis. Localized disease can sometimes be treated with topical or intralesional glucocorticoids; more active cases can usually be controlled with systemic glucocorticoids. Patients with severe, treatment-resistant disease may require more aggressive interventions as described above for patients with severe PV.

PARANEOPLASTIC PEMPHIGUS

Paraneoplastic pemphigus (PNP) is an autoimmune acantholytic mucocutaneous disease associated with an occult or confirmed neoplasm. Patients with PNP typically show painful mucosal erosive lesions in association with papulosquamous and/or lichenoid eruptions that often progress to blisters. Palm and sole involvement is common in these patients and raises the possibility that prior reports of neoplasia-associated erythema multiforme actually may have represented unrecognized cases of PNP. Biopsies of lesional skin from these patients show varying combinations of acantholysis, keratinocyte necrosis, and vacuolar-interface dermatitis. Direct immunofluorescence microscopy of patient skin shows deposits of IgG and complement on the surface of keratinocytes and (variably) similar immunoreactants in the epidermal basement membrane zone. Patients with PNP have IgG autoantibodies against cytoplasmic proteins that are members of the plakin family (e.g., desmoplakins I and II, bullous pemphigoid antigen 1, envoplakin, periplakin, and plectin) and cell-surface proteins that are members of the cadherin family (e.g., Dsg3 and Dsg1). Passive transfer studies have shown that autoantibodies from patients with PNP are pathogenic.

The predominant neoplasms associated with PNP are non-Hodgkin's lymphoma, chronic lymphocytic leukemia, thymoma, spindle cell tumors, Waldenström's macroglobulinemia, and Castleman's disease; the latter is particularly common among children with PNP. In addition to severe skin lesions, many patients with PNP develop life-threatening bronchiolitis obliterans. PNP is generally resistant to conventional therapies (i.e., those used to treat PV); rare patients may improve (or even remit) following ablation or removal of underlying neoplasms.

BULLOUS PEMPHIGOID

Bullous pemphigoid (BP) is a polymorphic autoimmune subepidermal blistering disease usually seen in the elderly. Initial lesions may consist of urticarial plaques; most patients eventually display tense blisters on either normal-appearing or erythematous skin (Fig. 55-2). The lesions are usually distributed over the lower abdomen, groin, and flexor surface of the extremities; oral mucosal lesions are found in some patients. Pruritus may be nonexistent or severe. As lesions evolve, tense blisters tend to rupture and be replaced by erosions with or without surmounting crust. Nontraumatized blisters heal without scarring. The major histocompatibility complex class II allele HLA-DQβ1*0301 is prevalent in patients with BP. Despite isolated reports, several studies have shown that patients with BP do not have an increased incidence of malignancy in comparison with appropriately age- and gender-matched controls.

Biopsies of early lesional skin demonstrate subepidermal blisters and histologic features that roughly correlate with the clinical character of the particular lesion under study. Lesions on normal-appearing skin generally show a sparse perivascular leukocytic infiltrate with some eosinophils; conversely, biopsies of inflammatory lesions typically show an eosinophil-rich infiltrate at sites of vesicle formation and in perivascular areas. In addition to eosinophils, cell-rich lesions also contain mononuclear

FIGURE 55-2 Bullous pemphigoid with tense vesicles and bullae on erythematous, urticarial bases. (*Courtesy of the Yale Resident's Slide Collection; with permission.*)

cells and neutrophils. It is not possible to distinguish BP from other subepidermal blistering diseases by routine histologic techniques alone.

Direct immunofluorescence microscopy of normal-appearing perilesional skin from patients with BP shows linear deposits of IgG and/or C3 in the epidermal basement membrane. The sera of ~70% of these patients contain circulating IgG autoantibodies that bind the epidermal basement membrane of normal human skin in indirect immunofluorescence microscopy. IgG from an even higher percentage of patients shows reactivity to the epidermal side of 1 M NaCl split skin [an alternative immunofluorescence microscopy test substrate used to distinguish circulating IgG anti-basement membrane autoantibodies in patients with BP from those in patients with similar, yet different, subepidermal blistering diseases (see below)]. In BP, circulating autoantibodies recognize 230- and 180-kDa hemidesmosome-associated proteins in basal keratinocytes [i.e., bullous pemphigoid antigen (BPAG)1 and BPAG2, respectively]. Autoantibodies against BPAG2 are thought to deposit in situ, activate complement, produce dermal mast cell degranulation, and generate granulocyte-rich infiltrates that cause tissue damage and blister formation.

BP may persist for months to years, with exacerbations or remissions. Although extensive involvement may result in widespread erosions and compromise cutaneous integrity, the mortality rate is relatively low. Nonetheless, deaths may occur in elderly and/or debilitated patients. The mainstay of treatment is systemic glucocorticoids. Patients with local or minimal disease can sometimes be controlled with topical glucocorticoids alone; patients with more extensive lesions generally respond to systemic glucocorticoids either alone or in combination with immunosuppressive agents. Patients will usually respond to prednisone, 0.75–1 mg/kg per day. In some instances, azathioprine (2–2.5 mg/kg per day), mycophenolate mofetil (20–35 mg/kg per day), or cyclophosphamide (1–2 mg/kg per day) are necessary adjuncts.

PEMPHIGOID GESTATIONIS

Pemphigoid gestationis (PG), also known as *herpes gestationis*, is a rare, nonviral, subepidermal blistering disease of pregnancy and the puerperium. PG may begin during any trimester of pregnancy or present shortly after delivery. Lesions are usually distributed over the abdomen, trunk, and extremities; mucous membrane lesions are rare. Skin lesions in these patients may be quite polymorphic and consist of erythematous urticarial papules and plaques, vesiculopapules, and/or frank bullae. Lesions are almost always very pruritic. Severe exacerbations of PG frequently occur after delivery, typically within 24–48 h. PG tends to recur in subsequent pregnancies, often beginning earlier during such gestations. Brief flare-ups of disease may occur with resumption of menses and may develop in patients later exposed to oral contraceptives. Occasionally, infants of affected mothers demonstrate transient skin lesions.

Biopsies of early lesional skin show teardrop-shaped subepidermal vesicles forming in dermal papillae in association with an eosinophil-rich leukocytic infiltrate. Differentiation of PG from other subepidermal bullous diseases by light microscopy is difficult. However, direct immunofluorescence microscopy of perilesional skin from PG patients reveals the immunopathologic hallmark of this disorder—linear deposits of C3 in epidermal basement membrane. These deposits develop as a consequence of complement activation produced by low titer IgG anti-basement membrane autoantibodies directed against BPAG2, the same hemidesmosome-associated protein that is targeted by autoantibodies in patients with BP—a subepidermal bullous disease that resembles PG clinically, histologically, and immunopathologically.

The goals of therapy in patients with PG are to prevent the development of new lesions, relieve intense pruritus, and care for erosions at sites of blister formation. Many patients require treatment with moderate doses of daily glucocorticoids (i.e., 20–40 mg prednisone) at some point in their course. Mild cases (or brief flare-ups) may be controlled by vigorous use of potent topical glucocorticoids. Infants born of mothers with PG appear to be at increased risk of being slightly premature or "small for dates." Current evidence suggests that there is no difference in the incidence of uncomplicated live births in PG patients treated with systemic glucocorticoids and in those managed more conservatively. If systemic glucocorticoids are administered, newborns are at risk for development of reversible adrenal insufficiency.

DERMATITIS HERPETIFORMIS

Dermatitis herpetiformis (DH) is an intensely pruritic, papulovesicular skin disease characterized by lesions symmetrically distributed over extensor surfaces (i.e., elbows, knees, buttocks, back, scalp, and posterior neck) (see Fig. 52-8). Primary lesions in this disorder consist of papules, papulovesicles, or urticarial plaques. Because pruritus is prominent, patients may present with excoriations and crusted papules but no observable primary lesions. Patients sometimes report that their pruritus has a distinctive burning or stinging component; the onset of such local symptoms reliably heralds the development of distinct clinical lesions 12–24 h later. Almost all DH patients have an associated, usually subclinical, gluten-sensitive enteropathy (Chap. 288), and >90% express the HLA-B8/DRw3 and HLA-DQw2 haplotypes. DH may present at any age, including childhood; onset in the second to fourth decades is most common. The disease is typically chronic.

Biopsy of early lesional skin reveals neutrophil-rich infiltrates within dermal papillae. Neutrophils, fibrin, edema, and microvesicle formation at these sites are characteristic of early disease. Older lesions may demonstrate nonspecific features of a subepidermal bulla or an excoriated papule. Because the clinical and histologic features of this disease can be variable and resemble other subepidermal blistering disorders, the diagnosis is confirmed by direct immunofluorescence microscopy of normal-appearing perilesional skin. Such studies demonstrate granular deposits of IgA (with or without complement components) in the papillary dermis and along the epidermal basement membrane zone. IgA deposits in the skin are unaffected by control of disease with medication; however, these immunoreactants may diminish in intensity or disappear in patients maintained for long periods on a strict gluten-free diet (see below). Patients with DH have granular deposits of IgA in their epidermal basement membrane zone and should be distinguished from individuals with linear IgA deposits at this site (see below).

Although most DH patients do not report overt gastrointestinal symptoms or have laboratory evidence of malabsorption, biopsies of small bowel usually reveal blunting of intestinal villi and a lymphocytic infiltrate in the lamina propria. As is true for patients with celiac disease, this gastrointestinal abnormality can be reversed by a gluten-free diet. Moreover, if maintained, this diet alone may control the skin disease and eventuate in clearance of IgA deposits from these patients' epidermal basement membrane zone. Subsequent gluten exposure in such patients alters the morphology of their small bowel, elicits a flare-up of their skin disease, and is associated with the reappearance of IgA in their epidermal basement membrane zone. As in patients with celiac disease, dietary gluten sensitivity in patients with DH is associated with IgA anti-endomysial autoantibodies that target tissue transglutaminase. Recent studies suggest that patients with DH also have high-avidity IgA autoantibodies against epidermal transglutaminase 3 and that the latter is co-localized with granular deposits of IgA in the papillary dermis of DH patients. Patients with DH also have an increased incidence of thyroid abnormalities, achlorhydria, atrophic gastritis, and antigastric parietal cell autoantibodies. These associations likely relate to the high frequency of the HLA-B8/DRw3 haplotype in these patients, since this marker is commonly linked to autoimmune disorders. The mainstay of treatment of DH is dapsone, a sulfone. Patients respond rapidly (24–48 h) to dapsone (50–200 mg/d) but require careful pretreatment evaluation and close follow-up to ensure that complications are avoided or controlled. All patients on >100 mg/d dapsone will have some hemolysis and methemoglobinemia. These are expected pharmacologic side effects of this agent. Gluten restriction can control DH and lessen dapsone requirements; this diet must rigidly exclude gluten to be of maximal benefit. Many months of dietary restriction may be necessary before a beneficial result is achieved. Good dietary counseling by a trained dietitian is essential.

LINEAR IgA DISEASE

Linear IgA disease, once considered a variant form of dermatitis herpetiformis, is actually a separate and distinct entity. Clinically, these patients may resemble individuals with DH, BP, or other subepidermal blistering diseases. Lesions typically consist of papulovesicles, bullae, and/or urticarial plaques predominantly on central or flexural sites. Oral mucosal involvement occurs in some patients. Severe pruritus resembles that seen in patients with DH. Patients with linear IgA disease do not have an increased frequency of the HLA-B8/DRw3 haplotype or an associated enteropathy and hence are not candidates for treatment with a gluten-free diet.

The histologic alterations in early lesions may be virtually indistinguishable from those in DH. However, direct immunofluorescence microscopy of normal-appearing perilesional skin reveals linear deposits of IgA (and often C3) in the epidermal basement membrane zone. Most patients with linear IgA disease demonstrate circulating IgA anti-basement membrane autoantibodies directed against neoepitopes in the proteolytically processed extracellular domain of BPAG2. These patients generally respond to treatment with dapsone, 50–200 mg/d.

EPIDERMOLYSIS BULLOSA ACQUISITA

EBA is a rare, noninherited, polymorphic, chronic, subepidermal blistering disease. (The inherited form is discussed in Chap. 357.) Patients with classic or noninflammatory EBA have blisters on noninflamed skin, atrophic scars, milia, nail dystrophy, and oral lesions. Because lesions generally occur at sites exposed to minor trauma, classic EBA is considered to be a mechanobullous disease. Other patients with EBA have widespread inflammatory, scarring, and bullous lesions that resemble severe BP. Inflammatory EBA may evolve into the classic, noninflammatory form of this disease. Rare patients present with lesions that predominate on mucous membranes. The HLA-DR2 haplotype is found with increased frequency in EBA patients. Recent studies suggest that EBA is often associated with inflammatory bowel disease (especially Crohn's disease).

The histology of lesional skin varies depending on the character of the lesion being studied. Noninflammatory bullae show subepidermal blisters with a sparse leukocytic infiltrate and resemble those in patients with porphyria cutanea tarda. Inflammatory lesions consist of neutrophil-rich subepidermal blisters. EBA patients have continuous deposits of IgG (and frequently C3 as well as other complement components) in a linear pattern within the epidermal basement membrane zone. Ultrastructurally, these immunoreactants are found in the sublamina densa region in association with anchoring fibrils. Approximately 50% of EBA patients have demonstrable circulating IgG anti-basement membrane autoantibodies directed against type VII collagen—the collagen species that comprises anchoring fibrils. Such IgG autoantibodies bind the dermal side of 1 M NaCl split skin (in contrast to IgG autoantibodies in patients with BP). Recent studies have shown that passive transfer of experimental or patient IgG directed against type VII collagen can produce lesions in mice that clinically, histologically, and immunopathologically resemble those seen in patients with inflammatory EBA.

Treatment of EBA is generally unsatisfactory. Some patients with inflammatory EBA may respond to systemic glucocorticoids, either alone or in combination with immunosuppressive agents. Other patients (especially those with neutrophil-rich inflammatory lesions) may respond to dapsone. The chronic, noninflammatory form of this disease is largely resistant to treatment, although some patients may respond to cyclosporine, azathioprine, or IV immunoglobulin (IVIg).

CICATRICIAL PEMPHIGOID

Cicatricial pemphigoid (CP) is a rare, acquired, subepithelial immunobullous disease characterized by erosive lesions of mucous membranes and skin that result in scarring of at least some sites of involvement. Common sites of involvement include the oral mucosa (especially the gingiva) and conjunctiva; other sites that may be affected include the nasopharyngeal, laryngeal, esophageal, and anogenital mucosa. Skin lesions (present in about one-third of patients) tend to predominate on the scalp, face, and upper trunk and generally consist of a few scattered erosions or tense blisters on an erythematous or urticarial base. CP is typically a chronic and progressive disorder. Serious complications may arise as a consequence of ocular, laryngeal, esophageal, or anogenital lesions. Erosive conjunctivitis may result in shortened fornices, symblephara, ankyloblepharon, entropion, corneal opacities, and (in severe cases) blindness. Similarly, erosive lesions of the larynx may cause hoarseness, pain, and tissue loss that, if unrecognized and untreated, may eventuate in complete destruction of the airway. Esophageal lesions may result in stenosis and/or strictures that may place patients at risk for aspiration. Strictures may also complicate anogenital involvement.

Biopsies of lesional tissue generally demonstrate subepithelial vesiculobullae and a mononuclear leukocytic infiltrate. Neutrophils and eosinophils may be seen in biopsies of early lesions; older lesions may demonstrate a scant leukocytic infiltrate and fibrosis. Direct immunofluorescence microscopy of perilesional tissue typically demonstrates deposits of IgG, IgA, and/or C3 in the epidermal basement membrane of these patients. Because many of these patients show no evidence of circulating anti-basement membrane autoantibodies, testing of perilesional skin is important diagnostically. Although CP was once thought to be a single nosologic entity, it is now largely regarded as a disease phenotype that may develop as a consequence of an autoimmune reaction against a variety of different molecules in epidermal basement membrane (e.g., BPAG2, laminin 5, type VII collagen, and other antigens yet to be completely defined). Recent studies suggest that CP patients with anti-laminin 5 autoantibodies have an increased relative risk for cancer. Treatment of CP is largely dependent upon sites of involvement. Due to potentially severe complications, patients with ocular, laryngeal, esophageal, and/or anogenital involvement require aggressive systemic treatment with dapsone, prednisone, or the latter in combination with another immunosuppressive agent (e.g., azathioprine, mycophenolate mofetil, or cyclophosphamide) or IVIg. Less threatening forms of the disease may be managed with topical or intralesional glucocorticoids.

AUTOIMMUNE SYSTEMIC DISEASES WITH PROMINENT CUTANEOUS FEATURES

DERMATOMYOSITIS

The cutaneous manifestations of dermatomyositis (Chap. 383) are often distinctive but at times may resemble those of systemic lupus erythematosus (SLE) (Chap. 313), scleroderma (Chap. 316), or other overlapping connective tissue diseases (Chap. 316). The extent and severity of cutaneous disease may or may not correlate with the extent and severity of the myositis. The cutaneous manifestations of dermatomyositis are similar whether the disease appears in children or the elderly, except that calcification of subcutaneous tissue is a common late sequela in childhood dermatomyositis.

The cutaneous signs of dermatomyositis may precede or follow the development of myositis by weeks to years. Cases lacking muscle involve-

FIGURE 55-3 Dermatomyositis. Periorbital violaceous erythema characterizes the classic heliotrope rash. (*Courtesy of James Krell, MD; with permission.*)

ment (i.e., dermatomyositis sine myositis) have also been reported. The most common manifestation is a purple-red discoloration of the upper eyelids, sometimes associated with scaling ("heliotrope" erythema; Fig. 55-3) and periorbital edema. Erythema on the cheeks and nose in a "butterfly" distribution may resemble the malar eruption of SLE. Erythematous or violaceous scaling patches are common on the upper anterior chest, posterior neck, scalp, and the extensor surfaces of the arms, legs, and hands. Erythema and scaling may be particularly prominent over the elbows, knees, and the dorsal interphalangeal joints. Approximately one-third of patients have violaceous, flat-topped papules over the dorsal interphalangeal joints that are pathognomonic of dermatomyositis (Gottron's sign or Gottron's papules; Fig. 55-4). These lesions can be contrasted with the erythema and scaling on the dorsum of the fingers in some patients with SLE, which spares the skin over the interphalangeal joints. Periungual telangiectasia may be prominent. Lacy or reticulated erythema may be associated with fine scaling on the extensor surfaces of the thighs and upper arms. Other patients, particularly those with long-standing disease, develop areas of hypopigmentation, hyperpigmentation, mild atrophy, and telangiectasia known as *poikiloderma*. Poikiloderma is rare in both SLE and scleroderma and thus can serve as a clinical sign that distinguishes dermatomyositis from these two diseases. Cutaneous changes may be similar in scleroderma and dermatomyositis and may include thickening and binding down of the skin of the hands (sclerodac-

FIGURE 55-4 Gottron's sign. Dermatomyositis often involves the hands as erythematous flat-topped papules over the knuckles (Gottron's sign). Periungual telangiectases are also evident.

and upper chest. These acute lesions, while sometimes evanescent, usually last for days and are often associated with exacerbations of systemic disease. Skin biopsy of acute lesions may show only a sparse dermal infiltrate of mononuclear cells and dermal edema. In some instances, cellular infiltrates around blood vessels and hair follicles are notable, as is hydropic degeneration of basal cells of the epidermis. Direct immunofluorescence microscopy of lesional skin frequently reveals deposits of immunoglobulin(s) and complement in the epidermal basement membrane zone. Treatment is aimed at control of systemic disease; photoprotection in this, as well as in other forms of LE, is very important.

Subacute cutaneous lupus erythematosus (SCLE) is characterized by a widespread photosensitive, nonscarring eruption. Most of these patients have SLE in which renal and central nervous system involvement is mild or absent. SCLE may present as a papulosquamous eruption that resembles psoriasis or annular lesions that resemble those seen in erythema multiforme. In the papulosquamous form, discrete erythematous papules arise on the back, chest, shoulders, extensor surfaces of the arms, and the dorsum of the hands; lesions are uncommon on the face, flexor surfaces of the arms, and below the waist. These slightly scaling papules tend to merge into large plaques, some with a reticulate appearance. The annular form involves the same areas and presents with erythematous papules that evolve into oval, circular, or polycyclic lesions. The lesions of SCLE are more widespread but have less tendency for scarring than do lesions of discoid LE. Skin biopsy reveals a dense mononuclear cell infiltrate around hair follicles and blood vessels in the superficial dermis, combined with hydropic degeneration of basal cells in the epidermis. Direct immunofluorescence microscopy of lesional skin reveals deposits of immunoglobulin(s) in the epidermal basement membrane zone in about half these cases. A particulate pattern of IgG deposition throughout the epidermis has recently been associated with SCLE. Most SCLE patients have anti-Ro autoantibodies. Local therapy alone is usually unsuccessful. Most patients require treatment with aminoquinoline antimalarials. Low-dose therapy with oral glucocorticoids is sometimes necessary. Photoprotective measures against both ultraviolet B and A wavelengths are very important.

Discoid lupus erythematosus (DLE, also called *chronic cutaneous LE*) is characterized by discrete lesions, most often found on the face, scalp, and/or external ears. The lesions are erythematous papules or plaques with a thick, adherent scale that occludes hair follicles (follicular plugging). When the scale is removed, its underside shows small excrescences that correlate with the openings of hair follicles (so called "carpet tacking"), a finding relatively specific for DLE. Long-standing lesions develop central atrophy, scarring, and hypopigmentation but frequently have erythematous, sometimes raised borders (Fig. 55-6). These lesions persist for years and tend to expand slowly. Only 5–10% of patients with DLE meet the American Rheumatism Association criteria for SLE. However, typical discoid lesions are frequently seen in patients with SLE. Biopsy of DLE lesions shows hyperkeratosis, follicular plugging, atrophy of the epidermis, hydropic degeneration of basal keratinocytes, and a mononuclear cell infiltrate adjacent to epidermal, adnexal, and microvascular basement membranes. Direct immunofluorescence microscopy demonstrates immunoglobulin(s) and complement deposits at the basement membrane zone in ~90% of cases. Treatment is focused on control of local cutaneous disease and consists mainly of photoprotection and topical or intralesional glucocorticoids. If local therapy is ineffective, use of aminoquinoline antimalarials may be indicated.

SCLERODERMA AND MORPHEA

The skin changes of scleroderma (Chap. 316) usually begin on the hands, feet, and face, with episodes of recurrent nonpitting edema. Sclerosis of the skin begins distally on the fingers (sclerodactyly) and spreads proximally, usually accompanied by resorption of bone of the fingertips, which may have punched out ulcers, stellate scars, or areas of hemorrhage (Fig. 55-7). The fingers may actually shrink in size and become sausage-shaped, and since the fingernails are usually unaffected, the nails may curve over the end of the fingertips. Periungual telangiectases are usually present, but periungual erythema is rare. In advanced cases, the extremities show contractures and calcinosis cutis. Facial involvement includes a smooth, unwrinkled brow, taut skin over the nose,

FIGURE 55-5 *A.* **Acute cutaneous lupus erythematosus** showing prominent, scaly, malar erythema. Involvement of other sun-exposed sites is also common. *B.* **Acute cutaneous LE** on the upper chest demonstrating brightly erythematous and slightly edematous papules and plaques. (*B, Courtesy of Robert Swerlick, MD; with permission.*)

tyly) as well as Raynaud's phenomenon. However, the presence of severe muscle disease, Gottron's papules, heliotrope erythema, and poikiloderma serve to distinguish patients with dermatomyositis. Skin biopsy of erythematous, scaling lesions of dermatomyositis may reveal only mild nonspecific inflammation but sometimes may show changes indistinguishable from those found in SLE, including epidermal atrophy, hydropic degeneration of basal keratinocytes, edema of the upper dermis, and a mild mononuclear cell infiltrate. Direct immunofluorescence microscopy of lesional skin is usually negative, although granular deposits of immunoglobulin(s) and complement in the epidermal basement membrane zone have been described in some patients. Treatment should be directed at the systemic disease. Topical glucocorticoids are sometimes useful; patients should avoid exposure to ultraviolet irradiation and use photoprotective measures such as broad-spectrum sunscreens.

LUPUS ERYTHEMATOSUS

The cutaneous manifestations of lupus erythematosus (LE) (Chap. 313) can be divided into acute, subacute, and chronic types. *Acute cutaneous LE* is characterized by erythema of the nose and malar eminences in a "butterfly" distribution (Fig. 55-5). The erythema is often sudden in onset, accompanied by edema and fine scale, and correlated with systemic involvement. Patients may have widespread involvement of the face as well as erythema and scaling of the extensor surfaces of the extremities

FIGURE 55-6 Discoid lupus erythematosus. Violaceous, hyperpigmented, atrophic plaques, often with evidence of follicular plugging, which may result in scarring, are characteristic of discoid lupus erythematosus (also called chronic cutaneous lupus erythematosus).

shrinkage of tissue around the mouth, and perioral radial furrowing (Fig. 55-8). Matlike telangiectases are often present, particularly on the face and hands. Involved skin feels indurated, smooth, and bound to underlying structures; hyperpigmentation and hypopigmentation are also often present. Raynaud's phenomenon, i.e., cold-induced blanching, cyanosis, and reactive hyperemia, is present in almost all patients and can precede development of scleroderma by many years. The combination of calcinosis cutis, Raynaud's phenomenon, esophageal dysmotility, sclerodactyly, and telangiectasia has been termed the *CREST syndrome*. Anticentromere antibodies have been reported in a very high percentage of patients with the CREST syndrome but in only a small minority of patients with scleroderma. Skin biopsy reveals thickening of the dermis and homogenization of collagen bundles. Direct immunofluorescence microscopy of lesional skin is usually negative.

Morphea is characterized by localized thickening and sclerosis of skin, usually affecting young adults or children. Morphea begins as erythematous or flesh-colored plaques that become sclerotic, develop central hypopigmentation, and demonstrate an erythematous border. In most cases, patients have one or a few lesions, and the disease is termed *localized morphea*. In some patients, widespread cutaneous lesions may occur, without systemic involvement. This form is called *generalized morphea*. Most patients with morphea do not have autoantibodies. Skin

FIGURE 55-8 Scleroderma often eventuates in development of an expressionless, mask-like facies.

biopsy of morphea is indistinguishable from that of scleroderma. Linear scleroderma is a limited form of disease that presents in a linear, band-like distribution and tends to involve deep as well as superficial layers of skin. Scleroderma and morphea are usually quite resistant to therapy. For this reason, physical therapy to prevent joint contractures and to maintain function is employed and is often helpful.

Diffuse fasciitis with eosinophilia is a clinical entity that can sometimes be confused with scleroderma. There is usually the sudden onset of swelling, induration, and erythema of the extremities frequently following significant physical exertion. The proximal portions of extremities (arms, forearms, thighs, legs) are more often involved than are the hands and feet. While the skin is indurated, it is usually not bound down as in scleroderma; contractures may occur early secondary to fascial involvement. The latter may also cause muscle groups to be separated and veins to appear depressed. These skin findings are accompanied by peripheral blood eosinophilia, increased erythrocyte sedimentation rate, and sometimes hypergammaglobulinemia. Deep biopsy of affected areas of skin reveals inflammation and thickening of the deep fascia overlying muscle. An inflammatory infiltrate composed of eosinophils and mononuclear cells is usually found. Patients with eosinophilic fasciitis appear to be at increased risk to develop bone marrow failure or other hematologic abnormalities. While the ultimate course of eosinophilic fasciitis is uncertain, many patients respond favorably to treatment with prednisone in doses ranging from 40–60 mg/d.

The *eosinophilia-myalgia syndrome*, a disorder reported in epidemic numbers in 1989 and linked to ingestion of L-tryptophan manufactured by a single company in Japan, is a multisystem disorder characterized by debilitating myalgias and absolute eosinophilia in association with varying combinations of arthralgias, pulmonary symptoms, and peripheral edema. In a later phase (i.e., 3–6 months after initial symptoms), these patients often develop localized sclerodermatous skin changes, weight loss, and/or neuropathy (Chap. 316). The precise cause of this syndrome, which may resemble other sclerotic skin conditions, is unknown. However, the implicated lots of L-tryptophan contained the contaminant 1,1-ethylidene bis[tryptophan]. This contaminant may be pathogenic or a marker for another substance that provokes the disorder.

FURTHER READINGS

ANHALT GJ: Paraneoplastic pemphigus. J Investig Dermatol Symp Proc 9:29, 2004

BRAVERMAN IM: Connective tissue diseases, in *Skin Signs of Systemic Disease*, 3d ed. Philadelphia, Saunders, 1998

MUTASIM DF et al: Immunobullous diseases. J Am Acad Dermatol 52:1029, 2005

FIGURE 55-7 Scleroderma showing acral sclerosis and focal digital ulcers.

PAYNE AS et al: Desmosomes and disease: Pemphigus and bullous impetigo. Curr Opin Cell Biol 16:536, 2004

SCHMIDT E, ZILLIKENS D: Autoimmune and inherited subepidermal blistering diseases: Advances in the clinic and the laboratory. Adv Dermatol 16:113, 2000

SONTHEIMER RD: Skin manifestations of systemic autoimmune connective tissue disease: Diagnostics and therapeutics. Best Pract Res Clin Rheumatol 18:429, 2004

UDEY MC, STANLEY JR: Pemphigus—diseases of antidesmosomal autoimmunity. JAMA 282:572, 1999

YANCEY KB, EGAN CA: Pemphigoid: Clinical, histologic, immunopathologic, and therapeutic considerations. JAMA 284:350, 2000

56 Cutaneous Drug Reactions

Jean-Claude Roujeau, Robert S. Stern,
Bruce U. Wintroub

Cutaneous reactions are among the most frequent adverse reactions to drugs. Every physician will see patients suffering from them. Most are benign, but a few can be life-threatening. Prompt recognition of severe reactions, drug withdrawal, and appropriate therapeutic interventions can minimize toxicity. This chapter focuses on adverse cutaneous reactions to drugs other than topical agents; it covers their incidence, patterns, and pathogenesis and provides some practical guidelines on treatment, assessment of causality, and future utilization of drugs.

USE OF PRESCRIPTION DRUGS IN THE UNITED STATES

In the United States more than 3 billion prescriptions for over 60,000 drug products, which include more than 2000 different active agents, are dispensed annually. Hospital inpatients alone annually receive about 120 million courses of drug therapy, and half of adult Americans receive prescription drugs on a regular outpatient basis. Many additional patients use over-the-counter medicines that may cause adverse cutaneous reactions.

INCIDENCE OF CUTANEOUS REACTIONS

Several large cohort studies established that acute cutaneous reaction to drugs affected about 3% of hospital inpatients. Reactions usually occur a few days to 4 weeks after initiation of therapy.

Many drugs of common use are associated with a 1–2% rate of "rashes" during premarketing clinical trials. The risk is often higher when medications are used in general unselected populations. The rate may reach 3–7% for amoxicillin, sulfamethoxazole, and many anticonvulsants (Table 56-1). It may be even higher with anti-HIV agents.

In addition to acute eruptions, a variety of skin diseases can be induced or exacerbated by prolonged utilization of drugs, e.g., pruritus, pigmentation, nail or hair disorders, psoriasis, and pemphigus. These chronic drug reactions are not frequent, but neither their incidence nor their impact on public health has been evaluated.

In a series of 48,005 inpatients over a 20-year period, morbilliform rash (91%) and urticaria (6%) were the most frequent skin reactions. Severe reactions are actually too rare to be detected in such cohorts. Their incidence has been estimated to be in the range of 1 in 10,000 to 1 in 1 million users. Even though they are rare, severe cutaneous reactions to drugs have an important impact on health and on the risk-versus-benefit evaluation of medicines because of significant mortality and sequelae.

Some populations are at increased risks of drug reactions: patients with collagen vascular diseases, bone marrow graft recipients, and those with acute Epstein-Barr virus infection. It has also been established that HIV infection increases the risk of drug allergy (Chap. 182). This was true for many drugs but has been evaluated mainly with sulfamethoxazole. Up to 40% of HIV-infected patients had skin reactions when treated with high doses, and about 15% reacted to the same dosage that induced 3–5% eruptions in non-HIV-infected populations. How HIV promotes allergy to certain medications has not yet been explained.

PATHOGENESIS OF DRUG REACTIONS

Untoward cutaneous responses to drugs can arise as a result of immunologic or nonimmunologic mechanisms. A variety of adverse reactions result from mechanisms that do not involve an immunologic process. Drug reactions are a public health problem because of their frequent occurrence, occasional severity, and impact on the use of medications. The skin is among the organs most often affected by adverse drug reactions. The list of conditions that can be triggered by medications includes nearly all dermatologic diseases. Many of these adverse reactions result from mechanisms that do not involve an immunologic process. Obvious examples are pigmentary changes related to accumulation in the dermis of amiodarone, antimalarials, minocycline, quinolones, alteration of hair follicles by cytostatics, and lipodystrophy associated with metabolic effects of anti-HIV medications. These side effects are mostly toxic, predictable, and often can be avoided at least in part by simple preventive measures.

IMMUNOLOGIC DRUG REACTIONS

For most acute drug eruptions, benign or severe, accumulated data suggest an immunologic basis. In the last 10 years drug-specific T cell clones were derived from the blood lymphocytes or from skin lesions of patients with a variety of drug allergies. Since these clones had been obtained after several stimulations in vitro with the drug, their relevance to explain the original manifestations of allergy can be questioned. Regardless, these T cell clones brought definite evidence that drugs can be recognized as antigens by human T cells, and that these T cells play a role in drug allergy. Specific clones were obtained with penicillin G, amoxicillin, cephalosporins, sulfamethoxazole, phenobarbital, carbamazepine, lamotrigine, i.e., many of the medications that are frequently a cause of drug eruptions. Both CD4 and CD8 clones were often obtained, whatever the clinical type of eruption.

Some clones produced a T_H0 profile of cytokines (simultaneous release of IL-4 and IFN-γ). A T_H2 orientation was frequent in CD4+ clones while CD8+ clones were usually T_H1 and often cytotoxic. Drug presentation to T cell was MHC-restricted, usually as expected by HLA class II for CD4+ cells and by HLA class I for CD8. But there were also less classic situations like HLA class II restricted cytotoxic CD4 clones. With many drugs, an original observation was that the drug could be presented to the TCR and activate a specific clone without prior processing by the antigen-presenting cell and through a noncovalent binding to the MHC or its embedded peptide. Actually, some specific TCR could recognize sulfamethoxazole presented either in covalent or

TABLE 56-1 CUTANEOUS REACTIONS TO DRUGS RECEIVED BY AT LEAST 1000 PATIENTS (BCDSP)[a]

Drug	Reactions, No.	Recipients, No.	Rate, %	95% Confidence Interval
Amoxicillin	63	1225	5.1	3.9–6.4
Ampicillin	215	4763	4.5	3.9–5.1
Co-trimoxazole	46	1235	3.7	2.7–4.8
Semisynthetic penicillins	41	1436	2.9	2.0–3.7
Red blood cells	67	3386	2.0	1.5–2.4
Penicillin G	68	4204	1.6	1.2–2.0
Cephalosporins	27	1781	1.5	0.9–2.1
Gentamicin	13	1277	1.0	0.5–1.6

[a]BCDSP, Boston Collaborative Drug Surveillance Program.
Source: Adapted from Bigby.

noncovalent bound form, but the former was the exception and the latter the rule. Since the noncovalent binding is reminiscent of the pharmacologic interaction between a drug and its receptor, the denomination of pharmoco-immune (p-i) concept has been proposed.

Once a drug has induced an immune response, the final phenotype of the reaction probably depends on the nature of effectors: cytotoxic (CD8+) T cells in blistering reactions, chemokines for reactions mediated by neutrophils or eosinophils, and collaboration with B cells for production of specific antibodies for urticarial reactions.

Immediate Reactions Immediate reactions depend on the release of mediators of inflammation by tissue mast cells or circulating basophilic leukocytes. These mediators include histamine, leukotrienes, prostaglandins, platelet-activating factor, enzymes, and proteoglycans. Drugs can trigger mediator release either directly ("anaphylactoid" reaction) or through IgE-specific antibodies. These reactions are usually manifest in the skin and gastrointestinal, respiratory, and cardiovascular systems (Chap. 311). Primary symptoms and signs include pruritus, urticaria, nausea, vomiting, cramps, bronchospasm, and laryngeal edema—and, occasionally, anaphylactic shock with hypotension and death. They occur within minutes of drug exposure. Nonsteroidal anti-inflammatory drugs (NSAIDs), including aspirin, and radiocontrast media are frequent causes of pharmacologically mediated anaphylactoid reactions, which can occur on first exposure. Penicillins and myorelaxants used in general anesthesia are the most frequent causes of IgE-dependent reactions to drugs, which require prior sensitization. Release of mediators is triggered when polyvalent drug protein conjugates cross-link IgE molecules fixed to sensitized cells. Certain routes of administration favor different clinical patterns (e.g., gastrointestinal effects from oral route, circulatory effects from intravenous route).

Immune Complex-Dependent Reactions Because the use of nonhuman sera is now uncommon, this mechanism is rarely relevant to adverse reactions seen today. Serum sickness is produced by tissue deposition of circulating immune complexes with consumption of complement. It is characterized by fever, arthritis, nephritis, neuritis, edema, and an urticarial, papular, or purpuric rash (Chap. 319). It was first described following administration of foreign sera; it may now occur with monoclonal antibodies. In classic serum sickness, symptoms develop 6 days or more after exposure to a drug, the latent period representing the time needed to synthesize antibody. Cephalosporin administration in febrile children may be associated with a clinically similar "serum sickness–like" reaction. The real mechanism of this reaction is unknown but is unrelated to complement activation.

Cutaneous or systemic vasculitis, a relatively rare cutaneous complication of drugs, may also be a result of immune complex deposition (Chap. 319).

Delayed Hypersensitivity Delayed hypersensitivity mechanisms directed by drug-specific T cells are probably the most important mechanisms in the etiology of the most common drug eruptions—morbilliform exanthems—and also of rare and severe forms such as hypersensitivity syndrome, acute generalized exanthematous pustulosis (AGEP), Stevens-Johnson syndrome (SJS), and toxic epidermal necrolysis (TEN). Drug-specific T cells have been detected in these types of drug eruptions.

Contrary to what has been believed for years, the antigen is more often the native drug itself than its metabolites. It remains to better understand why the stimulation of T cells by medications leads to reactions that are clinically so diverse. Some answers were provided by the study of effector cells obtained at the site of skin lesions. Drug-specific cytotoxic T cells have been detected in the skin lesions of fixed drug eruptions and of TEN. In TEN, blisters that result from accumulation of interstitial fluid under the necrotic epidermis contain T lymphocytes that are able to kill autologous lymphocytes and keratinocytes in a drug-specific, HLA-restricted, and perforin/granzyme-mediated pathway.

Drug-specific clones producing CXCL8, a neutrophil-attracting chemokine, were obtained from skin tests of patients with AGEP, a neutrophil-mediated drug reaction.

One may therefore assume that the final pattern of drug eruptions results both from the nature of effectors—cytotoxic T cells in blistering reactions, chemokines in reactions mediated by neutrophils or eosinophils—and from the intensity of stimulation and response.

Genetic Factors and Cutaneous Drug Reactions Specific genetically determined defects in the ability of an individual to detoxify toxic reactive drug metabolites predispose such individuals to the development of drug toxicity. It has also been suspected that a slow acetylator phenotype increases the risk of rash from sulfonamides. However, in two large prospective cohorts of HIV-infected patients treated with sulfonamides, no association of drug eruption with acetylation genotype was found.

Recent literature shows that genetic factors may be important predictors of severe drug reactions. Hypersensitivity to the anti-HIV medication abacavir was strongly associated with HLA B*5701. In Taiwan, within a homogeneous Han Chinese population, a 100% association was observed between SJS or TEN related to carbamazepine and HLA B*1502. In the same population, another 100% association was found between SJS, TEN, or hypersensitivity syndrome/drug reaction with eosinophilia and systemic symptoms (DRESS) related to allopurinol and HLA B*5801. These observations have important theoretical implications. By pointing to HLA genes, they strongly support a key role for immune mechanisms. However, the strong associations found in Taiwan have not been observed in other countries with more heterogenous populations. Therefore, widespread practical applications of these findings are not yet possible.

CLINICAL PRESENTATION OF CUTANEOUS DRUG REACTIONS

NONIMMUNE CUTANEOUS REACTIONS

Exacerbation or Induction of Dermatologic Diseases A variety of agents can exacerbate preexisting diseases or sometimes induce a disease that may or may not disappear after withdrawal of the inducing medication. For example, NSAIDs, lithium, beta blockers, and angiotensin-converting enzyme (ACE) inhibitors can exacerbate plaque psoriasis, while antimalarials can worsen pustular psoriasis. Acne may be induced by glucocorticoids, androgens, and lithium. Minocycline and thiazide diuretics may exacerbate subacute systemic lupus erythematosus, and pemphigus can be induced by D-penicillamine, captopril, and other ACE inhibitors. The hypothesis that a drug may be responsible should always be considered, especially in cases with atypical clinical presentation, unusual age of onset, or unexpected evolution.

Photosensitivity Eruptions Photosensitivity eruptions are usually most marked in sun-exposed areas but may extend to sun-protected areas. The mechanism is almost always phototoxicity. Phototoxic reactions resemble sunburn and can occur with first exposure to a drug. Their severity depends on the tissue level of the drug, its efficiency as a photosensitizer, and the extent of exposure to the activating wavelengths of ultraviolet light (Chap. 57).

Common orally administered photosensitizing drugs include many fluoroquinolones and cycline antibiotics. Other drugs less frequently encountered are chlorpromazine, thiazides, and several NSAIDs (ibuprofen, naproxen, piroxicam). Because UV-A and visible light, which trigger these reactions, are not easily absorbed by nonopaque sunscreens and are transmitted through window glass, photosensitivity reactions may be difficult to block.

Photosensitivity reactions abate with removal of either the drug or ultraviolet radiation, use of high-potency sunscreens that block UV-A light, and treating the reaction as one would a sunburn. Rarely, individuals develop persistent reactivity to light, necessitating long-term avoidance of sun exposure.

Pigmentation Changes Drugs, either systemic or topical, may cause a variety of pigmentary changes in the skin. Oral contraceptives may induce melasma. Long-term minocycline or pefloxacin may cause blue-gray pigmentation, while amiodarone causes a more purple coloration. Long-term high-dose phenothiazine results in gray-brown pigmentation of sun-exposed areas. Numerous cancer chemotherapeutic agents may be associated with pigmentation, e.g., bleomycin, busulfan, daunorubicin, cyclophosphamide, hydroxyurea, and methotrexate. Pigmentation changes may also occur in mucous membranes (busulfan), nails (zidovudine), hair, and teeth.

Warfarin Necrosis of Skin This rare reaction usually occurs between the third and tenth days of therapy with warfarin derivatives, usually in women. The more common sites are breasts, thighs, and buttocks. Lesions are sharply demarcated, erythematous, indurated, and purpuric and may resolve or progress to form large, irregular, hemorrhagic bullae with eventual necrosis and slow-healing eschar formation.

Development of the syndrome is unrelated to drug dose, and the course is not altered by discontinuation of the drug after onset of the eruption. Warfarin reactions are associated with protein C deficiency. Warfarin anticoagulation in heterozygotes for protein C deficiency causes a precipitous fall in circulating levels of protein C, permitting hypercoagulability and thrombosis in the cutaneous microvasculature, with consequent areas of necrosis. Similar reactions have been associated with heparin. Heparin-induced necrosis may have clinically similar features but is probably due to heparin-induced platelet aggregation with subsequent occlusion of blood vessels.

Warfarin-induced cutaneous necrosis is treated with vitamin K and heparin. Treatment with protein C concentrates may also be helpful.

Drug-Induced Hair Disorders · DRUG-INDUCED HAIR LOSS Medications may affect hair follicles at two different phases of their cycle. *Anagen effluvium* occurs within days of drug administration, whereas in *telogen effluvium*, the delay is 2–4 months. Both present as diffuse nonscarring alopecia most often reversible after discontinuation of the responsible agent.

The prevalence and severity of alopecia depend on the drug as well as on individual predisposition. A considerable number of drugs have been reported to induce hair loss. These include antineoplastic agents (alkylating agents, bleomycin, vinca alkaloids, platinum compounds), anticonvulsants (carbamazepine, valproate), antihypertensive drugs (beta blockers), antidepressants, antithyroid drugs, interferons (IFNs), oral contraceptives, and hypolipidemics.

HIRSUTISM Hirsutism is an excessive growth of coarse hair with masculine characteristics in a female, most often on the lateral aspects of face and back. Hirsutism results from androgenic stimulation of hormone-sensitive hair follicles.

Anabolic steroids, oral contraceptives of the nonsteroid progesterone type, testosterone, and corticotropin can induce hirsutism.

HYPERTRICHOSIS Hypertrichosis differs from hirsutism by being located mainly on the forehead and temporal regions. It is usually reversible. Drugs responsible for hypertrichosis include anti-inflammatory drugs, glucocorticoids, vasodilators (diazoxide, minoxidil), diuretics (acetazolamide), anticonvulsants (phenytoin), immunosuppressive agents, psoralens, and zidovudine.

Changes in hair color or structure are uncommon adverse effects from medications. Hair discoloration may occur with chloroquine, IFN-α, chemotherapeutic agents, and tyrosine kinase inhibitors. Changes in hair structure have been observed in patients given EGFR inhibitors.

Drug-Induced Nail Disorders These usually involve several or all 20 nails and need months to resolve after withdrawal of the offending agent. The pathogenesis is most often toxic. Drug-induced nail changes include Beau's line (transversal depression of the nail plate), onycholysis (detachment of the distal part of the nail plate), onychomadesis (detachment of the proximal part of the nail plate), pigmentation, and paronychia (inflammation of periungual skin).

ONYCHOLYSIS Onycholysis may occur as a consequence of phototoxic reactions, particularly with tetracyclines, fluoroquinolones, phenothiazines, and psoralens, as well as in persons taking NSAIDs, captopril, retinoids, sodium valproate, and many chemotherapeutic agents such as anthracyclines or taxanes including paclitaxel and docetaxel. The risk of onycholysis in patients receiving cytotoxic drugs can be increased by exposure to sunlight.

ONYCHOMADESIS Onychomadesis is caused by temporary arrest of nail matrix mitotic activity. Common drugs reported to induce onychomadesis include carbamazepine, lithium, retinoids, and chemotherapeutic agents such as cyclophosphamide and vincristine.

PARONYCHIA Paronychia and multiple pyogenic granuloma with progressive and painful periungual abscess of fingers and toes are a side effect of systemic retinoids, lamivudine, indinavir, and anti-EGFR monoclonal antibodies (cetuximab, gefitinib).

NAIL DISCOLORATION Some drugs, including anthracyclines, taxanes, fluorouracil, and zidovudine, may induce nail bed hyperpigmentation through melanocyte stimulation. It appears to be reversible and dose-dependent.

Pruritus Pruritus is a common symptom of most drug eruptions, but it may also occur without skin lesions as the only manifestation of drug intolerance. Severe pruritus may occur in up to 50% of African patients treated with antimalarials and lead to poor compliance. It is much rarer in Caucasians.

IMMUNE CUTANEOUS REACTIONS: BENIGN

Maculopapular Eruptions Morbilliform or maculopapular eruptions are the most common of all drug-induced reactions, often start on the trunk or areas of pressure or trauma, and consist of erythematous macules and papules that are frequently symmetric and may become confluent. Involvement of mucous membranes is unusual, with the exception of scaly lips; the eruption may be associated with moderate to severe pruritus and fever. Diagnosis is rarely assisted by laboratory testing. Skin biopsy is useless because it shows normal skin or very mild and nonspecific changes. A viral exanthem is the principal differential diagnostic consideration, especially in children. Absence of enanthems, absence of symptoms in ears, nose, and throat and upper respiratory tract, and polymorphism of the skin lesions support a drug rather than a viral eruption.

Maculopapular reactions usually develop within 1 week of initiation of therapy and last less than 2 weeks. Occasionally these eruptions may decrease or fade with continued use of the responsible drug. Since the eruption may also worsen, the suspect drug should be discontinued unless it is essential. Oral antihistamines, emollients, and soothing baths may help relieve pruritus. Short courses of potent topical glucocorticoids can reduce inflammation and symptoms. Systemic glucocorticoid treatment is rarely indicated.

Urticaria/Angioedema *Urticaria* is the second most frequent type of cutaneous reaction to drugs. However, "drug allergy" explains no more than 10–20% of acute urticaria cases. It is a skin reaction characterized by pruritic, red wheals of varying size. Individual lesions rarely last more than 24 h. Deep edematous dermal and subcutaneous tissues are known as *angioedema*. Angioedema may involve mucous membranes. Urticaria and angioedema may be part of a life-threatening anaphylactic reaction.

Drug-induced urticaria may be caused by three mechanisms: an IgE-dependent mechanism, circulating immune complexes (serum sickness), and nonimmunologic activation of effector pathways. IgE-dependent urticarial reactions usually occur within 36 h of drug exposure but can occur within minutes. Immune complex–induced urticaria associated with serum sickness usually occurs 6–12 days after first exposure. In this syndrome, the urticarial eruption may be accompanied by fever, hematuria, arthralgias, hepatic dysfunction, and neurologic symptoms.

Certain drugs, such as NSAIDs, ACE inhibitors, angiotensin II antagonists, and radiographic dyes, may induce urticarial reactions, angioedema, and anaphylaxis in the absence of drug-specific antibody. Although ACE inhibitors, aspirin, penicillin, and blood products are the most frequent causes of urticarial eruptions, urticaria has been observed in association with nearly all drugs. Drugs may also cause chronic urticaria, which lasts more than 6 weeks. Aspirin frequently exacerbates this problem.

The treatment of urticaria or angioedema depends on the severity of the reaction and the rate at which it is evolving. In severe cases, with respiratory or cardiovascular compromise, epinephrine is the mainstay of therapy, but its effect is reduced in patients using beta blockers. Treatment with systemic glucocorticoids, sometimes administered IV, is helpful. In addition to drug withdrawal, for patients with only cutaneous symptoms and without symptoms of angioedema or anaphylaxis, oral antihistamines are usually sufficient.

Fixed Drug Eruptions   These reactions are characterized by one or more sharply demarcated, erythematous lesions, sometimes leading to a blister. Hyperpigmentation results after resolution of the acute inflammation. With rechallenge, the lesion recurs in the same (i.e., fixed) location. Lesions often involve the lips, hands, legs, face, genitalia, and oral mucosa and cause a burning sensation. Most patients have multiple lesions. Fixed drug eruptions have been associated with phenolphthalein, sulfonamides, cyclines, dipyrone, NSAIDs, and barbiturates. Patch testing has been used in Europe to help establish the etiology.

IMMUNE CUTANEOUS REACTIONS: SEVERE

Vasculitis   Cutaneous necrotizing vasculitis often presents as palpable purpuric lesions that may be generalized or limited to the lower extremities or other dependent areas (Chap. 319). Urticarial lesions, ulcers, and hemorrhagic blisters also occur. Vasculitis may involve other organs, including the liver, kidney, brain, and joints. Drugs are an infrequent cause of vasculitis. Infection and collagen vascular disease are responsible for the majority of cases.

Propylthiouracil induces a cutaneous vasculitis that is accompanied by leukopenia and splenomegaly. Direct immunofluorescent changes in these lesions suggest immune-complex deposition. Drugs implicated in vasculitis include allopurinol, thiazides, sulfonamides, other antimicrobials, and several NSAIDs. The presence of eosinophils in the perivascular infiltrate of skin biopsy may indicate a higher probability of a drug etiology.

Pustular Eruptions   AGEP is a rare reaction pattern, often associated with exposure to drugs. Usually beginning on the face or intertriginous areas, small nonfollicular pustules overlying erythematous and edematous skin may coalesce and lead to superficial ulceration. Differentiating this eruption from TEN in its initial stages may be difficult. A skin biopsy is important and shows scattered pustules in the upper part of the epidermis instead of the full-thickness necrosis that characterizes TEN. Fever is present with elevated neutrophil counts, and sepsis is often suspected. Acute pustular psoriasis is the principal differential diagnostic consideration. AGEP often begins within a few days of initiating drug treatment, most notably antibiotics. For other associated drugs, diltiazem, chloroquine, hydroxychloroquine or terbinafine, AGEP begins later: 7–14 days after initiation of treatment.

Hypersensitivity Syndrome   Initially described with phenytoin, hypersensitivity syndrome—a multiorgan drug-induced reaction—is also known as *DRESS* and *drug-induced hypersensitivity syndrome* (*DIHS*). It presents as a widespread erythematous eruption that may become purpuric or lichenoid and is accompanied by many of the following features: fever, facial and periorbital edema, tender generalized lymphadenopathy, leukocytosis (often with atypical lymphocytes and eosinophils), hepatitis, and sometimes nephritis or pneumonitis. The cutaneous reaction usually begins 2–8 weeks after the drug is started and lasts longer than mild eruptions after drug cessation. Symptoms may persist for several weeks, especially hepatitis. The eruption recurs with rechallenge, and cross-reactions among aromatic anticonvulsants, including phenytoin, carbamazepine, and barbiturates, are frequent. Other drugs causing this syndrome include lamotrigine, minocycline, dapsone, allopurinol, and sulfonamides, as well as abacavir and zalcitabine in HIV-infected patients. Reactivation of herpes viruses, especially of herpes virus 6, has been reported to be frequent in this syndrome. The role of virus infection is still unclear; it may contribute to long-lasting manifestations such as hepatitis or encephalitis. Mortality as high as 10% has been reported. In life-threatening situations such as pneumonitis or nephritis, systemic glucocorticoids (prednisone, 0.5–1.0 mg/kg) seem to reduce symptoms. Topical high-potency glucocorticoids may also be helpful. In all cases, rapid withdrawal of the suspected drug is required.

Stevens-Johnson Syndrome and Toxic Epidermal Necrolysis   *SJS* and *TEN* are terms that, most believe, describe the same usually drug-induced disorder, which is characterized by blisters and epidermal detachment resulting from epidermal necrosis in the absence of substantial dermal inflammation. The term *SJS* is now used to describe cases with blisters developing on dusky or purpuric macules in which total body surface area blistering and eventual detachment is <10%. The term *SJS/TEN* is used to describe cases with 10–30% detachment, and *TEN* is used to describe cases with >30% detachment. Erythema multiforme major is now considered by most to be different from SJS, characterized by typical "target" lesions and resulting from a reaction to infection, most commonly from herpes simplex virus.

Patients with SJS, SJS/TEN, or TEN initially present with acute symptoms, painful skin lesions, fever >39°C (102.2°F), sore throat, and visual impairment resulting from mucous membrane and ocular lesions. Intestinal and pulmonary involvements are associated with a poor prognosis, as are a greater extent of epidermal detachment and older age. About 10% and 30% of SJS- and TEN-affected persons die from their disease, respectively. Drugs that most commonly cause SJS or TEN are anti-infectious sulfonamides, nevirapine, allopurinol, lamotrigine, aromatic anticonvulsants, and oxicam NSAIDs. At this time SJS or TEN have no treatment of proven efficacy. The best results come from early diagnosis, immediate discontinuation of any suspected drug, and supportive therapy, paying close attention to ocular complications, often in burn units or intensive care units.

DRUGS OF SPECIAL INTEREST

ALLOPURINOL

Together with sulfonamides and antiepileptics, allopurinol is one of the "usual suspects" that induce frequently mild maculopapular eruptions (in at least 3% of users) and may also cause more severe reactions including hypersensitivity/DRESS and SJS/TEN. Because of increasing utilization it is one of the most frequent causes of life-threatening reactions.

ANTI-HIV MEDICATIONS

In clinical trials, combinations of highly active antiretroviral treatments were frequently associated with ≥10% "drug eruptions." Two drugs, nevirapine and abacavir, have been associated with specific risks.

Nevirapine has both a high risk of maculopapular eruptions and a very high risk (about 1 in 1000) of SJS or TEN. Progressive escalation of daily doses has been shown to decrease the risk of mild eruption but does not abrogate the risk of severe reactions.

Abacavir is associated with a 4–5% risk of a hypersensitivity reaction, which is remarkable because of the association of symptoms suggesting a type I reaction (dyspnea, diarrhea, low blood pressure, shock on rechallenge) and signs of delayed hypersensitivity (rash, late onset, hepatitis). The risk is lower in patients of African ancestry and strongly correlated with HLAB*5701.

PENICILLIN

The utilization rate of penicillin has decreased markedly since it has been the subject of many investigations and a model for "drug allergy." Incidence of cutaneous reactions is about 1%. About 85% of cutaneous reactions to penicillin are morbilliform, and about 10% are urticaria or angioedema. Anaphylaxis and serum sickness appear to be due to IgE antibodies in serum.

Delayed reactions, mainly maculopapular eruptions, are much more common with aminopenicillins, involving 4–7% of users. The question of cross-reactivity between β-lactam antibiotics and preventing the risk of anaphylaxis is discussed below ("Management of a Patient with a Drug Eruption").

NONSTEROIDAL ANTI-INFLAMMATORY DRUGS

Most NSAIDs, including aspirin, cause immediate allergy-like symptoms in susceptible individuals. Approximately 1% of persons experience urticaria or angioedema, and about half as many (0.5%) experience rhinosinusitis and asthma.

Urticaria/angioedema may be delayed up to 24 h and may occur at any age. The rhinosinusitis-asthma syndrome generally develops within 1 h of drug administration. Recurrences are frequent and can be complicated by nasal and sinus infection, polyposis, bloody discharge, and nasal eosinophilia. In many individuals with this syndrome, asthma that can be life-threatening eventually ensues whenever NSAIDs are subsequently ingested. Proof of the association of symptoms and NSAID use requires either clear-cut history of symptoms following drug ingestion or an oral challenge. That procedure must be conducted only in a hospital setting by experienced personnel. Cross-reactivity between NSAIDs that inhibit cyclooxygenase (COX) 1 is common, while reactivity to COX-2 inhibitors is less frequent. The reaction is pharmacologic, and patients who are sensitive to NSAIDs cannot be identified by assessment of IgE antibody to aspirin, lymphocyte sensitization, or in vitro immunologic testing.

Other reactions can also occur with NSAIDs, including phototoxicity with many agents, a pattern of pseudoporphyria being often related to naproxen, hypersensitivity/DRESS (oxicam derivatives, COX-2 inhibitors), and SJS or TEN (phenylbutazone, oxicam derivatives, diclofenac).

RADIOCONTRAST MEDIA

Large numbers of patients are exposed to radiocontrast agents. High-osmolality radiocontrast media were about five times more likely to induce urticaria (1%) or anaphylaxis than were newer low-osmolality media. Severe reactions are rare with either type of contrast media. About one-third of those with mild reactions to previous exposure re-react on re-exposure. In most cases, these reactions are probably not immunologic. Pretreatment with prednisone and diphenhydramine reduces reaction rates. Persons with a reaction to a high-osmolality contrast media should be given low-osmolality media if later contrast studies are required.

ANTICONVULSANTS

Along with sulfonamide antibiotics, phenobarbital, phenytoin, and carbamazepine among the older anticonvulsants, and lamotrigine among the newer, are associated with many types of severe reactions and a high incidence of less severe reactions, particularly in children. These drugs have among the highest risk of SJS, TEN, and hypersensitivity syndrome in immunologically normal patients. The aromatic anticonvulsants can induce a pseudolymphoma syndrome and induce gingival hyperplasia.

SULFONAMIDES

Antibacterial sulfonamides have a rather high risk of causing cutaneous eruptions and are among the drugs most frequently implicated in SJS and TEN. The combination of sulfamethoxazole and trimethoprim frequently induces adverse cutaneous reactions in patients with AIDS (Chap. 182). Desensitization is often successful in AIDS patients with morbilliform eruptions but is not recommended in AIDS patients who manifested erythroderma or a bullous reaction in response to their earlier sulfonamide exposure.

Reaction rates are much lower with nonantibiotic sulfonamides, including diuretics or antidiabetic agents. Cross-reactivity between antibiotic and nonantibiotic sulfonamides is, at most, infrequent.

VANCOMYCIN

Vancomycin causes two unusual but recognizable cutaneous reactions: linear IgA bullous dermatosis (a transient blistering eruption) and *red man syndrome*. Red man syndrome occurs during rapid IV infusion of vancomycin. This is thought to be a histamine-related anaphylactoid reaction characterized by flushing, diffuse maculopapular eruption, hypotension, and, in rare cases, cardiac arrest.

AGENTS USED IN CANCER CHEMOTHERAPY

Since many agents used in cancer chemotherapy inhibit cell division, rapidly proliferating elements of the skin, including hair, mucous membranes, and appendages, are sensitive to their effects. As a result, stomatitis and alopecia are among the most frequent dose-dependent side effects of chemotherapy. Various nail abnormalities have been described: onycholysis, dystrophy, Beau's lines, white lines, and pigmentation. Sterile cellulitis and phlebitis and ulceration of pressure areas occur with many of these agents. Also reported is acral erythema, which begins with dysesthesia followed by redness and a painful edematous eruption of the palms and soles; it is caused by cytarabine, doxorubicin, methotrexate, and 5-fluorouracil. Urticaria, angioedema, and exfoliative dermatitis also have been seen, as has local and diffuse hyperpigmentation.

Hypersensitivity to carboplatin or cisplatin is not rare (with an incidence of 10–20%) among patients receiving multiple treatments with these drugs. It is probably IgE mediated. Moderate to severe reactions including respiratory distress and hypotension are also observed in 10–20% of patients receiving paclitaxel regardless of premedication with glucocorticoids and histamine H(1) and H(2) antagonists.

GLUCOCORTICOIDS

Both systemic and topical glucocorticoids cause a variety of skin changes, including acneiform eruptions, atrophy, striae, and other stigmata of Cushing's syndrome, and in sufficiently high doses can retard wound healing. Patients using glucocorticoids are at higher risk for bacterial, yeast, and fungal skin infections that may be misinterpreted as drug eruptions but are instead drug side effects. Allergy to glucocorticoids may also occur either as contact dermatitis to topical formulations or as systemic reactions, including anaphylaxis.

BIOLOGIC THERAPIES

These include cytokines and monoclonal antibodies.

Injection-site reactions are the most frequent adverse event. The severity varies from mild redness to deep inflammation and necrosis. In most cases the treatment can be continued and the severity of reactions will decrease with time.

Like all foreign proteins, monoclonal antibodies may induce urticaria, angioedema, anaphylactic reactions, and serum sickness.

Alopecia is a common complication of IFN-α. A nonspecific highly pruritic "dermatitis" is frequent in patients receiving IFN and ribavirin for hepatitis C.

Induction or exacerbation of various immune-mediated disorders, especially lupus erythematosus, has been reported with many biologicals (interleukin 2, IFN-α, anti–tumor necrosis factor α).

Granulocyte colony-stimulating factor may induce various neutrophilic dermatoses, including Sweet's syndrome and pyoderma gangrenosum, and can exacerbate psoriasis.

Cetuximab is a member of a new family of antineoplastic agents that inhibit the EGF receptor. These molecules induce acneiform eruptions after a mean interval of 10 days in a majority of patients. The severity of the eruption was shown to correlate with a better anticancer effect. Systemic antibiotics and topical anti-acne treatments are helpful.

Although not usually classified as adverse drug reactions, skin infections and skin cancer could become a major concern with long-term use of immune-modifying biologicals.

ANTIMALARIAL AGENTS

Antimalarial agents are used as therapy for several skin diseases, including the skin manifestations of lupus and polymorphous light eruption, but they can also induce cutaneous reactions. The most frequent is pruritus, which occurs in up to 50% of African patients receiving chloroquine and may be severe enough to lead to discontinuation of treatment.

Pigmentation disturbances, including black pigmentation of the face, mucous membranes, and pretibial and subungual areas, occur

TABLE 56-2 CLINICAL AND LABORATORY FINDINGS ASSOCIATED WITH MORE SERIOUS DRUG-INDUCED CUTANEOUS CLINICAL FINDINGS

Cutaneous
   Confluent erythema
   Facial edema or central facial involvement
   Skin pain
   Palpable purpura
   Skin necrosis
   Blisters or epidermal detachment
   Positive Nikolsky's sign
   Mucous membrane erosions
   Urticaria
   Swelling of tongue
General
   High fever [temperature >40°C (>104°F)]
   Enlarged lymph nodes
   Arthralgias or arthritis
   Shortness of breath, wheezing, hypotension
Laboratory results
   Eosinophil count >1000/μL
   Lymphocytosis with atypical lymphocytes
   Abnormal liver function tests

Source: Adapted from Roujeau and Stern.

with antimalarials. Quinacrine (mepacrine) causes generalized, cutaneous yellow discoloration. Less frequent reactions include pustular eruptions (AGEP) and hypersensitivity/DRESS.

MANAGEMENT OF A PATIENT WITH A DRUG ERUPTION

There are four main questions to be answered when seeing an eruption:

1. Is it a severe eruption or the onset of a form that may become severe?
2. Is it a drug reaction?
3. Which drug(s) are suspected, and which should be withdrawn?
4. What is recommended for future use of drugs?

EARLY DIAGNOSIS OF SEVERE ERUPTIONS

Many patients who experience a severe skin reaction complain that the diagnosis has been delayed, sometimes for several days. Initially, most eruptions look nonspecific. Of special importance is the rapid recognition of reactions that may become serious or life-threatening. Table 56-2 lists clinical and laboratory features that, if present, suggest the reaction may be serious. Table 56-3 provides key features of the most serious adverse cutaneous reactions. Intensity of symptoms and rapid progression of signs should raise the suspicion of a severe eruption. Any doubt should lead to consultation with a dermatologist and/or referral of the patient to a specialized center.

CONFIRMATION OF DRUG REACTION

The probability of drug etiology varies with the pattern of the reaction. Only fixed drug eruptions are always drug-induced. Maculopapular eruptions are usually viral in children and drug-induced in adults. Among severe reactions, attribution to drugs varies from 10–20% for anaphylaxis and vasculitis to 70–90% for AGEP, DRESS, SJS, or TEN. Skin biopsy helps in characterizing the reaction but does not indicate drug causality. Blood counts and liver and renal function tests are important for evaluating organ involvement. The association of mild elevation of liver enzymes and high eosinophil count is frequent but not specific for a drug reaction. Blood tests that could identify an alternative cause, antinuclear antibody tests, and serology or polymerase chain reaction for infections may be of great importance for final assessment of etiology.

WHICH DRUG(S) TO SUSPECT AND WITHDRAW

Most cases of drug eruptions occur during the first course of treatment with a new medication, after a delay that varies with the type of reaction. A notable exception is IgE-mediated urticaria and anaphylaxis that need presensitization and develop a few minutes to a few hours after rechallenge. Characteristic time lags between onset of treatment and reaction are 4–14 days for maculopapular eruptions, 7–21 days for SJS/TEN, and 14–48 days for DRESS. Medications introduced for the first time in the relevant time frame are prime suspects. Two other important elements to suspect causality at this stage are (1) previous experience with the drug in the population and (2) alternative etiologic candidates.

TABLE 56-3 CLINICAL FEATURES OF SELECTED SEVERE CUTANEOUS REACTIONS OFTEN INDUCED BY DRUGS

Diagnosis	Mucosal Lesions	Typical Skin Lesions	Frequent Signs and Symptoms	Alternative Causes Not Related to Drugs
Stevens-Johnson syndrome	Erosions usually at ≥two sites	Small blisters on dusky purpuric macules or atypical targets; rare areas of confluence; detachment ≤10% of body surface area	Most cases involve fever	10–20% cause not determined
Toxic epidermal necrolysis[a]	Erosions usually at ≥two sites	Individual lesions like those seen in Stevens-Johnson syndrome; confluent erythema; outer layer of epidermis separates readily from basal layer with lateral pressure; large sheet of necrotic epidermis; total detachment of >30% of body surface area	Nearly all cases involve fever, "acute skin failure," leukopenia	10–20% cause not determined
Hypersensitivity syndrome	Infrequent	Severe exanthematous rash (may become purpuric), exfoliative dermatitis	30–50% of cases involve fever, lymphadenopathy, hepatitis, nephritis, carditis, eosinophilia, atypical lymphocytes	Cutaneous lymphoma
Acute generalized exanthematous pustulosis	About 20% erosions mouth, tongue	Initially nonfollicular small pustules overlying edematous erythema, sometimes leading to superficial ulcers	Fever, burning, pruritus, facial swelling, leukocytosis, hypocalcemia	Infection
Serum sickness or reactions resembling serum sickness	Absent	Morbilliform lesions, sometimes with urticaria	Fever, arthralgias	Infection
Anticoagulant-induced necrosis	Infrequent	Erythema then purpura and necrosis, especially of fatty areas	Pain in affected areas	Disseminated intravascular coagulopathy, septicemia
Angioedema	Often involved	Urticaria or swelling of central part of face	Respiratory distress, cardiovascular collapse	Insect stings, foods

[a]Overlap of Stevens-Johnson syndrome and toxic epidermal necrolysis with features of both and attachment of 10 to 30% of body surface area may occur.

Source: Adapted from Roujeau and Stern.

The decision to continue or discontinue any medication will depend on the severity of the reaction, the severity of the primary disease, degree of suspicion of causality, and feasibility of an alternative safer treatment. In many instances when a decision of "treating through" an eruption has been made, the rash disappears in a few days. This was seen in patients with AIDS treated for opportunistic infections with antibacterial sulfonamides. The decision to treat through an eruption should, however, remain the exception and withdrawal of every suspect drug the general rule. On the other hand, drugs that are not suspected and are important for the patient, e.g., antidiabetic or antihypertensive agents, generally should not be withdrawn. This approach prevents reluctance to future utilization of these agents.

RECOMMENDATION FOR FUTURE USE OF DRUGS

The aims are (1) to prevent the recurrence of the drug eruption and (2) not to compromise future treatments by contraindicating otherwise useful medications.

Begin with thorough assessment of drug causality. Drug causality is evaluated based on timing of the reaction, evaluation of other possible causes, effect of drug withdrawal or continuation, and knowledge of medications that have been associated with the observed reaction. Combination of these criteria leads to considering the causality as definite, probable, possible, or unlikely.

A drug with "unlikely" causality or that has been continued when the reaction improved or reintroduced without a reaction can be administered safely.

A drug with a "definite" or "probable" causality should be contraindicated, and a warning card given to the patient.

A drug with a "possible" causality may be submitted to further investigations depending on the expected need for future treatment.

The usefulness of drug tests is still debated. Many in vitro tests have been developed. They include lymphocyte proliferation assays, measuring the production of cytokines by patient lymphocytes in presence of medication, lymphocyte toxicity tests, and basophil degranulation assays. The predictive value of these tests has not been validated in any large series of affected patients, and these tests are research and not clinical tools.

In patients with history suggesting immediate IgE-mediated reactions to penicillin, skin testing with major and minor determinants of penicillins or cephalosporins has proved useful for identifying patients at risk of anaphylactic reactions to these agents. However, skin tests themselves carry a small risk of anaphylaxis. Negative skin tests do not totally rule out IgE-mediated reactivity, but the risk of anaphylaxis in response to penicillin administration in patients with negative skin tests is about 1% while about two-thirds of patients with a positive skin test experience an allergic response on rechallenge.

For patients with late drug reactions, the clinical usefulness of skin tests is more questionable. At least one of a combination of several tests (prick, patch, and intradermal) is positive in 50–70% of patients with a reaction "definitely" attributed to a single medication. This low sensitivity probably contributes to the fact that readministration of drugs that had been tested negative resulted in up to 17% eruptions.

CROSS-SENSITIVITY

Because of the possibility of cross-sensitivity among chemically related drugs, many physicians recommend avoidance of not only the medication that induced the reaction but also all drugs of the same group.

There are two types of cross-sensitivity. Reactions that depend on a pharmacologic interaction may recur with all drugs that target the same pathway, whether structurally similar or not. This is the case with angioedema caused by NSAIDs and ACE inhibitors. In this situation, the risk of recurrence varies from drug to drug in a particular class; however, avoidance of all drugs in the class is usually recommended. The other cross-sensitivity manifests in the risk that structurally related drugs are cross-recognized by the immune system. This is a real problem with aromatic antiepileptics (barbiturates, phenytoin, carbamazepine), with up to 50% reaction to a second drug in patients who reacted to one. For other drugs, in vitro as well as in vivo data have suggested that cross-reactivity existed only between compounds with very similar chemical structures. Sulfamethoxazole-specific lymphocytes may occasionally recognize a few other antibacterial sulfonamides but not diuretics, antidiabetic drugs, or anti-COX2 NSAIDs with a sulfonamide group.

Recent data suggest that although the risk of a drug eruption to another drug was increased in persons with a prior reaction, "cross-sensitivity" was probably not the explanation. As an example, persons with a history of an allergic-like reaction to penicillin were at higher risk to develop a reaction to antibacterial sulfonamides than to cephalosporin.

These data suggest that the list of drugs to avoid after a drug reaction should be limited to the causative one(s) and to a few very similar medications.

Because of growing evidence that some severe cutaneous reactions to drugs are associated with HLA genes, it is probably wise to recommend that first-degree family members of patients with severe cutaneous reactions also should avoid these causative medications.

Desensitization can be considered in those with history of reaction to a medication that must be used again. Efficacy of such procedures has been demonstrated in cases of immediate reaction to penicillin and positive skin tests, anaphylactic reactions to platinum chemotherapy, and delayed reactions to sulfonamides in patients with AIDS. Various protocols are available, including oral and parenteral approaches. Oral desensitization appears to have a lower risk of serious anaphylactic reactions. However, desensitization carries the risk of anaphylaxis regardless of how it is performed. After desensitization, many patients experience non-life-threatening reactions during therapy with the culprit drug.

REPORTING

Any severe reaction to drugs should be notified to a regulatory agency or to pharmaceutical companies. Because severe reactions are too rare to be detected in premarketing clinical trials, spontaneous reports are of critical importance for early detection of unexpected life-threatening events. To be useful, the report should contain enough details to permit ascertainment of severity and drug causality. This permits recognition of similar cases that may be reported from several different sources.

FURTHER READINGS

AUQUIER-DUNANT A et al: Severe cutaneous adverse reactions. Correlations between clinical patterns and causes of erythema multiforme majus, Stevens-Johnson syndrome, and toxic epidermal necrolysis: Results of an international prospective study. Arch Dermatol 138:1019, 2002

BAHRAMI S et al: Tissue eosinophilia as an indicator of drug-induced cutaneous small-vessel vasculitis. Arch Dermatol 142:155, 2006

BIGBY M: Rates of cutaneous reactions to drugs. Arch Dermatol 137:765, 2001

BREATHNACH SM: Adverse cutaneous reactions to drugs. Clin Med 2:15, 2002

ELIASZEWICZ M et al: Prospective evaluation of risk factors of cutaneous drug reactions to sulfonamides in patients with AIDS. J Am Acad Dermatol 47:40, 2002

HUNG SI et al: HLAB*5801 allele as a genetic marker for severe cutaneous reactions caused by allopurinol. Proc Natl Acad Sci USA 102:4134, 2005

LEE CW et al: Rapid inpatient/outpatient desensitization for chemotherapy hypersensitivity: Standard protocol effective in 57 patients for 255 courses. Gynecol Oncol 99:393, 2005

MESSAAD D et al: Drug provocation tests in patients with a history suggesting an immediate drug hypersensitivity reaction. Ann Intern Med 140:I30, 2004

PICHLER WJ: Delayed drug hypersensitivity reactions. Ann Intern Med 139:683, 2003

ROUJEAU JC: Immune mechanisms in drug allergy. Allergology Internat J 55:27, 2006

ROUJEAU JC, STERN RS: Severe adverse cutaneous reactions to drugs. N Engl J Med 331:1272, 1994

WYATT AJ et al: Cutaneous reactions to chemotherapy and their management. Am J Clin Dermatol 7:45, 2006

57 Photosensitivity and Other Reactions to Light

David R. Bickers

PART 2

Cardinal Manifestations and Presentation of Diseases

SOLAR RADIATION

Sunlight is the most visible and obvious source of comfort in the environment. The sun provides the beneficial effects of warmth and vitamin D synthesis; however, acute and chronic sun exposure also have pathologic consequences. Few effects of sun exposure beyond those affecting the skin have been identified, but cutaneous exposure to sunlight is the major cause of human skin cancer and can exert immunosuppressive effects as well.

The sun's energy reaching the earth's surface is limited to components of the ultraviolet (UV), the visible, and portions of the infrared spectra. The cutoff at the short end of the UV is at ~290 nm; this is due primarily to stratospheric ozone formed by highly energetic ionizing radiation, thereby preventing penetration to the earth's surface of the shorter, more energetic, potentially more harmful wavelengths of solar radiation. Indeed, concern about destruction of the ozone layer by chlorofluorocarbons released into the atmosphere has led to international agreements to reduce production of these chemicals.

Measurements of solar flux indicate that there is a twentyfold regional variation in the amount of energy at 300 nm that reaches the earth's surface. This variability relates to seasonal effects; the path of sunlight transmission through ozone and air; the altitude (4% increase for each 300 m of elevation); the latitude (increasing intensity with decreasing latitude); and the amount of cloud cover, fog, and pollution.

The major components of the photobiologic action spectrum capable of affecting human skin include the UV and visible wavelengths between 290 and 700 nm. In addition, the wavelengths beyond 700 nm in the infrared spectrum primarily emit heat and under certain circumstances may exacerbate the pathologic effects of energy in the UV and visible spectra.

The UV spectrum reaching the earth represents <10% of total incident solar energy and is arbitrarily divided into two major segments, UV-B and UV-A, comprising the wavelengths from 290–400 nm. UV-B consists of wavelengths between 290 and 320 nm. This portion of the photobiologic action spectrum is the most efficient in producing redness or erythema in human skin and hence is sometimes known as the "sunburn spectrum." UV-A represents those wavelengths between 320 and 400 nm and is ~1000-fold less efficient in producing skin redness than is UV-B.

The wavelengths between 400 and 700 nm are visible to the human eye. The photon energy in the visible spectrum is not capable of damaging human skin in the absence of a photosensitizing chemical. Without the absorption of energy by a molecule there can be no photosensitivity. Thus the *absorption spectrum* of a molecule is defined as the range of wavelengths absorbed by it, whereas the *action spectrum* for an effect of incident radiation is defined as the range of wavelengths that evoke the response.

Photosensitivity occurs when a photon-absorbing chemical (chromophore) present in the skin absorbs incident energy, becomes excited, and transfers the absorbed energy to various structures or to oxygen.

UV RADIATION (UVR) AND SKIN STRUCTURE AND FUNCTION

Skin consists of two major compartments: the outer epidermis, a stratified squamous epithelium, and the underlying dermis rich in matrix proteins such as collagen and elastin. Both of these compartments are susceptible to damage from sun exposure. The epidermis and the dermis contain several chromophores capable of absorbing incident solar energy including nucleic acids, proteins, and lipids. The outermost epidermal layer, the stratum corneum, is a major absorber of UV-B, and <10% of incident UV-B wavelengths penetrate through the epi-

dermis to the dermis. Approximately 3% of radiation below 300 nm, 20% of radiation below 360 nm, and 33% of short visible radiation reaches the basal cell layer in untanned human skin. In contrast, UV-A readily penetrates to the dermis and is capable of altering structural and matrix proteins that contribute to photoaging of chronically sun-exposed skin, particularly in individuals of light complexion.

Molecular Targets for UVR-Induced Skin Effects   Epidermal DNA, predominantly in keratinocytes and in Langerhans cells (LCs), which are dendritic antigen-presenting cells, absorbs UV-B and undergoes structural changes including the formation of cyclobutane dimers and 6,4-photoproducts. These structural changes are potentially mutagenic and can be repaired by mechanisms that result in their recognition and excision and the reestablishment of normal base sequences. The efficient repair of these structural aberrations is crucial, since individuals with defective DNA repair are at high risk for the development of cutaneous cancer. For example, patients with xeroderma pigmentosum (XP), an autosomal recessive disorder, are characterized by variably deficient repair of UV-induced photoproducts, and their skin phenotype often manifests the dry, leathery appearance of prematurely photoaged skin as well as basal cell and squamous cell carcinomas and melanoma in the first two decades of life. Studies in mice using knockout gene technology have verified the importance of functional genes regulating these repair pathways in preventing the development of UV-induced cancer. Furthermore, incorporation of a bacterial DNA repair enzyme, T4N5 endonuclease, into liposomes in a product applied to skin of patients with XP selectively removes cyclobutane pyrimidine dimers and reduces the degree of solar damage and skin cancer. DNA damage in LCs may contribute to the known immunosuppressive effects of UV-B (see "Immunologic Effects," below).

Cutaneous Optics and Chromophores   Chromophores are endogenous or exogenous chemical components that can absorb physical energy. Endogenous chromophores are of two types: (1) chemicals that are normal components of skin, including nucleic acids, proteins, lipids, and 7-dehydrocholesterol, the precursor of vitamin D; and (2) chemicals, such as porphyrins, synthesized elsewhere in the body that circulate in the bloodstream and diffuse into the skin. Normally, only trace amounts of porphyrins are present in the skin, but in selected diseases known as the porphyrias (Chap. 352), increased amounts are released into the circulation from the bone marrow and the liver and are transported to the skin, where they absorb incident energy both in the Soret band, around 400 nm (short visible), and to a lesser extent in the red portion of the visible spectrum (580–660 nm). This results in the generation of reactive oxygen species that can mediate structural damage to the skin, manifest as erythema, edema, urticaria, or blister formation.

Acute Effects of Sun Exposure   The acute effects of skin exposure to sunlight include sunburn and vitamin D synthesis. Molecular targets for UVR in addition to DNA include molecular oxygen leading to the generation of reactive oxygen species (ROS), cell membranes, and urocanic acid.

SUNBURN   This painful skin condition is caused predominantly by UV-B. Generally speaking, an individual's ability to tolerate sunlight is inversely proportional to the degree of melanin pigmentation. Melanin, a complex tyrosine polymer, is synthesized in specialized epidermal dendritic cells known as melanocytes and is packaged into *melanosomes* that are transferred via dendritic process into *keratinocytes*, thereby providing photoprotection and simultaneously darkening the skin. Sun-induced melanogenesis is a consequence of increased tyrosinase activity in melanocytes that in turn is a consequence of a human gene, the melanocortin1 receptor (*MCIR*), that accounts for the wide variation in human skin and hair color. Human *MCIR* encodes a 317-amino-acid G-coupled receptor (melanocortin receptor) that binds α-melanocyte-stimulating hormone. This leads to increased intracellular cyclic AMP and protein kinase A, followed by increased transcription of microphthalmia transcription factor

TABLE 57-1	SKIN TYPE AND SUNBURN SENSITIVITY (FITZPATRICK CLASSIFICATION)
Type	**Description**
I	Always burn, never tan
II	Always burn, sometimes tan
III	Sometimes burn, sometimes tan
IV	Sometimes burn, always tan
V	Never burn, sometimes tan
VI	Never burn, always tan

(MITF) that regulates melanogenesis. *MCIR* mutations account for population differences in skin color, ability to tan, and cancer susceptibility. The Fitzpatrick classification of human skin is a function of the efficiency of the epidermal-melanin unit and can usually be ascertained by asking an individual two questions: (1) Do you burn after sun exposure? and (2) Do you tan after sun exposure? The answers to these questions permit division of the population into six skin types varying from type I (always burn, never tan) to type VI (never burn, always tan) (Table 57-1).

Sunburn is due to vasodilatation of dermal blood vessels. There is a lag in time between skin exposure to sunlight and the development of visible redness (usually 4–12 h), suggesting that an epidermal chromophore causes delayed production and/or release of vasoactive mediator(s), or cytokines, that diffuse to the dermal vasculature to evoke vasodilatation.

The action spectrum for sunburn erythema includes the UV-B and UV-A. Photons in the UV-B are at least 1000-fold more efficient than photons in the UV-A in evoking the response. However, UV-A may contribute to sunburn erythema at midday when much more UV-A than UV-B is present in the solar spectrum. UV-induced activation of nuclear factor-κB (NF-κB)-dependent gene transactivation can augment release of several proinflammatory cytokines including interleukin (IL) 1B, 1L-6, IL-8, vascular endothelial growth factor, prostaglandin E$_2$, and tumor necrosis factor α. Local accumulation of these cytokines occurs in sunburned skin, providing chemotactic factors that attract neutrophils and macrophages. It is of interest that nonsteroidal anti-inflammatory drugs (NSAIDs) can reduce sunburn erythema, perhaps by blocking I-κB kinase 2, the enzyme essential for nuclear translocation of cytosolic NF-κB.

VITAMIN D PHOTOCHEMISTRY Cutaneous exposure to UV-B causes photolysis of epidermal 7-dehydrocholesterol converting it to pre-vitamin D$_3$, which then undergoes a temperature-dependent isomerization to form the stable hormone vitamin D$_3$. This compound then diffuses to the dermal vasculature and circulates systemically where it is converted to the functional hormone 1,25-dihydroxyvitamin D$_3$[1,25(OH)$_2$D$_3$]. Vitamin D metabolites from the circulation or those produced in the skin itself can augment epidermal differentiation signaling. Controversy exists regarding the importance of sun exposure in vitamin D homeostasis. At present, it is important to emphasize that the use of sunscreens does not substantially diminish vitamin D levels. Since aging also substantially decreases the ability of human skin to photocatalytically produce vitamin D$_3$, the widespread use of sunscreens that filter out UV-B has led to concern that vitamin D deficiency may become a significant clinical problem in the elderly.

Chronic Effects of Sun Exposure: Nonmalignant The clinical features of photodamaged sun-exposed skin consist of wrinkling, blotchiness, and telangiectasia and a roughened, irregular, "weather-beaten" leathery appearance. Whether this photoaging represents accelerated chronologic aging or a separate and distinct process is not clear.

Within chronically sun-exposed epidermis, there is thickening (acanthosis) and morphologic heterogeneity within the basal cell layer. Higher but irregular melanosome content may be present in some keratinocytes, indicating prolonged residence of the cells in the basal cell layer. These structural changes may help to explain the leathery texture and the blotchy discoloration of sun-damaged skin.

UV-A is important in the pathogenesis of photoaging in human skin, and ROS are likely involved. The dermis and its connective tissue matrix are the major site for sun-associated chronic damage, manifest as solar elastosis, a massive increase in thickened irregular masses of abnormal elastic fibers. Collagen fibers are also abnormally clumped in the deeper dermis of sun-damaged skin. The chromophore(s), the action spectra, and the specific biochemical events orchestrating these changes are only partially understood, although UV-A seems to be primarily involved. Chronologically aged, sun-protected skin and photoaged skin share important molecular features including connective tissue damage and elevated matrix metalloproteinases (MMPs). MMPs are enzymes involved in the degradation of the extracellular matrix, and UV-A induces MMP-1 and MMP-3 mRNA expression, leading to enhanced collagen breakdown. In addition, UV-A reduces type I procollagen mRNA expression.

Chronic Effects of Sun Exposure: Malignant One of the major known consequences of chronic skin exposure to sunlight is nonmelanoma skin cancer. The two types of nonmelanoma skin cancer are *basal cell carcinoma* (BCC) and *squamous cell carcinoma* (SCC; Chap. 83). There are three major steps for cancer induction: initiation, promotion, and progression. Exposure of human skin to sunlight results in *initiation*, a step whereby structural (mutagenic) changes in DNA evoke an irreversible alteration in the target cell (*keratinocyte*) that begins the tumorigenic process. Exposure to a tumor initiator such as UV-B is believed to be a necessary but not sufficient step in the malignant process, since initiated skin cells not exposed to tumor promoters do not generally develop tumors. The second stage in tumor development is *promotion*, a multistep process whereby chronic exposure to sunlight evokes epigenetic changes that culminate in the clonal expansion of initiated cells and cause the development, over many years, of premalignant growths known as *actinic keratoses*, a minority of which may progress to form skin cancer. Based on extensive studies it seems clear that UV-B is a *complete carcinogen*, meaning that it can act as both a tumor initiator and a promoter.

The third and final step in the malignant process is *malignant conversion* of benign precursors into malignant lesions, a process thought to require additional genetic alterations in already transformed cells. Skin carcinogenesis is thought to be caused by the accumulation of mutations in the tumor-suppressor gene *p53* as a result of UV-induced DNA damage. Indeed both human and murine UV-induced skin cancers have unique *p53* mutations (C → T and CC → TT transitions) that are present in the majority of these lesions. Studies have shown that sunscreens can substantially reduce the frequency of these signature mutations in *p53* and can dramatically inhibit the induction of tumors. The *p53* mutations are present in sun-exposed normal human skin, in actinic keratoses, and in nonmelanoma skin cancers including BCC and SCC.

BCCs also manifest mutations in the tumor-suppressor gene known as *patched*, which results in activation of hedgehog signaling, and enhanced activity of *smoothened*, which in turn causes downstream activation of transcription factors that augment cell proliferation. Thus, these tumors can manifest mutations in both p53 and in *patched*.

Sun exposure causes nonmelanoma cancers and melanoma of the skin, although the evidence is far more direct for its role in nonmelanoma (BCC and SCC) than in melanoma. Approximately 80% of nonmelanoma skin cancers develop on exposed body areas, including the face, the neck, and the hands. Major risk factors include male sex, childhood sun exposures, older age, fair skin, and residence at latitudes closer to the equator. Whites of darker complexions (e.g., Hispanics) have one-tenth the risk of developing such cancers compared to fair-skinned individuals. Blacks are at substantially reduced risk for all forms of skin cancer. More than 1.3 million individuals in the United States develop nonmelanoma skin cancer annually, and the lifetime risk for a fair-skinned individual to develop such a neoplasm is estimated at ~15%. A consensus exists that the incidence of nonmelanoma skin cancer in the population is increasing at the rate of 2–3% per year, for unknown reasons. One potential explanation is the widespread use of indoor tanning. It is estimated that 30 million people tan indoors in the United States annually, including >2 million adolescents.

The relationship of sun exposure to melanoma development is less clear-cut, but suggestive evidence supports an association. The strongest risk factors for melanoma include positive family history for melanoma, multiple dysplastic nevi, and prior melanoma. Melanomas occasionally develop by the teenage years, indicating that the latent period for tumor growth is less than that of nonmelanoma skin cancer. Melanomas are among the most rapidly increasing of all human malignancies (Chap. 83). Epidemiologic studies of immigrant populations of similar ethnic stock indicate that individuals born in one area or who migrate to the same locale before age 10 have higher age-specific melanoma rates than individuals arriving later. It is thus reasonable to conclude that life in a sunny climate from birth or early childhood increases the risk of melanoma. In general, risk does not correlate with cumulative sun exposure but may relate to the duration and extent of exposure in childhood. Epidemiologic studies have shown that indoor tanning is a risk factor for melanoma.

Meta-analysis of 17 case-control studies in patients with melanoma concluded that the protective effect of sunscreens against this type of tumor could not be substantiated, but this is likely due to failure to control for confounding factors such as sunscreen stability and frequency of application. Since no prospective studies are available to address this issue, it seems reasonable to recommend that patients at risk for melanoma utilize photoprotection such as sun avoidance, high sun protective factor (SPF) sunscreens, and protective clothing.

Immunologic Effects   Exposure to solar radiation causes local (inhibition of immune responses to antigens applied at the irradiated site) and systemic (inhibition of immune responses to antigens applied at remote unirradiated sites) immunosuppression. The action spectrum for UV-induced immunosuppression closely mimics the absorption spectrum of DNA. Pyrimidine dimers in LCs may inhibit antigen presentation. The absorption spectrum of epidermal urocanic acid closely mimics the action spectrum for UV-B-induced immunosuppression. *Trans-cis* isomerization of urocanic acid in the stratum corneum leads to its systemic absorption and consequent immunosuppressive effects. Furthermore administration of modest doses of UV-B to human skin reduces the degree of allergic sensitization to the potent contact allergen, dinitrochlorobenzene. This is associated with ROS-induced depletion of epidermal LCs.

Higher doses of UV-radiation evoke diminished immunologic responses to antigens introduced either epicutaneously or intracutaneously at sites distant from the irradiated site. These suppressed responses are also associated with the induction of antigen-specific suppressor T lymphocytes and may be mediated by as yet undefined factors that are released from epidermal cells at the irradiated site. One important consequence of chronic sun exposure and the concomitant immunosuppression is enhanced risk of skin cancer. Perhaps the most graphic demonstration of the role of immunosuppression in enhancing the risk of nonmelanoma skin cancer has come from studies of patients receiving organ transplantation who are on chronic immunosuppressive antirejection drug regimens. More than 50% of transplant patients develop BCCs and SCCs, and these cancers are the most common malignancy arising in immunosuppressed solid-organ transplant recipients. Human papilloma viruses (HPVs) may also play a role in the increased risk of SCCs in these patients since tumors display an HPV DNA carriage rate of almost 80%. These patients require close periodic monitoring and rigorous photoprotection using sunscreens, protective clothing, and sun avoidance.

PHOTOSENSITIVITY DISEASES

The diagnosis of photosensitivity requires a careful history to define the duration of the signs and symptoms, the length of time between exposure to sunlight and the development of subjective complaints, and visible changes in the skin. The age of onset can also be a helpful clue; for example, the acute photosensitivity of erythropoietic protoporphyria almost always begins in childhood, whereas the chronic photosensitivity

TABLE 57-2	CLASSIFICATION OF PHOTOSENSITIVITY DISEASES
Type	**Disease**
Genetic	Erythropoietic porphyria
	Erythropoietic protoporphyria
	Porphyria cutanea tarda—familial
	Variegate porphyria
	Hepatoerythropoietic porphyria
	Albinism
	Xeroderma pigmentosum
	Rothmund-Thompson disease
	Bloom syndrome
	Cockayne's disease
	Kindler syndrome
	Phenylketonuria
Metabolic	Porphyria cutanea tarda—sporadic
	Hartnup disease
	Kwashiorkor
	Pellagra
	Carcinoid syndrome
Phototoxic	
Internal	Drugs
External	Drugs, plants, food
Photoallergic	
Immediate	Solar urticaria
Delayed	Drug photoallergy
	Persistent light reaction/chronic actinic dermatitis
Neoplastic and degenerative	Photoaging
	Actinic keratosis
	Melanoma and nonmelanoma skin cancer
Idiopathic	Polymorphous light eruption
	Hydroa aestivale
	Actinic prurigo
Photoaggravated	Lupus erythematosus
	Systemic
	Subacute cutaneous
	Discoid
	Dermatomyositis
	Herpes simplex
	Lichen planus actinicus
	Acne vulgaris (aestivale)

of porphyria cutanea tarda (PCT) typically begins in the fourth and fifth decades. A history of exposure to topical and systemic drugs and chemicals may provide important clues. Many classes of drugs can cause photosensitivity on the basis of either phototoxicity or photoallergy. Fragrances such as musk ambrette that were previously present in numerous cosmetic products are also potent photosensitizers.

Examination of the skin may also offer important clues. Anatomic areas that are naturally protected from direct sunlight such as the hairy scalp, the upper eyelids, the retroauricular areas, and the infranasal and submental regions may be spared, whereas exposed areas show characteristic features of the pathologic process. These anatomic localization patterns are often helpful, but not infallible, in making the diagnosis. For example, airborne contact sensitizers that are blown onto the skin may produce dermatitis that can be difficult to distinguish from photosensitivity, despite the fact that such material may trigger skin reactivity in areas shielded from direct sunlight.

Many dermatologic conditions may be caused or aggravated by sunlight (Table 57-2). The role of light in evoking these responses may be dependent on genetic abnormalities ranging from well-described defects in DNA repair that occur in XP to the inherited abnormalities in heme synthesis that characterize the porphyrias. In certain photosensitivity diseases, the chromophore has been identified, whereas in the majority, the energy-absorbing agent is unknown.

Polymorphous Light Eruption   After sunburn, the most common type of photosensitivity disease is *polymorphous light eruption* (PLE), the mechanism of which is unknown. Many affected individuals never seek medical attention because the condition is often transient, becoming manifest each spring with initial sun exposure but then subsiding spontaneously with continuing exposure, a phenomenon known as "hardening." The major manifestations of PLE include pruritic (often intensely so) erythematous papules that may coalesce into plaques in a patchy distribution on exposed areas of the trunk and forearms. The face is usually less seriously involved.

The diagnosis can be confirmed by skin biopsy and by performing phototest procedures in which skin is exposed to multiple erythema doses of UV-A and UV-B. The action spectrum for PLE is usually within these portions of the solar spectrum.

Treatment of this PLE includes the use of sunscreens and the induction of hardening by the cautious administration of artificial UV-B (broad-band or narrow-band) and/or UV-A radiation for 2–3 weeks prior to initial sun exposure.

Phototoxicity and Photoallergy   These photosensitivity disorders are related to the topical or systemic administration of drugs and other chemicals. Both reactions require the absorption of energy by a drug or chemical resulting in the production of an excited-state photosensitizer that can transfer its absorbed energy to a bystander molecule or to molecular oxygen, thereby generating tissue-destructive chemical species, including ROS.

Phototoxicity is a nonimmunologic reaction caused by drugs and chemicals, a few of which are listed in Table 57-3. The usual clinical manifestations include erythema resembling a sunburn reaction that quickly desquamates, or "peels," within several days. In addition, edema, vesicles, and bullae may occur.

Photoallergy is much less common and is distinct in that this is an immunopathologic process. The excited-state photosensitizer may create highly unstable haptenic free radicals that bind covalently to macromolecules to form a functional antigen capable of evoking a delayed hypersensitivity response. Some of the drugs and chemicals that produce photoallergy are listed in Table 57-4. The clinical manifestations typically differ from those of phototoxicity in that an intensely pruritic eczematous dermatitis tends to predominate and evolves into lichenified, thickened, "leathery" changes in sun-exposed areas. A small subset (perhaps 5–10%) of patients with photoallergy may develop a persistent exquisite hypersensitivity to light even when the offending drug or chemical is identified and eliminated, a condition known as *persistent light reaction*.

A very uncommon type of persistent photosensitivity is known as *chronic actinic dermatitis*. These patients are typically elderly men with a long history of preexisting allergic contact dermatitis or photosensitivity. They are usually exquisitely sensitive to UV-B, UV-A, and visible wavelengths.

Diagnostic confirmation of phototoxicity and photoallergy can often be obtained using phototest procedures. In patients with suspected phototoxicity, determining the minimal erythema dose (MED) while the patient is exposed to a suspected agent and then repeating the MED after discontinuation of the agent may provide a clue to the causative drug or chemical. Photopatch testing can be performed to confirm the diagnosis of photoallergy. This is a simple variant of ordinary patch testing in which a series of known photoallergens is applied to the skin in duplicate and one set is irradiated with a suberythema dose of UV-A. Development of eczematous changes at sites exposed to sensitizer and light is a positive result. The characteristic abnormality in patients with persistent light reaction is a diminished threshold to erythema evoked by UV-B. Patients with chronic actinic dermatitis usually manifest a broad spectrum of UV hyperresponsiveness and require meticulous photoprotection including avoiding sun exposure, high (>30) SPF sunscreens, and in severe cases systemic immunosuppression, preferably with azathioprine (1–2 mg/kg per day).

The management of drug photosensitivity involves first and foremost the elimination of exposure to the chemical agents responsible for the reaction and minimization of sun exposure. The acute symptoms of phototoxicity may be ameliorated by cool, moist compresses, topical glucocorticoids, and systemically administered NSAIDs. In severely affected individuals, a rapidly tapered course of systemic glucocorticoids may be useful. Judicious use of analgesics may be necessary.

Photoallergic reactions require a similar management approach. Furthermore, patients with persistent light reaction and chronic actinic dermatitis must be meticulously protected against light exposure. In selected patients in whom chronic systemic high-dose glucocorticoids pose unacceptable risks, it may be necessary to employ immunosuppressive drugs such as azathioprine, cyclophosphamide, cyclosporine, or mycophenolate mofetil.

Porphyria   The porphyrias (Chap. 352) are a group of diseases that have in common inherited or acquired derangements in the synthesis of heme. Heme is an iron-chelated tetrapyrrole or porphyrin, and the nonmetal chelated porphyrins are potent photosensitizers that absorb light intensely in both the short (400–410 nm) and the long (580–650 nm) portions of the visible spectrum.

Heme cannot be reutilized and must be continuously synthesized, and the two body compartments with the largest capacity for its production are the bone marrow and the liver. Accordingly, the porphyrias originate in one or the other of these organs, with the end result of excessive endogenous production of potent photosensitizing porphyrins. The porphyrins circulate in the bloodstream and diffuse into the skin, where they absorb solar energy, become photoexcited, generate ROS, and evoke cutaneous photosensitivity. The mechanism of porphyrin photosensitization is known to be photodynamic, or oxygen-dependent, and is mediated by ROS such as singlet oxygen and superoxide anions.

Porphyria cutanea tarda is the most common type of human porphyria and is associated with decreased activity of the enzyme uroporphyrinogen decarboxylase associated with a number of gene mutations. There are two basic types of PCT: (1) the sporadic or acquired type, generally seen in individuals ingesting ethanol or receiving estrogens; and (2) the inherited type, in which there is autosomal dominant transmission of deficient enzyme activity. Both forms are associated with increased hepatic iron stores.

In both types of PCT, the predominant feature is a chronic photosensitivity characterized by increased fragility of sun-exposed skin, particularly areas subject to repeated trauma such as the dorsa of the hands, the

TABLE 57-4	PHOTOALLERGIC DRUGS	
	Topical	Systemic
6-Methylcoumarin	+	
Aminobenzoic acid and esters	+	
Bithionol	+	
Chlorpromazine		+
Diclofenac		+
Fluoroquinolones		+
Halogenated salicylanilides	+	
Hypericin (St John's Wort)	+	+
Musk ambrette	+	
Piroxicam		+
Promethazine		+
Sulfonamides		+
Sulfonylureas		+

TABLE 57-3	PHOTOTOXIC DRUGS	
	Topical	Systemic
Amiodarone		+
Dacarbazine		+
Fluoroquinolones		+
5-Fluorouracil	+	+
Furosemide		+
Nalidixic acid		+
Phenothiazines		+
Psoralens	+	+
Retinoids	+/−	+
Sulfonamides		+
Sulfonylureas		+
Tetracyclines		+
Thiazides		+
Vinblastine		+

forearms, the face, and the ears. The predominant skin lesions are vesicles and bullae that rupture, producing moist erosions, often with a hemorrhagic base, that heal slowly with crusting and purplish discoloration of the affected skin. Hypertrichosis, mottled pigmentary change, and scleroderma-like induration are associated features. Biochemical confirmation of the diagnosis can be obtained by measurement of urinary porphyrin excretion, plasma porphyrin assay, and by assay of erythrocyte and/or hepatic uroporphyrinogen decarboxylase. Multiple mutations of the uroporphyrinogen decarboxylase gene have been identified in human populations, including exon skipping and base substitutions. Some patients with PCT have associated mutations in the *HFE* gene linked to hemochromatosis. This could contribute to the iron overload seen in PCT, although iron status as measured by serum ferritin, iron levels, and transferrin saturation is no different from that in PCT patients without *HFE* mutations. Prior hepatitis C virus infection appears to be an independent risk factor for PCT.

Treatment of PCT consists of repeated phlebotomies to diminish the excessive hepatic iron stores and/or intermittent low doses of the antimalarial drugs chloroquine and hydroxychloroquine. Long-term remission of the disease can be achieved if the patient eliminates exposure to porphyrinogenic agents.

Erythropoietic protoporphyria originates in the bone marrow and is due to a decrease in the mitochondrial enzyme ferrochelatase secondary to numerous gene mutations. The major clinical features include an acute photosensitivity characterized by subjective burning and stinging of exposed skin that often develops during or just after exposure. There may be associated skin swelling and, after repeated episodes, a waxlike scarring.

The diagnosis is confirmed by demonstration of elevated levels of free erythrocyte protoporphyrin. Detection of increased plasma protoporphyrin helps to differentiate lead poisoning and iron-deficiency anemia, in both of which elevated erythrocyte protoporphyrin levels occur in the absence of cutaneous photosensitivity and of elevated plasma protoporphyrin levels.

Treatment consists of reducing sun exposure and the oral administration of the carotenoid β-carotene, which is an effective scavenger of free radicals. This drug increases tolerance to sun exposure in many affected individuals, although it has no effect on deficient ferrochelatase.

An algorithm for managing patients with photosensitivity is illustrated in **Fig. 57-1**.

PHOTOPROTECTION

Since photosensitivity of the skin results from exposure to sunlight, it follows that absolute avoidance of the sun would eliminate these disorders. Unfortunately, contemporary life-styles make this an impractical alternative for most individuals, and this has led to a search for better approaches to photoprotection.

Natural photoprotection is provided by structural proteins in the epidermis, particularly keratins and melanin. The amount of melanin and its distribution in cells is genetically regulated, and individuals of darker complexion (skin types IV–VI) are at decreased risk for the development of acute sunburn and cutaneous malignancy.

Other forms of photoprotection include clothing and sunscreens. Clothing constructed of tightly woven sun-protective fabrics, irrespective of color, affords substantial protection. Wide-brimmed hats, long sleeves, and trousers all reduce direct exposure. Sunscreens are now considered to be over-the-counter drugs and category I ingredients are recognized by the U.S. Food and Drug Administration (FDA) as monographed and safe and effective. These are listed in **Table 57-5**. Sunscreens are rated for their photoprotective effect by their SPF. The SPF is simply a ratio of the time required to produce sunburn erythema with and without sunscreen application. The monograph stipulates that sunscreens must be rated on a scale ranging from minimal (SPF ≮2 and ≯12) to moderate (SPF ≮12 and ≯30) to high (SPF ≥30, labeled as 30+). No SPF number >30 can be placed on the label.

In addition to light absorption, a critical determinant of the sustained photoprotective effect of sunscreens is their water-resistance.

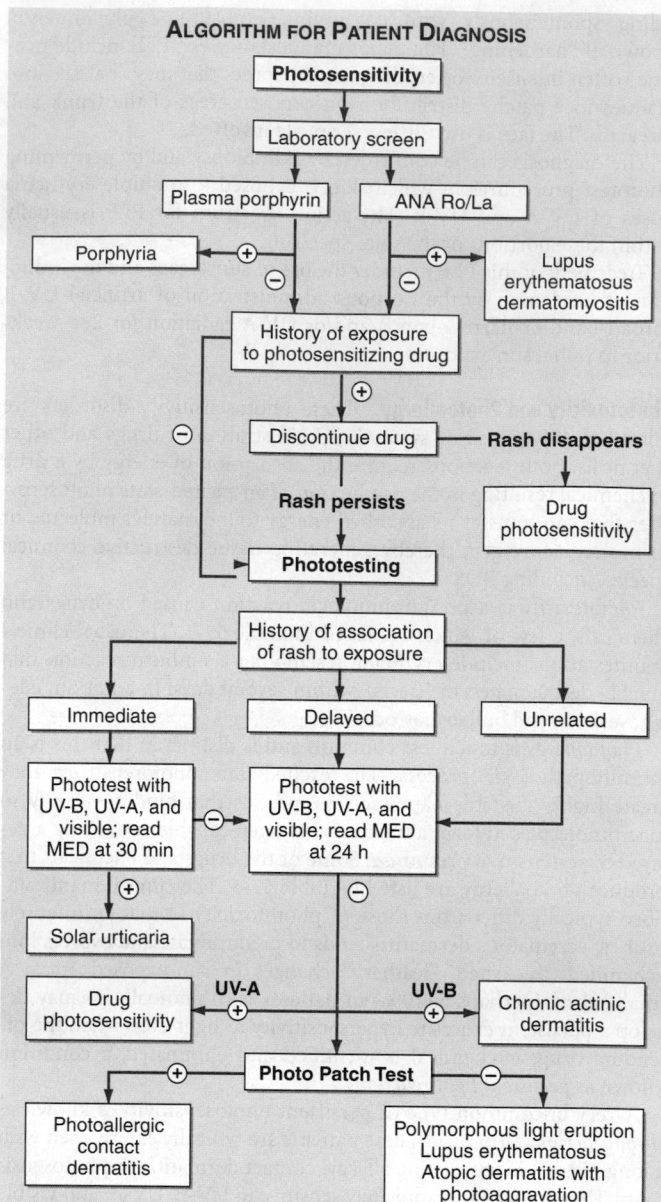

FIGURE 57-1 An algorithm for the diagnosis of a patient with photosensitivity.

TABLE 57-5	FDA CATEGORY 1 MONOGRAPHED SUNSCREEN INGREDIENTS[a]
Ingredients	**Maximum Concentration, %**
p-Aminobenzoic acid (PABA)	15
Avobenzone	3
Cinoxate	3
Dioxybenzone (benzophenone-8)	3
Ecamsule[b]	15
Homosalate	15
Menthyl anthranilate	5
Octocrylene	10
Octyl methoxycinnamate	7.5
Octyl salicylate	5
Oxybenzone (benzophenone-3)	6
Padimate O (octyl dimethyl PABA)	8
Phenylbenzimidazole sulfonic acid	4
Sulisobenzone (benzophenone-4)	10
Titanium dioxide	25
Trolamine salicylate	12
Zinc oxide	25

[a]FDA, U.S. Food and Drug Administration.
[b]Recently approved by the FDA.

The FDA monograph has also defined strict testing criteria for sunscreens making this claim.

Some degree of photoprotection can also be achieved by limiting the time of exposure during the day. Since the majority of an individual's total lifetime sun exposure may occur by the age of 18, it is important to educate parents and young children about the hazards of sunlight. Simply eliminating exposure at midday will substantially reduce lifetime UV-B exposure.

PHOTOTHERAPY AND PHOTOCHEMOTHERAPY

UV can also be used therapeutically. The administration of UV-B alone or in combination with topically applied agents can induce remissions of psoriasis and atopic dermatitis.

Photochemotherapy in which topically applied or systemically administered psoralens are combined with UV-A (PUVA) is also effective in treating psoriasis and in the early stages of cutaneous T cell lymphoma and vitiligo. Psoralens are tricyclic furocoumarins that, when intercalated into DNA and exposed to UV-A, form adducts with pyrimidine bases and eventually form DNA cross-links. These structural changes are thought to decrease DNA synthesis and relate to the improvement that occurs in psoriasis. The reason that PUVA photochemotherapy is effective in cutaneous T cell lymphoma is not clear.

In addition to its effects on DNA, PUVA photochemotherapy also stimulates epidermal thickening and melanin synthesis; the latter provides the rationale for its use in the depigmenting disease vitiligo. Oral 8-methoxypsoralen and UV-A appear to be most effective in this regard, but as many as 100 treatments extending over 12–18 months may be required to promote satisfactory repigmentation.

Not surprisingly the major side effects of long-term UV-B phototherapy and PUVA photochemotherapy mimic those seen in individuals with chronic sun exposure and include skin dryness, actinic keratoses, and an increased risk of skin cancer. Despite these risks, the therapeutic index of these modalities continues to be excellent.

FURTHER READINGS

LIM HW et al: Sunlight, tanning booths, and vitamin D. J Am Acad Dermatol 52:868, 2005

MILLER AJ, MIHM MC JR: Melanoma. N Engl J Med 355:51, 2006

MORISON WL: Photosensitivity. N Engl J Med 350:111, 2004

SCHADE N et al: Ultraviolet B radiation–induced immunosuppression: Molecular mechanisms and cellular alterations. Photochem Photobiol Sci 3:699, 2005

WONG TH, REES JL: The relation between melanocortin I receptor variation and generation of phenotypic diversity in the cutaneous response to ultraviolet radiation. Peptides 26:1965, 2005

SECTION 10 HEMATOLOGIC ALTERATIONS

58 Anemia and Polycythemia
John W. Adamson, Dan L. Longo

HEMATOPOIESIS AND THE PHYSIOLOGIC BASIS OF RED CELL PRODUCTION

Hematopoiesis is the process by which the formed elements of the blood are produced. The process is regulated through a series of steps beginning with the pluripotent hematopoietic stem cell. Stem cells are capable of producing red cells, all classes of granulocytes, monocytes, platelets, and the cells of the immune system. The precise molecular mechanism—either intrinsic to the stem cell itself, or through the action of extrinsic factors—by which the stem cell becomes committed to a given lineage is not fully defined. However, experiments in mice suggest that erythroid cells come from a common erythroid/megakaryocyte progenitor that does not develop in the absence of expression of the GATA-1 and FOG-1 (friend of GATA-1) transcription factors (Chap. 68). Following lineage commitment, hematopoietic progenitor and precursor cells come increasingly under the regulatory influence of growth factors and hormones. For red cell production, erythropoietin (EPO) is the regulatory hormone. EPO is required for the maintenance of committed erythroid progenitor cells that, in the absence of the hormone, undergo programmed cell death (*apoptosis*). The regulated process of red cell production is *erythropoiesis*, and its key elements are illustrated in Fig. 58-1.

In the bone marrow, the first morphologically recognizable erythroid precursor is the pronormoblast. This cell can undergo 4–5 cell divisions that result in the production of 16–32 mature red cells. With increased EPO production, or the administration of EPO as a drug, early progenitor cell numbers are amplified and, in turn, give rise to increased numbers of erythrocytes. The regulation of EPO production itself is linked to O_2 availability.

In mammals, O_2 is transported to tissues bound to the hemoglobin contained within circulating red cells. The mature red cell is 8 μm in diameter, anucleate, discoid in shape, and extremely pliable in order to

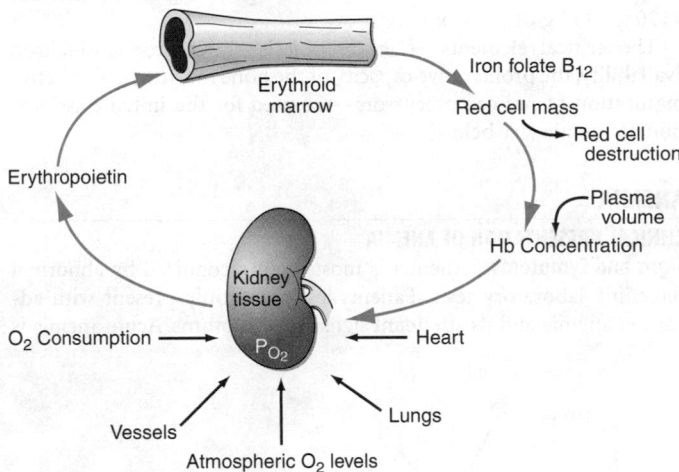

FIGURE 58-1 The physiologic regulation of red cell production by tissue oxygen tension. Hb, hemoglobin.

traverse the microcirculation successfully; its membrane integrity is maintained by the intracellular generation of ATP. Normal red cell production results in the daily replacement of 0.8–1% of all circulating red cells in the body, since the average red cell lives 100–120 days. The organ responsible for red cell production is called the *erythron*. The erythron is a dynamic organ made up of a rapidly proliferating pool of marrow erythroid precursor cells and a large mass of mature circulating red blood cells. The size of the red cell mass reflects the balance of red cell production and destruction. The physiologic basis of red cell production and destruction provides an understanding of the mechanisms that can lead to anemia.

The physiologic regulator of red cell production, the glycoprotein hormone EPO, is produced and released by peritubular capillary lining cells within the kidney. These cells are highly specialized epithelial-like cells. A small amount of EPO is produced by hepatocytes. The fundamental stimulus for EPO production is the availability of O_2 for tissue metabolic needs. Impaired O_2 delivery to the kidney can result from a decreased red cell mass (*anemia*), impaired O_2 loading of the hemoglobin molecule or a high O_2 affinity mutant hemoglobin (*hypoxemia*), or, rarely, impaired blood flow to the kidney (renal artery stenosis). EPO governs the day-to-day production of red cells, and ambient levels of the hormone can be measured in the plasma by sensitive immunoassays—the normal level being 10–25 U/L. When the hemoglobin concentration falls below 100–120 g/L (10–12 g/dL), plasma EPO levels increase in proportion to the severity of the anemia (Fig. 58-2). In circulation, EPO has a half-clearance time of 6–9 h. EPO acts by binding to specific receptors on the surface of marrow erythroid precursors, inducing them to proliferate and to mature. With EPO stimulation, red cell production can increase four- to fivefold within a 1- to 2-week period but only in the presence of adequate nutrients, especially iron. The functional capacity of the erythron, therefore, requires normal renal production of EPO, a functioning erythroid marrow, and an adequate supply of substrates for hemoglobin synthesis. A defect in any of these key components can lead to anemia. Generally, anemia is recognized in the laboratory when a patient's hemoglobin level or hematocrit is reduced below an expected value (the normal range). The likelihood and severity of anemia are defined based on the deviation of the patient's hemoglobin/hematocrit from values expected for age- and sex-matched normal subjects. The hemoglobin concentration in adults has a Gaussian distribution. The mean hematocrit value for adult males is 47% (± SD 7) and that for adult females is 42% (± 5). Any single hematocrit or hemoglobin value carries with it a likelihood of associated anemia. Thus, a hematocrit of ≤39% in an adult male or <35% in an adult female has only about a 25% chance of being normal. Suspected low hemoglobin or hematocrit values are more easily interpreted if previous values for the same patient are known for comparison. The World Health Organization (WHO) defines anemia as a hemoglobin level < 130 g/L (13 g/dL) in men and <120 g/L (12 g/dL) in women.

The critical elements of erythropoiesis—EPO production, iron availability, the proliferative capacity of the bone marrow, and effective maturation of red cell precursors—are used for the initial classification of anemia (see below).

ANEMIA

CLINICAL PRESENTATION OF ANEMIA

Signs and Symptoms   Anemia is most often recognized by abnormal screening laboratory tests. Patients less commonly present with advanced anemia and its attendant signs and symptoms. Acute anemia is nearly always due to blood loss or hemolysis. If blood loss is mild, enhanced O_2 delivery is achieved through changes in the O_2-hemoglobin dissociation curve mediated by a decreased pH or increased CO_2 (*Bohr effect*). With acute blood loss, hypovolemia dominates the clinical picture and the hematocrit and hemoglobin levels do not reflect the volume of blood lost. Signs of vascular instability appear with acute losses of 10–15% of the total blood volume. In such patients, the issue is not anemia but hypotension and decreased organ perfusion. When >30% of the blood volume is lost suddenly, patients are unable to compensate with the usual mechanisms of vascular contraction and changes in regional blood flow. The patient prefers to remain supine and will show postural hypotension and tachycardia. If the volume of blood lost is >40% (i.e., >2 L in the average-sized adult), signs of hypovolemic shock including confusion, dyspnea, diaphoresis, hypotension, and tachycardia appear (Chap. 101). Such patients have significant deficits in vital organ perfusion and require immediate volume replacement.

With acute hemolytic disease, the signs and symptoms depend on the mechanism that leads to red cell destruction. Intravascular hemolysis with release of free hemoglobin may be associated with acute back pain, free hemoglobin in the plasma and urine, and renal failure. Symptoms associated with more chronic or progressive anemia depend on the age of the patient and the adequacy of blood supply to critical organs. Symptoms associated with moderate anemia include fatigue, loss of stamina, breathlessness, and tachycardia (particularly with physical exertion). However, because of the intrinsic compensatory mechanisms that govern the O_2-hemoglobin dissociation curve, the gradual onset of anemia—particularly in young patients—may not be associated with signs or symptoms until the anemia is severe [hemoglobin <70–80 g/L (7–8 g/dL)]. When anemia develops over a period of days or weeks, the total blood volume is normal to slightly increased and changes in cardiac output and regional blood flow help compensate for the overall loss in O_2-carrying capacity. Changes in the position of the O_2-hemoglobin dissociation curve account for some of the compensatory response to anemia. With chronic anemia, intracellular levels of 2,3-bisphosphoglycerate rise, shifting the dissociation curve to the right and facilitating O_2 unloading. This compensatory mechanism can only maintain normal tissue O_2 delivery in the face of a 20–30 g/L (2–3 g/dL) deficit in hemoglobin concentration. Finally, further protection of O_2 delivery to vital organs is achieved by the shunting of blood away from organs that are relatively rich in blood supply, particularly the kidney, gut, and skin.

Certain disorders are commonly associated with anemia. Chronic inflammatory states (e.g., infection, rheumatoid arthritis) are associated with mild to moderate anemia, whereas lymphoproliferative disorders, such as chronic lymphocytic leukemia and certain other B cell neoplasms, may be associated with autoimmune hemolysis.

APPROACH TO THE PATIENT:
Anemia

The evaluation of the patient with anemia requires a careful history and physical examination. Nutritional history related to drugs or alcohol intake and family history of anemia should always be assessed. Certain geographic backgrounds and ethnic origins are associated with an increased likelihood of an inherited disorder of the hemoglobin molecule or intermediary metabolism. Glucose-6-phosphate dehydrogenase (G6PD) deficiency and certain hemoglobinopathies are seen more commonly in those of Middle Eastern or African origin, including African Americans who have a high frequency of G6PD deficiency. Other information that may be useful includes exposure to certain toxic agents or drugs and symptoms related to other disorders commonly associated with anemia. These include symptoms and signs such as bleeding, fatigue, malaise, fever, weight loss, night sweats, and other systemic symptoms. Clues to the mechanisms of anemia may be provided on physical examination by findings of infection, blood in the stool, lymphadenopathy, splenomegaly, or petechiae. Splenomegaly and lymphade-

FIGURE 58-2 Erythropoietin levels in response to anemia. When the hemoglobin level falls to 120 g/L (12 g/dL), plasma erythropoietin levels increase logarithmically. In the presence of renal disease or chronic inflammation, EPO levels are typically lower than expected for a particular level of anemia. As individuals age, the level of EPO needed to sustain normal hemoglobin levels appears to increase. (*From Hillman et al.*)

TABLE 58-1 LABORATORY TESTS IN ANEMIA DIAGNOSIS

I. Complete blood count (CBC)
  A. Red blood cell count
    1. Hemoglobin
    2. Hematocrit
    3. Reticulocyte count
  B. Red blood cell indices
    1. Mean cell volume (MCV)
    2. Mean cell hemoglobin (MCH)
    3. Mean cell hemoglobin concentration (MCHC)
    4. Red cell distribution width (RDW)
  C. White blood cell count
    1. Cell differential
    2. Nuclear segmentation of neutrophils
  D. Platelet count
  F. Cell morphology
    1. Cell size
    2. Hemoglobin content
    3. Anisocytosis
    4. Poikilocytosis
    5. Polychromasia

II. Iron supply studies
  A. Serum iron
  B. Total iron-binding capacity
  C. Serum ferritin
III. Marrow examination
  A. Aspirate
    1. M/E ratio[a]
    2. Cell morphology
    3. Iron stain
  B. Biopsy
    1. Cellularity
    2. Morphology

[a]M/E ratio, ratio of myeloid to erythroid precursors.

TABLE 58-3 CHANGES IN NORMAL HEMOGLOBIN/HEMATOCRIT VALUES WITH AGE AND PREGNANCY

Age/Sex	Hemoglobin g/dL	Hematocrit %
At birth	17	52
Childhood	12	36
Adolescence	13	40
Adult man	16 (±2)	47 (±6)
Adult woman (menstruating)	13 (±2)	40 (±6)
Adult woman (postmenopausal)	14 (±2)	42 (±6)
During pregnancy	12 (±2)	37 (±6)

Source: From Hillman et al.

is important, and clinical laboratories often provide a description of both the red and white cells, a white cell differential count, and the platelet count. In patients with severe anemia and abnormalities in red blood cell morphology and/or low reticulocyte counts, a bone marrow aspirate or biopsy may be important to assist in the diagnosis. Other tests of value in the diagnosis of specific anemias are discussed in chapters on specific disease states.

The components of the CBC also help in the classification of anemia. *Microcytosis* is reflected by a lower than normal MCV (<80), whereas high values (>100) reflect *macrocytosis*. The MCH and MCHC reflect defects in hemoglobin synthesis (*hypochromia*). Automated cell counters describe the red cell volume distribution width (RDW). The MCV (representing the peak of the distribution curve) is insensitive to the appearance of small populations of macrocytes or microcytes. An experienced laboratory technician will be able to identify minor populations of large or small cells or hypochromic cells before the red cell indices change.

Peripheral Blood Smear The peripheral blood smear provides important information about defects in red cell production. As a complement to the red cell indices, the blood smear also reveals variations in cell size (*anisocytosis*) and shape (*poikilocytosis*). The degree of anisocytosis usually correlates with increases in the RDW or the range of cell sizes. Poikilocytosis suggests a defect in the maturation of red cell precursors in the bone marrow or fragmentation of circulating red cells. The blood smear may also reveal *polychromasia*—red cells that are slightly larger than normal and grayish blue in color on the Wright-Giemsa stain. These cells are reticulocytes that have been prematurely released from the bone marrow, and their color represents residual amounts of ribosomal RNA. These cells appear in circulation in response to EPO stimulation or to architectural damage of the bone marrow (fibrosis, infiltration of the marrow by malignant cells, etc.) that results in their disordered release from the marrow. The appearance of nucleated red cells, Howell-Jolly bodies, target cells, sickle cells, and others may provide clues to specific disorders (Figs. 58-3 to 58-11).

nopathy suggest an underlying lymphoproliferative disease, while petechiae suggest platelet dysfunction. Past laboratory measurements may be helpful to determine a time of onset.

In the anemic patient, physical examination may demonstrate a forceful heartbeat, strong peripheral pulses, and a systolic "flow" murmur. The skin and mucous membranes may be pale if the hemoglobin is <80–100 g/L (8–10 g/dL). This part of the physical examination should focus on areas where vessels are close to the surface such as the mucous membranes, nail beds, and palmar creases. If the palmar creases are lighter in color than the surrounding skin when the hand is hyperextended, the hemoglobin level is usually <80 g/L (8 g/dL).

LABORATORY EVALUATION Table 58-1 lists the tests used in the initial workup of anemia. A routine complete blood count (CBC) is required as part of the evaluation and includes the hemoglobin, hematocrit, and red cell indices: the mean cell volume (MCV) in femtoliters, mean cell hemoglobin (MCH) in picograms per cell, and mean concentration of hemoglobin per volume of red cells (MCHC) in grams per liter (non-SI: grams per deciliter). The red cell indices are calculated as shown in Table 58-2, and the normal variations in the hemoglobin and hematocrit with age are shown in Table 58-3. A number of physiologic factors affect the CBC including age, sex, pregnancy, smoking, and altitude. High-normal hemoglobin values may be seen in men and women who live at altitude or smoke heavily. Hemoglobin elevations due to smoking reflect normal compensation due to the displacement of O_2 by CO in hemoglobin binding. Other important information is provided by the reticulocyte count and measurements of iron supply including *serum iron*, *total iron-binding capacity* (TIBC; an indirect measure of the transferrin level), and *serum ferritin*. Marked alterations in the red cell indices usually reflect disorders of maturation or iron deficiency. A careful evaluation of the peripheral blood smear

TABLE 58-2 RED BLOOD CELL INDICES

Index	Normal Value
Mean cell volume (MCV) = (hematocrit × 10)/(red cell count × 10^6)	90 ± 8 fL
Mean cell hemoglobin (MCH) = (hemoglobin × 10)/(red cell count × 10^6)	30 ± 3 pg
Mean cell hemoglobin concentration = (hemoglobin × 10)/hematocrit, or MCH/MCV	33 ± 2%

FIGURE 58-3 Normal blood smear (Wright's stain). High-power field showing normal red cells, a neutrophil, and a few platelets. (*From Hillman et al.*)

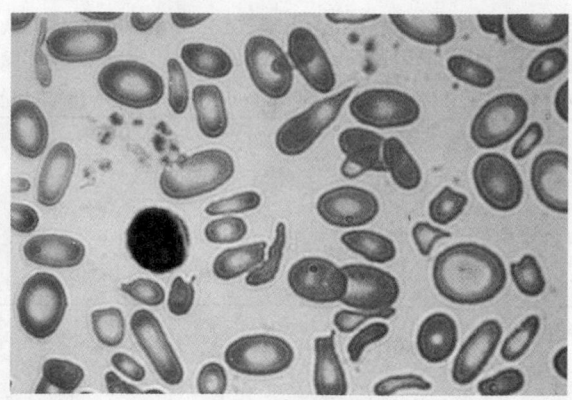

FIGURE 58-4 Severe iron-deficiency anemia. Microcytic and hypochromic red cells smaller than the nucleus of a lymphocyte associated with marked variation in size (anisocytosis) and shape (poikilocytosis). (*From Hillman et al.*)

FIGURE 58-5 Macrocytosis. Red cells are larger than a small lymphocyte and well hemoglobinized. Often macrocytes are oval-shaped (macroovalocytes).

FIGURE 58-6 Howell-Jolly bodies. In the absence of a functional spleen, nuclear remnants are not culled from the red cells and remain as small homogeneously staining blue inclusions on Wright stain. (*From Hillman et al.*)

FIGURE 58-7 Red cell changes in myelofibrosis. The left panel shows a teardrop-shaped cell. The right panel shows a nucleated red cell. These forms are seen in myelofibrosis with extramedullary hematopoiesis.

FIGURE 58-8 Target cells. Target cells have a bull's-eye appearance and are seen in thalassemia and in liver disease. (*From Hillman et al.*)

FIGURE 58-9 Red cell fragmentation. Red cells may become fragmented in the presence of foreign bodies in the circulation such as mechanical heart valves or in the setting of thermal injury. (*From Hillman et al.*)

Reticulocyte Count An accurate reticulocyte count is key to the initial classification of anemia. Normally, reticulocytes are red cells that have been recently released from the bone marrow. They are identified by staining with a supravital dye that precipitates the ribosomal RNA (Fig. 58-12). These precipitates appear as blue or black punctate spots. This residual RNA is metabolized over the first 24–36 h of the reticulocyte's lifespan in circulation. Normally, the reticulocyte count ranges from 1–2% and reflects the daily replacement of 0.8–1.0% of the circulating red cell population. A reticulocyte count provides a reliable measure of red cell production.

In the initial classification of anemia, the patient's reticulocyte count is compared with the expected reticulocyte response. In general, if the EPO and erythroid marrow responses to moderate anemia [hemoglobin < 100 g/L (10 g/dL)] are intact, the red cell production rate increases to two to three times normal within 10 days following the onset of anemia. In the face of established anemia, a reticulocyte response less than two to three times normal indicates an inadequate marrow response.

In order to use the reticulocyte count to estimate marrow response, two corrections are necessary. The first correction adjusts

FIGURE 58-10 Uremia. The red cells in uremia may acquire numerous, regularly spaced, small spiny projections. Such cells, called burr cells or echinocytes, are readily distinguishable from irregularly spiculated acanthocytes shown in Fig. 58-11.

FIGURE 58-11 Spur cells. Spur cells are recognized as distorted red cells containing several irregularly distributed thornlike projections. Cells with this morphologic abnormality are also called acanthocytes. (*From Hillman et al.*)

FIGURE 58-12 Reticulocytes. Methylene blue stain demonstrates residual RNA in newly made red cells. (*From Hillman et al.*)

the reticulocyte count based on the reduced number of circulating red cells. With anemia, the percentage of reticulocytes may be increased while the absolute number is unchanged. To correct for this effect, the reticulocyte percentage is multiplied by the ratio of the patient's hemoglobin or hematocrit to the expected hemoglobin/hematocrit for the age and gender of the patient (Table 58-4). This provides an estimate of the reticulocyte count corrected for anemia. In order to convert the corrected reticulocyte count to an index of marrow production, a further correction is required, depending on whether some of the reticulocytes in circulation have been released from the marrow prematurely. For this second correction, the peripheral blood smear is examined to see if there are polychromatophilic macrocytes present. These cells, representing

TABLE 58-4	CALCULATION OF RETICULOCYTE PRODUCTION INDEX

Correction #1 for anemia:
  This correction produces the corrected reticulocyte count
  In a person whose reticulocyte count is 9%, hemoglobin 7.5 g/dL, hematocrit 23%, the absolute reticulocyte count = 9 × (7.5/15) [or × (23/45)]= 4.5%
Correction #2 for longer life of prematurely released reticulocytes in the blood:
  This correction produces the reticulocyte production index
  In a person whose reticulocyte count is 9%, hemoglobin 7.5 gm/dL, hematocrit 23%, the reticulocyte production index

$$= 9 \times \frac{(7.5/15)(\text{hemoglobin correction})}{2 \ (\text{maturation time correction})} = 2.25$$

prematurely released reticulocytes, are referred to as "shift" cells, and the relationship between the degree of shift and the necessary shift correction factor is shown in Fig. 58-13. The correction is necessary because these prematurely released cells survive as reticulocytes in circulation for >1 day, thereby providing a falsely high estimate of daily red cell production. If polychromasia is increased, the reticulocyte count, already corrected for anemia, should be divided again by a factor of 2 to account for the prolonged reticulocyte maturation time. The second correction factor varies from 1–3 depending on the severity of anemia. In general, a correction of 2 is commonly used. An appropriate correction is shown in Table 58-4. If polychromatophilic cells are not seen on the blood smear, the second correction is not required. The now doubly corrected reticulocyte count is the *reticulocyte production index*, and it provides an estimate of marrow production relative to normal.

Premature release of reticulocytes is normally due to increased EPO stimulation. However, if the integrity of the bone marrow release process is lost through tumor infiltration, fibrosis, or other disorders, the appearance of nucleated red cells or polychromatophilic macrocytes should still invoke the second reticulocyte correction. The shift correction should always be applied to a patient with anemia and a very high reticulocyte count to provide a true index of effective red cell production. Patients with severe chronic hemolytic anemia may increase red cell production as much as six- to sevenfold. This measure alone, therefore, confirms the fact that the patient has an appropriate EPO response, a normally functioning bone marrow, and sufficient iron available to meet the de-

FIGURE 58-13 Correction of the reticulocyte count. In order to use the reticulocyte count as an indicator of effective red cell production, the reticulocyte number must be corrected based on the level of anemia and the circulating life span of the reticulocytes. Erythroid cells take ~4.5 days to mature. At normal hematocrit levels, they are released to the circulation with ~1 day left as reticulocytes. However, with different levels of anemia, erythroid cells are released from the marrow prematurely. Most patients come to clinical attention with hematocrits in the mid-20s and thus a correction factor of 2 is commonly used because the observed reticulocytes will live for 2 days in the circulation before losing their RNA.

TABLE 58-5   NORMAL MARROW RESPONSE TO ANEMIA

Hematocrit	Production Index	Reticulocytes (incl corrections)	Marrow M:E Ratio
45	1	1	3:1
35	2.0–3.0	4.8%/3.8/2.5	2:1–1:1
25	3.0–5.0	14%/8/4.0	1:1–1:2
15	3.0–5.0	30%/10/4.0	1:1–1:2

mands for new red cell formation. Table 58-5 demonstrates the normal marrow response to anemia. If the reticulocyte production index is <2 in the face of established anemia, a defect in erythroid marrow proliferation or maturation must be present.

Tests of Iron Supply and Storage   The laboratory measurements that reflect the availability of iron for hemoglobin synthesis include the serum iron, the TIBC, and the percent transferrin saturation. The percent transferrin saturation is derived by dividing the serum iron level (× 100) by the TIBC. The normal serum iron ranges from 9–27 μmol/L (50–150 μg/dL), while the normal TIBC is 54–64 μmol/L (300–360 μg/dL); the normal transferrin saturation ranges from 25–50%. A diurnal variation in the serum iron leads to a variation in the percent transferrin saturation. The serum ferritin is used to evaluate total-body iron stores. Adult males have serum ferritin levels that average ~100 μg/L, corresponding to iron stores of ~1 g. Adult females have lower serum ferritin levels averaging 30 μg/L, reflecting lower iron stores (300 mg). A serum ferritin level of 10–15 μg/L represents depletion of body iron stores. However, ferritin is also an acute-phase reactant and, in the presence of acute or chronic inflammation, may rise severalfold above baseline levels. As a rule, a serum ferritin > 200 μg/L means there is at least some iron in tissue stores.

Bone Marrow Examination   A bone marrow aspirate and smear or a needle biopsy may be useful in the evaluation of some patients with anemia. In patients with hypoproliferative anemia and normal iron status, a bone marrow is indicated. Marrow examination can diagnose primary marrow disorders such as myelofibrosis, a red cell maturation defect, or an infiltrative disease (Figs. 58-14 to 58-16). The increase or decrease of one cell lineage (myeloid vs. erythroid) compared to another is obtained by a differential count of nucleated cells in a bone marrow smear [the myeloid/erythroid (M/E) ratio]. A patient with a hypoproliferative anemia (see below) and a reticulocyte production index < 2 will demonstrate an M/E ratio of 2 or 3:1. In contrast, patients with hemolytic disease and a production index > 3 will have an M/E ratio of at least 1:1. Maturation disorders are identified from the discrepancy between the M/E ratio and the reticulocyte production index (see below). Either the marrow smear or biopsy can be stained for the presence of iron stores or iron in developing red cells. The storage iron is in the form of ferritin or *hemosiderin*. On carefully prepared bone marrow smears, small ferritin granules can normally be seen under oil immersion in 20–40% of developing erythroblasts. Such cells are called *sideroblasts*.

OTHER LABORATORY MEASUREMENTS   Additional laboratory tests may be of value in confirming specific diagnoses. For details of these tests and how they are applied in individual disorders, see Chaps. 98 to 102.

DEFINITION AND CLASSIFICATION OF ANEMIA
Initial Classification of Anemia   The functional classification of anemia has three major categories. These are: (1) marrow production defects (*hypoproliferation*), (2) red cell maturation defects (*ineffective erythropoiesis*), and (3) decreased red cell survival (*blood loss/hemolysis*). The classification is shown in Fig. 58-17. A hypoproliferative anemia is typically seen with a low reticulocyte production index together with little or no change in red cell morphology (a normocytic, normochromic anemia) (Chap. 98). Maturation disorders typically have a slight to moderately elevated reticulocyte production index that is ac-

FIGURE 58-14 Normal bone marrow. This is a low-power view of a section of a normal bone marrow biopsy stained with hematoxylin and eosin (H&E). Note that the nucleated cellular elements account for ~40–50% and the fat (clear areas) accounts for ~50–60% of the area. (*From Hillman et al.*)

FIGURE 58-15 Erythroid hyperplasia. This marrow shows an increase in the fraction of cells in the erythroid lineage as might be seen when a normal marrow compensates for acute blood loss or hemolysis. The M/E ratio is about 1:1. (*From Hillman et al.*)

FIGURE 58-16 Myeloid hyperplasia. This marrow shows an increase in the fraction of cells in the myeloid or granulocytic lineage as might be seen in a normal marrow responding to infection. The M/E ratio is >3:1. (*From Hillman et al.*)

companied by either macrocytic (Chap. 100) or microcytic (Chaps. 98, 99) red cell indices. Increased red blood cell destruction secondary to hemolysis results in an increase in the reticulocyte production index to at least three times normal (Chap. 101), provided sufficient iron is available. Hemorrhagic anemia does not typically result in production indices of more than 2.0–2.5 times normal because of the limitations placed on expansion of the erythroid marrow by iron availability.

In the first branch point of the classification of anemia, a reticulocyte production index > 2.5 indicates that hemolysis is most likely. A reticulocyte production index < 2 indicates either a hypoproliferative anemia or maturation disorder. The latter two possibilities can often

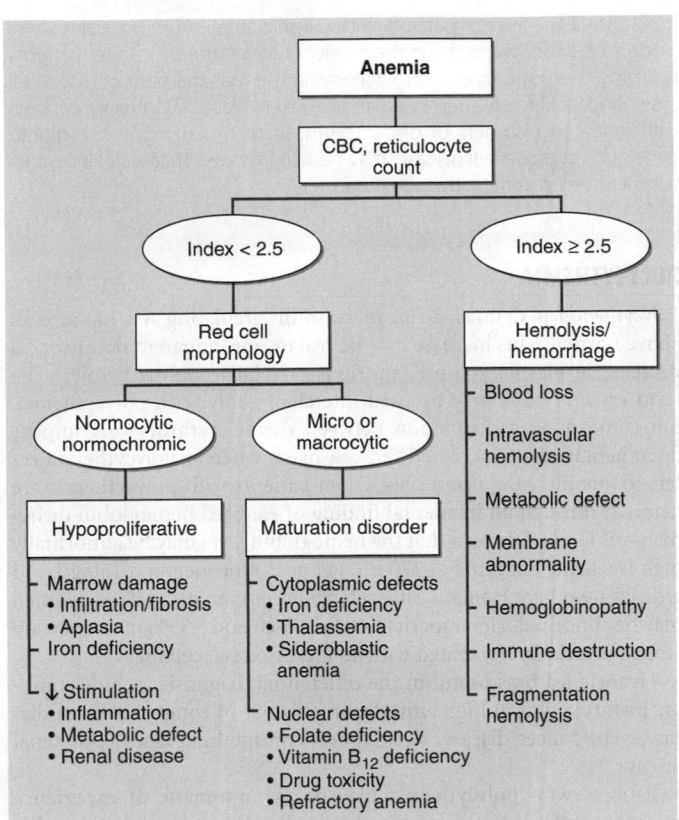

FIGURE 58-17 The physiologic classification of anemia. CBC, complete blood count.

be distinguished by the red cell indices, by examination of the peripheral blood smear, or by a marrow examination. If the red cell indices are normal, the anemia is almost certainly hypoproliferative in nature. Maturation disorders are characterized by ineffective red cell production and a low reticulocyte production index. Bizarre red cell shapes—macrocytes or hypochromic microcytes—are seen on the peripheral blood smear. With a hypoproliferative anemia, no erythroid hyperplasia is noted in the marrow, whereas patients with ineffective red cell production have erythroid hyperplasia and an M/E ratio < 1:1.

Hypoproliferative Anemias At least 75% of all cases of anemia are hypoproliferative in nature. A hypoproliferative anemia reflects absolute or relative marrow failure in which the erythroid marrow has not proliferated appropriately for the degree of anemia. The majority of hypoproliferative anemias are due to mild to moderate iron deficiency or inflammation. A hypoproliferative anemia can result from marrow damage, iron deficiency, or inadequate EPO stimulation. The last may reflect impaired renal function, suppression of EPO production by inflammatory cytokines such as interleukin 1, or reduced tissue needs for O_2 from metabolic disease such as hypothyroidism. Only occasionally is the marrow unable to produce red cells at a normal rate, and this is most prevalent in patients with renal failure. With diabetes mellitus or myeloma, the EPO deficiency may be more marked than would be predicted by the degree of renal insufficiency. In general, hypoproliferative anemias are characterized by normocytic, normochromic red cells, although microcytic, hypochromic cells may be observed with mild iron deficiency or long-standing chronic inflammatory disease. The key laboratory tests in distinguishing between the various forms of hypoproliferative anemia include the serum iron and iron-binding capacity, evaluation of renal and thyroid function, a marrow biopsy or aspirate to detect marrow damage or infiltrative disease, and serum ferritin to assess iron stores. Occasionally, an iron stain of the marrow will be needed to determine the pattern of iron distribution. Patients with the anemia of acute or chronic inflammation show a distinctive pattern of serum iron (low), TIBC (normal or low), percent

transferrin saturation (low), and serum ferritin (normal or high). These changes in iron values are brought about by hepcidin, the iron regulatory hormone that is increased in inflammation (Chap. 98). A distinct pattern of results is noted in mild to moderate iron deficiency (low serum iron, high TIBC, low percent transferrin saturation, low serum ferritin) (Chap. 98). Marrow damage by drugs, such as the antiretrovirals used to treat HIV infection, infiltrative disease such as leukemia or lymphoma, or marrow aplasia can usually be diagnosed from the peripheral blood and bone marrow morphology. With infiltrative disease or fibrosis, a marrow biopsy is required.

Maturation Disorders The presence of anemia with an inappropriately low reticulocyte production index, macro- or microcytosis on smear, and abnormal red cell indices suggests a maturation disorder. Maturation disorders are divided into two categories: nuclear maturation defects, associated with macrocytosis and abnormal marrow development, and cytoplasmic maturation defects, associated with microcytosis and hypochromia usually from defects in hemoglobin synthesis. The inappropriately low reticulocyte production index is a reflection of the ineffective erythropoiesis that results from the destruction within the marrow of developing erythroblasts. Bone marrow examination shows erythroid hyperplasia.

Nuclear maturation defects result from vitamin B_{12} or folic acid deficiency, drug damage, or myelodysplasia. Drugs that interfere with cellular DNA metabolism, such as methotrexate or alkylating agents, can produce a nuclear maturation defect. Alcohol, alone, is also capable of producing macrocytosis and a variable degree of anemia, but this is usually associated with folic acid deficiency. Measurements of folic acid and vitamin B_{12} are key not only in identifying the specific vitamin deficiency but also because they reflect different pathogenetic mechanisms.

Cytoplasmic maturation defects result from severe iron deficiency or abnormalities in globin or heme synthesis. Iron deficiency occupies an unusual position in the classification of anemia. If the iron-deficiency anemia is mild to moderate, erythroid marrow proliferation is decreased and the anemia is classified as hypoproliferative. However, if the anemia is severe and prolonged, the erythroid marrow will become hyperplastic despite the inadequate iron supply, and the anemia will be classified as ineffective erythropoiesis with a cytoplasmic maturation defect. In either case, an inappropriately low reticulocyte production index, microcytosis, and a classic pattern of iron values make the diagnosis clear and easily distinguish iron deficiency from other cytoplasmic maturation defects such as the thalassemias. Defects in heme synthesis, in contrast to globin synthesis, are less common and may be acquired or inherited (Chap. 352). Acquired abnormalities are usually associated with myelodysplasia, may lead to either a macro- or microcytic anemia, and are frequently associated with mitochondrial iron loading. In these cases, iron is taken up by the mitochondria of the developing erythroid cell but not incorporated into heme. The iron-encrusted mitochondria surround the nucleus of the erythroid cell, forming a ring. Based on the distinctive finding of so-called ringed sideroblasts on the marrow iron stain, patients are diagnosed as having a sideroblastic anemia—almost always reflecting myelodysplasia. Again, studies of iron parameters are helpful in the differential diagnosis and management of these patients.

Blood Loss/Hemolytic Anemia In contrast to anemias associated with an inappropriately low reticulocyte production index, hemolysis is associated with red cell production indices ≥2.5 times normal. The stimulated erythropoiesis is reflected in the blood smear by the appearance of increased numbers of polychromatophilic macrocytes. A marrow examination is rarely indicated if the reticulocyte production index is increased appropriately. The red cell indices are typically normocytic or slightly macrocytic, reflecting the increased number of reticulocytes. Acute blood loss is not associated with an increased reticulocyte production index because of the time required to increase EPO production and, subsequently, marrow proliferation. Subacute blood loss may be associated with modest reticulocytosis. Anemia from chronic blood loss presents more often as iron deficiency than with the picture of increased red cell production.

The evaluation of blood loss anemia is usually not difficult. Most problems arise when a patient presents with an increased red cell production index from an episode of acute blood loss that went unrecognized. The cause of the anemia and increased red cell production may not be obvious. The confirmation of a recovering state may require observations over a period of 2–3 weeks, during which the hemoglobin concentration will be seen to rise and the reticulocyte production index fall.

Hemolytic disease, while dramatic, is among the least common forms of anemia. The ability to sustain a high reticulocyte production index reflects the ability of the erythroid marrow to compensate for hemolysis and, in the case of extravascular hemolysis, the efficient recycling of iron from the destroyed red cells to support red cell production. With intravascular hemolysis, such as paroxysmal nocturnal hemoglobinuria, the loss of iron may limit the marrow response. The level of response depends on the severity of the anemia and the nature of the underlying disease process.

Hemoglobinopathies, such as sickle cell disease and the thalassemias, present a mixed picture. The reticulocyte index may be high but is inappropriately low for the degree of marrow erythroid hyperplasia (Chap. 99).

Hemolytic anemias present in different ways. Some appear suddenly as an acute, self-limited episode of intravascular or extravascular hemolysis, a presentation pattern often seen in patients with autoimmune hemolysis or with inherited defects of the Embden-Meyerhof pathway or the glutathione reductase pathway. Patients with inherited disorders of the hemoglobin molecule or red cell membrane generally have a lifelong clinical history typical of the disease process. Those with chronic hemolytic disease, such as hereditary spherocytosis, may actually present not with anemia but with a complication stemming from the prolonged increase in red cell destruction such as symptomatic bilirubin gallstones or splenomegaly. Patients with chronic hemolysis are also susceptible to aplastic crises if an infectious process interrupts red cell production.

The differential diagnosis of an acute or chronic hemolytic event requires the careful integration of family history, the pattern of clinical presentation and—whether the disease is congenital or acquired—by a careful examination of the peripheral blood smear. Precise diagnosis may require more specialized laboratory tests, such as hemoglobin electrophoresis or a screen for red cell enzymes. Acquired defects in red cell survival are often immunologically mediated and require a direct or indirect antiglobulin test or a cold agglutinin titer to detect the presence of hemolytic antibodies or complement-mediated red cell destruction.

℞ ANEMIA

An overriding principle is to initiate treatment of mild to moderate anemia only when a specific diagnosis is made. Rarely, in the acute setting, anemia may be so severe that red cell transfusions are required before a specific diagnosis is made. Whether the anemia is of acute or gradual onset, the selection of the appropriate treatment is determined by the documented cause(s) of the anemia. Often, the cause of the anemia may be multifactorial. For example, a patient with severe rheumatoid arthritis who has been taking anti-inflammatory drugs may have a hypoproliferative anemia associated with chronic inflammation as well as chronic blood loss associated with intermittent gastrointestinal bleeding. In every circumstance, it is important to evaluate the patient's iron status fully before and during the treatment of any anemia. **Transfusion is discussed in Chap. 107; iron therapy is discussed in Chap. 98; treatment of megaloblastic anemia is discussed in Chap. 100; treatment of other entities is discussed in their respective chapters (sickle cell anemia, Chap. 99; hemolytic anemias, Chap. 101; aplastic anemia and myelodysplasia, Chap. 102).**

Therapeutic options for the treatment of anemias have expanded dramatically during the past 25 years. Blood component therapy is available and safe. Recombinant EPO as an adjunct to anemia management has transformed the lives of patients with chronic renal failure on dialysis and made some improvements in the quality of life of anemic cancer patients receiving chemotherapy. Improvements in the management of sickle cell crises and sickle cell anemia have also taken place. Eventually, patients with inherited disorders of globin synthesis or mutations in the globin gene, such as sickle cell disease, may benefit from the successful introduction of targeted genetic therapy (Chap. 65).

POLYCYTHEMIA

Polycythemia is defined as an increase in circulating red blood cells above normal. This increase may be real or only apparent because of a decrease in plasma volume (spurious or relative polycythemia). The term *erythrocytosis* may be used interchangeably with polycythemia, but some draw a distinction between them; erythrocytosis implies documentation of increased red cell mass, whereas polycythemia refers to any increase in red cells. Often patients with polycythemia are detected through an incidental finding of elevated hemoglobin or hematocrit levels. Concern that the hemoglobin level may be abnormally high is usually triggered at 170 g/L (17 g/dL) for men and 150 g/L (15 g/dL) for women. Hematocrit levels >50% in men or >45% in women may be abnormal. Hematocrits >60% in men and >55% in women are almost invariably associated with an increased red cell mass.

Historic features useful in the differential diagnosis include smoking history; living at high altitude; or a history of congenital heart disease, peptic ulcer disease, sleep apnea, chronic lung disease, or renal disease.

Patients with polycythemia may be asymptomatic or experience symptoms related to the increased red cell mass or an underlying disease process that leads to increased red cell production. The dominant symptoms from increased red cell mass are related to hyperviscosity and thrombosis (both venous and arterial), because the blood viscosity increases logarithmically at hematocrits >55%. Manifestations range from digital ischemia to Budd-Chiari syndrome with hepatic vein thrombosis. Abdominal thromboses are particularly common. Neurologic symptoms such as vertigo, tinnitus, headache, and visual disturbances may occur. Hypertension is often present. Patients with *polycythemia vera* may have aquagenic pruritus and symptoms related to hepatosplenomegaly. Patients may have easy bruising, epistaxis, or bleeding from the gastrointestinal tract. Patients with hypoxemia may develop cyanosis on minimal exertion or have headache, impaired mental acuity, and fatigue.

The physical examination usually reveals a ruddy complexion. Splenomegaly favors polycythemia vera as the diagnosis (Chap. 103). The presence of cyanosis or evidence of a right-to-left shunt suggests congenital heart disease presenting in the adult, particularly tetralogy of Fallot or Eisenmenger syndrome (Chap. 229). Increased blood viscosity raises pulmonary artery pressure; hypoxemia can lead to increased pulmonary vascular resistance. Together these factors can produce cor pulmonale.

Polycythemia can be spurious (related to a decrease in plasma volume; Gaisbock's syndrome), primary, or secondary in origin. The secondary causes are all associated with increases in EPO levels: either a physiologically adapted appropriate elevation based on tissue hypoxia (lung disease, high altitude, CO poisoning, high-affinity hemoglobinopathy) or an abnormal overproduction (renal cysts, renal artery stenosis, tumors with ectopic EPO production). A rare familial form of polycythemia is associated with normal EPO levels but hyperresponsive EPO receptors due to mutations.

APPROACH TO THE PATIENT:
Polycythemia

As shown in Fig. 58-18, the first step is to document the presence of an increased red cell mass using the principle of isotope dilution by administering ^{51}Cr-labeled autologous red blood cells to the patient and sampling blood radioactivity over a 2-h period. If the red

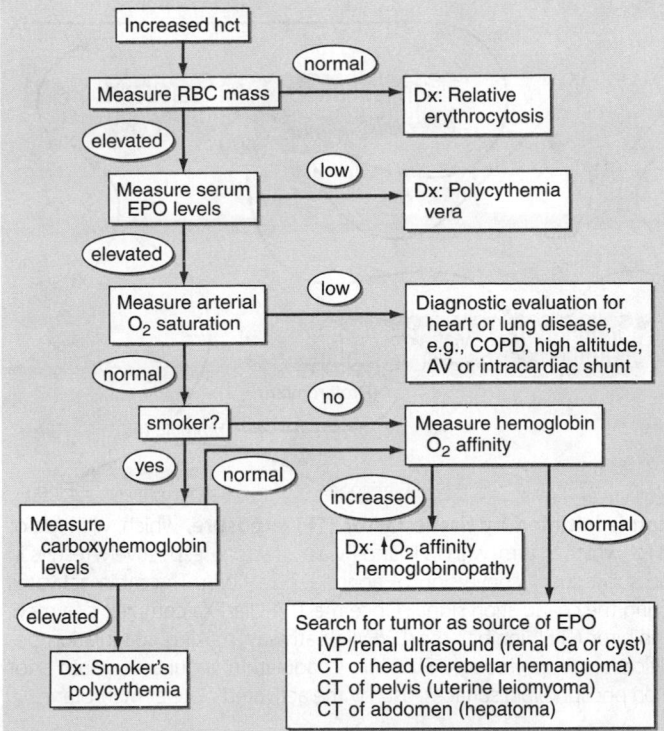

FIGURE 58-18 An approach to diagnosing patients with polycythemia. RBC, red blood cell; EPO, erythropoietin; COPD, chronic obstructive pulmonary disease; AV, atrioventricular; IVP, intravenous pyelogram; hct, hematocrit.

cell mass is normal (<36 mL/kg in men, <32 mL/kg in women), the patient has spurious polycythemia. If the red cell mass is increased (>36 mL/kg in men, >32 mL/kg in women), serum EPO levels should be measured. If EPO levels are low or unmeasurable, the

patient most likely has polycythemia vera. Ancillary tests that support this diagnosis include elevated white blood cell count, increased absolute basophil count, and thrombocytosis. A mutation in *JAK-2* (Val617Phe), a key member of the cytokine intracellular signaling pathway, can be found in 70–95% of patients with polycythemia vera.

If serum EPO levels are elevated, one attempts to distinguish whether the elevation is a physiologic response to hypoxia or is related to autonomous production. Patients with low arterial O_2 saturation (<92%) should be further evaluated for the presence of heart or lung disease, if they are not living at high altitude. Patients with normal O_2 saturation who are smokers may have elevated EPO levels because of CO displacement of O_2. If carboxyhemoglobin (COHb) levels are high, the diagnosis is smoker's polycythemia. Such patients should be urged to stop smoking. Those who cannot stop smoking require phlebotomy to control their polycythemia. Patients with normal O_2 saturation who do not smoke either have an abnormal hemoglobin that does not deliver O_2 to the tissues (evaluated by finding elevated O_2-hemoglobin affinity) or have a source of EPO production that is not responding to the normal feedback inhibition. Further workup is dictated by the differential diagnosis of EPO-producing neoplasms. Hepatoma, uterine leiomyoma, and renal cancer or cysts are all detectable with abdominopelvic CT scans. Cerebellar hemangiomas may produce EPO, but they nearly always present with localizing neurologic signs and symptoms rather than polycythemia-related symptoms.

ACKNOWLEDGMENT
Dr. Robert S. Hillman wrote this chapter in the 14th edition, and elements of his chapter were retained here.

FURTHER READINGS

HILLMAN RS et al: *Hematology in Clinical Practice*, 4th ed. New York, McGraw-Hill, 2005

59 Bleeding and Thrombosis
Barbara A. Konkle

The human hemostatic system provides a natural balance between procoagulant and anticoagulant forces. The procoagulant forces include platelet adhesion and aggregation and fibrin clot formation; anticoagulant forces include the natural inhibitors of coagulation and fibrinolysis. Under normal circumstances, hemostasis is regulated to promote blood flow; however, it is also prepared to clot blood rapidly to arrest blood flow and prevent exsanguination. After bleeding is successfully halted, the system remodels the damaged vessel to restore normal blood flow. The major components of the hemostatic system, which function in concert, are (1) platelets and other formed elements of blood, such as monocytes and red cells; (2) plasma proteins (the coagulation and fibrinolytic factors and inhibitors); and (3) the vessel wall itself.

STEPS OF NORMAL HEMOSTASIS

PLATELET PLUG FORMATION

On vascular injury, platelets adhere to the site of injury, usually the denuded vascular intimal surface. Platelet adhesion is mediated primarily by von Willebrand factor (vWF), a large multimeric protein present in both plasma and in the extracellular matrix of the subendothelial vessel wall, which serves as the primary "molecular glue," providing sufficient strength to withstand the high levels of shear stress that would tend to detach them with the flow of blood. Platelet adhesion is

also facilitated by direct binding to subendothelial collagen through specific platelet membrane collagen receptors.

Platelet adhesion results in subsequent platelet activation and aggregation. This process is enhanced and amplified by humoral mediators in plasma (e.g., epinephrine, thrombin); mediators released from activated platelets (e.g., adenosine diphosphate, serotonin); and vessel wall extracellular matrix constituents that come in contact with adherent platelets (e.g., collagen, vWF). Activated platelets undergo the release reaction, during which they secrete contents that further promote aggregation and inhibit the naturally anticoagulant endothelial cell factors. During platelet aggregation (platelet-platelet interaction), additional platelets are recruited from the circulation to the site of vascular injury, leading to the formation of an occlusive platelet thrombus. The platelet plug is anchored and stabilized by the developing fibrin mesh.

The platelet glycoprotein (Gp) IIb/IIIa ($\alpha_{IIb}\beta_3$) complex is the most abundant receptor on the platelet surface. Platelet activation converts the normally inactive GpIIb/IIIa receptor into an active receptor, enabling binding to fibrinogen and vWF. Because the surface of each platelet has about 50,000 GpIIb/IIIa fibrinogen binding sites, numerous activated platelets recruited to the site of vascular injury can rapidly form an occlusive aggregate by means of a dense network of intercellular fibrinogen bridges. Since this receptor is the key mediator of platelet aggregation, it has become an effective target for antiplatelet therapy.

FIBRIN CLOT FORMATION

Plasma coagulation proteins (*clotting factors*) normally circulate in plasma in their inactive forms. The sequence of coagulation protein reactions that culminate in the formation of fibrin was originally described as a *waterfall* or a *cascade*. Two pathways of blood coagulation have been described in the past: the so-called extrinsic, or tissue factor, pathway and the so-called intrinsic, or contact activation, pathway. We now know that coagulation is normally initiated through tissue factor (TF) exposure and activation through the classic *extrinsic pathway*, but with critically important amplification through elements of the classic *intrinsic pathway*, as illustrated in **Fig. 59-1**. These reactions take place on phospholipid surfaces, usually the activated platelet surface. Coagulation testing in the laboratory can reflect other influences due to the artificial nature of the in vitro systems used (see below).

The immediate trigger for coagulation is vascular damage that exposes blood to TF that is constitutively expressed on the surfaces of subendothelial cellular components of the vessel wall, such as smooth-muscle cells and fibroblasts. TF is also present in circulating microparticles, presumably shed from cells including monocytes and platelets. TF binds the serine protease factor VIIa; the complex activates factor X to factor Xa. Alternatively, the complex can indirectly activate factor X by initially converting factor IX to factor IXa, which then activates factor X. The participation of factor XI in hemostasis is not dependent on its activation by factor XIIa but rather on its positive feedback activation by thrombin. Thus, factor XIa functions in the propagation and amplification, rather than in the initiation, of the coagulation cascade.

Factor Xa, which can be formed through the actions of either the tissue factor/factor VIIa complex or factor IXa (with factor VIIIa as a cofactor), converts prothrombin to thrombin, the pivotal protease of the coagulation system. The essential cofactor for this reaction is factor Va. Like the homologous factor VIIIa, factor Va is produced by thrombin-induced limited proteolysis of factor V. Thrombin is a multifunctional enzyme that converts soluble plasma fibrinogen to an insoluble fibrin matrix. Fibrin polymerization involves an orderly process of intermolecular associations (**Fig. 59-2**). Thrombin also activates factor XIII (fibrin-stabilizing factor) to factor XIIIa, which covalently cross-links and thereby stabilizes the fibrin clot.

The assembly of the clotting factors on activated cell membrane surfaces greatly accelerates their reaction rates and also serves to localize blood clotting to sites of vascular injury. The critical cell membrane components, acidic phospholipids, are not normally exposed on resting cell membrane surfaces. However, when platelets, monocytes, and endothelial cells are activated by vascular injury or inflammatory stimuli, the procoagulant head groups of the membrane anionic phospholipids become translocated to the surfaces of these cells or released as part of microparticles, making them available to support and promote the plasma coagulation reactions.

ANTITHROMBOTIC MECHANISMS

Several physiologic antithrombotic mechanisms act in concert to prevent clotting under normal circumstances. These mechanisms operate to preserve blood fluidity and limit blood clotting to specific focal sites of vascular injury. Endothelial cells have many antithrombotic effects. They produce prostacyclin, nitric oxide, and ectoADPase/CD39, which act to inhibit platelet binding, secretion, and aggregation. Endothelial cells produce anticoagulant factors including heparan proteoglycans, antithrombin, TF pathway inhibitor, and thrombomodulin. They also activate fibrinolytic mechanisms through the production of tissue plasminogen activator 1, urokinase, plasminogen activator inhibitor, and annexin-2. The sites of action of the major physiologic antithrombotic pathways are shown in **Fig. 59-3**.

Antithrombin (or antithrombin III) is the major plasma protease inhibitor of thrombin and the other clotting factors in coagulation.

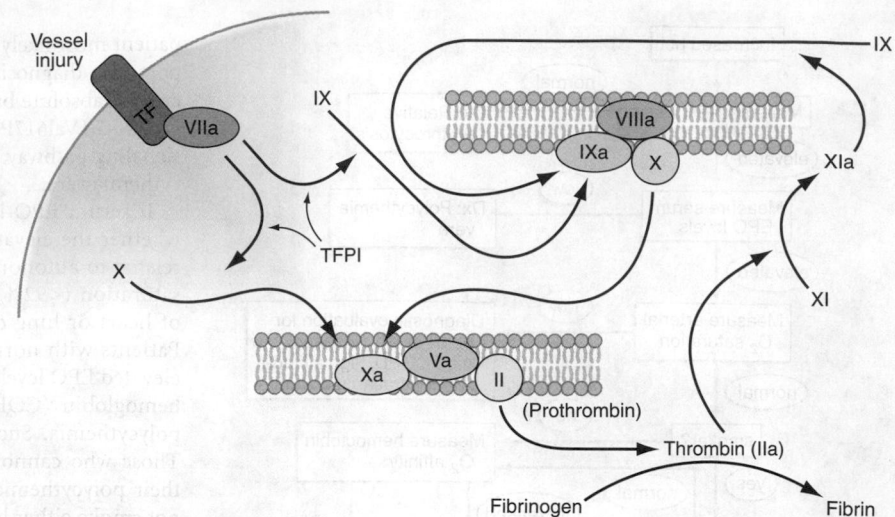

FIGURE 59-1 Coagulation is initiated by tissue factor (TF) exposure, which, with factor (F)VIIa, activates FIX and FX, which in turn, with FVIII and FV as cofactors, respectively, results in thrombin formation and subsequent conversion of fibrinogen to fibrin. Thrombin activates FXI, FVIII, and FV, amplifying the coagulation signal. Once the TF/FVIIa/FXa complex is formed, tissue factor pathway inhibitor (TFPI) inhibits the TF/FVIIa pathway, making coagulation dependent on the amplification loop through FIX/FVIII. Coagulation requires calcium (not shown) and takes place on phospholipid surfaces, usually the activated platelet membrane.

Antithrombin neutralizes thrombin and other activated coagulation factors by forming a complex between the active site of the enzyme and the reactive center of antithrombin. The rate of formation of these inactivating complexes increases by a factor of several thousand in the presence of heparin. Antithrombin inactivation of thrombin and other activated clotting factors occurs physiologically on vascular surfaces, where glycosaminoglycans, including heparan sulfates, are present to catalyze these reactions. Inherited quantitative or qualitative deficiencies of antithrombin lead to a lifelong predisposition to venous thromboembolism.

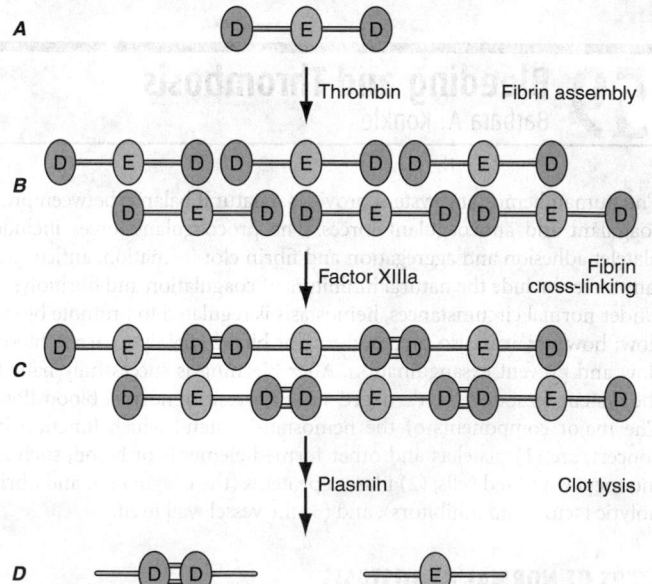

FIGURE 59-2 Fibrin formation and dissolution. A. Fibrinogen is a trinodular structure consisting of 2 D domains and 1 E domain. Thrombin activation results in an ordered lateral assembly of protofibrils **(B)** with noncovalent associations. FXIIIa cross-links the D domains on adjacent molecules **(C).** Fibrin and fibrinogen (not shown) lysis by plasmin occurs at discrete sites and results in intermediary fibrin(ogen) degradation products (not shown). D-Dimers are the product of complete lysis of fibrin, maintaining the cross-linked D domains.

FIGURE 59-3 Sites of action of the four major physiologic antithrombotic pathways: antithrombin (AT); protein C/S (PC/PS); tissue factor pathway inhibitor (TFPI); and the fibrinolytic system, consisting of plasminogen, plasminogen activator (PA), and plasmin. PT, prothrombin; Th, thrombin; FDP, fibrin(ogen) degradation products. [Modified from BA Konkle, AI Schafer, in DP Zipes et al (eds): Braunwald's Heart Disease, 7th ed. Philadelphia, Saunders, 2005.]

Protein C is a plasma glycoprotein that becomes an anticoagulant when it is activated by thrombin. The thrombin-induced activation of protein C occurs physiologically on thrombomodulin, a transmembrane proteoglycan binding site for thrombin on endothelial cell surfaces. The binding of protein C to its receptor on endothelial cells places it in proximity to the thrombin-thrombomodulin complex, therefore enhancing its activation efficiency. Activated protein C acts as an anticoagulant by cleaving and inactivating activated factors V and VIII. This reaction is accelerated by a cofactor, protein S, which, like protein C, is a glycoprotein that undergoes vitamin K–dependent posttranslational modification. Quantitative or qualitative deficiencies of protein C or protein S, or resistance to the action of activated protein C by a specific mutation at its target cleavage site in factor Va (Factor V Leiden), lead to hypercoagulable states.

Tissue factor pathway inhibitor (TFPI) is a plasma protease inhibitor that regulates the TF-induced extrinsic pathway of coagulation. TFPI inhibits the TF/FVIIa/FXa complex, essentially turning off the TF/FVIIa initiation of coagulation, which then becomes dependent on the "amplification loop" via FXI and FVIII activation by thrombin. TFPI is bound to lipoprotein and can also be released by heparin from endothelial cells, where it is bound to glycosaminoglycans, and from platelets. The heparin-mediated release of TFPI may play a role in the anticoagulant effects of unfractionated and low-molecular-weight heparins.

THE FIBRINOLYTIC SYSTEM

Any thrombin that escapes the inhibitory effects of the physiologic anticoagulant systems is available to convert fibrinogen to fibrin. In response, the endogenous fibrinolytic system is then activated to dispose of intravascular fibrin and thereby maintain or reestablish the patency of the circulation. Just as thrombin is the key protease enzyme of the coagulation system, plasmin is the major protease enzyme of the fibrinolytic system, acting to digest fibrin to fibrin degradation products. The general scheme of fibrinolysis is shown in Fig. 59-4.

FIGURE 59-4 A schematic diagram of the fibrinolytic system. Tissue plasminogen activator (tPA) is released from endothelial cells, binds the fibrin clot, and activates plasminogen to plasmin. Excess fibrin is degraded by plasmin to distinct degradation products (FDPs). Any free plasmin is complexed with α₂-antiplasmin (α₂PI).

The plasminogen activators, tissue type plasminogen activator (tPA) and the urokinase type plasminogen activator (uPA), cleave the Arg560-Val561 bond of plasminogen to generate the active enzyme plasmin. The lysine-binding sites of plasmin (and plasminogen) permit it to bind to fibrin, so that physiologic fibrinolysis is "fibrin specific." Both plasminogen (through its lysine-binding sites) and tPA possess specific affinity for fibrin and thereby bind selectively to clots. The assembly of a ternary complex, consisting of fibrin, plasminogen, and tPA, promotes the localized interaction between plasminogen and tPA and greatly accelerates the rate of plasminogen activation to plasmin. Moreover, partial degradation of fibrin by plasmin exposes new plasminogen and tPA binding sites in carboxy-terminus lysine residues of fibrin fragments to enhance these reactions further. This creates a highly efficient mechanism to generate plasmin focally on the fibrin clot, which then becomes plasmin's substrate for digestion to fibrin degradation products.

Plasmin cleaves fibrin at distinct sites of the fibrin molecule leading to the generation of characteristic fibrin fragments during the process of fibrinolysis (Fig. 59-2). The sites of plasmin cleavage of fibrin are the same as those in fibrinogen. However, when plasmin acts on covalently cross-linked fibrin, D-dimers are released; hence, D-dimers can be measured in plasma as a relatively specific test of fibrin (rather than fibrinogen) degradation. D-Dimer assays can be used as sensitive markers of blood clot formation, and some have been validated for clinical use to exclude the diagnosis of deep venous thrombosis (DVT) and pulmonary embolism in selected populations.

Physiologic regulation of fibrinolysis occurs primarily at two levels: (1) plasminogen activator inhibitors (PAIs), specifically PAI1 and PAI2, inhibit the physiologic plasminogen activators; and (2) α₂ antiplasmin inhibits plasmin. PAI1 is the primary inhibitor of tPA and uPA in plasma. α₂ antiplasmin is the main inhibitor of plasmin in human plasma, inactivating any nonfibrin clot–associated plasmin.

APPROACH TO THE PATIENT:
Bleeding and Thrombosis

CLINICAL PRESENTATION Disorders of hemostasis may be either inherited or acquired. A detailed personal and family history is key in determining the chronicity of symptoms and the likelihood of the disorder being inherited and it provides clues to underlying conditions that have contributed to the bleeding or thrombotic state. In addition, the history can give clues as to the etiology by determining (1) the bleeding (mucosal and/or joint) or thrombosis (arterial and/or venous) site, and (2) whether an underlying bleeding or clotting tendency was enhanced by another medical condition or the introduction of medications or dietary supplements.

History of Bleeding A history of bleeding is the most important predictor of bleeding risk. In evaluating a patient for a bleeding disorder, a history of at-risk situations, including the response to past surgeries, should be assessed. Does the patient have a history of spontaneous or trauma/surgery-induced bleeding? Spontaneous hemarthroses are a hallmark of moderate and severe factors VIII and IX deficiency and, in rare circumstances, of other clotting factor deficiencies. Mucosal bleeding symptoms are more suggestive of underlying platelet disorders or von Willebrand disease (vWD), termed *disorders of primary hemostasis or platelet plug formation*. Disorders affecting primary hemostasis are shown in Table 59-1.

The development of bruises (ecchymoses) after trauma is normal; however, an exaggerated response to trauma may be an indication of an underlying bleeding disorder. Ecchymoses presenting without known trauma, particularly on the trunk, and especially large ecchymoses, >2 in. in diameter, may be a sign of an underlying bleeding disorder. The introduction of medications or nutritional supplements with platelet inhibitory activity often enhance bruising and bleeding in a patient with an underlying bleeding disorder. Easy bruising can also be a sign of medical conditions in which there is no identifiable coagulopathy; instead, the conditions are caused by an abnormality of blood vessels or their supporting tissues. In Ehlers-Danlos syndrome there may be posttraumatic bleeding and a history of joint hyperextensibility. Cushing's syndrome, chronic steroid use, and aging result in changes in skin and subcutaneous tissue, and subcutaneous bleeding occurs in response to minor trauma. The latter has been termed *senile purpura*.

Epistaxis is a common symptom, particularly in children and in dry climates, and may not reflect an underlying bleeding disorder. However, it is the most common symptom in hereditary hemorrhagic telangiectasia and in boys with vWD. Clues that epistaxis is a symptom of an underlying bleeding disorder include lack of seasonal variation and bleeding that requires medical evaluation or treatment, including cauterization. Bleeding with eruption of primary teeth is seen in children with more severe bleeding disorders, such as moderate and severe hemophilia. It is uncommon in children with mild bleeding disorders. Patients with disorders of primary hemostasis (platelet adhesion) do have increased bleeding after dental cleanings and other procedures that involve gum manipulation.

Menorrhagia is defined quantitatively as a loss of >80 cc of blood per cycle, based on blood loss required to produce iron-deficiency anemia. A complaint of heavy menses is subjective and has a poor correlation with excessive blood loss. Predictors of menorrhagia include bleeding resulting in iron-deficiency anemia or a need for blood transfusion, excessive pad or tampon use, menses lasting longer than 8 days, passage of clots, bleeding through protection, or flooding at night. Menorrhagia is a common symptom in women with underlying bleeding disorders and is reported in the majority of women with vWD and factor XI deficiency and in symptomatic carriers of hemophilia A. Women with underlying bleeding disorders are more likely to have other bleeding symptoms, including bleeding after dental extractions, postoperative bleeding, and postpartum bleeding, and are much more likely to have menorrhagia beginning at menarche than women with menorrhagia due to other causes.

Postpartum hemorrhage is a common symptom in women with underlying bleeding disorders. This occurs most commonly in the first 48 h after delivery, but it may also be manifest by prolonged or excessive bleeding after discharge from the hospital. Women with a history of postpartum hemorrhage have a high risk of recurrence with subsequent pregnancies. Rupture of ovarian cysts with intraabdominal hemorrhage has also been reported in women with underlying bleeding disorders.

Tonsillectomy is a major hemostatic challenge, as intact hemostatic mechanisms are essential to prevent excessive bleeding from the tonsillar bed. Bleeding may occur early after surgery or after approximately 7 days postoperatively, with loss of the eschar at the operative site. Similar delayed bleeding is seen after colonic polyp resection by

TABLE 59-1   PRIMARY HEMOSTATIC (PLATELET PLUG) DISORDERS

Defects of Platelet Adhesion
  von Willebrand disease
  Bernard-Soulier syndrome (absence of dysfunction of GpIb-IX-V)
Defects of Platelet Aggregation
  Glanzmann's thrombasthenia (absence or dysfunction of GpIIbIIIa)
  Afibrinogenemia
Defects of Platelet Secretion
  Decreased cyclooxygenase activity
    Drug-induced (aspirin, nonsteroidal anti-inflammatory agents)
    Inherited
  Granule storage pool defects
    Inherited
    Acquired
  Nonspecific drug effects
  Uremia
  Platelet coating (e.g., paraprotein, penicillin)
Defect of platelet coagulant activity
  Scott's syndrome

cautery. Gastrointestinal (GI) bleeding and hematuria are usually due to underlying pathology and procedures to identify and treat the bleeding site should be undertaken, even in patients with known bleeding disorders. vWD, particularly types 2 and 3, has been associated with angiodysplasia of the bowel and GI bleeding.

Hemarthroses and spontaneous muscle hematomas are characteristic of moderate or severe congenital factor VIII or IX deficiency. They can also be seen in moderate and severe deficiencies of fibrinogen, prothrombin, and of factors V, VII, and X. Spontaneous hemarthroses occur rarely in other bleeding disorders except for severe vWD, with associated FVIII levels <5%. Muscle and soft tissue bleeds are also common in acquired FVIII deficiency. Bleeding into a joint results in severe pain and swelling, as well as loss of function, but is rarely associated with discoloration from bruising around the joint. Life-threatening sites of bleeding include bleeding into the oropharynx, where bleeding can obstruct the airway, into the central nervous system, and into the retroperitoneum. Central nervous system bleeding is the major cause of bleeding-related deaths in patients with severe congenital factor deficiencies.

Prohemorrhagic Effects of Medications and Dietary Supplements
Aspirin and other nonsteroidal anti-inflammatory drugs (NSAIDs) that inhibit cyclooxygenase 1 impair primary hemostasis and may exacerbate bleeding from another cause or even unmask a previously occult mild bleeding disorder such as vWD. All NSAIDs, however, can precipitate gastrointestinal bleeding, which may be more severe in patients with underlying bleeding disorders. The aspirin effect on platelet function as assessed by aggregometry can persist for up to 7 days, although it has frequently returned to normal by 3 days after the last dose. The effect of other NSAIDs is shorter, as the inhibitor effect is reversed when the drug is removed.

Many herbal supplements can impair hemostatic function (Table 59-2). Some have been more convincingly associated with a bleeding risk than others. Fish oil or concentrated omega 3 fatty acid supplements impair platelet activation. They alter platelet biochemistry to produce more PGI3, a more potent platelet inhibitor than prostacyclin (PGI2), and more thromboxane A3, a less potent platelet activator than thromboxane A2. In fact, diets naturally rich in omega 3 fatty acids can result in a prolonged bleeding time and abnormal platelet aggregation studies, but the actual associated bleeding risk is unclear. Vitamin E appears to inhibit protein kinase C–mediated platelet aggregation and nitric oxide production. In patients with unexplained bruising or bleeding, it is prudent to review any new medications or supplements and discontinue those that may be associated with bleeding.

Underlying Systemic Diseases That Cause or Exacerbate a Bleeding Tendency Acquired bleeding disorders are commonly secondary to, or associated with, systemic disease. The clinical evaluation of a patient with a bleeding tendency must therefore include a thorough

| TABLE 59-2 | HERBAL SUPPLEMENTS ASSOCIATED WITH INCREASED BLEEDING |

Herbs with Potential Anti-Platelet Activity
Ginkgo (*Ginkgo biloba L.*)
Garlic (*Allium sativum*)
Bilberry (*Vaccinium myrtillus*)
Ginger (*Gingiber officinale*)
Dong quai (*Angelica sinensis*)
Feverfew (*Tanacetum parthenium*)
Asian Ginseng (*Panax ginseng*)
American Ginseng (*Panax quinquefolius*)
Siberian ginseng/eleuthero (*Eleuterococcus senticosus*)
Tumeric (*Circuma longa*)
Meadowsweet (*Filipendula ulmaria*)
Willow (*Salix* spp.)
Coumarin-Containing Herbs
Motherworth (*Leonurus cardiaca*)
Chamomile (*Matricaria recutita, Chamaemelum mobile*)
Horse chestnut (*Aesculus hippocastanum*)
Red clover (*Trifolium pratense*)
Fenugreek (*Trigonella foenum-graecum*)

assessment for evidence of underlying disease. Bruising or mucosal bleeding may be the presenting complaint in liver disease, severe renal impairment, hypothyroidism, paraproteinemias or amyloidosis, and conditions causing bone marrow failure. All coagulation factors are synthesized in the liver and hepatic failure results in combined factor deficiencies. This is often compounded by thrombocytopenia from splenomegaly due to portal hypertension. Coagulation factors II, VII, IX, X and proteins C, S, and Z are dependent on vitamin K for posttranslational modification. Although Vitamin K is required in both procoagulant and anticoagulant processes, the phenotype of vitamin K deficiency or the warfarin effect on coagulation is bleeding.

The normal blood platelet count is 150,000–450,000/μL. Thrombocytopenia results from decreased production, increased destruction, and/or sequestration. Although the bleeding risk varies somewhat by the reason for the thrombocytopenia, bleeding rarely occurs in isolated thrombocytopenia at counts <50,000/μL and usually not until <10,000–20,000/μL. Coexisting coagulopathies, as seen in liver failure or disseminated coagulation; infection; platelet-inhibitory drugs; and underlying medical conditions can all increase the risk of bleeding in the thrombocytopenic patient. Most procedures can be performed in patients with a platelet count of 50,000/μL. The level needed for major surgery will depend on the type of surgery and the patients' underlying medical state, although a count of approximately 80,000/μL is likely sufficient.

History of Thrombosis   The risk of thrombosis, like that of bleeding, is influenced by both genetic and environmental influences. The major risk factor for arterial thrombosis is atherosclerosis, while those for venous thrombosis are immobility, surgery, underlying medical conditions such as malignancy, medications such as hormonal therapy, obesity, and genetic predispositions. Factors that increase risks for venous and both venous and arterial thromboses are shown in Table 59-3.

The most important point in a history related to venous thrombosis is whether the thrombotic event was idiopathic (meaning there was no clear precipitating factor) or was a precipitated event. In patients without underlying malignancy, having an idiopathic event is the strongest predictor of recurrence of venous thromboembolism. In patients who have a vague history of thrombosis, a history of being treated with warfarin suggests a past DVT. Age is an important risk factor for venous thrombosis; the risk of DVT increases per decade, with an approximate incidence of 1/100,000 per year in early childhood to 1/200 per year among octogenarians. Family history is helpful in determining if there is a genetic predisposition and how strong that predisposition appears to be.

A genetic thrombophilia that confers a relatively small increased risk, such as being a heterozygote for the prothrombin G20210A or factor V Leiden mutation, may be a relatively minor determinant of

| TABLE 59-3 | RISK FACTORS FOR THROMBOSIS |

Venous	Venous and Arterial
Inherited	**Inherited**
Factor V Leiden	Homocystinuria
Prothrombin G20210A	Dysfibrinogenemia
Antithrombin deficiency	
Protein C deficiency	**Mixed (Inherited and acquired)**
Protein S deficiency	Hyperhomocysteinemia
Elevated FVIII	
	Acquired
Acquired	Malignancy
Age	Antiphospholipid antibody syndrome
Previous thrombosis	Hormonal therapy
Immobilization	Polycythemia vera
Major surgery	Essential thrombocythemia
Pregnancy & puerperium	Paroxysmal nocturnal hemoglobinuria
Hospitalization	Thrombotic thrombocytopenic
Obesity	purpura
Infection	Heparin-induced thrombocytopenia
APC resistance, nongenetic	Disseminated intravascular coagulation
Unknown[a]	
Elevated factor II, IX, XI	
Elevated TAFI levels	
Low levels of TFPI	

[a]Unknown whether risk is inherited or acquired.
Note: APC, activated protein C; TAFI, thrombin-activatable fibrinolysis inhibitor; TFPI, tissue factor pathway inhibitor.

risk in an elderly individual undergoing a high risk surgical procedure. As shown in Fig. 59-5, a thrombotic event often has more than one contributing factor. Predisposing factors must be carefully assessed to determine the risk of recurrent thrombosis, and with consideration of the patient's bleeding risk, determine the length of anticoagulation. Similar consideration should be given to determining the need to test the patient and family members for genetic thrombophilias.

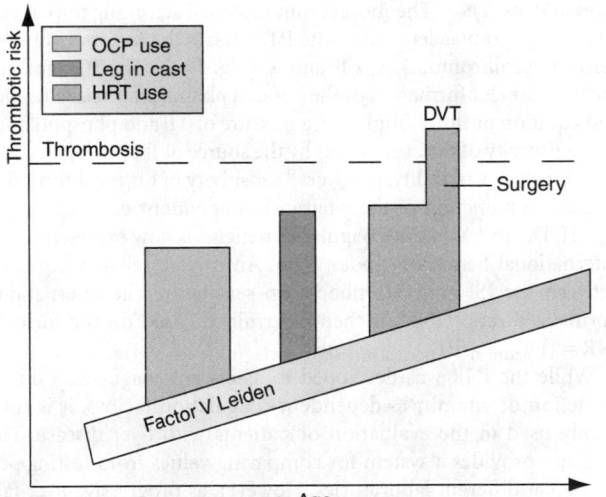

FIGURE 59-5 Thrombotic risk over time. Shown schematically is an individual's thrombotic risk over time. An underlying Factor V Leiden mutation provides a "theoretically" constant increased risk. The thrombotic risk increases with age and, intermittently, with oral contraceptive (OCP) or hormone replacement (HRT) use; other events may increase the risk further. At some point the cumulative risk may increase to the threshold for thrombosis and result in deep venous thrombosis (DVT). Note: The magnitude and duration of risk portrayed in the figure is meant for example only and may not precisely reflect the relative risk determined by clinical study. [From BA Konkle, A Schafer, in DP Zipes et al (eds): Braunwald's Heart Disease, 7th ed. Philadelphia, Saunders, 2005; modified with permission from FR Rosendaal: Venous thrombosis: A multicausal disease. Lancet 353:1167, 1999.]

LABORATORY EVALUATION Careful history taking and clinical examination are essential components in the assessment of bleeding and thrombotic risk. The use of laboratory tests of coagulation complement, but cannot substitute for, clinical assessment. No test provides a global assessment of hemostasis. The bleeding time has been used to assess bleeding risk; however, it does not predict bleeding risk with surgery and is not recommended for this indication. The PFA-100, an instrument that measures platelet-dependent coagulation under flow conditions, is more sensitive and specific for platelet disorders and vWD than the bleeding time; however, it is not sensitive enough to rule out underlying mild bleeding disorders. Also, it has not been evaluated prospectively to determine its utility in predicting bleeding risk, although such studies are underway.

For routine preoperative and preprocedure testing, an abnormal prothrombin time (PT) may detect liver disease or vitamin K deficiency that had not been previously appreciated. Studies have not confirmed the usefulness of an activated partial thromboplastin time (aPTT) in preoperative evaluations in patients with a negative bleeding history. The primary use of coagulation testing should be to confirm the presence and type of bleeding disorder in a patient with a suspicious clinical history.

Because of the nature of coagulation assays, proper sample acquisition and handling is critical to obtaining valid results. In patients with abnormal coagulation assays who have no bleeding history, repeat studies with attention to these factors frequently results in normal values. Most coagulation assays are performed in sodium citrate anticoagulated plasma that is recalcified for the assay. Because the anticoagulant is in liquid solution and needs to be added to blood in proportion to the plasma volume, incorrectly filled or inadequately mixed blood collection tubes will give erroneous results. Vacutainer tubes should be filled to >90% of the recommended fill, which is usually denoted by a line on the tube. An elevated hematocrit (>55%) can result in a false value due to a decreased plasma to anticoagulant ratio.

Screening Assays   The most commonly used screening tests are the PT, aPTT, and platelet count. The PT assesses the factors I (fibrinogen), II (prothrombin), V, VII and X (**Fig. 59-6**). The PT measures the time for clot formation of the citrated plasma after recalcification and addition of thromboplastin, a mixture of TF and phospholipids. The sensitivity of the assay varies by the source of thromboplastin. To adjust for this variability, the overall sensitivity of different thromboplastins to reduction of the vitamin K–dependent clotting factors II, VII, IX, and X in anticoagulated patients is now expressed as the International Sensitivity Index (ISI). An inverse relationship exists between the ISI and thromboplastin sensitivity. The international normalized ratio (INR) is then determined based on the formula: INR = $(PT_{patient}/PT_{normal\ mean})^{ISI}$.

While the INR was developed to assess anticoagulation due to reduction of vitamin K–dependent coagulation factors, it is commonly used in the evaluation of patients with liver disease. This measure provides a system for comparing values from testing performed at different laboratories. However, as progressive liver failure is associated with variable changes in coagulation factors, the degree of prolongation of either the PT or the INR only roughly predicts the bleeding risk. Thrombin generation has been shown to be normal in many patients with mild to moderate liver dysfunction. As the PT only measures one aspect of hemostasis affected by liver dysfunction, we likely overestimate the bleeding risk of a mildly elevated INR in this setting.

The aPTT assesses the intrinsic and common coagulation pathways, factors XI, IX, VIII, X, V, II, fibrinogen, and also prekallikrein, high molecular weight kininogen and factor XII (Fig. 59-6). The aPTT reagent contains phospholipids derived from either animal or vegetable sources that function as a platelet substitute in the coagulation pathways and includes an activator of the intrinsic co-

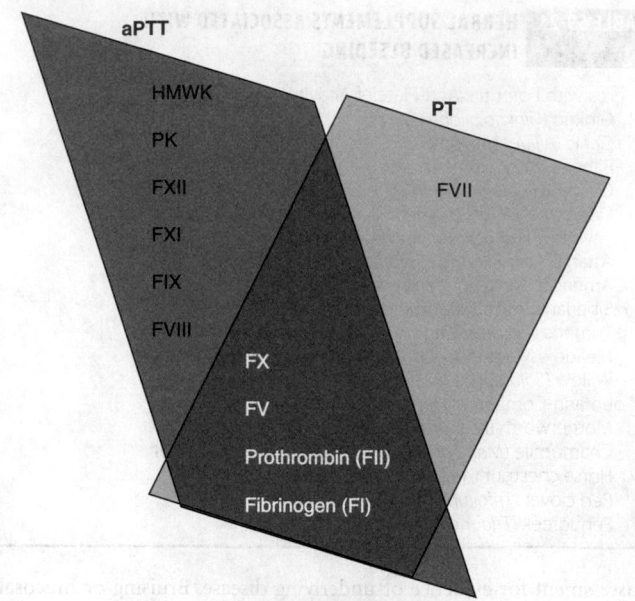

FIGURE 59-6 Coagulation factor activity tested in the activated partial thromboplastin time (aPTT) in red and prothrombin time (PT) in green, or both. HMWK, high-molecular-weight kininogen; PK, prekallikrein; F, factor.

agulation system, such as ellagic acid or the particulate activators kaolin, celite, or micronized silica.

The phospholipid composition of aPTT reagents varies, which influences the sensitivity of individual reagents to clotting factor deficiencies and to inhibitors such as heparin and lupus anticoagulants. Thus, aPTT results will vary from one laboratory to another, and the normal range in the laboratory where the testing occurs should be used in the interpretation. Local laboratories can relate their aPTT values to therapeutic heparin anticoagulation by correlating aPTT values with direct measurements of heparin activity (anti-Xa or protamine titration assays) in samples from heparinized patients, although correlation between these assays is often poor. The aPTT reagent will vary in sensitivity to individual factor deficiencies and usually becomes prolonged with individual factor deficiencies of 30–50%. The relationship between defects in secondary hemostasis (fibrin formation) and coagulation test abnormalities is shown in Table 59-4.

Mixing Studies   Mixing studies are used to evaluate a prolonged aPTT or, less commonly PT, to distinguish between a factor deficiency and an inhibitor. In this assay, normal plasma and patient plasma are mixed in a 50:50 ratio, and the aPTT or PT is determined immediately and after incubation at 37°C for varying times, typically 30, 60, and/or 120 min. With isolated factor deficiencies, the aPTT will correct with mixing and stay corrected with incubation. With aPTT prolongation due to a lupus anticoagulant, the mixing and incubation will show no correction. In acquired neutralizing factor antibodies, such as an acquired factor VIII inhibitor, the initial assay may or may not correct immediately after mixing but will prolong or remain prolonged with incubation at 37°C. Failure to correct with mixing can also be due to the presence of other inhibitors or interfering substances such as heparin, fibrin split products, and paraproteins.

Specific Factor Assays   Decisions to proceed with specific clotting factor assays will be influenced by the clinical situation and the results of coagulation screening tests. Precise diagnosis and effective management of inherited and acquired coagulation deficiencies necessitate quantitation of the relevant factors. When bleeding is severe, specific assays are often urgently required to guide appropriate therapy. Individual factor assays are usually performed as modifications of the mixing study, where the patient's plasma is

TABLE 59-4 HEMOSTATIC DISORDERS AND COAGULATION TEST ABNORMALITIES

Prolonged activated partial thromboplastin time (aPTT)
   No clinical bleeding – ↓ factors XII, high-molecular-weight kininogen, protein kinase
   Variable, but usually mild, bleeding – ↓ factor XI, mild ↓ FVIII and FIX
   Frequent, severe bleeding – severe deficiencies of FVIII and FIX
   Heparin
Prolonged prothrombin time (PT)
   Factor VII deficiency
   Vitamin K deficiency – early
   Warfarin anticoagulation
Prolonged aPTT and PT
   Factor II, V or X deficiency
   Vitamin K deficiency – late
   Direct thrombin inhibitors
Prolonged thrombin time
   Heparin or heparin-like inhibitors
   Mild or no bleeding – dysfibrinogenemia
   Frequent, severe bleeding – afibrinogenemia
Prolonged PT and/or aPTT not correct with mixing with normal plasma
   Bleeding – specific factor inhibitor
   No symptoms, or clotting and/or pregnancy loss – lupus anticoagulant
   Disseminated intravascular coagulation
   Heparin or direct thrombin inhibitor
Abnormal clot solubility
   Factor XIII deficiency
   Inhibitors or defective cross-linking
Rapid clot lysis
   Deficiency of α_2-antiplasmin or plasminogen activator inhibitor 1
   Treatment with fibrinolytic therapy

mixed with plasma deficient in the factor being studied. This will correct all factor deficiencies to >50%, thus making prolongation of clot formation due to a factor deficiency dependent on the factor missing from the added plasma.

Testing for Antiphospholipid Antibodies

Antibodies to phospholipids (cardiolipin) or phospholipid-binding proteins (β_2-microglobulin and others) are detected by ELISA. When these antibodies interfere with phospholipid-dependent coagulation tests, they are termed *lupus anticoagulants*. The aPTT has variable sensitivity to lupus anticoagulants, depending in part on the aPTT reagents used. An assay utilizing a sensitive reagent has been termed an *LA-PTT*. The dilute Russell Viper Venom test (dRVVT) and the tissue thromboplastin time (TTI) are modifications of standard tests with the phospholipid reagent decreased, thus increasing the sensitivity to antibodies that interfere with the phospholipid component. The tests, however, are not specific for lupus anticoagulants, as factor deficiencies or other inhibitors also result in prolongation. Documentation of a lupus anticoagulant requires not only prolongation of a phospholipid-dependent coagulation test but also lack of correction when mixed with normal plasma and correction with the addition of activated platelet membranes or certain phospholipids, e.g., hexagonal phase.

Other Coagulation Tests

The thrombin time and the reptilase time measure fibrinogen conversion to fibrin and are prolonged when the fibrinogen level is low (usually <80–100 mg/dL); qualitatively abnormal, as seen in inherited or acquired dysfibrinogenemias; or when fibrin/fibrinogen degradation products interfere. The thrombin time, but not the reptilase time, is prolonged in the presence of heparin. Measurement of anti-factor Xa plasma inhibitory activity is a test frequently used to assess low-molecular-weight heparin (LMWH) activity or as a direct measurement of unfractionated heparin (UFH) activity. Heparin in the patient sample inhibits the enzymatic conversion of an Xa-specific chromogenic substrate to colored product by factor Xa. Standard curves are created using multiple concentrations of UFH and LMWH and are used to calculate the concentration of anti-Xa activity in the patient plasma.

Laboratory Testing for Thrombophilia

Laboratory assays to detect thrombophilic states include molecular diagnostic, immunologic and functional assays. These assays vary in their sensitivity and specificity for the condition being tested. Furthermore, acute thrombosis, acute illnesses, inflammatory conditions, pregnancy, and medications affect levels of many coagulation factors and their inhibitors. Antithrombin is decreased by heparin and in the setting of acute thrombosis. Protein C and S levels may be increased in the setting of acute thrombosis and are decreased by warfarin. Antiphospholipid antibodies are frequently transiently positive in acute illness. As thrombophilia evaluations are usually performed to assess the need to extend anticoagulation, testing should be performed in a steady state, remote from the acute event. In most instances warfarin anticoagulation can be stopped after the initial 3–6 months of treatment, and testing is performed at least 3 weeks later. Furthermore, sensitive markers of coagulation activation, notably the D-dimer assay and the thrombin generation test, hold promise as predictors, when elevated, of recurrent thrombosis when measured at least 1 month from discontinuation of warfarin, although further study is needed to better support this application.

Measures of Platelet Function

The bleeding time has been used to assess bleeding risk; however, it has not been found to predict bleeding risk with surgery, and it is not recommended for use for this indication. The PFA-100 and similar instruments that measure platelet-dependent coagulation under flow conditions are generally more sensitive and specific for platelet disorders and vWD than the bleeding time; however, data are insufficient to support their use to predict bleeding risk or monitor response to therapy. When they are used in the evaluation of a patient with bleeding symptoms, abnormal results, as with the bleeding time, require specific testing, such as vWF assays and/or platelet aggregation studies. Since all of these "screening" assays may miss patients with mild bleeding disorders, further studies are needed to define their role in hemostasis testing.

For classic platelet aggregometry, various agonists are added to the patient's platelet-rich plasma, and platelet agglutination and aggregation are observed. Tests of platelet secretion in response to agonists can also be measured. These tests are affected by many factors, including numerous medications, and the association between minor defects in aggregation or secretion in these assays and bleeding risk is not clearly established.

ACKNOWLEDGMENT

Robert I. Handin, MD, contributed this chapter in the 16th edition and some material from that chapter have been retained here.

FURTHER READINGS

BAUER KA: Management of thrombophilia. J Thromb Haemost 1:1429, 2003

BOCKENSTEDT PL: Laboratory methods in hemostasis, in *Thrombosis and Hemorrhage*, 3d ed, J Loscalzo, AI Schafer (eds). Philadelphia, Lippincott Williams & Wilkins, 2003, pp 363–423

COLMAN RW et al: Overview of hemostasis, in *Hemostasis and Thrombosis*, 5th ed, RW Colman et al (eds). Philadelphia, Lippincott Williams & Wilkins, 2006, pp 3–16

HEIT JA: The epidemiology of venous thromboembolism in the community: Implications for prevention and management. J Thromb Thrombol 21:23, 2006

KONKLE BA: Clinical approach to the bleeding patient, in *Hemostasis and Thrombosis*, 5th ed, RW Colman et al (eds). Philadelphia, Lippincott Williams & Wilkins, 2006, pp 1147–1158

ORTEL TL: The antiphospholipid syndrome: What are we really measuring? How do we measure it? And how do we treat it? J Thromb Thrombol 21:79, 2006

ROBERTS HR et al: A cell-based model of thrombin generation. Sem Thromb Hemost 32(Suppl 1):32, 2006

60 Enlargement of Lymph Nodes and Spleen

Patrick H. Henry, Dan L. Longo

This chapter is intended to serve as a guide to the evaluation of patients who present with enlargement of the lymph nodes (*lymphadenopathy*) or the spleen (*splenomegaly*). Lymphadenopathy is a rather common clinical finding in primary care settings, whereas palpable splenomegaly is less so.

LYMPHADENOPATHY

Lymphadenopathy may be an incidental finding in patients being examined for various reasons, or it may be a presenting sign or symptom of the patient's illness. The physician must eventually decide whether the lymphadenopathy is a normal finding or one that requires further study, up to and including biopsy. Soft, flat, submandibular nodes (<1 cm) are often palpable in healthy children and young adults, and healthy adults may have palpable inguinal nodes of up to 2 cm, which are considered normal. Further evaluation of these normal nodes is not warranted. In contrast, if the physician believes the node(s) to be abnormal, then pursuit of a more precise diagnosis is needed.

APPROACH TO THE PATIENT:
Lymphadenopathy

Lymphadenopathy may be a primary or secondary manifestation of numerous disorders, as shown in Table 60-1. Many of these disorders are infrequent causes of lymphadenopathy. In primary care practice, more than two-thirds of patients with lymphadenopathy have nonspecific causes or upper respiratory illnesses (viral or bacterial), and <1% have a malignancy. In one study, 84% of patients referred for evaluation of lymphadenopathy had a "benign" diagnosis. The remaining 16% had a malignancy (lymphoma or metastatic adenocarcinoma). Of the patients with benign lymphadenopathy, 63% had a nonspecific or reactive etiology (no causative agent found), and the remainder had a specific cause demonstrated, most commonly infectious mononucleosis, toxoplasmosis, or tuberculosis. Thus, the vast majority of patients with lymphadenopathy will have a nonspecific etiology requiring few diagnostic tests.

CLINICAL ASSESSMENT The physician will be aided in the pursuit of an explanation for the lymphadenopathy by a careful medical history, physical examination, selected laboratory tests, and perhaps an excisional lymph node biopsy.

The *medical history* should reveal the setting in which lymphadenopathy is occurring. Symptoms such as sore throat, cough, fever, night sweats, fatigue, weight loss, or pain in the nodes should be sought. The patient's age, sex, occupation, exposure to pets, sexual behavior, and use of drugs such as diphenylhydantoin are other important historic points. For example, children and young adults usually have benign (i.e., nonmalignant) disorders, such as viral or bacterial upper respiratory infections, infectious mononucleosis, toxoplasmosis, and, in some countries, tuberculosis, which account for the observed lymphadenopathy. In contrast, after age 50 the incidence of malignant disorders increases and that of benign disorders decreases.

The *physical examination* can provide useful clues such as the extent of lymphadenopathy (localized or generalized), size of nodes, texture, presence or absence of nodal tenderness, signs of inflammation over the node, skin lesions, and splenomegaly. A thorough ear, nose, and throat (ENT) examination is indicated in adult patients with cervical adenopathy and a history of tobacco use. Localized or regional adenopathy implies involvement of a single anatomic area. Generalized adenopathy has been defined as involvement of three or

TABLE 60-1   DISEASES ASSOCIATED WITH LYMPHADENOPATHY

1. Infectious diseases
    a. Viral—infectious mononucleosis syndromes (EBV, CMV), infectious hepatitis, herpes simplex, herpesvirus-6, varicella-zoster virus, rubella, measles, adenovirus, HIV, epidemic keratoconjunctivitis, vaccinia, herpesvirus-8
    b. Bacterial—streptococci, staphylococci, cat-scratch disease, brucellosis, tularemia, plague, chancroid, melioidosis, glanders, tuberculosis, atypical mycobacterial infection, primary and secondary syphilis, diphtheria, leprosy
    c. Fungal—histoplasmosis, coccidioidomycosis, paracoccidioidomycosis
    d. Chlamydial—lymphogranuloma venereum, trachoma
    e. Parasitic—toxoplasmosis, leishmaniasis, trypanosomiasis, filariasis
    f. Rickettsial—scrub typhus, rickettsialpox, Q fever
2. Immunologic diseases
    a. Rheumatoid arthritis
    b. Juvenile rheumatoid arthritis
    c. Mixed connective tissue disease
    d. Systemic lupus erythematosus
    e. Dermatomyositis
    f. Sjögren's syndrome
    g. Serum sickness
    h. Drug hypersensitivity—diphenylhydantoin, hydralazine, allopurinol, primidone, gold, carbamazepine, etc.
    i. Angioimmunoblastic lymphadenopathy
    j. Primary biliary cirrhosis
    k. Graft-vs.-host disease
    l. Silicone-associated
    m. Autoimmune lymphoproliferative syndrome
3. Malignant diseases
    a. Hematologic—Hodgkin's disease, non-Hodgkin's lymphomas, acute or chronic lymphocytic leukemia, hairy cell leukemia, malignant histiocytosis, amyloidosis
    b. Metastatic—from numerous primary sites
4. Lipid storage diseases—Gaucher's, Niemann-Pick, Fabry, Tangier
5. Endocrine diseases—hyperthyroidism
6. Other disorders
    a. Castleman's disease (giant lymph node hyperplasia)
    b. Sarcoidosis
    c. Dermatopathic lymphadenitis
    d. Lymphomatoid granulomatosis
    e. Histiocytic necrotizing lymphadenitis (Kikuchi's disease)
    f. Sinus histiocytosis with massive lymphadenopathy (Rosai-Dorfman disease)
    g. Mucocutaneous lymph node syndrome (Kawasaki's disease)
    h. Histiocytosis X
    i. Familial mediterranean fever
    j. Severe hypertriglyceridemia
    k. Vascular transformation of sinuses
    l. Inflammatory pseudotumor of lymph node
    m. Congestive heart failure

Note: EBV, Epstein-Barr virus; CMV, cytomegalovirus.

more noncontiguous lymph node areas. Many of the causes of lymphadenopathy (Table 60-1) can produce localized *or* generalized adenopathy, so this distinction is of limited utility in the differential diagnosis. Nevertheless, generalized lymphadenopathy is frequently associated with nonmalignant disorders such as infectious mononucleosis [Epstein-Barr virus (EBV) or cytomegalovirus (CMV)], toxoplasmosis, AIDS, other viral infections, systemic lupus erythematosus (SLE), and mixed connective tissue disease. Acute and chronic lymphocytic leukemias and malignant lymphomas also produce generalized adenopathy in adults.

The site of localized or regional adenopathy may provide a useful clue about the cause. Occipital adenopathy often reflects an infection of the scalp, and preauricular adenopathy accompanies conjunctival infections and cat-scratch disease. The most frequent site of regional adenopathy is the neck, and most of the causes are benign—upper respiratory infections, oral and dental lesions, infectious mononucleosis, other viral illnesses. The chief malignant causes include metastatic cancer from head and neck, breast, lung, and thyroid primaries. Enlargement of supraclavicular and scalene nodes is always abnormal. Because these nodes drain regions of the lung and retroperitoneal space, they can reflect lymphomas, other cancers, or infectious processes arising in these areas. Virchow's node is an enlarged left supraclavicular node infiltrated with metastatic cancer from a gastrointestinal primary. Metastases to supraclavicular nodes also occur from lung, breast, testis, or ovarian cancers. Tuberculosis, sarcoidosis, and toxoplasmosis are nonneoplastic causes of supraclavicular adenopathy. Axillary adenopathy is usually due to injuries or localized infections of the ipsilateral upper extremity. Malignant causes include melanoma or lymphoma and, in women, breast cancer. Inguinal lymphadenopathy is usually secondary to infections or trauma of the lower extremities and may accompany sexually transmitted diseases such as lymphogranuloma venereum, primary syphilis, genital herpes, or chancroid. These nodes may also be involved by lymphomas and metastatic cancer from primary lesions of the rectum, genitalia, or lower extremities (melanoma).

The size and texture of the lymph node(s) and the presence of pain are useful parameters in evaluating a patient with lymphadenopathy. Nodes <1.0 cm^2 in area (1.0 cm × 1.0 cm or less) are almost always secondary to benign, nonspecific reactive causes. In one retrospective analysis of younger patients (9–25 years) who had a lymph node biopsy, a maximum diameter of >2 cm served as one discriminant for predicting that the biopsy would reveal malignant or granulomatous disease. Another study showed that a lymph node size of 2.25 cm^2 (1.5 cm × 1.5 cm) was the best size limit for distinguishing malignant or granulomatous lymphadenopathy from other causes of lymphadenopathy. Patients with node(s) ≤1.0 cm^2 should be observed after excluding infectious mononucleosis and/or toxoplasmosis unless there are symptoms and signs of an underlying systemic illness.

The texture of lymph nodes may be described as soft, firm, rubbery, hard, discrete, matted, tender, movable, or fixed. Tenderness is found when the capsule is stretched during rapid enlargement, usually secondary to an inflammatory process. Some malignant diseases such as acute leukemia may produce rapid enlargement and pain in the nodes. Nodes involved by lymphoma tend to be large, discrete, symmetric, rubbery, firm, mobile, and nontender. Nodes containing metastatic cancer are often hard, nontender, and nonmovable because of fixation to surrounding tissues. The coexistence of splenomegaly in the patient with lymphadenopathy implies a systemic illness such as infectious mononucleosis, lymphoma, acute or chronic leukemia, SLE, sarcoidosis, toxoplasmosis, cat-scratch disease, or other less common hematologic disorders. The patient's story should provide helpful clues about the underlying systemic illness.

Nonsuperficial presentations (thoracic or abdominal) of adenopathy are usually detected as the result of a symptom-directed diagnostic workup. Thoracic adenopathy may be detected by routine chest radiography or during the workup for superficial adenopathy. It may also be found because the patient complains of a cough or wheezing from airway compression; hoarseness from recurrent laryngeal nerve involvement; dysphagia from esophageal compression; or swelling of the neck, face, or arms secondary to compression of the superior vena cava or subclavian vein. The differential diagnosis of mediastinal and hilar adenopathy includes primary lung disorders and systemic illnesses that characteristically involve mediastinal or hilar nodes. In the young, mediastinal adenopathy is associated with infectious mononucleosis and sarcoidosis. In endemic regions, histoplasmosis can cause unilateral paratracheal lymph node involvement that mimics lymphoma. Tuberculosis can also cause unilateral adenopathy. In older patients, the differential diagnosis includes primary lung cancer (especially among smokers), lymphomas, metastatic carcinoma (usually lung), tuberculosis, fungal infection, and sarcoidosis.

Enlarged intraabdominal or retroperitoneal nodes are usually malignant. Although tuberculosis may present as mesenteric lymphadenitis, these masses usually contain lymphomas or, in young men, germ cell tumors.

LABORATORY INVESTIGATION The laboratory investigation of patients with lymphadenopathy must be tailored to elucidate the etiology suspected from the patient's history and physical findings. One study from a family practice clinic evaluated 249 younger patients with "enlarged lymph nodes, not infected" or "lymphadenitis." No laboratory studies were obtained in 51%. When studies were performed, the most common were a complete blood count (CBC) (33%), throat culture (16%), chest x-ray (12%), or monospot test (10%). Only eight patients (3%) had a node biopsy, and half of those were normal or reactive. The CBC can provide useful data for the diagnosis of acute or chronic leukemias, EBV or CMV mononucleosis, lymphoma with a leukemic component, pyogenic infections, or immune cytopenias in illnesses such as SLE. Serologic studies may demonstrate antibodies specific to components of EBV, CMV, HIV, and other viruses; *Toxoplasma gondii*; *Brucella*; etc. If SLE is suspected, then antinuclear and anti-DNA antibody studies are warranted.

The chest x-ray is usually negative, but the presence of a pulmonary infiltrate or mediastinal lymphadenopathy would suggest tuberculosis, histoplasmosis, sarcoidosis, lymphoma, primary lung cancer, or metastatic cancer and demands further investigation.

A variety of imaging techniques (CT, MRI, ultrasound, color Doppler ultrasonography) have been employed to differentiate benign from malignant lymph nodes, especially in patients with head and neck cancer. CT and MRI are comparably accurate (65–90%) in the diagnosis of metastases to cervical lymph nodes. Ultrasonography has been used to determine the long (L) axis, short (S) axis, and a ratio of long to short axis in cervical nodes. An L/S ratio of <2.0 has a sensitivity and a specificity of 95% for distinguishing benign and malignant nodes in patients with head and neck cancer. This ratio has greater specificity and sensitivity than palpation or measurement of either the long or the short axis alone.

The indications for lymph node biopsy are imprecise, yet it is a valuable diagnostic tool. The decision to biopsy may be made early in a patient's evaluation or delayed for up to 2 weeks. Prompt biopsy should occur if the patient's history and physical findings suggest a malignancy; examples include a solitary, hard, nontender cervical node in an older patient who is a chronic user of tobacco; supraclavicular adenopathy; and solitary or generalized adenopathy that is firm, movable, and suggestive of lymphoma. If a primary head and neck cancer is suspected as the basis of a solitary, hard cervical node, then a careful ENT examination should be performed. Any mucosal lesion that is suspicious for a primary neoplastic process should be biopsied first. If no mucosal lesion is detected, an excisional biopsy of the largest node should be performed. Fine-needle aspiration should not be performed as the first diagnostic procedure. Most diagnoses require more tissue than such aspiration can provide, and it often delays a definitive diagnosis. Fine-needle aspiration should be reserved for thyroid nodules and for confirmation of relapse in patients whose primary diagnosis is known. If the primary physician is uncertain about whether to proceed to biopsy, consultation with a hematologist or medical oncologist should be helpful. In primary care practices, <5% of lymphadenopathy patients will require a biopsy. That percentage will be considerably larger in referral practices, i.e., hematology, oncology, or ENT.

Two groups have reported algorithms that they claim will identify more precisely those lymphadenopathy patients who should have a biopsy. Both reports were retrospective analyses in referral practices. The first study involved patients 9–25 years of age who had a node biopsy performed. Three variables were identified that predicted those young patients with peripheral lymphadenopathy who should undergo biopsy; lymph node size >2 cm in diameter and abnormal chest x-ray had positive predictive values, whereas recent ENT symptoms had negative predictive values. The second study evaluated 220 lymphadenopathy patients in a hematology unit and identified five variables [lymph node size, location (supraclavicular or nonsupraclavicular), age (>40 years or <40 years), texture (nonhard or hard), and tenderness] that were utilized in a mathematical model to identify those patients requiring a biopsy. Positive predictive value was found for age >40 years, supraclavicular location, node size >2.25 cm², hard texture, and lack of pain or tenderness. Negative predictive value was evident for age <40 years, node size <1.0 cm², nonhard texture, and tender or painful nodes. Ninety-one percent of those who required biopsy were correctly classified by this model. Since both of these studies were retrospective analyses and one was limited to young patients, it is not known how useful these models would be if applied prospectively in a primary care setting.

Most lymphadenopathy patients do not require a biopsy, and at least half require no laboratory studies. If the patient's history and physical findings point to a benign cause for lymphadenopathy, then careful follow-up at a 2- to 4-week interval can be employed. The patient should be instructed to return for reevaluation if the node(s) increase in size. Antibiotics are not indicated for lymphadenopathy unless strong evidence of a bacterial infection is present. Glucocorticoids should not be used to treat lymphadenopathy because their lympholytic effect obscures some diagnoses (lymphoma, leukemia, Castleman's disease) and they contribute to delayed healing or activation of underlying infections. An exception to this statement is the life-threatening pharyngeal obstruction by enlarged lymphoid tissue in Waldeyer's ring that is occasionally seen in infectious mononucleosis.

SPLENOMEGALY

STRUCTURE AND FUNCTION OF THE SPLEEN

The spleen is a reticuloendothelial organ that has its embryologic origin in the dorsal mesogastrium at about 5 weeks' gestation. It arises in a series of hillocks, migrates to its normal adult location in the left upper quadrant (LUQ), and is attached to the stomach via the gastrolienal ligament and to the kidney via the lienorenal ligament. When the hillocks fail to unify into a single tissue mass, accessory spleens may develop in around 20% of persons. The function of the spleen has been elusive. Galen believed it was the source of "black bile" or melancholia, and the word *hypochondria* (literally, beneath the ribs) and the idiom "to vent one's spleen" attest to the beliefs that the spleen had an important influence on the psyche and emotions. In humans its normal physiologic roles seem to be the following:

1. Maintenance of quality control over erythrocytes in the red pulp by removal of senescent and defective red blood cells. The spleen accomplishes this function through a unique organization of its parenchyma and vasculature (**Fig. 60-1**).
2. Synthesis of antibodies in the white pulp.
3. The removal of antibody-coated bacteria and antibody-coated blood cells from the circulation.

An increase in these normal functions may result in splenomegaly.

The spleen is composed of *red pulp* and *white pulp*, which are Malpighi's terms for the red blood–filled sinuses and reticuloendothelial cell–lined cords and the white lymphoid follicles arrayed within the red pulp matrix. The spleen is in the portal circulation. The reason for this is unknown but may relate to the fact that lower blood pressure allows less rapid flow and minimizes damage to normal erythrocytes. Blood flows into the spleen at a rate of about 150 mL/min through the splenic artery, which ultimately ramifies into central arterioles. Some blood goes from the arterioles to capillaries and then to splenic veins and out of the spleen, but the majority of blood from central arterioles flows into the macrophage-lined sinuses and cords. The blood entering the sinuses reenters the circulation through the splenic venules, but the blood entering the cords is subjected to an inspection of sorts.

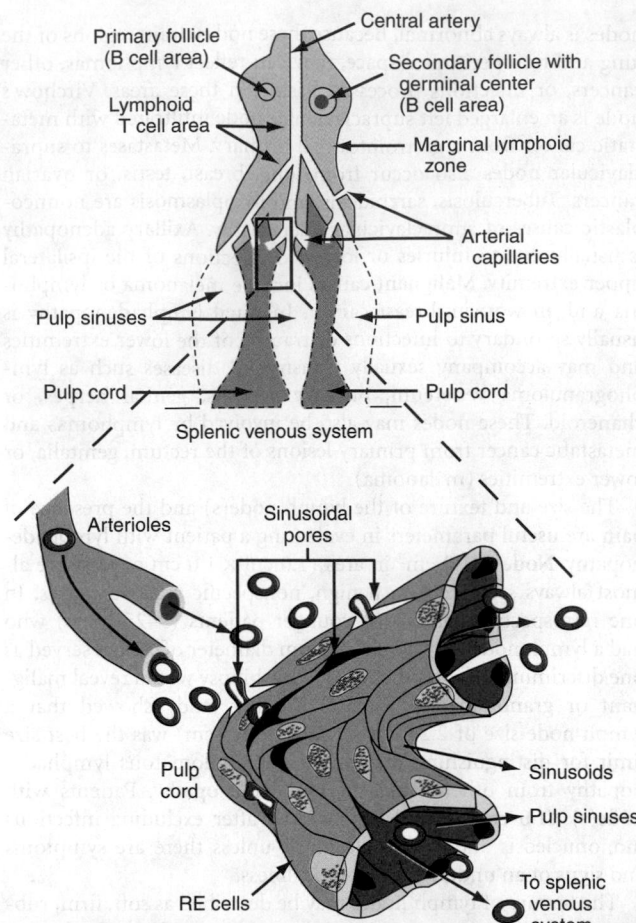

FIGURE 60-1 Schematic spleen structure. The spleen comprises many units of red and white pulp centered around small branches of the splenic artery, called *central arteries*. White pulp is lymphoid in nature and contains B cell follicles, a marginal zone around the follicles, and T cell–rich areas sheathing arterioles. The red pulp areas include pulp sinuses and pulp cords. The cords are dead ends. In order to regain access to the circulation, red blood cells must traverse tiny openings in the sinusoidal lining. Stiff, damaged, or old red cells cannot enter the sinuses. *(Top portion of figure from CA Janeway et al: Immunobiology, 5th ed., New York, Garland, 2001; bottom portion of figure from RS Hillman, KA Ault: Hematology in Clinical Practice, 4th ed. New York, McGraw-Hill, 2005.)*

In order to return to the circulation, the blood cells in the cords must squeeze through slits in the cord lining to enter the sinuses that lead to the venules. Old and damaged erythrocytes are less deformable and are retained in the cords, where they are destroyed and their components recycled. Red cell inclusion bodies such as parasites (Chap. 203 and **e18**), nuclear residua (Howell-Jolly bodies, Fig. 58-6), or denatured hemoglobin (Heinz bodies) are pinched off in the process of passing through the slits, a process called *pitting*. The culling of dead and damaged cells and the pitting of cells with inclusions appear to occur without significant delay since the blood transit time through the spleen is only slightly slower than in other organs.

The spleen is also capable of assisting the host in adapting to its hostile environment. It has at least three adaptive functions: (1) clearance of bacteria and particulates from the blood, (2) the generation of immune responses to certain pathogens, and (3) the generation of cellular components of the blood under circumstances in which the marrow is unable to meet the needs (i.e., extramedullary hematopoiesis). The latter adaptation is a recapitulation of the blood-forming function the spleen plays during gestation. In some animals, the spleen also serves a role in the vascular adaptation to stress because it stores red blood cells (often hemoconcentrated to higher hematocrits than normal) under normal circumstances and contracts under the influence of β-adrenergic stimulation to provide the animal with an autotransfusion and improved oxygen-carrying capacity. However, the normal human spleen does not sequester or store red blood cells and does not contract in response to sympathetic stimuli. The normal human spleen contains approximately one-third of the total body platelets and a significant number of marginated neutrophils. These sequestered cells are available when needed to respond to bleeding or infection.

APPROACH TO THE PATIENT:
Splenomegaly

CLINICAL ASSESSMENT The most common *symptoms* produced by diseases involving the spleen are pain and a heavy sensation in the LUQ. Massive splenomegaly may cause early satiety. Pain may result from acute swelling of the spleen with stretching of the capsule, infarction, or inflammation of the capsule. For many years it was believed that splenic infarction was clinically silent, which at times is true. However, Soma Weiss, in his classic 1942 report of the self-observations by a Harvard medical student on the clinical course of subacute bacterial endocarditis, documented that severe LUQ and pleuritic chest pain may accompany thromboembolic occlusion of splenic blood flow. Vascular occlusion, with infarction and pain, is commonly seen in children with sickle cell crises. Rupture of the spleen, from either trauma or infiltrative disease that breaks the capsule, may result in intraperitoneal bleeding, shock, and death. The rupture itself may be painless.

A palpable spleen is the major *physical sign* produced by diseases affecting the spleen and suggests enlargement of the organ. The normal spleen is said to weigh <250 g, decreases in size with age, normally lies entirely within the rib cage, has a maximum cephalo-caudad diameter of 13 cm by ultrasonography or maximum length of 12 cm and/or width of 7 cm by radionuclide scan, and is usually not palpable. However, a palpable spleen was found in 3% of 2200 asymptomatic, male, freshman college students. Follow-up at 3 years revealed that 30% of those students still had a palpable spleen without any increase in disease prevalence. Ten-year follow-up found no evidence for lymphoid malignancies. Furthermore, in some tropical countries (e.g., New Guinea) the incidence of splenomegaly may reach 60%. Thus, the presence of a palpable spleen does not always equate with presence of disease. Even when disease is present, splenomegaly may not reflect the primary disease but rather a reaction to it. For example, in patients with Hodgkin's disease, only two-thirds of the palpable spleens show involvement by the cancer.

Physical examination of the spleen utilizes primarily the techniques of palpation and percussion. Inspection may reveal fullness in the LUQ that descends on inspiration, a finding associated with a massively enlarged spleen. Auscultation may reveal a venous hum or friction rub.

Palpation can be accomplished by bimanual palpation, ballotment, and palpation from above (Middleton maneuver). For bimanual palpation, which is at least as reliable as the other techniques, the patient is supine with flexed knees. The examiner's left hand is placed on the lower rib cage and pulls the skin toward the costal margin, allowing the fingertips of the right hand to feel the tip of the spleen as it descends while the patient inspires slowly, smoothly, and deeply. Palpation is begun with the right hand in the left lower quadrant with gradual movement toward the left costal margin, thereby identifying the lower edge of a massively enlarged spleen. When the spleen tip is felt, the finding is recorded as centimeters below the left costal margin at some arbitrary point, i.e., 10–15 cm, from the midpoint of the umbilicus or the xiphisternal junction. This allows other examiners to compare findings or the initial examiner to determine changes in size over time. Bimanual palpation in the right lateral decubitus position adds nothing to the supine examination.

Percussion for splenic dullness is accomplished with any of three techniques described by Nixon, Castell, or Barkun:

1. *Nixon's method*: The patient is placed on the right side so that the spleen lies above the colon and stomach. Percussion begins at the lower level of pulmonary resonance in the posterior axillary line and proceeds diagonally along a perpendicular line toward the lower midanterior costal margin. The upper border of dullness is normally 6–8 cm above the costal margin. Dullness >8 cm in an adult is presumed to indicate splenic enlargement.
2. *Castell's method*: With the patient supine, percussion in the lowest intercostal space in the anterior axillary line (8th or 9th) produces a resonant note if the spleen is normal in size. This is true during expiration or full inspiration. A dull percussion note on full inspiration suggests splenomegaly.
3. *Percussion of Traube's semilunar space*: The borders of Traube's space are the sixth rib superiorly, the left midaxillary line laterally, and the left costal margin inferiorly. The patient is supine with the left arm slightly abducted. During normal breathing, this space is percussed from medial to lateral margins, yielding a normal resonant sound. A dull percussion note suggests splenomegaly.

Studies comparing methods of percussion and palpation with a standard of ultrasonography or scintigraphy have revealed sensitivity of 56–71% for palpation and 59–82% for percussion. Reproducibility among examiners is better for palpation than percussion. Both techniques are less reliable in obese patients or patients who have just eaten. Thus, the physical examination techniques of palpation and percussion are imprecise at best. It has been suggested that the examiner perform percussion first and, if positive, proceed to palpation; if the spleen is palpable, then one can be reasonably confident that splenomegaly exists. However, not all LUQ masses are enlarged spleens; gastric or colon tumors and pancreatic or renal cysts or tumors can mimic splenomegaly.

The presence of an enlarged spleen can be more precisely determined, if necessary, by liver-spleen radionuclide scan, CT, MRI, or ultrasonography. The latter technique is the current procedure of choice for routine assessment of spleen size (normal = a maximum cephalocaudad diameter of 13 cm) because it has high sensitivity and specificity and is safe, noninvasive, quick, mobile, and less costly. Nuclear medicine scans are accurate, sensitive, and reliable but are costly, require greater time to generate data, and utilize immobile equipment. They have the advantage of demonstrating accessory splenic tissue. CT and MRI provide accurate determination of spleen size, but the equipment is immobile and the procedures are expensive. MRI appears to offer no advantage over CT. Changes in spleen structure such as mass lesions, infarcts, inhomogeneous infiltrates, and cysts are more readily assessed by CT, MRI, or ultrasonography. None of these techniques is very reliable in the detection of patchy infiltration (e.g., Hodgkin's disease).

DIFFERENTIAL DIAGNOSIS Many of the diseases associated with splenomegaly are listed in Table 60-2. They are grouped according to the presumed basic mechanisms responsible for organ enlargement:

1. Hyperplasia or hypertrophy related to a particular splenic function such as reticuloendothelial hyperplasia (work hypertrophy) in diseases such as hereditary spherocytosis or thalassemia syndromes that require removal of large numbers of defective red blood cells; immune hyperplasia in response to systemic infection (infectious mononucleosis, subacute bacterial endocarditis) or to immunologic diseases (immune thrombocytopenia, SLE, Felty's syndrome).
2. Passive congestion due to decreased blood flow from the spleen in conditions that produce portal hypertension (cirrhosis, Budd-Chiari syndrome, congestive heart failure).
3. Infiltrative diseases of the spleen (lymphomas, metastatic cancer, amyloidosis, Gaucher's disease, myeloproliferative disorders with extramedullary hematopoiesis).

TABLE 60-2 DISEASES ASSOCIATED WITH SPLENOMEGALY GROUPED BY PATHOGENIC MECHANISM

Enlargement Due to Increased Demand for Splenic Function

Reticuloendothelial system hyperplasia (for removal of defective erythrocytes)
  Spherocytosis
  Early sickle cell anemia
  Ovalocytosis
  Thalassemia major
  Hemoglobinopathies
  Paroxysmal nocturnal hemoglobinuria
  Pernicious anemia
Immune hyperplasia
  Response to infection (viral, bacterial, fungal, parasitic)
    Infectious mononucleosis
    AIDS
    Viral hepatitis
    Cytomegalovirus
    Subacute bacterial endocarditis
    Bacterial septicemia
    Congenital syphilis
    Splenic abscess
    Tuberculosis
    Histoplasmosis
    Malaria
    Leishmaniasis
    Trypanosomiasis
    Ehrlichiosis
  Disordered immunoregulation
    Rheumatoid arthritis (Felty's syndrome)
    Systemic lupus erythematosus
    Collagen vascular diseases
    Serum sickness
    Immune hemolytic anemias
    Immune thrombocytopenias
    Immune neutropenias
    Drug reactions
    Angioimmunoblastic lymphadenopathy
    Sarcoidosis
    Thyrotoxicosis (benign lymphoid hypertrophy)
    Interleukin 2 therapy
Extramedullary hematopoiesis
  Myelofibrosis
  Marrow damage by toxins, radiation, strontium
  Marrow infiltration by tumors, leukemias, Gaucher's disease

Enlargement Due to Abnormal Splenic or Portal Blood Flow

Cirrhosis
Hepatic vein obstruction
Portal vein obstruction, intrahepatic or extrahepatic
Cavernous transformation of the portal vein
Splenic vein obstruction
Splenic artery aneurysm
Hepatic schistosomiasis
Congestive heart failure
Hepatic echinococcosis
Portal hypertension (any cause including the above): "Banti's disease"

Infiltration of the Spleen

Intracellular or extracellular depositions
  Amyloidosis
  Gaucher's disease
  Niemann-Pick disease
  Tangier disease
  Hurler's syndrome and other mucopolysaccharidoses
  Hyperlipidemias
Benign and malignant cellular infiltrations
  Leukemias (acute, chronic, lymphoid, myeloid, monocytic)
  Lymphomas
  Hodgkin's disease
  Myeloproliferative syndromes (e.g., polycythemia vera, essential thrombocytosis)
  Angiosarcomas
  Metastatic tumors (melanoma is most common)
  Eosinophilic granuloma
  Histiocytosis X
  Hamartomas
  Hemangiomas, fibromas, lymphangiomas
  Splenic cysts

Unknown Etiology

Idiopathic splenomegaly
Berylliosis
Iron-deficiency anemia

---

ease, myeloproliferative disorders). Similarly, the platelet count may be normal, decreased when there is enhanced sequestration or destruction of platelets in an enlarged spleen (congestive splenomegaly, Gaucher's disease, immune thrombocytopenia), or increased in the myeloproliferative disorders such as polycythemia vera.

The CBC may reveal cytopenia of one or more blood cell types, which should suggest *hypersplenism*. This condition is characterized by splenomegaly, cytopenia(s), normal or hyperplastic bone marrow, and a response to splenectomy. The latter characteristic is less precise because reversal of cytopenia, particularly granulocytopenia, is sometimes not sustained after splenectomy. The cytopenias result from increased destruction of the cellular elements secondary to reduced flow of blood through enlarged and congested cords (congestive splenomegaly) or to immune-mediated mechanisms. In hypersplenism, various cell types usually have normal morphology on the peripheral blood smear, although the red cells may be spherocytic due to loss of surface area during their longer transit through the enlarged spleen. The increased marrow production of red cells should be reflected as an increased reticulocyte production index, although the value may be less than expected due to increased sequestration of reticulocytes in the spleen.

The need for additional laboratory studies is dictated by the differential diagnosis of the underlying illness of which splenomegaly is a manifestation.

The differential diagnostic possibilities are much fewer when the spleen is "massively enlarged," palpable more than 8 cm below the left costal margin or its drained weight is ≥1000 g (Table 60-3). The vast majority of such patients will have non-Hodgkin's lymphoma, chronic lymphocytic leukemia, hairy cell leukemia, chronic myelogenous leukemia, myelofibrosis with myeloid metaplasia, or polycythemia vera.

LABORATORY ASSESSMENT The major laboratory abnormalities accompanying splenomegaly are determined by the underlying systemic illness. Erythrocyte counts may be normal, decreased (thalassemia major syndromes, SLE, cirrhosis with portal hypertension), or increased (polycythemia vera). Granulocyte counts may be normal, decreased (Felty's syndrome, congestive splenomegaly, leukemias), or increased (infections or inflammatory dis-

SPLENECTOMY

Splenectomy is infrequently performed for diagnostic purposes, especially in the absence of clinical illness or other diagnostic tests that suggest underlying disease. More often splenectomy is performed for symptom control in patients with massive splenomegaly, for disease control in patients with traumatic splenic rupture, or for correction of cytopenias in patients with hypersplenism or immune-mediated destruction of one or more cellular blood elements. Splenectomy is necessary for staging of patients with Hodgkin's disease only in those with clinical stage I or II disease in whom radiation therapy alone is contemplated as the treatment. Noninvasive staging of the spleen in Hodgkin's disease is not a sufficiently reliable basis for treatment decisions because one-third of normal-sized spleens will be involved with Hodgkin's disease and one-third of enlarged spleens will be tumor-free. Although splenectomy in chronic myelogenous leukemia does not affect the natural history of disease, removal of the massive spleen usually makes patients significantly more comfortable and simplifies their management by significantly reducing transfusion requirements. Splenectomy is an effective secondary or tertiary treatment for two chronic B cell leukemias, hairy cell leukemia and prolymphocytic leukemia, and for the very rare splenic mantle cell or marginal zone lymphoma. Splenectomy in these diseases may be associated with significant tumor regression in bone marrow and other sites of disease.

TABLE 60-3 DISEASES ASSOCIATED WITH MASSIVE SPLENOMEGALY[a]

Chronic myelogenous leukemia	Gaucher's disease
Lymphomas	Chronic lymphocytic leukemia
Hairy cell leukemia	Sarcoidosis
Myelofibrosis with myeloid metaplasia	Autoimmune hemolytic anemia
Polycythemia vera	Diffuse splenic hemangiomatosis

[a]The spleen extends greater than 8 cm below left costal margin and/or weighs more than 1000 g.

Similar regressions of systemic disease have been noted after splenic irradiation in some types of lymphoid tumors, especially chronic lymphocytic leukemia and prolymphocytic leukemia. This has been termed the *abscopal effect*. Such systemic tumor responses to local therapy directed at the spleen suggest that some hormone or growth factor produced by the spleen may affect tumor cell proliferation, but this conjecture is not yet substantiated. A common therapeutic indication for splenectomy is traumatic or iatrogenic splenic rupture. In a fraction of patients with splenic rupture, peritoneal seeding of splenic fragments can lead to *splenosis*—the presence of multiple rests of spleen tissue not connected to the portal circulation. This ectopic spleen tissue may cause pain or gastrointestinal obstruction, as in endometriosis. A large number of hematologic, immunologic, and congestive causes of splenomegaly can lead to destruction of one or more cellular blood elements. In the majority of such cases, splenectomy can correct the cytopenias, particularly anemia and thrombocytopenia. In a large series of patients seen in two tertiary care centers, the indication for splenectomy was diagnostic in 10% of patients, therapeutic in 44%, staging for Hodgkin's disease in 20%, and incidental to another procedure in 26%. Perhaps the only contraindication to splenectomy is the presence of marrow failure, in which the enlarged spleen is the only source of hematopoietic tissue.

The absence of the spleen has minimal long-term effects on the hematologic profile. In the immediate postsplenectomy period, leukocytosis (up to 25,000/μL) and thrombocytosis (up to 1×10^6/μL) may develop, but within 2–3 weeks, blood cell counts and survival of each cell lineage are usually normal. The chronic manifestations of splenectomy are marked variation in size and shape of erythrocytes (anisocytosis, poikilocytosis) and the presence of Howell-Jolly bodies (nuclear remnants), Heinz bodies (denatured hemoglobin), basophilic stippling, and an occasional nucleated erythrocyte in the peripheral blood. When such erythrocyte abnormalities appear in a patient whose spleen has not been removed, one should suspect splenic infiltration by tumor that has interfered with its normal culling and pitting function.

The most serious consequence of splenectomy is increased susceptibility to bacterial infections, particularly those with capsules such as *Streptococcus pneumoniae*, *Haemophilus influenzae*, and some gramnegative enteric organisms. Patients under age 20 years are particularly susceptible to overwhelming sepsis with *S. pneumoniae*, and the overall actuarial risk of sepsis in patients who have had their spleens removed is about 7% in 10 years. The case-fatality rate for pneumococcal sepsis in splenectomized patients is 50–80%. About 25% of patients without spleens will develop a serious infection at some time in their life. The frequency is highest within the first 3 years after splenectomy. About 15% of the infections are polymicrobial, and lung, skin, and blood are the most common sites. No increased risk of viral infection has been noted in patients who have no spleen. The susceptibility to bacterial infections relates to the inability to remove opsonized bacteria from the bloodstream and a defect in making antibodies to T cell–independent antigens such as the polysaccharide components of bacterial capsules. Pneumococcal vaccine (23-valent polysaccharide vaccine) should be administered to all patients 2 weeks before elective splenectomy. The Advisory Committee on Immunization Practices recommends that even splenectomized patients receive pneumococcal vaccine with a repeat vaccination 5 years later. Efficacy has not been proven in this setting, and the recommendation discounts the possibility that administration of the vaccine may actually lower the titer of specific pneumococcal antibodies. A more effective pneumococcal conjugate vaccine that involves T cells in the response is now available (Prevenar, 7-valent). The vaccine to *Neisseria meningitidis* should also be given to patients in whom elective splenectomy is planned. Although efficacy data for *Haemophilus influenzae* type b vaccine are not available for older children or adults, it may be given to patients who have had a splenectomy.

Splenectomized patients should be educated to consider any unexplained fever as a medical emergency. Prompt medical attention with evaluation and treatment of suspected bacteremia may be life-saving. Routine chemoprophylaxis with oral penicillin can result in the emergence of drug-resistant strains and is not recommended.

In addition to an increased susceptibility to bacterial infections, splenectomized patients are also more susceptible to the parasitic disease babesiosis. The splenectomized patient should avoid areas where the parasite *Babesia* is endemic (e.g., Cape Cod, MA).

Surgical removal of the spleen is an obvious cause of hyposplenism. Patients with sickle cell disease often suffer from autosplenectomy as a result of splenic destruction by the numerous infarcts associated with sickle cell crises during childhood. Indeed, the presence of a palpable spleen in a patient with sickle cell disease after age 5 suggests a coexisting hemoglobinopathy, e.g., thalassemia or hemoglobin C. In addition, patients who receive splenic irradiation for a neoplastic or autoimmune disease are also functionally hyposplenic. The term *hyposplenism* is preferred to *asplenism* in referring to the physiologic consequences of splenectomy because asplenia is a rare, specific, and fatal congenital abnormality in which there is a failure of the left side of the coelomic cavity (which includes the splenic anlagen) to develop normally. Infants with asplenia have no spleens, but that is the least of their problems. The right side of the developing embryo is duplicated on the left so there is liver where the spleen should be, there are two right lungs, and the heart comprises two right atria and two right ventricles.

FURTHER READINGS

BARKUN AN et al: The bedside assessment of splenic enlargement. Am J Med 91:512, 1991

GRAVES SA et al: Does this patient have splenomegaly? JAMA 270:2218, 1993

KRAUS MD et al: The spleen as a diagnostic specimen: A review of ten years' experience at two tertiary care institutions. Cancer 91:2001, 2001

MCINTYRE OR, EBAUGH FG JR: Palpable spleens: Ten year follow-up. Ann Intern Med 90:130, 1979

PANGALIS GA et al: Clinical approach to lymphadenopathy. Semin Oncol 20:570, 1993

Recommended Adult Immunization Schedule—United States, October 2005–September 2006. MMWR 54(40):Q1, 2005

WILLIAMSON HA JR: Lymphadenopathy in a family practice: A descriptive study of 240 cases. J Fam Pract 20:449, 1985

61 Disorders of Granulocytes and Monocytes

Steven M. Holland, John I. Gallin

Leukocytes, the major cells comprising inflammatory and immune responses, include neutrophils, T and B lymphocytes, natural killer (NK) cells, monocytes, eosinophils, and basophils. These cells have specific functions, such as antibody production by B lymphocytes or destruction of bacteria by neutrophils, but in no single infectious disease is the exact role of the cell types completely established. Thus, whereas neutrophils are classically thought to be critical to host defense against bacteria, they may also play important roles in defense against viral infections.

The blood delivers leukocytes to the various tissues from the bone marrow, where they are produced. Normal blood leukocyte counts are $4.3–10.8 \times 10^9$/L, with neutrophils representing 45–74% of the cells, bands 0–4%, lymphocytes 16–45%, monocytes 4–10%, eosinophils 0–7%, and basophils 0–2%. Variation among individuals and among different ethnic groups can be substantial with lower leukocyte numbers for certain African-American ethnic groups. The various leukocytes are derived from a common stem cell in the bone marrow. Three-

FIGURE 61-1 Schematic events in neutrophil production, recruitment, and inflammation. The four cardinal signs of inflammation (rubor, tumor, calor, dolor) are indicated, as are the interactions of neutrophils with other cells and cytokines. PMN, polymorphonuclear leukocytes; G-CSF, granulocyte colony-stimulating factor; IL, interleukin; TNF-α, tumor necrosis factor α.

fourths of the nucleated cells of bone marrow are committed to the production of leukocytes. Leukocyte maturation in the marrow is under the regulatory control of a number of different factors, known as colony-stimulating factors (CSFs) and interleukins (ILs). Because an alteration in the number and type of leukocytes is often associated with disease processes, total white blood count (WBC) (cells per μL) and differential counts are informative. This chapter focuses on neutrophils, monocytes, and eosinophils. Lymphocytes and basophils are discussed in Chaps. 308 and 311, respectively.

NEUTROPHILS

MATURATION

Important events in neutrophil life are summarized in Fig. 61-1. In normal humans, neutrophils are produced only in the bone marrow. The minimum number of stem cells necessary to support hematopoiesis is estimated to be 400–500 at any one time. Human blood monocytes, tissue macrophages, and stromal cells produce CSFs, hormones required for the growth of monocytes and neutrophils in the bone marrow. The hematopoietic system not only produces enough neutrophils ($\sim 1.3 \times 10^{11}$ cells per 80-kg person per day) to carry out physiologic functions but also has a large reserve stored in the marrow, which can be mobilized in response to inflammation or infection. An increase in the number of blood neutrophils is called *neutrophilia*, and the presence of immature cells is termed a *shift to the left*. A decrease in the number of blood neutrophils is called *neutropenia*.

Neutrophils and monocytes evolve from pluripotent stem cells under the influence of cytokines and CSFs (Fig. 61-2). The proliferation phase through the metamyelocyte takes about 1 week, while the maturation phase from metamyelocyte to mature neutrophil takes another week. The myeloblast is the first recognizable precursor cell and is followed by the *promyelocyte*. The promyelocyte evolves when the classic lysosomal granules, called the *primary*, or *azurophil*, granules are produced. The primary granules contain hydrolases, elastase, myeloperoxidase, cathepsin G, cationic proteins, and bactericidal/permeability-increasing protein, which is important for killing gram-negative bacteria. Azurophil granules also contain *defensins*, a family of cysteine-rich polypeptides with broad antimicrobial activity against bacteria, fungi, and certain enveloped viruses. The promyelocyte divides to produce the *myelocyte*, a cell responsible for the synthesis of the *specific*, or *secondary*,

granules, which contain unique (specific) constituents such as lactoferrin, vitamin B_{12}–binding protein, membrane components of the reduced nicotinamide-adenine dinucleotide phosphate (NADPH) oxidase required for hydrogen peroxide production, histaminase, and receptors for certain chemoattractants and adherence-promoting factors (CR3) as well as receptors for the basement membrane component, laminin. The secondary granules do not contain acid hydrolases and therefore are not classic lysosomes. Packaging of secondary granule contents during myelopoiesis is controlled by CCAAT/enhancer binding protein-ε. Secondary granule contents are readily released extracellularly, and their mobilization is important in modulating inflammation. During the final stages of maturation, no cell division occurs, and the cell passes through the metamyelocyte stage and then to the band neutrophil with a sausage-shaped nucleus (Fig. 61-3). As the band cell matures, the nucleus assumes a lobulated configuration. The nucleus of neutrophils normally contains up to four segments (Fig. 61-4). Excessive segmentation (more than five nuclear lobes) may be a manifestation of folate or vitamin B_{12} deficiency (see Fig. 100-4) and the congenital neutropenia syndrome of warts, hypogammaglobulinemia, infections, and myelokathexis (WHIM) described below. The Pelger-Hüet anomaly (Fig. 61-5), an infrequent dominant benign inherited trait, results in neutrophils with distinctive bilobed nuclei that must be distinguished from band forms. Acquired

Cell	Stage	Surface Markers[a]	Characteristics
	MYELOBLAST	CD33, CD13, CD15	Prominent nucleoli
	PROMYELOCYTE	CD33, CD13, CD15	Large cell Primary granules appear
	MYELOCYTE	CD33, CD13, CD15, CD14, CD11b	Secondary granules appear
	METAMYELOCYTE	CD33, CD13, CD15, CD14, CD11b	Kidney bean–shaped nucleus
	BAND FORM	CD33, CD13, CD15, CD14, CD11b CD10, CD16	Condensed, band–shaped nucleus
	NEUTROPHIL	CD33, CD13, CD15, CD14, CD11b CD10, CD16	Condensed, multilobed nucleus

[a]CD= Cluster Determinant; ● Nucleolus; ● Primary granule; ♦ Secondary granule.

FIGURE 61-2 Stages of neutrophil development shown schematically. G-CSF (granulocyte colony-stimulating factor) and GM-CSF (granulocyte-macrophage colony-stimulating factor) are critical to this process. Identifying cellular characteristics and specific cell-surface markers are listed for each maturational stage.

FIGURE 61-3 Neutrophil band with Döhle body. The neutrophil with a sausage-shaped nucleus in the center of the field is a band form. Döhle bodies are discrete, blue-staining nongranular areas found in the periphery of the cytoplasm of the neutrophil in infections and other toxic states. They represent aggregates of rough endoplasmic reticulum.

bilobed nuclei, pseudo Pelger-Huet anomaly, can occur with acute infections or in myelodysplastic syndromes. The physiologic role of the normal multilobed nucleus of neutrophils is unknown, but it may allow great deformation of neutrophils during migration into tissues at sites of inflammation.

In severe acute bacterial infection, prominent neutrophil cytoplasmic granules, called *toxic granulations*, are occasionally seen. Toxic granulations are immature or abnormally staining azurophil granules. Cytoplasmic inclusions, also called *Döhle bodies* (Fig. 61-3), can be seen during infection and are fragments of ribosome-rich endoplasmic reticulum. Large neutrophil vacuoles are often present in acute bacterial infection and probably represent pinocytosed (internalized) membrane.

Neutrophils are heterogeneous in function. Monoclonal antibodies have been developed that recognize only a subset of mature neutrophils. The meaning of neutrophil heterogeneity is not known.

The morphology of eosinophils and basophils is shown in **Fig. 61-6.**

MARROW RELEASE AND CIRCULATING COMPARTMENTS

Specific signals, including IL-1, tumor necrosis factor α (TNF-α), the CSFs, complement fragments, and chemokines, mobilize leukocytes from the bone marrow and deliver them to the blood in an unstimulated state. Under normal conditions, ~90% of the neutrophil pool is in the bone marrow, 2–3% in the circulation, and the remainder in the tissues (Fig. 61-7).

The circulating pool exists in two dynamic compartments: one freely flowing and one marginated. The freely flowing pool is about one-half the neutrophils in the basal state and is composed of those cells that are in the blood and not in contact with the endothelium. Marginated leukocytes are those that are in close physical contact with the endothelium (Fig. 61-8). In the pulmonary circulation, where an extensive capillary bed (~1000 capillaries per alveolus) exists, margination occurs because the capillaries are about the same size as a mature neutrophil. Therefore, neutrophil fluidity and deformability are neces-

FIGURE 61-4 Normal granulocyte. The normal granulocyte has a segmented nucleus with heavy, clumped chromatin; fine neutrophilic granules are dispersed throughout the cytoplasm.

FIGURE 61-5 Pelger-Hüet anomaly. In this benign disorder, the majority of granulocytes are bilobed. The nucleus frequently has a spectacle-like, or "pince-nez," configuration.

FIGURE 61-6 Normal eosinophil and basophil. The eosinophil contains large, bright orange granules and usually a bilobed nucleus. The basophil contains large purple-black granules that fill the cell and obscure the nucleus.

sary to make the transit through the pulmonary bed. Increased neutrophil rigidity and decreased deformability lead to augmented neutrophil trapping and margination in the lung. In contrast, in the systemic postcapillary venules, margination is mediated by the interaction of specific cell-surface molecules called *selectins*. Selectins are glycoproteins expressed on neutrophils and endothelial cells, among others, that cause a low-affinity interaction, resulting in "rolling" of the neutrophil along the endothelial surface. On neutrophils, the molecule L-selectin [cluster determinant (CD) 62L] binds to glycosylated proteins on endothelial cells [e.g., glycosylation-dependent cell adhesion molecule (GlyCAM1) and CD34]. Glycoproteins on neutrophils, most importantly sialyl-Lewis^x (SLe^x, CD15s), are targets for binding of selectins expressed on endothelial cells [E-selectin (CD62E) and P-selectin (CD62P)] and other leukocytes. In response to chemotactic stimuli from injured tissues (e.g., complement product C5a, leukotriene B$_4$, IL-8) or bacterial products [e.g., N-formylmethionyl-leucylphenylalanine (f-metleuphe)], neutrophil adhesiveness increases, and the cells "stick" to the endothelium through *integrins*. The integrins are leukocyte glycoproteins that exist as complexes of a common CD18 β chain with CD11a (LFA-1), CD11b (called Mac-1, CR3, or the C3bi receptor), and CD11c (called p150, 95 or CR4). CD11a/CD18 and CD11b/CD18 bind to specific endothelial receptors [intercellular adhesion molecules (ICAM) 1 and 2].

On cell stimulation, L-selectin is shed from neutrophils, and E-selectin increases in the blood, presumably because it is shed from endothelial cells; receptors for chemoattractants and opsonins are mobilized; and the phagocytes orient toward the chemoattractant source in the extravascular space, increase their motile activity (chemokinesis), and migrate directionally (chemotaxis) into tissues. The process of migration into tissues is called *diapedesis* and involves the crawling of neutrophils between postcapillary endothelial cells that open junctions between ad-

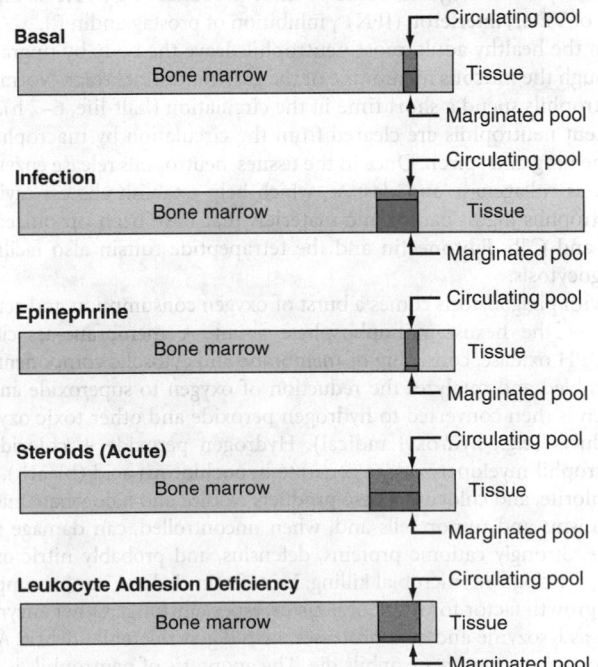

FIGURE 61-7 Schematic neutrophil distribution and kinetics between the different anatomic and functional pools.

FIGURE 61-8 Neutrophil travel through the pulmonary capillaries is dependent on neutrophil deformability. Neutrophil rigidity (e.g., caused by C5a) enhances pulmonary trapping and response to pulmonary pathogens in a way that is not so dependent on cell-surface receptors. Intraalveolar chemotactic factors, such as those caused by certain bacteria (e.g., *Streptococcus pneumoniae*) lead to diapedesis of neutrophils from the pulmonary capillaries into the alveolar space. Neutrophil interaction with the endothelium of the systemic postcapillary venules is dependent on molecules of attachment. The neutrophil "rolls" along the endothelium using selectins: neutrophil CD15s (sialyl-Lewis^x) binds to CD62E (E-selectin) and CD62P (P-selectin) on endothelial cells; CD62L (L-selectin) on neutrophils binds to CD34 and other molecules (e.g., GlyCAM-1) expressed on endothelium. Chemokines or other activation factors stimulate integrin-mediated "tight adhesion": CD11a/CD18 (LFA-1) and CD11b/CD18 (Mac-1, CR3) bind to CD54 (ICAM-1) and CD102 (ICAM-2) on the endothelium. Diapedesis occurs between endothelial cells: CD31 (PECAM-1) expressed by the emigrating neutrophil interacts with CD31 expressed at the endothelial cell-cell junction.

jacent cells to permit leukocyte passage. Diapedesis involves platelet/endothelial cell adhesion molecule (PECAM) 1 (CD31), which is expressed on both the emigrating leukocyte and the endothelial cells. The endothelial responses (increased blood flow from increased vasodilation and permeability) are mediated by anaphylatoxins (e.g., C3a and C5a) as well as vasodilators such as histamine, bradykinin, serotonin, nitric oxide, vascular endothelial growth factor (VEGF), and prostaglandins E and I. Cytokines regulate some of these processes [e.g., TNF-α induction of VEGF, interferon (IFN) γ inhibition of prostaglandin E].

In the healthy adult, most neutrophils leave the body by migration through the mucous membrane of the gastrointestinal tract. Normally, neutrophils spend a short time in the circulation (half-life, 6–7 h). Senescent neutrophils are cleared from the circulation by macrophages in the lung and spleen. Once in the tissues, neutrophils release enzymes, such as collagenase and elastase, which help establish abscess cavities. Neutrophils ingest pathogenic materials that have been opsonized by IgG and C3b. Fibronectin and the tetrapeptide tuftsin also facilitate phagocytosis.

With phagocytosis comes a burst of oxygen consumption and activation of the hexose-monophosphate shunt. A membrane-associated NADPH oxidase, consisting of membrane and cytosolic components, is assembled and catalyzes the reduction of oxygen to superoxide anion, which is then converted to hydrogen peroxide and other toxic oxygen products (e.g., hydroxyl radical). Hydrogen peroxide + chloride + neutrophil myeloperoxidase generate hypochlorous acid (bleach), hypochlorite, and chlorine. These products oxidize and halogenate microorganisms and tumor cells and, when uncontrolled, can damage host tissue. Strongly cationic proteins, defensins, and probably nitric oxide also participate in microbial killing. Lactoferrin chelates iron, an important growth factor for microorganisms, especially fungi. Other enzymes, such as lysozyme and acid proteases, help digest microbial debris. After 1–4 days in tissues, neutrophils die. The apoptosis of neutrophils is also cytokine-regulated; granulocyte colony-stimulating factor (G-CSF) and IFN-γ prolong their life span. Under certain conditions, such as in de-

layed-type hypersensitivity, monocyte accumulation occurs within 6–12 h of initiation of inflammation. Neutrophils, monocytes, microorganisms in various states of digestion, and altered local tissue cells make up the inflammatory exudate, pus. Myeloperoxidase confers the characteristic green color to pus and may participate in turning off the inflammatory process by inactivating chemoattractants and immobilizing phagocytic cells.

Neutrophils respond to certain cytokines [IFN-γ, granulocyte-macrophage colony-stimulating factor (GM-CSF), IL-8] and produce cytokines and chemotactic signals [TNF-α, IL-8, macrophage inflammatory protein (MIP) 1] that modulate the inflammatory response. In the presence of fibrinogen, f-met leu phe or leukotriene B$_4$ induces IL-8 production by neutrophils, providing autocrine amplification of inflammation. *Chemokines* (*chemo*attractant cytokines) are small proteins produced by many different cell types, including endothelial cells, fibroblasts, epithelial cells, neutrophils, and monocytes, that regulate neutrophil, monocyte, eosinophil, and lymphocyte recruitment and activation. Chemokines transduce their signals through heterotrimeric G protein–linked receptors that have seven cell membrane–spanning domains, the same type of cell-surface receptor that mediates the response to the classic chemoattractants f-metleuphe and C5a. Four major groups of chemokines are recognized based on the cysteine structure near the N terminus: C, CC, CXC, and CXXXC. The CXC cytokines such as IL-8 mainly attract neutrophils; CC chemokines such as MIP-1 attract lymphocytes, monocytes, eosinophils, and basophils; the C chemokine lymphotactin is T cell tropic; the CXXXC chemokine fractalkine attracts neutrophils, monocytes, and T cells. These molecules and their receptors not only regulate the trafficking and activation of inflammatory cells, but specific chemokine receptors serve as co-receptors for HIV infection (Chap. 182) and have a role in atherogenesis.

NEUTROPHIL ABNORMALITIES

A defect in the neutrophil life cycle can lead to dysfunction and compromised host defenses. Inflammation is often depressed, and the clinical result is often recurrent with severe bacterial and fungal infections. Aphthous ulcers of mucous membranes (gray ulcers without pus) and gingivitis and periodontal disease suggest a phagocytic cell disorder. Patients with congenital phagocyte defects can have infections within the first few days of life. Skin, ear, upper and lower respiratory tract, and bone infections are common. Sepsis and meningitis are rare. In some disorders the frequency of infection is variable, and patients can go for months or even years without major infection. Aggressive management of these congenital diseases has extended the life span of patients well beyond 30 years.

Neutropenia   The consequences of absent neutrophils are dramatic. Susceptibility to infectious diseases increases sharply when neutrophil counts fall below 1000 cells/μL. When the absolute neutrophil count (ANC; band forms and mature neutrophils combined) falls to <500 cells/μL, control of endogenous microbial flora (e.g., mouth, gut) is impaired; when the ANC is <200/μL, the inflammatory process is absent. Neutropenia can be due to depressed production, increased peripheral destruction, or excessive peripheral pooling. A falling neutrophil count or a significant decrease in the number of neutrophils below steady-state levels, together with a failure to increase neutrophil counts in the setting of infection or other challenge, requires investigation. Acute neutropenia, such as that caused by cancer chemotherapy, is more likely to be associated with increased risk of infection than neutropenia of long duration (months to years) that reverses in response to infection or carefully controlled administration of endotoxin (see "Laboratory Diagnosis," below).

Some causes of inherited and acquired neutropenia are listed in Table 61-1. The most common neutropenias are iatrogenic, resulting from the use of cytotoxic or immunosuppressive therapies for malignancy or control of autoimmune disorders. These drugs cause neutropenia because they result in decreased production of rapidly growing progenitor (stem) cells of the marrow. Certain antibiotics such as chloramphenicol, trimethoprim-sulfamethoxazole, flucytosine, vidarabine, and the antiretroviral drug zidovudine may cause neutropenia by inhibiting proliferation of myeloid precursors. The marrow suppression is generally dose-related and dependent on continued administration of the drug. Recombinant human G-CSF usually reverses this form of neutropenia.

Another important mechanism for iatrogenic neutropenia is the effect of drugs that serve as immune haptens and sensitize neutrophils or neutrophil precursors to immune-mediated peripheral destruction. This form of drug-induced neutropenia can be seen within 7 days of exposure to the drug; with previous drug exposure, resulting in preexisting antibodies, neutropenia may occur a few hours after administration of the drug. Although any drug can cause this form of neutropenia, the most frequent causes are commonly used antibiotics, such as sulfa-containing compounds, penicillins, and cephalosporins. Fever and eosinophilia may also be associated with drug reactions, but often these signs are not present. Drug-induced neutropenia can be severe, but discontinuation of the sensitizing drug is sufficient for recovery, which is usually seen within 5–7 days and is complete by 10 days. Readministration of the sensitizing drug should be avoided, since abrupt neutropenia will often result. For this reason, diagnostic challenge should be avoided.

Autoimmune neutropenias caused by circulating antineutrophil antibodies are another form of acquired neutropenia that results in increased destruction of neutrophils. Acquired neutropenia may also be seen with viral infections, including infection with HIV. Acquired neutropenia may be cyclic in nature, occurring at intervals of several weeks. Acquired cyclic or stable neutropenia may be associated with an expansion of large granular lymphocytes (LGLs), which may be T cells, NK cells, or NK-like cells. Patients with LGL lymphocytosis may have moderate blood and bone marrow lymphocytosis, neutropenia, polyclonal hypergammaglobulinemia, splenomegaly, rheumatoid arthritis, and absence of lymphadenopathy. Such patients may have a chronic and relatively stable course. Recurrent bacterial infections are frequent. Benign and malignant forms of this syndrome occur. In some patients, a spontaneous regression has occurred even after 11 years, suggesting an immunoregulatory defect as the basis for at least one form of the disorder. Glucocorticoids, cyclosporine, IFN-α, and nucleosides such as 2-chlorodeoxyadenosine each have induced remission.

Hereditary Neutropenias Hereditary neutropenias are rare and may manifest in early childhood as a profound constant neutropenia or agranulocytosis. Congenital forms of neutropenia include Kostmann's syndrome (neutrophil count <100/μL), which is often fatal due to mutations in the anti-apoptosis gene HAX-1; severe chronic neutropenia (neutrophil count of 300–1500/μL) due to mutations in neutrophil elastase; hereditary cyclic neutropenia, or, more appropriately, cyclic hematopoiesis, also due to mutations in neutrophil elastase; the cartilage-hair hypoplasia syndrome due to mutations in the mitochondrial RNA-processing endoribonuclease RMRP; Shwachman Diamond syndrome associated with pancreatic insufficiency due to mutations in the Shwachman-Bodian-Diamond syndrome gene *SBDS*; the WHIM [*w*arts, *h*ypogammaglobulinemia, *i*nfections, *m*yelokathexis (retention of WBCs in the marrow)] syndrome, characterized by neutrophil hypersegmentation and bone marrow myeloid arrest due to mutations in the chemokine receptor CXCR4; and neutropenias associated with other immune defects, such as X-linked agammaglobulinemia, Wiskott-Aldrich syndrome, and CD40 ligand deficiency. Mutations in the G-CSF receptor can develop in severe congenital neutropenia and are linked to leukemia.

Maternal factors can be associated with neutropenia in the newborn. Transplacental transfer of IgG directed against antigens on fetal neutrophils can result in peripheral destruction. Drugs (e.g., thiazides) ingested during pregnancy can cause neutropenia in the newborn by either depressed production or peripheral destruction.

In Felty's syndrome—the triad of rheumatoid arthritis, splenomegaly, and neutropenia (Chap. 314)—spleen-produced antibodies can shorten neutrophil life span, while LGLs can attack marrow neutrophil precursors. Splenectomy may increase neutrophil count in Felty's syndrome and lower serum neutrophil-binding IgG. Some Felty's syndrome patients also have neutropenia associated with an increased number of LGLs. Splenomegaly with peripheral trapping and destruction of neutrophils is also seen in lysosomal storage diseases and in portal hypertension.

Neutrophilia Neutrophilia results from increased neutrophil production, increased marrow release, or defective margination (Table 61-2). The most important acute cause of neutrophilia is infection.

TABLE 61-1 CAUSES OF NEUTROPENIA

Decreased Production
Drug-induced—alkylating agents (nitrogen mustard, busulfan, chlorambucil, cyclophosphamide); antimetabolites (methotrexate, 6-mercaptopurine, 5-flucytosine); noncytotoxic agents [antibiotics (chloramphenicol, penicillins, sulfonamides), phenothiazines, tranquilizers (meprobamate), anticonvulsants (carbamazepine), antipsychotics (clozapine), certain diuretics, anti-inflammatory agents, antithyroid drugs, many others]
Hematologic diseases—idiopathic, cyclic neutropenia, Chédiak-Higashi syndrome, aplastic anemia, infantile genetic disorders (see text)
Tumor invasion, myelofibrosis
Nutritional deficiency—vitamin B_{12}, folate (especially alcoholics)
Infection—tuberculosis, typhoid fever, brucellosis, tularemia, measles, infectious mononucleosis, malaria, viral hepatitis, leishmaniasis, AIDS

Peripheral Destruction
Antineutrophil antibodies and/or splenic or lung trapping
Autoimmune disorders—Felty's syndrome, rheumatoid arthritis, lupus erythematosus
Drugs as haptens—aminopyrine, α-methyldopa, phenylbutazone, mercurial diuretics, some phenothiazines
Wegener's granulomatosis

Peripheral Pooling (Transient Neutropenia)
Overwhelming bacterial infection (acute endotoxemia)
Hemodialysis
Cardiopulmonary bypass

TABLE 61-2 CAUSES OF NEUTROPHILIA

Increased Production
Idiopathic
Drug-induced—glucocorticoids, G-CSF
Infection—bacterial, fungal, sometimes viral
    Inflammation—thermal injury, tissue necrosis, myocardial and pulmonary infarction, hypersensitivity states, collagen vascular diseases
    Myeloproliferative diseases—myelocytic leukemia, myeloid metaplasia, polycythemia vera
Increased Marrow Release
Glucocorticoids
Acute infection (endotoxin)
Inflammation—thermal injury
Decreased or Defective Margination
Drugs—epinephrine, glucocorticoids, nonsteroidal anti-inflammatory agents
Stress, excitement, vigorous exercise
Leukocyte adhesion deficiency type 1 (integrin β chain, CD18); leukocyte adhesion deficiency type 2 (selectin ligand, CD15s, sialyl-Lewis^{x})
Miscellaneous
Metabolic disorders—ketoacidosis, acute renal failure, eclampsia, acute poisoning
Drugs—lithium
Other—metastatic carcinoma, acute hemorrhage or hemolysis

TABLE 61-3 **TYPES OF GRANULOCYTE AND MONOCYTE DISORDERS**

Function	Cause of Indicated Dysfunction		
	Drug-Induced	**Acquired**	**Inherited**
Adherence-aggregation	Aspirin, colchicine, alcohol, glucocorticoids, ibuprofen, piroxicam	Neonatal state, hemodialysis	Leukocyte adhesion deficiency types 1 and 2
Deformability		Leukemia, neonatal state, diabetes mellitus, immature neutrophils	
Chemokinesis-chemotaxis	Glucocorticoids (high dose), auranofin, colchicine (weak effect), phenylbutazone, naproxen, indomethacin, interleukin 2	Thermal injury, malignancy, malnutrition, periodontal disease, neonatal state, systemic lupus erythematosus, rheumatoid arthritis, diabetes mellitus, sepsis, influenza virus infection, herpes simplex virus infection, acrodermatitis enteropathica, AIDS	Chédiak-Higashi syndrome, neutrophil-specific granule deficiency, hyper IgE–recurrent infection (Job's) syndrome (in some patients), Down syndrome, α-mannosidase deficiency, severe combined immunodeficiency, Wiskott-Aldrich syndrome
Microbicidal activity	Colchicine, cyclophosphamide, glucocorticoids (high dose), TNF-α blocking antibodies	Leukemia, aplastic anemia, certain neutropenias, tuftsin deficiency, thermal injury, sepsis, neonatal state, diabetes mellitus, malnutrition, AIDS	Chédiak-Higashi syndrome, neutrophil-specific granule deficiency, chronic granulomatous disease, defects in IFN-γ/IL-12 axis

Neutrophilia from acute infection represents both increased production and increased marrow release. Increased production is also associated with chronic inflammation and certain myeloproliferative diseases. Increased marrow release and mobilization of the marginated leukocyte pool are induced by glucocorticoids. Release of epinephrine, as with vigorous exercise, excitement, or stress, will demarginate neutrophils in the spleen and lungs and double the neutrophil count in minutes. Cigarette smoking can increase neutrophil counts into the abnormal range. Leukocytosis with cell counts of 10,000–25,000/μL occurs in response to infection and other forms of acute inflammation and results from both release of the marginated pool and mobilization of marrow reserves. Persistent neutrophilia with cell counts of ≥30,000–50,000/μL is called a *leukemoid reaction*, a term often used to distinguish this degree of neutrophilia from leukemia. In a leukemoid reaction, the circulating neutrophils are usually mature and not clonally derived.

Abnormal Neutrophil Function Inherited and acquired abnormalities of phagocyte function are listed in Table 61-3. The resulting diseases are best considered in terms of the functional defects of adherence, chemotaxis, and microbicidal activity. The distinguishing features of the important inherited disorders of phagocyte function are shown in Table 61-4.

DISORDERS OF ADHESION Two main types of leukocyte adhesion deficiency (LAD) have been described, LAD 1 and LAD 2. Both are autosomal recessive traits and result in the inability of neutrophils to exit the circulation to sites of infection, leading to leukocytosis and increased susceptibility to infection (Fig. 61-8). Patients with LAD 1 have mutations in CD18, the common component of the integrins LFA-1, Mac-1, and p150,95, leading to a defect in tight adhesion between neutrophils and the endothelium. The heterodimer formed by CD18/CD11b (Mac-1) is also the receptor for the complement-derived opsonin C3bi (CR3). The *CD18* gene is located on distal chromosome 21q. The severity of the defect determines the severity of clinical disease. Complete lack of expression of the leukocyte integrins results in a severe phenotype in which inflammatory stimuli do not increase the expression of leukocyte integrins on neutrophils or activated T and B cells. Neutrophils (and monocytes) from patients with LAD 1 adhere poorly to endothelial cells and protein-coated surfaces and exhibit defective spreading, aggregation, and chemotaxis. Patients with LAD 1 have recurrent bacterial infections involving the skin, oral and genital mucosa, and respiratory and intestinal tracts; persistent leukocytosis (neutrophil counts of 15,000–20,000/μL) because cells do not marginate; and, in severe cases, a history of delayed separation of the umbilical stump. Infections, especially of the skin, may become necrotic with progressively enlarging borders, slow healing, and development

of dysplastic scars. The most common bacteria are *Staphylococcus aureus* and enteric gram-negative bacteria. LAD 2 is caused by an abnormality of fucosylation of SLe^x (CD15s), the ligand on neutrophils that interacts with selectins on endothelial cells and is responsible for neutrophil rolling along the endothelium. Infection susceptibility in LAD 2 appears to be less severe than in LAD 1. LAD 2 is also known as *congenital disorder of glycosylation IIc* (CDGIIc).

DISORDERS OF NEUTROPHIL GRANULES The most common neutrophil defect is myeloperoxidase deficiency, a primary granule defect inherited as an autosomal recessive trait; the incidence is ~1 in 2000 persons. Isolated myeloperoxidase deficiency is not associated with clinically compromised defenses, presumably because other defense systems such as hydrogen peroxide generation are amplified. Microbicidal activity of neutrophils is delayed but not absent. Myeloperoxidase deficiency may make other acquired host defense defects more serious. An acquired form of myeloperoxidase deficiency occurs in myelomonocytic leukemia and acute myeloid leukemia.

Chédiak-Higashi syndrome (CHS) is a rare disease with autosomal recessive inheritance due to defects in the lysosomal transport protein LYST, encoded by the gene *CHS1* at 1q42. This protein is required for normal packaging and disbursement of granules. Neutrophils (and all cells containing lysosomes) from patients with CHS characteristically have large granules (Fig. 61-9) making it a systemic disease. Patients with CHS have nystagmus, partial oculocutaneous albinism, and an increased number of infections resulting from many bacterial agents. Some CHS patients develop an "accelerated phase" in childhood with a hemophagocytic syndrome and an aggressive lymphoma requiring bone marrow transplantation. CHS neutrophils and monocytes have impaired chemotaxis and abnormal rates of microbial killing due to slow rates of fusion of the lysosomal granules with phagosomes. NK cell function is also impaired. CHS patients may develop a severe disabling peripheral neuropathy in adulthood that can lead to bed confinement.

Specific granule deficiency is a rare autosomal recessive disease in which the production of secondary granules and their contents, as well as the primary granule component defensins, is defective. The defect in bacterial killing leads to severe bacterial infections. One type of specific granule deficiency is due to a mutation in the CCAAT/enhancer binding protein-ε, a regulator of expression of granule components.

CHRONIC GRANULOMATOUS DISEASE Chronic granulomatous disease (CGD) is a group of disorders of granulocyte and monocyte oxidative metabolism. Although CGD is rare, with an incidence of 1 in 200,000 individuals, it is an important model of defective neutrophil oxidative metabolism. Most often CGD is inherited as an X-linked recessive trait; 30% of patients inherit the disease in an autosomal recessive pattern.

TABLE 61-4 INHERITED DISORDERS OF PHAGOCYTE FUNCTION: DIFFERENTIAL FEATURES

Clinical Manifestations	Cellular or Molecular Defects	Diagnosis
Chronic Granulomatous Diseases (70% X-linked, 30% Autosomal Recessive)		
Severe infections of skin, ears, lungs, liver, and bone with catalase-positive microorganisms such as *S. aureus*, *Burkholderia cepacia*, *Aspergillus* spp., *Chromobacterium violaceum*; often hard to culture organism; excessive inflammation with granulomas, frequent lymph node suppuration; granulomas can obstruct GI or GU tracts; gingivitis, aphthous ulcers, seborrheic dermatitis	No respiratory burst due to the lack of one of four NADPH oxidase subunits in neutrophils, monocytes, and eosinophils	NBT or DHR test; no superoxide and H_2O_2 production by neutrophils; immunoblot for NADPH oxidase components; genetic detection
Chédiak-Higashi Syndrome (Autosomal Recessive)		
Recurrent pyogenic infections, especially with *S. aureus*; many patients get lymphoma-like illness during adolescence; periodontal disease; partial oculocutaneous albinism, nystagmus, progressive peripheral neuropathy, mental retardation in some patients	Reduced chemotaxis and phagolysosome fusion, increased respiratory burst activity, defective egress from marrow, abnormal skin window; defect in LYST	Giant primary granules in neutrophils and other granule-bearing cells (Wright's stain); genetic detection
Specific Granule Deficiency (Autosomal Recessive)		
Recurrent infections of skin, ears, and sinopulmonary tract; delayed wound healing; decreased inflammation; bleeding diathesis	Abnormal chemotaxis, impaired respiratory burst and bacterial killing, failure to up-regulate chemotactic and adhesion receptors with stimulation, defect in transcription of granule proteins; defect in C/EBPε	Lack of secondary (specific) granules in neutrophils (Wright's stain), no neutrophil-specific granule contents (i.e., lactoferrin), no defensins, platelet α granule abnormality; genetic detection
Myeloperoxidase Deficiency (Autosomal Recessive)		
Clinically normal except in patients with underlying disease such as diabetes mellitus; then candidiasis or other fungal infections	No myeloperoxidase due to pre- and post-translational defects	No peroxidase in neutrophils; genetic detection
Leukocyte Adhesion Deficiency		
Type 1: Delayed separation of umbilical cord, sustained neutrophilia, recurrent infections of skin and mucosa, gingivitis, periodontal disease	Impaired phagocyte adherence, aggregation, spreading, chemotaxis, phagocytosis of C3bi-coated particles; defective production of CD18 subunit common to leukocyte integrins	Reduced phagocyte surface expression of the CD18-containing integrins with monoclonal antibodies against LFA-1 (CD18/CD11a), Mac-1 or CR3 (CD18/CD11b), p150,95 (CD18/CD11c); genetic detection
Type 2: Mental retardation, short stature, Bombay (hh) blood phenotype, recurrent infections, neutrophilia	Impaired phagocyte rolling along endothelium	Reduced phagocyte surface expression of Sialyl-Lewis^x, with monoclonal antibodies against CD15s; genetic detection
Phagocyte Activation Defects (X-linked and Autosomal Recessive)		
NEMO deficiency: mild hypohidrotic ectodermal dysplasia; broad based immune defect: pyogenic and encapsulated bacteria, viruses, *Pneumocystis*, mycobacteria; X-linked	Impaired phagocyte activiation by IL-1, IL-18, TLR, CD40, TNF-α leading to problems with inflammation and antibody production	Poor in vitro response to endotoxin; lack of NF-κB activation; genetic detection
IRAK4 deficiency: susceptibility to pyogenic bacteria such as staphylococci, streptococci, clostridia; resistant to mycobacteria; autosomal recessive	Impaired phagocyte activation by endotoxin through TLR and other pathways; TNF-α signaling preserved	Poor in vitro response to endotoxin; lack of NF-κB activation by endotoxin; genetic detection
Hyper IgE–Recurrent Infection Syndrome (Autosomal Dominant) (Job's Syndrome)		
Eczematoid or pruritic dermatitis, "cold" skin abscesses, recurrent pneumonias with *S. aureus* with bronchopleural fistulae and cyst formation, mild eosinophilia, mucocutaneous candidiasis, characteristic facies, restrictive lung disease, scoliosis, delayed primary dental deciduation	Reduced chemotaxis in some patients, reduced suppressor T cell activity	Clinical features, involving lungs, skeleton, and immune system; serum IgE > 2000 IU/mL
Mycobacteria Susceptibility (Autosomal Dominant and Recessive Forms)		
Severe local or disseminated infections with bacille Calmette-Guérin (BCG), nontuberculous mycobacteria, salmonella, histoplasmosis, poor granuloma formation	Inability to kill intracellular organisms due to low IFN-γ production; mutations in IFN-γ receptors, IL-12 receptor, IL-12 p40, STAT-1, NEMO	Low or very high levels of IFN-γ receptor 1; functional assays of cytokine production and response; genetic detection

Abbreviations: GI, gastrointestinal; GU, genitourinary; NADPH, nicotinamide-adenine dinucleotide phosphate; NBT, nitroblue tetrazolium (dye test); DHR, dihydrorhodamine (oxidation test); LYST, lysosomal transport protein; C/EBPε, CCAAT/enhancer binding protein-ε; NEMO, NF-κB essential modulator; TLR, Toll-like receptor; IL, interleukin; TNF, tumor necrosis factor; IRAK4, IL-1 receptor–associated kinase protein-ε, NEMO 4; IFN, interferon.

Mutations in the genes for the four proteins that assemble at the plasma membrane account for all patients with CGD. Two proteins (a 91-kDa protein, abnormal in X-linked CGD, and a 22-kDa protein, absent in one form of autosomal recessive CGD) form the heterodimer cytochrome b-558 in the plasma membrane. Two other proteins (47 and 67 kDa, abnormal in the other autosomal recessive forms of CGD) are cytoplasmic in origin and interact with the cytochrome after cell activation to form NADPH oxidase, required for hydrogen peroxide production. Leukocytes from patients with CGD have severely diminished hydrogen peroxide production. The genes involved in each of the defects have been

FIGURE 61-9 Chédiak-Higashi syndrome. The granulocytes contain huge cytoplasmic granules formed from aggregation and fusion of azurophilic and specific granules. Large abnormal granules are found in other granule-containing cells throughout the body.

cloned and sequenced and the chromosome locations identified. Patients with CGD characteristically have increased numbers of infections due to catalase-positive microorganisms (organisms that destroy their own hydrogen peroxide). When patients with CGD become infected, they often have extensive inflammatory reactions, and lymph node suppuration is common despite the administration of appropriate antibiotics. Aphthous ulcers and chronic inflammation of the nares are often present. Granulomas are frequent and can obstruct the gastrointestinal or genitourinary tracts. The excessive inflammation probably reflects failure to inhibit the synthesis or degradation of chemoattractants and antigens, leading to persistent neutrophil accumulation. Impaired killing of intracellular microorganisms by macrophages may lead to persistent cell-mediated immune activation and granuloma formation. Autoimmune complications such as immune thrombocytopenic purpura and juvenile rheumatoid arthritis are also increased in CGD. In addition, discoid lupus is more common in X-linked carriers.

DISORDERS OF PHAGOCYTE ACTIVATION Phagocytes depend on cell-surface stimulation to induce signals that evoke multiple levels of the inflammatory response, including cytokine synthesis, chemotaxis, and antigen presentation. Mutations affecting the major pathway that signals through NF-κB have been noted in patients with a variety of infection susceptibility syndromes. If the defects are at a very late stage of signal transduction, in the protein critical for NF-κB activation known as the NF-κB essential modulator (NEMO), then affected males develop ectodermal dysplasia and severe immune deficiency with susceptibility to bacteria, fungi, mycobacteria, and viruses. If the defect in NF-κB activation is closer to the signaling source, in the IL-1 receptor–associated kinase 4 (IRAK4), then children have a marked susceptibility to pyogenic infections early in life but develop resistance to infection later.

MONONUCLEAR PHAGOCYTES

The mononuclear phagocyte system is composed of monoblasts, promonocytes, and monocytes, in addition to the structurally diverse tissue macrophages that make up what was previously referred to as the reticuloendothelial system. Macrophages are long-lived phagocytic cells capable of many of the functions of neutrophils. They are also secretory cells that participate in many immunologic and inflammatory processes distinct from neutrophils. Monocytes leave the circulation by diapedesis more slowly than neutrophils and have a half-life in the blood of 12–24 h.

After blood monocytes arrive in the tissues, they differentiate into macrophages ("big eaters") with specialized functions suited for specific anatomic locations. Macrophages are particularly abundant in capillary walls of the lung, spleen, liver, and bone marrow, where they function to remove microorganisms and other noxious elements from the blood. Alveolar macrophages, liver Kupffer cells, splenic macrophages, peritoneal macrophages, bone marrow macrophages, lymphatic macrophages, brain microglial cells, and dendritic macrophages all have specialized functions. Macrophage-secreted products include lysozyme, neutral proteases, acid hydrolases, arginase, complement components, enzyme inhibitors (plasmin, α_2-macroglobulin), binding proteins (transferrin, fibronectin, transcobalamin II), nucleosides, and cytokines (TNF-α; IL-1, -8, -12, -18). IL-1 (Chaps. 17 and 308) has many functions, including initiating fever in the hypothalamus, mobilizing leukocytes from the bone marrow, and activating lymphocytes and neutrophils. TNF-α is a pyrogen that duplicates many of the

actions of IL-1 and plays an important role in the pathogenesis of gram-negative shock (Chap. 265). TNF-α stimulates production of hydrogen peroxide and related toxic oxygen species by macrophages and neutrophils. In addition, TNF-α induces catabolic changes that contribute to the profound wasting (cachexia) associated with many chronic diseases.

Other macrophage-secreted products include reactive oxygen and nitrogen metabolites, bioactive lipids (arachidonic acid metabolites and platelet-activating factors), chemokines, CSFs, and factors stimulating fibroblast and vessel proliferation. Macrophages help regulate the replication of lymphocytes and participate in the killing of tumors, viruses, and certain bacteria (*Mycobacterium tuberculosis* and *Listeria monocytogenes*). Macrophages are key effector cells in the elimination of intracellular microorganisms. Their ability to fuse to form giant cells that coalesce into granulomas in response to some inflammatory stimuli is important in the elimination of intracellular microbes and is under the control of IFN-γ. Nitric oxide induced by IFN-γ is an important effector against intracellular parasites, including tuberculosis and *Leishmania*.

Macrophages play an important role in the immune response (Chap. 308). They process and present antigen to lymphocytes and secrete cytokines that modulate and direct lymphocyte development and function. Macrophages participate in autoimmune phenomena by removing immune complexes and other substances from the circulation. Polymorphisms in macrophage receptors for immunoglobulin (FcγRII) determine susceptibility to some infections and autoimmune diseases. In wound healing, they dispose of senescent cells, and they contribute to atheroma development. Macrophage elastase mediates development of emphysema from cigarette smoking.

DISORDERS OF THE MONONUCLEAR PHAGOCYTE SYSTEM

Many disorders of neutrophils extend to mononuclear phagocytes. Thus, drugs that suppress neutrophil production in the bone marrow can cause monocytopenia. Transient monocytopenia occurs after stress or glucocorticoid administration. Monocytosis is associated with tuberculosis, brucellosis, subacute bacterial endocarditis, Rocky Mountain spotted fever, malaria, and visceral leishmaniasis (kala azar). Monocytosis also occurs with malignancies, leukemias, myeloproliferative syndromes, hemolytic anemias, chronic idiopathic neutropenias, and granulomatous diseases such as sarcoidosis, regional enteritis, and some collagen vascular diseases. Patients with LAD, hyperimmunoglobulin E–recurrent infection (Job's) syndrome, CHS, and CGD all have defects in the mononuclear phagocyte system.

Monocyte cytokine production or response is impaired in some patients with disseminated nontuberculous mycobacterial infection who are not infected with HIV. Genetic defects in the pathways regulated by IFN-γ and IL-12 lead to impaired killing of intracellular bacteria, mycobacteria, salmonellae, and certain viruses (**Fig. 61-10**).

Certain viral infections impair mononuclear phagocyte function. For example, influenza virus infection causes abnormal monocyte chemotaxis. Mononuclear phagocytes can be infected by HIV using CCR5, the chemokine receptor that acts as a co-receptor with CD4 for HIV. T lymphocytes produce IFN-γ, which induces FcR expression and phagocytosis and stimulates hydrogen peroxide production by mononuclear phagocytes and neutrophils. In certain diseases, such as AIDS, IFN-γ production may be deficient, while in other diseases, such as T cell lymphomas, excessive release of IFN-γ may be associated with erythrophagocytosis by splenic macrophages.

Autoinflammatory diseases are characterized by abnormal cytokine regulation leading to excess inflammation in the absence of infection. These diseases can mimic infectious or immunodeficient syndromes. Gain-of-function mutations in the TNF-α receptor cause TNF-α receptor–associated periodic syndrome (TRAPS), which is characterized by recurrent fever in the absence of infection, due to persistent stimulation of the TNF-α receptor (Chap. 323). Diseases with abnormal IL-1 regulation leading to fever include familial Mediterranean fever due to mutations in *pyrin*. Mutations in *cold-induced autoinflammatory syndrome 1* lead to neonatal onset multisystem autoinflammatory disease, familial

FIGURE 61-10 Lymphocyte-macrophage interactions underlying resistance to mycobacteria and other intracellular parasites such as *Salmonella*. Mycobacteria infect macrophages, leading to the production of IL-12, which activates T or NK cells through its receptor, leading to production of IL-2 and IFN-γ. IFN-γ acts through its receptor on macrophages to upregulate TNF-α and IL-12 and kill intracellular parasites. Mutant forms of the cytokines and receptors shown in large type have been found in severe cases of nontuberculous mycobacterial infection and salmonellosis.

cold urticaria, and Muckle-Wells syndrome. Pyoderma gangrenosum, acne, and sterile pyogenic arthritis is caused by mutations in CD2BP1. In contrast to these syndromes of overexpression of proinflammatory cytokines, blockade of TNF-α by the antagonists infliximab, etanercept, and adalimumab has been associated with severe infections due to tuberculosis, nontuberculous mycobacteria, and fungi (Chap. 323).

Monocytopenia occurs with acute infections, with stress, and after treatment with glucocorticoids. Monocytopenia also occurs in aplastic anemia, hairy cell leukemia, acute myeloid leukemia, and as a direct result of myelotoxic drugs.

EOSINOPHILS

Eosinophils and neutrophils share similar morphology, many lysosomal constituents, phagocytic capacity, and oxidative metabolism. Eosinophils express a specific chemoattractant receptor and respond to a specific chemokine, eotaxin. Little is known about the role of eosinophils. Eosinophils are much longer lived than neutrophils, and unlike neutrophils, tissue eosinophils can recirculate. During most infections, eosinophils are not important. However, in invasive helminthic infections, such as hookworm, schistosomiasis, strongyloidiasis, toxocariasis, trichinosis, filariasis, echinococcosis, and cysticercosis, the eosinophil plays a central role in host defense. Eosinophils are associated with bronchial asthma, cutaneous allergic reactions, and other hypersensitivity states.

The distinctive feature of the red-staining (Wright's stain) eosinophil granule is its crystalline core consisting of an arginine-rich protein (major basic protein) with histaminase activity, important in host defense against parasites. Eosinophil granules also contain a unique eosinophil peroxidase that catalyzes the oxidation of many substances by hydrogen peroxide and may facilitate killing of microorganisms.

Eosinophil peroxidase, in the presence of hydrogen peroxide and halide, initiates mast cell secretion in vitro and thereby promotes inflammation. Eosinophils contain cationic proteins, some of which bind to heparin and reduce its anticoagulant activity. Eosinophil-derived neurotoxin and eosinophil cationic protein are ribonucleases that can kill respiratory syncytial virus. Eosinophil cytoplasm contains Charcot-Leyden crystal protein, a hexagonal bipyramidal crystal first

observed in a patient with leukemia and then in sputum of patients with asthma; this protein is lysophospholipase and may function to detoxify certain lysophospholipids.

Several factors enhance the eosinophil's function in host defense. T cell–derived factors enhance the ability of eosinophils to kill parasites. Mast cell–derived eosinophil chemotactic factor of anaphylaxis (ECFa) increases the number of eosinophil complement receptors and enhances eosinophil killing of parasites. Eosinophil CSFs (e.g., IL-5) produced by macrophages increase eosinophil production in the bone marrow and activate eosinophils to kill parasites.

EOSINOPHILIA

Eosinophilia is the presence of >500 eosinophils per μL of blood and is common in many settings besides parasite infection. Significant tissue eosinophilia can occur without an elevated blood count. A common cause of eosinophilia is allergic reaction to drugs (iodides, aspirin, sulfonamides, nitrofurantoin, penicillins, and cephalosporins). Allergies such as hay fever, asthma, eczema, serum sickness, allergic vasculitis, and pemphigus are associated with eosinophilia. Eosinophilia also occurs in collagen vascular diseases (e.g., rheumatoid arthritis, eosinophilic fasciitis, allergic angiitis, and periarteritis nodosa) and malignancies (e.g., Hodgkin's disease; mycosis fungoides; chronic myeloid leukemia; and cancer of the lung, stomach, pancreas, ovary, or uterus), as well as in Job's syndrome and CGD. Eosinophilia is commonly present in the helminthic infections. IL-5 is the dominant eosinophil growth factor. Therapeutic administration of the cytokines IL-2 and GM-CSF frequently leads to transient eosinophilia. The most dramatic hypereosinophilic syndromes are Loeffler's syndrome, tropical pulmonary eosinophilia, Loeffler's endocarditis, eosinophilic leukemia, and idiopathic hypereosinophilic syndrome (50,000–100,000/μL).

The idiopathic hypereosinophilic syndrome represents a heterogeneous group of disorders with the common feature of prolonged eosinophilia of unknown cause and organ system dysfunction, including the heart, central nervous system, kidneys, lungs, gastrointestinal tract, and skin. The bone marrow is involved in all affected individuals, but the most severe complications involve the heart and central nervous system. Clinical manifestations and organ dysfunction are highly variable. Eosinophils are found in the involved tissues and likely cause tissue damage by local deposition of toxic eosinophil proteins such as eosinophil cationic protein and major basic protein. In the heart, the pathologic changes lead to thrombosis, endocardial fibrosis, and restrictive endomyocardiopathy. The damage to tissues in other organ systems is similar. Some cases are due to mutations involving the platelet-derived growth factor receptor, and these are extremely sensitive to the tyrosine kinase inhibitor imatinib. Glucocorticoids, hydroxyurea, and IFN-α each have been used successfully, as have therapeutic antibodies against IL-5. Cardiovascular complications are managed aggressively.

The *eosinophilia-myalgia syndrome* is a multisystem disease, with prominent cutaneous, hematologic, and visceral manifestations, that frequently evolves into a chronic course and can occasionally be fatal. The syndrome is characterized by eosinophilia (eosinophil count >1000/μL) and generalized disabling myalgias without other recognized causes. Eosinophilic fasciitis, pneumonitis, and myocarditis; neuropathy culminating in respiratory failure; and encephalopathy may occur. The disease is caused by ingesting contaminants in L-tryptophan–containing products. Eosinophils, lymphocytes, macrophages, and fibroblasts accumulate in the affected tissues, but their role in pathogenesis is unclear. Activation of eosinophils and fibroblasts and the deposition of eosinophil-derived toxic proteins in affected tissues may contribute. IL-5 and transforming growth factor β have been implicated as potential mediators. Treatment is withdrawal of products containing L-tryptophan and the administration of glucocorticoids. Most patients recover fully, remain stable, or show slow recovery, but the disease can be fatal in up to 5% of patients.

EOSINOPENIA

Eosinopenia occurs with stress, such as acute bacterial infection, and after treatment with glucocorticoids. The mechanism of eosinopenia of acute bacterial infection is unknown but is independent of endogenous glucocorticoids, since it occurs in animals after total adrenalectomy. There is no known adverse effect of eosinopenia.

HYPERIMMUNOGLOBULIN E–RECURRENT INFECTION SYNDROME

The hyperimmunoglobulin E–recurrent infection syndrome, or Job's syndrome, is a rare multisystem disease in which the immune system, bone, teeth, lung, and skin are affected. Abnormal chemotaxis is a variable feature. The molecular basis for this syndrome is still not known, but some cases show clear autosomal dominant transmission with linkage to 4q. Patients with this syndrome have characteristic facies with broad nose, kyphoscoliosis and osteoporosis, and eczema. The primary teeth erupt normally but do not deciduate, often requiring extraction. Patients develop recurrent sinopulmonary and cutaneous infections that tend to be much less inflamed than appropriate for the degree of infection and have been referred to as "cold abscesses." A high degree of suspicion is required to diagnose infections in these patients, who may appear well despite extensive disease. The cold abscesses have been considered a reflection of too few phagocytes arriving too late, perhaps due to a lymphocyte factor inhibiting chemotaxis. However, the chemotactic defect in these patients is variable, and the fundamental basis for the impaired defenses is complex and poorly defined.

LABORATORY DIAGNOSIS AND MANAGEMENT

Initial studies of WBC and differential and often a bone marrow examination may be followed by assessment of bone marrow reserves (steroid challenge test), marginated circulating pool of cells (epinephrine challenge test), and marginating ability (endotoxin challenge test) (Fig. 61-7). In vivo assessment of inflammation is possible with a Rebuck skin window test or an in vivo skin blister assay, which measures the ability of leukocytes and inflammatory mediators to accumulate locally in the skin. In vitro tests of phagocyte aggregation, adherence, chemotaxis, phagocytosis, degranulation, and microbicidal activity (for *S. aureus*) may help pinpoint cellular or humoral lesions. Deficiencies of oxidative metabolism are detected with either the nitroblue tetrazolium (NBT) dye test or the dihydrorhodamine (DHR) oxidation test. These tests are based on the ability of products of oxidative metabolism to alter the oxidation states of reporter molecules so that they can be detected microscopically (NBT) or by flow cytometry (DHR). Qualitative studies of superoxide and hydrogen peroxide production may further define neutrophil oxidative function.

Patients with leukopenias or leukocyte dysfunction often have delayed inflammatory responses. Therefore, clinical manifestations may be minimal despite overwhelming infection, and unusual infections must always be suspected. Early signs of infection demand prompt, aggressive culturing for microorganisms, use of antibiotics, and surgical drainage of abscesses. Prolonged courses of antibiotics are often required. In patients with CGD, prophylactic antibiotics (trimethoprim-sulfamethoxazole) and antifungals (itraconazole) markedly diminish the frequency of life-threatening infections. Short courses of glucocorticoids may relieve gastrointestinal or genitourinary tract obstruction by granulomas in patients with CGD. Recombinant human IFN-γ, which nonspecifically stimulates phagocytic cell function, reduces the frequency of infections in patients with CGD by 70% and reduces the severity of infection. This effect of IFN-γ in CGD is additive to the effect of prophylactic antibiotics. The recommended dose is 50 μg/m^2 subcutaneously three times weekly. IFN-γ has also been used successfully in the treatment of leprosy, nontuberculous mycobacteria, and visceral leishmaniasis.

Rigorous oral hygiene reduces but does not eliminate the discomfort of gingivitis, periodontal disease, and aphthous ulcers; chlorhexidine mouthwash and tooth brushing with a hydrogen peroxide–sodium bicarbonate paste helps many patients. Oral antifungal agents (fluconazole or itraconazole) have reduced mucocutaneous candidiasis in patients with Job's syndrome. Androgens, glucocorticoids, lithium, and immunosuppressive therapy have been used to restore myelopoiesis in patients with neutropenia due to impaired production. Recombinant G-CSF is useful in the management of certain forms of neutropenia due to depressed neutrophil production, especially those related to cancer chemotherapy. Patients with chronic neutropenia with evidence of a good bone marrow reserve need not receive prophylactic antibiotics. Patients with chronic or cyclic neutrophil counts < 500/μL may benefit from prophylactic antibiotics and G-CSF during periods of neutropenia. Oral trimethoprim-sulfamethoxazole (160/800 mg) twice daily can prevent infection. Increased numbers of fungal infections are not seen in patients with CGD on this regimen. Oral quinolones such as levofloxacin and ciprofloxacin are alternatives.

In the setting of cytotoxic chemotherapy with severe, persistent neutropenia, trimethoprim-sulfamethoxazole prevents *Pneumocystis jiroveci* pneumonia. These patients, and patients with phagocytic cell dysfunction, should avoid heavy exposure to airborne soil, dust, or decaying matter (mulch, manure), which are often rich in *Nocardia* and the spores of *Aspergillus* and other fungi. Restriction of activities or social contact has no proven role in reducing risk of infection.

Cure of some congenital phagocyte defects is possible by bone marrow transplantation (Chap. 108). However, complications of bone marrow transplantation are still serious, and with rigorous medical care many patients with phagocytic disorders can go for years without a life-threatening infection. The identification of specific gene defects in patients with LAD 1, CGD, and other immunodeficiencies has led to gene therapy trials in a number of genetic white cell disorders.

FURTHER READINGS

HORWITZ MS et al: Neutrophil elastase in cyclic and severe congenital neutropenia. Blood 109:1817, 2007

KLION AD et al: Approaches to the treatment of hypereosinophilic syndromes: A workshop summary report. J Allergy Clin Immunol 117:1292, 2006

NATHAN C: Neutrophils and immunity: Challenges and opportunities. Nat Rev Immunol 6:173, 2006

PUEL A et al: Heritable defects of the human TLR signalling pathways. J Endotoxin Res 11:220, 2005

ROSENZWEIG SD, HOLLAND SM: Phagocyte immunodeficiencies and their infections. J Allergy Clin Immunol 113:620, 2004

SEGAL BH et al: Genetic, biochemical, and clinical features of chronic granulomatous disease. Medicine (Baltimore) 79:170, 2000

62 Principles of Human Genetics
J. Larry Jameson, Peter Kopp

IMPACT OF GENETICS ON MEDICAL PRACTICE

The beginning of the new millennium was marked by the announcement that the vast majority of the human genome had been sequenced. This milestone in the exploration of the human genome was preceded by numerous conceptual and technological advances. They include, among others, the elucidation of the DNA double-helix structure, the discovery of restriction enzymes and the polymerase chain reaction (PCR), the development and automatization of DNA sequencing, and the generation of genetic and physical maps by the Human Genome Project (HGP). The consequences of this wealth of knowledge for the practice of medicine are profound. To date, the most significant impact of genetics has been to enhance our understanding of disease etiology and pathogenesis. However, genetics is rapidly playing a more prominent role in the diagnosis, prevention, and treatment of disease (Chap. 64). Genetic approaches have proven invaluable for the detection of infectious pathogens and are used clinically to identify agents that are difficult to culture such as mycobacteria, viruses, and parasites. In many cases, molecular genetics has improved the feasibility and accuracy of diagnostic testing and is beginning to open new avenues for therapy, including gene and cellular therapy (Chaps. 65 and 67). Molecular genetics has already significantly changed the treatment of human disease. Peptide hormones, growth factors, cytokines, and vaccines can now be produced in large amounts using recombinant DNA technology. Targeted modification of these peptides provides the practitioner with improved therapeutic tools, as illustrated by genetically modified insulin analogues with more favorable kinetics. There is hope that a better understanding of the genetic basis of human disease will also have an increasing impact on disease prevention.

Genetics has traditionally been viewed through the window of relatively rare single-gene diseases. Taken together, these disorders account for ~10% of pediatric admissions and childhood mortality. It is, however, increasingly apparent that virtually every medical condition, maybe with the exception of simple trauma, has a genetic component. As is often evident from a patient's family history, many common disorders such as hypertension, heart disease, asthma, diabetes mellitus, and mental illnesses are significantly influenced by the genetic background. These polygenic or multifactorial (complex) disorders involve the contributions of many different genes, as well as environmental factors, that can modify disease risk (Chap. 64). A major current challenge is to elucidate the genetic components that contribute to the pathogenesis of complex disorders. The recent publication of a comprehensive catalogue of human single-nucleotide polymorphism (SNP) haplotypes, the HapMap Project, provides an essential resource for genome-wide association studies (see below).

Cancer has a genetic basis since it results from acquired somatic mutations in genes controlling growth, apoptosis, and cellular differentiation (Chap. 79). In addition, the development of many cancers is associated with a hereditary predisposition. The prevalence of genetic diseases, combined with their severity and chronic nature, imposes a great financial, social, and emotional burden on society.

Genetics has historically focused on chromosomal and metabolic disorders, reflecting the long-standing availability of techniques to diagnose these conditions. For example, conditions such as trisomy 21 (Down syndrome) or monosomy X (Turner syndrome) can be diagnosed using cytogenetics (Chap. 63). Likewise, many metabolic disorders (e.g., phenylketonuria, familial hypercholesterolemia) are diagnosed using biochemical analyses. Recent advances in DNA diagnostics have ex-

tended the field of genetics to include virtually all medical specialties. In cardiology, for example, the molecular basis of inherited cardiomyopathies and ion channel defects that predispose to arrhythmias is being defined (Chaps. 226 and 231). In neurology, genetics has unmasked the pathophysiology of a startling number of neurodegenerative disorders (Chap. 360). Hematology has evolved dramatically, from its incipient genetic descriptions of hemoglobinopathies to the current understanding of the molecular basis of red cell membrane defects, clotting disorders, and thrombotic disorders (Chaps. 99 and 110).

New concepts derived from genetic studies can sometimes clarify the pathogenesis of disorders that were previously opaque. For example, although many different genetic defects can cause peripheral neuropathies, disruption of the normal folding of the myelin sheaths is frequently a common final pathway (Chap. 379). Several genetic causes of obesity appear to converge on a physiologic pathway that involves products of the proopiomelanocortin polypeptide and the MC4R receptor, thus identifying a key mechanism for appetite control (Chap. 74). A similar phenomenon is emerging for genetically distinct forms of Alzheimer's disease, several of which lead to the formation of neurofibrillary tangles (Chap. 365). The identification of defective genes often leads to the detection of cellular pathways involved in key physiologic processes. Examples include identification of the cystic fibrosis conductance regulator (*CFTR*) gene; the Duchenne muscular dystrophy (*DMD*) gene, which encodes dystrophin; and the fibroblast growth factor receptor-3 (*FGFR3*) gene, which is responsible for achondroplastic dwarfism. Similarly, transgenic (over)expression, and targeted gene "knock-out" and "knock-in" models help to unravel the physiologic function of genes.

The astounding rate at which new genetic information is being generated creates a major challenge for physicians, health care providers, and basic investigators. The terminology and techniques used for discovery evolve continuously. Much genetic information presently resides in computer databases or is being published in basic science journals. Databases provide easy access to the expanding information about the human genome, genetic disease, and genetic testing (Table 62-1). For example, several thousand monogenic disorders are summarized in a large, continuously evolving compendium, referred to as the *Online Mendelian Inheritance in Man* (OMIM) catalogue (Table 62-1). The ongoing refinement of bioinformatics is simplifying the access to this seemingly daunting onslaught of new information.

CHROMOSOMES AND DNA REPLICATION
Organization of DNA into Chromosomes • *SIZE OF THE HUMAN GENOME*

The human genome is divided into 23 different chromosomes, including 22 autosomes (numbered 1–22) and the X and Y sex chromosomes. Adult cells are *diploid*, meaning they contain two homologous sets of 22 autosomes and a pair of sex chromosomes. Females have two X chromosomes (XX), whereas males have one X and one Y chromosome (XY). As a consequence of meiosis, germ cells (sperm or oocytes) are haploid and contain one set of 22 autosomes and one of the sex chromosomes. At the time of fertilization, the diploid genome is reconstituted by pairing of the homologous chromosomes from the mother and father. With each cell division (mitosis), chromosomes are replicated, paired, segregated, and divided into two daughter cells (Chap. 63).

The human genome is estimated to contain ~30,000–40,000 genes, a smaller number than initially predicted, that are divided among the 23 chromosomes. A *gene* is a functional unit that is regulated by transcription (see below) and encodes a RNA product, which is most commonly, but not always, translated into a protein that exerts activity within or outside the cell. Historically, genes were identified because they conferred specific traits that are transmitted from one generation to the next. Increasingly, they are characterized based on expression in

TABLE 62-1 SELECTED DATABASES RELEVANT FOR GENOMICS AND GENETIC DISORDERS

Site	URL	Comment
National Center for Biotechnology Information (NCBI)	http://www.ncbi.nlm.nih.gov/	Molecular biology information, public databases, computational biology. Software for analyzing genome data. Extensive links to other databases, genome resources, and tutorials
National Human Genome Research Institute	http://www.genome.gov/	Web links providing information about the human genome sequence, genomes of other organisms, and genomic research
Ensembl Genome browser	http://www.ensembl.org/	Maps and sequence information of eukaryotic genomes
Online Mendelian Inheritance in Man	http://www.ncbi.nlm.nih.gov/omim/	Online compendium of Mendelian disorders and human genes causing genetic disorders
Office of Biotechnology Activities National Institutes of Health	www4.od.nih.gov/oba/	Information about recombinant DNA and gene transfer
		Medical, ethical, legal, and social issues raised by genetic testing
		Medical, ethical, legal, and social issues raised by xenotransplantation
American College of Medical Genetics	http://www.acmg.net/	Extensive links to other databases relevant for the diagnosis, treatment, and prevention of genetic disease
Cancer Genome Anatomy Project (CGAP)	http://cgap.nci.nih.gov/	Information about gene expression profiles of normal, precancer, and cancer cells
GenLink	http://www.genlink.wustl.edu	Multimedia database resource for human genetics and telomere research
GeneTests	http://www.genetests.org/	International directory of genetic testing laboratories and prenatal diagnosis clinics Reviews and educational materials
Genomes Online Database (GOLD)	http://www.genomesonline.org/	Information on published and unpublished genomes
HUGO Gene Nomenclature	http://www.gene.ucl.ac.uk/nomenclature	Gene names and symbols
MITOMAP, a human mitochondrial genome database	http://www.mitomap.org/	A compendium of polymorphisms and mutations of the human mitochondrial DNA
Mitochondrial disorders	http://www.neuro.wustl.edu/neuromuscular/mitosyn.html	Overview on clinical syndromes associated with mtDNA mutations
DNA repeat sequences & disease	http://www.neuro.wustl.edu/neuromuscular/mother/dnarep.htm	Overview on clinical syndromes associated with DNA repeats
Online Mendelian Inheritance in Animals (OMIA)	http://omia.angis.org.au/	Online compendium of Mendelian disorders in animals
The Jackson Laboratory	http://www.jax.org/	Information about murine models and the mouse genome
International HapMap Project	http://www.hapmap.org/	Catalogue of haplotypes in different ethnic groups relevant for association studies and pharmacogenomics
Nuclear Receptor Signaling Atlas	http://nursa.org	Atlas of nuclear receptors, coregulators, and ligands
Dolan DNA Learning Center, Cold Spring Harbor Laboratories	http://www.dnalc.org/	Educational material about selected genetic disorders, DNA, eugenics, and genetic origin
The Online Metabolic and Molecular Bases of Inherited Disease (OMMBID)	http://genetics.accessmedicine.com	Online version of the comprehensive text on The Metabolic and Molecular Bases of Inherited Disease, 8e

Note: Databases are evolving constantly. Pertinent information may be found by using links listed in the few selected databases. Instructions for the use of genome-related databases have been published [Nat Genet 32(Suppl):1–79, 2002].

various tissues. The number of genes greatly underestimates the complexity of genetic expression, as single genes can generate multiple spliced mRNA products, which are translated into proteins that are subject to complex posttranslational modification, such as phosphorylation. *Proteomics,* the study of the proteome using technologies of large-scale protein separation and identification, is an emerging field focused on protein variation and function. Similarly, the field of *metabolomics* aims at determining the composition and modifications of the *metabolome,* the complement of low-molecular-weight molecules, many of which participate in various metabolic functions. These analyses, which are heavily dependent on bioinformatics, reveal that physiologic or pathologic alterations have myriad effects on the proteome and the metabolome and emphasize that these processes involve *modular networks* rather than *linear pathways.*

Human DNA consists of ~3 billion base pairs (bp) of DNA per haploid genome. DNA length is normally measured in units of 1000 bp (kilobases, kb) or 1,000,000 bp (megabases, Mb). Not all DNA encodes genes. In fact, genes account for only ~10–15% of DNA. Much of the remaining DNA consists of highly repetitive sequences, the function of which is poorly understood. These repetitive DNA regions, along with nonrepetitive sequences that do not encode genes, may serve a structural role in the packaging of DNA into chromatin, i.e., DNA bound to histone proteins, and chromosomes (Fig. 62-1). If only 10% of DNA is expressed and there are 30,000 genes, the average gene would be ~10 kb in length. Although many genes are about this size, the range is quite broad. For example, some genes are only a few hundred bp, whereas others, such as the *DMD* gene, are extraordinarily large (2 Mb).

STRUCTURE OF DNA Each gene is composed of a linear polymer of DNA. DNA is a double-stranded helix composed of four different bases: adenine (A), thymidine (T), guanine (G), and cytosine (C). Adenine is paired to thymidine, and guanine is paired to cytosine, by hydrogen bond interactions that span the double helix. DNA has several remarkable features that make it ideal for the transmission of genetic information. It is relatively stable, at least in comparison to RNA or proteins. The double-stranded nature of DNA and its feature of strict base-pair complementarity permit faithful replication during cell division. As described below, complementarity also allows the transmission of genetic information from DNA → RNA → protein (Fig. 62-2). Messenger RNA (mRNA) is encoded by the so-called sense or coding strand of the DNA double helix and is translated into proteins by ribosomes.

The presence of four different bases provides surprising genetic diversity. In the protein-coding regions of genes, the DNA bases are arranged into codons, a triplet of bases that specifies a particular amino acid. It is possible to arrange the four bases into 64 different triplet codons (4^3). Each codon specifies 1 of the 20 different amino acids, or a regulatory signal, such as initiation and stop of translation. Because there are more codons than amino acids, the genetic code is degenerate; that is, most amino acids can be specified by several different codons. By arranging the codons in different combinations and in various lengths, it is possible to generate the tremendous diversity of primary protein structure.

FIGURE 62-1 Structure of chromatin and chromosomes. Chromatin is composed of double-strand DNA that is wrapped around histone and nonhistone proteins forming nucleosomes. The nucleosomes are further organized into solenoid structures. Chromosomes assume their characteristic structure, with short (p) and long (q) arms at the metaphase stage of the cell cycle.

Replication of DNA and Mitosis

Genetic information in DNA is transmitted to daughter cells under two different circumstances: (1) somatic cells divide by mitosis, allowing the diploid (2n) genome to replicate itself completely in conjunction with cell division; and (2) germ cells (sperm and ova) undergo meiosis, a process that enables the reduction of the diploid (2n) set of chromosomes to the haploid state (1n) (Chap. 63).

Prior to mitosis, cells exit the resting, or G_0 state, and enter the cell cycle (Chap. 80). After traversing a critical checkpoint in G_1, cells undergo DNA synthesis (S phase), during which the DNA in each chromosome is replicated, yielding two pairs of sister chromatids ($2n \rightarrow 4n$). The process of DNA synthesis requires stringent fidelity in order to avoid transmitting errors to subsequent generations of cells. Genetic abnormalities of DNA mismatch/repair include xeroderma pigmentosum, Bloom syndrome, ataxia telangiectasia, and hereditary nonpolyposis colon cancer (HNPCC), among others. Many of these disorders strongly predispose to neoplasia because of the rapid acquisition of additional mutations (Chap. 79). After completion of DNA synthesis, cells enter G_2 and progress through a second checkpoint before entering mitosis. At this stage, the chromosomes condense and are aligned along the equatorial plate at metaphase. The two identical sister chromatids, held together at the centromere, divide and migrate to opposite poles of the cell (see Fig. 63-3). After formation of a nuclear membrane around the two separated sets of chromatids, the cell divides and two daughter cells are formed, thus restoring the diploid (2n) state.

Assortment and Segregation of Genes during Meiosis

Meiosis occurs only in germ cells of the gonads. It shares certain features with mitosis but involves two distinct steps of cell division that reduce the chromosome number to the haploid state. In addition, there is active recombination that generates genetic diversity. During the first cell division, two sister chromatids ($2n \rightarrow 4n$) are formed for each chromosome pair and there is an exchange of DNA between homologous paternal and maternal chromosomes. This process involves the formation of *chiasmata*, structures that correspond to the DNA segments that cross over between the maternal and paternal homologues (Fig. 62-3). Usually there is at least one crossover on each chromosomal arm; recombination occurs more frequently in female meiosis than in male meiosis. Subsequently, the chromosomes segregate randomly. Because there are 23 chromosomes, there exist 2^{23} (>8 million) possible combinations of chromosomes. Together with the genetic exchanges that occur during recombination, chromosomal segregation generates tremendous diversity, and each gamete is genetically unique. The process of recom-

FIGURE 62-2 Flow of genetic information. Multiple extracellular signals activate intracellular signal cascades that result in altered regulation of gene expression through the interaction of transcription factors with regulatory regions of genes. RNA polymerase transcribes DNA into RNA that is processed to mRNA by excision of intronic sequences. The mRNA is translated into a polypeptide chain to form the mature protein after undergoing posttranslational processing. HAT, histone acetyl transferase; CBP, CREB-binding protein; CREB, cyclic AMP response element–binding protein; CRE, cyclic AMP responsive element; CoA, Co activator; TAF, TBP-associated factors; GTF, general transcription factors; TBP, TATA-binding protein; TATA, TATA box; RE, response element; NH_2, aminoterminus; COOH, carboxyterminus.

FIGURE 62-3 Crossing-over and genetic recombination. During chiasma formation, either of the two sister chromatids on one chromosome pairs with one of the chromatids of the homologous chromosome. Genetic recombination occurs through crossing-over and results in recombinant and nonrecombinant chromosome segments in the gametes. Together with the random segregation of the maternal and paternal chromosomes, recombination contributes to genetic diversity and forms the basis of the concept of linkage.

bination, and the independent segregation of chromosomes, provide the foundation for performing linkage analyses, whereby one attempts to correlate the inheritance of certain chromosomal regions (or linked genes) with the presence of a disease or genetic trait (see below).

After the first meiotic division, which results in two daughter cells (2*n*), the two chromatids of each chromosome separate during a second meiotic division to yield four gametes with a haploid state (1*n*). When the egg is fertilized by sperm, the two haploid sets are combined, thereby restoring the diploid state (2*n*) in the zygote.

REGULATION OF GENE EXPRESSION

Mechanisms that regulate gene expression play a critical role in the function of genes. The transcription of genes is controlled primarily by *transcription factors* that bind to DNA sequences in the regulatory regions of genes. As described below, mutations in transcription factors cause a significant number of genetic disorders. Gene expression is also influenced by *epigenetic events*, such as X-inactivation and imprinting, processes in which DNA methylation or histone modifications are associated with gene silencing. Several genetic disorders, such as Prader-Willi syndrome (neonatal hypotonia, developmental delay, obesity, short stature, and hypogonadism) and Albright hereditary osteodystrophy (resistance to parathyroid hormone, short stature, brachydactyly, resistance to other hormones in certain subtypes), exhibit the consequences of genomic imprinting. Most studies of gene expression have focused on the regulatory DNA elements of genes that control transcription. However, it should be emphasized that gene expression requires a series of steps, including mRNA processing, protein translation, and posttranslational modifications, all of which are actively regulated (Fig. 62-2).

The new field of *functional genomics* is based on the concept that understanding alterations of gene expression under various physiologic and pathologic conditions provides insight into the underlying processes, and by revealing certain gene expression profiles, this knowledge may be of diagnostic and therapeutic relevance. The large-scale study of expression profiles, which takes advantage of microarray technologies, is also referred to as *transcriptomics* because the complement of mRNAs transcribed by the cellular genome is called the *transcriptome*.

Structure of Genes A gene product is usually a protein but can occasionally consist of RNA that is not translated (e.g., microRNAs). *Exons* refer to the portion of genes that are eventually spliced together to form mRNA. *Introns* refer to the spacing regions between the exons that are spliced out of precursor RNAs during RNA processing (Fig. 62-2).

The gene locus also includes regions that are necessary to control its expression. The regulatory regions most commonly involve sequences upstream (5′) of the transcription start site, although there are also examples of control elements within introns or downstream of the coding regions of a gene. The upstream regulatory regions are also referred to as the *promoter*. The minimal promoter usually consists of a TATA box (which binds TATA-binding protein, TBP) and initiator sequences that enhance the formation of an active transcription complex. A gene may generate various transcripts through the use of alternative promoters and/or alternative splicing of exons, mechanisms that contribute to the enormous diversity of proteins and their functions. Transcriptional termination signals reside downstream, or 3′, of a gene. Specific sequences, such as the AAUAAA sequence at the 3′ end of the mRNA, designate the site for polyadenylation (poly-A tail), a process that influences mRNA transport to the cytoplasm, stability, and translation efficiency. A rigorous test of the regulatory region boundaries involves expressing a gene in a transgenic animal to determine whether the isolated DNA flanking sequences are sufficient to recapitulate the normal developmental, tissue-specific, and signal-responsive features of the endogenous gene. This has been accomplished for only a few genes; there are many examples in which large genomic fragments only partially reconstitute normal gene regulation in vivo, implying the presence of distant regulatory sequences. Genome-wide analyses of selected transcription factor binding sites, such as for the estrogen receptor, reveal that the majority of regulatory sites are very distant from the transcription start sites of genes. A detailed understanding of mechanisms that regulate genes is also relevant for gene therapy strategies that require normal gene regulation (Chap. 65).

The number of DNA sequences and transcription factors that regulate transcription is much greater than originally anticipated. Most genes contain at least 15–20 discrete regulatory elements within 300 bp of the transcription start site. This densely packed promoter region often contains binding sites for ubiquitous transcription factors such as CAAT box/enhancer binding protein (C/EBP), cyclic AMP response element–binding (CREB) protein, selective promoter factor 1 (Sp-1), or activator protein 1 (AP-1). However, factors involved in cell-specific expression may also bind to these sequences. For example, basic helix-loop-helix (bHLH) proteins bind to E-boxes in the promoters of myogenic genes, and steroidogenic factor 1 (SF-1) binds to a specific recognition site in the regulatory region of multiple steroidogenic enzyme genes. Key regulatory elements may also reside at a large distance from the proximal promoter. The globin and the immunoglobulin genes, for example, contain *locus control regions* that are several kilobases away from the structural sequences of the gene. Specific groups of transcription factors that bind to these promoter and enhancer sequences provide a combinatorial code for regulating transcription. In this manner, relatively ubiquitous factors interact with more restricted factors to allow each gene to be expressed and regulated in a unique manner that is dependent on developmental state, cell type, and numerous extracellular stimuli. As described below, the transcription factors that bind to DNA actually represent only the first level of regulatory control. Other proteins—*coactivators* and *co-repressors*—interact with the DNA-binding transcription factors to generate large regulatory complexes. These complexes are subject to control by numerous cell-signaling pathways, including phosphorylation, acetylation, sumoylation, and ubiquitinylation. Ultimately, the recruited transcription factors interact with, and stabilize, components of the basal transcription complex that assembles at the site of the TATA box

FIGURE 62-4 Point mutations causing β-thalassemia as example of allelic heterogeneity. The β-globin gene is located in the globin gene cluster. Point mutations can be located in the promoter, the CAP site, the 5'-untranslated region, the initiation codon, each of the three exons, the introns, or the polyadenylation signal. Many mutations introduce missense or nonsense mutations, whereas others cause defective RNA splicing. Not shown here are deletion mutations of the β-globin gene or larger deletions of the globin locus that can also result in thalassemia. ▼, Promoter mutations; *, CAP site; ●, 5'UTR; ①, Initiation codon; ◆, Defective RNA processing; ✦, Missense and nonsense mutations; Ⓐ, Poly A signal.

and initiator region. This basal transcription factor complex consists of >30 different proteins. Gene transcription occurs when RNA polymerase begins to synthesize RNA from the DNA template.

Mutations can occur in all domains of a gene (Fig. 62-4). A point mutation occurring within the coding region leads to an amino acid substitution if the codon is altered. Point mutations that introduce a premature stop codon result in a truncated protein. Large deletions may affect a portion of a gene or an entire gene, whereas small deletions and insertions alter the reading frame if they do not represent a multiple of three bases. These "frameshift" mutations lead to an entirely altered carboxy terminus. Mutations occurring in regulatory or intronic regions may result in altered expression or splicing of genes. Examples are shown in Fig. 62-5.

Transcriptional Activation and Repression Every gene is controlled uniquely, whether in its spatial or temporal pattern of expression or in its response to extracellular signals. It is estimated that transcription factors account for ~30% of expressed genes. A growing number of identified genetic diseases involve transcription factors (Table 62-2). The MODY (maturity-onset diabetes of the young) disorders are representative of this group of diseases; mutations in several different islet cell–specific transcription factors cause various forms of MODY (Chap. 338).

Transcriptional activation can be divided into three main mechanisms:

1. Events that alter chromatin structure can enhance the access of transcription factors to DNA. For example, histone acetylation generally opens chromatin structure and is correlated with transcriptional activation.
2. Posttranslational modifications of transcription factors, such as phosphorylation, can induce the assembly of active transcription complexes. As an example, phosphorylation of CREB protein on serine 133 induces a con-

formational change that allows the recruitment of CREB-binding protein (CBP), a factor that integrates the actions of many transcription factors, including proteins, with histone acetyltransferase activity.

3. Transcriptional activators can displace a repressor protein. This mechanism is particularly common during development when the pattern of transcription factor expression changes dynamically.

Of course, these mechanisms are not mutually exclusive, and most genes are activated by some combination of these events.

Suppression of gene expression is as important as gene activation in the control of cell differentiation and function. Some mechanisms of repression are the corollary of activation. For example, repression is often associated with histone deacetylation or protein dephosphorylation. For nuclear hormone receptors, transcriptional silencing involves the recruitment of repression complexes that contain histone deacetylase activity. Aberrant expression of repressor proteins is sometimes associated with neoplasia. The t(15;17) chromosomal translocation that occurs in promyelocytic leukemia fuses the *PML* gene to a portion of the retinoic acid receptor α (*RAR* α) gene (Table 62-2). This event causes unregulated transcriptional repression in a manner that precludes normal cellular differentiation. The addition of the RAR ligand, retinoic acid, activates the receptor, thereby relieving repression and allowing cells to differentiate and ultimately undergo apoptosis. This mechanism has therapeutic importance as the addition of retinoic acid to treatment regimens induces a higher remission rate in patients with promyelocytic leukemia (Chap. 104). Methylation of promoter regions is frequently found in neoplasms and silences gene expression.

CLONING AND SEQUENCING DNA

A description of recombinant DNA techniques, the methodology used for the manipulation, analysis, and characterization of DNA segments, is beyond the scope of this chapter. As these methods are wide-

FIGURE 62-5 A. Examples of mutations. The coding strand is shown with the encoded amino acid sequence. **B.** Chromatograms of sequence analyses after amplification of genomic DNA by polymerase chain reaction.

TABLE 62-2 **SELECTED EXAMPLES OF DISEASES CAUSED BY MUTATIONS AND REARRANGEMENTS IN TRANSCRIPTION FACTOR CLASSES**

Transcription Factor Class	Example	Associated Disorder
Nuclear receptors	Androgen receptor	Complete or partial androgen insensitivity (recessive missense mutations) Spinobulbar muscular atrophy (CAG repeat expansion)
Zinc finger proteins	WT1	WAGR syndrome: Wilm's tumor, aniridia, genitourinary malformations, mental retardation
Basic helix-loop-helix	MITF	Waardenburg syndrome type 2A
Homeobox	IPF1	Maturity onset of diabetes mellitus type 4 (heterozygous mutation/haploinsufficiency) Pancreatic agenesis (homozygous mutation)
Leucine zipper	Retina leucine zipper (NRL)	Autosomal dominant retinitis pigmentosa
High mobility group (HMG) proteins	SRY	Sex-reversal
Forkhead	HNF4α, HNF1α, HNF1β	Maturity-onset of diabetes mellitus types 1, 3, 5
Paired box	PAX3	Waardenburg syndrome types 1 and 3
T-box	TBX5	Holt-Oram syndrome (thumb anomalies, atrial or ventricular septum defects, phocomelia)
Cell cycle control proteins	P53	Li-Fraumeni syndrome, other cancers
Coactivators	CREB binding protein (CBP)	Rubinstein-Taybi syndrome
General transcription factors	TATA-binding protein (TBP)	Spinocerebellar ataxia 17 (CAG expansion)
Transcription elongation factor	VHL	Von Hippel–Lindau syndrome (renal cell carcinoma, pheochromocytoma, pancreatic tumors, hemangioblastomas) Autosomal dominant inheritance, somatic inactivation of second allele (Knudson two-hit model)
Runt	CBFA2	Familial thrombocytopenia with propensity to acute myelogenous leukemia
Chimeric proteins due to translocations	PML—RAR	Acute promyelocytic leukemia t(15;17)(q22;q11.2-q12) translocation

Note: Selected abbreviations include: SRY, sex determining region Y; HNF, hepatocyte nuclear factor; CREB (cAMP responsive element binding) binding protein; VHL, Von Hippel–Lindau; PML, promyelocytic leukemia; RAR, retinoic acid receptor.

ly used in genetics and molecular diagnostics, however, it is useful to review briefly some of the fundamental principles of cloning and DNA sequencing.

Cloning of Genes *Cloning* refers to the creation of a recombinant DNA molecule that can be propagated indefinitely. The ability to clone genes and cDNAs therefore provides a permanent and renewable source of these reagents. Cloning is essential for DNA sequencing, nucleic acid hybridization studies, expression of recombinant proteins, and other recombinant DNA procedures.

The cloning of DNA involves the insertion of a DNA fragment into a cloning vector, followed by the propagation of the recombinant DNA in a host cell. The most straightforward cloning strategy involves inserting a DNA fragment into bacterial plasmids. Plasmids are small, autonomously replicating, circular DNA molecules that propagate separately from the chromosome in bacterial cells. The process of DNA insertion relies heavily on the use of restriction enzymes, which cleave DNA at highly specific sequences (usually 4–6 bp in length). Restriction enzymes generate complementary, cohesive sequences at the ends of the DNA fragment, which allow them to be efficiently ligated to the plasmid vector. Because plasmids contain genes that confer resistance to antibiotics, their presence in the host cell can be used for selection and DNA amplification.

A variety of vectors (e.g., plasmids, phage, bacterial, or yeast artificial chromosomes) are used for cloning. Many of these are used for creating *libraries*, a term that refers to a collection of DNA clones. A genomic library represents an array of clones derived from genomic DNA. These overlapping DNA fragments represent the entire genome

and can ultimately be arranged according to their linear order. cDNA libraries reflect clones derived from mRNA, typically from a particular tissue source. Thus, a cDNA library from the heart contains copies of mRNA expressed specifically in cardiac myocytes, in addition to those that are expressed ubiquitously. For this reason, a heart cDNA library will be enriched with cardiac-specific gene products and will differ from cDNA libraries generated from liver or pituitary mRNAs. As an example of the complexity of a genomic library, consider that the human genome contains 3×10^9 bp and the average genomic insert in a λ phage library is ~10^4 bp. Therefore, it requires at least 3×10^5 clones to represent all genomic DNA. Specific clones are isolated from the several hundred thousand clones by using DNA hybridization.

With completion of the HGP, all human genes have been cloned and sequenced. As a result, many of these cloning procedures are now unnecessary or greatly facilitated by the extensive information concerning DNA markers and the sequence of DNA (see below).

Nucleic Acid Hybridization Nucleic acid *hybridization* is a fundamental principle in molecular biology that takes advantage of the fact that the two complementary strands of nucleic acids bind, or *hybridize*, to one another with very high specificity. The goal of hybridization is to detect specific nucleic acid (DNA or RNA) sequences in a complex background of other sequences. This technique is used for Southern blotting, Northern blotting, and for screening libraries (see above). Further adaptation of hybridization techniques has led to the development of microarray DNA chips.

SOUTHERN BLOT Southern blotting is used to analyze whether genes have been deleted or rearranged. It is also used to detect restriction fragment length polymorphisms (RFLPs). Genomic DNA is digested with restriction endonucleases and separated by gel electrophoresis. Individual fragments can then be transferred to a membrane and detected after hybridization with specific radioactive DNA probes. Because single base-pair mismatches can disrupt the hybridization of short DNA probes (oligonucleotides), a variation of the Southern blot, termed *oligonucleotide-specific hybridization* (OSH), uses short oligonucleotides to distinguish normal from mutant genes.

NORTHERN BLOT Northern blots are used to analyze patterns and levels of gene expression in different tissues. In a Northern blot, mRNA is separated on a gel and transferred to a membrane, and specific transcripts are detected using radiolabeled DNA as a probe. This technique has been largely supplanted by more sensitive and comprehensive methods such as reverse transcriptase (RT)–PCR and gene expression arrays on DNA chips (see below).

MICROARRAY TECHNOLOGY A comprehensive approach to genome-scale studies consists of *microarrays*, or *DNA chips*. These microarrays consist of thousands of synthetic nucleic acid sequences aligned on thin glass or silicon surfaces. Fluorescently labeled test sample DNA or RNA is hybridized to the chip, and a computerized scanner detects sequence matches. Microarrays allow the detection of variations in DNA sequence and are used for mutational analysis and genotyping. Alternatively, the expression pattern of large numbers of mRNA transcripts can be determined by hybridization of RNA samples to cDNA or genomic microarrays. This method has tremendous potential in the era of functional genomics and permits comprehensive analyses of gene expression profiles. As one example, microarrays can be used to develop genetic fingerprints of different types of malignancies, providing information useful for classification, pathophysiology, prognosis, and treatment.

The Polymerase Chain Reaction The PCR, introduced in 1985, has revolutionized the way DNA analyses are performed and has become a cornerstone of molecular biology and genetic analysis. In essence, PCR provides a rapid way of amplifying specific DNA fragments in vitro. Exquisite specificity is conferred by the use of PCR primers, which are designed for a given DNA sequence. The geometric amplification of the DNA after multiple cycles yields remarkable sensitivity. As a result, PCR can be used to amplify DNA from very small samples, including single cells. These properties also allow DNA amplification from a variety of tissue sources including blood samples, biopsies, surgical or autopsy specimens, or cells from hair or saliva. PCR can also be used to study mRNA. In this case, the enzyme RT is first used to convert the RNA to DNA, which can then be amplified by PCR. This procedure, commonly known as *RT-PCR*, is useful as a quantitative measure of gene expression.

PCR provides a key component of molecular diagnostics. It provides a strategy for the rapid amplification of DNA (or mRNA) to search for mutations by a wide array of techniques, including DNA sequencing. PCR is also used for the amplification of highly polymorphic di- or trinucleotide repeat sequences or the genotyping of SNPs, which allow various polymorphic alleles to be traced in genetic linkage or association studies. PCR is increasingly used to diagnose various microbial pathogens.

DNA Sequencing DNA sequencing is now an automated procedure. Although many protocols exist, the most commonly used strategy currently uses the capillary electrophoresis-based Sanger method in which dideoxynucleotides are used to randomly terminate DNA polymerization at each of the four bases (A,G,T,C). After separating the array of terminated DNA fragments using high-resolution gel or capillary electrophoresis, it is possible to deduce the DNA sequence by examining the progression of fragment lengths generated in each of the four nucleotide reactions. The use of fluorescently labeled dideoxynucleotides allows automated detection of the different bases and direct computer analysis of the DNA sequence (Fig. 62-5). Significant efforts are underway to develop faster, more cost-effective DNA sequencing technologies. These include the use of pyrosequencing chemistries; whole-genome sequencing using solid-phase sequencing; mass spectrometry; detection of fluorescently labeled bases in flow cytometry; direct reading of the DNA sequence by scanning, tunneling, or atomic force microscopy; and sequence analysis using DNA chips.

TRANSGENIC MICE AS MODELS OF GENETIC DISEASE
Several organisms have been studied extensively as genetic models, including *Mus musculus* (mouse), *Drosophila melanogaster* (fruit fly), *Caenorhabditis elegans* (nematode), *Saccharomyces cerevisiae* (baker's yeast), and *Escherichia coli* (colonic bacterium). The ability to use these evolutionarily distant organisms as genetic models that are relevant to human physiology reflects a surprising conservation of genetic pathways and gene function. Trans-

genic mouse models have been particularly valuable, because many human and mouse genes exhibit similar structure and function, and because manipulation of the mouse genome is relatively straightforward compared to those of other mammalian species.

Transgenic strategies in mice can be divided into two main approaches: (1) expression of a gene by random insertion into the genome, and (2) deletion or targeted mutagenesis of a gene by homologous recombination with the native endogenous gene (knockout, knock-in) (Fig. 62-6; Table 62-3). Transgenic mice are generated by pronuclear injection of foreign DNA into fertilized mouse oocytes and subsequent transfer into the oviduct of pseudopregnant foster mothers.

Transgenic expression of genes can be useful for studying disorders that are sensitive to gene dosage. Overexpression of *PMP22*, for example, mimics a common duplication of this gene in type IA Charcot-Marie-Tooth disease (Chap. 379). Duplication of the *PMP22* gene results in high levels of expression of peripheral myelin protein 22, and this dosage effect is responsible for the demyelinating neuropathy. Expression of the Y chromosome–specific gene, *SRY*, in XX females demonstrates that *SRY* is sufficient to induce the formation of testes. This finding confirms the pathogenic role of *SRY* translocations to the X chromosome in sex-reversed XX females. Huntington disease is an autosomal dominant disorder caused by expansion of a CAG trinucleotide repeat that encodes a polyglutamine tract. Targeted deletion of the Huntington disease (*HD*) gene does not induce the neurologic disorder. On the other hand, transgenic expression of the entire gene or of the first exon containing the sequence encoding the expanded polyglutamine repeat is sufficient to cause many features of the neurologic disorder, indicating a gain-of-function property for the expanded polyglutamine-containing protein. Transgenic strategies can also be used as a precursor to gene therapy. Expression of dystrophin, the pro-

Prepare DNA transgene

Inject transgene into male pronucleus of fertilized ovum

Implant ovum into pseudopregnant female

Test tail DNA of F1 generation for transgene

Breed to homozygosity

Prepare targeting construct

Select for homologous recombination in embryonic stem (ES) cells

Introduce selected ES cells into blastocyst and implant

Mixed coat color in chimeric mice

Breed to homozygosity

FIGURE 62-6 Transgenic mouse models. *Left.* Transgenic mice are generated by pronuclear injection of foreign DNA into fertilized mouse oocytes and subsequent transfer into the oviduct of pseudopregnant foster mothers. ***Right.*** For targeted mutagenesis (gene knock-out/knock-in), embryonic stem (ES) cells are transfected with the targeted (mutagenized) transgene. The transgene undergoes homologous recombination with the wild-type gene. After selection, positive ES cells are introduced into blastocysts and implanted into foster mothers. Chimeric mice can be identified based on the mixed coat color of the offspring. Heterozygous mice are bred to obtain mice homozygous for the mutant allele.

TABLE 62-3 GENETICALLY MODIFIED ANIMALS

Commonly Used Description	Technical Principle	Remarks
Transgenic	Pronuclear injection of transgene	Commonly used Genomic DNA or cDNA constructs Random integration of transgene Variable copy numbers of transgene Variable expression in each individual founder Gain-of-function models due to overexpression using tissue-specific promoters Loss-of-function models using anti-sense and dominant negative transgenes Inducible expression possible (Tetracycline, ecdysone) Applicable to several species
(Targeted) Knock-out	Substitution of functional gene with inactive gene by homologous recombination in embryonic stem cells	Predominantly used in mice Tissue-specific knock-out possible (Cre/lox) Absence of phenotype possible due to redundancy
(Targeted) Knock-in	Introduction of subtle mutation(s) into gene by substitution of endogenous gene with gene carrying a specific mutation. Homologous recombination in embryonic stem cells	Predominantly used in mice Can accurately model human disease
Forward genetics	Mutations created randomly by ENU (N-ethyl-N-nitrourea)	Selection of phenotype followed by genetic characterization Useful for identifying novel genes
Congenic strains	Mating of an inbred *donor* strain with a disease phenotype with an inbred *recipient* strain in order to define the genomic region responsible for the disorder	Useful for mapping disease-causing genes
Cloning	Introduction of nucleus into enucleated eggs (nuclear transfer)	Successful in several mammalian species including sheep (Dolly), mice, cows, monkeys Cloning of genetically identical individuals May affect life-span Ethical concerns

tein that is deleted in Duchenne muscular dystrophy, partially corrects the disorder in a mouse model of Duchenne's. Targeted expression of oncogenes has been valuable to study mechanisms of neoplasia and to generate immortalized cell lines. For example, expression of the simian virus 40 (SV40) large T antigen under the direction of the insulin promoter induces the formation of islet cell tumors.

The creation of gene knock-out and knock-in models takes advantage of the fact that a segment of DNA can be substituted by another that is identical (homologous), or nearly identical, by recombination. This permits integration of deletions that disrupt the gene (knock-out) or selected mutations (knock-in) into the target gene of choice. The transgene is introduced into embryonic stem (ES) cells by transfection and, after selection of cells with an integrated transgene, the positive ES cells are introduced into blastocysts and implanted into foster mothers. Chimeric mice can be identified based on the mixed coat color of the offspring. Heterozygous mice are bred to obtain mice homozygous for the mutant allele. This is particularly useful for genes that would be lethal if deleted universally or during early development. The list of genes that have been modified by this approach is very large.

Many of these knock-outs do not have an apparent phenotype, either because of redundant functions of the other genes or because the phenotype is subtle. For example, deletion of the hypoxanthine phosphoribosyltransferase (HPRT) gene (*Hprt*) does not cause characteristic features of Lesch-Nyhan syndrome in mice because of their reliance on adenine phosphoribosyltransferase (APRT) in the purine salvage pathway. Deletion of the retinoblastoma (*Rb*) gene encoding p105 does not lead to retinoblastoma or other tumors that characterize the human syndrome. However, mice with combinatorial deletion of several Rb-related proteins exhibit features similar to the human disorder. These examples underscore the fact that the functions of genes, and their interactions with genetic background and the environment, are not necessarily identical in mice and humans. On the other hand, the deletion of many genes pro-

vides a remarkably faithful model of human disorders. In addition to clarifying pathophysiology, these models facilitate the development of therapies, both genetic and pharmaceutical.

Many variations of these basic approaches now exist that allow genes to be expressed or deleted in specific cell types, at different times during development, or at varying levels. Consequently, transgenic technology has emerged as a powerful strategy for defining the physiologic effects of deleting or overexpressing a gene, as well as providing unique genetic models for dissecting pathophysiology or testing therapies. In addition to transgenic animal models, naturally occurring mutations in mice and other species continue to provide fundamental insights into human disease. A compendium of natural and transgenic animal models is provided in continuously evolving databases (Table 62-1).

IMPLICATIONS OF THE HUMAN GENOME PROJECT

The HGP was initiated in the mid-1980s as an ambitious effort to characterize the human genome, culminating in a complete DNA sequence. The initial main goals were (1) creation of genetic maps, (2) development of physical maps, and (3) determination of the complete human DNA sequence. Some analogies help in appreciating the scope of the HGP. The 23 pairs of human chromosomes encode ~30,000–40,000 genes. The total length of DNA is ~3 billion bp, which is nearly 1000-fold greater than that of the *E. coli* genome. If the human DNA sequence were printed out, it would correspond to about 120 volumes of *Harrison's Principles of Internal Medicine*.

The Genetic Map Given the size and complexity of the human genome, initial efforts aimed at developing genetic maps to provide orientation and to delimit where a gene of interest may be located. A *genetic map* describes the order of genes and defines the position of a gene relative to other loci on the same chromosome. It is constructed by assessing how frequently two markers are inherited together (i.e., *linked*) by association studies. Distances of the genetic map are expressed in recombination units, or centiMorgans (cM). One cM corresponds to a recombination frequency of 1% between two polymorphic markers; 1 cM corresponds to ~1 Mb of DNA (Fig. 62-3). Any polymorphic sequence variation can be useful for mapping purposes. Examples of polymorphic markers include variable number of tandem repeats (VNTRs), RFLPs, microsatellite repeats, and SNPs; the latter two methods are now used predominantly because of the high density of markers and because they are amenable to automated procedures.

The Physical Map Cytogenetics and chromosomal banding techniques provide a relatively low-resolution microscopic view of genetic loci. Physical maps indicate the position of a locus or gene in absolute values. Sequence-tagged sites (STSs) are used as a standard unit for physical mapping and serve as sequence-specific landmarks for arranging overlapping cloned fragments in the same order as they occur in the genome. These overlapping clones allow the characterization of contiguous DNA sequences, commonly referred to as *contigs*. This approach led to high-resolution physical maps by cloning the whole genome into overlapping fragments and has been essential for the identification of disease-causing genes by positional cloning.

SNPs
(612,977)

Known Genes
(1260)

Chromosome 7

p22.3 p22.1 p21.3 p21.1 p15.3 p15.1 p14.3 p14.1 p13 p12.3 p12.1 p11.2 q11.21 q11.22 q11.23 q21.11 q21.13 q21.3 q22.1 q22.3 q31.1 q31.31 q31.33 q32.1 q33 q34 q35 q36.1 q36.3

116.90 Mb   116.94 Mb   116.98 Mb   117.02 Mb   117.06 Mb

← 200 Kb →

CFTR Gene

← 20 Kb →

SNPs

■ Intronic   ■ Splice site

■ Coding region, synonymous   ■ Coding region, non-synonymous   ■ Coding region, frameshift

FIGURE 62-7 Chromosome 7 is shown with the density of single nucleotide polymorphisms (SNPs) and genes above. A 200-kb region in 7q31.2 containing the *CFTR* gene is shown below. The *CFTR* gene contains 27 exons. More than 1420 mutations in this gene have been found in patients with cystic fibrosis. A 20-kb region encompassing exons 4–9 is shown in further amplified in order to illustrate the SNPs in this region.

Recent insights into the structure of the normal human genome show that certain blocks of DNA sequences, often containing numerous genes, can be duplicated one or several times. This *copy number variation* (CNV), which tends to vary in a specific manner among different populations, is associated with hot spots of chromosomal rearrangements and is thought to play an important role in normal human variation and in genetic disease.

The identification of the ~10 million SNPs estimated to occur in the human genome has generated a catalogue of common genetic variants that occur in human beings from distinct ethnic backgrounds (Fig. 62-7). SNPs that are in close proximity are inherited together, i.e., they are linked, and are referred to as *haplotypes*, hence the name HapMap (Fig. 62-8). The HapMap describes the nature and location of these SNP haplotypes and how they are distributed among individuals within and among populations. The HapMap information is greatly facilitating genome-wide association studies designed to elucidate the complex interactions among multiple genes and lifestyle factors in multifactorial disorders (see below). Moreover, haplotype analyses may become useful to assess variations in responses to medications (*pharmacogenomics*) and environmental factors, as well as the prediction of disease predisposition.

The Human DNA Sequence The complete DNA sequence of each chromosome provides the highest resolution physical map. The primary focus of the HGP was to obtain DNA sequence for the entire human genome as well as model organisms. Although the prospect of

Recombination
Multiple generations →

SNP	1	2	3	4	5	6	7	8	9	10	11	12	13	14	15	16
Haplotype 1	A	A	G	T	C	A	G	G	C	A	C	T	C	A	A	G
Haplotype 2	G	G	T	C	A	G	A	T	C	A	C	T	C	A	A	G
Haplotype 3	A	A	G	T	C	A	G	G	T	G	G	C	A	G	C	T
Haplotype 4	G	G	T	C	A	G	A	T	C	A	G	C	A	G	C	T
Haplotype 5	A	A	G	T	C	A	A	T	C	A	C	T	C	A	A	G
Haplotype 6	G	G	T	C	A	G	G	G	T	G	C	T	C	A	A	G

Tag SNP G $\frac{G}{T}$ $\frac{C}{T}$ $\frac{A}{G}$

FIGURE 62-8 The origin of haplotypes is due to repeated recombination events occurring in multiple generations. Over time, this leads to distinct haplotypes. These haplotype blocks can often be characterized by genotyping selected Tag single nucleotide polymorphisms, an approach that now facilitates performing genome-wide association studies.

determining the complete sequence of the human genome seemed daunting several years ago, technical advances in DNA sequencing and bioinformatics led to the completion of a draft human sequence in June 2000, well in advance of the original goal year of 2003. High-quality reference sequences, completed in 2003, further closed gaps and reduced remaining ambiguities, and the HGP announced the completion of the DNA sequence for the last of the human chromosomes in May 2006. In addition to the human genome, the whole genomes of >2000 organisms have been sequenced partially or completely [Genomes Online Database (GOLD); Table 62-1]. They include, among others, eukaryotes such as man and mouse; *S. cerevisiae*, *C. elegans*, and *D. melanogaster*; bacteria (e.g., *E. coli*); and archeae, viruses, organelles (mitochondriae, chloroplasts), and plants (e.g., *Arabidopsis thaliana*). This information, together with technological advances and refinement of computational bioinformatics, has led to a fast-paced transition from the study of single genes to whole genomes. The current directions arising from the HGP include, among others, (1) the comparison of entire genomes (*comparative genomics*), (2) the study of large-scale expression of RNAs (*functional genomics)* and proteins (*proteomics*) in order to detect differences between various tissues in health and disease, (3) the characterization of the variation among individuals by establishing catalogues of sequence variations and SNPs (HapMap project), and (4) the identification of genes that play critical roles in the development of polygenic and multifactorial disorders.

Ethical Issues   Implicit in the HGP is the idea and hope that identifying disease-causing genes can lead to improvements in diagnosis, treatment, and prevention. It is estimated that most individuals harbor several serious recessive genes. However, completion of the human genome sequence, determination of the association of genetic defects with disease, and studies of genetic variation raise many new issues with implications for the individual and mankind. The controversies concerning the cloning of mammals and the establishment of human ES cells underscore the relevance of these questions. Moreover, the information gleaned from genotypic results can have quite different impacts, depending on the availability of strategies to modify the course of disease. For example, the identification of mutations that cause multiple endocrine neoplasia (MEN) type 2 or hemochromatosis allows specific interventions for affected family members. On the other hand, at present, the identification of an Alzheimer or Huntington disease gene does not alter therapy and outcomes. In addition, the progress in this area is unpredictable, as underscored by the finding that angiotensin II receptor blockers may slow disease progression in Marfan syndrome.

Genetic test results can generate anxiety in affected individuals and family members, and there is the possibility of discrimination on the basis of the test results. Most genetic disorders are likely to fall into an intermediate category where the opportunity for prevention or treatment is significant but limited (Chap. 64). For these reasons, the scientific components of the HGP have been paralleled by efforts to examine ethical and legal implications as new issues arise. About 5% of the HGP budget has been allocated to studies addressing the ethical, legal, and social implications associated with the increasing knowledge about the human genome and the genetic basis of disease.

Many issues raised by the genome project are familiar, in principle, to medical practitioners. For example, an asymptomatic patient with increased low-density lipoprotein (LDL) cholesterol, high blood pressure, or a strong family history of early myocardial infarction is known to be at increased risk of coronary heart disease. In such cases, it is clear that the identification of risk factors and an appropriate intervention are beneficial. Likewise, patients with phenylketonuria, cystic fibrosis, or sickle cell anemia are often identified as having a genetic disease early in life. These precedents can be helpful for adapting policies that relate to genetic information. We can anticipate similar efforts, whether based on genotypes or other markers of genetic predisposition, to be applied to many disorders. One confounding aspect of the rapid expansion of information is that our ability to make clinical decisions often lags behind initial insights into genetic mechanisms of disease. For example, when genes that predispose to breast cancer, such as *BRCA1*, are described, they generate tremendous public interest in the potential to predict disease, but many years of clinical research are still required to rigorously establish genotype and phenotype correlations.

Whether related to informed consent, participation in research, or the management of a genetic disorder that affects an individual or their families, there is a great need for more information about fundamental principles of genetics. The pervasive nature of the role of genetics in medicine makes it imperative for physicians and other health care professionals to become more informed about genetics and to provide advice and counseling in conjunction with trained genetic counselors (Chap. 64). The application of screening and prevention strategies will therefore require intensive patient and physician education, changes in health care financing, and legislation to protect patient's rights.

TRANSMISSION OF GENETIC DISEASE

Origins and Types of Mutations   A *mutation* can be defined as any change in the primary nucleotide sequence of DNA regardless of its functional consequences. Some mutations may be lethal, others are less deleterious, and some may confer an evolutionary advantage. Mutations can occur in the germline (sperm or oocytes); these can be transmitted to progeny. Alternatively, mutations can occur during embryogenesis or in somatic tissues. Mutations that occur during development lead to *mosaicism*, a situation in which tissues are composed of cells with different genetic constitutions. If the germline is mosaic, a mutation can be transmitted to some progeny but not others, which sometimes leads to confusion in assessing the pattern of inheritance. Somatic mutations that do not affect cell survival can sometimes be detected because of variable phenotypic effects in tissues (e.g., pigmented lesions in McCune-Albright syndrome). Other somatic mutations are associated with neoplasia because they confer a growth advantage to cells. Epigenetic events, heritable changes that do not involve changes in gene sequence (e.g., altered DNA methylation), may influence gene expression or facilitate genetic damage. With the exception of triplet nucleotide repeats, which can expand (see below), mutations are usually stable.

Mutations are structurally diverse—they can involve the entire genome, as in triploidy (one extra set of chromosomes), or gross numerical or structural alterations in chromosomes or individual genes (Chap. 63). Large deletions may affect a portion of a gene or an entire gene, or, if several genes are involved, they may lead to a *contiguous gene syndrome*. Unequal crossing-over between homologous genes can result in fusion gene mutations, as illustrated by color blindness (Chap. 29). Mutations involving single nucleotides are referred to as *point mutations* (Fig. 62-5). Substitutions are called *transitions* if a purine is replaced by another purine base (A ↔ G) or if a pyrimidine is replaced by another pyrimidine (C ↔ T). Changes from a purine to a pyrimidine, or vice versa, are referred to as *transversions*. If the DNA sequence change occurs in a coding region and alters an amino acid, it is called a *missense mutation*. Depending on the functional consequences of such a missense mutation, amino acid substitutions in different regions of the protein can lead to distinct phenotypes. *Polymorphisms* are sequence variations that have a frequency of at least 1%. Usually, they do not result in a perceptible phenotype. Often they consist of single base-pair substitutions that do not alter the protein coding sequence because of the degenerate nature of the genetic code (synonymous polymorphism), although it is possible that some might alter mRNA stability, translation, or the amino acid sequence (nonsynonymous polymorphism) (Fig. 62-7). These types of base substitutions are encountered frequently during genetic testing and must be distinguished from true mutations that alter protein expression or function. Small nucleotide deletions or insertions cause a shift of the codon reading frame (*frameshift*). Most commonly, reading frame alterations result in an abnormal protein segment of variable length before termination of translation occurs at a stop codon (*nonsense mutation*) (Fig. 62-5). Mutations in intronic sequences or in exon junctions may destroy or create splice donor or splice acceptor sites. Mutations may also be found in the regulatory sequences of genes, resulting in reduced gene transcription.

MUTATION RATES As noted before, mutations represent an important cause of genetic diversity as well as disease. Mutation rates are difficult to determine in humans because many mutations are silent and because testing is often not adequate to detect the phenotypic consequences. Mutation rates vary in different genes but are estimated to occur at a rate of ~10^{-10}/bp per cell division. Germline mutation rates (as opposed to somatic mutations) are relevant in the transmission of genetic disease. Because the population of oocytes is established very early in development, only ~20 cell divisions are required for completed oogenesis, whereas spermatogenesis involves ~30 divisions by the time of puberty and 20 cell divisions each year thereafter. Consequently, the probability of acquiring new point mutations is much greater in the male germline than the female germline, in which rates of aneuploidy are increased (Chap. 63). Thus, the incidence of new point mutations in spermatogonia increases with paternal age (e.g., achondrodysplasia, Marfan syndrome, neurofibromatosis). It is estimated that about 1 in 10 sperm carries a new deleterious mutation. The rates for new mutations are calculated most readily for autosomal dominant and X-linked disorders and are ~10^{-5}–10^{-6}/locus per generation. Because most monogenic diseases are relatively rare, new mutations account for a significant fraction of cases. This is important in the context of genetic counseling, as a new mutation can be transmitted to the affected individual but does not necessarily imply that the parents are at risk to transmit the disease to other children. An exception to this is when the new mutation occurs early in germline development, leading to *gonadal mosaicism*.

UNEQUAL CROSSING-OVER Normally, DNA recombination in germ cells occurs with remarkable fidelity to maintain the precise junction sites for the exchanged DNA sequences (Fig. 62-3). However, mispairing of homologous sequences leads to unequal crossover, with gene duplication on one of the chromosomes and gene deletion on the other chromosome. A significant fraction of growth hormone (*GH*) gene deletions, for example, involve unequal crossing-over (Chap. 333). The *GH* gene is a member of a large gene cluster that includes a growth hormone variant gene as well as several structurally related chorionic somatomammotropin genes and pseudogenes (highly homologous but functionally inactive relatives of a normal gene). Because such gene clusters contain multiple homologous DNA sequences arranged in tandem, they are particularly prone to undergo recombination and, consequently, gene duplication or deletion. On the other hand, duplication of the *PMP22* gene because of unequal crossing-over results in increased gene dosage and type IA Charcot-Marie-Tooth disease. Unequal crossing-over resulting in deletion of *PMP22* causes a distinct neuropathy called *hereditary liability to pressure palsy* (Chap. 379).

Glucocorticoid-remediable aldosteronism (GRA) is caused by a rearrangement involving the genes that encode aldosterone synthase (*CYP11B2*) and steroid 11β-hydroxylase (*CYP11B1*), normally arranged in tandem on chromosome 8q. These two genes are 95% identical, predisposing to gene duplication and deletion by unequal crossing-over. The rearranged gene product contains the regulatory regions of 11β-hydroxylase fused to the coding sequence of aldosterone synthetase. Consequently, the latter enzyme is expressed in the adrenocorticotropic hormone (ACTH)-dependent zona fasciculata of the adrenal gland, resulting in overproduction of mineralocorticoids and hypertension (Chap. 336).

Gene conversion refers to a nonreciprocal exchange of homologous genetic information; it is probably more common than generally recognized. In human genetics, gene conversion has been used to explain how an internal portion of a gene is replaced by a homologous segment copied from another allele or locus; these genetic alterations may range from a few nucleotides to a few thousand nucleotides. As a result of gene conversion, it is possible for short DNA segments of two chromosomes to be identical, even though these sequences are distinct in the parents. A practical consequence of this phenomenon is that nucleotide substitutions can occur during gene conversion between related genes, often altering the function of the gene. In disease states, gene conversion often involves intergenic exchange of DNA between a gene and a related pseudogene. For example, the 21-hydroxylase gene (*CYP21A2*) is adjacent to a nonfunctional pseudogene (*CYP21A1P*). Many of the nucleotide substitutions that are found in the *CYP21A2* gene in patients with congenital adrenal hyperplasia correspond to sequences that are present in the *CYP21A1P* pseudogene, suggesting gene conversion as a mechanism of mutagenesis. In addition, mitotic gene conversion has been suggested as a mechanism to explain revertant mosaicism in which an inherited mutation is "corrected" in certain cells. For example, patients with autosomal recessive generalized atrophic benign epidermolysis bullosa have acquired reverse mutations in one of the two mutated *COL17A1* alleles, leading to clinically unaffected patches of skin.

INSERTIONS AND DELETIONS Though many instances of insertions and deletions occur as a consequence of unequal crossing-over, there is also evidence for internal duplication, inversion, or deletion of DNA sequences. The fact that certain deletions or insertions appear to occur repeatedly as independent events suggests that specific regions within the DNA sequence predispose to these errors. For example, certain regions of the *DMD* gene appear to be hot spots for deletions. Some regions within the human genome are rearrangement hot spots and lead to CNVs (see above).

ERRORS IN DNA REPAIR Because mutations caused by defects in DNA repair accumulate as somatic cells divide, these types of mutations are particularly important in the context of neoplastic disorders (Chap. 80). Several genetic disorders involving DNA repair enzymes underscore their importance. Patients with xeroderma pigmentosum have defects in DNA damage recognition or in the nucleotide excision and repair pathway (Chap. 83). Exposed skin is dry and pigmented and is extraordinarily sensitive to the mutagenic effects of ultraviolet irradiation. More than 10 different genes have been shown to cause the different forms of xeroderma pigmentosum. This finding is consistent with the earlier classification of this disease into different complementation groups in which normal function is rescued by the fusion of cells derived from two different forms of xeroderma pigmentosum.

Ataxia telangiectasia causes large telangiectatic lesions of the face, cerebellar ataxia, immunologic defects, and hypersensitivity to ionizing radiation (Chap. 368). The discovery of the ataxia telangiectasia mutated (*ATM*) gene reveals that it is homologous to genes involved in DNA repair and control of cell cycle checkpoints. Mutations in the *ATM* gene give rise to defects in meiosis as well as increasing susceptibility to damage from ionizing radiation. Fanconi's anemia is also associated with an increased risk of multiple acquired genetic abnormalities. It is characterized by diverse congenital anomalies and a strong predisposition to develop aplastic anemia and acute myelogenous leukemia (Chap. 104). Cells from these patients are susceptible to chromosomal breaks caused by a defect in genetic recombination. At least eight different complementation groups have been identified, and several loci and genes associated with Fanconi's anemia have been mapped or cloned. HNPCC (Lynch syndrome) is characterized by autosomal dominant transmission of colon cancer, young age (<50 years) of presentation, predisposition to lesions in the proximal large bowel, and associated malignancies such as uterine cancer and ovarian cancer. HNPCC is caused by mutations in one of several different mismatch repair (MMR) genes including MutS homologue 2 (*MSH2*), MutL homologue 1 (*MLH1*), and *MSH6* (Chap. 87). These enzymes are involved in the detection of nucleotide mismatches and in the recognition of slipped-strand trinucleotide repeats. Germline mutations in these genes lead to microsatellite instability and a high mutation rate in colon cancer. Genetic screening tests for this disorder are now being used for families considered to be at risk (Chap. 64). Recognition of HNPCC allows early screening with colonoscopy and the implementation of prevention strategies using nonsteroidal anti-inflammatory drugs.

DIPYRIMIDINE AND CPG SEQUENCES Certain DNA sequences are particularly susceptible to mutagenesis. Successive pyrimidine residues (e.g., T-T or C-C) are subject to the formation of ultraviolet light–induced photoadducts. If these pyrimidine dimers are not repaired by the nucleotide excision repair pathway, mutations will be introduced after DNA synthesis. The dinucleotide C-G, or CpG, is also a hot spot for a specific type of mutation. In this case, methylation of the cytosine is associated with an enhanced rate of deamination to uracil, which is then replaced with thymine. This C → T transition (or G → A on the opposite strand) accounts for at least one-third of point mutations associated with polymorphisms and mutations. Many of the *MSH2* mutations in HNPCC, for example, involve CpG sequences. In addition to the fact that certain types of mutations (C → T or G → A) are relatively common, the nature of the genetic code also results in overrepresentation of certain amino acid substitutions.

UNSTABLE DNA SEQUENCES *Trinucleotide repeats* may be unstable and expand beyond a critical number. Mechanistically, the expansion is thought to be caused by unequal recombination and slipped mispairing. A premutation represents a small increase in trinucleotide copy number. In subsequent generations, the expanded repeat may increase further in length and result in an increasingly severe phenotype, a process called *dynamic mutation* (see below for discussion of anticipation). Trinucleotide expansion was first recognized as a cause of the fragile X syndrome, one of the most common causes of mental retardation. Other disorders arising from a similar mechanism include Huntington disease (Chap. 365), X-linked spinobulbar muscular atrophy (Chap. 369), and myotonic dystrophy (Chap. 382). Malignant cells are also characterized by genetic instability, indicating a breakdown in mechanisms that regulate DNA repair and the cell cycle.

Functional Consequences of Mutations Functionally, mutations can be broadly classified as gain-of-function and loss-of-function mutations. Gain-of-function mutations are typically dominant, i.e., they result in phenotypic alterations when a single allele is affected. Inactivating mutations are usually recessive, and an affected individual is homozygous or compound heterozygous (e.g., carrying two different mutant alleles of the same gene) for the disease-causing mutations. Alternatively, mutation in a single allele can result in *haploinsufficiency*, a situation in which one normal allele is not sufficient to maintain a normal phenotype. Haploinsufficiency is a commonly observed mechanism in diseases associated with mutations in transcription factors (Table 62-2). Remarkably, the clinical features among patients with an identical mutation in a transcription factor often vary significantly. One mechanism underlying this variability consists in the influence of modifying genes. Haploinsufficiency can also affect the expression of rate-limiting enzymes. For example, haploinsufficiency in enzymes involved in heme synthesis can cause porphyrias (Chap. 352).

An increase in dosage of a gene product may also result in disease, as illustrated by the duplication of the *DAX1* gene in dosage-sensitive sex-reversal (Chap. 343). Mutation in a single allele can also result in loss of function due to a dominant-negative effect. In this case, the mutated allele interferes with the function of the normal gene product by one of several different mechanisms: (1) a mutant protein may interfere with the function of a multimeric protein complex, as illustrated by mutations in type 1 collagen (*COL1A1*, *COL1A2*) genes in osteogenesis imperfecta (Chap. 357); (2) a mutant protein may occupy binding sites on proteins or promoter response elements, as illustrated by thyroid hormone resistance, a disorder in which inactivated thyroid hormone receptor binds to target genes and functions as an antagonist of normal receptors (Chap. 335); or (3) a mutant protein can be cytotoxic as in α_1 antitrypsin deficiency (Chap. 254) or autosomal dominant neurohypophyseal diabetes insipidus (Chap. 334), in which the abnormally folded proteins are trapped within the endoplasmic reticulum and ultimately cause cellular damage.

Genotype and Phenotype · ALLELES, GENOTYPES, AND HAPLOTYPES An observed trait is referred to as a *phenotype*; the genetic information defining the phenotype is called the *genotype*. Alternative forms of a gene or a genetic marker are referred to as *alleles*. Alleles may be polymorphic variants of nucleic acids that have no apparent effect on gene expression or function. In other instances, these variants may have subtle effects on gene expression, thereby conferring the adaptive advantages associated with genetic diversity. On the other hand, allelic variants may reflect mutations in a gene that clearly alter its function. The common Glu6Val (E6V) sickle cell mutation in the β-*globin* gene and the ΔF508 deletion of phenylalanine (F) in the *CFTR* gene are examples of allelic variants of these genes that result in disease. Because each individual has two copies of each chromosome (one inherited from the mother and one inherited from the father), he or she can have only two alleles at a given locus. However, there can be many different alleles in the population. The normal or common allele is usually referred to as *wild type*. When alleles at a given locus are identical, the individual is *homozygous*. Inheriting identical copies of a mutant allele occurs in many autosomal recessive disorders, particularly in circumstances of consanguinity. If the alleles are different on the maternal and the paternal copy of the gene, the individual is *heterozygous* at this locus (Fig. 62-5). If two different mutant alleles are inherited at a given locus, the individual is said to be a *compound heterozygote*. *Hemizygous* is used to describe males with a mutation in an X chromosomal gene or a female with a loss of one X chromosomal locus.

Genotypes describe the specific alleles at a particular locus. For example, there are three common alleles (E2, E3, E4) of the apolipoprotein E (*APOE*) gene. The genotype of an individual can therefore be described as *APOE3/4* or *APOE4/4* or any other variant. These designations indicate which alleles are present on the two chromosomes in the *APOE* gene at locus 19q13.2. In other cases, the genotype might be assigned arbitrary numbers (e.g., 1/2) or letters (e.g., B/b) to distinguish different alleles.

A *haplotype* refers to a group of alleles that are closely linked together at a genomic locus (Fig. 62-8). Haplotypes are useful for tracking the transmission of genomic segments within families and for detecting evidence of genetic recombination, if the crossover event occurs between the alleles (Fig. 62-3). As an example, various alleles at the histocompatibility locus antigen (HLA) on chromosome 6p are used to establish haplotypes associated with certain disease states. For example, 21-hydroxylase deficiency, complement deficiency, and hemochromatosis are each associated with specific HLA haplotypes. It is now recognized that these genes lie in close vicinity to the HLA locus, which explains why HLA associations were identified even before the disease genes were cloned and localized. In other cases, specific HLA associations with diseases such as ankylosing spondylitis (HLA-B27) or type 1 diabetes mellitus (HLA-DR4) reflect the role of specific HLA allelic variants in susceptibility to these autoimmune diseases. The recent characterization of common SNP haplotypes in four populations from different parts of the world through the HapMap project is providing a novel tool for association studies designed to detect genes involved in the pathogenesis of complex disorders (Table 62-1). The presence or absence of certain haplotypes may also become relevant for the customized choice of medical therapies (pharmacogenomics) or for preventative strategies.

ALLELIC HETEROGENEITY *Allelic heterogeneity* refers to the fact that different mutations in the same genetic locus can cause an identical or similar phenotype. For example, many different mutations of the β-globin locus can cause β-thalassemia (Table 62-4) (Fig. 62-4). In essence, allelic heterogeneity reflects the fact that many different mutations are capable of altering protein structure and function. For this reason, maps of inactivating mutations in genes usually show a near-random distribution. Exceptions include: (1) a founder effect, in which a particular mutation that does not affect reproductive capacity can be traced to a single individual; (2) "hot spots" for mutations, in which the nature of the DNA sequence predisposes to a recurring mutation; and (3) localization of mutations to certain domains that are particularly critical for protein function. Allelic heterogeneity creates a practical problem for genetic testing because one must often examine the entire genetic locus for mutations, as these can differ in each pa-

TABLE 62-4 SELECTED EXAMPLES OF LOCUS HETEROGENEITY AND PHENOTYPIC HETEROGENEITY

Phenotypic Heterogeneity

Gene, Protein	Phenotype	Inheritance	OMIM
LMNA, Lamin A/C	Emery–Dreifuss muscular dystrophy (AD)	AD	181350
	Familial partial lipodystrophy Dunnigan	AD	151660
	Hutchinson-Gilford progeria	AD	176670
	Atypical Werner syndrome	AD	150330
	Dilated cardiomyopathy	AD	115200
	Early-onset atrial fibrillation	AD	607554
	Emery–Dreifuss muscular dystrophy (AR)	AR	604929
	Limb-girdle muscular dystrophy type 1B	AR	159001
	Charcot-Marie-Tooth type 2B1	AR	605588
KRAS	Noonan syndrome	AD	163950
	Cardio-facio-cutaneous syndrome	AD	115150

Locus Heterogeneity

Phenotype	Gene	Chromosomal Location	Protein
Familial hypertrophic cardiomyopathy			
Genes encoding sarcomeric proteins	MYH7	14q12	Myosin heavy chain beta
	TNNT2	1q2	Troponin-T2
	TPM1	15q22.1	Tropomyosin alpha
	MYBPC3	11p11q	Myosin binding protein C
	TNNI3	19q13.4	Troponin 1
	MYL2	12q23-24.3	Myosin light chain 2
	MYL3	3p	Myosin light chain 3
	TTN	2q24.3	Cardiac titin
	ACTC	15q11	Cardiac alpha actin
	MYH6	14q1	Myosin heavy chain alpha
	MYLK2	20q13.3	Myosin light-peptide kinase
	CAV3	3p25	Caveolin 3
Genes encoding nonsarcomeric proteins	MTT1	Mitochondrial	tRNA isoleucine
	MTTG	Mitochondrial	tRNA glycine
	PRKAG2	7q35-q36	AMP-activated protein kinase γ2 subunit
	DMPK	19q13.2-13.3	Myotonin protein kinase (myotonic dystrophy)
	FRDA	9q13	Frataxin (Friedreich ataxia)
Polycystic kidney disease	PKD1	16p13.3-13.12	Polycystin 1 (AD)
	PKD2	4q21.-23	Polycystin 2 (AD)
	PKHD1	6p21.1-p12	Fibrocystin (AR)
Noonan syndrome	PTPN11	12q24.1	Protein-tyrosine phosphatase 2c
	KRAS	12p12.1	KRAS

Note: AD, autosomal dominant; AR, autosomal recessive.

tient. For example, there are >1400 reported mutations in the *CFTR* gene (Fig. 62-7). The mutational analysis initially focuses on a panel of mutations that are particularly frequent (often taking the ethnic background of the patient into account), but a negative result does not exclude the presence of a mutation elsewhere in the gene. One should also be aware that mutational analyses generally focus on the coding region of a gene without considering regulatory and intronic regions. Because disease-causing mutations may be located outside the coding regions, negative results should be interpreted with caution.

PHENOTYPIC HETEROGENEITY *Phenotypic heterogeneity* occurs when more than one phenotype is caused by allelic mutations (e.g., different mutations in the same gene) (Table 62-4). For example, laminopathies are monogenic multisystem disorders that result from mutations in the *LMNA* gene, which encodes the nuclear lamins A and C. Twelve autosomal dominant and four autosomal recessive disorders are caused by mutations in the *LMNA* gene. They include several forms of lipodystrophies, Emery-Dreifuss muscular dystrophy, progeria syndromes, a form of neuronal Charcot-Marie-Tooth disease (type 2B1), and a group of overlapping syndromes. Remarkably, hierarchical cluster analysis has revealed that the phenotypes vary depending on the position of the mutation. Similarly, identical mutations in the *FGFR2* gene can result in very distinct phenotypes: Crouzon syndrome (craniofacial synostosis), or Pfeiffer syndrome (acrocephalopolysyndactyly).

LOCUS OR NONALLELIC HETEROGENEITY AND PHENOCOPIES *Nonallelic or locus heterogeneity* refers to the situation in which a similar disease phenotype results from mutations at different genetic loci. This often occurs when more than one gene product produces different subunits of an interacting complex or when different genes are involved in the same genetic cascade or physiologic pathway. For example, osteogenesis imperfecta can arise from mutations in two different procollagen genes (*COL1A1* or *COL1A2*) that are located on different chromosomes (Chap. 357). The effects of inactivating mutations in these two genes are similar because the protein products comprise different subunits of the helical collagen fiber. Similarly, muscular dystrophy syndromes can be caused by mutations in various genes, consistent with the fact that it can be transmitted in an X-linked (Duchenne or Becker), autosomal dominant (limb-girdle muscular dystrophy type 1), or autosomal recessive (limb-girdle muscular dystrophy type 2) manner (Chap. 382). Mutations in the X-linked *DMD* gene, which encodes dystrophin, are the most common cause of muscular dystrophy. This feature reflects the large size of the gene as well as the fact that the phenotype is expressed in hemizygous males because they have only a single copy of the X chromosome. Dystrophin is associated with a large protein complex linked to the membrane-associated cytoskeleton in muscle. Mutations in several different components of this protein complex can also cause muscular dystrophy syndromes. Although the phenotypic features of some of these disorders are distinct, the phenotypic spectrum caused by mutations in different genes overlaps, thereby leading to nonallelic heterogeneity. It should be noted that mutations in dystrophin also cause allelic heterogeneity. For example, mutations in the *DMD* gene can cause either Duchenne or the less severe Becker muscular dystrophy, depending on the severity of the protein defect.

Recognition of nonallelic heterogeneity is important for several reasons: (1) the ability to identify disease loci in linkage studies is reduced by including patients with similar phenotypes but different genetic disorders; (2) genetic testing is more complex because several different genes need to be considered along with the possibility of different mutations in each of the candidate genes; and (3) novel information is gained about how genes or proteins interact, providing unique insights into molecular physiology.

Phenocopies refer to circumstances in which nongenetic conditions mimic a genetic disorder. For example, features of toxin- or drug-induced neurologic syndromes can resemble those seen in Huntington disease, and vascular causes of dementia share phenotypic features with familial forms of Alzheimer dementia (Chap. 365). Children born with activating mutations of the thyroid-stimulating hormone receptor (TSH-R) exhibit goiter and thyrotoxicosis similar to that seen in neonatal Graves' disease, which is caused by the transfer of maternal autoantibodies to the fetus (Chap. 335). As in nonallelic heterogeneity, the presence of phenocopies has the potential to confound linkage studies and genetic testing. Patient history and subtle differences in phenotype can often provide clues that distinguish these disorders from related genetic conditions.

VARIABLE EXPRESSIVITY AND INCOMPLETE PENETRANCE The same genetic mutation may be associated with a phenotypic spectrum in different

CHAPTER 62 Principles of Human Genetics

affected individuals, thereby illustrating the phenomenon of *variable expressivity*. This may include different manifestations of a disorder variably involving different organs (e.g., MEN), the severity of the disorder (e.g., cystic fibrosis), or the age of disease onset (e.g., Alzheimer dementia). MEN-1 illustrates several of these features. Families with this autosomal dominant disorder develop tumors of the parathyroid gland, endocrine pancreas, and the pituitary gland (Chap. 345). However, the pattern of tumors in the different glands, the age at which tumors develop, and the types of hormones produced vary among affected individuals, even within a given family. In this example, the phenotypic variability arises, in part, because of the requirement for a second mutation in the normal copy of the *MEN1* gene, as well as the large array of different cell types that are susceptible to the effects of *MEN1* gene mutations. In part, variable expression reflects the influence of modifier genes, or genetic background, on the effects of a particular mutation. Even in identical twins, in whom the genetic constitution is essentially the same, one can occasionally see variable expression of a genetic disease.

Interactions with the environment can also influence the course of a disease. For example, the manifestations and severity of hemochromatosis can be influenced by iron intake (Chap. 351), and the course of phenylketonuria is affected by exposure to phenylalanine in the diet (Chap. 358). Other metabolic disorders, such as hyperlipidemias and porphyria, also fall into this category. Many mechanisms, including genetic effects and environmental influences, can therefore lead to variable expressivity. In genetic counseling, it is particularly important to recognize this variability, as one cannot always predict the course of disease, even when the mutation is known.

Penetrance refers to the proportion of individuals with a mutant genotype that express the phenotype. If all carriers of a mutant express the phenotype, penetrance is complete, whereas it is said to be *incomplete* or *reduced* if some individuals do not have any features of the phenotype. Dominant conditions with incomplete penetrance are characterized by skipping of generations with unaffected carriers transmitting the mutant gene. For example, hypertrophic obstructive cardiomyopathy (HCM) caused by mutations in the *myosin-binding protein C* gene is a dominant disorder with clinical features in only a subset of patients who carry the mutation (Chap. 231). Patients who have the mutation but no evidence of the disease can still transmit the disorder to subsequent generations. In many conditions with postnatal onset, the proportion of gene carriers who are affected varies with age. Thus, when describing penetrance, one has to specify age. For example, for disorders such as Huntington disease or familial amyotrophic lateral sclerosis, which present late in life, the rate of penetrance is influenced by the age at which the clinical assessment is performed. *Imprinting* can also modify the penetrance of a disease (see below). For example, in patients with Albright hereditary osteodystrophy, mutations in the Gsα subunit (*GNAS1* gene) are expressed clinically only in individuals who inherit the mutation from their mother (Chap. 347).

SEX-INFLUENCED PHENOTYPES   Certain mutations affect males and females quite differently. In some instances, this is because the gene resides on the X or Y sex chromosomes (X-linked disorders and Y-linked disorders). As a result, the phenotype of mutated X-linked genes will be expressed fully in males but variably in heterozygous females, depending on the degree of X-inactivation and the function of the gene. For example, most heterozygous female carriers of factor VIII deficiency (hemophilia A) are asymptomatic because sufficient factor VIII is produced to prevent a defect in coagulation (Chap. 110). On the other hand, some females heterozygous for the X-linked lipid storage defect caused by α-galactosidase A deficiency (Fabry disease) experience mild manifestations of painful neuropathy, as well as other features of the disease (Chap. 355). Because only males have a Y chromosome, mutations in genes such as *SRY*, which causes male-to-female sex-reversal, or *DAZ* (deleted in azoospermia), which causes abnormalities of spermatogenesis, are unique to males (Chap. 343).

Other diseases are expressed in a sex-limited manner because of the differential function of the gene product in males and females. Activat-ing mutations in the luteinizing hormone receptor cause dominant male-limited precocious puberty in boys (Chap. 340). The phenotype is unique to males because activation of the receptor induces testosterone production in the testis, whereas it is functionally silent in the immature ovary. Biallelic inactivating mutations of the follicle-stimulating hormone (FSH) receptor cause primary ovarian failure in females because the follicles do not develop in the absence of FSH action. In contrast, affected males have a more subtle phenotype, because testosterone production is preserved (allowing sexual maturation) and spermatogenesis is only partially impaired (Chap. 340). In congenital adrenal hyperplasia, most commonly caused by 21-hydroxylase deficiency, cortisol production is impaired and ACTH stimulation of the adrenal gland leads to increased production of androgenic precursors (Chap. 336). In females, the increased androgen level causes ambiguous genitalia, which can be recognized at the time of birth. In males, the diagnosis may be made on the basis of adrenal insufficiency at birth, because the increased adrenal androgen level does not alter sexual differentiation, or later in childhood, because of the development of precocious puberty. Hemochromatosis is more common in males than in females, presumably because of differences in dietary iron intake and losses associated with menstruation and pregnancy in females (Chap. 351).

Chromosomal Disorders   Chromosomal or cytogenetic disorders are caused by numerical or structural aberrations in chromosomes. Deviations in chromosome number are common causes of abortions, developmental disorders, and malformations. *Contiguous gene syndromes*, i.e., large deletions affecting several genes, have been useful for identifying the location of new disease-causing genes. Because of the variable size of gene deletions in different patients, a systematic comparison of phenotypes and locations of deletion breakpoints allows positions of particular genes to be mapped within the critical genomic region. For discussion of disorders of chromosome number and structure, see Chap. 63.

Monogenic Mendelian Disorders   Monogenic human diseases are frequently referred to as *Mendelian disorders* because they obey the principles of genetic transmission originally set forth in Gregor Mendel's classic work. The continuously updated OMIM catalogue lists several thousand of these disorders and provides information about the clinical phenotype, molecular basis, allelic variants, and pertinent animal models (Table 62-1). The mode of inheritance for a given phenotypic trait or disease is determined by pedigree analysis. All affected and unaffected individuals in the family are recorded in a pedigree using standard symbols (Fig. 62-9). The principles of allelic segregation, and the transmission of alleles from parents to children, are illustrated in Fig. 62-10. One dominant (A) allele and one recessive (a) allele can display three Mendelian modes of inheritance: autosomal dominant, autosomal recessive, and X-chromosomal. About 65% of human monogenic disorders are autosomal dominant, 25% are autosomal recessive, and 5% are X-linked. Genetic testing is now available for many of these disorders and plays an increasingly important role in clinical medicine (Chap. 64).

AUTOSOMAL DOMINANT DISORDERS   Autosomal dominant disorders assume particular relevance because mutations in a single allele are sufficient to cause the disease. In contrast to recessive disorders, in which disease pathogenesis is relatively straightforward because there is loss of gene function, dominant disorders can be caused by various disease mechanisms, many of which are unique to the function of the genetic pathway involved.

In autosomal dominant disorders, individuals are affected in successive generations; the disease does not occur in the offspring of unaffected individuals. Males and females are affected with equal frequency because the defective gene resides on one of the 22 autosomes (Fig. 62-11A). Autosomal dominant mutations alter one of the two alleles at a given locus. Because the alleles segregate randomly at meiosis, the probability that an offspring will be affected is 50%. Unless there is a new germline mutation, an affected individual has an af-

FIGURE 62-9 **Standard pedigree symbols.**

fected parent. Children with a normal genotype do not transmit the disorder. Due to differences in penetrance or expressivity (see above), the clinical manifestations of autosomal dominant disorders may be variable. Because of these variations, it is sometimes challenging to determine the pattern of inheritance.

It should be recognized, however, that some individuals acquire a mutated gene from an unaffected parent. De novo germline mutations occur more frequently during later cell divisions in gametogenesis, which explains why siblings are rarely affected. As noted before, new germline mutations occur more frequently in fathers of advanced age. For example, the average age of fathers with new germline mutations that cause Marfan's syndrome is ~37 years, whereas fathers who transmit the disease by inheritance have an average age of ~30 years.

AUTOSOMAL RECESSIVE DISORDERS In recessive disorders, the mutated alleles result in a complete or partial loss of function. They frequently involve enzymes in metabolic pathways, receptors, or proteins in signaling cascades. In an autosomal recessive disease, the affected individual, who can be of either sex, is a homozygote or compound heterozygote for a single-gene defect. With a few important exceptions, autosomal recessive diseases are rare and often occur in the context of parental consanguinity. The relatively high frequency of certain recessive disorders, such as sickle cell anemia, cystic fibrosis, and thalassemia, is partially explained by a selective biologic advantage for the heterozygous state (see below). Though heterozygous carriers of a defective allele are usually clinically normal, they may display subtle differences in phenotype that only become apparent with more precise

FIGURE 62-10 **Segregation of alleles.** Segregation of genotypes in the offspring of parents with one dominant (A) and one recessive (a) allele. The distribution of the parental alleles to their offspring depends on the combination present in the parents. Filled symbols = affected individuals.

FIGURE 62-11 **Dominant, recessive, X-linked, and mitochondrial (matrilinear) inheritance.**

testing or in the context of certain environmental influences. In sickle cell anemia, for example, heterozygotes are normally asymptomatic. However, in situations of dehydration or diminished oxygen pressure, sickle cell crises can also occur in heterozygotes (Chap. 99).

In most instances, an affected individual is the offspring of heterozygous parents. In this situation, there is a 25% chance that the offspring will have a normal genotype, a 50% probability of a heterozygous state, and a 25% risk of homozygosity for the recessive alleles (Figs. 62-10, 62-11B). In the case of one unaffected heterozygous and one affected homozygous parent, the probability of disease increases to 50% for each child. In this instance, the pedigree analysis mimics an autosomal dominant mode of inheritance (*pseudodominance*). In contrast to autosomal dominant disorders, new mutations in recessive alleles are rarely manifest because they usually result in an asymptomatic carrier state.

X-LINKED DISORDERS Males have only one X chromosome; consequently, a daughter always inherits her father's X chromosome in addition to one of her mother's two X chromosomes. A son inherits the Y chromosome from his father and one maternal X chromosome. Thus, the characteristic features of X-linked inheritance are (1) the absence of father-to-son transmission, and (2) the fact that all daughters of an affected male are obligate carriers of the mutant allele (Fig. 62-11C). The risk of developing disease due to a mutant X-chromosomal gene differs in the two sexes. Because males have only one X chromosome, they are hemizygous for the mutant allele; thus, they are more likely to develop the mutant phenotype, regardless of whether the mutation is dominant or recessive. A female may be either heterozygous or homozygous for the mutant allele, which may be dominant or recessive. The terms *X-linked dominant* or *X-linked recessive* are therefore only applicable to expression of the mutant phenotype in women. In addition, the expression of X-chromosomal genes is influenced by X chromosome inactivation (see below).

Y-LINKED DISORDERS The Y chromosome has a relatively small number of genes. One such gene, the sex-region determining Y factor (*SRY*), which encodes the testis-determining factor (*TDF*), is crucial for normal male development. Normally there is infrequent exchange of sequences on the Y chromosome with the X chromosome. The *SRY* region is adjacent to the pseudoautosomal region, a chromosomal segment on the X and Y chromosomes with a high degree of homology. A crossing-over occasionally involves the *SRY* region with the distal tip of the X chromosome during meiosis in the male. Translocations can result in XY females with the Y chromosome lacking the *SRY* gene or XX males harboring the *SRY* gene on one of the X chromosomes (Chap. 343). Point mutations in the *SRY* gene may also result in individuals with an XY genotype and an incomplete female phenotype. Most of these mutations occur de novo. Men with oligospermia/azoospermia frequently have microdeletions on the long arm of the Y chromosome that involve one or more of the azoospermia factor (*AZF*) genes.

Exceptions to Simple Mendelian Inheritance Patterns • MITOCHONDRIAL DISORDERS

Mendelian inheritance refers to the transmission of genes encoded by DNA contained in the nuclear chromosomes. In addition, each mitochondrion contains several copies of a small circular chromosome. The mitochondrial DNA (mtDNA) is ~16.5 kb and encodes transfer and ribosomal RNAs and 13 proteins that are components of the respiratory chain involved in oxidative phosphorylation and ATP generation. The mitochondrial genome does not recombine and is inherited through the maternal line because sperm does not contribute significant cytoplasmic components to the zygote. A noncoding region of the mitochondrial chromosome, referred to as D-loop, is highly polymorphic. This property, together with the absence of mtDNA recombination, makes it a valuable tool for studies tracing human migration and evolution, and it is also used for specific forensic applications.

Inherited mitochondrial disorders are transmitted in a matrilineal fashion; all children from an affected mother will inherit the disease, but it will not be transmitted from an affected father to his children (Fig. 62-11*D*). Alterations in the mtDNA affecting enzymes required for oxidative phosphorylation lead to reduction of ATP supply, generation of free radicals, and induction of apoptosis. Several syndromic disorders arising from mutations in the mitochondrial genome are known in humans and they affect both protein-coding and tRNA genes (Table 62-1 and Table 62-5). The broad clinical spectrum often involves (cardio)myopathies and encephalopathies because of the high dependence of these tissues on oxidative phosphorylation. The age of onset and the clinical course are highly variable because of the unusual mechanisms of mtDNA transmission, which replicates independently from nuclear DNA. During cell replication, the proportion of wild-type and mutant mitochondria can drift among different cells and tissues. The resulting heterogeneity in the proportion of mitochondria with and without a mutation is referred to as *heteroplasmia* and underlies the phenotypic variability that is characteristic of mitochondrial diseases.

Acquired somatic mutations in mitochondria are thought to be involved in several age-dependent degenerative disorders affecting predominantly muscle and the peripheral and central nervous system (e.g., Alzheimer's and Parkinson's disease). Establishing that a mtDNA alteration is causal for a clinical phenotype is challenging because of the high degree of polymorphism in mtDNA and the phenotypic variability characteristic of these disorders. Certain pharmacologic treatments may have an impact on mitochondria and/or their function.

TABLE 62-5 SELECTED MITOCHONDRIAL DISEASES

Disease/Syndrome	OMIM #
MELAS syndrome: mitochondrial myopathy with encephalopathy, lactacidosis, and stroke	540000
Leber's optic atrophy: hereditary optical neuropathy	535000
Kearns-Sayre syndrome (KSS): ophthalmoplegia, pigmental degeneration of the retina, cardiomyopathy	530000
MERRF syndrome: myoclonic epilepsy and ragged-red fibers	545000
Neurogenic muscular weakness with ataxia and retinitis pigmentosa (NARP)	551500
Progressive external ophthalmoplegia (CEOP)	258470
Pearson syndrome (PEAR): bone marrow and pancreatic failure	557000
Autosomal dominant inherited mitochondrial myopathy with mitochondrial deletion (ADMIMY)	157640
Somatic mutations in cytochrome *b* gene: exercise intolerance, lactic acidosis, complex III deficiency, muscle pain, ragged-red fibers	516020

For example, treatment with the antiretroviral compound azidothymidine (AZT) causes an acquired mitochondrial myopathy through depletion of muscular mtDNA.

MOSAICISM Mosaicism refers to the presence of two or more genetically distinct cell lines in the tissues of an individual. It results from a mutation that occurs during embryonic, fetal, or extrauterine development. The developmental stage at which the mutation arises will determine whether germ cells and/or somatic cells are involved. Chromosomal mosaicism results from non-disjunction at an early embryonic mitotic division, leading to the persistence of more than one cell line, as exemplified by some patients with Turner syndrome (Chap. 343). Somatic mosaicism is characterized by a patchy distribution of genetically altered somatic cells. The McCune-Albright syndrome, for example, is caused by activating mutations in the stimulatory G protein α ($G_s\alpha$) that occur early in development (Chap. 347). The clinical phenotype varies depending on the tissue distribution of the mutation; manifestations include ovarian cysts that secrete sex steroids and cause precocious puberty, polyostotic fibrous dysplasia, café-au-lait skin pigmentation, growth hormone–secreting pituitary adenomas, and hypersecreting autonomous thyroid nodules (Chap. 341).

X-INACTIVATION, IMPRINTING, AND UNIPARENTAL DISOMY According to traditional Mendelian principles, the parental origin of a mutant gene is irrelevant for the expression of the phenotype. There are, however, important exceptions to this rule. *X-inactivation* prevents the expression of most genes on one of the two X-chromosomes in every cell of a female. Gene inactivation also occurs on selected chromosomal regions of autosomes. This phenomenon, referred to as *genomic imprinting*, leads to inheritable preferential expression of one of the parental alleles. It is of pathophysiologic importance in disorders where the transmission of disease is dependent on the sex of the transmitting parent and, thus, plays an important role in the expression of certain genetic disorders. Two classic examples are the Prader-Willi syndrome and Angelman syndrome (Chap. 63). Prader-Willi syndrome is characterized by diminished fetal activity, obesity, hypotonia, mental retardation, short stature, and hypogonadotropic hypogonadism. Deletions of the paternal copy of the Prader-Willi locus located on the short arm of chromosome 15 result in a contiguous gene syndrome involving missing paternal copies of the *necdin* and *SNRPN* genes, among others. In contrast, patients with Angelman syndrome, characterized by mental retardation, seizures, ataxia, and hypotonia, have deletions involving the maternal copy of this region on chromosome 15. These two syndromes may also result from *uniparental disomy*. In this case, the syndromes are not caused by deletions on chromosome 15 but by the inheritance of either two maternal chromosomes (Prader-Willi syndrome) or two paternal chromosomes (Angelman syndrome).

Imprinting and the related phenomenon of allelic exclusion may be more common than currently documented, as it is difficult to examine

TABLE 62-6 SELECTED TRINUCLEOTIDE REPEAT DISORDERS

Disease	Locus	Repeat	Triplet Length (Normal/Disease)	Inheritance	Gene Product
X-chromosomal spinobulbar muscular atrophy (SBMA)	Xq11-q12	CAG	11–34/40–62	XR	Androgen receptor
Fragile X-syndrome (FRAXA)	Xq27.3	CGG	6–50/200–300	XR	FMR-1 protein
Fragile X-syndrome (FRAXE)	Xq28	GCC	6–25/>200	XR	FMR-2 protein
Dystrophia myotonica (DM)	19q13.2-q13.3	CTG	5–30/200–1000	AD, variable penetrance	Myotonin protein kinase
Huntington disease (HD)	4p16.3	CAG	6–34/37–180	AD	Huntingtin
Spinocerebellar ataxia type 1 (SCA1)	6p21.3-21.2	CAG	6–39/40–88	AD	Ataxin 1
Spinocerebellar ataxia type 2 (SCA2)	12q24.1	CAG	15–31/34–400	AD	Ataxin 2
Spinocerebellar ataxia type 3 (SCA3); Machado Joseph disease (MD)	14q21	CAG	13–36/55–86	AD	Ataxin 3
Spinocerebellar ataxia type 6 (SCA6, CACNAIA)	19p13.1-13.2	CAG	4–16/20–33	AD	Alpha 1A voltage-dependent L-type calcium channel
Spinocerebellar ataxia type 7 (SCA7)	3p21.1-p12	CAG	4–19/37 to >300	AD	Ataxin 7
Spinocerebellar ataxia type 12 (SCA12)	5q31	CAG	6–26/66–78	AD	Protein phosphatase 2A
Dentorubral pallidoluysiane atrophy (DRPLA)	12p	CAG	7–23/49–75	AD	Atrophin 1
Friedreich ataxia (FRDA1)	9q13-21	GAA	7–22/200–900	AR	Frataxin

Note: AD, autosomal dominant; AR, autosomal recessive; XR, X-linked recessive.

levels of mRNA expression from the maternal and paternal alleles in specific tissues or in individual cells. Genomic imprinting, or uniparental disomy, is involved in the pathogenesis of several other disorders and malignancies (Chap. 63). For example, hydatidiform moles contain a normal number of diploid chromosomes, but they are all of paternal origin. The opposite situation occurs in ovarian teratomata, with 46 chromosomes of maternal origin. Expression of the imprinted gene for insulin-like growth factor II (IGF-II) is involved in the pathogenesis of the cancer-predisposing Beckwith-Wiedemann syndrome (BWS) (Chap. 79). These children show somatic overgrowth with organomegalies and hemihypertrophy, and they have an increased risk of embryonal malignancies such as Wilm's tumor. Normally, only the paternally derived copy of the IGF-II gene is active and the maternal copy is inactive. Imprinting of the IGF-II gene is regulated by H19, which encodes an RNA transcript that is not translated into protein. Disruption or lack of H19 methylation leads to a relaxation of IGF-II imprinting and expression of both alleles.

Meiotically and mitotically heritable changes in gene expression not associated with DNA sequence alterations are referred to as epigenetic effects. These changes involve DNA methylation, histone modifications, and RNA-mediated silencing, resulting in gene repression without a change in the coding sequence. Epigenetic alterations are increasingly recognized to play a role in human diseases such as cancer, mental retardation, hematologic disorders, and possibly in aging. For example, de novo methylation of CpG islands, regions of >500 bp in size with a GC content >55% in promoter regions that are normally unmethylated, is a hallmark of human cancers. Inhibitors of enzymes controlling epigenetic modifications such as histone deacetylases and DNA methyltransferases reverse gene silencing and represent a promising new group of antineoplastic agents.

SOMATIC MUTATIONS Cancer can be defined as a genetic disease at the cellular level (Chap. 79). Cancers are monoclonal in origin, indicating that they have arisen from a single precursor cell with one or several mutations in genes controlling growth (proliferation or apoptosis) and/or differentiation. These acquired somatic mutations are restricted to the tumor and its metastases and are not found in the surrounding normal tissue. The molecular alterations include dominant gain-of-function mutations in oncogenes, recessive loss-of-function mutations in tumor-suppressor genes and DNA repair genes, gene amplification, and chromosome rearrangements. Rarely, a single mutation in certain genes may be sufficient to transform a normal cell into a malignant cell. In most cancers, however, the development of a malignant phenotype requires several genetic alterations for the gradual progression from a normal cell to a cancerous cell, a phenomenon termed multistep carcinogenesis (Chaps. 79, 80). Most human tumors express telo-

merase, an enzyme formed of a protein and an RNA component, which adds telomere repeats at the ends of chromosomes during replication. This mechanism impedes shortening of the telomers, which is associated with senescence in normal cells, and is associated with enhanced replicative capacity in cancer cells. Telomerase inhibitors may provide a novel strategy for treating advanced human cancers.

In many cancer syndromes, there is an inherited predisposition to tumor formation. In these instances, a germline mutation is inherited in an autosomal dominant fashion inactivating one allele of an autosomal tumor-suppressor gene. If the second allele is inactivated by a somatic mutation or by epigenetic silencing in a given cell, this will lead to neoplastic growth (Knudson two-hit model). Thus, the defective allele in the germline is transmitted in a dominant mode, though tumorigenesis results from a biallelic loss of the tumor-suppressor gene in an affected tissue. The classic example to illustrate this phenomenon is retinoblastoma, which can occur as a sporadic or hereditary tumor. In sporadic retinoblastoma, both copies of the retinoblastoma (RB) gene are inactivated through two somatic events. In hereditary retinoblastoma, one mutated or deleted RB allele is inherited in an autosomal dominant manner and the second allele is inactivated by a subsequent somatic mutation. This two-hit model applies to other inherited cancer syndromes such as MEN-1 (Chap. 345) and neurofibromatosis type 2 (Chap. 374).

NUCLEOTIDE REPEAT EXPANSION DISORDERS Several diseases are associated with an increase in the number of nucleotide repeats above a certain threshold (Table 62-6). The repeats are sometimes located within the coding region of the genes, as in Huntington disease or the X-linked form of spinal and bulbar muscular atrophy (SBMA, Kennedy syndrome). In other instances, the repeats probably alter gene regulatory sequences. If an expansion is present, the DNA fragment is unstable and tends to expand further during cell division. The length of the nucleotide repeat often correlates with the severity of the disease. When repeat length increases from one generation to the next, disease manifestations may worsen or be observed at an earlier age; this phenomenon is referred to as anticipation. In Huntington disease, for example, there is a correlation between age of onset and length of the triplet codon expansion (Chap. 360). Anticipation has also been documented in other diseases caused by dynamic mutations in trinucleotide repeats (Table 62-6). The repeat number may also vary in a tissue-specific manner. In myotonic dystrophy, the CTG repeat may be tenfold greater in muscle tissue than in lymphocytes (Chap. 382).

Complex Genetic Disorders The expression of many common diseases such as cardiovascular disease, hypertension, diabetes, asthma, psychiatric disorders, and certain cancers is determined by a combination of ge-

CHAPTER 62

Principles of Human Genetics

TABLE 62-7   GENES AND LOCI INVOLVED IN MONO- AND POLYGENIC FORMS OF DIABETES

Disorder	Genes or Susceptibility Locus	Chromosomal Location	Other Factors
Monogenic forms of diabetes			
MODY 1	HNF4α (hepatocyte nuclear factor 4α)	20q12-q13.1	AD inheritance
MODY 1	GCK (glucokinase)	7p15-p13	
MODY 1	HNF1α (hepatocyte nuclear factor 1α)	12q24.2	
MODY 1	IPF1 (insulin receptor substrate)	13q12.1	
MODY 5 (renal cysts, diabetes)	HNF1β (hepatocyte nuclear factor 1β)	17cen-q21.3	
MODY 6	NeuroD1 (neurogenic differention factor 1)	2q32	
Diabetes mellitus type 2; loci and genes linked and/or associated with susceptibility for diabetes mellitus type 2	**Genes and loci identified by linkage/association studies**		
	CPN10 (Calpain-10)	2q37.3	Diet
	HNF4α (hepatocyte nuclear factor 4α)	20q12-q13.1	Energy expenditure
	PTPN1 (protein-tyrosine phosphatase)	20q13.1-q13.2	Obesity
	PKLR (liver pyruvate kinase)	1q21	
	CASQ1 (calsequestrin 1)	1q21	
	APM1 (adiponectin)	3q27	
	TCF7L2 (transcription factor 7-like 2)	10q25.3	
	1q21-23	1q21-23	
	2q	2q	
	3q22-27	3q22-27	
	8p21-23	8p21-23	
	11q	11q	
	12q24	12q24	
	15	15	
	18p11	18p11	
	20q	20q	
	20p	20p	
	Selected candidate genes with possible contribution		
	PPARγ (Peroxisome proliferator receptor γ)	3p25	
	KCNJ11(ATP-sensitive K channel Kir6.2)	11p15.1	
	ABCC8 (ATP-binding cassette, subfamily c, member 8)	11p15.1	
	Insulin VNTR	11p15	
	IRS-1 (insulin receptor substrate)	2q36	
	PGC1α (PPAR γ coactivatory α)	4p15.1	
	ENPP1 (ectonucleotide pyrophosphatase/phosphodiesterase 1)	6q22-23	

Note: MODY, maturity onset diabetes of the young; AD, autosomal dominant; VNTR, variable number of tandem repeats.

netic background, environmental factors, and lifestyle. A trait is called *polygenic* if multiple genes contribute to the phenotype or *multifactorial* if multiple genes are assumed to interact with environmental factors. Genetic models for these complex traits need to account for genetic heterogeneity and interactions with other genes and the environment. Complex genetic traits may be influenced by modifying genes that are not linked to the main gene involved in the pathogenesis of the trait. This type of gene-gene interaction, or *epistasis*, plays an important role in polygenic traits that require the simultaneous presence of variations in multiple genes to result in a pathologic phenotype.

Type 2 diabetes mellitus provides a paradigm for considering a multifactorial disorder, as genetic, nutritional, and lifestyle factors are intimately interrelated in disease pathogenesis (Table 62-7) (Chap. 338). The identification of genetic variations and environmental factors that either predispose to or protect against disease is essential for predicting disease risk, designing preventive strategies, and developing novel therapeutic approaches. The study of rare monogenic diseases may provide insight into some of genetic and molecular mechanisms important in the pathogenesis of complex diseases. For example, the identification of the hepatocyte nuclear factor α (HNFα) in maturity-onset of diabetes type 4 defined it as a *candidate gene* in the pathogenesis of diabetes mellitus type 2 (Tables 62-2 and 62-8). Genome scans have identified various loci that may be associated with susceptibility to development of diabetes mellitus in certain populations. Efforts to identify susceptibility genes require very large sample sizes, and positive results may depend on ethnicity, ascertainment criteria, and statistical analysis. Association studies analyzing the potential influence of (biologically functional) SNPs and SNP haplotypes on a particular phenotype are a promising approach for the detection of involved genes.

Linkage and Association Studies   There are two primary strategies for mapping genes that cause or increase susceptibility to human disease: (1) classic linkage can be performed based on a known genetic model

or, when the model is unknown, by studying pairs of affected relatives; or (2) disease genes can be mapped using allelic association studies (Table 62-8).

GENETIC LINKAGE   *Genetic linkage* refers to the fact that genes are physically connected, or linked, to one another along the chromosomes. Two fundamental principles are essential for understanding the concept of linkage: (1) when two genes are close together on a chromosome, they are usually transmitted together, unless a recombination event separates them (Figs. 62-3, 62-8); and (2) the odds of a crossover, or recombination event, between two linked genes is proportional to the distance that separates them. Thus, genes that are further apart are more likely to undergo a recombination event than genes that are very close together. The detection of chromosomal loci that segregate with a disease by linkage can be used to identify the gene responsible for the disease (*positional cloning*) and to predict the odds of disease gene transmission in genetic counseling.

Polymorphisms are essential for linkage studies because they provide a means to distinguish the maternal and paternal chromosomes in an individual. On average, 1 out of every 1000 bp varies from one person to the next. Although this degree of variation seems low (99.9% identical), it means that >3 million sequence differences exist between any two unrelated individuals and the probability that the sequence at such loci will differ on the two homologous chromosomes is high (often >70–90%). These sequence variations include VNTRs, short tandem repeats (STRs), and SNPs. Most STRs, also called *polymorphic microsatellite markers*, consist of di-, tri-, or tetranucleotide repeats that can be measured readily using PCR (Fig. 62-12). Characterization of SNPs, using DNA chips, provides an important new tool for comprehensive analyses of genetic variation, linkage, and association studies. Although these sequence variations usually have no apparent functional consequences, they provide much of the basis for variation in genetic traits.

TABLE 62-8 **GENETIC APPROACHES FOR IDENTIFYING DISEASE GENES**

Method	Indications and Advantages	Limitations
Linkage Studies		
Classical linkage analysis (parametric methods)	Analysis of monogenic traits Suitable for genome scan Control population not required Useful for multifactorial disorders in isolated populations	Difficult to collect large informative pedigrees Difficult to obtain sufficient statistical power for complex traits
Allele-sharing methods (nonparametric methods) Affected sib and relative pair analyses Sib pair analysis	Suitable for identification of susceptibility genes in polygenic and multifactorial disorders Suitable for genome scan Control population not required if allele frequencies are known Statistical power can be increased by including parents and relatives	Difficult to collect sufficient number of subjects Difficult to obtain sufficient statistical power for complex traits Reduced power compared to classical linkage, but not sensitive to specification of genetic mode
Association Studies		
Case-control studies Linkage disequilibrium Transmission disequilibrium test (TDT) Whole-genome association studies	Suitable for identification of susceptibility genes in polygenic and multifactorial disorders Suitable for testing specific allelic variants of known candidate loci Facilitated by HapMap data, making whole-genome studies more feasible Does not necessarily need relatives	Requires large sample size and matched control population False-positive results in the absence of suitable control population Candidate gene approach does not permit to detect novel genes and pathways Whole-genome association studies very expensive

In order to identify a chromosomal locus that segregates with a disease, it is necessary to characterize polymorphic DNA markers from affected and unaffected individuals of one or several pedigrees. One

can then assess whether certain marker alleles cosegregate with the disease. Markers that are closest to the disease gene are less likely to undergo recombination events and therefore receive a higher linkage score. Linkage is expressed as a lod (logarithm of odds) score—the ratio of the probability that the disease and marker loci are linked rather than unlinked. Lod scores of +3 (1000:1) are generally accepted as supporting linkage, whereas a score of −2 is consistent with the absence of linkage.

An example of the use of linkage analysis is shown in Fig. 62-12. In this case, the gene for the autosomal dominant disorder MEN-1 is known to be located on chromosome 11q13. Using positional cloning, the *MEN1* gene was identified and shown to encode menin, a tumor suppressor. Affected individuals inherit a mutant form of the *MEN1* gene, predisposing them to certain types of tumors (parathyroid, pituitary, pancreatic islet) (Chap. 345). In the tissues that develop a tumor, a "second hit" occurs in the normal copy of the *MEN1* gene. This somatic mutation may be a point mutation, a microdeletion, or loss of a chromosomal fragment (detected as loss of heterozygosity, LOH). Within a given family, linkage to the *MEN1* gene locus can be assessed without necessarily knowing

FIGURE 62-12 CAG repeat length and linkage analysis in multiple endocrine neoplasia (MEN) type 1. *Upper panel.* Detection of different alleles using polymorphic microsatellite markers. The example depicts a CAG trinucleotide repeat. PCR with primers flanking the polymorphic region results in products of variable length, depending on the number of CAG repeats. After characterization of the alleles in the parents, transmission of the paternal and maternal alleles can be determined. *Lower panel.* Genotype analysis using microsatellite markers in a family with MEN-1. Two microsatellite markers, A and B, are located in close proximity to the *MEN1* gene on chromosome 11q13. For each individual, the A and B alleles have been determined. Based on this analysis, the genotype A3,B4 is linked to the disease because it occurs in the two affected individuals I-1 and II-1 but not in unaffected siblings. Because the disease allele is linked to A3,B4 within the affected family, it is likely that the individual III-1 is a carrier of the mutated *MEN1* gene. Although III-5 also has the A3,B4 genotype, she has inherited the allele from her unaffected father (II-4), who is not related to the original family. The A3,B4 genotype is only associated with MEN-1 in the original family, but not in the general population. Therefore, individual III-5 is not at risk for developing the disease.

the specific mutation in the *MEN1* gene. Using polymorphic STRs that are close to the *MEN1* gene, one can assess transmission of the different *MEN1* alleles and compare this pattern to development of the disorder to determine which allele is associated with risk of MEN-1. In the pedigree shown, the affected grandfather in generation I carries alleles 3 and 4 on the chromosome with the mutated *MEN1* gene and alleles 2 and 2 on his other chromosome 11. Consistent with linkage of the 3/4 genotype to the *MEN1* locus, his son in generation II is affected, whereas his daughter (who inherits the 2/2 genotype from her father) is unaffected. In the third generation, transmission of the 3/4 genotype indicates risk of developing MEN-1, assuming that no genetic recombination between the 3/4 alleles and the *MEN1* gene has occurred. After a specific mutation in the *MEN1* gene is identified within a family, it is possible to track transmission of the mutation itself, thereby eliminating uncertainty caused by recombination.

ALLELIC ASSOCIATION, LINKAGE DISEQUILIBRIUM, AND HAPLOTYPES *Allelic association* refers to a situation in which the frequency of an allele is significantly increased or decreased in individuals affected by a particular disease in comparison to controls. Linkage and association differ in several aspects. Genetic linkage is demonstrable in families or sibships. Association studies, on the other hand, compare a population of affected individuals with a control population. Association studies can be performed as case-control studies that include unrelated affected individuals and matched controls, or as family-based studies that compare the frequencies of alleles transmitted or not transmitted to affected children.

Allelic association studies are particularly useful for identifying susceptibility genes in complex diseases. When alleles at two loci occur more frequently in combination than would be predicted (based on known allele frequencies and recombination fractions), they are said to be in *linkage disequilibrium*. In **Fig. 62-13**, a mutation, Z, has occurred at a susceptibility locus where the normal allele is Y. The mutation is in close proximity to a genetic polymorphism with allele A or B. With time, the chromosomes carrying the A and Z alleles accumulate and represent 10% of the chromosomes in the population. The fact that the disease susceptibility gene, Z, is found preferentially, or exclusively, in association with the A allele illustrates linkage disequilibrium. Though not all chromosomes carrying the A allele carry the disease gene, the A allele is associated with an increased risk because of its possible association with the Z allele. This model implies that it may be possible in the future to identify Z directly to provide a more accurate prediction of disease susceptibility. Evidence for linkage disequilibrium can be helpful in mapping disease genes because it suggests that the two loci, in this case A and Z, are tightly linked.

Detecting the genetic factors contributing to the pathogenesis of common complex disorders remains a great challenge. In many instances, these are low-penetrance alleles, i.e., variations that individually only have a subtle effect on disease development, and they can only be identified by unbiased genome-wide association studies. Most variants are in noncoding or regulatory sequences but do not alter protein structure. The analysis of complex disorders is further complicated by ethnic differences in disease prevalence, differences in allele frequencies in known susceptibility genes among different populations, locus and allelic heterogeneity, gene-gene and gene-environment interactions, and the possibility of phenocopies. The HapMap Project is now making genome-wide association studies for the characterization of complex disorders more realistic. Adjacent SNPs are inherited together as blocks, and these blocks can be identified by genotyping selected marker SNPs, so-called *Tag SNPs*, thereby reducing cost and workload (Fig. 62-8). The availability of this information permits the characterization of a limited number of SNPs to identify the set of haplotypes present in an individual, e.g., in cases and controls. This, in turn, permits genome-wide association studies by searching for associations of certain haplotypes with a disease phenotype of interest, an essential step for unraveling the genetic factors contributing to complex disorders.

POPULATION GENETICS In population genetics, the focus changes from alterations in an individual's genome to the distribution pattern of different genotypes in the population. In a case where there are only two alleles, A and a, the frequency of the genotypes will be $p^2 + 2pq + q^2 = 1$, with p^2 corresponding to the frequency of AA, $2pq$ to the frequency of Aa, and q^2 to aa. When the frequency of an allele is known, the frequency of the genotype can be calculated. Alternatively, one can determine an allele frequency, if the genotype frequency has been determined.

Allele frequencies vary among ethnic groups and geographical regions. For example, heterozygous mutations in the *CFTR* gene are relatively common in populations of European origin but are rare in the African population. Allele frequencies may vary because certain allelic variants confer a selective advantage. For example, heterozygotes for the sickle cell mutation, which is particularly common in West Africa, are more resistant to malarial infection because the erythrocytes of heterozygotes provide a less favorable environment for *Plasmodium* parasites. Though homozygosity for the sickle cell gene is associated with severe anemia and sickle crises (Chap. 99), heterozygotes have a higher probability of survival because of the reduced morbidity and mortality from malaria; this phenomenon has led to an increased frequency of the mutant allele. Recessive conditions are more prevalent in geographically isolated populations because of the more restricted gene pool.

APPROACH TO THE PATIENT:
Inherited Disorders

For the practicing clinician, the family history remains an essential step in recognizing the possibility of a hereditary component. When taking the history, it is useful to draw a detailed pedigree of the first-degree relatives (e.g., parents, siblings, and children), since they share 50% of genes with the patient. Standard symbols for pedigrees are depicted in Fig. 62-9. The family history should include information about ethnic background, age, health status, and (infant) deaths. Next, the physician should explore whether there is a family history of the same or related illnesses to the current problem. An inquiry focused on commonly occurring disorders such as cancers, heart disease, and diabetes mellitus should follow. Because of the possibility of age-dependent expressivity and penetrance, the family history will need intermittent updating. If the findings suggest a genetic disorder, the clinician will have to assess whether some of the patient's relatives may be at risk of carrying or transmitting the disease. In this circumstance, it is useful to confirm and extend the pedigree based on input from several family members. This information may form the basis for carrier detection, genetic

Wild-type: Polymorphic alleles
A = 40%; B = 60%
Wild-type allele Y = 100%

Linkage disequilibrium: Allele A is associated with the mutation Z in 10%. B is never associated with the mutation Z, unless a recombination has occurred between the two loci.

FIGURE 62-13 Linkage disequilibrium.

counseling, early intervention, and prevention of a disease in relatives of the index patient (Chap. 64).

In instances where a diagnosis at the molecular level may be relevant, the physician will have to identify an appropriate laboratory that can perform the test. Genetic testing is becoming more readily available through commercial laboratories. For uncommon disorders, the test may only be performed in a specialized research laboratory. Approved laboratories offering testing for inherited disorders can be identified in continuously updated on-line resources (GeneTests; Table 62-1). If genetic testing is considered, the patient and the family should be informed about the potential implications of positive results, including psychological distress and the possibility of discrimination. The patient or caretakers should be informed about the meaning of a negative result, technical limitations, and the possibility of false-negative and inconclusive results. For these reasons, genetic testing should only be performed after obtaining *informed consent*. Published ethical guidelines address the specific aspects that should be considered when testing children and adolescents. Genetic testing should usually be limited to situations in which the results may have an impact on the medical management.

IDENTIFYING THE DISEASE-CAUSING GENE

Genomic medicine aims to enhance the quality of medical care through the use of genotypic analysis (DNA testing) to identify genetic predisposition to disease, to select more specific pharmacotherapy, and to design individualized medical care based on genotype. Genotype can be deduced by analysis of protein (e.g., hemoglobin, apoprotein E), mRNA, or DNA. However, technological advances have made DNA analysis particularly useful because it can be readily applied to all but the largest genes (Fig. 62-14).

DNA testing is performed by mutational analysis or linkage studies in individuals at risk for a genetic disorder known to be present in a family. Mass screening programs require tests of high sensitivity and specificity to be cost-effective. Prerequisites for the success of genetic screening programs include the following: that the disorder is potentially serious; that it can be influenced at a presymptomatic stage by changes in behavior, diet, and/or pharmaceutical manipulations; and that the screening does not result in any harm or discrimination. Screening in Jewish populations for the autosomal recessive neurodegenerative storage disease Tay-Sachs has reduced the number of affected individuals. In contrast, screening for sickle cell trait/disease in African Americans has led to unanticipated problems of discrimination by health insurers and employers. Mass screening programs harbor additional potential problems. For example, screening for the most common genetic alteration in cystic fibrosis, the ΔF508 mutation with a frequency of ~70% in northern Europe, is feasible and seems to be effective. One has to keep in mind, however, that there is pronounced allelic heterogeneity and that the disease can be caused by >1400 other mutations. The search for these less common mutations would substantially increase costs but not the effectiveness of the screening program as a whole. Occupational screening programs aim to detect individuals with increased risk for certain professional activities (e.g., α_1 antitrypsin deficiency and smoke or dust exposure).

Mutational Analyses DNA sequence analysis is increasingly used as a diagnostic tool and has significantly enhanced diagnostic accuracy. It is used for determining carrier status and for prenatal testing in monogenic disorders (Chap. 64). Numerous techniques are available for the detection of mutations (Table 62-9). In a very broad sense, one can distinguish between techniques that allow for screening the absence or presence of known mutations (screening mode) or techniques that definitively characterize mutations. Analyses of large alterations in the genome are possible using classic methods such as cytogenetics, fluorescent in situ hybridization (FISH), and Southern blotting (Chap. 63), as well as more sensitive novel techniques that search for multiple single exon deletions or duplications.

More discrete sequence alterations rely heavily on the use of the PCR, which allows rapid gene amplification and analysis. Moreover, PCR makes it possible to perform genetic testing and mutational analysis with small amounts of DNA extracted from leukocytes or even from single cells, buccal cells, or hair roots. Screening for point mutations can be performed by numerous methods (Table 62-9); most are based on the recognition of mismatches between nucleic acid duplexes, electrophoretic separation of single- or double-stranded DNA, or sequencing of DNA fragments amplified by PCR. DNA sequencing can be performed directly on PCR products or on fragments cloned into plasmid vectors amplified in bacterial host cells.

RT-PCR may be useful to detect absent or reduced levels of mRNA expression due to a mutated allele. Protein truncation tests (PTT) can be used to detect the broad array of mutations that result in premature termination of a polypeptide during its synthesis. The isolated cDNA is transcribed and translated in vitro, and the proteins are analyzed by gel electrophoresis. Comparison of electrophoretic mobility with the wild-type protein allows detection of truncated mutants.

The majority of traditional diagnostic methods are gel-based. Novel technologies for the analysis of mutations, genotyping, large-scale sequencing, and mRNA expression profiles are in rapid development. DNA chip technologies allow hybridization of DNA or RNA to hundreds of thousands of probes simultaneously. Microarrays are being used clinically for mutational analysis of several human disease genes, as well as for the identification of viral sequence variations. Together with the knowledge gained from the HGP, these technologies provide the foundation to expand from a focus on single genes to analyses at the scale of the genome. Faster and cheaper sequencing technologies are under development, and it has been anticipated that sequencing the whole genome of an individual for a cost of ≤$1000 will become a reality within this decade. The availability of comprehensive individual sequence information is expected to have a significant impact on medical care and preventative strategies, but it also raises ethical and legal concerns how such information may be used by insurers and employers.

A general algorithm for the approach to mutational analysis is outlined in Fig. 62-14. The importance of a detailed clinical phenotype cannot be overemphasized. This is the step where one should also consider the possibility of genetic heterogeneity and phenocopies. If obvious candidate genes are suggested by the phenotype, they can be analyzed directly. After identification of a mutation, it is essential to demonstrate that it segregates with the phenotype. The functional characterization of novel mutations is labor inten-

FIGURE 62-14 Approach to genetic disease.

TABLE 62-9 METHODS USED FOR THE DETECTION OF MUTATIONS

Method	Principle	Type of Mutation Detected
Commonly Used Techniques		
Cytogenetic analysis	Unique visual appearance of various chromosomes	Numerical or structural abnormalities in chromosomes
Fluorescent in situ hybridization (FISH)	Hybridization to chromosomes with fluorescently labeled probes	Numerical or structural abnormalities in chromosomes
Southern blot	Hybridization with genomic probe or cDNA probe after digestion of high molecular DNA	Large deletion, insertion, rearrangement, expansions of triplet repeat, amplification
Polymerase chain reaction (PCR)	Amplification of DNA segment	Expansion of triplet repeats, variable number of tandem repeats (VNTR), gene rearrangements, translocations; prepare DNA for other mutation methods
Reverse transcriptase PCR (RT-PCR)	Reverse transcription, amplification of DNA segment → absence or reduction of mRNA transcription	Analyze expressed mRNA (cDNA) sequence; detect loss of expression
DNA sequencing	Direct sequencing of PCR products. Sequencing of DNA segments cloned into plasmid vectors	Point mutations, small deletions and insertions
Restriction fragment polymorphism (RFLP)	Detection of altered restriction pattern of genomic DNA (Southern blot) or PCR products	Point mutations, small deletions and insertions
Other Techniques		
Single-strand conformational polymorphism (SSCP)	PCR of DNA segment: Mutations result in conformational change and altered mobility	Point mutations, small deletions and insertions
Denaturing gradient gel electrophoresis (DGGE)	PCR of DNA segment: Mutations result in conformational change and altered mobility	Point mutations, small deletions and insertions
RNAse cleavage	Cleavage of mismatch between mutated and wild-type sequence	Point mutations, small deletions and insertions
Oligonucleotide specific hybridization (OSH)	Hybridization of PCR products to wild-type or mutated oligonucleotides immobilized on chips or slides	Point mutations, small deletions and insertions
Microarrays	Hybridization of PCR products to wild-type or mutated oligonucleotides	Point mutations, small deletions and insertions. Genotyping of SNPs
Protein truncation test (PTT)	Transcription/translation of cDNA isolated from tissue sample	Mutations leading to premature truncations
Pyrosequencing	Clonal amplification of single DNA fragments on microparticles followed by massive parallel sequencing	Sequencing of whole genomes of microorganisms, resequencing of amplicons
Multiplex ligation-dependent probe amplification (MLPA)	Quantification of PCR-generated amplicons reflecting the number of copies of a specific DNA sequence	Copy number variations

sive and may require analyses in vitro or in transgenic models in order to document the relevance of the genetic alteration.

Prenatal diagnosis of numerous genetic diseases in instances with a high risk for certain disorders is now possible by direct DNA analysis. *Amniocentesis* involves the removal of a small amount of amniotic fluid, usually at 16 weeks of gestation. Cells can be collected and submitted for karyotype analyses, FISH, and mutational analysis of selected genes. The main indications for amniocentesis include advanced maternal age above age 35, abnormal serum triple marker test (α-fetoprotein, β human chorionic gonadotropin, pregnancy-associated plasma protein A, or unconjugated estriol), a family history of chromosomal abnormalities, or a Mendelian disorder amenable to genetic testing. Prenatal diagnosis can also be performed by *chorionic villus sampling* (CVS), in which a small amount of the chorion is removed by a transcervical or transabdominal biopsy. Chromosomes and DNA obtained from these cells can be submitted for cytogenetic and mutational analyses. CVS can be performed earlier in gestation (weeks 9–12) than amniocentesis, an aspect that may be of relevance when termination of pregnancy is a consideration. Later in pregnancy, beginning at about 18 weeks of gestation, percutaneous umbilical blood sampling (PUBS) permits collection of fetal blood for lymphocyte culture and analysis. In combination with in vitro fertilization (IVF) techniques, it is even possible to perform genetic diagnoses in a single cell removed from the four- to eight-cell embryo or to analyze the first polar body from an oocyte. Preconceptual diagnosis thereby avoids therapeutic abortions but is extremely costly and labor intensive. Lastly, it has to be emphasized that excluding a specific disorder by any of these approaches is never equivalent to the assurance of having a normal child.

Mutations in certain cancer susceptibility genes, such as *BRCA1* and *BRCA2*, may identify individuals with an increased risk for the development of malignancies and result in risk-reducing interventions. The detection of mutations is an important diagnostic and prognostic tool in leukemias and lymphomas. The demonstration of the presence or absence of mutations and polymorphisms is also relevant for the rapidly evolving field of pharmacogenomics, including the identification of differences in drug treatment response or metabolism as a function of genetic background. For example, the thiopurine drugs 6-mercaptopurine and azathioprine are commonly used cytotoxic and immunosuppressive agents. They are metabolized by thiopurine methyltransferase (TPMT), an enzyme with variable activity associated with genetic polymorphisms in 10% of Caucasians and complete deficiency in about 1/300 individuals. Patients with intermediate or deficient TPMT activity are at risk for excessive toxicity, including fatal myelosuppression. Characterization of these polymorphisms allows mercaptopurine doses to be modified based on TPMT genotype. Pharmacogenomics may increasingly permit individualized drug therapy, improve drug effectiveness, reduce adverse side effects, and provide cost-effective pharmaceutical care.

FURTHER READINGS

ALTSHULER D et al: for The International HapMap Consortium: A haplotype map of the human genome. Nature 437:1299, 2005

GUTTMACHER AE, COLLINS FS: Realizing the promise of genomics in biomedical research. JAMA 294:1399, 2005

——— et al: The family history—more important than ever. N Engl J Med 351:2333, 2004

ROCKMAN MV, KRUGLYAK L: Genetics of global gene expression. Nat Rev Genet 7:862, 2006

RODEN DM et al: Pharmacogenomics: Challenges and opportunities. Ann Intern Med 145:749, 2006

SERVICE RF: Gene sequencing. The race for the $1000 genome. Science 311:1544, 2006

WOLFSBERG TG et al: A user's guide to the human genome. Nat Genet 35(Suppl 1): 2003

63 Chromosome Disorders
Terry Hassold, Stuart Schwartz

In humans, the normal diploid number of chromosomes is 46, consisting of 22 pairs of autosomal chromosomes (numbered 1–22 in decreasing size) and one pair of sex chromosomes (XX in females and XY in males). The genome is estimated to contain between 30,000 and 40,000 genes. Even the smallest autosome contains between 200 and 300 genes. Not surprisingly, duplications or deletions of chromosomes, or even small chromosome segments, have profound consequences on normal gene expression, leading to severe developmental and physiologic abnormalities.

Deviations in number or structure of the 46 human chromosomes are astonishingly common, despite severe deleterious consequences. Chromosomal disorders occur in an estimated 10–25% of all pregnancies. They are the leading cause of fetal loss and, among pregnancies surviving to term, the leading known cause of birth defects and mental retardation.

In recent years, the practice of cytogenetics has shifted from conventional cytogenetic methodology to a union of cytogenetic and molecular techniques. Formerly the province of research laboratories, fluorescence in situ hybridization (FISH) and related molecular cytogenetic technologies have been incorporated into everyday practice in clinical laboratories. As a result, there is an increased appreciation of the importance of "subtle" constitutional cytogenetic abnormalities, such as microdeletions and imprinting disorders, as well as previously recognized translocations and disorders of chromosome number.

VISUALIZING CHROMOSOMES

CONVENTIONAL CYTOGENETIC ANALYSIS

In theory, chromosome preparations can be obtained from any actively dividing tissue by causing the cells to arrest in metaphase, the stage of the cell cycle when chromosomes are maximally condensed. In practice, only a small number of tissues are used for routine chromosome analysis: amniocytes or chorionic villi for prenatal testing and blood, bone marrow, or skin fibroblasts for postnatal studies. Samples of blood, bone marrow, and chorionic villi can be processed using short-term culture techniques that yield results in 1–3 days. Analysis of other tissue types typically involves long-term cell culture, requiring 1–3 weeks of processing before cytogenetic analysis is possible.

Cells are isolated at metaphase or prometaphase and treated chemically or enzymatically to reveal chromosome "bands" (Fig. 63-1). Analysis of the number of chromosomes in the cell and the distribution of bands on individual chromosomes allow the identification of numerical or structural abnormalities. This strategy is useful for characterizing the normal chromosome complement and determining the incidence and types of major chromosome abnormalities.

Each human chromosome contains two specialized structures: a centromere and two telomeres. The centromere, or primary constriction, divides the chromosome into short (p) and long (q) arms and is responsible for the segregation of chromosomes during cell division. The telomeres, or chromosome ends, "cap" the p and q arms and are important for allowing DNA replication at the ends of the chromosomes. Prior to DNA replication, each chromosome consists of a single chromatid copy of the DNA double helix. After DNA replication and continuing until the time of cell division (including metaphase, when chromosomes are typically visualized), each chromosome consists of two identical sister chromatids (Fig. 63-1).

MOLECULAR CYTOGENETICS

The introduction of FISH methodologies in the late 1980s revolutionized the field of cytogenetics. In principle, FISH is similar to other DNA-DNA hybridization methodologies. The probe is labeled with a hapten, such as biotin or digoxigenin, to allow detection with a fluorophore (e.g., FITC or rhodamine). After the hybridization step, the specimen is counter-stained and the preparations are visualized with a fluorescence microscope.

FIGURE 63-1 A. An idealized human chromosome, showing the centromere (cen), long (q) and short (p) arms, and telomeres (tel). **B.** A G-banded human karyotype from a normal (46,XX) female.

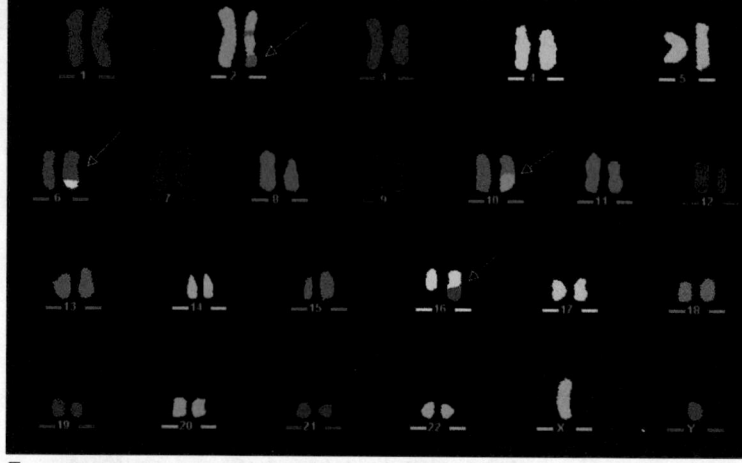

PART 3 Genetics and Disease

FIGURE 63-2 Examples of different applications of fluorescence in situ hybridization (FISH) to human metaphase and interphase preparations. **A, B.** Aneuploidy detection: Interphase FISH using chromosome 13 (green) and chromosome 21 (red) unique sequence probes on interphase cells from direct amniotic fluid preparations. In "A" (a normal cell), two signals for both chromosomes 13 and 21 are seen; in "B," three signals for chromosome 21 are seen, indicating trisomy 21 in the fetus. **C.** Aneuploidy detection: Two-color FISH with telomere probes from the short arm (green) and the long arm (red) of chromosome 8. Hybridization with these probes shows fluorescence of both probes to three separate chromosomes, indicating the presence of trisomy 8 in this individual. **D.** Microdeletion detection: Two-color FISH is used to detect a microdeletion of chromosome 22 associated with velocardiofacial (VCF) syndrome. A probe for ARSA (a locus on the distal portion of chromosome 22, visualized as a green signal) is observed on both chromosomes 22. However, a probe for TUPLE1 (a locus within the VCF region of chromosome 22, visualized in red) hybridizes to only the normal chromosome. **E.** Characterization of structural rearrangements: M-FISH (multicolor FISH) is used to detect a complex chromosome rearrangement involving a translocation between chromosome 6 and 16, as well as a translocation and inversion involving chromosomes 2 and 10.

Types of FISH Probes A variety of probes are available for use with FISH, including chromosome-specific paints (chromosome libraries), repetitive probes, and single-copy probes (Fig. 63-2). Chromosome libraries hybridize to sequences that span the entirety of the chromosome from which they are derived and, as a result, they can be used to "paint" individual chromosomes.

Repetitive probes recognize amplified DNA sequences present in chromosomes. The most common are α-satellite DNA probes that are complementary to DNA sequences found at the centromeric regions of all human chromosomes. A vast number of *single-copy probes* are now available as a result of the human genome project. These probes can be as small as 1 kb, though normally they are much larger and are packaged into cosmids (40 kb), bacterial artificial chromosomes (BACs) or P1 clones (100–200 kb), or yeast artificial chromosomes (YACs) (1–2 Mb). Many are available commercially, including probes for a variety of microdeletion syndromes and for subtelomeric regions of individual chromosomes.

Applications of FISH The majority of FISH applications involve hybridization of one or two probes of interest as an adjunctive procedure to conventional chromosomal banding techniques. In this regard, FISH can be utilized to identify specific chromosomes, characterize de novo duplications or deletions, and clarify subtle chromosomal rearrangements. Its greatest utilization, however, is in the detection of microdeletions (see below). Though conventional cytogenetic studies can detect some microdeletions, initial detection and/or confirmation with FISH is essential. In fact, since appropriate FISH probes have become available, detection of microdeletion syndromes has increased significantly.

In addition to metaphase FISH, cells can be analyzed at a variety of stages. Interphase analysis, for example, can be used to make a rapid diagnosis in instances when metaphase chromosome preparations are not yet available (e.g., amniotic fluid interphase analysis). Interphase analysis also increases the number of cells available for examination, allows for investigation of nuclear organization, and provides results when cells do not progress to metaphase. One specialized type of interphase analysis involves the application of FISH to paraffin-embedded sections, thereby preserving the architecture of the tissue.

The use of interphase FISH has increased recently, especially for analyses of amniocentesis samples. These studies are performed on uncultured amniotic fluid, typically using DNA probes specific for the chromosomes most commonly identified in trisomies (chromosomes 13, 18, 21, and the X and Y). These studies can be performed rapidly (24–72 h) and will ascertain about 60% of the abnormalities detected prenatally. Another area in which interphase analysis is routinely utilized is cancer cytogenetics (Chap. 79). Many site-specific translocations are associated with specific types of malignancies. For example, there are probes available for both the Abelson (Abl) oncogene and breakpoint cluster region (bcr) involved in chronic myelogenous leukemia (CML); these probes are labeled in red and green, respectively; the fusion of these genes in CML combines the fluorescent colors and appears as a yellow hybridization signal.

In addition to standard metaphase and interphase FISH analyses, a number of enhanced techniques have been developed for specific types of analysis, including multicolor FISH techniques, reverse painting, comparative genomic hybridization, and fiber FISH. *Spectral karyotyping* (SKY) and multicolor FISH (m-FISH) techniques use combinatorially labeled probes that create a unique color for individual chromosomes. This technology is useful in the identification of unknown chromosome material (such as markers of duplications) but is most commonly used with the complex rearrangements seen in cancer specimens.

Fiber FISH is a technique in which chromosomes are mechanically stretched, using a variety of different methods. It provides a higher resolution of analysis than conventional FISH.

Comparative genomic hybridization (CGH) is a method that can be used only when DNA is available from a specimen of interest. The entire DNA specimen from the sample of interest is labeled in one color (e.g., green), and the normal control DNA specimen is indicated by another color (e.g., red). These are mixed in equal amounts and hybridized to normal metaphase chromosomes. The red-to-green ratio is analyzed by a computer program, which determines where the DNA of interest may have gains or losses of material. This technique is useful in the analysis of tumors, particularly in those cases where cytogenetic analysis is not possible.

An extension of CGH promises to yield another major advance for examining human chromosomes. Specifically, the development of CGH "arrays" uses protocols that are similar to standard CGH, except that test DNA is hybridized to DNAs that are spread on arrays, rather than hybridized to normal chromosomes. Depending on the type of array (most are constructed utilizing either BACs or oligonucleotides), the resolution can be up to 150 kb, far greater than for standard chromosome analysis. This technology has been used to study cryptic chromosomal imbalances in patients with mental retardation and multiple congenital anomalies, as well as in prenatal diagnosis. It has also been used to detect microdeletions and microduplications in cancer and in previously unidentified genomic disorders. Although this technology is still in development, its use is anticipated to increase in the near term.

INDICATIONS FOR CYTOGENETIC ANALYSIS

Primary indications for karyotypic analysis vary according to the developmental stage/age of the conceptus/individual under investigation. One especially important application is in prenatal diagnosis (particularly for pregnancies involving older women), assaying for chromosomal abnormalities in either chorionic villi of first-trimester fetuses or amniotic fluid of second-trimester fetuses. Tissue specimens from spontaneously aborted fetuses or stillbirths can also be examined for chromosome abnormalities. Interphase cytogenetics (using FISH) is increasingly being used to study individual blastomeres of preimplantation embryos (with in vitro fertilization–derived pregnancies). This makes it possible to detect aneuploid or structurally unbalanced embryos or, in the case of sex-linked disorders, to identify male conceptuses; such embryos would not be used to initiate pregnancies.

Among infants and children, peripheral blood is examined, most often in individuals with specific phenotypic abnormalities. For example, karyotypic analysis can be used for the confirmation or exclusion of a specific chromosomal syndrome (e.g., trisomy 21); in patients with unexplained psychomotor retardation with or without dysmorphic features; in cases of monogenic disorders associated with mental retardation and/or dysmorphic features; and with abnormalities of sexual differentiation and development.

In adults, peripheral blood can be examined in patients with infertility or recurrent miscarriages, since chromosome abnormalities can lead to meiotic arrest or to genetically unbalanced gametes. An important branch of cytogenetics is concerned with analyses of bone marrow, unstimulated peripheral blood, and lymph nodes of tumors, as chromosomal abnormalities are a common correlate of leukemia, lymphoma, and solid tumors (Chap. 79).

CYTOGENETIC TESTING IN PRENATAL DIAGNOSIS

The vast majority of prenatal diagnostic studies are performed to rule out a chromosomal abnormality, but cells may also be propagated for biochemical studies or molecular analyses of DNA. Three procedures are used to obtain samples for prenatal diagnosis: amniocentesis, chorionic villus sampling (CVS), and fetal blood sampling. Amniocentesis is the most common procedure and is routinely performed at 15–17 weeks of gestation. On some occasions, early amniocentesis at 12–14 weeks is performed to expedite results, although less fluid is obtained at this time. Early amniocentesis carries a greater risk of spontaneous abortion or fetal injury but provides results at an earlier stage of pregnancy.

The vast majority of amniocenteses are performed in the context of advanced maternal age, the best-known correlate of trisomy (see below). Additional reasons for amniocentesis referral include an abnormal "triple- or quad-marker assay" and/or detection of ultrasound abnormalities. In this assay, levels of human chorionic gonadotropin, α-fetoprotein, and unconjugated estriol (and, in the quad assay, inhibin) in the maternal serum are quantified and used to adjust the maternal age-predicted risk of a trisomy 21 or trisomy 18 fetus. Specific ultrasound abnormalities, when detected at midtrimester, can also be associated with chromosomal defects. When a nonspecific ultrasound abnormality is present, the estimated risk of a chromosomal defect is ~16%. Associations of chromosomal abnormalities and specific types of abnormal ultrasound findings are listed in Table 63-1.

CVS is the second most common procedure for genetic prenatal diagnosis. Because this procedure is routinely performed at about 10–12 weeks of gestation, it allows for an earlier detection of abnormalities and a safer pregnancy termination, if desired. CVS is a relatively safe procedure (spontaneous abortions, <0.5–1%). Because there is an increased association of limb defects when the procedure is performed earlier (<10 weeks of gestation), CVS is applicable during a narrow time frame of gestation. CVS involves the use of a catheter inserted transvaginally; ~25 mg of villi are aspirated from the chorion frondosum (the fetal portion of the placenta). By adding colchicine directly to the rapidly dividing cytotrophoblasts, results can be obtained within 24–48 h. Findings from these procedures should be confirmed

TABLE 63-1	**FREQUENCY OF CHROMOSOME ABNORMALITIES, IDENTIFIED ON THE BASIS OF ABNORMAL ULTRASOUND FINDINGS**	
	Chromosomal Abnormalities (Frequency)	
Ultrasound Finding	**Average, %**	**Range in Different Studies, %**
Abnormal ultrasound (nonspecific)	16	13–35
Omphalocele	39	26–54
Cystic hygroma	68	46–78
Congenital heart disease	30	8–40
Choroid plexus cyst	5	4–10

by analyses of cultured mesenchymal cells, as they are more reliably derived from the fetus.

Percutaneous umbilical blood sampling (PUBS) is a method for obtaining fetal blood during the second and third trimesters of pregnancy. PUBS is usually performed when ultrasound abnormalities are detected late in the second trimester. PUBS is also used when cytogenetic results from amniocentesis need clarification, such as in the detection of mosaicism.

CHROMOSOME ABNORMALITIES

CHROMOSOMES IN CELL DIVISION

To understand the etiology of chromosome abnormalities, it is important to review the movement of chromosomes during cell division. In somatic tissues, chromosomes are replicated during the S-phase of the cell cycle, so that each replicated chromosome consists of two identical sister chromatids. When the cell enters mitosis, each of the 46 chromosomes align on the metaphase plate, with the centromeres co-oriented toward opposite spindle poles (Fig. 63-3). At anaphase the sister chromatids separate, with each of the daughter cells receiving one sister chromatid from each of the 46 chromosomes.

Chromosome segregation is more complicated in germ cell division, since the number of chromosomes must be reduced from 46 to 23 in the mature sperm and eggs. This is accomplished by two rounds of division—meiosis I and meiosis II (Fig. 63-3). In meiosis I, homologous chromosomes pair and exchange genetic material, then align on the metaphase plate, and finally separate from one another. Thus, by the end of meiosis I, only 23 of the original 46 chromosomes are represented in each of the two daughter cells. Meiosis II quickly follows meiosis I and is essentially a "haploid mitosis," involving separation of the sister chromatids in each of the 23 chromosomes.

Although the fundamentals of meiosis are the same in males and females, there are important distinctions, particularly in the timing of meiotic divisions. In males, meiosis begins with puberty and continues throughout the individual's lifetime. In females, meiosis begins prenatally, with oocytes proceeding through the first stages of meiosis I but arresting at mid-prophase. At the time of birth, the first meiotic division is suspended in oocytes. Only after ovulation many years later do oocytes complete meiosis I and proceed to the metaphase stage of meiosis II; if fertilized, the oocyte then completes the second meiotic division. Thus, in females, the first meiotic division takes at least 10–15 years and as many as 40–45 years to complete. Maternal age–related increases in the incidence of trisomy are likely the consequence of this protracted process of cell division.

INCIDENCE AND TYPES OF CHROMOSOME ABNORMALITIES

Errors in meiosis, or in early cleavage divisions, occur with extraordinary frequency. At least 10–25% of all pregnancies, for example, involve chromosomally abnormal conceptions. A large proportion of these terminate in the earliest stages of pregnancy, many of which go unrecognized. Nevertheless, even among clinically recognized pregnancies, nearly 10% of fetuses are chromosomally unbalanced. For the three types of clinically recognized pregnancies—spontaneous abortions, stillbirths, and livebirths—the frequencies of different chromosomal abnormalities are summarized in Table 63-2. The most common abnormalities are numerical, involving fetuses with additional (trisomy) or missing (monosomy) chromosomes, or those with one (triploidy) or two (tetraploidy) additional sets of chromosomes. Structural chromosome abnormalities are much less common, although several of the most important clinical chromosomal disorders involve structural rearrangements (see below).

By far the most common abnormality is trisomy, which is identified in ~25% of spon-

FIGURE 63-3 Chromosome segregation in meiosis. A. In meiosis I, each of the 23 pairs of chromosomes finds its "partner," or homologue, and exchanges genetic material (recombines) with it. At metaphase, each homologous pair aligns on the equatorial plate; at anaphase, each member of the homologous pair segregates from its partner. Thus, at the end of meiosis I, each daughter cell contains 23 chromosomes, with each chromosome consisting of two sister chromatids. **B.** In meiosis II, each chromosome aligns on the metaphase plate, and at anaphase, each of the two sister chromatids divides from the other. Thus, at the end of meiosis II, each daughter cell (e.g., the oocyte or spermatocyte) contains 23 chromosomes, with each chromosome consisting of one sister chromatid. In mitosis, the chromosomes behave exactly as they do in meiosis II, except that somatically dividing cells contain 46 chromosomes, not the 23 that are present in the meiosis II cell.

taneous abortions and 0.3% of newborns. Trisomies for all chromosomes have now been identified in embryos or fetuses, but there is considerable variation in frequency for various chromosomes. For example, trisomy 16 is extraordinarily common, accounting for about one-third of all trisomies in spontaneous abortions, whereas trisomies 1, 5, 11, and 19 have been identified less often. Available evidence suggests two reasons for this variation: (1) some chromosomes (e.g., chromosome 16) are more likely to segregate abnormally or undergo nondisjunction during meiosis than are others; and (2) the potential for development varies widely among different trisomic conditions, with some being eliminated very early in gestation, others surviving to the time of clinical pregnancy recognition, and some (e.g., trisomies 13, 18, and 21 and sex chromosome trisomies) being compatible with survival to term.

TABLE 63-2	**FREQUENCY AND DISTRIBUTION OF CHROMOSOME ABNORMALITIES IN DIFFERENT TYPES OF CLINICALLY RECOGNIZABLE PREGNANCIES**			
	Frequency of Abnormality			
Chromosome Abnormality	**Spontaneous Abortion**	**Stillbirth**	**Livebirth**	**Probability of Surviving to Term, %**
Trisomy, all	25.1	4.0	0.3	5
+13, 18, 21	4.5	2.7	0.14	15
+16	7.5	—	—	0
Sex chromosome monosomy (45,X)	8.7	0.1	0.01	1
Triploidy	6.4	0.2	—	0
Tetraploidy	2.4	—	—	0
Structural abnormality	2.0	0.8	0.3	45
Total abnormalities	50.0	5.1	0.6	5

CHROMOSOMAL SYNDROMES

While most chromosomally abnormal conceptions perish in utero, several conditions are compatible with survival to term. The best-characterized of these are numerical abnormalities, involving loss or gain of individual chromosomes, and abnormalities resulting from unbalanced translocations. FISH and other molecular studies have led to the identification of two "new" types of chromosome abnormalities, commonly referred to as *microdeletion syndromes* and *imprinting syndromes*.

NUMERICAL ABNORMALITIES

Virtually all types of numerical abnormalities are eliminated prenatally, so that only those involving small, gene-poor autosomes or the sex chromosomes are identified with any frequency among live-borns. Clinically, the most important of these is trisomy 21, the most frequent cause of Down syndrome. Depending on the maternal age structure of the population and the utilization of prenatal testing, the incidence of trisomy 21 ranges from 1/600 to 1/1000 live births, making it the most common chromosome abnormality in live-born individuals. Like most trisomies, the incidence of trisomy 21 is highly correlated with maternal age, increasing from about 1/1500 live births for women 20 years of age to 1/30 for women ≥45 years.

In addition to trisomy 21, only two other autosomal trisomies, 13 and 18, occur with any frequency in livebirths. Incidence rates for trisomies 13 and 18 in livebirths are 1/20,000 and 1/10,000, respectively. Unlike trisomy 21, which is associated with near-normal life expectancy, both trisomies 13 and 18 are associated with death in infancy, typically occurring during the first year of life.

Three sex chromosome trisomies—the 47,XXX, 47,XXY (Klinefelter syndrome), and 47,XYY conditions—are quite common, with each occurring in about 1/2000 newborns. Of all the trisomic conditions, these three have the fewest phenotypic complications. In fact, with the exception of infertility in Klinefelter syndrome (Chap. 343), it is likely that most individuals with such trisomic conditions would go undetected. The additional Y chromosome in the 47,XYY condition is small and contains only a few genes. Most Y-linked genes are involved in testicular development or spermatogenesis. Thus, dosage imbalance of Y-linked genes has relatively little effect on other developmental processes. The 47,XYY genotype is associated with increased height. Its role in antisocial behavior, postulated initially because of an increased prevalence among some penalized populations, is unclear.

For the 47,XXX and 47,XXY conditions, the situation is different—the X chromosome contains >1000 genes, many of them essential for normal development. How, then, are 47,XXX and 47,XXY individuals spared from the catastrophic consequences of dosage imbalance? The answer lies in the biology of X chromosome gene expression. In normal females, one of the chromosomes undergoes *X inactivation* in somatic cells. The inactivation of the paternal or maternal X chromosome occurs randomly in each somatic cell and thereby serves as a mechanism of dosage compensation, ensuring that males and females have equal expression of most X-linked genes. The inactivation process occurs at the blastocyst stage of development; prior to this, both X chromosomes are active. In addition, not all X-linked genes are inactivated. Some genes on the X chromosome "escape" the inactivating mechanism and are expressed from both X chromosomes. In disorders such as Klinefelter syndrome, some genes may be expressed from both X chromosomes, resulting in its phenotypic features.

As a rule, monosomic conditions are incompatible with fetal development and, consequently, autosomal monosomies are only rarely identified in spontaneous abortions and are not found among live-born individuals. In fact, the only monosomy compatible with live birth is the 45,X condition, which causes Turner syndrome. The 45,X chromosome constitution occurs with surprisingly high frequency, present in at least 1–2% of all pregnancies. More than 99% of all 45,X conceptions are spontaneously aborted. Thus, live-born individuals with a 45,X chromosome constitution represent a rare group of survivors. The 45,X phenotype is mild, presumably because the second copy of many X chromosomal genes is normally inactivated. Nonetheless, Turner syndrome causes gonadal dysgenesis, resulting in infertility and failure to

TABLE 63-3 STUDIES OF THE PARENT AND MEIOTIC/MITOTIC STAGE OF ORIGIN OF HUMAN TRISOMIES AND SEX CHROMOSOME MONOSOMY

	Origin, %				
	Paternal		Maternal		
	I	II	I	II	Mitotic
Trisomy					
2	28	—	54	13	6
7	—	—	17	26	57
15	—	15	76	9	—
16	—	1	96	3	—
18	—	—	33	56	11
21	3	5	67	22	2
22	3	—	94	3	—
XXY	46	—	38	14	3
XXX	—	6	60	16	18
Monosomy					
X[a]	80		20		

[a]Results pertain to nonmosaic 45,X individuals.

undergo secondary sexual development, along with a number of other phenotypic features (Chap. 343). Several other structural abnormalities of the X chromosome such as deletions, isochromosome X, or ring chromosomes can cause Turner syndrome. Mosaicism, including 45,X/45,XX, 45X/45,XXX, 45,X/45,XY, and others, also occurs (see below) and contributes to the phenotypic spectrum in Turner syndrome.

Because numerical abnormalities originate in meiosis (Table 63-3), affected individuals have missing or extra chromosomes in all cells. In a small proportion of cases, a mitotic nondisjunctional event occurs at an early stage in an individual with an initially normal chromosome constitution. Alternatively, a "normalizing" mitotic nondisjunctional event may result in a normal chromosome complement in some cells of an embryo. In either case, the embryo is a mosaic, with some cells bearing a normal chromosome constitution and others an aneuploid number of chromosomes. The phenotypic consequences are difficult to predict because they depend on the timing of nondisjunction and the distribution of normal and abnormal cells in different tissues. Nevertheless, mosaicism may lead to clinical abnormalities indistinguishable from those of nonmosaic individuals; for example, nearly 5% of all cases of Down syndrome involve individuals with mosaic trisomy 21, and about 15% of individuals with Turner syndrome are mosaic for various sex chromosomal constitutions as described above.

The Origin and Etiology of Numerical Abnormalities Over the past decade, a number of studies have used DNA polymorphisms to investigate the origin of different types of chromosome abnormalities (Fig. 63-4). The most thoroughly investigated types have been numerical abnormalities (Table 63-3). Sex chromosome monosomy usually results from loss of the paternal sex chromosome, regardless of whether the conception is live-born or spontaneously aborted.

Trisomies show remarkable variation in parental origin. For example, paternal nondisjunction is responsible for nearly 50% of 47,XXY but only 5–10% of cases of trisomies 13, 14, 15, 21, and 22; it is rarely, if ever, the source of the additional chromosome in trisomy 16. Similarly, there is considerable variability in the meiotic stage of origin. For example, all cases of trisomy 16 may be due to meiosis I errors, whereas for trisomy 21, one-third of cases are associated with meiosis II errors, and for trisomy 18, the majority of cases are apparently due to meiosis II nondisjunction. In spite of this variation in parental and meiotic origin, nondisjunction at maternal meiosis I appears to be the most common source of trisomy.

Maternal Age and Trisomy The association between increasing maternal age and trisomy is the most important etiologic factor in con-

FIGURE 63-4 Use of DNA technology to determine the origin of chromosome abnormalities. A. Analysis of a chromosome 21–specific DNA polymorphism demonstrates that the trisomic individual received two chromosomes 21 from his mother and one from his father; thus, the extra chromosome 21 resulted from an error in oogenesis. **B.** Inheritance of a chromosome 15–specific DNA polymorphism in an individual with Prader-Willi syndrome (PWS). The affected individual has received two maternal, but no paternal, chromosomes 15; thus, the individual is said to have maternal uniparental disomy 15, a common cause of PWS.

genital chromosomal disorders. Among women under the age of 25, ~2% of all clinically recognized pregnancies are trisomic; by the age of 36, however, this figure increases to 10% and by the age of 42, to >33% (Fig. 63-5). This association between maternal age and trisomy is exerted without respect to race, geography, or socioeconomic factors and likely affects segregation of all chromosomes.

Despite the importance of increasing age, little is known about the mechanism by which aging leads to abnormal chromosomal segrega-

FIGURE 63-5 Estimated maternal age–adjusted rates of trisomy among all clinically recognized pregnancies (e.g., spontaneous abortions, stillbirths, and livebirths). Among women in their forties, over 25% of all pregnancies are estimated to involve a trisomic conception; the vast majority of these spontaneously abort, with only trisomies 13, 18, and 21 and sex chromosome trisomies surviving to term with any appreciable frequency.

tion. As noted above, it is thought to originate in maternal meiosis I owing to the protracted time to completion (often ≥40 years) in females, and recent studies suggest that it may be associated with alterations in meiotic crossing-over. In trisomy 21, for example, crossover patterns appear to be similarly abnormal in younger and older mothers of trisomic conceptions. Thus, it has been suggested that two distinct steps, or "hits," may be involved in maternal age–related nondisjunction. The first hit, which is age independent, involves the establishment of a "vulnerable" crossover configuration in the fetal oocyte; the second hit, which is age dependent, involves abnormal processing of the vulnerable bivalent structure at metaphase I. If this model is correct, it suggests that the nondisjunctional process is the same in younger and older women, but it occurs more frequently with aging, possibly because of age-dependent degradation of meiotic proteins.

STRUCTURAL CHROMOSOME ABNORMALITIES

Structural rearrangements involve breakage and reunion of chromosomes. Although less common than numerical abnormalities, they present additional challenges from a genetic counseling standpoint. This is because structural abnormalities, unlike numerical abnormalities, can be present in "balanced" form in clinically normal individuals but transmitted in "unbalanced" form to progeny, thereby resulting in a hereditary form of chromosome abnormality.

Rearrangements may involve exchanges of material between different chromosomes (translocations) or loss, gain, or rearrangements of individual chromosomes (e.g., deletions, duplications, inversions, rings, or isochromosomes). Of particular clinical importance are *translocations*, which involve two basic types: Robertsonian and reciprocal. Robertsonian rearrangements are a special class of translocation, in which the long arms of two acrocentric chromosomes (chromosomes 13, 14, 15, 21, and 22) join together, generating a fusion chromosome that contains virtually all of the genetic material of the original two chromosomes. If the Robertsonian translocation is present in unbalanced form, a monosomic or trisomic conception ensues. For example, ~3% of Down syndrome cases are attributable to unbalanced Robertsonian translocations, most often involving chromosomes 14 and 21. In this instance, the affected individual has 46 chromosomes, including one structurally normal chromosome 14, two structurally normal chromosomes 21, and one fusion 14/21 chromosome. This effect leads to a normal diploid dosage for chromosome 14 and to a triplication of chromosome 21, thus resulting in Down syndrome. Similarly, a small proportion of individuals with trisomy 13 syndrome are clinically affected because of an unbalanced Robertsonian translocation.

Reciprocal translocations involve mutual exchanges between any two chromosomes. In this circumstance, the phenotypic consequences associated with unbalanced translocations depend on the location of the breakpoints, which dictate the amount of material that has been "exchanged" between the two chromosomes. Because most reciprocal translocations involve unique sets of breakpoints, it is difficult to predict the phenotypic consequences in any one situation. In general, severity is determined by the amount of excess or missing chromosome material in individuals with unbalanced translocations.

In addition to rearrangements between chromosomes, there are several examples of intrachromosome structural abnormalities. The most common and deleterious of these involve loss of chromosome material due to deletions. The two best-characterized deletion syndromes, Wolf-Hirschhorn syndrome and cri-du-chat syndrome, result from loss of relatively small chromosomal segments on chromosomes 4p and 5p, respectively. Nonetheless, each is associated with multiple congenital anomalies, developmental delays, profound retardation, and reduced lifespan.

Microdeletion Syndromes The term *contiguous gene syndrome* refers to genetic disorders that mimic a combination of single-gene disorders. They result from the deletion of a small number of tightly clustered genes. Because some are too small to be detected cytogenetically, they are termed *microdeletions*. The application of molecular tech-

TABLE 63-4 **SOME COMMONLY IDENTIFIED MICRODELETION AND MICRODUPLICATION SYNDROMES**

Syndrome	Cytogenetic Location	Principal Features	Imprinting Effects
Langer-Giedion syndrome	8q24.1 (del)	Sparse hair, bulbous nose, variable mental retardation	No
WAGR complex	11p13 (del)	Wilms' tumor, aniridia, genito-urinary disorders, mental retardation	No
Beckwith-Wiedemann syndrome	11p15 (dup)	Macrosomia, macroglossia, omphalocoele	Yes, occasionally associated with "paternal uniparental disomy" (see text)
Retinoblastoma	13q14.11 (del)	Retinoblastoma due to homozygous loss of functional RB allele	No obvious effect, although abnormal RB allele more likely to be paternal
Prader-Willi syndrome	15q11-13 (del)	Obesity, hypogonadism, mental retardation	Yes, prototypic imprinting disorder (see text)
Angelman syndrome	15q11-13 (del)	Ataxic gait	With Prader-Willi syndrome, prototypic imprinting disorder (see text)
α-Thalassemia and mental retardation	16p13.3 (del)	α-Thalassemia and mental retardation, due to deletion of distal 16p, including α-globin locus	No
Smith-Magenis syndrome	17p11.2 (del)	Brachycephaly, midface hypoplasia, mental retardation	No
Miller-Dieker syndrome	17p13 (del)	Dysmorphic facies, lissencephaly	No
Charcot-Marie-Tooth syndrome type 1A	17p11.2 (dup)	Progressive neuropathy due to microduplication	No
DiGeorge syndrome/ velocardiofacial syndrome	22q11 (del)	Abnormalities of third and fourth branchial arches	No

niques has led to the identification of at least 18 of these microdeletion syndromes (Table 63-4). Some of the more common ones include the Wilms' tumor–aniridia complex (WAGR), Miller Dieker syndrome (MDS), and velocardiofacial (VCF) syndrome. WAGR is characterized by mental retardation and involvement of multiple organs, including kidney (Wilm's tumor), eye (aniridia), and the genitourinary system. The cytogenetic abnormality involves a deletion of a part of the short arm of chromosome 11 (11p13), which typically is detectable on well-banded chromosome preparations. In MDS, a disorder characterized by mental retardation, dysmorphic faces, and lissencephaly, the deletion involves chromosome 17 (17p13). Using FISH, 17p deletions have been detected in >90% of patients with MDS as well as in 20% of cases of isolated lissencephaly.

Deletions involving the long arm of chromosome 22 (22q11) are the most common microdeletions identified to date, present in ~1/3000 newborns. VCF syndrome, the most commonly associated syndrome, consists of learning disabilities or mild mental retardation, palatal defects, a hypoplastic aloe nasi and long nose, and congenital heart defects (conotruncal defect). Some individuals with 22q11 deletion are more severely affected and present with DiGeorge syndrome, which involves abnormalities in the development of the third and fourth branchial arches leading to thymic hypoplasia, parathyroid hypoplasia, and conotruncal heart defects. In ~30% of these cases, a deletion at 22q11 can be detected with high-resolution banding; by combing conventional cytogenetics, FISH, and molecular detection techniques (i.e., Southern blotting or polymerase chain reaction analyses), these rates improve to >90%. Additional studies have demonstrated a surprisingly high frequency of 22q11 deletions in individuals with nonsyndromic conotruncal defects. Approximately 10% of individuals with a 22q11 deletion inherited it from a parent with a similar deletion.

Smith-Magenis syndrome involves a microdeletion localized to the proximal region of the short arm of chromosome 17 (17p11.2). Affected individuals have mental retardation, dysmorphic facial features, delayed speech, peripheral neuropathy, and behavior abnormalities. Most of these deletions can be detected with cytogenetic analysis, although FISH is available to confirm these findings. In contrast, William syndrome, a chromosome 7 (7q11.23) microdeletion, cannot be diagnosed with stan-

dard or high-resolution analysis; it is only detectable utilizing FISH or other molecular methods. William syndrome involves a deletion of the elastin gene and is characterized by mental retardation, dysmorphic features, a gregarious personality, premature aging, and congenital heart disease (usually supravalvular aortic stenosis).

In addition to microdeletion syndromes, there is now at least one well-described microduplication syndrome, Charcot-Marie-Tooth type 1A (CMT1A). This is a nerve conduction disease previously thought to be transmitted as a simple autosomal dominant disorder. Recent molecular studies have demonstrated that affected individuals are heterozygous for duplication of a small region of chromosome 17 (17p11.2–12). Although it is not yet clear why increased gene dosage would result in CMT1A, the inheritance pattern is explained by the fact that one-half of the offspring of affected individuals inherit the duplication-carrying chromosome.

IMPRINTING DISORDERS

Two other microdeletion syndromes, Prader-Willi syndrome (PWS) and Angelman syndrome (AS), exhibit parent-of-origin, or "imprinting," effects. For many years, it has been known that cytogenetically detectable deletions of chromosome 15 occur in a proportion of patients with PWS, as well as in those with AS. This seemed curious, as the clinical manifestations of the two syndromes are very dissimilar. PWS is characterized by obesity, hypogonadism, and mild to moderate mental retardation, whereas AS is associated with microcephaly, ataxic gait, seizures, inappropriate laughter, and severe mental retardation. New insight into the pathogenesis of these disorders has been provided by the recognition that parental origin of the deletion determines which phenotype ensues: if the deletion is paternal, the result is PWS, whereas if the deletion is maternal, the result is AS (Fig. 63-2).

This scenario is complicated further by the recognition that not all individuals with PWS or AS carry the chromosome 15 deletion. For such individuals, the parental origin of the chromosome 15 region is again the important determinant. In PWS, for example, nondeletion patients invariably have two maternal and no paternal chromosomes 15 [maternal uniparental disomy (UPD)], whereas for some nondeletion AS patients the reverse is true (paternal UPD). This indicates that at least some genes on chromosome 15 are differently expressed, depending on which parent contributed the chromosome. Additionally, this means that normal fetal development requires the presence of one maternal and one paternal copy of chromosome 15.

Approximately 70% of PWS cases are due to paternal deletions of 15q11-q13, whereas 25% are due to maternal UPD, and about 5% are caused by mutations in a chromosome 15 imprinting center. In AS, 75% of cases are due to maternal deletions, and only 2% are due to paternal UPD. The remaining cases are presumably caused by imprinting mutations (5%), or mutations in the *UBE3A* gene, which is associated with AS. The UPD cases are mostly caused by meiotic nondisjunction resulting in trisomy 15, subsequently followed by a normalizing mitotic nondisjunction event ("trisomy rescue") resulting in two normal chromosomes 15, both from the same parent. *UBE3A* is the only maternally imprinted gene known in the critical region of chromosome 15. However, several paternally imprinted genes, or expressed-sequence tags (ESTs), have been identified, including *ZNF127*, *IPW*, *SNRPN*, *SNURF*, *PAR1*, and *PAR5*.

Chromosomal regions that behave in the manner observed in PWS and AS are said to be *imprinted*. This phenomenon is involved in differential expression of certain genes on different chromosomes. Chromosome 11 is one of these with an imprinted region, since it is known that a small proportion of individuals with the Beckwith-Wiedemann overgrowth syndrome have two paternal but no maternal copies of this chromosome.

ACQUIRED CHROMOSOME ABNORMALITIES IN CANCER

In addition to the constitutional cytogenetic chromosomal abnormalities that are present at birth, somatic chromosomal changes can be acquired later in life and are often associated with malignant conditions. As with constitutional abnormalities, somatic changes can include the net loss of chromosomal material (due to a deletion or loss of a chromosome), net gain of material (duplication or gain of a chromosome), and relocation of DNA sequences (translocation). Cytogenetic changes have been particularly well studied in (1) leukemias, e.g., Philadelphia chromosome translocation in CML [t(9;22)(q34.1;q11.2)]; and (2) lymphomas, e.g., translocations of *MYC* in Burkitt's [t(8;14)(q24; q32)]. These and other translocations are useful for diagnosis, classification, and prognosis. Analyses of cytogenetic changes are also useful in certain solid tumors. For example, a complex karyotype with Wilms' tumor, diploidy in medulloblastoma, and Her-2/neu amplification in breast cancer are poor prognostic signs. For detailed discussion of cancer genetics, see Chap. 79.

FURTHER READINGS

DAVE BJ, SANGER WG: Role of cytogenetics and molecular cytogenetics in the diagnosis of genetic imbalances. Semin Pediatr Neurol 14(1):2, 2007

JIANG F, KATZ RL: Use of interphase fluorescence in situ hybridization as a powerful diagnostic tool in cytology. Diagn Mol Pathol 11:47, 2002

LEE C et al: Multicolor fluorescence in situ hybridization in clinical cytogenetic diagnostics. Curr Opin Pediatr 13:550, 2002

MENTEN B et al: Emerging patterns of cryptic chromosomal imbalance in patients with idiopathic mental retardation and multiple congenital anomalies: A new series of 140 patients and review of published reports. J Med Genet 43:625, 2006

NASMYTH K: Segregating sister genomes: The molecular biology of chromosome separation. Science 297:559, 2002

RICKMAN L et al: Prenatal detection of unbalanced chromosomal rearrangements by array CGH. J Med Genet 43: 353, 2006

RIMOIN DL et al (eds): *Emery and Rimoin's Principles and Practice of Medical Genetics*, 4th ed. Philadelphia, Churchill Livingstone, 2001

SHARP AJ et al: Discovery of previously unidentified genomic disorders from the duplication architecture of the human genome. Nat Genet 38:1038, 2006

64 The Practice of Genetics in Clinical Medicine
Susan Miesfeldt, J. Larry Jameson

IMPLICATIONS OF MOLECULAR GENETICS FOR INTERNAL MEDICINE

The field of medical genetics has traditionally focused on chromosomal abnormalities (Chap. 63) and Mendelian disorders (Chap. 62). However, there is genetic susceptibility to many common adult-onset diseases, including atherosclerosis, cardiac disorders, asthma, hypertension, autoimmune diseases, diabetes mellitus, macular degeneration, Alzheimer's disease, psychiatric disorders, and many forms of cancer. Genetic contributions to these common disorders involve more than the ultimate expression of an illness; these genes can also influence the severity of infirmity, effect of treatment, and progression of disease.

The primary care clinician is now faced with the role of recognizing and counseling patients at risk for a number of genetically influenced illnesses. Among the greater than 20,000 genes in the human genome, it is estimated that each of us harbors several potentially deleterious mutations. Fortunately, many of these alterations are recessive and clinically silent. An even greater number, however, represent genetic variants that alter disease susceptibility, severity, or response to therapy.

Genetic medicine is changing the way diseases are classified, enhancing our understanding of pathophysiology, providing practical information concerning drug metabolism and therapeutic responses, and allowing for individualized screening and health care management programs. In view of these changes, the physician must integrate personal medical history, family history, and diagnostic molecular testing into the overall care of individual patients and their families. Surveys indicate that patients still turn to their primary care internist for guidance about genetic disorders, even though they may be seeing other specialists. The internist has an important role in educating patients about the indications, benefits, risks, and limitations of genetic testing in the management of a number of diverse diseases. This is a difficult task, as scientific advances in genetic medicine have outpaced the translation of these discoveries into standards of clinical care.

COMMON ADULT-ONSET GENETIC DISORDERS
MULTIFACTORIAL INHERITANCE

The risk for many adult-onset disorders reflects the combined effects of genetic factors at multiple loci that may function independently or in combination with other genes or environmental factors. Our understanding of the genetic basis of these disorders is incomplete, despite the clear recognition of genetic susceptibility. In type 2 diabetes mellitus, for example, the concordance rate in monozygotic twins ranges between 50 and 90%. Diabetes or impaired glucose tolerance occurs in 40% of siblings and in 30% of the offspring of an affected individual. Despite the fact that diabetes affects 5% of the population and exhibits a high degree of heritability, only a few genetic mutations (most of which are rare) that might account for the familial nature of the disease have been identified. They include certain mitochondrial DNA disorders (Chap. 62), mutations in a cascade of genes that control pancreatic islet cell development and function (*HNF4α, HNF1α, IPF1, TCF7L2, glucokinase*), insulin receptor mutations, and others (Chap. 338). Superimposed on this genetic background are environmental influences such as diet, exercise, pregnancy, and medications.

Identifying susceptibility genes associated with multifactorial adult-onset disorders is a formidable task. Nonetheless, a reasonable goal for these types of diseases is to identify genes that increase (or decrease) disease risk by a factor of two or more. For common diseases such as diabetes or heart disease, this level of risk has important implications for health. In much the same way that cholesterol is currently used as a biochemical marker of cardiovascular risk, we can anticipate the development of genetic panels with similar predictive power. The advent of DNA-sequencing chips represents an important technical advance that promises to make large-scale testing more feasible (Chap. 62). Whether to perform a genetic test for a particular inherited adult-onset disorder, such as hemochromatosis, multiple endocrine neoplasia (MEN) type 1, prolonged QT syndrome, or Huntington disease, is a complex decision; it depends on the clinical features of the disorder, the desires of the patient and family, and whether the results of genetic testing will alter medical decision-making or treatment (see below).

Population Screening Mass genetic screening programs require tests of high enough sensitivity and specificity to be cost-effective. An effective screening program should fulfill the following criteria: that the tested disorder is prevalent and serious; that it can be influenced presymptomatically through lifestyle changes, screening, or medications;

and that identification of risk does not result in undue discrimination or harm. Screening individuals of Jewish descent for the autosomal recessive neurodegenerative disorder Tay-Sachs disease has resulted in a dramatic decline in the incidence of this syndrome in the United States. On the other hand, screening for sickle cell disease or trait in the African-American population has sometimes resulted in insurance and employment discrimination.

Mass screening for complex genetic disorders can result in potential problems. For example, cystic fibrosis is most commonly associated with alterations in ΔF508. This variant accounts for 30–80% of mutant alleles depending on the ethnic group. Nevertheless, cystic fibrosis is associated with pronounced genetic heterogeneity with more than 1000 disease-related mutations. The American College of Medical Genetics recommends a panel of 23 alleles, including the ΔF508 allele, for routine diagnostic and carrier testing. Analysis for the less common cystic fibrosis–associated mutations would greatly impact the cost of testing without significantly influencing the effectiveness of mass screening. Nevertheless, the individual who carries one of the less common cystic fibrosis–associated alterations will not benefit if testing is limited to a routine panel.

Occupational health screening programs hold promise but also raise concerns about employment discrimination. These concerns were brought to light in 2001 when it was discovered that a railroad company was testing its employees, without consent, for a rare genetic condition that results in susceptibility to carpal tunnel syndrome. The Equal Employment Opportunity Commission argued that the tests were unlawful under the Americans with Disabilities Act.

THE FAMILY HISTORY

When two or more first-degree relatives are affected with asthma, cardiovascular disease, type 2 diabetes, breast cancer, colon cancer, or melanoma, the relative risk ranges from two- to fivefold, underscoring the importance of family history for these prevalent disorders. Pending further advances in genetic testing, the key to assessing the inherited risk for common adult-onset diseases rests in the collection and interpretation of a detailed personal and family medical history in conjunction with a directed physical examination. For example, a history of multiple family members with early-onset coronary artery disease, glucose intolerance, and hypertension should suggest increased risk for genetic, and perhaps environmental, predisposition to metabolic syndrome (Chap. 236). Individual patients with this family history should be monitored for the possible development of hypertension, diabetes, and hyperlipidemia. They should be counseled about the importance of avoiding additional risk factors such as obesity and cigarette smoking.

Family history should be recorded in the form of a pedigree. At a minimum, pedigrees should convey health-related data on all first-degree relatives and selected second-degree relatives, including grandparents. When pedigrees appear to suggest an inherited disease, they should be extended to include additional family members. The determination of risk for an asymptomatic individual will vary depending on the size of the pedigree, the number of unaffected relatives, and the types of diagnoses, as well as the ages of disease onset within the family. For example, a woman with two first-degree relatives with breast cancer is at greater risk for a Mendelian disorder if she has a total of three female first-degree relatives than if she has a total of ten female first-degree relatives. Additional variables that should be documented in the pedigree include the presence or absence of nonhereditary risk factors among those affected with diseases, and the finding of multiple diseases in an individual patient. For instance, a woman with a history of both colon cancer and endometrial cancer is at risk for hereditary nonpolyposis colon cancer (HNPCC) regardless of her family history.

When assessing the personal and family history, the physician should be alert to a younger age of disease onset than is usually seen in the general population. A 30-year-old with acute myocardial infarction should be considered at risk for a hereditary trait, even if there is no family history of premature coronary artery disease (Chap. 235). The absence of the nonhereditary risk factors typically associated with

a disease also raises the prospect of genetic causation. A personal or family history of deep-vein thrombosis, in the absence of known environmental or medical risk factors, suggests a hereditary thrombotic disorder (Chap. 111). The physical examination also may provide important clues about the risk for a specific inherited disorder. A patient presenting with xanthomas at a young age should prompt consideration of familial hypercholesterolemia. Some adult-onset disease-causing mutations are more prevalent in certain ethnic groups. For instance, >2% of the Ashkenazi population carry one of three specific mutations in the *BRCA1* or *BRCA2* genes. The prevalence of the factor V Leiden allele ranges from 3 to 7% in Caucasians but is much lower in Africans or Asians.

Recall of family history is often inaccurate. This is especially so when the history is remote and families become more dispersed geographically. It can be helpful to ask patients to fill out family history forms before or after their visits, as this provides them with an opportunity to contact relatives. Attempts should be made to confirm the illnesses reported in the family history before making important and, in certain circumstances, irreversible management decisions. This process is often labor intensive and ideally involves interviews of additional family members or reviewing medical records, autopsy reports, and death certificates.

Although many inherited disorders will be suggested by the clustering of relatives with the same or related conditions, it is important to note that *disease penetrance* is incomplete for most multifactorial genetic disorders. As a result, the pedigree obtained in such families may not exhibit a clear Mendelian inheritance pattern, as not all family members carrying the disease-associated alleles will manifest a clinical disorder. Furthermore, genes associated with some of these disorders often exhibit *variable expression* of disease. For example, the breast cancer–associated gene *BRCA1* can predispose to several different malignancies in the same family, including cancers of the breast, ovary, and prostate (Chap. 79). For common diseases such as breast cancer, some family members without the disease-causing mutation may also develop breast cancer, representing another confounding variable in the pedigree analysis.

Some of the aforementioned features of the family history are illustrated in Fig. 64-1. In this example, the proband, a 36-year-old woman (IV-1), has a strong history of breast and ovarian cancer on the paternal side of her family. The early age of onset, as well as the co-occurrence of breast and ovarian cancer in this family, suggests the

FIGURE 64-1 A 36-year-old woman (*arrow*) seeks consultation because of her family history of cancer. The patient expresses concern that the multiple cancers in her relatives imply an inherited predisposition to develop cancer. The family history is recorded and records of the patient's relatives confirm the reported diagnoses.

possibility of an inherited mutation in *BRCA1* or *BRCA2*. It is unclear though—without genetic testing—whether her father inherited such a mutation and transmitted it to her. After appropriate genetic counseling of the proband and her family, one approach to DNA analysis in this family is to test the cancer-affected 42-year-old living cousin for the presence of a *BRCA1* or *BRCA2* mutation. If a mutation is found, then it is possible to test for this particular alteration in the proband and other family members, if they so desire. In the example shown, if the proband's father has the *BRCA1* mutation, there is a 50:50 probability that the mutation was transmitted to her, and genetic testing can be used to establish the absence or presence of this alteration.

GENETIC TESTING FOR ADULT-ONSET DISORDERS

A critical first step before initiating genetic testing is to ensure that the correct clinical diagnosis has been made, whether based on family history, characteristic physical findings, or biochemical testing. Careful clinical assessment can define the *phenotype*, thereby preventing unnecessary testing and directing testing toward the most probable candidate genes (Fig. 64-2). For patients identified by population-based screening (e.g., diabetes, hypercholesterolemia), testing might involve known candidate genes, or genome-wide linkage studies (HapMap) of the population could be used as part of a research study to identify susceptibility alleles. For patients with a strong family history (e.g., breast cancer, hemochromatosis), testing often includes known candidate genes, or traditional linkage analyses within pedigrees can identify disease-causing genes. Once candidate genes are known, mutational analyses can be performed after pretest genetic counseling (see below).

Many disorders exhibit the feature of *locus heterogeneity*, which refers to the fact that mutations in different genes can cause phenotypically similar disorders. For example, osteogenesis imperfecta (Chap. 357), long QT syndrome (Chap. 226), muscular dystrophy (Chap. 382), homocystinuria (Chap. 358), retinitis pigmentosa (Chap. 29), and hereditary predisposition to colon cancer (Chap. 87) or breast cancer (Chap. 86) can each be caused by mutations in distinct genes. The pattern of disease transmission, clinical course, and treatment may differ significantly, depending on the specific gene affected. In these cases, the choice of which genes to test is often determined by unique clinical and family history features, the relative prevalence of mutations in various genes, or test availability.

METHODOLOGIC APPROACHES TO GENETIC TESTING

Genetic testing is performed in much the same way as other specialized laboratory tests. In the United States, genetic testing laboratories

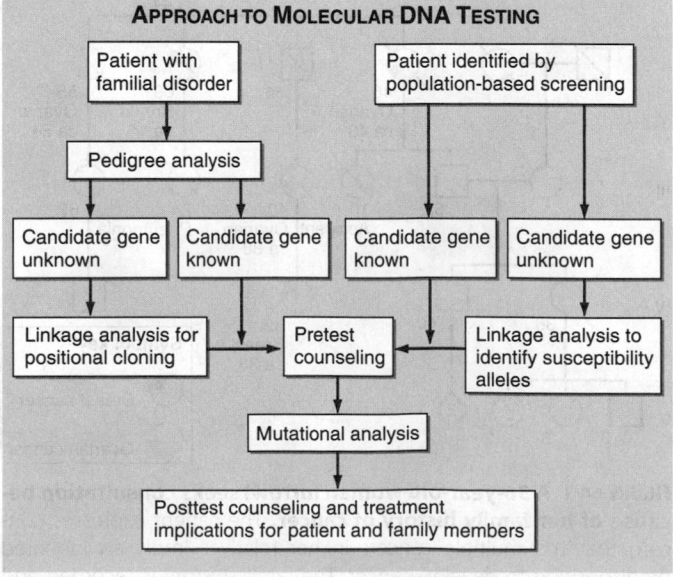

APPROACH TO MOLECULAR DNA TESTING

FIGURE 64-2 Approach to identifying a disease-causing gene.

are CLIA (Clinical Laboratory Improvement Act) approved to ensure that they meet quality and proficiency standards. A useful source for various genetic tests is *www.genetests.org*.

DNA testing is most commonly performed by DNA sequence analysis for mutations, although genotype can also be deduced through the study of RNA or protein (e.g., apoprotein E, hemoglobin, immunohistochemistry). The determination of DNA sequence alterations relies heavily on the use of polymerase chain reaction (PCR), which allows rapid amplification and analysis of the gene of interest. In addition, PCR enables genetic testing on minimal amounts of DNA extracted from a wide range of tissue sources including leukocytes, fibroblasts, epithelial cells in saliva or hair, and archival tissues. Amplified DNA can be analyzed directly by DNA sequencing or it can be hybridized to DNA chips or blots to detect the presence of normal and mutant DNA sequences. Direct DNA sequencing is increasingly used for prenatal diagnosis as well as for determination of hereditary disease susceptibility. Analyses of large alterations in the genome are possible using cytogenetics, fluorescent in situ hybridization (FISH), or Southern blotting (Chap. 63).

Protein truncation tests (PTTs) are used to detect mutations that result in the premature termination of a polypeptide occurring during protein synthesis. In this assay, the isolated complementary DNA (cDNA) is transcribed and translated in vitro, and the protein is analyzed by gel electrophoresis. The truncated (mutant) gene product is readily identified as its electrophoretic mobility differs from that of the normal protein. This test is used most commonly for analyses of large genes with significant genetic heterogeneity such as *DMD*, *APC*, and the *BRCA* genes.

Like all laboratory tests, there are limitations to the accuracy and interpretation of genetic tests. In addition to technical errors, genetic tests are sometimes designed to detect only the most common mutations. In this case, a negative result must be qualified by the possibility that the individual may have a mutation that is not included in the test. In addition, a negative result does not mean that there is not a mutation in some other gene that causes a similar inherited disorder.

In addition to molecular testing for established disease, genetic testing for susceptibility to chronic disease is being increasingly integrated into the practice of medicine. In most cases, however, the discovery of disease-associated genes has greatly outpaced studies that assess clinical outcomes and the impact of interventions. Until such evidence-based studies are available, predictive molecular testing must be approached with caution and should be offered only to patients who have been adequately counseled and have provided informed consent. In the majority of cases, genetic testing should be offered only to individuals with a suggestive personal or family medical history or in the context of a clinical trial.

Predictive genetic testing falls into two distinct categories. *Presymptomatic testing* applies to diseases where a specific genetic alteration is associated with a near 100% likelihood of developing disease. In contrast, *predisposition testing* predicts a risk for disease that is less than 100%. For example, presymptomatic testing is available for those at risk for Huntington's disease, whereas predisposition testing is considered for those at risk for hereditary breast cancer. It is important to note that, for the majority of adult-onset, multifactorial genetic disorders, testing is purely predictive. Test results cannot reveal with confidence whether, when, or how the disease will manifest itself. For example, not everyone with the apolipoprotein E allele (ε4) will develop Alzheimer's disease, and individuals without this genetic marker can still develop the disorder (Chap. 365).

Molecular analysis is generally more informative if testing is initiated in a symptomatic family member, since the identification of a mutation can direct the testing of other at-risk family members (whether they are symptomatic or not). In the absence of additional familial or environmental risk factors, individuals who test negative for the mutation found in the affected family member can be informed that they are at general population risk for that particular disease. Furthermore, they can be reassured that they are not at risk for passing on the mutation to their children. On the other hand, asymptomatic family members who test positive for the known mutation must be informed that they are at increased risk for disease development and for transmitting the alteration to their children.

Clinicians providing pretest counseling and education should assess the patient's ability to cope with test results. Individuals who demonstrate signs and symptoms of emotional distress should have their psychosocial needs addressed before proceeding with molecular testing. Generally, genetic testing should not be offered at a time of personal crisis or acute illness within the family. Patients will derive more benefit from test results if they are emotionally able to comprehend and absorb the information. It is important to assess patients' preconceived notions of their personal likelihood of disease in preparing pretest educational strategies. Often, patients harbor unwarranted fear or denial of their likelihood of genetic risk.

Genetic testing has the potential of affecting the way individual family members relate to one another, both negatively and positively. As a result, patients addressing the option of molecular testing must consider how test results might impact their relationships with relatives, partners, spouses, and friends. In families with a known genetic mutation, those who test positive must consider the impact of their carrier status on their present and future lifestyles; those who test negative may manifest *survivor guilt*. Family members are likely to differ in their emotional and social responses to the same information. Counseling should also address the potential consequences of test results on relationships with a spouse or child. Parents who are found to have a disease-associated mutation often express considerable anxiety and despair as they address the issue of risk to their children.

When a condition does not manifest until adulthood, clinicians will be faced with the question of whether at-risk children should be offered molecular testing and, if so, at what age. Although the matter is debated, several professional organizations have cautioned that genetic testing for adult-onset disorders should not be offered to children. Many of these conditions are not preventable; consequently, such information can pose significant psychosocial risk to the child. In addition, there is concern that testing during childhood violates a child's right to make an informed decision regarding testing upon reaching adulthood. On the other hand, testing should be offered in childhood for disorders that may manifest early in life, especially when management options are available. For example, children at risk for familial adenomatous polyposis (FAP), associated with alterations in the *APC* gene, may develop polyps as early as their teens, and progression to an invasive cancer can occur by their twenties. Likewise, children at risk for MEN type 2, which is caused by mutations in the *RET* proto-oncogene, may develop medullary thyroid cancer early in childhood, and the issue of prophylactic thyroidectomy should be addressed with the parents of children with documented mutations (Chap. 345).

INFORMED CONSENT
When the issue of testing is addressed, patients should be strongly encouraged to involve other relatives in the decision-making process, as molecular diagnostics will likely have an impact on the entire family. Informed consent for molecular testing begins with detailed education and counseling (Fig. 64-3). The patient must fully understand the risks, benefits, and limitations of undergoing the analysis. Informed consent should include a written document, drafted clearly and concisely in a language and format that is comprehensible to the patient, who should be made aware of the disposition of test results. Informed consent should also include a discussion of the mechanics of testing. Most molecular testing for hereditary disease involves DNA-based analysis of peripheral blood. In the majority of circumstances, test results should be given only to the individual, in person, and with a support person in the room.

Because molecular testing of an asymptomatic individual often allows prediction of future risk, the patient should understand any potential long-term medical, psychological, and social implications of this decision. In the United States, legislation affecting this area is still evolving, and it is important to explore with the patient the potential impact that test results may have on employment and future health, as well as disability and life insurance coverage.

Patients should understand that alternatives to molecular analysis remain available if they decide not to proceed with this option. They

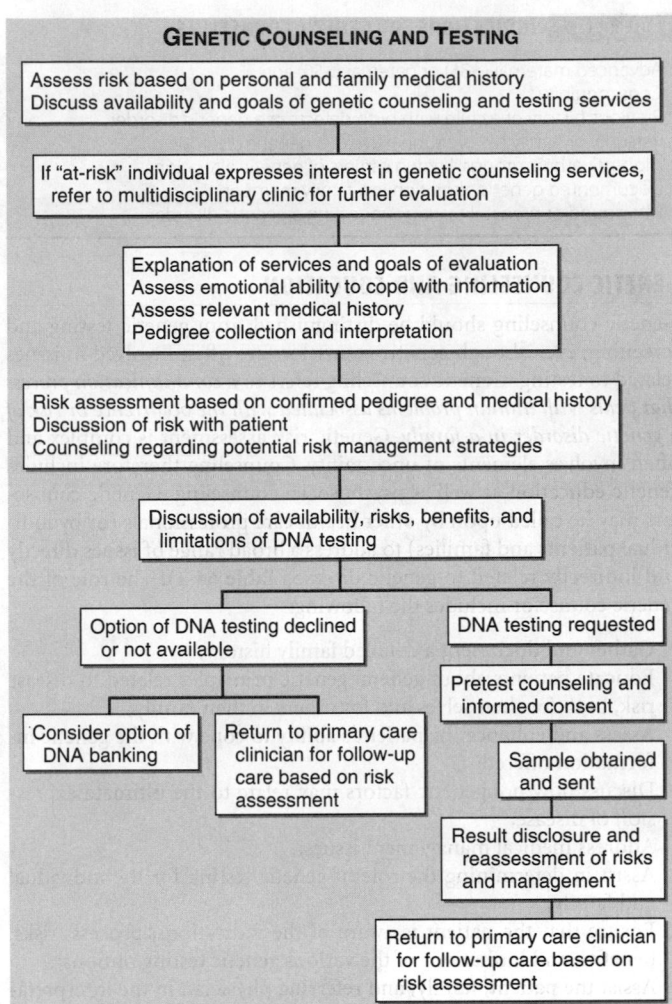

GENETIC COUNSELING AND TESTING

Assess risk based on personal and family medical history
Discuss availability and goals of genetic counseling and testing services

If "at-risk" individual expresses interest in genetic counseling services, refer to multidisciplinary clinic for further evaluation

Explanation of services and goals of evaluation
Assess emotional ability to cope with information
Assess relevant medical history
Pedigree collection and interpretation

Risk assessment based on confirmed pedigree and medical history
Discussion of risk with patient
Counseling regarding potential risk management strategies

Discussion of availability, risks, benefits, and limitations of DNA testing

Option of DNA testing declined or not available → Consider option of DNA banking / Return to primary care clinician for follow-up care based on risk assessment

DNA testing requested
Pretest counseling and informed consent
Sample obtained and sent
Result disclosure and reassessment of risks and management
Return to primary care clinician for follow-up care based on risk assessment

FIGURE 64-3 Algorithm for genetic counseling in association with genetic testing.

should also be notified that testing is available in the future if they are not currently prepared to undergo analysis. The option of DNA banking should be presented so that samples are readily available for future use by family members, if needed.

FOLLOW-UP CARE AFTER TESTING
Depending on the nature of the genetic disorder, posttest interventions may include (1) cautious surveillance and appropriate health care screening, (2) specific medical interventions, (3) chemoprevention, (4) risk avoidance, and (5) referral to support services. For example, patients with known pathologic mutations in *BRCA1* or *BRCA2* are offered intensive screening as well as the option of prophylactic mastectomy and oophorectomy. In addition, such women may be eligible for preventive treatment with tamoxifen, or enrollment in a chemoprevention clinical trial. In contrast, those at known risk for Huntington's disease are offered continued follow-up and supportive services, including physical and occupational therapy, and social services or support groups, as indicated. Specific interventions will change as translational research continues to enhance our understanding of these genetic diseases and as more is learned about the functions of the gene products involved.

Individuals who test negative for a mutation in a disease-associated gene identified in an affected family member must be reminded that they may still be at risk for the disease. This is of particular importance for common diseases such as diabetes mellitus, cancer, and coronary artery disease. For example, a woman who finds that she does not carry the disease-associated mutation in *BRCA2* previously discovered in her family must be reminded that she still requires the same breast cancer screening recommended for the general population.

TABLE 64-1	INDICATIONS FOR GENETIC COUNSELING
Advanced maternal (>35) or paternal (>50) age	
Consanguinity	
Previous history of a child with birth defects or a genetic disorder	
Personal or family history suggestive of a genetic disorder	
High-risk ethnic groups; known carriers of genetic alterations	
Documented genetic alteration in a family member	
Ultrasound or prenatal testing suggesting a genetic disorder	

GENETIC COUNSELING AND EDUCATION

Genetic counseling should be distinguished from genetic testing and screening, even though genetic counselors are often involved in issues related to testing. Genetic counseling refers to *a communication process that deals with human problems associated with the occurrence or risk of a genetic disorder in a family*. Genetic risk assessment is complex and often involves elements of uncertainty. Counseling therefore includes genetic education as well as psychosocial counseling. Genetic counselors may be called upon by other health care professionals (or by individual patients and families) to address a broad range of issues directly and indirectly related to genetic disease (Table 64-1). The role of the genetic counselor includes the following:

- Gather and document a detailed family history;
- Educate patients about general genetic principles related to disease risk, both for themselves and for others in their family;
- Assess and enhance the patient's ability to cope with the genetic information offered;
- Discuss how nongenetic factors may relate to the ultimate expression of disease;
- Address medical management issues;
- Assist in determining the role of genetic testing for the individual and family;
- Ensure that the patient is aware of the indications, process, risks, benefits, and limitations of the various genetic testing options;
- Assist the patient, family, and referring physician in the interpretation of the test results; and
- Refer the patient and other at-risk family members for additional medical and support services, if necessary.

The complexity of genetic counseling and the broad scope of genetic diseases have led to the development of specialized, multidisciplinary clinics designed to provide broad-based support and medical care for those at risk and their family members. Such specialty clinics are well established in the areas of cancer and neurodegenerative disorders. The multidisciplinary teams are often composed of medical geneticists, specialist physicians, genetic counselors, nurses, psychologists, social workers, and biomedical ethicists who work together to consider difficult diagnostic, treatment, and testing decisions. Such a format also provides primary care physicians with invaluable support and assistance as they follow and treat at-risk patients.

The approach to genetic counseling has important ethical, social, and financial implications. Philosophies related to genetic counseling vary widely by country and center. In North American centers, for example, counseling is generally offered in a nondirective manner, wherein patients learn to understand how their values factor into a particular medical decision. Nondirective counseling is particularly appropriate when there are no data demonstrating a clear benefit associated with a particular intervention or when an intervention is considered experimental. For example, nondirective genetic counseling is employed when a person is deciding whether to undergo genetic testing for Huntington's disease (Chap. 365). At this time, there is no clear benefit (in terms of medical outcome) to an at-risk individual undergoing genetic testing for this disease, as its course cannot be altered by therapeutic interventions. However, testing can have an important impact on this individual's perception of the future and his or her interpersonal relationships and plans for reproduction. Therefore, the decision to pursue testing rests on the individual's belief system and values. On the other hand, a more directive approach is appropriate when a condition can be treated. In a family with FAP, colon cancer screening and prophylactic colectomy should be recommended for known *APC* mutation carriers. The counselor and clinician following this family must ensure that the at-risk family members have access to the resources necessary to adhere to these recommendations.

Genetic education is central to an individual's ability to make an informed decision regarding testing options and treatment. Although genetic counselors represent one source of genetic education, other health care providers also need to contribute to patient education. Patients at risk for genetic disease should understand fundamental medical genetic principles and terminology relevant to their situation. This includes the concept of genes, how they are transmitted, and how they confer hereditary disease risk. An adequate knowledge of patterns of inheritance will allow patients to understand the probability of disease risk for themselves and other family members. It is also important to impart the concepts of disease penetrance and expression. For most complex adult-onset genetic disorders, asymptomatic patients should be advised that a positive test result does not always translate into future disease development. In addition, the role of nongenetic factors, such as environmental exposures, must be discussed in the context of multifactorial disease risk and disease prevention. Finally, patients should understand the natural history of the disease as well as the potential options for intervention, including screening, prevention, and—in certain circumstances—pharmacologic treatment or prophylactic surgery.

THERAPEUTIC INTERVENTIONS BASED ON GENETIC RISK FOR DISEASE

Specific treatments are now available for an increasing number of genetic disorders, whether identified through population-based screening or directed testing (Table 64-2). Although the strategies for therapeutic interventions are best developed for childhood hereditary metabolic diseases, these principles are making their way into the diagnosis and

TABLE 64-2	EXAMPLES OF GENETIC TESTING AND POSSIBLE INTERVENTIONS		
Genetic Disorder	**Inheritance**	**Genes**	**Interventions**
Oncologic			
Hereditary nonpolyposis colon cancer	AD	*MSH2, MLH1, MSH6, PMS1, PMS2, TGFBR2*	Early endoscopic screening
Familial adenomatous polyposis	AD	*APC*	Early endoscopic screening Nonsteroidal anti-inflammatory drugs Colectomy
Familial breast and ovarian cancer	AD	*BRCA1, BRCA2*	Estrogen receptor antagonists Early screening by exams and mammography Consideration of prophylactic surgery
Familial melanoma	AD	*CDKN2A*	Avoidance of UV light Screening and biopsies
Basal cell nevus syndrome	AD	*PTCH*	Avoidance of UV light Screening and biopsies

(continued)

Genetic Disorder	Inheritance	Genes	Interventions
Hematologic			
Factor V Leiden	AD	*F5*	Avoidance of thrombogenic risk factors and oral contraceptives
Hemophilia A	XL	*F8C*	Factor VIII replacement
Hemophilia B	XL	*F9*	Factor IX replacement Possible gene therapy
Glucose 6-PO4 dehydrogenase deficiency	XL	*G6PD*	Avoidance of oxidant drugs
Cardiovascular			
Hypertrophic cardiomyopathy	AD	*MYH7, MYBPC3, TMSA, TNNT2, TPM1*	Echocardiographic screening Early pharmacologic intervention Myomectomy
Long QT syndrome	AD	*KCNQ1, SCN5A, HERG, MiRP1, KCNE1, KCNE2*	Electrocardiographic screening Early pharmacologic intervention Implantable cardioverter defibrillator devices
Marfan syndrome	AD	*FBN1*	Echocardiographic screening Prophylactic beta blockers
Gastrointestinal			
Familial Mediterranean fever	AR	*MEFV*	Colchicine treatment
Hemochromatosis	AR	*HFE*	Phlebotomy
Pulmonary			
α_1 Antitrypsin deficiency	AR	*PI*	Avoidance of smoking Avoidance of occupational and environmental toxins
Primary pulmonary hypertension	AD	*BMPR2*	Treatment with pulmonary vasodilators
Renal			
Polycystic kidney disease	AD	*PKHD1, PKHD2*	Prevention of hypertension Prevention of urinary tract infections Kidney transplantation
Nephrogenic diabetes insipidus	XL, AR	*AVPR2, AQP2*	Fluid replacement Thiazides, amiloride
Endocrine			
Neurohypophyseal diabetes insipidus	AD	*AVP*	Replace vasopressin
Maturity-onset diabetes of the young	AD	Multiple genes	Screen and treat for diabetes
Familial hypocalciuric hypercalcemia	AD	*CASR*	Avoidance of parathyroidectomy
Kallmann syndrome	XL	*KAL*	Induction of puberty with hormone replacement
Multiple endocrine neoplasia type 2	AD	*RET*	Prophylactic thyroidectomy Screening for pheochromocytoma and hyperparathyroidism
21-hydroxylase deficiency	AR	*CYP21*	Glucocorticoid and mineralocorticoid treatment
Neurologic			
Malignant hyperthermia	AD	*RYR1*	Avoidance of precipitating anesthetics
Hyperkalemic periodic paralysis	AD	*SCN4A*	Acetazolamide
Adrenoleukodystrophy	XL	*ABCD1*	Possible bone marrow transplant for severe childhood CNS form
Duchenne and Becker muscular dystrophy	XL	*DMD*	Corticosteroids Possible future myoblast transfer
Familial Parkinson disease	AD	*SNCA, PARK2*	Amantadine, anticholinergics, levodopa, monoamine oxidase B inhibitors
Wilson disease	AR	*ATP7B*	Zinc, trientene

Abbreviations: AD, autosomal dominant; AR, autosomal recessive; CNS, central nervous system; XL, X-linked.

management of adult-onset disorders. Hereditary hemochromatosis illustrates many of the issues raised by the availability of genetic screening in the adult population. For instance, it is relatively common (approximately 1 in 200 individuals of northern European descent are homozygous), and its complications are potentially preventable through phlebotomy (Chap. 351). The identification of the *HFE* gene, mutations of which are associated with this syndrome, has sparked interest in the use of DNA-based testing for presymptomatic diagnosis of the disorder. However, up to one-third of individuals who are homozygous for the *HFE* mutation do not have evidence of iron overload. Consequently, in the absence of a positive family history, current recommendations include phenotypic screening for evidence of iron overload followed by genetic testing. Whether genetic screening for hemochromatosis will someday be coupled to assessment of phenotypic expression awaits further studies. In contrast to the issue of population screening, it is important to test and counsel other family members when the diagnosis of hemochromatosis has been made in a proband. Testing allows the physician to exclude family members who are not at risk. It also permits presymptomatic detection of iron overload and the institution of treatment (phlebotomy) before the development of organ damage.

Preventive measures and therapeutic interventions are not restricted to metabolic disorders. Identification of familial forms of long QT syn-

CHAPTER 64

The Practice of Genetics in Clinical Medicine

drome, associated with ventricular arrhythmias, allows early electrocardiographic testing and the use of prophylactic antiarrhythmic therapy, overdrive pacemakers, or defibrillators (Chap. 226). Individuals with familial hypertrophic cardiomyopathy can be screened by ultrasound, treated with beta blockers or other drugs, and counseled about the importance of avoiding strenuous exercise and dehydration (Chap. 231). Likewise, individuals with Marfan syndrome can be treated with beta blockers and monitored for the development of aortic aneurysms (Chap. 242). Individuals with α_1 antitrypsin deficiency can be strongly counseled to avoid cigarette smoking and exposure to environmental pulmonary and hepatotoxins. Various host genes influence the pathogenesis of certain infectious diseases in humans, including HIV (Chap. 182). The factor V Leiden allele increases risk of thrombosis (Chap. 59). Approximately 3% of the worldwide population is heterozygous for this mutation. Moreover, it is found in up to 25% of patients with recurrent deep-vein thrombosis or pulmonary embolism. Women who are heterozygous or homozygous for this allele should therefore avoid the use of oral contraceptives and receive heparin prophylaxis after surgery or trauma.

The field of pharmacogenomics seeks to identify genes that alter drug metabolism or confer susceptibility to toxic drug reactions. Pharmacogenomics permits individualized drug therapy, resulting in improved treatment outcomes, reduced toxicities, and more cost-effective pharmaceutical care. Examples include succinylcholine sensitivity, thiopurine methyltransferase (TPMT) deficiency, malignant hyperthermia, dihydropyrimidine dehydrogenase deficiency, the porphyrias, and glucose-6-phosphase dehydrogenase (G6PD) deficiency.

As noted above, the identification of genes that increase the risk of specific types of neoplasia is rapidly changing the management of many cancers. Identifying family members with mutations that predispose to FAP or hereditary nonpolyposis colon cancer (HNPCC) can lead to recommendations of early cancer screening or prophylactic surgery (Chap. 87). Similar principles apply to familial forms of melanoma, basal cell carcinoma, and cancers of the breast, ovary, and thyroid gland. It should be recognized, however, that most cancers harbor several distinct genetic abnormalities by the time they acquire invasive or metastatic potential (Chaps. 79 and 80). Consequently, the major impact of genetic testing in these cases is to allow more intensive clinical screening, as it remains very challenging to predict disease penetrance, expression, or clinical course.

Although genetic diagnosis of these and other disorders is only beginning to be used in the clinical setting, predictive testing holds the promise of allowing earlier and more targeted interventions that can reduce morbidity and mortality. We can expect the availability of genetic tests to expand. A critical challenge for physicians and other health care providers is to keep pace with these advances in genetic medicine and to implement testing judiciously.

FURTHER READINGS

CLAYTON EW: Ethical, legal, and social implications of genomic medicine. N Engl J Med 349:562, 2003

COLLINS FS, WATSON JD: Genetic discrimination: Time to act. Science 302:745, 2003

ENSENAUER RE: Genetic testing: Practical, ethical, and counseling considerations. Mayo Clin Proc 80:63, 2005

GUTTMACHER AE, COLLINS FS: Genomic medicine—a primer. N Engl J Med 347:1512, 2002

HARPER PS: *Practical Genetic Counselling*, 5th ed. Oxford, Butterworth Heinmann, 1998

MCCANDLESS SE et al: The burden of genetic disease on inpatient care in a children's hospital. Am J Hum Genet 74:121, 2004

WOLFBERG AJ: Genes on the web—Direct-to-consumer marketing of genetic testing. N Engl J Med 355:543, 2006

65 Gene Therapy in Clinical Medicine
Katherine A. High

Gene transfer is a novel area of therapeutics in which the active agent is a nucleic acid sequence rather than a protein or small molecule. Because delivery of naked DNA or RNA to a cell is an inefficient process, most gene transfer is carried out using a vector, or gene delivery vehicle. These vehicles have generally been engineered from viruses by deleting some or all of the viral genome and replacing it with the therapeutic gene of interest under the control of a suitable promoter (Table 65-1). Gene transfer strategies can be described in terms of three essential elements: (1) a vector, (2) a gene to be delivered, and

TABLE 65-1 CHARACTERISTICS OF GENE DELIVERY VEHICLES

Features	Retroviral	Lentiviral	Adenoviral	AAV	Human Foamy Virus	HSV-1	SV-40	Alpha-Viruses
Viral genome	RNA	RNA	DNA	DNA	RNA	DNA	DNA	RNA
Cell division requirement	Yes	G1 phase	No	No	No	No	No	No
Packaging limitation	8 kb	8 kb	8–30 kb	5 kb	8.5 kb	40–150 kb	5 kb	5 kb
Immune responses to vector	Few	Few	Extensive	Few	Few	Few in recombinant virus	Few	Few
Genome integration	Yes	Yes	Poor	Poor	Yes	No	Poor	No
Long-term expression	Yes	Yes	No	Yes	Yes	No	No	No
Main advantages	Persistent gene transfer in dividing cells	Persistent gene transfer in transduced tissues	Highly effective in transducing various tissues	Elicits few inflammatory responses, nonpathogenic	Persistent gene expression in both dividing and nondividing cells	Large packaging capacity with persistent gene transfer	Wide host cell range; lack of immunogenicity	Limited immune responses against the vector
Main disadvantages	Theoretical risk of insertional mutagenesis (occurred in 3 cases)	Might induce oncogenesis in some cases	Viral capsid elicits strong immune responses	Limited packaging capacity	In need of a stable packaging system	Residual cytotoxicity with neuron specificity	Limited packaging capacity	Transduced gene expression is transient

Note: AAV, adeno-associated virus; HSV, herpes simplex virus; SV, sarcoma virus.

(3) a relevant target cell to which the DNA or RNA is delivered. The series of steps in which the donated DNA enters the target cell and begins expression is referred to as *transduction*. Gene delivery can take place in vivo, in which the vector is directly injected into the patient or, in the case of hematopoietic and some other target cells, ex vivo, with removal of the target cells from the patient, followed by return of the modified autologous cells after gene transfer in the laboratory. The latter approach offers opportunities to integrate gene transfer techniques with cellular therapies (Chap. 67).

Gene transfer technology is still under development and protocols are experimental. Gene therapy is one of the most complex therapeutic modalities yet attempted, and each new disease represents a therapeutic problem for which dosing, safety, and efficacy must be defined. Nonetheless, gene transfer remains one of the most powerful concepts in modern molecular medicine and has the potential to address a host of diseases for which there are currently no cures or, in some cases, no available treatment. Over 5000 subjects have been enrolled in gene transfer studies, and serious adverse events have been rare. Gene therapies are being developed for a wide variety of disease entities (Fig. 65-1).

GENE TRANSFER FOR GENETIC DISEASE

Gene transfer strategies for genetic disease generally involve gene addition therapy. This approach most commonly involves transfer of the missing gene to a physiologically relevant target cell. However, other strategies are possible, including supplying a gene that achieves a similar biologic effect through an alternative pathway (e.g., factor VIIa for hemophilia A); supplying an antisense oligonucleotide to splice out a mutant exon if the sequence is not critical to the function of the protein (as has been done with the dystrophin gene in Duchenne muscular dystrophy); or downregulating a harmful response through an siRNA. Two distinct strategies are used to achieve long-term gene expression: one is to transduce stem cells with an integrating vector, so that all progeny cells will carry the donated gene; the other is to transduce long-lived cells, such as skeletal muscle or neural cells. In the case of long-lived cells, integration into the target cell genome is unnecessary, provided the donated DNA can be stabilized in an episomal form.

Immunodeficiency Disorders: Proof of Principle Early attempts to provide gene replacement into hematopoietic stem cells (HSCs) were stymied by the relatively low transduction efficiency of retroviral vec-

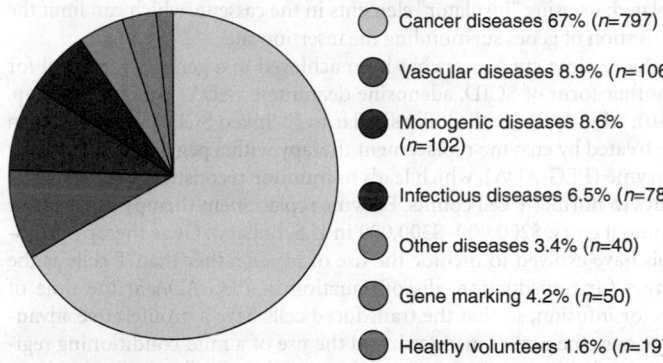

Cancer diseases 67% (*n*=797)

Vascular diseases 8.9% (*n*=106)

Monogenic diseases 8.6% (*n*=102)

Infectious diseases 6.5% (*n*=78)

Other diseases 3.4% (*n*=40)

Gene marking 4.2% (*n*=50)

Healthy volunteers 1.6% (*n*=19)

FIGURE 65-1 Indications in gene therapy clinical trials. The chart divides clinical gene transfer studies by disease classification. A majority of trials have addressed cancer, with monogenic disorders and cardiovascular diseases the next largest categories. (*Reproduced with permission from J Gene Med. New Jersey, Wiley, 2006.*)

tors, which require dividing target cells for integration. Because HSCs are normally quiescent, they are a formidable transduction target. However, identification of cytokines that induced cell division without promoting differentiation of stem cells, along with technical improvements in the isolation and transduction of HSCs, led to modest but real gains in transduction efficiency.

The first convincing therapeutic effect from gene transfer occurred with X-linked severe combined immunodeficiency disease (SCID), which results from mutations in the gene (*IL2RG*) encoding the γc subunit of a cytokine receptor required for normal development of T and NK cells (Chap. 310). Affected infants present in the first few months of life with overwhelming infections and/or failure to thrive. In this disorder, it was recognized that the transduced cells, even if few in number, would have a proliferative advantage compared to the nontransduced cells, which lack receptors for the cytokines required for lymphocyte development and maturation. Complete reconstitution of the immune system, including documented responses to standard childhood vaccinations, clearing of infections, and remarkable gains in growth occurred in most of the treated children. However, two developed a syndrome similar to T cell acute lymphocytic leukemia, with splenomegaly, rising white counts, and the emergence of a single clone of T cells. In these children, the retroviral vector had integrated within a gene, *LMO-2* (LIM only-2), which encodes a component of a transcription factor complex involved in hematopoietic development. Insertion of the retroviral long terminal repeat is thought to increase the expression of *LMO-2*.

The X-linked SCID studies were a watershed event in the evolution of gene therapy. They demonstrated conclusively that gene therapy could cure disease; of the 16 infants eventually treated in these trials, 15 achieved correction of the immunodeficiency disorder. Unfortunately, 3 later developed a leukemia-like disorder, but 12 are alive and free of complications at time periods ranging up to 7 years after initial treatment. These studies also demonstrated that insertional mutagenesis leading to cancer was more than a hypothetical possibility. As a result of the experience in these trials, all protocols using integrating vectors in hematopoietic cells must include a plan for monitoring sites of insertion and clonal proliferation. Strategies to overcome this complication have included employing a "suicide" gene cassette in the vector, so that errant clones can be quickly

	Non-Viral Vectors			
Features	**Transposon/ Transposase System**	**Liposomes**	**Naked DNA**	**Site-Specific Integrase**
Viral genome	N/A	N/A	N/A	N/A
Cell division requirement	No	No	No	No
Packaging limitation	Undetermined, probably large	Undetermined, probably large	Undetermined, probably large	Undetermined, probably large
Immune responses to vector	No	No	No	No
Genome integration	Yes	No	No	Yes
Long-term expression	Yes	No	No	Undetermined
Main advantages	Transfects many cell types with long-term gene expression	Transfects many cell types. Large holding capacity to enable a high number of base pairs	Efficient in gene transfer; limited immunogenicity	Specific integration site
Main disadvantages	Early stage in development	Expensive to produce	Transient and low-level expression	Early stage in development

ablated; or using "insulator" elements in the cassette, which can limit the activation of genes surrounding the insertion site.

More clear-cut success has been achieved in a gene therapy trial for another form of SCID, adenosine deaminase (ADA) deficiency (Chap. 310). ADA-SCID is clinically similar to X-linked SCID, although it can be treated by enzyme replacement therapy with a pegylated form of the enzyme (PEG-ADA), which leads to immune reconstitution but not always to normal T cell counts. Enzyme replacement therapy is expensive (annual costs: $200,000–$300,000 in U.S. dollars). Gene therapy protocols have evolved to include the use of HSCs rather than T cells as the target for transduction; discontinuation of PEG-ADA at the time of vector infusion, so that the transduced cells have a proliferative advantage over the non-transduced; and the use of a mild conditioning regimen to facilitate engraftment of the transduced cells. There have been no complications in the six children treated on this protocol, with a median follow-up of >4 years. Based on current data, the efficacy of gene transfer for ADA-SCID is convincing, but longer term follow-up will be required to determine whether this approach is sufficiently safe to be routinely recommended as an alternative to PEG-ADA.

Other diseases likely to be amenable to transduction of HSCs include Wiskott-Aldrich syndrome (trials underway), chronic granulomatous disease, sickle cell disease, and thalassemia.

Long-Term Expression in Genetic Disease: In Vivo Gene Transfer with Recombinant Adeno-Associated Viral (AAV) Vectors Recombinant AAV vectors have emerged as attractive gene delivery vehicles for genetic disease. Engineered from a small replication-defective DNA virus, they are devoid of viral coding sequences and trigger very little immune response in experimental animals. They are capable of transducing non-dividing target cells, and the donated DNA is stabilized primarily in an episomal form, thus minimizing risks associated with insertional mutagenesis. Because the vector has a tropism for certain long-lived cell types, such as skeletal muscle, the central nervous system (CNS), and hepatocytes, long-term expression can be achieved even in the absence of integration.

Clinical trials using recombinant AAV vectors are now ongoing for muscular dystrophies, α_1-antitrypsin deficiency, lipoprotein lipase deficiency, hemophilia B, and a form of congenital blindness called Leber's congenital amaurosis. Hemophilia is often considered a promising disease model for gene transfer, as the gene product does not require precise regulation of expression and biologically active clotting factors can be synthesized in a variety of tissue types, permitting latitude in choice of target tissue. Moreover, raising circulating factor levels from <1% (levels seen in those severely affected) into the range of 5% greatly improves the phenotype of the disease. Preclinical studies with recombinant AAV vectors infused into skeletal muscle or liver have resulted in long-term (>5 years) expression of factor VIII or factor IX in the hemophilic dog model. Administration to skeletal muscle of an AAV vector expressing factor IX in patients with hemophilia was safe and resulted in long-term expression as measured by muscle biopsy, but circulating levels never rose >1% for sustained periods, and a large number of IM injections (>80–100) was required to access a large muscle mass. Intravascular vector delivery has been employed to access large areas of skeletal muscle in animal models of hemophilia and will likely be tested in upcoming trials. Administration of an AAV vector expressing factor IX to the liver in humans with hemophilia resulted in therapeutic circulating levels at the highest dose tested, but expression at these levels (>5%) lasted for only 6–10 weeks before declining to baseline (<1%). A memory T cell response to viral capsid, present in humans but not in other animal species (which are not natural hosts for the virus), may be a contributing factor in the loss of expression. Fortunately, triggering of the memory T cell response appears tissue-specific, and it is possible that introduction of the vector into immunoprivileged sites, such as the CNS (e.g., for Parkinson's disease) or the retina, will avoid this complication.

Leber's congenital amaurosis (LCA) is a form of retinal degenerative disease, characterized by severe early-onset blindness. This disease, not currently treatable, is caused by mutations in several different genes; ~15% of cases of LCA are due to a mutation in a gene, *RPE65*, encoding a retinal pigment epithelial protein. In dogs with a null mutation in *RPE65*, sight has been restored after subretinal injection of an AAV vector expressing *RPE65*. Transgene expression appears to be stable, with the first animals treated >5 years ago continuing to manifest electrophysiologic and behavioral evidence of visual function. As is the case for X-linked SCID, gene transfer must occur relatively early in life to achieve correction of the genetic disease, although the exact limitations imposed by age await clinical studies. AAV-RPE65 trials have now been approved in both the United States and Great Britain. Other inherited retinal degenerative disorders may also be amenable to correction by gene transfer, as are certain complex acquired disorders such as age-related macular degeneration, which affects several million people worldwide. The neovascularization that occurs in age-related macular degeneration can be inhibited by expression of vascular endothelial growth factor (VEGF) inhibitors such as angiostatin, or through the use of RNAi-mediated knockdown of VEGF. Early-phase trials of siRNAs that target VEGF RNA are underway, but these require repeated intravitreal injection of the siRNAs; an AAV vector–mediated approach might allow long-term knockdown of VEGF.

GENE THERAPY FOR CANCER

The majority of clinical gene transfer experience has been in subjects with cancer (Fig. 65-1). As a general rule, a feature that distinguishes gene therapies from conventional cancer therapeutics is that the former are less toxic, in some cases because they are delivered locally (e.g., intratumoral injections), and in other cases because they are targeted specifically to elements of the tumor (immunotherapies, anti-angiogenic approaches).

Cancer gene therapies can be divided into local and systemic approaches (Table 65-2). Some of the earliest cancer gene therapy trials focused on local delivery of a prodrug or a suicide gene that would increase sensitivity of tumor cells to cytotoxic drugs. A frequently used strategy has been intratumoral injection of an adenoviral vector expressing the thymidine kinase (*TK*) gene. Cells that take up and express the *TK* gene can be killed after the administration of gancyclovir, which is phosphorylated to a toxic nucleoside by *TK*. Because cell division is required for the toxic nucleoside to affect cell viability, this strategy was initially used in aggressive brain tumors (glioblastoma multiforme) where the cycling tumor cells were affected but the nondividing normal neurons were not. More recently, this approach has been explored for locally recurrent prostate, breast, and colon tumors, among others.

Another local approach uses adenoviral-mediated expression of the tumor suppressor p53, which is mutated in a wide variety of cancers. This strategy has shown complete and partial responses in squamous cell carcinoma of the head and neck, esophageal cancer, and non-small cell lung cancer after direct intratumoral injection of the vector. Response rates (~15%) are comparable to those of other single agents. The use of oncolytic viruses that selectively replicate in tumor cells but not in normal cells has also shown promise in squamous cell carcinoma of the head and neck and in other solid tumors. This approach is based on the observation that deletion of certain viral genes abolishes their ability to replicate in normal cells but not in tumor cells. An advantage of this strategy is that the replicating vector can proliferate and spread within the tumor, facilitating eventual tumor clearance. However, physical limitations to viral spread, including fibrosis, intermixed normal cells, basement membranes, and necrotic areas within the tu-

TABLE 65-2	GENE THERAPY STRATEGIES IN CANCER

Local/regional approaches
   Suicide gene/prodrug
   Suppressor oncogene
   Oncolytic virus
Systemic response
   Chemoprotection
   Immunomodulation
   Anti-angiogenesis

mor, may reduce clinical efficacy. Oncolytic viruses are licensed and available in some countries, but not in the United States.

Because metastatic disease rather than uncontrolled growth of the primary tumor is the source of mortality for most cancers, there has been considerable interest in developing systemic gene therapy approaches. One strategy has been to promote more efficient recognition of tumor cells by the immune system. Approaches have included transduction of tumor cells with immune-enhancing genes encoding cytokines, chemokines, or co-stimulatory molecules. Sustained clinical responses provide evidence that the transduced cells can act as a vaccine. In a related approach, patient lymphocytes have been transduced with genes encoding a T cell receptor–like molecule, with a tumor antigen–binding domain fused to an intracellular signaling domain to allow T cell activation, thereby converting normal lymphocytes into cells capable of recognizing and destroying tumor cells. A third immunotherapy approach relies on ex vivo manipulation of dendritic cells to enhance the presentation of tumor antigens. These immunologic approaches may be of particular value in treating minimal residual disease after other anticancer modalities.

Gene transfer strategies have also been developed for inhibiting tumor angiogenesis. These have included constitutive expression of angiogenesis inhibitors such as angiostatin and endostatin; use of siRNA to reduce levels of VEGF or VEGF receptor; and combined approaches in which autologous T cells are genetically modified to recognize antigens specific to tumor vasculature. These studies are still in early-phase testing.

Another novel systemic approach is the use of gene transfer to protect normal cells from the toxicities of chemotherapy. The most extensively studied of these approaches has been transduction of hematopoietic cells with genes encoding resistance to chemotherapeutic agents, including the multidrug resistance gene *MDR1* or the gene encoding O^6-methylguanine DNA methyltransferase (*MGMT*). Ex vivo transduction of hematopoietic cells, followed by autologous transplantation, is being investigated as a strategy for allowing administration of higher doses of chemotherapy than would otherwise be tolerated.

GENE THERAPY FOR VASCULAR DISEASE

The third major category addressed by gene transfer studies is cardiovascular disease. The most extensive experience has been in trials designed to increase blood flow to either skeletal (critical limb ischemia) or cardiac muscle (angina/myocardial ischemia). Initial treatment options for both of these groups include mechanical revascularization or medical management, but a subset of patients are not candidates for, or fail, these approaches. These patients have formed the first cohorts for evaluation of gene transfer to achieve therapeutic angiogenesis. The major transgene used has been VEGF, attractive because of its specificity for endothelial cells; other transgenes have included fibroblast growth factor (FGF) and hypoxia-inducible factor 1, α subunit (HIF-1α). The design of most of the trials has included direct IM (or myocardial) injection of either a plasmid or an adenoviral vector expressing the transgene. Both of these vectors are likely to result in only short-term expression of VEGF. This strategy may be adequate, however, as there is no need for continued transgene expression once the new vessels have formed. Direct injection favors local expression, which should help to avoid systemic effects such as retinal neovascularization or new vessel formation in a nascent tumor. Initial trials of adeno-VEGF or plasmid-VEGF injection have resulted in improvement over baseline in terms of frequency of claudication/angina or amounts of nitroglycerin consumption. Study designs including placebo control groups and more objective endpoints (exercise duration at 3 or 6 months, rest and stress cardiac perfusion scans, and regional wall motion assessed by nonfluoroscopic electroanatomic mapping) continue to suggest a beneficial effect of gene transfer, although definitive conclusions will require larger studies. Continuing areas of investigation include choice of the optimal vector (adenoviral vs. plasmid), the optimal transgene (VEGF, HIF-1α, FGF, etc.), the optimal method of delivery in cardiac indications (intracoronary vs. direct myocardial), ideal objective endpoints, and whether concurrent administration of cytokines to mobilize endothelial progenitor cells will augment the therapeutic effect.

TABLE 65-3	TAKING HISTORY FROM SUBJECTS ENROLLED IN GENE TRANSFER STUDIES

Elements of History for Subjects Enrolled in Gene Transfer Trials

1. What vector was administered? Is it predominantly integrating [retroviral, lentiviral, herpesvirus (latency and reactivation)], or non-integrating (plasmid, adenoviral, AAV)?
2. What was the route of administration of the vector?
3. What was the target tissue?
4. What gene was transferred in? A disease-related gene? A marker?
5. Were there any adverse events noted after gene transfer?

Screening Questions for Long-Term Follow-Up in Gene Transfer Subjects[a]

1. Has a new malignancy been diagnosed?
2. Has a new neurologic/ophthalmologic disorder, or exacerbation of a preexisting disorder, been diagnosed?
3. Has a new autoimmune or rheumatologic disorder been diagnosed?
4. Has a new hematologic disorder been diagnosed?

[a]Factors influencing long-term risk include: integration of the vector into the genome; vector persistence without integration; and transgene-specific effects.

OTHER DISEASES

The power and versatility of gene transfer approaches are such that there are few serious disease entities for which gene transfer therapies are *not* under development. Besides those already discussed, other areas of interest include gene therapies for HIV and for neurodegenerative disorders. The latter include studies in patients with Parkinson's disease, where AAV vectors expressing enzymes required for enhanced production of dopamine, or of the inhibitory neurotransmitter γ-aminobutyric acid, have been introduced into affected areas of the brain (striatum, subthalamic nucleus) by stereotactic neurosurgery. In Alzheimer's disease, an ex vivo approach in which autologous fibroblasts are transduced with a retroviral vector expressing nerve growth factor, then reimplanted into the basal forebrain, has slowed the rate of cognitive decline in a small Phase I study.

SUMMARY

The development of new classes of therapeutics typically takes two to three decades; monoclonal antibodies and recombinant proteins are recent examples. Gene therapeutics, which entered clinical testing in the early 1990s, are well along in the course of development, and are likely to become increasingly important as a therapeutic modality in the twenty-first century. A central question to be addressed is the long-term safety of gene transfer, and regulatory agencies have mandated a 15-year follow-up for subjects enrolled in gene therapy trials (Table 65-3). Realization of the therapeutic benefits of the Human Genome Project, and of new discoveries such as RNAi, will depend on continued progress in gene transfer technology.

ACKNOWLEDGMENT
I would like to thank Valder Arruda, MD, PhD, for his review of the manuscript.

FURTHER READINGS

HACEIN-BEY-ABINA S et al: LMO2-associated clonal T cell proliferation in two patients after gene therapy for SCID-XI. Science 302:415, 2003

LIN E, NEMUNAITIS J: Oncolytic viral therapies. Cancer Gene Ther 11:643, 2004

MANNO CS et al: Successful transduction of liver in hemophilia by AAV-Factor IX and limitations imposed by the host immune response. Nat Med 12:342, 2006

SADELAIN M et al: Targeting tumours with genetically enhanced T lymphocytes. Nat Rev Cancer 3:35, 2003

SHAH PB, LOSORDO DW: Non-viral vectors for gene therapy: Clinical trials in cardiovascular disease. Adv Genet 54:339, 2005

SKARLATOS SI: New programs for gene- and cell-based therapies at NHLBI. Clin Pharmacol Ther 82:334, 2007

Gene Therapy Clinical Trials Worldwide. J Gene Med, New Jersey, Wiley, 2006 *www.abedia.com/wiley/indications.php*

CHAPTER 65 Gene Therapy in Clinical Medicine

66 Stem Cell Biology
Minoru S. H. Ko

Stem cell biology is a relatively new field that explores the characteristics and possible clinical applications of the different types of pluripotential cells that serve as the progenitors of more differentiated cell types. In addition to potential therapeutic applications (Chap. 67), patient-derived stem cells can also provide disease models and a means to test drug effectiveness.

IDENTIFICATION, ISOLATION, AND DERIVATION OF STEM CELLS
Resident Stem Cells   The definition of stem cells remains elusive. Stem cells were originally postulated as *unspecified* or *undifferentiated* cells that provide a source of renewal of skin, intestine, and blood cells throughout the lifespan. These *resident stem cells* are now identified in a variety of organs, i.e., epithelia of the skin and digestive system, bone marrow, blood vessels, brain, skeletal muscle, liver, testis, and pancreas, based on their specific locations, morphology, and biochemical markers.

Isolated Stem Cells   Unequivocal identification of stem cells requires the separation and purification of cells, usually based on a combination of specific cell-surface markers. These *isolated stem cells*, e.g., hematopoietic stem (HS) cells, can be studied in detail and used in clinical applications, such as bone marrow transplantation (Chap. 68). However, the lack of specific cell-surface markers for other types of stem cells has made it difficult to isolate them in large quantities. This challenge has been partially addressed in animal models by genetically marking different cell types with green fluorescence protein driven by cell-specific promoters. Alternatively, putative stem cells have been isolated from a variety of tissues as side population (SP) cells using fluorescence-activated cell sorting after staining with Hoechst 33342 dye. However, the SP phenotype should be used with caution as it may not be function for stem cells.

Cultured Stem Cells   It is desirable to culture and expand stem cells in vitro to obtain a sufficient quantity for analysis and potential therapeutic use. Although the derivation of stem cells in vitro has been a major obstacle in stem cell biology, the number and types of *cultured stem cells* have increased progressively (Table 66-1). The cultured stem cells derived from resident stem cells are often called *adult stem cells* to indicate their adult origins and to distinguish them from *embryonic stem* (ES) and *embryonic germ* (EG) *cells*. However, considering the presence of embryo-derived tissue-specific stem cells, e.g., trophoblast stem (TS) cells, and the possible derivation of similar cells from embryo/fetus, e.g., neural stem (NS) cells, it is more appropriate to use the term, *tissue stem cells*.

Successful derivation of cultured stem cells (both embryonic and tissue stem cells) often requires the identification of necessary growth factors and culture conditions, mimicking the microenvironment or *niche* of the resident stem cells. For example, the derivation of mouse TS cells, once considered impossible, became possible by using FGF4, a ligand known to be expressed by cells adjacent to the developing trophoblast in vivo. Therefore, it may be possible to culture other resident stem cells (e.g., intestinal stem cells) or isolated stem cells (e.g., HS cells) by studying the factors that constitute their normal niche.

SELF-RENEWAL AND PROLIFERATION OF STEM CELLS
Symmetric and Asymmetric Cell Division   The most widely accepted stem cell definition is a cell with a unique capacity to produce unaltered daughter cells (*self-renewal*) and to generate specialized cell types (*potency*). Self-renewal can be achieved in two ways. *Asymmetric cell division* produces one daughter cell that is identical to the parental cell and one daughter cell that is different from the parental cell and is a progenitor or differentiated cell. Asymmetric cell division does not increase the number of stem cells. *Symmetric cell division* produces two identical daughter cells. For stem cells to proliferate in vitro, they must divide symmetrically. Self-renewal alone cannot define stem cells, because any established cell line, e.g., HeLa cells or NIH3T3 cells, proliferate by symmetric cell division.

Unlimited Expansion In Vitro   Resident stem cells are often quiescent and divide infrequently. However, once the stem cells are successfully cultured in vitro, they often acquire the capacity to divide continuously and the ability to proliferate beyond the normal limit of passages typical of primary cultured cells (sometimes called *immortality*). These features are primarily seen in ES cells, but have also been demonstrated for NS cells, MS cells, MAPCs, maGSCs (adult-derived tissue stem cells), and USSCs (newborn-derived tissue stem cells), thereby enhancing the potential of these cells for therapeutic use (Table 66-1).

Stability of Genotype and Phenotype   The capacity to actively proliferate is associated with the potential accumulation of chromosomal abnormalities and mutations. Mouse ES cells have been extensively used to produce gene-targeted animals and are known to maintain their euploid karyotype and genome integrity. In contrast, human ES cells appear to be more susceptible to mutations after long-term culture. Another limitation is the possible formation of tumors after transplanting actively dividing stem cells. Mouse ES cells can form teratomas when injected into immunosuppressed animals.

POTENCY AND DIFFERENTIATION OF STEM CELLS
Developmental Potency   The term *potency* is used to indicate a cell's ability to differentiate into specialized cell types. The current lack of knowledge about the molecular nature of potency requires the experimental manipulation of stem cells to demonstrate their potency. For example, in vivo testing can be done by injecting stem cells into mouse blastocysts or immunosuppressed adult mice and determining how many different cell types are formed from the injected cells. In vitro testing can be done by differentiating cells in various culture conditions to determine how many different cell types are formed from the cells. The in vivo assays are not applicable to human stem cells. The formal demonstration of self-renewal and potency is performed by demonstrating that a single cell possesses such abilities in vitro (*clonality*). Cultured stem cells are tentatively grouped according to their potency (Fig. 66-1).

From Totipotency to Unipotency   *Totipotent cells* can form an entire organism autonomously. Only a fertilized egg (zygote) possesses this feature. *Pluripotent cells* (e.g., ES cells) can form almost all the body's cell lineages (endoderm, mesoderm, and ectoderm), including germ cells. *Multipotent cells* (e.g., HS cells) can form multiple cell lineages but cannot form all of the body's cell lineages. *Oligopotent cells* (e.g., NS cells) can form more than one cell lineage but are more restricted than multipotent cells. Oligopotent cells are sometimes called *progenitor cells* or *precursor cells*; however, these terms are often more strictly used to define partially differentiated or lineage-committed cells (e.g., myeloid progenitor cells) that can divide into different cell types but lack self-renewing capacity. *Unipotent cells* or *monopotent cells*, e.g., spermatogonial stem (SS) cells, can form a single differentiated cell lineage. Terminally differentiated cells, such as fibroblast cells, also have a capacity to proliferate (which may be called self-renewal) but maintain the same cell type (e.g., no potency to form another cell type) and are not, therefore, considered unipotent cells.

Nuclear Reprogramming   Development naturally progresses from totipotent fertilized eggs to pluripotent epiblast cells, to multipotent cells, and finally to terminally differentiated cells. According to Wad-

TABLE 66-1 TYPES OF CULTURED STEM CELLS

Name	Source, Derivation, Maintenance, and Properties
Embryonic stem cells (ES, ESC)	ES cells can be derived by culturing blastocysts or immuno-surgically isolated inner cell mass (ICM) from blastocysts on a feeder layer of MEFs with LIF (m) or without LIF (h). ES cells are to originate from the epiblast (m, h). ES cells grow as tightly adherent multicellular colonies with a population doubling time of ~12 h (m), maintain a stable euploid karyotype even after extensive culture and manipulation, can differentiate into a variety of cell types in vitro, and can contribute to all cell types, including functional sperm and oocytes, when injected into a blastocyst (m). ES cells form relatively flat, compact colonies with the population doubling time of 35–40 h (h).
Embryonic germ cells (EG, EGC)	EG cells can be derived by culturing primordial germ cells (PGCs) from embryos at E8.5–E12.5 on a feeder layer of MEFs with FGF2 and LIF (m). EG cells can be derived by culturing gonadal tissues from 5–11 week post-fertilization embryo/fetus on a feeder layer of MEFs with FGF2, forskolin, and LIF (h). EG cells show essentially the same pluripotency as ES cells when injected into mouse blastocysts (m). The only known difference is the imprinting status of some genes (e.g., Igf2r): Imprinting is normally erased during germline development, and thus, the imprinting status of in EG cells is different from that of ES cells.
Trophoblast stem cells (TS, TSC)	TS cells can be derived by culturing trophectoderm cells of E3.5 blastocysts, extraembryonic ectoderm of E6.5 embryos, and chorionic ectoderm of E7.5 embryos on a feeder layer of MEFs with FGF4 (m). TS cells can differentiate into trophoblast giant cells in vitro (m). TS can contribute exclusively to all trophoblast subtypes when injected into blastocysts (m).
Extraembryonic endoderm cells (XEN)	XEN cells can be derived by culturing the ICM in non-ES cell culture condition (m). XEN cells can contribute only to the parietal endoderm lineage when injected into a blastocyst (m).
Embryonic carcinoma cells (EC)	EC cells can be derived from teratocarcinoma—a type of cancer that most commonly develops in the testes. EC cells rarely show pluripotency in vitro, but they can contribute to all cell types when injected into blastocysts. EC cells often have an aneuploid karyotype and other genome alterations.
Mesenchymal stem cells (MS, MSC)	MS cells can be derived from bone marrow, muscle, adipose tissue, peripheral blood, and umbilical cord blood (m, h). MS cells can differentiate into mesenchymal cell types, including adipocytes, osteocytes, chondrocytes, and myocytes (m, h).
Multipotent adult stem cells (MAPC)	MAPCs can be derived by culturing bone marrow mononuclear cells, after depleting CD45+ and GlyA+ cells, with FCS, EGF, and PDGF-BB (h). MAPCs are very rare cells that are present within MSC cultures from postnatal bone marrow (m, h). MAPCs can also be isolated from postnatal muscle and brain (m). MAPCs can be cultured for >120 population doublings. MAPCs can differentiate into all tissues in vivo when injected into a mouse blastocyst, and can differentiate into various cell lineages of mesodermal, ectodermal, and endodermal origin in vitro (m).
Spermatogonial stem cells (SS, SSC)	SS cells can be derived by culturing newborn testis on STS-feeder cells with GDNF (m). SS cells can reconstitute long-term spermatogenesis after transplantation into recipient testes and restore fertility.
Germline stem cells (GS, GSC)	GS cells can be derived from neonatal testis (m). GS cells can differentiate into three germlayers in vitro and contribute to a variety of tissues, including germline, when injected into blastocysts.
Multipotent adult germline stem cells (maGSC)	maGSC can be derived from adult testis (m). maGSC can differentiate into three germlayers in vitro and can contribution to a variety of tissues, including germline, when injected into blastocysts.
Neural stem cells (NS, NSC)	NS cells can be derived from fetal and adult brain (subventricular zone, ventricular zone, and hippocampus) and cultured as a heterogeneous cell population of monolayer or floating cell clusters called neurospheres. NS cells can differentiate into neuron and glia in vivo and in vitro. Recently, the culture of pure population of symmetrically dividing adherent NS cells became possible in the presence of FGF2 and EGF.
Unrestricted somatic stem cells (USSC)	USSCs are rare cells derived from newborn cord blood (h). USSCs can be derived by culturing the mononuclear fraction of cord blood in the presence of 30% FCS and 10^{-7} M dexamethasone. USSCs can differentiate into a variety of cell types in vitro and can contribute a variety of cells types in in vivo transplantation experiments in rat, mouse, and sheep (h). USSCs are CD45- adherent cells and can be expanded to 10^{15} cells without losing pluripotency (h).

Note: m, mouse; h, human; FGF, fibroblast growth factor; FCS, fetal calf serum; EGF, epidermal growth factor; PDGF, platelet-derived growth factor; GDNF, glial cell line–derived neurotrophic factor; LIF, leukemia inhibitory factor; MEF, mouse embryonic fibroblast.

transplantation, or nuclear transfer (NT), procedures (often called "cloning"), where the nucleus of a differentiated cell is transferred into an enucleated oocyte. Although this is an error-prone procedure and the success rate is very low, live animals have been produced using adult somatic cells as donors in sheep, mouse, and other mammals. In mice, it has been demonstrated that ES cells derived from blastocysts made by somatic cell NT are indistinguishable from normal ES cells. NT can potentially be used to produce *patient-specific ES cells* carrying a genome identical to that of the patient. However, the successful implementation of this procedure has not been reported in humans. Setting aside technical and ethical issues, the limited supply of human oocytes will be a major problem for clinical applications of NT. Alternatively, successful nuclear reprogramming of somatic cells by fusing them with ES cells has been demonstrated in mouse and human. However, it is not yet clear how ES-derived DNA can be removed from hybrid cells. More direct nuclear reprogramming of somatic cells by transfecting specific genes or by exposing the cells to ES cell extracts is the subject of current research.

Stem Cell Plasticity or Transdifferentiation The prevailing paradigm in developmental biology is that once cells are differentiated, their phenotypes are stable. However, a number of reports have shown that tissue stem cells, which are thought to be lineage-committed multipotent cells, possess the capacity to differentiate into cell types outside their lineage restrictions (called *transdifferentiation*). For example, HS cells may be converted into neurons as well as germ cells. This feature may provide a means to use tissue stem cells derived directly from a patient for therapeutic purposes, thereby eliminating the need to use embryonic stem cells or elaborate procedures such as nuclear reprogramming a patient's somatic cells. However, more strict criteria and rigorous validation are required to establish tissue stem cell plasticity. For example, observations of transdifferentiation may reflect cell fusion, contamination with progenitor cells from other cell lineages, or persistence of pluripotent embryonic cells in adult organs. Therefore, the assignment of potency to each cultured stem cell in Fig. 66-1 should be taken with caution. Whether transdifferentiation exists and can be used for therapeutic purposes remains to be determined conclusively.

Directed Differentiation of Stem Cells Pluripotent stem cells (e.g., ES cells) can differentiate into multiple cell types, but in culture they normally differentiate into heterogeneous cell populations in a stochastic manner. However, for therapeutic uses, it is desirable to direct stem cells into specific cell types (e.g., insulin-secreting beta cells). This is an active area of stem cell research, and protocols are being developed to achieve this goal. In any of these directed cell differentiation systems, the cell phenotype must be evaluated critically. Interestingly, it has been reported that mouse ES cells can differentiate in vitro into oocytes as well as sperm, which are capable of fertilizing an oocyte to produce live offspring.

dington's epigenetic landscape, this is analogous to a ball moving down a slope. The reversal of the terminally differentiated cells to totipotent or pluripotent cells (called *nuclear reprogramming*) can thus be seen as an uphill gradient that never occurs in normal conditions. However, nuclear reprogramming has been achieved using *nuclear*

Stage Potency	Preimplantation	Embryonic, fetal	Postnatal	Adult
Totipotent	Zygote[m,h]			
Pluripotent	ES[m,h]	EG[m,h]	GS[m] USSC[h] MAPC[m,h]	EC[m,h] maGSC[m] MAPC[m,h]
Multipotent				MS[m,h]
Oligopotent	TS[m]			NS[m,h]
Unipotent	XEN[m]			SSC[m]
Terminally differentiated cells				

FIGURE 66-1 Potency and source developmental stage of cultured stem cells. For abbreviations of stem cells, see Table 66-1. Note that stem cells are often abbreviated with or without "cells," e.g., ES cells or ESCs for embryonic stem cells. m, mouse; h, human.

MOLECULAR CHARACTERIZATION OF STEM CELLS

Genomics and Proteomics In addition to standard molecular biological approaches, genomics and proteomics have been extensively applied to the analysis of stem cells. For example, DNA microarray analyses have revealed the expression levels of essentially all genes and identified specific markers for some stem cells. Similarly, the protein profiles of stem cells have been assessed by using mass spectrophotometry. These methodologies are beginning to provide a novel means to characterize and classify various stem cells and the molecular mechanisms that give them their unique characteristics.

Stemness This term has been used to designate the essential molecular characteristics of stem cells. It is also used to indicate common genetic programs shared among ES cells and tissue stem cells (HS and NS cells). A number of common genes, such as stress-response genes, have been identified, but the lack of commonality among different studies raises concerns about the validity of this concept.

Pivotal Genes Involved in ES Cell Regulation Recent work has begun to identify genes involved in the regulation of stem cell function. For example, three genes—*Pou5f1* (Oct3/4), *Nanog*, and *Sox2*—govern key gene regulatory pathways/networks for the maintenance of self-renewal and pluripotency of mouse and human ES cells. Similarly, it has been shown that the interaction and balance among three transcription factors—*Pou5f1*, *Cdx2*, and *Gata6*—determine the fate of mouse ES cells: upregulation of *Cdx2* differentiates ES cells into trophoblast cells, whereas upregulation of *Gata6* differentiates ES cells into primitive endoderm. These types of analyses should provide molecular clues about the function of stem cells and lead to a more effective means to manipulate stem cells for future therapeutic use.

FURTHER READINGS

CERVERA RP, STOJKOVIC M: Human embryonic stem cell derivation and nuclear transfer: Impact on regenerative therapeutics and drug discovery. Clin Pharmacol Ther 82(3):310, 2007

DEPARTMENT OF HEALTH AND HUMAN SERVICES: Regenerative Medicine 2006. August 2006. http://stemcells.nih.gov/info/scireport

KO MSH, MCLAREN A: Epigenetics of germ cells, stem cells, and early embryos. Dev Cell 10:161, 2006

LANZA R et al (eds): Handbook of Stem Cells, vols 1 and 2. London, Elsevier Academic Press, 2004

MARSHAK DR et al (eds): Stem Cell Biology, New York, Cold Spring Harbor Laboratory Press, 2001

ODORICO J et al (eds): Human Embryonic Stem Cells. New York, BIOS Scientific Publishers, 2005

67 Applications of Stem Cell Biology in Clinical Medicine

John A. Kessler

Organ damage and the resultant inflammatory responses initiate a series of repair processes, including stem cell proliferation, migration, and differentiation, often in combination with angiogenesis and remodeling of the extracellular matrix. Endogenous stem cells in tissues such as liver and skin have a remarkable ability to regenerate the organs, whereas heart and brain have a much more limited capability for self-repair. Under rare circumstances, circulating stem cells may contribute to regenerative responses by migrating into a tissue and differentiating into organ-specific cell types. The goal of stem cell therapies is to promote cell replacement in organs that are damaged beyond their ability for self-repair.

SOURCES OF STEM CELLS FOR TISSUE REPAIR

Different types of stem cells include embryonic stem (ES) cells, umbilical cord blood stem cells, organ-specific somatic stem cells (e.g., neural stem cells for treatment of the brain), and somatic stem cells capable of generating cell types specific for the target rather than the donor organ (e.g., bone marrow mesenchymal stem cells for cardiac repair) (Chap. 66). ES cells self-renew endlessly so that a single cell line with carefully characterized traits can generate large numbers of cells that can be immunologically matched with potential transplant recipients. However, little is currently known about the mechanisms that govern differentiation of these cells or processes that limit their unbridled proliferation. Human ES cells are difficult to culture and grow slowly. ES cells tend to develop abnormal karyotypes and have the potential to form teratomas if they are not committed to the desired cell types before transplantation. The study of human ES cells has been controversial, and their use in clinical applications would be unacceptable to some patients and physicians despite their enormous potential. Somatic cell nuclear transfer ("therapeutic cloning") represents an alternative method for creating ES cell lines that are genetically identical to the patient. It may also be possible to derive pluripotent stem cells from spermatogonia in the adult human testis, providing another strategy for obtaining genetically identical stem cells.

Umbilical cord blood stem/progenitor cells are associated with less graft-versus-host disease compared to marrow stem cells. They have less HLA restriction than adult marrow stem cells, and they are less likely to be contaminated with herpesvirus. However, it is unclear how many different cell types these cells can generate, and methods for differentiating them into nonhematopoietic phenotypes are largely lacking. The quantity of cells from any single source can also be limiting.

Organ-specific multipotent stem cells are already somewhat specialized and may be easier to induce into desired cell types. These cells could potentially be obtained from the patient and amplified in culture, thereby circumventing the problems associated with immune rejection. Multipotent stem cells are relatively easy to harvest from bone marrow (Chap. 68) but are more difficult to isolate from other tissues, such as heart and brain. Substantial efforts have therefore been devoted to obtaining more pluripotent stem cell populations, such as bone marrow mesenchymal stem cells (MSCs) or adipose stem cells, for use in regenerative strategies. Tissue culture evidence suggests that these stem cell populations are able to generate a variety of cell types, including myocytes, chondrocytes, tendon cells, osteoblasts, cardiomyocytes, adipocytes, hepatocytes, and neurons, through a process known as transdifferentiation. However, it is unclear how effectively these differentiated cells integrate into organs, survive, and function after transplantation in vivo. Early studies of bone marrow–derived stem cells transplanted into heart, liver, and other organs suggested that the cells had differentiated into organ-specific cell types. Subsequent studies, however, revealed that the stem cells had fused with cells resident in the organs. Further studies will be necessary to determine whether transdifferentiation of MSCs or other stem cell populations occurs at a high enough frequency to be useful for stem cell replacement therapy.

Regardless of the source of the stem cells used in regenerative strategies, a number of generic problems must be overcome for the development of successful clinical applications. These include development of methods for reliably generating large numbers of specific cell types, minimizing the risk of tumor formation or proliferation of inappropriate cell types, ensuring the viability and function of the engrafted cells, overcoming immune rejection when autografts are not used, and facilitating revascularization of the regenerated tissue. Each organ system will also pose tissue-specific problems for stem cell therapies.

STRATEGIES FOR STEM CELL REPLACEMENT

Stem cell transplantation is not a new concept and it is already part of established medical practice. Hematopoietic stem cells (HSCs) (Chap. 68) are responsible for the long-term repopulation of all blood elements in bone marrow transplant recipients. HSC transplantation is now the gold standard against which other stem cell transplantation therapies will be measured. Transplantation of differentiated cells is also a clinical reality, as donated organs (e.g., liver, kidney) and tissues (i.e., cornea, eye, skin) are often used to replace damaged tissues. However, the clinical need for transplantable tissues and organs far outweighs the available supply, and organ transplantation has limited potential for some tissues such as the brain. Stem cells offer the possibility of a renewable source of cell replacement for virtually all organs.

At least three different therapeutic concepts for cell replacement have been considered (Fig. 67-1): (1) injection of stem cells directly into the damaged organ or into the circulation, allowing them to "home" into the damaged tissue; (2) in vitro differentiation of stem cells followed by transplantation into a damaged organ—e.g., pancreatic islet cells could be generated from stem cells prior to transplantation into patients with diabetes, whereas cardiomyocytes could be generated to treat ischemic heart disease; and (3) stimulation of endogenous stem cells to facilitate repair—e.g., administration of appropriate growth factors to amplify numbers of endogenous stem/progenitor cells or direct them to differentiate into the desired cell types. In addition to these strategies for cell replacement, the ex vivo or in situ generation of tissues provides an alternative means of tissue engineering (Chap. 69). Stem cells are also excellent vehicles for cellular gene therapy (Chap. 65).

DISEASE-SPECIFIC STEM CELL APPROACHES

ISCHEMIC HEART DISEASE AND CARDIOMYOCYTE REGENERATION

Because of the high prevalence of ischemic heart disease, extensive efforts have been devoted to cell replacement of cardiomyocytes. Historically, the adult heart has been viewed as a terminally differentiated organ without the capacity for regeneration. However, the heart has the ability to achieve low levels of cardiomyocyte regeneration as well as revascularization. This regeneration is likely accomplished by cardi-

FIGURE 67-1 Strategies for transplantation of stem cells. 1. Undifferentiated or partially differentiated stem cells may be injected directly in the target organ or intravenously. 2. Stem cells may be differentiated ex vivo prior to injection into the target organ. 3. Growth factors or other drugs may be injected to stimulate endogenous stem cell populations.

ac stem cells resident in the heart, and possibly by cells originating in the bone marrow. If such cells could be characterized, isolated, and amplified ex vivo, they might provide an ideal source of stem cells for therapeutic use. For effective myocardial repair, cells must be delivered either systemically or locally, and the cells must survive, engraft, and differentiate into functional cardiomyocytes that couple mechanically and electrically with the recipient myocardium. The optimal method for cell delivery is not yet clear, and various experimental studies have employed intramyocardial, transendocardial, intravenous, and intracoronary injections. In experimental myocardial infarction, functional improvements have been achieved after transplantation of a variety of different cell types, including ES cells, bone marrow stem cells, endothelial stem cells, and adipose stem cells. Bone marrow stem cells in particular have been examined in clinical trials of human ischemic heart disease. These have largely been small, nonrandomized studies that typically combine cell treatment with conventional therapies. Although the fate of the cells and mechanisms by which they altered cardiac function are open questions, these studies have shown small but measurable improvement in cardiac function and, in some cases, reduction in infarct size. The preponderance of evidence suggests that the functional benefits are not derived from direct generation of cardiomyocytes but rather from indirect effects of the stem cells on resident cells. This may reflect the release of soluble growth factors, induction of angiogenesis, or some other mechanism.

DIABETES MELLITUS

The success of islet cell and pancreas transplantation provides proof of concept for a cell-based approach for type I diabetes. However, the demand for donor pancreata far exceeds the number available, and maintenance of long-term graft survival remains a problem. The search for a renewable source of stem cells capable of regenerating pancreatic islets has therefore been intensive.

Pancreatic β cell turnover occurs in the normal pancreas, although the source of the new β cells is controversial. Attempts to promote endogenous regenerative processes have not yet been successful, but this remains a potentially viable approach. A number of different cell types are candidates for use in stem cell replacement, including ES cells, hepatic progenitor cells, pancreatic ductal progenitor cells, and bone marrow stem cells. Successful therapy will depend on developing a source of cells that can be amplified and have the ability to synthesize, store, and release insulin when it is required, primarily in response to changes in the glucose level. The proliferative capacity of the replacement cells must be tightly regulated to avoid excessive expansion of β cell numbers with the consequent development of hyperinsulinemia/hypoglycemia, and the cells must avoid immune rejection. Although ES cells can be differentiated into cells that produce insulin, these cells have relatively low insulin content and a high rate of apoptosis, and they generally lack the capacity to normalize blood glucose in diabetic animals. Thus, ES cells have not yet been useful for the large-scale production of differentiated islet cells.

During embryogenesis, the pancreas, liver, and gastrointestinal tract are all derived from the anterior endoderm, and transdifferentiation of the pancreas to liver and vice versa has been observed in certain pathologic conditions. Multipotential stem cells also reside within gastric glands and intestinal crypts. Thus, hepatic, pancreatic, and/or gastrointestinal precursor cells may be candidates for cell-based therapy of diabetes.

NERVOUS SYSTEM

Neural cells have been differentiated from a variety of stem cell populations. Human ES cells can be induced to generate neural stem cells, and these cells can give rise to neurons, oligodendroglia, and astrocytes. These neural stem cells have been transplanted into the rodent brain with formation of appropriate cell types and no tumor formation. Multipotent stem cells present in the adult brain can also generate all of the major neural cell types, but highly invasive procedures would be necessary to obtain autologous cells. Fetal neural stem cells derived from miscarriages or abortuses are an alternative, and a clinical trial of fetal neural stem cells in Batten disease is commencing. Transdifferentiation of bone marrow and adipose stem cells into neural stem cells, and vice versa, has been reported, and clinical trials of such cells have begun for a number of neurologic disorders. Clinical trials of a conditionally immortalized human cell line and of human umbilical cord blood cells in stroke are also planned. Neurologic disorders that have already been targeted for stem cell therapies include spinal cord injury, amyotrophic lateral sclerosis, stroke, traumatic brain injury, Batten disease, and Parkinson's disease. In Parkinson's disease, the major motor features result from the loss of a single cell population, dopaminergic neurons within the substantia nigra pars compacta. Two clinical trials of fetal nigral transplantation failed to meet their primary endpoint and were complicated by the development of dyskinesia. Transplantation of stem cell–derived dopamine-producing cells offers a number of potential advantages over fetal transplants, including the ability of stem cells to migrate and disperse within tissue, the potential for engineering regulatable release of dopamine, and the ability to engineer cells to produce factors that will enhance cell survival. Nevertheless, the experience with fetal transplants points out the difficulties that may be encountered.

At least some of the neurologic dysfunction after spinal cord injury reflects demyelination, and both ES cells and marrow-derived stem cells are able to facilitate remyelination after experimental spinal cord injury. Clinical trials of marrow-derived stem cells have already begun, and this may be the first disease targeted for the clinical use of ES cells. Marrow-derived stem cells are also being used in the treatment of stroke, traumatic brain injury, and amyotrophic lateral sclerosis (ALS), where possible benefits are more likely to be indirect trophic effects or remyelination rather than neuron replacement. At present, no population of transplanted stem cells has been shown to generate neurons that extend axons over long distances to form synaptic connections (such as would be necessary for replacement of upper motor neurons in ALS, stroke, or other disorders).

LIVER

Transplantation is currently the only successful treatment for end-stage liver diseases, but this approach is limited by the shortage of liver grafts. Clinical trials of hepatocyte transplantation demonstrate that it can potentially substitute for organ transplantation, but the paucity of available cells also limits this strategy. Potential sources of stem cells include endogenous liver stem cells (such as oval cells), ES cells, bone marrow cells, and umbilical cord blood cells. Although a series of studies in humans as well as animals suggested that transplanted bone marrow stem cells can generate hepatocytes, this phenomenon largely reflects the fusion of the transplanted cells with endogenous liver cells, giving the erroneous appearance of new hepatocytes. ES cells have been differentiated into hepatocytes and transplanted in animal models of liver failure without formation of teratomas.

OTHER ORGAN SYSTEMS AND THE FUTURE

The use of stem cells in regenerative medicine has been studied for many other organ systems and cell types, including skin, eye, cartilage, bone, kidney, lung, endometrium, vascular endothelium, smooth muscle, striated muscle, and others. In fact, the potential for stem cell regeneration of damaged organs and tissues is virtually limitless. However, numerous obstacles must be overcome before stem cell therapies can become a widespread clinical reality. Only HSCs have been adequately characterized by surface markers to allow unambiguous identification, a prerequisite for reliable clinical applications. The pathways for differentiating stem cells into specific cellular phenotypes are still unknown, the migration of transplanted cells is uncontrolled, and the response of the cells to the environment of diseased organs is unpredictable. Future strategies may employ the coadministration of scaffolding, artificial extracellular matrix, and/or growth factors to orchestrate differentiation of stem cells and their organization into appropriate constituents of the organ. Imaging techniques are needed to visualize stem cells in vivo after transplantation into humans. Fortunately, stem cells can be engineered before transplantation to contain contrast agents that may make this feasible. The potential for tumor formation and the problems associated with immune rejection are significant impediments. Many strategies for cell replacement already include vasoactive endothelial growth factor (VEGF) coadministration to foster vascularization, which is required for survival and function of the transplant. Some stem cells have been engineered to have an inducible suicide gene so that the cells can be eradicated in the event of tumor formation or some other complication. The potential for stem cell therapies to revolutionize medical care is extraordinary, and disorders such as myocardial infarction, diabetes, Parkinson's disease and many others are attractive targets. However, such stem cell–based therapies are at a very early stage of development, and perfection of techniques for clinical transplantation of predictable, well-characterized cells will be a difficult and lengthy undertaking.

ETHICAL ISSUES

Stem cell therapies raise contentious ethical issues that must be addressed in parallel with the scientific and medical opportunities. Our society has great diversity in religious beliefs, concepts of individual rights, tolerance for uncertainty and risk, and boundaries for how scientific interventions should be used to alter the outcome of disease. In the United States, the federal government has authorized research using human ES lines in existence before August 2001 but has restricted the use of federal funds for developing new human ES lines. However, these existing lines develop abnormalities with time in culture and are contaminated with mouse proteins. These findings have sparked renewed debate about the need to develop new human ES cell lines.

In considering ethical issues associated with the use of stem cells, it is helpful to draw from experience with other scientific advances, such as organ transplantation, recombinant DNA technology, implantation of mechanical devices, neuroscience and cognitive research, in vitro fertilization, and prenatal genetic testing. From these and other precedents, we learn the importance of understanding and testing fundamental biology in the laboratory setting and in animal models before applying new techniques in carefully controlled clinical trials. When these trials occur, they must include full informed consent and have careful oversight by external review groups.

Ultimately, medical interventions will be scientifically feasible but ethically or socially unacceptable to some members of a society. Stem cell research raises questions about the definition of human life, and it has raised deep fears about our ability to balance issues of justice and safety with the needs of critically ill patients. Health care providers and experts with backgrounds in ethics, law, and sociology must help guard against the premature or inappropriate application stem cell therapies, and the inappropriate use of vulnerable population groups. On the other hand, these therapies offer important new strategies for the treatment of otherwise irreversible disorders. An open dialogue between the scientific community, physicians, patients, and their advocates, lawmakers, and the lay population is important to raise and address ethical issues and to balance the benefits and risks associated with stem cell transfer.

ACKNOWLEDGMENTS

The author acknowledges the contributions of David Bodine, J. Larry Jameson, and Ron McKay to this chapter in the 16th edition.

FURTHER READINGS

COMMITTEE ON THE BIOLOGICAL AND BIOMEDICAL APPLICATIONS OF STEM CELL RESEARCH et al: Stem Cells and the Future of Regenerative Medicine. Washington, D.C., National Academies Press, 2002

HOLLAND S et al: The Human Embryonic Stem Cell Debate: Science, Ethics and Public Policy. Cambridge, MA, MIT Press, 2001

LANZA R et al (eds): Essentials of Stem Cell Biology. San Diego, Elsevier Academic Press, 2006

MIMEAULT M et al: Stem cells: A revolution in therapeutics-recent advances in stem cell biology and their therapeutic applications in regenerative medicine and cancer therapies. Clin Pharmacol Ther 82(3):252, 2007

NATIONAL INSTITUTES OF HEALTH: Stem cell information page. URL: *http://stemcells.nih.gov/index.asp*.

PUCEAT M, BALLIS A: Embryonic stem cells: From bench to bedside. Clin Pharmacol Ther 82(3):337, 2007

SUGARMAN J: Ethics and stem cell therapeutics for cardiovascular disease. Prog Cardiovasc Dis 50(1):1, 2007

VATS A et al: Stem cells. Lancet 366:592, 2005

68 Hematopoietic Stem Cells
David T. Scadden, Dan L. Longo

All of the cell types in the peripheral blood and some cells in every tissue of the body are derived from hematopoietic (*hemo*: blood; *poiesis*: creation) stem cells. If the hematopoietic stem cell is damaged and can no longer function (e.g., due to the nuclear accident at Chernobyl), a person would survive 2–4 weeks in the absence of extraordinary support measures. With the clinical use of hematopoietic stem cells, tens of thousands of lives are saved each year (Chap. 108). Stem cells produce tens of billions of blood cells daily from a stem cell pool that is estimated to be only in the hundreds of thousands. How stem cells do this, how they persist for many decades despite the production demands, and how they may be better used in clinical care are important issues in medicine.

The study of blood cell production has become a paradigm for how other tissues may be organized and regulated. Basic research in hematopoiesis that includes defining stepwise molecular changes accompanying functional changes in maturing cells, aggregating cells into functional subgroups, and demonstrating hematopoietic stem cell regulation by a specialized microenvironment are concepts worked out in hematology, but they offer models for other tissues. Moreover, these concepts may not be restricted to normal tissue function but extend to malignancy. Stem cells are rare cells among a heterogeneous population of cell types, and their behavior is assessed mainly in experimental animal models involving reconstitution of hematopoiesis. Thus, much of what we know about stem cells is imprecise and based on inferences from genetically manipulated animals.

CARDINAL FUNCTIONS OF HEMATOPOIETIC STEM CELLS

All stem cell types have two cardinal functions: self-renewal and differentiation (Fig. 68-1). Stem cells exist to generate, maintain, and repair tissues. They function successfully if they can replace a wide variety of shorter-lived mature cells over prolonged periods. The process of self-renewal (see below) assures that a stem cell population can be sustained over time. Without self-renewal, the stem cell pool could exhaust over time and tissue maintenance would not be possible. The process of differentiation provides the effectors of tissue function: mature cells. Without proper differentiation, the integrity of tissue function would be compromised and organ failure would ensue.

In the blood, mature cells have variable average life spans, ranging from 7 h for mature neutrophils to a few months for red blood cells to many years for memory lymphocytes. However, the stem cell pool is the

FIGURE 68-1 Signature characteristics of the stem cell. Stem cells have two essential features: the capacity to differentiate into a variety of mature cell types and the capacity for self-renewal. Intrinsic factors associated with self-renewal include expression of Bmi-1, Gfi-1, PTEN, STAT5, Tel/Atv6, p21, p18, MCL-1, Mel-18, RAE28, and HoxB4. Extrinsic signals for self-renewal include Notch, Wnt, SHH, and Tie2/Ang-1. Based mainly on murine studies, hematopoietic stem cells express the following cell surface molecules: CD34, Thy-1 (CD90), c-Kit receptor (CD117), CD133, CD164, and c-Mpl (CD110, also known as the thrombopoietin receptor).

central, durable source of all blood and immune cells, maintaining a capacity to produce a broad range of cells from a single cell source and yet keeping itself vigorous over decades of life. As an individual stem cell divides, it has the capacity to accomplish one of three division outcomes: two stem cells, two cells destined for differentiation, or one stem cell and one differentiating cell. The former two outcomes are the result of symmetric cell division, whereas the latter indicates a different outcome for the two daughter cells—an event termed *asymmetric cell division*. The relative balance for these types of outcomes may change during development and under particular kinds of demands on the stem cell pool.

DEVELOPMENTAL BIOLOGY OF HEMATOPOIETIC STEM CELLS

During development, blood cells are produced at different sites. Initially, the yolk sac provides oxygen-carrying red blood cells, and then several sites of intraembryonic blood cell production become involved. These intraembryonic sites engage in sequential order, moving from the genital ridge at a site where the aorta, gonadal tissue, and mesonephros are emerging to the fetal liver and then, in the second trimester, to the bone marrow and spleen. As the location of stem cells changes, the relative abundance of cells they produce also changes, progressively increasing in the complexity of cell types from those simply carrying oxygen to platelets supporting a more complex vasculature to the cells of innate immunity and finally to the cells of adaptive immunity. Stem cell proliferation remains high, even in the bone marrow, until shortly after birth, when it appears to dramatically decline. The cells in the bone marrow are thought to arrive by the bloodborne transit of cells from the fetal liver after calcification of the long bones has begun. The presence of stem cells in the circulation is not unique to a time window in development. Rather, hematopoietic stem cells appear to circulate throughout life. The time that cells spend freely circulating appears to be brief (measured in minutes in the mouse), but the cells that do circulate are functional and can be used for transplantation. The number of stem cells that circulate can be increased in a number of ways to facilitate harvest and transfer to the same or a different host.

MOBILITY OF HEMATOPOIETIC STEM CELLS

Cells entering and exiting the bone marrow do so through a series of molecular interactions. Circulating stem cells (through CD162 and CD44) engage the lectins P- and E-selectin on the endothelial surface to slow the movement of the cells to a rolling phenotype. Stem cell integrins are then activated and accomplish firm adhesion between the stem cell and vessel wall, with a particularly important role for stem cell VCAM-1 engaging endothelial VLA-4. The chemokine CXCL12 (SDF1) interacting with stem cell CXCR4 receptors also appears to be important in the process of stem cells getting from the circulation to where they engraft in the bone marrow. This is particularly true in the developmental move from fetal liver to bone marrow; however, the role for this molecule in adults appears to be more related to retention of stem cells in the bone marrow rather the process of getting them there. Interrupting that retention process through either specific molecular blockers of the CXCR4/CXCL12 interaction, cleavage of CXCL12, or downregulation of the receptor can all result in the release of stem cells into the circulation. This process is an increasingly important aspect of recovering stem cells for therapeutic use as it has permitted the harvesting process to be done by leukapheresis rather than bone marrow punctures in the operating room. Refining our knowledge of how stem cells get into and out of the bone marrow may improve our ability to obtain stem cells and make them more efficient at finding their way to the specific sites for blood cell production, the so-called stem cell niche.

HEMATOPOIETIC STEM CELL MICROENVIRONMENT

The concept of a specialized microenvironment, or stem cell niche, was first proposed to explain why cells derived from the bone marrow of one animal could be used in transplantation and again be found in the bone marrow of the recipient. This niche is more than just a housing site for stem cells, however. It is an anatomic location where regulatory signals are provided that allow the stem cells to thrive, to expand if needed, and to provide varying amounts of descendant daughter cells. In addition, unregulated growth of stem cells may be problematic based on their undifferentiated state and self-renewal capacity. Thus, the niche must also regulate the number of stem cells produced. In this manner, the niche has the dual functions of serving as a site of nurture but imposing limits for stem cells: in effect, acting as both a nest and a cage.

The niche for blood stem cells changes with each of the sites of blood production during development, but for most of human life it is located in the bone marrow. Within the bone marrow, at least two niche sites have been proposed: on trabecular bone surfaces and in the perivascular space. Stem cells may be found in both places by histologic analysis, and functional regulation has been shown at the bone surface. Specifically, bone-forming mesenchymal cells, osteoblasts, participate in hematopoietic stem cell function, affecting their location, proliferation, and number. The basis for this interaction is through a number of molecules mediating location, such as the chemokine CXCL12 (SDF1) and N-cadherin, through proliferation signals mediated by angiopoietin 1, and signaling to modulate self-renewal or survival by factors such as Notch ligands, kit ligand, and Wnts. Other bone components, such as the extracellular matrix glycoprotein, os-

teopontin, and the high ionic calcium found at trabecular surfaces, contribute to the unique microenvironment, or stem cell niche, on trabecular bone. This physiology has practical applications. First, medications altering niche components may have an effect on stem cell function. This has now been shown for a number of compounds, and some are being clinically tested. Second, it is now possible to assess whether the niche participates in disease states and to examine whether targeting the niche with medications may alter the outcome of certain diseases.

EXCESS CAPACITY OF HEMATOPOIETIC STEM CELLS

In the absence of disease, one never runs out of hematopoietic stem cells. Indeed, serial transplantation studies in mice suggest that sufficient stem cells are present to reconstitute several animals in succession, with each animal having normal blood cell production. The fact that allogeneic stem cell transplant recipients also never run out of blood cells in their life span, which can extend for decades, argues that even the limiting numbers of stem cells provided to them are sufficient. How stem cells respond to different conditions to increase or decrease their mature cell production remains poorly understood. Clearly, negative feedback mechanisms affect the level of production of most of the cells, leading to the normal tightly regulated blood cell counts. However, many of the regulatory mechanisms that govern production of more mature progenitor cells do not apply or apply differently to stem cells. Similarly, most of the molecules shown to be able to change the size of the stem cell pool have little effect on more mature blood cells. For example, the growth factor erythropoietin, which stimulates red blood cell production from more mature precursor cells, has no effect on stem cells. Similarly, granulocyte colony-stimulating factor drives the rapid proliferation of granulocyte precursors but does not affect cell cycling of stem cells. Rather, it changes the location of stem cells by indirect means, altering molecules such as CXCL12 that tether stem cells to their niche. Molecules shown to be important for altering the proliferation of stem cells, such as the cyclin-dependent kinase inhibitor p21Cip1, have little or no effect on progenitor proliferation. Hematopoietic stem cells have governing mechanisms that are distinct from the cells they generate.

HEMATOPOIETIC STEM CELL DIFFERENTIATION

Hematopoietic stem cells sit at the base of a branching hierarchy of cells culminating in the many mature cell types that compose the blood and immune system (Fig. 68-2). The maturation steps leading to terminally differentiated and functional blood cells take place both as a consequence of intrinsic changes in gene expression and niche-directed and cytokine-directed changes in the cells. Our knowledge of the details remains incomplete (see *http://stemcell.princeton.edu/* for a comprehensive listing of gene expression in stem cells). As stem cells mature to progenitors, precursors, and, finally, mature effector cells, they undergo a series of functional changes. These include the obvious acquisition of functions defining mature blood cells, such as phagocytic capacity or hemoglobinization. They also include the progressive loss of plasticity, i.e., the ability to become other cell types. For example, the myeloid progenitor can make all cells in the myeloid series but none in the lymphoid series. As common myeloid progenitors mature, they become precursors for either monocytes and granulocytes or erythrocytes and megakaryocytes, but not both. Some amount of reversibility of this process may exist early in the differentiation cascade, but that is lost beyond a distinct stage. As cells differentiate, they may also lose proliferative capacity (Fig. 68-3). Mature granulocytes are incapable of proliferation and only increase in number by increased production from precursors. Lymphoid cells retain the capacity to proliferate but have linked their proliferation to the recognition of particular proteins or peptides by specific antigen receptors on their surface. In most tissues the proliferative cell population is a more immature progenitor population. In general, cells within the highly proliferative progenitor cell compartment are also relatively short-lived, making their way through the differentiation process in a defined molecular program involving the sequential activation of particular sets

Stem Cells   Progenitor Cells   Lineage Committed Precursors   Mature Cells

FIGURE 68-2 Hierarchy of hematopoietic differentiation. *Stem cells* are multipotent cells that are the source of all descendant cells and have the capacity to provide either long-term (measured in years) or short-term (measured in months) cell production. *Progenitor cells* have a more limited spectrum of cells they can produce and are generally a short-lived, highly proliferative population also known as transient amplifying cells. *Precursor cells* are cells committed to a single blood cell lineage but with a continued ability to proliferate; they do not have all the features of a fully mature cell. *Mature cells* are the ter-minally differentiated product of the differentiation process and are the effector cells of specific activities of the blood and immune system. Progress through the pathways is mediated by alterations in gene expression. The regulation of the differentiation by soluble factors and cell-cell communications within the bone marrow niche are still being defined. The transcription factors that characterize particular cell transitions are illustrated on the arrows; the soluble factors that contribute to the differentiation process are in blue. SCF, stem cell factor; EPO, erythropoietin; TPO, thrombopoietin.

of genes. For any particular cell type, the differentiation program is difficult to speed up. The time it takes for hematopoietic progenitors to become mature cells is ~10–14 days in humans, evident clinically by the interval between cytotoxic chemotherapy and blood count recovery in patients.

SELF-RENEWAL

The hematopoietic stem cell must balance its three potential fates: apoptosis, self-renewal, and differentiation. The proliferation of cells is generally not associated with the ability to undergo a self-renewing division except among memory T and B cells and among stem cells. Self-renewal capacity gives way to differentiation as the only option after cell division when cells leave the stem cell compartment, until they have the opportunity to become memory lymphocytes. In addition to this self-renewing capacity, stem cells have an additional feature characterizing their proliferation machinery. Stem cells in most mature adult tissues are deeply quiescent. In the hematopoietic system, stem cells are also highly cytokine-resistant, remaining dormant even when cytokines drive bone marrow progenitors to proliferation rates measured in hours, not days. Stem cells, in contrast, are thought to divide at inter-vals measured in months to years, at least as estimated in nonhuman primates. This deep quiescence is difficult to overcome in vitro, limiting the ability to effectively expand human hematopoietic stem cells. The process may be controlled by particularly high levels of expression of cyclin-dependent kinase inhibitors that restrict entry of stem cells into cell cycle, blocking the G1-S transition. Modifying the levels of molecules such as p21Cip1 and p18INK4c in the laboratory has resulted in increased stem cell proliferation and number in mice and in some limited human cell studies. Exogenous signals from the niche also appear to enforce quiescence, including the activation of the tyrosine kinase receptor Tie2 on stem cells by angiopoietin 1 on osteoblasts.

The regulation of stem cell proliferation also appears to change with age. In mice, the cyclin-dependent kinase inhibitor p16INK4a accumulates in stem cells in older animals and is associated with a change in five different stem cell functions, including cell cycling. Lowering expression of p16INK4a in older animals improves stem cell cycling and capacity to reconstitute hematopoiesis in adoptive hosts, making them similar to younger animals. Mature cell numbers are unaffected. Therefore, molecular events governing the specific functions of stem cells are being gradually made clear and offer the potential of new ap-

FIGURE 68-3 Relative function of cells in the hematopoietic hierarchy. The boxes represent distinct functional features of cells in the myeloid (*upper box*) versus lymphoid (*lower box*) lineages.

proaches to changing stem cell function for therapy. One critical stem cell function that remains poorly defined is the molecular regulation of self-renewal.

For medicine, self-renewal is perhaps the most important function of stem cells because it is critical in regulating the number of stem cells. Stem cell number is a key limiting parameter for both autologous and allogeneic stem cell transplantation. Were we to have the ability to use fewer stem cells or expand limited numbers of stem cells ex vivo, it might be possible to reduce the morbidity and expense of stem cell harvests and enable use of other stem cell sources. Specifically, umbilical cord blood is a rich source of stem cells. However, the volume of cord blood units is extremely small, and therefore the total number of hematopoietic stem cells that can be obtained is generally only sufficient to transplant an individual of <40 kg. This limitation restricts what would otherwise be an extremely promising source of stem cells. Two features of cord blood stem cells are particularly important. (1) They are derived from a diversity of individuals that far exceeds the adult donor pool and therefore can overcome the majority of immunologic cross-matching obstacles. (2) Cord blood stem cells have a large number of T cells associated with them, but (paradoxically) they appear to be associated with a lower incidence of graft-versus-host disease when compared with similarly mismatched stem cells from other sources. If stem cell expansion by self-renewal could be achieved, the number of cells available might be sufficient for use in larger adults. An alternative approach to this problem is to improve the efficiency of engraftment of donor stem cells. Graft engineering is exploring methods of adding cell components that may enhance engraftment. Furthermore, at least some data suggest that depletion of host NK (natural killer) cells may lower the number of stem cells necessary to reconstitute hematopoiesis.

Some limited understanding of self-renewal exists and, intriguingly, implicates gene products that are associated with the chromatin state, a high-order organization of chromosomal DNA that influences transcription. These include members of the polycomb family, a group of zinc finger–containing transcriptional regulators that interact with the chromatin structure, contributing to the accessibility of groups of genes for transcription. Certain members, including Bmi-1 and Gfi-1, are important in enabling hematopoietic stem cell self-renewal through modification of cell cycle regulators such as the cyclin-dependent kinase inhibitors. In the absence of either of these genes, hematopoietic stem cells decline in number and function. In contrast, dysregulation of *Bmi-1* has been associated with leukemia; it may promote leukemic stem cell self-renewal when it is overexpressed. Other transcription regulators have also been associated with self-renewal,

particularly homeobox, or "hox," genes. These transcription factors are named for their ability to govern large numbers of genes, including those determining body patterning in invertebrates. HoxB4 is capable of inducing extensive self-renewal of stem cells through its DNA-binding motif. Other members of the hox family of genes have been noted to affect normal stem cells, but they are also associated with leukemia. External signals that may influence the relative self-renewal versus differentiation outcomes of stem cell cycling include the Notch ligands and specific Wnt ligands. Intracellular signal transducing intermediates are also implicated in regulating self-renewal but, interestingly, are not usually associated with the pathways activated by Notch or Wnt receptors. They include PTEN, an inhibitor of the AKT pathway, and STAT5, both of which are usually downstream of activated growth factor receptors and necessary for normal stem cell functions, including self-renewal, at least in mouse models. The connections between these molecules remain to be defined, and their role in physiologic regulation of stem cell self-renewal is still poorly understood.

CANCER IS SIMILAR TO AN ORGAN WITH SELF-RENEWING CAPACITY

The relationship of stem cells to cancer is an important evolving dimension of adult stem cell biology. Cancer may share principles of organization with normal tissues. Cancer might have the same hierarchical organization of cells with a base of stemlike cells capable of the signature stem-cell features, self-renewal and differentiation. These stemlike cells might be the basis for perpetuation of the tumor and represent a slowly dividing, rare population with distinct regulatory mechanisms, including a relationship with a specialized microenvironment. A subpopulation of self-renewing cells in cancer has been defined. A more sophisticated understanding of the stem-cell organization of cancers may lead to improved strategies for attacking the many common and difficult-to-treat types of malignancies that have been relatively refractory to interventions aimed at dividing cells.

Does the concept of cancer stem cells provide insight into the cellular origin of cancer? The fact that some cells within a cancer have stem cell–like properties does not necessarily mean that the cancer arose in the stem cell itself. Rather, more mature cells could have acquired the self-renewal characteristics of stem cells. Any single genetic event is unlikely to be sufficient to enable full transformation of a normal cell to a frankly malignant one. Rather, cancer is a multistep process, and for the multiple steps to accumulate, the cell of origin must be able to persist for prolonged periods. It must also be able to generate large numbers of daughter cells. The normal stem cell has these properties and, by virtue of its having intrinsic self-renewal capability, may be more readily converted to a malignant phenotype. This hypothesis has been tested experimentally in the hematopoietic system. Taking advantage of the cell-surface markers that distinguish hematopoietic cells of varying maturity, stem cells, progenitors, precursors, and mature cells can be isolated. Powerful transforming gene constructs were placed in these cells, and it was found that the cell with the greatest potential to produce a malignancy was indeed the stem cell. This does not prove that stem cells give rise to all tumors, but it does suggest that stem cells may be susceptible to malignant conversion and may be the population of greatest interest in developing strategies to protect against, monitor, or treat nascent malignancy.

WHAT ELSE CAN HEMATOPOIETIC STEM CELLS DO?

Some experimental data have suggested that hematopoietic stem cells or other cells mobilized into the circulation by the same factors that mobilize hematopoietic stem cells are capable of playing a role in healing the vascular and tissue damage associated with stroke and myocardial infarction. These data are controversial, and the applicability of a stem-cell approach to nonhematopoietic conditions remains experimental. However, the application of the evolving knowledge of hematopoietic stem cell biology may lead to wide-ranging clinical uses.

The stem cell therefore represents a true dual-edged sword. It has tremendous healing capacity and is essential for life. Uncontrolled, it can threaten the life it maintains. Understanding how stem cells function, the signals that modify their behavior, and the tissue niches that modulate stem cell responses to injury and disease are critical for more effectively developing stem cell–based medicine. That aspect of medicine will include the use of the stem cells and the use of drugs to target stem cells to enhance repair of damaged tissues. It will also include the careful balance of interventions to control stem cells where they may be dysfunctional or malignant.

69 Tissue Engineering
Jennifer Anderson, Joseph P. Vacanti

The origins of tissue engineering date to the sixteenth century when complex skin flaps were used to replace the nose. Modern tissue engineering combines the disciplines of materials sciences and life sciences to replace a diseased or damaged organ with a living, functional substitute. The most common tissue engineering approach combines cells and matrices to produce a living structure (Fig. 69-1). These strategies also include the use of scaffolding, cells, and growth factors to shape new tissues. The term *regenerative medicine* has emerged as a concept inclusive of tissue engineering and stem cell therapy (Chap. 67).

CELLULAR COMPONENTS OF TISSUE ENGINEERING
The foundation of tissue engineering is the combination of a three-dimensional scaffold with live and functional cells. Cells used in tissue engineering should be easily accessible and capable of proliferation while maintaining their differentiated function. There are three possible sources for cells: autologous, allogenic, and xenogenic. *Autologous cells* are isolated directly from the patient. They have the advantage of avoiding immune-mediated rejection. However, a potential limitation is that they may not be available or able to proliferate to the required tissue mass. *Allogenic cells* are harvested from a donor other than the patient. They have the advantage of being more readily available, but the immune system must be modulated to avoid rejection. *Xenogenic cells,* or those from a different species, may also be used but also risk immune rejection or transmission of animal pathogens.

Although cells such as fibroblasts and smooth-muscle cells proliferate rapidly, other cells proliferate slowly or lose their tissue-specific function when cultured, thereby limiting their use. In addition, cellular characteristics may depend on their location within the body. For example, the cell-to-cell interactions and function of endothelial cells in the pulmonary microvasculature are different from those in the blood-brain barrier. The microenvironment of the cell, including the presence of other cell types, soluble factors, and the presence of physical or mechanical forces may also alter the function of a transplanted cell.

Stem cells provide a promising cell source because they are capable of rapid proliferation and they can be induced to differentiate into multiple cell lineages (Chaps. 66 and 67). Human embryonic stem cells are capable of differentiating into endoderm, mesoderm, or ectoderm tissue types. Multipotent adult stem cells have been found in multiple mature tissues including the bone marrow, brain, heart, and liver. In addition to being able to differentiate into numerous lineages, adult stem cells generate a relatively muted immune response.

SCAFFOLDS
A scaffold provides a three-dimensional framework to support the tissue or organ-specific cells. The scaffold not only provides mechanical support, but it must also supply critical nutrients and transport metabolites to and from the developing tissue. Important scaffold properties vary depending on the tissue but typically include specific

FURTHER READINGS
CHUTE JP: Stem cell homing. Curr Opin Hematol 13:399, 2006
JORDAN CT: The leukemic stem cell. Best Pract Res Clin Haematol 20:13, 2007
LAIOSA CV et al: Determinants of lymphoid-myeloid lineage diversification. Annu Rev Immunol 24:705, 2006
MIKKOLA HK, ORKIN SH: The journey of developing hematopoietic stem cells. Development 133:3733, 2006
SCADDEN DT: The stem cell niche as an entity of action. Nature 441:1075, 2006

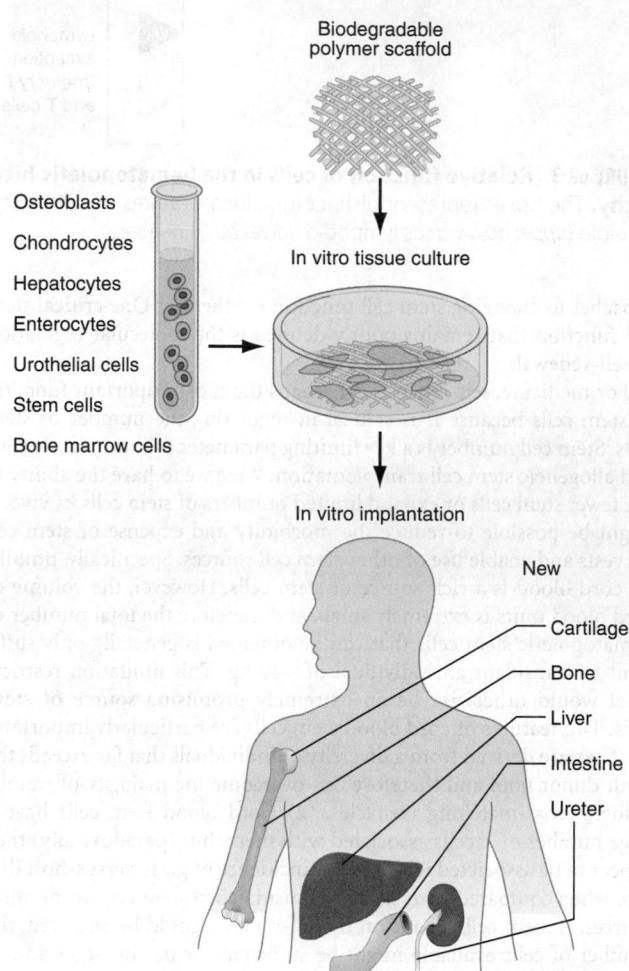

FIGURE 69-1 Schematic of basic principles of tissue engineering. [From Langer R, Vacanti J: Tissue engineering. Science 260:1993 (Fig. 1), with permission.]

biomechanical properties, porosity, biocompatibility, and appropriate surface characteristics for cell adhesion and differentiation.

Scaffolds can be natural materials or synthetic polymers and are typically biodegradable. Natural materials such as collagen and alginates are biocompatible. However, it is difficult to control their mechanical properties, and they may generate an immune reaction. Synthetic polymers such as polyglycolic acid and polyethylene, on the other hand, can be tailored to provide more acceptable mechanical properties but are associated with a strong inflammatory response. Nonbiodegradable synthetic polymers such as polytetrafluoroethylene and polyethylene provide well-defined mechanical and structural properties. However, their long-term presence in the body can lead to a chronic inflammatory response, which results in poor tissue quality. Polylactic acid and polyglycolic acid are examples of biodegradable polymers. Although the degradation of these materials can be partially

PART 4 Regenerative Medicine

TABLE 69-1 FDA-APPROVED TISSUE-ENGINEERED PRODUCTS

Name of Product	Brief Description
Alloderm (LifeCell)	Acellular dermal matrix for tissue repair
Apligraf (Organogenesis)	Living skin equivalent approved for the treatment of venous leg ulcers and diabetic foot ulcers
Carticel (Genzyme Biosurgery)	Autologous chondrocytes approved for cartilage repair
Dermagraft (Smith and Nephew)	Living skin equivalent approved for full-thickness diabetic foot ulcers
Durasis (Cook Surgical Products)	Porcine small-intestine submucosa for replacement of dura mater
Epicel (Genzyme Biosurgery)	Living skin equivalent approved for burn patients
OrCel (Ortec)	Living skin equivalent approved for burn patients
Surgisis (Cook Surgical Products)	Porcine small-intestine submucosa for dermal wounds and reinforcement of weakened tissue

TABLE 69-2 TISSUE-ENGINEERING PRODUCTS IN CLINICAL TRIALS

TRC (Aastrom)	Autologous adult bone marrow cells for bone grafting
LiverX2000 (Algenix)	Extracorporeal liver assist device
Encapsulated proliferated islet (Amcyte)	Encapsulated islet cells
Myocell (Bioheart)	Encapsulated cells for myocardial infarction
BioSeed-C, BioSeed-Oral Bone (Biotissue Technologies)	Autologous tissue repair for bone and cartilage
E-matrix (Encelle)	Repair or regeneration of diseased or damaged tissue
MarkII (Excorp)	Extracorporeal liver assist device
ICX-PRO, ICX-TRC (Intercytex)	Wound repair and hair regeneration
HuCNS-SC (Stem Cell Inc)	Human central nervous system stem cells
NT-501 (Neurotech SA)	Encapsulated cell technology for long-term delivery of therapeutic factors to retina
Procord (Proneuron)	Autologous activated macrophage therapy for patients with acute complete spinal cord injury
ChondroCelect (Tigenix)	Autologous chondrocyte implantation
Spheramine (Titan Pharmaceutical)	Retinal pigment epithelial cells in micro-carriers to provide continuous source of dopamine in the brain
ELAD (Vigagen)	Extracorporeal liver assist device

controlled, nonuniform degradation and varying degradation rates in different anatomic locations represent challenges.

The surface properties of the materials used for the scaffold are important for adhesion, migration, and cell differentiation. Ongoing research is focused on tethering growth factors or peptide sequences to the surface of the scaffold to improve adhesion and migration.

BIOREACTORS

Initially, cells used in tissue engineering were cultured in static conditions. Improvements in bioreactor technology more closely approximate physiologic parameters for tissue growth. By modulating rates of flow and mixing, the transfer of nutrients, gases, metabolites, and regulatory molecules can be maximized. Mechanical stimuli can also impact the newly forming tissue. For example, tissue-engineered blood vessels exposed to shear stress in a pulsatile flow bioreactor have greater burst strength and collagen content than those not exposed to shear stress.

TISSUE ENGINEERING SUCCESSES

Several tissue-engineered skin substitutes have been approved by the U.S. Food and Drug Administration (FDA) and in use for >10 years (Table 69-1). One of these products uses neonatal dermal fibroblasts isolated from human foreskins cultured on a scaffold of polylactide coglycolide. The polymer scaffold gradually degrades in the presence of water. A bilayer skin substitute has also been developed: dermal fibroblasts are cultured in a collagen solution and then coated with several layers of keratinocytes. Cartilage tissue engineering is also showing promise; autologous chondrocytes from a healthy portion of the patient's joint are expanded in culture and then implanted into the site of injury. Other scaffold-based products are based on processed animal submucosa or dura. In addition to these FDA-approved products, numerous tissue-engineered products are currently in clinical trials (Table 69-2). Engineered tissues being actively investigated include bone, mandible, teeth, cartilage, skin, cornea, bladder, urethra, small-diameter blood vessels, and the pulmonary artery.

CHALLENGES TO TISSUE ENGINEERING

The greatest success in tissue engineering to date has been in tissues such as skin and cartilage where the requirements for nutrients and oxygen are relatively low. Due to oxygen diffusion limitations, the maximal thickness of an engineered tissue is 150–200 μm if there is not an intrinsic capillary network. Strategies used to overcome this limitation include transplantation of the tissue directly into the patient's vasculature or trying to induce angiogenesis by incorporating growth factors such as vascular endothelial cell growth factor into the scaffold. A more recent approach involves the creation of an intrinsic network of vascular channels immediately adjacent to the engineered tissue. A combination of microelectro mechanical systems (MEMS) fabrication technology and computational models of fractal branching allows the construction of an intrinsic microvascular network scaffold within a biocompatible polymer. This preformed capillary-like network can be seeded with cells and ultimately sustains the growth and function of complex three-dimensional tissues.

Immune rejection of allogenic cells is another major obstacle. The use of immunosuppressive drugs is not considered an optimal solution to this problem. One potential solution is to develop "universal donor" cells by masking the histocompatibility proteins on the cell surface.

Off-the-shelf availability will need to be addressed for tissue engineering products to be used widely. Ideally, products should be reproducible and available at a wide variety of hospitals, including those without sophisticated facilities for cell culture and cell proliferation.

FURTHER READINGS

AHSAN T, NEREM RM: Bioengineered tissues: The science, the technology, and the industry. Orthod Craniofacial Res 8:134, 2005

LAVIK E, LANGER R: Tissue engineering: Current state and perspectives. Appl Microbiol Biotechnol 65:1, 2004

LYSAGHT MJ, HAZLEHURST AL: Tissue engineering: The end of the beginning. Tissue Engineering 10:12, 2004

SHEIH SJ, VACANTI JP: State-of-the-art tissue engineering: From tissue engineering to organ building. Surgery 137:1, 2005

YOW KH et al: Tissue engineering of vascular conduits. Br J Surg 93(6):652, 2006

70 Nutritional Requirements and Dietary Assessment

Johanna Dwyer

Nutrients are substances that must be supplied by the diet because they are not synthesized in the body in sufficient amounts. Nutrient requirements for groups of healthy persons have been determined experimentally. For good health we require energy-providing nutrients (protein, fat, and carbohydrate), vitamins, minerals, and water. Specific nutrient requirements include 9 essential amino acids, several fatty acids, 4 fat-soluble vitamins, 10 water-soluble vitamins, and choline. Several inorganic substances, including 4 minerals, 7 trace minerals, 3 electrolytes, and the ultratrace elements, also must be supplied in the diet.

The required amounts of the essential nutrients differ by age and physiologic state. Conditionally essential nutrients are not required in the diet but must be supplied to individuals who do not synthesize them in adequate amounts, such as those with genetic defects, those having pathologic states with nutritional implications, and developmentally immature infants. Many organic phytochemicals and zoochemicals present in foods have health effects. For example, dietary fiber has beneficial effects on gastrointestinal function. Other bioactive food constituents or contaminants such as lead may have negative health effects.

ESSENTIAL NUTRIENT REQUIREMENTS

ENERGY

For weight to remain stable, energy intake must match energy output. The major components of energy output are resting energy expenditure (REE) and physical activity; minor sources include the energy cost of metabolizing food (thermic effect of food or specific dynamic action) and shivering thermogenesis (e.g., cold-induced thermogenesis). The average energy intake is about 2800 kcal/d for American men and about 1800 kcal/d for American women, although these estimates vary with body size and activity level. Formulas for estimating REE are useful for assessing the energy needs of an individual whose weight is stable. Thus, for males, REE = 900 + 10w, and for females, REE = 700 + 7w, where w is weight in kilograms. The calculated REE is then adjusted for physical activity level by multiplying by 1.2 for sedentary, 1.4 for moderately active, or 1.8 for very active individuals. The final figure provides a rough estimate of total caloric needs in a state of energy balance. Formulas to provide more precise estimates of energy requirements are provided by the Food and Nutrition Board, Institute of Medicine, National Academy of Sciences in recent reports on dietary reference intakes. For further discussion of energy balance in health and disease, see Chap. 72.

PROTEIN

Dietary protein consists of both essential and other amino acids that are required for protein synthesis. The nine essential amino acids are histidine, isoleucine, leucine, lysine, methionine/cystine, phenylalanine/tyrosine, threonine, tryptophan, and valine. All amino acids can be used for energy, and certain amino acids (e.g., alanine) can also be used for gluconeogenesis. When energy intake is inadequate, protein intake must be increased, since ingested amino acids are diverted into pathways of glucose synthesis and oxidation. In extreme energy deprivation, protein-calorie malnutrition may ensue (Chap. 72).

For adults, the recommended dietary allowance (RDA) for protein is about 0.6 g/kg desirable body weight per day, assuming that energy needs are met and that the protein is of relatively high biologic value. Current recommendations for a healthy diet call for at least 10–14% of calories from protein. Biologic value tends to be highest for animal proteins, followed by proteins from legumes (beans), cereals (rice, wheat, corn), and roots. Combinations of plant proteins that complement one another in biologic value or combinations of animal and plant proteins can increase biologic value and lower total protein requirements.

Protein needs increase during growth, pregnancy, lactation, and rehabilitation after malnutrition. Tolerance to normal amounts of dietary protein is decreased in renal insufficiency and liver failure, precipitating encephalopathy in patients with cirrhosis of the liver.

FAT AND CARBOHYDRATE

Fats are a concentrated source of energy and constitute on average 34% of calories in U.S. diets. For optimal health, saturated fat and trans-fat should be limited to <10% of calories, and polyunsaturated fats to <10% of calories, with monounsaturated fats constituting the remainder of fat intake. At least 55% of total calories should be derived from carbohydrates. The brain requires about 100 g/d of glucose for fuel; other tissues use about 50 g/d. Some tissues (e.g., brain and red blood cells) rely on glucose supplied either exogenously or from muscle proteolysis. Over time, some adaptations in carbohydrate needs are possible in other tissues during hypocaloric states (Chap. 339).

WATER

For adults, 1.0–1.5 mL water per kcal of energy expenditure is sufficient under usual conditions to allow for normal variations in physical activity, sweating, and solute load of the diet. Water losses include 50–100 mL/d in the feces, 500–1000 mL/d by evaporation or exhalation, and, depending on the renal solute load, ≥1000 mL/d in the urine. If external losses increase, intakes must increase accordingly to avoid underhydration. Fever increases water losses by approximately 200 mL/d per °C; diarrheal losses vary but may be as great as 5 L/d with severe diarrhea. Heavy sweating and vomiting also increase water losses. When renal function is normal and solute intakes are adequate, the kidneys can adjust to increased water intake by excreting up to 18 L/d of excess water (Chap. 334). However, obligatory urine outputs can compromise hydration status when there is inadequate intake or when losses increase in disease or kidney damage.

Infants have high requirements for water because of their large ratio of surface area to volume, the limited capacity of the immature kidney to handle high renal solute loads, and their inability to communicate their thirst. During pregnancy, 30 mL/d additional water is needed. During lactation, milk production increases water requirements by approximately 1000 mL/d, or 1 mL for each mL of milk produced. Special attention must be paid to the water needs of the elderly, who have reduced total body water and blunted thirst sensation, and may be taking diuretics.

OTHER NUTRIENTS

See Chap. 71 for a detailed description of vitamins and trace minerals.

DIETARY REFERENCE INTAKES AND RECOMMENDED DIETARY ALLOWANCES

Fortunately, human life and well-being can be maintained within a fairly wide range for most nutrients. However, the capacity for adaptation is not infinite—too much of a nutrient, as well as too little, may have adverse effects on health. Therefore, quantitative benchmark recommendations on nutrient intakes have been developed to guide clinical practice. These estimates are collectively referred to as the *dietary reference intakes* (DRIs). The DRIs supplant but include the *recommended dietary allowances* (RDAs), the single reference values used in the United States since 1989. DRIs include the *estimated average requirement* (EAR) of a nutrient, as well as three other reference values used for dietary planning for individuals: the RDA or, if it cannot be established, the *adequate intake* (AI), and the tolerable *upper level* (UL). The current DRIs for vitamins and elements are provided in Tables 70-1 and 70-2, respectively.

TABLE 70-1 DIETARY REFERENCE INTAKES: RECOMMENDED INTAKES FOR INDIVIDUALS—VITAMINS

Life-Stage Group	Vitamin, μg/d					Thia-mine, mg/d	Ribo-flavin, mg/d	Niacin, mg/d[e]	Vitamin B6, mg/d	Folate, μg/d[f]	Vitamin B12, μg/d	Panto-thenic Acid, mg/d	Biotin, μg/d	Choline, mg/d[g]
	A[a]	C	D[b,c]	E[d]	K									
Infants														
0–6 mo	400	40	5	4	2.0	0.2	0.3	2	0.1	65	0.4	1.7	5	125
7–12 mo	500	50	5	5	2.5	0.3	0.4	4	0.3	80	0.5	1.8	6	150
Children														
1–3 y	**300**	**15**	5	**6**	30	**0.5**	**0.5**	**6**	**0.5**	**150**	**0.9**	2	8	200
4–8 y	**400**	**25**	5	**7**	55	**0.6**	**0.6**	**8**	**0.6**	**200**	**1.2**	3	12	250
Males														
9–13 y	**600**	**45**	5	**11**	60	**0.9**	**0.9**	**12**	**1.0**	**300**	**1.8**	4	20	375
14–18 y	**900**	**75**	5	**15**	75	**1.2**	**1.3**	**16**	**1.3**	**400**	**2.4**	5	25	550
19–30 y	**900**	**90**	5	**15**	120	**1.2**	**1.3**	**16**	**1.3**	**400**	**2.4**	5	30	550
31–50 y	**900**	**90**	5	**15**	120	**1.2**	**1.3**	**16**	**1.3**	**400**	**2.4**	5	30	550
51–70 y	**900**	**90**	10	**15**	120	**1.2**	**1.3**	**16**	**1.7**	**400**	**2.4**[h]	5	30	550
>70 y	**900**	**90**	15	**15**	120	**1.2**	**1.3**	**16**	**1.7**	**400**	**2.4**[h]	5	30	550
Females														
9–13 y	**600**	**45**	5	**11**	60	**0.9**	**0.9**	**12**	**1.0**	**300**	**1.8**	4	20	375
14–18 y	**700**	**65**	5	**15**	75	**1.0**	**1.0**	**14**	**1.2**	**400**[i]	**2.4**	5	25	400
19–30 y	**700**	**75**	5	**15**	90	**1.1**	**1.1**	**14**	**1.3**	**400**[i]	**2.4**	5	30	425
31–50 y	**700**	**75**	5	**15**	90	**1.1**	**1.1**	**14**	**1.3**	**400**[i]	**2.4**	5	30	425
51–70 y	**700**	**75**	10	**15**	90	**1.1**	**1.1**	**14**	**1.5**	**400**	**2.4**[h]	5	30	425
>70 y	**700**	**75**	15	**15**	90	**1.1**	**1.1**	**14**	**1.5**	**400**	**2.4**[h]	5	30	425
Pregnancy														
≤18 y	**750**	**80**	5	**15**	75	**1.4**	**1.4**	**18**	**1.6**	**600**[j]	**2.6**	6	30	450
19–30 y	**770**	**85**	5	**15**	90	**1.4**	**1.4**	**18**	**1.9**	**600**[j]	**2.6**	6	30	450
31–50 y	**770**	**85**	5	**15**	90	**1.4**	**1.4**	**18**	**1.9**	**600**[j]	**2.6**	6	30	450
Lactation														
≤18 y	**1200**	**115**	5	**19**	75	**1.4**	**1.6**	**17**	**2.0**	**500**	**2.8**	7	35	550
19–30 y	**1300**	**120**	5	**19**	90	**1.4**	**1.6**	**17**	**2.0**	**500**	**2.8**	7	35	550
31–50 y	**1300**	**120**	5	**19**	90	**1.4**	**1.6**	**17**	**2.0**	**500**	**2.8**	7	35	550

Note: This table presents recommended dietary allowances (RDAs) in **bold type** and adequate intakes (AIs) in ordinary type. RDAs and AIs may both be used as goals for individual intake. RDAs are set to meet the needs of almost all individuals (97 to 98%) in a group. For healthy breastfed infants, the AI is the mean intake. The AI for other life stage and gender groups is believed to cover needs of all individuals in the group, but lack of data or uncertainty in the data prevent being able to specify with confidence the percentage of individuals covered by this intake.

[a]As retinol activity equivalents (RAEs). 1 RAE = 1 μg retinol, 12 μg β-carotene, 24 μg α-carotene, or 24 μg β-cryptoxanthin. To calculate RAEs from retinol equivalents (REs) of provitamin A carotenoids in foods, divide the REs by 2. For preformed vitamin A in foods or supplements and for provitamin A carotenoids in supplements, 1 RE = 1 RAE.

[b]As calciferol. 1 μg calciferol = 40 IU vitamin D.

[c]In the absence of adequate exposure to sunlight.

[d]As α-tocopherol. α-Tocopherol includes RRR-α-tocopherol, the only form of α-tocopherol that occurs naturally in foods, and the 2R-stereoisomeric forms of α-tocopherol (RRR-, RSR-, RRS-, and RSS-α-tocopherol) that occur in fortified foods and supplements. It does not include the 2S-stereoisomeric forms of α-tocopherol (SRR-, SSR-, SRS-, and SSS-α-tocopherol), also found in fortified foods and supplements.

[e]As niacin equivalents (NE). 1 mg of niacin = 60 mg of tryptophan; 0–6 months = preformed niacin (not NE).

[f]As dietary folate equivalents (DFEs). 1 DFE = 1 μg food folate = 0.6 μg of folic acid from fortified food or as a supplement consumed with food = 0.5 μg of a supplement taken on an empty stomach.

[g]Although AIs have been set for choline, there are few data to assess whether a dietary supply of choline is needed at all stages of the life cycle, and it may be that the choline requirement can be met by endogenous synthesis at some of these stages.

[h]Because 10 to 30% of older people may malabsorb food-bound B12, it is advisable for those >50 years to meet their RDA mainly by consuming foods fortified with B12 or a supplement containing B12.

[i]In view of evidence linking inadequate folate intake with neural tube defects in the fetus, it is recommended that all women capable of becoming pregnant consume 400 μg from supplements or fortified foods in addition to intake of food folate from a varied diet.

[j]It is assumed that women will continue consuming 400 μg from supplements or fortified food until their pregnancy is confirmed and they enter prenatal care, which ordinarily occurs after the end of the periconceptional period—the critical time for formation of the neural tube.

Source: Food and Nutrition Board, Institute of Medicine—National Academy of Sciences Dietary Reference Intakes, 2000, 2002, reprinted with permission. Courtesy of the National Academy Press, Washington, DC. *http://www.nap.edu*

ESTIMATED AVERAGE REQUIREMENT

When florid manifestations of the classic dietary deficiency diseases such as rickets, scurvy, xerophthalmia, and protein-calorie malnutrition were common, nutrient adequacy was inferred from the absence of their clinical signs. Later, it was determined that biochemical and other changes were evident long before the clinical deficiency became apparent. Consequently, criteria of nutrient adequacy are now based on biologic markers when they are available. Priority is given to sensitive biochemical, physiologic, or behavioral tests that reflect early changes in regulatory processes or maintenance of body stores of nutrients. Current definitions focus on the amount of a nutrient that minimizes the risk of chronic degenerative diseases.

The EAR is the amount of a nutrient estimated to be adequate for half of the healthy individuals of a specific age and sex. The types of evidence and criteria used to establish nutrient requirements vary by nutrient, age, and physiologic group. The EAR is not useful clinically for estimating nutrient adequacy in individuals because it is a medi-an requirement for a group; 50% of individuals in a group fall below the requirement and 50% fall above it. Thus, a person with a usual intake at the EAR has a 50% risk of an inadequate intake. For these reasons, other standards, described below, are more useful for clinical purposes.

RECOMMENDED DIETARY ALLOWANCES

The RDA is the nutrient-intake goal for planning diets of individuals; it is used in the MyPyramid food guide of the U.S. Department of Agriculture (USDA), therapeutic diets, and descriptions of the nutritional content of processed foods and dietary supplements. The nutrient content in a food is stated by weight or as a percentage of the daily value (DV), a variant of the RDA that, for an adult, represents the highest RDA for an adult consuming 2000 kcal/d.

The RDA is the average daily dietary intake level that meets the nutrient requirements of nearly all healthy persons of a specific sex, age, life stage, or physiologic condition (such as pregnancy or lactation).

The RDA is defined statistically as 2 standard deviations (SD) above the EAR to ensure that the needs of most individuals are met.

The risk of dietary inadequacy increases as intake falls further below the RDA. However, the RDA is an overly generous criterion for evaluating nutrient adequacy. For example, by definition the RDA exceeds the actual requirements of all but about 2 to 3% of the population. Therefore, many people whose intake falls below the RDA may still be getting enough of the nutrient.

ADEQUATE INTAKE

It is not possible to set an RDA for some nutrients that do not have an established EAR. In this circumstance, the AI is based on observed, or experimentally determined, approximations of nutrient intakes in healthy people. In the DRIs established to date, AIs rather than RDAs are proposed for infants up to age 1 year, as well as for calcium, chromium, vitamin D, fluoride, manganese, pantothenic acid, biotin, choline, sodium, chloride, potassium, and water for persons of all ages.

TOLERABLE UPPER LEVELS OF NUTRIENT INTAKE

Healthy individuals derive no established benefit from consuming nutrient levels above the RDA or AI. Excessive nutrient intake can disturb body functions and cause acute, progressive, or permanent disabilities. The tolerable UL is the highest level of chronic nutrient intake (usually daily) that is unlikely to pose a risk of adverse health effects for most of the population. Data on the adverse effects of large amounts of many nutrients are unavailable or too limited to establish a UL. Therefore, the lack of a UL does *not* mean that the risk of adverse effects from high intake is nonexistent. Individual nutrients in foods that most people eat rarely reach levels that exceed the UL. However, nutritional supplements provide more concentrated amounts of nutrients per

dose and, as a result, pose a greater potential risk of toxicity. Nutrient supplements are labeled with "Supplement Facts" that express the amount of nutrient in absolute units or as the percent of the DV provided per recommended serving size. Total nutrient consumption, including both food and supplements, should not exceed RDA levels.

FACTORS ALTERING NUTRIENT NEEDS

The DRIs are affected by age, sex, rate of growth, pregnancy, lactation, physical activity, composition of diet, coexisting diseases, and drugs. When only slight differences exist between the requirements for nutrient sufficiency and excess, dietary planning becomes more difficult.

PHYSIOLOGIC FACTORS

Growth, strenuous physical activity, pregnancy, and lactation increase needs for energy and several essential nutrients, including water. Energy needs rise during pregnancy, due to the demands of fetal growth, and during lactation, because of the increased energy required for milk production. Energy needs decrease with loss of lean body mass, the major determinant of REE. Because both health and physical activity tend to decline with age, energy needs in older persons, especially those over 70, tend to be less than those of younger persons.

DIETARY COMPOSITION

Dietary composition affects the biologic availability and utilization of nutrients. For example, the absorption of iron may be impaired by high amounts of calcium or lead; non-heme iron uptake may be impaired by the lack of ascorbic acid and amino acids in the meal. Protein utilization by the body may be decreased when essential amino acids are not present in sufficient amounts. Animal foods, such as

| TABLE 70-2 | DIETARY REFERENCE INTAKES: RECOMMENDED INTAKES FOR INDIVIDUALS—ELEMENTS |

Life-Stage Group	Cal-cium, mg/d	Chro-mium, μg/d	Copper, μg/d	Fluo-ride, mg/d	Iodine, μg/d	Iron, mg/d	Magne-sium, mg/d	Manga-nese, mg/d	Molyb-denum, μg/d	Phos-phorus mg/d	Sele-nium, μg/d	Zinc, mg/d
Infants												
0–6 mo	210	0.2	200	0.01	110	0.27	30	0.003	2	100	15	2
7–12 mo	270	5.5	220	0.5	130	**11**	75	0.6	3	275	20	**3**
Children												
1–3 y	500	11	**340**	0.7	**90**	**7**	**80**	1.2	**17**	**460**	**20**	**3**
4–8 y	800	15	**440**	1	**90**	**10**	**130**	1.5	**22**	**500**	**30**	**5**
Males												
9–13 y	1300	25	**700**	2	**120**	**8**	**240**	1.9	**34**	**1250**	**40**	**8**
14–18 y	1300	35	**890**	3	**150**	**11**	**410**	2.2	**43**	**1250**	**55**	**11**
19–30 y	1000	35	**900**	4	**150**	**8**	**400**	2.3	**45**	**700**	**55**	**11**
31–50 y	1000	35	**900**	4	**150**	**8**	**420**	2.3	**45**	**700**	**55**	**11**
51–70 y	1200	30	**900**	4	**150**	**8**	**420**	2.3	**45**	**700**	**55**	**11**
>70 y	1200	30	**900**	4	**150**	**8**	**420**	2.3	**45**	**700**	**55**	**11**
Females												
9–13 y	1300	21	**700**	2	**120**	**8**	**240**	1.6	**34**	**1250**	**40**	**8**
14–18 y	1300	24	**890**	3	**150**	**15**	**360**	1.6	**43**	**1250**	**55**	**9**
19–30 y	1000	25	**900**	3	**150**	**18**	**310**	1.8	**45**	**700**	**55**	**8**
31–50 y	1000	25	**900**	3	**150**	**18**	**320**	1.8	**45**	**700**	**55**	**8**
51–70 y	1200	20	**900**	3	**150**	**8**	**320**	1.8	**45**	**700**	**55**	**8**
>70 y	1200	20	**900**	3	**150**	**8**	**320**	1.8	**45**	**700**	**55**	**8**
Pregnancy												
≤18 y	1300	29	**1000**	3	**220**	**27**	**400**	2.0	**50**	**1250**	**60**	**12**
19–30 y	1000	30	**1000**	3	**220**	**27**	**350**	2.0	**50**	**700**	**60**	**11**
31–50 y	1000	30	**1000**	3	**220**	**27**	**360**	2.0	**50**	**700**	**60**	**11**
Lactation												
≤18 y	1300	44	**1300**	3	**290**	**10**	**360**	2.6	**50**	**1250**	**70**	**13**
19–30 y	1000	45	**1300**	3	**290**	**9**	**310**	2.6	**50**	**700**	**70**	**12**
31–50 y	1000	45	**1300**	3	**290**	**9**	**320**	2.6	**50**	**700**	**70**	**12**

Note: This table presents recommended dietary allowances (RDAs) in **bold type** and adequate intakes (AIs) in ordinary type. RDAs and AIs may both be used as goals for individual intake. RDAs are set to meet the needs of almost all individuals (97 to 98%) in a group. For healthy breastfed infants, the AI is the mean intake. The AI for other life stage and gender groups is believed to cover needs of all individuals in the group, but lack of

data or uncertainty in the data prevent being able to specify with confidence the percentage of individuals covered by this intake.

Source: Food and Nutrition Board, Institute of Medicine—National Academy of Sciences Dietary Reference Intakes, 2000, 2002, reprinted with permission. Courtesy of the National Academy Press, Washington, DC. http://www.nap.edu

milk, eggs, and meat, have high biologic values with most of the needed amino acids present in adequate amounts. Plant proteins in corn (maize), soy, and wheat have lower biologic values and must be combined with other plant or animal proteins to achieve optimal utilization by the body.

ROUTE OF ADMINISTRATION

The RDAs apply only to oral intakes. When nutrients are administered parenterally, similar values can sometimes be used for amino acids, carbohydrates, fats, sodium, chloride, potassium, and most of the vitamins, since their intestinal absorption is nearly 100%. However, the oral bioavailability of most mineral elements may be only half that obtained by parenteral administration. For some nutrients that are not readily stored in the body, or cannot be stored in large amounts, timing of administration may also be important. For example, amino acids cannot be used for protein synthesis if they are not supplied together; instead they will be used for energy production.

DISEASE

Specific dietary deficiency diseases include protein-calorie malnutrition; iron, iodine, and vitamin A deficiency; megaloblastic anemia due to vitamin B_{12} or folic acid deficiency; vitamin D–deficiency rickets; scurvy due to lack of ascorbic acid; beriberi due to lack of thiamine; and pellagra due to lack of niacin and protein (Chaps. 71 and 72). Each deficiency disease is characterized by imbalances at the cellular level between the supply of nutrients or energy and the body's nutritional needs for growth, maintenance, and other functions. Imbalances in nutrient intakes are recognized as risk factors for certain chronic degenerative diseases, such as saturated and trans-fat and cholesterol in coronary artery disease; sodium in hypertension; obesity in hormone-dependent endometrial and breast cancers; and ethanol in alcoholism. However, the etiology and pathogenesis of these disorders are multifactorial, and diet is only one of many risk factors. Osteoporosis, for example, is associated with calcium deficiency as well as risk factors related to environment (e.g., smoking, sedentary lifestyle), physiology (e.g., estrogen deficiency), genetic determinants (e.g., defects in collagen metabolism), and drug use (chronic steroids) (Chap. 348).

DIETARY ASSESSMENT

In clinical situations, nutritional assessment is an iterative process that involves (1) screening for malnutrition; (2) assessing food and dietary supplement intake, and establishing the absence or presence of malnutrition and its possible causes; and (3) planning for the most appropriate nutritional therapy. Some disease states affect the bioavailability, requirements, utilization, or excretion of specific nutrients. In these circumstances, specific measurements of various nutrients may be required to ensure adequate replacement (Chap. 72).

Most health care facilities have a nutrition screening process in place for identifying possible malnutrition after hospital admission. Nutritional screening is required by the Joint Commission on Accreditation of Healthcare Organizations (JCAHO), but there are no universally recognized or validated standards. The factors that are usually assessed include abnormal weight for height or body mass index (e.g., BMI <18.5 or >25); reported weight change (involuntary loss or gain of >5 kg in the past 6 months) (Chap. 41); diagnoses with known nutritional implications (metabolic disease, any disease affecting the gastrointestinal tract, alcoholism, and others); present therapeutic dietary prescription; chronic poor appetite; presence of chewing and swallowing problems or major food intolerances; need for assistance with preparing or shopping for food, eating, or other aspects of self care; and social isolation. Reassessment of nutrition status should occur periodically in hospitalized patients—at least once every week.

A more complete dietary assessment is indicated for patients who exhibit a high risk of malnutrition based on nutrition screening. The type of assessment varies with the clinical setting, severity of the patient's illness, and stability of his or her condition.

ACUTE CARE SETTINGS

Acute care settings, anorexia, various diseases, test procedures, and medications can compromise dietary intake. Under such circumstances, the goal is to identify and avoid inadequate intake and ensure appropriate alimentation. Dietary assessment focuses on what patients are currently eating, whether they are able and willing to eat, and whether they experience any problems with eating. Dietary intake assessment is based on information from observed intakes; medical record; history; clinical examination; and anthropometric, biochemical, and functional status. The objective is to gather enough information to establish the likelihood of malnutrition due to poor dietary intake or other causes and to assess whether nutritional therapy is indicated.

Simple observations may suffice to suggest inadequate oral intake. These include dietitians' and nurses' notes, the amount of food eaten on trays, frequent tests and procedures that are likely to cause meals to be skipped, nutritionally inadequate diet orders such as clear liquids or full liquids for more than a few days, fever, gastrointestinal distress, vomiting, diarrhea, a comatose state, and diseases or treatments that involve any part of the alimentary tract. Acutely ill patients with diet-related diseases such as diabetes require assessment because an inappropriate diet may exacerbate these conditions and adversely affect other therapies. Abnormal biochemical values [serum albumin levels <35 g/L (<3.5 mg/dL); serum cholesterol levels <3.9 mmol/L (<150 mg/dL)] are nonspecific but may also indicate a need for further nutritional assessment.

Most therapeutic diets offered in hospitals are calculated to meet individual nutrient requirements and the RDA. However, there are exceptions including clear liquids, some full liquid diets, and test diets, which are inadequate for several nutrients and should not be used, if possible, for more than 24 h. As much as half of the food served to hospitalized patients is not eaten, so it cannot be assumed that the intakes of hospitalized patients are adequate. Dietary assessment should compare how much and what food the patient has consumed with the diet that has been provided. Major deviations in intakes of energy, protein, fluids, or other nutrients of special concern for the patient's illness should be noted and corrected.

Nutritional monitoring is especially important for patients who are very ill and who have extended lengths of stay. Patients who are fed by special enteral and parenteral routes also require special nutritional assessment and monitoring by physicians with training in nutrition support and/or dietitians with certification in nutrition support (Chap. 73).

AMBULATORY SETTINGS

The aim of dietary assessment in the outpatient setting is to determine whether the patient's usual diet is a health risk in itself or if it contributes to existing chronic disease-related problems. Dietary assessment also provides the basis for planning a diet that fulfills therapeutic goals while ensuring patient adherence. The outpatient dietary assessment should review the adequacy of present and usual food intakes, including vitamin and mineral supplements, medications, and alcohol, as all of these may affect the patient's nutritional status. The assessment should focus on the dietary constituents that are most likely to be involved or compromised by a specific diagnosis, as well as any comorbidities that are present. More than one day's intake should be reviewed to provide a better representation of the usual diet.

There are many ways to assess the adequacy of the patient's habitual diet. These include a food guide, a food exchange list, a diet history, or a food frequency questionnaire. A commonly used food guide for healthy persons is the USDA's food pyramid, which is useful as a basis for identifying inadequate intakes of essential nutrients, as well as likely excesses in fat, saturated fat, sodium, sugar, and alcohol (Table 70-3). The guide is available online (*www.MyPyramid.gov*) and can be tailored to the needs of persons of different ages and life stages by varying the number of servings. The process of reviewing the guide with patients helps to identify food groups eaten in excess of recommendations or in insufficient quantities and helps them to transition to healthier dietary patterns. For those prescribed therapeutic diets, assessment against prescriptions stated as food exchange lists may be useful. These include, for example, the American Diabetes Association food exchange lists for diabetes, or the American Dietetic Association food exchange lists for renal disease.

TABLE 70-3 MY PYRAMID: THE USDA FOOD GUIDE PYRAMID FOR HEALTHY PERSONS

Servings and Examples of Standard Portion Sizes	Lower: 1600 kcal	Moderate: 2200 kcal	Higher: 2800 kcal
Fruits, cups	1.5	2	2.5
Vegetables, cups	2	3	3.5
Grains, oz eq	5	7	10
(1 slice bread, 1 cup ready to eat cereal, 0.5 cup cooked rice, pasta, cooked cereal)			
Meat and beans, oz eq	5	6	7
(1 oz lean meat, poultry, or fish; 1 egg, 1 Tbsp. peanut butter, 0.25 cup cooked dry beans, or 0.5 oz nuts or seeds)			
Milk, cups	3	3	3
(1 cup milk or yogurt, 1.5 oz natural or 2 oz processed cheese)			
Oils, tsp	5	6	8
Discretionary calorie allowance, kcal (remaining calories after accounting for all of the above)	132	290	426

Abbreviation: oz eq, ounce equivalent.
Source: Data from United States Department of Agriculture. http://www.MyPyramid.com

71 Vitamin and Trace Mineral Deficiency and Excess

Robert M. Russell, Paolo M. Suter

Vitamins and trace minerals are required constituents of the human diet since they are either inadequately synthesized or not synthesized in the human body. Only small amounts of these substances are needed for carrying out essential biochemical reactions (e.g., acting as coenzymes or prosthetic groups). Overt vitamin or trace mineral deficiencies are rare in Western countries due to a plentiful, varied, and inexpensive food supply; however, multiple nutrient deficiencies may appear together in persons who are chronically ill or alcoholic. Moreover, subclinical vitamin and trace mineral deficiencies, as diagnosed by laboratory testing, are quite common in the normal population—especially in the geriatric age group.

Famine, emergency-affected and displaced populations, and refugees are at increased risk for protein-energy malnutrition and classic micronutrient deficiencies (vitamin A, iron, iodine), as well as for thiamine (beriberi), riboflavin, vitamin C (scurvy), and niacin (pellagra) overt deficiencies.

Body stores of vitamins and minerals vary tremendously. For example, vitamin B_{12} and vitamin A stores are large, and an adult may not become deficient for 1 or more years after being on a depleted diet. However, folate and thiamine may become depleted within weeks when eating a deficient diet. Therapeutic modalities can deplete essential nutrients from the body; for example, hemodialysis removes water-soluble vitamins, which must be replaced by supplementation.

There are several roles for vitamins and trace minerals in diseases: (1) deficiencies of vitamins and minerals may be caused by disease states such as malabsorption; (2) both deficiency and excess of vitamins and minerals can cause disease in and of themselves (e.g., vitamin A intoxication and liver disease); and (3) vitamins and minerals in high doses may be used as drugs (e.g., niacin for hypercholesterolemia). The hematologic-related vitamins and minerals (Chaps. 98, 100) are considered only briefly in this chapter, as are the bone-related vitamins and minerals (vitamin D, calcium, phosphorus; Chap. 346), since they are covered elsewhere (Tables 71-1, 71-2, and Fig. 71-1).

NUTRITIONAL STATUS ASSESSMENT

Full nutritional status assessment is reserved for seriously ill patients and those at very high nutritional risk when the cause of malnutrition is still uncertain after initial clinical evaluation and dietary assessment. It involves multiple dimensions, including documentation of dietary intake, anthropometric measurements, biochemical measurements of blood and urine, clinical examination, health history, and functional status. For further discussion of nutritional assessment, see Chap. 72.

GLOBAL CONSIDERATIONS

New nutrient-based terminologies with dietary reference intakes have been developed not only in North America, but in the United Kingdom and Europe, and by the World Health Organization/Food and Agricultural Organization of the United Nations (WHO/FAO). These different standards have many similarities in their basic concepts, definitions, and levels of nutrients recommended, but there are some differences, owing to assumptions made, functional criteria chosen, the timeliness of the evidence reviewed, and expert judgment.

FURTHER READINGS

GIBSON RS: *Principles of Nutritional Assessment*, 2d ed. Oxford University Press, London, 2005

MURPHY SP et al: Multivitamin-multimineral supplements' effect on total nutrient intake. Am J Clin Nutr 85(1): 280S, 2007

SHILS ME et al (eds): *Modern Nutrition in Health and Disease*, 10th ed. Philadelphia, Lippincott Williams and Wilkins, 2005

VITAMINS

THIAMINE (VITAMIN B₁)

Thiamine was the first B vitamin to be identified and is therefore also referred to as vitamin B_1. Thiamine functions in the decarboxylation of α-ketoacids, such as pyruvate α-ketoglutarate, and branched-chain amino acids and thus is a source of energy generation. In addition, thiamine pyrophosphate acts as a coenzyme for a transketolase reaction that mediates the conversion of hexose and pentose phosphates. It has also been postulated that thiamine plays a role in peripheral nerve conduction, although the exact chemical reactions underlying this function are unknown.

Food Sources The median intake of thiamine in the United States from food alone is 2 mg/d. Primary food sources for thiamine include yeast, organ meat, pork, legumes, beef, whole grains, and nuts. Milled rice or grains contain little thiamine, if any. Thiamine deficiency is therefore more common in cultures that rely heavily on a rice-based diet. Tea, coffee (regular and decaffeinated), raw fish, and shellfish contain thiaminases, which can destroy the vitamin. Thus, drinking large amounts of tea or coffee can theoretically lower thiamine body stores.

Deficiency Most dietary deficiency of thiamine worldwide is the result of poor dietary intake. In Western countries, the primary causes of thiamine deficiency are alcoholism and chronic illness, such as cancer. Alcohol interferes directly with the absorption of thiamine and with the synthesis of thiamine pyrophosphate. Thiamine should always be replenished when refeeding a patient with alcoholism, as carbohydrate repletion without adequate thiamine can precipitate acute thiamine deficiency. Other at-risk populations are women with prolonged hyperemesis gravidarum and anorexia, patients with an overall poor nutritional status on parenteral glucose, and patients on chronic diuretic therapy due to increased urinary thiamine losses. Maternal thiamine deficiency can lead to infantile beriberi in breast-fed children. Thiamine deficiency should also be considered in the setting of motor vehicle accidents associated with head injury.

Thiamine deficiency in its early stage induces anorexia and nonspecific symptoms (e.g., irritability, decrease in short-term memory). Prolonged thiamine deficiency causes beriberi, which is classically categorized as wet or dry, although there is considerable overlap. In either

TABLE 71-1   **PRINCIPAL CLINICAL FINDINGS OF VITAMIN MALNUTRITION**

Nutrient	Clinical Finding	Dietary Level per Day Associated with Overt Deficiency in Adults	Contributing Factors to Deficiency
Thiamine	Beriberi: neuropathy, muscle weakness and wasting, cardiomegaly, edema, ophthalmoplegia, confabulation	<0.3 mg/1000 kcal	Alcoholism, chronic diuretic use, hyperemesis
Riboflavin	Magenta tongue, angular stomatitis, seborrhea, cheilosis	<0.6 mg	—
Niacin	Pellagra: pigmented rash of sun-exposed areas, bright red tongue, diarrhea, apathy, memory loss, disorientation	<9.0 niacin equivalents	Alcoholism, vitamin B_6 deficiency, riboflavin deficiency, tryptophan deficiency
Vitamin B_6	Seborrhea, glossitis convulsions, neuropathy, depression, confusion, microcytic anemia	<0.2 mg	Alcoholism, isoniazid
Folate	Megaloblastic anemia, atrophic glossitis, depression, ↑ homocysteine	<100 μg/d	Alcoholism, sulfasalazine, pyrimethamine, triamterene
Vitamin B_{12}	Megaloblastic anemia, loss of vibratory and position sense, abnormal gait, dementia, impotence, loss of bladder and bowel control, ↑ homocysteine, ↑ methylmalonic acid	<1.0 μg/d	Gastric atrophy (pernicious anemia), terminal ileal disease, strict vegetarianism, acid reducing drugs (e.g., H_2 blockers)
Vitamin C	Scurvy: petechiae, ecchymosis, coiled hairs, inflamed and bleeding gums, joint effusion, poor wound healing, fatigue	<10 mg/d	Smoking, alcoholism
Vitamin A	Xerophthalmia, nightblindness, Bitot's spots, follicular hyperkeratosis, impaired embryonic development, immune dysfunction	<300 μg/d	Fat malabsorption, infection, measles, alcoholism, protein-energy malnutrition
Vitamin D	Rickets: skeletal deformation, rachitic rosary, bowed legs; osteomalacia	<2.0 μg/d	Aging, lack of sunlight exposure, fat malabsorption, deeply pigmented skin
Vitamin E	Peripheral neuropathy, spinocerebellar ataxia, skeletal muscle atrophy, retinopathy	Not described unless underlying contributing factor is present	Occurs only with fat malabsorption, or genetic abnormalities of vitamin E metabolism/transport
Vitamin K	Elevated prothrombin time, bleeding	<10 μg/d	Fat malabsorption, liver disease, antibiotic use

form of beriberi, patients may complain of pain and paresthesia. *Wet beriberi* presents primarily with cardiovascular symptoms, due to impaired myocardial energy metabolism and dysautonomia, and can occur after 3 months of a thiamine-deficient diet. Patients present with an enlarged heart, tachycardia, high-output congestive heart failure, peripheral edema, and peripheral neuritis. Patients with *dry beriberi* present with a symmetric peripheral neuropathy of the motor and sensory systems with diminished reflexes. The neuropathy affects the legs most markedly, and patients have difficulty rising from a squatting position.

Alcoholic patients with chronic thiamine deficiency may also have central nervous system (CNS) manifestations known as *Wernicke's encephalopathy*, consisting of horizontal nystagmus, ophthalmoplegia (due to weakness of one or more extraocular muscles), cerebellar ataxia, and mental impairment (Chap. 387). When there is an additional loss of memory and a confabulatory psychosis, the syndrome is known as *Wernicke-Korsakoff syndrome*. Despite the typical clinical picture and history, Wernicke-Korsakoff syndrome is underdiagnosed.

The laboratory diagnosis of thiamine deficiency is usually made by a functional enzymatic assay of transketolase activity measured before and after the addition of thiamine pyrophosphate. A >25% stimulation by the addition of thiamine pyrophosphate (an activity coefficient of 1.25) is taken as abnormal. Thiamine or the phosphorylated esters of thiamine in serum or blood can also be measured by high-performance liquid chromatography (HPLC) to detect deficiency.

℞ THIAMINE DEFICIENCY

In acute thiamine deficiency with either cardiovascular or neurologic signs, 100 mg/d of thiamine should be given parenterally for 7 days, followed by 10 mg/d orally until there is complete recovery. Cardiovascular improvement occurs within 24 h, and ophthalmoplegic improvement occurs within 24 h. Other manifestations gradually clear, although psychosis in Wernicke-Korsakoff syndrome may be permanent or persist for several months.

Toxicity   Although anaphylaxis has been reported after high doses of thiamine, no adverse effects have been recorded from either food or

supplements at high doses. Thiamine supplements may be bought over the counter in doses of up to 50 mg/d.

RIBOFLAVIN (VITAMIN B_2)
Riboflavin is important for the metabolism of fat, carbohydrate, and protein, reflecting its role as a respiratory coenzyme and an electron donor. Enzymes that contain flavin adenine dinucleotide (FAD) or flavin-mononucleotide (FMN) as prosthetic groups are known as *flavoenzymes* (e.g., succinic acid dehydrogenase, monoamine oxidase, glutathione reductase). FAD is a cofactor for methyltetrahydrofolate reductase and therefore modulates homocysteine metabolism. The vitamin also plays a role in drug and steroid metabolism, including detoxification reactions.

Although much is known about the chemical and enzymatic reactions of riboflavin, the clinical manifestations of riboflavin deficiency are nonspecific and similar to those of other B vitamin deficiencies. Riboflavin deficiency is manifested principally by lesions of the mucocutaneous surfaces of the mouth and skin (Table 71-1). In addition to the mucocutaneous lesions, corneal vascularization, anemia, and personality changes have been described with riboflavin deficiency.

Deficiency and Excess   Riboflavin deficiency is almost always due to dietary deficiency. Milk, other dairy products, and enriched breads and cereals are the most important dietary sources of riboflavin in the United States, although lean meat, fish, eggs, broccoli, and legumes are also good sources. Riboflavin is extremely sensitive to light, and milk should be stored in containers that protect against photodegradation. Laboratory diagnosis of riboflavin deficiency can be made by measurement of red blood cell or urinary riboflavin concentrations or by measurement of erythrocyte glutathione reductase activity, with and without added FAD. Because the capacity of the gastrointestinal tract to absorb riboflavin is limited (~20 mg if given in one oral dose), riboflavin toxicity has not been described.

NIACIN (VITAMIN B_3)
The term *niacin* refers to nicotinic acid and nicotinamide and their biologically active derivatives. Nicotinic acid and nicotinamide serve as precursors of two coenzymes, nicotinamide adenine dinucleotide (NAD) and NAD phosphate (NADP), which are important in numer-

ous oxidation and reduction reactions in the body. In addition, NAD and NADP are active in adenine diphosphate–ribose transfer reactions involved in DNA repair and calcium mobilization.

Metabolism and Requirements   Nicotinic acid and nicotinamide are absorbed well from the stomach and small intestine. Niacin bioavailability is high from beans, milk, meat, and eggs; bioavailability from cereal grains is lower. Since flour is enriched with the "free" niacin (i.e., non-coenzyme form), bioavailability is excellent. Median intakes of niacin in the United States considerably exceed the recommended dietary allowance (RDA).

The amino acid tryptophan can be converted to niacin with an efficiency of 60:1 by weight. Thus, the RDA for niacin is expressed in niacin equivalents. A lower conversion of tryptophan to niacin occurs in vitamin B6 and/or riboflavin deficiencies, or in the presence of isoniazid. The urinary excretion products of niacin include 2-pyridone and 2-methyl nicotinamide, measurements of which are used in diagnosis of niacin deficiency.

Deficiency   Niacin deficiency causes *pellagra*, which is mostly found among people eating corn-based diets in parts of China, Africa, and India. Pellagra in North America is found mainly among alcoholics; in patients with congenital defects of intestinal and kidney absorption of tryptophan (Hartnup disease; Chap. 358); and in patients with carcinoid syndrome (Chap. 344), where there is increased conversion of tryptophan to serotonin. In the setting of famine or population displacement, the occurrence of pellagra results from the absolute lack of niacin but also the deficiency of micronutrients required for the conversion of tryptophan to niacin (e.g., iron, riboflavin, and pyridoxine). The early symptoms of pellagra include loss of appetite, generalized weakness and irritability, abdominal pain, and vomiting.

Bright red glossitis then ensues, followed by a characteristic skin rash that is pigmented and scaling, particularly in skin areas exposed to sunlight. This rash is known as *Casal's necklace* because it forms a ring around the neck; it is seen in advanced cases. Vaginitis and esophagitis may also occur. Diarrhea (in part due to proctitis and in part due to malabsorption), depression, seizures, and dementia are also part of the pellagra syndrome—the four *D*s: *d*ermatitis, *d*iarrhea, and *d*ementia leading to *d*eath.

℞ PELLAGRA

Treatment of pellagra consists of oral supplementation of 100–200 mg of nicotinamide or nicotinic acid three times daily for 5 days. High doses of nicotinic acid (2 g/d in a time-release form) are used for the treatment of elevated cholesterol and triglyceride levels and/or low high-density lipoprotein (HDL) cholesterol level (Chap. 350).

Toxicity   Prostaglandin-mediated flushing due to binding of the vitamin to a G protein–coupled receptor has been observed at daily doses as low as 50 mg of niacin when taken as a supplement or as therapy for dyslipidemia. There is no evidence of toxicity from niacin derived from food sources. Flushing always starts in the face and may be accompanied by skin dryness, itching, paresthesia, and headache. Premedication with aspirin may alleviate these symptoms. Flushing is subject to tachyphylaxis and often improves with time. Nausea, vomiting, and abdominal pain also occur at similar doses of niacin. Hepatic toxicity is the most serious toxic reaction due to niacin and may present as jaundice with elevated aspartate aminotransferase (AST) and alanine aminotransferase (ALT) levels. A few cases of fulminant hepatitis requiring liver transplantation have been reported at doses of

TABLE 71-2   DEFICIENCIES AND TOXICITIES OF METALS

Element	Deficiency	Toxicity	Tolerable Upper (Dietary) Intake Level
Boron	No biologic function determined	Developmental defects, male sterility, testicular atrophy	20 mg/d (extrapolated from animal data)
Calcium	Reduced bone mass, osteoporosis	Renal insufficiency (milk-alkalai syndrome), nephrolithiasis, impaired iron absorption	2500 mg/d (milk-alkalai)
Copper	Anemia, growth retardation, defective keratinization and pigmentation of hair, hypothermia, degenerative changes in aortic elastin, osteopenia, mental deterioration	Nausea, vomiting, diarrhea, hepatic failure, tremor, mental deterioration, hemolytic anemia, renal dysfunction	10 mg/d (liver toxicity)
Chromium	Impaired glucose tolerance	Occupational: renal failure, dermatitis, pulmonary cancer	ND
Fluoride	↑ Dental caries	Dental and skeletal fluorosis, osteosclerosis	10 mg/d (fluorosis)
Iodine	Thyroid enlargement, ↓ T4, cretinism	Thyroid dysfunction, acne-like eruptions	1100 μg/d (thyroid dysfunction)
Iron	Muscle abnormalities, kilonychia, pica, anemia, ↓ work performance, impaired cognitive development, premature labor, ↑ perinatal maternal mortality	Gastrointestinal effects (nausea, vomiting, diarrhea, constipation), iron overload with organ damage, acute systemic toxicity	45 mg/d of elemental iron (GI side effects)
Manganese	Impaired growth and skeletal development, reproduction, lipid and carbohydrate metabolism; upper body rash	General: Neurotoxicity, Parkinson-like symptoms Occupational: Encephalitis-like syndrome, Parkinson-like syndrome, psychosis, pneumoconiosis	11 mg/d (neurotoxicity)
Molybdenum	Severe neurologic abnormalities	Reproductive and fetal abnormalities	2 mg/d extrapolated from animal data
Selenium	Cardiomyopathy, heart failure, striated muscle degeneration	General: Alopecia, nausea, vomiting, abnormal nails, emotional lability, peripheral neuropathy, lassitude, garlic odor to breath, dermatitis Occupational: Lung and nasal carcinomas, liver necrosis, pulmonary inflammation	400 μg/d (hair, nail changes)
Phosphorous	Rickets (osteomalacia), proximal muscle weakness, rhabdomyolysis, paresthesia, ataxia, seizure, confusion, heart failure, hemolysis, acidosis	Hyperphosphatemia	4000 mg/d
Zinc	Growth retardation, ↓ taste and smell, alopecia, dermatitis, diarrhea, immune dysfunction, failure to thrive, gonadal atrophy, congenital malformations	General: Reduced copper absorption, gastritis, sweating, fever, nausea, vomiting Occupational: Respiratory distress, pulmonary fibrosis	40 mg/d (impaired copper metabolism)

Note: ND, not determined; GI, gastrointestinal.

3–9 g/d. Other toxic reactions include glucose intolerance, hyperuricemia, macular edema, and macular cysts. The upper limit for daily niacin intake has been set at 35 mg. However, this upper limit does not pertain to the therapeutic use of niacin.

PYRIDOXINE (VITAMIN B$_6$)

Vitamin B$_6$ refers to a family of compounds including pyridoxine, pyridoxal, pyridoxamine, and their 5′-phosphate derivatives. 5′-Pyridoxal phosphate (PLP) is a cofactor for more than 100 enzymes involved in amino acid metabolism. Vitamin B$_6$ is also involved in heme and neurotransmitter synthesis and in the metabolism of glycogen, lipids, steroids, sphingoid bases, and several vitamins, including the conversion of tryptophan to niacin.

Dietary Sources Plants contain vitamin B$_6$ in the form of pyridoxine, whereas animal tissues contain PLP and pyridoxamine phosphate. The vitamin B$_6$ contained in plants is less bioavailable than that from animal tissues. Rich food sources of vitamin B$_6$ include legumes, nuts, wheat bran, and meat, although it is present in all food groups.

Deficiency Symptoms of vitamin B$_6$ deficiency include epithelial changes, as seen frequently with other B vitamin deficiencies. In addition, severe vitamin B$_6$ deficiency can lead to peripheral neuropathy, abnormal electroencephalograms, and personality changes including depression and confusion. In infants, diarrhea, seizures, and anemia have been reported. Microcytic, hypochromic anemia is due to diminished hemoglobin synthesis, since the first enzyme involved in heme biosynthesis (aminolevulinate synthase) requires PLP as a cofactor (Chap. 98). In some case reports, platelet dysfunction has also been reported. Since vitamin B$_6$ is necessary for the conversion of homocysteine to cystathionine, it is possible that chronic low-grade vitamin B$_6$ deficiency may result in hyperhomocysteinemia and increased risk of cardiovascular disease (Chaps. 235, 358). Independent of homocysteine, low levels of circulating vitamin B$_6$ have also been associated with inflammation and elevated C-reactive protein levels.

Certain medications such as isoniazid, L-dopa, penicillamine, and cycloserine interact with PLP due to a reaction with carbonyl groups. Pyridoxine should be given concurrently with isoniazid to avoid neuropathy. The increased ratio of AST (or SGOT) to ALT (or SGPT) seen in alcoholic liver disease reflects the relative vitamin B$_6$ dependence of ALT. Vitamin B$_6$ dependency syndromes that require pharmacologic doses of vitamin B$_6$ are rare; they include cystathionine β-synthase deficiency, pyridoxine-responsive (primarily sideroblastic) anemias, and gyrate atrophy with chorioretinal degeneration due to decreased activity of the mitochondrial enzyme ornithine aminotransferase. In these situations, 100–200 mg/d of oral vitamin B$_6$ is required for treatment.

High doses of vitamin B$_6$ have been used to treat carpal tunnel syndrome, premenstrual syndrome, schizophrenia, autism, and diabetic neuropathy but have not been found to be effective.

Vitamin	Active derivative or cofactor form	Principal function
Thiamine (B$_1$)	Thiamine pyrophosphate	Coenzyme for cleavage of carbon-carbon bonds; amino acid and carbohydrate metabolism
Riboflavin (B$_2$)	Flavin mononucleotide (FMN) and flavin adenine dinucleotide (FAD)	Cofactor for oxidation, reduction reactions, and covalently attached prosthetic groups for some enzymes
Niacin	Nicotinamide adenine dinucleotide phosphate (NADP) and nicotinamide adenine dinucleotide (NAD)	Coenzymes for oxidation and reduction reactions
Vitamin B$_6$	Pyridoxal phosphate	Cofactor for enzymes of amino acid metabolism
Folate	Polyglutamate forms of (5, 6, 7, 8) tetrahydrofolate with carbon unit attachments	Coenzyme for one carbon transfer in nucleic acid and amino acid metabolism
Vitamin B$_{12}$	Methylcobalamine Adenosylcobalamin	Coenzyme for methionine synthase and L-methylmalonyl-CoA mutase

FIGURE 71-1 The structures and principal functions of vitamins associated with human disorders.

Vitamin	Active derivative or cofactor form	Principal function
Vitamin C	Ascorbic acid and dehydrascorbic acid	Participation as a redox ion in many biological oxidation and hydrogen transfer reactions
Vitamin A (β-Carotene) (Retinol)	Retinol, retinaldehyde, and retinoic acid	Formation of rhodopsin (vision) and glycoproteins (epithelial cell function); also regulates gene transcription
Vitamin D	1, 25-Dihydroxyvitamin D	Maintenance of blood calcium and phosphorous levels; antiproliferative hormone
Vitamin E	Tocopherols and tocotrienols	Antioxidants
Vitamin K	Vitamin K hydroquinone	Cofactor for posttranslation carboxylation of many proteins including essential clotting factors

FIGURE 71-1 (*Continued*) The structures and principal functions of vitamins associated with human disorders.

The laboratory diagnosis of vitamin B_6 deficiency is generally made on the basis of low plasma PLP values (<20 nmol/L). Treatment of vitamin B_6 deficiency is 50 mg/d; higher doses of 100–200 mg/d are given if vitamin B_6 deficiency is related to medication use. Vitamin B_6 should not be given with L-dopa, since the vitamin interferes with the action of this drug.

Toxicity The safe upper limit for vitamin B_6 has been set at 100 mg/d, although no adverse effects have been associated with high intakes of vitamin B_6 from food sources only. When toxicity occurs, it causes a severe sensory neuropathy, leaving patients unable to walk. Some cases of photosensitivity and dermatitis have also been reported.

FOLATE, VITAMIN B_{12}
See Chap. 90.

VITAMIN C
Both ascorbic acid and its oxidized product dehydroascorbic acid are biologically active. Actions of vitamin C include antioxidant activity, promotion of nonheme iron absorption, carnitine biosynthesis, the conversion of dopamine to norepinephrine, and the synthesis of many peptide hormones. Vitamin C is also important for connective tissue metabolism and cross-linking (proline hydroxylation), and it is a component of many drug-metabolizing enzyme systems, particularly the mixed-function oxidase systems.

Absorption and Dietary Sources Almost complete absorption of vitamin C occurs if <100 mg is administered in a single dose; however, only 50% or less is absorbed at doses >1 g. Enhanced degradation and fecal and urinary excretion of vitamin C occur at higher intake levels.

Good dietary sources of vitamin C include citrus fruits, green vegetables (especially broccoli), tomatoes, and potatoes. Consumption of five servings of fruits and vegetables a day provides vitamin C in excess of the RDA, 90 mg/d for males and 75 mg/d for females. In addition, approximately 40% of the U.S. population consumes vitamin C as a dietary supplement in which "natural forms" of vitamin C are no more bioavailable than synthetic forms. Smoking, hemodialysis, pregnancy, and stress (e.g., infection, trauma) appear to increase vitamin C requirements.

Deficiency Vitamin C deficiency causes scurvy. In the United States, this is seen primarily among the poor and elderly, in alcoholics who consume <10 mg/d of vitamin C, and also in individuals consuming macrobiotic diets. In addition to generalized fatigue, symptoms of scurvy primarily reflect impaired formation of mature connective tissue and include bleeding into skin (petechiae, ecchymoses, perifollicular hemorrhages); inflamed and bleeding gums; and manifestations of bleeding into joints, the peritoneal cavity, pericardium, and the adrenal glands. In children, vitamin C deficiency may cause impaired bone growth. Laboratory diagnosis of vitamin C deficiency is made on the basis of low plasma or leukocyte levels.

Administration of vitamin C (200 mg/d) improves the symptoms of scurvy within a matter of several days. High-dose vitamin C supplementation (e.g., 1–2 g/d) might slightly decrease the symptoms and duration of upper respiratory tract infections. Vitamin C supplementation has also been reported to be useful in Chédiak-Higashi syndrome (Chap. 61) and osteogenesis imperfecta (Chap. 357). Diets high in vitamin C have been claimed to lower the incidence of certain cancers, particularly esophageal and gastric cancers. If proved, this effect may be due to the fact that vitamin C can prevent the conversion of nitrites and secondary amines to carcinogenic nitrosamines. However, one intervention study from China did not show vitamin C to be protective.

Toxicity Taking >2 g of vitamin C in a single dose may result in abdominal pain, diarrhea, and nausea. Since vitamin C may be metabolized to oxalate, it is feared that chronic, high-dose vitamin C supplementation could result in an increased prevalence of kidney stones. However, this has not been borne out in several trials, except in patients with preexisting renal disease. Thus, it is reasonable to advise patients with a past history of kidney stones to not take large doses of vitamin C. There is also an unproven but possible risk that chronic high doses of vitamin C could promote iron overload in patients taking supplemental iron. High doses of vitamin C can induce hemolysis in patients with glucose-6-phosphate dehydrogenase deficiency, and doses >1 g/d can cause false-negative guaiac reactions as well as interfere with tests for urinary glucose.

BIOTIN

Biotin is a water-soluble vitamin that plays a role in gene expression, gluconeogenesis, and fatty acid synthesis and serves as a CO_2 carrier on the surface of both cytosolic and mitochondrial carboxylase enzymes. The vitamin also functions in the catabolism of specific amino acids (e.g., leucine). Excellent food sources of biotin include organ meat such as liver or kidney, soy, beans, yeast, and egg yolks; however, egg white contains the protein avidin, which strongly binds the vitamin and reduces its bioavailability.

Biotin deficiency due to low dietary intake is rare; rather, deficiency is due to inborn errors of metabolism. Biotin deficiency has been induced by experimental feeding of egg white diets and in patients with short bowels who received biotin-free parenteral nutrition. In the adult, biotin deficiency results in mental changes (depression, hallucinations), paresthesia, anorexia, and nausea. A scaling, seborrheic, and erythematous rash may occur around the eyes, nose, and mouth as well as on the extremities. In infants, biotin deficiency presents as hypotonia, lethargy, and apathy. In addition, the infant may develop alopecia and a characteristic rash that includes the ears. The laboratory diagnosis of biotin deficiency can be established based on a decreased urinary concentration or an increased urinary excretion of 3-hydroxyisovaleric acid after a leucine challenge. Treatment requires pharmacologic doses of biotin, using up to 10 mg/d. No toxicity is known.

PANTOTHENIC ACID (VITAMIN B$_5$)

Pantothenic acid is a component of coenzyme A and phosphopantetheine, which are involved in fatty acid metabolism and the synthesis of cholesterol, steroid hormones, and all compounds formed from isoprenoid units. In addition, pantothenic acid is involved in the acetylation of proteins. The vitamin is excreted in the urine, and the laboratory diagnosis of deficiency is made on the basis of low urinary vitamin levels.

The vitamin is ubiquitous in the food supply. Liver, yeast, egg yolks, whole grains, and vegetables are particularly good sources. Human pantothenic acid deficiency has been demonstrated only in experimental feeding of diets low in pantothenic acid or by giving a specific pantothenic acid antagonist. The symptoms of pantothenic acid deficiency are nonspecific and include gastrointestinal disturbance, depression, muscle cramps, paresthesia, ataxia, and hypoglycemia. Pantothenic acid deficiency is believed to have caused the burning feet syndrome seen in prisoners of war during World War II. No toxicity of this vitamin has been reported.

CHOLINE

Choline is a precursor for acetylcholine, phospholipids, and betaine. Choline is necessary for the structural integrity of cell membranes, cholinergic neurotransmission, lipid and cholesterol metabolism, methyl-group metabolism, and transmembrane signaling. Recently, a recommended adequate intake was set at 550 mg/d for adult males and 425 mg/d for adult females, although certain genetic polymorphisms can increase an individual's requirement for choline. Choline is thought to be a "conditionally essential" nutrient, in that de novo synthesis occurs in the liver and is less than the vitamin's utilization only under certain stress conditions (e.g., alcoholic liver disease). The dietary requirement of choline depends on the status of other methyl-group donors (folate, vitamin B$_{12}$, and methionine) and thus varies widely. Choline is widely distributed in food (e.g., egg yolk, wheat germ, organ meat, milk) in the form of lecithin (phosphatidylcholine). Choline deficiency has occurred in patients receiving parenteral nutrition devoid of choline. Deficiency results in fatty liver, elevated transaminase levels, and skeletal muscle damage with high creatine phosphokinase values. The diagnosis of choline deficiency is currently made on the basis of low plasma levels, although nonspecific conditions (e.g., heavy exercise) may suppress plasma levels.

Toxicity from choline results in hypotension, cholinergic sweating, diarrhea, salivation, and a fishy body odor. The upper limit for choline has been set at 3.5 g/d. Therapeutically, choline has been suggested for patients with dementia and for patients at high risk of cardiovascular disease, due to its ability to lower cholesterol and homocysteine levels. However, such benefits have yet to be documented. Choline- and betaine-restricted diets are of therapeutic value in trimethylaminuria (fish odor syndrome).

FLAVONOIDS

Flavonoids constitute a large family of polyphenols that contribute to the aroma, taste, and color of fruits and vegetables. Major groups of dietary flavonoids include anthocyanidins in berries; catechins in green tea and chocolate; flavonols (e.g., quercitin) in broccoli, kale, leeks, onion, and the skins of grapes and apples; and isoflavones (e.g., genistein) in legumes. Isoflavones have a low bioavailability and are partially metabolized by the intestinal flora. The dietary intake of flavonoids is estimated to be between 10 and 100 mg/d, although this is almost certainly an underestimate due to the lack of knowledge of their concentrations in many foods. Several flavonoids have been shown to have antioxidant activity and to affect cell signaling. From observational epidemiologic studies and from limited clinical human and animal studies, flavonoids have been postulated to play a role in the prevention of several chronic diseases, including neurodegenerative disease, diabetes, and osteoporosis. The ultimate importance and usefulness of their compounds against human disease have yet to be demonstrated.

VITAMIN A

Vitamin A, in the strictest sense, refers to retinol. However, the oxidized metabolites, retinaldehyde and retinoic acid, are also biologically active compounds. The term *retinoids* includes all molecules (including synthetic molecules) that are chemically related to retinol. Retinaldehyde (11-*cis*) is the essential form of vitamin A that is required for normal vision, whereas retinoic acid is necessary for normal morphogenesis, growth, and cell differentiation. Retinoic acid does not function in vision and, in contrast to retinol, is not involved in reproduction. Vitamin A also plays a role in iron utilization, humoral immunity, T cell–mediated immunity, natural killer cell activity, and phagocytosis. Vitamin A is commercially available in esterified forms (e.g., acetate, palmitate) since it is more stable as an ester.

There are more than 600 carotenoids in nature, and approximately 50 of these can be metabolized to vitamin A. β-Carotene is the most prevalent carotenoid in the food supply that has provitamin A activity. In humans, significant fractions of carotenoids are absorbed intact and are stored in liver and fat. It is now estimated that 12 μg or greater of dietary β-carotene is equivalent to 1 μg of retinol, whereas 24 μg or greater of other dietary provitamin A carotenoids (e.g., cryptoxanthin, α-carotene) is equivalent to 1 μg of retinol.

Metabolism   The liver contains approximately 90% of the vitamin A reserves and secretes vitamin A in the form of retinol, which is bound to retinol-binding protein. Once this has occurred, the retinol-binding protein complex interacts with a second protein, transthyretin. This trimolecular complex functions to prevent vitamin A from being filtered by the kidney glomerulus, to protect the body against the toxicity of retinol and to allow retinol to be taken up by specific cell-surface receptors that recognize retinol-binding protein. A certain amount of vitamin A enters peripheral cells even if it is not bound to retinol-binding protein. After retinol is internalized by the cell, it becomes bound to a series of cellular retinol-binding proteins, which function as sequestering and transporting agents as well as co-ligands for enzymatic reactions. Certain cells also contain retinoic acid–binding proteins, which have sequestering functions but also shuttle retinoic acid to the nucleus and enable its metabolism.

Retinoic acid is a ligand for certain nuclear receptors that act as transcription factors. Two families of receptors (RAR and RXR receptors) are active in retinoid-mediated gene transcription. Retinoid receptors regulate transcription by binding as dimeric complexes to specific DNA sites, the retinoic acid response elements, in target genes (Chap. 332). The receptors can either stimulate or repress gene expression in response to their ligands. RAR binds all-*trans* retinoic acid and 9-*cis* retinoic acid, whereas RXR binds only 9-*cis* retinoic acid.

The retinoid receptors play an important role in controlling cell proliferation and differentiation. Retinoic acid is useful in the treatment of promyelocytic leukemia (Chap. 104) and is also used in the treatment of cystic acne because it inhibits keratinization, decreases sebum secretion, and possibly alters the inflammatory reaction (Chap. 53). RXRs dimerize with other nuclear receptors to function as coregulators of genes responsive to retinoids, thyroid hormone, and calcitriol. RXR agonists induce insulin sensitivity experimentally, perhaps because RXR is a cofactor for the peroxisome-proliferator-activated receptors (PPARs), which are targets for the thiazolidinedione drugs such as rosiglitazone and troglitazone (Chap. 338).

Dietary Sources The retinol activity equivalent (RAE) is used to express the vitamin A value of food. One RAE is defined as 1 μg of retinol (0.003491 mmol), 12 μg of β-carotene, and 24 μg of other provitamin A carotenoids. In older literature, vitamin A was often expressed in international units (IU), with 1 RAE being equal to 3.33 IU of retinol and 20 IU of β-carotene, but these units are no longer in current scientific use.

Liver, fish, and eggs are excellent food sources for preformed vitamin A; vegetable sources of provitamin A carotenoids include dark green and deeply colored fruits and vegetables. Moderate cooking of vegetables enhances carotenoid release for uptake in the gut. Carotenoid absorption is also aided by some fat in a meal. Infants are particularly susceptible to vitamin A deficiency because neither breast nor cow's milk supplies enough vitamin A to prevent deficiency. In developing countries, chronic dietary deficit is the main cause of vitamin A deficiency and is exacerbated by infection. In early childhood, low vitamin A status results from inadequate intakes of animal food sources and edible oils, both of which are expensive, coupled with seasonal unavailability of vegetables and fruits, and lack of marketed fortified food products. Concurrent zinc deficiency can interfere with the mobilization of vitamin A from liver stores. Alcohol interferes with the conversion of retinol to retinaldehyde in the eye by competing for alcohol (retinol) dehydrogenase. Drugs that interfere with the absorption of vitamin A include mineral oil, neomycin, and cholestyramine.

Deficiency Vitamin A deficiency is endemic where diets are chronically poor, especially in Southern Asia, Sub-Saharan Africa, some areas of Latin America, and the Western Pacific, including parts of China. Vitamin A status is usually assessed by measuring serum retinol [normal range, 1.05–3.50 μmol/L (30–100 μg/dL)] or blood spot retinol or by tests of dark adaptation. Stable isotopic or invasive liver biopsy methods exist to estimate total body stores of vitamin A. Based on deficient serum retinol [<0.70 μmol/L (20 μg/dL)], there are more than 125 million preschool-age children with vitamin A deficiency, among whom ~4 million have an ocular manifestation of deficiency termed *xerophthalmia*. This condition includes milder stages of night blindness and conjunctival xerosis (dryness) with Bitot's spots (white patches of keratinized epithelium appearing on the sclera) as well as rare, potentially blinding corneal ulceration and necrosis. Keratomalacia (softening of the cornea) leads to corneal scarring that blinds at least a quarter of a million children each year and is associated with a fatality rate of 4–25%. However, vitamin A deficiency at any stage poses an increased risk of mortality from diarrhea, dysentery, measles, malaria, and respiratory disease. Vitamin A deficiency can compromise barrier and innate and acquired immune defenses to infection. Vitamin A supplementation can markedly reduce risk of child mortality (23–34%, on average) where deficiency is widely prevalent. About 10% of pregnant women in undernourished settings also develop night blindness, assessed by history, during the latter half of pregnancy and this moderate vitamin A deficiency is associated with an increased risk of maternal infection and mortality.

℞ **VITAMIN A DEFICIENCY**

Any stage of xerophthalmia should be treated with 60 mg of vitamin A in oily solution, usually contained in a soft-gel capsule. The same dose is repeated 1 and 14 days later. Doses should be reduced by half for patients 6–11 months of age. Mothers with night blindness or Bitot's spots should be given vitamin A orally, either 3 mg daily or 7.5 mg twice a week for 3 months. These regimens are efficacious, and they are less expensive and more widely available than injectable water-miscible vitamin A. A common approach to prevention is to supplement young children living in high-risk areas with 60 mg every 4–6 months, with a half-dose given to infants 6–11 months of age.

Uncomplicated vitamin A deficiency rarely occurs in industrialized countries. One high-risk group, extremely low-birth-weight infants (<1000 g), is likely to be vitamin A–deficient and should be supplemented with 1500 μg (or RAE) of vitamin A, three times a week for 4 weeks. Severe measles in any society can lead to secondary vitamin A deficiency. Children hospitalized with measles should receive two 60-mg doses of vitamin A on two consecutive days. Vitamin A deficiency most often occurs in patients with malabsorptive diseases (e.g., celiac sprue, short-bowel syndrome), who have abnormal dark adaptation or symptoms of night blindness without other ocular changes. Typically, such patients are treated for 1 month with 15 mg/d of a water-miscible preparation of vitamin A. This is followed by a lower maintenance dose with the exact amount determined by monitoring serum retinol.

There are no specific deficiency signs or symptoms that result from carotenoid deficiency. It was postulated that β-carotene would be an effective chemopreventive agent for cancer because numerous epidemiologic studies had shown that diets high in β-carotene were associated with lower incidences of cancers of the respiratory and digestive systems. However, intervention studies in smokers found that treatment with high doses of β-carotene actually resulted in more lung cancers than did treatment with placebo. Non–provitamin A carotenoids, such as lutein and zeaxanthin, have been suggested to protect against macular degeneration. The non–provitamin A carotenoid lycopene has been proposed to protect against prostate cancer. However, the effectiveness of these agents has not been proven by intervention studies, and the mechanisms underlying these purported biologic actions are unknown.

Toxicity Acute toxicity of vitamin A was first noted in Arctic explorers who ate polar bear liver and has also been seen after administration of 150 mg in adults or 100 mg in children. Acute toxicity is manifested by increased intracranial pressure, vertigo, diplopia, bulging fontanels in children, seizures, and exfoliative dermatitis; it may result in death. In children being treated for vitamin A deficiency according to the protocols outlined above, transient bulging of fontanels occurs in 2% of infants, and transient nausea, vomiting, and headache occur in 5% of preschoolers. Chronic vitamin A intoxication is largely a concern in industrialized countries and has been seen in normal adults who ingest 15 mg/d and children who ingest 6 mg/d of vitamin A over a period of several months. Manifestations include dry skin, cheilosis, glossitis, vomiting, alopecia, bone demineralization and pain, hypercalcemia, lymph node enlargement, hyperlipidemia, amenorrhea, and features of pseudotumor cerebri with increased intracranial pressure and papilledema. Liver fibrosis with portal hypertension and bone demineralization may result from chronic vitamin A intoxication. When vitamin A is provided in excess to pregnant women, congenital malformations have included spontaneous abortions, craniofacial abnormalities, and valvular heart disease. In pregnancy, the daily dose of vitamin A should not exceed 3 mg. Commercially available retinoid derivatives are also toxic, including 13-*cis*-retinoic acid, which has been associated with birth defects. As a result, contraception should be continued for at least 1 year, and possibly longer, in women who have taken 13-*cis* retinoic acid.

High doses of carotenoids do not result in toxic symptoms but should be avoided in smokers due to an increased risk of lung cancer. Carotenemia, which is characterized by a yellowing of the skin (creases of the palms and soles) but not the sclerae, may be present after ingestion of >30 mg of β-carotene daily. Hypothyroid patients are particularly susceptible to the development of carotenemia due to impaired breakdown of carotene to vitamin A. Reduction of carotenes from the diet results in the disappearance of skin yellowing and carotenemia over a period of 30–60 days.

VITAMIN D

See Chap. 346, Fig. 71-1, and Table 71-1.

VITAMIN E

Vitamin E is a collective name for all stereoisomers of tocopherols and tocotrienols, although only the 2R tocopherols meet human requirements. Vitamin E acts as a chain-breaking antioxidant and is an efficient pyroxyl radical scavenger, which protects low-density lipoproteins (LDLs) and polyunsaturated fats in membranes from oxidation. A network of other antioxidants (e.g., vitamin C, glutathione) and enzymes maintains vitamin E in a reduced state. Vitamin E also inhibits prostaglandin synthesis and the activities of protein kinase C and phospholipase A_2.

Absorption and Metabolism   After absorption, vitamin E is taken up from chylomicrons by the liver, and a hepatic α tocopherol transport protein mediates intracellular vitamin E transport and incorporation into very low-density lipoprotein (VLDL). The transport protein has particular affinity for the RRR isomeric form of α tocopherol; thus this natural isomer has the most biologic activity.

Requirement   Vitamin E is widely distributed in the food supply and is particularly high in sunflower oil, safflower oil, and wheat germ oil; γ tocotrienols are notably present in soybean and corn oils. Vitamin E is also found in meats, nuts, and cereal grains, and small amounts are present in fruits and vegetables. Vitamin E pills containing doses of 50–1000 mg are ingested by a large fraction of the U.S. population. The RDA for vitamin E is 15 mg/d (34.9 µmol or 22.5 IU) for all adults. Diets high in polyunsaturated fats may necessitate a slightly higher requirement for vitamin E.

Dietary deficiency of vitamin E does not exist. Vitamin E deficiency is seen in only severe and prolonged malabsorptive diseases, such as celiac disease, or after small-intestinal resection. Children with cystic fibrosis or prolonged cholestasis may develop vitamin E deficiency characterized by areflexia and hemolytic anemia. Children with abetalipoproteinemia cannot absorb or transport vitamin E and become deficient quite rapidly. A familial form of isolated vitamin E deficiency also exists; it is due to a defect in the α tocopherol transport protein. Vitamin E deficiency causes axonal degeneration of the large myelinated axons and results in posterior column and spinocerebellar symptoms. Peripheral neuropathy is initially characterized by areflexia, with progression to an ataxic gait, and by decreased vibration and position sensations. Ophthalmoplegia, skeletal myopathy, and pigmented retinopathy may also be features of vitamin E deficiency. Either vitamin E or selenium deficiency in the host has been shown to increase certain viral mutations and, therefore, virulence. The laboratory diagnosis of vitamin E deficiency is made on the basis of low blood levels of α tocopherol (<5 µg/mL, or <0.8 mg of α tocopherol per gram of total lipids).

℞ VITAMIN E DEFICIENCY

Symptomatic vitamin E deficiency should be treated with 800–1200 mg of α tocopherol per day. Patients with abetalipoproteinemia may need as much as 5000–7000 mg/d. Children with symptomatic vitamin E deficiency should be treated with 400 mg/d orally of water-miscible esters; alternatively, 2 mg/kg per d may be administered intramuscularly. Vitamin E in high doses may protect against oxygen-induced retrolental fibroplasia and bronchopulmonary dysplasia, as well as intraventricular hemorrhage of prematurity. Vitamin E has been suggested to increase sexual performance, to treat intermittent claudication, and to slow the aging process, but evidence for these properties is lacking. When given in combination with other antioxidants, vitamin E may help to prevent macular degeneration. High doses (60–800 mg/d) of vitamin E have been shown in controlled trials to improve parameters of immune function and to reduce colds in nursing home residents, but intervention studies using vitamin E to prevent cardiovascular disease or cancer have not shown efficacy and, at doses >400 mg/d, may even increase all-cause mortality.

Toxicity   All forms of vitamin E are absorbed and could contribute to toxicity. High doses of vitamin E (>800 mg/d) may reduce platelet aggregation and interfere with vitamin K metabolism and are therefore contraindicated in patients taking warfarin. Nausea, flatulence, and diarrhea have been reported at doses >1 g/d.

VITAMIN K

There are two natural forms of vitamin K: vitamin K_1, also known as *phylloquinone*, from vegetable and animal sources, and vitamin K_2, or *menaquinone*, which is synthesized by bacterial flora and found in hepatic tissue. Phylloquinone can be converted to menaquinone in some organs.

Vitamin K is required for the posttranslational carboxylation of glutamic acid, which is necessary for calcium binding to γ-carboxylated proteins such as prothrombin (factor II); factors VII, IX, and X; protein C; protein S; and proteins found in bone (osteocalcin) and vascular smooth muscle (e.g., matrix Gla protein). However, the importance of vitamin K for bone mineralization and prevention of vascular calcification is not known. Warfarin-type drugs inhibit γ-carboxylation by preventing the conversion of vitamin K to its active hydroquinone form.

Dietary Sources   Vitamin K is found in green leafy vegetables such as kale and spinach, and appreciable amounts are also present in margarine and liver. Vitamin K is present in vegetable oils and is particularly rich in olive, canola, and soybean oils. The average daily intake by Americans is estimated to be approximately 100 µg/d.

Deficiency   The symptoms of vitamin K deficiency are due to hemorrhage, and newborns are particularly susceptible because of low fat stores, low breast milk levels of vitamin K, sterility of the infantile intestinal tract, liver immaturity, and poor placental transport. Intracranial bleeding, as well as gastrointestinal and skin bleeding, can occur in vitamin K–deficient infants 1–7 days after birth. Thus, vitamin K (1 mg IM) is given prophylactically at the time of delivery.

Vitamin K deficiency in adults may be seen in patients with chronic small-intestinal disease (e.g., celiac disease, Crohn's disease), in those with obstructed biliary tracts, or after small-bowel resection. Broad-spectrum antibiotic treatment can precipitate vitamin K deficiency by reducing gut bacteria, which synthesize menaquinones, and by inhibiting the metabolism of vitamin K. In patients with warfarin therapy, the antiobesity drug orlistat can lead to INR changes due to vitamin K malabsorption. The diagnosis of vitamin K deficiency is usually made on the basis of an elevated prothrombin time or reduced clotting factors, although vitamin K may also be measured directly by HPLC. Vitamin K deficiency is treated using a parenteral dose of 10 mg. For patients with chronic malabsorption, 1–2 mg/d of vitamin K should be given orally, or 1–2 mg/week can be taken parenterally. Patients with liver disease may have an elevated prothrombin time because of liver cell destruction as well as vitamin K deficiency. If an elevated prothrombin time does not improve on vitamin K therapy, it can be deduced that it is not the result of vitamin K deficiency.

Toxicity   Toxicity from dietary phylloquinones and menaquinones has not been described. High doses of vitamin K can impair the actions of oral anticoagulants.

MINERALS

Table 71-2.

CALCIUM

See Chap. 346.

ZINC

Zinc is an integral component of many metalloenzymes in the body; it is involved in the synthesis and stabilization of proteins, DNA, and

RNA and plays a structural role in ribosomes and membranes. Zinc is necessary for the binding of steroid hormone receptors and several other transcription factors to DNA. Zinc is absolutely required for normal spermatogenesis, fetal growth, and embryonic development.

Absorption The absorption of zinc from the diet is inhibited by dietary phytate, fiber, oxalate, iron, and copper, as well as by certain drugs including penicillamine, sodium valproate, and ethambutol. Meat, shellfish, nuts, and legumes are good sources of bioavailable zinc, whereas zinc in grains and legumes is less available for absorption.

Deficiency Mild zinc deficiency has been described in many diseases, including diabetes mellitus, HIV/AIDS, cirrhosis, alcoholism, inflammatory bowel disease, malabsorption syndromes, and sickle cell disease. In these diseases, mild chronic zinc deficiency can cause stunted growth in children, decreased taste sensation (hypogeusia), and impaired immune function. Severe chronic zinc deficiency has been described as a cause of hypogonadism and dwarfism in several Middle Eastern countries. In these children, hypopigmented hair is also part of the syndrome. Acrodermatitis enteropathica is a rare autosomal recessive disorder characterized by abnormalities in zinc absorption. Clinical manifestations include diarrhea, alopecia, muscle wasting, depression, irritability, and a rash involving the extremities, face, and perineum. The rash is characterized by vesicular and pustular crusting with scaling and erythema. Occasional patients with Wilson's disease have developed zinc deficiency as a consequence of penicillamine therapy (Chap. 354).

The diagnosis of zinc deficiency is usually made by a serum zinc level of <12 μmol/L (<70 μg/dL). Pregnancy and birth control pills may cause a slight depression in serum zinc levels, and hypoalbuminemia from any cause can result in hypozincemia. In acute stress situations, zinc may be redistributed from serum into tissues. Zinc deficiency may be treated with 60 mg elemental zinc, orally twice a day. Zinc gluconate lozenges (13 mg elemental zinc every 2 h while awake) have been reported to reduce the duration and symptoms of the common cold in adults, but studies are conflicting.

Zinc deficiency is prevalent in many developing countries and usually coexists with other micronutrient deficiencies (especially iron). Zinc (20 mg/d) may be an effective adjunctive therapeutic strategy for diarrheal disease in children.

Toxicity Acute zinc toxicity after oral ingestion causes nausea, vomiting, and fever. Zinc fumes from welding may also be toxic and cause fever, respiratory distress, excessive salivation, sweating, and headache. Chronic large doses of zinc may depress immune function and cause hypochromic anemia as a result of copper deficiency.

COPPER

Copper is an integral part of numerous enzyme systems including amine oxidases, ferroxidase (ceruloplasmin), cytochrome-*c* oxidase, superoxide dismutase, and dopamine hydroxylase. Copper is also a component of ferroprotein, a transport protein involved in the basolateral transfer of iron during absorption from the enterocyte. As such, copper plays a role in iron metabolism, melanin synthesis, energy production, neurotransmitter synthesis, and CNS function; the synthesis and cross-linking of elastin and collagen; and the scavenging of superoxide radicals. Dietary sources of copper include shellfish, liver, nuts, legumes, bran, and organ meats.

Deficiency Dietary copper deficiency is relatively rare, although it has been described in premature infants who are fed milk diets and in infants with malabsorption (Table 71-2). Copper-deficiency anemia has been reported in patients with malabsorptive diseases and nephrotic syndrome and in patients treated for Wilson's disease with chronic high doses of oral zinc, which can interfere with copper absorption. Menkes kinky hair syndrome is an X-linked metabolic disturbance of copper metabolism characterized by mental retardation, hypocupremia, and decreased circulating ceruloplasmin (Chap. 357). It is caused by mutations in the copper-transporting *ATP7A* gene. Children with this disease often die within 5 years because of dissecting aneurysms or cardiac rupture. Aceruloplasminemia is a rare autosomal recessive disease characterized by tissue iron overload, mental deterioration, microcytic anemia, and low serum iron and copper concentrations.

The diagnosis of copper deficiency is usually made on the basis of low serum levels of copper (<65 μg/dL) and low ceruloplasmin levels (<20 mg/dL). Serum levels of copper may be elevated in pregnancy or stress conditions since ceruloplasmin is an acute-phase reactant and 90% of circulating copper is bound to ceruloplasmin.

Toxicity Copper toxicity is usually accidental (Table 71-2). In severe cases, kidney failure, liver failure, and coma may ensue. In Wilson's disease, mutations in the copper transporting *ATP7B* gene lead to accumulation of copper in the liver and brain, with low blood levels due to decreased ceruloplasmin (Chap. 354).

SELENIUM

Selenium, in the form of selenocysteine, is a component of the enzyme glutathione peroxidase, which serves to protect proteins, cell membranes, lipids, and nucleic acids from oxidant molecules. As such, selenium is being actively studied as a chemopreventive agent against certain cancers, such as prostate. Selenocysteine is also found in the deiodinase enzymes, which mediate the deiodination of thyroxine to triiodothyronine (Chap. 335). Rich dietary sources of selenium include seafood, muscle meat, and cereals, although the selenium content of cereal is determined by the soil concentration. Countries with low soil concentrations include parts of Scandinavia, China, and New Zealand. *Keshan disease* is an endemic cardiomyopathy found in children and young women residing in regions of China where dietary intake of selenium is low (<20 μg/d). Concomitant deficiencies of iodine and selenium may worsen the clinical manifestations of cretinism. Chronic ingestion of high amounts of selenium leads to selenosis characterized by hair and nail brittleness and loss, garlic breath odor, skin rash, myopathy, irritability, and other abnormalities of the nervous system.

CHROMIUM

Chromium potentiates the action of insulin in patients with impaired glucose tolerance, presumably by increasing insulin receptor–mediated signaling, although its usefulness in treating type II diabetes is uncertain. In addition, improvement in blood lipid profiles has been reported in some patients. The usefulness of chromium supplements in muscle building is not substantiated. Rich food sources of chromium include yeast, meat, and grain products. Chromium in the trivalent state is found in supplements and is largely nontoxic; however, chromium-6 is a product of stainless steel welding and is a known pulmonary carcinogen, as well as a cause of liver, kidney, and CNS damage.

MAGNESIUM

See Chap. 346.

FLUORIDE, MANGANESE, AND ULTRATRACE ELEMENTS

An essential function for fluoride in humans has not been described, although it is useful for the maintenance of structure in teeth and bone. Adult fluorosis results in mottled and pitted defects in tooth enamel as well as brittle bone (skeletal fluorosis).

Manganese and molybdenum deficiencies have been reported in patients with rare genetic abnormalities and in a few patients receiving prolonged total parenteral nutrition. Several manganese-specific enzymes have been identified (e.g., manganese superoxide dismutase). Deficiencies of manganese have been reported to result in bone demineralization, poor growth, ataxia, disturbances in carbohydrate and lipid metabolism, and convulsions.

Ultratrace elements are defined as those needed in amounts <1 mg/d. Essentiality has not been established for most ultratrace elements, although selenium, chromium, and iodine are clearly essential (Chap. 335). *Molybdenum* is necessary for the activity of sulfite and xanthine oxidase, and molybdenum deficiency may result in skeletal and brain lesions.

FURTHER READINGS

BONAA KH et al: Homocysteine lowering and cardiovascular events after acute myocardial infarction. N Engl J Med 354:1578, 2006

DAY E et al: Thiamine for Wernicke-Korsakoff Syndrome in people at risk from alcohol abuse. Cochrane Database Syst Rev CD004033, 2004

LICHTENSTEIN AH, RUSSELL RM: Essential nutrients in a healthy diet: Food or supplements? JAMA 294:1, 2005

MILLER ER et al: Meta-analysis: High-dosage vitamin E supplementation may increase all-cause mortality. Ann Intern Med 142:37, 2005

MORRIS MC et al: Dietary folate and vitamin B12 intake and cognitive decline among community-dwelling older persons. Arch Neurol 62:641, 2005

MURPHY SP et al: Multivitamin-multimineral supplements' effect on total nutrient intake. Am J Clin Nutr 85(1):280S, 2007

PENNISTON KL, TANUMIHARDJO: The acute and chronic toxic effects of vitamin A. Am J Clin Nutr 83:191, 2006

PRENTICE RL: Clinical trials and observational studies to assess the chronic disease benefits and risks of multivitamin-multimineral supplements. Am J Clin Nutr 85(1):308S, 2007

TOUVIER M et al: Dual association of beta-carotene with risk of tobacco-related cancers in a cohort of French women. J Natl Cancer Inst 97:1338, 2005

VERMEER C et al: Beyond deficiency: Potential benefits of increased intakes of vitamin K for bone and vascular health. Eur J Nutr 43:325, 2004

72 Malnutrition and Nutritional Assessment
Douglas C. Heimburger

Malnutrition can arise from primary or secondary causes, with the former resulting from inadequate or poor-quality food intake and the latter from diseases that alter food intake or nutrient requirements, metabolism, or absorption. Primary malnutrition occurs mainly in developing countries and under conditions of war or famine. Secondary malnutrition, the main form encountered in industrialized countries, was largely unrecognized until the early 1970s, when it became appreciated that persons with adequate food supplies can become malnourished as a result of acute or chronic diseases that alter nutrient intake or metabolism. Various studies have shown that protein-energy malnutrition (PEM) affects one-third to one-half of patients on general medical and surgical wards in teaching hospitals. The consistent finding that nutritional status influences patient prognosis underscores the importance of preventing, detecting, and treating malnutrition.

PROTEIN-ENERGY MALNUTRITION

The two major types of PEM are *marasmus* and *kwashiorkor*. These conditions are compared in Table 72-1. Marasmus and kwashiorkor can occur singly or in combination, as *marasmic kwashiorkor*. Kwashiorkor can occur rapidly, whereas marasmus is the end result of a gradual wasting process that passes through stages of underweight, then mild, moderate, and severe cachexia.

MARASMUS

The end stage of cachexia, marasmus is a state in which virtually all available body fat stores have been exhausted due to starvation. Conditions that produce marasmus in developed countries tend to be chronic and indolent, such as cancer, chronic pulmonary disease, and anorexia nervosa. Marasmus is easy to detect because of the patient's starved appearance. The diagnosis is based on severe fat and muscle wastage resulting from prolonged calorie deficiency. Diminished skin-fold thickness reflects the loss of fat reserves; reduced arm muscle circumference with temporal and interosseous muscle wasting reflects the catabolism of protein throughout the body, including vital organs such as the heart, liver, and kidneys.

The laboratory findings in marasmus are relatively unremarkable. The creatinine-height index (the 24-h urinary creatinine excretion compared with normal values based on height) is low, reflecting the loss of muscle mass. Occasionally, the serum albumin level is reduced, but it stays above 2.8 g/dL in uncomplicated cases. Despite a morbid appearance, immunocompetence, wound healing, and the ability to handle short-term stress are reasonably well preserved in most patients with marasmus.

Marasmus is a chronic, fairly well-adapted form of starvation rather than an acute illness; it should be treated cautiously, in an attempt to reverse the downward trend gradually. Although nutritional support is necessary, overly aggressive repletion can result in severe, even life-threatening metabolic imbalances such as hypophosphatemia and cardiorespiratory failure. When possible, oral or enteral nutritional support is preferred; treatment started slowly allows readaptation of metabolic and intestinal functions (Chap. 73).

KWASHIORKOR

In contrast to marasmus, kwashiorkor in developed countries occurs mainly in connection with acute, life-threatening illnesses such as trauma and sepsis, and chronic illnesses that involve acute-phase in-

TABLE 72-1 COMPARISON OF MARASMUS AND KWASHIORKOR

	Marasmus	Kwashiorkor[a]
Clinical setting	↓ Energy intake	↓ Protein intake during stress state
Time course to develop	Months or years	Weeks
Clinical features	Starved appearance	Well-nourished appearance
	Weight <80% standard for height	Easy hair pluckability[b]
	Triceps skinfold <3 mm	Edema
	Mid-arm muscle circumference <15 cm	
Laboratory findings	Creatinine-height index <60% standard	Serum albumin <2.8 g/dL
		Total iron-binding capacity <200 μg/dL
		Lymphocytes <1500/μL
		Anergy
Clinical course	Reasonably preserved responsiveness to short-term stress	Infections
		Poor wound healing, decubitus ulcers, skin breakdown
Mortality	Low unless related to underlying disease	High
Diagnostic criteria	Triceps skinfold <3 mm	Serum albumin <2.8 g/dL
	Mid-arm muscle circumference <15 cm	At least one of the following:
		Poor wound healing, decubitus ulcers, or skin breakdown
		Easy hair pluckability[b]
		Edema

[a]The findings used to diagnose kwashiorkor must be unexplained by other causes.
[b]Tested by *firmly* pulling a lock of hair from the top (not the sides or back), grasping with the thumb and forefinger. An average of three or more hairs removed easily and painlessly is considered abnormal hair pluckability.

flammatory responses. The physiologic stress produced by these illnesses increases protein and energy requirements at a time when intake is often limited. A classic scenario for kwashiorkor is the acutely stressed patient who receives only 5% dextrose solutions for periods as brief as 2 weeks. Although the etiologic mechanisms are not clear, the protein-sparing response normally seen in starvation is blocked by the stressed state and by carbohydrate infusion.

In its early stages, the physical findings of kwashiorkor are few and subtle. Fat reserves and muscle mass are initially unaffected, giving the deceptive appearance of adequate nutrition. Signs that support the diagnosis of kwashiorkor include easy hair pluckability, edema, skin breakdown, and poor wound healing. The major *sine qua non* is severe reduction of levels of serum proteins such as albumin (<2.8 g/dL) and transferrin (<150 mg/dL) or iron-binding capacity (<200 μg/dL). Cellular immune function is depressed, reflected by lymphopenia (<1500 lymphocytes/μL in adults and older children) and lack of response to skin test antigens (anergy).

The prognosis of adult patients with full-blown kwashiorkor is not good, even with aggressive nutritional support. Surgical wounds often dehisce (fail to heal), pressure sores develop, gastroparesis and diarrhea can occur with enteral feeding, the risk of gastrointestinal bleeding from stress ulcers is increased, host defenses are compromised, and death from overwhelming infection may occur despite antibiotic therapy. Unlike treatment in marasmus, aggressive nutritional support is indicated to restore better metabolic balance rapidly (Chap. 73). Although kwashiorkor in children is less foreboding, perhaps because a lesser degree of stress is required to precipitate the disorder, it is still a serious condition.

MARASMIC KWASHIORKOR

Marasmic kwashiorkor, the combined form of PEM, develops when the cachectic or marasmic patient experiences acute stress such as surgery, trauma, or sepsis, superimposing kwashiorkor onto chronic starvation. An extremely serious, life-threatening situation can occur because of the high risk of infection and other complications. It is important to determine the major component of PEM so that the appropriate nutritional plan can be developed. If kwashiorkor predominates, the need for vigorous nutritional therapy is urgent; if marasmus predominates, feeding should be more cautious.

PHYSIOLOGIC CHARACTERISTICS OF HYPOMETABOLIC AND HYPERMETABOLIC STATES

The metabolic characteristics and nutritional needs of hypermetabolic patients who are stressed from injury, infection, or chronic inflammatory illness differ from those of hypometabolic patients who are unstressed but chronically starved. In both cases, nutritional support is important, but misjudgments in selecting the appropriate approach may have disastrous consequences.

The hypometabolic patient is typified by the relatively unstressed but mildly catabolic and chronically starved individual who, with time, will develop marasmus. The hypermetabolic patient stressed from injury or infection is catabolic (experiencing rapid breakdown of body mass) and is at high risk for developing kwashiorkor, if nutritional needs are not met and/or the illness does not resolve quickly. As summarized in Table 72-2, the two states are distinguished by differing perturbations of metabolic rate, rates of protein breakdown (proteolysis), and rates of gluconeogenesis. These differences are mediated by proinflammatory cytokines and counterregulatory hormones—tumor necrosis factor, interleukins 1 and 6, C-reactive protein, catecholamines (epinephrine and norepinephrine), glucagon, and cortisol—that are relatively reduced in hypometabolic patients and increased in hypermetabolic patients. Although insulin levels are also elevated in stressed patients, insulin resistance in the target tissues prevents insulin-mediated anabolic actions.

METABOLIC RATE

In starvation and semistarvation, the resting metabolic rate falls between 10% and 30% as an adaptive response to energy restriction, slowing the rate of weight loss. By contrast, resting metabolic rate rises

TABLE 72-2 PHYSIOLOGIC CHARACTERISTICS OF HYPOMETABOLIC AND HYPERMETABOLIC STATES

Physiologic Characteristics	Hypometabolic, Nonstressed Patient (Cachectic, Marasmic)	Hypermetabolic, Stressed Patient (Kwashiorkor Risk[a])
Cytokines, catecholamines, glucagon, cortisol, insulin	↓	↑
Metabolic rate, O₂ consumption	↓	↑
Proteolysis, gluconeogenesis	↓	↑
Ureagenesis, urea excretion	↓	↑
Fat catabolism, fatty acid utilization	↑	↑
Adaptation to starvation	Normal	Abnormal

[a]These changes characterize the stressed, kwashiorkor-risk patient seen in developed countries; they differ in some respects from the characteristics of primary kwashiorkor seen in developing countries.

in the presence of physiologic stress in proportion to the degree of the insult. It may increase by about 10% after elective surgery, 20–30% after bone fractures, 30–60% with severe infections such as peritonitis or gram-negative septicemia, and as much as 110% after major burns.

If the metabolic rate (energy requirement) is not matched by energy intake, weight loss results—slowly in hypometabolism and quickly in hypermetabolism. Losses of up to 10% of body weight are unlikely to be detrimental; however, losses greater than this in acutely ill hypermetabolic patients may be associated with rapid deterioration in body function.

PROTEIN CATABOLISM

The rate of endogenous protein breakdown (catabolism) to supply energy needs normally falls during uncomplicated energy deprivation. After about 10 days of total starvation, the unstressed individual loses about 12–18 g/d protein (equivalent to approximately 2 oz of muscle tissue or 2–3 g of nitrogen). By contrast, in injury and sepsis, protein breakdown accelerates in proportion to the degree of stress, to 30–60 g/d after elective surgery, 60–90 g/d with infection, 100–130 g/d with severe sepsis or skeletal trauma, and >175 g/d with major burns or head injuries. These losses are reflected by proportional increases in the excretion of urea nitrogen, the major byproduct of protein breakdown.

GLUCONEOGENESIS

The major aim of protein catabolism during a state of starvation is to provide the glucogenic amino acids (especially alanine and glutamine) that serve as substrates for endogenous glucose production (gluconeogenesis) in the liver. In the hypometabolic/starved state, protein breakdown for gluconeogenesis is minimized, especially as ketones derived from fatty acids become the substrate preferred by certain tissues. In the hypermetabolic/stress state, gluconeogenesis increases dramatically and in proportion to the degree of the insult, to increase the supply of glucose (the major fuel of reparation). Glucose is the only fuel that can be utilized by hypoxic tissues (anaerobic glycolysis), white blood cells, and newly generated fibroblasts. Infusions of glucose partially offset a negative energy balance but do not significantly suppress the high rates of gluconeogenesis in the catabolic patient. Hence, adequate supplies of protein are needed to replace the amino acids utilized for this metabolic response.

In summary, the hypometabolic patient is adapted to starvation and conserves body mass by reducing the metabolic rate and using fat as the primary fuel (rather than glucose and its precursor amino acids). The hypermetabolic patient also uses fat as a fuel but rapidly breaks down body protein to produce glucose, causing loss of muscle and organ tissue and endangering vital body functions.

MICRONUTRIENT MALNUTRITION

The same illnesses and reductions in nutrient intake that lead to PEM often produce deficiencies of vitamins and minerals as well (Chap. 71).

Deficiencies of nutrients that are stored in small amounts (such as the water-soluble vitamins) are lost through external secretions, such as zinc in diarrhea fluid or burn exudate, and are probably more common than generally recognized.

Deficiencies of vitamin C, folic acid, and zinc are reasonably common in sick patients. Signs of scurvy such as corkscrew hairs on the lower extremities are frequently found in chronically ill and/or alcoholic patients. The diagnosis can be confirmed with plasma vitamin C levels. Folic acid intakes and blood levels are often less than optimal, even among healthy persons; when illness, alcoholism, poverty, or poor dentition is present, deficiencies are common. Low blood zinc levels are prevalent in patients with malabsorption syndromes such as inflammatory bowel disease. Patients with zinc deficiency often exhibit poor wound healing, pressure ulcer formation, and impaired immunity. Thiamine deficiency is a common complication of alcoholism, but its manifestations are often prevented by therapeutic doses of thiamine in patients treated for alcohol abuse.

Patients with low plasma vitamin C levels usually respond to the doses found in multivitamin preparations, but patients with deficiencies should be supplemented with 250–500 mg/d. Folic acid is absent from some oral multivitamin preparations; patients with deficiencies should be supplemented with about 1 mg/d. Patients with zinc deficiencies resulting from large external losses sometimes require oral daily supplementation with 220 mg of zinc sulfate one to three times daily. For these reasons, laboratory assessments of the micronutrient status of patients at high risk are desirable.

Hypophosphatemia develops in hospitalized patients with remarkable frequency and generally results from rapid intracellular shifts of phosphate in cachectic or alcoholic patients receiving intravenous glucose (Chap. 46). The adverse clinical sequelae are numerous; some, such as acute cardiopulmonary failure, can be life-threatening.

NUTRITIONAL ASSESSMENT

Because interactions between illness and nutrition are complex, many physical and laboratory findings reflect both underlying disease and nutritional status. Therefore, the nutritional evaluation of a patient requires an integration of the history, physical examination, anthropometrics, and laboratory studies. This approach helps both to detect nutritional problems and to avoid concluding that isolated findings indicate nutritional problems when they do not. For example, hypoalbuminemia caused by an underlying illness does not necessarily indicate malnutrition.

NUTRITIONAL HISTORY

A nutritional history is directed toward identifying underlying mechanisms that put patients at risk for nutritional depletion or excess. These mechanisms include inadequate intake, impaired absorption, decreased utilization, increased losses, and increased requirements of nutrients.

Individuals with the characteristics listed in Table 72-3 are at particular risk for nutritional deficiencies.

PHYSICAL EXAMINATION

Physical findings that suggest vitamin, mineral, and protein-energy deficiencies and excesses are outlined in Table 72-4. Most of the phys-

---

TABLE 72-3	THE HIGH-RISK PATIENT

Underweight (body mass index <18.5) and/or recent loss of ≥10% of usual body weight
Poor intake: anorexia, food avoidance (e.g., psychiatric condition), or NPO status for more than about 5 days
Protracted nutrient losses: malabsorption, enteric fistulae, draining abscesses or wounds, renal dialysis
Hypermetabolic states: sepsis, protracted fever, extensive trauma or burns
Alcohol abuse or use of drugs with antinutrient or catabolic properties: steroids, antimetabolites (e.g., methotrexate), immunosuppressants, antitumor agents
Impoverishment, isolation, advanced age

---

ical findings are not specific for individual nutrient deficiencies, and they must be integrated with the historic, anthropometric, and laboratory findings. For example, the finding of follicular hyperkeratosis on the back of the arms is a fairly common, normal finding. On the other hand, if it is widespread in a person who consumes little fruit and vegetables and smokes regularly (increasing ascorbic acid requirements), vitamin C deficiency is likely. Similarly, easily pluckable hair may be a consequence of chemotherapy, but in a hospitalized patient who has poorly healing surgical wounds and hypoalbuminemia, it suggests kwashiorkor.

ANTHROPOMETRICS

Anthropometric measurements provide information on body muscle mass and fat reserves. The most practical and commonly used measurements are body weight, height, triceps skinfold (TSF), and mid-arm muscle circumference (MAMC). Body weight is one of the most useful nutritional parameters to follow in patients who are acutely or chronically ill. Unintentional weight loss during illness often reflects loss of lean body mass (muscle and organ tissue), especially if it is rapid and not caused by diuresis. This can be an ominous sign since it indicates use of vital body protein stores as a metabolic fuel. The reference standard for normal body weight, body mass index (BMI, or weight in kilograms divided by height, in meters, squared), is discussed in Chap 75. BMIs <18.5 are considered underweight, 18.5–24.9 are normal, 25–29.9 are overweight, and ≥30 are obese.

Measurement of skinfold thickness is useful for estimating body fat stores, because about 50% of body fat is normally located in the subcutaneous region. Skinfold thicknesses can also permit discrimination of fat mass from muscle mass. The TSF is a convenient site that is generally representative of the body's overall fat level. A thickness of <3 mm suggests virtually complete exhaustion of fat stores. The MAMC, often used to estimate skeletal muscle mass, is calculated as follows:

$$\text{MAMC (cm)} = \text{upper arm circumference (cm)} - [0.314 \times \text{TSF (mm)}]$$

LABORATORY STUDIES

A number of laboratory tests used routinely in clinical medicine can yield valuable information about a patient's nutritional status if a slightly different approach to their interpretation is used. For example, abnormally low serum albumin levels, total iron-binding capacity, and anergy may have a distinct explanation, but collectively they may represent kwashiorkor. In the clinical setting of a hypermetabolic, acutely ill patient who is edematous and has easily pluckable hair and inadequate protein intake, the diagnosis of kwashiorkor is clear-cut. Commonly used laboratory tests for assessing nutritional status are outlined in Table 72-5. The table also provides tips to help avoid assigning nutritional significance to tests that may be abnormal for non-nutritional reasons.

Assessment of Circulating (Visceral) Proteins The serum proteins most used to assess nutritional status include albumin, total iron-binding capacity (or transferrin), thyroxine-binding prealbumin (or transthyretin), and retinol-binding protein. Because they have differing synthesis rates and half-lives—the half-life of serum albumin is about 21 days whereas those of prealbumin and retinol-binding protein are about 2 days and 12 h, respectively—some of these proteins reflect changes in nutritional status more quickly than others. However, rapid fluctuations can also make shorter-half-life proteins less reliable.

Levels of circulating proteins are influenced by their rates of synthesis and catabolism, "third spacing" (loss into interstitial spaces), and, in some cases, external loss. Although an adequate intake of calories and protein is necessary to achieve optimal circulating protein levels, serum protein levels generally do not reflect protein intake. For example, a drop in the serum level of albumin or transferrin often accompanies significant physiologic stress (e.g., from infection

TABLE 72-4 PHYSICAL FINDINGS OF NUTRITIONAL DEFICIENCIES

Clinical Findings	Possible Deficiency[a]	Possible Excess
Hair, Nails		
Corkscrew hairs and unemerged coiled hairs	Vitamin C	
Easily pluckable hair	Protein	
Flag sign (transverse depigmentation of hair)	Protein	
Sparse hair	Protein, biotin, zinc	Vitamin A
Transverse ridging of nails	Protein	
Skin		
Cellophane appearance	Protein	
Cracking (flaky paint or crazy pavement dermatosis)	Protein	
Follicular hyperkeratosis	Vitamins A, C	
Petechiae (especially perifollicular)	Vitamin C	
Purpura	Vitamins C, K	
Pigmentation, scaling of sun-exposed areas	Niacin	
Poor wound healing, decubitus ulcers	Protein, vitamin C, zinc	
Scaling	Vitamin A, essential fatty acids, biotin	Vitamin A
Yellow pigmentation sparing sclerae (benign)	Zinc (hyperpigmented)	Carotene
Eyes		
Night blindness	Vitamin A	
Papilledema		Vitamin A
Perioral		
Angular stomatitis	Riboflavin, pyridoxine, niacin	
Cheilosis (dry, cracking, ulcerated lips)	Riboflavin, pyridoxine, niacin	
Oral		
Atrophic lingual papillae (slick tongue)	Riboflavin, niacin, folate, vitamin B_{12}, protein, iron	
Glossitis (scarlet, raw tongue)	Riboflavin, niacin, pyridoxine, folate, vitamin B_{12}	
Hypogeusesthesia, hyposmia	Zinc	
Swollen, retracted, bleeding gums (if teeth present)	Vitamin C	
Bones, Joints		
Beading of ribs, epiphyseal swelling, bowlegs	Vitamin D	
Tenderness, subperiosteal hemorrhage in children	Vitamin C	
Neurologic		
Confabulation, disorientation	Thiamine (Korsakoff psychosis)	
Drowsiness, lethargy, vomiting		Vitamin A
Dementia	Niacin, vitamin B_{12}, folate	
Headache		Vitamin A
Ophthalmoplegia	Thiamine, phosphorus	
Peripheral neuropathy (e.g., weakness, paresthesias, ataxia, foot drop, and decreased tendon reflexes, fine tactile sense, vibratory sense, and position sense)	Thiamine, pyridoxine, vitamin B_{12}	Pyridoxine
Tetany	Calcium, magnesium	
Other		
Edema	Protein, thiamine	
Heart failure	Thiamine ("wet" beriberi), phosphorus	
Hepatomegaly	Protein	Vitamin A
Parotid enlargement	Protein (consider also bulimia)	
Sudden heart failure, death	Vitamin C	

[a]In this table, "protein deficiency" is used to signify kwashiorkor.

or injury) and is not necessarily an indication of malnutrition or poor intake. A low serum albumin level in a burned patient with both hypermetabolism and increased dermal losses of protein may not indicate malnutrition. On the other hand, adequate nutritional support of the patient's calorie and protein needs is critical for returning circulating proteins to normal levels as stress resolves. Thus low values by themselves do not define malnutrition, but they often point to increased risk of malnutrition because of the hypermetabolic stress state. As long as significant physiologic stress persists, serum protein levels remain low, even with aggressive nutritional support. However, if the levels do not rise after the underlying illness improves, the patient's protein and calorie needs should be reassessed to ensure that intake is sufficient.

Assessment of Vitamin and Mineral Status The use of laboratory tests to confirm suspected micronutrient deficiencies is desirable because the physical findings for these are often equivocal or nonspecific. Low blood micronutrient levels can predate more serious clinical manifestations and may also indicate drug-nutrient interactions.

ESTIMATING ENERGY AND PROTEIN REQUIREMENTS
A patient's basal energy expenditures (BEE, measured in kilocalories per day) can be estimated from height, weight, age, and gender using the Harris-Benedict equations:

$$\text{Men: BEE} = 66.47 + 13.75W + 5.00H - 6.76A$$

$$\text{Women: BEE} = 655.10 + 9.56W + 1.85H - 4.68A$$

where W is weight in kg; H is height in cm, and A is age in years. After solving these equations, total energy requirements are estimated by multiplying the BEE by a factor that accounts for the stress of illness. Multiplying by 1.1–1.4 yields a range 10–40% above basal that estimates the 24-h energy expenditure of the majority of patients. The lower value (1.1) is used for patients without evidence of significant physiologic stress; the higher value (1.4) is appropriate for patients with marked stress such as sepsis or trauma. The result is used as a 24-h energy goal for feeding.

When it is important to have a more accurate assessment of energy expenditure, it can be measured at the bedside using indirect calorimetry. This technique is useful in patients who are believed to be hypermetabolic from sepsis or trauma and whose body weights cannot be obtained accurately. Indirect calorimetry can also be useful in patients having difficulty weaning from a ventilator, as their energy needs should not be exceeded to avoid excessive CO_2 production. Patients at the extremes of weight (e.g., obese persons) and/or age are good candidates as well, because the Harris-Benedict equations were developed from measurements in adults with roughly normal body weights.

Because urea is a major byproduct of protein catabolism, the amount of urea nitrogen excreted each day can be used to estimate the rate of protein catabolism and to determine if protein intake is adequate to offset it. Total protein loss and protein balance can be calculated from the urinary urea nitrogen (UUN) as follows:

$$\text{Protein catabolic rate (g/d)} = [24\text{-h UUN (g)} + 4] \times 6.25 \text{ (g protein/g nitrogen)}$$

The value of 4 g added to the UUN represents a liberal estimate of the unmeasured nitrogen lost in the urine (e.g., creatinine and uric acid), sweat, hair, skin, and feces. When protein intake is low (e.g., less

TABLE 72-5 LABORATORY TESTS FOR NUTRITIONAL ASSESSMENT

Test (Normal Values)	Nutritional Use	Causes of Normal Value Despite Malnutrition	Other Causes of Abnormal Value
Serum albumin (3.5–5.5 g/dL)	2.8–3.5: Compromised protein status <2.8: Possible kwashiorkor Increasing value reflects positive protein balance	Dehydration Infusion of albumin, fresh frozen plasma, or whole blood	**Low** Common: Infection and other stress, especially with poor protein intake Burns, trauma Congestive heart failure Fluid overload Severe liver disease Uncommon: Nephrotic syndrome Zinc deficiency Bacterial stasis/overgrowth of small intestine
Serum prealbumin, also called transthyretin (20–40 mg/dL; lower in prepubertal children)	10–15 mg/dL: Mild protein depletion 5–10 mg/dL: Moderate protein depletion <5 mg/dL: Severe protein depletion Increasing value reflects positive protein balance	Chronic renal failure	Similar to serum albumin
Serum total iron binding capacity (TIBC) 240–450 µg/dL	<200: Compromised protein status, possible kwashiorkor Increasing value reflects positive protein balance More labile than albumin	Iron deficiency	**Low** Similar to serum albumin **High** Iron deficiency
Prothrombin time 12.0–15.5 sec	Prolongation: vitamin K deficiency		**Prolonged** Anticoagulant therapy (warfarin) Severe liver disease
Serum creatinine 0.6–1.6 mg/dL	<0.6: Muscle wasting due to prolonged energy deficit Reflects muscle mass		**High** Despite muscle wasting: Renal failure Severe dehydration
24-h urinary creatinine 500–1200 mg/d (standardized for height and sex)	Low value: muscle wasting due to prolonged energy deficit	>24-h collection Decreasing serum creatinine	**Low** Incomplete urine collection Increasing serum creatinine Neuromuscular wasting
24-h urinary urea nitrogen (UUN) <5 g/d (depends on level of protein intake)	Determine level of catabolism (as long as protein intake is ≥10 g below calculated protein loss or <20 g total, but at least 100 g carbohydrate is provided) 5–10 g/d = mild catabolism or normal fed state 10–15 g/d = moderate catabolism >15 g/d = severe catabolism Estimate protein balance Protein balance = protein intake – protein loss where protein loss (protein catabolic rate) = [24-h UUN (g) + 4] × 6.25 Adjustments required in burn patients and others with large nonurinary nitrogen losses and in patients with fluctuating BUN levels (e.g., renal failure)		
Blood urea nitrogen (BUN) 8–23 mg/dL	<8: Possibly inadequate protein intake 12–23: Possibly adequate protein intake >23: Possibly excessive protein intake If serum creatinine is normal, use BUN If serum creatinine is elevated, use BUN/creatinine ratio (normal range is essentially the same as for BUN)		**Low** Severe liver disease Anabolic state Syndrome of inappropriate antidiuretic hormone **High** Despite poor protein intake: Renal failure (use BUN/creatinine ratio) Congestive heart failure Gastrointestinal hemorrhage

than about 20 g/d), the equation indicates both the patient's protein requirement and the severity of the catabolic state (Table 72-5). More substantial protein intakes can raise the UUN because some of the ingested (or infused) protein is catabolized and converted to UUN. Thus at lower protein intakes the equation is useful for estimating *requirements*, and at higher protein intakes it is useful for assessing protein *balance*.

Protein balance (g/d) = Protein intake – Protein catabolic rate

FURTHER READINGS

AMERICAN SOCIETY FOR PARENTERAL AND ENTERAL NUTRITION: *The science and practice of nutrition support: A case-based core curriculum.* Dubuque, Kendall/Hunt, 2001. Available online at: www.nutritioncare.org

BAKER H: Nutrition in the elderly: Hypovitaminosis and its implications. Geriatrics 62(8):22, 2007

CHAPMAN IM: Nutritional disorders in the elderly. Med Clin North Am 90(5):887, 2006

HEIMBURGER DC, ARD JD (eds): *Handbook of Clinical Nutrition,* 4th ed. Philadelphia, Mosby Elsevier, 2006

SHILS ME et al (eds): *Modern Nutrition in Health and Disease,* 10th ed. Baltimore, Lippincott Williams & Wilkins, 2005

73 Enteral and Parenteral Nutrition Therapy

Bruce R. Bistrian, David F. Driscoll

The ability to provide specialized nutritional support (SNS) represents a major advance in medical therapy. Nutritional support, via either enteral or parenteral routes, is used in two main settings: (1) to provide adequate nutritional intake during the recuperative phase of illness or injury, when the patient's ability to ingest or absorb nutrients is impaired, and (2) to support the patient during the systemic response to inflammation, injury, or infection during an extended critical illness. SNS is also used in patients with permanent loss of intestinal length or function. In addition, an increasing number of elderly patients living in nursing homes and chronic care facilities receive enteral feeding, usually as a consequence of inadequate nutritional intake.

Enteral refers to feeding via a tube placed into the gut to deliver liquid formulas containing all essential nutrients. *Parenteral* refers to the infusion of complete nutrient solutions into the bloodstream via a peripheral vein or, more commonly, by central venous access to meet nutritional needs. Enteral feeding is generally the preferred route because of benefits derived from maintaining the digestive, absorptive, and immunologic barrier functions of the gastrointestinal tract. Small-bore pliable tubes have largely replaced large-bore rubber tubes, making placement easier and more acceptable to patients. Infusion pumps have also improved the delivery of nutrient solutions.

For short-term use, enteral tubes can be placed via the nose into the stomach, duodenum, or jejunum. For long-term use, these sites can be accessed through the abdominal wall using endoscopic, radiologic, or surgical procedures. Intestinal tolerance of tube feeding may be limited during acute illness by gastric retention or diarrhea. Parenteral feeding has greater risk of infection, reflecting the need for venous access, and a greater propensity for inducing hyperglycemia. However, these risks can generally be managed successfully by SNS teams. For the postoperative patient with preexisting malnutrition, or in trauma patients who were previously well nourished, SNS is strikingly cost-effective. In the most critically ill patient in the intensive care unit, SNS can dramatically enhance survival. Although enteral nutrition (EN) can be provided by most health care teams caring for hospitalized patients, safe and effective parenteral nutrition (PN) usually requires specialized teams.

APPROACH TO THE PATIENT:
Requirements for Specialized Nutritional Support

INDICATIONS FOR SPECIALIZED NUTRITIONAL SUPPORT Although at least 15–20% of patients in acute care hospitals have evidence of significant malnutrition, only a small fraction will benefit from SNS. For others, wasting is an inevitable component of a terminal disease and the course of the disease will not be altered by SNS. The decision to use SNS should be based on the likelihood that preventing protein-calorie malnutrition (PCM) will increase the likelihood of recovery, reduce infection rates, improve healing, or otherwise shorten the hospital stay. In the case of the elderly or chronically ill patient for whom full recovery is not anticipated, the decision to feed is usually based on whether SNS will extend the duration and quality of life. The decision-making process used to decide when to use SNS is depicted in Fig. 73-1.

The first step in deciding to administer SNS is to consider the nutritional implications of the disease process. Is the condition or its treatment likely to impair food intake and absorption for a prolonged period of time? For example, a well-nourished individual can tolerate approximately 7 days of starvation while experiencing a systemic response to inflammation (SRI). The second step is to determine if the patient is already significantly malnourished to the degree that critical functions such as wound healing, immune function, or ventilatory function are impaired (Chap. 72). An unintentional weight loss of >10% during the previous 6 months or a weight/height <90% of standard, when associated with physiologic impairment, represents significant PCM. Weight loss >20% of usual or <80% of standard reflects severe PCM. The presence or absence of SRI should be noted, since inflammation, injury, and infection increase the rate of lean tissue loss. SRI also has pathophysiologic effects that influence nutritional responses such as fluid retention and hyperglycemia, as well as impairment of anabolic responses to nutritional support.

Once it is determined that a patient is already or at risk of becoming malnourished, the next step is to decide whether SNS will impact positively on the patient's response to disease. In the end stages of many chronic illnesses with accompanying PCM, particularly those due to cancer or terminal neurologic disorders, nutrition may not reverse the PCM or improve quality of life. While the provision of food and water is part of basic medical care, nutrition delivered by tube or catheter, either enterally or parenterally, is associated with risk and discomfort. Thus, SNS should be recommended only when potential benefits exceed risks, and should be undertaken with the consent of the patient. Like other life support measures, enteral or parenteral therapy is difficult to withdraw once started. Initiating nutrition support may be appropriate before a final prognosis can be determined, but this should not preclude its subsequent withdrawal. If preventing or treating PCM with SNS is appropriate, nutritional requirements and the method of delivery should be determined. The optimal route depends on the degree of gut function and somewhat on the available technical resources.

The timing of nutritional support is based on evaluation of the preexisting nutritional status, the presence and extent of SRI, and the anticipated clinical course. SRI is identified by the standard clinical signs of leukocytosis, tachycardia, tachypnea, and/or temperature elevation or depression. Although the degree of hypoalbuminemia provides an estimate of SRI severity, normal serum albumin levels will not be restored by adequate nutritional support until the SRI remits, even though nutritional benefits can be achieved by adequate feeding.

The SRI can be graded as severe, moderate, or mild. Examples of severe SRI include sepsis or other inflammatory conditions like pancreatitis requiring ICU care, multiple trauma with an Injury Severity Score > 20–25 or APACHE II > 25, closed head injury with a Glasgow Coma Scale < 8, or major third-degree burns of >40% of body surface area. Moderate SRI includes less severe infections, injuries, or inflammatory conditions like pneumonia, major surgery, acute hepatic or renal insufficiency, and exacerbations of ulcerative colitis or regional enteritis requiring hospitalization. PCM should also be defined as severe, moderate, or minimal as assessed by weight/height, percent recent weight loss, and body mass index. The body mass index in relation to nutritional status is listed in Table 73-1. A patient with a severe SRI requires early feeding within the first several days of care because the condition is likely to produce inadequate spontaneous intake over the next 7 days. A moderate SRI, as commonly seen during a postoperative period without oral intake that exceeds 5 days, benefits from adequate feeding by day 5–7 if the patient was initially well nourished. If severely malnourished, candidates for elective major surgery benefit from preoperative nutritional repletion for 5–7 days. However, this is not often possible. Thus, early postoperative feeding is indicated. Patients with a moderate SRI and moderate PCM also benefit from earlier feeding within the first several days.

EFFICACY OF SNS IN DIFFERENT DISEASE STATES Efficacy studies have shown that malnourished patients undergoing major thoracoabdominal surgery benefit from SNS. Critical illness requiring ICU care including major burns, major trauma, severe sepsis, closed

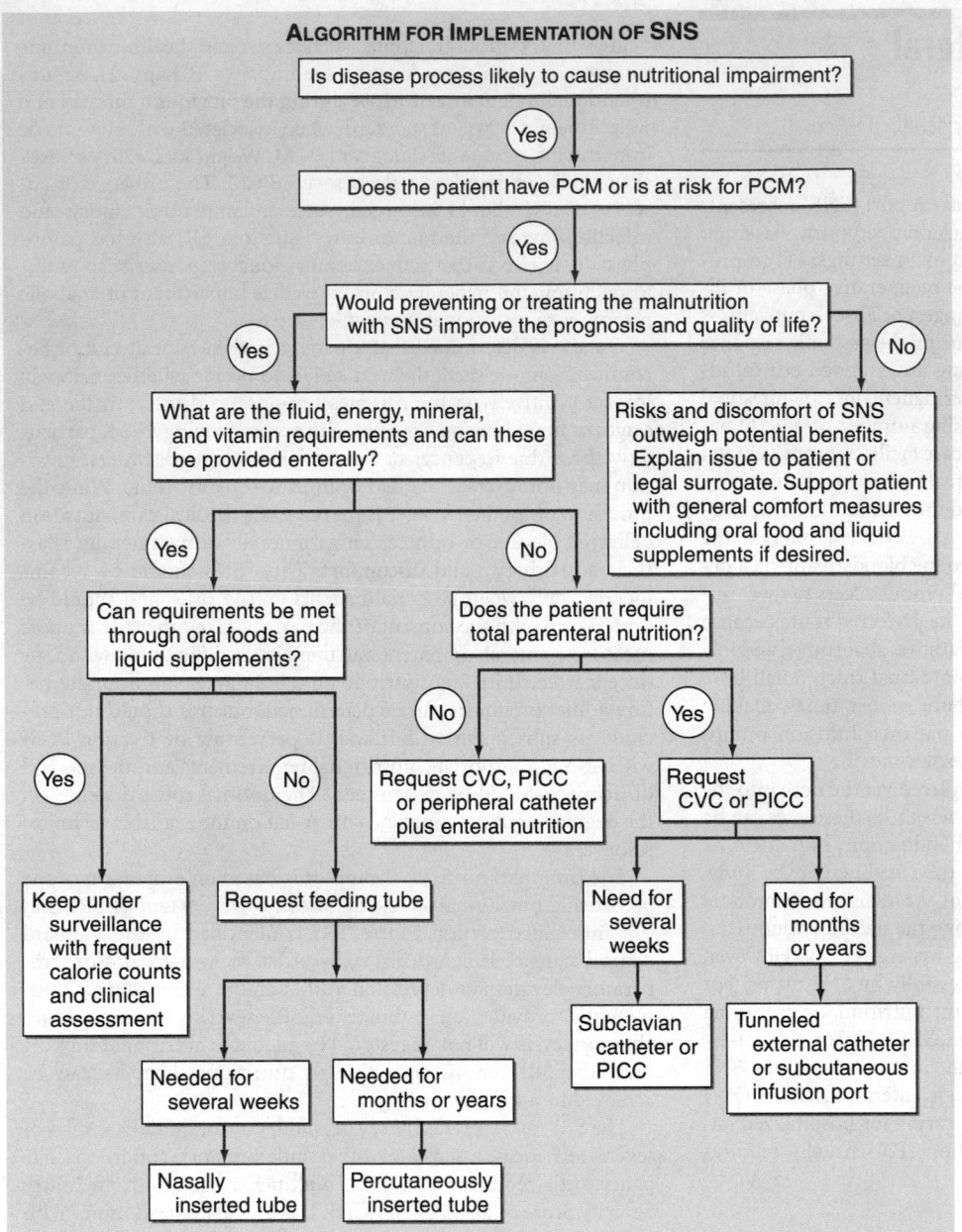

FIGURE 73-1 Decision-making for the implementation of specialized nutrition support (SNS). CVC, central venous catheter; PICC, peripherally inserted central catheter. *(Adapted from previous chapter by Lyn Howard, MD.)*

and exercise capacity and higher mortality rates. However, there is little convincing evidence that SNS as caloric supplementation improves nutrition or pulmonary function. PCM is also common in the course of cancer and HIV disease, although less so in the latter with the advent of highly active antiretroviral therapy. When PCM develops as a consequence of SRI in these conditions, there is limited likelihood of substantial efficacy or benefit from SNS. However, when PCM develops as a consequence of gastrointestinal dysfunction, SNS can be effective. Although no randomized trials have been performed for SNS provided for hyperemesis gravidarum, there is considerable clinical evidence that it improves pregnancy outcomes.

RISKS AND BENEFITS OF SPECIALIZED NUTRITION SUPPORT The risks are determined primarily by patient factors such as state of alertness, swallowing competence, the route of delivery, underlying conditions, and the experience of the supervising clinical team. The safest and least costly approach is to avoid SNS by close attention to oral food intake, by adding an oral liquid supplement, or in certain chronic conditions by using medications to stimulate appetite. Nutrient intake monitoring by frequent calorie counts or oral formula selection is best performed by a nutritionist.

Enteral tube feeding is often required in patients with anorexia, impaired swallowing, or bowel disease. The bowel and its associated digestive organs derive 70% of their required nutrients directly from food in the lumen. Arginine, glutamine, short-chain fatty acids, long-chain omega 3 fatty acids, and nucleotides available in some specialty enteral formulas are particularly important for maintaining immunity. Enteral feeding also supports gut function by stimulating splanchnic blood flow, neuronal activity, IgA antibody release, and secretion of gastrointestinal hormones that stimulate gut trophic activity. These factors

head injury, and severe pancreatitis [positive CT scan and Acute Physiology and Chronic Health Evaluation II (APACHE II) > 10] all benefit by early SNS, as indicated by reduced mortality and morbidity. In critical illness, initiation of SNS within 24 h of injury or ICU admission is associated with a ~50% reduction in mortality. Patients with nitrogen accumulation disorders of renal and hepatic failure have a likelihood of PCM of >50% and at least a moderate SRI. Improvements in morbidity, including infection rates, encephalopathy, liver or renal function, and length of hospital stay have been found with SNS. Inflammatory bowel disease—including Crohn's disease particularly, and, to a lesser degree, ulcerative colitis—often produce PCM. In the outpatient setting, SNS in Crohn's disease can improve nutritional status, quality of life, and the likelihood of remission. With pulmonary disease in the critically ill, SNS improves ventilatory status, and in acute lung injury the use of omega 3 fats as a component of SNS improves gas exchange and respiratory dynamics and reduces the need for mechanical ventilation. Low body weight in chronic obstructive pulmonary disease is associated with diminished pulmonary status

TABLE 73-1	BODY MASS INDEX (BMI) AND NUTRITIONAL STATUS
BMI	**Nutritional Status**
>30 kg/m²	Obese
>25–30 kg/m²	Overweight
20–25 kg/m²	Normal
<18.5 kg/m²	Moderate malnutrition
<16 kg/m²	Severe malnutrition
<13 kg/m²	Lethal in males
<11 kg/m²	Lethal in females

From D Driscoll, B Bistrian: Parenteral and enteral nutrition in the intensive care unit, in *Intensive Care Medicine*, R Irwin, J Rippe (eds). Lippincott Williams & Wilkins, Philadelphia, 2003.

support the gut as an immunologic barrier against enteric pathogens. For these reasons, some luminal nutrition should be provided, even when PN is required to provide most of the nutritional support. The combination of some enteral feeding either by mouth or by enteral tube with parenteral feeding often shortens the transition to full enteral feeding, which can generally be used when >50% of requirements can be met enterally. Substantial nutritional benefit can be achieved by providing ~50% of energy needs for periods of up to 10 days, if protein and other essential nutrient requirements are met. For longer periods of time, it may be preferable to provide 75–80% of energy needs, rather than full feeding, if this improves gastrointestinal tolerance, glycemic control, and avoidance of excess fluid administration.

In the past, bowel rest through PN was the cornerstone of treatment for many severe gastrointestinal disorders. However, the value of providing even minimal amounts of EN is now widely accepted. The development of protocols to facilitate more widespread use of EN include initiation within 24 h of ICU admission; aggressive use of the head-upright position; postpyloric and nasojejunal feeding tubes; prokinetic agents; more rapid increases in feeding rates; tolerance of higher gastric residuals; and nurse-administered algorithms. PN alone is generally necessary only for severe gut dysfunction due to prolonged ileus, obstruction, or severe hemorrhagic pancreatitis. In the critically ill, feeding adequately by PN beginning within the first 24 h of care improves mortality and is more effective than delayed EN. Early feeding of the critically ill in the ICU is associated with a 50% reduction in mortality, but there is also a 50% increase in infection risk. Much of the increase in morbidity related to PN and EN is due to hyperglycemia, which can be significantly reduced by insulin therapy. The level of glycemia necessary to accomplish this goal, whether <110 mg/dL or only <150 mg/dL, is not yet defined.

Although PN was initially relatively expensive, its components are often less expensive than specialty enteral formulas. Percutaneous placement of a central venous catheter into the subclavian or internal jugular vein with advancement into the superior vena cava can be accomplished at the bedside by trained personnel using sterile techniques. Peripherally inserted central catheters can also be placed within the lumen in the central vein, but this technique is usually more appropriate for non-ICU patients. The subclavian or internal jugular lines can be changed over a wire, but this carries a greater risk of pneumothorax or serious vascular damage. The peripherally inserted catheters are subject to position-related flow, and the catheter cannot be changed over a wire. Inserting a nasogastric tube is a bedside procedure, but many critically ill patients have impaired gastric emptying that increases the risk of aspiration pneumonia. This risk can be reduced by feeding directly into the jejunum beyond the ligament of Treitz. This usually requires fluoroscopic guidance or endoscopic placement. In patients who have planned laparotomies or other conditions likely to require a prolonged need for SNS, it is advantageous to place a jejunal feeding tube at the time of surgery.

Although most SNS is delivered in hospitals, some patients require it on a long-term basis. If they have a safe environment and a willingness to learn the self-care techniques, SNS can be administered at home. The clinical outcomes of patients with severe intestinal disorders treated with home PN or EN are summarized in Table 73-2. PN infused at home is usually cycled overnight to give greater daytime freedom. Other important considerations in determining the appropriateness of home PN or EN are that the patient's prognosis is longer than several months and that the therapy benefits quality of life.

DISEASE-SPECIFIC NUTRITIONAL SUPPORT SNS is basically a support therapy and is primary therapy only for the treatment or prevention of malnutrition. Certain conditions require modification of nutritional support because of organ or system impairment. For instance, in nitrogen accumulation disorders, protein intake may need to be reduced. However, in renal disease, except for brief periods of several days, protein intakes should approach requirement levels of at least 0.8 g/kg or higher up to 1.2 g/kg as long as the

TABLE 73-2 SUMMARY OF OUTCOMES FOR PATIENTS ON HOME PARENTERAL AND ENTERAL NUTRITION (HPEN)

Diagnosis	Number in Group	Age in Years	% Survival[a] on Therapy	Therapy Status, % at 1 year[b] Full Oral Nutrition	Continued on HPEN Rx	Died	Rehabilitation[c] Status, % in 1st year C	P	M	Complications[d] per Patient-Year HPEN	NonHPEN
Home Parenteral Nutrition											
Crohn's disease	562	36	96	70	25	2	60	38	2	0.9	1.1
Ischemic bowel disease	331	49	87	27	48	19	53	41	6	1.4	1.1
Motility disorder	299	45	87	31	44	21	49	39	12	1.3	1.1
Congenital bowel defect	172	5	94	42	47	9	63	27	11	2.1	1.0
Hyperemesis gravidarum	112	28	100	100	0	0	83	16	1	1.5	3.5
Chronic pancreatitis	156	42	90	82	10	5	60	38	2	1.2	2.5
Radiation enteritis	145	58	87	28	49	22	42	49	9	0.8	1.1
Chronic adhesive obstructions	120	53	83	47	34	13	23	68	10	1.7	1.4
Cystic fibrosis	51	17	50	38	13	36	24	66	16	0.8	3.7
Cancer	2122	44	20	26	8	63	29	57	14	1.1	3.3
AIDS	280	33	10	13	6	73	8	63	29	1.6	3.3
Home Enteral Nutrition											
Neurologic disorders of swallowing	1134	65	55	19	25	48	5	24	71	0.3	0.9
Cancer	1644	61	30	30	6	59	21	59	21	0.4	2.7

[a]Survival rates on therapy are values at 1 year, calculated by the life table method. This will differ from the percentage listed as died under Therapy Status, since all patients with known end points are considered in this latter measure. The ratio of observed versus expected deaths is equivalent to a Standard Mortality Ratio.

[b]Not shown are those patients who were back in hospital or who had changed therapy type by 12 months.

[c]Rehabilitation is designated complete (C), partial (P), or minimal (M), relative to the patient's ability to sustain normal age-related activity.

[d]Complications refer only to those complications that resulted in rehospitalization.

Source: Derived from North American HPEN Registry.

Table taken from previous chapter by Lyn Howard, MD.

blood urea nitrogen does not exceed 100 mg/dL. If this is not possible, then dialysis or hemofiltration should be considered to allow better feeding. In hepatic failure, intakes of 1.2–1.4 g/kg up to the optimal 1.5 g/kg should be attempted, as long as encephalopathy due to protein intolerance is not encountered. In the presence of protein intolerance, formulas containing 33–50% branched-chain amino acids are available at the 1.2–1.4-g/kg level. Cardiac patients, and many severely stressed patients, often benefit from fluid and sodium restriction to levels of 1000 mL of total parenteral nutrition (TPN) formula and 5–20 meq of sodium per day. In patients with severe chronic PCM characterized by severe weight loss and tissue wasting, TPN must be instituted gradually because of the profound antinatriuresis, antidiuresis, and intracellular accumulation of potassium, magnesium, and phosphorus. This is usually accomplished by limiting fluid intakes initially to about 1000 mL containing modest carbohydrate content of 10–20% dextrose, low sodium, and ample potassium, magnesium, and phosphorus, with careful assessment of fluid and electrolyte status. Protein need not be restricted.

THE DESIGN OF INDIVIDUAL REGIMENS

FLUID REQUIREMENTS

The normal daily requirement for fluid is 30 mL/kg of body weight from all sources (IV infusions, per tube, or oral intake), plus any replacement of abnormal losses such as an osmotic diuresis, nasogastric drainage, wound output, or diarrheal/ostomy losses. Electrolyte and mineral losses can be estimated or measured and also need to be replaced (Table 73-3). Fluid restriction may be necessary in patients with fluid overload, and fluid inputs can be limited to 1200 mL/d if urine is the only significant fluid output. When severe fluid overload occurs, the optimal PN solution for central venous administration is a concentrated 1-L solution of 7% crystalline amino acids (70 g) and 21% dextrose (210 g), which provides an amount of nitrogen and glucose that is effective at protein-sparing.

Patients requiring PN or EN in the acute care setting generally have some element of associated hormonal adaptations (e.g., increased secretion of antidiuretic hormone, aldosterone, insulin, glucagon, or cortisol) that cause fluid retention and hyperglycemia. Weight gain in the critically ill, whether receiving SNS or not, is invariably the consequence of fluid retention, since lean tissue accretion is minimal in the acute phase of illness. Because excess fluid removal can be difficult, limiting fluid intake to allow for balanced intake and output is more effective.

ENERGY REQUIREMENTS

Total energy expenditure comprises resting energy expenditure (two-thirds) plus activity energy expenditure (one-third) (Chap. 72). Resting energy expenditure includes the calories necessary for basal metabolism at bed rest. Activity energy expenditure represents one-fourth to one-third of the total, and the thermal effect of feeding is about 10% of the total energy expenditure. For normally nourished healthy individuals, the total energy expenditure is about 30–35 kcal/kg. Although critical illness increases resting energy expenditure, only in initially

well-nourished individuals with the highest systemic inflammatory response, such as that from severe multiple trauma, burns, closed head injury, or sepsis, do total energy expenditures reach 40–45 kcal/kg. The chronically ill patient with lean tissue loss has reduced basal energy expenditure, and inactivity which results in a total energy expenditure of about 20–25 kcal/kg. About 95% of such patients need <30 kcal/kg to achieve energy balance. Because providing about 50% of measured energy expenditure as SNS is at least equally efficacious for the first 10 days of critical illness, actual measurement of energy expenditure is not generally necessary in the early period of SNS. However, in patients who remain critically ill beyond several weeks, in the severely malnourished for whom estimates of energy expenditure are unreliable, or in those who are difficult to wean from ventilators, it is reasonable to actually measure energy expenditure and to aim for energy balance with SNS.

Insulin resistance is associated with increased gluconeogenesis and reduced glucose utilization, predisposing a patient to hyperglycemia. This is aggravated in patients receiving exogenous carbohydrate from SNS. Normalization of blood glucose levels by insulin infusion in critically ill patients receiving SNS reduces morbidity and mortality. In mild or moderately malnourished patients, a reasonable goal is to provide metabolic support to improve protein synthesis and maintain metabolic homeostasis. Hypocaloric nutrition providing only about 1000 kcal/d and 70 g protein for up to 10 days requires less fluid and reduces the likelihood of poor glycemic control. Energy content can be advanced to 20–25 kcal/kg with 1.5 g protein/kg as conditions permit and definitely during the second week of SNS. Patients with multiple trauma, closed head injury, and severe burns often have much higher energy expenditures, but there is little evidence that providing more than 30 kcal/kg has additional benefit, and it risks hyperglycemia.

Generally, because glucose is an essential tissue fuel, glucose and amino acids are provided parenterally until the level of resting energy expenditure is reached. At this point, adding fat becomes beneficial, since more parenteral glucose stimulates de novo lipogenesis by the liver—an energy-inefficient process. Polyunsaturated long-chain triglycerides are the chief ingredient in most parenteral fat emulsions and the majority of the fat in enteral feeding formulas. These vegetable oil–based emulsions provide essential fatty acids. Enteral feeding formulas have fat content that ranges from 3% of calories up to as much as 50% of calories, while parenteral fat comes in separate containers as 10, 20, and 30% emulsions that can be infused separately or mixed by the pharmacy under controlled conditions as all-in-one or total nutrient admixture with glucose, amino acids, lipid, electrolytes, vitamins, and minerals. Although parenteral fat is required at only about 3% of energy requirements to meet essential fatty acid requirements, when provided as an all-in-one mixture of carbohydrate, fat, and protein, 2–3% fat in the TPN mixtures, representing about 20–30% of calories as fat, is provided to ensure emulsion stability. If given separately, parenteral fat should not be provided at rates exceeding 0.11 g/kg body weight per h or about 100 g over 12 h—equivalent to 1 L of 10% parenteral fat and 500 mL of 20% parenteral fat.

Medium-chain triglycerides, which contain saturated fatty acids with chain lengths of 6, 8, 10, or 12 carbons, are provided in a number of enteral feeding formulas because they are absorbed preferentially. Fish oil contains polyunsaturated fatty acids of the omega 3 family, which have been shown to improve immune function and reduce the inflammatory response. Parenteral emulsions containing medium-chain triglycerides, olive oil, and fish oil are available in Europe and Japan but not yet in the United States.

Carbohydrates are provided as hydrous glucose providing 3.4 kcal/g in PN formulas. In enteral formulas, glucose is the carbohydrate source in so-called monomeric diets. These diets provide protein as amino acids and fat in minimal amounts (3%) to meet essential fatty acid requirements. Monomeric formulas are designed to optimize absorption in the seriously compromised gut. These formulas, like the im-

TABLE 73-3 ENTERIC FLUID VOLUMES AND THEIR ELECTROLYTE CONTENT[a]

	L/d	Na	K	Cl	HCO$_3$	H
Oral intake	2–3					
Enteric secretions						
Saliva	1–2	15	30	15	50	—
Gastric juice	1.5–2	50–70	5–15	90–120	0	70–100
Bile	0.5–1.5	120–150	5–15	80–120	30–50	—
Pancreatic	0.5–1	100–140	10	70–100	60–110	—
Small intestine	1–2	80–140	10–20	80–120	20–40	—

[a]All in mEq/L.
Source: Adapted from previous chapter by Lyn Howard, MD, in *Harrison's Principles of Internal Medicine*.

mune-enhancing diets, are quite expensive. In polymeric diets, the carbohydrate source is usually an osmotically less active polysaccharide, protein is usually soy or casein protein, and fat is present in amounts from 25 to 50%. Such formulas are usually well tolerated by patients with normal intestinal length, and some are acceptable for oral consumption.

PROTEIN OR AMINO ACID REQUIREMENTS

Although the recommended dietary allowance for protein is 0.8 g/kg per d, maximal rates of repletion occur with 1.5 g/kg in the malnourished. In the severely catabolic patient, this higher level minimizes protein loss. In patients requiring SNS in the acute care setting, at least 1 g/kg is recommended, with greater amounts up to 1.5 g/kg as volume, renal, and hepatic tolerances allow. The standard parenteral and enteral formulas contain protein of high biologic value and meet the requirements for the eight essential amino acids. In protein-intolerant conditions such as renal and hepatic failure, modified amino acid formulas should be considered. In hepatic failure, higher branched-chain amino acid–enriched formulas appear to improve outcomes. Conditionally essential amino acids like arginine and glutamine may also have some benefit in supplemental amounts.

Protein (nitrogen) balance provides a measure of feeding efficacy of PN or EN. It is calculated as protein intake/6.25 because proteins are on average 16% nitrogen (N), minus the 24-h urine urea N (UUN) plus 4 g N, which reflects other N losses. In the critically ill, a mild negative balance of 2–4 g N/d is usually achievable with a similarly mild positive balance in the recuperating patient. Each g N represents approximately 30 g lean tissue.

MINERAL AND VITAMIN REQUIREMENTS

Parenteral electrolyte, vitamin, and trace mineral requirements are summarized in Tables 73-4, 73-5, and 73-6. Electrolyte modifications are necessary with substantial gastrointestinal losses from nasogastric drainage or intestinal losses from fistulas, diarrhea or ostomy outputs. Such losses also imply extra calcium, magnesium, and zinc losses. Excessive urine or potassium losses with amphotericin, or magnesium losses with cisplatin or in renal failure, necessitate adjustments in sodium, potassium, magnesium, phosphorus, and acid-base balance. Vitamin and trace element requirements are met by the daily provision of a complete parenteral vitamin supplement and trace elements for PN, and with the provision of adequate amounts of enteral feeding formulas that contain these micronutrients.

PARENTERAL NUTRITION

INFUSION TECHNIQUE AND PATIENT MONITORING

Parenteral feeding through a peripheral vein is limited by osmolality and volume constraints. Solutions that contain more than 3% amino acids and 5% glucose (290 kcal/L) are poorly tolerated peripherally. Parenteral fat (20%) can be given to increase the calories delivered. The total volume required to provide a marginal protein intake of 60 g and 1680 total kcal is 2.5 L. However, the risk of significant morbidity and mortality from incompatibilities of calcium and phosphate salts is greatest in these low-osmolality, low-glucose regimens. Parenteral feeding via a peripheral vein is generally intended as a supplement to oral feeding and is not optimal for the critically ill. Peripheral parenteral nutrition may benefit from small amounts of heparin at 1000 U/L and co-infusion with parenteral fat to reduce osmolality, but volume constraints still limit the value of this therapy. Peripherally inserted central catheters (PICCs) can be used for the short term to provide concentrated glucose parenteral solutions of 20–25% dextrose and 4–7% amino acids, while avoiding some of the complications of catheter placement via a large central vein. With PICC lines, however, flow can be position-related, and the lines cannot be exchanged over a wire for infection monitoring. For these reasons, in the critically ill, centrally placed catheters are preferred. The subclavian approach is best tolerated by the patient and is the easiest to dress. The jugular approach is less likely to lead to a pneumothorax. The femoral approach is discouraged because of the greater risk of catheter infection. For long-term feeding in the home, tunneled catheters and implanted ports reduce infection risk and are more acceptable to patients. However, tunneled catheters require placement in the operating room.

Catheters are made of silastic, polyurethane, or polyvinyl chloride. Silastic catheters are less thrombogenic and are best for tunneled catheters. Polyurethane is best for temporary catheters. Dressing changes with dry gauze at regular intervals should be performed by nurses skilled in catheter care to avoid infection. Chlorhexidine solution is more effective than alcohol or iodine compounds. Appropriate monitoring for patients receiving PN is summarized in Table 73-7.

TABLE 73-5 PARENTERAL MULTIVITAMIN REQUIREMENTS FOR ADULTS

Vitamin	Recently Revised Value
Vitamin A	3300 IU
Thiamin (B₁)	6 mg
Riboflavin (B₂)	3.6 mg
Niacin (B₃)	40 mg
Folic acid	600 µg
Pantothenic acid	15 mg
Pyridoxine (B₆)	6 mg
Cyanocobalamin (B₁₂)	5 µg
Biotin	60 µg
Ascorbic acid (C)	200 mg
Vitamin D	200 IU
Vitamin E	10 IU
Vitamin K[a]	150 µg

[a]A product is available that does not contain vitamin K. Vitamin K supplementation is recommended at 2–4 mg/week in patients not receiving oral anticoagulation therapy if using this product.

TABLE 73-6 PARENTERAL TRACE METAL SUPPLEMENTATION FOR ADULTS[a]

Trace Mineral	Intake
Zinc	2.5–4 mg/d, an additional 10–15 mg/d per L of stool or ileostomy output
Copper	0.5–1.5 mg/d, possibility of retention in biliary tract obstruction
Manganese	0.1–0.3 mg/d, possibility of retention in biliary tract obstruction
Chromium	10–15 µg/d
Selenium	20–100 µg/d, necessary for long-term PN, optional for short-term TPN
Molybdenum	20–120 µg/d, necessary for long-term PN, optional for short-term PN
Iodine	75–150 µg/d, necessary for long-term PN, optional for short-term PN

[a]Commercial products are available that have the first four, first five, and all seven of these metals in recommended amounts.

Note: PN, parenteral nutrition; TPN, total parenteral nutrition.

TABLE 73-4 USUAL DAILY ELECTROLYTE ADDITIONS TO PARENTERAL NUTRITION

Electrolyte	Parenteral Equivalent of RDA	Usual Intake
Sodium		1–2 meq/kg + replacement, but can be as low as 5–40 meq/d
Potassium		40–100 meq/d + replacement of unusual losses
Chloride		As needed for acid-base balance, but usually 2:1 to 1:1 with acetate
Acetate		As needed for acid-base balance
Calcium	10 meq	10–20 meq/d
Magnesium	10 meq	8–16 meq/d
Phosphorus	30 mmol	20–40 mmol

TABLE 73-7 MONITORING THE PATIENT ON PARENTERAL NUTRITION

Clinical Data Monitored Daily

General sense of well-being
Strength as evidenced in getting out of bed, walking, resistance exercise as appropriate
Vital signs including temperature, blood pressure, pulse, and respiratory rate
Fluid balance: weight at least several times weekly, fluid intake (parenteral and enteral) vs fluid output (urine, stool, gastric drainage, wound, ostomy)
Parenteral nutrition delivery equipment: tubing, pump, filter, catheter, dressing
Nutrient solution composition

Laboratory Daily

Finger-stick glucose	Three times daily until stable
Blood glucose, Na, K, Cl, HCO$_3$, BUN	Daily until stable and fully advanced, then twice weekly
Serum creatinine, albumin, PO$_4$, Ca, Mg, Hb/Hct, WBC	Baseline, then twice weekly
INR	Baseline, then weekly
Micronutrient tests	As indicated

Note: Hb, hemoglobin; Hct, hematocrit; INR, international normalized ratio; WBC, white blood cell count.
Source: Adapted from chapter by Lyn Howard, MD, in HPIM, 16e.

COMPLICATIONS

Mechanical The insertion of a central venous catheter should be performed by trained and experienced personnel using aseptic techniques to limit the major common complications of pneumothorax and inadvertent arterial puncture or injury. Catheter position should be radiographically confirmed to be in the superior vena cava distal to the junction with the jugular or subclavian vein and not directly against the vessel wall. Thrombosis related to the catheter may occur at the site of entry into the vein and extend to encase the catheter. Catheter infection predisposes to thrombosis, as does the systemic inflammatory response. The addition of 6000 U of heparin in the daily parenteral formula in hospitalized patients with temporary catheters reduces the risk of fibrin sheath formation and catheter infection. Temporary catheters that develop a thrombus should be removed and, based on clinical findings, treated with anticoagulants. Thrombolytic therapy can be considered for patients with permanent catheters depending on the ease of replacement and presence of alternate, reasonably acceptable venous access sites. Low-dose warfarin therapy of 1 mg/d reduces the risk of thrombosis in permanent catheters used for home PN, but full anticoagulation may be required in patients who have recurrent thrombosis related to permanent catheters. A recent U.S. Food and Drug Administration mandate to reformulate parenteral multivitamins to include vitamin K at a dose of 150 μg daily may affect the efficacy of low-dose warfarin therapy. There is a "no vitamin K" version available for patients receiving this therapy. Catheters can become mechanically occluded and may also become occluded by fibrin at the tip, or by fat, minerals, or drugs intraluminally. These occlusions can be managed with low-dose alteplase for fibrin, with indwelling 70% alcohol for fat, with 0.1 N hydrochloric acid for mineral precipitates, and with either 0.1 N hydrochloric acid or 0.1 N sodium hydroxide for drugs, depending on their pH.

Metabolic The most common problems related to PN are fluid overload and hyperglycemia (Table 73-8). Hypertonic dextrose stimulates a much higher insulin level than meal feeding. Because insulin is a potent antinatriuretic and antidiuretic hormone, hyperinsulinemia leads to sodium and fluid retention. In the absence of gastrointestinal losses or renal dysfunction, net fluid retention is likely when total fluid intake exceeds 2000 mL/d. Close monitoring of body weight, as well as fluid intake and output, is necessary to prevent this complication. In the absence of significant renal impairment, the sodium content of the urine is likely to be <10 meq/L. Providing sodium in limited amounts of 40 meq/d and the use of both glucose and fat in the PN mixture to lower total glucose and sodium will help reduce fluid retention. The elevated insulin also increases the intracellular transport of potassium, magnesium, and phosphorus, which can precipitate a dangerous refeeding syndrome if the total glucose content of the PN solution is advanced too quickly in severely malnourished patients. It is generally best to start PN with <200 g glucose/d to assess glucose tolerance. Regular insulin can be added to the PN formula to establish glycemic control, and the insulin doses can be increased proportionately as the glucose is advanced. As a general rule, patients with insulin-dependent diabetes require about twice their usual home insulin doses when they are receiving TPN at 20–25 kcal/kg, largely as a consequence of parenteral glucose administration and some loss of insulin to the TPN container. As a rough estimate, the amount of insulin can be provided in a similar proportion to the amount of calories provided as TPN relative to full feeding, and the insulin can be placed in the TPN formula. Subcutaneous regular insulin can be provided to improve glucose control as assessed by measurements of blood glucose every 6 h. About two-

TABLE 73-8 SELECTED METABOLIC DISTURBANCES AND THEIR CORRECTION

Disturbance	Cause	Corrective Action with PN
Hyponatremia	Increased total body water or decreased total body sodium	Decrease free water or increase sodium
Hypernatremia	Occurs commonly with excessive isotonic or hypertonic fluid followed by diuretic administration with free water clearance; can also occur with dehydration and normal total body sodium	Increase free water to produce net positive fluid balance maintaining sodium and chloride balance
Hypokalemia	Inadequate intake relative to need	Use supplements
	Excessive diuresis, tubular dysfunction	Use supplements
	Magnesium deficiency	Increase PN magnesium
	Metabolic alkalosis	Correct alkalosis
	Hyperinsulinemia	Maintain constant PN, increase potassium
Hyperkalemia	Excessive provision	Reduce supplements
	Metabolic acidosis	Evaluate alkalosis, treat with PN acetate salt and decrease potassium
	Renal deterioration	Evaluate patient and adjust PN as indicated
Hypocalcemia	Reciprocal response to phosphorus repletion	Increase calcium
	Critical illness effect	Increase calcium
	Severe malabsorption	Supplement calcium
Hypercalcemia	Excessive administration or pathologic (cancer, hyperparathyroidism)	Reduce or eliminate calcium
Hypomagnesemia	Increased requirements due to diuretic use, alcoholism, malabsorption, malnutrition	Supplement magnesium
	Critical illness	Supplement magnesium
Hypophosphatemia	Inadequate intake relative to needs related to malnutrition, alcohol use	Supplement phosphorus
	Increased calcium intake	Use supplements
Hyperphosphatemia	Excessive administration or worsening renal function	Reduce phosphorus
Azotemia	Excessive amino acid infusion or worsening renal function	Reduce amino acid level but consider renal replacement therapy if cannot provide 1 g protein per kg for prolonged periods

Note: PN, parenteral nutrition.

thirds of the total 24-h amount can be added to the next day's order, with subcutaneous insulin supplements as needed. Advances in TPN concentration should be made when reasonable glucose control is established, and the insulin dose adjusted proportionately to the calories added as glucose and amino acids. These are general rules, and they are conservative. Given the adverse clinical impact of hyperglycemia, it may be necessary to use continuous insulin therapy as a separate infusion with a standard protocol to initially establish control. Once established, this insulin dose can be added to the PN formula. Acid-base imbalance is also common during PN therapy. Amino acid formulas are buffered, but critically ill patients are prone to metabolic acidosis, often due to renal tubular impairment. The use of sodium and potassium acetate salts in the PN formula may address this problem. Bicarbonate salts should not be used because they are incompatible with TPN formulations. Nasogastric drainage produces a hypochloremic alkalosis that can be managed by attention to chloride balance. Occasionally, hydrochloric acid may be required for a more rapid response or when diuretic therapy limits the ability to provide substantial sodium chloride. Up to 100 meq/L and up to 150 meq of hydrochloric acid per day may be placed in a fat-free PN formula.

Infectious Infections of the central access catheter rarely occur in the first 72 h. Fever during this period is usually from infection elsewhere or another cause. Fever that develops during PN can be addressed by checking the catheter site and, if the site looks clean, exchanging the catheter over a wire with cultures taken through the catheter and at the catheter tip. If these cultures are negative, as they are most of the time, the new catheter can continue to be used. If a culture is positive for a relatively nonpathogenic bacteria like *Staphylococcus epidermidis*, consider a second exchange over a wire with repeat cultures or replace the catheter depending on the clinical circumstances. If cultures are positive for more pathogenic bacteria, or for fungi like *Candida albicans*, it is generally best to replace the catheter at a new site. Whether antibiotic treatment is required is a clinical decision, but *C. albicans* grown from the blood culture in a patient receiving PN should always be treated because the consequences of failure to treat can be dire.

Catheter infections can be minimized by dedicating the feeding catheter to PN, without blood sampling or medication administration. Central catheter infections are a serious complication with an attributed mortality of 12–25%. Infections in central venous catheters dedicated to feeding should occur less frequently than 3 per 1000 catheter-days. Home PN catheters that become infected may be treated through the catheter without removal of the catheter, particularly if the offending organism is *S. epidermidis*. Clearing of the biofilm and fibrin sheath by local treatment of the catheter with indwelling alteplase may increase the likelihood of eradication. Antibiotic lock therapy with high concentrations of antibiotic, with or without heparin in addition to systemic therapy, may improve efficacy. Sepsis with hypotension should precipitate catheter removal in either the temporary or permanent PN setting.

ENTERAL NUTRITION

TUBE PLACEMENT AND PATIENT MONITORING

The types of enteral feeding tubes, methods of insertion, their clinical uses, and potential compli-

cations are outlined in Table 73-9. The different types of enteral formulas are listed in Table 73-10. Patients receiving EN are at risk for many of the same metabolic complications as those who receive PN and should be monitored in the same manner. EN can be a source of similar problems, but not to the same degree, because the insulin response to EN is about half of that seen with PN. Enteral feeding formulas have fixed electrolyte compositions that are generally modest in sodium and somewhat higher in potassium content. Acid-base disturbances can be addressed to a more limited extent with EN. Acetate salts can be added to the formula to treat chronic metabolic acidosis. Calcium chloride can be added to treat mild chronic metabolic alkalosis. Medications and other additives to enteral feeding formulas can clog the tubes (e.g., calcium chloride may interact with casein-based formulas to produce insoluble calcium caseinate products) and may reduce the efficacy of some drugs (e.g., phenytoin). Since small-bore tubes are easily displaced, tube position should be checked at intervals by aspirating and measuring the pH of the gut fluid (<4 in the stomach, >6 in the jejunum).

COMPLICATIONS

Aspiration The debilitated patient with poor gastric emptying and impairment of swallowing and cough is at risk for aspiration; this is particularly true for those who are mechanically ventilated. Tracheal suctioning induces coughing and gastric regurgitation, and cuffs on endotracheal or tracheostomy tubes seldom protect against aspiration. Preventive measures include elevating the head of the bed to 30 degrees,

TABLE 73-9 ENTERAL FEEDING TUBES

Type/Insertion Technique	Clinical Uses	Potential Complications
Nasogastric Tube		
External measurement: nostril, ear, xiphisternum; tube stiffened by ice water or stylet; position verified by injecting air and auscultating, or by x-ray	Short-term clinical situation (weeks) or longer periods with intermittent insertion; bolus feeding simpler, but continuous drip with pump better tolerated	Aspiration; ulceration of nasal and esophageal tissues, leading to stricture
Nasoduodenal Tube		
External measurement: nostril, ear, anterior superior iliac spine; tube stiffened by stylet and passed through pylorus under fluoroscopy or with endoscopic loop	Short-term clinical situations where gastric emptying impaired or proximal leak suspected; requires continuous drip with pump	Spontaneous pulling back into stomach (position verified by aspirating content, pH > 6); diarrhea common, fiber-containing formulas may help
Gastrostomy Tube		
Percutaneous placement endoscopically, radiologically, or surgically; after tract established, can be converted to a gastric "button"	Long-term clinical situations, swallowing disorders, or impaired small-bowel absorption requiring continuous drip	Aspiration; irritation around tube exit site; peritoneal leak; balloon migration and obstruction of pylorus
Jejunostomy Tube		
Percutaneous placement endoscopically or radiologically via pylorus or endoscopically or surgically directly into the jejunum	Long-term clinical situations where gastric emptying impaired; requires continuous drip with pump; direct endoscopic placement (PEJ) is the most comfortable for patient	Clogging or displacement of tube; jejunal fistula if large-bore tube used; diarrhea from dumping; irritation of surgical anchoring suture
Combined Gastrojejunostomy Tube		
Percutaneous placement endoscopically, radiologically, or surgically; intragastric arm for continuous or intermittent gastric suction; jejunal arm for enteral feeding	Used for patients with impaired gastric emptying and at high risk for aspiration or patients with acute pancreatitis or proximal leaks	Clogging: especially of small bore jejunal tube

Note: All small tubes are at risk for clogging, especially if used for crushed medications. In long-term enteral patients, gastrostomy and jejunostomy tubes can be exchanged for a low-profile "button" once the tract is established.
Source: Adapted from chapter in *Harrison's Principles of Internal Medicine*, 16e, by Lyn Howard, MD.

TABLE 73-10 ENTERAL FORMULAS

Composition Characteristics	Clinical Indications
Standard Enteral Formula	

1. Complete dietary products (+)[a]
  a. Caloric density 1 kcal/mL
  b. Protein ~14% cals, caseinates, soy, lactalbumin
  c. CHO ~60% cals, hydrolyzed corn starch, maltodextrin, sucrose
  d. Fat ~30% cals, corn, soy, safflower oils
  e. Recommended daily intake of all minerals and vitamins in >1500 kcal/d
  f. Osmolality (mosmol/kg): ~300
	Suitable for most patients requiring tube feeding; some can be used orally

Modified Enteral Formulas	
1. Caloric density 1.5–2 kcal/mL (+)	Fluid-restricted patients
2. a. High protein ~20–25% protein (+)	Critically ill patients
b. Hydrolyzed protein to small peptides (+)	Impaired absorption
c. ↑ Arginine, glutamine, nucleotides, ω3 fat (+++)	Immune-enhancing diets
d. ↑ Branched-chain amino acids, ↓ aromatic amino acids (+++)	Liver failure patients intolerant of 0.8 g/kg protein
e. Low protein of high biologic value	Renal failure patient for brief periods if critically ill
3. a. Low fat, partial MCT substitution (+)	Fat malabsorption
b. ↑ Fat >40% cals (++)	Pulmonary failure with CO_2 retention on standard formula, limited utility
c. ↑ Fat from MUFA (++)	Improvement in glycemic index control in diabetes
d. ↑ Fat from ω3 and ↓ ω6 linoleic acid (+++)	Improved ventilation in ARDS
4. Fiber provided as soy polysaccharide (+)	Improved laxation

Cost: + inexpensive; ++ moderately expensive; +++ very expensive.

Note: ARDS, acute respiratory distress syndrome; CHO, carbohydrate; MCT, medium-chain triglyceride; MUFA, mononounsaturated fatty acids; ω3 or ω6, polyunsaturated fat with first double bond at carbon 3 (fish oils) or carbon 6 (vegetable oils).

Source: Adapted from chapter in *Harrison's Principles of Internal Medicine,* 16e, by Lyn Howard, MD.

using nurse-directed algorithms for formula advancement, combining enteral with parenteral feeding, and using post–ligament of Treitz feeding. Tube feeding should not be discontinued for gastric residuals of <300 mL unless there are other signs of gastrointestinal intolerance such as nausea, vomiting, or abdominal distention. Continuous feeding using pumps is better tolerated intragastrically and is essential for feeding into the jejunum. For small-bowel feeding, residuals are not assessed but abdominal pain and distention should be monitored.

Diarrhea Enteral feeding often leads to diarrhea, especially if bowel function is compromised by disease or drugs, particularly broad-spectrum antibiotics. Diarrhea may be controlled by the use of a continuous drip, with a fiber-containing formula, or by adding an antidiarrheal agent to the formula. However, *Clostridium difficile*, which is a common cause of diarrhea in patients being tube fed, should be ruled out before using antidiarrheal agents. H2 blockers may also assist in reducing the net fluid presented to the colon. Diarrhea associated with enteral feeding does not necessarily imply inadequate absorption of nutrients other than water and electrolytes. Amino acids and glucose are particularly well absorbed in the upper small bowel except in the most diseased or shortest bowel. Since luminal nutrients exert trophic effects on the gut mucosa, it is often appropriate to persist with tube feeding, despite the diarrhea, even when this necessitates supplemental parenteral fluid support.

ACKNOWLEDGMENT

The authors acknowledge the contributions of Lyn Howard, MD, the author in earlier editions of HPIM, to material in this chapter.

FURTHER READINGS

AUGUST D et al: Evidence-based approach to optimal management of HPEN access. J Parenter Enteral Nutr 30:S5, 2006

BISTRIAN B, McCOWEN K: Nutritional support in the adult intensive care unit: Key controversies. Crit Care Med 34:1525, 2006

CENTERS FOR DISEASE CONTROL AND PREVENTION: Reduction in central line–associated bloodstream infections among patients in intensive care units—Pennsylvania, April 2001–March 2005. MMWR 54:1013, 2005

DEBAVEYE Y, VAN DEN BERGHE G: Risks and benefits of nutritional support during critical illness. Annu Rev Nutr 26:513, 2006

KORETZ RL et al: Does enteral nutrition affect clinical outcome? A systematic review of the randomized trials. Am J Gastroenterol 102(2):412, 2007

MILNE A et al: Meta-analysis: Protein and energy supplementation in older people. Ann Intern Med 144:37, 2006

PLANK LD, HILL GL: Energy balance in critical illness. Proc Nutr Soc 62:545, 2003

SIMPSON F, DOIG GS: Parenteral vs. enteral nutrition in the critically ill patient: A meta-analysis of trials using the intention to treat principle. Intensive Care Med 31:12, 2005

VAN DEN BERGHE G et al: Intensive insulin therapy in the critically ill patients. N Engl J Med 345:1359, 2001

74 Biology of Obesity
Jeffrey S. Flier, Eleftheria Maratos-Flier

In a world where food supplies are intermittent, the ability to store energy in excess of what is required for immediate use is essential for survival. Fat cells, residing within widely distributed adipose tissue depots, are adapted to store excess energy efficiently as triglyceride and, when needed, to release stored energy as free fatty acids for use at other sites. This physiologic system, orchestrated through endocrine and neural pathways, permits humans to survive starvation for as long as several months. However, in the presence of nutritional abundance and a sedentary lifestyle, and influenced importantly by genetic endowment, this system increases adipose energy stores and produces adverse health consequences.

DEFINITION AND MEASUREMENT

Obesity is a state of excess adipose tissue mass. Although often viewed as equivalent to increased body weight, this need not be the case—lean but very muscular individuals may be overweight by numerical standards without having increased adiposity. Body weights are distributed continuously in populations, so that choice of a medically meaningful distinction between lean and obese is somewhat arbitrary. Obesity is therefore more effectively defined by assessing its linkage to morbidity or mortality.

Although not a direct measure of adiposity, the most widely used method to gauge obesity is the *body mass index* (BMI), which is equal to weight/height^2 (in kg/m^2) (Fig. 74-1). Other approaches to quantifying obesity include anthropometry (skin-fold thickness), densitometry (underwater weighing), CT or MRI, and electrical impedance. Using data from the Metropolitan Life Tables, BMIs for the midpoint of all heights and frames among both men and women range from 19–26 kg/m^2; at a similar BMI, women have more body fat than men. Based on data of substantial morbidity, a BMI of 30 is most commonly used as a threshold for obesity in both men and women. Large-scale epidemiologic studies suggest that all-cause, metabolic, cancer, and cardiovascular morbidity begin to rise (albeit at a slow rate) when BMIs are ≥ 25, suggesting that the cut-off for obesity should be low-

FIGURE 74-1 Nomogram for determining body mass index. To use this nomogram, place a ruler or other straight edge between the body weight (without clothes) in kilograms or pounds located on the left-hand line and the height (without shoes) in centimeters or inches located on the right-hand line. The body mass index is read from the middle of the scale and is in metric units. (*Copyright 1979, George A. Bray, M.D.; used with permission.*)

Labels within figure:
Weight — kg lb
Body Mass Index [kg/m²]
WOMEN RELATIVE RISK — VERY HIGH / HIGH / MODERATE / LOW / VERY LOW
MEN RELATIVE RISK — VERY HIGH / HIGH / MODERATE / LOW / VERY LOW
Height — cm in.

ered. Most authorities use the term *overweight* (rather than obese) to describe individuals with BMIs between 25 and 30. A BMI between 25 and 30 should be viewed as medically significant and worthy of therapeutic intervention, especially in the presence of risk factors that are influenced by adiposity, such as hypertension and glucose intolerance.

The distribution of adipose tissue in different anatomic depots also has substantial implications for morbidity. Specifically, intraabdominal and abdominal subcutaneous fat have more significance than subcutaneous fat present in the buttocks and lower extremities. This distinction is most easily made clinically by determining the waist-to-hip ratio, with a ratio >0.9 in women and >1.0 in men being abnormal. Many of the most important complications of obesity, such as insulin resistance, diabetes, hypertension, hyperlipidemia, and hyperandrogenism in women, are linked more strongly to intraabdominal and/or upper body fat than to overall adiposity (Chap. 236). The mechanism underlying this association is unknown but may relate to the fact that intraabdominal adipocytes are more lipolytically active than those from other depots. Release of free fatty acids into the portal circulation has adverse metabolic actions, especially on the liver. Whether adipokines and cytokines secreted by visceral adipocytes play an additional role in systemic complications of obesity is an area of active investigation.

PREVALENCE

Data from the National Health and Nutrition Examination Surveys (NHANES) show that the percent of the American adult population with obesity (BMI > 30) has increased from 14.5% (between 1976 and 1980) to 30.5% (between 1999 and 2000). As many as 64% of U.S. adults ≥20 years of age were overweight (defined as BMI > 25) between the years of 1999 and 2000. Extreme obesity (BMI ≥40) has also increased and affects 4.7% of the population. The increasing prevalence of medically significant obesity raises great concern. Obesity is more common among women and in the poor; the prevalence in children is also rising at a worrisome rate.

PHYSIOLOGIC REGULATION OF ENERGY BALANCE

Substantial evidence suggests that body weight is regulated by both endocrine and neural components that ultimately influence the effector arms of energy intake and expenditure. This complex regulatory system is necessary because even small imbalances between energy intake and expenditure will ultimately have large effects on body weight. For example, a 0.3% positive imbalance over 30 years would result in a 9-kg (20-lb) weight gain. This exquisite regulation of energy balance cannot be monitored easily by calorie-counting in relation to physical activity. Rather, body weight regulation or dysregulation depends on a complex interplay of hormonal and neural signals. Alterations in stable weight by forced overfeeding or food deprivation induce physiologic changes that resist these perturbations: with weight loss, appetite increases and energy expenditure falls; with overfeeding, appetite falls and energy expenditure increases. This latter compensatory mechanism frequently fails, however, permitting obesity to develop when food is abundant and physical activity is limited. A major regulator of these adaptive responses is the adipocyte-derived hormone leptin, which acts through brain circuits (predominantly in the hypothalamus) to influence appetite, energy expenditure, and neuroendocrine function (see below).

Appetite is influenced by many factors that are integrated by the brain, most importantly within the hypothalamus (Fig. 74-2). Signals that impinge on the hypothalamic center include neural afferents, hormones, and metabolites. Vagal inputs are particularly important, bringing information from viscera, such as gut distention. Hormonal signals include leptin, insulin, cortisol, and gut peptides. Among the latter are ghrelin, which is made in the stomach and stimulates feeding, and peptide YY (PYY) and cholecystokinin, which are made in the small intestine and signal to the brain through direct action on hypothalamic control centers and/or via the vagus nerve. Metabolites, including glucose, can influence appetite, as seen by the effect of hypoglycemia to induce hunger; however, glucose is not normally a major regulator of appetite. These diverse hormonal, metabolic, and neural signals act by influencing the expression and release of various hypothalamic peptides [e.g., neuropeptide Y (NPY), Agouti-related peptide (AgRP), α-melanocyte-stimulating hormone (α-MSH), and melanin-concentrating hormone (MCH)] that are integrated with serotonergic, catecholaminergic, endocannabinoid,

FIGURE 74-2 The factors that regulate appetite through effects on central neural circuits. Some factors that increase or decrease appetite are listed. NPY, neuropeptide Y; MCH, melanin-concentrating hormone; AgRP, Agouti-related peptide; MSH, melanocyte-stimulating hormone; CART, cocaine- and amphetamine-related transcript; GLP-1, glucagon-related peptide-1; CCK, cholecystokinin.

and opioid signaling pathways (see below). Psychological and cultural factors also play a role in the final expression of appetite. Apart from rare genetic syndromes involving leptin, its receptor, and the melanocortin system, specific defects in this complex appetite control network that influence common cases of obesity are not well defined.

Energy expenditure includes the following components: (1) resting or basal metabolic rate; (2) the energy cost of metabolizing and storing food; (3) the thermic effect of exercise; and (4) adaptive thermogenesis, which varies in response to chronic caloric intake (rising with increased intake). Basal metabolic rate accounts for ~70% of daily energy expenditure, whereas active physical activity contributes 5–10%. Thus, a significant component of daily energy consumption is fixed.

Genetic models in mice indicate that mutations in certain genes (e.g., targeted deletion of the insulin receptor in adipose tissue) protect against obesity, apparently by increasing energy expenditure. Adaptive thermogenesis occurs in *brown adipose tissue* (BAT), which plays an important role in energy metabolism in many mammals. In contrast to white adipose tissue, which is used to store energy in the form of lipids, BAT expends stored energy as heat. A mitochondrial *uncoupling protein* (UCP-1) in BAT dissipates the hydrogen ion gradient in the oxidative respiration chain and releases energy as heat. The metabolic activity of BAT is increased by a central action of leptin, acting through the sympathetic nervous system, which heavily innervates this tissue. In rodents, BAT deficiency causes obesity and diabetes; stimulation of BAT with a specific adrenergic agonist (β_3 agonist) protects against diabetes and obesity. Although BAT exists in humans (especially neonates), its physiologic role is not yet established. Homologues of UCP-1 (UCP-2 and -3) may mediate uncoupled mitochondrial respiration in other tissues.

THE ADIPOCYTE AND ADIPOSE TISSUE

Adipose tissue is composed of the lipid-storing adipose cell and a stromal/vascular compartment in which cells including preadipocytes and macrophages reside. Adipose mass increases by enlargement of adipose cells through lipid deposition, as well as by an increase in the number of adipocytes. Obese adipose tissue is also characterized by increased numbers of infiltrating macrophages. The process by which adipose cells are derived from a mesenchymal preadipocyte involves an orchestrated series of differentiation steps mediated by a cascade of specific transcription factors. One of the key transcription factors is *peroxisome proliferator-activated receptor γ* (PPARγ), a nuclear receptor that binds the thiazolidinedione class of insulin-sensitizing drugs used in the treatment of type 2 diabetes (Chap. 338).

Although the adipocyte has generally been regarded as a storage depot for fat, it is also an endocrine cell that releases numerous mole-

FIGURE 74-3 Factors released by the adipocyte that can affect peripheral tissues. PAI, plasminogen activator inhibitor; TNF, tumor necrosis factor; RBP4, retinal binding protein 4.

cules in a regulated fashion (Fig. 74-3). These include the energy balance–regulating hormone leptin, cytokines such as tumor necrosis factor (TNF) α and interleukin (IL)-6, complement factors such as factor D (also known as *adipsin*), prothrombotic agents such as plasminogen activator inhibitor I, and a component of the blood pressure regulating system, angiotensinogen. Adiponectin, an abundant adipose-derived protein whose levels are reduced in obesity, enhances insulin sensitivity and lipid oxidation and it has vascular protective effects, whereas resistin and RBP4, whose levels are increased in obesity, may induce insulin resistance. These factors, and others not yet identified, play a role in the physiology of lipid homeostasis, insulin sensitivity, blood pressure control, coagulation, and vascular health, and are likely to contribute to obesity-related pathologies.

ETIOLOGY OF OBESITY

Though the molecular pathways regulating energy balance are beginning to be illuminated, the causes of obesity remain elusive. In part, this reflects the fact that obesity is a heterogeneous group of disorders. At one level, the pathophysiology of obesity seems simple: a chronic excess of nutrient intake relative to the level of energy expenditure. However, due to the complexity of the neuroendocrine and metabolic systems that regulate energy intake, storage, and expenditure, it has been difficult to quantitate all the relevant parameters (e.g., food intake and energy expenditure) over time in human subjects.

Role of Genes versus Environment Obesity is commonly seen in families, and the heritability of body weight is similar to that for height. Inheritance is usually not Mendelian, however, and it is difficult to distinguish the role of genes and environmental factors. Adoptees more closely resemble their biologic than adoptive parents with respect to obesity, providing strong support for genetic influences. Likewise, identical twins have very similar BMIs whether reared together or apart, and their BMIs are much more strongly correlated than those of dizygotic twins. These genetic effects appear to relate to both energy intake and expenditure.

Whatever the role of genes, it is clear that the environment plays a key role in obesity, as evidenced by the fact that famine prevents obesity in even the most obesity-prone individual. In addition, the recent increase in the prevalence of obesity in the United States is far too rapid to be due to changes in the gene pool. Undoubtedly, genes influence the susceptibility to obesity in response to specific diets and availability of nutrition. Cultural factors are also important—these relate to both availability and composition of the diet and to changes in the level of physical activity. In industrial societies, obesity is more common among poor women, whereas in underdeveloped countries, wealthier women are more often obese. In children, obesity correlates to some degree with time spent watching television. Although the role of diet composition in obesity continues to generate controversy, it appears that high-fat diets may promote obesity, especially when combined with diets rich in simple (as opposed to complex) carbohydrates.

Additional environmental factors may contribute to the increasing obesity prevalence. Both epidemiologic correlations and experimental data suggest that sleep deprivation leads to increased obesity. Less well

FIGURE 74-4 The physiologic system regulated by leptin. Rising or falling leptin levels act through the hypothalamus to influence appetite, energy expenditure, and neuroendocrine function and through peripheral sites to influence systems such as the immune system.

supported in humans are potential changes in gut flora with capacity to alter energy balance and a possible role for obesigenic viral infections.

Specific Genetic Syndromes For many years obesity in rodents has been known to be caused by a number of distinct mutations distributed through the genome. Most of these single-gene mutations cause both hyperphagia and diminished energy expenditure, suggesting a physiologic link between these two parameters of energy homeostasis. Identification of the *ob* gene mutation in genetically obese (ob/ob) mice represented a major breakthrough in the field. The ob/ob mouse develops severe obesity, insulin resistance, and hyperphagia, as well as efficient metabolism (e.g., it gets fat even when ingesting the same number of calories as lean litter mates). The product of the *ob* gene is the peptide leptin, a name derived from the Greek root *leptos*, meaning thin. Leptin is secreted by adipose cells and acts primarily through the hypothalamus. Its level of production provides an index of adipose energy stores (Fig. 74-4). High leptin levels decrease food intake and increase energy expenditure. Another mouse mutant, db/db, which is resistant to leptin, has a mutation in the leptin receptor and develops a similar syndrome. The *OB* gene is present in humans and expressed in fat. Several families with morbid, early-onset obesity caused by inactivating mutations in either leptin or the leptin receptor have been described, thus demonstrating the biologic relevance of leptin in humans. The obesity in these individuals begins shortly after birth, is severe, and is accompanied by neuroendocrine abnormalities. The most prominent of these is hypogonadotropic hypogonadism, which is reversed by lep-

tin replacement. Central hypothyroidism and growth retardation are seen in the mouse model, but their occurrence in leptin-deficient humans is less clear. To date, there is no evidence to suggest that mutations or polymorphisms in the leptin or leptin receptor genes play a prominent role in common forms of obesity.

Mutations in several other genes cause severe obesity in humans (Table 74-1); each of these syndromes is rare. Mutations in the gene encoding proopiomelanocortin (POMC) cause severe obesity through failure to synthesize α-MSH, a key neuropeptide that inhibits appetite in the hypothalamus. The absence of POMC also causes secondary adrenal insufficiency due to absence of adrenocorticotropic hormone (ACTH), as well as pale skin and red hair due to absence of α-MSH. Proenzyme convertase 1 (PC-1) mutations are thought to cause obesity by preventing synthesis of α-MSH from its precursor peptide, POMC. α-MSH binds to the type 4 melanocortin receptor (MC4R), a key hypothalamic receptor that inhibits eating. Heterozygous loss-of-function mutations of this receptor account for as much as 5% of severe obesity. These five genetic defects define a pathway through which leptin (by stimulating POMC and increasing α-MSH) restricts food intake and limits weight (Fig. 74-5).

In addition to these human obesity genes, studies in rodents reveal several other molecular candidates for hypothalamic mediators of human obesity or leanness. The *tub* gene encodes a hypothalamic peptide of unknown function; mutation of this gene causes late-onset obesity. The *fat* gene encodes carboxypeptidase E, a peptide-processing enzyme; mutation of this gene is thought to cause obesity by disrupting production of one or more neuropeptides. AgRP is coexpressed with NPY in arcuate nucleus neurons. AgRP antagonizes α-MSH action at MC4 receptors, and its overexpression induces obesity. In contrast, a mouse deficient in the peptide MCH, whose administration causes feeding, is lean.

A number of complex human syndromes with defined inheritance are associated with obesity (Table 74-2). Although specific genes are undefined at present, their identification will likely enhance our understanding of more common forms of human obesity. In the Prader-Willi syndrome, obesity coexists with short stature, mental retardation, hypogonadotropic hypogonadism, hypotonia, small hands and feet, fish-shaped mouth, and hyperphagia. Most patients have a chromosome 15 deletion, and reduced expression of the signaling protein necdin may be an important cause of defective hypothalamic neural development in this disorder (Chap. 63). Bardet-Biedl syndrome

TABLE 74-1	**SOME OBESITY GENES IN HUMANS AND MICE**			
Gene	**Gene Product**	**Mechanism of Obesity**	**In Human**	**In Rodent**
Lep (ob)	Leptin, a fat-derived hormone	Mutation prevents leptin from delivering satiety signal; brain perceives starvation	Yes	Yes
LepR (db)	Leptin receptor	Same as above	Yes	Yes
POMC	Proopiomelanocortin, a precursor of several hormones and neuropeptides	Mutation prevents synthesis of melanocyte-stimulating hormone (MSH), a satiety signal	Yes	Yes
MC4R	Type 4 receptor for MSH	Mutation prevents reception of satiety signal from MSH	Yes	Yes
AgRP	Agouti-related peptide, a neuropeptide expressed in the hypothalamus	Overexpression inhibits signal through MC4R	No	Yes
PC-1	Prohormone convertase 1, a processing enzyme	Mutation prevents synthesis of neuropeptide, probably MSH	Yes	No
Fat	Carboxypeptidase E, a processing enzyme	Same as above	No	Yes
Tub	Tub, a hypothalamic protein of unknown function	Hypothalamic dysfunction	No	Yes
TrkB	TrkB, a neurotrophin receptor	Hyperphagia due to uncharacterized hypothalamic defect	Yes	Yes

FIGURE 74-5 A central pathway through which leptin acts to regulate appetite and body weight. Leptin signals through proopiomelanocortin (POMC) neurons in the hypothalamus to induce increased production of α-melanocyte-stimulating hormone (α-MSH), requiring the processing enzyme PC-1 (proenzyme convertase 1). α-MSH acts as an agonist on melanocortin-4 receptors to inhibit appetite, and the neuropeptide AgRp (Agouti-related peptide) acts as an antagonist of this receptor. Mutations that cause obesity in humans are indicated by the solid green arrows.

(BBS) is a genetically heterogeneous disorder characterized by obesity, mental retardation, retinitis pigmentosa, renal and cardiac malformations, polydactyly, and hypogonadotropic hypogonadism. At least eight genetic loci have been identified, and BBS may involve defects in ciliary function.

Other Specific Syndromes Associated with Obesity · *CUSHING'S SYNDROME* Although obese patients commonly have central obesity, hypertension, and glucose intolerance, they lack other specific stigmata of Cushing's syndrome (Chap. 336). Nonetheless, a potential diagnosis of Cushing's syndrome is often entertained. Cortisol production and urinary metabolites (17OH steroids) may be increased in simple obesity. Unlike in Cushing's syndrome, however, cortisol levels in blood and urine in the basal state and in response to corticotropin-releasing hormone (CRH) or ACTH are normal; the overnight 1-mg dexamethasone suppression test is normal in 90%, with the remainder being normal on a standard 2-day low-dose dexamethasone suppression test. Obesity may be associated with excessive local reactivation of cortisol in fat by 11β-hydroxysteroid dehydrogenase 1, an enzyme that converts inactive cortisone to cortisol.

HYPOTHYROIDISM The possibility of hypothyroidism should be considered, but it is an uncommon cause of obesity; hypothyroidism is easily ruled out by measuring thyroid-stimulating hormone (TSH). Much of the weight gain that occurs in hypothyroidism is due to myxedema (Chap. 335).

INSULINOMA Patients with insulinoma often gain weight as a result of overeating to avoid hypoglycemic symptoms (Chap. 339). The increased substrate plus high insulin levels promote energy storage in fat. This can be marked in some individuals but is modest in most.

CRANIOPHARYNGIOMA AND OTHER DISORDERS INVOLVING THE HYPOTHALAMUS Whether through tumors, trauma, or inflammation, hypothalamic dysfunction of systems controlling satiety, hunger, and energy expenditure can cause varying degrees of obesity (Chap. 333). It is uncommon to identify a discrete anatomic basis for these disorders. Subtle hypothalamic dysfunction is probably a more common cause of obesity than can be documented using currently available imaging techniques. Growth hormone (GH), which exerts lipolytic activity, is diminished in obesity and is increased with weight loss. Despite low GH levels, insulin-like growth factor (IGF) I (somatomedin) production is normal, suggesting that GH suppression is a compensatory response to increased nutritional supply.

Pathogenesis of Common Obesity Obesity can result from increased energy intake, decreased energy expenditure, or a combination of the two. Thus, identifying the etiology of obesity should involve measurements of both parameters. However, it is nearly impossible to perform direct and accurate measurements of energy intake in free-living individuals, and the obese, in particular, often underreport intake. Measurements of chronic energy expenditure have only recently become available using doubly labeled water or metabolic chamber/rooms. In subjects at stable weight and body composition, energy intake equals expenditure. Consequently, these techniques allow assessment of energy intake in free-living individuals. The level of energy expenditure differs in established obesity, during periods of weight gain or loss, and in the pre- or postobese state. Studies that fail to take note of this phenomenon are not easily interpreted.

TABLE 74-2 A COMPARISON OF SYNDROMES OF OBESITY—HYPOGONADISM AND MENTAL RETARDATION

Feature	Syndrome				
	Prader-Willi	**Laurence-Moon-Biedl**	**Ahlstrom**	**Cohen**	**Carpenter**
Inheritance	Sporadic; two-thirds have defect	Autosomal recessive	Autosomal recessive	Probably autosomal recessive	Autosomal recessive
Stature	Short	Normal; infrequently short	Normal; infrequently short	Short or tall	Normal
Obesity	Generalized Moderate to severe Onset 1–3 yrs	Generalized Early onset, 1–2 yrs	Truncal Early onset, 2–5 yrs	Truncal Mid-childhood, age 5	Truncal, gluteal
Craniofacies	Narrow bifrontal diameter Almond-shaped eyes Strabismus V-shaped mouth High-arched palate	Not distinctive	Not distinctive	High nasal bridge Arched palate Open mouth Short philtrum	Acrocephaly Flat nasal bridge High-arched palate
Limbs	Small hands and feet Hypotonia	Polydactyly	No abnormalities	Hypotonia Narrow hands and feet	Polydactyly Syndactyly Genu valgum
Reproductive status	1° Hypogonadism	1° Hypogonadism	Hypogonadism in males but not in females	Normal gonadal function or hypogonadotrophic hypogonadism	2° Hypogonadism
Other features	Enamel hypoplasia Hyperphagia Temper tantrums Nasal speech			Dysplastic ears Delayed puberty	
Mental retardation	Mild to moderate		Normal intelligence	Mild	Slight

There is continued interest in the concept of a body weight "set point." This idea is supported by physiologic mechanisms centered around a sensing system in adipose tissue that reflects fat stores and a receptor, or "adipostat," that is in the hypothalamic centers. When fat stores are depleted, the adipostat signal is low, and the hypothalamus responds by stimulating hunger and decreasing energy expenditure to conserve energy. Conversely, when fat stores are abundant, the signal is increased, and the hypothalamus responds by decreasing hunger and increasing energy expenditure. The recent discovery of the *ob* gene, and its product leptin, and the *db* gene, whose product is the leptin receptor, provides important elements of a molecular basis for this physiologic concept (see above).

What Is the Status of Food Intake in Obesity? (Do the Obese Eat More Than the Lean?)

This question has stimulated much debate, due in part to the methodologic difficulties inherent in determining food intake. Many obese individuals believe that they eat small quantities of food, and this claim has often been supported by the results of food intake questionnaires. However, it is now established that average energy expenditure increases as individuals get more obese, due primarily to the fact that metabolically active lean tissue mass increases with obesity. Given the laws of thermodynamics, the obese person must therefore eat more than the average lean person to maintain their increased weight. It may be the case, however, that a subset of individuals who are predisposed to obesity have the capacity to become obese initially without an absolute increase in caloric consumption.

What Is the State of Energy Expenditure in Obesity?

The average total daily energy expenditure is higher in obese than lean individuals when measured at stable weight. However, energy expenditure falls as weight is lost, due in part to loss of lean body mass and to decreased sympathetic nerve activity. When reduced to near-normal weight and maintained there for a while, (some) obese individuals have lower energy expenditure than (some) lean individuals. There is also a tendency for those who will develop obesity as infants or children to have lower resting energy expenditure rates than those who remain lean.

The physiologic basis for variable rates of energy expenditure (at a given body weight and level of energy intake) is essentially unknown. A mutation in the human β_3-adrenergic receptor may be associated with increased risk of obesity and/or insulin resistance in certain (but not all) populations. Homologues of the BAT uncoupling protein, named UCP-2 and UCP-3, have been identified in both rodents and humans. UCP-2 is expressed widely, whereas UCP-3 is primarily expressed in skeletal muscle. These proteins may play a role in disordered energy balance.

One newly described component of thermogenesis, called *nonexercise activity thermogenesis* (NEAT), has been linked to obesity. It is the thermogenesis that accompanies physical activities other than volitional exercise, such as the activities of daily living, fidgeting, spontaneous muscle contraction, and maintaining posture. NEAT accounts for about two-thirds of the increased daily energy expenditure induced by overfeeding. The wide variation in fat storage seen in overfed individuals is predicted by the degree to which NEAT is induced. The molecular basis for NEAT and its regulation is unknown.

Leptin in Typical Obesity

The vast majority of obese persons have increased leptin levels but do not have mutations of either leptin or its receptor. They appear, therefore, to have a form of functional "leptin resistance." Data suggesting that some individuals produce less leptin per unit fat mass than others or have a form of relative leptin deficiency that predisposes to obesity are at present contradictory and unsettled. The mechanism for leptin resistance, and whether it can be overcome by raising leptin levels, is not yet established. Some data suggest that leptin may not effectively cross the blood-brain barrier as levels rise. It is also apparent from animal studies that leptin signaling inhibitors, such as SOCS3 and PTP1b, are involved in the leptin-resistant state.

PATHOLOGIC CONSEQUENCES OF OBESITY

(See also Chap. 75) Obesity has major adverse effects on health. Obesity is associated with an increase in mortality, with a 50–100% increased

risk of death from all causes compared to normal-weight individuals, mostly due to cardiovascular causes. Obesity and overweight together are the second leading cause of preventable death in the United States, accounting for 300,000 deaths per year. Mortality rates rise as obesity increases, particularly when obesity is associated with increased intraabdominal fat (see above). Life expectancy of a moderately obese individual could be shortened by 2–5 years, and a 20- to 30-year-old male with a BMI > 45 may lose 13 years of life. It is also apparent that the degree to which obesity affects particular organ systems is influenced by susceptibility genes that vary in the population.

Insulin Resistance and Type 2 Diabetes Mellitus

Hyperinsulinemia and insulin resistance are pervasive features of obesity, increasing with weight gain and diminishing with weight loss (Chap. 236). Insulin resistance is more strongly linked to intraabdominal fat than to fat in other depots. The molecular link between obesity and insulin resistance in tissues such as fat, muscle, and liver has been sought for many years. Major factors under investigation include: (1) insulin itself, by inducing receptor downregulation; (2) free fatty acids, known to be increased and capable of impairing insulin action; (3) intracellular lipid accumulation; and (4) various circulating peptides produced by adipocytes, including the cytokines TNF-α and IL-6, RBP4, and the "adipokines" adiponectin and resistin, which are produced by adipocytes, have altered expression in obese adipocytes, and are capable of modifying insulin action. Despite nearly universal insulin resistance, most obese individuals do not develop diabetes, suggesting that the onset of diabetes requires an interaction between obesity-induced insulin resistance and other factors that predispose to diabetes, such as impaired insulin secretion (Chap. 338). Obesity, however, is a major risk factor for diabetes, and as many as 80% of patients with type 2 diabetes mellitus are obese. Weight loss and exercise, even of modest degree, are associated with increased insulin sensitivity and often improve glucose control in diabetes.

Reproductive Disorders

Disorders that affect the reproductive axis are associated with obesity in both men and women. Male hypogonadism is associated with increased adipose tissue, often distributed in a pattern more typical of females. In men >160% ideal body weight, plasma testosterone and sex hormone–binding globulin (SHBG) are often reduced, and estrogen levels (derived from conversion of adrenal androgens in adipose tissue) are increased (Chap. 340). Gynecomastia may be seen. However, masculinization, libido, potency, and spermatogenesis are preserved in most of these individuals. Free testosterone may be decreased in morbidly obese men whose weight is >200% ideal body weight.

Obesity has long been associated with menstrual abnormalities in women, particularly in women with upper body obesity (Chap. 341). Common findings are increased androgen production, decreased SHBG, and increased peripheral conversion of androgen to estrogen. Most obese women with oligomenorrhea have the polycystic ovarian syndrome (PCOS), with its associated anovulation and ovarian hyperandrogenism; 40% of women with PCOS are obese. Most nonobese women with PCOS are also insulin-resistant, suggesting that insulin resistance, hyperinsulinemia, or the combination of the two are causative or contribute to the ovarian pathophysiology in PCOS in both obese and lean individuals. In obese women with PCOS, weight loss or treatment with insulin-sensitizing drugs often restores normal menses. The increased conversion of androstenedione to estrogen, which occurs to a greater degree in women with lower body obesity, may contribute to the increased incidence of uterine cancer in postmenopausal women with obesity.

Cardiovascular Disease

The Framingham Study revealed that obesity was an independent risk factor for the 26-year incidence of cardiovascular disease in men and women [including coronary disease, stroke, and congestive heart failure (CHF)]. The waist/hip ratio may be the best predictor of these risks. When the additional effects of hypertension and glucose intolerance associated with obesity are included, the adverse impact of obesity is even more evident. The effect of obesity on cardiovascular mortality in women may be seen at BMIs as low as 25. Obesity, especially abdominal obesity, is associated with an atherogenic lipid profile; with increased low-density lipoprotein (LDL) cholesterol, very low density lipoprotein, and triglyceride; and with decreased high-density lipoprotein cholesterol and decreased levels of the vascular protective adipokine adiponectin (Chap. 350). Obesity is also associated with hypertension. Measurement of blood pressure in the obese requires use of a larger cuff size to avoid artifactual increases. Obesity-induced hypertension is associated with increased peripheral resistance and cardiac output, increased sympathetic nervous system tone, increased salt sensitivity, and insulin-mediated salt retention; it is often responsive to modest weight loss.

Pulmonary Disease Obesity may be associated with a number of pulmonary abnormalities. These include reduced chest wall compliance, increased work of breathing, increased minute ventilation due to increased metabolic rate, and decreased functional residual capacity and expiratory reserve volume (Chap. 246). Severe obesity may be associated with obstructive sleep apnea and the "obesity hypoventilation syndrome" with attenuated hypoxic and hypercapnic ventilatory responses (Chap. 258). Sleep apnea can be obstructive (most common), central, or mixed and is associated with hypertension. Weight loss (10–20 kg) can bring substantial improvement, as can major weight loss following gastric bypass or restrictive surgery. Continuous positive airway pressure has been used with some success.

Gallstones Obesity is associated with enhanced biliary secretion of cholesterol, supersaturation of bile, and a higher incidence of gallstones, particularly cholesterol gallstones (Chap. 305). A person 50% above ideal body weight has about a sixfold increased incidence of symptomatic gallstones. Paradoxically, fasting increases supersaturation of bile by decreasing the phospholipid component. Fasting-induced cholecystitis is a complication of extreme diets.

Cancer Obesity in males is associated with higher mortality from cancer, including cancer of the esophagus, colon, rectum, pancreas, liver, and prostate; obesity in females is associated with higher mortality from cancer of the gallbladder, bile ducts, breasts, endometrium, cervix, and ovaries. Some of the latter may be due to increased rates of conversion of androstenedione to estrone in adipose tissue of obese individuals. It was recently estimated that obesity accounts for 14% of cancer deaths in men and 20% in women in the United States.

Bone, Joint, and Cutaneous Disease Obesity is associated with an increased risk of osteoarthritis, no doubt partly due to the trauma of added weight bearing and joint malalignment. The prevalence of gout may also be increased (Chap. 327). Among the skin problems associated with obesity is acanthosis nigricans, manifested by darkening and thickening of the skin folds on the neck, elbows, and dorsal interphalangeal spaces. Acanthosis reflects the severity of underlying insulin resistance and diminishes with weight loss. Friability of skin may be increased, especially in skin folds, enhancing the risk of fungal and yeast infections. Finally, venous stasis is increased in the obese.

FURTHER READINGS

FAROOQI IS, O'RAHILLY S: Genetics of obesity. Philos Trans R Soc Lond B Biol Sci 361:1095, 2006

FLIER JS: Obesity wars: Molecular progress confronts an expanding epidemic. Cell 116:337, 2004

KERSHAW EE, FLIER JS: Adipose tissue as an endocrine organ. J Clin Endocrinol Metab 89:2548, 2004

MORTON GJ et al: Central nervous system control of food intake and body weight. Nature 443:289, 2006

MURPHY KG et al: Gut peptides in the regulation of food intake and energy homeostasis. Endocr Rev 27:719, 2006

OGDEN CL et al: The epidemiology of obesity. Gastroenterology 132(6):2087, 2007

OGDEN CL et al: Prevalence of overweight and obesity in the United States, 1999–2004. JAMA 295:1549, 2006

75 Evaluation and Management of Obesity

Robert F. Kushner

Over 66% of U.S. adults are currently categorized as overweight or obese, and the prevalence of obesity is increasing rapidly throughout most of the industrialized world. Based on statistics from the World Health Organization, overweight and obesity may soon replace more traditional public health concerns such as undernutrition and infectious diseases as the most significant contributors to ill health. Children and adolescents are also becoming more obese, indicating that the current trends will accelerate over time. Obesity is associated with an increased risk of multiple health problems, including hypertension, type 2 diabetes, dyslipidemia, degenerative joint disease, and some malignancies. Thus, it is important for physicians to routinely identify, evaluate, and treat patients for obesity and associated comorbid conditions.

EVALUATION

The U.S. Preventive Services Task Force recommends that physicians screen all adult patients for obesity and offer intensive counseling and behavioral interventions to promote sustained weight loss. This recommendation is consistent with previously released guidelines from the National Heart, Lung, and Blood Institute (NHLBI) and a number of medical societies. The five main steps in the evaluation of obesity are described below and include (1) focused obesity-related history, (2) physical examination to determine the degree and type of obesity, (3) comorbid conditions, (4) fitness level, and (5) the patient's readiness to adopt lifestyle changes.

The Obesity-Focused History Information from the history should address the following six questions:

- What factors contribute to the patient's obesity?
- How is the obesity affecting the patient's health?
- What is the patient's level of risk from obesity?
- What are the patient's goals and expectations?
- Is the patient motivated to begin a weight management program?
- What kind of help does the patient need?

Although the vast majority of obesity can be attributed to behavioral features that affect diet and physical activity patterns, the history may suggest secondary causes that merit further evaluation. Disorders to consider include polycystic ovarian syndrome, hypothyroidism, Cushing's syndrome, and hypothalamic disease. Drug-induced weight gain should also to be considered. Common causes include antidiabetes agents (insulin, sulfonylureas, thiazolidinediones); steroid hormones; psychotropic agents; mood stabilizers (lithium); antidepressants (tricyclics, monoamine oxidase inhibitors, paraxetine, mirtazapine); and antiepileptic drugs (valproate, gabapentin, carbamazepine). Other medications such as nonsteroidal anti-inflammatory drugs and calcium-channel blockers may cause peripheral edema, but they do not increase body fat.

The patient's current diet and physical activity patterns may reveal factors that contribute to the development of obesity in addition to identifying behaviors to target for treatment. This type of historical information is best obtained by using a questionnaire in combination with an interview.

TABLE 75-1 BODY MASS INDEX (BMI) TABLE

BMI	19	20	21	22	23	24	25	26	27	28	29	30	31	32	33	34	35
Height, inches								Body Weight, pounds									
58	91	96	100	105	110	115	119	124	129	134	138	143	148	153	158	162	167
59	94	99	104	109	114	119	124	128	133	138	143	148	153	158	163	168	173
60	97	102	107	112	118	123	128	133	138	143	148	153	158	163	168	174	179
61	100	106	111	116	122	127	132	137	143	148	153	158	164	169	174	180	185
62	104	109	115	120	126	131	136	142	147	153	158	164	169	175	180	186	191
63	107	113	118	124	130	135	141	146	152	158	163	169	175	180	186	191	197
64	110	116	122	128	134	140	145	151	157	163	169	174	180	186	192	197	204
65	114	120	126	132	138	144	150	156	162	168	174	180	186	192	198	204	210
66	118	124	130	136	142	148	155	161	167	173	179	186	192	198	204	210	216
67	121	127	134	140	146	153	159	166	172	178	185	191	198	204	211	217	223
68	125	131	138	144	151	158	164	171	177	184	190	197	203	210	216	223	230
69	128	135	142	149	155	162	169	176	182	189	196	203	209	216	223	230	236
70	132	139	146	153	160	167	174	181	188	195	202	209	216	222	229	236	243
71	136	143	150	157	165	172	179	186	193	200	208	215	222	229	236	243	250
72	140	147	154	162	169	177	184	191	199	206	213	221	228	235	242	250	258
73	144	151	159	166	174	182	189	197	204	212	219	227	235	242	250	257	265
74	148	155	163	171	179	186	194	202	210	218	225	233	241	249	256	264	272
75	152	160	168	176	184	192	200	208	216	224	232	240	248	256	264	272	279
76	156	164	172	180	189	197	205	213	221	230	238	246	254	263	271	279	287

BMI	36	37	38	39	40	41	42	43	44	45	46	47	48	49	50	51	52	53	54
58	172	177	181	186	191	196	201	205	210	215	220	224	229	234	239	244	248	253	258
59	178	183	188	193	198	203	208	212	217	222	227	232	237	242	247	252	257	262	267
60	184	189	194	199	204	209	215	220	225	230	235	240	245	250	255	261	266	271	276
61	190	195	201	206	211	217	222	227	232	238	243	248	254	259	264	269	275	280	285
62	196	202	207	213	218	224	229	235	240	246	251	256	262	267	273	278	284	289	295
63	203	208	214	220	225	231	237	242	248	254	259	265	270	278	282	287	293	299	304
64	209	215	221	227	232	238	244	250	256	262	267	273	279	285	291	296	302	308	314
65	216	222	228	234	240	246	252	258	264	270	276	282	288	294	300	306	312	318	324
66	223	229	235	241	247	253	260	266	272	278	284	291	297	303	309	315	322	328	334
67	230	236	242	249	255	261	268	274	280	287	293	299	306	312	319	325	331	338	344
68	236	243	249	256	262	269	276	282	289	295	302	308	315	322	328	335	341	348	354
69	243	250	257	263	270	277	284	291	297	304	311	318	324	331	338	345	351	358	365
70	250	257	264	271	278	285	292	299	306	313	320	327	334	341	348	355	362	369	376
71	257	265	272	279	286	293	301	308	315	322	329	338	343	351	358	365	372	379	386
72	265	272	279	287	294	302	309	316	324	331	338	346	353	361	368	375	383	390	397
73	272	280	288	295	302	310	318	325	333	340	348	355	363	371	378	386	393	401	408
74	280	287	295	303	311	319	326	334	342	350	358	365	373	381	389	396	404	412	420
75	287	295	303	311	319	327	335	343	351	359	367	375	383	391	399	407	415	423	431
76	295	304	312	320	328	336	344	353	361	369	377	385	394	402	410	418	426	435	443

BMI and Waist Circumference Three key anthropometric measurements are important to evaluate the degree of obesity—weight, height, and waist circumference. The body mass index (BMI), calculated as weight (kg)/height (m)^2, or as weight (lbs)/height (inches)$^2 \times$ 703, is used to classify weight status and risk of disease (Tables 75-1 and 75-2). BMI is used since it provides an estimate of body fat and is related to risk of disease. Lower BMI thresholds for overweight and obesity have been proposed for the Asia-Pacific region since this population appears to be at-risk at lower body weights for glucose and lipid abnormalities.

Excess abdominal fat, assessed by measurement of waist circumference or waist-to-hip ratio, is independently associated with higher risk for diabetes mellitus and cardiovascular disease. Measurement of the waist circumference is a surrogate for visceral adipose tissue and should be performed in the horizontal plane above the iliac crest. Cut points that define higher risk for men and women based on ethnicity have been proposed by the International Diabetes Federation (Table 75-3).

TABLE 75-2 CLASSIFICATION OF WEIGHT STATUS AND RISK OF DISEASE

	BMI (kg/m^2)	Obesity Class	Risk of Disease
Underweight	<18.5		
Healthy weight	18.5–24.9		
Overweight	25.0–29.9		Increased
Obesity	30.0–34.9	I	High
Obesity	35.0–39.9	II	Very high
Extreme Obesity	≥40	III	Extremely high

Source: Adapted from National Institutes of Health, National Heart, Lung, and Blood Institute: *Clinical Guidelines on the Identification, Evaluation, and Treatment of Overweight and Obesity in Adults.* U.S. Department of Health and Human Services, Public Health Service, 1998.

TABLE 75-3 ETHNIC-SPECIFIC VALUES FOR WAIST CIRCUMFERENCE

Ethnic Group	Waist Circumference
Europeans	
Men	>94 cm (37 in)
Women	>80 cm (31.5 in)
South Asians and Chinese	
Men	>90 cm (35 in)
Women	>80 cm (31.5 in)
Japanese	
Men	>85 cm (33.5 in)
Women	>90 cm (35 in)
Ethnic south and central Americans	Use south Asian recommendations until more specific data are available.
Sub-Saharan Africans	Use European data until more specific data are available.
Eastern Mediterranean and Middle East (Arab) populations	Use European data until more specific data are available.

Source: From KGMM Alberti et al for the IDF Epidemiology Task Force Consensus Group: The metabolic syndrome—a new worldwide definition. Lancet 366:1059, 2005.

Physical Fitness Several prospective studies have demonstrated that physical fitness, reported by questionnaire or measured by a maximal treadmill exercise test, is an important predictor of all-cause mortality independent of BMI and body composition. These observations highlight the importance of taking an exercise history during examination as well as emphasizing physical activity as a treatment approach.

Obesity-Associated Comorbid Conditions The evaluation of comorbid conditions should be based on presentation of symptoms, risk factors, and index of suspicion. All patients should have a fasting lipid panel (total, LDL, and HDL cholesterol and triglyceride levels) and blood glucose measured at presentation along with blood pressure determination. Symptoms and diseases that are directly or indirectly related to obesity are listed in Table 75-4. Although individuals vary, the number and severity of organ-specific comorbid conditions usually rise with increasing levels of obesity. Patients at very high absolute risk include the following: established coronary heart disease; presence of other atherosclerotic diseases such as peripheral arterial disease, abdominal aortic aneurysm, and symptomatic carotid artery disease; type 2 diabetes; and sleep apnea.

Assessing the Patient's Readiness to Change An attempt to initiate lifestyle changes when the patient is not ready usually leads to frustration and may hamper future weight-loss efforts. Assessment includes patient motivation and support, stressful life events, psychiatric status, time availability and constraints, and appropriateness of goals and expectations. Readiness can be viewed as the balance of two opposing forces: (1) motivation, or the patient's desire to change; and (2) resistance, or the patient's resistance to change.

A helpful method to begin a readiness assessment is to "anchor" the patient's interest and confidence to change on a numerical scale. Using this technique, the patient is asked to rate his or her level of interest and confidence on a scale from 0 to 10, with 0 being not so important (or confident) and 10 being very important (or confident) to lose weight at this time. This exercise helps to establish readiness to change and also serves as a basis for further dialogue.

℞ OBESITY

THE GOAL OF THERAPY The primary goal of treatment is to improve obesity-related comorbid conditions and reduce the risk of developing future comorbidities. Information obtained from the history, physical examination, and diagnostic tests is used to determine risk and develop a treatment plan (Fig. 75-1). The decision of how aggressively to treat the patient, and which modalities to use, is determined by the patient's risk status, expectations, and available resources. Therapy for obesity always begins with lifestyle management and may include pharmacotherapy or surgery, depending on BMI risk category (Table 75-5). Setting an initial weight-loss goal of 10% over 6 months is a realistic target.

LIFESTYLE MANAGEMENT Obesity care involves attention to three essential elements of lifestyle: dietary habits, physical activity, and behavior modification. Because obesity is fundamentally a disease of energy imbalance, all patients must learn how and when energy is consumed (diet), how and when energy is expended (physical activity), and how to incorporate this information into their daily life (behavior therapy). Lifestyle management has been shown to result in a modest (typically 3–5 kg) weight loss compared to no treatment or usual care.

Diet Therapy The primary focus of diet therapy is to reduce overall calorie consumption. The NHLBI guidelines recommend initiating treatment with a calorie deficit of 500–1000 kcal/d compared to the patient's habitual diet. This reduction is consistent with a goal of losing approximately 1–2 lb per week. This calorie deficit can be accomplished by suggesting substitutions or alternatives to the diet. Examples include choosing smaller portion sizes, eating more fruits and vegetables, consuming more whole-grain cereals, selecting leaner cuts of meat and skimmed dairy products, reducing fried foods and other added fats and oils, and drinking water instead of caloric beverages. It is important that the dietary counseling remains patient-centered and that the goals are practical, realistic, and achievable.

The macronutrient composition of the diet will vary depending on the patient's preference and medical condition. The 2005 U.S. Department of

TABLE 75-4 OBESITY-RELATED ORGAN SYSTEMS REVIEW

Cardiovascular	Respiratory
Hypertension	Dyspnea
Congestive heart failure	Obstructive sleep apnea
Cor pulmonale	Hypoventilation syndrome
Varicose veins	Pickwickian syndrome
Pulmonary embolism	Asthma
Coronary artery disease	**Gastrointestinal**
Endocrine	Gastroesophageal reflux disease
Metabolic syndrome	Nonalcoholic fatty liver disease
Type 2 diabetes	Cholelithiasis
Dyslipidemia	Hernias
Polycystic ovarian syndrome	Colon cancer
Musculoskeletal	**Genitourinary**
Hyperuricemia and gout	Urinary stress incontinence
Immobility	Obesity-related glomerulopathy
Osteoarthritis (knees and hips)	Hypogonadism (male)
Low back pain	Breast and uterine cancer
Carpal tunnel syndrome	Pregnancy complications
Psychological	**Neurologic**
Depression/low self-esteem	Stroke
Body image disturbance	Idiopathic intracranial hypertension
Social stigmatization	Meralgia paresthetica
Integument	Dementia
Striae distensae	
Stasis pigmentation of legs	
Lymphedema	
Cellulitis	
Intertrigo, carbuncles	
Acanthosis nigricans	
Acrochordon (skin tags)	
Hidradenitis suppurativa	

Agriculture Dietary Guidelines for Americans (Chap. 70), which focus on health promotion and risk reduction, can be applied to treatment of the overweight or obese patient. The recommendations include maintaining a diet rich in whole grains, fruits, vegetables, and dietary fiber; consuming two servings (8 oz) of fish high in omega 3 fatty acids per week; decreasing sodium to <2300 mg/d; consuming 3 cups of milk (or equivalent low-fat or fat-free dairy products) per day; limiting cholesterol to <300 mg/d; and keeping total fat between 20 and 35% of daily calories and saturated fats to <10% of daily calories. Application of these guidelines to specific calorie goals can be found on the website www.mypyramid.gov. The revised Dietary Reference Intakes for Macronutrients released by the Institute of Medicine recommends 45–65% of calories from carbohydrates, 20–35% from fat, and 10–35% from protein. The guidelines also recommend daily fiber intake of 38 g (men) and 25 g (women) for persons over 50 years of age and 30 g (men) and 21 g (women) for those under 50.

Since portion control is one of the most difficult strategies for patients to manage, the use of pre-prepared products, such as meal replacements, is a simple and convenient suggestion. Examples include frozen entrees, canned beverages and bars. Use of meal replacements in the diet has been shown to result in a 7–8% weight loss.

A current area of controversy is the use of low-carbohydrate, high-protein diets for weight loss. These diets are based on the concept that carbohydrates are the primary cause of obesity and lead to insulin resistance. Most low-carbohydrate diets (e.g., South Beach, Zone, and Sugar Busters!) recommend a carbohydrate level of approximately 40–46% of energy. The Atkins diet contains 5–15% carbohydrate, depending on the phase of the diet. Several randomized, controlled trials of these low-carbohydrate diets have demonstrated greater weight loss at 6 months with improvement in coronary heart disease risk factors, including an increase in HDL cholesterol and a decrease in triglyceride levels. Weight loss between groups did not remain statistically significant at 1 year; however, low-carbohydrate diets appear to be at least as effective as low-fat diets in inducing weight loss for up to 1 year.

Another dietary approach to consider is the concept of energy density, which refers to the number of calories (energy) a food contains per unit of weight. People tend to ingest a constant volume of food, regardless of caloric or macronutrient content. Adding water or fiber to a food decreases its energy density by increasing weight without affecting caloric content. Examples of foods with low-energy density include soups, fruits, vegetables, oatmeal, and lean meats. Dry foods and high-fat foods such as pret-

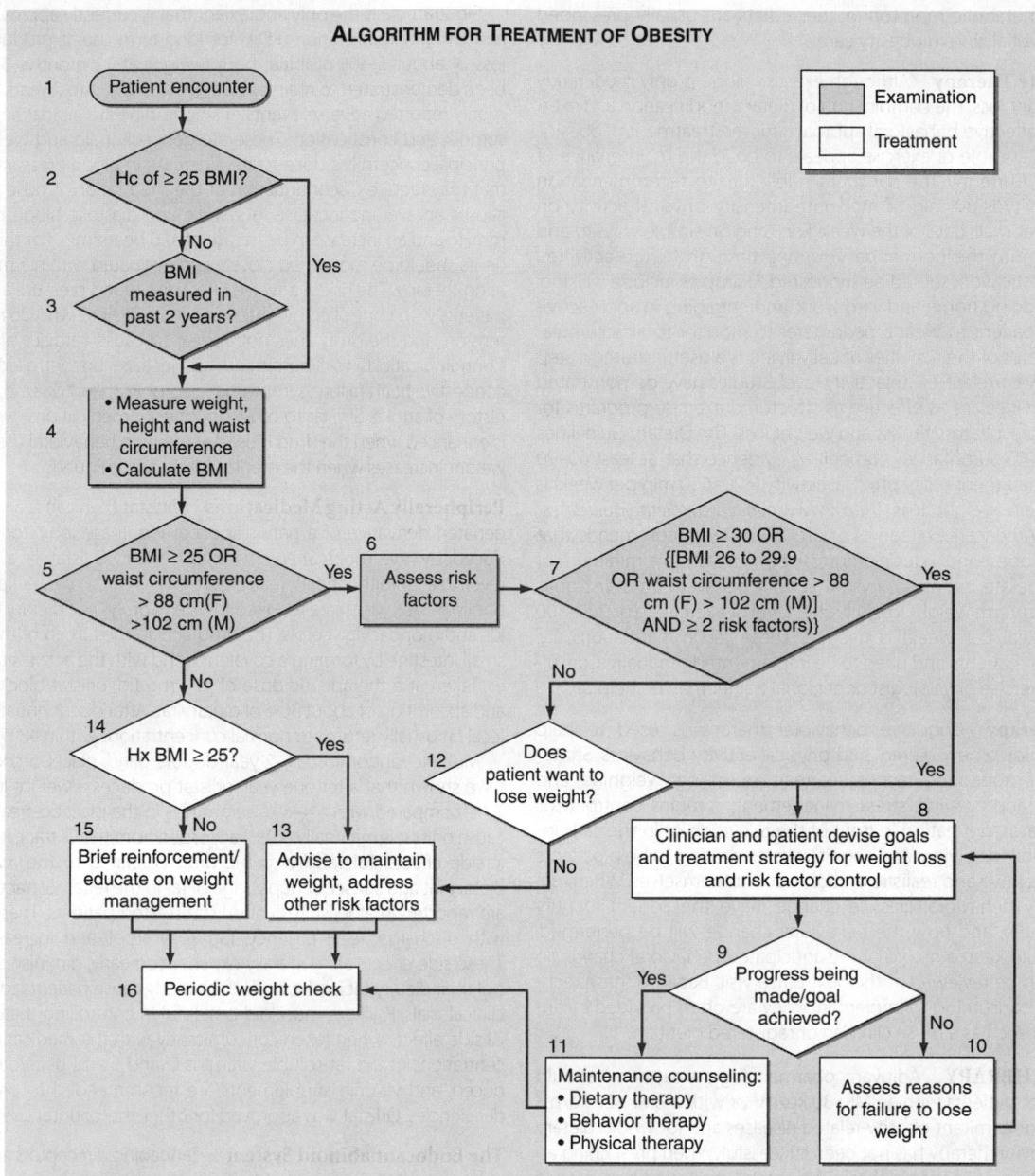

FIGURE 75-1 Treatment algorithm. This algorithm applies only to the assessment for overweight and obesity and subsequent decisions on that assessment. It does not reflect any initial overall assessment for other conditions that the physician may wish to perform. Ht, height; Hx, history; Wt, weight. *(From National, Heart, Lung, and Blood Institute: Clinical guidelines on the identification, evaluation, and treatment of overweight and obesity in adults: The evidence report. Washington, DC, US Department of Health and Human Services, 1998.)*

zels, cheese, egg yolks, potato chips, and red meat have a high-energy density. Diets containing low-energy dense foods have been shown to control hunger and result in decreased caloric intake and weight loss.

Occasionally, very-low-calorie diets (VLCDs) are prescribed as a form of aggressive dietary therapy. The primary purpose of a VLCD is to promote a rapid and significant (13–23 kg) short-term weight loss over a 3–6 month period. These propriety formulas typically supply ≤800 kcal, 50–80 g protein, and 100% of the recommended daily intake for vitamins and minerals. According to a review by the National Task Force on the Prevention and Treatment of Obesity, indications for initiating a VLCD include well-motivated individuals who are moderately to severely obese (BMI >30), have failed at more conservative approaches to weight loss, and have a medical condition that would be immediately improved with rapid weight loss. These conditions include poorly controlled type 2 diabetes, hypertriglyceridemia, obstructive sleep apnea, and symptomatic peripheral edema. The risk for gallstone formation increases exponentially at rates of weight loss >1.5 kg/week (3.3 lb/week). Prophylaxis against gallstone formation with ursodeoxycholic acid, 600 mg/d, is effective in reducing this risk. Because of the

TABLE 75-5 A GUIDE TO SELECTING TREATMENT

Treatment	BMI Category				
	25–26.9	27–29.9	30–35	35–39.9	≥40
Diet, exercise, behavior therapy	With comorbidities	With comorbidities	+	+	+
Pharmacotherapy		With comorbidities	+	+	+
Surgery				With comorbidities	+

Source: From National Heart, Lung, and Blood Institute, North American Association for the Study of Obesity (2000).

PART 5 Nutrition

need for close metabolic monitoring, these diets are usually prescribed by physicians specializing in obesity care.

Physical Activity Therapy Although exercise alone is only moderately effective for weight loss, the combination of dietary modification and exercise is the most effective behavioral approach for the treatment of obesity. The most important role of exercise appears to be in the maintenance of the weight loss. Currently, the *minimum* public health recommendation for physical activity is 30 min of moderate intensity physical activity on most, and preferably all, days of the week. Focusing on simple ways to add physical activity into the normal daily routine through leisure activities, travel, and domestic work should be suggested. Examples include walking, using the stairs, doing home and yard work, and engaging in sport activities. Asking the patient to wear a pedometer to monitor total accumulation of steps as part of the activities of daily living is a useful strategy. Step counts are highly correlated with activity level. Studies have demonstrated that lifestyle activities are as effective as structured exercise programs for improving cardiorespiratory fitness and weight loss. The Dietary Guidelines for Americans 2005 summarizes compelling evidence that at least 60–90 min of daily moderate-intensity physical activity (420–630 min per week) is needed to sustain weight loss (*http://www.health.gov/dietaryguidelines/dga2005/*). The American College of Sports Medicine recommends that overweight and obese individuals progressively increase to a minimum of 150 min of moderate intensity physical activity per week as a first goal. However, for long-term weight loss, a higher level of exercise (e.g., 200–300 min or ≥2000 kcal per week) is needed. These recommendations are daunting to most patients and need to be implemented gradually. Consultation with an exercise physiologist or personal trainer may be helpful.

Behavioral Therapy Cognitive behavioral therapy is used to help change and reinforce new dietary and physical activity behaviors. Strategies include self-monitoring techniques (e.g., journaling, weighing, and measuring food and activity); stress management; stimulus control (e.g., using smaller plates, not eating in front of the television or in the car); social support; problem solving; and cognitive restructuring to help patients develop more positive and realistic thoughts about themselves. When recommending any behavioral lifestyle change, have the patient identify what, when, where, and how the behavioral change will be performed. The patient should keep a record of the anticipated behavioral change so that progress can be reviewed at the next office visit. Because these techniques are time-consuming to implement, they are often provided by ancillary office staff such as a nurse clinician or registered dietitian.

PHARMACOTHERAPY Adjuvant pharmacologic treatments should be considered for patients with a BMI >30 kg/m^2 or with a BMI >27 kg/m^2 who also have concomitant obesity-related diseases and for whom dietary and physical activity therapy has not been successful. When prescribing an antiobesity medication, patients should be actively engaged in a lifestyle program that provides the strategies and skills needed to effectively use the drug since this support increases total weight loss.

There are several potential targets of pharmacologic therapy for obesity. The most thoroughly explored treatment is suppression of appetite via centrally active medications that alter monoamine neurotransmitters. A second strategy is to reduce the absorption of selective macronutrients from the gastrointestinal (GI) tract, such as fat. These two mechanisms form the basis for all currently prescribed antiobesity agents. A third target, selective blocking of the endocannabinoid system, has recently been identified.

Centrally Acting Anorexiant Medications Appetite-suppressing drugs, or anorexiants, affect satiety—the absence of hunger after eating—and hunger—a biologic sensation that initiates eating. By increasing satiety and decreasing hunger, these agents help patients reduce caloric intake without a sense of deprivation. The target site for the actions of anorexiants is the ventromedial and lateral hypothalamic regions in the central nervous system (Chap. 74). Their biological effect on appetite regulation is produced by augmenting the neurotransmission of three monoamines: norepinephrine; serotonin [5-hydroxytryptamine (5-HT)]; and, to a lesser degree, dopamine. The classic sympathomimetic adrenergic agents (benzphetamine, phendimetrazine, diethylpropion, mazindol, and phentermine) function by stimulating norepinephrine release or by blocking its reuptake. In contrast, sibutramine (Meridia) functions as a serotonin and norepinephrine reuptake inhibitor. Unlike other previously used anorexiants, sibutramine is not pharmacologically related to amphetamine and has no addictive potential.

Sibutramine is the only anorexiant that is currently approved by the Food and Drug Administration (FDA) for long-term use. It produces an average loss of about 5–9% of initial body weight at 12 months. Sibutramine has been demonstrated to maintain weight loss for up to 2 years. The most commonly reported adverse events of sibutramine are headache, dry mouth, insomnia, and constipation. These are generally mild and well-tolerated. The principal concern is a dose-related increase in blood pressure and heart rate that may require discontinuation of the medication. A dose of 10–15 mg/d causes an average increase in systolic and diastolic blood pressure of 2–4 mmHg and an increase in heart rate of 4–6 beats/min. For this reason, all patients should be monitored closely and evaluated within 1 month after initiating therapy. The risk of adverse effects on blood pressure are no greater in patients with controlled hypertension than in those who do not have hypertension, and the drug does not appear to cause cardiac valve dysfunction. Contraindications to sibutramine use include uncontrolled hypertension, congestive heart failure, symptomatic coronary heart disease, arrhythmias, or history of stroke. Similar to other antiobesity medications, weight reduction is enhanced when the drug is used along with behavioral therapy, and body weight increases when the medication is discontinued.

Peripherally Acting Medications Orlistat (Xenical) is a synthetic hydrogenated derivative of a naturally occurring lipase inhibitor, lipostatin, produced by the mold *Streptomyces toxytricini*. Orlistat is a potent, slowly reversible inhibitor of pancreatic, gastric, and carboxylester lipases and phospholipase A2, which are required for the hydrolysis of dietary fat into fatty acids and monoacylglycerols. The drug acts in the lumen of the stomach and small intestine by forming a covalent bond with the active site of these lipases. Taken at a therapeutic dose of 120 mg tid, orlistat blocks the digestion and absorption of about 30% of dietary fat. After discontinuation of the drug, fecal fat usually returns to normal concentrations within 48–72 h.

Multiple randomized, 1–2 year double-blind, placebo-controlled studies have shown that after one year, orlistat produces a weight loss of about 9–10%, compared with a 4–6% weight loss in the placebo-treated groups. Because orlistat is minimally (<1%) absorbed from the GI tract, it has no systemic side effects. Tolerability to the drug is related to the malabsorption of dietary fat and subsequent passage of fat in the feces. GI tract adverse effects are reported in at least 10% of orlistat-treated patients. These include flatus with discharge, fecal urgency, fatty/oily stool, and increased defecation. These side effects are generally experienced early, diminish as patients control their dietary fat intake, and infrequently cause patients to withdraw from clinical trials. Psyllium mucilloid is helpful in controlling the orlistat-induced GI side effects when taken concomitantly with the medication. Serum concentrations of the fat-soluble vitamins D and E and β–carotene may be reduced, and vitamin supplements are recommended to prevent potential deficiencies. Orlistat was approved for other-the-counter use in 2007.

The Endocannabinoid System Cannabinoid receptors and their endogenous ligands have been implicated in a variety of physiologic functions, including feeding, modulation of pain, emotional behavior, and peripheral lipid metabolism. Cannabis and its main ingredient, Δ^9-tetrahydrocannabinol (THC), is an exogenous cannabinoid compound. Two endocannabinoids have been identified, anandamide and 2-arachidonyl glyceride. Two cannabinoid receptors have been identified: CB_1 (abundant in the brain) and CB_2 (present in immune cells). The brain endocannabinoid system is thought to control food intake through reinforcing motivation to find and consume foods with high incentive value and to regulate actions of other mediators of appetite. The first selective cannabinoid CB_1 receptor antagonist, rimonabant, was discovered in 1994. The medication antagonizes the orexigenic effect of THC and suppresses appetite when given alone in animal models. Several large prospective, randomized controlled trials have demonstrated the effectiveness of rimonabant as a weight-loss agent. Taken as a 20 mg dose, subjects lost an average of 6.5 kg (14.32 lb) compared to 1.5 kg (3.3 lb) for placebo at 1 year. Concomitant improvements were seen in waist circumference and cardiovascular risk factors. The most common reported side effects include depression, anxiety, and nausea. FDA approval of Rimonabant is still pending.

SURGERY Bariatric surgery can be considered for patients with severe obesity (BMI ≥40 kg/m^2) or those with moderate obesity (BMI ≥35 kg/m^2) associated with a serious medical condition. Surgical weight loss functions by reducing caloric intake and, depending on the procedure, macronutrient absorption.

Weight-loss surgeries fall into one of two categories: restrictive and restrictive-malabsorptive (**Fig. 75-2**). Restrictive surgeries limit the amount of food the stomach can hold and slow the rate of gastric emptying. The vertical

FIGURE 75-2 Bariatric surgical procedures. Examples of operative interventions used for surgical manipulation of the gastrointestinal tract. **A.** Laparoscopic gastric band (LAGB). **B.** The Roux-en-Y gastric bypass. **C.** Biliopancreatic diversion with duodenal switch. **D.** Biliopancreatic diversion. (*From ML Kendrick, GF Dakin. Surgical approaches to obesity. Mayo Clin Proc 815:518, 2006; with permission.*)

banded gastroplasty (VBG) is the prototype of this category but is currently performed on a very limited basis due to lack of effectiveness in long-term trials. Laparoscopic adjustable silicone gastric banding (LASGB) has replaced the VBG as the most commonly performed restrictive operation. The first banding device, the lap-band, was approved for use in the United States in 2001. In contrast to previous devices, the diameter of this band is adjustable by way of its connection to a reservoir that is implanted under the skin. Injection or removal of saline into the reservoir tightens or loosens the band's internal diameter, thus changing the size of the gastric opening.

The three restrictive-malabsorptive bypass procedures combine the elements of gastric restriction and selective malabsorption. These procedures include Roux-en-Y gastric bypass (RYGB), biliopancreatic diversion (BPD), and biliopancreatic diversion with duodenal switch (BPDDS) (Fig. 75-2). RYGB is the most commonly performed and accepted bypass procedure. It may be performed with an open incision or laparoscopically.

Although no recent randomized controlled trials compare weight loss after surgical and nonsurgical interventions, data from meta-analyses and large databases, primarily obtained from observational studies, suggest that bariatric surgery is the most effective weight-loss therapy for those with clinically severe obesity. These procedures generally produce a 30–35% average total body weight loss that is maintained in nearly 60% of patients at 5 years. In general, mean weight loss is greater after the combined restrictive-malabsorptive procedures compared to the restrictive procedures. An abundance of data supports the positive impact of bariatric surgery on obesity-related morbid conditions, including diabetes mellitus, hypertension, obstructive sleep apnea, dyslipidemia, and nonalcoholic fatty liver disease.

Surgical mortality from bariatric surgery is generally <1% but varies with the procedure, patient's age and comorbid conditions, and experience of the surgical team. The most common surgical complications include stomal stenosis or marginal ulcers (occurring in 5–15% of patients) that present as prolonged nausea and vomiting after eating or inability to advance the diet to solid foods. These complications are typically treated by endoscopic balloon dilatation and acid suppression therapy, respectively. For patients who undergo LASGB, there are no intestinal absorptive abnormalities other than mechanical reduction in gastric size and outflow. Therefore, selective deficiencies occur uncommonly unless eating habits become unbalanced. In contrast, the restrictive-malabsorptive procedures increase risk for micronutrient deficiencies of vitamin B_{12}, iron, folate, calcium, and vitamin D. Patients with restrictive-malabsorptive procedures require lifelong supplementation with these micronutrients.

FURTHER READINGS

Bray GA, Greenway FL: Pharmacologic treatment of the overweight patient. Pharmacol Rev 59:151, 2007

Bray GA, Ryan DH: Drug treatment of the overweight patient. Gastroenterology 132(6):2239, 2007

Buchwald H et al: Bariatric surgery: A systematic review and meta-analysis. JAMA 292:1724, 2004

DeMaria EJ: Bariatric surgery for morbid obesity. N Engl J Med 356:2176, 2007

Haslam DW, James WPT: Obesity. Lancet 366:1197, 2005

Kushner RF: Roadmaps for clinical practice: Case studies in disease prevention and health promotion—assessment and management of adult obesity: A primer for physicians. Chicago, American Medical Association, 2003. (Available online at *www.ama-assn.org/ama/pub/category/10931.html*)

McTigue KM et al: Screening and interventions for obesity in adults: Summary of the evidence for the U.S. Preventive Services Task Force. Ann Intern Med 139:933, 2003. (Appendix tables available at *www.annals.org*)

National Heart, Lung, and Blood Institute, North American Association for the Study of Obesity: Practical guide: Identification, evaluation, and treatment of overweight and obesity in adults. Bethesda, MD, National Institutes of Health pub number 00-4084, Oct. 2000. Available online: *http://www.nhlbi.nih.gov/guidelines/obesity/practgde.htm*

Padwal R et al: Long-term pharmacotherapy for overweight and obesity: A systematic review and meta-analysis of randomized controlled trials. Int J Obesity 27:1437, 2003

Wadden TA et al: Lifestyle modification for the management of obesity. Gastroenterology 132(6):2226, 2007

76 Eating Disorders
B. Timothy Walsh

Anorexia nervosa and bulimia nervosa are characterized by severe disturbances of eating behavior. The salient feature of *anorexia nervosa* (AN) is a refusal to maintain a minimally normal body weight. *Bulimia nervosa* (BN) is characterized by recurrent episodes of binge eating followed by abnormal compensatory behaviors, such as self-induced vomiting. AN and BN are distinct clinical syndromes but share certain features in common. Both disorders occur primarily among previously healthy young women who become overly concerned with body shape and weight. Many patients with BN have past histories of anorexia nervosa, and many patients with AN engage in binge eating and purging behavior. In the current diagnostic system, the critical distinction between AN and BN depends on body weight: patients with AN are, by definition, significantly underweight, whereas patients with BN have body weights in the normal range or above.

Binge eating disorder (BED) is a more recently described syndrome characterized by repeated episodes of binge eating, similar to those of BN, in the absence of inappropriate compensatory behavior. Patients with BED are typically middle-aged men or women with significant obesity. They have an increased frequency of anxiety and depression compared to similarly obese patients without BED. It is not established that patients with BED are at increased risk for medical complications or that they require specific treatment interventions.

ANOREXIA NERVOSA

EPIDEMIOLOGY

Among women, the lifetime prevalence of the full syndrome of AN is approximately 1%. AN is much less common in males. AN is more prevalent in cultures where food is plentiful and in which being thin is associated with attractiveness. Individuals who pursue interests that place a premium on thinness, such as ballet and modeling, are at greater risk. The incidence of AN has increased in recent decades.

ETIOLOGY

The etiology of AN is unknown but appears to involve a combination of psychological, biologic, and cultural risk factors. Risk factors, such as sexual or physical abuse and a family history of mood disturbance, are best viewed as nonspecific risk factors that increase vulnerability to a range of psychiatric disorders, including AN.

Patients who develop AN are inclined to be more obsessional and perfectionist than their peers. The disorder often begins as a diet not distinguishable at the outset from those undertaken by many adolescents and young women. As weight loss progresses, the fear of gaining weight grows; dieting becomes stricter; and psychological, behavioral, and medical aberrations increase. Eating disorders, including AN, may develop among individuals with type 1 diabetes mellitus and are associated with poorer glycemic control and an increased frequency of complications (Chap. 338).

Numerous physiologic disturbances, including abnormalities in a variety of neurotransmitter systems, have been described in AN (see below). It is difficult to distinguish neurochemical, metabolic, and hormonal changes that may have a role in the initiation or perpetuation of the syndrome from those that are secondary to the disorder. The resolution of most of these abnormalities with weight restoration argues against an etiologic role.

Genetic factors contribute to the risk of development of AN, as its incidence is greater in families with one affected member and the concordance in monozygotic twins is greater than in dizygotic twins. However, specific genes have not been identified.

CLINICAL FEATURES

AN typically begins in mid to late adolescence, sometimes in association with a stressful life event such as leaving home for school (Table 76-1). The disorder occasionally develops in early puberty, before menarche, but seldom begins after age 40. Despite being underweight, patients with AN are irrationally afraid of gaining weight, often out of a concern that weight gain will get "out of control." They also exhibit a distortion of body image, which may express itself in several ways. For example, despite being emaciated, patients with AN may believe that their body as a whole, or some part of their body, is too fat. Further weight loss is viewed by the patient as a fulfilling accomplishment, while weight gain is seen as a personal failure. Patients with AN rarely complain of hunger or fatigue and often exercise extensively. Despite the denial of hunger, one-quarter to one-half of patients with AN engage in eating binges. Patients tend to become socially withdrawn and increasingly committed to work or study, dieting, and exercise. As weight loss progresses, thoughts of food dominate mental life and idiosyncratic rules develop around eating. Patients with AN may obsessively collect cookbooks and recipes and be drawn to food-related occupations.

Physical Features Patients with AN typically have few physical complaints but may note cold intolerance. Gastrointestinal motility is diminished, leading to reduced gastric emptying and constipation. Some women who develop AN after menarche report that their menses ceased before significant weight loss occurred. Weight and height should be measured to allow calculation of body mass index (BMI; kg/m^2). Vital signs may reveal bradycardia, hypotension, and mild hypothermia. Soft, downy hair growth (lanugo) sometimes occurs, and alopecia may be seen. Salivary gland enlargement, which is associated with starvation as well as with binge eating and vomiting, may make the face appear surprisingly full in contrast to the marked general wasting. Acrocyanosis of the digits is common, and peripheral edema can be seen in the absence of hypoalbuminemia, particularly when the patient begins to regain weight. Consumption of large amounts of vegetables containing vitamin A can result in a yellow tint to the skin (*hypercarotenemia*), which is especially notable on the palms.

Laboratory Abnormalities Mild normochromic, normocytic anemia is frequent, as is mild to moderate leukopenia, with a disproportionate reduction of polymorphonuclear leukocytes. Dehydration may result in slightly increased levels of blood urea nitrogen and creatinine. Serum transaminase levels may increase, especially during the early phases of refeeding. The level of serum proteins is usually normal. Blood sugar is often low and serum cholesterol may be moderately elevated. Hypokalemic alkalosis suggests self-induced vomiting or the use

---

TABLE 76-1 COMMON CHARACTERISTICS OF ANOREXIA NERVOSA AND BULIMIA NERVOSA

	Anorexia Nervosa[a]	Bulimia Nervosa
Clinical Characteristics		
Onset	Mid-adolescence	Late adolescence/early adulthood
Female:male	10:1	10:1
Lifetime prevalence in women	1%	1–3%
Weight	Markedly decreased	Usually normal
Menstruation	Absent	Usually normal
Binge eating	25–50%	Required for diagnosis
Mortality	~5% per decade	Low
Physical and Laboratory Findings[a]		
Skin/extremities	Lanugo	
	Acrocyanosis	
	Edema	
Cardiovascular	Bradycardia	
	Hypotension	
Gastrointestinal	Salivary gland enlargement	Salivary gland enlargement
	Slow gastric emptying	Dental erosion
	Constipation	
	Elevated liver enzymes	
Hematopoietic	Normochromic, normocytic anemia	
	Leukopenia	
Fluid/Electrolyte	Increased BUN, creatinine	Hypokalemia
	Hypokalemia	Hypochloremia
		Alkalosis
Endocrine	Hypoglycemia	
	Low estrogen or testosterone	
	Low LH and FSH	
	Low-normal thyroxine	
	Normal TSH	
	Increased cortisol	
Bone	Osteopenia	

[a]Patients with the binge-eating/purging subtype of anorexia nervosa may also exhibit the physical and laboratory findings associated with bulimia nervosa.

Abbreviations: BUN, blood urea nitrogen; LH, luteinizing hormone; FSH, follicle stimulating hormone; TSH, thyroid stimulating hormone.

of diuretics. Hyponatremia is common and may result from excess fluid intake and disturbances in the secretion of antidiuretic hormone.

Endocrine Abnormalities The regulation of virtually every endocrine system is altered in AN, but the most striking changes occur in the reproductive system. Amenorrhea is hypothalamic in origin and reflects diminished production of gonadotropin-releasing hormone (GnRH). When exogenous GnRH is administered in a pulsatile manner, pituitary responses of luteinizing hormone (LH) and follicle-stimulating hormone (FSH) are normalized, indicating the absence of a primary pituitary abnormality. The resulting gonadotropin deficiency causes low plasma estrogen in women and reduced testosterone in men. The hypothalamic GnRH pulse generator is exquisitely sensitive, particularly in women, to body weight, stress, and exercise, each of which may contribute to *hypothalamic amenorrhea* in AN (Chap. 341).

Serum leptin levels are markedly reduced in AN as a result of undernutrition and decreased body fat mass. The reduction in leptin appears to be the primary factor responsible for the disturbances of the hypothalamic-pituitary-gonadal axis, and to be an important mediator of the other neuroendocrine abnormalities characteristic of AN (Chap. 74).

Serum cortisol and 24-h urine free cortisol levels are generally elevated but without characteristic clinical signs of cortisol excess. Thyroid function tests resemble the pattern seen in euthyroid sick syndrome (Chap. 335). Thyroxine (T_4) and free T_4 levels are usually in the low-normal range, triiodothyronine (T_3) levels are reduced, and reverse T_3 (rT_3) is elevated. The level of thyroid-stimulating hormone (TSH) is normal or partially suppressed. Growth hormone is increased, but insulin-like growth factor 1 (IGF-1), which is produced mainly by the liver, is reduced, as in other conditions of starvation. Diminished bone density is routinely observed in AN and reflects the effects of multiple nutritional deficiencies, reduced gonadal steroids, and increased cortisol. The degree of bone density reduction is proportional to the length of the illness, and patients are at risk for the development of symptomatic fractures. The occurrence of AN during adolescence may lead to the premature cessation of linear bone growth and a failure to achieve expected adult height.

Cardiac Abnormalities Cardiac output is reduced, and congestive heart failure occurs rarely during rapid refeeding. The electrocardiogram usually shows sinus bradycardia, reduced QRS voltage, and nonspecific ST-T-wave abnormalities. Some patients develop a prolonged QT_c interval, which may predispose to serious arrhythmias, particularly when electrolyte abnormalities also are present.

DIAGNOSIS

The diagnosis of AN is based on the presence of characteristic behavioral, psychological, and physical attributes (Table 76-2). Widely accepted diagnostic criteria are provided by the American Psychiatric Association's *Diagnostic and Statistical Manual of Mental Disorders* (DSM-IV). These criteria include weight <85% of that expected for age and height, which is roughly equivalent to a BMI of 18.5 kg/m^2 for adult women. This weight criterion is somewhat arbitrary, so that a patient who meets all other diagnostic criteria but weighs between 85 and 90% of expected would still merit the diagnosis of AN. The current diagnostic criteria require that women with AN not have spontaneous menses, but occasional patients with the characteristics and complications of AN describe regular menstruation. Two mutually exclusive subtypes of AN are specified in DSM-IV. Patients whose weight loss

TABLE 76-2 DIAGNOSTIC FEATURES OF ANOREXIA NERVOSA

Refusal to maintain body weight at or above a minimally normal weight for age and height. (This includes a failure to achieve weight gain expected during a period of growth leading to an abnormally low body weight.)
Intense fear of weight gain or becoming fat.
Distortion of body image (e.g., feeling fat despite an objectively low weight or minimizing the seriousness of low weight).
Amenorrhea. (This criterion is met if menstrual periods occur only following hormone—e.g., estrogen—administration.)

is maintained primarily by caloric restriction, perhaps augmented by excessive exercise, are considered to have the "restricting" subtype of AN. The "binge eating/purging" subtype is characterized by binge eating and self-induced vomiting and/or laxative abuse. Patients with the binge/purge subtype are more prone to develop electrolyte imbalances, are more emotionally labile, and are more likely to have other problems with impulse control, such as drug abuse.

The diagnosis of AN can usually be made confidently in a patient with a history of weight loss accomplished by restrictive dieting and excessive exercise, accompanied by a marked reluctance to gain weight. Patients with AN often deny that they have a serious problem and may be brought to medical attention by concerned family or friends. In atypical presentations, other causes of significant weight loss in previously healthy young people should be considered, including inflammatory bowel disease, gastric outlet obstruction, diabetes mellitus, central nervous system (CNS) tumors, or neoplasm (Chap. 41).

PROGNOSIS

The course and outcome of AN are highly variable. One-quarter to one-half of patients eventually recover fully, with few psychological or physical sequelae. However, many patients have persistent difficulties with weight maintenance, depression, and eating disturbances, including BN. The development of obesity following AN is rare. The long-term mortality of AN is among the highest associated with any psychiatric disorder. Approximately 5% of patients die per decade of follow-up, primarily due to the physical effects of chronic starvation or by suicide.

Virtually all of the physiologic abnormalities associated with AN are observed in other forms of starvation and markedly improve or disappear with weight gain. A worrisome exception is the reduction in bone mass, which may not recover fully, particularly when AN occurs during adolescence when peak bone mass is normally achieved.

℞ ANOREXIA NERVOSA

Because of the profound physiologic and psychological effects of starvation, there is a broad consensus that weight restoration to at least 90% of predicted weight is the primary goal in the treatment of AN. Unfortunately, because most patients resist this goal, the management of AN is often accompanied by frustration for the patient, the family, and the physician. Patients typically exaggerate their food intake and minimize their symptoms. Some patients resort to subterfuge to make their weights appear higher, for example, by water-loading before they are weighed. In attempting to engage the patient in treatment, it may be useful for the physician to elicit the patient's physical concerns (e.g., about osteoporosis, weakness, or fertility) and, provide education about the importance of normalizing nutritional status in order to address those concerns. The physician should reassure the patient that weight gain will not be permitted to get "out of control" but simultaneously emphasize that weight restoration is medically and psychologically imperative.

The intensity of the initial treatment, including the need for hospitalization, is determined by the patient's current weight, the rapidity of recent weight loss, and the severity of medical and psychological complications (Fig. 76-1). Hospitalization should be strongly considered for patients weighing <75% of expected, even if the results of routine blood studies are within normal limits. Acute medical problems, such as severe electrolyte imbalances, should be identified and addressed. Nutritional restoration can almost always be successfully accomplished by oral feeding, and parenteral methods are rarely required. For severely underweight patients, sufficient calories (approximately 1200–1800 kcal/d) should be provided initially in divided meals as food or liquid supplements to maintain weight and to permit stabilization of fluid and electrolyte balance. Calories can then be gradually increased to achieve a weight gain of 1–2 kg (2–4 lb) per week, typically requiring an intake of 3000–4000 kcal/d. Meals must be supervised, ideally by personnel who are firm regarding the necessity of food consumption, empathic regarding the challenges entailed, and reassuring about the patient's eventual recovery. Patients have great psychological difficulty complying with the need for increased caloric consumption, and the assistance of psychiatrists or psychologists experienced in the treatment of AN is usually necessary.

Less severely affected patients may be treated in a partial hospitalization program where medical and psychiatric supervision is available and

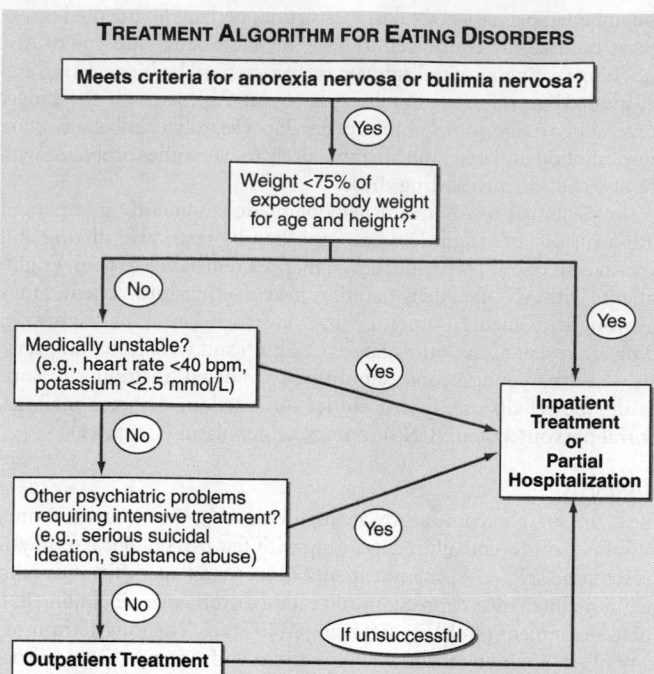

TREATMENT ALGORITHM FOR EATING DISORDERS

FIGURE 76-1 An algorithm for basic treatment decisions regarding patients with anorexia nervosa or bulimia nervosa. Based on the American Psychiatric Association's practice guidelines for the treatment of patients with eating disorders. *Although outpatient management may be considered for patients with anorexia nervosa weighing more than 75% of expected, there should be a low threshold for using more intensive interventions if the weight loss has been rapid or if current weight is <80% of expected.

several meals can be monitored each day. Outpatient treatment may suffice for mildly ill patients. Weight must be monitored at frequent intervals, and explicit goals agreed on for weight gain, with the understanding that more intensive treatment will be required if the level of care initially employed is not successful. For younger patients, the active involvement of the family in treatment is crucial regardless of the treatment venue.

Psychiatric treatment focuses primarily on two issues. First, patients require much emotional support during the period of weight gain. Patients often intellectually agree with the need to gain weight, but strenuously resist increases in caloric intake, and often surreptitiously discard food that is provided. Second, patients must learn to base their self-esteem not on the achievement of an inappropriately low weight, but on the development of satisfying personal relationships and the attainment of reasonable academic and occupational goals. While this is often possible, some patients with AN develop other serious emotional and behavioral symptoms such as depression, self-mutilation, obsessive-compulsive behavior, and suicidal ideation. These symptoms may require additional therapeutic interventions, in the form of psychotherapy, medication, or hospitalization.

Medical complications occasionally occur during refeeding. Especially in the early stages of treatment, severely malnourished patients may develop a "refeeding syndrome" characterized by hypophosphatemia, hypomagnesemia, and cardiovascular instability. Acute gastric dilatation has been described when refeeding is rapid. As in other forms of malnutrition, fluid retention and peripheral edema may occur, but they generally do not require specific treatment in the absence of cardiac, renal, or hepatic dysfunction. Transient modest elevations in serum liver enzyme levels occasionally occur. Multivitamins should be given, and an adequate intake of vitamin D (400 IU/d) and calcium (1500 mg/d) should be provided to minimize bone loss.

No psychotropic medications are of established value in the treatment of AN; tricyclic antidepressants are contraindicated when there is prolongation of the QT_c interval. The alterations of cortisol and thyroid hormone metabolism do not require specific treatment and are corrected by weight gain. Estrogen treatment appears to have minimal impact on bone density in underweight patients, and the small benefit of bisphosphonate treatment

appears to be outweighed by the potential risks of such agents in young women.

BULIMIA NERVOSA

EPIDEMIOLOGY

In women, the full syndrome of BN occurs with a lifetime prevalence of 1–3%. Variants of the disorder, such as occasional binge eating or purging, are much more common and occur in 5–10% of young women. The frequency of BN among men is less than one-tenth of that among women. The prevalence of BN increased dramatically in the early 1970s and 1980s but may have leveled off or declined somewhat in recent years.

ETIOLOGY

As with AN, the etiology of BN is likely to be multifactorial. Patients who develop BN describe a higher-than-expected prevalence of childhood and parental obesity, suggesting that a predisposition toward obesity may increase vulnerability to this eating disorder. The marked increase in the number of cases of BN during the past 25 years and the rarity of BN in underdeveloped countries suggest that cultural factors are important. Several biologic abnormalities in patients with BN may perpetuate this disorder once it has begun. These include abnormalities of CNS serotonergic function, which is involved in eating behavior, and disruption of peripheral satiety mechanisms, including the release of cholecystokinin (CCK) from the small intestine.

CLINICAL FEATURES

The typical patient presenting for treatment of BN is a woman of normal weight in her mid-twenties who reports binge eating and purging 5–10 times a week for 5–10 years (Table 76-3). The disorder usually begins in late adolescence or early adulthood during or following a diet, often in association with depressed mood. The self-imposed caloric restriction leads to increased hunger and to overeating. In an attempt to avoid weight gain, the patient induces vomiting, takes laxatives or diuretics, or engages in some other form of compensatory behavior. During binges, patients with this disorder tend to consume large amounts of sweet foods with a high fat content, such as dessert items. The most frequent compensatory behaviors are self-induced vomiting and laxative abuse, but a wide variety of techniques have been described, including the omission of insulin injections by individuals with type 1 diabetes mellitus. Initially, patients may experience a sense of satisfaction that appealing food can be eaten without weight gain. However, as the disorder progresses, patients perceive diminished control over eating. Binges increase in size and frequency and are provoked by a variety of stimuli, such as transient depression, anxiety, or a sense that too much food has been consumed in a normal meal. Between binges, patients restrict caloric intake, which increases hunger and sets the stage for the next binge. Typically, patients with BN are ashamed of their behavior and endeavor to keep their disorder hidden from family and friends. Like patients with AN, those with BN place an unusual emphasis on weight and shape as a basis for their self-esteem. Many patients with BN have mild symptoms of depression. Some patients exhibit serious mood and behavioral disturbances, such as suicide attempts, sexual promiscuity, and drug and alcohol abuse. Although vomiting may be

TABLE 76-3	DIAGNOSTIC FEATURES OF BULIMIA NERVOSA

Recurrent episodes of binge eating, which is characterized by the consumption of a large amount of food in a short period of time and a feeling that the eating is out of control.
Recurrent inappropriate behavior to compensate for the binge eating, such as self-induced vomiting.
The occurrence of both the binge eating and the inappropriate compensatory behavior at least twice weekly, on average, for 3 months.
Overconcern with body shape and weight.

Note: If the diagnostic criteria for anorexia nervosa are simultaneously met, only the diagnosis of anorexia nervosa is given.

triggered initially by manual stimulation of the gag reflex, most patients with BN develop the ability to induce vomiting at will. Rarely, patients resort to the regular use of syrup of ipecac. Laxatives and diuretics are frequently taken in impressive quantities, such as 30 or 60 laxative pills on a single occasion. The resulting fluid loss produces dehydration and a feeling of emptiness but has little impact on caloric balance.

The physical abnormalities associated with BN primarily result from the purging behavior. Painless bilateral salivary gland hypertrophy (sialadenosis) may be noted. A scar or callus on the dorsum of the hand may develop due to repeated trauma from the teeth among patients who manually stimulate the gag reflex. Recurrent vomiting and the exposure of the lingual surfaces of the teeth to stomach acid lead to loss of dental enamel and eventually to chipping and erosion of the front teeth. Laboratory abnormalities are surprisingly infrequent, but hypokalemia, hypochloremia, and hyponatremia are observed occasionally. Repeated vomiting may lead to alkalosis, whereas repeated laxative abuse may produce a mild metabolic acidosis. Serum amylase may be slightly elevated due to an increase in the salivary isoenzyme.

Serious physical complications resulting from BN are rare. Oligomenorrhea and amenorrhea are more frequent than among women without eating disorders. Arrhythmias occasionally occur secondary to electrolyte disturbances. Tearing of the esophagus and rupture of the stomach have been reported and constitute life-threatening events. Some patients who chronically abuse laxatives or diuretics develop transient peripheral edema when this behavior ceases, presumably due to high levels of aldosterone secondary to persistent fluid and electrolyte depletion.

DIAGNOSIS

The critical diagnostic features of BN are repeated episodes of binge eating followed by inappropriate and abnormal behaviors aimed at avoiding weight gain (Table 76-3). The diagnosis of BN requires a candid history from the patient detailing frequent, large eating binges followed by the purposeful use of inappropriate mechanisms to avoid weight gain. Most patients with BN who present for treatment are distressed by their inability to control their eating behavior but are able to provide such details if queried in a supportive and nonjudgmental fashion.

As in AN, there are two subtypes of BN. Patients with the "purging" subtype utilize compensatory behaviors that directly rid the body of calories or fluids (e.g., self-induced vomiting, laxative, or diuretic abuse), whereas those with the "nonpurging" subtype attempt to compensate for binges by fasting or by excessive exercise. Patients with the nonpurging subtype tend to be heavier and are less prone to fluid and electrolyte disturbances.

PROGNOSIS

The prognosis of BN is much more favorable than that of AN. Mortality is low, and full recovery occurs in approximately 50% of patients within 10 years. Approximately 25% of patients have persistent symptoms of BN over many years. Few patients progress from BN to AN.

Rx BULIMIA NERVOSA

BN can usually be treated on an outpatient basis (Fig. 76-1). Cognitive behavioral therapy (CBT) is a short-term (4–6 months) psychological treatment that focuses on the intense concern with shape and weight, the persistent dieting, and the binge eating and purging that characterize this disorder. Patients are directed to monitor the circumstances, thoughts, and emotions associated with binge/purge episodes, to eat regularly, and to challenge their assumptions linking weight to self-esteem. CBT produces symptomatic remission in 25–50% of patients.

Numerous double-blind, placebo-controlled trials have documented that antidepressant medications are useful in the treatment of BN but are probably somewhat less effective than CBT. Although efficacy has been established for virtually all chemical classes of antidepressants, only the selective serotonin reuptake inhibitor fluoxetine (Prozac) has been approved for use in BN by the U.S. Food and Drug Administration. Antidepressant medications are helpful even for patients with BN who are not depressed, and the dose of fluoxetine recommended for BN (60 mg/d) is higher than that typically used to treat depression. These observations suggest that different mechanisms may underlie the utility of these medications in BN and in depression.

A subset of patients does not respond to CBT, antidepressant medication, or their combination. More intensive forms of treatment, including hospitalization, may be required.

FURTHER READINGS

AMERICAN PSYCHIATRIC ASSOCIATION: Practice guidelines for the treatment of patients with eating disorders, third edition. Am J Psychiatry, 2006

CHAN JL, MANTZOROS CS: Role of leptin in energy-deprivation states: Normal human physiology and clinical implications for hypothalamic amenorrhoea and anorexia nervosa. Lancet 366:74, 2005

KATZMAN DK: Medical complications in adolescents with anorexia: A review of the literature. Int J Eat Disord 37(Suppl):S52, 2005

KESKI-RAHKONEN A et al: Epidemiology and course of anorexia nervosa in the community. Am J Psychiatry 164(8):1259, 2007

KLEIN DA, WALSH BT: Eating disorders: Clinical features and pathophysiology. Physiol Behav 81:359, 2004

MEHLER PS: Clinical practice. Bulimia nervosa. N Engl J Med 349:875, 2003

SYSKO R, WALSH BT: A critical evaluation of the efficacy of self-help interventions for the treatment of bulimia nervosa and binge-eating disorder. Int J Eat Disord Oct 5 2007, epub ahead of print

YAGER J, ANDERSEN AE: Clinical practice. Anorexia nervosa. N Engl J Med 353:1481, 2005

SECTION 1   **NEOPLASTIC DISORDERS**

77   Approach to the Patient with Cancer
Dan L. Longo

The application of current treatment techniques (surgery, radiation therapy, chemotherapy, and biological therapy) results in the cure of nearly two of three patients diagnosed with cancer. Nevertheless, patients experience the diagnosis of cancer as one of the most traumatic and revolutionary events that has ever happened to them. Independent of prognosis, the diagnosis brings with it a change in a person's self-image and in his or her role in the home and workplace. The prognosis of a person who has just been found to have pancreatic cancer is the same as the prognosis of the person with aortic stenosis who develops the first symptoms of congestive heart failure (median survival, ~8 months). However, the patient with heart disease may remain functional and maintain a self-image as a fully intact person with just a malfunctioning part, a diseased organ ("a bum ticker"). By contrast, the patient with pancreatic cancer has a completely altered self-image and is viewed differently by family and anyone who knows the diagnosis. He or she is being attacked and invaded by a disease that could be anywhere in the body. Every ache or pain takes on desperate significance. Cancer is an exception to the coordinated interaction among cells and organs. In general, the cells of a multicellular organism are programmed for collaboration. Many diseases occur because the specialized cells fail to perform their assigned task. Cancer takes this malfunction one step further. Not only is there a failure of the cancer cell to maintain its specialized function, but it also strikes out on its own; the cancer cell competes to survive using natural mutability and natural selection to seek advantage over normal cells in a recapitulation of evolution. One consequence of the traitorous behavior of cancer cells is that the patient feels betrayed by his or her body. The cancer patient feels that he or she, and not just a body part, is diseased.

THE MAGNITUDE OF THE PROBLEM

No nationwide cancer registry exists; therefore, the incidence of cancer is estimated on the basis of the National Cancer Institute's Surveillance, Epidemiology, and End Results (SEER) database, which tabulates cancer incidence and death figures from nine sites, accounting for about 10% of the U.S. population, and from population data from the U.S. Census Bureau. In 2007, 1.445 million new cases of invasive cancer (766,860 men, 678,060 women) were diagnosed and 559,650 persons (289,550 men, 270,100 women) died from cancer. The percent distribution of new cancer cases and cancer deaths by site for men and women are shown in Table 77-1. Cancer incidence has been declining by about 2% each year since 1992.

The most significant risk factor for cancer overall is age; two-thirds of all cases were in those over age 65. Cancer incidence increases as the third, fourth, or fifth power of age in different sites. For the interval between birth and age 39, 1 in 72 men and 1 in 51 women will develop cancer; for the interval between ages 40 and 59, 1 in 12 men and 1 in 11 women will develop cancer; and for the interval between ages 60 and 79, 1 in 3 men and 1 in 5 women will develop cancer. Overall, men have a 45% risk of developing cancer at some time during their lives; women have a 37% lifetime risk.

Cancer is the second leading cause of death behind heart disease. Deaths from heart disease have declined 45% in the United States

since 1950 and continue to decline. Cancer has overtaken heart disease as the number one cause of death in persons under age 85 years (Fig. 77-1). After a 70-year period of increases, cancer deaths began to decline in 1997 (Fig. 77-2). The five leading causes of cancer deaths are shown for various populations in Table 77-2. Along with the decrease in incidence has come an increase in survival for cancer patients. The 5-year survival for white patients was 39% in 1960–1963 and 68% in 1996–2002. Cancers are more often deadly in blacks; the 5-year survival was 57% for the 1996–2002 interval. Incidence and mortality vary among racial and ethnic groups (Table 77-3). The basis for these differences is unclear.

CANCER AROUND THE WORLD

In 2002, 11 million new cancer cases and 7 million cancer deaths were estimated worldwide. When broken down by region of the world, ~45% of cases were in Asia, 26% in Europe, 14.5% in North America, 7.1% in Central/South America, 6% in Africa, and 1% in Australia/New Zealand (Fig. 77-3). Lung cancer is the most common cancer and the most common cause of cancer death in the world. Its incidence is highly variable, affecting only 2 per 100,000 African women but as many as 61 per 100,000 North American men. Breast cancer is the second most common cancer worldwide; however, it ranks fifth as a cause of death behind lung, stomach, liver, and colorectal cancer. Among the eight most common forms of cancer, lung (2-fold), breast (3-fold), prostate (2.5-fold), and colorectal (3-fold) cancers are more common in more developed countries than in less developed countries. By contrast, liver (2-fold), cervical (2-fold), and esophageal (2- to 3-fold) cancers are more common in less developed

TABLE 77-1   DISTRIBUTION OF CANCER INCIDENCE AND DEATHS FOR 2007

Male			Female		
Sites	**%**	**Number**	**Sites**	**%**	**Number**
Cancer Incidence					
Prostate	29	218,890	Breast	26	178,480
Lung	15	114,760	Lung	15	98,620
Colorectal	10	79,130	Colorectal	11	74,630
Bladder	7	50,040	Endometrial	6	39,080
Lymphoma	4	34,200	Lymphoma	4	28,990
Melanoma	4	33,910	Melanoma	4	26,030
Kidney	4	31,590	Thyroid	4	25,480
Leukemia	3	24,800	Ovary	3	22,430
Oral cavity	3	24,180	Kidney	3	19,600
Pancreas	2	18,830	Leukemia	3	19,440
All others	18	136,530	All others	21	145,280
All sites	100	776,860	All sites	100	678,060
Cancer Deaths					
Lung	31	89,510	Lung	26	70,880
Prostate	9	27,050	Breast	15	40,460
Colorectal	9	26,000	Colorectal	10	26,180
Pancreas	6	16,840	Pancreas	6	16,530
Leukemia	4	12,320	Ovary	6	15,280
Liver	4	11,280	Leukemia	4	9470
Esophagus	4	10,900	Lymphoma	3	9060
Bladder	3	9630	Endometrial	3	7400
Lymphoma	3	9600	CNS	2	5590
Kidney	3	8080	Liver	2	5500
All others	24	68,340	All others	23	63,750
All sites	100	289,550	All sites	100	270,100

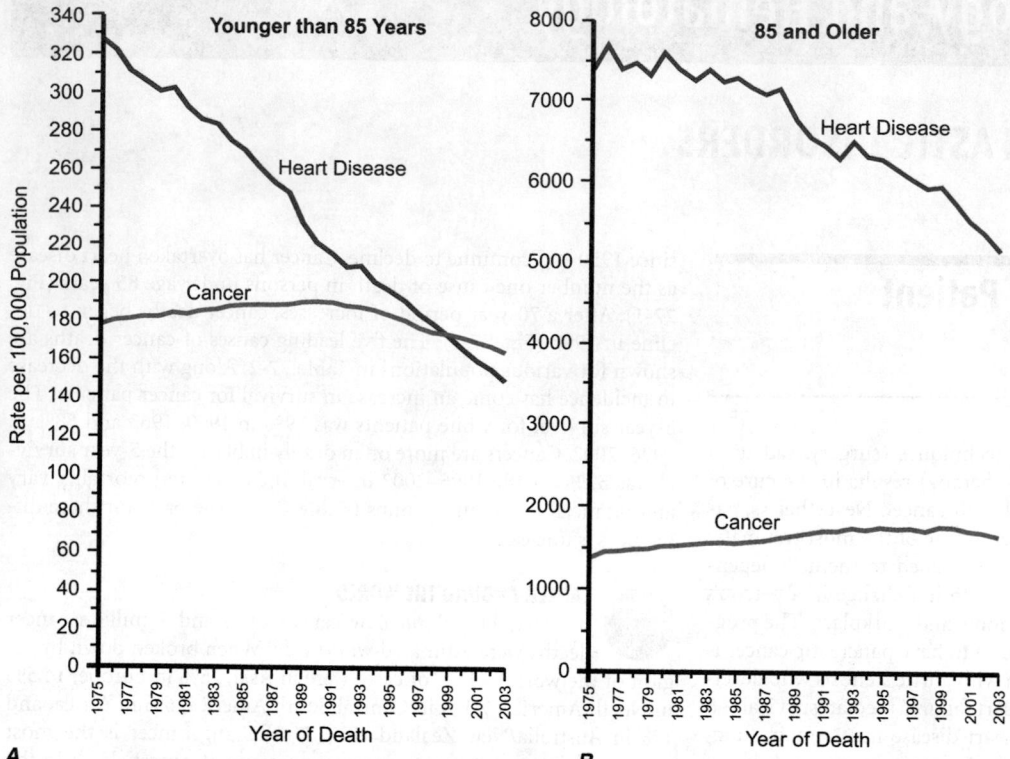

FIGURE 77-1 Death rates for heart disease and cancer among people younger and older than age 85. **A.** In people younger than 85 years, cancer has overtaken heart disease as the largest cause of death. **B.** In people over 85 years, heart disease is by far the major cause of death. *(From Jemal et al.)*

countries. Stomach cancer incidence is similar in more and less developed countries but is much more common in Asia than North America or Africa. The most common cancers in Africa are cervical, breast, and liver cancers. It has been estimated that nine modifiable risk factors are responsible for more than one-third of cancers worldwide. These include smoking, alcohol consumption, obesity, physical inactivity, low fruit and vegetable consumption, unsafe sex, air pollution, indoor smoke from household fuels, and contaminated injections.

PATIENT MANAGEMENT

Important information is obtained from every portion of the routine history and physical examination. The duration of symptoms may reveal the chronicity of disease. The past medical history may alert the physician to the presence of underlying diseases that may affect the choice of therapy or the side effects of treatment. The social history may reveal occupational exposure to carcinogens or habits, such as smoking or alcohol consumption, that may influence the course of disease and its treatment. The family history may suggest an underlying familial cancer predisposition and point out the need to begin surveillance or other preventive therapy for unaffected siblings of the patient. The review of systems may suggest early symptoms of metastatic disease or a paraneoplastic syndrome.

DIAGNOSIS

The diagnosis of cancer relies most heavily on invasive tissue biopsy and should never be made without obtaining tissue; no noninvasive diagnostic test is sufficient to define a disease process as cancer. Although in rare clinical settings (e.g., thyroid nodules) fine-needle aspiration is an acceptable diagnostic procedure, the diagnosis generally depends on obtaining adequate tissue to permit careful evaluation of the histology of the tumor, its grade, and its invasiveness and to yield further molecular diagnostic information, such as the expression of cell-surface markers or intracellular proteins that typify a particular cancer, or the presence of a molecular marker, such as the t(8;14) translocation of Burkitt's lymphoma. Increasing evidence links the expression of certain genes with the

prognosis and response to therapy (Chaps. 79, 80).

Occasionally a patient will present with a metastatic disease process that is defined as cancer on biopsy but has no apparent primary site of disease. Efforts should be made to define the primary site based on age, sex, sites of involvement, histology and tumor markers, and personal and family history. Particular attention should be focused on ruling out the most treatable causes (Chap. 95).

Once the diagnosis of cancer is made, the management of the patient is best undertaken as a multidisciplinary collaboration among the primary care physician, medical oncologists, surgical oncologists, radiation oncologists, oncology nurse specialists, pharmacists, social workers, rehabilitation medicine specialists, and a number of other consulting professionals working closely with each other and with the patient and family.

DEFINING THE EXTENT OF DISEASE AND THE PROGNOSIS

The first priority in patient management after the diagnosis of cancer is established and shared with the patient is to determine the extent of disease. The curability of a tumor usually is inversely proportional to the tumor burden. Ideally, the tumor will be diagnosed before symptoms develop or as a consequence of screening efforts (Chap. 78). A very high proportion of such patients can be cured. However, most patients with cancer present with symptoms related to the cancer, caused either by mass effects of the tumor or by alterations associated with the production of cytokines or hormones by the tumor.

For most cancers, the extent of disease is evaluated by a variety of noninvasive and invasive diagnostic tests and procedures. This process is called *staging*. There are two types. *Clinical staging* is based on physical examination, radiographs, isotopic scans, CT scans, and other imaging procedures; *pathologic staging* takes into account information obtained during a surgical procedure, which might include intraoperative palpation, resection of regional lymph nodes and/or tissue adjacent to the tumor, and inspection and biopsy of organs commonly involved in disease spread. Pathologic staging includes histologic examination of all tissues removed during the surgical procedure. Surgical procedures performed may include a simple lymph node biopsy or more extensive procedures such as thoracotomy, mediastinoscopy, or laparotomy. Surgical staging may occur in a separate procedure or may be done at the time of definitive surgical resection of the primary tumor.

Knowledge of the predilection of particular tumors for spread to adjacent or distant organs helps direct the staging evaluation.

Information obtained from staging is used to define the extent of disease either as localized, as exhibiting spread outside of the organ of origin to regional but not distant sites, or as metastatic to distant sites. The most widely used system of staging is the TNM (tumor, node, metastasis) system codified by the International Union Against Cancer and the American Joint Committee on Cancer (AJCC). The TNM classification is an anatomically based system that categorizes the tumor on the basis of the size of the primary tumor lesion (T1–4, where a higher number indicates a tumor of larger size), the presence of nodal involvement (usually N0 and N1 for the absence and presence, respectively, of involved nodes, although some tumors have more elaborate

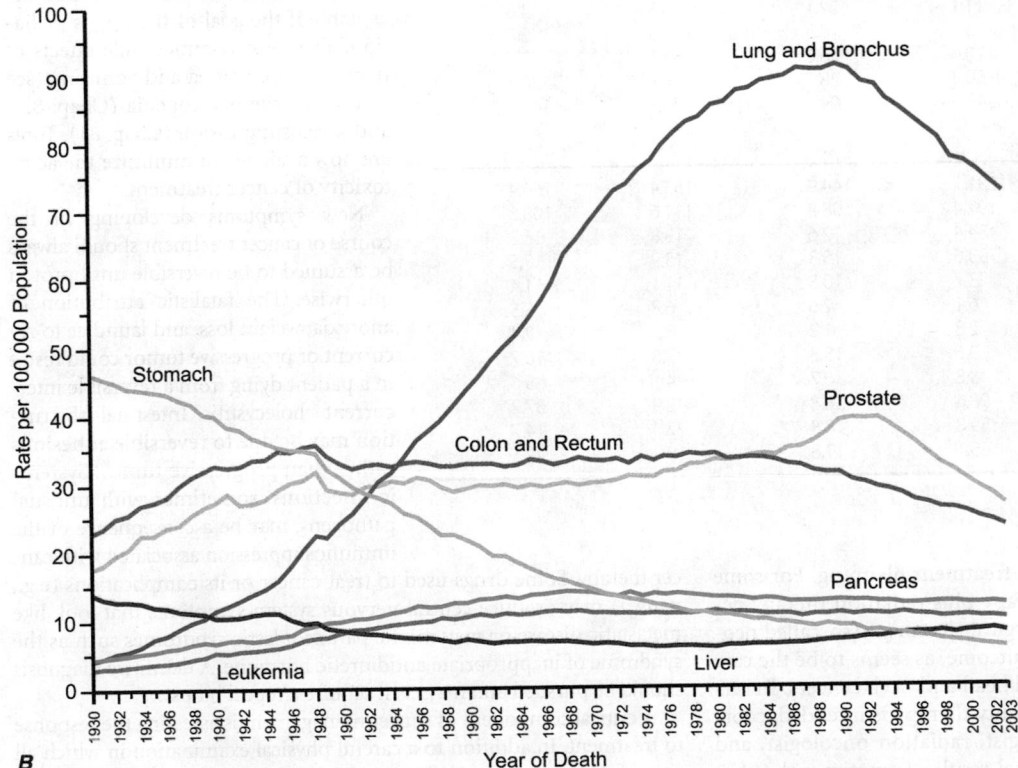

FIGURE 77-2 Sixty-year trend in cancer death rates for (**A**) women and (**B**) men, by site in the United States, 1930–2003. Rates are per 100,000 age-adjusted to the 2000 U.S. standard population. (*From Jemal et al.*)

Obstetricians (FIGO) classification for gynecologic cancers, and the Ann Arbor classification for Hodgkin's disease.[1]

Certain tumors cannot be grouped on the basis of anatomic considerations. For example, hematopoietic tumors such as leukemia, myeloma, and lymphoma are often disseminated at presentation and do not spread like solid tumors. For these tumors, other prognostic factors have been identified (Chaps. 104–106).

In addition to tumor burden, a second major determinant of treatment outcome is the physiologic reserve of the patient. Patients who are bedridden before developing cancer are likely to fare worse, stage for stage, than fully active patients. Physiologic reserve is a determinant of how a patient is likely to cope with the physiologic stresses imposed by the cancer and its treatment. This factor is difficult to assess directly. Instead, surrogate markers for physiologic reserve are used, such as the patient's age or Karnofsky performance status (Table 77-4). Older patients and those with a Karnofsky performance status <70 have a poor prognosis unless the poor performance is a reversible consequence of the tumor.

Increasingly, biologic features of the tumor are being related to prognosis. The expression of particular oncogenes, drug-resistance genes, apoptosis-related genes, and genes involved in metastasis are being found to influence response to therapy and prognosis. The presence of selected cytogenetic abnormalities may influence survival. Tumors with higher growth fractions, as assessed by expression of proliferation-related markers such as proliferating cell nuclear antigen (PCNA), behave more aggressively than tumors with lower growth fractions. Information obtained from studying the tumor itself will increasingly be used to influence treatment decisions. Host genes involved in drug metabolism can influence the safety and efficacy of particular treatments.

systems of nodal grading), and the presence of metastatic disease (M0 and M1 for the absence and presence, respectively, of metastases). The various permutations of T, N, and M scores (sometimes including tumor histologic grade G) are then broken into stages, usually designated by the roman numerals I through IV. Tumor burden increases and curability decreases with increasing stage. Other anatomic staging systems are used for some tumors, e.g., the Dukes classification for colorectal cancers, the International Federation of Gynecologists and

MAKING A TREATMENT PLAN

From information on the extent of disease and the prognosis and in conjunction with the patient's wishes, it is determined whether the treatment approach should be curative or palliative in intent. Cooperation among the various professionals involved in cancer treat-

[1]The AJCC *Manual for Staging Cancer*, 5th edition, can be obtained from the AJCC at 55 East Erie Street, Chicago, IL, 60611.

PART 6

Oncology and Hematology

TABLE 77-2 THE FIVE LEADING PRIMARY TUMOR SITES FOR PATIENTS DYING OF CANCER BASED ON AGE AND SEX IN 2004

Rank		All Ages	Age, years				
			Under 20	20–39	40–59	60–79	>80
1	M	Lung	Leukemia	Leukemia	Lung	Lung	Lung
	F	Lung	Leukemia	Breast	Breast	Lung	Lung
2	M	Prostate	CNS	CNS	Colorectal	Colorectal	Prostate
	F	Breast	CNS	Cervix	Lung	Breast	Colorectal
3	M	Colorectal	Bone sarcoma	Colorectal	Pancreas	Prostate	Colorectal
	F	Colorectal	Endocrine	Leukemia	Colorectal	Colorectal	Breast
4	M	Pancreas	Endocrine	Lymphoma	Liver	Pancreas	Bladder
	F	Pancreas	Soft tissue sarcoma	Colorectal	Ovary	Pancreas	Pancreas
5	M	Leukemia	Soft tissue sarcoma	Lung	Esophagus	Leukemia	Pancreas
	F	Ovary	Bone sarcoma	CNS	Pancreas	Ovary	Lymphoma

Note: M, male; F, female.

TABLE 77-3 CANCER INCIDENCE AND MORTALITY IN RACIAL AND ETHNIC GROUPS, U.S., 1999–2003

Site		White	Black	Asian/Pacific Islander	American Indian	Hispanic
Incidence per 100,000 Population						
All	M	555	639.8	385.5	359.9	444.1
	F	421.1	383.8	303.3	305	327.2
Breast		130.8	111.5	91.2	74.4	92.6
Colorectal	M	63.7	70.2	52.6	52.7	52.4
	F	45.9	53.5	38.0	41.9	37.3
Kidney	M	18	18.5	9.8	20.9	16.9
	F	9.3	9.5	4.9	10	9.4
Liver	M	7.2	11.1	22.1	14.5	14.8
	F	2.7	3.6	8.3	6.5	5.8
Lung	M	88.8	110.6	56.6	55.5	52.7
	F	56.2	50.3	28.7	33.8	26.7
Prostate		156	243	104	70.7	141.1
Deaths per 100,000 Population						
All	M	239.2	331	144.9	153.4	166.4
	F	163.4	192.4	98.8	111.6	108.8
Breast		25.4	34.4	12.6	13.8	16.3
Colorectal	M	23.7	33.6	15.3	15.9	17.5
	F	16.4	23.7	10.5	11.1	11.4
Kidney	M	6.2	6.1	2.6	6.8	5.5
	F	2.8	2.8	1.2	3.3	2.4
Liver	M	6.3	9.6	15.5	7.8	10.7
	F	2.8	3.8	6.7	4	5
Lung	M	73.8	98.4	38.8	42.9	37.2
	F	42	39.8	18.8	27	14.7
Prostate		26.7	65.1	11.8	18	22.1

Note: M, male; F, female.

ment is of the utmost importance in treatment planning. For some cancers, chemotherapy or chemotherapy plus radiation therapy delivered before the use of definitive surgical treatment (so-called neo-adjuvant therapy) may improve the outcome, as seems to be the case for locally advanced breast cancer and head and neck cancers. In certain settings in which combined modality therapy is intended, coordination among the medical oncologist, radiation oncologist, and surgeon is crucial to achieving optimal results. Sometimes the chemotherapy and radiation therapy need to be delivered sequentially, and other times concurrently. Surgical procedures may precede or follow other treatment approaches. It is best for the treatment plan either to follow a standard protocol precisely or else to be part of an ongoing clinical research protocol evaluating new treatments. Ad hoc modifications of standard protocols are likely to compromise treatment results.

The choice of treatment approaches was formerly dominated by the local culture in both the university and the practice settings. However, it is now possible to gain access electronically to standard treatment protocols and to every approved clinical research study

in North America through a personal computer interface with the Internet.[2]

The skilled physician also has much to offer the patient for whom curative therapy is no longer an option. Often a combination of guilt and frustration over the inability to cure the patient and the pressure of a busy schedule greatly limit the time a physician spends with a patient who is receiving only palliative care. Resist these forces. In addition to the medicines administered to alleviate symptoms (see below), it is important to remember the comfort that is provided by holding the patient's hand, continuing regular examinations, and taking time to talk.

MANAGEMENT OF DISEASE AND TREATMENT COMPLICATIONS

Because cancer therapies are toxic (Chap. 81), patient management involves addressing complications of both the disease and its treatment as well as the complex psychosocial problems associated with cancer. In the short term during a course of curative therapy, the patient's functional status may decline. Treatment-induced toxicity is less acceptable if the goal of therapy is palliation. The most common side effects of treatment are nausea and vomiting (see below), febrile neutropenia (Chap. 82), and myelosuppression (Chap. 81). Tools are now available to minimize the acute toxicity of cancer treatment.

New symptoms developing in the course of cancer treatment should always be assumed to be reversible until proven otherwise. The fatalistic attribution of anorexia, weight loss, and jaundice to recurrent or progressive tumor could result in a patient dying from a reversible intercurrent cholecystitis. Intestinal obstruction may be due to reversible adhesions rather than progressive tumor. Systemic infections, sometimes with unusual pathogens, may be a consequence of the immunosuppression associated with cancer therapy. Some drugs used to treat cancer or its complications (e.g., nausea) may produce central nervous system symptoms that look like metastatic disease or may mimic paraneoplastic syndromes such as the syndrome of inappropriate antidiuretic hormone. A definitive diagnosis should be pursued and may even require a repeat biopsy.

A critical component of cancer management is assessing the response to treatment. In addition to a careful physical examination in which all sites of disease are physically measured and recorded in a flow chart by date, response assessment usually requires periodic repeating of imaging

---

[2]The National Cancer Institute maintains a database called PDQ (Physician Data Query) that is accessible on the Internet under the name CancerNet at *wwwicic.nci.nih.gov/health.htm*. Information can be obtained through a facsimile machine using CancerFax by dialing 301-402-5874. Patient information is also provided by the National Cancer Institute in at least three formats: on the Internet via CancerNet at *wwwicic.nci.nih.gov/patient.htm*, through the CancerFax number listed above, or by calling 1-800-4-CANCER. The quality control for the information provided through these services is rigorous.

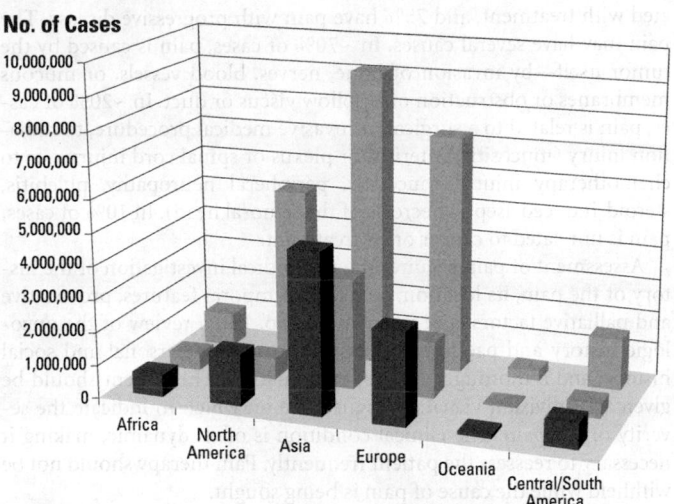

No. of Cases

Geographic Region

■ Incidence (n = 10,864,499) ■ Mortality (n = 6,724,931) ■ Prevalence (n = 24,576,453)

FIGURE 77-3 Worldwide overall annual cancer incidence, mortality and 5-year prevalence for the period of 1993–2001. (*From Kamangar et al.*)

tests that were abnormal at the time of staging. If imaging tests have become normal, repeat biopsy of previously involved tissue is performed to document complete response by pathologic criteria. Biopsies are not usually required if there is macroscopic residual disease. A *complete response* is defined as disappearance of all evidence of disease, and a *partial response* as >50% reduction in the sum of the products of the perpendicular diameters of all measurable lesions. The determination of partial response may also be based on a 30% decrease in the sums of the longest diameters of lesions (Response Evaluation Criteria in Solid Tumors, or RECIST, criteria). *Progressive disease* is defined as the appearance of any new lesion or an increase of >25% in the sum of the products of the perpendicular diameters of all measurable lesions (or an increase of 20% in the sums of the longest diameters by RECIST). Tumor shrinkage or growth that does not meet any of these criteria is considered *stable disease*. Some sites of involvement (e.g., bone) or patterns of involvement (e.g., lymphangitic lung or diffuse pulmonary infiltrates) are considered unmeasurable. No response is complete without biopsy documentation of their resolution, but partial responses may exclude their assessment unless clear objective progression has occurred.

Tumor markers may be useful in patient management in certain tumors. Response to therapy may be difficult to gauge with certainty. However, some tumors produce or elicit the production of markers that can be measured in the serum or urine and, in a particular patient, rising and falling levels of the marker are usually associated with increasing or decreasing tumor burden, respectively. Some clinically useful tumor markers are shown in Table 77-5. Tumor markers are not in themselves specific enough to permit a diagnosis of malignancy to be made, but once a malignancy has been diagnosed and shown

to be associated with elevated levels of a tumor marker, the marker can be used to assess response to treatment.

The recognition and treatment of depression are important components of management. The incidence of depression in cancer patients is ~25% overall and may be greater in patients with greater debility. This diagnosis is likely in a patient with a depressed mood (dysphoria) and/or a loss of interest in pleasure (anhedonia) for at least 2 weeks. In addition, three or more of the following symptoms are usually present: appetite change, sleep problems, psychomotor retardation or agitation, fatigue, feelings of guilt or worthlessness, inability to concentrate, and suicidal ideation. Patients with these symptoms should receive therapy. Medical therapy with a serotonin reuptake inhibitor such as fluoxetine (10–20 mg/d), sertraline (50–150 mg/d), or paroxetine (10–20 mg/d) or a tricyclic antidepressant such as amitriptyline (50–100 mg/d) or desipramine

TABLE 77-4 KARNOFSKY PERFORMANCE INDEX

Performance Status	Functional Capability of the Patient
100	Normal; no complaints; no evidence of disease
90	Able to carry on normal activity; minor signs or symptoms of disease
80	Normal activity with effort; some signs or symptoms of disease
70	Cares for self; unable to carry on normal activity or do active work
60	Requires occasional assistance but is able to care for most needs
50	Requires considerable assistance and frequent medical care
40	Disabled; requires special care and assistance
30	Severely disabled; hospitalization is indicated although death is not imminent
20	Very sick; hospitalization necessary; active supportive treatment is necessary
10	Moribund, fatal processes progressing rapidly
0	Dead

TABLE 77-5 TUMOR MARKERS

Tumor Markers	Cancer	Non-Neoplastic Conditions
Hormones		
Human chorionic gonadotropin	Gestational trophoblastic disease, gonadal germ cell tumor	Pregnancy
Calcitonin	Medullary cancer of the thyroid	
Catecholamines	Pheochromocytoma	
Oncofetal Antigens		
Alphafetoprotein	Hepatocellular carcinoma, gonadal germ cell tumor	Cirrhosis, hepatitis
Carcinoembryonic antigen	Adenocarcinomas of the colon, pancreas, lung, breast, ovary	Pancreatitis, hepatitis, inflammatory bowel disease, smoking
Enzymes		
Prostatic acid phosphatase	Prostate cancer	Prostatitis, prostatic hypertrophy
Neuron-specific enolase	Small cell cancer of the lung, neuroblastoma	
Lactate dehydrogenase	Lymphoma, Ewing's sarcoma	Hepatitis, hemolytic anemia, many others
Tumor-Associated Proteins		
Prostate-specific antigen	Prostate cancer	Prostatitis, prostatic hypertrophy
Monoclonal immunoglobulin	Myeloma	Infection, MGUS[a]
CA-125	Ovarian cancer, some lymphomas	Menstruation, peritonitis, pregnancy
CA 19-9	Colon, pancreatic, breast cancer	Pancreatitis, ulcerative colitis
CD30	Hodgkin's disease, anaplastic large cell lymphoma	—
CD25	Hairy cell leukemia, adult T cell leukemia/lymphoma	—

[a]MGUS, monoclonal gammopathy of uncertain significance.

CHAPTER 77 Approach to the Patient with Cancer

(75–150 mg/d) should be tried, allowing 4–6 weeks for response. Effective therapy should be continued at least 6 months after resolution of symptoms. If therapy is unsuccessful, other classes of antidepressants may be used. In addition to medication, psychosocial interventions such as support groups, psychotherapy, and guided imagery may be of benefit.

Many patients opt for unproven or unsound approaches to treatment when it appears that conventional medicine is unlikely to be curative. Those seeking such alternatives are often well educated and may be early in the course of their disease. Unsound approaches are usually hawked on the basis of unsubstantiated anecdotes and not only cannot help the patient but may be harmful. Physicians should strive to keep communications open and nonjudgmental, so that patients are more likely to discuss with the physician what they are actually doing. The appearance of unexpected toxicity may be an indication that a supplemental therapy is being taken.[3]

LONG-TERM FOLLOW-UP/LATE COMPLICATIONS

At the completion of treatment, sites originally involved with tumor are reassessed, usually by radiography or imaging techniques, and any persistent abnormality is biopsied. If disease persists, the multidisciplinary team discusses a new salvage treatment plan. If the patient has been rendered disease-free by the original treatment, the patient is followed regularly for disease recurrence. The optimal guidelines for follow-up care are not known. For many years, a routine practice has been to follow the patient monthly for 6–12 months, then every other month for a year, every 3 months for a year, every 4 months for a year, every 6 months for a year, and then annually. At each visit, a battery of laboratory and radiographic and imaging tests were obtained on the assumption that it is best to detect recurrent disease before it becomes symptomatic. However, where follow-up procedures have been examined, this assumption has been found to be untrue. Studies of breast cancer, melanoma, lung cancer, colon cancer, and lymphoma have all failed to support the notion that asymptomatic relapses are more readily cured by salvage therapy than symptomatic relapses. In view of the enormous cost of a full battery of diagnostic tests and their manifest lack of impact on survival, new guidelines are emerging for less frequent follow-up visits, during which the history and physical examination are the major investigations performed.

As time passes, the likelihood of recurrence of the primary cancer diminishes. For many types of cancer, survival for 5 years without recurrence is tantamount to cure. However, important medical problems can occur in patients treated for cancer and must be examined (**Chap. e13**). Some problems emerge as a consequence of the disease and some as a consequence of the treatment. An understanding of these disease- and treatment-related problems may help in their detection and management.

Despite these concerns, most patients who are cured of cancer return to normal lives.

SUPPORTIVE CARE

In many ways, the success of cancer therapy depends on the success of the supportive care. Failure to control the symptoms of cancer and its treatment may lead patients to abandon curative therapy. Of equal importance, supportive care is a major determinant of quality of life. Even when life cannot be prolonged, the physician must strive to preserve its quality. Quality-of-life measurements have become common endpoints of clinical research studies. Furthermore, palliative care has been shown to be cost-effective when approached in an organized fashion. A credo for oncology could be to cure sometimes, to extend life often, and to comfort always.

Pain   Pain occurs with variable frequency in the cancer patient: 25–50% of patients present with pain at diagnosis, 33% have pain associated with treatment, and 75% have pain with progressive disease. The pain may have several causes. In ~70% of cases, pain is caused by the tumor itself—by invasion of bone, nerves, blood vessels, or mucous membranes or obstruction of a hollow viscus or duct. In ~20% of cases, pain is related to a surgical or invasive medical procedure, to radiation injury (mucositis, enteritis, or plexus or spinal cord injury), or to chemotherapy injury (mucositis, peripheral neuropathy, phlebitis, steroid-induced aseptic necrosis of the femoral head). In 10% of cases, pain is unrelated to cancer or its treatment.

Assessment of pain requires the methodical investigation of the history of the pain, its location, character, temporal features, provocative and palliative factors, and intensity (Chap. 12); a review of the oncologic history and past medical history as well as personal and social history; and a thorough physical examination. The patient should be given a 10-division visual analogue scale on which to indicate the severity of the pain. The clinical condition is often dynamic, making it necessary to reassess the patient frequently. Pain therapy should not be withheld while the cause of pain is being sought.

A variety of tools are available with which to address cancer pain. About 85% of patients will have pain relief from pharmacologic intervention. However, other modalities, including antitumor therapy (such as surgical relief of obstruction, radiation therapy, and strontium-89 or samarium-153 treatment for bone pain), neurostimulatory techniques, regional analgesia, or neuroablative procedures are effective in an additional 12% or so. Thus, very few patients will have inadequate pain relief if appropriate measures are taken. A specific approach to pain relief is detailed in Chap. 11.

Nausea   Emesis in the cancer patient is usually caused by chemotherapy (Chap. 81). Its severity can be predicted from the drugs used to treat the cancer. Three forms of emesis are recognized on the basis of their timing with regard to the noxious insult. *Acute emesis*, the most common variety, occurs within 24 h of treatment. *Delayed emesis* occurs 1–7 days after treatment; it is rare, but, when present, usually follows cisplatin administration. *Anticipatory emesis* occurs before administration of chemotherapy and represents a conditioned response to visual and olfactory stimuli previously associated with chemotherapy delivery.

Acute emesis is the best understood form. Stimuli that activate signals in the chemoreceptor trigger zone in the medulla, the cerebral cortex, and peripherally in the intestinal tract lead to stimulation of the vomiting center in the medulla, the motor center responsible for coordinating the secretory and muscle contraction activity that leads to emesis. Diverse receptor types participate in the process, including dopamine, serotonin, histamine, opioid, and acetylcholine receptors. The serotonin receptor antagonists ondansetron and granisetron are the most effective drugs against highly emetogenic agents, but they are expensive.

As with the analgesia ladder, emesis therapy should be tailored to the situation. For mildly and moderately emetogenic agents, prochlorperazine, 5–10 mg PO or 25 mg PR, is effective. Its efficacy may be enhanced by administering the drug before the chemotherapy is delivered. Dexamethasone, 10–20 mg IV, is also effective and may enhance the efficacy of prochlorperazine. For highly emetogenic agents such as cisplatin, mechlorethamine, dacarbazine, and streptozocin, combinations of agents work best and administration should begin 6–24 h before treatment. Ondansetron, 8 mg PO every 6 h the day before therapy and IV on the day of therapy, plus dexamethasone, 20 mg IV before treatment, is an effective regimen. Addition of oral aprepitant (a substance P/neurokinin 1 receptor antagonist) to this regimen (125 mg on day 1, 80 mg on days 2 and 3) further decreases the risk of both acute and delayed vomiting. Like pain, emesis is easier to prevent than to alleviate.

Delayed emesis may be related to bowel inflammation from the therapy and can be controlled with oral dexamethasone and oral metoclopramide, a dopamine receptor antagonist that also blocks serotonin receptors at high dosages. The best strategy for preventing anticipatory emesis is to control emesis in the early cycles of therapy to prevent the conditioning from taking place. If this is unsuccessful, pro-

---

[3]Information about unsound methods may be obtained from the National Council Against Health Fraud, Box 1276, Loma Linda, CA 92354, or from the Center for Medical Consumers and Health Care Information, 237 Thompson Street, New York, NY 10012.

phylactic antiemetics the day before treatment may help. Experimental studies are evaluating behavior modification.

Effusions Fluid may accumulate abnormally in the pleural cavity, pericardium, or peritoneum. Asymptomatic malignant effusions may not require treatment. Symptomatic effusions occurring in tumors responsive to systemic therapy usually do not require local treatment but respond to the treatment for the underlying tumor. Symptomatic effusions occurring in tumors unresponsive to systemic therapy may require local treatment in patients with a life expectancy of at least 6 months.

Pleural effusions due to tumors may or may not contain malignant cells. Lung cancer, breast cancer, and lymphomas account for ~75% of malignant pleural effusions. Their exudative nature is usually gauged by an effusion/serum protein ratio of ≥0.5 or an effusion/serum lactate dehydrogenase ratio of ≥0.6. When the condition is symptomatic, thoracentesis is usually performed first. In most cases, symptomatic improvement occurs for <1 month. Chest tube drainage is required if symptoms recur within 2 weeks. Fluid is aspirated until the flow rate is <100 mL in 24 h. Then either 60 units of bleomycin or 1 g of doxycycline is infused into the chest tube in 50 mL of 5% dextrose in water; the tube is clamped; the patient is rotated on four sides, spending 15 min in each position; and, after 1–2 h, the tube is again attached to suction for another 24 h. The tube is then disconnected from suction and allowed to drain by gravity. If <100 mL drains over the next 24 h, the chest tube is pulled, and a radiograph taken 24 h later. If the chest tube continues to drain fluid at an unacceptably high rate, sclerosis can be repeated. Bleomycin may be somewhat more effective than doxycycline but is very expensive. Doxycycline is usually the drug of first choice. If neither doxycycline nor bleomycin is effective, talc can be used.

Symptomatic pericardial effusions are usually treated by creating a pericardial window or by stripping the pericardium. If the patient's condition does not permit a surgical procedure, sclerosis can be attempted with doxycycline and/or bleomycin.

Malignant ascites is usually treated with repeated paracentesis of small volumes of fluid. If the underlying malignancy is unresponsive to systemic therapy, peritoneovenous shunts may be inserted. Despite the fear of disseminating tumor cells into the circulation, widespread metastases are an unusual complication. The major complications are occlusion, leakage, and fluid overload. Patients with severe liver disease may develop disseminated intravascular coagulation.

Nutrition Cancer and its treatment may lead to a decrease in nutrient intake of sufficient magnitude to cause weight loss and alteration of intermediary metabolism. The prevalence of this problem is difficult to estimate because of variations in the definition of cancer cachexia, but most patients with advanced cancer experience weight loss and decreased appetite. A variety of both tumor-derived factors (e.g., bombesin, adrenocorticotropic hormone) and host-derived factors (e.g., tumor necrosis factor, interleukins 1 and 6, growth hormone) contribute to the altered metabolism, and a vicious cycle is established in which protein catabolism, glucose intolerance, and lipolysis cannot be reversed by the provision of calories.

It remains controversial how to assess nutritional status and when and how to intervene. Efforts to make the assessment objective have included the use of a prognostic nutritional index based on albumin levels, triceps skin fold thickness, transferrin levels, and delayed-type hypersensitivity skin testing. However, a simpler approach has been to define the threshold for nutritional intervention as >10% unexplained body weight loss, serum transferrin level <1500 mg/L (150 mg/dL), and serum albumin <34 g/L (3.4 g/dL).

The decision is important, because it appears that cancer therapy is substantially more toxic and less effective in the face of malnutrition. Nevertheless, it remains unclear whether nutritional intervention can alter the natural history. Unless some pathology is affecting the absorptive function of the gastrointestinal tract, enteral nutrition provided orally or by tube feeding is preferred over parenteral supplementation. How-

ever, the risks associated with the tube may outweigh the benefits. Megestrol acetate, a progestational agent, has been advocated as a pharmacologic intervention to improve nutritional status. Research in this area may provide more tools in the future as cytokine-mediated mechanisms are further elucidated.

Psychosocial Support The psychosocial needs of patients vary with their situation. Patients undergoing treatment experience fear, anxiety, and depression. Self-image is often seriously compromised by deforming surgery and loss of hair. Women who receive cosmetic advice that enables them to look better also feel better. Loss of control over how one spends time can contribute to the sense of vulnerability. Juggling the demands of work and family with the demands of treatment may create enormous stresses. Sexual dysfunction is highly prevalent and needs to be discussed openly with the patient. An empathetic health care team is sensitive to the individual patient's needs and permits negotiation where such flexibility will not adversely affect the course of treatment.

Cancer survivors have other sets of difficulties. Patients may have fears associated with the termination of a treatment they associate with their continued survival. Adjustments are required to physical losses and handicaps, real and perceived. Patients may be preoccupied with minor physical problems. They perceive a decline in their job mobility and view themselves as less desirable workers. They may be victims of job and/or insurance discrimination. Patients may experience difficulty reentering their normal past life. They may feel guilty for having survived and may carry a sense of vulnerability to colds and other illnesses. Perhaps the most pervasive and threatening concern is the ever-present fear of relapse (the Damocles syndrome).

Patients in whom therapy has been unsuccessful have other problems related to the end of life.

Death and Dying The most common causes of death in patients with cancer are infection (leading to circulatory failure), respiratory failure, hepatic failure, and renal failure. Intestinal blockage may lead to inanition and starvation. Central nervous system disease may lead to seizures, coma, and central hypoventilation. About 70% of patients develop dyspnea preterminally. However, many months usually pass between the diagnosis of cancer and the occurrence of these complications, and during this period the patient is severely affected by the possibility of death. The path of unsuccessful cancer treatment usually occurs in three phases. First, there is optimism at the hope of cure; when the tumor recurs, there is the acknowledgment of an incurable disease, and the goal of palliative therapy is embraced in the hope of being able to live with disease; finally, at the disclosure of imminent death, another adjustment in outlook takes place. The patient imagines the worst in preparation for the end of life and may go through stages of adjustment to the diagnosis. These stages include denial, isolation, anger, bargaining, depression, acceptance, and hope. Of course, patients do not all progress through all the stages or proceed through them in the same order or at the same rate. Nevertheless, developing an understanding of how the patient has been affected by the diagnosis and is coping with it is an important goal of patient management.

It is best to speak frankly with the patient and the family regarding the likely course of disease. These discussions can be difficult for the physician as well as for the patient and family. The critical features of the interaction are to reassure the patient and family that everything that can be done to provide comfort will be done. They will not be abandoned. Many patients prefer to be cared for in their homes or in a hospice setting rather than a hospital. The American College of Physicians has published a book called *Home Care Guide for Cancer: How to Care for Family and Friends at Home* that teaches an approach to successful problem-solving in home care. With appropriate planning, it should be possible to provide the patient with the necessary medical care as well as the psychological and spiritual support that will prevent the isolation and depersonalization that can attend in-hospital death.

The care of dying patients may take a toll on the physician. A "burnout" syndrome has been described that is characterized by fatigue, disengagement from patients and colleagues, and a loss of self-fulfillment. Efforts at stress reduction, maintenance of a balanced life, and setting realistic goals may combat this disorder.

End-of-Life Decisions   Unfortunately, a smooth transition in treatment goals from curative to palliative may not be possible in all cases because of the occurrence of serious treatment-related complications or rapid disease progression. Vigorous and invasive medical support for a reversible disease or treatment complication is assumed to be justified. However, if the reversibility of the condition is in doubt, the patient's wishes determine the level of medical care. These wishes should be elicited before the terminal phase of illness and reviewed periodically. Information about advance directives can be obtained from the American Association of Retired Persons, 601 E Street, NW, Washington, DC 20049, 202-434-2277 or Choice in Dying, 250 West 57th Street, New York, NY 10107, 212-366-5540. A full discussion of end-of-life management is in Chap. 11.

78 Prevention and Early Detection of Cancer

Otis W. Brawley, Barnett S. Kramer

Improved understanding of carcinogenesis has allowed cancer prevention and early detection (also known as cancer control) to expand beyond the identification and avoidance of carcinogens. Specific interventions to prevent cancer in those at risk, and more sensitive and specific screening for early detection of cancer are the goals.

Carcinogenesis is not simply an event but a process, a continuum of discrete cellular changes over time resulting in more autonomous cellular processes. Prevention concerns the identification and manipulation of the genetic, biologic, and environmental factors in the causal pathway of cancer.

EDUCATION AND HEALTHFUL HABITS

Public education on the avoidance of identified risk factors for cancer and encouraging healthy habits contributes to cancer prevention and control. The physician is a powerful messenger in this education campaign. The patient-physician encounter provides an opportunity to teach patients about the hazards of smoking, the features of a healthy lifestyle (including diet and exercise), use of proven cancer screening methods, and sun avoidance.

Smoking Cessation   Tobacco smoking is the most modifiable risk factor for cardiovascular disease, pulmonary disease, and cancer. Smokers have a 33% lifetime risk of dying prematurely from a tobacco-related cancer, cardiovascular, or pulmonary disease. Tobacco use causes more deaths from cardiovascular disease than from cancer. Lung cancer and cancers of the larynx, oropharynx, esophagus, kidney, bladder, pancreas, and stomach are all tobacco-related.

The degree of smoke exposure, meaning the number of cigarettes smoked per day as well as the level of inhalation of cigarette smoke, is correlated with risk of lung cancer mortality. Light- and low-tar cigarettes are not safer because smokers tend to inhale them more frequently and deeply.

Those who stop smoking have a 30–50% lower 10-year lung cancer mortality rate compared to those who continue smoking, despite the fact that some carcinogen-induced gene mutations persist for years after smoking cessation. Smoking cessation and avoidance have the potential to save more lives than any other public health activity.

FURTHER READINGS

GRUNBERG SM, HESKETH PJ: Control of chemotherapy-induced emesis. N Engl J Med 329:1790, 1993

JEMAL A et al: Cancer statistics, 2007. CA Cancer J Clin 57:43, 2007

KAMANGAR F et al: Patterns of cancer incidence, mortality, and prevalence across five continents: Defining priorities to reduce cancer disparities in different geographic regions of the world. J Clin Oncol 24:2137, 2006

LEVY MH: Pharmacologic treatment of cancer pain. N Engl J Med 335:1124, 1996

THERASSE P et al: New guidelines to evaluate response to treatment in solid tumors. J Natl Cancer Inst 92:205, 2000

U.S. DEPARTMENT OF HEALTH AND HUMAN SERVICES: *Clinical Practice Guideline Number 9, Management of Cancer Pain.* U.S. Department of Health and Human Services, Agency for Health Care Policy and Research publication no. 94-0592, 1994

WALSH D et al: The symptoms of advanced cancer: Relationship to age, gender, and performance status in 1000 patients. Support Care Cancer 8:175, 2000

The risk of tobacco smoke is not limited to the smoker. Environmental tobacco smoke, known as second hand or passive smoke, causes lung cancer and other cardiopulmonary diseases in nonsmokers.

Tobacco prevention is a pediatric issue. Over 80% of adult American smokers began smoking before the age of 18. Nearly 20% of Americans aged 12–18 have smoked a cigarette in the past month. Counseling of adolescents and young adults is critical to prevent smoking. A physician's simple advice to not start smoking or to quit smoking can be of benefit. Physicians should query patients on tobacco use on every office visit, record the answer with the vital signs, and ask smokers if they would like assistance in quitting.

Current approaches to smoking cessation recognize that smoking is an addiction (Chap. 390). The smoker who is quitting goes through a process with identifiable stages that include contemplation of quitting, an action phase in which the smoker quits, and a maintenance phase. Smokers who quit completely are more likely to be successful than those who gradually reduce the number of cigarettes smoked or change to lower tar or nicotine cigarettes. More than 90% of the Americans who have successfully quit smoking did so on their own without participation in an organized cessation program, but cessation programs are helpful for some smokers. The Community Intervention Trial for Smoking Cessation (COMMIT) was a 4-year program; it demonstrated that light smokers (<25 cigarettes per day) were more likely to benefit from simple cessation messages and cessation programs. Quit rates were 30.6% in the intervention group and 27.5% in the control group. The COMMIT interventions were not successful in heavy smokers (>25 cigarettes per day). Heavy smokers may need an intensive broad-based cessation program that includes counseling, behavioral strategies, and pharmacologic adjuncts, such as nicotine replacement (gum, patches, sprays, lozenges, and inhalers) and bupropion.

Cigar smoking has increased in the past decade. The health risks of cigars are similar to those of cigarettes. Smoking one or two cigars daily doubles the risk for oral and esophageal cancers; three or four cigars daily increases the risk of oral cancers more than eightfold and esophageal cancer fourfold. The risks of occasional use are unknown.

Smokeless tobacco is the fastest growing part of the tobacco industry and represents a substantial health risk. Chewing tobacco is a carcinogen linked to dental caries, gingivitis, oral leukoplakia, and oral cancer. The systemic effects of smokeless tobacco may increase risks for other cancers. Esophageal cancer is linked to carcinogens in tobacco being dissolved in saliva, swallowed, and coming into contact with the esophagus.

Physical Activity   Physical activity is associated with a decreased risk of colon and breast cancer. A variety of mechanisms have been proposed. However, such studies are prone to confounding factors such as recall bias, association of exercise with other health-related practices, and effects of preclinical cancers on exercise habits (reverse causality). Recommending adults to engage in at least 30 min of vigorous activity for ≥3 days a week is good health advice, though its effects on cancer incidence are unproven.

Diet Modification   International epidemiologic studies suggest that diets high in fat are associated with increased risk for cancers of the breast, colon, prostate, and endometrium. These cancers have their highest incidence and mortalities in western culture where fat comprises an average of 40–45% of the total calories consumed. In populations at low risk for these cancers, fat accounts for <20% of dietary calories.

Despite correlations, dietary fat has not been proven to cause cancer. Case-control and cohort epidemiologic studies give conflicting results. In addition, diet is a highly complex exposure to many nutrients and chemicals. Low-fat diets are associated with many dietary changes beyond simple subtraction of fat. Other lifestyle changes are also associated with adherence to a low-fat diet. The Women's Intervention Nutrition Study (WINS) evaluated the effects of low-fat diet on breast cancer recurrence in previously treated postmenopausal breast cancer patients. Breast cancer patients, mean age 62 years, were randomly assigned to a standard diet (40% fat) or a low-fat diet (26% fat). At 5 years, breast cancer had recurred in 9.8% of women in the low-fat diet group compared to 12.4% of women on the standard diet.

In observational studies, dietary fiber lowers the risk of colonic polyps and invasive cancer of the colon. However, cancer protective effects of increasing fiber and lowering dietary fat have not been proven in the context of a prospective clinical trial. The putative protective mechanisms are complex and speculative. Fiber binds oxidized bile acids and generates soluble fiber products, such as butyrate, that may have differentiating properties. Fiber does not increase bowel transit times. High-fiber diets could lower the risk of breast and prostate cancer by absorbing and inactivating dietary estrogenic and androgenic cancer promoters. However, two large prospective cohort studies of >100,000 health professionals showed no association between fruit and vegetable intake and risk of cancer.

The Polyp Prevention Trial randomly assigned 2000 elderly persons, who had polyps removed, to a low-fat, high-fiber diet versus routine diet for 4 years. No differences were noted in polyp formation.

The U.S. National Institutes of Health Women's Health Initiative, launched in 1994, is a long-term clinical trial enrolling >100,000 women aged 45–69. It placed women in 22 intervention groups. Participants received calcium/vitamin D supplementation, hormone-replacement therapy, and counseling to increase exercise, eat a low-fat diet, and cease smoking. The study showed that while dietary fat intake was significantly lower in the diet intervention group, invasive breast cancers were not reduced over an 8-year follow-up period compared to the control group. The difference in dietary fat averaged ~10% between the two groups. Scientific evidence does not currently establish the anticarcinogenic value of vitamin, mineral, or nutritional supplements in amounts greater than those provided by a balanced diet. However, consuming at least five servings of fruits and vegetables a day decreases dietary fat and increases fiber; such a diet may lower the risk of cardiovascular disease even if it does not influence cancer.

Energy Balance   Risk of cancer increases as body mass index increases over 25 kg/m². Obesity increases risks for cancers of the colon, breast (female postmenopausal), endometrium, kidney (renal cell), and esophagus, although causality is not established.

Relative risks of colon cancer are increased in obesity by 1.5–2.0 for men and 1.2–1.5 for women. Obese postmenopausal women have a 30–50% increased risk of breast cancer. A hypothesis for the association is that adipose tissue serves as a depot for aromatase that facilitates estrogen production. Adiposity is also associated with poorer survival and increased risk of recurrence after treatment.

Sun Avoidance   Nonmelanoma skin cancers (basal cell and squamous cell) are induced by cumulative exposure to ultraviolet (UV) radiation. Intermittent acute sun exposure and sun damage have been linked to melanoma. Sunburns, especially in childhood and adolescence, are associated with increased risk of melanoma in adulthood. Reduction of sun exposure through use of protective clothing and changing patterns of outdoor activities can reduce skin cancer risk. Sunscreens decrease the risk of actinic keratoses, the precursor to squamous cell skin cancer, but melanoma risk may be increased. Sunscreens prevent burning, but they may encourage more prolonged exposure to the sun and may not filter out wavelengths of energy that cause melanoma.

Educational interventions to help individuals accurately assess their risk of developing skin cancer have some impact. Self examination for skin pigment characteristics associated with melanoma, such as freckling, may be useful in identifying people at high risk. Those who recognize themselves as being at risk tend to be more compliant with sun-avoidance recommendations. Risk factors for melanoma include a propensity to sunburn, a large number of benign melanocytic nevi, and atypical nevi.

CANCER CHEMOPREVENTION

Chemoprevention involves the use of specific natural or synthetic chemical agents to reverse, suppress, or prevent carcinogenesis before the development of invasive malignancy.

Cancer develops through an accumulation of genetic and epigenetic changes that are potential points of intervention to prevent cancer. The initial changes are termed *initiation*. The alteration can be inherited or acquired through the action of physical, infectious, or chemical carcinogens. Like most human diseases, cancer arises from an interaction between genetics and environmental exposures (Table 78-1). Influences that cause the initiated cell to progress through the carcinogenic process and change

TABLE 78-1 SUSPECTED CARCINOGENS	
Carcinogens[a]	**Associated Cancer or Neoplasm**
Alkylating agents	Acute myeloid leukemia, bladder cancer
Androgens	Prostate cancer
Aromatic amines (dyes)	Bladder cancer
Arsenic	Cancer of the lung, skin
Asbestos	Cancer of the lung, pleura, peritoneum
Benzene	Acute myelocytic leukemia
Chromium	Lung cancer
Diethylstilbestrol (prenatal)	Vaginal cancer (clear cell)
Epstein-Barr virus	Burkitt's lymphoma, nasal T cell lymphoma
Estrogens	Cancer of the endometrium, liver, breast
Ethyl alcohol	Cancer of the liver, esophagus, head and neck
Helicobacter pylori	Gastric cancer, gastric MALT lymphoma
Hepatitis B or C virus	Liver cancer
Human immunodeficiency virus	Non-Hodgkin's lymphoma, Kaposi's sarcoma, squamous cell carcinomas (especially of the urogenital tract)
Human papilloma virus	Cervix cancer, head and neck cancer
Human T cell lymphotropic virus type I (HTLV-I)	Adult T cell leukemia/lymphoma
Immunosuppressive agents (azathioprine, cyclosporine, glucocorticoids)	Non-Hodgkin's lymphoma
Nitrogen mustard gas	Cancer of the lung, head and neck, nasal sinuses
Nickel dust	Cancer of the lung, nasal sinuses
Phenacetin	Cancer of the renal pelvis and bladder
Polycyclic hydrocarbons	Cancer of the lung, skin (especially squamous cell carcinoma of scrotal skin)
Schistosomiasis	Bladder cancer (squamous cell)
Sunlight (ultraviolet)	Skin cancer (squamous cell and melanoma)
Tobacco (including smokeless)	Cancer of the upper aerodigestive tract, bladder
Vinyl chloride	Liver cancer (angiosarcoma)

[a]Agents that are thought to act as cancer initiators and/or promoters.

phenotypically are termed *promoters*. Promoters include hormones such as androgens, linked to prostate cancer, and estrogen, linked to breast and endometrial cancer. The distinction between an initiator and promoter is sometimes arbitrary; some components of cigarette smoke are "complete carcinogens," acting as both initiators and promoters. Cancer can be prevented or controlled through interference with the factors that cause cancer initiation, promotion, or progression. Compounds of interest in chemoprevention often have antimutagenic, antioxidant, anti-inflammatory, antiproliferative, or pro-apoptotic activity (or a combination).

Chemoprevention of Cancers of the Upper Aerodigestive Tract Smoking causes diffuse epithelial injury in the head, neck, esophagus, and lung. Patients cured of squamous cell cancers of the lung, esophagus, head, and neck are at risk (as high as 5% per year) of developing second cancers of the upper aerodigestive tract. Cessation of cigarette smoking does not markedly decrease the cured cancer patient's risk of second malignancy, even though it does lower the cancer risk in those who have never developed a malignancy. Smoking cessation may halt the early stages of the carcinogenic process (such as metaplasia), but it may have no effect on late stages of carcinogenesis. This "field carcinogenesis" hypothesis for upper aerodigestive tract cancer has made "cured" patients an important population for chemoprevention of second malignancies.

Oral leukoplakia, a premalignant lesion commonly found in smokers, has been used as an intermediate marker allowing demonstration of chemopreventive activity in smaller shorter duration, randomized, placebo-controlled trials. Response was associated with upregulation of retinoic acid receptor-β (RAR-β). Therapy with high, relatively toxic doses of isoretinoin (13-*cis*-retinoic acid) causes regression of oral leukoplakia. However, the lesions recur when the therapy is withdrawn, suggesting the need for chronic administration. More tolerable doses of isoretinoin have not proven beneficial in the prevention of head and neck cancer. Isoretinoin also failed to prevent second malignancies in patients cured of early-stage non-small cell lung cancer; mortality rates were actually increased in current smokers.

Premalignant lesions in the oropharyngeal area have also responded to retinol, α-tocopherol (vitamin E), and selenium. Further study to define the activity of these drugs is ongoing.

Several large-scale trials have assessed agents in the chemoprevention of lung cancer in patients at high risk. In the α-tocopherol/β-carotene (ATBC) Lung Cancer Prevention Trial participants were male smokers, age 50–69 at entry. Participants had smoked an average of one pack of cigarettes per day for 35.9 years. Participants received α-tocopherol, β-carotene, and/or placebo in a randomized, 2 × 2 factorial design. After median follow-up of 6.1 years, lung cancer incidence and mortality were statistically significantly increased in those receiving β-carotene. α-Tocopherol had no effect on lung cancer mortality, and no evidence suggested interaction between the two drugs. Patients receiving α-tocopherol had a higher incidence of hemorrhagic stroke.

The β-Carotene and Retinol Efficacy Trial (CARET) involved 17,000 American smokers and workers with asbestos exposure. Entrants were randomly assigned to one of four arms and received β-carotene, retinol, and/or placebo in a 2 × 2 factorial design. This trial also demonstrated harm from β-carotene: a lung cancer rate of 5 per 1000 subjects per year for those taking placebo and of 6 per 1000 subjects per year for those taking β-carotene.

The ATBC and CARET results demonstrate the importance of testing chemoprevention hypotheses thoroughly before their widespread implementation as the results contradict a number of observational studies. In the ATBC trial, those taking α-tocopherol had a one-third reduction in the incidence of prostate cancer, compared to those not taking α-tocopherol. The Physicians' Health Trial showed no change in the risk of lung cancer for those taking β-carotene; fewer of its participants were smokers than those in the ATBC and CARET studies.

Chemoprevention of Colon Cancer Many of the current colon cancer prevention trials are based on the premise that most colorectal cancers develop from adenomatous polyps. These trials use adenoma recurrence or disappearance as a surrogate endpoint for colon cancer

prevention. Early clinical trial results suggest that nonsteroidal anti-inflammatory drugs (NSAIDs), such as piroxicam, sulindac, and aspirin, may prevent adenoma formation or cause regression of adenomatous polyps. The mechanism of action of NSAIDs is unknown, but they are presumed to work through the cyclooxygenase pathway. In the Physicians' Health Trial, aspirin had no effect on colon cancer incidence, although the 6-year assessment period may not have been long enough to evaluate this endpoint definitively. A number of studies suggest that NSAID use is associated with a lower risk of adenomatous polyps and invasive cancer. However, prospective trials have not shown that NSAIDs prevent colon cancer.

Cyclooxygenase-2 (COX-2) inhibitors may be even more effective. In a placebo-controlled trial, high-dose celecoxib reduced the recurrence of colorectal polyps in patients with familial adenomatous polyposis. The effect on colon cancer occurrence is unknown. Trials for prevention of sporadic colorectal cancers with COX-2 inhibitors were initiated but have been complicated by the association of these drugs with cardiovascular disease.

Epidemiologic studies suggest that diets high in calcium lower colon cancer risk. Calcium binds bile and fatty acids, which cause proliferation of colonic epithelium. It is hypothesized that calcium reduces intraluminal exposure to these compounds. Calcium supplementation decreases the risk of adenomatous polyp recurrence by ~20%. Trials of calcium with cancer-incidence endpoints are underway.

The Women's Health Initiative demonstrated that postmenopausal women taking premarin plus progestin have a 44% lower risk of colorectal cancer compared to women taking placebo. Of >16,600 women randomized and followed for a median of 5.6 years, 43 invasive colorectal cancers occurred in the hormone group and 72 in the placebo group. The positive effect on colon cancer is mitigated by the modest increase in cardiovascular and breast cancer risks associated with combined estrogen plus progestin therapy. Colorectal cancers diagnosed in women taking estrogen and progestin were in more advanced stage than those in women taking placebo.

A case-control study suggested that statins decrease the incidence of colorectal cancer. However, a meta-analysis of statin use showed no protective effect of statins on overall cancer incidence or death.

Chemoprevention of Breast Cancer Hormonal manipulation is being tested in the primary prevention of breast cancer. Tamoxifen is an antiestrogen with partial estrogen agonistic activity in some tissues, such as endometrium and bone. One of its actions is to upregulate transforming growth factor β, which decreases breast cell proliferation. In randomized placebo-controlled trials to assess tamoxifen as adjuvant therapy for breast cancer, tamoxifen reduced the number of new breast cancers in the opposite breast by more than a third. In a randomized placebo-controlled prevention trial involving >13,000 women at high risk, tamoxifen decreased the risk of developing breast cancer by 49% (from 43.4 to 22.0 per 1000 women) after a median follow-up of nearly 6 years. The International Breast Cancer Intervention Study (IBIS-I) trial had similar findings. In both studies tamoxifen also reduced bone fractures; a small increase in risk of endometrial cancer, stroke, pulmonary emboli, and deep vein thrombosis was noted. Tamoxifen has been approved by the U.S. Food and Drug Administration for reduction of breast cancer in women at high risk for the disease (1.66% risk at 5 years based on the Gail risk model: *http://www.nci.nih.gov/cancertopics/pdq/genetics/breast-and-ovarian/healthprofessional#Section_66*).

A trial comparing tamoxifen with another selective estrogen receptor modulator, raloxifene, showed that raloxifene is comparable to tamoxifen in cancer prevention. Raloxifene is associated with more noninvasive breast cancer than tamoxifen; the drugs are similar in risks of other cancers, fractures, ischemic heart disease, and stroke. Because the aromatase inhibitors are even more effective than tamoxifen in adjuvant breast cancer therapy, it is hoped that they also are more effective in breast cancer prevention. However, no data are available on this point.

Chemoprevention of Prostate Cancer Finasteride is a 5-α-reductase inhibitor. It inhibits conversion of testosterone to dihydrotestosterone

(DHT), a potent stimulator of prostate cell proliferation. The Prostate Cancer Prevention Trial randomly assigned men ≥55 years at average risk of prostate cancer to finasteride or placebo. After 7 years of therapy, the incidence of prostate cancer was 18.4% in the finasteride arm and 24.8% in the placebo arm, a statistically significant difference. However, the finasteride group had more patients with tumors of Gleason score 7 and higher compared to the placebo arm (6.4% vs 5.1%). The clinical significance of this finding, if any, is unknown.

Selenium is being tested as a prostate cancer preventive based on laboratory studies, epidemiologic data, and a small randomized skin cancer prevention trial that showed a significantly decreased number of prostate cancers in men taking selenium. In the placebo group, 16 prostate cancers were diagnosed versus 4 in the treatment group among the 843 men who began the study with a serum prostate specific antigen level <4 ng/mL.

The ATBC study cited above showed in secondary analysis that the risk of prostate cancer was reduced 33% in men taking α-tocopherol (99 cases in those on the drug; 151 cases on placebo). A prospective randomized trial to assess these drugs is ongoing.

Vaccines and Cancer Prevention A number of infectious agents cause cancer. Hepatitis B and C are linked to liver cancer, some human papilloma virus (HPV) strains are linked to cervical and head and neck cancer, and *Helicobacter pylori* is associated with gastric cancer and lymphoma. Vaccines to protect against these agents may reduce the risk of their associated cancers.

The hepatitis B vaccine is effective in preventing hepatitis and hepatomas due to chronic hepatitis B infection. Public health officials are encouraging widespread administration of the hepatitis B vaccine, especially in Asia, where the disease is epidemic.

A four-valent HPV vaccine (Gardasil) is 100% effective at preventing infection with any of the four component strains (6, 11, 16, 18). The vaccine is recommended for girls and women ages 9–26 years. Reduction in these HPV types could prevent >70% of the cervical cancers worldwide.

SURGICAL PREVENTION OF CANCER

Some organs in some individuals are at such high risk of developing cancer that surgical removal of the organ at risk is recommended. Women with severe cervical dysplasia are treated with conization and occasionally even hysterectomy. Colectomy is used to prevent colon cancer in patients with familial polyposis or ulcerative colitis.

Prophylactic bilateral mastectomy is chosen for breast cancer prevention among women with genetic predisposition to breast cancer. In a prospective series of 139 women with *BRCA1* and *BRCA2* mutations, 76 chose to undergo prophylactic mastectomy and 63 chose close surveillance. At 3 years, no cases of breast cancer had been diagnosed in those opting for surgery, but eight in the surveillance group had developed breast cancer. A larger retrospective cohort study reported that prophylactic mastectomy could reduce risk of breast cancer by 90%. The effect of the procedure on mortality is unknown. Observational studies are prone to a variety of biases associated with the choice to undergo prophylactic surgery; thus, such studies can give an overestimate of the magnitude of benefit.

Surgery is also used to manage hormonal cancers. Orchiectomy is an effective method of androgen deprivation in prostate cancer, and oophorectomy is effective in hormone-dependent breast cancer.

CANCER SCREENING

Screening is a means of detecting disease early in asymptomatic individuals, with the goal of decreasing morbidity and mortality. While screening can potentially save lives and has been shown to do so in cervical, colon, and probably breast cancer, it is also subject to a number of biases that can suggest a benefit when actually there is none. Biases can even mask net harm. Early detection does not in itself confer benefit. To be of value, screening must detect disease earlier, and treatment of earlier disease must yield a better outcome than treatment at the onset of symptoms. Cause-specific mortality, rather than survival after diagnosis, is the preferred endpoint (see below).

Because screening is done on asymptomatic, healthy persons, it should offer substantial likelihood of benefit that outweighs harm. Screening tests and their appropriate use should be carefully evaluated before their use is widely encouraged in screening programs, as a matter of public policy.

Screening examinations, tests, or procedures are usually not diagnostic of cancer but instead indicate that a cancer may be present. The diagnosis is then made following a workup that includes a biopsy and pathologic confirmation.

A number of genes have been identified that predispose for a disease, and many more will be identified in the near future. Testing for these genes can define a high-risk population. The ability to predict the development of a particular cancer may some day present therapeutic options as well as ethical dilemmas. It may eventually allow for early intervention to prevent a cancer or limit its severity. People at high risk may be ideal candidates for chemoprevention and screening; however, efficacy of these interventions in the high-risk population should be investigated. Currently, persons at high risk for a particular cancer can engage in intensive screening. While this course is clinically prudent, it is not known if it saves lives in these populations.

The Accuracy of Screening A screening test's accuracy or ability to discriminate disease is described by four indices: sensitivity, specificity, positive predictive value, and negative predictive value (Table 78-2). *Sensitivity*, also called the true positive rate, is the proportion of persons with the disease testing positive in the screen (i.e., the ability of the test to detect disease when it is present). *Specificity*, or 1-false positive rate, is the proportion of persons who do not have the disease and test negative in the screening test (i.e., the ability of a test to correctly identify that the disease is not present). The *positive predictive value* is the proportion of persons that test positive who actually have the disease. Similarly, *negative predictive value* is the proportion testing negative who do not have the disease. The sensitivity and specificity of a test are relatively independent of the underlying prevalence (or risk) of the disease in the population screened, but the predictive values depend strongly on the prevalence of the disease.

Screening is most beneficial, efficient, and economical when the target disease is common in the population being screened. To be valuable, the screening test should have a high specificity; sensitivity need not be very high.

Potential Biases of Screening Tests The common biases of screening are lead time, length-biased sampling, and selection. These biases can

TABLE 78-2 ASSESSMENT OF THE VALUE OF A DIAGNOSTIC TEST[a]

	Condition Present	Condition Absent
Positive test	a	b
Negative test	c	d

a = true positive
b = false positive
c = false negative
d = true negative

Sensitivity	The proportion of persons with the condition who test positive: $a/(a + c)$
Specificity	The proportion of persons without the condition who test negative: $d/(b + d)$
Positive predictive value (PPV)	The proportion of persons with a positive test who have the condition: $a/(a + b)$
Negative predictive value	The proportion of persons with a negative test who do not have the condition: $d/(c + d)$

Prevalence, sensitivity, and specificity determine PPV

$$PPV = \frac{prevalence \times sensitivity}{(prevalence \times sensitivity) + (1 - prevalence)(1 - specificity)}$$

[a]For diseases of low prevalence, such as cancer, poor specificity has a dramatic adverse effect on PPV such that only a small fraction of positive tests are true positives.

TABLE 78-3 SCREENING RECOMMENDATIONS FOR ASYMPTOMATIC NORMAL-RISK SUBJECTS[a]

Test or Procedure	USPSTF	ACS	CTFPHC
Sigmoidoscopy	Fair evidence to recommend	≥50, every 5 years	Fair evidence to consider
Fecal occult blood testing	≥50, good evidence for every 1–2 years	≥50, every year	Good evidence, age ≥50
Colonoscopy	No direct evidence	≥50, every 10 years	No direct evidence
Digital rectal examination	No recommendation	No recommendation	No recommendation
Prostate-specific antigen	Insufficient evidence to recommend	M: ≥50, every year	Recommendation against
Pap test	F: 18–65, every 1–3 years	F: with uterine cervix, beginning 3 years after first intercourse or by age 21. Yearly for standard Pap; every 2 years with liquid test.	Fair evidence to include in examination of sexually active women
Pelvic examination	No recommendation, advise adnexal palpation during exam for other reasons	F: 18–40, every 1–3 years with Pap test; >40, every year	Not considered
Breast self-examination	No recommendation	≥20, monthly	Fair evidence to exclude
Breast clinical examination	Insufficient evidence as a stand-alone without mammography	F: 20–40, every 3 years; >40, yearly	F: 50–69, every 1–2 years
Mammography	F: 40–75, every 1–2 years (fair evidence)	F: ≥40, every year	F: 50–69, every 1–2 years
Complete skin examination	Insufficient evidence for or against	Periodic exam	Poor evidence to include or exclude

[a]Summary of the screening procedures recommended for the general population by U.S. Preventive Services Task Force (USPSTF), the American Cancer Society (ACS), and the Canadian Task Force on Prevention Health Care (CTFPHC). These recommendations refer to asymptomatic persons who have no risk factors, other than age or gender, for the targeted condition.

Note: F, female; M, male.

make a screening test seem beneficial when actually it is not (or even causes net harm). Whether beneficial or not, screening can create the false impression of an epidemic by increasing the number of cancers diagnosed. It can also produce a shift in proportion of patients diagnosed at an early stage that improves survival statistics without reducing mortality (i.e., the number of deaths from a given cancer relative to the number of those at risk for the cancer). In such a case, the *apparent* duration of survival (measured from date of diagnosis) increases without lives being saved or life expectancy changed.

Lead-time bias occurs when a test does not influence the natural history of the disease; the patient is merely diagnosed at an earlier date. When lead-time bias occurs, survival *appears* increased, but life is not really prolonged. The screening test only prolongs the time the subject is aware of the disease and spends as a patient.

Length-biased sampling occurs when slow-growing, less aggressive cancers are detected during screening. Cancers diagnosed due to the onset of symptoms between scheduled screenings are on average more aggressive, and treatment outcomes are not as favorable. An extreme form of length bias sampling is termed *overdiagnosis*, the detection of "pseudo disease." The reservoir of some undetected slow-growing tumors is large. Many of these tumors fulfill the histologic criteria of cancer but will never become clinically significant or cause death. This problem is compounded by the fact that the most common cancers appear most frequently at ages when competing causes of death are more frequent.

Selection bias must be considered in assessing the results of any screening effort. The population most likely to seek screening may differ from the general population to which the screening test might be applied. The individuals screened may have volunteered because of a particular risk factor not found in the general population, such as a strong family history. In general, volunteers for studies are more health conscious and likely to have a better prognosis or lower mortality rate, irrespective of the screening result. This is termed the *healthy volunteer effect*.

Potential Drawbacks of Screening Risks associated with screening include harm caused by the screening intervention itself, harm due to the further investigation of persons with positive tests (both true and false positives), and harm from the treatment of persons with a true-positive result, even if life is extended by treatment. The diagnosis and treatment of cancers that would never have caused medical problems can lead to the harm of unnecessary treatment and give patients the anxiety of a cancer diagnosis. The psychosocial impact of cancer screening can also be substantial when applied to the entire population.

Assessment of Screening Tests Good clinical trial design can offset some biases of screening and demonstrate the relative risks and bene-

fits of a screening test. A randomized, controlled screening trial with cause-specific mortality as the endpoint provides the strongest support for a screening intervention. Overall survival should also be reported to detect an adverse effect of screening and treatment on other disease outcomes (e.g., cardiovascular disease). In a randomized trial, two like populations are randomly established. One is given the medical standard of care (which may be no screening at all) and the other receives the screening intervention being assessed. The two populations are compared over time. Efficacy for the population studied is established when the group receiving the screening test has a better cause-specific mortality rate than the control group. Studies showing a reduction in the incidence of advanced-stage disease, an improved survival, or a stage shift are weaker (and possibly misleading) evidence of benefit. These latter criteria are necessary but not sufficient to establish the value of a screening test.

Although a randomized, controlled screening trial provides the strongest evidence to support a screening test, it is not perfect. Unless the trial is population-based, it does not remove the question of generalizability to the target population. Screening trials generally involve thousands of persons and last for years. Less definitive study designs are therefore often used to estimate the effectiveness of screening practices. After a randomized controlled clinical trial, in descending order of strength, evidence may be derived from the findings of internally controlled trials using intervention allocation methods other than randomization (e.g., allocation by birth date, date of clinic visit); the findings of cohort or case-control analytic observational studies; the results of multiple time series study with or without the intervention; the opinions of respected authorities based on clinical experience, descriptive studies, or consensus reports of experts (the weakest form of evidence because even experts can be misled by biases).

Screening for Specific Cancers Widespread screening for cervical, colon, and likely breast cancer is beneficial for certain age groups. A number of organizations have considered whether or not to endorse routine use of certain screening tests. Because these groups have not used the same criteria to judge whether a screening test should be endorsed, they have arrived at different recommendations. The U.S. Preventive Services Task Force (USPSTF), the Canadian Task Force on Preventive Health Care, and the American Cancer Society (ACS) publish screening guidelines (Table 78-3). Special surveillance of those at high risk for a specific cancer because of a family history or a genetic risk factor may be prudent, but few studies have assessed the influence on mortality.

BREAST CANCER Breast self-examination, clinical breast examination by a care giver, and mammography have been advocated as useful

screening tools. Only screening mammography alone and screening mammography with clinical examination have been evaluated in randomized controlled trials. MRI is being assessed and is more accurate than mammography in women at high risk due to genetic predisposition or in women with very dense breast tissue.

A number of trials have suggested that annual or biennial screening with mammography or mammography plus clinical breast examination in normal-risk women over the age of 50 decreases breast cancer mortality. Each trial has been criticized for design flaws. In most trials, breast cancer mortality rate is decreased by 20–30%. Experts disagree on whether average-risk women age 40–49 should receive regular screening (Table 78-3). The significance of the screening effect in women aged 40–49 depends on the statistical test used. An analysis of eight large randomized trials showed no benefit from mammography screening for women aged 40–49 when assessed 5–7 years after trial entry. However, a small benefit emerged 10–12 years after study entry. What proportion of this benefit is due to screening after these women turned 50 is not known. In randomized screening studies of women aged 50–69, the mortality decline begins about 5 years after initiation of screening. Nearly half of women aged 40–49 screened annually will have false-positive mammograms necessitating further evaluation, often including biopsy. The risk of false-positive testing should be discussed with the patient.

No study of breast self-examination has shown it to decrease mortality; however, it is recommended as prudent by many organizations. A substantial fraction of breast cancers are first detected by patients. Self-examination leads to increased biopsy rate without reducing breast cancer mortality.

Genetic screening for *BRCA1* and *BRCA2* mutations and other markers of breast cancer risk has identified a group of women at high risk for breast cancer. Unfortunately when to begin and the optimal frequency of screening have not been defined. Mammography is less sensitive at detecting breast cancers in women carrying *BRCA1* and *-2* mutations, possibly because such cancers occur in younger women, in whom mammography is known to be less sensitive. MRI screening may be more effective.

CERVICAL CANCER Screening with Papanicolaou smears decreases cervical cancer mortality. The cervical cancer mortality rate has fallen substantially since the widespread use of the Pap smear. Most screening guidelines recommend regular Pap testing for all women who are or have been sexually active for 3 years or have reached the age of 21. With the onset of sexual activity comes the risk of sexual transmission of HPV, the most common etiologic factor for cervical cancer. The recommended interval for Pap screening varies from 1–3 years. At age 30, women who have had three normal test results in a row may get screened every 2–3 years. An upper age limit at which screening ceases to be effective is not known, but women ≥70 years with no abnormal results in the previous 10 years may choose to stop screening.

COLORECTAL CANCER Fecal occult blood testing (FOBT), digital rectal examination (DRE), rigid and flexible sigmoidoscopy, radiographic barium contrast studies, and colonoscopy have been considered for colorectal cancer screening. Annual FOBT could reduce colorectal cancer mortality by a third. The sensitivity for fecal occult blood is increased if specimens are re-hydrated before testing, but at the cost of lower specificity. The false-positive rate for rehydrated FOBT is high; 1–5% of persons tested have a positive test. Only 2–10% of those with occult blood in the stool have cancer and 20–30% have adenomas. The high false-positive rate of FOBT dramatically increases the number of colonoscopies performed.

Two case-control studies suggest that regular screening of those >50 years with sigmoidoscopy decreases mortality. This type of study is prone to selection biases. A quarter to a third of polyps can be discovered with the rigid sigmoidoscope; half are found with a 35-cm flexible scope and two-thirds to three-quarters are found with a 60-cm scope. Diagnosis of adenomatous polyps by sigmoidoscopy should lead to evaluation of the entire colon with colonoscopy and/or barium enema. The most efficient interval for screening sigmoidoscopy is unknown, but 5 years is often recommended. Case-control studies suggest that intervals of up to 15 years may confer benefit.

One-time colonoscopy detects ~25% more advanced lesions (polyps > 10 mm, villous adenomas, adenomatous polyps with high-grade dysplasia, invasive cancer) than one-time FOBT with sigmoidoscopy. Colonoscopy is well suited to screening subjects at high risk, such as those with ulcerative colitis or family predisposition. Perforation rates are 3/1000 for colonoscopy and 1/1000 for sigmoidoscopy. Debate continues on whether colonoscopy is too expensive and invasive for widespread use as a screening tool in standard-risk populations. DRE and barium enema are both insensitive as screening tools.

LUNG CANCER Chest x-ray and sputum cytology have been evaluated in randomized lung cancer screening trials. No reduction in lung cancer mortality has been seen, although all the controlled trials have had low statistical power. Even screening of high-risk subjects (smokers) has not proven beneficial. Spiral CT can diagnose lung cancers at early stages; however, false-positive rates are high. Spiral CT screening increases the number of lesions detected and increases the number of diagnostic and therapeutic procedures. However, its capacity to save lives is unproven.

OVARIAN CANCER Adnexal palpation, transvaginal ultrasound, and serum CA-125 assay have been considered for ovarian cancer screening. These tests alone and in combination do not have sufficiently high sensitivity or specificity to be recommended for routine screening of ovarian cancer. The risks and costs associated with the high number of false-positive results is an impediment to routine use of these modalities for screening. Most expert panels have concluded that routine screening for ovarian cancer is not indicated for standard-risk women or those with single affected family members, but might be worthwhile in families with genetic ovarian cancer syndromes.

PROSTATE CANCER The most common prostate cancer screening modalities are DRE and serum prostate-specific antigen (PSA) assay. Newer serum tests, such as measurement of bound to free serum PSA, have yet to be fully evaluated. An emphasis on PSA screening has caused prostate cancer to become the most common non-skin cancer diagnosed in American males. This disease is prone to lead-time bias, length bias, and overdiagnosis, and substantial debate rages among experts as to whether it is effective. Some experts are concerned that prostate cancer screening, more than screening for other cancers, may cause net harm. Prostate cancer screening clearly detects many asymptomatic cancers, but the ability to distinguish tumors that are lethal but still curable from those that pose little or no threat to health is limited. Men over age 50 have a high prevalence of indolent, clinically insignificant prostate cancers. No trial has yet demonstrated the benefit of prostate cancer screening and treatment.

The placebo arm of the Prostate Cancer Prevention Trial showed that rigorous screening of low-risk men for 7 years leads to the diagnosis of prostate cancer in >12% of patients. In addition, 15% of men who had normal DRE and PSA levels after 7 years were found to have prostate cancer on biopsy despite the normal screening tests. Thus, screening missed more disease than it found and >27% of normal-risk men in their late 60s were found to have prostate cancer.

The effectiveness of treatments for low-stage prostate cancer are under study. However, both surgery and radiation therapy may cause significant morbidity, such as impotence and urinary incontinence. Comparison of radical prostatectomy to "watchful waiting" in clinically diagnosed (not screen-detected) prostate cancers showed a small decrease in prostate cancer death rate in the surgery arm. One life was saved for every 18–20 men treated with radical prostatectomy. Urinary incontinence and sexual impotence were more common in the surgery arm. One current screening recommendation is that men over age 50 be offered screening and allowed to make a choice after being informed of potential risks and benefits (Table 78-3). A man should have a life expectancy of at least 10 years to be eligible for screening. The USPSTF has found insufficient evidence to recommend prostate cancer screening.

ENDOMETRIAL CANCER Transvaginal ultrasound and endometrial sampling have been advocated as screening tests for endometrial cancer. Benefit from routine screening has not been shown. Transvaginal ultrasound and endometrial sampling are indicated for workup of vaginal bleeding in postmenopausal women but are not considered as screening tests in symptomatic women.

SKIN CANCER Visual examination of all skin surfaces by the patient or by a health care provider is used in screening for basal and squamous cell cancers and melanoma. No prospective randomized study has been performed to look for a mortality decrease. Observational epidemiologic evidence from Scotland and Australia suggests that screening programs have caused a stage shift in melanomas diagnosed. Screening may reinforce sun avoidance and other skin cancer prevention behaviors.

FURTHER READINGS

BACH PB et al: Computed tomography screening and lung cancer outcomes. JAMA 297:953, 2007

BARRETT-CONNOR E et al: Effects of raloxifene on cardiovascular events and breast cancer in postmenopausal women. N Engl J Med 355:125, 2006

FISHER B et al: Tamoxifen for prevention of breast cancer: report of the National Surgical Adjuvant Breast and Bowel Project P-1 Study. J Natl Cancer Inst 90:1371, 1998

FREEDLAND SJ, PARTIN AW: Prostate-specific antigen: Update 2006. Urology 67:458, 2006

HUMPHREY LL et al: Breast cancer screening: A summary of the evidence for the U.S. Preventive Services Task Force. Ann Intern Med 137:347, 2002

PRENTICE RL et al: Low-fat dietary pattern and risk of invasive breast cancer. The Women's Health Initiative randomized controlled dietary modification trial. JAMA 295:629, 2006

WINAWER SJ et al: Guidelines for colonoscopy surveillance after polypectomy: A consensus update by the Multi-Society Task Force on Colorectal Cancer and the American Cancer Society. Gastroenterology 130:1872, 2006

WEBSITES

The Canadian Taskforce on Preventive Health Care
http://www.ctfphc.org/
The National Cancer Institute Cancernet
http://cancernet.nci.nih.gov/

79 Cancer Genetics
Pat J. Morin, Jeffrey M. Trent, Francis S. Collins, Bert Vogelstein

CANCER IS A GENETIC DISEASE

Cancer arises through a series of somatic alterations in DNA that result in unrestrained cellular proliferation. Most of these alterations involve actual sequence changes in DNA (i.e., mutations). They may arise as a consequence of random replication errors, exposure to carcinogens (e.g., radiation), or faulty DNA repair processes. While most cancers arise sporadically, familial clustering of cancers occurs in certain families that carry a germline mutation in a cancer gene.

HISTORICAL PERSPECTIVE

The idea that cancer progression is driven by sequential somatic mutations in specific genes has only gained general acceptance in the past 25 years. Before the advent of the microscope, cancer was believed to be composed of aggregates of mucus or other noncellular matter. By the middle of the nineteenth century, it became clear that tumors were masses of cells and that these cells arose from the normal cells of the tissue in which the cancer originated. However, the molecular basis for the uncontrolled proliferation of cancer cells was to remain a mystery for another century. During that time, a number of theories for the origin of cancer were postulated. The great biochemist Otto Warburg proposed the combustion theory of cancer, which stipulated that cancer was due to abnormal oxygen metabolism: while normal cells required oxygen, cancer cells could survive in its absence. In addition, some believed that all cancers were caused by viruses, and that cancer was in fact a contagious disease.

In the end, observations of cancer occurring in chimney sweeps, studies of x-rays, and the overwhelming data demonstrating cigarette smoke as a causative agent in lung cancer, together with Ames's work on chemical mutagenesis, were sufficient to convince many that cancer originated through changes in DNA. Although the viral theory of cancer did not prove to be generally accurate, the study of retroviruses led to the discovery of the first human *oncogenes* in the mid to late 1970s. Soon after, the study of families with genetic predisposition to cancer was instrumental in the discovery of *tumor-suppressor genes*. The field that studies the type of mutations, as well as the consequence of these mutations in tumor cells, is now known as *cancer genetics*.

THE CLONAL ORIGIN AND MULTISTEP NATURE OF CANCER

Nearly all cancers originate from a single cell; this clonal origin is a critical discriminating feature between neoplasia and hyperplasia. Multiple cumulative mutational events are invariably required for the progression from normal to fully malignant phenotype. The process can be seen as Darwinian microevolution in which, at each successive step, the mutated cells gain a growth advantage resulting in an increased representation relative to their neighbors (**Fig. 79-1**). It is believed that five to ten accumulated mutations are necessary for a cell to progress from the normal to the fully malignant phenotype.

We are beginning to understand the precise nature of the genetic alterations responsible for some malignancies and to get a sense of the order in which they occur. The best studied example is colon cancer, in which analyses of DNA from tissues extending from normal colon epithelium through adenoma to carcinoma have identified some of the genes mutated in the process (**Fig. 79-2**). Similar progression models are being elucidated for other malignancies.

GENERAL CLASSES OF CANCER GENES

There are two major classes of cancer genes. The first class comprises genes that directly affect cell growth either positively (*oncogenes*) or

FIGURE 79-1 Multistep clonal development of malignancy. In this diagram a series of five cumulative mutations (T1, T2, T4, T5, T6), each with a modest growth advantage acting alone, eventually results in a malignant tumor. Note that not all such alterations result in progression; for example, the T3 clone is a dead end. The actual number of cumulative mutations necessary to transform from the normal to the malignant state is unknown in most tumors. (*After P Nowell, Science 194:23, 1976, with permission.*)

FIGURE 79-2 Progressive somatic mutational steps in the development of colon carcinoma. The accumulation of alterations in a number of different genes results in the progression from normal epithelium through adenoma to full-blown carcinoma. Genetic Instability (microsatellite or chromosomal) accelerates the progression by increasing the likelihood of mutation at each step. Patients with familial polyposis are already one step into this pathway, since they inherit a germline alteration of the *APC* gene. TGF, transforming growth factor.

negatively (*tumor-suppressor genes*). These genes exert their effects on tumor growth through their ability to control cell division (cell birth) or cell death (apoptosis). Oncogenes are tightly regulated in normal cells. In cancer cells, oncogenes acquire mutations that relieve this control and lead to increased activity of the gene product. This mutational event typically occurs in a single allele of the oncogene and acts in a dominant fashion. In contrast, the normal function of tumor-suppressor genes is to restrain cell growth, and this function is lost in cancer. Because of the diploid nature of mammalian cells, both alleles must be inactivated to completely lose the function of a tumor-suppressor gene, leading to a recessive mechanism at the cellular level. From these ideas and studies on the inherited form of retinoblastoma, Knudson and others formulated the *two-hit hypothesis*, which in its modern version states that both copies of a tumor-suppressor gene must be inactivated in cancer.

The second class of cancer genes, the *caretakers*, does not directly affect cell growth but rather affects the ability of the cell to maintain the integrity of its genome. Cells with deficiency in these genes have an increased rate of mutations in all the genes, including oncogenes and tumor-suppressor genes. This "mutator" phenotype was first hypothesized by Loeb to explain how the multiple mutational events required for tumorigenesis can occur in the lifetime of an individual. A mutation phenotype has now been observed in cancer at both the nucleotide sequence and chromosomal levels.

MECHANISMS OF TUMOR-SUPPRESSOR INACTIVATION

The two major types of somatic lesions observed in tumor-suppressor genes during tumor development are *point mutations* and *large deletions*. Point mutations in the coding region of tumor-suppressor genes will frequently lead to truncated protein products or otherwise nonfunctional proteins. Similarly, deletions lead to the loss of a functional product and sometimes encompass the entire gene or even the entire chromosome arm, leading to loss of heterozygosity (LOH) in the tumor DNA compared to the corresponding normal tissue DNA (Fig. 79-3). LOH in tumor DNA is considered a hallmark for the presence of a tumor-suppressor gene at a particular locus, and LOH studies have been useful in the positional cloning of many tumor-suppressor genes. Gene silencing, which occurs in conjunction with hypermethylation of the promoter, is another mechanism of tumor-suppressor gene inactivation. Silencing is an epigenetic change rather than a sequence alteration.

FAMILIAL CANCER SYNDROMES

A small fraction of cancers occur in patients with a genetic predisposition. In these families, the affected individuals have a predisposing loss-of-function mutation in one allele of a tumor-suppressor gene or caretaker gene. The tumors in these patients show a loss of the remaining normal allele as a result of somatic events (point mutations or deletions), in agreement with the Knudson hypothesis (Fig. 79-3). Thus, most cells of

an individual with an inherited loss-of-function mutation in a tumor-suppressor gene are functionally normal, and only the rare cells that develop a mutation in the remaining normal allele will exhibit uncontrolled growth. The normal function of tumor suppressors is to restrain growth, to promote differentiation (gatekeeper genes), or to preserve genome integrity (caretaker genes).

Roughly 100 syndromes of familial cancer have been reported, although many are rare. The majority are inherited as autosomal dominant traits, although some of those associated with DNA repair abnormalities (xeroderma pigmentosum, Fanconi's anemia, ataxia telangiectasia) are autosomal recessive. Table 79-1 shows a number of cancer predisposition syndromes and the responsible genes. The current paradigm states that the genes mutated in familial syndromes can also be targets for somatic mutations in sporadic (noninherited) tumors. The study of cancer syndromes has thus provided invaluable insights into the mechanisms of progression for many tumor types. This section examines the case of inherited colon cancer in detail, but the same general lessons can be applied to all the cancer syndromes listed in Table 79-1.

Familial adenomatous polyposis (FAP) is a dominantly inherited colon cancer syndrome due to germline mutations in the adenomatous polyposis coli (*APC*) tumor-suppressor gene on chromosome 5. Patients with this syndrome develop hundreds to thousands of adenomas in the colon. Each of these adenomas has lost the normal remaining allele of *APC* but has not yet accumulated the required additional mutations to generate fully malignant cells (Fig. 79-2). However, out of these thousands of benign adenomas, several will invariably acquire further abnormalities and a subset will even develop into fully malignant cancers. *APC* is thus considered to be a gatekeeper for colon tumorigenesis; Fig. 79-4 shows germline and somatic mutations found

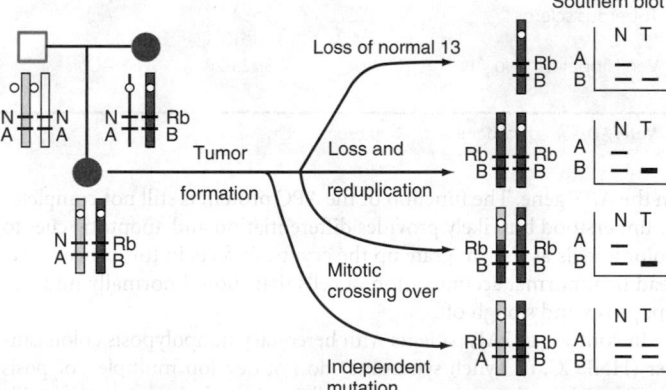

FIGURE 79-3 Diagram of possible mechanisms for tumor formation in an individual with hereditary (familial) retinoblastoma. On the left is shown the pedigree of an affected individual who has inherited the abnormal (Rb) allele from her affected mother. The four chromosomes of her two parents are drawn to indicate their origin. Just below the retinoblastoma locus a polymorphic marker is also analyzed in this family. The patient is AB at this locus, like her mother, whereas her father is AA. Thus the B allele must be on the chromosome carrying the retinoblastoma disease gene. Tumor formation results when the normal allele (N), which this patient inherited from her father, is inactivated. On the right are shown four possible ways in which this could occur. In each case, the resulting chromosome 13 arrangement is shown, as well as the results of a Southern blot comparing normal tissue with tumor tissue. Note that in the first three situations the normal allele (A) has been lost in the tumor tissue, which is referred to as loss of heterozygosity (LOH). (*From TD Gelehrter and FS Collins, in Principles of Medical Genetics, Baltimore, Williams and Wilkins, 1990, with permission.*)

TABLE 79-1   CANCER PREDISPOSITION SYNDROMES AND ASSOCIATED GENES

Syndrome	Gene	Chromosome	Inheritance	Tumors
Ataxia telangiectasia	ATM	11q22-q23	AR	Breast cancer
Autoimmune lymphoproliferative syndrome	FAS	10q24	AD	Lymphomas
	FASL	1q23		
Bloom syndrome	BLM	15q26.1	AR	Cancer of all types
Cowden syndrome	PTEN	10q23	AD	Breast, thyroid
Familial adenomatous polyposis	APC	5q21	AD	Intestinal adenoma, colorectal cancer
Familial melanoma	p16INK4	9p21	AD	Melanoma, pancreatic cancer
Familial Wilms tumor	WT1	11p13	AD	Pediatric kidney cancer
Hereditary breast/ovarian cancer	BRCA1	17q21	AD	Breast, ovarian, colon, prostate
	BRCA2	13q12.3		
Hereditary diffuse gastric cancer	CDH1	16q22	AD	Stomach cancers
Hereditary multiple exostoses	EXT1	8q24	AD	Exostoses, chondrosarcoma
	EXT2	11p11-12		
Hereditary prostate cancer	HPC1	1q24-25	AD	Prostate carcinoma
Hereditary retinoblastoma	RB1	13q14.2	AD	Retinoblastoma, osteosarcoma
Hereditary nonpolyposis colon cancer (HNPCC)	MSH2	2p16	AD	Colon, endometrial, ovarian, stomach, small bowel, ureter carcinoma
	MLH1	3p21.3		
	MSH6	2p16		
	PMS2	7p22		
Hereditary papillary renal carcinoma	MET	7q31	AD	Papillary renal tumor
Juvenile polyposis	SMAD4	18q21	AD	Gastrointestinal, pancreatic cancers
Li-Fraumeni	TP53	17p13.1	AD	Sarcoma, breast cancer
Multiple endocrine neoplasia type 1	MEN1	11q13	AD	Parathyroid, endocrine, pancreas, and pituitary
Multiple endocrine neoplasia type 2a	RET	10q11.2	AD	Medullary thyroid carcinoma, pheochromocytoma
Neurofibromatosis type 1	NF1	17q11.2	AD	Neurofibroma, neurofibrosarcoma, brain tumor
Neurofibromatosis type 2	NF2	22q12.2	AD	Vestibular schwannoma, meningioma, spine
Nevoid basal cell carcinoma syndrome (Gorlin's syndrome)	PTCH	9q22.3	AD	Basal cell carcinoma, medulloblastoma, jaw cysts
Tuberous sclerosis	TSC1	9q34	AD	Angiofibroma, renal angiomyolipoma
	TSC2	16p13.3		
Von Hippel–Lindau	VHL	3p25-26	AD	Kidney, cerebellum, pheochromocytoma

Note: AD, autosomal dominant; AR, autosomal recessive.

While most autosomal dominant inherited cancer syndromes are due to mutations in tumor-suppressor genes (Table 79-1), there are a few interesting exceptions. Multiple endocrine neoplasia type II, a dominant disorder characterized by pituitary adenomas, medullary carcinoma of the thyroid, and (in some pedigrees) pheochromocytoma, is due to gain-of-function mutations in the protooncogene *RET* on chromosome 10. Similarly, gain-of-function mutations in the tyrosine kinase domain of the *MET* oncogene lead to hereditary papillary renal carcinoma. Interestingly, loss-of-function mutations in the *RET* gene cause a completely different disease, Hirschsprung's disease [aganglionic megacolon (Chaps. 291 and 345)].

Although the Mendelian forms of cancer have taught us much about the mechanisms of growth control, most forms of cancer do not follow simple patterns of inheritance. In many instances (e.g., lung cancer), a strong environmental contribution is at work. Even in such circumstances, however, some individuals may be more genetically susceptible to developing cancer, given the appropriate exposure, due to the presence of modifier alleles.

GENETIC TESTING FOR FAMILIAL CANCER

The discovery of cancer susceptibility genes raises the possibility of DNA testing to predict the risk of cancer in individuals of affected families. An algorithm for cancer risk assessment and decision-making in high-risk families using genetic testing is shown in **Fig. 79-6**. Once a mutation is discovered in a family, subsequent testing of asymptomatic family members can be crucial in patient management. A negative gene test in these individuals can prevent years of anxiety in the knowledge that their cancer risk is no higher than that of the general population. On the other hand, a positive test may lead to alteration of clinical management, such as increased frequency of cancer screening and, when feasible and appropriate, prophylactic surgery. Potential negative consequences of a positive test result include psychological distress (anxiety, depression) and discrimination (insurance, employment). Testing should therefore not be conducted without counseling before and after disclosure of the test result. In addition, the decision to test should depend on whether effective interventions exist for the particular type of cancer to be tested. Despite these caveats, genetic cancer testing for some cancer syndromes already appears to have greater benefits than risks, and many companies now offer testing for various genes associated with the predisposition to breast cancer (*BRCA1* and *BRCA2*), melanoma (*p16INK4*), and colon cancer (*APC* and the HNPCC genes).

Because of the inherent problems of genetic testing such as cost, specificity, and sensitivity, it is not yet appropriate to offer these tests to the general population. However, testing may be appropriate in some subpopulations with a known increased risk, even without a defined family history. For example, two mutations in the breast cancer susceptibility gene *BRCA1*, 185delAG and 5382insC, exhibit a sufficiently high frequency in the Ashkenazi Jewish population that genetic testing of an individual of this ethnic group may be warranted.

in the *APC* gene. The function of the APC protein is still not completely understood but likely provides differentiation and apoptotic cues to colonic cells as they migrate up the crypts. Defects in this process may lead to abnormal accumulation of cells that should normally undergo apoptosis and slough off.

In contrast to FAP, patients with hereditary nonpolyposis colon cancer (HNPCC, or Lynch syndrome) do not develop multiple polyposis but instead develop only one or a small number of adenomas that rapidly progress to cancer. HNPCC is commonly defined by family history, with at least three individuals over at least two generations developing colon or endometrial cancer, and with at least one individual diagnosed before the age of 50. Most HNPCC is due to mutations in one of four DNA mismatch repair genes (Table 79-1), which are components of a repair system that is normally responsible for correcting errors in freshly replicated DNA. Germline mutations in *MSH2* and *MLH1* account for >60% of HNPCC cases, while mutations in *MSH6* and *PMS2* are much less frequent. When a somatic mutation inactivates the remaining wild-type allele of a mismatch repair gene, the cell develops a hypermutable phenotype characterized by profound genomic instability, especially for the short repeated sequences called *microsatellites*. This microsatellite instability (MIN) favors the development of cancer by increasing the rate of mutations in many genes, including oncogenes and tumor-suppressor genes (Fig. 79-2). These genes can thus be considered caretakers. **Figure 79-5** shows an example of the instability in allele sizes for dinucleotide repeats in the cancers of HNPCC patients.

FIGURE 79-4 Germline and somatic mutations in the tumor-suppressor gene APC. *APC* encodes a 2843-amino-acid protein with 6 major domains: an oligomerization region (O), armadillo repeats (ARM), 15-amino-acid repeats (15 AA), 20-amino-acid repeats (20 AA), a basic region, and a domain involved in binding EB1 and the *Drosophila* discs large homologue (E/D). Shown are the positions within the *APC* gene of a total of 650 somatic and 826 germline mutations (from the APC database at *http://p53.free.fr*). The vast majority of these mutations result in the truncation of the APC protein. Germline mutations are found to be relatively evenly distributed up to codon 1600 except for 2 mutation hotspots at amino acids 1061 and 1309, which together account for one-third of the mutations found in familial adenomatous polyposis (FAP) families. Somatic *APC* mutations in colon tumors cluster in an area of the gene known as the *mutation cluster region* (MCR). The location of the MCR suggests that the 20-amino-acid domain plays a crucial role in tumor suppression. Note that loss of the second functional *APC* allele in tumors from FAP families often occurs through loss of heterozygosity.

It is important that genetic test results be communicated to families by trained genetic counselors. To ensure that the families clearly understand its advantages and disadvantages and the impact it may have on their management and psyche, genetic testing should never be done before counseling. Significant expertise is needed to communicate the results of genetic testing to families. For example, one common mistake is to misinterpret the result of negative genetic tests. For many cancer predisposition genes, the sensitivity of genetic testing is only ≤70% (i.e., of

FIGURE 79-5 Demonstration of microsatellite instability in normal and tumor tissue from hereditary nonpolyposis colon cancer (HNPCC) patients. In each case the lane marked T contains DNA from a tumor, and the lane marked N contains DNA from normal tissue of the same patient. The marker (*D2S123*, located on chromosome 2) is a microsatellite composed of a tandem repeat of the dinucleotide CA, which varies in length from chromosome to chromosome. Normally, however, the length of the repeat is stable in somatic tissues. In this example, a polymerase chain reaction analysis has been applied to genomic DNA, and new alleles for the marker are apparent in tumors 1, 2, 5, and 7. Because the tumor tissue is defective in DNA mismatch repair, clonal abnormalities in copying of the CA repeat have arisen. Errors are also occurring in functional genes, eventually resulting in the malignant phenotype. (*From LA Aaltonen et al, Clues to the pathogenesis of familial colorectal cancer. Science 260:812, 1993, with permission; Copyright 1993 AAAS.*)

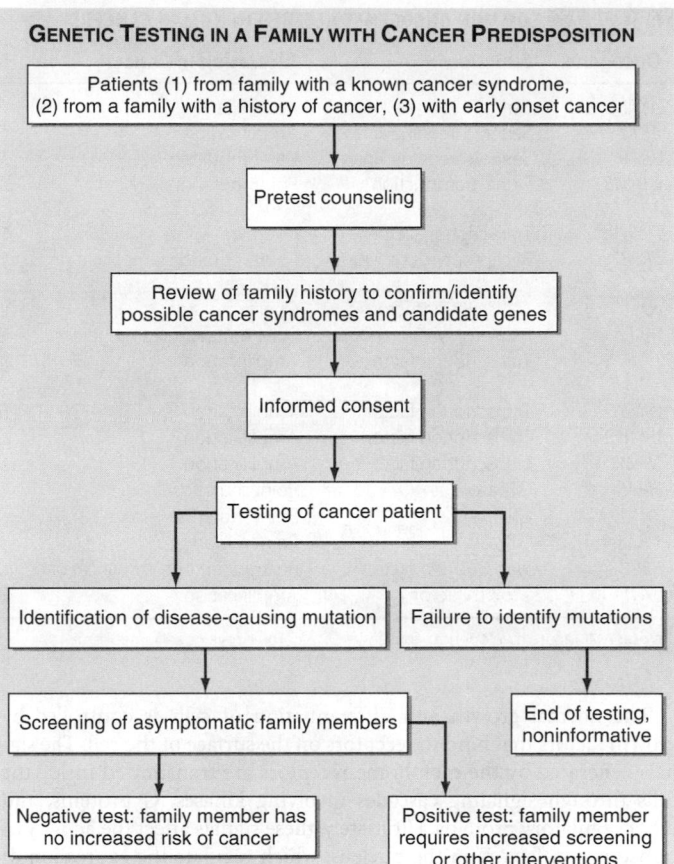

FIGURE 79-6 Algorithm for genetic testing in a family with cancer predisposition. The key step is the identification of a mutation in a cancer patient, which allows testing of asymptomatic family members. Asymptomatic family members who test positive may require increased screening or surgery, whereas others are at no greater risk for cancer than the general population.

100 kindreds tested, disease-causing mutations can be identified in only 70). Therefore, such testing should in general begin with an affected member of the kindred (the youngest family member still alive who has had the cancer of interest). If a mutation is not identified in this individual, then the test should be reported as noninformative (Fig. 79-6) rather than negative (because it is possible that the mutation in this individual is not detectable by standard genetic assays for purely technical reasons). On the other hand, if a mutation can be identified in this individual, then testing of other family members can be performed, and the sensitivity of such subsequent tests will be 100% (because the mutation in the family is in this case known to be detectable by the assay methods used).

ONCOGENES IN HUMAN CANCER

Oncogenes of the kind found in human cancers were initially discovered through their presence in the genome of retroviruses capable of causing cancers in chickens, mice, and rats. The cellular homologues of these viral genes are often targets of mutation or aberrant regulation in human cancer. Whereas many oncogenes were discovered because of their presence in retroviruses, other oncogenes, particularly those involved in translocations characteristic of particular leukemias and lymphomas, were isolated through genomic approaches. Investigators cloned the sequences surrounding the chromosomal translocations observed cytogenetically and then deduced the nature of the genes that were the targets of these translocations (see below). Some of these were oncogenes known from retroviruses [like *ABL*, involved in chronic myelogenous leukemia (CML)], while others were new (like *BCL2*, involved in B cell lymphoma). In the normal cellular environment, protooncogenes have crucial roles in cell proliferation and differentiation. Table 79-2 is a partial list of oncogenes known to be involved in human cancer.

TABLE 79-2 **COMMON ONCOGENES ALTERED IN HUMAN CANCERS**

Oncogene	Function	Alteration in Cancer	Neoplasm
AKT1	Serine/threonine kinase	Amplification	Gastric carcinoma
AKT2	Serine/threonine kinase	Amplification	Ovarian, breast, pancreas cancer
BRAF	Serine/threonine kinase	Point mutation	Melanoma, lung, colorectal cancer
CTNNB1	Signal transduction	Point mutation	Colon, prostate, melanoma, skin, others
FOS	Transcription factor	Overexpression	Osteosarcomas
ERBB2	Receptor tyrosine kinase	Point mutation, amplification	Breast, ovary, stomach, neuroblastoma
JUN	Transcription factor	Overexpression	Lung cancer
MET	Receptor tyrosine kinase	Point mutation, rearrangement	Osteocarcinoma, kidney, glioma
MYB	Transcription factor	Amplification	AML, CML, colon cancer, melanoma
C-MYC	Transcription factor	Amplification	Breast, colon, gastric, lung
L-MYC	Transcription factor	Amplification	Lung carcinoma, bladder
N-MYC	Transcription factor	Amplification	Neuroblastoma, lung cancer
HRAS	GTPase	Point mutation	Colon, lung, pancreas
KRAS	GTPase	Point mutation	Melanoma, colorectal cancer, AML
NRAS	GTPase	Point mutation	Various carcinomas, melanoma
REL	Transcription factor	Rearrangement, amplification	Lymphomas
WNT1	Growth factor	Amplification	Retinoblastoma

Note: AML, acute myelogenous leukemia; CML, chronic myelogenous leukemia.

The normal growth and differentiation of cells is controlled by growth factors that bind to receptors on the surface of the cell. The signals generated by the membrane receptors are transmitted inside the cells through signaling cascades involving kinases, G proteins, and other regulatory proteins. Ultimately, these signals affect the activity of transcription factors in the nucleus, which regulate the expression of genes crucial in cell proliferation, cell differentiation, and cell death. Oncogene products have been found to function at critical steps in these pathways (Chap. 80), and inappropriate activation of these pathways can lead to tumorigenesis.

MECHANISMS OF ONCOGENE ACTIVATION

Mechanisms that upregulate (or activate) cellular oncogenes fall into three broad categories: point mutation, DNA amplification, and chromosomal rearrangement.

Point Mutation Point mutation is a common mechanism of oncogene activation. For example, mutations in one of the *RAS* genes (*HRAS*, *KRAS*, or *NRAS*) are present in up to 85% of pancreatic cancers and 50% of colon cancers but are relatively uncommon in other cancer types. Remarkably—and in contrast to the diversity of mutations found in tumor-suppressor genes (Fig. 79-4)—most of the activated *RAS* genes contain point mutations in codons 12, 13, or 61 (which convey resistance to GAP, a protein that interacts with RAS and inactivates it through substitution of the GTP cofactor with GDP). The restricted pattern of mutation compared to tumor-suppressor genes reflects the fact that gain-of-function mutations of oncogenes are more difficult to attain than simple inactivation. Indeed, inactivation of a gene can be attained through the introduction of a stop codon anywhere in the coding sequence, whereas activations require precise substitutions at residues that normally downregulate the activity of the encoded protein. The specificity of oncogene mutations provides specific diagnostic opportunities, as it is much simpler to find mutations at specified positions than it is when mutations can be scattered throughout the gene (as in tumor-suppressor genes).

DNA Amplification The second mechanism for activation of oncogenes is DNA sequence amplification, leading to overexpression of the gene product. This increase in DNA copy number may cause cytologically recognizable chromosome alterations referred to as *homogeneous staining regions* (HSRs), if integrated within chromosomes, or *double minutes* (dmins), if extrachromosomal in nature. The recognition of DNA amplification is accomplished through various cytogenetic tech-

niques such as comparative genomic hybridization (CGH) and fluorescence in situ hybridization (FISH), which allow the visualization of chromosomal aberrations using fluorescent dyes. With these techniques, the entire genome can be surveyed for gains and losses of DNA sequences, thus pinpointing chromosomal regions likely to contain genes important in the development or progression of cancer. Noncytogenetic, molecular techniques for identifying amplifications have more recently become available.

Numerous genes have been reported to be amplified in cancer. Several genes, including *NMYC* and *LMYC*, were identified through their presence within the amplified DNA sequences of a tumor and had homology to known oncogenes. Because the region amplified often extends to hundreds of thousands of base pairs, more than one oncogene may be amplified in some cancers (particularly sarcomas). Genes simultaneously amplified in many cases include *MDM2*, *GLI*, *CDK4*, and *SAS*. Demonstration of amplification of a cellular gene is often a predictor of poor prognosis. For example, *ERBB2/HER2* and *NMYC* are often amplified in aggressive breast cancers and neuroblastoma, respectively.

Chromosomal Rearrangement Chromosomal alterations provide important clues to the genetic changes in cancer. The chromosomal alterations in human solid tumors such as carcinomas are heterogeneous and complex and likely reflect selection for the loss of tumor-suppressor genes on the involved chromosome. In contrast, the chromosome alterations in myeloid and lymphoid tumors are often simple translocations, i.e., reciprocal transfers of chromosome arms from one chromosome to another. Consequently, many detailed and informative chromosome analyses have been performed on hematopoietic cancers. The breakpoints of recurring chromosome abnormalities usually occur at the site of cellular oncogenes. Table 79-3 lists representative examples of recurring chromosome alterations in malignancy and the

TABLE 79-3 **REPRESENTATIVE ONCOGENES AT CHROMOSOMAL TRANSLOCATIONS**

Gene (Chromosome)	Translocation	Malignancy
ABL (9q34.1)–BCR (22q11)	(9;22)(q34;q11)	Chronic myelogenous leukemia
ATF1 (12q13)–EWS (22q12)	(12;22)(q13;q12)	Malignant melanoma of soft parts (MMSP)
BCL1 (11q13.3)–IgH (14q32)	(11;14)(q13;q32)	Mantle cell lymphoma
BCL2 (18q21.3)–IgH (14q32)	(14;18)(q32;q21)	Follicular lymphoma
FLI1 (11q24)–EWS (22q12)	(11;22)(q24;q12)	Ewing's sarcoma
LCK (1p34)–TCRB (7q35)	(1;7)(p34;q35)	T cell acute lymphocytic leukemia (ALL)
MYC (8q24)–IgH (14q32)	(8;14)(q24;q32)	Burkitt's lymphoma, B cell ALL
WT1 (11p13)–EWS (22q12)	(11;22)(p13;q12)	Desmoplastic small round cell tumor (DSRCT)
PAX3 (2q35)–FKHR/ALV(13q14)	(2;13)(q35;q14)	Alveolar rhabdomyosarcoma
PAX7 (1p36)–KHR/ALV(13q14)	(1;13)(p36;q14)	Alveolar rhabdomyosarcoma
RET (10q11.2)	(10;17)(q11.2;q23)	Papillary thyroid carcinomas

Source: From R Hesketh: *The Oncogene and Tumour Suppressor Gene Facts Book*, 2d ed. San Diego, Academic Press, 1997; with permission.

associated gene(s) rearranged or deregulated by the chromosomal rearrangement. Translocations are particularly common in lymphoid tumors, probably because these cell types normally rearrange their DNA to generate antigen receptors. Indeed, antigen receptor genes are commonly involved in the translocations, implying that an imperfect regulation of receptor gene rearrangement may be involved in the pathogenesis. An example is Burkitt's lymphoma, a B cell tumor characterized by a reciprocal translocation between chromosomes 8 and 14. Molecular analysis of Burkitt's lymphomas demonstrated that the breakpoints occurred within or near the *MYC* locus on chromosome 8 and within the immunoglobulin heavy chain locus on chromosome 14, resulting in the transcriptional activation of *MYC*. Enhancer activation by translocation, although not universal, appears to play an important role in malignant progression. In addition to transcription factors and signal transduction molecules, translocation may result in the overexpression of cell cycle regulatory proteins such as cyclins and of proteins that regulate cell death such as bcl-2.

The first reproducible chromosome abnormality detected in human malignancy was the Philadelphia chromosome detected in CML. This cytogenetic abnormality is generated by reciprocal translocation involving the *ABL* oncogene, a tyrosine kinase on chromosome 9, being placed in proximity to the *BCR* (breakpoint cluster region) on chromosome 22. Figure 79-7 illustrates the generation of the translocation and its protein product. The consequence of expression of the *BCR-ABL* gene product is the activation of signal transduction pathways leading to cell growth independent of normal external signals. Imatinib, a drug that specifically blocks the activity of *BCR-ABL* has shown remarkable efficacy with little toxicity in patients with CML. Knowledge of genetic alterations in cancer can lead to mechanism-based design and development of cancer drugs.

CHROMOSOMAL INSTABILITY IN SOLID TUMORS

Solid tumors are generally highly aneuploid, containing an abnormal number of chromosomes; these chromosomes also exhibit structural alterations such as translocations, deletions, and amplifications. Again, colon cancer has proven to be a particularly useful model for the study of chromosomal instability (CIN). As described above, some familial cases are characterized by the presence of MIN. Interestingly, MIN and CIN appear to be mutually exclusive in colon cancer, suggesting that they represent alternative mechanisms for the generation of a mutator phenotype in this cancer (Fig. 79-2). Other cancer types rarely exhibit MIN but almost always exhibit CIN. Normal cells possess several cell cycle checkpoints, often defined as quality-control requirements that have to be met before subsequent events are allowed to take place. The spindle checkpoint, which ensures proper chromosome attachment to the mitotic spindle before allowing the sister

chromatids to separate, has been shown to be deficient in certain cancers. The genes that, when mutated, may cause CIN have in general not yet been identified, although a few candidates mutated in a small number of tumors have been discovered. The identification of the cause of CIN in tumors will likely be a formidable task, considering that several hundred genes are thought to control the mitotic checkpoint and other cellular processes assuring proper chromosome segregation. Regardless of the mechanisms underlying CIN, the measurement of the number of chromosomal alterations present in tumors is now possible with both cytogenetic and molecular techniques, and several studies have shown that this information can be useful for prognostic purposes.

VIRUSES IN HUMAN CANCER

Certain human malignancies are associated with viruses. Examples include Burkitt's lymphoma (Epstein-Barr virus), hepatocellular carcinoma (hepatitis virus), cervical cancer [human papillomavirus (HPV)], and T cell leukemia (retroviruses). The mechanisms of action of these viruses are varied but always involve activation of growth-promoting pathways or inhibition of tumor-suppressor products in the infected cells. For example, HPV proteins E6 and E7 bind and inactivate cellular tumor suppressors p53 and pRB, respectively. Viruses are not sufficient for cancer development but constitute one alteration in the multistep process of cancer.

EPIGENETIC REGULATION OF GENE EXPRESSION IN CANCER

An *epigenetic modification* refers to a change in the genome, heritable by cell progeny, that does not involve a change in the DNA sequence. The inactivation of the second X chromosome in female cells is an example of an epigenetic mechanism that prevents gene expression from the inactivated chromosome. During embryologic development, regions of chromosomes from one parent are silenced and gene expression proceeds from the chromosome of the other parent. For most genes, expression occurs from both alleles or randomly from one allele or the other. The preferential expression of a particular gene exclusively from the allele contributed by one parent is called *parental imprinting* and is thought to be regulated by covalent modifications of chromatin protein and DNA (often methylation) of the silenced allele.

The role of epigenetic control mechanisms in the development of human cancer is unclear. However, a general decrease in the level of DNA methylation has been noted as a common change in cancer. In addition, numerous genes, including some tumor-suppressor genes, appear to become hypermethylated and silenced during tumorigenesis. *VHL* and *p16INK4* are well-studied examples of tumor-suppressor genes that are silenced through methylation in human cancers. Overall, epigenetic mechanisms may be responsible for reprogramming the expression of a large number of genes in cancer and, together with the mutation of specific genes, are likely to be crucial in the development of human malignancies.

GENE EXPRESSION AND MUTATIONAL PROFILING IN CANCER

The tumorigenesis process, driven by alterations in tumor suppressors, oncogenes, and epigenetic regulation, is accompanied by changes in gene expression. The advent of powerful new techniques such as microarrays and serial analysis of gene expression (SAGE) has allowed the study of gene expression in neoplastic cells on a scale never before accomplished. Indeed, it is now possible to identify expression levels of thousands of genes expressed in normal and cancer tissues. Figure 79-8 shows a typical cDNA array experiment examining gene expression in cancer. This global knowledge of gene expression allows the identification of differentially expressed genes and, in principle, the understanding of the complex molecular circuitry regulating normal and neoplastic behaviors. Such studies have led to molecular profiling of tumors, which has suggested general methods for distinguishing tumors of various biologic behaviors (molecular classification), elucidating pathways relevant to the development of tumors, and identifying molecular targets for the detection and therapy of cancer. The first practical applications of this technology have suggested that global

FIGURE 79-7 Specific translocation seen in chronic myelogenous leukemia (CML). The Philadelphia chromosome (Ph) is derived from a reciprocal translocation between chromosomes 9 and 22 with the breakpoint joining the sequences of the *ABL* oncogene with the *BCR* gene. The fusion of these DNA sequences allows the generation of an entirely novel fusion protein with modified function. (*Courtesy of ER Fearon and KR Cho; with permission.*)

Normal   Cancer

Tissues

Genes

Prepare
cDNA, label

Data analysis from
multiple arrays

Hybridize

Capture
image

FIGURE 79-8 A cDNA array experiment. RNA is prepared from cells, reverse transcribed to cDNA, and labeled with fluorescent dyes (typically green for normal cells and red for cancer cells). The fluorescent probes are mixed and hybridized to the cDNA array. Each spot on the array is a cDNA fragment that represents a different gene. The image is then captured with a fluorescence camera; red spots indicate higher expression in tumor compared with reference while green spots represent the opposite. Yellow signals indicate equal expression levels in normal and tumor specimens. After clustering analysis of multiple arrays, the results are typically represented graphically using Treeview software, which shows, for each sample, a color-coded representation of gene expression for every gene on the array.

gene expression profiling can provide prognostic information not evident from other clinical or laboratory tests. The National Cancer Institute, in conjunction with the National Center for Biotechnology Information, has undertaken the Cancer Genome Anatomy Project (CGAP) (*http://cgap.nci.nih.gov/*) to collect data on gene expression in normal and malignant tissues and make it available on the Internet.

In addition, with the completion of the Human Genome Project and advances in sequencing technologies, large-scale mutational profiling of the cancer genome has become possible. Hundreds of genes from a given pathway (MAPK pathway, for example) or from a gene

family can be systematically sequenced in a large number of cancers in order to identify genes that are crucial to human oncogenesis. This approach has been used to identify several novel targets in various cancers. For example, *B-RAF* mutations were identified in a large fraction of melanomas and *PIK3CA* mutations were identified in large fractions of colon, breast, and hepatocellular cancers. Most recently, this approach has been applied to an unbiased set of genes including about two-thirds of all those known to encode proteins. Hundreds of genes not previously implicated in cancers were shown to be altered in breast and colorectal cancers.

THE FUTURE

A revolution in cancer genetics has occurred in the past 25 years. Identification of cancer genes has led to a better understanding of the tumorigenesis process and has had important repercussions on all fields of biology. In spite of these spectacular advances, however, there has been little overall improvement in cancer death rates. It is hoped that, as the molecular mechanisms of cancer initiation and development continue to be elucidated, novel therapies based on pathophysiology rather than empiricism will emerge. Time will tell whether these strategies will rely on novel combinations or dosing schedules of conventional drugs or will be based on new approaches such as those involving gene therapy or immunotherapy. In addition, a better understanding of the molecular pathways and genetic alterations in cancer cells may lead to the development of sensitive strategies for early detection of cancer.

FURTHER READINGS

GARBER JE, OFFIT K: Hereditary cancer predisposition syndromes. J Clin Oncol 23:276, 2005

GOLUB TR et al: Molecular classification of cancer: Class discovery and class prediction by gene expression monitoring. Science 286:531, 1999

JALLEPALLI PV, LENGAUER C: Chromosome segregation and cancer: Cutting through the mystery. Nat Rev Cancer 1:109, 2001

LOEB LA: Mutator phenotype may be required for multistage carcinogenesis. Cancer Res 51:3075, 1991

MUNGER K: Disruption of oncogene/tumor suppressor networks during human carcinogenesis. Cancer Invest 20:71, 2002

PARSONS DW et al: Colorectal cancer: Mutations in a signaling pathway. Nature 436:792, 2005

STRAUSBERG RL et al: In silico analysis of cancer through the Cancer Genome Anatomy Project. Trends Cell Biol 11:S66, 2001

VOGELSTEIN B, KINZLER KW: The multistep nature of cancer. Trends Genet 9:138, 1993

80 Cancer Cell Biology and Angiogenesis
Robert G. Fenton, Dan L. Longo

Two characteristic features define a cancer: unregulated cell growth and tissue invasion/metastasis. Unregulated cell growth without invasion is a feature of *benign neoplasms*, or new growths. Cancer is a synonym for *malignant neoplasm*. Cancers of epithelial tissues are called *carcinomas*; cancers of nonepithelial (mesenchymal) tissues are called *sarcomas*. Cancers arising from hematopoietic or lymphoid cells are called *leukemias* or *lymphomas*.

Cancer is a genetic disease. The malignant phenotype often requires mutations in several different genes that regulate cell proliferation, survival, DNA repair, motility, invasion, and angiogenesis (**Table 80-1**). Cancer-causing mutations often activate signal transduction pathways leading to aberrant cell proliferation and perturbations of tissue-specific differentiation programs. The normal cell has protective mecha-

nisms that lead to the repair of DNA damage that occurs during DNA synthesis and mitosis and in response to environmental mutagens; these repair pathways are often abnormal in cancer cells. When a normal cell has sustained too much damage to repair, the cell activates a suicide pathway to prevent damage to the organ. These cell death pathways are also commonly altered in cancer cells, leading to the survival of damaged cells that would normally die. Cancer cells often exist under conditions of low oxygen tension (hypoxia) and nutrient deprivation, and selective pressure leads to the outgrowth of neoplastic variants that can survive under these conditions through the upregulation of a series of hypoxia-inducible genes (see below). The acquisition of novel phenotypic characteristics includes those that facilitate invasion and metastasis, such as the ability to break through basement membranes, migrate through the extracellular matrix and into the vascular compartment, and generate new blood vessels to support colonization in remote sites. The accumulation of genetic lesions may lead through an identifiable progression of altered phenotypes as is noted in colon cancer: hyperplasia → adenoma → dysplasia → carcinoma in situ → invasive carcinoma. Premalignant changes have also been identified in prostate, breast, and pancreatic cancers.

TABLE 80-1 PHENOTYPIC CHARACTERISTICS OF MALIGNANT CELLS

Deregulated cell proliferation: Loss of negative regulators (suppressor oncogenes, i.e., Rb, p53), and increased positive regulators (oncogenes, i.e., *Ras, Myc*). Leads to aberrant cell cycle control and includes loss of normal checkpoint responses.

Failure to differentiate: Arrest at a stage prior to terminal differentiation. May retain stem cell properties. (Frequently observed in leukemias due to transcriptional repression of developmental programs by the gene products of chromosomal translocations.)

Loss of normal apoptosis pathways: Inactivation of p53, increases in Bcl-2 family members. This defect enhances the survival of cells with oncogenic mutations and genetic instability and allows clonal expansion and diversification within the tumor without activation of physiologic cell death pathways.

Genetic instability: Defects in DNA repair pathways leading to either single or oligo-nucleotide mutations, (as in microsatellite instability, MIN) or more commonly chromosomal instability (CIN) leading to aneuploidy. Caused by loss of function of p53, BRCA1/2, mismatch repair genes, and others.

Loss of replicative senescence: Normal cells stop dividing after 25–50 population doublings. Arrest is mediated by the Rb, p16^{INK4a}, and p53 pathways. Further replication leads to telomere loss, with crisis. Surviving cells often harbor gross chromosomal abnormalities.

Increased angiogenesis: Due to increased gene expression of proangiogenic factors (VEGF, FGF, IL-8) by tumor or stromal cells, or loss of negative regulators (endostatin, tumstatin, thrombospondin).

Invasion: Loss of cell-cell contacts (gap junctions, cadherens) and increased production of matrix metalloproteinases (MMPs). Often takes the form of epithelial-to-mesenchymal transition (EMT) with anchored epithelial cells becoming more like motile fibroblasts.

Metastasis: Spread of tumor cells to lymph nodes or distant tissue sites. Limited by the ability of tumor cells to survive in a foreign environment.

Evasion of the immune system: Downregulation of MHC class I and II molecules; induction of T cell tolerance; inhibition of normal dendritic cell and/or T cell function; antigenic loss variants and clonal heterogeneity.

Note: VEGF, vascular endothelial growth factor; FGF, fibroblast growth factor; IL, interleukin.

CANCER CELL BIOLOGY

The treatment of most human cancers with conventional cytoreductive agents has been unsuccessful due to the Gompertzian-like growth kinetics of solid tumors (i.e., tumor growth is exponential in small tumors, with increasing doubling times as tumors expand; since conventional chemotherapeutic agents target proliferating cells, noncycling cells in large tumors are relatively resistant). Genetic instability is inherent in most cancer cells and predisposes to the development of intrinsic and acquired drug resistance. Thus, although tumors arise from a single cell (i.e., they are clonal), large tumors become very heterogeneous with multiple related subclones, some of which will be resistant to specific therapies, leading to the selection of progressively more resistant tumors as treatment progresses. Since a 1-cm tumor often contains 10^9 cells, and patients typically present to their physicians with 10^{10}–10^{11} tumor cells, the obstacle to curative treatment becomes more understandable. Rationally designed, target-based therapeutic agents, directed against the specific molecular derangements that distinguish malignant from nonmalignant cells, have become possible with advances in the understanding of oncogene and tumor-suppressor pathways. This chapter describes the convergence of scientific, pharmacologic, and medical knowledge that has led to the targeted therapy of cancer.

THERAPEUTIC APPROACHES TO CELL CYCLE ABNORMALITIES IN CANCER

The mechanism of cell division is substantially the same in all dividing cells and has been conserved throughout evolution. The process assures that the cell accurately duplicates its contents, especially its chromosomes. The cell cycle is divided into four phases. During M-phase, the replicated chromosomes are separated and packaged into two new nuclei by mitosis and the cytoplasm is divided between the two daughter cells by cytokinesis. The other three phases of the cell cycle are called *interphase*: G_1 (gap 1), during which the cell determines its readiness to commit to DNA synthesis; S (DNA synthesis), during which the genetic material is replicated and no re-replication is per-

mitted; and G_2 (gap 2), during which the fidelity of DNA replication is assessed and errors are corrected.

Deregulation of the molecular mechanisms controlling cell cycle progression is a hallmark of cancer. Progression from one phase of the cell cycle to the next is controlled by the orderly activation of cyclin-dependent kinases (CDKs) that are regulated by signaling events that couple a cell's physiologic response to its extracellular milieu. In normal cells, specific molecular signals, called *checkpoints*, prevent progression into the next phase of the cell cycle until all requisite physiologic processes are complete. Cancer cells often have defective cell cycle checkpoints. The transition through G_1 into S-phase is a critical regulator of cell proliferation, and the phosphorylation state of the retinoblastoma tumor-suppressor protein (pRB) at the restriction point in late G_1 determines whether a cell will enter S-phase. The complex of CDK4 or CDK6 with D type cyclins forms a G_1-specific kinase whose activity is regulated by growth factors, nutrients, and cell-cell and cell-matrix interactions. Subsequent formation of an active CDK2/cyclin E complex results in full phosphorylation of pRB, relieving its inhibitory effects on the S-phase-regulating transcription factor E2F/DP1, and permitting the activation of genes required for S-phase (such as dihydrofolate reductase, thymidine kinase, ribonucleotide reductase, and DNA polymerase). The activity of CDK/cyclin complexes can be blocked by CDK-inhibitors including p21$^{Cip1/Waf1}$, p16^{Ink4a}, and p27^{Kip1}, which block S-phase progression by preventing the phosphorylation of pRB.

Genetic lesions that render the retinoblastoma pathway nonfunctional are thought to occur in all human cancers. Loss of function of pRB as guardian of the G_1 restriction point enables cancer cells to enter a mitotic cycle without the normal input from external signals. Current therapeutic efforts to reverse the derangements of the retinoblastoma pathway have taken two main approaches. All kinases require the binding of ATP (and substrate) to the enzyme active site, followed by transfer of the γ-phosphate to serine, threonine, or tyrosine residues of the substrate. Flavopiridol was the first relatively selective CDK inhibitor identified, with Ki or IC$_{50}$s in the 40- to 400-nM range. Although flavopiridol was initially thought to prevent tumor cell proliferation by inhibition of cell cycle CDKs, it is now clear that regulation of cellular transcription elongation by the CDK7/cyclin H and CDK9/cyclin T1 complexes may be the critical target of flavopiridol. Phase II clinical trials of flavopiridol are in progress; responses have been reported in chronic lymphocytic leukemia after a dosing schedule was defined to optimize the pharmacokinetics of the drug. Laboratory efforts are focused on the development of novel classes of CDK inhibitors capable of specifically targeting individual CDK/cyclin complexes. A second therapeutic endeavor to regain control of pRB function involves reversing the epigenetic silencing of p16^{Ink4a} gene and is discussed below.

p53, the "guardian of the genome," is a sequence-specific transcription factor whose activity is regulated through tight control of p53 protein levels. Normally, levels of p53 are kept low by its association with the mdm2 oncogene product, which binds p53 and shuttles it out of the nucleus for proteolytic degradation. p53 levels are regulated by two checkpoint pathways that are activated in response to DNA damage or oncogene-induced cell proliferation (**Fig. 80-1**). The loss of p53 function abrogates these checkpoints and enables tumor cells to escape cell cycle arrest, senescence, or apoptosis despite accumulation of mutations and aberrant passage through the cell cycle.

Acquired mutation in p53 is the most common genetic alteration found in human cancer (>50%); germline mutation in p53 is the causative genetic lesion of the Li-Fraumeni familial cancer syndrome. In many tumors, one p53 allele on chromosome 17p is deleted and the other is mutated. The mutations often abrogate the DNA binding function of p53 that is required for its transcription factor activity and tumor-suppressor functions, and also result in high intracellular levels of p53 protein. Inactivation of the p53 pathway compromises cell cycle arrest, attenuates apoptosis induced by DNA damage or other stimuli, and predisposes cells to chromosome instability. This genomic instability greatly increases the probability that p53 null cells will acquire additional mutations and become malignant. *In summary, it is likely*

FIGURE 80-1 Induction of p53 by the DNA damage and oncogene checkpoints. In response to noxious stimuli, p53 and mdm2 are phosphorylated by the ataxia telangiectasia mutated (ATM) and related ATR serine/threonine kinases, as well as the immediated downstream checkpoint kinases, Chk1 and Chk2. This causes dissociation of p53 from mdm2, leading to increased p53 protein levels and transcription of genes leading to cell cycle arrest (p21$^{Cip1/Waf1}$) or apoptosis (e.g., the proapoptotic Bcl-2 family members Noxa and Puma). Inducers of p53 include hypoxia, DNA damage (caused by ultraviolet radiation, gamma irradiation, or chemotherapy), ribonucleotide depletion, and telomere shortening. A second mechanism of p53 induction is activated by oncogenes such as *Myc*, which promote aberrant G$_1$/S transition. This pathway is regulated by a second product of the Ink4a locus, p19^{ARF}, which is encoded by an *alternative reading frame* of the same stretch of DNA that codes for p16^{Ink4a}. Levels of ARF are upregulated by *Myc* and E2F, and ARF binds to mdm2 and rescues p53 from its inhibitory effect. This *oncogene checkpoint* leads to the death or senescence (an irreversible arrest in G1 of the cell cycle) of renegade cells that attempt to enter S phase without appropriate physiologic signals. Senescent cells have been identified in patients whose premalignant lesions harbor activated oncogenes, for instance, dysplastic nevi that encode an activated form of BRAF (see below), demonstrating that induction of senescence is a protective mechanism that operates in humans to prevent the outgrowth of neoplastic cells.

that all human cancers have genetic alterations that inactivate the Rb and p53 tumor-suppressor pathways.

Tumors expressing mutant p53 are more resistant to radiation therapy and chemotherapy than tumors with wild-type p53. If the transcriptional functions of the mutant p53 could be reestablished in tumor cells, massive apoptosis might ensue, whereas normal cells would be protected because they express very low levels of wild-type p53. Investigators have screened chemical libraries for compounds that inhibit tumor cell growth in a mutant p53-dependent manner. One compound entered cells and induced mutant p53 to adopt an active conformation such that p53-dependent transcriptional activation was restored and apoptosis was selectively induced. This compound also had anti-tumor activity in murine xenograft models. Other investigators have identified a low-molecular-weight, cell-permeable compound that inhibits the apoptotic functions of wild-type p53 found in normal host cells. This compound protected mice from the toxic effects of radiation therapy and chemotherapy, including bone marrow suppression, gastrointestinal dysfunction, and hair loss. Taken together, these approaches provide proof of principle for the pharmacologic manipulation of p53 function (mutant or wild-type) that could greatly enhance therapeutic efficacy while decreasing toxicity.

Knowledge of the molecular events governing cell cycle regulation has led to the development of viruses that replicate selectively in tumor cells with defined genetic lesions. Such "oncolytic" viruses include adenoviruses designed to replicate in tumor cells that lack functional p53 or have defects in the pRB pathway. The former group includes an adenovirus mutant in which the viral p55 protein (which binds and inhibits p53) was deleted; this virus selectively replicates in tumor cells lacking p53 function. This virus has shown efficacy in phase II clinical trials of head and neck tumors, especially when combined with 5-fluorouracil and cisplatin (50% partial or complete response). The complexities of virus-host interactions (i.e., immune response against replicating virus) will require further refinements of this novel technology before the clinical utility of this approach can be fully realized.

TELOMERASE

DNA polymerase is unable to replicate the tips of chromosomes, resulting in the loss of DNA at the specialized ends of chromosomes (called *telomeres*) with each replication cycle. At birth, human telomeres are 15- to 20-kb pairs long and are composed of tandem repeats of a six-nucleotide sequence (TTAGGG) that associate with specialized telomere-binding proteins to form a T-loop structure that protects the ends of chromosomes from being mistakenly recognized as damaged. The loss of telomeric repeats with each cell division cycle causes gradual telomere shortening, leading to growth arrest (called *replicative senescence*) when one or more critically short telomeres triggers a p53-regulated DNA-damage checkpoint response. Cells can bypass this growth arrest if pRB and p53 are nonfunctional, but cell death ensues when the unprotected ends of chromosomes precipitate chromosome fusions or other catastrophic DNA rearrangements (termed *crisis*). *The ability to bypass telomere-based growth limitations is thought to be a critical step in the evolution of most malignancies.* This occurs by the reactivation of telomerase expression in cancer cells. Telomerase is an enzyme that adds TTAGGG repeats onto the 3′ ends of chromosomes. It contains a catalytic subunit with reverse transcriptase activity (hTERT) and an RNA component that provides the template for telomere extension. Most normal somatic cells do not express sufficient telomerase to prevent telomere attrition with each cell division. Exceptions include stem cells (such as those found in hematopoietic tissues, gut and skin epithelium, and germ cells) that require extensive cell division to maintain tissue homeostasis. More than 90% of human cancers express high levels of telomerase that prevent telomere exhaustion and allow indefinite cell proliferation. In vitro experiments indicate that inhibition of telomerase activity leads to tumor cell apoptosis. Major efforts are underway to develop methods to inhibit telomerase activity in cancer cells. The reverse transcriptase activity of telomerase is a prime target for small-molecule pharmaceuticals. The protein component of telomerase (hTERT) can act as a tumor-associated antigen recognized by antigen-specific cytotoxic T lymphocytes (CTL) that lyse human melanoma, prostate, lung, breast, and colon cancer cells in vitro. Clinical trials of telomerase vaccines are underway.

SIGNAL TRANSDUCTION PATHWAYS AS THERAPEUTIC TARGETS IN CANCER CELLS

Since the discovery that the v-*src* oncogene has protein tyrosine kinase activity, the central role of tyrosine phosphorylation in cellular responses to growth factors has become apparent. Many tyrosine kinases act at the apex of signaling pathways and are transmembrane proteins (receptor tyrosine kinases, RTK) or are associated with structures at the plasma membrane (*Src*-, Janus-, and *Fak*-family kinases). RTKs are transmembrane glycoproteins that undergo dimerization upon ligand binding, with activation of their cytoplasmic tyrosine kinase domains by proximity-induced trans-phosphorylation of the activation loop. Tyrosine residues of the receptor or adaptor proteins (such as IRS-1 or Shc) are phosphorylated and act as docking sites for proteins containing SH2 (Src-homology 2) or PTB (phosphotyrosine binding) domains, thus initiating multiple signal transduction pathways (Fig. 80-2). Normally, tyrosine kinase activity is short-lived and reversed by protein tyrosine phosphatases (PTP). However, in many human cancers, tyrosine kinases or components of their downstream pathways are activated by mutation, gene amplification, or chromosomal translocations. Because these pathways regulate proliferation, survival, migration, and angiogenesis, they have been identified as important targets for cancer therapeutics.

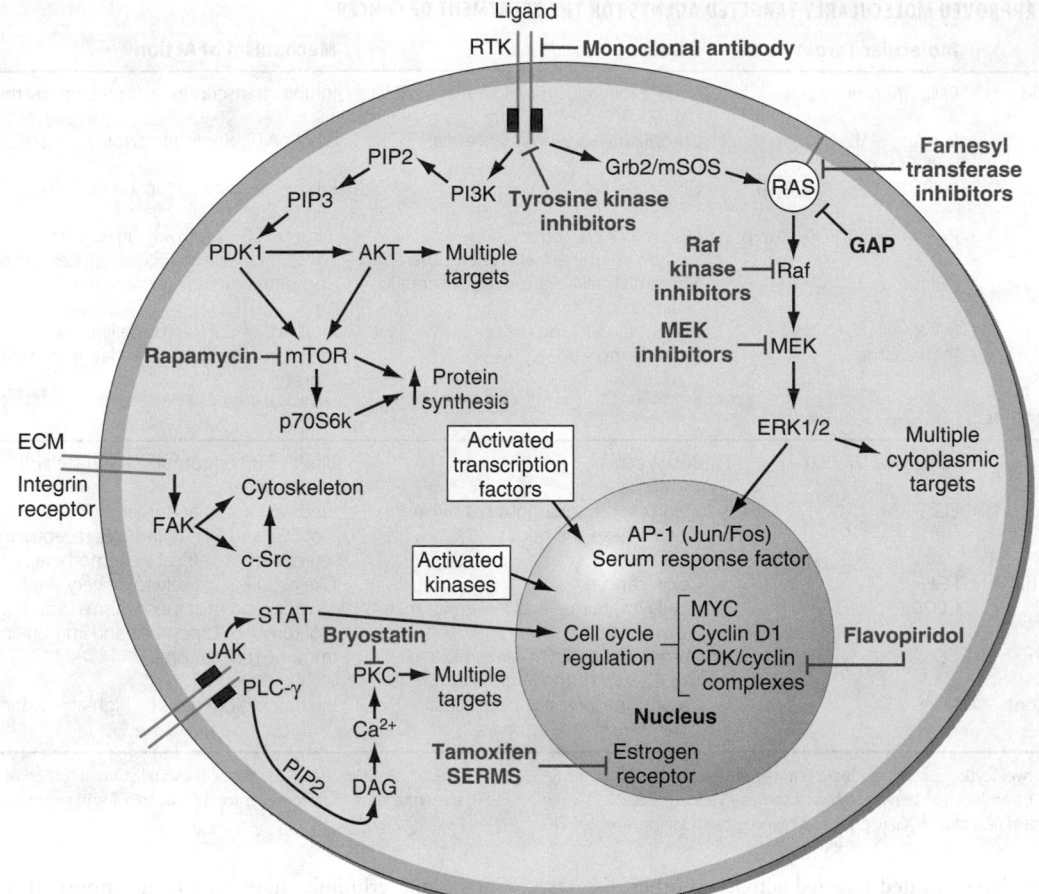

FIGURE 80-2 Therapeutic targeting of signal transduction pathways in cancer cells. Three major signal transduction pathways are activated by receptor tyrosine kinases (RTK). 1. The protooncogene Ras is activated by the Grb2/mSOS guanine nucleotide exchange factor, which induces an association with Raf and activation of downstream kinases (MEK and ERK1/2). 2. Activated PI3K phosphorylates the membrane lipid PIP_2 to generate PIP_3, which acts as a membrane-docking site for a number of cellular proteins including the serine/threonine kinases PDK1 and Akt. PDK1 has numerous cellular targets including Akt and mTOR. Akt phosphorylates target proteins that promote resistance to apoptosis and enhance cell cycle progression, while mTOR and its target p70S6K upregulate protein synthesis to potentiate cell growth. 3. Activation of PLC-γ leads the formation of diacylglycerol (DAG) and increased intracellular calcium, with activation of multiple isoforms of PKC and other enzymes regulated by the calcium/calmodulin system. Other important signaling pathways involve non-RTKs that are activated by cytokine or integrin receptors. Janus kinases (JAK) phosphorylate STAT (signal transducer and activator of transcription) transcription factors, which translocate to the nucleus and activate target genes. Integrin receptors mediate cellular interactions with the extracellular matrix (ECM), inducing activation of FAK (focal adhesion kinase) and c-Src, which activate multiple downstream pathways, including modulation of the cell cytoskeleton. Many activated kinases and transcription factors migrate into the nucleus where they regulate gene transcription, thus completing the path from extracellular signals, such as growth factors, to a change in cell phenotype, such as induction of differentiation or cell proliferation. The nuclear targets of these processes include transcription factors (e.g., Myc, AP-1, and serum response factor) and the cell cycle machinery (CDKs and cyclins). Inhibitors of many of these pathways have been developed for the treatment of human cancers. Examples of inhibitors that are currently being evaluated in clinical trials are shown in purple.

TARGETING Bcr-Abl WITH IMATINIB: PROOF OF PRINCIPLE

The protein product of the Philadelphia chromosome occurs in all patients with chronic myeloid leukemia (CML) and in ~30% of patients with adult acute lymphoid leukemia (ALL) and encodes the fusion protein Bcr-Abl. Although the c-*Abl* protooncogene is a nuclear protein whose kinase activity is tightly regulated as a part of the DNA damage response pathway (and actually induces growth arrest), the Bcr-Abl fusion protein is largely cytoplasmic with a constitutively activated tyrosine kinase domain. The deregulated tyrosine kinase activity of Bcr-Abl is required for its transforming activity. *The Abl tyrosine kinase inhibitor, imatinib mesylate (Gleevec), has validated the concept of a molecularly targeted approach to cancer treatment.*

Imatinib is a low-molecular-weight competitive inhibitor of the ATP binding site of Bcr-Abl, c-Abl, platelet-derived growth factor receptor (PDGFR), and c-Kit; hence it is not absolutely specific for the *Bcr-Abl* oncogene product (Table 80-2). Clinical studies have demonstrated remarkable activity of this agent in CML. In phase II studies of 532 chronic phase CML patients in whom interferon treatment had failed, 95% obtained a hematologic complete response, with only 9% relapse after a median follow-up of 18 months. With longer follow-up, 75% of patients treated with imatinib in chronic phase remain in remission after nearly 4 years. Imatinib was also active in CML blast crisis with a 52% response rate, although the responses were short-lived (78% relapse within 1 year). Relapse during treatment with imatinib was associated with reactivation of the tyrosine kinase either by amplification of the *Bcr-Abl* locus leading to increased levels of Bcr-Abl protein or, more commonly, by point mutations within the Bcr-Abl kinase domain that decreased imatinib binding without loss of Bcr-Abl kinase activity. These data constitute genetic proof that the target of imatinib is the Bcr-Abl tyrosine kinase, and that Bcr-Abl kinase activity is still required by imatinib-resistant cells. Two drugs have been developed (dasatinib and nilotinib) that are potent inhibitors against most imatinib resistant mutants; these compounds have demonstrated significant activity in patients with imatinib-resistant CML.

TABLE 80-2	FDA-APPROVED MOLECULARLY TARGETED AGENTS FOR THE TREATMENT OF CANCER		
Drug	**Molecular Target**	**Disease**	**Mechanism of Action**
All-*trans* retinoic acid (ATRA)	PML-RARα oncogene	Acute promyelocytic leukemia M3 AML; t(15;17)	Inhibits transcriptional repression by the PML-RARα
Imatinib (Gleevec)	Bcr-Abl, c-Abl, c-Kit, PDGFR-α/β,	Chronic myelogenous leukemia; GIST	Blocks ATP binding to tyrosine kinase active site.
Sunitinib (Sutent)	c-Kit, VEGFR-2, PDGFR-β, Flt-3	GIST; renal cell cancer	Inhibits activated c-Kit and PDGFR in GIST; inhibits VEGFR in RCC.
Sorafinib (Nexavar)	RAF, VEGFR-2, PDGFR-α/β, Flt-3, c-Kit	RCC; may have activity in melanoma when combined with chemotherapy	Targets VEGFR pathways in RCC. Possible activity against BRAF in melanoma, colon cancer, and others.
Erlotinib (Tarceva)	EGFR	Non-small cell lung cancer; pancreatic cancer	Competitive inhibitor of the ATP binding site of the EGFR.
Gefitinb (Iressa)	EGFR	Non-small cell lung cancer	Inhibitor of EGFR tyrosine kinase.
Bortezomib (Velcade)	Proteasome	Multiple myeloma	Inhibits proteolytic degradation of multiple cellular proteins.
Monoclonal Antibodies			
Trastuzumab (Herceptin)	HER2/neu (ERBB2)	Breast cancer	Binds HER2 on tumor cell surface and induces receptor internalization.
Cetuximab (Erbitux)	EGFR	Colon cancer, squamous cell carcinoma of the head and neck	Binds extracellular domain of EGFR and blocks binding of EGF and TGF-α; induces receptor internalization. Potentiates the efficacy chemotherapy and radiotherapy.
Panitumomab (Vectibix)	EGFR	Colon cancer	Like cetuximab; likely to be very similar in clinical activity
Rituximab (Rituxan)	CD20	B cell lymphomas and leukemias that express CD20	Multiple potential mechanisms including direct induction of tumor cell apoptosis and immune mechanisms.
Alemtuzumab (Campath)	CD52	Chronic lymphocytic leukemia and CD52-expressing lymphoid tumors	Immune mechanisms
Bevacizumab (Avastin)	VEGF	Colon, lung, breast cancers; data pending in other tumors	Inhibits angiogenesis by high-affinity binding to VEGF.

Note: PML-RARα, promyelocytic leukemia–retinoic acid receptor-alpha; AML, acute myeloid leukemia; t(15;17), translocation between chromosomes 15 and 17; VEGFR, vascular endothelial growth factor receptor; PDGFR, platelet-derived growth factor receptor; Flt- 3, fms-like tyrosine kinase-3; GIST, gastrointestinal stromal tumor; RCC, renal cell cancer; EGFR, epidermal growth factor receptor; TGF-α, transforming growth factor alpha.

Imatinib has also demonstrated targeted activity in other diseases, including gastrointestinal stromal tumors (GIST), rare mesenchymal tumors of the GI tract (stomach and small intestine). The pathogenic molecular event for most patients with this disease is mutation of the proto-oncogene c-*Kit*, leading to the constitutive activation of this receptor tyrosine kinase without the binding of its physiologic ligand, stem cell factor. About 10% of GISTs encode activating mutations of the PDGFRα instead of c-*Kit*. GISTs are thought to arise from or share a common stem cell with the interstitial cells of Cajal, which give rise to the myenteric plexus of the GI tract. Imatinib, which inhibits the c-Kit kinase domain, has demonstrated significant activity (>50% partial responses usually lasting 1–2 years) in this chemotherapy-refractory tumor. Resistance to imatinib develops due to secondary mutations in c-Kit, and many of these tumors are susceptible to treatment with the multitargeted TK inhibitor sunitinib that has activity against c-Kit as well as the PDGF and vascular endothelial growth factor (VEGF) receptors. Sunitinib is approved by the U.S. Food and Drug Administration for treatment of patients with imatinib-resistant GIST or who are intolerant of imatinib (Table 80-2). Interestingly, tumors with mutations in exon 11 of c-Kit's juxtamembrane region are particularly sensitive to imatinib, whereas those with exon 9 mutations (extracellular domain) respond better to sunitinib than imatinib. In the future, primary therapy for GIST may be determined by the specific molecular defect in c-Kit. Patients with chronic myelomonocytic leukemia (CMML, a myeloproliferative disorder) often harbor a Tel-PDGFR translocation that results in constitutive activation of the PDGFR kinase domain exclusively in the leukemic cells. Imatinib inhibits this kinase and has demonstrated significant activity in this disease. *These examples extend the proof of principle that targeting of signaling pathways in cancer cells can be highly efficacious with minimal toxicity, even when the drug does not have absolute target specificity.* Imatinib has become the paradigm of targeted drug development in other diseases.

TARGETING OTHER RECEPTOR TYROSINE KINASES

Epidermal growth factor receptor (EGFR) mutations define a novel subset of lung cancers. Clinical studies of two high-affinity competitive inhibitors of the ATP binding site in the EGFR kinase domain, ge-

fitinib and erlotinib, have provided important insights into the pathogenesis of different subsets of patients with non-small cell lung cancer (NSCLC). Phase III studies led to FDA approval after ~10–20% of advanced-stage patients treated with single-agent gefitinib or erlotinib had objective tumor responses. Responders tended to have adenocarcinoma or bronchoalveolar histology (not squamous or large cell), and were never-smokers, women, and of Eastern Asian origin. DNA sequence analysis of the *EGFR* gene isolated from the tumors of responding patients (mostly nonsmokers) demonstrated that most had acquired mutations of the kinase domain that led to increased tyrosine kinase activity. Frequently, patients with mutated alleles also had evidence of *EGFR* gene amplification by fluorescence in situ hybridization (FISH). These tumors exhibited euploid chromosome content, in contrast to tumors from smokers, which were most often aneuploid and harbored mutations in the K-*Ras* oncogene. In fact, mutated K-*Ras*, which occurs to the exclusion of EGFR mutation, appears to define a subset of patients with low likelihood of response to EGFR inhibitors. Thus the model has been proposed that the pathogenesis of NSCLC in never-smokers occurs through a novel pathway that is dependent on activated EGFR, and that tumors are *addicted* to this oncogene, rendering them highly susceptible to its inhibition (see Fig. 80-7). No EGFR kinase domain mutations have yet been found in tumors other than NSCLC. *Thus, these studies define a novel oncogenic pathway for an important human cancer, and provide a mechanism to identify subsets of patients likely to respond to the targeted therapy.* The wild-type EGFR is expressed by many other human cancers, and in colon cancer and head and neck cancers, targeting of the EGFR with a monoclonal antibody (cetuximab) has demonstrated improved survival when combined with chemotherapy or radiation therapy.

HER2/*neu* is a target in human breast cancer. The gene encoding HER2/*neu*, a member of the EGFR family, is amplified in ~20% of breast cancers. Tumors that overexpress HER2/*neu* are less responsive to chemotherapy, and patients with these tumors have a reduced survival compared with patients with normal levels of HER2/*neu*. Trastuzumab (Herceptin) is a humanized monoclonal antibody that binds HER2/*neu* on the surface of tumor cells and induces internalization of the receptor, thereby reducing the level of surface expression. This leads to inhibition of cell cycle progression and renders cancer cells more susceptible to the induction of apoptosis. Phase III clinical trials demonstrated that combining trastuzumab with chemotherapy significantly improved response rates and overall survival in patients with metastatic HER2-positive disease, leading to FDA approval. In addition, five randomized trials demonstrated that the addition of trastuzumab to chemotherapy in the adjuvant setting for patients with HER2-positive disease reduces the risk of recurrence by nearly 50%. These studies emphasize the critical pathogenic role of HER2-overexpression in a subset of breast cancer patients.

The PDGFR and its ligand, platelet-derived growth factor (PDGF), are overexpressed in many glioblastomas and in subsets of melanoma, ovarian, pancreatic, gastric, lung, and prostate cancers. Overexpression of the hepatocyte growth factor receptor c-MET has been observed in many human cancers and correlates with a poor prognosis, perhaps due to its role in invasion and metastasis. Small-molecule inhibitors of these RTKs are being developed for clinical use. As described below, the vascular endothelial growth factor receptor (VEGFR), TIE, and EPH RTK families have been identified as important therapeutic targets for inhibition of angiogenesis.

Signaling Pathways Downstream of RTKs: Ras and PI3K

Several oncogene and tumor-suppressor gene products are components of signal transduction pathways that emanate from RTK activation (Fig. 80-2). The most extensively studied are the Ras/mitogen-activated protein (MAP) kinase pathway and the phosphatidylinositol-3-kinase (PI3K) pathway, both of which regulate multiple processes in cancer cells, including cell cycle progression, resistance to apoptotic signals, angiogenesis, and cell motility. The development of inhibitors of these pathways is an important avenue of anticancer drug development.

Mutation of the *Ras* protooncogene occurs in 20% of human cancers and results in loss of the response of oncogenic Ras to GTPase-activating proteins (GAPs). The constitutively activated, GTP-bound Ras activates downstream effectors including the MAP kinase and PI3K/Akt pathways. Cancers of the pancreas, colon, and lung and AML harbor frequent *Ras* mutations, with the K-*Ras* allele affected more commonly (85%) than N-*Ras* (15%); H-*Ras* mutations are uncommon in human cancers. In addition, *Ras* activity in tumor cells can be increased by other mechanisms, including upregulation of RTK activity and mutation of GAP proteins (e.g., *NF1* mutations in type I neurofibromatosis). Ras proteins localize to the inner plasma membrane and require posttranslational modifications, including addition of a farnesyl lipid moiety to the cysteine residue of the carboxy-terminal CAAX-box motif. Inhibition of RAS farnesylation by rationally designed farnesyltransferase inhibitors (FTIs) demonstrated encouraging efficacy in preclinical models, most of which utilized oncogenic forms of H-Ras. Despite this, clinical trials of FTIs in patients whose tumors harbor *Ras* mutations have been disappointing, although some activity has been seen in AML. Upon further study, it appears that in the presence of FTIs, lipid modification of the K- and N-Ras proteins occurs by addition of a distinct lipid (geranylgeranyl) through the action of geranylgeranyl transferase-I (GGT-I), which results in restoration of Ras function. Thus, while FTIs are likely to have antitumor activity in select human cancers, their mechanism of action appears to occur by in-

FIGURE 80-3 Oncogene addiction and synthetic lethality: keys to discovery of new anti-cancer drugs. Panel **A.** Normal cells receive environmental signals that activate signaling pathways (pathways A, B, and C) that together promote G1 to S phase transition and passage through the cell cycle. Inhibition of one pathway (such as pathway A by a targeted inhibitor) has no significant effect due to redundancy provided by pathways B and C. In cancer cells, oncogenic mutations lead over time to dependency on the activated pathway, with loss of significant input from pathways B and C. The dependency or addiction of the cancer cell to pathway A makes it highly vulnerable to inhibitors that target components of this pathway. Clinically relevant examples include Bcr-Abl (CML), amplified HER2/*neu* (breast cancer), overexpressed or mutated EGF receptors (lung cancer), and mutated *BRAF* (melanoma). Panel **B.** Genes are said to have a synthetic lethal relationship when mutation of either gene alone is tolerated by the cell, but mutation of both genes leads to lethality. Thus, in the example, mutant *gene a* and *gene b* have a synthetic lethal relationship, implying that the loss of one gene makes the cell dependent on the function of the other gene. In cancer cells, loss of function of a tumor-suppressor gene (wild-type designated *gene A;* mutant designated *gene a*) may render the cancer cells dependent on an alternative pathway of which *gene B* is a component. As shown in the figure, if an inhibitor of *gene B* can be identified, this can cause death of the cancer cell, without harming normal cells (which maintain wild-type function for *gene A*). High-throughput screens can now be performed using isogenic cell line pairs in which one cell line has a defined defect in a tumor-suppressor pathway. Compounds can be identified that selectively kill the mutant cell line; targets of these compounds have a synthetic lethal relationship to the tumor-suppressor pathway, and are potentially important targets for future therapeutics. Note that this approach allows discovery of drugs that indirectly target deleted tumor-suppressor genes and hence greatly expands the list of physiologically relevant cancer targets.

hibition of farnesylation of proteins other than Ras, perhaps RhoB or Rheb (an activator of mTOR). Oncologists anxiously await the development of bona fide Ras-targeted therapeutics.

Effector pathways downstream of Ras are also targets of anticancer drug efforts. Activation of the Raf serine/threonine kinase is induced by binding to Ras and leads to activation of the MAP kinase pathway (Fig. 80-2). Two-thirds of melanomas and 10% of colon cancers harbor activating mutations in the *BRAF* oncogene, leading to constitutive activation of the downstream MAP/ERK kinase (MEK) and extracellular signal-regulated kinases (ERK1/2). This results in the phosphorylation of ERK's cytoplasmic and nuclear targets and alters the pattern of normal cellular gene expression. Inhibitors of Raf kinases (e.g., sorafinib) have entered clinical trials; their activity against tumors expressing mutant *BRAF* have been disappointing as single agents, but they appear to increase the activity of chemotherapy in some cases. Sorafinib also has significant activity against VEGFRs, and this may account for its clinical activity observed in highly vascular renal cell cancers (see below). Cells harboring mutant *BRAF* are highly sensitive to MEK inhibition, providing another example of "oncogene addiction" (Fig. 80-3).

PI3K is a heterodimeric lipid kinase that catalyses the conversion of phosphatidylinositol bisphosphate (PIP$_2$) to phosphatidylinositol trisphosphate (PIP$_3$), which acts as a plasma membrane docking site for proteins that contain a pleckstrin homology (PH) domain. These include the serine/threonine kinases Akt and PDK1 that are key downstream effectors of PI3K action (Fig. 80-2). The PI3K pathway is activated in 30–40% of human cancers and is thought to play a critical role in tumor cell survival, proliferation, growth, and glucose utilization. Amplification or activating point mutation of the gene encoding the catalytic subunit of PI3K (p110) is observed in 20–30% of breast, colon, brain, gastric, and ovarian cancers, and amplification of the *Akt2* gene occurs in breast, ovarian, and pancreatic cancers. The tumor suppressor PTEN (phosphatase with tensin homology), a lipid phosphatase that acts as an off signal for PI3K by dephosphorylating PIP_3, is mutated in many human cancers, leading to unchecked activity of the PI3K pathway. Akt promotes cell survival by activation of the transcription factor nuclear factor of κB (NFκB); it also enhances cell cycle progression by inhibition of glycogen synthetase kinase 3β (GSK3β) and FOXO transcription factors, thus preventing inactivation of Myc, β-catenin, cyclin D1, and cyclin E, and blocking upregulation of p27^{Kip1} and Bim (an apoptosis-inducing protein). Furthermore, the growth of cancer cells requires the activation of two downstream kinases, mammalian target of rapamycin (mTOR) and p70S6K, whose activities promote the translation of cellular mRNAs. Targeted interruption of the PI3K pathway is being attempted at multiple levels. Inhibitors of mTOR, including rapamycin and its more soluble ester derivative temsirolimus (tem), selectively kill human tumor cell lines with PTEN mutations and upregulated PI3K pathway activity. Early clinical data indicate that tem has activity in renal cell cancer, perhaps by blocking the translation of the transcription factor hypoxia-inducible factor (HIF)-1α mRNA, a mediator of cellular responses to hypoxia, which requires mTOR activity for efficient translation.

RTKs activate other signaling pathways. Activation of phospholipase C-γ(PLC) results in the hydrolysis of PIP_2 into diacylglycerol (DAG) and IP_3. DAG together with calcium ion (Ca^{2+}) activates protein kinase C (PKC), a family of serine/threonine-specific protein ki-

nases with different activation requirements, subcellular locations, and substrates in different cell types. PKC is the target of tumor-promoting phorbol esters, and its activation can modulate cell proliferation, differentiation, and tumorigenesis. The PKC inhibitor bryostatin 1 has reached phase II clinical trials and thus far has demonstrated only minimal antitumor activity. However, an antisense oligonucleotide directed against PKC and a number of small molecule inhibitors that demonstrate greater selectivity for PKC isoforms are undergoing clinical evaluation.

ALTERATIONS IN GENE TRANSCRIPTION IN CANCER CELLS: ROLE OF EPIGENETIC CHANGES

Chromatin structure regulates the hierarchical order of sequential gene transcription that governs differentiation and tissue homeostasis. Disruption of chromatin remodeling leads to aberrant gene expression and can induce proliferation of undifferentiated cells, leading to cancer. *Epigenetics* is defined as changes that alter the pattern of gene expression that persist across at least one cell division, but are not caused by changes in the DNA code. Epigenetic changes include alterations of chromatin structure mediated by methylation of cytosine residues in CpG dinucleotides, modification of histones by acetylation or methylation, or changes in higher-order chromosome structure (**Fig. 80-4**). The transcriptional regulatory regions of active genes often contain a high frequency of CpG dinucleotides (referred to as *CpG islands*), which under normal circumstances remain unmethylated. Expression of these genes is controlled by transient association with repressor or activator proteins that regulate transcriptional activation. However, hypermethylation of promoter regions is a common mechanism by which tumor-suppressor loci are epigenetically silenced in cancer cells.

FIGURE 80-4 Epigenetic regulation of gene expression in cancer cells. Tumor-suppressor genes are often epigenetically silenced in cancer cells. In the upper portion, a CpG island within the promoter and enhancer regions of the gene has been methylated, resulting in the recruitment of methyl-cytosine binding proteins (MeCP) and complexes with histone deacetylase (HDAC) activity. Chromatin is in a condensed, nonpermissive conformation that inhibits transcription. Clinical trials are under way utilizing the combination of demethylating agents such as 5-aza-2′-deoxycytidine plus HDAC inhibitors, which together confer

an open, permissive chromatin structure (*lower portion*). Transcription factors bind to specific DNA sequences in promoter regions and, through protein-protein interactions, recruit coactivator complexes containing histone acetyl transferase (HAT) activity. This enhances transcription initiation by RNA polymerase II and associated general transcription factors. The expression of the tumor-suppressor gene commences, with phenotypic changes that may include growth arrest, differentiation, or apoptosis.

Thus one allele may be inactivated by mutation or deletion (as occurs in loss of heterozygosity), while expression of the other allele is epigenetically silenced. The mechanisms that target suppressor oncogenes for this form of gene silencing are unknown.

Acetylation of the amino terminus of the core histones H3 and H4 induces an open chromatin conformation that promotes transcription initiation. Histone acetylases are components of coactivator complexes recruited to promoter/enhancer regions by sequence-specific transcription factors during the activation of genes (Fig. 80-4). Histone deacetylases (HDACs; at least 17 are encoded in the human genome) are recruited to genes by transcriptional repressors and prevent the initiation of gene transcription. Methylated cytosine residues in promoter regions become associated with methyl-cytosine–binding proteins that recruit protein complexes with HDAC activity. The balance between permissive and inhibitory chromatin structure is therefore largely determined by the activity of transcription factors in modulating the "histone code" and the methylation status of the genetic regulatory elements of genes.

The pattern of gene transcription is aberrant in all human cancers, and in many cases, epigenetic events are responsible. Unlike genetic events that alter DNA primary structure (e.g., deletions), epigenetic changes are potentially reversible and appear amenable to therapeutic intervention. In many human cancers, including pancreatic cancer and multiple myeloma, the p16^{Ink4a} promoter is inactivated by methylation, thus permitting the unchecked activity of CDK4/cyclin D and rendering pRB nonfunctional. In sporadic forms of renal, breast, and colon cancer, the von Hippel–Lindau (*VHL*), breast cancer 1 (*BRCA1*), and serine/threonine kinase 11 (*STK11*) genes, respectively, are epigenetically silenced. Other targeted genes include the p15^{Ink4b} CDK inhibitor, glutathione-S-transferase (which detoxifies reactive oxygen species), and the E-cadherin molecule (important for junction formation between epithelial cells). Epigenetic silencing can occur in premalignant lesions and can affect genes involved in DNA repair, thus predisposing to further genetic damage. Examples include MLH1 (mut L homologue) in hereditary nonpolyposis colon cancer (HNPCC, also called Lynch syndrome), which is critical for repair of mismatched bases that occur during DNA synthesis, and 0^6-methylguanine-DNA methyltransferase, which removes alkylated guanine adducts from DNA and is often silenced in colon, lung, and lymphoid tumors.

Many human leukemias have chromosomal translocations that code for novel fusion proteins with enzymatic activities that alter chromatin structure. The PML-RAR fusion protein, generated by the t(15;17) observed in most cases of acute promyelocytic leukemia (APL), binds to promoters containing retinoic acid response elements and recruits HDAC to these promoters, effectively inhibiting gene expression. This arrests differentiation at the promyelocyte stage and promotes tumor cell proliferation and survival. Treatment with pharmacologic doses of all-*trans* retinoic acid (ATRA), the ligand for RARα, results in the release of HDAC activity and the recruitment of coactivators, which overcomes the differentiation block. This induced differentiation of APL cells has greatly improved treatment of these patients and has provided a treatment paradigm for the reversal of epigenetic changes in cancer. However, for other leukemia-associated fusion proteins, such as AML-ETO and the MLL fusion proteins seen in AML and ALL, no ligand is known. Therefore, efforts are ongoing to determine the structural basis for interactions between translocation fusion proteins and chromatin remodeling proteins, and to use this information to rationally design small molecules that will disrupt specific protein-protein associations. Drugs that block the enzymatic activity of HDAC are being developed. A number of different chemical classes of HDAC inhibitors have demonstrated antitumor activity in clinical studies against cutaneous T cell lymphoma (e.g., vorinostat) and some solid tumors. HDAC inhibitors may target cancer cells via a number of mechanisms including upregulation of death receptors (DR4/5, FAS, and their ligands) and p21$^{Cip1/Waf1}$, as well as inhibition of cell cycle checkpoints.

Major therapeutic efforts are also under way to reverse the hypermethylation of CpG islands that characterizes many solid tumors. Drugs that induce DNA demethylation, such as 5-aza-2'-deoxycytidine, can lead to reexpression of silenced genes in cancer cells with restoration of function. However, 5-aza-2'-deoxycytidine has limited aqueous solubility and is myelosuppressive. Other inhibitors of DNA methyltransferases are in development. In ongoing clinical trials, inhibitors of DNA methylation are being combined with HDAC inhibitors. The hope is that by reversing coexisting epigenetic changes, the deregulated patterns of gene transcription in cancer cells will be at least partially reversed.

Aberrant signal transduction pathways activate a number of transcription factors that promote tumor cell proliferation and survival. These include signal transducer and activator of transcription (STAT)-3 and STAT5, NFκB, β-catenin (a component of the APC tumor-suppressor pathway), the heterodimer of c-Jun and Fos known as AP1, and c-Myc. The ability to target these transcription factors therapeutically does not currently exist. However, structural and molecular approaches may make it possible to identify small molecules that would inhibit protein-protein interactions needed for transcription factor dimerization or interaction with coactivator proteins. A small-molecule inhibitor has been developed that blocks the association of Myc with its partner Max, thereby inhibiting Myc-induced transformation. Many transcription factors are activated by phosphorylation, which can be prevented by tyrosine- or serine/threonine kinase inhibitors. The transcription factor NFκB is a heterodimer composed of p65 and p50 subunits that associate with an inhibitor, IκB, in the cell cytoplasm. In response to growth factor or cytokine signaling, a multi-subunit kinase called IKK (IκB-kinase) phosphorylates IκB and directs its degradation by the ubiquitin/proteasome system. NFκB, free of its inhibitor, translocates to the nucleus and activates target genes, many of which promote the survival of tumor cells. Novel drugs called *proteasome inhibitors* block the proteolysis of IκB, thereby preventing NFκB activation. For unexplained reasons, this is selectively toxic to tumor cells. Further studies have indicated that the antitumor effects of proteasome inhibitors are more complicated and involve the inhibition of the degradation of multiple cellular proteins. Proteasome inhibitors [bortezomib (Velcade)] have shown very significant activity in patients with multiple myeloma, including partial and complete remissions. Inhibitors of IKK are also in development, with the hope of more selectively blocking the degradation of IκB, thus "locking" NFκB in an inhibitory complex and rendering the cancer cell more susceptible to apoptosis-inducing agents.

Estrogen receptors (ERs) and androgen receptors, members of the steroid hormone family of nuclear receptors, are targets of inhibition by drugs used to treat breast and prostate cancers, respectively. Tamoxifen, a partial agonist and antagonist of ER function, can mediate tumor regression in metastatic breast cancer and can prevent disease recurrence in the adjuvant setting, saving thousands of lives each year. Tamoxifen binds to the ER and modulates its transcriptional activity, inhibiting activity in the breast but promoting activity in bone and uterine epithelium. Selective estrogen receptor modulators (SERMs) have been developed with the hope of a more beneficial modulation of ER activity, i.e., antiestrogenic activity in the breast, uterus, and ovary, but estrogenic for bone, brain, and cardiovascular tissues. Aromatase inhibitors, which block the conversion of androgens to estrogens in breast and subcutaneous fat tissues, have demonstrated improved clinical efficacy compared with tamoxifen and are often used as first-line therapy in patients with ER-positive disease (Chap. 86).

APOPTOSIS

Tissue homeostasis requires a balance between the death of aged, terminally differentiated cells and their renewal by proliferation of committed progenitors. Genetic damage to growth-regulating genes of stem cells could lead to catastrophic results for the host as a whole. However, genetic events causing activation of oncogenes or loss of tumor suppressors, which would be predicted to lead to unregulated cell proliferation, instead activate signal transduction pathways that block aberrant cell proliferation. These pathways can lead to programmed cell death (*apoptosis*) or irreversible growth arrest (*senescence*). Much as a pano-

FIGURE 80-5 Therapeutic strategies to overcome aberrant survival pathways in cancer cells. **1.** The extrinsic pathway of apoptosis can be selectively induced in cancer cells by TRAIL (the ligand for death receptors 4 and 5) or by agonistic monoclonal antibodies. **2.** Inhibition of antiapoptotic Bcl-2 family members with antisense oligonucleotides or inhibitors of the BH_3-binding pocket will promote formation of Bak- or Bax-induced pores in the mitochondrial outer membrane. **3.** Epigenetic silencing of APAF-1, caspase-8, and other proteins can be overcome using demethylating agents and inhibitors of histone deacetylases. **4.** Inhibitor of apoptosis proteins (IAP) blocks activation of caspases; small-molecule inhibitors of IAP function (mimicking SMAC action) should lower the threshold for apoptosis. **5.** Signal transduction pathways originating with activation of receptor tyrosine kinase receptors (RTKs) or cytokine receptors promote survival of cancer cells by a number of mechanisms. Inhibiting receptor function with monoclonal antibodies, such as trastuzumab or cetuximab, or inhibiting kinase activity with small-molecular inhibitors can block the pathway. **6.** The Akt kinase phosphorylates many regulators of apoptosis to promote cell survival; inhibitors of Akt may render tumor cells more sensitive to apoptosis-inducing signals; however, the possibility of toxicity to normal cells may limit the therapeutic value of these agents. **7** and **8.** Activation of the transcription factor NFκB (composed of p65 and p50 subunits) occurs when its inhibitor, IκB, is phosphorylated by IκB-kinase (IKK), with subsequent degradation of IκB by the proteasome. Inhibition of IKK activity should selectively block the activation of NFκB target genes, many of which promote cell survival. Inhibitors of proteasome function are FDA approved and may work in part by preventing destruction of IκB, thus blocking NFκB nuclear localization. NFκB is unlikely to be the only target for proteasome inhibitors.

ply of intra- and extracellular signals impinge upon the core cell cycle machinery to regulate cell division, so too these signals are transmitted to a core enzymatic machinery that regulates cell death and survival.

Apoptosis is induced by two main pathways (Fig. 80-5). The extrinsic pathway of apoptosis is activated by cross-linking members of the tumor necrosis factor (TNF) receptor superfamily, such as CD95 (Fas) and death receptors DR4 and DR5, by their receptors, Fas ligand or TRAIL (TNF-related apoptosis-inducing ligand), respectively. This induces the association of FADD (Fas-associated death domain) and procaspase-8 to death domain motifs of the receptors. Caspase-8 is activated and then cleaves and activates effector caspases-3 and -7, which then target cellular constituents (including caspase-activated DNAse, cytoskeletal proteins, and a number of regulatory proteins), inducing the morphologic

appearance characteristic of apoptosis. The intrinsic pathway of apoptosis is initiated by the release of cytochrome c and SMAC (second mitochondrial activator of caspases) from the mitochondrial intermembrane space in response to a variety of noxious stimuli, including DNA damage, loss of adherence to the extracellular matrix (ECM), oncogene-induced proliferation, and growth factor deprivation. Upon release into the cytoplasm, cytochrome c associates with dATP, procaspase-9, and the adaptor protein APAF-1, leading to the sequential activation of caspase-9 and effector caspases. SMAC binds to and blocks the function of inhibitor of apoptosis proteins (IAPs), negative regulators of caspase activation.

The release of apoptosis-inducing proteins from the mitochondria is regulated by pro- and antiapoptotic members of the Bcl-2 family. Antiapoptotic members (e.g., Bcl-2, Bcl-XL, and Mcl-1) associate with the mitochondrial outer membrane via their carboxy termini, exposing to the cytoplasm a hydrophobic binding pocket composed of Bcl-2 homology (BH) domains 1, 2, and 3 that is crucial for their activity. Perturbations of normal physiologic processes in specific cellular compartments lead to the activation of BH3-only proapoptotic family members (such as Bad, Bim, Bid, Puma, Noxa, and others) that can alter the conformation of the outer-membrane proteins Bax and Bak, which then oligomerize to form pores in the mitochondrial outer membrane resulting in cytochrome c release. If BH3-only proteins are sequestered by Bcl-2, Bcl-XL, or Mcl-1, pores do not form and apoptosis-inducing proteins are not released from the mitochondrion. The relative levels of expression of antiapoptotic Bcl-2 family members compared to the levels of proapoptotic BH3-only proteins at the mitochondrial membrane determines the activation state of the intrinsic pathway. The mitochondrion must therefore be recognized not only as an organelle with vital roles in intermediary metabolism and oxidative phosphorylation but also as a central regulatory structure of the apoptotic process.

The evolution of tumor cells to a more malignant phenotype requires the acquisition of genetic changes that subvert apoptosis pathways and promote cancer cell survival and resistance to anticancer therapies. However, because of their deranged physiology, cancer cells may be more vulnerable than normal cells to therapeutic interventions that target the apoptosis pathways that cancer cells are very dependent upon. For instance, overexpression of Bcl-2 as a result of the t(14;18) translocation contributes to follicular lymphoma. Upregulation of Bcl-2 expression is also observed in prostate, breast, and lung cancers and melanoma. Targeting of antiapoptotic Bcl-2 family members has been accomplished by the identification of several low-molecular-weight compounds that bind to the hydrophobic pockets of either Bcl-2 or Bcl-XL and block their ability to associate with death-inducing BH3-only proteins. These compounds inhibit the antiapoptotic activities of Bcl-2 and Bcl-XL at nanomolar concentrations and will soon be entering clinical trials, first as single agents and then in combination with cytotoxic agents.

Preclinical studies targeting death receptors DR4 and -5 have demonstrated that recombinant, soluble, human TRAIL or humanized monoclonal antibodies with agonist activity against DR4 or -5 can induce apoptosis of tumor cells while sparing normal cells. The mechanisms for this selectivity may include expression of decoy receptors or elevated levels of intracellular inhibitors (such as FLIP, which competes with caspase-8 for FADD) by normal cells but not tumor cells. Synergy has been shown between TRAIL-induced apoptosis and chemotherapeutic agents. For instance, some colon cancers encode mutated Bax protein as the result of mismatch repair (MMR) defects and are resistant to TRAIL. However, upregulation of Bak by chemotherapy restores the ability of TRAIL to activate the mitochondrial pathway of apoptosis. In early phase clinical trials, agonistic antibodies for DR4 and -5 and recombinant TRAIL trimers have led to the stabilization of tumor growth with a few cases of tumor shrinkage; however, studies have not yet shown that clinical activity correlates with activation of the extrinsic pathway of apoptosis.

Many of the signal transduction pathways perturbed in cancer promote tumor cell survival (Fig. 80-5). These include activation of the PI3K/Akt pathway, increased levels of the NFκB transcription factor, and epigenetic silencing of genes such as APAF-1 and caspase-8. Each of these pathways is a target for therapeutic agents that, in addition to affecting cancer cell proliferation or gene expression, may render cancer cells more susceptible to apoptosis, thus promoting synergy when combined with other chemotherapeutic agents.

Some tumor cells resist drug-induced apoptosis by expression of one or more members of the ABC family of ATP-dependent efflux pumps that mediate the multidrug resistance (MDR) phenotype. The prototype, P-glycoprotein (PGP), spans the plasma membrane 12 times and has two ATP-binding sites. Hydrophobic drugs (e.g., anthracyclines and vinca alkaloids) are recognized by PGP as they enter the cell and are pumped out. Numerous clinical studies have failed to demonstrate that drug resistance can be overcome using inhibitors of PGP. However, ABC transporters have different substrate specificities, and inhibition of a single family member may not be sufficient to overcome the MDR phenotype. A more rational targeting of specific transporters expressed by distinct tumor types may lead to increased efficacy.

METASTASIS: DETERMINING RISK AND DEVELOPING THERAPEUTIC STRATEGIES

The three major features of tissue invasion are cell adhesion to the basement membrane, local proteolysis of the membrane, and movement of the cell through the rent in the membrane and the ECM. Malignant cells that gain access to the circulation must then repeat those steps at a remote site, find a hospitable niche in a foreign tissue, and induce the growth of new blood vessels. There are currently few drugs that directly target the process of metastasis. Metalloproteinase inhibitors (see "Tumor Angiogenesis," below) represent an initial attempt to inhibit the migration of tumor cells into blood and lymphatic vessels. The rate-limiting step for metastasis is the ability for tumor cells to survive and expand in the novel microenvironment of the metastatic site, and multiple host-tumor interactions determine the ultimate outcome (**Fig. 80-6**).

The metastatic phenotype may be a characteristic of all cells constituting the primary tumor; however, it is likely that variants with metastatic potential arise due to genetic and epigenetic events that characterize tumor progression (Fig. 80-6). A number of candidate metastasis-suppressor genes have been identified. The loss of function of these genes enhances metastasis, and although the molecular mechanisms are in many cases uncertain, one common theme is an enhancing of the ability of the metastatic tumor cells to overcome the many apoptosis signals they encounter during the metastatic process. Gene expression profiling is being used to study the metastatic process with the goal of identifying signatures characteristic of primary tumors that have a high propensity to metastasize, leading to a more rational basis for the use of adjuvant chemotherapy.

Bone metastases are extremely painful, cause fractures of weight-bearing bones, can lead to hypercalcemia, and are a major cause of morbidity for cancer patients. Osteoclasts and their monocyte–derived precursors express the surface receptor RANK (receptor activator of NFκB), which is required for terminal differentiation and activation of osteoclasts. Osteo-

FIGURE 80-6 Oncogene signaling pathways are activated during tumor progression and promote metastatic potential. This figure shows a cancer cell that has undergone epithelial to mesenchymal transition (EMT) under the influence of several environmental signals. Critical components include activated transforming growth factor beta (TGF-β) and the hepatocyte growth factor (HGF)/c-Met pathways, as well as changes in the expression of adhesion molecules that mediate cell-cell and cell-extracellular matrix interactions. Important changes in gene expression are mediated by the Snail and Twist family of transcriptional repressors (whose expression is induced by the oncogenic pathways), leading to reduced expression of E-cadherin, a key component of adherens junctions between epithelial cells. This, in conjunction with upregulation of N-cadherin, a change in the pattern of expression of integrins (which mediate cell-extracellular matrix associations that are important for cell motility), and a switch in intermediate filament expression from cytokeratin to vimentin, results in the phenotypic change from adherent highly organized epithelial cells to motile and invasive cells with a fibroblast or mesenchymal morphology. EMT is thought to be an important step leading to metastasis in some human cancers. Host stromal cells, including tumor-associated fibroblasts and macrophages, play an important role in modulating tumor cell behavior through secretion of growth factors and proangiogenic cytokines, and matrix metalloproteinases that degrade the basement membrane. VEGF-A, -C, and -D are produced by tumor cells and stromal cells in response to hypoxia or oncogenic signals, and induce production of new blood vessels and lymphatic channels through which tumor cells metastasize to lymph nodes or tissues.

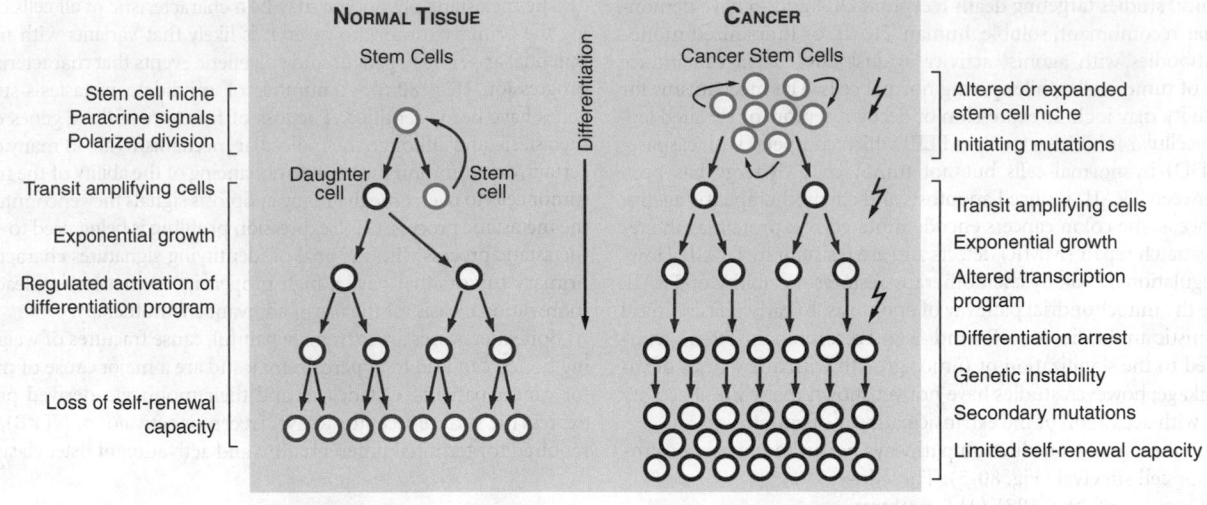

NORMAL TISSUE	CANCER

FIGURE 80-7 Cancer stem cells play a critical role in the initiation, progression, and resistance to therapy of malignant neoplasms. In normal tissues (*left*), homeostasis is maintained by asymmetric division of stem cells leading to one progeny cell that will differentiate, and one cell that will maintain the stem cell pool. This occurs within highly specific niches unique to each tissue, such as in close apposition to osteoblasts in bone marrow, or at the base of crypts in the colon. Here, paracrine signals from stromal cells, such as sonic hedgehog or Notch-ligands, as well as upregulation of β-catenin and telomerase, help to maintain stem cell features of unlimited self-renewal while preventing differentiation or cell death. This occurs in part through upregulation of the transcriptional repressor Bmi-1 and inhibition of the $p16^{Ink4a}$/Arf and p53 pathways. Daughter cells leave the stem cells niche and enter a proliferative phase (referred to as *transit-amplifying cells*) for a specified number of cell divisions, during which time a developmental program is activated, eventually giving rise to fully differentiated cells that have lost proliferative potential. Cell renewal equals cell death and homeostasis is maintained. In this hierarchal system, only stem cells are long-lived. Recent evidence has led to the hypothesis that cancers harbor stem cells that make up a small fraction (i.e., 0.001–1%) of all cancer cells. These cells share several features with normal stem cells, including an undifferentiated phenotype, unlimited self-renewal potential, a capacity for some degree of differentiation; however, due to initiating mutations (mutations are indicated by lightning bolts), they are no longer regulated by environmental cues. The cancer stem cell pool is expanded, and rapidly proliferating progeny, through additional mutations, may attain stem cell properties, although most of this population is thought to have a limited proliferative capacity. Differentiation programs are dysfunctional due to reprogramming of the pattern of gene transcription by oncogenic signaling pathways. Within the cancer transit-amplifying population, genomic instability generates aneuploidy and clonal heterogeneity as cells attain a fully malignant phenotype with metastatic potential. The cancer stem cell hypothesis has led to the idea that current cancer therapies may be effective at killing the bulk of tumor cells, but do not kill tumor stem cells, leading to a regrowth of tumors that is manifested as tumor recurrence or disease progression. Research is in progress to identify unique molecular features of cancer stem cells that can lead to their direct targeting by novel therapeutic agents.

blasts and other stromal cells express RANK ligand, as both a membrane-bound and soluble cytokine. Osteoprotegerin (OPG), a soluble receptor for RANK ligand produced by stromal cells, acts as a decoy receptor to inhibit RANK activation. The relative balance of RANK ligand and OPG determines the activation state of RANK on osteoclasts. Many tumors increase osteoclast activity by secretion of substances such as parathyroid hormone (PTH), PTH-related peptide, interleukin (IL)-1, or Mip1, that perturb the homeostatic balance of bone remodeling by increasing RANK signaling. One example is multiple myeloma, where tumor cell–stromal cell interactions activate osteoclasts and inhibit osteoblasts, leading to the development of multiple lytic bone lesions. Inhibition of RANK ligand by IV administration of recombinant OPG or the extracellular domain of RANK linked to an immunoglobulin Fc-receptor (RANK-Fc) can prevent further bone destruction. Bisphosphonates are also effective inhibitors of osteoclast function that are used in the treatment of cancer patients with bone metastases.

NEW CONCEPTS IN THE DEVELOPMENT OF CANCER THERAPEUTICS

CANCER STEM CELLS

It has long been recognized that only a small proportion of the cells within a tumor are capable of initiating colonies in vitro or of forming tumors at high efficiency when injected into immunocompromised NOD/SCID mice. Current work indicates that human acute and chronic myeloid leukemias (AML and CML) have a small population of cells (<1%) that have properties of stem cells, such as unlimited self-renewal and the capacity to cause leukemia when serially transplanted in mice. These cells have an undifferentiated phenotype (Thy1⁻CD34⁺CD38⁻, and negative for other differentiation markers) and resemble normal stem cells in many ways, but are no longer under homeostatic control (Fig. 80-7). Solid tumors may also contain a population of stem cells. Cancer stem cells, like their normal counterparts, have unlimited proliferative capacity and paradoxically traverse the cell cycle at a very slow rate; cancer growth occurs largely due to expansion of the stem cell pool, the unregulated proliferation of the transit amplifying population, and failure of apoptosis pathways (Fig. 80-7). Slow cell cycle progression, plus high levels of expression of anti-apoptotic Bcl-2 family members and drug efflux pumps of the MDR family, render cancer stem cells less vulnerable to cancer chemotherapy or radiation therapy. Implicit in the cancer stem cell hypothesis is the idea that failure to cure most human cancers is due to the fact that current therapeutic agents do not kill the stem cells. If cancer stem cells can be identified and isolated, then aberrant signaling pathways that distinguish these cells from normal tissue stem cells can be identified and targeted. Oncologists eagerly await a new class of agent that may directly attack the cells that drive tumor growth.

ONCOGENE ADDICTION AND SYNTHETIC LETHALITY

The concepts of oncogene addiction and synthetic lethality have spurred new drug development targeting oncogene and tumor-suppressor pathways. As discussed earlier in this chapter and outlined in Fig. 80-3, cancer cells become physiologically dependent upon signaling pathways containing activated oncogenes; this can effect proliferation (i.e., mutated Ras, BRAF, overexpressed Myc, or activated tyrosine kinases), survival (overexpression of Bcl-2 or NFκB), cell metabolism (as occurs when HIF-1α and Akt increase dependence on glycolysis), and perhaps angiogenesis (production of VEGF, e.g., renal cell cancer). In such cases, targeted inhibition of the pathway can lead to specific killing of the cancer cells. However, targeting defects in tumor-suppressor genes has been much more difficult, since the target of the mutation is often deleted. However, identifying genes that have a synthetic lethal relationship to tumor-suppressor pathways may allow targeting of proteins required uniquely by the tumor cells (Fig. 80-3, panel B). Several examples of this have been identified. For instance, the von Hippel–Landau tumor-suppressor-protein is inactivated in 60% of renal cell cancers, leading to overexpression of HIF-1α and the subsequent activation of downstream genes that promote angiogenesis, proliferation, survival, and altered glucose metabolism. HIF-1α mRNA has a complex 5′-terminus that indirectly requires the activity of mTOR (via activation of p70S6K and inhibition of 4E-BP) for efficient protein translation. Inhibitors of mTOR block HIF-1α translation and have significant clinical activity in renal cell cancer. In this case, mTOR is synthetic lethal to VHL loss (Fig. 80-3), and its inhibition results in selective killing of cancer cells. Conceptually, this provides a framework for genetic screens to identify other synthetic lethal combinations involving known tumor-suppressor genes, and development of novel therapeutic agents to target dependent pathways.

In summary, our expanding knowledge of the genetic and molecular abnormalities in cancer cells, and their phenotypic correlates, has led to the development and FDA approval of a number of targeted pharmaceutical agents for the treatment of cancer (Table 80-2). This list will expand to include inhibitors of pathways currently under investigation and those yet to be discovered, yielding novel therapeutics with greater efficacy with less toxicity.

TUMOR ANGIOGENESIS

The growth of primary and metastatic tumors to larger than a few millimeters requires the recruitment of neighboring blood vessels and vascular endothelial cells to support their metabolic requirements. The diffusion limit for oxygen in tissues is ~100 μm. A critical element in the growth of primary tumors and formation of metastatic sites is the *angiogenic switch*: the ability of the tumor to promote the formation of new capillaries from preexisting host vessels. The angiogenic switch is a phase in tumor development when the dynamic balance of pro- and antiangiogenic factors is tipped in favor of vessel formation by the effects of the tumor on its immediate environment. Stimuli for tumor angiogenesis include hypoxia, inflammation, and genetic lesions in oncogenes or tumor suppressors that alter tumor cell gene expression. Angiogenesis consists of several steps, including the stimulation of endothelial cells (ECs) by growth factors, the degradation of the ECM by proteases, proliferation of ECs and migration into the tumor, and the eventual formation of new capillary tubes.

Tumor blood vessels are not normal; they have chaotic architecture and blood flow. Due to an imbalance of angiogenic regulators such as VEGF and angiopoietins (see below), tumor vessels are tortuous and dilated with an uneven diameter, excessive branching, and shunting.

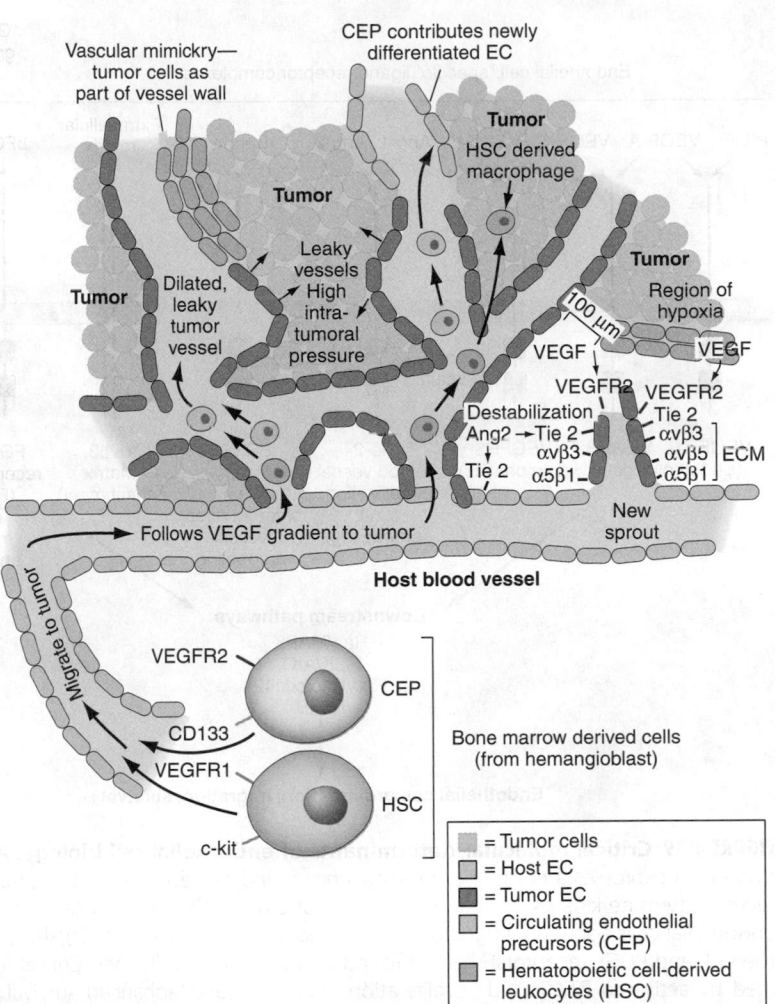

FIGURE 80-8 Tumor angiogenesis is a complex process involving many different cell types that must proliferate, migrate, invade, and differentiate in response to signals from the tumor microenvironment. Endothelial cells (ECs) sprout from host vessels in response to VEGF, bFGF, Ang2, and other proangiogenic stimuli. Sprouting is stimulated by VEGF/VEGFR2, Ang2/Tie-2, and integrin/extracellular matrix (ECM) interactions. Bone marrow–derived circulating endothelial precursors (CEPs) migrate to the tumor in response to VEGF and differentiate into ECs, while hematopoietic stem cells differentiate into leukocytes, including tumor-associated macrophages that secrete angiogenic growth factors and produce MMPs that remodel the ECM and release bound growth factors. Tumor cells themselves may directly form parts of vascular channels within tumors. The pattern of vessel formation is haphazard: vessels are tortuous, dilated, leaky, and branch in random ways. This leads to uneven blood flow within the tumor, with areas of acidosis and hypoxia (which stimulate release of angiogenic factors) and high intratumoral pressures that inhibit delivery of therapeutic agents.

Tumor blood flow is variable, with areas of hypoxia and acidosis leading to the selection of variants that are resistant to hypoxia-induced apoptosis (often due to the loss of p53 expression). Tumor vessel walls have numerous openings, widened interendothelial junctions, and discontinuous or absent basement membrane; this contributes to the high vascular permeability of these vessels and, together with lack of functional intratumoral lymphatics, causes interstitial hypertension within the tumor (which also interferes with the delivery of therapeutics to the tumor; Figs. 80-8, 80-9, and 80-10). Tumor blood vessels lack perivascular cells such as pericytes and smooth-muscle cells that normally regulate flow in response to tissue metabolic needs.

Unlike normal blood vessels, the vascular lining of tumor vessels is not a homogeneous layer of ECs but often consists of a mosaic of ECs and tumor cells; the concept of cancer cell–derived vascular channels, which may be lined by ECM secreted by the tumor cells, is referred to

Endothelial cell "specific" ligand/receptor complexes

Generalized growth factor receptors

FIGURE 80-9 Critical molecular determinants of endothelial cell biology. Angiogenic endothelium expresses a number of receptors not found on resting endothelium. These include receptor tyrosine kinases (RTK) and integrins that bind to the extracellular matrix and mediate endothelial cells adhesion, migration, and invasion. Endothelial cells (ECs) also express RTK (i.e., the FGF and PDGF receptors) that are found on many other cell types. Critical functions mediated by activated RTK include proliferation, migration, and enhanced survival of endothelial cells, as well as regulation of the recruitment of perivascular cells and bloodborne circulating endothelial precursors and hematopoietic stem cells to the tumor. Intracellular signaling via EC-specific RTK utilizes molecular pathways that may be targets for future antiangiogenic therapies.

as *vascular mimickry*. It is unclear whether tumor cells actually form structural elements of vascular channels or represent tumor cells in transit into or out of the vessel. However, the former is supported by evidence that in some human colon cancers, tumor cells can comprise up to 15% of vessel walls. The ECs of angiogenic blood vessels are unlike quiescent ECs found in adult vessels, where only 0.01% of ECs are dividing. During tumor angiogenesis, ECs are highly proliferative and express a number of plasma membrane proteins that are characteristic of activated endothelium, including growth factor receptors and adhesion molecules such as integrins.

MECHANISMS OF TUMOR VESSEL FORMATION

Tumors utilize a number of mechanisms to promote their vascularization, and in each case they subvert normal angiogenic processes to suit this purpose (Fig. 80-8). Primary or metastatic tumor cells sometimes arise in proximity to host blood vessels and grow around these vessels, parasitizing nutrients by coopting the local blood supply. However, most tumor blood vessels arise by the process of *sprouting*, in which tumors secrete trophic angiogenic molecules, the most potent being VEGF, that induce the proliferation and migration of host ECs into the tumor. Sprouting in normal and pathogenic angiogenesis is regulated by three families of transmembrane RTKs expressed on ECs and their ligands (VEGFs, angiopoietins, ephrins; Fig. 80-9), which are produced by tumor cells, inflammatory cells, or stromal cells in the tumor microenvironment.

When tumor cells arise in or metastasize to an avascular area, they grow to a size limited by hypoxia and nutrient deprivation. Hypoxia, a key regulator of tumor angiogenesis, causes the transcriptional in-

duction of the gene encoding VEGF by a process that involves stabilization of HIF-1α. Under normoxic conditions, HIF-1α levels are maintained at a low level by proteasome-mediated destruction regulated by a ubiquitin E3-ligase encoded by the VHL tumor-suppressor locus. However, under hypoxic conditions, HIF-1α is not hydroxylated and association with VHL does not occur; therefore HIF-1 levels increase, and target genes including VEGF, nitric oxide synthetase (NOS), and Ang2 are induced. Loss of the *VHL* genes, as occurs in familial and sporadic renal cell carcinomas, results in HIF-1α stabilization and induction of VEGF. Most tumors have hypoxic regions due to poor blood flow, and tumor cells in these areas stain positive for HIF-1α expression; in renal cancers with *VHL* deletion, all of the tumor cells express high levels of HIF-1α, and VEGF-induced angiogenesis leads to high microvascular density (hence the term *hypernephroma*).

VEGF and its receptors are required for *vasculogenesis* (the de novo formation of blood vessels from differentiating endothelial cells, as occurs during embryonic development) and angiogenesis under normal (wound healing, corpus luteum formation) and pathologic processes (tumor angiogenesis, inflammatory conditions such as rheumatoid arthritis). VEGF-A is a heparin-binding glycoprotein with at least four isoforms (splice variants) that regulates blood vessel formation by binding to the RTKs VEGFR1 and VEGFR2, which are expressed on all ECs in addition to a subset of hematopoietic cells (Fig. 80-8). VEGFR2 regulates EC proliferation, migration, and survival, while VEGFR1 may act as an antagonist of R1 in ECs but is probably also important for angioblast differentiation during embryogenesis. Tumor vessels appear to be more dependent on VEGFR signaling for growth and survival than normal ECs. While VEGF signaling is a critical initiator of angiogenesis, this is a complex process regulated by additional signaling pathways (Fig. 80-9). The angiopoietin, Ang1, produced by stromal cells, binds to the EC RTK Tie-2 and promotes the interaction of ECs with the ECM and perivascular cells, such as pericytes and smooth-muscle cells, to form tight, non-leaky vessels. PDGF and basic fibroblast growth factor (bFGF) help to recruit these perivascular cells. Ang1 is required for maintaining the quiescence and stability of mature blood vessels and prevents the vascular permeability normally induced by VEGF and inflammatory cytokines.

For tumor cell–derived VEGF to initiate sprouting from host vessels, the stability conferred by the Ang1/Tie2 pathway must be perturbed; this occurs by the secretion of Ang2 by ECs that are undergoing active remodeling. Ang2 binds to Tie2 and is a competitive inhibitor of Ang1 action: under the influence of Ang2, preexisting blood vessels become more responsive to remodeling signals, with less adherence of ECs to stroma and associated perivascular cells and more responsiveness to VEGF. Therefore, Ang2 is required at early stages of tumor angiogenesis for destabilizing the vasculature by making host ECs more sensitive to angiogenic signals. Since tumor ECs are blocked by Ang2, there is no stabilization by the Ang1/Tie2 interaction, and tumor blood vessels are leaky, hemorrhagic, and have poor association of ECs with underlying stroma. Sprouting tumor ECs express high levels of the transmembrane protein ephrin-B2 and its receptor, the RTK EPH whose signaling appears to work with the angiopoietins during vessel remodeling. During embryogenesis, EPH receptors are ex-

A. Normal blood vessel

Hierarchical branching

Low IP
Normoxic
Physiologic pH

Even blood distribution

Lumen

EC

BM

Pericytes

Tight junctions between EC
Well-formed BM
Pericyte coverage
Normal permeability

B. Tumor blood vessel

Tortuous vessels

High IP
High VEGF
Hypoxia
Acidosis

Haphazard blood flow

Lumen

EC

BM

Tumor cells

Loss of EC junction complexes
Irregular or no BM
Absent (or few) pericyte
Increased permeability

C. Treatment with bevacizamab (Early)

Normalization of vessels

Low IP
Less hypoxia
Less acidosis

Improved blood flow

Lumen

EC

BM

STET

Pericytes

More efficient delivery of chemotherapy and oxygen
Reduced permeability

D. Treatment with bevacizamab (Late)

Collapse of tumor vasculature

Lumen

EC

BM

Tumor cells

Death of EC due to loss of VEGF survival signals (plus chemotherapy or radiotherapy)
Apoptosis of tumor due to starvation and/or effects of chemotherapy.

FIGURE 80-10 Normalization of tumor blood vessels due to inhibition of VEGF signaling.
A. Blood vessels in normal tissues exhibit a regular hierarchical branching pattern that delivers blood to tissues in a spatially and temporally efficient manner to meet the metabolic needs of the tissue (top). At the microscopic level, tight junctions are maintained between endothelial cells (EC), which are adherent to a thick and evenly distributed basement membrane (BM). Pericytes form a surrounding layer that provides trophic signals to the EC and helps maintain proper vessel tone. Vascular permeability is regulated, interstitial fluid pressure is low, and oxygen tension and pH are physiologic. **B.** Tumors have abnormal vessels with tortuous branching and dilated, irregular interconnecting branches, causing uneven blood flow with areas of hypoxia and acidosis. This harsh environment selects genetic events that result in resistant tumor variants, such as the loss of p53. High levels of VEGF (secreted by tumor cells) disrupt gap junction communication, tight junctions, and adherens junctions between EC via src-mediated phosphorylation of proteins such as connexin 43, zonula occludens-1, VE-cadherin, and α/β-catenins. Tumor vessels have thin, irregular BM, and pericytes are sparse or absent. Together, these molecular abnormalities result in a vasculature that is permeable to serum macromolecules, leading to high tumor interstitial pressure, which can prevent the delivery of drugs to the tumor cells. This is made worse by the binding and activation of platelets at sites of exposed BM, with release of stored VEGF and microvessel clot formation, creating more abnormal blood flow and regions of hypoxia. **C.** In experimental systems, treatment with bevacizumab or blocking antibodies to VEGFR2 leads to changes in the tumor vasculature that has been termed *vessel normalization*. During the first week of treatment, abnormal vessels are eliminated or pruned (dotted lines), leaving a more normal branching pattern. ECs partially regain features such as cell-cell junctions, adherence to a more normal BM, and pericyte coverage. These changes lead to a decrease in vascular permeability, reduced interstitial pressure, and a transient increase in blood flow within the tumor. Note that in murine models, this normalization period lasts only for ~5–6 days. **D.** After continued anti-VEGF/VEGFR therapy (which is often combined with chemo- or radiotherapy), ECs die, leading to tumor cell death (either due to direct effects of the chemotherapy or lack of blood flow).

pressed on the endothelium of primordial venous vessels while the transmembrane ligand ephrin-B2 is expressed by cells of primordial arteries; the reciprocal expression may regulate differentiation and patterning of the vasculature.

A number of ubiquitously expressed host molecules play critical roles in normal and pathologic angiogenesis. Proangiogenic cytokines, chemokines, and growth factors secreted by stromal cells or inflammatory cells make important contributions to neovascularization, including bFGF, transforming growth factor-α (TGF-α), TNF-α, and IL-8. In contrast to normal endothelium, angiogenic endothelium overexpresses specific members of the integrin family of ECM-binding proteins that mediate EC adhesion, migration, and survival. Specifically, expression of integrins $\alpha_v\beta_3$, $\alpha_v\beta_5$, and $\alpha_5\beta_1$ mediate spreading and migration of ECs and are required for angiogenesis induced by VEGF and bFGF, which in turn can upregulate EC integrin expression. The $\alpha_v\beta_3$ integrin physically associates with VEGFR2 in the plasma membrane and promotes signal transduction from each receptor to promote EC proliferation (via focal adhesion kinase, src, PI3K, and other pathways) and survival (by inhibition of p53 and increasing the Bcl-2/Bax expression ratio). In addition, $\alpha_v\beta_3$ forms cell surface complexes with matrix metalloproteinases (MMPs), zinc-requiring proteases that cleave ECM proteins, leading to enhanced EC migration and the release of heparin-binding growth factors including VEGF and bFGF. EC adhesion molecules can be upregulated (i.e., by VEGF, TNF-α) or downregulated (by TGF-β); this, together with chaotic blood flow explains poor leukocyte-endothelial interactions in tumor blood vessels and may help tumor cells avoid immune surveillance.

Cells derived from hematopoietic progenitors in the host bone marrow contribute to tumor angiogenesis in a process linked to the secretion of VEGF and PlGF (placenta-derived growth factor) by tumor cells and their surrounding stroma. VEGF promotes the mobilization and recruitment of circulating endothelial cell precursors (CEPs) and hematopoietic stem cells (HSCs) to tumors where they co-localize and appear to cooperate in neovessel formation. CEPs express VEGFR2, while HSCs express VEGFR1, a receptor for VEGF and PlGF. Both CEPs and HSCs are derived from a common precursor, the hemangioblast. CEPs are thought to differentiate into ECs, whereas the role of HSC-derived cells (such as tumor-associated macrophages) may be to secrete angiogenic factors required for sprouting and stabilization of ECs (VEGF, bFGF, angiopoietins) and to activate MMPs, resulting in ECM remodeling and growth factor release. In mouse tumor models and in human cancers, increased numbers of CEPs and subsets of

TABLE 80-3 RANDOMIZED PHASE III CLINICAL TRIALS DEMONSTRATING THE EFFICACY OF BEVACIZUMAB IN COMBINATION WITH CHEMOTHERAPY FOR THE TREATMENT OF ADVANCED CANCERS

Tumor Type	Stage of Disease	Previous Treatment	Number of Patients	Chemotherapy Regimen	Outcome
Colon cancer	Metastatic	No	813	Irinotecan + 5-FU/LV ± bevacizumab	Increased OS (20.3 vs 15.6 months), PFS (10.6 vs 6.2 months), and RR (44.8 vs 34.8%)
Colon cancer	Metastatic	Second line; previous irinotecan/5-FU	829	FOLFOX ± bevacizumab	Increased OS (12.9 vs 10.8 months), PFS (7.2 vs 4.8 months), RR (21.8 vs 9.2%).
Non-small cell lung cancer (excluding squamous histology)	Metastatic	No	878	Carboplatinum + paclitaxel ± bevacizumab	Increased OS (12.5 vs 10.2 months), PFS (6.4 vs 4.5 months), RR (27.2 vs 10.0%).
Breast cancer	Recurrent or metastatic	No	722	Paclitaxel ± bevacizumab	Increased PFS (11.0 vs 6.2 months), RR (28 vs 14%).

Note: 5-FU, 5-fluorouracil; LV, leucovoran; OS, overall survival; PFS, progression-free survival; RR, response rate; FOLFOX, folinic acid (LV), 5-FU, and oxaliplatinum.

VEGFR-expressing HSCs can be detected in the circulation, which may correlate with increased levels of serum VEGF. It is not yet known whether levels of these cells have prognostic value or if changes during treatment correlate with inhibition of tumor angiogenesis. Whether CEPs and VEGFR1-expressing HSCs are required to maintain the long-term integrity of established tumor vessels is also unknown.

Lymphatic vessels also exist within tumors. Development of tumor lymphatics is associated with expression of VEGFR3 and its ligands VEGF-C and VEGF-D. The role of these vessels in tumor cell metastasis to regional lymph nodes remains to be determined, since, as discussed above, interstitial pressures within tumors are high and most lymphatic vessels may exit in a collapsed and nonfunctional state. However, VEGF-C levels correlate significantly with metastasis to regional lymph nodes in lung, prostate, and colorectal cancers,

ANTIANGIOGENIC THERAPY

Understanding the molecular mechanisms that regulate tumor angiogenesis may provide unique opportunities for cancer treatment. Acquired drug resistance of tumor cells due to their high intrinsic mutation rate is a major cause of treatment failure in human cancers. ECs comprising the tumor vasculature are genetically stable and do not share genetic changes with tumor cells; the EC apoptosis pathways are therefore intact. Each EC of a tumor vessel helps provide nourishment to many tumor cells, and although tumor angiogenesis can be driven by a number of exogenous proangiogenic stimuli, experimental data indicate that at least in some tumor types, blockade of a single growth factor (e.g., VEGF) may inhibit tumor-induced vascular growth. Angiogenesis inhibitors function by targeting the critical molecular pathways involved in EC proliferation, migration, and/or survival, many of which are unique to the activated endothelium in tumors. Inhibition of growth factor and adhesion-dependent signaling pathways can induce EC apoptosis with concomitant inhibition of tumor growth. Different types of tumors use distinct molecular mechanisms to activate the angiogenic switch. Therefore, it is doubtful that a single antiangiogenic strategy will suffice for all human cancers; rather, a number of agents will be needed, each responding to distinct programs of angiogenesis used by different human cancers.

Four randomized phase III clinical trials have demonstrated that the addition of bevacizumab (Avastin; a humanized monoclonal antibody that binds and inhibits VEGF) to chemotherapy results in significantly improved response rates, progression-free survival, and overall survival when compared to treatment with chemotherapy alone (Table 80-3). This effect was shown in the first-line treatment of patients with advanced colon, lung, and breast cancers, and in the second-line treatment of colon cancer. However, not all trials have been positive; in previously treated breast cancer, the addition of bevacizumab to capecitabine (an oral fluoropyrimidine) did not increase efficacy, and in previously untreated pancreatic cancer, bevacizumab did not enhance the efficacy of gemcitabine.

Several general principles have arisen from these studies. Bevacizumab appears to potentiate the effects of many different types of active chemotherapeutic regimens used to treat a variety of different tumor types. No phase III trials have demonstrated single-agent activity for bevacizumab; colon and lung cancer trials have demonstrated a lack of activity when used alone. An exception may be renal cell cancer (RCC), a tumor that is specifically dependent upon VEGF as the result of deletion of the VHL tumor suppressor and activation of the HIF-1α transcription factor (see above). A randomized phase II study of single-agent bevacizumab given at low or high dose compared to placebo in patients with advanced RCC demonstrated a significant prolongation of time to disease progression, a finding that merits further study.

The mechanisms by which bevacizumab enhances the activity of chemotherapy and possibly radiotherapy have been studied (Table 80-4). Inhibition of VEGF, especially in the early stages of treatment, has been postulated to result in the normalization of blood flow in tumors (Fig. 80-10). When given in combination with chemotherapy, this may enhance the delivery of cytotoxic agents to the tumor, where death of tumor cells and proliferating endothelial cells may result. As antiangiogenic therapy continues, growth of new tumor vessels is inhibited, leading to nutritional deprivation and death of tumor cells.

Bevacizumab is administered IV every 2–3 weeks (its half-life is nearly 20 days) and is generally well tolerated. Hypertension has been noted in most trials that utilize inhibitors of VEGF receptors, but only 10% of patients require treatment with anti-hypertensive agents and this rarely requires discontinuation of therapy. A mechanism for the hypertension may be a bevacizumab-induced decrease in vessel production of nitric oxide, resulting in vasoconstriction and increased blood pressure. Rare but serious side effects of bevacizumab include an increased risk of arterial thromboembolic events including stroke and myocardial infarction, usually in patients over the age of 65 with a history of cardiovascular disease. An increased risk of hemorrhage was noted in lung cancer patients with a squamous histology and large central tumors near the major mediastinal blood vessels. Cavitation of the

TABLE 80-4 MECHANISMS OF BEVACIZUMAB ACTION

1. Inhibition of VEGF-dependent signaling pathways required for the proliferation and survival of endothelial cells within the tumor vasculature. This may enhance the direct toxic effects of chemotherapy on tumor endothelial cells.
2. Inhibition of vascular permeability, decreasing interstitial pressure in tumors, and promoting delivery of therapeutic drugs and oxygen (a process termed *vessel normalization*).
3. Prevention of neoangiogenesis between cycles of chemotherapy, blocking tumor regrowth.
4. Inhibition of the recruitment of proangiogenic bone marrow–derived cells (including circulating endothelial precursors and monocytes) to the tumor vasculature.
5. Blocking potential direct effects of VEGF on tumors that have been reported to express VEGFR2, e.g., colon and pancreatic cancer cells.
6. Reversing the inhibitory activity of VEGF on dendritic cells, thereby promoting antitumor immunity.

Note: VEGF(R), vascular endothelial growth factor (receptor).

Ang 1

Ang 2

Novel inhibitors

VEGF

Anti-VEGF MoAb

VEGFR2

Kinase domain

Tie2 receptor

Stromal cell

Novel inhibitors

EPH receptor

Enhanced binding to ECM, vessel stabilization

Specific kinase inhibitors

Proliferation survival migration

Ephrin-B2

Anti-integrin MoAb, RGD peptides

$\alpha_v\beta_3$
$\alpha_v\beta_5$
$\alpha_5\beta_1$

Nucleus

Extracellular matrix (ECM)

Microtubules

Endothelial cell

MMPs (invasion, growth factor release)

MMP inhibitors

2-Methoxy estradiol

FIGURE 80-11 Knowledge of the molecular events governing tumor angiogenesis has led to a number of therapeutic strategies to block tumor blood vessel formation. The successful therapeutic targeting of VEGF is described in the text. Other endothelial cell–specific receptor tyrosine kinase pathways (e.g., angiopoietin/Tie2 and ephrin/EPH) are likely targets for the future. Ligation of the $\alpha_v\beta_3$ integrin is required for EC survival. Integrins are also required for EC migration and are important regulators of matrix metalloproteinase (MMP) activity, which modulates EC movement through the ECM as well as release of bound growth factors. Targeting of integrins includes development of blocking antibodies, small peptide inhibitors of integrin signaling, and arg-gly-asp-containing peptides that prevent integrin:ECM binding. Peptides derived from normal proteins by protealytic cleavage, including endostatin and tumstatin, inhibit angiogenesis by mechanisms that include interfering with integrin function. Signal transduction pathways that are dysregulated in tumor cells indirectly regulate EC function. Inhibition of EGF-family receptors, whose signaling activity is upregulated in a number of human cancers (e.g., breast, colon, and lung cancers), results in downregulation of VEGF and IL-8, while increasing expression of the antiangiogenic protein thrombospondin-1. The Ras/MAPK, PI3K/Akt, and Src kinase pathways constitute important anti-tumor targets that also regulate the proliferation and survival of tumor-derived EC. The discovery that EC from normal tissues express tissue-specific "vascular addressins" on their cell surface suggests that targeting specific EC subsets may be possible.

tumor with vessel rupture and massive hemoptysis lead to the exclusion of squamous cell cancers from treatment with bevacizumab. This potentially fatal side effect may actually reflect an increased activity of bevacizumab plus chemotherapy in squamous cell cancers. Other serious complications include bowel perforations that have been observed in 1–3% of patients (mainly those with colon and ovarian cancers).

Important questions remain concerning the clinical use of bevacizumab. Do patients develop resistance to this agent? Although patients with advanced colon, lung, and breast cancers benefit from treatment with bevacizumab-containing regiments, few patients are cured and most will relapse and die of their disease. While resistance of cancer cells to chemotherapeutic agents is expected, it is unclear to what extent the relapses reflect resistance to bevacizumab (if at all). Preclinical studies have demonstrated that inhibition of VEGF-mediated angiogenic pathways can select for tumor variants that utilize other angiogenic mechanisms, such as the secretion of the proangiogenic chemokine IL-8, which is a downstream mediator of the EGFR pathway. This has led to studies in which bevacizumab has been combined with cetuximab or erlotinib (inhibitors of EGFR signaling), and pre-

liminary phase II studies have shown efficacy of these combinations in heavily pretreated patients with colon and lung cancers.

The bevacizumab experience suggests that inhibition of the VEGF pathway will be most efficacious when combined with agents that directly target tumor cells. This also appears to be the case in the development of small-molecule inhibitors (SMI) that target VEGF receptor tyrosine kinase activity but are also inhibitory to other kinases that are expressed by tumor cells and important for their proliferation and survival. Sunitinib, FDA approved for the treatment of GIST (see above and Table 80-2), has activity directed against mutant c-Kit receptors, but also targets VEGFR and PDGFR, and has shown significant antitumor activity against metastatic RCC, presumably on the basis of its antiangiogenic activity. Similarly, sorafenib, originally developed as a Raf kinase inhibitor but with potent activity against VEGF and PDGF receptors, increases progression-free survival in RCC. Thus, agents that target both angiogenesis and tumor-specific signaling pathways may have greater efficacy against a broad range of cancers. A caveat is that RCC and GIST are highly dependent upon single signaling pathways (VEGF and c-Kit, respectively) whereas most solid tumors use a panoply of interconnected proliferation and survival pathways that are redundant and likely to be less amenable to single-agent targeting.

The success in targeting tumor angiogenesis has led to enhanced enthusiasm for the development of drugs that target other aspects of the angiogenic process; some of these therapeutic approaches are outlined in **Fig. 80-11**.

FURTHER READINGS

BILD AH et al: Oncogenic pathway signatures in human cancers as a guide to targeted therapies. Nature 439:353, 2006

DAI Y, GRANT S: Targeting multiple arms of the apoptotic regulatory machinery. Cancer Res 67:2908, 2007

FERRARA N, KERBEL RS: Angiogenesis as a therapeutic target. Nature 438:967, 2005

FINKEL T et al: The common biology of cancer and ageing. Nature 448:767, 2007

HUBER MA et al: Molecular requirements for epithelial-mesenchymal transition during tumor progression. Curr Opin Cell Biol 17:548, 2005

KAELIN JR WG: The concept of synthetic lethality in the context of anticancer therapy. Nat Rev Cancer 5:686, 2005

PANARES RL, GARCIA AA: Bevacizumab in the management of solid tumors. Expert Rev Anticancer Ther 7:434, 2007

SHARMA SV et al: Epidermal growth factor receptor mutations in lung cancer. Nat Rev Cancer 7:169, 2007

SHERBENOU DW, DRUCKER BJ: Applying the discovery of the Philadelphia chromosome. J Clin Invest 117:2068, 2007

VOUSDEN KH, LANE DP: p53 in health and disease. Nat Rev Mol Cell Biol 8:275, 2007

81 Principles of Cancer Treatment

Edward A. Sausville, Dan L. Longo

The goal of cancer treatment is first to eradicate the cancer. If this primary goal cannot be accomplished, the goal of cancer treatment shifts to palliation, the amelioration of symptoms, and preservation of quality of life while striving to extend life. The dictum *primum non nocere* is not the guiding principle of cancer therapy. When cure of cancer is possible, cancer treatments may be undertaken despite the certainty of severe and perhaps life-threatening toxicities. Every cancer treatment has the potential to cause harm, and treatment may be given that produces toxicity with no benefit. The therapeutic index of many interventions is quite narrow, and most treatments are given to the point of toxicity. Conversely, when the clinical goal is palliation, careful attention to minimizing the toxicity of potentially toxic treatments becomes a significant goal. Irrespective of the clinical scenario, the guiding principle of cancer treatment should be *primum succerrere*, "first hasten to help." Radical surgical procedures, large-field hyperfractionated radiation therapy, high-dose chemotherapy, and maximum tolerable doses of cytokines such as interleukin (IL) 2 are all used in certain settings where 100% of the patients will experience toxicity and side effects from the intervention and only a fraction of the patients will experience benefit. One of the challenges of cancer treatment is to use the various treatment modalities alone and together in a fashion that maximizes the chances for patient benefit.

Cancer treatments are divided into four main types: surgery, radiation therapy (including photodynamic therapy), chemotherapy (including hormonal therapy and molecularly targeted therapy), and biologic therapy (including immunotherapy and gene therapy). The modalities are often used in combination, and agents in one category can act by several mechanisms. For example, cancer chemotherapy agents can induce differentiation, and antibodies (a form of immunotherapy) can be used to deliver radiation therapy. Surgery and radiation therapy are considered local treatments, though their effects can influence the behavior of tumor at remote sites. Chemotherapy and biologic therapy are usually systemic treatments. *Oncology*, the study of tumors including treatment approaches, is a multidisciplinary effort with surgical-, radiotherapy-, and internal medicine–related areas of expertise. Treatments for patients with hematologic malignancies are often shared by hematologists and medical oncologists.

In many ways, cancer mimics an organ attempting to regulate its own growth. However, cancers have not set an appropriate limit on how much growth should be permitted. Normal organs and cancers share the property of having (1) a population of cells in cycle and actively renewing and (2) a population of cells not in cycle. In cancers, cells that are not dividing are heterogeneous; some have sustained too much genetic damage to replicate but have defects in their death pathways that permit their survival, some are starving for nutrients and oxygen, and some are out of cycle but poised to be recruited back into cycle and expand if needed (i.e., reversibly growth–arrested). Severely damaged and starving cells are unlikely to kill the patient. The problem is that the cells that are reversibly not in cycle are capable of replenishing tumor cells physically removed or damaged by radiation and chemotherapy. These include *cancer stem cells*, whose properties are being elucidated. The stem cell fraction may define new targets for therapies that will retard their ability to reenter the cell cycle.

Tumors follow a Gompertzian growth curve (**Fig. 81-1**); the growth fraction of a neoplasm starts at 100% with the first transformed cell and declines exponentially over time until at the time of diagnosis, with a tumor burden of $1–5 \times 10^9$ tumor cells, the growth fraction is usually 1–4%. Thus, peak growth rate occurs before the tumor is detectable. A key feature of a successful tumor is the ability to stimulate the development of a new supporting stroma through angiogenesis and production of proteases to allow invasion through basement membranes and normal tissue barriers (Chap. 80). Specific cellular mechanisms promote entry or withdrawal of tumor cells from the cell

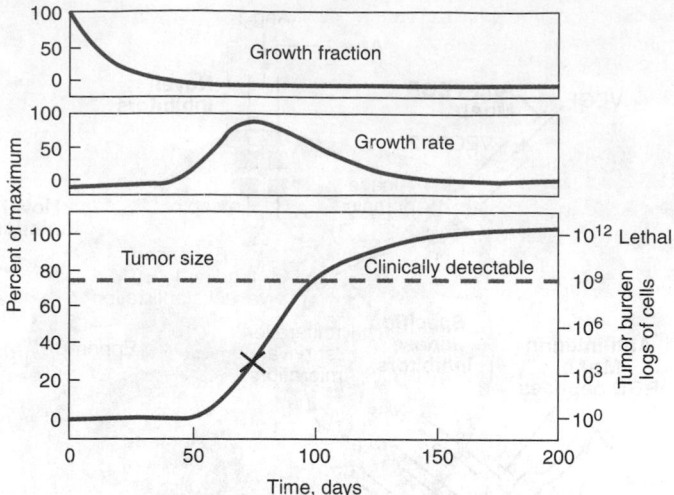

FIGURE 81-1 Gompertzian tumor growth. The growth fraction of a tumor declines exponentially over time (*top*). The growth rate of a tumor peaks before it is clinically detectable (*middle*). Tumor size increases slowly, goes through an exponential phase, and slows again as the tumor reaches the size at which limitation of nutrients or auto- or host regulatory influences can occur. The maximum growth rate occurs at 1/e, the point at which the tumor is about 37% of its maximum size (marked with an X). Tumor becomes detectable at a burden of about 10^9 (1 cm³) cells and kills the patient at a tumor cell burden of about 10^{12} (1 kg). Efforts to treat the tumor and reduce its size can result in an increase in the growth fraction and an increase in growth rate.

cycle. For example, when a tumor recurs after surgery or chemotherapy, frequently its growth is accelerated and the growth fraction of the tumor is increased. This pattern is similar to that seen in regenerating organs. Partial resection of the liver results in the recruitment of cells into the cell cycle, and the resected liver volume is replaced. Similarly, chemotherapy-damaged bone marrow increases its growth to replace cells killed by chemotherapy. However, cancers do not recognize a limit on their expansion. Monoclonal gammopathy of uncertain significance may be an example of a clonal neoplasm with intrinsic features that stop its growth before a lethal tumor burden is reached. A fraction of patients with this disorder go on to develop fatal multiple myeloma, but probably this occurs because of the accumulation of additional genetic lesions. Elucidation of the mechanisms that regulate this "organ-like" behavior of tumors may provide additional clues to cancer control and treatment.

PRINCIPLES OF CANCER SURGERY

Surgery is used in cancer prevention, diagnosis, staging, treatment (for both localized and metastatic disease), palliation, and rehabilitation.

PROPHYLAXIS

Cancer can be prevented by surgery in people who have premalignant lesions resected (e.g., premalignant lesions of skin, colon, cervix) and in those who are at increased risk of cancer from either an underlying disease (colectomy in those with pancolonic involvement with ulcerative colitis), the presence of genetic lesions (colectomy for familial polyposis, thyroidectomy for multiple endocrine neoplasia type 2, bilateral mastectomy or oophorectomy for familial breast or ovarian cancer syndromes), or a developmental anomaly (orchiectomy in those with an undescended testis). In some cases, prophylactic surgery is more radical than the surgical procedures used to treat the cancer after it develops. The assessment of risk involves many factors and should be undertaken with care before advising a patient to undergo such a major procedure. For breast cancer prevention, many experts use a 20% risk of developing breast cancer over the next 5 years as a threshold. However, patient fears play a major role in defining candidates for cancer prevention surgery. Counseling and education may not be enough to allay the fears of someone who has lost close family members to a malignancy.

DIAGNOSIS

The underlying principle in cancer diagnosis is to obtain as much tissue as safely possible. Owing to tumor heterogeneity, pathologists are better able to make the diagnosis when they have more tissue to examine. In addition to light-microscopic inspection of a tumor for pattern of growth, degree of cellular atypia, invasiveness, and morphologic features that aid in the differential diagnosis, sufficient tissue is of value in searching for genetic abnormalities and protein expression patterns, such as hormone receptor expression in breast cancers, that may aid in differential diagnosis or provide information about prognosis or likely response to treatment. Histologically similar tumors may have very different gene expression patterns when assessed by such techniques as microarray analysis using gene chips, with important differences in response to treatment. Such testing requires that the tissue be handled properly (e.g., immunologic detection of proteins is more effective in fresh-frozen tissue rather than in formalin-fixed tissue). Coordination among the surgeon, pathologist, and primary care physician is essential to ensure that the amount of information learned from the biopsy material is maximized.

These goals are best met by an *excisional biopsy* in which the entire tumor mass is removed with a small margin of normal tissue surrounding it. If an excisional biopsy cannot be performed, *incisional biopsy* is the procedure of second choice. A wedge of tissue is removed, and an effort is made to include the majority of the cross-sectional diameter of the tumor in the biopsy to minimize sampling error. The biopsy techniques that involve cutting into tumor carry with them a risk of facilitating the spread of the tumor. *Core-needle biopsy* usually obtains considerably less tissue, but this procedure often provides enough information to plan a definitive surgical procedure. *Fine-needle aspiration* generally obtains only a suspension of cells from within a mass. This procedure is minimally invasive, and if positive for cancer it may allow inception of systemic treatment when metastatic disease is evident, or it can provide a basis for planning a more meticulous and extensive surgical procedure.

STAGING

As noted in Chap. 77, an important component of patient management is defining the extent of disease. Radiographic and other imaging tests can be helpful in defining the clinical stage; however, pathologic staging requires defining the extent of involvement by documenting the histologic presence of tumor in tissue biopsies obtained through a surgical procedure. Axillary lymph node sampling in breast cancer and lymph node sampling at laparotomy for lymphomas and testicular, colon, and other intraabdominal cancers may provide crucial information for treatment planning and may determine the extent and nature of primary cancer treatment.

TREATMENT

Surgery is the most effective means of treating cancer. Today about 40% of cancer patients are cured by surgery. Unfortunately, a large fraction of patients with solid tumors (perhaps 60%) have metastatic disease that is not accessible for removal. However, even when the disease is not curable by surgery alone, the removal of tumor can obtain important benefits, including local control of tumor, preservation of organ function, debulking that permits subsequent therapy to work better, and staging information on extent of involvement. Cancer surgery aiming for cure is usually planned to excise the tumor completely with an adequate margin of normal tissue (the margin varies with the tumor and the anatomy), touching the tumor as little as possible to prevent vascular and lymphatic spread, and minimizing operative risk. Extending the procedure to resect draining lymph nodes obtains prognostic information, but such resections alone generally do not improve survival.

Increasingly, laparoscopic approaches are being used to address primary abdominal and pelvic tumors. Lymph node spread may be assessed using the sentinel node approach, in which the first draining

lymph node a spreading tumor would encounter is defined by injecting a dye into the tumor site at operation and then resecting the first node to turn blue. The sentinel node assessment is continuing to undergo clinical evaluation but appears to provide reliable information without the risks (lymphedema, lymphangiosarcoma) associated with resection of all the regional nodes. Advances in adjuvant chemotherapy and radiation therapy following surgery have permitted a substantial decrease in the extent of primary surgery necessary to obtain the best outcomes. Thus, lumpectomy with radiation therapy is as effective as modified radical mastectomy for breast cancer, and limb-sparing surgery followed by adjuvant radiation therapy and chemotherapy has replaced radical primary surgical procedures involving amputation and disarticulation for childhood rhabdomyosarcomas. More limited surgery is also being employed to spare organ function, as in larynx and bladder cancer. The magnitude of operations necessary to optimally control and cure cancer has also been diminished by technical advances; for example, the circular anastomotic stapler has allowed narrower (<2 cm) margins in colon cancer without compromise of local control rates, and many patients who would have had colostomies are able to maintain normal anatomy.

In some settings—e.g., bulky testicular cancer or stage III breast cancer—surgery is not the first treatment modality employed. After an initial diagnostic biopsy, chemotherapy and/or radiation therapy is delivered to reduce the size of the tumor and clinically control undetected metastatic disease. Such therapy is followed by a surgical procedure to remove residual masses; this is called *neoadjuvant therapy*. Because the sequence of treatment is critical to success and is different from the standard surgery-first approach, coordination among the surgical oncologist, radiation oncologist, and medical oncologist is crucial.

Surgery may be curative in a subset of patients with metastatic disease. Patients with lung metastases from osteosarcoma may be cured by resection of the lung lesions. In patients with colon cancer who have fewer than five liver metastases restricted to one lobe and no extrahepatic metastases, hepatic lobectomy may produce long-term disease-free survival in 25% of selected patients. Surgery can also be associated with systemic antitumor effects. In the setting of hormonally responsive tumors, oophorectomy and/or adrenalectomy may control estrogen production, and orchiectomy may reduce androgen production; both have effects on metastatic tumor growth. If resection of the primary lesion takes place in the presence of metastases, acceleration of metastatic growth may occur, perhaps based on the removal of a source of angiogenesis inhibitors and mass-related growth regulators in the tumor.

In selecting a surgeon or center for primary cancer treatment, consideration must be given to the volume of cancer surgeries undertaken by the site. Studies in a variety of cancers have shown that increased annual procedure volume appears to correlate with outcome. In addition, facilities with extensive support systems—e.g., for joint thoracic and abdominal surgical teams with cardiopulmonary bypass, if needed—may allow resection of certain tumors that would otherwise not be possible.

PALLIATION

Surgery is employed in a number of ways for supportive care: insertion of central venous catheters, control of pleural and pericardial effusions and ascites, caval interruption for recurrent pulmonary emboli, stabilization of cancer-weakened weight-bearing bones, and control of hemorrhage, among others. Surgical bypass of gastrointestinal, urinary tract, or biliary tree obstruction can alleviate symptoms and prolong survival. Surgical procedures may provide relief of otherwise intractable pain or reverse neurologic dysfunction (cord decompression). Splenectomy may relieve symptoms and reverse hypersplenism. Intrathecal or intrahepatic therapy relies on surgical placement of appropriate infusion portals. Surgery may correct other treatment-related toxicities such as adhesions or strictures.

REHABILITATION

Surgical procedures are also valuable in restoring a cancer patient to full health. Orthopedic procedures may be necessary to assure proper ambulation. Breast reconstruction can make an enormous impact on the patient's perception of successful therapy. Plastic and reconstructive surgery can correct the effects of disfiguring primary treatment.

PRINCIPLES OF RADIATION THERAPY

PHYSICAL PROPERTIES AND BIOLOGIC EFFECTS

Exposure to ionizing radiation is constant. Radiation comes from the sun and other cosmic sources, the ground, the air we breathe, the food we ingest, and from within our bodies. Radiation therapy uses radiation to treat cancer. Radiation is a physical form of treatment that damages any tissue in its path; its selectivity for cancer cells may be due to defects in a cancer cell's ability to repair sublethal DNA and other damage. Radiation causes breaks in DNA and generates free radicals from cell water that may damage cell membranes, proteins and organelles. Radiation damage is dependent on oxygen; hypoxic cells are more resistant. Augmentation of oxygen is the basis for radiation sensitization. Sulfhydryl compounds interfere with free radical generation and may act as radiation protectors.

Most radiation-induced cell damage is due to the formation of hydroxyl radicals:

$$\text{Ionizing radiation} + H_2O \rightarrow H_2O^+ + e^-$$

$$H_2O^+ + H_2O \rightarrow H_3O^+ + OH^\cdot$$

$$OH^\cdot \rightarrow \text{cell damage}$$

The dose-response curve for cells has both linear and exponential components. The linear component is from double-stranded DNA breaks produced by single hits. The exponential component represents breaks produced by multiple hits (Fig. 81-2). Plotting the fraction of surviving cells against doses of x-rays or gamma radiation, the curve has a shoulder that reflects the cell's repair of sublethal damage, followed by a linear portion reflecting greater cell kill with larger doses. The features that make a particular cell more sensitive or more resistant to the biologic effects of radiation are not completely defined.

Although radiation can interfere with many cellular processes, many experts feel that a cell must undergo a double-strand DNA break from radiation in order to be killed. The factors that influence tumor cell killing include the D_0 of the tumor (the dose required to deliver an average of one lethal hit to all the cells in a population), the D_q of the tumor (the threshold dose—a measure of the cell's ability to repair sublethal damage), hypoxia, tumor mass, growth fraction, and cell cycle time and phase (cells in late G_1 and S are more resistant). Rate of clinical response is not predictive; some cells do not die after radiation exposure until they attempt to replicate.

Therapeutic radiation is delivered in three ways: (1) *teletherapy*, with beams of radiation generated at a distance and aimed at the tumor within the patient; (2) *brachytherapy*, with encapsulated sources of radiation implanted directly into or adjacent to tumor tissues; and (3) *systemic therapy*, with radionuclides targeted in some fashion to a site of tumor. Teletherapy is the most commonly used form of radiation therapy.

Radiation from any source decreases in intensity as a function of the square of the distance from the source (inverse square law). Thus, if the radiation source is 5 cm above the skin surface and the tumor is 5 cm below the skin surface, the intensity of radiation in the tumor will be $5^2/10^2$, or 25% of the intensity at the skin. By contrast, if the radiation source is moved to 100 cm from the patient, the intensity of radiation in the tumor will be $100^2/105^2$, or 91% of the intensity at the skin. Teletherapy maintains intensity over a larger volume of target tissue by increasing the source-to-surface distance. In brachytherapy, the source-to-surface distance is small; thus, the effective treatment volume is small.

X-rays and gamma rays are the forms of radiation most commonly used to treat cancer. They are both electromagnetic, nonparticulate waves that cause the ejection of an orbital electron when absorbed. This orbital electron ejection is called *ionization*. X-rays are generated by linear accelerators; gamma rays are generated from decay of atomic nuclei in radioisotopes such as cobalt and radium. These waves behave biologically as packets of energy, called *photons*. Particulate forms of radiation are also used in certain circumstances. Electron beams have a very low tissue penetrance and are used to treat skin conditions such as mycosis fungoides. Neutron beams may be somewhat more effective than x-rays in treating salivary gland tumors. However, aside from these specialized uses, particulate forms of radiation such as neutrons, protons, and negative mesons, which should do more tissue damage because of their higher linear energy transfer and be less dependent on oxygen, have not yet found wide applicability to cancer treatment.

A number of parameters influence the damage done to tissue by radiation. Hypoxic cells are relatively resistant. Nondividing cells are more resistant than dividing cells. In addition to these biologic parameters, physical parameters of the radiation are also crucial. The energy of the radiation determines its ability to penetrate tissue. Low-energy orthovoltage beams (150–400 kV) scatter when they strike the body, much like light diffuses when it strikes particles in the air. Such beams result in more damage to adjacent normal tissues and less radiation delivered to the tumor. Megavoltage radiation (>1 MeV) has very low lateral scatter; this produces a skin-sparing effect, more homogeneous distribution of the radiation energy, and greater deposit of the energy

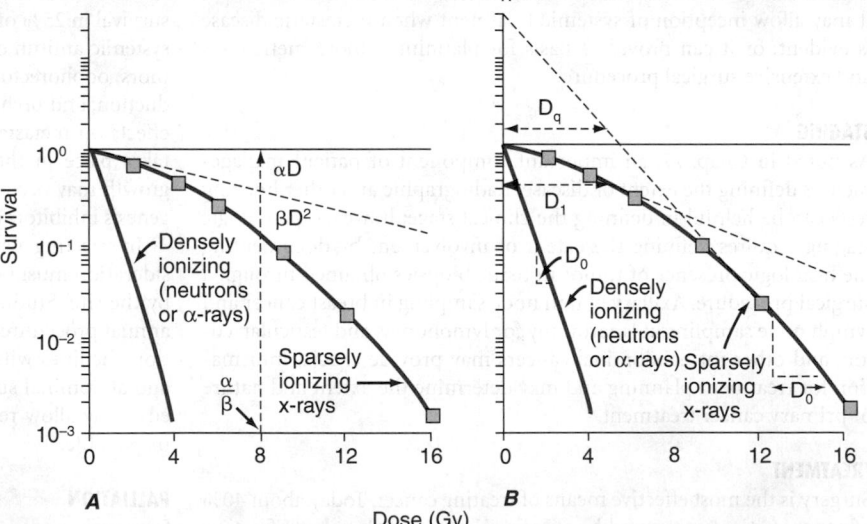

FIGURE 81-2 Shape of survival curve for mammalian cells exposed to radiation. The fraction of cells surviving is plotted on a logarithmic scale against dose on a linear scale. For alpha particles or low-energy neutrons (said to be densely ionizing), the dose-response curve is a straight line from the origin (i.e., survival is an exponential function of dose). The survival curve can be described by just one parameter, the slope. For x-rays or gamma rays (said to be sparsely ionizing), the dose-response curve has an initial linear slope, followed by a shoulder; at higher doses the curve tends to become straight again. **A.** The experimental data are fitted to a linear-quadratic function. There are two components of cell killing: one is proportional to dose (αD), while the other is proportional to the square of the dose (βD^2). The dose at which the linear and quadratic components are equal is the ratio α/β. The linear-quadratic curve bends continuously but is a good fit to experimental data for the first few decades of survival. **B.** The curve is described by the initial slope (D_1), the final slope (D_0), and a parameter that represents the width of the shoulder, either n or D_q. (*From EJ Hall: Radiobiology for the Radiologist, 5th ed. Philadelphia, Lippincott Williams & Wilkins, 2000; with permission.*)

in the tumor, or *target volume*. The tissues that the beam passes through to get to the tumor are called the *transit volume*. The maximum dose in the target volume is often the cause of complications to tissues in the transit volume, and the minimum dose in the target volume influences the likelihood of tumor recurrence. Dose homogeneity in the target volume is the goal.

Radiation is quantitated on the basis of the amount of radiation absorbed in the patient; it is not based on the amount of radiation generated by the machine. The *rad* (radiation *a*bsorbed *d*ose) is defined as 100 erg of energy per gram of tissue. The International System (SI) unit for rad is the Gray (Gy); 1 Gy = 100 rad. Radiation dose is measured by placing detectors at the body surface or calculating the dose based on radiating phantoms that resemble human form and substance. Radiation dose has three determinants: total absorbed dose, number of fractions, and time. A frequent error is to omit the number of fractions and the duration of treatment. This is analogous to saying that a runner completed a race in 20 s; without knowing how far he or she ran, the result is difficult to interpret. The time could be very good for a 200-m race or very poor for a 100-m race. Thus, a typical course of radiation therapy should be described as 4500 cGy delivered to a particular target (e.g., mediastinum) over 5 weeks in 180-cGy fractions. Most curative radiation treatment programs are delivered once a day, 5 days a week in 150- to 200-cGy fractions.

Compounds that incorporate into DNA and alter its stereochemistry (e.g., halogenated pyrimidines, cisplatin) augment radiation effects. Hydroxyurea, another DNA synthesis inhibitor, also potentiates radiation effects. Compounds that deplete thiols (e.g., buthionine sulfoximine) can also augment radiation effects. Hypoxia is a major factor that interferes with radiation effects.

APPLICATION TO PATIENTS

Teletherapy Radiation therapy can be used alone or together with chemotherapy to produce cure of localized tumors and control of the primary site of disease in tumors that have disseminated. Therapy is planned based on the use of a simulator with the treatment field or fields designed to accommodate an individual patient's anatomic features. Individualized treatment planning employs lead shielding tailored to shape the field and limit the radiation exposure of normal tissue. Often the radiation is delivered from two or three different positions. Conformal three-dimensional treatment planning permits the delivery of higher doses of radiation to the target volume without increasing complications in the transit volume.

Radiation therapy is a component of curative therapy for a number of diseases, including breast cancer, Hodgkin's disease, head and neck cancer, prostate cancer, and gynecologic cancers. Radiation therapy can also palliate disease symptoms in a variety of settings: relief of bone pain from metastatic disease, control of brain metastases, reversal of spinal cord compression and superior vena caval obstruction, shrinkage of painful masses, and opening of threatened airways. In high-risk settings, radiation therapy can prevent the development of leptomeningeal disease and brain metastases in acute leukemia and lung cancer.

Brachytherapy Brachytherapy involves placing a sealed source of radiation into or adjacent to the tumor and withdrawing the radiation source after a period of time precisely calculated to deliver a chosen dose of radiation to the tumor. This approach is often used to treat brain tumors and cervical cancer. The difficulty with brachytherapy is the short range of radiation effects (the inverse square law) and the inability to shape the radiation to fit the target volume. Normal tissue may receive toxic exposure to the radiation, with attendant radiation enteritis or cystitis in cervix cancer or brain injury in brain tumors.

Radionuclides and Radioimmunotherapy Nuclear medicine physicians or radiation oncologists may administer radionuclides with therapeutic effects. Iodine 131 is used to treat thyroid cancer since iodine is naturally taken up preferentially by the thyroid; it emits gamma rays that destroy the normal thyroid as well as the tumor. Strontium 89 and samarium 153 are two radionuclides that are preferentially taken up in bone, particularly sites of new bone formation. Both are capable of controlling bone metastases and the pain associated with them, but the dose-limiting toxicity is myelosuppression.

Monoclonal antibodies and other ligands can be attached to radioisotopes by conjugation (for nonmetal isotopes) or by chelation (for metal isotopes), and the targeting moiety can result in the accumulation of the radionuclide preferentially in tumor. Iodine 131–labeled anti-CD20 and yttrium 90–labeled anti-CD20 are active in B cell lymphoma, and other labeled antibodies are being evaluated. Thyroid uptake of labeled iodine is blocked by cold iodine. Dose-limiting toxicity is myelosuppression.

Photodynamic Therapy Some chemical structures (porphyrins, phthalocyanines) are selectively taken up by cancer cells by mechanisms not fully defined. When light, usually delivered by a laser, is shone on cells containing these compounds, free radicals are generated and the cells die. Hematoporphyrins and light are being used with increasing frequency to treat skin cancer; ovarian cancer; and cancers of the lung, colon, rectum, and esophagus. Palliation of recurrent locally advanced disease can sometimes be dramatic and last many months.

TOXICITY

Though radiation therapy is most often administered to a local region, systemic effects, including fatigue, anorexia, nausea, and vomiting, may develop that are related in part to the volume of tissue irradiated, dose fractionation, radiation fields, and individual susceptibility. Bone is among the most radioresistant organs, radiation effects being manifested mainly in children through premature fusion of the epiphyseal growth plate. By contrast, the male testis, female ovary, and bone marrow are the most sensitive organs. Any bone marrow in a radiation field will be eradicated by therapeutic irradiation. Organs with less need for cell renewal, such as heart, skeletal muscle, and nerves, are more resistant to radiation effects. In radiation-resistant organs, the vascular endothelium is the most sensitive component. Organs with more self-renewal as a part of normal homeostasis, such as the hematopoietic system and mucosal lining of the intestinal tract, are more sensitive. Acute toxicities include mucositis, skin erythema (ulceration in severe cases), and bone marrow toxicity. Often these can be alleviated by interruption of treatment.

Chronic toxicities are more serious. Radiation of the head and neck region often produces thyroid failure. Cataracts and retinal damage can lead to blindness. Salivary glands stop making saliva, which leads to dental caries and poor dentition. Taste and smell can be affected. Mediastinal irradiation leads to a threefold increased risk of fatal myocardial infarction. Other late vascular effects include chronic constrictive pericarditis, lung fibrosis, viscus stricture, spinal cord transection, and radiation enteritis. A serious late toxicity is the development of second solid tumors in or adjacent to the radiation fields. Such tumors can develop in any organ or tissue and occur at a rate of about 1% per year beginning in the second decade after treatment. Some organs vary in susceptibility to radiation carcinogenesis. A woman who receives mantle field radiation therapy for Hodgkin's disease at age 25 has a 30% risk of developing breast cancer by age 55 years. This is comparable in magnitude to genetic breast cancer syndromes. Women treated after age 30 have little or no increased risk of breast cancer. No data suggest that a threshold dose of therapeutic radiation exists below which the incidence of second cancers is decreased. High rates of second tumors occur in people who receive as little as 1000 cGy.

PRINCIPLES OF CHEMOTHERAPY

Medical oncology is the subspecialty of internal medicine that cares for and designs treatment approaches to patients with cancer, in conjunction with surgical and radiation oncologists. The core skills of the medical oncologist include the use of drugs that may have a beneficial effect on the natural history of the patient's illness or favorably influence the patient's quality of life. In general, the curability of a tumor is inversely related to tumor volume and directly related to drug dose.

Chemotherapy agents may be used for the treatment of active, clinically apparent cancer. Table 81-1, *A* lists those tumors considered curable by conventionally available chemotherapeutic agents when used to address disseminated or metastatic cancers. If a tumor is localized to a single site, serious consideration of surgery or primary radiation therapy should be given, as these treatment modalities may be curative as local treatments. Chemotherapy may be employed after the failure of these modalities to eradicate a local tumor or as part of multimodality approaches to offer primary treatment to a clinically localized tumor. In this event, it can allow organ preservation when given with radiation, as in the larynx or other upper airway sites; or sensitize tumors to radiation when given, for example, to patients concurrently receiving radiation for lung or cervix cancer (Table 81-1, *B*). Chemotherapy can be administered as an adjuvant, i.e., in addition to surgery (Table 81-1, *C*) or radiation, after all clinically apparent disease has been removed. This use of chemotherapy may have curative potential in breast and colorectal neoplasms, as it attempts to eliminate clinically unapparent tumor that may have already disseminated. As noted above, small tumors frequently have high growth fractions and therefore may be intrinsically more susceptible to the action of antiproliferative agents. Chemotherapy is routinely used in "conventional" dose regimens. In general, these doses produce reversible acute side effects, primarily consisting of transient myelosuppression with or without gastrointestinal toxicity (usually nausea), which are readily managed. High-dose chemotherapy regimens are predicated on the observation that the dose-response curve for many anticancer agents is rather steep, and increased dose can produce markedly increased therapeutic effect, although at the cost of potentially life-threatening complications that require intensive support, usually in the form of hematopoietic stem cell support from the patient (*autologous*) or from donors matched for histocompatibility loci (*allogeneic*). High-dose regimens have definite curative potential in defined clinical settings (Table 81-1, *D*).

Karnofsky was among the first to champion the evaluation of a chemotherapeutic agent's benefit by carefully quantitating its effect on tumor size and using these measurements to objectively decide the basis for further treatment of a particular patient or further clinical evaluation of a drug's potential. A partial response (PR) is defined conventionally as a decrease by at least 50% in a tumor's bidimensional area; a complete response (CR) connotes disappearance of all tumor; progression of disease signifies an increase in size of existing lesions by >25% from baseline or best response or development of new lesions; and "stable" disease fits into none of the above categories. Newer evaluation systems utilize unidimensional measurement, but the intent is similar in rigorously defining evidence for the activity of the agent in assessing its value to the patient.

If cure is not possible, chemotherapy may be undertaken with the goal of palliating some aspect of the tumor's effect on the host. Common tumors that may be meaningfully addressed with palliative intent are listed in Table 81-1, *E*. Usually, tumor-related symptoms may manifest as pain, weight loss, or some local symptom related to the tumor's effect on normal structures. Patients treated with palliative intent should be aware of their diagnosis and the limitations of the proposed treatments, have access to supportive care, and have suitable "performance status," according to assessment algorithms such as the one developed by Karnofsky or by the Eastern Cooperative Oncology Group (ECOG). ECOG performance status 0 (PS0) patients are without symptoms; PS1 patients have mild symptoms not requiring treatment; PS2, symptoms requiring some treatment; PS3, disabling symptoms, but allowing ambulation for >50% of the day; PS4, ambulation <50% of the day. Only PS0, PS1, and PS2 patients are generally considered suitable for palliative (noncurative) treatment. If there is curative potential, even poor-performance status patients may be treated, but their prognosis is usually inferior to that of good-performance patients treated with similar regimens.

An important perspective the primary care provider may bring to patients and their families facing incurable cancer is that, given the limited value of chemotherapeutic approaches at some point in the natural history, *palliative care* or *hospice-based* approaches, with meticulous and ongoing attention to symptom relief and with family, psychological, and spiritual support, should receive prominent attention as a valuable therapeutic plan (Chap. 11). Optimizing the quality of life rather than attempting to extend it becomes a valued intervention. Patients facing the impending progression of disease in a life-threatening way frequently choose to undertake toxic treatments of little to no potential value, and support provided by the primary caregiver in accessing palliative and hospice-based options can be critical in providing a basis for patients to make sensible choices.

CANCER DRUGS: OVERVIEW AND PRINCIPLES FOR USE

Cancer drug treatments are of four broad types. *Conventional chemotherapy agents* were historically derived by the empirical observation that these "small molecules" (generally with molecular weight <1500 Da) could cause major regression of experimental tumors growing in animals. These agents mainly target DNA structure or segregation of DNA as chromosomes in mitosis. *Targeted agents* refer to small molecules or "biologicals" (generally macromolecules such as antibodies or cytokines) designed and developed to interact with a defined molecular target important in either maintaining the malignant state or selectively expressed by the tumor cells. As described in Chapter 80, successful tumors have activated biochemical pathways that lead to uncontrolled proliferation through the action of, e.g., oncogene products, loss of cell cycle inhibitors, or loss of cell death regulation, and have acquired the capacity to replicate chromosomes indefinitely, invade, metastasize, and evade the immune system. Targeted therapies seek to capitalize on the biology behind the aberrant cellular behavior

---

TABLE 81-1 **CURABILITY OF CANCERS WITH CHEMOTHERAPY**

A. Advanced cancers with possible cure
Acute lymphoid and acute myeloid leukemia (pediatric/adult)
Hodgkin's disease (pediatric/adult)
Lymphomas—certain types (pediatric/adult)
Germ cell neoplasms
  Embryonal carcinoma
  Teratocarcinoma
  Seminoma or dysgerminoma
  Choriocarcinoma
Gestational trophoblastic neoplasia
Pediatric neoplasms
  Wilm's tumor
  Embryonal rhabdomyosarcoma
  Ewing's sarcoma
  Peripheral neuroepithelioma
  Neuroblastoma
Small-cell lung carcinoma
Ovarian carcinoma

B. Advanced cancers possibly cured by chemotherapy and radiation
Squamous carcinoma (head and neck)
Squamous carcinoma (anus)
Breast carcinoma
Carcinoma of the uterine cervix
Non-small cell lung carcinoma (stage III)
Small-cell lung carcinoma

C. Cancers possibly cured with chemotherapy as adjuvant to surgery
Breast carcinoma
Colorectal carcinoma[a]
Osteogenic sarcoma
Soft tissue sarcoma

D. Cancers possibly cured with "high-dose" chemotherapy with stem cell support
Relapsed leukemias, lymphoid and myeloid
Relapsed lymphomas, Hodgkin's and non-Hodgkin's
Chronic myeloid leukemia
Multiple myeloma

E. Cancers responsive with useful palliation, but not cure, by chemotherapy
Bladder carcinoma
Chronic myeloid leukemia
Hairy cell leukemia
Chronic lymphocytic leukemia
Lymphoma—certain types
Multiple myeloma
Gastric carcinoma
Cervix carcinoma
Endometrial carcinoma
Soft tissue sarcoma
Head and neck cancer
Adrenocortical carcinoma
Islet-cell neoplasms
Breast carcinoma
Colorectal carcinoma
Renal carcinoma

F. Tumor poorly responsive in advanced stages to chemotherapy
Pancreatic carcinoma
Biliary-tract neoplasms
Thyroid carcinoma
Carcinoma of the vulva
Non-small cell lung carcinoma
Prostate carcinoma
Melanoma
Hepatocellular carcinoma

[a]Rectum also receives radiation therapy.

as a basis for therapeutic effects. *Hormonal therapies* (the first form of targeted therapy) capitalize on the biochemical pathways underlying estrogen and androgen function and action as a therapeutic basis for approaching patients with tumors of breast, prostate, uterus, and ovarian origin. *Biologic therapies* are often macromolecules that have a particular target (e.g., antigrowth factor or cytokine antibodies) or may have the capacity to orchestrate or regulate the host immune response to kill tumor cells. Thus, biologic therapies include not only antibodies but cytokines and gene therapies.

The usefulness of any drug is governed by the extent to which a given dose causes a useful result (therapeutic effect; in the case of anticancer agents, toxicity to tumor cells) as opposed to a toxic effect. The *therapeutic index* is the degree of separation between toxic and therapeutic doses. Really useful drugs have large therapeutic indices, and this usually occurs when the drug target is expressed in the disease-causing compartment as opposed to the normal compartment. Classically, selective toxicity of an agent for an organ is governed by the expression of an agent's target or by differential accumulation into or elimination from compartments where toxicity is experienced or ameliorated, respectively. Currently used chemotherapeutic agents have the unfortunate property that their targets are present in both normal and tumor tissues. Therefore, they have relatively narrow therapeutic indices.

Following demonstration of activity in animal models, conventional chemotherapeutic agents are further evaluated to define an optimal schedule of administration and arrive at a drug formulation designed for a given route and schedule. Safety testing in two species on an analogous schedule of administration defines the starting dose for a phase I trial in humans. This is established as a fraction, usually one-sixth to one-tenth, of the dose just causing easily reversible toxicity in the more sensitive animal species. Escalating doses of the drug are then given during the human phase I trial until reversible toxicity is observed. Dose-limiting toxicity (DLT) defines a dose that conveys greater toxicity than would be acceptable in routine practice, allowing definition of a lower maximal tolerated dose (MTD). The occurrence of toxicity is, if possible, correlated with plasma drug concentrations. The MTD or a dose just lower than the MTD is usually the dose suitable for phase II trials, where a fixed dose is administered to a relatively homogeneous set of patients with a particular tumor type in an effort to define whether the drug causes regression of tumors. An "active" agent conventionally has PR rates of at least 20–25% with reversible non-life-threatening side effects, and it may then be suitable for study in phase III trials to assess efficacy in comparison to standard or no therapy.

Response, defined as tumor shrinkage, is but the most immediate indicator of drug effect. To be clinically valuable, responses must translate into clinical benefit. This is conventionally established by a beneficial effect on overall survival, or at least an increased time to further progression of disease. Active efforts are being made to quantitate effects of anticancer agents on quality of life. Cancer drug clinical trials conventionally use a toxicity grading scale where grade I toxicities do not require treatment, grade II often require symptomatic treatment but are not life-threatening, grade III toxicities are potentially life-threatening if untreated, grade IV toxicities are actually life-threatening, and grade V toxicities are those that result in the patient's death.

Development of targeted agents should proceed quite differently. While Phase I–III trials are still conducted, molecular analysis of human tumors more precisely defines targets expressed in a patient's tumor and should allow patient selection to enrich all trial phases with patients potentially responsive to the agent by virtue of expressing the target in the tumor. Clinical trials may be designed that assess the behavior of the drug in relation to its target. Ideally, the plasma concentration that affects the drug target is known, so escalation to MTD may not be necessary. Rather, the correlation of host toxicity while achieving an "optimal biologic dose" becomes a more relevant endpoint for Phase I and early Phase II trials with targeted agents.

Valuable cancer drug treatment strategies using conventional chemotherapy agents, targeted agents, hormonal treatments, or biologicals have one of two valuable outcomes. They can induce cancer cell death, resulting in tumor shrinkage with corresponding improvement

in patient survival, or increase the time until the disease progresses. Another potential outcome is to induce cancer cell *differentiation* or dormancy with loss of tumor cell replicative potential and reacquisition of phenotypic properties resembling normal cells. Blocking tumor cell differentiation may be a key feature in the pathogenesis of certain leukemias.

Cell death is a closely regulated process. *Necrosis* refers to cell death induced, for example, by physical damage with the hallmarks of cell swelling and membrane disruption. *Apoptosis*, or programmed cell death, refers to a highly ordered process whereby cells respond to defined stimuli by dying, and it recapitulates the necessary cell death observed during the ontogeny of the organism. *Anoikis* refers to the death of epithelial cells after removal from the normal milieu of substrate, particularly from cell-to-cell contact. Cancer chemotherapeutic agents can cause both necrosis and apoptosis. Apoptosis is characterized by chromatin condensation (giving rise to "apoptotic bodies"); cell shrinkage; and, in living animals, phagocytosis by surrounding stromal cells without evidence of inflammation. This process is regulated either by signal transduction systems that promote a cell's demise after a certain level of insult is achieved, or in response to specific cell-surface receptors that mediate cell death signals. Modulation of apoptosis by manipulation of signal transduction pathways has emerged as a basis for understanding the actions of drugs and designing new strategies to improve their use.

A general view of how cancer treatments work is that the interaction of a chemotherapeutic drug with its target induces a "cascade" of further signaling steps. These signals ultimately lead to cell death by triggering an "execution phase" where proteases, nucleases, and endogenous regulators of the cell death pathway are activated (**Fig. 81-3**).

Targeted agents differ from chemotherapy agents in that they do not indiscriminately cause macromolecular lesions but regulate the action of particular pathways. For example, the $p210^{bcr-abl}$ fusion protein tyrosine kinase drives chronic myeloid leukemia (CML), and HER-2/neu stimulates the proliferation of certain breast cancers. The tumor has been described as "addicted" to the function of these molecules in the sense that without the pathway's continued action, the tumor cell cannot survive. In this way, targeted agents may alter the "threshold" tumors have for undergoing apoptosis without actually creating any molecular lesions such as direct DNA strand breakage or altered membrane function.

While apoptotic mechanisms are important in regulating cellular proliferation and the behavior of tumor cells in vitro, in vivo it is unclear whether all of the actions of chemotherapeutic agents to cause cell death can be attributed to apoptotic mechanisms. However, changes in molecules that regulate apoptosis are correlated with clinical outcomes (e.g., *bcl2* overexpression in certain lymphomas conveys poor prognosis; pro-apoptotic *bax* expression is associated with a better outcome after chemotherapy for ovarian carcinoma). A better understanding of the relationship of cell death and cell survival mechanisms is needed.

Resistance to chemotherapy drugs has been postulated to arise either from cells not being in the appropriate phase of the cell cycle to allow drug lethality, or from decreased uptake, increased efflux, metabolism of the drug, or alteration of the target, e.g., by mutation or overexpression. Indeed, p170PGP (p170 P-glycoprotein; *mdr* gene product) was recognized from experiments with cells growing in tissue culture as mediating the efflux of chemotherapeutic agents in resistant cells. Certain neoplasms, particularly hematopoietic tumors, have an adverse prognosis if they express high levels of p170PGP, and modulation of this protein's function has been attempted by a variety of strategies.

Chemotherapeutic agents where drugs acting by different mechanisms were combined (e.g., an alkylating agent plus an antimetabolite plus a mitotic spindle blocker) proved to be more effective than single agents. Particular combinations were chosen to emphasize drugs whose individual toxicities to the host were, if possible, distinct. As agents emerge with novel mechanisms of action, combinations of drugs and targeted agents may maximize the chances of affecting critical pathways in the tumor.

FIGURE 81-3 Integration of cell death responses. Cell death through an apoptotic mechanism requires active participation of the cell. In response to interruption of growth factor (GF) or propagation of certain cytokine death signals (e.g., tumor necrosis factor receptor, TNF-R), there is activation of "upstream" cysteine aspartyl proteases (caspases), which then directly digest cytoplasmic and nuclear proteins, resulting in activation of "downstream" caspases; these cause activation of nucleases, resulting in the characteristic DNA fragmentation that is a hallmark of apoptosis. Chemotherapy agents that create lesions in DNA or alter mitotic spindle function seem to activate aspects of this process by damage ultimately conveyed to the mitochondria, perhaps by activating the transcription of genes whose products can produce or modulate the toxicity of free radicals. In addition, membrane damage with activation of sphingomyelinases results in the production of ceramides that can have a direct action at mitochondria. The antiapoptotic protein bcl2 attenuates mitochondrial toxicity, while proapoptotic gene products such as bax antagonize the action of bcl2. Damaged mitochondria release cytochrome C and apoptosis-activating factor (APAF), which can directly activate caspase 9, resulting in propagation of a direct signal to other downstream caspases through protease activation. Apoptosis-inducing factor (AIF) is also released from the mitochondrion and then can translocate to the nucleus, bind to DNA, and generate free radicals to further damage DNA. An additional proapoptotic stimulus is the bad protein, which can heterodimerize with bcl2 gene family members to antagonize apoptosis. Importantly, though, bad protein function can be retarded by its sequestration as phospho-bad through the 14-3-3 adapter proteins. The phosphorylation of bad is mediated by the action of the AKT kinase in a way that defines how growth factors that activate this kinase can retard apoptosis and promote cell survival.

CHEMOTHERAPEUTIC AGENTS USED FOR CANCER TREATMENT

Table 81-2 lists commonly used cancer chemotherapy agents and pertinent clinical aspects of their use. The drugs and schedules listed are examples that have proved tolerable and useful; the specific doses that may be used in a particular patient may vary somewhat with the particular treatment protocol, or plan, of treatment. Significant variation from these dose ranges should be carefully verified to avoid or anticipate toxicity. Not included in Table 81-2 are hormone receptor–directed agents, as the side effects are generally those expected from the interruption or augmentation of hormonal effect, and doses used in most cases are those that adequately saturate the intended hormone receptor. The drugs listed may be usefully grouped into three general categories: those affecting DNA, those affecting microtubules, and molecularly targeted agents.

Direct DNA-Interactive Agents DNA replication occurs during the synthesis or S-phase of the cell cycle, with chromosome segregation of the replicated DNA occurring in the M, or mitosis, phase. The G1 and

G2 "gap phases" precede S and M, respectively. Historically, chemotherapeutic agents have been divided into "phase-nonspecific" agents, which can act in any phase of the cell cycle, and "phase-specific" agents, which require the cell to be at a particular cell cycle phase to cause greatest effect. Once the agent has acted, cells may progress to "checkpoints" in the cell cycle where the drug-related damage may be assessed and either repaired or allowed to initiate apoptosis. An important function of certain tumor-suppressor genes such as p53 may be to modulate checkpoint function.

FORMATION OF COVALENT DNA ADDUCTS Alkylating agents as a class are cell cycle phase-nonspecific agents. They break down, either spontaneously or after normal organ or tumor cell metabolism, to reactive intermediates that covalently modify bases in DNA. This leads to cross-linkage of DNA strands or the appearance of breaks in DNA as a result of repair efforts. "Broken" or cross-linked DNA is intrinsically unable to complete normal replication or cell division; in addition, it is a potent activator of cell cycle checkpoints and further activates cell-signaling pathways that can precipitate apoptosis. As a class, alkylating agents share similar toxicities: myelosuppression, alopecia, gonadal dysfunction, mucositis, and pulmonary fibrosis. They differ greatly in a spectrum of normal organ toxicities. As a class they share the capacity to cause "second" neoplasms, particularly leukemia, many years after use, particularly when used in low doses for protracted periods.

Cyclophosphamide is inactive unless metabolized by the liver to 4-hydroxy-cyclophosphamide, which decomposes into an alkylating species, as well as to chloroacetaldehyde and acrolein. The latter causes chemical cystitis; therefore, excellent hydration must be maintained while using cyclophosphamide. If severe, the cystitis may be effectively treated by mesna (2-mercaptoethanesulfonate). Liver disease impairs drug activation. Sporadic interstitial pneumonitis leading to pulmonary fibrosis can accompany the use of cyclophosphamide, and high doses used in conditioning regimens for bone marrow transplant can cause cardiac dysfunction. Ifosfamide is a cyclophosphamide analogue also activated in the liver, but more slowly, and it requires coadministration of mesna to prevent bladder injury. Central nervous system (CNS) effects, including somnolence, confusion, and psychosis, can follow ifosfamide use; the incidence appears related to low body surface area or the presence of nephrectomy.

Several alkylating agents are less commonly used. Nitrogen mustard (mechlorethamine) is the prototypic agent of this class, decomposing rapidly in aqueous solution to potentially yield a bifunctional carbonium ion. It must be administered shortly after preparation into a rapidly flowing intravenous line. It is a powerful vesicant, and infiltration may be symptomatically ameliorated by infiltration of the affected site with 1/6 M thiosulfate. Even without infiltration, aseptic thrombophlebitis is frequent. It can be used topically as a dilute solution in cutaneous lymphomas, with a notable incidence of hypersensitivity reactions. It causes moderate nausea after intravenous administration.

Chlorambucil causes predictable myelosuppression, azoospermia, nausea, and pulmonary side effects. Busulfan can cause profound

TABLE 81-2 COMMONLY USED CANCER CHEMOTHERAPY AGENTS

Drug	Examples of Usual Doses	Toxicity	Interactions, Issues
Direct DNA-Interacting Agents			
Alkylators			

Cyclophosphamide	400–2000 mg/m² IV
	100 mg/m² PO qd
		Marrow (relative platelet sparing)
		Cystitis
		Common alkylator[a]
		Cardiac (high dose)
			Liver metabolism required to activate to
			  phosphoramide mustard + acrolein
			Mesna protects against "high-dose" bladder
			  damage

Mechlorethamine	6 mg/m² IV day 1 and day 8	Marrow Vesicant Nausea	Topical use in cutaneous lymphoma
Chlorambucil	1–3 mg/m² qd PO	Marrow Common alkylator[a]	
Melphalan	8 mg/m² qd × 5, PO	Marrow (delayed nadir) GI (high dose)	Decreased renal function delays clearance
Carmustine (BCNU)	200 mg/m² IV 150 mg/m² PO	Marrow (delayed nadir) GI, liver (high dose) Renal	
Lomustine (CCNU)	100–300 mg/m² PO	Marrow (delayed nadir)	
Ifosfamide	1.2 g/m² per day qd × 5 + mesna	Myelosuppressive Bladder Neurologic Metabolic acidosis Neuropathy	Isomeric analogue of cyclophosphamide More lipid soluble Greater activity vs testicular neoplasms and sarcomas Must use mesna
Procarbazine	100 mg/m² per day qd ×14	Marrow Nausea Neurologic Common alkylator[a]	Liver and tissue metabolism required Disulfiran-like effect with ethanol Acts as MAOI HBP after tyrosinase-rich foods
Dacarbazine (DTIC)	375 mg/m² IV day 1 and day 15	Marrow Nausea Flulike	Metabolic activation
Temozolomide	150–200 mg/m² qd × 5 q28d or 75 mg/m² qd × 6–7 weeks	Nausea/vomiting Headache/fatigue Constipation	Infrequent myelosuppression
Altretamine (formerly hexamethyl-melamine)	260 mg/m² per day qd ×14–21 as 4 divided oral doses	Nausea Neurologic (mood swing) Neuropathy Marrow (less)	Liver activation Barbiturates enhance/cimetidine diminishes

Cisplatin	20 mg/m² qd ×5 IV 1 q3–4 weeks or
	  100–200 mg/m² per dose IV q3–4
	  weeks
		Nausea
		Neuropathy
		Auditory
		Marrow platelets > WBCs
		Renal Mg²⁺, Ca²⁺
			Maintain high urine flow; osmotic diuresis,
			  monitor intake/output K⁺, Mg²⁺
			Emetogenic—prophylaxis needed
			Full dose if CrCl > 60 mL/min and tolerate fluid
			  push

Carboplatin	365 mg/m² IV q3–4 weeks as adjusted
	  for CrCl
		Marrow platelets > WBCs
		Nausea
		Renal (high dose)
			Reduce dose according to CrCl: to AUC of 5–7
			  mg/mL per min [AUC = dose/(CrCl + 25)]

Oxaliplatin	130 mg/m² q3 weeks over 2 h or
	  85 mg/m² q2 weeks
		Nausea
		Anemia
			Acute reversible neurotoxicity; chronic sensory
			  neurotox cumulative with dose; reversible
			  laryngopharyngeal spasm

Antitumor antibiotics			

Bleomycin	15–25 mg/d qd ×5 IV bolus or
	  continuous IV
		Pulmonary
		Skin effects
		Raynaud's
		Hypersensitivity
			Inactivate by bleomycin hydrolase (decreased
			  in lung/skin)
			O₂ enhances pulmonary toxicity
			Cisplatin-induced decrease in CrCl may increase
			  skin/lung toxicity
			Reduce dose if CrCl < 60 mL/min

Actinomycin D	10–15 μg/kg per day qd ×5 IV bolus	Marrow Nausea Mucositis Vesicant Alopecia	Radiation recall
Mitomycin C	6–10 mg/m² q6 weeks	Marrow Vesicant Hemolytic-uremic syndrome Lung CV—heart failure	Treat superficial bladder cancers by intravesical infusion Delayed marrow toxicity Cumulative marrow toxicity

Etoposide (VP16-213)	100–150 mg/m² IV qd ×3–5d
	  or 50 mg/m² PO qd ×21d
	  or up to 1500 mg/m² per dose (high
	  dose with stem cell support)
		Marrow (WBCs > platelet)
		Alopecia
		Hypotension
		Hypersensitivity (rapid IV)
		Nausea
		Mucositis (high dose)
			Hepatic metabolism—renal 30%
			Reduce doses with renal failure
			Schedule-dependant (5 day better than 1 day)
			Late leukemogenic
			Accentuate antimetabolite action

(continued)

PART 6

Oncology and Hematology

TABLE 81-2 COMMONLY USED CANCER CHEMOTHERAPY AGENTS (CONTINUED)

Drug	Examples of Usual Doses	Toxicity	Interactions, Issues
Topotecan	20 mg/m² IV q3–4 weeks over 30 min or 1.5–3 mg/m² q3–4 weeks over 24 h or 0.5 mg/m² per day over 21 days	Marrow Mucositis Nausea Mild alopecia	Reduce dose with renal failure No liver toxicity
Irinotecan (CPT II)	100–150 mg/m² IV over 90 min q3–4 weeks or 30 mg/m² per day over 120 h	Diarrhea: "early onset" with cramping, flushing, vomiting; "late onset" after several doses Marrow Alopecia Nausea Vomiting Pulmonary	Prodrug requires enzymatic clearance to active drug "SN 38" Early diarrhea likely due to biliary excretion Late diarrhea, use "high-dose" loperamide (2 mg q2–4 h)
Doxorubicin and daunorubicin	45–60 mg/m² dose q3–4 weeks or 10–30 mg/m² dose q week or continuous-infusion regimen	Marrow Mucositis Alopecia Cardiovascular acute/chronic Vesicant	Heparin aggregate; coadministration increases clearance Acetaminophen, BCNU increase liver toxicity Radiation recall
Idarubicin	10–15 mg/m² IV q 3 weeks or 10 mg/m² IV qd ×3	Marrow Cardiac (less than doxorubicin)	None established
Epirubicin	150 mg/m² IV q3 weeks	Marrow Cardiac	None established
Mitoxantrone	12 mg/m² qd ×3 or 12–14 mg/m² q3 weeks	Marrow Cardiac (less than doxorubicin) Vesicant (mild) Blue urine, sclerae, nails	Interacts with heparin Less alopecia, nausea than doxorubicin Radiation recall

Indirect DNA-Interacting Agents

Antimetabolites

Drug	Examples of Usual Doses	Toxicity	Interactions, Issues
Deoxycoformycin	4 mg/m² IV every other week	Nausea Immunosuppression Neurologic Renal	Excretes in urine Reduce dose for renal failure Inhibits adenosine deaminase
6-Mercaptopurine	75 mg/m² PO or up 500 mg/m² PO (high dose)	Marrow Liver Nausea	Variable bioavailability Metabolize by xanthine oxidase Decrease dose with allopurinol Increased toxicity with thiopurine methyltransferase deficiency
6-Thioguanine	2–3 mg/kg per day for up to 3–4 weeks	Marrow Liver Nausea	Variable bioavailability Increased toxicity with thiopurine methyltransferase deficiency
Azathioprine	1–5 mg/kg per day	Marrow Nausea Liver	Metabolizes to 6MP, therefore reduce dose with allopurinol Increased toxicity with thiopurine methyltransferase deficiency
2-Chlorodeoxyaden-osine	0.09 mg/kg per day qd ×7 as continuous infusion	Marrow Renal Fever	Notable use in hairy cell leukemia
Hydroxyurea	20–50 mg/kg (lean body weight) PO qd or 1–3 g/d	Marrow Nausea Mucositis Skin changes Rare renal, liver, lung, CNS	Decrease dose with renal failure Augments antimetabolite effect
Methotrexate	15–30 mg PO or IM qd ×3–5 or 30 mg IV days 1 and 8 or 1.5–12 g/m² per day (with leucovorin)	Marrow Liver/lung Renal tubular Mucositis	Rescue with leucovorin Excreted in urine Decrease dose in renal failure NSAIDs increase renal toxicity
5-Fluorouracil	375 mg/m² IV qd ×5 or 600 mg/m² IV days 1 and 8	Marrow Mucositis Neurologic Skin changes	Toxicity enhanced by leucovorin Dihydropyrimidine dehydrogenase deficiency increases toxicity Metabolizes in tissues
Capecitabine	665 mg/m² bid continuous; 1250 mg/m² bid 2 weeks on/ 1 off; 829 mg/m² bid 2 weeks on/ 1 off + 60 mg/d leucovorin	Diarrhea Hand-foot syndrome	Prodrug of 5FU due to intratumoral metabolism
Cytosine arabinoside	100 mg/m² per day qd ×7 by continuous infusion or 1–3 g/m² dose IV bolus	Marrow Mucositis Neurologic (high dose) Conjunctivitis (high dose) Noncardiogenic pulmonary edema	Enhances activity of alkylating agents Metabolizes in tissues by deamination
Azacytidine	750 mg/m² per week or 150–200 mg/m² per day ×5–10 (bolus) or (continuous IV)	Marrow Nausea Liver Neurologic Myalgia	Use limited to leukemia Altered methylation of DNA alters gene expression

(continued)

TABLE 81-2 **COMMONLY USED CANCER CHEMOTHERAPY AGENTS (CONTINUED)**

Drug	Examples of Usual Doses	Toxicity	Interactions, Issues
Gemcitabine	1000 mg/m² IV weekly ×7	Marrow Nausea Hepatic Fever/"flu syndrome"	
Fludarabine phosphate	25 mg/m² IV qd ×5	Marrow Neurologic Lung	Dose reduction with renal failure Metabolized to F-ara converted to F-ara ATP in cells by deoxycytidine kinase
Asparaginase	25,000 IU/m² q3–4 weeks or 6000 IU/m² per day qod for 3–4 weeks or 1000–2000 IU/m² for 10–20 days	Protein synthesis Clotting factors Glucose Albumin Hypersensitivity CNS Pancreatitis Hepatic	Blocks methotrexate action
Pemetrexed	200 mg/m² q3 weeks	Anemia Neutropenia Thrombocytopenia	Supplement folate/B$_{12}$ Caution in renal failure
Antimitotic agents			
Vincristine	1–1.4 mg/m² per week	Vesicant Marrow Neurologic GI: ileus/constipation; bladder hypotoxicity; SIADH Cardiovascular	Hepatic clearance Dose reduction for bilirubin >1.5 mg/dL Prophylactic bowel regimen
Vinblastine	6–8 mg/m² per week	Vesicant Marrow Neurologic (less common but similar spectrum to other vincas) Hypertension Raynaud's	Hepatic clearance Dose reduction as with vincristine
Vinorelbine	15–30 mg/m² per week	Vesicant Marrow Allergic/bronchospasm (immediate) Dyspnea/cough (subacute) Neurologic (less prominent but similar spectrum to other vincas)	Hepatic clearance
Paclitaxel	135–175 mg/m² per 24-h infusion or 175 mg/m² per 3-h infusion or 140 mg/m² per 96-h infusion or 250 mg/m² per 24-h infusion plus G-CSF	Hypersensitivity Marrow Mucositis Alopecia Sensory neuropathy CV conduction disturbance Nausea—infrequent	Premedicate with steroids, H$_1$ and H$_2$ blockers Hepatic clearance Dose reduction as with vincas
Docetaxel	100 mg/m² per 1-h infusion q3 weeks	Hypersensitivity Fluid retention syndrome Marrow Dermatologic Sensory neuropathy Nausea infrequent Some stomatitis	Premedicate with steroids, H$_1$ and H$_2$ blockers
Estramustine phosphate	14 mg/kg per day in 3–4 divided doses with water >2 h after meals Avoid Ca²⁺-rich foods	Nausea Vomiting Diarrhea CHF Thrombosis Gynecomastia	
NAB-Paclitaxel (protein bound)	260 mg/m² q3 weeks	Neuropathy Anemia Neutropenia Thrombocytopenia	Caution in hepatic insufficiency
Molecularly Targeted Agents			
Imatinib	400 mg/d, continuous	Nausea Periorbital edema	Myelosuppression not frequent in solid tumor indications
Tretinoin	45 mg/m² per day until complete response + anthrocycline-based regimen in APL	Teratogenic Cutaneous	APL differentiation syndrome: pulmonary dysfunction/infiltrate, pleural/pericardial effusion, fever
Bexarotene	300–400 mg/m² per day, continuous	Hypercholesterolemia Hypertriglyceridemia Cutaneous Teratogenic	Central hypothyroidism

(continued)

TABLE 81-2 COMMONLY USED CANCER CHEMOTHERAPY AGENTS (CONTINUED)

Drug	Examples of Usual Doses	Toxicity	Interactions, Issues
Gemtuzumab ozogamicin	9 mg/m^2 over 2 h q2 weeks, usually followed by chemotherapy or marrow transplant	Neutropenia Thrombocytopenia Hepatic	Postinfusion syndrome: fever, chills, hypotension Rare hepatic venoocclusive disease Mucositis uncommon
Denileukin diftitox	9–18 μg/kg per day × 5 d q 3 wk	Nausea/vomiting Chills/fever Asthenia Hepatic	Acute hypersensitivity: hypotension, vasodilation, rash, chest tightness Vascular leak: hypotension, edema, hypoalbuminemia, thrombotic events (MI, DVT, CVA)
Gefitinib	250 mg PO per day	Rash Diarrhea	In U.S., only with prior documented benefit
Erlotinib	150 mg PO per day	Rash Diarrhea	1 h before, 2 h after meals
Dasatinib	70 mg PO bid	Liver changes Rash Neutropenia Thrombocytopenia	
Sorafenib	400 mg PO bid	Diarrhea Hand-foot syndrome Other rash	
Sunitinib	50 mg PO qd for 4 of 6 weeks	Fatigue Diarrhea Neutropenia	
Miscellaneous			
Arsenic trioxide	0.16 mg/kg per day up to 50 days in APL	↑QT$_c$ Peripheral neuropathy Musculoskeletal pain Hyperglycemia	APL differentiation syndrome (see under tretinoin)

^{a}Common alkylator: alopecia, pulmonary, infertility, plus teratogenesis.

Note: APL, acute promyelocytic leukemia; AUC, area under the curve; CHF, congestive heart failure; CNS, central nervous system; CrCl, creatinine clearance; CV, cardiovascular; CVA, cerebrovascular accident; DVT, deep venous thrombosis; G-CSF, granulocyte colony-stimulating factor; GI, gastrointestinal; HBP, high blood pressure; MAOI, monoamine oxidase inhibitors; MI, myocardial infarction; 6MP, 6-mercaptopurine; NSAIDs, nonsteroidal anti-inflammatory drugs; SIADH, syndrome of inappropriate antidiuretic hormone; WBCs, white blood cells.

myelosuppression, alopecia, and pulmonary toxicity but is relatively "lymphocyte sparing." Its routine use in treatment of CML has been curtailed in favor of imatinib (Gleevec) or dasatinib, but it is still employed in transplant preparation regimens. Melphalan shows variable oral bioavailability and undergoes extensive binding to albumin and α$_1$-acidic glycoprotein. Mucositis appears more prominently; however, it has prominent activity in multiple myeloma.

Nitrosoureas break down to carbamoylating species that not only cause a distinct pattern of DNA base pair–directed toxicity but also can covalently modify proteins. They share the feature of causing relatively delayed bone marrow toxicity, which can be cumulative and long-lasting. Streptozotocin is unique in that its glucose-like structure conveys specific toxicity to the islet cells of the pancreas (for whose derivative tumor types it is prominently indicated) as well as causing renal toxicity in the form of Fanconi syndrome, including amino aciduria, glycosuria, and renal tubular acidosis. Methyl CCNU (lomustine) causes direct glomerular as well as tubular damage, cumulatively related to dose and time of exposure.

Procarbazine is metabolized in the liver and possibly in tumor cells to yield a variety of free radical and alkylating species. In addition to myelosuppression, it causes hypnotic and other CNS effects, including vivid nightmares. It can cause a disulfiram-like syndrome on ingestion of ethanol. Altretamine (formerly hexamethylmelamine) and thiotepa can chemically give rise to alkylating species, although the nature of the DNA damage has not been well characterized in either case. Thiotepa can be used for intrathecal treatment of neoplastic meningitis. Dacarbazine (DTIC) is activated in the liver to yield the highly reactive methyl diazonium cation. It causes only modest myelosuppression 21–25 days after a dose but causes prominent nausea on day 1. Temozolomide is structurally related to dacarbazine but was designed to be activated by nonenzymatic hydrolysis in tumors and is bioavailable orally.

Cisplatin was discovered fortuitously by observing that bacteria present in electrolysis solutions could not divide. Only the *cis* diamine configuration is active as an antitumor agent. It is hypothesized that in the intracellular environment, a chloride is lost from each position, being replaced by a water molecule. The resulting positively charged species is an efficient bifunctional interactor with DNA, forming Pt-based cross-links. Cisplatin requires administration with adequate hydration, including forced diuresis with mannitol to prevent kidney damage; even with the use of hydration, gradual decrease in kidney function is common, along with noteworthy anemia. Hypomagnesemia frequently attends cisplatin use and can lead to hypocalcemia and tetany. Other common toxicities include neurotoxocity with stocking-and-glove sensorimotor neuropathy. Hearing loss occurs in 50% of patients treated with conventional doses. Cisplatin is intensely emetogenic, requiring prophylactic antiemetics. Myelosuppression is less evident than with other alkylating agents. Chronic vascular toxicity (Raynaud's phenomenon, coronary artery disease) is a more unusual toxicity. Carboplatin displays less nephro-, oto-, and neurotoxicity. However, myelosuppression is more frequent, and as the drug is exclusively cleared through the kidney, adjustment of dose for creatinine clearance must be accomplished through use of various dosing nomograms. Oxaliplatin is a platinum analog with noteworthy activity in colon cancers refractory to other treatments. It is prominently neurotoxic.

ANTITUMOR ANTIBIOTICS AND TOPOISOMERASE POISONS Antitumor antibiotics are substances produced by bacteria that in nature appear to provide a chemical defense against other hostile microorganisms. As a class they bind to DNA directly and can frequently undergo electron transfer reactions to generate free radicals in close proximity to DNA, leading to DNA damage in the form of single-strand breaks or cross-links. Topoisomerase poisons include natural products or semisynthetic species derived ultimately from plants, and they modify enzymes that regulate the capacity of DNA to unwind to allow normal replication or transcription. These include topoisomerase I, which creates single-strand breaks that then rejoin following the passage of the other DNA strand through the break. Topoisomerase II creates double-strand breaks through which another segment of DNA duplex passes before rejoining. DNA damage from these agents can occur in any cell cycle phase, but cells tend to arrest in S-phase or G_2 of the cell cycle in cells with p53 and Rb pathway lesions as the result of defective checkpoint mechanisms in cancer cells. Owing to the role of topoisomerase I in the procession of the replication fork, topoisomerase I poisons cause lethality if the topoisomerase I–induced lesions are made in S-phase.

Doxorubicin can intercalate into DNA, thereby altering DNA structure, replication, and topoisomerase II function. It can also undergo reduction reactions by accepting electrons into its quinone ring system, with the capacity to undergo reoxidation to form reactive oxygen radicals after reoxidation. It causes predictable myelosuppression, alopecia, nausea, and mucositis. In addition, it causes acute cardiotoxicity in the form of atrial and ventricular dysrhythmias, but these are rarely of clinical significance. In contrast, cumulative doses >550 mg/m² are associated with a 10% incidence of chronic cardiomyopathy. The incidence of cardiomyopathy appears to be related to schedule (peak serum concentration), with low dose, frequent treatment, or continuous infusions better tolerated than intermittent higher dose exposures. Cardiotoxicity has been related to iron-catalyzed oxidation and reduction of doxorubicin, and not to topoisomerase action. Cardiotoxicity is related to peak plasma dose; thus, lower doses and continuous infusions are less likely to cause heart damage. Doxorubicin's cardiotoxicity is increased when given together with trastuzumab (Herceptin), the anti-HER-2/neu antibody. Radiation recall or interaction with concomitantly administered radiation to cause local site complications is frequent. The drug is a powerful vesicant, with necrosis of tissue apparent 4–7 days after an extravasation; therefore it should be administered into a rapidly flowing intravenous line. Dexrazoxane is an antidote to doxorubicin-induced extravasation. Doxorubicin is metabolized by the liver, so doses must be reduced by 50–75% in the presence of liver dysfunction. Daunorubicin is closely related to doxorubicin and was actually introduced first into leukemia treatment, where it remains part of curative regimens and has been shown preferable to doxorubicin owing to less mucositis and colonic damage. Idarubicin is also used in acute myeloid leukemia treatment and may be preferable to daunorubicin in activity. Encapsulation of daunorubicin into a liposomal formulation has attenuated cardiac toxicity and antitumor activity in Kaposi's sarcoma and ovarian cancer.

Bleomycin refers to a mixture of glycopeptides that have the unique feature of forming complexes with Fe^{2+} while also bound to DNA. Oxidation of Fe^{2+} gives rise to superoxide and hydroxyl radicals. The drug causes little, if any, myelosuppression. The drug is cleared rapidly, but augmented skin and pulmonary toxicity in the presence of renal failure has led to the recommendation that doses be reduced by 50–75% in the face of a creatinine clearance <25 mL/min. Bleomycin is not a vesicant and can be administered intravenously, intramuscularly, or subcutaneously. Common side effects include fever and chills, facial flush, and Raynaud's phenomenon. Hypertension can follow rapid intravenous administration, and the incidence of anaphylaxis with early preparations of the drug has led to the practice of administering a test dose of 0.5–1 unit before the rest of the dose. The most feared complication of bleomycin treatment is pulmonary fibrosis, which increases in incidence at >300 cumulative units administered and is minimally responsive to treatment (e.g., glucocorticoids). The earliest indicator of an adverse effect is a decline in the DL_{CO}, although cessation of drug immediately upon documentation of a decrease in DL_{CO} may not prevent further decline in pulmonary function. Bleomycin is inactivated by a bleomycin hydrolase, whose concentration is diminished in skin and lung. Because bleomycin-dependent electron transport is dependent on O_2, bleomycin toxicity may become apparent after exposure to transient very high PI_{O2}. Thus, during surgical procedures, patients with prior exposure to bleomycin should be maintained on the lowest PI_{O2} consistent with maintaining adequate tissue oxygenation.

Mitomycin C undergoes reduction of its quinone function to generate a bifunctional DNA alkylating agent. It is a broadly active antineoplastic agent with a number of unpredictable toxicities, including delayed bronchospasm 12–14 h after dosing and a chronic pulmonary

fibrosis syndrome more frequent at doses of 50–60 mg/m². Cardiomyopathy has been described, particularly in a setting of prior radiation therapy. A hemolytic/uremic syndrome carries an ultimate mortality rate of 25–50% and is poorly treated by conventional component support and exchange transfusion. Mitomycin is a notable vesicant and causes substantial nausea and vomiting. It can be used for intravesical instillation for curative treatment of superficial transitional bladder carcinomas and, with radiation therapy, for curative treatment of anal carcinoma.

Mitoxantrone is a synthetic compound that was designed to recapitulate features of doxorubicin but with less cardiotoxicity. It is quantitatively less cardiotoxic (comparing the ratio of cardiotoxic to therapeutically effective doses) but is still associated with a 10% incidence of cardiotoxicity at cumulative doses of >150 mg/m². It also causes alopecia. Cases of acute promyelocytic leukemia (APL) have arisen shortly after exposure of patients to mitoxantrone, particularly in the adjuvant treatment of breast cancer. While chemotherapy-associated leukemia is generally of the acute myeloid type, APL arising in the setting of prior mitoxantrone treatment had the typical t(15;17) chromosome translocation associated with APL, but the breakpoints of the translocation appeared to be at topoisomerase II sites that would be preferred sites of mitoxantrone action, clearly linking the action of the drug to the generation of the leukemia.

Etoposide was synthetically derived from the plant product podophyllotoxin; it binds directly to topoisomerase II and DNA in a reversible ternary complex. It stabilizes the covalent intermediate in the enzyme's action where the enzyme is covalently linked to DNA. This "alkali-labile" DNA bond was historically a first hint that an enzyme such as a topoisomerase might exist. The drug therefore causes a prominent G_2 arrest, reflecting the action of a DNA damage checkpoint. Prominent clinical effects include myelosuppression, nausea, and transient hypotension related to the speed of administration of the agent. Etoposide is a mild vesicant but is relatively free from other large-organ toxicities. When given at high doses or very frequently, topoisomerase II inhibitors may cause acute leukemia associated with chromosome 11q23 abnormalities in up to 1% of exposed patients.

Camptothecin was isolated from extracts of a Chinese tree and had notable antileukemia activity. Early clinical studies with the sodium salt of the hydrolyzed camptothecin lactone showed evidence of toxicity with little antitumor activity. Identification of topoisomerase I as the target of camptothecins and the need to preserve lactone structure allowed additional efforts to identify active members of this series. Topoisomerase I is responsible for unwinding the DNA strand by introducing single-strand breaks and allowing rotation of one strand about the other. In S-phase, topoisomerase I–induced breaks that are not promptly resealed lead to progress of the replication fork off the end of a DNA strand. The DNA damage is a potent signal for induction of apoptosis. Camptothecins promote the stabilization of the DNA linked to the enzyme in a so-called cleavable complex, analogous to the action of etoposide with topoisomerase II. Topotecan is a camptothecin derivative approved for use in gynecologic tumors and small cell lung cancer. Toxicity is limited to myelosuppression and mucositis. CPT-11, or irinotecan, is a camptothecin with evidence of activity in colon carcinoma. In addition to myelosuppression, it causes a secretory diarrhea related to the toxicity of a metabolite called SN-38. The diarrhea can be treated effectively with loperamide or octreotide.

Indirect Effectors of DNA Function: Antimetabolites A broad definition of antimetabolites would include compounds with structural similarity to precursors of purines or pyrimidines, or compounds that interfere with purine or pyrimidine synthesis. Antimetabolites can cause DNA damage indirectly, through misincorporation into DNA, abnormal timing or progression through DNA synthesis, or altered function of pyrimidine and purine biosynthetic enzymes. They tend to convey greatest toxicity to cells in S-phase, and the degree of toxicity increases with duration of exposure. Common toxic manifestations include stomatitis, diarrhea, and myelosuppression. Second malignancies are not associated with their use.

Methotrexate inhibits dihydrofolate reductase, which regenerates reduced folates from the oxidized folates produced when thymidine monophosphate is formed from deoxyuridine monophosphate. Without reduced folates, cells die a "thymine-less" death. N5-tetrahydrofolate or N5-formyltetrahydrofolate (leucovorin) can bypass this block and rescue cells from methotrexate, which is maintained in cells by polyglutamylation. The drug and other reduced folates are transported into cells by the folate carrier, and high concentrations of drug can bypass this carrier and allow diffusion of drug directly into cells. These properties have suggested the design of "high-dose" methotrexate regimens with leucovorin rescue of normal marrow and mucosa as part of curative approaches to osteosarcoma in the adjuvant setting and hematopoietic neoplasms of children and adults. Methotrexate is cleared by the kidney via both glomerular filtration and tubular secretion, and toxicity is augmented by renal dysfunction and drugs such as salicylates, probenecid, and nonsteroidal anti-inflammatory agents that undergo tubular secretion. With normal renal function, 15 mg/m^2 leucovorin will rescue 10^{-8} to 10^{-6} M methotrexate in three to four doses. However, with decreased creatinine clearance, doses of 50–100 mg/m^2 are continued until methotrexate levels are $<5 \times 10^{-8}$ M. In addition to bone marrow suppression and mucosal irritation, methotrexate can cause renal failure itself at high doses owing to crystallization in renal tubules; therefore, high-dose regimens require alkalinization of urine with increased flow by hydration. Methotrexate can be sequestered in third-space collections and leech back into the general circulation, causing prolonged myelosuppression. Less frequent adverse effects include reversible increases in transaminases and hypersensitivity-like pulmonary syndrome. Chronic low-dose methotrexate can cause hepatic fibrosis. When administered to the intrathecal space, methotrexate can cause chemical arachnoiditis and CNS dysfunction.

Pemetrexed is a novel folate-directed antimetabolite. It is "multitargeted" in that it inhibits the activity of several enzymes, including thymidylate synthetase, dihydrofolate reductase, and glycinamide ribonucleotide formyltransferase, thereby affecting the synthesis of both purine and pyrimidine nucleic acid precursors. To avoid significant toxicity to the normal tissues, patients receiving pemetrexed should also receive low-dose folate and vitamin B12 supplementation. Pemetrexed has notable activity against certain lung cancers and, in combination with cisplatin, also against mesotheliomas.

5-Fluorouracil (5FU) represents an early example of "rational" drug design in that it originated from the observation that tumor cells incorporate radiolabeled uracil more efficiently into DNA than normal cells, especially gut. 5FU is metabolized in cells to 5′FdUMP, which inhibits thymidylate synthetase (TS). In addition, misincorporation can lead to single-strand breaks, and RNA can aberrantly incorporate FUMP. 5FU is metabolized by dihydropyrimidine dehydrogenase, and deficiency of this enzyme can lead to excessive toxicity from 5FU. Oral bioavailability varies unreliably, but orally administered analogues of 5FU such as capecitabine have been developed that allow at least equivalent activity to many parenteral 5FU-based approaches to refractory cancers. Intravenous administration of 5FU leads to bone marrow suppression after short infusions but to stomatitis after prolonged infusions. Leucovorin augments the activity of 5FU by promoting formation of the ternary covalent complex of 5FU, the reduced folate, and TS. Less frequent toxicities include CNS dysfunction, with prominent cerebellar signs, and endothelial toxicity manifested by thrombosis, including pulmonary embolus and myocardial infarction.

Cytosine arabinoside (ara-C) is incorporated into DNA after formation of ara-CTP, resulting in S-phase–related toxicity. Continuous infusion schedules allow maximal efficiency, with uptake maximal at 5–7 μM. Ara-C can be administered intrathecally. Adverse effects include nausea, diarrhea, stomatitis, chemical conjunctivitis, and cerebellar ataxia. Gemcitabine is a cytosine derivative that is similar to ara-C in that it is incorporated into DNA after anabolism to the triphosphate, rendering DNA susceptible to breakage and repair synthesis, which differs from that in ara-C in that gemcitabine-induced lesions are very inefficiently removed. In contrast to ara-C, gemcitabine appears to have useful activity in a variety of solid tumors, with limited nonmyelosuppressive toxicities. 6-Thioguanine and 6-mercaptopurine (6MP) are used in the treatment of acute lymphoid leukemia. Although administered orally, they display variable bioavailability. 6MP is metabolized by xanthine oxidase and therefore requires dose reduction when used with allopurinol.

Fludarabine phosphate is a prodrug of F-adenine arabinoside (F-ara-A), which in turn was designed to diminish the susceptibility of ara-A to adenosine deaminase. F-ara-A is incorporated into DNA and can cause delayed cytotoxicity even in cells with low growth fraction, including chronic lymphocytic leukemia and follicular B cell lymphoma. CNS and peripheral nerve dysfunction and T cell depletion leading to opportunistic infections can occur in addition to myelosuppression. 2-Chlorodeoxyadenosine is a similar compound with activity in hairy cell leukemia. 2-Deoxycoformycin inhibits adenosine deaminase, with resulting increase in dATP levels. This causes inhibition of ribonucleotide reductase as well as augmented susceptibility to apoptosis, particularly in T cells. Renal failure and CNS dysfunction are notable toxicities in addition to immunosuppression. Hydroxyurea inhibits ribonucleotide reductase, resulting in S-phase block. It is orally bioavailable and useful for the acute management of myeloproliferative states.

Asparaginase is a bacterial enzyme that causes breakdown of extracellular asparagine required for protein synthesis in certain leukemic cells. This effectively stops tumor cell DNA synthesis, as DNA synthesis requires concurrent protein synthesis. The outcome of asparaginase action is therefore very similar to the result of the small-molecule antimetabolites. As asparaginase is a foreign protein, hypersensitivity reactions are common, as are effects on organs such as pancreas and liver that normally require continuing protein synthesis. This may result in decreased insulin secretion with hyperglycemia, with or without hyperamylasemia and clotting function abnormalities. Close monitoring of clotting functions should accompany use of asparaginase. Paradoxically, owing to depletion of rapidly turning over anticoagulant factors, thromboses particularly affecting the CNS may also be seen with asparaginase.

Mitotic Spindle Inhibitors Microtubules are cellular structures that form the mitotic spindle, and in interphase cells they are responsible for the cellular "scaffolding" along which various motile and secretory processes occur. Microtubules are composed of repeating noncovalent multimers of a heterodimer of α and subunits of the protein tubulin. Vincristine binds to the tubulin dimer with the result that microtubules are disaggregated. This results in the block of growing cells in M-phase; however, toxic effects in G$_1$ and S-phase are also evident. Vincristine is metabolized by the liver, and dose adjustment in the presence of hepatic dysfunction is required. It is a powerful vesicant, and infiltration can be treated by local heat and infiltration of hyaluronidase. At clinically used intravenous doses, neurotoxicity in the form of glove-and-stocking neuropathy is frequent. Acute neuropathic effects include jaw pain, paralytic ileus, urinary retention, and the syndrome of inappropriate antidiuretic hormone secretion. Myelosuppression is not seen. Vinblastine is similar to vincristine, except that it tends to be more myelotoxic, with more frequent thrombocytopenia and also mucositis and stomatitis. Vinorelbine is a vinca alkaloid that appears to have differences in resistance patterns in comparison to vincristine and vinblastine; it may be administered orally.

The taxanes include paclitaxel and docetaxel. These agents differ from the vinca alkaloids in that the taxanes stabilize microtubules against depolymerization. The "stabilized" microtubules function abnormally and are not able to undergo the normal dynamic changes of microtubule structure and function necessary for cell cycle completion. Taxanes are among the most broadly active antineoplastic agents for use in solid tumors, with evidence of activity in ovarian cancer, breast cancer, Kaposi's sarcoma, and lung tumors. They are administered intravenously, and paclitaxel requires use of a Cremophor-containing vehicle that can cause hypersensitivity reactions. Premedication with dexamethasone (20 mg orally or intravenously 12 and 6 h before treatment) and diphenhydramine (50 mg) and cimetidine (300 mg), both 30 min before treatment, decreases but does not eliminate the risk of hypersensitivity reactions to the paclitaxel vehicle. Docetaxel uses a polysorbate 80 formulation, which can cause fluid retention in addition to hypersensitivity reactions, and dexamethasone premedication with or without antihistamines is frequently used. A protein-bound formulation of paclitaxel (called *nab-paclitaxel*) has at least equivalent antineoplastic activity and decreased risk of hypersensitivity reactions. Paclitaxel may also cause hypersensitivity reactions, myelosuppression, neurotoxicity in the form of glove-and-stocking numbness, and paresthesia. Cardiac rhythm disturbances were observed in phase I and II trials, most commonly asymptomatic bradycardia but also, much more rarely, varying degrees of heart block. These have not emerged as clinically significant in the majority of patients. Docetaxel causes comparable degrees of myelosuppression and neuropathy. Hypersensitivity reactions, including bronchospasm, dyspnea, and hypotension, are less frequent but occur to some degree in up to 25% of patients. Fluid retention appears to result from a vascular leak syndrome that can aggravate preexisting effusions. Rash can complicate docetaxel administration, appearing prominently as a pruritic maculopapular rash affecting the forearms, but it has also been associated with fingernail ridging, breakdown, and skin discoloration. Stomatitis appears to be somewhat more frequent than with paclitaxel.

Estramustine was originally synthesized as a mustard derivative that might be useful in neoplasms that possessed estrogen receptors. However, no evidence of interaction with DNA was observed. Surprisingly, the drug caused metaphase arrest, and subsequent study revealed that it binds to microtubule-associated proteins, resulting in abnormal microtubule function. Estramustine binds to estramustine-binding proteins (EMBPs), which are notably present in prostate tumor tissue. The drug is used as an oral formulation in patients with prostate cancer. Gastrointestinal and cardiovascular adverse effects related to the estrogen moiety occur in up to 10% of patients, including worsened heart failure and thromboembolic phenomena. Gynecomastia and nipple tenderness can also occur.

Hormonal Agents   The family of steroid hormone receptor–related molecules has emerged as prominent targets for small molecules useful in cancer treatment. When bound to their cognate ligands, these receptors can alter gene transcription and, in certain tissues, induce apoptosis. The pharmacologic effect is a mirror or parody of the normal effects of the agent acting in nontransformed tissue, although the effects on tumors are mediated by indirect effects in some cases.

Glucocorticoids are generally given in "pulsed" high doses in leukemias and lymphomas, where they induce apoptosis in tumor cells. Cushing's syndrome or inadvertent adrenal suppression on withdrawal from high-dose glucocorticoids can be significant complications, along with infections common in immunosuppressed patients, in particular *Pneumocystis* pneumonia, which classically appears a few days after completing a course of high-dose glucocorticoids.

Tamoxifen is a partial estrogen receptor antagonist; it has a tenfold greater antitumor activity in breast cancer patients whose tumors express estrogen receptors than in those who have low or no levels of expression. Side effects include a somewhat increased risk of estrogen-related cardiovascular complications, such as thromboembolic phenomena, and a small increased incidence of endometrial carcinoma, which appears after chronic use (usually >5 years). Progestational agents—including medroxyprogesterone acetate, androgens including fluoxymesterone (Halotestin) and, paradoxically, estrogens—have approximately the same degree of activity in primary hormonal treatment of breast cancers that have elevated expression of estrogen receptor protein. Estrogen is not used often owing to prominent cardiovascular and uterotropic activity.

Aromatase refers to a family of enzymes that catalyze the formation of estrogen in various tissues, including the ovary and peripheral adipose tissue and some tumor cells. Aromatase inhibitors are of two types, the irreversible steroid analogs such as exemestane and the reversible inhibitors such as anastrozole or letrozole. Anastrozole is superior to tamoxifen in the adjuvant treatment of breast cancer in postmenopausal patients with estrogen receptor–positive tumors. Letrozole treatment affords benefit following tamoxifen treatment.

Adverse effects of aromatase inhibitors may include an increased risk of osteoporosis.

Prostate cancer is classically treated by androgen deprivation. Diethylstilbestrol (DES) acting as an estrogen at the level of the hypothalamus to downregulate hypothalamic luteinizing hormone (LH) production results in decreased elaboration of testosterone by the testicle. For this reason, orchiectomy is equally as effective as moderate-dose DES, inducing responses in 80% of previously untreated patients with prostate cancer but without the prominent cardiovascular side effects of DES, including thrombosis and exacerbation of coronary artery disease. In the event that orchiectomy is not accepted by the patient, testicular androgen suppression can also be effected by luteinizing hormone–releasing hormone (LHRH) agonists such as leuprolide and goserelin. These agents cause tonic stimulation of the LHRH receptor, with the loss of its normal pulsatile activation resulting in decreased output of LH by the anterior pituitary. Therefore, as primary hormonal manipulation in prostate cancer, one can choose orchiectomy or leuprolide, but not both. The addition of androgen receptor blockers, including flutamide or bicalutamide, is of uncertain additional benefit in extending overall response duration; the combined use of orchiectomy or leuprolide plus flutamide is referred to as *total androgen blockade*.

Tumors that respond to a primary hormonal manipulation may frequently respond to second and third hormonal manipulations. Thus, breast tumors that had previously responded to tamoxifen have, on relapse, notable response rates to withdrawal of tamoxifen itself or to subsequent addition of an aromatase inhibitor or progestin. Likewise, initial treatment of prostate cancers with leuprolide plus flutamide may be followed after disease progression by response to withdrawal of flutamide. These responses may result from the removal of antagonists from mutant steroid hormone receptors that have come to depend on the presence of the antagonist as a growth-promoting influence.

Additional strategies to treat refractory breast and prostate cancers that possess steroid hormone receptors may also address adrenal capacity to produce androgens and estrogens, even after orchiectomy or oophorectomy, respectively. Thus, aminoglutethimide or ketoconazole can be used to block adrenal synthesis by interfering with the enzymes of steroid hormone metabolism. Administration of these agents requires concomitant hydrocortisone replacement and additional glucocorticoid doses administered in the event of physiologic stress.

Humoral mechanisms can also result in complications of an underlying malignancy. Adrenocortical carcinomas can cause Cushing's syndrome as well as syndromes of androgen or estrogen excess. Mitotane can counteract these by decreasing synthesis of steroid hormones. Islet cell neoplasms can cause debilitating diarrhea, treated with the somatostatin analogue octreotide. Prolactin-secreting tumors can be effectively managed by the dopaminergic agonist bromocriptine.

TARGETED THERAPIES

A better understanding of cancer cell biology has suggested many new targets for cancer drug discovery and development. These include the products of oncogenes and tumor-suppressor genes, regulators of cell death pathways, mediators of cellular immortality such as telomerase, and molecules responsible for microenvironmental molding such as proteases or angiogenic factors. The essential difference in the development of agents that would target these processes is that the basis for discovery of the candidate drug is the a priori importance of the target in the biology of the tumor, rather than the initial detection of drug candidates based on the phenomenon of tumor cell regression in tissue culture or in animals. The following examples reflect the rapidly evolving clinical research activity in this area. **Figure 81-4** summarizes how FDA-approved targeted agents act.

Hematopoietic Neoplasms   Imatinib targets the ATP binding site of the p210$^{bcr-abl}$ protein tyrosine kinase that is formed as the result of the chromosome 9,22 translocation producing the Philadelphia chromosome in CML. Imatinib is superior to interferon plus chemotherapy in

FIGURE 81-4 Site of action of targeted agents. Signals proceeding from growth factor–related receptor tyrosine kinases (RTKs) such as EGF-R, erbB2, or c-kit can be interrupted by lapatinib, erlotinib, gefitinib, and imatinib, acting at the ATP binding site; or by cetuximab, trastuzumab, or panitumomab. Tyrosine kinases (TKs) that are not directly stimulated by growth factors such as p210 bcr-abl or src can be inhibited by imatinib, dasatinib, or nilotinib. Signals projected downstream from growth factor receptors can be affected by the multitargeted kinase inhibitor sorafenib, acting on c-raf, and, upon arrival at the nucleus, affect gene expression, which can be affected by the targeted transcriptional modulators vorinostat (targeting histone deacetylase), azacytidine derivatives (targeting DNA methyltransferase), or retinoid receptor modulators all-*trans*-retinoic acid (ATRA) or bexarotene. Cytokine receptors (CkRs) are one stimulus for degradation of the inhibitory subunit of the NFκB transcription factor by the proteosome. Bortezomib inhibits this process and can prevent activation of NFκB-dependent genes, among other growth-related effects. Sorafenib and sunitinib, acting as inhibitors of VEGF receptors, can modulate tumor blood vessel function through their action on endothelial cells, while bevacizumab targets the same process by combining with VEGF itself.

the initial treatment of the chronic phase of this disorder. It has lesser activity in the blast phase of CML, where the cells may have acquired additional mutations in p210$^{bcr-abl}$ itself or other genetic lesions. Its side effects are relatively tolerable in most patients and include hepatic dysfunction, diarrhea, and fluid retention. Rarely, patients receiving imatinib have decreased cardiac function, which may persist after discontinuation of the drug. The quality of response to imatinib enters into the decision about when to refer patients with CML for consideration of transplant approaches. Nilotinib is a tyrosine protein kinase inhibitor with a similar spectrum of activity to imatinib, but with increased potency and perhaps better tolerance by certain patients. Dasatinib, another inhibitor of the p210$^{bcr-abl}$ oncoproteins, is active in certain mutant variants of p210$^{bcr-abl}$ that are refractory to imatinib and arise during therapy with imatinib or are present de novo. Dasatinib also has inhibitory action against kinases belonging to the src tyrosine protein kinase family; this activity may contribute to its effects in hematopoietic tumors and suggest a role in solid tumors where src kinases are active. Only the T315I mutant is resistant to dasatinib; a new class of inhibitors called aurora kinase inhibitors is in development to address this problem.

All-*trans*-retinoic acid (ATRA) targets the PML-retinoic acid receptor (RAR) α fusion protein, which is the result of the chromosome 15,17 translocation pathogenic for most forms of APL. Administered orally, it causes differentiation of the neoplastic promyelocytes to mature granulocytes and attenuates the rate of hemorrhagic complications. Adverse effects include headache with or without pseudotumor cerebri and gastrointestinal and cutaneous toxicities. Another active

retinoid is the synthetic retinoid X receptor ligand bexarotene, which has activity in cutaneous T cell lymphoma.

Bortezomib is an inhibitor of the proteasome, the multi-subunit assembly of protease activities responsible for the selective degradation of proteins important in regulating activation of transcription factors, including NFκB and proteins regulating cell cycle progression. It has activity in multiple myeloma and certain lymphomas. Adverse effects include neuropathy, orthostatic hypotension with or without hyponatremia, and reversible thrombocytopenia.

Vorinostat is an inhibitor of histone deacetylases, responsible for maintaining the proper orientation of histones on DNA, with resulting capacity for transcriptional readiness. Acetylated histones allow entry of transcription factors and therefore increased expression of genes that are selectively repressed in tumors. The result can be differentiation with the emergence of a more normal cellular phenotype, or cell cycle arrest with expression of endogenous regulators of cell cycle progression. Vorinostat is approved for clinical use in cutaneous T cell lymphoma, with dramatic skin clearing and very few side effects.

DNA methyltransferase inhibitors including 5-azacytidine and 2'-deoxy-5-azacytidine can also increase transcription of genes "silenced" during the pathogenesis of a tumor by causing demethylation of the methylated cytosines that are acquired as an "epigenetic" (i.e., after the DNA is replicated) modification of DNA. These drugs were originally considered antimetabolites but have clinical value in myelodysplastic syndromes and certain leukemias when administered at low doses. Combinations of DNA methyltransferase inhibitors and histone deacetylase inhibitors may offer new approaches to reregulate chromatin function.

Targeted toxins utilize macromolecules such as antibodies or cytokines with high affinity for defined tumor cell surface molecules, such as a leukemia differentiation antigen, to which a therapeutic antibody can deliver a covalently linked potent cytotoxin (e.g., gemtuzumab ozogamicin, a drug linked to anti-CD33), or a growth factor such as IL-2 to deliver a toxin (in the form of diphtheria toxin in denileukin diftitox) to cells bearing the IL-2 receptor. The value of such targeted approaches is that in addition to maximizing the therapeutic index by differential expression of the target in tumor (as opposed to nonrenewable normal cells), selection of patients for clinical use can capitalize on assessing the target in the tumor.

Solid Tumors Small-molecule epidermal growth factor (EGF) antagonists act at the ATP binding site of the EGF receptor tyrosine kinase. In early clinical trials, gefitinib showed evidence of responses in a small fraction of patients with non-small cell lung cancer. Side effects were generally acceptable, consisting mostly of rash and diarrhea. Gefitinib was found to have antitumor activity mainly in the subset of patients with tumors containing activating mutations in the EGF receptor. Often patients who developed resistance to gefitinib have acquired additional mutations in the enzyme, similar to what was seen in imatinib-resistant CML. Erlotinib is another EGF receptor tyrosine kinase antagonist with somewhat superior activity to gefitinib in clinical trials in non-small cell lung cancer. Even patients with wild-type EGF receptors may benefit from erlotinib treatment. Lapitinib is a combined EGF receptor and erbB2 tyrosine kinase antagonist with activity in breast cancers refractory to anti-erbB2 antibodies.

In addition to the p210$^{bcr-abl}$ kinase, imatinib also has activity against the c-kit tyrosine kinase, activated in gastrointestinal stromal sarcoma, and the platelet derived growth factor receptor (PDGF-R), activated by translocation in certain sarcomas. Imatinib has found clinical utility in these neoplasms previously refractory to chemotherapeutic approaches.

"Multitargeted" kinase antagonists are small-molecule ATP site-directed antagonists that inhibit more than one protein kinase. Drugs of this type with prominent activity against the vascular endothelial growth factor receptor (VEGF-R) tyrosine kinase have activity in renal cell carcinoma. Sorafenib is a VEGF-R antagonist with activity against the *raf* serine-threonine protein kinase as well. Sunitinib has anti-VEGF-R as well as anti-PDGF-R and anti-c-kit activity. It causes prominent responses as well as stabilization of disease in renal cell cancers and gastrointestinal stromal tumors. Side effects for both agents are mostly acceptable, with fatigue and diarrhea encountered with both agents. The "hand-foot syndrome" with erythema and desquamation of the distal extremities, in some cases requiring dose modification, may be seen with sorafenib. Temsirolimus, an mTOR inhibitor, has activity in renal and breast cancer. It produces some hyperlipidemia (10%), myelosuppression (10%), and rare lung toxicity.

ACUTE COMPLICATIONS OF CANCER CHEMOTHERAPY

Myelosuppression The common cytotoxic chemotherapeutic agents almost invariably affect bone marrow function. Titration of this effect determines the MTD of the agent on a given schedule. The normal kinetics of blood cell turnover influence the sequence and sensitivity of each of the formed elements. Polymorphonuclear leukocytes (PMNs; $t_{1/2} = 6$–8 h), platelets ($t_{1/2} = 5$–7 days), and red blood cells (RBCs; $t_{1/2} = 120$ days) respectively have most, less, and least susceptibility to usually administered cytotoxic agents. The nadir count of each cell type in response to classes of agents is characteristic. Maximal neutropenia occurs 6–14 days after conventional doses of anthracyclines, antifolates, and antimetabolites. Alkylating agents differ from each other in the timing of cytopenias. Nitrosoureas, DTIC, and procarbazine can display delayed marrow toxicity, first appearing 6 weeks after dosing.

Complications of myelosuppression result from the predictable sequelae of the missing cells' function. *Febrile neutropenia* refers to the clinical presentation of fever (one temperature ≥38.5°C or three readings ≥38°C but ≤38.5°C per 24 h) in a neutropenic patient with an uncontrolled neoplasm involving the bone marrow or, more usually, in a patient undergoing treatment with cytotoxic agents. Mortality from uncontrolled infection varies inversely with the neutrophil count. If the nadir neutrophil count is >1000/μL, there is little risk; if <500/μL, risk of death is markedly increased. Management of febrile neutropenia has conventionally included empirical coverage with antibiotics for the duration of neutropenia (Chap. 82). Selection of antibiotics is governed by the expected association of infections with certain underlying neoplasms; careful physical examination (with scrutiny of catheter sites, dentition, mucosal surfaces, and perirectal and genital orifices by gentle palpation); chest x-ray; and Gram stain and culture of blood, urine, and sputum (if any) to define a putative site of infection. In the absence of any originating site, a broadly acting β-lactam with anti-*Pseudomonas* activity, such as ceftazidime, is begun empirically. The addition of vancomycin to cover potential cutaneous sites of origin (until these are ruled out or shown to originate from methicillin-sensitive organisms) or metronidazole or imipenem for abdominal or other sites favoring anaerobes reflects modifications tailored to individual patient presentations. The coexistence of pulmonary compromise raises a distinct set of potential pathogens, including *Legionella*, *Pneumocystis*, and fungal agents that may require further diagnostic evaluations such as bronchoscopy with bronchoalveolar lavage. Febrile neutropenic patients can be stratified broadly into two prognostic groups. The first, with expected short duration of neutropenia and no evidence of hypotension or abdominal or other localizing symptoms, may be expected to do well even with oral regimens, e.g., ciprofloxacin or moxifloxacin, or amoxicillin plus clavulinic acid. A less favorable prognostic group are patients with expected prolonged neutropenia, evidence of sepsis, and end-organ compromise, particularly pneumonia. These patients clearly require tailoring of their antibiotic regimen to their underlying presentation, with frequent empirical addition of antifungal agents if fever persists for 7 days without identification of an adequately treated organism or site.

Transfusion of granulocytes has no role in the management of febrile neutropenia, owing to their exceedingly short half-life, mechanical fra-

TABLE 81-3 INDICATIONS FOR THE CLINICAL USE OF G-CSF OR GM-CSF

Preventive Uses
With the first cycle of chemotherapy (so-called primary CSF administration)
  Not needed on a routine basis
  Use if the probability of febrile neutropenia is ≥20%
  Use if patient has preexisting neutropenia or active infection
  Age >65 treated for lymphoma with curative intent or other tumor treated by similar regimens
  Poor performance status
  Extensive prior chemotherapy
  Dose-dense regimens in a clinical trial or with strong evidence of benefit
With subsequent cycles if febrile neutropenia has previously occurred (so-called secondary CSF administration)
  Not needed after short duration neutropenia without fever
  Use if patient had febrile neutropenia in previous cycle
  Use if prolonged neutropenia (even without fever) delays therapy
Therapeutic Uses
Afebrile neutropenic patients
  No evidence of benefit
Febrile neutropenic patients
  No evidence of benefit
  May feel compelled to use in the face of clinical deterioration from sepsis, pneumonia, or fungal infection, but benefit unclear
In bone marrow or peripheral blood stem cell transplantation
  Use to mobilize stem cells from marrow
  Use to hasten myeloid recovery
In acute myeloid leukemia
  G-CSF of minor or no benefit
  GM-CSF of no benefit and may be harmful
In myelodysplastic syndromes
  Not routinely beneficial
  Use intermittently in subset with neutropenia and recurrent infection
What Dose and Schedule Should Be Used?
G-CSF: 5 μg/kg per day subcutaneously
GM-CSF: 250 μg/m² per day subcutaneously
Peg-filgrastim: one dose of 6 mg 24 h after chemotherapy
When Should Therapy Begin and End?
When indicated, start 24–72 h after chemotherapy
Continue until absolute neutrophil count is 10,000/μL
Do not use concurrently with chemotherapy or radiation therapy

Note: G-CSF, granulocyte colony-stimulating factor; GM-CSF, granulocyte-macrophage colony-stimulating factor.
Source: From the American Society of Clinical Oncology.

gility, and clinical syndromes of pulmonary compromise with leukostasis after their use. Instead, colony-stimulating factors (CSFs) are used to augment bone marrow production of PMNs. Early-acting factors such as IL-1, IL-3, and stem cell factor, have not been as useful clinically as late-acting, lineage-specific factors such as G-CSF (granulocyte colony-stimulating factor) or GM-CSF (granulocyte-macrophage colony-stimulating factor), erythropoietin (EPO), thrombopoietin, IL-6, and IL-11. CSFs may easily become overused in oncology practice. The settings in which their use has been proved effective are limited. G-CSF, GM-CSF, EPO, and IL-11 are currently approved for use. The American Society of Clinical Oncology has developed practice guidelines for the use of G-CSF and GM-CSF (Table 81-3).

Primary prophylaxis (i.e., shortly after completing chemotherapy to reduce the nadir) of G-CSF to patients receiving cytotoxic regimens is associated with a 20% incidence of febrile neutropenia. "Dose-dense" regimens, where cycling of chemotherapy is intended to be completed without delay of administered doses, may also benefit, but such patients should be on a clinical trial. Administration of G-CSF in these circumstances has reduced the incidence of febrile neutropenia in several studies by about 50%. Most patients, however, receive regimens that do not have such a high risk of expected febrile neutropenia, and therefore most patients initially should not receive G-CSF or GM-CSF. Special circumstances—such as a documented history of febrile neutropenia with the regimen in a particular patient or categories of patient at increased risk, such as patients > age 65 with aggressive lymphoma treated with curative chemotherapy regimens; extensive compromise of marrow by prior radiation or chemotherapy; or active, open wounds or deep-seated infection—may support primary treatment with G-CSF or GM-CSF. Administration of G-CSF or GM-CSF to afebrile neutropenic patients or to patients with low-risk febrile neutropenia is not recommended, and patients receiving concomitant chemoradiation treatment, particularly those with thoracic neoplasms, likewise are not generally recommended for treatment. In contrast, administration of G-CSF to high-risk patients with febrile neutropenia and evidence of organ compromise including sepsis syndrome, invasive fungal infection, concurrent hospitalization at the time fever develops, pneumonia, profound neutropenia ($<0.1 \times 10^9$/L), or age >65 years is reasonable.

Secondary prophylaxis refers to the administration of CSFs in patients who have experienced a neutropenic complication from a prior cycle of chemotherapy; dose reduction or delay may be a reasonably considered alternative. G-CSF or GM-CSF is conventionally started 24–72 h after completion of chemotherapy and continued until a PMN count of 10,000/μL is achieved, unless a "depot" preparation of G-CSF such as peg-filgrastim is used, where one dose is administered at least 14 days before the next scheduled administration of chemotherapy. Also, patients with myeloid leukemias undergoing induction therapy may have a slight reduction in the duration of neutropenia if G-CSF is commenced after completion of therapy and may be of particular value in elderly patients, but the influence on long-term outcome has not been defined. GM-CSF probably has a more restricted utility than G-CSF, with its use currently limited to patients after autologous bone marrow transplants, although proper head-to-head comparisons with G-CSF have not been conducted in most instances. GM-CSF may be associated with more systemic side effects.

Dangerous degrees of thrombocytopenia do not frequently complicate the management of patients with solid tumors receiving cytotoxic chemotherapy (with the possible exception of certain carboplatin-containing regimens), but they are frequent in patients with certain hematologic neoplasms where marrow is infiltrated with tumor. Severe bleeding related to thrombocytopenia occurs with increased frequency at platelet counts <20,000/μL and is very prevalent at counts <5000/μL.

The precise "trigger" point at which to transfuse patients is being evaluated in a randomized study. This issue is important not only because of the costs of frequent transfusion, but unnecessary platelet transfusions expose the patient to the risks of allosensitization and loss of value from subsequent transfusion owing to rapid platelet clearance, as well as the infectious and hypersensitivity risks inherent in any transfusion. Prophylactic transfusions to keep platelets >20,000/μL are reasonable in patients with leukemia who are stressed by fever or concomitant medical conditions (the threshold for transfusion is 10,000/μL in patients with solid tumors and no other bleeding diathesis or physiologic stressors such as fever or hypotension, a level that might also be reasonably considered for leukemia patients who are thrombocytopenic but not stressed or bleeding). In contrast, patients with myeloproliferative states may have functionally altered platelets despite normal platelet counts, and transfusion with normal donor platelets should be considered for evidence of bleeding in these patients. Careful review of medication lists to prevent exposure to nonsteroidal antiinflammatory agents and maintenance of clotting factor levels adequate to support near-normal prothrombin and partial thromboplastin time tests are important in minimizing the risk of bleeding in the thrombocytopenic patient.

Certain cytokines in clinical investigation have shown an ability to increase platelets (e.g., IL-6, IL-1, thrombopoietin), but clinical benefit and safety are not yet proven. IL-11 (oprelvekin) is approved for use in the setting of expected thrombocytopenia, but its effects on platelet counts are small, and it is associated with side effects such as headache, fever, malaise, syncope, cardiac arrhythmias, and fluid retention.

Anemia associated with chemotherapy can be managed by transfusion of packed RBCs. Transfusion is not undertaken until the hemoglobin falls to <80 g/L (8 g/dL) or if compromise of end-organ function occurs or an underlying condition (e.g., coronary artery disease) calls for maintenance of hemoglobin >90 g/L (9 g/dL). Patients who are to receive therapy for >2 months on a "stable" regimen and who are likely to require continuing transfusions are also candidates for EPO to maintain hemoglobin of 90–100 g/L (9–10 g/dL). In the setting of adequate iron stores and serum EPO levels <100 ng/mL, EPO, 150 U three times a week, can produce a slow increase in hemoglobin over about 2 months of administration. Depot formulations can be administered less frequently. It is unclear whether higher hemoglobin levels, up to 110–120 g/L (11–12 g/dL), are associated with improved quality of life to a degree that justifies the more intensive EPO use. Efforts to achieve levels at or above 120 g/L (12 g/dL) have been associated with increased thromboses and mortality. EPO may rescue hypoxic cells from death and contribute to tumor radioresistance. This may be a disadvantage in cancer but a great advantage in the setting of heart attacks and strokes.

Nausea and Vomiting   The most common side effect of chemotherapy administration is nausea, with or without vomiting. Nausea may be acute (within 24 h of chemotherapy), delayed (>24 h), or anticipatory of the receipt of chemotherapy. Patients may be likewise stratified for their risk of susceptibility to nausea and vomiting, with increased risk in young, female, heavily pretreated patients without a history of alcohol or drug use but with a history of motion or morning sickness. Antineoplastic agents vary in their capacity to cause nausea and vomiting. Highly emetogenic drugs (>90%) include mechlorethamine, streptozotocin, DTIC, cyclophosphamide at >1500 mg/m^2, and cisplatin; moderately emetogenic drugs (30–90% risk) include carboplatin, cytosine arabinoside (>1 mg/m^2), ifosfamide, conventional-dose cyclophosphamide, and anthracyclines; low-risk (10–30%) agents include fluorouracil, taxanes, etoposide, and bortezomib, with minimal risk (<10%) afforded by treatment with antibodies, bleomycin, busulfan, fludarabine, and vinca alkaloids. *Emesis* is a reflex caused by stimulation of the vomiting center in the medulla. Input to the vomiting center comes from the chemoreceptor trigger zone (CTZ) and afferents from the peripheral gastrointestinal tract, cerebral cortex, and heart. The different emesis "syndromes" require distinct management approaches. In addition, a conditioned reflex may contribute to anticipatory nausea arising after repeated cycles of chemotherapy. Accordingly, antiemesis agents differ in their locus and timing of action. Combining agents from different classes or the sequential use of different classes of agent is the cornerstone of successful management of chemotherapy-induced nausea and vomiting. Of great importance are the prophylactic administration of agents and such psychological techniques as the maintenance of a supportive milieu, counseling, and relaxation to augment the action of antiemetic agents.

Serotonin antagonists (5HT3) and neurokine (NK1) receptor antagonists are useful in "high-risk" chemotherapy regimens. The combination acts at both peripheral gastrointestinal as well as CNS sites that control nausea and vomiting. For example, the 5HT3 blocker dolasetron (Anzamet), 100 mg IV or p.o.; dexamethasone, 12 mg; and the NK1 antagonist aprepitant, 125 mg p.o., are combined on the day of administration of severely emetogenic regimens, with repetition of dexamethasone (8 mg) and aprepitant (80 mg) on days 2 and 3 for delayed nausea. Alternate 5HT3 antagonists include ondansetron (Zofran), given as 0.15 mg/kg intravenously for three doses just before and at 4 and 8 h after chemotherapy; palonosetron (Aloxi) at 0.25 mg over 30 s, 30 min prechemotherapy; and granisetron (Kytril,) given as a single dose of 0.01 mg/kg just before chemotherapy. Emesis from moderately emetic chemotherapy regimens may be prevented with a 5HT3 antagonist and dexamethasone alone for patients not receiving doxorubicin and cyclophosphamide combinations; the latter combination requires the 5HT3/dexamethasone/aprepitant on day 1 but aprepitant alone on days 2 and 3. Emesis from low-emetic-risk regimens may be prevented with 8 mg of dexamethasone alone, or with non-5HT3, non-NK1 antagonist approaches including the following.

Antidopaminergic phenothiazines act directly at the CTZ and include prochlorperazine (Compazine), 10 mg intramuscularly or intravenously, 10–25 mg orally or 25 mg per rectum every 4–6 h for up to four doses; and thiethylperazine (Torecan), 10 mg by potentially all the above routes every 6 h. Haloperidol (Haldol) is a butyrophenone dopamine antagonist given at 0.5–1.0 mg intramuscularly or orally every 8 h. Antihistamines such as diphenhydramine (Benadryl) have little intrinsic antiemetic capacity but are frequently given to prevent or treat dystonic reactions that can complicate use of the antidopaminergic agents. Lorazepam (Ativan) is a short-acting benzodiazepine that provides an anxiolytic effect to augment the effectiveness of a variety of agents when used at 1–2 mg intramuscularly, intravenously, or orally every 4–6 h. Metoclopramide (Reglan) acts on peripheral dopamine receptors to augment gastric emptying and is used in high doses for highly emetogenic regimens (1–2 mg/kg intravenously 30 min before chemotherapy and every 2 h for up to three additional doses as needed); intravenous doses of 10–20 mg every 4–6 h as needed or 50 mg orally 4 h before and 8 and 12 h after chemotherapy are used for moderately emetogenic regimens.

5-9-Tetrahydrocannabinol (Marinol) is a rather weak antiemetic compared to other available agents, but it may be useful for persisting nausea and is used orally at 10 mg every 3–4 h as needed.

Diarrhea Regimens that include fluorouracil infusions and/or irinotecan may produce severe diarrhea. Similar to the vomiting syndromes, chemotherapy-induced diarrhea may be immediate or can occur in a delayed fashion up to 48–72 h after the drugs. Careful attention to maintained hydration and electrolyte repletion, intravenously if necessary, along with antimotility treatments such as "high-dose" loperamide, commenced with 4 mg at the first occurrence of diarrhea, with 2 mg repeated every 2 h until 12 h without loose stools. Octreotide (100–150 μg), a somatostatin analog, or opiate-based preparations may be considered for patients not responding to loperamide.

Mucositis Irritation and inflammation of the mucous membranes particularly afflicting the oral and anal mucosa, but potentially involving the gastrointestinal tract, may accompany cytotoxic chemotherapy. Mucositis is due to damage to the proliferating cells at the base of the mucosal squamous epithelia or in the intestinal crypts. Topical therapies, including anesthetics and barrier-creating preparations, may provide symptomatic relief in mild cases. Palifermin or keratinocyte growth factor, a member of the fibroblast growth factor family, is effective in preventing severe mucositis in the setting of high-dose chemotherapy with stem cell transplantation for hematologic malignancies. It may also prevent mucositis from radiation.

Alopecia Chemotherapeutic agents vary widely in causing alopecia, with anthracyclines, alkylating agents, and topoisomerase inhibitors reliably causing near-total alopecia when given at therapeutic doses. Antimetabolites are more variably associated with alopecia. Psychological support and the use of cosmetic resources are to be encouraged, and "chemo caps" that reduce scalp temperature to decrease the degree of alopecia should be discouraged, particularly during treatment with curative intent of neoplasms such as leukemia or lymphoma, or in adjuvant breast cancer therapy. The richly vascularized scalp can certainly harbor micrometastatic or disseminated disease.

Gonadal Dysfunction and Pregnancy Cessation of ovulation and azoospermia reliably result from alkylating agent– and topoisomerase poison–containing regimens. The duration of these effects varies with age and sex. Males treated for Hodgkin's disease with mechlorethamine- and procarbazine-containing regimens are effectively sterile, whereas fertility usually returns after regimens that include cisplatin, vinblastine, or etoposide and after bleomycin for testicular cancer. Sperm banking before treatment may be considered to support patients likely to be sterilized by treatment. Females experience amenorrhea with anovulation after alkylating agent therapy; they are likely to recover normal menses if treatment is completed before age 30 but unlikely to recover menses after age 35. Even those who regain menses usually experience premature menopause. As the magnitude and extent of decreased fertility can be difficult to predict, patients should be counseled to maintain effective contraception, preferably by barrier means, during and after therapy. Resumption of efforts to conceive

should be considered in the context of the patient's likely prognosis. Hormone replacement therapy should be undertaken in women who do not have a hormonally responsive tumor. For those patients who have had a hormone-sensitive tumor primarily treated by a local modality, conventional practice would counsel against hormone replacement, but this issue is under investigation.

Chemotherapy agents have variable effects on the success of pregnancy (Chap. 7). All agents tend to have increased risk of adverse outcomes when administered during the first trimester, and strategies to delay chemotherapy, if possible, until after this milestone should be considered if the pregnancy is to continue to term. Patients in their second or third trimester can be treated with most regimens for the common neoplasms afflicting women in their childbearing years, with the exception of antimetabolites, particularly antifolates, which have notable teratogenic or fetotoxic effects throughout pregnancy. The need for anticancer chemotherapy per se is infrequently a clear basis to recommend termination of a concurrent pregnancy, although each treatment strategy in this circumstance must be tailored to the individual needs of the patient. Chronic effects of cancer treatment are reviewed in Chap. e13.

BIOLOGIC THERAPY

The goal of biologic therapy is to manipulate the host-tumor interaction in favor of the host. Theoretically, biologic approaches should reflect a bell-shaped dose-response curve where the maximum biologic effect is less than the MTD. However, empirical trial and error has led to the discovery that a number of biologic treatment approaches may produce antitumor effects, but nearly all of them are most active at their MTD. As a class, biologic therapies may be distinguished from molecularly targeted agents in that many biologic therapies require an active response (e.g., reexpression of silenced genes, or antigen expression) on the part of the tumor cell or on the part of the host (e.g., immunologic effects) to allow therapeutic effect. This may be contrasted with the more narrowly defined antiproliferative or apoptotic response that is the ultimate goal of molecularly targeted agents discussed above. However, there is much commonality in the strategies to evaluate and use molecularly targeted and biologic therapies.

IMMUNE MEDIATORS OF ANTITUMOR EFFECTS

The very existence of a cancer in a person is testimony to the failure of the immune system to deal effectively with the cancer. Tumors have a variety of means of avoiding the immune system: (1) they are often only subtly different from their normal counterparts; (2) they are capable of downregulating their major histocompatibility complex antigens, effectively masking them from recognition by T cells; (3) they are inefficient at presenting antigens to the immune system; (4) they can cloak themselves in a protective shell of fibrin to minimize contact with surveillance mechanisms; and (5) they can produce a range of soluble molecules, including potential immune targets, that can distract the immune system from recognizing the tumor cell or can kill the immune effector cells. Some of the cell products initially polarize the immune response away from cellular immunity (shifting from T_H1 to T_H2 responses; Chap. 308) and ultimately lead to defects in T cells that prevent their activation and cytotoxic activity. Cancer treatment further suppresses host immunity. A variety of strategies are being tested to overcome these barriers.

Cell-Mediated Immunity The strongest evidence that the immune system can exert clinically meaningful antitumor effects comes from allogeneic bone marrow transplantation. Adoptively transferred T cells from the donor expand in the tumor-bearing host, recognize the tumor as being foreign, and can mediate impressive antitumor effects (graft-versus-tumor effects). Three types of experimental interventions are being developed to take advantage of the ability of T cells to kill tumor cells.

1. Allogeneic T cells are transferred to cancer-bearing hosts in three major settings: in the form of allogeneic bone marrow transplantation, as pure lymphocyte transfusions following bone marrow re-

covery after allogeneic bone marrow transplantation, and as pure lymphocyte transfusions following immunosuppressive (but not myeloablative) therapy (so-called minitransplants). In each of these settings, the effector cells are donor T cells that recognize the tumor as being foreign, probably through minor histocompatibility differences. The main risk of such therapy is the development of graft-versus-host disease because of the minimal difference between the cancer and the normal host cells. This approach has been highly effective in certain hematologic cancers.

2. Autologous T cells are removed from the tumor-bearing host, manipulated in several ways in vitro, and given back to the patient. The two major classes of autologous T cell manipulation are (a) to develop tumor antigen–specific T cells and expand them to large numbers over many weeks ex vivo before administration, and (b) to activate the cells with polyclonal stimulators such as anti-CD3 and anti-CD28 after a short period ex vivo and try to expand them in the host after adoptive transfer with stimulation by IL-2, for example. Short periods removed from the patient permit the cells to overcome the tumor-induced T cell defects, and such cells traffic and home to sites of disease better than cells that have been in culture for many weeks. Individual centers have successful experiences with one or the other approach but not both, and whether one is superior to the other is not known.

3. Tumor vaccines are aimed at boosting T cell immunity. The finding that mutant oncogenes that are expressed only intracellularly can be recognized as targets of T cell killing greatly expanded the possibilities for tumor vaccine development. No longer is it difficult to find something different about tumor cells. However, major difficulties remain in getting the tumor-specific peptides presented in a fashion to prime the T cells. Tumors themselves are very poor at presenting their own antigens to T cells at the first antigen exposure (*priming*). Priming is best accomplished by professional antigen-presenting cells (dendritic cells). Thus, a number of experimental strategies are aimed at priming host T cells against tumor-associated peptides. Vaccine adjuvants such as GM-CSF appear capable of attracting antigen-presenting cells to a skin site containing a tumor antigen. Such an approach has been documented to eradicate microscopic residual disease in follicular lymphoma and give rise to tumor-specific T cells. Purified antigen-presenting cells can be pulsed with tumor, its membranes, or particular tumor antigens and delivered as a vaccine. Tumor cells can be transfected with genes that attract antigen-presenting cells. Other ideas are also being tested. In a variation on the theme of adoptive transfer, the tumor vaccine may be given to the normal bone marrow and lymphoid cell donor of an allogeneic transplant so that the donor immune system has more cells capable of recognizing the tumor specifically. Vaccines against viruses that cause cancers are safe and effective. Hepatitis B vaccine prevents hepatocellular carcinoma and a tetravalent human papilloma virus vaccine prevents infection by virus types currently accounting for 70% of cervical cancer. These vaccines are ineffective at treating patients who have developed a virus-induced cancer. Investigational vaccines have shown preliminary evidence of activity against multiple myeloma, certain lymphomas, and melanomas.

Antibodies In general, antibodies are not very effective at killing cancer cells. Because the tumor seems to influence the host toward making antibodies rather than generating cellular immunity, it is inferred that antibodies are easier for the tumor to fend off. Many patients can be shown to have serum antibodies directed at their tumors, but these do not appear to influence disease progression. However, the ability to grow very large quantities of high-affinity antibody directed at a tumor by the hybridoma technique has led to the application of antibodies to the treatment of cancer.

Clinical antitumor efficacy has been obtained using antibodies where the antigen-combining regions are grafted onto human immunoglobulin gene products (chimerized or humanized), or derive de novo from mice bearing human immunoglobulin gene loci. Such humanized antibodies against the CD20 molecule expressed on B cell lymphomas (rituximab) and against the HER-2/neu receptor overex-

pressed on epithelial cancers, especially breast cancer (trastuzumab), have become reliable tools in the oncologist's armamentarium. Each used alone can cause tumor regression (rituximab more than trastuzumab), and both appear to potentiate the effects of combination chemotherapy given just after antibody administration. Antibodies to CD52 are active in chronic lymphoid leukemia and T cell malignancies. EGF-R–directed antibodies (such as cetuximab and panitumomab) have activity in colorectal cancer refractory to chemotherapy, particularly when utilized to augment the activity of an additional chemotherapy program, and in the primary treatment of head and neck cancers treated with radiation therapy. The mechanism of action is unclear. Direct effects on the tumor may mediate an antiproliferative effect as well as stimulate the participation of host mechanisms involving immune cell or complement-mediated response to tumor cell–bound antibody. Alternatively, the antibody may alter the release of paracrine factors promoting tumor cell survival.

The anti-VEGF antibody bevacizumab shows little evidence of antitumor effect when used alone, but when combined with chemotherapeutic agents it improves the magnitude of tumor shrinkage and time to disease progression in colorectal, lung, and breast cancer. The mechanism for the effect is unclear and may relate to the capacity of the antibody to alter delivery and tumor uptake of the active chemotherapeutic agent.

Side effects include infusion–related hypersensitivity reactions, usually limited to the first infusion, which can be managed with glucocorticoid and/or antihistamine prophylaxis. In addition, distinct syndromes have emerged with different antibodies. Anti-EGF-R antibodies produce an acneiform rash that poorly responds to steroid cream treatment. Trastuzumab (anti-HER-2) can inhibit cardiac function, particularly in those patients with prior exposure to anthracyclines. Bevacizumab has a number of side effects of medical significance, including hypertension, proteinuria, hemorrhage, and gastrointestinal perforations with or without prior surgeries.

Conjugation of antibodies to drugs and toxins is discussed above; conjugates of antibodies with isotopes, photodynamic agents, and other killing moieties may also be effective. Radioconjugates targeting CD20 on lymphomas have been approved for use [ibritumomab tiuxetan (Zevalin), using yttrium-90 or ^{131}I-tositumomab]. Other conjugates are associated with problems that have not yet been solved (e.g., antigenicity, instability, poor tumor penetration).

Cytokines There are >70 separate proteins and glycoproteins with biologic effects in humans: interferon (IFN) α, β, γ; IL-1 through -29 (so far); the tumor necrosis factor (TNF) family [including lymphotoxin, TNF-related apoptosis-inducing ligand (TRAIL), CD40 ligand, and others]; and the chemokine family. Only a fraction of these has been tested against cancer; only IFN-α and IL-2 are in routine clinical use.

About 20 different genes encode IFN-α, and their biologic effects are indistinguishable. Interferon induces the expression of many genes, inhibits protein synthesis, and exerts a number of different effects on diverse cellular processes. Its antitumor effects appear to be antagonized in vitro by thymidine, suggesting that de novo thymidylate synthesis is also affected. The two recombinant forms that are commercially available are IFN-α2a and -α2b. In general, interferon antitumor effects are dose-related, and IFN is most effective at its MTD. Interferon is not curative for any tumor but can induce partial responses in follicular lymphoma, hairy cell leukemia, CML, melanoma, and Kaposi's sarcoma. It has been used in the adjuvant setting in stage II melanoma, multiple myeloma, and follicular lymphoma, with uncertain effects on survival. It produces fever, fatigue, a flulike syndrome, malaise, myelosuppression, and depression and can induce clinically significant autoimmune disease.

IL-2 must exert its antitumor effects indirectly through augmentation of immune function. Its biologic activity is to promote the growth and activity of T cells and natural killer (NK) cells. High doses of IL-2 can produce tumor regression in certain patients with metastatic melanoma and renal cell cancer. About 2–5% of patients may experience complete remissions that are durable, unlike any other treatment for these tumors. IL-2 is associated with myriad clinical side effects: intravascular volume depletion, capillary leak syndrome, adult respiratory distress syndrome, hypotension, fever, chills, skin rash, and impaired renal and liver function. Patients may require blood pressure support and intensive care to manage the toxicity. However, once the agent is stopped, most of the toxicities reverse completely within 3–6 days.

GENE THERAPIES

No gene therapy has been approved for routine clinical use. Several strategies are under evaluation, including the use of viruses that cannot replicate to express genes that can allow the action of drugs or directly inhibit cancer cell growth, viruses that can actually replicate but only in the context of the tumor cell, or viruses that can express antigens in the context of the tumor and therefore provoke a host-mediated immune response. Key issues in the success of these approaches will be in defining safe viral vector systems that escape host immune function and effectively target the tumor or tumor cell milieu. Other gene therapy strategies would utilize therapeutic oligonucleotides to target the expression of genes important in the maintenance of tumor cell viability.

ACKNOWLEDGMENTS

Stephen M. Hahn, MD, and Eli Glatstein, MD, contributed a chapter on radiation therapy in the prior edition, and some of their material has been incorporated into this chapter.

FURTHER READINGS

AMERICAN SOCIETY OF CLINICAL ONCOLOGY: 2006 Update of recommendations for the use of white blood cell growth factors: An evidence-based clinical practice guideline. J Clin Oncol 24:3187, 2006

———: Guideline for antiemetics in oncology: Update 2006. J Clin Oncol 24:2932, 2006

CHABNER BA, LONGO DL (eds): *Cancer Chemotherapy and Biotherapy: Principles and Practice*, 4th ed. Philadelphia, Lippincott Williams & Wilkins, 2006

FOLKMAN J: Angiogenesis: An organizing principle for drug discovery? Nat Rev Drug Discov 6:273, 2007

KRAUSE DS, VAN ETTEN RA: Tyrosine kinases as targets for cancer therapy. N Engl J Med 353:17, 2005

82 Infections in Patients with Cancer
Robert Finberg

Infections are a common cause of death and an even more common cause of morbidity in patients with a wide variety of neoplasms. Autopsy studies show that most deaths from acute leukemia and half of deaths from lymphoma are caused directly by infection. With more intensive chemotherapy, patients with solid tumors have also become more likely to die of infection. Fortunately, an evolving approach to prevention and treatment of infectious complications of cancer has decreased rates of infection-associated mortality and will probably continue to do so. This accomplishment has resulted from three major steps:

1. The concept of "early empirical" antibiotics reduced mortality rates among patients with leukemia and bacteremia from 84% in 1965 to 44% in 1972. With better availability (and early use) of broad-spectrum antibiotics, this figure has recently dropped to 20–36%.
2. "Empirical" antifungal therapy has lowered the incidence of disseminated fungal infection; in trial settings, mortality rates now range from 7 to 21%. An antifungal agent is administered—on the

basis of likely fungal infection—to neutropenic patients who, after 4–7 days of antibiotic therapy, remain febrile but have no positive cultures.
3. Use of antibiotics for afebrile neutropenic patients as broad-spectrum prophylaxis against infections promises to decrease both mortality and morbidity even further.

A physical predisposition to infection in patients with cancer (Table 82-1) can be a result of the neoplasm's production of a break in the skin. For example, a squamous cell carcinoma may cause local invasion of the epidermis, which allows bacteria to gain access to the subcutaneous tissue and permits the development of cellulitis. The artificial closing of a normally patent orifice can also predispose to infection: Obstruction of a ureter by a tumor can cause urinary tract infection, and obstruction of the bile duct can cause cholangitis. Part of the host's normal defense against infection depends on the continuous emptying of a viscus; without emptying, a few bacteria present as a result of bacteremia or local transit can multiply and cause disease.

A similar problem can affect patients whose lymph node integrity has been disrupted by radical surgery, particularly patients who have had radical node dissections. A common clinical problem following radical mastectomy is the development of cellulitis (usually caused by

TABLE 82-1	DISRUPTION OF NORMAL BARRIERS THAT MAY PREDISPOSE TO INFECTIONS IN PATIENTS WITH CANCER				
Type of Defense	**Specific Lesion**	**Cells Involved**	**Organism**	**Cancer Association**	**Disease**
Physical barrier	Breaks in skin	Skin epithelial cells	Staphylococci, streptococci	Head and neck, squamous cell carcinoma	Cellulitis, extensive skin infection
Emptying of fluid collections	Occlusion of orifices: ureters, bile duct, colon	Luminal epithelial cells	Gram-negative bacilli	Renal, ovarian, biliary tree, metastatic diseases of many cancers	Rapid, overwhelming bacteremia; urinary tract infection
Lymphatic function	Node dissection	Lymph nodes	Staphylococci, streptococci	Breast cancer surgery	Cellulitis
Splenic clearance of microorganisms	Splenectomy	Splenic reticuloendothelial cells	*Streptococcus pneumoniae, Haemophilus influenzae, Neisseria meningitidis, Babesia, Capnocytophaga canimorsus*	Hodgkin's disease, leukemia, idiopathic thrombocytopenic purpura	Rapid, overwhelming sepsis
Phagocytosis	Lack of granulocytes	Granulocytes (neutrophils)	Staphylococci, streptococci, enteric organisms, fungi	Hairy cell, acute myelocytic, and acute lymphocytic leukemias	Bacteremia
Humoral immunity	Lack of antibody	B cells	*S. pneumoniae, H. influenzae, N. meningitidis*	Chronic lymphocytic leukemia, multiple myeloma	Infections with encapsulated organisms, sinusitis, pneumonia
Cellular immunity	Lack of T cells	T cells and macrophages	*Mycobacterium tuberculosis, Listeria*, herpesviruses, fungi, other intracellular parasites	Hodgkin's disease, leukemia, T cell lymphoma	Infections with intracellular bacteria, fungi, parasites

TABLE 82-2 VACCINATION OF CANCER PATIENTS RECEIVING CHEMOTHERAPY

	Use in Indicated Patients		
Vaccine	Intensive Chemotherapy	Hodgkin's Disease	Hematopoietic Stem Cell Transplantation
Diphtheria-tetanus[a]	Primary series and boosters as necessary	No special recommendation	12, 14, and 24 months after transplantation
Poliomyelitis[b]	Complete primary series and boosters	No special recommendation	12, 14, and 24 months after transplantation
Haemophilus influenzae type b conjugate	Primary series and booster for children	Immunization before treatment and booster 3 months afterward	12, 14, and 24 months after transplantation
Hepatitis A	Not routinely recommended	Not routinely recommended	Not routinely recommended
Hepatitis B	Complete series	No special recommendation	12, 14, and 24 months after transplantation
23-Valent pneumococcal polysaccharide[c]	Every 5 years	Immunization before treatment and booster 3 months afterward	12 and 24 months after transplantation
4-Valent meningococcal conjugate[d]	Should be administered to splenectomized patients and patients living in endemic areas, including college students in dormitories	Should be administered to splenectomized patients and patients living in endemic areas, including college students in dormitories	Should be administered to splenectomized patients and patients living in endemic areas, including college students in dormitories
Influenza	Seasonal immunization	Seasonal immunization	Seasonal immunization
Measles/mumps/rubella	Contraindicated	Contraindicated during chemotherapy	After 24 months in patients without graft-versus-host disease
Varicella-zoster virus	Contraindicated[e]	Contraindicated	Contraindicated

[a]The Td (tetanus-diphtheria) combination is currently recommended for adults. Pertussis vaccines have not been recommended for people >6 years of age in the past. However, recent data indicate that the Tdap (tetanus–diphtheria–acellular pertussis) product is both safe and efficacious in adults.
[b]Live-virus vaccine is contraindicated; inactivated vaccine should be used.
[c]The seven-serotype pneumococcal conjugate vaccine is currently recommended only for children. It is anticipated that future vaccines will include more serotypes and will be recommended for adults.
[d]Currently licensed for people 11–55 years of age.
[e]Contact the manufacturer for more information on use in children with acute lymphocytic leukemia.

streptococci or staphylococci) because of lymphedema and/or inadequate lymph drainage. In most cases, this problem can be addressed by local measures designed to prevent fluid accumulation and breaks in the skin, but antibiotic prophylaxis has been necessary in refractory cases.

A life-threatening problem common to many cancer patients is the loss of the reticuloendothelial capacity to clear microorganisms after splenectomy. Splenectomy may be performed as part of the management of hairy cell leukemia, chronic lymphocytic leukemia (CLL), and chronic myelocytic leukemia (CML) and in Hodgkin's disease. Even after curative therapy for the underlying disease, the lack of a spleen predisposes such patients to rapidly fatal infections. The loss of the spleen through trauma similarly predisposes the normal host to overwhelming infection for life after splenectomy. The splenectomized patient should be counseled about the risks of infection with certain organisms, such as the protozoan *Babesia* (Chap. 204) and *Capnocytophaga canimorsus* (formerly dysgonic fermenter 2, or DF-2), a bacterium carried in the mouths of animals (Chaps. 140 and e14). Since encapsulated bacteria (*Streptococcus pneumoniae, Haemophilus influenzae,* and *Neisseria meningitidis*) are the organisms most commonly associated with postsplenectomy sepsis, splenectomized persons should be vaccinated (and revaccinated; Table 82-2 and Chap. 116) against the capsular polysaccharides of these organisms. Many clinicians recommend giving splenectomized patients a small supply of antibiotics effective against *S. pneumoniae, N. meningitidis,* and *H. influenzae* to avert rapid, overwhelming sepsis in the event that they cannot present for medical attention immediately after the onset of fever or other symptoms of bacterial infection. A few amoxicillin/clavulanic acid tablets are a reasonable choice for this purpose.

The level of suspicion of infections with certain organisms should depend on the type of cancer diagnosed (Table 82-3). Diagnosis of multiple myeloma or CLL should alert the clinician to the possibility of hypogammaglobulinemia. While immunoglobulin replacement therapy can be effective, in most cases prophylactic antibiotics are a cheaper, more convenient method of eliminating bacterial infections in CLL patients with hypogammaglobulinemia. Patients with acute lymphocytic leukemia (ALL), patients with non-Hodgkin's lymphoma, and all cancer patients treated with high-dose glucocorticoids (or glucocorticoid-containing chemotherapy regimens) should receive antibiotic prophylaxis for *Pneumocystis* infection (Table 82-3) for the duration of their chemotherapy. In addition to exhibiting susceptibility to certain infectious organisms, patients with cancer are likely to manifest their infections in characteristic ways.

SYSTEM-SPECIFIC SYNDROMES

SKIN-SPECIFIC SYNDROMES

Skin lesions are common in cancer patients, and the appearance of these lesions may permit the diagnosis of systemic bacterial or fungal

TABLE 82-3 INFECTIONS ASSOCIATED WITH SPECIFIC TYPES OF CANCER

Cancer	Underlying Immune Abnormality	Organisms Causing Infection
Multiple myeloma	Hypogammaglobulinemia	*Streptococcus pneumoniae, Haemophilus influenzae, Neisseria meningitidis*
Chronic lymphocytic leukemia	Hypogammaglobulinemia	*S. pneumoniae, H. influenzae, N. meningitidis*
Acute myelocytic or lymphocytic leukemia	Granulocytopenia, skin and mucous-membrane lesions	Extracellular gram-positive and gram-negative bacteria, fungi
Hodgkin's disease	Abnormal T cell function	Intracellular pathogens (*Mycobacterium tuberculosis,* Listeria, Salmonella, Cryptococcus, *Mycobacterium avium*)
Non-Hodgkin's lymphoma and acute lymphocytic leukemia	Glucocorticoid chemotherapy, T and B cell dysfunction	*Pneumocystis*
Colon and rectal tumors	Local abnormalities[a]	*Streptococcus bovis* (bacteremia)
Hairy cell leukemia	Abnormal T cell function	Intracellular pathogens (*M. tuberculosis,* Listeria, Cryptococcus, *M. avium*)

[a]The reason for this association is not well defined.

A

B

FIGURE 82-1 *A.* **Papules related to *Escherichia coli*** bacteremia in a neutropenic patient with acute lymphocytic leukemia. *B.* The same lesion the following day.

infection. While cellulitis caused by skin organisms such as *Streptococcus* or *Staphylococcus* is common, neutropenic patients—i.e., those with <500 functional polymorphonuclear leukocytes (PMNs)/μL—and patients with impaired blood or lymphatic drainage may develop infections with unusual organisms. Innocent-looking macules or papules may be the first sign of bacterial or fungal sepsis in immunocompromised patients (Fig. 82-1). In the neutropenic host, a macule progresses rapidly to ecthyma gangrenosum, a usually painless, round, necrotic lesion consisting of a central black or gray-black eschar with surrounding erythema. Ecthyma gangrenosum, which is located in nonpressure areas (as distinguished from necrotic lesions associated with lack of circulation), is often associated with *Pseudomonas aeruginosa* bacteremia (Chap. 145) but may be caused by other bacteria.

Candidemia (Chap. 196) is also associated with a variety of skin conditions and commonly presents as a maculopapular rash. Punch biopsy of the skin may be the best method for diagnosis.

Cellulitis, an acute spreading inflammation of the skin, is most often caused by infection with group A *Streptococcus* or *Staphylococcus aureus*, virulent organisms normally found on the skin (Chap. 119). Although cellulitis tends to be circumscribed in normal hosts, it may spread rapidly in neutropenic patients. A tiny break in the skin may lead to spreading cellulitis, which is characterized by pain and erythema; in the affected patients, signs of infection (e.g., purulence) are often lacking. What might be a furuncle in a normal host may require amputation because of uncontrolled infection in a patient presenting with leukemia. A dramatic response to an infection that might be trivial in a normal host can mark the first sign of leukemia. Fortunately, granulocytopenic patients are likely to be infected with certain types of organisms (Table 82-4); thus the selection of an antibiotic regimen is

somewhat easier than it might otherwise be (see "Antiviral Therapy," below). It is essential to recognize cellulitis early and to treat it aggressively. Patients who are neutropenic or have previously received antibiotics for other reasons may develop cellulitis with unusual organisms (e.g., *Escherichia coli*, *Pseudomonas*, or fungi). Early treatment, even of innocent-looking lesions, is essential to prevent necrosis and loss of tissue. Debridement to prevent spread may sometimes be necessary early in the course of disease, but it can often be performed after chemotherapy, when the PMN count increases.

Sweet's syndrome, or *febrile neutrophilic dermatosis*, was originally described in women with elevated white blood cell (WBC) counts. The disease is characterized by the presence of leukocytes in the lower dermis, with edema of the papillary body. Ironically, this disease now is usually seen in neutropenic patients with cancer, most often in association with acute leukemia but also in association with a variety of other malignancies. Sweet's syndrome usually presents as red or bluish-red papules or nodules that may coalesce and form sharply bordered plaques. The edema may suggest vesicles, but on palpation the lesions are solid, and vesicles probably never arise in this disease. The lesions are most common on the face, neck, and arms. On the legs, they may be confused with erythema nodosum. The development of lesions is often accompanied by high fevers and an elevated erythrocyte sedimentation rate. Both the lesions and the temperature elevation respond dramatically to glucocorticoid administration. Treatment begins with high doses of glucocorticoids (60 mg/d of prednisone) followed by tapered doses over the next 2–3 weeks.

Data indicate that *erythema multiforme* with mucous membrane involvement is often associated with herpes simplex virus (HSV) infection and is distinct from Stevens-Johnson syndrome, which is associated with drugs and tends to have a more widespread distribution. Since cancer patients are both immunosuppressed (and therefore susceptible to herpes infections) and heavily treated with drugs (and therefore subject to Stevens-Johnson syndrome), both of these conditions are common in this population.

Cytokines, which are used as adjuvants or primary treatments for cancer, can themselves cause characteristic rashes, further complicating the differential diagnosis. This phenomenon is a particular problem in bone marrow transplant recipients (Chap. 126), who, in addition to having the usual chemotherapy-, antibiotic-, and cytokine-induced rashes, are plagued by graft-versus-host disease.

CATHETER-RELATED INFECTIONS

Because IV catheters are commonly used in cancer chemotherapy and are prone to infection (Chap. 125), they pose a major problem in the care of patients with cancer. Some catheter-associated infections can be treated with antibiotics, while in others the catheter must be re-

TABLE 82-4	ORGANISMS LIKELY TO CAUSE INFECTIONS IN GRANULOCYTOPENIC PATIENTS
Gram-positive cocci	Enterobacter spp.
Staphylococcus epidermidis	*Serratia* spp.
Staphylococcus aureus	*Acinetobacter* spp.[a]
Viridans *Streptococcus*	*Citrobacter* spp.
Enterococcus faecalis	Gram-positive bacilli
Streptococcus pneumoniae	Diphtheroids
Gram-negative bacilli	JK bacillus[a]
Escherichia coli	Fungi
Klebsiella spp.	*Candida* spp.
Pseudomonas aeruginosa	*Aspergillus* spp.
Non-*aeruginosa Pseudomonas* spp.[a]	

[a]Often associated with intravenous catheters.

TABLE 82-5 **APPROACH TO CATHETER INFECTIONS IN IMMUNOCOMPROMISED PATIENTS**

Clinical Presentation	Catheter Removal	Antibiotics	Comments
Evidence of Infection, Negative Blood Cultures			
Exit-site erythema	Not necessary if infection responds to treatment	Usually begin treatment for gram-positive cocci.	Coagulase-negative staphylococci are most common.
Tunnel-site erythema	Required	Treat for gram-positive cocci pending culture results.	Failure to remove the catheter may lead to complications.
Blood Culture–Positive Infections			
Coagulase-negative staphylococci	Line removal optimal but may be unnecessary if patient is clinically stable and responds to antibiotics	Usually start with vancomycin. (Linezolid, quinupristin/dalfopristin, and daptomycin are all appropriate.)	If there are no contraindications to line removal, this course of action is optimal. If the line is removed, antibiotics may not be necessary.
Other gram-positive cocci (e.g., *Staphylococcus aureus*, *Enterococcus*); gram-positive rods (*Bacillus*, *Corynebacterium* spp.)	Recommended	Treat with antibiotics to which the organism is sensitive, with duration based on the clinical setting.	The incidence of metastatic infections following *S. aureus* infection (and the difficulty of treating enterococcal infection make line removal the recommended course of action. In addition, gram-positive rods do not respond readily to antibiotics alone.
Gram-negative bacteria	Recommended	Use an agent to which the organism is shown to be sensitive.	Organisms like *Stenotrophomonas*, *Pseudomonas*, and *Burkholderia* are notoriously hard to treat.
Fungi	Recommended	—	Fungal infections of catheters are extremely difficult to treat.

moved (Table 82-5). If the patient has a "tunneled" catheter (which consists of an entrance site, a subcutaneous tunnel, and an exit site), a red streak over the subcutaneous part of the line (the tunnel) is grounds for immediate removal of the catheter. Failure to remove catheters under these circumstances may result in extensive cellulitis and tissue necrosis.

More common than tunnel infections are exit-site infections, often with erythema around the area where the line penetrates the skin. Most authorities (Chap. 129) recommend treatment (usually with vancomycin) for an exit-site infection caused by a coagulase-negative *Staphylococcus*. Treatment of coagulase-positive staphylococcal infection is associated with a poorer outcome, and it is advisable to remove the catheter if possible. Similarly, many clinicians remove catheters associated with infections due to *P. aeruginosa* and *Candida* species, since such infections are difficult to treat and bloodstream infections with these organisms are likely to be deadly. Catheter infections caused by *Burkholderia cepacia*, *Stenotrophomonas* spp., *Agrobacterium* spp., and *Acinetobacter baumannii* as well as *Pseudomonas* spp. other than *aeruginosa* are likely to be very difficult to eradicate with antibiotics alone. Similarly, isolation of *Bacillus*, *Corynebacterium*, and *Mycobacterium* spp. should prompt removal of the catheter.

GASTROINTESTINAL TRACT–SPECIFIC SYNDROMES

Upper Gastrointestinal Tract Disease • INFECTIONS OF THE MOUTH
The oral cavity is rich in aerobic and anaerobic bacteria (Chap. 157) that normally live in a commensal relationship with the host. The antimetabolic effects of chemotherapy cause a breakdown of host defenses, leading to ulceration of the mouth and the potential for invasion by resident bacteria. Mouth ulcerations afflict most patients receiving chemotherapy and have been associated with viridans streptococcal bacteremia. The use of keratinocyte growth factor (palifermin) in a daily dose of 60 μg/kg for 3 days before chemotherapy and total-body irradiation is of proven value in preventing mucosal ulceration after stem cell transplantation. Fluconazole is clearly effective in the treatment of both local infections (thrush) and systemic infections (esophagitis) due to *Candida albicans*. Newer azoles (such as voriconazole) are similarly effective.

Noma (*cancrum oris*), commonly seen in malnourished children, is a penetrating disease of the soft and hard tissues of the mouth and adjacent sites, with resulting necrosis and gangrene. It has a counterpart in immunocompromised patients and is thought to be due to invasion of the tissues by *Bacteroides*, *Fusobacterium*, and other normal inhabitants of the mouth. Noma is associated with debility, poor oral hygiene, and immunosuppression.

Viruses, particularly HSV, are a prominent cause of morbidity in immunocompromised patients, in whom they are associated with severe mucositis. The use of acyclovir, either prophylactically or therapeutically, is of value.

ESOPHAGEAL INFECTIONS The differential diagnosis of esophagitis (usually presenting as substernal chest pain upon swallowing) includes herpes simplex and candidiasis, both of which are readily treatable.

Lower Gastrointestinal Tract Disease Hepatic candidiasis (Chap. 196) results from seeding of the liver (usually from a gastrointestinal source) in neutropenic patients. It is most common in patients being treated for acute leukemia and usually presents symptomatically around the time the neutropenia resolves. The characteristic picture is that of persistent fever unresponsive to antibiotics; abdominal pain and tenderness or nausea; and elevated serum levels of alkaline phosphatase in a patient with hematologic malignancy who has recently recovered from neutropenia. The diagnosis of this disease (which may present in an indolent manner and persist for several months) is based on the finding of yeasts or pseudohyphae in granulomatous lesions. Hepatic ultrasound or CT may reveal bull's-eye lesions. In some cases, MRI reveals small lesions not visible by other imaging modalities. The pathology (a granulomatous response) and the timing (with resolution of neutropenia and an elevation in granulocyte count) suggest that the host response to *Candida* is an important component of the manifestations of disease. In many cases, although organisms are visible, cultures of biopsied material may be negative. The designation *hepatosplenic candidiasis* or *hepatic candidiasis* is a misnomer because the disease often involves the kidneys and other tissues; the term *chronic disseminated candidiasis* may be more appropriate. Because of the risk of bleeding with liver biopsy, diagnosis is often based on imaging studies (MRI, CT). Amphotericin B is traditionally used for therapy (often for several months, until all manifestations of disease have disappeared), but fluconazole may be useful for outpatient therapy. The use of other antifungal agents and combination therapy is less well studied.

Typhlitis *Typhlitis* (also referred to as necrotizing colitis, neutropenic colitis, necrotizing enteropathy, ileocecal syndrome, and cecitis) is a clinical syndrome of fever and right-lower-quadrant tenderness in an immunosuppressed host. This syndrome is classically seen in neutropenic patients after chemotherapy with cytotoxic drugs. It may be more common among children than among adults and appears to be much more common among patients with acute myelocytic leukemia (AML) or ALL than among those with other types of cancer; a similar syndrome has been reported in patients infected with HIV type 1. Physical examination reveals right-lower-quadrant tenderness, with or without rebound tenderness. Associated diarrhea (often bloody) is common, and the diagnosis can be confirmed by the finding of a thickened cecal wall on CT, MRI, or ultrasonography. Plain films may reveal a right-lower-quadrant mass, but CT with contrast or MRI is a much more sensitive means of making the diagnosis. Although surgery is sometimes attempted to avoid perforation from ischemia, most cases resolve with medical therapy alone. The disease is sometimes associated with positive blood cultures (which usually yield aerobic gram-negative bacilli), and therapy is recommended for a broad spectrum of bacteria (particularly gram-negative bacilli, which are likely to be found in the bowel flora). Surgery is indicated in the case of perforation.

***Clostridium difficile*–Induced Diarrhea**   Patients with cancer are predisposed to the development of *C. difficile* diarrhea (Chap. 123) as a consequence of chemotherapy alone. Thus, they may have positive toxin tests before receiving antibiotics. Obviously, such patients are also subject to *C. difficile*–induced diarrhea as a result of antibiotic pressure. *C. difficile* should always be considered as a possible cause of diarrhea in cancer patients who have received antibiotics.

CENTRAL NERVOUS SYSTEM–SPECIFIC SYNDROMES
Meningitis   The presentation of meningitis in patients with lymphoma or CLL, patients receiving chemotherapy (particularly with glucocorticoids) for solid tumors, and patients who have received bone marrow transplants suggests a diagnosis of cryptococcal or listerial infection. As noted previously, splenectomized patients are susceptible to rapid, overwhelming infection with encapsulated bacteria (including *S. pneumoniae*, *H. influenzae*, and *N. meningitidis*). Similarly, patients who are antibody-deficient (such as patients with CLL, those who have received intensive chemotherapy, or those who have undergone bone marrow transplantation) are likely to have infections caused by these bacteria. Other cancer patients, however, because of their defective cellular immunity, are likely to be infected with other pathogens (Table 82-3).

Encephalitis   The spectrum of disease resulting from viral encephalitis is expanded in immunocompromised patients. A predisposition to infections with intracellular organisms similar to those encountered in patients with AIDS (Chap. 182) is seen in cancer patients receiving (1) high-dose cytotoxic chemotherapy, (2) chemotherapy affecting T cell function (e.g., fludarabine), or (3) antibodies that eliminate T cells (e.g., anti-CD3) or cytokine activity. Infection with varicella-zoster virus (VZV) has been associated with encephalitis that may be caused by VZV-related vasculitis. Chronic viral infections may also be associated with dementia and encephalitic presentations, and a diagnosis of progressive multifocal leukoencephalopathy should be considered when a patient who has received chemotherapy presents with dementia (Table 82-6). Other abnormalities of the central nervous system (CNS) that may be confused with infection include normal-pressure hydrocephalus and vasculitis resulting from CNS irradiation. It may be possible to differentiate these conditions by MRI.

Brain Masses   Mass lesions of the brain most often present as headache with or without fever or neurologic abnormalities. Infections associated with mass lesions may be caused by bacteria (particularly *Nocardia*), fungi (particularly *Cryptococcus* or *Aspergillus*), or parasites (*Toxoplasma*). Epstein-Barr virus (EBV)–associated lymphoproliferative disease may also present as single or multiple mass lesions of the brain. A biopsy may be required for a definitive diagnosis.

PULMONARY INFECTIONS
Pneumonia (Chap. 251) in immunocompromised patients may be difficult to diagnose because conventional methods of diagnosis depend on the presence of neutrophils. Bacterial pneumonia in neutropenic patients may present without purulent sputum—or, in fact, without

TABLE 82-6	DIFFERENTIAL DIAGNOSIS OF CENTRAL NERVOUS SYSTEM INFECTIONS IN PATIENTS WITH CANCER	
	Underlying Predisposition	
Findings on CT or MRI	**Prolonged Neutropenia**	**Defects in Cellular Immunity[a]**
Mass lesions	*Aspergillus* brain abscess *Nocardia* brain abscess *Cryptococcus* brain abscess	Toxoplasmosis EBV-LPD
Diffuse encephalitis	PML (J-C virus)	Infection with VZV, CMV, HSV, HHV-6, J-C virus (PML), *Listeria*

[a]High-dose glucocorticoid therapy, cytotoxic chemotherapy.
Abbreviations: CMV, cytomegalovirus; EBV-LPD, Epstein-Barr virus lymphoproliferative disease; HHV-6, human herpesvirus type 6; HSV, herpes simplex virus; PML, progressive multifocal leukoencephalopathy; VZV, varicella-zoster virus.

any sputum at all—and may not produce physical findings suggestive of chest consolidation (rales or egophony).

In granulocytopenic patients with persistent or recurrent fever, the chest x-ray pattern may help to localize an infection and thus to determine which investigative tests and procedures should be undertaken and which therapeutic options should be considered (Table 82-7). The difficulties encountered in the management of pulmonary infiltrates relate in part to the difficulties of performing diagnostic procedures on the patients involved. When platelet counts can be increased to adequate levels by transfusion, microscopic and microbiologic evaluation of the fluid obtained by endoscopic bronchial lavage is often diagnostic. Lavage fluid should be cultured for *Mycoplasma*, *Chlamydophila*, *Legionella*, *Nocardia*, more common bacterial pathogens, and fungi. In addition, the possibility of *Pneumocystis* pneumonia should be considered, especially in patients with ALL or lymphoma who have not received prophylactic trimethoprim-sulfamethoxazole (TMP-SMX). The characteristics of the infiltrate may be helpful in decisions about further diagnostic and therapeutic maneuvers. Nodular infiltrates suggest fungal pneumonia (e.g., that caused by *Aspergillus* or *Mucor*). Such lesions may best be approached by visualized biopsy procedures.

Aspergillus spp. (Chap. 197) can colonize the skin and respiratory tract or cause fatal systemic illness. Although *Aspergillus* may cause aspergillomas in a previously existing cavity or may produce allergic bronchopulmonary aspergillosis, the major problem posed by this genus in neutropenic patients is invasive disease due to *A. fumigatus* or *A. flavus*. The organisms enter the host following colonization of the respiratory tract, with subsequent invasion of the blood vessels. The disease is likely to present as a thrombotic or embolic event because of the organisms' ability to invade blood vessels. The risk of infection with *Aspergillus* correlates directly with the duration of neutropenia. In prolonged neutropenia, positive surveillance cultures for colonization of the nasopharynx with *Aspergillus* may predict the development of disease.

TABLE 82-7	DIFFERENTIAL DIAGNOSIS OF CHEST INFILTRATES IN IMMUNOCOMPROMISED PATIENTS	
	Cause of Pneumonia	
Infiltrate	**Infectious**	**Noninfectious**
Localized	Bacteria, *Legionella*, mycobacteria	Local hemorrhage or embolism, tumor
Nodular	Fungi (e.g., *Aspergillus* or *Mucor*), *Nocardia*	Recurrent tumor
Diffuse	Viruses (especially CMV), *Chlamydophila*, *Pneumocystis*, *Toxoplasma gondii*, mycobacteria	Congestive heart failure, radiation pneumonitis, drug-induced lung injury, diffuse alveolar hemorrhage (described after BMT)

Abbreviations: BMT, bone marrow transplantation; CMV, cytomegalovirus.

Patients with *Aspergillus* infection often present with pleuritic chest pain and fever, which are sometimes accompanied by cough. Hemoptysis may be an ominous sign. Chest x-rays may reveal new focal infiltrates or nodules. Chest CT may reveal a characteristic halo consisting of a mass-like infiltrate surrounded by an area of low attenuation. The presence of a "crescent sign" on a chest x-ray or a chest CT scan, in which the mass progresses to central cavitation, is characteristic of invasive *Aspergillus* infection but may develop as the lesions are resolving.

In addition to causing pulmonary disease, *Aspergillus* may invade through the nose or palate, with deep sinus penetration. The appearance of a discolored area in the nasal passages or on the hard palate should prompt a search for invasive *Aspergillus*. This situation is likely to require surgical debridement. Catheter infections with *Aspergillus* usually require both removal of the catheter and antifungal therapy.

Diffuse interstitial infiltrates suggest viral, parasitic, or *Pneumocystis* pneumonia. If the patient has a diffuse interstitial pattern on chest x-ray, it may be reasonable to institute empirical treatment with TMP-SMX (for *Pneumocystis*) and a quinolone (for *Chlamydophila*, *Mycoplasma*, and *Legionella*) or an erythromycin derivative (e.g., azithromycin) while considering invasive diagnostic procedures. Noninvasive procedures, such as staining of sputum smears for *Pneumocystis*, serum cryptococcal antigen tests, and urine testing for *Legionella* antigen, may be helpful. In transplant recipients who are seropositive for cytomegalovirus (CMV), a determination of CMV load in the serum should be considered. Viral load studies (which allow physicians to quantitate viruses) have superseded simple measurement of serum IgG, which merely documents prior exposure to virus. Infections with viruses that cause only upper respiratory symptoms in immunocompetent hosts, such as respiratory syncytial virus (RSV), influenza viruses, and parainfluenza viruses, may be associated with fatal pneumonitis in immunocompromised hosts. An attempt at early diagnosis by nasopharyngeal aspiration should be considered so that appropriate treatment can be instituted.

Bleomycin is the most common cause of chemotherapy-induced lung disease. Other causes include alkylating agents (such as cyclophosphamide, chlorambucil, and melphalan), nitrosoureas [carmustine (BCNU), lomustine (CCNU), and methyl-CCNU], busulfan, procarbazine, methotrexate, and hydroxyurea. Both infectious and noninfectious (drug- and/or radiation-induced) pneumonitis can cause fever and abnormalities on chest x-ray; thus, the differential diagnosis of an infiltrate in a patient receiving chemotherapy encompasses a broad range of conditions (Table 82-7). Since the treatment of radiation pneumonitis (which may respond dramatically to glucocorticoids) or drug-induced pneumonitis is different from that of infectious pneumonia, a biopsy may be important in the diagnosis. Unfortunately, no definitive diagnosis can be made in ~30% of cases, even after bronchoscopy.

Open-lung biopsy is the "gold standard" of diagnostic techniques. Biopsy via a visualized thoracostomy can replace an open procedure in many cases. When a biopsy cannot be performed, empirical treatment can be undertaken with a quinolone or erythromycin (or an erythromycin derivative such as azithromycin) and TMP-SMX (in the case of diffuse infiltrates) or with amphotericin B or other antifungal agents (in the case of nodular infiltrates). The risks should be weighed carefully in these cases. If inappropriate drugs are administered, empirical treatment may prove toxic or ineffective; either of these outcomes may be riskier than biopsy.

CARDIOVASCULAR INFECTIONS

Patients with Hodgkin's disease are prone to persistent infections by *Salmonella*, sometimes (and particularly often in elderly patients) affecting a vascular site. The use of IV catheters deliberately lodged in the right atrium is associated with a high incidence of bacterial endocarditis, presumably related to valve damage followed by bacteremia. Nonbacterial thrombotic endocarditis has been described in association with a variety of malignancies (most often solid tumors) and may follow bone marrow transplantation as well. The presentation of an embolic event with a new cardiac murmur suggests this diagnosis. Blood cultures are negative in this disease of unknown pathogenesis.

ENDOCRINE SYNDROMES

Infections of the endocrine system have been described in immunocompromised patients. *Candida* infection of the thyroid may be difficult to diagnose during the neutropenic period. It can be defined by indium-labeled WBC scans or gallium scans after neutrophil counts increase. CMV infection can cause adrenalitis with or without resulting adrenal insufficiency. The presentation of a sudden endocrine anomaly in an immunocompromised patient may be a sign of infection in the involved end organ.

MUSCULOSKELETAL INFECTIONS

Infection that is a consequence of vascular compromise, resulting in gangrene, can occur when a tumor restricts the blood supply to muscles, bones, or joints. The process of diagnosis and treatment of such infection is similar to that in normal hosts, with the following caveats:

1. *In terms of diagnosis,* a lack of physical findings resulting from a lack of granulocytes in the granulocytopenic patient should make the clinician more aggressive in obtaining tissue rather than relying on physical signs.

2. *In terms of therapy,* aggressive debridement of infected tissues may be required, but it is usually difficult to operate on patients who have recently received chemotherapy, both because of a lack of platelets (which results in bleeding complications) and because of a lack of WBCs (which may lead to secondary infection). A blood culture positive for *Clostridium perfringens*—an organism commonly associated with gas gangrene—can have a number of meanings (Chap. 135). Bloodstream infections with intestinal organisms such as *Streptococcus bovis* and *C. perfringens* may arise spontaneously from lower gastrointestinal lesions (tumor or polyps); alternatively, these lesions may be harbingers of invasive disease. The clinical setting must be considered in order to define the appropriate treatment for each case.

RENAL AND URETERAL INFECTIONS

Infections of the urinary tract are common among patients whose ureteral excretion is compromised (Table 82-1). *Candida*, which has a predilection for the kidney, can invade either from the bloodstream or in a retrograde manner (via the ureters or bladder) in immunocompromised patients. The presence of "fungus balls" or persistent candiduria suggests invasive disease. Persistent funguria (with *Aspergillus* as well as *Candida*) should prompt a search for a nidus of infection in the kidney.

Certain viruses are typically seen only in immunosuppressed patients. BK virus (polyomavirus hominis 1) has been documented in the urine of bone marrow transplant recipients and, like adenovirus, may be associated with hemorrhagic cystitis. BK-induced cystitis usually remits with decreasing immunosuppression. Anecdotal reports have described the treatment of infections due to adenovirus and BK virus with cidofovir.

ABNORMALITIES THAT PREDISPOSE TO INFECTION (Table 82-1)

THE LYMPHOID SYSTEM

It is beyond the scope of this chapter to detail how all the immunologic abnormalities that result from cancer or from chemotherapy for cancer lead to infections. Disorders of the immune system are discussed in other sections of this book. As has been noted, patients with antibody deficiency are predisposed to overwhelming infection with encapsulated bacteria (including *S. pneumoniae, H. influenzae,* and *N. meningitidis*). Infections that result from the lack of a functional cellular immune system are described in Chap. 182. It is worth mentioning, however, that patients undergoing intensive chemotherapy for any form of cancer will have not only defects due to granulocytopenia but also lymphocyte dysfunction, which may be profound. Thus, these patients—especially those receiving glucocorticoid-containing regimens or drugs that inhibit T cell activation or cytokine induction—should be given prophylaxis for *Pneumocystis* pneumonia.

THE HEMATOPOIETIC SYSTEM

Initial studies in the 1960s revealed a dramatic increase in the incidence of infections (fatal and nonfatal) among cancer patients with a granulocyte count of <500/μL. More recent studies have cited a figure of 48.3 infections per 100 neutropenic patients (<1000 granulocytes/μL) with hematologic malignancies and solid tumors, or 46.3 infections per 1000 days at risk.

Neutropenic patients are unusually susceptible to infection with a wide variety of bacteria; thus, antibiotic therapy should be initiated promptly to cover likely pathogens if infection is suspected. Indeed, early initiation of antibacterial agents is mandatory to prevent deaths. These patients are susceptible to gram-positive and gram-negative organisms found commonly on the skin and in the bowel (Table 82-4). Because treatment with narrow-spectrum agents leads to infection with organisms not covered by the antibiotics used, the initial regimen should target pathogens likely to be initial causes of bacterial infection in neutropenic hosts (Fig. 82-2).

℞ INFECTIONS IN CANCER PATIENTS

ANTIBACTERIAL THERAPY Hundreds of antibacterial regimens have been tested for use in patients with cancer. The major risk of infection is related to the degree of neutropenia seen as a consequence of either the disease or the therapy. Many of the relevant studies involved small populations in which the outcomes were generally good, and most lacked the statistical power to detect differences among the regimens studied. Each febrile neutropenic patient should be approached as a unique problem, with particular attention given to previous infections and recent antibiotic exposures. Several general guidelines are useful in the initial treatment of neutropenic patients with fever (Fig. 82-2):

1. In the initial regimen, it is necessary to use antibiotics active against both gram-negative and gram-positive bacteria (Table 82-4).
2. An aminoglycoside or an antibiotic without good activity against gram-positive organisms (e.g., ciprofloxacin or aztreonam) alone is not adequate in this setting.
3. The agents used should reflect both the epidemiology and the antibiotic resistance pattern of the hospital.
4. If the pattern of resistance justifies its use, a single third-generation cephalosporin constitutes an appropriate initial regimen in many hospitals.
5. Most standard regimens are designed for patients who have not previously received prophylactic antibiotics. The development of fever in a patient who has received antibiotics affects the choice of subsequent therapy, which should target resistant organisms and organisms known to cause infections in patients being treated with the antibiotics already administered.
6. Randomized trials have indicated the safety of oral antibiotic regimens in the treatment of "low-risk" patients with fever and neutropenia. Outpatients who are expected to remain neutropenic for <10 days and who have no concurrent medical problems (such as hypotension, pulmonary compromise, or abdominal pain) can be classified as low risk and treated with a broad-spectrum oral regimen.
7. Several large-scale studies indicate that prophylaxis with a fluoroquinolone (ciprofloxacin or levofloxacin) decreases morbidity and mortality rates among afebrile patients who are anticipated to have neutropenia of long duration.

The initial antibacterial regimen should be refined on the basis of culture results (Fig. 82-2). Blood cultures are the most relevant on which to base therapy; surface cultures of skin and mucous membranes may be misleading. In the case of gram-positive bacteremia or another gram-positive infection, it is important that the antibiotic be optimal for the organism isolated. Although it is not desirable to leave the patient unprotected, the addition of more and more antibacterial agents to the regimen is not appropriate unless there is a clinical or microbiologic reason to do so. Planned progressive therapy (the serial, empirical addition of one drug after another without culture data) is not efficacious in most settings and may have unfortunate consequences. Simply adding another antibiotic for fear that a gram-negative infection is present is a dubious practice. The synergy exhibited by β-lactams and aminoglycosides against certain gram-negative organisms (especially *P. aeruginosa*) provides the rationale

FIGURE 82-2 Algorithm for the diagnosis and treatment of febrile neutropenic patients.

for using two antibiotics in this setting, but recent analyses suggest that efficacy is not enhanced by the addition of aminoglycosides, while toxicity may be increased. Mere "double coverage," with the addition of a quinolone or another antibiotic that is not likely to exhibit synergy, has not been shown to be of benefit and may cause additional toxicities and side effects. Cephalosporins can cause bone marrow suppression, and vancomycin is associated with neutropenia in some healthy individuals (Chap. 127). Furthermore, the addition of multiple cephalosporins may induce β-lactamase production by some organisms; cephalosporins and double β-lactam combinations should probably be avoided altogether in *Enterobacter* infections.

ANTIFUNGAL THERAPY Fungal infections in cancer patients are most often associated with neutropenia. Neutropenic patients are predisposed to the development of invasive fungal infections, most commonly those due to *Candida* and *Aspergillus* species and occasionally those caused by *Fusarium*, *Trichosporon*, and *Bipolaris*. Cryptococcal infection, which is common among patients taking immunosuppressive agents, is uncommon among neutropenic patients receiving chemotherapy for AML. Invasive candidal disease is usually caused by *C. albicans* or *C. tropicalis* but can be caused by *C. krusei*, *C. parapsilosis*, and *C. glabrata*.

For decades it has been common clinical practice to add amphotericin B to antibacterial regimens if a neutropenic patient remains febrile despite 4–7 days of treatment with antibacterial agents. The rationale for the empirical addition of amphotericin B is that it is difficult to culture fungi before they cause disseminated disease and that mortality rates from disseminated fungal infections in granulocytopenic patients are high. Before the introduction of newer azoles into clinical practice, amphotericin B was the mainstay of antifungal therapy. The insolubility of amphotericin B has resulted in the marketing of several lipid formulations that are less toxic than the amphotericin B deoxycholate complex. However, because of the high cost of the lipid preparations, their use at many centers is reserved for patients who fail to respond to standard amphotericin B. Since the side effects of the formulations differ, unnecessary switching from one to another is not recommended.

Although fluconazole is efficacious in the treatment of infections due to many *Candida* spp., its use against serious fungal infections in immunocompromised patients is limited by its narrow spectrum: it has no activity against *Aspergillus* or against several non-*albicans Candida* spp. The release of newer broad-spectrum azoles (such as voriconazole and posaconazole) has provided another option for the treatment of *Aspergillus* infection (including CNS infection, in which amphotericin B has usually failed). In fact,

TABLE 82-8   ANTIVIRAL AGENTS ACTIVE AGAINST HERPESVIRUSES

Agent	Description	Spectrum	Toxicity	Other Issues
Acyclovir	Inhibits HSV polymerase	HSV, VZV (± CMV, EBV)	Rarely has side effects; crystalluria can occur at high doses	Long history of safety; original antiviral agent
Famciclovir	Prodrug of penciclovir (a guanosine analogue)	HSV, VZV (± CMV)	Associated with cancer in rats	Longer effective half-life than acyclovir
Valacyclovir	Prodrug of acyclovir; better absorption	HSV, VZV (± CMV)	Associated with thrombotic microangiopathy in one study of immunocompromised patients	Better oral absorption and longer effective half-life than acyclovir; can be given as a single daily dose for prophylaxis
Ganciclovir	More potent polymerase inhibitor; more toxic than acyclovir	HSV, VZV, CMV, HHV-6	Bone marrow suppression	Neutropenia may respond to G-CSF or GM-CSF
Valganciclovir	Prodrug of ganciclovir; better absorption	HSV, VZV, CMV, HHV-6	Bone marrow suppression	—
Cidofovir	Nucleotide analogue of cytosine	HSV, VZV, CMV; good in vitro activity against adenovirus and others	Nephrotoxic marrow suppression	Given IV once a week
Foscarnet	Phosphonoformic acid; inhibits viral DNA polymerase	HSV, VZV, CMV, HHV-6	Nephrotoxic; electrolyte abnormalities common	IV only

Abbreviations: ±, agent has some activity but not enough for the treatment of infections; CMV, cytomegalovirus; EBV, Epstein-Barr virus; G-CSF, granulocyte colony-stimulating factor; GM-CSF, granulocyte-macrophage colony-stimulating factor; HHV, human herpesvirus; HSV, herpes simplex virus; VZV, varicella-zoster virus.

experience indicates that these drugs may well supplant amphotericin B as the mainstay of treatment because of their lesser toxicity and better penetration into cerebrospinal fluid and other sites. Clinicians should be aware that the spectrum of each azole is somewhat different and that no drug can be assumed to be efficacious against all fungi. For example, while voriconazole is active against *Pseudallescheria boydii*, amphotericin B is not; however, voriconazole has no activity against *Mucor*. Recent studies suggest a role for posaconazole as a prophylactic agent in patients with prolonged neutropenia. **For a full discussion of antifungal therapy, see Chap. 191.**

Echinocandins (such as caspofungin) are useful in the treatment of infections caused by azole-resistant *Candida*. Studies in progress are assessing the use of these agents in combinations to determine whether treatment with multiple antifungal agents leads to better outcomes.

ANTIVIRAL THERAPY   The availability of a variety of agents active against herpes-group viruses, including some new agents with a broader spectrum of activity, has heightened focus on the treatment of viral infections, which pose a major problem in cancer patients. Viral diseases caused by the herpes group are prominent. Serious (and sometimes fatal) infections due to HSV and CMV are well documented, and VZV infections may be fatal to patients receiving chemotherapy. The roles of human herpesvirus (HHV) 6, HHV-7, and HHV-8 (Kaposi's sarcoma herpesvirus) in cancer pa-

tients are being defined (Chap. 175). While clinical experience is most extensive with acyclovir, which can be used therapeutically or prophylactically, a number of derivative drugs offer advantages over this agent **(Table 82-8)**.

In addition to the herpes group, several respiratory viruses (especially RSV) may cause serious disease in cancer patients. While vaccination with influenza vaccine is recommended (see below), it may be ineffective in this patient population. The availability of antiviral drugs with activity against influenza viruses gives the clinician additional options for the treatment of these patients **(Table 82-9)**.

OTHER THERAPEUTIC MODALITIES   Another way to address the problems of the febrile neutropenic patient is to replenish the neutrophil population. Although granulocyte transfusions are efficacious in the treatment of refractory gram-negative bacteremia, they do not have a documented role in prophylaxis. Because of the expense, the risk of leukoagglutinin reactions (which has probably been decreased by improved cell-separation procedures), and the risk of transmission of CMV from unscreened donors (which has been reduced by the use of filters), granulocyte transfusion is reserved for patients unresponsive to antibiotics. This modality is efficacious for documented gram-negative bacteremia refractory to antibiotics, particularly in situations where granulocyte numbers will be depressed for only a short period. The demonstrated usefulness of granulocyte colony-stimulating factor (G-CSF) in mobilizing neutrophils and advances in preservation techniques may make this option more useful than in the past.

A variety of cytokines, including G-CSF and granulocyte-macrophage colony-stimulating factor, enhance granulocyte recovery after chemotherapy and consequently shorten the period of maximal vulnerability to fatal infections. The role of these cytokines in routine practice is still a matter of some debate. Most authorities recommend their use only when neutropenia is both severe and prolonged. The cytokines themselves may have adverse effects, including fever, hypoxemia, and pleural effusions or serositis in other areas (Chap. 308). Since there is little evidence that their routine administration lessens the risk of death and since they are still expensive, the use of these cytokines has not become the standard of care in all centers. The role of other cytokines (such as macrophage colony-stimulating factor for monocytes or interferon-γ) in preventing or treating infections in granulocytopenic patients is under investigation.

TABLE 82-9   OTHER ANTIVIRAL AGENTS USEFUL IN THE TREATMENT OF INFECTIONS IN CANCER PATIENTS

Agent	Description	Spectrum	Toxicity	Other Issues
Amantadine, rimantadine	Interfere with uncoating	Influenza A only	5–10% fewer CNS effects with rimantadine	May be given prophylactically
Zanamivir	Neuraminidase inhibitor	Influenza A and B	Usually well tolerated	Inhalation only
Oseltamivir	Neuraminidase inhibitor	Influenza A and B	Usually well tolerated	PO dosing
Pleconaril	Blocks enterovirus binding and uncoating	90% of enteroviruses, 80% of rhinoviruses	Generally well tolerated	Decreases duration of meningitis; available for compassionate use only
Interferons	Cytokines with broad spectrum of activity	Used locally for warts, systemically for hepatitis	Fever, myalgias, bone marrow suppression	Not shown to be helpful in CMV infection; use limited by toxicity
Ribavirin	Purine analogue (precise mechanism of action unknown)	Broad theoretical spectrum; documented use against RSV, Lassa fever virus, and hepatitis viruses (with interferon)	IV form causes anemia	Given by aerosol for RSV infection (efficacy in doubt); approved for use in children with heart/lung disease

Abbreviations: CMV, cytomegalovirus; CNS, central nervous system; RSV, respiratory syncytial virus.

Once neutropenia has resolved, patients are not at increased risk of infection. However, depending on what drugs they receive, patients who continue on chemotherapeutic protocols remain at high risk for certain diseases. Any patient receiving more than a maintenance dose of glucocorticoids (including many treatment regimens for diffuse lymphoma) should also receive prophylactic TMP-SMX because of the risk of *Pneumocystis* infection; those with ALL should receive such prophylaxis for the duration of chemotherapy.

PREVENTION OF INFECTION IN CANCER PATIENTS

EFFECT OF THE ENVIRONMENT

Outbreaks of fatal *Aspergillus* infection have been associated with construction projects and materials in several hospitals. The association between spore counts and risk of infection suggests the need for a high-efficiency air-handling system in hospitals that care for large numbers of neutropenic patients. The use of laminar-flow rooms and prophylactic antibiotics has decreased the number of infectious episodes in severely neutropenic patients. However, because of the expense of such a program and the failure to show that it dramatically affects mortality rates, most centers do not routinely use laminar flow to care for neutropenic patients. Some centers use "reverse isolation," in which health care providers and visitors to a patient who is neutropenic wear gowns and gloves. Since most of the infections these patients develop are due to organisms that colonize the patients' own skin and bowel, the validity of such schemes is dubious, and limited clinical data do not support their use. Hand washing by all staff caring for neutropenic patients should be required to prevent the spread of resistant organisms.

The presence of large numbers of bacteria (particularly *P. aeruginosa*) in certain foods, especially fresh vegetables, has led some authorities to recommend a special "low-bacteria" diet. A diet consisting of cooked and canned food is satisfactory to most neutropenic patients and does not involve elaborate disinfection or sterilization protocols. However, there are no studies to support even this type of dietary restriction. Counseling of patients to avoid leftovers, deli foods, and unpasteurized dairy products is recommended.

PHYSICAL MEASURES

Although few studies address this issue, patients with cancer are predisposed to infections resulting from anatomic compromise (e.g., lymphedema resulting from node dissections after radical mastectomy). Surgeons who specialize in cancer surgery can provide specific guidelines for the care of such patients, and patients benefit from common-sense advice about how to prevent infections in vulnerable areas.

IMMUNOGLOBULIN REPLACEMENT

Many patients with multiple myeloma or CLL have immunoglobulin deficiencies as a result of their disease, and all allogeneic bone marrow transplant recipients are hypogammaglobinemic for a period after transplantation. However, current recommendations reserve intravenous immunoglobulin (IVIg) replacement therapy for those patients with severe (<400 mg/dL), prolonged hypogammaglobulinemia. Antibiotic prophylaxis has been shown to be cheaper and efficacious in preventing infections in most CLL patients with hypogammaglobulinemia. Routine use of IVIg replacement is not recommended.

SEXUAL PRACTICES

The use of condoms is recommended for severely immunocompromised patients. Any sexual practice that results in oral exposure to feces is not recommended. Neutropenic patients should be advised to avoid any practice that results in trauma, as even microscopic cuts may result in bacterial invasion and fatal sepsis.

ANTIBIOTIC PROPHYLAXIS

Several studies indicate that the use of oral fluoroquinolones prevents infection and decreases mortality rates among severely neutropenic patients. Fluconazole prevents *Candida* infections when given prophylactically to patients receiving bone marrow transplants. The use of broader-spectrum antifungal agents (e.g., posaconazole) appears to be more efficacious. Prophylaxis for *Pneumocystis* is mandatory for patients with ALL and for all cancer patients receiving glucocorticoid-containing chemotherapy regimens.

VACCINATION OF CANCER PATIENTS

In general, patients undergoing chemotherapy respond less well to vaccines than do normal hosts. Their greater need for vaccines thus leads to a dilemma in their management. Purified proteins and inactivated vaccines are almost never contraindicated and should be given to patients even during chemotherapy. For example, all adults should receive diphtheria-tetanus toxoid boosters at the indicated times as well as seasonal influenza vaccine. However, if possible, vaccination should not be undertaken concurrent with cytotoxic chemotherapy. If patients are expected to be receiving chemotherapy for several months and vaccination is indicated (for example, influenza vaccination in the fall), the vaccine should be given midcycle—as far apart in time as possible from the antimetabolic agents that will prevent an immune response. The meningococcal and pneumococcal polysaccharide vaccines should be given to patients before splenectomy, if possible. The *H. influenzae* type b conjugate vaccine should be administered to all splenectomized patients.

In general, live virus (or live bacterial) vaccines should not be given to patients during intensive chemotherapy because of the risk of disseminated infection. Recommendations on vaccination are summarized in Table 82-2.

FURTHER READINGS

Bohlius J et al: Granulopoiesis-stimulating factors to prevent adverse effects in the treatment of malignant lymphoma. Cochrane Database Syst Rev 3:CD003189, 2004

Gafter-Gvili A et al: Antibiotic prophylaxis for bacterial infections in afebrile neutropenic patients following chemotherapy. Cochrane Database Syst Rev 4:CD004386, 2005

Hall K et al: Diagnosis and management of long-term central venous catheter infections. J Vasc Interv Radiol 15:327, 2004

Paul M et al: Empirical antibiotic monotherapy for febrile neutropenia: Systematic review and meta-analysis of randomized controlled trials. J Antimicrob Chemother 57:176, 2006

Ullmann AJ et al: Posaconazole or fluconazole for prophylaxis in severe graft-versus-host disease. N Engl J Med 356:335, 2007

83 Cancer of the Skin
Arthur J. Sober, Hensin Tsao, Carl V. Washington

MELANOMA

Pigmented lesions are among the most common findings on skin examination. The challenge is to distinguish cutaneous melanomas, which may be lethal, from the remainder, which with rare exceptions are benign. Examples of malignant and benign pigmented lesions are shown in Fig. 83-1.

EPIDEMIOLOGY

Melanomas originate from neural crest-derived melanocytes; pigment cells present normally in the epidermis and sometimes in the dermis. This tumor affects around 62,000 individuals per year in the United States, resulting in 7910 deaths. Melanoma is the fifth most common cancer in men (5% of cancers) and the sixth most common in women (4% of cancers). The tumor can affect adults of all ages, even young

FIGURE 83-1 Atypical and malignant pigmented lesions. The most common melanoma is superficial spreading melanoma (not pictured). **A.** Acral lentiginous melanoma is the most common melanoma in blacks, Asians, and Hispanics and occurs as an enlarging hyperpigmented macule or plaque on the palms and soles. Lateral pigment diffusion is present. **B.** Nodular melanoma most commonly manifests itself as a rapidly growing, often ulcerated or crusted black nodule. **C.** Lentigo maligna melanoma occurs on sun-exposed skin as a large, hyperpigmented macule or plaque with irregular borders and variable pigmentation. **D.** Dysplastic nevi are irregularly pigmented and shaped nevomelanocytic lesions which may be associated with familial melanoma.

individuals (starting in the mid-teens); has distinct clinical features that make it detectable at a time when cure by surgical excision is possible; and is located on the skin surface, where it is visible. The incidence has increased dramatically (6% per year from 1973 to 1980, then 3% per year). Current lifetime risk ratio is 1:53 in males and 1:78 in females. The reason for this increase is uncertain but may involve increased recreational sun exposure, especially early in life. Individuals of similar ethnic background who immigrate after childhood to areas of high sun exposure (e.g., Israel and Australia) have lower melanoma rates than individuals of similar age who were either born in those countries or immigrated before age 10. The individuals most susceptible to development of melanoma are those with fair complexions, red or blond hair, blue eyes, and freckles and who tan poorly and sunburn easily. Other factors associated with increased risk include a family history of melanoma (~1 in 10 melanoma patients have a family member with melanoma), the presence of a clinically atypical mole (dysplastic nevus) or a giant congenital melanocytic nevus, the presence of a higher than average number of ordinary melanocytic nevi, and immunosuppression (Table 83-1). Individuals with 50 or more moles ≥2 mm in size have a 64-fold increased risk. About 30% of melanomas

TABLE 83-1	RISK FACTORS FOR CUTANEOUS MELANOMA

High risk (>50-fold increase in risk)
  Persistently changing mole
  Clinically atypical moles in patient with two family members with
    melanoma
  Adulthood (vs. childhood)
  >50 nevi ≥2 mm in diameter
Intermediate risk (~10-fold increase in risk)
  Family history of melanoma
  Sporadic clinically atypical moles
  Congenital nevi (?)
  White ethnicity (vs. black or East Asian ethnicity)
  Personal history of prior melanoma
Low risk (2- to 4-fold increase in risk)
  Immunosuppression
  Sun sensitivity or excess exposure to sun

Source: Adapted from AR Rhodes et al: JAMA 258:3146, 1987.

arise in a nevus. Some individuals with multiple primary melanomas and/or a strong family history have heritable mutations in the *CDKN2A* gene. Melanoma is relatively rare in heavily pigmented peoples. Dark-skinned populations (such as those of India and Puerto Rico), blacks, and East Asians have rates 10–20 times lower than lighter-skinned whites. In keeping with the role of sun exposure, the incidence is inversely correlated with the latitude of residence; at any latitude, darker-skinned persons have the lowest incidence. Melanoma is rare in children under age 10.

CLINICAL CHARACTERISTICS

There are four types of cutaneous melanoma (Table 83-2). In three of these—*superficial spreading melanoma, lentigo maligna melanoma,* and *acral lentiginous melanoma*—the lesion has a period of superficial (so-called radial) growth during which it increases in size but does not penetrate deeply. It is during this period that the melanoma is most capable of being cured by surgical excision. The fourth type—*nodular melanoma*—does not have a recognizable radial growth phase and usually presents as a deeply invasive lesion, capable of early metastasis. When tumors begin to penetrate deeply into the skin, they are in the so-called vertical growth phase. Melanomas with a radial growth phase are characterized by irregular and sometimes notched borders, variation in pigment pattern, and variation in color. An increase in size or change in color is noted by the patient in 70% of early lesions. Bleeding, ulceration, and pain are late signs and are of little help in early recognition. Superficial spreading melanoma is the most frequent variant observed in the white population. Melanomas arising in dysplastic nevi (see below) are usually of this type. The back is the most common site for melanoma in men. In women, the back and the lower leg (from knee to ankle) are common sites. Nodular melanomas are dark brown-black to blue-black nodules. Lentigo maligna melanoma is usually confined to chronically sun-damaged, sun-exposed sites (face, neck, back of hands) in older individuals. Acral lentiginous melanoma occurs on the palms, soles, nail beds, and mucous membranes. While this type occurs in whites, it is most frequent (along with nodular melanoma) in blacks and East Asians.

A fifth type of melanoma, the *desmoplastic melanoma,* is recognized. This tumor type is associated with a fibrotic response to the tumor, neural invasion, and a higher tendency to local recurrence. Occasionally, melanomas can be amelanotic, in which case the diagnosis is established histologically after biopsy of a new or changing skin nodule or because of a suspicion of a basal cell carcinoma (see below).

PROGNOSTIC FACTORS

The most important prognostic factor is the stage at the time of presentation. Fortunately, most melanomas are diagnosed in clinical stages I and II. The revised American Joint Committee on Cancer (AJCC) staging system for melanoma is based on microscopic primary tumor depth (Breslow's thickness), presence of ulceration, evidence of nodal involvement, and presence of metastatic disease to internal sites (Table 83-3). Certain anatomic sites may affect the prognosis. The favorable

TABLE 83-2 **CLINICAL FEATURES OF MALIGNANT MELANOMA**

Type	Site	Average Age at Diagnosis, Years	Duration of Known Existence, Years	Color
Lentigo maligna melanoma	Sun-exposed surfaces, particularly malar region of cheek and temple	70	5–20[a] or longer	In flat portions, shades of brown and tan predominant, but whitish gray occasionally present; in nodules, shades of reddish brown, bluish gray, bluish black
Superficial spreading melanoma	Any site (more common on upper back and, in women, on lower legs)	40–50	1–7	Shades of brown mixed with bluish red (violaceous), bluish black, reddish brown, and often whitish pink, and the border of lesion is at least in part visibly and/or palpably elevated
Nodular melanoma	Any site	40–50	Months to less than 5 years	Reddish blue (purple) or bluish black; either uniform in color or mixed with brown or black
Acral lentiginous melanoma	Palm, sole, nail bed, mucous membrane	60	1–10	In flat portions, dark brown predominantly; in raised lesions (plaques) brown-black or blue black predominantly

[a]During much of this time, the precursor stage, lentigo maligna, is confined to the epidermis.

Source: Adapted from AJ Sober, in *Pathophysiology of Dermatologic Diseases*, NA Soter, HP Baden (eds). New York, McGraw-Hill, 1984.

sites appear to be the forearm and leg (excluding feet), while unfavorable sites include scalp, hands, feet, and mucous membranes. In general, women with stage I or II disease have a better survival than men, perhaps in part because of earlier diagnosis; women frequently have melanomas on the lower leg, where self-recognition is more likely and prognosis is better. Older individuals, especially men over 60, have poorer prognoses. This finding has been explained in part by a tendency toward later diagnosis (and thus thicker tumors) in men and by a higher proportion in men of acral melanomas (palmar-plantar), which have a poorer prognosis. Melanoma may recur after many years. About 10–15% of first-time recurrences develop >5 years after treatment of the original lesion. The time to recurrence varies inversely with tumor thickness. An alternative prognostic scheme for clinical stages I and II melanoma, proposed by Clark, is based on the anatomic level of invasion in the skin. Level I is intraepidermal (in situ); level II penetrates the papillary dermis; level III spans the papillary dermis; level IV penetrates the reticular dermis; and level V penetrates into the subcutaneous fat. The 5-year survival for these stages averages 100, 95, 82, 71, and 49%, respectively.

NATURAL HISTORY

Melanomas may spread by the lymphatic channels or the bloodstream. The earliest metastases are often to regional lymph nodes. Lymphadenectomy may control early regional disease. Liver, lung, bone, and brain are common sites of hematogenous spread, but unusual sites, such as the anterior chamber of the eye, may also be involved. Once metastatic disease is established, cure is unlikely.

MANAGEMENT

The entire cutaneous surface, including the scalp and mucous membranes, should be examined in each patient. Bright room illumination is important, and a 7× to 10× hand lens is helpful for evaluating variation in pigment pattern. A history of relevant risk factors should be elicited. Any suspicious lesions should be biopsied, evaluated by a specialist, or recorded by chart and/or photography for follow-up. Examination of the lymph nodes and palpation of the abdominal viscera are part of the staging examination for suspected melanoma. The patient should be advised to have other family members screened if either melanoma or clinically atypical moles (dysplastic nevi) are present. The detection of early melanoma in relatives has been reported.

Melanoma prevention is based on protection from the sun. Routine use of a broad spectrum UV-A/UV-B sunblock with sun protection factor ≥15, use of protective clothing, and avoiding intense midday ultraviolet exposure should be recommended. The patient should be educated in the clinical features of melanoma and advised to report any growth or other change in a pigmented lesion. Patient education brochures are available from the American Cancer Society, the American Academy of Dermatology, the National Cancer Institute, and the Skin Cancer Foundation. Self-examination at 6- to 8-week intervals may enhance the likelihood of detecting change. The importance of routine follow-up visits for melanoma patients and patients with clinically atypical moles (dysplastic nevi) should be emphasized, as these visits may facilitate early detection of new primary tumors.

TABLE 83-3 **PROGNOSIS OF MELANOMA BY THICKNESS (BRESLOW) AND REVISED AJCC STAGES: 5-YEAR SURVIVAL RATES**

AJCC Stage	Thickness, mm	Ulceration	Nodal Disease	Distant Metastases
0	In situ	N/A	No	No
IA	<1	No	No	No
IB	<1	Yes	No	No
	1.01–2.0	No	No	No
IIA	1.01–2.0	Yes	No	No
	2.01–4.0	No	No	No
IIB	2.01–4.0	Yes	No	No
	>4.0	No	No	No
IIC	>4.0	Yes	No	No
IIIA	Any	No	Yes	No
			1 node w/microscopic disease	No
			2–3 nodes w/microscopic disease	No
IIIB	Any	Yes	1 node w/microscopic disease	No
	Any	Yes	2–3 nodes w/microscopic disease	No
	Any	No	1 node w/macroscopic disease	No
	Any	No	2–3 nodes w/macroscopic disease	No
	Any	Any	In transit or satellite disease w/out nodal disease	No
IIIC	Any	Yes	1 node w/macroscopic disease	No
		Yes	2–3 nodes w/macroscopic disease	No
		Any	≥4 metastatic or matted nodes, or in transit mets/satellites or metastatic nodes	No
IV	Any	Any	Any	Yes

Note: AJCC, American Joint Commission for Cancer.

Precursor Lesions Clinically atypical moles, also termed *dysplastic nevi*, occur in certain families affected by melanoma. In some families, melanomas occur nearly exclusively in

PART 6 Oncology and Hematology

TABLE 83-4 CLINICAL FEATURES DISTINGUISHING ATYPICAL MOLES FROM BENIGN ACQUIRED NEVI

Clinical Feature	Clinically Atypical Moles	Benign Acquired Nevi
Color	Variable mixtures of tan, brown, black, or red/pink within a single nevus; nevi may look very different from each other	Uniformly tan or brown
Shape	Irregular borders; pigment may fade off into surrounding skin; macular portion at the edge of the nevus	Round; sharp, clear-cut borders between the nevus and the surrounding skin; may be flat or elevated
Size	Usually >6 mm in diameter; may be >10 mm; occasionally <6 mm	Usually <6 mm in diameter
Number	Often very many (>100), but occasionally may be only one	In a typical adult, 10 to 40 are scattered over the body; perhaps 15% of patients have no nevi
Location	Sun-exposed areas; the back is the most common site, but dysplastic nevi may also be seen on the scalp, breasts, and buttocks	Generally on the sun-exposed surfaces of the skin above the waist; the scalp, breasts, and buttocks are rarely involved

Source: Modified from RJ Friedman et al: CA—A Cancer J Clinicians 33(3):130, 1985.

the individuals with dysplastic nevi. In other families, the nevi may not be present in all individuals with an increased risk of melanoma. The melanomas may arise in clinically atypical moles or in normal skin (in the latter situation the moles act as markers of increased risk). Individuals with clinically atypical moles and a strong family history of melanoma have been reported to have a >50% lifetime risk for developing melanoma. Table 83-4 lists the features that are characteristic of clinically atypical moles and that differentiate them from benign acquired nevi. The number of clinically atypical moles may vary from one to several hundred. Clinically atypical moles usually differ from each other in appearance. The borders are often hazy and indistinct, and the pigment pattern is more highly varied than that in benign acquired nevi. Of the 90% of melanoma patients whose disease is regarded as sporadic (i.e., who lack a family history of melanoma), ~40% have clinically atypical moles, as compared with an estimated 5–10% of the population at large. Further studies to determine the background frequency of clinically atypical moles are required, once greater unanimity exists regarding their clinical and histopathologic features. The observation that sporadic melanomas can arise in association with a clinically atypical mole makes this the most important precursor for melanoma. Less frequent precursors include the giant congenital melanocytic nevus. Congenital melanocytic nevi are present at birth or appear in the neonatal period (tardive form). The *giant melanocytic nevus*, also called the bathing trunk, cape, or garment nevus, is a rare malformation that affects perhaps 1 in 30,000 to 1 in 100,000 individuals. These nevi are usually >20 cm in diameter and may cover more than half the body surface. Giant nevi often occur in association with multiple small congenital nevi. The borders are sharp, and hair may be present. The lesions are usually dark brown and may have darker and lighter areas. Pigment is haphazardly displayed. The surface is smooth to rugose or cerebriform and may vary from one portion of the lesion to another.

A lifetime risk of melanoma development of 6% has been estimated. The risk is greatest before age 5 and next greatest between ages 5 and 10. Early detection of melanoma is difficult in these lesions because of the deep dermal or subcutaneous origin of primary melanoma and because of the large and varied surface of the nevus. Prophylactic excision early in life can be accomplished by staged removal with coverage by split-thickness skin grafts. Surgery cannot remove all at-risk nevus cells as some may penetrate into the muscles or central nervous system below the nevus. At present there are no uni-

form management guidelines for giant congenital nevi. The *small- to medium-sized congenital melanocytic nevus*, which affects approximately 1% of persons, usually presents as a raised dark- to medium-brown lesion with a smooth or papillomatous surface. The border is sharp, and lesions may be oriented along lines of skin cleavage. Follicular hyper- and hypopigmentation may coexist in a salt-and-pepper configuration. The lesion may have an excess of thick, coarse hairs. The risk of melanoma developing in these lesions is not known but appears to be relatively small. The management of small- to medium-sized congenital melanocytic nevi remains controversial. Melanomas in small congenital melanocytic nevi appear to occur after puberty, unlike melanomas that arise in giant congenital nevi and tend to occur much earlier in life. Melanomas can also arise in benign dermal and compound moles. Overall, it has been estimated that for a 20-year-old individual, the lifetime risk of any selected mole transforming into melanoma by age 80 years is approximately 0.03% (1 in 3,164) for men and 0.009% (1 in 10,800) for women.

Differential Diagnosis The aim of differential diagnosis is to distinguish benign pigmented lesions from melanoma and its precursor. If melanoma is a consideration, then biopsy is appropriate. Some benign look-alikes may be removed in the process of trying to detect authentic melanoma. Table 83-5 summarizes the distinguishing features of benign lesions that may be confused with melanoma. Early detection of melanoma may be facilitated by applying the "ABCD rules": A—asymmetry, benign lesions are usually symmetrical; B—border irregularity, most nevi have clear-cut borders; C—color variegation, benign lesions usually have uniform light or dark pigment; D—diameter >6 mm (the size of a pencil eraser). Of these criteria, the weakest is diameter >6

TABLE 83-5 PIGMENTED LESIONS THAT MUST BE DISTINGUISHED FROM CUTANEOUS MELANOMA AND ITS PRECURSORS

Blue nevus	Gunmetal or cerulean blue, blue-gray. Stable over time. One-half occur on dorsa of hands and feet. Lesions are usually single, small, 3 mm to <1 cm. Must be distinguished from nodular melanoma.
Compound nevus	Round or oval shape, well-demarcated, smooth-bordered. May be dome-shaped or papillomatous; colors range from flesh colored to very dark brown, with individual nevi being relatively homogeneous in color.
Hemangioma	Dome-shaped reddish, purple, blue nodule. Compression with a glass microscope slide may result in blanching. Must be distinguished from nodular melanoma.
Junctional nevus	Flat to barely raised brown lesion. Sharp border. Fine pigmentary stippling visible, especially upon magnification.
Lentigo Juvenile Solar	Flat, uniformly medium or dark brown lesion with sharp border. Solar lentigines are acquired lesions on sites of chronic solar exposure (face and backs of hands). Lesions are 2 mm to ≥1 cm. Solar lentigines have reticulate pigmentation upon magnification.
Pigmented basal cell carcinoma	Papular border. May have central ulceration. Usually on a sun-exposed surface in an older patient. Patient usually has dark brown eyes and dark brown or black hair.
Pigmented dermatofibroma	Lesion is not well demarcated visually, is firm, and dimples downward when compressed laterally. Usually on extremities. Usually <6 mm.
Seborrheic keratosis	Rough, sharp-bordered lesions that feel waxy and "stuck on"; range in color from flesh to tan, to dark brown. Presence of keratin plugs in surface is helpful for discriminating especially dark lesions from melanoma.
Subungual hematoma	Maroon (red-brown) coloration. As lesion grows out from nail fold, a curving clear area is seen.
Tattoo (medical or traumatic)	In medical tattoo, lesions are small pigmentary dots, often blue or green, which make a regular pattern (rectangle). Traumatic tattoos are irregular, and pigmentation may appear black.

mm since a significant fraction of melanomas are now diagnosed with diameters <6 mm. In addition, the above features are less helpful in the recognition of nodular melanomas, which may be symmetrical and have uniform colors. "Different" has been substituted for "diameter" by some. Addition of an "E" for evolution has been proposed as other features may become more significant if the lesion is changing.

Biopsy   Any pigmented cutaneous lesion that has changed in size or shape or has other features suggestive of malignant melanoma is a candidate for biopsy. The recommended technique is an excisional biopsy, as that facilitates pathologic assessment of the lesion, permits accurate measurement of thickness if the lesion is melanoma, and constitutes treatment if the lesion is benign. For large lesions or lesions on anatomic sites where excisional biopsy may not be feasible (such as the face, hands, or feet), an incisional biopsy through the most nodular or darkest area of the lesion is acceptable; this should include the vertical growth phase of the primary tumor, if present. Incisional biopsy does not appear to facilitate the spread of melanoma.

Staging   Once the diagnosis of malignant melanoma has been confirmed, the tumor must be staged to determine prognosis and treatment. The history should probe for evidence of metastatic disease, such as malaise, weight loss, headaches, visual difficulty, or bone pain. The physical examination should be directed especially to the skin, regional draining lymph nodes, central nervous system, liver, and spleen. In the absence of signs or symptoms of metastasis, few laboratory or radiologic tests are indicated for staging purposes. No tests or scans are routinely indicated unless the history or physical examination suggests metastasis to a specific organ. Once signs of metastasis exist, favored sites of spread, such as the liver, lungs, bone, and brain, should be evaluated. Patients are classified into four stages (Table 83-3).

℞ MELANOMA

SURGICAL MANAGEMENT   For a newly diagnosed cutaneous melanoma, wide surgical excision of the lesion with a margin of normal skin is necessary to remove all malignant cells and minimize possible local recurrence. The appropriate width of the margin is a source of controversy. A World Health Organization trial that prospectively randomized between 1- and 3-cm margins in 612 patients with thin malignant melanomas (≤2 mm thick) reported that the narrower margin resulted in higher rates of local recurrence but no difference in rates of nodal or distant metastases, disease-free survival, or overall survival. Another large randomized trial comparing 2- or 4-cm surgical margins for intermediate-thickness lesions (1–4 mm thick) also found no significant differences in overall survival. The following margins can be recommended for primary melanoma: in situ: 0.5 cm; invasive up to 1 mm thick: 1.0 cm; >1 mm: 2.0 cm. For lesions on the face, hands, and feet, strict adherence to these margins must give way to individual considerations about the constraints of surgery and minimization of morbidity. In all instances, however, inclusion of subcutaneous fat in the surgical specimen facilitates adequate thickness measurement and assessment of surgical margins by the pathologist.

Sentinel Node Biopsy   Sentinel node biopsy (SLNB) has replaced elective regional nodal dissection for the evaluation of regional nodal status. The initial draining node(s) from the primary site is/are identified by injecting a blue dye and a radioisotope around the primary site. The initial draining node(s) is/are then identified by inspection of the nodal basin for the blue stained node and/or the node with high uptake of the radioisotope. The identified nodes are removed and subjected to careful histopathologic processing with serial section hematoxylin and eosin stains as well as immunohistochemical stains that identify melanocytes. Sentinel lymph node examination is a valuable staging tool, and in the instance of a negative biopsy, SLNB may obviate the need for complete nodal dissection. Patients with lesions <0.75 mm thick have an excellent prognosis and are not candidates for SLNB unless other high-risk features are present (ulceration, shave biopsy with base involved, etc.). At the other extreme, patients with lesions >4 mm thick have such a high risk for distant metastases that controlling nodal disease may not alter the ultimate clinical outcome. A subset of patients with lesions of intermediate thickness may have a survival benefit from regional node dissection. SLNB is of value in selecting patients who may benefit from adjuvant therapy. Survival benefit of SLNB remains to be proven.

ADJUVANT THERAPY FOR NODAL DISEASE   For patients who are free of disease but at high risk for metastases, adjuvant therapy that complements surgery is needed to destroy occult micrometastases, prolong disease-free survival, and improve the cure rate. Many strategies have been tried unsuccessfully. However, adjuvant interferon (IFN) α2b may be capable of improving disease-free and overall survival in patients with nodal metastases (stage III disease). The U.S. Food and Drug Administration has approved a high-dose IFN adjuvant protocol consisting of 20 million units per square meter intravenously 5 days a week for 4 weeks followed by 10 million units per square meter subcutaneously three times a week for 11 months. In a large fraction of patients, these doses of IFN are associated with severe toxicity, including a flulike illness and decline in performance status. The toxicity in most patients reverses promptly with lower doses and when therapy is stopped.

TREATMENT OF METASTATIC DISEASE   Melanoma can metastasize to any internal organ, the brain being a particularly common site. Metastatic melanoma is generally incurable, with survival in patients with visceral metastases generally <1 year. Thus, the goal of treatment is usually palliation. Patients with soft tissue and nodal metastases fare better than those with liver and brain metastases. Metastases limited to regional nodes (AJCC stage III disease) warrant a therapeutic lymph node dissection. Surgical excision of a single metastasis to the lung or to a surgically accessible brain site can prolong survival. Stereotactic radiosurgery has been successful in the treatment of isolated brain metastases. Radiation therapy can provide local palliation for recurrent tumors or metastases. Patients who have advanced regional disease limited to a limb may benefit from hyperthermic limb perfusion with melphalan. High complete response rates have been reported, and responses are associated with significant palliation of symptoms.

A number of drugs and biological therapies have demonstrated minimal antitumor activity (15–20% partial response rates) in metastatic melanoma, including dacarbazine (DTIC); the nitrosoureas carmustine (BCNU), lomustine (CCNU), and semustine (methyl-CCNU); platinum analogues such as cisplatin and carboplatin; vinca alkaloids such as vincristine, vinblastine, and vindesine; the taxanes paclitaxel and docetaxel; IFN-α; and interleukin 2 (IL-2). Although limited in efficacy, single-agent dacarbazine is still considered the standard treatment. Ongoing trials are attempting to define superior combinations. IL-2 produces response rates similar to those seen with cytotoxic agents; however, active doses usually cause greater toxicity than chemotherapy. Response rates of >50% have been observed with IL-2 for intracutaneous and subcutaneous disease.

Melanoma can express cell-surface antigens that may be recognized by host immune cells. These melanoma-associated antigens alone or in combination may make it possible to develop vaccination strategies against melanoma. Such strategies include the use of purified tumor proteins as immunogens and the use of genetically altered tumor cells to elicit a T cell response. Alternative experimental approaches include efforts to expand tumor-specific T cells (either obtained from the tumor as tumor-infiltrating lymphocytes or harvested from the peripheral blood after vaccination) in vitro and transfer them into patients in large numbers. In addition, monoclonal antibodies to tumor antigens are being evaluated. Agents directed against the cell cycle pathways are also currently in trial. All of these experimental approaches will need considerable further development before being applicable on a wide scale. Advances in treating metastatic disease may also prove applicable in the adjuvant setting.

The absence of curative therapy for patients with metastatic melanoma underscores the importance of early detection and prevention as strategies to decrease melanoma mortality. Patients with stage 4 melanoma are best treated by medical oncologists with expertise in treating patients with advanced disease. Clinical trials should be considered as an option for this patient group.

NONMELANOMA SKIN CANCER

Nonmelanoma skin cancer (NMSC) is the most common cancer in the United States, with an estimated annual incidence of >1.5 million

FIGURE 83-2 Cutaneous neoplasms. A. Non-Hodgkin's lymphoma involves the skin with typical violaceous, "plum-colored" nodules. **B.** Squamous cell carcinoma is seen here as a hyperkeratotic crusted and somewhat eroded plaque on the lower lip. Sun-exposed skin such as the head, neck, hands, and arms are other typical sites of involvement. **C.** Actinic keratoses consists of hyperkeratotic erythematous papules and patches on sun-exposed skin. They arise in middle-aged to older adults and have some potential for malignant transformation. **D.** Metastatic carcinoma to the skin is characterized by inflammatory, often ulcerated dermal nodules. **E.** Mycosis fungoides is a cutaneous T cell lymphoma, and plaque stage lesions are seen in this patient. **F.** Keratoacanthoma is a low-grade squamous cell carcinoma that presents as an exophytic nodule with central keratinous debris. **G.** This basal cell carcinoma shows central ulceration and a pearly, rolled, telangiectatic tumor border.

cases. Basal cell carcinomas (BCCs) account for 70–80% of NMSCs. Squamous cell carcinomas (SCCs), while representing only ~20% of NMSC, are more significant because of their ability to metastasize (Fig. 83-2); they account for most of the 2400 deaths annually. Incidence rates have risen dramatically over the past decade.

ETIOLOGY

The causes of BCC and SCC are multifactorial. Cumulative exposure to sunlight, principally the ultraviolet B (UV-B) spectrum, is the most significant factor. Emerging data suggest that ultraviolet A radiation may be more carcinogenic than previously believed. Other factors associated with a higher incidence of skin cancer are male sex, older age, Celtic descent, a fair complexion, a tendency to sunburn easily, and an outdoor occupation. The incidence of these tumors increases with decreasing latitude. Most tumors develop on sun-exposed areas of the head and neck. Tumors are more common on the left side of the body in the United States but on the right side in England, presumably owing to asymmetric exposure during driving. As the earth's ozone shield continues to thin, further increases in the incidence of skin cancer are anticipated. In certain geographic areas, exposure to arsenic in well water or from industrial sources may significantly increase the risk of BCC and SCC. Skin cancer in affected individuals may be seen with or without other cutaneous markers of chronic arsenism (e.g., arsenical keratoses). Less common is exposure to the cyclic aromatic hydrocarbons in tar, soot, or shale. The risk of lip or oral SCC is increased with cigarette smoking. Human papillomaviruses and UV radiation may act as cocarcinogens.

Host factors associated with a high risk of skin cancer include immunosuppression induced by disease or drugs. Transplant recipients receiving chronic immunosuppressive therapy are particularly prone to SCC. The frequency of skin cancer is proportional to the duration of immunosuppression and the extent of sun exposure both before and after transplantation. Skin cancer is not uncommon in patients infected with HIV, and it may be more aggressive in this setting. Other factors include ionizing radiation, thermal burn scars, and chronic ulcerations. Several heritable conditions are associated with skin cancer (e.g., albinism, xeroderma pigmentosum, and basal cell nevus syndrome). Mutations in the tumor suppressor *patch* gene have been implicated in the development of BCC.

CLINICAL PRESENTATION

NMSCs are often asymptomatic, but nonhealing ulceration, bleeding, or pain can occur in advanced lesions.

Basal Cell Carcinoma BCC is a malignancy arising from epidermal basal cells. The least invasive of BCC subtypes, *superficial BCC*, classically consists of truncal erythematous, scaling plaques that slowly enlarge. This BCC subtype may be confused with benign inflammatory dermatoses, especially nummular eczema and psoriasis. BCC can also present as a small, slow-growing pearly nodule, often with small telangiectatic vessels on its surface (*nodular BCC*). The occasional presence of melanin in this variant of nodular BCC (*pigmented BCC*) may lead to confusion clinically with melanoma. *Morpheaform (fibrosing) BCC* and *micronodular BCC*, the most invasive subtypes, manifest as solitary, flat or slightly depressed, indurated, whitish or yellowish plaques. Borders are typically indistinct, a feature associated with a greater potential for extensive subclinical spread.

Squamous Cell Carcinoma Primary *cutaneous SCC* is a malignant neoplasm of keratinizing epidermal cells. SCC can grow rapidly and metastasize. The clinical features of SCC vary widely. Commonly, SCC appears as an ulcerated erythematous nodule or superficial erosion on the skin or lower lip, but it may present as a verrucous papule or plaque. Overlying telangiectasias are uncommon. The margins of this tumor may be ill-defined, and fixation to underlying structures may occur. Cutaneous SCC may develop anywhere on the body but usually arises on sun-damaged skin. A related neoplasm, keratoacanthoma, typically appears as a dome-shaped papule with a central keratotic crater, expands rapidly, and commonly regresses without therapy. This lesion can be difficult to differentiate from SCC.

Actinic keratoses and *cheilitis*, both premalignant forms of SCC, present as hyperkeratotic papules on sun-exposed areas. The potential for malignant degeneration in untreated lesions ranges from 0.25 to 20%. *Bowen's disease*, an in situ form of SCC, presents as a scaling, erythematous plaque. Treatment of premalignant and in situ lesions reduces the subsequent risk of invasive disease.

NATURAL HISTORY

Basal Cell Carcinoma The natural history of BCC is that of a slowly enlarging, locally invasive neoplasm. The degree of local destruction and risk of recurrence vary with the size, duration, location, and histologic subtype of the tumor; presence of recurrent disease; and various patient characteristics. Location on the central face, ears, or scalp may portend a higher risk. Small nodular, pigmented, cystic, or superficial BCCs respond well to most treatments. Large lesions and micronodular and morpheaform subtypes may be more aggressive. The metastatic potential of BCC has been estimated to be 0.0028–0.1%. Persons with either BCC or SCC have an increased risk of developing subsequent skin cancers, estimated to be up to 40% in 5 years.

Squamous Cell Carcinoma The natural history of SCC depends on both tumor and host characteristics. Tumors arising on actinically damaged skin have a lower metastatic potential than those on protected surfaces. The metastatic frequency of cutaneous SCC, reported at 0.3–5.2%, occurs most frequently in regional draining lymph nodes. Tumors occurring on the lower lip and ear have metastatic potentials approaching 13 and 11%, respectively. The metastatic potential of SCC arising in scars, chronic ulcerations, and genital or mucosal surfaces is higher. The overall metastatic rate for recurrent tumors may approach 30%. Large, poorly differentiated, deep tumors, with perineural or lymphatic invasion, often behave aggressively. Multiple tumors with rapid growth and aggressive behavior can be a therapeutic challenge in immunosuppressed patients.

℞ NONMELANOMA SKIN CANCER

BASAL CELL CARCINOMA The most frequently employed treatment modalities for BCC include electrodesiccation and curettage (ED&C), excision, cryosurgery, radiation therapy, laser therapy, Mohs micrographic surgery (MMS), topical 5-fluorouracil, and topical immunomodulators. The mode of therapy chosen depends on tumor characteristics, patient age, medical status, preferences of the patient, and other factors. ED&C remains the method most commonly employed by dermatologists. This method is selected for low-risk tumors (e.g., a small primary tumor of a less aggressive subtype in a favorable location). Excision, which offers the advantage of histologic control, is usually selected for more aggressive tumors or those in high-risk locations or, in many instances, for aesthetic reasons. Cryosurgery employing liquid nitrogen may be used for certain low-risk tumors but requires specialized equipment (cryoprobes) to be effective for advanced neoplasms. Radiation therapy, while not used as often, offers an excellent chance for cure in many cases of BCC. It is useful in patients not considered surgical candidates and as a surgical adjunct in high-risk tumors. Younger patients may not be good candidates for radiation therapy because of the risks of long-term carcinogenesis and radiodermatitis. Despite rapidly advancing technology in laser development, their long-term efficacy in treating infiltrative or recurrent lesions is still unknown. On the other hand, MMS, a specialized type of surgical excision that permits the best histologic control and preservation of uninvolved tissue, is associated with cure rates >98%. It is the preferred modality for lesions that are recurrent, in a high-risk location, or large and ill-defined and where maximal tissue conservation is critical (e.g., the eyelids). Topical 5-fluorouracil therapy should be limited to superficial BCC. New topicals, the immunomodulators, show promise in their efficacy at treating superficial and even nodular BCCs. Imiquimod, a relatively well-tolerated cream, has successfully undergone phase III clinical trials. Intralesional chemotherapy (5-fluorouracil and INF) and photodynamic therapy (which employs selective activation of a photoactive drug by visible light) have been used successfully in patients

TABLE 83-6 OTHER NONMELANOMA CUTANEOUS MALIGNANCIES

Tumor Type	Most Common Location	Recurrence Rate,[a] %	Metastatic Rate, %
Atypical fibroxanthoma	Head and neck	21	4
Merkel cell carcinoma	Head and neck	40	75
Dermatofibrosarcoma protuberans	Trunk	50	1
Sebaceous carcinoma	Eyelid	12	30
Microcystic adnexal carcinoma	Face	50	1 case
Porocarcinoma	Extremity	20	10
Eccrine carcinoma	Head and neck	36	11
Angiosarcoma	Head and neck	75	75

[a]Recurrence rates are the highest reported and were established prior to widespread use of Mohs micrographic surgery.

with numerous tumors. A topical endonuclease (T4N5 liposome lotion) has been shown to repair DNA and may decrease the rate of NMSC in xeroderma pigmentosum.

SQUAMOUS CELL CARCINOMA The therapy of cutaneous SCC should be based on an analysis of risk factors influencing the biologic behavior of the tumor. These include the size, location, and degree of histologic differentiation of the tumor as well as the age and physical condition of the patient. Surgical excision, MMS, and radiation therapy are standard methods of treatment. Cryosurgery and ED&C have been used successfully for premalignant lesions and small primary tumors. Metastases are treated with lymph node dissection, irradiation, or both. 13-*cis*-retinoic acid (1 mg orally every day) plus INF-α (3 million units subcutaneously or intramuscularly every day) may produce a partial response in most patients. Systemic chemotherapy combinations that include cisplatin may also be palliative in some patients.

PREVENTION

As the vast majority of skin cancers are related to chronic UV radiation exposure, patient and physician education could dramatically reduce their incidence. Emphasis should be placed on preventive measures beginning early in life. Patients must understand that damage from UV-B begins early, despite the fact that cancers develop years later. Regular use of sunscreens and protective clothing should be encouraged. Avoidance of tanning salons and midday (10 A.M.–2 P.M.) sun exposure is recommended. Precancerous and in situ lesions should be treated early. Early detection of small tumors affords simpler treatment modalities with higher cure rates and lower morbidity. In patients with a history of skin cancer, long-term follow-up for the detection of recurrence, metastasis, and new skin cancers should be emphasized. Chemoprophylaxis using synthetic retinoids is useful in controlling new lesions in some patients with multiple tumors.

OTHER NONMELANOMA CUTANEOUS MALIGNANCIES

Neoplasms of cutaneous adnexa and sarcomas of fibrous, mesenchymal, fatty, and vascular tissues make up 1–2% of NMSC (Table 83-6). Some can portend a poor prognosis such as *Merkel cell carcinoma*, which is a neural crest-derived, highly aggressive malignancy that exhibits a metastatic rate of 75% and a 5-year survival rate of 30–40%. Others, such as the human herpes virus 8-induced, HIV-related *Kaposi's sarcoma*, exhibit a more indolent course. The marked decrease in incidence of this tumor parallels the institution of the highly active antiretroviral therapy.

ACKNOWLEDGMENT

Katarina G. Chiller, MD, and Howard K. Koh, MD, contributed to this chapter in the 16th edition and material from that chapter is included here.

FURTHER READINGS

AMERICAN CANCER SOCIETY: Website at *www.cancer.org*

548 Balch CM et al: Prognostic factors analysis of 17,600 melanoma patients: Validation of the American Joint Committee on Cancer melanoma staging system. J Clin Oncol 19:3622, 2001

Balch CM et al: Final version of the AJCC staging system for cutaneous melanoma. J Clin Oncol 19:3635, 2001

Drake LA et al: Guidelines of care of basal cell carcinoma. J Am Acad Dermatol 26:117, 1992

——— et al: Guidelines of care for cutaneous squamous cell carcinoma. J Am Acad Dermatol 28:628, 1993

Geisse JK et al: Imiquimod 5% cream for the treatment of superficial basal cell carcinoma: A double-blind, randomized, vehicle-controlled study. J Am Acad Dermatol 47:390, 2002

Johnson TM et al: Staging workup, sentinel node biopsy, and follow-up tests for melanoma: Update of current concepts, Arch Dermatol 140:107, 2004

Morton DL et al: Sentinel-node biopsy on nodal observation in melanoma. N Engl J Med 355:1307, 2006

Petrella T et al: Single agent interleukin-2 in the treatment of metastatic melanoma: A systematic review. Cancer Treat Rev 2007 [epub ahead of print] PMID: 17562357

Rigel DS et al: ABCDE: An evolving concept in the early diagnosis of melanoma. Arch Dermatol 141:1032, 2005

Tsao H et al: Management of cutaneous melanoma. N Engl J Med 351:998, 2004

84 Head and Neck Cancer
Everett E. Vokes

Epithelial carcinomas of the head and neck arise from the mucosal surfaces in the head and neck area and typically are squamous cell in origin. This category includes tumors of the paranasal sinuses, the oral cavity, and the nasopharynx, oropharynx, hypopharynx, and larynx. Tumors of the salivary glands differ from the more common carcinomas of the head and neck in etiology, histopathology, clinical presentation, and therapy. Thyroid malignancies are described in Chap. 335.

INCIDENCE AND EPIDEMIOLOGY

The number of new cases of head and neck cancers in the United States was 40,500 in 2006, accounting for about 3% of adult malignancies. The worldwide incidence exceeds half a million cases annually. In North America and Europe, the tumors usually arise from the oral cavity, oropharynx, or larynx, whereas nasopharyngeal cancer is more common in the Mediterranean countries and in the Far East.

ETIOLOGY AND GENETICS

Alcohol and tobacco use are the most common risk factors for head and neck cancer in the United States. Smokeless tobacco is an etiologic agent for oral cancers. Other potential carcinogens include marijuana and occupational exposures such as nickel refining, exposure to textile fibers, and woodworking.

Dietary factors may contribute. The incidence of head and neck cancer is highest in people with the lowest consumption of fruits and vegetables. Certain vitamins, including carotenoids, may be protective if included in a balanced diet. Supplements of retinoids such as *cis*-retinoic acid have not been shown to prevent head and neck cancers (or lung cancer) and may increase the risk in active smokers.

Some head and neck cancers may have a viral etiology. The DNA of human papillomavirus (HPV) has been detected in the tissue of oral and tonsil cancers, and may predispose to oral and tonsillar cancer in the absence of tobacco and alcohol use. These patients can present at a somewhat younger age. The incidence of HPV-related head and neck cancer may be increasing. Epstein-Barr virus (EBV) infection is associated with nasopharyngeal cancer. Nasopharyngeal cancer occurs endemically in some countries of the Mediterranean and Far East, where EBV antibody titers can be measured to screen high-risk populations. Nasopharyngeal cancer has also been associated with consumption of salted fish.

No specific risk factors or environmental carcinogens have been identified for salivary gland tumors.

HISTOPATHOLOGY, CARCINOGENESIS, AND MOLECULAR BIOLOGY

Squamous cell head and neck cancers can be divided into well-differentiated, moderately well-differentiated, and poorly differentiated categories. Poorly differentiated tumors have a worse prognosis than well-differentiated tumors. For nasopharyngeal cancers, the less common differentiated squamous cell carcinoma is distinguished from nonkeratinizing and undifferentiated carcinoma (lymphoepithelioma) that contains infiltrating lymphocytes.

Salivary gland tumors can arise from the major (parotid, submandibular, sublingual) or minor salivary glands (located in the submucosa of the upper aerodigestive tract). Most parotid tumors are benign, but half of submandibular and sublingual gland tumors and most minor salivary gland tumors are malignant. Malignant tumors include mucoepidermoid and adenoidcystic carcinomas and adenocarcinomas.

The mucosal surface of the entire pharynx is exposed to alcohol- and tobacco-related carcinogens and is at risk for the development of a premalignant or malignant lesion, such as erythroplakia or leukoplakia (hyperplasia, dysplasia), that can progress to invasive carcinoma. Alternatively, multiple synchronous or metachronous cancers can develop. In fact, over time patients with early-stage head and neck cancer are at greater risk of dying from a second malignancy than from a recurrence of the primary disease.

Second head and neck malignancies are usually not therapy-induced; they reflect the exposure of the upper aerodigestive mucosa to the same carcinogens that caused the first cancer. These second primaries develop in the head and neck area, the lung, or the esophagus. Rarely, patients can develop a radiation therapy–induced sarcoma after having undergone prior radiotherapy for a head and neck cancer.

Chromosomal deletions and other alterations, most frequently involving chromosomes 3p, 9p, 17p, and 13q, have been identified in both premalignant and malignant head and neck lesions, as have mutations in tumor suppressor genes, such as the p53 gene. Amplification of oncogenes is less common, but overexpression of PRAD-1/bcl-1 (cyclin D1), bcl-2, transforming growth factor β, and the epidermal growth factor receptor (EGFR) have been described. EGFR overexpression has been shown to be very common, and its extent seems to be of prognostic importance.

Resected tumor specimens with histopathologically negative margins ("complete resection") can have residual tumor cells with persistent p53 mutations at the margins. Thus, a tumor-specific p53 mutation can be detected in some phenotypically "normal" surgical margins, indicating residual disease. Patients with such submicroscopic marginal involvement may have a worse prognosis than patients with truly negative margins.

CLINICAL PRESENTATION AND DIFFERENTIAL DIAGNOSIS

Most head and neck cancers occur after age 50, although these cancers can appear in younger patients, including those without known risk factors. The manifestations vary according to the stage and primary site of the tumor. Patients with nonspecific signs and symptoms in the head and neck area should be evaluated with a thorough otolaryngologic exam, particularly if symptoms persist longer than 2–4 weeks.

Cancer of the nasopharynx typically does not cause early symptoms. However, on occasion it may cause unilateral serous otitis media due to obstruction of the eustachian tube, unilateral or bilateral nasal obstruction, or epistaxis. Advanced nasopharyngeal carcinoma causes neuropathies of the cranial nerves.

Carcinomas of the oral cavity present as nonhealing ulcers, changes in the fit of dentures, or painful lesions. Tumors of the tongue base or oropharynx can cause decreased tongue mobility and alterations in speech. Cancers of the oropharynx or hypopharynx rarely cause early symptoms, but they may cause sore throat and/or otalgia.

Hoarseness may be an early symptom of laryngeal cancer, and persistent hoarseness requires referral to a specialist for indirect laryngoscopy and/or radiographic studies. If a head and neck lesion treated initially with antibiotics does not resolve in a short period, further workup is indicated; to simply continue the antibiotic treatment may be to lose the chance of early diagnosis of a malignancy.

Advanced head and neck cancers in any location can cause severe pain, otalgia, airway obstruction, cranial neuropathies, trismus, odynophagia, dysphagia, decreased tongue mobility, fistulas, skin involvement, and massive cervical lymphadenopathy, which may be unilateral or bilateral. Some patients have enlarged lymph nodes even though no primary lesion can be detected by endoscopy or biopsy; these patients are considered to have carcinoma of unknown primary (Fig. 84-1). If the enlarged nodes are located in the upper neck and the tumor cells are of squamous cell histology, the malignancy probably arose from a mucosal surface in the head or neck. Tumor cells in supraclavicular lymph nodes may also arise from a primary site in the chest or abdomen.

The physical examination should include inspection of all visible mucosal surfaces and palpation of the floor of mouth and tongue and of the neck. In addition to tumors themselves, leukoplakia (a white mucosal patch) or erythroplakia (a red mucosal patch) may be observed; these "premalignant" lesions can represent hyperplasia, dysplasia, or carcinoma in situ. All visible or palpable lesions should be biopsied. Further examination should be performed by a specialist. Additional staging procedures include CT of the head and neck to identify the extent of the disease. Patients with lymph node involvement should have chest radiography and a bone scan to screen for distant metastases. The definitive staging procedure is an endoscopic examination under anesthesia, which may include laryngoscopy, esophagoscopy, and bronchoscopy; during this procedure, multiple biopsy samples are obtained to establish a primary diagnosis, define the extent of primary disease, and identify any additional premalignant lesions or second primaries.

Head and neck tumors are classified according to the TNM system of the American Joint Committee on Cancer. This classification varies according to the specific anatomic subsite (Tables 84-1 and 84-2). Distant metastases are found in <10% of patients at initial diagnosis, but in autopsy series, microscopic involvement of the lungs, bones, or liver is more common, particularly in patients with advanced neck lymph node disease. Modern imaging techniques may increase the number of patients with clinically detectable distant metastases in the future.

In patients with lymph node involvement and no visible primary, the diagnosis should be made by lymph node excision. If the results indicate squamous cell carcinoma, a panendoscopy should be performed, with biopsy of all suspicious-appearing areas and directed biopsies of common primary sites, such as the nasopharynx, tonsil, tongue base, and pyriform sinus.

EVALUATION OF A PATIENT WITH CERVICAL ADENOPATHY

FIGURE 84-1 Evaluation of a patient with cervical adenopathy without a primary mucosal lesion; a diagnostic workup. FNA, fine-needle aspiration.

TABLE 84-1	TNM CLASSIFICATION FOR HEAD AND NECK CANCER (EXCEPT NASOPHARYNGEAL)	
Primary Tumor Site		
T Grade	Oropharynx	Hypopharynx
T1	0–2 cm	0–2 cm
T2	2.1–4 cm	>1 site, 2–4 cm
T3	>4 cm	>4 cm
T4a	Larynx, muscle of tongue, medial pterygoid, hard palate, mandible invasion	Thyroid/cricoid cartilage, hyoid bone, thyroid gland, esophagus, or central compartment soft tissue invasion
T4b	Lateral pterygoid muscle, pterygoid plates, lateral nasopharynx, or skull base or encases carotid artery invasion	Invasion of prevertebral fascia, encases carotid artery, or involves mediastinal structures
Regional Lymph Nodes (N)		
NX	Regional lymph nodes cannot be assessed	
N0	No regional lymph node metastasis	
N1	Unilateral metastasis in lymph node(s), ≤6 cm in greatest dimension, above the supraclavicular fossa	
N2	Bilateral metastasis in lymph node(s), ≤6 cm in greatest dimension, above the supraclavicular fossa	
N3	Metastasis in a lymph node(s) >6 cm and/or to supraclavicular fossa	
	N3a > 6 cm	
	N3b Extension to the supraclavicular fossa	
MX	Distant metastasis cannot be assessed	
M0	No distant metastasis	
M1	Distant metastasis	

Stage Grouping

Stage 0	Tis	N0	M0
Stage I	T1	N0	M0
Stage II	T2	N0	M0
Stage III	T3	N0	M0
	T1	N1	M0
	T2	N1	M0
	T3	N1	M0
Stage IVA	T4a	N0	M0
	T4a	N1	M0
	T1	N2	M0
	T2	N2	M0
	T3	N2	M0
	T4a	N2	M0
Stage IVB	T4b	Any N	M0
	Any T	N3	M0
Stage IVC	Any T	Any N	M1

TABLE 84-2 DEFINITION OF TNM–NASOPHARYNX

Primary Tumor (T)		Stage Grouping			
TX	Cannot be assessed	Stage 0	Tis	N0	M0
T0	No evidence	Stage I	T1	N0	M0
Tis	Carcinoma in situ	Stage IIA	T2a	N0	M0
T1	Tumor confined to the nasopharynx	Stage IIB	T1	N1	M0
T2	Tumor extends to soft tissues		T2	N1	M0
	T2a Tumor extends to the oropharynx and/or nasal cavity w/o parapharyngeal extension		T2a	N1	M0
	T2b Any tumor with parapharyngeal extension		T2b	N1	M0
T3	Tumor involves bony structures and/or paranasal sinuses		T2b	N1	M0
T4	Tumor with intracranial extension and/or involvement of cranial nerves, infratemporal fossa, hypopharynx, orbit, or masticator space	Stage III	T1	N2	M0
			T2a	N2	M0
Regional Lymph Nodes (N)			T2b	N2	M0
	The distribution and the prognostic impact of regional lymph node spread from nasopharynx cancer, particularly of the undifferentiated type, are different from those of other head and neck mucosal cancers and justify the use of a different N classification scheme.		T3	N0	M0
NX	Regional lymph nodes cannot be assessed		T3	N1	M0
N0	No regional lymph node metastasis		T3	N2	M0
N1	Unilateral metastasis in lymph node(s), ≤6 cm in greatest dimension, above the supraclavicular fossa		T4	N0	M0
N2	Bilateral metastasis in lymph node(s), ≤6 cm in greatest dimension, above the supraclavicular fossa		T4	N1	M0
N3	Metastasis in lymph node(s), >6 cm and/or to supraclavicular fossa		T4	N2	M0
N3a	Greater than 6 cm in dimension		Any T	N3	M0
N3b	Extension to the supraclavicular fossa		Any T	Any N	M1

℞ HEAD AND NECK CANCER

Patients with head and neck cancer can be categorized into three clinical groups: those with localized disease, those with locally or regionally advanced disease, and those with recurrent and/or metastatic disease. Comorbidities associated with tobacco and alcohol abuse can affect treatment outcome and define long-term risks for patients who are cured of their disease.

LOCALIZED DISEASE Nearly one-third of patients have localized disease; that is, T1 or T2 (stage I or stage II) lesions without detectable lymph node involvement or distant metastases. These lesions are treated with curative intent by surgery or radiation therapy. The choice of modality differs according to anatomic location and institutional expertise. Radiation therapy is often preferred for laryngeal cancer to preserve voice function, and surgery is preferred for small lesions in the oral cavity to avoid the long-term complications of radiation, such as xerostomia and dental decay. Overall 5-year survival is 60–90%. Most recurrences occur within the first 2 years following diagnosis and are usually local.

LOCALLY OR REGIONALLY ADVANCED DISEASE Locally or regionally advanced disease—disease with a large primary tumor and/or lymph node metastases—is the stage of presentation for >50% of patients. Such patients can also be treated with curative intent, but not with surgery or radiation therapy alone. Combined modality therapy including surgery, radiation therapy, and chemotherapy is most successful. Concomitant chemotherapy and radiation therapy appears to be the most effective approach. It can be administered either as a primary treatment for patients with unresectable disease, to pursue an organ preserving approach, or in the postoperative setting for intermediate-stage resectable tumors.

Induction Chemotherapy In this strategy, patients receive chemotherapy [usually cisplatin and fluorouracil (5-FU)] before surgery and radiation therapy. Most patients who receive three cycles show tumor reduction, and the response is clinically "complete" in up to half. This "sequential" multimodality therapy allows for organ preservation in patients with laryngeal and hypopharyngeal cancer, and it has been shown to result in higher cure rates compared with radiotherapy alone when drug combinations including cisplatin, 5-FU, and a taxane are used.

Concomitant Chemoradiotherapy With the concomitant strategy, chemotherapy and radiation therapy are given simultaneously rather than sequentially. Because most patients with head and neck cancer develop recurrent disease in the head and neck area, this approach is aimed at killing radiation-resistant cancer cells with chemotherapy. In addition, chemotherapy can enhance cell killing by radiation therapy. Toxicity (especially mucositis, grade 3 or 4 in 70–80%) is increased with concomitant chemoradiotherapy. However, metaanalyses of randomized trials document an improvement in 5-year survival of 8% with concomitant chemotherapy and radiation therapy. Results seem even more favorable when more active combinations of drugs are used but have not yet been validated in randomized trials. Five-year survival is 34–50%. In addition, concomitant chemoradiotherapy produces better laryngectomy-free survival (organ preservation) than radiation therapy alone in patients with advanced larynx cancer. The use of radiation therapy together with cisplatin has produced markedly improved survival in patients with advanced nasopharyngeal cancer.

The success of concomitant chemoradiotherapy in patients with unresectable disease has led to the testing of a similar approach in patients with resected disease as a postoperative therapy. Concomitant chemoradiotherapy produces a significant improvement over postoperative radiation therapy alone for patients whose tumors demonstrate higher risk features, such as spread beyond nodes, involvement of multiple lymph nodes, or positive margins following surgery.

Monoclonal antibody to the EGFR (cetuximab) increases survival rates when administered during radiotherapy. EGFR blockade results in radiation sensitization and has milder side effects than traditional chemotherapy agents. The integration of cetuximab into current standard chemoradiotherapy regimens is under investigation.

RECURRENT AND/OR METASTATIC DISEASE Ten percent of patients present with metastatic disease, and over half of patients with locoregionally advanced disease have recurrence, 20% outside the head and neck region. Patients with recurrent and/or metastatic disease are, with few exceptions, treated with palliative intent. Some patients may require local or regional radiation therapy for pain control, but most are given chemotherapy. Response rates to chemotherapy average only 30–50%; the duration of response averages only 3 months, and the median survival time is 6–8 months. Therefore, chemotherapy provides transient symptomatic benefit. Drugs with single-agent activity in this setting include methotrexate, 5-FU, cisplatin, paclitaxel, and docetaxel. Combinations of cisplatin with 5-FU, carboplatin with 5-FU, and cisplatin or carboplatin with paclitaxel or docetaxel are frequently used

EGFR-directed therapies, including monoclonal antibodies (e.g., cetuximab) and tyrosine kinase inhibitors (TKI) of the EGFR signaling pathway (e.g., erlotinib or gefitinib) have single-agent activity of approximately 10%. Side effects are usually limited to an acneiform rash and diarrhea (for the TKIs). Their impact on survival times when combined with traditional agents or in combination with other novel agents such as antiangiogenic compounds is under investigation.

CHEMOPREVENTION

β-Carotene and *cis*-retinoic acid can lead to the regression of leukoplakia. However, *cis*-retinoic acid does not reduce the incidence of second primaries.

TREATMENT COMPLICATIONS

Complications from treatment of head and neck cancer are usually correlated to the extent of surgery and exposure of normal tissue structures to radiation. Currently, the extent of surgery has been limited or completely replaced by chemotherapy and radiation therapy as the primary approach. Acute complications of radiation include mucositis and dysphagia. Long-term complications include xerostomia, loss of taste, decreased tongue mobility, second malignancies, dysphagia, and neck fibrosis. The complications of chemotherapy vary with the regimen used but usually include myelosuppression, mucositis, nausea and vomiting, and nephrotoxicity (with cisplatin).

The mucosal side effects of therapy can lead to malnutrition and dehydration. Many centers address issues of dentition before starting treatment, and some place feeding tubes to assure control of hydration and nutrition intake. About 50% of patients develop hypothyroidism from the treatment; thus, thyroid function should be monitored.

SALIVARY GLAND TUMORS

Most benign salivary gland tumors are treated with surgical excision, and patients with invasive salivary gland tumors are treated with surgery and radiation therapy. Neutron radiation may be particularly effective. These tumors may recur regionally; adenoidcystic carcinoma has a tendency to recur along the nerve tracks. Distant metastases may occur as late as 10–20 years after the initial diagnosis. For metastatic disease, therapy is given with palliative intent, usually chemotherapy with doxorubicin and/or cisplatin.

FURTHER READINGS

ADELSTEIN DJ et al: An intergroup phase III comparison of standard radiation therapy and two schedules of concurrent chemoradiotherapy in patients with unresectable squamous cell head and neck cancer. J Clin Oncol 21:92, 2003

BERNIER J et al: Postoperative irradiation with or without concomitant chemotherapy for locally advanced head and neck cancer. N Engl J Med 350:1945, 2004

BONNER JA et al: Radiotherapy plus cetuximab for squamous-cell carcinoma of the head and neck. N Engl J Med 354:567, 2006

BROCKSTEIN B, VOKES EE: Concurrent chemoradiotherapy for head and neck cancer. Semin Oncol 31:786, 2004

COHEN EE et al: The expanding role of systemic therapy in head and neck cancer. J Clin Oncol 22:1743, 2004

FORASTIERE AA et al: Concurrent chemotherapy and radiotherapy for organ preservation in advanced laryngeal cancer. N Engl J Med 349:2091, 2003

PFISTER DG et al: American Society of Clinical Oncology clinical practice guideline for the use of larynx-preservation strategies in the treatment of laryngeal cancer. J Clin Oncol 24:3693, 2006

SEIWERT TY et al: The chemoradiation paradigm in head and neck cancer. Nat Clin Pract Oncol 4:145, 2007

SLEBOS RJ et al: Gene expression differences associated with human papillomavirus status in head and neck squamous cell carcinoma. Clin Cancer Res 12:701, 2006

VOKES E et al: Weekly carboplatin and paclitaxel followed by concomitant TFHX chemoradiotherapy: Curative and organ preserving therapy for advanced head and neck cancer. J Clin Oncol 21:320, 2003

85 Neoplasms of the Lung
John D. Minna, Joan H. Schiller

THE MAGNITUDE OF THE PROBLEM

In 2007, primary carcinoma of the lung affected 114,760 males and 98,620 females in the United States; 86% die within 5 years of diagnosis, making it the leading cause of cancer death in both men and women. The incidence of lung cancer peaks between ages 55 and 65 years. Lung cancer accounts for 29% of all cancer deaths (31% in men, 26% in women). Lung cancer is responsible for more deaths in the United States each year than breast cancer, colon cancer, and prostate cancer combined; more women die each year of lung cancer than of breast cancer. The age-adjusted lung cancer death rate in males is decreasing, but in females it is stable or still increasing. These death rates are related to smoking; smoking cessation efforts begun 40 years ago in men are largely responsible for the change in incidence and death rates. However, women started smoking in substantial numbers about 10–15 years later than men; smoking cessation efforts need to increase for women. The 5-year overall lung cancer survival rate (15%) has nearly doubled in the past 30 years. The improvement is due to advances in combined-modality treatment with surgery, radiotherapy, and chemotherapy. The International Agency for Research on Cancer estimates that there will be over 1.18 million deaths from lung cancer worldwide in 2007, which will rise to 10 million deaths per year by 2030. This represents one lung cancer case for every 3 million cigarettes smoked. Thus, primary carcinoma of the lung is a major health problem with a generally grim prognosis.

PATHOLOGY

The term *lung cancer* is used for tumors arising from the respiratory epithelium (bronchi, bronchioles, and alveoli). Mesotheliomas, lymphomas, and stromal tumors (sarcomas) are distinct from epithelial lung cancer. Four major cell types make up 88% of all primary lung neoplasms according to the World Health Organization classification (Table 85-1). These are *squamous* or *epidermoid carcinoma*, *small cell* (also called *oat cell*) *carcinoma*, *adenocarcinoma* (including bronchioloalveolar), and *large cell carcinoma*. The remainder include undifferentiated carcinomas, carcinoids, bronchial gland tumors (including adenoid cystic carcinomas and mucoepidermoid tumors), and rarer tumor types. The various cell types have different natural histories and responses to therapy, and thus a correct histologic diagnosis by an experienced pathologist is the first step to correct treatment. In the past 25 years, adenocarcinoma has replaced squamous cell carcinoma as the most frequent histologic subtype, and the incidence of small cell carcinoma is on the decline.

Major treatment decisions are made on the basis of whether a tumor is classified as a small cell lung carcinoma (SCLC) or as one of the non-small cell lung cancer (NSCLC) varieties (squamous, adenocarcinoma, large cell carcinoma, bronchioloalveolar carcinoma, and mixed ver-

TABLE 85-1   FREQUENCY, AGE-ADJUSTED INCIDENCE, AND SURVIVAL RATES FOR DIFFERENT HISTOLOGIC TYPES OF LUNG CANCER[a]

Histologic Type of Thoracic Malignancy	Frequency, %	Age-Adjusted Rate	5-Year Survival Rate (All Stages)
Adenocarcinoma (and all subtypes)	32	17	17
Bronchioloalveolar carcinoma	3	1.4	42
Squamous cell (epidermoid) carcinoma	29	15	15
Small cell carcinoma	18	9	5
Large cell carcinoma	9	5	11
Carcinoid	1.0	0.5	83
Mucoepidermoid carcinoma	0.1	<0.1	39
Adenoid cystic carcinoma	<0.1	<0.1	48
Sarcoma and other soft tissue tumors	0.1	0.1	30
All others and unspecified carcinomas	11.0	6	NA
Total	100	52	14

[a]Data on histology frequency and age-adjusted incidence rates per 100,000 U.S. population are from 60,514 cases of invasive lung cancer involving all races and both sexes obtained from the data for 1983–1987 of the Surveillance, Epidemiology, and End Results (SEER) Program of the National Cancer Institute; 5-year relative survival rates for all stages, all races, and both sexes are from the SEER data on 87,128 carcinomas, 1978–1986. NA, not available.
Source: Summarized from Travis et al: Cancer 75:191, 1995.

sions of these). The histologic distinctions between SCLC and NSCLC include the following: SCLC has scant cytoplasm, small hyperchromatic nuclei with fine chromatin pattern and indistinct nucleoli with diffuse sheets of cells, while NSCLC has abundant cytoplasm, pleomorphic nuclei with coarse chromatin pattern, prominent nucleoli, and glandular or squamous architecture. Among the molecular distinctions, SCLC displays neuroendocrine properties absent in NSCLCs, production of specific peptide hormones [such as adrenocorticotropic hormone (ACTH), arginine vasopressin (AVP), atrial natriuretic factor (ANF), gastrin-releasing peptide (GRP)] and differences in oncogene and tumor-suppressor gene changes (SCLCs have *RB* mutations in 90% and *p16* abnormalities in 10% but never have *KRAS* or *EGFR* mutations, while NSCLCs have *RB* mutations in only 20%, *p16* changes in 50%, *KRAS* mutations in 30%, and *EGFR* mutations in ~10%). Both types have frequent *p53* mutations (>70% in SCLC and >50% in NSCLC), 3p allele loss (>90% in both), telomerase expression (>90% in both), and tumor-acquired promoter methylation in multiple genes (>80% in both, often involving the same genes, including *RASSF1A*). SCLCs are initially very responsive to combination chemotherapy (>70% responses, with 30% complete responses) and to radiotherapy (>90% responses); however, most SCLCs ultimately relapse. By contrast, NSCLCs have objective tumor shrinkage following radiotherapy in 30–50% of cases and response to combination chemotherapy in 20–35% of cases. At presentation, SCLCs usually have already spread such that surgery is unlikely to be curative and, given their responsiveness to chemotherapy, are managed primarily by chemotherapy with or without radiotherapy. Chemotherapy clearly provides symptom relief and survival advantage. By contrast, NSCLCs that are clinically localized at the time of presentation may be cured with either surgery or radiotherapy. The beneficial role of chemotherapy in NSCLC is in palliation of symptoms and improving survival modestly.

Although it is important to differentiate whether a tumor is SCLC or NSCLC for both prognostic and therapeutic reasons, it is less important to identify the histologic subtypes of NSCLC. Stage for stage, the histology of NSCLC is not an important prognostic factor, and in the past the different subtypes of NSCLC were rarely treated differently. However, lung adenocarcinomas (often with bronchioloalveolar features) may be responsive to therapy aimed at the epidermal growth factor receptor (EGFR) (see below). In addition, patients with squamous cell carcinoma may not be appropriate candidates for antiangiogenic therapy due to an increased risk of bleeding (see below).

Eighty-five percent of patients with lung cancer of all histologic types are current or former cigarette smokers. Of the annual 213,380 new cases of lung cancer, ~50% develop in former smokers. With increased success in smoking cessation efforts, the number of former smokers will grow, and these individuals will be important candidates for early detection and chemoprevention efforts.

All histologic types of lung cancer are due to smoking. However, lung cancer can also occur in individuals who have never smoked. By far the most common form of lung cancer arising in lifetime nonsmokers, in women, and in young patients (<45 years) is adenocarcinoma. However, in nonsmokers with adenocarcinoma involving the lung, the possibility of other primary sites should be considered. Squamous and small cell cancers usually present as central masses with endobronchial growth, while adenocarcinomas and large cell cancers tend to present as peripheral nodules or masses, frequently with pleural involvement. Squamous and large cell cancers cavitate in 10–20% of cases. Bronchioloalveolar carcinoma (BAC) is a subtype of adenocarcinoma that grows along the alveoli without invasion and can present radiographically as a single mass; as a diffuse, multinodular lesion; as a fluffy infiltrate; and on screening CT scans as a "ground glass" opacity. The male to female ratio is 1:1, and while BAC can be associated with smoking, it is often found in nonsmokers. Histologically pure BAC is relatively rare. More common is adenocarcinoma with BAC features. BAC may present in a mucinous form, which tends to be multicentric, and a nonmucinous form, which tends to be solitary. Many of the EGFR mutations found in nonsmoking lung cancers occur in adenocarcinomas with BAC histologic features.

ETIOLOGY

Most lung cancers are caused by carcinogens and tumor promoters inhaled via cigarette smoking. The prevalence of smoking in the United States is 28% for males and 25% for females, age 18 years or older; 38% of high school seniors smoke. The relative risk of developing lung cancer is increased about thirteenfold by active smoking and about 1.5-fold by long-term passive exposure to cigarette smoke. Chronic obstructive pulmonary disease, which is also smoking-related, further increases the risk of developing lung cancer. The lung cancer death rate is related to the total amount (often expressed in "cigarette pack-years") of cigarettes smoked, such that the risk is increased 60- to 70-fold for a man smoking two packs a day for 20 years as compared with a nonsmoker. Conversely, the chance of developing lung cancer decreases with cessation of smoking but may never return to the nonsmoker level. The increase in lung cancer rate in women is also associated with a rise in cigarette smoking. Women have a higher relative risk per given exposure than men (~1.5-fold higher). This sex difference may be due to a greater susceptibility to tobacco carcinogens in women, although the data are controversial.

About 15% of lung cancers occur in individuals who have never smoked. The majority of these are found in women. The reason for this sex difference is not known but may be related to hormonal factors.

Efforts to get people to stop smoking are mandatory. However, smoking cessation is extremely difficult, because the smoking habit represents a powerful addiction to nicotine (Chap. 390). Smoking addiction is both biologic and psychosocial. Different methods are available to help motivated smokers give up the habit, including counseling, behavioral therapy, nicotine replacement (gum, patch, sublingual spray, inhaler), and antidepressants (such as bupropion). However, one year after starting such smoking cessation aids, the methods are successful in only 20–25% of individuals. Preventing people from starting to smoke is thus very important, and this primary prevention effort needs to be targeted to children since most cigarette smoking addiction occurs during the teenage years.

Radiation is another environmental cause of lung cancer. People exposed to high levels of radon or receiving thoracic radiation therapy have a higher than normal incidence of lung cancer, particularly if they smoke.

BIOLOGY AND MOLECULAR PATHOGENESIS

Molecular genetic studies have shown the acquisition by lung cancer cells of a number of genetic lesions, including activation of dominant oncogenes and inactivation of tumor-suppressor or recessive oncogenes (Chaps. 79 and 80). In fact, lung cancer cells may have to accumulate a large number (perhaps ≥20) of such lesions. A small subpopulation (perhaps <1%) of cells within a tumor are responsible for the full malignant behavior of the tumor;—these are referred to as *cancer stem cells*. As part of this concept, the large bulk of the cells in a cancer are "offspring" of these cancer stem cells and, while clonally related to the cancer stem cell subpopulation, by themselves cannot regenerate the full malignant phenotype such as metastatic disease and unlimited replicative potential. These cancer stem cells are very important to identify since successful treatment of the tumor will require eradication of this stem cell component. These cancer stem cells may be more resistant to chemotherapy than the bulk of the tumor. Features that distinguish cancer stem cells from the remaining tumor cells have not been defined and validated.

Activation of Dominant Oncogenes Changes in dominant oncogenes include point mutations in the coding regions of the *RAS* family of oncogenes (particularly in the *KRAS* gene in adenocarcinoma of the lung); mutations in the tyrosine kinase domain of the EGFR found in adenocarcinomas from nonsmokers (~10% in the United States with rates >50% in nonsmoking East Asian patients); occasional mutations in *BRAF* and *PIK3CA* or activation of the PIK3CA/AKT/mTor pathway; amplification, rearrangement, and/or loss of transcriptional control of *myc* family oncogenes (c-, N-, and L-*myc*; changes in c-*myc* are found in non-small cell cancers, while changes in all *myc* family members are found in SCLC); overexpression of bcl-2 and other antiapoptotic proteins; overexpression of other EGFR family members such as Her-2/neu, and ERBB3; and activated expression of the telomerase gene in >90% of lung cancers. Genome-wide approaches are identifying other amplified or mutated dominant oncogenes that could be important new therapeutic targets.

Inactivation of Tumor-Suppressor Genes A large number of tumor-suppressor genes (recessive oncogenes) have been identified that are inactivated during the pathogenesis of lung cancer. This usually occurs by a tumor-acquired inactivating mutation of one allele [seen, for example, in the *p53* and retinoblastoma (*RB*) tumor-suppressor gene] or tumor-acquired inactivation of expression by tumor-acquired promoter DNA methylation (seen, for example, in the case of the *p16* and *RASSF1A* tumor-suppressor genes), which is then coupled with physical loss of the other parental allele ("loss of heterozygosity"). This leaves the tumor cell with only the functionally inactive allele and thus loss of function of the growth-regulatory tumor-suppressor gene. Genome-wide approaches have identified many such genes involved in lung cancer pathogenesis, including *p53*, *RB*, *RASSF1A*, *SEMA3B*, *SEMA3F*, *FUS1*, *p16*, *LKB1*, *RARβ*, and *FHIT*. Several tumor-suppressor genes on chromosome 3p appear to be involved in nearly all lung cancers. Allelic loss for this region occurs very early in lung cancer pathogenesis, including in histologically normal smoking-damaged lung epithelium.

Autocrine Growth Factors The large number of genetic and epigenetic lesions shows that lung cancer, like other common epithelial malignancies, arises as a multistep process that is likely to involve both carcinogens causing mutation ("initiation") and tumor promoters. Prevention can be directed at both processes. Lung cancer cells produce many peptide hormones and express receptors for these hormones. They can promote tumor cell growth in an "autocrine" fashion.

Highly carcinogenic derivatives of nicotine are formed in cigarette smoke. Lung cancer cells of all histologic types (and the cells from which they are derived) express nicotinic acetylcholine receptors. Nicotine activates signaling pathways in tumor and normal cells that block apoptosis. Thus, nicotine itself could be directly involved in lung cancer pathogenesis both as a mutagen and tumor promoter.

Inherited Predisposition to Lung Cancer While an inherited predisposition to develop lung cancer is not common, several features suggest a potential for familial association. People with inherited mutations in *RB* (patients with retinoblastomas living to adulthood) and *p53* (Li-Fraumeni syndrome) genes may develop lung cancer. First-degree relatives of lung cancer probands have a two- to threefold excess risk of lung cancer or other cancers, many of which are not smoking-related. An as yet unidentified gene in chromosome region 6q23 was found to segregate in families at high risk of developing lung cancer of all histologic types. Finally, certain polymorphisms of the P450 enzyme system (which metabolizes carcinogens) or chromosome fragility (*mutagen sensitivity*) genotypes are associated with the development of lung cancer. The use of any of these inherited differences to identify persons at very high risk of developing lung cancer would be useful in early detection and prevention efforts.

Therapy Targeted at Molecular Abnormalities A detailed understanding of the molecular pathogenesis should be applicable to new methods of early diagnosis, prevention, and treatment of lung cancer. Two examples of this translation involve EGFR and vascular endothelial growth factor (VEGF). EGFR belongs to the ERBB (HER) family of protooncogenes, including EGFR (ERBB1), Her2/neu (ERBB2), HER3 (ERBB3), and HER4 (ERBB4), cell-surface receptors consisting of an extracellular ligand-binding domain, a transmembrane structure, and an intracellular tyrosine kinase (TK) domain. The binding of ligand to receptor activates receptor dimerization and TK autophosphorylation, initiating a cascade of intracellular events, leading to increased cell

proliferation, angiogenesis, metastasis, and a decrease in apoptosis (Chap. 80). Overexpression of EGFR protein or amplification of the *EGFR* gene has been found in as many as 70% of NSCLCs.

Activating/oncogenic mutations (usually a missense or a small deletion mutation) in the TK domain of EGFR have been identified. These are found most commonly in women, East Asians, patients who have never smoked, and those with adenocarcinoma and BAC histology. This is also the group of patients who are most likely to have dramatic responses to drugs that inhibit TK activation [tyrosine kinase inhibitors (TKIs)]. EGFR mutations are almost never found in cancers other than lung cancer, nor in lung cancers that have *KRAS* mutations. These EGFR mutations, often associated with amplification of the *EGFR* gene, usually confer sensitivity of these lung cancers to EGFR TKIs (such as gefitinib or erlotinib), resulting in clinically beneficial tumor responses that unfortunately are still not permanent. In many cases the development of EGFR TKI resistance is associated with the development of another mutation in the *EGFR* gene (*T790M* mutation), or amplification of the *c-met* oncogene. However, other drugs with EGFR TKI activity are in development to which the lung cancers with these resistance mutations will respond as are drugs targeting c-met or its pathways.

The discovery of EGFR mutation/amplification driving lung cancer growth and the dramatic response of these tumors to oral EGFR TKI therapy has prompted a widespread search for other drugs "targeted" against oncogenic changes in lung cancer. An important example of another such target is VEGF, which, while not mutated, is inappropriately produced by lung cancers and stimulates tumor angiogenesis (Chap. 80). VEGF is often overexpressed in lung cancer, and the resulting increase in tumor microvessel density correlates with poor prognosis. A monoclonal antibody to the VEGF ligand, bevacizumab, has significant antitumor effects when used with chemotherapy in lung cancer (see below).

Molecular Profiles Predict Survival and Response Just as the presence of EGFR TK domain mutations and amplification is an excellent predictor of response to EGFR TKIs, molecular predictors of response to standard chemotherapy and other new targeted agents are being sought. Lung cancers can be molecularly typed at the time of diagnosis to yield information that predicts survival and defines agents to which the tumor is most likely to respond. One example is the identification of alterations in lung cancer DNA repair pathways that may predict resistance to chemotherapy. Patients whose tumors exhibit low activity of the excision-repair-cross complementation group 1 (ERCC1) proteins typically have a worse prognosis as they are unable to repair DNA adducts in the tumor. However, retrospective analysis shows that when treated with cisplatin, patients with tumors expressing low levels of ERCC1 activity appear to do better, as they are unable to repair DNA adducts caused by cisplatin, while patients with high ERCC1 activity actually do worse with cisplatin-based chemotherapy. Although these protein or gene expression "signatures" have yet to be validated in large prospective studies, it is possible that such information will allow future therapy to be tailored to the characteristics of each patient's tumor. Mass spectroscopy-based proteomic studies have identified unique protein patterns in the serum of patients, one of which allows for early diagnosis, while another can predict sensitivity or resistance to drugs. However, such methods have not been validated and may be difficult to implement in a patient care setting.

CLINICAL MANIFESTATIONS

Lung cancer gives rise to signs and symptoms caused by local tumor growth, invasion or obstruction of adjacent structures, growth in regional nodes through lymphatic spread, growth in distant metastatic sites after hematogenous dissemination, and remote effects of tumor products (paraneoplastic syndromes) (Chaps. 96 and 97).

Although 5–15% of patients with lung cancer are identified while they are asymptomatic, usually as a result of a routine chest radiograph or through the use of screening CT scans, most patients present with some sign or symptom. Central or endobronchial growth of the primary tumor may cause cough, hemoptysis, wheeze and stridor, dyspnea, and postobstructive pneumonitis (fever and productive cough). Peripheral growth of the primary tumor may cause pain from pleural or chest wall involvement, dyspnea on a restrictive basis, and symptoms of lung abscess resulting from tumor cavitation. Regional spread of tumor in the thorax (by contiguous growth or by metastasis to regional lymph nodes) may cause tracheal obstruction, esophageal compression with dysphagia, recurrent laryngeal nerve paralysis with hoarseness, phrenic nerve paralysis with elevation of the hemidiaphragm and dyspnea, and sympathetic nerve paralysis with Horner's syndrome (enophthalmos, ptosis, miosis, and ipsilateral loss of sweating). Malignant pleural effusion often leads to dyspnea. *Pancoast's* (or *superior sulcus tumor*) *syndrome* results from local extension of a tumor growing in the apex of the lung with involvement of the eighth cervical and first and second thoracic nerves, with shoulder pain that characteristically radiates in the ulnar distribution of the arm, often with radiologic destruction of the first and second ribs. Often Horner's syndrome and Pancoast's syndrome coexist. Other problems of regional spread include *superior vena cava syndrome* from vascular obstruction; pericardial and cardiac extension with resultant tamponade, arrhythmia, or cardiac failure; lymphatic obstruction with resultant pleural effusion; and lymphangitic spread through the lungs with hypoxemia and dyspnea. In addition, BAC can spread transbronchially, producing tumor growing along multiple alveolar surfaces with impairment of gas exchange, respiratory insufficiency, dyspnea, hypoxemia, and sputum production.

Extrathoracic metastatic disease is found at autopsy in >50% of patients with squamous carcinoma, 80% of patients with adenocarcinoma and large cell carcinoma, and >95% of patients with small cell cancer. Lung cancer metastases may occur in virtually every organ system. Common clinical problems related to metastatic lung cancer include brain metastases with headache, nausea, and neurologic deficits; bone metastases with pain and pathologic fractures; bone marrow invasion with cytopenias or leukoerythroblastosis; liver metastases causing liver dysfunction, biliary obstruction, anorexia, and pain; lymph node metastases in the supraclavicular region and occasionally in the axilla and groin; and spinal cord compression syndromes from epidural or bone metastases. Adrenal metastases are common but rarely cause adrenal insufficiency.

Paraneoplastic syndromes are common in patients with lung cancer and may be the presenting finding or first sign of recurrence. In addition, paraneoplastic syndromes may mimic metastatic disease and, unless detected, lead to inappropriate palliative rather than curative treatment. Often the paraneoplastic syndrome may be relieved with successful treatment of the tumor. In some cases, the pathophysiology of the paraneoplastic syndrome is known, particularly when a hormone with biologic activity is secreted by a tumor (Chap. 96). However, in many cases the pathophysiology is unknown. Systemic symptoms of anorexia, cachexia, weight loss (seen in 30% of patients), fever, and suppressed immunity are paraneoplastic syndromes of unknown etiology. *Endocrine syndromes* are seen in 12% of patients: hypercalcemia and hypophosphatemia resulting from the ectopic production by squamous tumors of parathyroid hormone (PTH) or, more commonly, PTH-related peptide; hyponatremia with the syndrome of inappropriate secretion of antidiuretic hormone or possibly atrial natriuretic factor by small cell cancer; and ectopic secretion of ACTH by small cell cancer. ACTH secretion usually results in additional electrolyte disturbances, especially hypokalemia, rather than the changes in body habitus that occur in Cushing's syndrome from a pituitary adenoma.

Skeletal–connective tissue syndromes include clubbing in 30% of cases (usually non-small cell carcinomas) and hypertrophic pulmonary osteoarthropathy in 1–10% of cases (usually adenocarcinomas), with periostitis and clubbing causing pain, tenderness, and swelling over the affected bones and a positive bone scan. *Neurologic-myopathic syndromes* are seen in only 1% of patients but are dramatic and include the myasthenic *Eaton-Lambert syndrome* and retinal blindness with small cell cancer, while peripheral neuropathies, subacute cerebellar degeneration, cortical degeneration, and polymyositis are seen with all lung cancer types. Many of these are caused by autoimmune responses such as the development of anti-voltage-gated calcium channel antibodies in the Eaton-Lambert syndrome (Chap. 97). Coagulation, thrombotic, or other hematologic manifestations occur in 1–8% of patients and include migratory venous thrombophlebitis (*Trousseau's syndrome*), nonbacterial thrombotic (marantic) endocarditis with arterial emboli, disseminated intravascular coagulation with hemorrhage, anemia, granulocytosis, and leukoerythroblastosis. Thrombotic disease complicating cancer is usually a poor prognostic sign. Cutaneous manifestations such as dermatomyositis and acanthosis nigricans are uncommon (1%), as are the renal manifestations of nephrotic syndrome or glomerulonephritis (≤1%).

DIAGNOSIS AND STAGING

SCREENING

Most patients with lung cancer present with advanced disease, raising the question of whether screening would detect these tumors at an earlier stage when they are theoretically more curable. The role of screening high-risk patients (for example current or former smokers >50 years of age) for early stage lung cancers is debated. Results from five randomized screening studies in the 1980s of chest x-rays with or without cytologic analysis of sputum did not show any impact on lung cancer–specific mortality from screening high-risk patients, although earlier-stage cancers were detected in the screened groups. These studies have been criticized for their design and statistical analyses, but they led to current recommendations not to use these tools to screen for lung cancer. However, low-dose, noncontrast, thin-slice, helical, or spiral CT has emerged as a possible new tool for lung cancer screening. Spiral CT is a scan in which only the pulmonary parenchyma is examined, thus negating the use of intravenous contrast and the necessity of a physician being present at the exam. The scan can usually be done quickly (within one breath) and involves low doses of radiation. In a nonrandomized study of current and former smokers from the Early Lung Cancer Action Project (ELCAP), low-dose CT was shown to be more sensitive than chest x-ray for detecting lung nodules and lung cancer in early stages. Survival from date of diagnosis is also long (10-year survival predicted to be 92% in screening-detected stage I NSCLC patients). Other nonrandomized CT screening studies of asymptomatic current or former smokers also found that early lung cancer cases were diagnosed more often with CT screening than predicted by standard incidence data. However, no decline in the number of advanced lung cancer cases or deaths from lung cancer was noted in the screened group. Thus, spiral CT appears to diagnose more lung cancer without improving lung cancer mortality. Concerns include the influence of lead-time bias, length-time bias, and over-diagnosis (cancers so slow-growing that they are unlikely to cause the death of the patient). Over-diagnosis is a well-established problem in prostate cancer screening, but it is surprising that some lung cancers are not fatal. However, many of the small adenocarcinomas found as "ground glass" opacities on screening CT appear to have such long doubling times (>400 days) that they may never harm the patient. While CT screening will detect lung cancer in 1–4% of the patients screened over a 5-year period, it also detects a substantial number of false-positive lung lesions (ranging from 25 to 75% in different series) that need follow-up and evaluation. The appropriate management of these small lesions is undefined. Unnecessary treatment of these patients may include thoracotomy and lung resection, thus adding to the cost, mortality, and morbidity of treatment. A large, randomized trial of CT screening for lung cancer (National Lung Cancer Screening Trial) involving ~55,000 individuals has completed accrual and will provide definitive data in the next several years on whether screening reduces lung cancer mortality. Until these results become available, routine CT screening for lung cancer cannot be recommended for any risk group. For those patients who want to be screened, physicians need to discuss the possible benefits and risks of such screening, including the risk of false-positive scans that could result in multiple follow-up CTs and possible biopsies for a malignancy that may not be life-threatening.

ESTABLISHING A DIAGNOSIS OF LUNG CANCER

Once signs, symptoms, or screening studies suggest lung cancer, a tissue diagnosis must be established. Tumor tissue can be obtained by a bronchial or transbronchial biopsy during fiberoptic bronchoscopy; by node biopsy during mediastinoscopy; from the operative specimen at the time of definitive surgical resection; by percutaneous biopsy of an enlarged lymph node, soft tissue mass, lytic bone lesion, bone marrow, or pleural lesion; by fine-needle aspiration of thoracic or extrathoracic tumor masses using CT guidance; or from an adequate cell block obtained from a malignant pleural effusion. In most cases, the pathologist should be able to make a definite diagnosis of epithelial malignancy and distinguish small cell from non-small cell lung cancer.

STAGING PATIENTS WITH LUNG CANCER

Lung cancer staging consists of two parts: first, a determination of the location of tumor (anatomic staging) and, second, an assessment of a patient's ability to withstand various antitumor treatments (physiologic staging). In a patient with NSCLC, *resectability* (whether the tumor can be entirely removed by a standard surgical procedure such as a lobectomy or pneumonectomy), which depends on the anatomic stage of the tumor, and *operability* (whether the patient can tolerate such a surgical procedure), which depends on the cardiopulmonary function of the patient, are determined.

Non-Small Cell Lung Cancer The TNM International Staging System should be used for cases of NSCLC, particularly in preparing patients for curative attempts with surgery or radiotherapy (Table 85-2). The various T (tumor size), N (regional node involvement), and M (presence or absence of distant metastasis) factors are combined to form different stage groups. At presentation, approximately one-third of patients have disease localized enough for a curative attempt with surgery or radiotherapy (patients with stage I or II disease and some with stage IIIA disease), one-third have distant metastatic disease (stage IV disease), and one-third have local or regional disease that may or may not be amenable to a curative attempt (some patients with stage IIIA disease and others with stage IIIB disease) (see below). This staging system provides useful prognostic information.

Small Cell Lung Cancer A simple two-stage system is used. In this system, *limited-stage disease* (seen in about 30% of all patients with SCLC) is defined as disease confined to one hemithorax and regional lymph nodes (including mediastinal, contralateral hilar, and usually ipsilateral supraclavicular nodes), while *extensive-stage disease* (seen in about 70% of patients) is defined as disease exceeding those boundaries. Clinical studies such as physical examination, x-rays, CT and bone scans, and bone marrow examination are used in staging. In part, the definition of limited-stage disease relates to whether the known tumor can be encompassed within a tolerable radiation therapy port. Thus, contralateral supraclavicular nodes, recurrent laryngeal nerve involvement, and superior vena caval obstruction can all be part of limited-stage disease. However, cardiac tamponade, malignant pleural effusion, and bilateral pulmonary parenchymal involvement generally qualify disease as extensive-stage because the organs within a curative radiation therapy port cannot safely tolerate curative radiation doses.

LUNG CANCER STAGING PROCEDURES

(Table 85-3) All patients with lung cancer should have a complete history and physical examination, with evaluation of all other medical problems, determination of performance status and history of weight loss, and a CT scan of the chest and abdomen with contrast. Positron emission tomography (PET) scans are sensitive in detecting both intrathoracic and metastatic disease. PET is useful in assessing the mediastinum and solitary pulmonary nodules. A standardized uptake value (SUV) of >2.5 is highly suspicious for malignancy. False negatives can be seen in

TABLE 85-2   TUMOR, NODE, METASTASIS INTERNATIONAL STAGING SYSTEM FOR LUNG CANCER

Stage	TNM Descriptors	5-Year Survival Rate, %	
		Clinical Stage	Surgical-Pathologic Stage
IA	T1 N0 M0	61	67
IB	T2 N0 M0	38	57
IIA	T1 N1 M0	34	55
IIB	T2 N1 M0	24	39
IIB	T3 N0 M0	22	38
IIIA	T3 N1 M0	9	25
	T1–2–3 N2 M0	13	23
IIIB	T4 N0–1–2 M0	7	<5
	T1–2–3–4 N3 M0	3	<3
IV	Any T any N M1	1	<1

Tumor (T) Status Descriptor

T0	No evidence of a primary tumor
TX	Primary tumor cannot be assessed, or tumor proven by the presence of malignant cells in sputum or bronchial washings but not visualized by imaging or bronchoscopy
TIS	Carcinoma in situ
T1	Tumor <3 cm in greatest dimension, surrounded by lung or visceral pleura, without bronchoscopic evidence of invasion more proximal than lobar bronchus (i.e., not in main bronchus)
T2	Tumor with any of following: >3 cm in greatest dimension; involves main bronchus, ≥2 cm distal to the carina; invades visceral pleura; associated with atelectasis or obstructive pneumonitis extending to hilum but does not involve entire lung
T3	Tumor of any size that directly invades any of the following: chest wall (including superior sulcus tumors), diaphragm, mediastinal pleura, parietal pericardium; or tumor in main bronchus <2 cm distal to carina but without involvement of carina; or associated atelectasis or obstructive pneumonitis of entire lung
T4	Tumor of any size that invades any of the following: mediastinum, heart, great vessels, trachea, esophagus, vertebral body, carina; or tumor with a malignant pleural or pericardial effusion,[a] or with satellite tumor nodule(s) within the ipsilateral primary-tumor lobe of the lung

Lymph Node (N) Involvement Descriptor

NX	Regional lymph nodes cannot be assessed
N0	No regional lymph node metastasis
N1	Metastasis to ipsilateral peribronchial and/or ipsilateral hilar lymph nodes, and intrapulmonary nodes involved by direct extension of the primary tumor
N2	Metastasis to ipsilateral mediastinal and/or subcarinal lymph node(s)
N3	Metastasis to contralateral mediastinal, contralateral hilar, ipsilateral or contralateral scalene, or supraclavicular lymph node(s)

Distant Metastasis (M) Descriptor

MX	Presence of distant metastasis cannot be assessed
M0	No distant metastasis
M1	Distant metastasis present[b]

[a]Most pleural effusions associated with lung cancer are due to tumor. However, in a few patients with multiple negative cytopathologic exams of a non-bloody, non-exudative pleural or pericardial effusion that clinical judgment dictates is not related to the tumor, the effusion should be excluded as a staging element and the patient's disease staged as T1, T2, or T3.

[b]Separate metastatic pulmonary tumor nodule(s) in the ipsilateral nonprimary tumor lobe(s) of the lung are classified as M1.

Source: Adapted from CF Mountain. Revisions in the International System for Staging of Lung Cancer. Chest 111:1710, 1997; with permission.

diabetes, in slow-growing tumors such as BAC, in concurrent infection such as tuberculosis, and in lesions <8 mm. False positives can also be seen in infections and granulomatous disease. Thus, PET should never be used alone to diagnose lung cancer, mediastinal involvement, or metastases. Instead, its primary function is to help guide a mediastinal biopsy for staging purposes and to help identify sites of metastatic disease. Fiberoptic bronchoscopy obtains material for pathologic examination

TABLE 85-3 PRETREATMENT STAGING PROCEDURES FOR PATIENTS WITH LUNG CANCER

All Patients

Complete history and physical examination
   Determination of performance status and weight loss
Complete blood count with platelet determination
Measurement of serum electrolytes, glucose, and calcium; renal and liver function tests
Electrocardiogram
Skin test for tuberculosis
Chest x-ray
CT scan of chest and abdomen
CT or MRI scan of brain and radionuclide scan of bone if any finding suggests the presence of tumor metastasis in these organs
Fiberoptic bronchoscopy with washings, brushings, and biopsy of suspicious lesions unless medically contraindicated or if it would not alter therapy (e.g., very late stage patient)
X-rays of suspicious bony lesions detected by scan or symptom
Barium swallow radiographic examination if esophageal symptoms exist
Pulmonary function studies and arterial blood gas measurements if signs or symptoms of respiratory insufficiency are present
Biopsy of accessible lesions suspicious for cancer if a histologic diagnosis is not yet made or if treatment or staging decisions would be based on whether or not a lesion contained cancer

Patients with Non-small Cell Lung Cancer Who Have No Contraindication[a] to Curative Surgery or Radiotherapy with or without Chemotherapy

All the above procedures, plus the following:
PET scan to evaluate mediastinum and detect metastatic disease
Pulmonary function tests and arterial blood gas measurements
Coagulation tests
CT or MRI scan of brain if symptoms suggestive
Cardiopulmonary exercise testing if performance status or pulmonary function tests are borderline
   If surgical resection is planned: surgical evaluation of the mediastinum at mediastinoscopy or at thoracotomy
   If the patient is a poor surgical risk or a candidate for curative radiotherapy: transthoracic fine-needle aspiration biopsy or transbronchial forceps biopsy of peripheral lesions if material from routine fiberoptic bronchoscopy is negative

Patients Presenting with Small Cell or Advanced Non-small Cell Lung Cancer

For proven small cell lung cancer, all the procedures under "All Patients," plus the following:
   CT or MRI scan of brain
   Bone marrow aspiration and biopsy (if peripheral blood counts abnormal)
For non-small cell lung cancer or cancer of unknown histology, all the procedures under "All Patients," plus the following:
   Fiberoptic bronchoscopy if indicated by hemoptysis, obstruction, pneumonitis, or no histologic diagnosis of cancer
   Biopsy of accessible lesions suspicious for tumor to obtain a histologic diagnosis or if therapy would be altered by finding of tumor
   Transthoracic fine-needle aspiration biopsy or transbronchial forceps biopsy of peripheral lesions if fiberoptic bronchoscopy is negative and no other material exists for a histologic diagnosis
   Diagnostic and therapeutic thoracentesis if a pleural effusion is present

[a]Patients with non-small cell lung cancer and extrathoracic metastatic disease, malignant pleural effusion, or intrathoracic disease beyond the bounds of a tolerable radiotherapy port.

Note: CT, computed tomography; PET, positron emission tomography.

and information on tumor size, location, degree of bronchial obstruction (i.e., assesses resectability), and recurrence.

Chest radiographs and CT scans are needed to evaluate tumor size and nodal involvement; old radiographs are useful for comparison. CT scans of the thorax and upper abdomen are of use in the preoperative staging of NSCLC to detect mediastinal nodes and pleural extension and occult abdominal disease (e.g., liver, adrenal), and in planning curative radiation therapy. However, mediastinal nodal involvement should be documented histologically if the findings will influence therapeutic decisions. Thus, sampling of lymph nodes via mediastinoscopy or thoracotomy to establish the presence or absence of N2 or

N3 nodal involvement is crucial in considering a curative surgical approach for patients with NSCLC with clinical stage I, II, or III disease, regardless of whether the PET is positive or negative. A preoperative mediastinoscopy may not need to be done in patients with normal-size nodes (by CT) that are PET-negative, as the discovery of micrometastases is unlikely to change the preoperative management of the disease, although lymph node sampling should be done intraoperatively. A standard nomenclature for referring to the location of lymph nodes involved with cancer has evolved (Fig. 85-1). Unless the CT-detected abnormalities are unequivocal, histology of suspicious extrathoracic lesions should be confirmed by procedures such as fine-needle aspiration if the patient would otherwise be considered for curative treatment. In SCLC, CT scans are used in the planning of chest radiation treatment and in the assessment of the response to chemotherapy and radiation therapy. Surgery or radiotherapy can make interpretation of conventional chest x-rays difficult; after treatment, CT scans can provide good evidence of tumor recurrence.

If signs or symptoms suggest involvement by tumor, brain CT or bone scans are performed, as well as radiography of any suspicious bony lesions. Any accessible lesions suspicious for cancer should be biopsied if involvement would influence treatment.

In patients presenting with a mass lesion on chest x-ray or CT scan and no obvious contraindications to a curative approach after the initial evaluation, the mediastinum must be investigated. Approaches vary among centers and include performing chest CT scan and mediastinoscopy (for right-sided tumors) or mediastinotomy (for left-sided lesions) on all patients and proceeding directly to thoracotomy for staging of the mediastinum. Patients who present with disease that is confined to the chest but not resectable, and who thus are candidates for neoadjuvant chemotherapy plus surgery or for curative radiotherapy with or without chemotherapy, should have additional tests done as indicated to evaluate specific symptoms. In patients presenting with NSCLC that is not curable, all the general staging procedures are done, plus fiberoptic bronchoscopy as indicated to evaluate hemoptysis, obstruction, or pneumonitis, as well as thoracentesis with cytologic examination (and chest tube drainage as indicated) if fluid is present. As a rule, a radiographic finding of an isolated lesion (such as an enlarged adrenal gland) should be confirmed as cancer by fine-needle aspiration before a curative attempt is rejected.

STAGING OF SMALL CELL LUNG CANCER

Pretreatment staging for patients with SCLC includes the initial general lung cancer evaluation with chest and abdominal CT scans (because of the high frequency of hepatic and adrenal involvement) as well as fiberoptic bronchoscopy with washings and biopsies to determine the tumor extent before therapy; brain CT scan (10% of patients have metastases); and radionuclide scans (bone) if symptoms or other findings suggest disease involvement in these areas. Bone marrow biopsies and aspirations are rarely performed given the low incidence of isolated bone marrow metastases. Chest and abdominal CT scans are very useful to evaluate and follow tumor response to therapy, and chest CT scans are helpful in planning chest radiotherapy ports.

If signs or symptoms of spinal cord compression or leptomeningitis develop at any time in lung cancer patients with disease of any histologic type, a spinal CT scan or MRI scan and examination of the cerebrospinal fluid cytology are performed. If malignant cells are detected, radiotherapy to the site of compression and intrathecal chemotherapy (usually with methotrexate) are given. In addition, a brain CT or MRI scan is performed to search for brain metastases, which often are associated with spinal cord or leptomeningeal metastases.

RESECTABILITY AND OPERABILITY

In patients with NSCLC, the following are major contraindications to curative surgery or radiotherapy alone: extrathoracic metastases; superior vena cava syndrome; vocal cord and, in most cases, phrenic nerve paralysis; malignant pleural effusion; cardiac tamponade; tumor within 2 cm of the carina (not curable by surgery but potentially curable by radiotherapy); metastasis to the contralateral lung; bilateral

Superior Mediastinal Nodes
- **1** Highest mediastinal
- **2** Upper paratracheal
- **3** Prevascular and retrotracheal
- **4** Lower paratracheal (including azygos nodes)

N2 = single digit, ipsilateral
N3 = single digit, contralateral or supraclavicular

Aortic Nodes
- **5** Subaortic (A-P window)
- **6** Para-aortic (ascending aorta or phrenic)

Inferior Mediastinal Nodes
- **7** Subcarinal
- **8** Paraesophageal (below carina)
- **9** Pulmonary ligament

N1 Nodes
- **10** Hilar
- **11** Interlobar
- **12** Lobar
- **13** Segmental
- **14** Subsegmental

FIGURE 85-1 Regional lymph node stations for lung cancer staging. *(Used by permission from CF Mountain, C Dresler: Chest 111:1718, 1997.)*

endobronchial tumor (potentially curable by radiotherapy); metastasis to the supraclavicular lymph nodes; contralateral mediastinal node metastases (potentially curable by radiotherapy); and involvement of the main pulmonary artery. Pleural effusions are generally considered malignant regardless of whether they are cytology positive, particularly if they are exudative, bloody, and have no other probable etiology. Most patients with SCLC have unresectable disease; however, if clinical findings suggest the potential for resection (most common with peripheral lesions), that option should be considered.

PHYSIOLOGIC STAGING

Patients with lung cancer often have cardiopulmonary and other problems related to chronic obstructive pulmonary disease as well as other medical problems. To improve their preoperative condition, correctable problems (e.g., anemia, electrolyte and fluid disorders, infections, and arrhythmias) should be addressed, smoking stopped, and appropriate chest physical therapy instituted. Since it is not always possible to predict whether a lobectomy or pneumonectomy will be required until the time of operation, a conservative approach is to restrict resectional surgery to patients who could potentially tolerate a pneumonectomy. In addition to nonambulatory performance status, a myocardial infarction within the past 3 months is a contraindication to thoracic surgery because 20% of patients will die of reinfarction. An infarction in the past 6 months is a relative contraindication. Other major contraindications include uncontrolled major arrhythmias, an FEV_1 (forced expiratory volume in 1 s) <1 L, CO_2 retention (resting P_{CO_2} >45 mmHg), DL_{CO} <40%, and severe pulmonary hypertension. Recommending surgery when the FEV_1 is 1.1–2.0 L or <80% predicted requires careful judgment, while an FEV_1 >2.5 L or >80% predicted usually permits a pneumonectomy. In patients with borderline lung function but a resectable tumor, cardiopulmonary exercise testing could be performed as part of the physiologic evaluation. This test allows an estimate of the maximal oxygen consumption ($\dot{V}_{O_2}$max). A $\dot{V}_{O_2}$max <15 mL/kg per min predicts for high risk of postoperative complications.

Rx LUNG CANCER

The overall treatment approach to patients with lung cancer is shown in **Table 85-4**. Patients should be encouraged to stop smoking, particularly if they will be undergoing surgery or radiation therapy. Those who do fare better than those who continue to smoke.

MANAGEMENT OF OCCULT AND STAGE 0 CARCINOMAS In the uncommon situation where malignant cells are identified in a sputum or bronchial washing specimen but the chest radiograph appears normal (TX tumor stage), the lesion must be localized. More than 90% can be localized by meticulous examination of the bronchial tree with a fiberoptic bronchoscope under general anesthesia and collection of a series of differential brushings and biopsies. Often, carcinoma in situ or multicentric lesions are found in these patients. Current recommendations are for the most conservative surgical resection, allowing removal of the cancer and conservation of lung parenchyma, even if the bronchial margins are positive for carcinoma in situ. The 5-year overall survival rate for these occult cancers is ~60%. Close follow-up of these patients is indicated because of the high incidence of second primary lung cancers (5% per patient per year). One approach to in situ or multicentric lesions uses systemically administered hematoporphyrin (which localizes to tumors and sensitizes them to light) followed by bronchoscopic phototherapy.

SOLITARY PULMONARY NODULE AND "GROUND GLASS" OPACITY Occasionally, when an x-ray or CT scan is done for another purpose, a patient will present with an incidental finding of an asymptomatic, solitary pulmonary nodule (SPN, defined as an x-ray density completely surrounded by normal aerated lung, with circumscribed margins, of any shape, usually 1–6 cm in greatest diameter). A decision to resect or follow the nodule must be made. Nodules of this size discovered in CT screening for lung cancer would also be of the size requiring a biopsy for tissue. Approximately 35% of all such lesions in adults are malignant, most being primary lung cancer, while <1% are malignant in nonsmokers <35 years of age. A complete history, including a smoking history, physical examination, routine laboratory tests, chest CT scan, fiberoptic bronchoscopy, and old chest x-rays or CT scans are obtained if available.

| TABLE 85-4 | SUMMARY OF TREATMENT APPROACH TO PATIENTS WITH LUNG CANCER |

Non-Small Cell Lung Cancer

Stages IA, IB, IIA, IIB, and some IIIA:
  Surgical resection for stages IA, IB, IIA, and IIB
  Surgical resection with complete-mediastinal lymph node dissection and consideration of neoadjuvant CRx for stage IIIA disease with "minimal N2 involvement" (discovered at thoracotomy or mediastinoscopy)
  Consider postoperative RT for patients found to have N2 disease
  Stage IB: discussion of risk/benefits of adjuvant CRx; not routinely given
  Stage II: Adjuvant CRx
Curative potential RT for "nonoperable" patients
Stage IIIA with selected types of stage T3 tumors:
  Tumors with chest wall invasion (T3): en bloc resection of tumor with involved chest wall and consideration of postoperative RT
  Superior sulcus (Pancoast's) (T3) tumors: preoperative RT (30–45 Gy) and CRx followed by en bloc resection of involved lung and chest wall with postoperative RT
  Proximal airway involvement (<2 cm from carina) without mediastinal nodes: sleeve resection if possible preserving distal normal lung or pneumonectomy
Stages IIIA "advanced, bulky, clinically evident N2 disease" (discovered preoperatively) and IIIB disease that can be included in a tolerable RT port:
  Curative potential concurrent RT + CRx if performance status and general medical condition are reasonable; otherwise, sequential CRx followed by RT, or RT alone
Stage IIIB disease with carinal invasion (T4) but without N2 involvement:
  Consider pneumonectomy with tracheal sleeve resection with direct reanastomosis to contralateral mainstem bronchus
Stage IV and more advanced IIIB disease:
  RT to symptomatic local sites
  CRx for ambulatory patients; consider CRx and bevacizumab for selected patients
  Chest tube drainage of large malignant pleural effusions
  Consider resection of primary tumor and metastasis for isolated brain or adrenal metastases

Small Cell Lung Cancer

Limited stage (good performance status): combination CRx + concurrent chest RT
Extensive stage (good performance status): combination CRx
Complete tumor responders (all stages): consider prophylactic cranial RT
Poor-performance-status patients (all stages):
  Modified-dose combination CRx
  Palliative RT

All Patients

RT for brain metastases, spinal cord compression, weight-bearing lytic bony lesions, symptomatic local lesions (nerve paralyses, obstructed airway, hemoptysis, intrathoracic large venous obstruction, in non-small cell lung cancer and in small cell cancer not responding to CRx)
Appropriate diagnosis and treatment of other medical problems and supportive care during CRx
Encouragement to stop smoking
Entrance into clinical trial, if eligible

Abbreviations: CRx, chemotherapy; RT, radiotherapy.

FIGURE 85-2 Algorithm for evaluation of a solitary pulmonary nodule (SPN). CXR, chest x-ray; CT, computed tomography; PET, positron emission tomography.

PET scans are useful in detecting lung cancers >7–8 mm in diameter. If no diagnosis is immediately apparent, the following risk factors would all argue strongly in favor of proceeding with resection to establish a histologic diagnosis: a history of cigarette smoking; age ≥35 years; a relatively large lesion; lack of calcification; chest symptoms; associated atelectasis, pneumonitis, or adenopathy; growth of the lesion revealed by comparison with old x-rays/CT scans; or a positive PET scan. At present, only two radiographic criteria are reliable predictors of the benign nature of an SPN: lack of growth over a period >2 years and certain characteristic patterns of calcification. Calcification alone does not exclude malignancy. However, a dense central nidus, multiple punctate foci, and "bull's eye" (granuloma) and "popcorn ball" (hamartoma) calcifications are all highly suggestive of a benign lesion. An algorithm for evaluating an SPN is shown in **Fig. 85-2**.

When old x-rays are not available, the PET scan is negative, and the characteristic calcification patterns are absent, the following approach is reasonable. Nonsmoking patients <35 years can be followed with serial CT every 3 months for 1 year and then yearly; if any significant growth is found, a histologic diagnosis is needed. For patients >35 years and all patients with a smoking history, a histologic diagnosis must be made, regardless of whether the lesion is PET positive or negative, since slow-growing cancers such as BAC can be PET negative. The sample for histologic diagnosis can be obtained either at the time of nodule resection or, if the patient is a poor operative risk, via video-assisted thoracic surgery (VATS) or transthoracic fine-needle biopsy. Some institutions use preoperative fine-needle aspiration on all such lesions; however, all positive lesions have to be resected, and negative cytologic findings in most cases have to be confirmed by histology on a resected specimen. Much has been made of sparing patients an operation; however, the high probability of finding a malignancy (particularly in smokers >35 years) and the excellent chance for surgical cure when the tumor is small both suggest an aggressive approach to these lesions.

Since the advent of screening CTs, small "ground-glass" opacities ("GGOs") have often been observed, particularly as the increased sensitivity of CTs enables detection of smaller lesions. Many of these GGOs, when biopsied, are found to be BAC. Some of the GGOs are semiopaque and referred to as "partial" GGOs, which are often more slowly growing, with atypical adenomatous hyperplasia histology, a lesion of unclear prognostic significance. By contrast, "solid" GGOs have a faster growth rate and usually are typical adenocarcinomas histologically.

NON-SMALL CELL LUNG CANCER   NSCLC Stages I and II

Surgery In patients with NSCLC stages IA, IB, IIA and IIB (Table 85-2) who can tolerate operation, the treatment of choice is pulmonary resection. If a complete resection is possible, the 5-year survival rate for N0 disease is about 60–80%, depending on the size of the tumor. The 5-year survival drops to about 50% when N1 (hilar node involvement) disease is present.

The extent of resection is a matter of surgical judgment based on findings at exploration. Clinical trials have shown that lobectomy is superior to wedge resection in reducing the rate of local recurrence. Pneumonectomy is reserved for patients with tumors involving multiple lobes or very central tumors and should only be performed in patients with excellent pulmonary reserve. In addition, patients undergoing a right-sided pneumonectomy after induction chemotherapy and radiation therapy (see below) have a high mortality rate and should be carefully selected before surgery. Wedge resection and segmentectomy (potentially by VATS) are reserved for patients with poor pulmonary reserve and small peripheral lesions.

Radiotherapy with Curative Intent

Patients with stage I or II disease who refuse surgery or are not candidates for pulmonary resection should be considered for radiation therapy with curative intent. The decision to administer high-dose radiotherapy is based on the extent of disease and the volume of the chest that requires irradiation. Patients with distant metastases, malignant pleural effusion, or cardiac involvement are not considered candidates for curative radiation treatment. The long-term survival for patients with all stages of lung cancer who receive radiation with curative intent is about 20%. In addition to being potentially curative, radiotherapy may increase the quality and length of life by controlling the primary tumor and preventing symptoms related to local recurrence in the lung.

Treatment with curative intent usually involves midplane doses of 60–64 Gy, while palliative thoracic radiation (see below) involves delivery of 30–45 Gy. The major dose-limiting concern is the amount of lung parenchyma and other organs in the thorax that are included in the treatment plan, including the spinal cord, heart, and esophagus. In patients with a major degree of underlying pulmonary disease, the treatment plan may have to be compromised because of the deleterious effects of radiation on pulmonary function.

The most common side effect of curative thoracic radiation is esophagitis. Other side effects include fatigue, radiation myelitis (rare), and radiation pneumonitis, which can sometimes progress to pulmonary fibrosis. The risk of radiation pneumonitis is proportional to the radiation dose and the volume of lung in the field. The full clinical syndrome (dyspnea, fever, and radiographic infiltrate corresponding to the treatment port) occurs in 5% of cases and is treated with glucocorticoids. Acute radiation esophagitis occurs during treatment but is usually self-limited, unlike spinal cord injury, which may be permanent and should be avoided by careful treatment planning. Brachytherapy (local radiotherapy delivered by placing radioactive "seeds" in a catheter in the tumor bed) provides a way to give a high local dose while sparing surrounding normal tissue.

NSCLC Stage IA

Patients with resected stage IA NSCLC receive no other therapy but are at a high risk of recurrence (~2–3% annually) or developing a second primary lung cancer. Thus, it is reasonable to follow these patients with CT scans for the first 5 years and consider entering them onto early detection and chemoprevention studies.

Adjuvant Chemotherapy for NSCLC Stages IB and II

A meta-analysis of more than 4300 patients showed a trend toward improved survival of ~5% at 5 years with cisplatin-based adjuvant therapy ($p = .08$). Subsequently, three randomized studies demonstrated no significant survival advantage despite the addition of more "modern" postoperative adjuvant chemotherapy regimens. However, since then at least three additional randomized trials and two meta-analyses showed a survival benefit in response to postoperative adjuvant-based therapy (**Table 85-5**). Consequently, adjuvant chemotherapy is now routinely recommended in NSCLC patients with a good performance status and stage IIA or IIB disease, though the beneficial effects are modest.

TABLE 85-5	RANDOMIZED STUDIES OF ADJUVANT CHEMOTHERAPY IN NSCLC					
Study	Treatment	Number of Patients	5-Year Survival (%)	Median Survival	Hazard Ratio (95% CI)	p Value
ECOG 3590 (II–IIIA)	Surgery → RT vs. Surgery + post-op concurrent RT + cis/ etoposide	242 246	39% 33%	39 months vs. 38 months	0.93 (0.74–1.18)	0.56
ALPI (I–IIIA)	Surgery alone vs. Surgery + post-op mitomycin/vindesine/ cisplatin	603 606	51% 43%	NR	0.96 (0.8–1.1)	0.59
Big Lung Trial (I–IIIB)	Surgery alone vs. Surgery + post-op chemotherapy[a]	189 192		33 months 34 months	1.02 (0.77–1.35)	0.90
IALT IB–IIIA	Surgery alone vs. Surgery + post-op Cis + VP16/vinca	405 361	40% 44.5%	NR	0.86 (0.76–0.98)	<0.03
UFT IA–IB	Surgery alone vs. Surgery + post-op UFT	488 469	85% 88%	—	0.71 (0.52–0.98)	0.04
CALGB IB (ASCO 06)	Surgery alone vs. Surgery + post-op carbo/paclitaxel	172 172	57% 59%	78 months 95 months	0.80 (0.60–1.07)	0.10
NCI-C IB–II	Surgery alone vs. Surgery + post-op Cis/vinorelbine	241 241	54% 69%	73 months 94 months	0.69 (0.52–0.91)	0.04
ANITA IB, II, IIIA	Surgery alone vs. Surgery + post-op Cis/vinorelbine	433 407	43% 51%	44 months 66 months	0.79 (50–88.5)	0.017

[a]Chemotherapy allowed: mitomycin, cisplatin, ifosfamide; mitomycin, vinblastine, cisplatin; cisplatin, vindesine; cisplatin, vinorelbine.

Note: RT, radiation therapy; NR, not reported; UFT, tegafur and uracil.

The role of adjuvant chemotherapy for stage IB disease is undefined. Subset analysis of all the randomized studies showed no benefit in patients with stage IB. In addition, one clinical trial focusing solely on IB disease and using carboplatin and paclitaxel (one of the most commonly used regimens for advanced disease) found a hazard ratio of 0.80 (20% reduction in death with adjuvant chemotherapy) that was not statistically significant. Thus, patients with stage IB NSCLC are not routinely given adjuvant therapy.

Adjuvant Radiotherapy for NSCLC Stages I–II After apparent complete resection, postoperative adjuvant radiation therapy does not improve survival and may actually be detrimental to survival in N0 and N1 disease.

Superior Sulcus or Pancoast Tumors Non-small cell carcinomas of the superior pulmonary sulcus producing *Pancoast's syndrome* appear to behave differently than lung cancers at other sites and are usually treated with combined radiotherapy and surgery. Patients with these carcinomas should have the usual preoperative staging procedures, including mediastinoscopy and CT and PET scans, to determine tumor extent and a neurologic examination (and sometimes nerve conduction studies) to document involvement or impingement of nerves in the region. If mediastinoscopy is negative, curative approaches may be used in treating Pancoast's syndrome despite its apparent locally invasive nature. The best results reported thus employed concurrent preoperative irradiation [30 Gy in 10 treatments] and cisplatin and etoposide, followed by an en bloc resection of the tumor and involved chest wall 3–6 weeks later; 65% of thoracotomy specimens showed either a complete response or minimal residual microscopic disease on pathologic evaluation. The 2-year survival rate was 55% for all eligible patients and 70% for patients who had a complete resection.

NSCLC with T3, N0 Disease (Stage IIB) The subset of T3, N0 disease (which does not present as Pancoast tumor) was initially considered stage III disease. However, it has a different natural history and treatment strategy than stage III N2 disease and is now considered as stage IIB. Patients with peripheral chest wall invasion should have resection of the involved ribs and underlying lung. Chest wall defects are then repaired with chest wall musculature or Marlex mesh and methylmethacrylate. Five-year survival rates as high as 35–50% have been found, and adjuvant chemotherapy is usually recommended.

NSCLC Stage III Treatment of locally advanced NSCLC is one of the most controversial issues in the management of lung cancer. Treatment options include a local therapy (surgery or radiation therapy) combined with systemic chemotherapy to control micrometastases. Interpretation of the results of clinical trials involving patients with locally advanced disease has been clouded by a number of issues, including changing diagnostic techniques, different staging systems, and heterogeneous patient populations with tumors that range from nonbulky stage IIIA (clinical N1 nodes with N2 nodes discovered only at the time of surgery, despite a negative mediastinoscopy) to bulky N2 nodes (enlarged adenopathy clearly visible on chest x-rays or multiple nodal level involvement) to clearly inoperable stage IIIB disease. Thus, a team approach involving pulmonary medicine, thoracic surgery, and medical and radiation oncology is essential for the management of these patients.

NSCLC Stage IIIA *Nonbulky IIIA* Surgery for N2 disease is a controversial area in the management of lung cancer. Patients with N2 disease can be divided into "minimal" disease (involvement of only one node with microscopic foci, usually discovered at thoracotomy or mediastinoscopy) and the more common "advanced" bulky disease, clinically obvious on CT scans and discovered preoperatively. Patients who have an incidental finding of N2 disease at the time of resection should receive adjuvant chemotherapy.

Bulky IIIA No evidence suggests that patients with "bulky," multilevel ipsilateral mediastinal nodes (N2) have improved survival with surgery and either pre- or postoperative chemotherapy compared to treatment with chemotherapy plus radiation therapy. This important issue was addressed in the multicenter randomized Intergroup 0139 Trial involving patients with pathologically staged N2 disease who received 45 Gy of induction radiation therapy plus two cycles of cisplatin and etoposide to "debulk" tumors. The patients were then randomly assigned to surgical resection of any residual tumor or to boost radiation therapy plus an additional two cycles of chemotherapy. Although a significant improvement in progression-free survival was observed at 5 years for those patients randomized to surgical resection (22% vs. 11%; $p = .017$), the difference in 5-year overall survival while favoring surgery (22% vs. 11%; $p = .10$) was not significant. This is important since treatment-related mortality was greater in the surgery arm (8% vs. 2%), with the majority of deaths occurring in patients undergoing pneumonectomy. Patients who had persistent N2 disease following neoadjuvant chemotherapy did particularly poorly, leading some oncologists to conclude that surgery for bulky IIIA disease should only be conducted in patients who have clearing of their mediastinal nodes following neoadjuvant therapy. The main role of neoadjuvant chemotherapy is to control micrometastatic disease, and if this macroscopically evident disease is not sensitive to chemotherapy, it is unlikely that the microscopic disease will be controlled. Thus, surgical removal of the primary tumor after such chemotherapy is probably fruitless. Likewise, neoadjuvant chemotherapy generally should not be used to render inoperable disease operable. One exception to this approach is T4, N0 or T4, N1 (stage IIIB, see below) disease for which preoperative chemotherapy may provide enough tumor debulking to allow otherwise unresectable disease to be resected. Chemotherapy may allow chest wall resection for direct extension of tumor, tracheal sleeve pneumonectomy, and sleeve lobectomy for lesions near the carina.

Bulky NSCLC Stage IIIA and Dry IIIB (IIIB without a Pleural Effusion) The presence of pathologically involved N2 nodes should be confirmed histologically because enlarged nodes detected by CT will be negative for cancer in ~30% of patients. Chemotherapy plus radiation therapy is the treatment of choice for patients with bulky stage IIIA or IIIB disease without pleural effusion (referred to as "dry IIIB"). Randomized studies demonstrate an improvement in median and long-term survival with chemotherapy followed by radiation therapy, compared with radiation therapy alone. Subsequent randomized trials have shown that administering chemotherapy and radiation therapy concurrently results in improved survival compared to sequential chemotherapy and radiation therapy, albeit with more side effects, such as fatigue, esophagitis, and neutropenia. Frequently, an additional two to three cycles of chemotherapy are also given. However, it is not clear whether these additional cycles should be administered before or after the chemoradiation, what the optimal drugs are, or whether doses should be attenuated during the radiation but given more frequently. (Lower doses of drugs may "sensitize" the tumor to radiation therapy but may not by themselves remove other microscopic disease.)

DISSEMINATED NON-SMALL CELL LUNG CANCER **Symptomatic Management of Metastatic Disease** Patients who present with or progress to metastatic NSCLC have a poor prognosis, as do patients with pleural effusions. Untreated, the median survival of both of these patient groups is roughly 4–6 months. They are often treated in the same way. Standard medical management, the judicious use of pain medications, the appropriate use of radiotherapy, and outpatient chemotherapy form the cornerstone of this management.

Palliative Radiation Therapy Patients whose primary tumor is causing urgent severe symptoms such as bronchial obstruction with pneumonitis, hemoptysis, upper airway or superior vena cava obstruction, brain or spinal cord compression, or painful bony metastases should have radiotherapy to the primary tumor to relieve these symptoms. Usually, radiation therapy is given as a course of 30–40 Gy over 2–4 weeks for palliative purposes. Radiation therapy provides relief of intrathoracic symptoms: hemoptysis, 84%; superior vena cava syndrome, 80%; dyspnea, 60%; cough, 60%; atelectasis, 23%; and vocal cord paralysis, 6%. Cardiac tamponade (treated with pericardiocentesis and radiation therapy to the heart), painful bony metastases (with relief in 66%), brain or spinal cord compression, and brachial plexus involvement may also be palliated with radiotherapy.

Brain metastases are often isolated sites of relapse in patients with adenocarcinoma of the lung otherwise controlled by surgery or radiotherapy. These are usually treated with radiation therapy and, in highly selected cases, with surgical resection. Usually, in addition to radiotherapy for brain metastases and cord compression, dexamethasone (25–100 mg/d in four divided doses) is also given and then rapidly tapered to the lowest dosage that relieves symptoms. Because of the high frequency of brain metastases, the use of prophylactic cranial irradiation (PCI, given to the whole brain before metastatic disease becomes manifest) has been considered. However, PCI is of no proven value. Screening asymptomatic patients with head CT scans to find such lesions before such metastases become clinically evident is also not proven beneficial.

Pleural effusions are common and are usually treated with thoracentesis. If they recur and are symptomatic, a pleurex catheter or chest tube drainage followed by pleurodesis with a sclerosing agent such as intrapleural talc, bleomycin, or tetracycline can be used. These sclerosing agents may be administered through the chest tube, or, in the case of talc, via thorascopic insufflation. In the former case, the chest cavity is completely drained. Xylocaine 1% is instilled (15 mL), followed by 50 mL normal saline. Then the sclerosing agent is dissolved in 100 mL normal saline, and this solution is injected through the chest tube. The chest tube is clamped for 4 h if tolerated, and the patient is rotated onto different sides to distribute the sclerosing agent. The chest tube is removed 24–48 h later, after drainage has become slight (usually <100 mL/24 h). While sclerosing agents have been widely used, an indwelling pleurex catheter is equivalent to chest tube drainage and better tolerated by patients. In this situation, the pleurex catheter is tunneled under the skin and can remain in place for weeks. The patient periodically drains the catheter into a specially designed bag, as needed.

Symptomatic endobronchial lesions that recur after surgery or radiotherapy or develop in patients with severely compromised pulmonary function are difficult to treat with conventional therapy. Neodymium-YAG (yttrium-aluminum-garnet) laser therapy administered through a flexible fiberoptic bronchoscope (usually under general anesthesia) can provide palliation in 80–90% of such patients even when the tumor has relapsed after radiotherapy. Local radiotherapy delivered by brachytherapy, photodynamic therapy using a photosensitizing agent, and endobronchial stents are other measures that can relieve airway obstruction from recurrent tumor.

Chemotherapy Chemotherapy palliates symptoms, improves the quality of life, and improves survival in newly diagnosed patients with stage IV NSCLC, particularly in patients with good performance status. Whereas the median survival for untreated patients is roughly 4–6 months, and 1-year survival is 5–10%, with combination chemotherapy the median survival is 8–10 months, 1-year survival is 30–35%, and 2-year survival 10–15%. Combination chemotherapy produces an objective tumor response in 20–30% of patients, although the response is complete in <5%. In addition, economic analysis has found chemotherapy to be cost-effective palliation for stage IV NSCLC. However, the use of chemotherapy for NSCLC requires clinical experience and careful judgment to balance potential benefits and toxicities for these patients.

Chemotherapy for previously untreated, good-performance-status patients typically consists of two drugs ("doublets"). Traditionally, one of the two drugs has been either cisplatin or carboplatin, and the other drug is a taxane (paclitaxel or docetaxel), gemcitabine, or a vinca alkaloid such as vinorelbine. No major difference in outcome has been observed between the standard chemotherapy doublets, although they differ in terms of schedule, side effects, and cost. Cytotoxic chemotherapy for first-line chemotherapy is typically administered for four to six cycles; no benefit has been shown for continuing the same chemotherapy beyond that point. After four to six cycles, chemotherapy is usually stopped and the patient observed closely for tumor progression, at which point second-line chemotherapy may be started if the patient's performance status remains good. Nausea with typical first-line regimens is usually mild, particularly when 5-HT3 serotonin antagonists are used as antiemetics. Hair loss depends on the choice of regimen and should be discussed with the patient. All regimens cause myelosuppression, but the incidence of neutropenic fevers, bleeding episodes, or anemia requiring transfusions is low. Growth-factor support is rarely needed. Elderly patients without significant comorbid conditions benefit from and tolerate chemotherapy much the same as their younger counterparts. However, patients with a poorer performance status seem to obtain less benefit.

Docetaxel and pemetrexed are second-line agents for patients who have progressive disease on first-line chemotherapy and still have a good performance status. Docetaxel improves progression-free survival and overall survival compared to best supportive care, and pemetrexed has roughly the same efficacy as docetaxel, but with fewer side effects.

VEGF Targeted Therapy Bevacizumab, a monoclonal antibody to VEGF, improves response rate, progression-free survival, and overall survival of patients with advanced disease when combined with chemotherapy (paclitaxel/carboplatin). Median, 1-year, and 2-year survival in response to chemotherapy plus bevacizumab was 12.3 months, 51%, and 23%, compared, respectively, to 10.3 months, 44%, and 15% with chemotherapy alone (hazard ratio 0.79, *p* = 0.003). A 1-year survival of >50% and a 2-year survival of >20% represents a significant improvement in long-term prognosis. The dose of bevacizumab administered on this trial was 15 mg/kg IV every 3 weeks. Bevacizumab side effects include bleeding, hypertension, and proteinuria, and the hemorrhagic side effects make this agent risky to use. Patients with squamous cancer cannot receive bevacizumab because of their tendency toward serious hemorrhagic side effects. Patients with brain metastases, hemoptysis, and bleeding disorders or who need anticoagulation are also not eligible to receive the agent. Despite these restrictions and careful patient selection, significant bleeding is noted in about 4% of patients.

EGFR Targeted Therapy Erlotinib is an oral inhibitor of the EGFR kinase that is used in second- and third-line therapy of NSCLC. Clinical responses have been seen in a large fraction of the small subset of patients with tumors bearing mutations in the EGFR. Prolonged survival with EGFR TKI treatment has also been observed in some patients whose tumors have amplification of the *EGFR* gene or overexpression of the receptor. Side effects of erlotinib differ from chemotherapy side effects of hair loss, nausea, and neutropenia, but they include acneiform skin rash and diarrhea. For patients whose tumors respond to EGFR TKI therapy, substantial clinical benefit is seen.

SMALL CELL LUNG CANCER SCLC is a chemotherapy-sensitive disease. Patients with limited stage disease have high response rates (60–80%) and a 10–30% complete response rate. The response rates in patients with extensive disease are somewhat lower (50%) and almost always partial responses. Tumor regressions usually occur quickly, within the first two cycles of treatment, and provide rapid palliation of tumor-related symptoms.

Chemotherapy significantly prolongs survival. Untreated, patients with limited-stage SCLC have a median survival of 12 weeks; the median survival with chemotherapy is 18 months, and long-term (>3 year) survival is 30–40%. The median survival of extensive-stage patients is 9 months; <5% of patients survive 2 years. Thus, although initially responsive, most patients with SCLC relapse, presumably due to the emergence of chemotherapy resistance.

Chemotherapy The chemotherapy combination most widely used for SCLC is etoposide plus cisplatin or carboplatin, given every 3 weeks on an

outpatient basis for four to six cycles. Increased dose intensity of chemotherapy adds toxicity without clear survival benefit. Appropriate supportive care (antiemetics, fluid support with cisplatin, monitoring of blood counts and blood chemistries, monitoring for signs of bleeding or infection, and, as required, use of hematopoietins) and adjustment of chemotherapy doses on the basis of nadir granulocyte counts are essential.

The prognosis of patients who relapse is poor. Patients who relapse >3 months since the completion of their initial chemotherapy (so-called chemosensitive disease) have a median survival of 4–5 months; patients who do not respond to initial chemotherapy or relapse within 3 months (chemorefractory disease) have a median survival of only 2–3 months. Patients with chemosensitive disease may be retreated with their initial regimen. Topotecan has modest activity as second-line therapy, or patients can be entered onto clinical trials testing new agents.

Considerations for Therapy of SCLC Limited-Stage Disease *Combined-Modality Chemoradiotherapy* Radiation therapy to the thorax is associated with a small but significant improvement in long-term survival for patients with limited-stage SCLC (5% at 3 years). Chemotherapy given concurrently with thoracic radiation is more effective than sequential chemoradiation but is associated with significantly more esophagitis and hematologic toxicity. In one randomized study, twice-daily hyperfractionated radiation was compared with a once-daily schedule; both were administered concurrently with four cycles of cisplatin and etoposide. Survival was significantly higher with the twice-daily regimen (median survival 23 months compared with 19 months; 5-year survival 26% compared with 16%), but the twice-daily regimen gave more grade 3 esophagitis and pulmonary toxicity. Patients should be carefully selected for concurrent chemoradiation therapy based on good performance status and pulmonary reserve.

PCI significantly decreases the development of brain metastases (which occur in about two-thirds of patients who do not receive PCI) and results in a small survival benefit (~5%) in patients who have obtained a complete response to induction chemotherapy. Deficits in cognitive ability following PCI are uncommon and often difficult to sort out from effects of chemotherapy or normal aging.

Radiation Therapy for Palliation Palliative radiation therapy is an important component of the management of SCLC patients. Cranial radiation often decreases the signs and symptoms of brain metastases. In the case of symptomatic, progressive lesions in the chest or at other critical sites, if radiotherapy has not yet been given to these areas, it may be administered in full doses (e.g., 40 Gy to the chest tumor mass).

Surgery Although surgical resection is not routinely recommended for SCLC, occasional patients meet the usual requirements for resectability (stage I or II disease with negative mediastinal nodes). Often this histologic diagnosis is made in some patients only on review of the resected surgical specimen. However, when such SCLC patients are discovered, they should receive standard SCLC chemotherapy. Retrospective series have reported high cure rates if postoperative chemotherapy is used, although it is unclear what the outcome would be with chemoradiation therapy alone, given the relatively low bulk disease of these patients.

LUNG CANCER PREVENTION

Deterring children from taking up smoking and helping young adults stop is likely to be the most effective lung cancer prevention. Smoking cessation programs are successful in 5–20% of volunteers; the poor efficacy is due to the addictive nature of nicotine use, which is as strong as addiction to heroin.

Chemoprevention is an experimental approach to reduce lung cancer risk; no benefit has yet been shown for chemoprevention. Two putative chemoprevention agents, vitamin E and β-carotene, actually increased the risk of lung cancer in heavy smokers.

BENIGN LUNG NEOPLASMS

The benign neoplasms of the lung, representing <5% of all primary tumors, include bronchial adenomas and hamartomas (90% of such lesions) and a group of very uncommon benign neoplasms (epithelial tumors such as bronchial papillomas, fibroepithelial polyps; mesenchymal tumors such as chondromas, fibromas, lipomas, hemangiomas, leiomyomas, pseudolymphomas; tumors of mixed origin such as teratomas; and other diseases such as endometriosis). The diagnostic and primary-treatment approach (surgery) is basically the same for all these neoplasms. They can present as central masses causing airway obstruction, cough, hemoptysis, and pneumonitis. The masses may or may not be visible on radiographs but are usually accessible to fiberoptic bronchoscopy. Alternatively, they can present without symptoms as SPNs and are evaluated accordingly. In all cases, the extent of surgery must be determined at operation, and a conservative procedure with appropriate reconstructions is usually performed.

BRONCHIAL ADENOMAS

Bronchial adenomas (80% are central) are slow-growing endobronchial lesions; they represent 50% of all benign pulmonary neoplasms. About 80–90% are carcinoids, 10–15% are adenocystic tumors (or cylindromas), and 2–3% are mucoepidermoid tumors. Adenomas present in patients 15–60 years old (average age 45) as endobronchial lesions and are often symptomatic for several years. Patients may have a chronic cough, recurrent hemoptysis, or obstruction with atelectasis, lobar collapse, or pneumonitis and abscess formation.

Bronchial adenomas of all types, because of their endobronchial and often central location, are usually visible by fiberoptic bronchoscopy. Because they are hypervascular, they can bleed profusely after bronchoscopic biopsy, and this problem should be anticipated. Bronchial adenomas must be considered as potentially malignant, thus requiring removal for symptom relief and because they can be locally invasive or recurrent, potentially can metastasize, and may produce paraneoplastic syndromes. Surgical excision is the primary treatment for all types of bronchial adenomas. The extent of surgery is determined at operation and should be as conservative as possible. Often bronchotomy with local excision, sleeve resection, segmental resection, or lobectomy is sufficient. Five-year survival rate after surgical resection is 95%, decreasing to 70% if regional nodes are involved. The treatment of metastatic pulmonary carcinoids is unclear because they can either be indolent or behave more like SCLC (Chap. 344). Assessment of the tempo and histology of the disease in the individual patient is necessary to determine if and when chemotherapy or radiotherapy is indicated.

CARCINOID AND OTHER NEUROENDOCRINE LUNG TUMORS

Neuroendocrine lung tumors represent a spectrum of pathologic entities, including typical carcinoid, atypical carcinoid, and large cell neuroendocrine cancer, as well as SCLC. SCLC and large cell neuroendocrine cancer are high-grade neuroendocrine tumors and in general should be treated as described for SCLC. By contrast, typical carcinoid and atypical carcinoids are low- and intermediate-grade tumors with different treatment approaches and in general are resistant to chemotherapy (Chap. 44). Carcinoids, like SCLCs, may secrete other hormones, such as ACTH or AVP, and can cause paraneoplastic syndromes that resolve on resection. Uncommonly, bronchial carcinoid metastases (usually to the liver) may produce the carcinoid syndrome, with cutaneous flush, bronchoconstriction, diarrhea, and cardiac valvular lesions, which SCLC does not do. Carcinoid tumors that have an unusually aggressive histologic appearance (referred to as *atypical carcinoids*) metastasize in 70% of cases to regional nodes, liver, or bone, compared with only a 5% rate of metastasis for carcinoids with typical histology. Large cell neuroendocrine cancer is a high-grade NSCLC with neuroendocrine features. These tumors are characterized by histologic features similar to small cell cancer, but they are formed by larger cells. The prognosis for patients with large cell neuroendocrine cancer is significantly worse than that for patients with atypical carcinoid and classic large cell cancer. Five-year survival is 21% for patients with large cell neuroendocrine cancer, 65% for atypical carcinoid, and 90% for typical carcinoid.

THYMOMAS

See **Chap. e12.**

HAMARTOMAS

Pulmonary hamartomas have a peak incidence at age 60 and are more frequent in men than in women. Histologically, they contain normal pulmonary tissue components (smooth muscle and collagen) in a disorganized fashion. They are usually peripheral, clinically silent, and benign in their behavior. Unless the radiographic findings are pathognomonic for hamartoma, with "popcorn" calcification, the lesions usually have to be resected for diagnosis, particularly if the patient is a smoker. VATS may minimize the surgical complications.

METASTATIC PULMONARY TUMORS

The lung is a frequent site of metastases from primary cancers outside the lung. Usually such metastatic disease is incurable. However, two special situations should be borne in mind. The first is the development of an SPN or a mass on chest x-ray in a patient known to have an extrathoracic neoplasm. This nodule may represent a metastasis or a new primary lung cancer. Because the natural history of lung cancer is often worse than that of other primary tumors, a single pulmonary nodule in a patient with a known extrathoracic tumor is approached as though the nodule is a primary lung cancer, particularly if the patient is >35 years and a smoker. If a vigorous search for other sites of active cancer proves negative, the nodule is surgically resected. Second, in some cases multiple metastatic pulmonary nodules can be resected with curative intent. This tactic is usually recommended if, after careful staging, it is found that (1) the patient can tolerate the contemplated pulmonary resection, (2) the primary tumor has been definitively and successfully treated (disease-free for >1 year), and (3) all known metastatic disease can be encompassed by the projected pulmonary resection. Patients with uncontrolled primary tumors and other extrapulmonary metastases are not considered. Primary tumors whose pulmonary metastases have been successfully resected for cure include osteogenic and soft tissue sarcomas; colon, rectal, uterine, cervix, and corpus tumors; head and neck, breast, testis, and salivary gland cancer; melanoma; and bladder and kidney tumors. Five-year survival rates of 20–30% have been found in selected series, and dramatic results have been achieved in patients with osteogenic sarcomas, where resection of pulmonary metastases (sometimes requiring several thoracotomies) is a standard curative treatment approach.

FURTHER READINGS

BLACK C et al: Population screening for lung cancer using computed tomography: Is there evidence of clinical effectiveness? A systematic review of the literature. Thorax 62:131, 2007

EBERHARDT W et al: Chemoradiation paradigm for the treatment of lung cancer. Nat Clin Pract Oncol 3:188, 2006

HAYES DN et al: Gene expression profiling reveals reproducible human lung adenocarcinoma subtypes in multiple independent patient cohorts. J Clin Oncol 24:5079, 2006

SATO M et al: Molecular genetics of lung cancer and translation to the clinic. J Thorac Oncol 2:327, 2007

STINNETT S et al: Role of chemotherapy for palliation in the lung cancer patient. J Support Oncol 5:19, 2007

SUBRAMANIAN J, GOVINDAN R: Lung cancer in never smokers: A review. J Clin Oncol 25:561, 2007

SUN S et al: Of molecules and cancer stem cells: Novel therapeutic strategies for lung cancer. J Clin Invest 117, 2007

WRIGHT G et al: Surgery for non-small cell lung cancer: Systematic review and meta-analysis of randomised controlled trials. Thorax 61:597, 2006

86 Breast Cancer
Marc E. Lippman

Breast cancer is a malignant proliferation of epithelial cells lining the ducts or lobules of the breast. In the year 2007, about 180,510 cases of invasive breast cancer and 40,910 deaths occurred in the United States. Epithelial malignancies of the breast are the most common cause of cancer in women (excluding skin cancer), accounting for about one-third of all cancer in women. As a result of improved treatment and earlier detection, mortality from breast cancer has begun to decrease substantially in the United States. This chapter will not consider rare malignancies presenting in the breast, such as sarcomas and lymphomas, but will focus on the epithelial cancers. Human breast cancer is a clonal disease; a single transformed cell—the product of a series of somatic (acquired) or germline mutations—is eventually able to express full malignant potential. Thus, breast cancer may exist for a long period as either a noninvasive disease or an invasive but nonmetastatic disease. These facts have significant clinical ramifications.

GENETIC CONSIDERATIONS Not more than 10% of human breast cancers can be linked directly to germline mutations. Several genes have been implicated in familial cases. The Li-Fraumeni syndrome is characterized by inherited mutations in the p53 tumor-suppressor gene, which lead to an increased incidence of breast cancer, osteogenic sarcomas, and other malignancies. Inherited mutations in *PTEN* have also been reported in breast cancer.

Another tumor-suppressor gene, *BRCA-1*, has been identified at the chromosomal locus 17q21; this gene encodes a zinc finger protein, and the product therefore may function as a transcription factor. The gene appears to be involved in gene repair. Women who inherit a mutated allele of this gene from either parent have at least a 60–80% lifetime chance of developing breast cancer and about a 33% chance of developing ovarian cancer. The risk is higher among women born after 1940, presumably due to promotional effects of hormonal factors. Men who carry a mutant allele of the gene have an increased incidence of prostate cancer and breast cancer. A fourth gene, termed *BRCA-2*, which has been localized to chromosome 13q12, is also associated with an increased incidence of breast cancer in men and women.

Germline mutations in *BRCA-1* and *BRCA-2* can be readily detected; patients with these mutations can be counseled appropriately. All women with strong family histories for breast cancer should be referred to genetic screening programs, particularly women of Ashkenazi Jewish descent who have a high likelihood of a specific *BRCA-1* mutation (deletion of adenine and guanine at position 185).

Even more important than the role these genes play in inherited forms of breast cancer may be their role in sporadic breast cancer. The p53 mutation is present in nearly 40% of human breast cancers as an acquired defect. Acquired mutations in *PTEN* occur in about 10% of the cases. *BRCA-1* mutation in sporadic primary breast cancer has not been reported. However, decreased expression of *BRCA-1* mRNA (possibly via gene methylation) and abnormal cellular location of the *BRCA-1* protein have been found in some breast cancers. Loss of heterozygosity of *BRCA-1* and *BRCA-2* suggests that tumor-suppressor activity may be inactivated in sporadic cases of human breast cancer. Finally, increased expression of a dominant oncogene plays a role in about a quarter of human breast cancer cases. The product of this gene, a member of the epidermal growth factor receptor superfamily, is called *erbB2* (HER-2, neu) and is overexpressed in these breast cancers due to gene amplification; this overexpression can contribute to transformation of human breast epithelium and is the target of effective systemic therapy in adjuvant and metastatic disease settings.

EPIDEMIOLOGY

Breast cancer is a hormone-dependent disease. Women without functioning ovaries who never receive estrogen-replacement therapy do not develop breast cancer. The female:male ratio is about 150:1. For most epithelial malignancies, a log-log plot of incidence versus age shows a single-component straight-line increase with every year of life. A similar plot for breast cancer shows two components: a straight-line increase with age but with a decrease in slope beginning at the age of menopause. The three dates in a woman's life that have a major impact on breast cancer incidence are age at menarche, age at first full-term pregnancy, and age at menopause. Women who experience menarche at age 16 have only 50–60% of the breast cancer risk of a woman having menarche at age 12; the lower risk persists throughout life. Similarly, menopause occurring 10 years before the median age of menopause (52 years), whether natural or surgically induced, reduces lifetime breast cancer risk by about 35%. Women who have a first full-term pregnancy by age 18 have a 30–40% lower risk of breast cancer compared with nulliparous women. Thus, length of menstrual life—particularly the fraction occurring before first full-term pregnancy—is a substantial component of the total risk of breast cancer. These three factors (menarche, age of first full-term pregnancy, and menopause) can account for 70–80% of the variation in breast cancer frequency in different countries. A meta-analysis has shown that duration of maternal nursing correlates with substantial risk reduction independent of either parity or age at first full-term pregnancy.

International variation in incidence has provided some of the most important clues on hormonal carcinogenesis. A woman living to age 80 in North America has one chance in nine of developing invasive breast cancer. Asian women have one-fifth to one-tenth the risk of breast cancer of women in North America or Western Europe. Asian women have substantially lower concentrations of estrogens and progesterone. These differences cannot be explained on a genetic basis because Asian women living in a western environment have sex steroid hormone concentrations and risks identical to those of their western counterparts. These migrant women and more notably their daughters also differ markedly in height and weight from Asian women in Asia; height and weight are critical regulators of age of menarche and have substantial effects on plasma concentrations of estrogens.

The role of diet in breast cancer etiology is controversial. While there are associative links between total caloric and fat intake and breast cancer risk, the exact role of fat in the diet is unproven. Increased caloric intake contributes to breast cancer risk in multiple ways: earlier menarche, later age at menopause, and increased postmenopausal estrogen concentrations reflecting enhanced aromatase activities in fatty tissues. Moderate alcohol intake also increases the risk by an unknown mechanism. Folic acid supplementation appears to modify risk in women who use alcohol but is not additionally protective in abstainers. Recommendations favoring abstinence from alcohol must be weighed against other social pressures and the possible cardioprotective effect of moderate alcohol intake.

Understanding the potential role of exogenous hormones in breast cancer is of extraordinary importance because millions of American women regularly use oral contraceptives and postmenopausal hormone replacement therapy. The most credible meta-analyses of oral contraceptive use suggest that these agents cause little if any increased risk of breast cancer. By contrast, oral contraceptives offer a substantial protective effect against ovarian epithelial tumors and endometrial cancers. Far more controversial are the data surrounding HRT in postmenopausal women. Data from the Women's Health Initiative (WHI) trial showed in a prospectively randomized design that conjugated equine estrogens plus progestins increased the risk of breast cancer and adverse cardiovascular events but with decreases in bone fractures and colorectal cancer. On balance there were more negative events with HRT. A parallel WHI trial with >12,000 women enrolled testing conjugated estrogens alone (in women who have had hysterectomies) showed no significant increase in breast cancer incidence. A meta-analysis of nonrandomized HRT studies suggests that most of the previously attributed benefit of HRT can be accounted for by higher socioeconomic status among users, which is presumably associated with better access to health care and healthier behaviors. Certain potential benefits of HRT, such as a putative protective effect on cognition with age, were not assessed in WHI. HRT is an area of rapid reevaluation, but it would appear (at least from breast cancer and cardiovascular disease vantage points) that there are serious concerns about long-term HRT use. HRT in women previously diagnosed with breast cancer increases recurrence rates.

In addition to the other factors, radiation is a risk factor in younger women. Women who have been exposed before age 30 to radiation in the form of multiple fluoroscopies (200–300 cGy) or treatment for Hodgkin's disease (>3600 cGy) have a substantial increase in risk of breast cancer, whereas radiation exposure after age 30 appears to have a minimal carcinogenic effect on the breast.

EVALUATION OF BREAST MASSES IN MEN AND WOMEN

Because the breasts are a common site of potentially fatal malignancy in women and because they frequently provide clues to underlying systemic diseases in both men and women, examination of the breast is an essential part of the physical examination. Unfortunately, internists frequently do not examine breasts in men, and, in women, they are apt to defer this evaluation to gynecologists. Because of the plausible association between early detection and improved outcome, it is the duty of every physician to distinguish breast abnormalities at the earliest possible stage and to institute a diagnostic workup. Women should be trained in breast self-examination (BSE). Although breast cancer in men is unusual, unilateral lesions should be evaluated in the same manner as in women, with the recognition that gynecomastia in men can sometimes begin unilaterally and is often asymmetric.

Virtually all breast cancer is diagnosed by biopsy of a nodule detected either on a mammogram or by palpation. Algorithms have been developed to enhance the likelihood of diagnosing breast cancer and reduce the frequency of unnecessary biopsy (Fig. 86-1).

THE PALPABLE BREAST MASS

Women should be strongly encouraged to examine their breasts monthly. A potentially flawed study from China has suggested that BSE does not alter survival, but given its safety, the procedure should still be encouraged. At worst, this practice increases the likelihood of

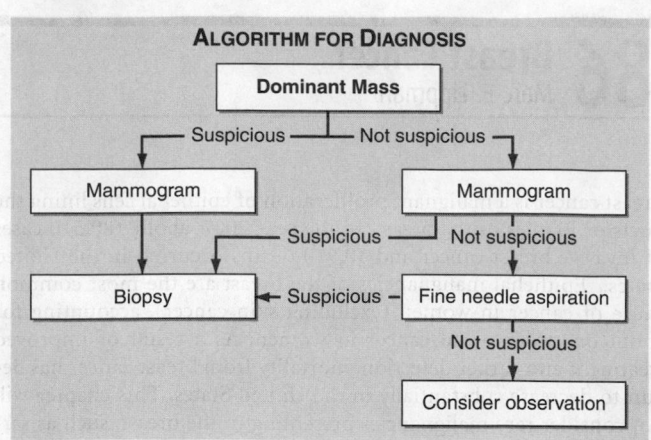

FIGURE 86-2 The "triple diagnosis" technique.

detecting a mass at a smaller size when it can be treated with more limited surgery. Breast examination by the physician should be performed in good light so as to see retractions and other skin changes. The nipple and areolae should be inspected, and an attempt should be made to elicit nipple discharge. All regional lymph node groups should be examined, and any lesions should be measured. Physical examination alone cannot exclude malignancy. Lesions with certain features are more likely to be cancerous (hard, irregular, tethered or fixed, or painless lesions). A negative mammogram in the presence of a persistent lump in the breast does not exclude malignancy. Palpable lesions require additional diagnostic procedures including biopsy.

In premenopausal women, lesions that are either equivocal or nonsuspicious on physical examination should be reexamined in 2–4 weeks, during the follicular phase of the menstrual cycle. Days 5–7 of the cycle are the best time for breast examination. A dominant mass in a postmenopausal woman or a dominant mass that persists through a menstrual cycle in a premenopausal woman should be aspirated by fine-needle biopsy or referred to a surgeon. If nonbloody fluid is aspirated, the diagnosis (cyst) and therapy have been accomplished together. Solid lesions that are persistent, recurrent, complex, or bloody cysts require mammography and biopsy, although in selected patients the so-called triple diagnostic techniques (palpation, mammography, aspiration) can be used to avoid biopsy (Figs. 86-1, 86-2, and 86-3). Ultrasound can be used in place of fine-needle aspiration to distinguish cysts from solid lesions. Not all solid masses are detected by ultrasound; thus, a palpable mass that is not visualized on ultrasound must be presumed to be solid.

Several points are essential in pursuing these management decision trees. First, risk-factor analysis is not part of the decision structure. No constellation of risk factors, by their presence or absence, can be used to exclude biopsy. Second, fine-needle aspiration should be used only in centers that have proven skill in obtaining such specimens and ana-

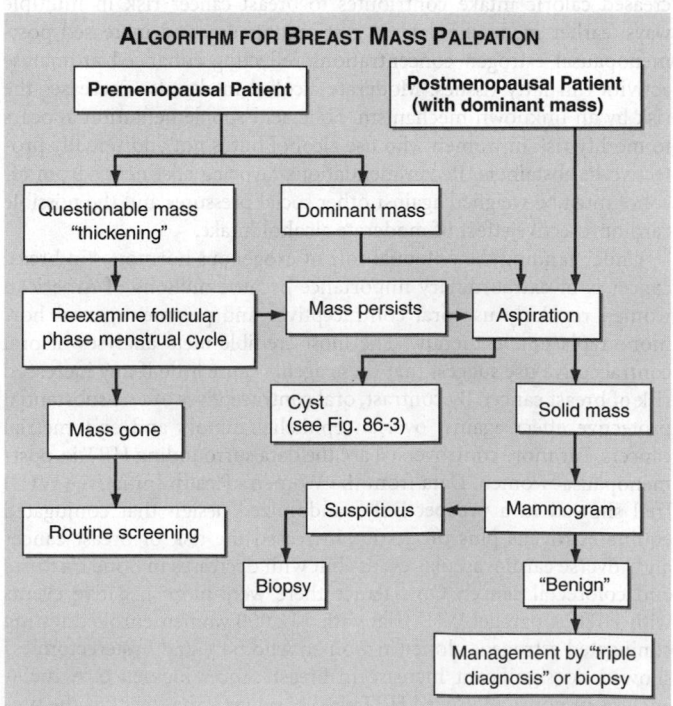

FIGURE 86-1 Approach to a palpable breast mass.

FIGURE 86-3 Management of a breast cyst.

lyzing them. The likelihood of cancer is low in the setting of a "triple negative" (benign-feeling lump, negative mammogram, and negative fine-needle aspiration), but it is not zero. The patient and physician must be aware of a 1% risk of false negatives. Third, additional technologies such as MRI, ultrasound, and sestamibi imaging cannot be used to exclude the need for biopsy, although in unusual circumstances they may provoke a biopsy.

THE ABNORMAL MAMMOGRAM

Diagnostic mammography should not be confused with *screening mammography*, which is performed after a palpable abnormality has been detected. Diagnostic mammography is aimed at evaluating the rest of the breast before biopsy is performed or occasionally is part of the triple-test strategy to exclude immediate biopsy.

Subtle abnormalities that are first detected by screening mammography should be evaluated carefully by compression or magnified views. These abnormalities include clustered microcalcifications, densities (especially if spiculated), and new or enlarging architectural distortion. For some nonpalpable lesions, ultrasound may be helpful either to identify cysts or to guide biopsy. If there is no palpable lesion and detailed mammographic studies are unequivocally benign, the patient should have routine follow-up appropriate to the patient's age.

If a nonpalpable mammographic lesion has a low index of suspicion, mammographic follow-up in 3–6 months is reasonable. Workup of indeterminate and suspicious lesions has been rendered more complex by the advent of stereotactic biopsies. Morrow and colleagues have suggested that these procedures are indicated for lesions that require biopsy but are likely to be benign—that is, for cases in which the procedure probably will eliminate additional surgery. When a lesion is more probably malignant, open biopsy should be performed with a needle localization technique. Others have proposed more widespread use of stereotactic core biopsies for nonpalpable lesions on economic grounds and because diagnosis leads to earlier treatment planning. However, stereotactic diagnosis of a malignant lesion does not eliminate the need for definitive surgical procedures, particularly if breast conservation is attempted. For example, after a breast biopsy with needle localization (i.e., local excision) of a stereotactically diagnosed malignancy, reexcision may still be necessary to achieve negative margins. To some extent, these issues are decided on the basis of referral pattern and the availability of the resources for stereotactic core biopsies. A reasonable approach is shown in Fig. 86-4.

BREAST MASSES IN THE PREGNANT OR LACTATING WOMAN

During pregnancy, the breast grows under the influence of estrogen, progesterone, prolactin, and human placental lactogen. Lactation is suppressed by progesterone, which blocks the effects of prolactin. Af-

ter delivery, lactation is promoted by the fall in progesterone levels, which leaves the effects of prolactin unopposed. The development of a dominant mass during pregnancy or lactation should never be attributed to hormonal changes. A dominant mass must be treated with the same concern in a pregnant woman as any other. Breast cancer develops in 1 in every 3000–4000 pregnancies. Stage for stage, breast cancer in pregnant patients is no different from premenopausal breast cancer in nonpregnant patients. However, pregnant women often have more advanced disease because the significance of a breast mass was not fully considered and/or because of endogenous hormone stimulation. Persistent lumps in the breast of pregnant or lactating women *cannot* be attributed to benign changes based on physical findings; such patients should be promptly referred for diagnostic evaluation.

BENIGN BREAST MASSES

Only about 1 in every 5–10 breast biopsies leads to a diagnosis of cancer, although the rate of positive biopsies varies in different countries and clinical settings. (These differences may be related to interpretation, medicolegal considerations, and availability of mammograms.) The vast majority of benign breast masses are due to "fibrocystic" disease, a descriptive term for small fluid-filled cysts and modest epithelial cell and fibrous tissue hyperplasia. However, fibrocystic disease is a histologic, not a clinical, diagnosis, and women who have had a biopsy with benign findings are at greater risk of developing breast cancer than those who have not had a biopsy. The subset of women with ductal or lobular cell proliferation (about 30% of patients), particularly the small fraction (3%) with atypical hyperplasia, have a fourfold greater risk of developing breast cancer than unbiopsied women, and the increase in the risk is about ninefold for women in this category who also have an affected first-degree relative. Thus, careful follow-up of these patients is required. By contrast, patients with a benign biopsy without atypical hyperplasia are at little risk and may be followed routinely.

SCREENING

Breast cancer is virtually unique among the epithelial tumors in adults in that screening (in the form of annual mammography) improves survival. Meta-analysis examining outcomes from every randomized trial of mammography conclusively shows a 25–30% reduction in the chance of dying from breast cancer with annual screening after age 50; the data for women between ages 40 and 50 are almost as positive. While controversy continues to surround the assessment of screening mammography, the preponderance of data strongly supports the benefits of screening mammography. New analyses of older randomized studies have suggested that screening may not work. While the design defects in some older studies cannot be retrospectively corrected, most experts, including panels of the American Society of Clinical Oncology and the American Cancer Society, continue to believe that screening conveys substantial benefit. Furthermore, the profound drop in breast cancer mortality seen over the past decade is unlikely to be solely attributable to improvements in therapy. It seems prudent to recommend annual mammography for women past the age of 40. Although no randomized study of BSE has ever shown any improvement in survival, its major benefit is identification of tumors appropriate for conservative local therapy. Better mammographic technology, including digitized mammography, routine use of magnified views, and greater skill in mammographic interpretation, combined with newer diagnostic techniques (MRI, magnetic resonance spectroscopy, positron emission tomography, etc.) may make it possible to identify breast cancers even more reliably and earlier. Screening by any technique other than mammography is not indicated; however, younger women who are *BRCA-1* or *BRCA-2* carriers may benefit from MRI screening where the higher sensitivity may outweigh the loss of specificity.

STAGING

Correct staging of breast cancer patients is of extraordinary importance. Not only does it permit an accurate prognosis, but in many cases therapeutic decision-making is based largely on the TNM (primary

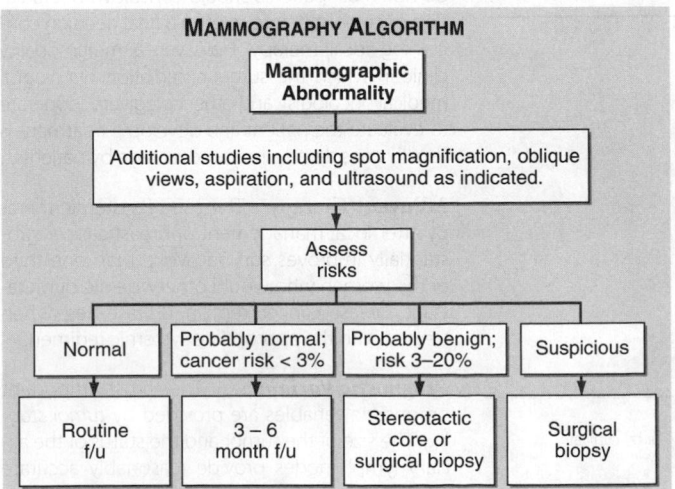

FIGURE 86-4 Approaches to abnormalities detected by mammogram. f/u, follow-up.

tumor, regional nodes, metastasis) classification (Table 86-1). Comparison with historic series should be undertaken with caution, as the staging has changed several times in the past 20 years. The current staging is complex and results in significant changes in outcome by stage as compared with prior staging systems.

℞ BREAST CANCER

PRIMARY BREAST CANCER Breast-conserving treatments, consisting of the removal of the primary tumor by some form of lumpectomy with

or without irradiating the breast, result in a survival that is as good as (or slightly superior to) that after extensive surgical procedures, such as mastectomy or modified radical mastectomy, with or without further irradiation. Postlumpectomy breast irradiation greatly reduces the risk of recurrence in the breast. While breast conservation is associated with a possibility of recurrence in the breast, 10-year survival is at least as good as that after more radical surgery. Postoperative radiation to regional nodes following mastectomy is also associated with an improvement in survival. Since radiation therapy can also reduce the rate of local or regional recurrence, it should be strongly considered following mastectomy for women with high-risk primary tumors (i.e., T2 in size, positive margins, positive nodes). At present, nearly one-third of women in the United States are managed by lumpectomy. Breast-conserving surgery is not suitable for all patients: it is not generally suitable for tumors >5 cm (or for smaller tumors if the breast is small), for tumors involving the nipple areola complex, for tumors with extensive intraductal disease involving multiple quadrants of the breast, for women with a history of collagen-vascular disease, and for women who either do not have the motivation for breast conservation or do not have convenient access to radiation therapy. However, these groups probably do not account for more than one-third of patients who are treated with mastectomy. Thus, a great many women still undergo mastectomy who could safely avoid this procedure and probably would if appropriately counseled.

An extensive intraductal component is a predictor of recurrence in the breast, and so are several clinical variables. Both axillary lymph node involvement and involvement of vascular or lymphatic channels by metastatic tumor in the breast are associated with a higher risk of relapse in the breast but are not contraindications to breast-conserving treatment. When these patients are excluded, and when lumpectomy with negative tumor margins is achieved, breast conservation is associated with a recurrence rate in the breast of substantially <10%. The survival of patients who have recurrence in the breast is somewhat worse than that of women who do not. Thus, recurrence in the breast is a negative prognostic variable for long-term survival. However, recurrence in the breast is not the *cause* of distant metastasis. If recurrence in the breast caused metastatic disease, then women treated with lumpectomy, who have a higher rate of recurrence in the breast, should have poorer survival than women treated with mastectomy, and they do not. Most patients should consult with a radiation oncologist before making a final decision concerning local therapy. However, a multimodality clinic in which the surgeon, radiation oncologist, medical oncologist, and other caregivers cooperate to evaluate the patient and develop a treatment is usually considered a major advantage by patients.

Adjuvant Therapy The use of systemic therapy after local management of breast cancer substantially improves survival. More than one-third of the women who would otherwise die of metastatic breast cancer remain disease-free when treated with the appropriate systemic regimen.

Prognostic Variables The most important prognostic variables are provided by *tumor staging*. The size of the tumor and the status of the axillary lymph nodes provide reasonably accurate information on the likelihood of tumor relapse. The relation of pathologic stage to 5-year survival is shown in **Table 86-2**. For most women, the need for adjuvant therapy can be readily defined

TABLE 86-1 STAGING OF BREAST CANCER

Primary Tumor (T)

T0	No evidence of primary tumor
TIS	Carcinoma in situ
T1	Tumor ≤2 cm
T1a	Tumor >0.1 cm but ≤0.5 cm
T1b	Tumor >0.5 but ≤1 cm
T1c	Tumor >1 cm but ≤2 cm
T2	Tumor >2 cm but ≤5 cm
T3	Tumor >5 cm
T4	Extension to chest wall, inflammation, satellite lesions, ulcerations

Regional Lymph Nodes (N)

PN0(i-)	No regional lymph node metastasis histologically, negative IHC
PN0(i+)	No regional lymph node metastasis histologically, positive IHC, no IHC cluster greater than 0.2 mm
PN0(mol-)	No regional lymph node metastasis histologically, negative molecular findings (RT-PCR)[a]
PN0(mol+)	No regional lymph node metastasis histologically, positive molecular findings (RT-PCR)[a]
PN1	Metastasis in one to three axillary lymph nodes, or in internal mammary nodes with microscopic disease detected by sentinal lymph node dissection but not clinically apparent
PN1mi	Micrometastasis (>0.2mm, none >2.0 mm)
PN1a	Metastasis in one to three axillary lymph nodes
PN1b	Metastasis in internal mammary nodes with microscopic disease detected by sentinel lymph node dissection but not *clinically apparent*[b]
PN1c	Metastasis in one to three axillary lymph nodes and in internal mammary lymph nodes with microscopic disease detected by sentinel lymph node dissection but not clinically apparent.[b] (If associated with greater than three positive axillary lymph nodes, the internal mammary nodes are classified as pN3b to reflect increased tumor burden.)
pN2	Metastasis in four to nine axillary lymph nodes, or in clinically apparent internal mammary lymph nodes in the *absence* of axillary lymph node metastasis
pN3	Metastasis in ten or more axillary lymph nodes, or in infraclavicular lymph nodes, or in clinically apparent[c] ipsilateral internal mammary lymph nodes in the *presence* of 1 or more positive axillary lymph nodes; or in more than 3 axillary lymph nodes with clinically negative microscopic metastasis in internal mammary lymph nodes; or in ipsilateral SCLNs

Distant Metastasis (M)

M0	No distant metastasis
M1	Distant metastasis (includes spread to ipsilateral supraclavicular nodes)

Stage Grouping

Stage 0	TIS	N0	M0
Stage I	T1	N0	M0
Stage IIA	T0	N1	M0
	T1	N1	M0
	T2	N0	M0
Stage IIB	T2	N1	M0
	T3	N0	M0
Stage IIIA	T0	N2	M0
	T1	N2	M0
	T2	N2	M0
	T3	N1, N2	M0
Stage IIIB	T4	Any N	M0
	Any T	N3	M0
Stage IIIC	Any T	N3	M0
Stage IV	Any T	Any N	M1

[a]RT-PCR, reverse transcriptase/polymerase chain reaction.
[b]Clinically apparent is defined as detected by imaging studies (excluding lymphoscintigraphy) or by clinical examination.
[c]T1 includes T1mic.
Source: Used with permission of the American Joint Committee on Cancer (AJCC), Chicago, Illinois. The original source for this material is the AJCC Cancer Staging Manual, Sixth Edition (2002) published by Springer-New York, www.springeronline.com.

TABLE 86-2	5-YEAR SURVIVAL RATE FOR BREAST CANCER BY STAGE
Stage	**5-Year Survival, %**
0	99
I	92
IIA	82
IIB	65
IIIA	47
IIIB	44
IV	14

Source: Modified from data of the National Cancer Institute—Surveillance, Epidemiology, and End Results (SEER).

on this basis alone. In the absence of lymph node involvement, involvement of microvessels (either capillaries or lymphatic channels) in tumors is nearly equivalent to lymph node involvement. The greatest controversy concerns women with intermediate prognoses. *There is rarely justification for adjuvant chemotherapy in most women with tumors <1 cm in size whose axillary lymph nodes are negative.* Detection of breast cancer cells either in the circulation or bone marrow is associated with an increased relapse rate. The most exciting development in this area is the use of gene expression arrays to analyze patterns of tumor gene expression. Several groups have independently defined gene sets that reliably predict disease-free and overall survival far more accurately than any single prognostic variable. Their value is now being assessed in prospective randomized trials. In addition, gene sets capable of predicting responses to endocrine therapy and specific chemotherapeutic drugs have also been described.

Estrogen and progesterone receptor status are of prognostic significance. Tumors that lack either or both of these receptors are more likely to recur than tumors that have them.

Several *measures of tumor growth rate* correlate with early relapse. S-phase analysis using flow cytometry is the most accurate measure. Indirect S-phase assessments using antigens associated with the cell cycle, such as PCNA (Ki67), are also valuable. Tumors with a high proportion (more than the median) of cells in S phase pose a greater risk of relapse; chemotherapy offers the greatest survival benefit for these tumors. Assessment of DNA content in the form of ploidy is of modest value, with nondiploid tumors having a somewhat worse prognosis.

Histologic classification of the tumor has also been used as a prognostic factor. Tumors with a poor nuclear grade have a higher risk of recurrence than tumors with a good nuclear grade. Semiquantitative measures such as the Elston score improve the reproducibility of this measurement.

Molecular changes in the tumor are also useful. Tumors that overexpress *erbB2* (HER-2/neu) or have a mutated p53 gene have a worse prognosis. Particular interest has centered on *erbB2* overexpression as measured by histochemistry or by fluorescence in situ hybridization. Tumors that overexpress *erbB2* are more likely to respond to higher doses of doxorubicin-containing regimens and predict those tumors that will respond to HER-2/neu antibodies (trastuzumab) (herceptin) and a Her-2/neu kinase inhibitor.

To grow, tumors must generate a neovasculature (Chap. 80). The presence of more microvessels in a tumor, particularly when localized in so-called "hot spots," is associated with a worse prognosis. This may assume even greater significance in light of blood vessel–targeting therapies such as bevacizumab (avastin).

Other variables that have also been used to evaluate prognosis include proteins associated with invasiveness, such as type IV collagenase, cathepsin D, plasminogen activator, plasminogen activator receptor, and the metastasis-suppressor gene *nm23*. None of these has been widely ac-

cepted as a prognostic variable for therapeutic decision-making. One problem in interpreting these prognostic variables is that most of them have not been examined in a study using a large cohort of patients.

Adjuvant Regimens Adjuvant therapy is the use of systemic therapies in patients whose known disease has received local therapy but who are at risk of relapse. Selection of appropriate adjuvant chemotherapy or hormone therapy is highly controversial in some situations. Meta-analyses have helped to define broad limits for therapy but do not help in choosing optimal regimens or in choosing a regimen for certain subgroups of patients. A summary of recommendations is shown in **Table 86-3**. In general, premenopausal women for whom any form of adjuvant systemic therapy is indicated should receive multidrug chemotherapy. The antiestrogen tamoxifen improves survival in premenopausal patients with positive estrogen receptors and should be added following completion of chemotherapy. Prophylactic castration may also be associated with a substantial survival benefit (primarily in estrogen receptor–positive patients) but is not widely used in this country.

Data on postmenopausal women are also controversial. The impact of adjuvant chemotherapy is quantitatively less clear-cut than in premenopausal patients, although survival advantages have been shown. The first decision is whether chemotherapy or endocrine therapy should be used. While adjuvant tamoxifen improves survival regardless of axillary lymph node status, the improvement in survival is modest for patients in whom multiple lymph nodes are involved. For this reason, it has been usual to give chemotherapy to postmenopausal patients who have no medical contraindications and who have more than one positive lymph node; tamoxifen is commonly given simultaneously or subsequently. For postmenopausal women for whom systemic therapy is warranted but who have a more favorable prognosis, tamoxifen may be used as a single agent. Large clinical trials have shown superiority for aromatase inhibitors over tamoxifen alone in the adjuvant setting. Unfortunately the optimal plan is unclear. Tamoxifen for 5 years followed by an aromatase inhibitor, the reverse strategy, or even switching to an aromatase inhibitor after 2–3 years of tamoxifen has been shown to be better than tamoxifen alone. No valid information currently permits selection among the three clinically approved aromatase inhibitors. Large clinical trials currently underway will help address these questions.

Most comparisons of adjuvant chemotherapy regimens show little difference among them, although small advantages for doxorubicin-containing regimens are usually seen.

One approach—so-called neoadjuvant chemotherapy—involves the administration of adjuvant therapy before definitive surgery and radiation

TABLE 86-3	SUGGESTED APPROACHES TO ADJUVANT THERAPY			
Age Group	**Lymph Node Status**[a]	**Endocrine Receptor (ER) Status**	**Tumor**	**Recommendation**
Premenopausal	Positive	Any	Any	Multidrug chemotherapy + tamoxifen if ER-positive + trastuzumab in HER-2/neu positive tumors
Premenopausal	Negative	Any	>2 cm, or 1–2 cm with other poor prognostic variables	Multidrug chemotherapy + tamoxifen if ER-positive + trastuzumab in HER-2/neu positive tumors
Postmenopausal	Positive	Negative	Any	Multidrug chemotherapy + trastuzumab in HER-2/neu positive tumors
Postmenopausal	Positive	Positive	Any	Aromatase inhibitors and tamoxifen with or without chemotherapy + trastuzumab in HER-2/neu positive tumors
Postmenopausal	Negative	Positive	>2 cm, or 1–2 cm with other poor prognostic variables	Aromatase inhibitors and tamoxifen + trastuzumab in HER-2/neu positive tumors
Postmenopausal	Negative	Negative	>2 cm, or 1–2 cm with other poor prognostic variables	Consider multidrug chemotherapy + trastuzumab in HER-2/neu positive tumors

[a]As determined by pathologic examination.

therapy. Because the objective response rates of patients with breast cancer to systemic therapy in this setting exceed 75%, many patients will be "downstaged" and may become candidates for breast-conserving therapy. However, overall survival has not been improved using this approach.

Other adjuvant treatments under investigation include the use of taxanes, such as paclitaxel and docetaxel, and therapy based on alternative kinetic and biologic models. In such approaches, high doses of single agents are used separately in relatively dose-intensive cycling regimens. Node-positive patients treated with doxorubicin-cyclophosphamide for four cycles followed by four cycles of a taxane have a substantial improvement in survival as compared with women receiving doxorubicin-cyclophosphamide alone, particularly in women with estrogen receptor–negative tumors. In addition, administration of the same drug combinations at the same dose but at more frequent intervals (q2 weeks with cytokine support as compared with the standard q3 weeks) is even more effective. Among the 25% of women whose tumors overexpress HER-2/neu, addition of trastuzumab given concurrently with a taxane and then for a year after chemotherapy produces significant improvement in survival. Though longer follow-up will be important, this is now the standard care for most women with HER-2/neu positive breast cancers. Cardiotoxicity, immediate and long-term, remains a concern, and further efforts to exploit nonanthracycline-containing regimens are being pursued. Very-high-dose therapy with stem cell transplantation in the adjuvant setting has not proved superior to standard dose therapy and should not be routinely used.

SYSTEMIC THERAPY OF METASTATIC DISEASE   Nearly half of patients treated for apparently localized breast cancer develop metastatic disease. Although a small number of these patients enjoy long remissions when treated with combinations of systemic and local therapy, most eventually succumb to metastatic disease. Soft tissue, bony, and visceral (lung and liver) metastases each account for approximately one-third of sites of initial relapses. However, by the time of death, most patients will have bony involvement. Recurrences can appear at any time after primary therapy. Half of all initial cancer recurrences occur >5 years after initial therapy.

Because the diagnosis of metastatic disease alters the outlook for the patient so drastically, it should rarely be made without biopsy. Every oncologist has seen patients with tuberculosis, gallstones, sarcoidosis, or other nonmalignant diseases misdiagnosed and treated as though they had metastatic breast cancer or even second malignancies such as multiple myeloma thought to be recurrent breast cancer. This is a catastrophic mistake and justifies biopsy for virtually every patient at the time of initial suspicion of metastatic disease.

The choice of therapy requires consideration of local therapy needs, the overall medical condition of the patient, and the hormone receptor status of the tumor, as well as clinical judgment. Because therapy of systemic disease is palliative, the potential toxicities of therapies should be balanced against the response rates. Several variables influence the response to systemic therapy. For example, the presence of estrogen and progesterone receptors is a strong indication for endocrine therapy. On the other hand, patients with short disease-free intervals, rapidly progressive visceral disease, lymphangitic pulmonary disease, or intracranial disease are unlikely to respond to endocrine therapy.

In many cases, systemic therapy can be withheld while the patient is managed with appropriate local therapy. Radiation therapy and occasionally surgery are effective at relieving the symptoms of metastatic disease, particularly when bony sites are involved. Many patients with bone-only or bone-dominant disease have a relatively indolent course. Under such circumstances, systemic chemotherapy has a modest effect, whereas radiation therapy may be effective for long periods. Other systemic treatments, such as strontium 89 and/or bisphosphonates, may provide a palliative benefit without inducing objective responses. Most patients with metastatic disease and certainly all who have bone involvement should receive concurrent bisphosphonates. Since the goal of therapy is to maintain well-being for as long as possible, emphasis should be placed on avoiding the most hazardous complications of metastatic disease, including pathologic fracture of the axial skeleton and spinal cord compression. New back pain in patients with cancer should be explored aggressively on an emergent basis; to wait for neurologic symptoms is a potentially catastrophic error. Metastatic involvement of endocrine organs can cause profound dysfunction, including adrenal insufficiency and hypopituitarism. Similarly, obstruction of the biliary tree or other impaired organ function may be better managed with a local therapy than with a systemic approach.

TABLE 86-4   ENDOCRINE THERAPIES FOR BREAST CANCER

Therapy	Comments

Castration
   Surgical
   LHRH agonists
	For premenopausal women

Antiestrogens	
Tamoxifen	Useful in pre- and postmenopausal women
"Pure" antiestrogens	Responses in tamoxifen-resistant and aromatase inhibitor resistant patients
Surgical adrenalectomy	Rarely employed second-line choice
Aromatase inhibitors	Low toxicity; now first choice for metastatic disease
High-dose progestogens	Common fourth-line choice after AIs, tamoxifen and fulvestrant
Hypophysectomy	Rarely used
Additive androgens or estrogens	Plausible fourth-line therapies; potentially toxic

Note: LHRH, luteinizing hormone–releasing hormone.

Endocrine Therapy   Normal breast tissue is estrogen-dependent. Both primary and metastatic breast cancer may retain this phenotype. The best means of ascertaining whether a breast cancer is hormone-dependent is through analysis of estrogen and progesterone receptor levels on the tumor. Tumors that are positive for the estrogen receptor and negative for the progesterone receptor have a response rate of ~30%. Tumors that have both receptors have a response rate approaching 70%. If neither receptor is present, the objective response rates are <10%. Receptor analyses provide information as to the correct ordering of endocrine therapies as opposed to chemotherapy. Because of their lack of toxicity and because some patients whose receptor analyses are reported as negative respond to endocrine therapy, an endocrine treatment should be attempted in virtually every patient with metastatic breast cancer. Potential endocrine therapies are summarized in **Table 86-4**. The choice of endocrine therapy is usually determined by toxicity profile and availability. In most patients, the initial endocrine therapy should be an aromatase inhibitor rather than tamoxifen. For the subset of women who are ER positive but also HER-2/neu positive, response rates to aromatase inhibitors are very substantially higher than to tamoxifen. Newer "pure" antiestrogens that are free of agonistic effects are also in clinical trial. Cases in which tumors shrink in response to tamoxifen withdrawal (as well as withdrawal of pharmacologic doses of estrogens) have been reported. Endogenous estrogen formation may be blocked by analogues of luteinizing hormone–releasing hormone in premenopausal women. Additive endocrine therapies, including treatment with progestogens, estrogens, and androgens, may also be tried in patients who respond to initial endocrine therapy; the mechanism of action of these latter therapies is unknown. Patients who respond to one endocrine therapy have at least a 50% chance of responding to a second endocrine therapy. It is not uncommon for patients to respond to two or three sequential endocrine therapies; however, combination endocrine therapies do not appear to be superior to individual agents, and combinations of chemotherapy with endocrine therapy are not useful. The median survival of patients with metastatic disease is approximately 2 years, and many patients, particularly older persons and those with hormone-dependent disease, may respond to endocrine therapy for 3–5 years or longer.

Chemotherapy   Unlike many other epithelial malignancies, breast cancer responds to multiple chemotherapeutic agents, including anthracyclines, alkylating agents, taxanes, and antimetabolites. Multiple combinations of these agents have been found to improve response rates somewhat, but they have had little effect on duration of response or survival. The choice among multidrug combinations frequently depends on whether adjuvant chemotherapy was administered and, if so, what type. While patients treated with adjuvant regimens such as cyclophosphamide, methotrexate, and fluorouracil (CMF regimens) may subsequently respond to the same combination in the metastatic disease setting, most oncologists use drugs to which the patients have not been previously exposed. Once patients have progressed after combination drug therapy, it is most common to treat them with single agents. Given the significant toxicity of most drugs, the use of a single effective agent will minimize toxicity by sparing the patient exposure to drugs that would be of little value. No method to select the drugs most efficacious for a given patient has been demonstrated to be useful.

Most oncologists use either an anthracycline or paclitaxel following failure with the initial regimen. However, the choice has to be balanced with individual needs. One randomized study has suggested docetaxel may be superior to paclitaxel. A nanoparticle formulation of paclitaxel (abraxane) has also shown promise.

The use of a humanized antibody to *erbB2* [trastuzumab (Herceptin)] combined with paclitaxel can improve response rate and survival for women whose metastatic tumors overexpress *erbB2*. The magnitude of the survival extension is modest in patients with metastatic disease. Similarly, the use of bevacizumab (avastin) has improved the response rate and response duration to paclitaxel. Objective responses in previously treated patients may also be seen with gemcitabine, capecitabine, navelbine, and oral etoposide.

High-Dose Chemotherapy Including Autologous Bone Marrow

Transplantation Autologous bone marrow transplantation combined with high doses of single agents can produce objective responses even in heavily pretreated patients. However, such responses are rarely durable and do not alter the clinical course for most patients with advanced metastatic disease.

STAGE III BREAST CANCER Between 10 and 25% of patients present with so-called locally advanced, or stage III, breast cancer at diagnosis. Many of these cancers are technically operable, whereas others, particularly cancers with chest wall involvement, inflammatory breast cancers, or cancers with large matted axillary lymph nodes, cannot be managed by surgery initially. Although no randomized trials have proved the efficacy of neoadjuvant chemotherapy, this approach has gained widespread use. More than 90% of patients with locally advanced breast cancer show a partial or better response to multidrug chemotherapy regimens that include an anthracycline. Early administration of this treatment reduces the bulk of the disease and frequently makes the patient a suitable candidate for salvage surgery and/or radiation therapy. These patients should be managed in multimodality clinics to coordinate surgery, radiation therapy, and systemic chemotherapy. Such approaches produce long-term disease-free survival in about 30–50% of patients.

BREAST CANCER PREVENTION Women who have one breast cancer are at risk of developing a contralateral breast cancer at a rate of approximately 0.5% per year. When adjuvant tamoxifen is administered to these patients, the rate of development of contralateral breast cancers is reduced. In other tissues of the body, tamoxifen has estrogen-like effects that are beneficial: preservation of bone mineral density and long-term lowering of cholesterol. However, tamoxifen has estrogen-like effects on the uterus, leading to an increased risk of uterine cancer (0.75% incidence after 5 years on tamoxifen). Tamoxifen also increases the risk of cataract formation. The Breast Cancer Prevention Trial (BCPT) revealed a >49% reduction in breast cancer among women with a risk of at least 1.66% taking the drug for 5 years. Raloxifene has shown similar breast cancer prevention potency but may have different effects on bone and heart. The two agents have been compared in a prospective randomized prevention trial (the STAR trial). The agents are approximately equivalent in preventing breast cancer with fewer thromboembolic events and endometrial cancers with raloxifene; however, raloxifene did not reduce noninvasive cancers as effectively as tamoxifen, so no clear winner has emerged.

NONINVASIVE BREAST CANCER Breast cancer develops as a series of molecular changes in the epithelial cells that lead to ever more malignant behavior. Increased use of mammography has led to more frequent diagnosis of noninvasive breast cancer. These lesions fall into two groups: ductal carcinoma in situ (DCIS) and lobular carcinoma in situ (lobular neoplasia). The management of both entities is controversial.

Ductal Carcinoma In Situ (DCIS) Proliferation of cytologically malignant breast epithelial cells within the ducts is termed *DCIS*. Atypical hyperplasia may be difficult to differentiate from DCIS. At least one-third of patients with untreated DCIS develop invasive breast cancer within 5 years. For many years, the standard treatment for this disease was mastectomy. However, treatment of this condition by lumpectomy and radiation therapy gives survival that is as good as the survival for invasive breast cancer treated by mastectomy. In one randomized trial, the combination of wide excision plus irradiation for DCIS caused a substantial reduction in the local recurrence rate as compared with wide excision alone with negative margins, though survival was identical in the two arms. No studies have compared either of these regimens to mastectomy. Addition of tamoxifen to any DCIS surgical/radiation therapy regimen further improves local control. Data for aromatase inhibitors in this setting are not available.

Several prognostic features may help to identify patients at high risk for local recurrence after either lumpectomy alone or lumpectomy with radiation therapy. These include extensive disease; age <40; and cytologic features such as necrosis, poor nuclear grade, and comedo subtype with overexpression of *erbB2*. Some data suggest that adequate excision with careful determination of pathologically clear margins is associated with a low recurrence rate. When surgery is combined with radiation therapy, recurrence (which is usually in the same quadrant) occurs with a frequency of ≤10%. Given the fact that half of these recurrences will be invasive, about 5% of the initial cohort will eventually develop invasive breast cancer. A reasonable expectation of mortality for these patients is about 1%, a figure that approximates the mortality rate for DCIS managed by mastectomy. Although this train of reasoning has not formally been proved valid, it is reasonable to recommend that patients who desire breast preservation, and in whom DCIS appears to be reasonably localized, be managed by adequate surgery with meticulous pathologic evaluation, followed by breast irradiation and tamoxifen. For patients with localized DCIS, axillary lymph node dissection is unnecessary. More controversial is the question of what management is optimal when there is any degree of invasion. Because of a significant likelihood (10–15%) of axillary lymph node involvement even when the primary lesion shows only microscopic invasion, it is prudent to do at least a level 1 and 2 axillary lymph node dissection for all patients with any degree of invasion; sentinel node biopsy may be substituted. Further management is dictated by the presence of nodal spread.

Lobular Neoplasia Proliferation of cytologically malignant cells within the lobules is termed *lobular neoplasia*. Nearly 30% of patients who have had adequate local excision of the lesion develop breast cancer (usually infiltrating ductal carcinoma) over the next 15–20 years. Ipsilateral and contralateral cancers are equally common. Therefore, lobular neoplasia may be a premalignant lesion that suggests an elevated risk of subsequent breast cancer, rather than a form of malignancy itself, and aggressive local management seems unreasonable. Most patients should be treated with tamoxifen for 5 years and followed with careful annual mammography and semiannual physical examinations. Additional molecular analysis of these lesions may make it possible to discriminate between patients who are at risk of further progression and require additional therapy and those in whom simple follow-up is adequate.

MALE BREAST CANCER Breast cancer is about 1/150th as frequent in men as in women; 1720 men developed breast cancer in 2006. It usually presents as a unilateral lump in the breast and is frequently not diagnosed promptly. Given the small amount of soft tissue and the unexpected nature of the problem, locally advanced presentations are somewhat more common. When male breast cancer is matched to female breast cancer by age and stage, its overall prognosis is identical. Although gynecomastia may initially be unilateral or asymmetric, any unilateral mass in a man over the age of 40 should receive a careful workup including biopsy. On the other hand, bilateral symmetric breast development rarely represents breast cancer and is almost invariably due to endocrine disease or a drug effect. It should be kept in mind, nevertheless, that the risk of cancer is much greater in men with gynecomastia; in such men, gross asymmetry of the breasts should arouse suspicion of cancer. Male breast cancer is best managed by mastectomy and axillary lymph node dissection (modified radical mastectomy). Patients with locally advanced disease or positive nodes should also be treated with irradiation. Approximately 90% of male breast cancers contain estrogen receptors, and approximately 60% of cases with metastatic disease respond to endocrine therapy. No randomized studies have evaluated adjuvant therapy for male breast cancer. Two historic experiences suggest that the disease responds well to adjuvant systemic therapy, and, if not medically contraindicated, the same criteria for the use of adjuvant therapy in women should be applied to men.

The sites of relapse and spectrum of response to chemotherapeutic drugs are virtually identical for breast cancers in either sex.

FOLLOW-UP OF BREAST CANCER PATIENTS

Despite the availability of sophisticated and expensive imaging techniques and a wide range of serum tumor marker tests, survival is not

TABLE 86-5 **BREAST CANCER SURVEILLANCE GUIDELINES**

Test	Frequency
Recommended	
History; eliciting symptoms; physical examination	q3–6 months × 3 years; q6–12 months × 2 years; then annually
Breast self-examination	Monthly
Mammography	Annually
Pelvic examination	Annually
Patient education about symptoms of recurrence	Ongoing
Coordination of care	Ongoing
Not Recommended	
Complete blood count	
Serum chemistry studies	
Chest radiographs	
Bone scans	
Ultrasound examination of the liver	
Computed tomography of chest, abdomen, or pelvis	
Tumor marker CA 15-3, CA 27-29	
Tumor marker CEA	

Source: Recommended Breast Cancer Surveillance Guidelines, ASCO Education Book, Fall, 1997.

influenced by early diagnosis of relapse. Surveillance guidelines are given in Table 86-5.

FURTHER READINGS

BREAST INTERNATIONAL GROUP (BIG) 1-98 COLLABORATIVE GROUP: A comparison of letrozole and tamoxifen in postmenopausal women with early breast cancer. N Engl J Med 353:2747, 2005

CITRON ML et al: Randomized trial of dose-dense versus conventionally scheduled and sequential versus concurrent combination chemotherapy as postoperative adjuvant treatment of node-positive primary breast cancer: First report of intergroup trial C9741/cancer and leukemia group B trial 9741. J Clin Oncol 21:1431, 2003

CLEATOR S et al: Triple-negative breast cancer: Therapeutic options. Lancet Oncol 8:235, 2007

EARLY BREAST CANCER TRIALISTS' COLLABORATIVE GROUP: Effects of chemotherapy and hormonal therapy for early breast cancer on recurrence and 15-year survival: An overview of the randomised trials. Lancet 365:1687, 2005

————: Effects of radiotherapy and of differences in the extent of surgery for early breast cancer on local recurrence and 15-year survival: An overview of the randomised trials. Lancet 366:2087, 2005

GIORDANO S et al: Breast cancer in men. Ann Intern Med 137:678, 2002

INGLE JN et al: Fulvestrant in women with advanced breast cancer after progression on prior aromatase inhibitor therapy: North central cancer treatment group trial N0032. J Clin Oncol 24:1052, 2006

JAKESZ R et al: Switching of postmenopausal women with endocrine-responsive early breast cancer to anastrozole after 2 years' adjuvant tamoxifen: Combined results of ABCSG trial 8 and ARNO 95 trial. Lancet 366:455, 2005

PARTRIDGE A, SCHAPIRA L: Pregnancy and breast cancer. Oncology 19:693, 2005

ROMOND EH et al: Trastuzumab plus adjuvant chemotherapy for operable HER2-positive breast cancer. N Engl J Med 353:1673, 2005

SANTEN RJ, MANSEL R: Benign breast disorders. N Engl J Med 353:275, 2005

SHAPIRO CL, WINER EL (eds): Late effects of treatment and survivorship issues in early-stage breast cancer. Sem Oncol 30:729, 2003

87 Gastrointestinal Tract Cancer
Robert J. Mayer

The gastrointestinal tract is the second most common noncutaneous site for cancer and the second major cause of cancer-related mortality in the United States.

ESOPHAGEAL CANCER

INCIDENCE AND ETIOLOGY

Cancer of the esophagus is a relatively uncommon but extremely lethal malignancy. The diagnosis was made in 15,560 Americans in 2007 and led to 13,940 deaths. Worldwide, the incidence of esophageal cancer varies strikingly. It occurs frequently within a geographic region extending from the southern shore of the Caspian Sea on the west to northern China on the east and encompassing parts of Iran, Central Asia, Afghanistan, Siberia, and Mongolia. High-incidence "pockets" of the disease are also present in such disparate locations as Finland, Iceland, Curaçao, southeastern Africa, and northwestern France. In North America and western Europe, the disease is more common in blacks than whites and in males than females; it appears most often after age 50 and seems to be associated with a lower socioeconomic status.

A variety of causative factors have been implicated in the development of the disease (Table 87-1). In the United States, esophageal cancer cases are either squamous cell carcinomas or adenocarcinomas. The etiology of squamous cell esophageal cancer is related to excess alcohol consumption and/or cigarette smoking. The relative risk increases with the amount of tobacco smoked or alcohol consumed, with these factors acting synergistically. The consumption of whiskey is linked to a higher incidence than the consumption of wine or beer. Squamous cell esophageal carcinoma has also been associated with the ingestion of nitrites, smoked opiates, and fungal toxins in pickled vegetables, as well as mucosal damage caused by such physical insults as long-term exposure to extremely hot tea, the ingestion of lye, radiation-induced strictures, and chronic achalasia. The presence of an esophageal web in association with glossitis and iron deficiency (i.e., Plummer-Vinson or Paterson-Kelly syndrome) and congenital hyperkeratosis and pitting of the palms and soles (i.e., tylosis palmaris et plantaris) have each been linked with squamous cell esophageal cancer, as have dietary deficiencies of molybdenum, zinc, and vitamin A.

TABLE 87-1 **SOME ETIOLOGIC FACTORS BELIEVED TO BE ASSOCIATED WITH ESOPHAGEAL CANCER**

Excess alcohol consumption
Cigarette smoking
Other ingested carcinogens
  Nitrates (converted to nitrites)
  Smoked opiates
  Fungal toxins in pickled vegetables
Mucosal damage from physical agents
  Hot tea
  Lye ingestion
  Radiation-induced strictures
  Chronic achalasia
Host susceptibility
  Esophageal web with glossitis and iron deficiency (i.e., Plummer-Vinson or Paterson-Kelly syndrome)
  Congenital hyperkeratosis and pitting of the palms and soles (i.e., tylosis palmaris et plantaris)
? Dietary deficiencies molybdenum, zinc, vitamin A
? Celiac sprue
Chronic gastric reflux (i.e., Barrett's esophagus) for adenocarcinoma

For unclear reasons, the incidence of squamous cell esophageal cancer has decreased somewhat in both the black and white population in the United States over the past 30 years, while the rate of adenocarcinoma has risen dramatically, particularly in white males. Adenocarcinomas arise in the distal esophagus in the presence of chronic gastric reflux and gastric metaplasia of the epithelium (Barrett's esophagus), which is more common in obese persons. Adenocarcinomas arise within dysplastic columnar epithelium in the distal esophagus. Even before frank neoplasia is detectable, aneuploidy and p53 mutations are found in the dysplastic epithelium. These adenocarcinomas behave clinically like gastric adenocarcinoma and now account for >60% of esophageal cancers.

CLINICAL FEATURES

About 10% of esophageal cancers occur in the upper third of the esophagus (cervical esophagus), 35% in the middle third, and 55% in the lower third. Squamous cell carcinomas and adenocarcinomas cannot be distinguished radiographically or endoscopically.

Progressive dysphagia and weight loss of short duration are the initial symptoms in the vast majority of patients. Dysphagia initially occurs with solid foods and gradually progresses to include semisolids and liquids. By the time these symptoms develop, the disease is usually incurable, since difficulty in swallowing does not occur until >60% of the esophageal circumference is infiltrated with cancer. Dysphagia may be associated with pain on swallowing (odynophagia), pain radiating to the chest and/or back, regurgitation or vomiting, and aspiration pneumonia. The disease most commonly spreads to adjacent and supraclavicular lymph nodes, liver, lungs, pleura, and bone. Tracheoesophageal fistulas may develop as the disease advances, leading to severe suffering. As with other squamous cell carcinomas, hypercalcemia may occur in the absence of osseous metastases, probably from parathormone-related peptide secreted by tumor cells (Chap. 96).

DIAGNOSIS

Attempts at endoscopic and cytologic screening for carcinoma in patients with Barrett's esophagus, while effective as a means of detecting high-grade dysplasia, have not yet been shown to improve the prognosis in individuals found to have a carcinoma. Routine contrast radiographs effectively identify esophageal lesions large enough to cause symptoms. In contrast to benign esophageal leiomyomas, which result in esophageal narrowing with preservation of a normal mucosal pattern, esophageal carcinomas show ragged, ulcerating changes in the mucosa in association with deeper infiltration, producing a picture resembling achalasia. Smaller, potentially resectable tumors are often poorly visualized despite technically adequate esophagograms. Because of this, esophagoscopy should be performed in all patients suspected of having an esophageal abnormality, to visualize the tumor and to obtain histopathologic confirmation of the diagnosis. Because the population of persons at risk for squamous cell carcinoma of the esophagus (i.e., smokers and drinkers) also has a high rate of cancers of the lung and the head and neck region, endoscopic inspection of the larynx, trachea, and bronchi should also be done. A thorough examination of the fundus of the stomach (by retroflexing the endoscope) is imperative as well. Endoscopic biopsies of esophageal tumors fail to recover malignant tissue in one-third of cases because the biopsy forceps cannot penetrate deeply enough through normal mucosa pushed in front of the carcinoma. Cytologic examination of tumor brushings complements standard biopsies and should be performed routinely. The extent of tumor spread to the mediastinum and para-aortic lymph nodes should be assessed by CT scans of the chest and abdomen and by endoscopic ultrasound. Positron emission tomography scanning provides a useful assessment of resectability, offering accurate information regarding spread to mediastinal lymph nodes.

℞ ESOPHAGEAL CANCER

The prognosis for patients with esophageal carcinoma is poor. Fewer than 5% of patients survive 5 years after the diagnosis; thus, management focuses on symptom control. Surgical resection of all gross tumor (i.e., total resection) is feasible in only 45% of cases, with residual tumor cells frequently present at the resection margins. Such esophagectomies have been associated with a postoperative mortality rate of 5–10% due to anastomotic fistulas, subphrenic abscesses, and respiratory complications. About 20% of patients who survive a total resection live 5 years. The efficacy of primary radiation therapy (5500–6000 cGy) for squamous cell carcinomas is similar to that of radical surgery, sparing patients perioperative morbidity but often resulting in less satisfactory palliation of obstructive symptoms. The evaluation of chemotherapeutic agents in patients with esophageal carcinoma has been hampered by ambiguity in the definition of "response" and the debilitated physical condition of many treated individuals. Nonetheless, significant reductions in the size of measurable tumor masses have been reported in 15–25% of patients given single-agent treatment and in 30–60% of patients treated with drug combinations that include cisplatin. Combination chemotherapy and radiation therapy as the initial therapeutic approach, either alone or followed by an attempt at operative resection, seems to be beneficial. When administered along with radiation therapy, chemotherapy produces a better survival outcome than radiation therapy alone. The use of preoperative chemotherapy and radiation therapy followed by esophageal resection appears to prolong survival as compared with controls in small, randomized trials, and some reports suggest that no additional benefit accrues when surgery is added if significant shrinkage of tumor has been achieved by the chemoradiation combination.

For the incurable, surgically unresectable patient with esophageal cancer, dysphagia, malnutrition, and the management of tracheoesophageal fistulas are major issues. Approaches to palliation include repeated endoscopic dilatation, the surgical placement of a gastrostomy or jejunostomy for hydration and feeding, and endoscopic placement of an expansive metal stent to bypass the tumor. Endoscopic fulguration of the obstructing tumor with lasers is the most promising of these techniques.

TUMORS OF THE STOMACH

GASTRIC ADENOCARCINOMA

Incidence and Epidemiology For unclear reasons, the incidence and mortality rates for gastric cancer have decreased markedly during the past 75 years. The mortality rate from gastric cancer in the United States has dropped in men from 28 to 5.8 per 100,000 persons, while in women the rate has decreased from 27 to 2.8 per 100,000. Nonetheless, 21,260 new cases of stomach cancer were diagnosed in the United States, and 11,210 Americans died of the disease in 2007. Gastric cancer incidence has decreased worldwide but remains high in Japan, China, Chile, and Ireland.

The risk of gastric cancer is greater among lower socioeconomic classes. Migrants from high- to low-incidence nations maintain their susceptibility to gastric cancer, while the risk for their offspring approximates that of the new homeland. These findings suggest that an environmental exposure, probably beginning early in life, is related to the development of gastric cancer, with dietary carcinogens considered the most likely factor(s).

Pathology About 85% of stomach cancers are adenocarcinomas, with 15% due to lymphomas and gastrointestinal stromal tumors (GIST) and leiomyosarcomas. Gastric adenocarcinomas may be subdivided into two categories: a *diffuse type*, in which cell cohesion is absent, so that individual cells infiltrate and thicken the stomach wall without forming a discrete mass; and an *intestinal type*, characterized by cohesive neoplastic cells that form glandlike tubular structures. The diffuse carcinomas occur more often in younger patients, develop throughout the stomach (including the cardia), result in a loss of distensibility of the gastric wall (so-called linitis plastica, or "leather bottle" appearance), and carry a poorer prognosis. Intestinal-type lesions are frequently ulcerative, more commonly appear in the antrum and lesser curvature of the stomach, and are often preceded by a prolonged precancerous process. While the incidence of diffuse carcinomas is similar in most populations, the intestinal type tends to predominate in the high-risk geographic regions and is less likely to be found in areas where the frequency of gastric cancer is declining. Thus, different etiologic factor(s) may be involved in these

TABLE 87-2 NITRATE-CONVERTING BACTERIA AS A FACTOR IN THE CAUSATION OF GASTRIC CARCINOMA[a]

Exogenous sources of nitrate-converting bacteria:
   Bacterially contaminated food (common in lower socioeconomic classes, who have a higher incidence of the disease; diminished by improved food preservation and refrigeration)
   ? *Helicobacter pylori* infection
Endogenous factors favoring growth of nitrate-converting bacteria in the stomach:
   Decreased gastric acidity
   Prior gastric surgery (antrectomy) (15- to 20-year latency period)
   Atrophic gastritis and/or pernicious anemia
   ? Prolonged exposure to histamine H_2-receptor antagonists

[a]Hypothesis: Dietary nitrates are converted to carcinogenic nitrites by bacteria.

two subtypes. In the United States, ~30% of gastric cancers originate in the distal stomach, ~20% arise in the midportion of the stomach, and ~37% originate in the proximal third of the stomach. The remaining 13% involve the entire stomach.

Etiology The long-term ingestion of high concentrations of nitrates in dried, smoked, and salted foods appears to be associated with a higher risk. The nitrates are thought to be converted to carcinogenic nitrites by bacteria (Table 87-2). Such bacteria may be introduced exogenously through the ingestion of partially decayed foods, which are consumed in abundance worldwide by the lower socioeconomic classes. Bacteria such as *Helicobacter pylori* may also contribute to this effect by causing chronic gastritis, loss of gastric acidity, and bacterial growth in the stomach. The effect of *H. pylori* eradication on the subsequent risk for gastric cancer in high-incidence areas is under investigation. Loss of acidity may occur when acid-producing cells of the gastric antrum have been removed surgically to control benign peptic ulcer disease or when achlorhydria, atrophic gastritis, and even pernicious anemia develop in the elderly. Serial endoscopic examinations of the stomach in patients with atrophic gastritis have documented replacement of the usual gastric mucosa by intestinal-type cells. This process of intestinal metaplasia may lead to cellular atypia and eventual neoplasia. Since the declining incidence of gastric cancer in the United States primarily reflects a decline in distal, ulcerating, intestinal-type lesions, it is conceivable that better food preservation and the availability of refrigeration to all socioeconomic classes have decreased the dietary ingestion of exogenous bacteria. *H. pylori* has not been associated with the diffuse, more proximal form of gastric carcinoma.

Several additional etiologic factors have been associated with gastric carcinoma. Gastric ulcers and adenomatous polyps have occasionally been linked, but data on a cause-and-effect relationship are unconvincing. The inadequate clinical distinction between benign gastric ulcers and small ulcerating carcinomas may, in part, account for this presumed association. The presence of extreme hypertrophy of gastric rugal folds (i.e., Ménétrier's disease), giving the impression of polypoid lesions, has been associated with a striking frequency of malignant transformation; such hypertrophy, however, does not represent the presence of true adenomatous polyps. Individuals with blood group A have a higher incidence of gastric cancer than persons with blood group O; this observation may be related to differences in the mucous secretion, leading to altered mucosal protection from carcinogens. A germline mutation in the E-cadherin gene, inherited in an autosomal dominant pattern and coding for a cell adhesion protein, has been linked to a high incidence of occult gastric cancers in young asymptomatic carriers. Duodenal ulcers are not associated with gastric cancer.

Clinical Features Gastric cancers, when superficial and surgically curable, usually produce no symptoms. As the tumor becomes more extensive, patients may complain of an insidious upper abdominal discomfort varying in intensity from a vague, postprandial fullness to a severe, steady pain. Anorexia, often with slight nausea, is very common but is not the usual presenting complaint. Weight loss may even-

tually be observed, and nausea and vomiting are particularly prominent with tumors of the pylorus; dysphagia and early satiety may be the major symptoms caused by diffuse lesions originating in the cardia. There are no early physical signs. A palpable abdominal mass indicates long-standing growth and predicts regional extension.

Gastric carcinomas spread by direct extension through the gastric wall to the perigastric tissues, occasionally adhering to adjacent organs such as the pancreas, colon, or liver. The disease also spreads via lymphatics or by seeding of peritoneal surfaces. Metastases to intraabdominal and supraclavicular lymph nodes occur frequently, as do metastatic nodules to the ovary (Krukenberg's tumor), periumbilical region ("Sister Mary Joseph node"), or peritoneal cul-de-sac (Blumer's shelf palpable on rectal or vaginal examination); malignant ascites may also develop. The liver is the most common site for hematogenous spread of tumor.

The presence of iron-deficiency anemia in men and of occult blood in the stool in both sexes mandates a search for an occult gastrointestinal tract lesion. A careful assessment is of particular importance in patients with atrophic gastritis or pernicious anemia. Unusual clinical features associated with gastric adenocarcinomas include migratory thrombophlebitis, microangiopathic hemolytic anemia, and acanthosis nigricans.

Diagnosis A double-contrast radiographic examination is the simplest diagnostic procedure for the evaluation of a patient with epigastric complaints. The use of double-contrast techniques helps to detect small lesions by improving mucosal detail. The stomach should be distended at some time during every radiographic examination, since decreased distensibility may be the only indication of a diffuse infiltrative carcinoma. Although gastric ulcers can be detected fairly early, distinguishing benign from malignant lesions radiographically is difficult. The anatomic location of an ulcer is not in itself an indication of the presence or absence of a cancer.

Gastric ulcers that appear benign by radiography present special problems. Some physicians believe that gastroscopy is not mandatory if the radiographic features are typically benign, if complete healing can be visualized by x-ray within 6 weeks, and if a follow-up contrast radiograph obtained several months later shows a normal appearance. However, we recommend gastroscopic biopsy and brush cytology for all patients with a gastric ulcer in order to exclude a malignancy. Malignant gastric ulcers must be recognized before they penetrate into surrounding tissues, because the rate of cure of early lesions limited to the mucosa or submucosa is >80%. Since gastric carcinomas are difficult to distinguish clinically or radiographically from gastric lymphomas, endoscopic biopsies should be made as deeply as possible, due to the submucosal location of lymphoid tumors.

The staging system for gastric carcinoma is shown in Table 87-3.

℞ GASTRIC ADENOCARCINOMA

Complete surgical removal of the tumor with resection of adjacent lymph nodes offers the only chance for cure. However, this is possible in less than a third of patients. A subtotal gastrectomy is the treatment of choice for patients with distal carcinomas, while total or near-total gastrectomies are required for more proximal tumors. The inclusion of extended lymph node dissection in these procedures appears to confer an added risk for complications without enhancing survival. The prognosis following complete surgical resection depends on the degree of tumor penetration into the stomach wall and is adversely influenced by regional lymph node involvement, vascular invasion, and abnormal DNA content (i.e., aneuploidy), characteristics found in the vast majority of American patients. As a result, the probability of survival after 5 years for the 25–30% of patients able to undergo complete resection is ~20% for distal tumors and <10% for proximal tumors, with recurrences continuing for at least 8 years after surgery. In the absence of ascites or extensive hepatic or peritoneal metastases, even patients whose disease is believed to be incurable by surgery should be offered resection of the primary lesion. Reduction of tumor bulk is the best form of palliation and may enhance the probability of benefit from subsequent therapy.

Gastric adenocarcinoma is a relatively radioresistant tumor, and adequate control of the primary tumor requires doses of external beam irradiation that exceed the tolerance of surrounding structures, such as bowel mucosa and spinal cord. As a result, the major role of radiation therapy in patients has been palliation of pain. Radiation therapy alone after a complete resection does not prolong survival. In the setting of surgically unresectable disease limited to the epigastrium, patients treated with 3500–4000 cGy did not live longer than similar patients not receiving radiotherapy; however, survival was prolonged slightly when 5-fluorouracil (5-FU) was given in combination with radiation therapy. In this clinical setting, the 5-FU may be functioning as a radiosensitizer.

The administration of combinations of cytotoxic drugs to patients with advanced gastric carcinoma has been associated with partial responses in 30–50% of cases; responders appear to benefit from treatment. Such drug combinations have generally included cisplatin combined with either epirubicin and infusional 5-FU or with irinotecan. Despite this encouraging response rate, complete remissions are uncommon, the partial responses are transient, and the overall influence of multidrug therapy on survival has been unclear. The use of adjuvant chemotherapy alone following the complete resection of a gastric cancer has only minimally improved survival. However, combination chemotherapy administered before and after surgery (*perioperative treatment*) as well as postoperative chemotherapy combined with radiation therapy reduces the recurrence rate and prolongs survival.

PRIMARY GASTRIC LYMPHOMA

Primary lymphoma of the stomach is relatively uncommon, accounting for <15% of gastric malignancies and ~2% of all lymphomas. The stomach is, however, the most frequent extranodal site for lymphoma, and gastric lymphoma has increased in frequency during the past 30 years. The disease is difficult to distinguish clinically from gastric adenocarcinoma; both tumors are most often detected during the sixth decade of life; present with epigastric pain, early satiety, and generalized fatigue; and are usually characterized by ulcerations with a ragged, thickened mucosal pattern demonstrated by contrast radiographs. The diagnosis of lymphoma of the stomach may occasionally be made through cytologic brushings of the gastric mucosa but usually requires a biopsy at gastroscopy or laparotomy. Failure of gastroscopic biopsies to detect lymphoma in a given case should not be interpreted as being conclusive, since superficial biopsies may miss the deeper lymphoid infiltrate. The macroscopic pathology of gastric lymphoma may also mimic adenocarcinoma, consisting of either a bulky ulcerated lesion localized in the corpus or antrum or a diffuse process spreading throughout the entire gastric submucosa and even extending into the duodenum. Microscopically, the vast majority of gastric lymphoid tumors are non-Hodgkin's lymphomas of B cell origin; Hodgkin's disease involving the stomach is extremely uncommon. Histologically, these tumors may range from well-differentiated, superficial processes [mucosa-associated lymphoid tissue (MALT)] to high-grade, large-cell lymphomas. Like gastric adenocarcinoma, infection with *H. pylori* increases the risk for gastric lymphoma in general and MALT lymphomas in particular. Gastric lymphomas spread initially to regional lymph nodes (often to Waldeyer's ring) and may then disseminate. Gastric lymphomas are staged like other lymphomas (Chap. 105).

℞ PRIMARY GASTRIC LYMPHOMA

Primary gastric lymphoma is a far more treatable disease than adenocarcinoma of the stomach, a fact that underscores the need for making the correct diagnosis. Antibiotic treatment to eradicate *H. pylori* infection has led

TABLE 87-3 STAGING SYSTEM FOR GASTRIC CARCINOMA

Stage	TNM	Features	No. of Cases, %	5-Year Survival, %
0	TisN0M0	Node negative; limited to mucosa	1	90
IA	T1N0M0	Node negative; invasion of lamina propria or submucosa	7	59
IB	T2N0M0	Node negative; invasion of muscularis propria	10	44
II	T1N2M0	Node positive; invasion beyond mucosa but within wall	17	29
	T2N1M0	*or*		
	T3N0M0	Node negative; extension through wall		
IIIA	T2N2M0	Node positive; invasion of muscularis propria or through wall	21	15
	T3N1-2M0			
IIIB	T4N0-1M0	Node negative; adherence to surrounding tissue	14	9
IV	T4N2M0	Node positive; adherence to surrounding tissue	30	3
		or		
	T1-4N0-2M1	Distant metastases		

Note: ACS, American Cancer Society.

Data from ACS

to regression of about 75% of gastric MALT lymphomas and should be considered before surgery, radiation therapy, or chemotherapy are undertaken in patients having such tumors. A lack of response to such antimicrobial treatment has been linked to a specific chromosomal abnormality, i.e., t(11;18). Responding patients should undergo periodic endoscopic surveillance because it remains unclear whether the neoplastic clone is eliminated or merely suppressed, although the response to antimicrobial treatment is quite durable. Subtotal gastrectomy, usually followed by combination chemotherapy, has led to 5-year survival rates of 40–60% in patients with localized high-grade lymphomas. The need for a major surgical procedure has been questioned, particularly in patients with preoperative radiographic evidence of nodal involvement, for whom chemotherapy [CHOP (cyclophosphamide, doxorubicin, vincristine, and prednisone)] plus rituximab is effective therapy. A role for radiation therapy is not defined because most recurrences develop at distant sites.

GASTRIC (NONLYMPHOID) SARCOMA

Leiomyosarcomas and GISTs make up 1–3% of gastric neoplasms. They most frequently involve the anterior and posterior walls of the gastric fundus and often ulcerate and bleed. Even those lesions that appear benign on histologic examination may behave in a malignant fashion. These tumors rarely invade adjacent viscera and characteristically do not metastasize to lymph nodes, but they may spread to the liver and lungs. The treatment of choice is surgical resection. Combination chemotherapy should be reserved for patients with metastatic disease. All such tumors should be analyzed for a mutation in the *c-kit* receptor. GISTs are unresponsive to conventional chemotherapy; ~50% of patients experience objective response and prolonged survival when treated with imatinib mesylate (Gleevec) (400–800 mg PO daily), a selective inhibitor of the *c-kit* tyrosine kinase. Many patients with GIST whose tumors have become refractory to imatinib subsequently benefit from sunitinib (Sutent), another inhibitor of the *c-kit* tyrosine kinase.

COLORECTAL CANCER

INCIDENCE

Cancer of the large bowel is second only to lung cancer as a cause of cancer death in the United States: 153,760 new cases occurred in 2007, and 52,180 deaths were due to colorectal cancer. The incidence rate has remained relatively unchanged during the past 30 years, while the mortality rate has decreased, particularly in females. Colorectal cancer generally occurs in persons ≥50 years.

POLYPS AND MOLECULAR PATHOGENESIS

Most colorectal cancers, regardless of etiology, arise from adenomatous polyps. A polyp is a grossly visible protrusion from the mucosal surface and may be classified pathologically as a nonneoplastic hamartoma (*juvenile polyp*), a hyperplastic mucosal proliferation (*hyperplastic polyp*), or an adenomatous polyp. Only adenomas are clearly premalignant, and only a minority of such lesions becomes cancer. Adenomatous polyps may be found in the colons of ~30% of middle-aged and ~50% of elderly people; however, <1% of polyps ever become malignant. Most polyps produce no symptoms and remain clinically undetected. Occult blood in the stool is found in <5% of patients with polyps.

A number of molecular changes are noted in adenomatous polyps, dysplastic lesions, and polyps containing microscopic foci of tumor cells (carcinoma in situ), which are thought to reflect a multistep process in the evolution of normal colonic mucosa to life-threatening invasive carcinoma. These developmental steps toward carcinogenesis include, but are not restricted to, point mutations in the K-*ras* protooncogene; hypomethylation of DNA, leading to gene activation; loss of DNA (*allelic loss*) at the site of a tumor-suppressor gene [the adenomatous polyposis coli (*APC*) gene] on the long arm of chromosome 5 (5q21); allelic loss at the site of a tumor-suppressor gene located on chromosome 18q [the deleted in colorectal cancer (*DCC*) gene]; and allelic loss at chromosome 17p, associated with mutations in the p53 tumor-suppressor gene (see Fig. 79-2). Thus, the altered proliferative pattern of the colonic mucosa, which results in progression to a polyp and then to carcinoma, may involve the mutational activation of an oncogene followed by and coupled with the loss of genes that normally suppress tumorigenesis. It remains uncertain whether the genetic aberrations always occur in a defined order. Based on this model, however, cancer is believed to develop only in those polyps in which most (if not all) of these mutational events take place.

Clinically, the probability of an adenomatous polyp becoming a cancer depends on the gross appearance of the lesion, its histologic features, and its size. Adenomatous polyps may be pedunculated (stalked) or sessile (flat-based). Cancers develop more frequently in sessile polyps. Histologically, adenomatous polyps may be tubular, villous (i.e., papillary), or tubulovillous. Villous adenomas, most of which are sessile, become malignant more than three times as often as tubular adenomas. The likelihood that any polypoid lesion in the large bowel contains invasive cancer is related to the size of the polyp, being negligible (<2%) in lesions <1.5 cm, intermediate (2–10%) in lesions 1.5–2.5 cm in size, and substantial (10%) in lesions >2.5 cm.

Following the detection of an adenomatous polyp, the entire large bowel should be visualized endoscopically or radiographically, since synchronous lesions are noted in about one-third of cases. Colonoscopy should then be repeated periodically, even in the absence of a previously documented malignancy, since such patients have a 30–50% probability of developing another adenoma and are at a higher-than-average risk for developing a colorectal carcinoma. Adenomatous polyps are thought to require >5 years of growth before becoming clinically significant; colonoscopy need not be carried out more frequently than every 3 years.

ETIOLOGY AND RISK FACTORS

Risk factors for the development of colorectal cancer are listed in Table 87-4.

Diet The etiology for most cases of large-bowel cancer appears to be related to environmental factors. The disease occurs more often in up-

TABLE 87-4 RISK FACTORS FOR THE DEVELOPMENT OF COLORECTAL CANCER

Diet: Animal fat
Hereditary syndromes (autosomal dominant inheritance)
   Polyposis coli
   Nonpolyposis syndrome (Lynch syndrome)
Inflammatory bowel disease
Streptococcus bovis bacteremia
Ureterosigmoidostomy
? Tobacco use

per socioeconomic populations who live in urban areas. Mortality from colorectal cancer is directly correlated with per capita consumption of calories, meat protein, and dietary fat and oil as well as elevations in the serum cholesterol concentration and mortality from coronary artery disease. Geographic variations in incidence are unrelated to genetic differences, since migrant groups tend to assume the large-bowel cancer incidence rates of their adopted countries. Furthermore, population groups such as Mormons and Seventh Day Adventists, whose lifestyle and dietary habits differ somewhat from those of their neighbors, have significantly lower-than-expected incidence and mortality rates for colorectal cancer. Colorectal cancer has increased in Japan since that nation has adopted a more "western" diet. At least three hypotheses have been proposed to explain the relationship to diet, none of which is fully satisfactory.

ANIMAL FATS One hypothesis is that the ingestion of animal fats found in red meats and processed meat leads to an increased proportion of anaerobes in the gut microflora, resulting in the conversion of normal bile acids into carcinogens. This provocative hypothesis is supported by several reports of increased amounts of fecal anaerobes in the stools of patients with colorectal cancer. Diets high in animal (but not vegetable) fats are also associated with high serum cholesterol, which is also associated with enhanced risk for the development of colorectal adenomas and carcinomas.

INSULIN RESISTANCE The large number of calories in "western" diets coupled with physical inactivity has been associated with a higher prevalence of obesity. Obese persons develop insulin resistance with increased circulating levels of insulin, leading to higher circulating concentrations of insulin-like growth factor type I (IGF-I). This growth factor appears to stimulate proliferation of the intestinal mucosa.

FIBER Contrary to prior beliefs, the results of randomized trials and case-controlled studies have failed to show any value for dietary fiber or diets high in fruits and vegetables in preventing the recurrence of colorectal adenomas or the development of colorectal cancer. The weight of epidemiologic evidence, however, implicates diet as being the major etiologic factor for colorectal cancer, particularly diets high in animal fat and in calories.

HEREDITARY FACTORS AND SYNDROMES

Up to 25% of patients with colorectal cancer have a family history of the disease, suggesting a hereditary predisposition. Inherited large-bowel cancers can be divided into two main groups: the well-studied but uncommon polyposis syndromes and the more common nonpolyposis syndromes (Table 87-5).

Polyposis Coli Polyposis coli (familial polyposis of the colon) is a rare condition characterized by the appearance of thousands of adenomatous polyps throughout the large bowel. It is transmitted as an autosomal dominant trait; the occasional patient with no family history probably developed the condition due to a spontaneous mutation. Polyposis coli is associated with a deletion in the long arm of chromosome 5 [including the *APC* (adenomatous polyposis coli) gene] in both neoplastic (somatic mutation) and normal (germline mutation) cells. The loss of this genetic material (i.e., allelic loss) results in the absence of tumor-suppressor genes whose protein products would normally inhibit neoplastic growth. The presence of soft tissue and bony tumors, congenital hypertrophy of the retinal pigment epithelium, mesenteric desmoid tumors, and ampullary cancers in addition to the colonic polyps characterizes a subset of polyposis coli known as *Gardner's syndrome*. The appearance of malignant tumors of the central nervous system accompanying polyposis coli defines *Turcot's syndrome*. The colonic polyps in all these conditions are rarely present before puberty but are generally evident in affected individuals by age 25. If the polyposis is not treated surgically, colorectal cancer will develop in almost all patients before age 40. Polyposis coli results from a defect in the colonic mucosa, leading to an abnormal proliferative pattern

TABLE 87-5 HEREDITABLE (AUTOSOMAL DOMINANT) GASTROINTESTINAL POLYPOSIS SYNDROMES

Syndrome	Distribution of Polyps	Histologic Type	Malignant Potential	Associated Lesions
Familial adenomatous polyposis	Large intestine	Adenoma	Common	None
Gardner's syndrome	Large and small intestines	Adenoma	Common	Osteomas, fibromas, lipomas, epidermoid cysts, ampullary cancers, congenital hypertrophy of retinal pigment epithelium
Turcot's syndrome	Large intestine	Adenoma	Common	Brain tumors
Nonpolyposis syndrome (Lynch syndrome)	Large intestine (often proximal)	Adenoma	Common	Endometrial and ovarian tumors
Peutz-Jeghers syndrome	Small and large intestines, stomach	Hamartoma	Rare	Mucocutaneous pigmentation; tumors of the ovary, breast, pancreas, endometrium
Juvenile polyposis	Large and small intestines, stomach	Hamartoma, rarely progressing to adenoma	Rare	Various congenital abnormalities

and impaired DNA repair mechanisms. Once the multiple polyps are detected, patients should undergo a total colectomy. The ileoanal anastomotic technique allows removal of the entire bowel while retaining the anal sphincter. Medical therapy with nonsteroidal anti-inflammatory drugs (NSAIDs) such as sulindac and cyclooxygenase-2 inhibitors such as celecoxib can decrease the number and size of polyps in patients with polyposis coli; however, this effect on polyps is only temporary, and NSAIDs are not proven to reduce the risk of cancer. Colectomy remains the primary therapy/prevention. The offspring of patients with polyposis coli, who often are prepubertal when the diagnosis is made in the parent, have a 50% risk for developing this premalignant disorder and should be carefully screened by annual flexible sigmoidoscopy until age 35. Proctosigmoidoscopy is a sufficient screening procedure because polyps tend to be evenly distributed from cecum to anus, making more-invasive and expensive techniques such as colonoscopy or barium enema unnecessary. Testing for occult blood in the stool is an inadequate screening maneuver. An alternative method for identifying carriers is testing DNA from peripheral blood mononuclear cells for the presence of a mutated *APC* gene. The detection of such a germline mutation can lead to a definitive diagnosis before the development of polyps.

Hereditary Nonpolyposis Colon Cancer Hereditary nonpolyposis colon cancer (HNPCC), also known as *Lynch syndrome*, is another autosomal dominant trait. It is characterized by the presence of three or more relatives with histologically documented colorectal cancer, one of whom is a first-degree relative of the other two; one or more cases of colorectal cancer diagnosed before age 50 in the family; and colorectal cancer involving at least two generations. In contrast to polyposis coli, HNPCC is associated with an unusually high frequency of cancer arising in the proximal large bowel. The median age for the appearance of an adenocarcinoma is <50 years, 10–15 years younger than the median age for the general population. Despite having a poorly differentiated histologic appearance, the proximal colon tumors in HNPCC have a better prognosis than sporadic tumors from patients of similar age. Families with HNPCC often include individuals with multiple primary cancers; the association of colorectal cancer with either ovarian or endometrial carcinomas is especially strong in women. It has been recommended that members of such families undergo biennial colonoscopy beginning at age 25 years, with intermittent pelvic ultrasonography and endometrial biopsy for afflicted women; such a screening strategy has not yet been validated. HNPCC is associated with germline mutations of several genes, particularly *hMSH2* on chromosome 2 and *hMLH1* on chromosome 3. These mutations lead to errors in DNA replication and are thought to result in DNA instability because of defective repair of DNA mismatches, resulting in abnormal cell growth and tumor development.

Testing tumor cells through molecular analysis of DNA or immunohistochemical staining of paraffin-fixed tissue for "microsatellite instability" (sequence changes reflecting defective mismatch repair) in patients under age 50 with colorectal cancer and a positive family history for colorectal or endometrial cancer may identify probands with HNPCC.

INFLAMMATORY BOWEL DISEASE

(Chap. 289) Large-bowel cancer is increased in incidence in patients with long-standing inflammatory bowel disease (IBD). Cancers develop more commonly in patients with ulcerative colitis than in those with granulomatous colitis, but this impression may result in part from the occasional difficulty of differentiating these two conditions. The risk of colorectal cancer in a patient with IBD is relatively small during the initial 10 years of the disease, but then it appears to increase at a rate of ~0.5–1% per year. Cancer may develop in 8–30% of patients after 25 years. The risk is higher in younger patients with pancolitis.

Cancer surveillance in patients with IBD is unsatisfactory. Symptoms such as bloody diarrhea, abdominal cramping, and obstruction, which may signal the appearance of a tumor, are similar to the complaints caused by a flare-up of the underlying disease. In patients with a history of IBD lasting ≥15 years who continue to experience exacerbations, the surgical removal of the colon can significantly reduce the risk for cancer and also eliminate the target organ for the underlying chronic gastrointestinal disorder. The value of such surveillance techniques as colonoscopy with mucosal biopsies and brushings for less-symptomatic individuals with chronic IBD is uncertain. The lack of uniformity regarding the pathologic criteria that characterize dysplasia and the absence of data that such surveillance reduces the development of lethal cancers have made this costly practice an area of controversy.

OTHER HIGH-RISK CONDITIONS

***Streptococcus bovis* Bacteremia** For unknown reasons, individuals who develop endocarditis or septicemia from this fecal bacterium have a high incidence of occult colorectal tumors and, possibly, upper gastrointestinal cancers as well. Endoscopic or radiographic screening appears advisable.

Tobacco Use Cigarette smoking is linked to the development of colorectal adenomas, particularly after >35 years of tobacco use. No biologic explanation for this association has yet been proposed.

PRIMARY PREVENTION

Several orally administered compounds have been assessed as possible inhibitors of colon cancer. The most effective class of chemopreventive agents is aspirin and other NSAIDs, which are thought to suppress cell proliferation by inhibiting prostaglandin synthesis. Regular aspirin use reduces the risk of colon adenomas and carcinomas as well as death from large-bowel cancer; such use also appears to diminish the likelihood for developing additional premalignant adenomas following treatment for a prior colon carcinoma. This effect of aspirin on colon carcinogenesis increases with the duration and dosage of drug use. Oral folic acid supplements and oral calcium supplements reduce the risk of adenomatous polyps and colorectal cancers in case-controlled studies. Antioxidant vitamins such as ascorbic acid, tocopherols, and β-carotene are ineffective at reducing the incidence of subsequent adenomas in patients who have undergone the removal of a colon adenoma. Estrogen-replacement therapy has been associated with a reduction in the risk of colorectal cancer in women, conceivably by an effect on bile acid synthesis and composition or by decreasing synthesis of IGF-I.

The otherwise unexplained reduction in colorectal cancer mortality in women may be a result of the widespread use of estrogen replacement in postmenopausal individuals.

SCREENING

The rationale for colorectal cancer screening programs is that earlier detection of localized, superficial cancers in asymptomatic individuals will increase the surgical cure rate. Such screening programs are important for individuals having a family history of the disease in first-degree relatives. The relative risk for developing colorectal cancer increases to 1.75 in such individuals and may be even higher if the relative was afflicted before age 60. The prior use of proctosigmoidoscopy as a screening tool was based on the observation that 60% of early lesions are located in the rectosigmoid. For unexplained reasons, however, the proportion of large-bowel cancers arising in the rectum has been decreasing during the past several decades, with a corresponding increase in the proportion of cancers in the more proximal descending colon. As such, the potential for rigid proctosigmoidoscopy to detect a sufficient number of occult neoplasms to make the procedure cost-effective has been questioned. Flexible, fiberoptic sigmoidoscopes permit trained operators to visualize the colon for up to 60 cm, which enhances the capability for cancer detection. However, this technique still leaves the proximal half of the large bowel unscreened.

Most programs directed at the early detection of colorectal cancers have focused on digital rectal examinations and fecal occult blood testing. The digital examination should be part of any routine physical evaluation in adults older than age 40, serving as a screening test for prostate cancer in men, a component of the pelvic examination in women, and an inexpensive maneuver for the detection of masses in the rectum. The development of the Hemoccult test has greatly facilitated the detection of occult fecal blood. Unfortunately, even when performed optimally, the Hemoccult test has major limitations as a screening technique. About 50% of patients with documented colorectal cancers have a negative fecal Hemoccult test, consistent with the intermittent bleeding pattern of these tumors. When random cohorts of asymptomatic persons have been tested, 2–4% have Hemoccult-positive stools. Colorectal cancers have been found in <10% of these "test-positive" cases, with benign polyps being detected in an additional 20–30%. Thus, a colorectal neoplasm will not be found in most asymptomatic individuals with occult blood in their stool. Nonetheless, persons found to have Hemoccult-positive stool routinely undergo further medical evaluation, including sigmoidoscopy, barium enema, and/or colonoscopy—procedures that are not only uncomfortable and expensive but also associated with a small risk for significant complications. The added cost of these studies would appear justifiable if the small number of patients found to have occult neoplasms because of Hemoccult screening could be shown to have an improved prognosis and prolonged survival. Prospectively controlled trials showed a statistically significant reduction in mortality from colorectal cancer for individuals undergoing annual screening. However, this benefit only emerged after >13 years of follow-up and was extremely expensive to achieve, since all positive tests (most of which were false-positive) were followed by colonoscopy. Moreover, these colonoscopic examinations quite likely provided the opportunity for cancer prevention through the removal of potentially premalignant adenomatous polyps since the eventual development of cancer was reduced by 20% in the cohort undergoing annual screening.

Screening techniques for large-bowel cancer in asymptomatic persons remain unsatisfactory. Compliance with any screening strategy within the general population is poor. At present, the American Cancer Society suggests fecal Hemoccult screening annually and flexible sigmoidoscopy every 5 years beginning at age 50 for asymptomatic individuals having no colorectal cancer risk factors. The American Cancer Society has also endorsed a "total colon examination" (i.e., colonoscopy or double-contrast barium enema) every 10 years as an alternative to Hemoccult testing with periodic flexible sigmoidoscopy. Colonoscopy has been shown to be superior to double-contrast barium enema and also to have a higher sensitivity for detecting villous or dysplastic adenomas or cancers than the strategy employing occult fecal blood testing and flexible sigmoidoscopy. Whether colonoscopy performed every 10 years beginning after age 50 will prove to be cost-effective and whether it may be supplanted as a screening maneuver by sophisticated radiographic techniques ("virtual colonoscopy") remains unclear. More effective techniques for screening are needed, perhaps taking advantage of the molecular changes that have been described in these tumors. Analysis of fecal DNA for multiple mutations associated with colorectal cancer is being tested.

CLINICAL FEATURES

Presenting Symptoms   Symptoms vary with the anatomic location of the tumor. Since stool is relatively liquid as it passes through the ileocecal valve into the right colon, cancers arising in the cecum and ascending colon may become quite large without resulting in any obstructive symptoms or noticeable alterations in bowel habits. Lesions of the right colon commonly ulcerate, leading to chronic, insidious blood loss without a change in the appearance of the stool. Consequently, patients with tumors of the ascending colon often present with symptoms such as fatigue, palpitations, and even angina pectoris and are found to have a hypochromic, microcytic anemia indicative of iron deficiency. Since the cancer may bleed intermittently, a random fecal occult blood test may be negative. As a result, the unexplained presence of iron-deficiency anemia in any adult (with the possible exception of a premenopausal, multiparous woman) mandates a thorough endoscopic and/or radiographic visualization of the entire large bowel (Fig. 87-1).

Since stool becomes more formed as it passes into the transverse and descending colon, tumors arising there tend to impede the passage of stool, resulting in the development of abdominal cramping, occasional obstruction, and even perforation. Radiographs of the abdomen often reveal characteristic annular, constricting lesions ("apple-core" or "napkin-ring") (Fig. 87-2).

Cancers arising in the rectosigmoid are often associated with hematochezia, tenesmus, and narrowing of the caliber of stool; anemia is an infrequent finding. While these symptoms may lead patients and their physicians to suspect the presence of hemorrhoids, the development of rectal bleeding and/or altered bowel habits demands a prompt digital rectal examination and proctosigmoidoscopy.

Staging, Prognostic Factors, and Patterns of Spread   The prognosis for individuals having colorectal cancer is related to the depth of tumor penetration into the bowel wall and the presence of both regional

FIGURE 87-1 Double-contrast air-barium enema revealing a sessile tumor of the cecum in a patient with iron-deficiency anemia and guaiac-positive stool. The lesion at surgery was a stage II adenocarcinoma.

FIGURE 87-2 Annular, constricting adenocarcinoma of the descending colon. This radiographic appearance is referred to as an "apple-core" lesion and is always highly suggestive of malignancy.

lymph node involvement and distant metastases. These variables are incorporated into the staging system introduced by Dukes and applied to a TNM classification method, in which T represents the depth of tumor penetration, N the presence of lymph node involvement, and M the presence or absence of distant metastases (Fig. 87-3). Superficial lesions that do not involve regional lymph nodes and do not penetrate through the submucosa (T_1) or the muscularis (T_2) are designated as *stage I* ($T_{1-2}N_0M_0$) disease; tumors that penetrate through the muscularis but have not spread to lymph nodes are *stage II* disease ($T_3N_0M_0$); regional lymph node involvement defines *stage III* ($T_xN_1M_0$) disease; and metastatic spread to sites such as liver, lung, or bone indicates *stage IV* ($T_xN_xM_1$) disease. Unless gross evidence of metastatic disease is present, disease stage cannot be determined accurately before surgical resection and pathologic analysis of the operative specimens. It is not clear whether the detection of nodal metastases by special immunohistochemical molecular techniques has the same prognostic implications as disease detected by routine light microscopy.

Most recurrences after a surgical resection of a large-bowel cancer occur within the first 4 years, making 5-year survival a fairly reliable indicator of cure. The likelihood for 5-year survival in patients with colorectal cancer is stage-related (Fig. 87-3). That likelihood has improved during the past several decades when similar surgical stages have been compared. The most plausible explanation for this improvement is more thorough intraoperative and pathologic staging. In particular, more exacting attention to pathologic detail has revealed that the prognosis following the resection of a colorectal cancer is not related merely to the presence or absence of regional lymph node involvement. Prognosis may be more precisely gauged by the number of involved

lymph nodes (one to three lymph nodes versus four or more lymph nodes). A minimum of 12 sampled lymph nodes is thought necessary to accurately define tumor stage. Other predictors of a poor prognosis after a total surgical resection include tumor penetration through the bowel wall into pericolic fat, poorly differentiated histology, perforation and/or tumor adherence to adjacent organs (increasing the risk for an anatomically adjacent recurrence), and venous invasion by tumor (Table 87-6). Regardless of the clinicopathologic stage, a preoperative elevation of the plasma carcinoembryonic antigen (CEA) level predicts eventual tumor recurrence. The presence of aneuploidy and specific chromosomal deletions, such as allelic loss in chromosome 18q (involving the *DCC* gene) in tumor cells, appears to predict a higher risk for metastatic spread, particularly in patients with stage II ($T_3N_0M_0$) disease. Conversely, the detection of microsatellite instability in tumor tissue indicates a more favorable outcome. In contrast to most other cancers, the prognosis in colorectal cancer is not influenced by the size of the primary lesion when adjusted for nodal involvement and histologic differentiation.

Cancers of the large bowel generally spread to regional lymph nodes or to the liver via the portal venous circulation. The liver represents the most frequent visceral site of metastasis; it is the initial site of distant spread in one-third of recurring colorectal cancers and is involved in more than two-thirds of such patients at the time of death. In general, colorectal cancer rarely spreads to the lungs, supraclavicular lymph nodes, bone, or brain without prior spread to the liver. A major exception to this rule occurs in patients having primary tumors in the distal rectum, from which tumor cells may spread through the paravertebral venous plexus, escaping the portal venous system and thereby reaching the lungs or supraclavicular lymph nodes without hepatic involvement. The median survival after the detection of distant metastases has ranged in the past from 6–9 months (hepatomegaly, abnormal liver chemistries) to 24–30 months (small liver nodule initially identified by elevated CEA level and subsequent CT scan), but effective systemic therapy is improving the prognosis.

℞ COLORECTAL CANCER

Total resection of tumor is the optimal treatment when a malignant lesion is detected in the large bowel. An evaluation for the presence of metastatic disease, including a thorough physical examination, chest radiograph, biochemical assessment of liver function, and measurement of the plasma CEA level, should be performed before surgery. When possible, a colonoscopy of the entire large bowel should be performed to identify synchronous neo-

Stage	I		II	III		IV
	T_1	T_2	T_3	N_1	N_2	M
Extent of tumor	No deeper than submucosa	Not through muscularis	Through muscularis	1-3 lymph node metastases	≥4 lymph node metastases	Distant metastases
5-year survival	>95%	>90%	70-85%	50-70%	25-60%	<5%
Stage at presentation — Colon	23%		31%	26%		20%
Stage at presentation — Rectal	34%		25%	26%		15%

Mucosa
Muscularis mucosa
Submucosa
Muscularis propria
Serosa
Fat
Lymph nodes

FIGURE 87-3 Staging and prognosis for patients with colorectal cancer.

TABLE 87-6   PREDICTORS OF POOR OUTCOME FOLLOWING TOTAL SURGICAL RESECTION OF COLORECTAL CANCER

Tumor spread to regional lymph nodes
Number of regional lymph nodes involved
Tumor penetration through the bowel wall
Poorly differentiated histology
Perforation
Tumor adherence to adjacent organs
Venous invasion
Preoperative elevation of CEA titer (>5.0 ng/mL)
Aneuploidy
Specific chromosomal deletion (e.g., allelic loss on chromosome 18q)

Note: CEA, carcinoembryonic antigen.

plasms and/or polyps. The detection of metastases should not preclude surgery in patients with tumor-related symptoms such as gastrointestinal bleeding or obstruction, but it often prompts the use of a less radical operative procedure. At the time of laparotomy, the entire peritoneal cavity should be examined, with thorough inspection of the liver, pelvis, and hemidiaphragm and careful palpation of the full length of the large bowel. Following recovery from a complete resection, patients should be observed carefully for 5 years by semiannual physical examinations and yearly blood chemistry measurements. If a complete colonoscopy was not performed preoperatively, it should be carried out within the first several postoperative months. Some authorities favor measuring plasma CEA levels at 3-month intervals because of the sensitivity of this test as a marker for otherwise undetectable tumor recurrence. Subsequent endoscopic or radiographic surveillance of the large bowel, probably at triennial intervals, is indicated, since patients who have been cured of one colorectal cancer have a 3–5% probability of developing an additional bowel cancer during their lifetime and a >15% risk for the development of adenomatous polyps. Anastomotic ("suture-line") recurrences are infrequent in colorectal cancer patients provided the surgical resection margins are adequate and free of tumor. The value of periodic CT scans of the abdomen, assessing for an early, asymptomatic indication of tumor recurrence, is an area of uncertainty, with some experts recommending the test be performed annually for the first three postoperative years.

Radiation therapy to the pelvis is recommended for patients with rectal cancer because it reduces the 20–25% probability of regional recurrences following complete surgical resection of stage II or III tumors, especially if they have penetrated through the serosa. This alarmingly high rate of local disease recurrence is believed to be due to the fact that the contained anatomic space within the pelvis limits the extent of the resection and because the rich lymphatic network of the pelvic side wall immediately adjacent to the rectum facilitates the early spread of malignant cells into surgically inaccessible tissue. The use of sharp rather than blunt dissection of rectal cancers (*total mesorectal excision*) appears to reduce the likelihood of local disease recurrence to ~10%. Radiation therapy, either pre- or postoperatively, reduces the likelihood of pelvic recurrences but does not appear to prolong survival. Preoperative radiotherapy is indicated for patients with large, potentially unresectable rectal cancers; such lesions may shrink enough to permit subsequent surgical removal. Radiation therapy is not effective in the primary treatment of colon cancer.

Systemic therapy for patients with colorectal cancer has become more effective. 5-FU remains the backbone of treatment for this disease. Partial responses are obtained in 15–20% of patients. The probability of tumor response appears to be somewhat greater for patients with liver metastases when chemotherapy is infused directly into the hepatic artery, but intraarterial treatment is costly and toxic and does not appear to appreciably prolong survival. The concomitant administration of folinic acid (leucovorin) improves the efficacy of 5-FU in patients with advanced colorectal cancer, presumably by enhancing the binding of 5-FU to its target enzyme, thymidylate synthase. A threefold improvement in the partial response rate is noted when folinic acid is combined with 5-FU; however, the effect on survival is marginal, and the optimal dose schedule remains to be defined. 5-FU is generally administered intravenously but may also be given orally in the form of capecitabine with seemingly similar efficacy.

Irinotecan (CPT-11), a topoisomerase 1 inhibitor, prolongs survival when compared to supportive care in patients whose disease has progressed on 5-FU. Furthermore, the addition of irinotecan to 5-FU and leucovorin (LV) improves response rates and survival of patients with metastatic disease. The

FOLFIRI regimen is as follows: irinotecan, 180 mg/m² as a 90-min infusion day 1; LV, 400 mg/m² as a 2-h infusion during irinotecan, immediately followed by 5-FU bolus, 400 mg/m² and 46-h continuous infusion of 2.4–3 g/m² every 2 weeks. Diarrhea is the major side effect from irinotecan. Oxaliplatin, a platinum analogue, also improves the response rate when added to 5-FU and LV as initial treatment of patients with metastatic disease. The *FOLFOX regimen* is the following: 2-h infusion of LV (400 mg/m² per day) followed by a 5-FU bolus (400 mg/m² per day) and 22-h infusion (1200 mg/m² per day) every 2 weeks, together with oxaliplatin, 85 mg/m² as a 2-h infusion on day 1. Oxaliplatin frequently causes a dose-dependent sensory neuropathy that usually resolves following the cessation of therapy. FOLFIRI and FOLFOX are equal in efficacy.

Monoclonal antibodies are also effective in patients with advanced colorectal cancer. Cetuximab (Erbitux) and panitumumab (Vectibix) are directed against the epidermal growth factor receptor (EGFR), a transmembrane glycoprotein involved in signaling pathways affecting growth and proliferation of tumor cells. Both cetuximab and panitumumab, when given alone, have been shown to benefit a small proportion of previously treated patients, and cetuximab appears to have therapeutic synergy with such chemotherapeutic agents as irinotecan, even in patients previously resistant to this drug; this suggests that cetuximab can reverse cellular resistance to cytotoxic chemotherapy. The use of both cetuximab and panitumumab can lead to an acne-like rash with the development and severity of the rash being correlated with the likelihood of antitumor efficacy. Inhibitors of the EGFR tyrosine kinase such as erlotinib (Tarceva) do not appear to be effective in colorectal cancer.

Bevacizumab (Avastin) is a monoclonal antibody directed against the vascular endothelial growth factor (VEGF) and is thought to act as an antiangiogenesis agent. The addition of bevacizumab to irinotecan-containing combinations and to FOLFOX improves the outcome observed with the chemotherapy alone. The use of bevacizumab can lead to hypertension, proteinuria, and an increased likelihood of thromboembolic events.

Patients with solitary hepatic metastases without clinical or radiographic evidence of additional tumor involvement should be considered for partial liver resection, because such procedures are associated with 5-year survival rates of 25–30% when performed on selected individuals by experienced surgeons.

The administration of 5-FU and LV for 6 months after resection of tumor in patients with stage III disease leads to a 40% decrease in recurrence rates and 30% improvement in survival. The likelihood of recurrence has been further reduced when oxaliplatin has been combined with 5-FU and LV (e.g. FOLFOX); unexpectedly, the addition of irinotecan to 5-FU and LV did not enhance outcome. Patients with stage II tumors do not appear to benefit from adjuvant therapy. In rectal cancer, the delivery of preoperative or postoperative combined modality therapy (5-FU plus radiation therapy) reduces the risk of recurrence and increases the chance of cure for patients with stages II and III tumors, with the preoperative approach being better tolerated. The 5-FU acts as a radiosensitizer when delivered together with radiation therapy. Life-extending adjuvant therapy is used in only about half of patients over age 65 years. This age bias is completely inappropriate as the benefits and tolerance of adjuvant therapy in patients age 65+ appear similar to those seen in younger individuals.

TUMORS OF THE SMALL INTESTINE

Small-bowel tumors comprise <3% of gastrointestinal neoplasms. Because of their rarity, a correct diagnosis is often delayed. Abdominal symptoms are usually vague and poorly defined, and conventional radiographic studies of the upper and lower intestinal tract often appear normal. Small-bowel tumors should be considered in the differential diagnosis in the following situations: (1) recurrent, unexplained episodes of crampy abdominal pain; (2) intermittent bouts of intestinal obstruction, especially in the absence of IBD or prior abdominal surgery; (3) intussusception in the adult; and (4) evidence of chronic intestinal bleeding in the presence of negative conventional contrast radiographs. A careful small-bowel barium study is the diagnostic procedure of choice; the diagnostic accuracy may be improved by infusing barium through a nasogastric tube placed into the duodenum (enteroclysis).

BENIGN TUMORS

The histology of benign small-bowel tumors is difficult to predict on clinical and radiologic grounds alone. The symptomatology of benign tumors is not distinctive, with pain, obstruction, and hemorrhage being the most frequent symptoms. These tumors are usually discovered during the fifth and sixth decades of life, more often in the distal rather than the proximal small intestine. The most common benign tumors are adenomas, leiomyomas, lipomas, and angiomas.

Adenomas These tumors include those of the islet cells and Brunner's glands as well as polypoid adenomas. *Islet cell adenomas* are occasionally located outside the pancreas; the associated syndromes are discussed in Chap. 344. *Brunner's gland adenomas* are not truly neoplastic but represent a hypertrophy or hyperplasia of submucosal duodenal glands. These appear as small nodules in the duodenal mucosa that secrete a highly viscous alkaline mucus. Most often, this is an incidental radiographic finding not associated with any specific clinical disorder.

Polypoid Adenomas About 25% of benign small-bowel tumors are polypoid adenomas (Table 87-5). They may present as single polypoid lesions or, less commonly, as papillary villous adenomas. As in the colon, the sessile or papillary form of the tumor is sometimes associated with a coexisting carcinoma. Occasionally, patients with Gardner's syndrome develop premalignant adenomas in the small bowel; such lesions are generally in the duodenum. Multiple polypoid tumors may occur throughout the small bowel (and occasionally the stomach and colorectum) in the Peutz-Jeghers syndrome. The polyps are usually hamartomas (juvenile polyps) having a low potential for malignant degeneration. Mucocutaneous melanin deposits as well as tumors of the ovary, breast, pancreas, and endometrium are also associated with this autosomal dominant condition.

Leiomyomas These neoplasms arise from smooth-muscle components of the intestine and are usually intramural, affecting the overlying mucosa. Ulceration of the mucosa may cause gastrointestinal hemorrhage of varying severity. Cramping or intermittent abdominal pain is frequently encountered.

Lipomas These tumors occur with greatest frequency in the distal ileum and at the ileocecal valve. They have a characteristic radiolucent appearance, are usually intramural and asymptomatic, but on occasion cause bleeding.

Angiomas While not true neoplasms, these lesions are important because they frequently cause intestinal bleeding. They may take the form of telangiectasia or hemangiomas. Multiple intestinal telangiectasias occur in a nonhereditary form confined to the gastrointestinal tract or as part of the hereditary Osler-Rendu-Weber syndrome. Vascular tumors may also take the form of isolated hemangiomas, most commonly in the jejunum. Angiography, especially during bleeding, is the best procedure for evaluating these lesions.

MALIGNANT TUMORS

While rare, small-bowel malignancies occur in patients with longstanding regional enteritis and celiac sprue as well as in individuals with AIDS. Malignant tumors of the small bowel are frequently associated with fever, weight loss, anorexia, bleeding, and a palpable abdominal mass. After ampullary carcinomas (many of which arise from biliary or pancreatic ducts), the most frequently occurring small-bowel malignancies are adenocarcinomas, lymphomas, carcinoid tumors, and leiomyosarcomas.

Adenocarcinomas The most common primary cancers of the small bowel are adenocarcinomas, accounting for ~50% of malignant tumors. These cancers occur most often in the distal duodenum and proximal jejunum, where they tend to ulcerate and cause hemorrhage or obstruction. Radiologically, they may be confused with chronic duodenal ulcer disease or with Crohn's disease if the patient has long-standing regional enteritis. The diagnosis is best made by endoscopy and biopsy under direct vision. Surgical resection is the treatment of choice.

Lymphomas Lymphoma in the small bowel may be primary or secondary. A diagnosis of a primary intestinal lymphoma requires histologic confirmation in a clinical setting in which palpable adenopathy and hepatosplenomegaly are absent and no evidence of lymphoma is seen on chest radiograph, CT scan, or peripheral blood smear or on bone marrow aspiration and biopsy. Symptoms referable to the small bowel are present, usually accompanied by an anatomically discernible lesion. Secondary lymphoma of the small bowel consists of involvement of the intestine by a lymphoid malignancy extending from involved retroperitoneal or mesenteric lymph nodes (Chap. 105).

Primary intestinal lymphoma accounts for ~20% of malignancies of the small bowel. These neoplasms are non-Hodgkin's lymphomas; they usually have a diffuse, large-cell histology and are of T cell origin. Intestinal lymphoma involves the ileum, jejunum, and duodenum, in decreasing frequency, a pattern that mirrors the relative amount of normal lymphoid cells in these anatomic areas. The risk of small-bowel lymphoma is increased in patients with a prior history of malabsorptive conditions (e.g., celiac sprue), regional enteritis, and depressed immune function due to congenital immunodeficiency syndromes, prior organ transplantation, autoimmune disorders, or AIDS.

The development of localized or nodular masses that narrow the lumen results in periumbilical pain (made worse by eating) as well as weight loss, vomiting, and occasional intestinal obstruction. The diagnosis of small-bowel lymphoma may be suspected from the appearance on contrast radiographs of patterns such as infiltration and thickening of mucosal folds, mucosal nodules, areas of irregular ulceration, or stasis of contrast material. The diagnosis can be confirmed by surgical exploration and resection of involved segments. Intestinal lymphoma can occasionally be diagnosed by peroral intestinal mucosal biopsy, but since the disease mainly involves the lamina propria, full-thickness surgical biopsies are usually required.

Resection of the tumor constitutes the initial treatment modality. While postoperative radiation therapy has been given to some patients following a total resection, most authorities favor short-term (three cycles) systemic treatment with combination chemotherapy. The frequent presence of widespread intraabdominal disease at the time of diagnosis and the occasional multicentricity of the tumor often make a total resection impossible. The probability of sustained remission or cure is ~75% in patients with localized disease but is ~25% in individuals with unresectable lymphoma. In patients whose tumors are not resected, chemotherapy may lead to bowel perforation.

A unique form of small-bowel lymphoma, diffusely involving the entire intestine, was first described in oriental Jews and Arabs and is referred to as *immunoproliferative small intestinal disease* (IPSID), *Mediterranean lymphoma*, or α-*heavy chain disease*. This is a B cell tumor. The typical presentation includes chronic diarrhea and steatorrhea associated with vomiting and abdominal cramps; clubbing of the digits may be observed. A curious feature in many patients with IPSID is the presence in the blood and intestinal secretions of an abnormal IgA that contains a shortened α-heavy chain and is devoid of light chains. It is suspected that the abnormal α chains are produced by plasma cells infiltrating the small bowel. The clinical course of patients with IPSID is generally one of exacerbations and remissions, with death frequently resulting from either progressive malnutrition and wasting or the development of an aggressive lymphoma. The use of oral antibiotics such as tetracycline appears to be beneficial in the early phases of the disorder, suggesting a possible infectious etiology. Combination chemotherapy has been administered during later stages of the disease, with variable results. Results are better when antibiotics and chemotherapy are combined.

Carcinoid Tumors Carcinoid tumors arise from argentaffin cells of the crypts of Lieberkühn and are found from the distal duodenum to the ascending colon, areas embryologically derived from the midgut. More than 50% of intestinal carcinoids are found in the distal ileum, with most congregating close to the ileocecal valve. Most intestinal carcinoids are asymptomatic and of low malignant potential, but invasion and metastases may occur, leading to the carcinoid syndrome (Chap. 344).

Leiomyosarcomas Leiomyosarcomas often are >5 cm in diameter and may be palpable on abdominal examination. Bleeding, obstruction, and perforation are common. Such tumors should be analyzed for the expression of mutant c-*kit* receptor (defining GIST), and in the presence of metastatic disease, justifying treatment with imatinib mesylate (Gleevec) or, in imatinib refractory patients, sunitinib (Sutent).

CANCERS OF THE ANUS

Cancers of the anus account for 1–2% of the malignant tumors of the large bowel. Most such lesions arise in the anal canal, the anatomic area extending from the anorectal ring to a zone approximately halfway between the pectinate (or dentate) line and the anal verge. Carcinomas arising proximal to the pectinate line (i.e., in the transitional zone between the glandular mucosa of the rectum and the squamous epithelium of the distal anus) are known as *basaloid*, *cuboidal*, or *cloacogenic* tumors; about one-third of anal cancers have this histologic pattern. Malignancies arising distal to the pectinate line have squamous histology, ulcerate more frequently, and constitute ~55% of anal cancers. The prognosis for patients with basaloid and squamous cell cancers of the anus is identical when corrected for tumor size and the presence or absence of nodal spread.

The development of anal cancer is associated with infection by human papillomavirus, the same organism etiologically linked to cervical cancer. The virus is sexually transmitted. The infection may lead to anal warts (condyloma accuminata), which may progress to anal intraepithelial neoplasia and on to squamous cell carcinoma. The risk for anal cancer is increased among homosexual males, presumably related to anal intercourse. Anal cancer risk is increased in both men and women with AIDS, possibly because their immunosuppressed state permits more severe papillomavirus infection. Anal cancers occur most commonly in middle-aged persons and are more frequent in women than men. At diagnosis, patients may experience bleeding, pain, sensation of a perianal mass, and pruritus.

Radical surgery (abdominal-perineal resection with lymph node sampling and a permanent colostomy) was once the treatment of choice for this tumor type. The 5-year survival rate after such a procedure was 55–70% in the absence of spread to regional lymph nodes and <20% if nodal involvement was present. An alternative therapeutic approach combining external beam radiation therapy with concomitant chemotherapy has resulted in biopsy-proven disappearance of all tumor in >80% of patients whose initial lesion was <3 cm in size. Tumor recurrences develop in <10% of these patients, meaning that ~70% of patients with anal cancers can be cured with nonoperative treatment. Surgery should be reserved for the minority of individuals who are found to have residual tumor after being managed initially with radiation therapy combined with chemotherapy.

FURTHER READINGS

CRUMP W et al: Lymphoma of the gastrointestinal tract. Semin Oncol 26:324, 1999

DEMETRI GD et al: Efficacy and safety of imatinib mesylate in advanced gastrointestinal stromal tumors. N Engl J Med 347:472, 2002

ENZINGER PC, MAYER RJ: Esophageal cancer. N Engl J Med 349:2241, 2003

HOHENBERGER P, GRETSCHEL S: Gastric cancer. Lancet 362:305, 2003

LYNCH HT, DE LA CHAPELLE A: Hereditary colorectal cancer. N Engl J Med 348:919, 2003

MEYERHARDT JA, MAYER RJ: Systemic therapy for colorectal cancer. N Engl J Med 352:476, 2005

ROSTRUM A et al: Nonsteroidal anti-inflammatory drugs and cyclooxygenase-2 inhibitors for primary prevention of colorectal cancer: A systematic review prepared for the US Preventive Services Task Force. Ann Intern Med 146:376, 2007

RYAN DP et al: Carcinoma of the anal canal. N Engl J Med 342:792, 2000

SPECHLER SJ: Barrett's esophagus. N Engl J Med 346:836, 2002

UEMURA N et al: *Helicobacter pylori* infection and the development of gastric cancer. N Engl J Med 345:784, 2001

WALSH JME, TERDIMAN JP: Colorectal cancer screening. JAMA 289:1288, 2003

WEITZ J et al: Colorectal cancer. Lancet 365:153, 2005

WOLAN BM et al: Adjuvant treatment of colorectal cancer. CA Cancer Clin J 57:168, 2007

---

88 Tumors of the Liver and Biliary Tree
Brian I. Carr

HEPATOCELLULAR CARCINOMA

INCIDENCE

Hepatocellular carcinoma (HCC) is one of the most common malignancies worldwide. The annual global incidence is about 1 million cases, with a male to female ratio of about 4:1. The incidence rate equals the death rate. In the United States, 19,160 new cases and 16,780 deaths were noted in 2007. The death rate in males in low-incidence countries such as the United States is 1.9 per 100,000 per year; in intermediate-incidence areas such as Austria and South Africa, annual death rates range from 5.1–20.0 per 100,000; and in high-incidence areas such as in Asia (China and Korea), death rates are as high as 23.1–150 per 100,000 per year (Table 88-1). The incidence of HCC in the United States is around 3 per 100,000 persons, with significant sex, ethnic, and geographic variations. These numbers are rapidly increasing and may be an underestimate. Around 4 million persons in the United States are chronic carriers of hepatitis C virus (HCV). About 10% of them, or 400,000, are likely to develop cirrhosis. Around 5% or 20,000 of these may develop HCC annually. Add to this the two other common predisposing factors—hepatitis B virus (HBV) and chronic alcohol consumption—and 60,000 new HCC cases annually seem possible. Future advances in HCC survival will likely depend on immunization strategies for HBV and HCV and earlier diagnosis by screening of patients at risk of HCC development.

TABLE 88-1	AGE-ADJUSTED INCIDENCE RATES FOR HEPATOCELLULAR CARCINOMA	
	Persons per 100,000 per Year	
Country	**Male**	**Female**
Argentina	6.0	2.5
Brazil, Recife	9.2	8.3
Brazil, Sao Paulo	3.8	2.6
Mozambique	112.9	30.8
South Africa, Cape: Black	26.3	8.4
South Africa, Cape: White	1.2	0.6
Senegal	25.6	9.0
Nigeria	15.4	3.2
Gambia	33.1	12.6
Burma	25.5	8.8
Japan	7.2	2.2
Korea	13.8	3.2
China, Shanghai	34.4	11.6
India, Bombay	4.9	2.5
India, Madras	2.1	0.7
Great Britain	1.6	0.8
France	6.9	1.2
Italy, Varese	7.1	2.7
Norway	1.8	1.1
Spain, Navarra	7.9	4.7

EPIDEMIOLOGY

Endemic hot spots occur in areas of China and sub-Saharan Africa, which are associated with both high endemic hepatitis B carrier rates and mycotoxin contamination of foodstuffs, stored grains, drinking water, and soil. Environmental factors are important; Japanese in Japan have a higher incidence than those living in Hawaii, who in turn have a higher incidence than those living in California.

ETIOLOGIC FACTORS

Chemical Carcinogens Probably the best-studied and most potent ubiquitous natural chemical carcinogen is a product of the *Aspergillus* fungus, called aflatoxin B_1. This mold and aflatoxin product can be found in stored grains in hot, humid places, where peanuts and rice are stored in unrefrigerated conditions. Aflatoxin contamination of foodstuffs correlates well with incidence rates in Africa and to some extent in China. In endemic areas of China, even farm animals such as ducks have HCC. The most potent carcinogens appear to be natural products of plants, fungi, and bacteria, such as bush trees containing pyrrollizidine alkaloids as well as tannic acid and safrole. Pollutants such as pesticides and insecticides are known rodent carcinogens.

Hepatitis Both case-control and cohort studies have shown a strong association between chronic hepatitis B carrier rates and increased incidence of HCC. In Taiwanese male postal carriers who were hepatitis B surface antigen (HBsAg)-positive, a 98-fold greater risk for HCC was found compared to HBsAg-negative individuals. The incidence of HCC in Alaskan natives is markedly increased related to a high prevalence of HBV infection. HBV-based HCC may arise from rounds of hepatic destruction with subsequent proliferation and not necessarily from frank cirrhosis. The increase in Japanese HCC incidence rates in the past three decades is thought to be from hepatitis C. A large-scale intervention study sponsored by the World Health Organization (WHO) is currently underway in Asia involving HBV vaccination of the newborn. HCC in African blacks is not associated with severe cirrhosis but is poorly differentiated and very aggressive. Despite uniform HBV carrier rates among the South African Bantu, there is a ninefold difference in HCC incidence between Mozambicans living along the coast and inland. These differences are attributed to the additional exposure to dietary aflatoxin B_1 and other carcinogenic mycotoxins. A typical interval between HCV-associated transfusion and subsequent HCC is ~30 years. HCV-associated HCC patients tend to have more frequent and advanced cirrhosis, but in HBV-associated HCC, only half the patients have cirrhosis; the remainder have chronic active hepatitis (Chap. 300).

Other Etiologic Conditions The 75–85% association of HCC with underlying cirrhosis has long been recognized, more typically with macronodular cirrhosis in Southeast Asia but also with micronodular cirrhosis (alcohol) in Europe and the United States (Chap. 302). It is still not clear whether cirrhosis itself is a predisposing factor to the development of HCC or whether the underlying causes of the cirrhosis are actually the carcinogenic factors. However, ~20 % of U.S. patients with HCC do not have underlying cirrhosis. Several underlying conditions are associated with an increased risk for cirrhosis-associated HCC (Table 88-2), including hep-

atitis, alcohol abuse, autoimmune chronic active hepatitis, cryptogenic cirrhosis, and nonalcoholic steatohepatitis (NASH). A less common association is with primary biliary cirrhosis and several metabolic diseases, including hemochromatosis, Wilson's disease, α_1-antitrypsin deficiency, tyrosinemia, porphyria cutanea tarda, glycogenesis types 1 and 3, citrullinemia, and orotic aciduria. The etiology of HCC in those 20% of patients who have no cirrhosis is unclear, and their HCC natural history not well-defined.

CLINICAL FEATURES

Symptoms in HCC patients include abdominal pain, weight loss, weakness, abdominal fullness and swelling, jaundice, and nausea (Table 88-3). Presenting signs and symptoms differ somewhat between high- and low-incidence areas. The most common symptom is abdominal pain in high-risk areas, especially in South African blacks; by contrast, only 40–50% of Chinese and Japanese patients present with abdominal pain. Abdominal swelling may occur as a consequence of ascites due to the underlying chronic liver disease or may be due to a rapidly expanding tumor. Occasionally, central necrosis or acute hemorrhage into the peritoneal cavity leads to death. In countries with an active surveillance program, HCC tends to be identified at an earlier stage when symptoms may be due only to the underlying disease. Jaundice is usually due to obstruction of the intrahepatic ducts by the underlying liver disease. Hematemesis may occur due to esophageal varices from the underlying portal hypertension. Bone pain is seen in 3–12% of patients, but necropsies show bone metastases in ~20% of patients. Patients may be asymptomatic.

Physical Signs Hepatomegaly is the most common physical sign, occurring in 50–90% of patients. Abdominal bruits are noted in 6–25%, and ascites occurs in 30–60% of patients. Ascites should be examined

TABLE 88-3 HEPATOCELLULAR CARCINOMA: CLINICAL PRESENTATION AT THE UNIVERSITY OF PITTSBURGH LIVER CANCER CENTER (n = 547)

	Number of Patients (%)
Symptom	
No symptom	129 (24)
Abdominal pain	219 (40)
Other (workup of anemia and various diseases)	64 (12)
Routine physical exam finding, elevated LFTs	129 (24)
Weight loss	112 (20)
Appetite loss	59 (11)
Weakness/malaise	83 (15)
Jaundice	30 (5)
Routine CT scan screening of known cirrhosis	92 (17)
Cirrhosis symptoms (ankle swelling, abdominal bloating, increased girth, pruritus, GI bleed)	98 (18)
Diarrhea	7 (1)
Tumor rupture	1
Patient characteristics	
Mean age (years)	56 ± 13
Male: Female	3:1
Ethnicity	
Caucasian	72%
Middle Eastern	10%
Asian	13%
African American	5%
Cirrhosis	81%
No cirrhosis	19%
Tumor characteristics	
Hepatic tumor numbers	
1	20%
2	25%
3 or more	65%
Portal vein invasion	75%
Unilobar	25%
Bilobar	75%

Note: LFTs, liver function tests; GI, gastrointestinal.

TABLE 88-2 RISK FACTORS FOR HEPATOCELLULAR CARCINOMA

Common	Unusual
Cirrhosis from any cause	Primary biliary cirrhosis
Hepatitis B or C chronic infection	Hemochromatosis
Ethanol chronic consumption	α_1 Antitrypsin deficiency
Nonalcoholic steatohepatitis (NASH)	Glycogen storage diseases
Aflatoxin B_1 or other mycotoxins	Citrullinemia
	Porphyria cutanea tarda
	Hereditary tyrosinemia
	Wilson's disease

by cytology. Splenomegaly is mainly due to portal hypertension. Weight loss and muscle wasting are common, particularly with rapidly growing or large tumors. Fever is found in 10–50% of patients, from unclear cause. The signs of chronic liver disease may be present, including jaundice, dilated abdominal veins, palmar erythema, gynecomastia, testicular atrophy, and peripheral edema. Budd-Chiari syndrome can occur due to HCC invasion of the hepatic veins; it should be suspected in patients with tense ascites and a large tender liver (Chap. 302).

Paraneoplastic Syndromes Most paraneoplastic syndromes in HCC are biochemical abnormalities without associated clinical consequences. They include hypoglycemia (also caused by end-stage liver failure), erythrocytosis, hypercalcemia, hypercholesterolemia, dysfibrinogenemia, carcinoid syndrome, increased thyroxin-binding globulin, changes in secondary sex characteristics (gynecomastia, testicular atrophy, and precocious puberty), and porphyria cutanea tarda. Mild hypoglycemia occurs in rapidly growing HCC as part of terminal illness, and profound hypoglycemia may occur, although the cause is unclear. Erythrocytosis occurs in 3–12% of patients, and hypercholesterolemia in 10–40%. A high percentage of patients have thrombocytopenia or leukopenia not caused by cancer infiltration of bone marrow, as in other tumor types.

STAGING

Although the TNM (primary *t*umor, regional *n*odes, *m*etastasis) staging system set up by the American Joint Commission for Cancers (AJCC) is sometimes used, the newer Cancer of the Liver Italian Program (CLIP) system is now popular as it takes cirrhosis into account, as does the Okuda system (Table 88-4). Other staging systems have been proposed and a consensus is needed. The best prognosis is stage I, solitary tumor <2 cm in diameter without vascular invasion. Adverse prognostic features include ascites, vascular invasion, and lymph node spread. Vascular invasion, in particular, has profound effects on prognosis and may be microscopic or macroscopic (visible on CT). Most large tumors have microscopic vascular invasion, so full staging can usually be made only after surgical resection. Stage III disease contains a mixture of lymph node–positive and –negative tumors. Stage III patients with positive lymph node disease have a poor prognosis, and few patients survive 1 year. The prognosis of stage IV is poor after either resection or transplantation, and 1-year survival is rare. A working staging system based entirely on clinical grounds that incorporates the contribution of the underlying liver disease was originally developed by Okuda et al. (Table 88-4). Patients with Okuda stage III have a dire prognosis, because they usually cannot be curatively resected and the condition of their liver typically precludes chemotherapy.

APPROACH TO THE PATIENT:
Hepatocellular Carcinoma

History and Physical The history is important in evaluating putative predisposing factors, including a history of hepatitis or jaundice, blood transfusion, or use of intravenous drugs. A family history of HCC or hepatitis should be sought, and a detailed social history taken to include job descriptions for industrial exposure to possible carcinogenic drugs as well as contraceptive hormones. Physical examination should include assessing stigmata of underlying liver disease such as jaundice, ascites, peripheral edema, spider nevi, palmar erythema, and weight loss. Evaluation of the abdomen for hepatic size, masses or ascites, hepatic nodularity and tenderness, and splenomegaly is needed, as is assessment of overall clinical performance status and psychosocial evaluation.

Serologic Assays α-Fetoprotein (AFP) is a serum tumor marker in HCC; however, it is only increased in about half of U.S. patients. The other widely used assay is that for des-γ-carboxy prothrombin (DCP), a protein induced by vitamin K absence (PIVKA-2). This protein is increased in as many as 80% of HCC patients but may also be elevated in patients with vitamin K deficiency; it is always elevated after use of warfarin. It may predict for portal vein invasion. In a patient presenting with either a new hepatic mass or other indications of recent hepatic decompensation, carcinoembryonic antigen (CEA), vitamin B_{12}, AFP, ferritin, PIVKA-2, and antimitochondrial Ab should be measured, and standard liver function tests should be performed, including prothrombin time (PT), partial thromboplastin time (PTT), albumin, transaminases, γ-glutamyl transpeptidase, and alkaline phosphatase. Decreases in platelet count and white blood cell count may reflect portal hypertension and associated hypersplenism. Hepatitis A, B, and C serology should be measured. If HBV or HCV serology is positive, quantitative measurements of HBV DNA or HCV RNA are needed.

Radiology An ultrasound examination of the liver is an excellent screening tool. The two characteristic vascular abnormalities are hypervascularity of the tumor mass (neovascularization or abnormal tumor-feeding arterial vessels) and thrombosis by tumor invasion of otherwise normal portal veins. To determine tumor size and extent and the presence of portal vein invasion accurately, a helical/triphasic CT scan of the abdomen and pelvis with fast contrast bolus technique should be performed to detect the vascular lesions typical of HCC. Portal vein invasion is normally detected as an obstruction and expansion of the vessel. A chest CT is used to exclude metastases. MRI can also provide detailed information, especially with the newer contrast agents. Ethiodol (Lipiodol) is an ethiodized oil emulsion retained by liver tumors that can be delivered by hepatic artery injection (5–15 mL) for CT imaging 1 week later. For small tumors, ethiodol injection is very helpful before biopsy because its histologic presence constitutes proof that the needle biopsied the mass under suspicion. A prospective comparison of triphasic CT, gadolinium-enhanced MRI, ultrasound, and fluorodeoxyglucose positron emission tomography (FDG-PET) scans demonstrated similar results for CT, MRI, and ultrasound; PET imaging was unsuccessful.

Pathologic Diagnosis Histologic proof of the presence of HCC is obtained through a core liver biopsy of the mass under ultrasound guidance as well as random biopsy of the underlying liver. Bleeding risk is increased compared to other cancers because (1) the tumors are hypervascular, and (2) patients often have thrombocytopenia and decreased clotting factors. Bleeding risk is further increased in the presence of ascites. Tracking of tumor has been an uncommon problem. Fine-needle aspirates may provide sufficient material for

---

TABLE 88-4	CLIP AND OKUDA STAGING SYSTEMS FOR HEPATOCELLULAR CARCINOMA

CLIP Classification

	Points		
Variables	**0**	**1**	**2**
i. Tumor number	Single	Multiple	—
Hepatic replacement by tumor (%)[a]	<50	<50	>50
ii. Child-Pugh score	A	B	C
iii. α-Fetoprotein level (ng/mL)	<400	≥400	—
iv. Portal vein thrombosis (CT)	No	Yes	—

CLIP stages (score = sum of points): CLIP 0, 0 points; CLIP 1, 1 point; CLIP 2, 2 points; CLIP 3, 3 points.

Okuda Classification

Tumor Size[a]		Ascites		Albumin (g/L)		Bilirubin (mg/dL)	
≥50%	<50	+	–	≤3	>3	≥3	<3
(+)	(–)	(+)	(–)	(+)	(–)	(+)	(–)

Okuda stages: stage 1, all (–); stage 2, 1 or 2 (+); stage 3, 3 or 4 (+).

[a]Extent of liver occupied by tumor.

Note: CLIP, Cancer of the Liver Italian Program.

diagnosis of cancer, but core biopsies are preferred. Tissue architecture must be examined to distinguish between HCC and metastatic adenocarcinoma; laparoscopic approaches can also be used. For patients suspected of having portal vein involvement, a core biopsy of the portal vein may be performed safely. If positive, this is regarded as an exclusion criterion for transplantation for HCC.

SCREENING HIGH-RISK POPULATIONS

Screening has not been shown to save lives. Prospective studies in high-risk populations showed that ultrasound was more sensitive than AFP elevations. An Italian study in patients with cirrhosis identified a yearly HCC incidence of 3% but showed no increase in the rate of detection of potentially curable tumors with aggressive screening. Prevention strategies including universal vaccination against hepatitis viruses are more likely to be effective than screening efforts. Despite absence of formal guidelines, most practitioners obtain 6-monthly AFP levels and perform CT (or ultrasound) when following high-risk patients (HBV carriers, HCV cirrhosis, family history of HCC).

℞ HEPATOCELLULAR CARCINOMA

Most HCC patients have two liver diseases, cirrhosis and HCC, each of which is an independent cause of death. The presence of cirrhosis usually places constraints on resection surgery, ablative therapies, and chemotherapy. Thus patient assessment and treatment planning have to take the severity of the nonmalignant liver disease into account. The clinical management choices for HCC can be complex **(Fig. 88-1)**. The natural history of HCC is highly variable. Patients presenting with advanced tumors (vascular invasion, symptoms, extrahepatic spread) have a median survival of ~4 months, with or without treatment. Treatment results from the literature are difficult to interpret. Survival is not always a measure of the efficacy of therapy because of the adverse effects on survival of the underlying liver disease. A multidisciplinary team, including a hepatologist, interventional radiologist, surgical oncologist, transplant surgeon, and medical oncologist, is important for the comprehensive management of HCC patients.

STAGES I AND II HCC Early-stage tumors are successfully treated using various techniques, including surgical resection, local ablation (thermal or radiofrequency), and local injection therapies (ethanol or acetic acid).

Because the majority of patients with HCC suffer from a field defect in the cirrhotic liver, they are at risk for subsequent multiple primary liver tumors. Many will also have significant underlying liver disease and may not tolerate major surgical loss of hepatic parenchyma; they may be eligible for orthotopic liver transplant (OLTX) in the future. An important principle in treating early-stage HCC is to use liver-sparing treatments and to focus on treatment of both the tumor and the cirrhosis.

Surgical Excision The risk of major hepatectomy is high (5–10% mortality) due to the underlying liver disease and the potential for liver failure. Preoperative portal vein occlusion can sometimes be performed to cause atrophy of the HCC-involved lobe and compensatory hypertrophy of the noninvolved liver, permitting safer resection. Intraoperative ultrasound is useful for planning the surgical approach. In cirrhotic patients, any major liver surgery can result in liver failure. The Child-Pugh classification of liver failure (Chap. 295) is a reliable prognosticator for tolerance of hepatic surgery, and only Child A patients should be considered for surgical resection. Child B and C patients with stages I and II HCC should be referred for OLTX if appropriate, as should patients with ascites or a recent history of variceal bleeding. Although open surgical excision is the most reliable, the patient may be better served with a laparoscopic approach to resection, using RFA or percutaneous ethanol injection (PEI). No adequate comparisons of these different techniques have been undertaken, and the choice of treatment is usually based on physician skill.

Local Ablation Strategies Radiofrequency ablation (RFA) uses heat to ablate tumors. The maximum size of the probe arrays allows for a 7-cm zone of necrosis, which would be adequate for a 3- to 4-cm tumor. The heat reliably kills cells within the zone of necrosis. Treatment of tumors close to the main portal pedicles can lead to bile duct injury and obstruction. This limits the tumors that are anatomically suited for this technique. RFA can be performed percutaneously with CT or ultrasound guidance, or by laparoscopy with ultrasound guidance.

Local Injection Therapy Numerous agents have been used for local injection into tumors, most commonly, ethanol (PEI). The relatively soft HCC within the hard background of cirrhotic liver allows for injection of large volumes of ethanol into the tumor without diffusion into the hepatic parenchyma or leakage out of the liver. PEI causes direct destruction of cancer cells, but it is not selective for cancer cells and will destroy normal cells in the vicinity. It usually requires multiple injections (average of three), in contrast to one for RFA. The maximum size of tumor reliably treated is 3 cm, even with multiple injections.

FIGURE 88-1 Treatment approach to patients with hepatocellular carcinoma. The initial clinical evaluation is aimed at assessing the extent of the tumor and the underlying functional compromise of the liver by cirrhosis. Patients are classified as having resectable disease, unresectable disease, or as transplantation candidates. Abbreviations: OLTX, orthotopic liver transplantation; TACE, transarterial chemoembolization; PEI, percutaneous ethanol injection; RFA, radiofrequency ablation; LN, lymph node. Child's A/B/C refers to the Child-Pugh classification of liver failure.

Liver Transplantation A viable option for stages I and II tumors in the setting of cirrhosis is OLTX, with survival approaching that for noncancer cases. OLTX for patients with a single lesion ≤ 5 cm or three or fewer nodules, each ≤ 3 cm (Milan criteria), resulted in excellent tumor-free survival (≥70% at 5 years). For advanced HCC, OLTX has been abandoned due to high tumor recurrence rates. Priority scoring for OLTX previously led to HCC patients waiting too long for their OLTX, resulting in some tumors becoming too advanced during the patient's wait for a donated liver. A variety of therapies were used as a "bridge" to OLTX, including RFA, PEI, and transarterial chemoembolization (TACE). These pretransplant treatments allow patients to remain on the waiting list longer, giving them greater opportunities to be transplanted. What remains unclear is whether this translates into prolonged survival after transplant. Further, it is not known whether patients who have had their tumor(s) treated preoperatively follow the recurrence pattern predicted by their tumor status at the time of transplant (i.e., post local ablative therapy), or if they follow the course set by their tumor parameters present before such treatment. The United Network for Organ Sharing (UNOS) point system for priority scoring of OLTX recipients now includes additional points for patients with HCC. The success of living related donor liver transplantation programs has also led to patients receiving transplantation earlier for HCC and often with greater than minimal tumors.

Adjuvant Therapy The role of adjuvant chemotherapy for patients after resection or OLTX remains unclear. No clear advantage in disease-free or overall survival has been found for either adjuvant or neoadjuvant approaches, though a meta-analysis of several trials revealed a significant improvement in disease-free and overall survival. Analysis of postoperative adjuvant systemic chemotherapy trials demonstrated no disease-free or overall survival advantage, but single studies of TACE and neoadjuvant ^{131}I-ethiodol have shown enhanced survival after resection.

STAGES III AND IV HCC Fewer surgical options exist for stage III tumors. In patients without cirrhosis, a major hepatectomy is feasible, although prognosis is poor. Patients with Child's A cirrhosis may be resected, but a lobectomy is associated with significant morbidity and mortality, and long-term prognosis is poor. Nevertheless, a small percentage of patients will achieve long-term survival, justifying an attempt at resection when feasible. Because of the advanced nature of these tumors, even successful resection can be followed by rapid recurrence. These patients are not considered candidates for transplantation because of the high tumor recurrence rates, unless their tumors can first be down-staged with neoadjuvant therapy. Decreasing the size of the primary tumor allows for less surgery, and the delay in surgery allows for extrahepatic disease to manifest on imaging studies and avoid unhelpful OLTX. The prognosis is poor for stage IV tumors, and no surgical treatment is recommended.

Systemic Chemotherapy A large number of controlled and uncontrolled clinical studies have been performed with most of the major classes of cancer chemotherapy. No single agent or combination of agents given systemically reproducibly leads to even a 25% response rate or has any effect on survival.

Regional Chemotherapy In contrast to the dismal results of systemic chemotherapy, a variety of agents given via the hepatic artery have activity in HCC confined to the liver (**Table 88-5**). Two randomized controlled trials have shown a survival advantage for TACE in a selected subset of patients. One used doxorubicin and the other used cisplatin. Despite the fact that increased hepatic extraction of chemotherapy has been shown for very few drugs, some drugs such as cisplatin, doxorubicin, mitomycin C, and possibly neocarzinostatin produce substantial objective responses when administered regionally. Few data are available on continuous hepatic arterial infusion for HCC, although pilot studies with cisplatin have shown encouraging responses. Because the reports have not usually stratified responses or survival based on TNM staging, it is difficult to know long-term prognosis in relation to tumor extent. Most of the studies on regional hepatic arterial chemotherapy also use an embolizing agent such as ethiodol, gelatin sponge particles (Gelfoam), starch (Spherex), or microspheres. Two products are composed of microspheres of defined size ranges—Embospheres (Biospheres) and Contour SE—using particles of 40–120, 100–300, 300–500, and 500–1000 μm in size. The optimal diameter of the particles for TACE has yet to be defined. Consistently higher objective response rates appear to be reported for arterial administration of drugs together with some form of he-

TABLE 88-5 SOME RANDOMIZED CLINICAL TRIALS INVOLVING TRANSHEPATIC ARTERY CHEMOEMBOLIZATION (TACE) FOR HEPATOCELLULAR CARCINOMA

Author	Year	Agents 1	Agents 2	Survival Effect
Kawaii	1992	Doxorubicin + embo	Embo	No
Chang	1994	Cisplatin + embo	Embo	No
Hatanaka	1995	Cisplatin, doxorubicin + embo	Same + ethiodol	No
Uchino	1993	Cisplatin, doxorubicin + oral FU	Same + tamoxifen	No
Lin	1988	Embo	Embo + IV FU	No
Yoshikawa	1994	Epirubicin + ethiodol (Lipiodol)	Epirubicin	No
Pelletier	1990	Doxorubicin + Gelfoam	None	No
Trinchet	1995	Cisplatin + Gelfoam	None	No
Bruix	1998	Coils and Gelfoam	None	No
Pelletier	1998	Cisplatin + ethiodol	None	No
Trinchet	1995	Cisplatin + Gelfoam	None	No
Pelletier	1998	Cisplatin + ethiodol	None	No
Lo	2002	Cisplatin + ethiodol	None	Yes
Llovet	2002	Doxorubicin + ethiodol	None	Yes

Note: embo, embolization; FU, fluorouracil.

patic artery occlusion compared with any form of systemic chemotherapy to date. The widespread use of some form of embolization in addition to chemotherapy has added to its toxicities. These include a frequent but transient fever, abdominal pain, and anorexia (all in >60% of patients). In addition, >20% of patients have increased ascites or transient elevation of transaminases. Cystic artery spasm and cholecystitis are also not uncommon. However, higher responses have also been obtained. The hepatic toxicities associated with embolization may be ameliorated by the use of degradable starch microspheres, with 50–60% response rates. A major problem in showing a survival advantage in patients responding to TACE is that many patients die of their underlying cirrhosis, not the tumor. However, improving patient quality of life is a legitimate goal of regional therapies.

Experimental Therapies Several therapies are being evaluated (**Table 88-6**). Epidermal growth factor (EGF) receptor antibodies and EGF receptor kinase inhibitors are in clinical trials, as are various anti-angiogenesis therapies. No effects on survival are yet reported. Oral sorafenib increases median survival from 6 to 9 months in advanced, unresectable HCC. Several forms of radiation therapy have been used in the treatment of HCC, including external beam and conformal radiation therapy. Radiation hepatitis remains a significant dose-limiting problem. The pure beta emit-

TABLE 88-6 SOME NOVEL MEDICAL TREATMENTS FOR HEPATOCELLULAR CARCINOMA

EGF receptor antibody
Erlotinib, Gefitinib
Kinase antagonists, Sorafenib
Vitamin K
IL-2
[131]I – ethiodol (Lipiodol)
[131]I – Ferritin
[90]Yttrium microspheres
[166]Holmium
Three-dimensional conformal radiation
Proton beam high-dose radiotherapy
Anti-angiogenesis strategies, Bevacizumab

Note: EGF, epidermal growth factor; IL, interleukin.

ter ^{90}yttrium attached to either glass or resin microspheres has been assessed in phase II trials of HCC and has encouraging survival effects with minimal toxicities. Randomized trials have yet to be performed. Vitamin K has been assessed in clinical trials at high dosage for its HCC-inhibitory actions. This idea is based on the characteristic biochemical defect in HCC of elevated plasma levels of immature prothrombin (DCP or PIVKA-2), due to a defect in the activity of prothrombin carboxylase, a vitamin K–dependent enzyme. Two vitamin K randomized controlled trials from Japan show decreased tumor occurrence. Patient participation in clinical trials aimed at assessing new therapies is encouraged.

SUMMARY
Most Common Modes of Patient Presentation

1. A patient with known history of hepatitis, jaundice, or cirrhosis, with an abnormality on ultrasound or CT scan, or rising AFP or DCP (PIVKA-2)
2. A patient with an abnormal liver function test as part of a routine examination
3. Radiologic workup for liver transplant for cirrhosis
4. Symptoms of HCC including cachexia, abdominal pain, or fever.

History and Physical Examination

1. Clinical jaundice, asthenia, itching (scratches), tremors, or disorientation
2. Hepatomegaly, splenomegaly, ascites, peripheral edema, skin signs of liver failure.

Clinical Evaluation

1. Blood tests: full blood count (splenomegaly), liver function tests, ammonia levels, electrolytes, α-fetoprotein and DCP (PIVKA-2), Ca^{2+} and Mg^{2+}; hepatitis B and C serology (and quantitative HBV DNA or HCV RNA, if either is positive); neurotensin (specific for fibrolamellar HCC)
2. Triphasic dynamic helical (spiral) CT scan of liver (if inadequate, then follow with an MRI); chest CT scan; upper and lower gastrointestinal endoscopy (for varices, bleeding, ulcers); and brain scan (only if symptoms suggest)
3. A core biopsy: of the tumor and separately of the underlying liver.

Therapy (See also Fig. 88-1)

1. HCC < 2 cm: RFA ablation, PEI, or resection
2. HCC > 2 cm, no vascular invasion: liver resection, RFA, or OLTX
3. Multiple unilobar tumors or tumor with vascular invasion: TACE
4. Bilobar tumors, no vascular invasion: TACE with OLTX for patients whose tumors have a response
5. Extrahepatic HCC or elevated bilirubin: Phase I and II studies.

OTHER PRIMARY LIVER TUMORS
FIBROLAMELLAR HCC (FL-HCC)

This rarer variant of HCC has a different biology than adult-type HCC. None of the known HCC causative factors seem important here. It is typically a disease of younger adults, often teenagers and predominantly females. It is AFP negative, but patients typically have elevated blood neurotensin levels, normal liver function tests, and no cirrhosis. Radiology is similar for HCC, except that characteristic adult-type portal vein invasion is less common. Although it is often multifocal in the liver, and therefore not resectable, metastases are common, especially to lungs and locoregional lymph nodes, but survival is often much better than with adult-type HCC. Resectable tumors are associated with 5-year survival of ≥50%. Patients often present with a huge liver or unexplained weight loss, fever, or elevated liver function tests on routine evaluations. These huge masses suggest slow growth. Surgical resection is the best management option, even for metastases, since these tumors respond much less well to chemotherapy than adult-type HCC. Although several series of OLTX for FL-HCC have been reported,

the patients usually to die from tumor recurrences, with a 2- to 5-year lag compared with OLTX for adult-type HCC. Anecdotal responses to gemcitabine plus cisplatin-TACE are reported.

EPITHELIOID HEMANGIOENDOTHELIOMA (EHE)

This rare vascular tumor of adults is also usually multifocal and can also be associated with prolonged survival, even in the presence of metastases, which are commonly in the lung. There is usually no underlying cirrhosis. Histologically, these tumors are usually of borderline malignancy and express factor VIII antigen, confirming their endothelial origin. OLTX may be associated with prolonged survival.

CHOLANGIOCARCINOMA (CCC)

CCC typically refers to mucin-producing adenocarcinomas (different from HCC) that arise from the bile ducts. They are grouped by their anatomic site of origin as intrahepatic, hilar (central, ~65% of CCCs), and peripheral (or distal, ~30% of CCCs). They arise on the basis of cirrhosis less frequently than HCC, excepting primary biliary cirrhosis. Nodular tumors arising at the bifurcation of the common bile duct are called *Klatskin tumors* and are often associated with a collapsed gallbladder, a finding that mandates visualization of the entire biliary tree. The approach to management of central and peripheral CCC is quite different. The incidence seems to be increasing in the United States. Although most CCCs have no obvious cause, several predisposing factors have been identified, including primary sclerosing cholangitis, an autoimmune disease (10–20% of PSC patients), and liver fluke in Asians, especially *Opisthorchis viverrini* and *Clonorchis sinensis*. CCC seems also to be associated with any cause of chronic biliary inflammation and injury, with alcoholic liver disease, choledocholithiasis, choledochal cysts (10%), and Caroli's disease. CCC most typically presents as painless jaundice, often with pruritus or weight loss, and acholic stools. Diagnosis is made by biopsy, percutaneously for peripheral liver lesions or, more commonly, via endoscopic retrograde cholangiopancreatography (ERCP) under direct vision for central lesions. The tumors often stain positively for cytokeratins 7, 8, and 19 and negatively for cytokeratin 20. However, histology alone cannot usually distinguish CCC from metastases from primary tumors of the colon or pancreas. Serologic tumor markers appear to be nonspecific, but CEA, CA 19-9, and CA-125 are often elevated in CCC patients and are useful for following response to therapy. Radiologic evaluation typically starts with ultrasound, which is useful in visualizing dilated bile ducts, and then proceeds with either MRI or magnetic resonance cholangiopancreatography (MRCP) or helical CT scans. Invasive ERCP is then needed to define the biliary tree and obtain a biopsy or is needed therapeutically to decompress an obstructed biliary tree with internal stent placement. If that fails, then percutaneous biliary drainage will be needed, with the biliary drainage flowing into an external bag. Central tumors often invade the porta hepatis, and locoregional lymph node involvement by tumor is frequent.

℞ CHOLANGIOCARCINOMA

Hilar CCC is resectable in ~30% of patients and usually involves bile duct resection and lymphadenectomy. Typical survival is around 24 months, with recurrences being mainly in the operative bed but with ~30% in the lungs and liver. Distal CCC, which involves the main ducts, is normally treated by resection of the extrahepatic bile ducts, often with pancreaticoduodenectomy. Survival is similar. Due to the high rates of locoregional recurrences or positive surgical margins, many patients get treated with postoperative adjuvant radiotherapy. Its effect on survival has not been assessed. Intraluminal brachyradiotherapy has also shown some promise. However, photodynamic therapy enhanced survival in one study. In this technique, sodium porfimer is injected IV and then subjected to intraluminal red light laser photoactivation. OLTX has been assessed for treatment of unresectable CCC, but 5-year survival was previously ~20%, so enthusiasm waned. However, neoadjuvant radiotherapy with sensitizing chemotherapy has shown better survival rates for CCC treated by OLTX from one institution; confirmation is needed. Multiple chemotherapeutic agents have been assessed for activity and survival in unresectable CCC. Most have been inactive. However, both systemic and hepatic arterial gemcitabine have shown promising results. The combination of this drug with others and with radiotherapy is being explored.

GALLBLADDER CANCER (GB Ca)

GB Ca has an even worse prognosis than CCC, with typical survival ~6 months or less. Women are affected much more commonly than men (4:1), unlike in HCC or CCC, and GB Ca is more common than CCC. Most patients have a history of gallstones, but very few patients with gallstones develop GB Ca (~0.2%). It presents similarly to CCC and is often diagnosed unexpectedly during gallstone or cholecystitis surgery. Presentation is typically that of chronic cholecystitis, chronic right upper quadrant pain and weight loss. Useful but nonspecific serum markers include CEA and CA 19-9. CT scans or MRCP typically reveal a gallbladder mass. The mainstay of treatment is surgical, either simple or radical cholecystectomy for stages I or II disease, respectively. Survival is nearly 100% at 5 years for stage I, and ranges from 60–90% at 5 years for stage II. More advanced GB Ca has worse survival, and many are unresectable. Adjuvant radiotherapy, used in the presence of local lymph node disease, has not been shown to enhance survival. Similar to CCC, chemotherapy is not useful in advanced or metastatic GB Ca.

CARCINOMA OF THE AMPULLA OF VATER

This tumor arises within 2 cm of the distal end of the common bile duct, and is mainly (90%) an adenocarcinoma. Locoregional lymph nodes are commonly involved (50%), and the liver is the most frequent site for metastases. The commonest clinical presentation is jaundice, and many patients also have pruritus, weight loss, and epigastric pain. Initial evaluation is performed with an abdominal ultrasound to assess vascular involvement, biliary dilatation, and liver lesions. This is followed by a CT scan, or MRI and especially MRCP. The most effective therapy is resection by pylorus-sparing pancreaticoduodenectomy, an aggressive procedure resulting in better survival rates than local resection. Survival rates are ~25% at 5 years in operable patients with involved lymph nodes and ~50% in patients without involved nodes. Unlike CCC, ~80% of patients are thought to be resectable at diagnosis. Adjuvant chemotherapy or radiotherapy has not been shown to be useful in enhancing survival. For metastatic tumors, chemotherapy is currently experimental.

TUMORS METASTATIC TO THE LIVER

These are predominantly from colon, pancreas, and breast primary tumors but can originate from any organ primary. Ocular melanomas are prone to liver metastasis. Tumor spread to the liver normally carries a poor prognosis for that tumor type. Colorectal and breast hepatic metastases were previously treated with continuous hepatic arterial infusion chemotherapy. However, more effective systemic drugs for these cancers, especially the addition of oxaliplatin to colorectal cancer regimens, have reduced the use of hepatic artery infusion therapy. In a large randomized study of systemic versus infusional plus systemic chemotherapy for resected colorectal metastases to the liver, the patients receiving infusional therapy had no survival advantage, mainly due to extrahepatic tumor spread. ^{90}Yttrium resin beads are approved in the United States for treatment of colorectal hepatic metastases. The role of this modality, either alone or in combination with chemotherapy, is being evaluated in many centers. Palliation may be obtained from chemoembolization, PEI, or RFA.

BENIGN LIVER TUMORS

Three common benign tumors occur and all are found predominantly in women. They are *hemangiomas, adenomas,* and *focal nodular hyperplasia* (FNH). FNH is typically benign, and usually no treatment is needed. Hemangiomas are the commonest and are entirely benign. Treatment is unnecessary unless their expansion causes symptoms. Adenomas are associated with contraceptive hormone use. They can cause pain and can bleed or rupture, causing acute problems. Their main interest for the physician is a low potential for malignant change and a 30% risk of bleeding. For this reason, considerable effort has gone into differentiating these three entities radiologically. Upon discovery of a liver mass, patients are usually advised to stop taking sex steroids, since adenoma regression may then occasionally occur. Adenomas can often be large masses ranging from 8–15 cm. Due to their size and definite, but low, malignant potential and potential for bleeding, adenomas are typically resected. The most useful diagnostic differentiating tool is a triphasic CT scan performed with HCC fast bolus protocol for arterial-phase imaging, together with subsequent delayed venous-phase imaging. Adenomas usually do not appear on the basis of cirrhosis, although both adenomas and HCCs are intensely vascular on the CT arterial phase and both can exhibit hemorrhage (40% of adenomas). However, adenomas have smooth, well-defined edges and enhance homogeneously, especially in the portal venous phase on delayed images, when HCCs no longer enhance. FNHs exhibit a characteristic central scar that is hypovascular on the arterial-phase and hypervascular on the delayed-phase CT images. MRI is even more sensitive in depicting the characteristic central scar of FNH.

FURTHER READINGS

FURUKAWA H et al: Living-donor liver transplantation for hepatocellular carcinoma. J Hepatobiliary Pancreat Surg 13:393, 2006

GOIN JE et al: Treatment of unresectable hepatocellular carcinoma with intrahepatic yttrium 90 microspheres. J Vasc Interv Radiol 16:161, 2005

LLOVET JM et al: A molecular signature to discriminate dysplastic nodules from early hepatocellular carcinoma. Gastroenterology 131:1758, 2006

PARIKH S, HYMAN D: Hepatocellular cancer: A guide for the internist. Am J Med 120:194, 2007

STEEL JL et al: Clinically meaningful changes in health-related quality of life in patients with hepatobiliary cancer. Ann Oncol 17:304, 2006

THORGEIRSSON S et al: Molecular prognostication of liver cancer: End of the beginning. J Hepatol 44:798, 2006

89 Pancreatic Cancer
Yu Jo Chua, David Cunningham

Over 90% of pancreatic cancers are ductal adenocarcinomas of the exocrine pancreas. These tumors occur twice as frequently in the pancreatic head compared to the rest of the organ, and tend to be aggressive, often presenting when locally inoperable or after distal metastases have occurred. Patients with pancreatic cancer have a poor prognosis, with a 5-year survival of only 5%. The discussion of pancreatic cancer here will be limited to ductal adenocarcinomas. Other types of pancreatic neoplasms include islet cell tumors and neuroendocrine tumors (Chap. 344).

INCIDENCE AND ETIOLOGY

Epidemiology   The lifetime risk of being diagnosed with pancreatic cancer in the United States is 1.27%. In the United States, it is estimated that approximately 37,170 people will be diagnosed with pancreatic cancer in 2007. Consistent with its associated poor prognosis, 33,370 are expected to die from this disease in the same year, making it the fourth leading cause of cancer-related death. The median age of diagnosis of pancreatic cancer is 72 years, with the peak incidence of diagnosis between the ages of 65 and 84; it is rarely diagnosed in those below the age of 50. The incidence is slightly higher in men than women, and it is also higher in African Americans than in Caucasians.

Etiology Cigarette smoking, obesity, and nonhereditary chronic pancreatitis appear to be risk factors for the development of pancreatic cancer. With smoking, the risk seems to increase with the number of cigarettes consumed and decreases with smoking cessation. Less clear, and sometimes conflicting associations, have been observed for other environmental factors such as diet, coffee and alcohol consumption, previous partial gastrectomy or cholecystectomy, and *Helicobacter pylori*. An epidemiologic association between diabetes mellitus and pancreatic cancer has also been demonstrated; however, it is uncertain if diabetes is a precedent of, or consequence of, pancreatic cancer.

GENETIC CONSIDERATIONS Five to 10% of patients with pancreatic cancer also have an affected first-degree relative, suggesting that in some cases genetic factors are involved. These patients seem to present earlier than sporadic cases. The risk of pancreatic cancer is increased in certain syndromes, whether directly or indirectly, such as hereditary chronic pancreatitis, Peutz-Jeghers syndrome, Von Hippel-Lindau syndrome, familial atypical multiple-mole melanoma syndrome, ataxia-telangiectasia, Gardner's syndrome [a variant of familial adenomatous polyposis (FAP)] and Lynch syndrome II, a subtype of hereditary nonpolyposis colorectal cancer (HNPCC). Heavy smokers who also have homozygous deletions of the gene for glutathione-S transferase T1 (GSTT1), a carcinogen metabolizing enzyme, may be at particular risk. Activating mutations in the K-*ras* oncogene are found in nearly all pancreatic cancer. Loss-of-function mutations in several tumor suppressor genes occur in this disease, including p53, *CDKN2A* gene (also called multiple tumor suppressor-1 gene, leading in many cases to loss of function of p16), *DPC4*, and *BRCA2*. A feature almost unique to pancreatic cancer is the combination of K-*ras* and *CDKN2A* mutations.

CLINICAL FEATURES

Presenting Features Common presenting features of pancreatic cancer include pain (present in >80% of patients with locally advanced or metastatic disease), obstructive jaundice, weight loss, and anorexia. Patients with jaundice may also have pruritus, pale stools, and dark urine; they often have tumors in the pancreatic head, and tend to be diagnosed earlier and with earlier stage disease. Other symptoms tend to be more insidious, so that in the absence of jaundice, the interval between onset and diagnosis can be prolonged. Pain, for example, is often more of a problem in patients with lesions in the body or tail of the pancreas where the primary tumor is more likely to become quite large or to invade adjacent structures (such as the splanchnic nerves) before becoming manifest; these patients frequently have inoperable disease. When present, pain is often felt as a dull ache in the upper abdomen and may radiate to the back, and characteristically may improve upon leaning forward. It may initially be intermittent, and may worsen with meals. These patients may suffer from marked weight loss, which may result from a combination of anorexia, early satiety, malabsorption or diarrhea/steatorrhea. Other less common presenting features include the diagnosis of glucose intolerance (particularly within 2 years of cancer diagnosis), previous pancreatitis, migratory superficial thrombophlebitis (Trousseau's syndrome), gastrointestinal hemorrhage from varices, and splenomegaly.

Physical Findings Patients with early disease may not have any significant abnormalities detectable on physical examination. Jaundice may be a presenting feature in some; in these patients a palpable, nontender gallbladder (Courvoisier's sign) may be palpated under the right costal margin. Patients with more advanced disease may have an abdominal mass, hepatomegaly, splenomegaly, or ascites. The left supraclavicular lymph node (Virchow's node) may be involved with tumor, or widespread peritoneal disease may be palpable on rectal examination in the pouch of Douglas.

Imaging Studies (Fig. 89-1) Ultrasound is often used as an initial investigation for patients with jaundice, or with less-specific symptoms such as upper abdominal discomfort, and is able to assess the biliary tract, gall bladder, pancreas, and liver. Computed tomography (CT) scanning is preferable to ultrasound even though it is more costly, as it is less operator-dependent, more reproducible, and less susceptible to interference from intestinal gas. The sensitivity and specificity of CT is markedly improved by the use of pancreatic protocol scanning on modern multislice scanners. CT may show a pancreatic mass, dilatation of the biliary system or pancreatic duct, or distal spread to the liver, regional lymph nodes, or peritoneum (and/or associated ascites). When helical CT is combined with the use of intravenous contrast, it may also help determine resectability by providing information on the involvement of important vascular structures such as the celiac axis, superior mesenteric or portal vessels. Endoscopic retrograde cholangiopancreatography (ERCP) is also widely used in the diagnosis of pancreatic cancer, particularly when CT and ultrasound fail to show a mass lesion, and may reveal either stricture or obstruction in either the pancreatic or common bile duct. ERCP can also be used to obtain brushings of a stricture for cytology or for placing stents in order to relieve obstructive jaundice. Endoscopic ultrasound (EUS) may be useful in the diagnosis of small lesions (<2–3 cm in diameter) and, in some cases, for local staging as well as evaluating invasion of major vascular structures. EUS-guided fine-needle aspiration may also be used to obtain cytology for confirming the diagnosis, particularly in patients with potentially operable disease (see below). While magnetic resonance imaging (MRI) does not offer any advantages over CT in the routine evaluation of patients with possible pancreatic cancer, magnetic resonance cholangiopancreatography (MRCP) may be better than CT for defining the anatomy of the pancreatic duct and biliary tree, being able to image the ducts both above and below a stricture. The sensitivity of MRCP is comparable to ERCP, but does not require contrast administration to the ductal system, so that there is less associated morbidity. MRCP may be useful when cannulation of the pancreatic duct by ERCP has been unsuccessful or may be difficult, such as when normal anatomy is changed by surgery. Positron-emission tomography with ^{18}F-fluoro-2deoxyglucose (FDG-PET) may be useful for excluding occult distal metastasis in patients with localized disease who are being worked up for surgery or in patients with unresectable localized disease being considered for chemoradiotherapy.

Tissue Diagnosis and Cytology Patients with disease that is potentially curable by surgery, and in whom a highly suspicious lesion is seen on imaging, are often taken directly to surgery without prior tissue confirmation of cancer. This is because of theoretical concerns that a percutaneous fine-needle aspiration may result in dissemination of cancer intraperitoneally or along the track of the biopsy needle. In addition, negative cytology may not be sufficient evidence to avoid surgery, particularly with small lesions. EUS-guided fine-needle aspiration is increasingly being used, even in patients with potentially resectable disease, as there is less risk of intraperitoneal spread of cancer. Other methods of obtaining specimens for cytological analysis include sampling of pancreatic juices or brushings of ductal lesions obtained by ERCP.

Serum Markers The most widely used serum marker in pancreatic cancer is cancer-associated antigen 19-9 (CA 19-9). It has a reported sensitivity and specificity of about 80–90%, and is suggestive, rather than confirmatory, of the diagnosis of pancreatic cancer. Serum levels of CA 19-9 can be elevated in patients with jaundice without pancreatic cancer present. The level of CA 19-9 may have prognostic implications, with very high levels sometimes found in patients with inoperable disease. In advanced disease, patients treated with chemotherapy who had high pretreatment levels of CA 19-9 have also been found to have a worse survival, whereas those patients whose levels of marker fell with treatment had a better outcome. In patients with cancers with elevated CA 19-9, serial evaluation of this marker is useful for monitoring re-

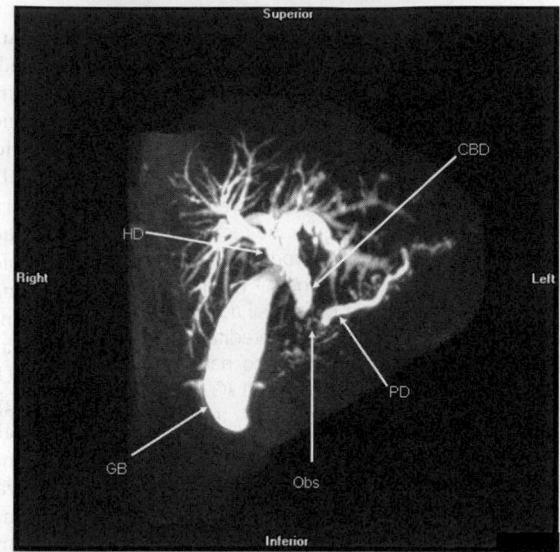

FIGURE 89-1 Carcinoma of the pancreas. A. Sonogram showing pancreatic carcinoma (P), dilated intrahepatic bile ducts (d), dilated portal vein (pv), and inferior vena cava (IVC). **B.** Computed tomography scan showing pancreatic carcinoma (*dark arrows*). **C.** Endoscopic retrograde showing abrupt cutoff of the duct of Wirsung (*arrow*). **D.** Magnetic resonance cholangiopancreatography showing obstruction (Obs) in the pancreatic duct (PD). The gallbladder (GB), hepatic duct (HD), and common bile duct (CBD) are labeled.

sponses to treatment. In patients with completely resected tumors, follow-up with CA 19-9 is useful for detecting recurrence.

Staging   In pancreatic cancer, which has a poor prognosis, the value of detailed clinical staging is limited. The most clinically relevant distinction to make is between patients with disease that may be resected with curative intent, and those with advanced disease in whom treatment is palliative (Table 89-1).

Surveillance in High-Risk Individuals   Routine screening for pancreatic cancer is not recommended due to a high false-positive rate of the available tests. However, screening may be reasonable in certain high-risk individuals, such as those with strong family histories, although the optimal timing, frequency, and method of screening is unknown.

One recommendation is to commence screening at the age of 35 in patients with hereditary pancreatitis, or 10 years before the age of the youngest diagnosis of pancreatic cancer in those with a significant family history using spiral CT, followed by EUS when CT results have been indeterminate.

℞ PANCREATIC CANCER

Symptoms and the associated impaired performance status are significant issues in the management of patients with pancreatic cancer, as they can have a marked negative impact on the ability to safely deliver chemotherapy or perform curative surgery. For example, patients with malabsorption secondary to pancreatic insufficiency may be treated with pancreatic enzyme supplementation. Indeed effective symptom management is as important a therapeutic goal as survival prolongation.

ADVANCED PANCREATIC CANCER   These patients have metastatic or locally advanced inoperable disease and are the majority with newly diagnosed disease. Debulking surgery or partial resections have no role, as these procedures are associated with the same risks as a curative resection but are unlikely to improve survival. Many patients may, however, benefit from endoscopic biliary or duodenal stenting, and some patients from nerve plexus blocks or ablation. Less frequently, intestinal bypass surgery is required.

The deoxycytidine analogue gemcitabine, given as a single agent (gemcitabine 1000 mg/m^2 weekly for 7 weeks followed by 1 week rest, then weekly for 3 weeks every 4 weeks thereafter), has been the preferred treatment for these patients since it was shown to yield clinical benefit (a composite parameter for evaluating symptomatic benefit of treatment used in some trials of this disease) and improved survival compared to 5-fluorouracil. The median survival observed with single-agent gemcitabine in randomized trials is about 6 months, with a 12-month survival of approximately 18%. Furthermore, two randomized trials have shown im-

TABLE 89-1	**STAGING OF PANCREATIC CARCINOMA**	
	Stage Grouping	**TNM Staging**[a]
Localized resectable	I	T1–2 N0 M0
	II	T3 N0 M0 or T1–3 N1 M0
Locally advanced	III	T4 N(any) M0
Metastatic	IV	T(any) N(any) M1

[a]TNM, tumor, nodes, metastasis.
Note: T1, tumor limited to pancreas, ≤2 cm; T2, tumor limited to pancreas, >2 cm; T3, tumor extends beyond the pancreas but without involvement of celiac axis or superior mesenteric artery; T4, tumor involves celiac axis or the superior mesenteric artery (unresectable primary tumor); N0, no regional lymph node metastasis (regional lymph nodes are the peripancreatic lymph nodes, including the lymph nodes along the hepatic artery, celiac axis and pyloric/splenic regions); N1, regional lymph node metastasis; M0, no distal metastasis; M1, distal metastasis.
Source: Modified from Greene, Page; with permission.

proved survival from the addition of either the oral fluoropyrimidine, capecitabine (gemcitabine 1000 mg/m² days 1, 8, and 15 plus capecitabine 1660 mg/m² days 1–21, repeated every 28 days), or the tyrosine kinase inhibitor of the epidermal growth factor receptor (EGFR), erlotinib (standard gemcitabine plus erlotinib 100 mg daily). The survival improvement observed with both of these combinations appears similar, and the addition of capecitabine to gemcitabine in this regimen does not appear to increase the toxicity above single-agent gemcitabine. Either combination should, therefore, be considered as options for treating these patients. Second-line treatment options in pancreatic cancer are limited although there may be an emerging role for oxaliplatin-based chemotherapy; fit patients who have failed first-line treatment should be offered entry into clinical trials. On-going clinical trials are evaluating the potential benefits of incorporating other novel targeted agents into the treatment of pancreatic cancer, usually together with gemcitabine.

In patients with locally advanced unresectable disease, external beam chemoradiotherapy may be useful, either as initial treatment or as consolidation after induction chemotherapy.

OPERABLE DISEASE Complete surgical resection in patients with localized disease (stage I or II disease), with distal metastases excluded by prior CT scan of the abdomen and pelvis, and CT of the chest or chest x-ray, is potentially curative. However, such surgery is only possible in 10–15% of patients, many of whom will suffer from recurrences of their disease. Indeed, the 5-year survival reported in randomized trials with surgery alone is approximately 10%, although modern series have improved on these results. Outcomes tend to be more favorable in patients with lymph node–negative disease, smaller tumors (less than 3 cm), negative resection margins and well-differentiated tumors. Despite a dismal long term outcome, these patients still have a better survival with surgery than with other palliative measures.

Surgery is usually preceded by laparoscopy in order to exclude peritoneal metastases not seen on other staging investigations. Pancreaticoduodenectomy, also known as the Whipple procedure, is the standard operation for cancers of the head or uncinate process of the pancreas. The procedure involves resection of the pancreatic head, duodenum, first 15 cm of the jejunum, common bile duct, and gallbladder, and a partial gastrectomy, with the pancreatic and biliary anastomosis placed 45 to 60 cm proximal to the gastrojejunostomy. Perioperative mortality rates have fallen to less than 5%, reflecting greater experience with the surgery and perioperative management of these patients. However, this type of surgery is highly specialized and should ideally only occur in dedicated centers with a high volume of these cases and specialized surgeons.

Adjuvant treatment for patients with curatively resected pancreatic cancer is controversial, with divergent treatment approaches preferred in the United States and in Europe, based on the results of different randomized trials conducted on both sides of the Atlantic. In the United States, fluoropyrimidine-based postoperative chemoradiotherapy followed by adjuvant chemotherapy is preferred. In Europe, because a large randomized trial (the European Study Group for Pancreatic Cancer 1 or ESPAC1 trial) showed a survival benefit for adjuvant chemotherapy with 5-fluorouracil (5FU) **(Fig. 89-2)**, this approach is more common practice.

No. at Risk	0	12	24	36	48	60
No CT —	142	89	41	18	11	7
CT —	147	99	56	38	22	11

FIGURE 89-2 Survival by adjuvant chemotherapy. Kaplan-Meier estimates of survival from the European Study Group for Pancreatic Cancer 1 (ESPAC1) trial for the comparison of adjuvant chemotherapy versus no adjuvant chemotherapy (CT) in patients with resected pancreatic cancer (hazard ratio for death, 0.71; 95% confidence interval, 0.55 to 0.92; p = .009). (*Reprinted with permission from JP Neoptolemos, DD Stocken, H Friess, et al: A randomized trial of chemoradiotherapy and chemotherapy after resection of pancreatic cancer. N Engl J Med 350:1200–1210, 2004. Copyright 2004, Massachusetts Medical Society.*)

FURTHER READINGS

ALEXAKIS N et al: Current standards of surgery for pancreatic cancer. Br J Surg 91:1410, 2004

BARUGOLA G et al: The determinant factors of recurrence following resection for ductal pancreatic cancer. JOP 8(Suppl 1):132, 2007

CHUA YJ, CUNNINGHAM D: Chemotherapy for advanced pancreatic cancer. Best Pract Res Clin Gastroenterol 20:327, 2006

DIMAGNO EP et al: AGA technical review on the epidemiology, diagnosis, and treatment of pancreatic ductal adenocarcinomas. American Gastroenterological Association. Gastroenterology 117:1464, 1999

GREENE FL, PAGE DL (eds.): *Exocrine Pancreas, AJCC Cancer Staging Manual*, 6th ed, New York, Springer, pp 157–164, 2002

NEOPTOLEMOS JP et al: A randomized trial of chemoradiotherapy and chemotherapy after resection of pancreatic cancer. N Engl J Med 350:1200, 2004

WILLETT CG et al: Locally advanced pancreatic cancer. J Clin Oncol 23:4538, 2005

90 Bladder and Renal Cell Carcinomas

Howard I. Scher, Robert J. Motzer

BLADDER CANCER

A transitional cell epithelium lines the urinary tract from the renal pelvis to the ureter, urinary bladder, and the proximal two-thirds of the urethra. Cancers can occur at any point: 90% of malignancies develop in the bladder, 8% in the renal pelvis, and the remaining 2% in the ureter or urethra. Bladder cancer is the fourth most common cancer in men and the thirteenth in women, with an estimated 67,160 new cases and 13,750 deaths in the United States predicted for the year

2007. The almost 5:1 ratio of incidence to mortality reflects the higher frequency of the less lethal superficial variants compared to the more lethal invasive and metastatic variants. The incidence is three times higher in men than in women, and twofold higher in whites than in blacks, with a median age at diagnosis of 65 years.

Once diagnosed, urothelial tumors exhibit polychronotropism—the tendency to recur over time and in new locations in the urothelial tract. As long as urothelium is present, continuous monitoring of the tract is required.

EPIDEMIOLOGY

Cigarette smoking is believed to contribute to up to 50% of the diagnosed urothelial cancers in men and up to 40% in women. The risk of developing a urothelial malignancy in male smokers is increased two- to fourfold relative to nonsmokers and continues for 10 years or longer after cessation. Other implicated agents include the aniline dyes, the drugs phenacetin and chlornaphazine, and external beam radiation. Chronic cyclophosphamide exposure may also increase risk, whereas vitamin A supplements appear to be protective. Exposure to *Schistosoma haematobium*, a parasite found in many developing countries, is associated with an increase in both squamous and transitional cell carcinomas of the bladder.

PATHOLOGY

Clinical subtypes are grouped into three categories: 75% are superficial, 20% invade muscle, and 5% are metastatic at presentation. Staging of the tumor within the bladder is based on the pattern of growth and depth of invasion: Ta lesions grow as exophytic lesions; carcinoma in situ (CIS) lesions start on the surface and tend to invade. The revised tumor, node, metastasis (TNM) staging system is illustrated in **Fig. 90-1**. About half of invasive tumors presented originally as superficial lesions that later progressed. Tumors are also rated by grade. Grade I lesions (highly differentiated tumors) rarely progress to a higher stage, whereas grade III tumors do.

More than 95% of urothelial tumors in the United States are transitional cell in origin. Pure squamous cancers with keratinization constitute 3%, adenocarcinomas 2%, and small cell tumors (with paraneoplastic syndromes) <1%. Adenocarcinomas develop primarily in the urachal remnant in the dome of the bladder or in the periurethral tissues; some assume a signet cell histology. Lymphomas and melanomas are rare. Of the transitional cell tumors, low-grade papillary lesions that grow on a central stalk are most common. These tumors are very friable, have a tendency to bleed, are at high risk for recurrence, and yet rarely progress to the more lethal invasive variety. In contrast, CIS is a high-grade tumor that is considered a precursor of the more lethal muscle-invasive disease.

FIGURE 90-1 Bladder staging. TNM, tumor, node, metastasis.

PATHOGENESIS

The multicentric nature of the disease and high rate of recurrence has led to the hypothesis of a field defect in the urothelium that results in a predisposition to cancer. Molecular genetic analyses suggest that the superficial and invasive lesions develop along distinct molecular pathways in which primary tumorigenic aberrations precede secondary changes associated with progression to a more advanced stage. Low-grade papillary tumors that do not tend to invade or metastasize harbor constitutive activation of the receptor-tyrosine kinase-Ras signal transduction pathway and a high frequency of fibroblast growth factor receptor 3 (FGFR3) mutations. In contrast, CIS and invasive tumors have a higher frequency of *TP53* and *RB* gene alternations. Within all clinical stages, including Tis, T1, and T2 or greater lesions, tumors with alterations in *p53*, *p21*, and/or *RB* have a higher probability of recurrence, metastasis, and death from disease.

CLINICAL PRESENTATION, DIAGNOSIS, AND STAGING

Hematuria occurs in 80–90% of patients and often reflects exophytic tumors. The bladder is the most common source of gross hematuria (40%), but benign cystitis (22%) is a more common cause than bladder cancer (15%) (Chap. 45). Microscopic hematuria is more commonly of prostate origin (25%); only 2% of bladder cancers produce microscopic hematuria. Once hematuria is documented, a urinary cytology, visualization of the urothelial tract by CT or intravenous pyelogram, and cystoscopy are recommended if no other etiology is found. Screening asymptomatic individuals for hematuria increases the diagnosis of tumors at an early stage but has not been shown to prolong life. After hematuria, irritative symptoms are the next most common presentation, which may reflect in situ disease. Obstruction of the ureters may cause flank pain. Symptoms of metastatic disease are rarely the first presenting sign.

The endoscopic evaluation includes an examination under anesthesia to determine whether a palpable mass is present. A flexible endoscope is inserted into the bladder, and bladder barbotage is performed. The visual inspection includes mapping the location, size, and number of lesions, as well as a description of the growth pattern (solid vs. papillary). An intraoperative video is often recorded. All visible tumors should be resected, and a sample of the muscle underlying the tumor should be obtained to assess the depth of invasion. Normal-appearing areas are biopsied at random to ensure no field defect. A notation is made as to whether a tumor was completely or incompletely resected. Selective catheterization and visualization of the upper tracts should be performed if the cytology is positive and no disease is visible in the bladder. Ultrasonography, CT, and/or MRI may help to determine whether a tumor extends to perivesical fat (T3) and to document nodal spread. Distant metastases are assessed by CT of the chest and abdomen, MRI, or radionuclide imaging of the skeleton.

℞ BLADDER CANCER

Management depends on whether the tumor invades muscle and whether it has spread to the regional lymph nodes and beyond. The probability of spread increases with increasing T stage.

SUPERFICIAL DISEASE At a minimum, the management of a superficial tumor is complete endoscopic resection with or without intravesical therapy. The decision to recommend intravesical therapy depends on the histologic subtype, number of lesions, depth of invasion, presence or absence of CIS, and antecedent history. Recurrences develop in upward of 50% of cases, of which 5–20% progress to a more advanced stage. In general, solitary papillary lesions are managed by transurethral surgery alone. CIS and recurrent disease are treated by transurethral surgery followed by intravesical therapy.

Intravesical therapies are used in two general contexts: as an adjuvant to a complete endoscopic resection to prevent recurrence or, less commonly, to eliminate disease that cannot be controlled by endoscopic resection alone. Intravesical treatments are advised for patients with recurrent disease, >40% involvement of the bladder surface by tumor, diffuse CIS, or T1 disease. The standard intravesical therapy, based on randomized comparisons, is bacillus Calmette-Guerin (BCG) in six weekly instillations, followed by monthly maintenance administrations for ≥1 year. Other agents with activity include mitomycin-C, interferon (IFN), and gemcitabine. The side effects of intravesical therapies include dysuria, urinary frequency, and, depending on the drug, myelosuppression or contact dermatitis. Rarely, intravesical BCG may produce a systemic illness associated with granulomatous infections in multiple sites that requires antituberculin therapy.

Following the endoscopic resection, patients are monitored for recurrence at 3-month intervals during the first year. Recurrence may develop anywhere along the urothelial tract, including the renal pelvis, ureter, or urethra. A consequence of the "successful" treatment of tumors in the bladder is an increase in the frequency of extravesical recurrences (e.g., urethra or ureter). Those with persistent disease or new tumors are generally considered for a second course of BCG or for intravesical chemotherapy with valrubicin or gemcitabine. In some cases cystectomy is recommended, although the specific indications vary. Tumors in the ureter or renal pelvis are typically managed by resection during retrograde examination or, in some cases, by instillation through the renal pelvis. Tumors of the prostatic urethra may require cystectomy if the tumor cannot be resected completely.

INVASIVE DISEASE The treatment of a tumor that has invaded muscle can be separated into control of the primary tumor and, depending on the pathologic findings at surgery, systemic chemotherapy. Radical cystectomy is the standard, although in selected cases a bladder-sparing approach is used; this approach includes complete endoscopic resection; partial cystectomy; or a combination of resection, systemic chemotherapy, and external beam radiation therapy. In some countries, external beam radiation therapy is considered standard. In the United States, its role is limited to those patients deemed unfit for cystectomy, those with unresectable local disease, or as part of an experimental bladder-sparing approach.

Indications for cystectomy include muscle-invading tumors not suitable for segmental resection; low-stage tumors unsuitable for conservative management (e.g., due to multicentric and frequent recurrences resistant to intravesical instillations); high-grade tumors (T1G3) associated with CIS; and bladder symptoms, such as frequency or hemorrhage, that impair quality of life.

Radical cystectomy is major surgery that requires appropriate preoperative evaluation and management. The procedure involves removal of the bladder and pelvic lymph nodes and creation of a conduit or reservoir for urinary flow. Grossly abnormal lymph nodes are evaluated by frozen section. If metastases are confirmed, the procedure is often aborted. In males, radical cystectomy includes the removal of the prostate, seminal vesicles, and proximal urethra. Impotence is universal unless the nerves responsible for erectile function are preserved. In females, the procedure includes removal of the bladder, urethra, uterus, fallopian tubes, ovaries, anterior vaginal wall, and surrounding fascia.

Previously, urine flow was managed by directing the ureters to the abdominal wall, where it was collected in an external appliance. Currently, most patients receive either a continent cutaneous reservoir constructed from detubularized bowel or an orthotopic neobladder. Some 70% of men receive a neobladder. With a continent reservoir, 65–85% of men will be continent at night and 85–90% during the day. Cutaneous reservoirs are drained by intermittent catheterization; orthotopic neobladders are drained more naturally. Contraindications to a neobladder include renal insufficiency, an inability to self-catheterize, or an exophytic tumor or CIS in the urethra. Diffuse CIS in the bladder is a relative contraindication based on the risk of a urethral recurrence. Concurrent ulcerative colitis or Crohn's disease may hinder the use of resected bowel.

A partial cystectomy may be considered when the disease is limited to the dome of the bladder, a margin of at least 2 cm can be achieved, there is no CIS in other sites, and the bladder capacity is adequate after the tumor

TABLE 90-1 SURVIVAL FOLLOWING SURGERY FOR BLADDER CANCER

Pathologic Stage	5-Year Survival, %	10-Year Survival, %
T2,N0	89	87
T3a,N0	78	76
T3b,N0	62	61
T4,N0	50	45
Any T,N1	35	34

has been removed. This occurs in 5–10% of cases. Carcinomas in the ureter or in the renal pelvis are treated with nephroureterectomy with a bladder cuff to remove the tumor.

The probability of recurrence following surgery is predicted on the basis of pathologic stage, presence or absence of lymphatic or vascular invasion, and nodal spread. Among those whose cancers recur, the recurrence develops in a median of 1 year (range 0.04–11.1 years). Long-term outcomes vary by pathologic stage and histology **(Table 90-1)**. The number of lymph nodes removed is also prognostic, whether or not the nodes contained tumor.

Chemotherapy (described below) has been shown to prolong the survival of patients with invasive disease, but only when combined with definitive treatment of the bladder by radical cystectomy or radiation therapy. Thus, for the majority of patients, chemotherapy alone is inadequate to clear the bladder of disease. Experimental studies are evaluating bladder preservation strategies by combining chemotherapy and radiation therapy in patients whose tumors were endoscopically removed.

METASTATIC DISEASE The primary goal of treatment for metastatic disease is to achieve complete remission with chemotherapy alone or with a combined-modality approach of chemotherapy followed by surgical resection of residual disease, as is done routinely for the treatment of germ cell tumors. One can define a goal in terms of cure or palliation on the basis of the probability of achieving a complete response to chemotherapy using prognostic factors, such as Karnofsky Performance Status (KPS) (<80%), and whether the pattern of spread is nodal or visceral (liver, lung, or bone). For those with zero, one, or two risk factors, the probability of complete remission is 38, 25, and 5%, respectively, and median survival is 33, 13.4, and 9.3 months, respectively. Patients who are functionally compromised or who have visceral disease or bone metastases rarely achieve long-term survival. The toxicities also vary as a function of risk, and treatment-related mortality rates are as high as 3–4% using some combinations in these poor-risk patient groups.

CHEMOTHERAPY A number of chemotherapeutic drugs have shown activity as single agents; cisplatin, paclitaxel, and gemcitabine are considered most active. Standard therapy consists of two-, three-, or four-drug combinations. Overall response rates of >50% have been reported using combinations such as methotrexate, vinblastine, doxorubicin, and cisplatin (M-VAC); cisplatin and paclitaxel (PT); gemcitabine and cisplatin (GC); or gemcitabine, paclitaxel, and cisplatin (GTC). M-VAC was considered standard, but the toxicities of neutropenia and fever, mucositis, diminished renal and auditory function, and peripheral neuropathy led to the development of alternative regimens. At present, GC is used more commonly than M-VAC, based on the results of a comparative trial of M-VAC versus GC that showed less neutropenia and fever, and less mucositis for the GC regimen. Anemia and thrombocytopenia were more common with GC. GTC is not more effective than GC.

Chemotherapy has also been evaluated in the neoadjuvant and adjuvant settings. In a randomized trial, patients receiving three cycles of neoadjuvant M-VAC followed by cystectomy had a significantly better median (6.2 years) and 5-year survival (57%) compared to cystectomy alone (median survival 3.8 years; 5-year survival 42%). Similar results were obtained in an international study of three cycles of cisplatin, methotrexate, and vinblastine (CMV) followed by either radical cystectomy or radiation therapy. The decision to administer adjuvant therapy is based on the risk of recurrence after cystectomy. Indications for adjuvant chemotherapy include the presence of nodal disease, extravesical tumor extension, or vascular invasion in the resected specimen. Another study of adjuvant therapy found that four cycles of CMV delayed recurrence, although an effect on survival was less clear. Additional trials are studying taxane- and gemcitabine-based combinations.

The management of bladder cancer is summarized in **Table 90-2**.

TABLE 90-2 MANAGEMENT OF BLADDER CANCER

Nature of Lesion	Management Approach
Superficial	Endoscopic removal, usually with intravesical therapy
Invasive disease	Cystectomy ± systemic chemotherapy (before or after surgery)
Metastatic disease	Curative or palliative chemotherapy (based on prognostic factors) ± surgery

CARCINOMA OF THE RENAL PELVIS AND URETER

About 2500 cases of renal pelvis and ureter cancer occur each year; nearly all are transitional cell carcinomas similar to bladder cancer in biology and appearance. This tumor is also associated with chronic phenacetin abuse and with Balkan nephropathy, a chronic interstitial nephritis endemic in Bulgaria, Greece, Bosnia-Herzegovina, and Romania.

The most common symptom is painless gross hematuria, and the disease is usually detected on intravenous pyelogram during the work-up for hematuria. Patterns of spread are like those in bladder cancer. For low-grade disease localized to the renal pelvis and ureter, nephroureterectomy (including excision of the distal ureter with a portion of the bladder) is associated with 5-year survival of 80–90%. More invasive or histologically poorly differentiated tumors are more likely to recur locally and to metastasize. Metastatic disease is treated with the chemotherapy used in bladder cancer, and the outcome is similar to that of metastatic transitional cell cancer of bladder origin.

RENAL CELL CARCINOMA

Renal cell carcinomas account for 90–95% of malignant neoplasms arising from the kidney. Notable features include resistance to cytotoxic agents, infrequent responses to biologic response modifiers such as interleukin (IL) 2, and a variable clinical course for patients with metastatic disease, including anecdotal reports of spontaneous regression.

EPIDEMIOLOGY

The incidence of renal cell carcinoma continues to rise and is now nearly 51,000 cases annually in the United States, resulting in 13,000 deaths. The male to female ratio is 2:1. Incidence peaks between the ages of 50–70, although this malignancy may be diagnosed at any age. Many environmental factors have been investigated as possible contributing causes; the strongest association is with cigarette smoking (accounting for 20–30% of cases). Risk is also increased for patients who have acquired cystic disease of the kidney associated with end-stage renal disease, and for those with tuberous sclerosis. Most cases are sporadic, although familial forms have been reported. One is associated with von Hippel-Lindau (VHL) syndrome, which predisposes to renal cell carcinomas, retinal hemangioma, hemangioblastoma of the spinal cord and cerebellum, and pheochromocytoma. Roughly 35% of individuals with VHL disease develop renal cell cancer. An increased incidence has also been reported for first-degree relatives.

PATHOLOGY AND GENETICS

Renal cell neoplasia represents a heterogeneous group of tumors with distinct histopathologic, genetic, and clinical features ranging from benign to high-grade malignant (Table 90-3). They are classified on the basis of morphology and histology. Categories include clear cell carcinoma (60% of cases), papillary tumors (5–15%), chromophobic tumors (5–10%), oncocytomas (5–10%), and collecting or Bellini duct tumors (<1%). Papillary tumors tend to be bilateral and multifocal. Chromophobic tumors have a more indolent clinical course, and oncocytomas are considered benign neoplasms. In contrast, Bellini duct carcinomas, which are thought to arise from the collecting ducts within the renal medulla, are very rare but very aggressive. They tend to affect younger patients.

TABLE 90-3 CLASSIFICATION OF EPITHELIAL NEOPLASMS ARISING FROM THE KIDNEY

Carcinoma Type	Growth Pattern	Cell of Origin	Cytogenetics
Clear cell	Acinar or sarcomatoid	Proximal tubule	3p–
Papillary	Papillary or sarcomatoid	Proximal tubule	+7, +17, –Y
Chromophobic	Solid, tubular, or sarcomatoid	Cortical collecting duct	Hypodiploid
Oncocytic	Tumor nests	Cortical collecting duct	Undetermined
Collecting duct	Papillary or sarcomatoid	Medullary collecting duct	Undetermined

Clear cell tumors, the predominant histology, are found in >80% of patients who develop metastases. Clear cell tumors arise from the epithelial cells of the proximal tubules and usually show chromosome 3p deletions. Deletions of 3p21–26 (where the *VHL* gene maps) are identified in patients with familial as well as sporadic tumors. *VHL* encodes a tumor-suppressor protein that is involved in regulating the transcription of vascular endothelial growth factor (VEGF), platelet-derived growth factor (PDGF), and a number of other hypoxia-inducible proteins. Inactivation of *VHL* leads to overexpression of these agonists of the VEGF and PDGF receptors, which promote tumor angiogenesis and tumor growth. Agents that inhibit proangiogenic growth factor activity show antitumor effects.

CLINICAL PRESENTATION

The presenting signs and symptoms include hematuria, abdominal pain, and a flank or abdominal mass. This classic triad occurs in 10–20% of patients. Other symptoms are fever, weight loss, anemia, and a varicocele (Table 90-4). The tumor can also be found incidentally on a radiograph. Widespread use of radiologic cross-sectional imaging procedures (CT, ultrasound, MRI) contributes to earlier detection, including incidental renal masses detected during evaluation for other medical conditions. The increasing number of incidentally discovered low-stage tumors has contributed to an improved 5-year survival for patients with renal cell carcinoma and increased use of nephron-sparing surgery (partial nephrectomy). A spectrum of paraneoplastic syndromes has been associated with these malignancies, including erythrocytosis, hypercalcemia, nonmetastatic hepatic dysfunction (Stauffer syndrome), and acquired dysfibrinogenemia. Erythrocytosis is noted at presentation in only about 3% of patients. Anemia, a sign of advanced disease, is more common.

The standard evaluation of patients with suspected renal cell tumors includes a CT scan of the abdomen and pelvis, chest radiograph, urine analysis, and urine cytology. If metastatic disease is suspected from the chest radiograph, a CT of the chest is warranted. MRI is useful in evaluating the inferior vena cava in cases of suspected tumor involvement or invasion by thrombus. In clinical practice, any solid

TABLE 90-4 SIGNS AND SYMPTOMS IN PATIENTS WITH RENAL CELL CANCER

Presenting Sign or Symptom	Incidence, %
Classic triad: hematuria, flank pain, flank mass	10–20
Hematuria	40
Flank pain	40
Palpable mass	25
Weight loss	33
Anemia	33
Fever	20
Hypertension	20
Abnormal liver function	15
Hypercalcemia	5
Erythrocytosis	3
Neuromyopathy	3
Amyloidosis	2
Increased erythrocyte sedimentation rate	55

renal masses should be considered malignant until proven otherwise; a definitive diagnosis is required. If no metastases are demonstrated, surgery is indicated, even if the renal vein is invaded. The differential diagnosis of a renal mass includes cysts, benign neoplasms (adenoma, angiomyolipoma, oncocytoma), inflammatory lesions (pyelonephritis or abscesses), and other primary or metastatic cancers. Other malignancies that may involve the kidney include transitional cell carcinoma of the renal pelvis, sarcoma, lymphoma, and Wilms' tumor. All of these are less common causes of renal masses than is renal cell cancer.

STAGING AND PROGNOSIS

Two staging systems used are the Robson classification and the American Joint Committee on Cancer (AJCC) staging system. According to the AJCC system, stage I tumors are <7 cm in greatest diameter and confined to the kidney, stage II tumors are ≥7 cm and confined to the kidney, stage III tumors extend through the renal capsule but are confined to Gerota's fascia (IIIa) or involve a single hilar lymph node (N1), and stage IV disease includes tumors that have invaded adjacent organs (excluding the adrenal gland) or involve multiple lymph nodes or distant metastases. The rate of 5-year survival varies by stage: >90% for stage I, 85% for stage II, 60% for stage III, and 10% for stage IV.

Rx RENAL CELL CARCINOMA

LOCALIZED TUMORS The standard management for stage I or II tumors and selected cases of stage III disease is radical nephrectomy. This procedure involves en bloc removal of Gerota's fascia and its contents, including the kidney, the ipsilateral adrenal gland, and adjacent hilar lymph nodes. The role of a regional lymphadenectomy is controversial. Extension into the renal vein or inferior vena cava (stage III disease) does not preclude resection even if cardiopulmonary bypass is required. If the tumor is resected, half of these patients have prolonged survival.

Nephron-sparing approaches via open or laparoscopic surgery may be appropriate for patients who have only one kidney, depending on the size and location of the lesion. A nephron-sparing approach can also be used for patients with bilateral tumors, accompanied by a radical nephrectomy on the opposite side. Partial nephrectomy techniques are being applied electively to resect small masses for patients with a normal contralateral kidney. Adjuvant therapy following this surgery does not improve outcome, even in cases with a poor prognosis.

ADVANCED DISEASE Surgery has a limited role for patients with metastatic disease. However, long-term survival may occur in patients who relapse after nephrectomy in a solitary site that can be removed. One indication for nephrectomy with metastases at initial presentation is to alleviate pain or hemorrhage of a primary tumor. Also, a cytoreductive nephrectomy before systemic treatment improves survival for carefully selected patients with stage IV tumors.

Metastatic renal cell carcinoma is highly refractory to chemotherapy and only infrequently responsive to cytokine therapy with IL-2 or IFN-α. IFN-α and IL-2 produce regressions in 10–20% of patients, but on occasion these responses are durable. IL-2 was approved on the observation of durable complete remission in a small proportion of cases.

The situation changed dramatically when two large-scale randomized trials established a role for antiangiogenic therapy in this disease as predicted by the genetic studies. These trials separately evaluated two orally administered antiangiogenic agents, sorafenib and sunitinib, that inhibited receptor tyrosine kinase signaling through the VEGF and PDGF receptors. Both showed efficacy as second-line treatment following progression during cytokine treatment, resulting in approval by regulatory authorities for the treatment of advanced renal cell carcinoma. A randomized phase 3 trial comparing sunitinib to IFN-α showed superior efficacy for sunitinib with an acceptable safety profile. The trial resulted in a change in the standard first-line treatment from IFN to sunitinib. Sunitinib is usually given orally at a dose of 50 mg/d for 4 weeks out of 6. Diarrhea is the main toxicity. Sorafenib is usually given orally at a dose of 400 mg bid. In addition to diarrhea, toxicities include rash, fatigue, and hand-foot syndrome. Temsirolimus, a mammalian target of rapamycin (mTOR) inhibitor, also has activity in previously treated patients. The usual dosage is 25 mg IV weekly.

The prognosis of metastatic renal cell carcinoma is variable. In one analysis, no prior nephrectomy, a KPS <80, low hemoglobin, high corrected calcium, and abnormal lactate dehydrogenase were poor prognostic factors. Patients with zero, one or two, and three or more factors had a median survival of 24, 12, and 5 months, respectively. These tumors may follow an unpredictable and protracted clinical course. It may be best to document progression before considering systemic treatment.

FURTHER READINGS

Black PC et al: Molecular markers of urothelial cancer and their use in the monitoring of superficial urothelial cancer. J Clin Oncol 24:5528, 2006

Brassell SA, Kamat AM: Contemporary intravesical treatment options for urothelial carcinoma of the bladder. J Natl Compr Canc Netw 4:1027, 2006

Cohen HT, McGovern FJ: Renal-cell carcinoma. N Engl J Med 353:2477, 2005

Huang WC et al: Chronic kidney disease after nephrectomy in patients with renal cortical tumours: A retrospective cohort study. Lancet Oncol 7:735, 2006

Mitra AP et al: Molecular pathways in invasive bladder cancer: New insights into mechanisms, progression, and target identification. J Clin Oncol 24:5552, 2006

Motzer RJ et al: Sunitinib in patients with metastatic renal cell carcinoma. JAMA 295:2516, 2006

Nelson EC et al: Renal cell carcinoma: Current status and emerging therapies. Cancer Treat Rev 33:299, 2007

Sugano K, Kakizoe T: Genetic alterations in bladder cancer and their clinical applications in molecular tumor staging. Nature Clin Pract 3:642, 2006

Winquist E et al: Neoadjuvant chemotherapy for transitional cell carcinoma of the bladder: A systematic review and meta-analysis. J Urol 171:561, 2004

91 Benign and Malignant Diseases of the Prostate

Howard I. Scher

Benign and malignant changes in the prostate increase with age. Autopsies of men in the eighth decade of life show hyperplastic changes in >90% and malignant changes in >70% of individuals. The high prevalence of these diseases among the elderly, who often have competing causes of morbidity and mortality, mandates a risk-adapted approach to diagnosis and treatment. This can be achieved by considering these diseases as a series of states. Each state represents a distinct clinical milestone for which intervention(s) may be recommended based on current symptoms or the risk of developing symptoms or death from disease within a given time frame (Fig. 91-1). For benign proliferative disorders, symptoms of urinary frequency, infection, and potential for obstruction are weighed against the side effects and complications of medical or surgical therapy. For prostate malignancies, the risks of developing the disease, symptoms, or death from cancer are balanced against the morbidities of the interventions recommended and preexisting comorbid conditions.

ANATOMY AND PATHOLOGY

The prostate is located in the pelvis and is surrounded by the rectum, the bladder, the periprostatic and dorsal vein complexes that are responsible for erectile function, and the urinary sphincter that is re-

FIGURE 91-1 Clinical states of prostate cancer. PSA, prostate-specific antigen.

sponsible for passive urinary control. The prostate is composed of branching tubuloalveolar glands arranged in lobules and surrounded by a stroma. The acinal unit includes an epithelial compartment made up of epithelial, basal, and neuroendocrine cells and a stromal compartment that includes fibroblasts and smooth-muscle cells. The compartments are separated by a basement membrane. Prostate-specific antigen (PSA) and acid phosphatase are produced in the epithelial cells. Both prostate epithelial cells and stromal cells express androgen receptors and depend on androgens for growth. Testosterone, the major circulating androgen, is converted by the enzyme 5α-reductase to dihydrotestosterone in the gland.

The periurethral portion of the gland increases in size during puberty and after the age of 55 due to the growth of nonmalignant cells in the transition zone of the prostate that surrounds the urethra. Most cancers develop in the peripheral zone, and cancers in this location can often be palpated during a digital rectal examination (DRE).

PROSTATE CANCER

In 2007 in the United States, ~218,890 prostate cancer cases were diagnosed, and 27,050 men died from prostate cancer. The absolute number of prostate cancer deaths has decreased in the past 5 years; this has been attributed by some to the widespread use of PSA-based detection strategies. However, screening has not been shown to improve survival in prospective randomized trials. The paradox of management is that although the disease remains the second leading cause of cancer deaths in men, only 1 man in 8 with prostate cancer will die of his disease.

EPIDEMIOLOGY

Epidemiologic studies show that the risk of being diagnosed with prostate cancer increases by a factor of 2 if one first-degree relative is affected and by 4 if two or more are affected. Current estimates are that 40% of early-onset and 5–10% of all prostate cancers are hereditary. Prostate cancer affects ethnic groups differently. Matched for age, African-American males compared to white males have both a greater number of prostatic intraepithelial neoplasia (PIN) lesions, which are precursors to cancer, and larger tumors, possibly related to the higher levels of testosterone seen in African-American males. PIN, the precursor of cancer, is typically multifocal and highly unstable. Polymorphic variants of the androgen receptor gene, the cytochrome P450 C17 gene, and the steroid 5α-reductase type II (*SRD5A2*) gene have also been implicated in the variations in incidence.

The incidence of autopsy-detected cancers is similar around the world, while the incidence of clinical disease varies. Thus, environmental factors may play a role. High consumption of dietary fats, such as α-linoleic acid, or the polycyclic aromatic hydrocarbons that form when red meats are cooked is believed to increase risk. Similar to breast cancer in Asian women, the risk of prostate cancer in Asian men increases when they move to Western environments. Protective factors include consumption of the isoflavinoid genistein (which inhibits 5α-reductase), cruciferous vegetables that contain the isothiocyanate sulforaphane, retinoids such as lycopene (in tomatoes), and inhibitors of cholesterol biosynthesis (e.g., statin drugs). The antioxidants α-tocopherol (vitamin E) and selenium may also reduce risk.

The development of a prostate cancer is a multistep process. One early change is hypermethylation of the GSTP1 gene promoter, which leads to loss of function of a gene that detoxifies carcinogens. A role for inflammation has been suggested based on the finding that many prostate cancers occur adjacent to a lesion termed *PIA (proliferative-inflammatory atrophy)*. This also suggests a role for oxidative damage.

DIAGNOSIS AND TREATMENT BY CLINICAL STATE

The disease continuum—from the appearance of a preneoplastic and invasive lesion localized to the prostate, to a metastatic lesion that results in symptoms and, ultimately, mortality from prostate cancer—can span decades. Management at all points is centered on competing risks that are defined by considering the disease as a series of clinical states (Fig. 91-1). The states are defined operationally, on the basis of whether or not a cancer diagnosis has been established and, for those already diagnosed, whether or not metastases are detectable on imaging studies and the measured level of testosterone in the blood. With this approach, an individual resides in only one state and remains in that state until he has progressed. At each assessment, the decision to offer treatment and the specific form of treatment is based on the risk posed by the cancer, relative to competing causes of mortality that may be present in that individual. It follows that the more advanced the disease, the greater the need for treatment. For those without a cancer diagnosis, the decision to undergo testing to detect a cancer is based on the probability that a clinically significant cancer may be present. For those with a prostate cancer diagnosis, the clinical state model considers the probability of developing symptoms or dying from disease. Thus, a patient with localized prostate cancer who has had all cancer removed surgically remains in the state of localized disease as long as the PSA remains undetectable. The time within a state becomes a measure of the efficacy of an intervention, though the effect may not be assessable for years. As many men with active cancer are not at risk for developing metastases, symptoms, or death, the states model allows a distinction between *cure*—the elimination of all cancer cells, the primary therapeutic objective when treating most cancers—and *cancer control*, in which the tempo of the illness is altered and symptoms controlled until the patient dies of other causes. These can be equivalent therapeutically from a patient standpoint if the patient has not experienced symptoms of the disease or the treatment needed to control it. Even when a recurrence is documented, immediate therapy is not always necessary. Rather, as at the time of diagnosis, the need for intervention is based on the tempo of the illness as it unfolds in the individual, relative to the risk-to-benefit ratio of the therapy being considered.

NO CANCER DIAGNOSIS

Prevention Several agents are under investigation for their potential to reduce the risk of clinically significant prostate cancer. Finasteride, a 5α-reductase inhibitor, has been tested in men ages ≥55 years in the Prostate Cancer Prevention Trial, a double-blind, randomized multicenter trial. The prostate cancer detection rate was 18.4% (803 of 4364) in the finasteride group and 24.4% (1147 of 4692) in the placebo group. Early concerns that the cancers detected in the finasteride group were high-grade [37% (280 of 757 cancers) vs. 22% (237 of 1068 cancers) for the placebo group] have been shown to be an artifact of the reduced volume of the malignant epithelial cells in finasteride-treated patients. No effect on survival was detected. Vitamin E and selenium are also being tested as preventive agents (the SELECT study).

Physical Examination The need to pursue a diagnosis of prostate cancer is based on symptoms, an abnormal DRE, or an elevated serum PSA. The urologic history should focus on symptoms of outlet obstruction, continence, potency, or change in ejaculatory pattern.

The DRE focuses on prostate size and consistency and abnormalities within or beyond the gland. Many cancers occur in the peripheral zone and can be palpated on DRE. Carcinomas are characteristically hard, nodular, and irregular, while induration may be due to benign prostatic hypertrophy (BPH) or to calculi or tumor. Overall, 20–25% of men with an abnormal DRE have cancer.

Prostate-Specific Antigen PSA is a kallikrein-like serine protease that causes liquefaction of seminal coagulum. It is produced by both nonmalignant and malignant epithelial cells. PSA is prostate-specific, not prostate cancer–specific, and serum PSA increases may occur from prostatitis, BPH, and prostate cancer. The performance of a prostate biopsy can increase PSA levels up to tenfold for 8–10 weeks. The serum PSA level is not affected by DRE. PSA circulates in the blood as an inactive complex

PART 6 Oncology and Hematology

with the protease inhibitors α_1-antichymotrypsin and β_2-macroglobulin, and it has an estimated half-life in serum of 2–3 days. Levels should be undetectable if the prostate has been removed. Immunohistochemical staining for PSA can be used to establish a prostate cancer diagnosis.

PSA testing was approved in 1994 for early detection of prostate cancer, but there is controversy on its use. The American Cancer Society recommends that physicians offer PSA testing and a DRE on an annual basis for men over age 50 with an anticipated survival of >10 years; this includes men up to age 76 years. For African Americans and men with a family history of prostate cancer, testing is advised to begin at age 45. The American Urologic Association recommendations are similar, with a proviso that the risks and benefits of the performance of these tests are not defined. The National Comprehensive Cancer Network advises testing at age 40, tailoring additional testing to the age-specific median. The American College of Physicians recommends that physicians "describe the potential benefits and known harms of screening" and to "individualize the decision to screen." PSA values may fluctuate for no apparent reason; thus, an isolated abnormal value should be confirmed before proceeding with further testing.

The PSA criteria used to recommend a diagnostic prostate biopsy have evolved over time. The goal is to increase the sensitivity of the test for younger men more likely to die of the disease and to reduce the frequency of detecting cancers of low malignant potential in elderly men more likely to die of other causes. Age-specific reference ranges reduce the upper limit of normal for younger men and increase it for older men. Different thresholds alter the sensitivity and specificity of detection. The threshold for performance of a biopsy was 4.0 ng/mL, which has been reduced to 2.6 ng/mL for men <60 by many groups based on the finding that nearly half of the men with PSAs who reached this level increased to 4 within a relatively short (4-year) time frame, and that, once diagnosed, nearly one-third had spread beyond the confines of the gland. Most PSA is complexed to α_1-chymotrypsin (ACT); only a small percentage is "free." To improve diagnostic accuracy for men with a PSA between 4 and 10, the risk of cancer is under 10% if the free PSA is >25% but as high as 56% for those with a free PSA <10%. PSA density measurements were developed to correct for the contribution of BPH to the total PSA level. PSA density is calculated by dividing the serum PSA by the prostate weight estimated from transrectal ultrasound (TRUS). Values <0.10 ng/mL per cm^3 are consistent with BPH, while those >0.15 suggest cancer. *PSA velocity* is the rate of change in PSA levels over time and is expressed most commonly as the PSA doubling time. It is particularly useful for men with seemingly normal values that are rising. For men with a PSA above 4, rates of rise >0.75 ng/mL per year suggest cancer, while for those with lower PSA levels, rates above 0.5 ng/mL per year should be used to advise a biopsy. As an example, an increase from 2.5 to 3.2 in a 1-year period would warrant further testing. Free and complexed PSA measurements are used when levels are between 4 and 10 ng/mL to decide whether a biopsy is needed. The level of free PSA is lower in men with cancer. The ratios of free to total, complexed to total, and free to complexed PSA have also been used. In one series, specificity improved by 20% by defining normal ranges as free/total >0.15, complexed/total <0.70, and free/complexed >0.25.

PSA-based detection strategies have changed the clinical spectrum of the disease. Now, 95–99% of newly diagnosed cancers are clinically localized, 40% are not palpable, and of these, 70% are pathologically organ-confined. The downside of widespread PSA screening is the detection and treatment of cancers with such a low malignant potential that they would not have shortened survival or produced symptoms during the patient's lifetime. The side effects of treatment, including impotence, incontinence, and bowel dysfunction, are unacceptable for these patients. Formal clinical trials to assess the value of screening on prostate cancer morbidity and mortality are ongoing. Until the results of these studies are available, men are advised to make an informed decision about whether to undergo testing.

A diagnostic algorithm based on the DRE and PSA findings is illustrated in **Fig. 91-2**. In general, a biopsy is recommended if the DRE or PSA is abnormal. Twenty-five percent of men with a PSA >4 ng/mL

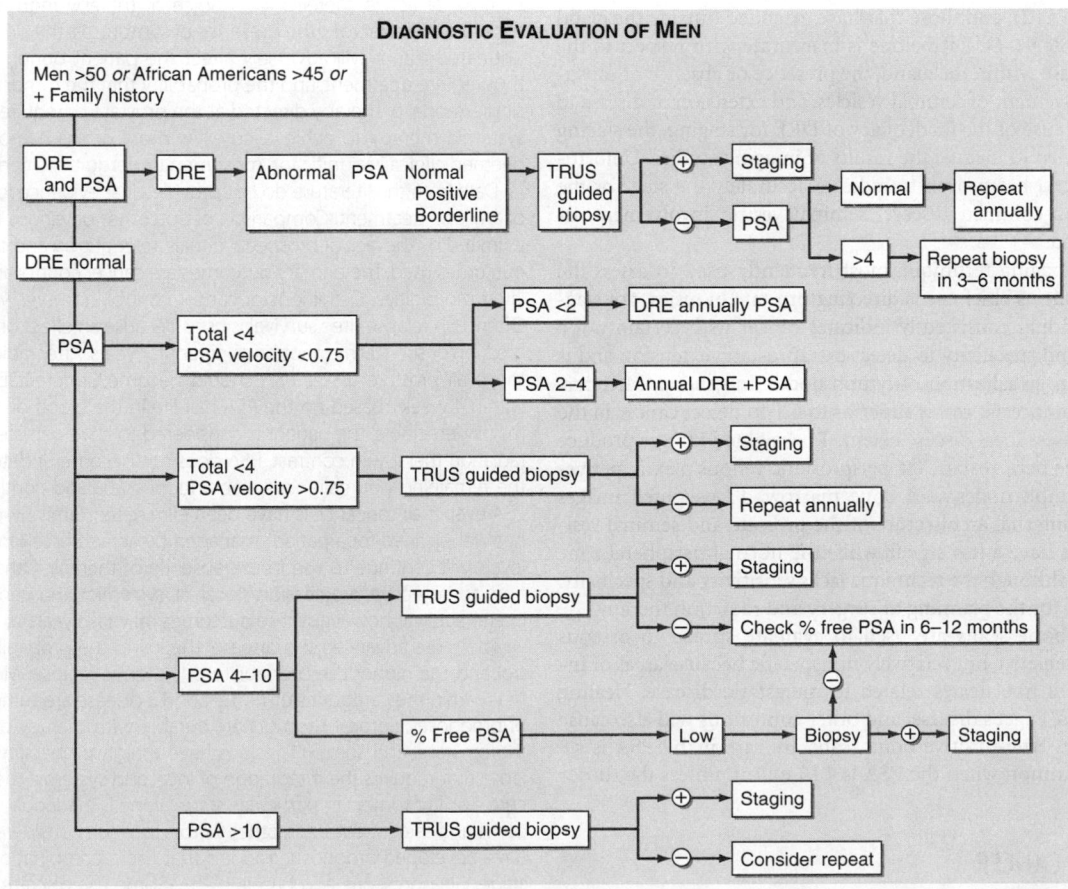

FIGURE 91-2 Algorithm for diagnostic evaluation of men based on digital rectal examination and prostate-specific antigen levels.

and an abnormal DRE have cancer, as do 17% of men with a PSA of 2.5–4.0 ng/mL and normal DRE.

Prostate Biopsy A diagnosis of cancer is established by a TRUS-guided needle biopsy. Direct visualization by ultrasound or MRI assures that all areas of the gland are sampled. A minimum of six separate cores, three from the right and three from the left, is advised, as is a separate biopsy of the transition zone if clinically indicated. More commonly, 12–14 cores are advised to increase the diagnostic yield. Patients with prostatitis should have a course of antibiotics before biopsy. Men with an abnormal PSA and negative biopsy are advised to undergo a repeat biopsy.

Each core of the biopsy is examined for the presence of cancer, and the amount of cancer is quantified based on the length of the tumor within the core and the percentage of the core involved.

Pathology The noninvasive proliferation of epithelial cells within ducts is termed *prostatic intraepithelial neoplasia*. PIN is a precursor of cancer, but not all PIN lesions develop into invasive cancers. Of the cancers identified, >95% are adenocarcinomas; the remainder are squamous or transitional cell tumors or, rarely, carcinosarcomas. Metastases to the prostate are rare, but in some cases colon cancers or transitional cell tumors of the bladder invade the gland by direct extension. When prostate cancer is diagnosed, a measure of histologic aggressiveness is assigned using the *Gleason grading system*, in which the dominant and secondary glandular histologic patterns are scored from 1 (well-differentiated) to 5 (undifferentiated) and summed to give a total score of 2–10 for each tumor. The most poorly differentiated area of tumor (i.e., the area with the highest histologic grade) often determines biologic behavior. The presence or absence of perineural invasion and extracapsular spread are also recorded.

Prostate Cancer Staging The TNM staging system includes categories for cancers that are palpable on DRE, those identified solely on the basis of an abnormal PSA (T1c), those that are palpable but clinically confined to the gland (T2), and those that have extended outside the gland (T3 and T4) (Table 91-1). DRE alone is inaccurate with respect to the extent of the disease within the gland, the presence or absence of capsular invasion, involvement of seminal vesicles, and extension of disease to lymph nodes. Because of the inadequacy of DRE for staging, the staging system was modified to include the results of imaging studies. Unfortunately, no single test has proven to indicate accurately the stage or presence of organ-confined disease, seminal vesicle involvement, or lymph node spread.

TRUS is the imaging technique most frequently used to assess the primary tumor, but its chief use is directing prostate biopsies, not staging. No TRUS finding consistently indicates cancer with certainty. CT lacks sensitivity and specificity to detect extraprostatic extension and is inferior to MRI in visualization of lymph nodes. In general, MRI performed with an endorectal coil is superior to CT to detect cancer in the prostate and to assess local disease extent. T1-weighted images produce a high signal in the periprostatic fat, periprostatic venous plexus, perivesicular tissues, lymph nodes, and bone marrow. T2-weighted images demonstrate the internal architecture of the prostate and seminal vesicles. Most cancers have a low signal, while the normal peripheral zone has a high signal, although the technique lacks sensitivity and specificity. MRI is also useful for the planning of surgery and radiation therapy.

Radionuclide bone scans are used to evaluate spread to osseous sites. This test is sensitive but relatively nonspecific because areas of increased uptake are not always related to metastatic disease. Healing fractures, arthritis, Paget's disease, and other conditions will also cause abnormal uptake. True-positive bone scans are rare if the PSA is <8 ng/mL and uncommon when the PSA is <10 ng/mL unless the tumor is high-grade.

℞ PROSTATE CANCER

CLINICALLY LOCALIZED DISEASE Localized prostate cancers are those that appear to be nonmetastatic after staging studies are performed.

TABLE 91-1 COMPARISON OF CLINICAL STAGE BY THE TNM CLASSIFICATION SYSTEM AND THE WHITMORE-JEWETT STAGING SYSTEM

TNM Stage	Description	Whitmore-Jewett Stage	Description
T1a	Nonpalpable, with 5% or less of resected tissue with cancer	A1	Well differentiated tumor on few chips from one lobe
T1b	Nonpalpable, with >5% of resected tissue with cancer	A2	Involvement more diffuse
T1c	Nonpalpable, detected due to elevated serum PSA		
T2a	Palpable, half of one lobe or less	BIN	Palpable, < one lobe, surrounded by normal tissue
T2b	Palpable, > half of one lobe but not both lobes	B1	Palpable, < one lobe
T2c	Palpable, involves both lobes	B2	Palpable, one entire lobe or both lobes
T3a	Palpable, unilateral extra-capsular extension	C1	Palpable, outside capsule, not into seminal vesicles
T3b	Palpable, bilateral extra-capsular extension		
T3c	Tumor invades seminal vesicle(s)	C2	Palpable, seminal vesicle involved
M1	Distant metastases	D	Metastatic disease

Source: Adapted from FF Schroder et al: TNM classification of prostate cancer. Prostate (Suppl) 4:129, 1992; and American Joint Committee on Cancer, 1992.

Patients with localized disease are managed by radical surgery, radiation therapy, or active surveillance. Choice of therapy requires the consideration of several factors: the presence of symptoms, the probability that the untreated tumor will adversely affect the patient during his lifetime and thus require treatment, and the probability that the tumor can be cured by single-modality therapy directed at the prostate or requires both local and systemic therapy to achieve cure. As most of the tumors detected are deemed clinically significant, most men undergo treatment.

Data from the literature do not provide clear evidence for the superiority of any one treatment. Comparison of outcomes of various forms of therapy is limited by the lack of prospective trials, referral bias, and differences in the outcomes used. The primary outcomes are cancer control and treatment-related morbidities. Definitions of cancer control, however, vary by modality. Often, PSA relapse–free survival is used because an effect on metastatic progression or survival may not be apparent for years. After radical surgery to remove all prostate tissue, PSA should become undetectable in the blood within 4 weeks, based on the PSA half-life in the blood of 3 days. If PSA remains detectable, the patient is considered to have persistent disease. After radiation therapy, in contrast, PSA does not become undetectable because the remaining nonmalignant elements of the gland continue to produce PSA even if all cancer cells have been eliminated. Similarly, cancer control is not well-defined for a patient managed by active surveillance because PSA levels will continue to rise in the absence of therapy. Other outcomes are time to objective progression (local or systemic) and cancer-specific and overall survival; however, these outcomes may take years to assess.

The more advanced the disease, the lower the probability of local control and the higher the probability of systemic relapse. More important is that within the categories of T1, T2, and T3 disease are tumors with a range of prognoses. Some T3 tumors are curable with therapy directed solely at the prostate, and some T1 lesions have a high probability of systemic relapse that requires the integration of local and systemic therapy to achieve cure. For T1c tumors in particular, stage alone is inadequate to predict outcome and select treatment; other factors must be considered. Many groups have developed prognostic models that use a combination of the initial T stage, Gleason score, and baseline PSA. Some use discrete cut points (PSA <10 or ≥10; Gleason score of ≤6, 7, or ≥8); others are nomograms that use PSA and Gleason score as continuous variables. These algorithms can be used to predict disease extent (organ-confined vs. non-organ-confined, node-negative or -positive) and the probability of success of treatment using a PSA-based definition specific to the local therapy under consideration. Specific nomograms have been developed for radical prostatectomy, external beam radiation therapy, and brachytherapy (seed implantation). These are being refined continually to incorporate other clinical parameters and biologic determinants. Surgical technique, radiation therapy delivery, and criteria for active surveillance continue to be refined and improved; the year of treatment affects outcomes independent of other factors. The improvements make treatment decisions a dynamic process.

The frequency of adverse events for the different treatment modalities varies with the modality used and the experience of the treating team. For example, following radical prostatectomy, incontinence rates range from 2 to 47% and impotence rates range from 25 to 89%. Part of the variability relates to how the complication is defined and whether the patient or physician is reporting the event. The time of the assessment is also important. After surgery, impotence is immediate but may reverse over time, while with radiation therapy impotence is not immediate but may develop over time. Of greatest concern to patients are the effects on continence, sexual potency, and bowel function.

Radical Prostatectomy The goal of radical prostatectomy is to excise the cancer completely with a clear margin, to maintain continence by preserving the external sphincter, and to preserve potency by preserving the autonomic nerves in the neurovascular bundle. Radical prostatectomy is advised for patients with a life expectancy of >10 years and is performed using a retropubic, perineal, or laparoscopic approach. Outcomes can be predicted using postoperative nomograms that consider pretreatment factors and the pathologic findings at surgery. PSA failure is defined as a value above 0.2 or 0.4 ng/mL, although the exact definition varies among series.

There is controversy over the definition of what constitutes "high risk" based on a predicted probability of success or failure. In these situations, nomograms and predictive models can only go so far. Exactly what probability of success or failure would lead a physician to recommend and a patient to seek alternative approaches is controversial. For example, it may be appropriate to recommend radical surgery for a younger patient with a low probability of cure.

Prostatectomy techniques continue to improve as the ability to determine whether the tumor is localized to the gland improves based on different biopsy algorithms and with imaging. The result is better case selection and better surgical planning, which in turn have led to more rapid recovery and higher rates of continence and potency. Factors associated with incontinence include older age and shorter urethra length. The specific surgical technique, open vs. laparoscopic vs. robotic, as well as the skill and experience of the surgeon are also factors for the preservation of neurovascular bundles and development of an anastomotic stricture. Surgical experience is also a factor. In a series treated at an academic center, 6% of patients had mild stress urinary incontinence (SUI) (requiring 1 pad/day), 2% moderate SUI (>1 pad/day), and 0.3% severe SUI (requiring an artificial urinary sphincter). At 1 year, 92% were completely continent. In contrast, the results in a Medicare population treated at multiple centers showed that at 3, 12, and 24 months following surgery, 58, 35, and 42% (respectively) wore pads in their underwear, and 24, 11, and 15% reported "a lot" of urine leakage.

Factors associated with recovery of erectile function include younger age, quality of erections before surgery, and the absence of damage to the neurovascular bundles. Erectile function returns in a median of 4–6 months if both bundles are preserved. Potency is reduced by half if at least one nerve bundle is sacrificed. In cases where cancer control requires the removal of both bundles, sural nerve grafts are being explored. Overall, with the availability of drugs such as sildenafil, intraurethral inserts of alprostadil, and intracavernosal injections of vasodilators, many patients recover satisfactory sexual function.

Neoadjuvant hormonal therapy has been explored in an attempt to improve the outcomes of surgery for high-risk patients. The results of several large trials testing 3 or 8 months of androgen depletion before surgery showed that serum PSA levels decreased by 96%, prostate volumes decreased by 34%, and margin positivity rates decreased from 41 to 17%. Unfortunately, hormones did not produce an improvement in PSA relapse–free survival. Thus, neoadjuvant hormonal therapy is not recommended.

Radiation Therapy Radiation therapy is given by external beam, by radioactive sources implanted into the gland, or by a combination.

External Beam Radiation Therapy Contemporary external beam radiation techniques now use three-dimensional conformal treatment plans with intensity-modulated radiation therapy (IMRT) to maximize the dose to the prostate and to minimize the exposure of the surrounding normal structures. The addition of IMRT has permitted further shaping of the dose, allowing the delivery of still higher doses to the prostate and a further reduction in normal tissue exposure. These advances have enabled the safe administration of doses >80 Gy, higher local control rates, and fewer side effects.

Cancer control after radiation therapy has been defined by various criteria, including a decline in PSA to <0.5 or 1 ng/mL, "nonrising" PSA values, and a negative biopsy of the prostate 2 years after completion of treatment. PSA relapse is defined as three consecutive rising PSA values from the nadir value, with the time to failure as a rise by 2 ng/mL or greater above the posttreatment nadir value.

Radiation dose is important. A PSA nadir of <1.0 ng/mL was observed in 90% of patients receiving 75.6 or 81.0 Gy vs. 76 and 56% of those receiving 70.2 Gy and 64.8 Gy, respectively. The positive biopsy rates at 2.5 years were 4% for those treated with 81 Gy vs. 27 and 36% for those receiving 75.6 or 70.2 Gy. The frequency of rectal complications relates directly to the volume of the anterior rectal wall receiving full-dose treatment.

Overall, radiation therapy is associated with a higher frequency of bowel complications (mainly diarrhea and proctitis) than surgery. Grade 3 rectal or urinary toxicities were seen in 2.1% of patients who received a median dose of 75.6 Gy. Grade 3 urethral strictures requiring dilatation developed in 1% of cases, all of whom had undergone a transurethral resection of the prostate (TURP). Pooled data show that the frequency of grade 3 and 4 toxicities is 6.9 and 3.5%, respectively, for patients who received >70 Gy. The frequency of erectile dysfunction is related to the quality of erections pretreatment, the dose administered, and the time of assessment. Postradiation erectile dysfunction is related to a disruption of the vascular supply and not the nerve fibers.

Neoadjuvant hormone therapy has also been studied in combination with radiation therapy. The aim is to decrease the size of the prostate and, consequently, to reduce the exposure of normal tissues to full-dose radiation, to increase local control rates, and to decrease the rate of systemic failure. Short-term hormone therapy can reduce toxicities and improve local control rates, but long-term treatment (2–3 years) is needed to prolong the time to PSA failure and lower the risk of metastatic disease. The impact on survival has been less clear.

Brachytherapy Brachytherapy is the direct implantation of radioactive sources into the prostate. It is based on the principle that the deposition of radiation energy in tissues decreases as a function of the square of the distance from the source (Chap. 81). The goal is to deliver intensive irradiation to the prostate, minimizing the exposure of the surrounding tissues. The current standard technique achieves a more homogeneous dose distribution by placing seeds according to a customized template based on CT and ultrasonographic assessment of the tumor and computer-optimized dosimetry. The implantation is performed transperineally, without an open procedure, with real-time imaging.

The improvements in brachytherapy techniques have resulted in fewer complications and a marked reduction in local failure rates. In a series of 197 patients followed for a median of 3 years, 5-year actuarial PSA relapse–free survival for patients with pretherapy PSA levels of 0–4, 4–10, and >10 ng/mL were 98, 90, and 89%, respectively. In a separate report of 201 patients who underwent posttreatment biopsies, 80% were negative, 17% were indeterminate, and 3% were positive. The results did not change with longer follow-up. Nevertheless, many physicians feel that implantation is best reserved for patients with good or intermediate prognostic features.

Brachytherapy is well tolerated, although most patients experience urinary frequency and urgency that can persist for several months. Incontinence has been seen in 2–4% of cases. Higher complication rates are observed in patients who have undergone a prior TURP or who have obstructive symptoms at baseline. Proctitis has been reported in <2% of patients.

Active Surveillance Active surveillance, described previously as *watchful waiting*, or *deferred therapy*, is a policy of monitoring the illness at fixed intervals with DREs, PSA measurements, and repeat biopsies of the prostate as indicated, but with no therapeutic intervention(s) until the tumor progresses. Progression can be based on PSA changes, local tumor growth, the development of symptoms, or metastatic disease. The practice evolved from studies of predominantly elderly men with well-differentiated tumors who demonstrated no clinically significant progression for protracted periods, during which a significant proportion died of intercurrent disease. In a structured literature review of patients treated by radical surgery, external beam radiation, or a deferred approach, the 10-year survival rates were 93% for radical prostatectomy, 74% for external beam radiation, and 84% for deferred treatment. Arguing against active surveillance are the results of a Swedish randomized trial of radical prostatectomy vs. active surveillance. With a median follow-up of 6.2 years, men treated by radical surgery had a lower risk of prostate cancer death relative to active surveillance patients (4.6% vs. 8.9%) and a lower risk of metastatic progression (hazard ratio 0.63).

Case selection is critical, and the criteria to select men who can safely choose active surveillance are under intense study. In a prostatectomy series, it was estimated that 10–15% of patients had "insignificant" cancers. Given the multifocality of the disease, a concern is the limited ability to predict pathologic findings on the basis of a needle biopsy, even when multiple cores are obtained. Nomograms to help predict which patients can safely be managed by active surveillance have been developed, and as their predictive accuracy improves, it can be anticipated that more patients will be candidates.

RISING PSA

This state consists of patients in whom the sole manifestation of disease is a rising PSA after surgery and/or radiation therapy. By definition, patients have no evidence of disease on scan. For these patients the central issue is whether the rise in PSA results from persistent disease in the primary site, systemic disease, or both. In theory, disease in the primary site may still be curable by additional local treatment; external beam radiation for patients who had undergone surgery, prostatectomy for patients who had undergone radiation therapy.

The decision to recommend radiation therapy after prostatectomy is often made on the basis of the pathologic findings at surgery, as imaging studies such as CT and bone scan are typically uninformative. Some recommend a Prostascint scan: imaging with a radiolabeled antibody to prostate-specific membrane antigen (PSMA), which is highly expressed on prostate epithelial cells, to help with this distinction. Antibody localization to the prostatic fossa suggests local recurrence; localization to extrapelvic sites predicts failure of radiation therapy. Others recommend that a biopsy of the urethrovesical anastomosis be obtained before considering radiation. Factors that predict for response to salvage radiation therapy are a positive surgical margin, lower Gleason grade, long interval from surgery to PSA failure, slow PSA doubling time, and low (<0.5–1.0 ng/mL) PSA value at the time of radiation treatment. Radiation therapy is generally not recommended if the PSA was persistently elevated after surgery, which usually indicates that the disease had spread outside of the area of the prostate bed and is unlikely to be controlled with radiation therapy.

For patients with a rising PSA after radiation therapy, salvage prostatectomy can be considered if the disease was "curable" at the outset, if persistent disease has been documented by a biopsy of the prostate, and if no metastatic disease is seen on imaging studies. Unfortunately, case selection is poorly defined in most series, and morbidities are significant. As currently performed, virtually all patients are impotent after salvage radical prostatectomy, and ~45% have either total urinary incontinence or stress incontinence. Major bleeding, bladder neck contractures, and rectal injury are not uncommon.

In many cases, the rise in PSA after surgery or radiation therapy indicates subclinical metastatic disease. In these cases, the need for treatment depends, in part, on the estimated probability that the patient will show evidence of metastatic disease on a scan and in what time frame. That immediate therapy is not always required was shown in a series where patients received no systemic therapy until metastatic disease was documented. Overall, the median time to metastatic progression was 8 years, and 63% of the patients with rising PSA values remained free of metastases at 5 years. Factors associated with progression included the Gleason grade of the primary tumor, time to recurrence, and PSA doubling times. For those with Gleason grade ≥8 tumors, the probability of metastatic pro-

gression was 37, 51, and 71% at 3, 5, and 7 years, respectively. If the time to recurrence was <2 years and PSA doubling time was long (>10 months), the proportion with metastatic disease at the same time intervals was 23, 32, and 53%, vs. 47, 69, and 79% if the doubling time was short (<10 months). A difficulty with predicting the course of disease in the rising PSA state is that most patients receive some form of therapy before the development of metastases. Nevertheless, predictive models continue to be refined. PSA doubling times are prognostic for survival. In one series, all patients who succumbed to disease had PSA doubling times of 3 months or less. Most physicians advise treatment when PSA doubling times are 12 months or less.

METASTATIC DISEASE: NONCASTRATE *Metastatic disease noncastrate* refers to patients with metastases visible on an imaging study and noncastrate levels of testosterone. The patient may be newly diagnosed or have a recurrence after treatment for localized disease. Symptoms of metastatic disease include pain from osseous spread, although many patients are asymptomatic despite extensive spread. Less common are symptoms related to marrow compromise (myelophthisis), coagulopathy, or spinal cord compression.

Standard treatment for noncastrate metastatic disease is to deplete androgens by medical or surgical means. Over 90% of male hormones originate in the testes; <10% are synthesized in the adrenal gland. Surgical orchiectomy is the "gold standard" approach but is least acceptable to patients. Medical therapies can be divided into agents that lower testosterone levels and antiandrogens that bind to the androgen receptor but do not signal **(Fig. 91-3)**.

Testosterone-Lowering Agents Medical therapies that lower testosterone levels include the gonadotropin-releasing hormone (GnRH) analogues, estrogens, and progestational agents. Estrogens such as diethylstilbestrol have fallen out of favor due to the risk of vascular complications such as fluid retention, phlebitis, emboli, and stroke. GnRH analogues (leuprolide acetate and goserelin acetate) initially produce a rise in luteinizing hormone and follicle-stimulating hormone followed by a downregulation of receptors in the pituitary gland, which effects a chemical castration. They were approved on the basis of randomized comparisons showing an improved safety profile (specifically, reduced cardiovascular toxicities) relative to diethylstilbestrol, with equivalent potency. The initial rise in testosterone may result in a clinical flare of the disease. These agents are therefore contraindicated in men with significant obstructive symptoms, cancer-related pain, or spinal cord compromise.

Agents that lower testosterone are associated with an androgen-depletion syndrome that includes hot flushes, weakness, fatigue, impotence, loss of muscle mass, changes in personality, anemia, depression, and a reduction in bone density. The bone changes can be prevented by treatment with bisphosphonates along with vitamin D and calcium supplementation. GnRH analogues also lead to an alteration in body composition and to glucose intolerance. Many taking them develop the metabolic syndrome.

FIGURE 91-3 Sites of action of different hormone therapies.

Antiandrogens Nonsteroidal antiandrogens such as flutamide, bicalutamide, and nilutamide block the binding of androgens to the receptor. When an antiandrogen is given alone, testosterone levels remain the same or increase. Compared to testosterone-lowering therapies, antiandrogens cause fewer hot flashes, less of an effect on libido, less muscle wasting, fewer personality changes, and less bone loss. Gynecomastia remains a significant problem but can be alleviated in part by tamoxifen.

Antiandrogens were approved initially to block the flare that results from GnRH analogue administration. They have also been studied as monotherapy and as part of a combined androgen blockade (also called maximal androgen blockade). Most reported randomized trials suggest that the cancer-specific outcomes are inferior when antiandrogens are used alone. Bicalutamide, even at 150 mg (three times the recommended dose), was associated with a shorter time to progression and inferior survival compared to surgical castration for patients with established metastatic disease. Nevertheless, some men may accept the trade-off of a potentially inferior cancer outcome for an improved quality of life.

Combined androgen blockade—the administration of an antiandrogen plus a GnRH analogue or surgical orchiectomy—was designed to inhibit both testicular and adrenal androgens at the outset. Cumulative results of randomized comparisons involving thousands of patients showed no advantage for combining an antiandrogen with surgical orchiectomy, while separate analyses of trials combining an antiandrogen with a GnRH analogue have shown a modest (<10%) survival advantage. Meta-analysis of all combined androgen blockade trials concluded that the approach was not more effective. In practice, most patients treated with a GnRH analogue receive an antiandrogen for the first 2–4 weeks of treatment to protect against the flare.

Intermittent Hormone Therapy Another way to reduce the side effects of androgen depletion is to administer hormones on an intermittent basis. This was proposed as a way to prevent the selection of cells that are resistant to androgen depletion. The hypothesis is that by allowing endogenous testosterone levels to rise, the cells that survive androgen depletion will induce a normal differentiation pathway. In this way, the surviving cells that are allowed to proliferate in the presence of androgen will retain sensitivity to subsequent androgen depletion. Applied in the clinic, androgen depletion is continued for 2–6 months beyond the point of maximal response. Once treatment is stopped, endogenous testosterone levels increase, and the symptoms associated with hormone treatment abate. PSA levels also begin to rise, and at some level treatment is restarted. With this approach, multiple cycles of regression and proliferation have been documented in individual patients. It is unknown whether the intermittent approach increases, decreases, or does not change the overall duration of sensitivity to androgen depletion. The preliminary reports suggest that the approach is safe, but long-term data are needed to assess the course in men with low PSA levels. A trial to address this question is ongoing.

Outcomes of Androgen Depletion The antiprostate cancer effects of the various androgen depletion strategies are similar, and the clinical course is predictable: an initial response, then a period of stability in which tumor cells are dormant and not proliferating, followed after a variable period of time by a rise in PSA and regrowth that is visible on a scan as a castration-resistant lesion. Androgen depletion is not curative because cells that survive castration are present when the disease is first diagnosed. Considered by disease manifestation, PSA levels return to normal in 60–70% of patients, and measurable disease regression occurs in 50%; improvements in bone scan occur in 25% of cases, but the majority remains stable. Duration of survival is inversely proportional to disease extent at the time androgen depletion is first started.

An active question is whether hormones should be given in the adjuvant setting after surgery or radiation treatment of the primary tumor or at the time that a PSA recurrence is documented, or to wait until metastatic disease or symptoms of disease are manifest. Trials in support of early therapy have often been underpowered relative to the reported benefit or have been criticized on methodologic grounds. One trial, although it showed a survival benefit for patients treated with radiation therapy and 3 years of androgen depletion relative to radiation alone, was criticized for the poor outcomes of the control group. Another showing a survival benefit for patients with positive lymph nodes who were randomized to immediate medical or surgical castration compared to observation ($p = .02$) was criticized because the confidence intervals around the 5- and 8-year survival distributions for

the two groups overlapped. A large randomized study comparing early to late hormone treatment (orchiectomy or GnRH analogue) in patients with locally advanced or asymptomatic metastatic disease showed that patients treated early were less likely to progress from M0 to M1 disease, to develop pain, and to die of prostate cancer. This trial was criticized because therapy was delayed "too long" in the late-treatment group. When patients treated by radical surgery, radiation therapy, or active surveillance were randomly assigned to receive bicalutamide, 150 mg, or placebo, hormone treatment produced a significant reduction in the proportion of patients who developed osseous metastases at 2 years (9% for bicalutamide; 13.8% for placebo). This result has not gained acceptance in part because too many "good-risk" patients were treated and because no effect on survival was demonstrated. These criticisms are valid; however, the net influence on survival from early hormone intervention is similar to that observed in patients with breast cancer, for which adjuvant hormonal therapy is routinely given.

METASTATIC DISEASE: CASTRATE Castration-resistant disease can manifest in many ways. For some it is a rise in PSA with no change in radiographs and no new symptoms. In others it is a rising PSA and progression in bone with or without symptoms of disease. Still others will show soft tissue disease with or without osseous metastases, and others have visceral spread. The prognosis, which is highly variable, can be predicted using nomograms designed for the castration-resistant disease state. The important point is that despite the failure of first-line hormone treatment, the majority of these tumors remain sensitive to second- and third-line hormonal treatments. Castration resistance does not indicate that the tumor is "hormone-refractory." The rising PSA is an indication of continued signaling through the androgen receptor axis.

The manifestations of disease in this patient group hinder the assessment of drugs and treatment standards because traditional measures of outcome such as tumor regression do not apply. Bone scans can be inaccurate for assessing changes in osseous disease, and no PSA-based outcome is a true surrogate for survival benefit. It is essential to define therapeutic objectives before initiating treatment, as there are defined standards of care for different disease manifestations. Therapeutic objectives need not be defined by survival only as useful endpoints also include relief of symptoms and delay of metastases or new symptoms of disease.

The management of patients with castrate metastatic disease requires first that the castrate status be documented. Patients receiving an antiandrogen alone, whose serum testosterone levels are elevated, should be treated first with a GnRH analogue or orchiectomy and observed for response. Patients on an antiandrogen in combination with a GnRH analogue should have the antiandrogen discontinued, as ~20% will respond to the selective discontinuation of the antiandrogen. Any withdrawal response occurs within weeks of stopping flutamide but may take 8–12 weeks with nilutamide and bicalutamide because of their long terminal half-lives. At the time of progression, a different antiandrogen can be given, as some tumors are not cross-resistant. An additional consideration in this setting is that significant androgen production persists in the adrenal gland and that one of the adaptive/selective changes, which occurs in the tumor itself, is the upregulation of adrenal synthetic enzymes, leading to autocrine signaling. High-dose ketoconazole, which inhibits adrenal androgen synthesis, is also often effective in these cases. Other hormones that may be active include estrogens, progestins, and glucocorticoids. Cytotoxic agents are considered when hormones are no longer effective, or the tempo of the illness suggests a more aggressive approach is needed.

Mitoxantrone was the first cytotoxic agent approved to provide palliation of pain secondary to castrate metastatic disease. The results established the important principle that systemic chemotherapy can provide palliation of pain in the absence of a survival benefit. In this trial, mitoxantrone-treated patients had a greater reduction in pain, less use of narcotics, and less fatigue. In 2004, docetaxel was established as the first-line standard cytotoxic drug for patients in this state, based on a trial showing that q3w docetaxel was superior to weekly therapy and to mitoxantrone. The results were confirmed in a second trial of estramustine/docetaxel vs. mitoxantrone. The addition of estramustine produced significant toxicity with no apparent improvement in survival and has been dropped from these regimens. Docetaxel and other microtubule targeted agents produce PSA declines in 50% of patients, measurable disease regression in 25%, and both an improvement in preexisting and prevention of future cancer-related pain.

Management of pain is a critical part of therapy. Optimal palliation requires assessing whether the symptoms and metastases are focal or diffuse and

TABLE 91-2 **AUA SYMPTOM INDEX**

Questions to Be Answered	Not at All	AUA Symptom Score (Circle 1 Number on Each Line)				
		Less than 1 Time in 5	Less than Half the Time	About Half the Time	More than Half the time	Almost Always
Over the past month, how often you have had a sensation of not emptying your bladder completely after you finished urinating?	0+	1	2	3	4	5
Over the past month, how often have you had to urinate again less than 2 h after you finished urinating?	0	1	2	3	4	5
Over the past month, how often have you found you stopped and started again several times when you urinated?	0	1	2	3	4	5
Over the past month, how often have you found it difficult to postpone urination?	0	1	2	3	4	5
Over the past month, how often have you had a weak urinary stream?	0	1	2	3	4	5
Over the past month, how often have you had to push or strain to begin urination?	0	1	2	3	4	5
Over the past month, how many times did you most typically get up to urinate from the time you went to bed at night until the time you got up in the morning?	(None)	(1 time)	(2 times)	(3 times)	(4 times)	(5 times)
Sum of 7 circled numbers (AUA Symptom Score): ____						

Note: AUA, American Urological Association.
Source: Barry MJ et al: J Urol 148:1549, 1992. Used with permission.

whether disease threatens the spinal cord, the cauda equina, or the base of the skull. Neurologic symptoms require emergency evaluation because loss of function may be permanent if not addressed quickly. Single sites of pain and areas of neurologic involvement are best treated with external beam radiation. As the disease is often diffuse, palliation at one site often is followed by the emergence of symptoms in a separate site that had not received radiation.

Given the bone-dominant pattern of prostate cancer spread, two bone-seeking radioisotopes, ^{89}Sr (Metastron) and ^{153}Sm-EDTMP (Quadramet), are approved for palliation of pain, although they have no effect on PSA or survival. Fewer patients treated with one of these isotopes developed new areas of pain or required additional radiation therapy compared to patients receiving external beam radiation therapy alone. Additionally, patients randomly assigned to a combination of ^{89}Sr and doxorubicin after induction chemotherapy had fewer skeletal events and longer survival than patients treated with doxorubicin alone. Confirmatory studies are ongoing. Addition of the bisphosphonate zoledronate to "standard therapy" in patients with castration-resistant disease resulted in fewer skeletal events relative to placebo. The skeletal events included microfractures, new pain, and need for radiation therapy. Bisphosphonates have a dual role: to protect against the bone loss associated with androgen depletion and to prevent skeletal events.

BENIGN DISEASE

SYMPTOMS

Benign proliferative disease may produce hesitancy, intermittent voiding, a diminished stream, incomplete emptying, and postvoid leakage. The severity of these symptoms can be quantitated with the self-administered American Urological Association Symptom Index (Table 91-2), although the degree of symptoms does not always relate to gland size. Resistance to urine flow reduces bladder compliance, leading to nocturia, urgency, and, ultimately, urinary retention. An episode of urinary retention may be precipitated by infection, tranquilizing drugs, antihistamines, and alcohol. Prostatitis often produces pain or induration. Typically, the symptoms remain stable over time and obstruction does not occur.

DIAGNOSTIC PROCEDURES AND TREATMENT

Asymptomatic patients do not require treatment regardless of the size of the gland, while those with an inability to urinate, gross hematuria, recurrent infection, or bladder stones may require surgery. In patients

with symptoms, uroflowmetry can identify those with normal flow rates who are unlikely to benefit from surgery and those with high postvoid residuals who may need other interventions. Pressure-flow studies detect primary bladder dysfunction. Cystoscopy is recommended if hematuria is documented and to assess the urinary outflow tract before surgery. Imaging of the upper tracts is advised for patients with hematuria, a history of calculi, or prior urinary tract problems.

Medical therapies for BPH include 5α-reductase inhibitors and α-adrenergic blockers. Finasteride (10 mg/d PO) and other 5α-reductase inhibitors that block the conversion of testosterone to dihydrotestosterone decrease prostate size, increase urine flow rates, and improve symptoms. They also lower baseline PSA levels by 50%, an important consideration when using PSA to guide biopsy recommendations. α-Adrenergic blockers such as terazosin (1–10 mg PO at bedtime) act by relaxing the smooth muscle of the bladder neck and increasing peak urinary flow rates. No data show that these agents influence the progression of the disease.

Surgical approaches include TURP, transurethral incision, or removal of the gland via a retropubic, suprapubic, or perineal approach. Also utilized are TULIP (transurethral ultrasound-guided laser-induced prostatectomy), stents, and hyperthermia.

FURTHER READINGS

LOBLAW DA et al: Initial hormonal management of androgen-sensitive metastatic, recurrent or progressive prostate cancer: 2006 update of an American Society of Clinical Oncology practice guideline. J Clin Oncol 25:1596, 2007

LOEB S, CATALONA WJ: Prostate-specific antigen in clinical practice. Cancer Letters 249:30, 2007

NELSON WG et al: Prostate cancer. N Engl J Med 349:366, 2003

SCHER HI, HELLER G: Clinical states in prostate cancer: Toward a dynamic model of disease progression. Urology 55:323, 2000

TANNOCK IM et al: Docetaxel plus prednisone or mitoxantrone plus prednisone for advanced prostate cancer. N Engl J Med 351:1502, 2004

THOMPSON IM et al: The influence of finasteride on the development of prostate cancer. N Engl J Med 349:215, 2003

THORPE A, NEAL D: Benign prostatic hyperplasia. Lancet 366:1359, 2003

YAO SL, DIPAOLA RS: Evidence-based approach to prostate cancer follow-up. Semin Oncol 30:390, 2003

92 Testicular Cancer
Robert J. Motzer, George J. Bosl

Primary germ cell tumors (GCTs) of the testis, arising by the malignant transformation of primordial germ cells, constitute 95% of all testicular neoplasms. Infrequently, GCTs arise from an extragonadal site, including the mediastinum, retroperitoneum, and, very rarely, the pineal gland. This disease is notable for the young age of the afflicted patients, the totipotent capacity for differentiation of the tumor cells, and its curability; about 95% of newly diagnosed patients are cured. Experience in the management of GCTs leads to improved outcome.

INCIDENCE AND EPIDEMIOLOGY

In 2007, 7920 new cases of testicular GCT were diagnosed in the United States; the incidence is decreasing after having increased slowly over the past 40 years. The tumor occurs most frequently in men between the ages of 20 and 40. A testicular mass in a male ≥50 years should be regarded as a lymphoma until proved otherwise. GCT is at least four to five times more common in white than in African-American males, and a higher incidence has been observed in Scandinavia and New Zealand than in the United States.

ETIOLOGY AND GENETICS

Cryptorchidism is associated with a severalfold higher risk of GCT. Abdominal cryptorchid testes are at a higher risk than inguinal cryptorchid testes. Orchiopexy should be performed before puberty, if possible. Early orchiopexy reduces the risk of GCT and improves the ability to save the testis. An abdominal cryptorchid testis that cannot be brought into the scrotum should be removed. About 2% of men with GCTs of one testis will develop a primary tumor in the other testis. Testicular feminization syndromes increase the risk of testicular GCT, and Klinefelter's syndrome is associated with mediastinal GCT.

An isochromosome of the short arm of chromosome 12 [i(12p)] is pathognomonic for GCT of all histologic types. Excess 12p copy number, either in the form of i(12p) or as increased 12p on aberrantly banded marker chromosomes, occurs in nearly all GCTs, but the gene(s) on 12p involved in the pathogenesis are not yet defined.

CLINICAL PRESENTATION

A painless testicular mass is pathognomonic for a testicular malignancy. More commonly, patients present with testicular discomfort or swelling suggestive of epididymitis and/or orchitis. In this circumstance, a trial of antibiotics is reasonable. However, if symptoms persist or a residual abnormality remains, then testicular ultrasound examination is indicated.

Ultrasound of the testis is indicated whenever a testicular malignancy is considered and for persistent or painful testicular swelling. If a testicular mass is detected, a radical inguinal orchiectomy should be performed. Because the testis develops from the gonadal ridge, its blood supply and lymphatic drainage originate in the abdomen and descend with the testis into the scrotum. An inguinal approach is taken to avoid breaching anatomic barriers and permitting additional pathways of spread.

Back pain from retroperitoneal metastases is common and must be distinguished from musculoskeletal pain. Dyspnea from pulmonary metastases occurs infrequently. Patients with increased serum levels of human chorionic gonadotropin (hCG) may present with gynecomastia. A delay in diagnosis is associated with a more advanced stage and possibly worse survival.

The staging evaluation for GCT includes a determination of serum levels of fetoprotein (AFP), hCG, and lactate dehydrogenase (LDH). After orchiectomy, a chest radiograph and a CT scan of the abdomen and pelvis should be performed. A chest CT scan is required if pulmonary nodules or mediastinal or hilar disease is suspected. Stage I disease is limited to the testis, epididymis, or spermatic cord. Stage II disease is limited to retroperitoneal (regional) lymph nodes. Stage III disease is disease outside the retroperitoneum, involving supradiaphragmatic nodal sites or viscera. The staging may be "clinical"—defined solely by physical examination, blood marker evaluation, and radiographs—or "pathologic"—defined by an operative procedure.

The regional draining lymph nodes for the testis are in the retroperitoneum, and the vascular supply originates from the great vessels (for the right testis) or the renal vessels (for the left testis). As a result, the lymph nodes that are involved first by a right testicular tumor are the interaortocaval lymph nodes just below the renal vessels. For a left testicular tumor, the first involved lymph nodes are lateral to the aorta (para-aortic) and below the left renal vessels. In both cases, further nodal spread is inferior, contralateral, and, less commonly, above the renal hilum. Lymphatic involvement can extend cephalad to the retrocrural, posterior mediastinal, and supraclavicular lymph nodes. Treatment is determined by tumor histology (seminoma versus nonseminoma) and clinical stage (Table 92-1).

PATHOLOGY

GCTs are divided into nonseminoma and seminoma subtypes. Nonseminomatous GCTs are most frequent in the third decade of life and can display the full spectrum of embryonic and adult cellular differentiation. This entity comprises four histologies: embryonal carcinoma, teratoma, choriocarcinoma, and endodermal sinus (yolk sac) tumor. Choriocarcinoma, consisting of both cytotrophoblasts and syncytiophoblasts, represents malignant trophoblastic differentiation and is invariably associated with secretion of hCG. Endodermal sinus tumor is the malignant counterpart of the fetal yolk sac and is associated with secretion of AFP. Pure embryonal carcinoma may secrete AFP or hCG, or both; this pattern is biochemical evidence of differentiation. Teratoma is composed of somatic cell types derived from two or more germ layers (ectoderm, mesoderm, or endoderm). Each of these histologies may be present alone or in combination with others. Nonseminomatous GCTs tend to metastasize early to sites such as the retroperitoneal lymph nodes and lung parenchyma. One-third of patients present with disease limited to the testis (stage I), one-third with retroperitoneal metastases (stage II), and one-third with more extensive supradiaphragmatic nodal or visceral metastases (stage III).

Seminoma represents about 50% of all GCTs, has a median age in the fourth decade, and generally follows a more indolent clinical

TABLE 92-1 GERM CELL TUMOR STAGING AND TREATMENT

Stage	Extent of Disease	Treatment	
		Seminoma	**Nonseminoma**
IA	Testis only, no vascular/lymphatic invasion (T1)	Radiation therapy	RPLND or observation
IB	Testis only, with vascular/lymphatic invasion (T2), or extension through tunica albuginea (T2), or involvement of spermatic cord (T3) or scrotum (T4)	Radiation therapy	RPLND
IIA	Nodes < 2 cm	Radiation therapy	RPLND or chemotherapy often followed by RPLND
IIB	Nodes 2–5 cm	Radiation therapy	RPLND +/− adjuvant chemotherapy or chemotherapy followed by RPLND
IIC	Nodes > 5 cm	Chemotherapy	Chemotherapy, often followed by RPLND
III	Distant metastases	Chemotherapy	Chemotherapy, often followed by surgery (biopsy or resection)

Note: RPLND, retroperitoneal lymph node dissection.

course. Most patients (70%) present with stage I disease, about 20% with stage II disease, and 10% with stage III disease; lung or other visceral metastases are rare. Radiation therapy is the treatment of choice in patients with stage I disease and stage II disease where the nodes are <5 cm in maximum diameter. When a tumor contains both seminoma and nonseminoma components, patient management is directed by the more aggressive nonseminoma component.

TUMOR MARKERS

Careful monitoring of the serum tumor markers AFP and hCG is essential in the management of patients with GCT, as these markers are important for diagnosis, as prognostic indicators, in monitoring treatment response, and in the detection of early relapse. Approximately 70% of patients presenting with disseminated nonseminomatous GCT have increased serum concentrations of AFP and/or hCG. While hCG concentrations may be increased in patients with either nonseminoma or seminoma histology, the AFP concentration is increased only in patients with nonseminoma. The presence of an increased AFP level in a patient whose tumor shows only seminoma indicates that an occult nonseminomatous component exists and the patient should be treated for nonseminomatous GCT. LDH levels are not as specific as AFP or hCG but are increased in 50–60% patients with metastatic nonseminoma and in up to 80% of patients with advanced seminoma.

AFP, hCG, and LDH levels should be determined before and after orchiectomy. Increased serum AFP and hCG concentrations decay according to first-order kinetics; the half-life is 24–36 h for hCG and 5–7 days for AFP. AFP and hCG should be assayed serially during and after treatment. The reappearance of hCG and/or AFP or the failure of these markers to decline according to the predicted half-life is an indicator of persistent or recurrent tumor.

Rx TESTICULAR CANCER

STAGE I NONSEMINOMA If, after an orchiectomy (for clinical stage I disease), radiographs and physical examination show no evidence of disease and serum AFP and hCG concentrations are either normal or declining to normal according to the known half-life, patients may be managed by either a nerve-sparing retroperitoneal lymph node dissection (RPLND) or surveillance. The retroperitoneal lymph nodes are involved by GCT (pathologic stage II) in 20–50% of these patients. The choice of surveillance or RPLND is based on the pathology of the primary tumor. If the primary tumor shows no evidence for lymphatic or vascular invasion and is limited to the testis (T1), then either option is reasonable. If lymphatic or vascular invasion is present or the tumor extends into the tunica, spermatic cord, or scrotum (T2 through T4), then surveillance should not be offered. Either approach should cure >95% of patients.

RPLND is the standard operation for removal of the regional lymph nodes of the testis (retroperitoneal nodes). The operation removes the lymph nodes ipsilateral to the primary site and the nodal groups adjacent to the primary landing zone. The standard (modified bilateral) RPLND removes all node-bearing tissue down to the bifurcation of the great vessels, including the ipsilateral iliac nodes. The major long-term effect of this operation is retrograde ejaculation and infertility. Nerve-sparing RPLND, usually accomplished by identification and dissection of individual nerve fibers, may avoid injury to the sympathetic nerves responsible for ejaculation. Normal ejaculation is preserved in ~90% of patients. Patients with pathologic stage I disease are observed, and only the <10% who relapse require additional therapy. If retroperitoneal nodes are found to be involved at RPLND, then a decision regarding adjuvant chemotherapy is made on the basis of the extent of retroperitoneal disease (see below).

Surveillance is an option in the management of clinical stage I disease when no vascular/lymphatic invasion is found (T1). Only 20–30% of patients have pathologic stage II disease, implying that most RPLNDs in this situation are not therapeutic. Surveillance and RPLND lead to equivalent long-term survival rates. Patient compliance is essential if surveillance is to be successful. Patients must be carefully followed with periodic chest radiography, physical examination, CT scan of the abdomen, and serum tumor marker determinations. The median time to relapse is about 7 months, and late relapses (>2 years) are rare. The 70–80% of patients who do not relapse require no

intervention after orchiectomy; treatment is reserved for those who do relapse. When the primary tumor is classified as T2 through T4 (extension beyond testis and epididymis or lymphatic/vascular invasion is identified), nerve-sparing RPLND is preferred. About 50% of these patients have pathologic stage II disease and are destined to relapse without the RPLND.

STAGE II NONSEMINOMA Patients with limited, ipsilateral retroperitoneal adenopathy (nodes usually ≤3 cm in largest diameter) and normal levels of AFP and hCG generally undergo a modified bilateral RPLND as primary management. Increased levels of either AFP or hCG or both imply metastatic disease outside the retroperitoneum; chemotherapy is used in this setting. The local recurrence rate after a properly performed RPLND is very low. Depending on the extent of disease, the postoperative management options include either surveillance or two cycles of adjuvant chemotherapy. Surveillance is the preferred approach for patients with resected "low-volume" metastases (tumor nodes ≤2 cm in diameter *and* <6 nodes involved) because the probability of relapse is one-third or less. For those who relapse, risk-directed chemotherapy is indicated (see below). Because relapse occurs in ≥50% of patients with "high-volume" metastases (>6 nodes involved, *or* any involved node >2 cm in largest diameter, *or* extranodal tumor extension), two cycles of adjuvant chemotherapy should be considered, as it results in cure in ≥98% of patients. Regimens consisting of etoposide (100 mg/m^2 daily on days 1–5) plus cisplatin (20 mg/m^2 daily on days 1–5) with or without bleomycin (30 units per day on days 2, 9, and 16) given at 3-week intervals are effective and well tolerated.

STAGES I AND II SEMINOMA Inguinal orchiectomy followed by retroperitoneal radiation therapy cures ~98% of patients with stage I seminoma. The dose of radiation therapy (2500–3000 cGy) is low and well tolerated, and the in-field recurrence rate is negligible. About 2% of patients relapse with supradiaphragmatic or systemic disease. Surveillance has been proposed as an option, and studies have shown that about 15% of patients relapse. The median time to relapse is 12–15 months, and late relapses (>5 years) may be more frequent than with nonseminoma. The relapse is usually treated with chemotherapy. Surveillance for clinical stage I seminoma is not recommended.

Nonbulky retroperitoneal disease (stage IIA and IIB) is also treated with radiation therapy. Prophylactic supradiaphragmatic fields are not used. Relapses in the anterior mediastinum are unusual. Approximately 90% of patients achieve relapse-free survival with retroperitoneal masses <5 cm in diameter. Because at least one-third of patients with bulkier disease relapse, initial chemotherapy is preferred for stage IIC disease.

CHEMOTHERAPY FOR ADVANCED GCT Regardless of histology, patients with stage IIC and stage III GCT are treated with chemotherapy. Combination chemotherapy programs based on cisplatin at doses of 100 mg/m^2 plus etoposide at doses of 500 mg/m^2 per cycle cure 70–80% of such patients, with or without bleomycin, depending on risk stratification (see below). A complete response (the complete disappearance of all clinical evidence of tumor on physical examination and radiography plus normal serum levels of AFP and hCG for ≥1 month) occurs after chemotherapy alone in ~60% of patients, and another 10–20% become disease-free with surgical resection of residual masses containing viable GCT. Lower doses of cisplatin result in inferior survival rates.

The toxicity of four cycles of the cisplatin/bleomycin/etoposide (BEP) regimen is substantial. Nausea, vomiting, and hair loss occur in most patients, although nausea and vomiting have been markedly ameliorated by modern antiemetic regimens. Myelosuppression is frequent, and symptomatic bleomycin pulmonary toxicity occurs in ~5% of patients. Treatment-induced mortality due to neutropenia with septicemia or bleomycin-induced pulmonary failure occurs in 1–3% of patients. Dose reductions for myelosuppression are rarely indicated. Long-term permanent toxicities include nephrotoxicity (reduced glomerular filtration and persistent magnesium wasting), ototoxicity, and peripheral neuropathy. When bleomycin is administered by weekly bolus injection, Raynaud's phenomenon appears in 5–10% of patients. Other evidence of small blood vessel damage is seen less often, including transient ischemic attacks and myocardial infarction.

RISK-DIRECTED CHEMOTHERAPY Because not all patients are cured and treatment may cause significant toxicities, patients are stratified into "good-risk" and "poor-risk" groups according to pretreatment clinical features. For good-risk patients, the goal is to achieve maximum efficacy with minimal toxicity. For poor-risk patients, the goal is to identify more effective therapy with tolerable toxicity.

TABLE 92-2 IGCCCG RISK CLASSIFICATION FOR ADVANCED GERM CELL TUMORS

Risk	Nonseminoma	Seminoma
Good	Gonadal or retroperitoneal primary site	Any primary site
	Absent nonpulmonary visceral metastases	Absent nonpulmonary visceral metastases
	AFP < 1000 ng/mL	
	Beta-hCG < 5000 mIU/mL	Any LDH, hCG
	LDH < 1.5 × upper limit or normal (ULN)	
Intermediate	Gonadal or retroperitoneal primary site	Any primary site
	Absent nonpulmonary visceral metastases	Presence of nonpulmonary visceral metastases
	AFP 1000–10,000 ng/mL	
	Beta-hCG 5000–50,000 mIU/mL	Any LDH, hCG
	LDH 1.5–10 × ULN	
Poor	Mediastinal primary site	No patients classified as poor prognosis
	Presence of nonpulmonary visceral metastases	
	AFP ≥ 10,000 ng/mL	
	Beta-hCG > 50,000 mIU/mL	
	LDH > 10 × ULN	

Note: AFP, α fetoprotein; hCG, human chorionic gonadotropin; LDH, lactate dehydrogenase.
Source: From International Germ Cell Cancer Consensus Group.

The International Germ Cell Cancer Consensus Group developed criteria to assign patients to three risk groups (good, intermediate, poor) **(Table 92-2)**. The marker cut-offs have been incorporated into the revised TNM (primary tumor, regional nodes, metastasis) staging of GCT. Hence, TNM stage groupings are now based on both anatomy (site and extent of disease) and biology (marker status and histology). Seminoma is either good or intermediate risk, based on the absence or presence of nonpulmonary visceral metastases. No poor-risk category exists for seminoma. Marker levels play no role in defining risk for seminoma. Nonseminomas have good-, intermediate-, and poor-risk categories based on the site of the primary tumor, the presence or absence of nonpulmonary visceral metastases, and marker levels.

For ~90% of patients with good-risk GCTs, four cycles of etoposide plus cisplatin (EP) or three cycles of BEP produce durable complete responses, with minimal acute and chronic toxicity. Pulmonary toxicity is absent when bleomycin is not used and is rare when therapy is limited to 9 weeks; myelosuppression with neutropenic fever is less frequent; and the treatment mortality rate is negligible. About 75% of intermediate-risk patients and 45% of poor-risk patients achieve durable complete remission with four cycles of BEP, and no regimen has proved superior. More effective therapy is needed.

POSTCHEMOTHERAPY SURGERY Resection of residual metastases after the completion of chemotherapy is an integral part of therapy. If the initial histology is nonseminoma and the marker values have normalized, all sites of residual disease should be resected. In general, residual retroperitoneal disease requires a modified bilateral RPLND. Thoracotomy (unilateral or bilateral) and neck dissection are less frequently required to remove residual mediastinal, pulmonary parenchymal, or cervical nodal disease. Viable tumor (seminoma, embryonal carcinoma, yolk sac tumor, or choriocarcinoma) will be present in 15%, mature teratoma in 40%, and necrotic debris and fibrosis in 45% of resected specimens. The frequency of teratoma or viable disease is highest in residual mediastinal tumors. If necrotic debris or mature teratoma is present, no further chemotherapy is necessary. If viable tumor is present but is completely excised, two additional cycles of chemotherapy are given.

If the initial histology is pure seminoma, mature teratoma is rarely present, and the most frequent finding is necrotic debris. For residual retroperitoneal disease, a complete RPLND is technically difficult owing to extensive postchemotherapy fibrosis. Observation is recommended when no radiographic abnormality exists on CT scan. Positive findings on a positron emission tomography (PET) scan correlate with viable seminoma in residua, and mandate surgical excision or biopsy.

SALVAGE CHEMOTHERAPY Of patients with advanced GCT, 20–30% fail to achieve a durable complete response to first-line chemotherapy. A combination of cisplatin, ifosfamide, and vinblastine (VelP) will cure about 25% of patients as a second-line therapy. Substitution of paclitaxel for vinblastine may be more effective in this setting. Patients are more likely to achieve a durable complete response if they had a testicular primary tumor and relapsed from a prior complete remission to first-line cisplatin-containing chemotherapy. In contrast, if the patient failed to achieve a complete response or has a primary mediastinal nonseminoma, then standard-dose salvage therapy is rarely beneficial. Treatment options for such patients include dose-intensive treatment, experimental therapies, and surgical resection.

Chemotherapy consisting of dose-intensive, high-dose carboplatin (≥1500 mg/m²) plus etoposide (≥1200 mg/m²), with or without cyclophosphamide, or ifosfamide, with peripheral blood stem cell support, induces a complete response in 25–40% of patients who have progressed after ifosfamide-containing salvage chemotherapy. About one-half of the complete responses will be durable. High-dose therapy is the treatment of choice and standard of care for this patient population. Paclitaxel is also active in previously treated patients and shows promise in high-dose combination programs. Cure is still possible in some relapsed patients.

EXTRAGONADAL GCT AND MIDLINE CARCINOMA OF UNCERTAIN HISTOGENESIS

The prognosis and management of patients with extragonadal GCT depends on the tumor histology and site of origin. All patients with a diagnosis of extragonadal GCT should have a testicular ultrasound examination. Nearly all patients with retroperitoneal or mediastinal seminoma achieve a durable complete response to BEP or EP. The clinical features of patients with primary retroperitoneal nonseminoma GCT are similar to those of patients with a primary of testis origin, and careful evaluation will find evidence of a primary testicular GCT in about two-thirds of cases. In contrast, a primary mediastinal nonseminomatous GCT is associated with a poor prognosis; one-third of patients are cured with standard therapy (four cycles of BEP). Patients with newly diagnosed mediastinal nonseminoma are considered to have poor-risk disease and should be considered for clinical trials testing regimens of possibly greater efficacy. In addition, mediastinal nonseminoma is associated with hematologic disorders, including acute myelogenous leukemia, myelodysplastic syndrome, and essential thrombocytosis unrelated to previous chemotherapy. These hematologic disorders are very refractory to treatment. Nonseminoma of any primary site may change into other malignant histologies such as embryonal rhabdomyosarcoma or adenocarcinoma. This is called malignant transformation. i(12p) has been identified in the transformed cell type, indicating GCT clonal origin.

A group of patients with poorly differentiated tumors of unknown histogenesis, midline in distribution, and not associated with secretion of AFP or hCG has been described; a few (10–20%) are cured by standard cisplatin-containing chemotherapy. i(12p) is present in ~25% of such tumors (the fraction that are cisplatin-responsive), confirming their origin from primitive germ cells. This finding is also predictive of the response to cisplatin-based chemotherapy and resulting long-term survival. These tumors are heterogeneous; neuroepithelial tumors and lymphoma may also present in this fashion.

FERTILITY

Infertility is an important consequence of the treatment of GCTs. Preexisting infertility or impaired fertility is often present. Azoospermia and/or oligospermia are present at diagnosis in at least 50% of patients with testicular GCTs. Ejaculatory dysfunction is associated with RPLND, and germ cell damage may result from cisplatin-containing chemotherapy. Nerve-sparing techniques to preserve the retroperitoneal sympathetic nerves have made retrograde ejaculation less likely in the subgroups of patients who are candidates for this operation. Spermatogenesis does recur in some patients after chemotherapy. However, because of the significant risk of impaired reproductive capacity, semen analysis and cryopreservation of sperm in a sperm bank should be recommended to all patients before treatment.

FURTHER READINGS

Bosl GJ et al: Testicular germ-cell cancer. N Engl J Med 337:242, 1997
———— et al: Cancer of the testis, in *Cancer: Principles and Practice of Oncology*, 7th ed, VT DeVita et al (eds). Philadelphia, Lippincott Williams & Wilkins, 2005, pp 1269–1294

Chaganti RSK, Houldsworth J: Genetics and biology of human male germ cell tumors. Cancer Res 60:1475, 2000

International Germ Cell Cancer Consensus Group: International Germ Cell Consensus Classification: A prognostic factor-based staging system for metastatic germ cell cancers. J Clin Oncol 15:594, 1997

Kondagunta GV et al: Etoposide and cisplatin chemotherapy for metastatic good-risk germ cell tumors. J Clin Oncol 23: 9290, 2005

Moore CJ et al: Management of difficult germ-cell tumors. Oncology 20:1565, 2006

Motzer R et al: Sequential dose-intensive paclitaxel, ifosfamide, carboplatin, and etoposide salvage therapy for germ cell tumor patients. J Clin Oncol 18:1173, 2000

Sonpaude G et al: Management of recurrent testicular germ cell tumors. Oncologist 12:51, 2007

93 Gynecologic Malignancies
Robert C. Young

OVARIAN CANCER

INCIDENCE AND EPIDEMIOLOGY

Ovarian cancer can develop from three distinctive cell types (germ cells, stromal cells, and epithelial cells), and each of these presents with distinctive features and outcomes and requires widely different management approaches. Epithelial ovarian cancer is the most common of the three and the leading cause of death from gynecologic cancer in the United States. In 2007, 22,430 new cases were diagnosed, and 15,280 women died from ovarian cancer. Epithelial ovarian cancer accounts for 5% of all cancer deaths in women in the United States; more women die of this disease than from cervical and endometrial cancer combined.

The age-specific incidence of the common epithelial type of ovarian cancer increases progressively and peaks in the eighth decade. Epithelial tumors, unlike germ cell and stromal tumors, are uncommon before the age of 40. Epidemiologic studies suggest higher incidences in women with a family history; in those who have been exposed to asbestos or talc; in industrialized nations; and in women with disordered ovarian function, including infertility, nulliparity, and frequent miscarriages. The use of ovulation-inducing drugs such as clomiphene has been implicated, but the studies have produced mixed results. Reduction in ovarian cancer risk is associated with pregnancy (each pregnancy reduces the ovarian cancer risk by about 10%), breast-feeding, and tubal ligation. Oral contraceptives reduce the risk of ovarian cancer in patients with a family history of cancer and in the general population. Many of these risk-reduction factors support the "incessant ovulation" hypothesis for ovarian cancer etiology, which implies that an aberrant repair process of the surface epithelium is central to ovarian cancer development. Estrogen replacement after menopause does not appear to increase the risk of ovarian cancer, although its use has declined substantially since the HRT trials demonstrated an increased cardiovascular risk.

Familial cases account for about 10% of all ovarian cancer. Compared to a lifetime risk of 1.6% in the general population, women with one affected first-degree relative have a 5% risk. In families with two or more affected first-degree relatives, the risk may exceed 50%. Two types of autosomal dominant familial cancers have been identified: (1) breast/ovarian cancer syndrome; and (2) the Lynch type II cancer family syndrome with nonpolyposis colorectal cancer, endometrial cancer, and ovarian cancer.

ETIOLOGY AND GENETICS

In women with hereditary breast/ovarian cancer, two susceptibility loci have been identified: *BRCA1*, located on chromosome 17q12-21, and *BRCA2*, on 13q12-13. Both are tumor-suppressor genes that produce nuclear proteins that interact with RAD 51, which effects genomic integrity. Both genes are large, and numerous mutations have been described; most are frameshift or nonsense mutations, and 86% produce truncated protein products. The implications of the many other mutations, including many missense mutations, are not known.

The cumulative risk of ovarian cancer with critical mutations of *BRCA1* or *-2* is 25%. Mutated genes can be inherited from either parent, so a complete family history is required. Men in such families have an increased risk of prostate cancer.

The Lynch type II syndrome is associated with an increased risk of ovarian cancer. Affected women often present at a younger age (<50 years). The predisposition results from germline mutations of mismatch repair genes (*MSH2*, *MLH1*, *MLH6*, *PMS1*, and *PMS2*). Because the risk of both endometrial and ovarian cancer is high, intensified screening and prophylactic surgery are often considered.

CLINICAL PRESENTATION AND DIFFERENTIAL DIAGNOSIS

Seventy percent of patients with ovarian cancer are first diagnosed when the disease has already spread beyond the true pelvis. The occurrence of abdominal pain, bloating, and urinary symptoms usually indicates advanced disease. Localized ovarian cancer is generally asymptomatic. However, progressive enlargement of a localized ovarian tumor can produce urinary frequency or constipation. Rarely, torsion of an ovarian mass causes acute abdominal pain or a surgical abdomen. In contrast to cervical or endometrial cancer, vaginal bleeding or discharge is rarely seen with early ovarian cancer. The diagnosis of early disease usually occurs with palpation of an asymptomatic adnexal mass during routine pelvic examination or as an incidental finding at surgery. However, most ovarian enlargements discovered on physical examination, especially in premenopausal women, are benign functional cysts that characteristically resolve over one to three menstrual cycles. Adnexal masses in premenarchal or postmenopausal women are more likely to be pathologic. A solid, irregular, fixed pelvic mass is usually ovarian cancer. Ultrasound studies usually show complex cysts with solid elements. Other causes of adnexal masses include pedunculated uterine fibroids, endometriosis, benign ovarian neoplasms, and inflammatory lesions of the bowel.

Evaluation of patients with suspected ovarian cancer should include measurement of CA-125. Between 80 and 85% of patients with epithelial ovarian cancer have levels of CA-125 ≥ 35 U/mL. Other malignant tumors can also elevate CA-125 levels, including cancers of the endometrium, cervix, fallopian tubes, pancreas, breast, lung, and colon. Certain nonmalignant conditions that can produce moderate elevations of CA-125 levels include pregnancy, endometriosis, pelvic inflammatory disease, and uterine fibroids. About 1% of normal females have serum CA-125 levels >35 U/mL. However, in postmenopausal women with an asymptomatic pelvic mass and CA-125 levels ≥65 U/mL, the test has a sensitivity of 97% and a specificity of 78%.

SCREENING

In contrast to patients who present with advanced disease, patients with early ovarian cancers (stages I and II) are commonly curable with conventional therapy. Thus, effective screening procedures would improve the cure rate in this disease. Although pelvic examination and CA-125 can occasionally detect early disease, these are relatively insensitive screening procedures. Transvaginal sonography is often used, but significant false-positive results are noted, particularly in premenopausal women. Doppler flow imaging coupled with transvaginal ultrasound may improve accuracy and reduce the high rate of false positives.

CA-125 has significant limitations as a screening test. Half of women with stages I and II ovarian cancer have normal CA-125 levels. Attempts have been made to improve the sensitivity and specificity by combinations of procedures, commonly transvaginal ultrasound and CA-125. In a screening study of 22,000 women, 42 had a positive screen and 11 had ovarian cancer (seven with advanced disease). In addition, eight women with a negative screen developed ovarian cancer. Thus, the false-positive rate would lead to a large number of unnecessary (i.e., negative) laparotomies if each positive screen resulted in a surgical exploration. In the United Kingdom, a large collaborative screening trial is underway to prospectively compare various screening techniques with controls. Until the results of such trials are available, the National Institutes of Health Consensus Conference recommended against screening for ovarian cancer among the general population without known risk factors for the disease. Although no evidence shows that screening saves lives, many physicians use annual pelvic examinations, transvaginal ultrasound, and CA-125 to screen women with a family history of ovarian cancer, Lynch type II, or breast/ovarian cancer syndrome.

Proteomic technologies have been used to identify patterns of proteins associated with early disease. Preliminary studies identified all 50 stage I patients with a sensitivity of 100%, a specificity of 95%, and a positive predictive value of 94%. However, difficulty in consistency of replicate samples, variability of results from different spectroscopy equipment, and the tendency of the artificial intelligence algorithms to overfit the data have limited its utility. Most proteins identified to date have been acute phase reactants, and extensive fractionation is necessary to identify unique cancer-specific proteins.

PATHOLOGY

Common epithelial tumors comprise most (85%) of the ovarian neoplasms. These may be benign (50%), malignant (33%), or tumors of low malignant potential (16%) (i.e., tumors of borderline malignancy). Epithelial tumors of low malignant potential have the cytologic features of malignancy but do not invade the ovarian stroma. More than 75% of borderline malignancies present in early stage and generally occur in the fourth or fifth decade of life. They usually have 10-year survival of 80–90%.

There are five major subtypes of common epithelial tumors: serous (50%); mucinous (25%), endometrioid (15%); clear cell (5%); and Brenner tumors (1%), the latter derived from the urothelium. Benign common epithelial tumors are almost always serous or mucinous and develop in women ages 20–60. They are frequently large (20–30 cm), bilateral, and cystic. Malignant epithelial tumors are usually seen in women over 40.

Although most ovarian tumors are epithelial, two other ovarian tumor types, stromal and germ cell tumors, are distinct in their cell of origin, have different clinical presentations and natural histories, and require different management (see below).

Metastasis to the ovary can occur from breast, colon, gastric, and pancreatic cancers. The Krukenberg tumor was classically described as bilateral ovarian masses from metastatic mucin-secreting gastrointestinal cancers.

STAGING AND PROGNOSTIC FACTORS

Laparotomy is the primary procedure used to establish the diagnosis and provide accurate staging. Less-invasive studies may help define the extent of spread, including chest x-rays, abdominal CT or MRI scans, and abdominal and pelvic sonography. Symptoms of bladder or renal dysfunction are evaluated by cystoscopy or intravenous pyelography.

A careful staging laparotomy with a total abdominal hysterectomy and bilateral salpingo-oophorectomy will establish the stage and extent of disease and allow for the cytoreduction of tumor masses in patients with advanced disease. Proper laparotomy requires a vertical incision of sufficient length to ensure adequate examination of the abdominal contents. The presence, amount, and cytology of any ascitic fluid should be noted. The primary tumor should be evaluated for rupture, excrescences, or dense adherence. Careful visual and manual inspection of the diaphragm and peritoneal surfaces is required. A partial omentectomy should be performed and the paracolic gutters inspected. Pelvic lymph nodes as well as para-aortic nodes in the region of the renal hilus should be biopsied. Since this surgical procedure defines stage, establishes prognosis, and determines the necessity for subsequent therapy, it should be performed by a surgeon with special expertise in ovarian cancer staging. Studies have shown that patients operated upon by gynecologic oncologists were properly staged 97% of the time, compared to 52 and 35% of cases staged by obstetricians/gynecologists and general surgeons, respectively. After staging, ~23% of women have stage I disease (cancer confined to the ovary or ovaries), 13% have stage II (disease confined to the true pelvis), 47% have stage III (disease spread into but confined to the abdomen), and 16% have stage IV disease (spread outside the pelvis and abdomen). The 5-year survival correlates with stage of disease: stage I, 90–95%; stage II, 70–80%; stage III, 25–50%; and stage IV, 1–5% (Table 93-1).

Prognosis in ovarian cancer is dependent not only on stage but on the extent of residual disease and histologic grade. Patients presenting with advanced disease but left without significant residual disease after surgery have a median survival of 39 months, compared to 17 months for those with suboptimal tumor resection.

If initial surgery does not produce minimal residual disease, a second cytoreductive surgery has been used after the first three cycles of chemotherapy; in one trial it was associated with a 6-month improvement in median duration of survival. Another randomized trial where more aggressive debulking surgery was initially carried out was unable to confirm this benefit.

Prognosis of epithelial tumors is also highly influenced by histologic grade but less so by histologic type. Although grading systems differ among pathologists, all grading systems show a better prognosis for well- or moderately differentiated tumors than for poorly differentiated histologies. Estimated 5-year survivals for patients by tumor grade are: well-differentiated, 88%; moderately differentiated, 58%; poorly differentiated, 27%.

The prognostic significance of pre- and postoperative CA-125 levels is uncertain. CA-125 levels generally reflect volume of disease, and high levels usually indicate unresectability and a poorer survival. Postoperative levels, if elevated, usually indicate residual disease. The rate of decline of CA-125 levels during initial therapy or the absolute level after one to three cycles of chemotherapy correlates with prognosis but is not sufficiently accurate to guide individual treatment decisions. Even when

TABLE 93-1 STAGING AND SURVIVAL IN GYNECOLOGIC MALIGNANCIES

Stage	Ovarian	5-Year Survival, %	Endometrial	5-Year Survival, %	Cervix	5-Year Survival, %
0	—		—		Carcinoma in situ	100
I	Confined to ovary	90	Confined to corpus	89	Confined to uterus	85
II	Confined to pelvis	70	Involves corpus and cervix	80	Invades beyond uterus but not to pelvic wall	65
III	Intraabdominal spread	15–20	Extends outside the uterus but not outside the true pelvis	30	Extends to pelvic wall and/or lower third of vagina, or hydronephrosis	35
IV	Spread outside abdomen	1–5	Extends outside the true pelvis or involves the bladder or rectum	9	Invades mucosa of bladder or rectum or extends beyond the true pelvis	7

CHAPTER 93 Gynecologic Malignancies

the CA-125 level falls to normal after surgery or chemotherapy, "second-look" laparotomy identifies residual disease in 60% of women.

Genetic and biologic factors may influence prognosis. Increased tumor levels of p53 are associated with a poorer prognosis in advanced disease. Epidermal growth factor receptors in ovarian cancer are associated with a decrease in disease-free survival, but the increased expression of HER-2/neu has given conflicting prognostic results. HER-2/neu is overexpressed in 20% of ovarian cancers, and responses have been seen to trastuzumab in this subset of patients.

Rx OVARIAN CANCER

The selection of therapy for patients with epithelial ovarian cancer depends on the stage, extent of residual tumor, and histologic grade. In general, patients are considered in three separate treatment groups: (1) those with early (stages I and II) ovarian cancer and microscopic or no residual disease, (2) patients with advanced (stage III) disease but minimal residual tumor (<1 cm) after initial surgery, and (3) patients with bulky residual tumor and advanced (stage III or IV) disease.

Patients with stage I disease, no residual tumor, and well or moderately differentiated tumors need no adjuvant therapy after definitive surgery, and 5-year survival exceeds 95%. For all other patients with early disease and those stage I patients with poor prognosis histologic grade, adjuvant platinum-based therapy is warranted. Large prospective randomized trials have demonstrated that adjuvant therapy improves disease-free and overall survival by 8% (82% vs. 74%, $p = .008$).

For patients with advanced (stage III) disease but with limited or no residual disease after definitive cytoreductive surgery (about half of all stage III patients), the primary therapy is platinum-based combination chemotherapy. Approximately 70% of women respond to initial combination chemotherapy, and 40–50% have a complete regression of disease. Unfortunately, only about half of these patients are free of disease if surgically restaged. Although a variety of combinations are active, a randomized prospective trial of paclitaxel and cisplatin compared to paclitaxel and carboplatin in patients with optimally resected advanced disease demonstrated equivalent disease-free and overall survivals but with significantly reduced toxicity with the carboplatin combination. This regimen of paclitaxel, 175 mg/m^2 by 3-h infusion, and carboplatin, dosed to an AUC (area under the curve) of 7.5, is the preferred treatment choice for patients with previously untreated advanced-stage disease.

Three randomized trials using intraperitoneal (IP) chemotherapy have demonstrated improved disease-free and overall survival compared to the intravenous administration of the same drugs. However, the increased toxicity (neuropathy, nephropathy, and catheter complications) is significant, and only about 40% of patients were able to receive full courses of therapy. Furthermore, the optimal dose and schedule of IP therapy has not been established, nor have any of the IP regimens been prospectively compared to the standard intravenous carboplatin-paclitaxel regimen. The ultimate role of IP therapy in the treatment of advanced ovarian cancer is unresolved.

Patients with advanced disease (stages III and IV) and bulky residual tumor are generally treated with intravenous paclitaxel-platinum combination, and while the overall prognosis is poorer, 5-year survival may reach 15–20%.

Historically, patients who had an excellent initial response to chemotherapy and no clinical evidence of disease had a second-look laparotomy. The second-look surgical procedure itself does not prolong overall survival, and outside of clinical trials its routine use is no longer recommended. Maintenance therapy may extend progression-free survival but has not improved overall survival.

Patients with advanced disease whose disease recurs after initial treatment are usually not curable but may benefit significantly from limited surgery to relieve intestinal obstruction, localized radiation therapy to relieve pressure or pain from mass lesions or metastasis, or palliative chemotherapy. The selection of chemotherapy for palliation depends on the initial regimen and evidence of drug resistance. Patients who had a complete regression of disease lasting ≥6 months often respond to reinduction with the same agents; patients relapsing within the first 6 months of initial therapy rarely do. Progestational agents, tamoxifen, or aromatase inhibitors produce responses in 5–15% of patients and have minimal side effects. Agents with >15% response rates in patients relapsing after initial combination chemotherapy include gemcitabine, topotecan, liposomal doxorubicin, and bevicizumab.

Bevicizumab is a monoclonal antibody that targets the vascular endothelial growth factor. Initial trials produced a 17% overall response rate in heavily pretreated patients. However, hypertension, thrombosis, and bowel perforations have been reported in some trials.

Patients with tumors of low malignant potential, even with advanced-stage disease, have longer survivals (80–90%) when managed with surgery alone. Radiation and chemotherapy do not improve outcome.

OVARIAN GERM CELL TUMORS

Fewer than 5% of all ovarian tumors are germ cell in origin. They include teratoma, dysgerminoma, endodermal sinus tumor, and embryonal carcinoma. Germ cell tumors of the ovary generally occur in younger women (75% of ovarian malignancies in women <30), display an unusually aggressive natural history, and are commonly cured with less-extensive nonsterilizing surgery and chemotherapy. Women cured of these malignancies are able to conceive and have normal children.

These neoplasms can be divided into three major groups: (1) benign tumors (usually dermoid cysts); (2) malignant tumors that arise from dermoid cysts; and (3) primitive malignant germ cell tumors, including dysgerminoma, yolk sac tumors, immature teratomas, embryonal carcinomas, and choriocarcinoma.

Dermoid cysts are teratomatous cysts usually lined by epidermis and skin appendages. They often contain hair, and calcified bone or teeth can sometimes be seen on conventional pelvic x-ray. They are almost always curable by surgical resection. Approximately 1% of these tumors have malignant elements, usually squamous cell carcinoma.

Malignant germ cell tumors are usually large (median—16 cm). Bilateral disease is rare except in dysgerminoma (10–15% bilaterality). Abdominal or pelvic pain in young women is the usual presenting symptom. Serum human chorionic gonadotropin (β-hCG) and α fetoprotein levels are useful in the diagnosis and management of these patients. Before the advent of chemotherapy, extensive surgery was routine, but it has now been replaced by careful evaluation of extent of spread, followed by resection of bulky disease and preservation of one ovary, the uterus, and the cervix, if feasible. This allows many affected women to preserve fertility. After surgical staging, 60–75% of women have stage I disease and 25–30% have stage III disease. Stages II and IV are infrequent.

Most of the malignant germ cell tumors are managed with chemotherapy after surgery. Regimens similar to those used in testicular cancer, such as BEP (bleomycin, etoposide, and cisplatin), with three or four courses given at 21-day intervals, have produced 95% long-term survival in patients with disease stages I–III. This regimen is the treatment of choice for all malignant germ cell tumors except grade I, stage I immature teratoma, where surgery alone is adequate, and perhaps early-stage dysgerminoma, where surgery and radiation therapy are used.

Dysgerminoma is the ovarian counterpart of testicular seminoma. The tumor is very sensitive to radiation therapy. The 5-year disease-free survival is 100% in early-stage patients and 61% in stage III disease. Unfortunately, the use of radiation therapy makes many patients infertile. BEP chemotherapy is equally or more effective and does not cause infertility. In incompletely resected patients with dysgerminoma treated with BEP, the 2-year disease-free survival is 95% and infertility is not observed. Combination chemotherapy (BEP) has replaced postoperative radiation therapy as the treatment of choice in women with ovarian dysgerminoma.

OVARIAN STROMAL TUMORS

Stromal tumors make up <10% of ovarian tumors. They are named for the stromal tissue involved: granulosa, theca, Sertoli, Leydig, and collagen-producing stromal cells. The granulosa and theca cell stromal cell tumors occur most frequently in the first three decades of life. Granulosa cell tumors frequently produce estrogen and cause menstrual abnormalities, bleeding, and precocious puberty. Endometrial carcinoma can be seen in 5% of these women, perhaps related to the persistent hyperestrogenism. Sertoli and Leydig cell tumors, when functional, produce androgens with resultant virilization or hirsutism. Some 75% of these stromal cell tumors present in stage I and can be cured with total abdominal hysterectomy and bilateral salpingo-oophorectomy. Stromal tumors generally grow slowly, and recurrences can occur 5–10 years after initial surgery; serum markers such as estradiol, inhibin, and müllerian inhibitory substance may be useful in monitoring patients. Neither radiation therapy nor chemotherapy has been documented to be consistently effective, and surgical management remains the primary treatment.

Ovarian stromal and germ cell tumors are sometimes components of complex genetic syndromes. Peutz-Jeghers syndrome (mucocutaneous pigmentation and intestinal polyps) is associated with ovarian sex cord stromal tumors and Sertoli cell tumors in men. Patients with gonadal dysgenesis (46XY genotype or mosaic for Y-containing cell lines) develop gonadoblastomas, and women with nevoid basal cell carcinomas have an increased risk of ovarian fibromas.

CARCINOMA OF THE FALLOPIAN TUBE

The fallopian tube is a very rare site of cancer in the female genital tract, although its epithelial surface far exceeds that of the ovary, where epithelial cancer is 20 times more common. Approximately 300 new cases occur yearly; 90% are papillary serous adenocarcinomas, with the remainder being mixed mesodermal, endometrioid, and transitional cell tumors. *BRCA1* and -*2* mutations are found in 16% of cases. The gross and microscopic characteristics and the spread of tumor are similar to those of ovarian cancer but can be distinguished if the tumor arises from the endosalpinx, where the tubal epithelium shows a transition between benign and malignant, and the ovaries and endometrium are normal or minimally involved. The differential diagnosis includes primary or metastatic ovarian cancer, chronic salpingitis, tuberculous salpingitis, salpingitis isthmica nodosa, and cautery artifact.

Unlike patients with ovarian cancer, patients often present with early symptoms, usually postmenopausal vaginal bleeding, pain, and leukorrhea. Surgical staging is similar to that used for ovarian cancer, and prognosis is related to stage and extent of residual disease. Patients with stages I and II disease are generally treated with surgery alone or with surgery and pelvic radiation therapy, although radiation therapy does not clearly improve 5-year survival (5-year survival, stage I: 74% vs. 75%; stage II: 43% vs. 48%). Patients with stages III and IV disease are treated with the same chemotherapy regimens used in advanced ovarian cancer; 5-year survival is similar (stage III, 20%; stage IV, 5%).

UTERINE CANCER

INCIDENCE AND EPIDEMIOLOGY

Carcinoma of the endometrium is the most common female pelvic malignancy. Approximately 39,080 new cases are diagnosed yearly, although in most (75%), tumor is confined to the uterine corpus at diagnosis, and therefore most can be cured. The 7400 deaths yearly make uterine cancer only the eighth leading cause of cancer death in females. It is primarily a disease of postmenopausal women, although 25% of cases occur in women ages <50 and 5% ages <40. The disease is common in Eastern Europe and the United States and uncommon in Asia.

Proliferation of the endometrium is under the control of estrogen, and prolonged exposure to unopposed estrogen from either endogenous or exogenous sources plays a central etiologic role. Risk factors for endometrial cancer include obesity, low fertility index, early menarche, late menopause, and chronic anovulation. Granulosa cell tumors of the ovary that secrete estrogen may present with synchronous endometrial cancers. Chronic unapposed estrogen replacement increases the risk, and women taking tamoxifen for breast cancer treatment or prevention have a twofold increased risk.

The Lynch syndrome occurs in families with an autosomal dominant mutation of mismatch repair genes *MLH1*, *MSH2*, *MSH6*, and *PMS2*, which predispose to nonpolyposis colon cancer as well as endometrial and ovarian cancer. The estimated lifetime risk for endometrial cancer is 40–60%, with a mean age around 50 years. Unlike colorectal cancer, endometrial cancer risk is not lower in *MSH6* mutation carriers. Most

women present with stage I disease, and the survival rate is generally good (5-year survival 88%). No unique endometrial screening strategies have been established for Lynch family gene carriers.

CLINICAL PRESENTATION

Endometrial carcinoma occurs most often in the sixth and seventh decades of life. Symptoms often include abnormal vaginal discharge (90%), abnormal postmenopausal bleeding (80%), and leukorrhea (10%). The risk of endometrial cancer associated with postmenopausal bleeding increases with advancing age (9% at age 50 vs. 60% at age 80). Evaluation of such patients should include a history and physical with pelvic examination followed by an endometrial biopsy or a fractional dilation and curettage. Outpatient procedures such as endometrial biopsy or aspiration curettage can be used but are definitive only when positive.

PATHOLOGY

Between 75 and 80% of all endometrial carcinomas are adenocarcinomas, and the prognosis depends on stage, histologic grade, and extent of myometrial invasion. Grade I tumors are highly differentiated adenocarcinomas, grade II tumors contain some solid areas, and grade III tumors are largely solid or undifferentiated. Adenocarcinoma with squamous differentiation is seen in 10% of patients; the most differentiated form is known as *adenoacanthoma*, and the poorly differentiated form is called *adenosquamous carcinoma*. Other less common pathologies include mucinous carcinoma (5%) and papillary serous carcinoma (<10%). This latter type has a natural history similar to ovarian carcinoma and should be managed in the same way. Rarer histologies include secretory (2%), ciliated, clear cell, and undifferentiated carcinomas.

STAGING

The staging of endometrial cancer requires surgery to establish the extent of disease and the depth of myometrial invasion. A total abdominal hysterectomy and bilateral salpingo-oophorectomy should be performed and peritoneal fluid sampled. Frozen sections of the uterine specimen are used to determine the histology and grade and depth of invasion. If indicated, pelvic and para-aortic lymphadenectomy is performed. After evaluation and staging, ~75% of patients are stage I, 13% are stage II, 9% are stage III, and 3% are stage IV. Five-year survival declines with advancing stage: stage I, 89%; stage II, 73%; stage III, 52%; and stage IV, 17% (Table 93-1).

℞ UTERINE CANCER

Patients with uncomplicated stage I endometrial carcinoma are effectively managed with total abdominal hysterectomy and bilateral salpingo-oophorectomy. Pre- or postoperative irradiation has been used, and although vaginal cuff recurrence is reduced, survival is not altered. In women with poor histologic grade, deep myometrial invasion, or extensive involvement of the lower uterine segment or cervix, intracavitary or external beam irradiation is warranted.

About 15% of women have endometrial carcinoma with extension to the cervix only (stage II), and management depends on the extent of cervical invasion. Superficial cervical invasion can be managed like stage I disease, but extensive cervical invasion requires radical hysterectomy or preoperative radiotherapy followed by extrafascial hysterectomy. Once disease is outside the uterus but still confined to the true pelvis (stage III), management generally includes surgery and irradiation. Patients who have involvement only of the ovary or fallopian tubes generally do well with such therapy (5-year survival of 80%). Other stage III patients with disease extending beyond the adnexa or those with serous carcinomas of the endometrium have a significantly poorer prognosis (5-year survival of 15%). Patients with positive para-aortic nodes (stage IIIC) or those with upper abdominal involvement (stage IV) have shown improved survival with platinum-based chemotherapy compared to whole-abdominal irradiation alone.

Patients with stage IV disease (outside the abdomen or invading the bladder or rectum) are treated palliatively with irradiation, surgery, and platinum-based chemotherapy. Progestational agents produce responses in ~10–20% of patients. Well-differentiated tumors respond most frequently, and response can be correlated with the level of progesterone receptor expression in the tumor. The commonly used progestational agents hydroxyprogesterone (Dilalutin), megestrol (Megace), and deoxyprogesterone (Provera) all produce similar response rates, and the antiestrogen tamoxifen (Nolvadex) produces responses in 10–25% of patients in a salvage setting.

Chemotherapy is not very successful in advanced endometrial carcinoma. The most active single agents with consistent response rates of ≥20% include cisplatin, carboplatin, doxorubicin, epirubicin, and paclitaxel. Combinations of drugs with or without progestational agents have generally produced response rates similar to single agents.

CERVIX CANCER

INCIDENCE AND EPIDEMIOLOGY

Carcinoma of the cervix was once the most common cause of cancer death in women, but over the past 40 years, the mortality rate has decreased by 50% due to widespread screening with the Pap smear. In 2007, ~11,150 new cases of invasive cervix cancer occurred, and >50,000 cases of carcinoma in situ were detected. There were 3670 deaths from the disease, and of those patients, ~85% had never had a Pap smear. Worldwide, cervical cancer is the third commonest cancer diagnosed, and it remains the major gynecologic cancer in underdeveloped countries. It is more common in lower socioeconomic groups, in women with early initial sexual activity and/or multiple sexual partners, and in smokers.

ETIOLOGY AND GENETICS

Venereal transmission of human papilloma virus (HPV) has an important etiologic role. Over 66 types of HPVs have been isolated, and many are associated with genital warts. Those types commonly associated with cervical carcinoma are 16, 18, 31, 33, 52, and 58, but 70% of cases are caused by HPV-16 and -18. These, along with many other types, are also associated with cervical intraepithelial neoplasia (CIN). The protein product of HPV-16, the E7 protein, binds and inactivates the tumor-suppressor gene Rb, and the E6 protein of HPV-18 has sequence homology to the SV40 large T antigen and the capacity to bind and inactivate the tumor-suppressor gene p53. E6 and E7 are both necessary and sufficient to cause cell transformation in vitro. These binding and inactivation events may explain the carcinogenic effects of the viruses (Chap. 178).

SCREENING AND PREVENTION

Vaccination against pathologic HPV appears to be an effective cervix cancer prevention strategy. Vaccines are made with inactivated virus-like particles that are noninfectious but highly immunogenic. The administration of a quadrivalent HPV vaccine against types 16, 18, 6, and 11 in a double-blind study of 2392 women completely prevented infection with the virus, and no cases of HPV-16–related CIN were seen in vaccinated women. This quadrivalent vaccine has been approved for use by the FDA for patients 9–26 years old and must be administered before HPV exposure to be effective. A second study with a bivalent vaccine (types 16 and 18) is underway. Both vaccines appear highly effective in preventing their particular HPV infections, and protection has persisted for at least 4.5 years after three injections over a 6-month period. Since not all oncogenic HPVs are targeted, patients will need to continue PAP smear surveillance.

Uncomplicated HPV infection in the lower genital tract can progress to CIN. This lesion precedes invasive cervical carcinoma and is classified as low-grade squamous intraepithelial lesion (SIL), high-grade SIL, and carcinoma in situ. Carcinoma in situ demonstrates cytologic evidence of neoplasia without invasion through the basement membrane and can persist unchanged for 10–20 years, but most of these eventually progress to invasive carcinoma.

The Pap smear is 90–95% accurate in detecting early lesions such as CIN but is less sensitive in detecting cancer when frankly invasive cancer or fungating masses are present. Inflammation, necrosis, and hemorrhage may produce false-positive smears, and colposcopic-directed biopsy is required when any lesion is visible on the cervix, regardless of Pap smear findings. The American Cancer Society recommends that women after onset of sexual activity, or >age 20, have two consecutive yearly smears. If negative, smears should be repeated every 3 years until age 65. The Pap smear can be reported as normal (includes benign, reactive, or reparative changes); atypical squamous cells of undetermined significance (ASCUS) or cannot exclude high-grade SIL (ASC-H); low- or high-grade CIN; or frankly malignant. Women with ASCUS, ASC-H, or low-grade CIN should have repeat smears in 3–6 months and be tested for HPV. Women with high-grade CIN or frankly malignant Pap smears should have colposcopic-directed cervical biopsy. Colposcopy is a technique using a binocular microscope and 3% acetic acid applied to the cervix in which abnormal areas appear white and can be biopsied directly. Cone biopsy is still required when endocervical tumor is suspected, colposcopy is inadequate, the biopsy shows microinvasive carcinoma, or when a discrepancy is noted between the Pap smear and the colposcopic findings. Cone biopsy alone is therapeutic for CIN in many patients, although a less radical electrocautery excision may be sufficient.

Approximately 70% of invasive cervix cancers are squamous cell tumors, 20–25% are adenocarcinomas, and 2–5% are adenosquamous with epithelial and glandular structures.

CLINICAL PRESENTATION AND STAGING

Patients with cervix cancer generally are asymptomatic, and the disease is detected on routine pelvic examination. Others present with abnormal bleeding or postcoital spotting that may increase to intermenstrual or prominent menstrual bleeding. Yellowish vaginal discharge, lumbosacral back pain, lower-extremity edema, and urinary symptoms may be present.

The staging of cervical carcinoma is clinical and generally completed with a pelvic examination under anesthesia with cystoscopy and proctoscopy. Chest x-rays, intravenous pyelograms, and CT are generally required, and MRI may be used to assess extracervical extension. Stage 0 is carcinoma in situ, stage I is disease confined to the cervix, stage II disease invades beyond the cervix but not to the pelvic wall or lower third of the vagina, stage III disease extends to the pelvic wall or lower third of the vagina or causes hydronephrosis, and stage IV is present when the tumor invades the mucosa of bladder or rectum or extends beyond the true pelvis (Fig. 93-1). Five-year survivals by stage are: stage I, 85%; stage II, 65%; stage III, 35%; and stage IV, 7% (Table 93-1).

℞ CERVIX CANCER

Carcinoma in situ (stage 0) can be managed successfully by cone biopsy or by abdominal hysterectomy. For stage I disease, results appear equivalent for either radical hysterectomy or radiation therapy. Patients with disease stages II–IV are primarily managed with external beam irradiation and intracavitary treatment or combined modality therapy. Retroperitoneal lymphadenectomy has no proven therapeutic role. Pelvic exenterations have become increasingly rare due to improved radiation control. However, they are sometimes performed for centrally recurrent or persistent disease.

In women with locally advanced disease (stages IIB–IVA), platinum-based chemotherapy given concomitantly with radiation therapy improves survival compared to radiation therapy alone. Cisplatin, 75 mg/m^2 over 4 h, followed by 5-fluorouracil (5-FU), 4 g given by 96-h infusion on days 1–5 of radiation therapy, is a common regimen. Two additional cycles of chemotherapy are given at 3-week intervals. Three randomized trials of platinum-based chemotherapy reduced the risk of recurrence by 30–50% across a wide spectrum of stages and presentations and were found to improve the survival rate in bulky stage I as well as locally advanced (stages IIB–IV) cervical cancer.

Chemotherapy has some palliative benefit in patients with unresectable advanced disease or recurrent disease. Active agents with ≥20% response rates include cisplatin, paclitaxel, vinorelbine, ifosfamide, and topotecan. The combination of topotecan and cisplatin has a modest survival advantage over cisplatin alone.

GESTATIONAL TROPHOBLASTIC NEOPLASIA

Gestational trophoblastic diseases are a group of related diseases that form a spectrum from benign hydatidiform mole to trophoblastic malignancy (placental-site trophoblastic tumor and choriocarcinoma). Malignant forms account for <1% of female gynecologic malignancies and can be cured with appropriate chemotherapy. Deaths from this disease have become rare in the United States.

EPIDEMIOLOGY

The incidence is about 1 per 1500 pregnancies in the United States and is nearly tenfold higher in Asia. Maternal age >45 years is a risk factor for hydatidiform mole as is a prior history of molar pregnancy. Choriocarcinoma occurs in ~1 in 25,000 pregnancies or 1 in 20,000 live births. Prior history of hydatidiform mole is a risk factor for choriocarcinoma. A woman with a previous molar pregnancy is 1000 times more likely to develop choriocarcinoma than a woman with a prior normal-term pregnancy.

PATHOLOGY AND ETIOLOGY

The trophoblastic neoplasms have been divided by morphology into complete or partial hydatidiform mole, invasive mole, placental-site trophoblastomas, and choriocarcinomas. Hydatidiform moles contain clusters of villi with hydropic changes, hyperplasia of the trophoblast, and the absence of fetal vessels. Invasive moles differ only by invasion into the uterine myometrium. Placental-site trophoblastic tumors are predominantly made up of cytotrophoblast cells arising from the placental implantation site. Choriocarcinomas consist of anaplastic trophoblastic tissue with both cytotrophoblastic and syncytiotrophoblastic elements and no identifiable villi.

Complete moles result from uniparental disomy in which loss of the maternal genes (23 autosomes plus X) occurs by unknown mechanisms and is followed by duplication of the paternal haploid genome (23 autosomes plus X). Uncommonly (5%), moles result from dispermic fertilization of an empty egg, resulting in either 46XY or 46XX genotype. Partial moles result from dispermic fertilization of an egg with retention of the maternal haploid set of chromosomes, resulting in diandric triploidy (Chap. 62).

CLINICAL PRESENTATION

Molar pregnancies are generally associated with first-trimester bleeding and excessive uterine size. About 45% of patients have ovarian theca-lutein cysts present on ultrasound. The β-hCG levels are generally markedly elevated. Fetal parts and heart sounds are not present. The diagnosis is generally made by the passage of grapelike clusters from the uterus, but ultrasound demonstration of the hydropic mole can be diagnostic. Patients suspected of a molar pregnancy require a chest film, careful pelvic examinations, and weekly serial monitoring of β-hCG levels.

℞ GESTATIONAL TROPHOBLASTIC NEOPLASIA

Patients with hydatidiform moles require suction curettage coupled with postevacuation monitoring of β-hCG levels. In most women (80%), the β-hCG titer progressively declines within 8–10 days of evacuation (serum half-life is 24–36 h). Patients should be monitored on a monthly basis and should not become pregnant for at least a year. Patients found to have invasive mole at curettage are generally treated with hysterectomy and chemotherapy. Approximately half of patients with choriocarcinoma develop

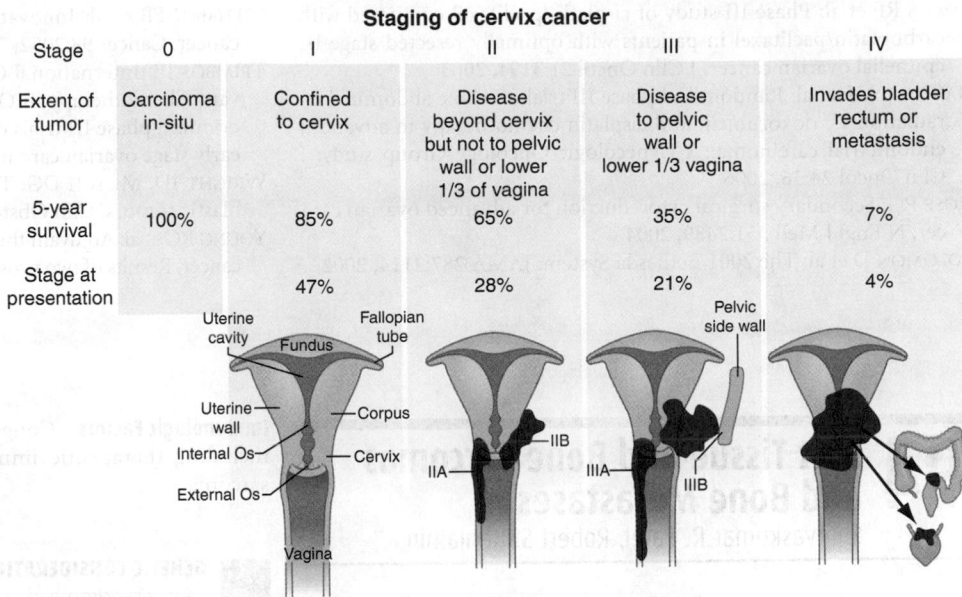

FIGURE 93-1 Anatomic display of the stages of cervix cancer defined by location, extent of tumor, frequency of presentation, and 5-year survival.

Stage	0	I	II	III	IV
Extent of tumor	Carcinoma in-situ	Confined to cervix	Disease beyond cervix but not to pelvic wall or lower 1/3 of vagina	Disease to pelvic wall or lower 1/3 vagina	Invades bladder rectum or metastasis
5-year survival	100%	85%	65%	35%	7%
Stage at presentation		47%	28%	21%	4%

Staging of cervix cancer

the malignancy after a molar pregnancy, and the other half develop the malignancy after abortion, ectopic pregnancy, or occasionally after a normal full-term pregnancy.

Chemotherapy is used for gestational trophoblastic neoplasia and often as chemoprophylaxis after molar evacuation to reduce postmolar tumors. It is also used in hydatidiform mole if β-hCG levels rise or plateau or if metastases develop. Patients with invasive mole or choriocarcinoma require chemotherapy. Several regimens are effective for low-risk patients, including methotrexate at 30 mg/m² intramuscularly on a weekly basis until β-hCG titers are normal. However, methotrexate (1 mg/kg) every other day for four doses, followed by leukovorin (0.1 mg/kg) intravenously 24 h after methotrexate, is associated with a cure rate of ≥90% and low toxicity. Intermittent courses are continued until the β-hCG titer becomes undetectable for 3 consecutive weeks; then patients are monitored monthly for a year.

Patients with high-risk tumors (high β-hCG levels, disease presenting ≥4 months after antecedent pregnancy, brain or liver metastasis, or failure of single-agent methotrexate) are initially treated with combination chemotherapy. EMA-CO (a cyclic non-cross-resistant combination of etoposide, methotrexate, and dactinomycin alternating with cyclophosphamide and vincristine); cisplatin, bleomycin, and vinblastine; and cisplatin, etoposide, and bleomycin are effective regimens. EMA-CO is now the regimen of choice for patients with high-risk disease because of excellent survival rates (>80%) and less toxicity. The use of etoposide carries a 1.5% lifetime risk of acute myeloid leukemia (sixteenfold relative risk) and other solid tumors. As a result, etoposide-containing regimens should be reserved for patients with high-risk features. Patients with brain or liver metastases are usually treated with local irradiation to metastatic sites in conjunction with chemotherapy. Long-term studies of patients cured of trophoblastic disease have not demonstrated an increased risk of maternal complications or fetal abnormalities with subsequent pregnancies.

FURTHER READINGS

CHAMPION V et al: Quality of life in long-term survivors of ovarian germ cell tumors: A gynecologic oncology group study. Gynecol Oncol 105:687, 2007

KOUTSKY LA: A controlled trial of a human papilloma virus type 16 vaccine. N Engl J Med 347:1645, 2002

LINDOR NM et al: Recommendations for the care of individuals with an inherited predisposition to Lynch Syndrome. JAMA 296:1507, 2006

MODUGNO F: Ovarian Cancer and High Risk Women Symposium Presenters. Ovarian cancer and high-risk women: Implications for prevention, screening and early detection. Gynecol Oncol 91:15, 2003

610 OZOLS RF et al: Phase III study of cisplatin/paclitaxel compared with carboplatin/paclitaxel in patients with optimally resected stage III epithelial ovarian cancer. J Clin Oncol 21:3194, 2003

RANDALL ME et al: Randomized phase III trial of whole abdominal irradiation vs. doxorubicin and cisplatin chemotherapy in advanced endometrial carcinoma: A Gynecologic Oncology Group study. J Clin Oncol 24:36, 2006

ROSE PG: Secondary surgical cytoreduction for advanced ovarian cancer. N Engl J Med 351:2489, 2004

SOLOMON D et al: The 2001 Bethesda System. JAMA 287:2114, 2002

STEHMAN FB et al: Innovations in the treatment of invasive cervical cancer. Cancer 98:2052, 2003

TRIMBOS JB: International Collaborative Neoplasm Trial I and Adjuvant Chemotherapy in Ovarian Neoplasm Trial: Two parallel randomized phase III trials of adjuvant chemotherapy in patients with early stage ovarian carcinoma. J Natl Cancer Inst 95:105, 2003

WRIGHT JD, MUTCH DG: Treatment of high-risk gestational trophoblastic tumors. Clin Obstet Gynecol 46:593, 2003

YOUNG RC et al: Adjuvant therapy in stage I and stage II epithelial ovarian cancer. Results of two prospective trials. N Engl J Med 327:1021, 1990

94 Soft Tissue and Bone Sarcomas and Bone Metastases

Shreyaskumar R. Patel, Robert S. Benjamin

Sarcomas are rare (<1% of all malignancies) mesenchymal neoplasms that arise in bone and soft tissues. These tumors are usually of mesodermal origin, although a few are derived from neuroectoderm, and they are biologically distinct from the more common epithelial malignancies. Sarcomas affect all age groups; 15% are found in children <15 years and 40% occur after age 55. Sarcomas are one of the most common solid tumors of childhood and are the fifth most common cause of cancer deaths in children. Sarcomas may be divided into two groups, those derived from bone and those derived from soft tissues.

SOFT TISSUE SARCOMAS

Soft tissues include muscles, tendons, fat, fibrous tissue, synovial tissue, vessels, and nerves. Approximately 60% of soft tissue sarcomas arise in the extremities, with the lower extremities involved three times as often as the upper extremities. Thirty percent arise in the trunk, the retroperitoneum accounting for 40% of all trunk lesions. The remaining 10% arise in the head and neck.

INCIDENCE

Approximately 9220 new cases of soft tissue sarcomas occurred in the United States in 2007. The annual age-adjusted incidence is 3.0 per 100,000 population, but the incidence varies with age. Soft tissue sarcomas constitute 0.7% of all cancers in the general population and 6.5% of all cancers in children.

EPIDEMIOLOGY

Malignant transformation of a benign soft tissue tumor is extremely rare, with the exception that malignant peripheral nerve sheath tumors (neurofibrosarcoma, malignant schwannoma) can arise from neurofibromas in patients with neurofibromatosis. Several etiologic factors have been implicated in soft tissue sarcomas.

Environmental Factors Trauma or previous injury is rarely involved, but sarcomas can arise in scar tissue resulting from a prior operation, burn, fracture, or foreign body implantation. Chemical carcinogens such as polycyclic hydrocarbons, asbestos, and dioxin may be involved in the pathogenesis.

Iatrogenic Factors Sarcomas in bone or soft tissues occur in patients who are treated with radiation therapy. The tumor nearly always arises in the irradiated field. The risk increases with time.

Viruses Kaposi's sarcoma (KS) in patients with HIV type 1, classic KS, and KS in HIV-negative homosexual men is caused by human herpes virus (HHV) 8 (Chap. 175). No other sarcomas are associated with viruses.

Immunologic Factors Congenital or acquired immunodeficiency, including therapeutic immunosuppression, increases the risk of sarcoma.

GENETIC CONSIDERATIONS Li-Fraumeni syndrome is a familial cancer syndrome in which affected individuals have germ-line abnormalities of the tumor-suppressor gene p53 and an increased incidence of soft tissue sarcomas and other malignancies, including breast cancer, osteosarcoma, brain tumor, leukemia, and adrenal carcinoma (Chap. 79). Neurofibromatosis 1 (NF-1, peripheral form, von Recklinghausen's disease) is characterized by multiple neurofibromas and café au lait spots. Neurofibromas occasionally undergo malignant degeneration to become malignant peripheral nerve sheath tumors. The gene for NF-1 is located in the pericentromeric region of chromosome 17 and encodes neurofibromin, a tumor-suppressor protein with GTPase-activating activity that inhibits Ras function (Chap. 374). Germ-line mutation of the *Rb-1* locus (chromosome 13q14) in patients with inherited retinoblastoma is associated with the development of osteosarcoma in those who survive the retinoblastoma and of soft tissue sarcomas unrelated to radiation therapy. Other soft tissue tumors, including desmoid tumors, lipomas, leiomyomas, neuroblastomas, and paragangliomas, occasionally show a familial predisposition.

Ninety percent of synovial sarcomas contain a characteristic chromosomal translocation t(X;18)(p11;q11) involving a nuclear transcription factor on chromosome 18 called *SYT* and two breakpoints on X. Patients with translocations to the second X breakpoint (*SSX2*) may have longer survival than those with translocations involving *SSX1*.

Insulin-like growth factor (IGF) type 2 is produced by some sarcomas and may act as an autocrine growth factor and as a motility factor that promotes metastatic spread. IGF-2 stimulates growth through IGF-1 receptors, but its effects on motility are through different receptors. If secreted in large amounts, IGF-2 may produce hypoglycemia (Chaps. 96, 339).

CLASSIFICATION

Approximately 20 different groups of sarcomas are recognized on the basis of the pattern of differentiation toward normal tissue. For example, rhabdomyosarcoma shows evidence of skeletal muscle fibers with cross-striations; leiomyosarcomas contain interlacing fascicles of spindle cells resembling smooth muscle; and liposarcomas contain adipocytes. When precise characterization of the group is not possible, the tumors are called *unclassified sarcomas*. All of the primary bone sarcomas can also arise from soft tissues (e.g., extraskeletal osteosarcoma). The entity *malignant fibrous histiocytoma* includes many tumors previously classified as fibrosarcomas or as pleomorphic variants of other sarcomas and is characterized by a mixture of spindle (fibrous) cells and round (histiocytic) cells arranged in a storiform pattern with frequent giant cells and areas of pleomorphism.

For purposes of treatment, most soft tissue sarcomas can be considered together. However, some specific tumors have distinct features. For example, *liposarcoma* can have a spectrum of behaviors. Pleomorphic liposarcomas and dedifferentiated liposarcomas behave like other high-grade sarcomas; in contrast, well-differentiated liposarcomas (better termed *atypical lipomatous tumors*) lack metastatic potential, and myxoid liposarcomas metastasize infrequently but, when they do, have a predilection for unusual metastatic sites containing fat, such as the retroperitoneum, mediastinum, and subcutaneous tissue. Rhabdomyosarcomas, Ewing's sarcoma, and other small-cell sarcomas tend to be more aggressive and are more responsive to chemotherapy than other soft tissue sarcomas.

Gastrointestinal stromal cell tumors (GISTs), previously classified as gastrointestinal leiomyosarcomas, are now recognized as a distinct entity within soft tissue sarcomas. Its cell of origin resembles the interstitial cell of Cajal, which controls peristalsis. The majority of malignant GISTs have activating mutations of the *c-kit* gene that result in ligand-independent phosphorylation and activation of the KIT receptor tyrosine kinase, leading to tumorigenesis.

DIAGNOSIS

The most common presentation is an asymptomatic mass. Mechanical symptoms referable to pressure, traction, or entrapment of nerves or muscles may be present. All new and persistent or growing masses should be biopsied, either by a cutting needle (core-needle biopsy) or by a small incision, placed so that it can be encompassed in the subsequent excision without compromising a definitive resection. Lymph node metastases occur in 5%, except in synovial and epithelioid sarcomas, clear-cell sarcoma (melanoma of the soft parts), angiosarcoma, and rhabdomyosarcoma, where nodal spread may be seen in 17%. The pulmonary parenchyma is the most common site of metastases. Exceptions are GISTs, which metastasize to the liver; myxoid liposarcomas, which seek fatty tissue; and clear-cell sarcomas, which may metastasize to bones. Central nervous system metastases are rare, except in alveolar soft part sarcoma.

Radiographic Evaluation   Imaging of the primary tumor is best with plain radiographs and MRI for tumors of the extremities or head and neck and by CT for tumors of the chest, abdomen, or retroperitoneal cavity. A radiograph and CT scan of the chest are important for the detection of lung metastases. Other imaging studies may be indicated, depending on the symptoms, signs, or histology.

STAGING AND PROGNOSIS

The histologic grade, relationship to fascial planes, and size of the primary tumor are the most important prognostic factors. The current American Joint Commission on Cancer (AJCC) staging system is shown in Table 94-1. Prognosis is related to the stage. Cure is common in the absence of metastatic disease, but a small number of patients with metastases can also be cured. Most patients with stage IV disease die within 12 months, but some patients may live with slowly progressive disease for many years.

Rx SOFT TISSUE SARCOMAS

AJCC stage I patients are adequately treated with surgery alone. Stage II patients are considered for adjuvant radiation therapy. Stage III patients may benefit from adjuvant chemotherapy. Stage IV patients are managed primarily with chemotherapy, with or without other modalities.

SURGERY   Soft tissue sarcomas tend to grow along fascial planes, with the surrounding soft tissues compressed to form a pseudocapsule that gives the sarcoma the appearance of a well-encapsulated lesion. This is invariably deceptive because "shelling out," or marginal excision, of such lesions results in a 50–90% probability of local recurrence. Wide excision with a negative margin, incorporating the biopsy site, is the standard surgical procedure for

TABLE 94-1   AJCC STAGING SYSTEM FOR SARCOMAS

Histologic Grade (G)	Tumor Size (T)	Node Status (N)	Metastases (M)
Well differentiated (G1)	≤5 cm (T1)	Not involved (N0)	Absent (M0)
Moderately differentiated (G2)	>5 cm (T2)	Involved (N1)	Present (M1)
Poorly differentiated (G3)	Superficial fascial involvement (Ta)		
Undifferentiated (G4)	Deep fascial involvement (Tb)		

Disease Stage	5-Year Survival, %
Stage I	98.8
A: G1,2; T1a,b; N0; M0	
B: G1,2; T2a; N0; M0	
Stage II	81.8
A: G1,2; T2b; N0; M0	
B: G3,4; T1; N0; M0	
C: G3,4; T2a; N0; M0	
Stage III G3,4; T2b; N0; M0	51.7
Stage IV	<20
A: any G; any T; N1; M0	
B: any G; any T; any N; M1	

local disease. The adjuvant use of radiation therapy and/or chemotherapy improves the local control rate and permits the use of limb-sparing surgery with a local control rate (85–90%) comparable to that achieved by radical excisions and amputations. Limb-sparing approaches are indicated except when negative margins are not obtainable, when the risks of radiation are prohibitive, or when neurovascular structures are involved so that resection will result in serious functional consequences to the limb.

RADIATION THERAPY   External beam radiation therapy is an adjuvant to limb-sparing surgery for improved local control. Preoperative radiation therapy allows the use of smaller fields and smaller doses but results in a higher rate of wound complications. Postoperative radiation therapy must be given to larger fields, as the entire surgical bed must be encompassed, and in higher doses to compensate for hypoxia in the operated field. Brachytherapy or interstitial therapy, in which the radiation source is inserted into the tumor bed, is comparable in efficacy (except in low-grade lesions), less time-consuming, and less expensive.

ADJUVANT CHEMOTHERAPY   Chemotherapy is the mainstay of treatment for Ewing's primitive neuroectodermal tumors (PNET) and rhabdomyosarcomas. Meta-analysis of 14 randomized trials revealed a significant improvement in local control and disease-free survival in favor of doxorubicin-based chemotherapy. Overall survival improvement was 4% for all sites and 7% for the extremity site. A chemotherapy regimen including an anthracycline and ifosfamide with growth factor support improved overall survival by 19% for high-risk (high-grade, ≥5 cm primary, or locally recurrent) extremity soft tissue sarcomas.

ADVANCED DISEASE   Metastatic soft tissue sarcomas are largely incurable, but up to 20% of patients who achieve a complete response become long-term survivors. The therapeutic intent, therefore, is to produce a complete remission with chemotherapy (<10%) and/or surgery (30–40%). Surgical resection of metastases, whenever possible, is an integral part of the management. Some patients benefit from repeated surgical excision of metastases. The two most active chemotherapeutic agents are doxorubicin and ifosfamide. These drugs show a steep dose-response relationship in sarcomas. Gemcitabine with or without docetaxel has become an established second-line regimen and is particularly active in patients with leiomyosarcomas. Dacarbazine also has some modest activity. Taxanes have selective activity in angiosarcomas, and vincristine, etoposide, and irinotecan are effective in rhadomyosarcomas and Ewing's sarcomas. Imatinib mesylate targets the KIT tyrosine kinase activity and is standard therapy for advanced/metastatic GISTs.

BONE SARCOMAS

INCIDENCE AND EPIDEMIOLOGY

Bone sarcomas are rarer than soft tissue sarcomas; they accounted for only 0.2% of all new malignancies and 2370 new cases in the United

States in 2007. Several benign bone lesions have the potential for malignant transformation. Enchondromas and osteochondromas can transform into chondrosarcoma; fibrous dysplasia, bone infarcts, and Paget's disease of bone can transform into either malignant fibrous histiocytoma or osteosarcoma.

CLASSIFICATION

Benign Tumors The common benign bone tumors include enchondroma, osteochondroma, chondroblastoma, and chondromyxoid fibroma, of cartilage origin; osteoid osteoma and osteoblastoma, of bone origin; fibroma and desmoplastic fibroma, of fibrous tissue origin; hemangioma, of vascular origin; and giant cell tumor, of unknown origin.

Malignant Tumors The most common malignant tumors of bone are plasma cell tumors (Chap. 106). The four most common malignant nonhematopoietic bone tumors are osteosarcoma, chondrosarcoma, Ewing's sarcoma, and malignant fibrous histiocytoma. Rare malignant tumors include chordoma (of notochordal origin), malignant giant cell tumor and adamantinoma (of unknown origin), and hemangioendothelioma (of vascular origin).

Musculoskeletal Tumor Society Staging System Sarcomas of bone are staged according to the Musculoskeletal Tumor Society staging system based on grade and compartmental localization. A Roman numeral reflects the tumor grade: stage I is low-grade, stage II is high-grade, and stage III includes tumors of any grade that have lymph node or distant metastases. In addition, the tumor is given a letter reflecting its compartmental localization. Tumors designated A are intracompartmental (i.e., confined to the same soft tissue compartment as the initial tumor), and tumors designated B are extracompartmental (i.e., extending into the adjacent soft tissue compartment or into bone). The tumor node metastasis (TNM) staging system is shown in Table 94-2.

OSTEOSARCOMA

Osteosarcoma, accounting for almost 45% of all bone sarcomas, is a spindle cell neoplasm that produces osteoid (unmineralized bone) or bone. About 60% of all osteosarcomas occur in children and adolescents in the second decade of life, and about 10% occur in the third decade of life. Osteosarcomas in the fifth and sixth decades of life are frequently secondary to either radiation therapy or transformation in a preexisting benign condition, such as Paget's disease. Males are affected 1.5–2 times as often as females. Osteosarcoma has a predilection for metaphyses of long bones; the most common sites of involvement are the distal femur, proximal tibia, and proximal humerus. The classification of osteosarcoma is complex, but 75% of osteosarcomas fall in the "classic" category, which include osteoblastic, chondroblastic, and fibroblastic osteosarcomas. The remaining 25% are classified as "variants" on the basis of (1) clinical characteristics, as in the case of osteosarcoma of the jaw, postradiation osteosarcoma, or Paget's osteosarcoma; (2) morphologic characteristics, as in the case of telangiectatic osteosarcoma, small cell osteosarcoma, or epithelioid osteosarcoma; or (3) location, as in parosteal or periosteal osteosarcoma. Diagnosis usually requires a synthesis of clinical, radiologic, and pathologic features. Patients typically present with pain and swelling of the affected area. A plain radiograph reveals a destructive lesion with a moth-eaten appearance, a spiculated periosteal reaction (sunburst appearance), and a cuff of periosteal new bone formation at the margin of the soft tissue mass (Codman's triangle). A CT scan of the primary tumor is best for defining bone destruction and the pattern of calcification, whereas MRI is better for defining intramedullary and soft tissue extension. A chest radiograph and CT scan are used to detect lung metastases. Metastases to the bony skeleton should be imaged by a bone scan. Almost all osteosarcomas are hypervascular. Angiography is not helpful for diagnosis, but it is the most sensitive test for assessing the response to preoperative chemotherapy. Pathologic diagnosis is established either with a core-needle biopsy, where feasible, or with an open biopsy with an appropriately placed incision that does not compromise future limb-sparing resection. Most osteosarcomas are high-grade. The most important prognostic factor for long-term survival is response to chemotherapy. Preoperative chemotherapy followed by limb-sparing surgery (which can be accomplished in >80% of patients) followed by postoperative chemotherapy is standard management. The effective drugs are doxorubicin, ifosfamide, cisplatin, and high-dose methotrexate with leucovorin rescue. The various combinations of these agents that have been used have all been about equally successful. Long-term survival rates in extremity osteosarcoma range from 60 to 80%. Osteosarcoma is radioresistant; radiation therapy has no role in the routine management. Malignant fibrous histiocytoma is considered a part of the spectrum of osteosarcoma and is managed similarly.

CHONDROSARCOMA

Chondrosarcoma, which constitutes ~20–25% of all bone sarcomas, is a tumor of adulthood and old age with a peak incidence in the fourth to sixth decades of life. It has a predilection for the flat bones, especially the shoulder and pelvic girdles, but can also affect the diaphyseal portions of long bones. Chondrosarcomas can arise de novo or as a malignant transformation of an enchondroma or, rarely, of the cartilaginous cap of an osteochondroma. Chondrosarcomas have an indolent natural history and typically present as pain and swelling. Radiographically, the lesion may have a lobular appearance with mottled or punctate or annular calcification of the cartilaginous matrix. It is difficult to distinguish low-grade chondrosarcoma from benign lesions by x-ray or histologic examination. The diagnosis is therefore influenced by clinical history and physical examination. A new onset of pain, signs of inflammation, and progressive increase in the size of the mass suggest malignancy. The histologic classification is complex, but most tumors fall within the classic category. Like other bone sarcomas, high-grade chondrosarcomas spread to the lungs. Most chondrosarcomas are resistant to chemotherapy, and surgical resection of primary or recurrent tumors, including pulmonary metastases, is the mainstay of therapy. This rule does not hold for two histologic variants. Dedifferentiated chondrosarcoma has a high-grade osteosarcoma or a malignant fibrous histiocytoma component that responds to chemo-

TABLE 94-2	STAGING SYSTEM FOR BONE SARCOMAS		
Primary tumor (T)	TX	Primary tumor cannot be assessed	
	T0	No evidence of primary tumor	
	T1	Tumor ≤8 cm in greatest dimension	
	T2	Tumor >8 cm in greatest dimension	
	T3	Discontinuous tumors in the primary bone site	
Regional lymph nodes (N)	NX	Regional lymph nodes cannot be assessed	
	N0	No regional lymph node metastasis	
	N1	Regional lymph node metastasis	
Distant metastasis (M)	MX	Distant metastasis cannot be assessed	
	M0	No distant metastasis	
	M1	Distant metastasis	
	M1a	Lung	
	M1b	Other distant sites	
Histologic grade (G)	GX	Grade cannot be assessed	
	G1	Well differentiated—low grade	
	G2	Moderately differentiated—low grade	
	G3	Poorly differentiated—high grade	
	G4	Undifferentiated—high grade (Ewing's is always classed G4)	

Stage Grouping

Stage IA	T1	N0	M0	G1,2 low grade
Stage IB	T2	N0	M0	G1,2 low grade
Stage IIA	T1	N0	M0	G3,4 high grade
Stage IIB	T2	N0	M0	G3,4 high grade
Stage III	T3	N0	M0	Any G
Stage IVA	Any T	N0	M1a	Any G
Stage IVB	Any T	N1	Any M	Any G
	Any T	Any N	M1b	Any G

therapy. Mesenchymal chondrosarcoma, a rare variant composed of a small cell element, also is responsive to systemic chemotherapy and is treated like Ewing's sarcoma.

EWING'S SARCOMA

Ewing's sarcoma, which constitutes ~10–15% of all bone sarcomas, is common in adolescence and has a peak incidence in the second decade of life. It typically involves the diaphyseal region of long bones and also has an affinity for flat bones. The plain radiograph may show a characteristic "onion peel" periosteal reaction with a generous soft tissue mass, which is better demonstrated by CT or MRI. This mass is composed of sheets of monotonous, small, round, blue cells and can be confused with lymphoma, embryonal rhabdomyosarcoma, and small-cell carcinoma. The presence of p30/32, the product of the *mic-2* gene (which maps to the pseudoautosomal region of the X and Y chromosomes) is a cell-surface marker for Ewing's sarcoma (and other members of a family of tumors called PNETs). Most PNETs arise in soft tissues; they include peripheral neuroepithelioma, Askin's tumor (chest wall), and esthesioneuroblastoma. Glycogen-filled cytoplasm detected by staining with periodic acid–Schiff is also characteristic of Ewing's sarcoma cells. The classic cytogenetic abnormality associated with this disease (and other PNETs) is a reciprocal translocation of the long arms of chromosomes 11 and 22, t(11;22), which creates a chimeric gene product of unknown function with components from the *fli-1* gene on chromosome 11 and *ews* on 22. This disease is very aggressive, and it is therefore considered a systemic disease. Common sites of metastases are lung, bones, and bone marrow. Systemic chemotherapy is the mainstay of therapy, often being used before surgery. Doxorubicin, cyclophosphamide or ifosfamide, etoposide, vincristine, and dactinomycin are active drugs. Local treatment for the primary tumor includes surgical resection, usually with limb salvage or radiation therapy. Patients with lesions below the elbow and below the mid-calf have a 5-year survival rate of 80% with effective treatment. Ewing's sarcoma is a curable tumor, even in the presence of obvious metastatic disease, especially in children <11 years old.

TUMORS METASTATIC TO BONE

Bone is a common site of metastasis for carcinomas of the prostate, breast, lung, kidney, bladder, and thyroid and for lymphomas and sarcomas. Prostate, breast, and lung primaries account for 80% of all bone metastases. Metastatic tumors of bone are more common than primary bone tumors. Tumors usually spread to bone hematogenously, but local invasion from soft tissue masses also occurs. In descending order of frequency, the sites most often involved are the vertebrae, proximal femur, pelvis, ribs, sternum, proximal humerus, and skull. Bone metastases may be asymptomatic or may produce pain, swelling, nerve root or spinal cord compression, pathologic fracture, or myelophthisis (replacement of the marrow). Symptoms of hypercalcemia may be noted in cases of bony destruction.

Pain is the most frequent symptom. It usually develops gradually over weeks, is usually localized, and often is more severe at night. When patients with back pain develop neurologic signs or symptoms, emergency evaluation for spinal cord compression is indicated (Chap. 270). Bone metastases exert a major adverse effect on quality of life in cancer patients.

Cancer in the bone may produce osteolysis, osteogenesis, or both. Osteolytic lesions result when the tumor produces substances that can directly elicit bone resorption (vitamin D–like steroids, prostaglandins, or parathyroid hormone–related peptide) or cytokines that can induce the formation of osteoclasts (interleukin 1 and tumor necrosis factor). Osteoblastic lesions result when the tumor produces cytokines that activate osteoblasts. In general, purely osteolytic lesions are best detected by plain radiography, but they may not be apparent until they are >1 cm. These lesions are more commonly associated with hypercalcemia and with the excretion of hydroxyproline-containing peptides indicative of matrix destruction. When osteoblastic activity is prominent, the lesions may be readily detected using radionuclide bone scanning (which is sensitive to new bone formation), and the radiographic appearance may show increased bone density or sclerosis. Osteoblastic lesions are associated with higher serum levels of alkaline phosphatase and, if extensive, may produce hypocalcemia. Although some tumors may produce mainly osteolytic lesions (e.g., kidney cancer) and others mainly osteoblastic lesions (e.g., prostate cancer), most metastatic lesions produce both types of lesion and may go through stages where one or the other predominates.

In older patients, particularly women, it may be necessary to distinguish metastatic disease of the spine from osteoporosis. In osteoporosis, the cortical bone may be preserved, whereas cortical bone destruction is usually noted with metastatic cancer.

℞ METASTATIC BONE DISEASE

Treatment of metastatic bone disease depends on the underlying malignancy and the symptoms. Some metastatic bone tumors are curable (lymphoma, Hodgkin's disease), and others are treated with palliative intent. Pain may be relieved by local radiation therapy. Hormonally responsive tumors are responsive to hormone inhibition (antiandrogens for prostate cancer, antiestrogens for breast cancer). Strontium 89 and samarium 153 are bone-seeking radionuclides that can exert antitumor effects and relieve symptoms. Bisphosphonates such as pamidronate may relieve pain and inhibit bone resorption, thereby maintaining bone mineral density and reducing risk of fractures in patients with osteolytic metastases from breast cancer and multiple myeloma. Careful monitoring of serum electrolytes and creatinine is recommended. Monthly administration prevents bone-related clinical events and may reduce the incidence of bone metastases in women with breast cancer. When the integrity of a weight-bearing bone is threatened by an expanding metastatic lesion that is refractory to radiation therapy, prophylactic internal fixation is indicated. Overall survival is related to the prognosis of the underlying tumor. Bone pain at the end of life is particularly common; an adequate pain relief regimen including sufficient amounts of narcotic analgesics is required. **The management of hypercalcemia is discussed in Chap. 347.**

FURTHER READINGS

BORDEN EC et al: Soft tissue sarcomas of adults: State of the translational science. Clin Cancer Res 9:1941, 2003

HELMAN LJ, MELTZER P: Mechanisms of sarcoma development. Nat Rev Cancer 3:685, 2003

MOCELLIN S et al: Adult soft tissue sarcomas: Conventional therapies and molecularly targeted approaches. Cancer Treat Rev 32:9, 2006

PISTERS PW et al: Evidence-based recommendations for local therapy for soft tissue sarcomas. J Clin Oncol 25:1003, 2007

SCURR M, JUDSON I: How to treat the Ewing's family of sarcomas in adult patients. Oncologist 11:65, 2006

VERWEIJ J et al: Progression-free survival in gastrointestinal stromal tumors with high-dose imatinib: Randomized trial. Lancet 364:1127, 2004

95 Carcinoma of Unknown Primary
Gauri R. Varadhachary, James L. Abbruzzese

Carcinoma of unknown primary (CUP) is a biopsy-proven (mainly epithelial) malignancy for which the anatomic site of origin remains unidentified after an intensive search. CUP is one of the 10 most frequently diagnosed cancers worldwide, accounting for approximately 3–5% of all cancer cases. Most investigators do not consider lymphomas, metastatic melanomas, and metastatic sarcomas that present without a known primary tumor to be CUP because these cancers have specific stage- and histology-based treatments that can guide management.

A standard workup for CUP includes a medical history; physical examination; and laboratory studies, including liver and renal function tests, hemogram, chest x-ray, CT scan of the abdomen and pelvis, mammography in women, and prostate-specific antigen (PSA) test in men. With the increasing availability of additional sophisticated imaging techniques and the emergence of targeted therapies that have been shown to be effective in several cancers, oncologists must decide on the extent of workup that is warranted. Specifically, they must consider how additional diagnostic procedures may affect the choice of therapy and the patient's survival and quality of life.

The reason tumors present as CUP remains unclear. One hypothesis is that the primary tumor either regresses after seeding the metastasis or remains so small that it is not detected. It is possible that CUP falls on the continuum of cancer presentation where the primary has been contained or eliminated by the natural body defenses. Alternatively, CUP may represent a specific malignant event that results in an increase in metastatic spread or survival relative to the primary. Whether the CUP metastases truly define a clone that is genetically and phenotypically unique to this diagnosis remains to be determined.

CUP BIOLOGY

No characteristics that are unique to CUP relative to metastases from known primaries have been identified. Abnormalities in chromosomes 1 and 12 and other complex abnormalities have been found. Aneuploidy has been described in 70% of CUP patients with metastatic adenocarcinoma or undifferentiated carcinoma. The overexpression of various genes, including *Ras, bcl-2* (40%), *her-2* (11%), and *p53* (26–53%), has been studied in CUP samples, but they seem to have no effect on response to therapy or survival. The extent of angiogenesis in CUP relative to that in metastases from known primaries has also been evaluated, but no consistent findings have emerged.

CLINICAL EVALUATION

Obtaining a thorough medical history from CUP patients is essential, paying particular attention to previous surgeries, removed lesions, and family medical history to assess potential hereditary cancers. Physical examination, including a digital rectal examination in men and breast and pelvic examinations in women, should be performed. Determining the patient's performance status, nutritional status, comorbid illnesses, and cancer-induced complications is essential since they may affect treatment planning.

Role of Serum Tumor Markers and Cytogenetics   Most tumor markers, including CEA, CA-125, CA 19-9, and CA 15-3, when elevated, are nonspecific and not helpful in determining the primary tumor site. Men who present with adenocarcinoma and osteoblastic metastasis should undergo a PSA test. Patients with an elevated PSA should be treated as having prostate cancer. In patients with undifferentiated or poorly differentiated carcinoma (especially with a midline tumor), elevated β-human chorionic gonadotropin (βhCG) and α fetoprotein (AFP) levels suggest the possibility of an extragonadal germ cell (testicular) tumor. Cytogenetic studies had a larger role in the past, although interpretation of these older studies can be challenging. In our opinion, with the availability of immunohistochemical stains, cytogenetic analyses are indicated only occasionally. We reserve them for undifferentiated neoplasms with inconclusive immunohistochemical stains and those for which a high suspicion of lymphoma exists.

Role of Imaging Studies   Chest x-rays are always obtained in CUP workups but are often negative, especially with low-volume disease. CT scans of the chest, abdomen, and pelvis can be used to help find the primary, evaluate the extent of disease, and select the most favorable biopsy site. Older studies suggested that the primary tumor site is detected in 20–35% of patients who undergo a CT scan of the abdomen and pelvis, although by current definition these patients would not be considered as having CUP. Older studies also suggest a latent primary tumor prevalence of 20%; with more sophisticated imaging, this prevalence is <10% today.

Mammography should be performed in all women who present with metastatic adenocarcinoma, especially in those with adenocarcinoma and isolated axillary adenopathy. MRI of the breast is a recognized follow-up modality in patients with suspected occult primary breast carcinoma (following negative mammography and sonography findings). The results of these imaging modalities can influence surgical management; a negative breast MRI result predicts a low tumor yield at mastectomy.

A conventional workup for a cervical CUP (neck lymphadenopathy with no known primary tumor) includes a CT scan or MRI and invasive studies, including indirect and direct laryngoscopy, bronchoscopy, and upper endoscopy. Ipsilateral (or bilateral) tonsillectomy (with histopathology) has been recommended for cervical CUP patients. ^{18}F-fluorodeoxyglucose (FDG) positron emission tomography (PET) scans are useful in this patient population and may help guide the biopsy; determine the extent of disease; facilitate the appropriate treatment, including planning radiation fields; and help with disease surveillance. Several studies have evaluated the utility of PET in patients with cervical CUP. These trials have included a small number of patients; primary tumors were identified in ~21–30%.

The diagnostic contribution of PET to the evaluation of noncervical CUP is controversial. PET or PET-CT helps to detect primary tumor in 20–35% of patients. PET-CT can be helpful for patients who are candidates for surgical intervention for solitary metastatic disease because the presence of disease outside the primary site will affect surgical consolidation planning.

Invasive studies, including upper endoscopy, colonoscopy, and bronchoscopy, should be limited to symptomatic patients or those with laboratory or pathologic abnormalities suggesting that these techniques will result in a high tumor yield.

PATHOLOGIC DIAGNOSIS OF CUP

A detailed pathologic examination of the most accessible biopsied tissue specimen is mandatory in CUP cases. Pathologic evaluation typically consists of hematoxylin-and-eosin stains and immunohistochemical tests. Electron microscopy is rarely used currently, although it may be selectively useful when making treatment decisions.

Light Microscopy Evaluation   Adequate tissue obtained by fine-needle aspiration or core-needle biopsy should first be stained with hematoxylin and eosin and subjected to light microscopic examination. On light microscopy, 60% of CUPs are found to be adenocarcinoma, and 5% are squamous cell carcinoma. The remaining 30% of lesions are diagnosed as poorly differentiated adenocarcinoma, poorly differentiated carcinoma, or poorly differentiated neoplasm. A small percentage of lesions are diagnosed as neuroendocrine cancers (2%), mixed tumors (adenosquamous, or sarcomatoid carcinomas), or undifferentiated neoplasm (Table 95-1).

Role of Immunohistochemical Analysis   Immunohistochemical stains are peroxidase-labeled antibodies against specific tumor antigens that are used to define tumor lineage. The number of available immunohistochemical stains is ever-increasing. However, in CUP cases, more is not necessarily better, and immunohistochemical stains should be used in conjunction with the patient's clinical presentation and imaging studies to select the best therapy. Communication between the cli-

TABLE 95-1	MAJOR HISTOLOGIES IN CUP
Histology	Proportion, %
Well to moderately differentiated adenocarcinoma	60
Squamous cell cancer	5
Poorly differentiated adenocarcinoma, poorly differentiated carcinoma	30
Neuroendocrine	2
Undifferentiated malignancy	3

TABLE 95-2	ADDITIONAL IMMUNOHISTOCHEMICAL STAINS USEFUL IN THE DIAGNOSIS OF CUP
Tissue Marker	Diagnosis
Estrogen and progesterone receptors	Breast cancer
BRST-1	Breast cancer
Gross cystic disease fibrous protein-15	Breast cancer
Thyroid transcription factor 1	Lung and thyroid cancer
Thyroglobulin	Thyroid cancer
Chromogranin, synaptophysin, neuron specific enolase	Neuroendocrine cancer
CDX-2	Gastrointestinal cancer
Calretinin, mesothelin	Mesothelioma
Leukocyte common antigen	Lymphoma
S-100, HMB-45	Melanoma
URO-III, thrombomodulin	Bladder cancer
α Fetoprotein	Hepatocellular cancer, germ cell cancer
β-Human chronic gonadotropin	Germ cell cancer
Prostate specific antigen	Prostate cancer

nician and pathologist is essential. No stain is 100% specific, and over-interpretation should be avoided. PSA and thyroglobulin tissue markers, which are positive in prostate and thyroid cancer, respectively, are the most specific of the current marker panel. However, these cancers rarely present as CUP, so the yield of these tests may be low. Fig. 95-1 delineates a simple algorithm for immunohistochemical staining in CUP cases. Table 95-2 lists additional tests that may be useful to further define the tumor lineage. A more comprehensive algorithm may improve the diagnostic accuracy but can make the process complex. With the use of immunohistochemical markers, electron microscopic analysis, which is time-consuming and expensive, is rarely needed.

There are 20 subtypes of cytokeratin (CK) intermediate filaments with different molecular weights and differential expression in various cell types and cancers. Monoclonal antibodies to specific CK subtypes have been used to help classify tumors according to their site of origin; commonly used CK stains in CUP are CK7 and CK20. CK7 is found in tumors of the lung, ovary, endometrium, and breast and not in those of the lower gastrointestinal tract, whereas CK20 is normally expressed in the gastrointestinal epithelium, urothelium, and Merkel's cells. CK20+/CK7– strongly suggest a primary tumor of the colon; 75–95% of colon tumors show this pattern of staining. CK20–/CK7+ suggests cancer of the lung, breast, ovary, endometrium, and pancreaticobiliary tract; some of these can also be CK20+. The nuclear CDX-2 transcription factor, which is the product of a homeobox gene necessary for intestinal organogenesis, is often used to aid in the diagnosis of gastrointestinal adenocarcinomas.

Thyroid transcription factor 1 (TTF-1) is a 38-kDa homeodomain-containing nuclear protein that plays a role in transcriptional activation during embryogenesis in the thyroid, diencephalon, and respiratory epithelium. TTF-1 nuclear staining is typically positive in lung and thyroid cancers. Approximately 68% of adenocarcinomas and 25% of squamous cell lung cancers stain positive for TTF-1, which helps differentiate a lung primary tumor from metastatic adenocarcinoma in a pleural effusion, the mediastinum, or the lung parenchyma.

Distinguishing pleural mesothelioma from lung adenocarcinoma can be challenging. Calretinin, Wilms' tumor gene-1 (WT-1), and mesothelin have been suggested as useful markers for mesothelioma.

Gross cystic disease fibrous protein-15, a 15-kDa monomer protein, is a marker of apocrine differentiation that is detected in 62–72% of breast carcinomas. UROIII, high-molecular-weight cytokeratin, thrombomodulin, and CK20 are the markers used to diagnose lesions of urothelial origin.

ROLE OF DNA MICROARRAY AND REVERSE TRANSCRIPTASE POLYMERASE CHAIN REACTION (RT-PCR) IN CUP

In the absence of a known primary, developing therapeutic strategies for CUP is challenging. The current diagnostic yield with imaging and immunochemistry is ~20–30% for CUP patients. The use of gene expression studies holds the promise of substantially increasing this yield. Gene expression profiles are most commonly generated using quantitative RT-PCR or DNA microarray.

Neural network programs have been used to develop predictive algorithms from the gene expression profiles. Typically, a training set of gene profiles from known cancers (preferably from metastatic sites) are used to train the software. The program can then be used to predict the origin of a test tumor, and presumably of true CUP. Comprehensive gene expression databases that have become available for common malignancies may also be useful in CUP. Investigators have used expression data from normal differentiated tissues to identify conserved expression profiles found in malignant tissue as a basis for predicting the tissue of origin. These approaches have been effective in blind testing against known primary cancers and their metastasis. However, because, by definition, the primary tumor site is not identifiable in CUP, validation of site prediction in this setting can be challenging, and any predictions currently must be supported by clinical and pathologic correlation. Prospective validation trials are currently evaluating the role of molecular studies in CUP.

Rx CARCINOMA OF UNKNOWN PRIMARY

GENERAL CONSIDERATIONS The treatment of CUP continues to evolve, albeit slowly. The median survival duration of most patients with disseminated CUP is ~6–10 months. Systemic chemotherapy is the primary treatment modality in most cases, but the careful integration of surgery, radiation therapy, and even periods of observation are important in the overall management of this condition (Figs. 95-2 and 95-3). Prognostic factors include performance status, site and number of metastases, response to chemotherapy, and serum lactate dehydrogenase (LDH) levels. Culine and colleagues developed a prognostic model using performance status and serum LDH levels, which allowed the assignment of patients into two subgroups with divergent outcomes. Future prospective trials using this prognostic model are warranted. Clinically, several CUP diagnoses fall into a favorable prog-

FIGURE 95-1 Approach to cytokeratin (CK7 and CK20) markers used in CUP.

FIGURE 95-2 Treatment algorithm for adenocarcinoma and poorly differentiated adenocarcinoma CUP. C, chemotherapy; IHC, immu-nohistochemistry; GI, gastrointestinal; CRT, chemoradiation; RT, radia-tion; PSA, prostate-specific antigen; MRI, magnetic resonance imaging.

nostic subset. Others, including those with disseminated CUP, have a more unfavorable prognosis.

TREATMENT OF FAVORABLE SUBSETS OF CUP   Women with Isolated Axillary Adenopathy   Women with isolated axillary adenopa-thy with adenocarcinoma or carcinoma should be treated for stage II or III breast cancer. These patients should undergo a breast MRI if mammogram and ultrasound are negative. Radiation therapy to the ipsilateral breast is indicated if the breast MRI is positive. Chemotherapy and/or hormonal therapy is indicated based on patient's age (premenopausal or postmeno-pausal), nodal disease bulk, and hormone receptor status (Chap. 86).

Women with Peritoneal Carcinomatosis   The term *primary peritoneal papillary serous carcinoma* (PPSC) has been used to describe CUP with carci-nomatosis with the pathologic and laboratory (elevated CA-125 antigen) characteristics of ovarian cancer but no ovarian primary tumor identified on transvaginal sonography or laparotomy. Studies suggest that ovarian can-cer and PPSC, which are both of mullerian origin, have similar gene expres-sion profiles. Similar to patients with ovarian cancer, patients with PPSC are candidates for cytoreductive surgery, followed by adjuvant taxane and plat-inum-based chemotherapy. In one retrospective study of 258 women with peritoneal carcinomatosis who had undergone cytoreductive surgery and chemotherapy, 22% of patients had a complete response to chemotherapy; the median survival duration was 18 months (range 11–24 months).

Poorly Differentiated Carcinoma with Midline Adenopathy   Men with poorly differentiated or undifferentiated carcinoma that presents as a mid-line adenopathy should be evaluated for extragonadal germ cell malignancy. They often experience a good response to treatment with platinum-based combination chemotherapy. Response rates of >50% have been noted, and 10–15% long-term survivors have been reported.

Neuroendocrine Carcinoma   Low-grade neuroendocrine carcinoma often has an indolent course, and treatment decisions are based on symp-toms and tumor bulk. Urine 5-HIAA and serum chromogranin may be ele-vated and can be followed as markers. Often the patient is treated with somatostatin analogues alone for hormone-related symptoms (diarrhea, flushing, nausea). Specific local therapies or systemic therapy would only be indicated if the patient is symptomatic with local pain secondary to sig-nificant growth of the metastasis or the hormone-related symptoms are not controlled with endocrine therapy. Patients with high-grade neuroen-docrine carcinoma are treated as having small cell lung cancer and are re-sponsive to chemotherapy; 20–25% show a complete response, and up to 10% patients survive more than 5 years.

Squamous Cell Carcinoma Presenting as Cervical Adenopathy   Pa-tients with early-stage squamous cell carcinoma involving the cervical lymph nodes are candidates for node dissection and radiation therapy, which can result in long-term survival. The role of chemotherapy in these patients is undefined, although chemoradiation therapy or induction chemotherapy is often used and is beneficial in bulky N2/N3 lymph node disease.

Solitary Metastatic Site   Patients with solitary metastases can also ex-perience good treatment outcomes. Some patients who present with lo-coregional disease are candidates for aggressive trimodality management; both prolonged disease-free interval and occasionally cure are possible.

FIGURE 95-3 Treatment algorithm for squamous cell CUP. CT, computed tomography; PET, positron emission tomography; RT, radia-tion; C, chemotherapy.

Men with Blastic Skeletal Metastases and Elevated PSA Blastic bone-only metastasis is a rare presentation, and elevated serum PSA or tumor staining with PSA may provide confirmatory evidence of prostate cancer in these patients. Those with elevated levels are candidates for hormonal therapy for prostate cancer, although it is important to rule out other primary tumors (lung most common).

MANAGEMENT OF DISSEMINATED CUP Patients who present with liver, brain, and adrenal metastatic disease usually have a poor prognosis. Beside primary peritoneal carcinoma, carcinomatosis presenting as CUP in other settings is not uncommon. Gastric, appendicular, colon, pancreas, and cholangiocarcinoma are all possible primaries, and imaging, endoscopy, and pathologic data help in the evaluation.

Traditionally, platinum-based combination chemotherapy regimens have been used to treat patients with CUP. In a phase II study by Hainsworth and colleagues, 55 mostly chemotherapy-naive patients were treated with paclitaxel, carboplatin, and oral etoposide every 3 weeks. The overall response rate was 47%, with median overall survival duration of 13.4 months. Briasoulis and colleagues reported similar response rates and survival durations in 77 patients with CUP who had been treated with paclitaxel and carboplatin. In this study, patients with nodal or pleural disease and women with peritoneal carcinomatosis had higher response rates and overall survival durations of 13 and 15 months, respectively. Studies incorporating newer agents, including gemcitabine, irinotecan, and targeted agents, are showing higher response rates. In a phase II randomized trial by Culine and colleagues, 80 patients were randomly assigned to receive gemcitabine with cisplatin or irinotecan with cisplatin; 78 patients were assessible for efficacy and toxicity. Objective responses were observed in 21 patients (55%) in the gemcitabine and cisplatin arm and in 15 patients (38%) in the irinotecan and cisplatin arm. The median survival was 8 months for gemcitabine and cisplatin and 6 months for irinotecan and cisplatin.

The role of second-line chemotherapy in CUP is poorly defined. Gemcitabine as a single agent has shown a partial response rate of 8%, and 25% of patients had minor responses or stable disease, with improved symptoms. Combination chemotherapy as a second- and third-line treatment may result in a slightly improved response.

Combination targeted therapy is being evaluated. Hainsworth and colleagues studied the combination of bevacizumab and erlotinib in 51 patients; 25% were chemotherapy-naive and had advanced bone or liver metastases, while the rest had been previously treated with 1 or 2 chemotherapy regimens. Responses were noted in 4 patients (8%), and 30 patients (59%) experienced stable disease or a minor response. The median overall survival was 8.9 months, with 42% of patients alive at 1 year.

Historically, patients with CUP have been treated with "global" regimens that work for a variety of primary cancers. With incremental improved responses over the past decade in known cancer types, we anticipate overall better response rates with newer regimens for selected CUP patients. With a more robust immunohistochemical panel (directed approach) and new molecular data, one may be able to create a more tailored algorithm for CUP patients.

SUMMARY

Patients with CUP should undergo a directed diagnostic search for the primary tumor on the basis of clinical and pathologic data. Subsets of patients have prognostically favorable disease, as defined by clinical or histologic criteria, and may substantially benefit from aggressive treatment and expect prolonged survival. However, for most patients who present with advanced CUP, the prognosis remains poor, with early resistance to available cytotoxic therapy. Research into the metastatic phenotype will help us improve our understanding of CUP tumor biology. Whether the CUP clone is a distinct molecular genotype-phenotype that is different from metastases of known primary tumors remains to be elucidated. The identification of specific CUP-related molecular and biochemical targets may help exploit therapeutic targeted agents for this entity.

FURTHER READINGS

ABBRUZZESE JL et al: The biology of unknown primary tumors. Semin Oncol 20:238, 1993

BUGAT R et al: Summary of the standards, options and recommendations for the management of patients with carcinoma of unknown primary site. Br J Cancer 89(Suppl 1):S59, 2003

CULINE S et al: Cisplatin in combination with either gemcitabine or irinotecan in carcinomas of unknown primary site: Results of a randomized phase II study—trial for the French Study Group on Carcinomas of Unknown Primary (GEFCAPI 01). J Clin Oncol 21:3479, 2003

DENNIS JL, OIEN KA: Hunting the primary: novel strategies for defining the origin of tumours. J Pathol 205:236, 2005

GRECO FA, HAINSWORTH JD: One-hour paclitaxel, carboplatin, and extended-schedule etoposide in the treatment of carcinoma of unknown primary site. Semin Oncol 24(6 Suppl 19):S19, 1997

KENDE AI et al: Expression of cytokeratins 7 and 20 in carcinomas of the gastrointestinal tract. Histopathology 42:137, 2003

LOBINS R, FLOYD J: Small cell carcinoma of unknown primary. Semin Oncol 34:39, 2007.

OLSON JA Jr et al: Magnetic resonance imaging facilitates breast conservation for occult breast cancer. Ann Surg Oncol 7:411, 2000

RUSTHOVEN KE et al: The role of fluorodeoxyglucose positron emission tomography in cervical lymph node metastases from an unknown primary tumor. Cancer 101:2641, 2004

VARADHACHARY GR et al: Diagnostic strategies for unknown primary cancer. Cancer 100:1776, 2004

96 Paraneoplastic Syndromes: Endocrinologic/Hematologic

J. Larry Jameson, Bruce E. Johnson

In addition to local tissue invasion and metastasis, neoplastic cells can produce a variety of peptides that that can stimulate hormonal, hematologic, dermatologic, or neurologic responses. *Paraneoplastic syndromes* refer to the disorders that accompany benign or malignant tumors but are not directly related to mass effects or invasion. Tumors of neuroendocrine origin, such as small cell lung carcinoma (SCLC) and carcinoids, produce a wide array of peptide hormones and are common causes of paraneoplastic syndromes. However, almost every type of malignancy has the potential to produce hormones or cytokines, or to induce immunologic responses. Careful studies of the prevalence of paraneoplastic syndromes indicate that they are more common than is generally appreciated. The signs, symptoms, and metabolic alterations associated with paraneoplastic disorders may be overlooked in the context of a malignancy and its treatment. Consequently, atypical clinical manifestations in a patient with cancer should prompt consideration of a paraneoplastic syndrome. The most common endocrinologic and hematologic syndromes associated with underlying neoplasia will be discussed here.

ENDOCRINE PARANEOPLASTIC SYNDROMES

Etiology Hormones can be produced from eutopic or ectopic sources. *Eutopic* refers to the expression of a hormone from its normal tissue of origin, whereas *ectopic* refers to hormone production from an atypical tissue source. For example, adrenocorticotropic hormone (ACTH) is expressed eutopically by the corticotrope cells of the anterior pituitary but it can be expressed ectopically in SCLC. Many hormones are produced at low levels from a wide array of tissues, in addition to the classic endocrine source. Thus, ectopic expression is often a quantitative change rather than an absolute change in tissue expression. Nevertheless, the term *ectopic expression* is firmly entrenched and conveys the abnormal physiology associated with neoplastic hormone production. In addition to high levels of hormones, ectopic expression is typically characterized by abnormal regulation of hormone production (e.g., defective feedback control) and peptide processing (resulting in large, unprocessed precursors).

A diverse array of molecular mechanisms has been suggested to cause ectopic hormone production, but this process remains incompletely understood. In rare instances, genetic rearrangements explain aberrant hormone expression. For example, translocation of the *parathyroid hormone (PTH)* gene resulted in high levels of PTH expression in an ovarian carcinoma, presumably because the genetic rearrangement brings the *PTH* gene under the control of ovary-specific regulatory elements. A related phenomenon is well documented in many forms of leukemia and lymphoma, in which somatic genetic rearrangements confer a growth advantage and alter cellular differentiation and function (Chap. 105). Although genetic rearrangements may cause selected cases of ectopic hormone production, this mechanism is probably unusual, as many tumors are associated with excessive production of numerous peptides. It is likely that cellular dedifferentiation underlies most cases of ectopic hormone production. In support of this idea, many cancers are poorly differentiated histologically, and certain tumor products, such as human chorionic gonadotropin (hCG), parathyroid hormone–related protein (PTHrP), and α fetoprotein, are characteristic of gene expression at earlier developmental stages. On the other hand, the propensity of certain cancers to produce particular hormones (e.g., squamous cell carcinomas produce PTHrP) suggests that dedifferentiation is partial or that selective pathways are derepressed. These expression profiles are likely to be driven by alterations in transcriptional repression, changes in DNA methylation, or other factors that govern cell differentiation. Consistent with this idea, many solid tumors harbor poorly differentiated "cancer stem cells," a subpopulation of cells that are capable of initiating new tumors.

In SCLC, the pathway of differentiation has been defined. The neuroendocrine phenotype is dictated in part by the basic-helix-loop-helix (bHLH) transcription factor human achaete-scute homologue 1 (hASH-1), which is expressed at abnormally high levels in SCLC associated with ectopic ACTH. The activity of hASH-1 is inhibited by hairy enhancer of split 1 (HES-1) and by Notch proteins, which are also capable of inducing growth arrest. Thus, abnormal expression of these developmental transcription factors appears to provide a link between cell proliferation and differentiation.

Ectopic hormone production would only be an epiphenomenon associated with cancer if it did not result in clinical manifestations. Excessive and unregulated production of hormones such as ACTH, PTHrP, or vasopressin can lead to substantial morbidity and can complicate the cancer treatment plan. Moreover, the paraneoplastic endocrinopathies are sometimes the presenting feature of underlying malignancy and may prompt the search for an unrecognized tumor.

A large number of paraneoplastic endocrine syndromes have been described, linking overproduction of particular hormones with specific types of tumors. However, certain recurring syndromes emerge from this group (Table 96-1). The most common paraneoplastic endocrine syndromes include hypercalcemia from overproduction of PTHrP and other factors, hyponatremia from excess vasopressin, and Cushing's syndrome from ectopic ACTH.

TABLE 96-1   PARANEOPLASTIC SYNDROMES CAUSED BY ECTOPIC HORMONE PRODUCTION

Paraneoplastic Syndrome	Ectopic Hormone	Typical Tumor Types[a]
Common		
Hypercalcemia of malignancy	Parathyroid hormone-related protein (PTHrP)	Squamous cell (head and neck, lung, skin), breast, genitourinary, gastrointestinal
	1,25 dihydroxyvitamin D	Lymphomas
	Parathyroid hormone (PTH) (rare)	Lung, ovary
	Prostaglandin E2 (PGE2) (rare)	Renal, lung
Syndrome of inappropriate antidiuretic hormone secretion (SIADH)	Vasopressin	Lung (squamous, small cell), gastrointestinal, genitourinary, ovary
Cushing's syndrome	Adrenocorticotropic hormone (ACTH)	Lung (small cell, bronchial carcinoid, adenocarcinoma, squamous), thymus, pancreatic islet, medullary thyroid carcinoma
	Corticotropin-releasing hormone (CRH) (rare)	Pancreatic islet, carcinoid, lung, prostate
	Ectopic expression of gastric inhibitory peptide (GIP), luteinizing hormone (LH)/ human chorionic gonadotropin (hCG), other G protein–coupled receptors (rare)	Macronodular adrenal hyperplasia
Less Common		
Non-islet cell hypoglycemia	Insulin-like growth factor (IGF-II)	Mesenchymal tumors, sarcomas, adrenal, hepatic, gastrointestinal, kidney, prostate
	Insulin (rare)	Cervix (small cell carcinoma)
Male feminization	hCG[b]	Testis (embryonal, seminomas), germinomas, choriocarcinoma, lung, hepatic, pancreatic islet
Diarrhea or intestinal hypermotility	Calcitonin[c]	Lung, colon, breast, medullary thyroid carcinoma
	Vasoactive intestinal peptide (VIP)	Pancreas, pheochromocytoma, esophagus
Rare		
Oncogenic osteomalacia	Phosphatonin [fibroblast growth factor 23 (FGF23)]	Hemangiopericytomas, osteoblastomas, fibromas, sarcomas, giant cell tumors, prostate, lung
Acromegaly	Growth hormone–releasing hormone (GHRH)	Pancreatic islet, bronchial and other carcinoids
	Growth hormone (GH)	Lung, pancreatic islet
Hyperthyroidism	Thyroid-stimulating hormone (TSH)	Hydatidiform mole, embryonal tumors, struma ovarii
Hypertension	Renin	Juxtaglomerula tumors, kidney, lung, pancreas, ovary

[a]Only the most common tumor types are listed. For most ectopic hormone syndromes, an extensive list of tumors has been reported to produce one or more hormones.

[b]hCG is produced eutopically by trophoblastic tumors. Certain tumors produce disproportionate amounts of the hCG α or hCG β subunits. High levels of hCG rarely cause hyperthyroidism because of weak binding to the TSH receptor.

[c]Calcitonin is produced eutopically by medullary thyroid carcinoma and is used as a tumor marker.

HYPERCALCEMIA CAUSED BY ECTOPIC PRODUCTION OF PTHrP
(See also Chap. 347)

Etiology Humoral hypercalcemia of malignancy (HHM) occurs in up to 20% of patients with cancer. HHM is most common in cancers of the lung, head and neck, skin, esophagus, breast, genitourinary tract, and in multiple myeloma and lymphomas. Several distinct humoral causes of HHM occur, most commonly overproduction of PTHrP. In addition to acting as a circulating humoral factor, bone metastases (e.g., breast, multiple myeloma) may produce PTHrP, leading to local osteolysis and hypercalcemia.

PTHrP is structurally related to PTH and it binds to the PTH receptor, explaining the similar biochemical features of HHM and hyperparathyroidism. PTHrP plays a key role in skeletal development and regulates cellular proliferation and differentiation in other tissues including skin, bone marrow, breast, and hair follicles. The mechanism of PTHrP induction in malignancy is incompletely understood; however, tumor-bearing tissues commonly associated with HHM normally produce PTHrP during development or cell renewal. Mutations in certain oncogenes, such as *Ras*, can activate PTHrP expression. In adult T cell lymphoma, the transactivating Tax protein produced by human T-cell lymphotropic virus I (HTLV-I) stimulates PTHrP promoter activity. Metastatic lesions to bone are more likely to produce PTHrP than are metastases in other tissues, suggesting that bone produces factors that enhance PTHrP production, or that PTHrP-producing metastases have a selective growth advantage in bone. Thus, PTHrP production can be stimulated by mutations in oncogenes, by altered expression of viral or cellular transcription factors, and by local growth factors.

Another relatively common cause of HHM is excess production of 1,25-dihydroxyvitamin D. Like granulomatous disorders associated with hypercalcemia, lymphomas can produce an enzyme that converts 25-hydroxyvitamin D to the more active 1,25-dihydroxyvitamin D, leading to enhanced gastrointestinal calcium absorption. Other causes of HHM include tumor-mediated production of osteolytic cytokines and inflammatory mediators.

Clinical Manifestations The typical presentation of HHM is a patient with a known malignancy who is found to be hypercalcemic on routine laboratory tests. Less often, hypercalcemia is the initial presenting feature of malignancy. Particularly when calcium levels are markedly increased [>3.5 mmol/L (>14 mg/dL)], patients may experience fatigue, mental status changes, dehydration, or symptoms of nephrolithiasis.

Diagnosis Features that favor HHM, as opposed to primary hyperparathyroidism, include known malignancy, recent onset of hypercalcemia, and very high serum calcium levels. Like hyperparathyroidism, hypercalcemia caused by PTHrP is accompanied by hypercalciuria and hypophosphatemia. Measurement of PTH is useful to exclude primary hyperparathyroidism; the PTH level should be suppressed in HHM. An elevated PTHrP level confirms the diagnosis, and it is increased in ~80% of hypercalcemic patients with cancer. 1,25-Dihydroxyvitamin D levels may be increased in patients with lymphoma.

℞ HUMORAL HYPERCALCEMIA OF MALIGNANCY

The management of HHM begins with removal of excess calcium in the diet, medications, or IV solutions. Oral phosphorus (e.g., 250 mg Neutra-Phos 3–4 times daily) should be given until serum phosphorus is >1.0 mmol/L (>3 mg/dL). Saline rehydration is used to dilute serum calcium and promote calciuresis. Forced diuresis with furosemide or other loop diuretics can enhance calcium excretion but provides relatively little value except in life-threatening hypercalcemia. When used, loop diuretics should be administered only after complete rehydration and with careful monitoring of fluid balance. Bisphosphonates such as pamidronate (30–90 mg IV), zolendronate (4–8 mg IV), or etidronate (7.5 mg/kg per day PO for 3–7 consecutive days) can reduce serum calcium within 1–2 days and suppress calcium release for several weeks. Bisphosphonate infusions can be repeated or oral bisphosphonates can be used for chronic treatment. Dialysis should be considered in severe hypercalcemia when saline hydration and bisphosphonate treatments are not possible or are too slow in onset. Previously used agents, such as calcitonin and mithramycin, have little utility now that bisphosphonates are available. Calcitonin (2–8 U/kg SC every 6–12 h) should be considered when rapid correction of severe hypercalcemia is needed. Hypercalcemia associated with lymphomas, multiple myeloma, or leukemia may respond to glucocorticoid treatment (e.g., prednisone 40–100 mg PO in four divided doses).

ECTOPIC VASOPRESSIN: TUMOR-ASSOCIATED SIADH
(See also Chap. 46)

Etiology Vasopressin is an antidiuretic hormone normally produced by the posterior pituitary gland. Ectopic vasopressin production by tumors is a common cause of the syndrome of inappropriate antidiuretic hormone (SIADH), occurring in at least half of patients with SCLC. Compensatory mechanisms, such as decreased thirst, suppression of aldosterone, and production of atrial natriuretic peptide (ANP), may mitigate the development of hyponatremia in patients who produce excessive vasopressin. Tumors with neuroendocrine features, such as SCLC and carcinoids, are the most common sources of ectopic vasopressin production, but it also occurs in other forms of lung cancer and with central nervous system (CNS) lesions, head and neck cancer, and genitourinary, gastrointestinal, and ovarian cancers. The mechanism of activation of the vasopressin gene in these tumors is unknown but often involves concomitant expression of the adjacent oxytocin gene, suggesting derepression of this locus.

Clinical Manifestations Most patients with ectopic vasopressin secretion are asymptomatic and are identified because of the presence of hyponatremia on routine chemistry testing. Symptoms may include weakness, lethargy, nausea, confusion, depressed mental status, and seizures. The severity of symptoms reflects the rapidity of onset as well as the extent of hyponatremia. Hyponatremia usually develops slowly but may be exacerbated by the administration of IV fluids or the institution of new medications. Thirst is typically suppressed.

Diagnosis The diagnostic features of ectopic vasopressin production are the same as those of other causes of SIADH (Chaps. 46 and 334). Hyponatremia and reduced serum osmolality occur in the setting of an inappropriately normal or increased urine osmolality. Urine sodium excretion is normal or increased unless volume depletion is present. Other causes of hyponatremia should be excluded, including renal, adrenal, or thyroid insufficiency. Physiologic sources of vasopressin stimulation (CNS lesions, pulmonary disease, nausea), adaptive circulatory mechanisms (hypotension, heart failure, hepatic cirrhosis), and medications, including many chemotherapeutic agents, should also be considered as possible causes of hyponatremia. Vasopressin assay is not usually necessary to make the diagnosis.

℞ ECTOPIC VASOPRESSIN: TUMOR-ASSOCIATED SIADH

Most patients with ectopic vasopressin production develop hyponatremia over several weeks or months. The disorder should be corrected gradually unless mental status is altered or there is risk of seizures. Treatment of the underlying malignancy may reduce ectopic vasopressin production but this response is slow, if it occurs at all. Fluid restriction to less than urine output, plus insensible losses, is often sufficient to partially correct hyponatremia. However, strict monitoring of the amount and types of liquids consumed or administered intravenously is required for fluid restriction to be effective. Salt tablets or saline are not helpful unless volume depletion is also present. Demeclocycline (150–300 mg orally three to four times daily) can be used to inhibit vasopressin action on the renal distal tubule but its onset of action is relatively slow (1–2 weeks). Conivaptan, a nonpeptide V$_2$-receptor antagonist, can be administered either PO (20–120 mg bid) or IV (10–40 mg), and is particularly effective when used in combination with fluid restriction in euvolemic hyponatremia. Severe hyponatremia (Na <

CHAPTER 96 Paraneoplastic Syndromes: Endocrinologic/Hematologic

115 meq/L) or mental status changes may require treatment with hypertonic (3%) or normal saline infusion together with furosemide, to enhance free water clearance. The rate of sodium correction should be slow (0.5–1 meq/L per h) to prevent rapid fluid shifts and the possible development of central pontine myelinolysis.

CUSHING'S SYNDROME CAUSED BY ECTOPIC ACTH PRODUCTION
(See also Chap. 336)

Etiology   Ectopic ACTH production accounts for 10–20% of Cushing's syndrome. The syndrome is particularly common in neuroendocrine tumors. SCLC (>50%) is by far the most common cause of ectopic ACTH, followed by thymic carcinoid (15%), islet cell tumors (10%), bronchial carcinoid (10%), other carcinoids (5%), and pheochromocytomas (2%). Ectopic ACTH production is caused by increased expression of the proopiomelanocortin (POMC) gene, which encodes ACTH, along with melanocyte-stimulating hormone (MSH), β lipotropin, and several other peptides. In many tumors, there is abundant but aberrant expression of the POMC gene from an internal promoter, proximal to the third exon, which encodes ACTH. However, because this product lacks the signal sequence necessary for protein processing, it is not secreted. Increased production of ACTH arises instead from less abundant, but unregulated, POMC expression from the same promoter site used in the pituitary. However, because the tumors lack many of the enzymes needed to process the POMC polypeptide, it is typically released as multiple large, biologically inactive fragments along with relatively small amounts of fully processed, active ACTH.

Rarely, corticotropin-releasing hormone (CRH) is produced by pancreatic islet tumors, SCLC, medullary thyroid cancer, carcinoids, or prostate cancer. When levels are high enough, CRH can cause pituitary corticotrope hyperplasia and Cushing's syndrome. Tumors that produce CRH sometimes also produce ACTH, raising the possibility of a paracrine mechanism for ACTH production.

A distinct mechanism for ACTH-independent Cushing's syndrome involves ectopic expression of various G protein–coupled receptors in the adrenal nodules. Ectopic expression of the gastric inhibitory peptide (GIP) receptor is the best-characterized example of this mechanism. In this case, meals induce GIP secretion, which inappropriately stimulates adrenal growth and glucocorticoid production.

Clinical Manifestations   The clinical features of hypercortisolemia are detected in only a small fraction of patients with documented ectopic ACTH production. Patients with ectopic ACTH syndrome generally exhibit less marked weight gain and centripetal fat redistribution, probably because the exposure to excess glucocorticoids is relatively short and because cachexia reduces the propensity for weight gain and fat deposition. The ectopic ACTH syndrome is associated with several clinical features that distinguish it from other causes of Cushing's syndrome (e.g., pituitary adenomas, adrenal adenomas, iatrogenic glucocorticoid excess). The metabolic manifestations of ectopic ACTH syndrome are dominated by fluid retention and hypertension, hypokalemia, metabolic alkalosis, glucose intolerance, and, often, steroid psychosis. The very high ACTH levels often cause increased pigmentation, and melanotrope-stimulating hormone (MSH) activity derived from the POMC precursor peptide is also increased. The extraordinarily high glucocorticoid levels in patients with ectopic sources of ACTH can lead to marked skin fragility and easy bruising. In addition, the high cortisol levels often overwhelm the renal 11β-hydroxysteroid dehydrogenase type II enzyme, which normally inactivates cortisol and prevents it from binding to renal mineralocorticoid receptors. Consequently, in addition to the excess mineralocorticoids produced by ACTH stimulation of the adrenal gland, high levels of cortisol exert activity through the mineralocorticoid receptor, leading to severe hypokalemia.

Diagnosis   The diagnosis of ectopic ACTH syndrome is usually not difficult in the setting of a known malignancy. Urine free cortisol levels fluctuate but are typically greater than two to four times normal and the plasma ACTH level is usually >22 pmol/L (>100 pg/mL). A suppressed ACTH level excludes this diagnosis and indicates an ACTH-independent cause of Cushing's syndrome (e.g., adrenal or exogenous glucocorticoid). In contrast to pituitary sources of ACTH, most ectopic sources of ACTH do not respond to glucocorticoid suppression. Therefore, high-dose dexamethasone (8 mg PO) suppresses 8:00 A.M. serum cortisol (50% decrease from baseline) in ~80% of pituitary ACTH-producing adenomas but fails to suppress ectopic ACTH in ~90% of cases. Bronchial and other carcinoids are well-documented exceptions to these general guidelines, as these ectopic sources of ACTH may exhibit feedback regulation indistinguishable from pituitary adenomas, including suppression by high-dose dexamethasone, and ACTH responsiveness to adrenal blockade with metyrapone. If necessary, petrosal sinus catheterization can be used to evaluate a patient with ACTH-dependent Cushing's syndrome when the source of ACTH is unclear. After CRH stimulation, a 3:1 petrosal sinus:peripheral ACTH ratio strongly suggests a pituitary ACTH source. Imaging studies are also useful in the evaluation of suspected carcinoid lesions, allowing biopsy and characterization of hormone production using special stains.

℞ CUSHING'S SYNDROME CAUSED BY ECTOPIC ACTH PRODUCTION

The morbidity associated with the ectopic ACTH syndrome can be substantial. Patients may experience depression or personality changes because of extreme cortisol excess. Metabolic derangements including diabetes mellitus and hypokalemia can worsen fatigue. Poor wound healing and predisposition to infections can complicate the surgical management of tumors, and opportunistic infections, caused by organisms such as *Pneumocystis carinii* and mycoses, are often the cause of death in patients with ectopic ACTH production. Depending on prognosis and treatment plans for the underlying malignancy, measures to reduce cortisol levels are often indicated. Treatment of the underlying malignancy may reduce ACTH levels but is rarely sufficient to reduce cortisol levels to normal. Adrenalectomy is not practical for most of these patients but should be considered if the underlying tumor is not resectable and the prognosis is otherwise favorable (e.g., carcinoid). Medical therapy with ketoconazole (200–400 mg PO bid), metyrapone (250–500 mg PO every 6 h), mitotane (3–6 g PO in four divided doses, tapered to maintain low cortisol production), or other agents that block steroid synthesis or action is often the most practical strategy for managing the hypercortisolism associated with ectopic ACTH production (Chap. 333). Glucocorticoid replacement should be provided to avoid adrenal insufficiency. Unfortunately, many patients will eventually progress despite medical blockade.

TUMOR-INDUCED HYPOGLYCEMIA CAUSED BY EXCESS PRODUCTION OF IGF-II
(See also Chap. 339)   Mesenchymal tumors, hemangiopericytomas, hepatocellular tumors, adrenal carcinomas, and a variety of other large tumors have been reported to produce excessive amounts of insulin-like growth factor type II (IGF-II) precursor, which binds weakly to insulin receptors and strongly to IGF-I receptors, leading to insulin-like actions. The gene encoding IGF-II resides on a chromosome 11p15 locus that is normally imprinted (that is, expression is exclusively from a single parental allele). Biallelic expression of the IGF-II gene occurs in a subset of tumors, suggesting loss of methylation and loss of imprinting as a mechanism for gene induction. In addition to increased IGF-II production, IGF-II bioavailability is increased due to complex alterations in circulating binding proteins. Increased IGF-II suppresses growth hormone (GH) and insulin, resulting in reduced IGF binding protein 3 (IGFBP-3), IGF-I, and acid-labile subunit (ALS). The reduction in ALS and IGFBP-3, which normally sequester IGF-II, causes it to be displaced to a small circulating complex that has greater access to insulin target tissues. For this reason, circulating IGF-II levels may not be markedly increased, despite causing hypoglycemia. In addition to IGF-II–mediated hypoglycemia, tumors may occupy enough of the liver to impair gluconeogenesis.

In most cases, the tumor causing hypoglycemia is clinically apparent and hypoglycemia develops in association with fasting. The diagnosis is made by documenting low serum glucose and suppressed insulin levels in association with symptoms of hypoglycemia. Serum IGF-II levels may not be increased (IGF-II assays may not detect IGF-II precursors). Increased IGF-II mRNA expression is found in most of these tumors. Any medications associated with hypoglycemia should be eliminated. Treatment of the underlying malignancy, if possible, may reduce the predisposition to hypoglycemia. Frequent meals and IV glucose, especially during sleep or fasting, are often necessary to prevent hypoglycemia. Glucagon, GH, and glucocorticoids have also been used to enhance glucose production.

HUMAN CHORIONIC GONADOTROPIN

hCG is composed of α and β subunits and can be produced as intact hormone, which is biologically active, or as uncombined biologically inert subunits. Ectopic production of intact hCG occurs most often in association with testicular embryonal tumors, germ cell tumors, extragonadal germinomas, lung cancer, hepatoma, and pancreatic islet tumors. Eutopic production of hCG occurs with trophoblastic malignancies. Low levels of hCG or its uncombined α or β subunits have been reported in a wide array of tumors. hCG α subunit production is particularly common in lung cancer and pancreatic islet cancer. In men, high hCG levels stimulate steroidogenesis and aromatase activity in testicular Leydig cells, resulting in increased estrogen production and the development of gynecomastia. Precocious puberty in boys or gynecomastia in men should prompt measurement of hCG and consideration of a testicular tumor or another source of ectopic hCG production. Most women are asymptomatic. hCG is easily measured. Treatment should be directed at the underlying malignancy.

ONCOGENIC OSTEOMALACIA

Hypophosphatemic oncogenic osteomalacia, also called tumor-induced osteomalacia (TIO), is characterized by markedly reduced serum phosphorus and renal phosphate wasting, leading to muscle weakness, bone pain, and osteomalacia. Serum calcium and PTH levels are normal and 1,25-dihydroxyvitamin D is low. Oncogenic osteomalacia is usually caused by benign mesenchymal tumors, such as hemangiopericytomas, fibromas, or giant cell tumors, often of the skeletal extremities or head. It has also been described in sarcomas and in patients with prostate and lung cancer. Resection of the tumor reverses the disorder, confirming its humoral basis. The circulating phosphaturic factor is called *phosphatonin*—a factor that inhibits renal tubular reabsorption of phosphate and renal conversion of 25-hydroxyvitamin D to 1,25-dihydroxyvitamin D. Phosphatonin has been identified as fibroblast growth factor 23 (FGF23). FGF23 levels are increased in some, but not all, patients with osteogenic osteomalacia. The disorder exhibits biochemical features similar to those seen with inactivating mutations in the *PHEX* gene, the cause of hereditary X-linked hypophosphatemia. The *PHEX* gene encodes a protease that activates FGF23. Treatment involves removal of the tumor, if possible, and supplementation with phosphate and vitamin D. Octreotide treatment reduces phosphate wasting in some patients with tumors that express somatostatin receptor subtype 2. Octreotide scans may also be useful to detect these tumors.

HEMATOLOGIC SYNDROMES

The elevation of granulocyte, platelet, and eosinophil counts in most patients with myeloproliferative disorders is caused by the proliferation of the myeloid elements due to the underlying disease rather than a paraneoplastic syndrome. The paraneoplastic hematologic syndromes in patients with solid tumors are less well characterized than the endocrine syndromes because the ectopic hormone(s) or cytokines responsible have not been identified in most of these tumors (Table 96-2). The extent of the paraneoplastic syndromes parallels the course of the cancer.

ERYTHROCYTOSIS

Ectopic production of erythropoietin by cancer cells causes most paraneoplastic erythrocytosis. The ectopically produced erythropoietin stimulates the production of red blood cells (RBC) in the bone mar-

TABLE 96-2 PARANEOPLASTIC HEMATOLOGIC SYNDROMES

Syndrome	Proteins	Cancers Typically Associated with Syndrome
Erythrocytosis	Erythropoietin	Renal cancers
		Hepatocarcinoma
		Cerebellar hemangioblastomas
Granulocytosis	G-CSF	Lung cancer
	GM-CSF	Gastrointestinal cancer
	IL-6	Ovarian cancer
		Genitourinary cancer
		Hodgkin's disease
Thrombocytosis	IL-6	Lung cancer
		Gastrointestinal cancer
		Breast cancer
		Ovarian cancer
		Lymphoma
Eosinophilia	IL-5	Lymphoma
		Leukemia
		Lung cancer
Thrombophlebitis	Unknown	Lung cancer
		Pancreatic cancer
		Gastrointestinal cancer
		Breast cancer
		Genitourinary cancer
		Ovarian cancer
		Prostate cancer
		Lymphoma

Note: G-CSF, granulocyte colony-stimulating factor; GM-CSF, granulocyte-macrophage CSF; IL, interleukin.

row and raises the hematocrit. Other lymphokines and hormones produced by cancer cells may stimulate erythropoietin release but have not been proven to cause erythrocytosis.

Most patients with erythrocytosis have an elevated hematocrit (>52% in men; >48% in women) that is detected on a routine blood count. Approximately 3% of patients with renal cell cancer, 10% of patients with hepatoma, and 15% of patients with cerebellar hemangioblastomas have erythrocytosis. In most cases the erythrocytosis is asymptomatic.

Patients with erythrocytosis due to a renal cell cancer, hepatoma, or CNS cancer should have measurement of red cell mass. If the red cell mass is elevated, the serum erythropoietin level should then be measured. Patients with an appropriate cancer, elevated erythropoietin levels, and no other explanation for erythrocytosis (e.g., hemoglobinopathy that causes increased O_2 affinity; Chap. 58) have the paraneoplastic syndrome.

℞ ERYTHROCYTOSIS

Successful resection of the cancer usually resolves the erythrocytosis. If the tumor cannot be resected or treated effectively with radiation therapy or chemotherapy, phlebotomy may control any symptoms related to erythrocytosis.

GRANULOCYTOSIS

Approximately 30% of patients with solid tumors have granulocytosis (granulocyte count > 8000/μL). In about half of patients with granulocytosis and cancer, the granulocytosis has an identifiable nonparaneoplastic etiology (infection, tumor necrosis, glucocorticoid administration, etc.). The other patients have proteins in urine and serum that stimulate the growth of bone marrow cells. Tumors and tumor cell lines from patients with lung, ovarian, and bladder cancers have been documented to produce granulocyte colony-stimulating factor (G-CSF), granulocyte-macrophage colony-stimulating factor (GM-CSF), and/or interleukin 6 (IL-6). However, the etiology of granulocytosis has not been characterized in most patients.

Patients with granulocytosis are nearly all asymptomatic, and the differential white blood cell count does not have a shift to immature forms of neutrophils. Granulocytosis occurs in 40% of patients with lung and gastrointestinal cancers, 20% of patients with breast cancer, 30% of patients with brain tumors and ovarian cancers, 20% of patients with Hodgkin's disease, and 10% of patients with renal cell carcinoma. Patients with advanced-stage disease are more likely to have granulocytosis than those with early-stage disease.

Paraneoplastic granulocytosis does not require treatment. The granulocytosis resolves when the underlying cancer is treated.

THROMBOCYTOSIS

Some 35% of patients with thrombocytosis (platelet count > 400,000/μL) have an underlying diagnosis of cancer. IL-6, a candidate molecule for the etiology of paraneoplastic thrombocytosis, stimulates the production of platelets in vitro and in vivo. Some patients with cancer and thrombocytosis have elevated levels of IL-6 in plasma. Another candidate molecule is thrombopoietin, a peptide hormone that stimulates megakaryocyte proliferation and platelet production. The etiology of thrombocytosis has not been established in most cases.

Patients with thrombocytosis are nearly all asymptomatic. Thrombocytosis is not clearly linked to thrombosis in patients with cancer. Thrombocytosis is present in 40% of patients with lung and gastrointestinal cancers, 20% of patients with breast, endometrial, and ovarian cancers, and 10% of patients with lymphoma. Patients with thrombocytosis are more likely to have advanced-stage disease and have a poorer prognosis than patients without thrombocytosis. Paraneoplastic thrombocytosis does not require treatment.

EOSINOPHILIA

Eosinophilia is present in ~1% of patients with cancer. Tumors and tumor cell lines from patients with lymphomas or leukemia may produce IL-5, which stimulates eosinophil growth. Activation of IL-5 transcription in lymphomas and leukemias may involve translocation of the long arm of chromosome 5, to which the genes for IL-5 and other cytokines map.

Patients with eosinophilia are typically asymptomatic. Eosinophilia is present in 10% of patients with lymphoma, 3% of patients with lung cancer, and occasional patients with cervical, gastrointestinal, renal, and breast cancer. Patients with markedly elevated eosinophil counts (>5000/μL) can develop shortness of breath and wheezing. A chest radiograph may reveal diffuse pulmonary infiltrates from eosinophil infiltration and activation in the lungs.

℞ EOSINOPHILIA

Definitive treatment is directed at the underlying malignancy: tumors should be resected or treated with radiation or chemotherapy. In most patients who develop shortness of breath related to eosinophilia, symptoms resolve with the use of oral or inhaled glucocorticoids.

THROMBOPHLEBITIS

Deep venous thrombosis and pulmonary embolism are the most common thrombotic conditions in patients with cancer. Migratory or recurrent thrombophlebitis may be the initial manifestation of cancer. Nearly 15% of patients who develop deep venous thrombosis or pulmonary embolism have a diagnosis of cancer (Chap. 111). The coexistence of peripheral venous thrombosis with visceral carcinoma, particularly pancreatic cancer, is called *Trousseau's syndrome*.

Pathogenesis Patients with cancer are predisposed to thromboembolism because they are often at bedrest or immobilized, and tumors may obstruct or slow blood flow. Chronic IV catheters also predispose to clotting. In addition, clotting may be promoted by release of procoagulants or cytokines from tumor cells or associated inflammatory cells, or by platelet adhesion or aggregation. The specific molecules that promote thromboembolism have not been identified.

In addition to cancer causing secondary thrombosis, primary thrombophilic diseases may be associated with cancer. For example, the antiphospholipid antibody syndrome is associated with a wide range of pathologic manifestations. About 20% of patients with this syndrome have cancers. Among patients with cancer and antiphospholipid antibodies, 35–45% develop thrombosis.

Clinical Manifestations Patients with cancer who develop deep venous thrombosis usually develop swelling or pain in the leg, and physical examination reveals tenderness, warmth, and redness. Patients who present with pulmonary embolism develop dyspnea, chest pain, and syncope, and physical examination shows tachycardia, cyanosis, and hypotension. Some 5% of patients with no history of cancer who have a diagnosis of deep venous thrombosis or pulmonary embolism will have a diagnosis of cancer within 1 year. The most common cancers associated with thromboembolic episodes include lung, pancreatic, gastrointestinal, breast, ovarian, and genitourinary cancers, lymphomas, and brain tumors. Patients with cancer who undergo surgical procedures requiring general anesthesia have a 20–30% risk of deep venous thrombosis.

Diagnosis The diagnosis of deep venous thrombosis in patients with cancer is made by impedance plethysmography or bilateral compression ultrasonography of the leg veins. Patients with a noncompressible venous segment have deep venous thrombosis. If compression ultrasonography is normal and a high clinical suspicion exists for deep venous thrombosis, venography should be done to look for a luminal filling defect. Elevation of D-dimer is not as predictive of deep venous thrombosis in patients with cancer as it is in patients without cancer.

Patients with symptoms and signs suggesting a pulmonary embolism should be evaluated with a chest radiograph, electrocardiogram, arterial blood gas analysis, and ventilation–perfusion scan. Patients with mismatched segmental perfusion defects have a pulmonary embolus. Patients with equivocal ventilation–perfusion findings should be evaluated as described above for deep venous thrombosis in their legs. If deep venous thrombosis is detected, they should be anticoagulated. If deep venous thrombosis is not detected, they should be considered for a pulmonary angiogram.

Patients without a diagnosis of cancer who present with an initial episode of thrombophlebitis or pulmonary embolus need no additional tests for cancer other than a careful history and physical examination. In light of the many possible primary sites, diagnostic testing in asymptomatic patients is wasteful. However, if the clot is refractory to standard treatment or is in an unusual site, or if the thrombophlebitis is migratory or recurrent, efforts to find an underlying cancer are indicated.

℞ THROMBOPHLEBITIS

Patients with cancer and a diagnosis of deep venous thrombosis or pulmonary embolism should be treated initially with IV unfractionated heparin or low-molecular-weight heparin for at least 5 days and warfarin started within 1 or 2 days. The warfarin dose should be adjusted so the international normalized ratio (INR) is 2–3. Patients with proximal deep venous thrombosis and a relative contraindication to heparin anticoagulation (hemorrhagic brain metastases or pericardial effusion) should be considered for placement of a filter in the inferior vena cava (Greenfield filter) to prevent pulmonary embolism. Warfarin should be administered for 3–6 months. An alternative approach is to use low-molecular-weight heparin for 6 months. Patients with cancer who undergo a major surgical procedure should be considered for heparin prophylaxis or pneumatic boots. Breast cancer patients undergoing chemotherapy and patients with implanted catheters should be considered for prophylaxis (1 mg/d warfarin).

Cutaneous paraneoplastic syndromes are discussed in Chap. 54. Neurologic paraneoplastic syndromes are discussed in Chap. 97.

FURTHER READINGS

AL-TOURAH AJ et al: Paraneoplastic erythropoietin-induced polycythemia associated with small lymphocytic lymphoma. J Clin Oncol 24:2388, 2006

DELELLIS RA, XIA L: Paraneoplastic endocrine syndromes: A review. Endocr Pathol 14:303, 2003

EMEL EA et al: Sensitivity of fibroblast growth factor 23 measurements in tumor-induced osteomalacia. J Clin Endocrinol Metab 91:2055, 2006

GABRILOVICH M et al: Paraneoplastic polymyositis associated with squamous cell carcinoma of the lung. Chest 129(6):1721, 2006

JAN DE BEUR SM: Tumor-induced osteomalacia. JAMA 294:1260, 2005

JONES PA, BAYLIN SB: The fundamental role of epigenetic events in cancer. Nat Rev Genet 3:415, 2002

STEWART AF: Clinical practice. Hypercalcemia associated with cancer. N Engl J Med 352:373, 2005

97 Paraneoplastic Neurologic Syndromes

Josep Dalmau, Myrna R. Rosenfeld

Paraneoplastic neurologic disorders (PNDs) are cancer-related syndromes that can affect any part of the nervous system (Table 97-1). They are remote effects of cancer, caused by mechanisms other than metastasis or by any of the complications of cancer such as coagulopathy, stroke, metabolic and nutritional conditions, infections, and side effects of cancer therapy. In 60% of patients the neurologic symptoms precede the cancer diagnosis. Overall, clinically disabling PNDs occur in 0.5–1% of all cancer patients, but they occur in 2–3% of patients with neuroblastoma or small cell lung cancer (SCLC), and in 30–50% of patients with thymoma or sclerotic myeloma.

PATHOGENESIS

Most PNDs are mediated by immune responses triggered by neuronal proteins (onconeuronal antigens) expressed by tumors. In PNDs of the central nervous system (CNS), many antibody-associated immune responses have been identified (Table 97-2). These antibodies usually react with the patient's tumor, and their detection in serum or cerebrospinal fluid (CSF) strongly predicts the presence of cancer. The target antigens are usually intracellular proteins with roles in neuronal development and function. Some of the antibodies react with epitopes located in critical protein domains, disrupting protein function and leading to neuronal apoptosis. In addition to onconeuronal antibodies, most PNDs of the CNS are associated with infiltrates of CD4+ and CD8+ T cells, microglial activation, gliosis, and variable neuronal loss. The infiltrating T cells are often in close contact with neurons undergoing degeneration, suggesting a primary pathogenic role. T cell–mediated cytotoxicity may contribute directly to cell death in these PNDs. Thus both humoral and cellular immune mechanisms participate in the pathogenesis of many PNDs. This complex immunopathogenesis may underlie the resistance of many of these conditions to therapy.

Neuronal cell-surface antigens can be the target of antibodies in some patients with paraneoplastic encephalitis. A few of these antigens have been identified, including the NR1/NR2 subunits of NMDA receptors (Fig. 97-1) and voltage-gated potassium channels (VGKC). These disorders are more responsive to immunotherapy than those associated with immune responses to intracellular antigens.

Only four of the antibodies listed in Table 97-2 have been shown to play a direct pathogenic role in PNDs; all produce distinctive disorders of the peripheral nervous system. These are: antibodies to P/Q-type voltage-gated calcium channels (VGCC) in patients with the Lambert-Eaton myasthenic syndrome (LEMS); antibodies to acetylcholine receptors in patients with myasthenia gravis; antibodies to VGKC in some patients with peripheral nerve hyperexcitability (neuromyotonia); and antibodies to ganglionic acetylcholine receptors in some patients with autonomic neuropathy. Common features of these four antibodies are that they target cell-surface molecules and that their passive transfer to animals reproduces the disorders. Plasma exchange or immunomodulation with intravenous immunoglobulin (IVIg) usually produces neurologic improvement. Each of these disorders can occur without cancer, and therefore detection of these antibodies does not predict the presence of cancer.

Other PNDs are likely immune-mediated, although their antigens are unknown. These include several syndromes of inflammatory neuropathies and myopathies. In addition, many patients with typical PND syndromes are antibody-negative.

For still other PNDs, the cause remains quite obscure. These include, among others, several neuropathies that occur in the terminal stages of cancer and a number of neuropathies associated with plasma cell dyscrasias or lymphoma without evidence of inflammatory infiltrates or deposits of immunoglobulin, cryoglobulin, or amyloid.

TABLE 97-1   PARANEOPLASTIC SYNDROMES OF THE NERVOUS SYSTEM

Syndromes of the brain, brainstem, and cerebellum
  Focal encephalitis
    Cortical encephalitis
    Limbic encephalitis
    Brainstem encephalitis
    Cerebellar dysfunction
    Autonomic dysfunction
  Paraneoplastic cerebellar degeneration
  Opsoclonus-myoclonus
Syndromes of the spinal cord
  Subacute necrotizing myelopathy
  Motor neuron dysfunction
  Myelitis
  Stiff-person syndrome
Syndromes of dorsal root ganglia
  Sensory neuronopathy
Multiple levels of involvement
  Encephalomyelitis,[a] sensory neuronopathy, autonomic dysfunction
Syndromes of peripheral nerve
  Chronic and subacute sensorimotor peripheral neuropathy
  Vasculitis of nerve and muscle
  Neuropathy associated with malignant monoclonal gammopathies
  Peripheral nerve hyperexcitability
  Autonomic neuropathy
Syndromes of the neuromuscular junction
  Lambert-Eaton myasthenic syndrome
  Myasthenia gravis
Syndromes of the muscle
  Polymyositis/dermatomyositis
  Acute necrotizing myopathy
Syndromes affecting the visual system
  Cancer-associated retinopathy (CAR)
  Melanoma-associated retinopathy (MAR)
  Uveitis (usually in association with encephalomyelitis)

[a]Includes cortical, limbic, or brainstem encephalitis, cerebellar dysfunction, myelitis.

APPROACH TO THE PATIENT:
Paraneoplastic Neurologic Disorders

The diagnosis and management of PNDs may be difficult for several reasons. First, it is common for symptoms to appear before the presence of a tumor is known. Second, the neurologic syndrome can evolve in a rapidly progressive fashion, producing a severe and usually irreversible neurologic deficit in a short period of time. There is evidence that prompt tumor control improves the course of PNDs. Therefore, the major concern of the physician is to recognize a disorder promptly as paraneoplastic in order to identify and treat the tumor.

PND OF THE CENTRAL NERVOUS SYSTEM AND DORSAL ROOT GANGLIA
When symptoms involve brain, spinal cord, or dorsal root ganglia, the suspicion of PND is usually based on a combination of clinical, radiologic, and CSF findings. In these cases, a biopsy of the affected tissue is often difficult to obtain, and although useful to rule out other disorders (e.g., metastasis, infection), neuropathologic findings are

PART 6

Oncology and Hematology

TABLE 97-2 PARANEOPLASTIC ANTINEURONAL ANTIBODIES, ASSOCIATED SYNDROMES AND CANCERS

Antibody	Syndrome	Associated Cancers
Anti-Hu (ANNA-1)	PEM (including cortical, limbic, brainstem encephalitis, cerebellar dysfunction, myelitis), PSN, autonomic dysfunction	SCLC, other neuroendocrine tumors
Anti-Yo (PCA-1)	PCD	Ovary and other gynecologic cancers, breast
Anti-Ri (ANNA-2)	PCD, brainstem encephalitis, opsoclonus-myoclonus	Breast, gynecological, SCLC
Anti-Tr	PCD	Hodgkin's lymphoma
Anti-Zic	PCD, encephalomyelitis	SCLC and other neuro-endocrine tumors
Anti-CV$_2$/CRMP5	PEM, PCD, chorea, peripheral neuropathy, uveitis	SCLC, thymoma, other
Anti-Ma proteins[a]	Limbic, hypothalamic, brainstem encephalitis (infrequently PCD)	Germ-cell tumors of testis, lung cancer, other solid tumors
Anti-NR1/NR2 subunits of NMDA receptor	Encephalitis with prominent psychiatric symptoms, seizures, hypoventilation	Ovarian teratoma
Anti-amphiphysin	Stiff-person syndrome, PEM	Breast, SCLC
Anti-VGCC[b]	LEMS, PCD	SCLC, lymphoma
Anti-AChR[b]	MG	Thymoma
Anti-VGKC[b]	Peripheral nerve hyperexcitability (neuromyotonia), limbic encephalitis	Thymoma, SCLC, others
Anti-recoverin	Cancer-associated retinopathy (CAR)	SCLC and other
Anti-bipolar cells of the retina	Melanoma-associated retinopathy (MAR)	Melanoma

[a]Patients with antibodies to Ma2 are usually men with testicular cancer. Patients with additional antibodies to other Ma proteins are men or women with a variety of solid tumors.
[b]These antibodies can occur with or without a cancer association.
Note: PEM: paraneoplastic encephalomyelitis; PCD, paraneoplastic cerebellar degeneration; PSN, paraneoplastic sensory neuronopathy; LEMS, Lambert-Eaton myasthenic syndrome; MG, myasthenia gravis; VGCC, voltage-gated calcium channel; AChR, acetylcholine receptor; VGKC, voltage-gated potassium channel; SCLC, small-cell lung cancer; NMDA, N-methyl-D-aspartate.

not specific for PND. Furthermore, there are no specific radiologic or electrophysiologic tests that are diagnostic of PND. The presence of antineuronal antibodies (Table 97-2) may help in the diagnosis with the following caveats: (1) antibodies are detected in only 60–70% of PNDs of the CNS; (2) antibodies may be present in both the serum and CSF, but in some patients only the CSF is positive (especially with antibodies to Tr and Ma proteins); (3) antibodies (usually at low titer) are present in a variable proportion of cancer patients without PND; (4) there is an imperfect correlation between antibody titers and the course of the neurologic disorder; (5) several antibodies may associate with a similar syndrome, with the antibody specificity often correlating with the tumor type (e.g., cerebellar degeneration is associated with anti-Tr antibodies if the tumor is Hodgkin's disease but with anti-Yo antibodies if the tumor is ovarian or breast cancer); and (6) several antibodies may be present in the serum or CSF of the same patient (e.g., anti-Hu and anti-CV$_2$/CRMP5).

MRI and CSF studies are important to rule out neurologic complications due to the direct spread of cancer, particularly metastatic and leptomeningeal disease. In most PNDs the MRI findings are nonspecific. Paraneoplastic limbic encephalitis is usually associated with characteristic MRI abnormalities in the mesial temporal lobes (see below), but similar findings can occur with other disorders [e.g., nonparaneoplastic limbic encephalitis with antibodies to VGKC, human herpesvirus (HHV) 6 encephalitis] (Fig. 97-2). The CSF profile of patients with PND of the CNS or dorsal root ganglia typically consists of mild to moderate pleocytosis (<200 mononuclear cells, predominantly lymphocytes), an increase in the protein concentration, intrathecal synthesis of IgG, and a variable presence of oligoclonal bands.

PND OF NERVE AND MUSCLE If symptoms involve peripheral nerve, neuromuscular junction, or muscle, the diagnosis of a specific PND is usually established on clinical, electrophysiologic, and pathologic grounds. The clinical history, accompanying symptoms (e.g., anorexia, weight loss), and type of syndrome dictate the studies and degree of effort needed to demonstrate a neoplasm. For ex-

A

B

FIGURE 97-1 Antibodies to NR1/NR2 subunits of the NMDA receptor in a patient with paraneoplastic encephalitis and ovarian teratoma. *Panel A* is a section of dentate gyrus of rat hippocampus immunolabeled (brown staining) with the patient's antibodies. The reactivity predominates in the molecular layer, which is highly enriched in dendritic processes. *Panel B* shows the antibody reactivity with cultures of rat hippocampal neurons; the intense green immunolabeling is due to the antibodies against the NR1/NR2 subunits of NMDA receptors.

FIGURE 97-2 Fluid-attenuated inversion recovery sequence MRI of a patient with limbic encephalitis and voltage-gated potassium channel antibodies. Note the abnormal hyperintensity involving the medial aspect of the temporal lobes.

ry infiltrates, neuronal loss, gliosis) beyond the symptomatic regions. Several clinicopathologic syndromes may occur alone or in combination: (1) *cortical encephalitis*, which may present as "epilepsia partialis continua"; (2) *limbic encephalitis*, characterized by confusion, depression, agitation, anxiety, severe short-term memory deficits, partial complex seizures, and dementia; the MRI usually shows unilateral or bilateral medial temporal lobe abnormalities, best seen with T2 and fluid-attenuated inversion recovery sequences, and occasionally enhancing with gadolinium; (3) *brainstem encephalitis,* resulting in eye movement disorders (nystagmus, opsoclonus, supranuclear or nuclear paresis), cranial nerve paresis, dysarthria, dysphagia, and central autonomic dysfunction; (4) *cerebellar gait and limb ataxia*; (5) *myelitis*, which may cause lower or upper motor neuron symptoms, myoclonus, muscle rigidity, and spasms; and (6) *autonomic dysfunction* as a result of involvement of the neuraxis at multiple levels, including hypothalamus, brainstem, and autonomic nerves (see autonomic neuropathy). Cardiac arrhythmias, postural hypotension, or central hypoventilation are frequent causes of death in patients with encephalomyelitis.

Paraneoplastic encephalomyelitis and focal encephalitis are usually associated with SCLC, but many other cancers have also been reported. Patients with SCLC and these syndromes usually have anti-Hu antibodies in serum and CSF. Anti-CV2/CRMP5 antibodies occur less frequently; some of these patients may develop chorea or uveitis. Antibodies to Ma proteins are associated with limbic, hypothalamic and brainstem encephalitis and occasionally with cerebellar symptoms (Fig. 97-3); some patients develop hypersomnia, cataplexy, and severe hypokinesia. MRI abnormalities are frequent, including those described with limbic encephalitis and variable

ample, the frequent association of LEMS with SCLC should lead to a chest and abdomen CT or body positron emission tomography (PET) scan and, if negative, periodic tumor screening for at least 3 years after the neurologic diagnosis. In contrast, the weak association of polymyositis with cancer calls into question the need for repeated cancer screenings in this situation. Serum and urine immunofixation studies should be considered in patients with peripheral neuropathy of unknown cause; detection of a monoclonal gammopathy suggests the need for additional studies to uncover a B cell or plasma cell malignancy. In paraneoplastic neuropathies, diagnostically useful antineuronal antibodies are limited to anti-CV2/CRMP5 and anti-Hu.

For any type of PND, if antineuronal antibodies are negative, the diagnosis relies on the demonstration of cancer and the exclusion of other cancer-related or independent neurologic disorders. Body PET scans often uncover tumors undetected by other tests.

SPECIFIC PARANEOPLASTIC NEUROLOGIC SYNDROMES (Table 97-3)

PARANEOPLASTIC ENCEPHALOMYELITIS AND FOCAL ENCEPHALITIS

The term *encephalomyelitis* describes an inflammatory process with multifocal involvement of the nervous system, including brain, brainstem, cerebellum, and spinal cord. It is often associated with dorsal root ganglia and autonomic dysfunction. For any given patient, the clinical manifestations are determined by the area or areas predominantly involved, but pathology almost always reveals abnormalities (inflamma-

TABLE 97-3 | ANTIBODY-ASSOCIATED PARANEOPLASTIC AND NONPARANEOPLASTIC SYNDROMES[a]

Syndrome	Antibodies		
	Paraneoplastic		Nonparaneoplastic
	Frequent	Infrequent	
Limbic encephalitis	Ma2, Hu, CV2/CRMP5, *anti-NR1/NR2 of NMDA receptor*	Tr, VGKC	VGKC
Cerebellar degeneration	Yo, Tr, P/Q VGCC, Hu, Zic, Ri, CV2/CRMP5, Ma1-2	*mGluR1; MAZ*	Gliadin, GAD
Hypothalamic, brainstem encephalitis	Ma2, Hu	CV2/CRMP5	
Encephalomyelitis	Hu, Zic	CV2/CRMP5, Ri, amphiphysin	
Chorea	CV2/CRMP5		
Opsoclonus-myoclonus	Ri	Hu, Ma2, Yo,	
Stiff-person syndrome	Amphiphysin	*Gephyrin*, Ri	GAD
PNH (neuromyotonia)	VGKC		VGKC
Myasthenia gravis	AChR		AChR, MuSK
LEMS	P/Q-type VGCC	*MysB*	P/Q-type VGCC
Sensory neuronopathy	Hu		
Axonal sensorimotor neuropathy	Hu, CV2/CRMP5		Monoclonal gammopathy (M protein)[b]
Autonomic neuropathy	Hu	CV2/CRMP5, ganglionic AChR	Ganglionic AChR
Predominant sensory demyelinating neuropathy		MAG, ganglioside antibodies: often present with Waldenström's macroglobulinemia	MAG, ganglioside antibodies, often present with MGUS
Paraneoplastic retinopathy	Recoverin (CAR), anti-bipolar cell antibodies (*MAR*), *anti-enolase*	*Tubby-like protein 1, PNR*	*Anti-enolase*

[a]Antibodies have been validated by more than one laboratory and/or the protein sequence of the target antigen is known.
[b]The M protein usually does not have specific antibody activity.
Note: *Italics* indicate that commercial testing for these antibodies is not available. PNH, peripheral nerve hyperexcitability; CAR, cancer-associated retinopathy; MAR, melanoma-associated retinopathy; PNR, photoreceptor-specific nuclear receptor; MGUS, monoclonal gammopathy of uncertain significance; VGKC, voltage-gated potassium channel; GAD, glutamic acid decarboxylase; AChR, acetylcholine receptor; LEMS, Lambert-Eaton myasthenic syndrome; VGCC, voltage-gated calcium channel; MAG, myelin-associated glycoprotein; NMDA, *N*-methyl-D-aspartate.

A   B   C

FIGURE 97-3 MRI and tumor of a patient with anti-Ma2-associated encephalitis. **Panels A** and **B** are fluid-attenuated inversion recovery MRI sequences showing abnormal hyperintensities in the medial temporal lobes, hypothalamus and upper brainstem. **Panel C** corresponds to a section of the patient's orchiectomy incubated with a specific marker (Oct4) of germ-cell tumors. The positive (brown) cells correspond to an intratubular germ-cell neoplasm.

involvement of the hypothalamus, basal ganglia, or upper brainstem. Antibodies to NR1/NR2 subunits of the NMDA receptor associate with a severe, potentially lethal, but treatment-responsive encephalitis. The affected patients are young women who develop combinations of psychiatric symptoms, seizures, dyskinesias, stupor and hypoventilation. The oncologic associations of these antibodies are shown in Table 97-2.

℞ ENCEPHALITIS AND ENCEPHALOMYELITIS

Most types of paraneoplastic encephalitis and encephalomyelitis respond poorly to treatment. Stabilization of symptoms or partial neurologic improvement may occasionally occur, particularly if there is a satisfactory response of the tumor to treatment. The roles of plasma exchange, IVIg, and immunosuppression have not been established. Approximately 30% of patients with anti-Ma2-associated encephalitis respond to treatment of the tumor (usually a germ-cell neoplasm of the testis) and immunotherapy. Two other syndromes that are responsive to treatment of the tumor and immunotherapy are the encephalitis that associates with antibodies to the NR1/NR2 subunits of NMDA receptors in patients with teratoma of the ovary, and the encephalitis that associates with VGKC antibodies in some patients with thymoma or SCLC.

PARANEOPLASTIC CEREBELLAR DEGENERATION

This disorder is often preceded by a prodrome that may include dizziness, oscillopsia, blurry or double vision, nausea, and vomiting. A few days or weeks later, dysarthria, gait and limb ataxia, and variable dysphagia can appear. The examination usually shows downbeating nystagmus and, rarely, opsoclonus. Brainstem dysfunction, upgoing toes, or a mild neuropathy may occur, but more often the symptoms and signs are restricted to the cerebellum. Early in the course, MRI studies are usually normal; later, the MRI typically reveals cerebellar atrophy. The disorder results from extensive degeneration of Purkinje cells, with variable involvement of other cerebellar cortical neurons, deep cerebellar nuclei, and spinocerebellar tracts. The tumors more frequently involved are SCLC, cancer of the breast and ovary, and Hodgkin's lymphoma.

Anti-Yo antibodies in patients with breast and gynecologic cancers and anti-Tr antibodies in patients with Hodgkin's lymphoma are the two paraneoplastic antibodies typically associated with prominent or pure cerebellar degeneration. Antibodies to P/Q-type VGCC occur in some patients with SCLC and cerebellar dysfunction; only some of these patients develop LEMS. Of note, a variable degree of cerebellar dysfunction can be associated with virtually any type of antibody-related PND of the CNS (Table 97-2).

℞ CEREBELLAR DEGENERATION

A number of single case reports have described neurologic improvement after tumor removal, plasma exchange, IVIg, cyclophosphamide, rituximab, or glucocorticoids. However, large series of patients with antibody-positive paraneoplastic cerebellar degeneration show that this disorder rarely improves with any treatment.

PARANEOPLASTIC OPSOCLONUS-MYOCLONUS SYNDROME

Opsoclonus is a disorder of eye movement characterized by involuntary, chaotic saccades that occur in all directions of gaze; it is frequently associated with myoclonus and ataxia. Opsoclonus-myoclonus may be cancer-related or idiopathic. When the cause is paraneoplastic, the tumors involved are usually cancer of the lung and breast in adults and neuroblastoma in children. The pathologic substrate of opsoclonus-myoclonus is unclear. Most SCLC patients do not have detectable antineuronal antibodies. A small subset of patients with ataxia, opsoclonus, and other eye movement disorders develop anti-Ri antibodies; in rare instances muscle rigidity, autonomic dysfunction, and dementia also occur. The tumor most frequently involved in anti-Ri-associated syndromes is breast cancer.

If the tumor is not successfully treated, the paraneoplastic opsoclonus-myoclonus syndrome in adults often progresses to encephalopathy, coma, and death. In addition to treating the tumor, symptoms may respond to immunotherapy (glucocorticoids, plasma exchange, and/or IVIg).

At least 50% of children with opsoclonus-myoclonus have an underlying neuroblastoma. Hypotonia, ataxia, behavioral changes, and irritability are frequent accompanying symptoms. Many patients harbor antibodies to neuronal cell surface antigens of unknown identity. Neurologic symptoms often improve with treatment of the tumor (including chemotherapy) and with glucocorticoids, adrenocorticotropic hormone (ACTH), plasma exchange, IVIg, and rituximab. Many patients are left with psychomotor retardation and behavioral and sleep problems.

PARANEOPLASTIC SYNDROMES OF THE SPINAL CORD

The number of reports of paraneoplastic spinal cord syndromes, such as *subacute motor neuronopathy* and *acute necrotizing myelopathy*, has decreased in recent years. This may represent a true decrease in incidence, due to improved and prompt oncologic interventions, or may be because of the identification of nonparaneoplastic etiologies.

Some patients with cancer develop *upper* or *lower motor neuron dysfunction* or both, resembling amyotrophic lateral sclerosis. It is unclear whether these disorders have a paraneoplastic etiology or simply coincide with the presence of cancer. There are isolated case reports of cancer patients with motor neuron dysfunction who had neurologic improvement after tumor treatment. A more than coincidental association occurs between lymphoma and motor neuron dysfunction. A search for lymphoma should be undertaken in patients with a motor neuron syndrome who are found to have a monoclonal protein in serum or CSF.

Paraneoplastic myelitis may present with upper or lower motor neuron symptoms, segmental myoclonus, and rigidity. This syndrome can appear as the presenting manifestation of encephalomyelitis and may be associated with SCLC and serum anti-Hu, anti-CV$_2$/CRMP5, or anti-amphiphysin antibodies.

Paraneoplastic myelopathy can also produce several syndromes characterized by prominent muscle stiffness and rigidity. The spectrum ranges from focal symptoms in one or several extremities (*stiff-limb syndrome* or *stiff-person syndrome*) to a disorder that also affects the brainstem (known as *encephalomyelitis with rigidity*) and likely has a different pathogenesis.

PARANEOPLASTIC STIFF-PERSON SYNDROME

This disorder is characterized by progressive muscle rigidity, stiffness, and painful spasms triggered by auditory, sensory, or emotional stimuli. Rigidity mainly involves the lower trunk and legs, but it can affect the upper extremities and neck. Symptoms improve with sleep and general anesthetics. Electrophysiologic studies demonstrate continuous motor unit activity. Antibodies associated with the stiff-person syndrome target proteins [glutamic acid decarboxylase (GAD), amphiphysin] involved in the function of inhibitory synapses utilizing γ-aminobutyric acid (GABA) or glycine as neurotransmitters. Paraneoplastic stiff-person syndrome and amphiphysin antibodies are often related to breast cancer. By contrast, antibodies to GAD may occur in some cancer patients but are much more frequently present in the nonparaneoplastic disorder.

℞ STIFF-PERSON SYNDROME

Optimal treatment of stiff-person syndrome requires therapy of the underlying tumor, glucocorticoids, and symptomatic use of drugs that enhance GABA-ergic transmission (diazepam, baclofen, sodium valproate, tiagabine, vigabatrin). A benefit of IVIg has been demonstrated for the nonparaneoplastic disorder but remains to be established for the paraneoplastic syndrome.

PARANEOPLASTIC SENSORY NEURONOPATHY OR DORSAL ROOT GANGLIONOPATHY

This syndrome is characterized by sensory deficits that may be symmetric or asymmetric, painful dysesthesias, radicular pain, and decreased or absent reflexes. All modalities of sensation and any part of the body including face and trunk can be involved. Specialized sensations such as taste and hearing can also be affected. Electrophysiologic studies show decreased or absent sensory nerve potentials with normal or near-normal motor conduction velocities. Symptoms result from an inflammatory, likely immune-mediated, process that targets the dorsal root ganglia, causing neuronal loss, proliferation of satellite cells, and secondary degeneration of the posterior columns of the spinal cord. The dorsal nerve roots, and less frequently the anterior nerve roots and peripheral nerves, may also be involved.

℞ SENSORY NEUROPATHY

This disorder often precedes or is associated with encephalomyelitis and autonomic dysfunction and has the same immunologic and oncologic associations, e.g., anti-Hu antibodies and SCLC. As with anti-Hu-associated encephalomyelitis, the therapeutic approach focuses on prompt treatment of the tumor. Glucocorticoids occasionally produce clinical stabilization or improvement. The benefit of IVIg and plasma exchange is not proved.

PARANEOPLASTIC PERIPHERAL NEUROPATHIES

These disorders may develop any time during the course of the neoplastic disease. Neuropathies occurring at late stages of cancer or lymphoma usually cause mild to moderate sensorimotor deficits due to axonal degeneration of unclear etiology. These neuropathies are often masked by concurrent neurotoxicity from chemotherapy and other cancer therapies. In contrast, the neuropathies that develop in the early stages of cancer often show a rapid progression, sometimes with a relapsing and remitting course, and evidence of inflammatory infiltrates and axonal loss or demyelination in biopsy studies. If demyelinating features predominate (Chap. 379), IVIg or glucocorticoids may improve symptoms. Occasionally anti-CV$_2$/CRMP5 antibodies are present; detection of anti-Hu suggests concurrent dorsal root ganglionitis.

Guillain-Barré syndrome and *brachial plexitis* have occasionally been reported in patients with lymphoma, but there is no clear evidence of a paraneoplastic association.

Malignant monoclonal gammopathies include: (1) multiple myeloma and sclerotic myeloma associated with IgG or IgA monoclonal proteins; and (2) Waldenström's macroglobulinemia, B cell lymphoma, and chronic B cell lymphocytic leukemia associated with IgM monoclonal proteins. These disorders may cause neuropathy by a variety of mechanisms, including compression of roots and plexuses by metastasis to vertebral bodies and pelvis, deposits of amyloid in peripheral nerves, and paraneoplastic mechanisms. The paraneoplastic variety has several distinctive features. Approximately half of patients with sclerotic myeloma develop a sensorimotor neuropathy with predominantly motor deficits, resembling a chronic inflammatory demyelinating neuropathy (Chap. 380); some patients develop elements of the POEMS syndrome (*p*olyneuropathy, *o*rganomegaly, *e*ndocrinopathy, *M* protein, *s*kin changes). Treatment of the plasmacytoma or sclerotic lesions usually improves the neuropathy. In contrast, the sensorimotor or sensory neuropathy associated with multiple myeloma rarely responds to treatment. Between 5 and 10% of patients with Waldenström's macroglobulinemia develop a distal symmetric sensorimotor neuropathy with predominant involvement of large sensory fibers. These patients may have IgM antibodies in their serum against myelin-associated glycoprotein and various gangliosides (Chap. 380). In addition to treating the Waldenström's macroglobulinemia, other therapies may improve the neuropathy, including plasma exchange, IVIg, chlorambucil, cyclophosphamide, fludarabine, or rituximab.

Vasculitis of the nerve and muscle causes a painful symmetric or asymmetric distal sensorimotor neuropathy with variable proximal weakness. It predominantly affects elderly men and is associated with an elevated erythrocyte sedimentation rate and increased CSF protein concentration. SCLC and lymphoma are the primary tumors involved. Pathology demonstrates axonal degeneration and T cell infiltrates involving the small vessels of the nerve and muscle. Immunosuppressants (glucocorticoids and cyclophosphamide) often result in neurologic improvement.

Peripheral nerve hyperexcitability (*neuromyotonia*, or *Isaacs' syndrome*) is characterized by spontaneous and continuous muscle fiber activity of peripheral nerve origin. Clinical features include cramps, muscle twitching (fasciculations or myokymia), stiffness, delayed muscle relaxation (pseudomyotonia), and spontaneous or evoked carpal or pedal spasms. The involved muscles may be hypertrophic, and some patients develop paresthesias and hyperhydrosis. CNS dysfunction, including mood changes, sleep disorder, or hallucinations, may occur. The electromyogram (EMG) shows fibrillations; fasciculations; and doublet, triplet, or multiplet single unit (myokymic) discharges that have a high intraburst frequency. An immune pathogenesis is suggested by the frequent presence of serum antibodies to VGKC. The disorder often occurs without cancer; if paraneoplastic, benign and malignant thymomas and SCLC are the usual tumors. Phenytoin, carbamazepine, and plasma exchange improve symptoms.

Paraneoplastic autonomic neuropathy usually develops as a component of other disorders, such as LEMS and encephalomyelitis. It may rarely occur as a pure or predominantly autonomic neuropathy with adrenergic or cholinergic dysfunction at the pre- or postganglionic levels. Patients can develop several life-threatening complications, such as gastrointestinal paresis with pseudoobstruction, cardiac dysrhythmias, and postural hypotension. Other symptoms include dry mouth, erectile dysfunction, anhidrosis, and sphincter dysfunction; abnormal pupillary responses may be found. The disorder has been reported to occur in association with several tumors, including SCLC, cancer of the pancreas or testis, carcinoid tumors, and lymphoma. Because autonomic symptoms can also be the presenting feature of encephalomyelitis, serum anti-Hu and anti-CV$_2$/CRMP5 antibodies should also be sought. Serum antibodies to ganglionic acetylcholine receptors have been reported in this syndrome, but they also occur without a cancer association. (See Chap. 370.)

LAMBERT-EATON MYASTHENIC SYNDROME

LEMS is discussed in Chap. 381.

MYASTHENIA GRAVIS

Myasthenia gravis is discussed in Chap. 381.

POLYMYOSITIS-DERMATOMYOSITIS

Polymyositis and dermatomyositis are discussed in detail in Chap. 383.

ACUTE NECROTIZING MYOPATHY

Patients with this syndrome develop myalgias and rapid progression of weakness involving the extremities and the pharyngeal and respiratory muscles, often resulting in death. Serum muscle enzymes are elevated, and muscle biopsy shows extensive necrosis with minimal or absent inflammation and sometimes deposits of complement. The disorder occurs as a paraneoplastic manifestation of a variety of cancers including SCLC and cancer of the gastrointestinal tract, breast, kidney, and prostate, among others. Glucocorticoids or treatment of the underlying tumor rarely control the disorder.

PARANEOPLASTIC VISUAL SYNDROMES

This group of disorders involves the retina and, less frequently, the uvea and optic nerves. The term *cancer-associated retinopathy* is used to describe paraneoplastic cone and rod dysfunction characterized by photosensitivity, progressive loss of vision and color perception, central or ring scotomas, night blindness, and attenuation of photopic and scotopic responses in the electroretinogram (ERG). The most commonly associated tumor is SCLC. Melanoma-associated retinopathy affects patients with metastatic cutaneous melanoma. Patients develop the acute onset of night blindness and shimmering, flickering, or pulsating photopsias that often progress to visual loss. The ERG demonstrates reduction in the b-wave amplitude. Paraneoplastic optic neuritis and uveitis are very uncommon and can develop in association with encephalomyelitis. Some patients with paraneoplastic uveitis harbor anti-CV$_2$/CRMP5 antibodies.

Some paraneoplastic retinopathies are associated with serum antibodies that specifically react with the subset of retinal cells undergoing degeneration, supporting an immune-mediated pathogenesis (Tables 97-2 and 97-3). Paraneoplastic retinopathies usually fail to improve with treatment, although rare responses to glucocorticoids, plasma exchange, and IVIg have been reported.

FURTHER READINGS

ANTOINE JC, CAMDESSANCHÉ JP: Peripheral nervous system involvement in patients with cancer. Lancet Neurol 6:75, 2007

BATALLER L et al: Autoimmune limbic encephalitis in 39 patients: Immunophenotypes and outcomes. J Neurol Neurosurg Psychiatry 78:381, 2007

DALMAU J et al: Paraneoplastic anti-N-methyl-D-aspartate receptor encephalitis associated with ovarian teratoma. Ann Neurol 61:25, 2007

MATHEW RM et al: Orchiectomy for suspected microscopic tumor in patients with anti-Ma2-associated encephalitis. Neurology 68:900, 2007

ROSENFELD MR, DALMAU J: Current therapies for neuromuscular manifestations of paraneoplastic syndromes. Curr Neurol Neurosci Rep 6:77, 2006

SECTION 2 — HEMATOPOIETIC DISORDERS

98 Iron Deficiency and Other Hypoproliferative Anemias
John W. Adamson

Anemias associated with normocytic and normochromic red cells and an inappropriately low reticulocyte response (reticulocyte index <2.0–2.5) are *hypoproliferative anemias*. This category includes early iron deficiency (before hypochromic microcytic red cells develop), acute and chronic inflammation (including many malignancies), renal disease, hypometabolic states such as protein malnutrition and endocrine deficiencies, and anemias from marrow damage. Marrow damage states are discussed in Chap. 102.

Hypoproliferative anemias are the most common anemias, and anemia associated with acute and chronic inflammation is the most common of these. The anemia of inflammation, like iron deficiency, is related in part to abnormal iron metabolism. The anemias associated with renal disease, inflammation, cancer, and hypometabolic states are characterized by an abnormal erythropoietin response to the anemia.

IRON METABOLISM

Iron is a critical element in the function of all cells, although the amount of iron required by individual tissues varies during development. At the same time, the body must protect itself from free iron, which is highly toxic in that it participates in chemical reactions that generate free radicals such as singlet O_2 or OH^-. Consequently, elaborate mechanisms have evolved that allow iron to be made available for physiologic functions while at the same time conserving this element and handling it in such a way that toxicity is avoided.

The major role of iron in mammals is to carry O_2 as part of hemoglobin. O_2 is also bound by myoglobin in muscle. Iron is a critical element in iron-containing enzymes, including the cytochrome system in mitochondria. Iron distribution in the body is shown in Table 98-1. Without iron, cells lose their capacity for electron transport and energy metabolism. In erythroid cells, hemoglobin synthesis is impaired, resulting in anemia and reduced O_2 delivery to tissue.

THE IRON CYCLE IN HUMANS

Figure 98-1 outlines the major pathways of internal iron exchange in humans. Iron absorbed from the diet or released from stores circulates in the plasma bound to *transferrin*, the iron transport protein. Trans-

TABLE 98-1 BODY IRON DISTRIBUTION

	Iron Content, mg	
	Adult Male, 80 kg	Adult Female, 60 kg
Hemoglobin	2500	1700
Myoglobin/enzymes	500	300
Transferrin iron	3	3
Iron stores	600–1000	0–300

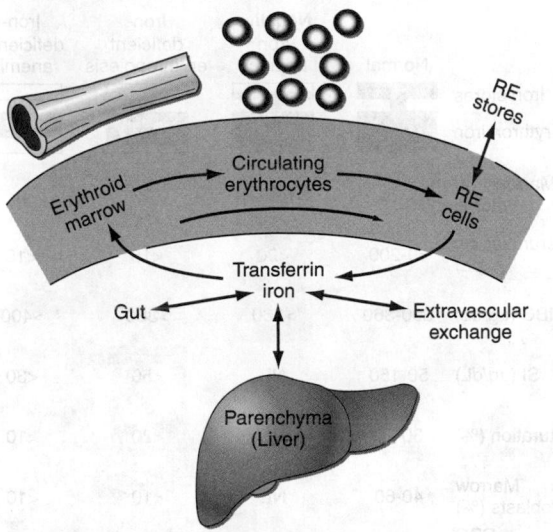

FIGURE 98-1 Internal iron exchange. Normally about 80% of iron passing through the plasma transferrin pool is recycled from broken-down red cells. Absorption of about 1 mg/d is required from the diet in men, 1.4 mg/d in women to maintain homeostasis. As long as transferrin saturation is maintained between 20–60% and erythropoiesis is not increased, iron stores are not required. However, in the event of blood loss, dietary iron deficiency, or inadequate iron absorption, up to 40 mg/d of iron can be mobilized from stores. RE, reticuloendothelial.

ferrin is a bilobed glycoprotein with two iron binding sites. Transferrin that carries iron exists in two forms—*monoferric* (one iron atom) or *diferric* (two iron atoms). The turnover (half-clearance time) of transferrin-bound iron is very rapid—typically 60–90 min. Because almost all of the iron transported by transferrin is delivered to the erythroid marrow, the clearance time of transferrin-bound iron from the circulation is affected most by the plasma iron level and the erythroid marrow activity. When erythropoiesis is markedly stimulated, the pool of erythroid cells requiring iron increases and the clearance time of iron from the circulation decreases. The half-clearance time of iron in the presence of iron deficiency is as short as 10–15 min. With suppression of erythropoiesis, the plasma iron level typically increases and the half-clearance time may be prolonged to several hours. Normally, the iron bound to transferrin turns over 10–20 times per day. Assuming a normal plasma iron level of 80–100 μg/dL, the amount of iron passing through the transferrin pool is 20–24 mg/d.

The iron-transferrin complex circulates in the plasma until it interacts with specific *transferrin receptors* on the surface of marrow erythroid cells. Diferric transferrin has the highest affinity for transferrin receptors; apotransferrin (transferrin not carrying iron) has very little affinity. While transferrin receptors are found on cells in many tissues within the body—and all cells at some time during development will display transferrin receptors—the cell having the greatest number of receptors (300,000 to 400,000/cell) is the developing erythroblast.

Once the iron-bearing transferrin interacts with its receptor, the complex is internalized via clathrin-coated pits and transported to an acidic endosome, where the iron is released at the low pH. The iron is then made available for heme synthesis while the transferrin-receptor complex is recycled to the surface of the cell, where the bulk of the transferrin is released back into circulation and the transferrin receptor reanchors into the cell membrane. At this point a certain amount of the transferrin receptor protein may be released into circulation and can be measured as soluble transferrin receptor protein. Within the erythroid cell, iron in excess of the amount needed for hemoglobin synthesis binds to a storage protein, *apoferritin*, forming *ferritin*. This mechanism of iron exchange also takes place in other cells of the body expressing transferrin receptors, especially liver parenchymal cells where the iron can be incorporated into heme-containing enzymes or stored. The iron incorporated into hemoglobin subsequently enters the circulation as new red cells are re-

leased from the bone marrow. The iron is then part of the red cell mass and will not become available for reutilization until the red cell dies.

In a normal individual, the average red cell life span is 120 days. Thus, 0.8–1.0% of red cells turn over each day. At the end of its life span, the red cell is recognized as senescent by the cells of the *reticuloendothelial (RE) system*, and the cell undergoes phagocytosis. Once within the RE cell, the hemoglobin from the ingested red cell is broken down, the globin and other proteins are returned to the amino acid pool, and the iron is shuttled back to the surface of the RE cell, where it is presented to circulating transferrin. It is the efficient and highly conserved recycling of iron from senescent red cells that supports steady state (and even mildly accelerated) erythropoiesis.

Since each milliliter of red cells contains 1 mg of elemental iron, the amount of iron needed to replace those red cells lost through senescence amounts to 16–20 mg/d (assuming an adult with a red cell mass of 2 L). Any additional iron required for daily red cell production comes from the diet. Normally, an adult male will need to absorb at least 1 mg of elemental iron daily to meet needs, while females in the childbearing years will need to absorb an average of 1.4 mg/d. However, to achieve a maximum proliferative erythroid marrow response to anemia, additional iron must be available. With markedly stimulated erythropoiesis, demands for iron are increased by as much as six- to eightfold. With extravascular hemolytic anemia, the rate of red cell destruction is increased, but the iron recovered from the red cells is efficiently reutilized for hemoglobin synthesis. In contrast, with intravascular hemolysis or blood loss anemia, the rate of red cell production is limited by the amount of iron that can be mobilized from stores. Typically, the rate of mobilization under these circumstances will not support red cell production more than 2.5 times normal. If the delivery of iron to the stimulated marrow is suboptimal, the marrow's proliferative response is blunted, and hemoglobin synthesis is impaired. The result is a hypoproliferative marrow accompanied by microcytic, hypochromic anemia.

While blood loss or hemolysis places a demand on the iron supply, conditions associated with inflammation interfere with iron release from stores and can result in a rapid decrease in the serum iron (see below).

NUTRITIONAL IRON BALANCE

The balance of iron in humans is tightly controlled and designed to conserve iron for reutilization. There is no regulated excretory pathway for iron, and the only mechanisms by which iron is lost from the body are blood loss (via gastrointestinal bleeding, menses, or other forms of bleeding) and the loss of epithelial cells from the skin, gut, and genitourinary tract. Normally, the only route by which iron comes into the body is via absorption from food or from medicinal iron taken orally. Iron may also enter the body through red-cell transfusions or injection of iron complexes. The margin between the amount of iron available for absorption and the requirement for iron in growing infants and the adult female is narrow; this accounts for the great prevalence of iron deficiency worldwide—currently estimated at one-half billion people.

The amount of iron required from the diet to replace losses averages about 10% of body iron content a year in men and 15% in women of childbearing age. Dietary iron content is closely related to total caloric intake (approximately 6 mg of elemental iron per 1000 calories). Iron bioavailability is affected by the nature of the foodstuff, with heme iron (e.g., red meat) being most readily absorbed. In the United States, the average iron intake in an adult male is 15 mg/d with 6% absorption; for the average female, the daily intake is 11 mg/d with 12% absorption. An individual with iron deficiency can increase iron absorption to about 20% of the iron present in a meat-containing diet but only 5–10% of the iron in a vegetarian diet. As a result, one-third of the female population in the United States has virtually no iron stores. Vegetarians are at an additional disadvantage because certain foodstuffs that include phytates and phosphates reduce iron absorption by about 50%. When ionizable iron salts are given together with food, the amount of iron absorbed is reduced. When the percentage of iron absorbed from individual food items is compared with the percentage for an equivalent amount of ferrous salt, iron in vegetables is only about one-twentieth as available, egg iron one-eighth, liver iron one-half, and heme iron one-half to two-thirds.

Infants, children, and adolescents may be unable to maintain normal iron balance because of the demands of body growth and lower dietary intake of iron. During the last two trimesters of pregnancy, daily iron requirements increase to 5–6 mg. That is the reason why iron supplements are strongly recommended for pregnant women in developed countries. Enthusiasm for supplementing foods such as bread and cereals with iron has waned in the face of concerns that the very prevalent hemochromatosis gene would result in an unacceptable risk of iron overload.

Iron absorption takes place largely in the proximal small intestine and is a carefully regulated process. For absorption, iron must be taken up by the luminal cell. That process is facilitated by the acidic contents of the stomach, which maintains the iron in solution. At the brush border of the absorptive cell, the ferric iron is converted to the ferrous form by a ferrireductase. Transport across the membrane is accomplished by divalent metal transporter 1 (DMT-1, also known as Nramp 2 or DCT-1). DMT-1 is a general cation transporter. Once inside the gut cell, iron may be stored as ferritin or transported through the cell to be released at the basolateral surface to plasma transferrin through the membrane-embedded iron exporter, ferroportin. The function of ferroportin is negatively regulated by hepcidin, the principal iron regulatory hormone. In the process of release, iron interacts with another ferroxidase, hephaestin, which oxidizes the iron to the ferric form for transferrin binding. Hephaestin is similar to ceruloplasmin, the copper-carrying protein.

Iron absorption is influenced by a number of physiologic states. Erythroid hyperplasia, for example, stimulates iron absorption, even in the face of normal or increased iron stores, and hepcidin levels are inappropriately low. The molecular mechanism underlying this relationship is not known. Thus, patients with anemias associated with high levels of ineffective erythropoiesis absorb excess amounts of dietary iron. Over time, this may lead to iron overload and tissue damage. In iron deficiency, hepcidin levels are low and iron is much more efficiently absorbed from a given diet; the contrary is true in states of secondary iron overload. The normal individual can reduce iron absorption in situations of excessive intake or medicinal iron intake; however, while the percentage of iron absorbed goes down, the absolute amount goes up. This accounts for the acute iron toxicity occasionally seen when children ingest large numbers of iron tablets. Under these circumstances, the amount of iron absorbed exceeds the transferrin binding capacity of the plasma, resulting in free iron that affects critical organs such as cardiac muscle cells.

IRON-DEFICIENCY ANEMIA

Iron deficiency is one of the most prevalent forms of malnutrition. Globally, 50% of anemia is attributable to iron deficiency and accounts for around 841,000 deaths annually worldwide. Africa and parts of Asia bear 71% of the global mortality burden; North America represents only 1.4% of the total morbidity and mortality associated with iron deficiency.

STAGES OF IRON DEFICIENCY

Iron-deficiency anemia is the condition in which there is anemia and clear evidence of iron lack. The progression to iron deficiency can be divided into three stages (Fig. 98-2). The first stage is *negative iron balance*, in which the demands for (or losses of) iron exceed the body's ability to absorb iron from the diet. This stage results from a number of physiologic mechanisms, including blood loss, pregnancy (in which the demands for red cell production by the fetus outstrip the mother's ability to provide iron), rapid growth spurts in the adolescent, or inadequate dietary iron intake. Blood loss in excess of 10–20 mL of red cells per day is greater than the amount of iron that the gut can absorb from a normal diet. Under these circumstances the iron deficit must be made up by mobilization of iron from RE storage sites. During this period, iron stores—reflected by the serum ferritin level or the appearance of stain-

FIGURE 98-2 Laboratory studies in the evolution of iron deficiency. Measurements of marrow iron stores, serum ferritin, and total iron-binding capacity (TIBC) are sensitive to early iron-store depletion. Iron-deficient erythropoiesis is recognized from additional abnormalities in the serum iron (SI), percent transferrin saturation, the pattern of marrow sideroblasts, and the red cell protoporphyrin level. Patients with iron-deficiency anemia demonstrate all the same abnormalities plus hypochromic microcytic anemia. *(From Hillman and Finch, with permission.)*

	Normal	Negative iron balance	Iron-deficient erythropoiesis	Iron-deficiency anemia
Marrow iron stores	1-3+	0-1+	0	0
Serum ferritin (µg/L)	50-200	<20	<15	<15
TIBC (µg/dL)	300-360	>360	>380	>400
SI (µg/dL)	50-150	NL	<50	<30
Saturation (%)	30-50	NL	<20	<10
Marrow sideroblasts (%)	40-60	NL	<10	<10
RBC protoporphyrin (µg/dL)	30-50	NL	>100	>200
RBC morphology	NL	NL	NL	Microcytic/hypochromic

able iron on bone marrow aspirations—decrease. As long as iron stores are present and can be mobilized, the serum iron, total iron-binding capacity (TIBC), and red cell protoporphyrin levels remain within normal limits. At this stage, red cell morphology and indices are normal.

When iron stores become depleted, the serum iron begins to fall. Gradually, the TIBC increases, as do red cell protoporphyrin levels. By definition, marrow iron stores are absent when the serum ferritin level is <15 µg/L. As long as the serum iron remains within the normal range, hemoglobin synthesis is unaffected despite the dwindling iron stores. Once the transferrin saturation falls to 15–20%, hemoglobin synthesis becomes impaired. This is a period of *iron-deficient erythropoiesis*. Careful evaluation of the peripheral blood smear reveals the first appearance of microcytic cells, and if the laboratory technology is available, one finds hypochromic reticulocytes in circulation. Gradually, the hemoglobin and hematocrit begin to fall, reflecting *iron-deficiency anemia*. The transferrin saturation at this point is 10–15%.

When moderate anemia is present (hemoglobin 10–13 g/dL), the bone marrow remains hypoproliferative. With more severe anemia (hemoglobin 7–8 g/dL), hypochromia and microcytosis become more prominent, target cells and misshapen red cells (poikilocytes) appear on the blood smear as cigar- or pencil-shaped forms, and the erythroid marrow becomes increasingly ineffective. Consequently, with severe prolonged iron-deficiency anemia, erythroid hyperplasia of the marrow develops, rather than hypoproliferation.

CAUSES OF IRON DEFICIENCY

Conditions that increase demand for iron, increase iron loss, or decrease iron intake or absorption can produce iron deficiency (Table 98-2).

CLINICAL PRESENTATION OF IRON DEFICIENCY

Certain clinical conditions carry an increased likelihood of iron deficiency. Pregnancy, adolescence, periods of rapid growth, and an intermittent history of blood loss of any kind should alert the clinician to possible iron deficiency. A cardinal rule is that the appearance of iron deficiency in an adult male means gastrointestinal blood loss until

TABLE 98-2	CAUSES OF IRON DEFICIENCY

Increased demand for iron and/or hematopoiesis
    rapid growth in infancy or adolescence
    pregnancy
    erythropoietin therapy
Increased iron loss
    chronic blood loss
    menses
    acute blood loss
    blood donation
    phlebotomy as treatment for polycythemia vera
Decreased iron intake or absorption
    inadequate diet
    malabsorption from disease (sprue, Crohn's disease)
    malabsorption from surgery (post-gastrectomy)
    acute or chronic inflammation

FIGURE 98-3 Serum ferritin levels as a function of sex and age. Iron store depletion and iron deficiency are accompanied by a fall in serum ferritin level below 20 μg/L. *(From Hillman et al, with permission.)*

proven otherwise. Signs related to iron deficiency depend on the severity and chronicity of the anemia in addition to the usual signs of anemia—fatigue, pallor, and reduced exercise capacity. *Cheilosis* (fissures at the corners of the mouth) and *koilonychia* (spooning of the fingernails) are signs of advanced tissue iron deficiency. The diagnosis of iron deficiency is typically based on laboratory results.

LABORATORY IRON STUDIES

Serum Iron and Total Iron-Binding Capacity   The serum iron level represents the amount of circulating iron bound to transferrin. The TIBC is an indirect measure of the circulating transferrin. The normal range for the serum iron is 50–150 μg/dL; the normal range for TIBC is 300–360 μg/dL. Transferrin saturation, which is normally 25–50%, is obtained by the following formula: serum iron × 100 ÷ TIBC. Iron-deficiency states are associated with saturation levels below 18%. In evaluating the serum iron, the clinician should be aware that there is a diurnal variation in the value. A transferrin saturation >50% indicates that a disproportionate amount of the iron bound to transferrin is being delivered to nonerythroid tissues. If this persists for an extended time, tissue iron overload may occur.

Serum Ferritin   Free iron is toxic to cells, and the body has established an elaborate set of protective mechanisms to bind iron in various tissue compartments. Within cells, iron is stored complexed to protein as ferritin or hemosiderin. Apoferritin binds to free ferrous iron and stores it in the ferric state. As ferritin accumulates within cells of the RE system, protein aggregates are formed as hemosiderin. Iron in ferritin or hemosiderin can be extracted for release by the RE cells, although hemosiderin is less readily available. Under steady-state conditions, the serum ferritin level correlates with total body iron stores; thus, the serum ferritin level is the most convenient laboratory test to estimate iron stores. The normal value for ferritin varies according to the age and gender of the individual (Fig. 98-3). Adult males have serum ferritin values averaging about 100 μg/L, while adult females have levels averaging 30 μg/L. As iron stores are depleted, the serum ferritin falls to <15 μg/L. Such levels are diagnostic of absent body iron stores.

Evaluation of Bone Marrow Iron Stores   Although RE cell iron stores can be estimated from the iron stain of a bone marrow aspirate or biopsy, the measurement of serum ferritin has largely supplanted bone marrow aspirates for determination of storage iron (Table 98-3). The serum ferritin level is a better indicator of iron overload than the marrow iron stain. However, in addition to storage iron, the marrow iron stain provides information about the effective delivery of iron to developing erythroblasts. Normally, when the marrow smear is stained for iron, 20–40% of developing erythroblasts—called *sideroblasts*—will have visible ferritin granules in their cytoplasm. This represents iron in excess of that needed for hemoglobin synthesis. In states in which release of iron from storage sites is blocked, RE iron will be detectable, and there will be few or no sideroblasts. In the myelodysplastic syndromes, mitochondrial dysfunction can occur, and accumulation of iron in mitochondria appears in a necklace fashion around the nucleus of the erythroblast. Such cells are referred to as *ringed sideroblasts*.

Red Cell Protoporphyrin Levels   Protoporphyrin is an intermediate in the pathway to heme synthesis. Under conditions in which heme synthesis is impaired, protoporphyrin accumulates within the red cell. This reflects an inadequate iron supply to erythroid precursors to support hemoglobin synthesis. Normal values are <30 μg/dL of red cells. In iron deficiency, values in excess of 100 μg/dL are seen. The most common causes of increased red cell protoporphyrin levels are absolute or relative iron deficiency and lead poisoning.

Serum Levels of Transferrin Receptor Protein   Because erythroid cells have the highest numbers of transferrin receptors on their surface of any cell in the body, and because transferrin receptor protein (TRP) is released by cells into the circulation, serum levels of TRP reflect the total erythroid marrow mass. Another condition in which TRP levels are elevated is absolute iron deficiency. Normal values are 4–9 μg/L determined by immunoassay. This laboratory test is becoming increasingly available and, along with the serum ferritin, has been proposed to distinguish between iron deficiency and the anemia of chronic inflammation (see below).

DIFFERENTIAL DIAGNOSIS

Other than iron deficiency, only three conditions need to be considered in the differential diagnosis of a hypochromic microcytic anemia (Table 98-4). The first is an inherited defect in globin chain synthesis: the thalassemias. These are differentiated from iron deficiency most readily by serum iron values; normal or increased serum iron levels and transferrin saturation are characteristic of the thalassemias.

The second condition is the anemia of chronic inflammation with inadequate iron supply to the erythroid marrow. The distinction between true iron-deficiency anemia and the anemia associated with chronic inflammation is among the most common diagnostic problems encountered by clinicians (see below). Usually the anemia of chronic inflammation is normocytic and normochromic. The iron

TABLE 98-3	IRON STORE MEASUREMENTS	
Iron Stores	**Marrow Iron Stain, 0–4+**	**Serum Ferritin, μg/L**
0	0	<15
1–300 mg	Trace to 1+	15–30
300–800 mg	2+	30–60
800–1000 mg	3+	60–150
1–2 g	4+	>150
Iron overload	—	>500–1000

TABLE 98-4 **DIAGNOSIS OF MICROCYTIC ANEMIA**

Tests	Iron Deficiency	Inflammation	Thalassemia	Sideroblastic Anemia
Smear	Micro/hypo	Normal micro/hypo	Micro/hypo with targeting	Variable
SI	<30	<50	Normal to high	Normal to high
TIBC	>360	<300	Normal	Normal
Percent saturation	<10	10–20	30–80	30–80
Ferritin (μg/L)	<15	30–200	50–300	50–300
Hemoglobin pattern	Normal	Normal	Abnormal	Normal

Note: SI, serum iron; TIBC, total iron-binding capacity.

values usually make the differential diagnosis clear, as the ferritin level is normal or increased and the percent transferrin saturation and TIBC are typically below normal.

Finally, the myelodysplastic syndromes represent the third and least common condition. Occasionally, patients with myelodysplasia have impaired hemoglobin synthesis with mitochondrial dysfunction, resulting in impaired iron incorporation into heme. The iron values again reveal normal stores and more than an adequate supply to the marrow, despite the microcytosis and hypochromia.

℞ IRON-DEFICIENCY ANEMIA

The severity and cause of iron-deficiency anemia will determine the appropriate approach to treatment. As an example, symptomatic elderly patients with severe iron-deficiency anemia and cardiovascular instability may require red cell transfusions. Younger individuals who have compensated for their anemia can be treated more conservatively with iron replacement. The foremost issue for the latter patient is the precise identification of the cause of the iron deficiency.

For the majority of cases of iron deficiency (pregnant women, growing children and adolescents, patients with infrequent episodes of bleeding, and those with inadequate dietary intake of iron), oral iron therapy will suffice. For patients with unusual blood loss or malabsorption, specific diagnostic tests and appropriate therapy take priority. Once the diagnosis of iron-deficiency anemia and its cause is made, there are three major therapeutic approaches.

RED CELL TRANSFUSION Transfusion therapy is reserved for individuals who have symptoms of anemia, cardiovascular instability, continued and excessive blood loss from whatever source, and require immediate intervention. The management of these patients is less related to the iron deficiency than it is to the consequences of the severe anemia. Not only do transfusions correct the anemia acutely, but the transfused red cells provide a source of iron for reutilization, assuming they are not lost through continued bleeding. Transfusion therapy will stabilize the patient while other options are reviewed.

ORAL IRON THERAPY In the asymptomatic patient with established iron-deficiency anemia, treatment with oral iron is usually adequate. Multiple preparations are available, ranging from simple iron salts to complex iron compounds designed for sustained release throughout the small intestine (Table 98-5). While the various preparations contain different amounts of iron, they are generally all absorbed well and are effective in treatment. Some come with other compounds designed to enhance iron absorption, such as ascorbic acid. It is not clear whether the benefits of such compounds justify their costs. Typically, for iron replacement therapy, up to 300 mg of elemental iron per day is given, usually as three or four iron tablets (each containing 50–65 mg elemental iron) given over the course of the day. Ideally, oral iron preparations should be taken on an empty stomach, since foods may inhibit iron absorption. Some patients with gastric disease or prior gastric surgery require special treatment with iron solutions, since the retention capacity of the stomach may be reduced. The retention capacity is necessary for dissolving the shell of the iron tablet before the release of iron. A dose of 200–300 mg of elemental iron per day should result in the absorption of iron up to 50 mg/d. This supports a red cell production level of two to three times normal in an individual with a normally functioning marrow and appropriate erythropoietin stimulus. However, as the hemoglobin level rises, erythropoietin stimula-

tion decreases, and the amount of iron absorbed is reduced. The goal of therapy in individuals with iron-deficiency anemia is not only to repair the anemia, but also to provide stores of at least 0.5–1.0 g of iron. Sustained treatment for a period of 6–12 months after correction of the anemia will be necessary to achieve this.

Of the complications of oral iron therapy, gastrointestinal distress is the most prominent and is seen in 15–20% of patients. Abdominal pain, nausea, vomiting, or constipation may lead to noncompliance. Although small doses of iron or iron preparations with delayed release may help somewhat, the gastrointestinal side effects are a major impediment to the effective treatment of a number of patients.

The response to iron therapy varies, depending on the erythropoietin (EPO) stimulus and the rate of absorption. Typically, the reticulocyte count should begin to increase within 4–7 days after initiation of therapy and peak at $1^{1}/2$ weeks. The absence of a response may be due to poor absorption, noncompliance (which is common), or a confounding diagnosis. A useful test in the clinic to determine the patient's ability to absorb iron is the *iron tolerance test*. Two iron tablets are given to the patient on an empty stomach, and the serum iron is measured serially over the subsequent 2 hours. Normal absorption will result in an increase in the serum iron of at least 100 μg/dL. If iron deficiency persists despite adequate treatment, it may be necessary to switch to parenteral iron therapy.

PARENTERAL IRON THERAPY Intravenous iron can be given to patients who are unable to tolerate oral iron; whose needs are relatively acute; or who need iron on an ongoing basis, usually due to persistent gastrointestinal blood loss. Parenteral iron use has been rising rapidly in the last several years with the recognition that recombinant erythropoietin therapy induces a large demand for iron—a demand that frequently cannot be met through the physiologic release of iron from RE sources. The safety of parenteral iron—particularly iron dextran—has been a concern. The serious adverse reaction rate to intravenous iron dextran is 0.7%. Fortunately, newer iron complexes are available in the United States, such as sodium ferric gluconate (Ferrlecit) and iron sucrose (Venofer), that have a much lower rate of adverse effects.

Parenteral iron is used in two ways: one is to administer the total dose of iron required to correct the hemoglobin deficit and provide the patient with at least 500 mg of iron stores; the second is to give repeated small doses of parenteral iron over a protracted period. The latter approach is common in dialysis centers, where it is not unusual for 100 mg of elemental iron to be given weekly for 10 weeks to augment the response to recombinant EPO therapy. The amount of iron needed by an individual patient is calculated by the following formula:

$$\text{Body weight (kg)} \times 2.3 \times (15\text{–patient's hemoglobin, g/dL}) + 500 \text{ or } 1000 \text{ mg (for stores).}$$

In administering intravenous iron dextran, anaphylaxis is a concern. Anaphylaxis is much rarer with the newer preparations. The factors that have correlated with an anaphylactic-like reaction include a history of multiple allergies or a prior allergic reaction to dextran (in the case of iron dextran). Generalized symptoms appearing several days after the infusion of a

TABLE 98-5 **ORAL IRON PREPARATIONS**

Generic Name	Tablet (Iron Content), mg	Elixir (Iron Content), mg in 5 mL
Ferrous sulfate	325 (65)	300 (60)
	195 (39)	90 (18)
Extended release	525 (105)	
Ferrous fumarate	325 (107)	
	195 (64)	100 (33)
Ferrous gluconate	325 (39)	300 (35)
Polysaccharide iron	150 (150)	100 (100)
	50 (50)	

large dose of iron can include arthralgias, skin rash, and low-grade fever. This may be dose-related, but it does not preclude the further use of parenteral iron in the patient. To date, patients with sensitivity to iron dextran have been safely treated with iron gluconate. If a large dose of iron is to be given (>100 mg), the iron preparation should be diluted in 5% dextrose in water or 0.9% NaCl solution. The iron solution can then be infused over a 60- to 90-min period (for larger doses) or at a rate convenient for the attending nurse or physician. While a test dose (25 mg) of parenteral iron dextran is recommended, in reality a slow infusion of a larger dose of parenteral iron solution will afford the same kind of early warning as a separately injected test dose. Early in the infusion of iron, if chest pain, wheezing, a fall in blood pressure, or other systemic symptoms occur, the infusion of iron should be stopped immediately.

OTHER HYPOPROLIFERATIVE ANEMIAS

In addition to mild to moderate iron-deficiency anemia, the hypoproliferative anemias can be divided into four categories: (1) chronic inflammation, (2) renal disease, (3) endocrine and nutritional deficiencies (hypometabolic states), and (4) marrow damage (Chap. 102). With chronic inflammation, renal disease, or hypometabolism, endogenous EPO production is inadequate for the degree of anemia observed. For the anemia of chronic inflammation, the erythroid marrow also responds inadequately to stimulation, due in part to defects in *iron reutilization*. As a result of the lack of adequate EPO stimulation, an examination of the peripheral blood smear will disclose only an occasional polychromatophilic ("shift") reticulocyte. In cases of iron deficiency or marrow damage, appropriate elevations in endogenous EPO levels are typically found, and shift reticulocytes will be present on the blood smear.

ANEMIA OF ACUTE AND CHRONIC INFLAMMATION/INFECTION (THE ANEMIA OF CHRONIC DISEASE)

The anemia of chronic disease—which encompasses inflammation, infection, tissue injury, and conditions (such as cancer) associated with the release of proinflammatory cytokines—is one of the most common forms of anemia seen clinically and probably the most important in the differential diagnosis of iron deficiency, since many of the features of the anemia are brought about by inadequate iron delivery to the marrow, despite the presence of normal or increased iron stores. This is reflected by a low serum iron, increased red cell protoporphyrin, a hypoproliferative marrow, transferrin saturation in the range of 15–20%, and a normal or increased serum ferritin. The serum ferritin values are often the most distinguishing feature between true iron-deficiency anemia and the iron-deficient erythropoiesis associated with inflammation. Typically, serum ferritin values increase threefold over basal levels in the face of inflammation. All of these changes are due to the effects of inflammatory cytokines and hepcidin, the key iron regulatory hormone, acting at several levels of erythropoiesis (Fig. 98-4).

Interleukin 1 (IL-1) directly decreases EPO production in response to anemia. IL-1, acting through accessory cell release of interferon γ (IFN-γ), suppresses the response of the erythroid marrow to EPO—an effect that can be overcome by EPO administration in vitro and in vivo. In addition, tumor necrosis factor (TNF), acting through the release of IFN-γ by marrow stromal cells, also suppresses the response to EPO. Hepcidin, made by the liver, is increased in inflammation and acts to suppress iron absorption and iron release from storage sites. The overall result is a chronic hypoproliferative anemia with classic changes in iron metabolism. The anemia is further compounded by a mild to moderate shortening in red cell survival.

With chronic inflammation, the primary disease will determine the severity and characteristics of the anemia. For instance, many patients with cancer also

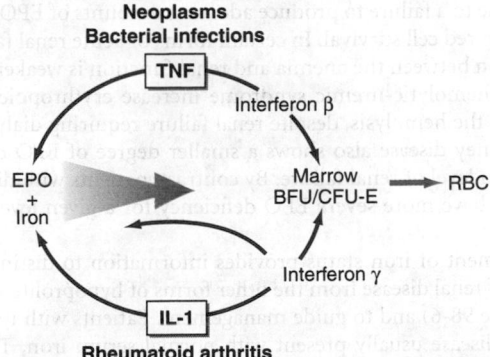

FIGURE 98-4 Suppression of erythropoiesis by inflammatory cytokines. Through the release of tumor necrosis factor (TNF) and interferon γ (IFN-γ), neoplasms and bacterial infections suppress erythropoietin (EPO) production and the proliferation of erythroid progenitors [erythroid burst-forming units and erythroid colony-forming units (BFU/CFU-E)]. The mediators in patients with vasculitis and rheumatoid arthritis include interleukin 1 (IL-1) and IFN-γ. The red arrows indicate sites of inflammatory cytokine inhibitory effects.

have anemia that is typically normocytic and normochromic. In contrast, patients with long-standing active rheumatoid arthritis or chronic infections such as tuberculosis will have a microcytic, hypochromic anemia. In both cases, the bone marrow is hypoproliferative, but the differences in red cell indices reflect differences in the availability of iron for hemoglobin synthesis. Occasionally, conditions associated with chronic inflammation are also associated with chronic blood loss. Under these circumstances, a bone marrow aspirate stained for iron may be necessary to rule out absolute iron deficiency. However, the administration of iron in this case will correct the iron deficiency component of the anemia and leave the inflammatory component unaffected.

The anemia associated with acute infection or inflammation is typically mild but becomes more pronounced over time. Acute infection can produce a fall in hemoglobin levels of 2–3 g/dL within 1 or 2 days; this is largely related to the hemolysis of red cells near the end of their natural life span. The fever and cytokines released exert a selective pressure against cells with more limited capacity to maintain the red cell membrane. In most individuals the mild anemia is reasonably well tolerated, and symptoms, if present, are associated with the underlying disease. Occasionally, in patients with preexisting cardiac disease, moderate anemia (hemoglobin 10–11 g/dL) may be associated with angina, exercise intolerance, and shortness of breath. The erythropoietic profile that distinguishes the anemia of inflammation from the other causes of hypoproliferative anemias is shown in Table 98-6.

ANEMIA OF RENAL DISEASE

Chronic renal failure is usually associated with a moderate to severe hypoproliferative anemia; the level of the anemia correlates with the severity of the renal failure. Red cells are typically normocytic and normochromic, and reticulocytes are decreased. The anemia is pri-

TABLE 98-6 DIAGNOSIS OF HYPOPROLIFERATIVE ANEMIAS

Tests	Iron Deficiency	Inflammation	Renal Disease	Hypometabolic States
Anemia	Mild to severe	Mild	Mild to severe	Mild
MCV (fL)	60–90	80–90	90	90
Morphology	Normo-microcytic	Normocytic	Normocytic	Normocytic
SI	<30	<50	Normal	Normal
TIBC	>360	<300	Normal	Normal
Saturation (%)	<10	10–20	Normal	Normal
Serum ferritin (μg/L)	<15	30–200	115–150	Normal
Iron stores	0	2–4+	1–4+	Normal

Note: MCV, mean corpuscular volume; SI, serum iron; TIBC, total iron-binding capacity.

marily due to a failure to produce adequate amounts of EPO and a reduction in red cell survival. In certain forms of acute renal failure, the correlation between the anemia and renal function is weaker. Patients with the hemolytic-uremic syndrome increase erythropoiesis in response to the hemolysis, despite renal failure requiring dialysis. Polycystic kidney disease also shows a smaller degree of EPO deficiency for a given level of renal failure. By contrast, patients with diabetes or myeloma have more severe EPO deficiency for a given level of renal failure.

Assessment of iron status provides information to distinguish the anemia of renal disease from the other forms of hypoproliferative anemia (Table 98-6) and to guide management. Patients with the anemia of renal disease usually present with normal serum iron, TIBC, and ferritin levels. However, those maintained on chronic hemodialysis may develop iron deficiency from blood loss through the dialysis procedure. Iron must be replenished in these patients to ensure an adequate response to EPO therapy (see below).

ANEMIA IN HYPOMETABOLIC STATES

Patients who are starving, particularly for protein, and those with a variety of endocrine disorders that produce lower metabolic rates, may develop a mild to moderate hypoproliferative anemia. The release of EPO from the kidney is sensitive to the need for O_2, not just O_2 levels. Thus, EPO production is triggered at lower levels of blood O_2 content in disease states (such as hypothyroidism and starvation) where metabolic activity, and thus O_2 demand, is decreased.

Endocrine Deficiency States The difference in the levels of hemoglobin between men and women is related to the effects of androgen and estrogen on erythropoiesis. Testosterone and anabolic steroids augment erythropoiesis; castration and estrogen administration to males decrease erythropoiesis. Patients who are hypothyroid or have deficits in pituitary hormones also may develop a mild anemia. Pathogenesis may be complicated by other nutritional deficiencies since iron and folic acid absorption can be affected by these disorders. Usually, correction of the hormone deficiency reverses the anemia.

Anemia may be more severe in Addison's disease, depending on the level of thyroid and androgen hormone dysfunction; however, anemia may be masked by decreases in plasma volume. Once such patients are given cortisol and volume replacement, the hemoglobin level may fall rapidly. Mild anemia complicating hyperparathyroidism may be due to decreased EPO production as a consequence of the renal effects of hypercalcemia or to impaired proliferation of erythroid progenitors.

Protein Starvation Decreased dietary intake of protein may lead to mild to moderate hypoproliferative anemia; this form of anemia may be prevalent in the elderly. The anemia can be more severe in patients with a greater degree of starvation. In marasmus, where patients are both protein- and calorie-deficient, the release of EPO is impaired in proportion to the reduction in metabolic rate; however, the degree of anemia may be masked by volume depletion and becomes apparent after refeeding. Deficiencies in other nutrients (iron, folate) may also complicate the clinical picture but may not be apparent at diagnosis. Changes in the erythrocyte indices on refeeding should prompt evaluation of iron, folate, and B_{12} status.

Anemia in Liver Disease A mild hypoproliferative anemia may develop in patients with chronic liver disease from nearly any cause. The peripheral blood smear may show spur cells and stomatocytes from the accumulation of excess cholesterol in the membrane from a deficiency of lecithin cholesterol acyltransferase. Red cell survival is shortened, and the production of EPO is inadequate to compensate. In alcoholic liver disease, nutritional deficiencies are common and complicate the management. Folate deficiency from inadequate intake, as well as iron deficiency from blood loss and inadequate intake, can alter the red cell indices.

HYPOPROLIFERATIVE ANEMIAS

Many patients with hypoproliferative anemias experience recovery of normal hemoglobin levels when the underlying disease is appropriately treated. For those in whom such reversals are not possible—such as patients with end-stage kidney disease, cancer, and chronic inflammatory diseases—symptomatic anemia requires treatment. The two major forms of treatment are transfusions and EPO.

TRANSFUSIONS Thresholds for transfusion should be altered based on the patient's symptoms. In general, patients without serious underlying cardiovascular or pulmonary disease can tolerate hemoglobin levels above 8 g/dL and do not require intervention until the hemoglobin falls below that level. Patients with more physiologic compromise may need to have their hemoglobin levels kept above 11 g/dL. A typical unit of packed red cells increases the hemoglobin level by 1 g/dL. Transfusions are associated with certain infectious risks (Chap. 107), and chronic transfusions can produce iron overload. Importantly, the liberal use of blood has been associated with increased morbidity and mortality, particularly in the intensive care setting. Therefore, in the absence of documented tissue hypoxia, a conservative approach to the use of red cell transfusions is preferable.

ERYTHROPOIETIN (EPO) EPO is particularly useful in anemias in which endogenous EPO levels are inappropriately low, such as the hypoproliferative anemias. Iron status must be evaluated and iron repleted to obtain optimal effects from EPO. In patients with chronic renal failure, the usual dose of EPO is 50–150 U/kg three times a week intravenously. Hemoglobin levels of 10–12 g/dL are usually reached within 4–6 weeks if iron levels are adequate; 90% of these patients respond. Once a target hemoglobin level is achieved, the EPO dose can be decreased. A fall in hemoglobin level occurring in the face of EPO therapy usually signifies the development of an infection or iron depletion. Aluminum toxicity and hyperparathyroidism can also compromise the EPO response. When an infection intervenes, it is best to interrupt the EPO therapy and rely on transfusion to correct the anemia until the infection is adequately treated. The dose needed to correct the anemia in patients with cancer is higher, up to 300 U/kg three times a week, and only about 60% of patients respond.

Longer-acting preparations of EPO can reduce the frequency of injections. Darbepoetin alfa, a molecularly modified EPO with additional carbohydrate, has a half-life in the circulation that is 3–4 times longer than epoetin alfa, permitting weekly or every other week dosing.

ACKNOWLEDGMENT
Dr. Robert S. Hillman was the author of this chapter in the 14th edition, and material from his chapter has been retained.

FURTHER READINGS

BAILIE GR et al: Parenteral iron use in the management of anemia in end-stage renal disease patients. Am J Kidney Dis 35:1, 2000

BRUGNARA C: Iron deficiency and erythropoiesis: New diagnostic approaches. Clin Chem 49:1573, 2003

FLEMING RE, BACON BR: Orchestration of iron homeostasis. N Engl J Med 352:1741, 2005

GANZ T: Hepcidin, a key regulator of iron metabolism and mediator of inflammation. Blood 102:783, 2003

HILLMAN RS et al: *Hematology in Clinical Practice*, 4th ed. New York, McGraw-Hill, 2005

STOLTZFUS RF: Iron deficiency: Global prevalence and consequences. Food Nutr Bull 24(Suppl 4):S99, 2003

THOMAS C et al: The diagnostic plot: A concept for identifying different states of iron deficiency and monitoring the response to epoetin therapy. Med Oncol 23:23, 2006

99 Disorders of Hemoglobin
Edward J. Benz, Jr.

Hemoglobin is critical for normal oxygen delivery to tissues; it is also present in erythrocytes in such high concentrations that it can alter red cell shape, deformability, and viscosity. Hemoglobinopathies are disorders affecting the structure, function, or production of hemoglobin. These conditions are usually inherited and range in severity from asymptomatic laboratory abnormalities to death in utero. Different forms may present as hemolytic anemia, erythrocytosis, cyanosis, or vasoocclusive stigmata.

PROPERTIES OF THE HUMAN HEMOGLOBINS

HEMOGLOBIN STRUCTURE

Different hemoglobins are produced during embryonic, fetal, and adult life (Fig. 99-1). Each consists of a tetramer of globin polypeptide chains: a pair of α-like chains 141 amino acids long and a pair of β-like chains 146 amino acids long. The major adult hemoglobin, HbA, has the structure $\alpha_2\beta_2$. HbF ($\alpha_2\gamma_2$) predominates during most of gestation, and HbA$_2$ ($\alpha_2\delta_2$) is minor adult hemoglobin. Embryonic hemoglobins need not be considered here.

Each globin chain enfolds a single heme moiety, consisting of a protoporphyrin IX ring complexed with a single iron atom in the ferrous state (Fe^{2+}). Each heme moiety can bind a single oxygen molecule; a molecule of hemoglobin can transport up to four oxygen molecules.

The amino acid sequences of the various globins are highly homologous to one another. Each has a highly helical *secondary structure*. Their globular *tertiary structures* can cause the exterior surfaces to be rich in polar (hydrophilic) amino acids that enhance solubility and the interior to be lined with nonpolar groups, forming a hydrophobic pocket into which heme is inserted. The tetrameric *quaternary structure* of HbA contains two $\alpha\beta$ dimers. Numerous tight interactions (i.e., $\alpha_1\beta_1$ contacts) hold the α and β chains together. The complete tetramer is held together by interfaces (i.e., $\alpha_1\beta_2$ contacts) between the α-like chain of one dimer and the non-α chain of the other dimer.

The hemoglobin tetramer is highly soluble but individual globin chains are insoluble. Unpaired globin precipitates, forming inclusions that damage the cell. Normal globin chain synthesis is balanced so that each newly synthesized α or non-α globin chain will have an available partner with which to pair.

Solubility and reversible oxygen binding are the key properties deranged in hemoglobinopathies. Both depend most on the hydrophilic surface amino acids, the hydrophobic amino acids lining the heme pocket, a key histidine in the F helix, and the amino acids forming the $\alpha_1\beta_1$ and $\alpha_1\beta_2$ contact points. Mutations in these strategic regions tend to be the ones that alter clinical behavior.

FIGURE 99-1 The globin genes. The α-like genes (α,ζ) are encoded on chromosome 16; the β-like genes ($\beta,\gamma,\delta,\varepsilon$) are encoded on chromosome 11. The ζ and ε genes encode embryonic globins.

FUNCTION OF HEMOGLOBIN

To support oxygen transport, hemoglobin must bind O$_2$ efficiently at the partial pressure of oxygen (P$_{O_2}$) of the alveolus, retain it, and release it to tissues at the P$_{O_2}$ of tissue capillary beds. Oxygen acquisition and delivery over a relatively narrow range of oxygen tensions depend on a property inherent in the tetrameric arrangement of heme and globin subunits within the hemoglobin molecule called *cooperativity* or *heme-heme interaction*.

At low oxygen tensions, the hemoglobin tetramer is fully deoxygenated (Fig. 99-2). Oxygen binding begins slowly as O$_2$ tension rises. However, as soon as some oxygen has been bound by the tetramer, an abrupt increase occurs in the slope of the curve. Thus, hemoglobin molecules that have bound some oxygen develop a higher oxygen affinity, greatly accelerating their ability to combine with more oxygen. This S-shaped oxygen equilibrium curve (Fig. 99-2), along which substantial amounts of oxygen loading *and unloading* can occur over a narrow range of oxygen tensions, is physiologically more useful than the high-affinity hyperbolic curve of individual monomers.

Oxygen affinity is modulated by several factors. The Bohr effect is the ability of hemoglobin to deliver more oxygen to tissues at low pH. It arises from the stabilizing action of protons on deoxyhemoglobin, which binds protons more readily than oxyhemoglobin because it is a weaker acid (Fig. 99-2). Thus, hemoglobin has a lower oxygen affinity at low pH. The major small molecule that alters oxygen affinity in humans is 2,3-bisphosphoglycerate (2,3-BPG, formerly 2,3-DPG), which lowers oxygen affinity when bound to hemoglobin. HbA has a reasonably high affinity for 2,3-BPG. HbF does not bind 2,3-BPG, so it tends to have a higher oxygen affinity in vivo. Hemoglobin also binds nitric oxide reversibly; this interaction may influence vascular tone, but its physiologic relevance remains unclear.

Proper oxygen transport depends on the tetrameric structure of the proteins, the proper arrangement of the charged amino acids, and interaction with protons or 2,3-BPG.

DEVELOPMENTAL BIOLOGY OF HUMAN HEMOGLOBINS

Red cells first appearing at about 6 weeks after conception contain the embryonic hemoglobins Hb Portland ($\zeta_2\gamma_2$), Hb Gower I ($\zeta_2\varepsilon_2$), and Hb Gower II ($\alpha_2\varepsilon_2$). At 10–11 weeks, fetal hemoglobin (HbF; $\alpha_2\gamma_2$) becomes predominant. The switch to nearly exclusive synthesis of adult hemoglobin (HbA; $\alpha_2\beta_2$) occurs at about 38 weeks (Fig. 99-1). Fetuses and newborns therefore require α-globin but not β-globin for normal gestation. Small amounts of HbF are produced during postnatal life. A few red cell clones called *F cells* are progeny of a small pool of immature committed erythroid precursors (BFU-e) that retain the ability to produce HbF. Profound erythroid stresses, such as severe hemolytic anemias, bone marrow transplant, or cancer chemotherapy, cause more of the F-potent BFU-e to be recruited. HbF levels thus tend to rise in some patients with sickle cell anemia or thalassemia. This phenomenon is also important because it probably explains the ability of hydroxyurea to increase levels of HbF in adults. Agents such as butyrate that inhibit histone deacetylase and modify chromatin structure can also activate fetal globin genes partially after birth.

GENETICS AND BIOSYNTHESIS OF HUMAN HEMOGLOBIN

The human hemoglobins are encoded in two tightly linked gene clusters; the α-like globin genes are clustered on chromosome 16, and the β-like genes on chromosome 11 (Fig. 99-1). The α-like cluster consists of two α-globin genes and a single copy of the ζ gene. The non-α gene cluster consists of a single ε gene, the Gγ and Aγ fetal globin genes, and the adult δ and β genes.

Important regulatory sequences flank each gene. Immediately upstream are typical promoter elements needed for the assembly of the transcription initiation complex. Sequences in the 5' flanking region of the γ and the β genes appear to be crucial for the correct developmental regulation of these genes, while elements that function like classic enhancers and silencers are in the 3' flanking regions. The locus control region (LCR) elements located far upstream appear to control the overall level of expression of each cluster. These elements achieve

FIGURE 99-2 Hemoglobin-oxygen dissociation curve. The hemoglobin tetramer can bind up to four molecules of oxygen in the iron-containing sites of the heme molecules. As oxygen is bound, 2,3-BPG and CO_2 are expelled. Salt bridges are broken, and each of the globin molecules changes its conformation to facilitate oxygen binding. Oxygen release to the tissues is the reverse process, salt bridges being formed and 2,3-BPG and CO_2 bound. Deoxyhemoglobin does not bind oxygen efficiently until the cell returns to conditions of higher pH, the most important modulator of O_2 affinity (Bohr effect). When acid is produced in the tissues, the dissociation curve shifts to the right, facilitating oxygen release and CO_2 binding. Alkalosis has the opposite effect, reducing oxygen delivery.

their regulatory effects by interacting with *trans*-acting transcription factors. Some of these factors are ubiquitous (e.g., Sp1 and YY1), while others are more or less limited to erythroid cells or hematopoietic cells (e.g., GATA-1, NFE-2, and EKLF). The LCR controlling the α-globin gene cluster is modulated by a SWI/SNF-like protein called *ATRX*; this protein appears to influence chromatin remodeling and DNA methylation. The association of α thalassemia with mental retardation and myelodysplasia in some families appears to be related to mutations in the ATRX pathway. This pathway also modulates genes specifically expressed during erythropoiesis, such as those that encode the enzymes for heme biosynthesis. Normal red blood cell (RBC) differentiation requires the coordinated expression of the globin genes with the genes responsible for heme and iron metabolism. RBC precursors contain a protein, α-hemoglobin stabilizing protein (AHSP), that enhances the folding and solubility of α globin, which is otherwise easily denatured, leading to insoluble precipitates. These precipitates play an important role in the thalassemia syndromes and certain unstable hemoglobin disorders. Polymorphic variation in the amounts and/or functional capacity of AHSP might explain some of the clinical variability seen in patients inheriting identical thalassemia mutations. AHSP may be a therapeutic target, particularly in syndromes of intermediate severity.

CLASSIFICATION OF HEMOGLOBINOPATHIES

There are five major classes of hemoglobinopathies (Table 99-1). *Structural hemoglobinopathies* occur when mutations alter the amino acid sequence of a globin chain, altering the physiologic properties of the variant hemoglobins and producing the characteristic clinical abnormalities. The most clinically relevant variant hemoglobins polymerize abnormally, as in sickle cell anemia, or exhibit altered solubility or oxygen-binding affinity. *Thalassemia syndromes* arise from mutations that impair production or translation of globin mRNA, leading to deficient globin chain biosynthesis. Clinical abnormalities are attributable to the inadequate supply of hemoglobin and the imbalances in the production of individual globin chains, leading to premature destruction of erythroblasts and RBC. *Thalassemic hemoglobin variants* combine features of thalassemia (e.g., abnormal globin biosynthesis) and of structural hemoglobinopathies (e.g., an abnormal amino acid sequence). *Hereditary persistence of fetal hemo-*

globin (HPFH) is characterized by synthesis of high levels of fetal hemoglobin in adult life. *Acquired hemoglobinopathies* include modifications of the hemoglobin molecule by toxins (e.g., acquired methemoglobinemia) and abnormal hemoglobin synthesis (e.g., high levels of HbF production in preleukemia and α thalassemia in myeloproliferative disorders).

EPIDEMIOLOGY

Hemoglobinopathies are especially common in areas in which malaria is endemic. This clustering of hemoglobinopathies is assumed to reflect a selective survival advantage for the abnormal RBC, which presumably provide a less hospitable environment during the obligate RBC stages of the parasitic life cycle. Very young children with α thalassemia are *more* susceptible to infection with the nonlethal *Plasmodium vivax*. Thalassemia might then favor a natural protection against infection with the more lethal *P. falciparum*.

Thalassemias are the most common genetic disorders in the world, affecting nearly 200 million people worldwide. About 15% of American blacks are silent carriers for α thalassemia; α-thalassemia trait (minor) occurs in 3% of American blacks and in 1–15% of persons of Mediterranean origin. β Thalassemia has a 10–15% incidence in individuals from the Mediterranean and Southeast Asia and 0.8% in American blacks. The number of severe cases of thalassemia in the United States is about 1000. Sickle cell disease is the most common structural hemoglobinopathy occurring in heterozygous form in ~8% of American blacks and in homozygous form in 1 in 400. Between 2 and 3% of American blacks carry a hemoglobin C allele.

INHERITANCE AND ONTOGENY

Hemoglobinopathies are autosomal co-dominant traits—compound heterozygotes who inherit a different abnormal mutant allele from

TABLE 99-1	CLASSIFICATION OF HEMOGLOBINOPATHIES

I. Structural hemoglobinopathies—hemoglobins with altered amino acid sequences that result in deranged function or altered physical or chemical properties
  A. Abnormal hemoglobin polymerization—HbS, hemoglobin sickling
  B. Altered O_2 affinity
    1. High affinity—polycythemia
    2. Low affinity—cyanosis, pseudoanemia
  C. Hemoglobins that oxidize readily
    1. Unstable hemoglobins—hemolytic anemia, jaundice
    2. M hemoglobins—methemoglobinemia, cyanosis
II. Thalassemias—defective biosynthesis of globin chains
  A. α Thalassemias
  B. β Thalassemias
  C. δβ, γδβ, αβ Thalassemias
III. Thalassemic hemoglobin variants—structurally abnormal Hb associated with co-inherited thalassemic phenotype
  A. HbE
  B. Hb Constant Spring
  C. Hb Lepore
IV. Hereditary persistence of fetal hemoglobin—persistence of high levels of HbF into adult life
V. Acquired hemoglobinopathies
  A. Methemoglobin due to toxic exposures
  B. Sulfhemoglobin due to toxic exposures
  C. Carboxyhemoglobin
  D. HbH in erythroleukemia
  E. Elevated HbF in states of erythroid stress and bone marrow dysplasia

each parent exhibit composite features of each. For example, patients inheriting sickle β thalassemia exhibit features of β thalassemia and sickle cell anemia. The α chain is present in HbA, HbA₂, and HbF; α-chain mutations thus cause abnormalities in all three. The α-globin hemoglobinopathies are symptomatic in utero and after birth because normal function of the α-globin gene is required throughout gestation and adult life. In contrast, infants with β-globin hemoglobinopathies tend to be asymptomatic until 3–9 months of age, when HbA has largely replaced HbF.

DETECTION AND CHARACTERIZATION OF HEMOGLOBINOPATHIES—GENERAL METHODS

Of the many methods available for hemoglobin analysis, electrophoretic techniques are used for routine clinical purposes. Electrophoresis at pH 8.6 on cellulose acetate membranes is especially simple, inexpensive, and reliable for initial screening. Agar gel electrophoresis at pH 6.1 in citrate buffer is often used as a complementary method because each method detects different variants. Comparison of results obtained in each system usually allows unambiguous diagnosis, but some important variants are electrophoretically silent. These mutant hemoglobins can usually be characterized by more specialized techniques such as isoelectric focusing and/or high-pressure liquid chromatography (HPLC).

Quantitation of the hemoglobin profile is often desirable. HbA₂ is frequently elevated in β-thalassemia trait and depressed in iron deficiency. HbF is elevated in HPFH, some β-thalassemia syndromes, and occasional periods of erythroid stress or marrow dysplasia. For characterization of sickle cell trait, sickle thalassemia syndromes, or HbSC disease, and for monitoring the progress of exchange transfusion therapy to lower the percentage of circulating HbS, quantitation of individual hemoglobins is also required. In most laboratories, quantitation is performed only if the test is specifically ordered.

Because some variants can comigrate with HbA or HbS (sickle hemoglobin), electrophoretic assessment should always be regarded as incomplete unless functional assays for hemoglobin sickling, solubility, or oxygen affinity are also performed, as dictated by the clinical presentation. The best sickling assays involve measurement of the degree to which the hemoglobin sample becomes insoluble, or gelated, as it is deoxygenated (i.e., sickle solubility test). Unstable hemoglobins are detected by their precipitation in isopropanol or after heating to 50°C. High-O₂ affinity and low-O₂ affinity variants are detected by quantitating the P₅₀, the partial pressure of oxygen at which the hemoglobin sample becomes 50% saturated with oxygen. Direct tests for the percent carboxyhemoglobin and methemoglobin, employing spectrophotometric techniques, can readily be obtained from most clinical laboratories on an urgent basis.

Complete characterization, including amino acid sequencing or gene cloning and sequencing, is available from several investigational laboratories around the world. Polymerase chain reaction (PCR), allele-specific oligonucleotide hybridization, and automated DNA sequencing allow identification of globin gene mutations in a few days.

Laboratory evaluation remains an adjunct, rather than the primary diagnostic aid. Diagnosis is best established by recognition of a characteristic history, physical findings, peripheral blood smear morphology, and abnormalities of the complete blood cell count (e.g., profound microcytosis with minimal anemia in thalassemia trait).

STRUCTURALLY ABNORMAL HEMOGLOBINS

SICKLE CELL SYNDROMES

The sickle cell syndromes are caused by a mutation in the β-globin gene that changes the sixth amino acid from glutamic acid to valine. HbS ($\alpha_2\beta_2^{6\ Glu\rightarrow Val}$) polymerizes reversibly when deoxygenated to

FIGURE 99-3 Pathophysiology of sickle cell crisis.

form a gelatinous network of fibrous polymers that stiffen the RBC membrane, increase viscosity, and cause dehydration due to potassium leakage and calcium influx (Fig. 99-3). These changes also produce the sickle shape. Sickled cells lose the pliability needed to traverse small capillaries. They possess altered sticky membranes (especially reticulocytes) that are abnormally adherent to the endothelium of small venules. These abnormalities provoke unpredictable episodes of microvascular vasoocclusion and premature RBC destruction (hemolytic anemia). Hemolysis occurs because the spleen destroys the abnormal RBC. The rigid adherent cells also clog small capillaries and venules, causing tissue ischemia, acute pain, and gradual end-organ damage. This venoocclusive component usually dominates the clinical course. Prominent manifestations include episodes of ischemic pain (i.e., painful crises) and ischemic malfunction or frank infarction in the spleen, central nervous system, bones, liver, kidneys, and lungs (Fig. 99-3).

Several sickle syndromes occur as the result of inheritance of HbS from one parent and another hemoglobinopathy, such as β thalassemia or HbC ($\alpha_2\beta_2^{6\ Glu\rightarrow Lys}$), from the other parent. The prototype disease, sickle cell anemia, is the homozygous state for HbS (Table 99-2).

Clinical Manifestations of Sickle Cell Anemia Most patients with sickling syndromes suffer from hemolytic anemia, with hematocrits from 15–30%, and significant reticulocytosis. Anemia was once thought to exert protective effects against vasoocclusion by reducing blood viscosity. However, natural history and drug therapy trials suggest that an *increase* in the hematocrit and feedback inhibition of reticulocytosis might be beneficial, even at the expense of increased blood viscosity. The role of adhesive reticulocytes in vasoocclusion might account for these paradoxical effects.

Granulocytosis is common. The white count can fluctuate substantially and unpredictably during and between painful crises, infectious episodes, and other intercurrent illnesses.

TABLE 99-2 CLINICAL FEATURES OF SICKLE HEMOGLOBINOPATHIES

Condition	Clinical Abnormalities	Hemoglobin Level g/L (g/dL)	MCV, fL	Hemoglobin Electrophoresis
Sickle cell trait	None; rare painless hematuria	Normal	Normal	Hb S/A:40/60
Sickle cell anemia	Vasoocclusive crises with infarction of spleen, brain, marrow, kidney, lung; aseptic necrosis of bone; gallstones; priapism; ankle ulcers	70–100 (7–10)	80–100	Hb S/A:100/0 Hb F:2–25%
S/β° thalassemia	Vasoocclusive crises; aseptic necrosis of bone	70–100 (7–10)	60–80	Hb S/A:100/0 Hb F:1–10%
S/β⁺ thalassemia	Rare crises and aseptic necrosis	100–140 (10–14)	70–80	Hb S/A:60/40
Hemoglobin SC	Rare crises and aseptic necrosis; painless hematuria	100–140 (10–14)	80–100	Hb S/A:50/0 Hb C:50%

Vasoocclusion causes protean manifestations. Intermittent episodes of vasoocclusion in connective and musculoskeletal structures produce painful ischemia manifested by acute pain and tenderness, fever, tachycardia, and anxiety. These recurrent episodes, called *painful crises*, are the most common clinical manifestation. Their frequency and severity vary greatly. Pain can develop almost anywhere in the body and may last from a few hours to 2 weeks. Repeated crises requiring hospitalization (>3 per year) correlate with reduced survival in adult life, suggesting that these episodes are associated with accumulation of chronic end-organ damage. Provocative factors include infection, fever, excessive exercise, anxiety, abrupt changes in temperature, hypoxia, or hypertonic dyes.

Repeated micro-infarction can destroy tissues having microvascular beds that promote sickling. Thus, the spleen is frequently lost within the first 18–36 months of life, causing susceptibility to infection, particularly by pneumococci. Acute venous obstruction of the spleen (*splenic sequestration crisis*), a rare occurrence in early childhood, may require emergency transfusion and/or splenectomy to prevent trapping of the entire arterial output in the obstructed spleen. Occlusion of retinal vessels can produce hemorrhage, neovascularization, and eventual detachments. Renal papillary necrosis invariably produces isosthenuria. More widespread renal necrosis leads to renal failure in adults, a common late cause of death. Bone and joint ischemia can lead to aseptic necrosis, especially of the femoral or humeral heads; chronic arthropathy; and unusual susceptibility to osteomyelitis, which may be caused by organisms, such as *Salmonella*, rarely encountered in other settings. The *hand-foot syndrome* is caused by painful infarcts of the digits and dactylitis. Stroke is especially common in children; a small subset tend to suffer repeated episodes. Stroke is less common in adults and is often hemorrhagic. A particularly painful complication in males is priapism, due to infarction of the penile venous outflow tracts; permanent impotence is a frequent consequence. Chronic lower leg ulcers probably arise from ischemia and superinfection in the distal circulation.

Acute chest syndrome is a distinctive manifestation characterized by chest pain, tachypnea, fever, cough, and arterial oxygen desaturation. It can mimic pneumonia, pulmonary emboli, bone marrow infarction and embolism, myocardial ischemia, or in situ lung infarction. Acute chest syndrome is thought to reflect in situ sickling within the lung producing pain and temporary pulmonary dysfunction. Often it is difficult or impossible to distinguish among other possibilities. Pulmonary infarction and pneumonia are the most frequent underlying or concomitant conditions in patients with this syndrome. Repeated episodes of acute chest pain correlate with reduced survival. Acutely, reduction in arterial oxygen saturation is especially ominous because it promotes sickling on a massive scale. Chronic acute or subacute pulmonary crises lead to pulmonary hypertension and cor pulmonale, an increasingly common cause of death as patients survive longer.

Sickle cell syndromes are remarkable for their clinical heterogeneity. Some patients remain virtually asymptomatic into or even through adult life, while others suffer repeated crises requiring hospitalization from early childhood. Patients with sickle thalassemia and sickle-HbE tend to have similar, slightly milder, symptoms, perhaps because of the ameliorating effects of production of other hemoglobins within the RBC. Hemoglobin SC disease, one of the more common variants of sickle cell anemia, is frequently marked by lesser degrees of hemolytic anemia and a greater propensity for the development of retinopathy and aseptic necrosis of bones. In most respects, however, the clinical manifestations resemble sickle cell anemia. Some rare hemoglobin variants actually aggravate the sickling phenomenon. The clinical variability in different patients inheriting the same disease-causing mutation (sickle hemoglobin) has made sickle cell disease the focus of efforts to identify modifying genetic polymorphisms in other genes that might account for the heterogeneity. To date, these genome screening efforts have not yielded modifying genes, other than those known to affect the hemoglobin profile directly: e.g., persistence of fetal hemoglobin in adult life, α thalassemia, or co-inheritance of other hemoglobin structural variants. The complexity of the data obtained

FIGURE 99-4 Sickle cell anemia. The elongated and crescent-shaped red blood cells seen on this smear represent circulating irreversibly sickled cells. Target cells and a nucleated red blood cell are also seen.

thus far undermines the expectation that genome-wide analysis will yield individualized profiles that predict a patient's clinical course.

Nevertheless, a number of interesting patterns have emerged from these modifying gene analyses. For example, genes affecting the inflammatory response or cytokine expression appear to be modifying candidates. Genes that affect transcriptional regulation of lymphocytes may be involved. Thus, it appears likely that key polymorphic changes in the patient's inflammatory response to the damages provoked by sickle red cells or in the response to chronic or recurrent infections may prove to be important for prognosticating the clinical severity of disease.

Clinical Manifestations of Sickle Cell Trait Sickle cell trait is usually asymptomatic. Anemia and painful crises are exceedingly rare. An uncommon but highly distinctive symptom is painless hematuria often occurring in adolescent males, probably due to papillary necrosis. Isosthenuria is a more common manifestation of the same process. Sloughing of papillae with urethral obstruction has been reported, as have isolated cases of massive sickling or sudden death due to exposure to high altitudes or extremes of exercise and dehydration.

Diagnosis Sickle cell syndromes are suspected on the basis of hemolytic anemia, RBC morphology (Fig. 99-4), and intermittent episodes of ischemic pain. Diagnosis is confirmed by hemoglobin electrophoresis and the sickling tests already discussed. Thorough characterization of the exact hemoglobin profile of the patient is important, because sickle thalassemia and hemoglobin SC disease have distinct prognoses or clinical features. Diagnosis is usually established in childhood, but occasional patients, often with compound heterozygous states, do not develop symptoms until the onset of puberty, pregnancy, or early adult life. Genotyping of family members and potential parental partners is critical for genetic counseling. Details of the childhood history establish prognosis and need for aggressive or experimental therapies. Factors associated with increased morbidity and reduced survival are more than three crises requiring hospitalization per year, chronic neutrophilia, a history of splenic sequestration or hand-foot syndrome, and second episodes of acute chest syndrome. Patients with a history of cerebrovascular accidents are at higher risk for repeated episodes and require especially close monitoring using Doppler carotid flow measurements. Patients with severe or repeated episodes of acute chest syndrome may need lifelong transfusion support, utilizing partial exchange transfusion, if possible.

℞ SICKLE CELL SYNDROMES

Patients with sickle cell syndromes require ongoing continuity of care. Familiarity with the pattern of symptoms provides the best safeguard against excessive use of the emergency room, hospitalization, and habituation to addictive narcotics. Additional preventive measures include regular slit-lamp examinations to monitor development of retinopathy; antibiotic prophylaxis appropriate for splenectomized patients during dental or other invasive procedures; and vigorous oral hydration during or in anticipation of periods of extreme exercise, exposure to heat or cold, emotional stress, or infection. Pneumococcal and *Haemophilus influenzae* vaccines are less effective in splenectomized individuals. Thus, patients with sickle cell anemia should be vaccinated early in life.

The management of acute painful crisis includes vigorous hydration, thorough evaluation for underlying causes (such as infection), and aggressive analgesia administered by a standing order and/or patient-controlled analgesia (PCA) pump. Morphine (0.1–0.15 mg/kg every 3–4 h) or meperidine (0.75–1.5 mg/kg every 2–4 h) should control severe pain. Meperidine should be used only for acute short-term pain control; as a chronic analgesic, it is unsuitable. Bone pain may respond as well to ketorolac (30–60 mg initial dose, then 15–30 mg every 6–8 h). Inhalation of nitrous oxide can provide short-term pain relief, but great care must be exercised to avoid hypoxia and respiratory depression. Nitrous oxide also elevates O_2 affinity, reducing O_2 delivery to tissues. Its use should be restricted to experts. Many crises can be managed at home with oral hydration and oral analgesia. Use of the emergency room should be reserved for especially severe symptoms or circumstances in which other processes, e.g., infection, are strongly suspected. Nasal oxygen should be employed as appropriate to protect arterial saturation. Most crises resolve in 1–7 days. Use of blood transfusion should be reserved for extreme cases: transfusions do not shorten the duration of the crisis.

No tests are definitive to diagnose acute painful crisis. Critical to good management is an approach that recognizes that most patients reporting crisis symptoms do indeed have crisis or another significant medical problem. Diligent diagnostic evaluation for underlying causes is imperative, even though these are found infrequently. In adults, the possibility of aseptic necrosis or sickle arthropathy must be considered, especially if pain and immobility become repeated or chronic at a single site. Nonsteroidal anti-inflammatory agents are often effective for sickle cell arthropathy.

Acute chest syndrome is a medical emergency that may require management in an intensive care unit. Hydration should be monitored carefully to avoid the development of pulmonary edema, and oxygen therapy should be especially vigorous for protection of arterial saturation. Diagnostic evaluation for pneumonia and pulmonary embolism should be especially thorough, since these may occur with atypical symptoms. Critical interventions are transfusion to maintain a hematocrit > 30, and emergency exchange transfusion if arterial saturation drops to <90%. As patients with sickle cell syndrome increasingly survive into their fifth and sixth decades, end-stage renal failure and pulmonary hypertension are becoming increasingly prominent causes of end-stage morbidity. A sickle cell cardiomyopathy and/or premature coronary artery disease may compromise cardiac function in later years. Sickle cell patients have received kidney transplants, but they often experience an increase in the frequency and severity of crises, possibly due to increased infection as a consequence of immunosuppression.

The most significant advance in the therapy of sickle cell anemia has been the introduction of hydroxyurea as a mainstay of therapy for patients with severe symptoms. Hydroxyurea (10–30 mg/kg per day) increases fetal hemoglobin and may also exert beneficial affects on RBC hydration, vascular wall adherence, and suppression of the granulocyte and reticulocyte counts; dosage is titrated to maintain a white cell count between 5000 and 8000 per μL. White cells and reticulocytes may play a major role in the pathogenesis of sickle cell crisis, and their suppression may be an important benefit of hydroxyurea therapy.

Hydroxyurea should be considered in patients experiencing repeated episodes of acute chest syndrome or with more than three crises per year requiring hospitalization. The utility of this agent for reducing the incidence of other complications (priapism, retinopathy) is under evaluation, as are the long-term side effects. Hydroxyurea offers broad benefits to most patients whose disease is severe enough to impair their functional status, and it may improve survival. HbF levels increase in most patients within a few months.

The antitumor drug, 5-azacytidine, was the first agent found to elevate HbF. It never achieved widespread use because of concerns about acute toxicity and carcinogenesis. However, low doses of the related agent, 5-deoxyazacytidine (decitabine) can elevate HbF with acceptable toxicity.

Bone marrow transplantation can provide definitive cures but is known to be effective and safe only in children. Prognostic features justifying bone marrow transplant are the presence of repeated crises early in life, a high neutrophil count, or the development of hand-foot syndrome. Children at risk for stroke can now be identified through the use of Doppler ultrasound techniques. Prophylactic exchange transfusion appears to substantially reduce the risk of stroke in this population. Children who do suffer a cerebrovascular accident should be maintained for at least 3–5 years on a program of vigorous exchange transfusion, as the risk of second strokes is extremely high.

Gene therapy for sickle cell anemia is being intensively pursued, but no safe measures are currently available. Agents blocking RBC dehydration or vascular adhesion, such as clotrimazole or magnesium, may have value as an adjunct to hydroxyurea therapy, pending the completion of ongoing trials. Combinations of clotrimazole and magnesium are being evaluated.

UNSTABLE HEMOGLOBINS

Amino acid substitutions that reduce solubility or increase susceptibility to oxidation produce unstable hemoglobins that precipitate, forming inclusion bodies injurious to the RBC membrane. Representative mutations are those that interfere with contact points between the α and β subunits [e.g., Hb Philly ($\beta^{35Tyr \rightarrow Phe}$)], alter the helical segments [e.g., Hb Genova ($\beta^{28Leu \rightarrow Pro}$)], or disrupt interactions of the hydrophobic pockets of the globin subunits with heme [e.g., Hb Köln ($\beta^{98Val \rightarrow Met}$)] (Table 99-3). The inclusions, called *Heinz bodies*, are clinically detectable by staining with supravital dyes such as crystal violet. Removal of these inclusions by the spleen generates pitted, rigid cells that have shortened life spans, producing hemolytic anemia of variable severity, sometimes requiring chronic transfusion support. Splenectomy may be needed to correct the anemia. Leg ulcers and premature gallbladder disease due to bilirubin load are frequent stigmata.

Unstable hemoglobins occur sporadically, often by spontaneous new mutations. Heterozygotes are often symptomatic because a significant Heinz body burden can develop even when the unstable variant accounts for a portion of the total hemoglobin. Symptomatic unstable hemoglobins tend to be β-globin variants, because sporadic mutations affecting only one of the four α globins would generate only 20–30% abnormal hemoglobin.

HEMOGLOBINS WITH ALTERED OXYGEN AFFINITY

High-affinity hemoglobins [e.g., Hb Yakima ($\beta^{99Asp \rightarrow His}$)] bind oxygen more readily but deliver less O_2 to tissues at normal capillary P_{O_2} levels (Fig. 99-2). Mild tissue hypoxia ensues, stimulating RBC production and erythrocytosis (Table 99-3). In extreme cases, the hematocrits can rise to 60–65%, increasing blood viscosity and producing typical symptoms (headache, somnolence, or dizziness). Phlebotomy may be required. Typical mutations alter interactions within the heme pocket or disrupt the Bohr effect or salt-bond site. Mutations that impair the interaction of HbA with 2,3-BPG can increase O_2 affinity because 2,3-BPG binding lowers O_2 affinity.

Low-affinity hemoglobins [e.g., Hb Kansas ($\beta^{102Asn \rightarrow Lys}$)] bind sufficient oxygen in the lungs, despite their lower oxygen affinity, to achieve nearly full saturation. At capillary oxygen tensions, they lose sufficient amounts of oxygen to maintain homeostasis at a low hematocrit (Fig. 99-2) (*pseudoanemia*). Capillary hemoglobin desaturation can also be sufficient to produce clinically apparent cyanosis. Despite these findings, patients usually require no specific treatment.

TABLE 99-3	REPRESENTATIVE ABNORMAL HEMOGLOBINS WITH ALTERED SYNTHESIS OR FUNCTION		
Designation	**Mutation**	**Population**	**Main Clinical Effects**[a]
Sickle or S	$\beta^{6Glu \rightarrow Val}$	African	Anemia, ischemic infarcts
C	$\beta^{6Glu \rightarrow Lys}$	African	Mild anemia; interacts with HbS
E	$\beta^{26Glu \rightarrow Lys}$	Southeast Asian	Microcytic anemia, splenomegaly, thalassemic phenotype
Köln	$\beta^{98Val \rightarrow Met}$	Sporadic	Hemolytic anemia, Heinz bodies when splenectomized
Yakima	$\beta^{99Asp \rightarrow His}$	Sporadic	Polycythemia
Kansas	$\beta^{102Asn \rightarrow Lys}$	Sporadic	Mild anemia
M. Iwata	$\alpha^{87His \rightarrow Tyr}$	Sporadic	Methemoglobinemia

[a]See text for details.

Methemoglobin is generated by oxidation of the heme iron moieties to the ferric state, causing a characteristic bluish-brown muddy color resembling cyanosis. Methemoglobin has such high oxygen affinity that virtually no oxygen is delivered. Levels >50–60% are often fatal.

Congenital methemoglobinemia arises from globin mutations that stabilize iron in the ferric state [e.g., HbM Iwata ($\alpha^{87His \rightarrow Tyr}$), Table 99-3] or from mutations that impair the enzymes that reduce methemoglobin to hemoglobin (e.g., methemoglobin reductase, NADP diaphorase). Acquired methemoglobinemia is caused by toxins that oxidize heme iron, notably nitrate and nitrite-containing compounds.

DIAGNOSIS AND MANAGEMENT OF PATIENTS WITH UNSTABLE HEMOGLOBINS, HIGH-AFFINITY HEMOGLOBINS, AND METHEMOGLOBINEMIA

Unstable hemoglobin variants should be suspected in patients with nonimmune hemolytic anemia, jaundice, splenomegaly, or premature biliary tract disease. Severe hemolysis usually presents during infancy as neonatal jaundice or anemia. Milder cases may present in adult life with anemia or only as unexplained reticulocytosis, hepatosplenomegaly, premature biliary tract disease, or leg ulcers. Because spontaneous mutation is common, family history of anemia may be absent. The peripheral blood smear often shows anisocytosis, abundant cells with punctate inclusions, and irregular shapes (i.e., poikilocytosis).

The two best tests for diagnosing unstable hemoglobins are the Heinz body preparation and the isopropanol or heat stability test. Many unstable Hb variants are electrophoretically silent. A normal electrophoresis does not rule out the diagnosis.

Severely affected patients may require transfusion support for the first 3 years of life, because splenectomy before age 3 is associated with a significantly higher immune deficit. Splenectomy is usually effective thereafter, but occasional patients may require lifelong transfusion support. Even after splenectomy, patients can develop cholelithiasis and leg ulcers. Splenectomy can also be considered in patients exhibiting severe secondary complications of chronic hemolysis, even if anemia is absent. Precipitation of unstable hemoglobins is aggravated by oxidative stress, e.g., infection, antimalarial drugs.

High-O$_2$ affinity hemoglobin variants should be suspected in patients with erythrocytosis. The best test for confirmation is measurement of the P$_{50}$. A high-O$_2$ affinity Hb causes a significant left shift (i.e., lower numeric value of the P$_{50}$); confounding conditions, e.g., tobacco smoking or carbon monoxide exposure, can also lower the P$_{50}$.

High-affinity hemoglobins are often asymptomatic; rubor or plethora may be telltale signs. When the hematocrit reaches to 55–60%, symptoms of high blood viscosity and sluggish flow (headache, lethargy, dizziness, etc.) may be present. These persons may benefit from judicious phlebotomy. Erythrocytosis represents an appropriate attempt to compensate for the impaired oxygen delivery by the abnormal variant. Overzealous phlebotomy may stimulate increased erythropoiesis or aggravate symptoms by thwarting this compensatory mechanism. The guiding principle of phlebotomy should be to improve oxygen delivery by reducing blood viscosity and increasing blood flow rather than restoration of a normal hematocrit. Modest iron deficiency may aid in control.

Low-affinity hemoglobins should be considered in patients with cyanosis or a low hematocrit with no other reason apparent after thorough evaluation. The P$_{50}$ test confirms the diagnosis. Counseling and reassurance are the interventions of choice.

Methemoglobin should be suspected in patients with hypoxic symptoms who appear cyanotic but have a Pa$_{O_2}$ sufficiently high that hemoglobin should be fully saturated with oxygen. A history of nitrite or other oxidant ingestions may not always be available; some exposures may be unapparent to the patient, and others may result from suicide attempts. The characteristic muddy appearance of freshly drawn blood can be a critical clue. The best diagnostic test is methemoglobin assay, which is usually available on an emergency basis.

Methemoglobinemia often causes symptoms of cerebral ischemia at levels >15%; levels >60% are usually lethal. Intravenous injection of 1 mg/kg of methylene blue is effective emergency therapy. Milder cases and follow-up of severe cases can be treated orally with methylene blue (60 mg three to four times each day) or ascorbic acid (300–600 mg/d).

THALASSEMIA SYNDROMES

The thalassemia syndromes are inherited disorders of α- or β-globin biosynthesis. The reduced supply of globin diminishes production of hemoglobin tetramers, causing hypochromia and microcytosis. Unbalanced accumulation of α and β subunits occurs because the synthesis of the unaffected globins proceeds at a normal rate. Unbalanced chain accumulation dominates the clinical phenotype. Clinical severity varies widely, depending on the degree to which the synthesis of the affected globin is impaired, altered synthesis of other globin chains, and co-inheritance of other abnormal globin alleles.

CLINICAL MANIFESTATIONS OF β-THALASSEMIA SYNDROMES

Mutations causing thalassemia can affect any step in the pathway of globin gene expression: transcription, processing of the mRNA precursor, translation, and posttranslational metabolism of the β-globin polypeptide chain. The most common forms arise from mutations that derange splicing of the mRNA precursor or prematurely terminate translation of the mRNA.

Hypochromia and microcytosis characterize all forms of β thalassemia because of the reduced amounts of hemoglobin tetramers (Fig. 99-5). In heterozygotes (β-thalassemia trait), this is the only abnormality seen. Anemia is minimal. In more severe homozygous states, unbalanced α- and β-globin accumulation causes accumulation of highly insoluble unpaired α chains. They form toxic inclusion bodies that kill developing erythroblasts in the marrow. Few of the proerythroblasts beginning erythroid maturation survive. The few resulting RBCs bear a burden of inclusion bodies that are detected in the spleen, shortening the RBC life span and producing severe hemolytic anemia. The resulting profound anemia stimulates erythropoietin release and compensatory erythroid hyperplasia, but the marrow response is sabotaged by ineffective erythropoiesis. Anemia persists. Erythroid hyperplasia can become exuberant and produce masses of extramedullary erythropoietic tissue in the liver and spleen.

Massive bone marrow expansion deranges growth and development. Children develop characteristic "chipmunk" facies due to maxillary marrow hyperplasia and frontal bossing. Thinning and pathologic fracture of long bones and vertebrae may occur due to cortical invasion by erythroid elements and profound growth retardation. Hemolytic anemia causes hepatosplenomegaly, leg ulcers, gallstones, and high-output congestive heart failure. The conscription of caloric resources to support erythropoiesis leads to inanition, susceptibility to infection, endocrine dysfunction, and in the most severe cases, death during the first decade of life. Chronic transfusions with RBCs improves oxygen delivery, suppresses the excessive ineffective erythropoiesis, and prolongs life, but the inevitable side effects, notably iron overload, usually prove fatal by age 30.

Severity is highly variable. Known modulating factors are those that ameliorate the burden of unpaired α-globin inclusions. Alleles associated with milder synthetic defects and co-inheritance of α-thalassemia trait reduce clinical severity by reducing accumulation of excess α

FIGURE 99-5 **β-Thalassemia intermedia.** Microcytic and hypochromic red blood cells are seen that resemble the red blood cells of severe iron deficiency anemia. Many elliptical and teardrop-shaped red blood cells are noted.

globin. HbF persists to various degrees in β thalassemias. γ-Globin gene chains can substitute for β chains, generating more hemoglobin and reducing the burden of α-globin inclusions. The terms β-*thalassemia major* and β-*thalassemia intermedia* are used to reflect the clinical heterogeneity. Patients with β-thalassemia major require intensive transfusion support to survive. Patients with β-thalassemia intermedia have a somewhat milder phenotype and can survive without transfusion. The terms β-*thalassemia minor* and β-*thalassemia trait* describe asymptomatic heterozygotes for β thalassemia.

TABLE 99-4 THE α THALASSEMIAS

Condition	Hemoglobin A, %	Hemoglobin H (β^4), %	Hemoglobin Level, g/L (g/dL)	MCV, fL
Normal	97	0	150 (15)	90
Silent thalassemia: $-\alpha/\alpha\alpha$	98–100	0	150 (15)	90
Thalassemia trait: $-\alpha/-\alpha$ homozygous α-thal-2[a] or $--/\alpha\alpha$ heterozygous α-thal-1[a]	85–95	Rare red blood cell inclusions	120–130 (12–13)	70–80
Hemoglobin H disease: $--/-\alpha$ heterozygous α-thal-1/α-thal-2	70–95	5–30	60–100 (6–10)	60–70
Hydrops fetalis: $--/--$ homozygous α-thal-1	0	5–10[b]	Fatal in utero or at birth	

[a]When both α alleles on one chromosome are deleted, the locus is called α-thal-1; when only a single α allele on one chromosome is deleted, the locus is called α-thal-2.
[b]90–95% of the hemoglobin is hemoglobin Barts (tetramers of γ chains).

α-THALASSEMIA SYNDROMES

The four classic α thalassemias, most common in Asians, are α-thalassemia-2 trait, in which one of the four α-globin loci is deleted; α-thalassemia-1 trait, with two deleted loci; HbH disease, with three loci deleted; and hydrops fetalis with Hb Bart's, with all four loci deleted (Table 99-4). Nondeletion forms of α thalassemia also exist.

α-*Thalassemia-2 trait* is an asymptomatic, silent carrier state. α-*Thalassemia-1 trait* resembles β-thalassemia minor. Offspring doubly heterozygous for α-thalassemia-2 and α-thalassemia-1 exhibit a more severe phenotype called *HbH disease*. Heterozygosity for a deletion that removes both genes from the same chromosome (*cis* deletion) is common in Asians and in those from the Mediterranean region, as is homozygosity for α-thalassemia-2 (*trans* deletion). Both produce asymptomatic hypochromia and microcytosis.

In *HbH disease*, HbA production is only 25–30% normal. Fetuses accumulate some unpaired β chains. In adults, unpaired β chains accumulate and are soluble enough to form β_4 tetramers called HbH. HbH forms few inclusions in erythroblasts and precipitates in circulating RBC. Patients with HbH disease have thalassemia intermedia characterized by moderately severe hemolytic anemia but milder ineffective erythropoiesis. Survival into mid-adult life without transfusions is common.

The homozygous state for the α-thalassemia-1 *cis* deletion (hydrops fetalis) causes total absence of α-globin synthesis. No physiologically useful hemoglobin is produced beyond the embryonic stage. Excess γ globin forms tetramers called *Hb Barts* (γ_4), which has a very high oxygen affinity. It delivers almost no O_2 to fetal tissues, causing tissue asphyxia, edema (hydrops fetalis), congestive heart failure, and death in utero. α-Thalassemia-2 trait is common (15–20%) among people of African descent. The *cis* α-thalassemia-1 deletion is almost never seen, however. Thus, α-thalassemia-2 and the *trans* form of α-thalassemia-1 are very common, but HbH disease and hydrops fetalis are almost never encountered.

It has been known for some time that some patients with myelodysplasia or erythroleukemia produce RBC clones containing HbH. This phenomenon is due to mutations in the ATRX pathway that affect the LCR of the α-globin gene cluster.

DIAGNOSIS AND MANAGEMENT OF THALASSEMIAS

The diagnosis of β-thalassemia major is readily made during childhood on the basis of severe anemia accompanied by the characteristic signs of massive ineffective erythropoiesis: hepatosplenomegaly, profound microcytosis, a characteristic blood smear (Fig. 99-5), and elevated levels of HbF, HbA₂, or both. Many patients require chronic hypertransfusion therapy designed to maintain a hematocrit of at least 27–30% so that erythropoiesis is suppressed. Splenectomy is required if the annual transfusion requirement (volume of RBCs per kilogram of body weight per year) increases by >50%. Folic acid supplements may be useful. Vaccination with Pneumovax in anticipation of eventual splenectomy is advised, as is close monitoring for infection, leg ulcers, and biliary tract disease. Many patients develop endocrine

deficiencies as a result of iron overload. Early endocrine evaluation is required for glucose intolerance, thyroid dysfunction, and delayed onset of puberty or secondary sexual characteristics.

Patients with β-thalassemia intermedia exhibit similar stigmata but can survive without chronic hypertransfusion. Management is particularly challenging because a number of factors can aggravate the anemia, including infection, onset of puberty, and development of splenomegaly and hypersplenism. Some patients may eventually benefit from splenectomy. The expanded erythron can cause absorption of excessive dietary iron and hemosiderosis, even without transfusion.

β-Thalassemia minor (i.e., thalassemia trait) usually presents as profound microcytosis and hypochromia with target cells, but only minimal or mild anemia. The mean corpuscular volume is rarely >75 fL; the hematocrit is rarely <30–33%. Hemoglobin electrophoresis classically reveals an elevated HbA₂ (3.5–7.5%), but some forms are associated with normal HbA₂ and/or elevated HbF. Genetic counseling and patient education are essential. Patients with β-thalassemia trait should be warned that their blood picture resembles iron deficiency and can be misdiagnosed. They should eschew empirical use of iron; yet iron deficiency can develop during pregnancy or from chronic bleeding.

Persons with α-thalassemia trait may exhibit mild hypochromia and microcytosis usually without anemia. HbA₂ and HbF levels are normal. Affected individuals usually require only genetic counseling. HbH disease resembles β-thalassemia intermedia, with the added complication that the HbH molecule behaves like moderately unstable hemoglobin. Patients with HbH disease should undergo splenectomy if excessive anemia or a transfusion requirement develops. Oxidative drugs should be avoided. Iron overload leading to death can occur in more severely affected patients.

PREVENTION

Antenatal diagnosis of thalassemia syndromes is now widely available. DNA diagnosis is based on PCR amplification of fetal DNA, obtained by amniocentesis or chorionic villus biopsy followed by hybridization to allele-specific oligonucleotides probes. The probes can be designed to detect simultaneously the subset of mutations that account for 95–99% of the α- or β-thalassemias that occur in a particular group.

THALASSEMIC STRUCTURAL VARIANTS

Thalassemic structural variants are characterized by both defective synthesis and abnormal structure.

HEMOGLOBIN LEPORE

Hb Lepore [$\alpha_2(\delta\beta)_2$] arises by an unequal crossover and recombination event that fuses the proximal end of the δ-gene with the distal end of the closely linked β-gene. The resulting chromosome contains only the fused δβ gene. The Lepore (δβ) globin is synthesized poorly because the fused gene is under the control of the weak δ-globin promoter. Hb Lepore alleles have a phenotype like β thalassemia, except for the added presence of 2–20% Hb Lepore. Compound heterozygotes for Hb Lepore and a classic β-thalassemia allele may also have severe thalassemia.

HEMOGLOBIN E

HbE (i.e., $\alpha_2\beta_2^{26Glu\rightarrow Lys}$) is extremely common in Cambodia, Thailand, and Vietnam. The gene has become far more prevalent in the United States as a result of immigration of Asian persons, especially in California, where HbE is the most common variant detected. HbE is mildly unstable but not enough to affect RBC life span significantly. The high frequency of the HbE gene may be a result of the thalassemia phenotype associated with its inheritance. Heterozygotes resemble individuals with mild β-thalassemia trait. Homozygotes have somewhat more marked abnormalities but are asymptomatic. Compound heterozygotes for HbE and a β-thalassemia gene can have β-thalassemia intermedia or β-thalassemia major, depending on the severity of the coinherited thalassemic gene.

The β^E allele contains a single base change in codon 26 that causes the amino acid substitution. However, this mutation activates a cryptic RNA splice site generating a structurally abnormal globin mRNA that cannot be translated from about 50% of the initial pre-mRNA molecules. The remaining 40–50% are normally spliced and generate functional mRNA that is translated into β^E-globin because the mature mRNA carries the base change that alters codon 26.

Genetic counseling of the persons at risk for HbE should focus on the interaction of HbE with β thalassemia rather than HbE homozygosity, a condition associated with asymptomatic microcytosis, hypochromia, and hemoglobin levels rarely <1 g/L (<10 g/dL).

HEREDITARY PERSISTENCE OF FETAL HEMOGLOBIN

HPFH is characterized by continued synthesis of high levels of HbF in adult life. No deleterious effects are apparent, even when all of the hemoglobin produced is HbF. These rare patients demonstrate convincingly that prevention or reversal of the fetal to adult hemoglobin switch would provide effective therapy for sickle cell anemia and β thalassemia.

ACQUIRED HEMOGLOBINOPATHIES

The two most important acquired hemoglobinopathies are carbon monoxide poisoning and methemoglobinemia (see above). Carbon monoxide has a higher affinity for hemoglobin than does oxygen; it can replace oxygen and diminish O_2 delivery. Chronic elevation of carboxyhemoglobin levels to 10 or 15%, as occurs in smokers, can lead to secondary polycythemia. Carboxyhemoglobin is cherry red in color and masks the development of cyanosis usually associated with poor O_2 delivery to tissues.

Abnormalities of hemoglobin biosynthesis have also been described in blood dyscrasias. In some patients with myelodysplasia, erythroleukemia, or myeloproliferative disorders, a mild form of HbH disease may also be seen. The abnormalities are not severe enough to alter the course of the underlying disease.

Rx TRANSFUSIONAL HEMOSIDEROSIS

Chronic blood transfusion can lead to blood-borne infection, alloimmunization, febrile reactions, and lethal iron overload (Chap. 107). A unit of packed RBCs contains 250–300 mg iron (1 mg/mL). The iron assimilated by a single transfusion of two units of packed RBCs is thus equal to a 1- to 2-year intake of iron. Iron accumulates in chronically transfused patients because no mechanisms exist for increasing iron excretion: an expanded erythron causes especially rapid development of iron overload because accelerated erythropoiesis promotes excessive absorption of dietary iron. Vitamin C should not be supplemented because it generates free radicals in iron excess states.

Patients who receive >100 units of packed RBCs usually develop hemosiderosis. The ferritin level rises, followed by early endocrine dysfunction (glucose intolerance and delayed puberty), cirrhosis, and cardiomyopathy. Liver biopsy shows both parenchymal and reticuloendothelial iron. The superconducting quantum-interference device (SQUID) is accurate at measuring hepatic iron but not widely available. Cardiac toxicity is often insidious. Early development of pericarditis is followed by dysrhythmia and pump failure. The onset of heart failure is ominous, often presaging death within a year (Chap. 351).

The decision to start long-term transfusion support should also prompt one to institute therapy with iron-chelating agents. Desferoxamine (Desferal) is for parenteral use. Its iron-binding kinetics require chronic slow infusion via a metering pump. The constant presence of the drug improves the efficiency of chelation and protects tissues from occasional releases of the most toxic fraction of iron—low-molecular-weight iron—which may not be sequestered by protective proteins.

Desferoxamine is relatively nontoxic. Occasional cataracts, deafness, and local skin reactions, including urticaria, occur. Skin reactions can usually be managed with antihistamines. Negative iron balance can be achieved, even in the face of a high transfusion requirement, but this alone does not prevent long-term morbidity and mortality in chronically transfused patients. Irreversible end-organ deterioration develops at relatively modest levels of iron overload, even if symptoms do not appear for many years thereafter. To enjoy a significant survival advantage, chelation must begin before 5–8 years of age in β-thalassemia major.

Deferasirox is a promising oral iron-chelating agent. Single daily doses of 20 or 30 mg deferasirox produced reductions in liver iron concentration comparable to desferoxamine in chronically transfused adult and pediatric patients. Deferasirox produces some elevations in liver enzymes and slight but persistent increases in serum creatinine, without apparent clinical consequence. Other toxicities are similar to those of desferoxamine. Its toxicity profile is acceptable, although long-term effects are still being evaluated.

EXPERIMENTAL THERAPIES

BONE MARROW TRANSPLANTATION, GENE THERAPY, AND MANIPULATION OF HbF

Bone marrow transplantation provides stem cells able to express normal hemoglobin; it has been used in a large number of patients with β thalassemia and a smaller number of patients with sickle cell anemia. Early in the course of disease, before end-organ damage occurs, transplantation is curative in 80–90% of patients. In highly experienced centers, the treatment-related mortality is <10%. Since survival into adult life is possible with conventional therapy, the decision to transplant is best made in consultation with specialized centers.

Gene therapy of thalassemia and sickle cell disease has proved to be an elusive goal. Uptake of gene vectors into the nondividing hematopoietic stem cells has been inefficient. Lentiviral-type vectors that can transduce nondividing cells may solve this problem.

Reestablishing high levels of fetal hemoglobin synthesis should ameliorate the symptoms of β thalassemia. Cytotoxic agents such as hydroxyurea and cytarabine promote high levels of HbF synthesis, probably by stimulating proliferation of the primitive HbF-producing progenitor cell population (i.e., F cell progenitors). Unfortunately, no regimen has yet been identified that ameliorates the clinical manifestations of β thalassemia. Butyrates stimulate HbF production, but only transiently. Pulsed or intermittent administration has been found to sustain HbF induction in the majority of patients with sickle cell disease. It is unclear whether butyrates will have similar activity in patients with β thalassemia.

APLASTIC AND HYPOPLASTIC CRISIS IN PATIENTS WITH HEMOGLOBINOPATHIES

Patients with hemolytic anemias sometimes exhibit an alarming decline in hematocrit during and immediately after acute illnesses. Bone marrow suppression occurs in almost everyone during acute inflammatory illnesses. In patients with short RBC life spans, suppression can affect RBC counts more dramatically. These hypoplastic crises are usually transient and self-correcting before intervention is required.

Aplastic crisis refers to a profound cessation of erythroid activity in patients with chronic hemolytic anemias. It is associated with a rapidly falling hematocrit. Episodes are usually self-limited. Aplastic crises are caused by infection with a particular strain of parvovirus, B19A. Children infected with this virus usually develop permanent immunity.

Aplastic crises do not often recur and are rarely seen in adults. Management requires close monitoring of the hematocrit and reticulocyte count. If anemia becomes symptomatic, transfusion support is indicated. Most crises resolve spontaneously within 1–2 weeks.

FURTHER READINGS

ATAGA KI, ORRINGA EP: Hypercoagulability in sickle cell disease: A curious paradox. Am J Med 115:721, 2003

DESIMONE J et al: Maintenance of elevated fetal hemoglobin levels by decitabine during dose interval treatment of sickle cell anemia. Blood 99:3905, 2002

NEUFELD EJ: Oral chelators deferasirox and deferiprone for transfusional iron overload in thalassemia major: New data, new questions. Blood 107:3436, 2006

QUEK L, THEIN SL: Molecular therapies in beta-thalassaemia. Br J Haematol 136:353, 2007

STEINBERG MH: Pathophysiologically based drug treatment of sickle cell disease. Trends Pharmacol Sci 27:204, 2006

SWITZER JA et al: Pathophysiology and treatment of stroke in sickle-cell disease: Present and future. Lancet Neurol 5:501, 2006

WARE RE et al: Predictors of fetal hemoglobin response in children with sickle cell anemia receiving hydroxyurea therapy. Blood 99:10, 2002

100 Megaloblastic Anemias
A. Victor Hoffbrand

The megaloblastic anemias are a group of disorders characterized by the presence of distinctive morphologic appearances of the developing red cells in the bone marrow. The cause is usually deficiency of either cobalamin (vitamin B_{12}) or folate, but megaloblastic anemia may arise because of genetic or acquired abnormalities affecting the metabolism of these vitamins or because of defects in DNA synthesis not related to cobalamin or folate (Table 100-1). Cobalamin and folate absorption and metabolism are described next and then the biochemical basis, clinical and laboratory features, causes, and treatment of megaloblastic anemia. The marrow is usually cellular, and the anemia is based on ineffective erythropoiesis.

COBALAMIN

Cobalamin (vitamin B_{12}) exists in a number of different chemical forms. All have a cobalt atom at the center of a corrin ring. In nature, the vitamin is mainly in the 2-deoxyadenosyl (ado) form, which is located in mitochondria. It is the cofactor for the enzyme methylmalonyl CoA mutase. The other major natural cobalamin is methylcobalamin, the form in human plasma and in cell cytoplasm. It is the cofactor for methionine synthase. There are also minor amounts of hydroxocobalamin to which methyl- and adocobalamin are rapidly converted by exposure to light.

Dietary Sources and Requirements Cobalamin is synthesized solely by microorganisms. Ruminants obtain cobalamin from the foregut, but the only source for humans is food of animal origin, e.g., meat, fish, and dairy products. Vegetables, fruits, and other foods of non-animal origin are free from cobalamin unless they are contaminated by bacteria. A normal Western diet contains between 5 and 30 μg of cobalamin daily. Adult daily losses (mainly in the urine and feces) are between 1 and 3 μg (~0.1% of body stores) and, as the body does not have the ability to degrade cobalamin, daily requirements are also about 1–3 μg. Body stores are of the order of 2–3 mg, sufficient for 3–4 years if supplies are completely cut off.

TABLE 100-1 CAUSES OF MEGALOBLASTIC ANEMIA

Cobalamin deficiency or abnormalities of cobalamin metabolism (see Tables 100-3, 100-4)

Folate deficiency or abnormalities of folate metabolism (see Table 100-5)

Therapy with antifolate drugs (e.g., methotrexate)

Independent of either cobalamin or folate deficiency and refractory to cobalamin and folate therapy:
  Some cases of acute myeloid leukemia, myelodysplasia
  Therapy with drugs interfering with synthesis of DNA [e.g., cytosine arabinoside, hydroxyurea, 6-mercaptopurine, azidothymidine (AZT)]
  Orotic aciduria (responds to uridine)
  Thiamine-responsive

Absorption Two mechanisms exist for cobalamin absorption. One is passive, occurring equally through buccal, duodenal, and ileal mucosa; it is rapid but extremely inefficient, <1% of an oral dose being absorbed by this process. The normal physiologic mechanism is active; it occurs through the ileum and is efficient for small (a few micrograms) oral doses of cobalamin and is mediated by gastric intrinsic factor (IF). Dietary cobalamin is released from protein complexes by enzymes in the stomach, duodenum, and jejunum; it combines rapidly with a salivary glycoprotein that belongs to the family of cobalamin-binding proteins known as haptocorrins (HCs). In the intestine, the haptocorrin is digested by pancreatic trypsin and the cobalamin transferred to IF.

IF is produced in the gastric parietal cells of the fundus and body of the stomach, and its secretion parallels that of hydrochloric acid. The IF-cobalamin complex passes to the ileum, where IF attaches to a specific receptor (cubilin) on the microvillus membrane of the enterocytes. Cubilin is also present in yolk sac and renal proximal tubular epithelium. Cubulin appears to traffic by means of amnionless (AMN), an endocytic receptor protein that directs sublocalization and endocytosis of cubulin with its ligand IF-cobalamin complex. The cobalamin-IF complex enters the ileal cell where IF is destroyed. After a delay of about 6 h, the cobalamin appears in portal blood attached to transcobalamin (TC) II.

Between 0.5 and 5.0 μg of cobalamin enters the bile each day. This binds to IF, and a major portion of biliary cobalamin is normally reabsorbed together with cobalamin derived from sloughed intestinal cells. Because of the appreciable amount of cobalamin undergoing enterohepatic circulation, cobalamin deficiency develops more rapidly in individuals who malabsorb cobalamin than it does in vegans, in whom reabsorption of biliary cobalamin is intact.

Transport Two main cobalamin transport proteins exist in human plasma; they both bind cobalamin—one molecule for one molecule. One HC, known as TC I, is closely related to other cobalamin-binding HCs in milk, gastric juice, bile, saliva, and other fluids. These HCs differ from each other only in the carbohydrate moiety of the molecule. TC I is derived primarily from the specific granules in neutrophils. Normally, it is about two-thirds saturated with cobalamin, which it binds tightly. TC I does not enhance cobalamin entry into tissues. Glycoprotein receptors on liver cells are involved in the removal of TC I from plasma, and TC I may have a role in the transport of cobalamin analogues to the liver for excretion in bile.

The other major cobalamin transport protein in plasma is TC II. This is synthesized by liver and by other tissues, including macrophages, ileum, and endothelium. It normally carries only 20–60 ng of cobalamin per liter of plasma and readily gives up cobalamin to marrow, placenta, and other tissues, which it enters by receptor-mediated endocytosis.

FOLATE

Dietary Folate Folic (pteroylglutamic) acid is a yellow, crystalline, water-soluble substance. It is the parent compound of a large family of natural folate compounds, which differ from it in three respects:

TABLE 100-2 BIOCHEMICAL REACTIONS OF FOLATE COENZYMES

Reaction	Coenzyme Form of Folate Involved	Single Carbon Unit Transferred	Importance
Formate activation	THF	–CHO	Generation of 10-formyl-THF
Purine synthesis			
Formation of glycinamide ribonucleotide	5,10-MethyleneTHF	–CHO	Formation of purines needed for DNA, RNA synthesis, but reactions probably not rate limiting
Formylation of amino-imidazolecarboxamide-ribonucleotide (AICAR)	10-Formyl (CHO)THF		
Pyrimidine synthesis			
Methylation of deoxyuridine monophosphate (dUMP) to thymidine monophosphate (dTMP)	5,10-MethyleneTHF	–CH₃	Rate limiting in DNA synthesis Oxidizes THF to DHF Some breakdown of folate at the C-9–N-10 bond
Amino acid interconversion			
Serine–glycine interconversion	THF	=CH₂	Entry of single carbon units into active pool
Homocysteine to methionine	5-Methyl(M)THF	–CH₃	Demethylation of 5-MTHF to THF; also requires cobalamin, flavine adenine dinucleotide, ATP, and adenosylmethionine
Forminoglutamic acid to glutamic acid in histidine catabolism	THF	–HN–CH=	

DHF, dihydrofolate; THF, tetrahydrofolate.

(1) they are partly or completely reduced to di- or tetrahydrofolate (THF) derivatives; (2) they usually contain a single carbon unit (Table 100-2), and (3) 70–90% of natural folates are folate-polyglutamates.

Most foods contain some folate. The highest concentrations are found in liver, yeast, spinach, other greens, and nuts (>100 μg/100 g). The total folate content of an average Western diet is ~250 μg daily, but the amount varies widely according to the type of food eaten and the method of cooking. Folate is easily destroyed by heating, particularly in large volumes of water. Total-body folate in the adult is ~10 mg, the liver containing the largest store. Daily adult requirements are ~100 μg, so stores are only sufficient for 3–4 months in normal adults and severe folate deficiency may develop rapidly.

Absorption Folates are absorbed rapidly from the upper small intestine. The absorption of folate polyglutamates is less efficient than for monoglutamates; on average, ~50% of food folate is absorbed. Polyglutamate forms are hydrolysed to the monoglutamate derivatives, either in the lumen of the intestine or within the mucosa. All dietary folates are converted to 5-methylTHF (5-MTHF) within the small-intestinal mucosa before entering portal plasma. The monoglutamates are actively transported across the enterocyte by a carrier-mediated mechanism. Pteroylglutamic acid at doses >400 μg is absorbed largely unchanged and converted to natural folates in the liver. Lower doses are converted to 5-MTHF during absorption through the intestine.

About 60–90 μg of folate enters the bile each day and is excreted into the small intestine. Loss of this folate, together with the folate of sloughed intestinal cells, accelerates the speed with which folate deficiency develops in malabsorption conditions.

Transport Folate is transported in plasma; about one-third is loosely bound to albumin and two-thirds unbound. In all body fluids (plasma, cerebrospinal fluid, milk, bile) folate is largely, if not entirely, 5-MTHF in the monoglutamate form. Two types of folate-binding protein are involved in entry of MTHF into cells. A high-affinity folate receptor takes folate into cells by endocytosis, is internalized by clathrin-coated pits or in a vesicle (caveola), which is then acidified, releasing folate. Folate is then carried by the membrane folate transporter into the cytoplasm. The high-affinity receptor is attached to the outer surface of the cell membrane by glycosyl phosphatidylinositol linkages. It may be involved in

transport of oxidized folates and folate breakdown products to the liver for excretion in bile. An independent low-affinity reduced-folate carrier also mediates uptake of physiologic folates into cells but also of methotrexate.

Biochemical Functions Folates (as the intracellular polyglutamate derivatives) act as coenzymes in the transfer of single-carbon units (Fig. 100-1 and Table 100-2). Two of these reactions are involved in purine and one in pyrimidine synthesis necessary for DNA and RNA replication. Folate is also a coenzyme for methionine synthesis, in which methylcobalamin is also involved in and in which THF is regenerated. THF is the acceptor of single carbon units newly entering the active pool via conversion of serine to glycine. Methionine, the other product of the methionine synthase reaction, is the precursor for *S*-adenosylmethionine (SAM), the universal methyl donor involved in >100 methyltransferase reactions (Fig. 100-1).

During thymidylate synthesis, 5,10-methylene-THF is oxidized to DHF (dihydrofolate). The enzyme DHF reductase converts this to THF. The drugs methotrexate, pyrimethamine, and (mainly in bacteria) trimethoprim inhibit DHF reductase and so prevent formation of active THF coenzymes from DHF. A small fraction of the folate coenzyme is not recycled during thymidylate synthesis but is degraded.

BIOCHEMICAL BASIS OF MEGALOBLASTIC ANEMIA

The common feature of all megaloblastic anemias is a defect in DNA synthesis that affects rapidly dividing cells in the bone marrow. All conditions that give rise to megaloblastic changes share in common a disparity in the rate of synthesis or availability of the four immediate precursors of DNA: the deoxyribonucleoside triphosphates (dNTPs): dA(adenine)TP and dG(guanine)TP (purines), dT(thymine)TP and dC(cytosine)TP (pyrimidines). In deficiencies of either folate or cobalamin, there is failure to convert deoxyuridine monophosphate (dUMP) to deoxythymidine monophosphate (dTMP), the precursor of dTTP (Fig. 100-1). This is because folate is needed as the coenzyme 5,10-methylene-THF polyglutamate for conversion of dUMP to dTMP; the availability of 5,10-methylene-THF is reduced in either cobalamin or folate deficiency. An alternative theory for megaloblastic anemia in cobalamin or folate deficiency is misincorporation of uracil into DNA because of a build-up of deoxyuridine triphosphate (dUTP) at the DNA replication fork as a consequence of the block in conversion of dUMP to dTMP.

Cobalamin-Folate Relations Folate is required for many reactions in mammalian tissues. Only two reactions in the body are known to require cobalamin. Methylmalonyl CoA isomerization, which requires adocobalamin, and the methylation of homocysteine to methionine requires both methylcobalamin and both 5-MTHF (Fig. 100-1). This reaction is the first step in the pathway by which 5-MTHF, which enters bone marrow and other cells from plasma, is converted into all the intracellular folate coenzymes. The coenzymes are all polyglutamated (the larger size aiding retention in the cell), but the enzyme folate polyglutamate synthase can use only THF, not MTHF, as substrate. In cobalamin deficiency, MTHF accumulates in plasma, while intracellular folate concentrations fall due to failure of formation of THF, the substrate on which folate polyglutamates are built. This has been termed *THF starvation*, or the *methylfolate trap*.

FIGURE 100-1 The role of folates in DNA synthesis and in formation on *S*-adenosylmethionine (SAM), which is involved in numerous methylation reactions. *[Reprinted from Hoffbrand AV et al (eds), Postgraduate Haematology, 5th ed, Blackwell Publishing, Oxford, UK 2005; with permission.]*

This theory explains the abnormalities of folate metabolism that occur in cobalamin deficiency [high serum folate, low cell folate, positive purine precursor aminomidazole carboxamide ribonucleotide (AICAR) excretion; Table 100-2] and also why the anemia of cobalamin deficiency will respond to folic acid in large doses.

CLINICAL FEATURES

Many symptomless patients are detected through the finding of a raised mean corpuscular volume (MCV) on a routine blood count. The main clinical features in more severe cases are those of anemia. Anorexia is usually marked and there may be weight loss, diarrhea, or constipation. Glossitis, angular cheilosis, a mild fever in the more severely anemic patients, jaundice (unconjugated), and reversible melanin skin hyperpigmentation may also occur with deficiency of either folate or cobalamin. Thrombocytopenia sometimes leads to bruising, and this may be aggravated by vitamin C deficiency or alcohol in malnourished patients. The anemia and low leukocyte count may predispose to infections, particularly of the respiratory or urinary tracts. Cobalamin deficiency has also been associated with impaired bactericidal function of phagocytes.

General Tissue Effects of Cobalamin and Folate Deficiencies • *EPITHELIAL SURFACES* After the marrow, the next most affected tissues are the epithelial cell surfaces of the mouth, stomach, and small intestine and the respiratory, urinary, and female genital tracts. The cells show macrocytosis, with increased numbers of multinucleate and dying cells. The deficiencies may cause cervical smear abnormalities.

COMPLICATIONS OF PREGNANCY The gonads are also affected, and infertility is common in both men and women with either deficiency. Maternal folate deficiency has been implicated as a cause of prematurity, and both folate and cobalamin deficiency have been implicated in recurrent fetal loss and neural tube defects, discussed below.

NEURAL TUBE DEFECTS Folic acid supplements at the time of conception and in the first 12 weeks of pregnancy reduce by ~70% the incidence of neural tube defects (NTDs) (anencephaly, meningomyelocele, encephalocele, and spina bifida) in the fetus. Most of this protective effect can be achieved by taking folic acid, 0.4 mg daily at the time of conception.

The incidence of cleft palate and harelip can also be reduced by prophylactic folic acid. There is no clear simple relationship between maternal folate status and these fetal abnormalities, although overall the lower the maternal folate, the greater the risk to the fetus. NTDs can also be caused by antifolate and antiepileptic drugs.

An underlying maternal folate metabolic abnormality has also been postulated. One abnormality has been identified: reduced activity of the enzyme 5,10-methylene-THF reductase (MTHFR) (Fig. 100-1) caused by a common 677C→T polymorphism in the *MTHFR* gene. In one study, the prevalence of this polymorphism was found to be higher in the parents of NTD fetuses and in the fetuses themselves: homozygosity for the TT mutation was found in 13% compared with 5% in control subjects. The polymorphism codes for a thermolabile form of MTHFR. The homozygous state results in a lower mean serum and red cell folate level compared with control subjects, as well as significantly higher serum homocysteine levels. Tests for mutations in other enzymes possibly associated with NTDs, e.g., methionine synthase or serine–glycine hydroxymethylase, have been negative.

Autoantibodies to folate receptors have, however, been detected in 9 of 12 women who were or had been pregnant with a fetus with a NTD, but in only 2 of 20 control women. Antiserum to folate receptors results in resorption or multiple developmental abnormalities in mouse embryos. It is possible, therefore, that the association of antibodies to maternal folate receptors and NTDs reflects a causal relation.

CARDIOVASCULAR DISEASE Children with severe homocystinuria (blood levels ≥100 μmol/L) due to deficiency of one of three enzymes, methionine synthase, MHTFR, or cystathionine synthase (Fig. 100-1), suffer from vascular disease, e.g., ischemic heart disease, cerebrovascular disease, or pulmonary embolus as teenagers or in young adulthood. Lesser degrees of raised serum homocysteine and low levels of serum folate have been found to be associated with cerebrovascular, peripheral vascular, and coronary heart disease and with deep vein thrombosis. Prospective randomized trials of lowering homocysteine levels with supplements of folic acid, vitamin B_{12}, and vitamin B_6 against placebo over a 5-year period in patients with vascular disease or diabetes have not, however, shown a reduction of major cardiovascular events, nor have these supplements reduced the risk of recurrent cardiovascular disease after an acute myocardial infarct. It is possible that these trials were not sufficiently powered to detect a small (e.g., 10%) benefit or that some other underlying factor is responsible for both the vascular damage and the raised homocysteine. Alternatively, the beneficial effects of lowering homocysteine were offset in these trials by the vitamins stimulating endothelial cell proliferation. The results of longer and larger trials are needed to resolve these uncertainties.

MALIGNANCY Prophylactic folic acid in pregnancy has been found to reduce the subsequent incidence of acute lymphoblastic leukemia (ALL) in childhood. A significant negative association has also been found with the *MTHFR* 677(C→T) polymorphism and leukemias with mixed lineage leukemia (MLL) translocations, but a positive association with hyperdiploidy in infants with ALL or acute myeloid leukemia or with childhood ALL. A second polymorphism in the *MHTFR* gene, A1298C, is also strongly associated with hyperdiploid leukemia. There are various positive and negative associations between polymorphisms in folate-dependent enzymes and the incidence of adult ALL. The C677T polymorphism is thought to lead to increased thymidine pools and "better quality" of DNA synthesis by shunting 1-carbon groups towards thymidine and purine synthesis. This may explain its reported association with a lower risk for colorectal cancer. Other tumors that have been associated with folate polymorphisms or status include follicular lymphoma, breast cancer, and gastric cancer.

NEUROLOGIC MANIFESTATIONS Cobalamin deficiency may cause a bilateral peripheral neuropathy or degeneration (demyelination) of the posterior and pyramidal tracts of the spinal cord and, less frequently, optic atrophy or cerebral symptoms.

The patient, more frequently male, presents with paresthesias, muscle weakness, or difficulty in walking and sometimes dementia, psychotic disturbances, or visual impairment. Long-term nutritional cobalamin deficiency in infancy leads to poor brain development and impaired intellectual development. Folate deficiency has been suggested to cause organic nervous disease but this is uncertain, although methotrexate injected into the cerebrospinal fluid may cause brain or spinal cord damage.

An important clinical problem is the nonanemic patient with neurologic or psychiatric abnormalities and a low or borderline serum cobalamin level. In such patients, it is necessary to try to establish whether or not there is significant cobalamin deficiency, e.g., by careful examination of the blood film, cobalamin absorption studies, tests for antibodies to IF or parietal cells, and serum methylmalonic acid (MMA) measurement if available. A trial of cobalamin therapy for at least 3 months will also usually be needed to determine whether the symptoms improve.

The biochemical basis for cobalamin neuropathy remains obscure. Its occurrence in the absence of methylmalonic aciduria in TC II deficiency suggests that the neuropathy is related to the defect in homocysteine-methionine conversion. Accumulation of *S*-adenosylhomocysteine in the brain, resulting in inhibition of transmethylation reactions, has been suggested.

Psychiatric disturbance is common in both folate and cobalamin deficiencies. This, like the neuropathy, has been attributed to a failure of the synthesis of SAM, which is needed in methylation of biogenic amines (e.g., dopamine) as well as of proteins, phospholipids, and neurotransmitters in the brain (Fig. 100-1). Associations between lower serum folate or cobalamin levels and higher homocysteine levels and the development of Alzheimer's disease have been reported. A 2-year double-blind placebo-controlled randomized clinical trial involving healthy subjects >65 years old given folate, cobalamin, and vitamin B_6 supplements showed no benefit on cognitive performance, whereas a 3-year (FACIT) study did show benefit.

HEMATOLOGIC FINDINGS

Peripheral Blood Oval macrocytes, usually with considerable anisocytosis and poikilocytosis, are the main feature (Fig. 100-2*A*). The MCV is usually >100 fL unless a cause of microcytosis (e.g., iron deficiency or thalassemia trait) is present. Some of the neutrophils are hypersegmented (more than five nuclear lobes). There may be leukopenia due to a reduction in granulocytes and lymphocytes, but this is usually >1.5 × 10^9/L; the platelet count may be moderately reduced, rarely to <40 × 10^9/L. The severity of all these changes parallels the degree of anemia. In the nonanemic patient, the presence of a few macrocytes and hypersegmented neutrophils in the peripheral blood may be the only indication of the underlying disorder.

Bone Marrow In the severely anemic patient, the marrow is hypercellular with an accumulation of primitive cells due to selective death by apoptosis of more mature forms. The erythroblast nucleus maintains a primitive appearance despite maturation and hemoglobinization of the cytoplasm. The cells are larger than normoblasts, and an increased number of cells with eccentric lobulated nuclei or nuclear fragments may be present (Fig. 100-2*B*). Giant and abnormally shaped metamyelocytes and enlarged hyperpolyploid megakaryocytes are characteristic. In less anemic patients, the changes in the marrow may be difficult to recognize. The terms *intermediate*, *mild*, and *early* have been used. The term *megaloblastoid* does not mean mildly megaloblastic. It is used to describe cells with both immature appearing nuclei and defective hemoglobinization and is usually seen in myelodysplasia.

Chromosomes Bone marrow cells, transformed lymphocytes, and other proliferating cells in the body show a variety of changes including random breaks, reduced contraction, spreading of the centromere, and exaggeration of secondary chromosomal constrictions and overprominent satellites. Similar abnormalities may be produced by antimetabolite drugs (e.g., cytosine arabinoside, hydroxyurea, and methotrexate) that either interfere with DNA replication or folate metabolism and that also cause megaloblastic appearances.

Ineffective Hemopoiesis There is an accumulation of unconjugated bilirubin in plasma due to the death of nucleated red cells in the marrow (ineffective erythropoiesis). Other evidence for this includes raised urine urobilinogen, reduced haptoglobins and positive urine hemosiderin, and a raised serum lactate dehydrogenase. A weakly positive direct antiglobulin test due to complement can lead to a false diagnosis of autoimmune hemolytic anemia.

CAUSES OF COBALAMIN DEFICIENCY

Cobalamin deficiency is usually due to malabsorption. The only other cause is inadequate dietary intake.

Inadequate Dietary Intake • *ADULTS* Dietary cobalamin deficiency arises in vegans who omit meat, fish, eggs, cheese, and other animal products from their diet. The largest group in the world consists of Hindus, and it is likely that many millions of Indians are at risk of deficiency of cobalamin on a nutritional basis. Subnormal serum cobalamin levels are found in up to 50% of randomly selected, young, adult Indian vegans, but the deficiency usually does not progress to megaloblastic anemia since the diet of most vegans is not totally lacking cobalamin and the enterohepatic circulation of cobalamin is intact. Dietary cobalamin deficiency may also arise rarely in nonvegetarian individuals who exist on grossly inadequate diets because of poverty or psychiatric disturbance.

FIGURE 100-2 A. The peripheral blood in severe megaloblastic anemia. **B.** The bone marrow in severe megaloblastic anemia. *[Reprinted from Hoffbrand AV et al (eds) Postgraduate Haematology, 5th ed, Blackwell Publishing, Oxford, UK 2005; with permission.]*

INFANTS Cobalamin deficiency has been described in infants born to severely cobalamin-deficient mothers. These infants develop megaloblastic anemia at about 3–6 months of age, presumably because they are born with low stores of cobalamin and because they are fed breast milk of low cobalamin content. The babies have also shown growth retardation, impaired psychomotor development, and other neurologic sequelae.

Gastric Causes of Cobalamin Malabsorption
See Tables 100-3 and 100-4.

PERNICIOUS ANEMIA Pernicious anemia (PA) may be defined as a severe lack of IF due to gastric atrophy. It is a common disease in north Europeans but occurs in all countries and ethnic groups. The overall incidence is about 120 per 100 000 population in the United Kingdom (UK). The ratio of incidence in men and women in Caucasians is ~1:1.6 and the peak age of onset is 60 years, with only 10% of patients being <40 years of age. However, in some ethnic groups, notably black individuals and Latin Americans, the age of onset of PA is generally lower. The disease occurs more commonly than by chance in close relatives and in persons with other organ-specific autoimmune diseases, e.g., thyroid diseases, vitiligo, hypoparathyroidism, and Addison's disease. It is also associated with hypogammaglobulinemia, with premature graying or blue eyes, and in persons of blood group A. An association with human leukocyte antigen (HLA) 3 has been reported in some but not all series and, in those with endocrine disease, with HLA-B8, -B12, and -BW15. The life expectancy is normal in women once regular treatment has begun. Men have a slightly subnormal life expectancy as a result of a higher incidence of carcinoma of the stomach than in control subjects. Gastric output of hydrochloric acid, pepsin, and IF are severely reduced. The serum gastrin level is raised, and serum pepsinogen I levels are low.

GASTRIC BIOPSY This usually shows atrophy of all layers of the body and fundus, with loss of glandular elements, an absence of parietal and chief cells and replacement by mucous cells, a mixed inflammatory cell infiltrate, and perhaps intestinal metaplasia. The infiltrate of plasma cells and lymphocytes contains an excess of CD4 cells. The antral mucosa is usually well preserved. *Helicobacter pylori* infection is infrequent in PA, but it has been suggested that *H. pylori* gastritis occurs at an early phase of atrophic gastritis and presents in younger patients as iron deficiency anemia but in older patients as PA. *H. pylori* is suggested to stimulate an autoimmune process directed against parietal cells, the *H. pylori* infection then being gradually replaced, in some individuals, by an autoimmune process.

TABLE 100-3	CAUSES OF COBALAMIN DEFICIENCY SUFFICIENTLY SEVERE TO CAUSE MEGALOBLASTIC ANEMIA
Nutritional	Vegans
Malabsorption	Pernicious anemia
Gastric causes	Congenital absence of intrinsic factor or functional abnormality
	Total or partial gastrectomy
Intestinal causes	Intestinal stagnant loop syndrome: jejunal diverticulosis, ileocolic fistula, anatomic blind loop, intestinal stricture, etc.
	Ileal resection and Crohn's disease
	Selective malabsorption with proteinuria
	Tropical sprue
	Transcobalamin II deficiency
	Fish tapeworm

TABLE 100-4	MALABSORPTION OF COBALAMIN MAY OCCUR IN THE FOLLOWING CONDITIONS BUT IS NOT USUALLY SUFFICIENTLY SEVERE AND PROLONGED TO CAUSE MEGALOBLASTIC ANEMIA
Gastric causes	
Simple atrophic gastritis (food cobalamin malabsorption)	
Zollinger–Ellison syndrome	
Gastric bypass surgery	
Use of proton pump inhibitors	
Intestinal causes	
Gluten-induced enteropathy	
Severe pancreatitis	
HIV infection	
Radiotherapy	
Graft-versus-host disease	
Deficiencies of cobalamin, folate, protein, ?riboflavin, ?nicotinic acid	
Therapy with colchicine, para-aminosalicylate, neomycin, slow-release potassium chloride, anticonvulsant drugs, metformin, phenformin, cytotoxic drugs	
Alcohol	

SERUM ANTIBODIES Two types of IF immunoglobulin G antibody may be found in the sera of patients with PA. One, the "blocking," or type I, antibody, prevents the combination of IF and cobalamin, whereas the "binding," or type II, antibody prevents attachment of IF to ileal mucosa. Type I occurs in the sera of ~55% of patients and type II in 35%. IF antibodies cross the placenta and may cause temporary IF deficiency in the newborn infant. Patients with PA also show cell-mediated immunity to IF. Type I antibody has been detected rarely in the sera of patients without PA but with thyrotoxicosis, myxedema, Hashimoto's disease, or diabetes mellitus and in relatives of PA patients. IF antibodies have also been detected in gastric juice in ~80% of PA patients. These gastric antibodies may reduce absorption of dietary cobalamin by combining with small amounts of remaining IF.

Parietal cell antibody is present in the sera of almost 90% of adult patients with PA but is frequently present in other subjects. Thus, it occurs in as many as 16% of randomly selected female subjects aged >60 years. The parietal cell antibody is directed against the α and β subunits of the gastric proton pump (H^+,K^+-ATPase).

Juvenile Pernicious Anemia

This usually occurs in older children and resembles PA of adults. Gastric atrophy, achlorhydria, and serum IF antibodies are all present, although parietal cell antibodies are usually absent. About one-half of these patients show an associated endocrinopathy such as autoimmune thyroiditis, Addison's disease, or hypoparathyroidism; in some, mucocutaneous candidiasis occurs.

Congenital Intrinsic Factor Deficiency or Functional Abnormality

The affected child usually presents with megaloblastic anemia in the first to third year of life; a few have presented as late as the second decade. The child has no demonstrable IF but has a normal gastric mucosa and normal secretion of acid. The inheritance is autosomally recessive. Parietal cell and IF antibodies are absent. Variants have been described in which the child is born with IF that can be detected immunologically but is unstable or functionally inactive.

Gastrectomy

Following total gastrectomy, cobalamin deficiency is inevitable, and prophylactic cobalamin therapy should be commenced immediately following the operation. After partial gastrectomy, 10–15% of patients also develop this deficiency. The exact incidence and time of onset are most influenced by the size of the resection and the preexisting size of cobalamin body stores.

Food Cobalamin Malabsorption

Failure of release of cobalamin from binding proteins in food is believed to be responsible for this condition, more common in the elderly. It is associated with low serum cobalamin levels, with or without raised serum levels of MMA and homocysteine. Typically, these patients have normal cobalamin absorption, as measured with crystalline cobalamin, but show malabsorption when a modified test using food-bound cobalamin is used. The frequency of progression to severe cobalamin deficiency and reasons for this progression are not clear.

Intestinal Causes of Cobalamin Malabsorption • *INTESTINAL STAGNANT LOOP SYNDROME*

Malabsorption of cobalamin occurs in a variety of intestinal lesions in which there is colonization of the upper small intestine by fecal organisms. This may occur in patients with jejunal diverticulosis, enteroanastomosis, or intestinal stricture or fistula or with an anatomic blood loop due to Crohn's disease, tuberculosis, or an operative procedure.

ILEAL RESECTION Removal of ≥1.2 m of terminal ileum causes malabsorption of cobalamin. In some patients following ileal resection, particularly if the ileocecal valve is incompetent, colonic bacteria may contribute further to the onset of cobalamin deficiency.

SELECTIVE MALABSORPTION OF COBALAMIN WITH PROTEINURIA (IMERSLUND SYNDROME: IMERSLUND-GRÄSBECK SYNDROME; CONGENITAL COBALAMIN MALABSORPTION; AUTOSOMAL RECESSIVE MEGALOBLASTIC ANEMIA, MGA1) This autosomally recessive disease is the most common cause of megaloblastic anemia due to cobalamin deficiency in infancy in Western countries. More than 200 cases have been reported, with familial clusters in Finland, Norway, the Middle East, and North Africa. The patients secrete normal amounts of IF and gastric acid but are unable to absorb cobalamin. In Finland, impaired synthesis, processing, or ligand binding of cubilin due to inherited mutations is found. In Norway, mutation of the gene for *AMN* has been reported. Other tests of intestinal absorption are normal. Over 90% of the patients show nonspecific proteinuria, but renal function is otherwise normal and renal biopsy has not shown any consistent renal defect. A few have shown aminoaciduria and congenital renal abnormalities, such as duplication of the renal pelvis.

TROPICAL SPRUE Nearly all patients with acute and subacute tropical sprue show malabsorption of cobalamin; this may persist as the principal abnormality in the chronic form of the disease, when the patient may present with megaloblastic anemia or neuropathy due to cobalamin deficiency. Absorption of cobalamin usually improves after antibiotic therapy and, in the early stages, folic acid therapy.

FISH TAPEWORM INFESTATION The fish tapeworm (*Diphyllobothrium latum*) lives in the small intestine of humans and accumulates cobalamin from food, rendering this unavailable for absorption. Individuals acquire the worm by eating raw or partly cooked fish. Infestation is common around the lakes of Scandinavia, Germany, Japan, North America, and Russia. Megaloblastic anemia or cobalamin neuropathy occurs only in those with a heavy infestation.

GLUTEN-INDUCED ENTEROPATHY Malabsorption of cobalamin occurs in ~30% of untreated patients (presumably those in whom the disease extends to the ileum). Cobalamin deficiency is not severe in these patients and is corrected with a gluten-free diet.

SEVERE CHRONIC PANCREATITIS In this condition, lack of trypsin is thought to cause dietary cobalamin attached to gastric non-IF (R) binder to be unavailable for absorption. It has also been proposed that in pancreatitis, the concentration of calcium ions in the ileum falls below the level needed to maintain normal cobalamin absorption.

HIV INFECTION Serum cobalamin levels tend to fall in patients with HIV infection and are subnormal in 10–35% of those with AIDS. Malabsorption of cobalamin not corrected by IF has been shown in some, but not all, patients with subnormal serum cobalamin levels. Cobalamin deficiency sufficiently severe to cause megaloblastic anemia or neuropathy is rare.

ZOLLINGER–ELLISON SYNDROME Malabsorption of cobalamin has been reported in the Zollinger–Ellison syndrome. It is thought that there is a failure to release cobalamin from R-binding protein due to inactivation of pancreatic trypsin by high acidity, as well as interference with IF binding of cobalamin.

RADIOTHERAPY Both total-body irradiation and local radiotherapy to the ileum (e.g., as a complication of radiotherapy for carcinoma of the cervix) may cause malabsorption of cobalamin.

GRAFT-VERSUS-HOST DISEASE This commonly affects the small intestine. Malabsorption of cobalamin due to abnormal gut flora, as well as damage to ileal mucosa, is frequent.

DRUGS The drugs that have been reported to cause malabsorption of cobalamin are listed in Table 100-4. Megaloblastic anemia due to these drugs is, however, rare.

Abnormalities of Cobalamin Metabolism • *CONGENITAL TRANSCOBALAMIN II DEFICIENCY OR ABNORMALITY*

Infants with TC II deficiency usually present with megaloblastic anemia within a few weeks of birth. Serum cobalamin and folate levels are normal, but the anemia responds to massive (e.g., 1 mg three times weekly) injections of cobalamin. Some cases show neurologic complications. The protein may be present but functionally inert. Genetic abnormalities found include mutations of an intra-exonic cryptic splice site, extensive deletion, single nucleotide deletion, nonsense mutation, and an RNA editing defect. Malabsorption of cobalamin occurs in all cases and serum immunoglobulins are usually reduced. Failure to institute adequate cobalamin therapy or treatment with folic acid may lead to neurologic damage.

CONGENITAL METHYLMALONIC ACIDEMIA AND ACIDURIA

The infants with this abnormality are ill from birth with vomiting, failure to thrive, severe metabolic acidosis, ketosis, and mental retardation. Anemia, if present, is normocytic and normoblastic. The condition may be due to a functional defect in either mitochondrial methylmalonyl CoA mutase or its cofactor adocobalamin. Mutations in the methylmalonyl CoA mutase are not responsive, or only poorly responsive, to treatment with cobalamin. A proportion of the infants with failure of adocobalamin synthesis respond to cobalamin in large doses. Some children have combined methylmalonic aciduria and homocystinuria due to defective formation of both cobalamin coenzymes. This usually presents in the first year of life with feeding difficulties, developmental delay, microcephaly, seizures, hypotonia, and megaloblastic anemia.

ACQUIRED ABNORMALITY OF COBALAMIN METABOLISM: NITROUS OXIDE INHALATION

Nitrous oxide irreversibly oxidizes methylcobalamin to an inactive precursor; this inactivates methionine synthase. Megaloblastic anemia has occurred in patients undergoing prolonged N_2O anesthesia (e.g., in intensive care units). A neuropathy resembling cobalamin neuropathy has also been described in dentists and anesthetists who are repeatedly exposed to N_2O. Methylmalonic aciduria does not occur as adocobalamin is not inactivated by N_2O.

CAUSES OF FOLATE DEFICIENCY (Table 100-5)

Nutritional Dietary folate deficiency is common. Indeed, in most patients with folate deficiency a nutritional element is present. Certain individuals are particularly prone to have diets containing inadequate amounts of folate (Table 100-5). In the United States and other countries where fortification of the diet with folic acid has been adopted, the prevalence of folate deficiency has dropped dramatically and is now almost restricted to high-risk groups with increased folate needs. Nutritional folate deficiency occurs in kwashiorkor and scurvy and in infants with repeated infections or who are fed solely on goats' milk, which has a low folate content.

Malabsorption Malabsorption of dietary folate occurs in tropical sprue and in gluten-induced enteropathy. In the rare congenital syndrome of selective malabsorption of folate, there is an associated defect of folate transport into the cerebrospinal fluid, and these patients show megaloblastic anemia, which responds to physiologic doses of folic acid given parenterally but not orally. They also show mental retardation, convulsions, and other central nervous system abnormalities. Minor degrees of malabsorption may also occur following jejunal resection or partial gastrectomy, in Crohn's disease, and in systemic infections but, in these conditions, if severe deficiency occurs, it is usually largely due to poor nutrition. Malabsorption of folate has been described in patients receiving salazopyrine, cholestyramine, and triamterene.

Excess Utilization or Loss • **PREGNANCY** Folate requirements are increased by 200–300 μg to ~400 μg daily in a normal pregnancy, partly because of transfer of the vitamin to the fetus, but mainly because of increased folate catabolism due to cleavage of folate coenzymes in rapidly proliferating tissues. Megaloblastic anemia due to this deficiency is prevented by prophylactic folic acid therapy. It occurred in 0.5% of pregnancies in the UK and other Western countries before prophylaxis with folic acid, but the incidence is much higher in countries where the general nutritional status is poor.

Dietary[a]
   Particularly in: old age, infancy, poverty, alcoholism, chronic invalids, and the psychiatrically disturbed; may be associated with scurvy or kwashiorkor
Malabsorption
   Major causes of deficiency
      Tropical sprue, gluten-induced enteropathy in children and adults, and in association with dermatitis herpetiformis, specific malabsorption of folate, intestinal megaloblastosis caused by severe cobalamin or folate deficiency
   Minor causes of deficiency
      Extensive jejunal resection, Crohn's disease, partial gastrectomy, congestive heart failure, Whipple's disease, scleroderma, amyloid, diabetic enteropathy, systemic bacterial infection, lymphoma, salazopyrine
Excess utilization or loss
   Physiologic
      Pregnancy and lactation, prematurity
   Pathologic
      Hematologic diseases: chronic hemolytic anemias, sickle cell anemia, thalassemia major, myelofibrosis
      Malignant diseases: carcinoma, lymphoma, leukemia, myeloma
      Inflammatory diseases: tuberculosis, Crohn's disease, psoriasis, exfoliative dermatitis, malaria
      Metabolic disease: homocystinuria
      Excess urinary loss: congestive heart failure, active liver disease
      Hemodialysis, peritoneal dialysis
Antifolate drugs[b]
   Anticonvulsant drugs (phenytoin, primidone, barbiturates), sulphasalazine
   Nitrofurantoin, tetracycline, anti-tuberculosis (less well documented)
Mixed causes
   Liver diseases, alcoholism, intensive care units

[a]In severely folate-deficient patients with causes other than those listed under Dietary, poor dietary intake is often present.
[b]Drugs inhibiting dihydrofolate reductase are discussed in the text.

PREMATURITY The newborn infant, whether full term or premature, has higher serum and red cell folate concentrations than the adult. However, the newborn infant's demand for folate has been estimated to be up to 10 times that of adults on a weight basis, and the neonatal folate level falls rapidly to the lowest values at about 6 weeks of age. The falls are steepest and are liable to reach subnormal levels in premature babies, a number of whom develop megaloblastic anemia responsive to folic acid at about 4–6 weeks of age. This occurs particularly in the smallest babies (<1500 g birth weight) and in those who have feeding difficulties or infections or who have undergone multiple exchange transfusions. In these babies, prophylactic folic acid should be given.

HEMATOLOGIC DISORDERS Folate deficiency frequently occurs in chronic hemolytic anemia, particularly in sickle cell disease, autoimmune hemolytic anemia, and congenital spherocytosis. In these and other conditions of increased cell turnover (e.g., myelofibrosis, malignancies) folate deficiency arises because it is not completely reutilized after performing coenzyme functions.

INFLAMMATORY CONDITIONS Chronic inflammatory diseases, such as tuberculosis, rheumatoid arthritis, Crohn's disease, psoriasis, exfoliative dermatitis, bacterial endocarditis, and chronic bacterial infections, cause deficiency by reducing the appetite and by increasing the demand for folate. Systemic infections may also cause malabsorption of folate. Severe deficiency is virtually confined to the patients with the most active disease and the poorest diet.

HOMOCYSTINURIA This is a rare metabolic defect in the conversion of homocysteine to cystathionine. Folate deficiency occurring in most of these patients may be due to excessive utilization because of compensatory increased conversion of homocysteine to methionine.

LONG-TERM DIALYSIS As folate is only loosely bound to plasma proteins, it is easily removed from plasma by dialysis. In patients with an-

PART 6 Oncology and Hematology

orexia, vomiting, infections, and hemolysis, folate stores are particularly likely to become depleted. Routine folate prophylaxis is now given.

CONGESTIVE HEART FAILURE, LIVER DISEASE Excess urinary folate losses of >100 µg per day may occur in some of these patients. The explanation appears to be release of folate from damaged liver cells.

Antifolate Drugs A large number of epileptics, who are receiving long-term therapy with phenytoin or primidone, with or without barbiturates, develop low serum and red cell folate levels. The exact mechanism is unclear. Alcohol may also be a folate antagonist, as patients who are drinking spirits may develop megaloblastic anemia that will respond to normal quantities of dietary folate or to physiologic doses of folic acid only if alcohol is withdrawn. Macrocytosis of red cells is associated with chronic alcohol intake even when folate levels are normal. Inadequate folate intake is the major factor in the development of deficiency in spirit-drinking alcoholics. Beer is relatively folate-rich in some countries, depending on the technique used for brewing.

The drugs that inhibit DHF reductase include methotrexate, pyrimethamine, and trimethoprim. Methotrexate has the most powerful action against the human enzyme, whereas trimethoprim is most active against the bacterial enzyme and is only likely to cause megaloblastic anemia when used in conjunction with sulphamethoxazole in patients with preexisting folate or cobalamin deficiency. The activity of pyrimethamine is intermediate. The antidote to these drugs is folinic acid (5-formyl-THF).

Congenital Abnormalities of Folate Metabolism Some infants with congenital defects of folate enzymes (e.g., cyclohydrolase or methionine synthase) have had megaloblastic anemia.

DIAGNOSIS OF COBALAMIN AND FOLATE DEFICIENCIES

The diagnosis of cobalamin or folate deficiency has traditionally depended on the recognition of the relevant abnormalities in the peripheral blood and analysis of the blood levels of the vitamins.

Serum Cobalamin This is measured by an automated enzyme-linked immunoadsorbent (ELISA) assay. Normal serum levels range 118–148 pmol/L (160–200 ng/L) to ~738 pmol/L (1000 ng/L). In patients with megaloblastic anemia due to cobalamin deficiency, the level is usually <74 pmol/L (100 ng/L). In general, the more severe the deficiency, the lower the serum cobalamin level. In patients with spinal cord damage due to the deficiency, levels are very low even in the absence of anemia. Values of between 74 and 148 pmol/L (100 and 200 ng/L) are regarded as borderline. They may occur, for instance, in pregnancy, in patients with megaloblastic anemia due to folate deficiency. The serum cobalamin level is generally considered to be sufficiently robust, cost-effective, and most convenient to rule out cobalamin deficiency in the vast majority of patients suspected of having this problem.

Serum Methylmalonate and Homocysteine In patients with cobalamin deficiency sufficient to cause anemia or neuropathy, the serum MMA level is raised. Sensitive methods for measuring MMA and homocysteine in serum have been introduced and recommended for the early diagnosis of cobalamin deficiency, even in the absence of hematologic abnormalities or subnormal levels of serum cobalamin. Serum MMA levels fluctuate, however, in patients with renal failure. Mildly elevated serum MMA and/or homocysteine levels occur in up to 30% of apparently healthy volunteers, with serum cobalamin levels up to 258 pmol/L (350 ng/L) and normal serum folate levels; 15% of elderly subjects, even with cobalamin levels >258 pmol/L (>350 ng/L), have this pattern of raised metabolite levels. These findings bring into question the exact cut-off points for normal MMA and homocysteine levels. It is also unclear at present whether these mildly raised metabolite levels have clinical consequences.

Serum homocysteine is raised in both early cobalamin and folate deficiency but may be raised in other conditions, e.g., chronic renal disease, alcoholism, smoking, pyridoxine deficiency, hypothyroidism, therapy with steroids, cyclosporine, and other drugs. Levels are also higher in serum than in plasma, in men than in premenopausal women, in women taking hormone replacement therapy, or in oral contraceptive users and in elderly persons and patients with several inborn errors of metabolism affecting enzymes in trans-sulfuration pathways of homocysteine metabolism. Thus, homocysteine levels are not used for diagnosis of cobalamin or folate deficiency.

Cobalamin Absorption Studies of cobalamin absorption have been widely used, but difficulty in obtaining radioactive cobalamin and of ensuring IF preparations are free of viruses have led to reduced availability. For the urinary excretion (Schilling) test the patient is fasted overnight. Radioactive cyanocobalamin is given orally. Then, 2 h later an IM injection of cyanocobalamin or hydroxocobalamin (1 mg) is given ("flushing dose"). A 24-h urine specimen is collected for determination of radioactivity; low excretion shows malabsorption; the oral dose is then given again after 48 h with IF. The results distinguish between gastric and intestinal causes of cobalamin malabsorption.

Serum Folate This is also measured by an ELISA technique. In most laboratories, the normal range is from 11 nmol/L (2.0 µg/L) to ~82 nmol/L (15 µg/L). The serum folate level is low in all folate-deficient patients. It also reflects recent diet. Because of this, serum folate may be low before there is hematologic or biochemical evidence of deficiency. Serum folate rises in severe cobalamin deficiency because of the block in conversion of MTHF to THF inside cells; raised levels have also been reported in the intestinal stagnant loop syndrome, due to absorption of bacterially synthesized folate.

Red Cell Folate The red cell folate assay is a valuable test of body folate stores. It is less affected than the serum assay by recent diet and traces of hemolysis. In normal adults, concentrations range 880–3520 µmol/L (160–640 µg/L) of packed red cells. Subnormal levels occur in patients with megaloblastic anemia due to folate deficiency but also in nearly two-thirds of patients with severe cobalamin deficiency. False-normal results may occur if the folate-deficient patient has received a recent blood transfusion or if the patient has a raised reticulocyte count.

℞ MEGALOBLASTIC ANEMIA

It is usually possible to establish which of the two deficiencies, folate or cobalamin, is the cause of the anemia and to treat only with the appropriate vitamin. In patients who enter hospital severely ill, however, it may be necessary to treat with both vitamins in large doses once blood samples have been taken for cobalamin and folate assays and a bone marrow biopsy has been performed (if deemed necessary). Transfusion is usually unnecessary and inadvisable. If it is essential, packed red cells should be given slowly, one or two units only, with the usual treatment for heart failure if present. Potassium supplements have been recommended to obviate the danger of the hypokalemia that has been recorded in some patients during the initial hematologic response. Occasionally, an excessive rise in platelets occurs after 1–2 weeks of therapy. Antiplatelet therapy, e.g., aspirin should be considered if the platelet count rises to >800 × 10^9/L.

TREATMENT OF COBALAMIN DEFICIENCY It is usually necessary to treat patients who have developed cobalamin deficiency with lifelong regular cobalamin injections. In the UK, the form used is hydroxocobalamin; in the United States, cyanocobalamin. In a few instances, the underlying cause of cobalamin deficiency can be permanently corrected, e.g., the fish tapeworm, tropical sprue, or an intestinal stagnant loop that is amenable to surgery. The indications for starting cobalamin therapy are a well-documented megaloblastic anemia or other hematologic abnormalities or neuropathy due to the deficiency. Patients with borderline serum cobalamin levels but no hematologic or other abnormality should be followed, e.g., at yearly intervals to make sure that the cobalamin deficiency does not progress. If malabsorption of cobalamin or rises in serum MMA levels have also been demonstrated, however, they should also be given regular maintenance cobalamin therapy. Cobalamin should be given routinely to all patients who have had a total gastrectomy or ileal resection.

Patients who have undergone gastric reduction for control of obesity or who are receiving long-term treatment with proton pump inhibitors should be screened and, if necessary, given cobalamin replacement.

Replenishment of body stores should be complete with six 1000-μg IM injections of hydroxocobalamin given at 3- to 7-day intervals. More frequent doses are usually used in patients with cobalamin neuropathy, but there is no evidence that these produce a better response. For maintenance therapy, 1000 μg hydroxocobalamin IM once every 3 months is satisfactory. Because of the poorer retention of cyanocobalamin, protocols generally use higher and more frequent doses, e.g., 1000 μg IM, monthly, for maintenance treatment.

Toxic reactions are extremely rare and are usually due to contamination in its preparation rather than to cobalamin itself. Because a small fraction of cobalamin can be absorbed passively through mucous membranes even when there is complete failure of physiological IF-dependent absorption, large daily oral doses (1000–2000 μg) of cyanocobalamin can be used in PA for replacement and maintenance of normal cobalamin status. Sublingual therapy has also been proposed for those in whom injections are difficult because of a bleeding tendency and may not tolerate oral therapy. If oral therapy is used, it is important to monitor compliance, particularly with elderly, forgetful patients.

TREATMENT OF FOLATE DEFICIENCY   Oral doses of 5–15 mg folic acid daily are satisfactory, as sufficient folate is absorbed from these extremely large doses even in patients with severe malabsorption. The length of time therapy must be continued depends on the underlying disease. It is customary to continue therapy for about 4 months, when all folate-deficient red cells will have been eliminated and replaced by new folate-replete populations.

Before large doses of folic acid are given, cobalamin deficiency must be excluded and, if present, corrected, otherwise cobalamin neuropathy may develop, despite a response of the anemia of cobalamin deficiency to folate therapy. Studies in the United States, however, suggest that there is no increase in the proportion of individuals with low serum cobalamin levels and no anemia since food fortification with folic acid, but it is unknown if there has been a change in incidence of cobalamin neuropathy.

Long-term folic acid therapy is required when the underlying cause of the deficiency cannot be corrected and the deficiency is likely to recur, for instance, in chronic dialysis or hemolytic anemias. It may also be necessary in gluten-induced enteropathy if this does not respond to a gluten-free diet. Where mild but chronic folate deficiency occurs, it is preferable to encourage improvement in the diet after correcting the deficiency with a short course of folic acid. In any patient receiving long-term folic acid therapy, it is important to measure the serum cobalamin level at regular (e.g., once yearly) intervals to exclude the coincidental development of cobalamin deficiency.

Folinic Acid (5-Formyl-THF)   This is a stable form of fully reduced folate. It is given orally or parenterally to overcome the toxic effects of methotrexate or other DHF reductase inhibitors.

PROPHYLACTIC FOLIC ACID   In many countries, food is fortified with folic acid (in grain or flour) to prevent neural tube defects. It is also used in chronic dialysis patients and in parenteral feeds. Prophylactic folic acid has been used to reduce homocysteine levels to prevent cardiovascular disease, but further data are needed to assess the benefit for this and for cognitive function in the elderly.

Pregnancy   Folic acid, 400 μg daily, should be given as a supplement before and throughout pregnancy. In women who have had a previous fetus with a neural tube defect, 5 mg daily is recommended when pregnancy is contemplated and throughout the subsequent pregnancy.

Infancy and Childhood   The incidence of folate deficiency is so high in the smallest premature babies during the first 6 weeks of life that folic acid

(e.g., 1 mg daily) should be given routinely to those weighing <1500 g at birth and to larger premature babies who require exchange transfusions or develop feeding difficulties, infections, or vomiting and diarrhea.

The World Health Organization currently recommends routine supplementation with iron and folic acid in children in countries where iron deficiency is common and child mortality, largely due to infectious diseases, is high. However, some studies suggest that where malaria rates are high, this approach may increase the incidence of severe illness and death. Even where malaria is rare, there appears to be no survival benefit.

MEGALOBLASTIC ANEMIA NOT DUE TO COBALAMIN OR FOLATE DEFICIENCY OR ALTERED METABOLISM

This may occur with many antimetabolic drugs (e.g.,. hydroxyurea, cytosine arabinoside, 6-mercaptopurine) that inhibit DNA replication. Antiviral nucleoside analogues used in treatment of HIV infection may also cause macrocytosis and megaloblastic marrow changes. In the rare disease orotic aciduria, two consecutive enzymes in purine synthesis are defective. The condition responds to therapy with uridine, which by-passes the block. In thiamine-responsive megaloblastic anemia, there is a genetic defect in the high-affinity thiamine transport (*SLC19A2*) gene. This causes defective RNA ribose synthesis through impaired activity of transketolase, a thiamine-dependent enzyme in the pentose cycle. This leads to reduced nucleic acid production. It may be associated with diabetes mellitus and deafness and the presence of many ringed sideroblasts in the marrow. The explanation is unclear for megaloblastic changes in the marrow in some patients with acute myeloid leukemia and myelodysplasia.

FURTHER READINGS

Bazzano LA et al: Effect of folic acid supplementation on risk of cardiovascular diseases. JAMA 296:2720, 2006

Bønaa KH et al: Homocysteine lowering and cardiovascular events after acute myocardial infarction. N Engl J Med 354:1578, 2006

Chan JCW et al: Pernicious anemia in Chinese: A study of 181 patients in a Hong Kong Hospital. Medicine 85:129, 2006

Durga J et al: Effect of 3-year folic acid supplementation on cognitive function in older adults in the FACIT trial: A randomized double-blind, controlled trial. Lancet 369:208, 2007

Hershko C et al: Variable hematologic presentation of autoimmune gastritis: Age-related progression from iron deficiency to cobalamin depletion. Blood 107:1673, 2006

Lonn E et al: Homocysteine lowering with folic acid and B vitamins in vascular disease. N Engl J Med 354:1567, 2006

McMahon JA et al: A controlled trial of homocysteine lowering and cognitive performance. N Engl J Med 354:2764, 2006

Mills JL et al: Low vitamin B$_{12}$ concentrations in patients without anemia: The effect of folic acid fortification of grain. Am J Clin Nutr 77:1474, 2003

Rothenberg SP et al: Autoantibodies against folate receptors in women with a pregnancy complicated by a neural tube defect. N Engl J Med 350:134, 2004

Sazawal S et al: Effects of routine prophylactic supplementation with iron and folic acid on admission to hospital and mortality in preschool child mortality in Southern Nepal: Community-based, cluster-randomized, placebo-controlled trial. Lancet 367:144, 2006

101 Hemolytic Anemias and Anemia Due to Acute Blood Loss

Lucio Luzzatto

DEFINITIONS

A finite life span is a distinct characteristic of red cells. Hence, a logical, time-honored classification of anemias comprises three groups: decreased production of red cells, increased destruction of red cells, and acute blood loss. Red cell destruction and acute loss, both associated with increased reticulocyte production, are covered in this chapter. Red cell production defects are discussed in Chaps. 98–100.

Physical loss of red cells from the bloodstream—which in most cases also means physical loss *from* the body—is fundamentally different from destruction of red cells *within* the body. Therefore the clinical aspects and the pathophysiology of anemia in these two groups of patients are quite different, and they will be considered separately.

HEMOLYTIC ANEMIAS

Anemias due to increased destruction of red cells, or hemolytic anemias (HAs), may be *inherited* or *acquired*. From the clinical point of view, they may be more *acute* or more *chronic*, and they may vary from mild to very severe. The site of hemolysis may be predominantly *intravascular* or *extravascular*. With respect to mechanisms, HAs may be due to *intracorpuscular* or *extracorpuscular* causes (Table 101-1); however, before reviewing the individual types of HAs, it is appropriate to consider what they have in common.

GENERAL CLINICAL AND LABORATORY FEATURES

The clinical presentation of a patient with anemia is greatly influenced by whether the onset is abrupt or gradual, and HA is no exception. A patient with autoimmune hemolytic anemia or with favism may be a medical emergency, whereas a patient with mild hereditary spherocytosis or with cold agglutinin disease may be diagnosed after years. This is due in large measure to the remarkable ability of the body to adapt to anemia when it is slowly progressing (Chap. 58).

What differentiates HA from other anemias is that the patient has signs and symptoms arising directly from hemolysis (Table 101-2). At the clinical level, the main sign is *jaundice;* in addition, the patient may report discoloration of the urine. In many cases of HA, the spleen is enlarged because it is a preferential site of hemolysis; in some cases the liver may be enlarged as well. In all severe congenital forms of HA, skeletal changes may be noted due to over-activity of the bone marrow (although they are never as severe as in thalassemia).

TABLE 101-1 CLASSIFICATION OF HEMOLYTIC ANEMIAS[a]

	Intracorpuscular Defects	Extracorpuscular Factors
Hereditary	Hemoglobinopathies Enzymopathies Membrane-cytoskeletal defects	Familial hemolytic uremic syndrome (HUS)
Acquired	Paroxysmal nocturnal hemoglobinuria (PNH)	Mechanical destruction (microangiopathic) Toxic agents Drugs Infectious Autoimmune

[a]There is a strong correlation between hereditary causes and intracorpuscular defects, because such defects are due to inherited mutations; the one exception is PNH, because the defect is due to an acquired somatic mutation. There is also a strong correlation between acquired causes and extracorpuscular factors; the one exception is familial HUS, because here an inherited abnormality allows excessive complement activation, with bouts of production of membrane attack complex capable of severely damaging normal cells.

TABLE 101-2 GENERAL FEATURES OF HEMOLYTIC DISORDERS

General examination	Jaundice, pallor
Other physical findings	Spleen may be enlarged; bossing of skull in severe congenital cases
Hemoglobin	From normal to severely reduced
MCV, MCH	Usually increased
Reticulocytes	Increased
Bilirubin	Increased (mostly unconjugated)
LDH	Increased (up to 10× normal with intravascular hemolysis)
Haptoglobin	Reduced to absent

Note: MCV, mean corpuscular volume; MCH, mean corpuscular hemoglobin; LDH, lactate dehydrogenase.

The laboratory features of HA are related to (1) hemolysis per se and (2) the erythropoietic response of the bone marrow. In the serum, hemolysis regularly produces an increased unconjugated bilirubin, increased lactate dehydrogenase (LDH), increased aspartate transaminase, and reduced haptoglobin. Urobilinogen will be increased in both urine and stool. If hemolysis is mainly intravascular, the telltale sign is hemoglobinuria, often associated with hemosiderinuria and an increase in serum hemoglobin; in contrast, the bilirubin level may be normal or only mildly elevated. The main sign of the erythropoietic response by the bone marrow is an increase in reticulocytes (a test all too often neglected in the initial workup of a patient with anemia). Usually the increase will be reflected in both the percentage of reticulocytes (the more commonly quoted figure) and the absolute reticulocyte count (the more definitive parameter). The increased number of reticulocytes is associated with an increased mean corpuscular volume (MCV) in the blood count. On the blood smear this is reflected in the presence of macrocytes; there is also polychromasia and sometimes nucleated red cells. In most cases a bone marrow aspirate is not necessary in the diagnostic workup; if it is done, it will show erythroid hyperplasia. In practice, once an HA is suspected, specific tests will usually be required for a definitive diagnosis of the specific type of HA.

GENERAL PATHOPHYSIOLOGY

The mature red cell is the product of a developmental pathway that brings the phenomenon of differentiation to an extreme. An orderly sequence of events produces synchronous changes whereby the gradual accumulation of a huge amount of hemoglobin in the cytoplasm (to a final level of 340 g/L, i.e., about 5 mM) goes hand in hand with the gradual loss of cellular organelles and of biosynthetic abilities. In the end the erythroid cell undergoes a process that has features of apoptosis, including nuclear pyknosis and actual loss of the nucleus. However, the final result is more altruistic than suicidal; the cytoplasmic body, instead of disintegrating, is now able to provide oxygen to all cells in the human organism for some remaining 120 days of the red cell "life" span.

As a result of this unique process of differentiation and maturation, intermediary metabolism is drastically curtailed in mature red cells (Fig. 101-1); for instance, cytochrome-mediated oxidative phosphorylation has been lost with the loss of mitochondria; therefore there is no backup to anaerobic glycolysis for the production of adenosine triphosphate (ATP). Also, the capacity of making protein has been lost with the loss of ribosomes. This places the cell's limited metabolic apparatus at risk because if any protein component deteriorates, it cannot be replaced as in most other cells; and in fact the activity of most enzymes gradually decreases as red cells age. Another consequence of the relative simplicity of red cells is that they have a very limited range of ways to manifest distress under hardship: in essence, any sort of metabolic failure will eventually lead either to structural damage to the membrane or to failure of the cation pump. In either case the life span of the red cell is reduced, which is the definition of a *hemolytic disorder*. If the rate of red cell destruction exceeds the capacity of the bone marrow to produce more red cells, the hemolytic disorder will manifest as *hemolytic anemia*.

Thus, the essential pathophysiologic process common to all HAs is an increased red cell turnover. The gold standard for proving that the

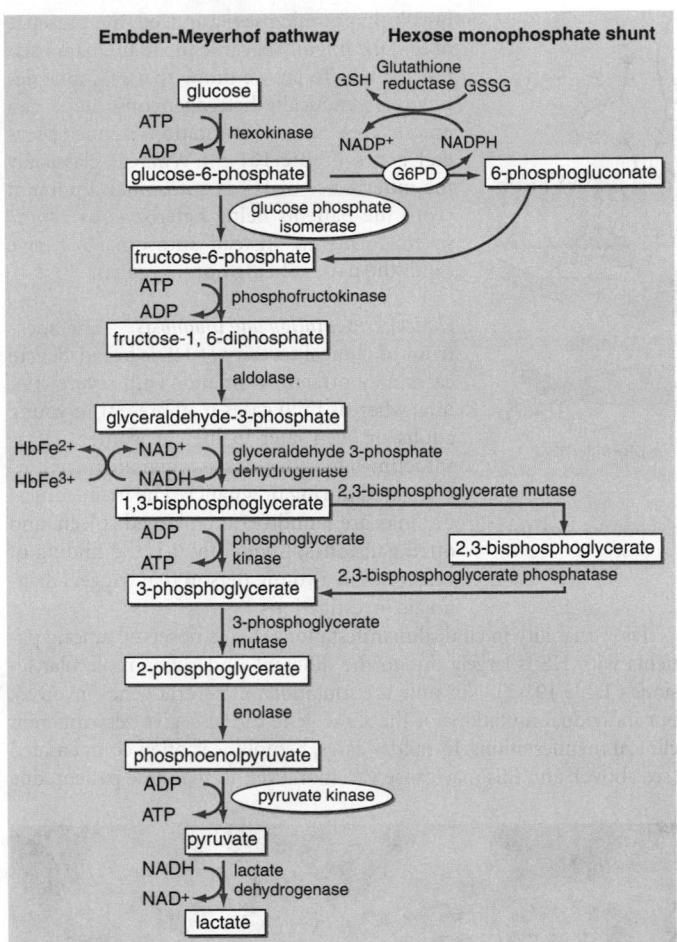

FIGURE 101-1 RBC metabolism. The Embden-Meyerhof pathway (glycolysis) generates ATP for energy and membrane maintenance. The generation of NADPH maintains hemoglobin in a reduced state. The hexose monophosphate shunt generates NADPH that is used to reduce glutathione, which protects the red cell against oxidant stress. Regulation of 2,3-bisphosphoglycerate levels is a critical determinant of oxygen affinity of hemoglobin. Enzyme deficiency states in order of prevalence: glucose-6-phosphate dehydrogenase (G6PD) >>> pyruvate kinase > glucose-6-phosphate isomerase > rare deficiencies of other enzymes in the pathway. The more common enzyme deficiencies are encircled.

life span of red cells is reduced (compared to the normal value of about 120 days) is a *red cell survival* study, which can be carried out by labeling the red cells with ^{51}Cr and measuring residual radioactivity over several days or weeks; however, this classic test is now available in very few centers and is rarely necessary. If the hemolytic event is transient, it does not usually cause any long-term consequences. However, if hemolysis is recurrent or persistent, the increased bilirubin production favors the formation of gallstones. If a considerable proportion of hemolysis takes place in the spleen, as is often the case, splenomegaly may become a prominent feature and hypersplenism may develop, with consequent neutropenia and/or thrombocytopenia.

The increased red cell turnover also has metabolic consequences. In normal subjects, the iron from effete red cells is very efficiently recycled by the body; however, with chronic intravascular hemolysis, the persistent hemoglobinuria will cause considerable iron loss, needing replacement. With chronic extravascular hemolysis, the opposite problem, iron overload, is more common, especially if the patient needs frequent blood transfusions. Chronic iron overload will cause secondary hemochromatosis; this will cause damage, particularly to the liver, eventually leading to cirrhosis, and to the heart muscle, eventually causing heart failure. The increased activity of the bone marrow

also entails an increased requirement for erythropoietic factors, particularly folic acid.

Compensated Hemolysis versus HA Red cell destruction is a potent stimulus for erythropoiesis, which is mediated by erythropoietin (EPO) produced by the kidney. This mechanism is so effective that in many cases the increased output of red cells from the bone marrow can fully balance an increased destruction of red cells. In such cases we say that hemolysis is *compensated*. The pathophysiology of compensated hemolysis is similar to that just described, except there is no anemia. This notion is important from the diagnostic point of view, because a patient with a hemolytic condition, even an inherited one, may present without anemia. It is also important from the point of view of management because compensated hemolysis may become "decompensated"—i.e., anemia may suddenly appear—in certain circumstances—for instance, pregnancy, folate deficiency, renal failure interfering with adequate EPO production, or an acute infection depressing erythropoiesis. Another general feature of chronic HA is seen when any intercurrent condition depresses erythropoiesis. When this happens, in view of the increased rate of red cell turnover, the effect will be predictably much more marked than in a person who does not have hemolysis. The most dramatic example is infection by parvovirus B19, which may cause a rather precipitous fall in hemoglobin, an occurrence sometimes referred to as *aplastic crisis*.

INHERITED HEMOLYTIC ANEMIAS

There are three essential components in the red cell: (1) hemoglobin, (2) the membrane-cytoskeleton complex, and (3) the metabolic machinery necessary to keep (1) and (2) in working order. Here we will discuss diseases of the latter two components. Diseases caused by abnormalities of hemoglobin are discussed in Chap. 99.

Hemolytic Anemias Due to Abnormalities of the Membrane-Cytoskeleton Complex The detailed architecture of the red cell membrane is complex, but its basic design is relatively simple (Fig. 101-2). The lipid bilayer, which incorporates phospholipids and cholesterol, is spanned by a number of proteins that have their hydrophobic transmembrane domains embedded in the membrane. Most of these proteins have hydrophilic domains extending toward both the outside and the inside of the cell. Other proteins are tethered to the membrane through a glycosylphosphatidylinositol (GPI) anchor, and they have only an extracellular domain. These proteins are arranged roughly perpendicular to or lying across the membrane; they include ion channels, receptors for complement components, receptors for other ligands, and some of unknown function. The most abundant of these proteins are glycophorins and the so-called band 3, an anion transporter. The extracellular domains of many of these proteins are heavily glycosylated, and they carry antigenic determinants that correspond to blood groups. Underneath the membrane, and tangential to it, is a network of other proteins that make up the cytoskeleton. The main cytoskeletal protein is spectrin, the basic unit of which is a dimer of α-spectrin and β-spectrin. The membrane is physically linked to the cytoskeleton by a third set of proteins (including ankyrin and the so-called band 4.1 and band 4.2), which thus connect these two structures intimately.

The membrane-cytoskeleton complex is indeed so integrated that, not surprisingly, an abnormality of almost any of its components will be disturbing or disruptive, causing structural failure, which results ultimately in hemolysis. These abnormalities are almost invariably inherited mutations, and thus diseases of the membrane-cytoskeleton complex belong to the category of inherited hemolytic anemias. Before the red cells lyse, they often exhibit more or less specific morphologic changes that alter the normal biconcave disc shape. Thus, the majority of the diseases in this group have been known for over a century as *hereditary spherocytosis* (HS) and *hereditary elliptocytosis* (HE). Their molecular basis has been elucidated.

HEREDITARY SPHEROCYTOSIS This is a relatively common type of hemolytic anemia, with an estimated frequency of at least 1 in 5000.

FIGURE 101-2 Diagram of red cell membrane/cytoskeleton. (For explanation see text.) *(From N Young et al: Clinical Hematology. Copyright Elsevier, 2006; with permission.)*

lysis in hypotonic media; indeed, the presence of *osmotic fragility* became the main diagnostic test for HS. Today we know that HS, thus defined, is genetically heterogeneous, i.e., it can arise from a variety of mutations in one of several genes (Table 101-3). Whereas classically the inheritance of HS is autosomal dominant (with the patients being heterozygous), some severe forms are instead autosomal recessive (with the patient being homozygous).

Clinical Presentation and Diagnosis   The spectrum of clinical severity of HS is broad. Severe cases may present in infancy with severe anemia, whereas mild cases may present in young adults or even later in life. In women, HS is sometimes first diagnosed when anemia is investigated during pregnancy. The main clinical findings are jaundice, an enlarged spleen, and often gallstones; frequently it is the finding of gallstones in a young person that triggers diagnostic investigations.

Its identification is credited to Minkowksy and Chauffard, who at the end of the 19th century reported families in whom HS was inherited as an autosomal dominant condition. From this seminal work, HS came to be defined as an inherited form of HA associated with the presence of spherocytes in the peripheral blood (Fig. 101-3A). In addition, in vitro studies revealed that the red cells were abnormally susceptible to

The variability in clinical manifestations that is observed among patients with HS is largely due to the different underlying molecular lesions (Table 101-3). Not only are mutations of several genes involved, but individual mutations of the same gene can also give very different clinical manifestations. In milder cases, hemolysis is often compensated (see above), and this may cause variation even in the same patient, due

FIGURE 101-3 Peripheral blood smear from patients with membrane-cytoskeleton abnormalities. *A.* Hereditary spherocytosis. ***B.*** Hereditary elliptocytosis, heterozygote. ***C.*** Elliptocytosis, with both alleles of the α-spectrin gene mutated. *[From L Luzzatto, in J Gribben and D Pravan (eds): Molecular Hematology, 2d edition. Oxford, Blackwell, 2005; with permission.]*

TABLE 101-3 INHERITED DISEASES OF THE RED CELL MEMBRANE-CYTOSKELETON

Gene	Chromosomal Location	Protein Produced	Disease(s) with Certain Mutations (Inheritance)	Comments
SPTA1	1q22-q23	α-Spectrin	HS (recessive) HE (dominant)	Rare. Mutations of this gene account for about 65% of HE. More severe forms may be due to coexistence of an otherwise silent mutant allele.
SPTB	14q23-q24.1	β-Spectrin	HS (dominant) HE (dominant)	Rare. Mutations of this gene account for ~30% of HE, including some severe forms.
ANK1	8p11.2	Ankyrin	HS (dominant)	May account for majority of HS.
SLC4A1	17q21	Band 3 (anion channel)	HS (dominant)	Mutations of this gene may account for ~25% of HS.
			Southeast Asian ovalocytosis (dominant)	Polymorphic mutation (deletion of 9 amino acids); clinically asymptomatic; protective against *Plasmodium falciparum*.
EPB41	1p33-p34.2	Band 4.1	HE (dominant)	Mutations of this gene account for about 5% of HE, mostly with prominent morphology but no hemolysis in heterozygotes; severe hemolysis in homozygotes.
EPB42	15q15-q21	Band 4.2	HS (recessive)	Mutations of this gene account for about 3% of HS.
RHAG	6p21.1-p11	Rhesus antigen	Chronic nonspherocytic hemolytic anemia	Very rare; associated with total loss of all Rh antigens.

Note: HS, hereditary spherocytosis; HE, hereditary elliptocytosis.

to the fact that intercurrent conditions (e.g., infection) cause decompensation. The anemia is usually normocytic, with the characteristic morphology that gives the disease its name. A characteristic feature is an increase in mean corpuscular hemoglobin concentration (MCHC): this is almost the only condition in which high MCHC is seen.

When there is a family history, it is usually easy to suspect the diagnosis, but there may be no family history for at least two reasons: (1) The patient may have a de novo mutation, i.e., a mutation that has taken place in a germ cell of one of his parents or early after zygote formation; and (2) the patient may have a recessive form of HS (Table 101-3). In most cases the diagnosis is confirmed on the basis of red cell morphology and a test for osmotic fragility, a modified version of which is called the "pink test." In some cases a definitive diagnosis can be obtained only by molecular studies demonstrating a mutation in one of the genes underlying HS. This is carried out only in laboratories with special expertise in this area.

℞ HEREDITARY SPHEROCYTOSIS

There is currently no treatment aimed at the cause of HS; no way has yet been found to correct the basic defect in the membrane-cytoskeleton structure. However, it has been apparent for a long time that the spleen plays a special role in HS, through a dual mechanism. On one hand, as in many other HAs, the spleen itself is a major site of destruction; on the other hand, transit through the splenic circulation makes the defective red cells more spherocytic and therefore accelerates their demise, even though lysis may take place elsewhere. For these reasons, splenectomy has long been regarded as a prime, almost obligatory therapeutic measure in HS. However, it also increases the risk of certain infections, and therefore current guidelines (not evidence-based) are as follows.

1. Avoid splenectomy in mild cases.
2. Delay splenectomy until at least 4 years of age, after the risk of severe sepsis has peaked.
3. Antipneumococcal vaccination before splenectomy is imperative, whereas penicillin prophylaxis postsplenectomy is controversial.
4. HS patients often may require cholecystectomy. It used to be considered mandatory to combine this procedure with splenectomy, but this may not be always necessary.

HEREDITARY ELLIPTOCYTOSIS HE is at least as heterogeneous as HS, both from the genetic (Table 101-3) and from the clinical point of view. Again it is the shape of the red cells that gives the name to these conditions, but there is no direct correlation between elliptocytic morphology and clinical severity. In fact, some mild or even asymptomatic cases may have nearly 100% elliptocytes, whereas in severe cases, all sorts of bizarre poikilocytes may predominate (Fig. 101-3B, C). Clinical features and recommended management are similar to those for HS. Although the spleen may not have the specific role it has in HS, in severe cases splenectomy may be beneficial. The prevalence of HE causing clinical disease is similar to that of HS. However, an asymptomatic form, referred to as *Southeast Asian ovalocytosis*, has a frequency of up to 7% in certain populations, presumably as a result of malaria selection.

STOMATOCYTOSIS This rare condition with autosomal dominant inheritance draws its name (mouth-like cells) from the fact that the normally round-shaped central pallor of red cells is replaced by a linear-shaped central pallor. Hemolysis is usually relatively mild. Splenectomy is contraindicated as it has been followed in a majority of cases by severe thromboembolic complications.

Enzyme Abnormalities When there is an important defect in the membrane or in the cytoskeleton, hemolysis is a direct consequence of the fact that the very structure of the red cell is abnormal. Instead, when one of the enzymes is defective, the consequences will depend on the precise role of that enzyme in the metabolic machinery of the red cell, which, in its first approximation, has two important functions: (1) to provide energy in the form of ATP, and (2) to prevent oxidative damage to hemoglobin and to other proteins.

ABNORMALITIES OF THE GLYCOLYTIC PATHWAY (Fig. 101-1) Since red cells, in the course of their differentiation, have sacrificed not only their nucleus and their ribosomes but also their mitochondria, they rely exclusively on the anaerobic portion of the glycolytic pathway for producing energy in the form of ATP. Most of the ATP is required by the red cell for cation transport against a concentration gradient across the membrane. If this fails, due to a defect of any of the enzymes of the glycolytic pathway, the result will be hemolytic disease.

Pyruvate Kinase Deficiency Abnormalities of the glycolytic pathway are all inherited and all rare (Table 101-4). Among them, deficiency of pyruvate kinase (PK) is the least rare, with an estimated prevalence of 1:10,000. The clinical picture is that of an HA that often presents in the newborn with neonatal jaundice; the jaundice persists and is usually associated with a very high reticulocytosis. The anemia is of variable severity; sometimes it is so severe as to require regular blood transfusions; sometimes it is mild, bordering on a nearly compensated hemolytic disorder. As a result, the diagnosis may be delayed, and in some cases it is made in young adults—for instance, in a woman during her first pregnancy, when the anemia may get worse. In part the delay in diagnosis is due to the fact that the anemia is remarkably well-tolerated because the metabolic block at the last step in glycolysis causes an increase in bisphosphoglycerate (or DPG), a major effector of the hemoglobin-oxygen dissociation curve. Thus, the oxygen delivery to the tissues is increased.

TABLE 101-4 RED CELL ENZYME ABNORMALITIES CAUSING HEMOLYSIS

	Enzyme (Acronym)	Chromo-somal Location	Prevalence of Enzyme Deficiency (Rank)	Clinical Manifestations Extra-Red Cell	Comments
Glycolytic pathway	Hexokinase (HK)	10q22	Very rare		Other isoenzymes known.
	Glucose 6-phosphate isomerase (G6PI)	19q31.1	Rare (4)	NM, CNS	
	Phosphofructokinase (PFK)	12q13	Very rare	Myopathy	
	Aldolase	16q22-24	Very rare		
	Triose phosphate isomerase (TPI)	12p13	Very rare	CNS (severe), NM	
	Glyceraldehyde 3-phosphate dehydro-genase (GAPD)	12p13.31–p13.1	Very rare	Myopathy	
	Diphosphoglycerate mutase (DPGM)	7q31-q34	Very rare		Erythrocytosis rather than hemolysis.
	Phosphoglycerate kinase (PGK)	Xq13	Very rare	CNS, NM	May benefit from splenectomy.
	Pyruvate kinase (PK)	1q21	Rare (2)		May benefit from splenectomy.
Redox	Glucose 6-phosphate dehydrogenase (G6PD)	Xq28	Common (1)	Very rarely granulocytes	In almost all cases only AHA from exogenous trigger.
	Glutathione synthase	20q11.2	Very rare	CNS	
	γ-Glutamylcysteine synthase	6p12	Very rare	CNS	
	Cytochrome b5 reductase	22q13.31–qter	Rare	CNS	Methemoglo-binemia rather than hemolysis.
Nucleotide metabo-lism	Adenylate kinase (AK)	9q34.1	Very rare	CNS	
	Pyrimidine 5'-nucleoti-dase (P5N)	3q11–q12	Rare (3)		May benefit from splenectomy.

Note: CNS, central nervous system; AHA, acquired hemolytic anemia.

℞ PYRUVATE KINASE DEFICIENCY

Management of PK deficiency is mainly supportive. In view of the marked increase in red cell turnover, oral folic acid supplements should be given constantly. Blood transfusion should be used as necessary, and iron chelation may have to be added if the blood transfusion requirement is high enough to cause iron overload. In these patients, who have more severe disease, splenectomy may be beneficial. There is a single case report of curative treatment of PK deficiency by bone marrow transplantation from an HLA-identical PK normal sib: this seems a viable option for severe cases when a sib donor is available.

Other Glycolytic Enzyme Abnormalities All of these defects are rare to very rare (Table 101-4), and all cause HA of varying degrees of severity. It is not unusual for the presentation to be in the guise of severe neonatal jaundice, which may require exchange transfusion; if the anemia is less severe, it may present later in life or may even remain asymptomatic and be detected incidentally when a blood count is done for unrelated reasons. The spleen is often enlarged. When other systemic manifestations occur, they involve the central nervous system, sometimes entailing severe mental retardation (particularly in the case of triose phosphate isomerase deficiency) or the neuromuscular system, or both. The *diagnosis* of HA is usually not difficult, thanks to the triad of normo-macrocytic anemia, reticulocytosis, and hyperbilirubinemia. Enzymopathies should be considered in the differential diagnosis of any chronic Coombs-negative HA. In most cases of glycolytic enzymopathies, the morphologic abnormalities of red cells characteristically seen in membrane disorders are absent. A definitive diagnosis can be made only by demonstrating the deficiency of an individual enzyme by quantitative assays carried out in only a few specialized laboratories. If a particular molecular abnormality is already known in the family, then of course one could test directly for that defect at the DNA level, bypassing the need for enzyme assays.

ABNORMALITIES OF REDOX METABOLISM

G6PD Deficiency Glucose 6-phosphate dehydrogenase (G6PD) is a housekeeping enzyme critical in the redox metabolism of all aerobic cells (Fig. 101-4). In red cells, its role is even more critical because it is the only source of reduced nicotinamide adenine dinucleotide phosphate (NADPH), which, directly and via reduced glutathione (GSH), defends these cells against oxidative stress. G6PD deficiency is a prime example of an HA due to interaction between an intracorpuscular and an extracorpuscular cause, because in the majority of cases hemolysis is triggered by an exogenous agent. Although in G6PD-deficient subjects there is a decrease in G6PD activity in most tissues, this is less marked than in red cells, and it does not seem to produce symptoms.

> **GENETIC CONSIDERATIONS** The *G6PD* gene is X-linked, and this has important implications. First, as males have only one *G6PD* gene (i.e., they are hemizygous for this gene), they must be either normal or G6PD-deficient. By contrast, females, having two *G6PD* genes, can be normal, deficient (homozygous), or intermediate (heterozygous). As a result of the phenomenon of X-chromosome inactivation, heterozygous females are genetic mosaics, with a highly variable ratio of G6PD-normal to G6PD-deficient cells and an equally variable degree of clinical expression; some heterozygotes can be just as affected as hemizygous males. The enzymatically active form of G6PD is either a dimer or a tetramer of a single protein subunit of 514 amino acids. G6PD-deficient subjects have been found invariably to have mutations in the coding region of the *G6PD* gene. Almost all of the 140 different mutations known are single missense point mutations, entailing single amino acid replacements in the G6PD protein. In most cases these mutations cause G6PD deficiency by decreasing the in vivo stability of the protein, and thus the physiologic decrease in G6PD

FIGURE 101-4 Diagram of redox metabolism in the red cell. G6P, glucose 6-phosphate; 6PG, 6-phosphogluconate; G6PD, glucose 6-phosphate dehydrogenase; GSH, reduced glutathione; GSSG, oxidized glutathione; Hb, hemoglobin; MetHb, methemoglobin; NADP, nicotinamide adenine dinucleotide phosphate; NADPH, reduced nicotinamide adenine dinucleotide phosphate.

activity that takes place with red cell ageing is greatly accelerated. In some cases an amino acid replacement can also affect the catalytic function of the enzyme.

Among the mutations, those underlying *chronic nonspherocytic hemolytic anemia* (CNSHA; see below) are a discrete subset. This much more severe clinical phenotype can be ascribed in some cases to adverse qualitative changes (for instance, a decreased affinity for the substrate, glucose 6-phosphate); or simply to the fact that the enzyme deficit is more extreme because it is more unstable. For instance, a cluster of mutations map at or near the dimer interface, and they prevent dimer formation.

TABLE 101-5 DRUGS THAT CARRY RISK OF CLINICAL HEMOLYSIS IN PERSONS WITH G6PD DEFICIENCY

	Definite Risk	Possible Risk	Doubtful Risk
Antimalarials	Primaquine Dapsone/chlorproguanil	Chloroquine	Quinine
Sulphonamides/sulphones	Sulphametoxazole Others Dapsone	Sulfasalazine Sulfadimidine	Sulfisoxazole Sulfadiazine
Antibacterial/antibiotics	Cotrimoxazole Nalidixic acid Nitrofurantoin Niridazole	Ciprofloxacin Norfloxacin	Chloramphenicol p-Aminosalicylic acid
Antipyretic/analgesics	Acetanilide Phenazopyridine (Pyridium)	Acetylsalicylic acid high dose (>3 g/d)	Acetylsalicylic acid <3 g/d Acetaminophen Phenacetin
Other	Naphthalene Methylene blue	Vitamin K analogues Ascorbic acid >1 g Rasburicase	Doxorubicin Probenecid

Epidemiology G6PD deficiency is widely distributed in tropical and subtropical parts of the world (Africa, Southern Europe, the Middle East, Southeast Asia, and Oceania) (Fig. 101-5) and wherever people from those areas have migrated; a conservative estimate is that at least 400 million people have a G6PD-deficiency gene. In several of these areas, the frequency of a G6PD-deficiency gene may be as high as 20% or more. It would be quite extraordinary for a trait that causes significant pathology to spread widely and reach high frequencies in many populations without conferring some biologic advantage. Indeed, G6PD is one of the best characterized examples of genetic polymorphisms in the human species. Clinical field studies and in vitro experiments strongly support the view that G6PD deficiency has been selected by *Plasmodium falciparum* malaria, by virtue of the fact that it confers a relative resistance against this highly lethal infection. Whether this protective effect is exerted mainly in hemizygous males or in females heterozygous for G6PD deficiency is still not clear. Different G6PD variants underlie G6PD deficiency in different parts of the world. Some of the more widespread variants are G6PD Mediterranean on the shores of the Mediterranean Sea, in the Middle East, and in India; G6PD A– in Africa and in Southern Europe; G6PD Vianchan and G6PD Mahidol in Southeast Asia; G6PD Canton in China; and G6PD Union worldwide. The heterogeneity of polymorphic G6PD variants is proof of their independent origin, and it supports the notion that they have been selected by a common environmental agent, in keeping with the concept of convergent evolution.

Clinical Manifestations The vast majority of people with G6PD deficiency remain clinically asymptomatic throughout their lifetime.

However, all of them have an increased risk of developing neonatal jaundice (NNJ) and a risk of developing acute HA when challenged by a number of oxidative agents. NNJ related to G6PD deficiency is very rarely present at birth: the peak incidence of clinical onset is between day 2 and day 3, and in most cases the anemia is not severe. However, NNJ can be very severe in some G6PD-deficient babies, especially in association with prematurity, infection, and/or environmental factors (such as naphthalene-camphor balls used in babies' bedding and clothing). In these cases, if inadequately managed, NNJ associated with G6PD deficiency can produce kernicterus and permanent neurologic damage.

Acute HA can develop as a result of three types of triggers: (1) fava beans, (2) infections, and (3) drugs (Table 101-5). Typically, a hemolytic attack starts with malaise, weakness, and abdominal or lumbar pain. After an interval of several hours to 2–3 days, the patient develops jaundice and often dark urine, due to hemoglobinuria (Table 101-6). The onset can be extremely abrupt, especially with favism in children. The anemia is moderate to extremely severe, usually normocytic and normochromic, and due partly to intravascular hemolysis; hence, it is associated with hemoglobinemia, hemoglobinuria, and low or absent plasma haptoglobin. The blood film shows anisocytosis, polychromasia, and spherocytes (Fig. 101-6). The most typical feature is the presence of bizarre poikilocytes with red cells that appear to have unevenly distributed hemoglobin (hemighosts) and red cells that appear to have had parts of them bitten away (bite cells or blister cells). A classic test, now rarely carried out, is supravital staining with methyl violet, which, if done promptly, reveals the presence of Heinz bodies, consisting of precipitates of denatured hemoglobin and regarded as a signature of oxidative damage to red cells (except for the rare occurrence of an unstable hemoglobin). LDH is high and so is the unconjugated bilirubin, indicating that there is also extravascular hemolysis. The most serious threat from acute HA in adults is the development of acute renal failure (exceedingly rare in children). Once the threat of acute anemia is over, and in the absence of comorbidity, full recovery from acute HA associated with G6PD deficiency is the rule.

A very small minority of subjects with G6PD deficiency have CNSHA of variable severity. The patient is always a male, usually with a history of NNJ, who may present with anemia or unexplained jaundice, or because of gallstones later in life. The spleen may be enlarged. The severity of anemia ranges from borderline to transfusion-dependent. The anemia is

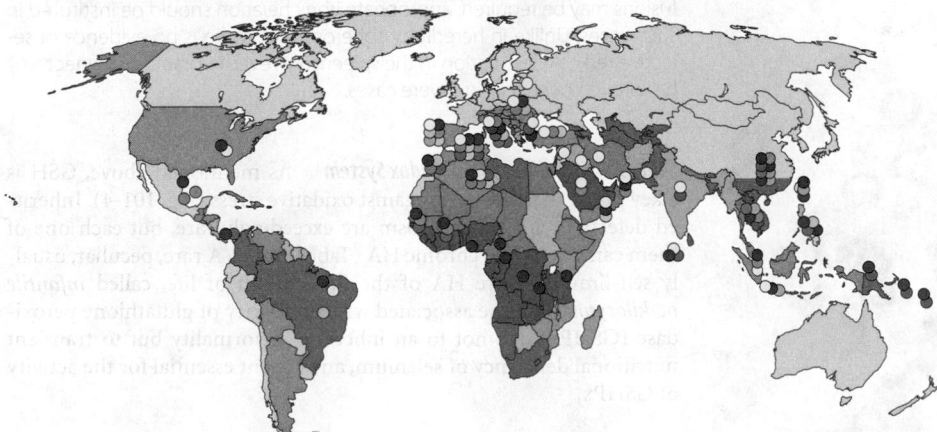

FIGURE 101-5 Epidemiology of G6PD deficiency throughout the world. The different shadings indicate increasingly high levels of prevalence, up to about 20%; the different colored symbols indicate individual genetic variants of G6PD, each one having a different mutation. [*From L Luzzatto et al in C Scriver et al (eds): The Metabolic & Molecular Bases of Inherited Disease, 8th edition. New York, McGraw-Hill, 2001.*]

TABLE 101-6 DISEASES/CLINICAL SITUATIONS WITH PREDOMINANTLY INTRAVASCULAR HEMOLYSIS

	Onset/Time Course	Main Mechanism	Appropriate Diagnostic Procedure	Comments
Mismatched blood transfusion	Abrupt	Nearly always ABO incompatibility	Repeat cross match	
Paroxysmal nocturnal hemoglobinuria (PNH)	Chronic with acute exacerbations	Complement (C)-mediated destruction of CD59(−) red cells	Flow cytometry to display a CD59(−) red cell population	Exacerbations due to C activation through any pathway
Paroxysmal cold hemoglobinuria (PCH)	Acute	Immune lysis of normal red cells	Test for Donath-Landsteiner antibody	Often triggered by viral infection
Septicemia	Very acute	Exotoxins produced by *Clostridium perfringens*	Blood cultures	Other organisms may be responsible
Microangiopathic	Acute or chronic	Red cell fragmentation	Red cell morphology on blood smear	Different causes ranging from endothelial damage to hemangioma to leaky prosthetic heart valve
March hemoglobinuria	Abrupt	Mechanical destruction	Targeted history taking	
Favism	Acute	Destruction of older fraction of G6PD-deficient red cells	G6PD assay	Triggered by ingestion of large dish of fava beans; but trigger can be infection or drug instead

usually normo-macrocytic, with reticulocytosis. Bilirubin and LDH are increased. Although hemolysis is, by definition, chronic in these patients, they are also vulnerable to acute oxidative damage, and therefore the same agents (see Table 101-5) that can cause acute HA in people with the ordinary type of G6PD deficiency will cause severe exacerbations in people with the severe form of G6PD deficiency. In some cases of CNSHA, the deficiency of G6PD is so severe in granulocytes that it becomes rate-limiting for their oxidative burst, with consequent increased susceptibility to bacterial infections.

Laboratory Diagnosis The suspicion of G6PD deficiency can be confirmed by semiquantitative methods often referred to as screening tests, which are suitable for population studies and can correctly classify male subjects, in the steady state, as G6PD-normal or G6PD-deficient. However, in clinical practice a diagnostic test is usually needed when the patient has had a hemolytic attack: this implies that the old-est, most G6PD-deficient red cells have been selectively destroyed, and young red cells, having higher G6PD activity, are being released into the circulation. Under these conditions, only a quantitative test can give a definitive result. In males this test will identify normal hemizygotes and G6PD-deficient hemizygotes; among females some heterozygotes will be missed, but those who are at most risk of hemolysis will be identified.

G6PD DEFICIENCY

The acute HA of G6PD deficiency is largely preventable by avoiding exposure to triggering factors of previously screened subjects. Of course, the practicability and cost-effectiveness of screening depends on the prevalence of G6PD deficiency in each individual community. Favism is entirely preventable by not eating fava beans. Prevention of drug-induced hemolysis is possible in most cases by choosing alternative drugs. When acute HA develops and once its cause is recognized, no specific treatment is needed in most cases. However, if the anemia is severe, it may be a medical emergency, especially in children, requiring immediate action, including blood transfusion. If acute renal failure develops, hemodialysis may be necessary, but if there is no previous kidney disease, full recovery is the rule. The management of NNJ associated with G6PD deficiency is no different from that of NNJ due to other causes.

In cases with CNSHA, if the anemia is not severe, regular folic acid supplements and regular hematologic surveillance will suffice. It will be important to avoid exposure to potentially hemolytic drugs, and blood transfusion may be indicated when exacerbations occur, mostly in concomitance with intercurrent infection. In rare patients, regular blood transfusions may be required; appropriate iron chelation should be instituted in such cases. Unlike in hereditary spherocytosis, there is no evidence of selective red cell destruction in the spleen: however, in practice splenectomy has proven beneficial in severe cases.

FIGURE 101-6 Peripheral blood smear from a 5-year-old G6PD-deficient boy with acute favism.

Other Abnormalities of the Redox System As mentioned above, GSH is a key player in the defense against oxidative stress (Fig. 101-4). Inherited defects of GSH metabolism are exceedingly rare, but each one of them can give rise to chronic HA (Table 101-4). A rare, peculiar, usually self-limited severe HA of the first month of life, called *infantile poikilocytosis*, may be associated with deficiency of glutathione peroxidase (GSHPx) due not to an inherited abnormality but to transient nutritional deficiency of selenium, an element essential for the activity of GSHPx.

PYRIMIDINE 5′-NUCLEOTIDASE (P5N) DEFICIENCY P5N is a key enzyme in the catabolism of nucleotides arising from the degradation of nucleic acids that takes place in the final stages of red cell maturation. How exactly its deficiency causes HA is not well understood, but a highly distinctive feature of this condition is a morphologic abnormality of the red cells known as *basophilic stippling*. The condition is rare, but it probably ranks third in frequency among red cell enzyme defects (after G6PD deficiency and PK deficiency). The anemia is lifelong, of variable severity, and may benefit from splenectomy.

Familial Hemolytic Uremic Syndrome (HUS)
This disorder is unique because, now that its basis has been elucidated, we can clearly see that hemolysis is due to an inherited defect, but this is external to red cells. HUS is defined as a microangiopathic hemolytic anemia with fragmented erythrocytes in the peripheral blood smear, thrombocytopenia (usually mild), and acute renal failure. An infection is usually the trigger of the syndrome, which tends to recur. When it does, the prognosis is serious. Although familial HUS is rare, studies of affected members from more than 100 families have revealed numerous mutations in any of three complement regulatory proteins: membrane cofactor protein, factor H, and factor I. It is thought that when complement is activated through the alternative pathway following damage to endothelial cells in the kidney, one of the results will be brisk hemolysis. Thus, the much more common Shiga toxin–related HUS can be regarded as a phenocopy of familial HUS.

ACQUIRED HEMOLYTIC ANEMIA

Mechanical Destruction of Red Cells
Although red cells are characterized by the remarkable deformability that enables them to squeeze through capillaries narrower than themselves thousands of times in their lifetime, there are at least two situations in which they succumb to shear, if not to wear and tear; the result is intravascular hemolysis resulting in hemoglobinuria. One situation, *march hemoglobinuria*, is acute and self-inflicted. Why a marathon runner may sometimes develop this complication and at another time does not is unclear (perhaps the footwear needs attention). A similar syndrome may develop after prolonged barefoot ritual dancing or vigorous bongo drumming. The other situation, which has been called *microangiopathic hemolytic anemia*, (Table 101-6) is chronic and iatrogenic; it takes place in patients with prosthetic heart valves, especially when paraprosthetic regurgitation is present. If the hemolysis consequent to mechanical trauma to the red cells is mild, and provided the supply of iron is adequate, it may be largely compensated. If more than mild anemia develops, reintervention to correct regurgitation may be required.

Toxic Agents and Drugs
A number of chemicals with oxidative potential, whether medicinal or not, can cause hemolysis even in people who are not G6PD-deficient (see above). Examples are hyperbaric oxygen (or 100% oxygen), nitrates, chlorates, methylene blue, dapsone, cisplatin, and numerous aromatic (cyclic) compounds. Other chemicals may be hemolytic through nonoxidative, largely unknown mechanisms; examples are arsine, stibine, copper, and lead. The HA caused by lead poisoning is characterized by basophilic stippling: it is in fact a phenocopy of that seen in P5N deficiency (see above), suggesting it is mediated at least in part by lead inhibiting this enzyme.

In these cases hemolysis appears to be mediated by a direct chemical action on red cells. But drugs can cause hemolysis through at least two other mechanisms. (1) A drug can behave as a hapten and induce antibody production. In rare subjects this happens, for instance, with penicillin. Upon a subsequent exposure, red cells are caught as innocent bystanders in the reaction between penicillin and antipenicillin antibodies. Hemolysis will subside as soon as penicillin administration is stopped. (2) A drug can trigger, perhaps through mimicry, the production of an antibody against a red cell antigen. The best-known example is methyldopa, an antihypertensive agent no longer in use, which in a small fraction of patients stimulated the production of the Rhesus antibody anti-e. In patients who have this antigen, the anti-e is a true autoantibody, which would then cause an autoimmune HA (see below). Usually HA would gradually subside once methyldopa was discontinued.

Nucleosides may also cause hemolysis by depletion of ATP. Ribavirin, a drug used in the treatment of hepatitis C, causes the destruction of red cells through this mechanism. Severe intravascular hemolysis can be caused by the venom of certain snakes (cobras and vipers), and HA can also follow spider bites.

Infection
By far the most frequent infectious cause of hemolytic anemia in endemic areas is malaria (Chap. 203). In other parts of the world, the most frequent cause is probably Shiga toxin–producing *Escherichia coli* O157:H7, now recognized as the main etiologic agent of HUS, more common in children than in adults (Chap. 143). Life-threatening intravascular hemolysis due to a toxin with lecithinase activity occurs with *Clostridium perfringens* sepsis (Table 101-6), particularly with open wounds, following septic abortion, or as a disastrous accident due to a contaminated blood unit. Occasionally HA is seen, especially in children, with sepsis or endocarditis from a variety of organisms.

Autoimmune Hemolytic Anemia (AIHA)
Except for countries where malaria is endemic, AIHA is the most common form of acquired hemolytic anemia. In fact, not quite appropriately, the two phrases are sometimes used synonymously.

PATHOPHYSIOLOGY AIHA is caused by an autoantibody directed against a red cell antigen, i.e., a molecule present on the surface of red cells. The autoantibody binds to the red cells. Once a red cell is coated by antibody, it will be destroyed by one or more mechanisms. In most cases the Fc portion of the antibody will be recognized by the Fc receptor of macrophages, and this will trigger erythrophagocytosis (Fig. 101-7). Thus, destruction of red cells will take place wherever macrophages are abundant—i.e., in the spleen, liver, and bone marrow. Because of the special anatomy of the spleen, this organ is particularly efficient in trapping antibody-coated red cells, and often this is the predominant site of red cell destruction. Although in severe cases even circulating monocytes can take part in this process, most of the phagocytosis-mediated red cell destruction takes place in the spleen and liver, and it is therefore called *extravascular hemolysis*. In some cases the nature of the antibody is such (usually an IgM antibody) that the antigen-antibody complex on the surface of red cells is able to activate complement (C). As a result, a large amount of membrane attack complex will form, and the red cells may be destroyed directly, known as *intravascular hemolysis*.

CLINICAL FEATURES The onset of AIHA is very often abrupt and can be dramatic. The hemoglobin level can drop, within days, to as low as 4 g/dL; the massive red cell removal will produce jaundice, and often the spleen will be enlarged. When this triad is present, the suspicion of AIHA must be high. When hemolysis is (in part) intravascular, the telltale sign will be hemoglobinuria, which the patient may report or for which the physician must test. The diagnostic test for AIHA is the antiglobulin test worked out in 1945 by R.R.A. Coombs and known since by his name. The beauty of this test is that it directly detects the pathogenetic mediator of the disease, i.e., the presence of antibody on the red cells themselves. When the test is positive, it clinches the diagnosis; when it is negative, the diagnosis is unlikely. However, the sensitivity of the Coombs test varies depending on the technology that is used, and in doubtful cases a repeat in a specialized lab is advisable; the term *Coombs-negative AIHA* is a last resort. In some cases the autoantibody has a defined identity: it may be specific for a Rhesus system antigen (often anti-e). In many cases it is regarded as "unspecific" because it reacts with virtually all types of red cells.

As in autoimmune diseases in general, the real cause of AIHA remains obscure. However, from the clinical point of view, an important feature is that AIHA can appear to be isolated, or it can develop as part of a more general autoimmune disease, particularly systemic lupus erythematosus (SLE), of which sometimes it may be the first manifestation. Therefore, when AIHA is diagnosed, a full screen for autoimmune disease is imperative. In some cases AIHA can be associated, on first presentation or subsequently, with autoimmune thrombocytopenia (Evans's syndrome).

℞ AUTOIMMUNE HEMOLYTIC ANEMIA

The first-line treatment of AIHA is glucocorticoids. A dose of prednisone of 1 mg/kg per day will cause a prompt remission in at least one-half of cases.

FIGURE 101-7 Mechanism of antibody-mediated immune destruction of red cells.
(From N Young et al: Clinical Hematology. Copyright Elsevier, 2006; with permission.)

Whereas some patients are apparently cured, relapses are not uncommon. For patients who do not respond, and for those who have relapsed, second-line treatment measures include long-term immunosuppression with low-dose prednisone, azathioprine, or cyclosporine. In patients whose AIHA has become chronic, and sometimes even earlier, splenectomy is a viable option: although it does not cure the disease, it can produce significant benefit by removing a major site of hemolysis, thus improving the anemia and/or reducing the need for immunosuppressive agents. Most of the management of AIHA is not evidence-based. However, the anti-CD20 antibody rituximab has produced responses. Anecdotal reports suggest response to intravenous immunoglobulin. In severe refractory cases, either auto- or allohematopoietic stem cell transplantation has been used, sometimes successfully.

Severe acute AIHA can be a medical emergency. The immediate treatment almost invariably includes transfusion of red cells. This may pose a special problem because if the antibody involved is "unspecific," all the blood units cross-matched will be incompatible. In these cases it is often correct, paradoxically, to transfuse incompatible blood, the rationale being that the transfused red cells will be destroyed no less but no more than the patient's own red cells, and in the meantime the patient stays alive. Clearly this rather unique situation requires good liaison and understanding between the clinical unit treating the patient and the blood transfusion/serology lab.

PAROXYSMAL COLD HEMOGLOBINURIA (PCH) PCH is a rather rare form of AIHA occurring mostly in children, usually triggered by a viral infection, usually self-limited, and characterized by involvement of the so-called Donath-Landsteiner antibody. In vitro this antibody has unique serologic features: it has anti-P specificity and binds to red cells only at a low temperature (optimally at 4°C), but when the temperature is shifted to 37°C, lysis of red cells takes place in the presence of complement. Consequently, in vivo there is intravascular hemolysis, resulting in hemoglobinuria. Clinically, the differential diagnosis must include other causes of hemoglobinuria (Table 101-2), but the presence of the Donath-Landsteiner antibody will prove PCH. Active supportive treatment, including blood transfusion, is needed to control the anemia; subsequently, recovery is the rule.

COLD AGGLUTININ DISEASE (CAD) This designation is used for a form of chronic AIHA that usually affects the elderly and has special clinical and pathologic features. First, the term *cold* refers to the fact that the autoanti-

body involved reacts with red cells poorly or not at all at 37°C, whereas it reacts strongly at lower temperatures.[1] As a result, hemolysis is more prominent the more the body is exposed to cold. The antibody is usually an IgM, usually has an anti-I specificity (the I antigen is present on the red cells of almost everyone), and may have a very high titer (1:100,000 or more has been observed). Second, the antibody is produced by an expanded clone of B lymphocytes, and sometimes its concentration in the plasma is high enough to show up as a spike in plasma protein electrophoresis—i.e., as a monoclonal gammopathy. Third, since the antibody is IgM, CAD is related to Waldenström macroglobulinemia (WM; Chap. 106), although in most cases the other clinical features of this disease are not present. Thus, CAD must be regarded as a form of WM, i.e., as a low-grade mature B-cell lymphoma that manifests at an earlier stage because the unique biologic properties of the IgM that it produces give the clinical picture of chronic HA.

In mild forms of CAD, avoidance of exposure to cold may be all that is needed to enable the patient to live with a reasonably comfortable quality of life, but in more severe forms the management of CAD is not easy. Blood transfusion is not very effective because donor red cells are I-positive and will be removed rapidly. Immunosuppressive/cytotoxic treatment with prednisone, azathioprine, or cyclophosphamide can reduce the antibody titer, but clinical efficacy is limited, and in view of the chronic nature of the disease, the side effects may prove unacceptable. Plasma exchange is a rational approach, but it is laborious and must be carried out, in some patients, at very frequent intervals. The picture may be changing, as in a recent study rituximab gave a response rate of 60%. Given the long clinical course of CAD, it remains to be seen with what periodicity this agent will need to be administered.

Paroxysmal Nocturnal Hemoglobinuria (PNH) PNH is an acquired chronic HA characterized by persistent intravascular hemolysis subject to recurrent exacerbations (Table 101-6; Fig. 101-8). In addition to hemolysis, there is often pancytopenia and a risk of venous thrombosis. This triad makes PNH a truly unique clinical condition; however, when not all of these three features are manifest on presentation, the diagnosis is often delayed, although it can be always made by appropriate laboratory investigations (see below).

PNH has about the same frequency in men and women, and it is encountered in all populations throughout the world, but it is a rare disease: its prevalence is 1–5 per million (it may be somewhat less rare in Southeast Asia and in the Far East). There is no evidence of inherited susceptibility. PNH has never been reported as a congenital disease, but it can present in small children or in people in their seventies, although most patients are young adults.

CLINICAL FEATURES The patient may seek medical attention because one morning she or he has passed "blood instead of urine." This distressing event may be regarded as the classical presentation; however, more frequently this symptom is not noticed or is suppressed. Indeed, the patient often presents simply as a problem in the differential diagnosis of *anemia*, whether symptomatic or discovered incidentally. Sometimes the anemia is associated from the outset with neutropenia or thrombocytopenia, or both. Some patients may present with recurrent attacks of severe abdominal pain, defying a specific diagnosis and eventually found to be caused by thrombosis. When thrombosis af-

---

[1]In the past, this type of antibody was called a cold antibody, whereas the antibodies causing the more common form of AIHA were called warm antibodies.

FIGURE 101-8 Consecutive urine samples from a patient with paroxysmal nocturnal hemoglobinuria (PNH). The variation in the severity of hemoglobinuria within hours is probably unique to this condition.

fects the hepatic veins, it may produce acute hepatomegaly and ascites, i.e., a full-fledged Budd-Chiari syndrome, which, in the absence of liver disease, ought to raise the suspicion of PNH.

The *natural history* of PNH can extend over decades. Without treatment, the median survival is ~8–10 years; in the past the commonest cause of death has been venous thrombosis followed by infection secondary to severe neutropenia and hemorrhage secondary to severe thrombocytopenia. PNH may evolve into aplastic anemia (AA), and PNH may manifest itself in patients who previously had AA. Rarely (estimated 1–2% of all cases), PNH may terminate in acute myeloid leukemia. On the other hand, full spontaneous recovery from PNH has been well documented, albeit rarely.

LABORATORY INVESTIGATIONS AND DIAGNOSIS The most consistent blood finding is anemia, which may range from mild to moderate to very severe. The anemia is usually normo-macrocytic, with unremarkable red cell morphology; if the MCV is high, it is usually largely accounted for by reticulocytosis, which may be quite marked (up to 20%, or up to 400,000/μL). The anemia may become microcytic if the patient is allowed to become iron-deficient as a result of chronic urinary blood loss through hemoglobinuria. Neutropenia and/or thrombocytopenia may or may not be present from the outset or may develop subsequently. Unconjugated bilirubin is mildly or moderately elevated, LDH is typically markedly elevated (values in the thousands are common), and haptoglobin is usually undetectable. All these findings make the diagnosis of HA compelling. Hemoglobinuria may be overt in a random urine sample; if it is not, it may be helpful to obtain serial urine samples, since hemoglobinuria can vary dramatically from day to day, and even from hour to hour (Fig. 101-8). The bone marrow is usually cellular with marked to massive erythroid hyperplasia, often with mild to moderate dyserythropoietic features (these do not justify confusing PNH with MDS). At some stage of the disease the marrow may become hypocellular or even frankly aplastic (see below).

The definitive diagnosis of PNH must be based on the demonstration that a substantial proportion of the patient's red cells have an increased susceptibility to complement (C), due to the deficiency on their surface of proteins (particularly CD59 and CD55) that normally protect the red cells from activated C. The sucrose hemolysis test is unreliable, and the acidified serum (Ham) test is carried out in few labs. The gold standard today is flow cytometry, which can be carried out on granulocytes as well as on red cells. A bimodal distribution of cells, with a discrete population that is CD59–, CD55–, is diagnostic of PNH. Usually this population is at least 5% of the total in the case of red cells and at least 20% of the total in the case of granulocytes.

PATHOPHYSIOLOGY Hemolysis in PNH is due to an intrinsic abnormality of the red cell, which makes it exquisitely sensitive to activated C, whether it is activated through the alternative pathway or through an antigen-antibody reaction. The former mechanism is mainly re-

sponsible for intravascular hemolysis in PNH. The latter mechanism explains why the hemolysis can be dramatically exacerbated in the course of a viral or bacterial infection. Hypersusceptibility to C is due to deficiency of several protective membrane proteins, of which CD59 is the most important because it hinders the insertion of C9 polymers into the membrane. The molecular basis for the deficiency of these proteins has been pinpointed not to a defect in any of the respective genes but rather to the shortage of a unique glycolipid molecule, GPI, which, through a peptide bond, anchors these proteins to the surface membrane of cells. The shortage of GPI is due in turn to a mutation in an X-linked gene, called *PIG-A*, required for an early step in GPI biosynthesis. In virtually each patient, the PIG-A mutation is different. This is not surprising, since these mutations are not inherited. Rather, each one takes place de novo in a hemopoietic stem cell (i.e., they are somatic mutations). As a result, the patient's marrow is a mosaic of mutant and nonmutant cells, and the peripheral blood always contains both PNH cells and normal (non PNH) cells. Thrombosis is one of the most immediately life-threatening complications of PNH and yet one of the least understood in its pathogenesis. It could be that deficiency of CD59 on the PNH platelet causes inappropriate platelet activation; however, other mechanisms are possible.

BONE MARROW FAILURE—RELATIONSHIP BETWEEN PNH AND AA It is not unusual that patients with firmly established PNH have a previous history of well-documented AA. On the other hand, sometimes a patient with PNH becomes less hemolytic and more pancytopenic and ultimately has the clinical picture of AA. Since AA is probably an organ-specific autoimmune disease in which T cells cause damage to hematopoietic stem cells, the same may be true of PNH, with the specific proviso that the damage spares PNH stem cells. Skewing of the T cell repertoire in patients with PNH supports this notion. In addition, in mouse models, PNH stem cells do not expand when the rest of the bone marrow is normal, and by high-sensitivity flow cytometry technology, very rare PNH cells harboring PIG-A mutations can be demonstrated in normal people. In view of these facts, it seems that an element of bone marrow failure (BMF) in PNH is the rule rather than the exception. An extreme view is that PNH is a form of AA in which BMF is masked by the massive expansion of the PNH clone that populates the patient's bone marrow. The mechanism whereby PNH stem cells escape the damage suffered by non-PNH stem cells is not yet known.

℞ PAROXYSMAL NOCTURNAL HEMOGLOBINURIA

Unlike other acquired HAs, PNH may be lifelong and most patients receive supportive treatment only, including transfusion of filtered red cells[2] whenever necessary. Folic acid supplements (at least 3 mg/d) are mandatory; the serum iron should be checked periodically and iron supplements administered as appropriate. Long-term glucocorticoids are not indicated because there is no evidence that they have any effect on chronic hemolysis, and their side effects are considerable and potentially dangerous. The only form of treatment that can provide a cure for PNH is allogeneic bone marrow transplantation (BMT); when an HLA-identical sibling is available, BMT should be offered to any young patient with severe PNH.

A major advance in the management of PNH has been the development of a humanized monoclonal antibody, eculizumab, directed against the complement protein C5 **(Fig. 101-9)**. By blocking the complement cascade downstream of C5, this antibody provides a medical intervention capable of controlling complement-dependent hemolysis in PNH. In an international multicenter placebo-controlled randomized trial on 87 patients who had been selected on grounds of having severe transfusion-dependent hemolysis, eculizumab completely abolished the need for blood transfusion in about one-half of the patients. Eculizumab administered intravenously at q2wk intervals also ameliorated the anemia in most patients and dramatically improved their quality of life.

---

[2]Now that filters with excellent removal of white cells are routinely used, the traditional washing of red cells, which aimed to avoid white cell reactions triggering hemolysis, is no longer necessary and considered wasteful.

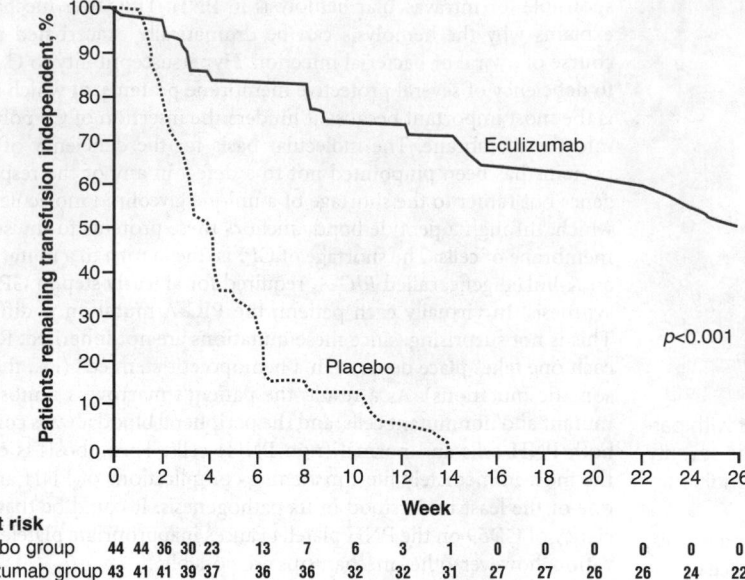

FIGURE 101-9 Therapeutic efficacy of an anti-C5 antibody on the anemia of paroxysmal nocturnal hemoglobinuria. *(From P Hillmen et al: N Engl J Med 355:1233, 2006; with permission.)*

For patients with PNH-AA syndrome, immunosuppressive treatment with antilymphocyte globulin (ALG or ATG) and cyclosporine A may be indicated. Although no formal trial has ever been conducted, this approach has helped particularly to relieve severe thrombocytopenia and/or neutropenia in patients in whom these were the main problem(s). By contrast, there is often little immediate effect on hemolysis. Thrombolytic therapy with tissue plasminogen activator may be indicated after severe thrombosis. Any patient who has had deep vein thrombosis at any site in the abdomen or in a limb should be on regular anticoagulant prophylaxis.

ANEMIA DUE TO ACUTE BLOOD LOSS

Blood loss causes anemia by two main mechanisms: first, by the direct loss of red cells; second, because if the loss of blood is protracted, it will gradually deplete the iron stores, eventually resulting in iron deficiency. Iron-deficiency anemia is discussed in Chap. 98.

Here we are concerned with *post-hemorrhagic anemia*, which follows *acute blood loss*. This can be *external* (as after trauma or due to postpartum hemorrhage) or *internal* (e.g., from bleeding in the gastrointestinal tract, rupture of the spleen, rupture of an ectopic pregnancy). In any of these cases—i.e., after the sudden loss of a large amount of blood—three clinical/pathophysiologic stages are noted.

1. At first, the dominant feature is hypovolemia, which poses a threat particularly to organs that normally have a high blood supply, such as the brain and the kidneys; therefore, loss of consciousness and acute renal failure are major threats. It is important to note that at this stage an ordinary blood count will not show anemia, as the hemoglobin concentration is not affected.
2. Next, as an emergency response, baroreceptors and stretch receptors will cause release of vasopressin and other peptides, and the body will shift fluid from the extravascular to the intravascular compartment, producing hemodilution. Thus, the hypovolemia gradually converts to anemia. The degree of anemia will reflect the amount of blood lost. If after 3 days the hemoglobin is, say, 7 g/dL, it means that about half of the entire blood volume had been lost.
3. Provided bleeding does not continue, the bone marrow response will gradually ameliorate the anemia if erythropoietin production, the erythroid progenitors, and iron supply are normal. Within about 2–3 days after acute hemorrhage, reticulocytes will increase in the blood and reach a maximum 7–10 days after the hemorrhage has been controlled. Reticulocyte counts of 20% may be achieved.

The diagnosis of acute post-hemorrhagic anemia (APHA) is usually straightforward, although sometimes internal bleeding episodes—after a traumatic injury or otherwise—may not be immediately obvious, even when large. Whenever an abrupt fall in hemoglobin has taken place, whatever history is given by the patient, APHA should be suspected. Supplementary history may have to be obtained by asking the appropriate questions, and appropriate investigations (e.g., a sonogram or an endoscopy) may have to be carried out. Internal bleeding may result in a rise in unconjugated bilirubin and a fall in serum haptoglobin.

℞ ANEMIA DUE TO BLOOD LOSS

With respect to treatment, a two-pronged approach is imperative. First, in many cases the blood lost needs to be replaced promptly. With many chronic anemias, finding and correcting the cause of the anemia is the first priority, and blood transfusion may not be even necessary, because the body is adapted to the anemia; with acute blood loss the reverse is true. Since the body is not adapted to the anemia, blood transfusion takes priority. Although fluorocarbon synthetic chemicals have shown promise, no "blood substitute" has yet become standard treatment. Second, while the emergency is being confronted, it is imperative to stop the hemorrhage and to eliminate its source.

ACKNOWLEDGMENT

H. Frank Bunn and Wendell Rosse contributed this chapter in the last edition and material from that chapter has been used here.

FURTHER READINGS

DACIE J: *The Haemolytic Anaemias*, 5 volumes. London, Churchill Livingstone, 1995

EBER S, LUX SE: Hereditary spherocytosis—defects in proteins that connect the membrane skeleton to the lipid bilayer. Semin Hematol 41:118, 2004

HEIER HE et al: Transfusion versus alternative treatment modalities in acute bleeding: A systematic review. Acta Anaesthesiol Scand 509:20, 2006

HILL A et al: Recent developments in the understanding and management of paroxysmal nocturnal hemoglobinuria. Br J Haematol 137:181, 2007

HILLMEN P, et al: The complement inhibitor eculizumab in paroxysmal nocturnal hemoglobinuria. N Engl J Med 355:1233, 2006

LUZZATTO L: Paroxysmal nocturnal hemoglobinuria, in *Clinical Hematology*, N Young, Gershon SL, High KA (eds). Philadelphia, Mosby, pp 326–339, 2006

ROSSE WF, HILLMEN P, SCHREIBER AD: Immune-mediated hemolytic anemia. *Hematology, Am Soc Hematol Educ Program* pp. 48–62, 2004

SHAPIRA Y et al: Erythropoietin can obviate the need for repeated heart valve replacement in high-risk patients with severe mechanical hemolytic anemia: Case reports and literature review. J Heart Valve Dis 10:431, 2001

102 Aplastic Anemia, Myelodysplasia, and Related Bone Marrow Failure Syndromes

Neal S. Young

The hypoproliferative anemias are normochromic, normocytic or macrocytic and are characterized by a low reticulocyte count. Deficient production of RBCs occurs with marrow damage and dysfunction, which may be secondary to infection, inflammation, and cancer. Hypoproliferative anemia is also a prominent feature of hematologic diseases that are described as bone marrow failure states; these include aplastic anemia, myelodysplasia (MDS), pure red cell aplasia (PRCA), and myelophthisis. Anemia in these disorders is often not a solitary or even the major hematologic finding. More frequent in bone marrow failure is pancytopenia: anemia, leukopenia, and thrombocytopenia. Low blood counts in the marrow failure diseases result from deficient hematopoiesis, as distinguished from blood count depression due to peripheral destruction of red cells (hemolytic anemias), platelets (idiopathic thrombocytopenic purpura or due to splenomegaly), and granulocytes (as in the immune leukopenias).

Hematopoietic failure syndromes are classified by dominant morphologic features of the bone marrow (Table 102-1). While practical distinction among these syndromes usually is clear, they can occur secondary to other diseases, and some processes are so closely related that the diagnosis may be complex. Patients may seem to suffer from two or three related diseases simultaneously, or one diagnosis may appear to evolve into another. Many of these syndromes share an immune-mediated mechanism of marrow destruction and some element of genomic instability resulting in a higher rate of malignant transformation.

APLASTIC ANEMIA

DEFINITION

Aplastic anemia is pancytopenia with bone marrow hypocellularity. Acquired aplastic anemia is distinguished from iatrogenic marrow aplasia, marrow hypocellularity after intensive cytotoxic chemotherapy for cancer. Aplastic anemia can also be constitutional: the genetic diseases Fanconi's anemia and dyskeratosis congenita, while frequently associated with typical physical anomalies and the development of

TABLE 102-1 DIFFERENTIAL DIAGNOSIS OF PANCYTOPENIA

Pancytopenia with Hypocellular Bone Marrow

Acquired aplastic anemia
Constitutional aplastic anemia (Fanconi's anemia, dyskeratosis congenita)
Some myelodysplasia
Rare aleukemic leukemia (AML)
Some acute lymphoid leukemia
Some lymphomas of bone marrow

Pancytopenia with Cellular Bone Marrow

Primary bone marrow diseases	Secondary to systemic diseases
Myelodysplasia	Systemic lupus erythematosus
Paroxysmal nocturnal hemoglobinuria	Hypersplenism
	B_{12}, folate deficiency
Myelofibrosis	Overwhelming infection
Some aleukemic leukemia	Alcohol
Myelophthisis	Brucellosis
Bone marrow lymphoma	Sarcoidosis
Hairy cell leukemia	Tuberculosis
	Leishmaniasis

Hypocellular Bone Marrow ± Cytopenia

Q fever
Legionnaires' disease
Anorexia nervosa, starvation
Mycobacteria

pancytopenia early in life, can also present as marrow failure in normal-appearing adults. Acquired aplastic anemia is often stereotypical in its manifestations, with the abrupt onset of low blood counts in a previously well young adult; seronegative hepatitis or a course of an incriminated medical drug may precede the onset. The diagnosis in these instances is uncomplicated. Sometimes blood count depression is moderate or incomplete, resulting in anemia, leukopenia, and thrombocytopenia in some combination. Aplastic anemia is related to both paroxysmal nocturnal hemoglobinuria (PNH; Chap. 101) and to MDS, and in some cases a clear distinction among these disorders may not be possible.

EPIDEMIOLOGY

The incidence of acquired aplastic anemia in Europe and Israel is two cases per million persons annually. In Thailand and China, rates of five to seven per million have been established. In general, men and women are affected with equal frequency, but the age distribution is biphasic, with the major peak in the teens and twenties and a second rise in the elderly.

ETIOLOGY

The origins of aplastic anemia have been inferred from several recurring clinical associations (Table 102-2); unfortunately, these relationships are not reliable in an individual patient and may not be etiologic. In addition, while most cases of aplastic anemia are idiopathic, little other than history separates these cases from those with a presumed etiology such as a drug exposure.

Radiation Marrow aplasia is a major acute sequela of radiation. Radiation damages DNA; tissues dependent on active mitosis are partic-

TABLE 102-2 CLASSIFICATION OF APLASTIC ANEMIA AND SINGLE CYTOPENIAS

Acquired	Inherited
Aplastic Anemia	
Secondary	Fanconi's anemia
Radiation	Dyskeratosis congenita
Drugs and chemicals	Shwachman-Diamond syndrome
Regular effects	Reticular dysgenesis
Idiosyncratic reactions	Amegakaryocytic thrombocytopenia
Viruses	Familial aplastic anemias
Epstein-Barr virus (infectious mononucleosis)	Preleukemia (monosomy 7, etc.)
Hepatitis (non-A, non-B, non-C hepatitis)	Nonhematologic syndrome (Down's, Dubowitz, Seckel)
Parvovirus B19 (transient aplastic crisis, PRCA)	
HIV-1 (AIDS)	
Immune diseases	
Eosinophilic fasciitis	
Hypoimmunoglobulinemia	
Thymoma/thymic carcinoma	
Graft-versus-host disease in immunodeficiency	
Paroxysmal nocturnal hemoglobinuria	
Pregnancy	
Idiopathic	
Cytopenias	
PRCA (see Table 102-4)	Congenital PRCA (Diamond-Blackfan anemia)
Neutropenia/Agranulocytosis	
Idiopathic	Kostmann's Syndrome
Drugs, toxins	Shwachman-Diamond syndrome
Pure white cell aplasia	Reticular dysgenesis
Thrombocytopenia	
Drugs, toxins	Amegakaryocytic thrombocytopenia
Idiopathic amegakaryocytic	Thrombocytopenia with absent radii

Note: PRCA, pure red cell aplasia.

ularly susceptible. Nuclear accidents can involve not only power plant workers but also employees of hospitals, laboratories, and industry (food sterilization, metal radiography, etc.), as well as innocents exposed to stolen, misplaced, or misused sources. While the radiation dose can be approximated from the rate and degree of decline in blood counts, dosimetry by reconstruction of the exposure can help to estimate the patient's prognosis and also to protect medical personnel from contact with radioactive tissue and excreta. MDS and leukemia, but probably not aplastic anemia, are late effects of radiation.

Chemicals Benzene is a notorious cause of bone marrow failure. Vast quantities of epidemiologic, clinical, and laboratory data link benzene to aplastic anemia, acute leukemia, and blood and marrow abnormalities. The occurrence of leukemia is roughly correlated with cumulative exposure, but susceptibility must also be important, as only a minority of even heavily exposed workers develop benzene myelotoxicity. The employment history is important, especially in industries where benzene is used for a secondary purpose, usually as a solvent. Benzene-related blood diseases have declined with regulation of industrial exposure. Although benzene is no longer generally available as a household solvent, exposure to its metabolites occurs in the normal diet and in the environment. The association between marrow failure and other chemicals is much less well substantiated.

Drugs (Table 102-3) Many chemotherapeutic drugs have marrow suppression as a major toxicity; effects are dose-dependent and will occur in all recipients. In contrast, idiosyncratic reactions to a large and diverse group of drugs may lead to aplastic anemia without a clear dose-response relationship. These associations rested largely on accumulated case reports until a large international study in Europe in the 1980s quantitated drug relationships, especially for nonsteroidal analgesics, sulfonamides, thyrostatic drugs, some psychotropics, penicil-

TABLE 102-3	SOME DRUGS AND CHEMICALS ASSOCIATED WITH APLASTIC ANEMIA

Agents that regularly produce marrow depression as major toxicity in commonly employed doses or normal exposures:
  Cytotoxic drugs used in cancer chemotherapy: *alkylating agents, antimetabolites, antimitotics,* some antibiotics

Agents that frequently but not inevitably produce marrow aplasia:
  Benzene

Agents associated with aplastic anemia but with a relatively low probability:
  Chloramphenicol
  Insecticides
  Antiprotozoals: *quinacrine* and chloroquine, mepacrine
  Nonsteroidal anti-inflammatory drugs (including *phenylbutazone,* indomethacin, ibuprofen, sulindac, aspirin)
  Anticonvulsants (*hydantoins, carbamazepine,* phenacemide, felbamate)
  Heavy metals (*gold,* arsenic, bismuth, mercury)
  Sulfonamides: some antibiotics, antithyroid drugs (methimazole, methylthiouracil, propylthiouracil), antidiabetes drugs (tolbutamide, chlorpropamide), carbonic anhydrase inhibitors (acetazolamide and methazolamide)
  Antihistamines (*cimetidine,* chlorpheniramine)
  D-Penicillamine
  Estrogens (in pregnancy and in high doses in animals)

Agents whose association with aplastic anemia is more tenuous:
  Other antibiotics (streptomycin, tetracycline, methicillin, mebendazole, trimethoprim/sulfamethoxazole, flucytosine)
  Sedatives and tranquilizers (chlorpromazine, prochlorperazine, piperacetazine, chlordiazepoxide, meprobamate, methyprylon)
  Allopurinol
  Methyldopa
  Quinidine
  Lithium
  Guanidine
  Potassium perchlorate
  Thiocyanate
  Carbimazole

Note: Terms set in italic show the most consistent association with aplastic anemia.

lamine, allopurinol, and gold. Not all associations necessarily reflect causation: a drug may have been used to treat the first symptoms of bone marrow failure (antibiotics for fever or the preceding viral illness) or provoked the first symptom of a preexisting disease (petechiae by nonsteroidal anti-inflammatory agents administered to the thrombocytopenic patient). In the context of total drug use, idiosyncratic reactions, while individually devastating, are rare events. Chloramphenicol, the most infamous culprit, reportedly produced aplasia in only about 1/60,000 therapy courses, and even this number is almost certainly an overestimate (risks are almost invariably exaggerated when based on collections of cases; although the introduction of chloramphenicol was perceived to have created an epidemic of aplastic anemia, its diminished use was not followed by a changed frequency of marrow failure). Risk estimates are usually lower when determined in population-based studies; furthermore, the low absolute risk is also made more obvious: even a ten- or twentyfold increase in risk translates, in a rare disease, to but a handful of drug-induced aplastic anemia cases among hundreds of thousands of exposed persons.

Infections Hepatitis is the most common preceding infection, and posthepatitis marrow failure accounts for about 5% of etiologies in most series. Patients are usually young men who have recovered from a bout of liver inflammation 1 to 2 months earlier; the subsequent pancytopenia is very severe. The hepatitis is seronegative (non-A, non-B, non-C, non-G) and possibly due to a novel, as yet undiscovered, virus. Fulminant liver failure in childhood also follows seronegative hepatitis, and marrow failure occurs at a high rate in these patients. Aplastic anemia can rarely follow infectious mononucleosis, and Epstein-Barr virus has been found in the marrow of a few patients, some without a suggestive preceding history. Parvovirus B19, the cause of transient aplastic crisis in hemolytic anemias and of some PRCAs (see below), does not usually cause generalized bone marrow failure. Mild blood count depression is frequent in the course of many viral and bacterial infections but resolves with the infection.

Immunologic Diseases Aplasia is a major consequence and the inevitable cause of death in *transfusion-associated graft-versus-host disease* (GVDH), which can occur after infusion of unirradiated blood products to an immunodeficient recipient. Aplastic anemia is strongly associated with the rare collagen vascular syndrome called *eosinophilic fasciitis,* which is characterized by painful induration of subcutaneous tissues (Chap. 316). Pancytopenia with marrow hypoplasia can also occur in systemic lupus erythematosus.

Pregnancy Aplastic anemia very rarely may occur and recur during pregnancy and resolve with delivery or with spontaneous or induced abortion.

Paroxysmal Nocturnal Hemoglobinuria An acquired mutation in the *PIG-A* gene in a hematopoietic stem cell is required for the development of PNH, but *PIG-A* mutations probably occur commonly in normal individuals. If the PIG-A mutant stem cell proliferates, the result is a clone of progeny deficient in glycosylphosphatidylinositol-linked cell surface membrane proteins (Chap. 101). Such PNH cells are now accurately enumerated using fluorescence-activated flow cytometry of CD55 or CD59 expression on granulocytes rather than Ham or sucrose lysis tests on red cells. Small clones of deficient cells can be detected in about half of patients with aplastic anemia at the time of presentation [and PNH cells are also seen in MDS (see below)]; frank hemolysis and thrombotic episodes occur in patients with large PNH clones (>50%). Functional studies of bone marrow from PNH patients, even those with mainly hemolytic manifestations, show evidence of defective hematopoiesis. Patients with an initial clinical diagnosis of PNH, especially younger individuals, may later develop frank marrow aplasia and pancytopenia; patients with an initial diagnosis of aplastic anemia may suffer from hemolytic PNH years after recovery of blood counts. One popular but unproven explanation for the aplastic anemia/PNH syndrome is selection of the deficient clones because they are favored for proliferation in the peculiar environment of immune-mediated marrow destruction.

Constitutional Disorders Fanconi's anemia, an autosomal recessive disorder, manifests as congenital developmental anomalies, progressive pancytopenia, and an increased risk of malignancy. Chromosomes in Fanconi's anemia are peculiarly susceptible to DNA cross-linking agents, the basis for a diagnostic assay. Patients with Fanconi's anemia typically have short stature, café au lait spots, and anomalies involving the thumb, radius, and genitourinary tract. At least 12 different genetic defects (all but one with an identified gene) have been defined; the most common, type A Fanconi's anemia, is due to a mutation in *FANCA*. Most of the Fanconi's anemia gene products form a protein complex that activates FANCD2 by monoubiquitination to play a role in the cellular response to DNA damage and especially interstrand cross-linking, a response that includes BRCA1, ATM, and NBS1.

Dyskeratosis congenita is characterized by mucous membrane leukoplasia, dystrophic nails, reticular hyperpigmentation, and the development of aplastic anemia during childhood. The X-linked variety is due to mutations in the *DKC1* (*dyskerin*) gene; the more unusual autosomal dominant type is due to mutation in *hTERC*, which encodes an RNA template, and *hTERT*, which encodes the catalytic reverse transcriptase, telomerase; these gene products cooperate in a repair complex to maintain telomere length. In Shwachman-Diamond syndrome, marrow failure is seen with pancreatic insufficiency and malabsorption; most patients have compound heterozygous mutations in *SBDS*, which has been implicated in RNA processing.

PATHOPHYSIOLOGY

Bone marrow failure results from severe damage to the hematopoietic cell compartment. In aplastic anemia, replacement of the bone marrow by fat is apparent in the morphology of the biopsy specimen (Fig. 102-1) and MRI of the spine. Cells bearing the CD34 antigen, a marker of early hematopoietic cells, are greatly diminished, and in functional studies, committed and primitive progenitor cells are virtually absent; in vitro assays have suggested that the stem cell pool is reduced to ≤1% of normal in severe disease at the time of presentation.

An intrinsic stem cell defect exists for the constitutional aplastic anemias: cells from patients with Fanconi's anemia exhibit chromosome damage and death on exposure to certain chemical agents. Telomeres are short in a large proportion of patients with aplastic anemia, and mutations in genes of the telomere repair complex (*TERC* and *TERT*) can be identified in some adults with apparently acquired marrow failure and without physical anomalies or typical family history.

Aplastic anemia does not appear to result from defective stroma or growth factor production.

Drug Injury Extrinsic damage to the marrow follows massive physical or chemical insults such as high doses of radiation and toxic chemicals. For the more common idiosyncratic reaction to modest doses of medical drugs, altered drug metabolism has been invoked as a likely mechanism. The metabolic pathways of many drugs and chemicals, especially if they are polar and have limited water solubility, involve enzymatic degradation to highly reactive electrophilic compounds;

FIGURE 102-1 **A.** Normal bone marrow biopsy. **B.** Normal bone marrow aspirate smear. The marrow is normally 30–70% cellular, and there is a heterogeneous mix of myeloid, erythroid, and lymphoid cells. **C.** Aplastic anemia biopsy. **D.** Marrow smear in aplastic anemia. The marrow shows replacement of hematopoietic tissue by fat and only residual stromal and lymphoid cells.

these intermediates are toxic because of their propensity to bind to cellular macromolecules. For example, derivative hydroquinones and quinolones are responsible for benzene-induced tissue injury. Excessive generation of toxic intermediates or failure to detoxify the intermediates may be genetically determined and apparent only on specific drug challenge; the complexity and specificity of the pathways imply multiple susceptibility loci and would provide an explanation for the rarity of idiosyncratic drug reactions.

Immune-Mediated Injury The recovery of marrow function in some patients prepared for bone marrow transplantation with antilymphocyte globulin (ALG) first suggested that aplastic anemia might be immune-mediated. Consistent with this hypothesis was the frequent failure of simple bone marrow transplantation from a syngeneic twin, without conditioning cytotoxic chemotherapy, which also argued both *against* simple stem cell absence as the cause and *for* the presence of a host factor producing marrow failure. Laboratory data support an important role for the immune system in aplastic anemia. Blood and bone marrow cells of patients can suppress normal hematopoietic progenitor cell growth, and removal of T cells from aplastic anemia bone marrow improves colony formation in vitro. Increased numbers of activated cytotoxic T cells are observed in aplastic anemia patients and usually decline with successful immunosuppressive therapy; cytokine measurements show a T_H1 immune response (interferon γ and tumor necrosis factor). Interferon and tumor necrosis factor induce Fas expression on CD34 cells, leading to apoptotic cell death; localization of activated T cells to bone marrow and local production of their soluble factors are probably important in stem cell destruction.

Early immune system events in aplastic anemia are not well understood. Analysis of T cell receptor expression suggests an oligoclonal, antigen-driven cytotoxic T cell response. Many different exogenous antigens appear capable of initiating a pathologic immune response, but at least some of the T cells may recognize true self-antigens. The rarity of aplastic anemia despite common exposures (medicines, hepatitis virus) suggests that genetically determined features of the immune response can convert a normal physiologic response into a sustained abnormal autoimmune process, including polymorphisms in histocompatibility antigens, cytokine genes, and genes that regulate T cell polarization and effector function.

CLINICAL FEATURES

History Aplastic anemia can appear with seeming abruptness or have a more insidious onset. Bleeding is the most common early symptom; a complaint of days to weeks of easy bruising, oozing from the gums, nose bleeds, heavy menstrual flow, and sometimes petechiae will have been noticed. With thrombocytopenia, massive hemorrhage is unusual, but small amounts of bleeding in the central nervous system can result in catastrophic intracranial or retinal hemorrhage. Symptoms of anemia are also frequent, including lassitude, weakness, shortness of breath, and a pounding sensation in the ears. Infection is an unusual first symptom in aplastic anemia (unlike in agranulocytosis, where pharyngitis, anorectal infection, or frank sepsis occur early). A striking feature of aplastic anemia is the restriction of symptoms to the hematologic system, and patients often feel and look remarkably well despite drastically reduced blood counts. Systemic complaints and weight loss should point to other etiologies of pancytopenia. Prior drug use, chemical exposure, and preceding viral illnesses must often be elicited with repeated questioning. A family history of hematologic diseases or blood abnormalities may indicate a constitutional etiology of marrow failure.

Physical Examination Petechiae and ecchymoses are typical, and retinal hemorrhages may be present. Pelvic and rectal examinations can often be deferred but, when performed, should be undertaken with great gentleness to avoid trauma; these will often show bleeding from the cervical os and blood in the stool. Pallor of the skin and mucous membranes is common except in the most acute cases or those already transfused. Infection on presentation is unusual but may occur if the patient has been symptomatic for a few weeks. Lymphadenopathy and splenomegaly are highly atypical of aplastic anemia. Café au lait spots and short stature suggest Fanconi's anemia; peculiar nails and leukoplakia suggest dyskeratosis congenita.

LABORATORY STUDIES

Blood The smear shows large erythrocytes and a paucity of platelets and granulocytes. Mean corpuscular volume (MCV) is commonly increased. Reticulocytes are absent or few, and lymphocyte numbers may be normal or reduced. The presence of immature myeloid forms suggests leukemia or MDS; nucleated red blood cells suggest marrow fibrosis or tumor invasion; abnormal platelets suggest either peripheral destruction or MDS.

Bone Marrow The bone marrow is usually readily aspirated but dilute on smear, and the fatty biopsy specimen may be grossly pale on withdrawal; a "dry tap" instead suggests fibrosis or myelophthisis. In severe aplasia the smear of the aspirated specimen shows only red cells, residual lymphocytes, and stromal cells; the biopsy (which should be >1 cm in length) is superior for determination of cellularity and shows mainly fat under the microscope, with hematopoietic cells occupying <25% of the marrow space; in the most serious cases the biopsy is virtually 100% fat. The correlation between marrow cellularity and disease severity is imperfect, in part because marrow cellularity declines physiologically with aging. Additionally, some patients with moderate disease by blood counts will have empty iliac crest biopsies, while "hot spots" of hematopoiesis may be seen in severe cases. If an iliac crest specimen is inadequate, cells may also be obtained by aspiration from the sternum. Residual hematopoietic cells should have normal morphology, except for mildly megaloblastic erythropoiesis; megakaryocytes are invariably greatly reduced and usually absent. Areas adjacent to the spicule should be searched for myeloblasts. Granulomas (in cellular specimens) may indicate an infectious etiology of the marrow failure.

Ancillary Studies Chromosome breakage studies of peripheral blood using diepoxybutane or mitomycin C should be performed on children and younger adults to exclude Fanconi's anemia. Genetic analysis

applicable to the constitutional marrow failure states is available in some laboratories. Chromosome studies of bone marrow cells are often revealing in MDS and should be negative in typical aplastic anemia. Flow cytometric assays have replaced the Ham test for the diagnosis of PNH. Serologic studies may show evidence of viral infection, such as Epstein-Barr virus and HIV. Posthepatitis aplastic anemia is typically seronegative. The spleen size should be determined by CT scanning or ultrasound if the physical examination of the abdomen is unsatisfactory. MRI may be helpful to assess the fat content of a few vertebrae in order to distinguish aplasia from MDS.

DIAGNOSIS

The diagnosis of aplastic anemia is usually straightforward, based on the combination of pancytopenia with a fatty, empty bone marrow. Aplastic anemia is a disease of the young and should be a leading diagnosis in the pancytopenic adolescent or young adult. When pancytopenia is secondary, the primary diagnosis is usually obvious from either history or physical examination: the massive spleen of alcoholic cirrhosis, the history of metastatic cancer or systemic lupus erythematosus, or miliary tuberculosis on chest radiograph (Table 102-1).

Diagnostic problems can occur with atypical presentations and among related hematologic diseases. While pancytopenia is most common, some patients with bone marrow hypocellularity have depression of only one or two of three blood lines, sometimes showing later progression to more recognizable aplastic anemia. The bone marrow in constitutional aplastic anemia is indistinguishable morphologically from the aspirate in acquired disease. The diagnosis can be suggested by family history, abnormal blood counts since childhood, or the presence of associated physical anomalies. Aplastic anemia may be difficult to distinguish from the hypocellular variety of MDS: MDS is favored by finding morphologic abnormalities, particularly of megakaryocytes and myeloid precursor cells, and typical cytogenetic abnormalities (see below).

PROGNOSIS

The natural history of severe aplastic anemia is rapid deterioration and death. Provision first of red blood cell and later of platelet transfusions and effective antibiotics are of some benefit, but few patients show spontaneous recovery. The major prognostic determinant is the blood count; severe disease is defined by the presence of two of three parameters: absolute neutrophil count <500/μL, platelet count <20,000/μL, and corrected reticulocyte count <1% (or absolute reticulocyte count <60,000/μL). Survival of patients who fulfill these criteria is about 20% at 1 year after diagnosis with only supportive care; patients with very severe disease, defined by an absolute neutrophil count <200/μL, fare even more poorly. Treatment has markedly improved survival in this disease.

℞ APLASTIC ANEMIA

Severe acquired aplastic anemia can be cured by replacement of the absent hematopoietic cells (and the immune system) by stem cell transplant, or it can be ameliorated by suppression of the immune system to allow recovery of the patient's residual bone marrow function. Hematopoietic growth factors have limited usefulness and glucocorticoids are of no value. Suspect exposures to drugs or chemicals should be discontinued; however, spontaneous recovery of severe blood count depression is rare, and a waiting period before beginning treatment may not be advisable unless the blood counts are only modestly depressed.

HEMATOPOIETIC STEM CELL TRANSPLANTATION This is the best therapy for the young patient with a fully histocompatible sibling donor (Chap. 108). Human leukocyte antigen (HLA) typing should be ordered as soon as the diagnosis of aplastic anemia is established in a child or younger adult. In transplant candidates, transfusion of blood from family members should be avoided so as to prevent sensitization to histocompatibility antigens; while transfusions in general should be minimized, limited numbers of blood products probably do not seriously affect outcome.

For allogeneic transplant from fully matched siblings, long-term survival rates for children are 80–90%. Transplant morbidity and mortality are increased among adults, due mainly to the higher risk of chronic GVHD and serious infections. Graft rejection was historically a major determinant of outcome in transplant for aplastic anemia, perhaps related to the underlying pathophysiology as well as to alloimmunization from transfusions (the latter now much improved by leukocyte depletion before blood product administration).

Most patients do not have a suitable sibling donor. Occasionally, a full phenotypic match can be found within the family and serve as well. Far more available are other alternative donors, either unrelated but histocompatible volunteers or closely but not perfectly matched family members. Survival using alternative donors is about half that of conventional sibling transplants but improving with higher-resolution HLA matching and more effective conditioning regimens and GVHD prophylaxis. Patients will be at risk for late complications, especially a higher rate of cancer, if radiation is used as a component of conditioning.

IMMUNOSUPPRESSION Used alone, ALG or antithymocyte globulin (ATG) induces hematologic recovery (independence from transfusion and a leukocyte count adequate to prevent infection) in about 50% of patients. The addition of cyclosporine to either ALG or ATG has further increased response rates to about 70% and especially improved outcomes for children and for severely neutropenic patients. Such combined treatment is now standard for patients with severe disease. An early robust hematologic response strongly correlates with long-term survival. Improvement in granulocyte number is generally apparent within 2 months of treatment. Most recovered patients continue to have some degree of blood count depression, the MCV remains elevated, and the bone marrow cellularity returns toward normal only very slowly, if at all. Relapse (recurrent pancytopenia) is frequent, often occurring as cyclosporine is discontinued; most, but not all, patients respond to reinstitution of immunosuppression, but some responders become dependent on continued cyclosporine administration. Development of MDS, with typical marrow morphologic or cytogenetic abnormalities, occurs in about 15% of treated patients, usually but not invariably associated with a return of pancytopenia, and some patients develop leukemia. A laboratory diagnosis of PNH can generally be made at the time of presentation of aplastic anemia by flow cytometry; recovered patients may have frank hemolysis if the PNH clone expands. Bone marrow examinations should be performed if there is an unfavorable change in blood counts.

Horse ATG is given at 40 mg/kg per day for 4 days; rabbit ALG is administered at 3.5 mg/kg per day for 5 days. For ATG, anaphylaxis is a rare but occasionally fatal complication; allergy can be tested by a skin-prick test with an undiluted solution and immediate observation; desensitization is feasible. ATG binds to peripheral blood cells; therefore, platelet and granulocyte numbers may fall further during active treatment. Serum sickness, a flu-like illness with a characteristic cutaneous eruption and arthralgia, often develops about 10 days after initiating treatment. Methylprednisolone, 1 mg/kg per day for 2 weeks, can ameliorate the immune consequences of heterologous protein infusion. Excessive or extended glucocorticoid therapy is associated with avascular joint necrosis. Cyclosporine is administered orally at an initial dose of 12 mg/kg per day in adults (15 mg/kg per day in children), with subsequent adjustment according to blood levels obtained every 2 weeks. Trough levels should be between 150 and 200 ng/mL. The most important side effects of chronic cyclosporine treatment are nephrotoxicity, hypertension, seizures, and opportunistic infections, especially *Pneumocystis carinii* (prophylactic treatment with monthly inhaled pentamidine is recommended).

Most patients with aplastic anemia lack a suitable marrow donor, and immunosuppression is the treatment of choice. Overall survival is equivalent with transplantation and immunosuppression. However, successful transplant cures marrow failure, while patients who recover adequate blood counts after immunosuppression remain at risk of relapse and malignant evolution. Because of excellent results in children and younger adults, allogeneic transplant should be performed if a suitable sibling donor is available. Increasing age and the severity of neutropenia are the most important factors weighing in the decision between transplant and immunosuppression in adults who have a matched family donor: older patients do better with ATG and cyclosporine, whereas transplant is preferred if granulocytopenia is profound. Some patients may prefer immunosuppression; transplant is used for failure to recover blood counts or occurrence of late complications.

Outcomes following both transplant and immunosuppression have improved with time. High doses of cyclophosphamide, without stem cell rescue, have been reported to produce durable hematologic recovery, without relapse or evolution to MDS, but this treatment can produce sustained severe fatal neutropenia and response is often delayed. New immunosuppressive drugs in clinical trial may further improve outcome.

OTHER THERAPIES The effectiveness of androgens has not been verified in controlled trials, but occasional patients will respond or even demonstrate blood count dependence on continued therapy. For patients with moderate disease or those with severe pancytopenia in whom immunosuppression has failed, a 3–4-month trial is appropriate. Hematopoietic growth factors, granulocyte colony-stimulating factor (G-CSF), granulocyte-macrophage CSF (GM-CSF), and interleukin 3 (IL-3) are not recommended as initial therapy for severe aplastic anemia, and even their role as adjuncts to immunosuppression is not well defined. Some patients may respond to combinations of growth factors after immunosuppression has failed.

SUPPORTIVE CARE Meticulous medical attention is required so that the patient may survive to benefit from definitive therapy or, having failed treatment, to maintain a reasonable existence in the face of pancytopenia. First and most important, infection in the presence of severe neutropenia must be aggressively treated by prompt institution of parenteral, broad-spectrum antibiotics, usually ceftazidime or a combination of an aminoglycoside, cephalosporin, and semisynthetic penicillin. Therapy is empirical and must not await results of culture, although specific foci of infection such as oropharyngeal or anorectal abscesses, pneumonia, sinusitis, and typhlitis (necrotizing colitis) should be sought on physical examination and with radiographic studies. When indwelling plastic catheters become contaminated, vancomycin should be added. Persistent or recrudescent fever implies fungal disease: *Candida* and *Aspergillus* are common, especially after several courses of antibacterial antibiotics, and a progressive course may be averted by timely initiation of antifungal therapy. Granulocyte transfusions using G-CSF–mobilized peripheral blood have appeared to be effective in the treatment of overwhelming or refractory infections in a few patients. Hand washing, the single best method of preventing the spread of infection, remains a neglected practice. Nonabsorbed antibiotics for gut decontamination are poorly tolerated and not of proven value. Total reverse isolation does not reduce mortality from infections.

Both platelet and erythrocyte numbers can be maintained by transfusion. Alloimmunization historically limited the usefulness of platelet transfusions and is now minimized by several strategies, including use of single donors to reduce exposure and physical or chemical methods to diminish leukocytes in the product; HLA-matched platelets are often effective in patients refractory to random donor products. Inhibitors of fibrinolysis such as aminocaproic acid have not been shown to relieve mucosal oozing; the use of low-dose glucocorticoids to induce "vascular stability" is unproven and not recommended. Whether platelet transfusions are better used prophylactically or only as needed remains unclear. Any rational regimen of prophylaxis requires transfusions once or twice weekly in order to maintain the platelet count >10,000/μL (oozing from the gut, and presumably also from other vascular beds, increases precipitously at counts <5000/μL). Menstruation should be suppressed either by oral estrogens or nasal follicle-stimulating hormone/luteinizing hormone (FSH/LH) antagonists. Aspirin and other nonsteroidal anti-inflammatory agents inhibit platelet function and must be avoided.

Red blood cells should be transfused to maintain a normal level of activity, usually at a hemoglobin value of 70 g/L (90 g/L if there is underlying cardiac or pulmonary disease); a regimen of 2 units every 2 weeks will replace normal losses in a patient without a functioning bone marrow. In chronic anemia, the iron chelators deferoxamine and deferasirox should be added at around the fiftieth transfusion in order to avoid secondary hemochromatosis.

PURE RED CELL APLASIA

Other, more restricted forms of marrow failure occur, in which only a single circulating cell type is affected and the aregenerative marrow shows corresponding absence or decreased numbers of specific precursor cells: aregenerative anemia as in PRCA (see below), thrombocytopenia with amegakaryocytosis (Chap. 109), and neutropenia without marrow myeloid cells in agranulocytosis (Chap. 61). In general, and in contrast to aplastic anemia and MDS, the unaffected lineages appear quantitatively and qualitatively normal. Agranulocytosis, the most frequent of these syndromes, is usually a complication of medical drug use (with agents similar to those related to aplastic anemia), either by a mechanism of direct chemical toxicity or by immune destruction. Agranulocytosis has an incidence similar to aplastic anemia but is especially frequent among the elderly and in women. The syndrome should resolve with discontinuation of exposure, but significant mortality is attached to neutropenia in the older and often previously unwell patient. Both pure white cell aplasia (agranulocytosis without incriminating drug exposure) and amegakaryocytic thrombocytopenia are exceedingly rare and, like PRCA, appear to be due to destructive antibodies or lymphocytes and can respond to immunosuppressive therapies. In all the single lineage failure syndromes, progression to pancytopenia or leukemia is unusual.

DEFINITION AND DIFFERENTIAL DIAGNOSIS

PRCA is characterized by anemia, reticulocytopenia, and absent or rare erythroid precursor cells in the bone marrow. The classification of PRCA is shown in Table 102-4. In adults, PRCA is acquired. An identical syndrome can occur constitutionally: Diamond-Blackfan anemia, or congenital PRCA, is diagnosed at birth or in early childhood and often responds to glucocorticoid treatment; a minority of patients have etiologic mutations in a ribosomal RNA processing gene called *RPS19*. Temporary red cell failure occurs in transient aplastic crisis of hemolytic anemias due to acute parvovirus infection (Chap. 177) and in transient erythroblastopenia of childhood, which affects normal children.

CLINICAL ASSOCIATIONS AND ETIOLOGY

PRCA has important associations with immune system diseases. A small minority of cases occur with a thymoma. More frequently, red cell aplasia can be the major manifestation of large granular lymphocytosis or may occur in chronic lymphocytic leukemia. Some patients may be hypogammaglobulinemic. As with agranulocytosis, PRCA can be due to an idiosyncratic reaction to a drug. Subcutaneous administration of erythropoietin can lead to PRCA mediated by neutralizing antibodies.

Like aplastic anemia, PRCA results from diverse mechanisms. Antibodies to red blood cell precursors are frequently present in the blood, but T cell inhibition is probably the more common immune mechanism. Cytotoxic lymphocyte activity restricted by histocompatibility locus or specific for human T cell leukemia/lymphoma virus I–infected cells, as well as natural killer cell activity inhibitory of erythropoiesis, have been demonstrated in particularly well-studied individual cases.

TABLE 102-4	CLASSIFICATION OF PURE RED CELL APLASIA

Self-limited
  Transient erythroblastopenia of childhood
  Transient aplastic crisis of hemolysis (acute B19 parvovirus infection)
Fetal red blood cell aplasia
  Nonimmune hydrops fetalis (in utero B19 parvovirus infection)
Hereditary pure red cell aplasia
  Congenital pure red cell aplasia (Diamond-Blackfan syndrome)
Acquired pure red cell aplasia
  Thymoma and malignancy
    Thymoma
    Lymphoid malignancies (and more rarely other hematologic diseases)
    Paraneoplastic to solid tumors
  Connective tissue disorders with immunologic abnormalities
    Systemic lupus erythematosus, juvenile rheumatoid arthritis, rheumatoid arthritis
    Multiple endocrine gland insufficiency
  Virus
    Persistent B19 parvovirus, hepatitis, adult T cell leukemia virus, Epstein-Barr virus
  Pregnancy
  Drugs
    Especially phenytoin, azathioprine, chloramphenicol, procainamide, isoniazid
    Erythropoietin
Idiopathic

Persistent Parvovirus B19 Infection Chronic parvovirus infection is an important, treatable cause of PRCA. This common virus causes a benign exanthem of childhood (fifth disease) and a polyarthralgia/arthritis syndrome in adults. In patients with underlying hemolysis (or any condition that increases demand for red blood cell production), parvovirus infection can cause a transient aplastic crisis and an abrupt but temporary worsening of the anemia due to failed erythropoiesis. In normal individuals, acute infection is resolved by production of neutralizing antibodies to the virus, but in the setting of congenital, acquired, or iatrogenic immunodeficiency, persistent viral infection may occur. The bone marrow shows red cell aplasia and the presence of giant pronormoblasts (Fig. 102-2), which is the cytopathic sign of B19 parvovirus infection. Viral tropism for human erythroid progenitor cells is due to its use of erythrocyte P antigen as a cellular receptor for entry. Direct cytotoxicity of virus causes anemia if demands on erythrocyte production are high; in normal individuals, the temporary cessation of red cell production is not clinically apparent, and skin and joint symptoms are mediated by immune complex deposition.

Rx PURE RED CELL APLASIA

History, physical examination, and routine laboratory studies may disclose an underlying disease or a suspect drug exposure. Thymoma should be sought by radiographic procedures. Tumor excision is indicated, but anemia does not necessarily improve with surgery. The diagnosis of parvovirus infection requires detection of viral DNA sequences in the blood (IgG and IgM antibodies are commonly absent). The presence of erythroid colonies has been considered predictive of response to immunosuppressive therapy in idiopathic PRCA.

Red cell aplasia is compatible with long survival with supportive care alone: a combination of erythrocyte transfusions and iron chelation. For persistent B19 parvovirus infection, almost all patients respond to intravenous immunoglobulin therapy (for example, 0.4 g/kg daily for 5 days), although relapse and retreatment may be expected, especially in patients with AIDS. The majority of patients with idiopathic PRCA respond favorably to immunosuppression. Most first receive a course of glucocorticoids. Also effective are cyclosporine, ATG, azathioprine, cyclophosphamide, and the monoclonal antibody daclizumab, an antibody to the IL-2 receptor. PRCA developing on erythropoietin therapy should be treated with immunosuppression and withdrawal of erythropoietin.

MYELODYSPLASIA

DEFINITION

The myelodysplasias (MDSs) are a heterogeneous group of hematologic disorders broadly characterized by cytopenias associated with a dysmorphic (or abnormal appearing) and usually cellular bone marrow, and by consequent ineffective blood cell production. A clinically useful nosology of these entities was first developed by the French-American-British Cooperative Group in 1983. Five entities were defined: refractory anemia (RA), refractory anemia with ringed sideroblasts (RARS), refractory anemia with excess blasts (RAEB), refractory anemia with excess blasts in transformation (RAEB-t), and chronic myelomonocytic leukemia (CMML). The World Health Organization classification (2002) recognizes that the distinction between RAEB-t and acute myeloid leukemia is arbitrary and groups them together as acute leukemia, notes that CMML behaves as a myeloproliferative disease, and separates refractory anemias with dysmorphic change restricted to erythroid lineage from those with multilineage changes (Table 102-5).

EPIDEMIOLOGY

Idiopathic MDS is a disease of the elderly; the mean age at onset is 68 years. There is a slight male preponderance. MDS is a relatively common form of bone marrow failure, with reported incidence rates of 35 to >100 per million persons in the general population and 120 to >500 per million in the elderly. MDS is rare in children, but monocytic leukemia can be seen. Therapy-related MDS is not age-related and may

A

B

C

D

FIGURE 102-2 Pathognomonic cells in marrow failure syndromes. A. Giant pronormoblast, the cytopathic effect of B19 parvovirus infection of the erythroid progenitor cell. **B.** Uninuclear megakaryocyte and microblastic erythroid precursors typical of the 5q– myelodysplasia syndrome. **C.** Ringed sideroblast showing perinuclear iron granules. **D.** Tumor cells present on a touch preparation made from the marrow biopsy of a patient with metastatic carcinoma.

but likely occur late in the sequence leading to leukemic transformation. Apoptosis of marrow cells is increased in MDS, presumably due to these acquired genetic alterations or possibly to an overlaid immune response. An immune pathophysiology has been suggested for trisomy 8 MDS, which often responds clinically to immunosuppressive therapy. Such patients have T cell activity directed to the cytogenetically aberrant clone. Sideroblastic anemia may be related to mutations in mitochondrial genes; ineffective erythropoiesis and disordered iron metabolism are the functional consequences of the genetic alterations.

CLINICAL FEATURES

Anemia dominates the early course. Most symptomatic patients complain of the gradual onset of fatigue and weakness, dyspnea, and pallor, but at least half the patients are asymptomatic and their MDS is discovered only incidentally on routine blood counts. Previous chemotherapy or radiation exposure is an important historic fact. Fever and weight loss should point to a myeloproliferative rather than myelodysplastic process. Children with Down syndrome are susceptible to MDS, and a family history may indicate a hereditary form of sideroblastic anemia or Fanconi's anemia.

The physical examination is remarkable for signs of anemia; about 20% of patients have splenomegaly. Some unusual skin lesions, including Sweet's syndrome (febrile neutrophilic dermatosis), occur with MDS. Autoimmune syndromes are not infrequent.

occur in as many as 15% of patients within a decade following intensive combined modality treatment for cancer. Rates of MDS have increased over time, due to the recognition of the syndrome by physicians and the aging of the population.

ETIOLOGY AND PATHOPHYSIOLOGY

MDS is caused by environmental exposures such as radiation and benzene; other risk factors have been reported inconsistently. Secondary MDS occurs as a late toxicity of cancer treatment, usually with a combination of radiation and the radiomimetic alkylating agents such as busulfan, nitrosourea, or procarbazine (with a latent period of 5–7 years) or the DNA topoisomerase inhibitors (2 years). Both acquired aplastic anemia following immunosuppressive treatment and Fanconi's anemia can evolve into MDS.

MDS is a clonal hematopoietic stem cell disorder leading to impaired cell proliferation and differentiation. Cytogenetic abnormalities are found in about half of patients, and some of the same specific lesions are also seen in frank leukemia; aneuploidy is more frequent than translocations. Both presenting and evolving hematologic manifestations result from the accumulation of multiple genetic lesions: loss of tumor suppressor genes, activating oncogene mutations, or other harmful alterations. Cytogenetic abnormalities are not random (loss of all or part of 5, 7, and 20, trisomy of 8) and may be related to etiology (11q23 following topoisomerase II inhibitors); chronic myelomonocytic leukemia is often associated with t(5;12) that creates a chimeric *tel-PDGFβ* gene. The type and number of cytogenetic abnormalities strongly correlate with the probability of leukemic transformation and survival. Mutations of N-*ras* (an oncogene), *p53* and *IRF-1* (tumor suppressor genes), *Bcl-2* (an antiapoptotic gene), and others have been reported in some patients

LABORATORY STUDIES

Blood Anemia is present in the majority of cases, either alone or as part of bi- or pancytopenia; isolated neutropenia or thrombocytopenia is more unusual. Macrocytosis is common, and the smear may be dimorphic with a distinctive population of large red blood cells. Platelets are also large and lack granules. In functional studies, they may show marked abnormalities, and patients may have bleeding symptoms despite seemingly adequate numbers. Neutrophils are hypogranulated; have hyposegmented, ringed, or abnormally segmented nuclei; contain Dohle bodies; and may be functionally deficient. Circulating myeloblasts usually correlate with marrow blast numbers, and their quantitation is important for classification and prognosis. The total white blood cell count is usually normal or low, except in chronic myelomonocytic leukemia. As in aplastic anemia, MDS can be associated with a clonal population of PNH cells.

Bone Marrow The bone marrow is usually normal or hypercellular, but in 20% of cases it is sufficiently hypocellular to be confused with aplasia. No single characteristic feature of marrow morphology distinguishes MDS, but the following are commonly observed: dyserythropoietic changes (especially nuclear abnormalities) and ringed sideroblasts in the erythroid lineage; hypogranulation and hyposegmentation in granulocytic precursors, with an increase in myeloblasts; and megakaryocytes showing reduced numbers or disorganized nuclei. Megaloblastic nuclei associated with defective hemoglobinization

TABLE 102-5 WORLD HEALTH ORGANIZATION CLASSIFICATION OF MYELODYSPLASTIC SYNDROMES

Disease	Frequency	Blood Findings	Bone Marrow Findings	Prognosis
Refractory anemia (RA)	5–10%	Anemia No or rare blasts	Erythroid dysplasia only <5% blasts <15% ringed sideroblasts	Protracted course Leukemic transformation in ~6%
Refractory anemia with ringed sideroblasts (RARS)	10–12%	Anemia No blasts	Erythroid dysplasia only ≥15% ringed sideroblasts <5% blasts	Protracted course Leukemia in ~1–2%
Refractory cytopenia with multilineage dysplasia (RCMD)	24%	Cytopenias (2 or 3 lineages) No or rare blasts No Auer rods <1 × 10^9/L monocytes	Dysplasia in ≥10% of cells in ≥2 lineages <5% blasts No Auer rods <15% ringed sideroblasts	Variable clinical course Leukemia in ~11%
RCMD with ringed sidero-blasts (RCMD-RS)	15%	Cytopenias (2 or 3 lineages) No or rare blasts No Auer rods <1 × 10^9/L monocytes	Dysplasia in ≥10% of cells in ≥2 lineages ≥15% ringed sideroblasts <5% blasts No Auer rods	
Refractory anemia with excess blasts-1 (RAEB-1)	40% (RAEB-1 +2)	Cytopenias <5% blasts No Auer rods <1 × 10^9/L monocytes	Unilineage or multilineage dysplasia 5–9% blasts No Auer rods	Progressive BM failure Leukemia in ~25%
Refractory anemia with excess blasts-2 (RAEB-2)		Cytopenias 5–19% blasts ±Auer rods <1 × 10^9/L monocytes	Unilineage or multilineage dysplasia 10–19% blasts ±Auer rods	Progressive BM failure Leukemia in ~33%
Myelodysplastic syndrome, unclassified (MDS-U)	Unknown	Cytopenias No or rare blasts No Auer rods	Dysplasia in myeloid or platelet lineage <5% blasts No Auer rods	Unknown
MDS with isolated del(5q)	Unknown	Anemia <5% blasts Platelets nl or increased	Nl or increased megakaryocytes with hypolobated nuclei <5% blasts No Auer rods Isolated del(5q)	Long survival

Note: BM, bone marrow.
Source: Extracted from Jaffe ES et al (eds): *Pathology and Genetics of Tumors of Haematopoietic and Lymphoid Tissues*. Lyon, IARC Press, 2001.

in the erythroid lineage are common. Prognosis strongly correlates with the proportion of marrow blasts. Cytogenetic analysis and fluorescent in situ hybridization can identify chromosomal abnormalities.

DIFFERENTIAL DIAGNOSIS
Deficiencies of vitamin B$_{12}$ or folate should be excluded by appropriate blood tests; vitamin B$_6$ deficiency can be assessed by a therapeutic trial of pyridoxine if the bone marrow shows ringed sideroblasts. Marrow dysplasia can be observed in acute viral infections, drug reactions, or chemical toxicity but should be transient. More difficult are the distinctions between hypocellular MDS and aplasia or between refractory anemia with excess blasts and early acute leukemia. The World Health Organization considers the presence of 20% blasts in the marrow as the criterion that separates acute myeloid leukemia from MDS.

PROGNOSIS
The median survival varies greatly from years for patients with 5q– or sideroblastic anemia to a few months in refractory anemia with excess blasts or severe pancytopenia associated with monosomy 7; an International Prognostic Scoring System (Table 102-6) assists in making predictions. Most patients die as a result of complications of pancytopenia and not due to leukemic transformation; perhaps one-third will succumb to other diseases unrelated to their MDS. Precipitous worsening of pancytopenia, acquisition of new chromosomal abnormalities on serial cytogenetic determination, and increase in the number of blasts are all poor prognostic indicators. The outlook in therapy-related MDS, regardless of type, is very poor, and most patients will progress within a few months to refractory acute myeloid leukemia.

℞ MYELODYSPLASIA

The therapy of MDS has been unsatisfactory. Only stem cell transplantation offers cure: survival rates of 50% at 3 years have been reported, but older patients are particularly prone to develop treatment-related mortality and morbidity. Results of transplant using matched unrelated donors are comparable, although most series contain younger and more highly selected cases.

MDS has been regarded as particularly refractory to cytotoxic chemotherapy regimens but is probably no more resistant to effective treatment than acute myeloid leukemia in the elderly, in whom drug toxicity is often fatal and remissions, if achieved, are brief.

TABLE 102-6 INTERNATIONAL PROGNOSTIC SCORING SYSTEM

Prognostic Variable	Score Value				
	0	0.5	1.0	1.5	2.0
Bone marrow blasts (%)	<5%	5–10%		11–20%	21–30%
Karyotype[a]	Good	Intermediate	Poor		
Cytopenia[b] (lineages affected)	0 or 1	2 or 3			

Risk Group Scores	Score
Low	0
Intermediate-1	0.5–1.0
Intermediate-2	1.5–2.0
High	≥2.5

[a]Good, normal, -Y, del(5q), del (20q); poor, complex (≥3 abnormalities) or chromosome 7 abnormalities; intermediate, all other abnormalities.
[b]Cytopenias defined as Hb <100 g/L, platelet count < 100,000/μL, absolute neutrophil count <1500/μL.

Low doses of cytotoxic drugs have been administered for their "differentiating" potential, and from this experience has emerged drug therapies based on pyrimidine analogues. Azacitidine is directly cytotoxic but also inhibits DNA methylation, thereby altering gene expression. Azacitidine improves blood counts and modestly improves survival in about 16% of MDS patients, compared to best supportive care. Azacitidine is administered subcutaneously at a dose of 75 mg/m^2, daily for 7 days, at 4-week intervals, for at least four cycles, although further cycles may be required to observe a response. Decitabine is closely related to azacitidine and more potent. Similar to azacitidine, about 20% of patients show responses in blood counts, with a duration of response of almost a year. Activity may be higher in more advanced MDS subtypes. Decitabine dose is 15 mg/m^2 by continuous intravenous infusion, every eight hours for three days, repeating the cycle every 6 weeks for at least four cycles. The major toxicity of both azacitidine and decitabine is myelosuppression, leading to worsened blood counts. Other symptoms associated with cancer chemotherapy frequently occur. Ironically, it has been difficult to establish that either agent acts in patients by a mechanism of DNA demethylation.

Thalidomide, a drug with many activities including antiangiogenesis and immunomodulation, has modest biologic activity in MDS. Lenalidomide, a thalidomide derivative with a more favorable toxicity profile, is particularly effective in reversing anemia in MDS patients with 5q– syndrome; not only do a high proportion of these patients become transfusion-independent with normal or near-normal hemoglobin levels, but their cytogenetics also become normal. Lenalidomide is administered orally, 10 mg daily. Most patients will improve within 3 months of initiating therapy. Toxicities include myelosuppression (worsening thrombocytopenia and neutropenia, necessitating blood count monitoring) and an increased risk of deep vein thrombosis and pulmonary embolism.

Other treatments for MDS include amifostine, an organic thiophosphonate that blocks apoptosis; it can improve blood counts but has significant toxicities. ATG and cyclosporine, as employed in aplastic anemia, also may produce sustained independence from transfusion, especially in younger MDS patients with more favorable International Prognostic Scoring System (IPSS) scores.

Hematopoietic growth factors can improve blood counts but, as in most other marrow failure states, have been most beneficial to patients with the least severe pancytopenia. G-CSF treatment alone failed to improve survival in a controlled trial. Erythropoietin alone or in combination with G-CSF can improve hemoglobin levels, but mainly in those with low serum erythropoietin levels who have no or only a modest need for transfusions.

The same principles of supportive care described for aplastic anemia apply to MDS. Despite improvements in drug therapy, many patients will be anemic for years. RBC transfusion support should be accompanied by iron chelation in order to prevent secondary hemochromatosis.

MYELOPHTHISIC ANEMIAS

Fibrosis of the bone marrow (see Fig. 103-2), usually accompanied by a characteristic blood smear picture called *leukoerythroblastosis*, can occur as a primary hematologic disease, called *myelofibrosis* or *myeloid metaplasia* (Chap. 103), and as a secondary process, called *myelophthisis*. Myelophthisis, or secondary myelofibrosis, is reactive. Fibrosis can be a response to invading tumor cells, usually an epithelial cancer of

breast, lung, a prostate origin or neuroblastoma. Marrow fibrosis may occur with infection of mycobacteria (both *Mycobacterium tuberculosis* and *M. avium*), fungi, or HIV, and in sarcoidosis. Intracellular lipid deposition in Gaucher disease and obliteration of the marrow space related to absence of osteoclast remodeling in congenital osteopetrosis also can produce fibrosis. Secondary myelofibrosis is a late consequence of radiation therapy or treatment with radiomimetic drugs. Usually the infectious or malignant underlying processes are obvious. Marrow fibrosis can also be a feature of a variety of hematologic syndromes, especially chronic myeloid leukemia, multiple myeloma, lymphomas, myeloma, and hairy cell leukemia.

The pathophysiology has three distinct features: proliferation of fibroblasts in the marrow space (myelofibrosis); the extension of hematopoiesis into the long bones and into extramedullary sites, usually the spleen, liver, and lymph nodes (myeloid metaplasia); and ineffective erythropoiesis. The etiology of the fibrosis is unknown but most likely involves dysregulated production of growth factors: platelet-derived growth factor and transforming growth factor β have been implicated. Abnormal regulation of other hematopoietins would lead to localization of blood-producing cells in nonhematopoietic tissues and uncoupling of the usually balanced processes of stem cell proliferation and differentiation. Myelofibrosis is remarkable for pancytopenia despite very large numbers of circulating hematopoietic progenitor cells.

Anemia is dominant in secondary myelofibrosis, usually normocytic and normochromic. The diagnosis is suggested by the characteristic leukoerythroblastic smear (see Fig. 103-1). Erythrocyte morphology is highly abnormal, with circulating nucleated red blood cells, teardrops, and shape distortions. White blood cell numbers are often elevated, sometimes mimicking a leukemoid reaction, with circulating myelocytes, promyelocytes, and myeloblasts. Platelets may be abundant and are often of giant size. Inability to aspirate the bone marrow, the characteristic "dry tap," can allow a presumptive diagnosis in the appropriate setting before the biopsy is decalcified.

The course of secondary myelofibrosis is determined by its etiology, usually a metastatic tumor or an advanced hematologic malignancy. Treatable causes must be excluded, especially tuberculosis and fungus. Transfusion support can relieve symptoms.

FURTHER READINGS

BAGBY GC, ALTER BP: Fanconi anemia. Semin Hematol 43:147, 2006

ESTEY E et al: Acute myeloid leukemia and myelodysplastic syndromes in older patients. J Clin Oncol 25:1908, 2007

FISCH P et al: Pure red cell aplasia. Br J Haematol 111:1010, 2000

LIPTON JM: Diamond Blackfan anemia: New paradigms for a "not so pure" inherited red cell aplasia. Semin Hematol 43:167, 2006

LIST A et al: Efficacy of lenalidomide in myelodysplastic syndromes. N Engl J Med 352:549, 2005

YOUNG NS, BROWN KE: Parvovirus B19. N Engl J Med 350:586, 2004
——— et al: Current concepts in the pathophysiology and treatment of aplastic anemia. Blood 108:2509, 2006

103 Polycythemia Vera and Other Myeloproliferative Diseases

Jerry L. Spivak

The World Health Organization (WHO) classification of the chronic myeloproliferative diseases includes seven disorders, some of which are rare or poorly characterized (Table 103-1) but all of which share an origin in a multipotent hematopoietic progenitor cell, overproduction of one or more of the formed elements of the blood without significant

dysplasia, a predilection to extramedullary hematopoiesis, myelofibrosis, and transformation at varying rates to acute leukemia. Within this broad classification, however, significant phenotypic heterogeneity exists. Some diseases, such as chronic myelogenous leukemia (CML), chronic neutrophilic leukemia (CNL) and chronic eosinophilic leukemia (CEL) express primarily a myeloid phenotype, while in others, such as polycythemia vera (PV), idiopathic myelofibrosis (IMF), and essential thrombocytosis (ET), erythroid or megakaryocytic hyperplasia predominates. The latter three disorders, in contrast to the former three, also appear capable of transforming into each other.

This phenotypic heterogeneity has a genetic basis; CML is the consequence of the balanced translocation between chromosomes 9 and

TABLE 103-1 WHO CLASSIFICATION OF CHRONIC MYELOPROLIFERATIVE DISORDERS

Chronic myelogenous leukemia, [Ph chromosome t(9;22)(q34;11), BCR/ABL-positive]
Chronic neutrophilic leukemia
Chronic eosinophilic leukemia (and the hypereosinophilic syndrome)
Polycythemia vera
Chronic idiopathic myelofibrosis (with extramedullary hematopoiesis)
Essential thrombocythemia
Chronic myeloproliferative disease, unclassifiable

22 [t(9;22)(q34;11)]; CNL has been associated with a t(15:19) translocation, and CEL with a deletion or balanced translocations involving the PDGFRα gene. By contrast, to a greater or lesser extent, PV, IMF, and ET are characterized by expression of a JAK2 mutation, V617F, which causes constitutive activation of this tyrosine kinase that is essential for the function of the erythropoietin and thrombopoietin receptors but not the granulocyte colony–stimulating factor receptor. This essential distinction is also reflected in the natural history of CML, CNL, and CEL, which is usually measured in years, and their high rate of transformation into acute leukemia. By contrast, the natural history of PV, IMF, and ET is usually measured in decades, and transformation to acute leukemia is uncommon in the absence of exposure to mutagenic agents. This chapter, therefore, will focus only on PV, IMF, and ET, because their clinical overlap is substantial and their clinical courses are distinctly different. Other chronic myeloproliferative disorders will be discussed in Chapter 104.

POLYCYTHEMIA VERA

Polycythemia vera (PV) is a clonal disorder involving a multipotent hematopoietic progenitor cell in which phenotypically normal red cells, granulocytes, and platelets accumulate in the absence of a recognizable physiologic stimulus. The most common of the chronic myeloproliferative disorders, PV occurs in 2 per 100,000 persons, sparing no adult age group and increasing with age to rates as high as 18/100,000. Familial transmission occurs but is infrequent. A slight overall male predominance has been observed, but women predominate within the reproductive age range.

ETIOLOGY

The etiology of PV is unknown. Although nonrandom chromosome abnormalities such as 20q, trisomy 8, and especially 9p, have been documented in up to 30% of untreated PV patients, unlike CML no consistent cytogenetic abnormality has been associated with the disorder. However, a mutation in the autoinhibitory, pseudokinase domain of the tyrosine kinase JAK2—which replaces valine with phenylalanine (V617F), causing constitutive activation of the kinase—appears to have a central role in the pathogenesis of PV.

JAK2 is a member of an evolutionarily well-conserved, nonreceptor tyrosine kinase family and serves as the cognate tyrosine kinase for the erythropoietin and thrombopoietin receptors. It also functions as an obligate chaperone for these receptors in the Golgi apparatus and is responsible for their cell-surface expression. The conformational change induced in the erythropoietin and thrombopoietin receptors following binding to erythropoietin or thrombopoietin leads to JAK2 autophosphorylation, receptor phosphorylation, and phosphorylation of proteins involved in cell proliferation, differentiation, and resistance to apoptosis. Transgenic animals lacking JAK2 die as embryos from severe anemia. Constitutive activation of JAK2 can explain the erythropoietin-independent erythroid colony formation, and the hypersensitivity of PV erythroid progenitor cells to erythropoietin and other hematopoietic growth factors, their resistance to apoptosis in vitro in the absence of erythropoietin, their rapid terminal differentiation, and their increase in Bcl-X$_L$ expression, all of which are characteristic in PV.

Importantly, the JAK2 gene is located on the short arm of chromosome 9, and loss of heterozygosity on chromosome 9p, due to uniparental disomy is the most common cytogenetic abnormality in PV. The segment of 9p involved contains the JAK2 locus; loss of heterozygosity in this region leads to homozygosity for the mutant JAK2 V617F. Over 90% of PV patients express this mutation, as do approximately 45% of IMF and ET patients. Homozygosity for the mutation occurs in approximately 30% of PV patients and 60% of IMF patients; homozygosity is rare in ET. Over time, a portion of PV JAK2 V617F heterozygotes become homozygotes, but usually not after 10 years of the disease. PV patients who do not express JAK2 V617F are not clinically different than those who do, nor do JAK2 V617F heterozygotes differ clinically from homozygotes. In general, patients who express JAK2 V617F are older than those who do not, but they do not have a longer duration of disease.

JAK2 V617F is the basis for many of the phenotypic and biochemical characteristics of PV, such as elevation of the leukocyte alkaline phosphatase (LAP) score and increased expression of the mRNA of PVR-1, a glycosylphosphatidylinositol (GPI)-linked membrane protein; however, it cannot solely account for the entire PV phenotype. First, PV patients with the same phenotype and documented clonal disease lack this mutation. Second, IMF patients have the same mutation but a different clinical phenotype. Third, familial PV can occur without the mutation, even when other members of the same family express it. Fourth, not all the cells of the malignant clone express JAK2 V617F. Fifth, JAK2 V617F has been observed in patients with long-standing idiopathic erythrocytosis. However, while JAK2 V617F alone may not be sufficient to cause PV, it is essential for the transformation of ET to PV, though not for its transformation to IMF.

CLINICAL FEATURES

Although splenomegaly may be the initial presenting sign in PV, most often the disorder is first recognized by the incidental discovery of a high hemoglobin or hematocrit. With the exception of aquagenic pruritus, no symptoms distinguish PV from other causes of erythrocytosis.

Uncontrolled erythrocytosis causes hyperviscosity, leading to neurologic symptoms such as vertigo, tinnitus, headache, visual disturbances, and transient ischemic attacks (TIAs). Systolic hypertension is also a feature of the red cell mass elevation. In some patients, venous or arterial thrombosis may be the presenting manifestation of PV. Any vessel can be affected, but cerebral, cardiac, or mesenteric vessels are most commonly involved. Intraabdominal venous thrombosis is particularly common in young women and may be catastrophic if a sudden and complete obstruction of the hepatic vein occurs. Indeed, PV should be suspected in any patient who develops hepatic vein thrombosis. Digital ischemia, easy bruising, epistaxis, acid-peptic disease, or gastrointestinal hemorrhage may occur due to vascular stasis or thrombocytosis. Erythema, burning, and pain in the extremities, a symptom complex known as erythromelalgia, is another complication of the thrombocytosis of PV. Given the large turnover of hematopoietic cells, hyperuricemia with secondary gout, uric acid stones, and symptoms due to hypermetabolism can also complicate the disorder.

The plasma erythropoietin level is a useful diagnostic test in patients with isolated erythrocytosis, because an elevated level excludes PV as the cause for the erythrocytosis.

DIAGNOSIS

When PV presents with erythrocytosis in combination with leukocytosis, thrombocytosis, or both, the diagnosis is apparent. However, when patients present with an elevated hemoglobin or hematocrit alone, or with thrombocytosis alone, the diagnostic evaluation is more complex because of the many diagnostic possibilities (Table 103-2). Furthermore, unless the hemoglobin level is ≥20 gm% (hematocrit ≥60%), it is not possible to distinguish PV from disorders causing plasma volume contraction. Uniquely in PV, an expanded plasma volume can mask an elevated red cell mass; thus, red cell mass and plasma volume determinations are mandatory to establish the presence of an absolute erythrocytosis and to distinguish this from relative erythrocytosis due to a reduction in plasma volume alone (also known as *stress* or *spurious erythrocytosis* or *Gaisböck's syndrome*). This is true even in with the discovery of the JAK2 V617F mutation, because not very patient with PV expresses this mutation, while

TABLE 103-2 CAUSES OF ERYTHROCYTOSIS

Relative erythrocytosis: Hemoconcentration secondary to dehydration, androgens, or tobacco abuse

Absolute erythrocytosis

Hypoxia
  Carbon monoxide intoxication
  High affinity hemoglobin
  High altitude
  Pulmonary disease
  Right-to-left shunts
  Sleep-apnea syndrome
  Neurologic disease

Renal disease
  Renal artery stenosis
    Focal sclerosing or membranous glomerulonephritis
    Renal transplantation

Tumors
  Hypernephroma
  Hepatoma
  Cerebellar hemangioblastoma
  Uterine fibromyoma
  Adrenal tumors
  Meningioma
  Pheochromocytoma

Drugs
  Androgens
  Recombinant erythropoietin

Familial (with normal hemoglobin function, Chuvash, erythropoietin receptor mutations)

Polycythemia vera

patients without PV do. Figure 58-18 illustrates a diagnostic algorithm for the evaluation of suspected erythrocytosis.

Once absolute erythrocytosis has been established, its cause must be determined. An elevated plasma erythropoietin level suggests either a hypoxic cause for erythrocytosis or autonomous erythropoietin production, in which case assessment of pulmonary function and an abdominal CT scan to evaluate renal and hepatic anatomy are appropriate. A normal erythropoietin level does not exclude a hypoxic cause for erythrocytosis. In PV, in contrast to hypoxic erythrocytosis, the arterial oxygen saturation is normal. However, a normal oxygen saturation does not exclude a high-affinity hemoglobin as a cause for erythrocytosis; documentation of previous hemoglobin levels and a family study are important.

Other laboratory studies that may aid in diagnosis include the red cell count, mean corpuscular volume, and red cell distribution width (RDW). Only three situations cause microcytic erythrocytosis: β-thalassemia trait, hypoxic erythrocytosis, and PV. With β-thalassemia trait the RDW is normal, whereas with hypoxic erythrocytosis and PV, the RDW is usually elevated due to iron deficiency. In many patients, the LAP level is also increased, as is the uric acid level. Elevated serum vitamin B$_{12}$ or B$_{12}$-binding capacity may be present. In patients with associated acid-peptic disease, occult gastrointestinal bleeding may lead to presentation with hypochromic, microcytic anemia.

A bone marrow aspirate and biopsy provide no specific diagnostic information since these may be normal or indistinguishable from ET or IMF, and unless there is a need to establish the presence of myelofibrosis or exclude some other disorder, these procedures need not be done. Although the presence of a cytogenetic abnormality such as trisomy 8 or 9 or 20q− in the setting of an expanded red cell mass supports a clonal etiology, no specific cytogenetic abnormality is associated with PV, and the absence of a cytogenetic marker does not exclude the diagnosis.

COMPLICATIONS

The major clinical complications of PV relate directly to the increase in blood viscosity associated with red cell mass elevation and indirectly to the increased turnover of red cells, leukocytes, and platelets with the attendant increase in uric acid and cytokine production. The latter appears to be responsible for the increase in peptic ulcer disease and for the pruritus associated with this disorder, although formal proof

for this has not been obtained. A sudden massive increase in spleen size can be associated with splenic infarction or progressive cachexia. Myelofibrosis appears to be part of the natural history of the disease but is a reactive, reversible process that does not itself impede hematopoiesis and by itself has no prognostic significance. In some patients, however, the myelofibrosis is accompanied by significant extramedullary hematopoiesis, hepatosplenomegaly, and transfusion-dependent anemia. The organomegaly can cause significant mechanical discomfort, portal hypertension, and cachexia. Although the incidence of acute nonlymphocytic leukemia is increased in PV, the incidence of acute leukemia in patients not exposed to chemotherapy or radiation is low, and the development of leukemia is related to older age but not disease duration, suggesting that the treatment exposure may be a more important risk factor than the disease itself.

Erythromelalgia is a curious syndrome of unknown etiology associated with thrombocytosis, primarily involving the lower extremities and manifested usually by erythema, warmth, and pain of the affected appendage and occasionally digital infarction. It occurs with a variable frequency in myeloproliferative disorder patients and is usually responsive to salicylates. Some of the central nervous system symptoms observed in patients with PV, such as ocular migraine, may represent a variant of erythromelalgia.

If left uncontrolled, erythrocytosis can lead to thrombosis involving vital organs such as the liver, heart, brain, or lungs. Patients with massive splenomegaly are particularly prone to thrombotic events because the associated increase in plasma volume masks the true extent of the red cell mass elevation as measured by the hematocrit or hemoglobin level. A "normal" hematocrit or hemoglobin level in a PV patient with massive splenomegaly should be considered indicative of an elevated red cell mass until proven otherwise.

℞ POLYCYTHEMIA VERA

PV is generally an indolent disorder whose clinical course is measured in decades, and its medical management should reflect its tempo. Thrombosis due to erythrocytosis is the most significant complication, and maintenance of the hemoglobin level at ≤140 g/L (14 g/dL; hematocrit <45%) in men and ≤120 g/L (12 g/dL; hematocrit <42%) in women is mandatory to avoid thrombotic complications. Phlebotomy serves initially to reduce hyperviscosity by bringing the red cell mass into the normal range. Periodic phlebotomies thereafter serve to maintain the red cell mass within the normal range and to induce a state of iron deficiency, which prevents an accelerated reexpansion of the red cell mass. In most PV patients, once an iron-deficient state is achieved, phlebotomy is usually only required at 3-month intervals. Neither phlebotomy nor iron deficiency increases the platelet count relative to the effect of the disease itself, and thrombocytosis is not correlated with thrombosis in PV, in contrast to the strong correlation between erythrocytosis and thrombosis in this disease. The use of salicylates as a tonic against thrombosis in PV patients is potentially harmful if the red cell mass is not controlled by phlebotomy. Anticoagulants are only indicated when a thrombosis has occurred and can be difficult to monitor owing to the artifactual imbalance between the test tube anticoagulant and plasma that occurs when blood from these patients is assayed for prothrombin or partial thromboplastin activity. Asymptomatic hyperuricemia (<10 mg%) requires no therapy, but allopurinol should be administered to avoid further elevation of the uric acid when chemotherapy is employed to reduce splenomegaly or leukocytosis or to treat pruritus. Generalized pruritus intractable to antihistamines or antidepressants such as doxepin can be a major problem in PV; hydroxyurea, interferon α (IFN-α), and psoralens with ultraviolet light in the A range (PUVA) therapy are other methods of palliation. Asymptomatic thrombocytosis requires no therapy unless the platelet count is sufficiently high to cause an acquired form of von Willebrand's disease due to proteolysis of high-molecular-weight vWF multimers. Symptomatic splenomegaly can be treated with IFN-α. Although the drug can be associated with significant side effects when used chronically, IFN-α reduces JAK2 V617F expression in PV patients, and its role in this disorder may be expanding. Anagrelide, a phosphodiesterase inhibitor, can reduce the platelet count and, if tolerated, is preferable to hydroxyurea because it lacks marrow toxicity. A reduction in platelet number may be necessary in the treatment of erythromelalgia or ocular migraine if salicylates are not effective or the platelet count is sufficiently high to cause an hemorrhagic diathesis. Alkylating agents and radioactive sodium phosphate (^{32}P) are leukemogenic in PV, and their use should be avoided. If a cytotoxic agent must be used, hydroxyurea is preferred, but this drug does not prevent either thrombosis or myelofibrosis in this disorder. Chemotherapy should be used for as short a time as possible. In some patients, massive splenomegaly unresponsive to reduction by hydroxyurea or IFN-α therapy and associated with intractable weight loss will require splenectomy. In some patients with end-stage disease, pulmonary hypertension may develop due to fibrosis and extramedullary hematopoiesis. Allogeneic bone marrow transplantation may be curative in young patients.

Most patients with PV can live long lives without functional impairment when their red cell mass is effectively managed with phlebotomy. Chemotherapy is never indicated to control the red cell mass unless venous access is inadequate.

CHRONIC IDIOPATHIC MYELOFIBROSIS

Chronic IMF (other designations include *agnogenic myeloid metaplasia* or *myelofibrosis with myeloid metaplasia*) is a clonal disorder of a multipotent hematopoietic progenitor cell of unknown etiology characterized by marrow fibrosis, extramedullary hematopoiesis, and splenomegaly. Chronic IMF is the least common chronic myeloproliferative disorder, and establishing this diagnosis in the absence of a specific clonal marker is difficult because myelofibrosis and splenomegaly are also features of both PV and CML. Furthermore, myelofibrosis and splenomegaly also occur in a variety of benign and malignant disorders (Table 103-3), many of which are amenable to specific therapies not effective in chronic IMF. In contrast to the other chronic myeloproliferative disorders and so-called acute or malignant myelofibrosis, which can occur at any age, chronic IMF primarily afflicts individuals in their sixth decade or later.

ETIOLOGY

The etiology of chronic IMF is unknown. Nonrandom chromosome abnormalities such as 9p, 20q–, 13q–, trisomy 8 or 9, or partial trisomy 1q are common, but no cytogenetic abnormality specific to the disease has been identified. The degree of myelofibrosis and the extent of extramedullary hematopoiesis are also not related. Fibrosis in this disorder is associated with overproduction of transforming growth factor β and tissue inhibitors of metalloproteinases, while osteosclerosis is associated with overproduction of osteoprotegerin, an osteoclast inhibitor. Marrow angiogenesis occurs due to increased production of vascular endothelial growth factor (VEGF). Importantly, fibroblasts in chronic IMF are polyclonal and not part of the neoplastic clone.

CLINICAL FEATURES

No signs or symptoms are specific for chronic IMF. Many patients are asymptomatic at presentation, and the disease is usually detected by the discovery of splenic enlargement and/or abnormal blood counts during a routine examination. However, in contrast to its companion myeloproliferative disorders, night sweats, fatigue, and weight loss may be presenting complaints. A blood smear shows the characteristic features of extramedullary hematopoiesis: teardrop-

FIGURE 103-1 Teardrop-shaped red blood cells indicative of membrane damage from passage through the spleen, a nucleated red blood cell, and immature myeloid cells indicative of extramedullary hematopoiesis are noted. This peripheral blood smear is related to any cause of extramedullary hematopoiesis.

shaped red cells, nucleated red cells, myelocytes, and promyelocytes; myeloblasts may also be present (Fig. 103-1). Anemia, usually mild initially, is the rule, while the leukocyte and platelet counts are either normal or increased, but either can be depressed. Mild hepatomegaly may accompany the splenomegaly but is unusual in the absence of splenic enlargement; isolated lymphadenopathy should suggest another diagnosis. Both serum lactate dehydrogenase and alkaline phosphatase levels can be elevated. The LAP score can be low, normal, or high. Marrow is usually inaspirable due to the myelofibrosis (Fig. 103-2), and bone x-rays may reveal osteosclerosis. Exuberant extramedullary hematopoiesis can cause ascites, portal, pulmonary or intracranial hypertension, intestinal or ureteral obstruction, pericardial tamponade, spinal cord compression, or skin nodules. Splenic enlargement can be sufficiently rapid to cause splenic infarction with fever and pleuritic chest pain. Hyperuricemia and secondary gout may ensue.

DIAGNOSIS

While the clinical picture described above is characteristic of chronic IMF, all of the clinical features described can also be observed in PV or CML. Massive splenomegaly commonly masks erythrocytosis in PV, and reports of intraabdominal thromboses in chronic IMF most likely represent instances of unrecognized PV. In some patients with chronic IMF, erythrocytosis has developed during the course of the disease. Furthermore, since many other disorders have features that overlap with chronic IMF but respond to distinctly different therapies, the diagnosis of chronic IMF is one of exclusion, which requires that the disorders listed in Table 103-3 be ruled out. A diagnostic algorithm has been proposed but does not distinguish one disease causing myeloid metaplasia from another.

The presence of teardrop-shaped red cells, nucleated red cells, myelocytes, and promyelocytes establishes the presence of extramedullary hematopoiesis, while the presence of leukocytosis, thrombocytosis with large and bizarre platelets, and circulating myelocytes suggests the presence of a myeloproliferative disorder as opposed to a secondary form of myelofibrosis (Table 103-3). Marrow is usually not aspirable due to increased marrow reticulin, but marrow biopsy will reveal a hypercellular marrow with trilineage hyperplasia and, in particular, increased numbers of megakaryocytes in clusters and with large, dysplastic nuclei. However, there are no characteristic morphologic abnormalities that distinguish IMF from the other chronic myeloproliferative disorders. Splenomegaly due to extramedullary hematopoiesis may be sufficiently massive to cause portal hypertension and variceal formation. In some patients, exuberant extramedullary hematopoiesis can dominate the

TABLE 103-3 DISORDERS CAUSING MYELOFIBROSIS

Malignant	Nonmalignant
Acute leukemia (lymphocytic, myelogenous, megakaryocytic)	HIV infection
Chronic myelogenous leukemia	Hyperparathyroidism
Hairy cell leukemia	Renal osteodystrophy
Hodgkin disease	Systemic lupus erythematosus
Idiopathic myelofibrosis	Tuberculosis
Lymphoma	Vitamin D deficiency
Multiple myeloma	Thorium dioxide exposure
Myelodysplasia	Gray platelet syndrome
Metastatic carcinoma	
Polycythemia vera	
Systemic mastocytosis	

FIGURE 103-2 This marrow section shows the marrow cavity replaced by fibrous tissue composed of reticulin fibers and collagen. When this fibrosis is due to a primary hematologic process, it is called *myelofibrosis*. When the fibrosis is secondary to a tumor or a granulomatous process, it is called *myelophthisis*.

clinical picture. An intriguing feature of chronic IMF is the occurrence of autoimmune abnormalities such as immune complexes, antinuclear antibodies, rheumatoid factor, or a positive Coombs' test. Whether these represent a host reaction to the disorder or are involved in its pathogenesis is unknown. Cytogenetic analysis of blood is useful both to exclude CML and for prognostic purposes, because complex karyotype abnormalities portend a poor prognosis in chronic IMF. For unknown reasons, the number of circulating CD34+ cells is markedly increased in chronic IMF (>15,000/μL) compared to the other chronic myeloproliferative disorders, unless they too develop myeloid metaplasia.

Importantly, approximately 45% of chronic IMF patients, like patients with its companion myeloproliferative disorders PV and ET, express the JAK2 V617F mutation, often as homozygotes. Such patients had a poorer survival in one retrospective study but not in another, where they were found to be older and to have higher hematocrits than those patients who were JAK2 V617F-negative.

COMPLICATIONS

Survival in chronic IMF varies according to specific clinical features (Table 103-4) but is shorter than in patients with PV or ET. The natural history of chronic IMF is one of increasing marrow failure with transfusion-dependent anemia and increasing organomegaly due to extramedullary hematopoiesis. As with CML, chronic IMF can evolve from a chronic phase to an accelerated phase with constitutional symptoms and increasing marrow failure. About 10% of patients develop an aggressive form of acute leukemia for which therapy is usually ineffective. Important prognostic factors for disease acceleration include anemia, leukocytosis, thrombocytopenia, the presence of circulating myeloblasts, older age, the presence of complex cytogenetic abnormalities, and constitutional symptoms such as unexplained fever, night sweats, or weight loss.

TABLE 103-4 RISK STRATIFICATION FOR IDIOPATHIC MYELOFIBROSIS

A. Prognostic factors[a]
Hemoglobin <10 gm%
White cell count < 4000/μL or > 30,000/μL

Number of prognostic factors	Risk group	Median survival (months)
0	Low	93
1–2	High	17

B. Prognostic factors[b]
Hemoglobin < 10 gm%
Constitutional symptoms
Blast cells > 1%

Number of prognostic factors	Risk group	Median survival (months)
0–1	Low	99
2–3	High	21

C. Prognostic factors[c]	Median survival (months)
Age <65 years Hemoglobin ≤10 gm%	
Karyotype: Normal	54
Abnormal	22
Age <65 years Hemoglobin >10 gm%	
Karyotype: Normal	180
Abnormal	72
Age >65 years Hemoglobin ≤10 gm%	
Karyotype: Normal	44
Abnormal	16
Age >65 years Hemoglobin >10 gm%	
Karyotype: Normal	70
Abnormal	78

[a]From B Dupriez et al. Blood 88:1013, 1996.
[b]From F Cervantes et al. Br J Haematol 102:684, 1998.
[c]From JT Reilly et al. Br J Haematol 98:96, 1997.

℞ CHRONIC IDIOPATHIC MYELOFIBROSIS

No specific therapy exists for chronic IMF. Anemia may be due to gastrointestinal blood loss and exacerbated by folic acid deficiency, and in rare instances, pyridoxine therapy has been effective. However, anemia is more often due to ineffective erythropoiesis uncompensated by extramedullary hematopoiesis in the spleen and liver. Neither recombinant erythropoietin nor androgens, such as Danazol, have proved consistently effective as therapy for anemia. Erythropoietin may worsen splenomegaly and will be ineffective if the serum erythropoietin level is >125 mU/L. A red cell splenic sequestration study can establish the presence of hypersplenism, for which splenectomy is indicated. Splenectomy may also be necessary if splenomegaly impairs alimentation and should be performed before cachexia sets in. In this situation, splenectomy should not be avoided because of concern over rebound thrombocytosis, loss of hematopoietic capacity, or compensatory hepatomegaly. However, for unexplained reasons, splenectomy increases the risk of blastic transformation. Splenic irradiation is, at best, temporarily palliative and associated with a significant risk of neutropenia and infection. Allopurinol can control significant hyperuricemia, and hydroxyurea has proved useful for controlling organomegaly in some patients. The role of IFN-α is still undefined and its side effects are more pronounced in the older individuals who are usually afflicted with this disorder. Glucocorticoids have been used to control constitutional symptoms and autoimmune complications and may ameliorate anemia alone or in combination with low dose thalidomide (50–100 mg/d). Allogeneic bone marrow transplantation is the only curative treatment and should be considered in younger patients; reduced-intensity conditioning regimens may permit hematopoietic cell transplantation to be extended to older individuals.

ESSENTIAL THROMBOCYTOSIS

Essential thrombocytosis (other designations include *essential thrombocythemia, idiopathic thrombocytosis, primary thrombocytosis, hemorrhagic thrombocythemia*) is a clonal disorder of unknown etiology involving a multipotent hematopoietic progenitor cell manifested clinically by overproduction of platelets without a definable cause. ET is an uncommon disorder, with an incidence of 1–2/100,000 and a distinct female predominance, in contrast to the other chronic myeloproliferative disorders. No clonal marker is available to consistently distinguish ET from the more common nonclonal, reactive forms of thrombocytosis (Table 103-5), making its diagnosis difficult. Once considered a disease of the elderly and responsible for significant morbidity due to hemorrhage or thrombosis, with the widespread use of electronic cell counters, it is now clear that ET can occur at any age in adults and often without symptoms or disturbances of hemostasis. There is an unexplained female predominance in contrast to the other chronic myeloproliferative disorders or the reactive forms of thrombocytosis where no sex difference exists. Because no specific clonal marker is available, clinical criteria have been proposed to distinguish ET from the other chronic myeloproliferative disorders, which may also present with thrombocytosis but have differing prognoses and therapy (Table 103-5). These criteria do not establish clonality; therefore, they

TABLE 103-5 CAUSES OF THROMBOCYTOSIS

Tissue inflammation: collagen vascular disease, inflammatory bowel disease
Malignancy
Infection
Myeloproliferative disorders: polycythemia vera, idiopathic myelofibrosis, essential thrombocytosis, chronic myelogenous leukemia
Myelodysplastic disorders: 5q-syndrome, idiopathic refractory sideroblastic anemia
Postsplenectomy or hyposplenism
Hemorrhage
Iron deficiency anemia
Surgery
Rebound: Correction of vitamin B_{12} or folate deficiency, post-ethanol abuse
Hemolysis
Familial: Thrombopoietin overproduction, constitutive Mpl activation

are truly useful only in identifying disorders such as CML, PV, or myelodysplasia, which can masquerade as ET, as opposed to actually establishing the presence of ET. Furthermore, as with "idiopathic" erythrocytosis, nonclonal benign forms of thrombocytosis exist (such as hereditary overproduction of thrombopoietin) that are not widely recognized because we currently lack adequate diagnostic tools.

ETIOLOGY

Megakaryocytopoiesis and platelet production depend upon thrombopoietin and its receptor, Mpl. As in the case of early erythroid and myeloid progenitor cells, early megakaryocytic progenitors require the presence of interleukin 3 (IL-3) and stem cell factor for optimal proliferation in addition to thrombopoietin. Their subsequent development is also enhanced by the chemokine stromal cell–derived factor 1 (SDF-1). However, megakaryocyte maturation and differentiation require thrombopoietin.

Megakaryocytes are unique among hematopoietic progenitor cells because reduplication of their genome is endomitotic rather than mitotic. In the absence of thrombopoietin, endomitotic megakaryocytic reduplication and, by extension, the cytoplasmic development necessary for platelet production are impaired. Like erythropoietin, thrombopoietin is produced in both the liver and the kidneys, and an inverse correlation exists between the platelet count and plasma thrombopoietic activity. Like erythropoietin, plasma levels of thrombopoietin are controlled largely by the size of its progenitor cell pool. In contrast to erythropoietin, but like its myeloid counterparts, granulocyte- and granulocyte-macrophage colony-stimulating factors, thrombopoietin not only enhances the proliferation of its target cells but also enhances the reactivity of their end-stage product, the platelet. In addition to its role in thrombopoiesis, thrombopoietin also enhances the survival of multipotent hematopoietic stem cells.

The clonal nature of ET was established by analysis of glucose-6-phosphate dehydrogenase isoenzyme expression in patients hemizygous for this gene, by analysis of X-linked DNA polymorphisms in informative women patients, and by the expression in patients of nonrandom, though variable, cytogenetic abnormalities. Although thrombocytosis is its principal manifestation, like the other chronic myeloproliferative disorders, a multipotent hematopoietic progenitor cell is involved in ET. Furthermore, a number of families have been described in which ET was inherited, in one instance as an autosomal dominant trait. In addition to ET, IMF and PV have also been observed in some kindreds.

CLINICAL FEATURES

Clinically, ET is most often identified incidentally when a platelet count is obtained during the course of a routine medical evaluation. Occasionally, review of previous blood counts will reveal that an elevated platelet count was present but overlooked for many years. No symptoms or signs are specific for ET, but these patients can have hemorrhagic and thrombotic tendencies expressed as easy bruising for the former and microvascular occlusions for the latter, such as erythromelalgia, ocular migraine, or TIAs. Physical examination is generally unremarkable except occasionally for mild splenomegaly. Massive splenomegaly is more indicative of another myeloproliferative disorder, in particular PV, IMF, or CML.

Anemia is unusual, but a mild neutrophilic leukocytosis is not. The blood smear is most remarkable for the number of platelets present, some of which may be very large. The LAP score is either normal or elevated. The large mass of circulating platelets may prevent the accurate measurement of serum potassium due to release of platelet potassium upon blood clotting. This type of hyperkalemia is a laboratory artifact and not associated with electrocardiographic abnormalities. Similarly, arterial oxygen measurements can be inaccurate unless thrombocythemic blood is collected on ice. The prothrombin and partial thromboplastin times are normal, while abnormalities of platelet function such as a prolonged bleeding time and impaired platelet aggregation can be present. However, in spite of much study, no platelet function abnormalities are characteristic of ET, and no platelet function test predicts the risk of clinically significant bleeding or thrombosis.

The elevated platelet count may hinder marrow aspiration, but marrow biopsy usually reveals megakaryocyte hyperplasia and hypertrophy, as well as an overall increase in marrow cellularity. If marrow reticulin is increased, another diagnosis should be considered. The absence of stainable iron demands an explanation because iron deficiency alone can cause thrombocytosis, and absent marrow iron in the presence of marrow hypercellularity is a feature of PV.

Nonrandom cytogenetic abnormalities occur in ET but are uncommon, and no specific or consistent abnormality is notable, even those involving chromosomes 3 and 1, where the genes for thrombopoietin and its receptor Mpl, respectively, are located.

DIAGNOSIS

Thrombocytosis is encountered in a broad variety of clinical disorders (Table 103-5) in many of which production of cytokines is increased. The absolute level of the platelet count is not a useful diagnostic aid for distinguishing between benign and clonal causes of thrombocytosis. About 50% of ET patients express the JAK2 V617F mutation. When JAK2 V617F is absent, cytogenetic evaluation is mandatory to determine if the thrombocytosis is due to CML or a myelodysplastic disorder such as the 5q– syndrome. Because the bcr-abl translocation can be present in the absence of the Ph chromosome, and because bcr-abl RT-PCR is associated with false-positive results, fluorescence in situ hybridization (FISH) analysis for bcr-abl is the preferred assay in patients with thrombocytosis in whom a cytogenetic study for the Ph chromosome is negative. Anemia and ringed sideroblasts are not features of ET, but they are features of idiopathic refractory sideroblastic anemia, and in some of these patients the thrombocytosis occurs in association with JAK2 V617F expression. Massive splenomegaly should suggest the presence of another myeloproliferative disorder, and in this setting a red cell mass determination should be performed because splenomegaly can mask the presence of erythrocytosis. Importantly, what appears to be ET can evolve into PV or IMF after a period of many years, revealing the true nature of the underlying myeloproliferative disorder.

COMPLICATIONS

Perhaps no other condition in clinical medicine has caused otherwise astute physicians to intervene inappropriately more often than thrombocytosis, particularly if the platelet count is $>1 \times 10^6/\mu L$. It is commonly believed that a high platelet count causes intravascular stasis and thrombosis; however, no controlled clinical study has ever established this association, and in patients younger than age 60, the incidence of thrombosis was not greater in patients with thrombocytosis than in age-matched controls.

To the contrary, very high platelet counts are associated primarily with hemorrhage due to acquired von Willebrand disease. This is not meant to imply that an elevated platelet count cannot cause symptoms in a patient with ET, but rather that the focus should be on the patient, not the platelet count. For example, some of the most dramatic neurologic problems in ET are migraine-related and respond only to lowering of the platelet count, while other symptoms such as erythromelalgia respond simply to platelet cyclooxygenase 1 inhibitors such as aspirin or ibuprofen, without a reduction in platelet number. Still others may represent an interaction between an atherosclerotic vascular system and a high platelet count, and others may have no relationship to the platelet count whatsoever. Recognition that PV can present with thrombocytosis as well as the discovery of previously unrecognized causes of hypercoagulability (Chap. 111) make the older literature on the complications of thrombocytosis unreliable.

℞ ESSENTIAL THROMBOCYTOSIS

Survival of patients with ET is not different than for the general population. An elevated platelet count in an asymptomatic patient without cardiovascular risk factors requires no therapy. Indeed, before any therapy is initiated in a patient with thrombocytosis, the cause of symptoms must be clearly identified as due to the elevated platelet count. When the platelet count rises above $1 \times 10^6/\mu L$, a substantial quantity of high-molecular-weight von

Willebrand multimers are removed from the circulation and destroyed by the platelets, resulting in an acquired form of von Willebrand disease. This can be identified by a reduction in ristocetin cofactor activity. In this situation, aspirin could promote hemorrhage. Bleeding in this situation usually responds to ε-aminocaproic acid, which can be given prophylactically before and after elective surgery. Plateletpheresis is at best a temporary and inefficient remedy that is rarely required. Importantly, ET patients treated with ^{32}P or alkylating agents are at risk of developing acute leukemia without any proof of benefit; combining either therapy with hydroxyurea increases this risk. If platelet reduction is deemed necessary on the basis of symptoms refractory to salicylates alone, IFN-α, the quinazoline derivative, anagrelide, or hydroxyurea can be used to reduce the platelet count, but none of these is uniformly effective nor without significant side effects. Hydroxyurea and aspirin are more effective than anagrelide and aspirin for prevention of TIAs but not more effective for the prevention of other types of arterial thrombosis and actually less effective for venous thrombosis. Normalizing the platelet count does not prevent either arterial or venous thrombosis. Risk of gastrointestinal bleeding is also higher when aspirin is combined with anagrelide.

As more clinical experience is acquired, ET is more benign than previously thought. Evolution to acute leukemia is more likely to be a conse-

quence of therapy than of the disease itself. In managing patients with thrombocytosis, the physician's first obligation is to do no harm.

FURTHER READINGS

BUSS DH et al: The incidence of thrombotic and hemorrhagic disorders in association with extreme thrombocytosis: An analysis of 129 cases. Am J Hematol 20:365, 1985

ELLIOT MA et al: Thrombosis and hemorrhage in polycythemia vera and essential thrombocythaemia. Br J Haematol 128:275, 2005

LEVINE RL, GILLILAND DG: JAK-2 mutations and their relevance to myeloproliferative disease. Curr Opin Hematol 14:43, 2007

REILLY JT: Idiopathic myelofibrosis: Pathogenesis to treatment. Hematol Oncol 24:56, 2006

SPIVAK JL: Polycythemia vera: Myths, mechanisms, and management. Blood 100:4272, 2002

VAINCHENKER W et al: A unique activating mutation in JAK2 (V617F) is at the origin of polycythemia vera and allows a new classification of myeloproliferative diseases. Hematology (Am Soc Hematol Educ Program):195, 2005

104 Acute and Chronic Myeloid Leukemia

Meir Wetzler, John C. Byrd, Clara D. Bloomfield

The myeloid leukemias are a heterogeneous group of diseases characterized by infiltration of the blood, bone marrow, and other tissues by neoplastic cells of the hematopoietic system. In 2006 the estimated number of new myeloid leukemia cases in the United States was 16,430. These leukemias comprise a spectrum of malignancies that, untreated, range from rapidly fatal to slowly growing. Based on their untreated course, the myeloid leukemias have traditionally been designated acute or chronic.

ACUTE MYELOID LEUKEMIA

INCIDENCE

The incidence of acute myeloid leukemia (AML) is ~3.7 per 100,000 people per year, and the age-adjusted incidence is higher in men than in women (4.6 versus 3.0). AML incidence increases with age; it is 1.9 in individuals <65 years and 18.6 in those >65. A significant increase in AML incidence has occurred over the past 10 years.

ETIOLOGY

Heredity, radiation, chemical and other occupational exposures, and drugs have been implicated in the development of AML. No direct evidence suggests a viral etiology.

Heredity Certain syndromes with somatic cell chromosome aneuploidy, such as trisomy 21 noted in Down syndrome, are associated with an increased incidence of AML. Inherited diseases with defective DNA repair, e.g., Fanconi anemia, Bloom syndrome, and ataxia telangiectasia, are also associated with AML. Congenital neutropenia (Kostmann syndrome) is a disease with mutations in the granulocyte colony-stimulating factor (G-CSF) receptor and, often, neutrophil elastase that may evolve into AML. Myeloproliferative syndromes may also evolve into AML (Chap. 103). Germ-line mutations of CCAAT/enhancer-binding protein α (C/EBP α), runt-related transcription factor 1 (RUNX1), and tumor protein p53 (TP53) have also been associated with a higher predisposition to AML in some series.

Radiation Survivors of the atomic bomb explosions in Japan had an increased incidence of myeloid leukemias that peaked 5–7 years after

exposure. Therapeutic radiation alone seems to add little risk of AML but can increase the risk in people also exposed to alkylating agents.

Chemical and Other Exposures Exposure to benzene, a solvent used in the chemical, plastic, rubber, and pharmaceutical industries, is associated with an increased incidence of AML. Smoking and exposure to petroleum products, paint, embalming fluids, ethylene oxide, herbicides, and pesticides, have also been associated with an increased risk of AML.

Drugs Anticancer drugs are the leading cause of therapy-associated AML. Alkylating agent–associated leukemias occur on average 4–6 years after exposure, and affected individuals have aberrations in chromosomes 5 and 7. Topoisomerase II inhibitor–associated leukemias occur 1–3 years after exposure, and affected individuals often have aberrations involving chromosome 11q23. Chloramphenicol, phenylbutazone, and, less commonly, chloroquine and methoxypsoralen can result in bone marrow failure that may evolve into AML.

CLASSIFICATION

The World Health Organization (WHO) classification (Table 104-1) includes different biologically distinct groups based on immunophenotype, clinical features, and cytogenetic and molecular abnormalities in addition to morphology. In contrast to the previously used French-American-British (FAB) schema, the WHO classification places limited reliance on cytochemistry. Since much of the recent literature and some ongoing studies use the FAB classification, a description of this system is also provided in Table 104-1. A major difference between the WHO and FAB systems is the blast cutoff for a diagnosis of AML as opposed to myelodysplastic syndrome (MDS); it is 20% in the WHO classification and 30% in the FAB. AML with 20–30% blasts as defined by the WHO classification can benefit from approved therapies for MDS (such as decitabine or 5-azacytidine) that were approved in the past by the Food and Drug Administration (FDA) for marketing based on trials using the FAB criteria.

Importantly, the WHO schema is the first leukemia classification system to consider genetic along with morphologic features to define different subsets of AML.

Immunophenotype and Relevance to the WHO Classification The immunophenotype of human leukemia cells can be studied by multiparameter flow cytometry after the cells are labeled with monoclonal antibodies to cell-surface antigens. This can be important for separating AML from acute lymphoblastic leukemia (ALL) and identifying some types of AML. For example, AML that is minimally differentiat-

TABLE 104-1   ACUTE MYELOID LEUKEMIA (AML) CLASSIFICATION SYSTEMS

World Health Organization Classification[a]

I. AML with recurrent genetic abnormalities
   AML with t(8;21)(q22;q22);*RUNX1/RUNX1T1*[b]
   AML with abnormal bone marrow eosinophils [inv(16)(p13q22) or t(16;16)(p13;q22);*CBFB/MYH11*]b
   Acute promyelocytic leukemia [AML with t(15;17)(q22;q12) (*PML/RARA*) and variants]b
   AML with 11q23 (*MLL*) abnormalities

II. AML with multilineage dysplasia
   Following a myelodysplastic syndrome or myelodysplastic syndrome/myeloproliferative disorder
   Without antecedent myelodysplastic syndrome

III. AML and myelodysplastic syndromes, therapy-related
   Alkylating agent–related
   Topoisomerase type II inhibitor–related
   Other types

IV. AML not otherwise categorized
   AML minimally differentiated
   AML without maturation
   AML with maturation
   Acute myelomonocytic leukemia
   Acute monoblastic and monocytic leukemia
   Acute erythroid leukemia
   Acute megakaryoblastic leukemia
   Acute basophilic leukemia
   Acute panmyelosis with myelofibrosis
   Myeloid sarcoma

French-American-British (FAB) Classification[c]	Incidence
M0: Minimally differentiated leukemia	5%
M1: Myeloblastic leukemia without maturation	20%
M2: Myeloblastic leukemia with maturation	30%
M3: Hypergranular promyelocytic leukemia	10%
M4: Myelomonocytic leukemia	20%
M4Eo: Variant: Increase in abnormal marrow eosinophils	
M5: Monocytic leukemia	10%
M6: Erythroleukemia (DiGuglielmo's disease)	4%
M7: Megakaryoblastic leukemia	1%

[a]ES Jaffe et al: *World Health Organization Classification of Tumours*. Lyon, IARC Press, 2001.
[b]Diagnosis is AML regardless of blast count.
[c]JM Bennett et al: Ann Intern Med 103:620, 1985.

ed (immature morphology and no lineage-specific cytochemical reactions) is diagnosed by flow-cytometric demonstration of the myeloid-specific antigens cluster designation (CD) 13 or 33. Similarly, acute megakaryoblastic leukemia can often be diagnosed only by expression of the platelet-specific antigens CD41 and/or CD61. While flow cytometry is useful, widely used, and, in some cases, essential for the diagnosis of AML, it is only supportive in establishing the different subtypes of AML through the WHO classification.

Clinical Features and Relevance to the WHO Classification The WHO classification considers clinical features in subdividing AML. For example, it identifies therapy-related AML as a separate entity and subclassifies this group based on the specific types of prior chemotherapy received. It also divides AML with multilineage dysplasia based upon the presence or absence of an antecedent MDS. These clinical features contribute to the prognosis of the specific type of AML.

Genetic Findings and Relevance to the WHO Classification The WHO classification is the first AML classification to incorporate genetic (chromosomal and molecular) information. Indeed, AML is first subclassified based on the presence or absence of specific recurrent genetic abnormalities. For example, AML FAB M3 is now designated *acute promyelocytic leukemia* (APL), based on the presence of either the t(15;17)(q22;q12) cytogenetic rearrangement or the *PML/RARα* product of the translocation. Thus, the WHO classification separates APL from

all other types of AML as a first step and forces the clinician to correctly identify the entity and tailor treatment(s) accordingly.

CHROMOSOMAL ANALYSES Chromosomal analysis of the leukemic cell provides the most important pretreatment prognostic information in AML. Two cytogenetic abnormalities have been invariably associated with specific morphologic features: t(15;17)(q22;q12) with APL and inv(16)(p13q22) with AML with abnormal bone marrow eosinophils. Many other chromosomal abnormalities have been associated primarily with one morphologic/immunophenotypic group, including t(8;21)(q22;q22) with slender Auer rods, expression of CD19, and abundance of normal eosinophils, and t(9;11)(p22;q23), as well as other translocations involving 11q23, with monocytic features. Many of the recurring chromosomal abnormalities in AML have been associated with specific clinical characteristics. More commonly associated with younger age are t(8;21) and t(15;17); with older age, del(5q) and del(7q). Myeloid sarcomas (see below) are associated with t(8;21) and disseminated intravascular coagulation (DIC) with t(15;17).

Molecular Classification Molecular study of many recurring cytogenetic abnormalities has revealed genes that may be involved in leukemogenesis; this information is increasingly being incorporated into the WHO classification. For instance, the t(15;17) encodes a chimeric protein, promyelocytic leukemia (Pml)/retinoic acid receptor α (Rarα), which is formed by the fusion of the retinoic acid receptor α (*RARα*) gene from chromosome 17 and the promyelocytic leukemia (*PML*) gene from chromosome 15. The *RARα* gene encodes a member of the nuclear hormone receptor family of transcription factors. After binding retinoic acid, *RARα* can promote expression of a variety of genes. The 15;17 translocation juxtaposes *PML* with *RARα* in a head-to-tail configuration that is under the transcriptional control of *PML*. Three different breakpoints in the *PML* gene lead to various fusion proteins. The Pml-Rarα fusion protein tends to suppress gene transcription and blocks differentiation of the cells. Pharmacologic doses of the Rarα ligand, all-*trans*-retinoic acid (tretinoin), relieve the block and promote differentiation (see below). Similar examples exist with a variety of other balanced translocations and inversions, including the t(8;21), t(9;11), t(6;9), and inv(16).

Molecular aberrations are also being identified that are useful for classifying risk of relapse in patients without cytogenetic abnormalities. A partial tandem duplication (PTD) of the *MLL* gene is found in 5–10% of patients with normal cytogenetics and results in short remission duration. FMS-like tyrosine kinase 3 (Flt3) is a tyrosine kinase receptor important in the development of myeloid and lymphoid lineages. Activating mutations of the gene *FLT3* are present in ~30% of adult AML patients due to internal tandem duplications (ITDs) in the juxtamembrane domain or mutations of the activating loop of the kinase. These occur more commonly in patients with normal karyotype. Continuous activation of Flt3 and downstream target kinases, including signal transducer and activator of transcription protein 5, Ras/mitogen-activated protein kinase, and phosphatidylinositol 3-kinase/Akt, provides increased proliferation and antiapoptotic signals to the myeloid progenitor cell. Presence of *FLT3* ITD in patients with normal cytogenetics predicts for short remission duration and inferior survival. Other molecular prognostic factors in patients with normal karyotype AML include mutations of the nucleophosmin gene (*NPM1*) and *C/EBPα* that are associated with improved treatment outcome. In contrast, overexpression of genes such as brain and acute leukemia, cytoplasmic (*BAALC*) predicts for poor outcome. Gene expression profiles to predict outcome in normal karyotype AML patients are under active investigation.

CLINICAL PRESENTATION

Symptoms Patients with AML most often present with nonspecific symptoms that begin gradually or abruptly and are the consequence of anemia, leukocytosis, leukopenia or leukocyte dysfunction, or thrombocytopenia. Nearly half have had symptoms for ≤3 months before the leukemia was diagnosed.

FIGURE 104-1 Morphology of AML cells. A. Uniform population of primitive myeloblasts with immature chromatin, nucleoli in some cells, and primary cytoplasmic granules. **B.** Leukemic myeloblast containing an Auer rod. **C.** Promyelocytic leukemia cells with prominent cytoplasmic primary granules. **D.** Peroxidase stain shows dark blue color characteristic of peroxidase in granules in AML.

Half mention fatigue as the first symptom, but most complain of fatigue or weakness at the time of diagnosis. Anorexia and weight loss are common. Fever with or without an identifiable infection is the initial symptom in ~10% of patients. Signs of abnormal hemostasis (bleeding, easy bruising) are noted first in 5% of patients. On occasion, bone pain, lymphadenopathy, nonspecific cough, headache, or diaphoresis is the presenting symptom.

Rarely patients may present with symptoms from a mass lesion located in the soft tissues, breast, uterus, ovary, cranial or spinal dura, gastrointestinal tract, lung, mediastinum, prostate, bone, or other organs. The mass lesion represents a tumor of leukemic cells and is called a *granulocytic sarcoma*, or *chloroma*. Typical AML may occur simultaneously, later, or not at all in these patients. This rare presentation is more common in patients with t(8;21).

Physical Findings Fever, splenomegaly, hepatomegaly, lymphadenopathy, sternal tenderness, and evidence of infection and hemorrhage are often found at diagnosis. Significant gastrointestinal bleeding, intrapulmonary hemorrhage, or intracranial hemorrhage occur most often in APL. Bleeding associated with coagulopathy may also occur in monocytic AML and with extreme degrees of leukocytosis or thrombocytopenia in other morphologic subtypes. Retinal hemorrhages are detected in 15% of patients. Infiltration of the gingivae, skin, soft tissues, or the meninges with leukemic blasts at diagnosis is characteristic of the monocytic subtypes and those with 11q23 chromosomal abnormalities.

Hematologic Findings Anemia is usually present at diagnosis and can be severe. The degree varies considerably, irrespective of other hematologic findings, splenomegaly, or duration of symptoms. The anemia is usually normocytic normochromic. Decreased erythropoiesis often results in a reduced reticulocyte count, and red blood cell (RBC) survival is decreased by accelerated destruction. Active blood loss also contributes to the anemia.

The median presenting leukocyte count is about 15,000/μL. Between 25 and 40% of patients have counts <5000/μL, and 20% have counts >100,000/μL. Fewer than 5% have no detectable leukemic cells in the blood. The morphology of the malignant cell varies in difference subsets. In AML the cytoplasm often contains primary (nonspecific) granules, and the nucleus shows fine, lacy chromatin with one or more nucleoli characteristic of immature cells. Abnormal rod-shaped granules called Auer rods are not uniformly present, but when they are, myeloid lineage is virtually certain (Fig 104-1). Poor neutrophil function may be noted by impaired phagocytosis and migration and morphologically by abnormal lobulation and deficient granulation.

Platelet counts <100,000/μL are found at diagnosis in ~75% of patients, and about 25% have counts <25,000/μL. Both morphologic and functional platelet abnormalities can be observed, including large and bizarre shapes with abnormal granulation and inability of platelets to aggregate or adhere normally to one another.

Pretreatment Evaluation Once the diagnosis of AML is suspected, a rapid evaluation and initiation of appropriate therapy should follow (Table 104-2). In addition to clarifying the subtype of leukemia, initial studies should evaluate the overall functional integrity of the major organ systems, including the cardiovascular, pulmonary, hepatic, and renal systems. Factors that have prognostic significance, either for achieving complete remission (CR) or for predicting the duration of CR, should also be assessed before initiating treatment. Leukemic cells should be obtained from all patients and cryopreserved for future use as new tests and therapeutics become available. All patients should be evaluated for infection.

Most patients are anemic and thrombocytopenic at presentation. Replacement of the appropriate blood components, if necessary, should begin promptly. Because qualitative platelet dysfunction or the presence of an infection may increase the likelihood of bleeding, evidence of hemorrhage justifies the immediate use of platelet transfusion, even if the platelet count is only moderately decreased.

TABLE 104-2 INITIAL DIAGNOSTIC EVALUATION AND MANAGEMENT OF ADULT PATIENTS WITH ACUTE MYELOID LEUKEMIA

History

Increasing fatigue or decreased exercise tolerance (anemia)
Excess bleeding or bleeding from unusual sites (DIC, thrombocytopenia)
Fevers or recurrent infections (granulocytopenia)
Headache, vision changes, nonfocal neurologic abnormalities (CNS leukemia or bleed)
Early satiety (splenomegaly)
Family history of AML (Fanconi, Bloom, or Kostmann syndromes or ataxia telangiectasia)
History of cancer (exposure to alkylating agents, radiation, topoisomerase II inhibitors)
Occupational exposures (radiation, benzene, petroleum products, paint, smoking, pesticides)

Physical Examination

Performance status (prognostic factor)
Ecchymosis and oozing from IV sites (DIC, possible acute promyelocytic leukemia)
Fever and tachycardia (signs of infection)
Papilledema, retinal infiltrates, cranial nerve abnormalities (CNS leukemia)
Poor dentition, dental abscesses
Gum hypertrophy (leukemic infiltration, most common in monocytic leukemia)
Skin infiltration or nodules (leukemia infiltration, most common in monocytic leukemia)
Lymphadenopathy, splenomegaly, hepatomegaly
Back pain, lower extremity weakness [spinal granulocytic sarcoma, most likely in t(8;21) patients]

Laboratory and Radiologic Studies

CBC with manual differential cell count
Chemistry tests (electrolytes, creatinine, BUN, calcium, phosphorus, uric acid, hepatic enzymes, bilirubin, LDH, amylase, lipase)
Clotting studies (prothrombin time, partial thromboplastin time, fibrinogen, D-dimer)
Viral serologies (CMV, HSV-1, varicella zoster)
RBC type and screen
HLA typing of patient, siblings, and parents for potential allogeneic SCT
Bone marrow aspirate and biopsy (morphology, cytogenetics, flow cytometry, molecular studies)
Cryopreservation of viable leukemia cells
Echocardiogram or heart scan
PA and lateral chest radiograph
Placement of central venous access device

Interventions for Specific Patients

Dental evaluation (for those with poor dentition)
Lumbar puncture (for those with symptoms of CNS involvement)
Screening spine MRI (for patients with back pain, lower extremity weakness, paresthesias)
Social work referral for patient and family psychosocial support

Counseling for All Patients

Provide patient with information regarding his/her disease, financial counseling, and support group contacts

Abbreviations: BUN, blood urea nitrogen; CBC, complete blood count; CMV, cytomegalovirus; CNS, central nervous system; DIC, disseminated intravascular coagulation; HLA, human leukocyte antigen; HSV, herpes simplex virus; LDH, lactate dehydrogenase; MRI, magnetic resonance imaging; PA, posteroanterior; RBC, red blood (cell) count; SCT, stem cell transplant.

About 50% of patients have a mild to moderate elevation of serum uric acid at presentation. Only 10% have marked elevations, but renal precipitation of uric acid and the nephropathy that may result is a serious but uncommon complication. The initiation of chemotherapy may aggravate hyperuricemia, and patients are usually started immediately on allopurinol and hydration at diagnosis. Rasburicase (recombinant uric oxidase) is also useful for treating uric acid nephropathy and often can normalize the serum uric acid level within hours with a single dose of treatment. The presence of high concentrations of lysozyme, a marker for monocytic differentiation, may be etiologic in renal tubular dysfunction, which could worsen other renal problems that arise during the initial phases of therapy.

PROGNOSTIC FACTORS

Many factors influence the likelihood of entering CR, the length of CR, and the curability of AML. CR is defined after examination of both blood and bone marrow. The blood neutrophil count must be ≥1000/μL and the platelet count ≥100,000/μL. Hemoglobin concentration is not considered in determining CR. Circulating blasts should be absent. While rare blasts may be detected in the blood during marrow regeneration, they should disappear on successive studies. Bone marrow cellularity should be >20% with trilineage maturation. The bone marrow should contain <5% blasts, and Auer rods should be absent. Extramedullary leukemia should not be present. For patients in morphologic CR, reverse transcriptase polymerase chain reaction (RT-PCR) to detect AML-associated molecular abnormalities and either metaphase cytogenetics or interphase cytogenetics by fluorescence in situ hybridization (FISH) to detect AML-associated cytogenetic aberrations are currently used to detect residual disease. Such detection of minimal residual disease may become a reliable discriminator between patients in CR who do or do not require additional and/or alternative therapies.

Age at diagnosis is among the most important risk factors. Advancing age is associated with a poorer prognosis, in part because of its influence on the patient's ability to survive induction therapy. Age also influences outcome because AML in older patients differs biologically. The leukemic cells in elderly patients more commonly express CD34 and the multidrug resistance 1 (MDR1) efflux pump that conveys resistance to natural product–derived agents such as the anthracyclines (see below). With each successive decade of age, a greater proportion of patients have more resistant disease. Chronic and intercurrent diseases impair tolerance to rigorous therapy; acute medical problems at diagnosis reduce the likelihood of survival. Performance status, independent of age, also influences ability to survive induction therapy and thus respond to treatment.

Chromosome findings at diagnosis are important independent prognostic factors. Patients with t(15;17) have a very good prognosis (approximately 85% cured), and those with t(8;21) and inv(16) a good prognosis (approximately 50% cured), while those with no cytogenetic abnormality have a moderately favorable outcome (approximately 40% cured). Patients with a complex karyotype, t(6;9), inv(3), or 7 have a very poor prognosis. This emphasizes the importance of cytogenetic as well as the previously discussed molecular assessment of the leukemia cells at diagnosis and relevance of storing samples for potential later use.

A prolonged symptomatic interval with cytopenias preceding diagnosis or a history of an antecedent hematologic disorder is another pretreatment clinical feature associated with a lower CR rate and shorter survival time. The CR rate is lower in patients who have had anemia, leukopenia, and/or thrombocytopenia for >3 months before the diagnosis of AML when compared to those without such a history. Responsiveness to chemotherapy declines as the duration of the antecedent disorder(s) increases. Secondary AML developing after treatment with cytotoxic agents for other malignancies is usually difficult to treat successfully.

A high presenting leukocyte count is an independent prognostic factor for attaining a CR. Among patients with hyperleukocytosis (>100,000/μL), early central nervous system bleeding and pulmonary leukostasis contribute to poor outcome with initial therapy.

In addition to pretreatment variables such as age, cytogenetics, and leukocyte count, several treatment factors correlate with prognosis in AML, including, most importantly, achievement of CR. In addition, patients who achieve CR after one induction cycle have longer CR durations than those requiring multiple cycles.

℞ ACUTE MYELOID LEUKEMIA

Treatment of the newly diagnosed patient with AML is usually divided into two phases, induction and postremission management (Fig. 104-2). The initial goal is to quickly induce CR. Once CR is obtained, further therapy must

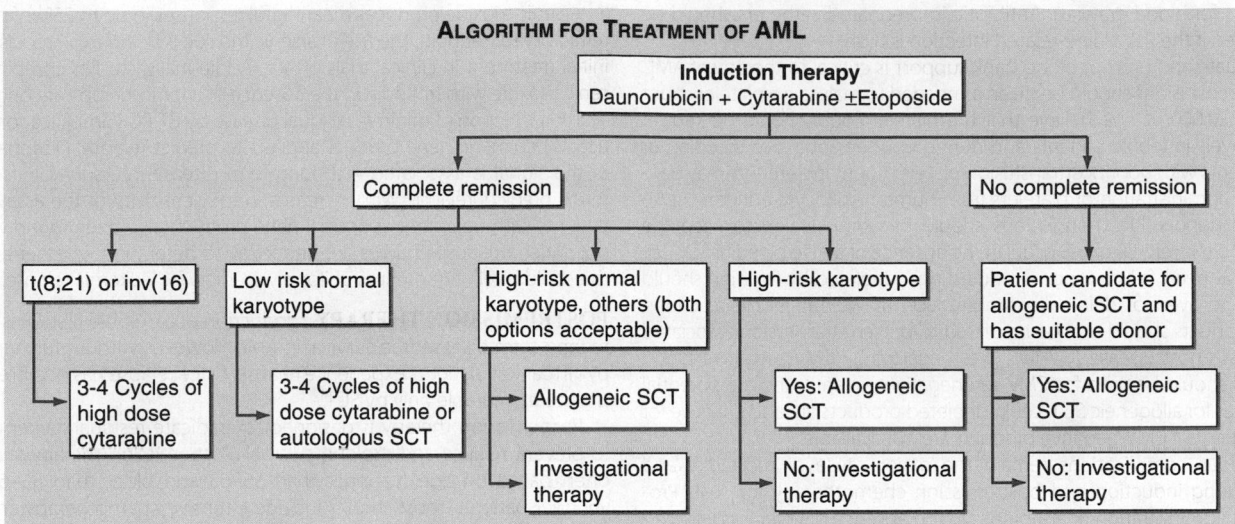

ALGORITHM FOR TREATMENT OF AML

Induction Therapy
Daunorubicin + Cytarabine ±Etoposide

Complete remission — **No complete remission**

t(8;21) or inv(16) | Low risk normal karyotype | High-risk normal karyotype, others (both options acceptable) | High-risk karyotype | Patient candidate for allogeneic SCT and has suitable donor

3-4 Cycles of high dose cytarabine | 3-4 Cycles of high dose cytarabine or autologous SCT | Allogeneic SCT / Investigational therapy | Yes: Allogeneic SCT / No: Investigational therapy | Yes: Allogeneic SCT / No: Investigational therapy

FIGURE 104-2 Flow chart for the therapy of newly diagnosed acute myeloid leukemia. For all forms of AML except acute promyelocytic leukemia (APL), standard therapy includes a 7-day continuous infusion of cytarabine (100–200 mg/m^2 per day) and a 3-day course of daunorubicin (45–60 mg/m^2 per day) or idarubicin (12–13 mg/m^2 per day) with or without 3 days of etoposide. Patients who achieve complete remission undergo postremission consolidation therapy, including sequential courses of high-dose cytarabine, autologous stem cell transplant (SCT), high-dose combination chemotherapy with allogeneic SCT, or novel therapies, based on their predicted risk of relapse (i.e., risk-stratified therapy). Patients with APL usually receive tretinoin together with anthracycline chemotherapy for remission induction and then consolidation chemotherapy (daunorubicin) followed by maintenance tretinoin, with or without chemotherapy. The role of cytarabine in APL induction and consolidation is controversial.

be used to prolong survival and achieve cure. The initial induction treatment and subsequent postremission therapy are often chosen based on the patient's age. The influence of intensifying therapy with traditional chemotherapy agents such as cytarabine and anthracyclines in younger patients (<60 years) appears to increase the cure rate of AML. In older patients the benefit of intensive therapy is controversial; novel therapies are being pursued.

INDUCTION CHEMOTHERAPY The most commonly used CR induction regimens (for patients other than those with APL) consist of combination chemotherapy with cytarabine and an anthracycline. Cytarabine is a cell cycle S-phase–specific antimetabolite that becomes phosphorylated intracellularly to an active triphosphate form that interferes with DNA synthesis. Anthracyclines are DNA intercalaters. Their primary mode of action is thought to be inhibition of topoisomerase II, leading to DNA breaks. Cytarabine is usually administered as a continuous intravenous infusion for 7 days. Anthracycline therapy generally consists of daunorubicin intravenously on days 1, 2, and 3 (the 7 and 3 regimen). Treatment with idarubicin for 3 days in conjunction with cytarabine by 7-day continuous infusion is at least as effective and may be superior to daunorubicin in younger patients. The addition of etoposide may improve the CR duration.

After induction chemotherapy, the bone marrow is examined to determine if the leukemia has been eliminated. If ≥5% blasts exist with ≥20% cellularity, the patient is usually re-treated with cytarabine and an anthracycline in doses similar to those given initially, but for 5 and 2 days, respectively. Our recommendation, however, is to change therapy in this setting. Patients who fail to attain CR after two induction courses should immediately proceed to an allogeneic stem cell transplant (SCT) if an appropriate donor exists. This approach is only applied to patients under the age of 70 with acceptable end-organ function.

With the 7 and 3 cytarabine/daunorubicin regimen outlined above, 65–75% of adults with de novo AML under the age of 60 years achieve CR. Two-thirds achieve CR after a single course of therapy, and one-third require two courses. About 50% of patients who do not achieve CR have a drug-resistant leukemia, and 50% do not achieve CR because of fatal complications of bone marrow aplasia or impaired recovery of normal stem cells. Higher induction treatment–related mortality and frequency of resistant disease have been observed with increasing age and in patients with prior hematologic disorders (MDS or myeloproliferative syndromes) or chemotherapy treatment for another malignancy.

High-dose cytarabine-based regimens have very high CR rates after a single cycle of therapy. When given in high doses, more cytarabine may enter the cells, saturate the cytarabine-inactivating enzymes, and increase the intracellular levels of 1-β-D-arabinofuranylcytosine-triphosphate, the active metabolite incorporated into DNA. Thus, higher doses of cytarabine may increase the inhibition of DNA synthesis and thereby overcome resistance to standard-dose cytarabine. In two randomized studies, high-dose cytarabine with an anthracycline produced CR rates similar to those achieved with standard 7 and 3 regimens. However, the CR duration was longer after high-dose cytarabine than after standard-dose cytarabine.

The hematologic toxicity of high-dose cytarabine-based induction regimens has typically been greater than that associated with 7 and 3 regimens. Toxicity with high-dose cytarabine includes myelosuppression, pulmonary toxicity, and significant and occasionally irreversible cerebellar toxicity. All patients treated with high-dose cytarabine must be closely monitored for cerebellar toxicity. Full cerebellar testing should be performed before each dose, and further high-dose cytarabine should be withheld if evidence of cerebellar toxicity develops. This toxicity occurs more commonly in patients with renal impairment and in those over age 60. The increased toxicity observed with high-dose cytarabine has limited the use of this therapy in elderly AML patients.

SUPPORTIVE CARE Measures geared to supporting patients through several weeks of granulocytopenia and thrombocytopenia are critical to the success of AML therapy. Patients with AML should be treated in centers expert in providing supportive measures.

Recombinant hematopoietic growth factors have been incorporated into clinical trials in AML. These trials have been designed to lower the infection rate after chemotherapy. Both G-CSF and granulocyte-macrophage colony-stimulating factor (GM-CSF) have reduced the median time to neutrophil recovery by an average of 5–7 days. This accelerated rate of neutrophil recovery, however, has not generally translated into significant reductions in infection rates or shortened hospitalizations. In most randomized studies, both G-CSF and GM-CSF have failed to improve the CR rate, disease-free survival, or overall survival. Although receptors for both G-CSF and GM-CSF are present on AML blasts, therapeutic efficacy is neither enhanced nor inhibited by these agents. The use of growth factors as supportive care for AML patients is controversial. We favor their use in elderly patients with complicated courses, those receiving intensive postremission regimens, patients with uncontrolled infections, or those participating in clinical trials.

Multilumen right atrial catheters should be inserted as soon as patients with newly diagnosed AML have been stabilized. They should be used thereafter for administration of intravenous medications and transfusions, as well as for blood drawing. Antibiotic-impregnated catheters should be considered if the risk of line-related infection is high.

Adequate and prompt blood bank support is critical to therapy of AML. Platelet transfusions should be given as needed to maintain a platelet count >10,000–20,000/μL. We believe that the platelet count should be kept at higher levels in febrile patients and during episodes of active bleeding or DIC. Patients with poor posttransfusion platelet count increments may benefit from administration of platelets from human leukocyte antigen (HLA)-matched donors. RBC transfusions should be administered to keep the hemoglobin level >80 g/L (8 g/dL) in the absence of active bleeding, DIC, or congestive heart failure. Blood products leukodepleted by filtration should be used to avert or delay alloimmunization as well as febrile reactions. Blood products should also be irradiated to prevent transfusion associated graft-versus-host disease (GVHD). Cytomegalovirus (CMV)-negative blood products should be used for CMV-seronegative patients who are potential candidates for allogeneic SCT. Leukodepleted products are also effective for these patients if CMV-negative products are not available.

Infectious complications remain the major cause of morbidity and death during induction and postremission chemotherapy for AML. Prophylactic administration of antibiotics in the absence of fever is controversial. Oral nystatin or clotrimazole is recommended to prevent localized candidiasis. For patients who are herpes simplex virus antibody titer–positive, acyclovir prophylaxis is effective in preventing reactivation of latent oral herpes infections.

Fever develops in most patients with AML, but infections are documented in only half of febrile patients. Early initiation of empirical broad-spectrum antibacterial and antifungal antibiotics has significantly reduced the number of patients dying of infectious complications (Chap. 82). An antibiotic regimen adequate to treat gram-negative organisms should be instituted at the onset of fever in a granulocytopenic patient after clinical evaluation, including a detailed physical examination with inspection of the indwelling catheter exit site and a perirectal examination, as well as procurement of cultures and radiographs aimed at documenting the source of fever. Specific antibiotic regimens should be based on antibiotic sensitivity data obtained from the institution at which the patient is being treated. Acceptable regimens include imipenem-cilastin; an antipseudomonal semisynthetic penicillin (e.g., piperacillin) combined with an aminoglycoside; a third-generation cephalosporin with antipseudomonal activity (i.e., ceftazidime or cefepime); or double β-lactam combinations (ceftazidime and piperacillin). Aminoglycosides should be avoided if possible in patients with renal insufficiency. For patients with known immediate-type hypersensitivity reactions to penicillin, aztreonam may be substituted for β-lactams. Aztreonam should be combined with an aminoglycoside or a quinolone antibiotic rather than used alone.

Empirical vancomycin is not given initially in the absence of suspected gram-positive infection or mucositis but should be initiated in neutropenic patients who remain febrile for 3 days; empirical systemic antifungal therapy is added at 7 days if fever persists. Voriconazole has been shown to be equivalent in efficacy and less toxic than amphotericin-B. Caspofungin or liposomal amphotericin are also considered for fungal infections not responsive to first-line therapy or when such therapy is not tolerated. Antibacterial and antifungal antibiotics should be continued until patients are no longer neutropenic, regardless of whether a specific source has been found for the fever.

TREATMENT OF PROMYELOCYTIC LEUKEMIA Tretinoin is an oral drug that induces the differentiation of leukemic cells bearing the t(15;17). APL is responsive to cytarabine and daunorubicin, but about 10% of patients treated with these drugs die from DIC induced by the release of granule components by dying tumor cells. Tretinoin does not produce DIC but produces another complication called the *retinoic acid syndrome*. Occurring within the first 3 weeks of treatment, it is characterized by fever, dyspnea, chest pain, pulmonary infiltrates, pleural and pericardial effusions, and hypoxia. The syndrome is related to adhesion of differentiated neoplastic cells to the pulmonary vasculature endothelium. Glucocorticoids, chemotherapy, and/or supportive measures can be effective for management of the retinoic acid syndrome. The mortality of this syndrome is about 10%.

Tretinoin (45 mg/m^2 per day orally until remission is documented) plus concurrent anthracycline chemotherapy appears to be among the safest and most effective treatments for APL. Unlike patients with other types of AML, patients with this subtype benefit from maintenance therapy with either tretinoin or chemotherapy.

Arsenic trioxide produces meaningful responses in up to 85% of patients refractory to tretinoin. The use of arsenic trioxide is being explored as part of initial treatment in clinical trials of APL. Additionally, studies combining arsenic trioxide with tretinoin in the absence of chemotherapy are ongoing.

The detection of minimal residual disease by RT-PCR amplification of the t(15;17) chimeric gene product appears to predict relapse. Disappearance of the signal is associated with long-term disease-free survival; its persistence predicts relapse. With increases in the sensitivity of the assay, some patients with persistent abnormal gene product have been found who do not suffer a relapse. Studies are underway to determine whether a critical threshold level of transcripts uniformly predicts for leukemia relapse.

POSTREMISSION THERAPY Induction of a durable first CR is critical to long-term disease-free survival in AML. However, without further therapy virtually all patients experience relapse. Once relapse has occurred, AML is generally curable only by SCT.

Postremission therapy is designed to eradicate residual leukemic cells to prevent relapse and prolong survival. Postremission therapy in AML is often based on age (younger than 55–65 and older than 55–65). For younger patients, most studies include intensive chemotherapy and allogeneic or autologous SCT. High-dose cytarabine is more effective than standard-dose cytarabine. The Cancer and Leukemia Group B (CALGB), for example, compared the duration of CR in patients randomly assigned postremission to four cycles of high (3 g/m^2, every 12 h on days 1, 3, and 5), intermediate (400 mg/m^2 for 5 days by continuous infusion), or standard (100 mg/m^2 per day for 5 days by continuous infusion) doses of cytarabine. A dose-response effect for cytarabine in patients with AML who were ≤60 years was demonstrated. High-dose cytarabine significantly prolonged CR and increased the fraction cured in patients with favorable [t(8;21) and inv(16)] and normal cytogenetics, but it had no significant effect on patients with other abnormal karyotypes. For older patients, exploration of attenuated intensive therapy that includes either chemotherapy or reduced intensity allogeneic SCT has been pursued. Postremission therapy is a setting for introduction of new agents **(Table 104-3)**.

Allogeneic SCT is used in patients <70 years old with an HLA-compatible donor who have high-risk cytogenetics. In the subset with normal cytogenetics and high-risk molecular features such as *FLT3* ITD, allogeneic SCT is best applied in the context of clinical trials, as the impact of aggressive therapy on outcome is unknown. Relapse following allogeneic SCT occurs in only a small fraction of patients, but toxicity is relatively high from treatment; complications include venoocclusive disease, GVHD, and infections. Autologous transplantation can be administered in young and older patients and uses the same preparative regimens. Patients subsequently receive their own stem cells collected while in remission. The toxicity is lower with autologous SCT (5% mortality rate), but the relapse rate is higher than with allogeneic SCT, and randomized studies have not demonstrated outcome superior to postremission conventional-dose chemotherapy. The increased relapse rate is due to the absence of the graft-versus-leuke-

TABLE 104-3	SELECTED NEW AGENTS UNDER STUDY FOR TREATMENT OF ADULTS WITH AML
Class of Drugs	**Example Agent(s)**
MDR1 modulators	Cyclosporine, LY335979
Demethylating agents	Decitabine, 5-azacytidine, zebularine
Histone deacetylase inhibitors	Suberoylanilide hydroxamic acid (SAHA), MS275, LBH589, valproic acid
Heavy metals	Arsenic trioxide, antimony
Farnesyl transferase inhibitors	R115777, SCH66336
FLT3 inhibitors	SU11248, PKC412, MLN518, CHIR-258
HSP-90 antagonists	17-allylaminogeldanamycin (17-AAG) or derivatives
BCR-ABL PDGFR/KIT inhibitors	Imatinib (ST1571, Gleevec), dasatinib, nilotinib
Telomerase inhibitor	GRN163L
Cell cycle inhibitors	Flavopiridol, CYC202 (R-Roscovitine), SNS-032
Nucleoside analogues	Clofarabine, troxacitabine
Humanized antibodies	Anti-CD33 (SGN33), anti-DR4, anti-DR5, anti-KiR
Toxin-conjugated antibodies	Gemtuzumab ozogamicin (Mylotarg)
Radiolabeled antibodies	Yttrium-90-labeled human M195

mia (GVL) effect seen with allogeneic SCT and possible contamination of the autologous stem cells with tumor cells. Purging tumor from the autologous stem cells has not lowered the relapse rate with autologous SCT.

Randomized trials comparing intensive chemotherapy and autologous and allogeneic SCT have shown improved duration of remission with allogeneic SCT compared to autologous SCT or chemotherapy alone. However, overall survival is generally not different; the improved disease control with allogeneic SCT is erased by the increase in fatal toxicity. While stem cells were previously harvested from the bone marrow, virtually all efforts currently collect these from the blood following mobilization regimens, including growth factors with or without chemotherapy. Prognostic factors may help select patients in first CR for whom transplant is most effective.

Our approach includes considering allogeneic SCT in first CR for patients with high-risk karyotypes. Patients with normal karyotypes who have other poor risk factors (e.g., an antecedent hematologic disorder, failure to attain remission with a single induction course, PTD of the MLL gene, ITD of the FLT3 gene, overexpression of BAALC) are also potential candidates. If a suitable HLA donor does not exist, novel therapeutic approaches are considered. Other novel transplant strategies, including reduced-intensity SCT, are being explored for consolidation of high-risk AML patients. Patients with t(8;21) and inv(16) are treated with repetitive doses of high-dose cytarabine, which offers a high frequency of cure without the morbidity of transplant. In AML patients with t(8;21) and inv(16), those with KIT mutations may be considered for novel investigational studies.

Autologous SCT is generally applied to AML patients only in the context of a clinical trial or when the risk of repetitive intensive chemotherapy represents a higher risk than the autologous SCT (e.g., in patients with severe platelet alloimmunization).

RELAPSE Once relapse occurs, patients are rarely cured with further standard-dose chemotherapy. Patients eligible for allogeneic SCT should receive transplants expeditiously at the first sign of relapse. Long-term disease-free survival is approximately the same (30–50%) with allogeneic SCT in first relapse or in second remission. Autologous SCT rescues about 20% of relapsed patients with AML who have chemosensitive disease. The most important factors predicting response at relapse are the length of the previous CR, whether initial CR was achieved with one or two courses of chemotherapy, and the type of postremission therapy.

Because of the poor outcome of patients in early first relapse (<12 months), it is justified (for patients without HLA-compatible donors) to explore innovative approaches, such as new drugs or immunotherapies (Table 104-3). Patients with longer first CR (>12 months) generally relapse with drug-sensitive disease and have a higher chance of attaining a CR. However, cure is uncommon, and treatment with novel approaches should be considered if SCT is not possible. One promising therapy is decitabine, a nucleoside analog that inhibits DNA methyltransferase and subsequently reverses aberrant methylation in AML cells. Interestingly, inhibiting DNA methyltransferase occurs at a much lower dose than previously used to produce a cytotoxic effect in AML. Low-dose decitabine yields CR in a small subset of patients with relapsed AML, including those with unfavorable karyotypes. New agents are needed.

For elderly patients (age >60) for whom clinical trials are not available, gemtuzumab ozogamicin (Mylotarg) is another alternative. This therapy is an antibody-targeted chemotherapy consisting of the humanized anti-CD33 antibody linked to calicheamicin, a potent antitumor antibiotic. The CR rate is ~30%. Its effectiveness in early relapsing (<6 months) or refractory AML patients is limited, possibly due to calicheamicin being a potent MDR1 substrate. Toxicity, including myelosuppression, infusion toxicity, and venoocclusive disease, can be observed with gemtuzumab ozogamicin. Pretreatment with glucocorticoids can diminish many of the infusion reactions associated with gemtuzumab ozogamicin. Studies are examining this treatment in combination with chemotherapy for both young and older patients with previously untreated AML.

CHRONIC MYELOGENOUS LEUKEMIA

INCIDENCE

The incidence of chronic myelogenous leukemia (CML) is 1.5 per 100,000 people per year, and the age-adjusted incidence is higher in men than in women (2.0 versus 1.2). The incidence of CML increases slowly with age until the middle forties, when it starts to rise rapidly.

CML incidence for males decreased slightly (4.4%) between 1997 and 2003 as compared to 1977–1997.

DEFINITION

The diagnosis of CML is established by identifying a clonal expansion of a hematopoietic stem cell possessing a reciprocal translocation between chromosomes 9 and 22. This translocation results in the head-to-tail fusion of the breakpoint cluster region (BCR) gene on chromosome 22q11 with the ABL (named after the abelson murine leukemia virus) gene located on chromosome 9q34. Untreated, the disease is characterized by the inevitable transition from a chronic phase to an accelerated phase and on to blast crisis in a median time of 4 years.

ETIOLOGY

No clear correlation with exposure to cytotoxic drugs has been found, and no evidence suggests a viral etiology. In the pre-imatinib era, cigarette smoking accelerated the progression to blast crisis and therefore adversely affected survival in CML. Atomic bomb survivors had an increased incidence; the development of a CML cell mass of $10,000/\mu L$ took 6.3 years. No increase in CML incidence was found in the survivors of the Chernobyl accident, suggesting that only large doses of radiation can induce CML.

PATHOPHYSIOLOGY

The product of the fusion gene resulting from the t(9;22) plays a central role in the development of CML. This chimeric gene is transcribed into a hybrid BCR/ABL mRNA in which exon 1 of ABL is replaced by variable numbers of 5' BCR exons. Bcr/Abl fusion proteins, $p210^{BCR/ABL}$, are produced that contain NH_2-terminal domains of Bcr and the COOH-terminal domains of Abl. A rare breakpoint, occurring within the 3' region of the BCR gene, yields a fusion protein of 230 kDa, $p230^{BCR/ABL}$. Bcr/Abl fusion proteins can transform hematopoietic progenitor cells in vitro. Furthermore, reconstituting lethally irradiated mice with bone marrow cells infected with retrovirus carrying the gene encoding the $p210^{BCR/ABL}$ leads to the development of a myeloproliferative syndrome resembling CML in 50% of the mice. Specific antisense oligomers to the BCR/ABL junction inhibit the growth of t(9;22)-positive leukemic cells without affecting normal colony formation.

The mechanism(s) by which $p210^{BCR/ABL}$ promotes the transition from the benign state to the fully malignant one is still unclear. Messenger RNA for BCR/ABL can occasionally be detected in normal individuals. However, attachment of the BCR sequences to ABL results in three critical functional changes: (1) the Abl protein becomes constitutively active as a tyrosine kinase (TK) enzyme, activating downstream kinases that prevent apoptosis; (2) the DNA-protein-binding activity of Abl is attenuated; and (3) the binding of Abl to cytoskeletal actin microfilaments is enhanced.

Disease Progression The events associated with transition to the acute phase, a common occurrence in the pre-imatinib era, were extensively studied. Chromosomal instability of the malignant clone, resulting, for example, in the acquisition of an additional t(9;22), trisomy 8, or 17p- (p53 loss), is a basic feature of CML. Acquisition of these additional genetic and/or molecular abnormalities is critical to the phenotypic transformation. Large deletions adjacent to the translocation breakpoint on the derivative 9 chromosome, detected by microsatellite polymerase chain reaction (PCR) or FISH, are associated with shorter survival times. Heterogeneous structural alterations of the p53 gene, as well as structural alterations and lack of protein production of the retinoblastoma gene and the catalytic component of telomerase, have been associated with disease progression in a subset of patients. Rare patients show alterations in the rat sarcoma viral oncogene homolog (RAS). Sporadic reports also document the presence of an altered MYC (named after the myelocytomatosis virus) gene. Progressive de novo DNA methylation at the BCR/ABL locus and hypomethylation of the LINE-1 retrotransposon promoter herald blastic transformation. Further, interleukin 1β may be involved in the progression of CML to the blastic phase. In addition, functional inactivation of the tumor suppressor protein phosphatase A2 may be required for blastic transformation. Finally, CML that develops resistance to imatinib is at an increased risk of progressing to accelerated/blast crisis. Multiple pathways to disease transformation exist, but the exact timing and relevance of each remain unclear.

CLINICAL PRESENTATION

Symptoms The clinical onset of the chronic phase is generally insidious. Accordingly, some patients are diagnosed while still asymptomatic, during health-screening tests; other patients present with fatigue, malaise, and weight loss or have symptoms resulting from splenic enlargement, such as early satiety and left upper quadrant pain or mass. Less common are features related to granulocyte or platelet dysfunction, such as infections, thrombosis, or bleeding. Occasionally, patients present with leukostatic manifestations due to severe leukocytosis or thrombosis such as vasoocclusive disease, cerebrovascular accidents, myocardial infarction, venous thrombosis, priapism, visual disturbances, and pulmonary insufficiency. Patients with p230$^{BCR/ABL}$-positive CML have a more indolent course.

Progression of CML is associated with worsening symptoms. Unexplained fever, significant weight loss, increasing dose requirement of the drugs controlling the disease, bone and joint pain, bleeding, thrombosis, and infections suggest transformation into accelerated or blastic phases. Fewer than 10–15% of newly diagnosed patients present with accelerated disease or with de novo blastic phase CML.

Physical Findings Minimal to moderate splenomegaly is the most common physical finding; mild hepatomegaly is found occasionally. Persistent splenomegaly despite continued therapy is a sign of disease acceleration. Lymphadenopathy and myeloid sarcomas are unusual except late in the course of the disease; when they are present, the prognosis is poor.

Hematologic Findings Elevated white blood cell counts (WBCs), with increases in both immature and mature granulocytes, are present at diagnosis. Usually <5% circulating blasts and <10% blasts and promyelocytes are noted with the majority of cells being myelocytes, metamyelocytes and band forms. Cycling of the counts may be observed in patients followed without treatment. Platelet counts are almost always elevated at diagnosis, and a mild degree of normocytic normochromic anemia is present. Leukocyte alkaline phosphatase is low in CML cells. Serum levels of vitamin B$_{12}$ and vitamin B$_{12}$–binding proteins are elevated. Phagocytic functions are usually normal at diagnosis and remain normal during the chronic phase. Histamine production secondary to basophilia is increased in later stages, causing pruritus, diarrhea, and flushing.

At diagnosis, bone marrow cellularity is increased, with an increased myeloid to erythroid ratio. The marrow blast percentage is generally normal or slightly elevated. Marrow or blood basophilia, eosinophilia, and monocytosis may be present. While collagen fibrosis in the marrow is unusual at presentation, significant degrees of reticulin stain–measured fibrosis are noted in about half of patients.

Disease acceleration is defined by the development of increasing degrees of anemia unaccounted for by bleeding or therapy; cytogenetic clonal evolution; or blood or marrow blasts between 10 and 20%, blood or marrow basophils ≥20%, or platelet count <100,000/μL. *Blast crisis* is defined as acute leukemia, with blood or marrow blasts ≥20%. Hyposegmented neutrophils may appear (Pelger-Huet anomaly). Blast cells can be classified as myeloid, lymphoid, erythroid, or undifferentiated, based on morphologic, cytochemical, and immunologic features. Occurrence of de novo blast crisis or following imatinib therapy is rare.

Chromosomal Findings The cytogenetic hallmark of CML, found in 90–95% of patients, is the t(9;22)(q34;q11.2). Originally, this was recognized by the presence of a shortened chromosome 22 (22q-), designated as the *Philadelphia chromosome*, that arises from the reciprocal t(9;22). Some patients may have complex translocations (designated as *variant translocations*) involving three, four, or five chromosomes (usually including chromosomes 9 and 22). However, the molecular consequences of these changes are similar to those resulting from the

typical t(9;22). All patients should have evidence of the translocation molecularly or by cytogenetics or FISH to make a diagnosis of CML.

PROGNOSTIC FACTORS

The clinical outcome of patients with CML is variable. Before imatinib mesylate, death was expected in 10% of patients within 2 years and in about 20% yearly thereafter, and the median survival time was ~4 years. Therefore, several prognostic models that identify different risk groups in CML were developed. The most commonly used staging systems have been derived from multivariate analyses of prognostic factors. The *Sokal index* identified percentage of circulating blasts, spleen size, platelet count, age, and cytogenetic clonal evolution as the most important prognostic indicators. This system was developed based on chemotherapy-treated patients. The *Hasford system* was developed on interferon (IFN) α–treated patients. It identified percentage of circulating blasts, spleen size, platelet count, age, and percentage of eosinophils and basophils as the most important prognostic indicators. This system differs from the Sokal index by ignoring clonal evolution and incorporating percentage of eosinophils and basophils. When applied to a data set of 272 patients treated with IFN-α, the Hasford system was better than the Sokal score for predicting survival time; it identified more low-risk patients but left only a small number of cases in the high-risk group. Preliminary results suggest that both the Sokal and the Hasford systems are applicable to imatinib-treated patients.

Rx CHRONIC MYELOGENOUS LEUKEMIA

The therapy of CML is changing rapidly because we have a proven curative treatment (allogeneic transplantation) that has significant toxicity and a new targeted treatment (imatinib) with excellent outcome based on 5-year follow-up data. Therefore, physician experience and patient preference must be factored into the treatment selection process. Discussion of both treatment options with a patient is indicated. The decision should focus on the outcomes, risks, and toxicities of the various approaches.

At present, the goal of therapy in CML is to achieve prolonged, durable, nonneoplastic, nonclonal hematopoiesis, which entails the eradication of any residual cells containing the *BCR/ABL* transcript. Hence the goal is complete molecular remission and cure. A proposed imatinib treatment algorithm for the newly diagnosed CML patient is presented in **Table 104-4**.

TABLE 104-4 IMATINIB TREATMENT MILESTONES FOR NEWLY DIAGNOSED CML PATIENTS

	Proposed Course of Action^a	
	Transplantation from an HLA-compatible (related or unrelated) donor, dasatinib, new drugs	Continue same^b or increase dose^c
Time, months	**Milestones**	
3	No complete hematologic remission	Complete hematologic remission^{b,d}
6	No cytogenetic remission	Any cytogenetic remission^c
12	Minor^e or no cytogenetic remission	Complete^{b,f} or partial^{c,g} cytogenetic remission
18	Partial, minor, or no cytogenetic remission	Complete cytogenetic remission^b
Anytime	Loss of previously achieved hematologic, cytogenetic, or molecular remission	

^{a}Nutritional Comprehensive Cancer Network, Chronic myelogenous leukemia.
^{b}Denotes that at the indicated milestones, patients should stay on the same dose.
^{c}Denotes that at the indicated milestones, for patients on 400 mg/d, one can either continue the same or increase the dose to a maximum of 600–800 mg, as tolerated.
^{d}Complete hematologic remission, WBC <10,000/μL, normal blood morphology, hemoglobin and platelet counts, and disappearance of splenomegaly.
^{e}Minor cytogenetic remission, 36–85% bone marrow metaphases with t(9;22).
^{f}Complete cytogenetic remission, no bone marrow metaphases with t(9;22).
^{g}Partial cytogenetic remission, 1–35% bone marrow metaphases with t(9;22).
Abbreviations: HLA, human leukocyte antigen; WBC, white blood cell count.

ALLOGENEIC SCT Allogeneic SCT is complicated by early mortality owing to the transplant procedure. Outcome of SCT depends on multiple factors including: (1) the patient (e.g., age and phase of disease); (2) the type of donor [e.g., syngeneic (monozygotic twins) or HLA-compatible allogeneic, related or unrelated]; (3) the preparative regimen (myeloablative or reduced intensity); (4) GVHD; and (5) posttransplantation treatment.

The Patient Patients should have acceptable end-organ function, be <70 years, and have a healthy, histocompatible donor. Furthermore, survival after SCT in the accelerated and blastic phases of the disease is significantly diminished and is associated with high rates of relapse. Bone marrow transplantation (BMT) early in the chronic phase (1–2 years from diagnosis) is superior to later BMT. In the imatinib era, allogeneic transplantation should be used when possible for patients with accelerated/blastic phases of the disease or those whose disease fails to respond or progresses on imatinib.

The Donor Transplantation from a family donor, who is either fully matched or mismatched at only one HLA locus, should be considered for any patient with CML who is a candidate for an HLA-related sibling transplant. Syngeneic BMT in patients with chronic-phase CML results in 7-year disease-free survival in 55% of patients, with a 30% relapse rate. BMT with an HLA-identical sibling in the chronic phase achieves 5-year disease-free survival in 40–70% of patients, with a 25% relapse rate. BMT from an HLA-matched unrelated donor in chronic phase <1 year from diagnosis and <30 years of age results in 5-year disease-free survival similar to matched-sibling donor transplantation. For all other groups, patients receiving BMT from unrelated donors have higher rates of graft failure and acute and chronic GVHD and prolonged convalescence after treatment, compared to those who receive allogeneic transplants from related donors.

Sex mismatch has an adverse effect on transplantation, with worse outcome associated with a female donor and male recipient. This has been attributed to GVHD against the male histocompatibility Y antigen.

Peripheral blood is now being studied as a source of hematopoietic progenitor cells; it may offer rapid engraftment and less risk for the donor. With unrelated donors, some studies demonstrated no difference in GVHD and improved disease-free survival when comparing peripheral blood to bone marrow stem cells. Using matched sibling donors in chronic-phase CML, marrow stem cells led to a higher cumulative incidence of relapse at 3 years, while peripheral blood stem cell recipients had a higher cumulative incidence of chronic GVHD. At the current time, some centers collect bone marrow and some peripheral blood from sibling donors for newly diagnosed chronic-phase CML patients. Patients with more advanced stages are offered peripheral blood SCT. Umbilical-cord blood may permit mismatched SCT with notably less GVHD; GVL effects do not appear to be impaired. A problem with cord blood is obtaining a sufficient number of progenitor cells to reconstitute hematopoiesis in an adult.

Preparative Regimens Myeloablative regimens have been studied by several groups. Cyclophosphamide plus total-body irradiation is comparable to busulphan plus cyclophosphamide in the 3-year probabilities of survival, relapse, event-free survival, speed of engraftment, and incidence of venooclusive disease of the liver. Significantly more patients in the total-body irradiation arm experienced major elevations of creatinine, acute GVHD, longer periods of fever, positive blood cultures, hospital admissions, and longer inpatient hospital stays. However, increased chronic GVHD, obstructive bronchiolitis, and alopecia were noted with busulphan. Measurement of busulphan levels revealed no significant association between busulphan levels and regimen-related toxicity, but low levels were associated with an increased risk of relapse. Intravenous busulphan allows better control of serum levels.

Reduced-intensity transplants in which the preparative regimen is aimed at eliminating host lymphocytes rather than bone marrow have been reported by numerous groups. No randomized trials comparing the two approaches have been published. Retrospective comparisons reveal that reduced-intensity conditioning regimens produce equivalent or acceptable results (in toxicity as well as outcome). Reduced toxicity with preserved antitumor efficacy is the goal, and therefore reduced-intensity transplantation is our recommendation.

Development and Type of GVHD Development of grade I GVHD (Chap. 108) decreases the risk of relapse compared to no GVHD. An even lower relapse rate was observed in patients with grade II GVHD but was accompanied by a substantially higher transplant-related mortality rate. The

decreased relapse rate may be caused by a GVL effect. Depletion of T lymphocytes from donor marrow can prevent GVHD but results in an increased risk of relapse, which exceeds the relapse rate after syngeneic SCT. Thus, T lymphocytes from the donor marrow mediate a significant antileukemic or GVL effect, and even syngeneic marrow may exhibit limited GVL activity in CML.

Posttransplantation Treatment *BCR/ABL* transcript levels have served as early predictors for hematologic relapse following transplantation. These should facilitate risk-adapted approaches with immunosuppression or TK inhibitor(s), or a combination of the two. Donor leukocyte infusions (without any preparative chemotherapy or GVHD prophylaxis) can induce hematologic and cytogenetic remissions in patients with CML who have relapsed after allogeneic SCT.

Imatinib can control CML that has recurred after allogeneic SCT but is sometimes associated with myelosuppression and recurrence of severe GVHD. Imatinib after allogeneic SCT is being studied for prevention of relapse in patients with advanced disease at the time of transplantation (i.e., patients at high risk for relapse), patients undergoing reduced-intensity transplants, or patients with slow reduction of *BCR/ABL* message following transplantation. Imatinib has also been combined with donor lymphocytes to induce rapid molecular remissions in CML patients with disease relapse after allogeneic SCT. Of interest are studies with newer TK inhibitors following transplantation for imatinib-resistant CML.

IMATINIB MESYLATE Imatinib mesylate (Gleevec) functions through competitive inhibition at the ATP binding site of the Abl kinase in the inactive conformation, which leads to inhibition of tyrosine phosphorylation of proteins involved in Bcr/Abl signal transduction. It shows specificity for Bcr/Abl, the receptor for platelet-derived growth factor, and Kit tyrosine kinases. Imatinib induces apoptosis in cells expressing Bcr/Abl.

In newly diagnosed CML, imatinib (400 mg/d) is more effective than IFN-α and cytarabine. The complete hematologic remission rate, at 18 months, of patients treated with imatinib was 97% compared to 69% in patients treated with IFN-α and cytarabine. Similarly, the complete cytogenetic remission rate was 76% with imatinib compared to 14% with IFN-α and cytarabine.

All imatinib-treated patients who achieved major molecular remission (26%), defined as ≥3 log reduction in *BCR/ABL* transcript level at 18 months compared to pretreatment level, were progression-free at 5 years. The progression-free survival (PFS) at 5 years for patients achieving complete cytogenetic remission but less pronounced molecular remission is 98%. The 5-year PFS for patients not achieving complete cytogenetic remission at 18 months was 87%. These results have led to a consensus that molecular responses can be used as a treatment goal in CML. Specific milestones have been developed for chronic-phase CML patients (Table 104-4). For example, chronic-phase CML patients who do not achieve any cytogenetic remission following six months of imatinib are unlikely to achieve major molecular remission and should be offered other treatment approaches.

Progression to accelerated/blastic phases of the disease was noted in 3% of patients treated with imatinib as compared to 8.5% of patients treated with IFN-α and cytarabine during the first year. Over time, the annual incidence of disease progression on imatinib decreased gradually to <1% during the fourth and fifth years, and no patient who achieved complete cytogenetic remission during the first year of imatinib treatment progressed to the accelerated/blastic phases of the disease.

Imatinib is administered orally. The main side effects are fluid retention, nausea, muscle cramps, diarrhea, and skin rashes. The management of these side effects is usually supportive. Myelosuppression is the most common hematologic side effect. Myelosuppression, while rare, may require holding drug and/or growth factor support. Doses <300 mg/d seem ineffective and may lead to development of resistance.

Four mechanisms of resistance to imatinib have been described to date. These are (1) gene amplification, (2) mutations at the kinase site, (3) enhanced expression of multidrug exporter proteins, and (4) alternative signaling pathways functionally compensating for the imatinib-sensitive mechanisms. All four mechanisms are being targeted in clinical trials.

BCR/ABL gene amplification and decreased intracellular imatinib concentrations are addressed by intensifying the therapy with higher (up to 800 mg/d) imatinib doses. Response in some patients has led to early intensification of imatinib dosage in newly diagnosed CML patients, resulting in improved major molecular remissions when retrospectively compared to controls treated with 400 mg/d. Randomized studies comparing 400 mg/d doses to 800 mg/d in newly diagnosed CML patients are ongoing.

Mutations at the kinase domain are being targeted by novel TK inhibitors that have a different conformation than imatinib, demonstrating activity against most imatinib-resistant mutations. Nilotinib (Tasigma), like imatinib, binds to the kinase domain in the inactive conformation. Dasatinib (Sprycel) binds to the kinase domain in the open conformation and also inhibits the SRC (sarcoma) family of kinases, addressing the last mechanism of resistance. CML with the T315I mutation is resistant to imatinib, nilotinib, and dasatinib.

Dasatinib is approved by the FDA for the treatment of all stages of CML with resistance or intolerance to prior therapy, including imatinib. Nilotinib will likely follow suit. Both are oral agents given twice daily, with toxicity profiles similar to imatinib with small but significant differences. Dasatinib was shown to cause pleural effusion in 22% of patients with 7% developing grade 3-4 toxicity. Nilotinib was associated with sudden death in six of approximately 550 CML patients. A suspected relationship to nilotinib was reported in two of these cases.

These new agents have changed the treatment algorithm of CML. For example, patients who do not achieve any cytogenetic remission at six months on imatinib will now be offered either dasatinib or SCT. IFN-α, though FDA-approved for CML, will only be offered if all other options have failed.

The encouraging results with imatinib have led clinicians to offer it as first-line therapy for newly diagnosed CML patients, including those who otherwise would have benefited from transplant (e.g., young patients with a matched sibling donor). Prior exposure to imatinib does not affect transplant outcome. However, delaying BMT for high-risk patients (Sokal/Hasford criteria) may result in disease progression. SCT after disease progression is associated with poorer outcome. Therefore, we recommend close monitoring of imatinib response, especially in these patients (Table 104-4).

INTERFERON   Before imatinib, when allogeneic SCT was not feasible, IFN-α therapy was the treatment of choice. Only longer follow-up of patients treated with imatinib will prove whether IFN-α will still have a role in the treatment of CML. Its mode(s) of action in CML is still unknown.

CHEMOTHERAPY   Initial management of patients with chemotherapy is currently reserved for rapid lowering of WBCs, reduction of symptoms, and reversal of symptomatic splenomegaly. Hydroxyurea, a ribonucleotide reductase inhibitor, induces rapid disease control. The initial dose is 1–4 g/d; the dose should be halved with each 50% reduction of the leukocyte count. Unfortunately, cytogenetic remissions with hydroxyurea are uncommon. Busulphan, an alkylating agent that acts on early progenitor cells, has a more prolonged effect. However, we do not recommend its use because of its serious side effects, which include unexpected, and occasionally fatal, myelosuppression in 5–10% of patients; pulmonary, endocardial, and marrow fibrosis; and an Addison-like wasting syndrome.

AUTOLOGOUS SCT   Autologous SCT could potentially cure CML if a means to select the residual normal progenitors, which coexist with their malignant counterparts, could be developed. As a source of autologous hematopoietic stem cells for transplantation, blood offers certain advantages over marrow (e.g., faster engraftment for the patient and no general anesthesia for the donor). Normal hematopoietic stem cells appear with increased frequency in the blood of patients with CML during the recovery phase after chemotherapy and G-CSF. A role for imatinib before stem cell collection to achieve minimal residual disease and following transplantation to maintain this status is currently being investigated. Specifically, several groups store peripheral blood stem cells from patients in major or complete molecular remissions. However, only a few cases have been transplanted following imatinib therapy. Therefore, such approaches should be performed only in clinical trials.

LEUKAPHERESIS AND SPLENECTOMY   Intensive leukapheresis may control the blood counts in chronic-phase CML; however, it is expensive and cumbersome. It is useful in emergencies where leukostasis-related complications such as pulmonary failure or cerebrovascular accidents are likely. It may also have a role in the treatment of pregnant women in whom it is important to avoid potentially teratogenic drugs.

Splenectomy was used in CML in the past because of the suggestion that evolution to the acute phase might occur in the spleen. However, this does not appear to be the case, and splenectomy is now reserved for symptomatic relief of painful splenomegaly unresponsive to imatinib or chemotherapy, or for significant anemia or thrombocytopenia associated with hypersplenism. Splenic radiation is used rarely to reduce the size of the spleen.

MINIMAL RESIDUAL DISEASE   The kinetics of *BCR/ABL* transcript elimination are currently replacing qualitative detection of the *BCR/ABL* message, in spite of a lack of standard acceptable methodology. A consensus panel has proposed ways to harmonize the different methods and to use a conversion factor so that individual laboratories will be able to express *BCR/ABL* transcript levels on an agreed upon scale.

Slow reduction of *BCR/ABL* transcripts following SCT correlates with the possibility of hematologic relapse. However, the definition of "slow reduction" depends on the preparative regimen (reduced-intensity versus fully myeloablative) and the selection of time-points to measure the transcript levels. While persistent RT-PCR positivity at 6 months was regarded as an indication for additional therapy in the past, current studies utilize periods between engraftment and day 100 for evaluating the clearance rate of *BCR/ABL* transcripts and recommending additional therapies. Large trials with longer follow-up are needed to establish consensus guidelines.

The randomized trial of imatinib versus IFN-α and cytarabine was the first to establish the concept of $\log_{10}$ reduction of *BCR/ABL* transcript from a standardized baseline for untreated patients. This measurement unit was developed instead of either the transcript numbers expressed per μg of leukocyte RNA or the ratio of *BCR/ABL* to a housekeeping gene on a log scale. In this randomized trial, patients who achieved $\geq$3 log reduction of BCR/ABL message had an extremely low probability of relapse, with a median follow-up of 60 months. It is unclear whether achieving complete molecular remission should still be the goal of treatment in this disease.

These studies also established the value and convenience of using peripheral blood instead of bone marrow testing as a means to assess disease status in patients who achieve complete cytogenetic responses. However, one still needs to consider following CML patients in complete cytogenetic remission and at least major molecular remission with annual cytogenetic bone marrow testing, as these patients are at risk of developing cytogenetic aberrations in t(9;22)-negative cells and secondary MDS/AML. These aberrations in the t(9;22)-negative cells are frequently transient, and their clinical significance is unclear. Such aberrations may occur in 7–10% of imatinib-treated patients. Development of MDS/AML is rare.

TREATMENT OF BLAST CRISIS   Treatments for primary blast crisis, including imatinib, are generally ineffective. Only 52% of patients treated with imatinib achieved hematologic remission (21% complete hematologic remission), and the median overall survival was 6.6 months. Patients who achieve complete hematologic remission or whose disease returns to a second chronic phase should be considered for allogeneic SCT. Other approaches include induction chemotherapy tailored to the phenotype of the blast cell followed by imatinib, with or without additional chemotherapy and SCT. Blast crisis following initial therapy with imatinib carries a dismal prognosis even if treated with dasatinib or nilotinib.

FURTHER READINGS

AML

FROHLING S et al: Genetics of myeloid malignancies: Pathogenetic and clinical implications. J Clin Oncol 23:6285, 2005

NATIONAL COMPREHENSIVE CANCER NETWORK: Acute myeloid leukemia. Clinical Practice Guidelines in Oncology, Version 1. 2006. *http://www.nccn.org/professionals/physician_gls/PDF/aml.pdf*

SANZ MA et al: Tricks of the trade for the appropriate management of newly diagnosed acute promyelocytic leukemia. Blood 105:3019, 2005

TALLMAN MS et al: Drug therapy for acute myeloid leukemia. Blood 106:1154, 2005

CML

CORTES J, KANTARJIAN H: New targeted approaches in chronic myeloid leukemia. J Clin Oncol 23:6316, 2005

HUGHES TP et al: Monitoring CML patients responding to treatment with tyrosine kinase inhibitors. Review and recommendations for 'harmonizing' current methodology for detecting BCR-ABL transcripts and kinase domain mutations and for expressing results. Blood 108:28, 2006

NATIONAL COMPREHENSIVE CANCER NETWORK: Chronic myelogenous leukemia. Clinical Practice Guidelines in Oncology, Version 1. 2007. *http://www.nccn.org/professionals/physician_gls/PDF/cml.pdf*

105 Malignancies of Lymphoid Cells
Dan L. Longo

Malignancies of lymphoid cells range from the most indolent to the most aggressive human malignancies. These cancers arise from cells of the immune system at different stages of differentiation, resulting in a wide range of morphologic, immunologic, and clinical findings. Insights on the normal immune system have allowed a better understanding of these sometimes confusing disorders.

Some malignancies of lymphoid cells almost always present as leukemia (i.e., primary involvement of bone marrow and blood), while others almost always present as lymphomas (i.e., solid tumors of the immune system). However, other malignancies of lymphoid cells can present as either leukemia or lymphoma. In addition, the clinical pattern can change over the course of the illness. This change is more often seen in a patient who seems to have a lymphoma and then develops the manifestations of leukemia over the course of the illness.

BIOLOGY OF LYMPHOID MALIGNANCIES: CONCEPTS OF THE WHO CLASSIFICATION OF LYMPHOID MALIGNANCIES

The classification of lymphoid cancers evolved steadily throughout the twentieth century. The distinction between leukemia and lymphoma was made early, and separate classification systems were developed for each. Leukemias were first divided into acute and chronic subtypes based on average survival. Chronic leukemias were easily subdivided into those of lymphoid or myeloid origin based on morphologic characteristics. However, a spectrum of diseases that were formerly all called *chronic lymphoid leukemia* has become apparent (Table 105-1). The acute leukemias were usually malignancies of blast cells with few identifying characteristics. When cytochemical stains became available, it was possible to divide these objectively into myeloid malignancies and acute leukemias of lymphoid cells. Acute leukemias of lymphoid cells have been subdivided based on morphologic characteristics by the French-American-British (FAB) group (Table 105-2). Using this system, lymphoid malignancies of small uniform blasts (e.g., typical childhood acute lymphoblastic leukemia) were called L1, lymphoid malignancies with larger and more variable size cells were called L2, and lymphoid malignancies of uniform cells with basophilic and sometimes vacuolated cytoplasm were called L3 (e.g., typical Burkitt's lymphoma cells). Acute leukemias of lymphoid cells have also been subdivided based on immunologic (i.e., T cell vs. B cell) and cytogenetic abnormalities (Table 105-2). Major cytogenetic subgroups include the t(9;22) (e.g., Philadelphia chromosome–positive acute lymphoblastic leukemia) and the t(8;14) found in the L3 or Burkitt's leukemia.

Non-Hodgkin's lymphomas were separated from Hodgkin's disease by recognition of the Sternberg-Reed cells early in the twentieth century. The histologic classification for non-Hodgkin's lymphomas has been one of the most contentious issues in oncology. Imperfect morphologic systems were supplanted by imperfect immunologic systems, and poor reproducibility of diagnosis has hampered progress. In 1999, the World Health Organization (WHO) classification of lymphoid malignancies was devised through a process of consensus development among international leaders in hematopathology and clinical

TABLE 105-2 CLASSIFICATION OF ACUTE LYMPHOID LEUKEMIA (ALL)

Immunologic Subtype	% of Cases	FAB Subtype	Cytogenetic Abnormalities
Pre-B ALL	75	L1, L2	t(9;22), t(4;11), t(1;19)
T cell ALL	20	L1, L2	14q11 or 7q34
B cell ALL	5	L3	t(8;14), t(8;22), t(2;8)

Note: FAB, French-American-British classification.

oncology. The WHO classification takes into account morphologic, clinical, immunologic, and genetic information and attempts to divide non-Hodgkin's lymphomas and other lymphoid malignancies into clinical/pathologic entities that have clinical and therapeutic relevance. This system is presented in Table 105-3. This system is clinically relevant and has a higher degree of diagnostic accuracy than those used previously. The possibilities for subdividing lymphoid malignancies are extensive. However, Table 105-3 presents in bold those malignancies that occur in at least 1% of patients. Specific lymphoma subtypes will be dealt with in more detail below. **Lymphomas associated with HIV infection are discussed in Chap. 182.**

GENERAL ASPECTS OF LYMPHOID MALIGNANCIES

ETIOLOGY AND EPIDEMIOLOGY
The relative frequency of the various lymphoid malignancies is shown in Fig. 105-1. Chronic lymphoid leukemia (CLL) is the most prevalent form of leukemia in western countries. It occurs most frequently in older adults and is exceedingly rare in children. In 2007, 15,340 new cases were diagnosed in the United States, but because of the prolonged survival associated with this disorder, the total prevalence is many times higher. CLL is more common in men than in women and more common in whites than in blacks. This is an uncommon malignancy in Asia. The etiologic factors for typical CLL are unknown.

In contrast to CLL, acute lymphoid leukemias (ALLs) are predominantly cancers of children and young adults. The L3 or Burkitt's leukemia occurring in children in developing countries seems to be associated with infection by the Epstein-Barr virus (EBV) in infancy. However, the explanation for the etiology of more common subtypes of ALL is much less certain. Childhood ALL occurs more often in higher socioeconomic subgroups. Children with trisomy 21 (Down's syndrome) have an increased risk for childhood acute lymphoblastic leukemia as well as acute myeloid leukemia. Exposure to high-energy radiation in early childhood increases the risk of developing T cell acute lymphoblastic leukemia.

The etiology of ALL in adults is also uncertain. ALL is unusual in middle-aged adults but increases in incidence in the elderly. However, acute myeloid leukemia is still much more common in older patients. Environmental exposures including certain industrial exposures, exposure to agricultural chemicals, and smoking might increase the risk of developing ALL as an adult. ALL was diagnosed in 5200 persons and AML in 13,410 persons in the United States in 2007.

The preponderance of evidence suggests that Hodgkin's disease is of B cell origin. The incidence of Hodgkin's disease appears fairly stable, with 8190 new cases diagnosed in 2007 in the United States. Hodgkin's disease is more common in whites than in blacks and more common in males than in females. A bimodal distribution of age at diagnosis has been observed, with one peak incidence occurring in patients in their twenties and the other in those in their eighties. Some of the late age peak may be attributed to confusion among entities with similar appearance such as anaplastic large cell lymphoma and T cell–rich B cell lymphoma. Patients in the younger age groups diagnosed in the United States largely have the nodular sclerosing subtype of Hodgkin's disease. Elderly patients, patients infected with HIV, and patients in third world countries more commonly have mixed-cellularity Hodgkin's disease or lymphocyte-depleted Hodgkin's disease. Infection by HIV is a risk factor for developing Hodgkin's disease. In addition, an association between infection by EBV and Hodgkin's disease has been suggested. A monoclonal or oligoclonal proliferation of EBV-

TABLE 105-1 LYMPHOID DISORDERS THAT CAN PRESENT AS "CHRONIC LEUKEMIA" AND BE CONFUSED WITH TYPICAL B CELL CHRONIC LYMPHOID LEUKEMIA

Follicular lymphoma	Prolymphocytic leukemia (B cell or T cell)
Splenic marginal zone lymphoma	
Nodal marginal zone lymphoma	Lymphoplasmacytic lymphoma
Mantle cell lymphoma	Sézary syndrome
Hairy cell leukemia	Smoldering adult T cell leukemia/lymphoma

TABLE 105-3 WHO CLASSIFICATION OF LYMPHOID MALIGNANCIES

B Cell	T Cell	Hodgkin's Disease
Precursor B cell neoplasm	Precursor T cell neoplasm	Nodular lymphocyte-pre-dominant Hodgkin's disease
Precursor B lymphoblastic leukemia/lymphoma (precursor B cell acute lymphoblastic leukemia)	**Precursor T lymphoblastic lymphoma/leukemia (precursor T cell acute lymphoblastic leukemia)**	
Mature (peripheral) B cell neoplasms	Mature (peripheral) T cell neoplasms	Classical Hodgkin's disease
B cell chronic lymphocytic leukemia/small lympho-cytic lymphoma	T cell prolymphocytic leukemia	Nodular sclerosis Hodgkin's disease
B cell prolymphocytic leukemia	T cell granular lymphocytic leukemia	Lymphocyte-rich clas-sic Hodgkin's disease
Lymphoplasmacytic lymphoma	Aggressive NK cell leukemia	Mixed-cellularity Hodgkin's disease
Splenic marginal zone B cell lym-phoma (± villous lymphocytes)	Adult T cell lymphoma/leukemia (HTLV-I+)	Lymphocyte-depletion Hodgkin's disease
Hairy cell leukemia	Extranodal NK/T cell lymphoma, nasal type	
Plasma cell myeloma/plasmacytoma	Enteropathy-type T cell lymphoma	
Extranodal marginal zone B cell lymphoma of MALT type	Hepatosplenic γδ T cell lymphoma	
Mantle cell lymphoma	Subcutaneous panniculitis-like T cell lymphoma	
Follicular lymphoma	**Mycosis fungoides/Sézary syndrome**	
Nodal marginal zone B cell lym-phoma (± monocytoid B cells)	Anaplastic large cell lymphoma, primary cutaneous type	
Diffuse large B cell lymphoma	**Peripheral T cell lymphoma, not otherwise specified (NOS)**	
Burkitt's lymphoma/Burkitt cell leukemia	**Angioimmunoblastic T cell lymphoma**	
	Anaplastic large cell lymphoma, primary systemic type	

Note: HTLV, human T cell lymphotropic virus; MALT, mucosa-associated lymphoid tissue; NK, natural killer; WHO, World Health Organization.
Malignancies in bold occur in at least 1% of patients.
Source: Adapted from Harris et al.

infected cells in 20–40% of the patients with Hodgkin's disease has led to proposals for this virus having an etiologic role in Hodgkin's disease. However, the matter is not settled definitively.

For unknown reasons, non-Hodgkin's lymphomas increased in frequency in the United States at the rate of 4% per year between 1950 and the late 1990s. The rate of increase in the past few years seems to be decreasing. About 63,190 new cases of non-Hodgkin's lymphoma were diagnosed in the United States in 2007. Non-Hodgkin's lymphomas are more frequent in the elderly and more frequent in men. Patients with both primary and secondary immunodeficiency states are predisposed to developing non-Hodgkin's lymphomas. These include patients with HIV infection; patients who have undergone organ transplantation; and patients with inherited immune deficiencies, the sicca syndrome, and rheumatoid arthritis.

The incidence of non-Hodgkin's lymphomas and the patterns of expression of the various subtypes differ geographically. T cell lymphomas are more common in Asia than in western countries, while certain subtypes of B cell lymphomas such as follicular lymphoma are more common in western countries. A specific subtype of non-Hodgkin's lymphoma known as the angiocentric nasal T/natural killer (NK) cell lymphoma has a striking geographic occurrence, being most frequent in Southern Asia and parts of Latin America. Another subtype of non-Hodgkin's lymphoma associated with infection by human T cell lymphotropic virus (HTLV) I is seen particularly in southern Japan and the Caribbean (Chap. 181).

A number of environmental factors have been implicated in the occurrence of non-Hodgkin's lymphoma, including infectious agents, chemical exposures, and medical treatments. Several studies have demonstrated an association between exposure to agricultural chemicals and an increased incidence in non-Hodgkin's lymphoma. Patients treated for Hodgkin's disease can develop non-Hodgkin's lymphoma; it is unclear whether this is a consequence of the Hodgkin's disease or its treatment. However, a number of non-Hodgkin's lymphomas are associated with infectious agents (Table 105-4). HTLV-I infects T cells and leads directly to the development of adult T cell lymphoma (ATL) in a small percentage of infected patients. The cumulative lifetime risk of developing lymphoma in an infected patient is 2.5%. The virus is transmitted by infected lymphocytes ingested by nursing babies of infected mothers, blood-borne transmission, or sexually. The median age of patients with ATL is ~56 years, emphasizing the long latency. HTLV-I is also the cause of tropical spastic paraparesis—a neurologic disorder that occurs somewhat more frequently than lymphoma and with shorter latency and usually from transfusion-transmitted virus (Chap. 181).

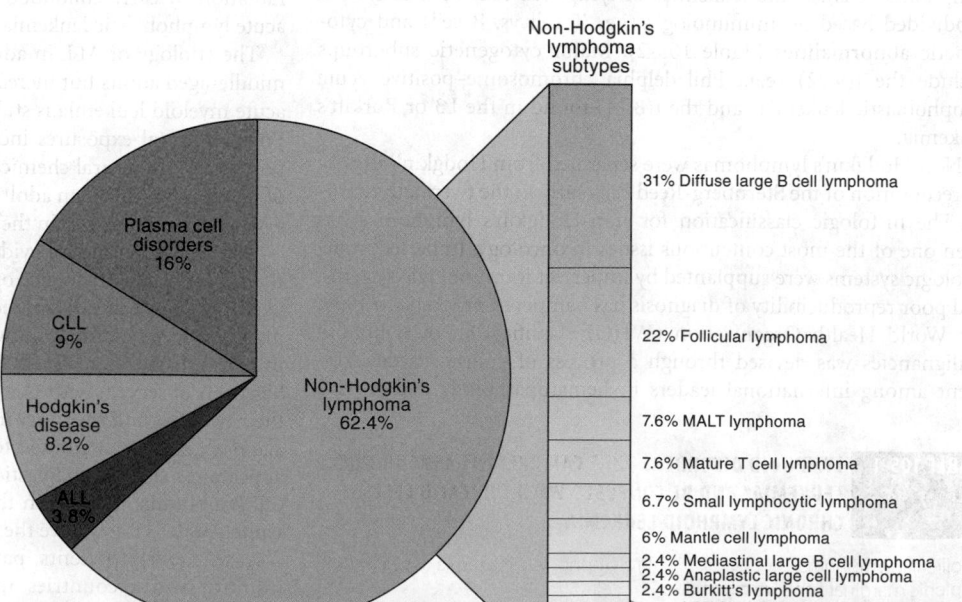

FIGURE 105-1 Relative frequency of lymphoid malignancies.

TABLE 105-4	INFECTIOUS AGENTS ASSOCIATED WITH THE DEVELOPMENT OF LYMPHOID MALIGNANCIES

Infectious Agent	Lymphoid Malignancy
Epstein-Barr virus	Burkitt's lymphoma
	Post–organ transplant lymphoma
	Primary CNS diffuse large B cell lymphoma
	Hodgkin's disease
	Extranodal NK/T cell lymphoma, nasal type
HTLV-I	Adult T cell leukemia/lymphoma
HIV	Diffuse large B cell lymphoma
	Burkitt's lymphoma
Hepatitis C virus	Lymphoplasmacytic lymphoma
Helicobacter pylori	Gastric MALT lymphoma
Human herpesvirus 8	Primary effusion lymphoma
	Multicentric Castleman's disease

Note: CNS, central nervous system; HTLV, human T cell lymphotropic virus; MALT, mucosa-associated lymphoid tissue, NK, natural killer.

TABLE 105-5	DISEASES OR EXPOSURES ASSOCIATED WITH INCREASED RISK OF DEVELOPMENT OF MALIGNANT LYMPHOMA

Inherited immunodeficiency disease	Autoimmune disease
Klinefelter's syndrome	Sjögren's syndrome
Chédiak-Higashi syndrome	Celiac sprue
Ataxia telangiectasia syndrome	Rheumatoid arthritis and
Wiscott-Aldrich syndrome	systemic lupus erythematosus
Common variable immuno-deficiency disease	Chemical or drug exposures
	Phenytoin
Acquired immunodeficiency diseases	Dioxin, phenoxyherbicides
Iatrogenic immunosuppression	Radiation
HIV-1 infection	Prior chemotherapy and
Acquired hypogammaglobulinemia	radiation therapy

EBV is associated with the development of Burkitt's lymphoma in Central Africa and the occurrence of aggressive non-Hodgkin's lymphomas in immunosuppressed patients in western countries. The majority of primary central nervous system (CNS) lymphomas are associated with EBV. EBV infection is strongly associated with the occurrence of extranodal nasal T/NK cell lymphomas in Asia and South America. Infection with HIV predisposes to the development of aggressive, B cell non-Hodgkin's lymphoma. This may be through overexpression of interleukin 6 by infected macrophages. Infection of the stomach by the bacterium *Helicobacter pylori* induces the development of gastric MALT (mucosa-associated lymphoid tissue) lymphomas. This association is supported by evidence that patients treated with antibiotics to eradicate *H. pylori* have regression of their MALT lymphoma. The bacterium does not transform lymphocytes to produce the lymphoma; instead, a vigorous immune response is made to the bacterium, and the chronic antigenic stimulation leads to the neoplasia. MALT lymphomas of the skin may be related to *Borrelia* sp. infections, those of the eyes to *Chlamydophila psittaci*, and those of the small intestine to *Campylobacter jejuni*.

Chronic hepatitis C virus infection has been associated with the development of lymphoplasmacytic lymphoma. Human herpesvirus 8 is associated with primary effusion lymphoma in HIV-infected persons and multicentric Castleman's disease, a diffuse lymphadenopathy associated with systemic symptoms of fever, malaise, and weight loss.

In addition to infectious agents, a number of other diseases or exposures may predispose to developing lymphoma (Table 105-5).

IMMUNOLOGY

All lymphoid cells are derived from a common hematopoietic progenitor that gives rise to lymphoid, myeloid, erythroid, monocyte, and megakaryocyte lineages. Through the ordered and sequential activation of a series of transcription factors, the cell first becomes committed to the lymphoid lineage and then gives rise to B and T cells. About 75% of all lymphoid leukemias and 90%

of all lymphomas are of B cell origin. A cell becomes committed to B cell development when it begins to rearrange its immunoglobulin genes. The sequence of cellular changes, including changes in cell-surface phenotype, that characterizes normal B cell development is shown in Fig. 105-2. A cell becomes committed to T cell differentiation upon migration to the thymus and rearrangement of T cell antigen receptor genes. The sequence of the events that characterize T cell development is depicted in Fig. 105-3.

Although lymphoid malignancies often retain the cell-surface phenotype of lymphoid cells at particular stages of differentiation, this information is of little consequence. The so-called stage of differentiation of a malignant lymphoma does not predict its natural history. For example, the clinically most aggressive lymphoid leukemia is Burkitt's

FIGURE 105-2 Pathway of normal B cell differentiation and relationship to B cell lymphomas. HLA-DR, CD10, CD19, CD20, CD21, CD22, CD5, and CD38 are cell markers used to distinguish stages of development. Terminal transferase (TdT) is a cellular enzyme. Immunoglobulin heavy chain gene rearrangement (HCR) and light chain gene rearrangement or deletion (κR or D, λR or D) occur early in B cell development. The approximate normal stage of differentiation associated with particular lymphomas is shown. ALL, acute lymphoid leukemia; CLL, chronic lymphoid leukemia; SL, small lymphocytic lymphoma.

T CELL DIFFERENTIATION

THYMUS

T CELL MALIGNANCIES

Stage I Prothymocyte — CD: 2, 7, 38, 71 — Majority of T cell ALL

Stage II Thymocyte — CD: 1, 2, 4, 7, 8, 38 — Minority of T-ALL Majority of T-LL

Stage III Thymocyte — CD: 2, 3, 4/8, 5, 6, 7; TCR — Minority of T-LL Rare T-ALL

PERIPHERAL BLOOD AND NODES

Mature T Helper Cell — CD: 2, 3, 4, 5, 6, 7; TCR — Majority of T-CLL, CTCL, Sezary Cell, NHL

Mature T Cytotoxic/ Suppressor Cell — CD: 2, 3, 4, 5, 6, 7; TCR — Minority of T-CLL, NHL

FIGURE 105-3 Pathway of normal T cell differentiation and relationship to T cell lymphomas. CD1, CD2, CD3, CD4, CD5, CD6, CD7, CD8, CD38, and CD71 are cell markers used to distinguish stages of development. T cell antigen receptors (TCR) rearrange in the thymus, and mature T cells emigrate to nodes and peripheral blood. ALL, acute lymphoid leukemia; T-ALL, T cell ALL; T-LL, T cell lymphoblastic lymphoma; T-CLL, T cell chronic lymphoid leukemia; CTCL, cutaneous T cell lymphoma; NHL, non-Hodgkin's lymphoma.

leukemia, which has the phenotype of a mature follicle center IgM-bearing B cell. Leukemias bearing the immunologic cell-surface phenotype of more primitive cells (e.g., pre-B ALL, CD10+) are less aggressive and more amenable to curative therapy than the "more mature" appearing Burkitt's leukemia cells. Furthermore, the apparent stage of differentiation of the malignant cell does not reflect the stage at which the genetic lesions that gave rise to the malignancy developed. For example, follicular lymphoma has the cell-surface phenotype of a follicle center cell, but its characteristic chromosomal translocation, the t(14;18), which involves juxtaposition of the antiapoptotic *bcl-2* gene next to the immunoglobulin heavy chain gene (see below), had to develop early in ontogeny as an error in the process of immunoglobulin gene rearrangement. Why the subsequent steps that led to transformation became manifest in a cell of follicle center differentiation is not clear.

The major value of cell-surface phenotyping is to aid in the differential diagnosis of lymphoid tumors that appear similar by light microscopy. For example, benign follicular hyperplasia may resemble follicular lymphoma; however, the demonstration that all the cells bear the same immunoglobulin light chain isotype strongly suggests the mass is a clonal proliferation rather than a polyclonal response to an exogenous stimulus.

Malignancies of lymphoid cells are associated with recurring genetic abnormalities. While specific genetic abnormalities have not been identified for all subtypes of lymphoid malignancies, it is presumed that they exist. Genetic abnormalities can be identified at a variety of levels including gross chromosomal changes (i.e., translocations, additions, or deletions); rearrangement of specific genes that may or may not be apparent from cytogenetic studies; and overexpression, underexpression, or mutation of specific oncogenes. Altered expression or mutation of specific proteins is particularly important. Many lymphomas contain balanced chromosomal translocations involving the anti-

gen receptor genes; immunoglobulin genes on chromosomes 2, 14, and 22 in B cells; and T cell antigen receptor genes on chromosomes 7 and 14 in T cells. The rearrangement of chromosome segments to generate mature antigen receptors must create a site of vulnerability to aberrant recombination. B cells are even more susceptible to acquiring mutations during their maturation in germinal centers; the generation of antibody of higher affinity requires the introduction of mutations into the variable region genes in the germinal centers. Other nonimmunoglobulin genes, e.g., *bcl-6*, may acquire mutations as well.

In the case of diffuse large B cell lymphoma, the translocation t(14; 18) occurs in ~30% of patients and leads to overexpression of the *bcl-2* gene found on chromosome 18. Some other patients without the translocation also overexpress the BCL-2 protein. This protein is involved in suppressing apoptosis—i.e., the mechanism of cell death most often induced by cytotoxic chemotherapeutic agents. A higher relapse rate has been observed in patients whose tumors overexpress the BCL-2 protein, but not in those patients whose lymphoma cells show only the translocation. Thus, particular genetic mechanisms have clinical ramifications.

Table 105-6 presents the best documented translocations and associated oncogenes for various subtypes of lymphoid malignancies. In some cases, such as the association of the t(14;18) in follicular lymphoma, the t(2;5) in anaplastic large T/null cell lymphoma, the t(8;14) in Burkitt's lymphoma, and the t(11;14) in mantle cell lymphoma, the great majority of tumors in patients with these diagnoses display these abnormalities. In other types of lymphoma where a minority of the patients have tumors expressing specific genetic abnormalities, the defects may have prognostic significance. No specific genetic abnormalities have been identified in Hodgkin's disease other than aneuploidy.

In typical B cell CLL, trisomy 12 conveys a poorer prognosis. In ALL in both adults and children, genetic abnormalities have important prognostic significance. Patients whose tumor cells display the t(9;22) have a much poorer outlook than patients who do not have this translocation. Other genetic abnormalities that occur frequently in adults with ALL include the t(4;11) and the t(8;14). The t(4;11) is associated with younger age, female predominance, high white cell counts, and L1 morphology. The t(8;14) is associated with older age, male predominance, frequent CNS involvement, and L3 morphology. Both are associated with a poor prognosis. In childhood ALL, hyperdiploidy has been shown to have a favorable prognosis.

TABLE 105-6	CYTOGENETIC TRANSLOCATION AND ASSOCIATED ONCOGENES OFTEN SEEN IN LYMPHOID MALIGNANCIES	
Disease	**Cytogenetic Abnormality**	**Oncogene**
CLL/small lymphocytic lymphoma	t(14;15)(q32;q13)	—
MALT lymphoma	t(11;18)(q21;q21)	API2/MALT, BCL-10
Precursor B cell acute lymphoid leukemia	t(9;22)(q34;q11) or variant	BCR/ABL
	t(4;11)(q21;q23)	AF4, ALLI
Precursor acute lymphoid leukemia	t(9;22)	BCR, ABL
	t(1;19)	E2A, PBX
	t(17;19)	HLF, E2A
	t(5;14)	HOX11L2, CTIP2
Mantle cell lymphoma	t(11;14)(q13;q32)	BCL-1, IgH
Follicular lymphoma	t(14;18)(q32;q21)	BCL-2, IgH
Diffuse large cell lymphoma	t(3;-)(q27;-)[a]	BCL-6
	t(17;-)(p13;-)	p53
Burkitt's lymphoma, Burkitt's leukemia	t(8;-)(q24;-)[a]	C-MYC
CD30+ Anaplastic large cell lymphoma	t(2;5)(p23;q35)	ALK
Lymphoplasmacytoid lymphoma	t(9;14)(p13;q32)	PAX5, IgH

[a]Numerous sites of translocation may be involved with these genes.

Note: CLL, chronic lymphoid leukemia; MALT, mucosa-associated lymphoid tissue; IgH, immunoglobulin heavy chain.

Gene profiling using array technology allows the simultaneous assessment of the expression of thousands of genes. This technology provides the possibility to identify new genes with pathologic importance in lymphomas, the identification of patterns of gene expression with diagnostic and/or prognostic significance, and the identification of new therapeutic targets. Recognition of patterns of gene expression is complicated and requires sophisticated mathematical techniques. Early successes using this technology in lymphoma include the identification of previously unrecognized subtypes of diffuse large B cell lymphoma whose gene expression patterns resemble either those of follicular center B cells or activated peripheral blood B cells. Patients whose lymphomas have a germinal center B cell pattern of gene expression have a considerably better prognosis than those whose lymphomas have a pattern resembling activated peripheral blood B cells. This improved prognosis is independent of other known prognostic factors. Similar information is being generated in follicular lymphoma and mantle cell lymphoma. The challenge remains to provide information from such techniques in a clinically useful time frame.

APPROACH TO THE PATIENT:
Lymphoid Cell Malignancies

Regardless of the type of lymphoid malignancy, the initial evaluation of the patient should include performance of a careful history and physical examination. These will help confirm the diagnosis, identify those manifestations of the disease that might require prompt attention, and aid in the selection of further studies to optimally characterize the patient's status to allow the best choice of therapy. It is difficult to overemphasize the importance of a carefully done history and physical examination. They might provide observations that lead to reconsidering the diagnosis, provide hints at etiology, clarify the stage, and allow the physician to establish rapport with the patient that will make it possible to develop and carry out a therapeutic plan.

For patients with ALL, evaluation is usually completed after a complete blood count, chemistry studies reflecting major organ function, a bone marrow biopsy with genetic and immunologic studies, and a lumbar puncture. The latter is necessary to rule out occult CNS involvement. At this point, most patients would be ready to begin therapy. In ALL, prognosis is dependent upon the genetic characteristics of the tumor, the patient's age, the white cell count, and the patient's overall clinical status and major organ function.

In CLL, the patient evaluation should include a complete blood count, chemistry tests to measure major organ function, serum protein electrophoresis, and a bone marrow biopsy. However, some physicians believe that the diagnosis would not always require a bone marrow biopsy. Patients often have imaging studies of the chest and abdomen looking for pathologic lymphadenopathy. Patients with typical B cell CLL can be subdivided into three major prognostic groups. Those patients with only blood and bone marrow involvement by leukemia but no lymphadenopathy, organomegaly, or signs of bone marrow failure have the best prognosis. Those with lymphadenopathy and organomegaly have an intermediate prognosis, and patients with bone marrow failure, defined as hemoglobin <100 g/L (10 g/dL) or platelet count <100,000/μL, have the worst prognosis. The pathogenesis of the anemia or thrombocytopenia is important to discern. The prognosis is adversely affected when either or both of these abnormalities are due to progressive marrow infiltration and loss of productive marrow. However, either or both may be due to autoimmune phenomena or to hypersplenism that can develop during the course of the disease. These destructive mechanisms are usually completely reversible (glucocorticoids for autoimmune disease; splenectomy for hypersplenism) and do not influence disease prognosis.

Two popular staging systems have been developed to reflect these prognostic groupings (Table 105-7). Patients with typical B cell CLL can have their course complicated by immunologic abnormalities including autoimmune hemolytic anemia, autoimmune thrombocytopenia, and hypogammaglobulinemia. Patients with hypogammaglobulinemia benefit from regular (monthly) γ globulin administration. Because of expense, γ globulin is often withheld until the patient experiences a significant infection. These abnormalities do not have a clear prognostic significance and should not be used to assign a higher stage.

Two other features may be used to assess prognosis in B cell CLL, but neither has yet been incorporated into a staging classification. At least two subsets of CLL have been identified based on the cytoplasmic expression of ZAP-70; expression of this protein, which is usually expressed in T cells, identifies a subgroup with poorer prognosis. A less powerful subsetting tool is CD38 expression. CD38+ tumors tend to have a poorer prognosis than CD38− tumors.

The initial evaluation of a patient with Hodgkin's disease or non-Hodgkin's lymphoma is similar. In both situations, the determination of an accurate anatomic stage is an important part of the evaluation. The staging system is the Ann Arbor staging system originally developed for Hodgkin's disease (Table 105-8).

TABLE 105-7 STAGING OF TYPICAL B CELL LYMPHOID LEUKEMIA

Stage	Clinical Features	Median Survival, Years
RAI System		
0: Low risk	Lymphocytosis only in blood and marrow	>10
I: Intermediate risk	Lymphocytosis + lymphadenopathy + splenomegaly ± hepatomegaly	7
II		
III: High risk	Lymphocytosis + anemia	1.5
IV	Lymphocytosis + thrombocytopenia	
Binet System		
A	Fewer than three areas of clinical lymphadenopathy; no anemia or thrombocytopenia	>10
B	Three or more involved node areas; no anemia or thrombocytopenia	7
C	Hemoglobin ≤10 g/dL and/or platelets <100,000/μL	2

TABLE 105-8 THE ANN ARBOR STAGING SYSTEM FOR HODGKIN'S DISEASE

Stage	Definition
I	Involvement of a single lymph node region or lymphoid structure (e.g., spleen, thymus, Waldeyer's ring)
II	Involvement of two or more lymph node regions on the same side of the diaphragm (the mediastinum is a single site; hilar lymph nodes should be considered "lateralized" and, when involved on both sides, constitute stage II disease)
III	Involvement of lymph node regions or lymphoid structures on both sides of the diaphragm
III₁	Subdiaphragmatic involvement limited to spleen, splenic hilar nodes, celiac nodes, or portal nodes
III₂	Subdiaphragmatic involvement includes paraaortic, iliac, or mesenteric nodes plus structures in III₁
IV	Involvement of extranodal site(s) beyond that designated as "E" More than one extranodal deposit at any location Any involvement of liver or bone marrow
A	No symptoms
B	Unexplained weight loss of >10% of the body weight during the 6 months before staging investigation Unexplained, persistent, or recurrent fever with temperatures >38°C during the previous month Recurrent drenching night sweats during the previous month
E	Localized, solitary involvement of extralymphatic tissue, excluding liver and bone marrow

TABLE 105-9	INTERNATIONAL PROGNOSTIC INDEX FOR NHL

Five clinical risk factors:
  Age ≥ 60 years
  Serum lactate dehydrogenase levels elevated
  Performance status ≥2 (ECOG) or ≤ 70 (Karnofsky)
  Ann Arbor stage III or IV
  >1 site of extranodal involvement
Patients are assigned a number for each risk factor they have
Patients are grouped differently based upon the type of lymphoma
For diffuse large B cell lymphoma:

0, 1 factor = low risk:	35% of cases; 5-year survival, 73%
2 factors = low-intermediate risk:	27% of cases; 5-year survival, 51%
3 factors = high-intermediate risk:	22% of cases; 5-year survival, 43%
4, 5 factors = high risk:	16% of cases; 5-year survival, 26%

For diffuse large B cell lymphoma treated with R-CHOP:

0 factor = very good:	10% of cases; 5-year survival, 94%
1, 2 factors = good:	45% of cases; 5-year survival, 79%
3, 4, 5 factors = poor:	45% of cases; 5-year survival, 55%

FIGURE 105-5 Acute lymphoblastic leukemia. The cells are heterogeneous in size, have round or convoluted nuclei, high nuclear/cytoplasmic ratio, and absence of cytoplasmic granules.

Evaluation of patients with Hodgkin's disease will typically include a complete blood count; erythrocyte sedimentation rate; chemistry studies reflecting major organ function; CT scans of the chest, abdomen, and pelvis; and a bone marrow biopsy. Neither a positron emission tomography (PET) scan nor a gallium scan is absolutely necessary for primary staging, but one performed at the completion of therapy allows evaluation of persisting radiographic abnormalities, particularly the mediastinum. Knowing that the PET scan or gallium scan is abnormal before treatment can help in this assessment. In most cases, these studies will allow assignment of anatomic stage and the development of a therapeutic plan.

In patients with non-Hodgkin's lymphoma, the same evaluation described for patients with Hodgkin's disease is usually carried out. In addition, serum levels of lactate dehydrogenase (LDH) and β$_2$-microglobulin and serum protein electrophoresis are often included in the evaluation. Anatomic stage is assigned in the same manner as used for Hodgkin's disease. However, the prognosis of patients with non-Hodgkin's lymphoma is best assigned using the International Prognostic Index (IPI) (Table 105-9). This is a powerful predictor of outcome in all subtypes of non-Hodgkin's lymphoma. Patients are assigned an IPI score based on the presence or absence of five adverse prognostic factors and may have none or all five of these adverse prognostic factors. Figure 105-4 shows the prognostic significance of this score in 1300 patients with all types of non-Hodgkin's lymphoma. With the addition of rituximab to CHOP, treatment outcomes have improved and the original IPI has lost some of its discrimination power. A revised IPI has been proposed that better predicts outcome of rituximab plus chemotherapy-based programs (Table 105-9). CT scans are routinely used in the evaluation of patients with all subtypes of non-Hodgkin's lymphoma, but PET and gallium scans are much more useful in aggressive

subtypes such as diffuse large B cell lymphoma than in more indolent subtypes such a follicular lymphoma or small lymphocytic lymphoma. While the IPI does divide patients with follicular lymphoma into subsets with distinct prognoses, the distribution of such patients is skewed toward lower-risk categories. A follicular lymphoma–specific IPI (FLIPI) has been proposed that replaces performance status with hemoglobin level [<120 g/L (<12 g/dL)] and number of extranodal sites with number of nodal sites (more than four). Low risk (zero or one factor) was assigned to 36% of patients, intermediate risk (two factors) to 37%, and poor risk (more than two factors) to 27% of patients.

CLINICAL FEATURES, TREATMENT, AND PROGNOSIS OF SPECIFIC LYMPHOID MALIGNANCIES

PRECURSOR CELL B CELL NEOPLASMS

Precursor B Cell Lymphoblastic Leukemia/Lymphoma The most common cancer in childhood is B cell ALL. Although this disorder can also present as a lymphoma in either adults or children, presentation as lymphoma is rare.

The malignant cells in patients with precursor B cell lymphoblastic leukemia are most commonly of pre-B cell origin. Patients typically present with signs of bone marrow failure such as pallor, fatigue, bleeding, fever, and infection related to peripheral blood cytopenias. Peripheral blood counts regularly show anemia and thrombocytopenia but might show leukopenia, a normal leukocyte count, or leukocytosis based largely on the number of circulating malignant cells (Fig. 105-5). Extramedullary sites of disease are frequently involved in patients who present with leukemia, including lymphadenopathy, hepato- or splenomegaly, CNS disease, testicular enlargement, and/or cutaneous infiltration.

The diagnosis is usually made by bone marrow biopsy, which shows infiltration by malignant lymphoblasts. Demonstration of a pre-B cell immunophenotype (Fig. 105-2) and, often, characteristic cytogenetic abnormalities (Table 105-6) confirm the diagnosis. An adverse prognosis in patients with precursor B cell ALL is predicted by a very high white cell count, the presence of symptomatic CNS disease, and unfavorable cytogenetic abnormalities. For example, t(9;22), frequently found in adults with B cell ALL, has been associated with a very poor outlook. The bcr/abl kinase inhibitors have improved the prognosis.

℞ PRECURSOR B CELL LYMPHOBLASTIC LEUKEMIA

The treatment of patients with precursor B cell ALL involves remission induction with combination chemotherapy, a consolidation phase that includes administration of high-dose systemic therapy and treatment to eliminate disease in the CNS, and a period of continuing therapy to prevent relapse and effect cure. The overall cure rate in children is 90%, while ~50% of adults are long-term disease-free survivors. This reflects the high proportion of adverse cytogenetic abnormalities seen in adults with precursor B cell ALL.

Precursor B cell lymphoblastic lymphoma is a rare presentation of precursor B cell lymphoblastic malignancy. These patients often have a rapid transformation to leukemia and should be treated as though they had presented with leukemia. The few patients who present with the disease confined to lymph nodes have a high cure rate.

FIGURE 105-4 Relationship of International Prognostic Index (IPI) to survival. Kaplan-Meier survival curves for 1300 patients with various kinds of lymphoma stratified according to the IPI.

TABLE 105-10 **CLINICAL CHARACTERISTICS OF PATIENTS WITH COMMON TYPES OF NON-HODGKIN'S LYMPHOMAS (NHL)**

Disease	Median Age, years	Frequency in Children	% Male	Stage I/II vs III/IV, %	B Symptoms, %	Bone Marrow Involvement, %	Gastrointestinal Tract Involvement, %	% Surviving 5 years
B cell chronic lymphocytic leukemia/small lymphocytic lymphoma	65	Rare	53	9 vs 91	33	72	3	51
Mantle cell lymphoma	63	Rare	74	20 vs 80	28	64	9	27
Extranodal marginal zone B cell lymphoma of MALT type	60	Rare	48	67 vs 33	19	14	50	74
Follicular lymphoma	59	Rare	42	33 vs 67	28	42	4	72
Diffuse large B cell lymphoma	64	~25% of childhood NHL	55	54 vs 46	33	16	18	46
Burkitt's lymphoma	31	~30% of childhood NHL	89	62 vs 38	22	33	11	45
Precursor T cell lymphoblastic lymphoma	28	~40% of childhood NHL	64	11 vs 89	21	50	4	26
Anaplastic large T/null cell lymphoma	34	Common	69	51 vs 49	53	13	9	77
Peripheral T cell non-Hodgkin's lymphoma	61	~5% of childhood NHL	55	20 vs 80	50	36	15	25

Note: MALT, mucosa-associated lymphoid tissue.

MATURE (PERIPHERAL) B CELL NEOPLASMS

B Cell Chronic Lymphoid Leukemia/Small Lymphocytic Lymphoma B cell CLL/small lymphocytic lymphoma represents the most common lymphoid leukemia, and when presenting as a lymphoma, it accounts for ~7% of non-Hodgkin's lymphomas. Presentation can be as either leukemia or lymphoma. The major clinical characteristics of B cell CLL/small lymphocytic lymphoma are presented in Table 105-10.

The diagnosis of typical B cell CLL is made when an increased number of circulating lymphocytes (i.e., $>4 \times 10^9$/L and usually $>10 \times 10^9$/L) is found (Fig. 105-6) that are monoclonal B cells expressing the CD5 antigen. Finding bone marrow infiltration by the same cells confirms the diagnosis. The peripheral blood smear in such patients typically shows many "smudge" or "basket" cells, nuclear remnants of cells damaged by the physical shear stress of making the blood smear. If cytogenetic studies are performed, trisomy 12 is found in 25–30% of patients. Abnormalities in chromosome 13 are also seen.

If the primary presentation is lymphadenopathy and a lymph node biopsy is performed, pathologists usually have little difficulty in making the diagnosis of small lymphocytic lymphoma based on morphologic findings and immunophenotype. However, even in these patients, 70–75% will be found to have bone marrow involvement and circulating monoclonal B lymphocytes are often present.

The differential diagnosis of typical B cell CLL is extensive (Table 105-1). Immunophenotyping will eliminate the T cell disorders and can often help sort out other B cell malignancies. For example, only mantle cell lymphoma and typical B cell CLL are usually CD5 positive. Typical B cell small lymphocytic lymphoma can be confused with other B cell disorders including lymphoplasmacytic lymphoma (i.e., the tissue manifestation of Waldenström's macroglobulinemia), nodal marginal zone B cell lymphoma, and mantle cell lymphoma. In addition, some small lymphocytic lymphomas have areas of large cells that can lead to confusion with diffuse large B cell lymphoma. An expert hematopathologist is vital for making this distinction.

Typical B cell CLL is often found incidentally when a complete blood count is done for another reason. However, complaints that might lead to the diagnosis include fatigue, frequent infections, and new lymphadenopathy. The diagnosis of typical B cell CLL should be considered in a patient presenting with an autoimmune hemolytic anemia or autoimmune thrombocytopenia. B cell CLL has also been associated with red cell aplasia. When this disorder presents as lymphoma, the most common abnormality is asymptomatic lymphadenopathy, with or without splenomegaly. The staging systems predict prognosis in patients with typical B cell CLL (Table 105-7). The evaluation of a new patient with typical B cell CLL/small lymphocytic lymphoma will include many of the studies (Table 105-11) that are used in patients with other non-Hodgkin's lymphomas. In addition, particular attention needs to be given to detecting immune abnormalities such as autoimmune hemolytic anemia, autoimmune thrombocytopenia, hypogammaglobulinemia, and red cell aplasia. Molecular analysis of immunoglobulin gene sequences in CLL has demonstrated that about half the patients have tumors expressing mutated immunoglobulin genes and half have tumors expressing unmutated or germ-line immunoglobulin sequences. Patients with unmutated immunoglobulins tend to have a more aggressive clinical course and are less responsive to therapy. Unfortunately, immunoglobulin gene sequencing is not routinely available. CD38 expression is said to be low in the better-

FIGURE 105-6 Chronic lymphocytic leukemia. The peripheral white blood cell count is high due to increased numbers of small, well-differentiated, normal-appearing lymphocytes. The leukemia lymphocytes are fragile, and substantial numbers of broken, smudged cells are usually also present on the blood smear.

TABLE 105-11 **STAGING EVALUATION FOR NON-HODGKIN'S LYMPHOMA**

Physical examination
Documentation of B symptoms
Laboratory evaluation
    Complete blood counts
    Liver function tests
    Uric acid
    Calcium
    Serum protein electrophoresis
    Serum β_2-microglobulin
Chest radiograph
CT scan of abdomen, pelvis, and usually chest
Bone marrow biopsy
Lumbar puncture in lymphoblastic, Burkitt's, and diffuse large B cell lymphoma with positive marrow biopsy
Gallium scan (SPECT) or PET scan in large cell lymphoma

Note: SPECT, single photon emission CT; PET, positron emission tomography.

prognosis patients expressing mutated immunoglobulin and high in poorer-prognosis patients expressing unmutated immunoglobulin, but this test has not been confirmed as a reliable means of distinguishing the two groups. ZAP-70 expression correlates with the presence of unmutated immunoglobulin genes, but the assay is not yet standardized and widely available.

℞ B CELL CHRONIC LYMPHOID LEUKEMIA/SMALL LYMPHOCYTIC LYMPHOMA

Patients whose presentation is typical B cell CLL with no manifestations of the disease other than bone marrow involvement and lymphocytosis (i.e., Rai stage O and Binet stage A; Table 105-7) can be followed without specific therapy for their malignancy. These patients have a median survival >10 years, and some will never require therapy for this disorder. If the patient has an adequate number of circulating normal blood cells and is asymptomatic, many physicians would not initiate therapy for patients in the intermediate stage of the disease manifested by lymphadenopathy and/or hepatosplenomegaly. However, the median survival for these patients is ~7 years, and most will require treatment in the first few years of follow-up. Patients who present with bone marrow failure (i.e., Rai stage III or IV or Binet stage C) will require initial therapy in almost all cases. These patients have a serious disorder with a median survival of only 1.5 years. It must be remembered that immune manifestations of typical B cell CLL should be managed independently of specific antileukemia therapy. For example, glucocorticoid therapy for autoimmune cytopenias and γ globulin replacement for patients with hypogammaglobulinemia should be used whether or not antileukemia therapy is given.

Patients who present primarily with lymphoma and have a low IPI score have a 5-year survival of ~75%, but those with a high IPI score have a 5-year survival of <40% and are more likely to require early therapy.

The most common treatments for patients with typical B cell CLL/small lymphocytic lymphoma have been chlorambucil or fludarabine, alone or in combination. Chlorambucil can be administered orally with few immediate side effects, while fludarabine is administered IV and is associated with significant immune suppression. However, fludarabine is by far the more active agent and is the only drug associated with a significant incidence of complete remission. The combination of rituximab (375–500 mg/m^2 day 1), fludarabine (25 mg/m^2 days 2–4 on cycle 1 and 1–3 in subsequent cycles), and cyclophosphamide (250 mg/m^2 with fludarabine) achieves complete responses in 69% of patients, and those responses are associated with molecular remissions in half of the cases. Half the patients experience grade III or IV neutropenia. For young patients presenting with leukemia requiring therapy, regimens containing fludarabine are the treatment of choice. Because fludarabine is an effective second-line agent in patients with tumors unresponsive to chlorambucil, the latter agent is often chosen in elderly patients who require therapy. Many patients who present with lymphoma will receive a combination chemotherapy regimen used in other lymphomas such as CVP (cyclophosphamide, vincristine, and prednisone) or CHOP (cyclophosphamide, doxorubicin, vincristine, and prednisone), although fludarabine-containing regimens may be preferable. Alemtuzimab (anti-CD52) is an antibody with activity in the disease, but it kills both B and T cells and is associated with more immune compromise than rituximab. Young patients with this disease can be candidates for bone marrow transplantation. Allogeneic bone marrow transplantation can be curative but is associated with a significant treatment-related mortality. Mini-transplants using immunosuppressive rather than myeloablative doses of preparative drugs are being studied (Chap. 108). The use of autologous transplantation in patients with this disorder has been discouraging.

Extranodal Marginal Zone B Cell Lymphoma of MALT Type Extranodal marginal zone B cell lymphoma of MALT type (MALT lymphoma) makes up ~8% of non-Hodgkin's lymphomas. This small cell lymphoma presents in extranodal sites. It was previously considered a small lymphocytic lymphoma or sometimes a pseudolymphoma. The recognition that the gastric presentation of this lymphoma was associated with *H. pylori* infection was an important step in recognizing it as a separate entity. The clinical characteristics of MALT lymphoma are presented in Table 105-10.

The diagnosis of MALT lymphoma can be made accurately by an expert hematopathologist based on a characteristic pattern of infiltration of small lymphocytes that are monoclonal B cells and CD5 negative. In some cases, transformation to diffuse large B cell lymphoma occurs, and both diagnoses may be made in the same biopsy. The differential diagnosis includes benign lymphocytic infiltration of extranodal organs and other small cell B cell lymphomas.

MALT lymphoma may occur in the stomach, orbit, intestine, lung, thyroid, salivary gland, skin, soft tissues, bladder, kidney, and CNS. It may present as a new mass, be found on routine imaging studies, or be associated with local symptoms such as upper abdominal discomfort in gastric lymphoma. Most MALT lymphomas are gastric in origin. At least two genetic forms of gastric MALT exist: one (accounting for ~50% of cases) characterized by t(11;18)(q21;q21) that juxtaposes the amino terminal of the *API2* gene with the carboxy terminal of the *MALT1* gene creating an API2/MALT1 fusion product, and the other characterized by multiple sites of genetic instability including trisomies of chromosomes 3, 7, 12, and 18. About 95% of gastric MALT lymphomas are associated with *H. pylori* infection, and those that are do not usually express t(11;18). The t(11;18) usually results in activation of NF-κB, which acts a survival factor for the cells. Lymphomas with t(11;18) translocations are genetically stable and do not evolve to diffuse large B cell lymphoma. By contrast, t(11;18)-negative MALT lymphomas often acquire *BCL6* mutations and progress to aggressive histology lymphoma. MALT lymphomas are localized to the organ of origin in ~40% of cases and to the organ and regional lymph nodes in ~30% of patients. However, distant metastasis can occur—particularly with transformation to diffuse large B cell lymphoma. Many patients who develop this lymphoma will have an autoimmune or inflammatory process such as Sjögren's syndrome (salivary gland MALT), Hashimoto's thyroiditis (thyroid MALT), *Helicobacter* gastritis (gastric MALT), *C. psittaci* conjunctivitis (ocular MALT), or *Borelia* skin infections (cutaneous MALT).

Evaluation of patients with MALT lymphoma follows the pattern (Table 105-11) for staging a patient with non-Hodgkin's lymphoma. In particular, patients with gastric lymphoma need to have studies performed to document the presence or absence of *H. pylori* infection. Endoscopic studies including ultrasound can help define the extent of gastric involvement. Most patients with MALT lymphoma have a good prognosis, with a 5-year survival of ~75%. In patients with a low IPI score, the 5-year survival is ~90%, while it drops to ~40% in patients with a high IPI score.

℞ MUCOSA-ASSOCIATED LYMPHOID TISSUE LYMPHOMA

MALT lymphoma is often localized. Local therapy such as radiation or surgery can effect cure, and this is one of the few times where surgery might be a reasonable primary therapy for a patient with non-Hodgkin's lymphoma. Patients with gastric MALT lymphomas who are infected with *H. pylori* can achieve remission in the majority of cases with eradication of the infection. These remissions can be durable, but molecular evidence of persisting neoplasia is frequent and the long-term outcome is uncertain. Patients who present with more extensive disease are most often treated with single-agent chemotherapy such as chlorambucil. Data on combination regimens that include rituximab are being generated, but its efficacy in other B cell tumors and low toxicity support its use. Coexistent diffuse large B cell lymphoma must be treated with combination chemotherapy (see below). The additional acquired mutations that mediate the histologic progression also convey *Helicobacter* independence to the growth.

Mantle Cell Lymphoma Mantle cell lymphoma makes up ~6% of all non-Hodgkin's lymphomas. This lymphoma was previously placed in a number of other subtypes. Its existence was confirmed by the recognition that these lymphomas have a characteristic chromosomal translocation, t(11;14), between the immunoglobulin heavy chain gene on chromosome 14 and the *bcl-1* gene on chromosome 11, and regularly overexpress the BCL-1 protein, also known as cyclin D1. Table 105-10 shows the clinical characteristics of mantle cell lymphoma.

The diagnosis of mantle cell lymphoma can be made accurately by an expert hematopathologist. As with all subtypes of lymphoma, an adequate biopsy is important. The differential diagnosis of mantle cell lymphoma includes other small cell B cell lymphomas. In particular, mantle cell lymphoma and small lymphocytic lymphoma share a characteristic expression of CD5. Mantle cell lymphoma usually has a slightly indented nucleus.

The most common presentation of mantle cell lymphoma is with palpable lymphadenopathy, frequently accompanied by systemic symptoms. Approximately 70% of patients will be stage IV at the time of diagnosis, with frequent bone marrow and peripheral blood involvement. Of the extranodal organs that can be involved, gastrointestinal involvement is particularly important to recognize. Patients who present with lymphomatosis polyposis in the large intestine usually have mantle cell lymphoma. Table 105-11 outlines the evaluation of patients with mantle cell lymphoma. Patients who present with gastrointestinal tract involvement often have Waldeyer's ring involvement, and vice versa. The 5-year survival for all patients with mantle cell lymphoma is ~25%, with only occasional patients who present with a high IPI score surviving 5 years and ~50% of patients with a low IPI score surviving 5 years.

℞ MANTLE CELL LYMPHOMA

Current therapies for mantle cell lymphoma are unsatisfactory. Patients with localized disease might be treated with combination chemotherapy followed by radiotherapy; however, these patients are exceedingly rare. For the usual presentation with disseminated disease, treatments have been unsatisfactory, with the minority of patients achieving complete remission. Aggressive combination chemotherapy regimens followed by autologous or allogeneic bone marrow transplantation are frequently offered to younger patients. For the occasional elderly, asymptomatic patient, observation followed by single-agent chemotherapy might be the most practical approach. An intensive combination chemotherapy regimen originally used in the treatment of acute leukemia, HyperC-VAD (cyclophosphamide, vincristine, doxorubicin, dexamethasone, cytarabine, and methotrexate), in combination with rituximab seems to be associated with better response rates—particularly in younger patients. CHOP plus rituximab has shown better response rates than CHOP alone, but long-term follow-up is lacking. Bortezomib induces transient partial responses in a minority of patients.

Follicular Lymphoma Follicular lymphomas make up 22% of non-Hodgkin's lymphomas worldwide and at least 30% of non-Hodgkin's lymphomas diagnosed in the United States. This type of lymphoma can be diagnosed accurately on morphologic findings alone and has been the diagnosis in the majority of patients in therapeutic trials for "low-grade" lymphoma in the past. The clinical characteristics of follicular lymphoma are presented in Table 105-10.

Evaluation of an adequate biopsy by an expert hematopathologist is sufficient to make a diagnosis of follicular lymphoma. The tumor is composed of small cleaved and large cells in varying proportions organized in a follicular pattern of growth (Fig. 105-7). Confirmation of B cell immunophenotype and the existence of the t(14;18) and abnormal expression of BCL-2 protein are confirmatory. The major differential diagnosis is between lymphoma and reactive follicular hyperplasia. The coexistence of diffuse large B cell lymphoma must be considered. Patients with follicular lymphoma are often subclassified into those with predominantly small cells, those with a mixture of small and large cells, and those with predominantly large cells. While this distinction cannot be made simply or very accurately, these subdivisions do have prognostic significance. Patients with follicular lymphoma with predominantly large cells have a higher proliferative fraction, progress more rapidly, and have a shorter overall survival with simple chemotherapy regimens.

The most common presentation for follicular lymphoma is with new, painless lymphadenopathy. Multiple sites of lymphoid involvement are typical, and unusual sites such as epitrochlear nodes are sometimes seen. However, essentially any organ can be involved, and extranodal presentations do occur. Most patients do not have fevers,

FIGURE 105-7 Follicular lymphoma. The normal nodal architecture is effaced by nodular expansions of tumor cells. Nodules vary in size and contain predominantly small lymphocytes with cleaved nuclei along with variable numbers of larger cells with vesicular chromatin and prominent nucleoli.

sweats, or weight loss, and an IPI score of 0 or 1 is found in ~50% of patients. Fewer than 10% of patients have a high (i.e., 4 or 5) IPI score. The staging evaluation for patients with follicular lymphoma should include the studies included in Table 105-11.

℞ FOLLICULAR LYMPHOMA

Follicular lymphoma is one of the malignancies most responsive to chemotherapy and radiotherapy. In addition, tumors in as many as 25% of the patients undergo spontaneous regression—usually transient—without therapy. In an asymptomatic patient, no initial treatment and watchful waiting can be an appropriate management strategy and is particularly likely to be adopted for older patients with advanced stage disease. For patients who do require treatment, single-agent chlorambucil or cyclophosphamide or combination chemotherapy with CVP or CHOP are most frequently used. With adequate treatment, 50–75% of patients will achieve a complete remission. While most patients relapse (median response duration is ~2 years), at least 20% of complete responders will remain in remission for >10 years. For the rare patient (15%) with localized follicular lymphoma, involved field radiotherapy produces long-term disease-free survival in the majority.

A number of therapies have been shown to be active in the treatment of patients with follicular lymphoma. These include cytotoxic agents such as fludarabine, and biologic agents such as interferon α, monoclonal antibodies with or without radionuclides, and lymphoma vaccines. In patients treated with a doxorubicin-containing combination chemotherapy regimen, interferon α given to patients in complete remission seems to prolong survival. The monoclonal antibody rituximab can cause objective responses in 35–50% of patients with relapsed follicular lymphoma, and radiolabeled antibodies appear to have response rates well in excess of 50%. The addition of rituximab to CHOP and other effective combination chemotherapy programs is beginning to show prolonged overall survival and a decreased risk of histologic progression. Trials with tumor vaccines have been encouraging. Both autologous and allogeneic hematopoietic stem cell transplantation yield high complete response rates in patients with relapsed follicular lymphoma, and long-term remissions can occur.

Patients with follicular lymphoma with a predominance of large cells have a shorter survival when treated with single-agent chemotherapy but seem to benefit from receiving an anthracycline-containing combination chemotherapy regimen plus rituximab. When their disease is treated aggressively, the overall survival for such patients is no lower than for patients with other follicular lymphomas, and the failure-free survival is superior.

Patients with follicular lymphoma have a high rate of histologic transformation to diffuse large B cell lymphoma (5–7% per year). This is recognized ~40% of the time during the course of the illness by repeat biopsy and is present in almost all patients at autopsy. This transformation is usually heralded by rapid growth of lymph nodes—often localized—and the development of systemic symptoms such as fevers, sweats, and weight loss. Although these patients have a poor prognosis, aggressive combination chemotherapy regimens can sometimes cause a complete remission in the diffuse large B cell lymphoma, at times leaving the patient with persisting follicular lymphoma.

Diffuse Large B Cell Lymphoma Diffuse large B cell lymphoma is the most common type of non-Hodgkin's lymphoma, representing ap-

FIGURE 105-8 Diffuse large B cell lymphoma. The neoplastic cells are heterogeneous but predominantly large cells with vesicular chromatin and prominent nucleoli.

proximately one-third of all cases. This lymphoma makes up the majority of cases in previous clinical trials of "aggressive" or "intermediate-grade" lymphoma. Table 105-10 shows the clinical characteristics of diffuse large B cell lymphoma.

The diagnosis of diffuse large B cell lymphoma can be made accurately by an expert hematopathologist (Fig. 105-8). Cytogenetic and molecular genetic studies are not necessary for diagnosis, but some evidence has accumulated that patients whose tumors overexpress the BCL-2 protein might be more likely to relapse than others. Patients with prominent mediastinal involvement are sometimes diagnosed as a separate subgroup having primary mediastinal diffuse large B cell lymphoma. This latter group of patients has a younger median age (i.e., 37 years) and a female predominance (66%). Subtypes of diffuse large B cell lymphoma, including those with an immunoblastic subtype and tumors with extensive fibrosis, are recognized by pathologists but do not appear to have important independent prognostic significance.

Diffuse large B cell lymphoma can present as either primary lymph node disease or at extranodal sites. More than 50% of patients will have some site of extranodal involvement at diagnosis, with the most common sites being the gastrointestinal tract and bone marrow, each being involved in 15–20% of patients. Essentially any organ can be involved, making a diagnostic biopsy imperative. For example, diffuse large B cell lymphoma of the pancreas has a much better prognosis than pancreatic carcinoma but would be missed without biopsy. Primary diffuse large B cell lymphoma of the brain is being diagnosed with increasing frequency. Other unusual subtypes of diffuse large B cell lymphoma such as pleural effusion lymphoma and intravascular lymphoma have been difficult to diagnose and associated with a very poor prognosis.

Table 105-11 shows the initial evaluation of patients with diffuse large B cell lymphoma. After a careful staging evaluation, ~50% of patients will be found to have stage I or II disease and ~50% will have widely disseminated lymphoma. Bone marrow biopsy shows involvement by lymphoma in ~15% of cases, with marrow involvement by small cells more frequent than by large cells.

℞ DIFFUSE LARGE B CELL LYMPHOMA

The initial treatment of all patients with diffuse large B cell lymphoma should be with a combination chemotherapy regimen. The most popular regimen in the United States is CHOP plus rituximab, although a variety of other anthracycline-containing combination chemotherapy regimens appear to be equally efficacious. Patients with stage I or nonbulky stage II can be effectively treated with three to four cycles of combination chemotherapy followed by involved field radiotherapy. The need for radiation therapy is unclear. Cure rates of 70–80% in stage II disease and 85–90% in stage I disease can be expected.

For patients with bulky stage II, stage III, or stage IV disease, six to eight cycles of CHOP plus rituximab are usually administered. A large randomized trial showed the superiority of CHOP combined with rituximab over CHOP alone in elderly patients. A frequent approach would be to administer four cycles of therapy and then reevaluate. If the patient has achieved a complete remission after four cycles, two more cycles of treatment might be given and then therapy discontinued. Using this approach, 70–80% of patients can be expected to achieve a complete remission, and 50–70% of

complete responders will be cured. The chances for a favorable response to treatment are predicted by the IPI. In fact, the IPI was developed based on the outcome of patients with diffuse large B cell lymphoma treated with CHOP-like regimens. For the 35% of patients with a low IPI score of 0–1, the 5-year survival is >70%, while for the 20% of patients with a high IPI score of 4–5, the 5-year survival is ~20%. The addition of rituximab to CHOP has improved each of those numbers by ~15%. A number of other factors, including molecular features of the tumor, levels of circulating cytokines and soluble receptors, and other surrogate markers, have been shown to influence prognosis. However, they have not been validated as rigorously as the IPI and have not been uniformly applied clinically.

Because a number of patients with diffuse large B cell lymphoma are either initially refractory to therapy or relapse after apparently effective chemotherapy, 30–40% of patients will be candidates for salvage treatment at some point. Alternative combination chemotherapy regimens can induce complete remission in as many as 50% of these patients, but long-term disease-free survival is seen in ≤10%. Autologous bone marrow transplantation is superior to salvage chemotherapy at usual doses and leads to long-term disease-free survival in ~40% of patients whose lymphomas remain chemotherapy-sensitive after relapse.

Burkitt's Lymphoma/Leukemia Burkitt's lymphoma/leukemia is a rare disease in adults in the United States, making up <1% of non-Hodgkin's lymphomas, but it makes up ~30% of childhood non-Hodgkin's lymphoma. Burkitt's leukemia, or L3 ALL, makes up a small proportion of childhood and adult acute leukemias. Table 105-10 shows the clinical features of Burkitt's lymphoma.

Burkitt's lymphoma can be diagnosed morphologically by an expert hematopathologist with a high degree of accuracy. The cells are homogeneous in size and shape (Fig. 105-9). Demonstration of a very high proliferative fraction and the presence of the t(8;14) or one of its variants, t(2;8) (c-myc and the λ light chain gene) or t(8;22) (c-myc and the κ light chain gene), can be confirmatory. Burkitt's cell leukemia is recognized by the typical monotonous mass of medium-sized cells with round nuclei, multiple nucleoli, and basophilic cytoplasm with cytoplasmic vacuoles. Demonstration of surface expression of immunoglobulin and one of the above-noted cytogenetic abnormalities is confirmatory.

Three distinct clinical forms of Burkitt's lymphoma are recognized; endemic, sporadic, and immunodeficiency-associated. Endemic and sporadic Burkitt's lymphomas occur frequently in children in Africa, and the sporadic form in western countries. Immunodeficiency-associated Burkitt's lymphoma is seen in patients with HIV infection.

Pathologists sometimes have difficulty distinguishing between Burkitt's lymphoma and diffuse large B cell lymphoma. In the past, a separate subgroup of non-Hodgkin's lymphoma intermediate between the two was recognized. When tested, this subgroup could not be diagnosed accurately. Distinction between the two major types of B cell aggressive non-Hodgkin's lymphoma can sometimes be made based on the extremely high proliferative fraction seen in patients with Burkitt's lymphoma (i.e., essentially 100% of tumor cells are in cycle) caused by c-myc deregulation.

FIGURE 105-9 Burkitt's lymphoma. The neoplastic cells are homogenous, medium-sized B cells with frequent mitotic figures, a morphologic correlate of high growth fraction. Reactive macrophages are scattered through the tumor and their pale cytoplasm in a background of blue-staining tumor cells give the tumor a so-called starry sky appearance.

Most patients in the United States with Burkitt's lymphoma present with peripheral lymphadenopathy or an intraabdominal mass. The disease is rapidly progressive and has a propensity to metastasize to the CNS. Initial evaluation should always include an examination of cerebral spinal fluid to rule out metastasis in addition to the other staging evaluations noted in Table 105-11. Once the diagnosis of Burkitt's lymphoma is suspected, a diagnosis must be made promptly and staging evaluation must be accomplished expeditiously. This is the most rapidly progressive human tumor, and any delay in initiating therapy can adversely affect the patient's prognosis.

℞ BURKITT'S LYMPHOMA

Treatment of Burkitt's lymphoma in both children and adults should begin within 48 h of diagnosis and involves the use of intensive combination chemotherapy regimens incorporating high doses of cyclophosphamide. Prophylactic therapy to the CNS is mandatory. Burkitt's lymphoma was one of the first cancers shown to be curable by chemotherapy. Today, cure can be expected in 70–80% of both children and young adults when effective therapy is administered precisely. Salvage therapy has been generally ineffective in patients failing the initial treatment, emphasizing the importance of the initial treatment approach.

Other B Cell Lymphoid Malignancies *B cell prolymphocytic leukemia* involves blood and marrow infiltration by large lymphocytes with prominent nucleoli. Patients typically have a high white cell count, splenomegaly, and minimal lymphadenopathy. The chances for a complete response to therapy are poor.

Hairy cell leukemia is a rare disease that presents predominantly in older males. Typical presentation involves pancytopenia, although occasional patients will have a leukemic presentation. Splenomegaly is usual. The malignant cells appear to have "hairy" projections on light and electron microscopy and show a characteristic staining pattern with tartrate-resistant acid phosphatase. Bone marrow is typically not able to be aspirated, and biopsy shows a pattern of fibrosis with diffuse infiltration by the malignant cells. Patients with this disorder are prone to unusual infections, including infection by *Mycobacterium avium intracellulare*, and to vasculitic syndromes. Hairy cell leukemia is responsive to chemotherapy with interferon α, pentostatin, or cladribine, with the latter being the usually preferred treatment. Clinical complete remissions with cladribine occur in the majority of patients, and long-term disease-free survival is frequent.

Splenic marginal zone lymphoma involves infiltration of the splenic white pulp by small, monoclonal B cells. This is a rare disorder that can present as leukemia as well as lymphoma. Definitive diagnosis is often made at splenectomy, which is also an effective therapy. This is an extremely indolent disorder, but when chemotherapy is required, the most usual treatment has been chlorambucil.

Lymphoplasmacytic lymphoma is the tissue manifestation of Waldenström's macroglobulinemia (Chap. 106). This type of lymphoma has been associated with chronic hepatitis C virus infection, and an etiologic association has been proposed. Patients typically present with lymphadenopathy, splenomegaly, bone marrow involvement, and occasionally peripheral blood involvement. The tumor cells do not express CD5. Patients often have a monoclonal IgM protein, high levels of which can dominate the clinical picture with the symptoms of hyperviscosity. Treatment of lymphoplasmacytic lymphoma can be aimed primarily at reducing the abnormal protein, if present, but will usually also involve chemotherapy. Chlorambucil, fludarabine, and cladribine have been utilized. The median 5-year survival for patients with this disorder is ~60%.

Nodal marginal zone lymphoma, also known as *monocytoid B cell lymphoma*, represents ~1% of non-Hodgkin's lymphomas. This lymphoma has a slight female predominance and presents with disseminated disease (i.e., stage III or IV) in 75% of patients. Approximately one-third of patients have bone marrow involvement, and a leukemic presentation occasionally occurs. The staging evaluation and therapy should use the same approach as used for patients with follicular lymphoma. Approximately 60% of the patients with nodal marginal zone lymphoma will survive 5 years after diagnosis.

PRECURSOR CELL T CELL MALIGNANCIES
Precursor T Cell Lymphoblastic Leukemia/Lymphoma Precursor T cell malignancies can present either as ALL or as an aggressive lymphoma. These malignancies are more common in children and young adults, with males more frequently affected than females.

Precursor T cell ALL can present with bone marrow failure, although the severity of anemia, neutropenia, and thrombocytopenia is often less than in precursor B cell ALL. These patients sometimes have very high white cell counts, a mediastinal mass, lymphadenopathy, and hepatosplenomegaly. Precursor T cell lymphoblastic lymphoma is most often found in young men presenting with a large mediastinal mass and pleural effusions. Both presentations have a propensity to metastasize to the CNS, and CNS involvement is often present at diagnosis.

℞ PRECURSOR T CELL LYMPHOBLASTIC LEUKEMIA/LYMPHOMA

Children with precursor T cell ALL seem to benefit from very intensive remission induction and consolidation regimens. The majority of patients treated in this manner can be cured. Older children and young adults with precursor T cell lymphoblastic lymphoma are also often treated with "leukemia-like" regimens. Patients who present with localized disease have an excellent prognosis. However, advanced age is an adverse prognostic factor. Adults with precursor T cell lymphoblastic lymphoma who present with high LDH levels or bone marrow or CNS involvement are often offered bone marrow transplantation as part of their primary therapy.

MATURE (PERIPHERAL) T CELL DISORDERS
Mycosis Fungoides Mycosis fungoides is also known as *cutaneous T cell lymphoma*. This lymphoma is more often seen by dermatologists than internists. The median age of onset is in the mid-fifties, and the disease is more common in males and in blacks.

Mycosis fungoides is an indolent lymphoma with patients often having several years of eczematous or dermatitic skin lesions before the diagnosis is finally established. The skin lesions progress from patch stage to plaque stage to cutaneous tumors. Early in the disease, biopsies are often difficult to interpret, and the diagnosis may only become apparent by observing the patient over time. In advanced stages, the lymphoma can spread to lymph nodes and visceral organs. Patients with this lymphoma may develop generalized erythroderma and circulating tumor cells, called *Sézary's syndrome*.

Rare patients with localized early stage mycosis fungoides can be cured with radiotherapy, often total-skin electron beam irradiation. More advanced disease has been treated with topical glucocorticoids, topical nitrogen mustard, phototherapy, psoralen with ultraviolet A (PUVA), electron beam radiation, interferon, antibodies, fusion toxins, and systemic cytotoxic therapy. Unfortunately, these treatments are palliative.

Adult T Cell Lymphoma/Leukemia Adult T cell lymphoma/leukemia is one manifestation of infection by the HTLV-I retrovirus. Patients can be infected through transplacental transmission, mother's milk, blood transfusion, and by sexual transmission of the virus. Patients who acquire the virus from their mother through breast milk are most likely to develop lymphoma, but the risk is still only 2.5% and the latency averages 55 years. Nationwide testing for HTLV-I antibodies and the aggressive implementation of public health measures could theoretically lead to the disappearance of adult T cell lymphoma/leukemia. Tropical spastic paraparesis, another manifestation of HTLV-I infection (Chap. 181), occurs after a shorter latency (1–3 years) and is most common in individuals who acquire the virus during adulthood from transfusion or sex.

The diagnosis of adult T cell lymphoma/leukemia is made when an expert hematopathologist recognizes the typical morphologic picture, a T cell immunophenotype (i.e., CD4 positive), and the presence in se-

FIGURE 105-10 Adult T cell leukemia/lymphoma. Peripheral blood smear showing leukemia cells with typical "flower-shaped" nucleus.

rum of antibodies to HTLV-I. Examination of the peripheral blood will usually reveal characteristic, pleomorphic abnormal CD4-positive cells with indented nuclei, which have been called "flower" cells (Fig. 105-10).

A subset of patients have a smoldering clinical course and long survival, but most patients present with an aggressive disease manifested by lymphadenopathy, hepatosplenomegaly, skin infiltration, pulmonary infiltrates, hypercalcemia, lytic bone lesions, and elevated LDH levels. The skin lesions can be papules, plaques, tumors, and ulcerations. Lung lesions can be either tumor or opportunistic infection in light of the underlying immunodeficiency in the disease. Bone marrow involvement is not usually extensive, and anemia and thrombocytopenia are not usually prominent. Although treatment by combination chemotherapy regimens can result in objective responses, true complete remissions are unusual, and the median survival of patients is ~7 months.

Anaplastic Large T/Null Cell Lymphoma Anaplastic large T/null cell lymphoma was previously usually diagnosed as undifferentiated carcinoma or malignant histiocytosis. Discovery of the CD30 (Ki-1) antigen and the recognition that some patients with previously unclassified malignancies displayed this antigen led to the identification of a new type of lymphoma. Subsequently, discovery of the t(2;5) and the resultant frequent overexpression of the anaplastic lymphoma kinase (ALK) protein confirmed the existence of this entity. This lymphoma accounts for ~2% of all non-Hodgkin's lymphomas. Table 105-10 shows the clinical characteristics of patients with anaplastic large T/null cell lymphoma.

The diagnosis of anaplastic large T/null cell lymphoma is made when an expert hematopathologist recognizes the typical morphologic picture and a T cell or null cell immunophenotype with CD30 positivity. Documentation of the t(2;5) and/or overexpression of ALK protein confirm the diagnosis. Some diffuse large B cell lymphomas can also have an anaplastic appearance but have the same clinical course or response to therapy as other diffuse large B cell lymphomas.

Patients with anaplastic large T/cell null cell lymphoma are typically young (median age, 33 years) and male (~70%). Some 50% of patients present in stage I/II, and the remainder with more extensive disease. Systemic symptoms and elevated LDH levels are seen in about one-half of patients. Bone marrow and the gastrointestinal tract are rarely involved, but skin involvement is frequent. Some patients with disease confined to the skin have a different and more indolent disorder that has been termed *cutaneous anaplastic large T/null cell lymphoma* and might be related to lymphomatoid papulosis.

Rx ANAPLASTIC LARGE T/NULL CELL LYMPHOMA

Treatment regimens appropriate for other aggressive lymphomas, such as diffuse large B cell lymphoma, should be utilized in patients with anaplastic large T/null cell lymphoma, with the exception that the B cell–specific antibody, rituximab, is omitted. Surprisingly, given the anaplastic appearance, this disorder has the best survival rate of any aggressive lymphoma. The 5-year survival is >75%. While traditional prognostic factors such as the IPI predict treatment outcome, overexpression of the ALK protein is an important prognostic factor, with patients overexpressing this protein having a superior treatment outcome.

Peripheral T Cell Lymphoma The peripheral T cell lymphomas make up a heterogeneous morphologic group of aggressive neoplasms that share a mature T cell immunophenotype. They represent ~7% of all cases of non-Hodgkin's lymphoma. A number of distinct clinical syndromes are included in this group of disorders. Table 105-10 shows the clinical characteristics of patients with peripheral T cell lymphoma.

The diagnosis of peripheral T cell lymphoma, or any of its specific subtypes, requires an expert hematopathologist, an adequate biopsy, and immunophenotyping. Most peripheral T cell lymphomas are CD4+, but a few will be CD8+, both CD4+ and CD8+, or have an NK cell immunophenotype. No characteristic genetic abnormalities have yet been identified, but translocations involving the T cell antigen receptor genes on chromosomes 7 or 14 may be detected. The differential diagnosis of patients suspected of having peripheral T cell lymphoma includes reactive T cell infiltrative processes. In some cases, demonstration of a monoclonal T cell population using T cell receptor gene rearrangement studies will be required to make a diagnosis.

The initial evaluation of a patient with a peripheral T cell lymphoma should include the studies in Table 105-11 for staging patients with non-Hodgkin's lymphoma. Unfortunately, patients with peripheral T cell lymphoma usually present with adverse prognostic factors, with >80% of patients having an IPI score ≥2 and >30% having an IPI score ≥4. As this would predict, peripheral T cell lymphomas are associated with a poor outcome, and only 25% of the patients survive 5 years after diagnosis. Treatment regimens are the same as those used for diffuse large B cell lymphoma (omitting rituximab), but patients with peripheral T cell lymphoma have a poorer response to treatment. Because of this poor treatment outcome, hematopoietic stem cell transplantation is often considered early in the care of young patients.

A number of specific clinical syndromes are seen in the peripheral T cell lymphomas. *Angioimmunoblastic T cell lymphoma* is one of the more common subtypes, making up ~20% of T cell lymphomas. These patients typically present with generalized lymphadenopathy, fever, weight loss, skin rash, and polyclonal hypergammaglobulinemia. In some cases, it is difficult to separate patients with a reactive disorder from those with true lymphoma.

Extranodal T/NK cell lymphoma of nasal type has also been called *angiocentric lymphoma* and was previously termed *lethal midline granuloma*. This disorder is more frequent in Asia and South America than in the United States and Europe. EBV is thought to play an etiologic role. Although most frequent in the upper airway, it can involve other organs. The course is aggressive, and patients frequently have the hemophagocytic syndrome. When marrow and blood involvement occur, distinction between this disease and leukemia might be difficult. Some patients will respond to aggressive combination chemotherapy regimens, but the overall outlook is poor.

Enteropathy-type intestinal T cell lymphoma is a rare disorder that occurs in patients with untreated gluten-sensitive enteropathy. Patients are frequently wasted and sometimes present with intestinal perforation. The prognosis is poor. *Hepatosplenic γδ T cell lymphoma* is a systemic illness that presents with sinusoidal infiltration of the liver, spleen, and bone marrow by malignant T cells. Tumor masses generally do not occur. The disease is associated with systemic symptoms and is often difficult to diagnosis. Treatment outcome is poor. *Subcutaneous panniculitis-like T cell lymphoma* is a rare disorder that is often confused with panniculitis. Patients present with multiple subcutaneous nodules, which progress and can ulcerate. Hemophagocytic syndrome is common. Response to therapy is poor. The development of the hemophagocytic syndrome (profound anemia, ingestion of erythrocytes by monocytes and macrophages) in the course of any peripheral T cell lymphoma is generally associated with a fatal outcome.

HODGKIN'S DISEASE
Classical Hodgkin's Disease Hodgkin's disease occurs in 8000 patients in the United States each year, and the disease does not appear to be increasing in frequency. Most patients present with palpable lymphadenopathy that is nontender; in most patients, these lymph nodes are in the neck, supraclavicular area, and axilla. More than half the patients will

FIGURE 105-11 Mixed cellularity Hodgkin's disease. A Reed-Sternberg cell is present near the center of the field; a large cell with a bilobed nucleus and prominent nucleoli giving an "owl's eyes" appearance. The majority of the cells are normal lymphocytes, neutrophils, and eosinophils that form a pleiomorphic cellular infiltrate.

have mediastinal adenopathy at diagnosis, and this is sometimes the initial manifestation. Subdiaphragmatic presentation of Hodgkin's disease is unusual and more common in older males. One-third of patients present with fevers, night sweats, and/or weight loss—B symptoms in the Ann Arbor staging classification (Table 105-8). Occasionally, Hodgkin's disease can present as a fever of unknown origin. This is more common in older patients who are found to have mixed-cellularity Hodgkin's disease in an abdominal site. Rarely, the fevers persist for days to weeks, followed by afebrile intervals and then recurrence of the fever. This pattern is known as *Pel-Ebstein fever*. Hodgkin's disease can occasionally present with unusual manifestations. These include severe and unexplained itching, cutaneous disorders such as erythema nodosum and ichthyosiform atrophy, paraneoplastic cerebellar degeneration and other distant effects on the CNS, nephrotic syndrome, immune hemolytic anemia and thrombocytopenia, hypercalcemia, and pain in lymph nodes on alcohol ingestion.

The diagnosis of Hodgkin's disease is established by review of an adequate biopsy specimen by an expert hematopathologist. In the United States, most patients have nodular sclerosing Hodgkin's disease, with a minority of patients having mixed-cellularity Hodgkin's disease. Lymphocyte-predominant and lymphocyte-depleted Hodgkin's disease are rare. Mixed-cellularity Hodgkin's disease or lymphocyte-depletion Hodgkin's disease are seen more frequently in patients infected by HIV (**Fig. 105-11**). The differential diagnosis of a lymph node biopsy suspicious for Hodgkin's disease includes inflammatory processes, mononucleosis, non-Hodgkin's lymphoma, phenytoin-induced adenopathy, and nonlymphomatous malignancies.

The staging evaluation for a patient with Hodgkin's disease would typically include a careful history and physical examination; complete blood count; erythrocyte sedimentation rate; serum chemistry studies including LDH; chest radiograph; CT scan of the chest, abdomen, and pelvis; and bone marrow biopsy. Many patients would also have a PET scan or a gallium scan. Although rarely utilized, a bipedal lymphangiogram can be helpful. PET and gallium scans are most useful to document remission. Staging laparotomies were once popular for most patients with Hodgkin's disease but are now done rarely because of an increased reliance on systemic rather than local therapy.

℞ CLASSICAL HODGKIN'S DISEASE

Patients with localized Hodgkin's disease are cured >90% of the time. In patients with good prognostic factors, extended-field radiotherapy has a high cure rate. Increasingly, patients with all stages of Hodgkin's disease are treated initially with chemotherapy. Patients with localized or good-prognosis disease receive a brief course of chemotherapy followed by radiotherapy to sites of node involvement. Patients with more extensive disease or those with B symptoms receive a complete course of chemotherapy. The most popular chemotherapy regimens used in Hodgkin's disease include doxorubicin, bleomycin, vinblastine, and dacarbazine (ABVD) and mechlorethamine, vincristine, procarbazine, and prednisone (MOPP), or combinations of the drugs in these two regimens. Today, most patients in the United States receive ABVD, but a weekly chemotherapy regimen administered for 12 weeks called *Stanford V* is becoming increasingly popular,

but includes radiation therapy, which has been associated with life-threatening late toxicities such as premature coronary artery disease and second solid tumors. In Europe a high-dose regimen called *BEACOPP* incorporating alkylating agents has become popular and might have a better response rate in very high risk patients. Long-term disease-free survival in patients with advanced disease can be achieved in >75% of patients who lack systemic symptoms and in 60–70% of patients with systemic symptoms.

Patients who relapse after primary therapy of Hodgkin's disease can frequently still be cured. Patients who relapse after initial treatment only with radiotherapy have an excellent outcome when treated with chemotherapy. Patients who relapse after an effective chemotherapy regimen are usually not curable with subsequent chemotherapy administered at standard doses. However, patients with a long initial remission can be an exception to this rule. Autologous bone marrow transplantation can cure half of patients who fail effective chemotherapy regimens.

Because of the very high cure rate in patients with Hodgkin's disease, long-term complications have become a major focus for clinical research. In fact, in some series of patients with early-stage disease, more patients died from late complications of therapy than from Hodgkin's disease itself. This is particularly true in patients with localized disease. The most serious late side effects include second malignancies and cardiac injury. Patients are at risk for the development of acute leukemia in the first 10 years after treatment with combination chemotherapy regimens that contain alkylating agents plus radiation therapy. The risk for development of acute leukemia appears to be greater after MOPP-like regimens than with ABVD. The risk of development of acute leukemia after treatment for Hodgkin's disease is also related to the number of exposures to potentially leukemogenic agents (i.e., multiple treatments after relapse) and the age of the patient being treated, with those >60 years at particularly high risk. The development of carcinomas as a complication of treatment for Hodgkin's disease has become a major problem. These tumors usually occur ≥10 years after treatment and are associated with use of radiotherapy. For this reason, young women treated with thoracic radiotherapy for Hodgkin's disease should institute screening mammograms 5–10 years after treatment, and all patients who receive thoracic radiotherapy for Hodgkin's disease should be discouraged from smoking. Thoracic radiation also accelerates coronary artery disease, and patients should be encouraged to minimize risk factors for coronary artery disease such as smoking and elevated cholesterol levels.

A number of other late side effects from the treatment of Hodgkin's disease are well known. Patients who receive thoracic radiotherapy are at very high risk for the eventual development of hypothyroidism and should be observed for this complication; intermittent measurement of thyrotropin should be made to identify the condition before it becomes symptomatic. Lhermitte's syndrome occurs in ~15% of patients who receive thoracic radiotherapy. This syndrome is manifested by an "electric shock" sensation into the lower extremities on flexion of the neck. Infertility is a concern for all patients undergoing treatment for Hodgkin's disease. In both women and men, the risk of permanent infertility is age-related, with younger patients more likely to recover fertility. In addition, treatment with ABVD rather than MOPP increases the chances to retain fertility.

Nodular Lymphocyte-Predominant Hodgkin's Disease Nodular lymphocyte-predominant Hodgkin's disease is now recognized as an entity distinct from classical Hodgkin's disease. Previous classification systems recognized that biopsies from a subset of patients diagnosed as having Hodgkin's disease contained a predominance of small lymphocytes and rare Reed-Sternberg cells. A subset of these patients have tumors with nodular growth pattern and a clinical course that varied from that of patients with classical Hodgkin's disease. This is an unusual clinical entity and represents <5% of cases of Hodgkin's disease.

Nodular lymphocyte-predominant Hodgkin's disease has a number of characteristics that suggest its relationship to non-Hodgkin's lymphoma. These include a clonal proliferation of B cells and a distinctive immunophenotype; tumor cells express J chain and display CD45 and epithelial membrane antigen (ema) and do not express two markers normally found on Sternberg-Reed cells, CD30 and CD15. This lymphoma tends to have a chronic, relapsing course and sometimes transforms to diffuse large B cell lymphoma.

The treatment of patients with nodular lymphocyte-predominant Hodgkin's disease is controversial. Some clinicians favor no treatment and merely close follow-up. In the United States, most physicians will treat localized disease with radiotherapy and disseminated disease with regimens utilized for patients with classical Hodgkin's disease. Regardless of the therapy utilized, most series report a long-term survival of >80%.

LYMPHOMA-LIKE DISORDERS

The most common condition that pathologists and clinicians might confuse with lymphoma is reactive, atypical lymphoid hyperplasia. Patients might have localized or disseminated lymphadenopathy and might have the systemic symptoms characteristic of lymphoma. Underlying causes include a drug reaction to phenytoin or carbamazepine. Immune disorders such as rheumatoid arthritis and lupus erythematosus, viral infections such as cytomegalovirus and EBV, and bacterial infections such as cat-scratch disease may cause adenopathy (Chap. 60). In the absence of a definitive diagnosis after initial biopsy, continued follow-up, further testing, and repeated biopsies, if necessary, are the appropriate approach rather than instituting therapy.

Specific conditions that can be confused with lymphoma include *Castleman's disease*, which can present with localized or disseminated lymphadenopathy; some patients have systemic symptoms. The disseminated form is often accompanied by anemia and polyclonal hypergammaglobulinemia, and the condition has been associated with overproduction of interleukin 6, possibly produced by human herpesvirus 8. Patients with localized disease can be treated effectively with local therapy, while the initial treatment for patients with disseminated disease is usually with systemic glucocorticoids.

Sinus histiocytosis with massive lymphadenopathy (*Rosai-Dorfman's disease*) usually presents with bulky lymphadenopathy in children or young adults. The disease is usually nonprogressive and self-limited, but patients can manifest autoimmune hemolytic anemia.

Lymphomatoid papulosis is a cutaneous lymphoproliferative disorder that is often confused with anaplastic large cell lymphoma involving the skin. The cells of lymphomatoid papulosis are similar to those seen in lymphoma and stain for CD30, and T cell receptor gene rearrangements are sometimes seen. However, the condition is characterized by waxing and waning skin lesions that usually heal, leaving small scars. In the absence of effective communication between the clinician and the pathologist regarding the clinical course in the patient, this disease will be misdiagnosed. Since the clinical picture is usually benign, misdiagnosis is a serious mistake.

ACKNOWLEDGMENT

James Armitage was a coauthor of this chapter in prior editions, and substantial material from those editions has been included here.

FURTHER READINGS

ANSEL SM, ARMITAGE JO: Management of Hodgkin lymphoma. Mayo Clin Proc 81:419, 2006

ARMITAGE JO et al: Lymphoma 2006: Classification and treatment. Oncology 20:231, 2006

BREPOELS L et al: PET and PET/CT for response evaluation in lymphoma: Current practice and developments. Leuk Lymphoma 48:270, 2007

HARRIS NL et al: World Health Organization classification of neoplastic diseases of the hematopoietic and lymphoid tissues: Report of the Clinical Advisory Committee Meeting, Airlie House, Virginia, November, 1997. J Clin Oncol 17:3835, 1999

SEHN LH et al: The revised International Prognostic Index (R-IPI) is a better predictor of outcome than the standard IPI for patients with diffuse large B-cell lymphoma treated with R-CHOP. Blood 109:1857, 2007

URBA WJ, LONGO DL: Hodgkin's disease. N Engl J Med 326:678, 1992

106 Plasma Cell Disorders
Nikhil C. Munshi, Dan L. Longo,
Kenneth C. Anderson

The *plasma cell disorders* are monoclonal neoplasms related to each other by virtue of their development from common progenitors in the B lymphocyte lineage. Multiple myeloma, Waldenström's macroglobulinemia, primary amyloidosis (Chap. 324), and the heavy chain diseases comprise this group and may be designated by a variety of synonyms such as *monoclonal gammopathies*, *paraproteinemias*, *plasma cell dyscrasias*, and *dysproteinemias*. Mature B lymphocytes destined to produce IgG bear surface immunoglobulin molecules of both M and G heavy chain isotypes with both isotypes having identical idiotypes (variable regions). Under normal circumstances, maturation to antibody-secreting plasma cells is stimulated by exposure to the antigen for which the surface immunoglobulin is specific; however, in the plasma cell disorders the control over this process is lost. The clinical manifestations of all the plasma cell disorders relate to the expansion of the neoplastic cells, to the secretion of cell products (immunoglobulin molecules or subunits, lymphokines), and to some extent to the host's response to the tumor. Normal development of B lymphocytes is discussed in Chap. 308.

There are three categories of structural variation among immunoglobulin molecules that form antigenic determinants, and these are used to classify immunoglobulins (Chap. 308). *Isotypes* are those determinants that distinguish among the main classes of antibodies of a given species and are the same in all normal individuals of that species. Therefore, isotypic determinants are, by definition, recognized by antibodies from a distinct species (heterologous sera) but not by antibodies from the same species (homologous sera). There are five heavy chain isotypes (M, G, A, D, E) and two light chain isotypes (κ, λ). *Allotypes* are distinct determinants that reflect regular small differences between individuals of the same species in the amino acid sequences of otherwise similar immunoglobulins. These differences are determined by allelic genes; by definition, they are detected by antibodies made in the same species. *Idiotypes* are the third category of antigenic determinants. They are unique to the molecules produced by a given clone of antibody-producing cells. Idiotypes are formed by the unique structure of the antigen-binding portion of the molecule.

Antibody molecules (Fig. 308-9) are composed of two heavy chains (mol wt ~ 50,000) and two light chains (mol wt ~ 25,000). Each chain has a constant portion (limited amino acid sequence variability) and a variable region (extensive sequence variability). The light and heavy chains are linked by disulfide bonds and are aligned so that their variable regions are adjacent to one another. This variable region forms the antigen recognition site of the antibody molecule; its unique structural features form a particular set of determinants, or idiotypes, that are reliable markers for a particular clone of cells because each antibody is formed and secreted by a single clone. Each chain is specified by distinct genes, synthesized separately, and assembled into an intact antibody molecule after translation. Because of the mechanics of the gene rearrangements necessary to specify the immunoglobulin variable regions (VDJ joining for the heavy chain, VJ joining for the light chain), a particular clone rearranges only one of the two chromosomes to produce an immunoglobulin molecule of only one light chain isotype and only one allotype (allelic exclusion). After exposure to antigen, the variable region may become associated with a new heavy chain isotype (class switch). Each clone of cells performs these sequential gene arrangements in a unique way. This results in each clone producing a unique immunoglobulin molecule. In most cells, light chains are synthesized in slight excess, are secreted as free light chains by plasma cells, and are cleared by the kidney, but <10 mg of such light chains is excreted per day.

FIGURE 106-1 Representative patterns of serum electrophoresis. The upper panel illustrates the normal pattern of serum protein on electrophoresis. Since there are many different immunoglobulins in the serum, their differing mobilities in an electric field produce a broad peak. In conditions associated with increases in polyclonal immuno-globulin, the broad peak is more prominent (middle panel). In mono-clonal gammopathies, the predominance of a product of a single cell produces a "church spire" sharp peak, usually in the γ globulin region (bottom panel).

Electrophoretic analysis of components of the serum proteins permits determination of the amount of immunoglobulin in the serum (Fig. 106-1). The immunoglobulins move heterogeneously in an electric field and form a broad peak in the gamma region. The γ globulin region of the electrophoretic pattern is usually increased in the sera of patients with plasma cell tumors. There is a sharp spike in this region called an *M component* (M for monoclonal). Less commonly, the M component may appear in the β_2 or α_2 globulin region. The antibody must be present at a concentration of at least 5 g/L (0.5 g/dL) to be detectable by this method. This corresponds to ~10^9 cells producing the antibody. Confirmation that such an M component is truly monoclonal relies on the use of immunoelectrophoresis that shows a single light and heavy chain type. Hence immunoelectrophoresis and electrophoresis provide qualitative and quantitative assessment of the M component, respectively. Once the presence of an M component has been confirmed, electrophoresis provides the more practical information for managing patients with monoclonal gammopathies. In a given patient, the amount of M component in the serum is a reliable measure of the tumor burden. This makes the M component an excellent tumor marker, yet it is not specific enough to be used to screen asymptomatic patients. In addition to the plasma cell disorders, M components may be detected in other lymphoid neoplasms such as chronic lymphocytic leukemia and lymphomas of B or T cell origin; nonlymphoid neoplasms such as chronic myeloid leukemia, breast cancer, and colon cancer; a variety of nonneoplastic conditions such as cirrhosis, sarcoidosis, parasitic diseases, Gaucher disease, and pyoderma gangrenosum; and a number of autoimmune conditions, including rheumatoid arthritis, myasthenia gravis, and cold agglutinin disease. At least two very rare skin diseases—lichen myxedematosus, or papular mucinosis, and necrobiotic xanthogranuloma—are associated with a monoclonal gammopathy. In papular mucinosis, highly cationic IgG is deposited in the dermis of patients. This organ specificity may reflect the specificity of the antibody for some antigenic component of the dermis. Necrobiotic xanthogranuloma is a histiocytic infiltration of the skin, usually of the face, that produces red or yellow nodules that can enlarge to plaques. Some 10% progress to myeloma.

The nature of the M component is variable in plasma cell disorders. It may be an intact antibody molecule of any heavy chain subclass, or it may be an altered antibody or fragment. Isolated light or heavy chains may be produced. In some plasma cell tumors such as extramedullary or solitary bone plasmacytomas, <$^1/_3$ of patients will have an M component. In ~20% of myelomas, only light chains are produced and in most cases are secreted in the urine as Bence Jones proteins. The frequency of myelomas of a particular heavy chain class is roughly proportional to the serum concentration, and therefore IgG myelomas are more common than IgA and IgD myelomas.

MULTIPLE MYELOMA

DEFINITION

Multiple myeloma represents a malignant proliferation of plasma cells derived from a single clone. The terms *multiple myeloma* and *myeloma* may be used interchangeably. The tumor, its products, and the host response to it result in a number of organ dysfunctions and symptoms of bone pain or fracture, renal failure, susceptibility to infection, anemia, hypercalcemia, and occasionally clotting abnormalities, neurologic symptoms, and manifestations of hyperviscosity.

ETIOLOGY

The cause of myeloma is not known. Myeloma occurred with increased frequency in those exposed to the radiation of nuclear warheads in World War II after a 20-year latency. A variety of chromosomal alterations have been found in patients with myeloma; 13q14 deletions, 17p13 deletions, and 11q abnormalities predominate. The most common translocations are t(11;14)(q13;q32) and t(4;14)(p16;q32), and evidence is strong that errors in switch recombination—the genetic mechanism to change antibody heavy chain isotype—participate in the transformation pathway. Overexpression of *myc* or *ras* genes has been noted in some cases. Mutations in p53 and Rb-1 have also been described, but no common molecular pathogenesis has yet emerged.

Myeloma has been seen more commonly than expected among farmers, wood workers, leather workers, and those exposed to petroleum products. The neoplastic event in myeloma may involve cells earlier in B cell differentiation than the plasma cell. Circulating B cells bearing surface immunoglobulin that share the idiotype of the M component are present in myeloma patients. Interleukin (IL) 6 may play a role in driving myeloma cell proliferation; a large fraction of myeloma cells exposed to IL-6 in vitro respond by proliferating. The IL-6 dependency of myeloma is controversial. It remains difficult to distinguish benign from malignant plasma cells on the basis of morphologic criteria in all but a few cases (Fig. 106-2).

INCIDENCE AND PREVALENCE

About 19,900 cases of myeloma were diagnosed in 2007, and 10,790 people died from the disease in the United States. Myeloma increases in incidence with age. The median age at diagnosis is 68 years; it is uncommon under age 40. The yearly incidence is around 4 per 100,000 and remarkably similar throughout the world.

FIGURE 106-2 Multiple myeloma (marrow). The cells bear characteristic morphologic features of plasma cells, round or oval cells with an eccentric nucleus composed of coarsely clumped chromatin, a densely basophilic cytoplasm, and a perinuclear clear zone (hof) containing the Golgi apparatus. Binucleate and multinucleate malignant plasma cells can be seen.

TABLE 106-1 CLINICAL FEATURES OF MULTIPLE MYELOMA

Clinical Finding	Underlying Cause and Pathogenetic Mechanism
Hypercalcemia, osteoporosis, pathologic fractures, lytic bone lesions, bone pain	Tumor expansion, production of osteoclast activating factor by tumor cells, osteoblast inhibitory factors
Renal failure	Hypercalcemia, light chain deposition, amyloidosis, urate nephropathy, drug toxicity (nonsteroidal anti-inflammatory agents, bisphosphonates), contrast dye
Easy fatigue—anemia	Bone marrow infiltration, production of inhibitory factors, hemolysis, decreased red cell production, decreased erythropoietin levels
Recurrent infections	Hypogammaglobulinemia, low CD4 count, decreased neutrophil migration
Neurologic symptoms	Hyperviscosity, cryoglobulinemia, amyloid deposits, hypercalcemia, nerve compression, anti-neuronal antibody, POEMS syndrome, therapy-related toxicity
Nausea and vomiting	Renal failure, hypercalcemia
Bleeding/clotting disorder	Interference with clotting factors, antibody to clotting factors, amyloid damage of endothelium, platelet dysfunction, antibody coating of platelet, therapy-related hypercoagulable defects

Note: POEMS, polyneuropathy, organomegaly, endocrinopathy, multiple myeloma, and skin changes.

Males are more commonly affected than females, and blacks have nearly twice the incidence of whites. Myeloma accounts for ~1% of all malignancies in whites and 2% in blacks; 13% of all hematologic cancers in whites and 33% in blacks.

The incidence of myeloma is highest in African-American and Pacific islanders; intermediate in Europeans and North American Caucasians; and lowest in developing countries including Asia. The higher incidence in more developed countries may result from the combination of a longer life expectancy and more frequent medical surveillance. Incidence of multiple myeloma in other ethnic groups including native Hawaiians, female Hispanics, American Indians from New Mexico, and Alaskan natives is higher relative to U.S. Caucasians in the same geographic area. Chinese and Japanese populations have a lower incidence than Caucasians. Immunoproliferative small intestinal disease with alpha heavy chain disease is most prevalent in the Mediterranean area. Despite these differences in prevalence, the characteristics, response to therapy, and prognosis of myeloma are similar worldwide.

PATHOGENESIS AND CLINICAL MANIFESTATIONS

(**Table 106-1**) Multiple myeloma (MM) cells bind via cell-surface adhesion molecules to bone marrow stromal cells (BMSCs) and extracellular matrix (ECM), which triggers MM cell growth, survival, drug resistance, and migration in the bone marrow milieu (**Fig. 106-3**). These effects are due both to direct MM cell–BMSC binding and to induction of various cytokines including IL-6, insulin-like growth factor-1 (IGF-1), vascular endothelial growth factor (VEGF), and stromal cell–derived growth factor (SDF)-1α. Growth, drug resistance, and migration are mediated via Ras/Raf/mitogen-activated protein kinase, PI3-K/Akt, and protein kinase C signaling cascades, respectively.

Bone pain is the most common symptom in myeloma, affecting nearly 70% of patients. The pain usually involves the back and ribs, and unlike the pain of metastatic carcinoma, which often is worse at night, the pain of myeloma is precipitated by movement. Persistent localized pain in a patient with myeloma usually signifies a pathologic fracture. The bone lesions of myeloma are caused by the proliferation of tumor cells, activation of osteoclasts that destroy bone, and suppression of osteoblasts that form new bone. The osteoclasts respond to osteoclast activating factors (OAF) made by the myeloma cells [OAF activity can be mediated by several cytokines, including IL-1, lymphotoxin, VEGF, receptor activator of NF-κB (RANK) ligand, macrophage inhibitory factor (MIP)-1α, and tumor necrosis factor (TNF)]. However, production of these factors decreases following administration of glucocorticoids or interferon (IFN) α. The bone lesions are lytic in nature and are rarely associated with osteoblastic new bone formation. Therefore, radioisotopic bone scanning is less useful in diagnosis than is plain radiography. The bony lysis results in substantial mobilization

FIGURE 106-3 Pathogenesis of multiple myeloma. Multiple myeloma cells interact with bone marrow stromal cells and extracellular matrix proteins via adhesion molecules, triggering adhesion-mediated signaling as well as cytokine production. This triggers cytokine-mediated signaling that provides growth, survival, and anti-apoptotic effects as well as development of drug resistance. HSP, heparin sulfate proteoglycan.

FIGURE 106-4 Bony lesions in multiple myeloma. The skull demonstrates the typical "punched out" lesions characteristic of multiple myeloma. The lesion represents a purely osteolytic lesion with little or no osteoblastic activity. *(Courtesy of Dr. Geraldine Schechter; with permission.)*

of calcium from bone, and serious acute and chronic complications of hypercalcemia may dominate the clinical picture (see below). Localized bone lesions may expand to the point that mass lesions may be palpated, especially on the skull (**Fig. 106-4**), clavicles, and sternum, and the collapse of vertebrae may lead to spinal cord compression.

The next most common clinical problem in patients with myeloma is susceptibility to bacterial infections. The most common infections are pneumonias and pyelonephritis, and the most frequent pathogens are *Streptococcus pneumoniae*, *Staphylococcus aureus*, and *Klebsiella pneumoniae* in the lungs and *Escherichia coli* and other gram-negative organisms in the urinary tract. In ~25% of patients, recurrent infections are the presenting features, and >75% of patients will have a serious infection at some time in their course. The susceptibility to infection has several contributing causes. First, patients with myeloma have diffuse hypogammaglobulinemia if the M component is excluded. The hypogammaglobulinemia is related to both decreased production and increased destruction of normal antibodies. Moreover, some patients generate a population of circulating regulatory cells in response to their myeloma that can suppress normal antibody synthesis. In the case of IgG myeloma, normal IgG antibodies are broken down more rapidly than normal because the catabolic rate for IgG antibodies varies directly with the serum concentration. The large M component results in fractional catabolic rates of 8–16% instead of the normal 2%. These patients have very poor antibody responses, especially to polysaccharide antigens such as those on bacterial cell walls. Most measures of T cell function in myeloma are normal, but a subset of CD4+ cells may be decreased. Granulocyte lysozyme content is low, and granulocyte migration is not as rapid as normal in patients with myeloma, probably the result of a tumor product. There are also a variety of abnormalities in complement functions in myeloma patients. All these factors contribute to the immune deficiency of these patients. Some commonly used therapeutic agents, e.g., dexamethasone, suppress immune responses and increase susceptibility to infection.

Renal failure occurs in nearly 25% of myeloma patients, and some renal pathology is noted in over half. Many factors contribute to this. Hypercalcemia is the most common cause of renal failure. Glomerular deposits of amyloid, hyperuricemia, recurrent infections, frequent use of nonsteroidal anti-inflammatory agents for pain control, use of iodinated contrast dye for imaging, bisphosphonate use, and occasional infiltration of the kidney by myeloma cells all may contribute to renal dysfunction. However, tubular damage associated with the excretion of light chains is almost always present. Normally, light chains are filtered, reabsorbed in the tubules, and catabolized. With the increase in the amount of light chains presented to the tubule, the tubular cells become overloaded with these proteins, and tubular damage results either

directly from light chain toxic effects or indirectly from the release of intracellular lysosomal enzymes. The earliest manifestation of this tubular damage is the adult Fanconi syndrome (a type 2 proximal renal tubular acidosis), with loss of glucose and amino acids, as well as defects in the ability of the kidney to acidify and concentrate the urine. The proteinuria is not accompanied by hypertension, and the protein is nearly all light chains. Generally, very little albumin is in the urine because glomerular function is usually normal. When the glomeruli are involved, nonselective proteinuria is also observed. Patients with myeloma also have a decreased anion gap [i.e., $Na^+ - (Cl^- + HCO_3^-)$] because the M component is cationic, resulting in retention of chloride. This is often accompanied by hyponatremia that is felt to be artificial (pseudohyponatremia) because each volume of serum has less water as a result of the increased protein. Renal dysfunction due to light chain deposition disease, light chain cast nephropathy, and amyloidosis is partially reversible with effective therapy. Myeloma patients are susceptible to developing acute renal failure if they become dehydrated.

Anemia occurs in ~80% of myeloma patients. It is usually normocytic and normochromic and related both to the replacement of normal marrow by expanding tumor cells and to the inhibition of hematopoiesis by factors made by the tumor. In addition, mild hemolysis may contribute to the anemia. A larger than expected fraction of patients may have megaloblastic anemia due to either folate or vitamin B_{12} deficiency. Granulocytopenia and thrombocytopenia are very rare. Clotting abnormalities may be seen due to the failure of antibody-coated platelets to function properly or to the interaction of the M component with clotting factors I, II, V, VII, or VIII. Deep venous thrombosis is also observed with use of thalidomide or lenalidomide in combination with dexamethasone. Raynaud's phenomenon and impaired circulation may result if the M component forms cryoglobulins, and hyperviscosity syndromes may develop depending on the physical properties of the M component (most common with IgM, IgG3, and IgA paraproteins). Hyperviscosity is defined on the basis of the relative viscosity of serum as compared with water. Normal relative serum viscosity is 1.8 (i.e., serum is normally almost twice as viscous as water). Symptoms of hyperviscosity occur at a level of 5–6, a level usually reached at paraprotein concentrations of ~40 g/L (4 g/dL) for IgM, 50 g/L (5 g/dL) for IgG3, and 70 g/L (7 g/dL) for IgA.

Although neurologic symptoms occur in a minority of patients, they may have many causes. Hypercalcemia may produce lethargy, weakness, depression, and confusion. Hyperviscosity may lead to headache, fatigue, visual disturbances, and retinopathy. Bony damage and collapse may lead to cord compression, radicular pain, and loss of bowel and bladder control. Infiltration of peripheral nerves by amyloid can be a cause of carpal tunnel syndrome and other sensorimotor mono- and polyneuropathies. Sensory neuropathy is also a side effect of thalidomide and bortezomib therapy.

Many of the clinical features of myeloma, e.g., cord compression, pathologic fractures, hyperviscosity, sepsis, and hypercalcemia, can present as medical emergencies. Despite the widespread distribution of plasma cells in the body, tumor expansion is dominantly within bone and bone marrow and, for reasons unknown, rarely causes enlargement of spleen, lymph nodes, or gut-associated lymphatic tissue.

DIAGNOSIS AND STAGING

The classic triad of myeloma is marrow plasmacytosis (>10%), lytic bone lesions, and a serum and/or urine M component. Bone marrow plasma cells are CD138+ and monoclonal. The most important differential diagnosis in patients with myeloma involves their separation from individuals with monoclonal gammopathies of uncertain significance (MGUS). MGUS are vastly more common than myeloma, occurring in 1% of the population over age 50 and in up to 10% individuals over age 75. The diagnostic criteria for MGUS, smoldering myeloma, and myeloma are described in **Table 106-2**. When bone marrow cells are exposed to radioactive thymidine in order to quantitate dividing cells, patients with MGUS always have a labeling index < 1%; patients with myeloma always have a labeling index > 1%. With long-term follow-up, ~1% per year of patients with MGUS go on to

TABLE 106-2 DIAGNOSTIC CRITERIA FOR MULTIPLE MYELOMA, MYELOMA VARIANTS, AND MONOCLONAL GAMMOPATHY OF UNKNOWN SIGNIFICANCE

Monoclonal gammopathy of undetermined significance (MGUS)
M protein in serum < 30 g/L
Bone marrow clonal plasma cells < 10%
No evidence of other B cell proliferative disorders
No myeloma-related organ or tissue impairment (no end organ damage, including bone lesions)[a]

Asymptomatic myeloma (smouldering myeloma)
M protein in serum ≥ 30 g/L *and/or*
Bone marrow clonal plasma cells ≥ 10%
No myeloma-related organ or tissue impairment (no end organ damage, including bone lesions)[a] or symptoms

Symptomatic multiple myeloma
M protein in serum and/or urine
Bone marrow (clonal) plasma cells[b] or plasmacytoma
Myeloma-related organ or tissue impairment (end organ damage, including bone lesions)

Nonsecretory myeloma
No M protein in serum and/or urine with immunofixation
Bone marrow clonal plasmacytosis ≥ 10% or plasmacytoma
Myeloma-related organ or tissue impairment (end organ damage, including bone lesions)[a]

Solitary plasmacytoma of bone
No M protein in serum and/or urine[c]
Single area of bone destruction due to clonal plasma cells
Bone marrow not consistent with multiple myeloma
Normal skeletal survey (and MRI of spine and pelvis if done)
No related organ or tissue impairment (no end organ damage other than solitary bone lesion)[a]

[a]Myeloma-related organ or tissue impairment (end organ damage) (ROTI): Calcium levels increased: serum calcium > 0.25 mmol/L above the upper limit of normal or > 2.75 mmol/L; renal insufficiency: creatinine > 173 mmol/L; anemia: hemoglobin 2 g/dL below the lower limit of normal or hemoglobin < 10 g/dL; bone lesions: lytic lesions or osteoporosis with compression fractures (MRI or CT may clarify); other: symptomatic hyperviscosity, amyloidosis, recurrent bacterial infections (>2 episodes in 12 months).
[b]If flow cytometry is performed, most plasma cells (>90%) will show a "neoplastic" phenotype.
[c]A small M component may sometimes be present.

develop myeloma. Non-IgG subtype, abnormal kappa/lambda free light chain ratio, and serum M protein > 15 g/L (1.5 g/dL) are associated with higher incidence of progression of MGUS to myeloma. Typically, patients with MGUS require no therapy. Their survival is ~2 years shorter than age-matched controls without MGUS. There are two important variants of myeloma, solitary bone plasmacytoma and extramedullary plasmacytoma. These lesions are associated with an M component in <30% of the cases, they may affect younger individuals, and both are associated with median survivals of ≥10 years. Solitary bone plasmacytoma is a single lytic bone lesion without marrow plasmacytosis. Extramedullary plasmacytomas usually involve the submucosal lymphoid tissue of the nasopharynx or paranasal sinuses without marrow plasmacytosis. Both tumors are highly responsive to local radiation therapy. If an M component is present, it should disappear after treatment. Solitary bone plasmacytomas may recur in other bony sites or evolve into myeloma. Extramedullary plasmacytomas rarely recur or progress.

The clinical evaluation of patients with myeloma includes a careful physical examination searching for tender bones and masses. Only a small minority of patients has an enlargement of the spleen and lymph nodes, the physiologic sites of antibody production. Chest and bone radiographs may reveal lytic lesions or diffuse osteopenia. MRI offers a sensitive means to document extent of bone marrow infiltration and cord or root compression in patients with pain syndromes. A complete blood count with differential may reveal anemia. Erythrocyte sedimentation rate is elevated. Rare patients (~2%) may have plasma cell leukemia with >2000 plasma cells/μL. This may be seen in disproportionate frequency in IgD (12%) and IgE (25%) myelomas. Serum calcium, urea nitrogen, creatinine, and uric acid levels may be elevated.

Protein electrophoresis and measurement of serum immunoglobulins and free light chains are useful for detecting and characterizing M spikes, supplemented by immunoelectrophoresis, which is especially sensitive for identifying low concentrations of M components not detectable by protein electrophoresis. A 24-h urine specimen is necessary to quantitate protein excretion, and a concentrated aliquot is used for electrophoresis and immunologic typing of any M component. Serum alkaline phosphatase is usually normal even with extensive bone involvement because of the absence of osteoblastic activity. It is also important to quantitate serum β_2-microglobulin (see below). Serum soluble IL-6 receptor levels and C-reactive protein may reflect physiologic IL-6 levels in the patient.

The serum M component will be IgG in 53% of patients, IgA in 25%, and IgD in 1%; 20% of patients will have only light chains in serum and urine. Dipsticks for detecting proteinuria are not reliable at identifying light chains, and the heat test for detecting Bence Jones protein is falsely negative in ~50% of patients with light chain myeloma. Fewer than 1% of patients have no identifiable M component; these patients usually have light chain myeloma in which renal catabolism has made the light chains undetectable in the urine. IgD myeloma may also present as light chain myeloma. About two-thirds of patients with serum M components also have urinary light chains. The light chain isotype may have an impact on survival. Patients secreting lambda light chains have a significantly shorter overall survival than those secreting kappa light chains. It is not clear whether this is due to some genetically important determinant of cell proliferation or because lambda light chains are more likely to cause renal damage and form amyloid than are kappa light chains. The heavy chain isotype may have an impact on patient management as well. About half of patients with IgM paraproteins develop hyperviscosity compared with only 2–4% of patients with IgA and IgG M components. Among IgG myelomas, it is the IgG3 subclass that has the highest tendency to form both concentration- and temperature-dependent aggregates, leading to hyperviscosity and cold agglutination at lower serum concentrations.

The various staging systems for patients with myeloma (Table 106-3) are functional systems for predicting survival and are based on a variety of clinical and laboratory tests, unlike the anatomic staging systems for solid tumors. The Durie-Salmon staging system is based on the hemoglobin, calcium, M component, and degree of skeletal involvement; the total-body tumor burden is estimated to be low (stage I), intermediate (stage II), or high (stage III), and the stages are further subdivided on the basis of renal function [A if serum creatinine <177 mol/L (<2 mg/dL), B if >177 (>2)]. Patients in stage IA have a median survival of >5 years and those in stage IIIB about 15 months. This staging system has been found not to predict prognosis after treatment with high-dose therapy or the novel targeted therapies that have emerged.

Serum β_2-microglobulin is a protein of 11,000 mol wt with homologies with the constant region of immunoglobulins that is the light chain of the class I major histocompatibility antigens (HLA-A, -B, -C) on the surface of every cell. Serum β_2-microglobulin is the single most powerful predictor of survival and can substitute for staging. Patients with β_2-microglobulin levels <0.004 g/L have a median survival of 43 months and those with levels >0.004 g/L only 12 months. Serum β_2-microglobulin and albumin levels are the basis for a three-stage International Staging System (ISS). It is also felt that once the diagnosis of myeloma is firm, histologic features of atypia may also exert an influence on prognosis. IL-6 may be an autocrine and/or paracrine growth factor for myeloma cells; elevated levels are associated with more aggressive disease. High labeling index and high levels of lactate dehydrogenase are also associated with poor prognosis.

Other factors that may influence prognosis are the number of cytogenetic abnormalities including hyperploidy, chromosome 13q and 17p deletion, t(4;14) and t(11;14); % plasma cells in the marrow; circulating plasma cells; performance status; as well as serum levels of soluble IL-6 receptor, C-reactive protein, hepatocyte growth factor, C-terminal cross-linked telopeptide of collagen I, transforming growth factor (TGF) β, and syndecan-1. Microarray profiling and comparative genomic hybridization have formed the basis for RNA- and DNA-

TABLE 106-3 MYELOMA STAGING SYSTEMS

Durie-Salmon Staging System

Stage	Criteria	Estimated Tumor Burden, $\times 10^{12}$ cells/m²
I	All of the following: 1. Hemoglobin >100 g/L (>10 g/dL) 2. Serum calcium <3 mmol/L (<12 mg/dL) 3. Normal bone x-ray or solitary lesion 4. Low M-component production a. IgG level <50 g/L (<5 g/dL) b. IgA level <30 g/L (<3 g/dL) c. Urine light chain <4 g/24 h	<0.6 (low)
II	Fitting neither I nor III	0.6–1.20 (intermediate)
III	One or more of the following: 1. Hemoglobin <85 g/L (<8.5 g/dL) 2. Serum calcium >3 mmol/L (>12 mg/dL) 3. Advanced lytic bone lesions 4. High M-component production a. IgG level >70 g/L (>7 g/dL) b. IgA level >50 g/L (>5 g/dL) c. Urine light chains >12 g/24 h	>1.20 (high)

Level	Stage	Median Survival, Months
Subclassification based on serum creatinine levels		
A < 177 μmol/L (<2 mg/dL)	IA	61
B > 177 μmol/L (>2 mg/dL)	IIA, B	55
	IIIA	30
	IIIB	15
International Staging System		
β_2M < 3.5, alb ≥ 3.5	I (28%)	62
β_2M < 3.5, alb < 3.5 *or* β_2M = 3.5–5.5	II (39%)	44
β_2M > 5.5	III (33%)	29

Note: β_2M, serum β_2-microglobulin in mg/L; alb, serum albumin in g/dL; (#), % patients presenting at each stage.

based prognostic staging systems, respectively. The ISS system is the most widely used method of assessing prognosis (Table 106-3).

℞ MULTIPLE MYELOMA

About 10% of patients with myeloma will have an indolent course demonstrating only very slow progression of disease over many years. Such patients only require antitumor therapy when the disease becomes symptomatic with development of anemia, hypercalcemia, progressive lytic bone lesions (including vertebral compression fractures), progressive rise in serum myeloma protein levels and/or Bence Jones proteinuria, or recurrent infections. Patients with solitary bone plasmacytomas and extramedullary plasmacytomas may be expected to enjoy prolonged disease-free survival after local radiation therapy to a dose of around 40 Gy. There is a low incidence of occult marrow involvement in patients with solitary bone plasmacytoma. Such patients are usually detected because their serum M component falls slowly or disappears initially only to return after a few months. These patients respond well to systemic chemotherapy.

Patients with symptomatic and/or progressive myeloma require therapeutic intervention. In general such therapy is of two sorts: systemic therapy to control the progression of myeloma, and symptomatic supportive care to prevent serious morbidity from the complications of the disease. Therapy can significantly prolong survival and improve the quality of life for myeloma patients.

The initial standard treatment for newly diagnosed myeloma is dependent on whether or not the patient is a candidate for high-dose chemotherapy with autologous stem cell transplant.

In patients who are transplant candidates, alkylating agents such as melphalan should be avoided since they damage stem cells, leading to decreased ability to collect stem cells for autologous transplant. High-dose pulsed glucocorticoids have been used either alone (dexamethasone 40 mg for 4 days every 2 weeks) or in combination VAD chemotherapy (vincristine, 0.4 mg/d in a 4-day continuous infusion; doxorubicin, 9 mg/m² per day in a 4-day continuous infusion; dexamethasone, 40 mg/d for 4 days per week for 3 weeks) for initial cytoreduction. However, two studies have combined thalidomide with dexamethasone as initial therapy for newly diagnosed multiple myeloma in transplant candidates and reported rapid responses in two-thirds of patients, while allowing for successful harvesting of peripheral blood stem cells for transplantation. A randomized phase III trial showed statistically significantly higher response rates for thalidomide (200 mg PO qhs) plus dexamethasone (40 mg for 4 days every 2 weeks) compared to dexamethasone alone, setting the stage for use of this combination as standard therapy in newly diagnosed patients. Initial therapy is continued until maximal cytoreduction. Importantly, novel agents bortezomib, a proteasome inhibitor, and lenalidomide, an immunomodulatory derivative of thalidomide, have similarly been combined with dexamethasone and obtained high response rates without compromising collection of stem cells for transplantation.

In patients who are not transplant candidates, therapy has consisted of intermittent pulses of an alkylating agent, L-phenylalanine mustard (L-PAM, melphalan) and prednisone administered for 4–7 days every 4–6 weeks. The usual doses of melphalan/prednisone (MP) are melphalan, 8 mg/m² per day, and prednisone, 25–60 mg/m² per day for 4 days. Doses may need adjustment due to unpredictable absorption and based on marrow tolerance. Patients responding to therapy generally have a prompt and gratifying reduction in bone pain, hypercalcemia, and anemia, and often have fewer infections. The serum M component lags substantially behind the symptomatic improvement, often taking 4–6 weeks to fall. This fall depends on the rate of tumor kill and the fractional catabolic rate of immunoglobulin, which in turn depends on the serum concentration (for IgG). Light chain excretion, with a functional half-life of ~6 h, may fall within the first week of treatment. However, since urine light chain levels may relate to renal tubular function, they are not a reliable measure of tumor cell kill. Calculations of tumor cell kill are made by extrapolation of the serum M component level and rely heavily on the assumption that every tumor cell produces immunoglobulin at a constant rate. About 60% of patients will achieve at least a 75% reduction in serum M component level and tumor cell mass in response to melphalan and prednisone. Although this is a tumor reduction of <1 log, clinical responses may last many months. The important feature of the level of the M protein is not how far or how fast it falls, but the rate of its increase after therapy. Efforts to improve the fraction of patients responding and the degree of response have involved adding other active agents to the treatment program. In patients >65 years, combining thalidomide with MP (MPT) obtains higher response rates and overall survival than MP alone, and MPT is the standard therapy for patients who are not transplant candidates.

Randomized studies comparing standard-dose therapy to high-dose melphalan therapy (HDT) with hematopoietic stem cell support have shown that HDT can achieve high overall response rates and prolonged progression-free and overall survival; however, few, if any, patients are cured. Although complete responses are rare (<5%) with standard-dose chemotherapy, HDT achieves 25–40% complete responses. In randomized studies, HDT produced better median event-free survival in four of five studies, higher complete response rate in four of five trials, and better overall survival in three of five studies. Two successive HDTs (tandem transplants) are more effective than single HDT in the subset of patients who do not achieve a complete or very good partial response to the first transplant. Allogeneic transplants may also produce high response rates, but treatment-related mortality may be as high as 40%. Non-myeloablative allogeneic transplantation is now under evaluation to reduce toxicity, while permitting an immune graft-vs.-myeloma effect.

There is no standard maintenance therapy to prolong time to progression. IFN-α has allowed modest benefit but has significant side effects. Oral prednisone maintenance therapy was effective in a single trial. Ongoing studies are evaluating maintenance thalidomide and lenalidomide to prolong progression-free survival post-transplant.

Relapsed myeloma can be treated with novel agents including lenalidomide and/or bortezomib. These agents target not only the tumor cell but also the tumor cell–bone marrow interaction and the bone marrow milieu. These agents in combination with dexamethasone can achieve up to 60% partial responses and 10–15% complete responses in patients with relapsed disease. The combination of bortezomib and liposomal doxorubicin is active in relapsed myeloma. Thalidomide, if not used as initial therapy, can achieve responses in refractory cases. High-dose melphalan and stem cell transplant, if not used earlier, also have activity in patients with refractory disease.

The median overall survival of patients with myeloma is 5–6 years, with subsets of patients surviving over 10 years. The major causes of death are progressive myeloma, renal failure, sepsis, or therapy-related acute leukemia or myelodysplasia. Nearly a quarter of patients die of myocardial infarction, chronic lung disease, diabetes, or stroke, all intercurrent illnesses related more to the age of the patient group than to the tumor.

Supportive care directed at the anticipated complications of the disease may be as important as primary antitumor therapy. The hypercalcemia generally responds well to bisphosphonates, glucocorticoid therapy, hydration, and natriuresis. Calcitonin may add to the inhibitory effects of glucocorticoids on bone resorption. Bisphosphonates (e.g., pamidronate 90 mg or zoledronate 4 mg once a month) reduce osteoclastic bone resorption and preserve performance status and quality of life, decrease bone-related complications, and may also have antitumor effects. Treatments aimed at strengthening the skeleton, such as fluorides, calcium, and vitamin D, with or without androgens, have been suggested but are not of proven efficacy. Iatrogenic worsening of renal function may be prevented by maintaining a high fluid intake to prevent dehydration and to help excrete light chains and calcium. In the event of acute renal failure, plasmapheresis is ~10 times more effective at clearing light chains than peritoneal dialysis; however, its role in reversing renal failure remains controversial. Importantly, reducing the protein load by effective antitumor therapy with agents such as bortezomib may result in functional improvement. Urinary tract infections should be watched for and treated early. Plasmapheresis may be the treatment of choice for hyperviscosity syndromes. Although the pneumococcus is a dreaded pathogen in myeloma patients, pneumococcal polysaccharide vaccines may not elicit an antibody response. Prophylactic administration of IV γ globulin preparations is used in the setting of recurrent serious infections. Chronic oral antibiotic prophylaxis is probably not warranted. Patients developing neurologic symptoms in the lower extremities, severe localized back pain, or problems with bowel and bladder control may need emergency MRI and radiation therapy for palliation. Most bone lesions respond to analgesics and chemotherapy, but certain painful lesions may respond most promptly to localized radiation. The anemia associated with myeloma may respond to erythropoietin along with hematinics (iron, folate, cobalamin). The pathogenesis of the anemia should be established and specific therapy instituted, where possible.

WALDENSTRÖM'S MACROGLOBULINEMIA

In 1948, Waldenström described a malignancy of lymphoplasmacytoid cells that secreted IgM. In contrast to myeloma, the disease was associated with lymphadenopathy and hepatosplenomegaly, but the major clinical manifestation was the hyperviscosity syndrome. The disease resembles the related diseases chronic lymphocytic leukemia, myeloma, and lymphocytic lymphoma. It originates from a post–germinal center B cell that has undergone somatic mutations and antigenic selection in the lymphoid follicle and has the characteristics of an IgM-bearing memory B cell. Waldenström's macroglobulinemia and IgM myeloma follow a similar clinical course, but therapeutic options are different. The diagnosis of IgM myeloma is usually reserved for patients with lytic bone lesions and predominant infiltration with CD138+ plasma cells in the bone marrow. Such patients are at greater risk of pathologic fractures than patients with Waldenström's macroglobulinemia.

The cause of macroglobulinemia is unknown. The disease is similar to myeloma in being slightly more common in men and occurring with increased incidence with age (median 64 years). There have been reports that the IgM in some patients with macroglobulinemia may have specificity for myelin-associated glycoprotein (MAG), a protein that has been associated with demyelinating disease of the peripheral nervous system and may be lost earlier and to a greater extent than the better known myelin basic protein in patients with multiple sclerosis. Sometimes patients with macroglobulinemia develop a peripheral neuropathy before the appearance of the neoplasm. There is speculation that the whole process begins with a viral infection that may elicit an antibody response that cross-reacts with a normal tissue component.

Like myeloma, the disease involves the bone marrow, but unlike myeloma, it does not cause bone lesions or hypercalcemia. Like myeloma, a serum M component is present in the serum in excess of 30 g/L (3 g/dL), but unlike myeloma, the size of the IgM paraprotein results in little renal excretion, and only ~20% of patients excrete light chains. Therefore, renal disease is not common. The light chain isotype is kappa in 80% of the cases. Patients present with weakness, fatigue, and recurrent infections, similar to myeloma patients, but epistaxis, visual disturbances, and neurologic symptoms such as peripheral neuropathy, dizziness, headache, and transient paresis are much more common in macroglobulinemia. Physical examination reveals adenopathy and hepatosplenomegaly, and ophthalmoscopic examination may reveal vascular segmentation and dilatation of the retinal veins characteristic of hyperviscosity states. Patients may have a normocytic, normochromic anemia, but rouleaux formation and a positive Coombs' test are much more common than in myeloma. Malignant lymphocytes are usually present in the peripheral blood. About 10% of macroglobulins are cryoglobulins. These are pure M components and are not the mixed cryoglobulins seen in rheumatoid arthritis and other autoimmune diseases. Mixed cryoglobulins are composed of IgM or IgA complexed with IgG, for which they are specific. In both cases, Raynaud's phenomenon and serious vascular symptoms precipitated by the cold may occur, but mixed cryoglobulins are not commonly associated with malignancy. Patients suspected of having a cryoglobulin based on history and physical examination should have their blood drawn into a warm syringe and delivered to the laboratory in a container of warm water to avoid errors in quantitating the cryoglobulin.

Rx WALDENSTRÖM'S MACROGLOBULINEMIA

Control of serious hyperviscosity symptoms such as an altered state of consciousness or paresis can be achieved acutely by plasmapheresis because 80% of the IgM paraprotein is intravascular. The median survival is ~50 months, similar to that of multiple myeloma. However, many individuals with Waldenström's macroglobulinemia have indolent disease that does not require therapy. Pretreatment parameters including older age, male sex, general symptoms, and cytopenias define a high-risk population. Fludarabine (25 mg/m² per day for 5 days every 4 weeks) or cladribine (0.1 mg/kg per day for 7 days every 4 weeks) are highly effective single agents. About 80% of patients respond to chemotherapy, and their median survival is >3 years. Rituximab (anti-CD20) can produce responses alone or combined with chemotherapy. As in multiple myeloma, bortezomib and lenalidomide also have activity.

POEMS SYNDROME

The features of this syndrome are *p*olyneuropathy, *o*rganomegaly, *e*ndocrinopathy, *m*ultiple myeloma, and *s*kin changes (POEMS). Patients usually have a severe, progressive sensorimotor polyneuropathy associated with sclerotic bone lesions from myeloma. Polyneuropathy occurs in ~1.4% of myelomas, but the POEMS syndrome is only a rare subset of that group. Unlike typical myeloma, hepatomegaly and lymphadenopathy occur in about two-thirds of patients, and splenomegaly is seen in one-third. The lymphadenopathy frequently resembles Castleman's disease histologically, a condition that has been linked to IL-6 overproduction. The endocrine manifestations include amenorrhea in women and impotence and gynecomastia in men. Hyperprolactinemia due to loss of normal inhibitory control by the hypothalamus may be associated with other central nervous system manifestations such as papilledema and elevated cerebrospinal fluid pressure and protein. Type 2 diabetes mellitus occurs in about one-third of patients. Hypothyroidism and adrenal insufficiency are occasionally noted. Skin changes are diverse: hyperpigmentation, hypertrichosis, skin thickening, and digital clubbing. Other manifestations include peripheral edema, ascites, pleural effusions, fever, and thrombocytosis.

The pathogenesis of the disease is unclear, but high circulating levels of the proinflammatory cytokines IL-1, IL-6, VEGF, and TNF have been documented and levels of the inhibitory cytokine TGF-β are lower than expected. Treatment of the myeloma may result in an improvement in the other disease manifestations.

Patients are often treated similarly to those with myeloma. Plasmapheresis does not appear to be of benefit in POEMS syndrome. Patients presenting with isolated sclerotic lesions may have resolution of neuropathic symptoms after local therapy for plasmacytoma with radiotherapy. Similar to multiple myeloma, novel agents as well as high-dose therapy with autologous stem cell transplant have been pursued in selected patients and have been associated with prolonged progression-free survival.

HEAVY CHAIN DISEASES

The heavy chain diseases are rare lymphoplasmacytic malignancies. Their clinical manifestations vary with the heavy chain isotype. Patients secrete a defective heavy chain that usually has an intact Fc fragment and a deletion in the Fd region. Gamma, alpha, and mu heavy chain diseases have been described, but no reports of delta or epsilon heavy chain diseases have appeared. Molecular biologic analysis of these tumors has revealed structural genetic defects that may account for the aberrant chain secreted.

GAMMA HEAVY CHAIN DISEASE (FRANKLIN'S DISEASE)

This disease affects individuals of widely different age groups and countries of origin. It is characterized by lymphadenopathy, fever, anemia, malaise, hepatosplenomegaly, and weakness. Its most distinctive symptom is palatal edema, resulting from involvement of nodes in Waldeyer's ring, and this may progress to produce respiratory compromise. The diagnosis depends on the demonstration of an anomalous serum M component [often <20 g/L (<2 g/dL)] that reacts with anti-IgG but not anti-light chain reagents. *The M component is typically present in both serum and urine.* Most of the paraproteins have been of the gamma$_1$ subclass, but other subclasses have been seen. The patients may have thrombocytopenia, eosinophilia, and nondiagnostic bone marrow. Patients usually have a rapid downhill course and die of infection; however, some patients have survived 5 years with chemotherapy.

ALPHA HEAVY CHAIN DISEASE (SELIGMANN'S DISEASE)

This is the most common of the heavy chain diseases. It is closely related to a malignancy known as *Mediterranean lymphoma*, a disease that affects young persons in parts of the world where intestinal parasites are common, such as the Mediterranean, Asia, and South America. The disease is characterized by an infiltration of the lamina propria of the small intestine with lymphoplasmacytoid cells that secrete truncated alpha chains. Demonstrating alpha heavy chains is difficult because the alpha chains tend to polymerize and appear as a smear instead of a sharp peak on electrophoretic profiles. Despite the polymerization, hyperviscosity is not a common problem in alpha heavy chain disease. Without J chain–facilitated dimerization, viscosity does not increase dramatically. Light chains are absent from serum and urine. The patients present with chronic diarrhea, weight loss, and malabsorption and have extensive mesenteric and paraaortic adenopathy. Respiratory tract involvement occurs rarely. Patients may vary widely in their clinical course. Some may develop diffuse aggressive histologies of malignant lymphoma. Chemotherapy may produce long-term remissions. Rare patients appear to have responded to antibiotic therapy, raising the question of the etiologic role of antigenic stimulation, perhaps by some chronic intestinal infection. Chemotherapy plus antibiotics may be more effective than chemotherapy alone. Immunoproliferative small intestinal disease (IPSID) is recognized as an infectious pathogen–associated human lymphoma that has association with *Campylobacter jejuni*. It involves mainly the proximal small intestine resulting in malabsorption, diarrhea, and abdominal pain. IPSID is associated with excessive plasma cell differentiation and produces truncated alpha heavy chain proteins lacking the light chains as well as the first constant domain. Early-stage IPSID responds to antibiotics (30–70% complete remission). Most untreated IPSID patients progress to lymphoplasmacytic and immunoblastic lymphoma.

MU HEAVY CHAIN DISEASE

The secretion of isolated mu heavy chains into the serum appears to occur in a very rare subset of patients with chronic lymphocytic leukemia. The only features that may distinguish patients with mu heavy chain disease are the presence of vacuoles in the malignant lymphocytes and the excretion of kappa light chains in the urine. The diagnosis requires ultracentrifugation or gel filtration to confirm the nonreactivity of the paraprotein with the light chain reagents, because some intact macroglobulins fail to interact with these serums. The tumor cells seem to have a defect in the assembly of light and heavy chains, because they appear to contain both in their cytoplasm. There is no evidence that such patients should be treated differently from other patients with chronic lymphocytic leukemia (Chap. 105).

FURTHER READINGS

GHOBRIAL IM et al: Waldenström macroglobulinaemia. Lancet Oncol 4:679, 2003

HAROUSSEAU JL, MOREAU P: Evolving role of stem cell transplantation in multiple myeloma. Clin Lymphoma Myeloma 6:89, 2005

HIDESHIMA T et al: Understanding multiple myeloma pathogenesis in the bone marrow to identify new therapeutic targets. Nature Rev Cancer 7:585, 2007

THE INTERNATIONAL MYELOMA WORKING GROUP: Criteria for the classification of monoclonal gammopathies, multiple myeloma and related disorders: A report of the International Myeloma Working Group. Br J Haematol 121:749, 2003

KUEHL WM, BERGSAGEL PL: Multiple myeloma: Evolving genetic events and host interactions. Nature Rev Cancer 2:175, 2002

KYLE RA, RAJKUMAR SV: Multiple myeloma. N Engl J Med 351:1860, 2004

——— et al: Prevalence of monoclonal gammopathy of undetermined significance. N Engl J Med 354:1362, 2006

——— et al: American Society of Clinical Oncology 2007 clinical practice guideline update on the role of bisphosphonates in multiple myeloma. J Clin Oncol 25:2464, 2007

MITSIADES CS et al: Focus on multiple myeloma. Cancer Cell 6:439, 2005

MUNSHI NC, ANDERSON KC: Plasma cell neoplasm, in *Principles and Practice of Oncology*, 7th ed, V DeVita, S Rosenberg, S Hellman (eds). Philadelphia, Lippincott–Raven Publishers, 2005

TREON SP et al: Update on treatment recommendations from the Third International Workshop on Waldenström's macroglobulinemia. Blood 107:3442, 2006

WAHNER-ROEDLER DL et al: Gamma-heavy chain disease: Review of 23 cases. Medicine 82:236, 2003

107 Transfusion Biology and Therapy

Jeffery S. Dzieczkowski, Kenneth C. Anderson

BLOOD GROUP ANTIGENS AND ANTIBODIES

The study of red blood cell (RBC) antigens and antibodies forms the foundation of transfusion medicine. Serologic studies initially characterized these antigens, but now the molecular composition and structure of many are known. Antigens, either carbohydrate or protein, are assigned to a blood group system based on the structure and similarity of the determinant epitopes. Other cellular blood elements and plasma proteins are also antigenic and can result in *alloimmunization*, the production of antibodies directed against the blood group antigens of another individual. These antibodies are called *alloantibodies*.

Antibodies directed against RBC antigens may result from "natural" exposure, particularly to carbohydrates that mimic some blood group antigens. Those antibodies that occur via natural stimuli are usually produced by a T cell–independent response (thus, generating no memory) and are IgM isotype. *Autoantibodies* (antibodies against autologous blood group antigens) arise spontaneously or as the result of infectious sequelae (e.g., from *Mycoplasma pneumoniae*) and are also often IgM. These antibodies are often clinically insignificant due to their low affinity for antigen at body temperature. However, IgM antibodies can activate the complement cascade and result in hemolysis. Antibodies that result from allogeneic exposure, such as transfusion or pregnancy, are usually IgG. IgG antibodies commonly bind to antigen at warmer temperatures and may hemolyze RBCs. Unlike IgM antibodies, IgG antibodies can cross the placenta and bind fetal erythrocytes bearing the corresponding antigen, resulting in hemolytic disease of the newborn, or *hydrops fetalis*.

Alloimmunization to leukocytes, platelets, and plasma proteins may also result in transfusion complications such as fevers and urticaria but generally does not cause hemolysis. Assay for these other alloantibodies is not routinely performed; however, they may be detected using special assays.

ABO ANTIGENS AND ANTIBODIES

The first blood group antigen system, recognized in 1900, was ABO, the most important in transfusion medicine. The major blood groups of this system are A, B, AB, and O. O type RBCs lack A or B antigens. These antigens are carbohydrates attached to a precursor backbone, may be found on the cellular membrane either as glycosphingolipids or glycoproteins, and are secreted into plasma and body fluids as glycoproteins. H substance is the immediate precursor on which the A and B antigens are added. This H substance is formed by the addition of fucose to the glycolipid or glycoprotein backbone. The subsequent addition of *N*-acetylgalactosamine creates the A antigen, while the addition of galactose produces the B antigen.

The genes that determine the A and B phenotypes are found on chromosome 9p and are expressed in a Mendelian codominant manner. The gene products are glycosyl transferases, which confer the enzymatic capability of attaching the specific antigenic carbohydrate. Individuals who lack the "A" and "B" transferases are phenotypically type "O," while those who inherit both transferases are type "AB." Rare individuals lack the H gene, which codes for fucose transferase, and cannot form H substance. These individuals are homozygous for the silent h allele (hh) and have Bombay phenotype (O_h).

The ABO blood group system is important because essentially all individuals produce antibodies to the ABH carbohydrate antigen that they lack. The naturally occurring anti-A and anti-B antibodies are termed *isoagglutinins*. Thus, type A individuals produce anti-B, while type B individuals make anti-A. Neither isoagglutinin is found in type AB individuals, while type O individuals produce both anti-A and anti-B. Thus, persons with type AB are "universal recipients" because they do not have antibodies against any ABO phenotype, while persons with type O blood can donate to essentially all recipients because their cells are not recognized by any ABO isoagglutinins. The rare individuals with Bombay phenotype produce antibodies to H substance (which is present on all red cells except those of hh phenotype) as well as to both A and B antigens and are therefore compatible only with other hh donors.

In most people, A and B antigens are secreted by the cells and are present in the circulation. Nonsecretors are susceptible to a variety of infections (e.g., *Candida albicans*, *Neisseria meningitidis*, *Streptococcus pneumoniae*, *Haemophilus influenzae*) as many organisms may bind to polysaccharides on cells. Soluble blood group antigens may block this binding.

Rh SYSTEM

The Rh system is the second most important blood group system in pretransfusion testing. The Rh antigens are found on a 30- to 32-kDa RBC membrane protein that has no defined function. Although >40 different antigens in the Rh system have been described, five determinants account for the vast majority of phenotypes. The presence of the D antigen confers Rh "positivity," while persons who lack the D antigen are Rh negative. Two allelic antigen pairs, E/e and C/c, are also found on the Rh protein. The three Rh genes, E/e, D, and C/c, are arranged in tandem on chromosome 1 and inherited as a haplotype, i.e., cDE or Cde. Two haplotypes can result in the phenotypic expression of two to five Rh antigens.

The D antigen is a potent alloantigen. About 15% of individuals lack this antigen. Exposure of these Rh-negative people to even small amounts of Rh-positive cells, by either transfusion or pregnancy, can result in the production of anti-D alloantibody.

OTHER BLOOD GROUP SYSTEMS AND ALLOANTIBODIES

More than 100 blood group systems are recognized, composed of more than 500 antigens. The presence or absence of certain antigens has been associated with various diseases and anomalies; antigens also act as receptors for infectious agents. Alloantibodies of importance in routine clinical practice are listed in Table 107-1.

Antibodies to *Lewis system* carbohydrate antigens are the most common cause of incompatibility during pretransfusion screening. The Lewis gene product is a fucosyl transferase and maps to chromosome 19. The antigen is not an integral membrane structure but is adsorbed to the RBC membrane from the plasma. Antibodies to Lewis antigens are usually IgM and cannot cross the placenta. Lewis antigens may be adsorbed onto tumor cells and may be targets of therapy.

I system antigens are also oligosaccharides related to H, A, B, and Le. I and i are not allelic pairs but are carbohydrate antigens that differ only in the extent of branching. The i antigen is an unbranched chain that is converted by the I gene product, a glycosyltransferase, into a branched chain. The branching process affects all the ABH antigens, which become progressively more branched in the first 2 years of life. Some patients with cold agglutinin disease or lymphomas can produce anti-I autoantibodies that cause RBC destruction. Occasional patients with mononucleosis or *Mycoplasma* pneumonia may develop cold agglutinins of either anti-I or anti-i specificity. Most adults lack i expression; thus, finding a donor for patients with anti-i is not difficult. Even though most adults express I antigen, binding is generally low at body temperature. Thus, administration of warm blood prevents isoagglutination.

The *P system* is another group of carbohydrate antigens controlled by specific glycosyltransferases. Its clinical significance is in rare cases of syphilis and viral infection that lead to paroxysmal cold hemoglobinuria. In these cases, an unusual autoantibody to P is produced that binds to RBCs in the cold and fixes complement upon warming. Antibodies with these biphasic properties are called *Donath-Landsteiner antibodies*. The P antigen is the cellular receptor of parvovirus B19 and also may be a receptor for *Escherichia coli* binding to urothelial cells.

The *MNSsU system* is regulated by genes on chromosome 4. M and N are determinants on glycophorin A, an RBC membrane protein, and S and s are determinants on glycophorin B. Anti-S and anti-s IgG antibodies may develop after pregnancy or transfusion and lead to hemolysis. Anti-U antibodies are rare but problematic; virtually every donor is incompatible because nearly all persons express U.

The *Kell* protein is very large (720 amino acids), and its secondary structure contains many different antigenic epitopes. The immunogenicity of Kell is third behind the ABO and Rh systems. The absence of the Kell precursor protein (controlled by a gene on X) is associated with acanthocytosis, shortened RBC survival, and a progressive form of muscular dystrophy that includes cardiac defects. This rare condition is called the *McLeod phenotype*. The K_x gene is linked to the 91-kDa component of

TABLE 107-1 RBC BLOOD GROUP SYSTEMS AND ALLOANTIGENS

Blood Group System	Antigen	Alloantibody	Clinical Significance
Rh (D, C/c, E/e)	RBC protein	IgG	HTR, HDN
Lewis (Le^a, Le^b)	Oligosaccharide	IgM/IgG	Rare HTR
Kell (K/k)	RBC protein	IgG	HTR, HDN
Duffy (Fy^a/Fy^b)	RBC protein	IgG	HTR, HDN
Kidd (Jk^a/Jk^b)	RBC protein	IgG	HTR (often delayed), HDN (mild)
I/i	Carbohydrate	IgM	None
MNSsU	RBC protein	IgM/IgG	Anti-M rare HDN, anti-S, -s, and -U HDN, HTR

Note: RBC, red blood cell; HDN, hemolytic disease of the newborn; HTR, hemolytic transfusion reaction.

the NADPH-oxidase on the X chromosome, deletion or mutation of which accounts for about 60% of cases of chronic granulomatous disease.

The *Duffy* antigens are codominant alleles, Fy^a and Fy^b, that also serve as receptors for *Plasmodium vivax*. More than 70% of persons in malaria-endemic areas lack these antigens, probably from selective influences of the infection on the population.

The *Kidd* antigens, Jk^a and Jk^b, may elicit antibodies transiently. A delayed hemolytic transfusion reaction that occurs with blood tested as compatible is often related to delayed appearance of anti-Jk^a.

PRETRANSFUSION TESTING

Pretransfusion testing of a potential recipient consists of the "type and screen." The "forward type" determines the ABO and Rh phenotype of the recipient's RBC by using antisera directed against the A, B, and D antigens. The "reverse type" detects isoagglutinins in the patient's serum and should correlate with the ABO phenotype, or forward type.

The alloantibody screen identifies antibodies directed against other RBC antigens. The alloantibody screen is performed by mixing patient serum with type O RBCs that contain the major antigens of most blood group systems and whose extended phenotype is known. The specificity of the alloantibody is identified by correlating the presence or absence of antigen with the results of the agglutination.

Cross-matching is ordered when there is a high probability that the patient will require a packed RBC (PRBC) transfusion. Blood selected for cross-matching must be ABO compatible and lack antigens for which the patient has alloantibodies. Nonreactive cross-matching confirms the absence of any major incompatibility and reserves that unit for the patient.

In the case of Rh-negative patients, every attempt must be made to provide Rh-negative blood components to prevent alloimmunization to the D antigen. In an emergency, Rh-positive blood can be safely transfused to an Rh-negative patient who lacks anti-D; however, the recipient is likely to become alloimmunized and produce anti-D. Rh-negative women of childbearing age who are transfused with products containing Rh-positive RBCs should receive passive immunization with anti-D (RhoGam or WinRho) to reduce or prevent sensitization.

BLOOD COMPONENTS

Blood products intended for transfusion are routinely collected as whole blood (450 mL) in various anticoagulants. Most donated blood is processed into components: PRBCs, platelets, and fresh-frozen plasma (FFP) or cryoprecipitate (Table 107-2). Whole blood is first separated into PRBCs and platelet-rich plasma by slow centrifugation. The platelet-rich plasma is then centrifuged at high speed to yield one unit of random donor (RD) platelets and one unit of FFP. Cryoprecipitate is produced by thawing FFP to precipitate the plasma proteins, then separated by centrifugation.

Apheresis technology is used for the collection of multiple units of platelets from a single donor. These single-donor apheresis platelets (SDAP) contain the equivalent of at least six units of RD platelets and have fewer contaminating leukocytes than pooled RD platelets.

Plasma may also be collected by apheresis. Plasma derivatives such as albumin, intravenous immunoglobulin, antithrombin, and coagulation factor concentrates are prepared from pooled plasma from many donors and are treated to eliminate infectious agents.

WHOLE BLOOD

Whole blood provides both oxygen-carrying capacity and volume expansion. It is the ideal component for patients who have sustained acute hemorrhage of ≥25% total blood volume loss. Whole blood is stored at 4°C to maintain erythrocyte via-

bility, but platelet dysfunction and degradation of some coagulation factors occurs. In addition, 2,3-bisphosphoglycerate levels fall over time, leading to an increase in the oxygen affinity of the hemoglobin and a decreased capacity to deliver oxygen to the tissues, a problem with all red cell storage. Whole blood is not readily available since it is routinely processed into components.

PACKED RED BLOOD CELLS

This product increases oxygen-carrying capacity in the anemic patient. Adequate oxygenation can be maintained with a hemoglobin content of 70 g/L in the normovolemic patient without cardiac disease; however, comorbid factors often necessitate transfusion at a higher threshold. The decision to transfuse should be guided by the clinical situation and not by an arbitrary laboratory value. In the critical care setting, liberal use of transfusions to maintain near-normal levels of hemoglobin may have unexpected negative effects on survival. In most patients requiring transfusion, levels of hemoglobin of 100 g/L are sufficient to keep oxygen supply from being critically low.

PRBCs may be modified to prevent certain adverse reactions. Leukocyte reduction of cellular blood products is increasingly common, and universal prestorage leukocyte reduction has been recommended. Prestorage filtration appears superior to bedside filtration as smaller amounts of cytokines are generated in the stored product. These PRBC units contain $<5 \times 10^6$ donor white blood cells (WBCs), and their use lowers the incidence of posttransfusion fever, cytomegalovirus (CMV) infections, and alloimmunization. Other theoretical benefits include less immunosuppression in the recipient and lower risk of infections. Plasma, which may cause allergic reactions, can be removed from cellular blood components by washing.

PLATELETS

Thrombocytopenia is a risk factor for hemorrhage, and platelet transfusion reduces the incidence of bleeding. The threshold for prophylactic platelet transfusion is 10,000/μL. In patients without fever or infections, a threshold of 5000/μL may be sufficient to prevent spontaneous hemorrhage. For invasive procedures, 50,000/μL platelets is the usual target level.

Platelets are given either as pools prepared from five to eight RDs or as SDAPs from a single donor. In an unsensitized patient without increased platelet consumption [splenomegaly, fever, disseminated intravascular coagulation (DIC)], six to eight units of RD platelets (about 1 unit per 10 kg body weight) are transfused, and each unit is anticipated to increase the platelet count 5000–10,000/μL. Patients who have received multiple transfusions may be alloimmunized to many HLA- and platelet-specific antigens and have little or no increase in their posttransfusion platelet counts. Patients who may require multiple transfusions are best served by receiving SDAP and leukocyte-reduced components to lower the risk of alloimmunization.

Refractoriness to platelet transfusion may be evaluated using the corrected count increment (CCI):

$$CCI = \frac{posttransfusion\ count - pretransfusion\ count}{number\ of\ platelets\ transfused \times 10^{11}} \times BSA$$

TABLE 107-2 CHARACTERISTICS OF SELECTED BLOOD COMPONENTS

Component	Volume, mL	Content	Clinical Response
PRBC	180–200	RBCs with variable leukocyte content and small amount of plasma	Increase hemoglobin 10 g/L and hematocrit 3%
Platelets	50–70	5.5×10^{10}/RD unit	Increase platelet count 5000–10,000/μL
	200–400	$\geq 3.0 \times 10^{11}$/SDAP product	CCI $\geq 10 \times 10^9$/L within 1 h and $\geq 7.5 \times 10^9$/L within 24 h posttransfusion
FFP	200–250	Plasma proteins—coagulation factors, proteins C and S, antithrombin	Increases coagulation factors about 2%
Cryoprecipitate	10–15	Cold-insoluble plasma proteins, fibrinogen, factor VIII, vWF	Topical fibrin glue, also 80 IU factor VIII

Note: PRBC, packed red blood cells; RBC, red blood cell; RD, random donor; SDAP, single-donor apheresis platelets; CCI, corrected count increment; FFP, fresh-frozen plasma; vWF, von Willebrand factor.

where BSA is body surface area measured in square meters. The platelet count performed 1 h after the transfusion is acceptable if the CCI is 10 $\times$ 10^9/mL, and after 18–24 h an increment of 7.5 $\times$ 10^9/mL is expected. Patients who have suboptimal responses are likely to have received multiple transfusions and have antibodies directed against class I HLA antigens. Refractoriness can be investigated by detecting anti-HLA antibodies in the recipient's serum. Patients who are sensitized will often react with 100% of the lymphocytes used for the HLA-antibody screen, and HLA-matched SDAPs should be considered for those patients who require transfusion. Although ABO-identical HLA-matched SDAPs provide the best chance for increasing the platelet count, locating these products is difficult. Platelet cross-matching is available in some centers. Additional clinical causes for a low platelet CCI include fever, bleeding, splenomegaly, DIC, or medications in the recipient.

FRESH-FROZEN PLASMA

FFP contains stable coagulation factors and plasma proteins: fibrinogen, antithrombin, albumin, as well as proteins C and S. Indications for FFP include correction of coagulopathies, including the rapid reversal of warfarin; supplying deficient plasma proteins; and treatment of thrombotic thrombocytopenic purpura. FFP should not be routinely used to expand blood volume. FFP is an acellular component and does not transmit intracellular infections, e.g., CMV. Patients who are IgA-deficient and require plasma support should receive FFP from IgA-deficient donors to prevent anaphylaxis (see below).

CRYOPRECIPITATE

Cryoprecipitate is a source of fibrinogen, factor VIII, and von Willebrand factor (vWF). It is ideal for supplying fibrinogen to the volume-sensitive patient. When factor VIII concentrates are not available, cryoprecipitate may be used since each unit contains approximately 80 units of factor VIII. Cryoprecipitate may also supply vWF to patients with dysfunctional (type II) or absent (type III) von Willebrand disease.

PLASMA DERIVATIVES

Plasma from thousands of donors may be pooled to derive specific protein concentrates, including albumin, intravenous immunoglobulin, antithrombin, and coagulation factors. In addition, donors who have high-titer antibodies to specific agents or antigens provide hyperimmune globulins, such as anti-D (RhoGam, WinRho), and antisera to hepatitis B virus (HBV), varicella-zoster virus, CMV, and other infectious agents.

ADVERSE REACTIONS TO BLOOD TRANSFUSION

Adverse reactions to transfused blood components occur despite multiple tests, inspections, and checks. Fortunately, the most common reactions are not life-threatening, although serious reactions can present with mild symptoms and signs. Some reactions can be reduced or prevented by modified (filtered, washed, or irradiated) blood components. When an adverse reaction is suspected, the transfusion should be stopped and reported to the blood bank for investigation.

Transfusion reactions may result from immune and nonimmune mechanisms. Immune-mediated reactions are often due to preformed donor or recipient antibody; however, cellular elements may also cause adverse effects. Nonimmune causes of reactions are due to the chemical and physical properties of the stored blood component and its additives.

Transfusion-transmitted viral infections are increasingly rare due to improved screening and testing. As the risk of viral infection is reduced, the relative risk of other reactions increases, such as hemolytic transfusion reactions and sepsis from bacterially contaminated components. More effort is being directed at improving pretransfusion quality assurance to further increase the safety of transfusion therapy. Infections, like any adverse transfusion reaction, must be brought to the attention of the blood bank for appropriate studies (Table 107-3).

IMMUNE-MEDIATED REACTIONS

Acute Hemolytic Transfusion Reactions
Immune-mediated hemolysis occurs when the recipient has preformed antibodies that lyse donor

TABLE 107-3 RISKS OF TRANSFUSION COMPLICATIONS

	Frequency, Episodes:Unit
Reactions	
Febrile (FNHTR)	1–4:100
Allergic	1–4:100
Delayed hemolytic	1:1000
TRALI	1:5000
Acute hemolytic	1:12,000
Fatal hemolytic	1:100,000
Anaphylactic	1:150,000
Infections[a]	
Hepatitis B	1:63,000
Hepatitis C	1:1,600,000
HIV-1	1:1,960,000
HIV-2	None reported
HTLV-I and -II	1:641,000
Malaria	1:4,000,000
Other complications	
RBC allosensitization	1:100
HLA allosensitization	1:10
Graft-versus-host disease	Rare

[a]Infectious agents rarely associated with transfusion, theoretically possible or of unknown risk include: Hepatitis A virus, parvovirus B-19, *Babesia microti* (babesiosis), *Borrelia burgdorferi* (Lyme disease), *Trypanosoma cruzi* (Chagas disease), and *Treponema pallidum*, human herpesvirus-8 and hepatitis G virus.

Note: FNHTR, febrile nonhemolytic transfusion reaction; TRALI, transfusion-related acute lung injury; HTLV, human T lymphotropic virus; RBC, red blood cell.

erythrocytes. The ABO isoagglutinins are responsible for the majority of these reactions, although alloantibodies directed against other RBC antigens, i.e., Rh, Kell, and Duffy, may result in hemolysis.

Acute hemolytic reactions may present with hypotension, tachypnea, tachycardia, fever, chills, hemoglobinemia, hemoglobinuria, chest and/or flank pain, and discomfort at the infusion site. Monitoring the patient's vital signs before and during the transfusion is important to identify reactions promptly. When acute hemolysis is suspected, the transfusion must be stopped immediately, intravenous access maintained, and the reaction reported to the blood bank. A correctly labeled posttransfusion blood sample and any untransfused blood should be sent to the blood bank for analysis. The laboratory evaluation for hemolysis includes the measurement of serum haptoglobin, lactate dehydrogenase (LDH), and indirect bilirubin levels.

The immune complexes that result in RBC lysis can cause renal dysfunction and failure. Diuresis should be induced with intravenous fluids and furosemide or mannitol. Tissue factor released from the lysed erythrocytes may initiate DIC. Coagulation studies including prothrombin time (PT), activated partial thromboplastin time (aPTT), fibrinogen, and platelet count should be monitored in patients with hemolytic reactions.

Errors at the patient's bedside, such as mislabeling the sample or transfusing the wrong patient, are responsible for the majority of these reactions. The blood bank investigation of these reactions includes examination of the pre- and posttransfusion samples for hemolysis and repeat typing of the patient samples; direct antiglobulin test (DAT), sometimes called the *direct Coombs test*, of the posttransfusion sample; repeating the cross-matching of the blood component; and checking all clerical records for errors. DAT detects the presence of antibody or complement bound to RBCs in vivo.

Delayed Hemolytic and Serologic Transfusion Reactions
Delayed hemolytic transfusion reactions (DHTRs) are not completely preventable. These reactions occur in patients previously sensitized to RBC alloantigens who have a negative alloantibody screen due to low antibody levels. When the patient is transfused with antigen-positive blood, an anamnestic response results in the early production of alloantibody that binds donor RBCs. The alloantibody is detectable 1–2 weeks following the transfusion, and the posttransfusion DAT may become positive due to circulating donor RBCs coated with antibody or complement. The transfused, alloantibody-coated erythrocytes are cleared

by the reticuloendothelial system. These reactions are detected most commonly in the blood bank when a subsequent patient sample reveals a positive alloantibody screen or a new alloantibody in a recently transfused recipient.

No specific therapy is usually required, although additional RBC transfusions may be necessary. Delayed serologic transfusion reactions are similar to DHTR, as the DAT is positive and alloantibody is detected; however, RBC clearance is not increased.

Febrile Nonhemolytic Transfusion Reaction   The most frequent reaction associated with the transfusion of cellular blood components is a febrile nonhemolytic transfusion reaction (FNHTR). These reactions are characterized by chills and rigors and a $\geq 1°C$ rise in temperature. FNHTR is diagnosed when other causes of fever in the transfused patient are ruled out. Antibodies directed against donor leukocyte and HLA antigens may mediate these reactions; thus, multiply transfused patients and multiparous women are felt to be at increased risk. Although antibodies may be demonstrated in the recipient's serum, investigation is not routinely done because of the mild nature of most FNHTR. The use of leukocyte-reduced blood products may prevent or delay sensitization to leukocyte antigens and thereby reduce the incidence of these febrile episodes. Cytokines released from cells within stored blood components may mediate FNHTR; thus, leukoreduction before storage may prevent these reactions. The incidence and severity of these reactions can be decreased in patients with recurrent reactions by premedicating with acetaminophen or other antipyretic agents.

Allergic Reactions   Urticarial reactions are related to plasma proteins found in transfused components. Mild reactions may be treated symptomatically by temporarily stopping the transfusion and administering antihistamines (diphenhydramine, 50 mg orally or intramuscularly). The transfusion may be completed after the signs and/or symptoms resolve. Patients with a history of allergic transfusion reaction should be premedicated with an antihistamine. Cellular components can be washed to remove residual plasma for the extremely sensitized patient.

Anaphylactic Reaction   This severe reaction presents after transfusion of only a few milliliters of the blood component. Symptoms and signs include difficulty breathing, coughing, nausea and vomiting, hypotension, bronchospasm, loss of consciousness, respiratory arrest, and shock. Treatment includes stopping the transfusion, maintaining vascular access, and administering epinephrine (0.5–1.0 mL of 1:1000 dilution subcutaneously). Glucocorticoids may be required in severe cases.

Patients who are IgA-deficient, <1% of the population, may be sensitized to this Ig class and are at risk for anaphylactic reactions associated with plasma transfusion. Individuals with severe IgA deficiency should therefore receive only IgA-deficient plasma and washed cellular blood components. Patients who have anaphylactic or repeated allergic reactions to blood components should be tested for IgA deficiency.

Graft-versus-Host Disease   Graft-versus-host disease (GVHD) is a frequent complication of allogeneic stem cell transplantation, in which lymphocytes from the donor attack and cannot be eliminated by an immunodeficient host. Transfusion-related GVHD is mediated by donor T lymphocytes that recognize host HLA antigens as foreign and mount an immune response, which is manifested clinically by the development of fever, a characteristic cutaneous eruption, diarrhea, and liver function abnormalities. GVHD can also occur when blood components that contain viable T lymphocytes are transfused to immunodeficient recipients or to immunocompetent recipients who share HLA antigens with the donor (e.g., a family donor). In addition to the aforementioned clinical features of GVHD, transfusion-associated GVHD (TA-GVHD) is characterized by marrow aplasia and pancytopenia. TA-GVHD is highly resistant to treatment with immunosuppressive therapies, including glucocorticoids, cyclosporine, antithymocyte globulin, and ablative therapy followed by allogeneic bone marrow transplantation. Clinical manifestations appear at 8–10 days, and death occurs at 3–4 weeks posttransfusion.

TA-GVHD can be prevented by irradiation of cellular components (minimum of 2500 cGy) before transfusion to patients at risk. Patients at risk for TA-GVHD include fetuses receiving intrauterine transfusions, selected immunocompetent (e.g., lymphoma patients) or immunocompromised recipients, recipients of donor units known to be from a blood relative, and recipients who have undergone marrow transplantation. Directed donations by family members should be discouraged (they are not less likely to transmit infection); lacking other options, the blood products from family members should always be irradiated.

Transfusion-Related Acute Lung Injury   This uncommon reaction results from the transfusion of donor plasma that contains high-titer anti-HLA antibodies that bind recipient leukocytes. The leukocytes aggregate in the pulmonary vasculature and release mediators that increase capillary permeability. The recipient develops symptoms of respiratory compromise and signs of noncardiogenic pulmonary edema, including bilateral interstitial infiltrates on chest x-ray. Treatment is supportive, and patients usually recover without sequelae. Testing the donor's plasma for anti-HLA antibodies can support this diagnosis. The implicated donors are frequently multiparous women, and transfusion of their plasma component should be avoided.

Posttransfusion Purpura   This reaction presents as thrombocytopenia 7–10 days after platelet transfusion and occurs predominantly in women. Platelet-specific antibodies are found in the recipient's serum, and the most frequently recognized antigen is HPA-1a found on the platelet glycoprotein IIIa receptor. The delayed thrombocytopenia is due to the production of antibodies that react to both donor and recipient platelets. Additional platelet transfusions can worsen the thrombocytopenia and should be avoided. Treatment with intravenous immunoglobulin may neutralize the effector antibodies, or plasmapheresis can be used to remove the antibodies.

Alloimmunization   A recipient may become alloimmunized to a number of antigens on cellular blood elements and plasma proteins. Alloantibodies to RBC antigens are detected during pretransfusion testing, and their presence may delay finding antigen-negative cross-match-compatible products for transfusion. Women of childbearing age who are sensitized to certain RBC antigens (i.e., D, c, E, Kell, or Duffy) are at risk for bearing a fetus with hemolytic disease of the newborn. Matching for D antigen is the only pretransfusion selection test to prevent RBC alloimmunization.

Alloimmunization to antigens on leukocytes and platelets can result in refractoriness to platelet transfusions. Once alloimmunization has developed, HLA-compatible platelets from donors who share similar antigens with the recipient may be difficult to find. Hence, prudent transfusion practice is directed at preventing sensitization through the use of leukocyte-reduced cellular components, as well as limiting antigenic exposure by the judicious use of transfusions and use of SDAPs.

NONIMMUNOLOGIC REACTIONS
Fluid Overload   Blood components are excellent volume expanders, and transfusion may quickly lead to volume overload. Monitoring the rate and volume of the transfusion and using a diuretic can minimize this problem.

Hypothermia   Refrigerated (4°C) or frozen (–18°C or below) blood components can result in hypothermia when rapidly infused. Cardiac dysrhythmias can result from exposing the sinoatrial node to cold fluid. Use of an in-line warmer will prevent this complication.

Electrolyte Toxicity   RBC leakage during storage increases the concentration of potassium in the unit. Neonates and patients in renal failure are at risk for hyperkalemia. Preventive measures, such as using fresh or washed RBCs, are warranted for neonatal transfusions because this complication can be fatal.

Citrate, commonly used to anticoagulate blood components, chelates calcium and thereby inhibits the coagulation cascade. Hypocalcemia, manifested by circumoral numbness and/or tingling sensation of the fingers and toes, may result from multiple rapid transfusions. Because citrate is quickly metabolized to bicarbonate, calcium infusion is seldom required in this setting. If calcium or any other intravenous infusion is necessary, it must be given through a separate line.

Iron Overload   Each unit of RBCs contains 200–250 mg of iron. Symptoms and signs of iron overload affecting endocrine, hepatic, and cardiac function are common after 100 units of RBCs have been transfused (total-body iron load of 20 g). Preventing this complication by using alternative therapies (e.g., erythropoietin) and judicious transfusion is preferable and cost effective. Deferoxamine and other chelating agents are available, but the response is often suboptimal.

Hypotensive Reactions   Transient hypotension may be noted among transfused patients who take angiotensin-converting enzyme (ACE) inhibitors. Since blood products contain bradykinin that is normally degraded by ACE, patients on ACE inhibitors may have increased bradykinin levels that cause hypotension. The blood pressure typically returns to normal without intervention.

Immunomodulation   Transfusion of allogeneic blood is immunosuppressive. Multiply transfused renal transplant recipients are less likely to reject the graft, and transfusion may result in poorer outcomes in cancer patients and increase the risk of infections. Transfusion-related immunomodulation is thought to be mediated by transfused leukocytes. Leukocyte-depleted cellular products may cause less immunosuppression, though controlled data have not been obtained and are unlikely to be obtained as the blood supply becomes universally leukocyte-depleted.

INFECTIOUS COMPLICATIONS

Nucleic acid amplification testing (NAT) began in 1999 to screen donated blood for the presence of HIV and hepatitis C virus (HCV) RNA. Since 2003 NAT has been used to detect West Nile virus (WNV) RNA in donated blood.

Viral Infections • HEPATITIS C VIRUS   Blood donations are tested for antibodies to HCV and HCV RNA. Fewer than 200 HCV RNA-positive, antibody-negative donors have been found. The risk of acquiring HCV through transfusion is now calculated to be approximately 1 in 2,000,000 units. Infection with HCV may be asymptomatic or lead to chronic active hepatitis, cirrhosis, and liver failure.

HUMAN IMMUNODEFICIENCY VIRUS TYPE 1   Donated blood is tested for antibodies to HIV-1, HIV-1 p24 antigen, and HIV RNA using NAT. Approximately a dozen seronegative donors have been shown to harbor HIV RNA. The risk of HIV-1 infection per transfusion episode is 1 in 2 million. Antibodies to HIV-2 are also measured in donated blood. No cases of HIV-2 infection have been reported in the United States since 1992.

HEPATITIS B VIRUS   Donated blood is screened for HBV using assays for hepatitis B surface antigen (HbsAg). NAT testing is not practical because of slow viral replication and lower levels of viremia. The risk of transfusion-associated HBV infection is 1 in 63,000 units, twentyfold greater than for HCV. Vaccination of individuals who require long-term transfusion therapy can prevent this complication.

OTHER HEPATITIS VIRUSES   Hepatitis A virus is rarely transmitted by transfusion; infection is typically asymptomatic and does not lead to chronic disease. Other transfusion-transmitted viruses—TTV, SEN-V, and GBV-C—do not cause chronic hepatitis or other disease states. Routine testing does not appear to be warranted.

WEST NILE VIRUS   Transfusion-transmitted WNV infections were documented in 2002. This RNA virus can be detected using NAT; routine screening began in 2003, and more than 1000 blood donors have tested positive. WNV infections range in severity from asymptomatic to fatal, with the older population at greater risk.

CYTOMEGALOVIRUS   This ubiquitous virus infects ≥50% of the general population and is transmitted by the infected "passenger" WBCs found in transfused PRBCs or platelet components. Cellular components that are leukocyte-reduced have a decreased risk of transmitting CMV, regardless of the serologic status of the donor. Groups at risk for CMV infections include immunosuppressed patients, CMV-seronegative transplant recipients, and neonates; these patients should receive leukocyte-depleted components or CMV seronegative products.

HUMAN T LYMPHOTROPIC VIRUS (HTLV) TYPE I   Assays to detect HTLV-I and -II are used to screen all donated blood. HTLV-I is associated with adult T cell leukemia/lymphoma and tropical spastic paraparesis in a small percentage of infected persons (Chap. 181). The risk of HTLV-I infection via transfusion is 1 in 641,000 transfusion episodes. HTLV-II is not clearly associated with any disease.

PARVOVIRUS B-19   Blood components and pooled plasma products can transmit this virus, the etiologic agent of erythema infectiosum, or fifth disease, in children. Parvovirus B-19 shows tropism for erythroid precursors and inhibits both erythrocyte production and maturation. Pure red cell aplasia, presenting either as acute aplastic crisis or chronic anemia with shortened RBC survival, may occur in individuals with an underlying hematologic disease, such as sickle cell disease or thalassemia (Chap. 102). The fetus of a seronegative woman is at risk for developing hydrops from this virus.

Bacterial Contamination   The relative risk of transfusion-transmitted bacterial infection has increased as the absolute risk of viral infections has dramatically decreased.

Most bacteria do not grow well at cold temperatures; thus, PRBCs and FFP are not common sources of bacterial contamination. However, some gram-negative bacteria can grow at 1° to 6°C. *Yersinia, Pseudomonas, Serratia, Acinetobacter* and *Escherichia* species have all been implicated in infections related to PRBC transfusion. Platelet concentrates, which are stored at room temperature, are more likely to contain skin contaminants such as gram-positive organisms, including coagulase-negative staphylococci. It is estimated that 1 in 1000–2000 platelet components is contaminated with bacteria. The risk of death due to transfusion-associated sepsis has been calculated at 1 in 17,000 for single-unit platelets derived from whole blood donation and 1 in 61,000 for apheresis product. Since 2004, blood banks have instituted methods to detect contaminated platelet components.

Recipients of transfusion contaminated with bacteria may develop fever and chills, which can progress to septic shock and DIC. These reactions may occur abruptly, within minutes of initiating the transfusion, or after several hours. The onset of symptoms and signs is often sudden and fulminant, which distinguishes bacterial contamination from an FNHTR. The reactions, particularly those related to gram-negative contaminants, are the result of infused endotoxins formed within the contaminated stored component.

When these reactions are suspected, the transfusion must be stopped immediately. Therapy is directed at reversing any signs of shock, and broad-spectrum antibiotics should be given. The blood bank should be notified to identify any clerical or serologic error. The blood component bag should be sent for culture and Gram stain.

Other Infectious Agents   Various parasites, including those causing malaria, babesiosis, and Chagas disease, can be transmitted by blood transfusion. Geographic migration and travel of donors shift the incidence of these rare infections. Other agents implicated in transfusion transmission include Lyme disease and variant Creutzfeldt-Jakob disease. These infections should be considered in the transfused patient in the appropriate clinical setting.

ALTERNATIVES TO TRANSFUSION

Alternatives to allogeneic blood transfusions that avoid homologous donor exposures with attendant immunologic and infectious risks remain attractive. Autologous blood is the best option when transfusion is anticipated. However, the cost:benefit ratio of autologous transfusion remains high. No transfusion is a zero-risk event; clerical errors and bacterial contamination remain potential complications even with autologous transfusions. Additional methods of autologous transfusion in the surgical patient include preoperative hemodilution, recovery of shed blood from sterile surgical sites, and postoperative drainage collection. Directed or designated donation from friends and family of the potential recipient has not been safer than volunteer donor component transfusions. Such directed donations may in fact place the recipient at higher risk for complications such as GVHD and alloimmunization.

Granulocyte and granulocyte-macrophage colony-stimulating factor are clinically useful to hasten leukocyte recovery in patients with leukopenia related to high-dose chemotherapy. Erythropoietin stimulates erythrocyte production in patients with anemia of chronic renal failure and other conditions, thus avoiding or reducing the need for transfusion. This hormone can also stimulate erythropoiesis in the autologous donor to enable additional donation.

FURTHER READINGS

BLAJCHMAN MA: The clinical benefits of the leukoreduction of blood products. J Trauma 60:S83, 2006

BRECHER ME, HAY SN: Bacterial contamination of blood components. Clin Micro Rev 18:195, 2005

———et al: *The Technical Manual*, 15th ed. Arlington, VA, American Association of Blood Banks, 2005

BUSCH MP et al: A new strategy for estimating risks of transfusion transmitted viral infections based on rates of detection of recently infected donors. Transfusion 45:254, 2005

RAGHAVANA M, MARIK PE: Anemia, allogeneic blood transfusion, and immunomodulation in the critically ill. Chest 127:295, 2005

SHEPPARD CA et al: Transfusion-related acute lung injury. Hematol Oncol Clin North Am 21:163, 2007

108 Hematopoietic Cell Transplantation

Frederick R. Appelbaum

Bone marrow transplantation was the original term used to describe the collection and transplantation of hematopoietic stem cells, but with the demonstration that the peripheral blood and umbilical cord blood are also useful sources of stem cells, *hematopoietic cell transplantation* has become the preferred generic term for this process. The procedure is usually carried out for one of two purposes: (1) to replace an abnormal but nonmalignant lymphohematopoietic system with one from a normal donor, or (2) to treat malignancy by allowing the administration of higher doses of myelosuppressive therapy than would otherwise be possible. The use of hematopoietic cell transplantation has been increasing, both because of its efficacy in selected diseases and because of increasing availability of donors. The International Bone Marrow Transplant Registry (*http://www.ibmtr.org*) estimates that about 50,000 transplants are performed each year.

THE HEMATOPOIETIC STEM CELL

Several features of the hematopoietic stem cell make transplantation clinically feasible, including its remarkable regenerative capacity, its ability to home to the marrow space following intravenous injection, and the ability of the stem cell to be cryopreserved. Transplantation of a single stem cell can replace the entire lymphohematopoietic system of an adult mouse. In humans, transplantation of a few percent of a donor's bone marrow volume regularly results in complete and sustained replacement of the recipient's entire lymphohematopoietic system, including all red cells, granulocytes, B and T lymphocytes, and platelets, as well as cells comprising the fixed macrophage population, including Kupffer cells of the liver, pulmonary alveolar macrophages, osteoclasts, Langerhans cells of the skin, and brain microglial cells. The ability of the hematopoietic stem cell to home to the marrow following intravenous injection is mediated, at least in part, by the interaction of cell-surface molecules, termed *selectins*, on bone marrow endothelial cells with ligands, termed *integrins*, on early hematopoietic cells. Human hematopoietic stem cells can survive freezing and thawing with little, if any, damage, making it possible to remove and store a portion of the patient's own bone marrow for later reinfusion following treatment of the patient with high-dose myelotoxic therapy.

CATEGORIES OF HEMATOPOIETIC CELL TRANSPLANTATION

Hematopoietic cell transplantation can be described according to the relationship between the patient and the donor and by the anatomic source of stem cells. In ~1% of cases, patients have identical twins who can serve as donors. With the use of syngeneic donors, there is no risk of graft-versus-host disease (GVHD) that often complicates allogeneic transplantation, and unlike the use of autologous marrow, there is no risk that the stem cells are contaminated with tumor cells.

Allogeneic transplantation involves a donor and recipient who are not immunologically identical. Following allogeneic transplantation, immune cells transplanted with the stem cells or developing from them can react against the patient, causing GVHD. Alternatively, if the immunosuppressive preparative regimen used to treat the patient before transplant is inadequate, immunocompetent cells of the patient can cause graft rejection. The risks of these complications are greatly influenced by the degree of matching between donor and recipient for antigens encoded by genes of the major histocompatibility complex.

The human leukocyte antigen (HLA) molecules are responsible for binding antigenic proteins and presenting them to T cells. The antigens presented by HLA molecules may derive from exogenous sources (e.g., during active infections) or may be endogenous proteins. If individuals are not HLA-matched, T cells from one individual will react strongly to the mismatched HLA, or "major antigens," of the second. Even if the individuals are HLA-matched, the T cells of the donor may react to differing endogenous, or "minor antigens," presented by the HLA of the recipient. Reactions to minor antigens tend to be less vigorous. The genes of major relevance to transplantation include HLA-A, -B, -C, and -D; they are closely linked and therefore tend to be inherited as haplotypes, with only rare crossovers between them. Thus, the odds that any one full sibling will match a patient are one in four, and the probability that the patient has an HLA-identical sibling is $1 - (0.75)^n$, where n equals the number of siblings.

With current techniques, the risk of graft rejection is 1–3%, and the risk of severe, life-threatening acute GVHD is ~15% following transplantation between HLA-identical siblings. The incidence of graft rejection and GVHD increases progressively with the use of family member donors mismatched for one, two, or three antigens. While survival following a one-antigen mismatched transplant is not markedly altered, survival following two- or three-antigen mismatched transplants is significantly reduced, and such transplants should be performed only as part of clinical trials.

Since the formation of the National Marrow Donor Program, it has become possible to identify HLA-matched unrelated donors for many patients. The genes encoding HLA antigens are highly polymorphic, and thus the odds of any two unrelated individuals being HLA-identical are extremely low, somewhat less than 1 in 10,000. However, by identifying and typing >7 million volunteer donors, HLA-matched donors can now be found for ~50% of patients for whom a search is initiated. It takes, on average, 3–4 months to complete a search and schedule and initiate an unrelated donor transplant. Results so far suggest that GVHD is somewhat increased and survival somewhat poorer with such donors than with HLA-matched siblings.

Autologous transplantation involves the removal and storage of the patient's own stem cells with subsequent reinfusion after the patient receives high-dose myeloablative therapy. Unlike allogeneic transplantation, there is no risk of GVHD or graft rejection with autologous transplantation. On the other hand, autologous transplantation lacks a graft-versus-tumor (GVT) effect, and the autologous stem cell product can be contaminated with tumor cells that could lead to relapse. A variety of techniques have been developed to "purge" autologous products of tumor cells. Some use antibodies directed at tumor-associated antigens plus complement, antibodies linked to toxins, or antibodies conjugated to immunomagnetic beads. In vitro incubation with certain chemotherapeutic agents such as 4-hydroperoxycyclophosphamide and long-term culture of bone marrow have also been shown to diminish tumor cell numbers in stem cell products. Another technique is positive selection of stem cells using antibodies to CD34, with subsequent column adherence or flow techniques to select normal stem cells while leaving tumor cells behind. All these approaches can reduce the number of tumor cells from 1000- to 10,000-fold and are clinically feasible; however, no prospective randomized trials have yet shown that any of these approaches results in a decrease in relapse rates or improvements in disease-free or overall survival.

Bone marrow aspirated from the posterior and anterior iliac crests has traditionally been the source of hematopoietic stem cells for transplantation. Typically, anywhere from 1.5 to 5×10^8 nucleated marrow cells per kilogram are collected for allogeneic transplantation. Several studies have found improved survival in the settings of both matched sibling and unrelated transplantation by transplanting higher numbers of bone marrow cells.

Hematopoietic stem cells circulate in the peripheral blood but in very low concentrations. Following the administration of certain hematopoietic growth factors, including granulocyte colony-stimulating factor (G-CSF) or granulocyte-macrophage colony-stimulating factor (GM-CSF), and during recovery from intensive chemotherapy, the concentration of hematopoietic progenitor cells in blood, as measured either by colony-forming units or expression of the CD34 antigen, increases markedly. This has made it possible to harvest adequate numbers of stem cells from the peripheral blood for transplantation. Donors are typically treated with 4 or 5 days of hematopoietic growth factor, following which stem cells are collected in one or two 4-h pheresis sessions. In the autologous setting, transplantation of $>2.5 \times 10^6$ CD34 cells per kilogram, a number easily collected in most circumstances, leads to rapid and sustained engraftment in virtually all cases. Compared to the use of autologous marrow, use of peripheral blood stem cells results in more rapid hematopoietic recovery, with granulocytes recovering to 500/μL by day 12 and platelets recovering to 20,000/μL by day 14. While this more rapid recovery diminishes the morbidity of transplantation, no studies show improved survival.

Hesitation in studying the use of peripheral blood stem cells for allogeneic transplantation was because peripheral blood stem cell products contain as much as one log more T cells than are contained in the typical marrow harvest; in animal models, the incidence of GVHD is related to the number of T cells transplanted. Nonetheless, clinical trials have shown that the use of growth factor–mobilized peripheral blood stem cells from HLA-matched family members leads to faster engraftment without an increase in acute GVHD. Chronic GVHD may be increased with peripheral blood stem cells, but in trials conducted so far, this has been more than balanced by reductions in relapse rates and nonrelapse mortality, with the use of peripheral blood stem cells resulting in improved overall survival.

Umbilical cord blood contains a high concentration of hematopoietic progenitor cells, allowing for its use as a source of stem cells for transplantation. Cord blood transplantation from family members has been explored in the setting where the immediate need for transplantation precludes waiting the 9 or so months generally required for the baby to mature to the point of donating marrow. Use of cord blood results in slower engraftment and peripheral count recovery than seen with marrow but a low incidence of GVHD, perhaps reflecting the low number of T cells in cord blood. Several banks have been developed to harvest and store cord blood for possible transplantation to unrelated patients from material that would otherwise be discarded. A summary of the first 562 unrelated cord blood transplants, facilitated by the New York Blood Center, reported engraftment in ~85% of patients but at a slower pace than seen with marrow. Severe GVHD was seen in 23% of patients. The risk of graft failure was related to the dose of cord blood cells per kilogram infused. The low cell content of most cord blood collections has limited the use of this approach for adult patients.

THE TRANSPLANT PREPARATIVE REGIMEN

The treatment regimen administered to patients immediately preceding transplantation is designed to eradicate the patient's underlying disease and, in the setting of allogeneic transplantation, immunosuppress the patient adequately to prevent rejection of the transplanted marrow. The appropriate regimen therefore depends on the disease setting and source of marrow. For example, when transplantation is performed to treat severe combined immunodeficiency and the donor is a histocompatible sibling, no treatment is required because no host cells require eradication and the patient is already too immunoincompetent to reject the transplanted marrow. For aplastic anemia, there is no large population of cells to eradicate, and high-dose cyclophosphamide plus antithymocyte globulin are sufficient to immunosuppress the patient adequately to accept the marrow graft. In the setting of thalassemia and sickle cell anemia, high-dose busulfan is frequently added to cyclophosphamide in order to eradicate hyperplastic host hematopoiesis. A variety of different regimens have been developed to treat malignant diseases. Most of these regimens include agents that have high activity against the tumor in question at conventional doses and have myelosuppression as their predominant dose-limiting toxicity. Therefore, these regimens commonly include busulfan, cyclophosphamide, melphalan, thiotepa, carmustine, etoposide, and total-body irradiation in various combinations.

Although high-dose treatment regimens have typically been used in transplantation, the understanding that much of the antitumor effect of transplantation derives from an immunologically mediated GVT response has led investigators to ask if less-intensive "nonmyeloablative" regimens might be effective and more tolerable. Evidence for a GVT effect comes from studies showing that posttransplant relapse rates are lowest in patients who develop acute and chronic GVHD, higher in those without GVHD, and higher still in recipients of T cell–depleted allogeneic or syngeneic marrow. The demonstration that complete remissions can be obtained in many patients who have relapsed posttransplant by simply administering viable lymphocytes from the original donor further strengthens the argument for a potent GVT effect. Accordingly, a variety of less-intensive nonmyeloablative regimens have been studied, ranging in intensity from the very minimum required to achieve engraftment (e.g., fludarabine plus 200 cGy total-body irradiation) to regimens of more immediate intensity (e.g., fludarabine plus melphalan). Studies to date document that engraftment can be readily achieved with less toxicity than seen with conventional transplantation. Furthermore, the severity of GVHD appears to be decreased because less tissue damage is done by the lower doses of drugs in the preparative regimen. Complete sustained responses have been documented in many patients, particularly those with more indolent hematologic malignancies. The role of nonmyeloablative transplants in any disease, however, has not been fully defined.

THE TRANSPLANT PROCEDURE

Marrow is usually collected from the donor's posterior and sometimes anterior iliac crests with the donor under general or spinal anesthesia. Typically, 10–15 mL/kg of marrow is aspirated, placed in heparinized media, and filtered through 0.3- and 0.2-mm screens to remove fat and bony spicules. The collected marrow may undergo further processing depending on the clinical situation, such as the removal of red cells to prevent hemolysis in ABO-incompatible transplants, the re-

moval of donor T cells to prevent GVHD, or attempts to remove possible contaminating tumor cells in autologous transplantation. Marrow donation is safe, with only very rare complications reported.

Peripheral blood stem cells are collected by leukophoresis after the donor has been treated with hematopoietic growth factors or, in the setting of autologous transplantation, sometimes after treatment with a combination of chemotherapy and growth factors. Stem cells for transplantation are generally infused through a large-bore central venous catheter. Such infusions are usually well tolerated, although occasionally patients develop fever, cough, or shortness of breath. These symptoms usually resolve with slowing of the infusion. When the stem cell product has been cryopreserved using dimethyl sulfoxide, patients more often experience short-lived nausea or vomiting due to the odor and taste of the cryoprotectant.

ENGRAFTMENT

Peripheral blood counts usually reach their nadir several days to a week posttransplant as a consequence of the preparative regimen, then cells produced by the transplanted stem cells begin to appear in the peripheral blood. The rate of recovery depends on the source of stem cells, the use of posttransplant growth factors, and the form of GVHD prophylaxis employed. If marrow is the source of stem cells, recovery to 100 granulocytes/μL occurs by day 16 and to 500/μL by day 22. Use of G-CSF–mobilized peripheral blood stem cells speeds the rate of recovery by ~1 week when compared to marrow. Use of a myeloid growth factor (G-CSF or GM-CSF) posttransplant can further accelerate recovery by 3–5 days, while use of methotrexate to prevent GVHD delays engraftment by a similar period. Following allogeneic transplantation, engraftment can be documented using fluorescence in situ hybridization of sex chromosomes if donor and recipient are sex-mismatched, HLA-typing if HLA-mismatched, or restriction fragment length polymorphism analysis if sex- and HLA-matched.

COMPLICATIONS FOLLOWING HEMATOPOIETIC CELL TRANSPLANT

Early Direct Chemoradiotoxicities   The transplant preparative regimens commonly used cause a spectrum of acute toxicities that vary according to the specific regimen but frequently result in nausea, vomiting, and mild skin erythema (Fig. 108-1). Regimens that include high-dose cyclophosphamide can result in hemorrhagic cystitis, which can usually be prevented by bladder irrigation or with the sulfhydryl compound mercaptoethanesulfonate (MESNA); rarely, acute hemorrhagic carditis is seen. Most preparative regimens will result in oral mucositis, which typically develops 5–7 days posttransplant and often requires

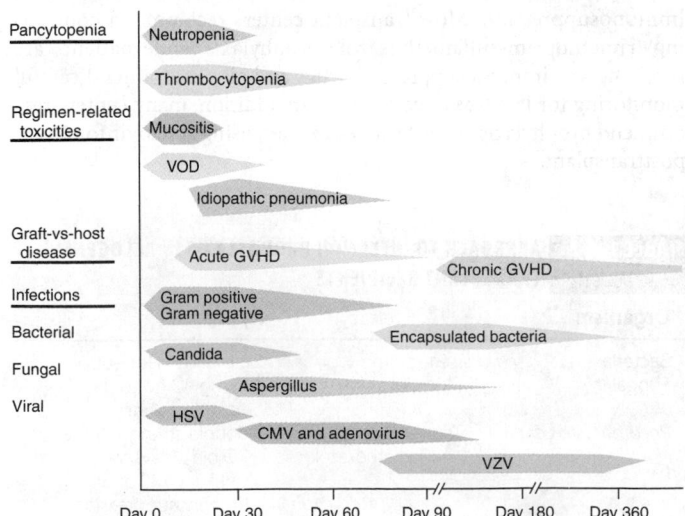

FIGURE 108-1 Major syndromes complicating marrow transplantation. VOD, venoocclusive disease; GVHD, graft-versus-host disease; HSV, herpes simplex virus; CMV, cytomegalovirus; VZV, varicella-zoster virus. The size of the shaded area roughly reflects the risk of the complication.

narcotic analgesia. Use of a patient-controlled analgesic pump provides the greatest patient satisfaction and results in a lower cumulative dose of narcotic. Patients begin losing their hair 5–6 days posttransplant and by 1 week are usually profoundly pancytopenic.

Approximately 10% of patients will develop venoocclusive disease of the liver, a syndrome resulting from direct cytotoxic injury to hepatic-venular and sinusoidal endothelium, with subsequent deposition of fibrin and the development of a local hypercoagulable state. This chain of events results in the clinical symptoms of tender hepatomegaly, ascites, jaundice, and fluid retention. These symptoms can develop any time during the first month posttransplant, with the peak incidence at day 16. Predisposing factors include prior exposure to intensive chemotherapy, pretransplant hepatitis of any cause, and use of more intense conditioning regimens. The mortality of venoocclusive disease is ~30%, with progressive hepatic failure culminating in a terminal hepatorenal syndrome. Both thrombolytic and antithrombotic agents, such as tissue plasminogen activator, heparin, and prostaglandin E, have been studied as therapy, but none has proven of consistent major benefit in controlled trials, and all have significant toxicity. Early studies with defibrotide, a polydeoxyribonucleotide, seem encouraging.

Although most pneumonias developing posttransplant are caused by infectious agents, in ~5% of patients a diffuse interstitial pneumonia will develop that is thought to be the result of direct toxicity of the preparative regimen. Bronchoalveolar lavage typically shows alveolar hemorrhage, and biopsies are typically characterized by diffuse alveolar damage, although some cases may have a more clearly interstitial pattern. High-dose glucocorticoids are often used as treatment, although randomized trials testing their utility have not been reported.

Late Direct Chemoradiotoxicities   Late complications of the preparative regimen include decreased growth velocity in children and delayed development of secondary sex characteristics. These complications can be partly ameliorated with the use of appropriate growth and sex hormone replacement. Most men become azoospermic, and most postpubertal women will develop ovarian failure, which should be treated. Thyroid dysfunction, usually well compensated, is sometimes seen. Cataracts develop in 10–20% of patients and are most common in patients treated with total-body irradiation and those who receive glucocorticoid therapy posttransplant for treatment of GVHD. Aseptic necrosis of the femoral head is seen in 10% of patients and is particularly frequent in those receiving chronic glucocorticoid therapy.

Graft-Versus-Host Disease   GVHD is the result of allogeneic T cells that were either transferred with the donor's stem cell inoculum or develop from it, reacting with antigenic targets on host cells. GVHD developing within the first 3 months posttransplant is termed *acute GVHD*, while GVHD developing or persisting beyond 3 months posttransplant is termed *chronic GVHD*. Acute GVHD most often first becomes apparent 2–4 weeks posttransplant and is characterized by an erythematous maculopapular rash; persistent anorexia or diarrhea, or both; and by liver disease with increased serum levels of bilirubin, alanine and aspartate aminotransferase, and alkaline phosphatase. Since many conditions can mimic acute GVHD, diagnosis usually requires skin, liver, or endoscopic biopsy for confirmation. In all these organs, endothelial damage and lymphocytic infiltrates are seen. In skin, the epidermis and hair follicles are damaged; in liver, the small bile ducts show segmental disruption; and in intestines, destruction of the crypts and mucosal ulceration may be noted. A commonly used rating system for acute GVHD is shown in Table 108-1. Grade I acute GVHD is of little clinical significance, does not affect the likelihood of survival, and does not require treatment. In contrast, grades II to IV GVHD are associated with significant symptoms and a poorer probability of survival, and they require aggressive therapy. The incidence of acute GVHD is higher in recipients of stem cells from mismatched or unrelated donors, in older patients, and in patients unable to receive full doses of drugs used to prevent the disease.

One general approach to the prevention of GVHD is the administration of immunosuppressive drugs early after transplant. Combina-

TABLE 108-1 CLINICAL STAGING AND GRADING OF ACUTE GRAFT-VERSUS-HOST DISEASE

Clinical Stage	Skin	Liver—Bilirubin, μmol/L (mg/dL)	Gut
1	Rash <25% body surface	34–51 (2–3)	Diarrhea 500–1000 mL/d
2	Rash 25–50% body surface	51–103 (3–6)	Diarrhea 1000–1500 mL/d
3	Generalized erythroderma	103–257 (6–15)	Diarrhea >1500 mL/d
4	Desquamation and bullae	>257 (> 15)	Ileus

Overall Clinical Grade	Skin Stage	Liver Stage	Gut Stage
I	1–2	0	0
II	1–3	1	1
III	1–3	2–3	2–3
IV	2–4	2–4	2–4

tions of methotrexate and either cyclosporine or tacrolimus are among the most effective and widely used regimens. Prednisone, anti–T cell antibodies, mycophenolate mofetil, and other immunosuppressive agents have also been or are being studied in various combinations. A second general approach to GVHD prevention is removal of T cells from the stem cell inoculum. While effective in preventing GVHD, T cell depletion is associated with an increased incidence of graft failure and of tumor recurrence posttransplant; as yet, little evidence suggests that T-cell depletion improves cure rates in any specific setting.

Despite prophylaxis, significant acute GVHD will develop in ~30% of recipients of stem cells from matched siblings and in as many as 60% of those receiving stem cells from unrelated donors. The disease is usually treated with glucocorticoids, antithymocyte globulin, or monoclonal antibodies targeted against T cells or T cell subsets.

Between 20 and 50% of patients surviving >6 months after allogeneic transplantation will develop chronic GVHD. The disease is more common in older patients, in recipients of mismatched or unrelated stem cells, and in those with a preceding episode of acute GVHD. The disease resembles an autoimmune disorder with malar rash, sicca syndrome, arthritis, obliterative bronchiolitis, and bile duct degeneration and cholestasis. Single-agent prednisone or cyclosporine is standard treatment at present, although trials of other agents are under way. In most patients, chronic GVHD resolves, but it may require 1–3 years of immunosuppressive treatment before these agents can be withdrawn without the disease recurring. Because patients with chronic GVHD are susceptible to significant infection, they should receive prophylactic trimethoprim-sulfamethoxazole, and all suspected infections should be investigated and treated aggressively.

Graft Failure While complete and sustained engraftment is usually seen posttransplant, occasionally marrow function either does not return or, after a brief period of engraftment, is lost. Graft failure after autologous transplantation can be the result of inadequate numbers of stem cells being transplanted, damage during ex vivo treatment or storage, or exposure of the patient to myelotoxic agents posttransplant. Infections with cytomegalovirus (CMV) or human herpes virus type 6 have also been associated with loss of marrow function. Graft failure after allogeneic transplantation can also be due to immunologic rejection of the graft by immunocompetent host cells. Immunologically based graft rejection is more common following use of less-immunosuppressive preparative regimens, in recipients of T cell–depleted stem cell products, and in patients receiving grafts from HLA-mismatched donors.

Treatment of graft failure usually involves removing all potentially myelotoxic agents from the patient's regimen and attempting a short trial of a myeloid growth factor. Persistence of lymphocytes of host origin in allogeneic transplant recipients with graft failure indicates immunologic rejection. Reinfusion of donor stem cells in such patients is usually unsuccessful unless preceded by a second immunosuppressive preparative regimen. Standard preparative regimens are generally tolerated poorly if administered within 100 days of a first transplant because of cumulative toxicities. However, use of regimens combining, for example, anti-CD3 antibodies with high-dose glucocorticoids, flu-

darabine plus low-dose total-body irradiation, or cyclophosphamide plus antithymocyte globulin have been effective in some cases.

Infection Posttransplant patients, particularly recipients of allogeneic transplantation, require unique approaches to the problem of infection. Early after transplantation, patients are profoundly neutropenic, and because the risk of bacterial infection is so great, most centers initiate antibiotic treatment once the granulocyte count falls to <500/μL. Fluconazole prophylaxis at a dose of 200–400 mg/kg per day reduces the risk of candidal infections. Patients seropositive for herpes simplex should receive acyclovir prophylaxis. One approach to infection prophylaxis is shown in Table 108-2. Despite these prophylactic measures, most patients will develop fever and signs of infection posttransplant. The management of patients who become febrile despite bacterial and fungal prophylaxis is a difficult challenge and is guided by individual aspects of the patient and by the institution's experience. The general problem of infection in the immunocompromised host is discussed in Chap. 126.

Once patients engraft, the incidence of bacterial infection diminishes; however, patients, particularly allogeneic transplant recipients, remain at significant risk of infection. During the period from engraftment until about 3 months posttransplant, the most common causes of infection are gram-positive bacteria, fungi (particularly *Aspergillus*) and viruses including CMV. CMV infection, which in the past was frequently seen and often fatal, can be prevented in seronegative patients by the use of seronegative blood products. The use of ganciclovir, either as prophylaxis beginning at the time of engraftment or initiated when CMV first reactivates as evidenced by development of antigenemia, can significantly reduce the risk of CMV disease in seropositive patients. Elimination of white blood cells from transfused blood products is another method to prevent CMV transmission. Foscarnet is effective for some patients who develop CMV antigenemia or infection despite the use of ganciclovir or who cannot tolerate the drug.

Pneumocystis jiroveci pneumonia, once seen in 5–10% of patients, can be prevented by treating patients with oral trimethoprim-sulfamethoxazole for 1 week pretransplant and resuming the treatment once patients have engrafted.

The risk of infection diminishes considerably beyond 3 months after transplant unless chronic GVHD develops, requiring continuous immunosuppression. Most transplant centers recommend continuing trimethoprim-sulfamethoxazole prophylaxis while patients are receiving any immunosuppressive drugs and also recommend careful monitoring for late CMV reactivation. In addition, many centers recommend prophylaxis against varicella zoster, using acyclovir for 1 year posttransplant.

TABLE 108-2 APPROACH TO INFECTION PROPHYLAXIS IN ALLOGENEIC TRANSPLANT RECIPIENTS

Organism		Approach
Bacterial	Ceftazidime	2 g IV q8h while neutropenic
Fungal	Fluconazole	400 mg PO qd to day 75 posttransplant
Pneumocystis carinii	Trimethoprim-sulfamethoxazole	1 double-strength tablet PO bid 2 days/week until day 180 or off immunosuppression
Viral		
Herpes simplex	Acyclovir	800 mg PO bid to day 30
Varicella zoster	Acyclovir	800 mg PO bid to day 365
Cytomegalovirus	Ganciclovir	5 mg/kg IV bid for 7 days, then 5 (mg/kg)/d 5 days/week to day 100

TREATMENT OF SPECIFIC DISEASES USING HEMATOPOIETIC CELL TRANSPLANTATION

℞ NONMALIGNANT DISEASES

IMMUNODEFICIENCY DISORDERS By replacing abnormal stem cells with cells from a normal donor, hematopoietic cell transplantation can cure patients of a variety of immunodeficiency disorders including severe combined immunodeficiency, Wiskott-Aldrich syndrome, and Chédiak-Higashi syndrome. The widest experience has been with severe combined immunodeficiency disease, where cure rates of 90% can be expected with HLA-identical donors and success rates of 50–70% have been reported using haplotype-mismatched parents as donors **(Table 108-3)**.

APLASTIC ANEMIA Transplantation from matched siblings after a preparative regimen of high-dose cyclophosphamide and antithymocyte globulin can cure up to 90% of patients <40 years with severe aplastic anemia. Results in older patients and in recipients of mismatched family member or unrelated marrow are less favorable; therefore, a trial of immunosuppressive therapy is generally recommended for such patients before considering transplantation. Transplantation is effective in all forms of aplastic anemia including, for example, the syndromes associated with paroxysmal nocturnal hemoglobinuria and Fanconi's anemia. Patients with Fanconi's anemia are abnormally sensitive to the toxic effects of alkylating agents and so less intensive preparative regimens must be used in their treatment (Chap. 102).

HEMOGLOBINOPATHIES Marrow transplantation from an HLA-identical sibling following a preparative regimen of busulfan and cyclophosphamide can cure 70–90% of patients with thalassemia major. The best outcomes can be expected if patients are transplanted before they develop hepatomegaly or portal fibrosis and if they have been given adequate iron chelation therapy. Among such patients, the probabilities of 5-year survival and disease-free survival are 95 and 90%, respectively. Although prolonged survival can be achieved with aggressive chelation therapy, transplantation is the only curative treatment for thalassemia. Transplantation is being studied as a curative approach to patients with sickle cell anemia. Two-year survival and disease-free survival rates of 90 and 80%, respectively, have been reported following matched sibling transplantation. Decisions about patient selection and the timing of transplantation remain difficult, but transplantation represents a reasonable option for younger pa-

tients who suffer repeated crises or other significant complications and who have not responded to other interventions (Chap. 99).

OTHER NONMALIGNANT DISEASES Theoretically, hematopoietic cell transplantation should be able to cure any disease that results from an inborn error of the lymphohematopoietic system. Transplantation has been used successfully to treat congenital disorders of white blood cells such as Kostmann's syndrome, chronic granulomatous disease, and leukocyte adhesion deficiency. Congenital anemias such as Blackfan-Diamond anemia can also be cured with transplantation. Infantile malignant osteopetrosis is due to an inability of the osteoclast to resorb bone, and since osteoclasts derive from the marrow, transplantation can cure this rare inherited disorder.

Hematopoietic cell transplantation has been used as treatment for a number of storage diseases caused by enzymatic deficiencies, such as Gaucher's disease, Hurler's syndrome, Hunter's syndrome, and infantile metachromatic leukodystrophy. Transplantation for these diseases has not been uniformly successful, but treatment early in the course of these diseases, before irreversible damage to extramedullary organs has occurred, increases the chance for success.

Transplantation is being explored as a treatment for severe acquired autoimmune disorders. These trials are based on studies demonstrating that transplantation can reverse autoimmune disorders in animal models and on the observation that occasional patients with coexisting autoimmune disorders and hematologic malignancies have been cured of both with transplantation.

℞ MALIGNANT DISEASES

ACUTE LEUKEMIA Allogeneic hematopoietic cell transplantation cures 15–20% of patients who do not achieve complete response from induction chemotherapy for acute myeloid leukemia (AML) and is the only form of therapy that can cure such patients. Cure rates of 30–35% are seen when patients are transplanted in second remission or in first relapse. The best results with allogeneic transplantation are achieved when applied during first remission, with disease-free survival rates averaging 55–60%. Chemotherapy alone can cure a portion of AML patients, and so the relative merits of transplanting all patients during first remission versus only transplanting very-high-risk patients and those who relapse continue to be discussed. Autologous transplantation is also able to cure a portion of patients with AML. The rates of disease recurrence with autologous transplantation are higher than those seen after allogeneic transplantation, and cure rates are somewhat less.

Similar to patients with AML, adults with acute lymphocytic leukemia who do not achieve a complete response to induction chemotherapy can be cured in 15–20% of cases with immediate transplantation. Cure rates improve to 30–50% in second remission, and therefore transplantation can be recommended for adults who have persistent disease after induction chemotherapy or who have subsequently relapsed. Transplantation in first remission results in cure rates around 55%. While transplantation appears to offer a clear advantage over chemotherapy for patients with high-risk disease, such as those with Philadelphia chromosome–positive disease, debate continues about whether adults with standard-risk disease should be transplanted in first remission or whether transplantation should be reserved until relapse. Autologous transplantation is associated with a higher relapse rate but a somewhat lower risk of nonrelapse mortality when compared to allogeneic transplantation. On balance, most experts recommend use of allogeneic stem cells if an appropriate donor is available.

CHRONIC LEUKEMIA Allogeneic hematopoietic cell transplantation is the only therapy shown to cure a substantial portion of patients with chronic myeloid leukemia (CML). Five-year disease-free survival rates are 15–20% for patients transplanted for blast crisis, 25–50% for accelerated-phase patients, and 60–70% for chronic phase patients, with cure rates as high as 80% at selected centers. Use of unrelated donors results in more GVHD and slightly worse survival than seen with matched siblings, although 3-year disease-free survival rates of 70% have been reported at some large centers. The timing of transplantation in CML has become more complicated with the introduction of imatinib mesylate, a remarkably effective, relatively nontoxic oral agent. Even though imatinib is not generally regarded as curative, given its favorable toxicity profile, most physicians favor its use as initial therapy for CML, with transplantation being reserved for those who fail to

TABLE 108-3 ESTIMATED 5-YEAR SURVIVAL RATES FOLLOWING TRANSPLANTATION[a]

Disease	Allogeneic, %	Autologous, %
Severe combined immunodeficiency	90	N/A
Aplastic anemia	90	N/A
Thalassemia	90	N/A
Acute myeloid leukemia		
First remission	55–60	50
Second remission	40	30
Acute lymphocytic leukemia		
First remission	50	40
Second remission	40	30
Chronic myeloid leukemia		
Chronic phase	70	ID
Accelerated phase	40	ID
Blast crisis	15	ID
Chronic lymphocytic leukemia	50	ID
Myelodysplasia	45	ID
Multiple myeloma	30	35
Non-Hodgkin's lymphoma		
First relapse/second remission	40	40
Hodgkin's disease		
First relapse/second remission	40	50
Breast cancer		
High-risk stage II	N/A	70
Stage IV	N/A	15

[a]These estimates are generally based on data reported by the International Bone Marrow Transplant Registry. The analysis has not been reviewed by their Advisory Committee.

Note: N/A, not applicable; ID, insufficient data.

achieve a complete cytogenetic response with imatinib, relapse after an initial response, or are intolerant of the drug (Chap. 104).

Allogeneic transplantation has been used to only a limited extent for chronic lymphocytic leukemia, in large part because of the chronic nature of the disease and because of the age profile of patients. With allogeneic transplantation, complete remissions have been achieved in the majority of patients so far reported, with disease-free survival rates of ~50% at 3 years. However, treatment-related mortality has been substantial, and further follow-up is needed. Encouraging results have been seen using reduced intensity preparative regimens before allogeneic transplantation.

MYELODYSPLASIA Between 40 and 50% of patients with myelodysplasia appear to be cured with allogeneic transplantation. Results are better among younger patients and those with less-advanced disease. However, some patients with myelodysplasia can live for extended periods without intervention, and so transplantation is generally recommended only for patients with disease categorized as intermediate risk I or greater according to the International Prognostic Scoring System (Chap. 102).

LYMPHOMA Patients with disseminated intermediate- or high-grade non-Hodgkin's lymphoma who have not been cured by first-line chemotherapy and are transplanted in first relapse or second remission can still be cured in 40–50% of cases. This represents a clear advantage over results obtained with conventional-dose salvage chemotherapy. It is unsettled whether patients with high-risk disease benefit from transplantation in first remission. Most experts favor the use of autologous rather than allogeneic transplantation for patients with intermediate or high grade non-Hodgkin's lymphoma, because fewer complications occur with this approach and survival appears equivalent. For patients with recurrent disseminated indolent non-Hodgkin's lymphoma, autologous transplantation results in high response rates and improved progression-free survival compared to salvage chemotherapy. However, late relapses are seen after transplantation. The role of autologous transplantation in the initial treatment of patients is under study. Nonmyeloablative preparative regimens followed by allogeneic transplantation result in high response rates in patients with indolent lymphomas, but the exact role of this approach remains to be defined.

The role of transplantation in Hodgkin's disease is similar to that in intermediate- and high-grade non-Hodgkin's lymphoma. With transplantation, 5-year disease-free survival is 20–30% in patients who never achieve a first remission with standard chemotherapy and up to 70% for those transplanted in second remission. Transplantation has no defined role in first remission in Hodgkin's disease.

MYELOMA Patients with myeloma who have progressed on first-line therapy can sometimes benefit from allogeneic or autologous transplantation. Autologous transplantation has been studied as part of the initial therapy of patients, and both disease-free survival as well as overall survival were improved with this approach in randomized trials. The use of autologous transplantation followed by nonmyeloablative allogeneic transplantation has shown encouraging results.

SOLID TUMORS Among women with metastatic breast cancer, 15–20% disease-free survival rates at 3 years have been reported, with better results seen in younger patients who have responded completely to standard-dose therapy before undergoing transplantation. Randomized trials have not shown superior survival for patients treated for metastatic disease with high-dose chemotherapy plus stem cell support. Randomized trials evaluating transplantation as treatment for primary breast cancer have yielded mixed results. No role for autologous transplantation has been established in the treatment of breast cancer.

Patients with testicular cancer who have failed first-line chemotherapy have been treated with autologous transplantation; ~10–20% of such patients apparently have been cured with this approach.

The use of high-dose chemotherapy with autologous stem cell support is being studied for several other solid tumors, including ovarian cancer, small cell lung cancer, neuroblastoma, and pediatric sarcomas. As in most other settings, the best results have been obtained in patients with limited amounts of disease and where the remaining tumor remains sensitive to conventional-dose chemotherapy. Few randomized trials of transplantation in these diseases have been completed.

Partial and complete responses have been reported following nonmyeloablative allogeneic transplantation for some solid tumors, most notably renal cell cancers. The GVT effect, well documented in the treatment of hematologic malignancies, may apply to selected solid tumors under certain circumstances.

POSTTRANSPLANT RELAPSE Patients who relapse following autologous transplantation sometimes respond to further chemotherapy, particularly if the remission following transplantation was long. More options are available for patients who relapse following allogeneic transplantation. Of particular interest are the response rates seen with infusion of unirradiated donor lymphocytes. Complete responses in as many as 75% of patients with chronic myeloid leukemia, 40% in myelodysplasia, 25% in AML, and 15% in myeloma have been reported. Major complications of donor lymphocyte infusions include transient myelosuppression and the development of GVHD. These complications depend on the number of donor lymphocytes given and the schedule of infusions, with less GVHD seen with lower dose, fractionated schedules.

FURTHER READINGS

APPELBAUM FR: Haematopoietic cell transplantation as immunotherapy. Nature 411:385, 2001

BARON F, STORB R: Hematopoietic stem cell transplantation after reduced-intensity conditioning for older adults with acute myeloid leukemia. Curr Opin Hematol 14:145, 2007

BENSINGER WI et al: Transplantation of bone marrow as compared with peripheral-blood cells from HLA-identical relatives in patients with hematologic cancers. N Engl J Med 344:175, 2001

COPELAN EA: Hematopoietic stem-cell transplantation. N Engl J Med 354:1813, 2006

PETERSDORF EW et al: Major-histocompatibility-complex class I alleles and antigens in hematopoietic-cell transplantation. N Engl J Med 345:1794, 2001

SECTION 3 — DISORDERS OF HEMOSTASIS

109 Disorders of Platelets and Vessel Wall

Barbara A. Konkle

Hemostasis is a dynamic process in which the platelet and the blood vessel wall play key roles. Platelets become activated upon adhesion to von Willebrand factor (vWF) and collagen in the exposed subendothelium after injury. Platelet activation is also mediated through shear forces imposed by blood flow itself, particularly in areas where the vessel wall is diseased, and is also affected by the inflammatory state of the endothelium. The activated platelet surface provides the major physiologic site for coagulation factor activation, which results in further platelet activation and fibrin formation. Genetic and acquired influences on the platelet and vessel wall, as well as on the coagulation and fibrinolytic systems, determine whether normal hemostasis, or bleeding or clotting symptoms, will result.

THE PLATELET

Platelets are released from the megakaryocyte, likely under the influence of flow in the capillary sinuses. The normal blood platelet count is 150,000–450,000/μL. The major regulator of platelet production is the hormone thrombopoietin (TPO), which is synthesized in the liver. Synthesis is increased with inflammation and specifically by interleukin 6. TPO binds to its receptor on platelets and megakaryocytes, by which it is removed from the circulation. Thus, a reduction in platelet and megakaryocyte mass increases the level of TPO, which then stimulates platelet production. Platelets circulate with an average life span of 7–10 days. Approximately one-third of the platelets reside in the spleen, and this number increases in proportion to splenic size, although the platelet count rarely decreases to <40,000/μL as the spleen enlarges. Platelets are physiologically very active but are anucleate, and thus they have limited capacity to synthesize new proteins.

Normal vascular endothelium contributes to preventing thrombosis by inhibiting platelet function (Chap. 59). When vascular endothelium is injured, these inhibitory effects are overcome, and platelets adhere to the exposed intimal surface primarily through vWF, a large multimeric protein present in both plasma and in the extracellular matrix of the subendothelial vessel wall. Platelet adhesion results in the generation of intracellular signals that lead to activation of the platelet glycoprotein (Gp) IIb/IIIa ($\alpha_{IIb}\beta_3$) receptor and resultant platelet aggregation.

Activated platelets undergo release of their granule contents, including nucleotides, adhesive proteins, growth factors, and procoagulants that serve to promote platelet aggregation and blood clot formation, and influence the environment of the forming clot. During platelet aggregation, additional platelets are recruited to the site of injury, leading to the formation of an occlusive platelet thrombus. The platelet plug is stabilized by the fibrin mesh that develops simultaneously as the product of the coagulation cascade.

THE VESSEL WALL

Endothelial cells line the surface of the entire circulatory tree, totaling 1–6×10^{13} cells, enough to cover a surface area equivalent to about six tennis courts. The endothelium is physiologically active, controlling vascular permeability, flow of biologically active molecules and nutrients, blood cell interactions with the vessel wall, the inflammatory response, and angiogenesis.

The endothelium normally presents an antithrombotic surface (Chap. 59) but rapidly becomes prothrombotic when stimulated, which promotes coagulation, inhibits fibrinolysis, and activates platelets. In many cases, endothelium-derived vasodilators are also platelet inhibitors (e.g., nitric oxide) and, conversely, endothelium-derived vasoconstrictors (e.g., endothelin) can also be platelet activators. The net effect of vasodilation and inhibition of platelet function is to promote blood fluidity, whereas the net effect of vasoconstriction and platelet activation is to promote hemostasis. Thus, blood fluidity and hemostasis are regulated by the balance of antithrombotic/prothrombotic and vasodilatory/vasoconstrictor properties of endothelial cells.

DISORDERS OF PLATELETS

THROMBOCYTOPENIA

Thrombocytopenia results from one or more of three processes: (1) decreased bone marrow production; (2) sequestration, usually in an enlarged spleen; and/or (3) increased platelet destruction. Disorders of production may be either inherited or acquired. In evaluating a patient with thrombocytopenia, a key step is to review the peripheral blood smear and to first rule out "pseudothrombocytopenia," particularly in a patient without an apparent cause for the thrombocytopenia. Pseudothrombocytopenia (Fig. 109-1B) is an in vitro artifact resulting from platelet agglutination via antibodies (usually IgG, but also IgM and IgA) when the calcium content is decreased by blood collection in ethylenediamine tetraacetic (EDTA), the anticoagulant present in tubes (purple top, often) used to collect blood for complete blood counts (CBCs). If a low platelet count is obtained in EDTA-anticoagulated blood, a blood smear can be evaluated and a platelet count determined in blood collected into sodium citrate (blue-top tube) or heparin (green-top tube), or ideally a smear of freshly obtained unanticoagulated blood, such as from a finger stick, can be examined.

APPROACH TO THE PATIENT:
Thrombocytopenia

The history and physical examination, results of the CBC, and review of the peripheral blood smear are all critical components in the initial evaluation of the thrombocytopenic patients (Fig. 109-2). The overall health of the patient and whether he/she is receiving drug treatment will influence the differential diagnosis. A healthy young adult with thrombocytopenia will have a much more limited differential diagnosis than an ill hospitalized patient who is receiving multiple medications. Except in unusual inherited disorders, decreased platelet production usually results from bone marrow disorders that also affect red blood cell (RBC) and/or white blood cell (WBC) production. Because myelodysplasia can present with isolated thrombocytopenia, the bone marrow should be examined in patients presenting with isolated thrombocytopenia who are older than 60 years. While inherited thrombocytopenia is rare, any prior platelet counts should be retrieved and a family history regarding thrombocytopenia obtained. A careful history of drug ingestion should be obtained, including nonprescription and herbal remedies, as drugs are the most common cause of thrombocytopenia.

The physical examination can document an enlarged spleen, evidence of chronic liver disease, and other underlying disorders. Mild to moderate splenomegaly may be difficult to appreciate in many individuals due to body habitus and/or obesity but can be easily assess by abdominal ultrasound. A platelet count of approximately 5000–10,000 is required to maintain vascular integrity in the microcirculation. When the platelet count is markedly decreased, petechiae first appear in areas of increased venous pressure, the ankles and feet in an ambulatory patient. Petechiae are pinpoint, nonblanching hemorrhages and are usually a sign of a decreased platelet number and not platelet dysfunction. Wet purpura, blood blisters that form on the oral mucosa, are thought to denote an increased risk of life-threatening hemorrhage in the thrombocytopenic patient. Excessive bruising is seen in disorders of both platelet number and function.

Infection-Induced Thrombocytopenia Many viral and bacterial infections result in thrombocytopenia and are the most common noniatrogenic cause of thrombocytopenia. This may or may not be associated with laboratory evidence of disseminated intravascular coagulation (DIC), which is most commonly seen in patients with systemic infections with gram negative bacteria. Infections can affect both platelet production and platelet survival. In addition, immune mechanisms can be at work, as in infectious mononucleosis and early HIV infection. Late in HIV infection, pancytopenia and decreased and dysplastic platelet production is more common. Immune-mediated thrombocytopenia (ITP2) in children usually follows a viral infection and almost always resolves spontaneously. This association of infection with ITP is less clear in adults.

Bone marrow examination is often requested for evaluation of occult infections. A study evaluating the role of bone marrow examination in fever of unknown origin in HIV-infected patients found that for 86% of patients, the same diagnosis was established by less-invasive techniques, notably blood culture. In some instances, however, the diagnosis can be made earlier; thus, a bone marrow examination and culture is recommended when the diagnosis is needed urgently or when other, less-invasive methods have been unsuccessful.

Drug-Induced Thrombocytopenia Many drugs have been associated with thrombocytopenia. A predictable decrease in platelet count occurs after treatment with many chemotherapeutic drugs due to bone marrow suppression (Chap. 81). Other commonly used drugs that cause isolated thrombocytopenia are listed in Table 109-1, but all drugs should be suspect in a patient with thrombocytopenia without an apparent cause and should be stopped, or substituted, if possible. A helpful website, Platelets on the Internet (*http://moon.ouhsc.edu/jgeorge*), lists drugs reported to have caused thrombocytopenia and the level of evidence supporting the association. Although not well studied, herbal and over-the-counter

FIGURE 109-1 Photomicrographs of peripheral blood smears. A. Normal peripheral blood. **B.** Platelet clumping in pseudothrombocytopenia. **C.** Abnormal large platelet in autosomal dominant macrothrombocytopenia. **D.** Schistocytes and decreased platelets in microangiopathic hemolytic anemia.

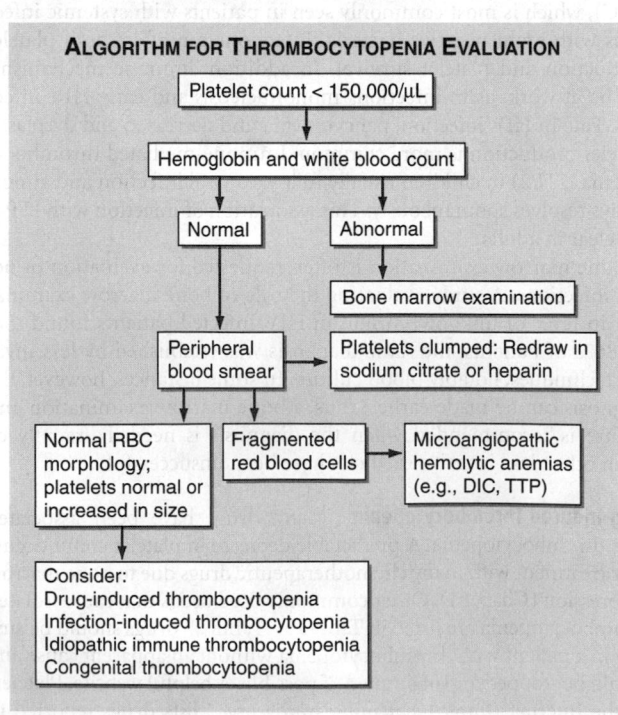

ALGORITHM FOR THROMBOCYTOPENIA EVALUATION

Platelet count < 150,000/μL

Hemoglobin and white blood count

Normal / Abnormal

Bone marrow examination

Peripheral blood smear

Platelets clumped: Redraw in sodium citrate or heparin

Normal RBC morphology; platelets normal or increased in size

Fragmented red blood cells

Microangiopathic hemolytic anemias (e.g., DIC, TTP)

Consider:
Drug-induced thrombocytopenia
Infection-induced thrombocytopenia
Idiopathic immune thrombocytopenia
Congenital thrombocytopenia

FIGURE 109-2 Algorithm for evaluating the thrombocytopenic patient.

preparations may also result in thrombocytopenia and should be discontinued in patients who are thrombocytopenic.

Classic drug-dependent antibodies are antibodies that react with specific platelet surface antigens and result in thrombocytopenia only when the drug is present. Many drugs are capable of inducing these antibodies, but for some reason they are more common with quinine and sulfonamides. Drug-dependent antibody binding can be demonstrated by laboratory assays, showing antibody binding in the presence of, but not without, the

TABLE 109-1 DRUGS DEFINITIVELY REPORTED TO CAUSE ISOLATED THROMBOCYTOPENIA[a]

Abciximab	Digoxin
Acetaminophen	Eptifibatide
Acyclovir	Hydrochlorothiazide
Aminosalicylic acid	Ibuprofen
Amiodarone	Levamisole
Amphotericin B	Octreotide
Ampicillin	Phenytoin
Carbamazepine	Quinine
Chlorpropamide	Rifampin
Danazol	Tamoxifen
Diatrizoate meglumine (Hypaque Meglumine)	Tirofiban
	Trimethoprim/sulfamethoxazole
Diclofenac	Vancomycin

[a]Drugs that preceded thrombocytopenia and full recovery occurred after drug discontinuation, but recurred with re-introduction of the drug, and other causes, including other drugs were excluded.

Source: Data from George and colleagues, http://moon.ouhsc.edu/jgeorge.

FIGURE 109-3 Time course of heparin-induced thrombocytopenia (HIT) development after heparin exposure. The timing of development after heparin exposure is a critical factor in determining the likelihood of HIT in a patient. HIT occurs early in heparin exposure only in the presence of preexisting heparin/platelet factor 4 (PF4) antibodies, which disappear from circulation by ~100 days following a prior exposure. Rarely, HIT may occur later after heparin exposure (termed *delayed-onset HIT*). In this setting, heparin/PF4 antibody testing is markedly positive. HIT can occur after exposure to either unfractionated heparin (UFH) or low-molecular-weight heparin (LMWH).

drug present in the assay. The thrombocytopenia typically occurs after a period of initial exposure (median length 21 days), or upon reexposure, and usually resolves in 7–10 days after drug withdrawal. The thrombocytopenia caused by the platelet GpIIbIIIa inhibitory drugs, such as abciximab, differs in that it may occur within 24 hours of initial exposure. This appears to be due to the presence of naturally occurring antibodies that cross-react with the drug bound to the platelet.

Heparin-Induced Thrombocytopenia   Drug-induced thrombocytopenia due to heparin differs from that seen with other drugs in two major ways. (1) The thrombocytopenia is not usually severe, with nadir counts rarely <20,000/μL. (2) Heparin-induced thrombocytopenia (HIT) is not associated with bleeding and, in fact, markedly increases the risk of thrombosis. HIT results from antibody formation to a complex of the platelet-specific protein platelet factor 4 (PF4) and heparin. The antiheparin/PF4 antibody can activate platelets through the FcγRIIa receptor and also likely activates endothelial cells. Many patients exposed to heparin develop antibodies to heparin/PF4, but do not appear to have adverse consequences. A fraction of those who develop antibodies will develop thrombocytopenia, and a portion of those (up to 50%) will develop HIT and thrombosis (HITT).

HIT can occur after exposure to low-molecular-weight heparin (LMWH), as well as unfractionated heparin (UFH), although it is about 10 times more common with the latter. Most patients develop HIT after exposure to heparin for 5–10 days (Fig. 109-3). It occurs before 5 days only in those who were exposed to heparin in the prior few weeks or months (< ~100 days) and have circulating antiheparin/PF4 antibodies. Rarely, thrombocytopenia and thrombosis begin several days after all heparin has been stopped (termed *delayed onset HIT*). The 4 "T"s have been recommended to be used in a diagnostic algorithm for HIT: *t*hrombocytopenia, *t*iming of platelet count drop, *t*hrombosis and other sequelae such as localized skin reactions, and o*t*her cause of thrombocytopenia not evident.

LABORATORY TESTING FOR HIT   HIT (antiheparin/PF4) antibodies can be detected using two types of assays. The most widely available is an enzyme-linked immunoassay (ELISA) with PF4/polyanion complex as the antigen. Since many patients develop antibodies but do not develop clinical HIT, the test has a low specificity for the diagnosis of HIT. This is especially true in patients who have undergone cardiopulmonary bypass surgery, where approximately 50% of patients develop these antibodies postoperatively. The other assay is a platelet activation assay that measures the ability of the patients' serum to activate platelets in the presence of heparin in a concentration-dependent manner. This test has lower sensitivity but higher specificity than the ELISA. However, HIT remains a clinical diagnosis. The main value in testing is in excluding the diagnosis with negative tests, particularly ELISA.

complication of HIT, even after heparin discontinuation, and can occur in both the venous and arterial systems. In patients diagnosed with HIT, imaging studies to evaluate the presence of thrombosis (at least lower-extremity duplex dopplers) are recommended. Patients requiring anticoagulation should be switched from heparin to an alternative anticoagulant. The direct thrombin inhibitors (DTIs) argatroban and lepirudin are effective in HITT. The DTI bivalirudin and the antithrombin-binding pentasaccharide fondaparinux appear to be effective but are not yet approved by the U.S. Food and Drug Administration (FDA) for this indication. Danaparoid, a mixture of glycosoaminoglycans with anti-Xa activity, has been used extensively for the treatment of HITT; it is no longer available in the United States but is in other countries. HIT antibodies cross-react with LMWH, and these preparations should not be used in the treatment of HIT.

Because of the high rate of thrombosis in patients with HIT, anticoagulation should be strongly considered, even in the absence of thrombosis. In patients with thrombosis, patients can be transitioned to warfarin, with treatment usually for 3–6 months. In patients without thrombosis, the duration of anticoagulation needed is undefined. An increased risk of thrombosis is present for at least 1 month after diagnosis; however, most thromboses occur early, and whether thrombosis occurs later if the patient is initially anticoagulated is unknown. Options include continuing anticoagulation until a few days after platelet recovery or for one month. Introduction of warfarin alone in the setting of HIT or HITT may precipitate thrombosis, particularly venous gangrene, presumably due to clotting activation and severely reduced levels of proteins C and S. Warfarin should only be started after alternative anticoagulation has been given for several days and the prothrombotic state has lessened.

Immune Thrombocytopenic Purpura (ITP)   Immune thrombocytopenic purpura (ITP; also termed *idiopathic thrombocytopenic purpura*) is an acquired disorder leading to immune-mediated destruction of platelets and possibly inhibition of platelet release from the megakaryocyte. In children it is usually an acute disease, most commonly following an infection, and with a self-limited course. In adults it usually runs a more chronic course. The exact nature of the immune dysfunction is generally not known. ITP is termed *secondary* if it is associated with an underlying disorder; autoimmune disorders, particularly systemic lupus erythematosis (SLE), and infections, such as HIV and hepatitis C, are common causes. The association of ITP with *Helicobacter pylori* infection is unclear.

ITP is characterized by mucocutaneous bleeding and a low, often very low, platelet count, with otherwise normal peripheral blood cells and smear. Patients usually present either with ecchymoses and petechiae, or with thrombocytopenia incidentally found on a routine CBC. Mucocutaneous bleeding, such as oral mucosa, gastrointestinal, or heavy menstrual bleeding, may be present. Rarely, life-threatening bleeding, including in the central nervous system, can occur. Wet purpura (blood blisters in the mouth) and retinal hemorrhages may herald life-threatening bleeding.

LABORATORY TESTING IN ITP   Laboratory testing for antibodies (serologic testing) is usually not helpful due to the low sensitivity and specificity of the tests. Bone marrow examination can be reserved for older adults (usually >60 years) or those who have other signs or laboratory abnormalities not explained by ITP, or in patients who do not respond to initial therapy. The peripheral blood smear may show large platelets, with otherwise normal morphology. Depending on the bleeding history, iron deficiency anemia may be present.

Laboratory testing is performed to evaluate for secondary causes of ITP and should include testing for HIV infection and hepatitis C (and other infections if indicated); serologic testing for SLE; serum protein electrophoresis and immunoglobulin levels to potentially detect hypogammaglobulinemia, IgA deficiency, or monoclonal gammopathies; and, if anemia is present, direct antiglobulin testing (Coombs test) to rule out combined autoimmune hemolytic anemia with ITP (Evans's syndrome).

℞ HEPARIN-INDUCED THROMBOCYTOPENIA

Early recognition is key in treatment of HIT, with prompt discontinuation of heparin and use of alternative anticoagulants. Thrombosis is a common

℞ IMMUNE THROMBOCYTOPENIC PURPURA

The treatment of ITP utilizes drugs that decrease reticuloendothelial uptake of the antibody-bound platelet and/or decrease antibody production.

However, the diagnosis of ITP does not necessarily mean that treatment must be instituted. Patients with platelet counts >30,000/μL appear not to have increased mortality related to the thrombocytopenia.

Initial treatment in patients without significant bleeding symptoms, severe thrombocytopenia (<5000/μL), or signs of impending bleeding (such as retinal hemorrhage or large oral mucosal hemorrhages) can be instituted as an outpatient using single agents. Traditionally this has been prednisone at 1 mg/kg, although $Rh_0(D)$ immune globulin therapy (WinRho SDF) at 50–75 μg/kg is also being used in this setting. $Rh_0(D)$ immune globulin must be used only in Rh+ patients as the mechanism of action is production of limited hemolysis, with antibody-coated cells "saturating" the Fc receptors, inhibiting Fc receptor function. Hemoglobin levels usually decrease (mean 1.7 g/dL), although severe intravascular hemolysis is a rare complication. Doses are reduced if given to anemic patients. Intravenous gamma globulin (IVIgG), which is pooled, primarily IgG antibodies, also blocks the Fc receptor system, but appears to work primarily through different mechanism(s). IVIgG has more efficacy than anti-$Rh_0(D)$ in post-splenectomized patients. IVIgG is dosed at 2 g/kg total, given in divided doses over 2–5 days. Side effects are usually related to the volume of infusion and infrequently include aseptic meningitis and renal failure. All immunoglobulin preparations are derived from human plasma and undergo treatment for viral inactivation.

For patients with severe ITP and/or symptoms of bleeding, hospital admission and combined modality therapy are given using high-dose glucocorticoids with IVIgG or anti-Rh_0D therapy, and, as needed, additional immunosuppressive agents. Rituximab, an anti-CD20 (B cell) antibody, has shown efficacy in the treatment of refractory ITP.

Splenectomy has been used for treatment of patients who relapse after glucocorticoids are tapered. Splenectomy remains an important treatment option; however, more patients than previously thought will go into a remission over time. Observation, if the platelet count is high enough, or intermittent treatment with anti-$Rh_0(D)$ or IVIgG may be a reasonable approach to see if the ITP will resolve. Vaccination against encapsulated organisms (especially pneumococcus, but also menningococcus and *Haemophilus influenzae*, depending on patient age and potential exposure) is recommended before splenectomy. Accessory spleen(s) are a very rare cause of relapse.

New drugs for ITP include TPO receptor agonists. This approach to treatment of ITP stems from the finding that many patients with ITP do not have increased TPO levels, as was previously hypothesized, nor do they all have increased platelet destruction. Two agents, one administered subcutaneously and another orally, have shown response in many patients with refractory ITP. Roles for these agents in ITP treatment are not fully defined.

Inherited Thrombocytopenia Thrombocytopenia is rarely inherited, either as an isolated finding or as part of a syndrome, and may be inherited in an autosomal dominant, autosomal recessive, or X-linked pattern. Many forms of autosomal dominant thrombocytopenia are now known to be associated with mutations in the nonmuscle myosin heavy chain *MYH9* gene. Interestingly, these include the May-Hegglin anomaly and Sebastian, Epstein's, and Fechtner syndromes, all of which have distinct distinguishing features. A common feature of these disorders is large platelets (Fig. 109-1*C*). Autosomal recessive disorders include congenital amegakaryocytic thrombocytopenia, thrombocytopenia with absent radii, and Bernard Soulier syndrome. The latter is primarily a functional platelet disorder due to absence of GPIb-IX-V, the vWF adhesion receptor. X-linked disorders include Wiskott-Aldrich syndrome and a dyshematopoietic syndrome resulting from a mutation in GATA-1, an important transcriptional regulator of hematopoiesis.

THROMBOTIC THROMBOCYTOPENIC PURPURA AND HEMOLYTIC UREMIC SYNDROME

Thrombotic thrombocytopenic microangiopathies are a group of disorders characterized by thrombocytopenia, a microangiopathic hemolytic anemia evident by fragmented RBCs (Fig. 109-1*D*) and laboratory evidence of hemolysis, and microvascular thrombosis. This includes thrombotic thrombocytopenic purpura (TTP) and hemolytic uremic syndrome (HUS), as well as syndromes complicating bone marrow transplantation, certain medications and infections, pregnan-

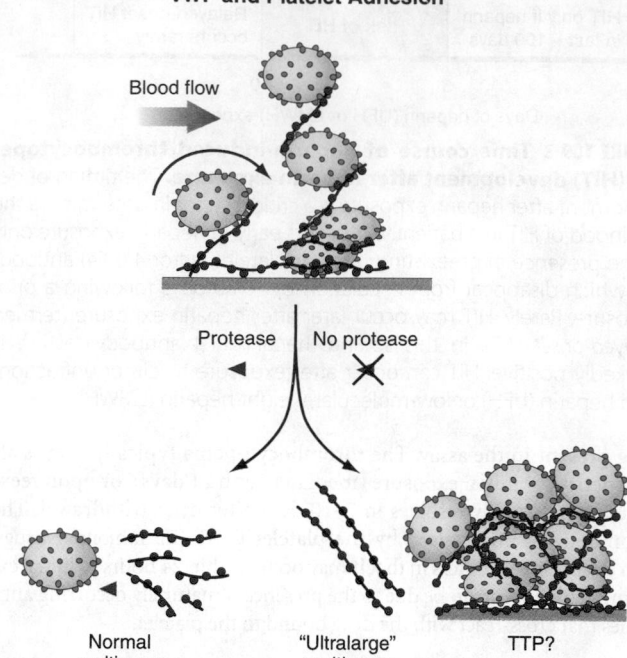

vWF and Platelet Adhesion

FIGURE 109-4 Pathogenesis of thrombotic thrombocytopenic purpura (TTP). Normally the ultra-high molecular-weight multimers of von Willebrand factor (vWF) produced by the endothelial cells are processed into smaller multimers by a plasma metalloproteinase called *ADAMTS13*. In TTP the activity of the protease is inhibited, and the ultra-high molecular-weight multimers of vWF initiate platelet aggregation and thrombosis. *(From Vesely et al., Copyright American Society of Hematology.)*

cy, and vasculitis. In DIC, while thrombocytopenia and microangiopathy are seen, a coagulopathy predominates, with consumption of clotting factors and fibrinogen resulting in an elevated prothrombin time (PT) and often activated partial thromboplastin time (aPTT). The PT and aPTT are characteristically normal in TTP or HUS.

Thrombotic Thrombocytopenic Purpura TTP and HUS were previously considered overlap syndromes. However, in the past few years the pathophysiology of inherited and idiopathic TTP has become better understood and clearly differs from HUS. TTP was first described in 1924 by Eli Moschcowitz and characterized by a pentad of findings that include microangiopathic hemolytic anemia, thrombocytopenia, renal failure, neurologic findings, and fever. The full-blown syndrome is less commonly seen now, probably due to earlier diagnosis. The introduction of treatment with plasma exchange markedly improved the prognosis in patients, with a decrease in mortality from 85–100% to 10–30%.

The pathogenesis of inherited (Upshaw-Schulman syndrome) and idiopathic TTP is related to a deficiency of, or antibodies to, a metalloprotease that cleaves vWF and ADAMTS13, respectively. vWF is normally secreted as ultra-large multimers, which are then cleaved by ADAMTS13. The persistence of ultra-large vWF molecules are thought to contribute to pathogenic platelet adhesion and aggregation (Fig. 109-4). This defect alone, however, is not sufficient to result in TTP as individuals with a congenital absence of ADAMTS13 develop TTP only episodically. Additional provocative factors have not been defined. The level of ADAMTS13 activity, as well as antibodies, can now be detected by laboratory assays. However, assays with sufficient sensitivity and specificity to direct clinical management have yet to be defined.

Idiopathic TTP appears to be more common in women than in men. No geographic or racial distribution has been defined. TTP is more common in patients with HIV infection and in pregnant women. Medication-related TTP may be secondary to antibody formation (ticlopidine and possibly clopidogrel) or direct endothelial toxicity (cyclosporine, mitomycin C, tacrolimus, quinine), although this is not always so clear, and fear of withholding treatment, as well as lack of other treatment alternatives, results in broad application of plasma exchange. However, withdrawal, or reduction in dose, of endothelial toxic agents may decrease the microangiopathy.

Rx THROMBOTIC THROMBOCYTOPENIC PURPURA

TTP is a devastating disease if not diagnosed and treated promptly. In patients presenting with new thrombocytopenia, with or without evidence of renal insufficiency and other elements of classic TTP, laboratory data should be obtained to rule out DIC and to evaluate for evidence of microangiopathic hemolytic anemia. Findings to support the TTP diagnosis include an increased lactate dehydrogenase and indirect bilirubin, decreased haptoglobin, and increased reticulocyte count, with a negative direct antiglobulin test. The peripheral smear should be examined for evidence of schistocytes (Fig. 109-1D). Polychromasia is usually also present due to the increased number of young red blood cells, and nucleated RBCs are often present, which is thought to be due to infarction in the microcirculatory system of the bone marrow.

Plasma exchange remains the mainstay of treatment of ITP. ADAMTS13 antibody–mediated TTP (idiopathic TTP) appears to respond best to plasma exchange. Plasma exchange is continued until the platelet count is normal and signs of hemolysis are resolved for at least 2 days. While never evaluated in clinical trial, the use of glucocorticoids seems a reasonable approach, but they should only be used as an adjunct to plasma exchange. Additionally, other immunomodulatory therapies have been reported to be successful in refractory or relapsing TTP, including rituximab, vincristine, cyclophosphamide, and splenectomy. The role of rituximab in the treatment of this disorder needs to be defined. A significant relapse rate is noted: 25–45% within 30 days of initial "remission" and 12–40% with late relapses. Relapses may be more frequent in patients with severe ADAMTS13 deficiency at presentation.

Hemolytic Uremic Syndrome   HUS is a syndrome characterized by acute renal failure, microangiopathic hemolytic anemia, and thrombocytopenia. It is seen predominantly in children and in most cases is preceded by an episode of diarrhea, often hemorrhagic in nature. *Escherichia coli* O157:H7 is the most frequent, although not only, etiologic serotype. HUS not associated with diarrhea (termed *DHUS*) is more heterogeneous in presentation and course. Some children who develop DHUS have been found to have mutations in genes encoding Factor H, a soluble complement regulator, and membrane cofactor protein that is mainly expressed in the kidney.

Rx HEMOLYTIC UREMIC SYNDROME

Treatment of HUS is primarily supportive. In D+HUS, many (~40%) children require at least some period of support with dialysis; however, the overall mortality is <5%. In D–HUS the mortality is higher, approximately 26%. Plasma infusion or plasma exchange has not been shown to alter the overall course. ADAMTS13 levels are generally reported to be normal in HUS, although occasionally they have been reported to be decreased. As ADAMTS13 assays improve, they may help in defining a subset that better fits a TTP diagnosis and may respond to plasma exchange.

THROMBOCYTOSIS

Thrombocytosis is almost always due to (1) iron deficiency; (2) inflammation, cancer, or infection (reactive thrombocytosis); or (3) an underlying myeloproliferative process [essential thrombocythemia or polycythemia vera (Chap. 103)] or, rarely, the 5q-myelodysplastic process (Chap. 102). Patients presenting with an elevated platelet count should be evaluated for underlying inflammation or malignancy, and iron deficiency should be ruled out. Thrombocytosis in response to acute or chronic inflammation has not been associated with an increased thrombotic risk. In fact, patients with markedly elevated platelet counts (>1.5 million), usually seen in the setting of a myeloproliferative disorder, have an increased risk of bleeding. This appears to be due, at

least in part, to acquired von Willebrand disease (vWD) due to platelet-vWF adhesion and removal.

QUALITATIVE DISORDERS OF PLATELET FUNCTION

Inherited Disorders of Platelet Function   Inherited platelet function disorders are thought to be relatively rare, although the prevalence of mild disorders of platelet function is unclear, in part because our testing for such disorders is suboptimal. Rare qualitative disorders include the autosomal recessive disorders Glanzmann's thrombasthenia (absence of the platelet GpIIbIIIa receptor) and Bernard Soulier syndrome (absence of the platelet GpIb-IX-V receptor). Both are inherited in an autosomal recessive fashion and present with bleeding symptoms in childhood.

Platelet storage pool disorder (SPD) is the classic autosomal dominant qualitative platelet disorder. This results from abnormalities of platelet granule formation. It is also seen as a part of inherited disorders of granule formation, such as Hermansky-Pudlak syndrome. Bleeding symptoms in SPD are variable but often mild. The most common inherited disorders of platelet function are disorders that prevent normal secretion of granule content. Few of the abnormalities have been dissected at the molecular level, but these are likely due to multiple abnormalities. They are usually described as *secretion defects*. Bleeding symptoms are usually mild in nature.

Rx INHERITED DISORDERS OF PLATELET DYSFUNCTION

Bleeding symptoms or prevention of bleeding in patients with severe dysfunction frequently requires platelet transfusion. Care is taken to limit the risk of alloimmunization by limiting exposure and using prestorage leukodepleted platelets for transfusion. Platelet disorders associated with milder bleeding symptoms frequently respond to desmopressin [1-deamino-8-D-arginine vasopressin (DDAVP)]. DDAVP increases plasma vWF and FVIII levels; whether it also has a direct effect on platelet function is unknown. Particularly for mucosal bleeding symptoms, antifibrinolytic therapy (epsilon-aminocaproic acid or tranexamic acid) is used alone or in conjunction with DDAVP or platelet therapy.

Acquired Disorders of Platelet Function   Acquired platelet dysfunction is common, usually due to medications, either intentionally, as with antiplatelet therapy, or unintentionally, as with high dose penicillins. Acquired platelet dysfunction occurs in uremia. This is likely multifactorial, but the resultant effect is defective adhesion and activation. The platelet defect is improved most by dialysis, but may also be improved by increasing the hematocrit to 27–32%, giving DDAVP (0.3 μg/kg), or use of conjugated estrogens. Platelet dysfunction also occurs with cardiopulmonary bypass due to the effect of the artificial circuit on platelets, and bleeding symptoms respond to platelet transfusion. Platelet dysfunction seen with underlying hematologic disorders can result from nonspecific interference by circulating paraproteins or intrinsic platelet defects in myeloproliferative and myelodysplastic syndromes.

VON WILLEBRAND DISEASE

vWD is the most common inherited bleeding disorder. Estimates from laboratory data suggest a prevalence of approximately 1%, but data based on symptomatic individuals suggest that it is closer to 0.1% of the population. vWF serves two roles: (1) as the major adhesion molecule that tethers the platelet to the exposed subendothelium; and (2) as the binding protein for FVIII, resulting in significant prolongation of the FVIII half-life in circulation. The platelet-adhesive function of vWF is critically dependent on the presence of large vWF multimers, while FVIII binding is not. Most of the symptoms of vWD are "platelet-like" except in more severe vWD when the FVIII is low enough to produce symptoms similar to those found in Factor VIII deficiency (hemophilia A).

vWD has been classified into three major types, with four subtypes of type 2 (Table 109-2). By far the most common type of vWD is type 1 disease, with a parallel decrease in vWF protein, vWF function, and

TABLE 109-2 LABORATORY DIAGNOSIS OF VON WILLEBRAND DISEASE

Type	aPTT	vWF Antigen	vWF Activity	FVIII Activity	Multimer
1	Nl or ↑	↓	↓	↓	Normal distribution, decreased in quantity
2A	Nl or ↑	↓	↓↓	↓	Loss of high and intermediate MW multimers
2B[a]	Nl or ↑	↓	↓↓	↓	Loss of high MW multimers
2M	Nl or ↑	↓	↓↓	↓	Normal distribution, decreased in quantity
2N	↑↑	Nl or ↓[b]	Nl or ↓[b]	↓↓	Normal distribution
3	↑↑	↓↓	↓↓	↓↓	Absent

[a]Usually also decreased platelet count.

[b]For type 2N, in the homozygous state, FVIII is very low; in the heterozygous state, only seen in conjunction with type 1 vWD.

Abbreviations: aPTT, activated partial thromboplastin time; vWF, von Willebrand factor; F, Factor; Nl, normal; MW, molecular weight.

FVIII levels, accounting for at least 80% of cases. Patients have predominantly mucosal bleeding symptoms, although postoperative bleeding can also be seen. Bleeding symptoms are very uncommon in infancy and usually manifest later in childhood with excessive bruising and epistaxis. Since these symptoms occur commonly in childhood, the clinician should particularly note bruising at sites unlikely to be traumatized and/or prolonged epistaxis requiring medical attention. Menorrhagia is a common manifestation of vWD. Menstrual bleeding resulting in anemia should warrant an evaluation for vWD and, if negative, functional platelet disorders. Frequently, mild type 1 vWD first manifests with dental extractions, particularly wisdom tooth extraction, or tonsillectomy.

Not all patients with low vWF levels have bleeding symptoms. Whether patients bleed or not will depend on the overall hemostatic balance they have inherited, along with environmental influences and the type of hemostatic challenges they experience. Although the inheritance of vWD is autosomal, many factors influence both vWF levels and bleeding symptoms. These have not all been defined but include blood type, thyroid hormone status, race, stress, exercise, and hormonal (both endogenous and exogenous) influences. Patients with type O blood have vWF protein levels about one-half those of patients with AB blood type; in fact, the normal range for patients with type O blood overlaps that usually considered diagnostic for vWD. A mildly decreased vWF level should perhaps be viewed more as a risk factor for bleeding than as an actual disease.

Patients with type 2 vWD have functional defects; thus, the vWF antigen measurement is significantly higher than the test of function. For types 2A, 2B, and 2M, vWF activity is decreased, measured as ristocetin cofactor or collagen binding activity. In type 2A vWD, the impaired function is due either to increased susceptibility to cleavage by ADAMTS13, resulting in loss of intermediate- and high-molecular weight (M.W.) multimers, or to decreased secretion of these multimers by the cell. Type 2B vWD results from gain of function mutations that result in increased spontaneous binding of vWF to platelets in circulation, with subsequent clearance of this complex by the reticuloendothelial system. The resulting vWF in the patients' plasma lacks the highest M.W. multimers, and the platelet count is usually modestly reduced. Type 2M results from a group of mutations that cause dysfunction of the molecule but do not affect multimer structure.

Type 2N vWD reflects mutations in vWF that preclude binding of FVIII. As FVIII is stabilized by binding to vWF, the FVIII in patients with type 2N vWD has a very short half-life, and the FVIII level is markedly decreased. This is sometimes termed *autosomal hemophilia*. Type 3 vWD, or severe vWD, describes patients with virtually no vWF antigen (usually <10%). Patients experience mucosal and joint postoperative symptoms as well as other bleeding symptoms. Some pa-

tients with type 3 vWD, particularly those with large vWF gene deletions, are at risk of developing antibodies to infused vWF.

Acquired vWD is a rare disorder, most commonly seen in patients with underlying lymphoproliferative disorders, including monoclonal gammopathies of undetermined significance (MGUS), multiple myeloma, and Waldenstrom's macroglobulinemia. It is seen most commonly in the setting of MGUS and should be suspected in patients, particularly elderly patients, with a new onset of severe mucosal bleeding symptoms.

Heyde's syndrome (aortic stenosis with gastrointestinal bleeding) is attributed to the presence of angiodysplasia of the gastrointestinal tract in patients with aortic stenosis. However, the shear stress on blood passing through the stenotic aortic valve appears to produce a change in vWF, making it susceptible to serum proteases. Consequently, large multimer forms are lost, leading to an acquired type 2 vWD, but return when the stenotic valve is replaced.

℞ VON WILLEBRAND DISEASE

The mainstay of treatment for type 1 vWD is 1-deamino-8-D-arginine vasopressin (DDAVP, or desmopressin), which results in release of vWF and FVIII from endothelial stores. DDAVP can be given intravenously or by an intranasal spray (1.5 mg/mL). The peak activity when given intravenously is approximately 30 min, while it is 2 h when given intranasally. The usual dose is 0.3 µg/kg intravenously or 2 squirts (1 in each nostril) for patients >50 kg (1 squirt for those <50 kg). It is recommended that patients with vWD be tested with DDAVP to assess their response before using it. In patients who respond well (increase in values of two- to fourfold), it can be used for procedures with minor-to-moderate risk of bleeding. Depending on the procedure, additional doses may be needed; it is usually given every 12–24 h. Less frequent dosing may result in less tachyphylaxis, which occurs when synthesis cannot compensate for the released stores. The major side effect of DDAVP is hyponatremia due to decreased free water clearance. This occurs most commonly in the very young and the very old, but fluid restriction should be advised for all patients for the 24 hours following each dose.

Some patients with types 2A and 2M vWD respond to DDAVP such that it can be used for minor procedures. For the other subtypes, for type 3 disease, and for major procedures requiring longer periods of normal hemostasis, vWF replacement can be given. Virally inactivated vWF-containing factor concentrates are thought to be safer than cryoprecipitate as the replacement product. Humate-P is the only FDA-approved product for this indication in the United States. Other concentrates have been studied in vWD, and a vWF concentrate is available in some countries in Europe.

Antifibrinolytic therapy, using either epsilon-aminocaproic acid or tranexamic acid, is an important therapy, either alone or in an adjunctive capacity, particularly for the prevention or treatment of mucosal bleeding. These agents are particularly useful in prophylaxis for dental procedures, with DDAVP for dental extractions and tonsillectomy, menorrhagia, and prostate procedures. It is contraindicated in the setting of upper urinary tract bleeding, due to the risk of ureteral obstruction.

DISORDERS OF THE VESSEL WALL

The vessel wall is an integral part of hemostasis, and separation of a fluid phase is artificial, particularly in disorders such as TTP or HIT that clearly involve the endothelium as well. Inflammation localized to the vessel wall, such as vasculitis, or inherited connective tissue disorders are abnormalities inherent to the vessel wall.

METABOLIC AND INFLAMMATORY DISORDERS

Acute febrile illnesses may result in vascular damage. This can result from immune complexes containing viral antigens or the viruses themselves. Certain pathogens, such as the rickettsiae causing Rocky Mountain spotted fever, replicate in endothelial cells and damage them. Vascular purpura may occur in patients with polyclonal gammopathies but more commonly in those with monoclonal gammopathies, including Waldenstrom's macroglobulinemia, multiple myeloma, and cryoglobulinemia. Patients with mixed cryoglobulinemia develop a more extensive maculopapular rash due to immune complex-mediated damage to the vessel wall.

Patients with scurvy (vitamin C deficiency) develop painful episodes of perifollicular skin bleeding as well as more systemic bleeding symptoms. Vitamin C is needed to synthesize hydroxyproline, an essential constituent of collagen. Patients with Cushing's syndrome or on chronic glucocorticoid therapy develop skin bleeding and easy bruising due to atrophy of supporting connective tissue. A similar phenomena is seen with aging, where, following minor trauma, blood spreads superficially under the epidermis. This has been termed *senile purpura*, and it is most common on skin that has been previously damaged by sun exposure.

Henoch-Schönlein, or anaphylactoid, purpura is a distinct, self-limited type of vasculitis that occurs in children and young adults. Patients have an acute inflammatory reaction with IgA and complement components in capillaries, mesangial tissues, and small arterioles, leading to increased vascular permeability and localized hemorrhage. The syndrome is often preceded by an upper respiratory infection, commonly with streptococcal pharyngitis, or is triggered by drug or food allergies. Patients develop a purpuric rash on the extensor surfaces of the arms and legs, usually accompanied by polyarthralgias or arthritis, abdominal pain, and hematuria from focal glomerulonephritis. All coagulation tests are normal, but renal impairment may occur. Glucocorticoids can provide symptomatic relief but do not alter the course of the illness.

INHERITED DISORDERS OF THE VESSEL WALL

Patients with inherited disorders of the connective tissue matrix, such as Marfan's syndrome, Ehlers-Danlos syndrome, and pseudoxanthoma elasticum, frequently report easy bruising. Inherited vascular abnormalities can result in increased bleeding. This is notably seen in hereditary hemorrhagic telangiectasia (HHT, or Osler-Weber-Rendu disease), a disorder where abnormal telangiectatic capillaries result in frequent bleeding episodes, primarily from the nose and gastrointestinal tract. Arteriovenous malformation (AVM) in the lung, brain, and liver may also occur in HHT. The telangiectasia can often be visualized on the oral and nasal mucosa. Two genes involved in the pathogenesis are *eng* (endoglin) on chromosome 9q33-34 (so-called HHT type 1), associated with pulmonary AVM in 40% of cases; and *alk1* (activin-receptor-like kinase 1) on chromosome 12q13, associated with a much lower risk of pulmonary AVM.

ACKNOWLEDGMENT
Robert Handin, MD, contributed this chapter in HPIM, 16e, and some materials from his chapter are included here.

FURTHER READINGS

AREPALLY GM, ORTEL TL: Clinical practice. Heparin-induced thrombocytopenia. N Engl J Med 355:809, 2006

ARMSTRONG E, KONKLE BA: Von Willebrand Disease, in *Clinical Hematology*, 1st ed, NS Young et al (eds). Philadelphia, Mosby Elsevier, 2006, pp 830–841

CINES DB, MCMILLAN R: Management of adult idiopathic thrombocytopenic purpura. Annu Rev Med 56:425, 2005

GEORGE JN: Clinical practice. Thrombotic thrombocytopenic purpura. N Engl J Med 354:1927, 2006

RAO AK et al: Inherited defects in platelet signaling mechanisms. Semin Thromb Hemostas 30:525, 2004

SADLER JE: New concepts in von Willebrand disease. Annu Rev Med 56:173, 2005

WARKENTIN TE: Heparin-induced thrombocytopenia. Disease-A-Month 51:141, 2005

110 Coagulation Disorders
Valder Arruda, Katherine A. High

Deficiencies of coagulation factors have been recognized for centuries. Patients with genetic deficiencies of plasma coagulation factors exhibit lifelong recurrent bleeding episodes into joints, muscles, and closed spaces, either spontaneously or following an injury. The most common inherited factor deficiencies are the hemophilias, X-linked diseases caused by deficiency of Factor (F) VIII (hemophilia A) or Factor IX (FIX, hemophilia B). Rare congenital bleeding disorders due to deficiencies of other factors, including FII (prothrombin), FV, FVII, FX, FXI, FXIII, and fibrinogen are usually inherited in an autosomal recessive manner (Table 110-1). Advances in characterization of the molecular bases of clotting factor deficiencies have contributed to a better understanding of the disease phenotypes and may allow more targeted therapeutic approaches through the development of small molecules, recombinant proteins, or cell and gene-based therapies.

Commonly used tests of hemostasis provide the initial screening for clotting factor activity (Fig. 110-1), and disease phenotype often correlates with the level of clotting activity. An isolated abnormal prothrombin time (PT) suggests FVII deficiency, whereas a prolonged activated partial thromboplastin time (aPTT) indicates most commonly hemophilia or FXI deficiency (Fig. 110-1). The prolongation of both PT and aPTT suggests deficiency of FV, FX, FII, or fibrinogen abnormalities. The addition of the missing factor to the subject's plasma at a range of doses will correct the abnormal clotting times; the result is expressed as percent of the activity observed in normal subjects.

Acquired deficiencies of plasma coagulation are more frequent than congenital disorders; the most common disorders include hemorrhagic diathesis of liver disease, disseminated intravascular coagulation (DIC), and vitamin K deficiency. In these disorders, blood coagulation is hampered by the deficiency of more than one clotting factor, and the bleeding episodes result from perturbation of both primary (e.g., platelet and vessel wall interactions) and secondary (coagulation) hemostasis.

TABLE 110-1 GENETIC AND LABORATORY CHARACTERISTICS OF INHERITED COAGULATION DISORDERS

Clotting Factor Deficiency	Inheritance	Prevalence in General Population	Laboratory Abnormality[a]			Minimum Hemostatic Levels	Treatment	Plasma Half-Life
			aPTT	PT	TT			
Fibrinogen	AR	1 in 1,000,000	+	+	+	100 mg/dL	Cryoprecipitate	2–4 d
Prothrombin	AR	1 in 2,000,000	+	+	–	20–30%	FFP/PCCs	3–4 d
Factor V	AR	1 in 1,000,000	+/–	+/–	–	15–20%	FFP	36 h
Factor VII	AR	1 in 500,000	–	+	–	15–20%	FFP/PCCs	4–6 h
Factor VIII	X-linked	1 in 5,000	+	–	–	30%	FVIII concentrates	8–12 h
Factor IX	X-linked	1 in 30,000	+	–	–	30%	FIX concentrates	18–24 h
Factor X	AR	1 in 1,000,000	+/–	+/–	–	15–20%	FFP/PCCs	40–60 h
Factor XI	AR	1 in 1,000,000	+	–	–	15–20%	FFP	40–70 h
Factor XII	AR	ND	+	–	–	[b]	[b]	60 h
HK	AR	ND	+	–	–	[b]	[b]	150 h
Prekallikrein	AR	ND	+	–	–	[b]	[b]	35 h
Factor XIII	AR	1 in 2,000,000	–	–	+/–	2–5%	Cryoprecipitate	11–14 d

[a]Values within normal range (–) or prolonged (+).
[b]No risk for bleeding, treatment is not indicated.
Abbreviations: HK, high-molecular weight kininogen; AR, autosomal recessive; aPTT, activated partial thromboplastin time; PT, prothrombin time; TT, thrombin time; ND, not determined; FFP, fresh frozen plasma; PCCs, prothrombin complex concentrates.

FIGURE 110-1 Coagulation cascade and laboratory assessment of clotting factor deficiency by activated partial prothrombin time (aPTT), prothrombin time (PT), and thrombin time (TT).

The development of antibodies to coagulation plasma proteins, clinically termed *inhibitors*, is a relatively rare problem that most often affects hemophilia A or B and FXI-deficient patients who receive repeated doses of the missing protein to control bleeding episodes. Inhibitors also occur among subjects without genetic deficiency of clotting factors—for example, in the postpartum setting, as a manifestation of underlying autoimmune or neoplastic disease, or idiopathically. Rare cases of inhibitors to thrombin or FV have been reported in patients receiving topical bovine thrombin preparation as a local hemostatic agent in complex surgeries. The diagnosis of inhibitors is based on the same tests as those used to diagnose inherited plasma coagulation factor deficiencies. However, the addition of the missing protein to the plasma of a subject with an inhibitor does not correct the abnormal aPTT and/or PT tests. This is the major laboratory difference between deficiencies and inhibitors. Additional tests are required to measure the specificity of the inhibitor and its titer.

The treatment of these bleeding disorders often requires replacement of the deficient protein using recombinant or purified plasma-derived products or fresh frozen plasma. Therefore, it is imperative to arrive at a proper diagnosis to optimize patient care without unnecessary exposure to the risks of bloodborne disease.

HEMOPHILIA

PATHOGENESIS AND CLINICAL MANIFESTATIONS

Hemophilia is an X-linked recessive hemorrhagic disease due to mutations in the *F8* gene (hemophilia A or classic hemophilia) or *F9* gene (hemophilia B). The disease affects 1 in 10,000 males worldwide, in all ethnic groups; hemophilia A represents 80% of all cases. Male subjects are clinically affected; women, who carry a single mutated gene, are generally asymptomatic. Family history of the disease is absent in approximately 30% of cases. In these cases, 80% of the mothers are carriers of the de novo mutated allele. More than 500 different mutations have been identified in the *F8* or *F9* genes. One of the most common hemophilia A mutations results from an inversion of the intron 22 sequence, which is present in 40% of cases of severe hemophilia A. Advances in molecular diagnosis now permit precise identification of mutations, allowing accurate diagnosis of women carriers of the hemophilia gene in affected families.

Clinically, hemophilia A and hemophilia B are indistinguishable. The disease phenotype correlates with the residual activity of FVIII or FIX and can be classified as severe (< 1%), moderate (1–5%), or mild (6–30%). In the severe and moderate forms, the disease is characterized by bleeding episodes into the joints (hemarthroses), soft tissues, and muscles after minor trauma or even spontaneously. Patients with mild disease experience infrequent bleeding that is usually secondary to trauma. Among those with residual FVIII or FIX activity >25% of normal, the disease is discovered only by bleeding after major trauma or during routine presurgery laboratory tests. Typically, the global tests of coagulation show only an isolated prolongation of the aPTT assay. Patients with hemophilia have normal bleeding times and platelet counts. The diagnosis is made after specific determination of FVIII or FIX clotting activity.

Early in life, bleeding may present after circumcision or rarely as intracranial hemorrhages. The disease is more evident when children begin to walk or crawl. In the severe form, the most common bleeding manifestations are the recurrent hemarthroses, which can affect every joint but mainly affect knees, elbows, ankles, shoulders, and hips. Acute hemarthroses are painful, and clinical signs are local swelling and erythema. To avoid pain, the patient may adopt a fixed position, which leads eventually to muscle contractures. Very young children unable to communicate verbally show irritability and a lack of movement of the affected joint. Chronic hemarthroses are debilitating, with synovial thickening and synovitis in response to the intraarticular blood. After a joint has been damaged, recurrent bleeding episodes result in the clinically recognized "target joint," which then establishes a vicious cycle of bleeding, resulting in progressive joint deformity that in critical cases requires surgery as the only therapeutic option. Hematomas into the muscle of distal parts of the limbs may lead to external compression of arteries, veins, or nerves, which can evolve to a compartment syndrome.

Bleeding into the oropharyngeal spaces, central nervous system, or the retroperitoneum is life-threatening and requires immediate therapy. Retroperitoneal hemorrhages can accumulate large quantities of blood along with formation of masses with calcification and inflammatory tissue reaction (pseudotumor syndrome), and they can also result in damage to the femoral nerve. Pseudotumors can also form in bones, especially long bones of the lower limbs. Hematuria is frequent among hemophilia patients, even in the absence of genitourinary pathology. It is often self-limited and may not require specific therapy.

℞ HEMOPHILIA

Without treatment, patients with severe hemophilia have a limited life expectancy. Advances in the blood fractionation industry during World War II resulted in the realization that plasma could be used to treat hemophilia, but the volumes required to achieve even modest elevation of circulating factor levels limits the utility of plasma infusion as an approach to disease management. The discovery in the 1960s that cryoprecipitate fraction of plasma was enriched for FVIII, in addition to the eventual purification of FVIII and FIX from plasma, led to the introduction of home infusion therapy with factor concentrates in the 1970s. The availability of factor concentrates resulted in a dramatic improvement in life expectancy and in quality of life for people with severe hemophilia. However, the contamination of the blood supply with hepatitis viruses and, subsequently, HIV resulted in widespread transmission of these bloodborne infections within the hemophilia population; complications of HIV and of hepatitis C are now the leading causes of death among US adults with severe hemophilia. The introduction of viral inactivation steps in the preparation of plasma-derived products in the mid-1980s greatly reduced the risk of HIV and hepatitis, and the risks were further reduced by the successful production of recombinant FVIII and FIX proteins, both licensed in the 1990s. It is uncommon for hemophilic patients born after 1985 to have contracted either hepatitis or HIV, and for these individuals, life expectancy is in the range of 65 years of age.

Factor replacement therapy for hemophilia can be provided either in response to a bleeding episode or as a prophylactic treatment. Primary prophylaxis is defined as a strategy for maintaining the missing clotting factor at levels ~1% or higher on a regular basis in order to prevent bleeds, especially the onset of hemarthroses. Hemophilic boys receiving regular infusions of FVIII (3 days/week) or FIX (2 days/week) can reach puberty without detectable joint abnormalities. Although highly recommended, this regimen is performed for <30% of patients because of the high cost, difficulties in accessing peripheral veins in young patients, and the potential infectious and thrombotic risks of long-term central vein catheters.

General considerations regarding the treatment of bleeds in hemophilia include (1) the need to begin the treatment as soon as possible because symptoms often precede objective evidence of bleeding; because of the superior efficacy of early therapeutic intervention, classic symptoms of bleeding into the joint in a reliable patient, headaches, or automobile or other accidents, require prompt replacement and further laboratory investigation; and (2) the need to avoid drugs that hamper platelet function such as aspirin or aspirin-containing drugs; to control pain, drugs such as ibuprofen or propoxyphene are preferred.

Factor VIII and Factor IX are dosed in units. One unit is by definition the amount of FVIII (100 ng/mL) or FIX (5 μg/mL) in 1 mL of normal plasma. One unit of FVIII per kilogram of body weight increases the plasma FVIII level by 2%. One can calculate the dose needed to increase FVIII levels to 100% in a 70-kg severe hemophilia patient (<1%) using the simple formula below. Thus, 3500 units of FVIII will raise the circulating level to 100%.

$$\text{FVIII dose (IU)} = \text{Target FVIII levels} - \text{FVIII baseline levels} \times \text{body weight (kg)} \times 0.5 \text{ unit/kg}$$

The doses for FIX replacement are different from those for FVIII, because FIX recovery postinfusion is usually only 50% of the predicted value. Therefore, the formula for FIX replacement is

$$\text{FIX dose (IU)} = \text{Target FIX levels} - \text{FIX baseline levels} \times \text{body weight (kg)} \times 1.0 \text{ unit/kg}$$

The FVIII half-life of 8–12 h requires injections twice a day to maintain therapeutic levels, whereas the FIX half-life is longer, ~24 h, so that once-a-day injection is sufficient. In specific situations such as postsurgery, continuous infusion of factor may be desirable because of its safety in achieving sustained factor levels at a lower total cost.

Cryoprecipitate is enriched with FVIII protein (each bag contains ~80 IU of FVIII) and was commonly used for the treatment of hemophilia A decades ago; it is still in use in some developing countries, but because of the risk of bloodborne diseases, this product should be avoided in hemophilia patients when factor concentrates are available.

Mild bleeds such as uncomplicated hemarthroses or superficial hematomas require initial therapy with factor levels of 30–50%. Additional doses to maintain levels of 15–25% for 2 or 3 days are indicated for severe hemarthroses, especially when these episodes affect the "target joint." Large hematomas, or bleeds into deep muscles, require factor levels of 50% or even higher if the clinical symptoms do not improve, and factor replacement may be required for a period of 1 week or longer. The control of serious bleeds, including those that affect the oropharyngeal spaces, central nervous system, and the retroperitoneum, require sustained protein levels of 50–100% for 7–10 days. Prophylactic replacement for surgery is aimed at achieving normal factor levels (100%) for a period of 7–10 days; replacement can then be tapered depending on the extent of the surgical wounds. Oral surgery is associated with extensive tissue damage, which usually requires factor replacement for 1–3 days coupled with oral antifibrinolytic drugs.

NON-TRANSFUSION THERAPY IN HEMOPHILIA   DDAVP (1-deamino-8-D-arginine vasopressin)   DDAVP is a synthetic vasopressin analogue that causes a transient rise in FVIII and von Willebrand factor (vWF), but not FIX, through a mechanism involving release from endothelial cells. Patients with moderate or mild hemophilia A should be tested to determine if they respond to DDAVP before a therapeutic application. DDAVP at doses of 0.3 μg/kg body weight infused over a 20-min period is expected to raise FVIII levels by two- to threefold over baseline, peaking between 30–60 min postinfusion. DDAVP does not improve FVIII levels in severe hemophilia A patients, as there are no stores to release. Repeated dosing of DDAVP results in tachyphylaxis because the mechanism is an increase in release rather than de novo synthesis of FVIII and vWF. More than three consecutive doses become ineffective and if further therapy is indicated, FVIII replacement is required to achieve hemostasis.

Antifibrinolytic Drugs   Bleeding in the gums, in the gastrointestinal tract, and during oral surgery requires the use of oral antifibrinolytic drugs such as ε-aminocaproic acid (EACA) or tranexamic acid to control local hemostasis. The duration of the treatment depending on the clinical indication is 1 week or longer. Tranexamic acid is given at doses of 25 mg/kg three to four times a day. EACA treatment requires a loading dose of 200 mg/kg (maximum of 10 g) followed by 100 mg/kg (maximum 30 g/d) every 6 h. These drugs are not indicated to control hematuria because of the risk of formation of an occlusive clot in the lumen of genitourinary tract structures.

COMPLICATIONS   Inhibitor Formation   The formation of alloantibodies to FVIII or FIX is currently the major complication of hemophilia treatment. The prevalence of inhibitors to FVIII is estimated at 5–10% of all cases and approximately 20% of severe hemophilia A patients. Inhibitors to FIX are detected in only 3–5% of all hemophilia B patients. The high-risk group for inhibitor formation includes severe deficiency (>80% of all cases of inhibitors), familial history of inhibitors, African descent, mutations in the FVIII or FIX gene resulting in deletion of large coding regions, or gross gene rearrangements. Inhibitors usually appear early in life, at a median of two years of age, and after 10 cumulative days of exposure.

The clinical diagnosis of inhibitor is suspected when patients do not respond to factor replacement at therapeutic doses. Inhibitors increase both morbidity and mortality in hemophilia. Because early detection of an inhibitor is critical to a successful correction of the bleeding or to eradication of the antibody, most hemophilia centers perform annual screening for inhibitors. The laboratory test required to confirm the presence of an inhibitor is an aPTT mixed with normal plasma. In most hemophilia patients, a 1:1 mix with normal plasma completely corrects the aPTT. In inhibitor patients, the aPTT on a 1:1 mix is abnormally prolonged, because the inhibitor neutralizes the FVIII clotting activity of the normal plasma. The Bethesda assay uses a similar principle and defines the specificity of the inhibitor and its titer. The results are expressed in Bethesda units (BU), in which 1 BU is the amount of antibody that neutralizes 50% of the FVIII or FIX present in normal plasma after 2 h of incubation at 37°C. Clinically, inhibitor patients are classified as low responders or high responders, which provides guidelines for optimal therapy. Therapy for inhibitor patients has two goals: the control of acute bleeding episodes and the eradication of the inhibitor. For the control of bleeding episodes, low responders, those with titers <5 BU, respond well to high doses of human or porcine FVIII (50–100 U/kg) with minimal or no increase in the inhibitor titers. However, high-responder patients—those with initial inhibitor titer >10 BU or an anamnestic response in the antibody titer to >10 BU even if low titer initially—do not respond to FVIII or FIX concentrates. The control of bleeding episodes in high-responder patients can be achieved by using concentrates enriched for prothrombin, FVII, FIX, FX [prothrombin complex concentrates (PCCs) or activated PCCs], and more recently by recombinant activated Factor VII (FVIIa) (Fig. 110-1). The rates of therapeutic success have been higher for FVIIa than for PCC or aPCC. For eradication of the inhibitory antibody, immunosuppression is not effective. The most effective strategy is immune tolerance induction (ITI) based on daily infusion of the missing protein until the inhibitor disappears, typically requiring periods longer than one year, with success rates in the range of 60%. Promising results have been obtained by adding anti-CD20 monoclonal antibody (rituximab) as a coadjuvant for the eradication of high levels of antibody in patients undergoing ITI.

Infectious Diseases   Hepatitis C virus (HCV) infection is the major cause of morbidity and the second leading cause of death in hemophilia patients exposed to older clotting factor concentrates. The vast majority of young patients treated with plasma-derived products from 1970 to 1985 became infected with HCV. It has been estimated that >80% of patients older than 20 years of age are HCV antibody positive as of 2006. The comorbidity of the underlying liver disease in hemophilia patients is clear when these individuals require invasive procedures; correction of both genetic and acquired (secondary to liver disease) deficiencies may be needed. Infection with HIV also swept the population of patients treated with plasma-derived concentrates two decades ago. Co-infection of HCV and HIV, present in almost 50% of hemophilia patients, is an aggravating factor for the evolution of liver disease. The response to HCV antiviral therapy in hemophilia is restricted to <30% of patients and is even poorer among those with both HCV and HIV infection. End-stage liver disease requiring organ transplantation may be curative for both the liver disease and for hemophilia.

Factor XI is a zymogen of an active serine protease (FXIa) in the intrinsic pathway of blood coagulation that activates FIX (Fig. 110-1). There are two pathways for the formation of FXIa. In an aPTT-based assay, the protease is the result of activation by FXIIa in conjunction with high-molecular-weight kininogen and kallikrein. Thrombin appears to be the physiologic activator of FXI. The generation of thrombin by the tissue-factor/Factor VIIa pathway activates FXI on the platelet surface, which contributes to additional thrombin generation after the clot has formed and thus augments resistance to fibrinolysis through a thrombin-activated fibrinolytic inhibitor (TAFI).

Factor XI deficiency is a rare bleeding disorder that occurs in the general population at a frequency of one in a million. However, the disease is highly prevalent among Ashkenazi and Iraqi Jewish populations, reaching a frequency of 6% as heterozygotes and 0.1–0.3% as homozygotes. More than 65 mutations in the *FXI* gene have been reported, whereas two to three mutations are found among affected Jewish populations.

Normal FXI clotting activity levels range from 70 to 150 U/dL. In heterozygous patients with moderate deficiency, FXI ranges from 20 to 70 U/dL, whereas in homozygous or double heterozygote patients, FXI levels are <1–20 U/dL. Patients with FXI levels <10% of normal have a high risk of bleeding, but the disease phenotype does not always correlate with residual FXI clotting activity. A family history is indicative of the risk of bleeding in the propositus. Clinically, the presence of mucocutaneous hemorrhages such as bruises, gum bleeding, epistaxis, hematuria, and menorrhagia are common, especially following trauma. This hemorrhagic phenotype suggests that tissues rich in fibrinolytic activity are more susceptible to FXI deficiency. Postoperative bleeding is common but not always present, even among patients with very low FXI levels.

℞ FACTOR XI DEFICIENCY

The treatment of FXI deficiency is based on the infusion of FFP at doses of 15–20 mL/kg to maintain trough levels ranging from 10 to 20%. Because FXI has a half-life of 40–70 h, the replacement therapy can be given on alternate days. The use of antifibrinolytic drugs is beneficial to control bleeds, with the exception of hematuria or bleeds in the bladder. The development of a FXI inhibitor was observed in 10% of severely FXI-deficient patients who received replacement therapy.

OTHER RARE BLEEDING DISORDERS

Collectively, the inherited disorders resulting from deficiencies of clotting factors other than FVIII, FIX, and FXI (Table 110-1) represent a group of rare bleeding diseases. The bleeding symptoms in these patients vary from asymptomatic (dysfibrinogenemia or FVII deficiency) to life-threatening (FX or FXIII deficiency). There is no pathognomonic clinical manifestation that suggests one specific disease, but overall, in contrast to hemophilia, hemarthrosis is a rare event, and bleeding in the mucosal tract or after umbilical cord clamping is common. Individuals heterozygous for plasma coagulation deficiencies are often asymptomatic. The laboratory assessment for the specific deficient factor following screening with general coagulation tests (Table 110-1) will establish the diagnosis.

Replacement therapy using fresh frozen plasma (FFP) or PCCs (containing prothrombin, FVII, FIX and FX) provides adequate hemostasis in response to bleeds or as prophylactic treatment. The use of PCCs should be carefully monitored and avoided in patients with underlying liver disease or those at high risk for thrombosis because of the risk of DIC.

FAMILIAL MULTIPLE COAGULATION DEFICIENCIES

Several bleeding disorders are characterized by the inherited deficiency of more than one plasma coagulation factor. To date, the genetic defects in two of these diseases have been characterized, and they provide new insights into the regulation of hemostasis by genes encoding proteins outside blood coagulation.

Combined Deficiency of FV and FVII Patients with combined FV and FVIII deficiency exhibit ~5% of residual clotting activity of each factor. Interestingly, the disease phenotype is a mild bleeding tendency, often following trauma. An underlying mutation has been identified in the endoplasmic reticulum/Golgi intermediate compartment (ERGIC-53) gene, a mannose-binding protein localized in the Golgi apparatus that functions as a chaperone for both FV and FVIII. In other families, mutations in the multiple coagulation factor deficiency 2 (MCFD2) gene have been defined; this gene encodes a protein that forms a Ca²⁺-dependent complex with ERGIC-53 and provides cofactor activity in the intracellular mobilization of both FV and FVIII.

Multiple Deficiencies of Vitamin K–Dependent Coagulation Factors Two enzymes involved in vitamin K metabolism have been associated with combined deficiency of all vitamin K–dependent proteins, including the procoagulant proteins prothrombin, VII, IX, and X and the anticoagulants protein C and protein S. Vitamin K is a fat-soluble vitamin that is a cofactor for carboxylation of the gamma carbon of the glutamic acid residues in the vitamin K dependent–factors, a critical step for calcium and phospholipid binding of these proteins (**Fig. 110-2**). The enzymes γ-glutamylcarboxylase and epoxide reductase are critical for the metabolism and regeneration of vitamin K. Mutations in the genes encoding the gamma-carboxylase (GGCX) or vitamin K epoxide reductase complex 1 (VKORC1) result in defective enzymes and thus in vitamin K–dependent factors with reduced activity, varying from 1 to 30% of normal. The disease phenotype is characterized by mild to severe bleeding episodes present from birth. Some patients respond to high doses of vitamin K. For severe bleeding, replacement therapy with FFP or PCCs may be necessary for achieving full hemostatic control.

DISSEMINATED INTRAVASCULAR COAGULATION

DIC is a clinicopathologic syndrome characterized by widespread intravascular fibrin formation in response to excessive blood protease activity that overcomes the natural anticoagulant mechanisms. DIC is associated with several underlying pathologies (**Table 110-2**). The most common causes are bacterial sepsis, malignant disorders such as solid tumors or acute promyelocytic leukemia (APL), and obstetric causes. DIC is diagnosed in almost half of pregnant women with abruptio placentae or with amniotic fluid embolism. Trauma, particularly to the brain, can also result in DIC. The exposure of blood to phospholipids from damaged tissue, hemolysis, and endothelial damage are all contributing factors to the development of DIC in this setting. Purpura fulminans is a severe form of DIC resulting from thrombosis of extensive areas of the skin; it affects predominantly young children following viral or bacterial infection, particularly those

FIGURE 110-2 The vitamin K cycle. Vitamin K is a cofactor for the formation of γ-carboxyglutamic acid residues on coagulation proteins. Vitamin K–dependent γ-glutamylcarboxylase, the enzyme that catalyzes the vitamin K epoxide reductase, regenerates reduced vitamin K. Warfarin blocks the action of the reductase and competitively inhibits the effects of vitamin K.

TABLE 110-2 COMMON CLINICAL CAUSES OF DISSEMINATED INTRAVASCULAR COAGULATION

Sepsis
  Bacterial
  Staphylococci, streptococci,
    pneumococci, meningo-
    cocci, gram-negative bacilli
  Viral
  Mycotic
  Parasitic
  Rickettsial
Trauma and tissue injury
  Brain injury (gunshot)
  Extensive burns
  Fat embolism
  Rhabdomyolysis

Vascular disorders
  Giant hemangiomas (Kasabach-
    Merrit syndrome)
  Large vessel aneurysms
    (e.g., aorta)
Obstetric complications
  Abruptio placentae
  Amniotic fluid embolism
  Dead fetus syndrome
  Septic abortion
Cancer
  Adenocarcinoma (prostate,
    pancreas, etc)
  Hematologic malignancies (acute
    promyelocytic leukemia)

Immunologic disorders
  Acute hemolytic transfusion
    reaction
  Organ or tissue transplant rejection
  Graft-versus-host disease

Drugs
  Fibrinolytic agents
  Aprotinin
  Warfarin (especially in neonates
    with protein C deficiency)
  Prothrombin complex
    concentrates
  Recreational drugs (amphetamines)
Envenomation
  Snake
  Insects

Liver disease
  Fulminant hepatic failure
  Cirrhosis
  Fatty liver of pregnancy

Miscellaneous
  Shock
  Respiratory distress syndrome
  Massive transfusion

with inherited or acquired hypercoagulability due to deficiencies of the components of the protein C pathway. Neonates homozygous for protein C deficiency also present high risk for purpura fulminans, with or without thrombosis of large vessels.

The central mechanism of DIC is the uncontrolled generation of thrombin by exposure of the blood to pathologic levels of tissue factor (Fig. 110-3). Simultaneous suppression of physiologic anticoagulant mechanisms and abnormal fibrinolysis further accelerate the process. Together these abnormalities contribute to systemic fibrin deposition in small and mid-sized vessels. The duration and intensity of the fibrin deposition can compromise the blood supply of many organs, especially the lung, kidney, liver, and brain, with consequent organ failure. The sustained activation of coagulation results in consumption of clotting factors and platelets, which in turn leads to systemic bleeding. This is further aggravated by secondary hyperfibrinolysis. Studies in animals demonstrate that the fibrinolytic system is indeed suppressed at the time of maximal activation of coagulation. Interestingly, in patients with APL, a severe hyperfibrinolytic state often occurs in addition to the coagulation activation. The release of several proinflammatory cytokines such as interleukin 6 and tumor necrosis factor α play central roles in mediating the coagulation defects in DIC and symptoms associated with systemic inflammatory response syndrome.

Clinical manifestations of DIC are related to the magnitude of the imbalance of hemostasis, to the underlying disease, or to both. The most common findings are bleeding ranging from oozing from venipuncture sites, petechiae, and ecchymoses to severe hemorrhage from the gastrointestinal tract or lung or into the central nervous system. In chronic DIC the bleeding symptoms are discreet and restricted to skin or mucosal surfaces. The hypercoagulability of DIC manifests as the occlusion of vessels in the microcirculation and resulting organ failure. Thrombosis of large vessels and cerebral embolism can also occur. Hemodynamic complications and shock are common among patients with acute DIC. The mortality ranges from 30 to >80% depending on the underlying disease, the severity of the DIC, and the age of the patient.

The diagnosis of clinically significant DIC is based on the presence of clinical and/or laboratory abnormalities of coagulation or thrombocytopenia. The laboratory diagnosis of DIC should prompt a search for the underlying disease if it is not already apparent. No single test establishes the diagnosis of DIC. The laboratory investigation should include coagulation tests [aPTT, PT, thrombin time (TT)] and markers of fibrin degradation products (FDP), in addition to platelet and red cell count and analysis of the blood smear. These tests should be repeated over a period of 6–8 h because an initially mild abnormality can changed dramatically in patients with severe DIC.

Common findings include the prolongation of PT and/or aPTT; platelet counts ≤ 100,000/mm³, or a rapid decline in platelet numbers; the presence of schistocytes (fragmented red cells) in the blood smear; and elevated levels of FDP. The most sensitive test for DIC is the FDP level. DIC is an unlikely diagnosis in the presence of normal levels of FDP. The D-dimer test is more specific for detection of fibrin (but not fibrinogen) degradation products and indicates that the cross-linked fibrin has been digested by plasmin. Because fibrinogen has a prolonged half-life, plasma levels diminish acutely only in severe cases of DIC. High-grade DIC is also associated with levels of antithrombin III or plasminogen activity <60% of normal.

Chronic DIC Low-grade, compensated DIC can occur in certain clinical situations, including giant hemangioma, metastatic carcinoma, or the dead fetus syndrome. Plasma levels of FDP or D-dimers are elevated. aPTT, PT, and fibrinogen values are within the normal range or high. Mild thrombocytopenia or normal platelet counts are also common findings. Red cell fragmentation is often detected but at a lower degree than in acute DIC.

Differential Diagnosis The differential diagnosis between DIC and severe liver disease is challenging and requires serial measurements of the laboratory parameters of DIC. Patients with severe liver disease are at risk for bleeding and manifest laboratory features including thrombocytopenia (due to platelet sequestration, portal hypertension, or hypersplenism), decreased synthesis of coagulation factors and natural anticoagulants, and elevated levels of FDP due to reduced hepatic clearance. However, in contrast to DIC, these laboratory parameters in liver disease do not change rapidly. Other important differential findings include the presence of portal hypertension or other clinical or laboratory evidence of underlying liver disease.

Microangiopathic disorders such as thrombotic thrombocytopenic purpura present an acute clinical onset of illness accompanied by throm-

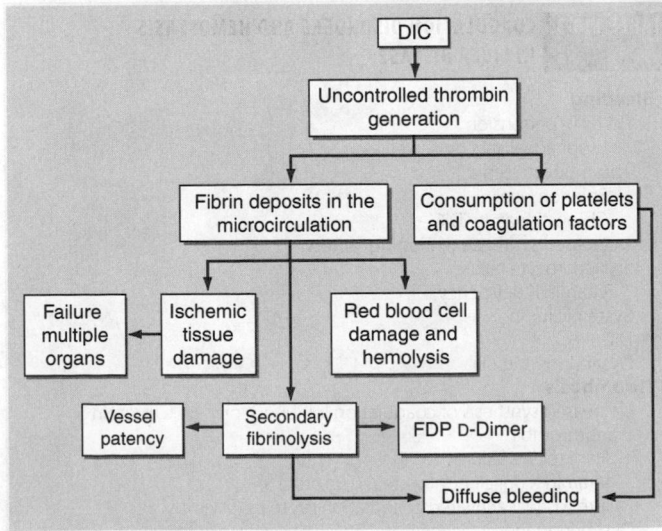

FIGURE 110-3 The pathophysiology of disseminated intravascular coagulation (DIC). Interactions between coagulation and fibrinolytic pathways result in bleeding and thrombosis in the microcirculation in patients with DIC.

bocytopenia, red cell fragmentation, and multiorgan failure. There is, however, no consumption of clotting factors or hyperfibrinolysis.

℞ DISSEMINATED INTRAVASCULAR COAGULATION

The morbidity and mortality associated with DIC are primarily related to the underlying disease rather than the complications of the DIC. The control or elimination of the underlying cause should therefore be the primary concern. Patients with severe DIC require control of hemodynamic parameters, respiratory support, and sometimes invasive surgical procedures. Attempts to treat DIC without accompanying treatment of the causative disease are likely to fail.

MANAGEMENT OF HEMORRHAGIC SYMPTOMS The control of bleeding in DIC patients with marked thrombocytopenia (platelet counts <10,000–20,000/mm³) and low levels of coagulation factors will require replacement therapy. The PT (>1.5 × normal) provides a good indicator of the severity of the clotting factor consumption. Replacement with FFP is indicated (1 unit of FFP increases most coagulation factors by 3% in an adult without DIC). Low levels of fibrinogen (<100 mg/dL) or brisk hyperfibrinolysis will require infusion of cryoprecipitate (plasma fraction enriched for fibrinogen, FVIII, and vWF). The replacement of 10 U of cryoprecipitate for every 2–3 U of FFP is sufficient to correct the hemostasis. The transfusion scheme must be adjusted according to the patient's clinical and laboratory evolution. Platelet concentrates at a dose of 1–2 U/10 kg body weight are sufficient for most DIC patients with severe thrombocytopenia.

Clotting factor concentrates are not recommended for control of bleeding in DIC because of the limited efficacy afforded by replacement of single factors (factor VIII or IX concentrates) and the high risk of products containing traces of activated blood proteases (PCCs), which further aggravates the disease.

REPLACEMENT OF COAGULATION OR FIBRINOLYSIS INHIBITORS Drugs to control coagulation such as heparin, antithrombin III (ATIII) concentrates, or antifibrinolytic drugs have all been tried in the treatment of DIC. Low doses of continuous infusion heparin (5–10 U/kg per h) may be effective in patients with low-grade DIC associated with solid tumor or APL or in a setting with recognized thrombosis. Heparin is also indicated for the treatment of purpura fulminans, during the surgical resection of giant hemangiomas, and during removal of a dead fetus. In acute DIC, the use of heparin is likely to aggravate bleeding. To date, the use of heparin in severe DIC patients is of no proven survival benefit.

The use of antifibrinolytic drugs, EACA, or tranexamic acid to prevent fibrin degradation by plasmin may reduce bleeding episodes in patients with DIC and confirmed hyperfibrinolysis. However, these drugs can increase the risk of thrombosis, and concomitant use of heparin is indicated. Patients with APL or those with chronic DIC associated with giant hemangiomas are among the few patients who may benefit from this therapy.

The use of protein C concentrates to treat purpura fulminans associated with acquired protein C deficiency or meningococcemia has been proved effective. The results from the replacement of ATIII in early phase studies are promising but require further study.

VITAMIN K DEFICIENCY

Vitamin K–dependent proteins are a heterogenous group, including clotting factor proteins and also proteins found in bone, lung, kidney, and placenta. Vitamin K mediates posttranslational modification of glutamate residues to γ-carboxylglutamate, a critical step for the activity of vitamin K–dependent proteins for calcium binding and proper assembly to phospholipid membranes (Fig. 110-2). Inherited deficiency of the functional activity of the enzymes involved in vitamin K metabolism, notably the GGCX or VKOR-1 (see above), results in bleeding disorders. The amount of vitamin K in the diet is often limiting for the carboxylation reaction, and thus recycling of the vitamin K is essential to maintain normal levels of vitamin K–dependent proteins. In adults, low dietary intake alone is seldom reason for severe vitamin K deficiency but may become common in association with the use of broad-spectrum antibiotics. Disease or surgical interventions

that affect the ability of the intestinal tract to absorb vitamin K, either through anatomic alterations or by changing the fat content of bile salts and pancreatic juices in the proximal small bowel, can result in significant reduction of vitamin K levels. Chronic liver diseases such as primary biliary cirrhosis also deplete vitamin K stores. Neonatal vitamin K deficiency and the resulting hemorrhagic disease of the newborn have been almost entirely eliminated by routine administration of vitamin K to all neonates. Prolongation of PT values is the most common and earliest finding in vitamin K–deficient patients due to reduction in prothrombin, FVII, FIX, and FX levels. FVII has the shortest half-life among these factors, which can prolong the PT before changes in the aPTT. Parenteral administration of vitamin K at a total dose of 10 mg is sufficient to restore normal levels of clotting factor within 8–10 h. In the presence of ongoing bleeding or a need for immediate correction before an invasive procedure, replacement with FFP or PCC is required. PCC should be avoided in patients with severe underlying liver disorders due to high risk of thrombosis. The reversal of excessive anticoagulant therapy with warfarin or warfarin-like drugs can be achieved by minimal doses of vitamin K (1 mg orally or by intravenous injection) for asymptomatic patients. This strategy can diminish the risk of bleeding while maintaining therapeutic anticoagulation for an underlying prothrombotic state.

COAGULATION DISORDERS ASSOCIATED WITH LIVER FAILURE

The liver is central to hemostasis because it is the site of synthesis and clearance of most procoagulant and natural anticoagulant proteins and of essential components of the fibrinolytic system. Liver failure is associated with a high risk of bleeding due to deficient synthesis of procoagulant factors and enhanced fibrinolysis. Thrombocytopenia is common in patients with liver disease and may be due to congestive splenomegaly (hypersplenism), or immune-mediated shortened platelet life span (primary biliary cirrhosis). In addition, several anatomic abnormalities secondary to underlying liver disease further promote the occurrence of hemorrhage (Table 110-3). Dysfibrinogenemia is a relatively common finding in patients with liver disease due to impaired fibrin polymeratization. The development of DIC concomitant to chronic liver disease is not uncommon and may enhance the risk for bleeding. Laboratory evaluation is mandatory for an optimal therapeutic strategy, either to control ongoing bleeding or to prepare the patients with liver disease for invasive procedures. Typically these patients present with prolonged PT, aPTT, and TT, depending on the degree of liver damage, thrombocytopenia, and normal or slight increase of FDP. Fibrinogen levels are diminished only in fulminant hepatitis, decompensated cirrhosis, or advanced

TABLE 110-3	COAGULATION DISORDERS AND HEMOSTASIS IN LIVER DISEASE

Bleeding
  Portal hypertension
    Esophageal varices
  Thrombocytopenia
    Splenomegaly
    Chronic or acute DIC
  Decreased synthesis of clotting factors
    Hepatocyte failure
    Vitamin K deficiency
  Systemic fibrinolysis
  DIC
  Dysfibrinogenemia
Thrombosis
  Decreased synthesis of coagulation inhibitors: protein C, protein S, antithrombin
    Hepatocyte failure
    Vitamin K deficiency (protein C, protein S)
  Failure to clear activated coagulation proteins (DIC)
  Dysfibrinogenemia
  Iatrogenic: Transfusion of prothrombin complex concentrates
    Antifibrinolytic agents: ε-aminocaproic acid (EACA), tranexamic acid

Note: DIC, disseminated intravascular coagulation.

liver disease, or in the presence of DIC. The presence of prolonged TT, normal fibrinogen, and FDP levels suggests dysfibrinogenemia. FVIII levels are often normal or elevated in patients with liver failure, and decreased levels suggest superimposing DIC. Because FV is only synthesized in the hepatocyte and is not a vitamin K–dependent protein, reduced levels of FV may be an indicator of hepatocyte failure. Normal levels of FV and low levels of FVII suggest vitamin K deficiency. Vitamin K levels may be reduced in patients with liver failure due to compromised storage in hepatocellular disease, changes in bile acids, or cholestasis that can diminish the absorption of vitamin K. Replacement of vitamin K may be desirable (10 mg given by slow intravenous injection) to improve hemostasis.

Treatment with FFP is the most effective way to correct hemostasis in patients with liver failure. Infusion of FFP (5–10 mL/kg; each bag contains ~200 mL) is sufficient to ensure 10–20% of normal levels of clotting factors but not correction of PT or aPTT. Even high doses of FFP (20 mL/kg) do not correct the clotting times in all patients. Monitoring for clinical symptoms and clotting times will determine if repeated doses are required 8–12 h after the first infusion. Platelet concentrates are indicated when platelet counts are <10,000–20,000/mm^3 to control an ongoing bleed or immediately before an invasive procedure if counts are <50,000/mm^3. Cryoprecipitate is indicated only when fibrinogen levels are <100 mg/mL; dosing is six bags for a 70-kg patient daily. As noted above, PCC infusion in patients with liver failure should be avoided due to the high risk of thrombotic complications. The safety of antifibrinolytic drugs to control bleeding in patients with liver failure is not yet well-defined and should be avoided.

ACQUIRED INHIBITORS OF COAGULATION FACTORS

An *acquired inhibitor* is an immune-mediated disease characterized by the presence of an autoantibody against a specific clotting factor. FVIII is the most common target of antibody formation, but inhibitors to prothrombin, FV, FIX, FX, and FXI are also reported. The disease occurs predominantly in older adults (median age of 60 years) but occasionally in pregnant or postpartum women with no previous history of bleeding. In 50% of patients with inhibitors, no underlying disease is identified at the time of diagnosis. In the remaining half, the causes are autoimmune diseases, malignancies (lymphomas, prostate cancer), dermatologic diseases, and pregnancy. Previous history of open surgery in which topical thrombin is used, especially preparations containing bovine FV, is sometimes associated. Bleeding episodes occur commonly into soft tissues and in the gastrointestinal

or urinary tracts and skin. In contrast to hemophilia, hemarthrosis is rare. Retroperitoneal hemorrhages and other life-threatening bleeding may appear suddenly. The overall mortality in untreated patients ranges from 8 to 22%, and most deaths occur within the first few weeks after presentation. The diagnosis is based on the prolonged aPTT with normal PT and TT. The aPTT remains prolonged after mixture of the test plasma with equal amounts of pooled normal plasma for 2 h at 37°C. The Bethesda assay using FVIII-deficient plasma as performed for inhibitor detection in hemophilia will confirm the diagnosis. Major bleeding is treated with high doses of human or porcine FVIII, PCC/PCCa, or recombinant FVIIa. High-dose intravenous gamma globulin and anti-CD20 monoclonal antibody (rituximab) have been reported to be effective in patients with autoantibodies to FVIII. In contrast to hemophilia, inhibitors in nonhemophilia patients are sometimes responsive to prednisone alone or in association with cytotoxic therapy (e.g., cyclophosphamide).

The presence of lupus anticoagulant can be associated with venous or arterial thrombotic disease. However, bleeding has also been reported in lupus anticoagulant; it is due to the presence of antibodies to prothrombin, which results in hypoprothrombinemia. Both disorders show a prolonged PTT that does not correct on mixing. To distinguish acquired inhibitors from lupus anticoagulants, the dilute Russell's viper venom test and the hexagonal-phase phospholipids test will be negative in patients with an acquired inhibitor and positive in patients with lupus anticoagulants. Moreover, lupus anticoagulant interferes with the clotting activity of many factors (FVIII, FIX, FXII, FXI), whereas acquired inhibitors are specific to a single factor.

FURTHER READINGS

Caldwell SH et al: Coagulation disorders and hemostasis in liver disease: Pathophysiology and critical assessment of current management. Hepatology 44:1039, 2006

Hoyer LW: Hemophilia A. N Engl J Med 330:39, 1994

Key NS, Negrier C: Coagulation factor concentrates: Past, present, and future. Lancet 370:439, 2007

Levi M, Opal SM: Coagulation abnormalities in critically ill patients. Critical Care 10:222, 2006

Mannucci PM, et al: Recessively inherited coagulation disorders. Blood 104:1243, 2004

Stafford DW: The vitamin K cycle. J Thromb Haemost 3:1873, 2005

111 Venous Thrombosis
F.R. Rosendaal, H.R. Büller

Venous thrombosis is the result of occlusive clot formation in the veins. It occurs mainly in the deep veins of the leg (deep vein thrombosis, DVT), from which parts of the clot frequently embolize to the lungs (pulmonary embolism, PE). Fewer than 5% of all venous thromboses occur at other sites (see "Thrombosis at Rare Sites," and "Superficial Thrombophlebitis," below). Venous thrombosis is common and often occurs spontaneously, but it also frequently accompanies medical and surgical conditions, both in the community and the hospital.

The symptoms of venous thrombosis are nonspecific, and therefore the clinical diagnosis is difficult and requires objective testing by imaging. Major complications of thrombosis include a disabling post-thrombotic syndrome and death due to fatal PE. Treatment with anticoagulants should be prompt and adequate.

Many risk factors for thrombosis are known, all of them related either to immobilization or to hypercoagulability. While it has no utility to assess the risk factor status after thrombosis has occurred, several acquired risk factors are so strong that they warrant prophylactic anticoagulation, in both those with and without a history of thrombosis. Detailed guidelines for primary prevention are available.

Venous thrombosis tends to recur. The risk factors for a first venous thrombosis are not the same as for recurrent venous thrombosis and to a large extent are unknown. Individuals from families with inherited thrombophilia tend to develop thrombosis at a young age and to have frequent recurrences.

EPIDEMIOLOGY
The incidence of a first venous thrombosis is 1–3 per 1000 persons per year. Around two-thirds manifest as DVT of the leg, and one-third as PE. Up to half of patients with PE have no signs of DVT. From 1–10% of venous thromboses prove fatal, with deaths predominantly, but not exclusively, among the elderly or in patients with severe underlying disease, notably cancer. The incidence of venous thrombosis is exponentially related to age, where a rule of 10 applies: in children the incidence is 1 per 100,000 per year; in young adults, 1 in 10,000 per year; in the middle-aged, 1 per 1000 per year; in the elderly the incidence is 1% per year, up to nearly 10% per year in the very oldest. The recurrence rate of venous thrombosis is 3–10% per year.

TABLE 111-1	RISK FACTORS FOR VENOUS THROMBOSIS	
Acquired	**Inherited**	**Mixed/Unknown**
Orthopedic surgery	Antithrombin deficiency	High levels of factor VIII
Neurosurgery	Protein C deficiency	High levels of factor IX
Major abdominal surgery	Protein S deficiency	High levels of factor XI
Major trauma	Factor V Leiden (FVL)	High levels of fibrinogen
Central venous catheters	Prothrombin 20210A	High levels of TAFI
Malignancy	Non-O blood group	Low levels of TFPI
Antiphospholipid syndrome	Dysfibrinogenemia	APC resistance in the absence
Puerperium	Factor XIII 34val	of FVL
Prolonged bed rest		Hyperhomocysteinemia
Pregnancy		High levels of PCI (PAI-3)
Obesity		
Plaster cast		
Oral contraceptives		
Hormonal replacement therapy		
Myeloproliferative disorders		
Polycythemia vera		
Long-haul travel		
Age		

Note: TAFI, thrombin activatable fibrinolysis inhibitor; TFPI, tissue factor pathway inhibitor; PCI, protein C inhibitor; PAI-3, plasminogen activator inhibitor-3; APC, activated protein C.

ETIOLOGY

The causes of thrombosis can be divided into those associated with immobilization, which are usually acquired, and those associated with hypercoagulability, which can be either genetic or acquired (Table 111-1). Venous thrombosis is a multicausal disease that occurs when several risk factors are present simultaneously in a particular combination. Often, long-term risk factors, e.g., genetic defects, are joined by short-term acquired factors (Fig. 111-1). While many factors simply add to the risk, contributing to an individual's "thrombosis potential," some factors may interact synergistically, when the combination adds more to the risk than the sum of the separate contributions of the risk factors (e.g., factor V Leiden and oral contraceptive use).

Several acquired risk factors are very strong, causing thrombosis in several percent of those afflicted, which implies a relative risk of ≥50. These are orthopedic, neurosurgical, and major abdominal interventions; major trauma with multiple fractures; central venous catheters; and metastasized cancer, particularly adenocarcinomas. Moderate risk factors are antiphospholipid antibody syndrome, puerperium, prolonged bedrest, and nonmetastasized cancers; pregnancy, oral contraceptive use, hormone replacement therapy, obesity, and long-distance travel are mild

risk factors, with a two- to fivefold increased risk.

Homozygous protein C or protein S deficiency leads to potentially fatal purpura fulminans directly after birth, while homozygous antithrombin deficiency is not compatible with life. These are exceedingly rare, except in communities with a high frequency of consanguinity. Heterozygous antithrombin deficiency and homozygous factor V Leiden are the strongest genetic risk factors, increasing the risk of thrombosis 20- to 50-fold. Heterozygous protein C and protein S deficiencies are moderate contributors to risk, with a relative risk of 10. Other genetic factors that are associated with venous thrombosis are either mild and increase the risk two- to fivefold (as is the case for factor V Leiden, prothrombin 20210A, and non-O blood groups) or have negligible effects on risk that are only of academic interest (MTHFR 677T, factor V HR2, FXIII val34leu, PAI-1 4G/5G).

Mildly increased risks are also present for abnormalities in the coagulation system of which the origin is unclear, such as elevated levels of procoagulant factors (fibrinogen, II, von Willebrand factor, VIII, IX, X, and XI) and an

Risk factors
— Overall thrombosis potential

Childhood disease

Use of oral contraceptives

Skiing accident leads to immobilization at age 30

Deep vein thrombosis at age 30

Deep vein thrombosis at age 50 with continued use of oral contraceptives and at advanced age by age and factor V Leiden alone

FIGURE 111-1 Models of thrombosis risk. In each panel, the figure shows the thrombosis (black) potential of each risk factor present during an individual's life and the resultant thrombosis potential (red). (*From FR Rosendaal: Venous thrombosis: A multicausal disease. Lancet 353:1167, 1999; with permission.*)

tifibrinolytic factors (TAFI), and low levels of anticoagulant factors (TFPI) (Table 111-1).

PROGNOSIS

Patients who have had a venous thrombosis have a high risk (3–10% per year) of another. Up to half of the recurrences after a first thrombosis in one leg occur in the other, indicating that systemic changes rather than residual local damage are associated with rethrombosis. Nevertheless, few of the established risk factors associated with a hypercoagulable state (such as factor V Leiden, prothrombin 20210A, and elevated levels of clotting factors VIII, IX, and XI) are associated with recurrence risk. Even the strongest prothrombotic abnormalities—antithrombin, protein C, and protein S deficiencies—increase the risk of recurrent thrombosis by 50% at most. The only two clear risk factors for recurrence are male sex (increasing risk three- to fourfold) and the absence of a clear precipitating factor at the first event (doubling recurrence risk); in other words, a first thrombosis following surgery or plaster cast is unlikely to recur.

Acquired risk factors, such as surgery, immobilization, and cancer, increase the risk of recurrent thrombosis—as they increase the risk of a first event.

PREVENTION

The presence of prothrombotic defects or a history of thrombosis does not usually lead to different preventative strategies, with the exception of the postpartum period, where anticoagulation seems indicated, particularly for antithrombin deficiency. Similarly, the decision for long-term or lifelong anticoagulation, i.e., beyond the period of increased risk, depends on the clinical presentation rather than on the presence of prothrombotic abnormalities. Before prescribing long-term anticoagulation, clinicians should be aware of the cumulative annual risk of major hemorrhage of 1–2%.

Patients with a history of thrombosis should not use estrogen-containing drugs, i.e., hormone replacement therapy is contraindicated and for contraception, mechanical methods are preferred.

Thrombophilia Testing Testing for prothrombotic abnormalities outside the setting of abundant familial thrombophilia serves no purpose. A positive test does not help in the diagnosis of thrombosis, nor does it predict the risk of recurrent thrombosis, nor, therefore, does it affect long-term preventive strategies.

HEREDITARY THROMBOPHILIA

Individuals from families with a hereditary tendency for venous thrombosis generally have a more severe thrombotic tendency than individuals not from such families. Even when the genetic defect is the same in the two groups, those with hereditary thrombophilia from affected families have their first thrombosis at a young age (20–35 years), few fail to develop thrombosis in their lifetime, and many have recurrent disease. Early studies on thrombotic risk associated with prothrombotic defects were based on such families and overestimated risks for all patients with thrombophilic defects. Generally, individuals from such families need not be treated differently than others, except (1) oral contraceptives containing estrogens should be discouraged in all, and (2) postpartum anticoagulant prophylaxis should be considered in those with prothrombotic defects. Long-term treatment can be considered after a first episode of thrombosis, but only in high-risk families, particularly those with antithrombin deficiency.

THROMBOSIS AT RARE SITES

One in 25 venous thromboses occurs in the arm, while other, even more rare locations are the brain (cerebral vein thrombosis), the digestive system (mesenteric vein thrombosis), and the liver (portal vein thrombosis, and hepatic vein thrombosis, also known as *Budd-Chiari syndrome*). Thrombosis of the arm is almost invariably associated with central venous catheters. Deteriorating liver function and portal hypertension may point to thrombosis in the hepatic or portal veins, neurologic defects to cerebral vein thrombosis, and severe abdominal

complaints to mesenteric vein thrombosis. In rare cases, DVT may be associated with embolic stroke, when a patent foramen ovale is present (paradoxical stroke). Although local abnormalities often play a role, a procoagulant state due to cancer or hereditary abnormalities increases the incidence of thrombosis in rare locations. In all these cases diagnosis is based on imaging, and treatment should consist of anticoagulation similar to that of more common forms of thrombosis, as well as treatment of local causes and consequences.

SUPERFICIAL THROMBOPHLEBITIS

A painful red string is a clear sign of superficial thrombophlebitis. This is the only type of venous thrombosis that can reliably be diagnosed without imaging techniques. Although research is limited, the causes of superficial thrombophlebitis appear similar to those of other forms of venous thrombosis, and extension to the deep vein occurs. Treatment options are a matter of debate and vary from anticoagulants to an expectant approach.

GLOBAL DATA

Venous thrombosis occurs in all ethnic groups, with possibly a somewhat higher incidence in Africans than in whites and Asians. Whereas acquired risk factors are largely identical in these large ethnic groups, the two most common genetic risk factors (factor V Leiden and prothrombin 20210A) are found only in whites. These are unique gain-of-function mutations with a very low mutation rate (i.e., they occurred only once). Loss-of-function mutations leading to deficiencies of antithrombin, protein C, and protein S do not differ much by ethnic group. Due to founder effects, prevalences of factor V Leiden and prothrombin 20210A may vary widely in ethnic subpopulations, i.e., in various European populations the prevalence of factor V Leiden varies between 1% (Italy) and 15% (southern Sweden). Acquired risk factors may vary by local circumstances, e.g., hyperhomocysteinemia due to differences in diet, reproductive factors due to number of pregnancies, and use of oral contraceptives. The literature on Africans and Asians is sparse.

DIAGNOSIS

The true prevalence of thrombosis in patients presenting with either clinically suspected DVT of the leg or PE is ~15–25%. Therefore, the diagnostic workup for both these diseases has two objectives: (1) to exclude the disease quickly and safely in as many patients as possible, preferably with noninvasive and easy-to-use and cost-effective methods; and (2) to confirm the presence of thrombosis in the remaining patients with an accurate imaging technique. The purpose of the first step is to withhold both unnecessary further diagnostic testing and anticoagulant treatment. Although the diagnostic workup of DVT and PE have much in common, they will be discussed separately.

Deep Vein Thrombosis The signs and symptoms of DVT, such as swelling, pain, redness, superficial venous dilatation, and Homan's sign (pain in the calf or behind the knee on dorsiflexion of the ankle), are nonspecific and consequently insufficient for ruling the disease in or out. The classic "gold standard" is contrast venography. Although very accurate, this method requires radiologic facilities and expertise and is invasive and sometimes uncomfortable for the patient. Ultrasonography, with noncompressibility of the vein as the sole criterion, has largely replaced contrast venography. The investigation is limited to the femoral vein in the groin and the popliteal vein in the popliteal fossa. This method has a very high sensitivity and specificity (95–100%) in symptomatic patients for proximal DVT. For isolated DVT in the calf veins the method is less accurate. This latter characteristic of compression ultrasonography explains the necessity of repeating the test after ~1 week in those patients with an initial normal test result in order to detect extending calf thrombi. However, the first objective of the diagnostic workup was to rule out DVT quickly and safely. For this purpose the combination of the assessment of clinical probability and the measurement of the D-dimer blood concentration has been shown to be very useful. The clinical probability can be best assessed by the

TABLE 111-2 **CLINICAL DECISION RULE FOR DIAGNOSING THROMBOSIS**

Decision rule for clinically suspected deep vein thrombosis (DVT)	Points
Active cancer (patient receiving treatment for cancer within the previous 6 months or currently receiving palliative treatment)	1
Paralysis, paresis, or recent plaster immobilization of the lower extremities	1
Recently bedridden for ≥3 days or major surgery within the previous 12 weeks requiring general or regional anesthesia	1
Localized tenderness along the distribution of the deep venous system	1
Entire leg swollen	1
Calf swelling at least 3 cm larger than that on the asymptomatic side (measured 10 cm below tibial tuberosity)	1
Pitting edema confined to the symptomatic leg	1
Collateral superficial veins (nonvaricose)	1
Previously documented deep vein thrombosis	1
Alternative diagnosis at least as likely as deep vein thrombosis	−2

Score <2: DVT unlikely
     ≥2: DVT likely

Decision rule for clinically suspected pulmonary embolism (PE)	Points
Clinical signs and symptoms of deep vein thrombosis (minimum of leg swelling and pain with palpation of the deep veins)	3
Alternative diagnosis less likely than pulmonary embolism	3
Heart rate > 100/min	1.5
Immobilization (>3 days) or surgery in the previous 4 weeks	1.5
Previous pulmonary embolism or deep vein thrombosis	1.5
Hemoptysis	1
Malignancy (receiving treatment, treated in the last 6 months or palliative)	1

Score ≤4: PE unlikely
     >4: PE likely

rule shown in Table 111-2, which results in a classification of either DVT likely or DVT unlikely. D-Dimer is a degradation product of cross-linked fibrin and therefore concentrations of D-dimer below a certain cut-off level are considered to indicate the absence of thrombosis. Elevations of D-dimer in patients > 70 years who do not have thrombosis make the test less useful in this population.

Withholding further diagnostic testing and anticoagulant treatment in those patients with an unlikely clinical probability and a normal D-dimer level, which constitutes 30–50% of all referred patients, is safe. The remaining patients need to undergo (repeated) compression ultrasonography. An alternative approach is to perform a whole-leg imaging test on the day of referral. The advantage of this approach is that it eliminates the need for a repeat test (and may even obviate the probability assessment and D-dimer testing). The major disadvantage is the detection and likely treatment of a substantial number of isolated calf DVTs that may otherwise have lysed spontaneously.

Pulmonary Embolism The signs and symptoms of PE, such as dyspnea, pleuritic chest pain, cough, and hemoptysis, are nonspecific and, as for DVT, insufficiently accurate to confirm or refute the diagnosis of PE. The classic gold standard is pulmonary angiography, which is an invasive method requiring expertise. Hence, very similar to the developments in the diagnosis of DVT, two (complementary) strategies have evolved. The first is the combination of the assessment of clinical probability and the measurement of the D-dimer blood level; the second is the introduction of spiral CT of the chest. The clinical probability can be categorized accurately using the rule developed for suspected PE (Table 111-2). In those with an unlikely probability, a D-dimer test should be performed and, if normal, the disease can be safely ruled out and no anticoagulant therapy is indicated. Depending on the referral pattern of patients, this combination rules out PE in 30–

60% of all referred patients. Those with either a likely clinical probability at presentation or an abnormal D-dimer (and unlikely probability) need to undergo an imaging test.

At present the most attractive method is the multi-slice spiral CT of the chest. This technique accurately detects pulmonary embolism and, if normal, has been shown to also safely rule out the presence of emboli. Another advantage is the possibility of detecting an alternative disease in the thorax in those in whom PE is excluded, which may provide an explanation for the presenting symptoms. Alternative diagnostic methods in the workup of suspected PE are perfusion-ventilation scintigraphy, ultrasonography of the legs, and pulmonary angiography. Although a normal perfusion scan adequately rules out PE and a high probability perfusion-ventilation scan adequately rules in PE, the major disadvantages are the high proportion of nondiagnostic test results (~50%) and therefore the need for additional (costly) testing, usually with pulmonary angiography.

The role of compression ultrasonography of the legs before angiography or spiral CT is limited, as only a small fraction of patients have abnormal results and it further complicates the workup.

℞ DEEP VEIN THROMBOSIS AND PULMONARY EMBOLISM

The objectives of anticoagulant treatment for DVT and PE are to minimize local extension of the disease in the acute phase and to reduce the risk of recurrence of the disease in the months to years after the initial episode. In addition, in DVT, treatment lowers the risk of the development of the postthrombotic syndrome (swelling, stasis dermatitis, ulceration, venous claudication); in PE, treatment reduces the risk of pulmonary hypertension.

A spectrum of treatment options is available. At one end an expectant approach is indicated with no treatment in the setting of minimal disease without a tendency to extend or recur (as is the case, for example, with small calf thrombi). At the other end is the DVT or PE that is massive, either with serious compromise of lung perfusion or with impending gangrene of the leg. In these circumstances, aggressive treatment with either thrombolysis or even surgical intervention may be required. However, the vast majority of patients with DVT or PE require treatment in the middle part of the spectrum, which consists of the use of anticoagulants, usually low-molecular-weight heparin (LMWH) and a vitamin K antagonist (VKA) such as warfarin. Although the treatments of DVT and PE have much in common, they will be discussed separately.

DEEP VEIN THROMBOSIS The standard treatment for DVT consists of an initial course of LMWH, given once or twice daily via SC injection at a dose of 100 U/kg, followed by a VKA. Unfractionated heparin given IV is an alternative for LMWH but is less and less used these days. LMWH does not require laboratory monitoring and is given in a fixed dose, usually adapted for body weight (categories). An alternative for the initial LMWH therapy is the short-acting synthetic pentasaccharide fondaparinux, which can be given as a once-a-day SC injection of 2.5 mg, without laboratory monitoring. Therapy with LMWH or fondaparinux should be started as soon as the diagnosis is confirmed or during the diagnostic workup if the clinical suspicion is high. VKA (warfarin) can be safely started at the same day and the dose is titrated according to the international normalized ratio (INR) with a target of 2.5 (range 2–3). LMWH therapy should be continued for at least 5 days and can be discontinued if the INR is >2 on two consecutive measurements at least 24 h apart. The recommendations for the duration of VKA treatment for a first episode of DVT are summarized in Table 111-3. For a first DVT secondary to a transient (reversible) risk factor, such as following surgery, after immobilization, or associated with oral contraceptive use, a treatment duration of 3 months with a VKA is recommended. For patients with a first episode of idiopathic DVT, the recommendation is to treat for 6–12 months. At present, evidence is insufficient to treat patients with a first episode of DVT and a documented thrombophilic abnormality differently from those with idiopathic thrombosis. Hence, the recommendation is also 6–12 months of VKA. A duration of 12 months is recommended for patients with a first episode of DVT with documented antiphospholipid antibodies or two or more thrombophilic abnormalities. The decision to continue VKA treatment after 6–12 months requires the balancing of the risks of recurrence and bleeding and should take the patient's preference into account. No strong recommendations exist about the treatment duration for a second episode of DVT, but minimally 12

TABLE 111-3 LONG-TERM TREATMENT WITH VITAMIN K ANTAGONISTS FOR DEEP VEIN THROMBOSIS (DVT) AND PULMONARY EMBOLISM (PE)

Patient Categories	Duration, months	Comments
First episode of DVT or PE secondary to a transient (reversible) risk factor	3	Recommendation applies to both proximal and calf vein thrombosis
First episode of idiopathic DVT or PE	6–12	Continuation of anticoagulant therapy after 6–12 months may be considered
First episode of DVT or PE with a documented thrombophilic abnormality	6–12	Continuation of anticoagulant therapy after 6–12 months may be considered
First episode of DVT or PE with documented antiphospholipid or two or more thrombophilic abnormalities	12	Continuation of anticoagulant therapy after 12 months may be considered

months are usually given and often treatment is continued longer. Again, this decision requires the balancing of risk and benefit.

The preferred intensity of VKA treatment for DVT is an INR between 2 and 3. Higher intensities are not more effective, whereas lower intensities are less effective with a similar bleeding risk. Although VKAs are generally used for long-term treatment, LMWH is preferred in patients with DVT and concomitant cancer. This treatment is associated with a lower risk of recurrent thrombosis than VKA and a similar risk of bleeding.

The role of thrombolytic therapy as well as surgical removal of the thrombus in the initial treatment of DVT is controversial; the current recommendations are to refrain from their use with the single exception of patients with massive, recent ileofemoral DVT at risk of limb gangrene.

Patients with DVT are at risk of developing the postthrombotic syndrome in the first years after the initial episode. This syndrome can range from mild, with some swelling and pain at the end of the day, to severe, with massive swelling and skin ulceration. Graduated elastic compression stockings to the knee with an ankle pressure of 30–40 mmHg fitted in the first weeks after the initial thrombosis and worn for 2 years reduce the risk of the postthrombotic syndrome by ~50%.

As a result of the introduction of LMWH for the initial treatment of DVT, most patients with DVT can be treated at home either entirely or after a short hospital stay. The LMWH can be self-injected or given by family members or visiting nurses.

PULMONARY EMBOLISM The initial treatment with LMWH followed by a VKA for patients with PE is identical to that for patients with DVT. The intensity and duration of VKA treatment is also no different (Table 111-3). An alternative for LMWH is unfractionated heparin, which is still often used. The main disadvantage of unfractionated heparin is the need for continuous IV infusion and the requirement of frequent laboratory monitoring and dose adjustments. In contrast, LMWH can be given in fixed doses adjusted only for body weight. Another alternative for the initial LMWH therapy is fondaparinux, which can be given as a 2.5-mg once-a-day SC injection, without laboratory monitoring.

The treatment with LWMH or fondaparinux followed by VKA is indicated for PE patients who are hemodynamically stable—the great majority of patients. However, for those patients with PE who are hemodynamically unstable (usually defined as a systolic blood pressure <90–100 mmHg), a course of thrombolytic therapy should be considered. When no contraindications for thrombolysis (such as recent surgery or a bleeding diathesis) exist, this therapy reduces the short-term risk of recurrent PE or death by ~50% as compared to heparin. Although streptokinase and urokinase have been used in patients with PE, the most widely applied regimen is recombinant tissue plasminogen activator r(tPA) (bolus of 10 mg IV, followed by 90 mg in 2 h).

A controversial area is the best therapy for PE patients who are hemodynamically stable, but who have echocardiographic evidence of right ventricular dysfunction (usually defined as paradoxical interventricular septal motion and right ventricular dilatation and impaired systolic function). Although these patients have a higher mortality risk compared to patients without right ventricular dysfunction, it is unclear whether more aggressive therapy (with thrombolytic therapy or catheter removal of thrombus) is beneficial in terms of mortality, recurrent PE, and major hemorrhage.

Another area of controversy is vena caval interruption, usually with caval filters. The current recommendation is that a filter, preferably removable, should be considered only for patients with a contraindication for anticoagulant therapy, as well as in those with recurrent PE despite adequate treatment.

FURTHER READINGS

PRANDONI P: Links between arterial and venous disease. J Intern Med 262:341, 2007

ROSENDAAL FR: Venous thrombosis, a multicausal disease. Lancet 353:1167, 1999

The Seventh ACCP Conference on Antithrombotic and Thrombolytic Therapy. Chest 126(3 Suppl):167S, 2004

112 Antiplatelet, Anticoagulant, and Fibrinolytic Drugs
Jeffrey I. Weitz

Arterial and venous thromboses are major causes of morbidity and mortality. Arterial thrombosis is the most common cause of acute myocardial infarction, ischemic stroke, and limb gangrene, whereas deep vein thrombosis leads to pulmonary embolism (PE), which can be fatal, and to the postphlebitic syndrome. Most arterial thrombi are superimposed on disrupted atherosclerotic plaque because plaque rupture exposes thrombogenic material in the plaque core to the blood. This material then triggers platelet aggregation and fibrin formation, which results in the generation of a platelet-rich thrombus that can temporarily or permanently occlude blood flow. In contrast to arterial thrombi, venous thrombi rarely form at sites of obvious vascular disruption. Although they can develop after surgical trauma to veins or secondary to indwelling venous catheters, venous thrombi usually originate in the valve cusps of the deep veins of the calf or in the muscular sinuses, where they are triggered by stasis. Sluggish blood flow in these veins reduces the oxygen supply to the avascular valve cusps. Endothelial cells lining these valve cusps become activated and express adhesion molecules on their surface. Tissue factor–bearing leukocytes and microparticles adhere to these activated cells and induce coagulation. Local thrombus formation is exacerbated by reduced clearance of activated clotting factors as a result of impaired blood flow. If the thrombi extend into more proximal veins of the leg, thrombus fragments can dislodge, travel to the lungs, and produce a PE.

Arterial and venous thrombi are composed of platelets and fibrin, but the proportions differ. Arterial thrombi are rich in platelets because of the high shear in the injured arteries. In contrast, venous thrombi, which form under low shear conditions, contain relatively few platelets and are predominantly composed of fibrin and trapped red cells. Because of the predominance of platelets, arterial thrombi appear white, whereas venous thrombi are red in color, reflecting the trapped red cells.

Antithrombotic drugs are used for prevention and treatment of thrombosis. Targeting the components of thrombi, these agents include (1) antiplatelet drugs, (2) anticoagulants, and (3) fibrinolytic agents (Fig. 112-1). With the predominance of platelets in arterial thrombi, strategies to inhibit or treat arterial thrombosis focus mainly

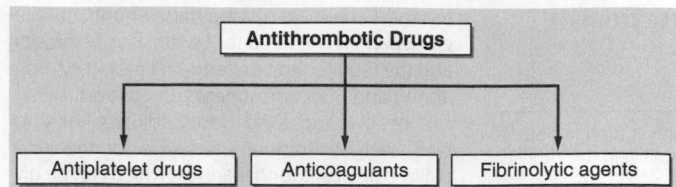

FIGURE 112-1 Classification of antithrombotic drugs.

on antiplatelet agents, although, in the acute setting, they often include anticoagulants and fibrinolytic agents. Anticoagulants are the mainstay of prevention and treatment of venous thromboembolism because fibrin is the predominant component of venous thrombi. Antiplatelet drugs are less effective than anticoagulants in this setting because of the limited platelet content of venous thrombi. Fibrinolytic therapy is used in selected patients with venous thromboembolism. For example, patients with massive or submassive PE can benefit from systemic or catheter-directed fibrinolytic therapy. The latter can also be used as an adjunct to anticoagulants for treatment of patients with extensive iliofemoral vein thrombosis.

ANTIPLATELET DRUGS

ROLE OF PLATELETS IN ARTERIAL THROMBOSIS

In healthy vasculature, circulating platelets are maintained in an inactive state by nitric oxide (NO) and prostacyclin released by endothelial cells lining the blood vessels. In addition, endothelial cells also express adenosine diphosphatase (ADPase) on their surface, which degrades ADP released from activated platelets. When the vessel wall is damaged, release of these substances is impaired and subendothelial matrix is exposed. Platelets adhere to exposed collagen, von Willebrand factor (vWF), and fibronectin via $\alpha_2\beta_1$, glycoprotein (GP) Ib-IX, and $\alpha_5\beta_1$ receptors, respectively, which are constitutively expressed on the

platelet surface. Adherent platelets undergo a change in shape, secrete ADP from their dense granules, and synthesize and release thromboxane A_2. Released ADP and thromboxane A_2, which are platelet agonists, activate ambient platelets and recruit them to the site of vascular injury (Fig. 112-2).

Disruption of the vessel wall also exposes tissue factor–expressing cells to the blood. Tissue factor initiates coagulation. Activated platelets potentiate coagulation by binding clotting factors and supporting the assembly of activation complexes that enhance thrombin generation. In addition to converting fibrinogen to fibrin, thrombin also serves as a potent platelet agonist and recruits more platelets to the site of vascular injury.

When platelets are activated, GPIIb/IIIa, the most abundant receptor on the platelet surface, undergoes a conformational change that enables it to bind fibrinogen. Divalent fibrinogen molecules bridge adjacent platelets together to form platelet aggregates. Fibrin strands, generated through the action of thrombin, then weave these aggregates together to form a platelet/fibrin mesh.

Antiplatelet drugs target various steps in this process. The commonly used drugs include aspirin, thienopyridines (clopidogrel and ticlopidine), dipyridimole, and GPIIb/IIIa antagonists.

ASPIRIN

The most widely used antiplatelet agent worldwide is aspirin. As a cheap and effective antiplatelet drug, aspirin serves as the foundation of most antiplatelet strategies.

MECHANISM OF ACTION Aspirin produces its antithrombotic effect by irreversibly acetylating and inhibiting platelet cyclooxygenase (COX)-1 (Fig. 112-3), a critical enzyme in the biosynthesis of thromboxane A_2. At high doses (~1 g/d), aspirin also inhibits COX-2, an inducible COX isoform found in endothelial cells and inflammatory cells. In endothelial cells, COX-2 initiates the synthesis of prostacyclin, a potent vasodilator and inhibitor of platelet aggregation.

FIGURE 112-2 Coordinated role of platelets and the coagulation system in thrombogenesis. Vascular injury simultaneously triggers platelet activation and aggregation and activation of the coagulation system. Platelet activation is initiated by exposure of subendothelial collagen and von Willebrand factor (vWF) onto which platelets adhere. Adherent platelets become activated and release ADP and thromboxane A_2, platelet agonists that activate ambient platelets and recruit them to the site of injury. When platelets are activated, glycoprotein IIb/IIIa on their surface undergoes a conformational change that enables it to ligate fibrinogen and mediate platelet aggregation. Coagulation is triggered by tissue factor exposed at the site of injury. Tissue factor triggers thrombin generation. As a potent platelet agonist, thrombin amplifies platelet recruitment to the site of injury. Thrombin also converts fibrinogen to fibrin, and the fibrin strands then weave the platelet aggregates together to form a platelet/fibrin thrombus.

FIGURE 112-3 Site of action of antiplatelet drugs. Aspirin inhibits thromboxane A_2 (TXA$_2$) synthesis by irreversibly acetylating cyclooxygenase-1 (COX-1). Reduced TXA$_2$ release attenuates platelet activation and recruitment to the site of vascular injury. Ticlopidine and clopidogrel irreversibly block P2Y$_{12}$, a key ADP receptor on the platelet surface. Therefore, these agents also attenuate platelet recruitment. Abciximab, eptifibatide, and tirofiban inhibit the final common pathway of platelet aggregation by blocking fibrinogen binding to activated glycoprotein (GP) IIb/IIIa.

COX-2 inhibitors were developed to block the production of inflammatory prostaglandins without affecting platelet function. The various COX-2 inhibitors differ in their selectivity for COX-2 relative to COX-1. By blocking prostacyclin synthesis without concomitant inhibition of thromboxane A_2 production, highly selective inhibitors of COX-2 increase the risk of cardiovascular events. Thus, long-term rofecoxib therapy increases the risk of myocardial infarction (MI) three- to fivefold, a finding that led to the withdrawal of this drug from the market.

INDICATIONS Aspirin is widely used for secondary prevention of cardiovascular events in patients with coronary artery, cerebrovascular, or peripheral vascular disease. Compared with placebo, aspirin produces a 25% reduction in the risk of cardiovascular death, MI, or stroke. Aspirin is also used for primary prevention in patients whose estimated annual risk of MI is >1%, a point where its benefits are likely to outweigh harms. This includes patients over the age of 40 with two or more major risk factors for cardiovascular disease or those over the age of 50 with one or more such risk factor. Aspirin is equally effective in men and women. In men, aspirin mainly reduces the risk of MI, while in women aspirin lowers the risk of stroke.

DOSAGES Aspirin is usually administered at doses of 75–325 mg once daily. Higher dose aspirin is not more effective than lower aspirin doses, and some analyses suggest reduced efficacy with higher doses. Because the side effects of aspirin are dose-related, daily aspirin doses of 75–100 mg are recommended for most indications. When rapid platelet inhibition is required, an initial aspirin dose of at least 160 mg should be given.

SIDE EFFECTS Most common side effects are gastrointestinal and range from dyspepsia to erosive gastritis or peptic ulcers with bleeding and perforation. These side effects are dose-related. Use of enteric-coated or buffered aspirin in place of plain aspirin does not eliminate the risk of gastrointestinal side effects. The overall risk of major bleeding with aspirin is 1–3% per year. The risk of bleeding is increased when aspirin is given in conjunction with anticoagulants, such as warfarin. When dual therapy is used, low-dose aspirin should be given (75–100 mg daily). Eradication of *Helicobacter pylori* infection and administration of proton pump inhibitors may reduce the risk of aspirin-induced gastrointestinal bleeding in patients with peptic ulcer disease.

Aspirin should not be administered to patients with a history of aspirin allergy characterized by bronchospasm. This problem occurs in ~0.3% of the general population but is more common in those with chronic urticaria or asthma, particularly in individuals with nasal polyps or chronic rhinitis. Hepatic and renal toxicity are observed with aspirin overdose.

ASPIRIN RESISTANCE Clinical aspirin resistance is defined as the failure of aspirin to protect patients from ischemic vascular events. This is not a helpful definition because it is made after the event occurs. Furthermore, it is not realistic to expect aspirin, which only blocks thromboxane A_2–induced platelet activation, to prevent all vascular events.

Aspirin resistance has also been described biochemically as failure of the drug to produce its expected inhibitory effects on tests of platelet function, such as thromboxane A_2 synthesis or arachidonic acid–induced platelet aggregation. However, the tests of platelet function used for diagnosis of biochemical aspirin resistance have not been well standardized. Furthermore, these tests are not proven to identify patients at risk of recurrent vascular events. In addition, resistance is not reversed by either giving higher doses of aspirin or adding other antiplatelet drugs. Thus, testing for aspirin resistance remains a research tool.

THIENOPYRIDINES

The thienopyridines include ticlopidine and clopidogrel, drugs that target $P2Y_{12}$, a key ADP receptor on platelets.

MECHANISM OF ACTION The thienopyridines are structurally related drugs that selectively inhibit ADP-induced platelet aggregation by irreversibly blocking $P2Y_{12}$ (Fig. 112-3). Ticlopidine and clopidogrel are both prodrugs that must be metabolized by the hepatic cytochrome P450 (CYP) enzyme system to acquire activity. Consequently, when given in usual doses, their onset of action is delayed for several days.

INDICATIONS Like aspirin, ticlopidine is more effective than placebo at reducing the risk of cardiovascular death, MI, and stroke in patients with atherosclerotic disease. Because of its delayed onset of action, ticlopidine is not recommended in patients with acute MI. Ticlopidine was used routinely as an adjunct to aspirin after coronary artery stenting and as an aspirin substitute in those intolerant to aspirin. Because clopidogrel is more potent than ticlopidine and has a better safety profile, clopidogrel has replaced ticlopidine.

When compared with aspirin in patients with recent ischemic stroke, MI, or peripheral arterial disease, clopidogrel reduced the risk of cardiovascular death, MI, and stroke by 8.7%. Therefore, clopidogrel is more effective than aspirin but is also more expensive. In some patients, clopidogrel and aspirin are combined to capitalize on their capacity to block complementary pathways of platelet activation. For example, the combination of aspirin plus clopidogrel is recommended for at least 4 weeks after implantation of a bare metal stent in a coronary artery and longer in those with a drug-eluting stent. Concerns about late in-stent thrombosis with drug-eluting stents have led some experts to recommend long-term use of clopidogrel plus aspirin for this indication.

The combination of clopidogrel and aspirin is also effective in patients with unstable angina. Thus, in 12,562 such patients, the risk of cardiovascular death, MI, or stroke was 9.3% in those randomized to the combination of clopidogrel and aspirin and 11.4% in those given aspirin alone. This 20% relative risk reduction with combination therapy was highly statistically significant. However, combining clopidogrel with aspirin increases the risk of major bleeding to about 2% per year. This bleeding risk persists even if the daily dose of aspirin is ≤100 mg. Therefore, the combination of clopidogrel and aspirin should only be used when there is a clear benefit. For example, this combination has not proven to be superior to clopidogrel alone in patients with acute ischemic stroke or to aspirin alone for primary prevention in those at risk for cardiovascular events.

DOSING Ticlopidine is given twice daily at a dose of 250 mg. The more potent clopidogrel is given once daily at a dose of 75 mg. Loading doses of clopidogrel are given when rapid ADP receptor blockade is desired. For example, patients undergoing coronary stenting are often given a loading dose of 300 mg, which effects inhibition of ADP-induced platelet aggregation in about 6 h. Loading doses of 600 or 900 mg produce an even more rapid effect.

SIDE EFFECTS The most common side effects of ticlopidine are gastrointestinal. More serious are the hematologic side effects, which include neutropenia, thrombocytopenia, and thrombotic thrombocytopenic purpura. These side effects usually occur within the first few months of starting treatment. Therefore, blood counts must be carefully monitored when initiating therapy with ticlopidine. Gastrointestinal and hematologic side effects are rare with clopidogrel.

THIENOPYRIDINE RESISTANCE There is between-subject variability in the capacity of the thienopyridines to inhibit ADP-induced platelet aggregation. This variability reflects, at least in part, genetic polymorphisms in the CYP isoenzymes involved in the metabolic activation of the drugs. For example, subjects with the *CYP2C19*2* allele exhibit decreased responsiveness to clopidogrel, as do those with reduced CYP3A4 activity. These findings raise the possibility that pharmacogenomic profiling may help identify clopidogrel-resistant patients. Point-of-care devices that assess the extent of platelet inhibition may also help to identify these patients. It is currently unknown, however, whether patients with biochemical evidence of clopidogrel resistance have a poorer outcome and whether administration of higher doses of clopidogrel to these patients overcomes this problem.

DIPYRIDAMOLE

Dipyridamole is a relatively weak antiplatelet agent on its own, but an extended-release formulation of dipyridamole combined with low-dose aspirin, a preparation known as *Aggrenox*, is used for prevention of stroke in patients with transient ischemic attacks.

MECHANISM OF ACTION   By inhibiting phosphodiesterase, dipyridamole blocks the breakdown of cAMP. Increased levels of cAMP reduce intracellular calcium and inhibit platelet activation. Dipyridamole also blocks the uptake of adenosine by platelets and other cells. This produces a further increase in local cAMP levels because the platelet adenosine A_2 receptor is coupled to adenylate cyclase (**Fig. 112-4**).

DOSING   Aggrenox is given twice daily. Each capsule contains 200 mg of extended-release dipyridamole and 25 mg of aspirin.

SIDE EFFECTS   Because dipyridamole has vasodilatory effects, it must be used with caution in patients with coronary artery disease. Gastrointestinal complaints, headache, facial flushing, dizziness, and hypotension can also occur. These symptoms often subside with continued use of the drug.

INDICATIONS   Dipyridamole plus aspirin was compared with aspirin or dipyridamole alone, or with placebo, in patients with an ischemic stroke or transient ischemic attack. The combination reduced the risk of stroke by 22.1% compared with aspirin and by 24.4% compared with dipyridamole. A second trial compared dipyridamole plus aspirin with aspirin alone for secondary prevention in patients with ischemic stroke. Vascular death, stroke, or MI occurred in 13% of patients given combination therapy and in 16% of those treated with aspirin alone. Based on these data, Aggrenox is often used for stroke prevention. However, because of its vasodilatory effects and the paucity of data supporting the use of dipyridamole in patients with symptomatic coronary artery disease, Aggrenox should not be used for stroke prevention in such patients.

GPIIB/IIIA RECEPTOR ANTAGONISTS

As a class, parenteral GPIIb/IIIa receptor antagonists have an established niche in patients with acute coronary syndromes. The three agents in this class are abciximab, eptifibatide, and tirofiban.

MECHANISM OF ACTION   A member of the integrin family of adhesion receptors, GPIIb/IIIa is found on the surface of platelets and megakaryocytes. With about 80,000 copies per platelet, GPIIb/IIIa is the most abundant receptor. Consisting of a non-covalently linked heterodimer, GPIIb/IIIa is inactive on resting platelets. When platelets are activated, inside-outside signal transduction pathways trigger a conformational activation of the receptor. Once activated, GPIIb/IIIa binds adhesive molecules, such as fibrinogen and, under high shear conditions, vWF. Binding is mediated by the Arg-Gly-Asp (RGD) sequence found on the α chains of fibrinogen and on vWF, and by the Lys-Gly-Asp (KGD) sequence located within a

FIGURE 112-4 Mechanism of action of dipyridamole. Dipyridamole increases levels of cyclic AMP in platelets by (1) blocking the reuptake of adenosine, and (2) inhibiting phosphodiesterase-mediated cyclic AMP degradation. By promoting calcium uptake, cyclic AMP reduces intracellular levels of calcium. This, in turn, inhibits platelet activation and aggregation.

unique dodecapeptide domain on the γ chains of fibrinogen. Once bound, fibrinogen and/or vWF bridge adjacent platelets together to induce platelet aggregation.

Although abciximab, eptifibatide, and tirofiban all target the GPIIb/IIIa receptor, they are structurally and pharmacologically distinct (**Table 112-1**). Abciximab is a Fab fragment of a humanized murine monoclonal antibody directed against the activated form of GPIIb/IIIa. Abciximab binds to the activated receptor with high affinity and blocks the binding of adhesive molecules. In contrast to abciximab, eptifibatide and tirofiban are synthetic small molecules. Eptifibatide is a cyclic heptapeptide that binds GPIIb/IIIa because it incorporates the KGD motif, whereas tirofiban is a nonpeptidic tyrosine derivative that acts as a RGD mimetic. Abciximab has a long half-life and can be detected on the surface of platelets for up to 2 weeks. Eptifibatide and tirofiban have shorter half-lives.

In addition to targeting the GPIIb/IIIa receptor, abciximab also inhibits the closely related $\alpha_v\beta_3$ receptor, which binds vitronectin, and $\alpha_M\beta_2$, a leukocyte integrin. In contrast, eptifibatide and tirofiban are specific for GPIIb/IIIa. Inhibition of $\alpha_v\beta_3$ and $\alpha_M\beta_2$ may endow abciximab with anti-inflammatory and/or antiproliferative properties that extend beyond platelet inhibition.

DOSING   All of the GPIIb/IIIa antagonists are given as an IV bolus followed by an infusion. Because they are cleared by the kidneys, the doses of eptifibatide and tirofiban must be reduced in patients with renal insufficiency.

SIDE EFFECTS   In addition to bleeding, thrombocytopenia is the most serious complication. Thrombocytopenia is immune-mediated and is

TABLE 112-1	FEATURES OF GPIIb/IIIa ANTAGONISTS		
Feature	**Abciximab**	**Eptifibatide**	**Tirofiban**
Description	Fab fragment of humanized mouse monoclonal antibody	Cyclical KGD-containing heptapeptide	Nonpeptidic RGD mimetic
Specific for GPIIb/IIIa	No	Yes	Yes
Plasma half-life	Short (min)	Long (2.5 h)	Long (2.0 h)
Platelet-bound half-life	Long (days)	Short (s)	Short (s)
Renal clearance	No	Yes	Yes

Note: KGD, Lys-Gly-Asp; RGD, Arg-Gly-Asp.

caused by antibodies directed against neoantigens on GPIIb/IIIa that are exposed upon antagonist binding. With abciximab, thrombocytopenia occurs in up to 5% of patients. Thrombocytopenia is severe in ~1% of these individuals. Thrombocytopenia is less common with the other two agents, occurring in ~1% of patients.

INDICATIONS   Abciximab and eptifibatide are used in patients undergoing percutaneous coronary interventions, particularly those with acute MI. Tirofiban is used in high-risk patients with unstable angina. Eptifibatide also can be used for this indication.

NEW ANTIPLATELET AGENTS
Thienopyridines that produce more predictable suppression of ADP-induced platelet aggregation are under investigation. Direct-acting reversible $P2Y_{12}$ antagonists have also been developed. These agents can be given orally or parenterally and have a rapid onset of action because they are not prodrugs. Finally, orally active inhibitors of the type 1 protease activated receptor (PAR-1), the major thrombin receptor on platelets, are also entering clinical trials.

ANTICOAGULANTS

There are both parenteral and oral anticoagulants. Currently available parenteral anticoagulants include heparin, low-molecular-weight heparin (LMWH), and fondaparinux, a synthetic pentasaccharide. The only available oral anticoagulants are the vitamin K antagonists, of which warfarin is the agent most often used in North America.

PARENTERAL ANTICOAGULANTS
Heparin   Heparin is a sulfated polysaccharide and is isolated from mammalian tissues rich in mast cells. Most commercial heparin is derived from porcine intestinal mucosa and is a polymer of alternating D-glucuronic acid and N-acetyl-D-glucosamine residues.

MECHANISM OF ACTION   Heparin acts as an anticoagulant by activating antithrombin (previously known as antithrombin III) and accelerating the rate at which antithrombin inhibits clotting enzymes, particularly thrombin and factor Xa. Antithrombin, the obligatory plasma cofactor for heparin, is a member of the serine protease inhibitor (serpin) superfamily. Synthesized in the liver and circulating in plasma at a concentration of 2.6 ± 0.4 µM, antithrombin acts as a suicide substrate for its target enzymes.

To activate antithrombin, heparin binds to the serpin via a unique pentasaccharide sequence that is found on one-third of the chains of commercial heparin (**Fig. 112-5**). The remainder of the heparin chains that lack this pentasaccharide sequence have little or no anticoagulant activity. Once bound to antithrombin, heparin induces a conformational change in the reactive center loop of antithrombin that renders it more readily accessible to its target proteases. This conformational change enhances the rate at which antithrombin inhibits factor Xa by at least two orders of magnitude but has little effect on the rate of thrombin inhibition by antithrombin. To catalyze thrombin inhibition, heparin serves as a template that binds antithrombin and thrombin simultaneously. Formation of this ternary complex brings the enzyme in close apposition to the inhibitor, thereby promoting the formation of a stable covalent thrombin-antithrombin complex.

Only pentasaccharide-containing heparin chains composed of at least 18 saccharide units (which correspond to a molecular weight of 5400) are of sufficient length to bridge thrombin and antithrombin together. With a mean molecular weight of 15,000, and a range of 5000–30,000, almost all of the chains of unfractionated heparin are long enough to effect this bridging function. Consequently, by definition, heparin has equal capacity to promote the inhibition of thrombin and factor Xa by antithrombin and is assigned an anti-factor Xa to anti-factor IIa (thrombin) ratio of 1:1.

Heparin causes the release of tissue factor pathway inhibitor (TFPI) from the endothelium. A factor Xa–dependent inhibitor of tissue factor–bound factor VIIa, TFPI may contribute to the antithrombotic activity of heparin. Longer heparin chains induce the release of more TFPI than shorter chains.

PHARMACOLOGY   Heparin must be given parenterally. It is usually administered SC or by continuous IV infusion. When used for therapeutic purposes, the IV route is most often employed. If heparin is given SC for treatment of thrombosis, the dose of heparin must be high enough to overcome the limited bioavailability associated with this method of delivery.

FIGURE 112-5 Mechanism of action of heparin, low-molecular-weight heparin (LMWH), and fondaparinux, a synthetic pentasaccharide. *A.* Heparin binds to antithrombin via its pentasaccharide sequence. This induces a conformational change in the reactive center loop of antithrombin that accelerates its interaction with factor Xa. To potentiate thrombin inhibition, heparin must simultaneously bind to antithrombin and thrombin. Only heparin chains composed of at least 18 saccharide units, which corresponds to a molecular weight of 5400, are of sufficient length to perform this bridging function. With a mean molecular weight of 15,000, all of the heparin chains are long enough to do this. ***B.*** LMWH has greater capacity to potentiate factor Xa inhibition by antithrombin than thrombin because, with a mean molecular weight of 4500–5000, at least half of the LMWH chains are too short to bridge antithrombin to thrombin. ***C.*** The pentasaccharide only accelerates factor Xa inhibition by antithrombin because the pentasaccharide is too short to bridge antithrombin to thrombin.

In the circulation, heparin binds to the endothelium and to plasma proteins other than antithrombin. Heparin binding to endothelial cells explains its dose-dependent clearance. At low doses, the half-life of heparin is short because it binds rapidly to the endothelium. With higher doses of heparin, the half-life is longer because heparin is cleared more slowly once the endothelium is saturated. Clearance is mainly extrarenal; heparin binds to macrophages, which internalize and depolymerize the long heparin chains and secrete shorter chains back into the circulation. Because of its dose-dependent clearance mechanism, the plasma half-life of heparin ranges from 30–60 min with bolus IV doses of 25 and 100 U/kg, respectively.

Once heparin enters the circulation, it binds to plasma proteins other than antithrombin, a phenomenon that reduces its anticoagulant activity. Some of the heparin-binding proteins found in plasma are acute-phase reactants whose levels are elevated in ill patients. Others, such as high-molecular-weight multimers of vWF, are released from activated platelets or endothelial cells. Activated platelets also release platelet factor 4 (PF4), a highly cationic protein that binds heparin with high affinity. The large amounts of PF4 found in the vicinity of platelet-rich arterial thrombi can neutralize the anticoagulant activity of heparin. This phenomenon may attenuate heparin's capacity to suppress thrombus growth.

Because the levels of heparin-binding proteins in plasma vary from person to person, the anticoagulant response to fixed or weight-adjusted doses of heparin is unpredictable. Consequently, coagulation monitoring is essential to ensure that a therapeutic response is obtained. This is particularly important when heparin is administered for treatment of established thrombosis because a subtherapeutic anticoagulant response may render patients at risk for recurrent thrombosis, whereas excessive anticoagulation increases the risk of bleeding.

MONITORING THE ANTICOAGULANT EFFECT   Heparin therapy can be monitored using the activated partial thromboplastin time (aPTT) or anti-factor Xa level. Although the aPTT is the test most often employed for this purpose, there are problems with this assay. aPTT reagents vary in their sensitivity to heparin, and the type of coagulometer used for testing can influence the results. Consequently, laboratories must establish a therapeutic aPTT range with each reagent-coagulometer combination by measuring the aPTT and anti-factor Xa level in plasma samples collected from heparin-treated patients. For most of the aPTT reagents and coagulometers in current use, therapeutic heparin levels are achieved with a two- to threefold prolongation of the aPTT.

Anti-factor Xa levels also can be used to monitor heparin therapy. With this test, therapeutic heparin levels range from 0.3–0.7 units/mL. Although this test is gaining in popularity, anti-factor Xa assays have yet to be standardized, and results can vary widely between laboratories.

Up to 25% of heparin-treated patients with venous thromboembolism require >35,000 units/d to achieve a therapeutic aPTT. These patients are considered heparin resistant. It is useful to measure anti-factor Xa levels in heparin-resistant patients because many will have a therapeutic anti-factor Xa level despite a subtherapeutic aPTT. This dissociation in test results occurs because elevated plasma levels of fibrinogen and factor VIII, both of which are acute-phase proteins, shorten the aPTT but have no effect on anti-factor Xa levels. Heparin therapy in patients who exhibit this phenomenon is best monitored using anti-factor Xa levels instead of the aPTT. Patients with congenital or acquired antithrombin deficiency and those with elevated levels of heparin-binding proteins may also need high doses of heparin to achieve a therapeutic aPTT or anti-factor Xa level. If there is good correlation between the aPTT and the anti-factor Xa levels, either test can be used to monitor heparin therapy.

DOSING   For prophylaxis, heparin is usually given in fixed doses of 5000 units SC two or three times daily. With these low doses, coagulation monitoring is unnecessary. In contrast, monitoring is essential when the drug is given in therapeutic doses. Fixed-dose or weight-based heparin nomograms are used to standardize heparin dosing and to shorten the time required to achieve a therapeutic anticoagulant response. At least two heparin nomograms have been validated in patients with venous thromboembolism and reduce the time required to achieve a therapeutic aPTT. Weight-adjusted heparin nomograms have also been evaluated in patients with acute coronary syndromes. After an IV heparin bolus of 5000 units or 70 units/kg, a heparin infusion rate of 12–15 units/kg per hour is usually administered. In contrast, weight-adjusted heparin nomograms for patients with venous thromboembolism use an initial bolus of 5000 units or 80 units/kg, followed by an infusion of 18 units/kg per hour. Thus, patients with venous thromboembolism appear to require higher doses of heparin to achieve a therapeutic aPTT than do patients with acute coronary syndromes. This may reflect differences in the thrombus burden. Heparin binds to fibrin, and the fibrin content of extensive deep vein thrombi is greater than that of small coronary thrombi.

LIMITATIONS   Heparin has pharmacokinetic and biophysical limitations (Table 112-2). The pharmacokinetic limitations reflect heparin's propensity to bind in a pentasaccharide-independent fashion to cells and plasma proteins. Heparin binding to endothelial cells explains its dose-dependent clearance, whereas binding to plasma proteins results in a variable anticoagulant response and can lead to heparin resistance.

The biophysical limitations of heparin reflect the inability of the heparin-antithrombin complex to (1) inhibit factor Xa when it is incorporated into the prothrombinase complex, the complex that converts prothrombin to thrombin; and (2) to inhibit thrombin bound to fibrin. Consequently, factor Xa bound to activated platelets within platelet-rich thrombi has the potential to generate thrombin, even in the face of heparin. Once this thrombin binds to fibrin, it too is protected from inhibition by the heparin-antithrombin complex. Clot-associated thrombin can then trigger thrombus growth by locally activating platelets and amplifying its own generation through feedback activation of factors V, VIII, and XI. Further compounding the problem is the potential for heparin neutralization by the high concentrations of PF4 released from activated platelets within the platelet-rich thrombus.

SIDE EFFECTS   The most common side effect of heparin is bleeding. Other complications include thrombocytopenia, osteoporosis, and elevated levels of transaminases.

Bleeding   The risk of heparin-induced bleeding increases with higher heparin doses. Concomitant administration of drugs that affect hemostasis, such as antiplatelet or fibrinolytic agents, increases the risk of bleeding, as does recent surgery or trauma. Heparin-treated patients with serious bleeding can be given protamine sulfate to neutralize the heparin. Protamine sulfate, a mixture of basic polypeptides isolated from salmon sperm, binds heparin with high affinity, and the resultant protamine-heparin complexes are then cleared. Typically, 1 mg of protamine sulfate neutralizes 100 units of heparin. Protamine sulfate is given IV. Anaphylactoid reactions to protamine sulfate can occur, and drug administration by slow IV infusion is recommended to reduce the risk.

TABLE 112-2   PHARMACOKINETIC AND BIOPHYSICAL LIMITATIONS OF HEPARIN

Limitations	Mechanism
Poor bioavailability at low doses	Binds to proteins in subcutaneous depot site
Dose-dependent clearance	Binds to macrophages
Variable anticoagulant response	Binds to plasma proteins whose levels vary from patient to patient
Reduced activity in the vicinity of platelet-rich thrombi	Neutralized by platelet factor 4 released from activated platelets
Limited activity against factor Xa incorporated in the prothrombinase complex and thrombin bound to fibrin	Reduced capacity of heparin-antithrombin complex to inhibit factor Xa bound to activated platelets and thrombin bound to fibrin

Thrombocytopenia Heparin can cause thrombocytopenia. Heparin-induced thrombocytopenia (HIT) is an antibody-mediated process that is triggered by antibodies directed against neoantigens on PF4 that are exposed when heparin binds to this protein. These antibodies, which are usually of the IgG isotype, bind simultaneously to the heparin-PF4 complex and to platelet Fc receptors. Such binding activates the platelets and generates platelet microparticles. Circulating microparticles are prothrombotic because they express anionic phospholipids on their surface and can bind clotting factors and promote thrombin generation.

The clinical features of HIT are illustrated in Table 112-3. Typically, HIT occurs 5–14 days after initiation of heparin therapy, but it can manifest earlier if the patient has received heparin within the past 3 months. It is rare for the platelet count to fall below 100,000/μL in patients with HIT, and even a 50% decrease in the platelet count from the pretreatment value should raise the suspicion of HIT in those receiving heparin. HIT is more common in surgical patients than in medical patients and, like many autoimmune disorders, occurs more frequently in females than in males.

HIT can be associated with thrombosis, either arterial or venous. Venous thrombosis, which manifests as DVT and/or PE, is more common than arterial thrombosis. Arterial thrombosis can manifest as ischemic stroke or acute MI. Rarely, platelet-rich thrombi in the distal aorta or iliac arteries can cause critical limb ischemia.

The diagnosis of HIT is established using enzyme-linked assays to detect antibodies against heparin-PF4 complexes or with platelet activation assays. Enzyme-linked assays are sensitive but can be positive in the absence of any clinical evidence of HIT. The most specific diagnostic test is the serotonin release assay. This test is performed by quantifying serotonin release when washed platelets loaded with labeled serotonin are exposed to patient serum in the absence or presence of varying concentrations of heparin. If the patient serum contains the HIT antibody, heparin addition induces platelet activation and serotonin release.

Management of HIT is outlined in Table 112-4. Heparin should be stopped in patients with suspected or documented HIT, and an alternative anticoagulant should be administered to prevent or treat thrombosis. The agents most often used for this indication are parenteral direct thrombin inhibitors, such as lepirudin, argatroban, or bivalirudin, or factor Xa inhibitors, such as fondaparinux or danaparoid.

Patients with HIT, particularly those with associated thrombosis, often have evidence of increased thrombin generation that can lead to consumption of protein C. If these patients are given warfarin without a concomitant parenteral anticoagulant to inhibit thrombin or thrombin generation, the further decrease in protein C levels induced by the vitamin K antagonist can trigger skin necrosis. To avoid this problem, patients with HIT should be treated with a direct thrombin inhibitor or fondaparinux until the platelet count returns to normal levels. At this point, low-dose warfarin therapy can be introduced, and the thrombin inhibitor can be discontinued when the anticoagulant response to warfarin has been therapeutic for at least 2 days.

Osteoporosis Treatment with therapeutic doses of heparin for >1 month can cause a reduction in bone density. This complication has been reported in up to 30% of patients given long-term heparin therapy, and symptomatic vertebral fractures occur in 2–3% of these individuals.

TABLE 112-4 MANAGEMENT OF HEPARIN-INDUCED THROMBOCYTOPENIA

Stop all heparin
Give an alternative anticoagulant, such as lepirudin, argatroban, bivalirudin, danaparoid, or fondaparinux
Do not give platelet transfusions
Do not give warfarin until the platelet count returns to its baseline level; if warfarin is administered, give vitamin K to restore the INR to normal
Evaluate for thrombosis, particularly deep vein thrombosis

Heparin causes bone loss both by decreasing bone formation and by enhancing bone resorption. Thus, heparin affects the activity of both osteoblasts and osteoclasts.

Elevated Levels of Transaminases Therapeutic doses of heparin frequently cause modest elevation in the serum levels of hepatic transaminases, without a concomitant increase in the level of bilirubin. The levels of transaminases rapidly return to normal when the drug is stopped. The mechanism of this phenomenon is unknown.

Low-Molecular-Weight Heparin Consisting of smaller fragments of heparin, LMWH is prepared from unfractionated heparin by controlled enzymatic or chemical depolymerization. The mean molecular weight of LMWH is 5000, one-third the mean molecular weight of unfractionated heparin. LMWH has advantages over heparin (Table 112-5) and has replaced heparin for most indications.

MECHANISM OF ACTION Like heparin, LMWH exerts its anticoagulant activity by activating antithrombin. With a mean molecular weight of 5000, which corresponds to about 17 saccharide units, at least half of the pentasaccharide-containing chains of LMWH are too short to bridge thrombin to antithrombin (Fig. 112-5). However, these chains retain the capacity to accelerate factor Xa inhibition by antithrombin because this activity is largely the result of the conformational changes in antithrombin evoked by pentasaccharide binding. Consequently, LMWH catalyzes factor Xa inhibition by antithrombin more than thrombin inhibition. Depending on their unique molecular weight distributions, LMWH preparations have anti-factor Xa to anti-factor IIa ratios ranging from 2:1–4:1.

PHARMACOLOGY Although usually given SC, LMWH also can be administered IV if a rapid anticoagulant response is needed. LMWH has pharmacokinetic advantages over heparin. These advantages reflect the fact that shorter heparin chains bind less avidly to endothelial cells, macrophages, and heparin-binding plasma proteins. Reduced binding to endothelial cells and macrophages eliminates the rapid, dose-dependent, and saturable mechanism of clearance that is a characteristic of unfractionated heparin. Instead, the clearance of LMWH is dose-independent and its plasma half-life is longer. Based on measurement of anti-factor Xa levels, LMWH has a plasma half-life of ~4 h. LMWH is cleared almost exclusively by the kidneys, and the drug can accumulate in patients with renal insufficiency.

LMWH exhibits about 90% bioavailability after SC injection. Because LMWH binds less avidly to heparin-binding proteins in plasma

TABLE 112-3 FEATURES OF HEPARIN-INDUCED THROMBOCYTOPENIA

Features	Details
Thrombocytopenia	Platelet count of ≤100,000/μL or a decrease in platelet count of ≥50%
Timing	Platelet count falls 5–10 days after starting heparin
Type of heparin	More common with unfractionated heparin than with low-molecular-weight heparin
Type of patient	More common in surgical patients than medical patients; more common in women than in men.
Thrombosis	Venous thrombosis more common than arterial thrombosis

TABLE 112-5 ADVANTAGES OF LMWH[a] OVER HEPARIN

Advantage	Consequence
Better bioavailability and longer half-life after SC injection	Can be given SC once or twice daily for both prophylaxis and treatment
Dose-independent clearance	Simplified dosing
Predictable anticoagulant response	Coagulation monitoring is unnecessary in most patients
Lower risk of heparin-induced thrombocytopenia	Safer than heparin for short- or long-term administration
Lower risk of osteoporosis	Safer than heparin for extended administration

[a]LMWH, low-molecular-weight heparin.

than heparin, LMWH produces a more predictable dose response, and resistance to LMWH is rare. With a longer half-life and more predictable anticoagulant response, LMWH can be given SC once or twice daily without coagulation monitoring, even when the drug is given in treatment doses. These properties render LMWH more convenient than unfractionated heparin. Capitalizing on this feature, studies in patients with venous thromboembolism have shown that home treatment with LMWH is as effective and safe as in-hospital treatment with continuous IV infusions of heparin. Outpatient treatment with LMWH streamlines care, reduces health care costs, and increases patient satisfaction.

MONITORING   In the majority of patients, LMWH does not require coagulation monitoring. If monitoring is necessary, anti-factor Xa levels must be measured because most LMWH preparations have little effect on the aPTT. Therapeutic anti-factor Xa levels with LMWH range from 0.5–1.2 units/mL when measured 3–4 h after drug administration. When LMWH is given in prophylactic doses, peak anti-factor Xa levels of 0.2–0.5 units/mL are desirable.

Indications for LMWH monitoring include renal insufficiency and obesity. LMWH monitoring in patients with a creatinine clearance of ≤50 mL/min is advisable to ensure that there is no drug accumulation. Although weight-adjusted LMWH dosing appears to produce therapeutic anti-factor Xa levels in patients who are overweight, this approach has not been extensively evaluated in those with morbid obesity. It may also be advisable to monitor the anticoagulant activity of LMWH during pregnancy because dose requirements can change, particularly in the third trimester. Monitoring should also be considered in high-risk settings, such as in patients with mechanical heart valves who are given LMWH for prevention of valve thrombosis, and when LMWH is used in treatment doses in infants or children.

DOSING   The doses of LMWH recommended for prophylaxis or treatment vary depending on the LMWH preparation. For prophylaxis, once-daily SC doses of 4000–5000 units are often used, whereas doses of 2500–3000 units are given when the drug is administered twice daily. For treatment of venous thromboembolism, a dose of 150–200 units/kg is given if the drug is administered once daily. If a twice-daily regimen is employed, a dose of 100 units/kg is given. In patients with unstable angina, LMWH is given SC on a twice-daily basis at a dose of 100–120 units/kg.

SIDE EFFECTS   The major complication of LMWH is bleeding. Meta-analyses suggest that the risk of major bleeding is lower with LMWH than with unfractionated heparin. HIT and osteoporosis are less common with LMWH than with unfractionated heparin.

Bleeding   Like the situation with heparin, bleeding with LMWH is more common in patients receiving concomitant therapy with antiplatelet or fibrinolytic drugs. Recent surgery, trauma, or underlying hemostatic defects also increase the risk of bleeding with LMWH.

Although protamine sulfate can be used as an antidote for LMWH, protamine sulfate incompletely neutralizes the anticoagulant activity of LMWH because it only binds the longer chains of LMWH. Because longer chains are responsible for catalysis of thrombin inhibition by antithrombin, protamine sulfate completely reverses the anti-factor IIa activity of LMWH. In contrast, protamine sulfate only partially reverses the anti-factor Xa activity of LMWH because the shorter pentasaccharide-containing chains of LMWH do not bind to protamine sulfate. Consequently, patients at high risk for bleeding may be more safely treated with continuous IV unfractionated heparin than with SC LMWH.

Thrombocytopenia   The risk of HIT is about fivefold lower with LMWH than with heparin. LMWH binds less avidly to platelets and causes less PF4 release. Furthermore, with lower affinity for PF4 than heparin, LMWH is less likely to induce the conformational changes in PF4 that trigger the formation of HIT antibodies.

LMWH should not be used to treat HIT patients because most HIT antibodies exhibit cross-reactivity with LMWH. This in vitro cross-reactivity is not simply a laboratory phenomenon because there are case reports of thrombosis when HIT patients are treated with LMWH.

Osteoporosis   The risk of osteoporosis is lower with long-term LMWH than with heparin. For extended treatment, therefore, LMWH is a better choice than heparin because of the lower risk of osteoporosis and HIT.

Fondaparinux   A synthetic analogue of the antithrombin-binding pentasaccharide sequence, fondaparinux differs from LMWH in several ways (Table 112-6). Fondaparinux is licensed for thromboprophylaxis in general surgical and high-risk orthopedic patients and as an alternative to heparin or LMWH for initial treatment of patients with established venous thromboembolism. It is likely that fondaparinux will also be approved for treatment of patients with acute coronary syndromes.

MECHANISM OF ACTION   As a synthetic analogue of the antithrombin-binding pentasaccharide sequence found in heparin and LMWH, fondaparinux has a molecular weight of 1728. Fondaparinux binds only to antithrombin (Fig. 112-5) and is too short to bridge thrombin to antithrombin. Consequently, fondaparinux catalyzes factor Xa inhibition by antithrombin and does not enhance the rate of thrombin inhibition.

PHARMACOLOGY   Fondaparinux exhibits complete bioavailability after SC injection. With no binding to endothelial cells or plasma proteins, the clearance of fondaparinux is dose independent and its plasma half-life is 17 h. The drug is given SC once daily. Because fondaparinux is cleared unchanged via the kidneys, it is contraindicated in patients with a creatinine clearance < 30 mL/min and should be used with caution in those with a creatinine clearance < 50 mL/min.

Fondaparinux produces a predictable anticoagulant response after administration in fixed doses because it does not bind to plasma proteins. The drug is given at a dose of 2.5 mg once daily for prevention of venous thromboembolism. For initial treatment of established venous thromboembolism, fondaparinux is given at a dose of 7.5 mg once daily. The dose can be reduced to 5 mg once daily for those weighing <50 kg and increased to 10 mg for those >100 kg. When given in these doses, fondaparinux is as effective as heparin or LMWH for initial treatment of patients with DVT or PE and produces similar rates of bleeding.

Fondaparinux is used at a dose of 2.5 mg once daily in patients with acute coronary syndromes. When this prophylactic dose of fondaparinux was compared with treatment doses of enoxaparin in patients with non-ST-segment elevation acute coronary syndromes, there was no difference in the rate of cardiovascular death, MI, or stroke at 9 days. However, the rate of major bleeding was 50% lower with fondaparinux than with enoxaparin, a difference that likely reflects the fact that the dose of fondaparinux was lower than that of enoxaparin. In acute coronary syndrome patients who require percutaneous coronary

TABLE 112-6   COMPARISON OF LMWH[a] AND FONDAPARINUX

Features	LMWH	Fondaparinux
Number of saccharide units	15–17	5
Catalysis of factor Xa inhibition	Yes	Yes
Catalysis of thrombin inhibition	Yes	No
Bioavailability after subcutaneous administration (%)	90	100
Plasma half-life (h)	4	17
Renal excretion	Yes	Yes
Induces release of tissue factor pathway inhibitor	Yes	No
Neutralized by protamine sulfate	Partially	No

[a]LMWH, low-molecular-weight heparin.

interventions, there is a risk of catheter thrombosis with fondaparinux, unless adjunctive heparin is given.

SIDE EFFECTS Fondaparinux does not cause HIT because it does not bind to PF4. In contrast to LMWH, there is no cross-reactivity of fondaparinux with HIT antibodies. Consequently, fondaparinux appears to be effective for treatment of HIT patients, although large clinical trials supporting its use are lacking.

The major side effect of fondaparinux is bleeding. There is no antidote for fondaparinux. Protamine sulfate has no effect on the anticoagulant activity of fondaparinux because it fails to bind to the drug. Recombinant activated factor VII reverses the anticoagulant effects of fondaparinux in volunteers, but it is unknown whether this agent will control fondaparinux-induced bleeding.

Parenteral Direct Thrombin Inhibitors Heparin and LMWH are indirect inhibitors of thrombin because their activity is mediated by antithrombin. In contrast, direct thrombin inhibitors do not require a plasma cofactor; instead, these agents bind directly to thrombin and block its interaction with its substrates. Approved parenteral direct thrombin inhibitors include lepirudin, argatroban, and bivalirudin (Table 112-7). Lepirudin and argatroban are licensed for treatment of patients with HIT, whereas bivalirudin is approved as an alternative to heparin in patients undergoing percutaneous coronary interventions, including those with HIT.

LEPIRUDIN A recombinant form of hirudin, lepirudin is a bivalent direct thrombin inhibitor that interacts with both the active site and exosite 1, the substrate binding site, on thrombin. For rapid anticoagulation, lepirudin is given by continuous IV infusion, but the drug can be given SC for thromboprophylaxis. Lepirudin has a plasma half-life of 60 min after IV infusion and is cleared by the kidneys. Consequently, lepirudin accumulates in patients with renal insufficiency. A high proportion of lepirudin-treated patients develop antibodies against the drug. Although these antibodies rarely cause problems, in a small subset of patients they can delay lepirudin clearance and enhance its anticoagulant activity. Serious bleeding has been reported in some of these patients.

Lepirudin is usually monitored using the aPTT, and the dose is adjusted to maintain an aPTT that is 1.5–2.5 times the control. The aPTT is not an ideal test for monitoring lepirudin therapy because the clotting time plateaus with higher drug concentrations. Although the ecarin clotting time provides a better index of lepirudin dose than the aPTT, the ecarin clotting time has yet to be standardized.

ARGATROBAN A univalent inhibitor that targets the active site of thrombin, argatroban is metabolized in the liver. Consequently, this drug must be used with caution in patients with hepatic insufficiency. Argatroban is not cleared via the kidneys, so this drug is safer than lepirudin for HIT patients with renal insufficiency.

Argatroban is administered by continuous IV infusion and has a plasma half-life of ~45 min. The aPTT is used to monitor its anticoagulant effect, and the dose is adjusted to achieve an aPTT 1.5–3 times the baseline value, but not to exceed 100 sec. Argatroban also prolongs the international normalized ratio (INR), a feature that can complicate the transitioning of patients to warfarin. This problem can be circumvented by using the levels of factor X to monitor warfarin in place of the INR. Alternatively, argatroban can be stopped for 2–3 h prior to INR determination.

BIVALIRUDIN A synthetic 20-amino-acid analogue of hirudin, bivalirudin is a divalent thrombin inhibitor. Thus, the N-terminal portion of bivalirudin interacts with the active site of thrombin, whereas its C-terminal tail binds to exosite 1, the substrate-binding domain on thrombin. Bivalirudin has a plasma half-life of 25 min, the shortest half-life of all the parenteral direct thrombin inhibitors. Bivalirudin is degraded by peptidases and is partially excreted via the kidneys. When given in high doses in the cardiac catheterization laboratory, the anti-

TABLE 112-7 COMPARISON OF THE PROPERTIES OF HIRUDIN, BIVALIRUDIN, AND ARGATROBAN

	Hirudin	Bivalirudin	Argatroban
Molecular mass	7000	1980	527
Site(s) of interaction with thrombin	Active site and exosite 1	Active site and exosite 1	Active site
Renal clearance	Yes	No	No
Hepatic metabolism	No	No	Yes
Plasma half-life (min)	60	25	45

coagulant activity of bivalirudin is monitored using the activated clotting time. With lower doses, its activity can be assessed using the aPTT.

Studies comparing bivalirudin with heparin suggest that bivalirudin produces less bleeding. This feature plus its short half-life make bivalirudin an attractive alternative to heparin in patients undergoing percutaneous coronary interventions. Bivalirudin also has been used successfully in HIT patients who require percutaneous coronary interventions.

ORAL ANTICOAGULANTS
Current oral anticoagulant practice dates back almost 60 years to when the vitamin K antagonists were discovered as a result of investigations into the cause of hemorrhagic disease in cattle. Characterized by a decrease in prothrombin levels, this disorder is caused by ingestion of hay containing spoiled sweet clover. Hydroxycoumarin, which was isolated from bacterial contaminants in the hay, interferes with vitamin K metabolism, thereby causing a syndrome similar to vitamin K deficiency.

Warfarin A water-soluble vitamin K antagonist initially developed as a rodenticide, warfarin is the coumarin derivative most often prescribed in North America. Like other vitamin K antagonists, warfarin interferes with the synthesis of the vitamin K–dependent clotting proteins, which include prothrombin (factor II) and factors VII, IX, and X. The synthesis of the vitamin K–dependent anticoagulant proteins, proteins C and S, is also reduced by vitamin K antagonists.

MECHANISM OF ACTION All of the vitamin K–dependent clotting factors possess glutamic acid residues at their N termini. A posttranslational modification adds a carboxyl group to the γ-carbon of these residues to generate γ-carboxyglutamic acid. This modification is essential for expression of the activity of these clotting factors because it permits their calcium-dependent binding to negatively charged phospholipid surfaces. The γ-carboxylation process is catalyzed by a vitamin K–dependent carboxylase. Thus, vitamin K from the diet is reduced to vitamin K hydroquinone by vitamin K reductase (Fig. 112-6). Vitamin K hydroquinone serves as a cofactor for the carboxylase enzyme, which in the presence of carbon dioxide replaces the hydrogen on the γ-carbon of glutamic acid residues with a carboxyl group. During this process, vitamin K hydroquinone is oxidized to vitamin K epoxide, which is then reduced to vitamin K by vitamin K epoxide reductase.

Warfarin inhibits vitamin K epoxide reductase (VKOR), thereby blocking the γ-carboxylation process. This results in the synthesis of vitamin K–dependent clotting proteins that are only partially γ-carboxylated. Warfarin acts as an anticoagulant because these partially γ-carboxylated proteins have reduced or absent biologic activity. The onset of action of warfarin is delayed until the newly synthesized clotting factors with reduced activity gradually replace their fully active counterparts.

The antithrombotic effect of warfarin depends on a reduction in the functional levels of factor X and prothrombin, clotting factors that have half-lives of 24 and 72 h, respectively. Because of the delay in achieving an antithrombotic effect, initial treatment with warfarin is supported by concomitant administration of a rapidly acting parenteral anticoagulant, such as heparin, LMWH, or fondaparinux, in patients with established thrombosis or at high risk for thrombosis.

PHARMACOLOGY Warfarin is a racemic mixture of R and S isomers. Warfarin is rapidly and almost completely absorbed from the gas-

FIGURE 112-6 Mechanism of action of warfarin. By blocking vitamin K epoxide reductase, warfarin inhibits vitamin K–dependent γ-carboxylation of factors II, VII, IX, and X. Dietary vitamin K is reduced to vitamin K hydroquinone (vitamin KH₂) by vitamin K reductase. Vitamin KH₂ serves as a cofactor for a vitamin K–dependent carboxylase that catalyzes the γ-carboxylation process, thereby converting prozymogens to zymogens capable of binding calcium and interacting with anionic phospholipid surfaces. During this process, vitamin KH₂ is oxidized to vitamin K epoxide, which is then reduced to vitamin K by vitamin K epoxide reductase.

trointestinal tract. Levels of warfarin in the blood peak about 90 min after drug administration. Racemic warfarin has a plasma half-life of 36–42 h, and >97% of circulating warfarin is bound to albumin. It is only the small fraction of unbound warfarin that is biologically active.

Warfarin accumulates in the liver where the two isomers are metabolized via distinct pathways. Oxidative metabolism of the more active S-isomer is effected by CYP2C9. Two relatively common variants, *CYP2C9*2* and *CYP2C9*3*, have reduced activity. Patients with these variants require lower maintenance dose of warfarin. Polymorphisms in VKORC1 can also influence the anticoagulant response to warfarin. These findings have prompted the recommendation that patients starting on warfarin should be tested for these polymorphisms and that this information should be incorporated into their warfarin dosing algorithms.

In addition to genetic factors, the anticoagulant effect of warfarin is influenced by diet, drugs, and various disease states. Fluctuations in dietary vitamin K intake affect the activity of warfarin. A wide variety of drugs can alter absorption, clearance, or metabolism of warfarin. Because of the variability in the anticoagulant response to warfarin, coagulation monitoring is essential to ensure that a therapeutic response is obtained.

MONITORING Warfarin therapy is most often monitored using the prothrombin time, a test that is sensitive to reductions in the levels of prothrombin, factor VII, and factor X. The test is performed by adding thromboplastin, a reagent that contains tissue factor, phospholipid, and calcium, to citrated plasma and determining the time to clot formation. Thromboplastins vary in their sensitivity to reductions in the levels of the vitamin K–dependent clotting factors. Thus, less sensitive thromboplastins will trigger the administration of higher doses of warfarin to achieve a target prothrombin time. This is problematic because higher doses of warfarin increase the risk of bleeding.

The INR was developed to circumvent many of the problems associated with the prothrombin time. To calculate the INR, the patient's prothrombin time is divided by the mean normal prothrombin time, and this ratio is then multiplied by the international sensitivity index (ISI), an index of the sensitivity of the thromboplastin used for prothrombin time determination to reductions in the levels of the vitamin K–dependent clotting factors. Highly sensitive thromboplastins have an ISI of 1.0. Most current thromboplastins have ISI values that range from 1.0–1.4.

Although the INR has helped to standardize anticoagulant practice, problems persist. The precision of INR determination varies depending on reagent-coagulometer combinations. This leads to variability in the INR results. Also complicating INR determination is unreliable reporting of the ISI by thromboplastin manufacturers. Furthermore, every laboratory must establish the mean normal prothrombin time with each new batch of thromboplastin reagent. To accomplish this, the prothrombin time must be measured in fresh plasma samples from at least 20 healthy volunteers using the same coagulometer that is used for patient samples.

For most indications, warfarin is administered in doses that produce a target INR of 2.0–3.0. An exception is patients with mechanical heart valves, where a target INR of 2.5–3.5 is recommended. Studies in atrial fibrillation demonstrate an increased risk of cardioembolic stroke when the INR falls to <1.7 and an increase in bleeding with INR values >4.5. These findings highlight the fact that vitamin K antagonists have a narrow therapeutic window. In support of this concept, a study in patients receiving long-term warfarin therapy for unprovoked venous thromboembolism demonstrated a higher rate of recurrent venous thromboembolism with a target INR of 1.5–1.9 compared with a target INR of 2.0–3.0.

DOSING Warfarin is usually started at a dose of 5–10 mg. The dose is then titrated to achieve the desired target INR. Because of its delayed onset of action, patients with established thrombosis or those at high risk for thrombosis are given concomitant treatment with a rapidly acting parenteral anticoagulant, such as heparin, LMWH, or fondaparinux. Initial prolongation of the INR reflects reduction in the functional levels of factor VII. Consequently, concomitant treatment with the parenteral anticoagulant should be continued until the INR has been therapeutic for at least two consecutive days. A minimum 5-day course of parenteral anticoagulation is recommended to ensure that the levels of prothrombin have been reduced into the therapeutic range with warfarin.

Because warfarin has a narrow therapeutic window, frequent coagulation monitoring is essential to ensure that a therapeutic anticoagulant response is obtained. Even patients with stable warfarin dose requirements should have their INR determined every 2–3 weeks. More frequent monitoring is necessary when new medications are introduced because so many drugs enhance or reduce the anticoagulant effects of warfarin.

SIDE EFFECTS Like all anticoagulants, the major side effect of warfarin is bleeding. A rare complication is skin necrosis. Warfarin crosses the placenta and can cause fetal abnormalities. Consequently, warfarin should not be used during pregnancy.

Bleeding At least half of the bleeding complications with warfarin occur when the INR exceeds the therapeutic range. Bleeding complications may be mild, such as epistaxis or hematuria, or more severe, such as retroperitoneal or gastrointestinal bleeding. Life-threatening intracranial bleeding can also occur.

To minimize the risk of bleeding, the INR should be maintained in the therapeutic range. In asymptomatic patients whose INR is between 3.5 and 4.5, warfarin should be withheld until the INR returns to the therapeutic range. If the INR is >4.5, a therapeutic INR can be achieved more rapidly by administration of low doses of sublingual vitamin K. A vitamin K dose of 1 mg is usually adequate for patients with an INR between 4.9 and 9, whereas 2–3 mg can be used for those with an INR > 9. Higher doses of vitamin K can be administered if more rapid reversal of the INR is required or if the INR is excessively high.

Patients with serious bleeding need more aggressive treatment. These patients should be given 10 mg of vitamin K by slow IV infusion. Additional vitamin K should be given until the INR is in the normal range. Treatment with vitamin K should be supplemented with fresh-frozen plasma as a source of the vitamin K–dependent clotting proteins. For life-threatening bleeds, or if patients cannot tolerate the volume load, recombinant factor VIIa or prothrombin complex concentrates can be used.

Warfarin-treated patients who experience bleeding when their INR is in the therapeutic range require investigation into the cause of the bleeding. Those with gastrointestinal bleeding often have underlying peptic ulcer disease or a tumor. Similarly, investigation of hematuria or uterine bleeding in patients with a therapeutic INR may unmask a tumor of the genitourinary tract.

Skin Necrosis A rare complication of warfarin, skin necrosis usually is seen 2–5 days after initiation of therapy. Well-demarcated erythematous lesions form on the thighs, buttocks, breasts, or toes. Typically, the center of the lesion becomes progressively necrotic. Examination of skin biopsies taken from the border of these lesions reveals thrombi in the microvasculature.

Warfarin-induced skin necrosis is seen in patients with congenital or acquired deficiencies of protein C or protein S. Initiation of warfarin therapy in these patients produces a precipitous fall in plasma levels of proteins C or S, thereby eliminating this important anticoagulant pathway before warfarin exerts an antithrombotic effect through lowering of the functional levels of factor X and prothrombin. The resultant procoagulant state triggers thrombosis. Why the thrombosis is localized to the microvasculature of fatty tissues is unclear.

Treatment involves discontinuation of warfarin and reversal with vitamin K, if needed. An alternative anticoagulant, such as heparin or LMWH, should be given in patients with thrombosis. Protein C concentrates or recombinant activated protein C can be given to protein C–deficient patients to accelerate healing of the skin lesions; fresh-frozen plasma may be of value for those with protein S deficiency. Occasionally, skin grafting is necessary when there is extensive skin loss.

Because of the potential for skin necrosis, patients with known protein C or protein S deficiency require overlapping treatment with a parenteral anticoagulant when initiating warfarin therapy. Warfarin should be started in low doses in these patients, and the parenteral anticoagulant should be continued until the INR is therapeutic for at least two to three consecutive days.

Pregnancy Warfarin crosses the placenta and can cause fetal abnormalities or bleeding. The fetal abnormalities include a characteristic embryopathy, which consists of nasal hypoplasia and stippled epiphyses. The risk of embryopathy is highest if warfarin is given in the first trimester of pregnancy. Central nervous system abnormalities can also occur with exposure to coumarins at any time during pregnancy. Finally, maternal administration of warfarin produces an anticoagulant effect in the fetus that can cause bleeding. This is of particular concern at delivery when trauma to the head during passage through the birth canal can lead to intracranial bleeding. Because of these potential problems, warfarin is contraindicated in pregnancy, particularly in the first and third trimesters. Instead, heparin, LMWH, or fondaparinux can be given during pregnancy for prevention or treatment of thrombosis.

Warfarin does not pass into the breast milk. Consequently, warfarin can safely be given to nursing mothers.

Special Problems Patients with a lupus anticoagulant or those who need urgent or elective surgery present special challenges. Although observational studies suggested that patients with thrombosis complicating the antiphospholipid antibody syndrome required higher intensity warfarin regimens to prevent recurrent thromboembolic events, two randomized trials showed that targeting an INR of 2.0–3.0 is as effective as higher intensity treatment and produces less bleeding. Monitoring warfarin therapy can be problematic in patients with antiphospholipid antibody syndrome if the lupus anticoagulant prolongs the baseline INR.

If patients receiving long-term warfarin treatment require an elective invasive procedure, warfarin can be stopped 5 days before the procedure to allow the INR to return to normal levels. Those at high risk for recurrent thrombosis can be bridged with once- or twice-daily SC injections of LMWH when the INR falls to <2.0. The last dose of LMWH should be given 12–24 h before the procedure, depending on whether LMWH is administered twice or once daily. After the procedure, treatment with warfarin can be restarted.

New Oral Anticoagulants New oral anticoagulants that target thrombin or factor Xa are under development. These drugs have a rapid onset of action and have half-lives that permit once- or twice-daily administration. Designed to produce a predictable level of anticoagulation, these new oral agents can be given in fixed doses without coagulation monitoring. Therefore, these drugs will be more convenient to administer than warfarin. The results of ongoing phase II and III clinical trials will determine the role of these new oral anticoagulants in the prevention and treatment of thrombosis.

FIBRINOLYTIC DRUGS

ROLE OF FIBRINOLYTIC THERAPY

Fibrinolytic drugs can be used to degrade thrombi and are administered systemically or can be delivered via catheters directly into the substance of the thrombus. Systemic delivery is used for treatment of acute MI, acute ischemic stroke, and most cases of massive PE. The goal of therapy is to produce rapid thrombus dissolution, thereby restoring antegrade blood flow. In the coronary circulation, restoration of blood flow reduces morbidity and mortality by limiting myocardial damage, whereas in the cerebral circulation, rapid thrombus dissolution decreases the neuronal death and brain infarction that produce irreversible brain injury. For patients with massive PE, the goal of thrombolytic therapy is to restore pulmonary artery perfusion.

Peripheral arterial thrombi and thrombi in the proximal deep veins of the leg are most often treated using catheter-directed thrombolytic therapy. Catheters with multiple side holes can be utilized to enhance drug delivery. In some cases, intravascular devices that fragment and extract the thrombus are used to hasten treatment. These devices can be used alone or in conjunction with fibrinolytic drugs.

MECHANISM OF ACTION

Currently approved fibrinolytic agents include streptokinase; acylated plasminogen streptokinase activator complex (anistreplase); urokinase; recombinant tissue-type plasminogen activator (rt-PA), which is also known as alteplase or activase; and two recombinant derivatives of rt-PA, tenecteplase and reteplase. All of these agents act by converting the proenzyme, plasminogen, to plasmin, the active enzyme (Fig. 112-7). Plasmin then degrades the fibrin matrix of thrombi and produces soluble fibrin degradation products.

Endogenous fibrinolysis is regulated at two levels. Plasminogen activator inhibitors, particularly the type 1 form (PAI-1), prevent excessive plasminogen activation by regulating the activity of t-PA and urokinase-type plasminogen activator (u-PA). Once plasmin is generated, it is regulated by plasmin inhibitors, the most important of which is α_2-antiplasmin. The plasma concentration of plasminogen is twofold higher than that of α_2-antiplasmin. Consequently, with pharmacologic doses of plasmino-

FIGURE 112-7 The fibrinolytic system and its regulation. Plasminogen activators convert plasminogen to plasmin. Plasmin then degrades fibrin into soluble fibrin degradation products. The system is regulated at two levels. Type 1 plasminogen activator inhibitor (PAI-1) regulates the plasminogen activators, whereas α_2-antiplasmin serves as the major inhibitor of plasmin.

gen activators, the concentration of plasmin that is generated can exceed that of α₂-antiplasmin. In addition to degrading fibrin, unregulated plasmin can also degrade fibrinogen and other clotting factors. This process, which is known as the *systemic lytic state*, reduces the hemostatic potential of the blood and increases the risk of bleeding.

The endogenous fibrinolytic system is geared to localize plasmin generation to the fibrin surface. Both plasminogen and t-PA bind to fibrin to form a ternary complex that promotes efficient plasminogen activation. In contrast to free plasmin, plasmin generated on the fibrin surface is relatively protected from inactivation by α₂-antiplasmin, a feature that promotes fibrin dissolution. Furthermore, C-terminal lysine residues exposed as plasmin degrades fibrin serve as binding sites for additional plasminogen and t-PA molecules. This creates a positive feedback that enhances plasmin generation. When used pharmacologically, the various plasminogen activators capitalize on these mechanisms to a lesser or greater extent.

Plasminogen activators that preferentially activate fibrin-bound plasminogen are considered fibrin-specific. In contrast, nonspecific plasminogen activators do not discriminate between fibrin-bound and circulating plasminogen. Activation of circulating plasminogen results in the generation of unopposed plasmin that can trigger the systemic lytic state. Alteplase and its derivatives are fibrin-specific plasminogen activators, whereas streptokinase, anistreplase, and urokinase are nonspecific agents.

STREPTOKINASE

Unlike other plasminogen activators, streptokinase is not an enzyme and does not directly convert plasminogen to plasmin. Instead, streptokinase forms a 1:1 stoichiometric complex with plasminogen. Formation of this complex induces a conformational change in plasminogen that exposes its active site (Fig. 112-8). This conformationally altered plasminogen then converts additional plasminogen molecules to plasmin.

Streptokinase has no affinity for fibrin, and the streptokinase-plasminogen complex activates both free and fibrin-bound plasminogen. Activation of circulating plasminogen generates sufficient amounts of plasmin to overwhelm α₂-antiplasmin. Unopposed plasmin not only degrades fibrin in the occlusive thrombus but also induces a systemic lytic state.

When given systemically to patients with acute MI, streptokinase reduces mortality. For this indication, the drug is usually given as an IV infusion of 1.5 million units over 30–60 min. Patients who receive streptokinase can develop antibodies against the drug, as can patients with prior streptococcal injection. These antibodies can reduce the effectiveness of streptokinase.

Allergic reactions occur in ~5% of patients treated with streptokinase. These may manifest as a rash, fever, chills, and rigors. Although anaphylactic reactions can occur, these are rare. Transient hypotension is common with streptokinase and has been attributed to plasmin-mediated release of bradykinin from kallikrein. The hypotension usually responds to leg elevation and administration of IV fluids and low-doses of vasopressors, such as dopamine or norepinephrine.

ANISTREPLASE

To generate this drug, streptokinase is combined with equimolar amounts of Lys-plasminogen, a plasmin-cleaved form of plasminogen with a Lys residue at its N terminus. The active site of Lys-plasminogen that is exposed upon combination with streptokinase is then masked with an anisoyl group. After IV infusion, the anisoyl group is slowly removed by deacylation, giving the complex a half-life of ~100 min. This allows drug administration via a single bolus infusion.

Although it is more convenient to administer, anistreplase offers few mechanistic advantages over streptokinase. Like streptokinase, anistreplase does not distinguish between fibrin-bound and circulating plasminogen. Consequently, it too produces a systemic lytic state. Likewise, allergic reactions and hypotension are just as frequent with anistreplase as they are with streptokinase.

When anistreplase was compared with alteplase in patients with acute MI, reperfusion was obtained more rapidly with alteplase than with anistreplase. Improved reperfusion was associated with a trend toward better

FIGURE 112-8 Mechanism of action of streptokinase. Streptokinase binds to plasminogen and induces a conformational change in plasminogen that exposes its active site. The streptokinase/plasmin(ogen) complex then serves as the activator of additional plasminogen molecules.

clinical outcomes and reduced mortality with alteplase. These results and the high cost of anistreplase have dampened the enthusiasm for its use.

UROKINASE

Urokinase is a two-chain serine protease derived from cultured fetal kidney cells with a molecular weight of 34,000. Urokinase converts plasminogen to plasmin directly by cleaving the Arg560-Val561 bond. Unlike streptokinase, urokinase is not immunogenic and allergic reactions are rare. Urokinase produces a systemic lytic state because it does not discriminate between fibrin-bound and circulating plasminogen.

Despite many years of use, urokinase has never been systemically evaluated for coronary thrombolysis. Instead, urokinase is often employed for catheter-directed lysis of thrombi in the deep veins or the peripheral arteries. Because of production problems, the availability of urokinase is limited.

ALTEPLASE

A recombinant form of single-chain t-PA, alteplase has a molecular weight of 68,000. Alteplase is rapidly converted into its two-chain form by plasmin. Although single- and two-chain forms of t-PA have equivalent activity in the presence of fibrin, in its absence, single-chain t-PA has tenfold lower activity.

Alteplase consists of five discrete domains (Fig. 112-9); the N-terminal A chain of two-chain alteplase contains four of these domains. Residues 4 through 50 make up the finger domain, a region that resembles the finger domain of fibronectin; residues 50 through 87 are homologous with epidermal growth factor, whereas residues 92 through 173 and 180 through 261, which have homology to the kringle domains of plasminogen, are designated as the first and second kringle, respectively. The fifth alteplase domain is the protease domain; it is located on the C-terminal B chain of two-chain alteplase.

The interaction of alteplase with fibrin is mediated by the finger domain and, to a lesser extent, by the second kringle domain. The affinity of alteplase for fibrin is considerably higher than that for fibrinogen. Consequently, the catalytic efficiency of plasminogen activation by alteplase is two to three orders of magnitude higher in the presence of fibrin than in the presence of fibrinogen. This phenomenon helps to localize plasmin generation to the fibrin surface.

Although alteplase preferentially activates plasminogen in the presence of fibrin, alteplase is not as fibrin-selective as was first predicted. Its fibrin specificity is limited because like fibrin, (DD)E, the major soluble degradation product of cross-linked fibrin, binds alteplase and plasminogen with high affinity. Consequently, (DD)E is as potent as fibrin as a stimula-

FIGURE 112-9 Domain structures of alteplase (t-PA), tenecteplase (TNK-t-PA), desmoteplase (b-PA), and reteplase (r-PA). The finger (F), epidermal growth factor (EGF), first and second kringles (K1 and K2, respectively), and protease (P) domains are illustrated. The glycosylation site (Y) on K1 has been repositioned in tenecteplase to endow it with a longer half-life. In addition, a tetra-alanine substitution in the protease domain renders tenecteplase resistant to PAI-1 inhibition. Desmoteplase differs from alteplase and tenecteplase in that it lacks a K2 domain. Reteplase is a truncated variant that lacks the F, EGF, and K1 domains.

tor of plasminogen activation by alteplase. Whereas plasmin generated on the fibrin surface results in thrombolysis, plasmin generated on the surface of circulating (DD)E degrades fibrinogen. Fibrinogenolysis results in the accumulation of fragment X, a high-molecular-weight clottable fibrinogen degradation product. Incorporation of fragment X into hemostatic plugs formed at sites of vascular injury renders them susceptible to lysis. This phenomenon may contribute to alteplase-induced bleeding.

A trial comparing alteplase with streptokinase for treatment of patients with acute MI demonstrated significantly lower mortality with alteplase than with streptokinase, although the absolute difference was small. The greatest benefit was seen in patients <75 years with anterior MI who presented <6 h after symptom onset.

For treatment of acute MI or acute ischemic stroke, alteplase is given as an IV infusion over 60–90 min. The total dose of alteplase usually ranges from 90–100 mg. Allergic reactions and hypotension are rare, and alteplase is not immunogenic.

TENECTEPLASE

Tenecteplase is a genetically engineered variant of t-PA and was designed to have a longer half-life than t-PA and to be resistant to inactivation by PAI-1. To prolong its half-life, a new glycosylation site was added to the first kringle domain (Fig. 112-9). Because addition of this extra carbohydrate side chain reduced fibrin affinity, the existing glycosylation site on the first kringle domain was removed. To render the molecule resistant to inhibition by PAI-1, a tetra-alanine substitution was introduced at residues 296–299 in the protease domain, the region responsible for the interaction of t-PA with PAI-1.

Tenecteplase is more fibrin-specific than t-PA. Although both agents bind to fibrin with similar affinity, the affinity of tenecteplase for (DD)E is significantly lower than that of t-PA. Consequently, (DD)E does not stimulate systemic plasminogen activation by tenecteplase to the same extent as t-PA. As a result, tenecteplase produces less fibrinogenolysis than t-PA.

For coronary thrombolysis, tenecteplase is given as a single IV bolus. In a large phase III trial that enrolled >16,000 patients, the 30-day

mortality rate with single-bolus tenecteplase was similar to that with accelerated dose t-PA. Although rates of intracranial hemorrhage were also similar with both treatments, patients given tenecteplase had fewer noncerebral bleeds and a reduced need for blood transfusions than those treated with t-PA. The improved safety profile of tenecteplase likely reflects its enhanced fibrin specificity.

RETEPLASE

Reteplase is a recombinant t-PA derivative and is a single-chain variant that lacks the finger, epidermal growth factor, and first kringle domains (Fig. 112-9). This truncated derivative has a molecular weight of 39,000. Reteplase binds fibrin more weakly than t-PA because it lacks the finger domain. Because it is produced in *Escherichia coli*, reteplase is not glycosylated. This endows it with a plasma half-life longer than that of t-PA. Consequently, reteplase is given as two IV boluses, which are separated by 30 min. Clinical trials have demonstrated that reteplase is at least as effective as streptokinase for treatment of acute MI, but the agent is not superior to t-PA.

NEW FIBRINOLYTIC AGENTS

Several new drugs are under investigation. These include desmoteplase (Fig. 112-9), a recombinant form of the full-length plasminogen activator isolated from the saliva of the vampire bat, and alfimeprase, a truncated form of fibrolase, an enzyme isolated from the venom of the southern copperhead snake. Desmoteplase, which is more fibrin-specific than t-PA, is being investigated for the treatment of acute ischemic stroke. With a potential for enhanced safety, desmoteplase may extend the window for treatment beyond 3 h. An ongoing phase III clinical trial is exploring this possibility. Alfimeprase is a metalloproteinase that degrades fibrin in a plasmin-independent fashion. Because of its unique mechanism of action, it was hoped that alfimeprase would provide more rapid degradation of thrombi. However, a phase III trial investigating the use of this agent in patients with peripheral arterial occlusion has been halted, at least temporarily. Therefore, the future of this drug is uncertain.

CONCLUSIONS AND FUTURE DIRECTIONS

Arterial and venous thromboses reflect a complex interplay among the vessel wall, platelets, the coagulation system, and the fibrinolytic pathways. Activation of coagulation also triggers inflammatory pathways that may contribute to thrombogenesis. A better understanding of the biochemistry of blood coagulation and advances in structure-based drug design have identified new targets and resulted in the development of novel antithrombotic drugs. Well-designed clinical trials have provided detailed information on which drugs to use and when to use them. Despite these advances, however, thromboembolic disorders remain a major cause of morbidity and mortality. Therefore, the search for better targets and more potent antiplatelet, anticoagulant, and fibrinolytic drugs continues.

FURTHER READINGS

KAMALI F: Genetic influences on the response to warfarin. Curr Opin Hematol 13:357, 2006

KEELING D et al: The management of heparin-induced thrombocytopenia. Br J Haematol 133:259, 2006

LIM W et al: Management of antiphospholipid antibody syndrome: A systematic review. JAMA 295:1050, 2006

MEADOWS TA, BHATT DL: Clinical aspects of platelet inhibitors and thrombus formation. Circ Res 100:1261, 2007

PALARETI G et al: D-Dimer testing to determine the duration of anticoagulation therapy. N Engl J Med 355:1780, 2006

SEGAL JB et al: Management of venous thromboembolism: A systematic review for a practice guideline. Ann Intern Med 146:211, 2007

SIMIONI P, TORMENE D: Inherited thrombophilia and venous thromboembolism. Semin Thromb Hemost 32:700, 2006

YUSUF S, MEHTA SR: Comparison of fondaparinux and enoxaparin in acute coronary syndromes. N Engl J Med 354:1464, 2006

113 Introduction to Infectious Diseases: Host–Pathogen Interactions

Lawrence C. Madoff, Dennis L. Kasper

Despite decades of dramatic progress in their treatment and prevention, infectious diseases remain a major cause of death and debility and are responsible for worsening the living conditions of many millions of people around the world. Infections frequently challenge the physician's diagnostic skill and must be considered in the differential diagnoses of syndromes affecting every organ system.

CHANGING EPIDEMIOLOGY OF INFECTIOUS DISEASES

With the advent of antimicrobial agents, some medical leaders believed that infectious diseases would soon be eliminated and become of historic interest only. Indeed, the hundreds of chemotherapeutic agents developed since World War II, most of which are potent and safe, include drugs effective not only against bacteria but also against viruses, fungi, and parasites. Nevertheless, we now realize that as we developed antimicrobial agents, microbes developed the ability to elude our best weapons and to counterattack with new survival strategies. Antibiotic resistance occurs at an alarming rate among all classes of mammalian pathogens. Pneumococci resistant to penicillin and enterococci resistant to vancomycin have become commonplace. Even *Staphylococcus aureus* strains resistant to vancomycin have appeared. Such pathogens present real clinical problems in managing infections that were easily treatable just a few years ago. Diseases once thought to have been nearly eradicated from the developed world—tuberculosis, cholera, and rheumatic fever, for example—have rebounded with renewed ferocity. Newly discovered and emerging infectious agents appear to have been brought into contact with humans by changes in the environment and by movements of human and animal populations. An example of the propensity for pathogens to escape from their usual niche is the alarming 1999 outbreak in New York of encephalitis due to West Nile virus, which had never previously been isolated in the Americas. In 2003, severe acute respiratory syndrome (SARS) was first recognized. This emerging clinical entity is caused by a novel coronavirus that may have jumped from an animal niche to become a significant human pathogen. By 2006, H5N1 avian influenza, having spread rapidly through poultry farms in Asia and having caused deaths in exposed humans, had reached Europe and Africa, heightening fears of a new influenza pandemic.

Many infectious agents have been discovered only in recent decades (Fig. 113-1). Ebola virus, human metapneumovirus, *Anaplasma phagocytophila* (the agent of human granulocytotropic ehrlichiosis), and retroviruses such as HIV humble us despite our deepening understanding of pathogenesis at the most basic molecular level. Even in developed countries, infectious diseases have made a resurgence. Between 1980 and 1996, mortality from infectious diseases in the United States increased by 64% to levels not seen since the 1940s.

The role of infectious agents in the etiology of diseases once believed to be noninfectious is increasingly recognized. For example, it is now widely accepted that *Helicobacter pylori* is the causative agent of peptic ulcer disease and perhaps of gastric malignancy. Human papillomavirus is likely to be the most important cause of invasive cervical cancer. Human herpesvirus type 8 is believed to be the cause of most cases of Kaposi's sarcoma. Epstein-Barr virus is a cause of certain lymphomas and may play a role in the genesis of Hodgkin's disease. The possibility certainly exists that other diseases of unknown cause, such as rheumatoid arthritis, sarcoidosis, or inflammatory bowel disease, have infectious etiologies. There is even evidence that atherosclerosis may have an infectious component. In contrast, there are data to suggest that decreased exposures to pathogens in childhood may be contributing to an increase in the observed rates of allergic diseases.

Medical advances against infectious diseases have been hindered by changes in patient populations. Immunocompromised hosts now constitute a significant proportion of the seriously infected population. Physicians immunosuppress their patients to prevent the rejection of transplants and to treat neoplastic and inflammatory diseases. Some infections, most notably that caused by HIV, immunocompromise the host in and of themselves. Lesser degrees of immunosuppression are associated with other infections, such as influenza and syphilis. Infectious agents that coexist peacefully with immunocompetent hosts wreak havoc in those who lack a complete immune system. AIDS has brought to prominence once-obscure organisms such as *Pneumocystis*, *Cryptosporidium parvum*, and *Mycobacterium avium*.

HOST FACTORS IN INFECTION

For any infectious process to occur, the pathogen and the host must first encounter each other. Factors such as geography, environment, and behavior thus influence the likelihood of infection. Although the initial encounter between a susceptible host and a virulent organism frequently results in disease, some organisms can be harbored in the host for years before disease becomes clinically evident. For a complete view, individual patients must be considered in the context of the population to which they belong. Infectious diseases do not often occur in isolation; rather, they spread through a group exposed from a point source (e.g., a contaminated water supply) or from one individual to another (e.g., via respiratory droplets). Thus, the clinician must be alert to infections prevalent in the community as a whole. A detailed history, including information on travel, behavioral factors, exposures to animals or potentially contaminated environments, and living and occupational conditions, must be elicited. For example, the likelihood of infection by *Plasmodium falciparum* can be significantly affected by altitude, climate, terrain, season, and even time of day. Antibiotic-resistant strains of *P. falciparum* are localized to specific geographic regions, and a seemingly minor alteration in a travel itinerary can dramatically influence the likelihood of acquiring chloroquine-resistant malaria. If such important details in the history are overlooked, inappropriate treatment may result in the death of the patient. Likewise, the chance of acquiring a sexually transmitted disease can be greatly affected by a relatively minor variation in sexual practices, such as the method used for contraception. Knowledge of the relationship between specific risk factors and disease allows the physician to influence a patient's health even before the development of infection by modification of these risk factors and—when a vaccine is available—by immunization.

Many specific host factors influence the likelihood of acquiring an infectious disease. Age, immunization history, prior illnesses, level of nutrition, pregnancy, coexisting illness, and perhaps emotional state all have some impact on the risk of infection after exposure to a potential pathogen. The importance of individual host defense mechanisms, either specific or nonspecific, becomes apparent in their absence, and

FIGURE 113-1 Map of the world showing examples of geographic locales where infectious diseases were noted to have emerged or resurged. *(Adapted from Addressing Emerging Infectious Disease Threats: A Prevention Strategy for the United States, Department of Health and Human Services, Centers for Disease Control and Prevention, 1994.)*

our understanding of these immune mechanisms is enhanced by studies of clinical syndromes developing in immunodeficient patients (Table 113-1). For example, the higher attack rate of meningococcal disease among people with deficiencies in specific complement proteins of the so-called membrane attack complex (see "Adaptive Immunity," below) than in the general population underscores the importance of an intact complement system in the prevention of meningococcal infection.

Medical care itself increases the patient's risk of acquiring an infection in several ways: (1) through contact with pathogens during hospitalization, (2) through breaching of the skin (with intravenous devices or surgical incisions) or mucosal surfaces (with endotracheal tubes or bladder catheters), (3) through introduction of foreign bodies, (4) through alteration of the natural flora with antibiotics, and (5) through treatment with immunosuppressive drugs.

Infection involves complicated interactions of microbe and host and inevitably affects both. In most cases, a pathogenic process consisting of several steps is required for the development of infections. Since the competent host has a complex series of barricades in place to prevent infection, the successful pathogen must use specific strategies at each of these steps. The specific strategies used by bacteria, viruses, and parasites (Chap. 114) have some remarkable conceptual similarities, but the strategic details are unique not only for each class of microorganism but also for individual species within a class.

THE IMMUNE RESPONSE

INNATE IMMUNITY

As they have co-evolved with microbes, higher organisms have developed mechanisms for recognizing and responding to microorganisms. Many of these mechanisms, referred to together as *innate immunity*, are evolutionarily ancient, having been conserved from insects to humans. In general, innate immune mechanisms exploit molecular patterns found specifically in pathogenic microorganisms. These "pathogen signatures" are recognized by host molecules that either directly interfere with the pathogen or initiate a response that does so. Innate immunity serves to protect the host without prior exposure to an infectious agent—i.e., before specific or adaptive immunity has had a chance to develop. Innate immunity also functions as a warning system that activates components of adaptive immunity early in the course of infection.

Toll-like receptors (TLRs) are instructive in illustrating how organisms are detected and send signals to the immune system. There are at least 11 TLRs, each specific to different biologic classes of molecules. For example, even minuscule amounts of lipopolysaccharide (LPS), a molecule found uniquely in gram-negative bacteria, are detected by LPS-binding protein, CD14, and TLR4 (see Fig. 114-3). The interaction of LPS with these components of the innate immune system prompts macrophages, via the transcriptional activator nuclear factor κB (NF-κB), to produce cytokines that lead to inflammation and enzymes that enhance the clearance of microbes. These initial responses serve not only to limit infection but also to initiate specific or adaptive immune responses.

ADAPTIVE IMMUNITY

Once in contact with the host immune system, the microorganism faces the host's tightly integrated cellular and humoral immune responses. Cellular immunity (Chap. 308), comprising T lymphocytes, macrophages, and natural killer cells, primarily recognizes and combats pathogens that proliferate intracellularly. Cellular immune mechanisms are important in immunity to all classes of infectious agents, including most viruses and many bacteria (e.g., *Mycoplasma, Chlamydophila, Listeria, Salmonella,* and *Mycobacterium*), parasites (e.g., *Trypanosoma, Toxoplasma,* and *Leishmania*), and fungi (e.g., *Histoplasma, Cryptococcus,* and *Coccidioides*). Usually, T lymphocytes are activated by macrophages and B lymphocytes, which present foreign antigens along with the host's own major histocompatibility complex antigen to the T cell receptor. Activated T cells may then act in several ways to fight infection. *Cytotoxic* T cells may directly attack and lyse host cells that express foreign antigens. *Helper* T cells stimulate the proliferation of B cells and the production of immunoglobulins. Antigen-presenting cells and T cells communicate with each other via a variety of signals, acting coordinately to instruct the immune system to respond in a specific fashion. T cells elaborate cytokines (e.g., interferon) that directly inhibit the growth of pathogens or stimulate killing by host macrophages and cytotoxic cells. Cytokines also augment the host's immunity by stimulating the inflammatory response (fever, the production of acute-phase serum components, and the proliferation of leukocytes). Cytokine stimulation does not always result in a favorable response in the host; septic shock (Chap. 265) and toxic shock syndrome (Chaps. 129 and 130) are among the conditions that are mediated by these inflammatory substances.

The immune system has also developed cells that specialize in controlling or downregulating immune responses. For example, T_{reg} cells, a subgroup of CD4+ T cells, prevent autoimmune responses by other T cells and are thought to be important in downregulating immune responses to foreign antigens. There appear to be both naturally occurring and acquired T_{reg} cells.

The reticuloendothelial system comprises monocyte-derived phagocytic cells that are located in the liver (Kupffer cells), lung (alveolar macrophages), spleen (macrophages and dendritic cells), kidney (mesangial cells), brain (microglia), and lymph nodes (macrophages and dendritic cells) and that clear circulating microorganisms. Although these tissue macrophages and polymorphonuclear leukocytes (PMNs) are capable of killing microorganisms without help, they function much more efficiently when pathogens are first *opsonized* (Greek, "to prepare for eating") by components of the complement system such as C3b and/or by antibodies.

Extracellular pathogens, including most encapsulated bacteria (those surrounded by a complex polysaccharide coat), are attacked by the humoral immune system, which includes antibodies, the complement cascade, and phagocytic cells. *Antibodies* are complex glycoproteins (also called *immunoglobulins*) that are produced by mature B lymphocytes, circulate in body fluids, and are secreted on mucosal surfaces. Antibodies specifically recognize and bind to foreign antigens. One of the most impressive features of the immune system is the ability to

TABLE 113-1 INFECTIONS ASSOCIATED WITH SELECTED DEFECTS IN IMMUNITY

Host Defect	Disease or Therapy Associated with Defect	Common Etiologic Agent of Infection
Nonspecific Immunity		
Impaired cough	Rib fracture, neuromuscular dysfunction	Bacteria causing pneumonia, aerobic and anaerobic oral flora
Loss of gastric acidity	Achlorhydria, histamine blockade	*Salmonella* spp., enteric pathogens
Loss of cutaneous integrity	Penetrating trauma, athlete's foot	*Staphylococcus* spp., *Streptococcus* spp.
	Burn	*Pseudomonas aeruginosa*
	Intravenous catheter	*Staphylococcus* spp., *Streptococcus* spp., gram-negative rods, coagulase-negative staphylococci
Implantable device	Heart valve	*Streptococcus* spp., coagulase-negative staphylococci, *Staphylococcus aureus*
	Artificial joint	*Staphylococcus* spp., *Streptococcus* spp., gram-negative rods
Loss of normal bacterial flora	Antibiotic use	*Clostridium difficile*, *Candida* spp.
Impaired clearance		
Poor drainage	Urinary tract infection	*Escherichia coli*
Abnormal secretions	Cystic fibrosis	Chronic pulmonary infection with *P. aeruginosa*
Inflammatory Response		
Neutropenia	Hematologic malignancy, cytotoxic chemotherapy, aplastic anemia, HIV infection	Gram-negative enteric bacilli, *Pseudomonas* spp., *Staphylococcus* spp., *Candida* spp.
Chemotaxis	Chédiak-Higashi syndrome, Job's syndrome, protein-calorie malnutrition	*S. aureus*, *Streptococcus pyogenes*, *Haemophilus influenzae*, gram-negative bacilli
	Leukocyte adhesion defects 1 and 2	Bacteria causing skin and systemic infections, gingivitis
Phagocytosis (cellular)	Systemic lupus erythematosus (SLE), chronic myelogenous leukemia, megaloblastic anemia	*Streptococcus pneumoniae*, *H. influenzae*
Splenectomy	—	*H. influenzae*, *S. pneumoniae*, other streptococci, *Capnocytophaga* spp., *Babesia microti*, *Salmonella* spp.
Microbicidal defect	Chronic granulomatous disease	Catalase-positive bacteria and fungi: staphylococci, *E. coli*, *Klebsiella* spp., *P. aeruginosa*, *Aspergillus* spp., *Nocardia* spp.
	Chédiak-Higashi syndrome	*S. aureus*, *S. pyogenes*
	Interferon γ receptor defect, interleukin 12 deficiency, interleukin 12 receptor defect	*Mycobacterium* spp., *Salmonella* spp.
Innate Immunity		
Complement system		
C3	Congenital liver disease, SLE, nephrotic syndrome	*S. aureus*, *S. pneumoniae*, *Pseudomonas* spp., *Proteus* spp.
C5	Congenital	*Neisseria* spp., gram-negative rods
C6, C7, C8	Congenital, SLE	*Neisseria meningitidis*, *N. gonorrhoeae*
Alternative pathway	Sickle cell disease	*S. pneumoniae*, *Salmonella* spp.
Toll-like receptor 4	Congenital	Gram-negative bacilli
Interleukin 1 receptor–associated kinase (IRAK) 4	Congenital	*S. pneumoniae*, *S. aureus*, other bacteria
Mannan-binding lectin	Congenital	*N. meningitidis*, other bacteria
Adaptive Immunity		
T lymphocyte deficiency/dysfunction	Thymic aplasia, thymic hypoplasia, Hodgkin's disease, sarcoidosis, lepromatous leprosy	*Listeria monocytogenes*, *Mycobacterium* spp., *Candida* spp., *Aspergillus* spp., *Cryptococcus neoformans*, herpes simplex virus, varicella-zoster virus
	AIDS	*Pneumocystis*, cytomegalovirus, herpes simplex virus, *Mycobacterium avium-intracellulare*, *C. neoformans*, *Candida* spp.
	Mucocutaneous candidiasis	*Candida* spp.
	Purine nucleoside phosphorylase deficiency	Fungi, viruses
B cell deficiency/dysfunction	Bruton's X-linked agammaglobulinemia	*S. pneumoniae*, other streptococci
	Agammaglobulinemia, chronic lymphocytic leukemia, multiple myeloma, dysglobulinemia	*H. influenzae*, *N. meningitidis*, *S. aureus*, *Klebsiella pneumoniae*, *E. coli*, *Giardia lamblia*, *Pneumocystis*, enteroviruses
	Selective IgM deficiency	*S. pneumoniae*, *H. influenzae*, *E. coli*
	Selective IgA deficiency	*G. lamblia*, hepatitis virus, *S. pneumoniae*, *H. influenzae*
Mixed T and B cell deficiency/dysfunction	Common variable hypogammaglobulinemia	*Pneumocystis*, cytomegalovirus, *S. pneumoniae*, *H. influenzae*, various other bacteria
	Ataxia-telangiectasia	*S. pneumoniae*, *H. influenzae*, *S. aureus*, rubella virus, *G. lamblia*
	Severe combined immunodeficiency	*S. aureus*, *S. pneumoniae*, *H. influenzae*, *Candida albicans*, *Pneumocystis*, varicella-zoster virus, rubella virus, cytomegalovirus
	Wiskott-Aldrich syndrome	Agents of infections associated with T and B cell abnormalities
	X-linked hyper-IgM syndrome	*Pneumocystis*, cytomegalovirus, *Cryptosporidium parvum*

generate an incredible diversity of antibodies capable of recognizing virtually every foreign antigen yet not reacting with self. In addition to being exquisitely specific for antigens, antibodies come in different structural and functional classes: IgG predominates in the circulation and persists for many years after exposure; IgM is the earliest specific antibody to appear in response to infection; secretory IgA is important in immunity at mucosal surfaces, while monomeric IgA appears in the serum; and IgE is important in allergic and parasitic diseases. Antibodies may directly impede the function of an invading organism, neutralize secreted toxins and enzymes, or facilitate the removal of the antigen (invading organism) by phagocytic cells. Immunoglobulins participate in cell-mediated immunity by promoting the antibody-dependent cellular cytotoxicity functions of certain T lymphocytes. Antibodies also promote the deposition of complement components on the surface of the invader.

The *complement* system (Chap. 308) consists of a group of serum proteins functioning as a cooperative, self-regulating cascade of enzymes that adhere to—and in some cases disrupt—the surface of invading organisms. Some of these surface-adherent proteins (e.g., C3b) can then act as opsonins for destruction of microbes by phagocytes. The later, "terminal" components (C7, C8, and C9) can directly kill some bacterial invaders (notably, many of the neisseriae) by forming a membrane attack complex and disrupting the integrity of the bacterial membrane, thus causing bacteriolysis. Other complement components, such as C5a, act as chemoattractants for PMNs (see below). Complement activation and deposition occur by either or both of two pathways: the *classic* pathway is activated primarily by immune complexes (i.e., antibody bound to antigen), and the *alternative* pathway is activated by microbial components, frequently in the absence of antibody. PMNs have receptors for both antibody and C3b, and antibody and complement function together to aid in the clearance of infectious agents.

PMNs, short-lived white blood cells that engulf and kill invading microbes, are first attracted to inflammatory sites by chemoattractants such as C5a, which is a product of complement activation at the site of infection. PMNs localize to the site of infection by adhering to cellular adhesion molecules expressed by endothelial cells. Endothelial cells express these receptors, called *selectins* (CD-62, ELAM-1), in response to inflammatory cytokines such as tumor necrosis factor α and interleukin 1. The binding of these selectin molecules to specific receptors on PMNs results in the adherence of the PMNs to the endothelium. Cytokine-mediated upregulation and expression of intercellular adhesion molecule 1 (ICAM 1) on endothelial cells then take place, and this latter receptor binds to β_2 integrins on PMNs, thereby facilitating diapedesis into the extravascular compartment. Once the PMNs are in the extravascular compartment, various molecules (e.g., arachidonic acids) further enhance the inflammatory process.

APPROACH TO THE PATIENT:
Infectious Diseases

The clinical manifestations of infectious diseases at presentation are myriad, varying from fulminant life-threatening processes to brief and self-limited conditions to indolent chronic maladies. A careful history is essential and must include details on underlying chronic diseases, medications, occupation, and travel. Risk factors for exposure to certain types of pathogens may give important clues to diagnosis. A sexual history may reveal risks for exposure to HIV and other sexually transmitted pathogens. A history of contact with animals may suggest numerous diagnoses, including rabies, Q fever, bartonellosis, *Escherichia coli* O157 infection, or cryptococcosis. Blood transfusions have been linked to diseases ranging from viral hepatitis to malaria to prion disease. A history of exposure to insect vectors (coupled with information about the season and geographic site of exposure) may lead to consideration of such diseases as Rocky Mountain spotted fever, other rickettsial diseases, tularemia, Lyme disease, babesiosis, malaria, trypanosomiasis, and numerous arboviral infections. Ingestion of contaminated liquids or foods may lead to enteric infection with *Salmonella*, *Listeria*, *Campylobacter*, amebas, cryptosporidia, or helminths. Since infectious diseases may involve many organ systems, a careful review of systems may elicit important clues as to the disease process.

The physical examination must be thorough, and attention must be paid to seemingly minor details, such as a soft heart murmur that might indicate bacterial endocarditis or a retinal lesion that suggests disseminated candidiasis or cytomegalovirus (CMV) infection. Rashes are extremely important clues to infectious diagnoses and may be the only sign pointing to a specific etiology (Chap. 18; **Chap. e5**). Certain rashes are so specific as to be pathognomonic—e.g., the childhood exanthems (measles, rubella, varicella), the target lesion of erythema migrans (Lyme disease), ecthyma gangrenosum (*Pseudomonas aeruginosa*), and eschars (rickettsial diseases). Other rashes, although less specific, may be exceedingly important diagnostic indicators. The prompt recognition of the early scarlatiniform and later petechial rashes of meningococcal infection or of the subtle embolic lesions of disseminated fungal infections in immunosuppressed patients can hasten life-saving therapy. Fever (Chaps. 17, 18, and 19) is a common manifestation of infection and may be its sole apparent indication. Sometimes the pattern of fever or its temporally associated findings may help refine the differential diagnosis. For example, fever occurring every 48–72 h is suggestive of malaria (Chap. 203). The elevation in body temperature in fever (through resetting of the hypothalamic setpoint mediated by cytokines) must be distinguished from elevations in body temperature from other causes such as drug toxicity (Chap. 19) or heat stroke (Chap. 17).

LABORATORY INVESTIGATIONS

Laboratory studies must be carefully considered and directed toward establishing an etiologic diagnosis in the shortest possible time, at the lowest possible cost, and with the least possible discomfort to the patient. Since mucosal surfaces and the skin are colonized with many harmless or beneficial microorganisms, cultures must be performed in a manner that minimizes the likelihood of contamination with this normal flora while maximizing the yield of pathogens. A sputum sample is far more likely to be valuable when elicited with careful coaching by the clinician than when collected in a container simply left at the bedside with cursory instructions. Gram's stains of specimens should be interpreted carefully and the quality of the specimen assessed. The findings on Gram's staining should correspond to the results of culture; a discrepancy may suggest diagnostic possibilities such as infection due to fastidious or anaerobic bacteria.

The microbiology laboratory must be an ally in the diagnostic endeavor. Astute laboratory personnel will suggest optimal culture and transport conditions or alternative tests to facilitate diagnosis. If informed about specific potential pathogens, an alert laboratory staff will allow sufficient time for these organisms to become evident in culture, even when the organisms are present in small numbers or are slow-growing. The parasitology technician who is attuned to the specific diagnostic considerations relevant to a particular case may be able to detect the rare, otherwise-elusive egg or cyst in a stool specimen. In cases where a diagnosis appears difficult, serum should be stored during the early acute phase of the illness so that a diagnostic rise in titer of antibody to a specific pathogen can be detected later. Bacterial and fungal antigens can sometimes be detected in body fluids, even when cultures are negative or are rendered sterile by antibiotic therapy. Techniques such as the polymerase chain reaction allow the amplification of specific DNA sequences so that minute quantities of foreign nucleic acids can be recognized in host specimens.

Rx INFECTIOUS DISEASES

Optimal therapy for infectious diseases requires a broad knowledge of medicine and careful clinical judgment. Life-threatening infections such as bacterial meningitis or sepsis, viral encephalitis, or falciparum malaria must be treated immediately, often before a specific causative organism is identified. Antimicrobial agents must be chosen empirically and must be active against the range of potential infectious agents consistent with the clinical scenario. In contrast, good clinical judgment sometimes dictates withholding of antimicrobial drugs in a self-limited process or until a specific diagnosis is made. The dictum *primum non nocere* should be adhered to, and it should be remembered that all antimicrobial agents carry a risk (and a cost) to the patient. Direct toxicity may be encountered—e.g., ototoxicity due to aminoglycosides, lipodystrophy due to antiretroviral agents, and hepatotoxicity due to antituberculous agents such as isoniazid and rifampin. Allergic reactions are common and can be serious. Since superinfection sometimes follows the eradication of the normal flora and colonization by a resistant organism, one invariant principle is that infectious disease therapy should be directed toward as narrow a spectrum of infectious agents as possible. Treatment specific for the pathogen should result in as little perturbation as possible of the host's microflora. Indeed, future therapeutic agents may act not by killing a microbe, but by interfering with one or more of its virulence factors.

With few exceptions, abscesses require surgical or percutaneous drainage for cure. Foreign bodies, including medical devices, must generally be removed in order to eliminate an infection of the device or of the adjacent tissue. Other infections, such as necrotizing fasciitis, peritonitis due to a perforated organ, gas gangrene, and chronic osteomyelitis, require surgery as the primary means of cure; in these conditions, antibiotics play only an adjunctive role.

The role of immunomodulators in the management of infectious diseases has received increasing attention. Glucocorticoids have been shown to be of benefit in the adjunctive treatment of bacterial meningitis and in therapy for *Pneumocystis* pneumonia in patients with AIDS. The use of these agents in other infectious processes remains less clear and in some cases (in cerebral malaria, for example) is detrimental. Activated protein C (drotrecogin alfa, activated) is the first immunomodulatory agent widely available for the treatment of severe sepsis. Its usefulness demonstrates the interrelatedness of the clotting cascade and systemic immunity. Other agents that modulate the immune response include prostaglandin inhibitors, specific lymphokines, and tumor necrosis factor inhibitors. Specific antibody therapy plays a role in the treatment and prevention of many diseases. Specific immunoglobulins have long been known to prevent the development of symptomatic rabies and tetanus. More recently, CMV immune globulin has been recognized as important not only in preventing the transmission of the virus during organ transplantation but also in treating CMV pneumonia in bone marrow transplant recipients. There is a strong need for well-designed clinical trials to evaluate each new interventional modality.

PERSPECTIVE

The genetic simplicity of many infectious agents allows them to undergo rapid evolution and to develop selective advantages that result in constant variation in the clinical manifestations of infection. Moreover, changes in the environment and the host can predispose new populations to a particular infection. The dramatic march of West Nile virus from a single focus in New York City in 1999 to locations throughout the North American continent by the summer of 2002 caused widespread alarm, illustrating the fear that new plagues induce in the human psyche. The intentional release of deadly spores of *Bacillus anthracis* via the U.S. Postal Service awakened many from a sense of complacency regarding biologic weapons.

"The terror of the unknown is seldom better displayed than by the response of a population to the appearance of an epidemic, particularly when the epidemic strikes without apparent cause." Edward H. Kass made this statement in 1977 in reference to the newly discovered Legionnaire's disease, but it could apply equally to SARS, H5N1 (avian) influenza, or any other new and mysterious disease. The potential for infectious agents to emerge in novel and unexpected ways requires that physicians and public health officials be knowledgeable, vigilant, and open-minded in their approach to unexplained illness. The emergence of antimicrobial-resistant pathogens (e.g., enterococci that are resistant to all known antimicrobial agents and cause infections that are essential-

ly untreatable) has led some to conclude that we are entering the "post-antibiotic era." Others have held to the perception that infectious diseases no longer represent as serious a concern to world health as they once did. The progress that science, medicine, and society as a whole have made in combating these maladies is impressive, and it is ironic that, as we stand on the threshold of an understanding of the most basic biology of the microbe, infectious diseases are posing renewed problems. We are threatened by the appearance of new diseases such as SARS, hepatitis C, and Ebola virus infection and by the reemergence of old foes such as tuberculosis, cholera, plague, and *Streptococcus pyogenes* infection. True students of infectious diseases were perhaps less surprised than anyone else by these developments. Those who know pathogens are aware of their incredible adaptability and diversity. As ingenious and successful as therapeutic approaches may be, our ability to develop methods to counter infectious agents so far has not matched the myriad strategies employed by the sea of microbes that surrounds us. Their sheer numbers and the rate at which they can evolve are daunting. Moreover, environmental changes, rapid global travel, population movements, and medicine itself—through its use of antibiotics and immunosuppressive agents—all increase the impact of infectious diseases. Although new vaccines, new antibiotics, improved global communication, and new modalities for treating and preventing infection will be developed, pathogenic microbes will continue to develop new strategies of their own, presenting us with an unending and dynamic challenge.

FURTHER READINGS

ARMSTRONG G et al: Trends in infectious disease mortality in the United States during the 20th century. JAMA 281:61, 1999

BARTLETT JG: Update in infectious diseases. Ann Intern Med 144:49, 2006

BLASER MJ: Introduction to bacteria and bacterial diseases, in *Principles and Practice of Infectious Diseases*, 6th ed, GL Mandell et al (eds). Philadelphia, Elsevier, 2005, p 2319

HENDERSON DA: Countering the posteradication threat of smallpox and polio. Clin Infect Dis 34:79, 2002

HOFFMAN J et al: Phylogenetic perspectives in innate immunity. Science 284:1313, 1999

HUNG DT et al: Small-molecule inhibitor of *Vibrio cholerae* virulence and intestinal colonization. Science 310:670, 2005

PROMED-MAIL: The Program for Monitoring Emerging Diseases. *www.promedmail.org*

PUCK JM: Primary immunodeficiency diseases. JAMA 278:1835, 1997

TYLER KL, NATHANSON N: Pathogenesis of viral infections, in *Fields Virology*, DM Knipe, PM Howley (eds). Philadelphia, Lippincott Williams & Wilkins, 2001, pp 199–244

WEISS ST: Eat dirt—the hygiene hypothesis and allergic diseases. N Engl J Med 347:930, 2002

114 Molecular Mechanisms of Microbial Pathogenesis
Gerald B. Pier

Over the past three decades, molecular studies of the pathogenesis of microorganisms have yielded an explosion of information about the various microbial and host molecules that contribute to the processes of infection and disease. These processes can be classified into several stages: microbial encounter with and entry into the host; microbial growth after entry; avoidance of innate host defenses; tissue invasion and tropism; tissue damage; and transmission to new hosts. *Virulence* is the measure of an organism's capacity to cause disease and is a function of the pathogenic factors elaborated by microbes. These factors

promote *colonization* (the simple presence of potentially pathogenic microbes in or on a host), *infection* (attachment and growth of pathogens and avoidance of host defenses), and *disease* (often, but not always, the result of activities of secreted toxins or toxic metabolites). In addition, the host's inflammatory response to infection greatly contributes to disease and its attendant clinical signs and symptoms.

MICROBIAL ENTRY AND ADHERENCE

ENTRY SITES
A microbial pathogen can potentially enter any part of a host organism. In general, the type of disease produced by a particular microbe is often a direct consequence of its route of entry into the body. The most common sites of entry are mucosal surfaces (the respiratory, alimentary, and urogenital tracts) and the skin. Ingestion, inhalation, and sexual contact are typical routes of microbial entry. Other portals of entry include sites

of skin injury (cuts, bites, burns, trauma) along with injection via natural (i.e., vector-borne) or artificial (i.e., needlestick) routes. A few pathogens, such as *Schistosoma* spp., can penetrate unbroken skin. The conjunctiva can serve as an entry point for pathogens of the eye.

Microbial entry usually relies on the presence of specific microbial factors needed for persistence and growth in a tissue. Fecal-oral spread via the alimentary tract requires a biology consistent with survival in the varied environments of the gastrointestinal tract (including the low pH of the stomach and the high bile content of the intestine) as well as in contaminated food or water outside the host. Organisms that gain entry via the respiratory tract survive well in small moist droplets produced during sneezing and coughing. Pathogens that enter by venereal routes often survive best on the warm moist environment of the urogenital mucosa and have restricted host ranges (e.g., *Neisseria gonorrhoeae*, *Treponema pallidum*, and HIV).

The biology of microbes entering through the skin is highly varied. Some organisms can survive in a broad range of environments, such as the salivary glands or alimentary tracts of arthropod vectors, the mouths of larger animals, soil, and water. A complex biology allows protozoan parasites such as *Plasmodium*, *Leishmania*, and *Trypanosoma* spp. to undergo morphogenic changes that permit transmission to mammalian hosts during insect feeding for blood meals. Plasmodia are injected as infective sporozoites from the salivary glands during mosquito feeding. *Leishmania* parasites are regurgitated as promastigotes from the alimentary tract of sandflies and are injected by bite into a susceptible host. Trypanosomes are ingested from infected hosts by reduviid bugs, multiply in the insects' gastrointestinal tract, and are released in feces onto the host's skin during subsequent feedings. Most microbes that land directly on intact skin are destined to die, as survival on the skin or in hair follicles requires resistance to fatty acids, low pH, and other antimicrobial factors on skin. Once it is damaged (and particularly if it becomes necrotic), the skin can be a major portal of entry and growth for pathogens and elaboration of their toxic products. Burn wound infections and tetanus are clear examples. After animal bites, pathogens resident in the animal's saliva gain access to the victim's tissues through the damaged skin. Rabies is the paradigm for this pathogenic process; rabies virus grows in striated muscle cells at the site of inoculation.

MICROBIAL ADHERENCE

Once in or on a host, most microbes must anchor themselves to a tissue or tissue factor; the possible exceptions are organisms that directly enter the bloodstream and multiply there. Specific ligands or adhesins for host receptors constitute a major area of study in the field of microbial pathogenesis. Adhesins comprise a wide range of surface structures, not only anchoring the microbe to a tissue and promoting cellular entry where appropriate but also eliciting host responses critical to the pathogenic process (Table 114-1). Most microbes produce multiple adhesins specific for multiple host receptors. These adhesins are often redundant, are serologically variable, and act additively or synergistically with other microbial factors to promote microbial sticking to host tissues. In addition, some microbes adsorb host proteins onto their surface and utilize the natural host protein receptor for microbial binding and entry into target cells.

Viral Adhesins (See also Chap. 161) All viral pathogens must bind to host cells, enter them, and replicate within them. Viral coat proteins serve as the ligands for cellular entry, and more than one ligand-receptor interaction may be needed; for example, HIV uses its envelope glycoprotein (gp) 120 to enter host cells by binding to both CD4 and one of two receptors for chemokines (designated CCR5 and CXCR4). Similarly, the measles virus H glycoprotein binds to both CD46 and the membrane-organizing protein moesin on host cells. The gB and gC proteins on herpes simplex virus bind to heparan sulfate; this adherence is not essential for entry but rather serves to concentrate virions close to the cell surface. This step is followed by attachment to mammalian cells mediated by the viral gD protein. Herpes simplex virus can use a number of eukaryotic cell surface receptors for entry, including the herpesvirus entry mediator (related to the tumor necrosis factor receptor); members of the immunoglobulin superfamily; two proteins called nectin-1 and nectin-2; and modified heparan sulfate.

Bacterial Adhesins Among the microbial adhesins studied in greatest detail are bacterial pili and flagella (Fig. 114-1). *Pili* or *fimbriae* are commonly used by gram-negative and gram-positive bacteria for attachment to host cells and tissues. In electron micrographs, these hairlike projections (up to several hundred per cell) may be confined to one end of the organism (polar pili) or distributed more evenly over the surface. An individual cell may have pili with a variety of functions. Most pili are made up of a major pilin protein subunit (molecular weight, 17,000–30,000) that polymerizes to form the pilus. Many strains of *Escherichia coli* isolated from urinary tract infections express mannose-binding type 1 pili, whose binding to the integral membrane glycoproteins called *uroplakins* that coat the cells in the bladder epithelium is inhibited by D-mannose. Other strains produce the Pap (pyelonephritis-associated) or P pilus adhesin that mediates binding to

TABLE 114-1 EXAMPLES OF MICROBIAL LIGAND-RECEPTOR INTERACTIONS

Microorganism	Type of Microbial Ligand	Host Receptor
Viral Pathogens		
Influenza virus	Hemagglutinin	Sialic acid
Measles virus		
Vaccine strain	Hemagglutinin	CD46/moesin
Wild-type strains	Hemagglutinin	Signaling lymphocytic activation molecule (SLAM)
Human herpesvirus type 6	?	CD46
Herpes simplex virus	Glycoprotein C	Heparan sulfate
HIV	Surface glycoprotein	CD4 and chemokine receptors (CCR5 and CXCR4)
Epstein-Barr virus	Envelope protein	CD21 (=CR2)
Adenovirus	Fiber protein	Coxsackie-adenovirus receptor (CAR)
Coxsackievirus	Viral coat proteins	CAR and major histocompatibility class I antigens
Bacterial Pathogens		
Neisseria spp.	Pili	Membrane cofactor protein (CD46)
Pseudomonas aeruginosa	Pili and flagella	Asialo-GM1
	Lipopolysaccharide	Cystic fibrosis transmembrane conductance regulator (CFTR)
Escherichia coli	Pili	Ceramides/mannose and digalactosyl residues
Streptococcus pyogenes	Hyaluronic acid capsule	CD44
Yersinia spp.	Invasin/accessory invasin locus	β_1 Integrins
Bordetella pertussis	Filamentous hemagglutinin	CR3
Legionella pneumophila	Adsorbed C3bi	CR3
Mycobacterium tuberculosis	Adsorbed C3bi	CR3; DC-SIGN[a]
Fungal Pathogens		
Blastomyces dermatitidis	WI-1	Possibly matrix proteins and integrins
Candida albicans	Int1p	Extracellular matrix proteins
Protozoal Pathogens		
Plasmodium vivax	Merozoite form	Duffy Fy antigen
Plasmodium falciparum	Erythrocyte-binding protein 175 (EBA-175)	Glycophorin A
Entamoeba histolytica	Surface lectin	N-Acetylglucosamine

[a]A novel dendritic cell–specific C-type lectin.

FIGURE 114-1 Bacterial surface structures. A and **B.** Traditional electron micrographic images of fixed cells of *Pseudomonas aeruginosa*. Flagella **(A)** and pili **(B)** projecting out from the bacterial poles can be seen. **C** and **D.** Atomic force microscopic image of live *P. aeruginosa* freshly planted onto a smooth mica surface. This technology reveals the fine, three-dimensional detail of the bacterial surface structures. *(Images courtesy of Dr. Martin Lee and Dr. Milan Bajmoczi, Harvard Medical School; with permission.)*

digalactose (gal-gal) residues on globosides of the human P blood groups. Both of these types of pili have proteins located at the tips of the main pilus unit that are critical to the binding specificity of the whole pilus unit. It is interesting that, although immunization with the mannose-binding tip protein (FimH) of type 1 pili prevents experimental *E. coli* bladder infections in mice and monkeys, a trial of this vaccine in humans was not successful. *E. coli* cells causing diarrheal disease express pilus-like receptors for enterocytes on the small bowel, along with other receptors termed *colonization factors*.

The type IV pilus, a common type of pilus found in *Neisseria* spp., *Moraxella* spp., *Vibrio cholerae*, *Legionella pneumophila*, *Salmonella enterica* serovar *typhi*, enteropathogenic *E. coli*, and *Pseudomonas aeruginosa*, mediates adherence of these organisms to target surfaces. These pili tend to have a relatively conserved amino-terminal region and a more variable carboxyl-terminal region. For some species (e.g., *N. gonorrhoeae*, *Neisseria meningitidis*, and enteropathogenic *E. coli*), the pili are critical for attachment to mucosal epithelial cells. For others, such as *P. aeruginosa*, the pili only partially mediate the cells' adherence to host tissues. Whereas interference with this stage of colonization would appear to be an effective antibacterial strategy, attempts to develop pilus-based vaccines for human diseases have not been highly successful to date.

Flagella are long appendages attached at either one or both ends of the bacterial cell (polar flagella) or distributed over the entire cell surface (peritrichous flagella). Flagella, like pili, are composed of a polymerized or aggregated basic protein. In flagella, the protein subunits form a tight helical structure and vary serologically with the species. Spirochetes such as *T. pallidum* and *Borrelia burgdorferi* have axial filaments similar to flagella running down the long axis of the center of the cell, and they "swim" by rotation around these filaments. Some bacteria can glide over a surface in the absence of obvious motility structures.

Other bacterial structures involved in adherence to host tissues include specific staphylococcal and streptococcal proteins that bind to human extracellular matrix proteins such as fibrin, fibronectin, fibrinogen, laminin, and collagen. Fibronectin appears to be a commonly used receptor for various pathogens; a particular amino acid sequence in fibronectin (Arg-Gly-Asp, or RGD) is critical for bacterial binding. Binding of the highly conserved *Staphylococcus aureus* surface protein clumping factor A (ClfA) to fibrinogen has been implicated in many aspects of pathogenesis. The conserved outer-core portion of the lipopolysaccharide (LPS) of *P. aeruginosa* mediates binding to the cystic fibrosis transmembrane conductance regulator (CFTR) on airway epithelial cells—an event that appears to be critical for normal host resistance to infection. A number of bacterial pathogens, including coagulase-negative staphylococci, *S. aureus*, and uropathogenic *E. coli* as well as *Yersinia pestis*, *Y. pseudotuberculosis*, and *Y. enterocolitica*, express a surface polysaccharide composed of poly N-acetylglucosamine. One function of this polysaccharide is to promote binding to materials used in catheters and other types of implanted devices; poly-N-acetylglucosamine may be a critical factor in the establishment of device-related infections by pathogens such as staphylococci and *E. coli*. High-powered imaging techniques (e.g., atomic force microscopy) have revealed that bacterial cells have a nonhomogeneous surface that is probably attributable to different concentrations of cell surface molecules, including microbial adhesins, at specific places on the cell surface (Fig114-1*D*).

Fungal Adhesins   Several fungal adhesins have been described that mediate colonization of epithelial surfaces, particularly adherence to structures like fibronectin, laminin, and collagen. The product of the *Candida albicans INT1* gene, Int1p, bears similarity to mammalian integrins that bind to extracellular matrix proteins. Transformation of normally nonadherent *Saccharomyces cerevisiae* with this gene allows these yeast cells to adhere to human epithelial cells. The agglutinin-like sequence (ALS) adhesins are large cell-surface glycoproteins mediating adherence of pathogenic *Candida* to host tissues. These adhesins are expressed under certain environmental conditions (often associated with stress) and are crucial for pathogenesis of fungal infections.

For several fungal pathogens that initiate infections after inhalation, the inoculum is ingested by alveolar macrophages, in which the fungal cells transform to pathogenic phenotypes.

Eukaryotic Pathogen Adhesins   Eukaryotic parasites use complicated surface glycoproteins as adhesins, some of which are lectins (proteins that bind to specific carbohydrates on host cells). For example, *Plasmodium vivax* binds (via Duffy-binding protein) to the Duffy blood group carbohydrate antigen Fy on erythrocytes. *Entamoeba histolytica* expresses two proteins that bind to the disaccharide galactose/N-acetylgalactosamine. Reports indicate that children with mucosal IgA antibody to one of these lectins are resistant to reinfection with virulent *E. histolytica*. A major surface glycoprotein (gp63) of *Leishmania* promastigotes is needed for these parasites to enter human macrophages—the principal target cell of infection. This glycoprotein promotes complement binding but inhibits complement lytic activity, allowing the parasite to use complement receptors for entry into macrophages; gp63 also binds to fibronectin receptors on macrophages. In addition, the pathogen can express a carbohydrate that mediates binding to host cells. Evidence suggests that, as part of hepatic granuloma formation, *Schistosoma mansoni* expresses a carbohydrate epitope related to the Lewis X blood group antigen that promotes adherence of helminthic eggs to vascular endothelial cells under inflammatory conditions.

HOST RECEPTORS

Host receptors are found both on target cells (e.g., epithelial cells lining mucosal surfaces) and within the mucous layer covering these cells. Microbial pathogens bind to a wide range of host receptors to establish infection (Table 114-1). Selective loss of host receptors for a pathogen may confer natural resistance to an otherwise susceptible population. For example, 70% of individuals in West Africa lack Fy antigens and are resistant to *P. vivax* infection. *S. enterica* serovar *typhi*, the etiologic agent of typhoid fever, uses CFTR to enter the gastrointestinal submucosa after being ingested. As homozygous mutations in *CFTR* are the cause of the life-shortening disease cystic fibrosis, heterozygote carriers (e.g., 4–5% of individuals of European ancestry) may have had a selective advantage due to decreased susceptibility to typhoid fever.

Numerous virus–target cell interactions have been described, and it is now clear that different viruses can use similar host-cell receptors for entry. The list of certain and likely host receptors for viral pathogens is long. Among the host membrane components that can serve as receptors for viruses are sialic acids, gangliosides, glycosaminoglycans, integrins and other members of the immunoglobulin superfamily, histocompatibility antigens, and regulators and receptors for complement components. A notable example of the effect of host receptors on the pathogenesis of infection comes from comparative binding studies of avian influenza A virus subtype H5N1 and influenza A virus strains expressing hemagglutinin subtype H1. The H1-subtype strains, which tend to be highly pathogenic and transmissible from human to human, bind to a receptor composed of two sugar molecules: sialic acid linked α-2-6 to galactose. This receptor is highly expressed in the airway epithelium. When virus is shed from this surface, its transmission via coughing and aerosol droplets is readily facilitated. In contrast, H5N1 avian influenza virus binds to sialic acid linked α-2-3 to galactose, and this receptor is highly expressed in pneumocytes in the alveoli. Alveolar infection is thought to underlie not only the high mortality rate associated with avian influenza but also the low human-to-human transmissibility rate of this strain, which is not readily transported to the airways (from which it could be expelled by coughing).

MICROBIAL GROWTH AFTER ENTRY

Once established on a mucosal or skin site, pathogenic microbes must replicate before causing full-blown infection and disease. Within cells, viral particles release their nucleic acids, which may be directly translated into viral proteins (positive-strand RNA viruses), transcribed from a negative strand of RNA into a complementary mRNA (negative-strand RNA viruses), or transcribed into a complementary strand of DNA (retroviruses); for DNA viruses, mRNA may be transcribed directly from viral DNA, either in the cell nucleus or in the cytoplasm. To grow, bacteria must acquire specific nutrients or synthesize them from precursors in host tissues. Many infectious processes are usually confined to specific epithelial surfaces—e.g., H1-subtype influenza to the respiratory mucosa, gonorrhea to the urogenital epithelium, and shigellosis to the gastrointestinal epithelium. While there are multiple reasons for this specificity, one important consideration is the ability of these pathogens to obtain from these specific environments the nutrients needed for growth and survival.

Temperature restrictions also play a role in limiting certain pathogens to specific tissues. Rhinoviruses, a cause of the common cold, grow best at 33°C and replicate in cooler nasal tissues but not as well in the lung. Leprosy lesions due to *Mycobacterium leprae* are found in and on relatively cool body sites. Fungal pathogens that infect the skin, hair follicles, and nails (dermatophyte infections) remain confined to the cooler, exterior, keratinous layer of the epithelium.

Many bacterial, fungal, and protozoal species grow in multicellular masses referred to as *biofilms*. These masses are biochemically and morphologically quite distinct from the free-living individual cells referred to as *planktonic cells*. Growth in biofilms leads to altered microbial metabolism, production of extracellular virulence factors, and decreased susceptibility to biocides, antimicrobial agents, and host defense molecules and cells. *P. aeruginosa* growing on the bronchial mucosa during chronic infection, staphylococci and other pathogens growing on implanted medical devices, and dental pathogens growing on tooth surfaces to form plaques represent several examples of microbial biofilm growth associated with human disease. Many other pathogens can form biofilms during in vitro growth, and it is increasingly accepted that this mode of growth contributes to microbial virulence and induction of disease.

AVOIDANCE OF INNATE HOST DEFENSES

As microbes have probably interacted with mucosal/epithelial surfaces since the emergence of multicellular organisms, it is not surprising that multicellular hosts have a variety of innate surface defense mechanisms that can sense when pathogens are present and contribute to their elimination. The skin is acidic and is bathed with fatty acids toxic to many microbes. Skin pathogens such as staphylococci must tolerate these adverse conditions. Mucosal surfaces are covered by a barrier composed of a thick mucous layer that entraps microbes and facilitates their transport out of the body by such processes as mucociliary clearance, coughing, and urination. Mucous secretions, saliva, and tears contain antibacterial factors such as lysozyme and antimicrobial peptides as well as antiviral factors such as interferons. Gastric acidity is inimical to the survival of many ingested pathogens, and most mucosal surfaces—particularly the nasopharynx, the vaginal tract, and the gastrointestinal tract—contain a resident flora of commensal microbes that interfere with the ability of pathogens to colonize and infect a host.

Pathogens that survive these factors must still contend with host endocytic, phagocytic, and inflammatory responses as well as with host genetic factors that determine the degree to which a pathogen can survive and grow. The growth of viral pathogens entering skin or mucosal epithelial cells can be limited by a variety of host genetic factors, including production of interferons, modulation of receptors for viral entry, and age- and hormone-related susceptibility factors; by nutritional status; and even by personal habits such as smoking and exercise.

ENCOUNTERS WITH EPITHELIAL CELLS

Over the past decade, many bacterial pathogens have been shown to enter epithelial cells (Fig. 114-2); the bacteria often use specialized surface structures that bind to receptors, with consequent internalization. However, the exact role and the importance of this process in infection and disease are not well defined for most of these pathogens. Bacterial entry into host epithelial cells is seen as a means for dissemination to adjacent or deeper tissues or as a route to sanctuary to avoid ingestion and killing by professional phagocytes. Epithelial cell entry appears, for instance, to be a critical aspect of dysentery induction by *Shigella*.

Curiously, the less virulent strains of many bacterial pathogens are more adept at entering epithelial cells than are more virulent strains; examples include pathogens that lack the surface polysaccharide capsule needed to cause serious disease. Thus, for *Haemophilus influenzae*, *Streptococcus pneumoniae*, *Streptococcus agalactiae* (group B *Streptococcus*), and *Streptococcus pyogenes*, isogenic mutants or variants lacking capsules enter epithelial cells better than the wild-type, encapsulated parental forms that cause disseminated disease. These observations have led to the proposal that epithelial cell entry may be primarily a manifestation of host defense, resulting in bacterial clearance by both shedding of epithelial cells containing internalized bacteria and initiation of a protective and nonpathogenic inflammatory response. However, a possible consequence of this process could be the opening of a hole in the epithelium, potentially allowing uningested organisms to enter the submucosa. This scenario has been documented in murine *S. enterica* serovar *typhimurium* infections and in experimental bladder infections with uropathogenic *E. coli*. In the latter system, bacterial pilus–mediated attachment to uroplakins induces exfoliation of the cells with attached bacteria. Subsequently, infection is produced by residual bacterial cells that invade the superficial bladder epithelium, where they can grow intracellularly into biofilm-like masses encased in an extracellular polysaccharide-rich matrix and surrounded by uroplakin. This mode of growth produces structures that have been referred to as *bacterial pods*. At low bacterial inocula, epithelial cell ingestion and subclinical inflammation are probably efficient means to eliminate pathogens; in contrast, at higher inocula, a proportion of surviving bacterial cells enter host tissue through the damaged mucosal surface and multiply, producing disease. Alternatively, failure of the appropriate epithelial cell response to a pathogen may allow the organism to survive on a mucosal surface where, if it avoids other host defenses, it can grow and cause a local infection. Along these lines, as

FIGURE 114-2 Entry of bacteria into epithelial cells. A. Internalization of *P. aeruginosa* by cultured human airway epithelial cells expressing wild-type cystic fibrosis transmembrane conductance regulator (CFTR), the cell receptor for bacterial ingestion. **B.** Entry of *P. aeruginosa* into murine tracheal epithelial cells after infection by the intranasal route.

noted above, *P. aeruginosa* is taken into epithelial cells by CFTR, a protein missing or nonfunctional in most severe cases of cystic fibrosis. The major clinical consequence is chronic airway-surface infection with *P. aeruginosa* in 80–90% of patients with cystic fibrosis. The failure of airway epithelial cells to ingest and promote the removal of *P. aeruginosa* via a properly regulated inflammatory response has been proposed as a key component of the hypersusceptibility of these patients to chronic airway infection with this organism.

ENCOUNTERS WITH PHAGOCYTES

Phagocytosis and Inflammation Phagocytosis of microbes is a major innate host defense that limits the growth and spread of pathogens. Phagocytes appear rapidly at sites of infection in conjunction with the initiation of inflammation. Ingestion of microbes by both tissue-fixed macrophages and migrating phagocytes probably accounts for the limited ability of most microbial agents to cause disease. A family of related molecules called *collectins, soluble defense collagens,* or *pattern-recognition molecules* are found in blood (mannose-binding lectins), in lung (surfactant proteins A and D), and most likely in other tissues as well and bind to carbohydrates on microbial surfaces to promote phagocyte clearance. Bacterial pathogens seem to be ingested principally by polymorphonuclear neutrophils (PMNs), while eosinophils are frequently found at sites of infection with protozoan or multicellular parasites. Successful pathogens, by definition, must avoid being cleared by professional phagocytes. One of several antiphagocytic

strategies employed by bacteria and by the fungal pathogen *Cryptococcus neoformans* is to elaborate large-molecular-weight surface polysaccharide antigens, often in the form of a capsule that coats the cell surface. Most pathogenic bacteria produce such antiphagocytic capsules. On occasion, proteins or polypeptides form capsule-like coatings on organisms such as *Bacillus anthracis*.

As activation of local phagocytes in tissues is a key step in initiating inflammation and migration of additional phagocytes into infected sites, much attention has been paid to microbial factors that initiate inflammation. Encounters with phagocytes are governed largely by the structure of the microbial constituents that elicit inflammation, and detailed knowledge of these structures for bacterial pathogens has contributed greatly to our understanding of molecular mechanisms of microbial pathogenesis (Fig. 114-3). One of the best-studied systems involves the interaction of LPS from gram-negative bacteria and the glycosylphosphatidylinositol (GPI)-anchored membrane protein CD14 found on the surface of professional phagocytes, including migrating and tissue-fixed macrophages and PMNs. A soluble form of CD14 is also found in plasma and on mucosal surfaces. A plasma protein, LPS-binding protein (LBP), transfers LPS to membrane-bound CD14 on myeloid cells and promotes binding of LPS to soluble CD14. Soluble CD14/LPS/LBP complexes bind to many cell types and may be internalized to initiate cellular responses to microbial pathogens. It has been shown that peptidoglycan and lipoteichoic acid from gram-positive bacteria and cell-surface products of mycobacteria and spirochetes can interact with CD14 (Fig. 114-3). Additional molecules, such as MD-2, also participate in the recognition of bacterial activators of inflammation.

GPI-anchored receptors do not have intracellular signaling domains. Instead, the mammalian Toll-like receptors (TLRs) transduce signals for cellular activation due to LPS binding. It has recently been shown that binding of microbial factors to TLRs to activate signal transduction occurs not on the cell surface, but rather in the phagosome of cells that have internalized the microbe. This interaction is probably due to the release of the microbial surface factor from the cell in the environment of the phagosome, where the liberated factor can bind to its cognate TLRs. TLRs initiate cellular activation through a series of signal-transducing molecules (Fig. 114-3) that lead to nuclear translocation of the transcription factor nuclear factor κB (NF-κB), a master-switch for production of important inflammatory cytokines such as tumor necrosis factor α (TNF-α) and interleukin (IL) 1.

Inflammation can be initiated not only with LPS and peptidoglycan but also with viral particles and other microbial products such as polysaccharides, enzymes, and toxins. Bacterial flagella activate inflammation by binding of a conserved sequence to TLR5. Some pathogens, including *Campylobacter jejuni, Helicobacter pylori,* and *Bartonella bacilliformis,* make flagella that lack this sequence and thus do not bind to TLR5. The result is a lack of efficient host response to infection. Bacteria also produce a high proportion of DNA molecules with unmethylated CpG residues that activate inflammation through TLR9. TLR3 recognizes double-strand RNA, a pattern-recognition molecule produced by many viruses during their replicative cycle. TLR1 and TLR6 associate with TLR2 to promote recognition of acylated microbial proteins and peptides.

The myeloid differentiation factor 88 (MyD88) molecule is a generalized adaptor protein that binds to the cytoplasmic domains of all known TLRs and also to receptors that are part of the IL-1 receptor (IL-1Rc) family. Numerous studies have shown that MyD88-mediated transduction of signals from TLRs and IL-1Rc is critical for innate resistance to infection. Mice lacking MyD88 are more susceptible than normal mice to infection with group B *Streptococcus, Listeria monocytogenes,* and *Mycobacterium tuberculosis.* However, it is now appreciated that some of the TLRs (e.g., TLR3 and TLR4) can activate signal transduction via an MyD88-independent pathway.

Additional Interactions of Microbial Pathogens and Phagocytes Other ways that microbial pathogens avoid destruction by phagocytes include production of factors that are toxic to phagocytes or that interfere with the chemotactic and ingestion function of phagocytes.

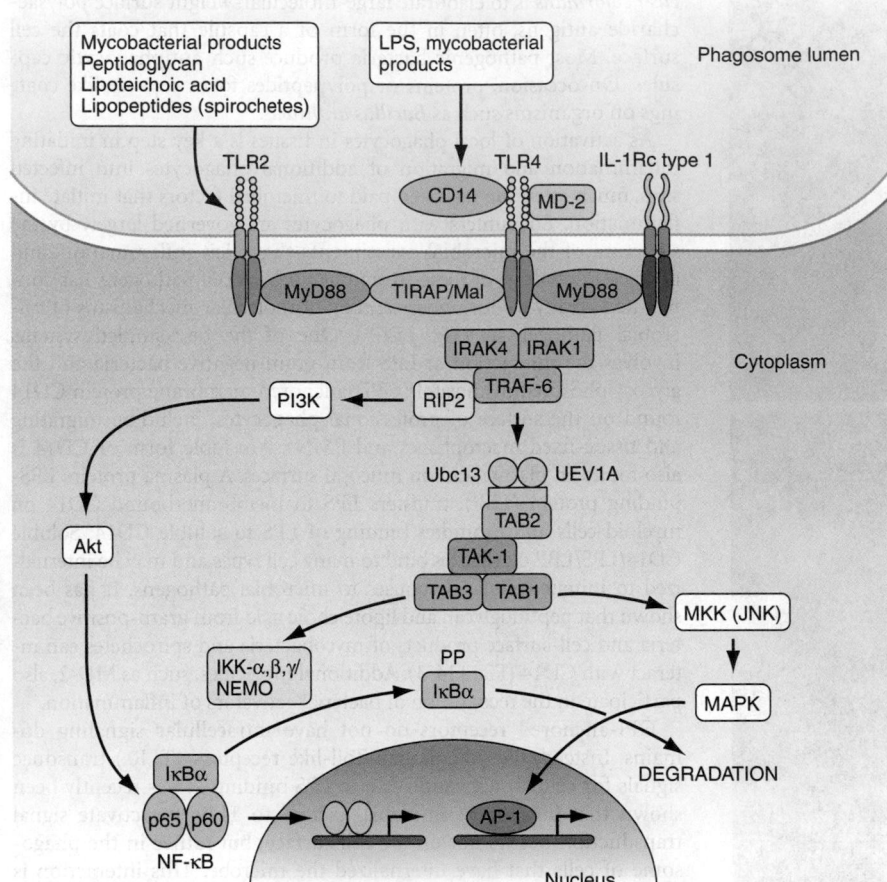

a process of internal degranulation, with the release of normally granule-sequestered toxic components into the phagocyte's cytoplasm. *E. histolytica*, an intestinal protozoan that causes amebic dysentery, can disrupt phagocyte membranes after direct contact via the release of protozoal phospholipase A and pore-forming peptides.

Microbial Survival inside Phagocytes Many important microbial pathogens use a variety of strategies to survive inside phagocytes (particularly macrophages) after ingestion. Inhibition of fusion of the phagocytic vacuole (the phagosome) containing the ingested microbe with the lysosomal granules containing antimicrobial substances (the lysosome) allows *M. tuberculosis*, *S. enterica* serovar *typhi*, and *Toxoplasma gondii* to survive inside macrophages. Some organisms, such as *L. monocytogenes*, escape into the phagocyte's cytoplasm to grow and eventually spread to other cells. Resistance to killing within the macrophage and subsequent growth are critical to successful infection by herpestype viruses, measles virus, poxviruses, *Salmonella*, *Yersinia*, *Legionella*, *Mycobacterium*, *Trypanosoma*, *Nocardia*, *Histoplasma*, *Toxoplasma*, and *Rickettsia*. *Salmonella* spp. use a master regulatory system, in which the *PhoP/PhoQ* genes control other genes, to enter and survive within cells; intracellular survival entails structural changes in the cell envelope LPS.

FIGURE 114-3 Cellular signaling pathways for production of inflammatory cytokines in response to microbial products. Various microbial cell-surface constituents interact with CD14, which in turn interacts in a currently unknown fashion with Toll-like receptors (TLRs). Some microbial factors do not need CD14 to interact with TLRs. Associating with TLR4 (and to some extent with TLR2) is MD-2, a cofactor that facilitates the response to lipopolysaccharide (LPS). Both CD14 and TLRs contain extracellular leucine-rich domains that become localized to the lumen of the phagosome upon uptake of bacterial cells; there, the TLRs can bind to microbial products. The TLRs are oligomerized, usually forming homodimers, and then bind to the general adaptor protein MyD88 via the C-terminal Toll/IL-1R (TIR) domains, which also bind to TIRAP (TIR domain-containing adaptor protein), a molecule that participates in the transduction of signals from TLR4. The MyD88/TIRAP complex activates signal-transducing molecules such as IRAK1 and IRAK4 (IL-1Rc-associated kinases 1 and 4); TRAF-6 (tumor necrosis factor receptor–associated factor 6); TAK-1 (transforming growth factor β–activating kinase 1); and TAB1, TAB2, and TAB3 (TAK1-binding proteins 1, 2, and 3). This signaling complex associates with the ubiquitin-conjugating enzyme Ubc13 and the Ubc-like protein UEV1A to catalyze the formation of a polyubiquitin chain on TRAF6. Polyubiquitination of TRAF6 activates TAK1, which, along with TAB2 (a protein that binds to lysine residue 63 in polyubiquitin chains via a conserved zinc-finger domain), phosphorylates the inducible kinase complex IKK-α, -β, and -γ. IKK-γ is also called NEMO [nuclear factor κB (NF-κB) essential modulator]. This large complex then phosphorylates the inhibitory component of NF-κB, IκBα, resulting in release of IκBα from NF-κB. Phosphorylated (PP) IκB is then degraded, and the two components of NF-κB, p50 and p65, translocate to the nucleus, where they bind to regulatory transcriptional sites on target genes, many of which encode inflammatory proteins. In addition to inducing NF-κB nuclear translocation, TAK1 also activates MAP kinase transducers such as the c-Jun N-terminal kinase (JNK) pathway, which can lead to nuclear translocation of the transcription factor AP1. Via the RIP2 protein, TRAF6 bound to IRAK can activate phosphatidylinositol-3 kinase (PI3K) and the regulatory protein Akt to dissociate NF-κB from IκBα, an event followed by translocation of the active NF-κB to the nucleus. (*Figure modified from an original produced by Dr. Terry Means and Dr. Douglas Golenbock.*)

TISSUE INVASION AND TISSUE TROPISM

TISSUE INVASION

Most viral pathogens cause disease by growth at skin or mucosal entry sites, but some pathogens spread from the initial site to deeper tissues. Virus can spread via the nerves (rabies virus) or plasma (picornaviruses) or within migratory blood cells (poliovirus, Epstein-Barr virus, and many others). Specific viral genes determine where and how individual viral strains can spread.

Bacteria may invade deeper layers of mucosal tissue via intracellular uptake by epithelial cells, traversal of epithelial cell junctions, or penetration through denuded epithelial surfaces. Among virulent *Shigella* strains and invasive *E. coli*, outer-membrane proteins are critical to epithelial cell invasion and bacterial multiplication. *Neisseria* and *Haemophilus* spp. penetrate mucosal cells by poorly understood mechanisms before dissemination into the bloodstream. Staphylococci and streptococci elaborate a variety of extracellular enzymes, such as hyaluronidase, lipases, nucleases, and hemolysins, that are probably important in breaking down cellular and matrix structures and allowing the bacteria access to deeper tissues and blood. Organisms that colonize the gastrointestinal tract can often translocate through the mucosa into the blood and, under circumstances in which host defenses are inadequate, cause bacteremia. *Y. enterocolitica* can invade the mucosa through the activity of the invasin protein. Some bacteria (e.g., *Brucella*) can be carried from a mucosal site to a distant site by phagocytic cells (e.g., PMNs) that ingest but fail to kill the bacteria.

Hemolysins, leukocidins, and the like are microbial proteins that can kill phagocytes that are attempting to ingest organisms elaborating these substances. For example, staphylococcal hemolysins inhibit macrophage chemotaxis and kill these phagocytes. Streptolysin O made by *S. pyogenes* binds to cholesterol in phagocyte membranes and initiates

Fungal pathogens almost always take advantage of host immuno-compromise to spread hematogenously to deeper tissues. The AIDS epidemic has resoundingly illustrated this principle: the immunodeficiency of many HIV-infected patients permits the development of life-threatening fungal infections of the lung, blood, and brain. Other than the capsule of *C. neoformans*, specific fungal antigens involved in tissue invasion are not well characterized. Both fungal and protozoal pathogens undergo morphologic changes to spread within a host. Yeast-cell forms of *C. albicans* transform into hyphal forms when invading deeper tissues. Malarial parasites grow in liver cells as merozoites and are released into the blood to invade erythrocytes and become trophozoites. *E. histolytica* is found as both a cyst and a trophozoite in the intestinal lumen, through which this pathogen enters the host, but only the trophozoite form can spread systemically to cause amebic liver abscesses. Other protozoal pathogens, such as *T. gondii*, *Giardia lamblia*, and *Cryptosporidium*, also undergo extensive morphologic changes after initial infection to spread to other tissues.

TISSUE TROPISM

The propensity of certain microbes to cause disease by infecting specific tissues has been known since the early days of bacteriology, yet the molecular basis for this propensity is understood somewhat better for viral pathogens than for other agents of infectious disease. Specific receptor-ligand interactions clearly underlie the ability of certain viruses to enter cells within tissues and disrupt normal tissue function, but the mere presence of a receptor for a virus on a target tissue is not sufficient for tissue tropism. Factors in the cell, route of viral entry, viral capacity to penetrate into cells, viral genetic elements that regulate gene expression, and pathways of viral spread in a tissue all affect tissue tropism. Some viral genes are best transcribed in specific target cells, such as hepatitis B genes in liver cells and Epstein-Barr virus genes in B lymphocytes. The route of inoculation of poliovirus determines its neurotropism, although the molecular basis for this circumstance is not understood.

The lesser understanding of the tissue tropism of bacterial and parasitic infections is exemplified by *Neisseria* spp. There is no well-accepted explanation of why *N. gonorrhoeae* colonizes and infects the human genital tract while the closely related species *N. meningitidis* principally colonizes the human oropharynx. *N. meningitidis* expresses a capsular polysaccharide, while *N. gonorrhoeae* does not; however, there is no indication that this property plays a role in the different tissue tropisms displayed by these two bacterial species. *N. gonorrhoeae* can use cytidine monophosphate *N*-acetylneuraminic acid from host tissues to add *N*-acetylneuraminic acid (sialic acid) to its lipooligosaccharide (LOS) O side chain, and this alteration appears to make the organism resistant to host defenses. Lactate, present at high levels on genital mucosal surfaces, stimulates sialylation of gonococcal LOS. Bacteria with sialic acid sugars in their capsules, such as *N. meningitidis*, *E. coli* K1, and group B streptococci, have a propensity to cause meningitis, but this generalization has many exceptions. For example, all recognized serotypes of group B streptococci contain sialic acid in their capsules, but only one serotype (III) is responsible for most cases of group B streptococcal meningitis. Moreover, both *H. influenzae* and *S. pneumoniae* can readily cause meningitis, but these organisms do not have sialic acid in their capsules.

TISSUE DAMAGE AND DISEASE

Disease is a complex phenomenon resulting from tissue invasion and destruction, toxin elaboration, and host response. Viruses cause much of their damage by exerting a cytopathic effect on host cells and inhibiting host defenses. The growth of bacterial, fungal, and protozoal parasites in tissue, which may or may not be accompanied by toxin elaboration, can also compromise tissue function and lead to disease. For some bacterial and possibly some fungal pathogens, toxin production is one of the best-characterized molecular mechanisms of pathogenesis, while host factors such as IL-1, TNF-α, kinins, inflammatory proteins, products of complement activation, and mediators derived from arachidonic acid metabolites (leukotrienes) and cellular degranulation (histamines) readily contribute to the severity of disease.

VIRAL DISEASE
See Chap. 170.

BACTERIAL TOXINS

Among the first infectious diseases to be understood were those due to toxin-elaborating bacteria. Diphtheria, botulism, and tetanus toxins are responsible for the diseases associated with local infections due to *Corynebacterium diphtheriae*, *Clostridium botulinum*, and *Clostridium tetani*, respectively. Enterotoxins produced by *E. coli*, *Salmonella*, *Shigella*, *Staphylococcus*, and *V. cholerae* contribute to diarrheal disease caused by these organisms. Staphylococci, streptococci, *P. aeruginosa*, and *Bordetella* elaborate various toxins that cause or contribute to disease, including toxic shock syndrome toxin 1 (TSST-1); erythrogenic toxin; exotoxins A, S, T, and U; and pertussis toxin. A number of these toxins (e.g., cholera toxin, diphtheria toxin, pertussis toxin, *E. coli* heat-labile toxin, and *P. aeruginosa* exotoxins A, S, and T) have adenosine diphosphate (ADP)-ribosyltransferase activity—i.e., the toxins enzymatically catalyze the transfer of the ADP-ribosyl portion of nicotinamide adenine diphosphate to target proteins and inactivate them. The staphylococcal enterotoxins, TSST-1, and the streptococcal pyogenic exotoxins behave as superantigens, stimulating certain T cells to proliferate without processing of the protein toxin by antigen-presenting cells. Part of this process involves stimulation of the antigen-presenting cells to produce IL-1 and TNF-α, which have been implicated in many of the clinical features of diseases like toxic shock syndrome and scarlet fever. A number of gram-negative pathogens (*Salmonella*, *Yersinia*, and *P. aeruginosa*) can inject toxins directly into host target cells by means of a complex set of proteins referred to as the type III secretion system. Loss or inactivation of this virulence system usually greatly reduces the capacity of a bacterial pathogen to cause disease.

ENDOTOXIN

The lipid A portion of gram-negative LPS has potent biologic activities that cause many of the clinical manifestations of gram-negative bacterial sepsis, including fever, muscle proteolysis, uncontrolled intravascular coagulation, and shock. The effects of lipid A appear to be mediated by the production of potent cytokines due to LPS binding to CD14 and signal transduction via TLRs, particularly TLR4. Cytokines exhibit potent hypothermic activity through effects on the hypothalamus; they also increase vascular permeability, alter the activity of endothelial cells, and induce endothelial-cell procoagulant activity. Numerous therapeutic strategies aimed at neutralizing the effects of endotoxin are under investigation, but so far the results have been disappointing. One drug, activated protein C (drotrecogin alfa, activated), was found to reduce mortality by ~20% during severe sepsis—a condition that can be induced by endotoxin during gram-negative bacterial sepsis.

INVASION

Many diseases are caused primarily by pathogens growing in tissue sites that are normally sterile. Pneumococcal pneumonia is mostly attributable to the growth of *S. pneumoniae* in the lung and the attendant host inflammatory response, although specific factors that enhance this process (e.g., pneumolysin) may be responsible for some of the pathogenic potential of the pneumococcus. Disease that follows bacteremia and invasion of the meninges by meningitis-producing bacteria such as *N. meningitidis*, *H. influenzae*, *E. coli* K1, and group B streptococci appears to be due solely to the ability of these organisms to gain access to these tissues, multiply in them, and provoke cytokine production leading to tissue-damaging host inflammation.

Specific molecular mechanisms accounting for tissue invasion by fungal and protozoal pathogens are less well described. Except for studies pointing to factors like capsule and melanin production by *C. neoformans* and (possibly) levels of cell wall glucans in some pathogenic fungi, the molecular basis for fungal invasiveness is not well defined. Melanism has been shown to protect the fungal cell against death caused by phagocyte factors such as nitric oxide, superoxide, and hypochlorite. Morphogenic variation and production of proteases (e.g., the *Candida* aspartyl proteinase) have been implicated in fungal invasion of host tissues.

If pathogens are effectively to invade host tissues (particularly the blood), they must avoid the major host defenses represented by complement and phagocytic cells. Bacteria most often avoid these defenses through their cell surface polysaccharides—either capsular polysaccharides or long O-side-chain antigens characteristic of the smooth LPS of gram-negative bacteria. These molecules can prevent the activation and/or deposition of complement opsonins or limit the access of phagocytic cells with receptors for complement opsonins to these molecules when they are deposited on the bacterial surface below the capsular layer. Another potential mechanism of microbial virulence is the ability of some organisms to present the capsule as an apparent self antigen through molecular mimicry. For example, the polysialic acid capsule of group B *N. meningitidis* is chemically identical to an oligosaccharide found on human brain cells.

Immunochemical studies of capsular polysaccharides have led to an appreciation of the tremendous chemical diversity that can result from the linking of a few monosaccharides. For example, three hexoses can link up in more than 300 different and potentially serologically distinct ways, while three amino acids have only six possible peptide combinations. Capsular polysaccharides, which have been used as effective vaccines against meningococcal meningitis as well as against pneumococcal and *H. influenzae* infections, may prove to be of value as vaccines against any organisms that express a nontoxic, immunogenic capsular polysaccharide. In addition, most encapsulated pathogens become virtually avirulent when capsule production is interrupted by genetic manipulation; this observation emphasizes the importance of this structure in pathogenesis.

HOST RESPONSE

The inflammatory response of the host is critical for interruption and resolution of the infectious process but also is often responsible for the signs and symptoms of disease. Infection promotes a complex series of host responses involving the complement, kinin, and coagulation pathways. The production of cytokines such as IL-1, TNF-α, and other factors regulated in part by the NF-κB transcription factor leads to fever, muscle proteolysis, and other effects, as noted above. An inability to kill or contain the microbe usually results in further damage due to the progression of inflammation and infection. In many chronic infections, degranulation of host inflammatory cells can lead to release of host proteases, elastases, histamines, and other toxic substances that can degrade host tissues. Chronic inflammation in any tissue can lead to the destruction of that tissue and to clinical disease associated with loss of organ function; an example is sterility from pelvic inflammatory disease caused by chronic infection with *N. gonorrhoeae*.

The nature of the host response elicited by the pathogen often determines the pathology of a particular infection. Local inflammation produces local tissue damage, while systemic inflammation, such as that seen during sepsis, can result in the signs and symptoms of septic shock. The severity of septic shock is associated with the degree of production of host effectors. Disease due to intracellular parasitism results from the formation of granulomas, wherein the host attempts to wall off the parasite inside a fibrotic lesion surrounded by fused epithelial cells that make up so-called multinucleated giant cells. A number of pathogens, particularly anaerobic bacteria, staphylococci, and streptococci, provoke the formation of an abscess, probably because of the presence of zwitterionic surface polysaccharides such as the capsular polysaccharide of *Bacteroides fragilis*. The outcome of an infection depends on the balance between an effective host response that eliminates a pathogen and an excessive inflammatory response that is associated with an inability to eliminate a pathogen and with the resultant tissue damage that leads to disease.

TRANSMISSION TO NEW HOSTS

As part of the pathogenic process, most microbes are shed from the host, often in a form infectious for susceptible individuals. However, the rate of transmissibility may not necessarily be high, even if the disease is severe in the infected individual, as transmissibility and virulence are not linked traits. Most pathogens exit via the same route by which they entered: respiratory pathogens by aerosols from sneezing or coughing or through salivary spread, gastrointestinal pathogens by fecal-oral spread, sexually transmitted diseases by venereal spread, and vector-borne organisms by either direct contact with the vector through a blood meal or indirect contact with organisms shed into environmental sources such as water. Microbial factors that specifically promote transmission are not well characterized. Respiratory shedding is facilitated by overproduction of mucous secretions, with consequently enhanced sneezing and coughing. Diarrheal toxins such as cholera toxin, *E. coli* heat-labile toxins, and *Shigella* toxins probably facilitate fecal-oral spread of microbial cells in the high volumes of diarrheal fluid produced during infection. The ability to produce phenotypic variants that resist hostile environmental factors (e.g., the highly resistant cysts of *E. histolytica* shed in feces) represents another mechanism of pathogenesis relevant to transmission. Blood parasites such as *Plasmodium* spp. change phenotype after ingestion by a mosquito—a prerequisite for the continued transmission of this pathogen. Venereally transmitted pathogens may undergo phenotypic variation due to the production of specific factors to facilitate transmission, but shedding of these pathogens into the environment does not result in the formation of infectious foci.

In summary, the molecular mechanisms used by pathogens to colonize, invade, infect, and disrupt the host are numerous and diverse. Each phase of the infectious process involves a variety of microbial and host factors interacting in a manner that can result in disease. Recognition of the coordinated genetic regulation of virulence factor elaboration when organisms move from their natural environment into the mammalian host emphasizes the complex nature of the host-parasite interaction. Fortunately, the need for diverse factors in successful infection and disease implies that a variety of therapeutic strategies may be developed to interrupt this process and thereby prevent and treat microbial infections.

FURTHER READINGS

CAMILLI A, BASSLER BL: Bacterial small-molecule signaling pathways. Science 311:1113, 2006

FINLAY BB, MCFADDEN G: Anti-immunology: Evasion of the host immune system by bacterial and viral pathogens. Cell 124:767, 2006

HAN J, ULEVITCH RJ: Limiting inflammatory responses during activation of innate immunity. Nat Immunol 6:1198, 2005

KAWAI T, AKIRA S: Innate immune recognition of viral infection. Nat Immunol 7:131, 2006

KNIREL YA et al: Structural features and structural variability of the lipopolysaccharide of *Yersinia pestis,* the cause of plague. J Endotoxin Res 12:3, 2006

MENDES-GIANNINI MJ et al: Interaction of pathogenic fungi with host cells: Molecular and cellular approaches. FEMS Immunol Med Microbiol 45:383, 2005

PIZARRO-CERDA J, COSSART P: Bacterial adhesion and entry into host cells. Cell 124:715, 2006

SPEAR PG et al: Different receptors binding to distinct interfaces on herpes simplex virus gD can trigger events leading to cell fusion and viral entry. Virology 344:17, 2006

TAKAHASHI K et al: The mannose-binding lectin: A prototypic pattern recognition molecule. Curr Opin Immunol 18:16, 2006

115 Approach to the Acutely Ill Infected Febrile Patient

Tamar F. Barlam, Dennis L. Kasper

The physician treating the acutely ill febrile patient must be able to recognize infections that require emergent attention. If such infections are not adequately evaluated and treated at initial presentation, the opportunity to alter an adverse outcome may be lost. In this chapter, the clinical presentations of and approach to patients with relatively common infectious disease emergencies are discussed. These infectious processes and their treatments are discussed in detail in other chapters. Noninfectious causes of fever are not covered in this chapter; information on the approach to fever of unknown origin, including that eventually shown to be of noninfectious etiology, is presented in Chap. 19.

APPROACH TO THE PATIENT:
Acute Febrile Illness

A physician must have a consistent approach to acutely ill patients. Even before the history is elicited and a physical examination performed, an immediate assessment of the patient's general appearance yields valuable information. The perceptive physician's subjective sense that a patient is septic or toxic often proves accurate. Visible agitation or anxiety in a febrile patient can be a harbinger of critical illness.

HISTORY   Presenting symptoms are frequently nonspecific. Detailed questions should be asked about the onset and duration of symptoms and about changes in severity or rate of progression over time. Host factors and comorbid conditions may enhance the risk of infection with certain organisms or of a more fulminant course than is usually seen. Lack of splenic function, alcoholism with significant liver disease, intravenous drug use, HIV infection, diabetes, malignancy, and chemotherapy all predispose to specific infections and frequently to increased severity. The patient should be questioned about factors that might help identify a nidus for invasive infection, such as recent upper respiratory tract infections, influenza, or varicella; prior trauma; disruption of cutaneous barriers due to lacerations, burns, surgery, or decubiti; and the presence of foreign bodies, such as nasal packing after rhinoplasty, barrier contraceptives, tampons, arteriovenous fistulas, or prosthetic joints. Travel, contact with pets or other animals, or activities that might result in tick exposure can lead to diagnoses that would not otherwise be considered. Recent dietary intake, medication use, social or occupational contact with ill individuals, vaccination history, recent sexual contacts, and menstrual history may be relevant. A review of systems should focus on any neurologic signs or sensorium alterations, rashes or skin lesions, and focal pain or tenderness and should also include a general review of respiratory, gastrointestinal, or genitourinary symptoms.

PHYSICAL EXAMINATION   A complete physical examination should be performed, with special attention to several areas that are sometimes given short shrift in routine examinations. Assessment of the patient's general appearance and vital signs, skin and soft tissue examination, and the neurologic evaluation are of particular importance.

The patient may appear either anxious and agitated or lethargic and apathetic. Fever is usually present, although elderly patients and compromised hosts [e.g., patients who are uremic or cirrhotic and those who are taking glucocorticoids or nonsteroidal anti-inflammatory drugs (NSAIDs)] may be afebrile despite serious underlying infection. Measurement of blood pressure, heart rate, and respiratory rate helps determine the degree of hemodynamic and metabolic compromise. The patient's airway must be evaluated to rule out the risk of obstruction from an invasive oropharyngeal infection.

The etiologic diagnosis may become evident in the context of a thorough skin examination (Chap. 18). Petechial rashes are typically seen with meningococcemia or Rocky Mountain spotted fever (RMSF); erythroderma is associated with toxic shock syndrome (TSS) and drug fever. The soft tissue and muscle examination is critical. Areas of erythema or duskiness, edema, and tenderness may indicate underlying necrotizing fasciitis, myositis, or myonecrosis. The neurologic examination must include a careful assessment of mental status for signs of early encephalopathy. Evidence of nuchal rigidity or focal neurologic findings should be sought.

DIAGNOSTIC WORKUP   After a quick clinical assessment, diagnostic material should be obtained rapidly and antibiotic and supportive treatment begun. Blood (for cultures; baseline complete blood count with differential; measurement of serum electrolytes, blood urea nitrogen, serum creatinine, and serum glucose; and liver function tests) can be obtained at the time an intravenous line is placed and before antibiotics are administered. Three sets of blood cultures should be performed for patients with possible acute endocarditis. Asplenic patients should have a blood smear examined to confirm the presence of Howell-Jolly bodies (indicating the absence of splenic function) and a buffy coat examined for bacteria; these patients can have >10^6 organisms per milliliter of blood (compared with 10^4/mL in patients with an intact spleen). Blood smears from patients at risk for severe parasitic disease, such as malaria or babesiosis, must be examined for the diagnosis and quantitation of parasitemia. Blood smears may also be diagnostic in ehrlichiosis.

Patients with possible meningitis should have cerebrospinal fluid (CSF) obtained before the initiation of antibiotic therapy. Focal findings, depressed mental status, or papilledema should be evaluated by brain imaging prior to lumbar puncture, which, in this setting, could initiate herniation. *Antibiotics should be administered before imaging but after blood for cultures has been drawn.* If CSF cultures are negative, blood cultures will provide the diagnosis in 50–70% of cases.

Focal abscesses necessitate immediate CT or MRI as part of an evaluation for surgical intervention. Other diagnostic procedures, such as cultures of wounds or scraping of skin lesions, should not delay the initiation of treatment for more than minutes. Once emergent evaluation, diagnostic procedures, and (if appropriate) surgical consultation (see below) have been completed, other laboratory tests can be conducted. Appropriate radiography, computed axial tomography, MRI, urinalysis, erythrocyte sedimentation rate (ESR) determination, and transthoracic or transesophageal echocardiography may all prove important.

℞ THE ACUTELY ILL PATIENT

In the acutely ill patient, empirical antibiotic therapy is critical and should be administered without undue delay. Increased prevalence of antibiotic resistance in community-acquired bacteria must be considered when antibiotics are selected. **Table 115-1** lists first-line treatments for infections considered in this chapter. In addition to the rapid initiation of antibiotic therapy, several of these infections require urgent surgical attention. Neurosurgical evaluation for subdural empyema or spinal epidural abscess, otolaryngologic surgery for possible mucormycosis, and cardiothoracic surgery for critically ill patients with acute endocarditis are as important as antibiotic therapy. For infections such as necrotizing fasciitis and clostridial myonecrosis, rapid surgical intervention supersedes other diagnostic or therapeutic maneuvers.

Adjunctive treatments may reduce morbidity and mortality and include dexamethasone for bacterial meningitis; intravenous immunoglobulin (IVIg) for TSS and necrotizing fasciitis caused by group A *Streptococcus*; low-dose hydrocortisone and fludrocortisone for septic shock; and drotrecogin alfa (activated), also known as recombinant human activated protein C, for meningococcemia and severe sepsis. Adjunctive therapies should usually be initiated within the first hours of treatment; however, dexamethasone for bacterial meningitis must be given before or at the time of the first dose of antibiotic.

TABLE 115-1 EMPIRICAL TREATMENT FOR COMMON INFECTIOUS DISEASE EMERGENCIES

Clinical Syndrome	Possible Etiologies	Treatment	Comments	See Chap.
Sepsis without a Clear Focus				
Septic shock	*Pseudomonas* spp., gram-negative enteric bacilli, *Staphylococcus* spp., *Streptococcus* spp.	Vancomycin (1 g q12h) **plus** Gentamicin (5 mg/kg per day) **plus either** Piperacillin/tazobactam (3.375 g q4h) **or** Cefepime (2 g q12h)	Adjust treatment when culture data become available. Drotrecogin alfa (activated)[a] or low-dose hydrocortisone and fludrocortisone[b] may improve outcome in patients with septic shock.	129, 130, 143, 145, 265
Overwhelming post-splenectomy sepsis	*Streptococcus pneumoniae*, *Haemophilus influenzae*, *Neisseria meningitidis*	Ceftriaxone (2 g q12h) **plus** Vancomycin (1 g q12h)	If a β-lactam–sensitive strain is identified, vancomycin can be discontinued.	265
Babesiosis	*Babesia microti* (U.S.), *B. divergens* (Europe)	**Either:** Clindamycin (600 mg tid) **plus** Quinine (650 mg tid) **or** Atovaquone (750 mg q12h) **plus** Azithromycin (500-mg loading dose, then 250 mg/d)	Atovaquone and azithromycin are as effective as clindamycin and quinine and are associated with fewer side effects. Treatment with doxycycline (100 mg bid[c]) for potential coinfection with *Borrelia burgdorferi* or *Ehrlichia* spp. may be prudent.	201, 204
Sepsis with Skin Findings				
Meningococcemia	*N. meningitidis*	Penicillin (4 mU q4h) **or** Ceftriaxone (2 g q12h)	Consider protein C replacement in fulminant meningococcemia.	136, 167
Rocky Mountain spotted fever (RMSF)	*Rickettsia rickettsii*	Doxycycline (100 mg bid)	If both meningococcemia and RMSF are being considered, use chloramphenicol alone (50–75 mg/kg per day in four divided doses) **or** ceftriaxone (2 g q12h) **plus** doxycycline (100 mg bid[c]) If RMSF is diagnosed, doxycycline is the proven superior agent.	
Purpura fulminans	*S. pneumoniae*, *H. influenzae*, *N. meningitidis*	Ceftriaxone (2 g q12h) **plus** Vancomycin (1 g q12h)	If a β-lactam–sensitive strain is identified, vancomycin can be discontinued.	136, 265
Erythroderma: toxic shock syndrome	Group A *Streptococcus*, *Staphylococcus aureus*	Vancomycin (1 g q12h) **plus** Clindamycin (600 mg q8h)	If a penicillin- or oxacillin-sensitive strain is isolated, those agents are superior to vancomycin (penicillin, 2 mU q4h; or oxacillin, 2 g q4h). The site of toxigenic bacteria should be debrided; IV immunoglobulin can be used in severe cases.[d]	129, 130
Sepsis with Soft Tissue Findings				
Necrotizing fasciitis	Group A *Streptococcus*, mixed aerobic/anaerobic flora	Penicillin (2 mU q4h) **plus** Clindamycin (600 mg q8h) **plus** Gentamicin (5 mg/kg per day)	Urgent surgical evaluation is critical. If community-acquired methicillin-resistant *S. aureus* is a concern, vancomycin (1 g q12h) can be substituted for penicillin while culture data are pending.	119, 130
Clostridial myonecrosis	*Clostridium perfringens*	Penicillin (2 mU q4h) **plus** Clindamycin (600 mg q8h)	Urgent surgical evaluation is critical.	135
Neurologic Infections				
Bacterial meningitis	*S. pneumoniae*, *N. meningitidis*	Ceftriaxone (2 g q12h) **plus** Vancomycin (1 g q12h)	If a β-lactam–sensitive strain is identified, vancomycin can be discontinued. If the patient is >50 years old or has comorbid disease, add ampicillin (2 g q4h) for *Listeria* coverage. Dexamethasone (10 mg q6h × 4 days) improves outcome in adult patients with meningitis (especially pneumococcal) and cloudy CSF, positive CSF Gram's stain, or a CSF leukocyte count >1000/μL.	376
Brain abscess, suppurative intracranial infections	*Streptococcus* spp., *Staphylococcus* spp., anaerobes, gram-negative bacilli	Vancomycin (1 g q12h) **plus** Metronidazole (500 mg q8h) **plus** Ceftriaxone (2 g q12h)	Urgent surgical evaluation is critical. If a penicillin- or oxacillin-sensitive strain is isolated, those agents are superior to vancomycin (penicillin, 4 mU q4h; or oxacillin, 2 g q4h).	376
Cerebral malaria	*Plasmodium falciparum*	Quinine (650 mg tid) **plus** Tetracycline (250 mg tid)	Do not use glucocorticoids.	201, 203

(continued)

TABLE 115-1 EMPIRICAL TREATMENT FOR COMMON INFECTIOUS DISEASE EMERGENCIES (CONTINUED)

Clinical Syndrome	Possible Etiologies	Treatment	Comments	See Chap.
Spinal epidural abscess	*Staphylococcus* spp., gram-negative bacilli	Vancomycin (1 g q12h) *plus* Ceftriaxone (2 g q24h)	Surgical evaluation is essential. If a penicillin- or oxacillin-sensitive strain is isolated, those agents are superior to vancomycin (penicillin, 4 mU q4h; or oxacillin, 2 g q4h).	372
Focal Infections				
Acute bacterial endocarditis	*S. aureus*, β-hemolytic streptococci, HACEK group,[e] *Neisseria* spp., *S. pneumoniae*	Ceftriaxone (2 g q12h) *plus* Vancomycin (1 g q12h)	Adjust treatment when culture data become available. Surgical evaluation is essential.	118

[a]Drotrecogin alfa (activated) is administered at a dose of 24 μg/kg per hour for 96 h. It has been approved for use in patients with severe sepsis and a high risk of death as defined by an Acute Physiology and Chronic Health Evaluation II (APACHE II) score of ≥25 and/or multiorgan failure.
[b]Hydrocortisone (50-mg IV bolus q6h) with fludrocortisone (50-μg tablet daily for 7 days) may improve outcomes of severe sepsis, particularly in the setting of relative adrenal insufficiency.

[c]Tetracyclines can be antagonistic in action to β-lactam agents. Adjust treatment as soon as the diagnosis is confirmed.
[d]The optimal dose of IV immunoglobulin has not been determined, but the median dose in observational studies is 2 g/kg (total dose administered over 1–5 days).
[e]*Haemophilus aphrophilus*, *H. paraphrophilus*, *H. parainfluenzae*, *Actinobacillus actinomycetemcomitans*, *Cardiobacterium hominis*, *Eikenella corrodens*, and *Kingella kingae*.

SPECIFIC PRESENTATIONS

The infections considered below according to common clinical presentation can have rapidly catastrophic outcomes, and their immediate recognition and treatment can be life-saving. Recommended empirical therapeutic regimens are presented in Table 115-1.

SEPSIS WITHOUT AN OBVIOUS FOCUS OF PRIMARY INFECTION

These patients initially have a brief prodrome of nonspecific symptoms and signs that progresses quickly to hemodynamic instability with hypotension, tachycardia, tachypnea, respiratory distress, and altered mental status. Disseminated intravascular coagulation (DIC) with clinical evidence of a hemorrhagic diathesis is a poor prognostic sign.

Septic Shock (See also Chap. 265) Patients with bacteremia leading to septic shock may have a primary site of infection (e.g., pneumonia, pyelonephritis, or cholangitis) that is not evident initially. Elderly patients with comorbid conditions, hosts compromised by malignancy and neutropenia, and patients who have recently undergone a surgical procedure or hospitalization are at increased risk for an adverse outcome. Gram-negative bacteremia with organisms such as *Pseudomonas aeruginosa* or *Escherichia coli* and gram-positive infection with organisms such as *Staphylococcus aureus* or group A streptococci can present as intractable hypotension and multiorgan failure. Treatment can usually be initiated empirically on the basis of the presentation (Table 265-3). Adjunctive therapy with either drotrecogin alfa (activated) or glucocorticoids should be considered for patients with severe sepsis.

Overwhelming Infection in Asplenic Patients (See also Chap. 265) Patients without splenic function are at risk for overwhelming bacterial sepsis. Asplenic adult patients succumb to sepsis at 58 times the rate of the general population; 50–70% of cases occur within the first 2 years after splenectomy, with a mortality rate of up to 80%, but the increased risk persists throughout life. In asplenia, encapsulated bacteria cause the majority of infections. Adults, who are more likely to have antibody to these organisms, are at lower risk than children. *Streptococcus pneumoniae* is the most common isolate, causing 50–70% of cases, but the risk of infection with *Haemophilus influenzae* or *Neisseria meningitidis* is also high. Severe clinical manifestations of infections due to *E. coli*, *S. aureus*, group B streptococci, *P. aeruginosa*, *Capnocytophaga*, *Babesia*, and *Plasmodium* have been described.

Babesiosis (See also Chap. 204) A history of recent travel to endemic areas raises the possibility of infection with *Babesia*. Between 1 and 4 weeks after a tick bite, the patient experiences chills, fatigue, anorexia, myalgia, arthralgia, shortness of breath, nausea, and headache; ecchymosis and/or petechiae are occasionally seen. The tick that most commonly transmits *Babesia*, *Ixodes scapularis*, also transmits *Borrelia burgdorferi* (the agent of Lyme disease) and *Ehrlichia*; co-infection can occur, resulting in more severe disease. Infection with the European species *Babesia divergens* is more frequently fulminant than that due to the U.S. species *Babesia microti*. *B. divergens* causes a febrile syndrome with hemolysis, jaundice, hemoglobinemia, and renal failure and is associated with a mortality rate of >50%. Severe babesiosis is especially common in asplenic hosts but does occur in hosts with normal splenic function, particularly at >60 years of age. Complications include renal failure, acute respiratory failure, and DIC.

Other Sepsis Syndromes Tularemia (Chap. 151) is seen throughout the United States but occurs primarily in Arkansas, Oklahoma, and Missouri. This disease is associated with wild rabbit, tick, and tabanid fly contact. The uncommon typhoidal form can be associated with gram-negative septic shock and a mortality rate of >30%. In the United States, plague (Chap. 152) occurs primarily in New Mexico, Arizona, and Colorado after contact with ground squirrels, prairie dogs, or chipmunks. Plague can occur with greater frequency outside the United States, especially in developing countries in Africa and Asia. The septic form is particularly rare and is associated with shock, multiorgan failure, and a 30% mortality rate. These rare infections should be considered in the appropriate epidemiologic setting. The Centers for Disease Control and Prevention lists tularemia and plague, along with anthrax, as important agents that might be used for bioterrorism (Chap. 214).

SEPSIS WITH SKIN MANIFESTATIONS

(See also Chap. 18) Maculopapular rashes may reflect early meningococcal or rickettsial disease but are usually associated with nonemergent infections. Exanthems are usually viral. Primary HIV infection commonly presents with a rash that is typically maculopapular and involves the upper part of the body but can spread to the palms and soles. The patient is usually febrile and can have lymphadenopathy, severe headache, dysphagia, diarrhea, myalgias, and arthralgias. Recognition of this syndrome provides an opportunity to prevent transmission and to institute treatment and monitoring early on.

Petechial rashes caused by viruses are seldom associated with hypotension or a toxic appearance, although severe measles can be an exception. In other settings, petechial rashes require more urgent attention.

Meningococcemia (See also Chap. 136) Almost three-quarters of patients with bacteremic *N. meningitidis* infection have a rash. Meningococcemia most often affects young children (i.e., those 6 months to 5 years old). In sub-Saharan Africa, the high prevalence of serogroup A meningococcal disease has been a threat to public health for more than a century. In addition, epidemic outbreaks occur every 8–12 years. In the United States, sporadic cases and outbreaks occur in daycare centers, schools (grade school through college), and army barracks. Household members of index cases are at 400–800 times greater risk of disease than the general population. Patients may exhibit fever, headache, nausea, vomiting, myalgias, changes in mental status, and meningismus. However, the rapidly progressive form of disease is not usually associated with meningitis. The rash is initially pink, blanching, and maculopapular, appearing on the trunk and extremities, but then becomes hemorrhagic, forming petechiae. Petechiae are first seen at the ankles, wrists, axillae, mucosal surfaces, and palpebral and bulbar conjunctiva, with subsequent spread to the lower extremities and trunk. A cluster of petechiae may be seen at pressure points—e.g., where a blood pressure cuff has been inflated. In rapidly progressive meningococcemia (10–20% of cases), the petechial rash quickly becomes purpuric (see Fig. 52-5), and patients develop DIC, multiorgan failure, and shock. Of these patients, 50–60% die, and survivors often require extensive debridement or amputation of gangrenous extremities. Hypotension with petechiae for <12 h is associated with significant mortality. The mortality rate can exceed 90% among patients without meningitis who have rash, hypotension, and a normal or low white blood cell (WBC) count and ESR. Cyanosis, coma, oliguria, metabolic acidosis, and elevated partial thromboplastin time are also associated with a fatal outcome. Correction of protein C deficiency may improve outcome. Antibiotics given in the office by the primary care provider before hospital evaluation and admission may improve prognosis; this observation suggests that early initiation of treatment may be life-saving.

Rocky Mountain Spotted Fever   (See also Chap. 167) RMSF is a tick-borne disease caused by *Rickettsia rickettsii* that occurs throughout North and South America. A history of known tick bite is common; however, if such a history is lacking, a history of travel or outdoor activity (e.g., camping in tick-infested areas) can be ascertained. For the first 3 days, headache, fever, malaise, myalgias, nausea, vomiting, and anorexia are present. By day 3, half of patients have skin findings. Blanching macules develop initially on the wrists and ankles and then spread over the legs and trunk. The lesions become hemorrhagic and are frequently petechial. The rash spreads to palms and soles later in the course. The centripetal spread is a classic feature of RMSF. However, 10–15% of patients with RMSF never develop a rash. The patient can be hypotensive and develop noncardiogenic pulmonary edema, confusion, lethargy, and encephalitis progressing to coma. The CSF contains 10–100 cells/µL, usually with a predominance of mononuclear cells. The CSF glucose level is often normal; the protein concentration may be slightly elevated. Renal and hepatic injury and bleeding secondary to vascular damage are noted. Untreated infection has a mortality rate of 30%.

Although RMSF is the most severe rickettsial disease, other rickettsial diseases cause significant morbidity and mortality worldwide. *Mediterranean spotted fever* caused by *Rickettsia conorii* is found in Africa, southwestern and south-central Asia, and southern Europe. Patients have fever, flu-like symptoms, and an inoculation eschar at the site of the tick bite. A maculopapular rash develops within 1–7 days, involving the palms and soles but sparing the face. Elderly patients or those with diabetes, alcoholism, uremia, or congestive heart failure are at risk for severe disease characterized by neurologic involvement, respiratory distress, and gangrene of the digits. Mortality rates associated with this severe form of disease approach 50%. *Epidemic typhus*, caused by *Rickettsia prowazekii*, is transmitted in louse-infested environments and emerges in conditions of extreme poverty, war, and natural disaster. Patients experience a sudden onset of high fevers, severe headache, cough, myalgias, and abdominal pain. A maculopapular rash develops (primarily on the trunk) in more than half of patients and can progress to petechiae and purpura. Serious signs include delirium, coma, seizures, noncardiogenic pulmonary edema, skin necrosis, and peripheral gangrene. Mortality rates approached 60% in the preantibiotic era and continue to exceed 10–15% in contemporary outbreaks. *Scrub typhus*, caused by *Orientia tsutsugamushi*—a separate genus in the family Rickettsiaceae—is transmitted by larval mites or chiggers and is one of the most common infections in southeastern Asia and the western Pacific. The organism is found in areas of heavy scrub vegetation (e.g., along riverbanks). Patients

present with fever and lymphadenopathy, may have an inoculation eschar, and may develop a maculopapular rash. Severe cases progress to pneumonia, meningoencephalitis, DIC, and renal failure. Mortality rates range from 1% to 35%.

If recognized in a timely fashion, rickettsial disease is very responsive to treatment. Doxycycline (100 mg twice daily for 3–14 days) is the treatment of choice for both adults and children. The newer macrolides and chloramphenicol may be suitable alternatives.

Purpura Fulminans   (See also Chaps. 136 and 265) Purpura fulminans is the cutaneous manifestation of DIC and presents as large ecchymotic areas and hemorrhagic bullae. Progression of petechiae to purpura, ecchymoses, and gangrene is associated with congestive heart failure, septic shock, acute renal failure, acidosis, hypoxia, hypotension, and death. Purpura fulminans has been associated primarily with *N. meningitidis* but, in splenectomized patients, may be associated with *S. pneumoniae* and *H. influenzae*. Several small studies have suggested that correction of the protein C deficiency evident in meningococcal purpura fulminans with drotrecogin alfa (activated) may dramatically improve outcome.

Ecthyma Gangrenosum   Septic shock caused by *P. aeruginosa* or *Aeromonas hydrophila* can be associated with ecthyma gangrenosum (see Fig. 145-1): hemorrhagic vesicles surrounded by a rim of erythema with central necrosis and ulceration. These gram-negative bacteremias are most common among patients with neutropenia, extensive burns, and hypogammaglobulinemia.

Other Emergent Infections Associated with Rash   *Vibrio vulnificus* and other noncholera *Vibrio* bacteremic infections (Chap. 149) can cause focal skin lesions and overwhelming sepsis in hosts with liver disease. After ingestion of contaminated shellfish, there is a sudden onset of malaise, chills, fever, and hypotension. The patient develops bullous or hemorrhagic skin lesions, usually on the lower extremities, and 75% of patients have leg pain. The mortality rate can be as high as 50–60%. *Capnocytophaga canimorsus* can cause septic shock in asplenic patients. Infection with this fastidious gram-negative rod typically presents after a dog bite as fever, chills, myalgia, vomiting, diarrhea, dyspnea, confusion, and headache. Findings can include an exanthem or erythema multiforme (see Fig. 52-9), cyanotic mottling or peripheral cyanosis, petechiae, and ecchymosis. About 30% of patients with this fulminant form die of overwhelming sepsis and DIC, and survivors may require amputation because of gangrene.

Erythroderma   TSS (Chaps. 129 and 130) is usually associated with erythroderma. The patient presents with fever, malaise, myalgias, nausea, vomiting, diarrhea, and confusion. There is a sunburn-type rash that may be subtle and patchy but is usually diffuse and is found on the face, trunk, and extremities. Erythroderma, which desquamates after 1–2 weeks, is more common in *Staphylococcus*-associated than in *Streptococcus*-associated TSS. Hypotension develops rapidly—often within hours—after the onset of symptoms. Multiorgan failure is seen. Early renal failure may precede hypotension and distinguishes this syndrome from other septic shock syndromes. Commonly there is no indication of a primary focal infection, although possible cutaneous or mucosal portals of entry for the organism can be ascertained when a careful history is taken. Colonization rather than overt infection of the vagina or a postoperative wound, for example, is typical with staphylococcal TSS, and the mucosal areas appear hyperemic but not infected. The diagnosis of TSS is defined by the clinical criteria of fever, rash, hypotension, and multiorgan involvement. The mortality rate is 5% for menstruation-associated TSS, 10–15% for nonmenstrual TSS, and 30–70% for streptococcal TSS.

Viral Hemorrhagic Fevers   Viral hemorrhagic fevers (Chaps. 189 and 190) are zoonotic illnesses caused by viruses that reside in either animal reservoirs or arthropod vectors. These diseases occur worldwide and are restricted to areas where the host species live.

They are caused by four major groups of viruses: Arenaviridae (e.g., Lassa fever in Africa), Bunyaviridae (e.g., Rift Valley fever in Africa or hantavirus hemorrhagic fever with renal syndrome in Asia), Filoviridae (e.g., Ebola and Marburg virus infections in Africa), and Flaviviridae (e.g., yellow fever in Africa and South America and dengue in Asia, Africa, and the Americas). Lassa fever as well as Ebola and Marburg virus infections are also transmitted from person to person. The vectors for most viral fevers are found in rural areas; dengue and yellow fever are important exceptions. After a prodrome of fever, myalgias, and malaise, patients develop evidence of vascular damage, petechiae, and local hemorrhage. Shock, multifocal hemorrhaging, and neurologic signs (e.g., seizures or coma) predict a poor prognosis. Although supportive care to maintain blood pressure and intravascular volume is key, ribavirin may be useful against Arenaviridae and Bunyaviridae. Dengue (Chap. 189) is the most common arboviral disease worldwide. More than a quarter of a million cases of dengue hemorrhagic fever occur each year, with 25,000 deaths. Patients have a triad of symptoms: hemorrhagic manifestations, evidence of plasma leakage, and platelet counts <100,000/μL. Mortality rates are 10–20%. If dengue shock syndrome develops, mortality can reach 40%. Immediate supportive care and volume-replacement therapy are life-saving.

SEPSIS WITH A SOFT TISSUE/MUSCLE PRIMARY FOCUS
See also Chap. 119.

Necrotizing Fasciitis   This infection may arise at a site of minimal trauma or postoperative incision and may also be associated with recent varicella, childbirth, or muscle strain. The most common causes of necrotizing fasciitis are group A streptococci alone (Chap. 130) and a mixed facultative and anaerobic flora (Chap. 119). Diabetes mellitus, peripheral vascular disease, and intravenous drug use are associated risk factors. Use of NSAIDs has been reported to allow progression of skin or soft tissue infections; however, prospective studies have not shown that NSAIDs increase the risk of disease or exacerbate established infection. The patient may have bacteremia and hypotension without other organ-system failure. Physical findings are minimal compared with the severity of pain and the degree of fever. The examination is often unremarkable except for soft tissue edema and erythema. The infected area is red, hot, shiny, swollen, and exquisitely tender. In untreated infection, the overlying skin develops blue-gray patches after 36 h, and cutaneous bullae and necrosis develop after 3–5 days. Necrotizing fasciitis due to a mixed flora, but not that due to group A streptococci, can be associated with gas production. Without treatment, pain decreases because of thrombosis of the small blood vessels and destruction of the peripheral nerves—an ominous sign. The mortality rate is 25–30% overall, >70% in association with TSS, and nearly 100% without surgical intervention. Life-threatening necrotizing fasciitis may also be due to *Clostridium perfringens* (Chap. 135); in this condition, the patient is extremely toxic and the mortality rate is high. Within 48 h, rapid tissue invasion and systemic toxicity associated with hemolysis and death ensue. The distinction between this entity and clostridial myonecrosis is made by muscle biopsy. Necrotizing fasciitis caused by community-acquired methicillin-resistant *S. aureus* (MRSA) was recently described. The MRSA-infected patients required extensive surgical debridement, but there were no deaths.

Clostridial Myonecrosis   (See also Chap. 135) Myonecrosis is often associated with trauma or surgery but can be spontaneous. The incubation period is usually 12–24 h long, and massive necrotizing gangrene develops within hours of onset. Systemic toxicity, shock, and death can occur within 12 h. The patient's pain and toxic appearance are out of proportion to physical findings. On examination, the patient is febrile, apathetic, tachycardic, and tachypneic and may express a feeling of impending doom. Hypotension and renal failure develop later, and hyperalertness is evident preterminally. The skin over the affected area is bronze-brown, mottled, and edematous. Bullous lesions with serosanguineous drainage and a mousy or sweet odor can be present. Crepitus can occur secondary to gas production in muscle tissue. The mortality

rate is >65% with spontaneous myonecrosis, which is often associated with *Clostridium septicum* and underlying malignancy. The mortality rates associated with trunk and limb infection are 63% and 12%, respectively, and any delay in surgical treatment increases the risk of death.

NEUROLOGIC INFECTIONS WITH OR WITHOUT SEPTIC SHOCK

Bacterial Meningitis   (See also Chap. 376) Bacterial meningitis is one of the most common infectious disease emergencies involving the central nervous system. Although hosts with cell-mediated immune deficiency (including transplant recipients, diabetic patients, elderly patients, and cancer patients receiving certain chemotherapeutic agents) are at particular risk for *Listeria monocytogenes* meningitis, most cases in adults are due to *S. pneumoniae* (30–50%) and *N. meningitidis* (10–35%). The classic presentation of headache, meningismus, and fever is seen in only one-half to two-thirds of patients. The elderly can present without fever or meningeal signs despite lethargy and confusion. Cerebral dysfunction is evidenced by confusion, delirium, and lethargy that can progress to coma. A fulminant presentation with sepsis and brain edema occurs in some cases; papilledema at presentation is unusual and suggests another diagnosis (e.g., an intracranial lesion). Focal signs, including cranial nerve palsies (IV, VI, VII), can be seen in 10–20% of cases; 50–70% of patients have bacteremia. A poor outcome is associated with coma, hypotension, meningitis due to *S. pneumoniae*, respiratory distress, a CSF glucose level of <0.6 mmol/L (<10 mg/dL), a CSF protein level of >2.5 g/L, a peripheral WBC count of <5000/μL, and a serum sodium level of <135 mmol/L.

Suppurative Intracranial Infections   (See also Chap. 376) In suppurative intracranial infections, rare intracranial lesions present along with sepsis and hemodynamic instability. Rapid recognition of the toxic patient with central neurologic signs is crucial to improvement of the dismal prognosis of these entities. *Subdural empyema* arises from the paranasal sinus in 60–70% of cases. Microaerophilic streptococci and staphylococci are the predominant etiologic organisms. The patient is toxic, with fever, headache, and nuchal rigidity. Of all patients, 75% have focal signs and 6–20% die. Despite improved survival rates, 15–44% of patients are left with permanent neurologic deficits. *Septic cavernous sinus thrombosis* follows a facial or sphenoid sinus infection; 70% of cases are due to staphylococci, and the remainder are due primarily to aerobic or anaerobic streptococci. A unilateral or retroorbital headache progresses to a toxic appearance and fever within days. Three-quarters of patients have unilateral periorbital edema that becomes bilateral and then progresses to ptosis, proptosis, ophthalmoplegia, and papilledema. The mortality rate is as high as 30%. *Septic thrombosis of the superior sagittal sinus* spreads from the ethmoid or maxillary sinuses and is caused by *S. pneumoniae*, other streptococci, and staphylococci. The fulminant course is characterized by headache, nausea, vomiting, rapid progression to confusion and coma, nuchal rigidity, and brainstem signs. If the sinus is totally thrombosed, the mortality rate exceeds 80%.

Brain Abscess   (See also Chap. 376) Brain abscess often occurs without systemic signs. Almost half of patients are afebrile, and presentations are more consistent with a space-occupying lesion in the brain; 70% of patients have headache, 50% have focal neurologic signs, and 25% have papilledema. Abscesses can present as single or multiple lesions resulting from contiguous foci or hematogenous infection, such as endocarditis. The infection progresses over several days from cerebritis to an abscess with a mature capsule. More than half of infections are polymicrobial, with an etiology consisting of aerobic bacteria (primarily streptococcal species) and anaerobes. Abscesses arising hematogenously are especially apt to rupture into the ventricular space, causing a sudden and severe deterioration in clinical status and high mortality. Otherwise, mortality is low but morbidity is high (30–55%). Patients presenting with stroke and a parameningeal infectious focus, such as sinusitis or otitis, may have a brain abscess, and physicians must maintain a high level of suspicion. Prognosis worsens in patients with a fulminant course, delayed diagnosis, abscess rupture into the ventricles, multiple abscesses, or abnormal neurologic status at presentation.

Cerebral Malaria (See also Chap. 203) This entity should be urgently considered if patients who have recently traveled to areas endemic for malaria present with a febrile illness and lethargy or other neurologic signs. Fulminant malaria is caused by *Plasmodium falciparum* and is associated with temperatures of >40°C (>104°F), hypotension, jaundice, adult respiratory distress syndrome, and bleeding. By definition, any patient with a change in mental status or repeated seizure in the setting of fulminant malaria has cerebral malaria. In adults, this nonspecific febrile illness progresses to coma over several days; occasionally, coma occurs within hours and death within 24 h. Nuchal rigidity and photophobia are rare. On physical examination, symmetric encephalopathy is typical, and upper motor neuron dysfunction with decorticate and decerebrate posturing can be seen in advanced disease. Unrecognized infection results in a 20–30% mortality rate.

Spinal Epidural Abscesses (See also Chap. 372) Patients with spinal epidural abscesses often present with back pain and develop neurologic deficits late in their course. At-risk patients include those with diabetes mellitus; intravenous drug use; chronic alcohol abuse; recent spinal trauma, surgery, or epidural anesthesia; and other comorbid conditions, such as HIV infection. The thoracic or lumbar spine is the most common location; cervical spine infections are associated with worse outcomes. Staphylococci are the most common etiologic agents. This diagnosis must immediately be considered in patients with a history of antecedent back pain and new neurologic symptoms. Almost 60% of patients have fever, and almost 90% have back pain. Paresthesia, bowel and bladder dysfunction, radicular pain, and weakness are frequent neurologic complaints, and examination of the patient may reveal abnormal reflexes and motor and sensory deficits. The ESR and leukocyte counts are usually elevated. Rapid recognition and treatment, which may include surgical drainage, can prevent or minimize permanent neurologic sequelae.

OTHER FOCAL SYNDROMES WITH A FULMINANT COURSE

Infection at virtually any primary focus (e.g., osteomyelitis, pneumonia, pyelonephritis, or cholangitis) can result in bacteremia and sepsis. TSS has been associated with focal infections such as septic arthritis, peritonitis, sinusitis, and wound infection. Rapid clinical deterioration and death can be associated with destruction of the primary site of infection, as is seen in endocarditis and in necrotizing infections of the oropharynx (in which edema suddenly compromises the airway).

Rhinocerebral Mucormycosis (See also Chap. 198) Patients with diabetes or malignancy are at risk for invasive rhinocerebral mucormycosis. Patients present with low-grade fever, dull sinus pain, diplopia, decreased mental status, decreased ocular motion, chemosis, proptosis, dusky or necrotic nasal turbinates, and necrotic hard-palate lesions that respect the midline. Without rapid recognition and intervention, the process continues on an inexorable invasive course, with high mortality.

Acute Bacterial Endocarditis (See also Chap. 118) This entity presents with a much more aggressive course than subacute endocarditis. Bacteria such as *S. aureus, S. pneumoniae, L. monocytogenes, Haemophilus* spp., and streptococci of groups A, B, and G attack native valves. Mortality rates range from 10% to 40%. The host may have comorbid conditions such as underlying malignancy, diabetes mellitus, intravenous drug use, or alcoholism. The patient presents with fever, fatigue, and malaise <2 weeks after onset of infection. On physical examination, a changing murmur and congestive heart failure may be noted. Hemorrhagic macules on palms or soles (*Janeway lesions*) sometimes develop. Petechiae, Roth's spots, splinter hemorrhages, and splenomegaly are unusual. Rapid valvular destruction, particularly of the aortic valve, results in pulmonary edema and hypotension. Myocardial

abscesses can form, eroding through the septum or into the conduction system and causing life-threatening arrhythmias or high-degree conduction block. Large friable vegetations can result in major arterial emboli, metastatic infection, or tissue infarction. Emboli can lead to stroke, changes in mental status, visual disturbances, aphasia, ataxia, headache, meningismus, brain abscess, cerebritis, spinal cord infarct with paraplegia, arthralgia, osteomyelitis, splenic abscess, septic arthritis, and hematuria. Older patients with *S. aureus* endocarditis are especially likely to present with nonspecific symptoms—a circumstance that delays diagnosis and worsens prognosis. Rapid intervention is crucial for a successful outcome.

Inhalational Anthrax (See also Chap. 214) Inhalational anthrax, the most severe form of disease caused by *Bacillus anthracis*, had not been reported in the United States for more than 25 years until the recent use of this organism as an agent of bioterrorism (Chap. 214). Patients presented with malaise, fever, cough, nausea, drenching sweats, shortness of breath, and headache. Rhinorrhea was unusual. All patients had abnormal chest roentgenograms at presentation. Pulmonary infiltrates, mediastinal widening, and pleural effusions were the most common findings. Hemorrhagic meningitis was seen in 38% of these patients. Survival was more likely when antibiotics were given during the prodromal period and if multidrug regimens were used. In the absence of urgent intervention with antimicrobial agents and supportive care, inhalational anthrax progresses rapidly to hypotension, cyanosis, and death.

Avian Influenza (H5N1) Infection (See also Chap. 180) Human cases of avian influenza were first reported in Hong Kong. Recent cases have occurred primarily in Southeast Asia, particularly Vietnam. However, evidence of a rapidly expanding geographic distribution of the virus throughout the world is of grave concern. Avian influenza should be considered in patients with severe respiratory tract illness, particularly if they have been exposed to poultry. To date, human-to-human transmission is rare. Patients present with high fever, an influenza-like illness, and lower respiratory tract symptoms. Watery diarrhea may develop and may precede respiratory symptoms. Dyspnea develops a median of 5 days after the onset of symptoms and can progress to respiratory distress syndrome, multiorgan failure, and death within 9–10 days after the onset of illness. Early antiviral treatment with neuraminidase inhibitors should be initiated along with aggressive supportive measures.

Hantavirus Pulmonary Syndrome (See also Chap. 189) Hantavirus pulmonary syndrome (HPS) has been documented in the United States (primarily the southwestern states), Canada, and South America. Most cases occur in rural areas and are associated with exposure to rodents. Patients present with a nonspecific viral prodrome of fever, malaise, myalgias, nausea, vomiting, and dizziness that may progress to pulmonary edema and respiratory failure. HPS causes myocardial depression and increased pulmonary vascular permeability; therefore, careful fluid resuscitation and use of pressor agents are crucial. Aggressive cardiopulmonary support during the first few hours of illness can be life-saving.

CONCLUSION

Acutely ill febrile patients with the syndromes discussed in this chapter require close observation, aggressive supportive measures, and—in most cases—admission to intensive care units. The most important task of the physician is to distinguish these patients from other infected febrile patients who will not progress to fulminant disease. The alert physician must recognize the acute infectious disease emergency and then proceed with appropriate urgency.

FURTHER READINGS

BEIGEL JH et al: Avian influenza A (H5N1) infection in humans. N Engl J Med 353:1374, 2005

DAROUICHE RO: Spinal epidural abscess. N Engl J Med 355:2012, 2006

HASHAM S et al: Necrotising fasciitis. BMJ 330:830, 2005

IDRO R et al: Pathogenesis, clinical features, and neurological outcome of cerebral malaria. Lancet Neurol 4:827, 2005

KYAW MH et al: Evaluation of severe infection and survival after splenectomy. Am J Med 119:276.e1, 2006

NGUYEN HB et al: Severe sepsis and septic shock: Review of the literature and emergency department management guidelines. Ann Emerg Med 48:28, 2006

OSBORN MK, STEINBERG JP: Subdural empyema and other suppurative complications of paranasal sinusitis. Lancet Infect Dis 7:62, 2007

STEPHENS DS et al: Epidemic meningitis, meningococcaemia, and *Neisseria meningitidis*. Lancet 369:2196, 2007

VAN DE BEEK D et al: Community-acquired bacterial meningitis in adults. N Engl J Med 354:44, 2006

WILLS BA et al: Comparison of three fluid solutions for resuscitation in dengue shock syndrome. N Engl J Med 353:877, 2005

116 Immunization Principles and Vaccine Use

Gerald T. Keusch, Kenneth J. Bart, Mark Miller

Vaccines play a special role in the health and security of nations. The World Health Organization (WHO) cites immunization and the provision of clean water as the two public health interventions that have had the greatest impact on the world's health, and the World Bank notes that vaccines are among the most cost-effective health interventions available. Over the past century, the integration of immunization into routine health care services in many countries has provided caregivers with some degree of control over disease-related morbidity and mortality, especially among infants and children.

Despite these extraordinary successes, vaccines and their constituents (e.g., the mercury compound thimerosal, formerly used as a preservative) have come under attack in some countries as causes of neurodevelopmental disorders, such as autism and attention-deficit hyperactivity disorder; diabetes; and a variety of allergic and autoimmune diseases. Although millions of lives are saved by vaccines each year and countless cases of postinfection disability are averted, some segments of the public are increasingly unwilling to accept any risk whatsoever of vaccine-associated complications (severe or otherwise), and resistance to vaccination is growing.

No medical procedure is absolutely risk-free, and the risk to the individual must always be balanced with benefits to the individual and to the population at large. This dichotomy poses two essential challenges for the medical and public health communities with respect to vaccines: (1) to create more effective and ever-safer vaccines, and (2) to educate patients and the general public more fully about the benefits as well as the risks of vaccine use. Because immunity to infectious diseases is acquired only by infection itself or by immunization, sustained vaccination programs for each birth cohort will continue to be necessary to control vaccine-preventable infectious diseases until and unless their etiologic agents can be eradicated from every region of the world.

An unwavering scientific and public health commitment to immunization is essential in countering public distrust and political pressure to legislate well-intentioned but ill-informed vaccine safety laws in response to the concerns of organized antivaccine advocacy groups. Ironically, it is the public health success of vaccines that has created a significant part of the problem: because the major fatal and disabling diseases of childhood are only rarely seen today in the United States, parents and young practitioners most likely will never have seen tetanus, diphtheria, *Haemophilus influenzae* disease, polio, or measles. Under these circumstances, the risks of immunization can easily (if erroneously) be perceived to outweigh the benefits, and this perception can be fueled by inaccurate information, poor science, and zealous advocacy. Caregivers must be prepared to educate parents about the importance of childhood immunization and to address their concerns effectively.

The medical community must also appreciate public concern about the sheer number of vaccines now licensed and the attendant fear that the more vaccines are administered, the more likely it is that complications and adverse immunologic consequences will occur. More than 50 biologic products are presently licensed in the United States, and dozens of antigens (many of them components of vaccine-combination products) are recommended for routine immunization of infants, children, adolescents, and adults (**Figs. 116-1** and **116-2**). Moreover, new vaccines are continually becoming available—e.g., human papillomavirus (HPV) vaccine for use in adolescent girls to prevent cervical cancer (Chap. 178) and a herpes simplex vaccine to prevent zoster (Chap. 173). Still other vaccines are used in special situations, including responses to outbreaks (e.g., polio), prophylaxis in travelers (e.g., yellow fever), and fulfillment of regional requirements (e.g., Japanese B encephalitis).

Of course, for many serious infectious agents, such as eukaryotic pathogens (protozoa and helminths) and HIV, effective and safe vaccines remain only a hope for the future. Current concern about the potential for a human pandemic of H5N1 avian influenza, against which a vaccine product is lacking, underscores the lag time between emerging public health needs and vaccine development programs.

The U.S. government's document *Healthy People 2010 Objectives for the Nation* includes a set of immunization indicators. The goals are for 80% of children to receive diphtheria–tetanus–acellular pertussis (DTaP), poliovirus, measles-mumps-rubella (MMR), *H. influenzae* type b (Hib), and hepatitis B vaccines and for 90% of adults to receive influenza and pneumococcal vaccines by 2010. Unfortunately, even these modest goals may not be attained in the United States.

IMPACT OF IMMUNIZATION

The epidemiologically appropriate use of vaccine resulted in the global eradication of smallpox, permitting the cessation of routine smallpox vaccination. Unfortunately, recent concerns about the potential use of smallpox virus for bioterrorism have led to renewed consideration of the need for routine smallpox immunization and for a new, effective, and much safer smallpox vaccine. Immunization has eliminated naturally transmitted poliomyelitis from the Western Hemisphere, Europe, and the western Pacific. However, polio has recrudesced in some countries in Africa, the Middle East, and parts of Asia because of interruption (for a variety of reasons) of immunization programs. Measles, which affected nearly 100% of children in the prevaccination era, has been effectively eliminated from most of the Western Hemisphere by widespread immunization; a global campaign to reduce measles mortality rates elsewhere is under way. The virtual elimination of rubella and congenital rubella syndrome, neonatal tetanus, and diphtheria in the United States is entirely due to vaccination. The introduction of Hib conjugate vaccines for immunization of infants has all but eliminated invasive Hib infections (including meningitis and pneumonia) among children <5 years of age. This vaccine both elicits durable immunity by the time maternal-derived antibodies dissipate and reduces nasopharyngeal carriage of Hib, thus diminishing the risk of transmission. The introduction of polyvalent pneumococcal polysaccharide conjugate vaccine is beginning to have a significant impact on serious invasive pneumococcal diseases, including otitis media. Vaccine has reduced the incidence of varicella by 70–87% in high-coverage areas. In short, vaccines work.

DEFINITIONS

The terms *vaccination* and *immunization* are often used interchangeably, although technically the former denotes the administration of a vaccine, whereas the latter refers to the induction or provision of immunity by any means, active or passive. Thus vaccination does not guarantee immunization, and immunization may not involve vaccine.

Recommended Immunization Schedule for Persons Aged 0–6 Years
UNITED STATES • 2007

Vaccine ▼ Age ▶	Birth	1 month	2 months	4 months	6 months	12 months	15 months	18 months	19–23 months	2–3 years	4–6 years
Hepatitis B [1]	HepB	HepB	HepB	see footnote 1	HepB	HepB	HepB	HepB	HepB Series	HepB Series	HepB Series
Rotavirus [2]			Rota	Rota	Rota						
Diphtheria, Tetanus, Pertussis [3]			DTaP	DTaP	DTaP		DTaP	DTaP			DTaP
Haemophilus influenzae type b [4]			Hib	Hib	*Hib* [4]	Hib	Hib	Hib	Hib		
Pneumococcal [5]			PCV	PCV	PCV	PCV	PCV			PCV / PPV	PCV / PPV
Inactivated Poliovirus			IPV	IPV	IPV	IPV	IPV	IPV			IPV
Influenza [6]					Influenza (Yearly)	Influenza (Yearly)	Influenza (Yearly)	Influenza (Yearly)	Influenza (Yearly)	Influenza (Yearly)	Influenza (Yearly)
Measles, Mumps, Rubella [7]						MMR	MMR				MMR
Varicella [8]						Varicella	Varicella				Varicella
Hepatitis A [9]						HepA (2 doses)	HepA (2 doses)	HepA (2 doses)	HepA (2 doses)	HepA Series	HepA Series
Meningococcal [10]										MPSV4	MPSV4

Range of recommended ages	Catch-up immunization	Certain high-risk groups

A

FIGURE 116-1 These schedules indicate the recommended ages for routine administration of currently licensed childhood vaccines, as of December 1, 2006, for children aged 0–6 and 7–18 years. Additional information is available at http://www.cdc.gov/nip/recs/child-schedule.htm. Any dose not administered at the recommended age should be administered at any subsequent visit, when indicated and feasible. Additional vaccines may be licensed and recommended during the year. Licensed combination vaccines may be used whenever any components of the combination are indicated and other components of the vaccine are not contraindicated and if approved by the Food and Drug Administration for that dose of the series. Providers should consult the respective Advisory Committee on Immunization Practices statement for detailed recommendations. Clinically significant adverse events that follow immunization should be reported to the Vaccine Adverse Event Reporting System (VAERS). Guidance about how to obtain and complete a VAERS form is available at http://www.vaers, hhs.gov or by telephone, 800-822-7967.

A. Recommended immunization schedule for persons aged 0–6 years—United States, 2006–2007. **1. Hepatitis B vaccine (HepB).** *(Minimum age: birth)* **At birth:** Administer monovalent HepB to all newborns before hospital discharge. If mother is hepatitis surface antigen (HBsAg)-positive, administer HepB and 0.5 mL of hepatitis B immune globulin (HBIG) within 12 hours of birth. If mother's HBsAg status is unknown, administer HepB within 12 hours of birth. Determine the HBsAg status as soon as possible and if HBsAg-positive, administer HBIG (no later than age 1 week). If mother is HBsAg-negative, the birth dose can only be delayed with physician's order and mother's negative HBsAg laboratory report documented in the infant's medical record. **After the birth dose:** The HepB series should be completed with either monovalent HepB or a combination vaccine containing HepB. The second dose should be administered at age 1–2 months. The final dose should be administered at age ≥24 weeks. Infants born to HBsAg-positive mothers should be tested for HBsAg and antibody to HBsAg after completion of ≥3 doses of a licensed HepB series, at age 9–18 months (generally at the next well-child visit). **4-month dose:** It is permissible to administer 4 doses of HepB when combination vaccines are administered after the birth dose. If monovalent HepB is used for doses after the birth dose, a dose at age 4 months is not needed. **2. Rotavirus vaccine (Rota).** *(Minimum age: 6 weeks)* Administer the first dose at age 6–12 weeks. Do not start the series later than age 12 weeks. Administer the final dose in the series by age 32 weeks. Do not administer a dose later than age 32 weeks. Data on safety and efficacy outside of these age ranges are insufficient. **3. Diphtheria and tetanus toxoids and acellular pertussis vaccine (DTaP).** *(Minimum age: 6 weeks)* The fourth dose of DTaP may be administered as early as age 12 months, provided 6 months have elapsed since the third dose. Administer the final dose in the series at age 4–6 years. **4. *Haemophilus influenzae* type b conjugate vaccine (Hib).** *(Minimum age: 6 weeks)* If PRP-OMP (Pedvax-HIB or ComVax [Merck]) is administered at ages 2 and 4 months, a dose at age 6 months is not required. TriHiBit (DTaP/Hib) combination products should not be used for primary immunization but can be used as boosters following any Hib vaccine in children aged ≥12 months. **5. Pneumococcal vaccine.** *(Minimum age: 6 weeks for pneumococcal conjugate vaccine [PCV]; 2 years for pneumococcal polysaccharide vaccine [PPV]).* Administer PCV at ages 24–59 months in certain high-risk groups. Administer PPV to children aged ≥2 years in certain high-risk groups. See MMWR 2000;49(No. RR-9):1–35. **6. Influenza vaccine.** *(Minimum age: 6 months for trivalent inactivated influenza vaccine [TIV]; 5 years for live, attenuated influenza vaccine [LAIV]).* All children aged 6–59 months and close contacts of all children aged 0–59 months are recommended to receive influenza vaccine. Influenza vaccine is recommended annually for children aged ≥59 months with certain risk factors, health-care workers, and other persons (including household members) in close contact with persons in groups at high risk. See MMWR 2006;55(No. RR-10):1–41. For healthy persons aged 5–49 years, LAIV may be used as an alternative to TIV. Children receiving TIV should receive 0.25 mL if aged 6–35 months or 0.5 mL if aged ≥3 years. Children aged <9 years who are receiving influenza vaccine for the first time should receive 2 doses (separated by ≥4 weeks for TIV and ≥6 weeks for LAIV). **7. Measles, mumps, and rubella vaccine (MMR).** *(Minimum age: 12 months)* Administer the second dose of MMR at age 4–6 years. MMR may be administered before age 4–6 years, provided ≥4 weeks have elapsed since the first dose and both doses are administered at age ≥12 months. **8. Varicella vaccine.** *(Minimum age: 12 months)* Administer the second dose of varicella vaccine at age 4–6 years. Varicella vaccine may be administered before age 4–6 years, provided that ≥3 months have elapsed since the first dose and both doses are administered at age ≥12 months. If second dose was administered ≥28 days following the first dose, the second dose does not need to be repeated.

(continued)

Recommended Immunization Schedule for Persons Aged 7–18 Years
UNITED STATES • 2007

Vaccine ▼ Age ▶	7–10 years	11–12 YEARS	13–14 years	15 years	16–18 years
Tetanus, Diphtheria, Pertussis [1]	see footnote 1	Tdap		Tdap	
Human Papillomavirus [2]	see footnote 2	HPV (3 doses)		HPV Series	
Meningococcal [3]	MPSV4	MCV4		MCV4 [3] / MCV4	
Pneumococcal [4]		PPV			
Influenza [5]		Influenza (Yearly)			
Hepatitis A [6]		HepA Series			
Hepatitis B [7]		HepB Series			
Inactivated Poliovirus [8]		IPV Series			
Measles, Mumps, Rubella [9]		MMR Series			
Varicella [10]		Varicella Series			

B

  ▨ Range of recommended ages   ▨ Catch-up immunization   ▨ Certain high-risk groups

FIGURE 116-1 (Continued)

9. Hepatitis A vaccine (HepA). *(Minimum age: 12 months)* HepA is recommended for all children aged 1 year (i.e., aged 12–23 months). The 2 doses in the series should be administered at least 6 months apart. Children not fully vaccinated by age 2 years can be vaccinated at subsequent visits. HepA is recommended for certain other groups of children, including in areas where vaccination programs target older children. See MMWR 2006;55(No. RR-7):1–23. **10. Meningococcal polysaccharide vaccine (MPSV4).** *(Minimum age: 2 years)* Administer MPSV4 to children aged 2–10 years with terminal complement deficiencies or anatomic or functional asplenia and certain other high-risk groups. See MMWR 2005;54(No. RR-7):1–21.

B. Recommended immunization schedule for persons aged 7–18 years—United States, 2006–2007. **1. Tetanus and diphtheria toxoids and acellular pertussis vaccine (Tdap).** *(Minimum age: 10 years for BOOSTRIX and 11 years for ADACEL)* Administer at age 11–12 years for those who have completed the recommended childhood DTP/DTaP vaccination series and have not received a tetanus and diphtheria toxoids vaccine (Td) booster dose. Adolescents aged 13–18 years who missed the 11–12 year Td/Tdap booster dose should also receive a single dose of Tdap if they have completed the recommended childhood DTP/DTaP vaccination series. **2. Human papillomavirus vaccine (HPV).** *(Minimum age: 9 years)* Administer the first dose of the HPV vaccine series to females at age 11–12 years. Administer the second dose 2 months after the first dose and the third dose 6 months after the first dose. Administer the HPV vaccine series to females at age 13–18 years if not previously vaccinated. **3. Meningococcal vaccine.** *(Minimum age: 11 years for meningococcal conjugate vaccine [MCV4]; 2 years for meningococcal polysaccharide vaccine [MPSV4]).* Administer MCV4 at age 11–12 years and to previously unvaccinated adolescents at high school entry (at approximately age 15 years). Administer MCV4 to previously unvaccinated college freshmen living in dormitories; MPSV4 is an acceptable alternative. Vaccination against invasive meningococcal disease is recommended for children and adolescents aged ≥2 years with terminal complement deficiencies or anatomic or functional asplenia

and certain other high-risk groups. See MMWR 2005;54(No. RR-7):1–21. Use MPSV4 for children aged 2–10 years and MCV4 or MPSV4 for older children. **4. Pneumococcal polysaccharide vaccine (PPV).** *(Minimum age: 2 years)* Administer for certain high-risk groups. See MMWR 1997;46(No. RR-8):1–24, and MMWR 2000;49(No. RR-9):1–35. **5. Influenza vaccine.** *(Minimum age: 6 months for trivalent inactivated influenza vaccine [TIV]; 5 years for live, attenuated influenza vaccine [LAIV]).* Influenza vaccine is recommended annually for persons with certain risk factors, health-care workers, and other persons (including household members) in close contact with persons in groups at high risk. See MMWR 2006;55 (No. RR-10):1–41. For healthy persons aged 5–49 years, LAIV may be used as an alternative to TIV. Children aged <9 years who are receiving influenza vaccine for the first time should receive 2 doses (separated by ≥4 weeks for TIV and ≥6 weeks for LAIV). **6. Hepatitis A vaccine (HepA).** *(Minimum age: 12 months)* The 2 doses in the series should be administered at least 6 months apart. HepA is recommended for certain other groups of children, including in areas where vaccination programs target older children. See MMWR 2006;55 (No. RR-7):1–23. **7. Hepatitis B vaccine (HepB).** *(Minimum age: birth)* Administer the 3-dose series to those who were not previously vaccinated. A 2-dose series of Recombivax HB is licensed for children aged 11–15 years. **8. Inactivated poliovirus vaccine (IPV).** *(Minimum age: 6 weeks)* For children who received an all-IPV or all-oral poliovirus (OPV) series, a fourth dose is not necessary if the third dose was administered at age ≥4 years. If both OPV and IPV were administered as part of a series, a total of 4 doses should be administered, regardless of the child's current age. **9. Measles, mumps, and rubella vaccine (MMR).** *(Minimum age: 12 months)* If not previously vaccinated, administer 2 doses of MMR during any visit, with ≥4 weeks between the doses. **10. Varicella vaccine.** *(Minimum age: 12 months)* Administer 2 doses of varicella vaccine to persons without evidence of immunity. Administer 2 doses of varicella vaccine to persons aged <13 years at least 3 months apart. Do not repeat the second dose, if administered ≥28 days after the first dose. Administer 2 doses of varicella vaccine to persons aged ≥13 years at least 4 weeks apart.

Recommended Adult Immunization Schedule
United States, October 2006–September 2007

Recommended adult immunization schedule, by vaccine and age group

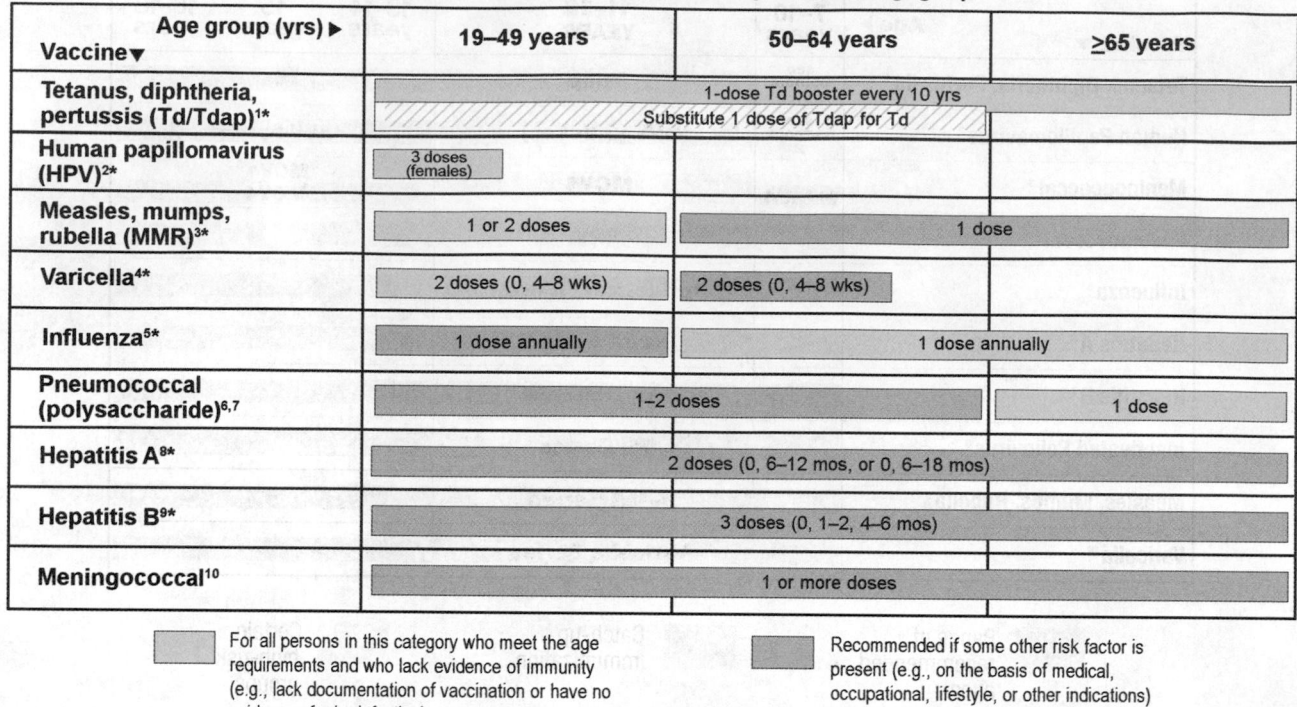

Age group (yrs) ▶ Vaccine ▼	19–49 years	50–64 years	≥65 years
Tetanus, diphtheria, pertussis (Td/Tdap)[1*]	1-dose Td booster every 10 yrs Substitute 1 dose of Tdap for Td		
Human papillomavirus (HPV)[2*]	3 doses (females)		
Measles, mumps, rubella (MMR)[3*]	1 or 2 doses	1 dose	
Varicella[4*]	2 doses (0, 4–8 wks)	2 doses (0, 4–8 wks)	
Influenza[5*]	1 dose annually	1 dose annually	
Pneumococcal (polysaccharide)[6,7]	1–2 doses		1 dose
Hepatitis A[8*]	2 doses (0, 6–12 mos, or 0, 6–18 mos)		
Hepatitis B[9*]	3 doses (0, 1–2, 4–6 mos)		
Meningococcal[10]	1 or more doses		

For all persons in this category who meet the age requirements and who lack evidence of immunity (e.g., lack documentation of vaccination or have no evidence of prior infection)

Recommended if some other risk factor is present (e.g., on the basis of medical, occupational, lifestyle, or other indications)

FIGURE 116-2 Recommended adult immunization schedule, by vaccine and age group—United States, 2006–2007. This schedule indicates the recommended age groups for routine administration of currently licensed vaccines for persons aged ≥19 years, as of October 1, 2006. Licensed combination vaccines may be used whenever any components of the combination are indicated and when the vaccine's other components are not contraindicated. For detailed recommendations on all vaccines, including those used primarily for travelers or that are issued during the year, consult the manufacturers' package inserts and the complete statements from the Advisory Committee on Immunization Practices (http://www.cdc.gov/nip/publications/acip-list.htm). Report all clinically significant postvaccination reactions to the Vaccine Adverse Event Reporting System (VAERS). Reporting forms and instructions on filing a VAERs report are available at http://vaers.hhs.gov or by telephone, 800-822-7967. Information on how to file a Vaccine Injury Compensation Program claim is available at http://www.hrsa.gov/vaccinecompensation or by telephone, 800-338-2382. To file a claim for vaccine injury, contact the U.S. Court of Federal Claims, 717 Madison Place, N.W., Washington, DC, 20005; telephone, 202-357-6400. Additional information about the vaccines in this schedule and contraindications for vaccination is also available at http://www.cdc.gov/nip or from the CDC-INFO Contact Center at 800-CDC-INFO (800-232-4636) in English and Spanish, 24 hours a day, 7 days a week.

1. Tetanus, diphtheria, and acellular pertussis (Td/Tdap) vaccination. Adults with uncertain histories of a complete primary vaccination series with diphtheria and tetanus toxoid–containing vaccines should begin or complete a primary vaccination series. A primary series for adults is 3 doses; administer the first 2 doses at least 4 weeks apart and the third dose 6–12 months after the second. Administer a booster dose to adults who have completed a primary series and if the last vaccination was received ≥10 years previously. Tdap or tetanus and diphtheria (Td) vaccine may be used; Tdap should replace a single dose of Td for adults aged <65 years who have not previously received a dose of Tdap (either in the primary series, as a booster, or for wound management). Only one of two Tdap products (Adacel [sanofi pasteur]) is licensed for use in adults. If the person is pregnant and received the last Td vaccination ≥10 years previously, administer Td during the second or third trimester; if the person received the last Td vaccination in <10 years, administer Tdap during the immediate postpartum period. A one-time administration of 1 dose of Tdap with an interval as short as 2 years from a previous Td vaccination is recom-

mended for postpartum women, close contacts of infants aged <12 months, and all healthcare workers with direct patient contact. In certain situations, Td can be deferred during pregnancy and Tdap substituted in the immediate postpartum period, or Tdap can be given instead of Td to a pregnant woman after an informed discussion with the woman (see www.cdc.gov/nip/publications/acip-list.htm). Consult the ACIP statement for recommendations for administering Td as prophylaxis in wound management (www.cdc.gov/mmwr/preview/mmwrhtml/00041645.htm). **2. Human papillomavirus (HPV) vaccination.** HPV vaccination is recommended for all women aged ≤ 26 years who have not completed the vaccine series. Ideally, vaccine should be administered before potential exposure to HPV through sexual activity; however, women who are sexually active should still be vaccinated. Sexually active women who have not been infected with any of the HPV vaccine types receive the full benefit of the vaccination. Vaccination is less beneficial for women who have already been infected with one or more of the four HPV vaccine types. A complete series consists of 3 doses. The second dose should be administered 2 months after the first dose; the third dose should be administered 6 months after the first dose. Vaccination is not recommended during pregnancy. If a woman is found to be pregnant after initiating the vaccination series, the remainder of the 3-dose regimen should be delayed until after completion of the pregnancy. **3. Measles, mumps, rubella (MMR) vaccination.** *Measles component:* adults born before 1957 can be considered immune to measles. Adults born during or after 1957 should receive ≥1 dose of MMR unless they have a medical contraindication, documentation of ≥1 dose, history of measles based on healthcare provider diagnosis, or laboratory evidence of immunity. A second dose of MMR is recommended for adults who (1) have been recently exposed to measles or in an outbreak setting; (2) have been previously vaccinated with killed measles vaccine; (3) have been vaccinated with an unknown type of measles vaccine during 1963–1967; (4) are students in postsecondary educational institutions; (5) work in a healthcare facility; or (6) plan to travel internationally. Withhold MMR or other measles-containing vaccines from HIV-infected persons with severe immunosuppression. *Mumps component:* adults born before 1957 can generally be considered immune to mumps. Adults born during or after 1957 should receive 1 dose of MMR unless they have a medical contraindication, history of mumps based on healthcare provider diagnosis, or laboratory evidence of immunity.

(continued)

FIGURE 116-2 (*Continued*)

A second dose of MMR is recommended for adults who (1) are in an age group that is affected during a mumps outbreak; (2) are students in post-secondary educational institutions; (3) work in a healthcare facility; or (4) plan to travel internationally. For unvaccinated healthcare workers born before 1957 who do not have other evidence of mumps immunity, consider giving 1 dose on a routine basis and strongly consider giving a second dose during an outbreak. *Rubella component:* administer 1 dose of MMR vaccine to women whose rubella vaccination history is unreliable or who lack laboratory evidence of immunity. For women of childbearing age, regardless of birth year, routinely determine rubella immunity and counsel women regarding congenital rubella syndrome. Do not vaccinate women who are pregnant or who might become pregnant within 4 weeks of receiving vaccine. Women who do not have evidence of immunity should receive MMR vaccine upon completion or termination of pregnancy and before discharge from the healthcare facility. **4. Varicella vaccination.** All adults without evidence of immunity to varicella should receive 2 doses of varicella vaccine. Special consideration should be given to those who (1) have close contact with persons at high risk for severe disease (e.g., healthcare workers and family contacts of immunocompromised persons) or (2) are at high risk for exposure or transmission (e.g., teachers of young children; child care employees; residents and staff members of institutional settings, including correctional institutions; college students; military personnel; adolescents and adults living in households with children; non-pregnant women of childbearing age; and international travelers). Evidence of immunity to varicella in adults includes any of the following: (1) documentation of 2 doses of varicella vaccine at least 4 weeks apart; (2) U.S.-born before 1980 (although for healthcare workers and pregnant women, birth before 1980 should not be considered evidence of immunity); (3) history of varicella based on diagnosis or verification of varicella by a healthcare provider (for a patient reporting a history of or presenting with an atypical case, a mild case, or both, healthcare providers should seek either an epidemiologic link with a typical varicella case or evidence of laboratory confirmation, if it was performed at the time of acute disease); (4) history of herpes zoster based on healthcare provider diagnosis; or (5) laboratory evidence of immunity or laboratory confirmation of disease. Do not vaccinate women who are pregnant or might become pregnant within 4 weeks of receiving the vaccine. Assess pregnant women for evidence of varicella immunity. Women who do not have evidence of immunity should receive dose 1 of varicella vaccine upon completion or termination of pregnancy and before discharge from the healthcare facility. Dose 2 should be administered 4–8 weeks after dose 1. **5. Influenza vaccination.** *Medical indications:* chronic disorders of the cardiovascular or pulmonary systems, including asthma; chronic metabolic diseases, including diabetes mellitus, renal dysfunction, hemoglobinopathies, or immuno-suppression (including immunosuppression caused by medications or HIV); any condition that compromises respiratory function or the handling of respiratory secretions or that can increase the risk of aspiration (e.g., cognitive dysfunction, spinal cord injury, or seizure disorder or other neuro-muscular disorder); and pregnancy during the influenza season. No data exist on the risk for severe or complicated influenza disease among persons with asplenia; however, influenza is a risk factor for secondary bacterial infections that can cause severe disease among persons with asplenia. *Occupational indications:* healthcare workers and employees of long-term-care and assisted living facilities. *Other indications:* residents of nursing homes and other long-term-care and assisted living facilities; persons likely to transmit influenza to persons at high risk (e.g., in-home household contacts and caregivers of children aged 0–59 months, or persons of all ages with high-risk conditions); and anyone who would like to be vaccinated. Healthy, nonpregnant persons aged 5–49 years without high-risk medical conditions who are not contacts of severely immunocompromised persons in special care units can receive either intranasally administered influenza vaccine (FluMist) or inactivated vaccine. Other persons should receive the inactivated vaccine. **6. Pneumococcal polysaccharide vaccination.** *Medical indications:* chronic disorders of the pulmonary system (excluding asthma); cardiovascular diseases; diabetes mellitus; chronic liver diseases, including liver disease as a result of alcohol abuse (e.g., cirrhosis); chronic renal failure or nephrotic syndrome; functional or anatomic asplenia (e.g., sickle cell disease or splenectomy [if elective splenectomy is planned, vacci-

nate at least 2 weeks before surgery]); immunosuppressive conditions (e.g., congenital immunodeficiency, HIV infection [vaccinate as close to diagnosis as possible when CD4 cell counts are highest], leukemia, lymphoma, multiple myeloma, Hodgkin disease, generalized malignancy, or organ or bone marrow transplantation); chemotherapy with alkylating agents, anti-metabolites, or high-dose, long-term corticosteroids; and cochlear implants. *Other indications:* Alaska Natives and certain American Indian populations and residents of nursing homes or other long-term–care facilities. **7. Revaccination with pneumococcal polysaccharide vaccine.** One-time revaccination after 5 years for persons with chronic renal failure or nephrotic syndrome; functional or anatomic asplenia (e.g., sickle cell disease or splenectomy); immunosuppressive conditions (e.g., congenital immunodeficiency, HIV infection, leukemia, lymphoma, multiple myeloma, Hodgkin disease, generalized malignancy, or organ or bone marrow transplantation); or chemotherapy with alkylating agents, antimetabolites, or high-dose, long-term corticosteroids. For persons aged ≥65 years, one-time revaccination if they were vaccinated ≥5 years previously and were aged <65 years at the time of primary vaccination. **8. Hepatitis A vaccination.** *Medical indications:* persons with chronic liver disease and persons who receive clotting factor concentrates. *Behavioral indications:* men who have sex with men and persons who use illegal drugs. *Occupational indications:* persons working with hepatitis A virus (HAV)–infected primates or with HAV in a research laboratory setting. *Other indications:* persons traveling to or working in countries that have high or intermediate endemicity of hepatitis A (a list of countries is available at *www.cdc.gov/travel/diseases.htm*) and any person who would like to obtain immunity. Current vaccines should be administered in a 2-dose schedule at either 0 and 6–12 months, or 0 and 6–18 months. If the combined hepatitis A and hepatitis B vaccine is used, administer 3 doses at 0, 1, and 6 months. **9. Hepatitis B vaccination.** *Medical indications:* persons with end-stage renal disease, including patients receiving hemodialysis; persons seeking evaluation or treatment for a sexually transmitted disease (STD); persons with HIV infection; persons with chronic liver disease; and persons who receive clotting factor concentrates. *Occupational indications:* healthcare workers and public-safety workers who are exposed to blood or other potentially infectious body fluids. *Behavioral indications:* sexually active persons who are not in a long-term, mutually monogamous relationship (i.e., persons with >1 sex partner during the previous 6 months); current or recent injection-drug users; and men who have sex with men. *Other indications:* household contacts and sex partners of persons with chronic hepatitis B virus (HBV) infection; clients and staff members of institutions for persons with developmental disabilities; all clients of STD clinics; international travelers to countries with high or intermediate prevalence of chronic HBV infection (a list of countries is available at *www.cdc.gov/travel/diseases.htm*); and any adult seeking protection from HBV infection. Settings where hepatitis B vaccination is recommended for all adults: STD treatment facilities; HIV testing and treatment facilities; facilities providing drug-abuse treatment and prevention services; healthcare settings providing services for injection-drug users or men who have sex with men; correctional facilities; end-stage renal disease programs and facilities for chronic hemodialysis patients; and institutions and nonresidential daycare facilities for persons with developmental disabilities. *Special formulation indications:* for adult patients receiving hemodialysis and other immunocompromised adults, 1 dose of 40 µg/mL (Recombivax HB) or 2 doses of 20 µg/mL (Engerix-B). **10. Meningococcal vaccination.** *Medical indications:* adults with anatomic or functional asplenia, or terminal complement component deficiencies. *Other indications:* first-year college students living in dormitories; microbiologists who are routinely exposed to isolates of *Neisseria meningitidis*; military recruits; and persons who travel to or live in countries in which meningococcal disease is hyperendemic or epidemic (e.g., the "meningitis belt" of sub-Saharan Africa during the dry season [December–June]), particularly if their contact with local populations will be prolonged. Vaccination is required by the government of Saudi Arabia for all travelers to Mecca during the annual Hajj. Meningococcal conjugate vaccine is preferred for adults with any of the preceding indications who are aged ≤ 55 years, although meningococcal polysaccharide vaccine (MPSV4) is an acceptable alternative. Revaccination after 5 years might be indicated for adults previously vaccinated with MPSV4 who remain at high risk for infection (e.g., persons residing in areas in which disease is epidemic).

The immune system, composed of a variety of cell types and soluble factors, is geared toward the recognition of and response to "foreign" substances termed *antigens*. Vaccines convey antigens from living or killed microorganisms (or protein or carbohydrate molecules derived from these antigens) to elicit immune responses that are generally protective but can occasionally backfire and cause harm to the recipient. Specific immune responses, which interrupt the infectious process, generally take the form of immunoglobulin proteins called *antibodies* and/or activated immune cells that recognize particular antigens from an infectious agent. Immunity is medically induced by active or passive immunization. *Active immunization*—i.e., the administration of a vaccine—induces immunity that is usually long-lasting and is sometimes life-long. In contrast, *passive immunization*—i.e., the administration of exogenously produced immune substances or of protective products made in animals—elicits temporary immunity that dissipates with the turnover of the administered protective substances. Used together, the two methods can produce a complementary effect; this is the case, for example, with the coadministration of hepatitis B vaccine and hepatitis B immune globulin. Caution is required, however: the combination of active and passive immunization can also interfere with the development of immunity—e.g., when measles vaccine is administered within 6 weeks of measles immunoglobulin.

When multiple species or serotypes of an organism exist and share common, cross-reactive antigens, vaccination may induce broad immunity to all or most of the related forms or may result in serotype-specific immunity against the immunizing strain alone. One of the virtues of whole-organism vaccines is their potential to contain all the protective antigens of the organism. This advantage is balanced by the possibility of adverse responses to reactive but nonprotective antigens present in the mix. Because the immune response is genetically controlled, all individuals cannot be expected to respond identically to the same vaccine. Additional vaccine constituents affect immunogenicity, efficacy, and safety and may render one formulation superior to another formulation of the same antigens (see "Adjuvants," below).

Approaches to Active Immunization   The two standard approaches to active immunization are (1) the use of live, generally attenuated infectious agents (e.g., measles virus); and (2) the use of inactivated agents (e.g., influenza virus), their constituents (e.g., *Bordetella pertussis*), or their products, which are now commonly obtainable through genetic engineering (e.g., hepatitis B vaccine). For many diseases (e.g., poliomyelitis), both live and inactivated vaccines have been employed, each offering advantages and disadvantages.

Live attenuated vaccines consisting of selected or genetically altered organisms that are avirulent or dramatically attenuated, yet remain immunogenic, typically generate long-lasting immunity. These vaccines are designed to cause a subclinical or mild illness and an immune response that mimics natural infection. They offer the advantage of microbial replication in vivo, which simulates natural infection; they may confer life-long protection with one dose; they can present all potential antigens, including those made only in vivo, thus overcoming immunogenetic restrictions in some hosts; and they can reach the local sites most relevant to the induction of protective immunity.

Nonliving vaccines typically require multiple doses and periodic boosters for the maintenance of immunity. The exceptions to this rule are the pure polysaccharide vaccines, whose effects cannot be boosted by additional exposures because polysaccharides do not elicit immunologic memory. Nonliving vaccines administered parenterally fail to induce mucosal immunity because they lack a delivery system that can effectively transport them to local mucosal antigen-processing cells. Nonetheless, nonliving parenteral vaccines can be extremely efficacious. For example, hepatitis A vaccine appears to be effective in nearly 100% of recipients. Currently available nonliving vaccines consist of inactivated whole organisms (e.g., plague vaccine), detoxified protein exotoxins (e.g., tetanus toxoid), recombinant protein antigens (e.g., hepatitis B vaccine), or carbohydrate antigens—either soluble purified capsular material (e.g., serotype-specific *Streptococcus pneumoniae*

polysaccharides) or polysaccharide conjugated to a protein carrier to induce a memory response (e.g., Hib polysaccharide conjugated to a suitable protein moiety).

Despite their many advantages, live vaccines are not always preferable. For example, after several decades of extensive use, live oral polio vaccine (OPV) is no longer recommended in the United States because of the rare but real risk of vaccine-associated polio due to reversion to virulence. However, the WHO continues to recommend OPV for use in the developing world because of lower costs and logistical advantages.

Approaches to Passive Immunization   Passive immunization is generally used to provide temporary immunity in a person exposed to an infectious disease who has not been actively immunized; this situation can arise when active immunization is unavailable (e.g., for respiratory syncytial virus) or when active immunization simply has not been implemented before exposure (e.g., for rabies). Passive immunization is used in the treatment of certain illnesses associated with toxins (e.g., diphtheria) as well as for some snake and spider bites and as a specific or nonspecific immunosuppressant [Rho(D) immune globulin and antilymphocyte globulin, respectively]. Three types of preparations can be used in passive immunization: (1) standard human immune serum globulin for IM or IV administration; (2) special immune serum globulins with a known content of antibody to specific agents (e.g., hepatitis B virus or varicellazoster immune globulin); and (3) specific animal antisera and antitoxins.

Postexposure Immunization   For certain infections, active or passive immunization soon after exposure can prevent or attenuate disease expression. Recommended postexposure immunization regimens are shown in Table 116-1. For example, giving either measles immune globulin within 6 days of exposure or measles vaccine within the first few days after exposure may prevent symptomatic infection. Nonimmune pregnant women exposed to rubella can minimize clinical illness by postexposure passive immunization; however, this measure may fail to prevent viremia and infection of the fetus and thus may be followed by the congenital rubella syndrome. Proper immunization for tetanus plays an important role in dirty-wound management. The need for active immunization—with or without passive immunization—depends on the wound's condition and the patient's immunization history. Tetanus is rare among persons with documented receipt of a primary series of tetanus toxoid doses. Tetanus immune globulin is helpful in patients with clinical tetanus, but survivors must be actively immunized since the disease does not stimulate protective levels of antitoxin antibody. Administration of rabies immune globulin plus rabies vaccine in the immediate postexposure period is highly effective in preventing disease. Similarly, for persons who have not been actively immunized, administration of hepatitis A immune globulin within 2 weeks of exposure to hepatitis A virus is likely to prevent clinical illness. Evidence also supports the efficacy of human hepatitis B immune globulin in preventing disease after exposure. While no high-titer preparation is available for postexposure protection against non-A, non-B hepatitis, standard human immune serum globulin is efficacious. VariZIG, a highly purified preparation of human antibody to varicella-zoster virus (VZV), is licensed in Canada for the prevention of varicella in nonimmune pregnant women who are exposed to infected individuals. At the time of this writing, this product is available in the United States from the Centers for Disease Control and Prevention (CDC) under an investigational new drug (IND) protocol or under an expanded-access program through the U.S. Food and Drug Administration.

THE IMMUNE RESPONSE

While many constituents of infectious microorganisms and their products (e.g., exotoxins) are or can be rendered immunogenic, only some stimulate protective immune responses that can prevent infection and/or clinical illness or (as in the case of rotavirus) can attenuate illness, providing protection against severe disease but not against infection or mild illness. The immune system is complex, and many factors—including antigen composition and presentation as well as host

TABLE 116-1 RECOMMENDED POSTEXPOSURE IMMUNIZATION WITH IMMUNOGLOBULIN PREPARATIONS IN THE UNITED STATES

Disease	Indicated	Comments
Measles	Yes	Standard human immune globulin is recommended for exposed infants and adults with normal immunocompetence (but with a contraindication to measles vaccine) and for immunocompromised patients exposed to measles (regardless of immunization status). Patients should be actively immunized 3–6 months after immunoglobulin administration. Recommended dose: 0.25–0.50 mL/kg (40–80 mg of IgG/kg) IM; 80 mg of IgG/kg for immunocompromised contact; maximum, 15 mL.
Rubella	No	Efficacy is unreliable; therefore, standard human immune globulin is recommended for administration only to antibody-negative pregnant women in the first trimester who have a documented rubella exposure and will not consider terminating the pregnancy. Recommended dose is 0.55 mL/kg (90 mg of IgG/kg) IM.
Tetanus	Yes	Human tetanus immune globulin (TIG) has replaced equine tetanus antitoxin because of the risk of serum sickness with equine serum. Recommended dose for postexposure prophylaxis is 250–500 units of TIG (10–20 mg of IgG/kg) IM. Recommended dose for treatment of tetanus is 3000–6000 units of TIG IM.
Rabies	Yes	Human rabies immune globulin (RIG) is preferred over equine rabies antiserum because of the risk of serum sickness with equine serum. RIG or antiserum is recommended for nonimmunized individuals with animal bites in whom rabies cannot be ruled out and with other exposures to known rabid animals. Recommended dose of RIG is 20 IU/kg (22 mg of IgG/kg). Recommended dose of antiserum is 40 IU/kg. Rabies vaccine is given as well at 0, 3, 7, 14, and 28 days.
Hepatitis A	Yes	Standard immune serum globulin is given in a single dose of 0.02–0.04 mL/kg or (for continuous exposure) in a dose up to 0.06 mL/kg every 5 months. Postexposure treatment with hepatitis A immune globulin has not been studied.
Varicella	Yes	VariZIG, a new Canadian purified human immune globulin containing high-titer IgG antibody to varicella-zoster virus, is intended for patients without evidence of immunity to varicella who are exposed to infection and who are at high risk for severe disease and complications. It is not currently licensed in the United States but instead has investigational new drug status. VariZIG may be obtained under expanded-access provisions for patients who meet the enrollment criteria and choose to participate. Maximal benefit requires administration within 96 h of exposure. The recommended dose is 125 units/10 kg of body weight, up to a maximum of 625 units.

ing B lymphocytes and/or effector T cells. Pure polysaccharide antigens, such as the first-generation pneumococcal vaccine, evoke immune responses that are independent of T cells and are not enhanced by repeated administration. However, conjugation of the same polysaccharide to a suitable protein converts the carbohydrate antigen into one that is T cell–dependent and able to induce immunologic memory and secondary responses to reexposure. Although levels of vaccine-induced antibodies may decline over time, revaccination or infection generally elicits a rapid (anamnestic) protective secondary response consisting of IgG antibodies, with little or no detectable IgM. Thus, a lack of measurable antibody in an immunized individual does not necessarily indicate secondary vaccine failure. Similarly, the mere presence of detectable antibodies after immunization does not ensure clinical protection: the level of circulating antibody may need to exceed a threshold value in order to mediate protection (e.g., 0.01 IU/mL for tetanus antitoxin).

Mucosal Immunity Some pathogens are confined to and replicate only at mucosal surfaces (e.g., *Vibrio cholerae*), whereas others first encounter the host at a mucosal surface before they invade systemically (e.g., influenza virus). A distinctive immunoglobulin, *secretory IgA*, is produced at mucosal surfaces and is adapted to resist degradation and to function at these sites. Vaccines may be specifically designed to induce secretory IgA and thereby to block the essential initial steps in disease pathogenesis that occur on mucosal surfaces. Given its complexity, mucosal immunology has become a separate branch of the field of immunology.

Measurement of the Immune Response Immune responses to vaccines are often gauged by the concentration of specific antibody in serum. Although seroconversion (i.e., transition from antibody-negative to antibody-positive status) serves as a dependable indicator of an immune response, it does not necessarily correlate with protection unless serum antibody is the critical mechanism in vivo and the levels achieved are sufficient (e.g., against measles). In some instances, serum antibody correlates with clinical protection but does not directly mediate it (e.g., vibriocidal serum antibodies in cholera).

Herd Immunity Successful vaccination protects immunized individuals from infection, thereby decreasing the percentage of susceptible persons within a population and reducing the possibility of infection transmission to others. At a definable prevalence of immunity, an infectious organism can no longer circulate freely among the remaining susceptibles. This indirect protection of unvaccinated (nonimmune) persons is called the *herd immunity effect*; through this effect, vaccination programs may confer societal benefits that exceed individual costs. The level of vaccine coverage needed to elicit herd immunity depends on the patterns of interaction among individuals within the population and the biology of the specific infectious agent. For example, measles virus and VZV have high transmission rates and require a higher level of vaccine coverage for herd immunity than do organisms with lower transmission rates, such as *S. pneumoniae*. Wherever herd immunity for poliomyelitis and measles has been induced with vaccines, transmission of infection has ceased; however, herd immunity may wane if immuni-

characteristics—are critical for stimulation of the desired immune responses (Chap. 308).

The Primary Response The primary response to a vaccine antigen includes an apparent latent period of several days before immune responses can be detected. Although the immune system is rapidly activated, it takes 7–10 days for activated B lymphocytes to produce enough antibody to be detected in the circulation. The primarily IgM antibodies seen initially are rapidly produced but have only a low affinity for the antigen. After the first week, high-affinity IgG antibodies begin to be produced in quantity; this switch from IgM to IgG production requires the participation of CD4+ T-helper lymphocytes—the "middle men" of the immune response. Because precursors for T cells mature within the thymus gland, antigens that stimulate T cells are referred to as *T* or *thymus-dependent* antigens. Circulating antigen-specific T lymphocytes that implement cell-mediated immune responses are identified in the peripheral bloodstream only after several days but begin to increase in number immediately after antigenic stimulation.

Activation of these responses typically requires co-recognition of the antigen by specific molecular species of HLA, the major histocompatibility complex, which is present on the surface of lymphocytes and macrophages. Some individuals cannot respond to one or more antigens, even when repeatedly exposed, because they do not have the genes for the particular HLA type involved in antigen recognition, processing, and presentation for an immune response. This situation is known as *primary vaccine failure*.

The Secondary Response Stronger and faster humoral or cell-mediated responses are elicited by a second exposure to the same antigen and are detectable within days of the "booster" dose. The secondary response depends on immunologic memory induced by the primary exposure and is characterized by a marked proliferation of IgG antibody–produczation programs are interrupted (as was the case for diphtheria in the former Soviet Union) or if a sufficient percentage of individuals refuse to be immunized because of a fear of vaccine-related adverse events (as occurred for pertussis in the United Kingdom and Japan). In either setting, the loss of herd immunity has led to renewed circulation of the organism and subsequent large outbreaks with serious consequences.

PRINCIPLES OF VACCINE USE

Route of Administration Microbes differ in their routes of infection, patterns of transmission, and predispositions for certain age groups. The route of vaccine administration (oral, intranasal, intradermal, transdermal, subcutaneous, or intramuscular) takes these factors into account in order to maximize protection and minimize adverse events. Vaccine development is more a pragmatic undertaking than an exact science, guided only in part by immunologic principles and shaped largely by the results of clinical trials. While vaccines can theoretically be given by any route, each vaccine has unique characteristics adapted to a particular route and, in practice, must be given by the licensed route, for which optimal immunogenicity and safety have been documented. For example, vaccines containing adjuvants are designed for injection into the muscle mass. Mucosal administration of vaccines designed for parenteral administration may not induce good systemic responses because such vaccines do not induce mucosal secretory IgA. Administration of hepatitis B vaccine into the gluteal rather than the deltoid muscle may fail to induce an adequate immune response, while SC rather than IM administration of DTaP vaccine increases the risk of adverse reactions. Injectable biologicals should be administered at sites where the likelihood of local, neural, vascular, or tissue injury is minimized.

Age Because age influences the response to vaccines, schedules for immunization are based on age-dependent responses determined empirically in clinical trials. The presence of high levels of maternal antibody and/or the immaturity of the immune system in the early months of life impairs the initial immune response to some vaccines (e.g., measles and pneumococcal polysaccharide vaccines) but not to others (e.g., hepatitis B vaccine). In the elderly, vaccine responses may be diminished because of the natural waning of the immune system, and larger amounts of an antigen may be required to produce the desired response (e.g., in vaccination against influenza). In contrast, in some age groups, the use of substandard amounts of antigen is sufficient for immunity induction and reduces the risk of adverse effects (e.g., a reduced dose of diphtheria toxoid for persons ≥7 years of age). Age-related adverse events are discussed in a later section.

Target Populations and Timing of Administration Disease attack rates differ across the human life span, and the timing of immunization must consider these variations along with the age-specific response to vaccines, the durability of the immune response, and the logistics for optimal identification and vaccination of the groups at risk. Aside from immunologic parameters, many factors are involved, including demographic features; thus, vaccination programs are really as much community as individual endeavors. Schedules for immunization are ultimately derived from careful consideration of the many relevant variables and may ultimately depend on the best opportunities to reach the target groups (e.g., infancy, school entry, puberty, college enrollment, military induction, entry into the workplace). Health care workers administering vaccines or caring for patients with vaccine-preventable diseases have a special responsibility to be adequately immunized themselves and to take all necessary precautions to minimize the risk of spreading infection (e.g., hand washing between immunizations or other interactions with patients). Catch-up immunization schedules for infants and children through the age of 18 years have been approved by the CDC (Fig. 116-3).

For common and highly communicable childhood diseases such as measles, the target population is the universe of susceptible individuals, and the time to immunize is as early in life as is feasible and effective. In the industrialized world, immunization with live-virus vaccine at 12–15 months of age has become the norm because the vaccine protects >95% of children immunized at this age and there is little measles morbidity or mortality among infants <1 year of age. In contrast, under crowded conditions in the developing world, measles remains a significant cause of death among young infants. For optimal benefit in this situation, it is necessary to immunize early enough to narrow the window of vulnerability between the rapid decline of maternal antibody 4–6 months after birth and the development of vaccine-induced active immunity; this choice must be made despite the less efficient immune response in children <1 year old.

Invasive infections due to Hib (meningitis, pneumonia, and epiglottitis) occur primarily in young children, with rates rising sharply after the disappearance of maternally derived antibody. First-generation Hib polysaccharide vaccines often failed when administered during infancy because very young children cannot respond to pure polysaccharides. This problem has been overcome by conjugating the capsular polysaccharide with a protein to create a T cell–dependent antigen, to which infants effectively respond.

In contrast, rubella is primarily a threat to the fetus rather than to infants and young children. The ideal strategy would be to immunize all women of reproductive age before they became pregnant. Because it is difficult to ensure this type of coverage, rubella is included in a combination vaccine with measles and mumps (MMR) that is administered during infancy and boosted at the age of 4–6 years. It is recommended that pregnant women be screened for rubella antibodies and that seronegative women be given rubella vaccine after delivery. Similar considerations apply to the use of the vaccine against HPV that was recently approved in the United States and is intended primarily to prevent cervical cancer in women. Accordingly, it is recommended that the vaccine be given at the age of 11–12 years (or as early as 9 years), so that all are immunized before becoming sexually active.

Some vaccines, such as the influenza and polyvalent pneumococcal polysaccharide products, were originally formulated to prevent pneumonia hospitalizations and deaths among the elderly. These products have been consistently underused, in large part because physicians and otherwise-healthy older individuals ignore the recommendations but also because vaccines continue to be thought of as interventions for infants and children. There is considerable debate about alternative strategies to reduce the burden of these diseases in the elderly by indirectly protecting them through childhood vaccination, which would reduce transmission. The development of new vaccines and the exploitation of new routes of administration may facilitate this approach; examples include the development of pneumococcal conjugate vaccines and the administration of influenza vaccine by the intranasal route, respectively. The pneumococcal conjugate vaccine has made it possible to immunize young infants at risk of pneumococcal pneumonia, meningitis, and otitis media, but whether immunity will persist or will need boosting in adulthood remains to be determined. What is clear is that the number of recommended vaccines and the strategies for their deployment are undergoing constant revision.

Adjuvants The immune response to some antigens is enhanced by the addition of adjuvants—nonspecific boosters of immune responses. Adjuvants include aluminum salts or, in the case of polysaccharides such as the polyribose phosphate oligosaccharide of Hib, a carrier protein to which the polysaccharide is conjugated. Adjuvants are essential to the efficacy of a number of inactivated vaccines, including diphtheria and tetanus toxoids, acellular pertussis vaccine, and hepatitis B vaccine; they also appear to be required for enhancement of the response to killed H5N1 avian influenza vaccines. The mechanism by which adjuvants enhance immunogenicity is not well defined but appears to relate to the ability of the adjuvant to activate antigen-presenting cells, frequently through stimulation of Toll-like receptors. Other reported mechanisms for adjuvant effects include rendering of soluble antigens into a particulate form, the mobilization of phagocytes to the site of antigen deposition, and the slowing down of antigen release in order to prolong stimulation of the immune response. Identification of new adjuvants that are safe, more effective, and inexpensive is a high priority for vaccine researchers and manufacturers.

Catch-up Immunization Schedule
for Persons Aged 4 Months–18 Years Who Start Late or Who Are More Than One Month Behind

The table below provides catch-up schedules and minimum intervals between doses for children whose vaccinations have been delayed. A vaccine series does not need to be restarted, regardless of the time that has elapsed between doses. Use the section appropriate for the child's age.

Vaccine	Minimum Age for Dose 1	Minimum Interval Between Doses			
		Dose 1 to Dose 2	Dose 2 to Dose 3	Dose 3 to Dose 4	Dose 4 to Dose 5
CATCH-UP SCHEDULE FOR PERSONS AGED 4 MONTHS – 6 YEARS					
Hepatitis B[1]	**Birth**	**4 weeks**	**8 weeks** (and 16 weeks after first dose)		
Rotavirus[2]	**6 wks**	**4 weeks**	**4 weeks**		
Diphtheria, Tetanus, Pertussis[3]	**6 wks**	**4 weeks**	**4 weeks**	**6 months**	**6 months**[3]
***Haemophilus influenzae* type b**[4]	**6 wks**	**4 weeks** if first dose administered at age <12 months **8 weeks (as final dose)** if first dose administered at age 12-14 months **No further doses needed** if first dose administered at age ≥ 15 months	**4 weeks**[4] if current age < 12 months **8 weeks (as final dose)**[4] if current age ≥ 12 months and second dose administered at age < 15 months **No further doses needed** if previous dose administered at age ≥ 15 months	**8 weeks (as final dose)** This dose only necessary for children aged 12 months–5 years who received 3 doses before age 12 months	
Pneumococcal[5]	**6 wks**	**4 weeks** if first dose administered at age <12 months and current age < 24 months **8 weeks (as final dose)** if first dose administered at age ≥ 12 months or current age 24–59 months **No further doses needed** for healthy children if first dose administered at age ≥ 24 months	**4 weeks** if current age < 12 months **8 weeks (as final dose)** if current age ≥ 12 months **No further doses needed** for healthy children if previous dose administered at age ≥ 24 months	**8 weeks (as final dose)** This dose only necessary for children aged 12 months–5 years who received 3 doses before age 12 months	
Inactivated Poliovirus[6]	**6 wks**	**4 weeks**	**4 weeks**	**4 weeks**[6]	
Measles, Mumps, Rubella[7]	**12 mos**	**4 weeks**			
Varicella[8]	**12 mos**	**3 months**			
Hepatitis A[9]	**12 mos**	**6 months**			
CATCH-UP SCHEDULE FOR PERSONS AGED 7–18 YEARS					
Tetanus, Diphtheria/ Tetanus, Diphtheria, Pertussis[10]	**7 yrs**[10]	**4 weeks**	**8 weeks** if first dose administered at age < 12 months **6 months** if first dose administered at age ≥ 12 months	**6 months** if first dose administered at age < 12 months	
Human Papillomavirus[11]	**9 yrs**	**4 weeks**	**12 weeks**		
Hepatitis A[9]	**12 mos**	**6 months**			
Hepatitis B[1]	**Birth**	**8 weeks** (and 16 weeks after first dose)			
Inactivated Poliovirus[6]	**6 wks**	**4 weeks**	**4 weeks**	**4 weeks**[6]	
Measles, Mumps, Rubella[7]	**12 mos**	**4 weeks**			
Varicella[8]	**12 mos**	**4 weeks** if first dose administered at age ≥ 13 years **3 months** if first dose administered at age < 13 years			

FIGURE 116-3 Catch-up immunization schedule for persons aged 4 months–18 years who start late or who are more than 1 month behind. 1. Hepatitis B vaccine (HepB). *(Minimum age: birth)* Administer the 3-dose series to those who were not previously vaccinated. A 2-dose series of Recombivax HB is licensed for children aged 11–15 years. **2. Rotavirus vaccine (Rota).** *(Minimum age: 6 weeks)* Do not start the series later than age 12 weeks. Administer the final dose in the series by age 32 weeks. Do not administer a dose later than age 32 weeks. Data on safety and efficacy outside of these age ranges are insufficient. **3. Diphtheria and tetanus toxoids and acellular pertussis vaccine (DTaP).** *(Minimum age: 6 weeks)* The fifth dose is not necessary if the fourth dose was administered at age ≥4 years. DTaP is not indicated for persons aged ≥7 years. **4. *Haemophilus influenzae* type b conjugate vaccine (Hib).** *(Minimum age: 6 weeks)* Vaccine is not generally recommended for children aged ≥5 years. If current age <12 months and the first 2 doses were PRP-OMP (PedvaxHIB or ComVax [Merck]), the third (and final) dose should be administered at age 12–15 months and at least 8 weeks after the second dose. If first dose was administered at age 7–11 months, administer 2 doses separated by 4 weeks plus a booster at age 12–15 months. **5. Pneumococcal conjugate vaccine (PCV).** *(Minimum age: 6 weeks)* Vaccine is not generally recommended for children aged ≥5 years. **6. Inactivated poliovirus vaccine (IPV).** *(Minimum age: 6 weeks)* For children who received an all-IPV or all-oral poliovirus (OPV) series, a fourth dose is not necessary if third dose was administered at age ≥4 years. If both OPV and IPV were administered as part of a series, a total of 4 doses should be administered, regardless of the child's current age. **7. Measles, mumps, and rubella vaccine (MMR).** *(Minimum age: 12 months)* The second dose of MMR is recommended routinely at age 4–6 years but may be administered earlier if desired. If not previously vaccinated, administer 2 doses of MMR during any visit with ≥4 weeks between the doses. **8. Varicella vaccine.** *(Minimum age: 12 months)* The second dose of varicella vaccine is recommended routinely at age 4–6 years but may be administered earlier if desired. Do not repeat the second dose in persons aged <13 years if administered ≥28 days after the first dose. **9. Hepatitis A vaccine (HepA).** *(Minimum age: 12 months)* HepA is recommended for certain groups of children, including in areas where vaccination programs target older children. See MMWR 2006;55(No. RR-7):1–23. **10. Tetanus and diphtheria toxoids vaccine (Td) and tetanus and diphtheria toxoids and acellular pertussis vaccine (Tdap).** *(Minimum ages: 7 years for Td, 10 years for BOOSTRIX, and 11 years for ADACEL)* Tdap should be substituted for a single dose of Td in the primary catch-up series or as a booster if age appropriate; use Td for other doses. A 5-year interval from the last Td dose is encouraged when Tdap is used as a booster dose. A booster (fourth) dose is needed if any of the previous doses were administered at age <12 months. Refer to ACIP recommendations for further information. See MMWR 2006;55(No. RR-3). **11. Human papillomavirus vaccine (HPV).** *(Minimum age: 9 years)* Administer the HPV vaccine series to females at age 13–18 years if not previously vaccinated.

CHAPTER 116

Immunization Principles and Vaccine Use

RECOMMENDATIONS FOR USE

Two or more vaccines should not be mixed in the same syringe in an effort to diminish the number of needle sticks unless such a practice is specifically endorsed by licensure. Disposable needles and syringes must be safely discarded to prevent inadvertent needle stick injury. While the importance of using a new syringe and needle for each vaccine recipient is obvious, reuse of contaminated equipment is a common reality in resource-poor settings. One-time-use, "auto-destruct" needles and syringes have been designed to prevent this practice, but their use adds to the cost of vaccine delivery.

Wherever effective primary health care systems ensure access to medical services for the majority and the population is educated about the need for and efficacy of vaccines, coverage rates for basic immunizations are usually high, regardless of the route of vaccine administration or the number of doses necessary. However, without systematic attention to the completion of multiple-dose vaccine schedules, coverage rates for second, third, and booster doses may drop off, and the efficacy of immunization may be significantly diminished.

RISK ASSESSMENT

Vaccines are considered safe when the risk of use is judged to be acceptable in relation to the benefits. For vaccines given to healthy individuals for diseases that are no longer common, acceptable risks are set at very low levels—indeed, far lower than for most medical products. However, "safety" does not and cannot ever mean "zero risk." The determination of safety is thus based on a scientific assessment of the data and a considered judgment of all the issues involved, including benefits and risks. Communities and individuals may differ, both among themselves and from health care professionals, in how they perceive the risks, benefits, and acceptability of vaccines and in how they judge the amount of uncertainty that is tolerable. Some parent advocacy groups, such as those that oppose mandatory vaccination, feel that no amount of risk is acceptable, especially for childhood vaccines.

SOURCES OF IMMUNIZATION RECOMMENDATIONS

Harmonized recommendations for vaccine use in the United States are developed by several professional groups. Schedules for immunization of children and adolescents and of adults are shown in Figs. 116-1 and 116-2, respectively. Vaccines recommended for special use are shown in Table 116-2.

As noted above, the number of licensed vaccines and the strategies for their best use change constantly as new products, new indications, and new information become available. The Advisory Committee on Immunization Practices (ACIP) regularly amends immunization recommendations to reflect the evolution of vaccines and vaccination policy in the United States. Changes for 2006 include the following points:

- to implement standing orders to administer hepatitis B vaccine—soon after birth and before hospital discharge—to all infants except those with documented hepatitis B–negative mothers;
- to target adults at high risk for hepatitis B vaccination;
- to use a new tetanus toxoid/reduced-dose diphtheria toxoid plus acellular pertussis combination vaccine (Tdap) formulated for adolescents and adults in place of Td;
- to provide meningococcal conjugate vaccine (MCV4) to all children at 11–12 years of age, to unvaccinated adolescents at age 15, and to all college freshmen living in dormitories;
- to administer hepatitis A vaccine to all children at 1 year of age;
- to administer three doses of the newly licensed rotavirus vaccine at 2, 4, and 6 months of age, with the first dose given by 12 weeks of age and the last by 32 weeks of age;
- to immunize children 6 months to 5 years of age with influenza vaccine and to expand routine use of the vaccine for their household contacts and out-of-home caregivers;
- to administer Tdap to protect health care personnel from pertussis and to reduce their potential to transmit nosocomial infections, as-

signing the highest priority to those who have direct contact with infants <1 year old; and
- to administer HPV vaccine routinely to girls at 11–12 years of age.

VACCINES FOR ROUTINE USE

Infants and Children   It is current practice for all children in the United States to receive DTaP, poliovirus, MMR, Hib, hepatitis B, and varicella vaccines and to receive pneumococcal conjugate, hepatitis A, and rotavirus vaccines in the absence of specific contraindications (Fig. 116-1; *www.cdc.gov/vaccines/vpd-vac/vaccines-list.htm*). Annual influenza seasonal vaccine is recommended for all children 6 months to 5 years old and to other children who have certain risk factors or who reside with persons with certain chronic disorders. In several European countries, meningococcal C conjugate vaccine is routinely recommended for children.

Teenagers   It is now recommended that all adolescents routinely receive quadrivalent meningococcal conjugate vaccine for serogroups A, C, Y, and W135 and the new-formulation Tdap vaccine. Girls should be given HPV vaccine, ideally at the age of 11–12 years but certainly before becoming sexually active (Fig. 116-1; *www.cdc.gov/vaccines/recs/schedules/teen-schedule.htm*).

Adults, Including College Students   (Fig. 116-2) Immunization recommendations for adults (≥18 years old) fall into four categories: (1) routine vaccines for all adults; (2) vaccines for high-risk exposure groups (health care and other institutional workers, prisoners, students, military personnel, travelers to endemic areas, injection drug users, and men who have sex with men); (3) vaccines for persons at high risk for severe outcomes of infection (pregnant women; the elderly; persons with chronic medical conditions, including diabetes, alcoholism, immunodeficiency, and renal, hepatic, respiratory, or cardiac disease); and (4) vaccines for household contacts of persons in group 3.

Because a substantial proportion of adults in the United States no longer have protective levels of antibodies to tetanus or diphtheria, all adults should receive routine booster doses of Td every 10 years. For those under age 65 years, one-time substitution of Tdap suitable for adults (Adacel, Sanofi-Pasteur) in place of the usual Td booster is recommended. Pregnant women who received their last Td booster >10 years previously may receive Td during the second or third trimester; those boosted <10 years previously (and as recently as 2 years before) should receive Tdap after delivery. Adults who have contact with infants <12 months of age should receive a single dose of Tdap—ideally at least 2 weeks before contact begins—if the most recent Td booster was ≥2 years earlier. If not previously immunized, adults require a primary immunizing course of Td. Young adults without laboratory evidence or a reliable history of past vaccination or disease should be immunized against measles, mumps, rubella, and varicella. A second dose of MMR vaccine is recommended for groups with a higher risk of exposure and for health care workers with certain other indications. Unless they have documented proof of immunity, rubella vaccine should be given to all nonpregnant women of childbearing age. Rubella-susceptible pregnant women should be vaccinated as early as possible in the postpartum period. Live-virus vaccines, such as MMR and varicella vaccines, are contraindicated in pregnant women and immunosuppressed individuals. Routine immunization against polio (with inactivated vaccine) is not recommended for adults unless they are at particular risk of exposure because of travel to the remaining endemic areas. College students, particularly freshmen living in dormitory settings, are at increased risk of meningococcal meningitis, as are military recruits; individuals in both of these groups should be offered the meningococcal polysaccharide or conjugate vaccine for serogroups A, C, Y, and W-135.

Current recommendations also include influenza vaccine for routine annual administration to individuals with chronic illness at any age, to persons living in the same household as chronically ill individuals, and to all adults >50 years of age. Polyvalent pneumococcal polysaccharide vaccine is similarly recommended for adults ≥65 years of age and for all chronically ill persons. Hepatitis B vaccine should be given to adults at high risk from clinical, occupational, behavioral, or

TABLE 116-2   SPECIAL VACCINES FOR INFANTS, CHILDREN, AND ADULTS

Vaccine	Vaccine Type	Route of Administration	Indications	Efficacy	Adverse Events
Anthrax	Inactivated avirulent bacteria	SC (6 doses primary plus annual booster)	For high risk of exposure (e.g., persons in contact with or involved in manufacture of animal hides, furs, bone meal, wool, goat hair) and military risk of biowarfare exposure	90% antibody response; efficacy uncertain	No serious adverse effects known
Tuberculosis (BCG)	Live bacteria (attenuated *Mycobacterium bovis*)	ID	Not generally recommended in U.S. because of low risk of TB and interference with PPD test. Consider for PPD-negative children in prolonged contact with ineffectively treated adult TB patients or those with drug-resistant TB and for health care workers in high-risk settings. Not for immunosuppressed individuals	Variable for adult pulmonary TB; best used to prevent childhood TB, meningitis, and miliary disease	Regional adenitis, disseminated BCG infection in immunocompromised hosts
Cholera	Killed whole bacteria	Oral	Travelers to endemic areas; however, not recommended for use by U.S. citizens because of extremely low risk. Not available in the U.S.	60–85%, short duration	Frequent fever and local reactions, pain, swelling
Plague	Inactivated bacteria	IM	Laboratory workers; foresters in endemic areas; ?travelers	90% antibody response; efficacy uncertain	10% local reactions; rare sterile abscess and hypersensitivity
Rabies	Inactivated virus grown in cell culture (human diploid cell or purified chick embryo cell) or grown in cell culture and adsorbed to aluminum phosphate	IM or ID	Preexposure immunization for travelers to high-risk countries, laboratory workers, and veterinarians or postexposure immunization following a bite from a proven or suspected rabies-infected animal	Virtually 100% for pre- or postexposure immunization	25% local reactions; 6% of patients receiving booster doses may develop immune complex reactions with arthropathy, arthritis, angioedema
Yellow fever	Live attenuated virus	SC	Travelers to endemic areas; laboratory workers	High	Rare associated neurologic complications (encephalitis, encephalopathy) or viscerotropic disease (fever; hypotension; respiratory, renal, or hepatic failure; lymphocytopenia; thrombocytopenia; and high risk of death)
Japanese B encephalitis	Inactivated virus	SC	Travelers to endemic areas	80–90%	Anaphylaxis/severe delayed allergic reactions common; recipients should be observed for 10 days
Typhoid	Purified Vi polysaccharide (not for children <2 years of age)	IM	Travelers (≥2 years old) to high-risk areas (southern Asia and other developing areas) except febrile patients	50–80%	Local reactions, mild
	Oral live attenuated Ty21a strain	Oral	Travelers (≥6 years old) to high-risk areas as above, except within 24 h of antibiotic ingestion or in febrile patients	50–80%	Nil

Note: SC, subcutaneous; BCG, bacille Calmette-Guérin; ID, intradermal; PPD, purified protein derivative; TB, tuberculosis.

Source: Recommendations of the Advisory Committee on Immunization Practices of the Centers for Disease Control and Prevention, American Academy of Pediatrics, American College of Physicians.

travel exposures, including patients undergoing hemodialysis, routine recipients of clotting factors, health care workers exposed to potentially infected blood or blood products, individuals living and working in institutions for the mentally handicapped, travelers to highly endemic countries, persons at excess risk for sexually transmitted diseases, injection drug users, and household contacts of known carriers of hepatitis B surface antigen. Hepatitis A vaccine is recommended for these same groups and for persons with clotting disorders or chronic liver disease. There are a number of other special-use vaccines whose administration is related to travel and occupational exposures (e.g., Japanese B encephalitis, typhoid fever, yellow fever, and rabies); specific recommendations for the use of these vaccines in the United States can be found at *www.cdc.gov/nip/recs/adult-schedule.htm*.

Simultaneous Administration of Multiple Vaccines   There are no contraindications to the simultaneous administration of multiple individual vaccines, although the use of licensed combination vaccines can significantly reduce the required number of injections during the first 2 years of life. Combination DTaP/Hib vaccine should not be used for primary immunization of infants because it results in a blunted, suboptimal response to Hib; the combination may be used for booster immunizations.

Simultaneous administration of the most widely used live and inactivated vaccines has not resulted in impaired antibody responses or in elevated rates of adverse reactions. In fact, this approach increases the likelihood that a child will ultimately be fully immunized. The simultaneous administration of vaccines is useful in any age group when the potential exists for exposure to multiple infectious diseases during travel to endemic countries. Live-virus vaccines may be given together on the same day; if this approach is not feasible, an interval of at least 30 days should be allowed to avoid interference in the response to one or another of the administered vaccine strains.

Because high doses of immune globulin can inhibit the efficacy of measles and rubella vaccines, an interval of at least 3 months is recommended between the administration of immune globulin and that of MMR vaccine or its components. However, postpartum vaccination of rubella-susceptible women should not be delayed because of the administration of anti-Rho(D) immune globulin or any other blood product during the last trimester or at delivery. Should the administration of an immune globulin preparation become necessary after vaccination, it should be postponed, if at all possible, for at least 14 days to allow time for vaccine-virus replication and development of immunity. In general, there is little interaction of immune globulin with inactivated vaccines, and postexposure passive prophylaxis can be given together with hepatitis B vaccine or tetanus toxoid, resulting in both immediate and long-lasting protection.

Adverse Events   Vaccines are generally very safe. Serious adverse events proven to be due to currently licensed vaccines are rare. Concerns about vaccine safety have at times become inflated in conjunction with complacency about the consequences of infections no longer routinely transmitted in the United States. As a result, some parents have refused to have their infants and children immunized.

An *adverse reaction* or *vaccine side effect* is an untoward vaccine effect that is extraneous to the vaccine's primary purpose (to produce immunity). An adverse event can be either a true vaccine reaction or an event whose occurrence is temporally related to a vaccine dose but is entirely unrelated to the vaccine itself. As vaccines are routinely administered through childhood, coincidental events are inevitable. Because our understanding of the underlying biologic mechanisms that cause adverse events remains limited, a few highly publicized claims—unsubstantiated by validated data or analysis—can easily heighten the suspicion that some or all vaccines routinely cause unacceptable adverse events. Antivaccine advocacy groups actively encourage the avoidance of immunization because they believe that vaccines cause certain disorders (e.g., autism). This situation presents a challenge to physicians and public health officials who must educate parents and practitioners about vaccine benefits and risks.

It is true that modern vaccines, while remarkably safe and effective, are associated with adverse events in some recipients and that these events range from frequent and mild to rare and serious or even life-threatening. The decision to recommend a vaccine involves an assessment of the risks of disease and its complications for those who remain unimmunized and the benefit-to-risk ratio of vaccination itself. Because these factors may change over time, the balance between societal benefits and individual risks must be continually evaluated. Valid and invalid contraindications to childhood immunization and appropriate precautions in the use of specific vaccines are reported by the CDC (Table 116-3); updated information can be found at *www.cdc.gov/vaccines/recs/vac-admin/ downloads/contraindications_guide.pdf*. A putative link between measles immunization and autism has been the subject of intense international controversy. The Institute of Medicine of the U.S. National Academies of Science has issued four recent reports whose findings (1) fail to support hypotheses that vaccines are associated with multiple sclerosis, neurodevelopmental disorders (e.g., autism), or immune dysfunction; (2) provide no evidence for a temporal association of these conditions with vaccination; and (3) elucidate no biologically plausible basis for the purported relationships.

An illuminating example is the case of Rotashield, a rhesus reassortant rotavirus vaccine, which was introduced for routine use in the United States in the late 1990s. Within 9 months of its introduction, cases of intussusception were reported by the CDC to be temporally associated with the administration of the initial vaccine dose. This report led first to the cessation of the vaccine's use and subsequently to its withdrawal from the market and the discontinuation of its production. The withdrawal of the vaccine in the United States made its use impossible in developing countries, where the risk of any increase in intussusception would have been dramatically outweighed by the benefit of decreased rotavirus mortality rates. It is now apparent that the susceptibility to intussception is age related, with virtually no events in children <90 days of age. Almost a decade later, a new rotavirus vaccine has been licensed

in the United States and recommended for routine use beginning at ≤2 months of age. In the interim, some 4–5 million infants have died of rotavirus diarrhea in the developing world; most of these deaths could have been prevented by the original rhesus rotavirus vaccine.

Vaccine components, including protective antigens, animal proteins introduced during vaccine production, and antibiotics or other preservatives or stabilizers, can certainly cause allergic reactions in some recipients. These reactions may be local or systemic, including urticaria and serious anaphylaxis. The most common extraneous allergen is egg protein derived from the growth of measles, mumps, influenza, and yellow fever viruses in embryonated eggs. Gelatin, used as a heat stabilizer, has been implicated in rare but severe allergic reactions. Local or systemic reactions (probably due to antigen-antibody complexes) can result from the too frequent administration of vaccines such as Td or rabies vaccine. Because live-virus vaccines can interfere with tuberculin test responses, necessary tuberculin testing should be done either on the day of immunization or at least 6 weeks later.

USE OF VACCINES IN SPECIAL CIRCUMSTANCES

Breast Feeding   Neither killed nor live vaccines affect the safety of breast feeding for either mother or infant. Breast-fed infants can be immunized on a normal schedule. Even premature infants can be immunized at their appropriate chronologic age. Seroconversion in response to hepatitis vaccine at birth may be impaired in some premature infants with birth weights of <2000 g. By a chronologic age of 1 month, however, premature infants—regardless of initial birth weight or gestational age—are as likely to respond adequately to vaccines as older and larger infants.

Occupational Exposure   Immunization recommendations for most occupational groups remain to be developed. Specific practices for the immunization of U.S. health care workers against hepatitis B are mandated by the Occupational Safety and Health Administration. Persons employed in caring for patients with chronic diseases can transmit influenza and should be vaccinated annually, independent of age. Rubella is transmitted to and from health care workers in medical facilities, particularly in pediatric practice. Health care workers who might transmit rubella to pregnant patients should be documented to be immune to rubella; susceptible individuals should be promptly immunized. Persons providing health care are also at greater risk from measles and varicella than the general public, and those who are likely to come into contact with measles- and varicella-infected patients should be documented to be immune or be immunized.

HIV Infection and Other Medical Conditions   Limited studies in HIV-infected individuals have found no increase in the risk of adverse events from the use of live or inactivated vaccines. It is not surprising that immune responses may not be as vigorous in immunocompromised individuals as in those with a normal immune system; therefore, persons known to be infected with HIV should be immunized with recommended vaccines in the same manner as individuals with a normal immune system and as early in the course of their disease as possible, before immune function becomes significantly impaired. If MMR immunization is indicated, HIV-infected patients may receive the standard attenuated vaccine; if polio vaccination is required, these patients and their household contacts should receive inactivated polio vaccine.

Albeit prudent, it is not necessary to test for HIV before making decisions about the immunization of asymptomatic individuals from known HIV risk groups. Live attenuated vaccines are contraindicated in other immunocompromised patients, including those with congenital immunodeficiency syndromes, those who have undergone splenectomy, and those who are receiving immunosuppressive therapy. Passive immunization with immunoglobulin preparations or antitoxins can be considered in individual cases, either as postexposure prophylaxis or as part of the treatment of established infection.

Travel   (See also Chap. 117) The International Sanitary Regulations allow countries to impose requirements for yellow fever and killed

TABLE 116-3 VALID AND INVALID CONTRAINDICATIONS TO VACCINATION

Vaccine	Valid Contraindication[a]	Invalid Contraindication
All vaccines in general	Serious allergic reactions (e.g., anaphylaxis) to a previous vaccine dose or a vaccine component *Precaution:* Moderate or severe concurrent illness with or without fever	Mild acute illness with or without fever Mild to moderate local reactions; low-grade or moderate fever after a previous dose Lack of previous physical examination in a well-appearing person Current antimicrobial therapy (except certain live bacterial vaccines) Convalescent phase of illness Premature birth (except hepatitis B in some circumstances) Recent exposure to infectious diseases History of penicillin allergy, other nonvaccine allergies; relatives with allergies; receiving desensitization treatment
DTaP[b]	Severe allergic reaction to a previous dose or a vaccine component Encephalopathy (e.g., coma, decreased level of consciousness, prolonged seizures) within 7 days of a previous dose of DTP or DTaP Progressive neurologic disorder, including infantile spasms, uncontrolled epilepsy, progressive encephalopathy: defer DTaP until neurologic status is clarified and stabilized *Precaution:* Fever of ≥40.5°C at ≤48 h after a previous dose of DTP or DTaP Collapse or shock-like state (i.e., hypotonic hyporesponsive episode ≤48 h after a previous dose of DTP or DTaP) Seizure ≤3 days after a previous dose of DTP or DTaP Persistent, inconsolable crying lasting ≥3 h/≤48 h after a previous dose of DTP or DTaP Moderate or severe acute illness with or without fever	Temperature of <40.5°C; fussiness; mild drowsiness after a prior dose of DTP or DTaP Family history of seizures, sudden infant death syndrome, or adverse event after DTP or DTaP Stable neurologic conditions (e.g., cerebral palsy, well-controlled convulsions, developmental delay)
DT, Td	Severe allergic reaction after a previous dose or to a vaccine component *Precaution:* Guillain-Barré syndrome ≤6 weeks after a previous dose of tetanus toxoid–containing vaccine Moderate or severe acute illness with or without fever	
IPV	Severe allergic reaction to a previous dose or a vaccine component *Precautions:* Pregnancy; moderate or severe acute illness with or without fever	
MMR	Severe allergic reaction to a previous dose or a vaccine component Pregnancy Known severe immunodeficiency (e.g., hematologic and solid tumors, congenital immunodeficiency, long-term immunosuppressive therapy, or severely symptomatic HIV infection) *Precautions:* Recent (≤11 months) receipt of antibody-containing blood products (specific interval depends on product); history of thrombocytopenia and thrombocytopenic purpura; moderate or severe acute illness with or without fever	Positive tuberculin skin test; simultaneous TB skin testing Breast-feeding Pregnancy of recipient's mother or other close or household contact; recipient is childbearing-age female or immunodeficient family member or household contact; asymptomatic or mildly symptomatic HIV infection; allergy to eggs
Hib	Severe allergic reaction to a previous dose or a vaccine component Age <6 weeks *Precaution:* Moderate or severe acute illness with or without fever	
Hepatitis B	Severe allergic reaction to a previous dose or a vaccine component *Precautions:* Infant weighing <2000 g; moderate or severe acute illness with or without fever	Pregnancy; autoimmune disease (e.g., systemic lupus erythematosus or rheumatoid arthritis)
Hepatitis A	Severe allergic reaction to a previous dose or a vaccine component *Precaution:* Pregnancy; moderate or severe acute illness with or without fever	
Varicella	Severe allergic reaction to a previous dose or a vaccine component Substantial suppression of cellular immunity Pregnancy *Precaution:* Recent (≤11 months) receipt of antibody-containing blood products (specific interval depends on product)	Pregnancy of recipient's mother or another close or household contact Immunodeficient family member or household contact; asymptomatic or mildly symptomatic HIV infection
Pneumococcal conjugate vaccines	Severe allergic reaction to a previous dose or a vaccine component *Precaution:* Moderate or severe acute illness with or without fever	
Influenza	Severe allergic reaction to a previous dose or a vaccine component, including egg protein *Precaution:* Moderate or severe acute illness with or without fever	Nonsevere (e.g., contact) allergy to latex or thimerosal; concurrent administration of warfarin or aminophylline
Pneumococcal polysaccharide vaccines	Severe allergic reaction to a previous dose or a vaccine component *Precaution:* Moderate or severe acute illness with or without fever	

[a]Events or conditions listed as precautions should be reviewed carefully. Benefits and risks of administering a specific vaccine to a person under these circumstances should be considered. If the risk from the vaccine is believed to outweigh the benefit, the vaccine should not be administered. If the benefit of vaccination is believed to outweigh the risk, the vaccine should be administered.

[b]Whether and when to administer DTaP to children with proven or suspected underlying neurologic disorders should be decided on a case-by-case basis.

Note: DTP, diphtheria and tetanus toxoids and whole-cell pertussis vaccine; DTaP, diphtheria and tetanus toxoids and acellular pertussis vaccine; DT, diphtheria and tetanus toxoids; Td, tetanus and reduced-dose diphtheria toxoids, adsorbed; IPV, inactivated polio vaccine; MMR, measles, mumps, and rubella vaccine; Hib, *Haemophilus influenzae* type b vaccine.

Source: General Recommendations on Immunization. MMWR 51(RR02): 1, 2002.

cholera vaccines as a condition for admission, even though the latter vaccine is not an effective public health tool. Travelers should know whether these vaccines are required for entry into the countries on their itinerary to avoid being turned back or immunized on the spot, with the inherent danger of unsafe injections in poor developing countries. Infants, children, and adults should have all routine immunizations updated before traveling, especially to developing countries, with particular attention to polio, measles, and DTaP or Tdap, depending on age. Immunity to hepatitis A and hepatitis B is advisable for travelers. Special-use vaccines (Table 116-2), including rabies, typhoid, Japanese B encephalitis, and plague vaccines, should be considered for those individuals who expect to go beyond the usual tourist routes or to spend extended periods in rural areas in disease-endemic regions. Most U.S. cities have travel clinics that maintain up-to-date epidemiologic information and can provide the appropriate vaccines. The CDC maintains a useful website for travelers (*www.cdc.gov/travel*).

CURRENT CONTROVERSIES

Even though vaccines are very safe and serious adverse events proven to be due to licensed vaccines are rare, the recent rise in the reporting of autism spectrum disorders has led some parents of affected children to claim that thimerosal—used as a preservative—is the cause of the problem. No study has yet implicated thimerosal or the vaccines in which it has been used as a likely cause of these disorders; however, fully 50% of cases before the Vaccine Injury Compensation Program concern autism allegedly due to mercury. In 1999, thimerosal was removed from single-dose formulations of recommended childhood vaccines in the United States; the exception is influenza vaccine, for which thimerosal-free preparations have been in short supply. There is no evidence that the frequency of autism diagnoses has changed since the discontinuation of thimerosal use, but further observation is necessary. It is important to resolve these controversies, particularly because it may be difficult to ensure product sterility in developing countries—where multidose vials of vaccine are most cost-effective—without the use of preservative.

Disparities in vaccine coverage among the majority and minority communities in the United States persist. Reasons for underimmunization include limited access to health care, lack of insurance, assignment of a low priority to preventive measures, and insufficient knowledge about vaccines and the importance of being vaccinated. The persistence of wild poliovirus in immunocompromised individuals and the reversion of live poliovirus vaccine to virulence in several communities have catalyzed debate about whether it really is possible to eradicate poliovirus from the world (thus allowing the cessation of immunization) or whether the best that can be hoped for is the worldwide elimination of clinical disease, with continued routine immunization to keep the risk low.

The addition of new, individually injectable vaccines to the childhood immunization schedule has heightened parental concerns about multiple injections at a single clinic visit. The continued development and testing of vaccine combinations aim to mitigate these concerns. Even when multiple injections are required, providers must make every effort to administer all indicated vaccines at each visit.

DELIVERY OF VACCINES

Over the past 25 years, considerable progress has been made to ensure that every child in the United States is fully immunized by the time of school entry. All 50 states now require immunization for school entry, and most have laws addressing attendance at preschools and day-care centers. Despite the dramatic impact of immunization and of other improvements in health care on the incidence of vaccine-preventable illness in the United States, many children still are not fully immunized, both in poor communities with inadequate health services and in affluent communities where parental concern about potential adverse events may exceed concern about now-uncommon diseases. The failure to vaccinate preschool children was largely responsible for the resurgence of measles in the United States in 1989–1991, with >55,000 cases and >130 measles-related deaths. Outbreaks of pertussis, mumps, and congenital rubella syndrome have occurred wherever immunization rates among preschool children are low. While indigenous transmission of polio, measles, and rubella has been eliminated in the United States, the risk of imported infection and spread to vaccine-naïve susceptible persons persists.

ACCESS TO IMMUNIZATION

Four major barriers to infant and childhood immunization have been identified within the health care system: (1) low public awareness and lack of public demand for immunization, (2) inadequate access to immunization services, (3) missed opportunities to administer vaccines, and (4) inadequate resources for public health and preventive programs. National outreach and educational campaigns promote parental awareness of the value of vaccination and encourage health care providers to use every opportunity to vaccinate the children in their care.

HANDLING OF VACCINES

Vaccines must be handled and stored with care. Attention to the entire "cold chain"—from storage, shelf life, reconstitution, and shelf life after reconstitution and opening—is essential to ensuring that clients receive potent vaccines. Vaccines should be kept at 2°–8°C and, with the exception of varicella vaccine and live attenuated influenza vaccine, should not be frozen. The latter two vaccines should be kept frozen at –15°C. Measles vaccine must be protected from light, which inactivates the virus.

STANDARDS FOR IMMUNIZATION PRACTICE

National standards of immunization for childhood, adolescent, and adult practice have been established to define common policies and practices for public health clinics and physicians' private offices (Table 116-4). These standards represent the most desirable immunization practices and highlight the need to distinguish between valid contraindications and conditions that are often considered to be but are not in fact contraindications (*www.cdc.gov/vaccines/recs/vac-admin/downloads/contraindications_guide.pdf*).

Among the valid contraindications applicable to all vaccines are a history of anaphylaxis or other serious allergic reactions to a vaccine or vaccine component and the presence of a moderate or severe illness, with or without fever. Infants who develop encephalopathy within 72 h of a dose of DTP or DTaP should not receive further doses; those who experience a "precaution" event should not normally receive further doses. Because of theoretical risks to the fetus, pregnant women should not receive MMR or varicella vaccine. Diarrhea, minor respiratory illness (with or without fever), mild to moderate local reactions to a previous dose of vaccine, the concurrent or recent use of antimicrobial agents, mild to moderate malnutrition, and the convalescent phase of an acute illness are not valid contraindications to routine immunization. Failure to vaccinate children because of these conditions is increasingly viewed as a missed opportunity for immunization.

CONTROL OF VACCINE-PREVENTABLE DISEASE

A continuing task of public health practice is to maintain individual and herd immunity, and the job is not over once a population is fully vaccinated. Rather, it is imperative to immunize each subsequent generation as long as the threat of the reintroduction of the disease from anywhere in the world persists. Ongoing surveillance and prompt reporting of disease to local or state health departments are essential to this goal, ensuring a continuing awareness of the possibility of vaccine-preventable illness. Nearly all vaccine-preventable diseases are notifiable, and individual case data are routinely forwarded to the CDC. These data are used to detect outbreaks or other unusual events that require investigation and to evaluate prevention and control policies, practices, and strategies.

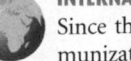 **INTERNATIONAL CONSIDERATIONS**
Since the establishment of the Expanded Programme on Immunization (EPI) by the WHO in 1981 and the involvement of UNICEF in the program's implementation, levels of coverage for the

TABLE 116-4 STANDARDS FOR IMMUNIZATION PRACTICE

Child and Adolescent Immunization Practice

1. Immunization services are readily available.
2. Vaccinations are coordinated with other health care services and provided in a "medical home" when possible.
3. Barriers to vaccination are identified and minimized.
4. Patient's costs are minimized.
5. Health care professionals review the vaccination and health status of patients at every encounter to determine which vaccines are indicated.
6. Health care professionals assess for and follow only medically accepted contraindications.
7. Parents/guardians and patients are educated about the benefits and risks of vaccination in a culturally appropriate manner and in easy-to-understand language.
8. Health care professionals follow appropriate procedures for vaccine storage and handling.
9. Up-to-date written vaccination protocols are accessible at all locations where vaccines are administered.
10. Persons who administer vaccines and staff who manage or support vaccine administration are knowledgeable and receive ongoing education.
11. Health care professionals simultaneously administer as many indicated vaccine doses as possible.
12. Vaccination records for patients are accurate, complete, and easily accessible.
13. Health care professionals report adverse events following vaccination promptly and accurately to the VAERS and are aware of the VICP.
14. All personnel who have contact with patients are appropriately vaccinated.
15. Systems are used to remind parents/guardians, patients, and health care professionals when vaccinations are due and to recall patients whose vaccinations are overdue.
16. Office- or clinic-based patient record reviews and vaccination coverage assessments are performed annually.
17. Health care professionals practice community-based approaches.

Adult Immunization Practice

1. Adult immunization services are readily available.
2. Barriers to receiving vaccines are identified and minimized.
3. Patient's out-of-pocket costs are minimized.
4. Health care professionals routinely review the vaccination status of patients.
5. Health care professionals assess for valid contraindications.
6. Patients are educated about risks and benefits of vaccination in easy-to-understand language.
7. Written vaccination protocols are available at all locations where vaccinations are administered.
8. Persons who administer vaccines are properly trained.
9. Health care professionals recommend simultaneous administration of all indicated vaccine doses.
10. Vaccination records for patients are accurate and easily accessible.
11. All personnel who have contact with patients are appropriately vaccinated.
12. Systems are developed and used to remind patients and health care professionals when vaccinations are due and to recall patients whose vaccinations are overdue.
13. Standing orders for vaccinations are employed.
14. Regular assessments of vaccination coverage levels are conducted in the provider's practice.
15. Patient-oriented and community-based approaches are used to reach target populations.

Note: VAERS, Vaccine Adverse Events Reporting System; VICP, Vaccine Injury Compensation Program.
Source: Centers for Disease Control and Prevention, in *Epidemiology and Prevention of Vaccine-Preventable Diseases*, 2006, Appendix H. These standards can be found at *www.cdc.gov/nip/publications*.

concerns remain about the adequacy of long-term strategies to ensure continuity, the impact of vaccine campaigns on the provision of routine services, and unsafe injection practices.

Because infectious diseases know no geographic or political boundaries, uncontrolled disease anywhere in the world poses a threat to the United States, even without bioterrorism. Vaccines offer the opportunity to effectively control and even eliminate some diseases through individual and herd protection. Vaccines also represent the best societal hope for stopping the pandemic of HIV infection throughout the world and for efficiently controlling malaria and tuberculosis. Issues of cost, liability, risk, and profitability limit the interest of the pharmaceutical industry in the development of vaccines for infectious diseases of the poor.

SOURCES OF INFORMATION ON IMMUNIZATION

- Official vaccine package circulars and Vaccine Administration Statements from the CDC
- Report of the Committee on Infectious Diseases of the American Academy of Pediatrics ("Red Book")
- Recommendations of the Advisory Committee on Immunization Practices, CDC
- Guide for Adult Immunization, American College of Physicians
- Health Information for International Travel (published yearly) and Advisory Memoranda on Travel (published periodically), CDC
- Control of Communicable Diseases in Man, American Public Health Association
- Technical Bulletin of the College of Obstetrics and Gynecology
- National Network for Immunization Information, Infectious Diseases Society of America/Pediatric Infectious Diseases Society/American Academy of Pediatrics/American Nurses Association

recommended basic children's vaccines (bacille Calmette-Guérin, poliomyelitis, DTP/DTaP, and measles) have risen from 5% to ~80% worldwide, although coverage does not necessarily translate into protective immunity. Each year, at least 2.7 million deaths from measles, neonatal tetanus, and pertussis and 200,000 cases of paralysis due to polio are prevented by immunization. Despite the successes of this program, many vaccine-preventable diseases remain prevalent in the developing world. Measles, for example, continues to kill an estimated 500,000 children each year, and diphtheria, whooping cough, polio, and neonatal tetanus still occur at unacceptably high rates. An estimated 20–35% of all deaths of children are due to vaccine-preventable diseases.

In addition to the antigens included in the EPI for routine use in the developing world, others (hepatitis B, Hib, Japanese B encephalitis, yellow fever, meningococcal, mumps, and rubella) are used regionally, depending on disease epidemiology and resources. The rationale for inclusion of hepatitis B vaccine in Africa and Asia is to prevent the subsequent development of hepatocellular carcinoma, which is strongly linked with the persistence of hepatitis B virus from early childhood. The delivery of vaccines in mass campaigns on national immunization days, superseding even civil wars and insurgencies, has resulted in the cessation of transmission of poliomyelitis in the Western Hemisphere, the western Pacific, and Europe and in the virtual elimination of clinical measles from the Western Hemisphere. Periodic vaccination campaigns complement routine infant and childhood vaccination services under the rubric "catch up, follow up, and keep up." Despite these successes,

FURTHER READINGS

BONHOEFFER J, HEININGER U: Immunization: Perception and evidence. Curr Opin Infect Dis 20:237, 2007

BROWN NJ et al: Vaccination, seizures and "vaccine damage." Curr Opin Neurol 20:181, 2007

BRUCE AYLWARD R et al: Risk management in a polio-free world. Risk Anal 26:1441, 2006

GOLDIE S: A public health approach to cervical cancer control: Considerations of screening and vaccination strategies. Int J Gynaecol Obstet 94(Suppl 1):S95, 2006

JACOBSON RM et al: Why is evidence-based medicine so harsh on vaccines? An exploration of the method and its natural biases. Vaccine 25:3165, 2007

KAUFMANN SH: The contribution of immunology to the rational design of novel antibacterial vaccines. Nat Rev Microbiol 5:491, 2007

KIMMEL SR et al: Addressing immunization barriers, benefits, and risks. J Fam Pract 56:S61, 2007

REELER AV: Anthropological perspectives on injections: A reivew. Bull World Health Organ 78:135, 2000

THOMPSON KM, TEBBENS RJ: Eradication versus control for poliomyelitis: An economic anlysis. Lancet 369:1363, 2007

VAN DER ZEIJST BA et al: On the design of national vaccination programmes. Vaccine 25:3143, 2007

CHAPTER 116

Immunization Principles and Vaccine Use

117 Health Advice for International Travel

Jay S. Keystone, Phyllis E. Kozarsky

According to the World Tourism Organization, the number of international tourist arrivals in 2004 reached an all-time record of 763 million. This number represents an increase over the 2003 figure of almost 11%—the highest and the only double-digit percentage increase since 1980, when these statistics were first collected. Not only are more people traveling; travelers are seeking more exotic and remote destinations. Studies show that 50–75% of short-term travelers to the tropics or subtropics report some health impairment. Most of these health problems are minor: only 5% require medical attention, and <1% require hospitalization. Although infectious agents contribute substantially to morbidity among travelers, these pathogens account for only ~1% of deaths in this population. Cardiovascular disease and injuries are the most frequent causes of death among travelers from the United States, accounting for 49% and 22% of deaths, respectively. Age-specific rates of death due to cardiovascular disease are similar among travelers and nontravelers. In contrast, rates of death due to injury (the majority from motor vehicle, drowning, or aircraft accidents) are several times higher among travelers. Figure 117-1 summarizes the monthly incidence of health problems during travel in developing countries.

GENERAL ADVICE

Health maintenance recommendations are based not only on the traveler's destination but also on assessment of risk, which is determined by health status, specific itinerary, and lifestyle during travel. Detailed information regarding country-specific risks and recommendations may be obtained from the Centers for Disease Control and Prevention (CDC) publication *Health Information for International Travel* (available at *www.cdc.gov/travel/yb/*).

Fitness for travel is an issue of growing concern in view of the increased numbers of elderly and chronically ill individuals journeying to exotic destinations (see "Travel and Special Hosts," below). Since most commercial aircraft are pressurized to 2500 m (8000 ft) above sea level (corresponding to a Pa_{O_2} of ~55 mmHg), individuals with serious cardiopulmonary problems or anemia should be evaluated before travel. In addition, those who have recently had surgery, a myocardial infarction, a cerebrovascular accident, or a deep-vein thrombosis may be at high risk for adverse events during flight. A summary of current recommendations regarding fitness to fly has been published by the Aerospace Medical Association Air Transport Medicine Committee (*www.asma.org/publications/*). A pretravel health assessment may be advisable for individuals considering particularly adventurous recreational activities, such as mountain climbing and scuba diving.

IMMUNIZATIONS FOR TRAVEL

Immunizations for travel fall into three broad categories: *routine* (childhood/adult boosters that are necessary regardless of travel), *required* (immunizations that are mandated by international regulations for entry into certain areas or for border crossings), and *recommended* (immunizations that are desirable because of travel-related risks). Vaccines commonly given to travelers are listed in Table 117-1.

Routine Immunizations • DIPHTHERIA, TETANUS, AND POLIO   Diphtheria (Chap. 131) continues to be a problem worldwide. Large outbreaks have occurred over the past decade in the independent states formerly encompassed by the Soviet Union. Serologic surveys show that tetanus (Chap. 133) antitoxin is lacking in many North Americans, especially in women over the age of 50. The risk of polio (Chap. 184) to the international traveler is extremely low, and wild-type poliovirus has been eradicated from the western hemisphere and Europe.

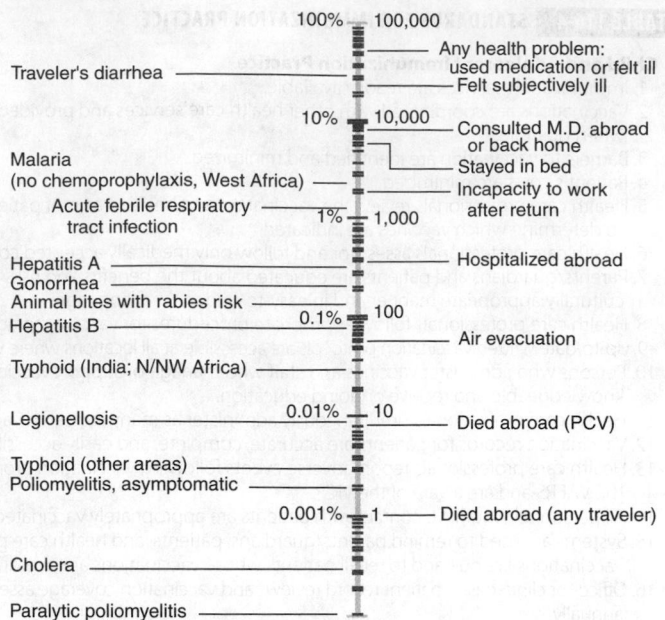

FIGURE 117-1   Incidence rate, per month, of health problems during a stay in developing countries. PCV, Peace Corps volunteer. *(From Steffen R, Lobel HO: Epidemiologic basis for the practice of travel medicine. J Wilderness Med 5:56, 1994. Reprinted with permission from Chapman and Hall, New York.)*

However, studies in the United States suggest that 12% of adult travelers are unprotected against at least one poliovirus serogroup. Foreign travel offers an ideal opportunity to have these immunizations updated. With the recent increase in pertussis in adults, the diphtheria-tetanus-acellular pertussis (Tdap) combination may replace the Td vaccine as a 10-year booster once an adult polio immunization has been administered.

MEASLES   Measles (rubeola) continues to be a major cause of morbidity and mortality in the developing world (Chap. 185). Several outbreaks of measles in the United States have been linked to imported cases. The group at highest risk consists of persons born after 1956 and vaccinated before 1980, in many of whom primary vaccination failed.

INFLUENZA   Influenza—possibly the most common vaccine-preventable infection in travelers—occurs year-round in the tropics and during the summer months in the southern hemisphere (coinciding with the winter months in the northern hemisphere). One prospective study showed that influenza developed in 1% of travelers to Southeast Asia per month of stay. Vaccination should be considered for all travelers to these regions, particularly those who are elderly or chronically ill. Travel-related influenza continues to occur during summer months in Alaska and the Northwest Territories of Canada among cruise-ship passengers and staff (Chap. 180).

PNEUMOCOCCAL INFECTION   Regardless of travel, pneumococcal vaccine should be administered routinely to the elderly and to persons at high risk of serious infection, including those with chronic heart, lung, or renal disease and those who have been splenectomized or have sickle cell disease (Chap. 128).

Required Immunizations • YELLOW FEVER   Documentation of vaccination against yellow fever (Chap. 189) may be required as a condition of entry into or passage through countries of sub-Saharan Africa and equatorial South America, where the disease is endemic or epidemic, or for entry into countries at risk of having the infection introduced. This vaccine is given only by state-authorized yellow fever centers, and its administration must be documented on an official International Certificate of Vaccination. A registry of U.S. clinics that provide the vac-

TABLE 117-1 VACCINES COMMONLY USED FOR TRAVEL

Vaccine	Primary Series	Booster Interval
Cholera, live oral (CVD 103 - HgR)	1 dose	6 months
Hepatitis A (Havrix), 1440 enzyme immunoassay U/mL	2 doses, 6–12 months apart, IM	None required
Hepatitis A (VAQTA, AVAXIM, EPAXAL)	2 doses, 6–12 months apart, IM	None required
Hepatitis A/B combined (Twinrix)	3 doses at 0, 1, and 6–12 months *or* 0, 7, and 21 days plus booster at 1 year, IM	None required *except* 12 months (once only, for accelerated schedule)
Hepatitis B (Engerix B): accelerated schedule	3 doses at 0, 1, and 2 months *or* 0, 7, and 21 days plus booster at 1 year, IM	12 months, once only
Hepatitis B (Engerix B or Recom-bivax): standard schedule	3 doses at 0, 1, and 6 months, IM	None required
Immune globulin (hepatitis A prevention)	1 dose IM	Intervals of 3–5 months, depending on initial dose
Japanese encephalitis (JEV, Biken)	3 doses, 1 week apart, SC	12–18 months (first booster), then 4 years
Meningococcus, quadrivalent [Menimmune (polysaccharide), Menactra (conjugate)]	1 dose SC	>3 years (optimum booster schedule not yet determined)
Rabies (HDCV), rabies vaccine absorbed (RVA), or purified chick embryo cell vaccine (PCEC)	3 doses at 0, 7, and 21 or 28 days, IM	None required except with exposure
Typhoid Ty21a, oral live attenuated (Vivotif)	1 capsule every other day × 4 doses	5 years
Typhoid Vi capsular polysaccharide, injectable (Typhim Vi)	1 dose IM	2 years
Yellow fever	1 dose SC	10 years

cine is available from the CDC (*www.cdc.gov/travel/*). Recent data suggest that fewer than 50% of travelers entering areas endemic for yellow fever are immunized. Severe adverse events associated with this vaccine have recently increased in incidence. First-time vaccine recipients may present with a syndrome characterized as either neurotropic (1 case per 150,000–250,000 doses) or viscerotropic (1 case per 200,000–300,000 doses; among persons >60 years of age, 1 case per 40,000–50,000). Advanced age and thymic disease seem to increase the risk for these adverse events (*www.cdc.gov/nip/publications/VIS/vis-yf.pdf*).

MENINGOCOCCAL MENINGITIS   Protection against meningitis (using one of the quadrivalent vaccines) is required for entry into Saudi Arabia during the Hajj (Chap. 136).

Recommended Immunizations • **HEPATITIS A AND B**   Hepatitis A (Chap. 298) is one of the most frequent vaccine-preventable infections of travelers. The risk is six times greater for travelers who stray from the usual tourist routes. The mortality rate for hepatitis A increases with age, reaching almost 3% among individuals over age 50. Of the four hepatitis A vaccines currently available in North America (two in the United States), all are interchangeable and have an efficacy rate of >95%.

Long-stay overseas workers appear to be at considerable risk for hepatitis B infection (Chap. 298). The recommendation that all travelers be immunized against hepatitis B before departure is supported by two recent studies showing that 17% of the assessed travelers who received health care abroad had some type of injection; according to the World Health Organization, nonsterile equipment is used for up to 75% of all injections given in the developing world. A combined hepatitis A and B vaccine is now available in the United States and has been approved for administration on a 3-week accelerated schedule. It seems prudent to consider immunization of all travelers against hepatitis A and B.

TYPHOID FEVER   The attack rate for typhoid fever (Chap. 146) is 1 case per 30,000 per month of travel to the developing world. However, the attack rates in India, Senegal, and North Africa are tenfold higher and are especially high among travelers to relatively remote destinations

and among VFRs (immigrants returning to their homelands to visit friends or relatives). Between 1994 and 1999 in the United States, 77% of imported cases involved the latter group. Both of the available vaccines—one oral (live) and the other injectable (polysaccharide)—have efficacy rates of ~70%. In some countries, a combined hepatitis A/typhoid vaccine is available.

MENINGOCOCCAL MENINGITIS   Although the risk of meningococcal disease among travelers has not been quantified, it is likely to be higher among travelers who live with poor indigenous populations in overcrowded conditions (Chap. 136). Either the older polysaccharide vaccine or the newer quadrivalent conjugate vaccine is recommended for persons traveling to sub-Saharan Africa during the dry season or to areas of the world where there are epidemics. The vaccine, which protects against serogroups A, C, Y, and W-135, has an efficacy rate of >90%.

JAPANESE ENCEPHALITIS   The risk of Japanese encephalitis (Chap. 189), an infection transmitted by mosquitoes in rural Asia and Southeast Asia, is ~1 case per 5000 travelers per month of stay in an endemic area. Most symptomatic infections among U.S. residents have involved military personnel or their families. The vaccine efficacy rate is >90%; serious allergic reactions occur only rarely. The vaccine is recommended for persons staying >1 month in rural endemic areas or for shorter periods if their activities (e.g., camping, bicycling, hiking) in these areas will increase exposure risk. A Vero cell vaccine may be licensed in the United States within the next 2 years.

CHOLERA   The risk of cholera (Chap. 149) is extremely low, with ~1 case per 500,000 journeys to endemic areas. Cholera vaccine, no longer available in the United States, was rarely recommended but was considered for aid and health care workers in refugee camps or in disaster-stricken/war-torn areas. A more effective oral cholera vaccine is available in other countries.

RABIES   Domestic animals, primarily dogs, are the major transmitters of rabies in developing countries (Chap. 188). Several studies have shown that the risk of rabies posed by a dog bite in an endemic area translates into 1–3.6 cases per 1000 travelers per month of stay. Countries where canine rabies is highly endemic include Mexico, the Philippines, Sri Lanka, India, Thailand, and Vietnam. The three vaccines available in the United States provide >90% protection. Rabies vaccine is recommended for long-stay travelers, particularly children, and persons who may be occupationally exposed to rabies in endemic areas. Even after receipt of a preexposure rabies vaccine series, two postexposure doses are required. Travelers who have had the preexposure series will not require rabies immune globulin (which is often unavailable in developing countries) if they are exposed to the disease.

PREVENTION OF MALARIA AND OTHER INSECT-BORNE DISEASES

It is estimated that more than 30,000 American and European travelers develop malaria each year (Chap. 203). The risk to travelers is highest in Oceania and sub-Saharan Africa (estimated at 1:5 and 1:50 per month of stay, respectively, among persons not using chemoprophylaxis); intermediate in malarious areas on the Indian subcontinent and in Southeast Asia (1:250–1:1000 per month); and low in South and Central America (1:2500–1:10,000 per month). Of the more than 1000 cases of malaria reported annually in the United States, 90% of those due to *Plasmodium falciparum* occur in travelers returning or immigrating from Africa and

Oceania. VFRs are at the highest risk of acquiring malaria. With the worldwide increase in chloroquine- and multidrug-resistant falciparum malaria, decisions about chemoprophylaxis have become more difficult. In addition, the spread of malaria due to primaquine- and chloroquine-resistant strains of *Plasmodium vivax* has added to the complexity of treatment. The case-fatality rate of falciparum malaria in the United States is 4%; however, in only one-third of patients who die is the diagnosis of malaria considered before death.

Several studies indicate that fewer than 50% of travelers adhere to basic recommendations for malaria prevention. Keys to the prevention of malaria include both personal protection measures against mosquito bites (especially between dusk and dawn) and malaria chemoprophylaxis. The former measures include the use of DEET-containing insect repellents, permethrin-impregnated bed-nets and clothing, screened sleeping accommodations, and protective clothing. A new insect repellent containing picaridin as an active ingredient appears to be quite efficacious and is available in the United States only in low-concentration formulations that require frequent reapplications. Thus, in regions where infections such as malaria are transmitted, DEET products (25–50%) are recommended, even for children and infants >2 months of age. Personal protection measures also help prevent other insect-transmitted illnesses, such as dengue fever (Chap. 189). Over the past decade, the incidence of dengue has increased, particularly in the Caribbean region, Latin America, and Southeast Asia. Dengue virus is transmitted by an urban-dwelling mosquito that bites primarily at dawn and dusk.

Table 117-2 lists the currently recommended drugs of choice for prophylaxis of malaria, by destination.

PREVENTION OF GASTROINTESTINAL ILLNESS

Diarrhea, the leading cause of illness in travelers (Chap. 122), is usually a short-lived, self-limited condition; however, 40% of affected individuals need to alter their scheduled activities, and another 20% are confined to bed. The most important determinant of risk is the destination. Incidence rates per 2-week stay have been reported to be as low as 8% in industrialized countries and as high as 55% in parts of Africa, Central and South America, and Southeast Asia. Infants and young adults are at particularly high risk. A recent review suggested that there is little correlation between dietary indiscretions and the occurrence of travelers' diarrhea. Earlier studies of U.S. students in Mexico showed that eating meals in restaurants and cafeterias or consuming food from street vendors was associated with increased risk.

Etiology (See also Table 122-3) The most frequently identified pathogens causing travelers' diarrhea are toxigenic *Escherichia coli* and enteroaggregative *E. coli* (Chap. 143), although in some parts of the world (notably northern Africa and Southeast Asia) *Campylobacter* infections (Chap. 148) appear to predominate. Other common causative organisms include *Salmonella* (Chap. 146), *Shigella* (Chap. 147), ro-

TABLE 117-2 MALARIA CHEMOSUPPRESSIVE REGIMENS ACCORDING TO GEOGRAPHIC AREA[a]

Geographic Area	Drug of Choice	Alternatives
Central America (north of Panama), Haiti, Dominican Republic, Iraq, Egypt, Turkey, northern Argentina, and Paraguay	Chloroquine	Mefloquine Doxycycline Atovaquone/ proguanil
South America including Panama (except northern Argentina and Paraguay); Asia (including Southeast Asia); Africa; and Oceania	Mefloquine Doxycycline Atovaquone-proguanil (Malarone)	Primaquine
Thai-Myanmar and Thai-Cambodian borders	Doxycycline Atovaquone-proguanil (Malarone)	

[a]See CDC's *Health Information for International Travel 2005–2006.*
Note: See also Chap. 203.

tavirus (Chap. 183), and norovirus (Chap. 183). The latter virus has caused numerous outbreaks on cruise ships. Except for giardiasis (Chap. 208), parasitic infections are uncommon causes of travelers' diarrhea. A growing problem for travelers is the development of antibiotic resistance among many bacterial pathogens. Examples include strains of *Campylobacter* resistant to quinolones and strains of *E. coli*, *Shigella*, and *Salmonella* resistant to trimethoprim-sulfamethoxazole.

Precautions Although the mainstay of prevention of travelers' diarrhea involves food and water precautions, the literature has repeatedly documented dietary indiscretions by 98% of travelers within the first 72 h after arrival at their destination. The maxim "Boil it, cook it, peel it, or forget it!" is easy to remember but apparently difficult to follow. General food and water precautions include eating foods piping hot; avoiding foods that are raw, poorly cooked, or sold by street vendors; and drinking only boiled or commercially bottled beverages, particularly those that are carbonated. Heating kills diarrhea-causing organisms, whereas freezing does not; therefore, ice cubes made from unpurified water should be avoided.

Self-Treatment (See also Table 122-5) As travelers' diarrhea often occurs despite rigorous food and water precautions, travelers should carry medications for self-treatment. An antibiotic is useful in reducing the frequency of bowel movements and duration of illness in moderate to severe diarrhea. The standard regimen is a 3-day course of a quinolone taken twice daily (or, in the case of some newer formulations, once daily). However, studies have shown that a single double dose of a quinolone may be equally effective. For diarrhea acquired in areas such as Thailand, where >90% of *Campylobacter* infections are quinolone resistant, azithromycin may be a better alternative. Rifaximin, a poorly absorbed rifampin derivative, is highly effective against noninvasive bacterial pathogens such as toxigenic and enteroaggregative *E. coli.*

The current approach to self-treatment of travelers' diarrhea is for the traveler to carry three once-daily doses of an antibiotic and to use as many doses as necessary to resolve the illness. If neither high fever nor blood in the stool accompanies the diarrhea, loperamide may be taken in combination with the antibiotic.

Prophylaxis Prophylaxis of travelers' diarrhea with bismuth subsalicylate is widely used but only ~60% effective. For certain individuals (e.g., athletes, persons with a repeated history of travelers' diarrhea, and persons with chronic diseases), a single daily dose of a quinolone or azithromycin or a once-daily rifaximin regimen during travel of <1 month's duration is 75–90% efficacious in preventing travelers' diarrhea.

Illness after Return Although extremely common, acute travelers' diarrhea is usually self-limited or amenable to antibiotic therapy. Persistent bowel problems after the traveler returns home have a less well-defined etiology and may require medical attention from a specialist. Infectious agents (e.g., *Giardia lamblia*, *Cyclospora cayetanensis*, *Entamoeba histolytica*) appear to be responsible for only a small proportion of cases with persistent bowel symptoms. By far the most frequent causes of persistent diarrhea after travel are postinfectious sequelae such as lactose intolerance or irritable bowel syndrome. A recent meta-analysis showed that postinfectious irritable bowel syndrome may occur in as many as 4–13% of cases. When no infectious etiology can be identified, a trial of metronidazole therapy for presumed giardiasis, a strict lactose-free diet for 1 week, or a several-week trial of high-dose hydrophilic mucilloid (plus lactulose for persons with constipation) relieves the symptoms of many patients.

PREVENTION OF OTHER TRAVEL-RELATED PROBLEMS

Travelers are at high risk for *sexually transmitted diseases* (Chap. 124). Surveys have shown that large numbers engage in casual sex, and there is a reluctance to use condoms consistently. An increasing number of travelers are being diagnosed with *schistosomiasis* (Chap. 212). Travelers should be cautioned to avoid bathing, swimming, or wading in freshwater lakes, streams, or rivers in parts of tropical South America, the Caribbean, Africa, and Southeast Asia. Prevention of *travel-associated injury* depends mostly on common-sense precautions. Riding on motorcycles (especially without helmets) and in overcrowded public vehicles is not recommended; individuals should not travel in developing countries by road after dark, particularly in rural areas. In addition to its association with motor vehicle accidents, excessive alcohol use has been a significant factor in drownings, assaults, and injuries. Travelers are cautioned to avoid walking barefoot because of the risk of hookworm and *Strongyloides* infections (Chap. 210) and snakebites (Chap. 391).

THE TRAVELER'S MEDICAL KIT

A traveler's medical kit is strongly advisable. The contents may vary widely, depending on the itinerary, duration of stay, style of travel, and local medical facilities. While many medications are available abroad (often over the counter), directions for their use may be nonexistent or in a foreign language, or a product may be outdated or counterfeit. For example, a recent multicountry study in Southeast Asia showed that a mean of 53% (range, 21–92%) of antimalarial products were counterfeit or contained inadequate amounts of active drug. In the medical kit, the short-term traveler should consider carrying an analgesic; an antidiarrheal agent and an antibiotic for self-treatment of travelers' diarrhea; antihistamines; a laxative; oral rehydration salts; a sunscreen with a skin-protection factor of at least 30; a DEET-containing insect repellent for the skin; an insecticide for clothing (permethrin); and, if necessary, an antimalarial drug. To these medications, the long-stay traveler might add a broad-spectrum general-purpose antibiotic (levofloxacin or azithromycin), an antibacterial eye and skin ointment, and a topical antifungal cream. Regardless of the duration of travel, a first-aid kit containing such items as scissors, tweezers, and bandages should be considered. A practical approach to self-treatment of infections in the long-stay traveler who carries a once-daily dose of antibiotics is to use 3 tablets "below the waist" (bowel and bladder infections) and 6 tablets "above the waist" (skin and respiratory infections).

TRAVEL AND SPECIAL HOSTS

PREGNANCY AND TRAVEL

(See also Chap. 7) A woman's medical history and itinerary, the quality of medical care at her destinations, and her degree of flexibility determine whether travel is wise during pregnancy. According to the American College of Obstetrics and Gynecology, the safest part of pregnancy in which to travel is between 18 and 24 weeks, when there is the least danger of spontaneous abortion or premature labor. Some obstetricians prefer that women stay within a few hundred miles of home after the 28th week of pregnancy in case problems arise. In general, however, healthy women may be advised that it is acceptable to travel.

Relative contraindications to international travel during pregnancy include a history of miscarriage, premature labor, incompetent cervix, or toxemia. General medical problems such as diabetes, heart failure, severe anemia, or a history of thromboembolic disease should also prompt the pregnant woman to postpone her travels. Finally, regions in which the pregnant woman and her fetus may be at excessive risk (e.g., those at high altitudes and those where live-virus vaccines are required or where multidrug-resistant malaria is endemic) are not ideal destinations during any trimester.

Malaria Malaria during pregnancy carries a significant risk of morbidity and death. Levels of parasitemia are highest and failure to clear the parasites after treatment is most frequent among primigravidae. Severe disease, with complications such as cerebral malaria, massive hemolysis, and renal failure, is especially likely in pregnancy. Fetal sequelae include spontaneous abortion, stillbirth, preterm delivery, and congenital infection.

Travelers' Diarrhea Pregnant travelers must be extremely cautious regarding their food and beverage intake. Dehydration due to travelers' diarrhea can lead to inadequate placental blood flow. Infections such as toxoplasmosis, hepatitis E, and listeriosis can also have serious sequelae in pregnancy.

The mainstay of therapy for travelers' diarrhea is rehydration. Loperamide may be used if necessary. For self-treatment, azithromycin may be the best option. Although quinolones are increasingly being used safely during pregnancy and rifaximin is poorly absorbed from the gastrointestinal tract, they are not approved for this indication.

Because of the major problems encountered when infants are given local foods and beverages, women are strongly encouraged to breast-feed when traveling with a neonate. A nursing mother with travelers' diarrhea should not stop breast-feeding but should increase her fluid intake.

Air Travel and High-Altitude Destinations Commercial air travel is not a risk to the healthy pregnant woman or to the fetus. The higher radiation levels reported at altitudes of >10,500 m (>35,000 ft) should pose no problem to the healthy pregnant traveler. Since each airline has a policy regarding pregnancy and flying, it is best to check with the specific carrier when booking reservations. Domestic air travel is usually permitted until the 36th week, whereas international air travel is generally curtailed after the 32nd week.

There are no known risks for pregnant women who travel to high-altitude destinations and stay for short periods. However, there are likewise no data on the safety of pregnant women at altitudes of >4500 m (15,000 ft).

THE HIV-INFECTED TRAVELER

(See also Chap. 182) The HIV-infected traveler is at special risk of serious infections due to a number of pathogens that may be more prevalent at travel destinations than at home. However, the degree of risk depends primarily on the state of the immune system at the time of travel. For persons whose CD4+ T cell counts are normal or >500/μL, no data suggest a greater risk during travel than for persons without HIV infection. Individuals with AIDS (CD4+ T cell counts of <200/μL) and others who are symptomatic need special counseling and should visit a travel medicine practitioner before departure, especially when traveling to the developing world.

Several countries now routinely deny entry to HIV-positive individuals, even though these restrictions do not appear to decrease rates of transmission of the virus. In general, HIV testing is required of those individuals who wish to stay abroad >3 months or who intend to work or study abroad. Some countries will accept an HIV serologic test done within 6 months of departure, whereas others will not accept a blood test done at any time in the traveler's home country. Border officials often have the authority to make inquiries of individuals entering a country and to check the medications they are carrying. If a drug such as zidovudine is identified, the person may be barred from entering the country. Information on testing requirements for specific countries is available from consular offices but is subject to frequent change.

Immunizations All of the HIV-infected traveler's routine immunizations should be up to date (Chap. 116). The response to immunization may be impaired at CD4+ T cell counts of <200/μL (and in some cases at even higher counts). Thus HIV-infected persons should be vaccinated as early as possible to ensure adequate immune responses to all vaccines. In patients receiving highly active antiretroviral therapy, at least 3 months must elapse before regenerated CD4+ T cells can be considered fully functional; therefore, in these patients, vaccinations should be delayed. However, when the risk of illness is high or the sequelae of illness are serious, immunization is recommended. In certain circumstances, it may be prudent to check the adequacy of the serum antibody response before departure.

Because of the increased risk of infections due to *Streptococcus pneumoniae* and other bacterial pathogens that cause pneumonia following influenza, pneumococcal polysaccharide and influenza vaccines should be administered. The estimated rates of response to influenza vaccine are >80% among persons with asymptomatic HIV infection and <50% among those with AIDS.

In general, live attenuated vaccines are contraindicated for persons with immune dysfunction. Because measles (rubeola) can be a severe and lethal infection in HIV-positive patients, these patients should receive the measles vaccine (or the combination measles-mumps-rubella vaccine) unless the CD4+ T cell count is <200/μL. Between 18% and 58% of symptomatic HIV-infected vaccinees develop adequate antibody titers, and 50–100% of asymptomatic HIV-infected persons seroconvert.

It is recommended that the live yellow fever vaccine not be given to HIV-infected travelers. Although the potential adverse effects of a live vaccine in an HIV-infected individual are always a consideration, there appear to have been no reported cases of illness in those who have inadvertently received this vaccine. Nonetheless, if the CD4+ T cell count is <200/μL, an alternative itinerary that poses no risk of exposure to yellow fever is recommended. If the traveler is passing through or traveling to an area where the vaccine is required but the disease risk is low, a physician's waiver should be issued.

A transient increase in viremia (lasting days to weeks) has been demonstrated in HIV-infected individuals following immunization against influenza, pneumococcal infection, and tetanus (Chap. 182). However, at this point, there is no evidence that this transient increase is detrimental.

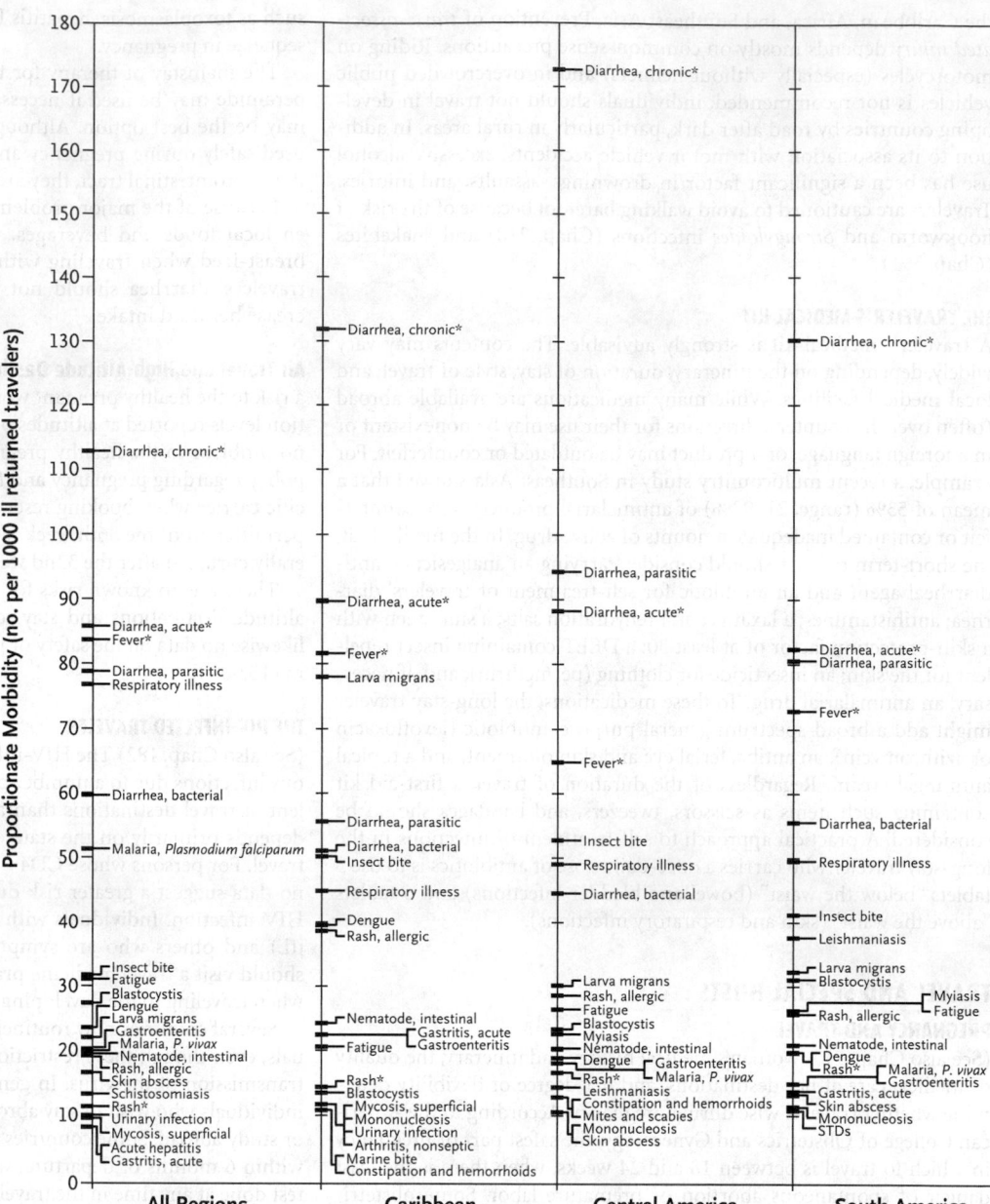

FIGURE 117-2 Proportionate morbidity among ill travelers returning from the developing world, according to region of travel. The proportions (not incidence rates) are shown for each of the top 22 specific diagnoses among all ill returned travelers within each region.

Gastrointestinal Illness Decreased levels of gastric acid, abnormal gastrointestinal mucosal immunity, other complications of HIV infection, and medications taken by HIV-infected patients make travelers' diarrhea especially problematic in these individuals. Travelers' diarrhea is likely to occur more frequently, be more severe, be accompanied by bacteremia, and be more difficult to treat. Although uncommon, *Cryptosporidium, Isospora belli, and Microsporidium* infections are associated with increased morbidity and mortality in AIDS patients.

The HIV-infected traveler must be careful to consume only appropriately prepared foods and beverages and may benefit from antibiotic prophylaxis for travelers' diarrhea. Sulfonamides (as used to prevent pneumocystosis) are ineffective because of widespread resistance.

Other Travel-Related Infections Data are lacking on the severity of many vector-borne diseases in HIV-infected individuals. Malaria is especially severe in asplenic persons and in those with AIDS. The HIV load doubles during malaria, with subsidence in ~8–9 weeks; the significance of this increase in viral load is unknown.

Visceral leishmaniasis (Chap. 205) has been reported in numerous HIV-infected travelers. Diagnosis may be difficult, given that splenomegaly and hyperglobulinemia are often lacking and serologic results are frequently negative. Sandfly bites may be prevented by evening use of insect repellents.

Certain respiratory illnesses, such as histoplasmosis and coccidioidomycosis, cause greater morbidity and mortality among patients with AIDS. Although tuberculosis is common among HIV-infected persons (especially in developing countries), its acquisition by the short-term HIV-infected traveler has not been reported as a major problem.

Medications Adverse events due to medications and drug interactions are common and raise complex issues for HIV-infected persons. Rates of cutaneous reaction (e.g., increased cutaneous sensitivity to sulfonamides) are unusually high among patients with AIDS. Since zidovudine is metabolized by hepatic glucuronidation, inhibitors of this process may elevate serum levels of the drug. Concomitant administration of the antimalarial drug mefloquine and the antiretroviral agent ritonavir may result in decreased plasma levels of ritonavir. In contrast, no significant influence of concomitant mefloquine administration on plasma levels of indinavir or nelfinavir was detected in two HIV-infected travelers. There is a strong theoretical concern that the

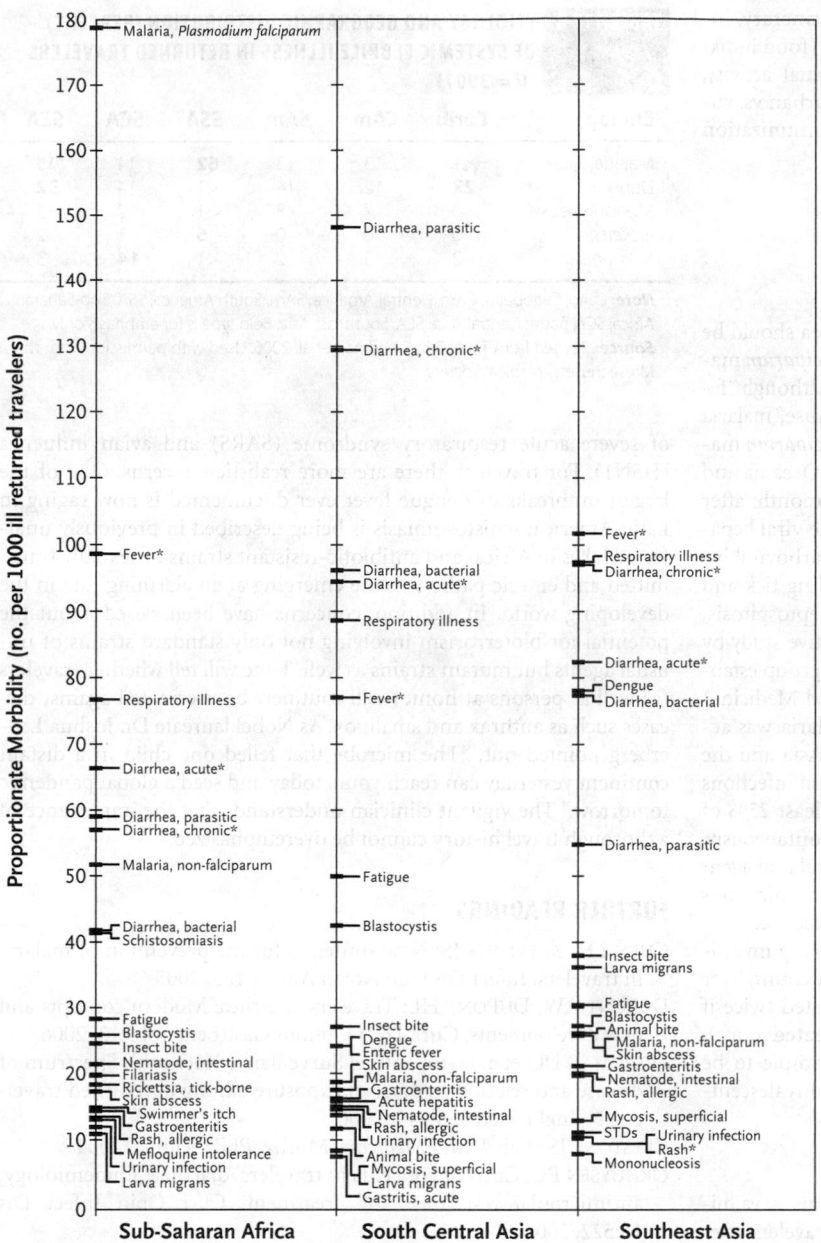

Proportionate Morbidity (no. per 1000 ill returned travelers)

Sub-Saharan Africa

- 180 — Malaria, *Plasmodium falciparum*
- 100 — Fever*
- 78 — Respiratory illness
- 68 — Diarrhea, acute*
- 60 — Diarrhea, parasitic
- 58 — Diarrhea, chronic*
- 52 — Malaria, non-falciparum
- 42 — Diarrhea, bacterial
- 41 — Schistosomiasis
- 31 — Fatigue
- 28 — Blastocystis
- 26 — Insect bite
- 24 — Nematode, intestinal
- 22 — Filariasis
- 21 — Rickettsia, tick-borne
- 19 — Skin abscess
- 16 — Swimmer's itch
- 15 — Gastroenteritis
- 13 — Rash, allergic
- 12 — Mefloquine intolerance
- 11 — Urinary infection
- 10 — Larva migrans

South Central Asia

- 147 — Diarrhea, parasitic
- 131 — Diarrhea, chronic*
- 98 — Diarrhea, bacterial
- 96 — Diarrhea, acute*
- 90 — Respiratory illness
- 78 — Fever*
- 51 — Fatigue
- 43 — Blastocystis
- 26 — Insect bite
- 25 — Dengue
- 24 — Enteric fever
- 22 — Skin abscess
- 21 — Malaria, non-falciparum
- 20 — Gastroenteritis
- 18 — Acute hepatitis
- 16 — Nematode, intestinal
- 14 — Rash, allergic
- 13 — Urinary infection
- 12 — Animal bite
- 11 — Mycosis, superficial
- 10 — Larva migrans
- 9 — Gastritis, acute

Southeast Asia

- 100 — Fever*
- 98 — Respiratory illness
- 96 — Diarrhea, chronic*
- 83 — Diarrhea, acute*
- 80 — Dengue
- 78 — Diarrhea, bacterial
- 56 — Diarrhea, parasitic
- 38 — Insect bite
- 37 — Larva migrans
- 31 — Fatigue
- 30 — Blastocystis
- 29 — Animal bite
- 28 — Malaria, non-falciparum
- 26 — Skin abscess
- 24 — Gastroenteritis
- 22 — Nematode, intestinal
- 21 — Rash, allergic
- 16 — Mycosis, superficial
- 14 — STDs
- 13 — Urinary infection
- 12 — Rash*
- 11 — Mononucleosis

FIGURE 117-2 (Continued) STDs, sexually transmitted diseases. Asterisks indicate syndromic diagnoses for which specific etiologies could not be assigned. (*Reprinted with permission from Freedman et al. © 2006 Massachusetts Medical Society.*)

antimalarial drugs lumefantrine (combined with artemisinin in Coartem and Riamet) and halofantrine may interact with HIV protease inhibitors and nonnucleoside reverse transcriptase inhibitors since the latter are known to be potent inhibitors of cytochrome P450.

CHRONIC ILLNESS, DISABILITY, AND TRAVEL

Chronic health problems need not prevent travel, but special measures can make the journey safer and more comfortable.

Heart Disease   Cardiovascular events are the main cause of deaths among travelers and of in-flight emergencies on commercial aircraft. Extra supplies of all medications should be kept in carry-on luggage, along with a copy of a recent electrocardiogram and the name and telephone number of the traveler's physician at home. Pacemakers are not affected by airport security devices, although electronic telephone checks of pacemaker function cannot be transmitted by international satellites. Travelers with electronic defibrillators should carry a note to that effect and ask for hand screening. A traveler may benefit from supplemental oxygen; since oxygen delivery systems are not standard, sup-

plementary oxygen should be ordered by the traveler's physician well before flight time. Travelers may benefit from aisle seating and should walk, perform stretching and flexing exercises, consider wearing support hose, and remain hydrated during the flight to prevent venous thrombosis and pulmonary embolism.

Chronic Lung Disease   Chronic obstructive pulmonary disease is one of the most common diagnoses in patients who require emergency-department evaluation for symptoms occurring during airline flights. The best predictor of the development of in-flight problems is the sea-level Pa_{O_2}. A Pa_{O_2} of at least 72 mmHg corresponds to an in-flight arterial Pa_{O_2} of ~55 mmHg when the cabin is pressurized to 2500 m (8000 ft). If the traveler's baseline Pa_{O_2} is <72 mmHg, the provision of supplemental oxygen should be considered. Contraindications to flight include active bronchospasm, lower respiratory infection, lower-limb deep-vein phlebitis, pulmonary hypertension, and recent thoracic surgery (within the preceding 3 weeks) or pneumothorax. Decreased outdoor activity at the destination should be considered if air pollution is excessive.

Diabetes Mellitus   Alterations in glucose control and changes in insulin requirements are common problems among patients with diabetes who travel. Changes in time zone, in the amount and timing of food intake, and in physical activity demand vigilant assessment of metabolic control. The traveler with diabetes should pack medication (including a bottle of regular insulin for emergencies), insulin syringes and needles, equipment and supplies for glucose monitoring, and snacks in carry-on luggage. Insulin is stable for ~3 months at room temperature but should be kept as cool as possible. The name and telephone number of the home physician and a card and bracelet listing the patient's medical problems and the type and dose of insulin used should accompany the traveler. In traveling eastward (e.g., from the United States to Europe), the morning insulin dose on arrival may need to be decreased. The blood glucose can then be checked during the day to determine whether additional insulin is required. For flights westward, with lengthening of the day, an additional dose of regular insulin may be required.

Other Special Groups   Other groups for whom special travel measures are encouraged include patients undergoing dialysis, those with transplants, and those with other disabilities. Up to 13% of travelers have some disability, but few advocacy groups and tour companies dedicate themselves to this growing population. Medication interactions are a source of serious concern for these travelers, and appropriate medical information should be carried, along with the home physician's name and telephone number. Some travelers taking glucocorticoids carry stress doses in case they become ill. Immunization of these immunocompromised travelers may result in less than adequate protection. Thus the traveler and the physician must carefully consider which destinations are appropriate.

PROBLEMS AFTER RETURN

The most common medical problems encountered by travelers after their return home are diarrhea, fever, respiratory illnesses, and skin diseases (**Fig. 117-2**). Frequently ignored problems are fatigue and emotional stress, especially in long-stay travelers. The approach to diagnosis requires some knowledge of geographic medicine, in particular the epidemiology and clinical presentation of infectious disorders. A geographic history should focus on the traveler's exact itinerary, including dates of arrival and departure; exposure history (food indiscretions, drinking-water sources, freshwater contact, sexual activity, animal contact, insect bites); location and style of travel (urban vs. rural, first-class hotel accommodation vs. camping); immunization history; and use of antimalarial chemosuppression.

DIARRHEA

See "Prevention of Gastrointestinal Illness," above.

FEVER

Fever in a traveler who has returned from a malarious area should be considered a medical emergency because death from *P. falciparum* malaria can follow an illness of only several days' duration. Although "fever from the tropics" does not always have a tropical cause, malaria should be the first diagnosis considered. The risk of *P. falciparum* malaria is highest among travelers returning from Africa or Oceania and among those who become symptomatic within the first 2 months after return. Other important causes of fever after travel include viral hepatitis (hepatitis A and E), typhoid fever, bacterial enteritis, arboviral infections (e.g., dengue fever), rickettsial infections (including tick and scrub typhus and Q fever), and—in rare instances—leptospirosis, acute HIV infection, and amebic liver abscess. A cooperative study by GeoSentinel (an emerging infectious disease surveillance group established by the CDC and the International Society of Travel Medicine) showed that, among 3907 febrile returned travelers, malaria was acquired most often from Africa, dengue from Southeast Asia and the Caribbean, typhoid fever from southern Asia, and rickettsial infections (tick typhus) from southern Africa (Table 117-3). In at least 25% of cases, no etiology can be found, and the illness resolves spontaneously. Clinicians should keep in mind that no present-day antimalarial agent guarantees protection from malaria and that some immunizations (notably, that against typhoid fever) are only partially protective.

When no specific diagnosis is forthcoming, the following investigations, where applicable, are suggested: complete blood count, liver function tests, thick/thin blood films for malaria (repeated twice if necessary), urinalysis, urine and blood cultures (repeated once), chest x-ray, and collection of an acute-phase serum sample to be held for subsequent examination along with a paired convalescent-phase serum sample.

SKIN DISEASES

Pyodermas, sunburn, insect bites, skin ulcers, and cutaneous larva migrans are the most common skin conditions affecting travelers after their return home. In those with persistent skin ulcers, a diagnosis of cutaneous leishmaniasis, mycobacterial infection, or fungal infection should be considered. Careful, complete inspection of the skin is important in detecting the rickettsial eschar in a febrile patient or the central breathing hole in a "boil" due to myiasis.

EMERGING INFECTIOUS DISEASES

In recent years, travel and commerce have fostered the worldwide spread of HIV infection, led to the reemergence of cholera as a global health threat, and created considerable fear about the possible spread

TABLE 117-3	ETIOLOGY AND GEOGRAPHIC DISTRIBUTION (PERCENT) OF SYSTEMIC FEBRILE ILLNESS IN RETURNED TRAVELERS (N = 3907)					
Etiology	Carib	CAm	SAm	SSA	SCA	SEA
Malaria	<1	13	13	**62**	14	13
Dengue	**23**	12	14	<1	14	**32**
Mononucleosis	7	7	8	1	2	3
Rickettsia	0	0	0	6	1	2
Salmonella	2	3	2	<1	**14**	3

Note: Carib, Caribbean; CAm, Central America; SAm, South America; SSA, Sub-Saharan Africa; SCA, South Central Asia; SEA, Southeast Asia. Bold type is for emphasis only.
Source: Revised from Table 2 in Freedman et al, 2006. Used with permission from the Massachusetts Medical Society.

of severe acute respiratory syndrome (SARS) and avian influenza (H5N1). For travelers, there are more realistic concerns. One of the largest outbreaks of dengue fever ever documented is now raging in Latin America; schistosomiasis is being described in previously unaffected lakes in Africa; and antibiotic-resistant strains of sexually transmitted and enteric pathogens are emerging at an alarming rate in the developing world. In addition, concerns have been raised about the potential for bioterrorism involving not only standard strains of unusual agents but mutant strains as well. Time will tell whether travelers (as well as persons at home) will routinely be vaccinated against diseases such as anthrax and smallpox. As Nobel laureate Dr. Joshua Lederberg pointed out, "The microbe that felled one child in a distant continent yesterday can reach yours today and seed a global pandemic tomorrow." The vigilant clinician understands that the importance of a thorough travel history cannot be overemphasized.

FURTHER READINGS

CHEN LH, KEYSTONE JS: New strategies for the prevention of malaria in travelers. Infect Dis Clin North Am 19:185, 2005

DUPONT AW, DUPONT HL: Travelers' diarrhea: Modern concepts and new developments. Curr Treat Options Gastroenterol 9:13, 2006

FREEDMAN DO et al (GeoSentinel Surveillance Network): Spectrum of disease and relation to place of exposure among ill returned travelers. N Engl J Med 354:119, 2006

KEYSTONE JS et al: *Travel Medicine*. Mosby, Philadelphia, 2004

OKHUYSEN PC: Current concepts in travelers' diarrhea: Epidemiology, antimicrobial resistance and treatment. Curr Opin Infect Dis 18:522, 2005

RYAN ET et al: Illness after international travel. N Engl J Med 347:505, 2002

SHLIM DR: Update in traveler's diarrhea. Infect Dis Clin North Am 19:137, 2005

SOHAIL MR, FISCHER PR: Health risks to air travelers. Infect Dis Clin North Am 19:67, 2005

WILSON ME, CHEN LH: Dermatologic infectious diseases in international travelers. Curr Infect Dis Rep 6:54, 2004

WEBSITES OF INTEREST: Chronic renal failure: *www.kidney.org*. Diabetes: *www.diabetesmonitor.com/other-14.htm*. Dialysis: *www.dialysisfinder.com*. Disability: *www.access-able.com*. HIV: *www.aegis.com*

118 Infective Endocarditis
Adolf W. Karchmer

The prototypic lesion of infective endocarditis, the *vegetation* (Fig. 118-1), is a mass of platelets, fibrin, microcolonies of microorganisms, and scant inflammatory cells. Infection most commonly involves heart valves (either native or prosthetic) but may also occur on the low-pressure side of the ventricular septum at the site of a defect, on the mural endocardium where it is damaged by aberrant jets of blood or foreign bodies, or on intracardiac devices themselves. The analogous process involving arteriovenous shunts, arterioarterial shunts (patent ductus arteriosus), or a coarctation of the aorta is called *infective endarteritis*.

Endocarditis may be classified according to the temporal evolution of disease, the site of infection, the cause of infection, or a predisposing risk factor such as injection drug use. While each classification criterion provides therapeutic and prognostic insight, none is sufficient alone. *Acute endocarditis* is a hectically febrile illness that rapidly damages cardiac structures, hematogenously seeds extracardiac sites, and, if untreated, progresses to death within weeks. *Subacute endocarditis* follows an indolent course; causes structural cardiac damage only slowly, if at all; rarely metastasizes; and is gradually progressive unless complicated by a major embolic event or ruptured mycotic aneurysm.

In developed countries, the incidence of endocarditis ranges from 2.6 to 7.0 cases per 100,000 population per year and remained relatively stable from 1950 to 2000. While rates of congenital heart diseases remain constant, other predisposing conditions in developed countries have shifted from chronic rheumatic heart disease to illicit IV drug use, degenerative valve disease, intracardiac devices, and health care–associated infection. The incidence of endocarditis is notably increased among the elderly. In reported series, 10–30% of endocarditis cases involve prosthetic valves. The risk of prosthesis infection is greatest during the first 6 months after valve replacement; gradually declines to a low, stable rate thereafter; and is similar for mechanical and bioprosthetic devices.

ETIOLOGY

Although many species of bacteria and fungi cause sporadic episodes of endocarditis, only a few bacterial species cause the majority of cases (Table 118-1). The pathogens vary somewhat with the clinical types of endocarditis, in part because of different portals of entry. The oral cavity, skin, and upper respiratory tract are the respective primary portals for the viridans streptococci, staphylococci, and HACEK organisms (*Haemophilus, Actinobacillus, Cardiobacterium, Eikenella,* and *Kingella*) causing community-acquired native valve endocarditis. *Streptococcus bovis* originates from the gastrointestinal tract, where it is associated with polyps and colonic tumors, and enterococci enter the bloodstream from the genitourinary tract. Health care–associated native valve endocarditis is the consequence of bacteremia arising from intravascular catheter infections, nosocomial wound and urinary tract infections, and chronic invasive procedures such as hemodialysis. Endocarditis complicates 6–25% of episodes of catheter-associated *Staphylococcus aureus* bacteremia; the higher rates are detected by careful transesophageal echocardiography (TEE) screening (see "Echocardiography," below).

Prosthetic valve endocarditis arising within 2 months of valve surgery is generally the result of intraoperative contamination of the prosthesis or a bacteremic postoperative complication. The nosocomial nature of these infections is reflected in their primary microbial causes: coagulase-negative staphylococci (CoNS), *S. aureus*, facultative gram-negative bacilli, diphtheroids, and fungi. The portals of entry and organisms causing cases beginning >12 months after surgery are similar to those in community-acquired native valve endocarditis. Epidemiologic evidence suggests that prosthetic valve endocarditis due to CoNS that presents 2–12 months after surgery often represents delayed-onset nosocomial infection. At least 85% of CoNS strains that cause prosthetic valve endocarditis within 12 months of surgery are methicillin-resistant; the rate of methicillin resistance decreases to 25% among CoNS strains causing prosthetic valve endocarditis that presents >1 year after valve surgery.

Transvenous pacemaker lead– and/or implanted defibrillator–associated endocarditis is usually nosocomial. The majority of episodes occur within weeks of implantation or generator change and are caused by *S. aureus* or CoNS.

Endocarditis occurring among injection drug users, especially when infection involves the tricuspid valve, is commonly caused by *S. aureus* strains, many of which are methicillin-resistant. Left-sided valve infections in addicts have a more varied etiology and involve abnormal valves, often ones damaged by prior episodes of endocarditis. A number of these cases are caused by *Pseudomonas aeruginosa* and *Candida* species, and sporadic cases are due to unusual organisms such as *Bacillus, Lactobacillus,* and *Corynebacterium* species. Polymicrobial endocarditis is more common among injection drug users than among patients who do not inject drugs. The presence of HIV in the former population does not significantly influence the causes of endocarditis.

From 5 to 15% of patients with endocarditis have negative blood cultures; in one-third to one-half of these cases, cultures are negative because of prior antibiotic exposure. The remainder of these patients are infected by fastidious organisms, such as nutritionally variant organisms (now designated *Granulicatella* and *Abiotrophia* species), HACEK organisms, and *Bartonella* species. Some fastidious organisms that cause endocarditis do so in characteristic epidemiologic settings (e.g., *Coxiella burnetii* in Europe, *Brucella* species in the Middle East). *Tropheryma whipplei* causes an indolent, culture-negative, afebrile form of endocarditis.

PATHOGENESIS

Unless it is injured, the endothelium is resistant to infection by most bacteria and to thrombus formation. Endothelial injury (e.g., at the site of impact of high-velocity blood jets or on the low-pressure side of a cardiac structural lesion) causes aberrant flow and allows either direct infection by virulent organisms or the development of an uninfected

FIGURE 118-1 Vegetations (*arrows*) due to viridans streptococcal endocarditis involving the mitral valve.

TABLE 118-1 ORGANISMS CAUSING MAJOR CLINICAL FORMS OF ENDOCARDITIS

	Native Valve Endocarditis		Prosthetic Valve Endocarditis at Indicated Time of Onset (Months) after Valve Surgery			Endocarditis in Injection Drug Users		
Organism	**Community-Acquired** (*n* = 683)	**Health Care–Associated** (*n* = 128)	**< 2** (*n* = 144)	**2–12** (*n* = 31)	**> 12** (*n* = 194)	**Right-Sided** (*n* = 346)	**Left-Sided** (*n* = 204)	**Total** (*n* = 675)[a]
Streptococci[b]	32	8	1	9	31	5	15	12
Pneumococci	1	—	—	—	—	—	—	—
Enterococci	8	16	8	12	11	2	24	9
Staphylococcus aureus	35	44[c]	22	12	18	77	23	57
Coagulase-negative staphylococci	4	15	33	32	11	—	—	—
Fastidious gram-negative coccobacilli (HACEK group)[d]	3	—	—	—	6	—	—	—
Gram-negative bacilli	3	5	13	3	6	5	13	7
Candida spp.	1	6	8	12	1	—	12	4
Polymicrobial/miscellaneous	6	1	3	6	5	8	10	7
Diphtheroids	—	—	6	—	3	—	—	0.1
Culture-negative	5	5	5	6	8	3	3	3

[a] The total number of cases is larger than the sum of right- and left-sided cases because the location of infection was not specified in some cases.

[b] Includes viridans streptococci; *Streptococcus bovis*; other non–group A, groupable streptococci; and *Abiotrophia* spp. (nutritionally variant, pyridoxal-requiring streptococci).

[c] Methicillin resistance is common among these *S. aureus* strains.

[d] Includes *Haemophilus* spp., *Actinobacillus actinomycetemcomitans*, *Cardiobacterium hominis*, *Eikenella* spp., and *Kingella* spp.

Note: Data are compiled from multiple studies.

platelet-fibrin thrombus—a condition called *nonbacterial thrombotic endocarditis* (NBTE). The thrombus subsequently serves as a site of bacterial attachment during transient bacteremia. The cardiac conditions most commonly resulting in NBTE are mitral regurgitation, aortic stenosis, aortic regurgitation, ventricular septal defects, and complex congenital heart disease. These conditions result from rheumatic heart disease (particularly in the developing world, where rheumatic fever remains prevalent), mitral valve prolapse, degenerative heart disease, and congenital malformations. NBTE also arises as a result of a hypercoagulable state; this phenomenon gives rise to the clinical entity of *marantic endocarditis* (uninfected vegetations seen in patients with malignancy and chronic diseases) and to bland vegetations complicating systemic lupus erythematosus and the antiphospholipid antibody syndrome.

Organisms that cause endocarditis generally enter the bloodstream from mucosal surfaces, the skin, or sites of focal infection. Except for more virulent bacteria (e.g., *S. aureus*) that can adhere directly to intact endothelium or exposed subendothelial tissue, microorganisms in the blood adhere to sites at NBTE. If resistant to the bactericidal activity of serum and the microbicidal peptides released locally by platelets, the organisms proliferate and induce a procoagulant state at the site by eliciting tissue factor from adherent monocytes or, in the case of *S. aureus*, from monocytes and from intact endothelium. Fibrin deposition combines with platelet aggregation, stimulated by tissue factor and independently by proliferating microorganisms, to generate an infected vegetation. The organisms that commonly cause endocarditis have surface adhesin molecules, collectively called microbial surface components recognizing adhesin matrix molecules (MSCRAMMs), that mediate adherence to NBTE sites or injured endothelium. Fibronectin-binding proteins present on many gram-positive bacteria, clumping factor (a fibrinogen- and fibrin-binding surface protein) on *S. aureus*, and glucans or FimA (a member of the family of oral mucosal adhesins) on streptococci facilitate adherence. Fibronectin-binding proteins are required for *S. aureus* invasion of intact endothelium; thus these surface proteins may facilitate infection of previously normal valves. In the absence of host defenses, organisms enmeshed in the growing platelet-fibrin vegetation proliferate to form dense microcolonies. Organisms deep in vegetations are metabolically inactive (nongrowing) and relatively resistant to killing by antimicrobial agents. Proliferating surface organisms are shed into the bloodstream continuously.

The pathophysiologic consequences and clinical manifestations of endocarditis—other than constitutional symptoms, which probably result from cytokine production—arise from damage to intracardiac structures; embolization of vegetation fragments, leading to infection or infarction of remote tissues; hematogenous infection of sites during bacteremia; and tissue injury due to the deposition of circulating immune complexes or immune responses to deposited bacterial antigens.

CLINICAL MANIFESTATIONS

The clinical syndrome of infective endocarditis is highly variable and spans a continuum between acute and subacute presentations. Native valve endocarditis (whether acquired in the community or in association with health care), prosthetic valve endocarditis, and endocarditis due to injection drug use share clinical and laboratory manifestations (Table 118-2). The causative microorganism is primarily responsible for the temporal course of endocarditis. β-Hemolytic streptococci, *S. aureus*, and pneumococci typically result in an acute course, although

TABLE 118-2 CLINICAL AND LABORATORY FEATURES OF INFECTIVE ENDOCARDITIS

Feature	Frequency, %
Fever	80–90
Chills and sweats	40–75
Anorexia, weight loss, malaise	25–50
Myalgias, arthralgias	15–30
Back pain	7–15
Heart murmur	80–85
New/worsened regurgitant murmur	10–40
Arterial emboli	20–50
Splenomegaly	15–50
Clubbing	10–20
Neurologic manifestations	20–40
Peripheral manifestations (Osler's nodes, subungual hemorrhages, Janeway lesions, Roth's spots)	2–15
Petechiae	10–40
Laboratory manifestations	
Anemia	70–90
Leukocytosis	20–30
Microscopic hematuria	30–50
Elevated erythrocyte sedimentation rate	>90
Elevated C-reactive protein level	>90
Rheumatoid factor	50
Circulating immune complexes	65–100
Decreased serum complement	5–40

S. aureus occasionally causes subacute disease. Endocarditis caused by *Staphylococcus lugdunensis* (a coagulase-negative species) or by enterococci may present acutely. Subacute endocarditis is typically caused by viridans streptococci, enterococci, CoNS, and the HACEK group. Endocarditis caused by *Bartonella* species and the agent of Q fever, *C. burnetii*, is exceptionally indolent.

The clinical features of endocarditis are nonspecific. However, these symptoms in a febrile patient with valvular abnormalities or a behavior pattern that predisposes to endocarditis (e.g., injection drug use) suggest the diagnosis, as do bacteremia with organisms that frequently cause endocarditis, otherwise-unexplained arterial emboli, and progressive cardiac valvular incompetence. In patients with subacute presentations, fever is typically low-grade and rarely exceeds 39.4°C (103°F); in contrast, temperatures of 39.4°–40°C (103°–104°F) are often noted in acute endocarditis. Fever may be blunted or absent in patients who are elderly or severely debilitated or who have marked cardiac or renal failure.

Cardiac Manifestations
Although heart murmurs are usually indicative of the predisposing cardiac pathology rather than of endocarditis, valvular damage and ruptured chordae may result in new regurgitant murmurs. In acute endocarditis involving a normal valve, murmurs are heard on presentation in only 30–45% of patients but ultimately are detected in 85%. Congestive heart failure develops in 30–40% of patients; it is usually a consequence of valvular dysfunction but occasionally is due to endocarditis-associated myocarditis or an intracardiac fistula. Heart failure due to aortic valve dysfunction progresses more rapidly than does that due to mitral valve dysfunction. Extension of infection beyond valve leaflets into adjacent annular or myocardial tissue results in perivalvular abscesses, which in turn may cause fistulae (from the root of the aorta into cardiac chambers or between cardiac chambers) with new murmurs. Abscesses may burrow from the aortic valve annulus through the epicardium, causing pericarditis. Extension of infection into paravalvular tissue adjacent to either the right or the noncoronary cusp of the aortic valve may interrupt the conduction system in the upper interventricular septum, leading to varying degrees of heart block. Although perivalvular abscesses arising from the mitral valve may potentially interrupt conduction pathways near the atrioventricular node or in the proximal bundle of His, such interruption occurs infrequently. Emboli to a coronary artery may result in myocardial infarction; nevertheless, embolic transmural infarcts are rare.

Noncardiac Manifestations
The classic nonsuppurative peripheral manifestations of subacute endocarditis are related to the duration of infection and, with early diagnosis and treatment, have become infrequent. In contrast, septic embolization mimicking some of these lesions (subungual hemorrhage, Osler's nodes) is common in patients with acute *S. aureus* endocarditis (Fig. 118-2). Musculoskeletal symptoms, including nonspecific inflammatory arthritis and back pain, usually remit promptly with treatment but must be distinguished from focal metastatic infection. Hematogenously seeded focal infection may involve any organ but most often is clinically evident in the skin, spleen, kidneys, skeletal system, and meninges. Arterial emboli are clinically apparent in up to 50% of patients. Vegetations >10 mm in diameter (as measured by echocardiography) and those located on the mitral valve are more likely to embolize than are smaller or nonmitral vegetations. Embolic events—often with infarction—involving the extremities, spleen, kidneys, bowel, or brain are often noted at presentation. With effective antibiotic treatment, the frequency of embolic events decreases from 13 per 1000 patient-days during the initial week to 1.2 per 1000 patient-days after the third week. Emboli occurring late during or after effective therapy do not in themselves constitute evidence of failed antimicrobial treatment. Neurologic symptoms, most often resulting from embolic strokes, occur in up to 40% of patients. Other neurologic complications include aseptic or purulent meningitis, intracranial hemorrhage due to hemorrhagic infarcts or ruptured mycotic aneurysms, seizures, and encephalopathy. (*Mycotic aneurysms* are focal dilations of arteries occurring at points in the ar-

FIGURE 118-2 Septic emboli with hemorrhage and infarction due to acute *Staphylococcus aureus* endocarditis. (*Used with permission of L. Baden.*)

tery wall that have been weakened by infection in the vasa vasorum or where septic emboli have lodged.) Microabscesses in brain and meninges occur commonly in *S. aureus* endocarditis; surgically drainable intracerebral abscesses are infrequent.

Immune complex deposition on the glomerular basement membrane causes diffuse hypocomplementemic glomerulonephritis and renal dysfunction, which typically improve with effective antimicrobial therapy. Embolic renal infarcts cause flank pain and hematuria but rarely cause renal dysfunction.

Manifestations of Specific Predisposing Conditions
In almost 50% of patients who have endocarditis associated with injection drug use, infection is limited to the tricuspid valve. These patients present with fever, faint or no murmur, and (in 75% of cases) prominent pulmonary findings related to septic emboli, including cough, pleuritic chest pain, nodular pulmonary infiltrates, and occasionally pyopneumothorax. Infection involving valves on the left side of the heart presents with the typical clinical features of endocarditis.

Health care–associated endocarditis (defined as that which is nosocomial, arises after recent hospitalization, or is a direct consequence of long-term indwelling devices) has typical manifestations if it is not associated with a retained intracardiac device. Endocarditis associated with flow-directed pulmonary artery catheters is often cryptic, with symptoms masked by comorbid critical illness, and is commonly diagnosed at autopsy. Transvenous pacemaker lead– and/or implanted defibrillator–associated endocarditis may be associated with obvious or cryptic generator pocket infection and results in fever, minimal murmur, and pulmonary symptoms due to septic emboli.

Late-onset prosthetic valve endocarditis presents with typical clinical features. Cases arising within 60 days of valve surgery (early onset) lack peripheral vascular manifestations, and typical symptoms may be obscured by comorbidity associated with recent surgery. In both early-onset and more delayed presentations, paravalvular infection is common and often results in partial valve dehiscence, regurgitant murmurs, congestive heart failure, or disruption of the conduction system.

DIAGNOSIS
The Duke Criteria
The diagnosis of infective endocarditis is established with certainty only when vegetations obtained at cardiac surgery, at autopsy, or from an artery (an embolus) are examined histologically and microbiologically. Nevertheless, a highly sensitive and specific diagnostic schema—known as the *Duke criteria*—has been developed on the basis of clinical, laboratory, and echocardiographic findings (Table 118-3). Documentation of two major criteria, of one major and three minor criteria, or of five minor criteria allows a clinical diagnosis of definite endocarditis. The diagnosis of endocarditis is rejected if an alternative

TABLE 118-3 THE DUKE CRITERIA FOR THE CLINICAL DIAGNOSIS OF INFECTIVE ENDOCARDITIS

Major Criteria

1. Positive blood culture
   - Typical microorganism for infective endocarditis from two separate blood cultures
     - Viridans streptococci, *Streptococcus bovis*, HACEK group, *Staphylococcus aureus*, or
     - Community-acquired enterococci in the absence of a primary focus, *or*
   - Persistently positive blood culture, defined as recovery of a microorganism consistent with infective endocarditis from:
     - Blood cultures drawn >12 h apart; *or*
     - All of three or a majority of four or more separate blood cultures, with first and last drawn at least 1 h apart
   - Single positive blood culture for *Coxiella burnetii* or phase I IgG antibody titer of >1:800
2. Evidence of endocardial involvement
   - Positive echocardiogram*a*
     - Oscillating intracardiac mass on valve or supporting structures or in the path of regurgitant jets or in implanted material, in the absence of an alternative anatomic explanation, *or*
     - Abscess, *or*
     - New partial dehiscence of prosthetic valve, *or*
   - New valvular regurgitation (increase or change in preexisting murmur not sufficient)

Minor Criteria

1. Predisposition: predisposing heart condition or injection drug use
2. Fever ≥38.0°C (≥100.4°F)
3. Vascular phenomena: major arterial emboli, septic pulmonary infarcts, mycotic aneurysm, intracranial hemorrhage, conjunctival hemorrhages, Janeway lesions
4. Immunologic phenomena: glomerulonephritis, Osler's nodes, Roth's spots, rheumatoid factor
5. Microbiologic evidence: positive blood culture but not meeting major criterion as noted previously*b* or serologic evidence of active infection with organism consistent with infective endocarditis

---

*a*Transesophageal echocardiography is recommended for assessing possible prosthetic valve endocarditis or complicated endocarditis.
*b*Excluding single positive cultures for coagulase-negative staphylococci and diphtheroids, which are common culture contaminants, and organisms that do not cause endocarditis frequently, such as gram-negative bacilli.
Note: HACEK, *Haemophilus* spp., *Actinobacillus actinomycetemcomitans*, *Cardiobacterium hominis*, *Eikenella corrodens*, *Kingella* species.
Source: Adapted from Li et al., with permission from the University of Chicago Press.

diagnosis is established, if symptoms resolve and do not recur with ≤4 days of antibiotic therapy, or if surgery or autopsy after ≤4 days of antimicrobial therapy yields no histologic evidence of endocarditis. Illnesses not classified as definite endocarditis or rejected are considered cases of possible infective endocarditis when either one major and one minor criterion or three minor criteria are identified. Requiring the identification of clinical features of endocarditis for classification as possible infective endocarditis increases the specificity of the schema without significantly reducing its sensitivity.

The roles of bacteremia and echocardiographic findings in the diagnosis of endocarditis are appropriately emphasized in the Duke criteria. The requirement for multiple positive blood cultures over time is consistent with the continuous low-density bacteremia characteristic of endocarditis (≤100 organisms/mL). Among patients with untreated endocarditis who ultimately have a positive blood culture, 95% of all blood cultures are positive; in 98% of these cases, one of the initial two sets of cultures yields the microorganism. The diagnostic criteria attach significance to the species of organism isolated from blood cultures. To fulfill a major criterion, the isolation of an organism that causes both endocarditis and bacteremia in the absence of endocarditis (e.g., *S. aureus*, enterococci) must take place repeatedly (i.e., persistent bacteremia) and in the absence of a primary focus of infection. Organisms that rarely cause endocarditis but commonly contaminate blood cultures (e.g., diphtheroids, CoNS) must be isolated repeatedly if their isolation is to serve as a major criterion.

Blood Cultures Isolation of the causative microorganism from blood cultures is critical not only for diagnosis but also for determination of antimicrobial susceptibility and planning of treatment. In the absence of prior antibiotic therapy, three blood culture sets (with two bottles per set), separated from each other by at least 1 h, should be obtained from different venipuncture sites over 24 h. If the cultures remain negative after 48–72 h, two or three additional blood culture sets should be obtained, and the laboratory should be consulted for advice regarding optimal culture techniques. Empirical antimicrobial therapy should not be administered initially to hemodynamically stable patients with subacute endocarditis, especially those who have received antibiotics within the preceding 2 weeks; thus, if necessary, additional blood culture sets can be obtained without the confounding effect of empirical treatment. Patients with acute endocarditis or with deteriorating hemodynamics who may require urgent surgery should be treated empirically immediately after three sets of blood cultures are obtained over several hours.

Non-Blood-Culture Tests Serologic tests can be used to implicate causally some organisms that are difficult to recover by blood culture: *Brucella*, *Bartonella*, *Legionella*, and *C. burnetii*. Pathogens can also be identified in surgically recovered vegetations or emboli by culture, by microscopic examination with special stains (i.e., the periodic acid–Schiff stain for *T. whipplei*), and by use of polymerase chain reaction (PCR) to recover unique microbial DNA or 16S rRNA that, when sequenced, allows identification of organisms.

Echocardiography Imaging with echocardiography allows anatomic confirmation of infective endocarditis, sizing of vegetations, detection of intracardiac complications, and assessment of cardiac function (**Fig. 118-3**). Transthoracic echocardiography (TTE) is noninvasive and exceptionally specific; however, it cannot image vegetations <2 mm in diameter, and in 20% of patients it is technically inadequate because of emphysema or body habitus. Thus, TTE detects vegetations in only 65% of patients with definite clinical endocarditis; i.e., it has a sensitivity of 65%. Moreover, TTE is not adequate for evaluating prosthetic valves or detecting intracardiac complications. TEE is safe and significantly more sensitive than TTE. It detects vegetations in >90% of patients with definite endocarditis; nevertheless, false-negative studies are noted in 6–18% of endocarditis patients. TEE is the optimal method for the diagnosis of prosthetic endocarditis or the detection of myocardial abscess, valve perforation, or intracardiac fistulae.

Experts favor echocardiographic evaluation of all patients with a clinical diagnosis of endocarditis; however, the test should not be used to screen patients with a low probability of endocarditis (e.g., patients with unexplained fever). An American Heart Association approach to the use of echocardiography for evaluation of patients with suspected endocarditis is illustrated in **Fig. 118-4**. A negative TEE when endocarditis is likely does not exclude the diagnosis but rather warrants repetition of the study in 7–10 days.

Other Studies Many laboratory studies that are not diagnostic—i.e., complete blood count, creatinine determination, liver function tests, chest radiography, and electrocardiography—are nevertheless important in the management of patients with endocarditis. The erythrocyte sedimentation rate, C-reactive protein level, and circulating immune complex titer are commonly increased in endocarditis (Table 118-2). Cardiac catheterization is useful primarily to assess coronary artery patency in older individuals who are to undergo surgery for endocarditis.

℞ INFECTIVE ENDOCARDITIS

ANTIMICROBIAL THERAPY It is difficult to eradicate bacteria from the avascular vegetation in infective endocarditis because this site is relatively deficient in host defenses and because the largely nongrowing, metabolically inactive bacteria are less easily killed by antibiotics. To cure endocarditis, all bacteria in the vegetation must be killed; therefore, therapy must be bactericidal and prolonged. Antibiotics are generally given

A

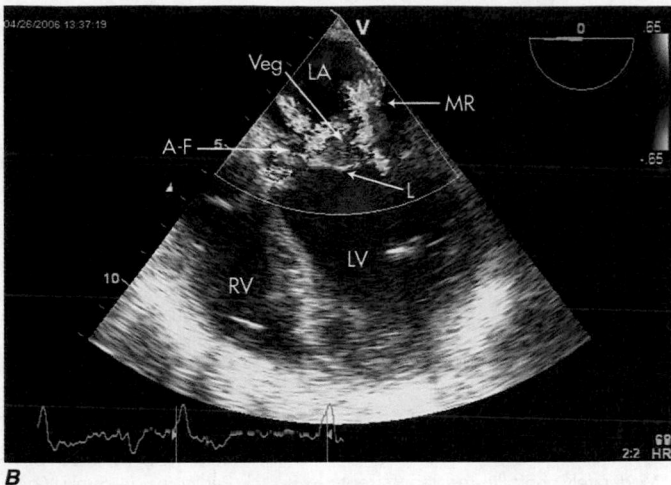
B

FIGURE 118-3 Imaging of a mitral valve infected with *Staphylococcus aureus* by low-esophageal four-chamber-view transesophageal echocardiography (TEE). **A.** Two-dimensional echocardiogram showing a large vegetation with an adjacent echolucent abscess cavity. **B.** Color-flow Doppler image showing severe mitral regurgitation through both the abscess-fistula and the central valve orifice. A, abscess; A-F, abscess-fistula; L, valve leaflets; LA, left atrium; LV, left ventricle; MR, mitral central valve regurgitation; RV, right ventricle; veg, vegetation. *(With permission of Andrew Burger, M.D.)*

parenterally and must reach high serum concentrations that will, through passive diffusion, lead to effective concentrations in the depths of the vegetation. The choice of effective therapy requires precise knowledge of the susceptibility of the causative microorganisms. The decision to initiate treatment before a cause is defined must balance the need to establish a microbiologic diagnosis against the potential progression of disease or the need for urgent surgery (see "Blood Cultures," above). The individual vulnerabilities of the patient should be weighed in the selection of therapy—

e.g., simultaneous infection at other sites (such as meningitis), allergies, end-organ dysfunction, interactions with concomitant medications, and risks of adverse events.

Although given for several weeks longer, the regimens recommended for the treatment of endocarditis involving prosthetic valves (except for staphylococcal infections) are similar to those used to treat native valve infection **(Table 118-4)**. Recommended doses and durations of therapy should be adhered to unless alterations are required by adverse events.

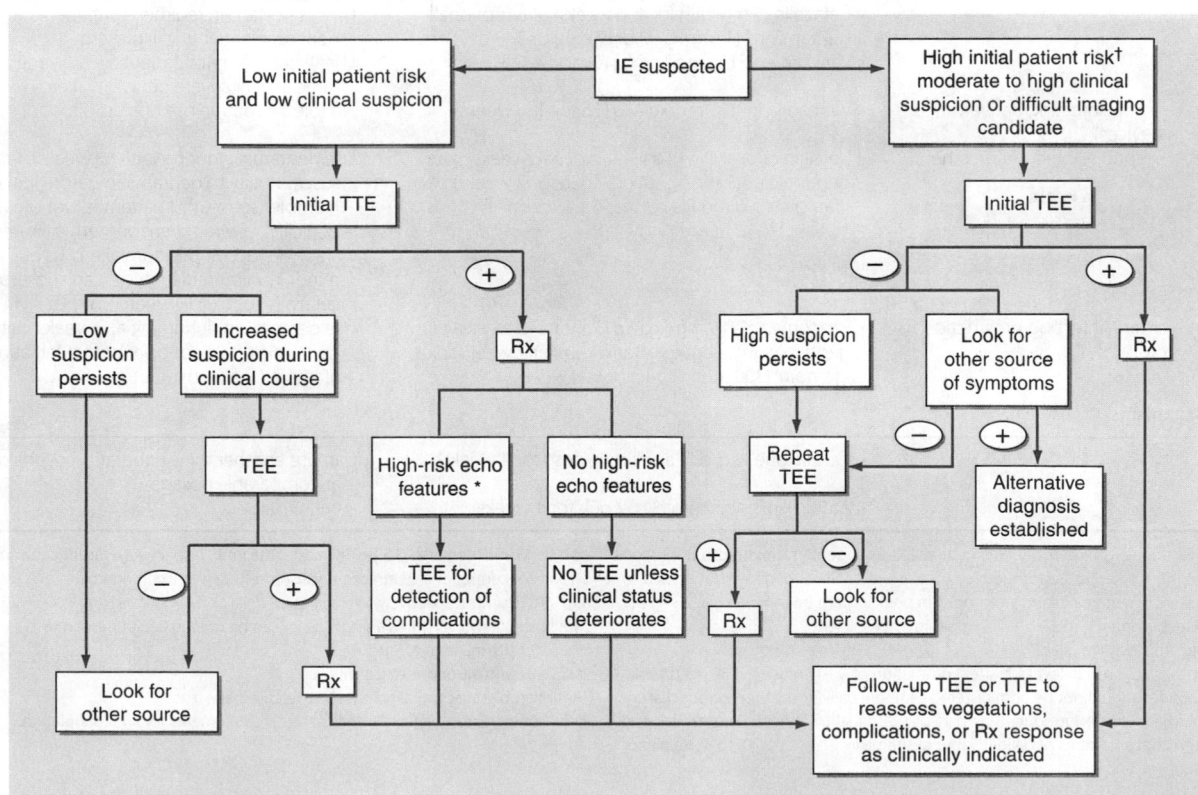

FIGURE 118-4 The diagnostic use of transesophageal and transtracheal echocardiography (TEE and TTE, respectively). †High initial patient risk for endocarditis as listed in Table 118-8 or evidence of intracardiac complications (new regurgitant murmur, new electrocardiographic conduction changes, or congestive heart failure). *High-risk echocardiographic features include large vegetations, valve insufficiency, paravalvular infection, or ventricular dysfunction. Rx indicates initiation of antibiotic therapy. *[Reproduced with permission from Diagnosis and Management of Infective Endocarditis and Its Complications (Circulation 1998; 98:2936-2948. © 1998 American Heart Association.)]*

TABLE 118-4 ANTIBIOTIC TREATMENT FOR INFECTIVE ENDOCARDITIS CAUSED BY COMMON ORGANISMS[a]

Organism	Drug (Dose, Duration)	Comments
Streptococci		
Penicillin-susceptible[b] streptococci, S. bovis	• Penicillin G (2–3 mU IV q4h for 4 weeks) • Ceftriaxone (2 g/d IV as a single dose for 4 weeks) • Vancomycin[c] (15 mg/kg IV q12h for 4 weeks) • Penicillin G (2–3 mU IV q4h) or ceftriaxone (2 g IV qd) for 2 weeks plus gentamicin[d] (3 mg/kg qd IV or IM, as a single dose[e] or divided into equal doses q8h for 2 weeks)	— Can use ceftriaxone in patients with nonimmediate penicillin allergy Use vancomycin in patients with severe or immediate β-lactam allergy Avoid 2-week regimen when risk of aminoglycoside toxicity is increased and in prosthetic valve or complicated endocarditis
Relatively penicillin-resistant[f] streptococci	• Penicillin G (4 mU IV q4h) or ceftriaxone (2 g IV qd) for 4 weeks plus gentamicin[d] (3 mg/kg qd IV or IM, as a single dose[e] or divided into equal doses q8h for 2 weeks) Vancomycin[c] as noted above for 4 weeks	Penicillin alone at this dose for 6 weeks or with gentamicin during initial 2 weeks preferred for prosthetic valve endocarditis caused by streptococci with penicillin MIC ≤0.1 μg/mL
Moderately penicillin-resistant[g] streptococci, nutritionally variant organisms, or Gemella morbillorum	• Penicillin G (4–5 mU IV q4h) or ceftriaxone (2 g IV qd) for 6 weeks plus gentamicin[d] (3 mg/kg qd IV or IM as a single dose[e] or divided into equal doses q8h for 6 weeks) • Vancomycin[c] as noted above for 4 weeks	Preferred for prosthetic valve endocarditis caused by streptococci with penicillin MICs of >0.1 μg/mL —
Enterococci[h]		
	• Penicillin G (4–5 mU IV q4h) plus gentamicin[d] (1 mg/kg IV q8h), both for 4–6 weeks • Ampicillin (2 g IV q4h) plus gentamicin[d] (1 mg/kg IV q8h), both for 4–6 weeks • Vancomycin[c] (15 mg/kg IV q12h) plus gentamicin[d] (1 mg/kg IV q8h), both for 4–6 weeks	Can use streptomycin (7.5 mg/kg q12h) in lieu of gentamicin if there is not high-level resistance to streptomycin — Use vancomycin plus gentamicin for penicillin-allergic patients, or desensitize to penicillin
Staphylococci		
Methicillin-susceptible, infecting native valves (no foreign devices)	• Nafcillin or oxacillin (2 g IV q4h for 4–6 weeks) plus (optional) gentamicin[d] (1 mg/kg IM or IV q8h for 3–5 days) • Cefazolin (2 g IV q8h for 4–6 weeks) plus (optional) gentamicin[d] (1 mg/kg IM or IV q8h for 3–5 days) • Vancomycin[c] (15 mg/kg IV q12h for 4–6 weeks)	Can use penicillin (4 mU q4h) if isolate is penicillin-susceptible (does not produce β-lactamase) Can use cefazolin regimen for patients with nonimmediate penicillin allergy Use vancomycin for patients with immediate (urticarial) or severe penicillin allergy
Methicillin-resistant, infecting native valves (no foreign devices)	• Vancomycin[c] (15 mg/kg IV q12h for 4–6 weeks)	No role for routine use of rifampin
Methicillin-susceptible, infecting prosthetic valves	• Nafcillin or oxacillin (2 g IV q4h for 6–8 weeks) plus gentamicin[d] (1 mg/kg IM or IV q8h for 2 weeks) plus rifampin[i] (300 mg PO q8h for 6–8 weeks)	Use gentamicin during initial 2 weeks; determine susceptibility to gentamicin before initiating rifampin (see text); if patient is highly allergic to penicillin, use regimen for methicillin-resistant staphylococci; if β-lactam allergy is of the minor, nonimmediate type, can substitute cefazolin for oxacillin/nafcillin
Methicillin-resistant, infecting prosthetic valves	• Vancomycin[c] (15 mg/kg IV q12h for 6–8 weeks) plus gentamicin[d] (1 mg/kg IM or IV q8h for 2 weeks) plus rifampin[i] (300 mg PO q8h for 6–8 weeks)	Use gentamicin during initial 2 weeks; determine gentamicin susceptibility before initiating rifampin (see text)
HACEK Organisms		
	• Ceftriaxone (2 g/d IV as a single dose for 4 weeks) • Ampicillin/sulbactam (3 g IV q6h for 4 weeks)	Can use another third-generation cephalosporin at comparable dosage —

[a]Doses are for adults with normal renal function. Doses of gentamicin, streptomycin, and vancomycin must be adjusted for reduced renal function. Ideal body weight is used to calculate doses of gentamicin and streptomycin per kilogram (men = 50 kg + 2.3 kg per inch over 5 feet; women = 45.5 kg + 2.3 kg per inch over 5 feet).
[b]MIC, ≤0.1 μg/mL.
[c]Desirable peak vancomycin level 1 h after completion of a 1-h infusion is 30–45 μg/mL.
[d]Aminoglycosides should not be administered as single daily doses for enterococcal endocarditis and should be introduced as part of the initial treatment. Target peak and trough serum concentrations of divided-dose gentamicin 1 h after a 20- to 30-min infusion or IM injection are ~3.5 μg/mL and ≤1 μg/mL, respectively; target peak and trough serum concentrations of streptomycin (timing as with gentamicin) are 20–35 μg/mL and <10 μg/mL, respectively.
[e]Netilmicin (4 mg/kg qd, as a single dose) can be used in lieu of gentamicin.
[f]MIC, >0.1 μg/mL and <0.5 μg/mL.
[g]MIC, ≥0.5 μg/mL and <8.0 μg/mL.
[h]Antimicrobial susceptibility must be evaluated; see text.
[i]Rifampin increases warfarin and dicumarol requirements for anticoagulation.

Organism-Specific Therapies *Streptococci* To select the optimal therapy for streptococcal endocarditis, the minimum inhibitory concentration (MIC) of penicillin for the causative isolate must be determined (Table 118-4). The 2-week penicillin/gentamicin or ceftriaxone/gentamicin regimens should not be used to treat complicated native valve infection or prosthetic valve endocarditis. The regimen recommended for relatively penicillin-resistant streptococci is advocated for treatment of endocarditis caused by organisms of group B, C, or G. Endocarditis caused by nutritionally variant organisms (*Granulicatella* or *Abiotrophia* species) and *Gemella morbillorum* is treated with the regimen for moderately penicillin-resistant streptococci, as is prosthetic valve endocarditis caused by these organisms or by streptococci with a penicillin MIC of >0.1 μg/mL (Table 118-4).

Enterococci Enterococci are resistant to oxacillin, nafcillin, and the cephalosporins and are only inhibited—not killed—by penicillin, ampicillin, teicoplanin (not available in the United States), and vancomycin. To kill enterococci requires the synergistic interaction of a cell wall–active antibiotic (penicillin, ampicillin, vancomycin, or teicoplanin) that is effective at achievable serum concentrations and an aminoglycoside (gentamicin or streptomycin) to which the isolate does not exhibit high-level resistance. An isolate's resistance to cell wall–active agents or its ability to replicate in the presence of gentamicin at ≥500 μg/mL or streptomycin at 1000–2000 μg/mL—a phenomenon called *high-level aminoglycoside resistance*—indicates that the ineffective antimicrobial agent cannot participate in the interaction to produce killing. High-level resistance to gentamicin predicts that tobramycin, netilmicin, amikacin, and kanamycin also will be ineffective. In fact, even when enterococci are not highly resistant to gentamicin, it is difficult to predict the ability of these other aminoglycosides to participate in synergistic killing; consequently, they should not in general be used to treat enterococcal endocarditis.

Enterococci causing endocarditis must be tested for high-level resistance to streptomycin and gentamicin, β-lactamase production, and susceptibility to penicillin and ampicillin (MIC ≤16 μg/mL) and to vancomycin (MIC ≤8 μg/mL). If the isolate produces β-lactamase, ampicillin/sulbactam or vancomycin can be used as the cell wall–active component; if the penicillin/ampicillin MIC is >16 μg/mL, vancomycin can be considered; and if the vancomycin MIC is >8 μg/mL, penicillin or ampicillin may be considered. In the absence of high-level resistance, gentamicin or streptomycin should be used as the aminoglycoside (Table 118-4). If there is high-level resistance to both these drugs, no aminoglycoside should be given; instead, an 8- to 12-week course of a single cell wall–active agent is suggested—or, for *E. faecalis*, high doses of ampicillin plus either ceftriaxone or cefotaxime. If this alternative therapy fails or the isolate is resistant to all of the commonly used agents, surgical treatment is advised. The role of newer agents potentially active against multidrug-resistant enterococci [quinupristin/dalfopristin (*E. faecium* only), linezolid, and daptomycin] in the treatment of endocarditis has not been established. Although the dose of gentamicin used to achieve bactericidal synergy in treating enterococcal endocarditis is smaller than that used in standard therapy, nephrotoxicity is not uncommon during treatment for 4–6 weeks. Regimens wherein the aminoglycoside component of treatment has been truncated at 2–3 weeks because of toxicity have been curative. Thus, discontinuation of the aminoglycoside is recommended when toxicity develops in patients with enterococcal endocarditis who have responded satisfactorily to therapy.

Staphylococci The regimens used to treat staphylococcal endocarditis (Table 118-4) are based not on coagulase production but rather on the presence or absence of a prosthetic valve or foreign device, the native valve(s) involved, and the resistance of the isolate to penicillin and methicillin. Penicillinase is produced by 95% of staphylococci; thus, all isolates should be considered penicillin-resistant until shown not to produce this enzyme. Similarly, methicillin resistance has become so prevalent among staphylococci, including *S. aureus*, that therapy should be initiated with a regimen for methicillin-resistant organisms and subsequently revised if the strain proves to be susceptible to methicillin. The addition of gentamicin (if the isolate is susceptible) to a β-lactam antibiotic to enhance therapy for native mitral or aortic valve endocarditis is optional. Its addition hastens eradication of bacteremia but does not improve survival rates. If added, gentamicin should be limited to the initial 3–5 days of therapy to minimize nephrotoxicity. Gentamicin generally is not added to the vancomycin regimen in this setting. The efficacy of linezolid or daptomycin as an alternative to vancomycin for left-sided, methicillin-resistant *S. aureus* (MRSA) endocarditis has not been established.

Methicillin-susceptible *S. aureus* endocarditis that is uncomplicated and limited to the tricuspid or pulmonic valve—a condition occurring almost exclusively in injection drug users—can often be treated with a 2-week course that combines oxacillin or nafcillin (but not vancomycin) with gentamicin. Prolonged fevers (≥5 days) during therapy suggest that these patients should receive standard therapy. Right-sided endocarditis caused by MRSA is treated for 4 weeks with standard doses of vancomycin or daptomycin (6 mg/kg as a single daily dose).

Staphylococcal prosthetic valve endocarditis is treated for 6–8 weeks with a multidrug regimen. Rifampin is an essential component because it kills staphylococci that are adherent to foreign material. Two other agents (selected on the basis of susceptibility testing) are combined with rifampin to prevent in vivo emergence of resistance. Because many staphylococci (particularly MRSA and *S. epidermidis*) are resistant to gentamicin, the utility of gentamicin or an alternative agent should be established before rifampin treatment is begun. If the isolate is resistant to gentamicin, another aminoglycoside or a fluoroquinolone (chosen in light of susceptibility results) or another active agent should be substituted for gentamicin.

Other Organisms In the absence of meningitis, endocarditis caused by *Streptococcus pneumoniae* with a penicillin MIC of ≤1.0 can be treated with IV penicillin (4 million units every 4 h), ceftriaxone (2 g/d as a single dose), or cefotaxime (at a comparable dosage). Infection caused by pneumococcal strains with a penicillin MIC of ≥2.0 should be treated with vancomycin. Until the strain's susceptibility to penicillin is established, therapy should consist of vancomycin plus ceftriaxone, especially if concurrent meningitis is suspected. *P. aeruginosa* endocarditis is treated with an antipseudomonal penicillin (ticarcillin or piperacillin) and high doses of tobramycin (8 mg/kg per day in three divided doses). Endocarditis caused by Enterobacteriaceae is treated with a potent β-lactam antibiotic plus an aminoglycoside. Corynebacterial endocarditis is treated with penicillin plus an aminoglycoside (if the organism is susceptible to the aminoglycoside) or with vancomycin, which is highly bactericidal for most strains. Therapy for *Candida* endocarditis consists of amphotericin B plus flucytosine and early surgery; long-term (if not indefinite) suppression with an oral azole is advised. Caspofungin treatment of *Candida* endocarditis has been effective in sporadic cases; nevertheless, the role of echinocandins in this setting has not been established.

Empirical Therapy In designing and executing therapy without culture data (i.e., before culture results are known or when cultures are negative), clinical and epidemiologic clues to etiology must be weighed, and both the pathogens associated with the specific endocarditis syndrome and the hazards of suboptimal therapy must be considered. Thus, empirical therapy for acute endocarditis in an injection drug user should cover MRSA and gram-negative bacilli. The initiation of treatment with vancomycin plus gentamicin immediately after blood is obtained for cultures covers these as well as many other potential causes. In the treatment of culture-negative episodes, marantic endocarditis must be excluded and fastidious organisms sought serologically. In the absence of confounding prior antibiotic therapy, it is unlikely that *S. aureus*, CoNS, or enterococcal infection will present with negative blood cultures. Thus, in this situation, these organisms are not the determinants of therapy for subacute endocarditis. Pending the availability of diagnostic data, blood culture–negative subacute native valve endocarditis is treated with ceftriaxone plus gentamicin; these two antimicrobial agents plus vancomycin should be used if prosthetic valves are involved.

Outpatient Antimicrobial Therapy Fully compliant patients who have sterile blood cultures, are afebrile during therapy, and have no clinical or echocardiographic findings that suggest an impending complication may complete therapy as outpatients. Careful follow-up and a stable home setting are necessary, as are predictable IV access and use of antimicrobial agents that are stable in solution.

Monitoring Antimicrobial Therapy The serum bactericidal titer—the highest dilution of the patient's serum during therapy that kills 99.9% of the standard inoculum of the infecting organism—is no longer recommended for assessment of standard regimens. However, in the treatment of endocarditis caused by unusual organisms, this measurement, although not standardized and difficult to interpret, may provide a patient-specific assessment of in vivo antibiotic effect. Serum concentrations of aminoglycosides and vancomycin should be monitored.

Antibiotic toxicities, including allergic reactions, occur in 25–40% of patients and commonly arise during the third week of therapy. Blood tests to detect renal, hepatic, and hematologic toxicity should be performed periodically.

In most patients, effective antibiotic therapy results in subjective improvement and resolution of fever within 5–7 days. Blood cultures should be repeated daily until sterile, rechecked if there is recrudescent fever, and performed again 4–6 weeks after therapy to document cure. Blood cultures become sterile within 2 days after the start of appropriate therapy when infection is caused by viridans streptococci, enterococci, or HACEK organisms. In *S. aureus* endocarditis, β-lactam therapy results in sterile cultures in 3–5 days, whereas positive cultures may persist for 7–9 days with vancomycin treatment. When fever persists for 7 days despite appropriate antibiotic therapy, patients should be evaluated for paravalvular abscess and for extracardiac abscesses (spleen, kidney) or complications (embolic events). Recrudescent fever raises the question of these complications but also of drug reactions or complications of hospitalization. Serologic abnormalities (e.g., in C-reactive protein level, erythrocyte sedimentation rate, rheumatoid factor) resolve slowly and do not reflect response to treatment. Vegetations become smaller with effective therapy, but at 3 months after cure half are unchanged and 25% are slightly larger.

SURGICAL TREATMENT Intracardiac and central nervous system complications of endocarditis are important causes of morbidity and death associated with this infection. In some cases, effective treatment for these complications requires surgery. Most of the clinical indications for surgical treatment of endocarditis are not absolute **(Table 118-5)**. The risks and benefits as well as the timing of surgical treatment must therefore be individualized **(Table 118-6)**.

Intracardiac Surgical Indications Most surgical interventions are warranted by intracardiac findings, detected most reliably by TEE. Because of the highly invasive nature of prosthetic valve endocarditis, as many as 40% of affected patients merit surgical treatment. In many patients, coincident rather than single intracardiac events necessitate surgery.

Congestive Heart Failure Moderate to severe refractory congestive heart failure caused by new or worsening valve dysfunction is the major indication for cardiac surgical treatment of endocarditis. Of patients with moderate to severe heart failure due to valve dysfunction who are treated medically, 60–90% die within 6 months. In this setting, surgical treatment improves outcome, with mortality rates of 20% in native valve endocarditis and 35–55% in prosthetic valve infection. Surgery can relieve functional stenosis due to large vegetations or restore competence to damaged regurgitant valves.

Perivalvular Infection This complication, which occurs in 10–15% of native valve and 45–60% of prosthetic valve infections, is suggested by persistent unexplained fever during appropriate therapy, new electrocardiographic conduction disturbances, and pericarditis. Extension can occur from any valve but is most common with aortic valve infection. TEE with color Doppler is the test of choice to detect perivalvular abscesses (sensitivity, ≥85%). Although occasional perivalvular infections are cured medically, surgery is warranted when fever persists, fistulae develop, prostheses are dehisced and unstable, and invasive infection relapses after appropriate treatment. Cardiac rhythm must be monitored since high-grade heart block may require insertion of a pacemaker.

Uncontrolled Infection Continued positive blood cultures or otherwise-unexplained persistent fevers (in patients with either blood culture–positive or –negative endocarditis) despite optimal antibiotic therapy

TABLE 118-5 INDICATIONS FOR CARDIAC SURGICAL INTERVENTION IN PATIENTS WITH ENDOCARDITIS

Surgery required for optimal outcome
Moderate to severe congestive heart failure due to valve dysfunction
Partially dehisced unstable prosthetic valve
Persistent bacteremia despite optimal antimicrobial therapy
Lack of effective microbicidal therapy (e.g., fungal or *Brucella* endocarditis)
S. aureus prosthetic valve endocarditis with an intracardiac complication
Relapse of prosthetic valve endocarditis after optimal antimicrobial therapy

Surgery to be strongly considered for improved outcome[a]
Perivalvular extension of infection
Poorly responsive *S. aureus* endocarditis involving the aortic or mitral valve
Large (>10-mm diameter) hypermobile vegetations with increased risk of embolism
Persistent unexplained fever (≥10 days) in culture-negative native valve endocarditis
Poorly responsive or relapsed endocarditis due to highly antibiotic-resistant enterococci or gram-negative bacilli

[a]Surgery must be carefully considered; findings are often combined with other indications to prompt surgery.

TABLE 118-6 TIMING OF CARDIAC SURGICAL INTERVENTION IN PATIENTS WITH ENDOCARDITIS

Timing	Indication for Surgical Intervention	
	Strong Supporting Evidence	Conflicting Evidence, but Majority of Opinions Favor Surgery
Emergent (same day)	Acute aortic regurgitation plus preclosure of mitral valve	
	Sinus of Valsalva abscess ruptured into right heart	
	Rupture into pericardial sac	
Urgent (within 1–2 days)	Valve obstruction by vegetation	Major embolus plus persisting large vegetation (>10 mm in diameter)
	Unstable (dehisced) prosthesis	
	Acute aortic or mitral regurgitation with heart failure (New York Heart Association class III or IV)	
	Septal perforation	
	Perivalvular extension of infection with/without new electrocardiographic conduction system changes	
	Lack of effective antibiotic therapy	
Elective (earlier usually preferred)	Progressive paravalvular prosthetic regurgitation	Staphylococcal PVE
	Valve dysfunction plus persisting infection after ≥7–10 days of antimicrobial therapy	Early PVE (≤2 months after valve surgery)
	Fungal (mold) endocarditis	Fungal endocarditis (*Candida* spp.)
		Antibiotic-resistant organisms

Abbreviation: PVE, prosthetic valve endocarditis.
Source: Adapted from L Olaison, G Pettersson: Infect Dis Clin North Am 16:453, 2002.

may reflect uncontrolled infection and may warrant surgery. Surgical treatment is also advised for endocarditis caused by organisms against which clinical experience indicates that effective antimicrobial therapy is lacking. This category includes infections caused by yeasts, fungi, *P. aeruginosa*, other highly resistant gram-negative bacilli, *Brucella* species, and probably *C. burnetii*.

S. aureus Endocarditis Mortality rates for *S. aureus* prosthetic valve endocarditis exceed 70% with medical treatment but are reduced to 25% with surgical treatment. In patients with intracardiac complications associated with *S. aureus* prosthetic valve infection, surgical treatment reduces the mortality rate twentyfold. Surgical treatment should be considered for patients with *S. aureus* native aortic or mitral valve infection who have TTE-demonstrable vegetations and remain septic during the initial week of therapy. Isolated tricuspid valve endocarditis, even with persistent fever, rarely requires surgery.

Prevention of Systemic Emboli Death and persisting morbidity due to emboli are largely limited to patients suffering occlusion of cerebral or coronary arteries. Echocardiographic determination of vegetation size and anatomy, although predictive of patients at high risk of systemic emboli, does not identify those patients in whom the benefits of surgery to prevent emboli clearly exceed the risks of the surgical procedure and an implanted prosthetic valve. Net benefits favoring surgery are most likely when the risk of embolism is high and other surgical benefits can be achieved simultaneously—e.g., repair of a moderately dysfunctional valve or debridement of a paravalvular abscess. Reduced overall risks of surgical intervention (e.g., use of vegetation resection and valve repair to avoid insertion of a prosthesis) make the benefit-to-risk ratio more favorable and this intervention more attractive.

Timing of Cardiac Surgery In general, when indications for surgical treatment of infective endocarditis are identified, surgery should not be delayed simply to permit additional antibiotic therapy, since this course of action increases the risk of death (Table 118-6). Delay is justified only when infection is controlled and congestive heart failure is fully compensated with medical therapy. After 14 days of recommended antibiotic therapy, excised valves are culture-negative in 99% and 50% of patients with strep-tococcal and *S. aureus* endocarditis, respectively. Recrudescent endocarditis involving a new implanted prosthetic valve follows surgery in 2% of patients with culture-positive native valve endocarditis and in 6–15% of patients with active prosthetic valve endocarditis. These risks are more acceptable than the high mortality rates that result when surgery is inappropriately delayed or not performed.

Among patients who have experienced a neurologic complication of endocarditis, further neurologic deterioration can occur as a consequence of cardiac surgery. The risk of significant neurologic exacerbation is related to the interval between the complication and the surgery. Whenever feasible, cardiac surgery should be delayed for 2–3 weeks after a nonhemorrhagic embolic stroke and for 4 weeks after a hemorrhagic embolic stroke. A ruptured mycotic aneurysm should be clipped and cerebral edema allowed to resolve before cardiac surgery.

Antibiotic Therapy after Cardiac Surgery Bacteria visible in Gram-stained preparations of excised valves do not necessarily indicate a failure of antibiotic therapy. Organisms have been detected on Gram's stain—or their DNA has been detected by PCR—in excised valves from 45% of patients who have successfully completed the recommended therapy for endocarditis. In only 7% of these patients are the organisms, most of which are unusual and antibiotic resistant, cultured from the valve. Despite the detection of organisms or their DNA, relapse of endocarditis after surgery is uncommon. Thus, for uncomplicated native valve infection caused by susceptible organisms in conjunction with negative valve cultures, the duration of preoperative plus postoperative treatment should equal the total duration of recommended therapy, with ~2 weeks of treatment administered after surgery. For endocarditis complicated by paravalvular abscess, partially treated prosthetic valve infection, or cases with culture-positive valves, a full course of therapy should be given postoperatively.

Extracardiac Complications Splenic abscess develops in 3–5% of patients with endocarditis. Effective therapy requires either image-guided percutaneous drainage or splenectomy. Mycotic aneurysms occur in 2–15% of endocarditis patients; half of these cases involve the cerebral arteries and present as headaches, focal neurologic symptoms, or hemorrhage. Cerebral aneurysms should be monitored by angiography. Some will resolve with effective antimicrobial therapy, but those that persist, enlarge, or leak should be treated surgically if possible. Extracerebral aneurysms present as local pain, a mass, local ischemia, or bleeding; these aneurysms are treated by resection.

OUTCOME

Older age, severe comorbid conditions, delayed diagnosis, involvement of prosthetic valves or the aortic valve, an invasive (*S. aureus*) or antibiotic-resistant (*P. aeruginosa*, yeast) pathogen, intracardiac complications, and major neurologic complications adversely impact outcome. Death and poor outcome often are related not to failure of antibiotic therapy but rather to the interactions of comorbidities and endocarditis-related end-organ complications. Overall survival rates for patients with native valve endocarditis caused by viridans streptococci, HACEK organisms, or enterococci (susceptible to synergistic therapy) are 85–90%. For *S. aureus* native valve endocarditis in patients who do not inject drugs, survival rates are 55–70%, whereas 85–90% of injection drug users survive this infection. Prosthetic valve endocarditis beginning within 2 months of valve replacement results in mortality rates of 40–50%, whereas rates are only 10–20% in later-onset cases.

PREVENTION

Antibiotic prophylaxis has been recommended by the American Heart Association in conjunction with selected procedures considered to entail a risk for bacteremia and endocarditis. The benefits of prophylaxis, however, are not established and in fact may be modest: only 50% of patients presenting with native valve endocarditis know that they have a predisposing valve lesion, most endocarditis cases do not follow a procedure, and 35% of cases are caused by organisms not targeted by

TABLE 118-7 ANTIBIOTIC REGIMENS FOR PROPHYLAXIS OF ENDOCARDITIS IN ADULTS WITH HIGH-RISK CARDIAC LESIONS^{a,b}

A. Standard oral regimen
   1. Amoxicillin 2.0 g PO 1 h before procedure
B. Inability to take oral medication
   1. Ampicillin 2.0 g IV or IM within 1 h before procedure
C. Penicillin allergy
   1. Clarithromycin or azithromycin 500 mg PO 1 h before procedure
   2. Cephalexin^c 2.0 g PO 1 h before procedure
   3. Clindamycin 600 mg PO 1 h before procedure
D. Penicillin allergy, inability to take oral medication
   1. Cefazolin^c or ceftriaxone^c 1.0 g IV or IM 30 min before procedure
   2. Clindamycin 600 mg IV or IM 1 h before procedure

^{a}Dosing for children: for amoxicillin, ampicillin, cephalexin, or cefadroxil, use 50 mg/kg PO; cefazolin, 25 mg/kg IV; clindamycin, 20 mg/kg PO, 25 mg/kg IV; clarithromycin, 15 mg/kg PO; gentamicin, 1.5 mg/kg IV or IM, and vancomycin, 20 mg/kg IV.
^{b}For high-risk lesions, see Table 118-8. Prophylaxis is not advised for other lesions.
^{c}Do not use cephalosporins in patients with immediate hypersensitivity (urticaria, angioedema, anaphylaxis) to penicillin.
Source: W Wilson et al: Circulation, published online 4/19/07.

prophylaxis. Dental treatments, the procedures most widely accepted as predisposing to endocarditis, are no more frequent during the 3 months preceding endocarditis than in uninfected matched controls. Furthermore, the frequency and magnitude of bacteremia associated with dental procedures and routine daily activities (e.g., tooth brushing and flossing) are similar. Because patients undergo dental procedures infrequently, exposure of endocarditis-vulnerable cardiac structures to bacteremia-causing oral cavity organisms is notably greater from routine daily activities than from dental care. It is estimated that annual exposure of heart valves to bacteremia-causing organisms may be 5.6 million times greater from routine daily activity than from a tooth extraction. The relation of gastrointestinal and genitourinary procedures to subsequent endocarditis is more tenuous than that of dental procedures.

Antibiotic prophylaxis, if 100% effective, likely prevents only a small number of cases of endocarditis; nevertheless, it is possible that rare cases are prevented. Weighing the potential benefits, potential adverse events, and costs associated with antibiotic prophylaxis, the expert committee of the American Heart Association has dramatically restricted the recommendations for antibiotic prophylaxis. Prophylactic antibiotics (Table 118-7) are advised only for those patients at highest risk for severe morbidity or death from endocarditis (Table 118-8). Prophylaxis is recommended only for dental procedures wherein there is manipulation of gingival tissue or the periapical region of the teeth or perforation of the oral mucosa (including surgery on the respiratory tract). Although prophylaxis is not advised for patients undergoing gastrointestinal or genitourinary tract procedures, it is recommended that effective treatment be given to these high-risk patients before or when they undergo procedures on an infected genitourinary tract or on infected skin and related soft tissue. Maintaining good dental hygiene is also advised. (For further details, see *http://www.americanheart.org/presenter.jhtml?identifier=3047083*.)

TABLE 118-8 HIGH-RISK CARDIAC LESIONS FOR WHICH ENDOCARDITIS PROPHYLAXIS IS ADVISED BEFORE DENTAL PROCEDURES

Prosthetic heart valves
Prior endocarditis
Unrepaired cyanotic congenital heart disease, including palliative shunts or conduits
Completely repaired congenital heart defects during the 6 months after repair
Incompletely repaired congenital heart disease with residual defects adjacent to prosthetic material
Valvulopathy developing after cardiac transplantation

Source: W Wilson et al: Circulation, published online 4/19/07.

BADDOUR LM et al: Diagnosis, antimicrobial therapy, and management of complications. A statement for healthcare professionals from the Committee on Rheumatic Fever, Endocarditis, and Kawasaki Disease, Council on Cardiovascular Disease in the Young, and the Councils on Clinical Cardiology, Stroke, and Cardiovascular Surgery and Anesthesia, American Heart Association. Circulation 111:e394, 2005

DURACK DT (ed): Infective endocarditis. Infect Dis Clin North Am 16:255, 2002

FOWLER VG JR et al: Endocarditis and intravascular infections, in *Principles and Practice of Infectious Diseases*, 6th ed, GL Mandell et al (eds). Philadelphia, Elsevier Churchill Livingstone, 2005, pp 975–1021

HORSTKOTTE D et al: Guidelines on prevention, diagnosis and treatment of infective endocarditis. Executive summary, The Task Force on Infective Endocarditis of the European Society of Cardiology. Eur Heart J 25:267, 2004

KARCHMER AW: Infective endocarditis, in *Heart Disease*, 8th ed, E Braunwald et al (eds). Philadelphia, Elsevier Saunders, 2007, in press

———, LONGWORTH DL: Infections of intracardiac devices. Cardiol Clin 21:253, 2003

LI JS et al: Proposed modifications to the Duke criteria for the diagnosis of infective endocarditis. Clin Infect Dis 30:633, 2000

MOREILLON P, QUE YA: Infective endocarditis. Lancet 363:139, 2004

MORRIS AJ et al: Bacteriological outcome after valve surgery for active infective endocarditis: Implications for duration of treatment after surgery (abstract). Clin Infect Dis 41:187, 2005

VIKRAM HR et al: Impact of valve surgery on 6-month mortality in adults with complicated, left-sided native valve endocarditis: A propensity analysis. JAMA 290:3207, 2003

WILSON W et al: Prevention of infective endocarditis. Guidelines from the American Heart Association. A guideline from the American Heart Association Rheumatic Fever, Endocarditis, and Kawasaki Disease Committee, Council on Cardiovascular Disease in the Young, and the Council on Clinical Cardiology, Council on Cardiovascular Surgery and Anesthesia, and the Quality of Care and Outcomes Research Interdisciplinary Working Group. Circulation, April 19, 2007 (epub ahead of print) (*http://www.americanheart.org/presenter.jhtml?identifier=3047083*)

119 Infections of the Skin, Muscle, and Soft Tissues

Dennis L. Stevens

ANATOMIC RELATIONSHIPS: CLUES TO THE DIAGNOSIS OF SOFT TISSUE INFECTIONS

Protection against infection of the epidermis depends on the mechanical barrier afforded by the stratum corneum, since the epidermis itself is devoid of blood vessels (**Fig. 119-1**). Disruption of this layer by burns or bites, abrasions, foreign bodies, primary dermatologic disorders (e.g., herpes simplex, varicella, ecthyma gangrenosum), surgery, or vascular or pressure ulcer allows penetration of bacteria to the deeper structures. Similarly, the hair follicle can serve as a portal either for components of the normal flora (e.g., *Staphylococcus*) or for extrinsic bacteria (e.g., *Pseudomonas* in hot-tub folliculitis). Intracellular infection of the squamous epithelium with vesicle formation may arise from cutaneous inoculation, as in infection with herpes simplex virus (HSV)

FIGURE 119-1 Structural components of the skin and soft tissue, superficial infections, and infections of the deeper structures. The rich capillary network beneath the dermal papillae plays a key role in the localization of infection and in the development of the acute inflammatory reaction.

type 1; from the dermal capillary plexus, as in varicella and infections due to other viruses associated with viremia; or from cutaneous nerve roots, as in herpes zoster. Bacteria infecting the epidermis, such as *Streptococcus pyogenes*, may be translocated laterally to deeper structures via lymphatics, an event that results in the rapid superficial spread of erysipelas. Later, engorgement or obstruction of lymphatics causes flaccid edema of the epidermis, another characteristic of erysipelas.

The rich plexus of capillaries beneath the dermal papillae provides nutrition to the stratum germinativum, and physiologic responses of this plexus produce important clinical signs and symptoms. For example, infective vasculitis of the plexus results in petechiae, Osler's nodes, Janeway lesions, and palpable purpura, which, if present, are important clues to the existence of endocarditis (Chap. 118). In addition, metastatic infection within this plexus can result in cutaneous manifestations of disseminated fungal infection (Chap. 196), gonococcal infection (Chap. 137), *Salmonella* infection (Chap. 146), *Pseudomonas* infection (i.e., ecthyma gangrenosum; Chap. 145), meningococcemia (Chap. 136), and staphylococcal infection (Chap. 129). The plexus also provides bacteria with access to the circulation, thereby facilitating local spread or bacteremia. The postcapillary venules of this plexus are a major site of polymorphonuclear leukocyte sequestration, diapedesis, and chemotaxis to the site of cutaneous infection.

Exaggeration of these physiologic mechanisms by excessive levels of cytokines or bacterial toxins causes leukostasis, venous occlusion, and pitting edema. Edema with purple bullae, ecchymosis, and cutaneous anesthesia suggests loss of vascular integrity and necessitates exploration of the deeper structures for evidence of necrotizing fasciitis or myonecrosis. An early diagnosis requires a high level of suspicion in instances of unexplained fever and of pain and tenderness in the soft tissue, even in the absence of acute cutaneous inflammation.

Table 119-1 indicates the chapters in which the infections described below are discussed in greater detail. Many of these infections are illustrated in the chapters cited or in **Chap. e5** (Atlas of Rashes Associated with Fever).

INFECTIONS ASSOCIATED WITH VESICLES

(Table 119-1) Vesicle formation due to infection is caused by viral proliferation within the epidermis. In varicella and variola, viremia precedes the onset of a diffuse centripetal rash that progresses from macules to vesicles, then to pustules, and finally to scabs over the course of 1–2 weeks. Vesicles of varicella have a "dewdrop" appearance and develop in crops randomly about the trunk, extremities, and face over 3–4 days. Herpes zoster occurs in a single dermatome; the ap-

TABLE 119-1   SKIN AND SOFT TISSUE INFECTIONS

Lesion, Clinical Syndrome	Infectious Agent	Chapter(s)
Vesicles		
Smallpox	Variola virus	214
Chickenpox	Varicella-zoster virus	173
Shingles (herpes zoster)	Varicella-zoster virus	173
Cold sores, herpetic whitlow, herpes gladiatorum	Herpes simplex virus	172
Hand-foot-and-mouth disease	Coxsackievirus A16	184
Orf	Parapoxvirus	176
Molluscum contagiosum	Pox-like virus	176
Rickettsialpox	*Rickettsia akari*	167
Blistering distal dactylitis	*Staphylococcus aureus* or *Streptococcus pyogenes*	129, 130
Bullae		
Staphylococcal scalded-skin syndrome	*S. aureus*	129
Necrotizing fasciitis	*S. pyogenes, Clostridium* spp., mixed aerobes and anaerobes	157
Gas gangrene	*Clostridium* spp.	135
Halophilic vibrio	*Vibrio vulnificus*	149
Crusted lesions		
Bullous impetigo/ecthyma	*S. aureus*	129
Impetigo contagiosa	*S. pyogenes*	130
Ringworm	Superficial dermatophyte fungi	199
Sporotrichosis	*Sporothrix schenckii*	199
Histoplasmosis	*Histoplasma capsulatum*	192
Coccidioidomycosis	*Coccidioides immitis*	193
Blastomycosis	*Blastomyces dermatitidis*	194
Cutaneous leishmaniasis	*Leishmania* spp.	205
Cutaneous tuberculosis	*Mycobacterium tuberculosis*	158
Nocardiosis	*Nocardia asteroides*	155
Folliculitis		
Furunculosis	*S. aureus*	129
Hot-tub folliculitis	*Pseudomonas aeruginosa*	145
Swimmer's itch	*Schistosoma* spp.	212
Acne vulgaris	*Propionibacterium acnes*	53
Papular and nodular lesions		
Fish-tank or swimming-pool granuloma	*Mycobacterium marinum*	160
Creeping eruption (cutaneous larva migrans)	*Ancylostoma braziliense*	209
Dracunculiasis	*Dracunculus medinensis*	211
Cercarial dermatitis	*Schistosoma mansoni*	212
Verruca vulgaris	Human papillomaviruses 1, 2, 4	178
Condylomata acuminata (anogenital warts)	Human papillomaviruses 6, 11, 16, 18	178
Onchocerciasis nodule	*Onchocerca volvulus*	211
Cutaneous myiasis	*Dermatobia hominis*	e35
Verruca peruana	*Bartonella bacilliformis*	153
Cat-scratch disease	*Bartonella henselae*	153
Lepromatous leprosy	*Mycobacterium leprae*	159
Secondary syphilis (papulosquamous, nodular, and condylomata lata lesions)	*Treponema pallidum*	162
Tertiary syphilis (nodular gummatous lesions)	*T. pallidum*	162
Ulcers with or without eschars		
Anthrax	*Bacillus anthracis*	214
Ulceroglandular tularemia	*Francisella tularensis*	151, 214
Bubonic plague	*Yersinia pestis*	152, 214
Buruli ulcer	*Mycobacterium ulcerans*	160
Leprosy	*M. leprae*	159
Cutaneous tuberculosis	*M. tuberculosis*	158
Chancroid	*Haemophilus ducreyi*	139
Primary syphilis	*T. pallidum*	162
Erysipelas	*S. pyogenes*	130
Cellulitis	*Staphylococcus* spp., *Streptococcus* spp., various other bacteria	Various
Necrotizing fasciitis		
Streptococcal gangrene	*S. pyogenes*	130
Fournier's gangrene	Mixed aerobic and anaerobic bacteria	157
Staphylococcal necrotizing fasciitis	Methicillin-resistant *S. aureus*	129
Myositis and myonecrosis		
Pyomyositis	*S. aureus*	129
Streptococcal necrotizing myositis	*S. pyogenes*	130
Gas gangrene	*Clostridium* spp.	135
Nonclostridial (crepitant) myositis	Mixed aerobic and anaerobic bacteria	157
Synergistic nonclostridial anaerobic myonecrosis	Mixed aerobic and anaerobic bacteria	157

pearance of vesicles is preceded by pain for several days. Zoster may occur in persons of any age but is most common among immunosuppressed individuals and elderly patients, whereas most cases of varicella occur in young children. Vesicles due to HSV are found on or around the lips (HSV-1) or genitals (HSV-2) but may appear on the head and neck of young wrestlers (herpes gladiatorum) or on the digits of health care workers (herpetic whitlow). Recurrent herpes labialis (HSV-1) and herpes genitalis commonly follow primary infection. Coxsackievirus A16 characteristically causes vesicles on the hands, feet, and mouth of children. Orf is caused by a DNA virus related to smallpox virus and infects the fingers of individuals who work around goats and sheep. Molluscum contagiosum virus induces flaccid vesicles on the skin of healthy and immunocompromised individuals. Although variola (smallpox) in nature was eradicated as of 1977, recent terrorist events have renewed interest in this devastating infection (Chap. 214). Viremia beginning after an incubation period of 12 days is followed by a diffuse maculopapular rash, with rapid evolution to vesicles, pustules, and then scabs. Secondary cases can occur among close contacts.

Rickettsialpox begins after mite-bite inoculation of *Rickettsia akari* into the skin. A papule with a central vesicle evolves to form a 1- to 2.5-cm painless crusted black eschar with an erythematous halo and proximal adenopathy. While more common in the northeastern United States and the Ukraine in 1940–1950, rickettsialpox has recently been described in Ohio, Arizona, and Utah. Blistering dactylitis is a painful, vesicular, localized *Staphylococcus aureus* or group A streptococcal infection of the pulps of the distal digits of the hands.

INFECTIONS ASSOCIATED WITH BULLAE
(Table 119-1) Staphylococcal scalded-skin syndrome (SSSS) in neonates is caused by a toxin (exfoliatin) from phage group II *S. aureus*. SSSS must be distinguished from toxic epidermal necrolysis (TEN), which occurs primarily in adults, is drug-induced, and is associated with a higher mortality rate. Punch biopsy with frozen section is useful in making this distinction since the cleavage plane is the stratum corneum in SSSS and the stratum germinativum in TEN (Fig. 119-1). Intravenous γ-globulin is a promising treatment for TEN. Necrotizing fasciitis and gas gangrene also induce bulla formation (see "Necrotizing Fasciitis," below). Halophilic vibrio infection can be as aggressive and fulminant as necrotiz-

ing fasciitis; a helpful clue in its diagnosis is a history of exposure to waters of the Gulf of Mexico or the Atlantic seaboard or (in a patient with cirrhosis) the ingestion of raw seafood. The etiologic organism (*Vibrio vulnificus*) is highly susceptible to tetracycline.

INFECTIONS ASSOCIATED WITH CRUSTED LESIONS

(Table 119-1) Impetigo contagiosa is caused by *S. pyogenes*, and bullous impetigo is due to *S. aureus*. Both skin lesions may have an early bullous stage but then appear as thick crusts with a golden-brown color. Epidemics of impetigo caused by methicillin-resistant *S. aureus* (MRSA) have been reported. Streptococcal lesions are most common among children 2–5 years of age, and epidemics may occur in settings of poor hygiene, particularly among children of lower socioeconomic status in tropical climates. It is important to recognize impetigo contagiosa because of its relationship to poststreptococcal glomerulonephritis. Rheumatic fever is not a complication of skin infection caused by *S. pyogenes*. Superficial dermatophyte infection (ringworm) can occur on any skin surface, and skin scrapings with KOH staining are diagnostic. Primary infections with dimorphic fungi such as *Blastomyces dermatitidis* and *Sporothrix schenckii* can initially present as crusted skin lesions resembling ringworm. Disseminated infection with *Coccidioides immitis* can also involve the skin, and biopsy and culture should be performed on crusted lesions in patients from endemic areas. Crusted nodular lesions caused by *Mycobacterium chelonei* have been described in HIV-seropositive patients. Treatment with clarithromycin looks promising.

FOLLICULITIS

(Table 119-1) Hair follicles serve as portals for a number of bacteria, although *S. aureus* is the most common cause of localized folliculitis. Sebaceous glands empty into hair follicles and ducts and, if blocked, form sebaceous cysts, which may resemble staphylococcal abscesses or may become secondarily infected. Infection of sweat glands (hidradenitis suppurativa) can also mimic infection of hair follicles, particularly in the axillae. Chronic folliculitis is uncommon except in acne vulgaris, where constituents of the normal flora (e.g., *Propionibacterium acnes*) may play a role.

Diffuse folliculitis occurs in two settings. Hot-tub folliculitis is caused by *Pseudomonas aeruginosa* in waters that are insufficiently chlorinated and maintained at temperatures of 37–40°C. Infection is usually self-limited, although bacteremia and shock have been reported. Swimmer's itch occurs when a skin surface is exposed to water infested with freshwater avian schistosomes. Warm water temperatures and alkaline pH are suitable for mollusks that serve as intermediate hosts between birds and humans. Free-swimming schistosomal cercariae readily penetrate human hair follicles or pores but quickly die and elicit a brisk allergic reaction, causing intense itching and erythema.

PAPULAR AND NODULAR LESIONS

(Table 119-1) Raised lesions of the skin occur in many different forms. *Mycobacterium marinum* infections of the skin may present as cellulitis or as raised erythematous nodules. Erythematous papules are early manifestations of cat-scratch disease (with lesions developing at the primary site of inoculation of *Bartonella henselae*) and bacillary angiomatosis (also caused by *B. henselae*). Raised serpiginous or linear eruptions are characteristic of cutaneous larva migrans, which is caused by burrowing larvae of dog or cat hookworms (*Ancylostoma braziliense*) and which humans acquire through contact with soil that has been contaminated with dog or cat feces. Similar burrowing raised lesions are present in dracunculiasis caused by migration of the adult female nematode *Dracunculus medinensis*. Nodules caused by *Onchocerca volvulus* measure 1–10 cm in diameter and occur mostly in persons bitten by *Simulium* flies in Africa. The nodules contain the adult worm encased in fibrous tissue. Migration of microfilariae into the eyes may result in blindness. Verruca peruana is caused by *Bartonella bacilliformis*, which is transmitted to humans by the sandfly *Phlebotomus*. This condition can take the form of single gigantic lesions (several centimeters in diameter) or multiple small lesions (several mil-

limeters in diameter). Numerous subcutaneous nodules may also be present in cysticercosis caused by larvae of *Taenia solium*. Multiple erythematous papules develop in schistosomiasis; each represents a cercarial invasion site. Skin nodules as well as thickened subcutaneous tissue are prominent features of lepromatous leprosy. Large nodules or gummas are features of tertiary syphilis, whereas flat papulosquamous lesions are characteristic of secondary syphilis. Human papillomavirus may cause singular warts (verruca vulgaris) or multiple warts in the anogenital area (condylomata acuminata). The latter are major problems in HIV-infected individuals.

ULCERS WITH OR WITHOUT ESCHARS

(Table 119-1) Cutaneous anthrax begins as a pruritic papule, which develops within days into an ulcer with surrounding vesicles and edema and then into an enlarging ulcer with a black eschar. Cutaneous anthrax may cause chronic nonhealing ulcers with an overlying dirty-gray membrane, although lesions may also mimic psoriasis, eczema, or impetigo. Ulceroglandular tularemia may have associated ulcerated skin lesions with painful regional adenopathy. Although buboes are the major cutaneous manifestation of plague, ulcers with eschars, papules, or pustules are also present in 25% of cases.

Mycobacterium ulcerans typically causes chronic skin ulcers on the extremities of individuals living in the tropics. *Mycobacterium leprae* may be associated with cutaneous ulcerations in patients with lepromatous leprosy related to Lucio's phenomenon, in which immune-mediated destruction of tissue bearing high concentrations of *M. leprae* bacilli occurs, usually several months after initiation of effective therapy. *Mycobacterium tuberculosis* may also cause ulcerations, papules, or erythematous macular lesions of the skin in both normal and immunocompromised patients.

Decubitus ulcers are due to tissue hypoxia secondary to pressure-induced vascular insufficiency and may become secondarily infected with components of the skin and gastrointestinal flora, including anaerobes. Ulcerative lesions on the anterior shins may be due to pyoderma gangrenosum, which must be distinguished from similar lesions of infectious etiology by histologic evaluation of biopsy sites. Ulcerated lesions on the genitals may be either painful (chancroid) or painless (primary syphilis).

ERYSIPELAS

(Table 119-1) Erysipelas is due to *S. pyogenes* and is characterized by an abrupt onset of fiery-red swelling of the face or extremities. The distinctive features of erysipelas are well-defined indurated margins, particularly along the nasolabial fold; rapid progression; and intense pain. Flaccid bullae may develop during the second or third day of illness, but extension to deeper soft tissues is rare. Treatment with penicillin is effective; swelling may progress despite appropriate treatment, although fever, pain, and the intense red color diminish. Desquamation of the involved skin occurs 5–10 days into the illness. Infants and elderly adults are most commonly afflicted, and the severity of systemic toxicity varies.

CELLULITIS

(Table 119-1) Cellulitis is an acute inflammatory condition of the skin that is characterized by localized pain, erythema, swelling, and heat. Cellulitis may be caused by indigenous flora colonizing the skin and appendages (e.g., *S. aureus* and *S. pyogenes*) or by a wide variety of exogenous bacteria. Because the exogenous bacteria involved in cellulitis occupy unique niches in nature, a thorough history (including epidemiologic data) provides important clues to etiology. When there is drainage, an open wound, or an obvious portal of entry, Gram's stain and culture provide a definitive diagnosis. In the absence of these findings, the bacterial etiology of cellulitis is difficult to establish, and in some cases staphylococcal and streptococcal cellulitis may have similar features. Even with needle aspiration of the leading edge or a punch biopsy of the cellulitis tissue itself, cultures are positive in only 20% of cases. This observation suggests that relatively low numbers of bacteria may cause cellulitis and that the expanding area of erythema within the skin may be a direct effect of extracellular toxins or of the soluble mediators of inflammation elicited by the host.

Bacteria may gain access to the epidermis through cracks in the skin, abrasions, cuts, burns, insect bites, surgical incisions, and intravenous catheters. Cellulitis caused by *S. aureus* spreads from a central localized infection, such as an abscess, folliculitis, or an infected foreign body (e.g., a splinter, a prosthetic device, or an intravenous catheter). MRSA is rapidly replacing methicillin-sensitive *S. aureus* (MSSA) as a cause of cellulitis in both inpatient and outpatient settings. In contrast, cellulitis due to *S. pyogenes* is a more rapidly spreading, diffuse process frequently associated with lymphangitis and fever. Recurrent streptococcal cellulitis of the lower extremities may be caused by organisms of group A, C, or G in association with chronic venous stasis or with saphenous venectomy for coronary artery bypass surgery. Streptococci also cause recurrent cellulitis among patients with chronic lymphedema resulting from elephantiasis, lymph node dissection, or Milroy's disease. Recurrent staphylococcal cutaneous infections are more common among individuals who have eosinophilia and elevated serum levels of IgE (Job's syndrome) and among nasal carriers of staphylococci. Cellulitis caused by *Streptococcus agalactiae* (group B *Streptococcus*) occurs primarily in elderly patients and those with diabetes mellitus or peripheral vascular disease. *Haemophilus influenzae* typically causes periorbital cellulitis in children in association with sinusitis, otitis media, or epiglottitis. It is unclear whether this form of cellulitis will (like meningitis) become less common as a result of the impressive efficacy of the *H. influenzae* type b vaccine.

Many other bacteria also cause cellulitis. Fortunately, these organisms occur in such characteristic settings that a good history provides useful clues to the diagnosis. Cellulitis associated with cat bites and, to a lesser degree, with dog bites is commonly caused by *Pasteurella multocida*, although in the latter case *Staphylococcus intermedius* and *Capnocytophaga canimorsus* (formerly DF-2) must also be considered. Sites of cellulitis and abscesses associated with dog bites and human bites also contain a variety of anaerobic organisms, including *Fusobacterium*, *Bacteroides*, aerobic and anaerobic streptococci, and *Eikenella corrodens*. *Pasteurella* is notoriously resistant to dicloxacillin and nafcillin but is sensitive to all other β-lactam antimicrobial agents as well as to quinolones, tetracycline, and erythromycin. Ampicillin/clavulanate, ampicillin/sulbactam, and cefoxitin are good choices for the treatment of animal or human bite infections. *Aeromonas hydrophila* causes aggressive cellulitis in tissues surrounding lacerations sustained in freshwater (lakes, rivers, and streams). This organism remains sensitive to aminoglycosides, fluoroquinolones, chloramphenicol, trimethoprim-sulfamethoxazole, and third-generation cephalosporins; it is resistant to ampicillin, however.

P. aeruginosa causes three types of soft tissue infection: ecthyma gangrenosum in neutropenic patients, hot-tub folliculitis, and cellulitis following penetrating injury. Most commonly, *P. aeruginosa* is introduced into the deep tissues when a person steps on a nail. Treatment includes surgical inspection and drainage, particularly if the injury also involves bone or joint capsule. Choices for empirical treatment while antimicrobial susceptibility data are awaited include an aminoglycoside, a third-generation cephalosporin (ceftazidime, cefoperazone, or cefotaxime), a semisynthetic penicillin (ticarcillin, mezlocillin, or piperacillin), or a fluoroquinolone (although drugs of the last class are not indicated for the treatment of children <13 years old).

Gram-negative bacillary cellulitis, including that due to *P. aeruginosa*, is most common among hospitalized, immunocompromised hosts. Cultures and sensitivity tests are critically important in this setting because of multidrug resistance (Chap. 145).

The gram-positive aerobic rod *Erysipelothrix rhusiopathiae* is most often associated with fish and domestic swine and causes cellulitis primarily in bone renderers and fishmongers. *E. rhusiopathiae* remains susceptible to most β-lactam antibiotics (including penicillin), erythromycin, clindamycin, tetracycline, and cephalosporins but is resistant to sulfonamides, chloramphenicol, and vancomycin. Its resistance to vancomycin, which is unusual among gram-positive bacteria, is of potential clinical significance since this agent is sometimes used in em-

pirical therapy for skin infection. Fish food containing the water flea *Daphnia* is sometimes contaminated with *M. marinum*, which can cause cellulitis or granulomas on skin surfaces exposed to the water in aquariums or injured in swimming pools. Rifampin plus ethambutol has been an effective therapeutic combination in some cases, although no comprehensive studies have been undertaken. In addition, some strains of *M. marinum* are susceptible to tetracycline or to trimethoprim-sulfamethoxazole.

NECROTIZING FASCIITIS

(Table 119-1) Necrotizing fasciitis, formerly called streptococcal gangrene, may be associated with group A *Streptococcus* or mixed aerobic-anaerobic bacteria or may occur as part of gas gangrene caused by *Clostridium perfringens*. Strains of MRSA that produce the Panton-Valentine leukocidin have been reported to cause necrotizing fasciitis. Early diagnosis may be difficult when pain or unexplained fever is the only presenting manifestation. Swelling then develops and is followed by brawny edema and tenderness. With progression, dark-red induration of the epidermis appears, along with bullae filled with blue or purple fluid. Later the skin becomes friable and takes on a bluish, maroon, or black color. By this stage, thrombosis of blood vessels in the dermal papillae (Fig. 119-1) is extensive. Extension of infection to the level of the deep fascia causes this tissue to take on a brownish-gray appearance. Rapid spread occurs along fascial planes, through venous channels and lymphatics. Patients in the later stages are toxic and frequently manifest shock and multiorgan failure.

Necrotizing fasciitis caused by mixed aerobic-anaerobic bacteria begins with a breach in the integrity of a mucous membrane barrier, such as the mucosa of the gastrointestinal or genitourinary tract. The portal can be a malignancy, diverticulum, hemorrhoid, anal fissure, or urethral tear. Other predisposing factors include peripheral vascular disease, diabetes mellitus, surgery, and penetrating injury to the abdomen. Leakage into the perineal area results in a syndrome called *Fournier's gangrene*, characterized by massive swelling of the scrotum and penis with extension into the perineum or the abdominal wall and legs.

Necrotizing fasciitis caused by *S. pyogenes* has increased in frequency and severity since 1985. It often begins deep at the site of a nonpenetrating minor trauma, such as a bruise or a muscle strain. Seeding of the site via transient bacteremia is likely, although most patients deny antecedent streptococcal infection. Alternatively, *S. pyogenes* may reach the deep fascia from a site of cutaneous infection or penetrating trauma. Toxicity is severe, and renal impairment may precede the development of shock. In 20–40% of cases, myositis occurs concomitantly, and, as in gas gangrene (see below), serum creatine phosphokinase levels may be markedly elevated. Necrotizing fasciitis due to mixed aerobic-anaerobic bacteria may be associated with gas in deep tissue, but gas usually is not present when the cause is *S. pyogenes* or MRSA. Prompt surgical exploration down to the deep fascia and muscle is essential. Necrotic tissue must be surgically removed, and Gram's staining and culture of excised tissue are useful in establishing whether group A streptococci, mixed aerobic-anaerobic bacteria, MRSA, or *Clostridium* species are present (see "Treatment," below).

MYOSITIS/MYONECROSIS

(Table 119-1) Muscle involvement can occur with viral infection (e.g., influenza, dengue, or coxsackievirus B infection) or parasitic invasion (e.g., trichinellosis, cysticercosis, or toxoplasmosis). Although myalgia can occur in most of these infections, severe muscle pain is the hallmark of pleurodynia (coxsackievirus B), trichinellosis, and bacterial infection. Acute rhabdomyolysis predictably occurs with clostridial and streptococcal myositis but may also be associated with influenza virus, echovirus, coxsackievirus, Epstein-Barr virus, and *Legionella* infections.

Pyomyositis is usually due to *S. aureus*, is common in tropical areas, and generally has no known portal of entry. Infection remains localized, and shock does not develop unless organisms produce toxic shock syndrome toxin 1 or certain enterotoxins and the patient lacks antibodies to the toxin produced by the infecting organisms. In contrast, *S. pyogenes* may induce primary myositis (referred to as *strepto-*

coccal necrotizing myositis) in association with severe systemic toxicity. Myonecrosis occurs concomitantly with necrotizing fasciitis in ~50% of cases. Both are part of the streptococcal toxic shock syndrome.

Gas gangrene usually follows severe penetrating injuries that result in interruption of the blood supply and introduction of soil into wounds. Such cases of traumatic gangrene are usually caused by the clostridial species *C. perfringens*, *C. septicum*, and *C. histolyticum*. Rarely, latent or recurrent gangrene can occur years after penetrating trauma; dormant spores that reside at the site of previous injury are most likely responsible. Spontaneous nontraumatic gangrene among patients with neutropenia, gastrointestinal malignancy, diverticulosis, or recent radiation therapy to the abdomen is caused by several clostridial species, of which *C. septicum* is the most commonly involved. The tolerance of this anaerobe to oxygen probably explains why it can initiate infection spontaneously in normal tissue anywhere in the body.

Synergistic nonclostridial anaerobic myonecrosis, also known as necrotizing cutaneous myositis and synergistic necrotizing cellulitis, is a variant of necrotizing fasciitis caused by mixed aerobic and anaerobic bacteria with the exclusion of clostridial organisms (see "Necrotizing Fasciitis," above).

DIAGNOSIS

This chapter has emphasized the physical appearance and location of lesions within the soft tissues as important diagnostic clues. The temporal progression of the lesions as well as the patient's travel history, animal exposure or bite history, age, underlying disease status, and lifestyle are

FIGURE 119-2 Computed tomography showing edema and inflammation of the left chest wall in a patient with necrotizing fasciitis and myonecrosis caused by group A *Streptococcus*.

also crucial considerations in the formulation of a narrowed differential diagnosis. However, even the astute clinician may find it challenging to diagnose all infections of the soft tissues by history and inspection alone. Soft tissue radiography, computed tomography (Fig. 119-2), and magnetic resonance imaging may be useful in determining the depth of infection and should be performed in patients with rapidly progressing lesions or evidence of systemic inflammatory response syndrome. These

TABLE 119-2 TREATMENT OF COMMON INFECTIONS OF THE SKIN

Diagnosis/Condition	Primary Treatment	Alternative Treatment	See Also Chap(s).
Animal bite (prophylaxis or early infection)[a]	Amoxicillin/clavulanate, 875/125 mg PO bid	Doxycycline, 100 mg PO bid	**e15**
Animal bite[a] (established infection)	Ampicillin/sulbactam, 1.5–3.0 g IV q6h	Clindamycin, 600–900 mg IV q8h *plus* Ciprofloxacin, 400 mg IV q12h *or* Cefoxitin, 2 g IV q6h	**e15**
Bacillary angiomatosis	Erythromycin, 500 mg PO qid	Doxycycline, 100 mg PO bid	153
Herpes simplex (primary genital)	Acyclovir, 400 mg PO tid for 10 days	Famciclovir, 250 mg PO tid for 5–10 days *or* Valacyclovir, 1000 mg PO bid for 10 days	172
Herpes zoster (immunocompetent host >50 years of age)	Acyclovir, 800 mg PO 5 times daily for 7–10 days	Famciclovir, 500 mg PO tid for 7–10 days *or* Valacyclovir, 1000 mg PO tid for 7 days	173
Cellulitis (staphylococcal or streptococcal)[b,c]	Nafcillin or oxacillin, 2 g IV q4–6h	Cefazolin, 1–2 g q8h *or* Ampicillin/sulbactam, 1.5–3.0 g IV q6h *or* Erythromycin, 0.5–1.0 g IV q6h *or* Clindamycin, 600–900 mg IV q8h	129, 130
MRSA skin infection[d]	Vancomycin, 1 g IV q12h	Linezolid, 600 mg IV q12h	129
Necrotizing fasciitis (group A streptococcal)[b]	Clindamycin, 600–900 mg IV q6–8h *plus* Penicillin G, 4 million units IV q4h	Clindamycin, 600–900 mg IV q6–8h *plus* Cephalosporin (first- or second-generation)	130
Necrotizing fasciitis (mixed aerobes and anaerobes)	Ampicillin, 2 g IV q4h *plus* Clindamycin, 600–900 mg IV q6–8h *plus* Ciprofloxacin, 400 mg IV q6–8h	Vancomycin, 1 g IV q6h *plus* Metronidazole, 500 mg IV q6h *plus* Ciprofloxacin, 400 mg IV q6–8h	157
Gas gangrene	Clindamycin, 600–900 mg IV q6–8h *plus* Penicillin G, 4 million units IV q4–6h	Clindamycin, 600–900 mg IV q6–8h *plus* Cefoxitin, 2 g IV q6h	135

[a]*Pasteurella multocida*, a species commonly associated with both dog and cat bites, is resistant to cephalexin, dicloxacillin, clindamycin, and erythromycin. *Eikenella corrodens*, a bacterium commonly associated with human bites, is resistant to clindamycin, penicillinase-resistant penicillins, and metronidazole but is sensitive to trimethoprim-sulfamethoxazole and fluoroquinolones.
[b]The frequency of erythromycin resistance in group A *Streptococcus* is currently ~5% in the United States but has reached 70–100% in some other countries. Most, but not all, erythromycin-resistant group A streptococci are susceptible to clindamycin. Approximately 90–95% of *Staphylococcus aureus* strains are sensitive to clindamycin.

[c]Severe hospital-acquired *S. aureus* infections or community-acquired *S. aureus* infections that are not responding to the β-lactam antibiotics recommended in this table may be caused by methicillin-resistant strains, requiring a switch to vancomycin or linezolid.
[d]Some strains of methicillin-resistant *S. aureus* (MRSA) remain sensitive to tetracycline and trimethoprim-sulfamethoxazole. Daptomycin (4 mg/kg IV q24h) or tigecycline (100-mg loading dose followed by 50 mg IV q12h) are alternative treatments for MRSA.

tests are particularly valuable for defining a localized abscess or detecting gas in tissue. Unfortunately, they may reveal only soft tissue swelling and thus are not specific for fulminant infections such as necrotizing fasciitis or myonecrosis caused by group A *Streptococcus* (Fig. 119-2), where gas is not found in lesions.

Aspiration of the leading edge or punch biopsy with frozen section may be helpful if the results are positive, but false-negative results occur in ~80% of cases. There is some evidence that aspiration alone may be superior to injection and aspiration with normal saline. Frozen sections are especially useful in distinguishing SSSS from TEN and are quite valuable in cases of necrotizing fasciitis. Open surgical inspection with debridement as indicated is clearly the best way to determine the extent and severity of infection and to obtain material for Gram's staining and culture. Such an aggressive approach is important and may be lifesaving if undertaken early in the course of fulminant infections where there is evidence of systemic toxicity.

Rx INFECTIONS OF THE SKIN, MUSCLE, AND SOFT TISSUES

A full description of the treatment of all the clinical entities described herein is beyond the scope of this chapter. As a guide to the clinician in selecting appropriate treatment, the antimicrobial agents useful in the most common and the most fulminant cutaneous infections are listed in **Table 119-2**.

Early and aggressive surgical exploration is essential in patients with suspected necrotizing fasciitis, myositis, or gangrene in order to (1) visualize the deep structures, (2) remove necrotic tissue, (3) reduce compartment pressure, and (4) obtain suitable material for Gram's staining and for aerobic and anaerobic cultures. Appropriate empirical antibiotic treatment for mixed aerobic-anaerobic infections could consist of ampicillin/sulbactam, cefoxitin, or the following combination: (1) clindamycin (600–900 mg intravenously every 8 h) or metronidazole (750 mg every 6 h) plus (2) ampicillin or ampicillin/sulbactam (2–3 g intravenously every 6 h) plus (3) gentamicin (1.0–1.5 mg/kg every 8 h). Group A streptococcal and clostridial infection of the fascia and/or muscle carries a mortality rate of 20–50% with penicillin treatment. In experimental models of streptococcal and clostridial necrotizing fasciitis/myositis, clindamycin has exhibited markedly superior efficacy, but no comparative trials have been performed in humans. Hyperbaric oxygen treatment may also be useful in gas gangrene

120 Osteomyelitis
Jeffrey Parsonnet

Osteomyelitis, an infection of bone, is caused most commonly by pyogenic bacteria and mycobacteria. As a useful framework for evaluating a patient and planning treatment, cases are classified on the basis of the causative agent; the route by which organisms gain access to bone; the duration of infection; the anatomic location of infection; and the local and systemic host factors that have a bearing on pathogenesis and outcome.

PATHOGENESIS AND PATHOLOGY

Microorganisms enter bone by hematogenous dissemination, by spread from a contiguous focus of infection, or by a penetrating wound. Trauma, ischemia, and foreign bodies enhance the susceptibility of bone to microbial invasion by exposing sites to which bacteria can bind and by impeding host defenses. Phagocytes attempt to contain the infection and, in the process, release enzymes that lyse bone. Bacteria escape host defenses by adhering tightly to damaged bone, by entering and persisting within osteoblasts, and by coating themselves and underlying surfaces with a protective polysaccharide-rich biofilm. Pus spreads into vascular channels, raising intraosseous pressure and impairing the flow of blood; as the untreated infection becomes chronic, ischemic necrosis of bone results in the separation

due to clostridial species. Antibiotic treatment should be continued until all signs of systemic toxicity have resolved, all devitalized tissue has been removed, and granulation tissue has developed (Chaps. 130, 135, and 157).

In summary, infections of the skin and soft tissues are diverse in presentation and severity and offer a great challenge to the clinician. This chapter provides an approach to diagnosis and understanding of the pathophysiologic mechanisms involved in these infections. More in-depth information is found in chapters on specific infections.

FURTHER READINGS

BISNO AI, STEVENS DL: Streptococcal infections in skin and soft tissues. N Engl J Med 334:240, 1996

BREMAN JG, HENDERSON DA: Diagnosis and management of smallpox. N Engl J Med 346:1300, 2002

CARPENTER CF, CHAMBERS HF: Daptomycin: Another novel agent for treating infections due to drug-resistant gram-positive pathogens. Clin Infect Dis 38:994, 2004

ELLIS-GROSSE EJ et al: The efficacy and safety of tigecycline in the treatment of skin and skin-structure infections: Results of 2 double-blind phase 3 comparison studies with vancomycin-aztreonam. Clin Infect Dis 41(Suppl 5):S341, 2005

FRIDKIN SK et al: Methicillin-resistant *Staphylococcus aureus* disease in three communities. N Engl J Med 352:1436, 2005

MILLER LG et al: Necrotizing fasciitis caused by community-associated methicillin-resistant *Staphylococcus aureus* in Los Angeles. N Engl J Med 352:1445, 2005

NORRBY-TEGLUND A, STEVENS DL: Novel therapies in streptococcal toxic shock syndrome: Attenuation of virulence factor expression and modulation of host response. Curr Opin Infect Dis 11:285, 1998

STEVENS DL: Streptococcal toxic shock syndrome associated with necrotizing fasciitis. Annu Rev Med 51:271, 2000

———: Necrotizing soft tissue infections. Curr Treat Opt Infect Dis 2:359, 2000

TALAN DA et al: Bacteriologic analysis of infected dog and cat bites. Emergency Medicine Animal Bite Infection Study Group. N Engl J Med 340:85, 1999

of large devascularized fragments (*sequestra*). When pus breaks through the cortex, subperiosteal or soft tissue abscesses form, and the elevated periosteum deposits new bone (an *involucrum*) around the sequestrum.

Microorganisms, infiltrates of neutrophils, and congested or thrombosed blood vessels are the principal histologic findings of acute osteomyelitis. The distinguishing feature of chronic osteomyelitis is necrotic bone, which is characterized by the absence of living osteocytes. Mononuclear cells predominate in chronic infections, and granulation and fibrous tissues replace bone that has been resorbed by osteoclasts. In the chronic stage, organisms may be too few to be seen on staining.

HEMATOGENOUS OSTEOMYELITIS

Hematogenous infection accounts for ~20% of cases of osteomyelitis and primarily affects children, in whom the long bones are infected, and older adults and IV drug users, in whom the spine is the most common site of infection.

ACUTE HEMATOGENOUS OSTEOMYELITIS

Infection usually involves a single bone, most commonly the tibia, femur, or humerus in children and vertebral bodies in injection drug users and older adults. Bacteria settle in the well-perfused metaphysis of growing bones, a network of venous sinusoids slows the flow of blood, and fenestrations in capillaries allow organisms to escape into the extravascular space. Because vascular anatomy changes with age, hematogenous infection of long bones is uncommon during adulthood and, when it occurs, usually involves the diaphysis.

On presentation, the child with osteomyelitis usually appears acutely ill, with fever, chills, localized pain and tenderness, and—in many cases—restriction of movement or difficulty bearing weight. Overlying erythema and swelling indicate extension of pus through the cortex. During infancy and after puberty, infection may spread through the epiphysis into the joint space. In children of other ages, extension of infection through the cortex results in involvement of joints if the metaphysis is intracapsular. Thus, septic arthritis of the elbow, shoulder, and hip may complicate osteomyelitis of the proximal radius, humerus, and femur, respectively. In children, the source of bacteremia is usually inapparent. A history is often obtained of recent blunt trauma to the area involved; presumably, this event results in a small intraosseous hematoma or vascular obstruction that predisposes to infection. Adults with hematogenous osteomyelitis may present either in the context of an infection elsewhere (e.g., the respiratory or urinary tract, a heart valve, or an intravascular catheter site) or without an obvious source of bacteremia.

Plain radiographs obtained early in the course of infection may show soft tissue swelling, but the first change in bone—a periosteal reaction—is not evident until at least 10 days after the onset of infection. Lytic changes can be detected only after 2–6 weeks, when 50–75% of bone density has been lost. Rarely, a well-circumscribed lytic lesion, or *Brodie's abscess*, is seen in a child who has been in pain for several months but has had no fever.

VERTEBRAL OSTEOMYELITIS

The vertebrae are the most common sites of hematogenous osteomyelitis in adults. Organisms reach the well-perfused vertebral body via spinal arteries and quickly spread from the end plate into the disk space and then to the adjacent vertebral body. Sources of bacteremia include the urinary tract (especially among men over age 50), dental abscesses, soft tissue infections, and contaminated IV lines, but the source of bacteremia is not evident in more than half of patients. Diabetes mellitus requiring insulin injection, a recent invasive medical procedure, hemodialysis, and injection drug use carry an increased risk of spinal infection. Many patients have a history of degenerative joint disease involving the spine, and some report an episode of trauma preceding the onset of infection. Penetrating injuries and surgical procedures involving the spine may cause nonhematogenous vertebral osteomyelitis or infection localized to a disk.

Most patients with vertebral osteomyelitis report neck or back pain; patients may describe atypical pain in the chest, the abdomen, or an extremity that is due to irritation of nerve roots. Symptoms are localized to the lumbar spine more often than to the thoracic spine (>50% vs. 35% of cases) or the cervical spine in pyogenic infections, but the thoracic spine is involved most commonly in tuberculous spondylitis (Pott's disease). More than 50% of patients experience a subacute illness in which a vague, dull pain gradually intensifies over 2–3 months. Fever is usually low-grade or absent, but some patients recall having had an episode of fever and chills prior to or at the onset of pain. An acute presentation with high fever and toxicity is less common and suggests ongoing bacteremia. Percussion over the involved vertebra elicits tenderness, and physical examination may reveal spasm of the paraspinal muscles and limitation of motion.

Laboratory findings at the time of presentation include a normal or modestly elevated white blood cell count, anemia, and, almost invariably, an increased erythrocyte sedimentation rate (ESR) and C-reactive protein (CRP) level. Blood cultures are positive only 20–50% of the time.

By the time the patient seeks medical attention, plain radiographs often show irregular erosions in the end plates of adjacent vertebral bodies and narrowing of the intervening disk space. This radiographic pattern is virtually diagnostic of bacterial infection because tumors and other diseases of the spine rarely cross the disk space. CT or MRI may demonstrate epidural, paraspinal, retropharyngeal, mediastinal, retroperitoneal, or psoas abscesses that originate in the spine.

A spinal epidural abscess may evolve suddenly or over several weeks; the classic clinical presentation is spinal pain progressing to radicular pain and/or weakness. Irreversible paralysis may result from failure to recognize epidural abscess before the development of neurologic deficits. MRI is the best procedure for detection of epidural abscess and should be performed in all cases of vertebral osteomyelitis accompanied by subjective weakness or objective neurologic abnormalities.

MICROBIOLOGY

More than 95% of cases of hematogenous osteomyelitis are caused by a single organism, with *Staphylococcus aureus* accounting for 50% of cases. Other common pathogens in children are group A streptococci and, during the neonatal period, group B streptococci and *Escherichia coli*. In adults, vertebral osteomyelitis is caused by *E. coli* and other enteric bacilli in ~25% of cases. *S. aureus*, *Pseudomonas aeruginosa*, *Serratia*, and *Candida albicans* infections are associated with injection drug use and may involve the sacroiliac, sternoclavicular, or pubic joints as well as the spine. *Salmonella* spp. and *S. aureus* are the major causes of long-bone osteomyelitis complicating sickle cell anemia and other hemoglobinopathies. Tuberculosis and brucellosis affect the spine more often than other bones. Other common sites of tuberculous osteomyelitis include the small bones of the hands and feet, the metaphyses of long bones, the ribs, and the sternum.

Unusual causes of hematogenous osteomyelitis include disseminated histoplasmosis, coccidioidomycosis, and blastomycosis in endemic areas. Immunocompromised persons may rarely develop osteomyelitis due to atypical mycobacteria, *Bartonella henselae*, or opportunistic fungi. Hematogenous osteomyelitis with *Mycobacterium bovis* has been reported following intravesicular instillation of bacille Calmette-Guérin (BCG) for cancer of the bladder. The etiology of chronic relapsing multifocal osteomyelitis, an inflammatory condition of children that is characterized by recurrent episodes of painful lytic lesions in multiple bones, has not been identified.

OSTEOMYELITIS SECONDARY TO A CONTIGUOUS FOCUS OF INFECTION

CLINICAL FEATURES

This broad category of osteomyelitis accounts for ~80% of all cases and occurs most commonly in adults. It includes infections introduced by penetrating injuries, such as bites, puncture wounds, and open fractures; by surgical procedures; and by direct extension of infection from adjacent soft tissues. Generalized vascular insufficiency and the presence of a foreign body are important predisposing factors and also make infection more difficult to cure.

Frequently, the diagnosis of this type of osteomyelitis is not made until the infection has already become chronic. The pain, fever, and inflammatory signs due to bony infection may be attributed to the original injury, to underlying bone or joint disease (such as degenerative arthritis), or to overlying soft tissue infection. Osteomyelitis may become apparent only weeks or months later, when a sinus tract develops, a surgical wound breaks down, or a fracture fails to heal. It may be impossible to distinguish radiographic abnormalities due to osteomyelitis from those due to the precipitating condition.

A special type of contiguous-focus osteomyelitis occurs in the setting of peripheral vascular disease and nearly always involves the small bones of the feet of adults with diabetes. This type of infection is a major cause of morbidity for patients with diabetes and results in many thousands of amputations per year. Diabetic neuropathy exposes the foot to frequent trauma and pressure sores, and the patient may be unaware of infection as it spreads into bone. Poor tissue perfusion impairs normal inflammatory responses and wound healing and creates a milieu that is conducive to anaerobic infections. It is often during the evaluation of a nonhealing ulcer, a swollen toe, or acute cellulitis that a radiograph provides the first evidence of osteomyelitis. If bone is palpable during examination of the base of an ulcer with a blunt surgical probe, osteomyelitis is likely.

MICROBIOLOGY

S. aureus is a pathogen in more than half of cases of contiguous-focus osteomyelitis. However, in contrast to hematogenous osteomyelitis,

TABLE 120-1 **DIAGNOSTIC IMAGING STUDIES FOR OSTEOMYELITIS**

Type of Study	Comments
Plain radiographs	Insensitive, especially in early osteomyelitis. May show periosteal elevation after 10 days, lytic changes after 2–6 weeks. Useful to look for anatomic abnormalities (e.g., fractures, bony variants, or deformities), foreign bodies, and soft tissue gas.
Three-phase bone scan (^{99m}Tc-MDP)	Characteristic finding in osteomyelitis: increased uptake in all three phases of scan. Highly sensitive (~95%) in acute infection; somewhat less sensitive if blood flow to bone is poor. Specificity moderate if plain films are normal, but poor in presence of neuropathic arthropathy, fractures, tumor, infarction.
Other radionuclide scans	Examples: ^{67}Ga-citrate, ^{111}In-labeled WBCs. ^{111}In-WBCs more specific than gallium but not always available. Often used in conjunction with bone scan because its greater specificity for inflammation than ^{99m}Tc-MDP helps to distinguish infectious from noninfectious processes. Lack of consensus over role; often supplanted by MRI when the latter is available.
Ultrasound	May detect subperiosteal fluid collection or soft tissue abscess adjacent to bone, but largely supplanted by CT and MRI.
CT	Limited role in acute osteomyelitis. In chronic osteomyelitis, excellent for detection of sequestra, cortical destruction, soft tissue abscesses, and sinus tracts. Use limited in the presence of a metallic foreign body.
MRI	As sensitive as ^{99m}Tc-MDP bone scan for acute osteomyelitis (~95%); detects changes in water content of marrow before disruption of cortical bone. High specificity (~87%), with better anatomic detail than nuclear studies. Procedure of choice for vertebral osteomyelitis because of high sensitivity for epidural abscess. Use may be limited by a metallic foreign body.

Abbreviations: MDP, monodiphosphonate; WBCs, white blood cells.

these infections are often polymicrobial and are more likely to involve gram-negative and anaerobic bacteria. Hence a mixture of staphylococci, streptococci, enteric organisms, and anaerobic bacteria may be isolated from a diabetic foot infection or pelvic osteomyelitis underlying a decubitus ulcer. Aerobic and anaerobic bacteria cause osteomyelitis following surgery or soft tissue infection of the oropharynx, paranasal sinuses, gastrointestinal tract, or female genital tract. A human bite may result in mixed infection of the hand, with anaerobes included among the etiologic agents. *S. aureus* is the principal cause of postoperative infections; coagulase-negative staphylococci are common pathogens after implantation of orthopedic appliances; and these organisms as well as gram-negative enteric bacilli, atypical mycobacteria, and *Mycoplasma* may cause sternal osteomyelitis after cardiac surgery. Infection with *P. aeruginosa* is frequently associated with puncture wounds of the foot, especially when a nail passes through a sneaker, and *Pasteurella multocida* infection commonly follows cat bites.

CHRONIC OSTEOMYELITIS

With prompt treatment, <5% of cases of acute hematogenous osteomyelitis progress to chronic osteomyelitis. Chronic infection is more likely to develop in contiguous-focus than in hematogenous osteomyelitis. The presence of a foreign body makes establishment of chronic infection especially likely.

A protracted clinical course, long periods of quiescence, and recurrent exacerbations are characteristic of chronic osteomyelitis. Sinus tracts between bone and skin may drain purulent material and occasionally pieces of necrotic bone. An increase in drainage, pain, or swelling signals an exacerbation, which is usually accompanied by increases in CRP level and ESR. Fever is unusual except when obstruction of a sinus tract leads to

soft tissue infection. Rare late complications include pathologic fractures, squamous cell carcinoma of the sinus tract, and amyloidosis.

DIAGNOSIS

Early diagnosis of acute osteomyelitis is critical because prompt antibiotic therapy may prevent necrosis of bone. The ESR and the CRP level are elevated in most cases of active osteomyelitis, including those in which constitutional symptoms and leukocytosis are lacking. These findings are not specific to osteomyelitis, however, and the ESR is occasionally normal in early infections. Baseline values are often useful in monitoring the efficacy of treatment.

A variety of radiologic tests are available for evaluation of osteomyelitis (Table 120-1). Evaluation usually begins with plain radiographs because of their ready availability, although they typically show no abnormalities during early infection. Three-phase bone scans (^{99}Tc-monodiphosphonate) offer high sensitivity but are often of low specificity, especially in the presence of underlying bone abnormalities. There is a lack of consensus over the optimal use of other radionuclide studies, and there is considerable variation between institutions in their use. Use of MRI (Fig. 120-1) is expanding because of its high sensitivity and specificity as well as its ability to demonstrate associated soft tissue abnormalities, but this modality is not available at all institutions.

The role of diagnostic imaging in chronic osteomyelitis is to detect active infection and delineate the extent of debridement necessary to remove necrotic bone and abnormal soft tissues. CT is more sensitive than plain films for the detection of sequestra, sinus tracts, and soft tissue abscesses. Both CT and ultrasound are useful for guiding percutaneous aspiration of subperiosteal and soft tissue fluid collections. Sequential technetium and gallium or indium scans may help determine whether infection is active and may distinguish infection from noninflammatory bone changes. MRI provides superior information about the anatomic extent of infection but does not always distinguish osteomyelitis from healing fractures and tumors. MRI is particularly useful in distinguishing cellulitis from osteomyelitis in the diabetic foot; however, no imaging modality consistently distinguishes infection from neuropathic osteopathy.

Appropriate samples for microbiologic studies should be obtained in all cases of suspected osteomyelitis before the initiation of antimicrobial therapy. Blood cultures are indicated in acute cases and are

FIGURE 120-1 Osteomyelitis of the thoracic spine demonstrated on a sagittal, fat-suppressed T1-weighted magnetic resonance image after the administration of IV gadolinium. At T8–T9, there is involvement of the adjacent vertebral bodies and intervening disk. Abnormally enhancing inflammatory tissue extends from the disk space anteriorly (*white arrow*) as well as posteriorly into the epidural space, compressing the thecal sac (*black arrow*).

| Organism | Suggested Regimen[a] | |
	Primary	Alternatives[b]
Staphylococcus aureus		
Penicillin-resistant, methicillin-sensitive (MSSA)	Nafcillin or oxacillin, 2 g IV q4h	Cefazolin, 1 g IV q8h; ceftriaxone, 1 g IV q24h; clindamycin, 900 mg IV q8h[c]
Penicillin-sensitive	Penicillin, 3–4 million U IV q4h	Cefazolin, ceftriaxone, clindamycin (as above)
Methicillin-resistant (MRSA)	Vancomycin, 15 mg/kg IV q12h; rifampin, 300 mg PO q12h (see text)	Clindamycin[c] (as above); linezolid, 600 mg IV or PO q12h[d]; daptomycin, 4–6 mg/kg IV q24h[d]
Streptococci (including *S. milleri*, β-hemolytic streptococci)	Penicillin (as above)	Cefazolin, ceftriaxone, clindamycin (as above)
Gram-negative aerobic bacilli		
Escherichia coli, other "sensitive" species	Ampicillin, 2 g IV q4h; cefazolin, 1 g IV q8h	Ceftriaxone, 1 g IV q24h; parenteral or oral fluoroquinolone (e.g., ciprofloxacin, 400 mg IV or 750 mg PO q12h)[e]
Pseudomonas aeruginosa	Extended-spectrum β-lactam agent (e.g., piperacillin, 3–4 g IV q4–6h; or ceftazidime, 2 g IV q12h) *plus* tobramycin, 5–7 mg/kg q24h[f]	May substitute parenteral or oral fluoroquinolone for β-lactam agents (if patient is allergic) or for tobramycin (in relation to nephrotoxicity)
Enterobacter spp., other "resistant" species	Extended-spectrum β-lactam agent IV or fluoroquinolone IV or PO[e] (as above)	
Mixed infections possibly involving anaerobic bacteria	Ampicillin/sulbactam, 1.5–3 g IV q6h; piperacillin/tazobactam, 3.375 g IV q6h	Carbapenem antibiotic or a combination of a fluoroquinolone plus clindamycin (as above) or metronidazole, 500 mg PO tid

[a]Duration of treatment is discussed in the text.

[b]Cephalosporins may be used for the treatment of patients allergic to penicillin whose reaction did not consist of anaphylaxis or urticaria (immediate-type hypersensitivity).

[c]Because of the possibility of inducible resistance, clindamycin must be used with caution for the treatment of strains resistant to erythromycin. Consult clinical microbiology laboratory.

[d]Experience is limited; there are anecdotal reports of efficacy.

[e]Oral fluoroquinolones must not be coadministered with divalent cations (calcium, magnesium, iron, aluminum), which block the drugs' absorption.

[f]Tobramycin levels and renal function must be monitored closely to minimize the risks of nephro- and ototoxicity.

positive in more than one-third of cases of hematogenous osteomyelitis in children and 25% of cases of vertebral osteomyelitis in adults. The presence of sepsis occasionally requires initiation of empirical therapy after blood samples alone have been obtained for culture. If blood cultures are negative, samples from needle aspiration of pus in bone or soft tissues or from a bone biopsy should be obtained for culture; in the case of vertebral osteomyelitis, these samples can usually be obtained percutaneously with the guidance of fluoroscopy or CT.

The results of culture of swabs of a sinus tract or the base of an ulcer correlate poorly with those of samples of the infected bone. For this reason, in cases of chronic osteomyelitis and contiguous-focus osteomyelitis, samples for aerobic and anaerobic culture should be obtained by percutaneous needle aspiration through uninfected tissue, percutaneous biopsy, or intraoperative biopsy at the time of surgical debridement. Coagulase-negative staphylococci and other organisms of low virulence should not automatically be disregarded as contaminants, especially in the presence of prosthetic materials. Special culture media may be necessary for the isolation of mycobacteria, fungi, and fastidious pathogens. In some cases, histopathologic examination of biopsy specimens may be the only way to confirm a diagnosis of osteomyelitis.

℞ TREATMENT

ANTIBIOTIC THERAPY (Table 120-2) Antibiotics should be administered only after appropriate specimens have been obtained for culture. Use of bactericidal agents has been recommended, although controlled data for this recommendation are lacking. Antibiotics should be given at a high dose; thus, for most agents, parenteral administration is required. Empirical therapy is guided by findings on Gram's staining of a specimen from the bone or abscess or is chosen to cover the most likely pathogens; such therapy should usually include high doses of an agent active against *S. aureus* (such as oxacillin, nafcillin, cefazolin, or vancomycin) or—if gram-negative organisms are likely to be involved—a third-generation cephalosporin, an aminoglycoside, or a fluoroquinolone. Empirical therapy should also include an agent active against anaerobes in the setting of a decubitus ulcer or diabetic foot infection.

Specific therapy is ultimately based on in vitro susceptibility testing of the organism(s) isolated from bone or blood. Outpatient parenteral antimicrobial therapy (OPAT) is appropriate for motivated and medically stable patients and represents a significant advance in management. Antibiotics that require infrequent dosing, such as ceftriaxone, ertapenem, daptomycin, and vancomycin, may facilitate home therapy, but these choices often have an overly broad spectrum of activity. Fortunately, many antibiotics can be given automatically by means of a portable infusion pump, which decreases the disruption otherwise caused by frequent administration of a drug. Use of a peripherally inserted central catheter (PICC line) also greatly facilitates outpatient drug administration. OPAT requires close coordination of nursing, pharmacy, and physician care, with clear delineations of responsibility for monitoring of safety and efficacy.

After administration of parenteral therapy for 5–10 days and after resolution of signs of active infection, oral antibiotics have been used with great success in children with hematogenous osteomyelitis. The doses of oral penicillins or cephalosporins required for the treatment of pediatric osteomyelitis are high, and adults may not tolerate such doses as well as children. With the exception of the fluoroquinolones, rifampin, and linezolid, few data support the use of oral antibiotics for adults with osteomyelitis. For treatment of infection due to Enterobacteriaceae, oral administration of a fluoroquinolone has been as successful as IV administration of β-lactam antibiotics. Caution should be exercised in the use of fluoroquinolones as the sole agents for treatment of infection due to *S. aureus* or *P. aeruginosa* because resistance may develop during therapy. Addition of oral rifampin (300 mg bid) to a fluoroquinolone has yielded encouraging results in infections due to *S. aureus*, but potential drug toxicity and drug interactions make this option desirable only for selected patients, such as those for whom parenteral therapy poses unacceptable logistical or financial hardship. Oral administration of metronidazole (500 mg every 8 h) results in high drug levels in serum and can take the place of IV regimens for the treatment of *Bacteroides* infections. The bacteriostatic drug linezolid (600 mg by mouth every 12 h) has been used successfully in uncontrolled studies involving moderate numbers of patients with infection caused by methicillin-resistant *S. aureus* (MRSA) and vancomycin-resistant enterococci, but data are currently insufficient to recommend the routine use of this agent. Data do not support the routine use of the serum minimal bactericidal concentration in guiding therapy.

Osteomyelitis caused by MRSA is a growing problem that poses unique challenges in terms of treatment. Vancomycin has historically been the drug of choice for MRSA osteomyelitis, but only because of a lack of acceptable alternatives. The drug is less effective than β-lactam agents in treating infections cause by methicillin-susceptible *S. aureus* (MSSA), and this low efficacy extends to infections caused by MRSA. Vancomycin should not be used for treatment of osteomyelitis caused by MSSA, and oral rifampin should be coadministered with vancomycin when the latter drug is used for MRSA infection unless there are compelling contraindications. Linezolid has performed reasonably well in uncontrolled studies of staphylococcal osteomyelitis. However, side effects and hematologic toxicity are common with this agent; thus, in the absence of controlled studies, its routine use is discouraged. Daptomycin, a bactericidal drug with favorable pharmacokinetics, has also been used successfully. Unfortunately, because resistance can develop during therapy (with resultant treatment failure), the routine use of this drug is not recommended. Trimethoprim-sulfamethoxazole, clindamycin, and tetracycline derivatives (doxycycline and minocycline) are often used—seemingly to good advantage—as "continuation therapy" for MRSA osteomyelitis after a course of a parenteral agent, but no controlled data are available to support this approach.

ACUTE HEMATOGENOUS OSTEOMYELITIS Early treatment of acute hematogenous osteomyelitis of childhood with 4–6 weeks of an appropriate antibiotic is usually successful; treatment for <3 weeks has resulted in a tenfold greater rate of failure. Surgical intervention in childhood cases is indicated for intraosseous or subperiosteal abscesses, concomitant septic arthritis, and lack of improvement of the acute signs of infection in 24–48 h. Acute hematogenous osteomyelitis of bones other than the spine in adults often requires surgical debridement.

VERTEBRAL OSTEOMYELITIS A 6- to 8-week course of treatment with an appropriate antibiotic is usually sufficient to cure vertebral osteomyelitis. Failure of the ESR to drop by two-thirds or more of its pretreatment level or of the CRP level to normalize is an indication for reevaluation and (possibly) longer treatment. Surgery is seldom necessary, even in cases of many months' duration, except in instances of spinal instability, new or progressive neurologic deficits, or large soft-tissue abscesses that cannot be drained percutaneously. All but small and asymptomatic epidural abscesses should be surgically drained. Patients should maintain bed rest until back pain has declined to the point at which ambulation is possible. Body casts are no longer used except for comfort.

CONTIGUOUS-FOCUS OSTEOMYELITIS Even when diagnosed early, contiguous-focus osteomyelitis usually requires surgery in addition to 4–6 weeks of appropriate antibiotic therapy because of underlying soft tissue infection or damage to bone from an injury or surgery. A 2-week course of antibiotics after thorough debridement and soft tissue coverage has yielded adequate results in the treatment of superficial osteomyelitis involving only the outer cortex of bone.

CHRONIC OSTEOMYELITIS The risks and benefits of aggressive therapy for chronic osteomyelitis should be weighed before any attempt is made to eradicate the infection. Some patients with extensive disease prefer to live with their infections rather than undergo multiple surgical procedures, take prolonged courses of antimicrobial therapy, and face the risk of loss of an extremity. Such persons often benefit from intermittent courses of oral antibiotics to suppress acute exacerbations.

Once the decision has been made to treat chronic osteomyelitis aggressively, the patient's nutritional and metabolic status should be optimized to expedite healing of soft tissues and bone. Antibiotic administration should be started several days before surgery to reduce inflammation if the etiology of the infection is known; if not, antibiotic therapy should be withheld until debridement. A 4- to 6-week course of appropriate antibiotic therapy is given postoperatively on the basis of the susceptibility pattern of organisms isolated from bone. A subsequent prolonged course of oral antibiotic therapy is often prescribed, especially in the setting of a foreign body, but controlled data for this approach are lacking. There are insufficient data to recommend either the routine use of hyperbaric oxygen or the use of antibiotic-impregnated methacrylate beads or other depots to deliver high levels of antibiotics to the bone. The success of therapy for chronic osteomyelitis still rests largely on the complete surgical removal of necrotic bone and abnormal soft tissues. In the past, the inability to repair large defects in bone and soft tissue limited the extent of debridement. Muscle flaps and skin grafts are now used routinely to cover large soft-tissue defects and to fill dead space, and bone grafts and vascularized bone transfer may restore a seriously compromised bone to a functional state.

In infections of recent fractures requiring internal fixators, such devices are often left in place and the infection is controlled by limited debridement and "suppressive" antibiotic therapy. Definitive surgical/antimicrobial therapy is delayed until bony union of the fracture has been achieved. If there is persistent nonunion of the fracture or loosening of the fixator, the appliance must be removed, the bone debrided, and an external fixator or a new internal fixator applied.

Osteomyelitis of the small bones of the feet in persons with vascular disease usually requires surgical treatment. The effectiveness of the surgery is limited by the blood supply to the site and the body's ability to heal the wound. Revascularization of the extremity is indicated if the vascular disease involves large arteries. In cases of decreased perfusion due to small-vessel disease, foot-sparing surgery may fail, and the best option is often suppressive therapy or amputation. The duration of antibiotic therapy depends on the surgical procedure performed. When the infected bone is removed entirely but residual infection of soft tissues remains, antibiotic therapy should be given for 2 weeks; if amputation eliminates infected bone and soft tissue, standard surgical prophylaxis is given; otherwise, postoperative antibiotics must be given for 4–6 weeks.

ACKNOWLEDGMENT

The substantial contributions of Dr. James H. Maguire to this chapter in previous editions are gratefully acknowledged.

FURTHER READINGS

DAROUICHE RO: Spinal epidural abscess. N Engl J Med 355:2012, 2006

KAIM AH et al: Imaging of chronic posttraumatic osteomyelitis. Eur Radiol 12:1193, 2002

KHATRI G et al: Effect of bone biopsy in guiding antimicrobial therapy for osteomyelitis complicating open wounds. Am J Med Sci 321:367, 2001

LEW DP, WALDVOGEL FA: Osteomyelitis. N Engl J Med 336:999, 1997

LIPSKY BA: Osteomyelitis of the foot in diabetic patients. Clin Infect Dis 25:1318, 1997

MCHENRY MC et al: Vertebral osteomyelitis: Long-term outcome for 253 patients from 7 Cleveland-area hospitals. Clin Infect Dis 34:1342, 2002

RISSING JP: Antimicrobial therapy for chronic osteomyelitis in adults: Role of the quinolones. Clin Infect Dis 25:1327, 1997

TICE AD et al: Outcomes of osteomyelitis among patients treated with outpatient parenteral antimicrobial therapy. Am J Med 114:723, 2003

TSUKAYAMA DT: Pathophysiology of posttraumatic osteomyelitis. Clin Orthop 360:22, 1999

ZARROUK V et al: Imaging does not predict the clinical outcome of bacterial osteomyelitis. Rheumatology 46:292, 2007

121 Intraabdominal Infections and Abscesses

Miriam J. Baron, Dennis L. Kasper

Intraperitoneal infections generally arise because a normal anatomic barrier is disrupted. This disruption may occur when the appendix, a diverticulum, or an ulcer ruptures; when the bowel wall is weakened by ischemia, tumor, or inflammation (e.g., in inflammatory bowel disease); or with adjacent inflammatory processes, such as pancreatitis or pelvic inflammatory disease, in which enzymes (in the former case) or organisms (in the latter) may leak into the peritoneal cavity. Whatever the inciting event, once inflammation develops and organisms usually contained within the bowel or another organ enter the normally sterile peritoneal space, a predictable series of events takes place. Intraabdominal infections occur in two stages: peritonitis and—if the patient survives this stage and goes untreated—abscess formation. The types of microorganisms predominating in each stage of infection are responsible for the pathogenesis of disease.

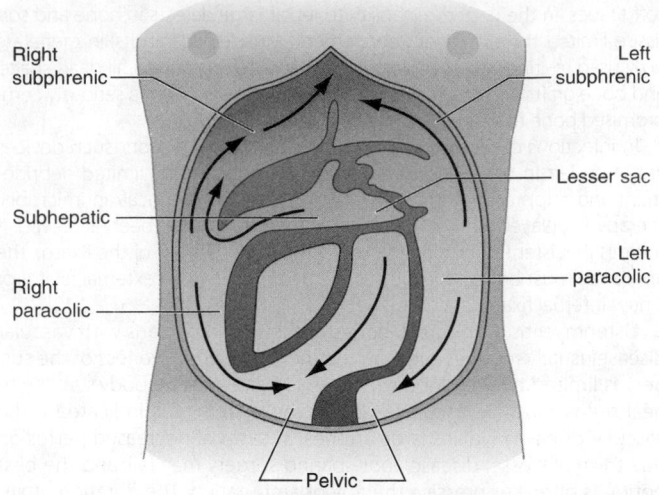

FIGURE 121-1 Diagram of the intraperitoneal spaces, showing the circulation of fluid and potential areas for abscess formation. Some compartments collect fluid or pus more often than others. These compartments include the pelvis (the lowest portion), the subphrenic spaces on the right and left sides, and Morrison's pouch, which is a posterosuperior extension of the subhepatic spaces and is the lowest part of the paravertebral groove when a patient is recumbent. The falciform ligament separating the right and left subphrenic spaces appears to act as a barrier to the spread of infection; consequently, it is unusual to find bilateral subphrenic collections. *[Reprinted with permission from B Lorber (ed): Atlas of Infectious Diseases, vol VII: Intra-abdominal Infections, Hepatitis, and Gastroenteritis. Philadelphia, Current Medicine, 1996, p 1.13.]*

PERITONITIS

Peritonitis is a life-threatening event that is often accompanied by bacteremia and sepsis syndrome (Chap. 265). The peritoneal cavity is large but is divided into compartments. The upper and lower peritoneal cavities are divided by the transverse mesocolon; the greater omentum extends from the transverse mesocolon and from the lower pole of the stomach to line the lower peritoneal cavity. The pancreas, duodenum, and ascending and descending colon are located in the anterior retroperitoneal space; the kidneys, ureters, and adrenals are found in the posterior retroperitoneal space. The other organs, including liver, stomach, gallbladder, spleen, jejunum, ileum, transverse and sigmoid colon, cecum, and appendix, are within the peritoneal cavity. The cavity is lined with a serous membrane that can serve as a conduit for fluids—a property exploited in peritoneal dialysis (Fig. 121-1). A small amount of serous fluid is normally present in the peritoneal space, with a protein content (consisting mainly of albumin) of <30 g/L and <300 white blood cells (WBCs, generally mononuclear cells) per microliter. In bacterial infections, leukocyte recruitment into the infected peritoneal cavity consists of an early influx of polymorphonuclear leukocytes (PMNs) and a prolonged subsequent phase of mononuclear cell migration. The phenotype of the infiltrating leukocytes during the course of inflammation is regulated primarily by resident-cell chemokine synthesis.

PRIMARY (SPONTANEOUS) BACTERIAL PERITONITIS

Peritonitis is either primary (without an apparent source of contamination) or secondary. The types of organisms found and the clinical presentations of these two processes are different. In adults, primary bacterial peritonitis (PBP) occurs most commonly in conjunction with cirrhosis of the liver (frequently the result of alcoholism). However, the disease has been reported in adults with metastatic malignant disease, postnecrotic cirrhosis, chronic active hepatitis, acute viral hepatitis, congestive heart failure, systemic lupus erythematosus, and lymphedema as well as in patients with no underlying disease. Al-

though PBP virtually always develops in patients with preexisting ascites, it is, in general, an uncommon event, occurring in ≤10% of cirrhotic patients. The cause of PBP has not been established definitively but is believed to involve hematogenous spread of organisms in a patient in whom a diseased liver and altered portal circulation result in a defect in the usual filtration function. Organisms multiply in ascites, a good medium for growth. The proteins of the complement cascade have been found in peritoneal fluid, with lower levels in cirrhotic patients than in patients with ascites of other etiologies. The opsonic and phagocytic properties of PMNs are diminished in patients with advanced liver disease.

The presentation of PBP differs from that of secondary peritonitis. The most common manifestation is fever, which is reported in up to 80% of patients. Ascites is found but virtually always predates infection. Abdominal pain, an acute onset of symptoms, and peritoneal irritation during physical examination can be helpful diagnostically, but the absence of any of these findings does not exclude this often-subtle diagnosis. Nonlocalizing symptoms (such as malaise, fatigue, or encephalopathy) without another clear etiology should also prompt consideration of PBP in a susceptible patient. It is vital to sample the peritoneal fluid of any cirrhotic patient with ascites and fever. The finding of >250 PMNs/μL is diagnostic for PBP, according to Conn (*http://jac.oxfordjournals.org/cgi/content/full/47/3/369*). This criterion does not apply to secondary peritonitis (see below). The microbiology of PBP is also distinctive. While enteric gram-negative bacilli such as *Escherichia coli* are most commonly encountered, gram-positive organisms such as streptococci, enterococci, or even pneumococci are sometimes found. In PBP, a single organism is typically isolated; anaerobes are found less frequently in PBP than in secondary peritonitis, in which a mixed flora including anaerobes is the rule. In fact, if PBP is suspected and multiple organisms including anaerobes are recovered from the peritoneal fluid, the diagnosis must be reconsidered and a source of secondary peritonitis sought.

The diagnosis of PBP is not easy. It depends on the exclusion of a primary intraabdominal source of infection. Contrast-enhanced CT is useful in identifying an intraabdominal source for infection. It may be difficult to recover organisms from cultures of peritoneal fluid, presumably because the burden of organisms is low. However, the yield can be improved if 10 mL of peritoneal fluid is placed directly into a blood culture bottle. Since bacteremia frequently accompanies PBP, blood should be cultured simultaneously. No specific radiographic studies are helpful in the diagnosis of PBP. A plain film of the abdomen would be expected to show ascites. Chest and abdominal radiography should be performed in patients with abdominal pain to exclude free air, which signals a perforation (Fig. 121-2).

℞ PRIMARY BACTERIAL PERITONITIS

Treatment for PBP is directed at the isolate from blood or peritoneal fluid. Gram's staining of peritoneal fluid often gives negative results in PBP. Therefore, until culture results become available, therapy should cover gram-negative aerobic bacilli and gram-positive cocci. Third-generation cephalosporins such as cefotaxime (2 g q8h, administered IV) provide reasonable initial coverage in moderately ill patients. Broad-spectrum antibiotics, such as penicillin/β-lactamase inhibitor combinations (e.g., piperacillin/tazobactam, 3.375 g q6h IV for adults with normal renal function) or ceftriaxone (2 g q24h IV), are also options. Empirical coverage for anaerobes is not necessary. After the infecting organism is identified, therapy should be narrowed to target the specific pathogen. Patients with PBP usually respond within 72 h to appropriate antibiotic therapy. Antimicrobial therapy can be administered for as little as 5 days if rapid improvement occurs and blood cultures are negative, but a course of up to 2 weeks may be required for patients with bacteremia and for those whose improvement is slow. Persistence of WBCs in the ascitic fluid after therapy should prompt a search for additional diagnoses.

Prevention PBP has a high rate of recurrence. Up to 70% of patients experience a recurrence within 1 year. Antibiotic prophylaxis reduces

FIGURE 121-2 **Pneumoperitoneum.** Free air under the diaphragm on an upright chest film suggests the presence of a bowel perforation and associated peritonitis. *(Image courtesy of Dr. John Braver; with permission.)*

this rate to <20%. Prophylactic regimens for adults with normal renal function include fluoroquinolones (ciprofloxacin, 750 mg weekly; norfloxacin, 400 mg/d) or trimethoprim-sulfamethoxazole (one double-strength tablet daily). However, long-term administration of broad-spectrum antibiotics in this setting has been shown to increase the risk of severe staphylococcal infections.

SECONDARY PERITONITIS

Secondary peritonitis develops when bacteria contaminate the peritoneum as a result of spillage from an intraabdominal viscus. The organisms found almost always constitute a mixed flora in which facultative gram-negative bacilli and anaerobes predominate, especially when the contaminating source is colonic. Early in the course of infection, when the host response is directed toward containment of the infection, exudate containing fibrin and PMNs is found. Early death in this setting is attributable to gram-negative bacillary sepsis and to potent endotoxins circulating in the bloodstream (Chap. 265). Gram-negative bacilli, particularly *E. coli*, are common bloodstream isolates, but *Bacteroides fragilis* bacteremia also occurs. The severity of abdominal pain and the clinical course depend on the inciting process. The organisms isolated from the peritoneum also vary with the source of the initial process and the normal flora at that site. Secondary peritonitis can result primarily from chemical irritation and/or bacterial contamination. For example, as long as the patient is not achlorhydric, a ruptured gastric ulcer will release low-pH gastric contents that will serve as a chemical irritant. The normal flora of the stomach comprises the same organisms found in the oropharynx (Chap. 157) but in lower numbers. Thus, the bacterial burden in a ruptured ulcer is negligible compared with that in a ruptured appendix. The normal flora of the colon below the ligament of Treitz contains ~10^{11} anaerobic organisms/g of feces but only 10^8 aerobes/g; therefore, anaerobic species account for 99.9% of the bacteria. Leakage of colonic contents (pH 7–8) does not cause significant chemical peritonitis, but infection is intense because of the heavy bacterial load.

Depending on the inciting event, local symptoms may occur in secondary peritonitis—for example, epigastric pain from a ruptured gastric ulcer. In appendicitis (Chap. 294), the initial presenting symptoms are often vague, with periumbilical discomfort and nausea followed in a number of hours by pain more localized to the right lower quadrant.

Unusual locations of the appendix (including a retrocecal position) can complicate this presentation further. Once infection has spread to the peritoneal cavity, pain increases, particularly with infection involving the parietal peritoneum, which is innervated extensively. Patients usually lie motionless, often with knees drawn up to avoid stretching the nerve fibers of the peritoneal cavity. Coughing and sneezing, which increase pressure within the peritoneal cavity, are associated with sharp pain. There may or may not be pain localized to the infected or diseased organ from which secondary peritonitis has arisen. Patients with secondary peritonitis generally have abnormal findings on abdominal examination, with marked voluntary and involuntary guarding of the anterior abdominal musculature. Later findings include tenderness, especially rebound tenderness. In addition, there may be localized findings in the area of the inciting event. In general, patients are febrile, with marked leukocytosis and a left shift of the WBCs to band forms.

While recovery of organisms from peritoneal fluid is easier in secondary than in primary peritonitis, a tap of the abdomen is rarely the procedure of choice in secondary peritonitis. An exception is in cases involving trauma, where the possibility of a hemoperitoneum may need to be excluded early. Emergent studies (such as abdominal CT) to find the source of peritoneal contamination should be undertaken if the patient is hemodynamically stable; unstable patients may require surgical intervention without prior imaging.

℞ SECONDARY PERITONITIS

Treatment for secondary peritonitis includes early administration of antibiotics aimed particularly at aerobic gram-negative bacilli and anaerobes (see below). Mild to moderate disease can be treated with many drugs covering these organisms, including broad-spectrum penicillin/β-lactamase inhibitor combinations (e.g., ticarcillin/clavulanate, 3.1 g q4–6h IV) or cefoxitin (2 g q4–6h IV). Patients in intensive care units should receive imipenem (500 mg q6h IV), meropenem (1 g q8h IV), or combinations of drugs, such as ampicillin plus metronidazole plus ciprofloxacin. The role of enterococci and *Candida* spp. in mixed infections is controversial. Secondary peritonitis usually requires both surgical intervention to address the inciting process and antibiotics to treat early bacteremia, to decrease the incidence of abscess formation and wound infection, and to prevent distant spread of infection. While surgery is rarely indicated in PBP in adults, it may be life-saving in secondary peritonitis.

Peritonitis may develop as a complication of abdominal surgeries. These infections may be accompanied by localizing pain and/or nonlocalizing symptoms such as fever, malaise, anorexia, and toxicity. As a nosocomial infection, postoperative peritonitis may be associated with organisms such as staphylococci, components of the gram-negative hospital microflora, and the microbes that cause PBP and secondary peritonitis, as described above.

PERITONITIS IN PATIENTS UNDERGOING CAPD

A third type of peritonitis arises in patients who are undergoing continuous ambulatory peritoneal dialysis (CAPD). Unlike PBP and secondary peritonitis, which are caused by endogenous bacteria, CAPD-associated peritonitis usually involves skin organisms. The pathogenesis of infection is similar to that of intravascular device–related infection, in which skin organisms migrate along the catheter, which both serves as an entry point and exerts the effects of a foreign body. Exit-site or tunnel infection may or may not accompany CAPD-associated peritonitis. Like PBP, CAPD-associated peritonitis is usually caused by a single organism. Peritonitis is, in fact, the most common reason for discontinuation of CAPD. Improvements in equipment design, especially the Y-set connector, have resulted in a decrease from one case of peritonitis per 9 months of CAPD to one case per 15 months.

The clinical presentation of CAPD peritonitis resembles that of secondary peritonitis in that diffuse pain and peritoneal signs are common. The dialysate is usually cloudy and contains >100 WBCs/μL, >50% of which are neutrophils. The most common organisms are *Staphylococcus* spp., which accounted for ~45% of cases in one recent series. Historically, coagulase-negative staphylococcal species were identified most commonly in these infections, but more recently these isolates have been decreasing in frequency. *Staphylococcus aureus* is more often involved among patients who are nasal carriers of the organism than among those who are not, and this organism is the most common pathogen in overt exit-site infections. Gram-negative bacilli and fungi such as *Candida* spp. are also found. Vancomycin-resistant enterococci and vancomycin-intermediate *S. aureus* have been reported to produce peritonitis in CAPD patients. The finding of more than one organism in dialysate culture should prompt evaluation for secondary peritonitis. As with PBP, culture of dialysate fluid in blood culture bottles improves the yield. To facilitate diagnosis, several hundred milliliters of removed dialysis fluid should be concentrated by centrifugation before culture.

℞ CAPD PERITONITIS

Empirical therapy for CAPD peritonitis should be directed at *S. aureus*, coagulase-negative *Staphylococcus*, and gram-negative bacilli until the results of cultures are available. Guidelines issued in 2005 suggest that agents should be chosen on the basis of local experience with resistant organisms. In some centers, a first-generation cephalosporin such as cefazolin (for gram-positive bacteria) and a fluoroquinolone or a third-generation cephalosporin such as ceftazidime (for gram-negative bacteria) may be reasonable; in areas with high rates of infection with methicillin-resistant *S. aureus*, vancomycin should be used instead of cefazolin, and gram-negative coverage may need to be broadened. Broad coverage including vancomycin should be particularly considered for toxic patients and for those with exit-site infections. Loading doses are administered intraperitoneally; doses depend on the dialysis method and the patient's renal function. Antibiotics are given either continuously (i.e., with each exchange) or intermittently (i.e., once daily, with the dose allowed to remain in the peritoneal cavity for at least 6 h). If the patient is severely ill, IV antibiotics should be added at doses appropriate for the patient's degree of renal failure. The clinical response to an empirical treatment regimen should be rapid; if the patient has not responded after 48 h of treatment, catheter removal should be considered.

TUBERCULOUS PERITONITIS
See Chap. 158.

INTRAABDOMINAL ABSCESSES

INTRAPERITONEAL ABSCESSES
Abscess formation is common in untreated peritonitis if overt gram-negative sepsis either does not develop or develops but is not fatal. In experimental models of abscess formation, mixed aerobic and anaerobic organisms have been implanted intraperitoneally. Without therapy directed at anaerobes, animals develop intraabdominal abscesses. As in humans, these experimental abscesses may stud the peritoneal cavity, lie within the omentum or mesentery, or even develop on the surface of or within viscera such as the liver.

Pathogenesis and Immunity There is often disagreement about whether an abscess represents a disease state or a host response. In a sense, it represents both: while an abscess is an infection in which viable infecting organisms and PMNs are contained in a fibrous capsule, it is also a process by which the host confines microbes to a limited space, thereby preventing further spread of infection. In any event, abscesses do cause significant symptoms, and patients with abscesses can be quite ill. Experimental work has helped to define both the host cells and the bacterial virulence factors responsible—most notably, in the case of *B. fragilis*. This organism, although accounting for only 0.5% of the normal colonic flora, is the anaerobe most frequently isolated from intraabdominal infections, is especially prominent in abscesses, and is the most common anaerobic bloodstream isolate. On clinical grounds, therefore, *B. fragilis* appears to be uniquely virulent. Moreover, *B. fragilis* acts alone to cause abscesses in animal models of intraabdominal infection, whereas most other *Bacteroides* species must act synergistically with a facultative organism to induce abscess formation.

Of the several virulence factors identified in *B. fragilis*, one is critical: the capsular polysaccharide complex (CPC) found on the bacterial surface. The CPC comprises at least eight distinct surface polysaccharides. Structural analysis of these polysaccharides has shown an unusual motif of oppositely charged sugars. Polysaccharides having these *zwitterionic* characteristics, such as polysaccharide A (PSA), evoke a host response in the peritoneal cavity that localizes bacteria into abscesses. *B. fragilis* and PSA have been found to adhere to primary mesothelial cells in vitro; this adherence, in turn, stimulates the production of tumor necrosis factor α (TNF-α) and intercellular adhesion molecule 1 (ICAM-1) by peritoneal macrophages. Although abscesses characteristically contain PMNs, the process of abscess induction depends on the stimulation of T lymphocytes by these unique zwitterionic polysaccharides. The stimulated CD4+ T lymphocytes secrete leukoattractant cytokines and chemokines. The alternative pathway of complement and fibrinogen also participate in abscess formation.

While antibodies to the CPC enhance bloodstream clearance of *B. fragilis*, CD4+ T cells are critical in immunity to abscesses. When administered subcutaneously, *B. fragilis* PSA has immunomodulatory characteristics and stimulates CD4+ T regulatory cells via an interleukin (IL) 2–dependent mechanism to produce IL-10. IL-10 downregulates the inflammatory response, thereby preventing abscess formation.

Clinical Presentation Of all intraabdominal abscesses, 74% are intraperitoneal or retroperitoneal and are not visceral. Most intraperitoneal abscesses result from fecal spillage from a colonic source, such as an inflamed appendix. Abscesses can also arise from other processes. They usually form within weeks of the development of peritonitis and may be found in a variety of locations—from omentum to mesentery, pelvis to psoas muscles, and subphrenic space to a visceral organ such as the liver, where they may develop either on the surface of the organ or within it. Periappendiceal and diverticular abscesses occur commonly. Diverticular abscesses are least likely to rupture. Infections of the female genital tract and pancreatitis are also among the more common causative events. When abscesses occur in the female genital tract—either as a primary infection (e.g., tuboovarian abscess) or as an infection extending into the pelvic cavity or peritoneum—*B. fragilis* figures prominently among the organisms isolated. *B. fragilis* is not found in large numbers in the normal vaginal flora. For example, it is encountered less commonly in pelvic inflammatory disease and endometritis without an associated abscess. In pancreatitis with leakage of damaging pancreatic enzymes, inflammation is prominent. Therefore, clinical findings such as fever, leukocytosis, and even abdominal pain do not distinguish pancreatitis itself from complications such as pancreatic pseudocyst, pancreatic abscess (Chap. 307), or intraabdominal collections of pus. Especially in cases of necrotizing pancreatitis, in which the incidence of local pancreatic infection may be as high as 30%, needle aspiration under CT guidance is performed to sample fluid for culture. Many centers prescribe preemptive antibiotics for patients with necrotizing pancreatitis. Imipenem is frequently used for this purpose since it reaches high tissue levels in the pancreas (although it is not unique in this regard). If needle aspiration yields infected fluid, most experts agree that surgery is superior to percutaneous drainage.

Diagnosis Scanning procedures have considerably facilitated the diagnosis of intraabdominal abscesses. Abdominal CT probably has the highest yield, although ultrasonography is particularly useful for the right upper quadrant, kidneys, and pelvis. Both indium-labeled WBCs and gallium tend to localize in abscesses and may be useful in finding a collection. Since gallium is taken up in the bowel, indium-labeled WBCs may have a slightly greater yield for abscesses near the bowel. Neither indium-labeled WBC nor gallium scans serve as a basis for a definitive diagnosis, however; both need to be followed by other, more specific studies, such as CT, if an area of possible abnormality is identified. Abscesses contiguous with or contained within diverticula are particularly difficult to diagnose with scanning procedures. Occasionally, a barium enema may detect a diverticular abscess not diagnosed by other procedures, although barium should not be injected if a perforation is sus-

FIGURE 121-3 Algorithm for the management of patients with intraabdominal abscesses using percutaneous drainage. Antimicrobial therapy should be administered concomitantly. [Reprinted with permission from B Lorber (ed): Atlas of Infectious Diseases, vol VII: Intra-abdominal Infections, Hepatitis, and Gastroenteritis. Philadelphia, Current Medicine, 1996, p 1.30, as adapted from OD Rotstein, RL Simmons, in SL Gorbach et al (eds): Infectious Diseases. Philadelphia, Saunders, 1992, p 668.]

pected. If one study is negative, a second study sometimes reveals a collection. Although exploratory laparotomy has been less commonly used since the advent of CT, this procedure still must be undertaken on occasion if an abscess is strongly suspected on clinical grounds.

℞ INTRAPERITONEAL ABSCESSES

An algorithm for the management of patients with intraabdominal (including intraperitoneal) abscesses is presented in **Fig. 121-3**. The treatment of intraabdominal infections involves the determination of the initial focus of infection, the administration of broad-spectrum antibiotics targeting the organisms involved, and the performance of a drainage procedure if one or more definitive abscesses have formed. Antimicrobial therapy, in general, is adjunctive to drainage and/or surgical correction of an underlying lesion or process in intraabdominal abscesses. Unlike the intraabdominal abscesses resulting from most causes, for which drainage of some kind is generally required, abscesses associated with diverticulitis usually wall off locally after rupture of a diverticulum, so that surgical intervention is not routinely required.

A number of agents exhibit excellent activity against aerobic gram-negative bacilli. Since mortality in intraabdominal sepsis is linked to gram-negative bacteremia, empirical therapy for intraabdominal infection always needs to include adequate coverage of gram-negative aerobic, facultative, and anaerobic organisms. Even if anaerobes are not cultured from clinical specimens, they still must be covered by the therapeutic regimen. Empirical antibiotic therapy should be the same as that discussed above for secondary peritonitis.

VISCERAL ABSCESSES

Liver Abscesses The liver is the organ most subject to the development of abscesses. In one study of 540 intraabdominal abscesses, 26% were visceral. Liver abscesses made up 13% of the total number, or 48% of all visceral abscesses. Liver abscesses may be solitary or multiple; they may arise from hematogenous spread of bacteria or from local spread from contiguous sites of infection within the peritoneal cavity. In the past, appendicitis with rupture and subsequent spread of infection was the most common source for a liver abscess. Currently, associated disease of the biliary tract is most common. Pylephlebitis (suppurative thrombosis of the portal vein), usually arising from infection in the pelvis but sometimes from infection elsewhere in the peritoneal cavity, is another common source for bacterial seeding of the liver.

Fever is the most common presenting sign of liver abscess. Some patients, particularly those with associated disease of the biliary tract, have symptoms and signs localized to the right upper quadrant, in-

cluding pain, guarding, punch tenderness, and even rebound tenderness. Nonspecific symptoms, such as chills, anorexia, weight loss, nausea, and vomiting, may also develop. Only 50% of patients with liver abscesses, however, have hepatomegaly, right-upper-quadrant tenderness, or jaundice; thus, half of patients have no symptoms or signs to direct attention to the liver. Fever of unknown origin (FUO) may be the only manifestation of liver abscess, especially in the elderly. Diagnostic studies of the abdomen, especially the right upper quadrant, should be a part of any FUO workup. The single most reliable laboratory finding is an elevated serum concentration of alkaline phosphatase, which is documented in 70% of patients with liver abscesses. Other tests of liver function may yield normal results, but 50% of patients have elevated serum levels of bilirubin, and 48% have elevated concentrations of aspartate aminotransferase. Other laboratory findings include leukocytosis in 77% of patients, anemia (usually normochromic, normocytic) in 50%, and hypoalbuminemia in 33%. Concomitant bacteremia is found in one-third of patients. A liver abscess is sometimes suggested by chest radiography, especially if a new elevation of the right hemidiaphragm is seen; other suggestive findings include a right basilar infiltrate and a right pleural effusion.

Imaging studies are the most reliable methods for diagnosing liver abscesses. These studies include ultrasonography, CT (**Fig. 121-4**), indium-labeled WBC or gallium scan, and MRI. More than one such study may be required. Organisms recovered from liver abscesses vary with the source. In liver infection arising from the biliary tree, enteric gram-negative aerobic bacilli and enterococci are common isolates. Unless previous surgery has been performed, anaerobes are not generally involved in liver abscesses arising from biliary infections. In contrast, in liver abscesses arising from pelvic and other intraperitoneal sources, a mixed flora including both aerobic and anaerobic species is common; *B. fragilis* is the species most frequently isolated. With hematogenous spread of infection, usually only a single organism is encountered; this species may be *S. aureus* or a streptococcal species such as *S. milleri*. Results of cultures obtained from drain sites are not reliable for defining the etiology of infections. Liver abscesses may also be caused by *Candida* spp.; such abscesses usually follow fungemia in patients receiving chemotherapy for cancer and often present when PMNs return after a period of neutropenia. Amebic liver abscesses are not an uncommon problem (Chap. 202). Amebic serologic testing gives positive results in >95% of cases; thus, a negative result helps to exclude this diagnosis.

℞ LIVER ABSCESSES (FIG. 121-3)

While drainage—either percutaneous (with a pigtail catheter kept in place) or surgical—is the mainstay of therapy for intraabdominal abscesses (in-

FIGURE 121-4 Multilocular liver abscess on CT scan. Multiple or multilocular abscesses are more common than solitary abscesses. [Reprinted with permission from B Lorber (ed): Atlas of Infectious Diseases, Vol VII: Intra-abdominal Infections, Hepatitis, and Gastroenteritis. Philadelphia, Current Medicine, 1996, Fig. 1.22.]

cluding liver abscesses), there is growing interest in medical management alone for pyogenic liver abscesses. The drugs used for empirical therapy include the same ones used in intraabdominal sepsis and secondary bacterial peritonitis. Usually, a diagnostic aspirate of abscess contents should be obtained before the initiation of empirical therapy, with antibiotic choices adjusted when the results of Gram's staining and culture become available. Cases treated without definitive drainage generally require longer courses of antibiotic therapy. When percutaneous drainage was compared with open surgical drainage, the average length of hospital stay for the former was almost twice that for the latter, although both the time required for fever to resolve and the mortality rate were the same for the two procedures. Mortality was appreciable despite treatment, averaging 15%. Several factors predict the failure of percutaneous drainage and therefore may favor primary surgical intervention. These factors include the presence of multiple, sizable abscesses; viscous abscess contents that tend to plug the catheter; associated disease (e.g., disease of the biliary tract) requiring surgery; or the lack of a clinical response to percutaneous drainage in 4–7 days.

Treatment of candidal liver abscesses often entails initial administration of amphotericin B or liposomal amphotericin, with subsequent fluconazole therapy (Chap. 196). In some cases, therapy with fluconazole alone (6 mg/kg daily) may be used—e.g., in clinically stable patients whose infecting isolate is susceptible to this drug.

Splenic Abscesses   Splenic abscesses are much less common than liver abscesses. The incidence of splenic abscesses has ranged from 0.14% to 0.7% in various autopsy series. The clinical setting and the organisms isolated usually differ from those for liver abscesses. The degree of clinical suspicion for splenic abscess needs to be high, as this condition is frequently fatal if left untreated. Even in the most recently published series, diagnosis was made only at autopsy in 37% of cases. While splenic abscesses may arise occasionally from contiguous spread of infection or from direct trauma to the spleen, hematogenous spread of infection is more common. Bacterial endocarditis is the most common associated infection (Chap. 118). Splenic abscesses can develop in patients who have received extensive immunosuppressive therapy (particularly those with malignancy involving the spleen) and in patients with hemoglobinopathies or other hematologic disorders (especially sickle cell anemia).

While ~50% of patients with splenic abscesses have abdominal pain, the pain is localized to the left upper quadrant in only half of these cases. Splenomegaly is found in ~50% of cases. Fever and leukocytosis are generally present; the development of fever preceded diagnosis by an average of 20 days in one series. Left-sided chest findings may include abnormalities to auscultation, and chest radiographic findings may include an infiltrate or a left-sided pleural effusion. CT scan of the abdomen has been the most sensitive diagnostic tool. Ultrasonography can yield the diagnosis but is less sensitive. Liver-spleen scan or gallium scan may also be useful. Streptococcal species are the most common bacterial isolates from splenic abscesses, followed by S. aureus—presumably reflecting the associated endocarditis. An increase in the prevalence of gram-negative aerobic isolates from splenic abscesses has been reported; these organisms often derive from a urinary tract focus, with associated bacteremia, or from another intraabdominal source. Salmonella species are seen fairly commonly, especially in patients with sickle cell hemoglobinopathy. Anaerobic species accounted for only 5% of isolates in the largest collected series, but the reporting of a number of "sterile abscesses" may indicate that optimal techniques for the isolation of anaerobes were not employed.

Rx SPLENIC ABSCESSES

Because of the high mortality figures reported for splenic abscesses, splenectomy with adjunctive antibiotics has traditionally been considered standard treatment and remains the best approach for complex, multilocular abscesses or multiple abscesses. However, percutaneous drainage has worked well for single, small (<3-cm) abscesses in some studies and may also be useful for patients with high surgical risk. Patients undergoing splenectomy should be vaccinated against encapsulated organisms (Streptococcus pneumoniae, Haemophilus influenzae, Neisseria meningitidis). The most important factor in successful treatment of splenic abscesses is early diagnosis.

Perinephric and Renal Abscesses   Perinephric and renal abscesses are not common: The former accounted for only ~0.02% of hospital admissions and the latter for ~0.2% in Altemeier's series of 540 intraabdominal abscesses. Before antibiotics became available, most renal and perinephric abscesses were hematogenous in origin, usually complicating prolonged bacteremia, with S. aureus most commonly recovered. Now, in contrast, >75% of perinephric and renal abscesses arise from a urinary tract infection. Infection ascends from the bladder to the kidney, with pyelonephritis occurring prior to abscess development. Bacteria may directly invade the renal parenchyma from medulla to cortex. Local vascular channels within the kidney may also facilitate the transport of organisms. Areas of abscess developing within the parenchyma may rupture into the perinephric space. The kidneys and adrenal glands are surrounded by a layer of perirenal fat that, in turn, is surrounded by Gerota's fascia, which extends superiorly to the diaphragm and inferiorly to the pelvic fat. Abscesses extending into the perinephric space may track through Gerota's fascia into the psoas or transversalis muscles, into the anterior peritoneal cavity, superiorly to the subdiaphragmatic space, or inferiorly to the pelvis. Of the risk factors that have been associated with the development of perinephric abscesses, the most important is concomitant nephrolithiasis obstructing urinary flow. Of patients with perinephric abscess, 20–60% have renal stones. Other structural abnormalities of the urinary tract, prior urologic surgery, trauma, and diabetes mellitus have also been identified as risk factors.

The organisms most frequently encountered in perinephric and renal abscesses are E. coli, Proteus spp., and Klebsiella spp. E. coli, the aerobic species most commonly found in the colonic flora, seems to have unique virulence properties in the urinary tract, including factors promoting adherence to uroepithelial cells. The urease of Proteus spp. splits urea, thereby creating a more alkaline and more hospitable environment for bacterial proliferation. Proteus spp. are frequently found in association with large struvite stones caused by the precipitation of magnesium ammonium sulfate in an alkaline environment. These stones serve as a nidus for recurrent urinary tract infection. While a single bacterial species is usually recovered from a perinephric or renal abscess, multiple species may also be found. If a urine culture is not contaminated with periurethral flora and is found to contain more than one organism, a perinephric abscess or renal abscess should be considered in the differential diagnosis. Urine cultures may also be polymicrobial in cases of bladder diverticulum.

Candida spp. can cause renal abscesses. This fungus may spread to the kidney hematogenously or by ascension from the bladder. The hallmark of the latter route of infection is ureteral obstruction with large fungal balls.

The presentation of perinephric and renal abscesses is quite nonspecific. Flank pain and abdominal pain are common. At least 50% of patients are febrile. Pain may be referred to the groin or leg, particularly with extension of infection. The diagnosis of perinephric abscess, like that of splenic abscess, is frequently delayed, and the mortality rate in some series is appreciable, although lower than in the past. Perinephric or renal abscess should be most seriously considered when a patient presents with symptoms and signs of pyelonephritis and remains febrile after 4 or 5 days of treatment. Moreover, when a urine culture yields a polymicrobial flora, when a patient is known to have renal stones, or when fever and pyuria coexist with a sterile urine culture, these diagnoses should be entertained.

Renal ultrasonography and abdominal CT are the most useful diagnostic modalities. If a renal or perinephric abscess is diagnosed, nephrolithiasis should be excluded, especially when a high urinary pH suggests the presence of a urea-splitting organism.

Rx PERINEPHRIC AND RENAL ABSCESSES

Treatment for perinephric and renal abscesses, like that for other intraabdominal abscesses, includes drainage of pus and antibiotic therapy directed at the organism(s) recovered. For perinephric abscesses, percutaneous drainage is usually successful.

Psoas Abscesses The psoas muscle is another location in which abscesses are encountered. Psoas abscesses may arise from a hematogenous source, by contiguous spread from an intraabdominal or pelvic process, or by contiguous spread from nearby bony structures (e.g., vertebral bodies). Associated osteomyelitis due to spread from bone to muscle or from muscle to bone is common in psoas abscesses. When Pott's disease was common, *Mycobacterium tuberculosis* was a frequent cause of psoas abscess. Currently, either *S. aureus* or a mixture of enteric organisms including aerobic and anaerobic gram-negative bacilli is usually isolated from psoas abscesses in the United States. *S. aureus* is most likely to be isolated when a psoas abscess arises from hematogenous spread or a contiguous focus of osteomyelitis; a mixed enteric flora is the most likely etiology when the abscess has an intraabdominal or pelvic source. Patients with psoas abscesses frequently present with fever, lower abdominal or back pain, or pain referred to the hip or knee. CT is the most useful diagnostic technique.

℞ PSOAS ABSCESSES

Treatment includes surgical drainage and the administration of an antibiotic regimen directed at the inciting organism(s).

Pancreatic Abscesses See Chap. 307.

ACKNOWLEDGMENT
The substantial contributions of Dori F. Zaleznik, MD, to this chapter in previous editions are gratefully acknowledged.

122 Acute Infectious Diarrheal Diseases and Bacterial Food Poisoning

Joan R. Butterton, Stephen B. Calderwood

Ranging from mild annoyances during vacations to devastating dehydrating illnesses that can kill within hours, acute gastrointestinal illnesses rank second only to acute upper respiratory illnesses as the most common diseases worldwide. In children <5 years old, attack rates range from 2–3 illnesses per child per year in developed countries to as high as 10–18 illnesses per child per year in developing countries. In Asia, Africa, and Latin America, acute diarrheal illnesses are not only a leading cause of morbidity in children—with an estimated 1 billion cases per year—but also a major cause of death. These illnesses are responsible for 4–6 million deaths per year, or a sobering total of 12,600 deaths per day. In some areas, >50% of childhood deaths are directly attributable to acute diarrheal illnesses. In addition, by contributing to malnutrition and thereby reducing resistance to other infectious agents, gastrointestinal illnesses may be indirect factors in a far greater burden of disease.

The wide range of clinical manifestations of acute gastrointestinal illnesses is matched by the wide variety of infectious agents involved, including viruses, bacteria, and parasitic pathogens (Table 122-1). This chapter discusses factors that enable gastrointestinal pathogens to cause disease, reviews host defense mechanisms, and delineates an approach to the evaluation and treatment of patients presenting with acute diarrhea. Individual organisms causing acute gastrointestinal illnesses are discussed in detail in subsequent chapters.

PATHOGENIC MECHANISMS

Enteric pathogens have developed a variety of tactics to overcome host defenses. Understanding the virulence factors employed by these organisms is important in the diagnosis and treatment of clinical disease.

FURTHER READINGS

CAMPILLO B et al: Epidemiology of severe hospital-acquired infections in patients with liver cirrhosis: Effect of long-term administration of norfloxacin. Clin Infect Dis 26:1066, 1998

GIBSON FC III et al: Cellular mechanism of intraabdominal abscess formation by *Bacteroides fragilis*. J Immunol 160:5000, 1998

JOHANSSEN EC, MADOFF LC: Infections of the liver and biliary system, in *Principles and Practice of Infectious Diseases*, 6th ed, GL Mandell et al (eds). Philadelphia, Elsevier Churchill Livingstone, 2005, pp 951–959

LEVISON ME, BUSH LM: Peritonitis and intraperitoneal abscesses, in *Principles and Practice of Infectious Diseases*, 6th ed, GL Mandell et al (eds). Philadelphia, Elsevier Churchill Livingstone, 2005, pp 927–945

PAPPAS PG et al: Guidelines for treatment of candidiasis. Clin Infect Dis 38:161, 2004

PIRAINO B et al: Peritoneal dialysis–related infections recommendations: 2005 update. Perit Dial Int 25:107, 2005

RAHIMIAN J et al: Pyogenic liver abscess: Recent trends in etiology and mortality. Clin Infect Dis 39:1654, 2004

SOLOMKIN JS et al: Guidelines for the selection of anti-infective agents for complicated intra-abdominal infections. Clin Infect Dis 37:997, 2003

TZIANABOS AO, KASPER DL: Anaerobic infections: General concepts, in *Principles and Practice of Infectious Diseases*, 6th ed, GL Mandell et al (eds). Philadelphia, Elsevier Churchill Livingstone, 2005, pp 2810–2816

TZIANABOS AO et al: T cells activated by zwitterionic molecules prevent abscesses induced by pathogenic bacteria. J Biol Chem 275:6733, 2000

VAN RULER O et al: Comparison of on-demand vs planned relaparotomy strategy in patients with severe peritonitis: A randomized trial. JAMA 298:865, 2007

Inoculum Size The number of microorganisms that must be ingested to cause disease varies considerably from species to species. For *Shigella*, enterohemorrhagic *Escherichia coli*, *Giardia lamblia*, or *Entamoeba*, as few as 10–100 bacteria or cysts can produce infection, while 10^5–10^8 *Vibrio cholerae* organisms must be ingested orally to cause disease. The infective dose of *Salmonella* varies widely, depending on the species, host, and food vehicle. The ability of organisms to overcome host defenses has important implications for transmission; *Shigella*, enterohemorrhagic *E. coli*, *Entamoeba*, and *Giardia* can spread by person-to-person contact, whereas under some circumstances *Salmonella* may have to grow in food for several hours before reaching an effective infectious dose.

Adherence Many organisms must adhere to the gastrointestinal mucosa as an initial step in the pathogenic process; thus, organisms that can compete with the normal bowel flora and colonize the mucosa have an important advantage in causing disease. Specific cell-surface proteins involved in attachment of bacteria to intestinal cells are important virulence determinants. *V. cholerae*, for example, adheres to the brush border of small-intestinal enterocytes via specific surface adhesins, including the toxin-coregulated pilus and other accessory colonization factors. Enterotoxigenic *E. coli*, which causes watery diarrhea, produces an adherence protein called *colonization factor antigen* that is necessary for colonization of the upper small intestine by the organism prior to the production of enterotoxin. Enteropathogenic *E. coli*, an agent of diarrhea in young children, and enterohemorrhagic *E. coli*, which causes hemorrhagic colitis and the hemolytic-uremic syndrome, produce virulence determinants that allow these organisms to attach to and efface the brush border of the intestinal epithelium.

Toxin Production The production of one or more exotoxins is important in the pathogenesis of numerous enteric organisms. Such toxins include *enterotoxins*, which cause watery diarrhea by acting directly on secretory mechanisms in the intestinal mucosa; *cytotoxins*, which cause destruction of mucosal cells and associated inflammatory diarrhea; and *neurotoxins*, which act directly on the central or peripheral nervous system.

TABLE 122-1 GASTROINTESTINAL PATHOGENS CAUSING ACUTE DIARRHEA

Mechanism	Location	Illness	Stool Findings	Examples of Pathogens Involved
Noninflammatory (entero-toxin)	Proximal small bowel	Watery diarrhea	No fecal leukocytes; mild or no increase in fecal lactoferrin	*Vibrio cholerae*, enterotoxigenic *Escherichia coli* (LT and/or ST), enteroaggregative *E. coli*, *Clostridium perfringens*, *Bacillus cereus*, *Staphylococcus aureus*, *Aeromonas hydrophila*, *Plesiomonas shigelloides*, rotavirus, norovirus, enteric adenoviruses, *Giardia lamblia*, *Cryptosporidium* spp., *Cyclospora* spp., microsporidia
Inflammatory (invasion or cytotoxin)	Colon or distal small bowel	Dysentery or inflammatory diarrhea	Fecal polymorphonuclear leukocytes; substantial increase in fecal lactoferrin	*Shigella* spp., *Salmonella* spp., *Campylobacter jejuni*, enterohemorrhagic *E. coli*, enteroinvasive *E. coli*, *Yersinia enterocolitica*, *Vibrio parahaemolyticus*, *Clostridium difficile*, ?*A. hydrophila*, ?*P. shigelloides*, *Entamoeba histolytica*
Penetrating	Distal small bowel	Enteric fever	Fecal mononuclear leukocytes	*Salmonella typhi*, *Y. enterocolitica*, ?*Campylobacter fetus*

Abbreviations: LT, heat-labile enterotoxin; ST, heat-stable enterotoxin. **Source:** After Guerrant and Steiner.

The prototypical enterotoxin is cholera toxin, a heterodimeric protein composed of one A and five B subunits. The A subunit contains the enzymatic activity of the toxin, while the B subunit pentamer binds holotoxin to the enterocyte surface receptor, the ganglioside G_{M1}. After the binding of holotoxin, a fragment of the A subunit is translocated across the eukaryotic cell membrane into the cytoplasm, where it catalyzes the ADP-ribosylation of a GTP-binding protein and causes persistent activation of adenylate cyclase. The end result is an increase of cyclic AMP in the intestinal mucosa, which increases Cl⁻ secretion and decreases Na⁺ absorption, leading to loss of fluid and the production of diarrhea.

Enterotoxigenic strains of *E. coli* may produce a protein called *heat-labile enterotoxin* (LT) that is similar to cholera toxin and causes secretory diarrhea by the same mechanism. Alternatively, enterotoxigenic strains of *E. coli* may produce *heat-stable enterotoxin* (ST), one form of which causes diarrhea by activation of guanylate cyclase and elevation of intracellular cyclic GMP. Some enterotoxigenic strains of *E. coli* produce both LT and ST.

Bacterial cytotoxins, in contrast, destroy intestinal mucosal cells and produce the syndrome of dysentery, with bloody stools containing inflammatory cells. Enteric pathogens that produce such cytotoxins include *Shigella dysenteriae* type 1, *Vibrio parahaemolyticus*, and *Clostridium difficile*. *S. dysenteriae* type 1 and Shiga toxin–producing strains of *E. coli* produce potent cytotoxins and have been associated with outbreaks of hemorrhagic colitis and hemolytic-uremic syndrome.

Neurotoxins are usually produced by bacteria outside the host and therefore cause symptoms soon after ingestion. Included are the staphylococcal and *Bacillus cereus* toxins, which act on the central nervous system to produce vomiting.

Invasion Dysentery may result not only from the production of cytotoxins but also from bacterial invasion and destruction of intestinal mucosal cells. Infections due to *Shigella* and enteroinvasive *E. coli* are characterized by the organisms' invasion of mucosal epithelial cells, intraepithelial multiplication, and subsequent spread to adjacent cells. *Salmonella* causes inflammatory diarrhea by invasion of the bowel mucosa but generally is not associated with the destruction of enterocytes or the full clinical syndrome of dysentery. *Salmonella typhi* and *Yersinia enterocolitica* can penetrate intact intestinal mucosa, multiply intracellularly in Peyer's patches and intestinal lymph nodes, and then disseminate through the bloodstream to cause enteric fever, a syndrome characterized by fever, headache, relative bradycardia, abdominal pain, splenomegaly, and leukopenia.

HOST DEFENSES

Given the enormous number of microorganisms ingested with every meal, the normal host must combat a constant influx of potential enteric pathogens. Studies of infections in patients with alterations in defense mechanisms have led to a greater understanding of the variety of ways in which the normal host can protect itself against disease.

Normal Flora The large numbers of bacteria that normally inhabit the intestine act as an important host defense by preventing colonization by potential enteric pathogens. Persons with fewer intestinal bacteria, such as infants who have not yet developed normal enteric colonization or patients receiving antibiotics, are at significantly greater risk of developing infections with enteric pathogens. The composition of the intestinal flora is as important as the number of organisms present. More than 99% of the normal colonic flora is made up of anaerobic bacteria, and the acidic pH and volatile fatty acids produced by these organisms appear to be critical elements in resistance to colonization.

Gastric Acid The acidic pH of the stomach is an important barrier to enteric pathogens, and an increased frequency of infections due to *Salmonella*, *G. lamblia*, and a variety of helminths has been reported among patients who have undergone gastric surgery or are achlorhydric for some other reason. Neutralization of gastric acid with antacids or H₂ blockers—a common practice in the management of hospitalized patients—similarly increases the risk of enteric colonization. In addition, some microorganisms can survive the extreme acidity of the gastric environment; rotavirus, for example, is highly stable to acidity.

Intestinal Motility Normal peristalsis is the major mechanism for clearance of bacteria from the proximal small intestine. When intestinal motility is impaired (e.g., by treatment with opiates or other antimotility drugs, anatomic abnormalities, or hypomotility states), the frequency of bacterial overgrowth and infection of the small bowel with enteric pathogens is increased. Some patients whose treatment for *Shigella* infection consists of diphenoxylate hydrochloride with atropine (Lomotil) experience prolonged fever and shedding of organisms, while patients treated with opiates for mild *Salmonella* gastroenteritis have a higher frequency of bacteremia than those not treated with opiates.

Immunity Both cellular immune responses and antibody production play important roles in protection from enteric infections. The wide spectrum of viral, bacterial, parasitic, and fungal gastrointestinal infections in patients with AIDS highlights the significance of cell-mediated immunity in protection from these pathogens. Humoral immunity is also important and consists of systemic IgG and IgM as well as secretory IgA. The mucosal immune system may be the first line of defense against many gastrointestinal pathogens. The binding of bacterial antigens to the luminal surface of M cells in the distal small bowel and the subsequent presentation of antigens to subepithelial lymphoid tissue lead to the proliferation of sensitized lymphocytes. These lymphocytes circulate and populate all of the mucosal tissues of the body as IgA-secreting plasma cells.

Genetic Determinants The mechanisms underlying genetic variation in host susceptibility remain poorly understood. People with blood group O show increased susceptibility to cholera, shigellosis, and norovirus infection. A polymorphism in the interleukin 8 gene is associated with increased risk of diarrhea from enteroaggregative *E. coli*.

APPROACH TO THE PATIENT:
Infectious Diarrhea or Bacterial Food Poisoning

The approach to the patient with possible infectious diarrhea or bacterial food poisoning is shown in Fig. 122-1.

HISTORY The answers to questions with high discriminating value can quickly narrow the range of potential causes of diarrhea and help determine whether treatment is needed. Important elements of the narrative history are detailed in Fig. 122-1.

PHYSICAL EXAMINATION The examination of patients for signs of dehydration provides essential information about the severity of the diarrheal illness and the need for rapid therapy. Mild dehydration is indicated by thirst, dry mouth, decreased axillary sweat, decreased urine output, and slight weight loss. Signs of moderate dehydration include an orthostatic fall in blood pressure, skin tenting, and sunken eyes (or, in infants, a sunken fontanelle). Signs of severe dehydration range from hypotension and tachycardia to confusion and frank shock.

DIAGNOSTIC APPROACH After the severity of illness is assessed, the clinician must distinguish between *inflammatory* and *noninflammatory* disease. Using the history and epidemiologic features of the case as guides, the clinician can then rapidly evaluate the need for further efforts to define a specific etiology and for therapeutic intervention. Examination of a stool sample may supplement the narrative history. Grossly bloody or mucoid stool suggests an inflammatory process. A test for fecal leukocytes (preparation of a thin smear of stool on a glass slide, addition of a drop of methylene blue, and examination of the wet mount) can suggest inflammatory disease in patients with diarrhea, although the predictive value of this test is still debated. A test for fecal lactoferrin, which is a marker of fecal leukocytes, is more sensitive and is available in latex agglutination and enzyme-linked immunosorbent assay formats. Causes of acute infectious diarrhea, categorized as inflammatory and noninflammatory, are listed in Table 122-1.

POST-DIARRHEA COMPLICATIONS Chronic complications may follow the resolution of an acute diarrheal episode. The clinician should inquire about prior diarrheal illness if the conditions listed in Table 122-2 are observed.

EPIDEMIOLOGY

Travel History Of the several million people who travel from temperate industrialized countries to tropical regions of Asia, Africa, and Central and South America each year, 20–50% experience a sudden onset of abdominal cramps, anorexia, and watery diarrhea; thus *traveler's diarrhea* is the most common travel-related illness (Chap. 117). The time of onset is usually 3 days to 2 weeks after the traveler's arrival in a tropical area; most cases begin within the first 3–5 days. The illness is generally self-limited, lasting 1–5 days. The high rate of diarrhea among travelers to underdeveloped areas is related to the ingestion of contaminated food or water.

The organisms that cause traveler's diarrhea vary considerably with location (Table 122-3). In all areas, enterotoxigenic and enteroaggregative *E. coli* are the most common isolates from persons with the classic secretory traveler's diarrhea syndrome.

FIGURE 122-1 Clinical algorithm for the approach to patients with community-acquired infectious diarrhea or bacterial food poisoning. Key to superscripts: **1.** Diarrhea lasting >2 weeks is generally defined as chronic; in such cases, many of the causes of acute diarrhea are much less likely, and a new spectrum of causes needs to be considered. **2.** Fever often implies invasive disease, although fever and diarrhea may also result from infection outside the gastrointestinal tract, as in malaria. **3.** Stools that contain blood or mucus indicate ulceration of the large bowel. Bloody stools without fecal leukocytes should alert the laboratory to the possibility of infection with Shiga toxin–producing enterohemorrhagic *Escherichia coli*. Bulky white stools suggest a small-intestinal process that is causing malabsorption. Profuse "rice-water" stools suggest cholera or a similar toxigenic process. **4.** Frequent stools over a given period can provide the first warning of impending dehydration. **5.** Abdominal pain may be most severe in inflammatory processes like those due to *Shigella, Campylobacter,* and necrotizing toxins. Painful abdominal muscle cramps, caused by electrolyte loss, can develop in severe cases of cholera. Bloating is common in giardiasis. An appendicitis-like syndrome should prompt a culture for *Yersinia enterocolitica* with cold enrichment. **6.** Tenesmus (painful rectal spasms with a strong urge to defecate but little passage of stool) may be a feature of cases with proctitis, as in shigellosis or amebiasis. **7.** Vomiting implies an acute infection (e.g., a toxin-mediated illness or food poisoning) but can also be prominent in a variety of systemic illnesses (e.g., malaria) and in intestinal obstruction. **8.** Asking patients whether anyone else they know is sick is a more efficient means of identifying a common source than is constructing a list of recently eaten foods. If a common source seems likely, specific foods can be investigated. See text for a discussion of bacterial food poisoning. **9.** Current antibiotic therapy or a recent history of treatment suggests *Clostridium difficile* diarrhea (Chap. 123). Stop antibiotic treatment if possible and consider tests for *C. difficile* toxins. Antibiotic use may increase the risk of other infections, such as salmonellosis. **10.** See text (and Chap. 117) for a discussion of traveler's diarrhea. (*After Guerrant and Steiner; RL Guerrant, DA Bobak: N Engl J Med 325:327, 1991; with permission.*)

TABLE 122-2 POST-DIARRHEA COMPLICATIONS OF ACUTE INFECTIOUS DIARRHEAL ILLNESS

Complication	Comments
Chronic diarrhea • Lactase deficiency • Small-bowel bacterial overgrowth • Malabsorption syndromes (tropical and celiac sprue)	Occurs in ~1% of travelers with acute diarrhea • Protozoa account for ~1/3 of cases
Initial presentation or exacerbation of inflammatory bowel disease	May be precipitated by traveler's diarrhea
Irritable bowel syndrome	Occurs in ~10% of travelers with traveler's diarrhea
Reiter's syndrome (reactive arthritis)	Particularly likely after infection with invasive organisms (*Shigella, Salmonella, Campylobacter*)
Hemolytic-uremic syndrome (hemolytic anemia, thrombocytopenia, and renal failure)	Follows infection with Shiga toxin–producing bacteria (*Shigella dysenteriae* type 1 and enterohemorrhagic *Escherichia coli*)

Location Day-care centers have particularly high attack rates of enteric infections. Rotavirus is most common among children <2 years old, with attack rates of 75–100% among those exposed. *G. lamblia* is more common among older children, with somewhat lower attack rates. Other common organisms, often spread by fecal-oral contact, are *Shigella, Campylobacter jejuni*, and *Cryptosporidium*. A characteristic feature of infection among children attending day-care centers is the high rate of secondary cases among family members.

Similarly, hospitals are sites in which enteric infections are concentrated. In medical intensive-care units and pediatric wards, diarrhea is

TABLE 122-3 EPIDEMIOLOGY OF TRAVELER'S DIARRHEA

Etiologic Agent	Approximate Percentage of Cases	Comments
Enterotoxigenic *Escherichia coli*	15–50	Single most important agent, particularly in summertime in semitropical areas; percentage of cases ranges from 15% in Asia to 50% in Latin America
Enteroaggregative *E. coli*	20–35	Emerging enteric pathogen of worldwide distribution
Shigella and enteroinvasive *E. coli*	10–25	Major causes of fever and dysentery
Salmonella	5–10	Causes fever and dysentery
Campylobacter jejuni	3–15	More common in winter in semitropical areas; more common in Asia
Aeromonas	5	Important in Thailand
Plesiomonas	5	Related to tropical travel and seafood consumption
Vibrio cholerae	0–10	Most common in India and Asia; also common in Central and South America
Rotavirus and norovirus	10–40	Latin America, Asia, and Africa; norovirus associated with seafood ingestion on cruise ships
Entamoeba histolytica	5	Particularly important in Mexico and Thailand
Giardia lamblia	<2	Zoonotic reservoirs in northern United States; affects hikers and campers who drink from freshwater streams; contaminates water supplies in Russia
Cryptosporidium	2	Affects travelers to Russia, Mexico, and Africa; causes large-scale urban outbreaks in United States
Cyclospora	<1	Affects travelers to Nepal, Haiti, and Peru; contaminates water or food
Unknown	20	Illness improves with antibacterial therapy, implicating bacterial diarrhea

Source: After Dupont.

one of the most common manifestations of nosocomial infections. *C. difficile* is the predominant cause of nosocomial diarrhea among adults in the United States. Viral pathogens, especially rotavirus, can spread rapidly in pediatric wards. Enteropathogenic *E. coli* has been associated with outbreaks of diarrhea in nurseries for newborns. One-third of elderly patients in chronic-care institutions develop a significant diarrheal illness each year; more than half of these cases are caused by cytotoxin-producing *C. difficile*. Antimicrobial therapy can predispose to pseudomembranous colitis by altering the normal colonic flora and allowing the multiplication of *C. difficile* (Chap. 123).

Age Most of the morbidity and mortality from enteric pathogens involves children <5 years of age. Breast-fed infants are protected from contaminated food and water and derive some protection from maternal antibodies, but their risk of infection rises dramatically when they begin to eat solid foods. Infants and younger children are more likely than adults to develop rotavirus disease, while older children and adults are more commonly infected with norovirus. Other organisms with higher attack rates among children than among adults include enterotoxigenic, enteropathogenic, and enterohemorrhagic *E. coli*; *C. jejuni*; and *G. lamblia*. In children, the incidence of *Salmonella* infections is highest among those <1 year of age, while the attack rate for *Shigella* infections is greatest among those 6 months to 4 years of age.

Bacterial Food Poisoning If the history and the stool examination indicate a noninflammatory etiology of diarrhea and there is evidence of a common-source outbreak, questions concerning the ingestion of specific foods and the time of onset of the diarrhea after a meal can provide clues to the bacterial cause of the illness. Potential causes of bacterial food poisoning are shown in Table 122-4.

Bacterial disease caused by an enterotoxin elaborated outside the host, such as that due to *Staphylococcus aureus* or *B. cereus*, has the shortest incubation period (1–6 h) and generally lasts <12 h. Most cases of staphylococcal food poisoning are caused by contamination from

TABLE 122-4 BACTERIAL FOOD POISONING

Incubation Period, Organism	Symptoms	Common Food Sources
1–6 H		
Staphylococcus aureus	Nausea, vomiting, diarrhea	Ham, poultry, potato or egg salad, mayonnaise, cream pastries
Bacillus cereus	Nausea, vomiting, diarrhea	Fried rice
8–16 H		
Clostridium perfringens	Abdominal cramps, diarrhea (vomiting rare)	Beef, poultry, legumes, gravies
B. cereus	Abdominal cramps, diarrhea (vomiting rare)	Meats, vegetables, dried beans, cereals
>16 H		
Vibrio cholerae	Watery diarrhea	Shellfish
Enterotoxigenic *Escherichia coli*	Watery diarrhea	Salads, cheese, meats, water
Enterohemorrhagic *E. coli*	Bloody diarrhea	Ground beef, roast beef, salami, raw milk, raw vegetables, apple juice
Salmonella spp.	Inflammatory diarrhea	Beef, poultry, eggs, dairy products
Campylobacter jejuni	Inflammatory diarrhea	Poultry, raw milk
Shigella spp.	Dysentery	Potato or egg salad, lettuce, raw vegetables
Vibrio parahaemolyticus	Dysentery	Mollusks, crustaceans

infected human carriers. Staphylococci can multiply at a wide range of temperatures; thus, if food is left to cool slowly and remains at room temperature after cooking, the organisms will have the opportunity to form enterotoxin. Outbreaks following picnics where potato salad, mayonnaise, and cream pastries have been served offer classic examples of staphylococcal food poisoning. Diarrhea, nausea, vomiting, and abdominal cramping are common, while fever is less so.

B. cereus can produce either a syndrome with a short incubation period—the *emetic* form, mediated by a staphylococcal type of enterotoxin—or one with a longer incubation period (8–16 h)—the *diarrheal* form, caused by an enterotoxin resembling *E. coli* LT, in which diarrhea and abdominal cramps are characteristic but vomiting is uncommon. The emetic form of *B. cereus* food poisoning is associated with contaminated fried rice; the organism is common in uncooked rice, and its heat-resistant spores survive boiling. If cooked rice is not refrigerated, the spores can germinate and produce toxin. Frying before serving may not destroy the preformed, heat-stable toxin.

Food poisoning due to *Clostridium perfringens* also has a slightly longer incubation period (8–14 h) and results from the survival of heat-resistant spores in inadequately cooked meat, poultry, or legumes. After ingestion, toxin is produced in the intestinal tract, causing moderately severe abdominal cramps and diarrhea; vomiting is rare, as is fever. The illness is self-limited, rarely lasting >24 h.

Not all food poisoning has a bacterial cause. Nonbacterial agents of short-incubation food poisoning include capsaicin, which is found in hot peppers, and a variety of toxins found in fish and shellfish (Chap. 391).

LABORATORY EVALUATION

Many cases of noninflammatory diarrhea are self-limited or can be treated empirically, and in these instances the clinician may not need to determine a specific etiology. Potentially pathogenic *E. coli* cannot be distinguished from normal fecal flora by routine culture, and tests to detect enterotoxins are not available in most clinical laboratories. In situations in which cholera is a concern, stool should be cultured on thiosulfate–citrate–bile salts–sucrose (TCBS) agar. A latex agglutination test has made the rapid detection of rotavirus in stool practical for many laboratories, while reverse-transcriptase polymerase chain reaction and specific antigen enzyme immunoassays have been developed for the identification of norovirus. At least three stool specimens should be examined for *Giardia* cysts or stained for *Cryptosporidium* if the level of clinical suspicion regarding the involvement of these organisms is high.

All patients with fever and evidence of inflammatory disease acquired outside the hospital should have stool cultured for *Salmonella*, *Shigella*, and *Campylobacter*. *Salmonella* and *Shigella* can be selected on MacConkey's agar as non-lactose-fermenting (colorless) colonies or can be grown on *Salmonella-Shigella* agar or in selenite enrichment broth, both of which inhibit most organisms except these pathogens. Evaluation of nosocomial diarrhea should initially focus on *C. difficile*; stool culture for other pathogens in this setting has an extremely low yield and is not cost-effective. Toxins A and B produced by pathogenic strains of *C. difficile* can be detected by rapid enzyme immunoassays and latex agglutination tests (Chap. 123). Isolation of *C. jejuni* requires inoculation of fresh stool onto selective growth medium and incubation at 42°C in a microaerophilic atmosphere. In many laboratories in the United States, *E. coli* O157:H7 is among the most common pathogens isolated from visibly bloody stools. Strains of this enterohemorrhagic serotype can be identified in specialized laboratories by serotyping but also can be identified presumptively in hospital laboratories as lactose-fermenting, indole-positive colonies of sorbitol nonfermenters (white colonies) on sorbitol MacConkey plates. Fresh stools should be examined for amebic cysts and trophozoites.

℞ INFECTIOUS DIARRHEA OR BACTERIAL FOOD POISONING

In many cases, a specific diagnosis is not necessary or not available to guide treatment. The clinician can proceed with the information obtained from the history, stool examination, and evaluation of dehydration severity. Empirical regimens for the treatment of traveler's diarrhea are listed in **Table 122-5**.

The mainstay of treatment is adequate rehydration. The treatment of cholera and other dehydrating diarrheal diseases was revolutionized by

---

TABLE 122-5 TREATMENT OF TRAVELER'S DIARRHEA ON THE BASIS OF CLINICAL FEATURES

Clinical Syndrome	Suggested Therapy
Watery diarrhea (no blood in stool, no fever), 1 or 2 unformed stools per day without distressing enteric symptoms	Oral fluids (Pedialyte, Lytren, or flavored mineral water) and saltine crackers
Watery diarrhea (no blood in stool, no fever), 1 or 2 unformed stools per day with distressing enteric symptoms	Bismuth subsalicylate (for adults): 30 mL or 2 tablets (262 mg/tablet) every 30 min for 8 doses; or loperamide[a]: 4 mg initially followed by 2 mg after passage of each unformed stool, not to exceed 8 tablets (16 mg) per day (prescription dose) or 4 caplets (8 mg) per day (over-the-counter dose); drugs can be taken for 2 days
Watery diarrhea (no blood in stool, no distressing abdominal pain, no fever), >2 unformed stools per day	Antibacterial drug[b] plus (for adults) loperamide[a] (see dose above)
Dysentery (passage of bloody stools) or fever (>37.8°C)	Antibacterial drug[b]
Vomiting, minimal diarrhea	Bismuth subsalicylate (for adults; see dose above)
Diarrhea in infants (<2 y old)	Fluids and electrolytes (Pedialyte, Lytren); continue feeding, especially with breast milk; seek medical attention for moderate dehydration, fever lasting >24 h, bloody stools, or diarrhea lasting more than several days
Diarrhea in pregnant women	Fluids and electrolytes; can consider attapulgite, 3 g initially, with dose repeated after passage of each unformed stool or every 2 h (whichever is earlier), for a total dosage of 9 g/d; seek medical attention for persistent or severe symptoms
Diarrhea despite trimethoprim-sulfamethoxazole prophylaxis	Fluoroquinolone—with loperamide[a] (see dose above) if no fever and no blood in stool, alone in cases of fever/dysentery
Diarrhea despite fluoroquinolone prophylaxis	Bismuth subsalicylate (see dose above) for mild to moderate disease; consult physician for moderate to severe disease or if disease persists

[a]Loperamide should not be used by patients with fever or dysentery; its use may prolong diarrhea in patients with infection due to *Shigella* or other invasive organisms.
[b]The recommended antibacterial drugs are as follows:
Travel to high-risk country other than Thailand:
Adults: (1) A fluoroquinolone such as ciprofloxacin, 750 mg as a single dose or 500 mg bid for 3 days; levofloxacin, 500 mg as a single dose or 500 mg qd for 3 days; or norfloxacin, 800 mg as a single dose or 400 mg bid for 3 days. (2) Azithromycin, 1000 mg as a single dose or 500 mg qd for 3 days. (3) Rifaximin, 200 mg tid or 400 mg bid for 3 days (not recommended for use in dysentery).
Children: Azithromycin, 10 mg/kg on day 1, 5 mg/kg on days 2 and 3 if diarrhea persists.

Alternative agent: furazolidone, 7.5 mg/kg per day in four divided doses for 5 days.
Travel to Thailand (with risk of fluoroquinolone-resistant *Campylobacter*):
Adults: Azithromycin (at above dose for adults). Alternative agent: a fluoroquinolone (at above doses for adults).
Children: Same as for children traveling to other areas (see above).
All patients should take oral fluids (Pedialyte, Lytren, or flavored mineral water) plus saltine crackers. If diarrhea becomes moderate or severe, if fever persists, or if bloody stools or dehydration develops, the patient should seek medical attention.
Source: After Dupont.

the promotion of oral rehydration solutions, the efficacy of which depends on the fact that glucose-facilitated absorption of sodium and water in the small intestine remains intact in the presence of cholera toxin. The use of oral rehydration solutions has reduced mortality due to cholera from >50% (in untreated cases) to <1%. The World Health Organization recommends a solution containing 3.5 g sodium chloride, 2.5 g sodium bicarbonate, 1.5 g potassium chloride, and 20 g glucose (or 40 g sucrose) per liter of water. Oral rehydration solutions containing rice or cereal as the carbohydrate source may be even more effective than glucose-based solutions, and the addition of L-histidine may reduce the frequency and volume of stool output. Patients who are severely dehydrated or in whom vomiting precludes the use of oral therapy should receive IV solutions such as Ringer's lactate.

Although most secretory forms of traveler's diarrhea—usually due to enterotoxigenic and enteroaggregative E. coli—can be treated effectively with rehydration, bismuth subsalicylate, or antiperistaltic agents, antimicrobial agents can shorten the duration of illness from 3–4 days to 24–36 h. Changes in diet have not been shown to have an impact on the duration of illness, while the efficacy of probiotics continues to be debated.

Antibiotic treatment for children who present with bloody diarrhea raises special concerns. Laboratory studies of enterohemorrhagic E. coli strains have demonstrated that a number of antibiotics induce replication of Shiga toxin–producing lambdoid bacteriophages, significantly increasing toxin production by these strains. Clinical studies have supported these laboratory results, and antibiotics are not recommended for the treatment of enterohemorrhagic E. coli infections in children.

PROPHYLAXIS

Improvements in hygiene to limit fecal-oral spread of enteric pathogens will be necessary if the prevalence of diarrheal diseases is to be significantly reduced in developing countries. Travelers can reduce their risk of diarrhea by eating only hot, freshly cooked food; by avoiding raw vegetables, salads, and unpeeled fruit; and by drinking only boiled or treated water and avoiding ice. Historically, few travelers to tourist destinations adhere to these dietary restrictions. However, an intensive hygienic effort in Jamaica involving government, hotel, and tourism agencies led to a decrease in the incidence of traveler's diarrhea by 72% from 1996 to 2002.

Bismuth subsalicylate is an inexpensive agent for the prophylaxis of traveler's diarrhea; it is taken at a dosage of 2 tablets (525 mg) four times a day. Treatment appears to be effective and safe for up to 3 weeks. Prophylactic antimicrobial agents, although effective, are not generally recommended for the prevention of traveler's diarrhea, ex-

cept when travelers are immunosuppressed or have other underlying illnesses that place them at high risk for morbidity from gastrointestinal infection. The risk of side effects and the possibility of developing an infection with a drug-resistant organism or with more harmful, invasive bacteria make it more reasonable to institute an empirical short course of treatment if symptoms develop. The recent availability of effective nonabsorbed antibiotics such as rifaximin may lead to new prophylactic options.

The possibility of exerting a major impact on the worldwide morbidity and mortality associated with diarrheal diseases has led to intense efforts to develop effective vaccines against the common bacterial and viral enteric pathogens. Recent research has yielded promising advances in the development of vaccines against rotavirus, *Shigella*, *V. cholerae*, *S. typhi*, and enterotoxigenic *E. coli*.

FURTHER READINGS

AL-ABRI SS et al: Traveller's diarrhoea. Lancet Infect Dis 5:349, 2005

BARTLETT JG: Clinical practice. Antibiotic-associated diarrhea. N Engl J Med 346:334, 2002

DUPONT HL: Travelers' diarrhea, in *Infections of the Gastrointestinal Tract*, 2d ed, MJ Blaser et al (eds). Philadelphia, Lippincott Williams & Wilkins, 2002, Chap 19

GUERRANT RL, STEINER TS: Principles and syndromes of enteric infection, in *Mandell, Douglas and Bennett's Principles and Practice of Infectious Diseases*, 5th ed, GL Mandell et al (eds). Philadelphia, Churchill Livingstone, 2000, Chap 81

KOO HL, DUPONT HL: Current and future developments in travelers' diarrhea therapy. Expert Rev Anti Infect Ther 4:417, 2006

MUSHER DM, MUSHER BL: Contagious acute gastrointestinal infections. N Engl J Med 351:2417, 2004

OKHUYSEN PC: Current concepts in travelers' diarrhea: Epidemiology, antimicrobial resistance and treatment. Curr Opin Infect Dis 18:522, 2005

SAZAWAL S et al: Efficacy of probiotics in prevention of acute diarrhoea: A meta-analysis of masked, randomised, placebo-controlled trials. Lancet Infect Dis 6:374, 2006

TAUXE RV et al: Foodborne disease, in *Mandell, Douglas and Bennett's Principles and Practice of Infectious Diseases*, 5th ed, GL Mandell et al (eds). Philadelphia, Churchill Livingstone, 2000, Chap 87

WONG CS et al: The risk of the hemolytic-uremic syndrome after antibiotic treatment of *Escherichia coli* O157:H7 infections. N Engl J Med 342:1930, 2000

123 Clostridium difficile–Associated Disease, Including Pseudomembranous Colitis

Dale N. Gerding, Stuart Johnson

DEFINITION

Clostridium difficile–associated disease (CDAD) is a unique colon infection that is acquired almost exclusively in association with antimicrobial use and the consequent disruption of the normal colonic flora. The most commonly diagnosed diarrheal illness acquired in the hospital, CDAD results from the ingestion of spores of *C. difficile* that vegetate, multiply, and secrete toxins, causing diarrhea and pseudomembranous colitis (PMC).

ETIOLOGY AND EPIDEMIOLOGY

C. difficile is an obligately anaerobic, gram-positive, spore-forming bacillus whose spores are found widely in nature, particularly in the environment of hospitals and chronic-care facilities. CDAD occurs most frequently in

hospitals and nursing homes where the level of antimicrobial use is high and the environment is contaminated by *C. difficile* spores.

Clindamycin, ampicillin, and cephalosporins were the first antibiotics associated with CDAD. The second- and third-generation cephalosporins, particularly cefotaxime, ceftriaxone, cefuroxime, and ceftazidime, are agents frequently responsible for this condition, and the fluoroquinolones (ciprofloxacin, levofloxacin, gatifloxacin, and moxifloxacin) are the most recent drug class to be implicated in hospital outbreaks. Penicillin/β-lactamase-inhibitor combinations such as ticarcillin/clavulanate and piperacillin/tazobactam pose significantly less risk. However, all antibiotics, including vancomycin and metronidazole (the agents most commonly used to treat CDAD), have been found to carry a risk of subsequent CDAD. Rare cases are reported in patients without prior antibiotic exposure.

C. difficile is acquired exogenously, most frequently in the hospital, and is carried in the stool of symptomatic and asymptomatic patients. The rate of fecal colonization is often ≥20% among adult patients hospitalized for >1 week; in contrast, the rate is 1–3% among community residents. The risk of *C. difficile* acquisition increases in proportion to length of hospital stay. Asymptomatic fecal carriage of *C. difficile* in healthy neonates is very common, with rates often exceeding 50% during the first 6 months of life, but associated disease in this population is rare. Spores of *C. difficile* are found on environmental surfaces (where the organism can persist for months) and on the hands of hospital personnel who fail to practice good hand hygiene. Hospital epidemics of CDAD have been attributed to a single *C. difficile* strain and to multiple strains present simultaneously. Other identified risk factors for CDAD include older age, greater severity of underlying illness, gastrointestinal surgery, use of electronic rectal thermometers, enteral tube feeding, and antacid treatment. Use of proton pump inhibitors may be a risk factor.

PATHOLOGY AND PATHOGENESIS

Spores of toxigenic *C. difficile* are ingested, survive gastric acidity, germinate in the small bowel, and colonize the lower intestinal tract, where they elaborate two large toxins: toxin A, an enterotoxin, and toxin B, a cytotoxin. These toxins initiate processes resulting in the disruption of epithelial-cell barrier function, diarrhea, and pseudomembrane formation. Toxin A is a potent neutrophil chemoattractant, and both toxins glucosylate the GTP-binding proteins of the Rho subfamily that regulate the actin cell cytoskeleton. Disruption of the cytoskeleton results in loss of cell shape, adherence, and tight junctions, with consequent fluid leakage. A third toxin, binary toxin CDT, was previously found in only ~6% of strains but is present in all isolates of the newly recognized epidemic strain (see "Global Considerations," below); this toxin is related to *C. perfringens* iota toxin. Its role in the pathogenesis of CDAD has not yet been defined.

The pseudomembranes of PMC are confined to the colonic mucosa and initially appear as 1- to 2-mm whitish-yellow plaques. The intervening mucosa appears unremarkable, but, as the disease progresses, the pseudomembranes coalesce to form larger plaques and become confluent over the entire colon wall (Fig. 123-1). The whole colon is usually involved, but 10% of patients have rectal sparing. Viewed microscopically, the pseudomembranes have a mucosal attachment point and contain necrotic leukocytes, fibrin, mucus, and cellular debris. The epithelium is eroded and necrotic in focal areas, with neutrophil infiltration of the mucosa.

Patients colonized with *C. difficile* were initially thought to be at high risk for CDAD. However, four prospective studies have shown that colonized patients actually have a decreased risk of subsequent CDAD. At least three events are proposed as essential for the develop-

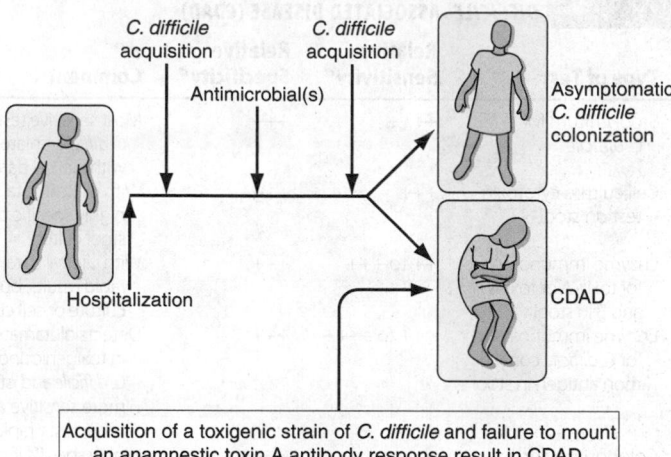

Pathogenesis model for *C. difficile* enteric disease

Acquisition of a toxigenic strain of *C. difficile* and failure to mount an anamnestic toxin A antibody response result in CDAD.

FIGURE 123-2 Pathogenesis model for hospital-acquired *Clostridium difficile*–associated diarrhea (CDAD). At least three events are integral to *C. difficile* pathogenesis. Exposure to antibiotics establishes susceptibility to infection. Once susceptible, the patient may acquire nontoxigenic (nonpathogenic) or toxigenic strains of *C. difficile* as a second event. Acquisition of toxigenic *C. difficile* may be followed by asymptomatic colonization or CDAD, depending on one or more additional events, including an inadequate host anamnestic IgG response to *C. difficile* toxin A.

ment of CDAD (Fig. 123-2). Exposure to antimicrobial agents is the first event and establishes susceptibility to *C. difficile* infection. The second event is exposure to toxigenic *C. difficile*. Given that the majority of patients do not develop CDAD after the first two events, a third event is clearly essential for its occurrence. Candidate third events include exposure to a *C. difficile* strain of particular virulence, exposure to antimicrobial agents especially likely to cause CDAD, and an inadequate host immune response. The host anamnestic serum IgG antibody response to toxin A of *C. difficile* is the most likely third event that determines which patients develop diarrhea and which patients remain asymptomatic. The majority of humans first develop antibody to *C. difficile* toxins when colonized asymptomatically during the first year of life. Infants are thought not to develop symptomatic CDAD because they lack suitable mucosal toxin receptors that develop later in life. In adulthood, serum levels of IgG antibody to toxin A increase more in response to infection in individuals who become asymptomatic carriers than in those who develop CDAD. For persons who develop CDAD, increasing levels of antitoxin A during treatment correlate with a lower risk of recurrence of CDAD.

GLOBAL CONSIDERATIONS

Rates and severity of CDAD in the United States, Canada, and Europe have increased markedly since the year 2000. Rates in U.S. hospitals tripled between 2000 and 2005. Hospitals in Montreal, Quebec, have reported rates four times higher than the 1997 baseline, with directly attributable mortality of 6.9% (increased from 1.5% previously). An epidemic strain, variously known as toxinotype III, REA type BI, PCR ribotype 027, and pulsed-field type NAP1, is thought to account for much of the increase in incidence and has been found in the United States, Canada, and Europe. The epidemic organism is characterized by (1) an ability to produce 16–23 times as much toxin A and toxin B as control strains in vitro; (2) the presence of a third toxin (binary toxin CDT); and (3) high-level resistance to all fluoroquinolones.

CLINICAL MANIFESTATIONS

Diarrhea is the most common manifestation caused by *C. difficile*. Stools are almost never grossly bloody and range from soft and unformed to watery or mucoid in consistency, with a characteristic odor. Patients may have as many as 20 bowel movements per day. Clinical and labora-

FIGURE 123-1 Autopsy specimen showing confluent pseudomembranes covering the cecum of a patient with pseudomembranous colitis. Note the sparing of the terminal ileum (*arrow*).

TABLE 123-1 RELATIVE SENSITIVITY AND SPECIFICITY OF DIAGNOSTIC TESTS FOR *CLOSTRIDIUM DIFFICILE*–ASSOCIATED DISEASE (CDAD)

Type of Test	Relative Sensitivity[a]	Relative Specificity[a]	Comment
Stool culture for *C. difficile*	++++	+++	Most sensitive test; specificity is ++++ if the *C. difficile* isolate tests positive for toxin; with clinical data, is diagnostic of CDAD
Cell culture cytotoxin test on stool	+++	++++	With clinical data, is diagnostic of CDAD; highly specific but not as sensitive as stool culture
Enzyme immunoassay for toxin A or toxins A and B in stool	++ to +++	+++	With clinical data, is diagnostic of CDAD; rapid results, but not as sensitive as stool culture or cell culture cytotoxin test
Enzyme immunoassay for *C. difficile* common antigen in stool	+++ to ++++	+++	Detects glutamate dehydrogenase found in toxigenic and nontoxigenic strains of *C. difficile* and other stool organisms; more sensitive and less specific than other tests; rapid results
Colonoscopy or sigmoidoscopy	+	++++	Highly specific if pseudomembranes are seen; insensitive compared with other tests

[a]According to both clinical and test-based criteria.
Note: ++++, >90%; +++, 71–90%; ++, 51–70%; +, ~50%.

tory findings include fever in 28% of cases, abdominal pain in 22%, and leukocytosis in 50%. When adynamic ileus (which is seen on x-ray in ~20% of cases) results in cessation of stool passage, the diagnosis of CDAD is frequently overlooked. A clue to the presence of unsuspected CDAD in these patients is unexplained leukocytosis, with ≥15,000 cells/μL. Such patients are at high risk for complications of *C. difficile* infection, particularly toxic megacolon and sepsis.

C. difficile diarrhea recurs after treatment in ~15–30% of cases, and this figure may be increasing. Recurrences may represent either relapses due to the same strain or reinfections with a new strain. Recurrence of clinical CDAD is likely to be a result of continued disruption of the normal fecal flora by the antibiotic used to treat CDAD.

DIAGNOSIS

The diagnosis of CDAD is based on a combination of clinical criteria: (1) diarrhea (≥3 unformed stools per 24 h for ≥2 days), with no other recognized cause; plus (2) toxin A or B detected in the stool, toxin-producing *C. difficile* detected by stool culture, or pseudomembranes seen in the colon. PMC is a more advanced form of CDAD and is visualized at endoscopy in only ~50% of patients with diarrhea who have a positive stool culture and toxin assay for *C. difficile* (Table 123-1). Endoscopy is a rapid diagnostic tool in seriously ill patients with suspected PMC and an acute abdomen, but a negative result in this examination does not rule out CDAD.

Despite the array of tests available for *C. difficile* and its toxins (Table 123-1), no single test has high sensitivity, high specificity, and rapid turnaround. The turnaround time for reporting of a positive result in the cell cytotoxicity test can be shortened to <24 h if cell cultures are examined at intervals as short as 4 h. However, this approach is labor intensive, and observation for 48 h is required for a conclusive test result. Most laboratory tests for toxins lack sensitivity. However, testing of multiple additional stool specimens is not recommended. Empirical treatment is appropriate if CDAD is strongly suspected on clinical grounds. Testing of asymptomatic patients is not recommended except for epidemiologic study purposes. In particular, so-called tests of cure following treatment are not recommended because many patients continue to harbor the organism and toxin after diarrhea has ceased and test results do not always predict recurrence of CDAD. Thus these results should not be used to restrict placement of patients in long-term-care or nursing home facilities.

℞ *CLOSTRIDIUM DIFFICILE*–ASSOCIATED DISEASE

PRIMARY CDAD When possible, discontinuation of any ongoing antimicrobial administration is recommended as the first step in treatment of CDAD. Earlier studies indicated that 15–23% of patients respond to this simple measure. However, with the advent of the current epidemic strain and the associated rapid clinical deterioration of some patients, prompt initiation of specific CDAD treatment has become the standard. General treatment guidelines include hydration and the avoidance of antiperistaltic agents and opiates, which may mask symptoms and possibly worsen disease. Nevertheless, antiperistaltic agents have been used safely with vancomycin or metronidazole for mild to moderate CDAD.

Although limited prospective randomized clinical trials showed no statistical differences among treatment agents for cessation of diarrhea (the primary outcome endpoint; Table 123-2), later observational studies suggest that response rates to metronidazole may have decreased. The clinical response rate for bacitracin is 10–20% lower than that for vancomycin; therefore, bacitracin use for first-line therapy is discouraged. All drugs, particularly vancomycin, should be given orally if possible. When IV metronidazole is administered, fecal bactericidal drug concentrations are achieved during acute diarrhea, and CDAD treatment has been successful; however, in the presence of adynamic ileus, IV metronidazole treatment of PMC has failed. In previous randomized trials, diarrhea response rates to oral therapy with vancomycin or metronidazole were ≥94%, but two recent observational studies found that metronidazole response rates had declined to 74% and 78%. Although the mean time to resolution of diarrhea is 2–4 days, the response to metronidazole may be much slower. Treatment should not be deemed a failure until a drug has been given for at least 6 days. On the basis of data for shorter courses of vancomycin (Table 123-2), it is recommended that metronidazole and vancomycin be given for at least 10 days, although no controlled comparisons are available. Although metronidazole is not approved for this indication by the U.S. Food and Drug Administration (FDA), most patients with mild to moderate illness respond to 500 mg given by mouth three times a day for 10 days; extension of the treatment period may be needed for slow responders. Because of the recent increase in metronidazole failures, patients treated with this drug should be monitored carefully for progressive defervescence (if fever is present), alleviation of abdominal pain and tenderness, decreases in the number of daily bowel movements, and decreases in the white blood cell (WBC) count. Clinical deterioration, with worsening signs and symptoms, or an unexplained increase in the WBC count during treatment are indications for a switch to vancomycin (usual dose, 125 mg orally four times a day). Although the use of vancomycin is discouraged for treatment of mildly to moderately ill patients, it is appropriate to use this agent for the initial treat-

TABLE 123-2 EXPECTED TREATMENT OUTCOMES BASED ON RANDOMIZED COMPARATIVE TRIALS OF ORAL THERAPY FOR *CLOSTRIDIUM DIFFICILE*–ASSOCIATED DISEASE

Treatment	Dose and Duration	Resolution of Diarrhea, %	Recurrence, %
Placebo or discontinuation of offending antibiotics	None	21	Unknown
Metronidazole	250 mg qid × 10 d	95	5
	250 mg qid × 10 d[a]	82	30
	500 mg tid × 10 d	94	17
Vancomycin	500 mg tid × 10 d	94	17
	500 mg qid × 10 d	100	15
	125 mg qid × 10 d[a]	91	19
	125 mg qid × 7 d	86	33
	125 mg qid × 5 d	75	Unknown
Teicoplanin	400 mg bid × 10 d	96	7
	100 mg bid × 10 d	96	8
Nitazoxanide	500 mg bid × 10 d	89	22
Fusidic acid	500 mg tid × 10 d	93	28
Bacitracin	25,000 U qid × 10 d	80	42

[a]Data from randomized trials reported in 2006.

ment of patients who appear seriously ill, particularly if they have a high WBC count (>15,000/μL); controlled clinical outcome data on vancomycin use against the epidemic strain are not available. A randomized prospective trial of the antiparasitic drug nitazoxanide showed that (although not approved by the FDA for this indication) it was at least as effective as metronidazole for the treatment of CDAD, providing a potential alternative to vancomycin and metronidazole.

RECURRENT CDAD Overall, ~15–30% of patients experience recurrences of CDAD, either as relapses caused by the original organism or as reinfections following treatment (Table 123-2). Recurrence rates are higher among patients ≥65 years old and among patients who remain in the hospital after the initial episode of CDAD. Patients who have a first recurrence of CDAD have a high rate of second recurrence (33–65%). In the first recurrence, re-treatment with metronidazole is comparable to treatment with vancomycin. Recurrent disease, once thought to be relatively mild, has been documented to pose a significant (11%) risk of serious complications (shock, megacolon, perforation, colectomy, or death within 30 days). There is no standard treatment for multiple recurrences, but long or repeated metronidazole courses should be avoided because of potential neurotoxicity. Approaches include the administration of vancomycin followed by the yeast *Saccharomyces boulardii*; the administration of vancomycin followed by synthetic fecal bacterial enema; and the intentional colonization of the patient with a nontoxigenic strain of *C. difficile*. None of these biotherapeutic approaches has been approved by the FDA for use in the United States. Other strategies include (1) the use of vancomycin in tapering doses or with pulse dosing every other day for 4–6 weeks and (2) sequential treatment with vancomycin (125 mg four times daily) followed by rifaximin (400 mg twice daily) for 14 days. IV immunoglobulin, which has also been used with some success, presumably provides antibodies to *C. difficile* toxins.

FULMINANT CDAD Fulminant (rapidly progressive and severe) CDAD presents the most difficult treatment challenge. Patients with fulminant disease often do not have diarrhea, and their illness mimics an acute surgical abdomen. Sepsis (hypotension, fever, tachycardia, leukocytosis) may result from severe CDAD. An acute abdomen (with or without toxic megacolon) may include signs of obstruction, ileus, colon-wall thickening, and ascites on abdominal CT, often with peripheral-blood leukocytosis (≥20,000 cells/μL). Whether or not the patient has diarrhea, the differential diagnosis of an acute abdomen, sepsis, or toxic megacolon should include CDAD if the patient has received antibiotics in the past 2 months. Cautious sigmoidoscopy or colonoscopy to visualize PMC and an abdominal CT examination are the best diagnostic tests in patients without diarrhea.

Medical management of fulminant CDAD is suboptimal because of the difficulty of delivering metronidazole or vancomycin to the colon by the oral route in the presence of ileus. Vancomycin (given via nasogastric tube and by retention enema) plus IV metronidazole have been used in uncontrolled studies with some success, but surgical colectomy may be life-saving if there is no response to medical management. The incidence of fulminant CDAD requiring colectomy appears to be increasing in the evolving epidemic.

PROGNOSIS
The mortality rate attributed to CDAD, previously found to be 0.6–3.5%, has reached 6.9% in recent outbreaks and is progressively higher with increasing age. Most patients recover, but recurrences are common.

PREVENTION AND CONTROL
Strategies for the prevention of CDAD are of two types: those aimed at preventing transmission of the organism to the patient and those aimed at reducing the risk of CDAD if the organism is transmitted. Transmission of *C. difficile* in clinical practice has been prevented by gloving of personnel, elimination of the use of contaminated electronic thermometers, and use of hypochlorite (bleach) solution for environmental decontamination of patients' rooms. Hand hygiene is critical; hand washing is recommended in CDAD outbreaks because alcohol hand gels are not sporicidal. CDAD outbreaks have been best controlled by restricting the use of specific antibiotics, such as clindamycin and second- and third-generation cephalosporins. Outbreaks of CDAD due to clindamycin-resistant strains have resolved promptly when clindamycin use was restricted.

FURTHER READINGS
HUBERT B et al: A portrait of the geographic dissemination of the *Clostridium difficile* North American pulsed-field type 1 strain and the epidemiology of *C. difficile*–associated disease in Quebec. Clin Infect Dis 44:238, 2007

JOHNSON S et al: Interruption of recurrent *Clostridium difficile*–associated diarrhea episodes by serial therapy with vancomycin and rifaximin. Clin Infect Dis 44:846, 2007

KYNE L et al: Association between antibody response to toxin A and protection against recurrent *Clostridium difficile* diarrhea. Lancet 357:189, 2001

—— et al: Asymptomatic carriage of *Clostridium difficile* and serum levels of IgG antibody against toxin A. N Engl J Med 342:390, 2000

LOO VG et al: A predominantly clonal multi-institutional outbreak of *Clostridium difficile*–associated diarrhea with high morbidity and mortality. N Engl J Med 353:2442, 2005

MCDONALD LC et al: *Clostridium difficile* infection in patients discharged from US short-stay hospitals, 1996-2003. Emerg Infect Dis 12:409, 2006

—— et al: An epidemic, toxin gene–variant strain of *Clostridium difficile*. N Engl J Med 353:2433, 2005

MCFARLAND LV: Alternative treatments for *Clostridium difficile* disease: What really works? J Med Microbiol 54:101, 2005

PEPIN J et al: The management and outcomes of a first recurrence of *Clostridium difficile* associated disease in Quebec. Clin Infect Dis 42:758, 2006

ZAR FA et al: A comparison of vancomycin and metronidazole for the treatment of *Clostridium difficile*–associated diarrhea, stratified by disease severity. Clin Infect Dis 45:302, 2007

124 Sexually Transmitted Infections: Overview and Clinical Approach
King K. Holmes

CLASSIFICATION AND EPIDEMIOLOGY

Worldwide, most adults acquire at least one sexually transmitted infection (STI), and many remain at risk for complications. Each year, for example, an estimated 6.2 million persons in the United States acquire a new genital human papillomavirus (HPV) infection, and many of these individuals are at risk for genital neoplasias. Certain STIs, such as syphilis, gonorrhea, HIV infection, hepatitis B, and chancroid, are most concentrated within "core populations" characterized by high rates of partner change, multiple concurrent partners, or "dense," highly connected sexual networks—e.g., involving prostitutes and their clients, some homosexual men, and persons involved in the use of illicit drugs, particularly crack cocaine and methamphetamine. Other STIs are distributed more evenly throughout societies. For example, chlamydial infections, genital infections with HPV, and genital herpes can spread widely, even in relatively low-risk populations.

In general, the product of three factors determines the initial rate of spread of any STI within a population: rate of sexual exposure of susceptible to infectious people, efficiency of transmission per exposure, and duration of infectivity of those infected. Accordingly, efforts to prevent and control STIs aim to decrease the rate of sexual exposure of susceptibles to infected persons (e.g., through individual counseling and efforts to change the norms of sexual behavior), to decrease the duration of infectivity (through early diagnosis and curative or suppressive treatment), and to decrease the efficiency of transmission (e.g., through promotion of condom use and safer sexual practices and recently through male circumcision).

TABLE 124-1 SEXUALLY TRANSMITTED AND SEXUALLY TRANSMISSIBLE MICROORGANISMS

Bacteria	Viruses	Other[a]
Transmitted in Adults Predominantly by Sexual Intercourse		
Neisseria gonorrhoeae	HIV (types 1 and 2)	Trichomonas vaginalis
Chlamydia trachomatis	Human T-cell lymphotropic virus type I	Phthirus pubis
Treponema pallidum	Herpes simplex virus type 2	
Haemophilus ducreyi	Human papillomavirus (multiple genotypes)	
Calymmatobacterium	Hepatitis B virus[b]	
granulomatis	Molluscum contagiosum virus	
Ureaplasma urealyticum		
Sexual Transmission Repeatedly Described but Not Well Defined or Not the Predominant Mode		
Mycoplasma hominis	Cytomegalovirus	Candida albicans
Mycoplasma genitalium	Human T-cell lymphotropic virus type II	Sarcoptes scabiei
Gardnerella vaginalis and	(?) Hepatitis C, D viruses	
other vaginal bacteria	Herpes simplex virus type 1	
Group B Streptococcus	(?) Epstein-Barr virus	
Mobiluncus spp.	Human herpesvirus type 8	
Helicobacter cinaedi		
Helicobacter fennelliae		
Transmitted by Sexual Contact Involving Oral-Fecal Exposure; of Declining Importance in Homosexual Men		
Shigella spp.	Hepatitis A virus	Giardia lamblia
Campylobacter spp.		Entamoeba histolytica

[a]Includes protozoa, ectoparasites, and fungi.
[b]Among U.S. patients for whom a risk factor can be ascertained, most hepatitis B virus infections are transmitted sexually or by injection drug use.

In all societies, STIs rank among the most common of all infectious diseases, with >30 infections now classified as predominantly sexually transmitted or as frequently sexually transmissible (Table 124-1). In developing countries, with three-quarters of the world's population and 90% of the world's STIs, such factors as population growth (especially in adolescent and young-adult age groups), rural-to-urban migration, wars, and poverty create exceptional vulnerability to disease resulting from risky sexual behaviors. During the 1990s, in China, Russia, the other states of the former Soviet Union, and South Africa, internal social structures changed rapidly as borders opened to the West, unleashing enormous new epidemics of HIV infection and other STIs. HIV has become the leading cause of death in some developing countries, and HPV and hepatitis B virus (HBV) remain important causes of cervical and hepatocellular carcinoma, respectively—two of the most common malignancies in the developing world. Sexually transmitted herpes simplex virus (HSV) infections now cause most genital ulcer disease throughout the world and an increasing proportion of cases of genital herpes in developing countries with generalized HIV epidemics, where the positive feedback loop between HSV and HIV transmission is a growing, intractable problem. Randomized trials of the efficacy of therapy against HSV-2 in preventing the acquisition or transmission of HIV infection will be completed in 2007–2008, and the outcome will help shape future efforts to prevent HIV infection. Globally, five curable STIs—gonorrhea, chlamydial infection, syphilis, chancroid, and trichomoniasis—caused ~350 million new infections annually in the mid-1990s. Up to 50% of women of reproductive age in developing countries have bacterial vaginosis (arguably acquired sexually). All six of these curable infections have been associated with increased risk of HIV transmission or acquisition.

In the United States, the prevalence of antibody to HSV-2 has begun to fall only recently (since the late 1990s), especially among adolescents and young adults; the decline is presumably due to delayed sexual debut, increased condom use, and lower rates of multiple (≥4) sex partners, as is well documented in the U.S. Youth Risk Behavior Surveillance System (YRBSS). Genital HPV remains the most common sexually transmitted pathogen in this country, infecting 60% of a cohort of initially HPV-negative, sexually active Washington state college women within 5 years in a study conducted from 1990 to 2000.

In industrialized countries, fear of HIV infection since the mid-1980s, coupled with widespread behavioral interventions and better-organized systems of care for the curable STIs, has helped curb the transmission of the latter diseases. Nonetheless, foci of hyperendemic transmission persist in the southeastern United States and in most large U.S. cities. Rates of gonorrhea and syphilis remain higher in the United States than in any other Western industrialized country. The remarkable resurgence of gonorrhea and syphilis among homosexual and bisexual men in many parts of the United States and Europe since the 1990s reflects increased risk-taking following the advent of potent antiretroviral therapy and has been accompanied by increasing HIV transmission in this group.

In the United States, the Centers for Disease Control and Prevention (CDC) has compiled reported rates of STIs since 1941. The incidence of reported gonorrhea peaked at 468 cases per 100,000 population in the mid-1970s, fell to a low of 112 cases per 100,000 in 2004, and rose slightly in 2005. Because of increased testing and more sensitive tests, the incidence of reported Chlamydia trachomatis infection has been increasing steadily since reporting began in 1984, reaching 333 cases per 100,000 in 2005. The incidence of primary and secondary syphilis per 100,000 peaked at 71 cases in 1946, fell rapidly to 3.9 cases in 1956, ranged from ~10 to 15 cases through 1987 (with markedly increased rates among homosexual men and African Americans), and then fell to a nadir of 2.1 cases in 2000–2001 (with rates falling most rapidly among heterosexual African Americans). Unfortunately, since 1996, with the introduction of highly active antiretroviral therapy and the increased use of "serosorting" (i.e., the avoidance by some homosexual men of unprotected sex with HIV-serodiscordant partners but not with HIV-seroconcordant partners, a strategy that provides no protection against STIs other than HIV infection), gonorrhea, syphilis, and chlamydial infection have had a remarkable resurgence among homosexual men in North America and Europe, and an outbreak of a rare type of chlamydial infection (lymphogranuloma venereum; LGV) that had virtually disappeared during the AIDS era has occurred.

MANAGEMENT OF COMMON SEXUALLY TRANSMITTED DISEASE (STD) SYNDROMES

Although other chapters discuss management of specific STIs, delineating treatment based on diagnosis of a specific infection, most patients are actually managed (at least initially) on the basis of presenting symptoms and signs and associated risk factors, even in industrialized countries. Table 124-2 lists some of the most common clinical STD syndromes and their microbial etiologies. Strategies for their management are outlined below. Chapters 181 and 182 address the management of infections with human retroviruses.

STD care and management begin with risk assessment and proceed to clinical assessment, diagnostic testing or screening, treatment, and prevention. Indeed, the routine care of any patient begins with risk assessment (e.g., for risk of heart disease, cancer). STD/HIV risk assessment is important in primary care, urgent care, and emergency care settings as well as in specialty clinics providing adolescent, prenatal, and family planning services. STD/HIV risk assessment guides interpretation of symptoms that could reflect an STD; decisions on screening or prophylactic/preventive treatment; risk reduction counseling and intervention (e.g., hepatitis B vaccination); and notification of partners of patients with known infections. Consideration of routine demographic data (e.g., gender, age, marital status, area of residence) is

TABLE 124-2 MAJOR STD SYNDROMES AND SEXUALLY TRANSMITTED MICROBIAL ETIOLOGIES

Syndrome	ST Microbial Etiologies
AIDS	HIV types 1 and 2
Urethritis: males	*Neisseria gonorrhoeae, Chlamydia trachomatis, Mycoplasma genitalium, Ureaplasma urealyticum* (?subspecies *urealyticum*), *Trichomonas vaginalis*, HSV
Epididymitis	*C. trachomatis, N. gonorrhoeae*
Lower genital tract infections: females	
Cystitis/urethritis	*C. trachomatis, N. gonorrhoeae*, HSV
Mucopurulent cervicitis	*C. trachomatis, N. gonorrhoeae, M. genitalium*
Vulvitis	*Candida albicans*, HSV
Vulvovaginitis	*C. albicans, T. vaginalis*
Bacterial vaginosis (BV)	BV-associated bacteria (see text)
Acute pelvic inflammatory disease	*N. gonorrhoeae, C. trachomatis*, BV-associated bacteria, *M. genitalium*, group B streptococci
Infertility	*N. gonorrhoeae, C. trachomatis*, BV-associated bacteria
Ulcerative lesions of the genitalia	HSV-1, HSV-2, *Treponema pallidum, Haemophilus ducreyi, C. trachomatis* (LGV strains), *Calymmatobacterium granulomatis*
Complications of pregnancy/puerperium	Several agents implicated
Intestinal infections	
Proctitis	*C. trachomatis, N. gonorrhoeae*, HSV, *T. pallidum*
Proctocolitis or enterocolitis	*Campylobacter* spp., *Shigella* spp., *Entamoeba histolytica*, other enteric pathogens
Enteritis	*Giardia lamblia*
Acute arthritis with urogenital infection or viremia	*N. gonorrhoeae* (e.g., DGI), *C. trachomatis* (e.g., Reiter's syndrome), HBV
Genital and anal warts	HPV (30 genital types)
Mononucleosis syndrome	CMV, HIV, EBV
Hepatitis	Hepatitis viruses, *T. pallidum*, CMV, EBV
Neoplasias	
Squamous cell dysplasias and cancers of the cervix, anus, vulva, vagina, or penis	HPV (especially types 16, 18, 31, 45)
Kaposi's sarcoma, body-cavity lymphomas	HHV-8
T cell leukemia	HTLV-I
Hepatocellular carcinoma	HBV
Tropical spastic paraparesis	HTLV-I
Scabies	*Sarcoptes scabiei*
Pubic lice	*Phthirus pubis*

Note: HSV, herpes simplex virus; LGV, lymphogranuloma venereum; DGI, disseminated gonococcal infection; HPV, human papillomavirus; CMV, cytomegalovirus; EBV, Epstein-Barr virus; HBV, hepatitis B virus; HTLV, human T-cell lymphotropic virus; HHV-8, human herpesvirus type 8.

a simple first step in STD/HIV risk assessment. For example, national guidelines now recommend routine screening of sexually active females ≤25 years of age for *C. trachomatis* infection. Table 124-3 provides a set of 10 STD/HIV risk-assessment questions that clinicians can pose verbally or that health care systems can adapt (with yes/no responses) into a routine self-administered questionnaire for use in clinics. The initial framing statement gives permission to discuss taboo topics.

Risk assessment is followed by clinical assessment (elicitation of information on specific current symptoms and signs of STDs). Confirmatory diagnostic tests (for persons with symptoms or signs) or screening tests (for those without symptoms or signs) may involve microscopic examination, culture, antigen detection tests, genetic probe or amplification tests, or serology. Initial syndrome-based treatment should cover the most likely causes. For certain syndromes, results of rapid tests can narrow the spectrum of this initial therapy (e.g., wet mount of vaginal fluid for women with vaginal discharge, Gram's stain of urethral discharge for men with urethral discharge, rapid plasma reagin test for genital ulcer). After the institution of treatment, STD management proceeds to the "4 C's" of prevention and control: contact tracing (see "Prevention and Control of STIs," below), ensuring

TABLE 124-3 TEN-QUESTION STD/HIV RISK ASSESSMENT

Framing Statement:
In order to provide the best care for you today and to understand your risk for certain infections, it is necessary for us to talk about your sexual behavior.

Screening Questions:
(1) Do you have any reason to think you might have a sexually transmitted disease? If so, what reason?
(2) For all adolescents <18 years old: Have you begun having any kind of sex yet?

STD History:
(3) Have you ever had any sexually transmitted diseases or any genital infections? If so, which ones?

Sexual Preference:
(4) Have you had sex with men, women, or both?

Injection Drug Use:
(5) Have you ever injected yourself ("shot up") with drugs? (If yes, have you ever shared needles or injection equipment?)
(6) Have you ever had sex with a gay or bisexual man or with anyone who had ever injected drugs?

Characteristics of Partner(s):
(7) Has your sex partner(s) had any sexually transmitted infections? If so, which ones?

STD Symptoms Checklist:
(8) Have you recently developed any of these symptoms?

For Men	**For Women**
(a) Discharge of pus (drip) from the penis	(a) Abnormal vaginal discharge (increased amount, abnormal odor, abnormal yellow color)
(b) Genital sores (ulcers) or rash	(b) Genital sores (ulcers), rash, or itching

Sexual Practices, Past 2 Months (for patients answering yes to any of the above questions, to guide examination and testing):
(9) Now I'd like to ask what parts of your body may have been sexually exposed to an STD (e.g., your penis, mouth, vagina, anus)?

Query about Interest in STD Screening Tests (for patients answering no to all of the above questions):
(10) Would you like to be tested for HIV or any other STDs today? (If yes, clinician can explore which STD and why.)

Source: Adapted from JR Curtis, KK Holmes, in KK Holmes et al (eds): *Sexually Transmitted Diseases*, 3d ed. New York, McGraw-Hill, 1999.

compliance with therapy, and counseling on risk reduction, including condom promotion and provision.

URETHRITIS IN MEN

Urethritis in men produces urethral discharge, dysuria, or both, usually without frequency of urination. Causes include *Neisseria gonorrhoeae, C. trachomatis, Mycoplasma genitalium, Ureaplasma urealyticum, Trichomonas vaginalis*, HSV, and perhaps adenovirus.

Until recently, *C. trachomatis* caused ~30–40% of cases of nongonococcal urethritis (NGU); however, the proportion of cases due to this organism may have declined in some populations served by effective chlamydial-control programs, and older men with urethritis appear less likely to have chlamydial infection. HSV and *T. vaginalis* each cause a small proportion of NGU cases in the United States. Recently, multiple studies have consistently implicated *M. genitalium* as a probable cause of many *Chlamydia*-negative cases. Fewer studies than in the past have implicated *Ureaplasma*; the ureaplasmas have been differentiated into *U. urealyticum* and *U. parvum*, and a few studies suggest that *U. urealyticum*—but not *U. parvum*—is associated with NGU. Coliform bacteria can cause urethritis in men who practice insertive anal intercourse. The initial diagnosis of urethritis in men currently includes specific tests only for *N. gonorrhoeae* and *C. trachomatis*. The following summarizes the approach to the patient with suspected urethritis:

1. *Establish the presence of urethritis.* If proximal-to-distal "milking" of the urethra does not express a purulent or mucopurulent discharge, even after the patient has not voided for several hours (or preferably overnight), a Gram's-stained smear of overt discharge or of an anterior urethral specimen obtained by passage of a small

urethrogenital swab 2–3 cm into the urethra usually reveals ≥5 neutrophils per 1000× field in areas containing cells; in gonococcal infection, such a smear usually reveals gram-negative intracellular diplococci as well. Alternatively, the centrifuged sediment of the first 20–30 mL of voided urine—ideally collected as the first morning specimen—can be examined for inflammatory cells, either by microscopy showing ≥10 leukocytes per high-power field or by the leukocyte esterase test. Patients with symptoms who lack objective evidence of urethritis may have functional rather than organic problems and generally do not benefit from repeated courses of antibiotics.

2. *Evaluate for complications or alternative diagnoses.* A brief history and examination will exclude epididymitis and systemic complications, such as disseminated gonococcal infection (DGI) and Reiter's syndrome. Although digital examination of the prostate gland seldom contributes to the evaluation of sexually active young men with urethritis, men with dysuria who lack evidence of urethritis as well as sexually inactive men with urethritis should undergo prostate palpation, urinalysis, and urine culture to exclude bacterial prostatitis and cystitis.

3. *Evaluate for gonococcal and chlamydial infection.* An absence of typical gram-negative diplococci on Gram's-stained smear of urethral exudate containing inflammatory cells warrants a preliminary diagnosis of NGU and should lead to testing of the urethral specimen for *C. trachomatis.* However, an increasing proportion of men with symptoms and/or signs of urethritis are simultaneously assessed for infection with *N. gonorrhoeae* and *C. trachomatis* by "multiplex" nucleic acid amplification tests (NAATs) of early-morning first-voided urine. Culture or NAAT for *N. gonorrhoeae* may be positive when Gram's staining is negative; certain strains of *N. gonorrhoeae* can result in negative urethral Gram's stains in up to 30% of cases of urethritis. Results of tests for gonococcal and chlamydial infection predict the patient's prognosis (with greater risk for recurrent NGU if neither chlamydiae nor gonococci are found than if either is detected) and can guide both the counseling given to the patient and the management of the patient's sexual partner(s).

4. *Treat urethritis promptly, while test results are pending.*

Table 124-4 summarizes the steps in management of sexually active men with urethral discharge and/or dysuria.

TABLE 124-4 MANAGEMENT OF URETHRAL DISCHARGE IN MEN

Usual causes	Usual initial evaluation
Chlamydia trachomatis	Demonstration of urethral discharge or pyuria
Neisseria gonorrhoeae	Exclusion of local or systemic complications
Mycoplasma genitalium	Urethral Gram's stain to confirm urethritis,
Ureaplasma urealyticum	detect gram-negative diplococci
Trichomonas vaginalis	Test for *N. gonorrhoeae, C. trachomatis*
Herpes simplex virus	

Initial Treatment for Patient and Partners

Treat gonorrhea (unless excluded):	plus	Treat chlamydial infection:
Ceftriaxone, 125 mg IM; *or* Cefpodoxime, 400 mg PO; *or* Cefixime, 400 mg PO*a*		Azithromycin, 1 g PO; *or* Doxycycline, 100 mg bid for 7 days

Management of Recurrence

Confirm objective evidence of urethritis. If patient was reexposed to untreated or new partner, repeat treatment of patient and partner.
If patient was not reexposed, consider infection with *T. vaginalis*b or doxycycline-resistant *M. genitalium* or *Ureaplasma,* and consider treatment with metronidazole, azithromycin, or both.

*a*Updates on the availability of cefixime can be obtained from the Centers for Disease Control and Prevention or state health departments.
*b*In men, the diagnosis of *T. vaginalis* infection requires culture (or nucleic acid amplification test, where available) of early-morning first-voided urine sediment or of a urethral swab specimen obtained before voiding.

URETHRITIS IN MEN

In practice, if Gram's stain does not reveal gonococci, urethritis is treated with a regimen effective for NGU, such as azithromycin (1.0 g PO in a single dose) or doxycycline (100 mg PO bid for 7 days). Both are effective, although azithromycin may give better results in *M. genitalium* infection. If gonococci are demonstrated by Gram's stain or if no diagnostic tests are performed to exclude gonorrhea definitively, treatment should include a single-dose regimen for gonorrhea (Chap. 137) plus azithromycin or doxycycline treatment for *C. trachomatis,* which frequently occurs as a urethral co-infection in men with gonococcal urethritis. Sexual partners should be tested for gonorrhea and chlamydial infection and should receive the same regimen given to the male index case. Patients with confirmed persistence or recurrence of urethritis after treatment should be re-treated with the initial regimen if they did not comply with the original treatment or were reexposed to an untreated partner. Otherwise, an intraurethral swab specimen and a first-voided urine sample should be tested for *T. vaginalis* (currently best done by culture, although NAATs appear to be more sensitive and are likely to become commercially available in the future). If compliance with initial treatment is confirmed and reexposure excluded, the recommended treatment is with metronidazole or tinidazole (2 g PO in a single dose) plus azithromycin (1 g PO in a single dose); the azithromycin component is especially important if this drug has not been given during initial therapy.

EPIDIDYMITIS

Acute epididymitis, almost always unilateral, produces pain, swelling, and tenderness of the epididymis, with or without symptoms or signs of urethritis. This condition must be differentiated from testicular torsion, tumor, and trauma. Torsion, a surgical emergency, usually occurs in the second or third decade of life and produces a sudden onset of pain, elevation of the testicle within the scrotal sac, rotation of the epididymis from a posterior to an anterior position, and absence of blood flow on Doppler examination or ^{99m}Tc scan. Persistence of symptoms after a course of therapy for epididymitis suggests the possibility of testicular tumor or of a chronic granulomatous disease, such as tuberculosis. In sexually active men under age 35, acute epididymitis is caused most frequently by *C. trachomatis* and less commonly by *N. gonorrhoeae* and is usually associated with overt or subclinical urethritis. Acute epididymitis occurring in older men or following urinary tract instrumentation is usually caused by urinary pathogens. Similarly, epididymitis in men who have practiced insertive rectal intercourse is often caused by Enterobacteriaceae. These men usually have no urethritis but do have bacteriuria.

EPIDIDYMITIS

Ceftriaxone (250 mg as a single dose IM) followed by doxycycline (100 mg PO twice daily for 10 days) constitutes effective treatment for epididymitis caused by *N. gonorrhoeae* or *C. trachomatis.* Fluoroquinolones are no longer recommended for treatment of gonorrhea in the United States because of the emergence of resistant strains of *N. gonorrhoeae,* especially (but not only) among homosexual men **(Fig. 124-1).** Levofloxacin (500 mg PO once daily for 10 days) is also effective for syndrome-based initial treatment of epididymitis when infection with Enterobacteriaceae is suspected; however, this regimen should probably be combined with effective therapy for possible gonococcal or chlamydial infection unless bacteriuria with Enterobacteriaceae is confirmed.

URETHRITIS AND THE URETHRAL SYNDROME IN WOMEN

C. trachomatis, N. gonorrhoeae, and occasionally HSV cause symptomatic urethritis—known as the urethral syndrome in women—that is characterized by "internal" dysuria (usually without urinary urgency or frequency), pyuria, and an absence of *Escherichia coli* and other uropathogens in urine at counts of ≥10²/mL. In contrast, the dysuria associated with vulvar herpes or vulvovaginal candidiasis (and perhaps with trichomoniasis) is often described as "external," being caused by painful contact of urine with the inflamed or ulcerated labia

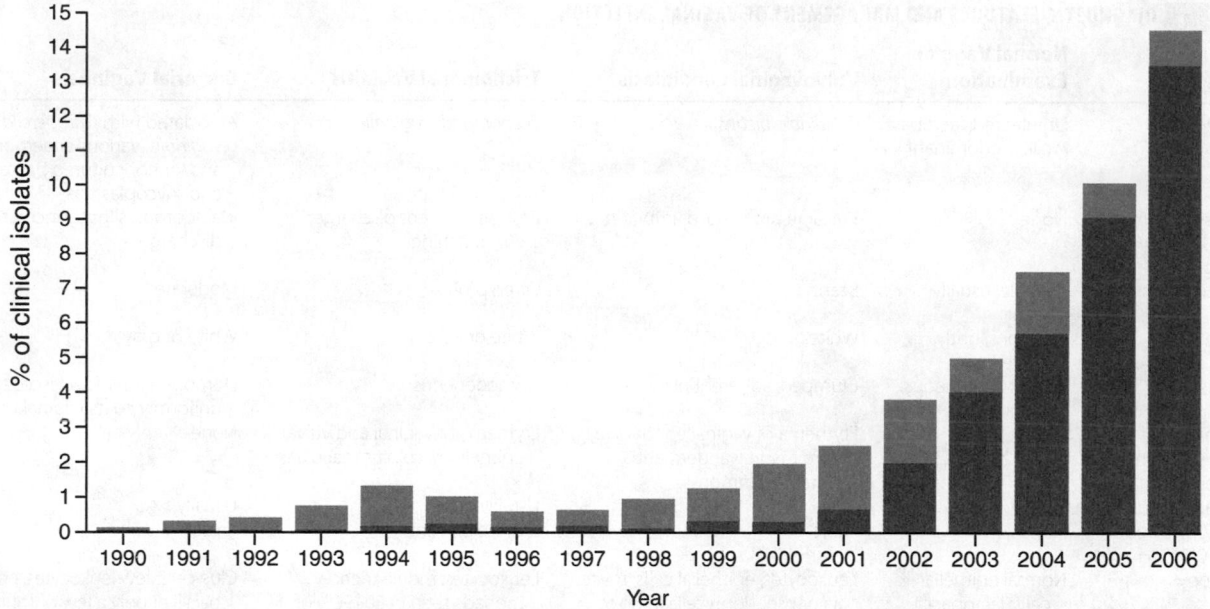

FIGURE 124-1 Percentage of *N. gonorrhoeae* isolates with intermediate resistance or resistance to ciprofloxacin, by year: Gonococcal Isolate Surveillance Project, United States, 1990–2006. Data for 2006 are preliminary (January–June only). ■, Intermediate resistance [ciprofloxacin minimum inhibitory concentrations (MICs) of 0.125–0.500 μg/mL]. ■, Resistance (ciprofloxacin MICs of ≥1.0 μg/mL). *(From Centers for Disease Control and Prevention: MMWR 56:332, 2007.)*

or introitus. Acute onset, association with urinary urgency or frequency, hematuria, or suprapubic bladder tenderness suggests bacterial cystitis. Among women with symptoms of acute bacterial cystitis, costovertebral pain and tenderness or fever suggests acute pyelonephritis. The management of bacterial urinary tract infection (UTI) is discussed in Chap. 282.

Signs of vulvovaginitis, coupled with symptoms of external dysuria, suggest vulvar infection (e.g., with HSV or *Candida albicans*). Among dysuric women without signs of vulvovaginitis, bacterial UTI must be differentiated from the urethral syndrome by assessment of risk, evaluation of the pattern of symptoms and signs, and specific microbiologic testing. An STI etiology of the urethral syndrome is suggested by young age, more than one current sexual partner, a new partner within the past month, a partner with urethritis, or coexisting mucopurulent cervicitis (see below). The finding of a single urinary pathogen, such as *E. coli* or *Staphylococcus saprophyticus*, at a concentration of $\geq 10^2$/mL in a properly collected specimen of midstream urine from a dysuric woman with pyuria indicates probable bacterial UTI, whereas pyuria with $<10^2$ conventional uropathogens per milliliter of urine ("sterile" pyuria) suggests acute urethral syndrome due to *C. trachomatis* or *N. gonorrhoeae*. Gonorrhea and chlamydial infection should be sought by specific tests (e.g., NAATs on the first 10 mL of voided urine). Among dysuric women with sterile pyuria caused by infection with *N. gonorrhoeae* or *C. trachomatis*, appropriate treatment alleviates dysuria.

VULVOVAGINAL INFECTIONS

Abnormal Vaginal Discharge If directly questioned about vaginal discharge during routine health checkups, many women acknowledge having nonspecific symptoms of vaginal discharge that do not correlate with objective signs of inflammation or with actual infection. However, unsolicited reporting of abnormal vaginal discharge does suggest bacterial vaginosis or trichomoniasis. Specifically, an abnormally increased amount or an abnormal odor of the discharge is associated with one or both of these conditions. Cervical infection with *N. gonorrhoeae* or *C. trachomatis* does not appear to cause an increased amount or abnormal odor of discharge, but cervicitis, like trichomoniasis, can include the production of an increased number of neutrophils in vaginal fluid, resulting in a yellow color. Vulvar conditions such as genital herpes or vulvovaginal candidiasis can cause vulvar pruritus, burning, irritation, or lesions as well as external dysuria (as urine passes over the inflamed vulva) or vulvar dyspareunia.

Certain vulvovaginal infections may have serious sequelae. Trichomoniasis, bacterial vaginosis, and vulvovaginal candidiasis have all been associated with increased risk of acquisition of HIV infection. Vaginal trichomoniasis and bacterial vaginosis early in pregnancy independently predict premature onset of labor. Bacterial vaginosis can also lead to anaerobic bacterial infection of the endometrium and salpinges. Vaginitis may be an early and prominent feature of toxic shock syndrome, and recurrent or chronic vulvovaginal candidiasis develops with increased frequency among women with systemic illnesses, such as diabetes mellitus or HIV-related immunosuppression (although only a very small proportion of women with recurrent vulvovaginal candidiasis in industrialized countries actually have a serious predisposing illness).

Thus vulvovaginal symptoms or signs warrant careful evaluation, including pelvic examination, simple rapid diagnostic tests, and appropriate therapy specific for the anatomic site and type of infection. Unfortunately, a survey in the United States indicated that clinicians seldom perform the tests required to establish the cause of such symptoms. Further, comparison of telephone and office management of vulvovaginal symptoms has documented the inaccuracy of the former, and comparison of evaluations by nurse-midwives with those by physician-practitioners showed that the practitioners' clinical evaluations correlated poorly both with the nurses' evaluations and with diagnostic tests. The diagnosis and treatment of the three most common types of vaginal infection are summarized in Table 124-5.

Inspection of the vulva and perineum may reveal tender genital ulcerations (typically due to HSV infection, occasionally due to chancroid) or fissures (typically due to vulvovaginal candidiasis) or discharge visible at the introitus before insertion of a speculum (suggestive of bacterial vaginosis or trichomoniasis). Speculum examination permits the clinician to discern whether the discharge in fact looks abnormal and whether any abnormal discharge in the vagina emanates from the cervical os (mucoid and, if abnormal, yellow) or from the vagina (not mucoid, since the vaginal epithelium does not produce mucus). Symptoms or signs of abnormal vaginal discharge should prompt testing of vaginal fluid for pH, for a fishy odor when mixed with 10% KOH, and for certain microscopic features when mixed with saline (motile trichomonads and/or "clue cells") and with

TABLE 124-5 DIAGNOSTIC FEATURES AND MANAGEMENT OF VAGINAL INFECTION

Feature	Normal Vaginal Examination	Vulvovaginal Candidiasis	Trichomonal Vaginitis	Bacterial Vaginosis
Etiology	Uninfected; lactobacilli predominant	*Candida albicans*	*Trichomonas vaginalis*	Associated with *Gardnerella vaginalis*, various anaerobic and/or noncultured bacteria, and mycoplasmas
Typical symptoms	None	Vulvar itching and/or irritation	Profuse purulent discharge; vulvar itching	Malodorous, slightly increased discharge
Discharge				
Amount	Variable; usually scant	Scant	Often profuse	Moderate
Color[a]	Clear or slightly white	White	White or yellow	White or gray
Consistency	Nonhomogeneous, floccular	Clumped; adherent plaques	Homogeneous	Homogeneous, low viscosity; uniformly coats vaginal walls
Inflammation of vulvar or vaginal epithelium	None	Erythema of vaginal epithelium, introitus; vulvar dermatitis, fissures common	Erythema of vaginal and vulvar epithelium; colpitis macularis	None
pH of vaginal fluid[b]	Usually ≤4.5	Usually ≤4.5	Usually ≥5.0	Usually >4.5
Amine ("fishy") odor with 10% KOH	None	None	May be present	Present
Microscopy[c]	Normal epithelial cells; lactobacilli predominant	Leukocytes, epithelial cells; mycelia or pseudomycelia in up to 80% of *C. albicans* culture-positive persons with typical symptoms	Leukocytes; motile trichomonads seen in 80–90% of symptomatic patients, less often in the absence of symptoms	Clue cells; few leukocytes; no lactobacilli or only a few outnumbered by profuse mixed flora, nearly always including *G. vaginalis* plus anaerobic species on Gram's stain (Nugent's score ≥7)
Other laboratory findings		Isolation of *Candida* spp.	Isolation of *T. vaginalis* or positive NAAT[d]	
Usual treatment	None	Azole cream, tablet, or suppository—e.g., miconazole 100-mg vaginal suppository or clotrimazole 100-mg vaginal tablet, once daily for 7 days Fluconazole, 150 mg orally (single dose)	Metronidazole or tinidazole, 2 g orally (single dose) Metronidazole, 500 mg PO bid for 7 days	Metronidazole, 500 mg PO bid for 7 days Clindamycin, 2% cream, one full applicator vaginally each night for 7 days
Usual management of sexual partner	None	None; topical treatment if candidal dermatitis of penis is detected	Examination for STD; treatment with metronidazole, 2 g PO (single dose)	Examination for STD; no treatment if normal

[a]Color of discharge is best determined by examination against the white background of a swab.
[b]pH determination is not useful if blood is present.
[c]To detect fungal elements, vaginal fluid is digested with 10% KOH prior to microscopic examination; to examine for other features, fluid is mixed (1:1) with physiologic saline.

Gram's stain is also excellent for detecting yeasts (less predictive of vulvovaginitis) and pseudomycelia or mycelin (strongly predictive of vulvovaginitis) and for distinguishing normal flora from the mixed flora seen in bacterial vaginosis, but it is less sensitive than the saline preparation for detection of *T. vaginalis*.
[d]NAAT, nucleic acid amplification test (where available).

10% KOH (pseudohyphae or hyphae indicative of vulvovaginal candidiasis). Additional objective laboratory tests useful for establishing the cause of abnormal vaginal discharge include Gram's staining to detect alterations in the vaginal flora; card tests for bacterial vaginosis, as described below; and a DNA probe test (the Affirm test) to detect *T. vaginalis* and *C. albicans* as well as the increased concentrations of *Gardnerella vaginalis* associated with bacterial vaginosis.

℞ VAGINAL DISCHARGE

Patterns of treatment for vaginal discharge vary widely. In developing countries, where clinics or pharmacies often dispense treatment based on symptoms alone without examination or testing, oral treatment with metronidazole—either as a 2-g single dose or as a 7-day regimen—provides reasonable coverage against both trichomoniasis and bacterial vaginosis, the usual causes of symptoms of vaginal discharge; metronidazole treatment of sex partners prevents reinfection of women with trichomoniasis, even though it does not help prevent the recurrence of bacterial vaginosis. Guidelines promulgated during the 1990s by the World Health Organization suggested treatment for cervical infection and for vulvovaginal candidiasis in women with symptoms of abnormal vaginal discharge; in retrospect, these recommendations were faulty, since these conditions seldom produce such symptoms.

In industrialized countries, clinicians treating symptoms and signs of abnormal vaginal discharge should at least differentiate between bacterial vaginosis and trichomoniasis, because optimal management of patients and partners differs for these two conditions (as discussed briefly below).

Vaginal Trichomoniasis (See also Chap. 208) Symptomatic trichomoniasis characteristically produces a profuse, yellow, purulent, homogeneous vaginal discharge and vulvar irritation, often with visible inflammation of the vaginal and vulvar epithelium and petechial lesions on the cervix (the so-called strawberry cervix, usually evident only by colposcopy). The pH of vaginal fluid usually rises to ≥5.0. In women with typical symptoms and signs of trichomoniasis, microscopic examination of vaginal discharge mixed with saline reveals motile trichomonads in most culture-positive cases. However, in the absence of symptoms or signs, culture is often required for detection of the organism. NAAT for *T. vaginalis* is as sensitive as or more sensitive than culture, and NAAT of urine has disclosed surprisingly high prevalences of this pathogen among men at several STD clinics in the United States. Treatment of asymptomatic as well as symptomatic cases reduces rates of transmission and prevents later development of symptoms.

℞ VAGINAL TRICHOMONIASIS

Only nitroimidazoles (e.g., metronidazole and tinidazole) consistently cure trichomoniasis. A single 2-g oral dose of metronidazole is effective and much less expensive than the alternatives. Tinidazole has a longer half-life than metronidazole and is useful in treating trichomoniasis that fails to respond to metronidazole. Treatment of male sexual partners—often facilitated by dispensing metronidazole to the female patient to give to her partner(s), with a warning about avoiding the concurrent use of alcohol—significantly reduces both the risk of reinfection and the reservoir of infection; treating the partner is the standard of care. Treatment with 0.75% metronidazole gel intravaginally, although moderately effective for bacterial vaginosis, is not reliable for vaginal trichomoniasis. Systemic use of metronidazole is not recommended during the first trimester of pregnancy but is considered safe thereafter. In a large randomized trial, metronidazole treatment of trichomoniasis during pregnancy did not reduce—and in fact actually increased—the frequency of perinatal morbidity.

Bacterial Vaginosis   This syndrome (formerly termed *nonspecific vaginitis, Haemophilus vaginitis, anaerobic vaginitis,* or *Gardnerella-associated vaginal discharge*) is characterized by symptoms of vaginal malodor and a slightly to moderately increased white discharge, which appears homogeneous, is low in viscosity, and evenly coats the vaginal mucosa. An interesting observation is that new genital HPV infection in young women is associated with increased subsequent risk of developing bacterial vaginosis. Other risk factors include multiple sexual partners and recent intercourse with a new partner, but metronidazole treatment of male partners has not reduced the rate of recurrence among affected women.

Among women with bacterial vaginosis, culture of vaginal fluid has shown markedly increased prevalences and concentrations of *G. vaginalis, Mycoplasma hominis,* and several anaerobic bacteria [e.g., *Mobiluncus* spp., *Prevotella* spp. (formerly *Bacteroides* spp.), and some *Peptostreptococcus* spp.] as well as an absence of hydrogen peroxide–producing *Lactobacillus* spp., which constitute most of the normal vaginal flora and perhaps help protect against certain cervical and vaginal infections. The use of broad-range polymerase chain reaction (PCR) amplification of 16S rDNA in vaginal fluid, with subsequent identification of specific bacterial species by various methods, has documented an even greater and unexpected bacterial diversity, including several unique species not previously cultivated [e.g., three species in the order Clostridiales that appear to be specific for bacterial vaginosis (Fig. 124-2)]. Also detected are DNA sequences related to *Atopobium vaginae,* an organism that is strongly associated with bacterial vaginosis, is resistant to metronidazole, and is associated with recurrent bacterial vaginosis after metronidazole treatment. Other species newly

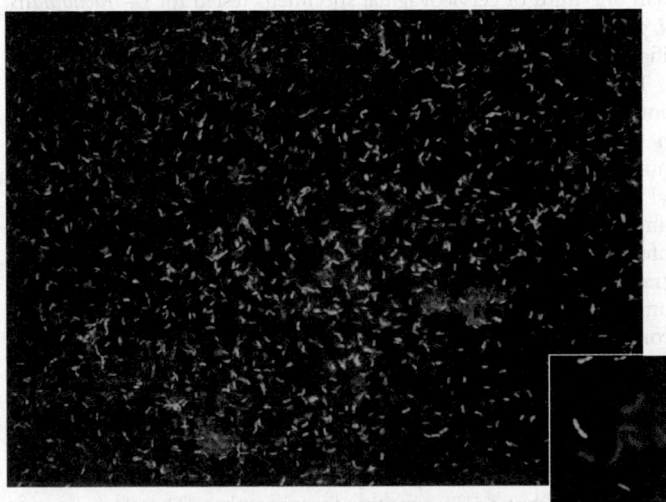

FIGURE 124-2 Broad-range PCR amplification of 16S rDNA in vaginal fluid from a woman with bacterial vaginosis shows a field of bacteria hybridizing with probes for bacterial vaginosis–associated bacterium 1 (BVAB1, visible as a thin, curved green rod) and for *Mobiluncus* (red). The inset shows that *Mobiluncus* (red) is larger than BVAB1 (green) but that the two have a similar morphology (curved rod). (*Reprinted with permission from DN Fredricks et al.*)

FIGURE 124-3 Wet mount of vaginal fluid showing typical clue cells from a woman with bacterial vaginosis. Note the obscured epithelial cell margins and the granular appearance attributable to many adherent bacteria (× 400). [*Photograph provided by Lorna K. Rabe, reprinted with permission from S Hillier et al, in KK Holmes et al (eds). Sexually Transmitted Diseases, 4th ed. New York, McGraw-Hill, 2008.*]

implicated in bacterial vaginosis include *Lactobacillus iners, Megasphaera, Leptotrichia, Eggerthella,* and *Dialister.*

Bacterial vaginosis is conventionally diagnosed clinically with the Amsel criteria, which include any three of the following four clinical abnormalities: (1) objective signs of increased white homogeneous vaginal discharge; (2) a vaginal discharge pH of >4.5; (3) liberation of a distinct fishy odor (attributable to volatile amines such as trimethylamine) immediately after vaginal secretions are mixed with a 10% solution of KOH; and (4) microscopic demonstration of "clue cells" (vaginal epithelial cells coated with coccobacillary organisms, which have a granular appearance and indistinct borders; Fig. 124-3) on a wet mount prepared by mixing vaginal secretions with normal saline in a ratio of ~1:1.

℞ BACTERIAL VAGINOSIS

The standard dosage of metronidazole for the treatment of bacterial vaginosis is 500 mg PO twice daily for 7 days. The single 2-g oral dose of metronidazole recommended for trichomoniasis produces somewhat lower short-term cure rates. Intravaginal treatment with 2% clindamycin cream [one full applicator (5 g containing 100 mg of clindamycin phosphate) each night for 7 nights] or with 0.75% metronidazole gel [one full applicator (5 g containing 37.5 mg of metronidazole) twice daily for 5 days] is also approved for use in the United States and does not elicit systemic adverse reactions. Oral clindamycin (300 mg bid for 7 days) and clindamycin ovules (100 g intravaginally once at bedtime for 3 days) have also been approved. Unfortunately, long-term recurrence (i.e., several months later) is distressingly common after either oral or intravaginal treatment. A randomized trial comparing this intravaginal gel containing 37.5 mg of metronidazole with a suppository containing 500 mg of metronidazole plus nystatin (the latter not marketed in the United States) showed significantly higher rates of recurrent bacterial vaginosis with the 37.5-mg regimen; this result suggests that higher metronidazole dosages may be important in topical intravaginal therapy. Treatment of male partners with metronidazole does not prevent recurrence of bacterial vaginosis.

A randomized trial of orally ingested lactobacilli found reduced rates of recurrent bacterial vaginosis; however, this result has not yet been either confirmed or refuted. A randomized multicenter trial in the United States found no benefit of repeated intravaginal inoculation of a vaginal peroxide-producing *Lactobacillus* species following treatment of bacterial vaginosis with metronidazole. A meta-analysis of 18 studies concluded that bacterial vaginosis during pregnancy substantially increased the risk of preterm delivery and of spontaneous abortion. However, most studies of topical intravaginal treatment of bacterial vaginosis with clindamycin during pregnancy have not reduced adverse pregnancy outcomes. Numerous trials of oral metronidazole treatment during pregnancy have given inconsistent results, and a 2007 Cochrane review concluded that antenatal treatment of women with bacterial vaginosis—even those with previous preterm delivery—did not reduce the risk of preterm delivery.

Vulvovaginal Pruritus, Burning, or Irritation Vulvovaginal candidiasis produces vulvar pruritus, burning, or irritation, generally without symptoms of increased vaginal discharge or malodor. Genital herpes can produce similar symptoms, with lesions sometimes difficult to distinguish from the fissures and inflammation caused by candidiasis. Signs of vulvovaginal candidiasis include vulvar erythema, edema, fissures, and tenderness. With candidiasis, a white scanty vaginal discharge sometimes takes the form of white thrush-like plaques or cottage cheese–like curds adhering loosely to the vaginal mucosa. *C. albicans* accounts for nearly all cases of symptomatic vulvovaginal candidiasis, which probably arise from endogenous strains of *C. albicans* that have colonized the vagina or the intestinal tract. Complicated vulvovaginal candidiasis includes cases that recur four or more times per year; are unusually severe; are caused by non-*albicans Candida* spp.; or occur in women with uncontrolled diabetes, debilitation, immunosuppression, or pregnancy.

The diagnosis of vulvovaginal candidiasis usually involves the demonstration of pseudohyphae or hyphae by microscopic examination of vaginal fluid mixed with saline or 10% KOH or subjected to Gram's staining. Microscopic examination is less sensitive than culture but correlates better with symptoms.

Rx VULVOVAGINAL PRURITUS, BURNING, OR IRRITATION

Symptoms and signs of vulvovaginal candidiasis warrant treatment, usually intravaginal administration of any of several imidazole antibiotics (e.g., miconazole or clotrimazole) for 3–7 days (Table 124-5). Over-the-counter marketing of such preparations has reduced the cost of care and made treatment more convenient for many women with recurrent yeast vulvovaginitis. However, most women who purchase these preparations do not have vulvovaginal candidiasis, while many do have other vaginal infections that require different treatment. Therefore, only women with classic symptoms of vulvar pruritus and a history of previous episodes of yeast vulvovaginitis documented by an experienced clinician should self-treat. Short-course topical intravaginal azole drugs are effective for the treatment of uncomplicated vulvovaginal candidiasis (e.g., clotrimazole, two 100-mg vaginal tablets daily for 3 days; or miconazole, a 1200-mg vaginal suppository as a single dose). Single-dose oral treatment with fluconazole (150 mg) is also effective and is preferred by many patients. Management of complicated cases (see above) and those that do not respond to the usual intravaginal or single-dose oral therapy often involves prolonged or periodic oral therapy; this situation is discussed extensively in the 2006 STD treatment guidelines published by the CDC. Treatment of sexual partners is not routinely indicated.

Other Causes of Vaginal Discharge or Vaginitis In the ulcerative vaginitis associated with staphylococcal toxic shock syndrome, *Staphylococcus aureus* should be promptly identified in vaginal fluid by Gram's stain and by culture. In desquamative inflammatory vaginitis, smears of vaginal fluid reveal neutrophils, massive vaginal epithelial-cell exfoliation with increased numbers of parabasal cells, and gram-positive cocci; this syndrome may respond to treatment with 2% clindamycin cream. Additional causes of vaginitis and vulvovaginal symptoms include retained foreign bodies (e.g., tampons), cervical caps, vaginal spermicides, vaginal antiseptic preparations or douches, vaginal epithelial atrophy (in postmenopausal women or during prolonged breast-feeding in the postpartum period), allergic reactions to latex condoms, vaginal aphthae associated with HIV infection or Behçet's syndrome, and vestibulitis (a poorly understood syndrome).

MUCOPURULENT CERVICITIS

Mucopurulent cervicitis (MPC) refers to inflammation of the columnar epithelium and subepithelium of the endocervix and of any con-

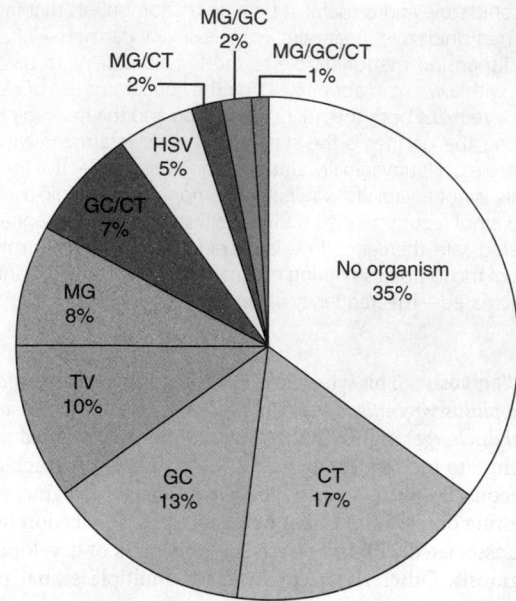

FIGURE 124-4 Organisms detected among female STD clinic patients with mucopurulent cervicitis (*n* = 167). GC, gonococcus; CT, *Chlamydia trachomatis*; MG, *Mycoplasma genitalium*; TV, *Trichomonas vaginalis*; HSV, herpes simplex virus. (*Courtesy of Dr. Lisa Manhart; with permission.*)

tiguous columnar epithelium that lies exposed in an ectopic position on the exocervix. MPC in women represents the "silent partner" of urethritis in men, being equally common and often caused by the same agents (*N. gonorrhoeae, C. trachomatis*, or—as shown by case-control studies—*M. genitalium*); however, MPC is more difficult than urethritis to recognize. As the most common manifestation of these serious bacterial infections in women, MPC can be a harbinger or sign of upper genital tract infection, also known as *pelvic inflammatory disease* (PID; see below). In pregnant women, MPC can lead to obstetric complications. In a prospective study in Seattle of 167 consecutive patients with MPC [defined on the basis of yellow endocervical mucopus or ≥30 polymorphonuclear leukocytes (PMNs)/1000× microscopic field] who were seen at STD clinics during the 1980s, slightly more than one-third of cervicovaginal specimens tested for *C. trachomatis, N. gonorrhoeae, M. genitalium*, HSV, and *T. vaginalis* revealed no identifiable etiology (**Fig. 124-4**).

The diagnosis of MPC rests on the detection of yellow mucopurulent discharge from the cervical os or of increased numbers of PMNs in Gram's-stained or Papanicolaou-stained smears of endocervical mucus. MPC due to *C. trachomatis* can also produce edematous cervical ectopy (see below) and endocervical bleeding upon gentle swabbing. Unlike the endocervicitis produced by gonococcal or chlamydial infection, cervicitis caused by HSV produces ulcerative lesions on the stratified squamous epithelium of the exocervix as well as on the columnar epithelium. Yellow cervical mucus on a white swab removed from the endocervix indicates the presence of PMNs. The mucus should be rolled thinly on a slide for Gram's staining. The presence of ≥20 PMNs/1000× microscopic field within strands of cervical mucus not contaminated by vaginal squamous epithelial cells or vaginal bacteria indicates endocervicitis (**Fig. 124-5**). Detection of intracellular gram-negative diplococci in carefully collected endocervical mucus is quite specific but ≤50% sensitive for gonorrhea. Therefore, specific and sensitive tests for *N. gonorrhoeae* as well as for *C. trachomatis* (e.g., NAATs) are also indicated in the evaluation of MPC.

Rx MUCOPURULENT CERVICITIS

Although the above criteria for MPC are neither highly specific nor highly predictive of gonococcal or chlamydial infection in some settings, the

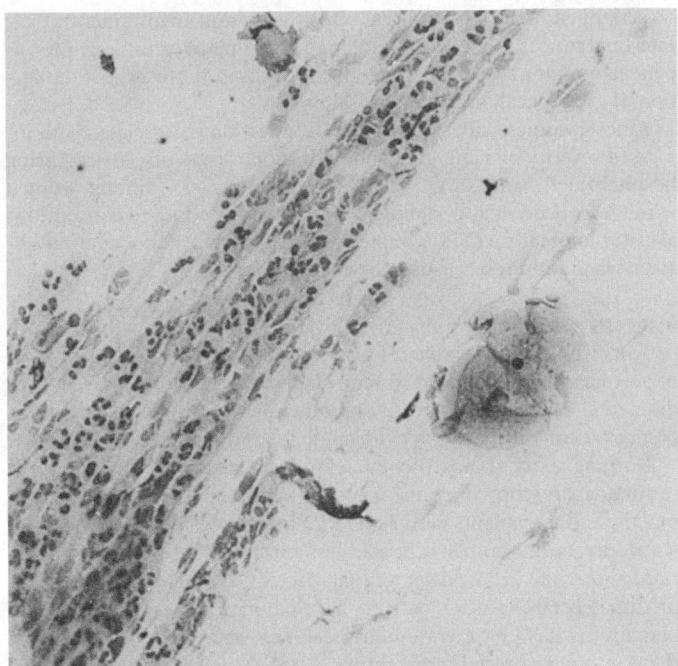

FIGURE 124-5 Gram's stain of cervical mucus, showing a strand of cervical mucus containing many polymorphonuclear leukocytes. This picture is typical of mucopurulent cervicitis. Note that leukocytes are not seen in areas of the slide containing vaginal epithelial cells, adjacent to the mucus strands.

2006 CDC guidelines call for consideration of empirical treatment for MPC, pending test results, in certain patients. Treatment with antibiotics active against *C. trachomatis* should be provided for women at increased risk for this common STI (risk factors: age <25 years, new or multiple sex partners, and unprotected sex), especially if follow-up connot be ensured and if a relatively insensitive diagnostic test (not a NAAT) is used. Concurrent therapy for gonorrhea is indicated if the prevalence of this infection is high (>5%) in the relevant patient population (e.g., young adults, a clinic with documented high prevalence). In this situation, therapy should include a single-dose regimen effective for gonorrhea plus treatment for chlamydial infection, as outlined in Table 124-4 for the treatment of urethritis. In settings where gonorrhea is much less common than chlamydial infection, initial therapy for chlamydial infection alone suffices, pending test results for gonorrhea. The etiology and potential benefit of treatment for endocervicitis not associated with gonorrhea or chlamydial infection have not been established. Although the antimicrobial susceptibility of *M. genitalium* is not yet well defined, the organism frequently persists after doxycycline therapy, and it currently seems reasonable to use azithromycin to treat possible *M. genitalium* infection in such cases. The sexual partner(s) of a woman with MPC should be examined and given a regimen similar to that chosen for the woman unless results of tests for gonorrhea or chlamydial infection in either partner warrant different therapy or no therapy.

CERVICAL ECTOPY

Cervical ectopy, often mislabeled "cervical erosion," is easily confused with infectious endocervicitis. Ectopy represents the presence of the one-cell-thick columnar epithelium extending from the endocervix out onto the visible ectocervix. In ectopy, the cervical os may contain clear or slightly cloudy mucus but usually not yellow mucopus. Colposcopy shows intact epithelium. Normally found during adolescence and early adulthood, ectopy gradually recedes through the second and third decades of life, as squamous metaplasia replaces the ectopic columnar epithelium. Oral contraceptive use favors the persistence or reappearance of ectopy, while smoking apparently accelerates squamous metaplasia. Cauterization of ectopy is not warranted. Ectopy may render the cervix more susceptible to infection with *N. gonorrhoeae*, *C. trachomatis*, or HIV.

PELVIC INFLAMMATORY DISEASE

The term *pelvic inflammatory disease* usually refers to infection that ascends from the cervix or vagina to involve the endometrium and/or fallopian tubes. Infection can extend beyond the reproductive tract to cause pelvic peritonitis, generalized peritonitis, perihepatitis, perisplenitis, or pelvic abscess. Rarely in young women, infection not related to STI extends secondarily to the pelvic organs (1) from adjacent foci of inflammation (e.g., appendicitis, regional ileitis, or diverticulitis), (2) as a result of hematogenous dissemination (e.g., of tuberculosis), or (3) as a complication of certain tropical diseases (e.g., schistosomiasis). Intrauterine infection can be primary (spontaneously occurring and usually sexually transmitted) or secondary to invasive intrauterine surgical procedures [e.g., dilatation and curettage, termination of pregnancy, insertion of an intrauterine device (IUD), or hysterosalpingography] or to parturition.

Etiology The agents most often implicated in acute PID include the primary causes of endocervicitis (e.g., *N. gonorrhoeae* and *C. trachomatis*) and organisms that can be regarded as components of an altered vaginal flora. In general, PID is most often caused by *N. gonorrhoeae* where there is a high incidence of gonorrhea—e.g., in developing countries and in indigent inner-city populations in the United States. In recent case-control studies, *M. genitalium* has also been significantly associated with histopathologic diagnoses of endometritis and with salpingitis.

Anaerobic and facultative organisms (especially *Prevotella* species, peptostreptococci, *E. coli*, *Haemophilus influenzae*, and group B streptococci) as well as genital mycoplasmas have been isolated from the peritoneal fluid or fallopian tubes in a varying proportion (typically one-fourth to one-third) of women with PID studied in the United States. The difficulty of determining the exact microbial etiology of an individual case of PID—short of using invasive procedures for specimen collection—has implications for the approach to empirical antimicrobial treatment of this infection.

Epidemiology In the United States, the estimated annual number of initial visits to physicians' offices for PID by women 15–44 years of age fell from an average of 400,000 during the 1980s to 250,000 in 1999 and then to 176,000 in 2005. Hospitalizations for acute PID in the United States also declined steadily throughout the 1980s and early 1990s but have remained fairly constant at 70,000–100,000 per year since 1995. Important risk factors for acute PID include the presence of endocervical infection or bacterial vaginosis, a history of salpingitis or of recent vaginal douching, and the use of an IUD (especially among nulliparous women, during the first few months after IUD insertion, and among women with multiple sex partners). Certain other iatrogenic factors, such as dilatation and curettage or cesarean section, can increase the risk of PID, especially among women with endocervical gonococcal or chlamydial infection or bacterial vaginosis. Symptoms of *N. gonorrhoeae*–associated and *C. trachomatis*–associated PID often begin during or soon after the menstrual period; this timing suggests that menstruation is a risk factor for ascending infection from the cervix and vagina. Experimental inoculation of the fallopian tubes of lower primates has shown that repeated exposure to *C. trachomatis* leads to the greatest degree of tissue inflammation and damage; thus, immunopathology probably contributes to the pathogenesis of chlamydial salpingitis. Women using oral contraceptives appear to be at decreased risk of symptomatic PID, and tubal sterilization reduces the risk of salpingitis by preventing intraluminal spread of infection into the tubes.

Clinical Manifestations • *ENDOMETRITIS: A CLINICAL PATHOLOGIC SYNDROME* A study of women with clinically suspected PID who were undergoing both endometrial biopsy and laparoscopy showed that those with endometritis alone differed from those who also had salpingitis in significantly less often having lower quadrant, adnexal, or cervical motion or abdominal rebound tenderness; fever; or elevated C-reactive protein levels. In addition, women with endometritis alone differed from those with neither endometritis nor salpingitis in more often having gonorrhea, chlamydial infection, and risk factors such as

CHAPTER 124

Sexually Transmitted Infections: Overview and Clinical Approach

douching or IUD use. Thus, women with endometritis alone were intermediate between those with neither endometritis nor salpingitis and those with salpingitis with respect to risk factors, clinical manifestations, cervical infection prevalence, and elevated C-reactive protein level. Women with endometritis alone are at lower risk of subsequent tubal occlusion and resulting infertility than are those with salpingitis.

SALPINGITIS   Symptoms of nontuberculous salpingitis classically evolve from a yellow or malodorous vaginal discharge caused by MPC and/or bacterial vaginosis to midline abdominal pain and abnormal vaginal bleeding caused by endometritis and then to bilateral lower abdominal and pelvic pain caused by salpingitis, with nausea, vomiting, and increased abdominal tenderness if peritonitis develops.

The abdominal pain in nontuberculous salpingitis is usually described as dull or aching. In some cases, pain is lacking or atypical, but active inflammatory changes are found in the course of an unrelated evaluation or procedure, such as a laparoscopic evaluation for infertility. Abnormal uterine bleeding precedes or coincides with the onset of pain in ~40% of women with PID, symptoms of urethritis (dysuria) occur in 20%, and symptoms of proctitis (anorectal pain, tenesmus, and rectal discharge or bleeding) are occasionally seen in women with gonococcal or chlamydial infection.

Speculum examination shows evidence of MPC (yellow endocervical discharge, easily induced endocervical bleeding) in the majority of women with gonococcal or chlamydial PID. Cervical motion tenderness is produced by stretching of the adnexal attachments on the side toward which the cervix is pushed. Bimanual examination reveals uterine fundal tenderness due to endometritis and abnormal adnexal tenderness due to salpingitis that is usually, but not necessarily, bilateral. Adnexal swelling is palpable in about one-half of women with acute salpingitis, but evaluation of the adnexae in a patient with marked tenderness is not reliable. The initial temperature is >38°C in only about one-third of patients with acute salpingitis. Laboratory findings include elevation of the erythrocyte sedimentation rate (ESR) in 75% of patients with acute salpingitis and elevation of the peripheral white blood cell count in up to 60%.

Unlike nontuberculous salpingitis, genital tuberculosis often occurs in older women, many of whom are postmenopausal. Presenting symptoms include abnormal vaginal bleeding, pain (including dysmenorrhea), and infertility. About one-quarter of these women have had adnexal masses. Endometrial biopsy shows tuberculous granulomas and provides optimal specimens for culture.

PERIHEPATITIS AND PERIAPPENDICITIS   Pleuritic upper abdominal pain and tenderness (usually localized to the right upper quadrant) develop in 3–10% of women with acute PID. Symptoms of perihepatitis arise during or after the onset of symptoms of PID and may overshadow lower abdominal symptoms, thereby leading to a mistaken diagnosis of cholecystitis. In perhaps 5% of cases of acute salpingitis, early laparoscopy reveals perihepatic inflammation ranging from edema and erythema of the liver capsule to exudate with fibrinous adhesions between the visceral and parietal peritoneum. When treatment is delayed and laparoscopy is performed late, dense "violin-string" adhesions can be seen over the liver; chronic exertional or positional right upper quadrant pain ensues when traction is placed on the adhesions. Although perihepatitis, also known as the *Fitz-Hugh–Curtis syndrome*, was for many years specifically attributed to gonococcal salpingitis, most cases are now attributed to chlamydial salpingitis. In patients with chlamydial salpingitis, serum titers of microimmunofluorescent antibody to *C. trachomatis* are typically much higher when perihepatitis is present than when it is absent.

Physical findings include right upper quadrant tenderness and usually include adnexal tenderness and cervicitis, even in patients whose symptoms do not suggest salpingitis. Results of liver function tests and right upper quadrant ultrasonography are nearly always normal. The presence of MPC and pelvic tenderness in a young woman with subacute pleuritic right upper quadrant pain and normal ultrasonography of the gallbladder points to a diagnosis of perihepatitis.

Periappendicitis (appendiceal serositis without involvement of the intestinal mucosa) has been found in ~5% of patients undergoing appendectomy for suspected appendicitis and can occur as a complication of gonococcal or chlamydial salpingitis.

Among women with salpingitis, HIV infection is associated with increased severity of salpingitis and with tuboovarian abscess requiring hospitalization and surgical drainage. Nonetheless, among women with HIV infection and salpingitis, the clinical reponse to conventional antimicrobial therapy (coupled with drainage of tuboovarian abscess, when found) has usually been satisfactory.

Diagnosis   Treatment appropriate for PID must not be withheld from patients who have an equivocal diagnosis; it is better to err on the side of overdiagnosis and overtreatment. On the other hand, it is essential to differentiate between salpingitis and other pelvic pathology, particularly surgical emergencies such as appendicitis and ectopic pregnancy.

Nothing short of laparoscopy definitively identifies salpingitis, but routine laparoscopy to confirm suspected salpingitis is generally impractical. Most patients with acute PID have lower abdominal pain of <3 weeks' duration, pelvic tenderness on bimanual pelvic examination, and evidence of lower genital tract infection (e.g., MPC). Approximately 60% of such patients have salpingitis at laparoscopy, and perhaps 10–20% have endometritis alone. Among the patients with these findings, a rectal temperature >38°C, a palpable adnexal mass, and elevation of the ESR to >15 mm/h also raise the probability of salpingitis, which has been found at laparoscopy in 68% of patients with one of these additional findings, 90% of patients with two, and 96% of patients with three. However, only 17% of all patients with laparoscopy-confirmed salpingitis have had all three additional findings.

In a woman with pelvic pain and tenderness, increased numbers of PMNs (30 per 1000× microscopic field in strands of cervical mucus) or leukocytes outnumbering epithelial cells in vaginal fluid (in the absence of trichomonal vaginitis, which also produces PMNs in vaginal discharge) increase the predictive value of a clinical diagnosis of acute PID, as do onset with menses, history of recent abnormal menstrual bleeding, presence of an IUD, history of salpingitis, and sexual exposure to a male with urethritis. Appendicitis or another disorder of the gut is favored by the early onset of anorexia, nausea, or vomiting; the onset of pain later than day 14 of the menstrual cycle; or unilateral pain limited to the right or left lower quadrant. Whenever the diagnosis of PID is being considered, serum assays for human β-chorionic gonadotropin should be performed; these tests are usually positive with ectopic pregnancy. Ultrasonography and MRI can be useful for the identification of tuboovarian or pelvic abscess. MRI of the tubes can also show increased tubal diameter, intratubal fluid, or tubal wall thickening in cases of salpingitis.

The primary and uncontested value of laparoscopy in women with lower abdominal pain is for the exclusion of other surgical problems. Some of the most common or serious problems that may be confused with salpingitis (e.g., acute appendicitis, ectopic pregnancy, corpus luteum bleeding, ovarian tumor) are unilateral. Unilateral pain or pelvic mass, although not incompatible with PID, is a strong indication for laparoscopy unless the clinical picture warrants laparotomy instead. Atypical clinical findings, such as the absence of lower genital tract infection, a missed menstrual period, a positive pregnancy test, or failure to respond to appropriate therapy, are other common indications for laparoscopy. Endometrial biopsy is relatively sensitive and specific for the diagnosis of endometritis, which correlates well with the presence of salpingitis.

Endocervical swab specimens should be examined by Gram's staining for PMNs and gram-negative diplococci and by NAATs for *N. gonorrhoeae* and *C. trachomatis*. The clinical diagnosis of PID made by expert gynecologists is confirmed by laparoscopy or endometrial biopsy in ~90% of women who also have cultures positive for *N. gonorrhoeae* or *C. trachomatis*. Even among women with no symptoms suggestive of acute PID who were attending an STD clinic or a gynecology clinic in Pittsburgh, endometritis was significantly associated with endocervical gonorrhea or chlamydial infection or with bacterial vaginosis, being detected in 26%, 27%, and 15% of women with these conditions, respectively.

Rx PELVIC INFLAMMATORY DISEASE

The 2006 CDC guidelines recommend initiation of empirical treatment for PID in sexually active young women and other women at risk for PID if they are experiencing pelvic or lower abdominal pain, if no other cause for the pain can be identified, and if pelvic examination reveals one or more of the following criteria for PID: cervical motion tenderness, uterine tenderness, or adnexal tenderness.

Women with suspected PID can be treated as either outpatients or inpatients. In the multicenter Pelvic Inflammatory Disease Evaluation and Clinical Health (PEACH) trial, 831 women with mild to moderately severe symptoms and signs of PID were randomized to receive either inpatient treatment with IV cefoxitin and doxycycline or outpatient treatment with a single IM dose of cefoxitin plus oral doxycycline. Short-term clinical and microbiologic outcomes and long-term outcomes were equivalent in the two groups. Nonetheless, hospitalization should be considered when (1) the diagnosis is uncertain and surgical emergencies such as appendicitis and ectopic pregnancy cannot be excluded, (2) the patient is pregnant, (3) pelvic abscess is suspected, (4) severe illness or nausea and vomiting preclude outpatient management, (5) the patient has HIV infection, (6) the patient is assessed as unable to follow or tolerate an outpatient regimen, or (7) the patient has failed to respond to outpatient therapy. Some experts also prefer to hospitalize adolescents with PID for initial therapy, although younger women do as well as older women on outpatient therapy.

Recommended combination regimens for ambulatory or parenteral management of PID are presented in **Table 124-6**. Women managed as outpatients should receive a combined regimen with broad activity, such as ceftriaxone to cover possible gonococcal infection followed by doxycycline to cover possible chlamydial infection. Metronidazole can be added, if tolerated, to enhance activity against anaerobes. Neither doxycycline nor the fluoroquinolones provide reliable coverage for gonococcal infection today. Although the 2006 CDC guidelines for ambulatory treatment of PID included the option of using an oral fluoroquinolone, with or without metronidazole, for 14 days, these guidelines are already outdated because of emerging gonococcal resistance to the fluoroquinolones. Although few methodologically sound clinical trials (especially with prolonged follow-up) have been conducted, one meta-analysis suggested a benefit of providing good coverage against anaerobes.

For hospitalized patients, the following two parenteral regimens have given nearly identical results in a multicenter randomized trial:

1. Doxycycline (100 mg twice daily, given IV or PO) plus cefotetan (2.0 g IV every 12 h) or cefoxitin (2.0 g IV every 6 h). Administration of these drugs should be continued by the IV route for at least 48 h after the patient's condition improves and then followed with oral doxycycline (100 mg twice daily) to complete 14 days of therapy.
2. Clindamycin (900 mg IV every 8 h) plus gentamicin (2.0 mg/kg IV or IM, followed by 1.5 mg/kg every 8 h) in patients with normal renal function. Once-daily dosing of gentamicin (with combination of the total daily dose into a single daily dose) has not been evaluated in PID but has been efficacious in other serious infections and could be substituted.

Treatment with these drugs should be continued for at least 48 h after the patient's condition improves and then followed with oral doxycycline (100 mg twice daily) or clindamycin (450 mg four times daily) to complete 14 days of therapy. In cases with tuboovarian abscess, clindamycin rather than doxycycline for continued therapy provides better coverage for anaerobic infection.

FOLLOW-UP Hospitalized patients should show substantial clinical improvement within 3–5 days. Women treated as outpatients should be clinically reevaluated within 72 h. A follow-up telephone survey of women seen in an emergency room and given a prescription for 10 days of oral doxycycline for PID found that 28% never filled the prescription and 41% stopped taking the medication early (after an average of 4.1 days), often because of persistent symptoms, lack of symptoms, or side effects. Women not responding favorably to ambulatory therapy should be hospitalized for parenteral therapy and further diagnostic evaluations, including a consideration of laparoscopy. Male sex partners should be evaluated and treated empirically for gonorrhea and chlamydial infection. After completion of

TABLE 124-6	COMBINATION ANTIMICROBIAL REGIMENS RECOMMENDED FOR OUTPATIENT TREATMENT OR FOR PARENTERAL TREATMENT OF PID	
Outpatient Regimens		**Parenteral Regimens**
Regimen A		Initiate parenteral therapy with either of the following regimens; continue parenteral therapy until 48 h after clinical improvement; then change to outpatient therapy, as described in the text.
Ofloxacin 400 mg PO bid for 14 days		
or		
Levofloxacin 500 mg PO once daily for 14 days		**Regimen A**
plus^a		Cefotetan 2 g IV q12h
Metronidazole 500 mg PO bid for 14 days		*or*
Regimen B		Cefoxitin 2 g IV q6h
Ceftriaxone 250 mg IM once		*plus*
plus		Doxycycline 100 mg IV or PO q12h
Doxycycline 100 mg PO bid for 14 days		**Regimen B**
plus^a		Clindamycin 900 mg IV q8h
Metronidazole 500 mg PO bid for 14 days		*plus*
		Gentamicin, loading dose of 2 mg/kg IV or IM, then maintenance dose of 1.5 mg/kg q8h

^aThe addition of metronidazole is recommended by some experts.

Source: Adapted from Centers for Disease Control and Prevention: MMWR Recomm Rep 55(RR-11):1, 2006.

treatment, tests for persistent or recurrent infection with *N. gonorrhoeae* or *C. trachomatis* should be performed if symptoms persist or recur or if the patient has not complied with therapy or has been reexposed to an untreated sex partner.

SURGERY Surgery is necessary for the treatment of salpingitis only in the face of life-threatening infection (such as rupture or threatened rupture of a tuboovarian abscess) or for drainage of an abscess. Conservative surgical procedures are usually sufficient. Pelvic abscesses can often be drained by posterior colpotomy, and peritoneal lavage can be used for generalized peritonitis.

Prognosis Late sequelae include infertility due to bilateral tubal occlusion, ectopic pregnancy due to tubal scarring without occlusion, chronic pelvic pain, and recurrent salpingitis. The overall postsalpingitis risk of infertility due to tubal occlusion in a large study in Sweden was 11% after one episode of salpingitis, 23% after two episodes, and 54% after three or more episodes. A University of Washington study found a sevenfold increase in the risk of ectopic pregnancy and an eightfold increase in the rate of hysterectomy after PID.

Prevention A randomized controlled trial designed to determine whether selective screening for chlamydial infection reduced the risk of subsequent PID showed that women randomized to undergo screening had a 56% lower rate of PID over the following year than did women receiving the usual care without screening. This report helped prompt U.S. national guidelines for risk-based chlamydial screening of young women to reduce the incidence of PID and the prevalence of post-PID sequelae, while also reducing sexual transmission of *C. trachomatis*.

ULCERATIVE GENITAL OR PERIANAL LESIONS

Genital ulceration reflects a set of important STIs, most of which sharply increase the risk of sexual acquisition and shedding of HIV. In a 1996 study of genital ulcers in 10 of the U.S. cities with the highest rates of primary syphilis, PCR testing of ulcer specimens demonstrated HSV in 62% of patients, *Treponema pallidum* in 13%, and *Haemophilus ducreyi* in 12–20%. Today, genital herpes probably represents an even higher proportion of genital ulcers in the United States and other industrialized countries.

 In Asia and Africa, chancroid (Fig. 124-6) was once considered the most common type of genital ulcer, followed in frequency by primary syphilis and then genital herpes. With increased efforts to control chancroid and syphilis, together with more frequent re-

FIGURE 124-6 Chancroid: multiple, painful, punched-out ulcers with undermined borders on the labia occurring after autoinoculation.

FIGURE 124-7 Lymphogranuloma venereum: striking tender lymph-adenopathy occurring at the femoral and inguinal lymph nodes, separated by a groove made by Poupart's ligament. This "sign-of-the-groove" is not considered specific for LGV; for example, lymphomas may present with this sign.

currences or persistence of genital herpes attributable to HIV infection, PCR testing of genital ulcers now clearly implicates genital herpes as the most common cause of genital ulceration in most developing countries. LGV (Fig. 124-7) and donovanosis (granuloma inguinale) continue to cause genital ulceration in developing countries. LGV virtually disappeared in industrialized countries during the first 20 years of the HIV pandemic, but outbreaks are again occurring in Europe (including the United Kingdom), in North America, and in Australia. In these outbreaks, LGV is usually causing anal and rectal disease in homosexual men, very often in association with HIV and/or hepatitis C virus infections. Other causes of genital ulcer include (1) candidiasis and traumatized genital warts—both readily recognized; (2) lesions due to genital involvement by more widespread dermatoses; and (3) cutaneous manifestations of systemic diseases, such as genital mucosal ulceration in Stevens-Johnson syndrome or Behçet's disease.

Diagnosis   Although most genital ulcerations cannot be diagnosed confidently on clinical grounds alone, clinical findings plus epidemiologic considerations (Table 124-7) can usually guide initial management (Table 124-8) pending results of further tests. Clinicians should order a rap-

id serologic test for syphilis in all cases of genital ulcer and a dark-field or direct immunofluorescence test (or PCR test, where available) for *T. pallidum* in all lesions except those highly characteristic of infection with HSV (i.e., those with herpetic vesicles). All patients presenting with genital ulceration should be counseled and tested for HIV infection.

Typical vesicles or pustules or a cluster of painful ulcers preceded by vesiculopustular lesions suggests genital herpes. These typical clinical manifestations make detection of the virus optional; however, many patients want confirmation of the diagnosis, and differentiation of HSV-1 from HSV-2 has prognostic implications, since the latter causes more frequent genital recurrences.

Painless, nontender, indurated ulcers with firm, nontender inguinal adenopathy suggest primary syphilis. If dark-field examination and a rapid serologic test for syphilis are initially negative and the patient will comply with follow-up and sexual abstinence, the performance of two more dark-field examinations on successive days before treatment is begun will improve the sensitivity of the diagnosis of syphilis, and repeated serologic testing for syphilis 1 or 2 weeks after treatment of seronegative primary syphilis usually demonstrates seroconversion.

"Atypical" or clinically trivial ulcers may be more common manifestations of genital herpes than classic vesiculopustular lesions. Specific tests for HSV in such lesions are therefore indicated (Chap. 172).

TABLE 124-7   CLINICAL FEATURES OF GENITAL ULCERS

Feature	Syphilis	Herpes	Chancroid	Lymphogranuloma Venereum	Donovanosis
Incubation period	9–90 days	2–7 days	1–14 days	3 days–6 weeks	1–4 weeks (up to 6 months)
Early primary lesions	Papule	Vesicle	Pustule	Papule, pustule, or vesicle	Papule
No. of lesions	Usually one	Multiple	Usually multiple, may coalesce	Usually one; often not detected, despite lymphadenopathy	Variable
Diameter	5–15 mm	1–2 mm	Variable	2–10 mm	Variable
Edges	Sharply demarcated, elevated, round, or oval	Erythematous	Undermined, ragged, irregular	Elevated, round, or oval	Elevated, irregular
Depth	Superficial or deep	Superficial	Excavated	Superficial or deep	Elevated
Base	Smooth, nonpurulent, relatively nonvascular	Serous, erythematous, nonvascular	Purulent, bleeds easily	Variable, nonvascular	Red and velvety, bleeds readily
Induration	Firm	None	Soft	Occasionally firm	Firm
Pain	Uncommon	Frequently tender	Usually very tender	Variable	Uncommon
Lymphadenopathy	Firm, nontender, bilateral	Firm, tender, often bilateral with initial episode	Tender, may suppurate, loculated, usually unilateral	Tender, may suppurate, loculated, usually unilateral	None; pseudobuboes

Source: From RM Ballard, in KK Holmes et al (eds): *Sexually Transmitted Diseases,* 4th ed. New York, McGraw-Hill, 2008.

TABLE 124-8 INITIAL MANAGEMENT OF GENITAL OR PERIANAL ULCER

Usual causes
Herpes simplex virus (HSV)
Treponema pallidum (primary syphilis)
Haemophilus ducreyi (chancroid)

Usual initial laboratory evaluation
Dark-field exam, direct FA, or PCR for *T. pallidum*; RPR or VDRL test for syphilis (if negative but primary syphilis suspected, repeat in 1 week); culture, direct FA, ELISA, or PCR for HSV; consider HSV-2-specific serology. In chancroid-endemic area: PCR or culture for *H. ducreyi*

Initial Treatment

Herpes confirmed or suspected (history or sign of vesicles):
Treat for genital herpes with acyclovir, valacyclovir, or famciclovir

Syphilis confirmed (dark-field, FA, or PCR showing *T. pallidum*, or RPR reactive):
Benzathine penicillin 2.4 million units IM once to patient, recent (e.g., within 3 months) seronegative partner(s), and all seropositive partners

Chancroid confirmed or suspected (diagnostic test positive, or HSV and syphilis excluded, and lesion persists):
Ciprofloxacin 500 mg PO as single dose *or*
Ceftriaxone 250 mg IM as single dose *or*
Azithromycin 1 g PO as single dose

Note: FA, fluorescent antibody; PCR, polymerase chain reaction; RPR, rapid plasma reagin; ELISA, enzyme-linked immunosorbent assay; HSV, herpes simplex virus; VDRL, Venereal Disease Research Laboratory.

Type-specific serologic tests for serum antibody to HSV-2, now commercially available, may give negative results, especially when patients present early with the initial episode of genital erpes or when HSV-1 is the cause of genital herpes (as is often the case today). Furthermore, a positive test for antibody to HSV-2 does not prove that the current lesions are herpetic, since nearly one-fourth of the general population of the United States (and no doubt a higher proportion of those at risk for other STIs) becomes seropositive for HSV-2 during early adulthood. Although even type-specific tests for HSV-2 that are commercially available in the United States are not 100% specific, a positive HSV-2 serology does enable the clinician to tell the patient that he or she has probably had genital herpes, should learn to recognize symptoms, should avoid sex during recurrences, and should consider use of condoms or suppressive antiviral therapy, both of which can reduce transmission to a sexual partner.

Demonstration of *H. ducreyi* by culture (or by PCR test, when available) is most useful when ulcers are painful and purulent, especially if inguinal lymphadenopathy with fluctuance or overlying erythema is noted; if chancroid is prevalent in the community; or if the patient has recently had a sexual exposure elsewhere in a chancroid-endemic area (e.g., a developing country). Enlarged, fluctuant lymph nodes should be aspirated for culture or PCR tests to detect *H. ducreyi* as well as for Gram's staining and culture to rule out the presence of other pyogenic bacteria.

When genital ulcers persist beyond the natural history of initial episodes of herpes (2–3 weeks) or of chancroid or syphilis (up to 6 weeks) and do not resolve with syndrome-based antimicrobial therapy, then—in addition to the usual tests for herpes, syphilis, and chancroid—biopsy is indicated to exclude donovanosis, carcinoma, and other nonvenereal dermatoses. HIV serology should also be undertaken, since chronic, persistent genital herpes is common in AIDS.

℞ ULCERATIVE GENITAL OR PERIANAL LESIONS

Immediate syndrome-based treatment for acute genital ulcerations (after collection of all necessary hdiagnostic specimens at the first visit) is often appropriate before all test results become available, because patients with typical initial or recurrent episodes of genital or anorectal herpes can benefit from prompt oral antiviral therapy (Chap. 172); because early treatment of sexually transmitted causes of genital ulcers decreases further transmission; and because some patients do not return for test results and treatment. The patient with nonvesicular ulcerative lesions who may not return for follow-up or may not discontinue sexual activity should receive initial treatment for syphilis, together with empirical therapy for chancroid if there has been an exposure in an area where chancroid occurs or if regional lymph node suppuration is evident. In resource-poor settings lacking ready access to diagnostic tests, this approach to syndromic treatment for syphilis and chancroid has helped bring these two diseases under control. Finally, empirical antimicrobial therapy may be indicated if ulcers persist and the diagnosis remains unclear after a week of observation despite attempts to diagnose herpes, syphilis, and chancroid.

PROCTITIS, PROCTOCOLITIS, ENTEROCOLITIS, AND ENTERITIS

Sexually acquired *proctitis*, with inflammation limited to the rectal mucosa (the distal 10–12 cm), results from direct rectal inoculation of typical STD pathogens. In contrast, inflammation extending from the rectum to the colon (*proctocolitis*), involving both the small and the large bowel (*enterocolitis*), or involving the small bowel alone (*enteritis*) can result from ingestion of typical intestinal pathogens through oral-anal exposure during sexual contact. Anorectal pain and mucopurulent, bloody rectal discharge suggest proctitis or proctocolitis. Proctitis commonly produces tenesmus (causing frequent attempts to defecate, but not true diarrhea) and constipation, whereas proctocolitis and enterocolitis more often cause true diarrhea. In all three conditions, anoscopy usually shows mucosal exudate and easily induced mucosal bleeding (i.e., a positive "wipe test"), sometimes with petechiae or mucosal ulcers. Exudate should be sampled for Gram's staining and other microbiologic studies. Sigmoidoscopy or colonoscopy shows inflammation limited to the rectum in proctitis or disease extending at least up into the sigmoid colon in proctocolitis.

The AIDS era brought an extraordinary shift in the clinical and etiologic spectrum of intestinal infections among homosexual men. The number of cases of the acute intestinal STIs described above fell as high-risk sexual behaviors became less common in this group. At the same time, the number of AIDS-related opportunistic intestinal infections increased rapidly, many associated with chronic or recurrent symptoms. The incidence of these infections has since fallen with increasingly effective antiretroviral therapy. Two species initially isolated in association with intestinal symptoms in homosexual men are now known as *Helicobacter cinaedi* and *Helicobacter fennelliae*, and both have subsequently been isolated from the blood of HIV-infected men with a syndrome of multifocal dermatitis and arthritis.

Acquisition of HSV, *N. gonorrhoeae*, or *C. trachomatis* (now again including LGV strains of *C. trachomatis*) during receptive anorectal intercourse causes most cases of infectious proctitis in women and homosexual men. Primary and secondary syphilis can also produce anal or anorectal lesions, with or without symptoms. Gonococcal or chlamydial proctitis typically involves the most distal rectal mucosa and the anal crypts and is clinically mild, without systemic manifestations. In contrast, primary proctitis due to HSV and proctocolitis due to the strains of *C. trachomatis* that cause LGV usually produce severe anorectal pain and often cause fever. Perianal ulcers and inguinal lymphadenopathy, most commonly due to HSV, can also occur in LGV or syphilis. Sacral nerve root radiculopathies, usually presenting as urinary retention, laxity of the anal sphincter, or constipation, may complicate primary herpetic proctitis. In LGV, rectal biopsy typically shows crypt abscesses, granulomas, and giant cells—findings resembling those in Crohn's disease; such findings should always prompt rectal culture and serology for LGV, which is a curable infection. Syphilis can also produce rectal granulomas, usually in association with infiltration by plasma cells or other mononuclear cells. Syphilis, LGV, and HSV infection involving the rectum can produce perirectal adenopathy that is sometimes mistaken for malignancy; syphilis, LGV, HSV infection, and chancroid involving the anus can produce inguinal adenopathy, because anal lymphatics drain to inguinal lymph nodes.

Diarrhea and abdominal bloating or cramping pain without anorectal symptoms and with normal findings on anoscopy and sigmoidoscopy occur with inflammation of the small intestine (enteritis) or with proximal colitis. In homosexual men without HIV infection, enteritis is often attributable to *Giardia lamblia*. Sexually acquired proctocolitis is most often due to *Campylobacter* or *Shigella* spp.

℞ PROCTITIS, PROCTOCOLITIS, ENTEROCOLITIS, AND ENTERITIS

Acute proctitis in persons who have practiced receptive anorectal intercourse is usually sexually acquired. Such patients should undergo anoscopy to detect rectal ulcers or vesicles and petechiae after swabbing of the rectal mucosa; to examine rectal exudates for PMNs and gram-negative diplococci; and to obtain rectal swab specimens for testing for rectal gonorrhea, chlamydial infection, herpes, and syphilis. Pending test results, patients with proctitis should receive empirical syndromic treatment—e.g., with ceftriaxone (a single IM dose of 125 mg for gonorrhea) plus doxycycline (100 mg PO twice daily for 7 days for possible chlamydial infection) plus treatment for herpes or syphilis if indicated.

PREVENTION AND CONTROL OF STIS

Prevention and control of STIs require the following:

1. Reduction of the average rate of sexual exposure to STIs through alteration of sexual risk behaviors and behavioral norms among both susceptible and infected persons in all population groups. The necessary changes include reduction in the total number of sexual partners and the number of concurrent sexual partners.
2. Reduction of the efficiency of transmission through the promotion of safer sexual practices, the use of condoms during casual or commercial sex, vaccination against HBV and HPV infection, male circumcision, and a growing number of other approaches (e.g., early detection and treatment of other STIs to reduce the efficiency of sexual transmission of HIV). We now know from longitudinal studies over the past decade that consistent condom use is associated with significant protection of both males and females against all STIs that have been examined, including HIV, HPV, and HSV infections as well as gonorrhea and chlamydial infection. The only exceptions are probably sexually transmitted *Phthirus pubis* and *Sarcoptes scabiei* infestations.
3. Shortening of the duration of infectivity of STIs through early detection and curative or suppressive treatment of patients and their sexual partners.

Financial and time constraints imposed by managed-care practice patterns, along with the reluctance of some clinicians to ask questions about stigmatized sexual behaviors, often curtail screening and prevention services. As outlined in Fig. 124-8, the success of clinicians' efforts to detect and treat STIs depends in part on societal efforts to teach young people how to recognize symptoms of STIs; to motivate those with symptoms to seek care promptly; and to make high-quality, appropriate care accessible, affordable, and acceptable, especially to the young indigent patients most likely to acquire an STI.

Since many infected individuals develop no symptoms or fail to recognize and report symptoms, clinicians should routinely perform an STI risk assessment for teenagers and young adults as a guide to selective screening. U.S. Preventive Services Task Force Guidelines recommend screening sexually active female patients ≤25 years of age for *C. trachomatis* whenever they present for health care (at least once a year); older women should be tested if they have more than one sexual partner, have begun a new sexual relationship since the previous test, or have another STI diagnosed. In the United States, widespread selective screening of young women for cervical *C. trachomatis* infection in some regions has been associated with a 50–60% drop in prevalence, and such screening also protects the individual woman from PID. Sensitive urine-based genetic amplification tests permit expansion of screening to men, teenage boys, and girls in settings where examination is not planned or is impractical (e.g., during pre-participation sports examinations or during initial medical evaluation of adolescent girls).

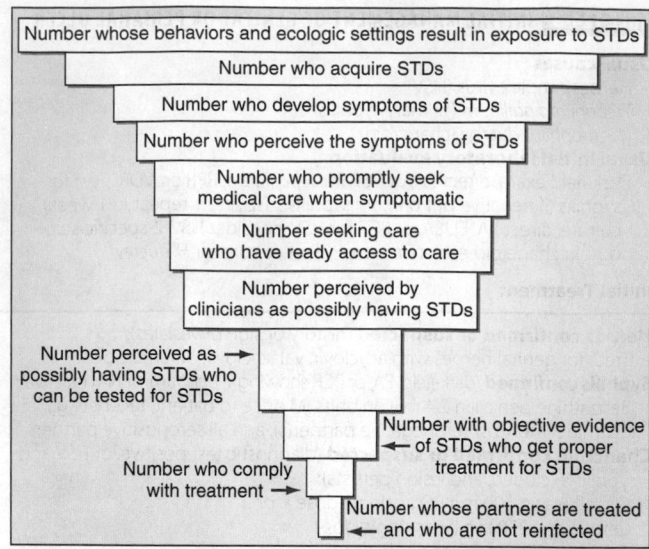

FIGURE 124-8 Critical control points for preventive and clinical interventions against sexually transmitted diseases (STDs). [*Adapted from HT Waller and MA Piot: Bull World Health Organ 41:75, 1969 and 43:1, 1970; and from "Resource allocation model for public health planning—a case study of tuberculosis control," Bull World Health Organ 84(Suppl), 1973.*]

Although gonorrhea is now substantially less common than chlamydial infection in industrialized countries, screening tests for *N. gonorrhoeae* are still appropriate for women and teenage girls attending STD clinics and for sexually active teens and young women from areas of high gonorrhea prevalence. Multiplex NAATs that combine screening for *N. gonorrhoeae* and *C. trachomatis* in a single low-cost assay now facilitate the prevention and control of both infections in populations at high risk.

All patients with newly detected STIs or at high risk for STIs according to routine risk assessment as well as all pregnant women should be encouraged to undergo serologic testing for syphilis and HIV infection, with appropriate HIV counseling before and after testing. Randomized trials have shown that risk-reduction counseling of patients with STIs significantly lowers subsequent risk of acquiring an STI; such counseling should now be considered a standard component of STI management. Preimmunization serologic testing for antibody to HBV is indicated for unvaccinated persons who are known to be at high risk, such as homosexually active men and injection drug users. In most young persons, however, it is more cost-effective to vaccinate against HBV without serologic screening. In 2006, the Advisory Committee on Immunization Practices (ACIP) of the CDC recommended the following: (1) Universal hepatitis B vaccination should be implemented for all unvaccinated adults in settings in which a high proportion of adults have risk factors for HBV infection (e.g., STD clinics, HIV testing and treatment facilities, drug-abuse treatment and prevention settings, health care settings targeting services to injection drug users or men who have sex with men, and correctional facilities). (2) In other primary care and specialty medical settings in which adults at risk for HBV infection receive care, health care providers should inform all patients about the health benefits of vaccination, the risk factors for HBV infection, and the persons for whom vaccination is recommended and should vaccinate adults who report risk factors for HBV infection as well as any adult who requests protection from HBV infection. To promote vaccination in all settings, health care providers should implement standing orders to identify adults recommended for hepatitis B vaccination, should administer HBV vaccination as part of routine clinical services, should not require acknowledgment of an HBV infection risk factor for adult vaccination, and should use available reimbursement mechanisms to remove financial barriers to hepatitis B vaccination.

In 2007, the ACIP recommended routine immunization of 9- to 26-year-old girls and women with the quadrivalent HPV vaccine (against

HPV types 6, 11, 16, and 18) approved by the U.S. Food and Drug Administration; the optimal age for recommended vaccination is 11–12 years because of the very high risk of HPV infection after sexual debut.

Partner notification is the process of identifying and informing partners of infected patients about possible exposure to an STI and of examining, testing, and treating partners as appropriate. In a series of 22 reports concerning partner notification during the 1990s, index patients with gonorrhea or chlamydial infection named a mean of 0.75–1.6 partners, of whom one-fourth to one-third were infected; those with syphilis named 1.8–6.3 partners, with one-third to one-half infected; and those with HIV infection named 0.76–5.31 partners, with up to one-fourth infected. Persons who transmit infection or who have recently been infected and are still in the incubation period usually have no symptoms or only mild symptoms and seek medical attention only when notified of their exposure. Therefore, the clinician must encourage patients to participate in partner notification, must ensure that exposed persons are notified, and must guarantee confidentiality to all involved. In the United States, local health departments often offer assistance in partner notification, treatment, and/or counseling. It seems both feasible and most useful to notify those partners exposed within the patient's likely period of infectiousness, which is often considered the preceding 1 month for gonorrhea, 1–2 months for chlamydial infection, and up to 3 months for early syphilis.

Persons with a new-onset STI always have a *source* contact who gave them the infection; in addition, they may have a *secondary* (*spread* or *exposed*) contact with whom they had sex after becoming infected. The identification and treatment of these two types of contacts have different objectives. Treatment of the source contact (often a casual contact) benefits the community by preventing further transmission; treatment of the recently exposed secondary contact (typically a spouse or another steady sexual partner) prevents both the development of serious complications (such as PID) in the partner and reinfection of the index patient. A survey of a random sample of U.S. physicians found that most instructed patients to abstain from sex during treatment, to use condoms, and to inform their sex partners after being diagnosed with gonorrhea, chlamydial infection, or syphilis; physicians sometimes gave the patients drugs for their partners. However, follow-up of the partners by physicians was infrequent. A randomized trial compared patients' delivery of therapy to partners exposed to gonorrhea or chlamydial infection with conventional notification and advice to partners to seek evaluation for STD; patients' delivery of partners' therapy (PDPT), also known as *expedited partner therapy* (EPT), significantly reduced combined rates of reinfection of the index patient with *N. gonorrhoeae* or *Chlamydia*.

State-by-state variations in regulations governing this approach have not been well defined, but the 2006 CDC STD treatment guidelines and the EPT final report of 2006 (*http://www.cdc.gov/std/treatment/EPTFinalReport2006.pdf*) describe its potential use. Currently, EPT is commonly used by many practicing physicians; it is not feasible in some settings and lacks clear legal sanctioning in some states.

In summary, clinicians and public health agencies share responsibility for the prevention and control of STIs. In the managed-care era, the role of primary care clinicians has become increasingly important in prevention as well as in diagnosis and treatment.

FURTHER READINGS

CENTERS FOR DISEASE CONTROL AND PREVENTION: Sexually transmitted diseases treatment guidelines, 2006. MMWR Recomm Rep 55(RR-11):1, 2006 (Erratum in MMWR Recomm Rep 55(36):997, 2006)

FREDRICKS DN et al: Molecular identification of bacteria associated with bacterial vaginosis. N Engl J Med 353:1899, 2005

FUTURE II GROUP: Quadrivalent vaccine against human papillomavirus to prevent high-grade cervical lesions. N Engl J Med 356:1915, 2007

GOLDEN MR et al: Effect of expedited treatment of sex partners on recurrent or persistent gonorrhea or chlamydial infection. N Engl J Med 352:676, 2005

HOLMES KK et al (eds): *Sexually Transmitted Diseases*, 4th ed. New York, McGraw-Hill, 2008

MANHART LE, HOLMES KK: Randomized controlled trials of individual-level, population-level, and multilevel interventions for preventing sexually transmitted infections: What has worked? J Infect Dis 191(Suppl 1):S7, 2005

MARKOWITZ LE et al: Quadrivalent human papillomavirus vaccine: Recommendations of the Advisory Committee on Immunization Practices (ACIP). MMWR Recomm Rep 56(RR-2):1, 2007

MAST EE et al: A comprehensive immunization strategy to eliminate transmission of hepatitis B virus infection in the United States: Recommendations of the Advisory Committee on Immunization Practices (ACIP) Part II: Immunization of adults. MMWR Recomm Rep 55(RR-16):1, 2006

WORKOWSKI KA: Sexually transmitted disease treatment guidelines. Clin Infect Dis 44(Suppl 3):S1, 2007

WORLD HEALTH ORGANIZATION: Sexually transmitted diseases diagnostics initiative. Geneva, WHO, 2001 (*http://www.who.int/std_diagnostics/news/SDI_founding_members.htm*)

SECTION 3 — CLINICAL SYNDROMES: HEALTH CARE–ASSOCIATED INFECTIONS

125 Health Care–Associated Infections

Robert A. Weinstein

The costs of hospital-acquired (nosocomial) and other health care–associated infections are great. It is estimated that these infections affect >2 million patients, cost $4.5 billion, and contribute to 88,000 deaths in U.S. hospitals annually. Efforts to lower infection risks have been challenged by the growing numbers of immunocompromised patients, antibiotic-resistant bacteria, fungal and viral superinfections, and invasive devices and procedures. Nevertheless, evidence-based guidelines for prevention and control are available (Table 125-1); according to some estimates, consistent application of these guidelines may reduce the risk of health care–associated infection by more than

one-third, and the growing viewpoint of consumer advocates is that almost all such infections are preventable. This chapter reviews health care–acquired and device-related infections and the basic surveillance, prevention, control, and treatment activities that have been developed to deal with these problems.

ORGANIZATION, RESPONSIBILITIES, AND INCREASING SCRUTINY OF INFECTION-CONTROL PROGRAMS

The standards of the Joint Commission on Accreditation of Healthcare Organizations require all accredited hospitals to have an active program for surveillance, prevention, and control of nosocomial infections. Education of physicians in infection control and health care epidemiology is required in infectious disease fellowship programs and is available by online courses. Diagnosis-related reimbursement has led hospital administrators to place increased emphasis on infection control. Federal concerns over "patient safety" have led to legislation that would limit re-

TABLE 125-1 SOURCES OF INFECTION-CONTROL GUIDANCE AND OVERSIGHT

Organization	Role	Major Constituents	Web Site
JCAHO	Regulatory	Hospitals, long-term-care facilities, laboratories	http://www.jcaho.org
CAP	Regulatory	Laboratories	http://www.cap.org
OSHA	Regulatory	Workers	http://www.osha.gov
CMS (formerly HCFA)	Regulatory	Medicare/Medicaid providers	http://www.cms.hhs.gov
CDC			
DHQP	Advisory	Health care facilities and personnel	http://www.cdc.gov/ncidod/hip/default.htm
HICPAC	Advisory	Health care facilities and personnel	http://www.cdc.gov/ncidod/hip/HICPAC/hicpac.htm
NIOSH	Advisory	Workers	http://www.cdc.gov/niosh/homepage.htm
AHRQ	Advisory	Broad (e.g., health care personnel)	http://www.ahrq.org
NQF	Advisory	Broad (e.g., health care personnel)	http://www.qualityforum.org
IOM	Advisory	Broad (e.g., health care personnel)	http://www.iom.edu
IDSA	Professional society	Infectious disease physicians/researchers	http://www.idsociety.org
SHEA	Professional society	Hospital epidemiologists	http://www.shea-online.org
APIC	Professional society	Infection-control practitioners	http://www.apic.org
MedQIC	Quality improvement	Broad (e.g., health care personnel)	http://www.medqic.org
IHI	Quality improvement	Broad (e.g., health care personnel)	http://www.ihi.org

Abbreviations: JCAHO, Joint Commission on Accreditation of Healthcare Organizations; CAP, College of American Pathologists; OSHA, Occupational Safety & Health Administration; CMS, Centers for Medicare & Medicaid Services; HCFA, Health Care Financing Administration; CDC, Centers for Disease Control and Prevention; DHQP, Division of Healthcare Quality Promotion; HICPAC, Healthcare Infection Control Practices Advisory Committee; NIOSH, National Institute for Occupational Safety and Health; AHRQ, Agency for Healthcare Research and Quality; NQF, National Quality Forum; IOM, Institute of Medicine; IDSA, Infectious Diseases Society of America; SHEA, Society for Healthcare Epidemiology of America, Inc.; APIC, Association for Professionals in Infection Control and Epidemiology, Inc.; MedQIC, Medicare Quality Improvement Community; IHI, Institute for Healthcare Improvement.

imbursement for hospital costs resulting from at least two (yet-to-be-determined) nosocomial infections. The patient safety movement has prompted major national efforts to improve, measure, and publicly report on processes of patient care (e.g., timely administration and appropriateness of perioperative antibiotic prophylaxis) and patient outcomes (e.g., surgical wound infection rates).

SURVEILLANCE

Traditionally, infection-control practitioners have surveyed inpatients for infections acquired in hospitals (defined as those neither present nor incubating at the time of admission). Surveillance involves review of microbiology laboratory results, "shoe-leather" epidemiology on nursing wards, and application of standardized definitions of infection. Some infection-control programs use computerized hospital databases for algorithm-driven electronic surveillance (e.g., of vascular catheter and surgical wound infections). Commercial health care information systems that facilitate these functions are considered "value-added" products.

Most hospitals aim surveillance at infections associated with a high level of morbidity or expense. Quality-improvement activities in infection control have led to increased surveillance of personnel compliance with infection-control policies (e.g., adherence to influenza vaccination recommendations). The growing number of states that require public reporting of processes for prevention of health care–associated infection and/or patient outcomes has added new complexity to what hospitals measure and how they measure it.

Results of surveillance are expressed as rates. In general, 5–10% of patients develop nosocomial infections—a rate that, as patient advocates emphasize, has remained unchanged for 20–30 years. However, such broad statistics have little value unless qualified by duration of risk, by site of infection, by patient population, and by exposure to risk factors. Meaningful denominators for infection rates include the number of patients exposed to a specific risk (e.g., patients using mechanical ventilators) or the number of intervention days (e.g., 1000 patient-days on a ventilator).

Temporal trends in rates should be reviewed, and rates should be compared with regional and national benchmarks. However, even comparison rates generated by the National Healthcare Safety Network (NHSN) have not been validated independently and represent a nonrandom sample of hospitals. [NHSN is the successor to the National Nosocomial Infections Surveillance System, a program of the Centers for Disease Control and Prevention (CDC) that collected data from more than 350 hospitals that use standardized definitions of nosocomial infections.] Interhospital comparisons may be misleading because of the wide range in risk factors and severity of underlying illnesses. Although systems for making adjustments for these factors either are rudimentary or have not been well validated, process measures (e.g., adherence to hand hygiene) do not usually require risk adjustment, and outcome measures (e.g., cardiac surgery wound infection rates) can identify hospitals with higher infection rates (e.g., in the top quartile) for further evaluation. Moreover, temporal analysis of an individual hospital's process and infection outcome rates helps to determine whether control measures are succeeding and where increased efforts should be focused.

EPIDEMIOLOGIC BASIS AND GENERAL MEASURES FOR PREVENTION AND CONTROL

Nosocomial infections follow basic epidemiologic patterns that can help to direct prevention and control measures. Nosocomial pathogens have reservoirs, are transmitted by predictable routes, and require susceptible hosts. Reservoirs and sources exist in the inanimate environment (e.g., tap water contaminated with *Legionella*) and in the animate environment (e.g., infected or colonized health care workers, patients, and hospital visitors). The mode of transmission usually is either cross-infection (e.g., indirect spread of pathogens from one patient to another on the inadequately cleaned hands of hospital personnel) or autoinoculation (e.g., aspiration of oropharyngeal flora into the lung along an endotracheal tube). Occasionally, pathogens (e.g., group A streptococci and many respiratory viruses) are spread from person to person via infectious droplets released by coughing or sneezing. Much less common—but often devastating in terms of epidemic risk—is true airborne spread of droplet nuclei (as in nosocomial chickenpox) or common-source spread by contaminated materials (e.g., contaminated intravenous fluids). Factors that increase host susceptibility include underlying conditions and the many medical-surgical interventions and procedures that bypass or compromise normal host defenses.

Through their programs, hospitals' infection-control committees must determine general and specific control measures. Given the prominence of cross-infection, hand hygiene is the single most important preventive measure in hospitals. Health care workers' rates of adherence to hand-hygiene recommendations are abysmally low (<50%). Reasons cited include inconvenience, time pressures, and skin damage from frequent washing. Sinkless alcohol rubs are quick and highly effective and actually improve hand condition since they contain emollients and allow the retention of natural protective oils that would be removed with repeated rinsing. Use of alcohol hand rubs between patient contacts is now recommended for all health care workers except when the hands are visibly soiled, in which case washing with soap and water is still required.

NOSOCOMIAL AND DEVICE-RELATED INFECTIONS

The fact that 25–50% or more of nosocomial infections are due to the combined effect of the patient's own flora and invasive devices highlights the importance of improvements in the use and design of such devices. Intensive education and "bundling" of evidence-based interventions (Table 125-2) can reduce infection rates through improved asepsis in handling and earlier removal of invasive devices, but the maintenance of such gains requires ongoing efforts. It is especially noteworthy that turnover or shortages of trained personnel jeopardize safe and effective patient care and have been associated with increased infection rates.

Urinary Tract Infections Urinary tract infections (UTIs) account for as many as 40–45% of nosocomial infections; up to 3% of bacteriuric patients develop bacteremia. Although UTIs contribute only 10–15% to prolongation of hospital stay and to extra costs, these infections are important reservoirs and sources for spread of antibiotic-resistant bacteria in hospitals. Almost all nosocomial UTIs are associated with preceding instrumentation or indwelling bladder catheters, which create a 3–10% risk of infection each day. UTIs generally are caused by pathogens that spread up the periurethral space from the patient's perineum or gastrointestinal tract—the most common pathogenesis in women—or via intraluminal contamination of urinary catheters, usually due to cross-infection by caregivers who are irrigating catheters or emptying drainage bags. Pathogens come occasionally from inadequately disinfected urologic equipment and rarely from contaminated supplies.

Hospitals should closely monitor essential performance measures for preventing nosocomial UTIs (Table 125-2). Sealed catheter–drainage tube junctions can help to prevent breaks in the system. Approaches to the prevention of UTIs also have included use of topical meatal antimicrobials, drainage bag disinfectants, and anti-infective catheters. None of the latter three measures is considered routine. In fact, a recent meta-analysis suggests that silver alloy–coated anti-infective catheters do not reduce the incidence of bacteriuria from that occurring with silicone catheters.

Administration of systemic antimicrobial agents for other purposes decreases the risk of UTI during the first 4 days of catheterization, after which resistant bacteria or yeasts emerge as pathogens. Selective decontamination of the gut is also associated with a reduced risk. Again, however, neither approach is routine.

Irrigation of catheters, with or without antimicrobial agents, may actually increase the risk of infection. A condom catheter for men without bladder obstruction may be more acceptable than an indwelling catheter, but the infection risks with the two types are similar unless the condom catheter is carefully maintained. The role of suprapubic catheters in preventing infection is not well defined.

Treatment of UTIs is based on the results of quantitative urine cultures (Chap. 282). The most common pathogens are *Escherichia coli*, nosocomial gram-negative bacilli, enterococci, and *Candida*. Several caveats apply in the treatment of institutionally acquired infection. First, in patients with chronic indwelling bladder catheters, especially those in long-term-care facilities, "catheter flora"—microorganisms living on encrustations within the catheter lumen—may differ from actual urinary tract pathogens. Therefore, for suspected infection in the setting of chronic catheterization (especially in women), it is useful to replace the bladder catheter and to obtain a freshly voided urine specimen. Second, as in all nosocomial infections, at the time treatment is initiated on the basis of a positive culture, it is useful to repeat the culture to verify the persistence of infection. Third, the frequency with which UTIs occur may lead to the erroneous assumption that this site alone is the source of infection in a febrile hospitalized patient. Fourth, recovery of *Staphylococcus aureus* from urine cultures may result from hematogenous seeding and may indicate an occult systemic infection. Finally, although *Candida* is now the most common pathogen in nosocomial UTIs in patients on intensive care units (ICUs), treatment of candiduria is often unsuccessful and is recommended only when there is upper-pole invasion, obstruction, neutropenia, or immunosuppression.

Pneumonia Pneumonia accounts for 15–20% of nosocomial infections but has been responsible for 24% of extra hospital days and 39% of extra costs—i.e., 6 days and the associated costs per episode. Almost all cases of bacterial nosocomial pneumonia are caused by aspiration of endogenous or hospital-acquired oropharyngeal (and occasionally gastric) flora. Nosocomial pneumonias are associated with more deaths than are infections at any other body site. However, attributable mortality for ventilator-associated pneumonia—the most common and lethal form of nosocomial pneumonia—is in the 6–14% range; this figure suggests that the risk of dying from nosocomial pneumonia is affected greatly by other factors, including comorbidities, inadequate antibiotic treatment, and the involvement of specific pathogens (particularly *Pseudomonas aeruginosa* and *Acinetobacter*). Surveillance and accurate diagnosis of pneumonia are often problematic in hospitals because many patients, especially those in the ICU, have abnormal chest roentgenographs, fever, and leukocytosis potentially attributable to multiple causes. Viral pneumonias, which are particularly important in pediatric and immunocompromised patients, are discussed in the virology section and in Chap. 251.

Risk factors for nosocomial pneumonia, particularly ventilator-associated pneumonia, include those events that increase colonization by potential pathogens (e.g., prior antimicrobial therapy, contaminat-

TABLE 125-2	EXAMPLES OF "BUNDLED INTERVENTIONS" TO PREVENT COMMON HEALTH CARE–ASSOCIATED INFECTIONS AND OTHER ADVERSE EVENTS

Prevention of Central Venous Catheter Infections

Educate personnel about catheter insertion and care.
Use chlorhexidine to prepare the insertion site.
Use maximum barrier precautions during catheter insertion.
Ask daily: Is the catheter needed?

Prevention of Ventilator-Associated Pneumonia and Complications

Elevate head of bed to 30–45 degrees.
Give "sedation vacation" and assess readiness to extubate daily.
Use peptic ulcer disease prophylaxis.
Use deep-vein thrombosis prophylaxis (unless contraindicated).

Prevention of Surgical-Site Infections

Administer prophylactic antibiotics within 1 h before surgery; discontinue within 24 h.
Limit any hair removal to the time of surgery; use clippers or do not remove hair at all.
Maintain normal perioperative glucose levels (cardiac surgery patients).[a]
Maintain perioperative normothermia (colorectal surgery patients).[a]

Prevention of Urinary Tract Infections

Place bladder catheters only when absolutely needed (e.g., to relieve obstruction), not solely for the provider's convenience.
Use aseptic technique for catheter insertion and urinary tract instrumentation.
Minimize manipulation or opening of drainage systems.
Remove bladder catheters as soon as is feasible.

[a] These components of care are supported by clinical trials and experimental evidence in the specified populations; they may prove valuable for other surgical patients as well.

Source: Adapted from information presented at the following websites: www.cdc.gov/ncidod/dhqp/gl_intravascular.html; www.cdc.gov/ncidod/dhqp/gl_hcpneumonia.html; www.cdc.gov/ncidod/dhqp/gl_surgicalsite.html; www.cdc.gov/ncidod/dhqp/gl_catheter_assoc.html; www.ihi.org; www.medqic.org/scip.

ed ventilator circuits or equipment, or decreased gastric acidity); those that facilitate aspiration of oropharyngeal contents into the lower respiratory tract (e.g., intubation, decreased levels of consciousness, or presence of a nasogastric tube); and those that reduce host defense mechanisms in the lung and permit overgrowth of aspirated pathogens (e.g., chronic obstructive pulmonary disease, old age, or upper abdominal surgery).

Control measures for pneumonia (Table 125-2) are aimed at the remediation of risk factors in general patient care (e.g., minimizing aspiration-prone supine positioning) and at meticulous aseptic care of respirator equipment (e.g., disinfecting or sterilizing all inline reusable components such as nebulizers, replacing tubing circuits at intervals of >48 h—rather than more frequently—to lessen the number of breaks in the system, and teaching aseptic technique for suctioning). The benefits of selective decontamination of the oropharynx and gut with nonabsorbable antimicrobial agents and/or use of short-course postintubation systemic antibiotics have been controversial. Among the logical preventive measures that require further investigation are the use of endotracheal tubes that provide channels for subglottic drainage of secretions and the use of noninvasive mechanical ventilation whenever feasible. It is noteworthy that reducing the rate of ventilator-associated pneumonia most often has not reduced overall ICU mortality; this fact suggests that this infection is a marker for patients with an otherwise-heightened risk of death.

The most likely pathogens for nosocomial pneumonia and treatment options are discussed in Chap. 251. Several considerations regarding diagnosis and treatment are worth emphasizing. Clinical criteria for diagnosis (e.g., fever, leukocytosis, development of purulent secretions, new or changing radiographic infiltrates, changes in oxygen requirement or ventilator settings) have high sensitivity but relatively low specificity. These criteria are most useful for selecting patients for bronchoscopic or nonbronchoscopic procedures that yield lower respiratory tract samples protected from upper-tract contamination; quantitative cultures of such specimens have diagnostic sensitivities in the range of 80%. Early-onset nosocomial pneumonia, which manifests within the first 4 days of hospitalization, is most often caused by community-acquired pathogens, such as *Streptococcus pneumoniae* and *Haemophilus* species. Late-onset pneumonias most commonly are due to *S. aureus*, *P. aeruginosa*, *Enterobacter* species, *Klebsiella pneumoniae*, or *Acinetobacter*—a pathogen of increasing concern in many ICUs. When invasive techniques are used to diagnose ventilator-associated pneumonia, the proportion of isolates accounted for by gram-negative bacilli decreases from 50–70% to 35–45%. Infection is polymicrobial in as many as 20–40% of cases. The role of anaerobic bacteria in ventilator-associated pneumonia is not well defined. A recent study suggested that 8 days is an appropriate duration of therapy for nosocomial pneumonia, with a longer duration (15 days in this study) when the pathogen is *Acinetobacter* or *P. aeruginosa*. Finally, in febrile patients (particularly those who have endotracheal and/or nasogastric tubes), more occult sources of respiratory tract infection, especially bacterial sinusitis and otitis media, should be considered.

Surgical Wound Infections Wound infections account for up to 20–30% of nosocomial infections but contribute up to 57% of extra hospital days and 42% of extra costs. The average wound infection has an incubation period of 5–7 days (longer than many postoperative stays), and many procedures are now performed on an outpatient basis. Thus the incidence of wound infections has become difficult to assess. These infections usually are caused by the patient's endogenous or hospital-acquired skin and mucosal flora and occasionally are due to airborne spread of skin squames that may be shed into the wound from members of the operating-room team. True airborne spread of infection through droplet nuclei is rare in operating rooms unless there is a "disseminator" (e.g., of group A streptococci or staphylococci) among the staff. In general, the most common risks for postoperative wound infection are related to the surgeon's technical skill, the patient's underlying diseases (e.g., diabetes mellitus, obesity) or advanced age, and inappropriate timing of antibiotic prophylaxis. Additional risk factors include the presence of drains, prolonged preoperative hospital stays, shaving of the operative site by razor the day before surgery, a long duration of surgery, and infection at remote sites (e.g., untreated UTI).

The substantial literature related to risk factors for surgical-site infections and the recognized morbidity and cost of these infections have led to national prevention efforts—the Surgical Infection Prevention (SIP) Project, the Institute for Healthcare Improvement (IHI) 100,000 Lives Campaign, and the Surgical Care Improvement Project (SCIP)—and to recommendations for "bundling" of evidence-based preventive measures (Table 125-2). Additional measures include attention to technical surgical issues and operating-room asepsis (e.g., avoiding open or prophylactic drains) and preoperative therapy for active infection. Reporting of surveillance results to surgeons has been associated with reductions in infection rates. The use of preoperative intranasal mupirocin to eliminate that reservoir for *S. aureus*, preoperative antiseptic bathing, and supplemental intra- and postoperative oxygen remain controversial because of conflicting study results.

The increasingly extensive review of infection rates by regulatory agencies and third-party payers emphasizes the importance of stratifying rates by patient-related risk factors and of developing meaningful systems for wound surveillance after the patient's discharge from the hospital or clinic (when >50% of infections first become apparent) or for use of surrogate markers of wound infection (e.g., prolonged postoperative antibiotic courses).

The epidemic of mad cow disease, centered in the United Kingdom, and associated human cases of variant Creutzfeldt-Jakob disease (Chap. 378) caused by disinfection-resistant prion agents have led to revised recommendations for decontaminating surgical instruments, especially those used for operations on the central nervous system or in patients with dementing illness of unknown etiology.

The process of diagnosing and treating wound infections begins with a careful assessment of the surgical site in the febrile postoperative patient. Clinical findings range from obvious cellulitis or abscess formation to subtler clues such as a sternal "click" following open heart surgery. Diagnosis of deeper organ-space infections or subphrenic abscesses requires a high index of suspicion and the use of CT or MRI. Diagnosis of infections of prosthetic devices, such as orthopedic implants, may be particularly difficult and often requires the use of interventional radiographic techniques to obtain periprosthetic specimens for culture. The most common pathogens in postoperative wound infections are *S. aureus*, coagulase-negative staphylococci, and enteric and anaerobic bacteria. In rapidly progressing postoperative infections, which manifest within 24–48 h of a surgical procedure, the level of suspicion regarding group A streptococcal or clostridial infection (Chaps. 130 and 135) should be high. Treatment of postoperative wound infections requires drainage or surgical excision of infected or necrotic material and antibiotic therapy aimed at the most likely or laboratory-confirmed pathogens.

Infections Related to Vascular Access and Monitoring Intravascular devices are common causes of local site infection and cause up to 50% of nosocomial bacteremias; central vascular catheters (CVCs) account for 80–90% of these infections. National estimates indicate that as many as 200,000 bloodstream infections associated with CVCs occur each year in the United States, with an attributable mortality of 12–25% and an estimated cost of $25,000 per episode; one-third to one-half of these episodes occur in ICUs. With increasing care of seriously ill patients in the community, vascular catheter–associated bloodstream infections acquired in outpatient settings may become as frequent as those acquired in hospitals. This possibility emphasizes the need to broaden surveillance activities.

Catheter-related bloodstream infections derive largely from the cutaneous microflora of the insertion site, with pathogens migrating extraluminally to the catheter tip, usually during the first week after insertion. In addition, contamination of hubs of CVCs or of the ports of "needleless" systems may lead to intraluminal infection over longer periods, particularly with surgically implanted or cuffed catheters. Intrinsic contamination of infusate, although rare, is the most common cause of epidemic device-related bloodstream infection; extrinsic contamination may cause up to half of endemic bacteremias related to arterial infusions used for hemodynamic monitoring. The most common pathogens isolated from vascular device–associated bacteremias include coagulase-negative staphylococci, *S. aureus* (with up to 50% or more of isolates in the United States resistant to methicillin), enterococci, nosocomial gram-negative bacilli, and *Candida*. Many pathogens, especially staphylococci, produce extracellular polysaccharide biofilms that facilitate attachment to catheters and provide sanctuary from antimicrobial agents. "Quorum-sensing" proteins help bacterial cells communicate during biofilm development.

Infections related to vascular catheters and monitoring devices may be the most preventable of nosocomial infections. Evidence-based bundles of control measures (Table 125-2) have been strikingly effective, eliminating all infections in one ICU study. Hospitals should periodically monitor adherence to these performance indicators. Use of antimicrobial- or antiseptic-impregnated CVCs does not appear necessary if the prevention bundle is fully implemented. Additional control measures for infections associated with vascular access include using a chlorhexidine-impregnated patch at the skin-catheter junction; avoiding the femoral site for catheterization because of higher risk of infection (most likely related to the density of the skin flora); moving peripheral catheters to a new site at specified intervals (e.g., every 72–96 h), which may be facilitated by use of an IV therapy team; and applying disposable transducers for pressure monitoring and aseptic technique for accessing transducers or other vascular ports. Improvements in composition of semitransparent access-site dressings and potential nursing benefits (ease of bathing and site inspection, protection of site from secretions) favor the use of such coverings. Unresolved issues include the best frequency for rotation of CVC sites (given that guidewire-assisted catheter changes at the same site do not lessen and may even increase infection risk); the appropriate role of mupirocin ointment, a topical antibiotic with excellent antistaphylococcal activity, in site care; the relative degrees of risk posed by peripherally inserted central catheters (PICC lines); and the risk-benefit of prophylactic use of heparin (to avoid catheter thrombi, which may be associated with increased risk of infection) or of vancomycin or alcohol (as catheter flushes or "locks"—i.e., concentrated anti-infective solutions instilled into the catheter lumen) for high-risk patients.

Vascular device–related infection is suspected on the basis of the appearance of the catheter site or the presence of fever or bacteremia without another source in patients with vascular catheters. The diagnosis is confirmed by the recovery of the same species of microorganism from peripheral-blood cultures (preferably two cultures drawn from peripheral veins by separate venipunctures) and from semiquantitative or quantitative cultures of the vascular catheter tip. Less commonly used diagnostic measures include differential time to positivity (>2 h) for blood drawn through the vascular access device compared with a sample from a peripheral vein or differences in quantitative cultures (a 5- to 10-fold or greater "step-up") for blood samples drawn simultaneously from a peripheral vein and from a CVC. When infusion-related sepsis is considered (e.g., because of the abrupt onset of fever or shock temporally related to infusion therapy), a sample of the infusate or blood product should be retained for culture.

Therapy for vascular access–related infection is directed at the pathogen recovered from the blood and/or infected site. Important considerations in treatment are the need for an echocardiogram (to evaluate the patient for bacterial endocarditis), the duration of therapy, and the need to remove potentially infected catheters. In one report, approximately one-fourth of patients with intravascular catheter–associated *S. aureus* bacteremia who were studied by transesophageal echocardiography had evidence of endocarditis; this test may be useful in determining the appropriate duration of treatment.

Detailed consensus guidelines for the management of intravascular catheter–related infections have been published and recommend catheter removal in most cases of bacteremia or fungemia due to nontunneled CVCs. When attempting to salvage a potentially infected catheter, some clinicians use the "antibiotic lock" technique, which may facilitate penetration of infected biofilms, in addition to systemic antimicrobial therapy. In one study of hemodialysis catheters, only about one-third of salvage attempts were successful, although delayed removal did not appear to increase the risk of complications.

Often, a potentially infected CVC may be exchanged over a guidewire. If cultures of the removed catheter tip are positive, the replacement catheter will be moved to a new site; if the tip cultures are negative, the replacement catheter may remain in the original site but may be at increased risk of subsequent infection due to this manipulation.

The authors of the consensus guidelines advise that the decision to remove a tunneled catheter or implanted device suspected of being the source of bacteremia or fungemia should be based on the severity of the patient's illness, the strength of the evidence that the device is infected, an assessment of the specific pathogens, and the presence of local or systemic complications. For patients with track-site infection, successful therapy without catheter removal is unusual. For patients with suppurative venous thrombophlebitis, excision of the affected vein is usually required.

ISOLATION TECHNIQUES

Written policies for the isolation of infectious patients are a standard component of infection-control programs. In 1996, the CDC revised its isolation guidelines to make them simpler; to recognize the importance of all body fluids, secretions, and excretions in the transmission of nosocomial pathogens; and to focus precautions on the major routes of infection transmission. These policies are currently being updated by the CDC to include integrated guidelines for control of multidrug-resistant organisms.

Standard precautions are designed for the care of all patients in hospitals and aim to reduce the risk of transmission of microorganisms from both recognized and unrecognized sources. These precautions include gloving as well as hand cleansing for potential contact with (1) blood; (2) all other body fluids, secretions, and excretions, whether or not they contain visible blood; (3) nonintact skin; and (4) mucous membranes. Depending on exposure risks, standard precautions also include use of masks, eye protection, and gowns.

Precautions for the care of patients with potentially contagious clinical syndromes (e.g., acute diarrhea) or with suspected or diagnosed colonization or infection with transmissible pathogens are based on probable routes of transmission: *airborne*, *droplet*, and *contact*. Sets of precautions may be combined for diseases that have more than one route of transmission (e.g., varicella).

Because some prevalent antibiotic-resistant pathogens, particularly vancomycin-resistant enterococci (VRE), may be present on *intact* skin of patients in hospitals, some experts recommend gloving for all contact with patients who are acutely ill and/or from high-risk units, such as ICUs. Wearing gloves does not replace the need for hand hygiene because hands occasionally become contaminated during wearing or removal of gloves. Some studies have suggested that use of gowns and gloves compared with routine care of patients (i.e., using neither of these barriers) decreases the risk of nosocomial infection; however, the benefit of gowning by personnel beyond that conferred by gloving and hand hygiene is controversial. Nevertheless, requiring increased precaution levels can improve the compliance of health care workers with isolation recommendations by 30%.

EPIDEMIC AND EMERGING PROBLEMS

Outbreaks and emerging pathogens are always big news but probably account for <5% of nosocomial infections. Concern about emerging pathogens often prompts authorities to require hospitals to develop contingency and response plans. The investigation and control of nosocomial epidemics require that infection-control personnel develop a case definition, confirm that an outbreak really exists (since many apparent epidemics are actually pseudo-outbreaks due to surveillance or laboratory artifacts), review aseptic practices and disinfectant use, determine the extent of the outbreak, perform an epidemiologic investigation to determine modes of transmission, work closely with microbiology personnel to culture for common sources or personnel carriers as appropriate and to type epidemiologically important isolates, and heighten surveillance to judge the effect of control measures. Control measures generally include reinforcing routine aseptic practices and hand hygiene during a search for compliance problems that may have fostered the outbreak, ensuring appropriate isolation of cases (and instituting cohort isolation and nursing if needed), and implementing further controls on the basis of the investigation's findings. Examples of some emerging and potential epidemic problems follow.

Viral Respiratory Infections: SARS and Influenza Infections caused by the severe acute respiratory syndrome (SARS)–associated coronavirus challenged health care systems globally in 2003 (Chap. 179). Basic infection-control measures helped to keep the worldwide case and death counts at ~8000 and ~800, respectively, although SARS was unforgiving of lapses in protocol adherence or laboratory biosafety. The epidemiology of SARS—spread largely in households once patients were ill or in hospitals—contrasts markedly with that of influenza (Chap. 180), which is often contagious a day before symptom onset, can spread rapidly in the community among nonimmune persons, and kills as many as 30,000 persons each year in the United States. Control of influenza has depended on (1) the use of effective vaccines, with increasingly broad recommendations for vaccination and emphasis on vaccination of health care workers; (2) the use of antiviral medications for early treatment and for prophylaxis as part of outbreak control, especially in high-risk settings like nursing homes or hospitals; and (3) infection control (surveillance and droplet precautions) for symptomatic patients.

Concerns about avian (H5N1) and pandemic influenza have led to recommendations for "respiratory hygiene and cough etiquette" and "source containment" (e.g., use of face masks and spatial separation) for outpatients with potentially infectious respiratory illnesses; to the concept of "social distancing" (e.g., closing community venues such as shopping malls) in the event of a pandemic; and to debate about the level of avian influenza respiratory protection required for health care workers—i.e., whether to use the higher-efficiency N95 respirators recommended for airborne isolation rather than the surgical masks used for droplet precautions.

Nosocomial Diarrhea A new, more virulent strain of *Clostridium difficile* has emerged in North America, and overall rates of *C. difficile*–associated diarrhea (Chap. 123) have increased in U.S. hospitals during the past few years. The potential role of exposure to newer fluoroquinolone antibiotics in driving these changes is being investigated. *C. difficile* control measures include judicious use of all antibiotics; heightened suspicion for "atypical" presentations (e.g., toxic megacolon or leukemoid reaction without diarrhea); and early diagnosis, treatment, and contact precautions.

Outbreaks of norovirus infection (Chap. 183) in U.S. and European health care facilities appear to be increasing in frequency, with the virus often introduced by ill visitors or health care workers. This pathogen should be suspected when nausea and vomiting are prominent aspects of bacterial culture–negative diarrheal syndromes. Contact precautions may need to be augmented by aggressive environmental cleaning (given the persistence of norovirus on inanimate objects) and active exclusion of ill staff and visitors.

Chickenpox Infection-control practitioners institute a varicella exposure investigation and control plan whenever health care workers either (1) are exposed to chickenpox (Chap. 173) in the community or through patients with initially unrecognized infections or (2) work during the 24 h before developing chickenpox. The names of exposed workers and patients are obtained; medical histories are reviewed, and (if necessary) serologic tests for immunity are conducted; physicians are notified of susceptible exposed patients; postexposure prophylaxis with varicella-zoster immune globulin (VZIG) is considered for immunocompromised or pregnant contacts (see Table 173-1); varicella vaccine is recommended or preemptive use of acyclovir is considered

as an alternative strategy in other susceptible persons; and susceptible exposed employees are furloughed during the at-risk period for disease (8–21 days or—if VZIG has been administered—28 days). Routine varicella vaccination of children and susceptible employees can markedly decrease risk and frequency of exposures.

Tuberculosis Important measures for the control of tuberculosis (Chap. 158) include prompt recognition, isolation, and treatment of cases; recognition of atypical presentations (e.g., lower-lobe infiltrates without cavitation); use of negative-pressure, 100% exhaust, private isolation rooms with closed doors and 6–12 or more air changes per hour; use of N95 "respirators" (approved by the National Institute for Occupational Safety and Health) by caregivers entering isolation rooms; possible use of high-efficiency particulate air filter units and/or ultraviolet lights for disinfecting air when other engineering controls are not feasible or reliable; and follow-up skin-testing of susceptible personnel who have been exposed to infectious patients before isolation. The use of new serologic tests, rather than skin tests, in the diagnosis of latent tuberculosis for infection control purposes is being studied.

Group A Streptococcal Infections The potential for an outbreak of group A streptococcal infection (Chap. 130) should be considered when even a single nosocomial case occurs. Most outbreaks involve surgical wounds and are due to the presence of an asymptomatic carrier in the operating room. Investigation can be confounded by carriage at extrapharyngeal sites such as the rectum and vagina. Health care workers in whom carriage has been linked to nosocomial transmission of group A streptococci are removed from the patient-care setting and are not permitted to return until carriage has been eliminated by antimicrobial therapy.

Fungal Infections Fungal spores are common in the environment, particularly on dusty surfaces. When dusty areas are disturbed during hospital repairs or renovation, the spores become airborne. Inhalation of spores by immunosuppressed (especially neutropenic) patients creates a risk of pulmonary and/or paranasal sinus infection and disseminated aspergillosis (Chap. 197). Routine surveillance among neutropenic patients for infections with filamentous fungi, such as *Aspergillus* and *Fusarium*, helps hospitals to determine whether they are facing unduly extensive environmental risks. As a matter of routine, hospitals should inspect and clean air-handling equipment, review all planned renovations with infection-control personnel and subsequently construct appropriate barriers, remove immunosuppressed patients from renovation sites, and consider the use of high-efficiency particulate air intake filters for rooms housing immunosuppressed patients.

Legionellosis Nosocomial *Legionella* pneumonia (Chap. 141) is most often due to contamination of potable water and predominantly affects immunosuppressed patients, particularly those receiving glucocorticoid medication. The risk varies greatly within and among geographic regions, depending on the extent of hospital hot-water contamination and on specific hospital practices (e.g., inappropriate use of nonsterile water in respiratory therapy equipment). Laboratory-based surveillance for nosocomial *Legionella* should be performed, and a diagnosis of legionellosis should probably be considered more often than it is. If cases are detected, environmental samples (e.g., tap water) should be cultured. If cultures yield *Legionella* and if typing of clinical and environmental isolates reveals a correlation, eradication measures should be pursued. An alternative approach is to periodically culture tap water in wards housing high-risk patients. If *Legionella* is found, a concerted effort should be made to culture samples from all patients with nosocomial pneumonia for *Legionella*.

Antibiotic-Resistant Bacteria Control of antibiotic resistance, particularly in outbreaks (Table 125-3), depends on close laboratory surveillance, with early detection of problems; on aggressive reinforcement of routine asepsis (e.g., hand hygiene); on implementation of barrier precautions for all colonized and/or infected patients; on use of patient-surveillance cultures to more fully ascertain the extent of patient

TABLE 125-3	CONTROLLING ANTIBIOTIC RESISTANCE: APPROACHES TO CONSIDER

Conduct surveillance for antibiotic resistance.

Perform molecular typing (e.g., pulsed-field gel electrophoresis) when rates increase.

For clonal expansion (e.g., single-strain outbreaks): Stress hand hygiene (alcohol hand rub and universal gloving); monitor adherence and give feedback.

For polyclonal expansion (e.g., multistrain outbreaks): Stress antibiotic prudence (consider antibiotic rotation for ICUs); monitor adherence and give feedback.

For continued problems: Obtain patient-surveillance cultures and isolate or provide cohort nursing for colonized/infected patients.

Control device-related infections.

Enlist administrative support proactively.

Source: Adapted from: RA Weinstein, Emerg Infect Dis 7:188, 2001; see also www.cdc.gov/ncidod/dhqp/pdf/ar/mdroGuideline2006.pdf.

colonization; and on timely initiation of an epidemiologic investigation when rates increase. Colonized personnel who are implicated in nosocomial transmission and patients who pose a threat may be decontaminated. In a few ICUs, selective decontamination of patients has been used successfully as a temporary emergency control measure for outbreaks of infection due to gram-negative bacilli. Other promising ICU control measures include daily bathing of patients with chlorhexidine and enforcement of environmental cleaning; in recent trials, each of these measures reduced cross-transmission of VRE. The value of "search-and-destroy" methods—i.e., the use of active surveillance cultures to detect and isolate the "resistance iceberg" of patients colonized with methicillin-resistant *S. aureus* (MRSA) or VRE—in non-outbreak settings has been controversial but is credited with elimination of nosocomial MRSA in the Netherlands and Denmark.

Currently, several antibiotic resistance problems are of particular health care concern. First, the emergence of community-acquired MRSA has been dramatic in many countries, with as many as 50% of community-acquired "staph infections" in some U.S. cities now caused by strains resistant to β-lactam antibiotics (Chap. 129). The potential incursion of these strains into hospitals and the resulting impact on control of nosocomial MRSA infections are of enormous concern. Second, in the ongoing global reemergence of nosocomial multidrug-resistant gram-negative bacilli, new problems include plasmid-mediated resistance to fluoroquinolones, metallo-β-lactamase-mediated resistance to carbapenems, and panresistant strains of *Acinetobacter*. Many of these multidrug-resistant strains are susceptible only to colistin, which has led to a "rediscovery" and renewed use of this drug. Finally, clinical infections with MRSA strains exhibiting high-level vancomycin resistance due to VRE-derived plasmids have been reported in several patients in the United States, often in the setting of prolonged or repeated treatment with vancomycin and/or VRE colonization. The detection of any of these current problems should trigger an epidemiologic investigation and aggressive infection-control measures.

Because the excessive use of broad-spectrum antibiotics underlies many resistance problems, aggressive antibiotic-control policies must be considered a cornerstone of resistance-control efforts. Recommendations for "antibiotic stewardship" are being promulgated by the Infectious Diseases Society of America. Although the efficacy of antibiotic-control measures in reducing rates of antimicrobial resistance has not been proven in prospective controlled trials, it seems worthwhile to restrict the use of particular agents to narrowly defined indications in order to limit selective pressure on the nosocomial flora.

Bioterrorism and Other "Surge-Event" Preparedness The horrific attack on the World Trade Center in New York City on September 11, 2001; the subsequent mailings of anthrax spores in the United States; and recently exposed terrorist plans and activities in the United Kingdom and elsewhere have made bioterrorism a prominent source of concern to hospital infection-control programs. The essentials for hospital preparedness (Table 125-4) entail education, internal and ex-

TABLE 125-4	HIGHLIGHTS OF HOSPITAL PREPAREDNESS FOR BIOTERRORISM AND OTHER "SURGE EVENTS"

Emergency Department: Educate (bioterrorism diagnoses, case definitions, and appropriate syndrome-based isolation precautions)

Laboratory: Identify protocols and laboratory safety procedures for agents of bioterrorism

Pharmacy: Develop medication and vaccine par stock, allocation, and delivery plans

Nursing: Assess bed and isolation surge capacity; help develop contingency plans to free bed space (e.g., early discharges)

Hospital Police: Plan for responsibilities as first responders and providers of risk assessment

Engineering/Buildings and Grounds: Evaluate air-handling systems and ensure familiarity with shutoffs and controls; educate about environmental decontamination

Outpatient Areas: Develop plans for delivery of prophylactic medications and/or vaccines

Public Health: Open lines of communication, education, and surveillance

The Community: Plan for infection-control practitioners to serve as liaisons for emergency departments, laboratories, and community providers

Administration: Perform resource assessment (e.g., medical supplies, transportation capabilities, potable water, sanitation facilities, provider backup, bed-space backup); oversee development of an incident command system

"Morale Officer": Keep staff functioning

ternal communication, and risk assessment. Up-to-date information on a variety of bioterrorism-associated issues is available from the CDC (see www.bt.cdc.gov).

EMPLOYEE HEALTH SERVICE ISSUES

An institution's employee health service is a critical component of its infection-control efforts. New employees should be processed through the service, where a contagious-disease history can be taken; evidence of immunity to a variety of diseases, such as hepatitis B, chickenpox, measles, mumps, and rubella, can be sought; immunizations for hepatitis B, measles, mumps, rubella, and varicella can be given as needed and a reminder about the need for yearly influenza immunization can be imparted; baseline and "booster" PPD (purified protein derivative of tuberculin) skin-testing or serologic testing for tuberculosis can be performed; and education about personal responsibility for infection control can be initiated. Evaluations of employees should be codified to meet the requirements of accrediting and regulatory agencies.

The employee health service must have protocols for dealing with workers who have been exposed to contagious diseases, such as those percutaneously or mucosally exposed to the blood of patients infected with HIV or hepatitis B or C virus. For example, postexposure HIV prophylaxis with a combination of two or three antiretroviral agents is recommended; free consultation is available from the CDC PEPLine (888-HIV-4911). Protocols are also needed for dealing with caregivers who have common contagious diseases (such as chickenpox, group A streptococcal infections, respiratory infections, and infectious diarrhea) and for those who have less common but high-visibility public health problems (such as chronic hepatitis B or C or HIV infection) for which exposure-control guidelines have been published by the CDC and by the Society for Healthcare Epidemiology of America.

FURTHER READINGS

Bratzler DW, Hunt DR: The Surgical Infection Prevention and Surgical Care Improvement Projects: National initiatives to improve outcomes for patients having surgery. Clin Infect Dis 43:322, 2006

Centers for Disease Control and Prevention: Environmental infection control guidelines. Recommendations of the Healthcare Infection Control Practices Advisory Committee. MMWR 52(RR10):1, 2003

———: Guideline for hand hygiene in health-care settings: Recommendations of the Healthcare Infection Control Practices Advisory Committee and the HICPAC/SHEA/APIC/IDSA Hand Hygiene Task Force. MMWR 51(RR-16):1, 2002

842 ———: Guidelines for preventing opportunistic infections among hematopoietic stem cell transplant recipients: Recommendations of CDC, the Infectious Diseases Society of America, and the American Society of Blood and Marrow Transplantation. MMWR 49(RR-10):1, 2000

HOTA B, WEINSTEIN RA: Basics work: Preventing infections in ICUs in developing countries. Crit Care Med 33:2133, 2005

MCKIBBEN L et al: Guidance on public reporting of healthcare-associated recommendations of the Healthcare Infection Control Practices Advisory Committee. Infect Control Hosp Epidemiol 26:580, 2005

MERMEL LA et al: Guidelines for the management of intravascular catheter–related infections. Clin Infect Dis 32:1249, 2001

STRAUSBAUGH LJ et al: Preventing transmission of multidrug-resistant bacteria in health care settings: A tale of two guidelines. Clin Infect Dis 42:828, 2006

WEINSTEIN RA et al: Infection control report cards—securing patient safety. N Engl J Med 353:225, 2005

———, BONTEN MJ: Controlling antibiotic resistant bacteria: What's an intensivist to do? Crit Care Med 33:2446, 2005

126 Infections in Transplant Recipients

Robert Finberg, Joyce Fingeroth

The evaluation of infections in transplant recipients involves consideration of both the donor and the recipient of the transplanted organ. Infections following transplantation are complicated by the use of drugs that are necessary to enhance the likelihood of survival of the transplanted organ but that also cause the host to be immunocompromised. Thus, what might have been a latent or asymptomatic infection in an immunocompetent donor or in the recipient prior to therapy can become a life-threatening problem when the recipient becomes immunosuppressed.

PRETRANSPLANTATION EVALUATION

A variety of organisms have been transmitted by organ transplantation (Table 126-1). Careful attention to the sterility of the medium used to process the organ combined with meticulous microbiologic evaluation reduces rates of transmission of bacteria that may be present or grow in the organ culture medium. From 2% to >20% of donor kidneys are estimated to be contaminated with bacteria—in most cases, with the organisms that colonize the skin or grow in the tissue culture medium used to bathe the donor kidney while it awaits implantation. The reported rate of bacterial contamination of transplanted stem cells (bone marrow, peripheral blood, cord blood) is as high as 17% but is most commonly ~1%. The use of enrichment columns and monoclonal-antibody depletion procedures results in a higher incidence of contamination. In one series of patients receiving contaminated products, 14% had fever or bacteremia, but none died. Results of cultures performed at the time of cryopreservation and at the time of thawing were helpful in guiding therapy for the recipient.

In many transplantation centers, transmission of infections that may be latent or clinically inapparent in the donor organ has resulted in the development of specific donor-screening protocols. In addition to ordering serologic studies focused on viruses such as herpes-group viruses [herpes simplex virus types 1 and 2 (HSV-1, HSV-2), varicella-zoster virus (VZV), cytomegalovirus (CMV), human herpesvirus (HHV) type 6, Epstein-Barr virus (EBV), and Kaposi's sarcoma–associated herpesvirus (KSHV)] as well as hepatitis B and C viruses, human immunodeficiency virus (HIV), human T cell lymphotropic virus type I, and

West Nile virus, donors should be screened for parasites such as *Toxoplasma gondii and Trypanosoma cruzi* (the latter particularly in Latin America). Clinicians caring for prospective organ donors should also consider assessing stool for parasites, should examine chest radiographs for evidence of granulomatous disease, and should perform purified protein derivative (PPD) skin testing or obtain blood for immune cell–based assays that detect active or latent *Mycobacterium tuberculosis* infection. An investigation of the donor's dietary habits (e.g., consumption of raw meat or fish or of unpasteurized dairy products), occupations or avocations (e.g., gardening or spelunking), and travel history (e.g., travel to areas with endemic fungi) is also mandatory. It is expected that the recipient will have been likewise assessed. Because of immune dysfunction resulting from chemotherapy or underlying chronic

---

TABLE 126-1 ORGANISMS TRANSMITTED BY ORGAN TRANSPLANTATION AND THEIR PRIMARY SITES OF REACTIVATION DISEASE[a]

	Blood	Lungs	Heart	Brain	Liver/Spleen	Skin
Viruses						
Cytomegalovirus[b]	+	+	±	±	+	±
Epstein-Barr virus[c]	+	+	±	±	+	±
Herpes simplex virus	+					+
Human herpesvirus type 6	+	+			+	+
Kaposi's sarcoma–associated herpesvirus	+	±			+	
Hepatitis B and C viruses	+				+	
Rabies virus[d]				+		
West Nile virus	+			+		
Fungi						
Candida albicans	+	+			+	+
Histoplasma capsulatum	+	+			+	+
Cryptococcus neoformans	+	+		+	±	+
Parasites						
Toxoplasma gondii[e]		+	+	+		
Strongyloides stercoralis[f,g]		+				
Trypanosoma cruzi[g]			+			
Plasmodium falciparum[g]	+					
Prion Diseases						
Creutzfeldt-Jakob disease (CJD)[h]				+		
Variant CJD/bovine spongiform encephalopathy[i]				+		

[a]+, well documented; ±, probably occurs.

[b]Cytomegalovirus reactivation is prone to occur in the transplanted organ. The same may be true for Kaposi's sarcoma–associated herpesvirus.

[c]Epstein-Barr virus reactivation usually presents as an extranodal proliferation of transformed B cells and can be present either as a diffuse disease or as a mass lesion in a single organ.

[d]Rabies virus has been transmitted through corneal transplants.

[e]*T. gondii* usually causes disease in the brain. In hematopoietic stem cell transplant recipients, acute pulmonary disease may also occur. Heart transplant recipients develop disease in the allograft.

[f]*Strongyloides* "hyperinfection" may present with pulmonary disease—often associated with gram-negative bacterial pneumonia.

[g]While transmission with organs has been described, it is unusual.

[h]CJD (sporadic and familial) has been transmitted with corneal transplants. Whether it can be transmitted with blood is not known.

[i]Variant CJD can be transmitted with transfused non-leukodepleted blood, posing a theoretical risk to transplant recipients.

TABLE 126-2	COMMON SOURCES OF INFECTIONS AFTER HEMATOPOIETIC STEM CELL TRANSPLANTATION		
	Period after Transplantation		
Infection Site	**Early (<1 Month)**	**Middle (1–4 Months)**	**Late (>6 Months)**
Disseminated	Aerobic gram-negative, gram-positive bacteria	*Nocardia* *Candida, Aspergillus*	Encapsulated bacteria (*Streptococcus pneumoniae, Haemophilus influenzae, Neisseria meningitidis*)
Skin and mucous membranes	HSV	HHV-6	VZV
Lungs	Aerobic gram-negative, gram-positive bacteria *Candida, Aspergillus* HSV	CMV, seasonal respiratory viruses *Pneumocystis* *Toxoplasma*	*Pneumocystis*
Gastrointestinal tract		CMV	
Kidney		BK virus, adenovirus	BK virus
Brain	HHV-6	HHV-6 *Toxoplasma*	*Toxoplasma* JC virus
Bone marrow	HHV-6		

Note: CMV, cytomegalovirus; HHV-6, human herpesvirus type 6; HSV, herpes simplex virus; VZV, varicella-zoster virus.

disease, however, direct testing of the recipient may prove less reliable. This chapter considers aspects of infection unique to various transplantation settings.

INFECTIONS IN HEMATOPOIETIC STEM CELL TRANSPLANT (HSCT) RECIPIENTS

Transplantation of hematopoietic stem cells from bone marrow or from peripheral or cord blood for cancer, immunodeficiency, or autoimmune disease results in a transient state of complete immunologic incompetence. Immediately after transplantation, both phagocytes and adaptive immune cells (T and B cells) are absent, and the host is extremely susceptible to infection. The reconstitution that follows transplantation has been likened to maturation of the immune system in neonates. The analogy does not entirely predict infections seen in HSCT recipients, however, because the new cells mature in an old host who has several latent infections already. Nevertheless, most infections occur in a predictable time frame after transplantation (Table 126-2).

BACTERIAL INFECTIONS

In the first month after hematopoietic stem cell transplantation, infectious complications are similar to those in granulocytopenic patients receiving chemotherapy for acute leukemia (Chap. 82). Because of the anticipated 1- to 3-week duration of neutropenia and the high rate of bacterial infection in this population, many centers give prophylactic antibiotics to patients upon initiation of myeloablative therapy. Quinolones decrease the incidence of gram-negative bacteremia among these patients. Bacterial infections are common in the first few days after hematopoietic stem cell transplantation. The organisms involved are predominantly those found on the skin or in IV catheters (*Staphylococcus aureus*, coagulase-negative staphylococci) and aerobic bacteria that colonize the bowel (*Escherichia coli*, *Klebsiella*, *Pseudomonas*). Beyond the first few days of neutropenia, infections with filamentous bacteria such as *Nocardia* become more common. Episodes of bacteremia due to encapsulated organisms mark the late posttransplantation period (>6 months after hematopoietic stem cell reconstitution). Chemotherapy and use of broad-spectrum antibiotics place HSCT patients at risk for diarrhea and colitis caused by *Clostridium difficile* overgrowth and toxin production.

FUNGAL INFECTIONS

Beyond the first week after transplantation, fungal infections become increasingly common, particularly among patients who have received broad-spectrum antibiotics. As in most granulocytopenic patients, *Candida* infections are most commonly seen in this setting. With increased use of prophylactic fluconazole, infections with resistant fungi—in partic-

ular, *Aspergillus* and other molds (*Fusarium, Scedosporium, Penicillium*)—have become more common, prompting some centers to replace fluconazole with agents such as caspofungin, voriconazole, and posaconazole. The role of antifungal prophylaxis with these different agents, in contrast to empirical treatment for suspected or documented infection, remains controversial (Chap. 82). In patients with graft-versus-host disease (GVHD) who require prolonged or indefinite courses of glucocorticoids and other immunosuppressive agents [e.g., cyclosporine, FK506 (tacrolimus), mycophenolate, rapamycin (sirolimus), antithymocyte globulin, or anti-CD52 antibody (alemtuzumab, an antilymphocyte and antimonocyte monoclonal antibody)], there is a high risk of fungal infection (usually with *Candida* or *Aspergillus*), even after engraftment and resolution of neutropenia. These patients are also at high risk for reactivation of latent fungal infection (histoplasmosis, coccidioidomycosis, blastomycosis) in areas where endemic fungi reside and if they have been involved in activities such as gardening or caving. Prolonged use of central venous catheters for parenteral nutrition (lipids) increases the risk of fungemia with *Malassezia*. Some centers administer prophylactic antifungal agents to these patients. Because of the high and prolonged risk of *Pneumocystis jiroveci* pneumonia (especially among patients being treated for hematologic malignancies), most patients receive maintenance prophylaxis with trimethoprim-sulfamethoxazole (TMP-SMX) starting 1 month after engraftment and continuing for at least 1 year.

PARASITIC INFECTIONS

The regimen just described for the fungal pathogen *Pneumocystis* may also protect patients seropositive for the parasite *T. gondii*, which may cause pneumonia or, more commonly, central nervous system (CNS) lesions. The advantages of maintaining HSCT recipients on daily TMP-SMX for 1 year after transplantation include some protection against *Listeria monocytogenes* and nocardial disease as well as late infections with *Streptococcus pneumoniae* and *Haemophilus influenzae*, which are a consequence of the inability of the immature immune system to respond to polysaccharide antigens.

VIRAL INFECTIONS

HSCT recipients are susceptible to infection with a variety of viruses, including primary and reactivation syndromes caused by most HHVs (Table 126-3) and acute infections caused by viruses that circulate in the community.

Herpes Simplex Virus Within the first 2 weeks after transplantation, most patients who are seropositive for HSV-1 excrete the virus from the oropharynx. The ability to isolate HSV declines with time. Administration of prophylactic acyclovir (or valacyclovir) to seropositive HSCT recipients has been shown to reduce mucositis and prevent HSV pneumonia (a rare condition reported almost exclusively in allogeneic HSCT recipients). Both esophagitis (usually due to HSV-1) and anogenital disease (commonly induced by HSV-2) may be prevented with acyclovir prophylaxis. For further discussion, see Chap. 172.

Varicella-Zoster Virus Reactivation of herpes zoster may occur within the first month but more commonly occurs several months after transplantation. Reactivation rates are ~40% for allogeneic recipients and 25% for autologous recipients. Localized zoster can spread rapidly in an immunosuppressed patient. Fortunately, disseminated disease can usually be controlled with high doses of acyclovir. Because of frequent dissemination among patients with skin lesions, acyclovir is given prophylactically in some centers to prevent severe disease. Low doses of acyclovir (400 mg orally, three times daily) appear to be effec-

TABLE 126-3 COMMON HERPESVIRUS SYNDROMES IN TRANSPLANT RECIPIENTS

Virus	Reactivation Disease
Herpes simplex virus type 1	Oral lesions
	Esophageal lesions
	Pneumonia (only in hematopoietic stem cell transplant recipients)
	Hepatitis
Herpes simplex virus type 2	Anogenital lesions
	Hepatitis
Varicella-zoster virus	Zoster (potentially disseminated)
Cytomegalovirus	Associated graft rejection
	Fever
	Bone marrow failure
	Pneumonitis
	Gastrointestinal disease
	Other
Epstein-Barr virus	B cell lymphoproliferative disease/lymphoma
	Oral hairy leukoplakia (rare)
Human herpesvirus type 6	Fever
	Delayed monocyte/platelet engraftment
	Encephalitis (controversial)
Human herpesvirus type 7	Undefined
Kaposi's sarcoma– associated virus	Kaposi's sarcoma
	Primary effusion lymphoma (rare)
	Multicentric Castleman's disease (rare)
	Marrow aplasia

tive in preventing reactivation of VZV. However, acyclovir can also suppress the development of VZV-specific immunity. Thus, its administration for only 6 months after transplantation does not prevent zoster from occurring when treatment is stopped. Some data suggest that administration of low doses of acyclovir for an entire year after transplantation is effective and may eliminate most cases of posttransplantation zoster. For further discussion, see Chap. 173.

Cytomegalovirus The onset of CMV disease (interstitial pneumonia, bone marrow suppression, graft failure, hepatitis/colitis) usually begins 30–90 days after transplantation, when the granulocyte count is adequate but immunologic reconstitution has not occurred. CMV disease rarely develops earlier than 14 days after transplantation and may become evident as late as 4 months after the procedure. It is of greatest concern in the second month after transplantation, particularly in allogeneic HSCT recipients. In cases in which the donor marrow is depleted of T cells (to prevent GVHD or eliminate a T cell tumor), the disease may be manifested earlier. The use of alemtuzumab to prevent GVHD in nonmyeloablative transplantation has been associated with an increase in CMV disease. Patients who receive ganciclovir for prophylaxis, preemptive treatment, or treatment (see below) may develop recurrent CMV infection even later than 4 months after transplantation, as treatment appears to delay the development of the normal immune response to CMV infection. Although CMV disease may present as isolated fever, granulocytopenia, thrombocytopenia, or gastrointestinal disease, the foremost cause of death from CMV infection in the setting of hematopoietic stem cell transplantation is pneumonia.

With the standard use of CMV-negative or filtered blood products, primary CMV infection should be a risk in allogeneic transplantation only when the donor is CMV-seropositive and the recipient is CMV-seronegative. Reactivation disease or superinfection with another strain from the donor is also common in CMV-positive recipients, and most seropositive patients who undergo hematopoietic stem cell transplantation excrete CMV, with or without clinical findings. Serious CMV disease is much more common among allogeneic than autologous recipients and is often associated with GVHD. In addition to pneumonia and marrow suppression (and, less often, graft failure), manifestations of CMV disease in HSCT recipients include fever with or without arthralgias, myalgias, hepatitis, and esophagitis. CMV ulcerations occur in both the lower and the upper gastrointestinal tract, and it may be difficult to distinguish diarrhea due to GVHD from that due to CMV infection. The finding of CMV in the liver of a patient with GVHD does not necessarily mean that CMV is responsible for hepatic enzyme abnormalities. It is interesting that the ocular and neurologic manifestations of CMV infections are uncommon in these patients.

Management of CMV disease in HSCT recipients includes strategies directed at prophylaxis and preemptive therapy (suppression of silent replication) and at treatment of disease. Prophylaxis results in a lower incidence of disease at the cost of treating many patients who otherwise would not require therapy. Because of the high fatality rate associated with CMV pneumonia in these patients and the difficulty of early diagnosis of CMV infection, prophylactic IV ganciclovir (or oral valganciclovir) has been used in some centers and has been shown to abort CMV disease during the period of maximal vulnerability (from engraftment to day 120 after transplantation). Ganciclovir also prevents HSV reactivation and reduces the risk of VZV reactivation; thus acyclovir prophylaxis should be discontinued when ganciclovir is administered. The foremost problem with the administration of ganciclovir relates to adverse effects, which include dose-related bone marrow suppression (thrombocytopenia, leukopenia, anemia, and pancytopenia). Because the frequency of CMV pneumonia is lower among autologous HSCT recipients (2–7%) than among allogeneic HSCT recipients (10–40%), prophylaxis in the former group will not become the rule until a less toxic oral antiviral agent becomes available. Promising new drugs that are now being assessed in clinical trials include maribavir, a benzimidazole ribonucleoside that inhibits a viral protein kinase activity (UL97).

Like prophylaxis, preemptive treatment, which targets patients with polymerase chain reaction (PCR) evidence of CMV entails the unnecessary treatment of many individuals (on the basis of a laboratory test that is not highly predictive of disease) with drugs that have adverse effects. Currently, because of the neutropenia associated with ganciclovir in HSCT recipients, a preemptive approach—that is, treatment of those patients in whose blood CMV is detected by an antigen or nucleic acid amplification test—is used at most centers. This approach is almost as effective as prophylaxis and causes less toxicity. Quantitative viral load assays, which are not dependent on circulating polymorphonuclear leukocytes, have supplanted antigen-based assays and are used by most centers. A positive test (or increasing viral load) prompts the initiation of preemptive therapy. When prophylaxis or preemptive therapy is stopped, late disease may occur, although by then the patient is often equipped with improved graft function and is better able to combat disease.

Treatment of CMV pneumonia in HSCT recipients (unlike that in other clinical settings) involves both IV immune globulin (IVIg) and ganciclovir. In patients who cannot tolerate ganciclovir, foscarnet is a useful alternative, although it may produce nephrotoxicity and electrolyte imbalance. When neither ganciclovir nor foscarnet is clinically tolerated, cidofovir can be used; however, its efficacy is less well established, and its side effects include nephrotoxicity. Case reports have suggested that the immunosuppressive agent leflunomide may be active in this setting, but controlled studies are lacking. Maribavir is under investigation for treatment as well as prophylaxis. Transfusion of CMV-specific T cells from the donor decreased viral load in a small series of patients; this result suggests that immunotherapy may play a role in the treatment of this disease in the future. For further discussion, see Chap. 175.

Human Herpesviruses 6 and 7 HHV-6, the cause of roseola in children, is a ubiquitous herpesvirus that reactivates (as determined by quantitative plasma PCR) in ~50% of HSCT recipients 2–4 weeks after transplantation. Reactivation is more common among patients requiring glucocorticoids for GVHD and among those receiving second transplants. Reactivation of HHV-6 (primarily type B) appears to be associated with delayed monocyte and platelet engraftment. Although encephalitis developing after transplantation has been associated with HHV-6 in cerebrospinal fluid (CSF), the causality of the association is not well defined. In several cases, plasma viremia was detected long before the onset of encephalitis; nevertheless, patients with encephalitis did tend to have very high viral loads in plasma at the time of CNS illness. HHV-6 DNA is sometimes found in lung samples after transplantation. However, its role in pneumonitis is also unclear. While HHV-6 has been shown to be susceptible to foscarnet (and possibly to ganciclovir) in vitro, the efficacy of antiviral treatment has not been well studied. Little is known about the related herpesvirus HHV-7 or its role in posttransplantation infection. For further discussion, see Chap. 175.

Epstein-Barr Virus Primary EBV infection can be fatal to HSCT recipients; EBV reactivation can cause EBV–B cell lymphoproliferative disease (EBV-LPD), which may also be fatal to patients taking immunosuppressive drugs. Latent EBV infection of B cells leads to several interesting phenomena in HSCT recipients. The marrow ablation that occurs as part of the HSCT procedure may sometimes eliminate latent EBV from the host. Infection can then be reacquired immediately after transplantation by transfer of infected donor B cells. Rarely, transplantation from a seronegative donor may result in cure. The recipient is then at risk for a second primary infection.

EBV-LPD can develop in the recipient's B cells (if any survive marrow ablation) but is more likely to be a consequence of outgrowth of infected donor cells. Both lytic and latent EBV replication are more likely during immunosuppression (e.g., they are associated with GVHD and the use of antibodies to T cells). Although less likely in autologous transplantation, reactivation can occur in T cell–depleted autologous recipients (e.g., patients being given antibodies to T cells for the treatment of a T cell lymphoma with marrow depletion). EBV-LPD, which can become apparent as early as 1–3 months after engraftment, can cause high fevers and cervical adenopathy resembling the symptoms of infectious mononucleosis but more commonly presents as an extranodal mass. The incidence of EBV-LPD among allogeneic HSCT recipients is 0.6–1%, which contrasts with figures of ~5% for renal transplant recipients and up to 20% for cardiac transplant patients. In all cases, EBV-LPD is more likely to occur with high-dose, prolonged immunosuppression, especially that caused by the use of antibodies to T cells, glucocorticoids, and calcineurin inhibitors (e.g., cyclosporine, FK506).

PCR can be used to monitor EBV production after hematopoietic stem cell transplantation. High or increasing viral loads predict an enhanced likelihood of developing EBV-LPD and should prompt rapid reduction of immunosuppression and search for a focus of disease. If reduction of immunosuppression does not have the desired effect, administration of a monoclonal antibody to CD20 (rituximab or others) for the treatment of B cell lymphomas that express this surface protein has elicited dramatic responses and currently constitutes first-line therapy for CD20-positive EBV-LPD. However, long-term suppression of new antibody responses accompanies therapy, and recurrences are not infrequent. Additional B cell–directed antibodies, including anti-CD22, are under study. The role of antivirals is uncertain because no available agents have been documented to have activity against the different forms of latent EBV infection. Preventing lytic replication in these patients would theoretically produce a statistical decrease in the frequency of latent disease by decreasing the number of virions available to cause additional infection. In case reports and small animal studies, ganciclovir and/or high-dose zidovudine together with other agents has been used to eradicate EBV-LPD and CNS lymphomas, another EBV-associated complication of transplantation. Both interferon and retinoic acid have been employed in the treatment of EBV-LPD, as has IVIg, but no large prospective studies have assessed the efficacy of any of these agents. Several additional drugs are undergoing preclinical evaluation. Standard chemotherapeutic regimens have been used as a last resort, even though patients' tolerance and long-term results have been disappointing. EBV-specific T cells generated from the donor have been used experimentally to prevent and to treat EBV-LPD in allogeneic recipients, and efforts are under way to increase the activity and specificity of ex vivo–generated T cells. For further discussion, see Chap. 174.

Human Herpesvirus 8 The EBV-related gammaherpesvirus KSHV, which is causally associated with Kaposi's sarcoma, with primary effusion lymphoma, and with multicentric Castleman's disease, has rarely resulted in disease in HSCT recipients, although some cases of virus-associated marrow aplasia have been reported in the peritransplantation period. The relatively low seroprevalence of KSHV in the population and the limited duration of profound T cell suppression after hematopoietic stem cell transplantation provide a probable explanation for the currently low incidence of KSHV disease. For further discussion, see Chap. 175.

Other (Nonherpes) Viruses The diagnosis of pneumonia in HSCT recipients poses some special problems. Because patients have undergone treatment with multiple chemotherapeutic agents and sometimes irradiation, their differential diagnosis should include—in addition to bacterial and fungal pneumonia—CMV pneumonitis, pneumonia of other viral etiologies, parasitic pneumonia, diffuse alveolar hemorrhage, and chemical- or radiation-associated pneumonitis. Since fungi and viruses [e.g., influenza A and B viruses, respiratory syncytial virus (RSV), parainfluenza virus (types 1, 2, and 3), metapneumoviruses, and adenoviruses] are also causes of pneumonia in this setting, it is important to diagnose CMV specifically (see "Cytomegalovirus," above). *M. tuberculosis* has been an uncommon cause of pneumonia among HSCT recipients in Western countries (accounting for <0.1–0.2% of cases) but is common in Hong Kong (5.5%) and in countries where the prevalence of tuberculosis is high. The recipient's exposure history is clearly critical in an assessment of posttransplantation infections.

Both RSV and parainfluenza viruses, particularly type 3, can cause severe or even fatal pneumonia in HSCT recipients. Infections with both of these agents sometimes occur as disastrous nosocomial epidemics. Preemptive treatment of upper airway infection and therapy for established lower tract invasion with aerosolized ribavirin and/or the anti-RSV monoclonal antibody palivizumab have been reported to lessen the severity of RSV disease in some studies. (Respigam, a polyclonal anti-RSV preparation, is no longer available.) However, no large prospective studies establishing the efficacy of these agents in HSCT recipients have been performed. Aerosolized ribavirin is difficult to administer. Antibody in particular may prove more active in immunocompromised hosts, but relevant evaluation is lacking.

Influenza also occurs in HSCT recipients and generally mirrors the presence of infection in the community. Progression to pneumonia is more common when infection occurs early after transplantation and when the recipient is lymphopenic. Several drugs are available for the treatment of influenza. Amantadine and rimantadine have limited effects, primarily reducing symptoms and shortening the duration of illness caused by sensitive strains of influenza A virus. The neuraminidase inhibitors oseltamivir (oral) and zanamivir (aerosolized) are active against both influenza A virus and influenza B virus and are a reasonable treatment option. Parenteral forms of neuraminidase inhibitors are undergoing clinical trials. An important preventive measure is immunization of household members, hospital staff members, and other frequent contacts.

Human metapneumovirus, a paramyxovirus, can sometimes cause severe pneumonia and respiratory failure in HSCT recipients; however, mild or even asymptomatic infection may be more common. At present, the overall contribution of human metapneumovirus to the burden of lower respiratory tract disease in HSCT recipients is unknown.

Adenovirus can be isolated from HSCT recipients at rates varying from 5 to 18%. Although hemorrhagic cystitis, pneumonia, gastroenteritis, and fatal disseminated infection have been reported, adenovirus infection, which (like CMV infection) usually occurs in the first or second month after transplantation, is often asymptomatic. A role for cidofovir therapy has been suggested, but the efficacy of this agent is unproven.

Infections with parvovirus B19 (presenting as anemia or occasionally as pancytopenia) and enteroviruses (sometimes fatal) can occur. Parvovirus infection may possibly respond to IVIg (Chap. 177). Intranasal pleconaril, a capsid-binding agent, is being studied for the treatment of enterovirus infection.

Rhinoviruses and coronaviruses are frequent co-pathogens in HSCT recipients; however, whether they independently contribute to significant pulmonary infection is not known. Rotaviruses are a common cause of gastroenteritis in these patients. The polyomavirus BK virus is found at high titers in the urine of patients who are profoundly immunosuppressed. BK viruria may be associated with hemorrhagic cystitis in these patients. Compared with the incidence among patients with impaired T cell function due to HIV infection, progressive multifocal leukoencephalopathy caused by the related JC virus is rare among HSCT recipients (Chap. 376). When transmitted by mosquitoes or by blood transfusion, West Nile virus can cause encephalitis and death after hematopoietic stem cell transplantation.

INFECTIONS IN SOLID ORGAN TRANSPLANT (SOT) RECIPIENTS

Morbidity and mortality among SOT recipients are reduced by the use of effective antibiotics. The organisms that cause acute infections in recipients of SOT are different from those that infect HSCT recipients because SOT recipients do not go through a period of neutropenia. As the transplantation procedure involves major surgery, however, SOT recipients are subject to infections at anastomotic sites and to wound infections. Compared with HSCT recipients, SOT patients are immunosuppressed for longer periods (often permanently). Thus they are susceptible to many of the same organisms as patients with chronically impaired T cell immunity (Chap. 82, especially Table 82-1).

During the early period (<1 month after transplantation), infections are most commonly caused by extracellular bacteria (staphylococci, streptococci, enterococci, *E. coli*, other gram-negative organisms), which often originate in surgical wound or anastomotic sites. The type of transplant largely determines the spectrum of infection.

In subsequent weeks, the consequences of the administration of agents that suppress cell-mediated immunity become apparent, and acquisition or reactivation of viruses and parasites (from the recipient or from the transplanted organ) can occur. CMV infection is often a problem, particularly in the first 6 months after transplantation and may present as severe systemic disease or as infection of the transplanted organ. HHV-6 reactivation (assessed by plasma PCR) occurs within the first 2–4 weeks after transplantation and may be associated with fever, leukopenia, and possibly encephalitis. Data suggest that replication of HHV-6 and HHV-7 may exacerbate CMV-induced disease. CMV is associated not only with generalized immunosuppression but also with organ-specific, rejection-related syndromes: glomerulopathy in kidney transplant recipients, bronchiolitis obliterans in lung transplant recipients, vasculopathy in heart transplant recipients, and the vanishing bile duct syndrome in liver transplant recipients. A complex interplay between increased CMV replication and enhanced graft rejection is well established: increasing immunosuppression leads to increased CMV replication, which is associated with graft rejection. For this reason, considerable attention has been focused on the diagnosis, prophylaxis, and treatment of CMV infection in SOT recipients. Early transmission of West Nile virus to transplant recipients from an organ donor has been reported; however, the risk of West Nile acquisition has been reduced by implementation of screening procedures.

Beyond 6 months after transplantation, infections characteristic of patients with defects in cell-mediated immunity—e.g., infections with *Listeria*, *Nocardia*, *Rhodococcus*, various fungi, and other intracellular pathogens—may be a problem. International patients and global travelers may experience reactivation of dormant infections with trypanosomes, *Leishmania*, *Plasmodium*, *Strongyloides*, and other parasites. Elimination of these late infections will not be possible until the patient develops specific tolerance to the transplanted organ in the absence of drugs that lead to generalized immunosuppression. Meanwhile, vigilance, prophylaxis/preemptive therapy (when indicated), and rapid diagnosis and treatment of infections can be lifesaving in SOT recipients, who, unlike most HSCT recipients, continue to be immunosuppressed.

SOT recipients are susceptible to EBV-LPD from as early as 2 months to many years after transplantation. The prevalence of this complication is increased by potent and prolonged use of T cell–suppressive drugs. Decreasing the degree of immunosuppression may in some cases reverse the condition. Among SOT patients, those with heart and lung transplants—who receive the most intensive immunosuppressive regimens—are most likely to develop EBV-LPD, particularly in the lungs. Although the disease usually originates in recipient B cells, several cases of donor origin, particularly in the transplanted organ, have been noted. High organ-specific content of B lymphoid tissues (e.g., bronchial-associated lymphoid tissue in the lung), anatomic factors (e.g., lack of access of host T cells to the transplanted organ because of disturbed lymphatics), and differences in major histocompatibility loci between the host T cells and the organ (e.g., lack of cell migration or lack of effective T cell/macrophage cooperation) may result in defective elimination of EBV-infected B cells. SOT recipients are also highly susceptible to the development of Kaposi's sarcoma and less frequently to the B cell proliferative disorders associated with KSHV, such as primary effusion lymphoma and multicentric Castleman's disease. Kaposi's sarcoma is much more common (in fact, 550–1000 times more common than in the general population), can develop very rapidly after transplantation, and can also occur in the allograft. However, because the seroprevalence of KSHV is very low in Western countries, Kaposi's sarcoma is not often observed.

KIDNEY TRANSPLANTATION
(See Table 126-4)

Early Infections Bacteria often cause infections that develop in the period immediately after kidney transplantation. There is a role for perioperative antibiotic prophylaxis, and many centers give cephalosporins to decrease the risk of postoperative complications. Urinary tract infections developing soon after transplantation are usually related to anatomic alterations resulting from surgery. Such early infections may require prolonged treatment (e.g., 6 weeks of antibiotic administration for pyelonephritis). Urinary tract infections that occur >6 months after transplantation may be treated for shorter periods because they do not seem to be associated with the high rate of pyelonephritis or relapse seen with infections that occur in the first 3 months.

Prophylaxis with TMP-SMX [1 double-strength tablet (800 mg of sulfamethoxazole, 160 mg of trimethoprim) per day] for the first 4–6 months after transplantation decreases the incidence of early and middle-period infections (see below, Table 126-4, and Table 126-5).

Middle-Period Infections Because of continuing immunosuppression, kidney transplant recipients are predisposed to lung infections characteristic of those in patients with T cell deficiency (i.e., infections

TABLE 126-4 COMMON INFECTIONS AFTER KIDNEY TRANSPLANTATION

Infection Site	Period after Transplantation		
	Early (<1 Month)	Middle (1–4 Months)	Late (>6 Months)
Urinary tract	Bacteria (*Escherichia coli*, *Klebsiella*, Enterobacteriaceae, *Pseudomonas*, *Enterococcus*) associated with bacteremia and pyelonephritis; *Candida*	CMV (fever, bone marrow suppression, hepatitis); BK virus (nephropathy, graft failure, vasculopathy)	Bacteria (late urinary tract infections usually not associated with bacteremia); BK virus (nephropathy, graft failure, generalized vasculopathy)
Lungs	Bacteria (*Legionella* in endemic settings)	CMV disease; *Pneumocystis*; *Legionella*	*Nocardia*; invasive fungi
Central nervous system		*Listeria* (meningitis); *Toxoplasma gondii*	CMV disease; *Listeria* (meningitis); *Cryptococcus* (meningitis); *Nocardia*

Note: CMV, cytomegalovirus.

TABLE 126-5 PROPHYLAXIS OF INFECTIONS IN TRANSPLANT RECIPIENTS

Risk Factor	Organism	Prophylactic Antibiotics	Examination(s)[a]
Travel to or residence in area with known risk of fungal infection	*Coccidioides, Histoplasma, Blastomyces*	Consider imidazoles	Chest radiography, antigen testing, serology
Latent viruses	HSV, VZV, EBV, CMV	Acyclovir after hematopoietic stem cell transplantation to prevent HSV and VZV; ganciclovir to prevent CMV in some settings	Serologic test for HSV, VZV, CMV, HHV-6, EBV, KSHV
Latent fungi and parasites	*Pneumocystis jiroveci, Toxoplasma gondii*	Trimethoprim-sulfamethoxazole (dapsone or atovaquone)	Serology for *Toxoplasma*
History of exposure to tuberculosis or latent tuberculosis	*Mycobacterium tuberculosis*	Isoniazid if recent conversion for positive chest imaging and/or no previous treatment	Chest imaging; PPD and/or cell-based assay

[a]Serologic examination, PPD testing, and interferon assays may be less reliable after transplantation.
Note: CMV, cytomegalovirus; EBV, Epstein-Barr virus; HHV-6, human herpesvirus type 6; HSV, herpes simplex virus; KSHV, Kaposi's sarcoma–associated herpesvirus; PPD, purified protein derivative; VZV, varicella-zoster virus.

with intracellular bacteria, mycobacteria, nocardiae, fungi, viruses, and parasites). The high mortality rates associated with *Legionella pneumophila* infection (Chap. 141) led to the closing of renal transplant units in hospitals with endemic legionellosis.

About 50% of all renal transplant recipients presenting with fever 1–4 months after transplantation have evidence of CMV disease; CMV itself accounts for the fever in more than two-thirds of cases and thus is the predominant pathogen during this period. CMV infection (Chap. 175) may also present as arthralgias, myalgias, or organ-specific symptoms. During this period, this infection may represent primary disease (in the case of a seronegative recipient of a kidney from a seropositive donor) or may represent reactivation disease or superinfection. Patients may have atypical lymphocytosis. Unlike immunocompetent patients, however, they often do not have lymphadenopathy or splenomegaly. Therefore, clinical suspicion and laboratory confirmation are necessary for diagnosis. The clinical syndrome may be accompanied by bone marrow suppression (particularly leukopenia). CMV also causes glomerulopathy and is associated with an increased incidence of other opportunistic infections. Because of the frequency and severity of disease, a considerable effort has been made to prevent and treat CMV infection in renal transplant recipients. An immune globulin preparation enriched with antibodies to CMV was used by many centers in the past in an effort to protect the group at highest risk for severe infection (seronegative recipients of seropositive kidneys). However, with the development of highly effective oral antiviral agents, CMV immune globulin is no longer used. Ganciclovir (valganciclovir) is beneficial when prophylaxis is indicated and for the treatment of serious CMV disease. One study showed a significant (50%) reduction in CMV disease and rejection at 6 months among patients who received prophylactic valacyclovir (an acyclovir congener) for the first 90 days after renal transplantation. Acyclovir (valacyclovir) is less efficacious but also less toxic than ganciclovir (valganciclovir). The availability of valganciclovir and valacyclovir has allowed most centers to move to oral prophylaxis for transplant recipients. Additional oral prophylactic agents, such as maribavir, are in clinical study.

Infection with the other herpes-group viruses may become evident within 6 months after transplantation or later. Early after transplantation, HSV may cause either oral or anogenital lesions that are usually responsive to acyclovir. Large ulcerating lesions in the anogenital area may lead to bladder and rectal dysfunction as well as predisposing to bacterial infection. VZV may cause fatal disseminated infection in nonimmune kidney transplant recipients, but in immune patients reactivation zoster usually does not disseminate outside the dermatome; thus disseminated VZV infection is a less fearsome complication in kidney transplantation than in hematopoietic stem cell transplanta-

tion. HHV-6 reactivation may take place and (although usually asymptomatic) may be associated with fever, rash, marrow suppression, or encephalitis.

EBV disease is more serious; it may present as an extranodal proliferation of B cells that invade the CNS, nasopharynx, liver, small bowel, heart, and other organs, including the transplanted kidney. The disease is diagnosed by the finding of a mass of proliferating EBV-positive B cells. The incidence of EBV-LPD is higher among patients who acquire EBV infection from the donor and among patients given high doses of cyclosporine, FK506, glucocorticoids, and anti–T cell antibodies. Disease may regress once immunocompetence is restored. KSHV infection can be transmitted with the donor kidney although it more often represents latent infection of the recipient. Kaposi's sarcoma often appears within 1 year after transplantation, although the range of onset is wide (1 month to ~20 years). Avoidance of immunosuppressive agents that inhibit calcineurin has been associated with less outgrowth of EBV and less CMV replication. The use of rapamycin (sirolimus) has led to regression of Kaposi's sarcoma.

The papovaviruses BK virus and JC virus (polyomavirus hominis types 1 and 2) have been cultured from the urine of kidney transplant recipients (as they have from that of HSCT recipients) in the setting of profound immunosuppression. High levels of BK virus replication detected by PCR in urine and blood are predictive of pathology, particularly in the setting of renal transplantation. Excretion of BK virus and BK viremia are associated with the development of ureteral strictures, polyomavirus-associated nephropathy (1–10% of renal transplant recipients), and (less commonly) generalized vasculopathy. Timely reduction of immunosuppression is critical and can reduce rates of graft loss related to polyomavirus-associated nephropathy from 90% to 10–30%. A possible role for treatment with cidofovir (given by the IV route and by bladder instillation), leflunomide, quinolones, and (most recently) lactoferrin has been reported, but the efficacy of these agents has not been substantiated through adequate clinical study. JC virus is associated with rare cases of progressive multifocal leukoencephalopathy. Adenoviruses may persist with continued immunosuppression in these patients, but disseminated disease like that which occurs in HSCT recipients is much less common.

Kidney transplant recipients are also subject to infections with other intracellular organisms. These patients may develop pulmonary infections with *Nocardia, Aspergillus,* and *Mucor* as well as infections with other pathogens in which the T cell/macrophage axis plays an important role. In patients without IV catheters, *L. monocytogenes* is a common cause of bacteremia ≥1 month after renal transplantation and should be seriously considered in renal transplant recipients presenting with fever and headache. Kidney transplant recipients may develop *Salmonella* bacteremia, which can lead to endovascular infections and require prolonged therapy. Pulmonary infections with *Pneumocystis* are common unless the patient is maintained on TMP-SMX prophylaxis. *Nocardia* infection (Chap. 155) may present in the skin, bones, and lungs or in the CNS, where it usually takes the form of single or multiple brain abscesses. Nocardiosis generally occurs ≥1 month after transplantation and may follow immunosuppressive treatment for an episode of rejection. Pulmonary findings are nonspecific: localized disease with or without cavities is most common, but the disease may disseminate. The diagnosis is made by culture of the organism from sputum or from the involved nodule. As with *Pneumocystis*, prophylaxis with TMP-SMX is often efficacious in the prevention of disease. The occurrence of *Nocardia* infections >2 years after transplantation suggests that a long-term prophylactic regimen may be justified.

Toxoplasmosis can occur in seropositive patients but is less common than in other transplant settings, usually developing in the first few months after kidney transplantation. Again, TMP-SMX is helpful in prevention. In endemic areas, histoplasmosis, coccidioidomycosis, and blastomycosis may cause pulmonary infiltrates or disseminated disease.

Late Infections Late infections (>6 months after kidney transplantation) may involve the CNS and include CMV retinitis as well as other CNS manifestations of CMV disease. Patients (particularly those whose immunosuppression has been increased) are at risk for subacute meningitis due to *Cryptococcus neoformans*. Cryptococcal disease may present in an insidious manner (sometimes as a skin infection before the development of clear CNS findings). *Listeria* meningitis may have an acute presentation and requires prompt therapy to avoid a fatal outcome.

Patients who continue to take glucocorticoids are predisposed to ongoing infection. "Transplant elbow" is a recurrent bacterial infection in and around the elbow that is thought to result from a combination of poor tensile strength of the skin of steroid-treated patients and steroid-induced proximal myopathy that requires patients to push themselves up with their elbows to get out of chairs. Bouts of cellulitis (usually caused by *S. aureus*) recur until patients are provided with elbow protection.

Kidney transplant recipients are susceptible to invasive fungal infections, including those due to *Aspergillus* and *Rhizopus*, which may present as superficial lesions before dissemination. Mycobacterial infection (particularly that with *Mycobacterium marinum*) can be diagnosed by skin examination. Infection with *Prototheca wickerhamii* (an achlorophyllic alga) has been diagnosed by skin biopsy. Warts caused by human papillomaviruses (HPVs) are a late consequence of persistent immunosuppression; imiquimod or other forms of local therapy are usually satisfactory.

Although BK virus replication and virus-associated disease can be detected far earlier, the median time to clinical diagnosis of polyomavirus-associated nephropathy is ~300 days, qualifying it as a late-onset disease. With establishment of better screening procedures (e.g., blood PCR), it is likely that this disease will be detected earlier (see "Middle-Period Infections," above).

HEART TRANSPLANTATION

Early Infections Sternal wound infection and mediastinitis are early complications of heart transplantation. An indolent course is common, with fever or a mildly elevated white blood cell count preceding the development of site tenderness or drainage. Clinical suspicion based on evidence of sternal instability and failure to heal may lead to the diagnosis. Common microbial residents of the skin (e.g., *S. aureus*, including methicillin-resistant strains, and *Staphylococcus epidermidis*) as well as gram-negative organisms (e.g., *Pseudomonas aeruginosa*) and fungi (e.g., *Candida*) are often involved. In rare cases, mediastinitis in heart transplant recipients can also be due to *Mycoplasma hominis* (Chap. 168). Since this organism requires an anaerobic environment for growth and may be difficult to see on conventional medium, the laboratory should be alerted that *M. hominis* infection is suspected. *M. hominis* mediastinitis has been cured with a combination of surgical debridement (sometimes requiring muscle-flap placement) and the administration of clindamycin and tetracycline. Organisms associated with mediastinitis may be cultured from accompanying pericardial fluid.

Middle-Period Infections *T. gondii* (Chap. 207) residing in the heart of a seropositive donor may be transmitted to a seronegative recipient. Thus serologic screening for *T. gondii* infection is important before and in the months after cardiac transplantation. Rarely, active disease can be introduced at the time of transplantation. The overall incidence of toxoplasmosis is so high in the setting of heart transplantation that some prophylaxis is always warranted. Although alternatives are available, the most frequently used agent is TMP-SMX, which prevents infection with *Pneumocystis* as well as with *Nocardia* and several other bacterial pathogens. CMV also has been transmitted by heart trans-

plantation. CNS infections can be caused by *Toxoplasma*, *Nocardia*, and *Aspergillus*. *L. monocytogenes* meningitis should be considered in heart transplant recipients with fever and headache.

CMV infection is associated with poor outcomes after heart transplantation. The virus is usually cultivable 1–2 months after transplantation, causes early signs and laboratory abnormalities (usually fever and atypical lymphocytosis or leukopenia and thrombocytopenia) at 2–3 months, and can produce severe disease (e.g., pneumonia) at 3–4 months. Seropositive recipients usually develop cultivable virus faster than patients whose primary CMV infection is a consequence of transplantation. Between 40 and 70% of patients develop symptomatic CMV disease in the form of (1) CMV pneumonia, the most likely form to be fatal; (2) CMV esophagitis and gastritis, sometimes accompanied by abdominal pain with or without ulcerations and bleeding; and (3) the CMV syndrome, consisting of CMV in the blood along with fever, leukopenia, thrombocytopenia, and hepatic enzyme abnormalities. Ganciclovir is efficacious in the treatment of CMV infection; prophylaxis with ganciclovir or possibly with other antiviral agents, as described for renal transplantation, may reduce the overall incidence of CMV-related disease. When prophylaxis is stopped, late-onset disease may occur. In fact, because of the expanded use of prophylaxis, this scenario is increasingly common, particularly in patients with ongoing GVHD.

Late Infections EBV infection usually presents as a lymphoma-like proliferation of B cells late after heart transplantation, particularly in patients maintained on intense immunosuppressive therapy. A subset of heart and heart-lung transplant recipients may develop early fulminant EBV-LPD (within 2 months). Treatment includes the reduction of immunosuppression (if possible), the use of glucocorticoid and calcineurin inhibitor–sparing regimens, and the consideration of therapy with anti–B cell antibodies (rituximab and possibly others). Immunomodulatory and antiviral agents continue to be studied, and aggressive chemotherapy is a last resort, as discussed earlier for HSCT recipients. KSHV-associated disease, including Kaposi's sarcoma and primary effusion lymphoma, has been reported in heart transplant recipients. Treatment with rapamycin (sirolimus) may prevent both rejection and outgrowth of KSHV-infected cells. Antitumor therapy is discussed in Chap. 81. Prophylaxis for *Pneumocystis* infection is required for these patients (see "Lung Transplantation, Late Infections," below).

LUNG TRANSPLANTATION

Early Infections It is not surprising that lung transplant recipients are predisposed to the development of pneumonia. The combination of ischemia and the resulting mucosal damage, together with accompanying denervation and lack of lymphatic drainage, probably contributes to the high rate of pneumonia (66% in one series). The prophylactic use of high doses of broad-spectrum antibiotics for the first 3–4 days after surgery may decrease the incidence of pneumonia. Gram-negative pathogens (Enterobacteriaceae and *Pseudomonas* species) are troublesome in the first 2 weeks after surgery (the period of maximal vulnerability). Pneumonia can also be caused by *Candida* (possibly as a result of colonization of the donor lung), *Aspergillus*, and *Cryptococcus*.

Mediastinitis may occur at an even higher rate among lung transplant recipients than among heart transplant recipients and most commonly develops within 2 weeks of surgery. In the absence of prophylaxis, pneumonitis due to CMV (which may be transmitted as a consequence of transplantation) usually presents between 2 weeks and 3 months after surgery, with primary disease occurring later than reactivation disease.

Middle-Period Infections The incidence of CMV infection, either reactivated or primary, is 75–100% if either the donor or the recipient is seropositive for CMV. CMV-induced disease appears to be most severe in recipients of lung and heart-lung transplants. Whether this severity relates to the mismatch in lung antigen-presenting and host immune cells or is attributable to other (nonimmunologic) factors is not known. More than half of lung transplant recipients with symptomatic

CMV disease have pneumonia. Difficulty in distinguishing the radiographic picture of CMV infection from other infections and organ rejection further complicates therapy. CMV can also cause bronchiolitis obliterans in lung transplants. The development of pneumonitis related to HSV has led to the prophylactic use of acyclovir. Such prophylaxis may also decrease rates of CMV disease, but ganciclovir is more active against CMV and is also active against HSV. The prophylaxis of CMV infection with IV ganciclovir—or increasingly with valganciclovir, the oral alternative—is recommended for lung transplant recipients. Antiviral alternatives are discussed in the earlier section on hematopoietic stem cell transplantation. Although the overall incidence of serious disease is decreased during prophylaxis, late disease may occur when prophylaxis is stopped—a pattern observed increasingly in recent years. With recovery from peritransplantation complications and, in many cases, a decrease in immunosuppression, the recipient is often better equipped to combat late infection.

Late Infections The incidence of *Pneumocystis* infection (which may present with a paucity of findings) is high among lung and heart-lung transplant recipients. Some form of prophylaxis for *Pneumocystis* pneumonia is indicated in all organ transplant situations (Table 126-5). Prophylaxis with TMP-SMX for 12 months after transplantation may be sufficient to prevent *Pneumocystis* disease in patients whose degree of immunosuppression is not increased.

As in other transplant recipients, infection with EBV may cause either a mononucleosis-like syndrome or EBV-LPD. The tendency of the B cell blasts to present in the lung appears to be greater after lung transplantation than after the transplantation of other organs. Reduction of immunosuppression and switching of regimens, as discussed in earlier sections, causes remission in some cases, but airway compression can be fatal and more rapid intervention may therefore become necessary. The approach to EBV-LPD is similar to that described in other sections.

LIVER TRANSPLANTATION
Early Infections As in other transplantation settings, early bacterial infections are a major problem after liver transplantation. Many centers administer systemic broad-spectrum antibiotics for the first 24 h or sometimes longer after surgery, even in the absence of documented infection. However, despite prophylaxis, infectious complications are common and are correlated with the duration of the surgical procedure and the type of biliary drainage. An operation lasting >12 h is associated with an increased likelihood of infection. Patients who have a choledochojejunostomy with drainage of the biliary duct to a Roux-en-Y jejunal bowel loop have more fungal infections than those whose bile is drained via a choledochocholedochostomy with anastomosis of the donor common bile duct to the recipient common bile duct.

Peritonitis and intraabdominal abscesses are common complications of liver transplantation. Bacterial peritonitis or localized abscesses may result from biliary leaks. Early leaks are even more common (incidence, ~17%) with live-donor liver transplants (LDLTs). Peritonitis in liver transplant recipients is often polymicrobial, commonly involving enterococci, aerobic gram-negative bacteria, staphylococci, anaerobes, *Candida*, or other invasive fungi. Only one-third of patients with intraabdominal abscesses have bacteremia. Abscesses within the first month after surgery may occur not only in and around the liver but also in the spleen, pericolic area, and pelvis. Treatment includes antibiotic administration and drainage as necessary.

Liver transplant patients have a high incidence of fungal infections, and the occurrence of fungal (often candidal) infection correlates with preoperative use of glucocorticoids, long duration of treatment with antibacterial agents, and posttransplantation use of immunosuppressive agents.

Middle-Period Infections The development of postsurgical biliary stricture predisposes patients to cholangitis. The incidence of strictures is increased in LDLT (~17% of liver transplant recipients); therefore, cholangitis is also more common among these patients. Transplant recipients who develop cholangitis may have high spiking fevers and rigors but often lack the characteristic signs and symptoms of classic cholangitis, including abdominal pain and jaundice. Although these findings may suggest graft rejection, rejection is typically accompanied by marked elevation of liver function enzymes. In contrast, in cholangitis in transplant recipients, results of liver function tests (with the possible exception of alkaline phosphatase levels) are often within the normal range. Definitive diagnosis of cholangitis in liver transplant recipients requires documentation of bacteremia or demonstration of aggregated neutrophils in bile duct biopsy specimens. Unfortunately, invasive studies of the biliary tract (either T-tube cholangiography or endoscopic retrograde cholangiopancreatography) may themselves lead to cholangitis. For this reason, many clinicians recommend an empirical trial of therapy with antibiotics covering gram-negative organisms and anaerobes before these procedures are undertaken as well as antibiotic coverage if they are eventually performed.

Reactivation of viral hepatitis is a common complication of liver transplantation (Chap. 298). Recurrent hepatitis B and C infections, for which transplantation may be performed, are problematic. To prevent hepatitis B virus reinfection, prophylaxis with an optimal antiviral agent or combination of agents (lamivudine, adefovir, entecavir) and hepatitis B immune globulin is currently recommended, although the optimal dose, route, and duration of therapy remain controversial. Success in preventing reinfection with hepatitis B virus has increased in recent years; in contrast, reinfection of the graft with hepatitis C virus occurs in all patients, with a variable time frame. Studies of aggressive pretransplantation treatment of selected recipients with antiviral agents and prophylactic/preemptive regimens are ongoing. However, early initiation of treatment for histologically documented disease with a combination of ribavirin and pegylated interferon has produced sustained responses at rates in the range of 25–40%.

As in other transplantation settings, reactivation disease with herpes-group viruses is common (Table 126-3). Herpesviruses can be transmitted in donor organs. Although CMV hepatitis occurs in ~4% of liver transplant recipients, it is usually not so severe as to require retransplantation. Without prophylaxis, CMV disease develops in the majority of seronegative recipients of organs from CMV-positive donors, but fatality rates are lower among liver transplant recipients than among lung or heart-lung transplant recipients. Disease due to CMV can also be associated with the vanishing bile duct syndrome after liver transplantation. Patients respond to treatment with ganciclovir; prophylaxis with oral forms of ganciclovir or high-dose acyclovir may decrease the frequency of disease. A role for HHV-6 reactivation in posttransplantation fever and leukopenia has been proposed, although the more severe sequelae described in hematopoietic stem cell transplantation are unusual. HHV-6 and HHV-7 appear to exacerbate CMV disease in this setting. EBV-LPD after liver transplantation shows a propensity for involvement of the liver, and such disease may be of donor origin. See previous sections for discussion of EBV infections in solid organ transplantation.

PANCREAS TRANSPLANTATION
Transplantation of the pancreas can be complicated by early bacterial and yeast infections. Most pancreatic transplants are drained into the bowel, whereas the remaining transplants (~20%) are drained into the bladder. A cuff of duodenum is used in the anastomosis between the pancreatic graft and either the gut or the bladder. Bowel drainage poses a risk of early abdominal and allograft infections with enteric bacteria and yeasts. These infections often result in loss of the graft. Bladder drainage causes a high rate of urinary tract infection and sterile cystitis; however, infection can usually be cured with appropriate antimicrobial agents. In both procedures, prophylactic antimicrobial agents are commonly used at the time of surgery. An alternative method—the transplantation of islet cells only—may eliminate the problems characteristically posed by wound and urinary tract sepsis in pancreatic transplant recipients.

Issues related to the development of CMV infection, EBV-LPD, and infections with opportunistic pathogens in patients receiving a pancreatic transplant are similar to those in other SOT recipients.

MISCELLANEOUS INFECTIONS IN SOLID ORGAN TRANSPLANTATION

Indwelling IV Catheter Infections
The prolonged use of indwelling IV catheters for administration of medications, blood products, and nutrition is common in diverse transplantation settings and poses a risk of local and bloodstream infections. Significant insertion-site infection is most commonly caused by *S. aureus*. Bloodstream infection most frequently develops within a week of catheter placement or in patients who become neutropenic. Coagulase-negative staphylococci are the most common isolates from the blood. For further discussion of differential diagnosis and therapeutic options, see Chap. 82.

Tuberculosis
The incidence of tuberculosis occurring within the first 12 months after solid organ transplantation is greater than that observed after hematopoietic stem cell transplantation (0.23–0.79%) and ranges broadly worldwide (1.2–15%), reflecting the prevalences of tuberculosis in local populations. Lesions suggesting prior tuberculosis on chest x-ray, older age, diabetes, chronic liver disease, GVHD, and intense immunosuppression are predictive of tuberculosis reactivation and development of disseminated disease in a host with latent disease. Tuberculosis has rarely been transmitted from the donor organ. In contrast to the low mortality rate among HSCT recipients, mortality rates among SOT patients are reported to be as high as 30%. Vigilance is indicated, as the presentation of disease is often extrapulmonary (gastrointestinal, genitourinary, central nervous, endocrine, musculoskeletal, laryngeal) and atypical, sometimes manifesting as a fever of unknown origin. A careful history and a direct evaluation of both the recipient and the donor prior to transplantation are optimal. Skin testing of the recipient with PPD may be unreliable because of chronic disease and/or immunosuppression, but newer cell-based assays that measure interferon and/or cytokine production may prove more sensitive in the future. Isoniazid toxicity has not been a significant problem except in the setting of liver transplantation. Therefore, appropriate prophylaxis should proceed. An assessment of the need to treat latent disease should include careful consideration of the possibility of a false-negative test result. Pending final confirmation of suspected tuberculosis, aggressive multidrug treatment in accordance with the guidelines of the Centers for Disease Control and Prevention (CDC), the Infectious Diseases Society of America, and the American Thoracic Society is indicated because of the high mortality rates among these patients. Altered drug metabolism (e.g., upon co-administration of rifampin and certain immunosuppressive agents) can be managed with careful monitoring of drug levels and appropriate dose adjustment. Close follow-up of hepatic enzymes is warranted, particularly during treatment with isoniazid, pyrazinamide, and/or rifampin. Drug-resistant tuberculosis is especially problematic in these individuals (Chap. 158).

Virus-Associated Malignancies
In addition to malignancy associated with gammaherpesvirus infection (EBV, KSHV) and simple warts (HPV), other tumors that are virus-associated or suspected of being virus-associated are more likely to develop in transplant recipients, particularly those who require long-term immunosuppression, than in the general population. The interval to tumor development is usually >1 year. Transplant recipients develop nonmelanoma skin or lip cancers that, in contrast to de novo skin cancers, have a high ratio of squamous cells to basal cells. HPV may play a major role in these lesions. Cervical and vulvar carcinomas, quite clearly associated with HPV, develop with

increased frequency in female transplant recipients. Among renal transplant recipients, rates of melanoma are modestly increased and rates of cancers of the kidney and bladder are increased.

VACCINATION OF TRANSPLANT RECIPIENTS

In addition to receiving antibiotic prophylaxis, transplant recipients should be vaccinated against likely pathogens (Table 126-6). In the case of HSCT recipients, optimal responses cannot be achieved until after immune reconstitution, despite previous immunization of both donor and recipient. Recipients of allogeneic HSCTs must be reimmunized if they are to be protected against pathogens. The situation is less clear-cut in the case of autologous transplantation. T and B cells in the peripheral blood may reconstitute the immune response if they are transferred in adequate numbers. However, cancer patients (particularly those with Hodgkin's disease, in whom vaccination has been extensively studied) who are undergoing chemotherapy do not respond normally to immunization, and titers of antibodies to infectious agents fall more rapidly than in healthy individuals. Therefore, even immunosuppressed patients who have not had HSCTs may need booster vaccine injections. If memory cells are specifically eliminated as part of a stem cell "cleanup" procedure, it will be necessary to reimmunize the recipient with a new primary series. Optimal times for immunizations of different transplant populations are being evaluated. Yearly immunization of household and other contacts (including health care personnel) against influenza benefits the patient by preventing local spread.

In the absence of compelling data as to optimal timing, it is reasonable to administer the pneumococcal and *H. influenzae* type b conjugate vaccines to both autologous and allogeneic HSCT recipients beginning 12 months after transplantation. A series that includes both the 7-valent pneumococcal conjugate vaccine and the 23-valent Pneumovax is now recommended (following CDC guidelines). The pneumococcal and *H. influenzae* type b vaccines are particularly important for patients who have undergone splenectomy. In addition, diphtheria, tetanus, acellular pertussis, and inactivated polio vaccines can all be given at these same intervals (12 months and, as required, 24 months after transplantation). *Neisseria meningitidis* polysaccharide (a new conjugate vaccine) is now available and will probably be recommended in the future. Some authorities recommend a new primary series for tetanus/diphtheria/pertussis and inactivated polio vaccine begin-

TABLE 126-6 VACCINATION FOR HEMATOPOIETIC STEM CELL TRANSPLANT (HSCT) OR SOLID ORGAN TRANSPLANT (SOT) RECIPIENTS

Vaccine	Type of Transplantation	
	HSCT	SOT[a]
Streptococcus pneumoniae, Haemophilus influenzae, Neisseria meningitidis	Immunize after transplantation (optimal timing not established) Use Prevnar Preimmunize donor (graft)[b] See CDC recommendations	Immunize before transplantation and every 5 years for Pneumovax (others not established) See CDC recommendations
Seasonal influenza	Vaccinate in the fall Vaccinate close contacts	Vaccinate in the fall Vaccinate close contacts
Poliomyelitis	Administer inactivated vaccine	Administer inactivated vaccine
Measles/mumps/rubella	Immunize 24 months after transplantation if patient does not have graft-versus-host disease	Immunize before transplantation with attenuated vaccine
Tetanus, diphtheria	Reimmunize after transplantation with primary series See CDC recommendations	Immunize before transplantation; give boosters at 10 years or as required; primary series not required
Hepatitis B and A	Reimmunize after transplantation See CDC recommendations	Immunize before transplantation as appropriate
Human papillomavirus	Recommendations pending	Recommendations pending

[a]Immunizations should be given before transplantation whenever possible.
[b]Studies indicate that it is possible to "immunize the graft" before transplantation.

ning 12 months after transplantation. Because of the risk of spread, household contacts of HSCT recipients (or of patients immunosuppressed as a result of chemotherapy) should receive only inactivated polio vaccine. Live-virus measles/mumps/rubella vaccine can be given to autologous HSCT recipients 24 months after transplantation and to most allogeneic HSCT recipients at the same point if they are not receiving maintenance therapy with immunosuppressive drugs and do not have ongoing GVHD. The risk of spread from a household contact is lower for MMR vaccine than for polio vaccine. Neither patients nor their household contacts should be vaccinated with vaccinia unless they have been exposed to the smallpox virus. Among patients who have active GVHD and/or are taking high maintenance doses of glucocorticoids, it may be prudent to avoid all live-virus vaccines. Vaccination to prevent hepatitis B and hepatitis A also seems advisable.

In the case of SOT recipients, administration of all the usual vaccines and of the indicated booster doses should be completed before immunosuppression, if possible, to maximize responses. For patients taking immunosuppressive agents, the administration of pneumococcal vaccine should be repeated every 5 years. No data are available for the meningococcal vaccine, but it is probably reasonable to administer it along with the pneumococcal vaccine. *H. influenzae* conjugate vaccine is safe and should be efficacious in this population; therefore, its administration before transplantation is recommended. Booster doses of this vaccine are not recommended for adults. SOT recipients who continue to receive immunosuppressive drugs should not receive live-virus vaccines. A person in this group who is exposed to measles should be given immune globulin. Similarly, an immunocompromised patient who is seronegative for varicella and who comes into contact with a person who has chickenpox should be given varicella-zoster immune globulin as soon as possible (and certainly within 96 h) or, if this is not possible, should be started immediately on a 10- to 14-day course of acyclovir therapy. Upon the discontinuation of treatment, clinical disease may still occur in a small number of patients; thus vigilance is indicated. Rapid re-treatment should limit the symptoms of disease. Household contacts of transplant recipients can receive live attenuated VZV vaccine, but vaccinees should avoid direct contact with the patient if a rash develops. Virus-like particle (VLP) vaccines (not live attenuated) have recently been licensed for the prevention of infection with several HPV serotypes most commonly implicated in cervical and anal carcinomas and in anogenital and laryngeal warts. For example, the tetravalent vaccine contains HPV serotypes 6, 11, 16, and 18. At present, no information is available about the safety, immunogenicity, or efficacy of this vaccine in transplant recipients.

Immunocompromised patients who travel may benefit from some but not all vaccines (Chaps. 116 and 117). In general, these patients should receive any killed or inactivated vaccine preparation appropriate to the area they are visiting; this recommendation includes the vaccines for Japanese encephalitis, hepatitis A and B, poliomyelitis, meningococcal infection, and typhoid. The live typhoid vaccines are not recommended for use in most immunocompromised patients, but inactivated or purified polysaccharide typhoid vaccine can be used. Live yellow fever vaccine should not be administered. On the other hand, primary immunization or boosting with the purified-protein hepatitis B vaccine is indicated if patients are likely to be exposed. Patients who will reside for >6 months in areas where hepatitis B is common (Africa, Southeast Asia, the Middle East, Eastern Europe, parts of South America, and the Caribbean) should receive hepatitis B vaccine. Inactivated hepatitis A vaccine should also be used in the appropriate setting (Chap. 116). A combined vaccine is now available that provides dual protection against hepatitis A and hepatitis B. If hepatitis A vaccine is not administered, travelers should consider receiving passive protection with immune globulin (the dose depending on the duration of travel in the high-risk area).

FURTHER READINGS

CORNELY OA et al: Posaconazole vs. fluconazole or itraconazole prophylaxis in patients with neutropenia. N Engl J Med 356:348, 2007

DYKEWICZ CA: Cytomegalovirus infection after liver transplantation: Summary of the guidelines for preventing opportunistic infections among hematopoietic stem cell transplant recipients. Clin Infect Dis 33:139, 2001

HIRSCH HH, SUTHANTHIRAN M: The natural history, risk factors and outcomes of polyomavirus BK–associated nephropathy after renal transplantation. Nat Clin Pract Nephrol 2:240, 2006

KOTTON CN et al: Prevention of infection in adult travelers after solid organ transplantation. Am J Transplant 5:8, 2004

MUNOZ P et al: *Mycobacterium tuberculosis* infection in recipients of solid organ transplants. Clin Infect Dis 40:581, 2005

ZERR DM et al: Clinical outcomes of human herpesvirus 6 reactivation after hematopoietic stem cell transplantation. Clin Infect Dis 40:932, 2005

SECTION 4   APPROACH TO THERAPY FOR BACTERIAL DISEASES

127   Treatment and Prophylaxis of Bacterial Infections

Gordon L. Archer, Ronald E. Polk

The development of vaccines and drugs that prevent and cure bacterial infections was one of the twentieth century's major contributions to human longevity and quality of life. Antibacterial agents are among the most commonly prescribed drugs of any kind worldwide. Used appropriately, these drugs are lifesaving. However, their indiscriminate use drives up the cost of health care, leads to a plethora of side effects and drug interactions, and fosters the emergence of bacterial resistance, rendering previously valuable drugs useless. The rational use of antibacterial agents depends on an understanding of (1) the drugs' mechanisms of action, spectrum of activity, pharmacokinetics, pharmacodynamics, toxicities, and interactions; (2) mechanisms underlying bacterial resistance; and (3) strategies that can be used by clinicians to limit resistance. In addition, patient-associated parameters, such as infection site, other drugs being taken, allergies, and immune and excretory status, are critically important to appropriate therapeutic decisions. This chapter provides specific data required for making an informed choice of antibacterial agent.

MECHANISMS OF ACTION

Antibacterial agents, like all antimicrobial drugs, are directed against unique targets not present in mammalian cells. The goal is to limit toxicity to the host and maximize chemotherapeutic activity affecting invading microbes only. *Bactericidal drugs* kill the bacteria that are within their spectrum of activity; *bacteriostatic drugs* only inhibit bacterial growth. While bacteriostatic activity is adequate for the treatment of most infections, bactericidal activity may be necessary for cure in patients with altered immune systems (e.g., neutropenia), protected infectious foci (e.g., endocarditis or meningitis), or specific infections (e.g., complicated *Staphylococcus aureus* bacteremia). The mechanisms of action of the antibacterial agents to be discussed in this section are summarized in Table 127-1 and are depicted in Fig. 127-1.

TABLE 127-1   MECHANISMS OF ACTION OF AND RESISTANCE TO MAJOR CLASSES OF ANTIBACTERIAL AGENTS

Letter for Fig. 127-1	Antibacterial Agent[a]	Major Cellular Target	Mechanism of Action	Major Mechanisms of Resistance
A	β-Lactams (penicillins and cephalosporins)	Cell wall	Inhibit cell-wall cross-linking	1. Drug inactivation (β-lactamase) 2. Insensitivity of target (altered penicillin-binding proteins) 3. Decreased permeability (altered gram-negative outer-membrane porins) 4. Active efflux
B	Vancomycin	Cell wall	Interferes with addition of new cell-wall subunits (muramyl pentapeptides)	Alteration of target (substitution of terminal amino acid of peptidoglycan subunit)
	Bacitracin	Cell wall	Prevents addition of cell-wall subunits by inhibiting recycling of membrane lipid carrier	Not defined
C	Macrolides (erythromycin)	Protein synthesis	Bind to 50S ribosomal subunit	1. Alteration of target (ribosomal methylation and mutation of 23S rRNA) 2. Active efflux
	Lincosamides (clindamycin)	Protein synthesis	Bind to 50S ribosomal subunit	Alteration of target (ribosomal methylation)
D	Chloramphenicol	Protein synthesis	Binds to 50S ribosomal subunit	1. Drug inactivation (chloramphenicol acetyltransferase) 2. Active efflux
E	Tetracycline	Protein synthesis	Binds to 30S ribosomal subunit	1. Decreased intracellular drug accumulation (active efflux) 2. Insensitivity of target
F	Aminoglycosides (gentamicin)	Protein synthesis	Bind to 30S ribosomal subunit	1. Drug inactivation (aminoglycoside-modifying enzyme) 2. Decreased permeability through gram-negative outer membrane 3. Active efflux
G	Mupirocin	Protein synthesis	Inhibits isoleucine tRNA synthetase	Mutation of gene for target protein or acquisition of new gene for drug-insensitive target
H	Quinupristin/dalfopristin (Synercid)	Protein synthesis	Binds to 50S ribosomal subunit	1. Alteration of target (ribosomal methylation: dalfopristin) 2. Active efflux (quinupristin) 3. Drug inactivation (quinupristin and dalfopristin)
I	Linezolid	Protein synthesis	Bind to 50S ribosomal subunit	Alteration of target (mutation of 23S rRNA)
J	Sulfonamides and trimethoprim	Cell metabolism	Competitively inhibit enzymes involved in two steps of folic acid biosynthesis	Production of insensitive targets [dihydropteroate synthetase (sulfonamides) and dihydrofolate reductase (trimethoprim)] that bypass metabolic block
K	Rifampin	Nucleic acid synthesis	Inhibits DNA-dependent RNA polymerase	Insensitivity of target (mutation of polymerase gene)
L	Metronidazole	Nucleic acid synthesis	Intracellularly generates short-lived reactive intermediates that damage DNA by electron transfer system	Not defined
M	Quinolones (ciprofloxacin)	DNA synthesis	Inhibit DNA gyrase (A subunit) and topoisomerase IV	1. Insensitivity of target (mutation of gyrase genes) 2. Decreased intracellular drug accumulation (active efflux)
	Novobiocin	DNA synthesis	Inhibits DNA gyrase (B subunit)	Not defined
N	Polymyxins (polymyxin B)	Cell membrane	Disrupt membrane permeability by charge alteration	Not defined
	Gramicidin	Cell membrane	Forms pores	Not defined
O	Daptomycin	Cell membrane	Forms channels that disrupt membrane potential	Not defined

[a]Compounds in parentheses are major representatives for the class.

INHIBITION OF CELL-WALL SYNTHESIS

One major difference between bacterial and mammalian cells is the presence in bacteria of a rigid wall external to the cell membrane. The wall protects bacterial cells from osmotic rupture, which would result from the cell's usual marked hyperosmolarity (by up to 20 atm) relative to the host environment. The structure conferring cell-wall rigidity and resistance to osmotic lysis in both gram-positive and gram-negative bacteria is peptidoglycan, a large, covalently linked sacculus that surrounds the bacterium. In gram-positive bacteria, peptidoglycan is the only layered structure external to the cell membrane and is thick (20–80 nm); in gram-negative bacteria, there is an outer membrane external to a very thin (1-nm) peptidoglycan layer.

Chemotherapeutic agents directed at any stage of the synthesis, export, assembly, or cross-linking of peptidoglycan lead to inhibition of bacterial cell growth and, in most cases, to cell death. Peptidoglycan is composed of (1) a backbone of two alternating sugars, N-acetylglucosamine and N-acetylmuramic acid; (2) a chain of four amino acids that extends down from the backbone (stem peptides); and (3) a peptide bridge that cross-links the peptide chains. Peptidoglycan is formed by the addition of subunits (a sugar with its five attached amino acids) that are assembled in the cytoplasm and transported through the cytoplasmic membrane to the cell surface. Subsequent cross-linking is driven by cleavage of the terminal stem-peptide amino acid.

Virtually all the antibiotics that inhibit bacterial cell-wall synthesis are bactericidal. That is, they eventually result in the cell's death due to osmotic lysis. However, much of the loss of cell-wall integrity following treatment with cell wall–active agents is due to the bacteria's own

Mechanisms of Action

GRAM-NEGATIVE | **GRAM-POSITIVE**

Mechanisms of Resistance

GRAM-NEGATIVE | **GRAM-POSITIVE**

② Detergent action on lipid gram ⊖ outer membrane.

③ Penetration of hydrophilic drugs through porin channels in gram ⊖ outer membrane.

④ Free diffusion through gram ⊕ cell envelope with binding to cell wall PG **or**

⑤ Binding to cell membrane PBP. Drug confined to space external to IM.

⑥ Diffusion or transport of drugs with intracellular target through IM.

⑦ Binding to ribosomal target for protein synthesis inhibition.

⑧ Antibiotic interaction with target protein leading to metabolic (DHFR, DHPS), protein synthetic (tRNA synthetase), or nucleic acid (DNA gyrase, RNA polymerase) abnormalities.

⑨ Direct interaction of reactive intermediates with nucleic acid.

⑩ Insertion into cell membrane, disrupting membrane potential.

① **Intrinsic resistance:** Inability of antibiotic to penetrate gram ⊖ envelope (e.g., vancomycin).

③ Mutant porin channels **decrease** antimicrobial **penetration**.

④ **Production of insensitive target** by acquired gene mediating production of altered peptidoglycan.

⑤a **Production of β-lactam-insensitive PBP target** by mutation of gene or acquisition of new gene.

⑤b **Inactivation** of β-lactam antibiotic by β-lactamases in periplasm (gram ⊖) or surrounding medium (gram ⊕).

⑥ **Active efflux** of drugs from cytoplasm or from gram ⊖ periplasm.

⑦a Decreased ribosomal binding due to **target site alteration**.

⑦b **Inactivation** of drug by chemical modification leading to decreased ribosomal interaction.

⑧ Mutation of target gene or acquisition of new gene producing a **drug-insensitive target** protein.

FIGURE 127-1 Mechanisms of action of and resistance to antibacterial agents. Black lines trace the routes of drug interaction with bacterial cells, from entry to target site. The letters in each figure indicate specific antibacterial agents or classes of agents, as shown in Table 127-1. The numbers correspond to mechanisms listed beneath each panel. 50s and 30s, large and small ribosome subunits; Ac, acetylation; Ad, adenylation; DHFR, dihydrofolate reductase; DHPS, dihydropteroate synthetase; IM, inner (cytoplasmic) membrane; LPS, lipopolysaccharide; OM, outer membrane; P, phosphorylation; PBP, penicillin-binding protein; PG, peptidoglycan.

cell-wall remodeling enzymes (autolysins) that cleave peptidoglycan bonds in the normal course of cell growth. In the presence of antibacterial agents that inhibit cell-wall growth, autolysis proceeds without normal cell-wall repair; weakness and eventual cellular lysis occur.

Antibacterial agents act to inhibit cell-wall synthesis in several ways, as described below.

BACITRACIN Bacitracin, a cyclic peptide antibiotic, inhibits the conversion to its active form of the lipid carrier that moves the water-soluble cytoplasmic peptidoglycan subunits through the cell membrane to the cell exterior.

GLYCOPEPTIDES Glycopeptides (vancomycin and teicoplanin) are high-molecular-weight antibiotics that bind to the terminal D-ala-nine–D-alanine component of the stem peptide while the subunits are external to the cell membrane but still linked to the lipid carrier. This binding sterically inhibits the addition of subunits to the peptidoglycan backbone.

β-LACTAM ANTIBIOTICS β-Lactam antibiotics (penicillins, cephalosporins, carbapenems, and monobactams; Table 127-2) are characterized by a four-membered β-lactam ring and prevent the cross-linking reaction called *transpeptidation*. The energy for attaching a peptide crossbridge from the stem peptide of one peptidoglycan subunit to another is derived from the cleavage of a terminal D-alanine residue from the subunit stem peptide. The cross-bridge amino acid is then attached to the penultimate D-alanine by transpeptidase enzymes. The β-lactam ring of the antibiotic forms an irreversible covalent acyl bond with the

TABLE 127-2 CLASSIFICATION OF β-LACTAM ANTIBIOTICS

Class	Route of Administration	
	Parenteral	**Oral**
Penicillins		
β-Lactamase–susceptible		
Narrow-spectrum	Penicillin G	Penicillin V
Enteric-active	Ampicillin	Amoxicillin, ampicillin
Enteric-active and antipseudomonal	Ticarcillin, piperacillin	None
β-Lactamase–resistant		
Antistaphylococcal	Oxacillin, nafcillin	Cloxacillin, dicloxacillin
Combined with β-lactamase inhibitors	Ticarcillin plus clavulanic acid, ampicillin plus sulbactam, piperacillin plus tazobactam	Amoxicillin plus clavulanic acid
Cephalosporins		
First-generation	Cefazolin, cephalothin, cephapirin	Cephalexin, cephradine, cefadroxil
Second-generation		
Haemophilus-active	Cefamandole, cefuroxime, cefonicid, ceforanide	Cefaclor, cefuroxime axetil, ceftibuten, cefdinir, cefprozil, cefpodoxime,[a] loracarbef
Bacteroides-active	Cefoxitin, cefotetan, cefmetazole	None
Third-generation		
Extended-spectrum	Ceftriaxone, cefotaxime, ceftizoxime	None
Extended-spectrum and antipseudomonal	Ceftazidime, cefepime	None
Carbapenems	Imipenem-cilastatin, meropenem, ertapenem	None
Monobactams	Aztreonam	None

[a]Some sources classify cefpodoxime as a third-generation oral agent because of a marginally broader spectrum.

transpeptidase enzyme (probably because of the antibiotic's steric similarity to the enzyme's D-alanine–D-alanine target), preventing the cross-linking reaction. Transpeptidases and similar enzymes involved in cross-linking are called *penicillin-binding proteins* (PBPs) because they all have active sites that bind β-lactam antibiotics.

INHIBITION OF PROTEIN SYNTHESIS

Most of the antibacterial agents that inhibit protein synthesis interact with the bacterial ribosome. The difference between the composition of bacterial and mammalian ribosomes gives these compounds their selectivity.

AMINOGLYCOSIDES Aminoglycosides (gentamicin, kanamycin, tobramycin, streptomycin, neomycin, and amikacin) are a group of structurally related compounds containing three linked hexose sugars. They exert a bactericidal effect by binding irreversibly to the 30S subunit of the bacterial ribosome and blocking initiation of protein synthesis. Uptake of aminoglycosides and their penetration through the cell membrane constitute an aerobic, energy-dependent process. Thus, aminoglycoside activity is markedly reduced in an anaerobic environment. *Spectinomycin*, an aminocyclitol antibiotic, also acts on the 30S ribosomal subunit but has a different mechanism of action from the aminoglycosides and is bacteriostatic rather than bactericidal.

MACROLIDES, KETOLIDES, AND LINCOSAMIDES *Macrolide antibiotics* (erythromycin, clarithromycin, and azithromycin) consist of a large lactone ring to which sugars are attached. *Ketolide antibiotics*, including telithromycin, replace the cladinose sugar on the macrolactone ring with a ketone group. These drugs bind specifically to the 50S portion of the bacterial ribosome and inhibit protein chain elongation. Although structurally unrelated to the macrolides, *lincosamides* (clindamycin and lincomycin) bind to a site on the 50S ribosome nearly identical to the binding site for macrolides.

STREPTOGRAMINS Streptogramins [quinupristin (streptogramin B) and dalfopristin (streptogramin A)], which are supplied as a combination in Synercid, are peptide macrolactones that also bind to the 50S ri-

bosomal subunit and block protein synthesis. Streptogramin B binds to a ribosomal site similar to the binding site for macrolides and lincosamides, whereas streptogramin A binds to a different ribosomal site, blocking the late phase of protein synthesis. The two streptogramins act synergistically to kill bacteria if the strain is susceptible to both components.

CHLORAMPHENICOL Chloramphenicol consists of a single aromatic ring and a short side chain. This antibiotic binds reversibly to the 50S portion of the bacterial ribosome at a site close to but not identical with the binding sites for the macrolides and lincosamides, inhibiting peptide bond formation.

LINEZOLID Linezolid is the only commercially available drug in the oxazolidinone class. Linezolid binds to the 50S ribosomal subunit and blocks the initiation of protein synthesis.

TETRACYCLINES AND GLYCYLCYCLINES Tetracyclines (tetracycline, doxycycline, and minocycline) and glycylcyclines (tigecycline) consist of four aromatic rings with various substituent groups. They interact reversibly with the bacterial 30S ribosomal subunit, blocking the binding of aminoacyl tRNA to the mRNA-ribosome complex. This mechanism is markedly different from that of the aminoglycosides, which also bind to the 30S subunit.

MUPIROCIN Mupirocin (pseudomonic acid) inhibits isoleucine tRNA synthetase by competing with bacterial isoleucine for its binding site on the enzyme and depleting cellular stores of isoleucine-charged tRNA.

INHIBITION OF BACTERIAL METABOLISM

The *antimetabolites* are all synthetic compounds that interfere with bacterial synthesis of folic acid. Products of the folic acid synthesis pathway function as coenzymes for the one-carbon transfer reactions that are essential for the synthesis of thymidine, all purines, and several amino acids. Inhibition of folate synthesis leads to cessation of bacterial cell growth and, in some cases, to bacterial cell death. The principal antibacterial antimetabolites are sulfonamides (sulfisoxazole, sulfadiazine, and sulfamethoxazole) and trimethoprim.

SULFONAMIDES Sulfonamides are structural analogues of *p*-aminobenzoic acid (PABA), one of the three structural components of folic acid (the other two being pteridine and glutamate). The first step in the synthesis of folic acid is the addition of PABA to pteridine by the enzyme dihydropteroic acid synthetase. Sulfonamides compete with PABA as substrates for the enzyme. The selective effect of sulfonamides is due to the fact that bacteria synthesize folic acid, while mammalian cells cannot synthesize the cofactor and must use exogenous supplies. However, the activity of sulfonamides can be greatly reduced by the presence of excess PABA or by the exogenous addition of end products of one-carbon transfer reactions (e.g., thymidine and purines). High concentrations of the latter substances may be present in some infections as a result of tissue and white cell breakdown, compromising sulfonamide activity.

TRIMETHOPRIM Trimethoprim is a diaminopyrimidine, a structural analogue of the pteridine moiety of folic acid. Trimethoprim is a competitive inhibitor of dihydrofolate reductase; this enzyme is responsible for reduction of dihydrofolic acid to tetrahydrofolic acid—the essential final component in the folic acid synthesis pathway. Like that of the sulfonamides, the activity of trimethoprim is compromised in the presence of exogenous thymine or thymidine.

INHIBITION OF NUCLEIC ACID SYNTHESIS OR ACTIVITY

Numerous antibacterial compounds have disparate effects on nucleic acids.

QUINOLONES The quinolones, including nalidixic acid and its fluorinated derivatives (ciprofloxacin, levofloxacin, and moxifloxacin), are synthetic compounds that inhibit the activity of the A subunit of the bacterial enzyme DNA gyrase as well as topoisomerase IV. DNA gyrase and topoisomerases are responsible for negative supercoiling of DNA—an essential conformation for DNA replication in the intact cell. Inhibition of the activity of DNA gyrase and topoisomerase IV is lethal to bacterial cells. The antibiotic *novobiocin* also interferes with the activity of DNA gyrase, but it interferes with the B subunit.

RIFAMPIN Rifampin, used primarily against *Mycobacterium tuberculosis*, is also active against a variety of other bacteria. Rifampin binds tightly to the B subunit of bacterial DNA-dependent RNA polymerase, thus inhibiting transcription of DNA into RNA. Mammalian-cell RNA polymerase is not sensitive to this compound.

NITROFURANTOIN Nitrofurantoin, a synthetic compound, causes DNA damage. The nitrofurans, compounds containing a single five-membered ring, are reduced by a bacterial enzyme to highly reactive, short-lived intermediates that are thought to cause DNA strand breakage, either directly or indirectly.

METRONIDAZOLE Metronidazole, a synthetic imidazole, is active only against anaerobic bacteria and protozoa. The reduction of metronidazole's nitro group by the bacterial anaerobic electron-transport system produces a transient series of reactive intermediates that are thought to cause DNA damage.

ALTERATION OF CELL-MEMBRANE PERMEABILITY

POLYMYXINS The polymyxins [polymyxin B and colistin (polymyxin E)] are cyclic, basic polypeptides. They behave as cationic, surface-active compounds that disrupt the permeability of both the outer and the cytoplasmic membranes of gram-negative bacteria.

GRAMICIDIN A Gramicidin A is a polypeptide of 15 amino acids that acts as an ionophore, forming pores or channels in lipid bilayers.

DAPTOMYCIN Insertion of daptomycin, a new bactericidal lipopeptide antibiotic, into the cell membrane of gram-positive bacteria forms a channel that causes depolarization of the membrane by efflux of intracellular ions, resulting in cell death.

MECHANISMS OF RESISTANCE

Some bacteria exhibit *intrinsic resistance* to certain classes of antibacterial agents (e.g., obligate anaerobic bacteria to aminoglycosides and gram-negative bacteria to vancomycin). In addition, bacteria that are ordinarily susceptible to antibacterial agents can acquire resistance. *Acquired resistance* is a major limitation to effective antibacterial chemotherapy. Resistance can develop by mutation of resident genes or by acquisition of new genes. New genes mediating resistance are usually spread from cell to cell by way of mobile genetic elements such as plasmids, transposons, and bacteriophages. The resistant bacterial populations flourish in areas of high antimicrobial use, where they enjoy a selective advantage over susceptible populations.

The major mechanisms used by bacteria to resist the action of antimicrobial agents are inactivation of the compound, alteration or overproduction of the antibacterial target through mutation of the target protein's gene, acquisition of a new gene that encodes a drug-insensitive target, decreased permeability of the cell envelope to the agent, failure to convert an inactive prodrug to its active derivative, and active efflux of

the compound from the periplasm or interior of the cell. Specific mechanisms of bacterial resistance to the major antibacterial agents are outlined below, summarized in Table 127-1, and depicted in Fig. 127-1.

β-LACTAM ANTIBIOTICS

Bacteria develop resistance to β-lactam antibiotics by a variety of mechanisms. Most common is the destruction of the drug by β-lactamases. The β-lactamases of gram-negative bacteria are confined to the periplasm, between the inner and outer membranes, while gram-positive bacteria secrete their β-lactamases into the surrounding medium. These enzymes have a higher affinity for the antibiotic than the antibiotic has for its target. Binding results in hydrolysis of the β-lactam ring. Genes encoding β-lactamases have been found in both chromosomal and extrachromosomal locations and in both gram-positive and gram-negative bacteria; these genes are often on mobile genetic elements. Many "advanced-generation" β-lactam antibiotics, such as ceftriaxone and cefepime, are stable in the presence of plasmid-mediated β-lactamases and are active against bacteria resistant to earlier-generation β-lactam antibiotics. However, extended-spectrum β-lactamases (ESBLs), either acquired on mobile genetic elements by gram-negative bacteria (e.g., *Klebsiella pneumoniae* and *Escherichia coli*) or present as stable chromosomal genes in other gram-negative species (e.g., *Enterobacter* spp.), have broad substrate specificity, hydrolyzing virtually all penicillins and cephalosporins. One strategy that has been devised for circumventing resistance mediated by β-lactamases is to combine the β-lactam agent with an inhibitor that avidly binds the inactivating enzyme, preventing its attack on the antibiotic. Unfortunately, the inhibitors (e.g., clavulanic acid, sulbactam, and tazobactam) do not bind all chromosomal β-lactamases (e.g., that of *Enterobacter*) and thus cannot be depended on to prevent the inactivation of β-lactam antibiotics by such enzymes. No β-lactam antibiotic or inhibitor has been produced that can resist all of the many β-lactamases that have been identified.

A second mechanism of bacterial resistance to β-lactam antibiotics is an alteration in PBP targets so that the PBPs have a markedly reduced affinity for the drug. While this alteration may occur by mutation of existing genes, the acquisition of new PBP genes (as in staphylococcal resistance to methicillin) or of new pieces of PBP genes (as in streptococcal, gonococcal, and meningococcal resistance to penicillin) is more important.

A final resistance mechanism is the coupling, in gram-negative bacteria, of a decrease in outer-membrane permeability with rapid efflux of the antibiotic from the periplasm to the cell exterior. Mutations of genes encoding outer-membrane protein channels called *porins* decrease the entry of β-lactam antibiotics into the cell, while additional proteins form channels that actively pump β-lactams out of the cell. Resistance of Enterobacteriaceae to some cephalosporins and resistance of *Pseudomonas* spp. to cephalosporins and piperacillin are the best examples of this mechanism.

VANCOMYCIN

Clinically important resistance to vancomycin was first described among enterococci in France in 1988. Vancomycin-resistant enterococci (VRE) have subsequently become disseminated worldwide. The genes encoding resistance are carried on plasmids that can transfer themselves from cell to cell and on transposons that can jump from plasmids to chromosomes. Resistance is mediated by enzymes that substitute D-lactate for D-alanine on the peptidoglycan stem peptide so that there is no longer an appropriate target for vancomycin binding. This alteration does not appear to affect cell-wall integrity, however. This type of acquired vancomycin resistance was confined for 14 years to enterococci—more specifically, to *Enterococcus faecium* rather than the more common pathogen *E. faecalis*. However, since 2002, *S. aureus* isolates that are highly resistant to vancomycin have been recovered from four patients in the United States. All of the isolates contain *vanA*, the gene that mediates vancomycin resistance in enterococci. In addition, since 1996, a few isolates of both *S. aureus* and *Staphylococcus epidermidis* that display a four- to eightfold reduction in susceptibility to vancomycin have been found worldwide, and many more isolates may contain subpopulations with reduced vancomycin susceptibility. These isolates have not acquired the genes that mediate vancomycin resistance in enterococci but are mutant bacteria with markedly thickened cell walls. These mutants were apparently selected in patients who were undergoing prolonged vancomycin therapy. The failure of vancomycin therapy in some patients infected with *S. aureus* or *S. epidermidis* strains exhibiting only intermediate susceptibility to this drug is thought to have resulted from this resistance.

AMINOGLYCOSIDES

The most common aminoglycoside resistance mechanism is inactivation of the antibiotic. Aminoglycoside-modifying enzymes, usually encoded on plasmids, transfer phosphate, adenyl, or acetyl residues from intracellular molecules to hydroxyl or amino side groups on the antibiotic. The modified antibiotic is less active because of diminished binding to its ribosomal target. Modifying enzymes that can inactivate any of the available aminoglycosides have been found in both gram-positive and gram-negative bacteria. A second aminoglycoside resistance mechanism, which has been identified predominantly in clinical isolates of *Pseudomonas aeruginosa*, is decreased antibiotic uptake, presumably due to alterations in the bacterial outer membrane.

MACROLIDES, KETOLIDES, LINCOSAMIDES, AND STREPTOGRAMINS

Resistance in gram-positive bacteria, which are the usual target organisms for macrolides, ketolides, lincosamides, and streptogramins, can be due to the production of an enzyme—most commonly plasmid-encoded—that methylates ribosomal RNA, interfering with binding of the antibiotics to their target. Methylation mediates resistance to erythromycin, clarithromycin, azithromycin, clindamycin, and streptogramin B. Resistance to streptogramin B converts quinupristin/dalfopristin from a bactericidal to a bacteriostatic antibiotic. Streptococci can also actively cause the efflux of macrolides, and staphylococci can cause the efflux of macrolides, clindamycin, and streptogramin A. Ketolides such as telithromycin retain activity against most isolates of *Streptococcus pneumoniae* that are resistant to macrolides. In addition, staphylococci can inactivate streptogramin A by acetylation and streptogramin B by either acetylation or hydrolysis. Finally, mutations in 23S ribosomal RNA that alter the binding of macrolides to their targets have been found in both staphylococci and streptococci.

CHLORAMPHENICOL

Most bacteria resistant to chloramphenicol produce a plasmid-encoded enzyme, chloramphenicol acetyltransferase, that inactivates the compound by acetylation.

TETRACYCLINES AND TIGECYCLINE

The most common mechanism of tetracycline resistance in gram-negative bacteria is a plasmid-encoded active-efflux pump that is inserted into the cytoplasmic membrane and extrudes antibiotic from the cell. Resistance in gram-positive bacteria is due either to active efflux or to ribosomal alterations that diminish binding of the antibiotic to its target. Genes involved in ribosomal protection are found on mobile genetic elements. A new parenteral tetracycline derivative (a glycylcycline), tigecycline, is active against tetracycline-resistant bacteria because it is not removed by efflux and can bind to altered ribosomes.

MUPIROCIN

Although the topical compound mupirocin was introduced into clinical use relatively recently, resistance is already becoming widespread in some areas. The mechanism appears to be either mutation of the target isoleucine tRNA synthetase so that it is no longer inhibited by the antibiotic or plasmid-encoded production of a form of the target enzyme that binds mupirocin poorly.

TRIMETHOPRIM AND SULFONAMIDES

The most prevalent mechanism of resistance to trimethoprim and the sulfonamides in both gram-positive and gram-negative bacteria is the acquisition of plasmid-encoded genes that produce a new, drug-insensitive target—specifically, an insensitive dihydrofolate reductase for trimethoprim and an altered dihydropteroate synthetase for sulfonamides.

QUINOLONES

The most common mechanism of resistance to quinolones is the development of one or more mutations in target DNA gyrases and topoisomerase IV that prevent the antibacterial agent from interfering with the enzymes' activity. Some gram-negative bacteria develop mutations that both decrease outer-membrane porin permeability and cause active drug efflux from the cytoplasm. Mutations that result in active quinolone efflux are also found in gram-positive bacteria.

RIFAMPIN

Bacteria rapidly become resistant to rifampin by developing mutations in the B subunit of RNA polymerase that render the enzyme unable to bind the antibiotic. The rapid selection of resistant mutants is the major limitation to the use of this antibiotic against otherwise-susceptible staphylococci and requires that the drug be used in combination with another antistaphylococcal agent.

LINEZOLID

Enterococci, streptococci, and staphylococci become resistant to linezolid in vitro by mutation of the 23S rRNA binding site. Clinical isolates of *E. faecium* and *E. faecalis* acquire resistance to linezolid readily by this mechanism, often during therapy, but linezolid-resistant staphylococcal and streptococcal isolates are rare.

MULTIPLE ANTIBIOTIC RESISTANCE

The acquisition by one bacterium of resistance to multiple antibacterial agents is becoming increasingly common. The two major mechanisms are the acquisition of multiple unrelated resistance genes and the development of mutations in a single gene or gene complex that mediate resistance to a series of unrelated compounds. The construction of multiresistant strains by acquisition of multiple genes occurs by sequential steps of gene transfer and environmental selection in areas of high-level antimicrobial use. In contrast, mutations in a single gene can conceivably be selected in a single step. Bacteria that are multiresistant by virtue of the acquisition of new genes include hospital-associated strains of gram-negative bacteria, enterococci, and staphylococci and community-acquired strains of salmonellae, gonococci, and pneumococci. Mutations that confer resistance to multiple unrelated antimicrobial agents occur in the genes encoding outer-membrane porins and efflux proteins of gram-negative bacteria. These mutations decrease bacterial intracellular and periplasmic accumulation of β-lactams, quinolones, tetracyclines, chloramphenicol, and aminoglycosides. Multiresistant bacterial isolates pose increasing problems in U.S. hospitals; strains resistant to all available antibacterial chemotherapy have already been identified.

PHARMACOKINETICS OF ANTIBIOTICS

The *pharmacokinetic profile* of an antibacterial agent refers to concentrations in serum and tissue versus time and reflects the processes of absorption, distribution, metabolism, and excretion. Important characteristics include peak and trough serum concentrations and mathematically derived parameters such as half-life, clearance, and distribution volume. Pharmacokinetic information is useful for estimating the appropriate antibacterial dose and frequency of administration, for adjusting dosages in patients with impaired excretory capacity, and for comparing one drug with another. In contrast, the *pharmacodynamic profile* of an antibiotic refers to the relationship between the pharmacokinetics of the antibiotic and its minimal inhibitory concentrations (MICs) for bacteria (see "Principles of Antibacterial Chemotherapy," below). **For further discussion of basic pharmacokinetic principles, see Chap. 5.**

ABSORPTION

Antibiotic *absorption* refers to the rate and extent of a drug's systemic bioavailability after oral, IM, or IV administration.

Oral Administration Most patients with infection are treated with oral antibacterial agents in the outpatient setting. Advantages of oral therapy over parenteral therapy include lower cost, generally fewer adverse effects (including complications of indwelling lines), and greater acceptance by patients. The percentage of an orally administered antibacterial agent that is absorbed (i.e., its *bioavailability*) ranges from as little as 10–20% (erythromycin and penicillin G) to nearly 100% [amoxicillin, clindamycin, metronidazole, doxycycline, trimethoprim-sulfamethoxazole (TMP-SMX), linezolid, and most fluoroquinolones]. These differences in bioavailability are not clinically important as long as drug concentrations at the site of infection are sufficient to inhibit or kill the pathogen. However, therapeutic efficacy may be compromised when absorption is reduced as a result of physiologic or pathologic conditions (such as the presence of food for some drugs or the shunting of blood away from the gastrointestinal tract in patients with hypotension), drug interactions (such as that of quinolones and metal cations), or noncompliance. The oral route is usually used for patients with relatively mild infections in whom absorption is not thought to be compromised by the preceding conditions. In addition, the oral route can often be used in more severely ill patients after they have responded to parenteral therapy.

Intramuscular Administration Although the IM route of administration usually results in 100% bioavailability, it is not as widely used in the United States as the oral and IV routes, in part because of the pain often associated with IM injections and the relative ease of IV access in the hospitalized patient. IM injection may be suitable for specific indications requiring an "immediate" and reliable effect (e.g., with long-acting forms of penicillin, including benzathine and procaine, and with single doses of ceftriaxone for acute otitis media or uncomplicated gonococcal infection).

Intravenous Administration The IV route is appropriate when oral antibacterial agents are not effective against a particular pathogen, when bioavailability is uncertain, or when larger doses are required than are feasible with the oral route. After IV administration, bioavailability is 100%; serum concentrations are maximal at the end of the infusion. For many patients in whom long-term antimicrobial therapy is required and oral therapy is not feasible, outpatient parenteral antibiotic therapy (OPAT), including the use of convenient portable pumps, may be cost-effective and safe. Alternatively, some oral antibacterial drugs (e.g., fluoroquinolones) are sufficiently active against Enterobacteriaceae to provide potency equal to that of parenteral therapy; oral use of such drugs may allow the patient to return home from the hospital earlier or to avoid hospitalization entirely.

DISTRIBUTION

To be effective, concentrations of an antibacterial agent must exceed the pathogen's MIC. Serum antibiotic concentrations usually exceed the MIC for susceptible bacteria, but since most infections are extravascular, the antibiotic must also distribute to the site of the infection. Concentrations of most antibacterial agents in interstitial fluid are similar to free-drug concentrations in serum. However, when the infection is located in a "protected" site where penetration is poor, such as cerebrospinal fluid (CSF), the eye, the prostate, or infected cardiac vegetations, high parenteral doses or local administration for prolonged periods may be required for cure. In addition, even though an antibacterial agent may penetrate to the site of infection, its activity may be antagonized by factors in the local environment, such as an unfavorable pH or inactivation by cellular degradation products. For example, since the activity of aminoglycosides is reduced at acidic pH, the acidic environment in many infected tissues may be partly responsible for the relatively poor efficacy of aminoglycoside monotherapy. In addition, the abscess milieu reduces the penetration and local activity of many antibacterial compounds, so that surgical drainage may be required for cure.

Most bacteria that cause human infections are located extracellularly. Intracellular pathogens such as *Legionella*, *Chlamydia*, *Brucella*, and *Salmonella* may persist or cause relapse if the antibacterial agent does not enter the cell. In general, β-lactams, vancomycin, and aminoglycosides penetrate cells poorly, whereas macrolides, ketolides, tetracyclines, metronidazole, chloramphenicol, rifampin, TMP-SMX, and quinolones penetrate cells well.

METABOLISM AND ELIMINATION

Like other drugs, antibacterial agents are disposed of by hepatic elimination (metabolism or biliary elimination), by renal excretion of the unchanged or metabolized form, or by a combination of the two processes. For most of the antibacterial drugs, metabolism leads to loss of in vitro activity, although some agents, such as cefotaxime, rifampin, and clarithromycin, have bioactive metabolites that may contribute to their overall efficacy.

The most practical application of information on the mode of excretion of an antibacterial agent is in adjusting dosage when elimination capability is impaired (Table 127-3). Direct, nonidiosyncratic toxicity from antibacterial drugs may result from failure to reduce the dosage given to patients with impaired elimination. For agents that are primarily cleared intact by glomerular filtration, drug clearance is correlated with creatinine clearance, and estimates of the latter can be used to guide dosage. For drugs whose elimination is primarily hepatic, no simple marker is useful for dosage adjustment in patients with liver disease. However, in patients with severe hepatic disease, residual metabolic capability is usually sufficient to preclude accumulation and toxic effects.

PRINCIPLES OF ANTIBACTERIAL CHEMOTHERAPY

The choice of an antibacterial compound for a particular patient and a specific infection involves more than just a knowledge of the agent's pharmacokinetic profile and in vitro activity. The basic tenets of chemotherapy, to be elaborated below, include the following: When appropriate, material containing the infecting organism(s) should be obtained before the start of treatment so that presumptive identifica-

TABLE 127-3 ANTIBACTERIAL DRUG DOSE ADJUSTMENTS IN PATIENTS WITH RENAL IMPAIRMENT

Antibiotic	Major Route of Excretion	Dosage Adjustment with Renal Impairment
Aminoglycosides	Renal	Yes
Azithromycin	Biliary	No
Cefazolin	Renal	Yes
Cefepime	Renal	Yes
Ceftazidime	Renal	Yes
Ceftriaxone	Renal/biliary	Modest reduction in severe renal impairment
Ciprofloxacin	Renal/biliary	Only in severe renal insufficiency
Clarithromycin	Renal/biliary	Only in severe renal insufficiency
Daptomycin	Renal	Yes
Erythromycin	Biliary	Only when given in high IV doses
Levofloxacin	Renal	Yes
Linezolid	Metabolism	No
Metronidazole	Biliary	No
Nafcillin	Biliary	No
Penicillin G	Renal	Yes (when given in high IV doses)
Piperacillin	Renal	Only with Cl_{cr} of <40 mL/min
Quinupristin/dalfopristin	Metabolism	No
Ticarcillin	Renal	Yes
Tigecycline	Biliary	No
TMP-SMX	Renal/biliary	Only in severe renal insufficiency
Vancomycin	Renal	Yes

Abbreviations: Cl_{cr}, creatinine clearance rate; TMP-SMX, trimethoprim-sulfamethoxazole.

tion can be made by microscopic examination of stained specimens and the organism can be grown for definitive identification and susceptibility testing. Awareness of local susceptibility patterns is useful when the patient is treated empirically. Once the organism is identified and its susceptibility to antibacterial agents is determined, the regimen with the narrowest effective spectrum should be chosen. The choice of antibacterial agent is guided by the pharmacokinetic and adverse-reaction profile of active compounds, the site of infection, the immune status of the host, and evidence of efficacy from well-performed clinical trials. If all other factors are equal, the least expensive antibacterial regimen should be chosen.

SUSCEPTIBILITY OF BACTERIA TO ANTIBACTERIAL DRUGS IN VITRO

Determination of the susceptibility of the patient's infecting organism to a panel of appropriate antibacterial agents is an essential first step in devising a chemotherapeutic regimen. Susceptibility testing is designed to estimate the susceptibility of a bacterial isolate to an antibacterial drug under standardized conditions. These conditions favor rapidly growing aerobic or facultative organisms and assess bacteriostasis only. Specialized testing is required for the assessment of bactericidal antimicrobial activity; for the detection of resistance among such fastidious organisms as obligate anaerobes, *Haemophilus* spp., and pneumococci; and for the determination of resistance phenotypes with variable expression, such as resistance to methicillin or oxacillin among staphylococci. Antimicrobial susceptibility testing is important when susceptibility is unpredictable, most often as a result of increasing acquired resistance among bacteria infecting hospitalized patients.

PHARMACODYNAMICS: RELATIONSHIP OF PHARMACOKINETICS AND IN VITRO SUSCEPTIBILITY TO CLINICAL RESPONSE

Bacteria have often been considered *susceptible* to an antibacterial drug if the achievable peak serum concentration exceeds the MIC by approximately fourfold. The *breakpoint* is the concentration of the antibiotic that separates susceptible from resistant bacteria (Fig. 127-2). When a majority of the isolates of a given bacterial species are inhibited at concentrations below the breakpoint, the species is considered to be within the spectrum of the antibiotic.

The pharmacodynamic profile of an antibiotic refers to the quantitative relationships between the time course of antibiotic concentrations in serum and tissue, in vitro susceptibility (MIC), and microbial response (inhibition of growth or rate of killing). Three pharmacodynamic parameters quantify these relationships: the ratio of the area under the plasma concentration vs. time curve to MIC (AUC/MIC), the ratio of the maximal serum concentration to the MIC (C_{max}/MIC),

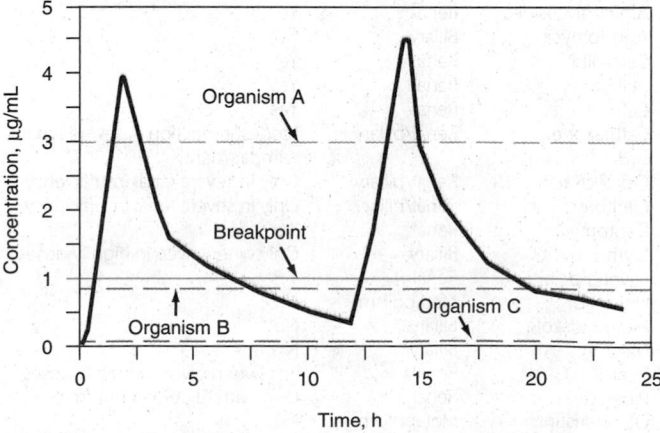

FIGURE 127-2 Relationship between pharmacokinetics of an antibiotic and susceptibility. Organism A is resistant, organism B is moderately susceptible, and organism C is very susceptible. Pharmacodynamic indices include the ratio of the peak serum concentration to MIC (C_{max}/MIC), the ratio of the area under the serum concentration vs. time curve to MIC (AUC/MIC), and the time that serum concentrations exceed the MIC ($t > $ MIC).

TABLE 127-4	PHARMACODYNAMIC INDICES OF MAJOR ANTIMICROBIAL CLASSES
Parameter Predicting Response	**Drug or Drug Class**
Time above the MIC	Penicillins, cephalosporins, carbapenems, aztreonam
24-h AUC/MIC	Aminoglycosides, fluoroquinolones, tetracyclines, vancomycin, macrolides, clindamycin, quinupristin/dalfopristin, tigecycline, daptomycin
Peak to MIC	Aminoglycosides, fluoroquinolones

Abbreviations: MIC, minimal inhibitory concentration; AUC, area under the concentration curve.

and the time during a dosing interval that plasma concentrations exceed the MIC ($t > $ MIC). The pharmacodynamic profile of an antibiotic class is characterized as either *concentration dependent* (fluoroquinolones, aminoglycosides), such that an increase in antibiotic concentration leads to a more rapid rate of bacterial death, or *time dependent* (β-lactams), such that the reduction in bacterial density is proportional to the time that concentrations exceed the MIC. For concentration-dependent antibiotics, the C_{max}/MIC or AUC/MIC ratio correlates best with the reduction in microbial density in vitro and in animal investigations. Dosing strategies attempt to maximize these ratios by the administration of a large dose relative to the MIC for anticipated pathogens, often at long intervals (relative to the serum half-life). Once-daily dosing of aminoglycoside antibiotics is the most practical consequence of these relationships. In contrast, dosage strategies for time-dependent antibiotics emphasize the administration of doses sufficient to maintain serum concentrations above the MIC for a critical portion of the dose interval. Response to β-lactam antibiotics, measured as the decline in bacterial density at the site of infection, is maximal when serum and tissue concentrations are maintained above the MIC for 30–50% of the dose interval. For example, the use of high-dose amoxicillin (90–100 mg/kg per day) in the treatment of acute otitis media increases not only the penetration of amoxicillin into the inner ear but also the duration of time that concentrations exceed the MIC for pneumococci. This approach provides effective therapy in most patients, including those whose pneumococcal isolates are penicillin resistant. The clinical implications of these pharmacodynamic relationships are in the early stages of investigation; their elucidation should eventually result in more rational antibacterial dosage regimens. Table 127-4 summarizes the pharmacodynamic properties of the major antibiotic classes.

STATUS OF THE HOST

Various host factors must be considered in the devising of antibacterial chemotherapy. The host's antibacterial *immune function* is of importance, particularly as it relates to opsonophagocytic function. Since the major host defense against acute, overwhelming bacterial infection is the polymorphonuclear leukocyte, patients with neutropenia must be treated aggressively and empirically with bactericidal drugs for suspected infection (Chap. 82). Likewise, patients who have deficient humoral immunity (e.g., those with chronic lymphocytic leukemia and multiple myeloma) and individuals with surgical or functional asplenia (e.g., those with sickle cell disease) should be treated empirically for infections with encapsulated organisms, especially the pneumococcus.

Pregnancy increases the risk of toxicity of certain antibacterial drugs for the mother (e.g., hepatic toxicity of tetracycline), affects drug disposition and pharmacokinetics, and—because of the risk of fetal toxicity—severely limits the choice of agents for treating infections. Certain antibacterial agents are contraindicated in pregnancy either because their safety has not been established (categories B and C) or because they are known to be toxic (categories D and X). Table 127-5 summarizes drug safety in pregnancy.

In patients with *concomitant viral infections*, the incidence of adverse reactions to antibacterial drugs may be unusually high. For example, persons with infectious mononucleosis and those infected with HIV experi-

TABLE 127-5 ANTIBACTERIAL DRUGS IN PREGNANCY

Antibacterial Drug	Toxicity in Pregnancy	Recommendation
Aminoglycosides	Possible 8th-nerve toxicity	Caution[a]
Chloramphenicol	Gray syndrome in newborn	Caution at term
Fluoroquinolones	Arthropathy in immature animals	Caution
Clarithromycin	Teratogenicity in animals	Contraindicated
Ertapenem	Decreased weight in animals	Caution
Erythromycin estolate	Cholestatic hepatitis	Contraindicated
Imipenem/cilastatin	Toxicity in some pregnant animals	Caution
Linezolid	Embryonic and fetal toxicity in rats	Caution
Meropenem	Unknown	Caution
Metronidazole	None known, but carcinogenic in rats	Caution
Nitrofurantoin	Hemolytic anemia in newborns	Caution; contraindicated at term
Quinupristin/dalfopristin	Unknown	Caution
Sulfonamides	Hemolysis in newborn with G6PD[b] deficiency; kernicterus in newborn	Caution; contraindicated at term
Tetracyclines/tigecycline	Tooth discoloration, inhibition of bone growth in fetus; hepatotoxicity	Contraindicated
Vancomycin	Unknown	Caution

[a]Use only for strong clinical indication in the absence of a suitable alternative.
[b]G6PD, glucose-6-phosphate dehydrogenase.

ence skin reactions more often to penicillins and folic acid synthesis inhibitors such as TMP-SMX, respectively.

In addition, the patient's age, sex, racial heritage, genetic background, and excretory status all determine the incidence and type of side effects that can be expected with certain antibacterial agents.

SITE OF INFECTION

The location of the infected site may play a major role in the choice and dose of antimicrobial drug. Patients with suspected *meningitis* should receive drugs that can cross the blood-CSF barrier; in addition, because of the relative paucity of phagocytes and opsonins at the site of infection, the agents should be bactericidal. Chloramphenicol, an older drug but occasionally useful in the treatment of meningitis, is bactericidal for common organisms causing meningitis (i.e., meningococci, pneumococci, and *Haemophilus influenzae*, but *not* enteric gram-negative bacilli), is highly lipid-soluble, and enters the CSF well. However, β-lactam drugs, the mainstay of therapy for most of these infections, do not normally reach high levels in CSF. Their efficacy is based on the increased permeability of the blood-brain and blood-CSF barriers to hydrophilic molecules during inflammation and the extreme susceptibility of most infectious organisms to even small amounts of β-lactam drug.

The vegetation, which is the major site of infection in *bacterial endocarditis*, is also a focus that is protected from normal host-defense mechanisms. Antibacterial therapy needs to be bactericidal, with the selected agent administered parenterally over a long period and at a dose that produces serum levels at least eight times higher than the minimal bactericidal concentration (MBC) for the infecting organism. Likewise, *osteomyelitis* involves a site that is resistant to opsonophagocytic removal of infecting bacteria; furthermore, avascular bone (sequestrum) represents a foreign body that thwarts normal host-defense mechanisms. *Chronic prostatitis* is exceedingly difficult to cure because most antibiotics do not penetrate through the capillaries serving the prostate, especially when acute inflammation is absent. *Intraocular infections*, especially endophthalmitis, are difficult to treat because retinal capillaries lacking fenestration hinder drug penetration into the vitreous from blood. Inflammation does little to disrupt this barrier. Thus, direct injection into the vitreous is necessary in many cases. Antibiotic penetration into *abscesses* is usually poor, and local conditions (e.g., low pH or the presence of enzymes that hydrolyze the drug) may further antagonize antibacterial activity.

In contrast, *urinary tract infections* (UTIs), when confined to the bladder, are relatively easy to cure, in part because of the higher concentration of most antibiotics in urine than in blood. Since blood is the usual reference fluid in defining susceptibility (Fig. 127-2), even organisms found to be resistant to achievable serum concentrations may be susceptible to achievable urine concentrations. For drugs that are used only for the treatment of UTIs, such as the urinary tract antiseptics nitrofurantoin and methenamine salts, achievable urine concentrations are used to determine susceptibility. Nitrofurantoin is often active against VRE and is a less expensive alternative to linezolid for the treatment of lower UTIs.

COMBINATION CHEMOTHERAPY

One of the tenets of antibacterial chemotherapy is that if the infecting bacterium has been identified, the most specific chemotherapy possible should be used. The use of a single agent with a narrow spectrum of activity against the pathogen diminishes the alteration of normal flora and thus limits the overgrowth of resistant nosocomial organisms (e.g., *Candida albicans*, enterococci, *Clostridium difficile*, or methicillin-resistant staphylococci), avoids the potential toxicity of multiple-drug regimens, and reduces cost. However, certain circumstances call for the use of more than one antibacterial agent. These are summarized below.

1. *Prevention of the emergence of resistant mutants.* Spontaneous mutations occur at a detectable frequency in certain genes encoding the target proteins for some antibacterial agents. The use of these agents can eliminate the susceptible population, select out resistant mutants at the site of infection, and result in the failure of chemotherapy. Resistant mutants are usually selected when the MIC of the antibacterial agent for the infecting bacterium is close to achievable levels in serum or tissues and/or when the site of infection limits the access or activity of the agent. Among the most common examples are rifampin for staphylococci, imipenem for *Pseudomonas*, and fluoroquinolones for staphylococci and *Pseudomonas*. Small-colony variants of staphylococci resistant to aminoglycosides also emerge during monotherapy with these antibiotics. A second antibacterial agent with a mechanism of action different from that of the first is added to prevent the emergence of these resistant mutants (e.g., imipenem plus an aminoglycoside or a fluoroquinolone for systemic *Pseudomonas* infections). However, since resistant mutants have emerged following combination chemotherapy, this approach clearly is not uniformly successful.

2. *Synergistic or additive activity.* Synergistic or additive activity involves a lowering of the MIC or MBC of each or all of the drugs tested in combination against a specific bacterium. In *synergy*, each agent is more active when combined with a second drug than it would be alone, and the drugs' combined activity is therefore greater than the sum of the individual activities of each drug. In an *additive relationship*, the combined activity of the drugs is equal to the sum of their individual activities. Among the best examples of a synergistic or additive effect, confirmed both in vitro and by animal studies, are the enhanced bactericidal activities of certain β-lactam/aminoglycoside combinations against enterococci, viridans streptococci, and *P. aeruginosa*. The synergistic or additive activity of these combinations has also been demonstrated against selected isolates of enteric gram-negative bacteria and staphylococci. The combination of trimethoprim and sulfamethoxazole has synergistic or additive activity against many enteric gram-negative bacteria. Most other antimicrobial combinations display indifferent activity (i.e., the combination is *no better* than the more active of the two agents alone), and some combinations (e.g., penicillin plus tetracycline against pneumococci) may be antagonistic (i.e., the combination is *worse* than either drug alone).

3. *Therapy directed against multiple potential pathogens.* For certain infections, either a mixture of pathogens is suspected or the patient is desperately ill with an as-yet-unidentified infection (see "Empirical Therapy," below). In these situations, the most important of the likely infecting bacteria must be covered by therapy until culture and susceptibility results become available. Examples of the former infections are intraabdominal or brain abscesses and infections of limbs in diabetic patients with microvascular disease. The latter situations include fevers in neutropenic patients, acute pneumonia from aspiration of oral flora by hospitalized patients, and septic shock or sepsis syndrome.

EMPIRICAL THERAPY

In many situations, antibacterial therapy is begun before a specific bacterial pathogen has been identified. The choice of agent is guided by the results of studies identifying the usual pathogens at that site or in that clinical setting, by pharmacodynamic considerations, and by the resistance profile of the expected pathogens in a particular hospital or geographic area. Situations in which empirical therapy is appropriate include the following:

1. *Life-threatening infection.* Any suspected bacterial infection in a patient with a life-threatening illness should be treated presumptively. Therapy is usually begun with more than one agent and is later tailored to a specific pathogen if one is eventually identified. Early therapy with an effective antimicrobial regimen has consistently been demonstrated to improve survival rates.
2. *Treatment of community-acquired infections.* In many situations, it is appropriate to treat non-life-threatening infections without obtaining cultures. These situations include outpatient infections such as community-acquired upper and lower respiratory tract infections, cystitis, cellulitis or local wound infection, urethritis, and prostatitis. However, if any of these infections recurs or fails to respond to initial therapy, every effort should be made to obtain cultures to guide re-treatment.

CHOICE OF ANTIBACTERIAL THERAPY

Infections for which specific antibacterial agents are among the drugs of choice are detailed in Table 127-6. No attempt has been made to include all of the potential situations in which antibacterial agents may be used. A more detailed discussion of specific bacteria and infections that they cause can be found elsewhere in this volume.

The choice of antibacterial therapy increasingly involves an assessment of the acquired resistance of major microbial pathogens to the antimicrobial agents available to treat them. Resistance rates are dynamic (Table 127-6), both increasing and decreasing in response to the environmental pressure applied by antimicrobial use. For example, a threefold increase in fluoroquinolone use in the community between 1995 and 2002 was associated with increasing rates of quinolone resistance in community-acquired strains of *S. pneumoniae, E. coli, Neisseria gonorrhoeae,* and *K. pneumoniae.* Fluoroquinolone resistance has also emerged rapidly among nosocomial isolates of *S. aureus* and *Pseudomonas* spp. as hospital use of this drug class has increased. In contrast, staphylococcal resistance to tetracyclines has decreased as the use of these antibiotics has declined. It is important to note that, in many cases, wide variations in worldwide antimicrobial-resistance trends may not be reflected in the values recorded at U.S. hospitals (e.g., for fluoroquinolone resistance in *N. gonorrhoeae*). Therefore, the most important factor in choosing initial therapy for an infection in which the susceptibility of the specific pathogen(s) is not known is information on local resistance rates. This information can be obtained from local clinical microbiology laboratories, state health departments, or publications of the Centers for Disease Control and Prevention (e.g., *Emerging Infectious Diseases* and *Morbidity and Mortality Weekly Report*).

ADVERSE REACTIONS

Adverse drug reactions are frequently classified by mechanism as either *dose-related* ("toxic") or *unpredictable*. Unpredictable reactions are either idiosyncratic or allergic. Dose-related reactions include aminoglycoside-induced nephrotoxicity, linezolid-induced thrombocytopenia, penicillin-induced seizures, and vancomycin-induced anaphylactoid reactions. Many of these reactions can be avoided by reducing dosage in patients with impaired renal function, limiting the duration of therapy, or reducing the rate of administration. Adverse reactions to antibacterial agents are a common cause of morbidity, requiring alteration in therapy and additional expense, and they occasionally result in death. The elderly, often those with the more severe infections, may be especially prone to certain adverse reactions. The most clinically relevant adverse reactions to common antibacterial drugs are listed in Table 127-7. For further discussion of adverse drug reactions, see Chap. 5.

DRUG INTERACTIONS

Antimicrobial drugs are a common cause of drug-drug interactions. Table 127-8 lists the most common and best-documented interactions of antibacterial agents with other drugs and characterizes the clinical relevance of these interactions. Coadministration of drugs paired in the tables does not necessarily result in clinically important adverse consequences. Recognition of the potential for an interaction before the administration of an antibacterial agent is crucial to the rational use of these drugs, since adverse consequences can often be prevented if the interaction is anticipated. Table 127-8 is intended only to heighten awareness of the potential for an interaction. Additional sources should be consulted to identify appropriate options. For further discussion of drug interactions, see Chap. 5.

MACROLIDES AND KETOLIDES

Erythromycin, clarithromycin, and telithromycin inhibit CYP3A4, the hepatic P450 enzyme that metabolizes many drugs, including cyclosporine, certain statins (lovastatin, simvastatin), theophylline, carbamazepine, warfarin, certain antineoplastic agents (e.g., vincristine, irinotecan), and ergot alkaloids. In ~10% of patients receiving digoxin, concentrations increase significantly when erythromycin or telithromycin is coadministered, and this increase may lead to digoxin toxicity. Azithromycin has little effect on the metabolism of other drugs. Many drugs (e.g., azole antifungal drugs, diltiazem, verapamil, and nefazodone) can also increase absorption or inhibit erythromycin metabolism. These effects are associated with prolongation of the QT interval and a fivefold increase in mortality rate. This example serves as a reminder that the true significance of drug-drug interactions may be subtle yet profound and that close attention to the evolving safety literature is important.

QUINUPRISTIN/DALFOPRISTIN

Quinupristin/dalfopristin is an inhibitor of CYP3A4. Its interactions with other drugs should be similar to those of erythromycin.

LINEZOLID

Linezolid is a monoamine oxidase inhibitor. Its concomitant administration with sympathomimetics (e.g., phenylpropanolamine) and with foods with high concentrations of tyramine should be avoided. Many case reports describe serotonin syndrome following coadministration of linezolid with selective serotonin reuptake inhibitors.

TETRACYCLINES

The most important interaction involving tetracyclines is reduced absorption when these drugs are coadministered with divalent and trivalent cations, such as antacids, iron compounds, or dairy products. Food also adversely affects absorption of most tetracyclines. Inducers of hepatic isoenzymes, such as phenytoin and rifampin, increase the clearance of doxycycline; although the clinical significance of this effect is unknown, use of an alternative antibiotic may be appropriate.

SULFONAMIDES

Sulfonamides, including TMP-SMX, increase the hypoprothrombinemic effect of warfarin by inhibition of its metabolism or by protein-binding displacement.

TABLE 127-6 INFECTIONS FOR WHICH SPECIFIC ANTIBACTERIAL AGENTS ARE AMONG THE DRUGS OF CHOICE

Agent	Infections	Common Pathogen(s) (Resistance Rate, %)[a]
Penicillin G	Syphilis, yaws, leptospirosis, groups A and B streptococcal infections, pneumococcal infections, actinomycosis, oral and periodontal infections, meningococcal meningitis and meningococcemia, viridans streptococcal endocarditis, clostridial myonecrosis, tetanus, anthrax, rat-bite fever, *Pasteurella multocida* infections, and erysipeloid (*Erysipelothrix rhusiopathiae*)	*Neisseria meningitidis*[b] (intermediate,[c] 15–30; resistant, 0; geographic variation) Viridans streptococci (intermediate, 15–30; resistant, 5–10) *Streptococcus pneumoniae* (intermediate, 23; resistant, 17)
Ampicillin, amoxicillin	Salmonellosis, acute otitis media, *Haemophilus influenzae* meningitis and epiglottitis, *Listeria monocytogenes* meningitis, *Enterococcus faecalis* UTI	*Escherichia coli* (37) *H. influenzae* (35) *Salmonella* spp.[b] (30–50; geographic variation) *Enterococcus* spp. (24)
Nafcillin, oxacillin	*Staphylococcus aureus* (non-MRSA) bacteremia and endocarditis	*S. aureus* (46; MRSA) *Staphylococcus epidermidis* (78; MRSE)
Piperacillin plus tazobactam	Intraabdominal infections (facultative enteric gram-negative bacilli plus obligate anaerobes); infections caused by mixed flora (aspiration pneumonia, diabetic foot ulcers); infections caused by *Pseudomonas aeruginosa*	*P. aeruginosa* (6)
Cefazolin	*E. coli* UTI, surgical prophylaxis, *S. aureus* (non-MRSA) bacteremia and endocarditis	*E. coli* (7) *S. aureus* (46; MRSA)
Cefoxitin, cefotetan	Intraabdominal infections and pelvic inflammatory disease	*Bacteroides fragilis* (12)
Ceftriaxone	Gonococcal infections, pneumococcal meningitis, viridans streptococcal endocarditis, salmonellosis and typhoid fever, hospital-acquired infections caused by nonpseudomonal facultative gram-negative enteric bacilli	*S. pneumoniae* (intermediate, 16; resistant, 0) *E. coli* and *Klebsiella pneumoniae* (1; ESBL producers)
Ceftazidime, cefepime	Hospital-acquired infections caused by facultative gram-negative enteric bacilli and *Pseudomonas*	*P. aeruginosa* (16) (See ceftriaxone for ESBL producers)
Imipenem, meropenem	Intraabdominal infections, hospital-acquired infections (non-MRSA), infections caused by *Enterobacter* spp. and ESBL-producing gram-negative bacilli	*P. aeruginosa* (6) *Acinetobacter* spp. (35)
Aztreonam	Hospital-acquired infections caused by facultative gram-negative bacilli and *Pseudomonas* in penicillin-allergic patients	*P. aeruginosa* (16)
Vancomycin	Bacteremia, endocarditis, and other serious infections due to MRSA; pneumococcal meningitis; antibiotic-associated pseudomembranous colitis[d]	*Enterococcus* spp. (24)
Daptomycin	VRE infections; MRSA bacteremia	UNK
Gentamicin, amikacin, tobramycin	Combined with a penicillin for staphylococcal, enterococcal, or viridans streptococcal endocarditis; combined with a β-lactam antibiotic for gram-negative bacteremia; pyelonephritis	Gentamicin: *E. coli* (6) *P. aeruginosa* (17) *Acinetobacter* spp. (32)
Erythromycin, clarithromycin, azithromycin	*Legionella*, *Campylobacter*, and *Mycoplasma* infections; CAP; group A streptococcal pharyngitis in penicillin-allergic patients; bacillary angiomatosis (*Bartonella henselae*); gastric infections due to *Helicobacter pylori*; *Mycobacterium avium-intracellulare* infections	*S. pneumoniae* (28) *Streptococcus pyogenes*[b] (0–10; geographic variation) *H. pylori*[b] (2–20; geographic variation)
Clindamycin	Severe, invasive group A streptococcal infections; infections caused by obligate anaerobes; infections caused by susceptible staphylococci	*S. aureus* (nosocomial = 58; CA-MRSA = 10[b])
Doxycycline, minocycline	Acute bacterial exacerbations of chronic bronchitis, granuloma inguinale, brucellosis (with streptomycin), tularemia, glanders, melioidosis, spirochetal infections caused by *Borrelia* (Lyme disease and relapsing fever; doxycycline), infections caused by *Vibrio vulnificus*, some *Aeromonas* infections, infections due to *Stenotrophomonas* (minocycline), plague, ehrlichiosis, chlamydial infections (doxycycline), granulomatous skin infections due to *Mycobacterium marinum* (minocycline), rickettsial infections, mild CAP, skin and soft tissue infections caused by gram-positive cocci (CA-MRSA infections, leptospirosis, syphilis, actinomycosis in the penicillin-allergic patient)	*S. pneumoniae* (17) MRSA (5)
Trimethoprim-sulfamethoxazole	Community-acquired UTI; *S. aureus* skin and soft tissue infections (CA-MRSA)	*E. coli* (19) MRSA (3)
Sulfonamides	Nocardial infections, leprosy (dapsone, a sulfone), and toxoplasmosis (sulfadiazine)	UNK
Ciprofloxacin, levofloxacin, moxifloxacin	CAP (levofloxacin and moxifloxacin); UTI; bacterial gastroenteritis; hospital-acquired gram-negative enteric infections; *Pseudomonas* infections (ciprofloxacin and levofloxacin)	*S. pneumoniae* (1) *E. coli* (13) *P. aeruginosa* (23) *Salmonella* spp. (10–50; geographic variation) *Neisseria gonorrhoeae*[b] (0–5, non–West Coast U.S.; 10–15, California and Hawaii; 20–70, Asia, England, Wales)
Rifampin	Staphylococcal foreign body infections, in combination with other antistaphylococcal agents; *Legionella* pneumonia	Staphylococci rapidly develop resistance during rifampin monotherapy.
Metronidazole	Obligate anaerobic gram-negative bacteria (*Bacteroides* spp.): abscess in lung, brain, or abdomen; bacterial vaginosis; antibiotic-associated *Clostridium difficile* disease	UNK
Linezolid	VRE; staphylococcal skin and soft tissue infection (CA-MRSA)	UNK
Polymyxin E (colistin)	Hospital-acquired infection due to gram-negative bacilli resistant to all other chemotherapy: *P. aeruginosa*, *Acinetobacter* spp., *Stenotrophomonas maltophilia*	UNK
Quinupristin/dalfopristin	VRE	Vancomycin-resistant *E. faecalis*[b] (100) Vancomycin-resistant *E. faecium* (10)
Mupirocin	Topical application to nares to eradicate *S. aureus* carriage	UNK

[a]Unless otherwise noted, resistance rates are based on all isolates tested in 2005 in the clinical microbiology laboratory at Virginia Commonwealth University Medical Center. The rates are consistent with those reported by the National Nosocomial Infections Surveillance System (Am J Infect Control 32:470, 2004).
[b]Data from recent literature sources.
[c]Intermediate resistance.

[d]Drug is given orally for this indication.
Abbreviations: CA-MRSA, community-acquired methicillin-resistant *S. aureus*; CAP, community-acquired pneumonia; MRSA, methicillin-resistant *S. aureus*; MRSE, methicillin-resistant *S. epidermidis*; UTI, urinary tract infection; VRE, vancomycin-resistant enterococci; ESBL, extended-spectrum β-lactamase; UNK, resistance rates unknown.

TABLE 127-7   MOST CLINICALLY RELEVANT ADVERSE REACTIONS TO COMMON ANTIBACTERIAL DRUGS

Drug	Adverse Event	Comments
β-Lactams	Allergies in ~1–4% of treatment courses	Cephalosporins cause allergy in 2–4% of penicillin-allergic patients. Aztreonam is safe in β-lactam–allergic patients.
	Nonallergic skin reactions	Ampicillin "rash" is common among patients with Epstein-Barr virus infection.
	Diarrhea, including *Clostridium difficile* colitis (Chap. 123)	—
Vancomycin	Anaphylactoid reaction ("red man syndrome")	Give as a 1- to 2-h infusion.
	Nephrotoxicity, ototoxicity, allergy, neutropenia	Rare
Aminoglycosides	Nephrotoxicity (generally reversible)	Greatest with prolonged therapy in the elderly or with preexisting renal insufficiency. Monitor serum creatinine every 2–3 days.
	Ototoxicity (often irreversible)	Risk factors similar to those for nephrotoxicity; both vestibular and hearing toxicities
Macrolides/ ketolides	Gastrointestinal distress	Most common with erythromycin
	Ototoxicity	High-dose IV erythromycin
	Cardiac toxicity	QTc prolongation and torsades de pointes, especially when inhibitors of erythromycin metabolism are given simultaneously
	Hepatic toxicity (telithromycin)	Warning added to prescribing information (July 2006)
	Respiratory failure in patients with myasthenia gravis (telithromycin)	Warning added to prescribing information (July 2006)
Clindamycin	Diarrhea, including *C. difficile* colitis	—
Sulfonamides	Allergic reactions	Rashes (more common in HIV-infected patients); serious dermal reactions, including erythema multiforme, Stevens-Johnson syndrome, toxic epidermal necrolysis
	Hematologic reactions	Uncommon; include agranulocytosis and granulocytopenia (more common in HIV-infected patients), hemolytic and megaloblastic anemia, thrombocytopenia
	Renal insufficiency	Crystalluria with sulfadiazine therapy
Fluoroquinolones	Diarrhea, including *C. difficile* colitis	—
	Contraindicated for general use in patients <18 years old and pregnant women	Appear safe in treatment of pulmonary infections in children with cystic fibrosis
	Central nervous system adverse effects (e.g., insomnia)	—
	Miscellaneous: allergies, tendon rupture, dysglycemias, QTc prolongation	Rare
Rifampin	Hepatotoxicity	Rare
	Orange discoloration of urine and body fluids	Common
	Miscellaneous: flu-like symptoms, hemolysis, renal insufficiency	Uncommon; usually related to intermittent administration
Metronidazole	Metallic taste	Common
Tetracyclines/ glycylcyclines	Gastrointestinal distress	Up to 20% with tigecycline
	Esophageal ulceration	Doxycycline (take in A.M. with fluids)
Linezolid	Myelosuppression	Follows long-term treatment
	Ocular and peripheral neuritis	Follow long-term treatment
Daptomycin	Distal muscle pain or weakness	Weekly creatine phosphokinase measurements, especially in patients also receiving statins

FLUOROQUINOLONES

There are two clinically important drug interactions involving fluoroquinolones. First, like tetracyclines, all fluoroquinolones are chelated by divalent and trivalent cations, with a consequential significant reduction in absorption. Second, ciprofloxacin inhibits the hepatic enzyme that metabolizes theophylline. Scattered case reports suggest that quinolones can also potentiate the effects of warfarin, but this ef-

fect has not been observed in most controlled trials.

RIFAMPIN

Rifampin is an excellent inducer of many cytochrome P450 enzymes and increases the hepatic clearance of a large number of drugs, including the following (with the indicated predictable outcomes): HIV-1 protease inhibitors (loss of viral suppression), oral contraceptives (pregnancy), warfarin (decreased prothrombin times), cyclosporine and prednisone (organ rejection or exacerbations of any underlying inflammatory condition), and verapamil and diltiazem (increased dosage requirements). Before rifampin is prescribed for any patient, a review of concomitant drug therapy is essential.

METRONIDAZOLE

Metronidazole can cause a disulfiram-like syndrome when alcohol is ingested. Thus, patients taking metronidazole should be instructed to avoid alcohol. Inhibition of the metabolism of warfarin by metronidazole leads to significant rises in prothrombin times.

PROPHYLAXIS OF BACTERIAL INFECTIONS

Antibacterial agents are occasionally indicated for use in patients who have no evidence of infection but who have been or are expected to be exposed to bacterial pathogens under circumstances that constitute a major risk of infection. The basic tenets of antimicrobial prophylaxis are as follows: (1) The risk or potential severity of infection should outweigh the risk of side effects from the antibacterial agent. (2) The antibacterial agent should be given for the shortest period necessary to prevent target infections. (3) The antibacterial agent should be given before the expected period of risk (e.g., within 1 h of incision before elective surgery) or as soon as possible after contact with an infected individual (e.g., prophylaxis for meningococcal meningitis).

Table 127-9 lists the major indications for antibacterial prophylaxis in adults. The table includes only those indications that are widely accepted, supported by well-designed studies, or recommended by expert panels. Prophylaxis is also used but is less widely accepted for recurrent cellulitis in conjunction with lymphedema, recurrent pneumococcal meningitis in conjunction with deficiencies in humoral immunity or CSF leaks, traveler's diarrhea, gram-negative sepsis in conjunction with neutropenia, and spontaneous bacterial peritonitis in conjunction with ascites. The use of antibacterial agents in children to prevent rheumatic fever and otitis media under certain circumstances is also common practice.

The major use of antibacterial prophylaxis is to prevent infections following surgical procedures. Antibacterial agents are administered just before the surgical procedure—and, for long operations, during the procedure as well—to ensure high drug concentrations in serum and tissues during surgery. The objective is to eradicate bacteria originating from the air of the operating suite, the skin of the surgical team, or the patient's own flora that may contaminate the wound. In all but colorectal surgical procedures, prophylaxis

TABLE 127-8 INTERACTIONS OF ANTIBACTERIAL AGENTS WITH OTHER DRUGS

Antibiotic	Interacts with	Potential Consequence (Clinical Significance[a])
Erythromycin/clarithromycin/ telithromycin	Theophylline	Theophylline toxicity (1)
	Carbamazepine	CNS depression (1)
	Digoxin	Digoxin toxicity (2)
	Triazolam/midazolam	CNS depression (2)
	Ergotamine	Ergotism (1)
	Warfarin	Bleeding (2)
	Cyclosporine/tacrolimus	Nephrotoxicity (1)
	Cisapride	Cardiac arrhythmias (1)
	Statins[b]	Rhabdomyolysis (2)
	Valproate	Valproate toxicity (2)
	Vincristine/vinblastine	Excess neurotoxicity (2)
Quinupristin/dalfopristin	Similar to erythromycin[c]	
Fluoroquinolones	Theophylline	Theophylline toxicity (2)[d]
	Antacids/sucralfate/iron	Subtherapeutic antibiotic levels (1)
Tetracycline	Antacids/sucralfate/iron	Subtherapeutic antibiotic levels (1)
Trimethoprim- sulfamethoxazole	Phenytoin	Phenytoin toxicity (2)
	Oral hypoglycemics	Hypoglycemia (2)
	Warfarin	Bleeding (1)
	Digoxin	Digoxin toxicity (2)
Metronidazole	Ethanol	Disulfiram-like reactions (2)
	Fluorouracil	Bone marrow suppression (1)
	Warfarin	Bleeding (2)
Rifampin	Warfarin	Clot formation (1)
	Oral contraceptives	Pregnancy (1)
	Cyclosporine/tacrolimus	Rejection (1)
	HIV-1 protease inhibitors	Increased viral load, resistance (1)
	Nonnucleoside reverse- transcriptase inhibitors	Increased viral load, resistance (1)
	Glucocorticoids	Loss of steroid effect (1)
	Methadone	Narcotic withdrawal symptoms (1)
	Digoxin	Subtherapeutic digoxin levels (1)
	Itraconazole	Subtherapeutic itraconazole levels (1)
	Phenytoin	Loss of seizure control (1)
	Statins	Hypercholesterolemia (1)
	Diltiazem	Subtherapeutic diltiazem levels (1)
	Verapamil	Subtherapeutic verapamil levels (1)

[a]1 = a well-documented interaction with clinically important consequences; 2 = an interaction of uncertain frequency but of potential clinical importance.

[b]Lovastatin and simvastatin are most affected; pravastatin and atorvastatin are less prone to clinically important effects.

[c]The macrolide antibiotics and quinupristin/dalfopristin inhibit the same human metabolic enzyme, CYP3A4, and similar interactions are anticipated.

[d]Ciprofloxacin only. Levofloxacin and moxifloxacin do not inhibit theophylline metabolism.

Note: New interactions are commonly reported after marketing. Consult the most recent prescribing information for updates.

Abbreviation: CNS, central nervous system.

is predominantly directed against staphylococci and cefazolin is the drug most commonly recommended. Prophylaxis is intended to prevent wound infection or infection of implanted devices, not all infections that may occur during the postoperative period (e.g., UTIs or pneumonia). Prolonged prophylaxis (beyond 24 h) merely alters the normal flora and favors infections with organisms resistant to the antibacterial agents used. A focus on appropriate surgical prophylaxis by the Centers for Medicare and Medicaid Services, coupled with national efforts by surgical societies, appears to be having a favorable impact on the appropriate use of antimicrobial drugs in the surgical setting, although additional improvements are needed.

DURATION OF THERAPY AND TREATMENT FAILURE

Until recently, there was little incentive to establish the most appropriate duration of treatment; patients were instructed to take a 7- or 10-day course of treatment for most common infections. A number of recent investigations have evaluated shorter durations of therapy, especially in patients with community-acquired pneumonia. Table 127-10 lists common bacterial infections for which treatment duration guidelines have been es-

tablished or for which there is sufficient clinical experience to establish treatment durations. The ultimate test of cure for a bacterial infection is the absence of relapse when therapy is discontinued. *Relapse* is defined as a recurrence of infection with the identical organism that caused the first infection. In general, therefore, the duration of therapy should be long enough to prevent relapse yet not excessive. Extension of therapy beyond the limit of effectiveness may increase the medication's side effects and encourage the selection of resistant bacteria. The art of treating bacterial infections lies in the ability to determine the appropriate duration of therapy for infections that are not covered by established guidelines. Re-treatment of infections for which therapy has failed usually requires a prolonged course (>4 weeks) with combinations of antibacterial agents.

MECHANISMS TO OPTIMIZE ANTIMICROBIAL USE

Antibiotic use is often not "rational," and it is easy to understand why. The diagnosis of bacterial infection is often uncertain, and patients may expect or demand antimicrobial agents in this tenuous situation. There is a bewildering array of drugs, each with claims of superiority over the competition. The rates of resistance for many bacterial pathogens are ever-changing, and even experts may not agree on the clinical significance of resistance in some pathogens. Investigations consistently report that ~50% of antibiotic use is in some way "inappropriate." Aside from the monetary cost of using unnecessary or overly expensive antibiotics, there are the more serious costs associated with excess morbidity from superinfections such as *C. difficile* disease, adverse drug reactions, drug interactions, and selection of resistant organisms. Although these costs are not yet well quantified, they add substantially to the overall costs of medical care.

At a time when fewer new antimicrobial drugs are entering the worldwide market than in the past, much has been written about the continued rise in rates of resistant microorganisms and its causes. The message seems clear: the use of existing and new antimicrobial agents must be more judicious and infection control more effective if we are to slow or reverse trends in resistance. The phrase *antimicrobial stewardship* is used to describe the new attitude toward antibacterial agents that must be adopted to preserve their usefulness. Appropriate stewardship requires that these drugs be used only when necessary, at the most appropriate dosage, and for the most appropriate duration. Increasing attention is being given to the relationships between differences in antibiotic consumption and differences in rates of resistance in different countries. While some newer antibacterial drugs undeniably represent important advances in therapy, many offer no advantage over older, less expensive agents. With rare exceptions, newer drugs are usually found to be no more effective than the comparison antibiotic in controlled trials, despite the "high prevalence of resistance" often touted to market the advantage of the new antibiotic over older therapies.

The following suggestions are intended to provide guidance through the antibiotic maze. First, objective evaluation of the merits of newer and older drugs is available. Online references such as the Johns Hopkins website (*hopkins-abxguide.org*) offer current and practical information regarding antimicrobial drugs and treatment regimens. Evidence-based practice guidelines for most infections are available from the Infectious Diseases

TABLE 127-9 PROPHYLAXIS OF BACTERIAL INFECTIONS IN ADULTS

Condition	Antibacterial Agent	Timing or Duration of Prophylaxis
Nonsurgical		
Cardiac lesions susceptible to bacterial endocarditis	Amoxicillin[a]	Before and after procedures causing bacteremia
Recurrent *S. aureus* infections	Mupirocin	5 days (intranasal)
Contact with patient with meningococcal meningitis	Rifampin Fluoroquinolone	2 days Single dose
Bite wounds[b]	Penicillin V or amoxicillin/clavulanic acid	3–5 days
Recurrent cystitis	Trimethoprim-sulfamethoxazole or a fluoroquinolone or nitrofurantoin	3 times per week for up to 1 year or after sexual intercourse
Surgical		
Clean (cardiac, vascular, neurologic, or orthopedic surgery)	Cefazolin (vancomycin)[c]	Before and during procedure
Ocular	Topical combinations and subconjunctival cefazolin	During and at end of procedure
Clean-contaminated (head and neck, high-risk gastroduodenal or biliary tract surgery; high-risk cesarean section; hysterectomy)	Cefazolin (or clindamycin for head and neck)	Before and during procedure
Clean-contaminated (vaginal or abdominal hysterectomy)	Cefazolin or cefoxitin or cefotetan	Before and during procedure
Clean-contaminated (high-risk genitourinary surgery)	Fluoroquinolone	Before and during procedure
Clean-contaminated (colorectal surgery or appendectomy)	Cefoxitin or cefotetan (add oral neomycin + erythromycin for colorectal)	Before and during procedure
Dirty[b] (ruptured viscus)	Cefoxitin or cefotetan ± gentamicin, clindamycin + gentamicin, or another appropriate regimen directed at anaerobes and gram-negative aerobes	Before and for 3–5 days after procedure
Dirty[b] (traumatic wound)	Cefazolin	Before and for 3–5 days after trauma

[a]Gentamicin should be added to the amoxicillin regimen for high-risk gastrointestinal and genitourinary procedures; vancomycin should be used in penicillin-allergic patients.

[b]In these cases, use of antibacterial agents actually constitutes treatment of infection rather than prophylaxis.

[c]Vancomycin is recommended only in institutions that have a high incidence of infection with methicillin-resistant staphylococci.

Society of America (*www.idsociety.org*). Second, clinicians should become comfortable using a few drugs recommended by independent experts and professional organizations and should resist the temptation to use a new drug unless the merits are clear. A new antibacterial agent with a "broader spectrum and greater potency" or a "higher serum concentration-to-MIC ratio" will not necessarily be more clinically efficacious. Third, clinicians

TABLE 127-10 DURATION OF THERAPY FOR BACTERIAL INFECTIONS

Duration of Therapy	Infections
Single dose	Gonococcal urethritis, streptococcal pharyngitis (penicillin G benzathine), primary and secondary syphilis (penicillin G benzathine)
3 days	Cystitis in young women, community- or travel-acquired diarrhea
3–10 days	Community-acquired pneumonia (3–5 days), community-acquired meningitis (pneumococcal or meningococcal), antibiotic-associated diarrhea (10 days), *Giardia* enteritis, cellulitis, epididymitis
2 weeks	*Helicobacter pylori*–associated peptic ulcer, neurosyphilis (penicillin IV), penicillin-susceptible viridans streptococcal endocarditis (penicillin plus aminoglycoside), disseminated gonococcal infection with arthritis, acute pyelonephritis, uncomplicated *S. aureus* catheter-associated bacteremia
3 weeks	Lyme disease, septic arthritis (nongonococcal)
4 weeks	Acute and chronic prostatitis, infective endocarditis (penicillin-resistant streptococcal)
>4 weeks	Acute and chronic osteomyelitis, *S. aureus* endocarditis, foreign-body infections (prosthetic-valve and joint infections), relapsing pseudomembranous colitis

should become familiar with local bacterial susceptibility profiles. It may not be necessary to use a new drug with "improved activity against *P. aeruginosa*" if that pathogen is rarely encountered or if it retains full susceptibility to older drugs. Fourth, a skeptical attitude toward manufacturers' claims is still appropriate. For example, rising rates of penicillin resistance in *S. pneumoniae* have been used to promote the use of broader-spectrum drugs, notably the fluoroquinolones. However, except in patients with meningitis, amoxicillin is still effective for infections caused by these "penicillin-resistant" strains. Finally, with regard to inpatient treatment with antibacterial drugs, a number of efforts to improve use are under study. The strategy of antibiotic "cycling" or rotation has not proved effective, but other strategies, such as heterogeneity or diversity of antibiotic use, may hold promise. Adoption of other evidence-based strategies to improve antimicrobial use may be the best way to retain the utility of existing compounds. For example, appropriate empirical treatment of the seriously ill patient with one or more broad-spectrum agents is important for improving survival rates, but therapy may often be simplified by switching to a narrower-spectrum agent or even an oral drug once the results of cultures and susceptibility tests become available. While there is an understandable temptation not to alter effective therapy, switching to a more specific agent once the patient's clinical condition has improved does not compromise outcome. A promising and active area of research includes the use of shorter courses of antimicrobial therapy. Many antibiotics that once were given for 7–10 days can be given for 3–5 days with no loss of efficacy and no increase in relapse rates (Table 127-10). Adoption of new guidelines for shorter-course therapy will not undermine the care of patients, many unnecessary complications and expenses will be avoided, and the useful life of these valuable drugs will perhaps be extended.

FURTHER READINGS

BARTLETT JG, PERL TM: The new *Clostridium difficile*—What does it mean? N Engl J Med 353:2503, 2005

COSGROVE SE, CARMELI Y: The impact of antimicrobial resistance on health and economic outcomes. Clin Infect Dis 36:1433, 2003

FISHMAN N: Antimicrobial stewardship. Am J Med 119:S53, 2006

GRUCHALLA RS, PIRMOHAMED M: Antibiotic allergy. N Engl J Med 354:601, 2006

JACOBY GA, MUNOZ-PRICE LS: The new β-lactamases. N Engl J Med 352:380, 2005

KOLLEF M: Appropriate empirical antibacterial therapy for nosocomial infections: Getting it right the first time. Drugs 63:2157, 2003

NAHUM GG et al: Antibiotic use in pregnancy and lactation: What is and is not known about teratogenic and toxic risks. Obstet Gynecol 107:1120, 2006

PETERSON LR: Penicillins for treatment of pneumococcal pneumonia: Does in vitro resistance really matter? Clin Infect Dis 42:224, 2006

POLK HC JR: Continuing refinements in surgical antibiotic prophylaxis. Arch Surg 140:1066, 2005

RAY WA et al: Oral erythromycin and the risk of sudden death from cardiac causes. N Engl J Med 351:1089, 2004

128 Pneumococcal Infections
Daniel M. Musher

Streptococcus pneumoniae (the pneumococcus) was recognized as a major cause of pneumonia in the 1880s. Although the name *Diplococcus pneumoniae* was originally assigned to the pneumococcus, the organism was renamed *Streptococcus pneumoniae* because, like other streptococci, it grows in chains in liquid medium. Widespread vaccination has reduced the incidence of pneumococcal infection, but this organism remains the principal bacterial cause of otitis media, acute purulent rhinosinusitis, pneumonia, and meningitis.

MICROBIOLOGY

Pneumococci are identified in the clinical laboratory as catalase-negative, gram-positive cocci that grow in pairs or chains and cause α-hemolysis on blood agar. More than 98% of pneumococcal isolates are susceptible to ethylhydrocupreine (optochin), and virtually all pneumococcal colonies are dissolved by bile salts.

Peptidoglycan and teichoic acid are the principal constituents of the pneumococcal cell wall, whose integrity depends on the presence of numerous peptide side chains cross-linked by the activity of enzymes such as trans- and carboxypeptidases. β-Lactam antibiotics inactivate these enzymes by covalently binding their active site. Unique to *S. pneumoniae* and present in all strains is C-substance ("cell-wall" substance), a polysaccharide consisting of teichoic acid with a phosphorylcholine residue. Surface-exposed choline residues serve as a site of attachment for potential virulence factors, such as pneumococcal surface protein A (PspA) and pneumococcal surface adhesin A (PsaA), which may prevent phagocytosis. Except for strains that cause conjunctivitis, nearly every clinical isolate of *S. pneumoniae* has a polysaccharide capsule, a structure that renders the bacteria virulent by preventing phagocytosis. All strains produce pneumolysin, a toxin that may cause many of the manifestations of pneumococcal infection.

There are 90 serologically distinct capsules of *S. pneumoniae*. Serotyping remains clinically relevant because the activity of available vaccines is based on stimulating antibody to specific capsular polysaccharides.

EPIDEMIOLOGY

S. pneumoniae colonizes the nasopharynx and, on any single occasion, can be isolated from 5–10% of healthy adults and from 20–40% of healthy children. Once adults are colonized, organisms are likely to persist for 4–6 weeks but may be present for as long as 6 months. Pneumococci spread from one individual to another by direct or droplet transmission as a result of close contact; transmission may be enhanced by crowding or poor ventilation. Day-care centers have been a site of spread, especially of penicillin-resistant strains of serotypes 6B, 14, 19F, and 23F. Outbreaks of pneumococcal disease occur among adults in crowded living conditions—e.g., in military barracks, prisons, and shelters for the homeless—as well as among susceptible populations in settings such as nursing homes. The risk of pneumococcal pneumonia is generally not increased by contact in schools or workplaces (including hospitals).

The incidence data provided below were obtained before widespread administration of pneumococcal conjugate vaccine to infants and children. (For the impact of widespread vaccination, see "Vaccination," below.) In the absence of vaccination (which alters natural history), invasive pneumococcal disease is, by far, most prevalent among children <2 years old. The incidence is low among older children and adults <65 years of age but then rises in older adults. The fatality rate is also highest at the extremes of age. One surveillance study in the late 1980s found incidences of pneumococcal bacteremia among infants, young adults, and persons ≥70 years of age to be 160, 5, and 70 cases per 100,000 population, respectively. Most cases of pneumococcal bacteremia in adults are due to pneumonia, and there are 3–4 cases of nonbacteremic pneumonia for every bacteremic case. Thus an estimated 20 cases of pneumococcal pneumonia per 100,000 young adults and 280 cases per 100,000 persons over the age of 70 occur annually. The disease is more frequent among men than among women. The incidence of pneumococcal bacteremia among adults exhibits a distinct midwinter peak and a striking dip in summer; in children, the incidence is relatively constant throughout the year except for a marked dip in midsummer. For reasons that are unclear but probably multifactorial, Native Americans, Native Alaskans, and African Americans are more susceptible to invasive pneumococcal disease than are Caucasians. Natives of the Pacific Rim region are likewise more susceptible.

PATHOGENETIC MECHANISMS

Infection results when pneumococci colonizing the nasopharynx are carried into anatomically contiguous areas (e.g., the eustachian tubes, the nasal sinuses) and bacterial clearance is hindered (e.g., by mucosal edema due to allergy or viral infection). Clearly, the resistance of pneumococci to phagocytosis is central to their capacity to cause infection. Pneumonia ensues when organisms are inhaled or aspirated into the bronchioles or alveoli and are not cleared—especially, for example, if mucus production is increased and/or ciliary action is damaged by viral infection or by cigarette smoke or other toxic substances. Viral infection may also inhibit clearance by upregulating pneumocyte receptors that bind pneumococci.

In normally sterile sites, such as the sinuses or the lungs, pneumococci activate complement, stimulating the production of cytokines that attract polymorphonuclear leukocytes (PMNs). The polysaccharide capsule, however, renders the pneumococci resistant to phagocytosis. In the absence of anticapsular antibody, a large bacterial inoculum and/or a compromise of phagocytic function allows the initiation of infection. Infection of the meninges, joints, bones, and peritoneal cavity may result from pneumococcal spread through the bloodstream, usually from a respiratory tract focus of infection. Unencapsulated pneumococci virtually never cause invasive disease, although they can cause conjunctivitis.

Symptoms of disease are largely attributable to the inflammatory response, which may cause pain by increasing pressure (as in sinusitis or otitis media) or may interfere with vital bodily functions by preventing oxygenation of blood (as in pneumonia) or by inhibiting blood flow (as in vasculitis due to meningitis). Cell-wall constituents of *S. pneumoniae*, especially peptidoglycan, activate complement by the alternative pathway; the reaction between cell-wall structures and antibody (present in all humans) also activates the classic complement pathway. The result is the release of C5a, a potent attractant for PMNs, into the surrounding medium. Peptidoglycan can also directly stimulate the release of proinflammatory cytokines such as interleukin (IL) 1β, tumor necrosis factor (TNF) α, and IL-6. All pneumococci generate pneumolysin, a toxin that damages ciliary cells and PMNs and also activates the classic complement pathway. Injection of pneumolysin into the lungs of experimental animals produces the histologic features of pneumonia; in mice, immunization with this substance or challenge with genetically engineered mutants that do not produce it is associated with a significant reduction in virulence.

HOST DEFENSE MECHANISMS

Mechanisms of host defense may be nonimmunologic or immunologic. Immunologic mechanisms may be natural (innate) or specific (humoral).

Nonimmunologic Mechanisms Nonimmunologic mechanisms that protect against pneumonia include filtration of air as it passes through the nasopharynx, the glottal reflex, laryngeal closure, the cough reflex, clearance of organisms from the lower airways by ciliated cells, and ingestion by pulmonary macrophages and PMNs of small bacterial inocula that manage to reach alveolar spaces. Respiratory virus infection, chronic pulmonary disease, or heart failure compromises these mechanisms, predisposing to the development of pneumococcal pneumonia.

Immunologic Mechanisms • *INNATE IMMUNITY* Innate immune mechanisms participate in clearance of pneumococci from the nasopharynx as well as in phagocytosis by PMNs and macrophages via the microbial pattern recognition receptor Toll-like receptor 2 (TLR2).

HUMORAL IMMUNITY Immunologically specific humoral mechanisms provide the best protection against pneumococcal infection. Most healthy adults have antibody to constituents of *S. pneumoniae*, such as PspA, PsaA, and the cell wall; however, there is no convincing evidence for an opsonic role of these antibodies, especially at their usual concentrations. Most healthy adults lack IgG antibody to the majority of pneumococcal capsular polysaccharides. Antibody appears after colonization, infection, or vaccination. In the first few weeks after colonization, nonspecific mechanisms probably protect the host from infection. Thereafter, newly developed anticapsular antibody provides a high degree of specific protection. Adults who are at risk of aspirating pharyngeal contents and/or who have diminished mechanisms of lower airway clearance are at risk of developing pneumonia before antibody is produced. Persons with a diminished capacity to form antibody probably remain susceptible as long as they are colonized.

The risk of serious pneumococcal infection is greatly increased in persons with conditions that compromise IgG synthesis and/or the phagocytic function of PMNs and macrophages. Most patients hospitalized for pneumococcal pneumonia have one or more of these conditions (Table 128-1). Once a pneumococcal infection has been initiated, the absence of a spleen predisposes to fulminant disease. The liver can remove opsonized (antibody-coated) pneumococci from the circulation; in the absence of antibody, however, only the slow passage of blood through the splenic sinuses and prolonged contact with reticuloendothelial cells in the cords of Billroth can result in bacterial clearance. Patients without spleens tend to develop overwhelming pneumococcal disease that rapidly progresses to death.

TABLE 128-1	CONDITIONS THAT COMMONLY PREDISPOSE TO PNEUMOCOCCAL INFECTION
Increased risk of exposure	Defective complement function
Day-care centers	Defective bacterial clearance[a]
Military training camps	Congenital asplenia, hyposplenia
Prisons	Splenectomy
Shelters for the homeless	Sickle cell disease
Respiratory infection, inflammation	Multifactorial conditions
Influenza, other viral respiratory infections	Infancy and aging
Air pollution	Chronic disease
Allergies	Prior hospitalization
Cigarette smoking	Alcoholism
Chronic obstructive pulmonary disease	Malnutrition
Other causes of chronic pulmonary inflammation or obstruction	HIV infection
	Chronic lung disease
	Glucocorticoid treatment
	Cirrhosis of the liver
Anatomical disruption of meninges (dural tear)	Renal insufficiency
Defective antibody formation	Diabetes mellitus
Common variable hypogamma-globulinemia	Anemia
	Coronary artery disease
Selective IgG subclass deficiency	Fatigue, stress, and/or exposure to cold
Multiple myeloma	
Chronic lymphocytic leukemia	
Lymphoma	

[a]The absence of a spleen predisposes to more fulminant infection (see text).

TABLE 128-2	MOST COMMON INFECTIONS CAUSED BY *STREPTOCOCCUS PNEUMONIAE* IN ADULTS
Site	**Infections**
Respiratory tract	Otitis media
	Acute sinusitis
	Tracheobronchitis
	Pneumonia
	Empyema
Central nervous system	Meningitis
	Brain abscess
Cardiac	Endocarditis
	Pericarditis
Soft tissue/skeletal	Septic arthritis
	Osteomyelitis
	Cellulitis
Other	Peritonitis
	Endometritis
	Primary bacteremia

SPECIFIC INFECTIONS CAUSED BY *S. PNEUMONIAE*

S. pneumoniae causes infections of the middle ear, sinuses, trachea, bronchi, and lungs (Table 128-2) by direct spread from the nasopharyngeal site of colonization. Infections of the central nervous system (CNS), heart valves, bones, joints, and peritoneal cavity usually arise by hematogenous spread. Peritoneal infection may also result from ascent via the fallopian tubes. The CNS may also be infected by drainage from nasopharyngeal lymphatics or veins or by contiguous spread of organisms (e.g., through a tear in the dura). Primary pneumococcal bacteremia—i.e., the presence of pneumococci in the blood with no apparent source—occurs commonly in children <2 years of age and accounts for a small percentage of all cases of pneumococcal bacteremia in adults; if no therapy is given, a source and/or a secondary site of infection may become apparent. Pleural infection results either from direct extension of pneumonia to the visceral pleura or from hematogenous bacterial spread from a pulmonary or extrapulmonary focus to the pleural space; the route usually cannot be determined in any individual case. Infections listed after meningitis in Table 128-2 are uncommon or rare.

Otitis Media and Sinusitis Otitis media and acute rhinosinusitis are similar in terms of pathogenesis. Bacteria are trapped in a normally sterile site when drainage is impaired, often as a result of viral infection, allergies, or exposure to pollutants (including cigarette smoke). In both disease states, *S. pneumoniae* is the most common or second most common isolate (after nontypable *Haemophilus influenzae*) from cultures of the infected site.

Pneumonia The distinctive symptoms and signs of pneumonia, whether due to the pneumococcus or to other bacteria, are (1) cough and sputum production, which reflect bacterial proliferation and the resulting inflammatory response in the alveoli; (2) fever; and (3) radiographic detection of an infiltrate.

PREDISPOSING CONDITIONS Pneumococcal pneumonia is most common at the extremes of age. Despite the undisputed role of *S. pneumoniae* as a major pathogenic bacterium for humans, the great majority of adults with pneumococcal pneumonia have underlying diseases that predispose them to infection. Otherwise-healthy military recruits involved in outbreaks of infection may be an exception to this rule; however, many of these individuals have been under extreme physical and/or psychological stress and/or have had an antecedent viral-type illness that may have reduced their normal host resistance. Infections with respiratory viruses, especially influenza virus, predispose to pneumococcal pneumonia. Other common predisposing conditions are alcoholism, malnutrition, chronic pulmonary disease of any kind (including asthma), cigarette smoking, HIV infection, diabetes mellitus, cirrhosis of the liver, anemia, prior hospitalization for any reason, renal insufficiency, and coronary artery disease (with or without recognized congestive heart failure). In elderly subjects, the predisposition is generally multifactorial.

FIGURE 128-1 A retrocardiac infiltrate in a patient with pneumococcal pneumonia. Right-lower-lobe consolidation is apparent in posterior-anterior *(left)* and lateral *(right)* views of the chest.

PRESENTING SYMPTOMS Patients often present with a clear exacerbation of a preexisting respiratory condition. They may have felt unwell for several days, with coryza or a nonproductive cough and low-grade fever, but they feel distinctly worse at the time of onset of pneumonia. Coughing, often productive of purulent sputum, becomes prominent. The temperature may rise to 38.9°–39.4°C (102°–103°F), although a substantial proportion of patients are afebrile at admission. In a small proportion of cases, the onset of disease follows a hyperacute pattern in which the patient suddenly has a single episode of shaking chills followed by sustained fever and a cough productive of blood-tinged sputum. In the elderly, the onset of disease may be especially insidious and may not suggest pneumonia at all. Such persons may have minimal cough, no sputum production, and no fever, instead appearing tired or confused. Nausea and vomiting or diarrhea occurs in up to 20% of cases of pneumococcal pneumonia. Symptoms of a new cardiac arrhythmia, myocardial ischemia, or an actual infarction occur in 10% of patients at a veterans' hospital who are admitted for pneumonia, and these manifestations may even predominate. The pneumonia may precipitate cardiogenic or noncardiogenic pulmonary edema. Pleuritic chest pain may result from extension of the inflammatory process to the visceral pleura; persistence of this pain, especially after the first day or two of treatment, raises concern about empyema (see "Complications," below). Clearly, the range of symptoms is sufficiently broad that no characteristic presentation distinguishes pneumococcal pneumonia from other types of bacterial pneumonia or from some types of nonbacterial pneumonia.

PHYSICAL FINDINGS Patients with pneumococcal pneumonia usually appear ill and have a grayish, anxious appearance that differs from that of persons with viral or mycoplasmal pneumonia. Temperature, pulse, and respiratory rate are typically elevated. Elderly patients may have only a slight temperature elevation or may be afebrile. Hypothermia may be documented instead of fever and is associated with increased morbidity and mortality. Pleuritic chest pain may cause diminished respiratory excursion (splinting) on the affected side. Dullness to percussion is noted in about half of cases, and vocal fremitus is increased over the area of consolidation. Breath sounds may be bronchial or tubular, and crackles are heard in most cases if enough air is being moved to generate them. Flatness to percussion at the lung base, absent fremitus, and lack of the expected degree of diaphragmatic motion suggest the presence of pleural fluid, which raises the possibility of empyema. The finding of a heart murmur—certainly if new—raises concern about endocarditis, a rare but serious complication. Hypoxia or the generalized response to pneumonia may cause the patient to be confused, but the appearance of confusion should also raise concern about meningitis. Obtundation or neck stiffness should lead to an immediate consideration of this complication.

RADIOGRAPHIC FINDINGS In patients sick enough to be hospitalized, pneumococcal pneumonia is limited to one lung segment in one-fourth of cases and to one lobe in another one-fourth, with multilobar disease in the remaining one-half. Air-space consolidation is the predominant finding and is detected in 80% of cases (Fig. 128-1). Air bronchogram (visualization of the air-filled bronchus against a background of alveolar consolidation) is evident in fewer than half of cases and is more common in bacteremic than in nonbacteremic disease. Rarely, pneumococcal pneumonia leads to a lung abscess. Although some pleural fluid may actually be present in half of cases, ≤20% of patients have a sufficient volume of fluid to allow aspiration, and in only a minority of these patients is empyema documented.

GENERAL LABORATORY FINDINGS Anemia (hemoglobin level, <10 g/dL) is documented in 25% of cases. The peripheral-blood white blood cell (WBC) count exceeds 12,000/μL in the great majority of patients with pneumococcal pneumonia. A low WBC count (<6000/μL) is found in 5–10% of persons hospitalized for pneumococcal pneumonia and is strongly associated with fatal disease. The serum bilirubin level is modestly elevated in one-third of cases; hypoxia, inflammatory changes in the liver, and breakdown of red blood cells in the lung are all thought to contribute to this increase. A serum albumin level of <2.5 g/dL in 30% of cases may indicate predisposing malnutrition or may be the result of sepsis. About 20% of patients have serum sodium concentrations of ≤130 meq/L, and another 20% have serum creatinine concentrations of ≥2 mg/dL. Abnormalities of pleural fluid in empyema are reviewed in Chap. 251.

DIFFERENTIAL DIAGNOSIS *S. pneumoniae* is the most common cause of so-called community-acquired pneumonia, but patients who present with this syndrome may actually have infection due to a broad array of microorganisms. The extensive list includes (but is not limited to) the following: *H. influenzae* or *Moraxella catarrhalis* in persons with little to predispose them other than chronic or acute inflammation of the air-

TABLE 128-3	CAUSES OF A PNEUMONIA SYNDROME LEADING TO HOSPITALIZATION OF ADULTS IN HOUSTON, TEXAS*a*	
Common	**Less Common**	
Streptococcus pneumoniae	*Moraxella catarrhalis*	
Haemophilus influenzae	*Staphylococcus aureus*	
Lung cancer	Pulmonary infarction	
Mycobacterium tuberculosis	*Klebsiella pneumoniae*	
Pneumocystis	*Cryptococcus, Histoplasma*	
Influenza (seasonal)	Respiratory syncytial virus	
	Microaerophilic and anaerobic mouth flora	
	Pseudomonas aeruginosa	
	Legionella species	
	Nontuberculous mycobacteria	
	Chlamydia pneumoniae	
	Nocardia species	
	Hamman-Rich syndrome, others	

*a*Pneumonia was defined as a syndrome consisting of fever, increased cough, sputum production, and an abnormal pulmonary shadow on chest x-ray.

FIGURE 128-2 Gram-stained sputum from a patient with pneumococcal pneumonia shows polymorphonuclear cells with no epithelial cells, indicating the origin of the sample in inflammatory exudate without contamination by saliva. Slightly pleomorphic gram-positive coccobacilli appear, generally in pairs. Displacement of stained proteinaceous background material outlines a capsule surrounding some of the organisms. When obtained from a patient with pneumonia, a sample like this one is highly specific in identifying the pneumococcus as the etiologic agent.

ways; *Staphylococcus aureus*, especially in persons who take glucocorticoids, who have influenza, or who have major anatomic disruption of the airways; *Streptococcus pyogenes*; *Neisseria meningitidis*; anaerobic and microaerophilic bacteria in persons who may have aspirated oropharyngeal contents; *Legionella*; *Pasteurella multocida* in dog or cat owners; gram-negative bacilli, especially in persons who have severely damaged lungs and are taking glucocorticoids; viruses, especially influenza virus (in season), adenovirus, or respiratory syncytial virus; *Mycobacterium tuberculosis*; fungi, including *Pneumocystis* (depending on epidemiologic factors and HIV infection status); *Mycoplasma*; *Chlamydia pneumoniae*, especially in older adults; and *Chlamydia psittaci* in bird owners. Many older men with lung cancer present with pneumonia, as do persons who have acute-onset inflammatory pulmonary conditions of uncertain etiology or those with pulmonary embolus and infarction. The breadth of this list vividly illustrates the deficiency of empirical therapy for community-acquired pneumonia (Table 128-3). Many of these diseases require evaluation, and the increasing availability of specific therapy makes a precise etiologic diagnosis desirable.

DIAGNOSTIC MICROBIOLOGY In patients with community-acquired pneumonia, a pneumococcal etiology is strongly suggested by the microscopic demonstration of large numbers of PMNs and slightly elongated gram-positive cocci in pairs and chains in the sputum. A sample such as the one shown in Fig. 128-2 is highly specific for pneumococcal infection of the lower airways. In the absence of such microscopic findings, the identification of pneumococci by culture is less specific, possibly reflecting colonization of the upper airways. Prior treatment with antibiotics can rapidly clear pneumococci from sputum. These factors need to be considered when sputum cultures from patients who appear to have pneumococcal pneumonia are said to yield only "normal mouth flora" and when the medical literature describes what appear to be poor results of sputum culture. A study of sputum Gram's stain and culture in patients with proven (bacteremic) pneumococcal pneumonia showed that about half of patients could not provide a sputum sample, provided a sample of poor quality, or had received antibiotics for >18 h; results in the remaining cases showed >80% sensitivity of microscopic examination of a Gram-stained sputum sample and 90% sensitivity of a sputum culture. Blood cultures yield *S. pneumoniae* in ~25% of patients hospitalized for pneumococcal pneumonia.

COMPLICATIONS Empyema is the most common complication of pneumococcal pneumonia, occurring in ~2% of cases. Some fluid appears in the pleural space in a substantial proportion of cases of pneumococcal pneumonia, but this parapneumonic effusion usually reflects an inflammatory response to infection that has been contained within the lung, and its presence is self-limited. When bacteria reach the pleural space—either hematogenously or as a result of contiguous spread, possibly across lymphatics of the visceral pleura—empyema results. The finding of frank pus, bacteria (by microscopic examination), or fluid with a pH

of ≤7.1 indicates the need for aggressive and complete drainage, preferably by prompt insertion of a chest tube, with verification by CT that fluid has been removed. Failure to drain most or all of the fluid indicates the need for additional treatment, including placement of other tube(s) (thoracostomy) or thoracotomy. Empyema is likely if fluid is present and fever and leukocytosis (even low-grade) persist after 4–5 days of appropriate antibiotic treatment for pneumococcal pneumonia. At this stage, thoracotomy is often needed for cure. Aggressive drainage is likely to reduce morbidity and mortality from empyema (Chap. 257).

Meningitis Except during outbreaks of meningococcal infection, *S. pneumoniae* is the most common cause of bacterial meningitis in adults. Because of the remarkable success of *H. influenzae* type b vaccine, *S. pneumoniae* now predominates among cases in infants and toddlers as well (but not among those in newborns); nevertheless, the incidence of pneumococcal meningitis among children has been dramatically reduced by use of the pediatric pneumococcal conjugate vaccine (see "Vaccination," below).

No distinctive clinical or laboratory features differentiate pneumococcal meningitis from other bacterial meningitides. Patients note the sudden onset of fever, headache, and stiffness or pain in the neck. Without treatment, there is a progression over 24–48 h to confusion and then obtundation. On physical examination, the patient looks acutely ill and has a rigid neck. In such cases, lumbar puncture should not be delayed for CT of the head unless papilledema or focal neurologic signs are evident. Typical findings in cerebrospinal fluid (CSF) consist of an increased WBC count (500–10,000 cells/μL) with ≥85% PMNs, an elevated protein level (100–500 mg/dL), and a decreased glucose level (<30 mg/dL). If antibiotics have not been given, large numbers of pneumococci are seen in Gram-stained CSF in virtually all cases, and specific therapy can be administered, although, because of its similar appearance, *Listeria* may be misidentified as the pneumococcus. If an effective antibiotic has already been given, the number of bacteria may be greatly decreased and microscopic examination of a Gram-stained specimen may yield negative results. In this situation, immunologic methods may detect pneumococcal capsule in the CSF in up to two-thirds of cases.

Other Syndromes The appearance of pneumococcal infection at other, ordinarily sterile body sites indicates hematogenous spread, usually during frank pneumonia or, in a small proportion of cases, from an inapparent focus of infection. A case of pneumococcal endocarditis is seen every few years at large tertiary-care hospitals. Purulent pericarditis, occurring as a separate entity or together with endocarditis, is even rarer. The name *Austrian's syndrome* is given to the concurrence of pneumococcal pneumonia, endocarditis, and meningitis. Septic arthritis can arise spontaneously in a natural or prosthetic joint or as a complication of rheumatoid arthritis. Osteomyelitis in adults tends to involve vertebral bones. Pneumococcal peritonitis occurs by one of three pathogenetic pathways: (1) hematogenous spread when ascites or other preexisting peritoneal disease is present; (2) local spread from a perforated viscus (usually appendicitis or perforated ulcer); or (3) transit via the fallopian tubes. Salpingitis may be recognized with or without accompanying peritonitis. Epidural and brain abscesses arise as a complication of sinusitis or mastoiditis. Cellulitis is also uncommon, developing most often in persons who have connective tissue diseases or HIV infection. The appearance of any of these unusual pneumococcal infections may suggest that tests for HIV infection should be undertaken. Finally, for reasons that are unclear, unencapsulated (but not encapsulated) pneumococci may cause sporadic or epidemic conjunctivitis.

℞ PNEUMOCOCCAL INFECTIONS

ANTIBIOTIC SUSCEPTIBILITY β-Lactam antibiotics, the cornerstone of therapy for serious pneumococcal infection, bind covalently to the active site and thereby block the action of enzymes (endo-, trans-, and carboxypeptidases) needed for cell-wall synthesis. Because these enzymes were identified by their reaction with radiolabeled penicillin, they are called *penicillin-binding proteins*. Until the late 1970s, virtually all clinical isolates of *S. pneumoniae* were susceptible to penicillin (i.e., were inhibited in vitro by concentrations of <0.06 μg/mL). Since then, an increasing number of isolates have shown some degree of resistance to penicillin. Resistance results when spontaneous mutation or acquisition of new genetic material alters penicillin-binding proteins in a manner that reduces their affinity for penicillin, thereby necessitating a higher concentration of penicillin for their saturation. The genetic information that renders pneumococci resistant to penicillin is acquired from oral streptococci and is transmitted along with genes that convey resistance to other antibiotics as well. Selection of antibiotic-resistant strains worldwide—especially in countries where antibiotics are available without prescription and in loci of high antibiotic use, such as day-care centers—greatly contributes to the prevalence of multidrug resistance.

At present, ~20% of pneumococcal isolates in the United States exhibit intermediate resistance to penicillin [minimal inhibitory concentration (MIC) 0.1–1.0 μg/mL], and 15% are resistant (MIC ≥2.0 μg/mL; **Fig. 128-3**). The rate of resistance is lower in countries that, by tradition, are conservative in their antibiotic use (e.g., Holland and Germany) and higher in countries where usage is more liberal (e.g., France). In Hong Kong and Korea, resistance rates approach 80%. These definitions of resistance, however, were based on drug levels achievable in CSF during treatment of meningitis, whereas levels reached in the bloodstream, lungs, and sinuses are actually much higher. Thus the MIC needs to be interpreted in light of the infection being treated. Pneumonia caused by a penicillin-resistant strain is likely to respond to conventional doses of β-lactam antibiotics, whereas meningitis may not. The recently revised definition of amoxicillin resistance (susceptible, MIC ≤2 μg/mL; intermediately resistant, MIC = 4 μg/mL; and resistant, MIC ≥8 μg/mL) is based on susceptibility to serum levels, with the assumption that no physician would knowingly treat meningitis with this oral medication. Pneumonia due to a pneumococcal strain with intermediate amoxicillin resistance is still likely to respond to treatment with this drug, whereas that due to a resistant strain may not. On the assumption that antibiotic concentrations in middle-ear

fluid or sinus cavities approach those in serum, similar inferences can be made about the treatment of otitis or sinusitis.

Penicillin-susceptible pneumococci are susceptible to all commonly used cephalosporins. Penicillin-intermediate strains tend to be resistant to all first- and many second-generation cephalosporins (of which cefuroxime retains the best efficacy), but most are susceptible to certain third-generation cephalosporins, including cefotaxime, ceftriaxone, cefepime, and the oral cefpodoxime. One-half of highly penicillin-resistant pneumococci are also resistant to cefotaxime, ceftriaxone, and cefepime, and nearly all are resistant to cefpodoxime. Just as in the case of penicillin, susceptibility to cefotaxime and ceftriaxone is defined on the basis of achievable CSF levels. Thus pneumonia caused by intermediately resistant strains (MIC = 2 μg/mL) still responds well to usual doses of these drugs, and pneumonia due to a resistant organism (MIC ≥4 μg/mL) is likely to respond. Meningitis due to intermediately resistant strains may not respond, and meningitis due to a resistant strain is likely not to respond to treatment with cefotaxime or ceftriaxone.

About one-quarter of all pneumococcal isolates in the United States are resistant to erythromycin and the newer macrolides, including azithromycin and clarithromycin, with much higher rates of resistance among penicillin-resistant strains. This resistance will certainly affect empirical therapy for bronchitis, sinusitis, and pneumonia. In the United States, the majority of macrolide-resistant pneumococci bear the so-called M phenotype (erythromycin MIC = 1–8 μg/mL) and are susceptible to clindamycin. In this case, resistance is mediated by an efflux pump mechanism; to some extent, M-type resistance can be overcome by clinically achievable levels of macrolides. In Europe, most macrolide resistance is due to a mutation in *ermB*, which confers high-level resistance not only to macrolides but also to clindamycin; >90% of pneumococcal isolates in the United States are susceptible to clindamycin. Rates of doxycycline resistance are similar to those observed for macrolides. One-third of pneumococcal isolates are resistant to trimethoprim-sulfamethoxazole. The newer fluoroquinolones remain effective against pneumococci; the rate of resistance is generally <2–3% in the United States but is higher elsewhere and may be much higher in closed environments where these drugs are heavily prescribed, such as nursing homes and assisted-living facilities. Ketolides (such as telithromycin) appear to be uniformly effective against pneumococci, as does vancomycin.

ANTIBIOTIC REGIMENS   Otitis Media   (Table 128-4) Current treatment recommendations for otitis media are based on the following points:

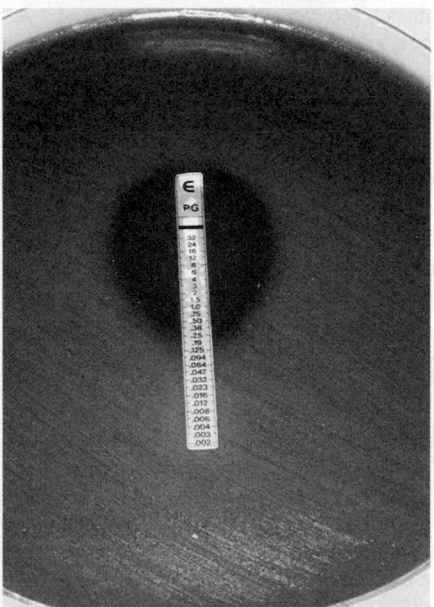

FIGURE 128-3 The e-strip method currently used by most laboratories to determine the susceptibility of *S. pneumoniae* to antibiotics. After the plate is streaked with a suspension of pneumococci, a strip impregnated with graded concentrations of the antibiotic under study (penicillin in the example shown) is placed on the surface, and the plate is incubated overnight at 37°C. The organism on the left is inhibited by a penicillin concentration of 0.016 μg/mL and is fully susceptible to this drug. The organism on the right is inhibited only by a penicillin concentration of 0.25 μg/mL and is intermediately resistant to this agent.

TABLE 128-4 REGIMENS FOR THE TREATMENT OF PNEUMOCOCCAL OTITIS MEDIA OR SINUSITIS[a]

Regimen	Drug, Dose	Duration	Comments
First-line	Amoxicillin, 1 g q8h[b]	Otitis: 3–5 days after clinical response, not to exceed 7 days total (see text) Sinusitis: 7–10 days after clinical response, not to exceed 2 weeks total	If this regimen fails, try a second-line regimen.
Second-line	Amoxicillin, 1 g q8h, plus clavulanic acid, 125 mg q8h[c] *or* Fluoroquinolone[d] *or* Telithromycin, 800 mg/d	Same as above	If this regimen fails, try the third-line regimen.
Third-line	Ceftriaxone, 1 g qd	Otitis: 3–5 days Sinusitis: Longer	If this regimen fails, consider complications. Consult an otolaryngologist and/or infectious disease specialist.

[a]Except as noted, doses are for adults. Treatment for otitis media or sinusitis is empirical, since aspiration of the involved area to establish an etiologic diagnosis is rarely undertaken, except under the conditions of a research protocol.
[b]Dose for infants and toddlers: 80–90 mg/kg per day in 2 or 3 divided doses.
[c]Give half as amoxicillin alone (500 mg) and half as amoxicillin (500 mg)/clavulanic acid (125 mg).
[d]Moxifloxacin, 400 mg/d; or levofloxacin, 500 mg/d.

(1) Acute otitis media is the most common diagnosis leading to an antibiotic prescription in the United States. (2) The diagnosis is often based on inadequate evidence for true middle-ear infection. (3) In proven cases, *S. pneumoniae* and *H. influenzae* are the most likely causes. (4) Because penetration into a closed space may be reduced, high serum levels of an effective antibiotic are required to treat otitis caused by intermediately or fully resistant pneumococci. (5) *S. pneumoniae* is more likely than *Haemophilus* and much more likely than *Moraxella* to cause progression to serious complications without specific therapy. (6) Antibiotics that are effective against pneumococci and yet resist β-lactamases tend to be very expensive compared with amoxicillin.

As a result of these considerations, the American Academies of Pediatrics and Family Practice recommend that clinicians apply due diligence in diagnosing otitis. In children 6 months to 2 years of age with nonsevere illness and an uncertain diagnosis and in children >2 years of age with nonsevere illness (even if the diagnosis seems certain), symptom-based therapy and observation may be used instead of antimicrobial therapy. When parents of children with otitis are given a prescription for an antibiotic but are instructed not to fill it unless the disease progresses, no antibiotic is given in many cases, yet rates of patient satisfaction are high. If otitis media is clearly diagnosed, high-dose amoxicillin is recommended (Table 128-4). If this regimen fails, highly penicillin-resistant pneumococci or β-lactamase-producing *Haemophilus* or *Moraxella* may be responsible; amoxicillin may be given at the same total dosage but with one-half of the dose in the form of amoxicillin/clavulanic acid. If this regimen fails, three doses of ceftriaxone at daily intervals are likely to be curative. A quinolone or ketolide may also be tried in adults. Patients must be monitored closely for a response. An otolaryngology consultation is recommended if all these treatments fail. Despite the detection (by molecular analysis) of pneumococcal DNA in middle-ear fluid, chronic serous otitis ("glue ear") is probably not due to active infection and does not require antibiotic therapy. Treatment for otitis is recommended for a total of 10 days in children <2 years of age but for only 5 days in children ≥2 years old who do not have complicated infections. A recent study reported identical rates of clinical and bacteriologic cure with a 10-day course of amoxicillin and a single dose of azithromycin (30 mg/kg).

Acute Sinusitis Just as the pathogenesis and microbial etiology of acute rhinosinusitis are similar to those of otitis media, so are the principles of diagnosis and treatment. The diagnosis is often empirical, and the less rigorously it is made, the more irrelevant antibiotics are likely to be. The estimated efficacy rate for amoxicillin/clavulanic acid, fluoroquinolones, and ceftriaxone (available for parenteral use only) is 90–92%, as opposed to 83–88% for amoxicillin, trimethoprim-sulfamethoxazole, and oral second- or

third-generation cephalosporins and 71–81% for macrolides and doxycycline. Treatment should be given for longer periods than are recommended for otitis media (perhaps 10–14 days), but the optimal duration is uncertain.

Pneumonia (Table 128-5) This section will deal primarily with the treatment of pneumococcal pneumonia. The broader issue of empirical therapy for community-acquired pneumonia is covered elsewhere (Chap. 251). Unless epidemiologic, clinical, and radiologic findings strongly favor another etiology, empirical therapy for pneumonia must include an agent that will be effective against *S. pneumoniae*, which remains the most likely causative agent of community-acquired pneumonia.

Outpatient Therapy Amoxicillin (1 g three times daily) effectively treats virtually all cases of pneumococcal pneumonia. Neither cefuroxime nor cefpodoxime offers any advantages over amoxicillin, and they are far more expensive. Telithromycin is likely to be equally effective. Moxifloxacin is also highly likely to be effective in the United States except in patients who come from a closed population where these drugs are used widely or who have themselves been treated recently with a quinolone. Clindamycin is effective in 90% of cases and doxycycline, azithromycin, or clarithromycin in 80%. Treatment failure resulting in bacteremic disease due to macrolide-resistant isolates has been amply documented in patients treated empirically with azithromycin. As noted above, rates of resistance to all these antibiotics are lower in some countries and much higher in others; high-dose amoxicillin remains the best option worldwide.

Inpatient Therapy Pneumococcal pneumonia is readily treatable with β-lactam antibiotics. The conventional dosages shown in Table 128-5 are acceptable against intermediately resistant strains and against many or

TABLE 128-5 REGIMENS FOR THE TREATMENT OF PNEUMOCOCCAL PNEUMONIA IN ADULTS[a]

Route, Drug	Dose, Schedule[b]
Oral Therapy	
Amoxicillin	1 g q8h
Quinolone, e.g., levofloxacin	500 mg q24h
Telithromycin	800 mg q24h
Parenteral Therapy	
Penicillin[c]	3–4 mU q4h
Ampicillin	1–2 g q6h
Ceftriaxone	1 g q12–24h
Cefotaxime	1–2 g q6–8h
Quinolone, e.g., gatifloxacin	400 mg q24h
Imipenem	500 mg q6h
Vancomycin[d]	500 mg q6h

[a]These regimens are recommended for treatment after a presumptive diagnosis of pneumococcal pneumonia is made on the basis of examination of a Gram-stained sputum sample or as a replacement for broader spectrum empirical therapy after a diagnosis of pneumococcal pneumonia is proven by culture. When a valid sputum specimen cannot be obtained, concern about other likely pathogens should prompt the selection of more all-inclusive therapeutic regimens. Readers are referred to guidelines for empirical treatment of community-acquired pneumonia.
[b]Therapy should continue for 5 days after defervescence, not to exceed 7–10 days total. A switch from parenteral to oral drug administration may be made as soon as the patient can tolerate oral medications.
[c]This regimen is listed more for historic than for practical reasons. The spectrum is overly narrow, although perfectly acceptable if a Gram-stained sputum specimen shows only pneumococci. However, the need for frequent administration, mandated by the short half-life of penicillin, renders this regimen impractical.
[d]Not proven to be effective by the extensive clinical experience that applies to the other regimens.

most fully resistant isolates. Recommended agents include ceftriaxone and cefotaxime. Ampicillin is also widely used, usually in the form of ampicillin/sulbactam. The likely efficacy of newer quinolones such as moxifloxacin, macrolides such as azithromycin, and clindamycin is discussed above. On the basis of in vitro considerations, vancomycin is likely to be uniformly effective against pneumococci; this drug or a quinolone should be used together with a third-generation cephalosporin for initial therapy in a patient who is likely to be infected with a highly antibiotic-resistant strain. Patients who have had a severe allergic reaction to penicillins or cephalosporins may be treated with a carbapenem (e.g., imipenem-cilastatin), a quinolone, or vancomycin. The failure of a patient to respond promptly should at least prompt consideration of drug resistance. Evidence for loculated infections (such as empyema) and/or other causes of fever should be sought and addressed appropriately.

Duration of Therapy The optimal duration of treatment for pneumococcal pneumonia is uncertain. Pneumococci begin to disappear from the sputum within several hours after the first dose of an effective antibiotic, and a single dose of procaine penicillin, which produces an effective antimicrobial level for 24 h, was curative in otherwise-healthy young adults in an era when all isolates were susceptible. Early in the antibiotic era, most physicians treated pneumococcal pneumonia for 5–7 days. In the absence of data suggesting a need for longer treatment, younger physicians tend to treat the infection for 10–14 days. In the opinion of this author, a few days of close observation and parenteral therapy followed by an oral antibiotic—with the entire course of treatment continuing for no more than 5 days after the patient becomes afebrile—may be the best approach for treating pneumococcal pneumonia, even in the presence of bacteremia. Cases with a second focus of infection (e.g., empyema or septic arthritis) require longer therapy.

Meningitis (Table 128-6) Pneumococcal meningitis should be treated initially with ceftriaxone plus vancomycin. Equivalent doses of cefotaxime or cefepime may be used in place of ceftriaxone. The cephalosporin will be effective against most—but not all—isolates and will readily penetrate the blood-brain barrier; all isolates will be susceptible to vancomycin, but this drug has a somewhat unpredictable capacity to cross the blood-brain barrier. If the isolate is shown to be susceptible or intermediately resistant, treatment can be continued with ceftriaxone, and vancomycin can be discontinued. If the organism is resistant, treatment with both drugs should be continued. A very few studies of experimental animals suggest benefits of the addition of rifampin, but in vitro studies indicate antagonism between this drug and ceftriaxone or vancomycin; in the absence of data to support the practice in humans, this author does not recommend that rifampin be added. Imipenem may be used in place of the cephalosporin in patients who have had life-threatening allergic reactions to β-lactam antibiotics. The total duration of therapy for pneumococcal meningitis is 10 days. A recent study demonstrated clear benefit from the addition of glucocorticoids (Chap. 376).

Endocarditis Pneumococcal endocarditis is associated with rapid destruction of heart valves. Pending results of susceptibility studies, treatment should be initiated with ceftriaxone or cefotaxime; if the prevalence of highly resistant strains increases, it might be prudent to add vancomycin until results of susceptibility studies are available. In vitro, aminoglycosides are somewhat synergistic and rifampin or quinolones are antagonistic with β-lactams against pneumococci; there is no clear evidence from in vivo studies that adding any of these antibiotics to the regimen is beneficial.

TABLE 128-6 TREATMENT OF PNEUMOCOCCAL MENINGITIS

Circumstance	Appropriate Course[a]
Diagnosis of pneumococcal meningitis; antibiotic susceptibility unknown	Treat with ceftriaxone, 2 g q12h, plus vancomycin, 500 mg q6h, until antibiotic susceptibility of organism is known.
Susceptibility results available	Continue treatment with ceftriaxone alone if organism is susceptible or intermediate; continue both ceftriaxone and vancomycin if organism is resistant.
Life-threatening penicillin allergy	Treat with imipenem, 500 mg q6h, rather than a β-lactam antibiotic.

[a]Treatment should be administered for 5–7 days after defervescence or for a total of 10 days.

TABLE 128-7 PROTECTIVE EFFICACY OF POLYVALENT PNEUMOCOCCAL POLYSACCHARIDE VACCINE[a]

Age, Years	No. of Subject Pairs	Years since Last Vaccination		
		<3	3–5	>5
<55	125	93	89	85
55–64	149	88	82	75
65–74	213	80	71	58
75–84	188	67	53	32
≥85	133	46	22	−13

[a]Results of a case-control study involving all cases of invasive pneumococcal disease in Connecticut during 7 years (1984–1990). Vaccinated subjects were matched with controls, and the rate of invasive pneumococcal disease was related to age and time since vaccination. The data, showing protective efficacy, suggest that, within 5 years of vaccination, protection rates decline with age—i.e., from ~90% in persons <65 years of age to <50% in persons ≥85 years old. Protection also declines with increasing time from vaccination to infection, and this decline is more prominent in older patients.
Source: Data adapted from ED Shapiro et al: N Engl J Med 325:1453, 1991; with permission.

OTHER THERAPEUTIC MODALITIES Addition of drotrecogin, an activated protein C preparation, may be beneficial in treating patients with severe pneumococcal sepsis. Glucocorticoids and agents that block the action of TNF-α, IL-1, or platelet-activating factor have conferred no benefit.

PREVENTION

Capsular Polysaccharide Vaccine The pneumococcal capsular polysaccharide vaccine administered to adults since the early 1980s contains 25 µg per dose of capsular polysaccharide from each of the 23 most prevalent serotypes of *S. pneumoniae*. Vaccination stimulates antibody to most serotypes in most recipients. One case-control study showed a protection rate of 85% lasting ≥5 years in adults <55 years old (Table 128-7). The level and duration of protection decreased with advancing age. Other studies have suggested an overall protection rate in the adult population of 50–70%. In high-risk subgroups (e.g., debilitated elderly persons and individuals with severe chronic lung disease), vaccine has not been shown conclusively to be effective. Persons who most need the vaccine because of poor IgG responses (e.g., those with lymphoma or AIDS) are likely not to respond at all. Nevertheless, the Advisory Committee on Immunization Practices of the Centers for Disease Control and Prevention has broadened its recommendations for pneumococcal vaccination to include all persons >2 years of age who are at substantially increased risk of developing pneumococcal infection and/or having a serious complication of such an infection. Perhaps most in need of vaccination are persons with anatomic or functional asplenia, who are at risk for overwhelming, life-threatening infections. Others who might fall within these recommendations are persons who (1) are over the age of 65; (2) have a CSF leak, diabetes mellitus, alcoholism, cirrhosis, chronic renal insufficiency, chronic pulmonary disease, or advanced cardiovascular disease; (3) have an immunocompromising condition associated with increased risk of pneumococcal disease (e.g., multiple myeloma, lymphoma, Hodgkin's disease, HIV infection, organ transplantation, or chronic glucocorticoid use); (4) are genetically at increased risk (e.g., Native Americans and Native Alaskans); or (5) live in environments where outbreaks are particularly likely to occur (e.g., nursing homes).

Recommendations regarding revaccination seem somewhat inconsistent. A single revaccination is advocated for persons over the age of 65 if >5 years have elapsed since the first vaccination. Since antibody levels decline and there is no anamnestic response, it seems more reasonable simply to recommend revaccination at 5-year intervals, especially in persons over the age of 65, who tend to have almost no adverse reaction to vaccination, and in splenectomized patients, who are most in need.

Protein-Conjugate Pneumococcal Vaccine Pneumococcal polysaccharide vaccine is not useful in children <2 years of age, whose immune system does not respond well to polysaccharide antigens. Conjugating

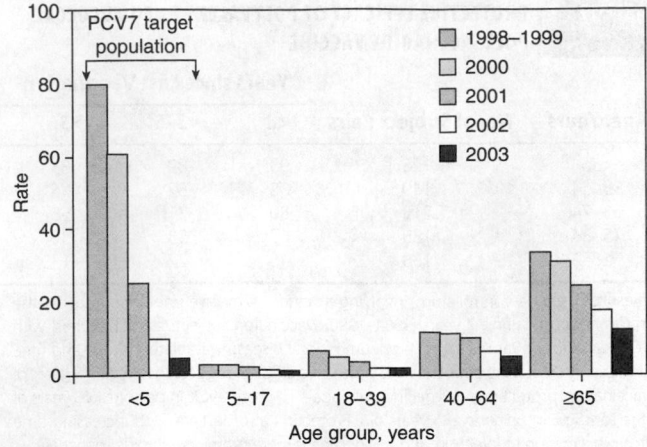

FIGURE 128-4 The rate of invasive pneumococcal disease per 100,000 population (*vertical axis*) is presented for each year since 2000 (*bars*) for different age groups (*horizontal axis*). Invasive pneumococcal disease is more common at the extremes of age. The incidence in all age groups has fallen steadily during the past 5 years. The observed reductions reflect direct effects and indirect ("herd") effects of widespread use of the 7-valent pneumococcal protein-conjugate vaccine (PCV7; see text). *(Adapted from Centers for Disease Control and Prevention, MMWR 54:893, 2005.)*

the polysaccharide to a protein yields an immunogen that is effective in infants and young children. Initial studies of a protein-conjugate pneumococcal vaccine consisting of capsular material from the seven serotypes most likely to cause disease in children (Prevnar) showed a 98% reduction in rates of bacteremia and meningitis and a 67% reduction in rates of otitis media due to vaccine serotypes. Since it was marketed in 2000, widespread use of this vaccine has caused a dramatic decline in the incidence of invasive pneumococcal disease among infants and children (Fig. 128-4). Colonization rates have also greatly decreased. In an Alaskan village, rates of carriage of vaccine strains decreased in children from 55% to 10% and in adults from 15% to 5%. Studies of protein conjugate vaccines that contain antigen from more than seven common infecting serotypes are nearing completion, with favorable results.

The incidence of invasive pneumococcal disease has also declined among unvaccinated children and among adults, to whom this vaccine is not even offered (Fig. 128-4). This decrease illustrates the "herd effect"—i.e., the impact of widespread vaccination on unvaccinated members of the population—and is probably attributable to the effects of the conjugate vaccine on nasopharyngeal carriage of vaccine serotypes. Another effect of the widespread use of this vaccine is the decreasing proportion of all pneumococcal disease that is due to antibiotic-resistant isolates, a trend that reflects the targeting of antibiotic-resistant strains by the vaccine. An unwanted effect of vaccination has been an increase in infections caused by serotypes that are not included in the vaccine (*replacement serotypes*), which, in fact, are increasingly expressing antibiotic resistance. Still, as noted above, the overall incidence of pneumococcal disease in all segments of the population has steadily declined. For further information, the reader is referred to the American Academy of Pediatrics *Red Book Online* (*http://aapredbook.aappublications.org*).

FURTHER READINGS

AMERICAN ACADEMY OF PEDIATRICS AND AMERICAN ACADEMY OF FAMILY PHYSICIANS CLINICAL PRACTICE GUIDELINE: Diagnosis and management of acute otitis media. Pediatrics 113:1451, 2004

CENTERS FOR DISEASE CONTROL AND PREVENTION: Direct and indirect effects of routine vaccination of children with 7-valent conjugate vaccine on incidence of invasive pneumococcal disease—United States 1998-2003. MMWR 54:893, 2005

FEDSON DS, MUSHER DM: Pneumococcal vaccine, in *Vaccines,* 4th ed, SA Plotkin, EA Mortimer Jr (eds). Philadelphia, Saunders, 2003

KARLOWSKY JA et al: Factors associated with relative rates of antimicrobial resistance among *Streptococcus pneumoniae* in the United States: Results from the TRUST Surveillance Program (1998-2002). Clin Infect Dis 36:963, 2003

LEXAU CA et al: Changing epidemiology of invasive pneumococcal disease among older adults in the era of pediatric pneumococcal conjugate vaccine. JAMA 294:2043, 2005

MANDELL LA et al: Update of practice guidelines for the management of community-acquired pneumonia in immunocompetent adults. Clin Infect Dis 37:1405, 2003

MUSHER DM: Pneumococcal vaccine—direct and indirect ("herd") effects (editorial). N Engl J Med 354:1522, 2006

————: *Streptococcus pneumoniae,* in *Principles and Practice of Infectious Diseases,* 6th ed, GL Mandell et al (eds). New York, Churchill Livingstone, 2004

———— et al: A fresh look at the definition of susceptibility of *Streptococcus pneumoniae* to beta-lactam antibiotics. Arch Intern Med 161:2538, 2001

TUOMANEN EI et al (eds): *The Pneumococcus.* Washington, DC, ASM Press, 2004

129 Staphylococcal Infections
Franklin D. Lowy

Staphylococcus aureus, the most virulent of the many staphylococcal species, has demonstrated its versatility by remaining a major cause of morbidity and mortality despite the availability of numerous effective antistaphylococcal antibiotics. *S. aureus* is a pluripotent pathogen, causing disease through both toxin-mediated and non-toxin-mediated mechanisms. This organism is responsible for both nosocomial and community-based infections that range from relatively minor skin and soft tissue infections to life-threatening systemic infections.

The "other" staphylococci, collectively designated *coagulase-negative staphylococci* (CoNS), are considerably less virulent than *S. aureus* but remain important pathogens in infections associated with prosthetic devices.

MICROBIOLOGY AND TAXONOMY

Staphylococci, gram-positive cocci in the family Micrococcaceae, form grapelike clusters on Gram's stain (Fig. 129-1). These organisms are catalase-positive (unlike streptococcal species), nonmotile, aerobic, and facultatively anaerobic. They are capable of prolonged survival on environmental surfaces in varying conditions.

More than 30 staphylococcal species are pathogenic. A simple strategy for identification of the more clinically important species is outlined in Fig. 129-2. Automated diagnostic systems, kits for biochemical characterization, and DNA-based assays are available for distinguishing among species. With few exceptions, *S. aureus* is distinguished from other staphylococcal species by its production of coagulase, a surface enzyme that converts fibrinogen to fibrin. Latex kits designed to detect both protein A and clumping factor also distinguish *S. aureus* from other staphylococcal species. *S. aureus* ferments mannitol, is positive for protein A, and produces DNAse. On blood agar plates, *S. aureus* tends to form golden β-hemolytic colonies; in contrast, CoNS produce small white nonhemolytic colonies.

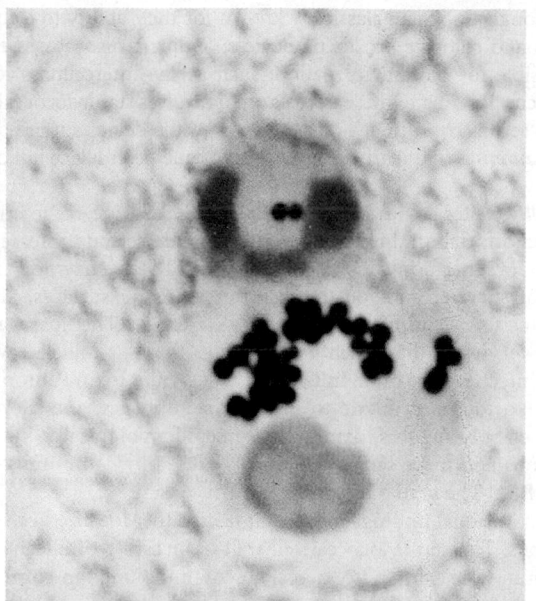

FIGURE 129-1 Gram's stain of *S. aureus* in a sputum sample with polymorphonuclear leukocytes. *(Reprinted with permission from FD Lowy: Staphylococcus aureus infections. N Engl J Med 339:520, 1998. © 1998 Massachusetts Medical Society. All rights reserved.)*

Determining whether multiple isolates (especially of CoNS) from a particular patient are the same or different is often an important factor in distinguishing contaminants from genuine pathogens. Determining whether multiple isolates from different patients are the same or different is relevant when there is concern that a nosocomial outbreak may have been due to a common point source (e.g., a contaminated medical instrument). Biochemical tests, often performed in conjunction with antimicrobial susceptibility testing, have been used as a relatively simple means of distinguishing among staphylococcal species or strains. More discriminating molecular typing methods, such as pulsed-field gel electrophoresis and sequence-based techniques, have also been used for this purpose.

FIGURE 129-2 Biochemical characterization of staphylococci: algorithm of biochemical tests used to discriminate among the clinically important staphylococci. Additional tests are necessary to identify all of the different species.

EPIDEMIOLOGY

S. aureus is a part of the normal human flora; ~25–50% of healthy persons may be persistently or transiently colonized. The rate of colonization is higher among insulin-dependent diabetics, HIV-infected patients, patients undergoing hemodialysis, and individuals with skin damage. The anterior nares are the most frequent site of human colonization, although the skin (especially when damaged), vagina, axilla, perineum, and oropharynx may also be colonized. These colonization sites serve as a reservoir of strains for future infections, and persons colonized with *S. aureus* are at greater risk of subsequent infection than are uncolonized individuals.

Overall, *S. aureus* is a leading cause of nosocomial infections. It is the most common cause of surgical wound infections and is second only to CoNS as a cause of primary bacteremia. Increasingly, nosocomial isolates are resistant to multiple drugs. In the community, *S. aureus* remains an important cause of skin and soft tissue infections, respiratory infections, and (among injection drug users) infective endocarditis. The increasing prevalence of home infusion therapy is another cause of community-acquired staphylococcal infections.

Most individuals who develop *S. aureus* infections are infected with their own colonizing strains. However, *S. aureus* may also be acquired from other people or from environmental exposures. Transmission most frequently results from transient colonization of the hands of hospital personnel, who then transfer strains from one patient to another. Spread of staphylococci in aerosols of respiratory or nasal secretions from heavily colonized individuals has also been reported.

In the past 10 years, numerous outbreaks of community-based infection caused by methicillin-resistant *S. aureus* (MRSA) in individuals with no prior medical exposure have been reported. These outbreaks have taken place in both rural and urban settings in widely separated regions throughout the world. The reports document a dramatic change in the epidemiology of MRSA infections. The outbreaks have occurred among such diverse groups as prisoners, athletes, Native Americans, and drug users. Risk factors common to these outbreaks include poor hygienic conditions, close contact, contaminated material, and damaged skin. The community-associated infections have been caused by a limited number of MRSA strains. In the United States, strain USA300 has been the predominant clone and is also responsible for an increasing number of nosocomial infections. Of concern has been the apparent capacity of community-acquired MRSA strains to cause serious disease in immunocompetent individuals. This ability may be due to the presence of different toxin-producing genes in these strains.

PATHOGENESIS

General Concepts *S. aureus* is a pyogenic pathogen known for its capacity to induce abscess formation at sites of both local and metastatic infections. This classic pathologic response to *S. aureus* defines the framework within which the infection will progress. The bacteria elicit an inflammatory response characterized by an initial intense polymorphonuclear leukocyte (PMN) response and the subsequent infiltration of macrophages and fibroblasts. Either the host cellular response (including the deposition of fibrin and collagen) contains the infection, or infection spreads to the adjoining tissue or the bloodstream.

In toxin-mediated staphylococcal disease, infection is not invariably present. For example, once toxin has been elaborated into food, staphylococcal food poisoning can develop in the absence of viable bacteria. In staphylococcal toxic shock syndrome (TSS), conditions allowing toxin elaboration at colonization sites (e.g., the presence of a superabsorbent tampon) suffice for initiation of clinical illness.

The *S. aureus* Genome The entire genome has been sequenced for numerous strains of *S. aureus*. Among the interesting revelations are (1) a high degree of nucleotide sequence similarity among the different strains; (2) acquisition of a relatively large amount of genetic information by horizontal transfer from other bacterial species; and (3) the presence of unique "pathogenicity" or "genomic" islands—mobile genetic elements that contain clusters of enterotoxin and exotoxin genes or antimicrobial resistance determinants. Among the genes in these islands are those carrying *mecA*, the gene responsible for methicillin resistance. Methicillin resistance–containing islands have been designated *staphylococcal cassette chromosome mecs* (SCC*mecs*) and range in size from ~20 to 60 kb. To date, five SCC*mecs* have been identified. Type 4 and type 5 SCC*mecs* have been associated with community-acquired MRSA strains.

A limited number of MRSA clones have been responsible for most community and hospital-associated infections worldwide. A comparison of these strains with those from earlier outbreaks (e.g., the phage 80/81 strains from the 1950s) has revealed preservation of the nucleotide sequence over time. This observation suggests that these strains possess determinants facilitating survival and spread.

Regulation of Virulence Gene Expression   In both toxin-mediated and non-toxin-mediated diseases due to *S. aureus*, the expression of virulence determinants associated with infection depends on a series of regulatory genes [e.g., accessory gene regulator (*agr*) and staphylococcal accessory regulator (*sar*)] that coordinately control the expression of many virulence genes. The regulatory gene *agr* is part of a quorum-sensing signal transduction pathway that senses and responds to bacterial density. Staphylococcal surface proteins are synthesized during the bacterial exponential growth phase in vitro. In contrast, many secreted proteins, such as α toxin, the enterotoxins, and assorted enzymes, are released during the postexponential growth phase.

It has been hypothesized that these regulatory genes serve a similar function in vivo. Successful invasion requires the sequential expression of these different bacterial elements. Bacterial adhesins are needed to initiate colonization of host tissue surfaces. The subsequent release of various enzymes enables the colony to obtain nutritional support and permits bacteria to spread to adjacent tissues. Studies with mutant strains in which these regulatory genes are inactivated show reduced virulence in several animal models of *S. aureus* infection.

Pathogenesis of Invasive S. aureus Infection   Staphylococci are opportunists. For these organisms to invade the host and cause infection, some or all of the following steps are necessary: inoculation and local colonization of tissue surfaces, invasion, evasion of the host response, and metastatic spread. The initiation of staphylococcal infection requires a breach in cutaneous or mucosal barriers. Colonizing strains or strains transferred from other individuals are inoculated into damaged skin, a wound, or the bloodstream.

Recurrences of *S. aureus* infections are common, apparently because of the capacity of these pathogens to survive, to persist in a quiescent state in various tissues, and then to cause recrudescent infections when suitable conditions arise.

NASAL COLONIZATION   The anterior nares is the principal site of staphylococcal colonization in humans. Colonization appears to involve the attachment of *S. aureus* to both nasal mucin and keratinized epithelial cells of the anterior nares. Other factors that may contribute to colonization include the influence of other resident nasal flora and their bacterial density, nasal mucosal damage (e.g., that resulting from inhalational drug use), and the antimicrobial properties of nasal secretions.

INOCULATION AND COLONIZATION OF TISSUE SURFACES   Staphylococci may be introduced into tissue as a result of minor abrasions, administration of medications such as insulin, or establishment of IV access with catheters. After their introduction into a tissue site, bacteria replicate and colonize the host tissue surface. A family of structurally related *S. aureus* surface proteins referred to as MSCRAMMs (microbial surface components recognizing adhesive matrix molecules) plays an important role as a mediator of adherence to these sites. MSCRAMMs such as clumping factor and collagen-binding protein enable the bacteria to colonize different tissue surfaces; these proteins contribute to the pathogenesis of invasive infections such as endocarditis and arthritis by facilitating the adherence of *S. aureus* to surfaces with exposed fibrinogen or collagen.

Although CoNS are classically known for their ability to elaborate a biofilm and colonize prosthetic devices, *S. aureus* also possesses genes responsible for biofilm formation, such as the intercellular adhesion (*ica*) locus. Binding to these devices often involves staphylococcal adherence to serum constituents that have coated the device surface. As a result, *S. aureus* is frequently isolated from biomedical-device infections.

INVASION   After colonization, staphylococci replicate at the initial site of infection, elaborating enzymes that include serine proteases, hyaluronidases, thermonucleases, and lipases. These enzymes facilitate bacterial survival and local spread across tissue surfaces, although their precise role in infections is not well defined. The lipases may facilitate survival in lipid-rich areas such as the hair follicles, where *S. aureus* infections are often initiated. The *S. aureus* toxin Panton-Valentine leukocidin is cytolytic to PMNs, macrophages, and monocytes. Strains elaborating this toxin have been epidemiologically linked with cutaneous and more serious infections caused by community-associated MRSA. The toxin's biologic role is uncertain.

Constitutional findings may result from either localized or systemic infections. The staphylococcal cell wall—consisting of alternating N-acetyl muramic acid and N-acetyl glucosamine units in combination with an additional cell wall component, lipoteichoic acid—can initiate an inflammatory response that includes the sepsis syndrome. Staphylococcal α toxin, which causes pore formation in various eukaryotic cells, can also initiate an inflammatory response with findings suggestive of sepsis.

EVASION OF HOST DEFENSE MECHANISMS   Evasion of host defense mechanisms is critical to invasion. Staphylococci possess an antiphagocytic polysaccharide microcapsule. Most human *S. aureus* infections are due to capsular types 5 and 8. The *S. aureus* capsule also plays a role in the induction of abscess formation. The capsular polysaccharides are characterized by a zwitterionic charge pattern (the presence of both negatively and positively charged molecules) that is critical to abscess formation. Protein A, an MSCRAMM unique to *S. aureus*, acts as an Fc receptor. It binds the Fc portion of IgG subclasses 1, 2, and 4, preventing opsonophagocytosis by PMNs. Both chemotaxis inhibitory protein of staphylococci (CHIPS, a secreted protein) and extracellular adherence protein (EAP, a surface protein) interfere with PMN migration to infection sites. The arginine catabolic mobile element (ACME), a cluster of genes unique to the USA300 clone, also may facilitate evasion.

An additional mechanism of *S. aureus* evasion is its capacity for intracellular survival. Both professional and nonprofessional phagocytes internalize staphylococci. Internalization by endothelial cells may provide a sanctuary that protects bacteria against the host's defenses. It also results in cellular changes, such as the expression of integrins and Fc receptors that may contribute to systemic manifestations of disease, including sepsis and vasculitis.

The intracellular environment favors the phenotypic expression of *S. aureus* small-colony variants. These menadione and hemin auxotrophic mutants are generally deficient in α toxin and can persist within endothelial cells. Small-colony variants are often selected after aminoglycoside therapy and are more commonly found in sites of persistent infections (e.g., chronic bone infections) and in respiratory secretions from patients with cystic fibrosis. These variants represent another mechanism for prolonged staphylococcal survival that may enhance the likelihood of recurrences. Finally, *S. aureus* can survive within PMNs and may use these cells to spread and to seed other tissue sites.

Host Response to S. aureus Infection   The primary host response to *S. aureus* infection is the recruitment of PMNs. These cells are attracted to infection sites by bacterial components such as formylated peptides or peptidoglycan as well as by the cytokines tumor necrosis factor (TNF) and interleukins (ILs) 1 and 6, which are released by activated macrophages and endothelial cells.

Although most individuals have antistaphylococcal antibodies, it is not clear that the antibody levels are qualitatively or quantitatively sufficient to protect against infection. Anticapsular and anti-MSCRAMM antibodies facilitate opsonization in vitro and have been protective against infection in several animal models.

Groups at Increased Risk of Infection Some diseases appear to entail multiple risk factors for *S. aureus* infection; diabetes, for example, combines an increased rate of *S. aureus* colonization and the use of injectable insulin with the possibility of impaired leukocyte function. Individuals with congenital or acquired qualitative or quantitative PMN defects are at increased risk of *S. aureus* infections; these include neutropenic patients (e.g., those receiving chemotherapeutic agents), individuals with defective intracellular staphylococcal killing (e.g., chronic granulomatous disease), and persons with Job's syndrome or Chédiak-Higashi syndrome. Other groups at risk include individuals with skin abnormalities and those with prosthetic devices.

Pathogenesis of Toxin-Mediated Disease *S. aureus* produces three types of toxin: cytotoxins, pyrogenic-toxin superantigens, and exfoliative toxins. Both epidemiologic and animal data suggest that antitoxin antibodies are protective against illness in TSS, staphylococcal food poisoning, and staphylococcal scalded-skin syndrome (SSSS). Illness develops after toxin synthesis and absorption and the subsequent toxin-initiated host response.

ENTEROTOXIN AND TOXIC SHOCK SYNDROME TOXIN 1 (TSST-1) The pyrogenic toxin superantigens are a family of small-molecular-size, structurally similar proteins that are responsible for two diseases: TSS and food poisoning. TSS results from the ability of enterotoxins and TSST-1 to function as T cell mitogens. In the normal process of antigen presentation, the antigen is first processed within the cell, and peptides are then presented in the major histocompatibility complex (MHC) class II groove, initiating a measured T cell response. In contrast, enterotoxins bind directly to the invariant region of MHC—outside the MHC class II groove. The enterotoxins can then bind T cell receptors via the vβ chain, resulting in a dramatic overexpansion of T cell clones (up to 20% of the total T cell population).

The consequence of this T cell expansion is a "cytokine storm," with the release of inflammatory mediators that include interferon (IFN) γ, IL-1, IL-6, TNF-α, and TNF-β. The resulting multisystem disease produces a constellation of findings that mimic those in endotoxin shock; however, the pathogenic mechanisms differ. It has been hypothesized that a contributing factor to TSS is the release of endotoxin from the gastrointestinal tract, which may synergistically enhance the toxin's effects.

A different region of the enterotoxin molecule is responsible for the symptoms of food poisoning. The enterotoxins are heat stable and can survive conditions that kill the bacteria. Illness results from the ingestion of preformed toxin. As a result, the incubation period is short (1–6 h). The toxin stimulates the vagus nerve and the vomiting center of the brain. It also appears to stimulate intestinal peristaltic activity.

EXFOLIATIVE TOXINS AND THE STAPHYLOCOCCAL SCALDED-SKIN SYNDROME The exfoliative toxins are responsible for SSSS. The toxins that produce disease in humans are of two serotypes: ETA and ETB. These toxins disrupt the desmosomes that link adjoining cells. Although the mechanism of this disruption remains uncertain, studies suggest that the toxins possess serine protease activity, which—through undefined mechanisms—triggers exfoliation. The result is a split in the epidermis at the granular level, and this event is responsible for the superficial desquamation of the skin that typifies this illness.

DIAGNOSIS

Staphylococcal infections are readily diagnosed by Gram's stain (Fig. 129-1) and microscopic examination of abscess contents or of infected tissue. Routine culture of infected material usually yields positive results, and blood cultures are sometimes positive even when infections are localized to extravascular sites. Polymerase chain reaction (PCR)–based assays have been applied to the rapid diagnosis of *S. aureus* infection and are increasingly used in clinical microbiology laboratories.

TABLE 129-1 COMMON ILLNESSES CAUSED BY *STAPHYLOCOCCUS AUREUS* **875**

Skin and Soft Tissue Infections
Folliculitis
Furuncle, carbuncle
Cellulitis
Impetigo
Mastitis
Surgical wound infections
Hidradenitis suppurativa
Musculoskeletal Infections
Septic arthritis
Osteomyelitis
Pyomyositis
Psoas abscess
Respiratory Tract Infections
Ventilator-associated or nosocomial pneumonia
Septic pulmonary emboli
Postviral pneumonia (e.g., influenza)
Empyema
Bacteremia and Its Complications
Sepsis, septic shock
Metastatic foci of infection (kidney, joints, bone, lung)
Infective endocarditis
Infective Endocarditis
Injection drug use–associated
Native-valve
Prosthetic-valve
Nosocomial
Device-Related Infections (e.g., intravascular catheters, prosthetic joints)
Toxin-Mediated Illnesses
Toxic shock syndrome
Food poisoning
Staphylococcal scalded-skin syndrome
Invasive Infections Associated with Community-Acquired MRSA
Necrotizing fasciitis
Waterhouse-Friderichsen syndrome
Necrotizing pneumonia
Purpura fulminans

To date, serologic assays have not proved useful for the diagnosis of staphylococcal infections. Determining whether patients with documented *S. aureus* bacteremia also have infective endocarditis or a metastatic focus of infection remains a diagnostic challenge (see "Bacteremia, Sepsis, and Infective Endocarditis," below).

CLINICAL SYNDROMES
(Table 129-1)

Skin and Soft Tissue Infections *S. aureus* causes a variety of cutaneous infections. Common predisposing factors include skin disease, skin damage (e.g., insect bites, minor trauma), injections (e.g., in diabetes, injection drug use), and poor personal hygiene. These infections are characterized by the formation of pus-containing blisters, which often begin in hair follicles and spread to adjoining tissues. *Folliculitis* is a superficial infection that involves the hair follicle, with a central area of purulence (pus) surrounded by induration and erythema. *Furuncles* (boils) are more extensive, painful lesions that tend to occur in hairy, moist regions of the body and extend from the hair follicle to become a true abscess with an area of central purulence. *Carbuncles* are most often located in the lower neck and are even more severe and painful, resulting from the coalescence of other lesions that extend to a deeper layer of the subcutaneous tissue. In general, furuncles and carbuncles are readily apparent, with pus often expressible or discharging from the abscess.

Mastitis develops in 1–3% of nursing mothers. The infection, which generally presents within 2–3 weeks after delivery, is characterized by findings that range from cellulitis to abscess formation. Systemic signs, such as fever and chills, are often present in more severe cases.

Other cutaneous *S. aureus* infections include impetigo, cellulitis, and hidradenitis suppurativa (recurrent follicular infections in regions such as the axilla). *S. aureus* is one of the most common causes of surgical wound infection.

It should be noted that many of these syndromes may also be due to group A streptococci or, less commonly, to other streptococcal species.

Musculoskeletal Infections   *S. aureus* is among the most common causes of bone infections—both those resulting from hematogenous dissemination and those arising from contiguous spread from a soft tissue site.

Hematogenous osteomyelitis in children most often involves the long bones. Infections present as fever and bone pain or with a child's reluctance to bear weight. The white blood cell count and erythrocyte sedimentation rate are often elevated. Blood cultures are positive in ~50% of cases. When necessary, bone biopsies for culture and histopathologic examination are usually diagnostic. Routine x-rays may be normal for up to 14 days after the onset of symptoms. ^{99m}Tc-phosphonate scanning often detects early evidence of infection. MRI is more sensitive than other techniques in establishing a radiologic diagnosis.

In adults, hematogenous osteomyelitis involving the long bones is less common. However, *vertebral osteomyelitis* is among the more common clinical presentations. Vertebral bone infections are most often seen in patients with endocarditis, those undergoing hemodialysis, diabetics, and injection drug users. These infections may present as intense back pain and fever but may also be clinically occult, presenting as chronic back pain and low-grade fever. *S. aureus* is the most common cause of epidural abscess, a complication that can result in neurologic compromise. Patients complain of difficulty voiding or walking and of radicular pain in addition to the symptoms associated with their osteomyelitis. Surgical intervention in this setting often constitutes a medical emergency. MRI most reliably establishes the diagnosis (Fig. 129-3).

Bone infections that result from contiguous spread tend to develop from soft tissue infections, such as those associated with diabetic or vascular ulcers, surgery, or trauma. Exposure of bone, a draining fistulous tract, failure to heal, or continued drainage suggests involvement of underlying bone. Bone involvement is established by bone culture and histopathologic examination (revealing, for example, evidence of PMN infiltration). Contamination of culture material from adjacent tissue can make the diagnosis of osteomyelitis difficult in the absence of pathologic confirmation. In addition, it is sometimes hard to distinguish radiologically between osteomyelitis and overlying soft tissue infection with underlying osteitis.

In both children and adults, *S. aureus* is the most common cause of *septic arthritis* in native joints. This infection is rapidly progressive and may be associated with extensive joint destruction if left untreated. It presents as intense pain on motion of the affected joint, swelling, and fever. Aspiration of the joint reveals turbid fluid, with >50,000 PMNs/μL and gram-positive cocci in clusters on Gram's stain (Fig. 129-1). In adults, arthritis may result from trauma, surgery, or hematogenous dissemination. The most commonly involved joints include the knees, shoulders, hips, and phalanges. Infection frequently develops in joints previously damaged by osteoarthritis or rheumatoid arthritis. Iatrogenic infections resulting from aspiration or injection of agents into the joint also occur. In these settings, the patient experiences increased pain and swelling in the involved joint in association with fever.

Pyomyositis is an unusual infection of skeletal muscles that is seen primarily in tropical climates but also occurs in immunocompromised and HIV-infected patients. Pyomyositis presents as fever, swelling, and pain overlying the involved muscle. Aspiration of fluid from the involved tissue reveals pus. Although a history of trauma may be associated with the infection, its pathogenesis is poorly understood.

Respiratory Tract Infections   Respiratory tract infections caused by *S. aureus* occur in selected clinical settings. *S. aureus* is a cause of serious infections in newborns and infants; these infections present as shortness of breath, fever, and respiratory failure. Chest x-ray may reveal pneumatoceles (shaggy, thin-walled cavities). Pneumothorax and empyema are recognized complications of this infection.

In adults, nosocomial *S. aureus* pulmonary infections are commonly seen in intubated patients in intensive care units. The clinical presentation is no different from that encountered in pulmonary infections of other bacterial etiologies. Patients produce increased volumes of purulent sputum and develop respiratory distress, fever, and new pulmonary infiltrates. Distinguishing bacterial pneumonia from respiratory failure of other causes or new pulmonary infiltrates in critically ill patients is often difficult and relies on a constellation of clinical, radiologic, and laboratory findings.

Community-acquired respiratory tract infections due to *S. aureus* most commonly follow viral infections or septic pulmonary emboli (e.g., in injection drug users). Influenza is the most common cause of the former type of presentation. Patients may present with fever, bloody sputum production, and midlung-field pneumatoceles or multiple, patchy pulmonary infiltrates. Diagnosis is made by sputum Gram's stain and culture. Blood cultures, although useful, are usually negative.

Bacteremia, Sepsis, and Infective Endocarditis   *S. aureus* bacteremia may be complicated by sepsis, endocarditis, vasculitis, or metastatic seeding (establishment of suppurative collections at other tissue sites). The frequency of metastatic seeding during bacteremia has been estimated to be as high as 31%. Among the more commonly seeded tissue sites are bones, joints, kidneys, and lungs.

Recognition of these complications by clinical and laboratory diagnostic methods alone is often difficult. Comorbid conditions that are frequently seen in association with *S. aureus* bacteremia and that increase the risk of complications include diabetes, HIV infection, and renal insufficiency. Other host factors associated with an increased risk of complications include presentation with community-acquired *S. aureus* bacteremia (except in injection drug users), lack of an identifiable primary focus, and the presence of prosthetic devices or material.

FIGURE 129-3 *S. aureus* **vertebral osteomyelitis involving the thoracic disk between T8 and T9 in a 63-year-old man. A.** The lower end plate is damaged (*arrow*), and there is an adjacent paraspinal mass (*arrowhead*). **B.** Sagittal T2-weighted magnetic resonance image of the spine, illustrating anterior wedging of the body of T8. *(Reprinted with permission from MA Artinian et al: Images in clinical medicine. Vertebral osteomyelitis. N Engl J Med 329:399, 1993. © 1993 Massachusetts Medical Society. All rights reserved.)*

Clinically, *S. aureus* sepsis presents in a manner similar to that documented for sepsis due to other bacteria. The well-described progression of hemodynamic changes—beginning with respiratory alkalosis and clinical findings of hypotension and fever—is commonly seen. The microbiologic diagnosis is established by positive blood cultures.

The overall incidence of *S. aureus* endocarditis has increased over the past 20 years. *S. aureus* is now the leading cause of endocarditis worldwide, accounting for 25–35% of cases. This increase is due, at least in part, to the increased use of intravascular devices; transesophageal echocardiography (TEE) studies found an infective endocarditis incidence of 25% among patients with *S. aureus* bacteremia and intravascular catheters. Other factors associated with an increased risk of endocarditis are injection drug use, hemodialysis, the presence of intravascular prosthetic devices, and immunosuppression. Despite the availability of effective antibiotics, mortality rates from these infections continue to range from 20 to 40%, depending on both the host and the nature of the infection. Complications of *S. aureus* endocarditis include cardiac valvular insufficiency, peripheral emboli, metastatic seeding, and central nervous system (CNS) involvement.

S. aureus is now a leading cause of endocarditis in many countries. *S. aureus* endocarditis is encountered in four clinical settings: (1) right-sided endocarditis in association with injection drug use, (2) left-sided native-valve endocarditis, (3) prosthetic-valve endocarditis, and (4) nosocomial endocarditis. In each of these settings, the diagnosis is established by recognition of clinical stigmata suggestive of endocarditis. These findings include cardiac manifestations, such as new or changing cardiac valvular murmurs; cutaneous evidence, such as vasculitic lesions, Osler's nodes, or Janeway lesions; evidence of right- or left-sided embolic disease; and a history suggesting a risk for *S. aureus* bacteremia. In the absence of antecedent antibiotic therapy, blood cultures are almost uniformly positive. Transthoracic echocardiography, while less sensitive than TEE, is less invasive and often establishes the presence of valvular vegetations.

Acute right-sided tricuspid valvular *S. aureus* endocarditis is most often seen in injection drug users. The classic presentation includes a high fever, a toxic clinical appearance, pleuritic chest pain, and the production of purulent (sometimes bloody) sputum. Chest x-rays reveal evidence of septic pulmonary emboli (small, peripheral, circular lesions that may cavitate with time). A high percentage of affected patients have no history of antecedent valvular damage. At the outset of their illness, patients may present with fever alone, without cardiac or other localizing findings. As a result, a high index of clinical suspicion is essential to the diagnosis.

Individuals with antecedent cardiac valvular damage more commonly present with left-sided native-valve endocarditis involving the previously affected valve. These patients tend to be older than those with right-sided endocarditis, their prognosis is worse, and their incidence of complications (including peripheral emboli, cardiac decompensation, and metastatic seeding) is higher.

S. aureus is one of the more common causes of prosthetic-valve endocarditis. This infection is especially fulminant in the early postoperative period and is associated with a high mortality rate. In most instances, medical therapy alone is not sufficient and urgent valve replacement is necessary. Patients are prone to develop valvular insufficiency or myocardial abscesses originating from the region of valve implantation.

The increased frequency of nosocomial endocarditis (15–30% of cases, depending on the series) reflects in part the increased use of intravascular devices. This form of endocarditis is most commonly caused by *S. aureus*. Because patients often are critically ill, are receiving antibiotics for various other indications, and have comorbid conditions, the diagnosis is not easily recognized.

Urinary Tract Infections Urinary tract infections (UTIs) are infrequently caused by *S. aureus*. In contrast with that of most other urinary pathogens, the presence of *S. aureus* in the urine suggests hematogenous dissemination. Ascending *S. aureus* infections occasionally result from instrumentation of the genitourinary tract.

Prosthetic Device–Related Infections *S. aureus* accounts for a large proportion of prosthetic device–related infections. These infections often involve intravascular catheters, prosthetic valves, orthopedic devices, peritoneal or intraventricular catheters, left-ventricular-assist devices, and vascular grafts. In contrast with the more indolent presentation of CoNS infections, *S. aureus* device-related infections often present more acutely, with both localized and systemic manifestations. The latter infections also tend to progress more rapidly. It is relatively common for a pyogenic collection to be present at the device site. Aspiration of these collections and performance of blood cultures are important components in establishing a diagnosis. *S. aureus* infections tend to occur more commonly soon after implantation unless the device is used for access (e.g., intravascular or hemodialysis catheters). In the latter instance, infections can occur at any time. As in most prosthetic-device infections, successful therapy usually involves removal of the device. Left in place, the device is a potential nidus for either persistent or recurrent infections.

Infections Associated with Community-Acquired MRSA The many unusual clinical presentations encountered in patients with community-associated MRSA infections include necrotizing fasciitis, necrotizing pneumonia, and sepsis with Waterhouse-Friderichsen syndrome or purpura fulminans. These life-threatening infections reflect the increased virulence of MRSA strains.

Toxin-Mediated Diseases • *TOXIC SHOCK SYNDROME* TSS was first recognized as a disease in children in 1978. The disease gained attention in the early 1980s, when a nationwide outbreak occurred among young, otherwise healthy, menstruating women. Epidemiologic investigation demonstrated that these cases were associated with menstruation and the use of a highly absorbent tampon that had recently been introduced to the market. Subsequent studies established the role of TSST-1 in these illnesses. Withdrawal of the tampon from the market resulted in a rapid decline in the incidence of this disease. However, menstrual and nonmenstrual cases continue to be reported.

The clinical presentation is similar in menstrual and nonmenstrual TSS, although the nature of the risk clearly differs. Evidence of clinical *S. aureus* infection is not a prerequisite. TSS results from the elaboration of an enterotoxin or the structurally related enterotoxin-like TSST-1. More than 90% of menstrual cases are caused by TSST-1, whereas a high percentage of nonmenstrual cases are caused by enterotoxins.

TSS begins with relatively nonspecific flulike symptoms. In menstrual cases, the onset usually comes 2 or 3 days after the start of menstruation. Patients present with fever, hypotension, and erythroderma of variable intensity. Mucosal involvement is common (e.g., conjunctival hyperemia). The illness can rapidly progress to symptoms that include vomiting, diarrhea, confusion, myalgias, and abdominal pain. These symptoms reflect the multisystemic nature of the disease, with involvement of the liver, kidneys, gastrointestinal tract, and/or CNS. Desquamation of the skin occurs during convalescence, usually 1–2 weeks after the onset of illness. Laboratory findings may include azotemia, leukocytosis, hypoalbuminemia, thrombocytopenia, and liver function abnormalities.

Diagnosis of TSS still depends on a constellation of findings rather than one specific finding (Table 129-2). Part of the case definition is the absence of laboratory evidence of other illnesses that are often included in the differential (e.g., Rocky Mountain spotted fever, rubeola, leptospirosis). Other diagnoses to be considered are drug toxicities, viral exanthems, sepsis, and Kawasaki disease. Illness occurs only in persons who lack antibody to TSST-1. Recurrences are possible if antibody fails to develop after the illness.

FOOD POISONING *S. aureus* is among the most common causes of food-borne outbreaks of infection in the United States. *S. aureus* food poisoning results from the inoculation of toxin-producing *S. aureus* into food by colonized food handlers. Toxin is then elaborated in such growth-promoting food as custards, potato salad, or processed meats. Even if the bacteria are killed by warming, the heat-stable toxin is not

TABLE 129-2 **CASE DEFINITION OF *S. AUREUS* TOXIC SHOCK SYNDROME**

1. Fever: temperature of ≥38.9°C (≥102°F)
2. Hypotension: systolic blood pressure of ≤90 mmHg, or orthostatic hypotension (orthostatic drop in diastolic blood pressure by ≥15 mmHg, orthostatic syncope, or orthostatic dizziness)
3. Diffuse macular rash with subsequent desquamation in 1 to 2 weeks after onset (including the palms and soles)
4. Multisystem involvement
   a. Hepatic: bilirubin or aminotransferase levels ≥2 times normal
   b. Hematologic: platelet count ≤100,000/μL
   c. Renal: blood urea nitrogen or serum creatinine level ≥2 times the normal upper limit
   d. Mucous membranes: vaginal, oropharyngeal, or conjunctival hyperemia
   e. Gastrointestinal: vomiting or diarrhea at onset of illness
   f. Muscular: severe myalgias or serum creatine phosphokinase level ≥2 times the upper limit
   g. Central nervous system: disorientation or alteration in consciousness without focal neurologic signs and in the absence of fever and hypotension
5. Negative serologic or other tests for measles, leptospirosis, and Rocky Mountain spotted fever as well as negative blood or cerebrospinal fluid cultures for organisms other than *S. aureus*

Source: M Wharton et al: Case definitions for public health surveillance. MMWR 39:1, 1990; with permission.

FIGURE 129-4 **Evidence of staphylococcal scalded-skin syndrome in a 6-year-old boy.** Nikolsky's sign, with separation of the superficial layer of the outer epidermal layer, is visible. *(Reprinted with permission from LA Schenfeld et al: Images in clinical medicine. Staphylococcal scalded skin syndrome. N Engl J Med 342:1178, 2000. © 2000 Massachusetts Medical Society. All rights reserved.)*

destroyed. The onset of illness is rapid, occurring within 1–6 h of ingestion. The illness is characterized by nausea and vomiting, although diarrhea, hypotension, and dehydration may also occur. The differential diagnosis includes diarrhea of other etiologies, especially that caused by similar toxins (e.g., the toxins elaborated by *Bacillus cereus*). The rapidity of onset, the absence of fever, and the epidemic nature of the presentation arouse suspicion of food poisoning. Symptoms generally resolve within 8–10 h. The diagnosis can be established by the demonstration of bacteria or the documentation of enterotoxin in the implicated food. Treatment is entirely supportive.

STAPHYLOCOCCAL SCALDED-SKIN SYNDROME SSSS most often affects newborns and children. The illness may vary from localized blister formation to exfoliation of much of the skin surface. The skin is usually fragile and often tender, with thin-walled, fluid-filled bullae. Gentle pressure results in rupture of the lesions, leaving denuded underlying skin (Nikolsky's sign; **Fig. 129-4**). The mucous membranes are usually spared. In more generalized infection, there are often constitutional symptoms, including fever, lethargy, and irritability with poor feeding. Significant amounts of fluid can be lost in more extensive cases. Illness usually follows localized infection at one of a number of possible sites. SSSS is much less common among adults but can follow infections caused by exfoliative toxin–producing strains.

PREVENTION
Prevention of the spread of *S. aureus* infections in the hospital setting involves hand washing and careful attention to appropriate isolation procedures. Through strict isolation practices, some Scandinavian countries have been remarkably successful at preventing the introduction and dissemination of MRSA in hospitals. Other countries, such as the United States and Great Britain, have been less successful.

The use of topical antimicrobial agents (e.g., mupirocin) to eliminate nasal colonization with *S. aureus* and to prevent subsequent infection has been investigated in a number of clinical settings. Elimination of nasal carriage of *S. aureus* has reduced the incidence of infections among patients undergoing hemodialysis and peritoneal dialysis. The prophylactic efficacy of topical mupirocin applied to the nares has been extensively investigated. While mupirocin eliminates nasal colonization with *S. aureus*, clinical trials to date have failed to demonstrate a subsequent reduction in the incidence of staphylococcal infections.

A capsular polysaccharide–protein conjugate vaccine and antibodies to the ligand-binding domains of several MSCRAMMs (e.g., clumping factor) are under investigation. While in vivo studies have been promising in either preventing or reducing the incidence of infections, none of these vaccines has yet been successful for either prophylaxis or therapy.

COAGULASE-NEGATIVE STAPHYLOCOCCAL INFECTIONS

CoNS, although considerably less virulent than *S. aureus*, are among the most common causes of prosthetic-device infections. Approximately half of the identified CoNS species have been associated with human infections. Of these species, *S. epidermidis* is the most common human pathogen overall; this component of the normal human flora is found on the skin (where it is the most abundant bacterial species) as well as in the oropharynx and vagina. *S. saprophyticus*, a novobiocin-resistant species, is a pathogen in UTIs.

PATHOGENESIS
Among CoNS, *S. epidermidis* is the species most commonly associated with prosthetic-device infections. Infection is a two-step process, with initial adhesion to the device followed by colonization. *S. epidermidis* is uniquely adapted to colonize these devices by its capacity to elaborate the extracellular polysaccharide (glycocalyx or slime) that facilitates formation of a protective biofilm on the device surface.

Implanted prosthetic material is often coated with host serum or tissue constituents such as fibrinogen or fibronectin. These molecules serve as potential bridging ligands, facilitating bacterial attachment to the device surface. A number of surface-associated proteins, such as autolysin (AtlE), fibrinogen-binding protein, and accumulation-associated protein (AAP), may play a role in attachment to either modified or unmodified prosthetic surfaces. The polysaccharide intercellular adhesin facilitates subsequent staphylococcal colonization and accumulation on the device surface. In *S. epidermidis*, *ica* genes are more commonly found in strains associated with device infections than in strains associated with colonization of mucosal surfaces. Biofilm appears to act as a barrier protecting bacteria from host defense mechanisms as well as from antibiotics, while providing a suitable environment for bacterial survival. Poly-γ-DL-glutamic acid is secreted by *S. epidermidis* and promotes protection against neutrophil phagocytosis.

Two additional staphylococcal species, *S. lugdunensis* and *S. schleiferi*, produce more serious infections (native-valve endocarditis and osteomyelitis) than do other CoNS. The basis for this enhanced virulence is not known, although both species appear to share more virulence determinants with *S. aureus* (e.g., clumping factor and lipase) than do other CoNS.

The capacity of *S. saprophyticus* to cause UTIs in young women appears to be related to its enhanced capacity to adhere to uroepithelial cells. A 160-kDa hemagglutinin/adhesin may contribute to this affinity.

DIAGNOSIS

While the detection of CoNS at sites of infection or in the bloodstream is not difficult by standard microbiologic culture methods, interpretation of these results is frequently problematic. Since these organisms are present in large numbers on the skin, they often contaminate cultures. It has been estimated that only 10–25% of blood cultures positive for CoNS reflect true bacteremia. Similar problems arise with cultures of other sites. Among the clinical findings suggestive of true bacteremia are fever, evidence of local infection (e.g., erythema or purulent drainage at the IV catheter site), leukocytosis, and systemic signs of sepsis. Laboratory findings suggestive of true bacteremia include multiple isolations of the same strain (i.e., the same species with the same antibiogram or a closely related DNA fingerprint) from separate cultures, growth of the strain within 48 h, and bacterial growth in both aerobic and anaerobic bottles.

CLINICAL SYNDROMES

CoNS cause diverse prosthetic device–related infections, including those that involve prosthetic cardiac valves and joints, vascular grafts, intravascular devices, and CNS shunts. In all of these settings, the clinical presentation is similar. The signs of localized infection are often subtle, the rate of disease progression is slow, and the systemic findings are often limited. Signs of infection, such as purulent drainage, pain at the site, or loosening of prosthetic implants, are sometimes evident. Fever is frequently but not always present, and there may be mild leukocytosis.

Infections that are not associated with prosthetic devices are infrequent, although native-valve endocarditis due to CoNS has accounted for ~5% of cases in some reviews. *S. lugdunensis* appears to be a more aggressive pathogen in this setting, causing greater mortality and rapid valvular destruction with abscess formation.

Rx STAPHYLOCOCCAL INFECTIONS

GENERAL PRINCIPLES OF THERAPY   Surgical incision and drainage of all suppurative collections constitute the most important therapeutic intervention for staphylococcal infections. The emergence of MRSA in the community has increased the importance of culturing all collections in order to identify pathogens and to determine antimicrobial susceptibility. Prosthetic-device infections are unlikely to be successfully managed unless the device is removed. In the limited number of situations in which removal is not possible or the infection is due to CoNS, an initial attempt at medical therapy without device removal may be warranted. Because of the well-recognized risk of complications associated with *S. aureus* bacteremia, therapy is generally prolonged (4–8 weeks) unless the patient is identified as being one of the small percentage of individuals who are at low risk for complications—e.g., immunocompetent patients and patients whose *S. aureus* infection is associated with a removable focus (such as an IV catheter) and whose device is promptly removed.

DURATION OF ANTIMICROBIAL THERAPY   Debate continues regarding the duration of therapy for bacteremic *S. aureus* infections. No carefully controlled, prospective study has addressed this question. A meta-analysis reviewing studies relevant to this issue concluded that insufficient information was available to determine which patients were candidates for short-course therapy (2 weeks rather than 4–8 weeks).

Among the findings associated with an increased risk of complicated bacteremia are persistently positive blood cultures 48–96 h after institution of therapy, acquisition of the infection in the community, a removable focus of infection (i.e., an intravascular catheter) that is not removed, and cutaneous or embolic manifestations of infection. In those immunocompetent patients for whom short-course therapy is planned, TEE to rule out endocarditis is warranted since neither clinical nor laboratory findings are adequate to detect cardiac involvement. In addition, an aggressive radiologic investigation to identify potential metastatic collections is indicated. All symptomatic sites must be carefully evaluated.

CHOICE OF ANTIMICROBIAL AGENTS   The choice of antimicrobial agents to treat both coagulase-positive staphylococcal and CoNS infections has become increasingly problematic because of the prevalence of multidrug-resistant strains. Data collected by the Centers for Disease Control and Prevention from intensive care units in the United States (1988–1998) show a dramatic increase in the number of isolates susceptible only to vancomycin. This trend is especially apparent with CoNS: >80% of nosocomial isolates are resistant to methicillin, and these MRSA strains are usually resistant to most other antibiotics as well. Because the selection of antimicrobial agents for the treatment of *S. aureus* infections is similar to that for CoNS infections, treatment options for these pathogens are discussed together and are summarized in **Table 129-3**.

As a result of the widespread dissemination of plasmids containing the enzyme penicillinase, few strains of staphylococci (<5%) remain susceptible to penicillin. However, against susceptible strains, penicillin remains the drug of choice. Penicillin-resistant isolates are treated with semisynthetic penicillinase-resistant penicillins (SPRPs), such as oxacillin or nafcillin. Methicillin, the first of the SPRPs, is now used infrequently. Cephalosporins are alternative therapeutic agents for these infections. Second- and third-generation cephalosporins do not have a therapeutic advantage over first-generation cephalosporins for the treatment of staphylococcal infections. The carbapenem imipenem has excellent activity against methicillin-sensitive *S. aureus* (MSSA) but not MRSA.

The isolation of MRSA was reported within 1 year of the introduction of methicillin. The prevalence of MRSA has since increased steadily. In many hospitals, 40–50% of *S. aureus* isolates are now resistant to methicillin. Resistance to methicillin indicates resistance to all SPRPs as well as all cephalosporins. Many MRSA isolates are also resistant to other antimicrobial families, including aminoglycosides, quinolones, and macrolides.

Production of a novel penicillin-binding protein (PBP 2a or 2′) is responsible for methicillin resistance. This protein is synthesized by the *mecA* gene, which (as stated above) is part of a large mobile genetic element—a pathogenicity or genomic island—called SCC*mec*. It is hypothesized that acquisition of this genetic material resulted from horizontal transfer from a related staphylococcal species, such as *S. sciuri*. Phenotypic expression of methicillin resistance may be constitutive (i.e., expressed in all organisms in a population) or heterogeneous (i.e., displayed by only a proportion of the total organism population). Detection of methicillin resistance in the clinical microbiology laboratory can be difficult if the strain expresses heterogeneous resistance. Therefore, susceptibility studies are routinely performed at reduced temperatures (≤35°C for 24 h), with increased concentrations of salt in the medium to enhance the expression of resistance. In addition to PCR-based techniques, a number of rapid methods for the detection of methicillin resistance have been developed.

Vancomycin remains the drug of choice for the treatment of MRSA infections. Because it is less bactericidal than the β-lactams, it should be used only after careful consideration in patients with a history of β-lactam allergies. In 1997, an *S. aureus* strain with reduced susceptibility to vancomycin (VISA) was reported from Japan. Subsequently, additional clinical isolates of VISA were reported from geographically disparate locations. These strains were all resistant to methicillin and many other antimicrobial agents. The VISA strains appear to evolve (under vancomycin selective pressure) from strains that are susceptible to vancomycin but are heterogeneous, with a small proportion of the bacterial population expressing the resistance phenotype. The mechanism of VISA resistance is due to an abnormal cell wall. Vancomycin is trapped by the abnormal peptidoglycan cross-linking and is unable to gain access to its target site.

In 2002, the first clinical isolate of fully vancomycin-resistant *S. aureus* was reported. Resistance in this and three subsequently reported clinical isolates was due to the presence of *vanA*, the gene responsible for expression of vancomycin resistance in enterococci. This observation suggested that resistance was acquired as a result of horizontal conjugal transfer from a vancomycin-resistant strain of *Enterococcus faecalis*. Several patients had both MRSA and vancomycin-resistant enterococci cultured from infection sites. The isolates remained susceptible to chloramphenicol, linezolid, minocycline, quinupristin/dalfopristin, and trimethoprim-sulfamethoxazole (TMP-SMX). The *vanA* gene is responsible for the synthesis of the dipeptide D-Ala-D-Lac in place of D-Ala-D-Ala. Vancomycin cannot bind to the altered peptide.

Alternatives to the β-lactams and vancomycin have less antistaphylococcal activity. Although the quinolones have reasonable in vitro activity against staphylococci, the frequency of fluoroquinolone resistance has in-

TABLE 129-3 ANTIMICROBIAL THERAPY FOR SERIOUS STAPHYLOCOCCAL INFECTIONS[a]

Sensitivity/ Resistance of Isolate	Drug of Choice	Alternative(s)	Comments
Sensitive to penicillin	Penicillin G (4 mU q4h)	Nafcillin (2 g q4h) or oxacillin (2 g q4h), cefazolin (2 g q8h), vancomycin (1 g q12h[b])	Fewer than 5% of isolates are sensitive to penicillin.
Sensitive to methicillin	Nafcillin or oxacillin (2 g q4h)	Cefazolin (2 g q8h[b]), vancomycin (1 g q12h[b])	Patients with penicillin allergy can be treated with a cephalosporin if the allergy does not involve an anaphylactic or accelerated reaction; vancomycin is the alternative. Desensitization to β-lactams may be indicated in selected cases of serious infection where maximal bactericidal activity is needed (e.g., prosthetic-valve endocarditis[c]). Type A β-lactamase may rapidly hydrolyze cefazolin and reduce its efficacy in endocarditis.
Resistant to methicillin	Vancomycin (1 g q12h[b])	TMP-SMX (TMP, 5 mg/kg q12h[b]), minocycline or doxycycline(100 mg PO q12h[b]), ciprofloxacin (400 mg q12h[b]), levofloxacin (500 mg q24h[b]), quinupristin/dalfopristin (7.5 mg/kg q8h), linezolid (600 mg q12h *except*: 400 mg q12h for uncomplicated skin infections); daptomycin (4–6 mg/kg q24h[b, c]) for bacteremia, endocarditis, and complicated skin infections; tigecycline (100 mg IV once, then 50 mg q12h) for skin and soft tissue infections; investigational drugs: oritavancin, dalbavancin, telavancin	Sensitivity testing is necessary before an alternative drug is used. Adjunctive drugs (those that should be used only in combination with other antimicrobial agents) include gentamicin (1 mg/kg q8h[b]), rifampin (300 mg PO q8h), and fusidic acid (500 mg q8h; not readily available in the United States). Quinupristin/dalfopristin is bactericidal against methicillin-resistant isolates unless the strain is resistant to erythromycin or clindamycin. The newer quinolones may retain in vitro activity against ciprofloxacin-resistant isolates; resistance may develop during therapy. The efficacy of adjunctive therapy is not well established in many settings. Both linezolid and quinupristin/dalfopristin have had in vitro activity against most VISA and VRSA strains. See footnote for treatment of prosthetic-valve endocarditis.[d]
Resistant to methicillin with intermediate or complete resistance to vancomycin[e]	Uncertain	Same as for methicillin-resistant strains; check antibiotic susceptibilities	Same as for methicillin-resistant strains; check antibiotic susceptibilities.
Not yet known (i.e., empirical therapy)	Vancomycin (1 g q12h)	—	Empirical therapy is given when the susceptibility of the isolate is not known. Vancomycin with or without an aminoglycoside is recommended for suspected community- or hospital-acquired *S. aureus* infections because of the increased frequency of methicillin-resistant strains in the community.

[a]Recommended dosages are for adults with normal renal and hepatic function. The route of administration is intravenous unless otherwise indicated.
[b]The dosage must be adjusted in patients with reduced creatinine clearance.
[c]Daptomycin cannot be used for pneumonia.
[d]For the treatment of prosthetic-valve endocarditis, the addition of gentamicin (1 mg/kg q8h) and rifampin (300 mg PO q8h) is recommended, with adjustment of the gentami-

cin dosage if the creatinine clearance rate is reduced.
[e]Vancomycin-resistant *S. aureus* isolates from clinical infections have been reported.
Source: Modified with permission of the *New England Journal of Medicine* (Lowy, 1998).
© 1998 Massachusetts Medical Society. All rights reserved.
Note: TMP-SMX, trimethoprim-sulfamethoxazole; VISA, vancomycin-intermediate *S. aureus*; VRSA, vancomycin-resistant *S. aureus*.

creased progressively, especially among methicillin-resistant isolates. MSSA strains have remained more susceptible to the fluoroquinolones than have methicillin-resistant strains. Of particular concern in MRSA is the possible emergence of quinolone resistance during therapy. Resistance to the quinolones is most commonly chromosomal and results from mutations of the topoisomerase IV or DNA gyrase genes, although multidrug efflux pumps may also contribute. While the newer quinolones exhibit increased in vitro activity against staphylococci, it is uncertain whether this increase translates into enhanced in vivo activity. Other antibiotics, such as minocycline and TMP-SMX, have been successfully used to treat MRSA infections in the face of vancomycin toxicity or intolerance.

Among the newer antistaphylococcal agents, the parenteral streptogramin quinupristin/dalfopristin displays bactericidal activity against all staphylococci, including VISA strains. This drug has been used successfully to treat serious MRSA infections. In cases of erythromycin or clindamycin resistance, quinupristin/dalfopristin is bacteriostatic against staphylococci.

Linezolid—the first member of a new drug family, the oxazolidinones—is bacteriostatic against staphylococci, has been well tolerated, and offers the advantage of comparable bioavailability after oral or parenteral administration. Cross-resistance with other inhibitors of protein synthesis has not been reported. Resistance to linezolid, although limited, has been reported. The efficacy of linezolid in the treatment of deep-seated infections such as osteomyelitis has not yet been established. There are insufficient data on the efficacy of either quinupristin/dalfopristin or linezolid for the treatment of infective endocarditis. Daptomycin, a new parenteral bactericidal agent with antistaphylococcal activity, is approved for the treatment of bacteremias (including right-sided endocarditis) and complicated skin infections. It is not effective in respiratory infections. This drug has a novel mechanism of action: it

disrupts the cytoplasmic membrane. Staphylococcal resistance to daptomycin has been reported. Tigecycline, a broad-spectrum minocycline analogue, has bacteriostatic activity against MRSA and is approved for use in skin and soft tissue infections as well as intraabdominal infections caused by *S. aureus*. A number of additional antistaphylococcal agents (e.g., dalbavancin, oritavancin, and ceftobiprole) are undergoing clinical trials.

Combinations of antistaphylococcal agents are sometimes used to enhance bactericidal activity in the treatment of serious infections such as endocarditis or osteomyelitis. In selected instances (e.g., right-sided endocarditis), drug combinations are also used to shorten the duration of therapy. Among the antimicrobial agents used in combinations are rifampin, aminoglycosides (e.g., gentamicin), and fusidic acid (which is not readily available in the United States). While these agents are not effective singly because of the frequent emergence of resistance, they have proved useful in combination with other agents because of their bactericidal activity against staphylococci.

In vitro studies have demonstrated synergy against staphylococci with the following combinations: (1) β-lactams and aminoglycosides; (2) vancomycin and gentamicin; (3) vancomycin, gentamicin, and rifampin (against CoNS); and (4) vancomycin and rifampin. In several instances, these in vitro observations have been supported by studies in the experimental animal model of endocarditis. There is limited information on combinations including newer agents such as daptomycin and tigecycline.

ANTIMICROBIAL THERAPY FOR SELECTED SETTINGS For uncomplicated skin and soft tissue infections, the use of oral antistaphylococcal agents is usually successful. For other infections, parenteral therapy is indicated.

S. aureus endocarditis is usually an acute, life-threatening infection. Thus prompt collection of blood for cultures must be followed immediately by empirical antimicrobial therapy. For S. aureus native-valve endocarditis, a combination of antimicrobial agents is often used. In a large prospective study, an SPRP combined with an aminoglycoside did not alter clinical outcome but did reduce the duration of S. aureus bacteremia. As a result, many clinicians begin therapy for life-threatening infections with a 3- to 5-day course of a β-lactam and an aminoglycoside (gentamicin, 1 mg/kg IV every 8 h). If a MRSA strain is isolated, vancomycin (30 mg/kg every 24 h, given in two equal doses up to a total of 2 g) is recommended. Patients are generally treated for 6 weeks.

In prosthetic-valve endocarditis, surgery in addition to antibiotic therapy is often necessary. The combination of a β-lactam agent—or, if the isolate is β-lactam-resistant, vancomycin (30 mg/kg every 24 h, given in two equal doses up to a total of 2 g)—with an aminoglycoside (gentamicin, 1 mg/kg IV every 8 h) and rifampin (300 mg orally or IV every 8 h) is recommended. This combination is used to avoid the possible emergence of rifampin resistance during therapy if only two drugs are used.

For hematogenous osteomyelitis or septic arthritis in children, a 4-week course of therapy is usually adequate. In adults, treatment is often more prolonged. For chronic forms of osteomyelitis, surgical debridement is necessary in combination with antimicrobial therapy. For joint infections, a critical component of therapy is the repeated aspiration or arthroscopy of the affected joint to prevent damage from leukocytes. The combination of rifampin with ciprofloxacin has been used successfully to treat prosthetic-joint infections, especially when the device cannot be removed. The efficacy of this combination may reflect enhanced activity against staphylococci in biofilms as well as the attainment of effective intracellular concentrations.

The choice of empirical therapy for staphylococcal infections depends in part on susceptibility data for the local geographic area. Increasingly, vancomycin (in combination with an aminoglycoside or rifampin for serious infections) is the drug of choice for both community- and hospital-acquired infections.

The increase in community-based MRSA skin and soft tissue infections has drawn attention to the need for initiation of appropriate empirical therapy. Oral agents that have been effective against these isolates include clindamycin, TMP-SMX, doxycycline, and linezolid. The antimicrobial susceptibility of isolates in different geographic regions has varied.

THERAPY FOR TOXIC SHOCK SYNDROME   Supportive therapy with reversal of hypotension is the mainstay of therapy for TSS. Both fluids and pressors may be necessary. Tampons or other packing material should be promptly removed. The role of antibiotics is less clear. Some investigators recommend a combination of clindamycin and a semisynthetic penicillin. Clindamycin is advocated because, as a protein synthesis inhibitor, it reduces toxin synthesis in vitro. A semisynthetic penicillin is suggested to eliminate any potential focus of infection as well as to eradicate persistent carriage that might increase the likelihood of recurrent illness. Anecdotal reports document the successful use of IV immunoglobulin to treat TSS. The role of glucocorticoids in the treatment of this disease is uncertain at present.

THERAPY FOR OTHER TOXIN-MEDIATED DISEASES   Therapy for staphylococcal food poisoning is entirely supportive. For SSSS, antistaphylococcal therapy targets the primary site of infection.

FURTHER READINGS

DIEP BA et al: Complete genome sequence of USA300, an epidemic clone of community-acquired meticillin-resistant *Staphylococcus aureus*. Lancet 367:731, 2006

FOWLER VG JR et al: *Staphylococcus aureus* endocarditis: A consequence of medical progress. JAMA 293:3012, 2005

——— et al: Role of echocardiography in evaluation of patients with *Staphylococcus aureus* bacteremia: Experience in 103 patients. J Am Coll Cardiol 30:1072, 1997

FRIDKIN SK et al: Methicillin-resistant *Staphylococcus aureus* disease in three communities. N Engl J Med 352:1436, 2005

GRUNDMANN H et al: Emergence and resurgence of meticillin-resistant *Staphylococcus aureus* as a public-health threat. Lancet 368:874, 2006

LOWY FD: Antimicrobial resistance: The example of *Staphylococcus aureus*. J Clin Invest 111:1265, 2003

MCCORMICK JK et al: Toxic shock syndrome and bacterial superantigens: An update. Annu Rev Microbiol 55:77, 2001

MORAN GJ et al: Methicillin-resistant *S. aureus* infections among patients in the emergency department. N Engl J Med 355:666, 2006

MYLOTTE JM, TAYARA A: *Staphylococcus aureus* bacteremia: Predictors of 30-day mortality in a large cohort. Clin Infect Dis 31:1170, 2000

SEYBOLD U et al: Emergence of community-associated methicillin-resistant *Staphylococcus aureus* USA300 genotype as a major cause of health care–associated blood stream infections. Clin Infect Dis 42:647, 2006

130 Streptococcal and Enterococcal Infections

Michael R. Wessels

Many varieties of streptococci are found as part of the normal flora colonizing the human respiratory, gastrointestinal, and genitourinary tracts. Several species are important causes of human disease. Group A *Streptococcus* (GAS, *S. pyogenes*) is responsible for streptococcal pharyngitis, one of the most common bacterial infections of school-age children, and for the postinfectious syndromes of acute rheumatic fever (ARF) and poststreptococcal glomerulonephritis (PSGN). Group B *Streptococcus* (GBS, *S. agalactiae*) is the leading cause of bacterial sepsis and meningitis in newborns and a major cause of endometritis and fever in parturient women. Enterococci are important causes of urinary tract infection, nosocomial bacteremia, and endocarditis. Viridans streptococci are the most common cause of bacterial endocarditis.

Streptococci are gram-positive, spherical to ovoid bacteria that characteristically form chains when grown in liquid media. Most streptococci that cause human infections are facultative anaerobes, although some are strict anaerobes. Streptococci are relatively fastidious organisms, requiring enriched media for growth in the laboratory. Clinicians and clinical microbiologists identify streptococci by several classification systems, including hemolytic pattern, Lancefield group, species name, and common or trivial name. Many streptococci associated with human infection produce a zone of complete (β) hemolysis around the bacterial colony when cultured on blood agar. The β-hemolytic streptococci can be classified by the Lancefield system, a serologic grouping based on the reaction of specific antisera with bacterial cell-wall carbohydrate antigens. With rare exceptions, organisms belonging to Lancefield groups A, B, C, and G are all β-hemolytic, and each is associated with characteristic patterns of human infection. Other streptococci produce a zone of partial (α) hemolysis, often imparting a greenish appearance to the agar. These α-hemolytic streptococci are further identified by biochemical testing and include *S. pneumoniae* (Chap. 128), an important cause of pneumonia, meningitis, and other infections, and several species referred to collectively as the *viridans streptococci*, which are part of the normal oral flora and are important agents of subacute bacterial endocarditis. Finally, some streptococci are nonhemolytic, a pattern sometimes called γ hemolysis. The classification of the major streptococcal groups causing human infections is outlined in Table 130-1. Among the organisms classified serologically as group D streptococci, the enterococci are now considered a separate genus on the basis of DNA homology studies. Thus species previously designated as *S. faecalis* and *S. faecium* have been renamed *Enterococcus faecalis* and *E. faecium*, respectively.

TABLE 130-1 CLASSIFICATION OF STREPTOCOCCI

Lancefield Group	Representative Species	Hemolytic Pattern	Typical Infections
A	S. pyogenes	β	Pharyngitis, impetigo, cellulitis, scarlet fever
B	S. agalactiae	β	Neonatal sepsis and meningitis, puerperal infection, urinary tract infection, diabetic ulcer infection, endocarditis
C, G	S. dysgalactiae subsp. equisimilis	β	Cellulitis, bacteremia, endocarditis
D	Enterococci: E. faecalis; E. faecium	Usually nonhemolytic	Urinary tract infection, nosocomial bacteremia, endocarditis
	Nonenterococci: S. bovis	Usually nonhemolytic	Bacteremia, endocarditis
Variable or nongroupable	Viridans streptococci: S. sanguis; S. mitis	α	Endocarditis, dental abscess, brain abscess
	Intermedius or milleri group: S. intermedius, S. anginosus, S. constellatus	Variable	Brain abscess, visceral abscess
	Anaerobic streptococci: Peptostreptococcus magnus	Usually nonhemolytic	Sinusitis, pneumonia, empyema, brain abscess, liver abscess

GROUP A STREPTOCOCCI

Lancefield's group A consists of a single species, *S. pyogenes*. As its species name implies, this organism is associated with a variety of suppurative infections. In addition, GAS can trigger the postinfectious syndromes of ARF (which is uniquely associated with *S. pyogenes* infection; Chap. 315) and PSGN (Chap. 277).

Worldwide, GAS infections and their postinfectious sequelae (primarily ARF and rheumatic heart disease) account for an estimated 500,000 deaths per year. Although data are incomplete, the incidence of all forms of GAS infection and that of rheumatic heart disease are thought to be tenfold higher in resource-limited countries than in developed countries (Fig. 130-1).

PATHOGENESIS

GAS elaborates a number of cell-surface components and extracellular products important in both the pathogenesis of infection and the human immune response. The cell wall contains a carbohydrate antigen that may be released by acid treatment. The reaction of such acid extracts with group A–specific antiserum is the basis for definitive identification of a streptococcal strain as *S. pyogenes*. The major surface protein of GAS is M protein, which occurs in more than 100 antigenically distinct types and is the basis for the serotyping of strains with specific antisera. The M protein molecules are fibrillar structures anchored in the cell wall of the organism that extend as hairlike projections away from the cell surface. The amino acid sequence of the distal or amino-terminal portion of the M protein molecule is quite variable, accounting for the antigenic variation of the different M types, while more proximal regions of the protein are relatively conserved. A newer technique for assignment of M type to GAS isolates uses the polymerase chain reaction to amplify the variable region of the M protein gene. DNA sequence analysis of the amplified gene segment can be compared with an extensive database [developed at the Centers for Disease Control and Prevention (CDC)] for assignment of M type. This method eliminates the need for typing sera, which are available in only a few reference laboratories. The presence of M protein on a GAS isolate correlates with its capacity to resist phagocytic killing in fresh human blood. This phenomenon appears to be due, at least in part, to the binding of plasma fibrinogen to M protein molecules on the streptococcal surface, which interferes with complement activation and deposition of opsonic complement fragments on the bacterial cell. This resistance to phagocytosis may be overcome by M protein–specific antibodies; thus individuals with antibodies to a given M type acquired as a result of prior infection are protected against subsequent infection with organisms of the same M type but not against that with different M types.

GAS also elaborates, to varying degrees, a polysaccharide capsule composed of hyaluronic acid. The production of large amounts of capsule by certain strains lends a characteristic mucoid appearance to the colonies. The capsular polysaccharide plays an important role in protecting GAS from ingestion and killing by phagocytes. In contrast to M protein, the hyaluronic acid capsule is a weak immunogen, and antibodies to hyaluronate have not been shown to be important in protective immunity. The presumed explanation is the apparent structural identity between streptococcal hyaluronic acid and the hyaluronic acid of mammalian connective tissues. The capsular polysaccharide may also play a role in GAS colonization of the pharynx by binding to CD44, a hyaluronic acid–binding protein expressed on human pharyngeal epithelial cells.

GAS produces a large number of extracellular products that may be important in local and systemic toxicity and in the spread of infection through tissues. These products include streptolysins S and O, toxins that damage cell membranes and account for the hemolysis produced by the organisms; streptokinase; DNases; protease; and pyrogenic exotoxins A, B, and C. The pyrogenic exotoxins, previously known as erythrogenic toxins, cause the rash of scarlet fever. Since the mid-1980s, pyrogenic exotoxin–producing strains of GAS have been linked to unusually severe invasive infections, including necrotizing fasciitis and the streptococcal toxic shock syndrome. Several extracellular

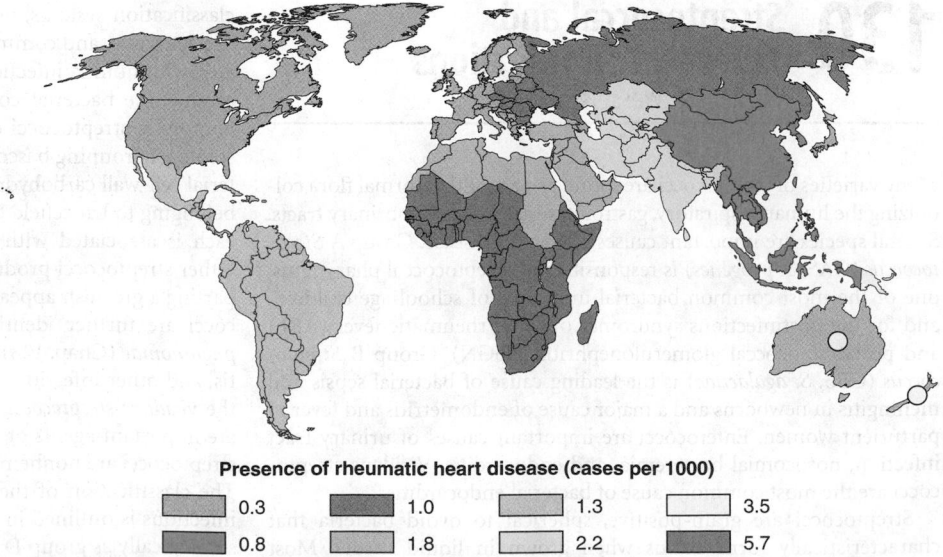

Presence of rheumatic heart disease (cases per 1000)

0.3	1.0	1.3	3.5
0.8	1.8	2.2	5.7

FIGURE 130-1 Prevalence of rheumatic heart disease in children 5–14 years old. The circles within Australia and New Zealand represent indigenous populations (and also Pacific Islanders in New Zealand). (*From Carapetis et al, 2005, with permission.*)

products stimulate specific antibody responses useful for serodiagnosis of recent streptococcal infection. Tests for these antibodies are used primarily for detection of preceding streptococcal infection in cases of suspected ARF or PSGN.

CLINICAL MANIFESTATIONS

Pharyngitis Although seen in patients of all ages, GAS pharyngitis is one of the most common bacterial infections of childhood, accounting for 20–40% of all cases of exudative pharyngitis in children; it is rare among those under the age of 3. Younger children may manifest streptococcal infection with a syndrome of fever, malaise, and lymphadenopathy without exudative pharyngitis. Infection is acquired through contact with another individual carrying the organism. Respiratory droplets are the usual mechanism of spread, although other routes, including food-borne outbreaks, have been well described.

The incubation period is 1–4 days. Symptoms include sore throat, fever and chills, malaise, and sometimes abdominal complaints and vomiting, particularly in children. Both symptoms and signs are quite variable, ranging from mild throat discomfort with minimal physical findings to high fever and severe sore throat associated with intense erythema and swelling of the pharyngeal mucosa and the presence of purulent exudate over the posterior pharyngeal wall and tonsillar pillars. Enlarged, tender anterior cervical lymph nodes commonly accompany exudative pharyngitis.

The differential diagnosis of streptococcal pharyngitis includes the many other bacterial and viral etiologies (Table 130-2). Streptococcal infection is an unlikely cause when symptoms and signs suggestive of viral infection are prominent (conjunctivitis, coryza, cough, hoarseness, or discrete ulcerative lesions of the buccal or pharyngeal mucosa). Because of the range of clinical presentations of streptococcal pharyngitis and the large number of other agents that can produce the same clinical picture, diagnosis of streptococcal pharyngitis on clinical grounds alone is not reliable.

The throat culture remains the diagnostic gold standard. Culture of a throat specimen that is properly collected (i.e., by vigorous rubbing of a sterile swab over both tonsillar pillars) and properly processed is the most sensitive and specific means of definitive diagnosis. A rapid diagnostic kit for latex agglutination or enzyme im-

TABLE 130-2 INFECTIOUS ETIOLOGIES OF ACUTE PHARYNGITIS

Organism	Associated Clinical Syndrome(s)
Viruses	
Rhinovirus	Common cold
Coronavirus	Common cold
Adenovirus	Pharyngoconjunctival fever
Influenza virus	Influenza
Parainfluenza virus	Cold, croup
Coxsackievirus	Herpangina, hand-foot-and-mouth disease
Herpes simplex virus	Gingivostomatitis (primary infection)
Epstein-Barr virus	Infectious mononucleosis
Cytomegalovirus	Mononucleosis-like syndrome
HIV	Acute (primary) infection syndrome
Bacteria	
Group A streptococci	Pharyngitis, scarlet fever
Group C or G streptococci	Pharyngitis
Mixed anaerobes	Vincent's angina
Arcanobacterium haemolyticum	Pharyngitis, scarlatiniform rash
Neisseria gonorrhoeae	Pharyngitis
Treponema pallidum	Secondary syphilis
Francisella tularensis	Pharyngeal tularemia
Corynebacterium diphtheriae	Diphtheria
Yersinia enterocolitica	Pharyngitis, enterocolitis
Yersinia pestis	Plague
Chlamydiae	
Chlamydia pneumoniae	Bronchitis, pneumonia
Chlamydia psittaci	Psittacosis
Mycoplasmas	
Mycoplasma pneumoniae	Bronchitis, pneumonia

TABLE 130-3 TREATMENT OF GROUP A STREPTOCOCCAL INFECTIONS

Infection	Treatment[a]
Pharyngitis	Benzathine penicillin G, 1.2 mU IM; *or* penicillin V, 250 mg PO tid or 500 mg PO bid × 10 days (Children <27 kg: Benzathine penicillin G, 600,000 units IM; *or* penicillin V, 250 mg PO bid or tid × 10 days)
Impetigo	Same as pharyngitis
Erysipelas/cellulitis	Severe: Penicillin G, 1–2 mU IV q4h
	Mild to moderate: Procaine penicillin, 1.2 mU IM bid
Necrotizing fasciitis/ myositis	Surgical debridement; *plus* penicillin G, 2–4 mU IV q4h; *plus* clindamycin,[b] 600–900 mg q8h
Pneumonia/empyema	Penicillin G, 2–4 mU IV q4h; *plus* drainage of empyema
Streptococcal toxic shock syndrome	Penicillin G, 2–4 mU IV q4h; *plus* clindamycin,[b] 600–900 mg q8h; *plus* intravenous immunoglobulin,[b] 2 g/kg as a single dose

[a] Penicillin allergy: Erythromycin (10 mg/kg PO qid up to a maximum of 250 mg per dose) may be substituted for oral penicillin. Alternative agents for parenteral therapy include first-generation cephalosporins—if the nature of the allergy is not an immediate hypersensitivity reaction (anaphylaxis or urticaria) or another potentially life-threatening manifestation (e.g., severe rash and fever)—or vancomycin.
[b] Efficacy unproven, but recommended by several experts. See text for discussion.

munoassay of swab specimens is a useful adjunct to throat culture. While precise figures on sensitivity and specificity vary, rapid diagnostic kits generally are >95% specific. Thus a positive result can be relied upon for definitive diagnosis and eliminates the need for throat culture. However, because rapid diagnostic tests are less sensitive than throat culture (relative sensitivity in comparative studies, 55–90%), a negative result should be confirmed by throat culture.

℞ GAS PHARYNGITIS

In the usual course of uncomplicated streptococcal pharyngitis, symptoms resolve after 3–5 days. The course is shortened little by treatment, which is given primarily to prevent suppurative complications and ARF. Prevention of ARF depends on eradication of the organism from the pharynx, not simply on resolution of symptoms, and requires 10 days of penicillin treatment (Table 130-3). Erythromycin may be substituted for penicillin in cases of penicillin allergy. Once-daily azithromycin is a more convenient but expensive alternative; a 5-day course is approved, but only limited data support equivalent efficacy to a standard 10-day course.

Resistance to erythromycin and other macrolides is common among isolates from several countries, including Spain, Italy, Finland, Japan, and Korea. Macrolide resistance may be becoming more prevalent elsewhere with the increasing use of this class of antibiotics. In areas with resistance rates exceeding 5–10%, macrolides should be avoided unless results of susceptibility testing are known. Follow-up culture after treatment is no longer routinely recommended but may be warranted in selected cases, such as those involving patients or families with frequent streptococcal infections or those occurring in situations in which the risk of ARF is thought to be high (e.g., when cases of ARF have recently been reported in the community).

COMPLICATIONS Suppurative complications of streptococcal pharyngitis have become uncommon with the widespread use of antibiotics for most symptomatic cases. These complications result from the spread of infection from the pharyngeal mucosa to deeper tissues by direct extension or by the hematogenous or lymphatic route and may include cervical lymphadenitis, peritonsillar or retropharyngeal abscess, sinusitis, otitis media, meningitis, bacteremia, endocarditis, and pneumonia. Local complications, such as peritonsillar or parapharyngeal abscess formation, should be considered in a patient with unusually severe or prolonged symptoms or localized pain associated with high fever and a toxic appearance. Nonsuppurative complications include ARF (Chap. 315) and PSGN (Chap. 277), both of which are thought to result from immune responses to streptococcal infection.

Penicillin treatment of streptococcal pharyngitis has been shown to reduce the likelihood of ARF but not that of PSGN.

Bacteriologic Treatment Failure and the Asymptomatic Carrier State Surveillance cultures have shown that up to 20% of individuals in certain populations may have asymptomatic pharyngeal colonization with GAS. There are no definitive guidelines for management of these asymptomatic carriers or of asymptomatic patients who still have a positive throat culture after a full course of treatment for symptomatic pharyngitis. A reasonable course of action is to give a single 10-day course of penicillin for symptomatic pharyngitis and, if positive cultures persist, not to re-treat unless symptoms recur. Studies of the natural history of streptococcal carriage and infection have shown that the risk both of developing ARF and of transmitting infection to others is substantially lower among asymptomatic carriers than among individuals with symptomatic pharyngitis. Therefore, overly aggressive attempts to eradicate carriage probably are not justified under most circumstances. An exception is the situation in which an asymptomatic carrier is a potential source of infection to others. Outbreaks of food-borne infection and nosocomial puerperal infection have been traced to asymptomatic carriers who may harbor the organisms in the throat, vagina, or anus or on the skin.

℞ ASYMPTOMATIC PHARYNGEAL COLONIZATION WITH GAS

When a carrier is transmitting infection to others, attempts to eradicate carriage are warranted. Data are limited on the best regimen to clear GAS after penicillin alone has failed. The combination of penicillin V (500 mg four times daily for 10 days) and rifampin (600 mg twice daily for the last 4 days) has been used to eliminate pharyngeal carriage. A 10-day course of oral vancomycin (250 mg four times daily) and rifampin (600 mg twice daily) has eradicated rectal colonization.

Scarlet Fever Scarlet fever consists of streptococcal infection, usually pharyngitis, accompanied by a characteristic rash (Fig. 130-2). The rash arises from the effects of one of three toxins, currently designated streptococcal pyrogenic exotoxins A, B, and C and previously known as erythrogenic or scarlet fever toxins. In the past, scarlet fever was thought to reflect infection of an individual lacking toxin-specific immunity with a toxin-producing strain of GAS. Susceptibility to scarlet fever was correlated with results of the Dick test, in which a small amount of erythrogenic toxin injected intradermally produced local erythema in susceptible individuals but elicited no reaction in those with specific immunity. Subsequent studies have suggested that development of the scarlet fever rash may reflect a hypersensitivity reaction requiring prior exposure to the toxin. For reasons that are not clear, scarlet fever has become less common in recent years, although strains of GAS that produce pyrogenic exotoxins continue to be prevalent in the population.

The symptoms of scarlet fever are the same as those of pharyngitis alone. The rash typically begins on the first or second day of illness over the upper trunk, spreading to involve the extremities but sparing the palms and soles. The rash is made up of minute papules, giving a characteristic "sandpaper" feel to the skin. Associated findings include circumoral pallor, "strawberry tongue" (enlarged papillae on a coated tongue, which later may become denuded), and accentuation of the rash in skin folds (Pastia's lines). Subsidence of the rash in 6–9 days is followed after several days by desquamation of the palms and soles. The differential diagnosis of scarlet fever includes other causes of fever and generalized rash, such as measles and other viral exanthems, Kawasaki disease, toxic shock syndrome, and systemic allergic reactions (e.g., drug eruptions).

Skin and Soft Tissue Infections GAS—and occasionally other streptococcal species—causes a variety of infections involving the skin, subcutaneous tissues, muscles, and fascia. While several clinical syndromes offer a useful means for classification of these infections, not all cases fit exactly into one category. The classic syndromes are general guides to predicting the level of tissue involvement in a particular patient, the probable clinical course, and the likelihood that surgical intervention or aggressive life support will be required.

IMPETIGO (PYODERMA) Impetigo, a superficial infection of the skin, is caused primarily by GAS and occasionally by other streptococci or *Staphylococcus aureus*. Impetigo is seen most often in young children, tends to occur during warmer months, and is more common in semitropical or tropical climates than in cooler regions. Infection is more common among children living under conditions of poor hygiene. Prospective studies have shown that colonization of unbroken skin with GAS precedes clinical infection. Minor trauma, such as a scratch or an insect bite, may then serve to inoculate organisms into the skin. Impetigo is best prevented, therefore, by attention to adequate hygiene. The usual sites of involvement are the face (particularly around the nose and mouth) and the legs, although lesions may occur at other locations. Individual lesions begin as red papules, which evolve quickly into vesicular and then pustular lesions that break down and coalesce to form characteristic honeycomb-like crusts (Fig. 130-3). Lesions are generally not painful, and patients do not appear ill. Fever is not a feature of impetigo and, if present, suggests either infection extending to deeper tissues or another diagnosis.

The classic presentation of impetigo usually poses little diagnostic difficulty. Cultures of impetiginous lesions often yield *S. aureus* as well as GAS. In almost all cases, streptococci are isolated initially and staphylococci appear later, presumably as secondary colonizing flora. In the past, penicillin was nearly always effective against these infections. However, an increasing frequency of penicillin treatment failure suggests that *S. aureus* may have become more prominent as a cause of impetigo. *Bullous impetigo* due to *S. aureus* is distinguished from typical streptococcal infection by more extensive, bullous lesions that break down and leave thin paper-like crusts instead of the thick amber crusts of streptococcal impetigo. Other skin lesions that may be confused with impetigo include herpetic lesions—either those of orolabial herpes simplex or those of chickenpox or zoster. Herpetic lesions can generally be distinguished by their appearance as more discrete, grouped vesicles and by a positive Tzanck test. In difficult cases, cultures of vesicular fluid should yield GAS in impetigo and the responsible virus in *Herpesvirus* infections.

FIGURE 130-2 Scarlet fever exanthem. Finely punctate erythema has become confluent (scarlatiniform); petechiae can occur and have a linear configuration within the exanthem in body folds (Pastia's lines). *(From Fitzpatrick, Johnson, Wolff: Color Atlas and Synopsis of Clinical Dermatology, 4th ed, New York, McGraw-Hill, 2001, with permission.)*

FIGURE 130-3 Impetigo contagiosa is a superficial streptococcal or *Staphylococcus aureus* infection consisting of honey-colored crusts and erythematous weeping erosions. Occasionally, bullous lesions may be seen. *(Courtesy of Mary Spraker, MD; with permission.)*

FIGURE 130-4 Erysipelas is a streptococcal infection of the superficial dermis and consists of well-demarcated, erythematous, edematous, warm plaques.

℞ STREPTOCOCCAL IMPETIGO

Treatment of streptococcal impetigo is the same as that for streptococcal pharyngitis. In view of evidence that *S. aureus* has become a relatively frequent cause of impetigo, empirical regimens should cover both streptococci and *S. aureus*. For example, either dicloxacillin or cephalexin can be given at a dose of 250 mg four times daily for 10 days. Topical mupirocin ointment is also effective. ARF is not a sequela to streptococcal skin infections, although PSGN may follow either skin or throat infection. The reason for this difference is not known. One hypothesis is that the immune response necessary for development of ARF occurs only after infection of the pharyngeal mucosa. In addition, the strains of GAS that cause pharyngitis are generally of different M protein types than those associated with skin infections; thus the strains that cause pharyngitis may have rheumatogenic potential, while the skin-infecting strains may not.

CELLULITIS Inoculation of organisms into the skin may lead to *cellulitis*: infection involving the skin and subcutaneous tissues. The portal of entry may be a traumatic or surgical wound, an insect bite, or any other break in skin integrity. Often, no entry site is apparent.

One form of streptococcal cellulitis, *erysipelas*, is characterized by a bright red appearance of the involved skin, which forms a plateau sharply demarcated from surrounding normal skin (Fig. 130-4). The lesion is warm to the touch, may be tender, and appears shiny and swollen. The skin often has a *peau d'orange* texture, which is thought to reflect involvement of superficial lymphatics; superficial blebs or bullae may form, usually 2–3 days after onset. The lesion typically develops over a few hours and is associated with fever and chills. Erysipelas tends to occur on the malar area of the face (often with extension over the bridge of the nose to the contralateral malar region) and the lower extremities. After one episode, recurrence at the same site—sometimes years later—is not uncommon.

Classic cases of erysipelas, with typical features, are almost always due to β-hemolytic streptococci, usually GAS and occasionally group C or G. Often, however, the appearance of streptococcal cellulitis is not sufficiently distinctive to permit a specific diagnosis on clinical grounds. The area involved may not be typical for erysipelas, the lesion may be less intensely red than usual and may fade into surrounding skin, and/or the patient may appear only mildly ill. In such cases, it is prudent to broaden the spectrum of empirical antimicrobial therapy to include other pathogens, particularly *S. aureus*, that can produce cellulitis with the same appearance. Staphylococcal infection should be suspected if cellulitis develops around a wound or an ulcer.

Streptococcal cellulitis tends to develop at anatomic sites in which normal lymphatic drainage has been disrupted, such as sites of prior cellulitis, the arm ipsilateral to a mastectomy and axillary lymph node dissection, a lower extremity previously involved in deep venous thrombosis or chronic lymphedema, or the leg from which a saphenous vein has been harvested for coronary artery bypass grafting. The organism may enter via a dermal breach some distance from the eventual site of clinical cellulitis. For example, some patients with recurrent leg cellulitis following saphenous vein removal stop having recurrent episodes only after treatment of tinea pedis on the affected extremity. Fissures in the skin presumably serve as a portal of entry for streptococci, which then produce infection more proximally in the leg at the site of previous injury. Streptococcal cellulitis may also involve recent surgical wounds. GAS is among the few bacterial pathogens that typically produce signs of wound infection and surrounding cellulitis within the first 24 h after surgery. These wound infections are usually associated with a thin exudate and may spread rapidly, either as cellulitis in the skin and subcutaneous tissue or as a deeper tissue infection (see below). Streptococcal wound infection or localized cellulitis may also be associated with *lymphangitis*, manifested by red streaks extending proximally along superficial lymphatics from the infection site.

℞ STREPTOCOCCAL CELLULITIS

See Table 130-3 and Chap. 119.

Deep Soft-Tissue Infections *Necrotizing fasciitis* (*hemolytic streptococcal gangrene*) involves the superficial and/or deep fascia investing the muscles of an extremity or the trunk. The source of the infection is either the skin, with organisms introduced into tissue through trauma (sometimes trivial), or the bowel flora, with organisms released during abdominal surgery or from an occult enteric source, such as a diverticular or appendiceal abscess. The inoculation site may be inapparent and is often some distance from the site of clinical involvement; e.g., the introduction of organisms via minor trauma to the hand may be associated with clinical infection of the tissues overlying the shoulder or chest. Cases associated with the bowel flora are usually polymicrobial, involving a mixture of anaerobic bacteria (such as *Bacteroides fragilis* or anaerobic streptococci) and facultative organisms (usually gram-negative bacilli). Cases unrelated to contamination from bowel organisms are most commonly caused by GAS alone or in combination with other organisms (most often *S. aureus*). Overall, GAS is implicated in ~60% of cases of necrotizing fasciitis. The onset of symptoms is usually quite acute and is marked by severe pain at the site of involvement, malaise, fever, chills, and a toxic appearance. The physical findings, particularly early on, may not be striking, with only minimal erythema of the overlying skin. Pain and tenderness are usually severe. In contrast, in more superficial cellulitis, the skin appearance is more abnormal, but pain and tenderness are only mild or moderate. As the infection progresses (often over several hours), the severity and extent of symptoms worsen, and skin changes become more evident, with the appearance of dusky or mottled erythema and edema. The marked tenderness of the involved area may evolve into anesthesia as the spreading inflammatory process produces infarction of cutaneous nerves.

Although myositis is more commonly due to *S. aureus* infection, GAS occasionally produces abscesses in skeletal muscles (*streptococcal myositis*), with little or no involvement of the surrounding fascia or overlying skin. The presentation is usually subacute, but a fulminant form has been described in association with severe systemic toxicity, bacteremia, and a high mortality rate. The fulminant form may reflect the same basic disease process seen in necrotizing fasciitis, but with the necrotizing inflammatory process extending into the muscles themselves rather than remaining limited to the fascial layers.

Rx DEEP SOFT-TISSUE INFECTIONS

Once necrotizing fasciitis is suspected, early surgical exploration is both diagnostically and therapeutically indicated. Surgery reveals necrosis and inflammatory fluid tracking along the fascial planes above and between muscle groups, without involvement of the muscles themselves. The process usually extends beyond the area of clinical involvement, and extensive debridement is required. Drainage and debridement are central to the management of necrotizing fasciitis; antibiotic treatment is a useful adjunct (Table 130-3), but surgery is life-saving.

Treatment for streptococcal myositis consists of surgical drainage—usually by an open procedure that permits evaluation of the extent of infection and ensures adequate debridement of involved tissues—and high-dose penicillin (Table 130-3).

Pneumonia and Empyema GAS is an occasional cause of pneumonia, generally in previously healthy individuals. The onset of symptoms may be abrupt or gradual. Pleuritic chest pain, fever, chills, and dyspnea are the characteristic manifestations. Cough is usually present but may not be prominent. Approximately one-half of patients with GAS pneumonia have an accompanying pleural effusion. In contrast to the sterile parapneumonic effusions typical of pneumococcal pneumonia, those complicating streptococcal pneumonia are almost always infected. The empyema fluid is usually visible by chest radiography on initial presentation, and its volume may increase rapidly. These pleural collections should be drained early, as they tend to become loculated rapidly, resulting in a chronic fibrotic reaction that may require thoracotomy for removal.

Bacteremia, Puerperal Sepsis, and Streptococcal Toxic Shock Syndrome GAS bacteremia is usually associated with an identifiable local infection. Bacteremia occurs rarely with otherwise uncomplicated pharyngitis, occasionally with cellulitis or pneumonia, and relatively frequently with necrotizing fasciitis. Bacteremia without an identified source raises the possibility of endocarditis, an occult abscess, or osteomyelitis. A variety of focal infections may arise secondarily from streptococcal bacteremia, including endocarditis, meningitis, septic arthritis, osteomyelitis, peritonitis, and visceral abscesses.

GAS is occasionally implicated in infectious complications of childbirth, usually endometritis and associated bacteremia. In the preantibiotic era, puerperal sepsis was commonly caused by GAS; currently, it is more often caused by GBS. Several nosocomial outbreaks of puerperal GAS infection have been traced to an asymptomatic carrier, usually someone present at delivery. The site of carriage may be the skin, throat, anus, or vagina.

Beginning in the late 1980s, several reports described patients with GAS infections associated with shock and multisystem organ failure. This syndrome was called the streptococcal toxic shock syndrome (TSS) because it shares certain features with staphylococcal TSS. In 1993, a case definition for streptococcal TSS was formulated (Table 130-4). The general features of the illness include fever, hypotension, renal impairment, and respiratory distress syndrome. Various types of rash have been described, but rash usually does not develop. Laboratory abnormalities include a marked shift to the left in the white blood cell differential, with many immature granulocytes; hypocalcemia; hy-

---

TABLE 130-4 PROPOSED CASE DEFINITION FOR THE STREPTOCOCCAL TOXIC SHOCK SYNDROME[a]

I. Isolation of group A streptococci (*Streptococcus pyogenes*)
  A. From a normally sterile site
  B. From a nonsterile site
II. Clinical signs of severity
  A. Hypotension *and*
  B. ≥2 of the following signs
    1. Renal impairment
    2. Coagulopathy
    3. Liver function impairment
    4. Adult respiratory distress syndrome
    5. A generalized erythematous macular rash that may desquamate
    6. Soft tissue necrosis, including necrotizing fasciitis or myositis; *or* gangrene

[a]An illness fulfilling criteria IA, IIA, and IIB is defined as a *definite* case. An illness fulfilling criteria IB, IIA, and IIB is defined as a *probable* case if no other etiology for the illness is identified.

Source: Modified from Working Group on Severe Streptococcal Infections: JAMA 269:390, 1993.

---

poalbuminemia; and thrombocytopenia, which usually becomes more pronounced on the second or third day of illness. In contrast to patients with staphylococcal TSS, the majority with streptococcal TSS are bacteremic. The most common associated infection is a soft tissue infection—necrotizing fasciitis, myositis, or cellulitis—although a variety of other associated local infections have been described, including pneumonia, peritonitis, osteomyelitis, and myometritis. Streptococcal TSS is associated with a mortality rate of ≥30%, with most deaths secondary to shock and respiratory failure. Because of its rapidly progressive and lethal course, early recognition of the syndrome is essential. Patients should receive aggressive supportive care (fluid resuscitation, pressors, and mechanical ventilation) in addition to antimicrobial therapy and, in cases associated with necrotizing fasciitis, surgical debridement. Exactly why certain patients develop this fulminant syndrome is not known. Early studies of the streptococcal strains isolated from these patients demonstrated a strong association with the production of pyrogenic exotoxin A. This association has been inconsistent in subsequent case series. Pyrogenic exotoxin A and several other streptococcal exotoxins act as superantigens to trigger release of inflammatory cytokines from T lymphocytes. Fever, shock, and organ dysfunction in streptococcal TSS may reflect, in part, the systemic effects of superantigen-mediated cytokine release.

Rx STREPTOCOCCAL TOXIC SHOCK SYNDROME

In light of the possible role of pyrogenic exotoxins or other streptococcal toxins in streptococcal TSS, treatment with clindamycin has been advocated by some authorities (Table 130-3), who argue that, through its direct action on protein synthesis, clindamycin is more effective in rapidly terminating toxin production than penicillin—a cell-wall agent. Support for this view comes from studies of an experimental model of streptococcal myositis, in which mice given clindamycin had a higher rate of survival than those given penicillin. Comparable data on the treatment of human infections are not available. Although clindamycin resistance in GAS is uncommon (<2% among U.S. isolates), it has been documented. Thus, if clindamycin is used for initial treatment of a critically ill patient, penicillin should be given as well until the antibiotic susceptibility of the streptococcal isolate is known.

Intravenous immunoglobulin has been used as adjunctive therapy for streptococcal TSS (Table 130-3). Pooled immunoglobulin preparations contain antibodies capable of neutralizing the effects of streptococcal toxins. Anecdotal reports and case series have suggested favorable clinical responses to intravenous immunoglobulin, but no prospective controlled trials have been reported.

Prevention No vaccine against GAS is commercially available. A formulation that consists of recombinant peptides containing epitopes of 26 M-protein types has undergone phase I and II testing in volunteers.

Early results indicate that the vaccine is well tolerated and elicits type-specific antibody responses.

Household contacts of individuals with invasive GAS infection (e.g., bacteremia, necrotizing fasciitis, or streptococcal TSS) are at greater risk of invasive infection than the general population. Asymptomatic pharyngeal colonization with GAS has been detected in up to 25% of persons with >4 h/d of same-room exposure to an index case. However, antibiotic prophylaxis is not routinely recommended for contacts of patients with invasive disease since such an approach (if effective) would require treatment of hundreds of contacts to prevent a single case.

STREPTOCOCCI OF GROUPS C AND G

Group C and group G streptococci are β-hemolytic bacteria that occasionally cause human infections similar to those caused by GAS. Strains that form small colonies on blood agar (<0.5 mm) are generally members of the *S. milleri* (*S. intermedius*, *S. anginosus*) group (see "Viridans Streptococci," below). Large-colony group C and G streptococci of human origin are now considered a single species, *S. dysgalactiae* subsp. *equisimilis*. They have been associated with pharyngitis, cellulitis and soft-tissue infections, pneumonia, bacteremia, endocarditis, and septic arthritis. Puerperal sepsis, meningitis, epidural abscess, intraabdominal abscess, urinary tract infection, and neonatal sepsis have also been reported. Group C or G streptococcal bacteremia most often affects elderly or chronically ill patients and, in the absence of obvious local infection, is likely to reflect endocarditis. Septic arthritis, sometimes involving multiple joints, may complicate endocarditis or develop in its absence. Distinct streptococcal species of Lancefield group C cause infections in domesticated animals, especially horses and cattle; some human infections are acquired through contact with animals or consumption of unpasteurized milk. These zoonotic organisms include *S. equi* subsp. *zooepidemicus* and *S. equi* subsp. *equi*.

℞ GROUP C OR G STREPTOCOCCAL INFECTION

Penicillin is the drug of choice for treatment of group C or G streptococcal infections. Antibiotic treatment is the same as for similar syndromes due to GAS (Table 130-3). Patients with bacteremia or septic arthritis should receive intravenous penicillin (2–4 mU every 4 h). All group C and G streptococci are sensitive to penicillin; nearly all are inhibited in vitro by concentrations of ≤0.03 μg/mL. Occasional isolates exhibit tolerance: although inhibited by low concentrations of penicillin, they are killed only by significantly higher concentrations. The clinical significance of tolerance is unknown. Because of the poor clinical response of some patients to penicillin alone, the addition of gentamicin (1 mg/kg every 8 h for patients with normal renal function) is recommended by some authorities for treatment of endocarditis or septic arthritis due to group C or G streptococci; however, combination therapy has not been shown to be superior to penicillin treatment alone. Patients with joint infections often require repeated aspiration or open drainage and debridement for cure; the response to treatment may be slow, particularly in debilitated patients and those with involvement of multiple joints. Infection of prosthetic joints almost always requires prosthesis removal in addition to antibiotic therapy.

GROUP B STREPTOCOCCI

Identified first as a cause of mastitis in cows, streptococci belonging to Lancefield's group B have since been recognized as a major cause of sepsis and meningitis in human neonates. GBS is also a frequent cause of peripartum fever in women and an occasional cause of serious infection in nonpregnant adults. Since the widespread institution of prenatal screening for GBS in the 1990s, the incidence of neonatal infection per 1000 live births has fallen from ~2–3 cases to ~1 case. During the same period, GBS infection in adults with underlying chronic illnesses has become more common; adults now account for a larger proportion of invasive GBS infections than do newborns.

Lancefield group B consists of a single species, *S. agalactiae*, which is definitively identified with specific antiserum to the group B cell wall–associated carbohydrate antigen. A streptococcal isolate can be classified presumptively as GBS on the basis of biochemical tests, including hydrolysis of sodium hippurate (in which 99% of isolates are positive), hydrolysis of bile esculin agar (in which 99–100% are negative), bacitracin susceptibility (in which 92% are resistant), and production of CAMP factor (in which 98–100% are positive). CAMP factor is a phospholipase produced by GBS that causes synergistic hemolysis with β lysin produced by certain strains of *S. aureus*. Its presence can be demonstrated by cross-streaking of the test isolate and an appropriate staphylococcal strain on a blood agar plate. GBS organisms causing human infections are encapsulated by one of nine antigenically distinct polysaccharides. The capsular polysaccharide is an important virulence factor. Antibodies to the capsular polysaccharide afford protection against GBS of the same (but not of a different) capsular type.

INFECTION IN NEONATES

Two general types of GBS infection in infants are defined by the age of the patient at presentation. *Early-onset infections* occur within the first week of life, with a median age of 20 h at onset. Approximately half of these infants have signs of GBS disease at birth. The infection is acquired during or shortly before birth from the colonized maternal genital tract. Surveillance studies have shown that 5–40% of women are vaginal or rectal carriers of GBS. Approximately 50% of infants delivered vaginally by carrier mothers become colonized, although only 1–2% of those colonized develop clinically evident infection. Prematurity and maternal risk factors (prolonged labor, obstetric complications, and maternal fever) are often involved. The presentation of early-onset infection is the same as that of other forms of neonatal sepsis. Typical findings include respiratory distress, lethargy, and hypotension. Essentially all infants with early-onset disease are bacteremic, one-third to one-half have pneumonia and/or respiratory distress syndrome, and one-third have meningitis.

Late-onset infections occur in infants 1 week to 3 months old (mean age at onset, 3–4 weeks). The infecting organism may be acquired during delivery (as in early-onset cases) or during later contact with a colonized mother, nursery personnel, or another source. Meningitis is the most common manifestation of late-onset infection and in most cases is associated with a strain of capsular type III. Infants present with fever, lethargy or irritability, poor feeding, and seizures. The various other types of late-onset infection include bacteremia without an identified source, osteomyelitis, septic arthritis, and facial cellulitis associated with submandibular or preauricular adenitis.

℞ GROUP B STREPTOCOCCAL INFECTION IN NEONATES

Penicillin is the agent of choice for all GBS infections. Empirical broad-spectrum therapy for suspected bacterial sepsis, consisting of ampicillin and gentamicin, is generally administered until culture results become available. If cultures yield GBS, many pediatricians continue to administer gentamicin, along with ampicillin or penicillin, for a few days until clinical improvement becomes evident. Infants with bacteremia or soft-tissue infection should receive penicillin at a dosage of 200,000 units/kg per day in divided doses; those with meningitis should receive 400,000 units/kg per day. Meningitis should be treated for at least 14 days because of the risk of relapse with shorter courses.

Prevention The incidence of GBS infection is unusually high among infants of women with risk factors: preterm delivery, early rupture of membranes (>24 h before delivery), prolonged labor, fever, or chorioamnionitis. Because the usual source of the organisms infecting a neonate is the mother's birth canal, efforts have been made to prevent GBS infections by the identification of high-risk carrier mothers and their treatment with various forms of antibiotic or immunoprophylaxis. Prophylactic administration of ampicillin or penicillin to such patients during delivery reduces the risk of infection in the newborn. This approach has been hampered by logistical difficulties in identifying colonized women before delivery; the results of vaginal cultures early in pregnancy are poor predictors of carrier status at delivery. The CDC recommends screening for anogenital colonization at 35–37 weeks of pregnancy by a swab culture of the lower vagina and anorectum; intrapartum chemoprophylaxis is recommended for culture-positive women and for women who, regardless of culture status, have previously given birth to an infant with GBS infection or have a history of GBS bacteriuria during pregnancy. Women whose culture status is unknown and who develop premature labor (<37 weeks), prolonged rupture of membranes (>18 h), or intrapartum fever should also receive intrapartum chemoprophylaxis. The recommended regimen for chemoprophylaxis is 5 million units of penicillin G followed by 2.5 million units every 4 h until delivery. Cefazolin is an alternative for women with a history of penicillin allergy who are thought not to be at high risk for anaphylaxis. For women with a history of immediate hypersensitivity, clindamycin or erythromycin may be substituted, but only if the colonizing isolate has been demonstrated to be susceptible. If susceptibility testing results are not available or indicate resistance, vancomycin should be used in this situation.

Treatment of all pregnant women who are colonized or have risk factors for neonatal infection will result in exposure of 15–25% of pregnant women and newborns to antibiotics, with the attendant risks of allergic reactions and selection for resistant organisms. Although still in the developmental stages, a GBS vaccine may ultimately offer a better solution to prevention. Because transplacental passage of maternal antibodies produces protective antibody levels in newborns, efforts are under way to develop a vaccine against GBS that can be given to childbearing-age women before or during pregnancy. Results of phase 1 clinical trials of GBS capsular polysaccharide–protein conjugate vaccines suggest that a multivalent conjugate vaccine would be safe and highly immunogenic.

INFECTION IN ADULTS

The majority of GBS infections in otherwise healthy adults are related to pregnancy and parturition. Peripartum fever, the most common manifestation, is sometimes accompanied by symptoms and signs of endometritis or chorioamnionitis (abdominal distention and uterine or adnexal tenderness). Blood and vaginal swab cultures are often positive. Bacteremia is usually transitory but occasionally results in meningitis or endocarditis. Infections in adults that are not associated with the peripartum period generally involve individuals who are elderly or have an underlying chronic illness, such as diabetes mellitus or a malignancy. Among the infections that develop with some frequency in adults are cellulitis and soft tissue infection (including infected diabetic skin ulcers), urinary tract infection, pneumonia, endocarditis, and septic arthritis. Other reported infections include meningitis, osteomyelitis, and intraabdominal or pelvic abscesses. Relapse or recurrence of invasive infection weeks to months after a first episode is documented in ~4% of cases.

℞ GROUP B STREPTOCOCCAL INFECTION IN ADULTS

GBS is less sensitive to penicillin than GAS, requiring somewhat higher doses. Adults with serious localized infections (pneumonia, pyelonephritis, abscess) should receive doses of ~12 million units of penicillin G daily; patients with endocarditis or meningitis should receive 18–24 million units per day in divided doses. Vancomycin is an acceptable alternative for penicillin-allergic patients.

ENTEROCOCCI AND NONENTEROCOCCAL GROUP D STREPTOCOCCI

ENTEROCOCCI

Lancefield group D includes the enterococci—organisms now classified in a separate genus from other streptococci—and nonenterococcal group D streptococci. Enterococci are distinguished from nonentero-

coccal group D streptococci by their ability to grow in the presence of 6.5% sodium chloride and by the results of other biochemical tests. The enterococcal species that are significant pathogens for humans are *E. faecalis* and *E. faecium*. Less commonly, similar infections are caused by *E. casseliflavus*, *E. durans*, *E. gallinarum*, or other enterococcal species. These organisms tend to affect patients who are elderly or debilitated, whose mucosal or epithelial barriers have been disrupted, or whose normal flora has been altered by antibiotic treatment. Urinary tract infections due to enterococci are quite common, particularly among patients who have received antibiotic treatment or undergone urinary tract instrumentation. Enterococci are a common cause of nosocomial bacteremia in patients with intravascular catheters and account for 10–20% of cases of bacterial endocarditis on both native and prosthetic valves. The presentation of enterococcal endocarditis is usually subacute but may be acute, with rapidly progressive valve destruction. Enterococci are frequently cultured from bile and are involved in infectious complications of biliary surgery and in liver abscesses. Moreover, enterococci are often isolated from polymicrobial infections arising from the bowel flora (e.g., intraabdominal abscesses), from abdominal surgical wounds, and from diabetic foot ulcers. While such mixed infections are frequently cured by antimicrobials not active against enterococci, specific therapy directed against enterococci is warranted when these organisms predominate or are isolated from blood cultures.

℞ ENTEROCOCCAL INFECTION

Unlike streptococci, enterococci are not reliably killed by penicillin or ampicillin alone at concentrations achieved clinically in the blood or tissues. Ampicillin reaches sufficiently high urinary concentrations to constitute adequate monotherapy for uncomplicated urinary tract infections. Because in vitro testing has shown evidence of synergistic killing of most enterococcal strains by the combination of penicillin or ampicillin with an aminoglycoside, combined therapy is recommended for enterococcal endocarditis and meningitis; the regimen is penicillin (3–4 million units every 4 h) or ampicillin (2 g every 4 h) plus moderate-dose gentamicin (1 mg/kg every 8 h for patients with normal renal function). Enterococcal endocarditis should be treated for at least 4 weeks and for 6 weeks if symptoms have been present for ≥3 months or if the infection involves a prosthetic valve. For nonendocarditis bacteremia and other serious enterococcal infections, it is not known whether the efficacy of a single β-lactam agent is improved by the addition of gentamicin, but many infectious disease specialists use combination therapy for such infections, especially in critically ill patients. Vancomycin, in combination with gentamicin, may be substituted for penicillin in allergic patients. Enterococci are resistant to all cephalosporins.

Antimicrobial susceptibility testing should be performed routinely on enterococcal isolates from serious infections, with therapy adjusted according to the results **(Table 130-5)**. Most enterococci are resistant to streptomycin, which should not be used unless in vitro testing indicates susceptibility. Although less widespread than streptomycin resistance, high-level resistance to gentamicin—with a minimum inhibitory concen-

TABLE 130-5 TREATMENT OPTIONS FOR ANTIBIOTIC-RESISTANT ENTEROCOCCAL INFECTIONS

Resistance Pattern	Recommended Therapy
β-Lactamase production	Gentamicin plus ampicillin/sulbactam, amoxicillin/clavulanate, imipenem, or vancomycin
β-Lactam resistance, but no β-lactamase production	Gentamicin plus vancomycin
High-level gentamicin resistance	Streptomycin-sensitive isolate: Streptomycin plus ampicillin or vancomycin Streptomycin-resistant isolate: No proven therapy (continuous-infusion ampicillin, prolonged treatment)
Vancomycin resistance	Ampicillin plus gentamicin
Vancomycin and β-lactam resistance	No uniformly bactericidal drugs; linezolid (all enterococci) or quinupristin/dalfopristin (*E. faecium* only)

tration (MIC) of >2000 µg/mL—is common. Gentamicin-resistant enterococci should be tested for streptomycin susceptibility, which they occasionally exhibit. If the isolate is resistant to all aminoglycosides, treatment with penicillin or ampicillin alone may be successful. Prolonged administration (i.e., for at least 6 weeks) of high-dose ampicillin (e.g., 12 g/d) is recommended for endocarditis due to these highly resistant enterococci.

Enterococci may be resistant to penicillins via two distinct mechanisms. The first is β-lactamase production (mediating resistance to penicillin and ampicillin), which has been reported for *E. faecalis* isolates from several locations in the United States and other countries. Because the amount of β-lactamase produced may be insufficient for detection by routine antibiotic susceptibility testing, isolates from serious infections should be screened specifically for β-lactamase production with a chromogenic cephalosporin or another method. For the treatment of β-lactamase–producing strains, vancomycin, ampicillin/sulbactam, amoxicillin/clavulanate, imipenem, or meropenem may be used in combination with gentamicin.

The second mechanism of penicillin resistance is not mediated by β-lactamase and may be due to altered penicillin-binding proteins. This intrinsic penicillin resistance is common among *E. faecium* isolates, which routinely are more resistant to β-lactam antibiotics than are isolates of *E. faecalis*. Moderately resistant enterococci (MICs of penicillin and ampicillin, 16–64 µg/mL) may be susceptible to high-dose penicillin or ampicillin plus gentamicin, but strains with MICs of ≥200 µg/mL must be considered resistant to clinically achievable levels of β-lactam antibiotics, including imipenem and meropenem. Vancomycin plus gentamicin is the recommended regimen for infections due to enterococci with high-level intrinsic resistance to β-lactams.

Vancomycin-resistant enterococci (VRE), first reported from clinical sources in the late 1980s, have become common in many hospitals. Three major vancomycin resistance phenotypes have been described: VanA, VanB, and VanC. The VanA phenotype is associated with high-level resistance to vancomycin and to teicoplanin, a related glycopeptide antibiotic not currently available in the United States. VanB and VanC strains are resistant to vancomycin but susceptible to teicoplanin, although teicoplanin resistance may develop during treatment in VanB strains. For enterococci resistant to both vancomycin and β-lactams, no established therapies provide uniformly bactericidal activity. Two newer agents active against VRE are quinupristin/dalfopristin and linezolid, which were approved for use in the United States in 1999 and 2000, respectively. Quinupristin/dalfopristin is a streptogramin combination with in vitro bacteriostatic activity against *E. faecium*, including VRE, but not against *E. faecalis* or other enterococcal species. Disadvantages of quinupristin/dalfopristin are its limited spectrum of activity against enterococcal species and its relatively frequent side effects of phlebitis and myalgia. Linezolid is an oxazolidinone antibiotic with good bacteriostatic activity against nearly all enterococci, including VRE. Limited clinical experience suggests that linezolid is at least as efficacious as quinupristin/dalfopristin, and linezolid is usually preferred because of its broader activity against all enterococci and the availability of both parenteral and oral formulations. Bone marrow toxicity (especially thrombocytopenia) and peripheral neuropathy are potential side effects. Two other antibiotics are active in vitro against VRE (both *E. faecalis* and *E. faecium*), although neither had been approved for treatment of these infections as of May 2006: daptomycin, a cyclic lipopeptide, and tigecycline, a glycylcycline related to tetracycline.

OTHER GROUP D STREPTOCOCCI

The main nonenterococcal group D streptococcal species that causes human infections is *S. bovis*. *S. bovis* endocarditis is often associated with neoplasms of the gastrointestinal tract—most frequently, a colon carcinoma or polyp—but is also reported in association with other bowel lesions. When occult gastrointestinal lesions are carefully sought, abnormalities are found in ≥60% of patients with *S. bovis* endocarditis. In contrast to the enterococci, nonenterococcal group D streptococci like *S. bovis* are reliably killed by penicillin as a single agent, and penicillin is the agent of choice for *S. bovis* infections.

VIRIDANS AND OTHER STREPTOCOCCI

VIRIDANS STREPTOCOCCI

Consisting of multiple species of α-hemolytic streptococci, the viridans streptococci are a heterogeneous group of organisms that are im-

portant agents of bacterial endocarditis (Chap. 118). Several species of viridans streptococci, including *S. salivarius*, *S. mitis*, *S. sanguis*, and *S. mutans*, are part of the normal flora of the mouth, where they live in close association with the teeth and gingiva. Some species contribute to the development of dental caries.

Previously known as *S. morbillorum*, *Gemella morbillorum* has been placed in a separate genus, along with *G. haemolysans*, on the basis of genetic-relatedness studies. These species resemble viridans streptococci with respect to habitat in the human host and associated infections.

The transient viridans streptococcal bacteremia induced by eating, tooth-brushing, flossing, and other sources of minor trauma, together with adherence to biologic surfaces, is thought to account for the predilection of these organisms to cause endocarditis (see Fig. 118-1). Viridans streptococci are also isolated, often as part of a mixed flora, from sites of sinusitis, brain abscess, and liver abscess.

Viridans streptococcal bacteremia occurs relatively frequently in neutropenic patients, particularly after bone marrow transplantation or high-dose chemotherapy for cancer. Some of these patients develop a sepsis syndrome with high fever and shock. Risk factors for viridans streptococcal bacteremia include chemotherapy with high-dose cytosine arabinoside, prior treatment with trimethoprim-sulfamethoxazole or a fluoroquinolone, treatment with antacids or histamine antagonists, mucositis, and profound neutropenia.

The *S. milleri* group (also referred to as the *S. intermedius* or *S. anginosus* group) includes three species that cause human disease: *S. intermedius*, *S. anginosus*, and *S. constellatus*. These organisms are often considered viridans streptococci, although they differ somewhat from other viridans streptococci in both their hemolytic pattern (they may be α-, β-, or nonhemolytic) and the disease syndromes they cause. This group commonly produces suppurative infections, particularly abscesses of brain and abdominal viscera, and infections related to the oral cavity or respiratory tract, such as peritonsillar abscess, lung abscess, and empyema.

℞ INFECTION WITH VIRIDANS STREPTOCOCCI

Isolates from neutropenic patients with bacteremia are often resistant to penicillin; thus these patients should be treated presumptively with vancomycin until the results of susceptibility testing become available. Viridans streptococci isolated in other clinical settings usually are sensitive to penicillin.

ABIOTROPHIA SPECIES (NUTRITIONALLY VARIANT STREPTOCOCCI)

Occasional isolates cultured from the blood of patients with endocarditis fail to grow when subcultured on solid media. These *nutritionally variant streptococci* require supplemental thiol compounds or active forms of vitamin B_6 (pyridoxal or pyridoxamine) for growth in the laboratory. The nutritionally variant streptococci are generally grouped with the viridans streptococci because they cause similar types of infections. However, they have been reclassified on the basis of 16S ribosomal RNA sequence comparisons into a separate genus, *Abiotrophia*, with two species: *A. defectivus* and *A. adjacens*.

℞ INFECTION WITH NUTRITIONALLY VARIANT STREPTOCOCCI

Treatment failure and relapse appear to be more common in cases of endocarditis due to nutritionally variant streptococci than in those due to the usual viridans streptococci. Thus the addition of gentamicin (1 mg/kg every 8 h for patients with normal renal function) to the penicillin regimen is recommended for endocarditis due to the nutritionally variant organisms.

OTHER STREPTOCOCCI

S. suis is an important pathogen in swine and has been reported to cause meningitis in humans, usually in individuals with occupational exposure to pigs. Strains of *S. suis* associated with human infections have generally reacted with Lancefield group R typing serum and sometimes with group D typing serum as well. Isolates may be α- or β-hemolytic and are sensitive to penicillin. *S. iniae*, a pathogen of fish, has been associated with infections in humans who have handled live or freshly killed fish. Cellulitis of the hand is the most common form of human infection, although bacteremia and endocarditis have been reported. *Anaerobic streptococci*, or *peptostreptococci*, are part of the normal flora of the oral cavity, bowel, and vagina. Infections caused by the anaerobic streptococci are discussed in Chap. 157.

FURTHER READINGS

BISNO AL et al: Practice guidelines for the diagnosis and management of group A streptococcal pharyngitis. Clin Infect Dis 35:113, 2002
———, STEVENS DL: Streptococcal infections of skin and soft tissues. N Engl J Med 334:240, 1996
CARAPETIS JR et al: The global burden of group A streptococcal diseases. Lancet Infect Dis 5:685, 2005
CENTERS FOR DISEASE CONTROL AND PREVENTION: Prevention of perinatal group B streptococcal disease. MMWR 51(RR-11):1, 2002

GASSAS A et al: Predictors of viridans streptococcal shock syndrome in bacteremic children with cancer and stem-cell transplant recipients. J Clin Oncol 22:1222, 2004
GIBBS RS et al: Perinatal infections due to group B streptococci. Obstet Gynecol 104:1062, 2004
JACKSON LA et al: Risk factors for group B streptococcal disease in adults. Ann Intern Med 123:415, 1995
KAUFFMAN CA: Therapeutic and preventative options for the management of vancomycin-resistant enterococcal infections. J Antimicrob Chemother 51(Suppl3):iii23, 2003
KAUL R et al: Intravenous immunoglobulin therapy for streptococcal toxic shock syndrome—a comparative observational study. The Canadian Streptococcal Study Group. Clin Infect Dis 28:800, 1999
THE PREVENTION OF INVASIVE GROUP A STREPTOCOCCAL INFECTIONS WORKSHOP PARTICIPANTS: Prevention of invasive group A streptococcal disease among household contacts of case patients and among postpartum and postsurgical patients: Recommendations from the Centers for Disease Control and Prevention. Clin Infect Dis 35:950, 2002

131 Diphtheria and Other Infections Caused by Corynebacteria and Related Species

William R. Bishai, John R. Murphy

DIPHTHERIA

Diphtheria is a nasopharyngeal and skin infection caused by *Corynebacterium diphtheriae*. Toxigenic strains of *C. diphtheriae* produce a protein toxin that causes systemic toxicity, myocarditis, and polyneuropathy. The toxin is associated with the formation of pseudomembranes in the pharynx during respiratory diphtheria. While toxigenic strains most frequently cause pharyngeal diphtheria, nontoxigenic strains commonly cause cutaneous disease. In the United States and Europe, diphtheria has been controlled in recent years with effective vaccination, although sporadic outbreaks have occurred. Diphtheria is still common in the Caribbean, Latin America, and the Indian subcontinent, where mass immunization programs are not enforced. Large epidemics have occurred in the independent states formerly encompassed by the Soviet Union. Additional outbreaks have been reported in Algeria, China, and Ecuador.

ETIOLOGY

C. diphtheriae is a gram-positive, unencapsulated, nonmotile, nonsporulating bacillus. *C. diphtheriae* organisms have a characteristic club-shaped bacillary appearance and typically form clusters of parallel rays (palisades) that are referred to as *Chinese characters*. In the specific laboratory media recommended for the cultivation of *C. diphtheriae*, tellurite, colistin, or nalidixic acid is responsible for selective isolation of the organism in the presence of other autochthonous pharyngeal microbes. Human isolates of *C. diphtheriae* may display nontoxigenic (*tox⁻*) or toxigenic (*tox⁺*) phenotypes. Corynebacteriophage beta carries the structural gene (*tox*) encoding diphtheria toxin, and a family of closely related corynebacteriophages are responsible for toxigenic conversion of *tox⁻ C. diphtheriae* to the *tox⁺* phenotype. Moreover, lysogenic conversion from a nontoxigenic to a toxigenic phenotype has been shown to occur in situ. Growth of toxigenic strains of *C. diphtheriae* under iron-limiting conditions leads to the optimal expression of diphtheria toxin, and these conditions are believed to be a mechanism of pathogenesis during human infection.

EPIDEMIOLOGY

C. diphtheriae is transmitted via the aerosol route, primarily during close contact. There are no significant reservoirs other than humans. The incubation period for respiratory diphtheria is 2–5 days; however, disease can develop as long as 10 days after exposure. Before the vaccine era, most individuals over the age of 10 were immune to *C. diphtheriae*; infants were protected by maternal IgG antibodies but became susceptible after ~6 months of age. Thus, the disease was seen primarily in children and nonimmune young adults. In temperate regions, respiratory diphtheria occurs year-round but is most common during winter months.

The development of diphtheria antitoxin and diphtheria toxoid vaccine led to the near-elimination of diphtheria in Western countries. The annual peak incidence rate was 191 cases per 100,000 population in the United States in 1921; in contrast, since 1980, the annual figure for the United States as a whole has been <5 cases. Nevertheless, pockets of colonization have persisted in North America, particularly in South Dakota, Ontario, and Washington state. Immunity induced by vaccination during childhood gradually decreases in adulthood. An estimated 30% of men 60–69 years old have antitoxin titers below the protective level. In addition to older age and lack of vaccination, risk factors for diphtheria outbreaks include alcoholism, low socioeconomic status, crowded living conditions, and Native American ethnic background. An outbreak that occurred in Seattle in 1972–1982 included 1100 cases, primarily manifesting as cutaneous disease. During the 1990s in the states of the former Soviet Union, a much larger diphtheria epidemic caused >150,000 cases and >5000 deaths. Clonally related toxigenic *C. diphtheriae* strains of the ET8 complex were associated with this outbreak. Given that the ET8 complex expressed a toxin against which the prevalent diphtheria toxoid vaccine was effective, the epidemic was attributed to failure of the public health infrastructure to effectively vaccinate the population. Beginning in 1998, the epidemic was controlled by mass vaccination programs. During the epidemic, the incidence rate was high among individuals from >15 years of age up to 50 years of age. Socioeconomic instability, migration, deteriorating public health programs, frequent vaccine shortages, delays in implementation of vaccination and of treatment in response to cases, and lack of public education and awareness were contributing factors in that outbreak.

Cutaneous diphtheria is usually a secondary infection that follows a primary skin lesion due to trauma, allergy, or autoimmunity. Most often, isolates from cases of cutaneous disease lack the *tox* gene and therefore do not express diphtheria toxin. In tropical regions, cutaneous diphtheria is more common than respiratory diphtheria. In contrast to respiratory disease, cutaneous diphtheria is not a reportable disease in United States.

Nontoxigenic strains of *C. diphtheriae* have also been associated with pharyngitis in Europe. Outbreaks have occurred among homosexual men and IV drug users.

PATHOGENESIS AND IMMUNOLOGY

Diphtheria toxin, produced by toxigenic strains of *C. diphtheriae*, is the primary virulence factor in clinical disease. The toxin is synthesized in precursor form; is released as a 535-amino-acid, single-chain protein; and has an LD_{50} of ~100 ng/kg of body weight. The toxin is produced in the pseudomembranous lesion and is taken up into the bloodstream, through which it is distributed to all organ systems. Once bound to its cell surface receptor (a heparin-binding, epidermal growth factor–like precursor), the toxin is internalized by receptor-mediated endocytosis and enters the cytosol from an acidified early endosomal compartment. In vitro, the toxin may be separated into two chains after digestion with serine proteases: the N-terminal A fragment and the C-terminal B fragment. Delivery of the A fragment into the eukaryotic cell cytosol results in irreversible inhibition of protein synthesis by NAD+-dependent ADP ribosylation of elongation factor 2. The eventual result is the death of the cell.

In 1926, Ramon at the Institut Pasteur found that formalinization of diphtheria toxin resulted in the production of diphtheria toxoid, which was nontoxic but highly immunogenic. Subsequent studies showed that immunization with diphtheria toxoid elicited antibodies that neutralized the toxin and prevented most manifestations of diphtheria. In the 1930s, mass immunization of children and susceptible adults commenced in the United States and Europe.

Individuals with an antitoxin titer of >0.01 unit/mL are at low risk of diphtheria disease. In populations where a majority of individuals have protective antitoxin titers, the carrier rate for toxigenic strains of *C. diphtheriae* decreases and the overall risk of diphtheria among susceptible individuals is reduced. Nevertheless, individuals with nonprotective titers may contract diphtheria through either travel or exposure to individuals who have recently returned from regions where the disease is endemic.

Characteristic pathologic findings of diphtheria include mucosal ulcers with a pseudomembranous coating composed of an inner band of fibrin and a luminal band of neutrophils. Initially white and firmly adherent, in advanced diphtheria the pseudomembranes turn gray and even green or black as necrosis progresses. Mucosal ulcers result from toxin-induced necrosis of the epithelium accompanied by edema, hyperemia, and vascular congestion of the submucosal base. A fibrinosuppurative exudate from the ulcer develops into the pseudomembrane. Ulcers and pseudomembranes in severe respiratory diphtheria may extend from the pharynx into medium-sized bronchial airways. Expanding and sloughing membranes may result in fatal airway obstruction.

APPROACH TO THE PATIENT:
Diphtheria

Although diphtheria is rare in the United States and other developed countries, this diagnosis should be considered in patients who have severe pharyngitis, particularly with difficulty swallowing, respiratory compromise, or signs of systemic disease including myocarditis or generalized weakness. In the differential diagnosis, the leading causes of pharyngitis that should be considered are respiratory viruses (rhinoviruses, influenza viruses, parainfluenza viruses, coronaviruses, and adenoviruses; ~25% of cases), group A streptococci (15–30%), group C streptococci (~5%), atypical bacteria such as *Mycoplasma pneumoniae* and *Chlamydophila pneumoniae* (15–20% in some series), and other viruses such as herpes simplex virus (~4%) and Epstein-Barr virus (EBV; <1% in infectious mononucleosis). Less common causes are acute HIV infection, infection with *Neisseria gonorrhoeae*, fusobacterial infection (e.g., Lemierre syndrome), and thrush due to *Candida albicans* or other *Candida* species. The presence of a pharyngeal pseudomembrane or an extensive exudate should prompt consideration of diphtheria (Fig. 131-1).

CLINICAL MANIFESTATIONS

Respiratory Diphtheria The clinical diagnosis of diphtheria is based on the constellation of sore throat; adherent tonsillar, pharyngeal, or nasal pseudomembranous lesions; and low-grade fever. In addition, diagnosis requires the isolation of *C. diphtheriae* or the histopathologic isolation of compatible gram-positive organisms. The Centers for Disease Control and Prevention (CDC) recognizes confirmed respiratory diphtheria (laboratory proven or epidemiologically linked to a culture-confirmed case) and probable respiratory diphtheria (clinically compatible but not laboratory proven or epidemiologically linked). Carriers are defined as individuals who have positive cultures for *C. diphtheriae* and either are asymptomatic or have symptoms but lack pseudomembranes. Most patients seek medical care for initial manifestations of sore throat and fever. Occasionally, weakness, dysphagia, headache, and voice change are the initial manifestations. Neck edema and difficulty breathing are seen in more advanced cases and carry a poor prognosis.

The systemic manifestations of diphtheria stem from the effects of diphtheria toxin and include weakness as a result of neurotoxicity and cardiac arrhythmias or congestive heart failure due to myocarditis. The pseudomembranous lesion is most often located in the tonsillopharyngeal region. Less commonly, the lesions are detected in the larynx, nares, and trachea or bronchial passages. Large pseudomembranes are associated with severe disease and a poor prognosis. A few patients develop massive swelling of the tonsils and present with "bull-neck" diph-

FIGURE 131-1 Respiratory diphtheria due to toxigenic *C. diphtheriae* producing exudative pharyngitis in a 47-year-old woman with neck edema and a pseudomembrane extending from the uvula to the pharyngeal wall. The characteristic white pseudomembrane is caused by diphtheria toxin–mediated necrosis of the respiratory epithelial layer, producing fibrinous coagulative exudate. Submucosal edema adds to airway narrowing. The pharyngitis is acute in onset, and respiratory obstruction from the pseudomembrane may occur in severe cases. Inoculation of pseudomembrane fragments or submembranous swabs onto Löffler's or tellurite selective medium reveals *C. diphtheriae*. (*Photograph by P. Strebel, MD, used by permission. From Kadirova et al.*)

FIGURE 131-2 Cutaneous diphtheria due to nontoxigenic *C. diphtheriae* on the lower extremity. *(From the Centers for Disease Control and Prevention.)*

theria, which results from massive edema of the submandibular and paratracheal region and is further characterized by foul breath, thick speech, and stridorous breathing. The diphtheritic pseudomembrane is gray or whitish and sharply demarcated. Unlike the exudative lesion associated with streptococcal pharyngitis, the pseudomembrane in diphtheria is tightly adherent to the underlying tissues. Attempts to dislodge the membrane may cause bleeding. Hoarseness suggests laryngeal diphtheria, in which laryngoscopy may be diagnostically helpful.

Cutaneous Diphtheria This is a variable dermatosis most often characterized by punched-out ulcerative lesions with necrotic sloughing or pseudomembrane formation (Fig. 131-2). The diagnosis requires cultivation of *C. diphtheriae* from lesions, which most commonly occur on the extremities. Patients usually seek medical attention because of nonhealing or enlarging skin ulcers, which may be associated with a preexisting wound or dermatoses such as eczema, psoriasis, and venous stasis disease. The lesions rarely exceed 5 cm.

Other Clinical Manifestations *C. diphtheriae* causes rare cases of endocarditis and septic arthritis, most often in patients with preexisting risk factors such as cardiac valvular disease, injection drug use, or cirrhosis.

COMPLICATIONS

Airway obstruction poses a significant early risk in patients presenting with advanced diphtheria. Pseudomembranes may slough and obstruct the airway or may advance to the larynx or into the tracheobronchial tree. Children are particularly prone to obstruction because of their small airways.

Polyneuropathy and myocarditis are late toxic manifestations of diphtheria. During the outbreak in the Kyrgyz Republic in 1995, myocarditis was seen in 22% and neuropathy in 5% of hospitalized patients. The mortality rate was 7% among patients with myocarditis as opposed to 2% among those without myocardial manifestations. The median time to death in hospitalized patients was 4.5 days. Myocarditis is typically associated with dysrhythmia of the conduction tract and dilated cardiomyopathy.

Neurologic manifestations may appear during the first or second week of illness, typically beginning with dysphagia and nasal dysarthria and progressing to other signs of cranial nerve involvement, including weakness of the tongue and facial numbness. Ciliary paralysis, which is typical, manifests as blurred vision due to paralysis of pupillary accommodation, with a preserved light reflex. Cranial neuropathy may be followed by respiratory and abdominal muscle weakness requiring artificial ventilation. Several weeks later—sometimes as cranial neuropathy is improving—a generalized sensorimotor polyneuropathy may appear, with prominent autonomic manifestations (including hypotension) in

some cases. The clinical syndrome and the findings on lumbar puncture of raised levels of protein without pleocytosis in cerebrospinal fluid resemble Guillain-Barré syndrome (Chap. 380). Pathologically, diphtheria neuropathy is a noninflammatory demyelinating disorder mediated by the exotoxin. Gradual improvement is the rule in patients who survive the acute phase.

Other complications of diphtheria include pneumonia, renal failure, encephalitis, cerebral infarction, and pulmonary embolism. Serum sickness can result from treatment with diphtheria antitoxin (see "Diphtheria Treatment," below).

DIAGNOSIS

The diagnosis of diphtheria is based on clinical signs and symptoms plus laboratory confirmation. Respiratory diphtheria should be considered in patients with sore throat, pharyngeal exudates, and fever. Other symptoms may include hoarseness, stridor, or palatal paralysis. The presence of a pseudomembrane should prompt consideration of diphtheria. Once a clinical diagnosis of diphtheria is made, diphtheria antitoxin should be administered as soon as possible.

Laboratory diagnosis is based either on cultivation of *C. diphtheriae* or toxigenic *C. ulcerans* from the site of infection or on the demonstration of local lesions with characteristic histopathology. *C. pseudodiphtheriticum*, a nontoxigenic organism, is a common component of the normal throat flora and does not pose a significant risk. Throat samples should be submitted to the laboratory for culture with the notation that diphtheria is being considered. This information should prompt cultivation on special selective medium and subsequent biochemical testing to differentiate *C. diphtheriae* from other nasopharyngeal commensal corynebacteria. All laboratory isolates of *C. diphtheriae*, including nontoxigenic strains, should be submitted to the CDC.

A diagnosis of cutaneous diphtheria requires laboratory confirmation since the lesions are not characteristic and are clinically indistinguishable from other dermatoses. Diphtheritic ulcers occasionally—but not consistently—have a punched-out appearance (Fig. 131-2). Patients in whom cutaneous diphtheria is identified should have the nasopharynx cultured for *C. diphtheriae*. The laboratory media for cutaneous diphtheria are the same as those used for respiratory diphtheria: Löffler's or Tinsdale's selective medium in addition to nonselective medium such as blood agar. As has been mentioned, respiratory diphtheria remains a notifiable disease in the United States, whereas cutaneous diphtheria is not.

℞ DIPHTHERIA

DIPHTHERIA ANTITOXIN Prompt administration of diphtheria antitoxin is critical in the management of respiratory diphtheria. The antitoxin—a horse antiserum—is effective in reducing the extent of local disease as well as the risk of complications of myocarditis and neuropathy. Rapid institution of antitoxin therapy is also associated with a significant reduction in mortality risk. Because diphtheria antitoxin cannot neutralize cell-bound toxin, prompt initiation is important. This product, which is no longer made commercially in the United States, is available from the CDC under an investigational new drug protocol and may be obtained by calling the Bacterial Vaccine Preventable Disease Branch of the National Immunization Program at 404-639-8257 between 8:00 A.M. and 4:30 P.M. U.S. Eastern time or at 770-488-7100 at other hours; the relevant website is *http://www.cdc.gov/nip/vaccine/dat/default.htm*. The current protocol for the use of antitoxin includes a test dose to rule out immediate-type hypersensitivity. Patients who exhibit hypersensitivity require desensitization before a full therapeutic dose of antitoxin is administered.

ANTIMICROBIAL THERAPY Antibiotics are used in the management of diphtheria primarily to prevent transmission to other susceptible contacts. Recommended options for the treatment of patients with respiratory diphtheria are as follows: (1) procaine penicillin G at a dosage of 600,000 units (for children, 12,500–25,000 U/kg) IM every 12 h until the patient can swallow comfortably, after which oral penicillin V is given at 125–250 mg four times daily to complete a 14-day course; or (2) erythromycin at a dosage of 500 mg IV every 6 h (for children, 40–50 mg/kg per day IV in two or four divided doses) until the patient can swallow comfortably, after which 500 mg is given PO four times daily to complete a 14-day course.

A clinical study in Vietnam found that penicillin was associated with a more rapid resolution of fever and a lower rate of bacterial resistance than erythromycin; however, relapses were more common with penicillin. Erythromycin therapy targets protein synthesis and thus offers the presumed benefit of stopping toxin synthesis more quickly than a cell wall–active β-lactam agent. Alternative agents for patients who are allergic to penicillin or cannot take erythromycin include rifampin and clindamycin. Eradication of *C. diphtheriae* should be documented at least 1 day after antimicrobial therapy is complete. A repeat throat culture 2 weeks later is recommended. For patients in whom the organism is not eradicated after a 14-day course of erythromycin or penicillin, an additional 10-day course followed by repeat culture is recommended.

Cutaneous diphtheria should be treated as described above for respiratory disease. Individuals infected with toxigenic strains should receive antitoxin. It is important to treat the underlying cause of the dermatoses in addition to the superinfection with *C. diphtheriae*.

Patients who recover from respiratory or cutaneous diphtheria should have antitoxin levels measured. If diphtheria antitoxin has been administered, this test should be performed 6 months later. Patients who recover from respiratory or cutaneous diphtheria should receive the appropriate vaccine (see "Prevention," below) to ensure the development of protective antibody titers, which does not occur in all cases.

MANAGEMENT Patients in whom diphtheria is suspected should be hospitalized in respiratory isolation rooms, with close monitoring of cardiac and respiratory function. A cardiac workup is recommended to assess the possibility of myocarditis. In patients with extensive pseudomembranes, consultation with an anesthesiologist or an ear, nose, and throat specialist is recommended because of the possibility that tracheostomy or intubation will be required. In some settings, pseudomembranes can be removed surgically. Treatment with glucocorticoids has not been shown to reduce the risk of myocarditis or polyneuropathy.

PROGNOSIS

Fatal pseudomembranous diphtheria typically occurs in patients with nonprotective antibody titers and in unimmunized patients. The pseudomembrane may increase in size from the time it is first noted. Risk factors for death include bullneck diphtheria; myocarditis with ventricular tachycardia; atrial fibrillation; complete heart block; an age of >60 years or <6 months; alcoholism; extensive pseudomembrane elongation; and laryngeal, tracheal, or bronchial involvement. Another important predictor of fatal outcome is the interval between local disease development and antitoxin administration. Cutaneous diphtheria has a low mortality rate and is rarely associated with myocarditis or peripheral neuropathy.

PREVENTION

Vaccination Sustained campaigns for vaccination of children and adequate boosting vaccination of adults are responsible for the exceedingly low incidence of diphtheria in most developed nations. At present, diphtheria toxoid vaccine is coadministered with tetanus (with or without acellular pertussis) vaccine. DTaP (full-level diphtheria and tetanus toxoids and acellular pertussis vaccine, adsorbed) is the currently recommended vaccine for children up to the age of 7; DTaP replaced DTP (diphtheria and tetanus toxoids and whole-cell pertussis vaccine) in 1997. Tdap is a tetanus toxoid, reduced diphtheria toxoid, and acellular pertussis vaccine formulated for adolescents and adults. Tdap was licensed for use in the United States in 2005 and is the recommended booster vaccine for children 11–12 years old and the recommended catch-up vaccine for children 7–10 and 13–18 years old. As of 2006, it is recommended that (1) adults 19–64 years old receive a single dose of Tdap if their last dose of Td (tetanus and reduced-dose diphtheria toxoids, adsorbed) was >10 years earlier and (2) intervals of <10 years be implemented for Tdap vaccination of health care workers, adults anticipating contact with infants, and adults not previously vaccinated for pertussis. Adults who have received acellular pertussis vaccines should continue to receive decennial Td booster vaccinations. The vaccination schedule is detailed in Chap. 116.

Prophylaxis of Contacts Close contacts of diphtheria cases should undergo throat culture to determine whether they are carriers. After samples for throat culture are obtained, antimicrobial prophylaxis should be considered for all close contacts, even those who are culture-negative. The options are 7–10 days of oral erythromycin or one dose of IM benzathine penicillin G (1.2 million units for persons ≥6 years old or 600,000 units for children <6 years old).

Contacts of diphtheria cases who have an uncertain immunization status should receive the appropriate diphtheria toxoid–containing vaccine. Tdap (rather than Td) is now recommended as the booster vaccine of choice for adults who have not recently received an acellular pertussis–containing vaccine. Carriers of *C. diphtheriae* in the community should be treated and vaccinated when identified.

NONDIPHTHERIAL CORYNEBACTERIA AND RELATED SPECIES

Nondiphtherial corynebacteria, which are also referred to as *diphtheroids* or *coryneforms*, are a widely diverse collection of bacteria that are taxonomically lumped together on the basis of their 16S rDNA signature nucleotides. The diversity of this group is exemplified by the wide range in guanine-plus-cytosine content (45–70%). Although frequently considered colonizers or contaminants, the nondiphtherial corynebacteria have been associated with invasive disease, particularly in immunocompromised patients. Specifically, for example, these organisms have been implicated in bacteremia, particularly in association with catheterization, endocarditis, prosthetic valve infection, meningitis, neurosurgical shunt infection, brain abscess, peritonitis (often in the setting of chronic ambulatory peritoneal dialysis), osteomyelitis, septic arthritis, urinary tract infection, empyema, and pneumonia. Patients infected with nondiphtherial corynebacteria usually have significant medical comorbidity or immunosuppression. Several of these organisms, including *C. jeikeium* and *C. urealyticum*, are associated with resistance to multiple antibiotics. The related organism *Rhodococcus equi* is associated with necrotizing pneumonia and granulomatous infection, particularly in immunocompromised individuals. Other related species that can cause infections in humans are *Actinomyces* (formerly *Corynebacterium*) *pyogenes* and *Arcanobacterium* (formerly *Corynebacterium*) *haemolyticum*.

MICROBIOLOGY AND LABORATORY DIAGNOSIS

These organisms are non-acid-fast, catalase-positive, aerobic or facultatively anaerobic bacilli. Their colonial morphologies vary widely; some species are small and α-hemolytic (similar to lactobacilli), whereas others form large white colonies (similar to yeasts). Many nondiphtherial coryneforms require special medium (e.g., Löffler's, Tinsdale's, or telluride medium) for growth.

EPIDEMIOLOGY

Humans are the natural reservoirs for several nondiphtherial coryneforms, including *C. xerosis*, *C. pseudodiphtheriticum*, *C. striatum*, *C. minutissimum*, *C. jeikeium*, *C. urealyticum*, and *A. haemolyticum*. Animal reservoirs are responsible for carriage of *A. pyogenes*, *C. ulcerans*, and *C. pseudotuberculosis*. Soil is the natural reservoir for *R. equi*.

C. pseudodiphtheriticum is part of the normal flora of the human pharynx and skin. *C. xerosis* is found on the skin, nasopharynx, and conjunctiva; *C. auris* in the external auditory canal; and *C. striatum* in the anterior nares and on the skin. *C. jeikeium* and *C. urealyticum* are found in the axilla, groin, and perineum, particularly in hospitalized patients. *C. ulcerans* and *C. pseudotuberculosis* infections have been associated with the consumption of raw milk from infected cattle.

Specific Nondiphtherial Coryneforms • *C. ulcerans* This organism causes a diphtheria-like illness and produces both diphtheria toxin and a dermonecrotic toxin. *C. ulcerans* is a commensal in horses and cattle and has been isolated from cow's milk. The organism causes exudative pharyngitis, primarily during summer months, in rural areas, and among individuals exposed to cattle. In contrast to diphtheria, *C. ulcerans* infection is considered a zoonosis, and person-to-person transmission has not been firmly established. Nevertheless, treatment with antitoxin and antibiotics should be initiated when respiratory *C. ulcerans* is identified, and a contact investigation (including throat cultures to determine the need for antimicrobial prophylaxis and vaccination with the appropriate diphtheria toxoid–containing vaccine for unimmunized human contacts) should be conducted. The organism grows on Löffler's, Tinsdale's, and telluride media as well as blood agar. In addition to exudative pharyngitis, cutaneous disease due to *C. ulcerans* has been reported. *C. ulcerans* is susceptible to a wide panel of antibiotics. Erythromycin and macrolides appear to be the first-line agents.

C. pseudotuberculosis (ovis)

Infections caused by *C. pseudotuberculosis* are rare and are reported almost exclusively from Australia. *C. pseudotuberculosis* causes suppurative granulomatous lymphadenitis and an eosinophilic pneumonia syndrome among individuals who handle horses, cattle, goats, and deer or who drink unpasteurized milk. The organism is an important veterinary pathogen, causing suppurative lymphadenitis, abscesses, and pneumonia, but is rarely a human pathogen. Successful treatment with erythromycin or tetracycline has been reported, with surgery also performed when indicated.

C. jeikeium (GROUP JK)

After a 1976 survey of diseases caused by nondiphtherial corynebacteria, CDC Group JK was recognized as an important opportunistic pathogen among neutropenic patients and later emerged in HIV-infected patients as an AIDS-associated opportunistic infection. This led to the organism's reclassification as a separate species, *C. jeikeium*. The predominant syndrome associated with *C. jeikeium* is sepsis, which can occur in conjunction with pneumonia, endocarditis, meningitis, osteomyelitis, or epidural abscess. Risk factors for *C. jeikeium* infection include hematologic malignancy, neutropenia from comorbid conditions, prolonged hospitalization, exposure to multiple antibiotics, and skin disruption. There is evidence that *C. jeikeium* is part of the normal flora of the inguinal, axillary, genital, and perirectal areas in hospitalized patients.

Broad-spectrum antimicrobial therapy appears to select for colonization. Originally described in the United States, *C. jeikeium* has also been reported in Europe. The gram-positive coccobacilli, which slightly resemble streptococci, grow as small, gray to white, glistening, nonhemolytic colonies on blood agar. *C. jeikeium* lacks urease and nitrate reductase and does not ferment most carbohydrates. It is resistant to most antibiotics tested except for vancomycin. Effective therapy involves removal of the source of infection, be it a catheter, a prosthetic joint, or a prosthetic valve. There have been efforts to prevent *C. jeikeium* infection by use of antibacterial soap in the care of high-risk patients in intensive care settings.

C. urealyticum (GROUP D2)

Identified as a urease-positive nondiphtherial *Corynebacterium* in 1972, *C. urealyticum* is an opportunistic cause of sepsis and urinary tract infection. This organism appears to be the etiologic agent of a severe urinary tract syndrome known as *alkaline-encrusted cystitis*: a chronic inflammatory bladder infection associated with deposition of ammonium magnesium phosphate on the surface and walls of ulcerating lesions in the bladder. In addition, *C. urealyticum* has been associated with pneumonia, peritonitis, endocarditis, osteomyelitis, and wound infection. It is similar to *C. jeikeium* in its resistance to most antibiotics except vancomycin, which has been used successfully in the treatment of severe infections.

C. minutissimum

Erythrasma is a cutaneous infection producing reddish-brown, macular, scaly, pruritic intertriginous patches. The dermatologic presentation under the Wood's lamp is of coral-red fluorescence. *C. minutissimum* appears to be a common cause of erythrasma, although there is evidence for a polymicrobial etiology in certain settings. In addition, this fluorescent microbe has been associated with bacteremia in patients with hematologic malignancy. Erythrasma responds to topical erythromycin, clarithromycin, clindamycin, or fusidic acid, although more severe infections may require oral macrolide therapy.

Other Nondiphtherial Corynebacteria

C. xerosis is a human commensal found in the conjunctiva, nasopharynx, and skin. This nontoxigenic organism is occasionally identified as a source of invasive infection in immunocompromised or postoperative patients and prosthetic joint recipients. *C. striatum* is found in the anterior nares and on the skin, face, and upper torso of normal individuals. Also nontoxigenic, this organism has been associated with invasive opportunistic infections in severely ill or immunocompromised patients. *C. amycolatum* is a new species isolated from human skin and is identified on the basis of a unique 16S ribosomal RNA sequence associated with opportunistic infection. *C. glucuronolyticum* is a new nonlipophilic species that causes male genitourinary tract infections such as prostatitis and urethritis. These infections may be successfully treated with a wide variety of antibacterial agents, including β-lactams, rifampin, aminoglycosides, or vancomycin; however, the organism appears to be resistant to fluoroquinolones, macrolides, and tetracyclines. *C. imitans* has been identified in Eastern Europe as a nontoxigenic cause of pharyngitis. *C. auris* has been isolated from children with otitis media and is susceptible to fluoroquinolones, rifampin, tetracycline, and vancomycin but resistant to penicillin G and variably susceptible to macrolides. *C. pseudodiphtheriticum* (*C. hofmannii*) is a nontoxigenic component of the normal human flora. Human infections—particularly endocarditis of either prosthetic or native valves and invasive pneumonia—have been identified only rarely. Although *C. pseudodiphtheriticum* may be isolated from the nasopharynx of patients with suspected diphtheria, it is part of the normal flora and does not produce diphtheria toxin. *C. propinquum*, a close relative of *C. pseudodiphtheriticum*, is part of CDC Group ANF-3 and is isolated from human respiratory tract specimens and blood. *C. afermentans* subspecies *lipophilum* belongs to CDC Group ANF-1 and has been isolated from human blood and abscess infections. *C. accolens* has been isolated from wound drainage, throat swabs, and sputum and is typically identified as a satellite of staphylococcal organisms; it has been associated with endocarditis. *C. bovis* is a veterinary commensal that has not been clearly identified as a cause of human disease. *C. aquaticum* is a water-associated organism that is occasionally isolated from patients using medical devices (e.g., for chronic ambulatory peritoneal dialysis or venous access).

Rhodococcus

Rhodococcus species are phylogenetically related to the corynebacteria. These gram-positive coccobacilli have been associated with tuberculosis-like infections in humans with granulomatous pathology. Although *R. equi* is best known, other species have been identified, including *R.* (also *Gordonia*) *bronchialis*, *R.* (also *Tsukamurella*) *aurantiacus*, *R. luteus*, *R. erythropolis*, *R. rhodochrous*, and *R. rubropertinctus*. *R. equi* has been recognized as a cause of pneumonia in horses since the 1920s; it causes related infections in cattle, sheep, and swine. *R. equi* is found in soil as an environmental microbe. The organisms vary in length; appear as spherical to long, curved, clubbed rods; and produce large, irregular mucoid colonies. *R. equi* does not ferment carbohydrates or liquefy gelatin and is often acid fast. An intracellular pathogen of macrophages, *R. equi* can cause granulomatous necrosis and caseation. The organism has been identified most commonly in pulmonary infections, but infections of brain, bone, and skin have also been reported. Most commonly, *R. equi* disease manifests as nodular cavitary pneumonia of the upper lobe—a picture similar to that seen in tuberculosis or nocardiosis. Most patients are immunocompromised, often with HIV infection. Subcutaneous nodular lesions have also been identified. The involvement of *R. equi* should be considered in any patient presenting with a tuberculosis-like syndrome. Infection due to *R. equi* has been treated successfully with antibiotics that penetrate intracellularly, including macrolides, clindamycin, rifampin, and trimethoprim-sulfamethoxazole. β-Lactam antibiotics have not been useful. The organism is routinely susceptible to vancomycin, which is considered the drug of choice.

Actinomyces pyogenes

A cause of seasonal leg ulcers in humans in rural Thailand, *A. pyogenes* is a well-known pathogen of cattle, sheep, goats, and pigs. A few human cases of sepsis, endocarditis, septic arthritis, pneumonia, meningitis, and empyema have been reported.

The agent is susceptible to β-lactams, tetracycline, aminoglycosides, and fluoroquinolones.

Arcanobacterium haemolyticum

A. haemolyticum was identified as an agent of wound infections in U.S. soldiers in the South Pacific during World War II. This organism appears to be a commensal of the human nasopharynx and skin but has been implicated as a cause of pharyngitis and chronic skin ulcers. In contrast to the much more common pharyngitis caused by *Streptococcus pyogenes*, *A. haemolyticum* pharyngitis is associated with a scarlatiniform rash on the trunk and proximal extremities in about half of cases; this illness is occasionally confused with toxic shock syndrome. Because *A. haemolyticum* pharyngitis primarily affects teenagers, it has been postulated that the rash-pharyngitis syndrome may represent copathogenicity or synergy with EBV or opportunistic secondary infection complicating EBV infection. *A. haemolyticum* has also been reported as a cause of bacteremia, soft tissue infection, osteomyelitis, and cavitary pneumonia, predominantly in the setting of underlying diabetes mellitus. The organism is susceptible to β-lactams, macrolides, fluoroquinolones, clindamycin, vancomycin, and doxycycline. Penicillin resistance has been reported.

FURTHER READINGS

CENTERS FOR DISEASE CONTROL AND PREVENTION: Availability of diphtheria antitoxin through an investigational new drug protocol. MMWR 53:413, 2004

———: Vaccine preventable deaths and the Global Immunization Vision and Strategy, 2006–2015. MMWR 55:511, 2006

DITTMANN S et al: Successful control of epidemic diphtheria in the states of the former Union of Soviet Socialist Republics: Lessons learned. J Infect Dis 181(Suppl 1):S10, 2000

HOLMES RK: Biology and molecular epidemiology of diphtheria toxin and the tox gene. J Infect Dis 181(Suppl 1):S156, 2000

KADIROVA R et al: Clinical characteristics and management of 676 hospitalized diphtheria cases, Kyrgyz Republic, 1995. J Infect Dis 181(Suppl 1):S110, 2000

KRETSINGER K et al: Preventing tetanus, diphtheria, and pertussis among adults: Use of tetanus toxoid, reduced diphtheria toxoid, and acellular pertussis vaccine; recommendations of the Advisory Committee on Immunization Practices (ACIP) and recommendation of ACIP, supported by the Healthcare Infection Control Practices Advisory Committee (HICPAC), for use of Tdap among health-care personnel. MMWR Recomm Rep 55(RR-17):1, 2006

MACGREGOR RR: *Corynebacterium diphtheriae*, in *Principles and Practice of Infectious Diseases*, 6th ed, GL Mandell et al (eds). Philadelphia, Elsevier Churchill Livingstone, 2005, pp 2457–2465

MCNEIL SA et al: Comparison of the safety and immunogenicity of concomitant and sequential administration of an adult formulation tetanus and diphtheria toxoids adsorbed combined with acellular pertussis (Tdap) vaccine and trivalent inactivated influenza vaccine in adults. Vaccine 25:3464, 2007; Epub 2007 Jan 9.

MEYER DK, REBOLI AC: Other coryneform bacteria and *Rhodococcus*, in *Principles and Practice of Infectious Diseases*, 6th ed, GL Mandell et al (eds). Philadelphia, Elsevier Churchill Livingstone, 2005, pp 2465–2478

PICHICHERO ME et al: Combined tetanus, diphtheria, and 5-component pertussis vaccine for use in adolescents and adults. JAMA 293:3003, 2005

132 Infections Caused by *Listeria monocytogenes*
Elizabeth L. Hohmann, Daniel A. Portnoy

Listeria monocytogenes is a food-borne pathogen that can cause serious infections, particularly in pregnant women and immunocompromised individuals. A ubiquitous saprophytic environmental bacterium, *L. monocytogenes* is also a pathogen with a broad host range. Humans are probably accidental hosts for this microorganism. *L. monocytogenes* is of interest not only to clinicians but also to basic scientists as a model intracellular pathogen that is used to study basic mechanisms of microbial pathogenesis and host immunity.

MICROBIOLOGY

L. monocytogenes is a facultatively anaerobic, nonsporulating, gram-positive rod that grows over a broad temperature range, including refrigeration temperatures. This organism is motile during growth at low temperatures but much less so at 37°C. The vast majority of cases of human listerial disease can be traced to serotypes 1/2a, 1/2b, and 4. *L. monocytogenes* is weakly β-hemolytic on blood agar, and (as detailed below) its β-hemolysin is an essential determinant of its pathogenicity.

PATHOGENESIS

Infections with *L. monocytogenes* follow ingestion of contaminated food that contains the bacteria at high concentrations. The conversion from environmental saprophyte to a pathogen involves the coordinate regulation of bacterial determinants of pathogenesis that mediate entry into cells, intracellular growth, and cell-to-cell spread. One essential determinant of *L. monocytogenes* pathogenesis is the transcriptional activator PrfA, which activates the majority of genes required for cell entry and intracellular parasitism. Many of the organism's pathogenic strategies can be examined experimentally in tissue culture models of infection; such a model is presented in Fig. 132-1. Like other enteric

FIGURE 132-1 Stages in the intracellular life cycle of *Listeria monocytogenes*. The central diagram depicts cell entry, escape from a vacuole, actin nucleation, actin-based motility, and cell-to-cell spread. Surrounding the diagram are representative electron micrographs from which it was derived. ActA, surface protein mediating nucleation of host actin filaments to propel bacteria intra- and intercellularly; LLO, listeriolysin O; PLCs, phospholipases C; Inl, internalin. See text for further details. (*Adapted with permission from LG Tilney and DA Portnoy: Actin filaments and the growth, movement, and spread of the intracellular bacterial parasite, Listeria monocytogenes. J Cell Biol 109:1597, 1989. © Rockefeller University Press.*)

pathogens, *L. monocytogenes* induces its own internalization by cells that are not normally phagocytic. Its entry into cells is mediated by host surface proteins classified as internalins. Internalin-mediated entry is important in the crossing of intestinal, blood-brain, and fetoplacental barriers, although how *L. monocytogenes* traffics from the intestine to the brain or fetus is only beginning to be investigated. In a pregnant guinea pig model of infection, *L. monocytogenes* was shown to traffic from maternal organs to the placenta; surprisingly, however, it also trafficked from the placenta back to maternal organs.

Perhaps the most important determinant of the pathogenesis of *L. monocytogenes* is its β-hemolysin, listeriolysin O (LLO). LLO is a pore-forming, cholesterol-dependent cytolysin. (Related cytolysins include streptolysin O, pneumolysin, and perfringolysin O, all of which are produced by extracellular pathogens.) LLO is largely responsible for mediating the rupture of the phagosomal membrane that forms after phagocytosis of *L. monocytogenes*. LLO probably acts by inserting itself into an acidifying phagosome, thereby preventing the vesicle's maturation. In addition, LLO acts as a translocation pore for one or both of the *L. monocytogenes* phospholipases that also contribute to vacuolar lysis. LLO synthesis and activity are controlled at multiple levels to ensure that its lytic activity is limited to acidic vacuoles and does not affect the cytosol. Mutations in LLO that influence its synthesis, cytosolic half-life, or pH optimum cause premature toxicity to infected cells. There is an inverse relationship between toxicity and virulence—i.e., the more cytotoxic the strain, the less virulent it is in animals.

Once in the cytosol, *L. monocytogenes* grows rapidly, with intracellular doubling times equivalent to those in rich media. One of the PrfA-regulated genes encodes a hexose-phosphate transporter that facilitates the growth of cytosolic bacteria on phosphorylated glucose derivatives of host origin.

Shortly after exposure to the mammalian-cell cytosol, *L. monocytogenes* produces ActA, another PrfA-regulated surface protein that mediates the nucleation of host actin filaments to propel the bacteria intra- and intercellularly. ActA mimics host proteins of the Wiskott-Aldrich syndrome protein (WASP) family by promoting the actin nucleation properties of the Arp2/3 complex. Thus, *L. monocytogenes* can enter the cytosol of almost any eukaryotic cell or cell extract and can exploit a conserved and essential actin-based motility system. Other pathogens as diverse as certain *Shigella*, *Mycobacterium*, *Rickettsia*, and *Burkholderia* spp. use a related pathogenic strategy that allows cell-to-cell spread without exposure to the extracellular milieu.

IMMUNE RESPONSE

The innate and acquired immune responses to *L. monocytogenes* have been studied extensively in mice. Shortly after IV injection, most bacteria are found in Kupffer cells in the liver, with some organisms in splenic macrophages. Listeriae that survive the bactericidal activity of initially infected macrophages grow in the cytosol and spread from cell to cell. In the liver, the result is infection of hepatocytes. Neutrophils are crucial to host defense during the first 24 h of infection, while influx of activated macrophages from the bone marrow is critical subsequently. Mice that survive sublethal infection clear the infection within a week, with consequent sterile immunity. Knockout mice have been used to show that interferon γ and tumor necrosis factor (TNF) are essential in controlling infection. While innate immunity is sufficient to control infection, the acquired immune response is required for sterile immunity. Immunity is cell-mediated; antibody plays no measurable role. The critical effector cells are cytotoxic (CD8+) T cells that recognize and lyse infected cells. The bacteria grow and spread from cell to cell. The host recognizes and lyses infected cells, and extracellular bacteria are killed by circulating activated phagocytes. A hallmark of the *L. monocytogenes* model is that killed vaccines do not provide protective immunity. The explanation for this fundamental observation is multifactorial, involving the generation of appropriate cytokines and the compartmentalization of bacterial proteins for antigen processing and presentation.

EPIDEMIOLOGY

L. monocytogenes usually enters the body via the gastrointestinal tract in foods. Listeriosis is most often sporadic, although outbreaks do occur. Recent annual incidences in the United States range from 2 to 9 cases per 1 million population. No epidemiologic or clinical evidence supports human-to-human transmission (other than vertical transmission from mother to fetus) or waterborne infection. In line with its survival and multiplication at refrigeration temperatures, *L. monocytogenes* is commonly found in processed and unprocessed foods of animal and plant origin, especially soft cheeses, delicatessen meats, hot dogs, milk, and cold salads. Because food supplies are increasingly centralized and normal hosts tolerate the organism well, outbreaks may not be immediately apparent; pulsed-field gel electrophoresis has proved useful in linking cases to specific foods. FoodNet, an active U.S. surveillance program, has demonstrated decreases in listeriosis incidence, although recent data from some European countries show a stable or increased number of cases, perhaps because of enhanced active surveillance. The U.S. Food and Drug Administration has a zero-tolerance policy for *L. monocytogenes* in ready-to-eat foods.

DIAGNOSIS

Symptoms of listerial infection overlap greatly with those of other infectious diseases. Timely diagnosis requires that the illness be considered in groups at risk: pregnant women; elderly persons; neonates; individuals immunocompromised by organ transplants, cancer, or treatment with TNF antagonists or glucocorticoids; and patients with a variety of chronic medical conditions, including alcoholism, diabetes, renal disease, rheumatologic illness, and iron overload. Meningitis in older adults (especially with parenchymal brain involvement or subcortical brain abscess) or a local outbreak of culture-negative febrile gastroenteritis should trigger consideration of *L. monocytogenes* infection. Listeriosis occasionally affects healthy, young, nonpregnant individuals. HIV-infected patients are at risk; however, listeriosis seems to be prevented by trimethoprim-sulfamethoxazole (TMP-SMX) prophylaxis targeting other AIDS-related infections. The diagnosis is typically made by culture of blood, cerebrospinal fluid (CSF), or amniotic fluid. *L. monocytogenes* may be confused with "diphtheroids" or pneumococci in gram-stained CSF or may be gram-variable and confused with *Haemophilus* spp. Serologic tests and polymerase chain reaction assays are not clinically useful diagnostic tools at present.

CLINICAL MANIFESTATIONS

Listerial infections present as several clinical syndromes, of which meningitis and septicemia are most common. Monocytosis is seen in infected rabbits but is not a hallmark of human infection.

Gastroenteritis Appreciated only since the outbreaks of the late 1980s, listerial gastroenteritis typically develops within 48 h of ingestion of a large inoculum of bacteria in contaminated foods such as milk, deli meats, and salads. Attack rates are high (50–100%). *L. monocytogenes* is neither sought nor found in routine fecal cultures, but its involvement should be considered in outbreaks when cultures for other likely pathogens are negative. Manifestations include fever, diarrhea, headache, and constitutional symptoms. The largest reported outbreak occurred in an Italian school system and included 1566 individuals; ~20% of patients were hospitalized, but only one person had a positive blood culture. Isolated gastrointestinal illness does not require antibiotic treatment. Surveillance studies show that 0.1–5% of healthy asymptomatic adults may have stool cultures positive for the organism.

Bacteremia *L. monocytogenes* septicemia presents with fever, chills, and myalgias/arthralgias and cannot be differentiated from septicemia involving other organisms. Meningeal symptoms, focal neurologic findings, or mental status changes may suggest the diagnosis. Bacteremia is documented in 70–90% of cancer patients with listeriosis. A nonspecific flulike illness with fever is a common presentation in pregnant women. Endocarditis of prosthetic and native valves is an uncommon complication, with reported fatality rates of 35–50% in case series. A lumbar puncture is often prudent, although not necessary, in pregnant women without central nervous system (CNS) symptoms.

Meningitis *L. monocytogenes* causes ~5–10% of all cases of community-acquired bacterial meningitis in adults in the United States. Case-fatality rates are reported to be 15–26% and do not appear to have changed over time. This diagnosis should be considered in all older or chronically ill adults with "aseptic" meningitis. The presentation is more frequently subacute (with illness developing over several days) than in meningitis of other bacterial etiologies, and nuchal rigidity and meningeal signs are less common. Photophobia is infrequent. Focal findings and seizures are common in some but not all series. The CSF profile in listerial meningitis most often shows white blood cell (WBC) counts in the range of 100–5000/μL (rarely higher); 75% of patients have WBC counts below 1000/μL, usually with a neutrophil predominance more modest than that in other bacterial meningitides. Low glucose levels and positive results on Gram's staining are found ~30–40% of the time.

Meningoencephalitis and Focal CNS Infection   *L. monocytogenes* can directly invade the brain parenchyma, producing either cerebritis or focal abscess. Approximately 10% of cases of CNS infection are macroscopic abscesses resulting from bacteremic seeding; the affected patients often have positive blood cultures. Concurrent meningitis can exist, but the CSF may appear normal. Abscesses can be misdiagnosed as metastatic or primary tumors and, in rare instances, occur in the cerebellum and the spinal cord. Invasion of the brainstem results in a characteristic severe rhombencephalitis, usually in otherwise healthy older adults. The presentation may be biphasic, with a prodrome of fever and headache followed by asymmetric cranial nerve deficits, cerebellar signs, and hemiparetic and hemisensory deficits. Respiratory failure can occur. The subacute course and the often minimally abnormal CSF findings may delay the diagnosis, which may be suggested by MRI images showing ring-enhancing lesions after gadolinium contrast and hyperintense lesions on diffusion-weighted imaging. MRI is superior to CT for the diagnosis of these infections.

Other Focal Infections   Focal infections of visceral organs; the eye; the pleural, peritoneal and pericardial spaces; and the bones and joints have all been reported.

Infection in Pregnancy and Neonatal Infection   Listeriosis in pregnancy is a severe and important infection. The usual presentation is a nonspecific acute or subacute febrile illness with myalgias, arthralgias, backache, and headache. Pregnant women with listeriosis are usually bacteremic. This syndrome should prompt blood cultures, especially in the absence of another reasonable explanation. Involvement of the CNS is rare in the absence of other risk factors. Preterm delivery is a common complication, and the diagnosis may be made only postpartum. As many as 70–90% of fetuses from infected women can become infected. Prepartum treatment of bacteremic women enhances the chances of delivery of a healthy infant. Women usually do well after delivery: maternal deaths are very rare, even when the diagnosis is made late in pregnancy or postpartum. Overall mortality rates for fetuses infected in utero approach 50% in some series; among live-born neonates treated with antibiotics, mortality rates are much lower (~20%). *Granulomatosis infantiseptica* is an overwhelming listerial fetal infection with miliary microabscesses and granulomas, most often in the skin, liver, and spleen. Less severe neonatal infection acquired in utero presents at birth. "Late-onset" neonatal illness typically develops ~10 days after delivery but can occur up to a month postpartum. Mothers of infants with late-onset disease are not ill.

℞ INFECTIONS CAUSED BY *LISTERIA MONOCYTOGENES*

No clinical trials have compared antimicrobial agents for the treatment of *L. monocytogenes* infections. Data obtained in studies conducted in vitro and in animals as well as observational clinical data indicate that ampicillin is the drug of choice, although penicillin is also highly active. Adults should receive IV ampicillin at high doses (2 g every 4 h), and most experts recommend the addition of gentamicin for synergy (1.0–1.7 mg/kg every 8 h). TMP-SMX, given IV, is the best alternative for the penicillin-allergic patient (15–20 mg of TMP/kg per day in divided doses every 6–8 h). The dosages recommended cover CNS infection and bacteremia (see below for duration); dosages must be reduced for patients with renal insufficiency. One small nonrandomized study supports a combination of ampicillin and TMP-SMX. Case reports document success with vancomycin, tetracycline, and erythromycin, although there are also reports of clinical failure with all three agents. Imipenem and the newer quinolones are possible alternative agents that have been efficacious in animal models, but clinical experience is very limited. Cephalosporins are *not* effective and should not be used. Neonates should receive ampicillin and gentamicin at doses based on weight.

The duration of therapy depends on the syndrome: 2 weeks for bacteremia, 3 weeks for meningitis, 6–8 weeks for brain abscess/encephalitis, and 4–6 weeks for endocarditis in both neonates and adults. Early-onset neonatal disease may be more severe and should be treated for >2 weeks.

COMPLICATIONS AND PROGNOSIS

About 50–70% of individuals who are promptly diagnosed and treated recover fully, but permanent neurologic sequelae are common in patients with brain abscess or rhombencephalitis. Of 100 live-born treated neonates in one series, 60% recovered fully, 24% died, and 13% had long-term neurologic or other complications.

PREVENTION

Healthy persons should take standard precautions to prevent foodborne illness: fully cooking meats, washing fresh vegetables, carefully cleaning utensils, and avoiding unpasteurized dairy products. In addition, persons at risk for listeriosis, including pregnant women, should avoid soft cheeses (although hard cheeses and yogurt are not problematic) and should avoid or thoroughly reheat ready-to-eat and delicatessen foods, even though the absolute risk they pose is relatively low.

FURTHER READINGS

BAKARDJIEV AI et al: *Listeria monocytogenes* traffics from maternal organs to the placenta and back. PLoS Pathog 2:e66, 2006
BORTOLUSSI R, MAILMAN TM: Listeriosis, in *Infectious Disease of the Fetus and Newborn Infant*, 6th ed, S Remington et al (eds). Philadelphia, Elsevier Saunders, 2005, p 465
HAMON M et al: *Listeria monocytogenes*: A multifaceted model. Nat Rev Microbiol 4:423, 2006
MYLONAKIS E et al: Listeriosis during pregnancy: A case series and review of 222 cases. Medicine (Baltimore) 81:260, 2002
OOI ST, LORBER B: Gastroenteritis due to *Listeria monocytogenes*. Clin Infect Dis 40:1327, 2005
PORTNOY DA (section ed): The listeriae, in *Gram-Positive Pathogens*, 2d edition, VA Fischetti et al (eds). Washington, DC, ASM Press, 2006, Section 4
TWETEN RK: Cholesterol-dependent cytolysins, a family of versatile pore-forming toxins. Infect Immun 73:6199, 2005
www.cdc.gov/foodnet/

133 Tetanus
Elias Abrutyn†

PART 7 Infectious Diseases

DEFINITION

Tetanus is a neurologic disorder, characterized by increased muscle tone and spasms, that is caused by tetanospasmin, a powerful protein toxin elaborated by *Clostridium tetani*. Tetanus occurs in several clinical forms, including generalized, neonatal, and localized disease.

ETIOLOGIC AGENT

C. tetani is an anaerobic, motile, gram-positive rod that forms an oval, colorless, terminal spore and thus assumes a shape resembling a tennis racket or drumstick. The organism is found worldwide in soil, in the inanimate environment, in animal feces, and occasionally in human feces. Spores may survive for years in some environments and are resistant to various disinfectants and to boiling for 20 min. Vegetative cells, however, are easily inactivated and are susceptible to several antibiotics, including metronidazole and penicillin.

Tetanospasmin is formed in vegetative cells under plasmid control. With autolysis, the single-chain toxin is released and cleaved to form a heterodimer consisting of a heavy chain (100 kDa), which mediates binding to and entry into nerve cells, and a light chain (50 kDa), which blocks neurotransmitter release. The genome of *C. tetani* has been sequenced. The amino acid structures of the two most powerful toxins known, botulinum toxin and tetanus toxin, are partially homologous.

EPIDEMIOLOGY

Tetanus occurs sporadically and almost always affects unimmunized persons; partially immunized persons and fully immunized individuals who fail to maintain adequate immunity with booster doses of vaccine may be affected as well.

Although tetanus is entirely preventable by immunization, the burden of disease worldwide is great. Tetanus is a notifiable disease in many countries, but reporting is known to be inaccurate and incomplete, particularly in developing countries. As a result, the World Health Organization considers the number of reported cases to be an underestimate and periodically undertakes case/death estimates to assess the burden of disease. In 2002 (the last year for which data are available), the *estimated* number of tetanus-related deaths in all age groups was 213,000, of which 180,000 (85%) were attributable to neonatal tetanus. In contrast, only 18,781 tetanus cases in total and 11,762 neonatal cases were actually *reported* for that year.

Tetanus is common in areas where soil is cultivated, in rural areas, in warm climates, during summer months, and among males. In countries without a comprehensive immunization program, tetanus occurs predominantly in neonates and other young children. It is noteworthy that international programs to eliminate neonatal tetanus have been in place for some time. In the United States and other nations with successful immunization programs, neonatal tetanus is rare (only three cases were reported in the United States during 1990–2004), and the disease affects other age groups (Fig. 133-1) and groups inadequately covered by immunization (such as nonwhites). The success of immunization in the United States is depicted in Fig. 133-2. Since 1976, fewer than 100 cases have been reported yearly. At present, the risk of tetanus in this country is highest among the elderly. A large-scale national serologic survey performed in 1988–1994 showed that 72% of Americans ≥6 years old had protective antibody levels. In contrast, only 30% of persons >70 years old were protected.

In the United States, most cases of tetanus follow an acute injury (puncture wound, laceration, abrasion, or other trauma). Tetanus may be acquired indoors or during outdoor activities (e.g., farming, gardening). The implicated injury may be major but can be so trivial that medical attention is not sought. In some cases, no injury or portal of entry can be identified. The disease may complicate chronic conditions such as skin ulcers, abscesses, and gangrene. Tetanus has also been associated with burns, frostbite, middle-ear infection, surgery, abortion, childbirth, body piercing, and drug abuse (notably "skin popping"). Recurrent tetanus has been reported.

PATHOGENESIS

Contamination of wounds with spores of *C. tetani* is probably a frequent occurrence. Germination and toxin production, however, take place only in wounds with low oxidation-reduction potential, such as those with devitalized tissue, foreign bodies, or active infection. *C. tetani* does not itself evoke inflammation, and the portal of entry retains a benign appearance unless coinfection with other organisms is present.

Toxin released in the wound binds to peripheral motor neuron terminals, enters the axon, and is transported to the nerve-cell body in the brainstem and spinal cord by retrograde intraneuronal transport. The toxin then migrates across the synapse to presynaptic terminals, where it blocks release of the inhibitory neurotransmitters glycine and γ-aminobutyric acid (GABA) from vesicles (see Fig. 134-1). The blocking of neurotransmitter release by tetanospasmin, a zinc metalloprotease, involves cleavage of synaptobrevin, a protein essential to proper function of the synaptic vesicle release apparatus. With diminished inhibition, the resting firing rate of the α motor neuron increases, producing rigidity. With lessened activity of reflexes that limit polysynaptic spread of impulses (a glycinergic activity), agonists and antagonists may be recruited rather than inhibited, with the consequent production of

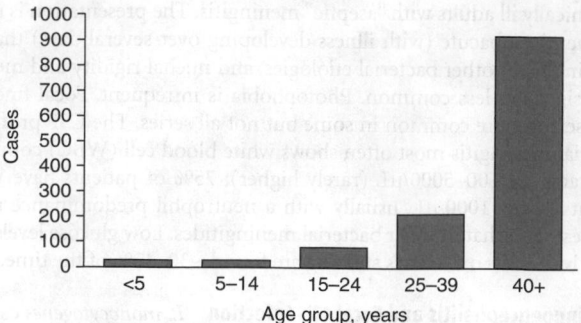

FIGURE 133-1 Tetanus: reported cases in the United States, by age group, 1980–2003; *N* = 1277. *(From Centers for Disease Control and Prevention, National Immunization Program. Tetanus and Tetanus Toxoid: Epidemiology and Prevention of Vaccine-Preventable Diseases. www.cdc.gov/nip/ed/vpd2006/Slides/chap06-tetanus9.ppt. Revised January 2006. Accessed 1/30/2007.)*

FIGURE 133-2 Impact of tetanus immunization in the United States, 1947–2005 (2005, provisional total). Tetanus vaccine became part of the routine childhood immunization schedule in the late 1940s. *(From Centers for Disease Control and Prevention, National Immunization Program. Tetanus and Tetanus Toxoid: Epidemiology and Prevention of Vaccine-Preventable Diseases. www.cdc.gov/nip/ed/vpd2006/Slides/chap06-tetanus9.ppt. Revised January 2006. Accessed 1/30/2007.)*

---

†Deceased. A contributor to HPIM since the 12th edition, Dr. Abrutyn passed away on February 22, 2007.

spasms. Toxin may also affect preganglionic sympathetic neurons in the lateral gray matter of the spinal cord and parasympathetic centers. Loss of inhibition of preganglionic sympathetic neurons may produce sympathetic hyperactivity and high circulating catecholamine levels. Tetanospasmin, like botulinum toxin, may block neurotransmitter release at the neuromuscular junction and produce weakness or paralysis, but this effect is clinically evident only in cephalic tetanus. Recovery requires sprouting of new nerve terminals.

In local tetanus, only the nerves supplying the affected muscles are involved. Generalized tetanus occurs when toxin released in the wound enters the lymphatics and bloodstream and is spread widely to distant nerve terminals; the blood-brain barrier blocks direct entry into the central nervous system. If it is assumed that intraneuronal transport times are equal for all nerves, short nerves are affected before long nerves: this fact explains the sequential involvement of nerves of the head, trunk, and extremities in generalized tetanus.

CLINICAL MANIFESTATIONS

Generalized tetanus, the most common form of the disease, is characterized by increased muscle tone and generalized spasms. The median time of onset after injury is 7 days; 15% of cases occur within 3 days and 10% after 14 days.

Typically, the patient first notices increased tone in the masseter muscles (trismus, or lockjaw). Dysphagia or stiffness or pain in the neck, shoulder, and back muscles appears concurrently or soon thereafter. The subsequent involvement of other muscles produces a rigid abdomen and stiff proximal limb muscles; the hands and feet are relatively spared. Sustained contraction of the facial muscles results in a grimace or sneer (risus sardonicus), and contraction of the back muscles produces an arched back (opisthotonos). Some patients develop paroxysmal, violent, painful, generalized muscle spasms that may cause cyanosis and threaten ventilation. These spasms occur repetitively and may be spontaneous or provoked by even the slightest stimulation. A constant threat during generalized spasms is reduced ventilation or apnea or laryngospasm. The severity of illness may be mild (muscle rigidity and few or no spasms), moderate (trismus, dysphagia, rigidity, and spasms), or severe (frequent explosive paroxysms). The patient may be febrile, although many patients have no fever; mentation is unimpaired. Deep tendon reflexes may be increased. Dysphagia or ileus may preclude oral feeding.

Autonomic dysfunction commonly complicates severe cases and is characterized by labile or sustained hypertension, tachycardia, dysrhythmia, hyperpyrexia, profuse sweating, peripheral vasoconstriction, and increased plasma and urinary catecholamine levels. Periods of bradycardia and hypotension may also be documented. Sudden cardiac arrest sometimes occurs, but its basis is unknown. Other complications include aspiration pneumonia, fractures, muscle rupture, deep-vein thrombophlebitis, pulmonary emboli, decubitus ulcer, and rhabdomyolysis.

Neonatal tetanus usually occurs as the generalized form and is usually fatal if left untreated. It develops in children born to inadequately immunized mothers, frequently after unsterile treatment of the umbilical cord stump. Its onset generally comes during the first 2 weeks of life.

Local tetanus is an uncommon form in which manifestations are restricted to muscles near the wound. The prognosis is excellent. *Cephalic tetanus*, a rare form of local tetanus, follows head injury or ear infection and involves one or more facial cranial nerves. The incubation period is a few days and mortality is high.

DIAGNOSIS

The diagnosis of tetanus is based entirely on clinical findings. Tetanus is unlikely if a reliable history indicates the completion of a primary vaccination series and the receipt of appropriate booster doses. Wounds should be cultured in suspected cases. However, *C. tetani* can be isolated from wounds of patients without tetanus and frequently cannot be recovered from wounds of those with tetanus. The leukocyte count may be

elevated. Cerebrospinal fluid examination yields normal results. Electromyograms may show continuous discharge of motor units and shortening or absence of the silent interval normally seen after an action potential. Nonspecific changes may be evident on the electrocardiogram. Muscle enzyme levels may be raised. Serum antitoxin levels of ≥0.1 IU/mL (as measured by enzyme-linked immunosorbent assay) are considered protective and make tetanus unlikely, although cases in patients with protective antitoxin levels have been reported.

The differential diagnosis includes conditions also producing trismus, such as alveolar abscess, strychnine poisoning, dystonic drug reactions (e.g., phenothiazines and metoclopramide), and hypocalcemic tetany. In addition, meningitis/encephalitis, rabies, and an acute intra-abdominal process (because of the rigid abdomen) might be considered. Markedly increased tone in central muscles (face, neck, chest, back, and abdomen), with superimposed generalized spasms and relative sparing of the hands and feet, strongly suggests tetanus.

℞ TETANUS

GENERAL MEASURES The goals of therapy are to eliminate the source of toxin, neutralize unbound toxin, and prevent muscle spasms while monitoring the patient's condition and providing support—especially respiratory support—until recovery. Patients should be admitted to a quiet room in an intensive care unit, where observation and cardiopulmonary monitoring can be maintained continuously but stimulation can be minimized. Protection of the airway is vital. Wounds should be explored, carefully cleansed, and thoroughly debrided.

ANTIBIOTIC THERAPY Although of unproven value, antibiotic therapy is administered to eradicate vegetative cells—the source of toxin. The use of penicillin (10–12 million units IV, given daily for 10 days) has been recommended, but metronidazole (500 mg every 6 h or 1 g every 12 h) is preferred by some experts on the basis of this drug's excellent antimicrobial activity and the absence of the GABA-antagonistic activity seen with penicillin. The drug of choice remains unclear: one nonrandomized clinical trial found a survival benefit with metronidazole, but another study failed to find a difference among benzathine penicillin, benzyl penicillin, and metronidazole. Clindamycin and erythromycin are alternatives for the treatment of penicillin-allergic patients. Additional specific antimicrobial therapy should be given for active infection with other organisms.

ANTITOXIN Given to neutralize circulating toxin and unbound toxin in the wound, antitoxin effectively lowers mortality; toxin already bound to neural tissue is unaffected. Human tetanus immune globulin (TIG) is the preparation of choice and should be given promptly. The dose is 3000–6000 units IM, usually in divided doses because the volume is large. The optimal dose is not known, however, and results from one study indicated that a 500-unit dose was as effective as higher doses. Pooled IVIg may be an alternative to TIG, but the specific antitoxin concentration in this formulation is not standardized. The value of administering antitoxin before wound manipulation or of injecting a dose proximal to the wound or infiltrating the wound is unclear. Additional doses are unnecessary because the half-life of antitoxin is long. Antibody does not penetrate the blood-brain barrier. Intrathecal administration should be considered experimental. Equine tetanus antitoxin (TAT) is not available in the United States but is used elsewhere. It is cheaper than human antitoxin, but the half-life is shorter and its administration commonly elicits a hypersensitivity reaction and serum sickness.

CONTROL OF MUSCLE SPASMS Many agents, alone and in combination, have been used to treat the muscle spasms of tetanus, which are painful and can threaten ventilation by causing laryngospasm or sustained contraction of ventilatory muscles.

 In some developing countries, cost, availability, and the ability to provide ventilatory support are important factors in the choice of therapy. The ideal therapeutic regimen would abolish spasmodic activity without causing oversedation and hypoventilation. Diazepam, a benzodiazepine and GABA agonist, is in wide use. The dose is titrated, and large doses (≥250 mg/d) may be required. Lorazepam, with a longer duration of action, and midazolam, with a short half-life, are other options. Barbiturates and chlorpromazine are considered second-line agents. Therapeutic paralysis with a nondepolarizing neuromuscular blocking agent and mechanical ventilation may be used for spasms unresponsive to medication or spasms that threaten ventilation. However, prolonged paralysis after discontinuation of therapy has been described. Other agents include propofol, which is expensive; dantrolene and intrathecal baclofen, which may allow shortening of the duration of therapeutic paralysis; succinylcholine, which has been associated with hyperkalemia; and magnesium sulfate. A recent double-blind, randomized, placebo-controlled clinical trial of magnesium sulfate in severe tetanus did not find a reduction in the need for ventilation or in mortality rate; however, use of midazolam and pipecuronium for treatment of muscle spasms and of verapamil for treatment of cardiovascular instability was reduced.

RESPIRATORY CARE Intubation or tracheostomy, with or without mechanical ventilation, may be required for hypoventilation due to oversedation or laryngospasm or for the avoidance of aspiration by patients with trismus, disordered swallowing, or dysphagia. The need for these procedures should be anticipated, and they should be undertaken electively and early.

AUTONOMIC DYSFUNCTION The optimal therapy for sympathetic overactivity has not been defined. Agents that have been considered include labetalol (an α- and β-adrenergic blocking agent that is recommended by some experts but that reportedly has caused sudden death), esmolol administered by continuous infusion (a beta blocker whose short half-life may be advantageous in the event of severe hypertension from unopposed α-adrenergic activity), clonidine (a central-acting antiadrenergic drug), verapamil, and morphine sulfate. Parenteral magnesium sulfate and continuous spinal or epidural anesthesia have been used but may be more difficult to administer and monitor. The relative efficacy of these modalities has yet to be determined. Hypotension or bradycardia may require volume expansion, use of vasopressors or chronotropic agents, or pacemaker insertion.

VACCINE Patients recovering from tetanus should be actively immunized (see below) because immunity is not induced by the small amount of toxin required to produce disease.

ADDITIONAL MEASURES Like all patients receiving ventilatory support, patients with tetanus require attention to hydration; nutrition; physiotherapy; prophylactic anticoagulation; bowel, bladder, and renal function; decubitus ulcer prevention; and treatment of intercurrent infection.

PREVENTION

Active Immunization All partially immunized and unimmunized adults should receive vaccine, as should those recovering from tetanus. The primary series for adults consists of three doses: the first and second doses are given 4–8 weeks apart, and the third dose is given 6–12 months after the second. A booster dose is required every 10 years and may be given at mid-decade ages—35, 45, and so on. Combined tetanus and diphtheria toxoid, adsorbed (Td, for adult use)—rather than single-antigen tetanus toxoid—is preferred for persons >7 years of age. Adsorbed vaccine is preferred because it produces more persistent antibody titers than fluid vaccine. Two combined tetanus/diphtheria/attenuated pertussis vaccines have recently been approved: one (ADACEL) for adults 19–64 years of age and the other (BOOSTRIX) for adolescents 11–18 years of age. The Advisory Committee on Immunization Practices has recommended a single dose of Tdap (ADACEL) for adults 19–64 years old who have not received Tdap.

Wound Management Proper wound management requires consideration of the need for (1) passive immunization with TIG and (2) active immunization with vaccine (Tdap or Td; Table 133-1). The dose of TIG for passive immunization of persons with wounds of average severity (250 units IM) produces a protective serum antibody level for at least 4–6 weeks; the appropriate dose of TAT, an equine-derived product, is 3000–6000 units. Vaccine and antibody should be administered at separate sites with separate syringes.

Neonatal Tetanus Preventive measures include maternal vaccination, even during pregnancy; efforts to increase the proportion of births that take place in the hospital; and the provision of training for nonmedical birth attendants.

TABLE 133-1 GUIDE TO TETANUS PROPHYLAXIS AND ROUTINE WOUND MANAGEMENT

History of Adsorbed Tetanus Toxoid (Doses)	Clean Minor Wound		All Other Wounds[a]	
	Tdap or Td[b]	TIG	Tdap or Td[b]	TIG
Unknown or <3	Yes	No	Yes	Yes
≥3	No[c]	No	No[d]	No

[a]Such as, but not limited to, wounds contaminated with dirt, feces, soil, and saliva; puncture wounds; avulsions; and wounds from missile or crushing injuries, burns, and frostbite.
[b]Tdap is preferred to Td for adults 19–64 years old who have never received Tdap. Td is preferred for adults who have received Tdap previously and is used when Tdap is not available. Td is also recommended for persons >64 years old. If TT and TIG are both used, TT adsorbed rather than TT for booster use only (fluid vaccine) should be used.
[c]Yes, if ≥10 years have elapsed since the last TT-containing vaccine dose.
[d]Yes, if ≥5 years have elapsed since the last TT-containing vaccine dose.
Note: Tdap, tetanus toxoid, reduced diphtheria toxoid, and acellular pertussis vaccine, adsorbed; DT, diphtheria and tetanus vaccine; DTP, diphtheria, tetanus, and pertussis vaccine; Td, tetanus-diphtheria toxoid, adsorbed; TIG, tetanus immune globulin; TT, tetanus toxoid.
Source: Modified from Centers for Disease Control and Prevention, 2006.

PROGNOSIS

The application of methods to monitor and support oxygenation has markedly improved the prognosis in tetanus. Mortality rates as low as 10% have been reported from units accustomed to handling such cases. In the United States in 2003, there were 20 cases and 2 deaths; no cases were in patients <18 years old, and 19 cases were ascribed to inadequate immunization. The outcome is poor in neonates and the elderly and in patients with a short incubation period, a short interval from the onset of symptoms to admission, or a short period from the onset of symptoms to the first spasm (period of onset). Outcome is also related to the extent of prior vaccination.

The course of tetanus extends over 4–6 weeks, and patients may require prolonged ventilator support. Increased tone and minor spasms can last for months, but recovery is usually complete.

FURTHER READINGS

ABRUTYN E, BERLIN JA: Intrathecal therapy of tetanus: A meta-analysis. JAMA 266:2262, 1991

AHMADSYAH I, SALIM A: Treatment of tetanus: An open study to compare the efficacy of procaine penicillin and metronidazole. BMJ 291:648, 1985

BLECK TP: *Clostridium tetani* (tetanus), in *Principles and Practice of Infectious Diseases*, 5th ed, GL Mandell et al (eds). New York, Churchill Livingstone, 2000, pp 2537–2543

CENTERS FOR DISEASE CONTROL AND PREVENTION: Preventing tetanus, diphtheria, and pertussis among adults: Use of tetanus toxoid, reduced diphtheria toxoid and acellular pertussis vaccine: Recommendations of the Advisory Committee on Immunization Practices (ACIP) and recommendation of ACIP, supported by the Healthcare Infection Control Practices Advisory Committee (HICPAC), for use of Tdap among health-care personnel. MMWR 55(RR17):1, 2006

CENTERS FOR DISEASE CONTROL AND PREVENTION: Tetanus—Puerto Rico, 2002. MMWR 51:613, 2002

———: Tetanus surveillance—United States, 1998–2000. Surveillance summaries, June 20, 2003. MMWR 52(SS-3):1, 2003

COOK TM et al: Tetanus: A review of the literature. Br J Anaesth 87:477, 2001

HSU SS et al: Tetanus in the emergency department: A current review. J Emerg Med 20:357, 2001

MCQUILLAN CM et al: Serologic immunity to diphtheria and tetanus in the United States. Ann Intern Med 136:660, 2002

THWAITES CL et al: Magnesium sulphate for the treatment of severe tetanus: A randomized controlled trial. Lancet 368:1436, 2006

134 Botulism
Elias Abrutyn[†]

DEFINITION

Botulism is a paralytic disease caused by potent protein neurotoxins elaborated by *Clostridium botulinum*. Illness begins with cranial nerve involvement and proceeds caudally to involve the extremities. Cases may be classified as (1) *food-borne botulism*, from ingestion of pre-formed toxin in food contaminated with *C. botulinum*; (2) *wound botulism*, from toxin produced in wounds contaminated with the organism; and (3) *intestinal botulism*, from ingestion of spores and production of toxin in the intestine of infants (infant botulism) or adults. Botulinum toxin, because of its extraordinary potency, has long been considered a threat as an agent of bioterrorism or biologic warfare that could be ac-quired by inhalation or ingestion (Chap. 214). Iatrogenic botulism can follow cosmetic or therapeutic use of toxin.

ETIOLOGIC AGENT

C. botulinum, a species encompassing a heterogeneous group of anaer-obic gram-positive organisms that form subterminal spores, is found in soil and marine environments throughout the world and elaborates the most potent bacterial toxin known. Organisms of types A through G have been distinguished by the antigenic specificities of their toxins; a classification system based on physiologic characteristics has also been described. Rare strains of other clostridial species—*C. butyricum* and *C. baratii*—have been found to produce toxin. *C. botulinum* strains with proteolytic activity can digest food and produce a spoiled appear-ance; nonproteolytic types leave the appearance of food unchanged.

Of the eight distinct toxin types described (A, B, C_1, C_2, D, E, F, and G), all except C_2 are neurotoxins; C_2 is a cytotoxin of unknown clinical significance. Botulinum neurotoxin, whether ingested, inhaled, or produced in the intestine or a wound, enters the vascular system and is transported to peripheral cholinergic nerve terminals, including neu-romuscular junctions, postganglionic parasympathetic nerve endings, and peripheral ganglia. The central nervous system is not involved. Steps in neurotoxin activity include binding, internalization in en-docytic vesicles, translocation to the cytosol, and proteolysis resulting in a blockage of the release of the neurotransmitter acetylcholine (Fig. 134-1). Cure follows sprouting of new nerve terminals.

Toxin types A, B, E, and (rarely) F cause disease in humans; type G (from *C. argentinense*) has been associated with sudden death, but not with neuroparalytic illness, in a few patients in Switzerland; and types C and D cause disease in animals.

EPIDEMIOLOGY

Human botulism occurs worldwide. In the United States, the geographic distribution of cases by toxin type parallels the distribution of organism types found in the environment. Type A predominates west of the Rocky Mountains; type B is generally distributed but is more common in the East; and type E is found in the Pacific Northwest, Alaska, and the Great Lakes area.

Food-borne botulism in the United States is associated primarily with home-canned food (particularly vegetables, fruit, and condiments) and less commonly with meat and fish. Type E outbreaks are frequently as-sociated with fish products. Commercial products occasionally cause outbreaks, some of which are attributable to improper handling after pur-chase. Outbreaks in restaurants, schools, and private homes have been traced to uncommon sources (commercial potpies, beef stew, turkey loaf, sautéed onions, baked potatoes, preserved green olives, bamboo shoots, and chopped garlic in oil). Food-borne botulism can occur when (1) food to be preserved is contaminated with spores, (2) preservation does not in-activate the spores but kills other putrefactive bacteria that might inhibit growth of *C. botulinum* and provides anaerobic conditions at a pH and

---

[†]Deceased. A contributor to HPIM since the 12th edition, Dr. Abrutyn passed away on February 22, 2007.

FIGURE 134-1 The synaptic vesicle release apparatus and the sites of action of botulinum toxins. Toxin acts to block neurotransmitter re-lease from the synaptic vesicle into the synaptic cleft. The site of action of tetanus toxin is also shown. *[From TP Bleck et al: In WM Scheld et al (eds): Infections of the Central Nervous System, 2d ed. New York, Raven Press, 1997; with permission.]*

temperature that allow germination and toxin production, and (3) food is not heated to a temperature that destroys toxin before being eaten.

CLINICAL MANIFESTATIONS

Food-Borne Botulism After ingestion of food containing toxin, illness varies from a mild condition for which no medical advice is sought to very severe disease that can result in death within 24 h. The incubation period is usually 18–36 h but, depending on toxin dose, can range from a few hours to several days. Symmetric descending paralysis is characteristic and can lead to respiratory failure and death. Cranial nerve involvement, which almost always marks the onset of symptoms, usually produces diplopia, dysarthria, dysphonia, and/or dysphagia. Weakness progresses, often rapidly, from the head to involve the neck, arms, thorax, and legs; occasionally, weakness is asymmetric. Nausea, vomiting, and abdominal pain may precede or follow the onset of paralysis. Dizziness, blurred vi-sion, dry mouth, and very dry, occasionally sore throat are common. Pa-tients are generally alert and oriented, but they may be drowsy, agitated, and anxious. Typically, they have no fever. Ptosis is frequent; the pupillary reflexes may be depressed, and fixed or dilated pupils are noted in half of patients. The gag reflex may be suppressed, and deep tendon reflexes may be normal or decreased. Sensory findings are usually absent. Paralytic ile-us, severe constipation, and urinary retention are common.

Wound Botulism Wound botulism occurs when the spores contami-nating a wound germinate and form vegetative organisms that pro-duce toxin. This rare condition resembles food-borne illness except that the incubation period is longer, averaging about 10 days, and gas-trointestinal symptoms are lacking. Wound botulism has been docu-mented after traumatic injury involving contamination with soil; in injection drug users, for whom black-tar heroin use has been identi-fied as a risk factor; and after cesarean delivery. The illness has oc-curred even after antibiotics have been given to prevent wound infection. When present, fever is probably attributable to concurrent infection with other bacteria. The wound may appear benign.

Intestinal Botulism In intestinal botulism, toxin is produced in and absorbed from the intestine after the germination of ingested spores. Intestinal botulism in infants (infant botulism) is the most common form of botulism. The severity ranges from mild illness with failure to thrive to fulminant severe paralysis with respiratory failure. Infant botulism may be one cause of sudden infant death. The identification of contaminated honey as one source of spores has led to the recom-

TABLE 134-1 FEATURES OF OUTBREAKS SUGGESTING DELIBERATE RELEASE OF BOTULINUM TOXIN[a]

- Outbreak of a large number of cases of acute flaccid paralysis with prominent bulbar palsies
- Outbreak with an unusual botulinum toxin type (i.e., type C, D, F, or G or type E toxin not associated with food of aquatic origin)
- Outbreak with a common geographic factor among cases (e.g., airport, work location) but without a common dietary exposure (i.e., features suggesting an aerosol attack)
- Multiple simultaneous outbreaks with no common source

[a]A careful travel and activity history, as well as a dietary history, should be taken in any suspected botulism outbreak. Patients should also be asked whether they know of other persons with similar symptoms.
Source: Reproduced with permission of the publisher from Arnon et al, 2002.

mendation that honey not be fed to children <12 months of age. Most cases, however, cannot be attributed to a particular food source. The factors permitting intestinal colonization with *C. botulinum* are not fully defined, but cases usually involve infants <6 months of age; susceptibility may decrease as the normal intestinal flora develops. Intestinal botulism involving adults is uncommon. The patient may have a history of gastrointestinal disease, gastrointestinal surgery, or recent antibiotic therapy. Toxin and organisms may be identified in the stool.

Bioterrorism and Biologic Warfare   (See also Chap. 214) Botulinum toxin could be dispersed as an aerosol (producing inhalational botulism) or as a contaminant in material to be ingested (producing food-borne botulism). Inhalational botulism resembles food-borne illness, but gastrointestinal symptoms are absent. Botulism follows adsorption of toxin from mucosal surfaces (gut, lung) and wounds, but the toxin does not penetrate intact skin. As a toxin-mediated illness, botulism is noncommunicable, and standard isolation precautions are sufficient. Features suggestive of an outbreak due to deliberate release of botulinum toxin are shown in Table 134-1.

DIAGNOSIS

A diagnosis of botulism must be considered in patients with symmetric descending paralysis who are afebrile and mentally intact. The bulbar musculature is involved initially, but sensory findings are absent and, early on, deep tendon reflexes remain intact. The differential diagnosis of botulism and distinguishing features are listed in Table 134-2. Depending on season and other epidemiologic factors, West Nile virus infection may also be a consideration.

The demonstration of toxin in serum by bioassay in mice is definitive, but this test may give negative results, particularly in wound and infant botulism. It is performed only by specific laboratories, which can be identified through regional public health authorities. Other assays are being developed and remain experimental. The demonstration of *C. botulinum* or its toxin in vomitus, gastric fluid, or stool is strongly suggestive of the diagnosis because intestinal carriage is rare. Isolation of the organism from food without toxin is insufficient grounds for the diagnosis. Wound cultures yielding the organism are suggestive of botulism. The edrophonium chloride (Tensilon) test for myasthenia gravis may be falsely positive in botulism but is usually less dramatically positive than in the former condition. Nerve conduction velocity is normal, but compound muscle action potentials on routine nerve stimulation studies are decreased with a supramaximal stimulus, and facilitation is evident after repetitive stimulation at high frequency. Single-fiber electromyography may be helpful. The white blood cell count and erythrocyte sedimentation rate are normal.

℞ BOTULISM

Patients should be hospitalized and monitored closely, both clinically and by spirometry, pulse oximetry, and measurement of arterial blood gases for incipient respiratory failure. Intubation and mechanical ventilation should be strongly considered when the vital capacity is <30% of predicted, especially when paralysis is progressing rapidly and hypoxemia with absolute or

TABLE 134-2 SELECTED MIMICS THAT MAY LEAD TO MISDIAGNOSIS OF BOTULISM

Condition	Features Distinguishing Condition from Botulism
Common Misdiagnoses	
Guillain-Barré syndrome[a] and its variants, especially Miller-Fisher variant	History of antecedent infection; paresthesias; often ascending paralysis; early areflexia; eventual CSF protein increase; EMG findings
Myasthenia gravis[a]	Recurrent paralysis; EMG findings; sustained response to anticholinesterase
Stroke[a]	Paralysis often asymmetric; abnormal CNS image
Intoxication with depressants (e.g., acute alcohol intoxication), organophosphates, carbon monoxide, or nerve gas	History of exposure; excessive drug levels detected in body fluids
Lambert-Eaton syndrome	Increased strength with sustained contraction; evidence of lung carcinoma; EMG findings similar to botulism
Tick paralysis	Paresthesias; ascending paralysis; tick attached to skin
Other Misdiagnoses	
Poliomyelitis	Antecedent febrile illness; asymmetric paralysis; CSF pleocytosis
CNS infections, especially of the brainstem	Mental status changes; CSF and EEG abnormalities
CNS tumor	Paralysis often asymmetric; abnormal CNS image
Streptococcal pharyngitis[b]	Absence of bulbar palsies; positive rapid antigen test result or throat culture
Psychiatric illness[a]	Normal EMG in conversion paralysis
Viral syndrome[a]	Absence of bulbar palsies and flaccid paralysis
Inflammatory myopathy[a]	Elevated creatine kinase level
Diabetic complications[a]	Sensory neuropathy; few cranial nerve palsies
Hyperemesis gravidarum[a]	Absence of bulbar palsies and acute flaccid paralysis
Hypothyroidism[a]	Abnormal thyroid function tests
Laryngeal trauma[a]	Absence of flaccid paralysis; dysphonia without flaccid paralysis
Overexertion[a]	Absence of bulbar palsies and acute flaccid paralysis

[a]Misdiagnoses made in a large outbreak of botulism (St. Louis ME et al: Botulism from chopped garlic: Delayed recognition of a major outbreak. Ann Intern Med 108:363, 1988).
[b]Pharyngeal erythema can occur in botulism.
Note: CNS, central nervous system; CSF, cerebrospinal fluid; EEG, electroencephalogram; EMG, electromyogram.
Source: Reproduced with permission of the publisher from Arnon et al, 2002.

relative hypercarbia is documented (Chap. 263). Serial measurements of the maximal static inspiratory pressure may be useful in predicting respiratory failure.

In food-borne illness, equine antitoxin should be administered as soon as possible after specimens are obtained for laboratory analysis. Treatment should not await laboratory analyses, which may take days. The previous trivalent antitoxin preparation (types A, B, and E) is no longer available. Instead, a bivalent preparation containing toxin types A and B and an investigational monovalent type E preparation can be obtained. The bivalent preparation is administered routinely; monovalent type E antitoxin is given in addition when exposure to type E toxin is suspected (after seafood ingestion, for example). In the United States, antitoxin as well as help with clinical management and laboratory confirmation are available at *any* time from state health departments or from the Centers for Disease Control and Prevention (CDC; emergency number, 770-488-7100). A limited supply of an investigational heptavalent antitoxin (types A through G) is maintained by the U.S. military for emergency use.

After testing for hypersensitivity to horse serum, antitoxin is given as recommended by the CDC; repeated doses are not considered necessary. Anaphylaxis and serum sickness are risks inherent in use of the equine product, and desensitization of allergic patients may be required. If there is no ileus, cathartics and enemas may be used to purge the gut of toxin; emetics or gastric lavage can also be used if the time since ingestion is brief (only a few hours). Neither the use of antibiotics to eliminate an intestinal source of possible continued toxin production nor the administration of guanidine hydrochloride and other drugs to reverse paralysis is of proven value.

Treatment of infant botulism requires supportive care and administration of human botulism immune globulin, which can be obtained by calling the California Department of Health Services at 510-231-7600 or by following the instructions at *www.infantbotulism.org*. Neither equine antitoxin nor antibiotics have been shown to be beneficial. In wound botulism, equine antitoxin is administered. The wound should be thoroughly explored and debrided, and an antibiotic such as penicillin should be given to eradicate *C. botulinum* from the site, even though the benefit of this therapy is unproven. Results of wound cultures should guide the use of other antibiotics.

Botulinum toxins are being employed for a variety of cosmetic and therapeutic purposes, and new uses are being evaluated. Generalized botulism-like weakness complicating therapy (iatrogenic botulism) has been reported but is rare.

PROGNOSIS

Type A disease is generally more severe than type B, and mortality rates from botulism are higher among patients above age 60 than among younger patients. With improved respiratory and intensive care, the case-fatality rate in food-borne illness has been reduced to ~7.5% and is low in infant botulism as well. Artificial respiratory support may be required for months in severe cases. Some patients experience residual weakness and autonomic dysfunction for as long as a year after disease onset.

PREVENTION

A pentavalent vaccine (types A through E) is available for use in highly exposed individuals. Spores are highly resistant to heat but can be inactivated by exposure to high temperature (116–121°C) and pressure, as in steam sterilizers or pressure cookers used in accordance with the manufacturer's instructions. Toxin is heat-labile and can be inactivated by exposure to a temperature of 85°C for 5 min. Newly identified cases should be reported immediately to public health authorities.

FURTHER READINGS

ARNON SS et al: Human botulism immune globulin for the treatment of infant botulism. N Engl J Med 354:462, 2006

———— et al: Botulinum toxin as a biological weapon, in *Bioterrorism: Guidelines for Medical and Public Health Management*, DA Henderson et al (eds). Chicago, AMA Press, 2002, pp 141–165

CAWTHORNE A et al: Botulism and preserved green olives. Emerg Infect Dis 11:781, 2005

CAYA JG et al: *Clostridium botulinum* and the clinical laboratorian: A detailed review of botulism, including biological warfare ramifications of botulinum toxin. Arch Pathol Lab Med 128:653, 2004

CENTERS FOR DISEASE CONTROL AND PREVENTION: Botulism from home-canned bamboo shoots—Nan Province, Thailand. MMWR 55:389, 2006

CHERTOW DS et al: Botulism in 4 adults following cosmetic injections with an unlicensed highly concentrated botulinum preparation. JAMA 206:2476, 2006

COOPER JG et al: *Clostridium botulinum*: An increasing complication of heroin misuse. Eur J Emerg Med 12:251, 2005

GUPTA A et al: Adult botulism type F in the United States, 1981-2002. Neurology 65:1694, 2005

LINDSTRÖM M, KORKEALA H: Laboratory diagnostics of botulism. Clin Microbiol Rev 19:298, 2006

MONTECUCCO C, MOLGO J: Botulinal neurotoxins: Revival of an old killer. Curr Opin Pharmacol 5:274, 2005

SOBEL J: Botulism. Clin Infect Dis 41:1167, 2005

135 Gas Gangrene and Other Clostridial Infections

Dennis L. Kasper, Lawrence C. Madoff

DEFINITION

Bacteria of the genus *Clostridium* are gram-positive, spore-forming, obligate anaerobes that are ubiquitous in nature. There are >60 recognized species of clostridia, many of which are generally considered saprophytic. Some of these species are pathogenic for humans and animals, particularly under conditions of lowered oxidation-reduction potential. Infections associated with these organisms range from localized wound contamination to overwhelming systemic disease. The four major disease categories for which clostridia are responsible are intestinal disorders, suppurative deep-tissue infections, skin and soft tissue infections, and bacteremia. Toxins play a major role in some of these syndromes. Colitis caused by *C. difficile* is discussed in Chap. 123.

ETIOLOGY

In humans, clostridia normally reside in the gastrointestinal tract and in the female genital tract, although they occasionally are isolated from the skin or the mouth. Of the known clostridial species, at least 30 have been isolated from human infections. Like several other pathogenic anaerobic bacterial species, clostridia are quite aerotolerant, but they do not grow on artificial media in the presence of oxygen. Clostridia characteristically produce abundant gas in artificial media and form subterminal endospores. *C. perfringens*, one of the most clinical-

ly important species, is encapsulated and nonmotile and rarely sporulates in artificial media; the spores can usually be destroyed by boiling. *C. tetani* and *C. botulinum* are discussed in detail in Chaps. 133 and 134, respectively.

Clostridia are present in the normal colonic flora at concentrations of 10^9–10^{10}/g. Of the ≥30 species that normally colonize humans, *C. ramosum* is the most abundant and is followed in frequency by *C. perfringens*. These organisms are universally present in soil at concentrations of up to 10^4/g. *C. perfringens* strains are classified (on the basis of their production of several lethal toxins) into five types, designated A through E. Type A predominates in fecal flora of humans as well as in soil, whereas the habitats of types B through E are thought to be the intestinal tracts of other animals. Although clostridia are gram-positive organisms, many species may appear to be gram-negative in clinical specimens or stationary-phase cultures. Therefore, the results of Gram's staining of cultures or clinical material should be interpreted with great care.

C. perfringens is the most common of the clostridial species isolated from tissue infections and bacteremias; next in frequency are *C. novyi* and *C. septicum*. In the category of enteric infections, *C. difficile* is an important cause of antibiotic-associated colitis, and *C. perfringens* is associated with food poisoning (type A) and enteritis necroticans (type C).

PATHOGENESIS

Despite the isolation of clostridial species from many serious traumatic wounds, the prevalence of severe infections due to these organisms is low. Two factors that appear to be essential to the development of severe disease are tissue necrosis and a low oxidation-reduction potential. *C. perfringens* requires ~14 amino acids and at least 6 additional growth factors for optimal growth. These nutrients are not found in appreciable concentrations in normal body fluids but are present in necrotic tissue. When *C. perfringens* grows in necrotic tissue, a zone of tissue damage due to the toxins elaborated by the organism allows progressive growth. In contrast, when only a few bacteria leak into the bloodstream from a small defect in the intestinal wall, the organisms do not have the opportunity to multiply rapidly because blood as a medium for growth is relatively deficient in certain amino acids and growth factors. Therefore, in a patient without tissue necrosis, bacteremia is usually benign.

C. perfringens possesses at least 17 possible virulence factors, including 12 active tissue toxins and enterotoxins. The enterotoxins include four major lethal toxins: α, β, ε, and ι. The α toxin is a phospholipase C (lecithinase) that splits lecithin into phosphorylcholine and diglyceride. It has been associated with gas gangrene and is known to be hemolytic, to destroy platelets and polymorphonuclear leukocytes (PMNs), and to cause widespread capillary damage. When injected IV, it causes massive intravascular hemolysis and damages liver mitochondria. The α toxin may be important in the initiation of muscle infections that can progress to gas gangrene. Experimentally, the higher the concentration of α toxin in the culture fluid, the smaller the dose of *C. perfringens* required to produce infection. The protective effect of antiserum is directly proportional to its content of α antitoxin. Studies suggest that θ toxin, a thiol-activated cytolysin that is also called *perfringolysin O* and is related to other cholesterol-dependent cytolysins such as listeriolysin and streptolysin O, may play an important role in pathogenesis by promoting vascular leukostasis, endothelial cell injury, and regional tissue hypoxia. The resulting perfusion defects extend the anaerobic environment and contribute to rapidly advancing tissue destruction. A characteristic pathologic finding in gas gangrene is the near absence of PMNs despite extensive tissue destruction. Experimental data indicate that both α and θ toxins are essential in the leukocyte aggregation that occurs at the margins of tissue injury instead of the expected infiltration of these cells into the area of damage. Genetically altered strains induce less leukocyte aggregation when α toxin is absent and none when θ toxin is missing. The other major toxins—β, ε, and ι—are known to increase capillary permeability.

CLINICAL MANIFESTATIONS
Intestinal Disorders • *FOOD POISONING*
C. perfringens, primarily type A, is the second or third most common cause of food poisoning in the United States (Chap. 122). The responsible toxin is thought to be a cytotoxin produced by >75% of strains isolated from cases of food-borne disease. The cytotoxin binds to a receptor on the small-bowel brush border and induces a calcium ion–dependent alteration in permeability. The associated loss of ions alters intracellular metabolism, resulting in cell death. Outbreaks generally have resulted from problems in the cooling and storage of food cooked in bulk. The food sources primarily involved are meat, meat products, and poultry. Generally, the implicated meats have been cooked, allowed to cool, and then recooked the following day, often in a stew or hash. Strains of *C. perfringens* that contaminate meat manage to survive initial cooking. During reheating, the organisms sporulate and germinate. The disease is associated with an attack rate that is often as high as 70%. Symptoms of food poisoning from type A strains develop 8–24 h after ingestion of foods heavily contaminated with the organism. The primary symptoms include epigastric pain, nausea, and watery diarrhea usually lasting 12–24 h. Fever and vomiting are uncommon. Molecular methods including ribotyping and pulsed-field gel electrophoresis have been used to detect fecal cytotoxin in outbreaks of food poisoning caused by *C. perfringens*.

C. perfringens has also been implicated in a more severe form of diarrhea than that of classic food poisoning. This more severe disease tends to occur in the elderly and has been associated with antibiotic use in hospitalized populations. In this form of disease, diarrhea is generally more profuse, of longer duration, and accompanied by abdominal pain. Blood and mucus have been detected in the feces of the affected patients. In one hospital-based study of a cluster of cases,

widespread environmental contamination with *C. perfringens* spores was documented.

ENTERITIS NECROTICANS Necrotizing enteritis (enteritis necroticans, or *pigbel*) is caused by β toxin produced by type C strains of *C. perfringens* following ingestion of a high-protein meal in conjunction with trypsin inhibitors (e.g., in sweet potatoes) by a susceptible host who has limited intestinal proteolytic activity. This disease has been reported among children and adults in New Guinea. A similar disease, *darmbrand*, was epidemic in Germany after World War II. Clinical features of pigbel include acute abdominal pain, bloody diarrhea, vomiting, shock, and peritonitis; 40% of patients die. Pathologic studies reveal an acute ulcerative process of the bowel restricted to the small intestine. The mucosa is lifted off the submucosa, with the formation of large denuded areas. Pseudomembranes composed of sloughed epithelium are common, and gas may dissect into the submucosa. The source of the organisms may be the patient's own intestinal flora; cultures of ingested pork have failed to yield the organism. Antibodies to the β toxin of *C. perfringens* have been of considerable benefit in changing the course of established disease. In a large-scale trial, children immunized with *C. perfringens* β toxoid were protected.

NEUTROPENIC ENTEROCOLITIS (TYPHLITIS) See Chaps. 82 and 157.

Suppurative Deep-Tissue Infections Clostridia are frequently recovered from various suppurative conditions in conjunction with other anaerobic and aerobic bacteria but can also be the only organisms isolated. These suppurative conditions, which exist with severe local inflammation but usually without the characteristic systemic signs induced by clostridial toxins, include intraabdominal sepsis, empyema, pelvic abscess, subcutaneous abscess, frostbite with gas gangrene, infection of a stump in an amputee, brain abscess, prostatic abscess, perianal abscess, conjunctivitis, infection of a renal cell carcinoma, and infection of an aortic graft.

Clostridia are isolated from approximately two-thirds of patients with intraabdominal infections resulting from intestinal perforation. *C. ramosum*, *C. perfringens*, and *C. bifermentans* are the most commonly isolated species. The presence of clostridial species does not affect the clinical presentation or outcome of these infections (Chap. 157).

An association has been made between malignancy and the isolation of *C. septicum* in the absence of a grossly contaminated deep traumatic wound; in this situation, *C. septicum* may cause spontaneous nontraumatic myonecrosis (Fig. 135-1). A major site for such a malignancy is the gastrointestinal tract, particularly the colon. An association with leukemia or with other solid tumors has also been noted, and one case of fatal myonecrosis has been reported in a patient with ovarian cancer. Some of these patients present with *C. septicum* bacteremia; these cases have a fulminant clinical course (discussed below). Others develop localized suppurative infection in the abdomen or the abdominal wall without bacteremia. Presumably, this infection arises from a silent perforation that leads to intraabdominal abscess formation.

Clostridia have been isolated from suppurative infections of the female genital tract, particularly tuboovarian and pelvic abscesses. The major species involved has been *C. perfringens*. Most of these suppurative infections are mild, with no evidence of uterine gangrene. *C. perfringens* has been isolated from as many as 20% of diseased gallbladders at surgery. One clinical syndrome, *emphysematous cholecystitis*, is caused by clostridial species at least 50% of the time. In this syndrome, gas forms in the biliary radicles and the wall of the gallbladder. Emphysematous cholecystitis is seen most often in diabetic patients. Although the mortality rate in this entity is higher than in more common forms of cholecystitis, there is no evidence of myonecrosis.

Clostridia are among the many organisms found in empyema fluid or isolated by transtracheal aspiration from patients with lung abscesses. There is no unique clinical clue to the presence of clostridia (as opposed to other organisms) in these infections. *C. perfringens* has been reported as a cause of empyema arising from aspiration pneumonia, pulmonary emboli, and infarction. However, the majority of cases of clostridial empyema are secondary to trauma.

FIGURE 135-1 Spontaneous nontraumatic clostridial myonecrosis (gas gangrene). A man in his 50s presented with severe pain in the right upper extremity. Over several hours, he developed progressive swelling and discoloration in that extremity (**A**), with hemorrhagic ecchymoses and bullae (**B**). Gram's stain of aspirate from bullous lesions revealed gram-positive bacilli (**C**). The patient underwent amputation of the extremity. Tissue Gram's stain (**D**) also showed gram-positive bacilli, and surgical cultures grew *C. septicum*. Subsequent evaluation of the patient led to the diagnosis of invasive colonic carcinoma. *(Images used with permission of Stephen Calderwood, MD, and www.idimages.org.)*

Skin and Soft Tissue Infections   Various categories of traumatic wound infections due to clostridia have been described: simple contamination, anaerobic cellulitis, fasciitis with or without systemic manifestations, and anaerobic myonecrosis.

SIMPLE CONTAMINATION   Clostridia are cultured most often from wounds in the absence of clinical signs of sepsis. As many as 30% of battle wounds are contaminated by clostridia without signs of suppuration, and 16% of penetrating abdominal wounds yield clostridia on culture despite treatment with cephalothin and kanamycin. In cases of trauma, clostridia are isolated with equal frequency from suppurative and well-healing wounds. Thus the diagnosis of clostridial infection should be based on clinical rather than bacteriologic criteria.

LOCALIZED INFECTION OF THE SKIN AND SOFT TISSUE WITHOUT SYSTEMIC SIGNS   This condition, originally referred to as *anaerobic cellulitis*, is a localized infection involving the skin and soft tissue and is due to clostridia alone or with other bacteria. There are no systemic signs of toxicity, although the infection may invade locally, producing necrosis. These infections tend to be relatively indolent, spreading slowly to contiguous areas. Localized infections are relatively free of pain and edema. Perhaps because of the lack of edema, gas that is limited to the wound and the immediately surrounding tissue may be more evident than in gas gangrene. In these localized infections, gas is never found intramuscularly. Cellulitis, perirectal abscesses, and diabetic foot ulcers are typical infections from which clostridial species can be isolated. If inadequately treated, these localized infections advance by extension through subcutaneous tissue and fascial planes into muscle and may produce severe systemic disease with signs of toxemia.

A localized form of suppurative myositis has been described in heroin addicts. These patients develop local pain and tenderness in discrete areas (particularly the thigh and forearm), with the subsequent appearance of fluctuance and crepitance that require surgical drainage. The unusual aspect of these infections is that they remain localized without systemic signs of toxicity. Moreover, the affected local areas are not necessarily sites of trauma or heroin injection. Pathologic examination reveals subcutaneous abscesses, purulent myositis, and fasciitis from which clostridia are recovered in pure culture; on occasion, mixed infections involving aerobes and anaerobes are found. Wound botulism has been reported in association with the injection of black tar heroin.

SPREADING CELLULITIS AND FASCIITIS WITH SYSTEMIC TOXICITY This condition involves diffuse spreading cellulitis and fasciitis, without myonecrosis and with only mild inflammation in muscle. Patients present with the abrupt onset of a syndrome that progresses rapidly (within hours) through the fascial planes. In cases with suppuration and gas in soft tissues as well as overwhelming toxemia, the infection is rapidly fatal. On physical examination there is subcutaneous crepitation but little localized pain. Surgery is of no proven value because there are no discretely involved tissues amenable to resection, as may be the case in myonecrosis. However, in rapidly advancing fasciitis, incision of the affected area is still the cornerstone of therapy. The initial local lesion may be quite innocuous and arises from an area involved by tumor or other infection and not by injury. The systemic toxic effects include hemolysis and injury of capillary membranes. Usually, this infection is fatal within 48 h, despite intensive therapy involving antitoxin and exchange transfusion. This syndrome is seen most commonly in patients with carcinoma, especially of the sigmoid or the cecum. Presumably, the tumor invades the fascia, and colonic contents leak into the abdominal wall. Patients present with extreme toxicity and occasionally with total-body crepitation. The syndrome differs from necrotizing fasciitis caused by other organisms in three respects: (1) rapid mortality, (2) rapid tissue invasion, and (3) the systemic effects of the toxin, typified by massive hemolysis.

GAS GANGRENE (CLOSTRIDIAL MYONECROSIS) Gas gangrene is characterized by rapid and extensive necrosis of muscle accompanied by gas formation and systemic toxicity and occurs when bacteria invade healthy muscle from adjacent traumatized muscle or soft tissue. The infection originates in a wound contaminated with clostridia. Although >30% of deep wounds are infected with clostridia, the incidence of clostridial myonecrosis is quite low. These infections occur in both military and civilian settings. An essential factor in the genesis of gas gangrene appears to be trauma, particularly involving deep muscle laceration. The entity of clostridial myonecrosis is relatively uncommon after simple, through-and-through bullet wounds without shattering of bone and is relatively common after shrapnel fragmentation wounds, particularly when deep muscle is involved. In civilian cases, gas gangrene can follow trauma, surgery, or IM injection. The trauma need not be severe; however, the wound must be deep, necrotic, and without communication to the surface. Indeed, seeding of muscle tissue by *C. septicum* from a gastrointestinal source—often a malignancy—may lead to spontaneous nontraumatic clostridial myonecrosis (Fig. 135-1).

The incubation period of gas gangrene is usually short: almost always <3 days and frequently <24 h. Some 80% of cases are caused by *C. perfringens*, while *C. novyi*, *C. septicum*, and *C. histolyticum* cause most of the remaining cases. Typically, gas gangrene begins with the sudden onset of pain in the region of the wound, which helps to differentiate it from spreading cellulitis. Once established, the pain increases steadily in severity but remains localized to the infected area and spreads only if the infection spreads. Soon after pain develops, local swelling and edema—accompanied by a thin, often hemorrhagic exudate—appear. Patients frequently develop marked tachycardia, but elevation in temperature may be only minimal. Gas usually is not obvious at this early stage and may be completely absent. Frothiness of the wound exudate may be noted. The skin is tense, white, often marbled with blue, and cooler than normal. The symptoms progress rapidly; swelling, edema, and toxemia increase, and a profuse serous discharge, which may have a peculiar sweetish smell, appears. Gram's staining of the wound exudate shows many gram-positive rods with relatively few inflammatory cells (Fig. 135-1*C*).

At surgery, muscle may appear pale because of the intensity of edema, but it does not contract when probed with a scalpel. When dissected, the muscle is beefy red and nonviable and can progress to become black, friable, and gangrenous. It is important to establish a diagnosis early, preferably by frozen-section biopsy of muscle.

Despite hypotension, renal failure, and (often) body crepitation, patients with myonecrosis frequently have a heightened awareness of their surroundings until just before death, when they lapse into toxic delirium and coma. In untreated cases, as the local wounds progress, the skin becomes bronzed; bullae appear, become filled with dark red fluid, and are accompanied by dark patches of cutaneous gangrene. Gas appears in later phases but may not be as obvious as in anaerobic cellulitis. Jaundice is rare in wound gas gangrene (in contrast to uterine infections) and, when it does appear, is almost invariably associated with hemoglobinuria, hemoglobinemia, and septicemia. Cases of clostridial myonecrosis without a history of trauma have been reported. These patients have bullous lesions and crepitation of the skin; they present with a rapidly worsening course that includes myonecrosis, especially of the extremities.

Bacteremia and Clostridial Sepsis The relatively common entity of transient clostridial bacteremia can arise in any hospitalized patient but is most common with a predisposing focus in the gastrointestinal tract, biliary tract, or uterus. Fever frequently resolves within 24–48 h without therapy. Despite the finding of clostridial bacteremia following septic abortions and the frequent isolation of clostridia from the lochia, most of the patients involved do not have evidence of sepsis. In one series of 60 patients with clostridial bacteremia, half had an infected site that could be associated with the bacteremia, while the other half had a totally unrelated illness, such as tuberculous pneumonia, meningitis, or benign gastroenteritis. By the time blood culture reports are returned, patients frequently are completely well and sometimes have been discharged. Therefore, when a blood culture is positive for clostridia, the patient must be assessed clinically rather than simply treated on the basis of the culture result.

Clostridial sepsis is an uncommon but almost invariably fatal illness following clostridial infection—primarily that of the uterus, colon, or biliary tract. This entity must be differentiated from transient clostridial bacteremia, which is much more common. *C. perfringens* causes the majority of cases of both sepsis and transient bacteremia. *C. septicum*, *C. sordellii*, and *C. novyi* account for most of the remainder of cases. *C. sordellii* sepsis with toxic shock syndrome has been associated with pregnancy and more recently with medically induced abortion. Clostridia account for 1–2.5% of all positive blood cultures in major hospital centers.

The majority of cases of clostridial sepsis originate from the female genital tract and follow septic abortion. Introduction of a foreign body is a common antecedent event. In the uterus, residual necrotic fetal and placental tissues and traumatized endometrium may allow the growth of clostridia. Only a small fraction of cases of septic abortion (1%) are followed by serious sepsis. In these instances, sepsis, fever, and chills begin 1–3 days after the attempted abortion. The initial signs are malaise, headache, severe myalgias, abdominal pain, nausea, vomiting, and occasionally diarrhea. Frequently, a bloody or brown vaginal discharge is noted. Patients may rapidly develop oliguria, hypotension, jaundice, and hemoglobinuria. The hemolysis, which is secondary to *C. perfringens* α toxin, causes a characteristic bronzing of the skin. As in myonecrosis, the mental status of severely ill patients is characterized by increased alertness and apprehension. Local examination of the pelvis reveals foul cervical discharge, occasionally with gas. Frequently, laceration marks around the cervix or perforation of the cervical segment is evident. If the infection involves the myometrium or has spread to the adnexa, extreme tenderness, guarding, and an adnexal mass may be found.

Laboratory studies in patients with sepsis reveal an elevated white blood cell count and may show pink, hemoglobin-tinged plasma. Anemia is proportional to the degree of hemolysis, and the hematocrit may be extremely low. Platelet counts may be reduced, and there is often evidence of disseminated intravascular coagulation (DIC). Oliguria or anuria, increasingly refractory hypotension, and hemorrhage and bruising may develop.

Clostridia may enter the bloodstream from the gastrointestinal or biliary tract. This occurrence is associated with ulcerative lesions or obstruction of the small or large intestine, necrotic or infiltrating malignancy, bowel surgery, or various abdominal catastrophes. The patient may present with an acute febrile illness, with chills and fever but no other signs of localized infection. Intravascular hemolysis occurs in

TABLE 135-1 TREATMENT OF CLOSTRIDIAL INFECTIONS[a]

Condition	Antibiotic Treatment	Penicillin Allergy	Adjunctive Treatment/Note
Contamination	None	—	—
Gas gangrene	Penicillin, 3–4 million units IV q4h, *plus* Clindamycin, 600 mg IV q6h	Chloramphenicol, metronidazole, imipenem, doxycycline (see text)[b]	Surgical debridement with wide excision is essential. Consider hyperbaric oxygen.
Clostridial sepsis	Penicillin, 3–4 million units IV q4h, *plus* Clindamycin, 600 mg IV q6h	Chloramphenicol, metronidazole, imipenem, doxycycline (see text)[b]	Transient bacteremia may be clinically insignificant.
Suppurative deep-tissue infections (e.g., abdominal wall, gynecologic)	Penicillin, 3–4 million units IV q4h, *plus* Gentamicin, 5 mg/kg IV q24h, *or* A third-generation cephalosporin (e.g., ceftriaxone, 2 g IV q12h)	As above, plus gentamicin or a quinolone	Empirical therapy should be given. Therapy should be based on Gram's stain and culture results when available.

[a]Treatment recommendations for *C. difficile* colitis, tetanus, and botulism are found in Chaps. 123, 133, and 134, respectively.
[b]Perform sensitivity testing; consider desensitization.

as many as half of such cases. Biliary or gastrointestinal symptoms, if present, may be the only clue to the etiology. Positive blood cultures provide the definitive clue to the diagnosis.

Patients with malignant disease can also develop rapidly fatal clostridial sepsis, particularly from a gastrointestinal focus. The most common species in this setting is *C. septicum*. Characteristic signs and symptoms include fever, tachycardia, hypotension, abdominal pain or tenderness, nausea, vomiting, and (preterminally) coma. The tachycardia may be out of proportion to the fever. Only ~20–30% of patients develop hemolysis. A striking feature of this syndrome is the rapidity of death, which frequently occurs in <12 h.

DIAGNOSIS

The diagnosis of clostridial disease, in association with positive cultures, must be based primarily on clinical findings. Because of the presence of clostridia in many wounds, their mere isolation from any site, including the blood, does not necessarily indicate severe disease. Smears of wound exudates, uterine scrapings, or cervical discharge may show abundant large gram-positive rods as well as other organisms. Cultures should be placed in selective media and incubated anaerobically for identification of clostridia. The diagnosis of clostridial myonecrosis can be established by frozen-section biopsy of muscle.

The urine of patients with severe clostridial sepsis may contain protein and casts, and some patients may develop severe uremia. Profound alterations of circulating erythrocytes are seen in severely toxemic patients. Patients have hemolytic anemia, which develops extremely rapidly, along with hemoglobinemia, hemoglobinuria, and elevated levels of serum bilirubin. Spherocytosis, increased osmotic and mechanical red blood cell fragility, erythrophagocytosis, and methemoglobinemia have been described. DIC may develop in patients with severe infection. In patients with severe sepsis, Wright's or Gram's staining of a smear of peripheral blood or buffy coat may demonstrate clostridia.

X-ray examination sometimes provides an important clue to the diagnosis by revealing gas in muscles, subcutaneous tissue, or the uterus. However, the finding of gas is not pathognomonic for clostridial infection. Other anaerobic bacteria, frequently mixed with aerobic organisms, may produce gas.

℞ CLOSTRIDIAL INFECTIONS

(Table 135-1) Traumatic wounds should be thoroughly cleansed and debrided. Traditionally, the antibiotic of choice for severe clostridial infection has been penicillin G (20 million units per day in adults). Penicillin G treatment of gas gangrene has become more controversial because of increasing resistance to this drug and data obtained from animal models of infection. In a mouse mod-

el of gas gangrene, antibiotics inhibiting toxin synthesis appeared to be preferable to cell wall–active drugs; clindamycin treatment enhanced survival more than therapy with penicillin; and the combination of clindamycin and penicillin was superior to penicillin alone. For severe clostridial sepsis, clindamycin may be used at a dose of 600 mg every 6 h in combination with high-dose penicillin (3–4 million units every 4 h). Although no clinical trials validate this choice, it is gaining acceptance in the infectious disease community.

In cases of penicillin sensitivity or allergy, other antibiotics should be considered, but all should be tested for in vitro activity because of the occasional isolation of resistant strains. Clostridia are frequently, but not universally, susceptible in vitro to cefoxitin, carbenicillin, chloramphenicol, clindamycin, metronidazole, doxycycline, imipenem, minocycline, tetracycline, third-generation cephalosporins, and vancomycin. For severe clostridial infections, sensitivity testing should be done before an antimicrobial agent with unpredictable activity is used. Simple contamination of a wound with clostridia should not be treated with antibiotics. Localized skin and soft tissue infection can be managed by debridement rather than with systemic antibiotics. Drugs are required when the process extends into adjacent tissue or when fever and systemic signs of sepsis are present. Surgery is a mainstay of therapy for gas gangrene. Amputation is often required for rapidly spreading infection involving a limb, as the process frequently fails to respond to antibiotics. Hysterectomy is required for uterine myonecrosis. Abdominal wall myonecrosis usually continues despite initial aggressive surgery and antibiotic therapy and requires repeated surgical debridement of all involved muscle.

Suppurative infections should be treated with antibiotics. Frequently, broad-spectrum antibiotics must be used because of the mixed flora involved in these infections. Aminoglycosides can be used for the aerobic gram-negative bacteria involved in mixed infections.

The use of a polyvalent gas gangrene antitoxin is still recommended by some authorities. At present, no such antitoxin is produced in the United States, and most centers have discontinued its use in the management of patients with suspected gas gangrene or clostridial postabortion sepsis because of questionable efficacy and the substantial risk of hypersensitivity to horse serum, from which the antitoxin is derived.

The use of hyperbaric oxygen in the treatment of gas gangrene is also controversial. Studies in humans are not well designed to answer questions on efficacy, but several knowledgeable authors believe that hyperbaric oxygen therapy has contributed to dramatic clinical improvement. Such therapy may, however, be associated with untoward effects due to oxygen toxicity and high atmospheric pressure. Some centers without hyperbaric chambers have reported acceptable mortality rates; thus expert surgical and medical management and control of complications are probably the most important factors in the treatment of gas gangrene. Fasciotomy should not be delayed for hyperbaric oxygen therapy.

ACKNOWLEDGMENTS

The authors acknowledge the contributions of Dori F. Zaleznik, MD, to this chapter in earlier editions.

FURTHER READINGS

Borriello SP: Clostridial disease of the gut. Clin Infect Dis 20:S242, 1995

Centers for Disease Control and Prevention: *Clostridium sordellii* toxic shock syndrome after medical abortion with mifepristone and intravaginal misoprostol—United States and Canada, 2001–2005. MMWR 54:724, 2005

Lorber B: Gas gangrene and other *Clostridium*-associated diseases, in *Principles and Practice of Infectious Diseases*, 6th ed, GL Mandell et al (eds). Philadelphia, Elsevier Churchill Livingstone, 2005, pp 2828–2838

908 MURRAY-LILLIBRIDGE K et al: Epidemiological findings and medical, legal, and public health challenges of an investigation of severe soft tissue infections and deaths among injecting drug users—Ireland, 2000. Epidemiol Infect 134:894, 2006

PRINSSEN HM et al: *Clostridium septicum* myonecrosis and ovarian cancer: A case report and review of literature. Gynecol Oncol 72:116, 1999

ROOD JI: Virulence genes of *Clostridium perfringens*. Annu Rev Microbiol 52:333, 1998

STEVENS DL, BRYANT AE: The role of clostridial toxins in the pathogenesis of gas gangrene. Clin Infect Dis 35:S93, 2002

WANG C et al: Hyperbaric oxygen for treating wounds: A systematic review of the literature. Arch Surg 138:272, 2003

SECTION 6   DISEASES CAUSED BY GRAM-NEGATIVE BACTERIA

136 Meningococcal Infections
Lee M. Wetzler

DEFINITION

Neisseria meningitidis is the etiologic agent of two life-threatening diseases: meningococcal meningitis and fulminant meningococcemia. More rarely, meningococci cause pneumonia, septic arthritis, pericarditis, urethritis, and conjunctivitis. Most cases are potentially preventable by vaccination.

ETIOLOGIC AGENT

Meningococci are gram-negative aerobic diplococci. Unlike the other neisseriae, they have a polysaccharide capsule. They are transmitted among humans—their only known habitat—via respiratory secretions. Colonization of the nasopharynx or pharynx is much more common than invasive disease.

MICROBIOLOGY AND CLASSIFICATION

On the basis of genome sequencing, *N. meningitidis* is categorized as a β-proteobacterium related to *Bordetella*, *Burkholderia*, *Kingella*, and *Methylomonas* and—more distantly—to *Vibrio*, *Haemophilus*, and *Escherichia coli*. Meningococci are traditionally classified by serologic typing systems based on structural differences in capsule (serogroup), major outer-membrane protein (OMP) porin (PorB, serotype), minor porin (PorA, serosubtype), and lipooligosaccharide (LOS, immunotype). Thus, for example, the meningococcal strain designation B:2b:P1.5:L3,7,9 reflects the serogroup (B), serotype (2b), serosubtype (P1.5), and immunotype (L3,7,9). Meningococci are also differentiated from the other Neisseriaceae by their pattern of sugar fermentation. *N. gonorrhoeae* ferments only glucose; *N. meningitidis* ferments glucose and maltose; and *N. lactamica* ferments glucose, maltose, and lactose.

Meningococci are classified into serogroups according to the antigenicity of their capsular polysaccharides, which reflects structural differences in these carbohydrates. Five serogroups (A, B, C, Y, and W-135; see below) are responsible for >90% of cases of meningococcal disease worldwide. One limitation of serogroup classification based on polysaccharide capsular structure is that the genes for capsule biosynthesis can be transferred from one strain to another, with consequent changes in the capsule structure of the recipient strain and therefore in its serogroup. Meningococcal serotypes and subtypes are defined by antigenic differences in specific OMPs. Thus, other methods for tracking meningococcal strains have become increasingly useful. Multilocus enzyme electrophoresis classifies bacteria into electrophoretic types (ETs), and variations in ET are not based on antigenic variations or alterations in outer-membrane component structures. Other techniques for establishing strain identity or nonidentity—i.e., pulsed-field gel electrophoresis of large DNA fragments and amplification of bacterial genomic sequences by polymerase chain reaction (PCR)—are based on the genetic make-up of the strain. These techniques are used for identification of the strains associated with outbreaks of disease. For example, the virulent III-1 clonal complex of serogroup A was first recognized in Nepal in 1983–1984; it spread to Mecca, then to sub-Saharan Africa, and subsequently to temperate Africa. The serogroup B ET-5 complex was first identified in Norway in the 1970s and later caused outbreaks in Europe, Cuba, and South and North America (most recently, in the Pacific Northwest). Serogroup C ET-24 (the ET-37 complex) has caused sporadic cases and outbreaks in Canada and the United States; in some analyses, it has been associated with high rates of mortality and morbidity.

EPIDEMIOLOGY

 Meningococcal disease occurs worldwide as isolated (sporadic) cases, institution- or community-based outbreaks, and large epidemics. Despite effective antibiotics and partially effective vaccines, *N. meningitidis* is still a leading global cause of meningitis and rapidly fatal sepsis, often in otherwise-healthy individuals.

N. meningitidis is unique among the major bacterial agents of meningitis in that it causes epidemic as well as endemic (sporadic) disease. In all, 300,000–500,000 cases of meningococcal disease occur worldwide each year—numbers that frequently are increased by large epidemics. The annual incidence of meningococcal disease is 1–2 cases per 100,000 population for sporadic disease, 5–10 cases per 100,000 for hypersporadic disease (localized outbreaks and case clusters), and 10–>1000 cases per 100,000 for pandemic and epidemic disease (e.g., serogroup A epidemics).

Serogroup A strains, which caused most of the large epidemics of meningococcal disease during the first half of the twentieth century, are now associated with recurring epidemics in sub-Saharan Africa (the African meningitis belt) and other locales in the developing world. In the largest meningococcal epidemic recorded, >300,000 cases and 30,000 deaths due to serogroup A *N. meningitidis* occurred in sub-Saharan Africa in 1996–1997. Serogroups B and C cause most cases of sporadic and epidemic meningococcal disease in industrialized countries. Since 1980, large serogroup B epidemics and/or outbreaks of serogroup A or C meningococcal disease have also occurred in Europe, the United States, Canada, China, Nepal, Mongolia, New Zealand, Cuba, Brazil, Chile, Saudi Arabia, and South Africa. In the United States and Canada during the 1990s, serogroup B was the most common cause of sporadic disease, while serogroup C was a more frequent cause of outbreaks. Serogroup Y has recently been isolated from almost one-third of cases of meningococcal disease in the United States. In general, patients with serogroup Y disease are older and more likely to be African American or to have a chronic underlying illness than are patients with disease caused by other serogroups. Serogroups Y and W-135 are isolated more often than the other serogroups from patients with pneumonia. In 2000, 2001, and 2002, worldwide epidemics of serogroup W-135 meningococcal disease occurred in association with the Muslim pilgrimage to Mecca (the Hajj) and in the meningitis belt of sub-Saharan Africa.

In the United States, the attack rate for sporadic meningococcal disease is ~1 case per 100,000 persons per year. Disease attack rates are highest among infants 3–9 months of age (10–15 cases per 100,000 infants per year). Attack rates are higher among children than among adults, and there is a second peak of incidence among teenagers, in whom outbreaks have often been tied to residence in barracks, dormitories, or other crowded conditions. This observation has prompted the recommendation that meningococcal polysaccharide-based vaccines (see below) be administered to incoming college freshmen to prevent outbreaks at colleges. Although the age-specific incidence is much lower among adults (<1 case per 100,000 persons per year), one-third to one-half of all cases of sporadic meningococcal disease occur in individuals ≥18 years of age. Peak disease incidence coincides with the winter peak of respiratory viral illnesses. During epidemics, disease incidence increases disproportionately among teenagers and young adults. In sub-Saharan Africa, epidemic outbreaks occur with the dry season and the coming of the dry dusty winds of the harmattan.

Meningococcal disease occurs more commonly among the household contacts of primary cases than in the general population. The secondary attack rate is 400–1000 per 100,000 household members. School-based clusters of cases have also been described; the attack rate among school contacts of cases has been estimated at 2–4 cases per 100,000 exposed individuals. In outbreaks on college campuses, attack rates have been highest among students living in dormitories. Most secondary cases occur within 2 weeks of the primary case, although some cases may develop as long as several months later. Secondary cases account for <2% of all cases reported each year in the United States.

Meningococcal colonization of the nasopharynx (asymptomatic carriage) can persist for months. In nonepidemic periods, ~10% of healthy individuals are colonized, as are up to 30% of persons living in relatively crowded conditions (e.g., in military barracks or college dormitories). Factors that predispose individuals to colonization with *N. meningitidis* include residence in the same household with a person who has meningococcal disease or is a carrier, household or institutional crowding, active or passive exposure to tobacco smoke, and a recent history of a viral upper respiratory infection. These factors have also been associated with an increased risk of meningococcal disease.

PATHOGENESIS

(Fig. 136-1) Meningococci that colonize the upper respiratory tract are internalized by nonciliated mucosal cells and may traverse them to enter the submucosa, from which they can make their way into the bloodstream. While meningococcal colonization of healthy humans is common, bloodstream infection is an infrequent event that is not essential for the organisms' survival and spread. The production of human disease has no obvious evolutionary advantage for either pathogen or host. Although some strains of *N. meningitidis* are thought to cause more severe disease in humans than do other strains, the basis for this difference is not understood. Meningococci may undergo important phenotypic changes when they adapt to growth in vivo; presumed virulence traits include the antiphagocytic capsular polysaccharide, an ability to sialylate LOS so that it mimics host-cell carbohydrate moieties and inhibits complement deposition, the secretion of IgA protease, and mechanisms for iron acquisition. However, there is little evidence that alteration in meningococcal components, putative toxins, or other secreted substances affects virulence. Moreover, the ET-5 strain of serogroup B *N. meningitidis* has been associated with high case-fatality rates in some populations but not in others. These points suggest that host factors, as opposed to bacterial components, are the main mediators of immune resistance and disease pathogenesis.

A meningococcal organism that enters the bloodstream from the nasopharynx and survives host defenses generally has one of two fates. If multiplication occurs slowly, the bacteria eventually may seed local sites, such as the meninges and/or (rarely) the joints or the pericardium. More rapid multiplication in the bloodstream is associated with the clinical features of meningococcemia [i.e., petechiae, purpura, disseminated intravascular coagulation (DIC), and shock], which usually causes symptoms before local sites become infected. Thus, compartmentalization of bacterial growth and host inflammation either in the blood or at a local site (usually the meninges) can occur.

Outer-Membrane Components Associated with Virulence Meningococcal strains are characterized by the expression of capsular polysaccha-

FIGURE 136-1 Meningococcal disease pathogenesis, susceptibility, and severity. After human-to-human transmission, environmental factors (smoking, co-infections), polymorphisms in innate immunity or other genes, and absence of mucosal antibodies may confer susceptibility to meningococcal invasion from the nasopharynx into the bloodstream. In individuals who lack bactericidal antibodies, terminal or alternative pathway complement-deficiency states and other genetic polymorphisms may influence the severity of the ensuing host response and the clinical presentation. Although each of these gene associations has been reported, most of them require confirmation in different ethnic groups. MBL, mannose-binding lectin; TNF, tumor necrosis factor; FcγRIIA, FCγRIIA R131 allele; PAI-1, plasminogen activator inhibitor 1; ACE-1, angiotensin-converting enzyme 1; IL, interleukin; IL-1Ra, interleukin 1 receptor antagonist.

ride and other outer-membrane structures, including LOS (endotoxin). Outer-membrane blebbing, meningococcal autolysis, molecular mimicry, genome plasticity, horizontal DNA exchange, and phase and/or antigenic variation are all important in meningococcal virulence.

CAPSULE The polysaccharide capsule is a major—if not *the* major—virulence factor of *N. meningitidis*. As stated above, meningococci isolated from the blood or cerebrospinal fluid (CSF) of patients with invasive meningococcal disease most often express capsules of serogroups A, B, C, Y, and W-135. Isolates from asymptomatic nasopharyngeal carriers are nongroupable or express B, Y, X, Z, or 29E capsular serogroups. Capsules impart antiphagocytic and antibactericidal properties to the meningococcus and thus enhance meningococcal survival during invasion of the bloodstream or CSF. Capsules also provide protective properties (e.g., preventing desiccation and phagocytic killing) and antiadherent properties; these properties promote meningococcal transmission, spread, and survival externally and within intracellular compartments such as phagocytic vacuoles.

Except in serogroup A, the major meningococcal capsular polysaccharides associated with invasive disease are composed of polymers of sialic acid (*N*-acetyl neuraminic acid, NANA) derivatives. The serogroup B capsule is composed of (α2→8)-linked NANA, the serogroup C capsule of (α2→9)-linked NANA, the serogroup Y capsule of alternating D-glucose and NANA, and the serogroup W-135 capsule of D-galactose and NANA. The differences in sialic acid capsule composition are derived from the distinct polysialyltransferases encoded by the fourth gene of the capsule biosynthesis operon, which is also used as a basis for capsule-specific PCR diagnosis. A four-gene operon encoding the capsule transport apparatus (ctr) is conserved among different serogroups and is also used in PCR diagnosis. The serogroup A capsule is composed of repeating units of (α)-linked *N*-acetyl-mannosamine-1-phosphate and is encoded by a four-gene biosynthesis cassette unique for this serogroup.

OUTER-MEMBRANE PROTEINS Meningococci isolated from sites of colonization or invasive disease are piliated. Pili are complex outer-membrane, protein-based organelles that facilitate adhesion—the first step in meningococcal–host cell interactions. Meningococci express two major OMP porins, PorA and PorB. Human opsonins and bactericidal antibodies induced during meningococcal disease have been shown to recognize PorA and PorB. Vaccines based on PorA-containing outer-membrane vesicles are under development. Another OMP, Opc, is involved in cell attachment and is also a target of bactericidal antibodies. Meningococci encounter iron-restricted environments during infection. The majority of host iron is presented intracellularly as hemoglobin and extracellularly as human transferrin and lactoferrin. Meningococci have evolved systems for acquisition of these iron-carrying molecules.

LIPOOLIGOSACCHARIDE Meningococcal LOS is structurally related to the lipopolysaccharide (LPS) expressed by many gram-negative bacilli. However, LOS does not have repeating O-antigen subunits of sugars. The lipid A moiety of LOS, which has been classically termed *endotoxin* (as opposed to the bacterial exotoxins), is the portion that mediates the induction of inflammatory cytokines often seen in disease. The effect of lipid A is due to an interaction with the innate immune receptor Toll-like receptor 4 (TLR4) in association with the membrane protein MD2. TLR4 and MD2 are found mainly on macrophages/monocytes, dendritic cells, and other phagocytes.

Rates of morbidity and mortality associated with meningococcal bacteremia and meningitis have been directly correlated with the amount of circulating meningococcal endotoxin. Whether this measure is an indication of overall bacterial load or is a direct pathogenic mechanism of disease is debatable. The ability of signaling through TLR4 by the lipid A moiety of LOS to induce production of inflammatory and proinflammatory cytokines from various immune cells suggests a direct relationship. However, other meningococcal outer-membrane components—e.g., meningococcal porins and lipoproteins (including the H8 lipoprotein)—induce immune cell activation via other TLRs, especially TLR2. A recently derived LOS⁻ meningococcal mutant was still able to induce significant production of proinflammatory cytokines [especially tumor necrosis factor α (TNF-α), interleukin (IL) 6, and IL-1β] by macrophages and cytokines. This observation suggests a potential role for these components in induction of meningococcal sepsis.

 Other Virulence Mechanisms The outer-membrane components of *N. meningitidis* (e.g., pili, LOS, Opa proteins, Opc, capsule) vary in expression or structure at high frequencies (10^{-2}–10^{-4} per cell per generation). Variation is the result of genetic switches that turn expression of a component on or off, regulate the amount of a component, or alter the structure of a component. Genetic events leading to phase and structural variation allow immune escape and create variability in the structures that are important in pathogenesis (on and off expression of attachment ligands, protection against serum killing, invasion determinants). The serogroup B capsule provides an example of how meningococci downregulate the human immune response through the expression of host-like antigens. The (α2→8)-linked polysialic acid capsule of serogroup B meningococci is identical to structures on the human neural cell adhesion molecule N-CAM. Meningococci are also characterized by frequent vesiculation (blebbing) of the outer membrane, and the amount of blebbing may vary between strains. Blebs contribute to the rapid initiation of the inflammatory and clotting cascades. They may also be related to the natural autolysis of meningococci that results in DNA release and facilitates genetic transformation.

Association of Virulence Mechanisms with Specific Meningococcal

Infections Specific disease manifestations of meningococcal infections have specific virulence and pathogenic mechanisms, as described below for fulminant meningococcemia and meningitis.

Fulminant Meningococcemia • *PURPURA FULMINANS* Fulminant

meningococcemia is perhaps the most rapidly lethal form of septic shock experienced by humans. It differs from most other forms of septic shock by the prominence of hemorrhagic skin lesions (petechiae, purpura; see Fig. 52-5) and the consistent development of DIC.

FIGURE 136-2 The pathogenesis of fibrin deposition in patients with fulminant meningococcemia. PAI-1, plasminogen activator inhibitor 1. (*Adapted from M Levi et al: Eur J Clin Invest 27:3, 1997.*)

The dominant proinflammatory molecule in the meningococcal cell wall is the endotoxin or LOS, and the outer membrane that contains it is poorly tethered to the underlying peptidoglycan. This structural peculiarity seems to account for the fact that meningococci shed LOS-containing membrane blebs as they grow. The bacteria can multiply to very high concentrations in the blood. The concentrations of endotoxin detected in the blood of patients with fulminant meningococcemia are 10- to 1000-fold higher than those found in the blood of patients with bacteremia due to other gram-negative bacteria. The bacteria and endotoxin-containing blebs stimulate monocytes, neutrophils, and endothelial cells, which then release cytokines and other mediators that can activate many distant targets, including other leukocytes, platelets, and endothelial cells. In addition, meningococci can invade the vascular endothelium. When activated, the endothelium produces molecules that can be procoagulant as well as adhesive for leukocytes.

Patients with fulminant meningococcemia usually have extremely high blood levels of both proinflammatory mediators—i.e., TNF-α, IL-1, interferon γ (IFN-γ), and IL-8—and anti-inflammatory mediators—i.e., IL-1 receptor antagonist (IL-1Ra), soluble IL-1 receptors, soluble TNF-α receptors, and IL-10. The plasma of patients with meningococcal shock can decrease the responses of normal leukocytes to stimuli such as LOS; the implication is that anti-inflammatory mediators predominate in the blood late in infection.

Procoagulant, antifibrinolytic forces are also active in the blood of patients with fulminant meningococcemia (Fig. 136-2). Monocytes express large amounts of tissue factor. Fibrinopeptide A and thrombin-antithrombin levels are high, reflecting active clotting, while antithrombin and fibrinogen levels are low. Although the tissue factor–regulated ("extrinsic") arm of coagulation predominates, the contact system (factors XII and XI, prekallikrein, high-molecular-weight kininogen) is also activated. Striking deficiencies of antithrombin and proteins C and S can occur; studies have found a strong negative correlation between protein C activity and both the size of purpuric skin lesions and the mortality rate. Plasminogen levels are decreased, while plasmin-antiplasmin complexes and plasminogen activator inhibitor 1 (PAI-1) levels in the blood are very high. PAI-1 levels have been correlated with mortality risk.

Fibrin deposition is therefore favored both by the procoagulant tendency (promoted through activation of tissue factor and deficiencies of proteins C and S and antithrombin) and by an antifibrinolytic tendency (favored by excessive PAI-1). Both platelets and leukocytes doubtless contribute to the formation of microthrombi and to the vascular injury that ensues. Thrombosis of small to mid-sized arteries can produce peripheral necrosis and gangrene, necessitating limb or digit amputation.

MENINGITIS Meningococcal bacteremia can result in the seeding of the meninges, pericardium, and large joints. Up to one-third of patients with meningococcal disease present with meningitis or other closed-space infections without signs of sepsis. How meningococci traverse the blood-brain barrier and enter the CSF or reach other closed sites is unclear. Meningococci have been shown to invade endothelial cells both experimentally and in vivo. The choroid plexus is also a potential site of meningococcal entry into the CSF. Meningococcal pili may bind CD46, a complement-regulatory protein that is expressed by the choroid plexus and meningeal epithelia. Upon meningococcal entry into the CSF, a vigorous local inflammatory response ensues, probably triggered by endotoxin-containing meningococcal membranes. Both bacterial growth and the inflammatory response occur within the CSF, where levels of endotoxin, IL-6, TNF-α, IL-1β, IL-1Ra, and IL-10 exceed the concentrations found in plasma by 100- to 1000-fold. The inflammatory response is largely confined to the subarachnoid space and contiguous structures. The inflammatory cytokines TNF-α and IL-1 released in meningococcal bacteremia may also enhance the permeability of the blood-brain barrier. Meningitis and other closed-space infections (e.g., arthritis, pericarditis) are the result of bacterial survival and multiplication at these sites. For example, meningitis and its sequelae are due to the induction of local inflammatory cytokines and other mediators (e.g., nitric oxide), leukocyte infiltration across the blood-brain barrier, breakdown of the blood-brain barrier with edema, release of metalloproteases, induction of cellular apoptosis, coagulation of vessels, and ischemia.

Patients who develop meningitis without meningococcemia may be individuals in whom meningococci do not grow rapidly in or have been cleared from the blood; may have antibodies or phagocytes that slow meningococcal growth; or may lack the (unknown) factors that allow *N. meningitidis* to multiply rapidly in vivo. If disease is recognized early, the prognosis of patients with meningococcal meningitis is substantially better than that of patients with fulminant meningococcemia.

HOST DEFENSE MECHANISMS

Preventing meningococcal growth in blood requires bactericidal and opsonic antibodies, complement, and phagocytes (Fig. 136-3). The major bactericidal antibodies are IgM and IgG, which (except for serogroup B) bind to the capsular polysaccharide. Immunity to meningococci is therefore serogroup specific. Antibodies to other surface (subcapsular) antigens may confer cross-serogroup protection. PorA, PorB, Opc, and LOS appear to be major targets of cross-reactivity and of serogroup B bactericidal antibodies. Infants are protected from meningococcal disease during the first months of life by passively transferred maternal IgG antibodies. As maternal antibody levels

FIGURE 136-3 Protection from meningococcal disease involves both antimeningococcal immunoglobulins and complement. Activation of complement by antimeningococcal IgM or IgG promotes bacterial lysis via the membrane attack complex (C5–C9), while C3b [produced by alternative, mannose-binding lectin (MBL), or classic pathway activation] and antimeningococcal IgG$_2$ cooperate to produce effective opsonophagocytosis. A neutrophil defect in binding IgG$_2$ (the FcγRIIA R131 allele) has been associated with more severe meningococcal disease. CR1, complement receptor 1; LOS, lipooligosaccharide.

wane, the attack rate increases, peaking at 3–9 months of age. Disease incidence declines as protective antibodies are induced by colonization with nonpathogenic bacteria that have cross-reactive antigens. In addition to *N. lactamica*, which frequently colonizes young children, some enteric bacteria have antigens that cross-react with those of meningococci. One theory relates the occurrence of some cases of meningococcal disease to the presence of high levels of IgA antibodies to meningococci, since these antibodies can block the bactericidal activity of IgM.

Complement is required for bactericidal activity and for efficient opsonophagocytosis. Individuals deficient in any of the late complement components (C5–C9) cannot assemble the membrane-attack complex (MAC) needed to kill *Neisseria*. Although the incidence of meningococcal disease is higher among those with late-complement-component deficiencies, these persons typically develop less severe disease than complement-sufficient individuals, do so at an older age, and tend to have disease due to uncommon serogroups (W-135, X, Y, Z, and 29E). Although only one-half of individuals with known late-complement-component deficiency ever experience meningococcal disease, some affected persons have several episodes. Deficiency of each of the terminal complement components is inherited in an autosomal recessive fashion. Properdin deficiency, in contrast, is X-linked; some affected males develop overwhelming meningococcal disease, an observation indicating that the alternative complement pathway is also needed for antimeningococcal host defense. Disease onset in properdin-deficient individuals typically occurs in the teens or twenties. There is also recent evidence that inherited differences in the mannose-binding lectin (MBL) pathway of complement activation may influence the risk of acquiring meningococcal disease in childhood. Alleles that decrease MBL synthesis have been associated with increased risk in the few studies reported to date.

Activation of the classic pathway of complement by antigen-antibody complexes or of the alternative pathway by LOS or capsular polysaccharide is important for producing and maintaining C3b (Fig. 136-3). Without C3b, neither bactericidal lysis nor phagocytosis can proceed effectively. When C3b is generated, meningococcal growth is probably checked by the MAC's bactericidal activity (induction of bacterial lysis) and by robust phagocytosis and opsonophagocytic killing of the bacterium due to complement deposition. Most IgG antibodies to the meningococcal polysaccharide are of the IgG$_2$ isotype; a phagocytic cell defect (the FcγRIIA R131 allele) that impairs the phagocytosis of IgG$_2$-coated particles has been associated with more severe meningococcal disease. This allele has also been associated with a more severe clinical course in patients with late-complement-component deficiency; thus effective phagocytosis may contribute to the relatively mild meningococcal disease usually observed in these individuals.

The results of studies of gene polymorphism–disease associations are summarized in Figs. 136-1 and 136-3. In individuals who lack bactericidal antibodies, protection from acquiring meningococcal bacteremia may be provided, at least in part, by innate immune mechanisms such as the MBL pathway for activating complement, complement factor C4b, and the TLR4 pathway for LOS recognition. Other genes may influence meningococcal survival in vivo [FcγIIA (CD32)], while still others seem to regulate the host inflammatory (IL-1β, IL-1Ra, TNF-α, angiotensin-converting enzyme) and clotting (PAI-1) responses to invading meningococci. Although many of these associations await confirmation in other populations of patients, in sum they point to important genetic influences on the acquisition and severity of meningococcal disease. This conclusion is supported by the overrepresentation of ABO blood group nonsecretors among patients with meningococcal disease and by the striking variability in meningococcal disease incidence among different racial groups.

CLINICAL MANIFESTATIONS

Upper Respiratory Tract Infections Although many patients who develop meningococcal meningitis or meningococcemia report having had throat soreness or other upper respiratory symptoms during the preceding week, it is uncertain whether these symptoms are due to infection with meningococci. Meningococcal pharyngitis is rarely diagnosed. Adult patients with *N. meningitidis* bacteremia more often have clinically apparent disease of the respiratory tract (pneumonia, sinusitis, tracheobronchitis, conjunctivitis) than do younger patients.

Meningococcemia Patients with meningococcal disease may have both meningococcemia and meningitis. These conditions have a wide clinical spectrum, with many overlapping features.

Approximately 10–30% of patients with meningococcal disease have meningococcemia without clinically apparent meningitis. Although meningococcal bacteremia may occasionally be transient and asymptomatic, in most individuals it is associated with fever, chills, nausea, vomiting, and myalgias. Prostration is common. The most distinctive feature is rash. Erythematous macules rapidly become petechial and, in severe cases, purpuric (see Fig. 52-5). Although the lesions are typically found on the trunk and lower extremities, they may also occur on the face, arms, and mucous membranes. The petechiae may coalesce into hemorrhagic bullae or may undergo necrosis and ulcerate. Patients with severe coagulopathy may develop ischemic extremities or digits, often with a sharp line of demarcation between normal and ischemic tissue.

In many patients with fulminant meningococcemia, the CSF may be normal and the CSF culture negative. Indeed, the absence of meningitis in a patient with meningococcemia is a poor prognostic sign; it suggests that the bacteria have multiplied so rapidly in the blood that meningeal seeding has not yet occurred or had time to elicit inflammation in the CSF. Most of these patients also lack evidence of an acute-phase response; i.e., the erythrocyte sedimentation rate is normal, and the C-reactive protein concentration in blood is low.

The *Waterhouse-Friderichsen syndrome* is a dramatic example of DIC-induced microthrombosis, hemorrhage, and tissue injury. Although overt adrenal failure is infrequently documented in patients with fulminant meningococcemia, patients may have partial adrenal insufficiency and be unable to mount the normal hypercortisolemic response to severe stress or cosyntropin stimulation. Almost all patients who die from fulminant meningococcemia have adrenal hemorrhages at autopsy.

Chronic meningococcemia (**Fig. 136-4**) is a rare syndrome of episodic fever, rash, and arthralgias that can last for weeks to months. The rash may be maculopapular; it is occasionally petechial. Splenomegaly may develop. If untreated or if treated with glucocorticoids, chronic meningococcemia may evolve into meningitis, fulminant meningococcemia, or (rarely) endocarditis.

Meningitis (See also Chap. 376) Common presenting symptoms of patients with meningococcal meningitis include nausea and vomiting,

headache, neck stiffness, lethargy, and confusion. The symptoms and signs of meningococcal meningitis cannot be distinguished from those elicited by other meningeal pathogens. Many patients with meningococcal meningitis have concurrent meningococcemia, however, and petechial or purpuric skin lesions (see Fig. 52-5) may suggest the correct diagnosis. CSF findings are consistent with those of purulent meningitis: hypoglycorrhachia, an elevated protein concentration, and a neutrophilic leukocytosis. A Gram's stain of CSF is usually positive (see "Diagnosis," below); when this finding is unaccompanied by CSF leukocytosis, the prognosis for normal recovery is often poor.

Other Manifestations Arthritis occurs in ~10% of patients with meningococcal disease. When arthritis develops during the first few days of the patient's illness, it usually reflects direct meningococcal invasion of the joint. Arthritis that begins later in the course is thought to be due to immune complex deposition. Primary meningococcal pneumonia occurs principally in adults, often in military populations, and is often due to serogroup Y. While meningococcal pericarditis is occasionally seen, endocarditis due to *N. meningitidis* is now exceedingly rare. Primary meningococcal conjunctivitis can be complicated by meningococcemia; systemic therapy is therefore warranted when this condition is diagnosed. Meningococcal urethritis has been reported in individuals who practice oral sex.

Complications Patients with meningococcal meningitis may develop cranial nerve palsies, cortical venous thrombophlebitis, and cerebral edema. Children may develop subdural effusions. Permanent sequelae can include mental retardation, deafness, and hemiparesis. The major long-term morbidity of fulminant meningococcemia is the loss of skin, limbs, or digits that results from ischemic necrosis and infarction.

DIAGNOSIS

Few clinical clues help the physician distinguish the patient with early meningococcal disease from patients with other acute systemic infections. The most useful clinical finding is the petechial or purpuric rash (see Fig. 52-5), but it must be differentiated from the petechial lesions seen with gonococcemia (see Fig. 137-2), Rocky Mountain spotted fever (see Fig. 167-1), hypersensitivity vasculitis (see Fig. 52-4), endemic typhus, and some viral infections. In one case series, one-half of the adults with meningococcal bacteremia had neither meningitis nor a rash.

The definitive diagnosis is established by recovering *N. meningitidis*, its antigens, or its DNA from normally sterile body fluids (e.g., blood, CSF, or synovial fluid) or from skin lesions. Meningococci grow best on Mueller-Hinton or chocolate blood agar at 35°C in an atmosphere that contains 5–10% CO_2. Specimens should be plated without delay. *N. meningitidis* bacteria are oxidase-positive, gram-negative diplococci that typically utilize maltose and glucose.

A Gram's stain of CSF reveals intra- or extracellular organisms in ~85% of patients with meningococcal meningitis. The latex agglutination test for meningococcal polysaccharides in the CSF is less sensitive. PCR amplification of DNA in buffy coat or CSF samples is more sensitive than either of these tests; like the latex agglutination test, PCR is unaffected by prior antibiotic therapy, as neither method requires viable organisms.

Throat or nasopharyngeal specimens should be cultured on Thayer-Martin medium, which suppresses the competing oral flora. Throat or nasopharyngeal cultures are recommended only for research or epidemiologic purposes, since a positive result merely confirms the carrier state and does not establish the existence of systemic disease.

FIGURE 136-4 Erythematous papular lesions are seen on the leg of this patient with chronic meningococcemia. (*Courtesy of Kenneth M. Kaye, MD, and Elaine T. Kaye, MD; with permission*).

℞ MENINGOCOCCAL INFECTIONS

(**Table 136-1**) A third-generation cephalosporin, such as cefotaxime or ceftriaxone, is preferred for initial therapy. One of these cephalosporins in combination with other agents may cover other bacteria (such as *Streptococcus pneumoniae* and *Haemophilus influenzae*) that can cause the same syndromes (Chap. 376). Penicillin G remains an acceptable alternative for

TABLE 136-1 ANTIBIOTIC TREATMENT, CHEMOPROPHYLAXIS, AND VACCINATIONS FOR INVASIVE MENINGOCOCCAL DISEASE

Antibiotic Treatment^a

1. Ceftriaxone 2 g IV q12h (100 mg/kg per day) or cefotaxime 2 g IV q4h
2. For penicillin-sensitive *N. meningitidis*: Penicillin G 18–24 million units per day in divided doses q4h (250,000 units/kg per day)
3. Chloramphenicol 75–100 mg/kg per day in divided doses q6h
4. Meropenem 1.0 g (children, 40 mg) IV q8h
5. In an outbreak setting in developing countries: Long-acting chloramphenicol in oil suspension (Tifomycin), single dose
   Adults: 3.0 g (6 mL)
   Children 1–15 years old: 100 mg/kg
   Children <1 year old: 50 mg/kg

Chemoprophylaxis^b

Rifampin (oral)
   Adults: 600 mg bid for 2 days
   Children ≥1 month old: 10 mg/kg bid for 2 days
   Children <1 month old: 5 mg/kg bid for 2 days
Ciprofloxacin (oral)
   Adults: 500 mg, 1 dose
Ofloxacin (oral)
   Adults: 400 mg, 1 dose
Ceftriaxone (IM)
   Adults: 250 mg, 1 dose
   Children <15 years old: 125 mg, 1 dose
Azithromycin (oral)
   500 mg, 1 dose

Vaccination^c

A, C, Y, W-135 vaccine (Memomune, Aventis Pasteur) or A, C vaccine
Single 0.5-mL subcutaneous injection
New C; A, C; and A, C, Y, W-135 meningococcal conjugate vaccines^d

^{a}Patients with meningococcal meningitis should receive antimicrobial therapy for at least 5 days.
^{b}Use is recommended for close contacts of cases or if ceftriaxone is not used for primary treatment.
^{c}At present, use is generally limited to the control of epidemics and to individuals with increased risk of meningococcal disease. Vaccine efficacy wanes after 3–5 years, and vaccine is not effective in recipients <2 years of age.
^{d}These vaccines appear to provide immunity in young children, a prolonged immune response, and herd immunity (decreased transmission and colonization).

confirmed invasive meningococcal disease in most countries. However, the prevalence of meningococci with reduced susceptibility to penicillin has been increasing, and high-level penicillin resistance has been reported. Other options include meropenem. In the patient who is allergic to β-lactam drugs, chloramphenicol is a suitable alternative; chloramphenicol-resistant meningococci have been reported from Vietnam and France. The newer fluoroquinolones gatifloxacin, moxifloxacin, and gemifloxacin have excellent in vitro activity against *N. meningitidis*, with measurable central nervous system (CNS) penetration, and appear promising in animal models. Patients with meningococcal meningitis should be given antimicrobial therapy for at least 5 days. While glucocorticoid therapy for meningitis in adults is controversial, many experts administer dexamethasone, beginning if possible before antibiotic therapy is initiated; the schedule is 10 mg IV given 15–20 min before the first antibiotic dose and then every 6 h for 4 days. The data regarding steroid use to diminish CNS inflammation are strongest for *H. influenzae* and *S. pneumoniae* meningitis, especially in children.

Patients with fulminant meningococcemia often experience diffuse leakage of fluid into extravascular spaces, shock, and multiple-organ dysfunction (Chaps. 264 and 265). Myocardial depression may be prominent. Supportive therapy, although never studied in randomized, placebo-controlled trials, is recommended. Standard measures include vigorous fluid resuscitation (often requiring several liters over the first 24 h), elective ventilation, and pressors. Some authorities recommend early hemodialysis or hemofiltration. Fresh-frozen plasma is often given to patients who are bleeding extensively or who have severely deranged clotting parameters. Many European experts have administered antithrombin III to such patients. Patients with fulminant meningococcemia in whom shock persists despite vigorous fluid resuscitation should receive supplemental glucocor-

ticoid treatment (hydrocortisone, 1 mg/kg every 6 h) pending tests of adrenal reserve.

Although it has not been formally tested in patients with fulminant meningococcemia, activated protein C (drotrecogin alfa, Xigris) is approved for use in patients with severe sepsis and dysfunction of more than one organ (APACHE II score > 25). Because of the pathophysiology, patients with meningococcemia may represent a group most likely to benefit from administration of activated protein C. The recommended dose is 24 μg/kg per hour, given as a continuous IV infusion for 96 h. Drotrecogin alfa is contraindicated when the peripheral-blood platelet count is <50,000/μL, however, and when there is active bleeding or a high risk of bleeding. Clotting parameters should be monitored closely while the drug is being infused; its administration should be discontinued 4–6 h before the performance of an invasive procedure. Drotrecogin alfa should not be used in patients with meningitis pending further evidence that it does not induce intracranial bleeding when the meninges are inflamed.

PROGNOSIS

When patients are first evaluated, the clinical features most strongly associated with a fatal outcome are shock, a purpuric or ecchymotic rash, a low or normal blood leukocyte count, an age of ≥60 years, and coma. The absence of meningitis, the presence of thrombocytopenia, low blood concentrations of antithrombin or proteins S and C, high blood levels of PAI-1, and a low erythrocyte sedimentation rate (or C-reactive protein level) have also been associated with increased mortality risk from meningococcal disease. It is possible that when meningitis symptoms are lacking, the patient may delay seeking medical therapy; this scenario could account for the increased mortality risk in asymptomatic meningitis. In contrast, the receipt of antibiotics before hospital admission has been associated with lower mortality rates in some studies.

PREVENTION

Meningococcal Polysaccharide Vaccines A single injection of quadrivalent meningococcal polysaccharide vaccine (serogroups A, C, W-135, and Y) immunizes ~80–95% of immunocompetent adults (Table 136-1). Children ≥3 months of age can be vaccinated to prevent serogroup A disease, but multiple doses are required; the vaccine is otherwise ineffective in children <2 years old. The duration of vaccine-induced immunity in adults is probably <5 years. There is currently no vaccine for serogroup B; its polysaccharide is a sialic acid homopolymer that is poorly immunogenic in humans. In addition to individuals with late-complement-component or properdin deficiency, persons with sickle cell anemia, asplenia, or splenectomy should receive the quadrivalent vaccine. Vaccination is also recommended for military recruits, pilgrims on the Hajj, and individuals traveling to sub-Saharan Africa during the dry months (June to December) or to other areas with epidemic meningococcal disease. The Advisory Committee on Immunization Practices of the Centers for Disease Control and Prevention (CDC) recommends vaccination of incoming college freshmen who will live in dormitories. In general, the vaccine should be given only to persons >2 years of age.

New meningococcal capsular oligosaccharide and polysaccharide conjugate vaccines (C; A and C; A, C, Y, and W-135) are being developed; some are currently undergoing clinical trials, and some are now in use in Europe and Canada. These vaccines are based on the approach used for the highly successful *H. influenzae* type b conjugate vaccines. Covalent linkage of the polysaccharide to a carrier protein converts the polysaccharide to a thymus-dependent antigen enhancing IgG anticapsular antibodies and memory B cells. Because levels of antibody in mucosal secretions are much higher after the administration of a conjugate vaccine than after vaccination with an unconjugated preparation, a major benefit of these vaccines may be the introduction of herd immunity. Memory response to meningococcal polysaccharide also appears to be an important effect of the conjugate vaccines. Meningococcal conjugate vaccines are not yet licensed in the United States. However, in the United Kingdom, serogroup C conjugate vaccines introduced in 2000 have had a marked impact on the incidence of serogroup C disease in the population vaccinated. If conjugate meningococcal vaccines prove to be capable of providing durable antibody or memory responses (particularly in infants and young children), their integration into the routine childhood immunization schedule would appear warranted. Vaccines for serogroup B meningococcal disease remain elusive; none of the group B vaccines studied in clinical trials has proven to be broadly effective, but these products have a role in the control of serogroup B epidemics. The identification of new meningococcal protective antigens and the development of better meningococcal vaccines are areas of continued research and hold promise for the prevention of diseases due to *N. meningitidis*.

In one new approach, *reverse vaccinology*, the sequenced genome of *N. meningitidis* is used to identify previously unrecognized OMPs that are common to all meningococcal strains and serogroups and that may be universal vaccinogen candidates. Thus far, a few promising candidates have been identified and are ready to undergo clinical trials.

Screening tests for complement-component deficiency should be conducted in patients who have a family history of meningococcal or disseminated gonococcal disease, especially in areas without epidemic or endemic meningococcal disease; in patients who have a recurrence; in patients whose first case occurs at ≥15 years of age; in patients with cases caused by serogroups other than A, B, or C; and in family members of patients found to have a complement deficiency.

Antimicrobial Chemoprophylaxis The attack rate for meningococcal disease among household or other close contacts of cases is >400-fold greater than that in the population as a whole. Close contacts of cases should receive chemoprophylaxis with rifampin, ciprofloxacin, ofloxacin, or azithromycin (Table 136-1). A single IM injection of ceftriaxone is also effective. Close contacts include persons who live in the same household, day-care center contacts, and anyone directly exposed to a patient's oral secretions. Casual contacts are not at increased risk. Chemoprophylaxis should be administered as soon as possible after the case is identified. Patients with meningococcal disease who have been treated with antibiotics other than ceftriaxone need some type of prophylaxis in order to eliminate meningococcal colonization in the oropharynx.

Isolation Precautions The CDC recommends that patients with meningococcal disease who are hospitalized be placed in respiratory isolation for the first 24 h.

Outbreak Control An organization- or community-based outbreak of meningococcal disease is defined as the occurrence of three or more cases within ≤3 months in persons who have a common affiliation or reside in the same area but who are not close contacts of one another; in addition, the primary disease attack rate must exceed 10 cases per 100,000 persons, and the case strains of *N. meningitidis* must be of the same molecular type. Mass vaccination should be considered when such outbreaks occur, and mass chemoprophylaxis may be used to control school- or other institution-based outbreaks. Consultation with public health authorities is recommended when such campaigns are contemplated.

ACKNOWLEDGMENT
The substantial contributions of David S. Stephens, MD, and Robert S. Munford, MD, to this chapter in previous editions are gratefully acknowledged.

FURTHER READINGS

BILUKHA O et al: Use of meningococcal vaccines in the United States. Pediatr Infect Dis J 26:371, 2007

GARDNER P: Clinical practice. Prevention of meningococcal disease. N Engl J Med 355:1466, 2006 (Erratum: N Engl J Med 356:536, 2007)

GIULIANI MM et al: A universal vaccine for serogroup B meningococcus. Proc Natl Acad Sci USA 103:10834, 2006

SCHNEIDER MC et al: Interactions between *Neisseria meningitidis* and the complement system. Trends Microbiol 15:233, 2007

SMIRNOVA I et al: Assay of locus-specific genetic load implicates rare Toll-like receptor 4 mutations in meningococcal susceptibility. Proc Natl Acad Sci USA 100:6075, 2003

SNAPE MD et al: Meningococcal polysaccharide-protein conjugate vaccines. Lancet Infect Dis 5:21, 2005

SNYDER LA et al: The majority of genes in the pathogenic *Neisseria* species are present in non-pathogenic *Neisseria lactamica*, including those designated as 'virulence genes.' BMC Genomics 7:128, 2006

STEPHENS DS et al: Epidemic meningitis, meningococcaemia, and *Neisseria meningitidis*. Lancet 369:2196, 2007

THOMPSON MJ et al: Clinical recognition of meningococcal disease in children and adolescents. Lancet 367:397, 2006

ZIMMER SM et al: Serogroup B meningococcal vaccines. Curr Opin Invest Drugs 7:733, 2006

137 Gonococcal Infections
Sanjay Ram, Peter A. Rice

DEFINITION

Gonorrhea is a sexually transmitted infection (STI) of epithelium and commonly manifests as cervicitis, urethritis, proctitis, and conjunctivitis. If untreated, infections at these sites can lead to local complications such as endometritis, salpingitis, tuboovarian abscess, bartholinitis, peritonitis, and perihepatitis in female patients; periurethritis and epididymitis in male patients; and ophthalmia neonatorum in newborns. Disseminated gonococcemia is an uncommon event whose manifestations include skin lesions, tenosynovitis, arthritis, and (in rare cases) endocarditis or meningitis.

MICROBIOLOGY

Neisseria gonorrhoeae is a gram-negative, nonmotile, non-spore-forming organism that grows singly and in pairs (i.e., as monococci and diplococci, respectively). Exclusively a human pathogen, the gonococcus contains, on average, three genome copies per coccal unit; this polyploidy permits a high level of antigenic variation and the survival of the organism in its host. Gonococci, like all other *Neisseria* species, are oxidase positive. They are distinguished from other neisseriae by their ability to grow on selective media and to utilize glucose but not maltose, sucrose, or lactose.

EPIDEMIOLOGY

The incidence of gonorrhea has declined significantly in the United States, but there were still ~325,000 newly reported cases in 2006. Gonorrhea remains a major public health problem worldwide, is a significant cause of morbidity in developing countries, and may play a role in enhancing transmission of HIV.

Gonorrhea predominantly affects young, nonwhite, unmarried, less educated members of urban populations. The number of reported cases probably represents half of the true number of cases—a discrepancy resulting from underreporting, self-treatment, and nonspecific treatment without a laboratory-proven diagnosis. The number of reported cases of gonorrhea in the United States rose from ~250,000 in the early 1960s to a high of 1.01 million in 1978. The peak recorded incidence of gonorrhea in modern times was reported in 1975, with 468 cases per 100,000 population in the United States. This peak was attributable to the interaction of several variables, including improved accuracy of diagnosis, changes in patterns of contraceptive use, and changes in sexual behavior. The incidence of the disease has since gradually declined and is currently estimated at 120 cases per 100,000, a figure that is still the highest among industrialized countries. A further decline in the overall incidence of gonorrhea in the United States over the past two decades may reflect increased condom use resulting from public health efforts to curtail HIV transmission. At present, the attack rate in the United States is highest among 15- to 19-year-old women and 20- to 24-year-old men; 40% of all reported cases occur in the preceding two groups together. From the standpoint of ethnicity, rates are highest among African Americans and lowest among persons of Asian or Pacific Island descent.

The incidence of gonorrhea is higher in developing countries than in industrialized nations. The exact incidence of any of the STIs is difficult to ascertain in developing countries because of limited surveillance and variable diagnostic criteria. Studies in Africa have clearly demonstrated that nonulcerative STIs such as gonorrhea (in addition to ulcerative STIs) are an independent risk factor for the transmission of HIV (Chap. 182).

Gonorrhea is transmitted from males to females more efficiently than in the opposite direction. The rate of transmission to a woman during a single unprotected sexual encounter with an infected man is ~40–60%. Oropharyngeal gonorrhea occurs in ~20% of women who practice fellatio with infected partners. Transmission in either direction by cunnilingus is rare.

In any population, there exists a small minority of individuals who have high rates of new-partner acquisition. These "core-group members" or "high-frequency transmitters" are vital in sustaining STI transmission at the population level. Another instrumental factor in sustaining gonorrhea in the population is the large number of infected individuals who are asymptomatic or have minor symptoms that are ignored. These persons, unlike symptomatic individuals, may not cease sexual activity and therefore continue to transmit the infection. This situation underscores the importance of contact tracing and empirical treatment of the sex partners of index cases.

PATHOGENESIS, IMMUNOLOGY, AND ANTIMICROBIAL RESISTANCE

Outer-Membrane Proteins • *PILI* Fresh clinical isolates of *N. gonorrhoeae* initially form piliated (fimbriated) colonies distinguishable on translucent agar. Pilus expression is rapidly switched off with unselected subculture because of rearrangements in pilus genes. This change is a basis for antigenic variation of gonococci. Piliated strains adhere better to cells derived from human mucosal surfaces and are more virulent in organ culture models and human inoculation experiments than nonpiliated variants. In a fallopian tube explant model, pili mediate gonococcal attachment to nonciliated columnar epithelial cells. This event initiates gonococcal phagocytosis and transport through these cells to intercellular spaces near the basement membrane or directly into the subepithelial tissue. CD46 (membrane cofactor protein) is present on urogenital epithelial cells in both men and women and has been determined to be a receptor for PilC; this subunit is located at the tip of the pilus molecule and is critical in mediating adherence. Pili are also essential for genetic competence and transformation of *N. gonorrhoeae*, which permit horizontal transfer of genetic material between different gonococcal lineages in vivo.

OPACITY-ASSOCIATED PROTEIN Another gonococcal surface protein that is important in adherence to epithelial cells is opacity-associated protein (Opa, formerly called protein II). Opa contributes to intergonococcal adhesion, which is responsible for the opaque nature of gonococcal colonies on translucent agar and the organism's adherence to a variety of eukaryotic cells, including polymorphonuclear leukocytes (PMNs). Certain Opa variants promote invasion of epithelial cells, and this effect has been linked with the ability of Opa to bind vitronectin, glycosaminoglycans, and several members of the carcinoembryonic antigen–related cell adhesion molecule (CEACAM) receptor family. *N. gonorrhoeae* Opa proteins that bind CEACAM 1, which is expressed by primary CD4+ T lymphocytes, suppress the activation and proliferation of these lymphocytes. This phenomenon may serve to explain the transient decrease in CD4+ T lymphocyte counts associated with gonococcal infection.

PORIN Porin (previously designated protein I) is the most abundant gonococcal surface protein, accounting for >50% of the organism's total outer-membrane protein. Porin molecules exist as trimers that provide anion-transporting aqueous channels through the otherwise-hydrophobic outer membrane. Porin shows stable interstrain antigenic variation and forms the basis for gonococcal serotyping. Two main serotypes have been identified: PorB.1A strains are often associated with disseminated gonococcal infection (DGI), while PorB.1B strains usually cause local genital infections only. DGI strains are generally resistant to the killing action of normal human serum and do not incite a significant local inflammatory response; therefore, they may not cause symptoms at genital sites. These characteristics may be related to the ability of PorB.1A strains to bind to complement-inhibitory molecules, resulting in a diminished inflammatory response. Porin can translocate to the cytoplasmic membrane of host cells—a process that could initiate gonococcal endocytosis and invasion.

OTHER OUTER-MEMBRANE PROTEINS Other notable outer-membrane proteins include H.8, a lipoprotein that is present in high concentration on the surface of all gonococcal strains and is an excellent target for antibody-based diagnostic testing. Transferrin-binding proteins (Tbp1 and Tbp2) and lactoferrin-binding protein are required for scavenging iron from transferrin and lactoferrin in vivo. Transferrin and iron have been shown to enhance the attachment of iron-deprived *N. gonorrhoeae* to human endometrial cells. IgA1 protease is produced by *N. gonorrhoeae* and may protect the organism from the action of mucosal IgA.

Lipooligosaccharide Gonococcal lipooligosaccharide (LOS) consists of a lipid A and a core oligosaccharide that lacks the repeating O-carbohydrate antigenic side chain seen in other gram-negative bacteria (Chap. 114). Gonococcal LOS possesses marked endotoxic activity and contributes to the local cytotoxic effect in a fallopian tube model. LOS core sugars undergo a high degree of phase variation under different conditions of growth; this variation reflects genetic regulation and expression of glycotransferase genes that dictate the carbohydrate structure of LOS. These phenotypic changes may affect interactions of *N. gonorrhoeae* with elements of the humoral immune system (antibodies and complement) and may also influence direct binding of organisms to both professional phagocytes and nonprofessional phagocytes (epithelial cells). For example, gonococci that are sialylated at their LOS sites bind complement factor H and inhibit the alternative pathway of complement. LOS sialylation may also decrease nonopsonic Opa-mediated association with neutrophils and inhibit the oxidative burst in PMNs. The unsialylated terminal lactosamine residue of LOS binds to an asialoglycoprotein receptor on male epithelial cells, which facilitates binding and subsequent gonococcal invasion of these cells.

Host Factors In addition to gonococcal structures that interact with epithelial cells, host factors seem to be important in mediating entry of gonococci into nonphagocytic cells. Activation of phosphatidylcholine-specific phospholipase C and acidic sphingomyelinase by *N. gonorrhoeae*, which results in the release of diacylglycerol and ceramide, is a requirement for the entry of *N. gonorrhoeae* into epithelial cells. Ceramide accumulation within cells leads to apoptosis, which may disrupt epithelial integrity and facilitate entry of gonococci into subepithelial tissue. Release of chemotactic factors as a result of complement activation contributes to inflammation, as does the toxic effect of LOS in provoking the release of inflammatory cytokines.

The importance of humoral immunity in host defenses against neisserial infections is best illustrated by the predisposition of persons deficient in terminal complement components (C5 through C9) to recurrent bacteremic gonococcal infections and to recurrent meningococcal meningitis or meningococcemia. Gonococcal porin induces T cell–proliferative responses in persons with urogenital gonococcal disease. A significant increase in porin-specific interleukin (IL) 4–producing CD4+ as well as CD8+ T lymphocytes is seen in individuals with mucosal gonococcal disease. A portion of these lymphocytes that show a porin-specific T_H2-type response could traffic to mucosal surfaces and play a role in immune protection against the disease. Few data clearly indicate that protective immunity is acquired from a previous gonococcal infection, although bactericidal and opsonophagocytic antibodies to porin and LOS may offer partial protection. On the other hand, women who are infected and acquire high levels of antibody to another outer-membrane protein, Rmp (reduction modifiable protein, formerly called protein III), may be especially likely to become reinfected with *N. gonorrhoeae* because Rmp antibodies block the effect of bactericidal antibodies to porin and LOS. Rmp shows little, if any, interstrain antigenic variation; therefore, Rmp antibodies potentially may block antibody-mediated killing of all gonococci. The mechanism of blocking has not been fully characterized, but Rmp antibodies noncompetitively inhibit binding of porin and LOS antibodies because of the proximity of these structures in the gonococcal outer membrane. In male volunteers who have no history of gonorrhea, the net effect of these events may influence the outcome of experimental challenge with *N. gonorrhoeae*. Because Rmp bears extensive homology to enterobacterial OmpA and meningococcal class 4 proteins, it is possible that these blocking antibodies result from prior exposure to cross-reacting proteins from these species and also play a role in first-time infection with *N. gonorrhoeae*.

Gonococcal Resistance to Antimicrobial Agents   It is no surprise that *N. gonorrhoeae*, with its remarkable capacity to alter its antigenic structure and adapt to changes in the microenvironment, has become resistant to numerous antibiotics. The first effective agents against gonorrhea were the sulfonamides, which were introduced in the 1930s and became ineffective within a decade. Penicillin was then employed as the drug of choice for the treatment of gonorrhea. By 1965, 42% of gonococcal isolates had developed low-level resistance to penicillin G. Resistance due to the production of penicillinase arose later.

Gonococci become fully resistant to antibiotics either by chromosomal mutations or by acquisition of R factors (plasmids). Two types of chromosomal mutations have been described. The first type, which is drug specific, is a single-step mutation leading to high-level resistance. The second type involves mutations at several chromosomal loci that combine to determine the level as well as the pattern of resistance. Strains with mutations in chromosomal genes were first observed in the late 1950s. As recently as 2004, chromosomal mutations accounted for resistance to penicillin, tetracycline, or both in ~12% of strains surveyed in the United States.

β-Lactamase (penicillinase)–producing strains of *N. gonorrhoeae* (PPNG) carrying plasmids with the Pc^r determinant had rapidly spread worldwide by the early 1980s. *N. gonorrhoeae* strains with plasmid-borne tetracycline resistance (TRNG) can mobilize some β-lactamase plasmids, and PPNG and TRNG occur together, sometimes along with strains exhibiting chromosomally mediated resistance (CMRNG). Penicillin, ampicillin, and tetracycline are no longer reliable for the treatment of gonorrhea and should not be used. Third-generation cephalosporins have remained highly effective as single-dose therapy for gonorrhea. Even though the minimal inhibitory concentrations (MICs) of ceftriaxone for certain strains may reach 0.015–0.125 mg/L (higher than the MICs of 0.0001–0.008 mg/L for fully susceptible strains), these levels are greatly exceeded in the blood, the urethra, and the cervix when the routinely recommended ceftriaxone and cefixime regimens are administered (see below). These regimens almost always result in an effective cure.

Quinolone-containing regimens were also recommended for treatment of gonococcal infections; the fluoroquinolones offered the advantage of antichlamydial activity when administered for 7 days. However, quinolone-resistant *N. gonorrhoeae* (QRNG) appeared soon after these agents were first used to treat gonorrhea; in the United States, quinolone-containing regimens are no longer routinely recommended for the treatment of gonorrhea.

 QRNG is particularly common in the Pacific Islands (including Hawaii) and Asia, where, in certain areas, all gonococcal strains are now resistant to quinolones. At present, QRNG is also common in parts of Europe and the Middle East. In the United States, QRNG has been identified in midwestern and eastern areas as well as in states on the Pacific coast, where resistant strains were first seen. Alterations in DNA gyrase and topoisomerase IV have been implicated as mechanisms of fluoroquinolone resistance.

Resistance to spectinomycin, which has been used in the past as an alternative agent, has been reported. Since this agent is usually not associated with resistance to other antibiotics, spectinomycin can be reserved for use against multiresistant strains of *N. gonorrhoeae*. Nevertheless, outbreaks caused by strains resistant to spectinomycin have been documented in Korea and England when the drug has been used for primary treatment of gonorrhea.

CLINICAL MANIFESTATIONS

Gonococcal Infections in Males   Acute urethritis is the most common clinical manifestation of gonorrhea in males. The usual incubation period after exposure is 2–7 days, although the interval can be longer and some men remain asymptomatic. Strains of the PorB.1A serotype tend to cause a greater proportion of cases of mild and asymptomatic urethritis than do PorB.1B strains. Urethral discharge and dysuria, usually without urinary frequency or urgency, are the major symptoms. The discharge initially is scant and mucoid but becomes profuse and purulent within a day or two. Gram's stain of the urethral discharge may reveal PMNs and gram-negative intracellular monococci and diplococci (Fig. 137-1). The clinical manifestations of gonococcal urethritis are usually more severe and overt than those of nongonococcal urethritis, including urethritis caused by *Chlamydia trachomatis* (Chap. 169); however, exceptions are common, and it is often impossible to differentiate the causes of urethritis on clinical grounds alone. The majority of cases of urethritis seen in the United States today are not caused by *N. gonorrhoeae* and/or *C. trachomatis*. Although a number of other organisms may be responsible, most cases do not have a specific etiologic agent identified.

Most symptomatic men with gonorrhea seek treatment and cease to be infectious. The remaining men, who are largely asymptomatic, accumulate in number over time and constitute about two-thirds of all infected men at any point in time. Together with men incubating the organism (who shed the organism but are asymptomatic), they serve as the source of spread of infection. Before the antibiotic era, symptoms of urethritis persisted for ~8 weeks. Epididymitis is now an uncommon complication, and gonococcal prostatitis occurs rarely, if at all. Other unusual local complications of gonococcal urethritis include edema of the penis due to dorsal lymphangitis or thrombophlebitis, submucous inflammatory "soft" infiltration of the urethral wall, periurethral abscess or fistulae, inflammation or abscess of Cowper's gland, and seminal vesiculitis. Balanitis may develop in uncircumcised men.

Gonococcal Infections in Females   •   *GONOCOCCAL CERVICITIS*   Mucopurulent cervicitis is the most common STI diagnosis in American women and may be caused by *N. gonorrhoeae*, *C. trachomatis*, and oth-

FIGURE 137-1 Gram's stain of urethral discharge from a male patient with gonorrhea shows gram-negative intracellular monococci and diplococci. *(From the Public Health Agency of Canada.)*

er organisms. Cervicitis may coexist with candidal or trichomonal vaginitis. *N. gonorrhoeae* primarily infects the columnar epithelium of the cervical os. Bartholin's glands occasionally become infected.

Women infected with *N. gonorrhoeae* usually develop symptoms. However, the women who either remain asymptomatic or have only minor symptoms may delay in seeking medical attention. These minor symptoms may include scant vaginal discharge issuing from the inflamed cervix (without vaginitis or vaginosis per se) and dysuria (often without urgency or frequency) that may be associated with gonococcal urethritis. Although the incubation period of gonorrhea is less well defined in women than in men, symptoms usually develop within 10 days of infection and are more acute and intense than those of chlamydial cervicitis.

The physical examination may reveal a mucopurulent discharge (mucopus) issuing from the cervical os. Because Gram's stain is not sensitive for the diagnosis of gonorrhea in women, specimens should be submitted for culture or a nonculture assay (see below). Edematous and friable cervical ectopy as well as endocervical bleeding induced by gentle swabbing are more often seen in chlamydial infection. Gonococcal infection may extend deep enough to produce dyspareunia and lower abdominal or back pain. In such cases, it is imperative to consider a diagnosis of pelvic inflammatory disease (PID) and to administer treatment for that disease (Chaps. 124 and 169).

N. gonorrhoeae may be recovered from the urethra and rectum of women with cervicitis, but these are rarely the only infected sites. Urethritis in women may produce symptoms of internal dysuria, which is often attributed to "cystitis." Pyuria in the absence of bacteriuria seen on Gram's stain of unspun urine, accompanied by urine cultures that fail to yield >10^5 colonies of bacteria usually associated with urinary tract infection, signifies the possibility of urethritis due to *C. trachomatis*. Urethral infection with *N. gonorrhoeae* may also occur in this context, but in this instance urethral cultures are usually positive.

GONOCOCCAL VAGINITIS The vaginal mucosa of healthy women is lined by stratified squamous epithelium and is rarely infected by *N. gonorrhoeae*. However, gonococcal vaginitis can occur in anestrogenic women (e.g., prepubertal girls and postmenopausal women), in whom the vaginal stratified squamous epithelium is often thinned down to the basilar layer, which can be infected by *N. gonorrhoeae*. The intense inflammation of the vagina makes the physical (speculum and bimanual) examination extremely painful. The vaginal mucosa is red and edematous, and an abundant purulent discharge is present. Infection in the urethra and in Skene's and Bartholin's glands often accompanies gonococcal vaginitis. Inflamed cervical erosion or abscesses in nabothian cysts may also occur. Coexisting cervicitis may result in pus in the cervical os.

Anorectal Gonorrhea Because the female anatomy permits the spread of cervical exudate to the rectum, *N. gonorrhoeae* is sometimes recovered from the rectum of women with uncomplicated gonococcal cervicitis. The rectum is the sole site of infection in only 5% of women with gonorrhea. Such women are usually asymptomatic but occasionally have acute proctitis manifested by anorectal pain or pruritus, tenesmus, purulent rectal discharge, and rectal bleeding. Among men who have sex with men (MSM), the frequency of gonococcal infection, including rectal infection, fell by ≥90% throughout the United States in the early 1980s, but a resurgence of gonorrhea among MSM has been documented in several cities since the 1990s. Gonococcal isolates from the rectum of MSM tend to be more resistant to antimicrobial agents than are gonococcal isolates from other sites. Gonococcal isolates with a mutation in *mtrR* (multiple transferable resistance repressor) or in the promoter region of the gene that encodes for this transcriptional repressor develop increased resistance to antimicrobial hydrophobic agents such as bile acids and fatty acids in feces and thus are found with increased frequency in MSM. This situation may have been responsible for higher rates of failure of treatment for rectal gonorrhea with older regimens consisting of penicillin or tetracyclines.

Pharyngeal Gonorrhea Pharyngeal gonorrhea is usually mild or asymptomatic, although symptomatic pharyngitis does occasionally occur with cervical lymphadenitis. The mode of acquisition is oral-genital sexual exposure, with fellatio being a more efficient means of transmission than cunnilingus. Most cases resolve spontaneously, and transmission from the pharynx to sexual contacts is rare. Pharyngeal infection almost always coexists with genital infection. Swabs from the pharynx should be plated directly onto gonococcal selective media. Pharyngeal colonization with *Neisseria meningitidis* needs to be differentiated from that with other *Neisseria* species.

Ocular Gonorrhea in Adults Ocular gonorrhea in an adult usually results from autoinoculation from an infected genital site. As in genital infection, the manifestations range from severe to occasionally mild or asymptomatic disease. The variability in clinical manifestations may be attributable to differences in the ability of the infecting strain to elicit an inflammatory response. Infection may result in a markedly swollen eyelid, severe hyperemia and chemosis, and a profuse purulent discharge. The massively inflamed conjunctiva may be draped over the cornea and limbus. Lytic enzymes from the infiltrating PMNs occasionally cause corneal ulceration and rarely cause perforation.

Prompt recognition and treatment of this condition are of paramount importance. Gram's stain and culture of the purulent discharge establish the diagnosis. Genital cultures should also be performed.

Gonorrhea in Pregnant Women, Neonates, and Children Gonorrhea in pregnancy can have serious consequences for both the mother and the infant. Recognition of gonorrhea early in pregnancy also identifies a population at risk for other STIs, particularly chlamydial infection and syphilis. The risks of salpingitis and PID—conditions associated with a high rate of fetal loss—are highest during the first trimester. Pharyngeal infection, most often asymptomatic, may be more common during pregnancy because of altered sexual practices. Prolonged rupture of the membranes, premature delivery, chorioamnionitis, funisitis (infection of the umbilical cord stump), and sepsis in the infant (with *N. gonorrhoeae* detected in the newborn's gastric aspirate during delivery) are common complications of maternal gonococcal infection at term. Other microorganisms and conditions, including *Mycoplasma hominis*, *Ureaplasma urealyticum*, *C. trachomatis*, and bacterial vaginosis, have been associated with similar complications.

The most common form of gonorrhea in neonates is ophthalmia neonatorum, which results from exposure to infected cervical secretions during parturition. Ocular neonatal instillation of a prophylactic agent (e.g., 1% silver nitrate eyedrops or ophthalmic preparations containing erythromycin or tetracycline) prevents ophthalmia neonatorum but is not effective for its treatment, which requires systemic antibiotics. The clinical manifestations are acute and usually begin 2–5 days after birth. An initial nonspecific conjunctivitis with a serosanguineous discharge is followed by tense edema of both eyelids, chemosis, and a profuse, thick, purulent discharge. Corneal ulcerations that result in nebulae or perforation may lead to anterior synechiae, anterior staphyloma, panophthalmitis, and blindness. Infections described at other mucosal sites in infants, including vaginitis, rhinitis, and anorectal infection, are likely to be asymptomatic. Pharyngeal colonization has been demonstrated in 35% of infants with gonococcal ophthalmia, and coughing is the most prominent symptom in these cases. Septic arthritis (see below) is the most common manifestation of systemic infection or DGI in the newborn. The onset usually comes at 3–21 days of age, and polyarticular involvement is common. Sepsis, meningitis, and pneumonia are seen in rare instances.

Any STI in children beyond the neonatal period raises the possibility of sexual abuse. Gonococcal vulvovaginitis is the most common manifestation of gonococcal infection in children beyond infancy. Anorectal and pharyngeal infections are common in these children and are frequently asymptomatic. The urethra, Bartholin's and Skene's glands, and the upper genital tract are rarely involved. All children with gonococcal infection should also be evaluated for chlamydial infection, syphilis, and possibly HIV infection.

FIGURE 137-2 Characteristic skin lesions in patients with proven gonococcal bacteremia. The lesions are in various stages of evolution. **A.** Very early petechia on finger. **B.** Early papular lesion, 7 mm in diameter, on lower leg. **C.** Pustule with central eschar resulting from early petechial lesion. **D.** Pustular lesion on finger. **E.** Mature lesion with central necrosis (black) on hemorrhagic base. **F.** Bullae on anterior tibial surface. *(Reprinted with permission from KK Holmes et al: Disseminated gonococcal infection. Ann Intern Med 74:979, 1971.)*

Gonococcal Arthritis (DGI) DGI or gonococcal arthritis results from gonococcal bacteremia. In the 1970s, DGI occurred in ~0.5–3% of persons with untreated gonococcal mucosal infection. The lower incidence of DGI at present is probably attributable to a decline in the prevalence of particular strains that are likely to disseminate. DGI strains resist the bactericidal action of human serum and generally do not incite inflammation at genital sites, probably because of limited generation of chemotactic factors. Strains recovered from DGI cases in the 1970s were often of the PorB.1A serotype, were highly susceptible to penicillin, and had special growth requirements (i.e., the AHU auxotype) that made the organism more fastidious and more difficult to isolate.

Menstruation is a risk factor for dissemination, and approximately two-thirds of cases of DGI are in women. In about half of affected women, symptoms of DGI begin within 7 days of onset of menses. Complement deficiencies, especially of the components involved in the assembly of the membrane attack complex (C5 through C9), predispose to neisserial bacteremia, and persons with more than one episode of DGI should be screened with an assay for total hemolytic complement activity.

The clinical manifestations of DGI have sometimes been classified into two stages: a bacteremic stage, which is less common today, and a joint-localized stage with suppurative arthritis. A clear-cut progression usually is not evident. Patients in the bacteremic stage have higher temperatures, and their fever is more frequently accompanied by chills. Painful joints are common and often occur in conjunction with tenosynovitis and skin lesions. Polyarthralgias usually include the knees, elbows, and more distal joints; the axial skeleton is generally spared. Skin lesions are seen in ~75% of patients and include papules and pustules, often with a hemorrhagic component (Fig. 137-2). Other manifestations of noninfectious dermatitis, such as nodular lesions, urticaria, and erythema multiforme, have been described. These lesions are usually on the extremities and number between 5 and 40. The differential diagnosis of the bacteremic stage of DGI includes reactive arthritis, acute rheumatoid arthritis, sarcoidosis, erythema nodosum, drug-induced arthritis, and viral infections (e.g., hepatitis B and acute HIV infection). The distribution of joint symptoms in reac-

tive arthritis differs from that in DGI (Fig. 137-3), as do the skin and genital manifestations (Chap. 318).

Suppurative arthritis involves one or two joints, most often (in decreasing order of frequency) the knees, wrists, ankles, and elbows; other joints are occasionally involved. Most patients who develop gonococcal septic arthritis do so without prior polyarthralgias or skin lesions; in the absence of symptomatic genital infection, this disease cannot be distinguished from septic arthritis caused by other pathogens. The differential diagnosis of acute arthritis in young adults is discussed in Chap. 328. Rarely, osteomyelitis complicates septic arthritis involving small joints of the hand.

Gonococcal endocarditis, although rare today, was a relatively common complication of DGI in the preantibiotic era, causing about one-quarter of reported cases of endocarditis. Another unusual complication of DGI is meningitis.

Gonococcal Infections in HIV-Infected Persons The association between gonorrhea and the acquisition of HIV has been demonstrated in several well-controlled studies, mainly in Kenya and Zaire. The nonulcerative STIs enhance the transmission of HIV by three- to fivefold, possibly because of increased viral shedding by persons with urethritis or cervicitis (Chap. 182). HIV has been detected by polymerase chain reaction (PCR) more commonly in ejaculates from HIV-positive men with gonococcal urethritis than in those from HIV-positive men with nongonococcal urethritis. PCR positivity diminishes twofold after appropriate therapy for urethritis. Not only does gonorrhea enhance the transmission of HIV; it may also increase the individual's risk for acquisition of HIV. A proposed mechanism is the significantly greater number of CD4+ T

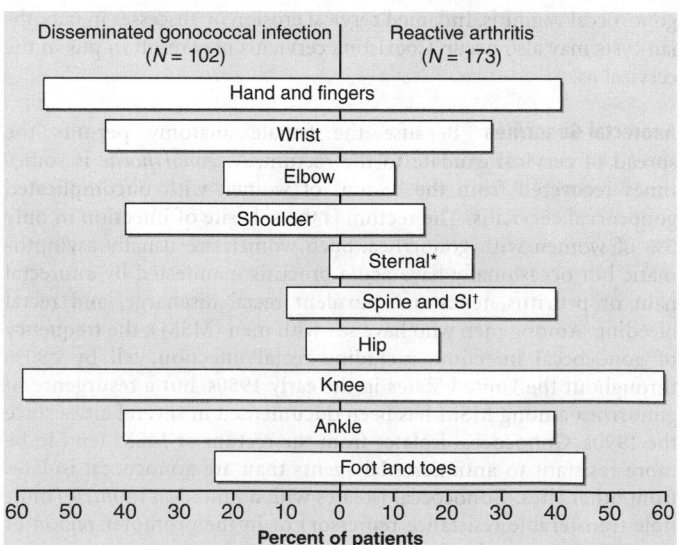

FIGURE 137-3 Distributions of joints with arthritis in 102 patients with disseminated gonococcal infection and 173 patients with reactive arthritis. *Includes the sternoclavicular joints. †SI, sacroiliac joint. *(Reprinted with permission from M Kousa et al: Frequent association of chlamydial infection with Reiter's syndrome. Sex Transm Dis 5:57, 1978.)*

lymphocytes and dendritic cells that can be infected by HIV in endocervical secretions of women with nonulcerative STIs than in those of women with ulcerative STIs.

LABORATORY DIAGNOSIS

A rapid diagnosis of gonococcal infection in men may be obtained by Gram's staining of urethral exudates (Fig. 137-1). The detection of gram-negative intracellular monococci and diplococci is usually highly specific and sensitive in diagnosing gonococcal urethritis in symptomatic males but is only ~50% sensitive in diagnosing gonococcal cervicitis. Samples should be collected with Dacron or rayon swabs. Part of the sample should be inoculated onto a plate of modified Thayer-Martin or other gonococcal selective medium for culture. It is important to process all samples immediately because gonococci do not tolerate drying. If plates cannot be incubated immediately, they can be held safely for several hours at room temperature in candle extinction jars prior to incubation. If processing is to occur within 6 h, transport of specimens may be facilitated by the use of nonnutritive swab transport systems such as Stuart or Amies medium. For longer holding periods (e.g., when specimens for culture are to be mailed), culture media with self-contained CO_2-generating systems (such as the JEMBEC or Gono-Pak systems) may be used. Specimens should also be obtained for the diagnosis of chlamydial infection.

PMNs are often seen in the endocervix on a Gram's stain, and an abnormally increased number (≥30 PMNs per field in five 1000× oil-immersion microscopic fields) establishes the presence of an inflammatory discharge. Unfortunately, the presence or absence of gram-negative intracellular monococci or diplococci in cervical smears does not accurately predict which patients have gonorrhea, and the diagnosis in this setting should be made by culture or another suitable nonculture diagnostic method. The sensitivity of a single endocervical culture is ~80–90%. If a history of rectal sex is elicited, a rectal wall swab (uncontaminated with feces) should be cultured. A presumptive diagnosis of gonorrhea cannot be made on the basis of gram-negative diplococci in smears from the pharynx, where other *Neisseria* species are components of the normal flora.

Nucleic acid probe tests are sometimes substituted for culture for the direct detection of *N. gonorrhoeae* in urogenital specimens. A common assay employs a nonisotopic chemiluminescent DNA probe that hybridizes specifically with gonococcal 16S ribosomal RNA; this assay is as sensitive as conventional culture techniques. A disadvantage of non-culture-based assays is that *N. gonorrhoeae* cannot be grown from the transport systems. Thus a culture-confirmatory test and formal antimicrobial susceptibility testing, if needed, cannot be performed. Nucleic acid amplification tests (NAATs), including Roche Amplicor, Gen-Probe APTIMA Combo2 (which also detects *Chlamydia*), and BD ProbeTec ET, offer an advantage: urine samples can be tested with a sensitivity similar to that obtained when urethral or cervical swab samples are assessed by culture and other non-NAATs.

Because of the legal implications, the preferred method for the diagnosis of gonococcal infection in children is a standardized culture. Two positive NAATs, each targeting a different nucleic acid sequence, may be substituted for culture of the cervix or the urethra as legal evidence of infection; however, cervical specimens are not recommended for prepubertal girls. Nonculture tests for gonococcal infection have not been approved by the U.S. Food and Drug Administration for use with specimens obtained from the pharynx and rectum of infected children. Cultures should be obtained from the pharynx and anus of both girls and boys, the vagina of girls, and the urethra of boys. For boys with a urethral discharge, a meatal specimen of the discharge is adequate for culture. Presumptive colonies of *N. gonorrhoeae* should be identified definitively by at least two independent methods.

Blood should be cultured in suspected cases of DGI. The use of Isolator blood culture tubes may enhance the yield. The probability of positive blood cultures decreases after 48 h of illness. Synovial fluid should be inoculated into blood culture broth medium and plated onto chocolate agar rather than selective medium because this fluid is not likely to be contaminated with commensal bacteria. Gonococci are infrequently recovered from early joint effusions containing <20,000 leukocytes/μL but may be recovered from effusions containing >80,000 leukocytes/μL. The organisms are seldom recovered from blood and synovial fluid of the same patient.

Rx GONOCOCCAL INFECTIONS

Treatment failure can lead to continued transmission and the emergence of antibiotic resistance. The importance of adequate treatment with a regimen that the patient will adhere to cannot be overemphasized. Thus highly effective single-dose regimens have been developed for uncomplicated gonococcal infections. The updated 2006 treatment guidelines for gonococcal infections from the Centers for Disease Control and Prevention are summarized in **Table 137-1**; the recommendations for uncomplicated gonorrhea apply to HIV-infected as well as HIV-uninfected patients.

Single-dose regimens of the third-generation cephalosporins ceftriaxone (given IM) and cefixime (given orally) are the mainstays of therapy for uncomplicated gonococcal infection of the urethra, cervix, rectum, or pharynx. Quinolone-containing regimens are no longer recommended in the United States as first-line treatment because of widespread resistance to these agents.

Because co-infection with *C. trachomatis* occurs frequently, initial treatment regimens must also incorporate an agent (e.g., azithromycin or doxycycline) that is effective against chlamydial infection. Pregnant women with gonorrhea, who should not take doxycycline, should receive concurrent treatment with a macrolide antibiotic for possible chlamydial infection. A single 1-g dose of azithromycin, which is effective therapy for uncomplicated chlamydial infections, results in an unacceptably low cure rate (93%) for gonococcal infections and should not be used alone. Spectinomycin has been an alternative regimen for the treatment of uncomplicated gonococcal infections in penicillin-allergic persons. However, spectinomycin is not available in the United States at this time. A single 2-g dose of azithromycin is effective against sensitive strains, but this drug is expensive, causes gastrointestinal distress, and is not recommended for routine or first-line treatment of gonorrhea.

Persons with uncomplicated infections who receive a recommended regimen do not need a test of cure. Cultures for *N. gonorrhoeae* should be performed if symptoms persist after therapy with an established regimen, and any gonococci isolated should be tested for antimicrobial susceptibility.

Symptomatic gonococcal pharyngitis is more difficult to eradicate than genital infection. Persons who cannot tolerate cephalosporins and those in whom quinolones are contraindicated may be treated with spectinomycin if it is available, but this agent results in a cure rate of ≤52%. Persons given spectinomycin should have a pharyngeal sample cultured 3–5 days after treatment as a test of cure. A single 2-g dose of azithromycin may be used in areas where rates of resistance to azithromycin are low.

Treatments for gonococcal epididymitis and PID are discussed in Chap. 124. Ocular gonococcal infections in older children and adults should be managed with a single dose of ceftriaxone combined with saline irrigation of the conjunctivae (both undertaken expeditiously), and patients should undergo a careful ophthalmologic evaluation that includes a slit-lamp examination.

DGI may require higher dosages and longer durations of therapy (Table 137-1). Hospitalization is indicated if the diagnosis is uncertain, if the patient has localized joint disease that requires aspiration, or if the patient cannot be relied on to comply with treatment. Open drainage is necessary only occasionally—e.g., for management of hip infections that may be difficult to drain percutaneously. Nonsteroidal anti-inflammatory agents may be indicated to alleviate pain and hasten improvement of affected joints. Gonococcal meningitis and endocarditis should be treated in the hospital with high-dose IV ceftriaxone (1–2 g every 12 h); therapy should continue for 10–14 days for meningitis and for at least 4 weeks for endocarditis. All persons who experience more than one episode of DGI should be evaluated for complement deficiency.

PREVENTION AND CONTROL

Condoms, if properly used, provide effective protection against the transmission and acquisition of gonorrhea as well as other infec-

TABLE 137-1 RECOMMENDED TREATMENT FOR GONOCOCCAL INFECTIONS: 2006 GUIDELINES OF THE CENTERS FOR DISEASE CONTROL AND PREVENTION (UPDATED IN 2007)

Diagnosis	Treatment of Choice
Uncomplicated gonococcal infection of the cervix, urethra, pharynx, or rectum[a]	
First-line regimens	Ceftriaxone (125 mg IM, single dose)
	or
	Cefixime (400 mg PO, single dose)
	plus
	Treatment for *Chlamydia* if chlamydial infection is not ruled out:
	Azithromycin (1 g PO, single dose)
	or
	Doxycycline (100 mg PO bid for 7 days)
Alternative regimens	Ceftizoxime (500 mg IM, single dose)
	or
	Cefotaxime (500 mg IM, single dose)
	or
	Spectinomycin (2 g IM, single dose)[b,c]
	or
	Cefotetan (1 g IM, single dose) plus probenecid (1 g PO, single dose)[b]
	or
	Cefoxitin (2 g IM, single dose) plus probenecid (1 g PO, single dose)[b]
Epididymitis	See Chap. 124
Pelvic inflammatory disease	See Chap. 124
Gonococcal conjunctivitis in an adult	Ceftriaxone (1 g IM, single dose)[d]
Ophthalmia neonatorum[e]	Ceftriaxone (25–50 mg/kg IV, single dose, not to exceed 125 mg)
Disseminated gonococcal infection[f]	
Initial therapy[g]	
Patient tolerant of β-lactam drugs	Ceftriaxone (1 g IM or IV q24h; recommended)
	or
	Cefotaxime (1 g IV q8h)
	or
	Ceftizoxime (1 g IV q8h)
Patients allergic to β-lactam drugs	Spectinomycin (2 g IM q12h)[c]
Continuation therapy	Cefixime (400 mg PO bid)
Meningitis or endocarditis	See text[h]

[a]True failure of treatment with a recommended regimen is rare and should prompt an evaluation for reinfection or consideration of an alternative diagnosis.

[b]Spectinomycin, cefotetan, and cefoxitin, which are alternative agents, currently are unavailable or in short supply in the United States.

[c]Spectinomycin may be ineffective for the treatment of pharyngeal gonorrhea.

[d]Plus lavage of the infected eye with saline solution (once).

[e]Prophylactic regimens are discussed in the text.

[f]Hospitalization is indicated if the diagnosis is uncertain, if the patient has frank arthritis with an effusion, or if the patient cannot be relied on to adhere to treatment.

[g]All initial regimens should be continued for 24–48 h after clinical improvement begins, at which time therapy may be switched to one of the continuation regimens to complete a full week of antimicrobial treatment. Treatment for chlamydial infection (as above) should be given if this infection has not been ruled out.

[h]Hospitalization is indicated to exclude suspected meningitis or endocarditis.

tions that are transmitted to and from genital mucosal surfaces. Spermicidal preparations used with a diaphragm or cervical sponges impregnated with nonoxynol 9 offer some protection against gonorrhea and chlamydial infection. However, the frequent use of preparations that contain nonoxynol 9 is associated with mucosal disruption that paradoxically may enhance the risk of HIV infection in the event of exposure. All patients should be instructed to refer sex partners for evaluation and treatment. All sex partners of persons with gonorrhea should be evaluated and treated for *N. gonorrhoeae* and *C. trachomatis* infections if their last contact with the patient took place within 60 days before the onset of symptoms or the diagnosis of infection in the patient. If the patient's last sexual encounter was >60 days before onset of symptoms or diagnosis, the patient's most recent sex partner should be treated. Partner-delivered medications or prescriptions for medications to treat gonorrhea and chlamydial infection diminish the likelihood of reinfection (or relapse) in the infected patient. In states where it is legal, this approach is an option for partner management. Patients should be instructed to abstain from sexual intercourse until therapy is completed and until they and their sex partners no longer have symptoms. Greater emphasis must be placed on prevention by public health education, individual patient counseling, and behavior modification. Sexually active persons, especially adolescents, should be offered screening for STIs. For males, a NAAT on urine or a urethral swab may be used for screening. Preventing the spread of gonorrhea may help reduce the transmission of HIV. No effective vaccine for gonorrhea is yet available, but efforts to test several candidates are under way.

ACKNOWLEDGMENTS

The authors acknowledge the contributions of Dr. King K. Holmes and Dr. Stephen A. Morse to the chapter on this subject in earlier editions.

FURTHER READINGS

CENTERS FOR DISEASE CONTROL AND PREVENTION: Gonococcal Isolate Surveillance Project (GISP); *www.cdc.gov/std/GISP/*

————: Update to CDC's sexually transmitted disease treatment guidelines 2006: Fluoroquinolones no longer recommended for treatment of gonococcal infections. MMWR 56(14):332, 2007

GAYDOS CA: Nucleic acid amplification tests for gonorrhea and *Chlamydia*: Practice and applications. Infect Dis Clin North Am 19:367, 2005

GOLDEN MR et al: Effect of expedited treatment of sex partners on recurrent or persistent gonorrhea or chlamydial infections. N Engl J Med 352:676, 2005

HOOK EW III, HOLMES KK: Gonococcal infections. Ann Intern Med 102:229, 1985

LAGA M et al: Non-ulcerative sexually transmitted diseases as risk factors for HIV-1 transmission in women: Results from a cohort study. AIDS 7:95, 1993

O'BRIEN JP et al: Disseminated gonococcal infection: A prospective analysis of 49 patients and a review of pathophysiology and immune mechanisms. Medicine (Baltimore) 62:395, 1983

138 *Moraxella* Infections
Daniel M. Musher

MORAXELLA CATARRHALIS

The gram-negative coccus *Moraxella catarrhalis* is a component of the normal bacterial flora of the upper airways and has been increasingly recognized as a cause of otitis media, sinusitis, and bronchopulmonary infection. Over the past several decades, this organism has been variously designated as *Micrococcus catarrhalis*, *Neisseria catarrhalis*, and *Branhamella catarrhalis*.

BACTERIOLOGY AND IMMUNITY
On Gram's staining, *M. catarrhalis* organisms appear as gram-negative cocci, sometimes occurring in pairs and having the side-by-side kidney-bean configuration of *Neisseria* (Fig. 138-1). These cocci tend to retain crystal violet during the decolorizing step and may be confused with *Staphylococcus aureus*. *Moraxella* colonies grow well on blood or chocolate agar but may be overlooked because of their resemblance to the *Neisseria* spp. that are major components of the normal pharyngeal flora. *Moraxella* is readily distinguishable from *Neisseria* spp. by biochemical tests.

Strains of *M. catarrhalis* show a surprising degree of homogeneity in terms of their outer-membrane proteins. Antibody to some of these proteins is generally present in serum of children >4 years old; however, colonizing or disease-causing isolates may survive in serum despite this naturally present antibody and complement. Bactericidal antibody emerges after natural infection and may be directed against one or more conserved outer-membrane proteins—a property of potential value in vaccine development. The presence of certain outer-membrane proteins is associated with virulence in mice, and antibody to these proteins may be protective. Antibody to lipooligosaccharide may also provide some degree of protection. These and other bacterial constituents are under investigation for use as vaccines.

EPIDEMIOLOGY
With repeated cultures and the use of selective media, *M. catarrhalis* can be isolated from the upper respiratory tract or saliva of >50% of healthy children and 3–7% of healthy adults. When conventional microbiologic techniques are used, *Moraxella* can be isolated from sputum of ~10% of persons who have chronic bronchitis and ~25% of those who have bronchiectasis in the absence of acute infection. Investigators in both the northern and southern hemispheres have reported a striking seasonal variation in the isolation of this organism from clinical specimens, with a peak in late winter/early spring and a nadir in late summer/early fall. Direct contact has not been shown to contribute to community-acquired infection, but nosocomial spread of infection has been documented occasionally.

CLINICAL MANIFESTATIONS
Otitis Media and Sinusitis *M. catarrhalis* is the third most common bacterial isolate from middle-ear fluid of children with otitis media, being surpassed only by *Streptococcus pneumoniae* and nontypable *Haemophilus influenzae*. This organism is also a prominent isolate from sinus cavities in acute and chronic sinusitis.

Purulent Tracheobronchitis and Pneumonia *M. catarrhalis* causes acute exacerbations of chronic bronchitis (increased production and/or purulence of sputum, which may be accompanied by fever and leukocytosis) and pneumonia. Acquisition of a new bacterial strain is often responsible. The great majority of infected persons are >50 years old and have a long history of cigarette smoking and underlying chronic obstructive pulmonary disease (COPD); many have lung cancer as well. In one study, 76% of affected persons had COPD (severe in many cases), and one-third of those with COPD had lung cancer; most patients also had clinical evidence of malnutrition. In one extensive series of cases, *M. catarrhalis* pneumonia did not occur in otherwise-healthy hosts. Recent prospective studies implicate this organism in ~10% of exacerbations of chronic bronchitis.

Symptoms of *M. catarrhalis* infection have been regarded as modest in severity. Both cough and the amount and purulence of sputum are usually increased above baseline. Chills are reported in one-quarter of patients, pleuritic pain in one-third, and malaise in 40%. Most patients have peak temperatures of <38.3°C (<101°F), and peripheral white blood cell counts are <10,000/µL in nearly one-quarter of cases. Microscopic examination of a high-quality sputum specimen after Gram's staining regularly reveals profuse organisms, and quantitative culture yields ~2×10^8 colony-forming units per milliliter. The radiologic appearance is variable; in one study, 43% of subjects had segmental or lobar infiltrates, and the remainder had a mixed pattern of subsegmental, segmental, interstitial, and diffuse involvement. These clinical, laboratory, and radiographic findings do not differ from those of pneumococcal or *Haemophilus* pneumonia in an older patient population. However, a far lesser degree of bloodstream invasion occurs in *M. catarrhalis* infection; in one series, none of 25 patients with *M. catarrhalis* pneumonia had bacteremia. Nevertheless, pneumonia due to *M. catarrhalis* is a marker for severe underlying disease: nearly half of patients die within 3 months of onset.

Other Syndromes Local extension causing empyema is very uncommon, and—as might be inferred from the low rate of bacteremia—metastatic complications of *M. catarrhalis* pneumonia, such as septic arthritis, are exceedingly rare. As of 1995, 58 cases of bacteremic infection due to *M. catarrhalis* had been reported, mainly in children <10 years old or adults >60 years old; most of these patients had severe underlying lung disease and/or were immunocompromised. The syndromes reported have included bacteremia with no apparent focus, pneumonia, endocarditis, and meningitis. A petechial or purpuric rash, reminiscent of that observed in meningococcal sepsis and associated with disseminated intravascular coagulation, has been described in a few cases.

DIAGNOSIS
Microscopic examination of Gram-stained sputum yields characteristic findings (Fig. 138-1). The presence of many polymorphonuclear leukocytes without epithelial cells indicates that the sputum sample is of good quality; since most patients with *Moraxella* infection have chronic lung disease, it is usually not difficult to obtain an acceptable specimen. Large numbers of *Moraxella* organisms are seen as gram-negative cocci, often lining up side by side and thus resembling pairs of kidneys.

FIGURE 138-1 Gram-stained sputum from a patient with acute purulent tracheobronchitis. Many polymorphonuclear neutrophils and a few macrophages are seen along with many gram-negative cocci (*Moraxella catarrhalis*), a few of which appear as pairs. Nearly all organisms are cell associated and probably have been taken up by phagocytes, consistent with the notion that *Moraxella* is a lower-grade pathogen than organisms that are found extracellularly in sputum specimens (e.g., *Streptococcus pneumoniae*).

TABLE 138-1	**THERAPY FOR INFECTION CAUSED BY MORAXELLA CATARRHALIS**

Drug(s)	Dose and Duration
Oral Therapy for Lower Respiratory Infection[a]	
Trimethoprim-sulfamethoxazole	160/800 mg qd for 5–7 days
Doxycycline	200 mg/d for 5–7 days
Azithromycin	500 mg/d for 5 days
Telithromycin	800 mg/d for 5–7 days
Amoxicillin/clavulanic acid	500 mg tid for 7 days
Ciprofloxacin	500 mg bid for 5 days
Cefuroxime	250–500 mg bid for 10 days
Cefpodoxime	200 mg bid for 10–14 days
Parenteral Therapy for Lower Respiratory Infection in Hospitalized Patients[b]	
Ampicillin/sulbactam	1.5/0.5 g q6h
Ceftriaxone	1 g/d
Cefotaxime	1 g q8h
Azithromycin	500 mg/d

[a]The same dosages apply for sinusitis, but some authorities treat for 10 days with macrolides, tetracyclines, and quinolones and for 14 days with β-lactam agents.
[b]After the patient's condition has stabilized, the regimen may be changed to oral medications at the indicated doses and durations.

℞ MORAXELLA INFECTIONS

M. catarrhalis is widely susceptible to most antibiotics used to treat lower respiratory tract infection (Table 138-1). Penicillin resistance first appeared in isolated strains in the mid-1970s and is now found in 94% of clinical isolates. This resistance is mediated by two closely related β-lactamases, BRO-1 and BRO-2. These enzymes are active against penicillin, ampicillin, and amoxicillin but less so against cephalosporins, especially third-generation cephalosporins; they also bind avidly to clavulanic acid and sulbactam. Thus a β-lactam/β-lactamase inhibitor combination such as amoxicillin/clavulanate offers excellent treatment. Second- and third-generation cephalosporins are effective alternatives. Isolates in the United States are also nearly uniformly susceptible to fluoroquinolones, newer macrolides, ketolides, and doxycycline; ~90% are susceptible to trimethoprim-sulfamethoxazole. A 5-day course of therapy has been shown to cure respiratory infection, although a longer course is required in sinusitis.

Treatment of sinusitis or otitis media is empirical, as appropriate specimens are usually obtained only in research studies. In the treatment of pneumonia during the period between the identification of gram-negative cocci in a Gram-stained specimen and the final identification of the organisms by culture, the severity of the condition and the potential presence of other infecting organisms should guide antibiotic selection. For example, an exacerbation of bronchitis caused by *M. catarrhalis* might be treated with doxycycline or an advanced macrolide. However, the microscopic identification of this organism in a patient with pneumonia may still lead to a preference for initial therapy (at least until culture results become available) with ampicillin/sulbactam, a third-generation cephalosporin, or a quinolone because of the possibility that resistant pneumococci are also present but have been overlooked by Gram's stain.

OTHER *MORAXELLA* SPECIES

Other *Moraxella* species are occasional causes of a wide range of infections, including bronchitis, pneumonia, empyema, endocarditis, meningitis, conjunctivitis, endophthalmitis, urinary tract infection, septic arthritis, and wound infection. In a report on all *Moraxella* isolates submitted to the Centers for Disease Control and Prevention between

TABLE 138-2	***MORAXELLA* SPECIES OTHER THAN *M. CATARRHALIS***		

Moraxella Species	Number of Isolates	Common Sites/ Clinical Association	Number (Percent) for Each Site
M. osloensis[a]	199	Blood	44 (22)
		CSF	18 (9)
		Urine	17 (9)
		Respiratory tract	24 (12)
M. nonliquefaciens	356	Blood	27 (8)
		CSF	6 (2)
		Respiratory tract	196 (55)
M. canis	74	Dog-bite wound	53 (72)
M-6	47	Blood, bone	15 (32)
M. lacunata	33	Conjunctivitis, keratitis	23 (70)
M. urethralis	28	Urine	16 (57)
		Genital tract	3 (11)
M. phenylpyruvica	73	Blood	19 (26)
		CSF	8 (11)
		Urine	12 (16)
M. atlantae	44	Blood	20 (45)
		CSF	5 (11)

[a]Some of these isolates would now be distinguished as a new species, *Moraxella lincolnii*.
Note: CSF, cerebrospinal fluid.
Source: Adapted from a summary of CDC experience (Graham et al).

1953 and 1980, certain clinical associations were apparent (Table 138-2). *M. osloensis* and *M. nonliquefaciens*, the most commonly isolated species, were cultured from various normally sterile body sites, including blood, cerebrospinal fluid, and joints. *M. osloensis* was the *Moraxella* species most frequently isolated from blood; *M. nonliquefaciens* tended to be isolated from the ears, nose, or throat (47%) or the sputum (8%) and has since been implicated as a cause of conjunctivitis and keratitis. *M. urethralis* was isolated most often from urine and the genital tract and probably represents the *Moraxella* species implicated previously in urethritis. More than half of isolates of *M. phenylpyruvica* and *M. atlantae* were obtained from normally sterile sites. One study found *Moraxella* spp., including *M. catarrhalis*, in 35% of infected cat-bite wounds and in 10% of infected dog-bite wounds. The clinical features of infections due to *Moraxella* spp. other than *M. catarrhalis* and the nature of the hosts in which they occur have not been fully characterized.

FURTHER READINGS

GRAHAM DR et al: Infections caused by *Moraxella*, *Moraxella urethralis*, *Moraxella*-like groups M-5 and M-6, and *Kingella kingae* in the United States, 1953–1980. Rev Infect Dis 12:423, 1990

IOANNIDIS JPA et al: Spectrum and significance of bacteremia due to *Moraxella catarrhalis*. Clin Infect Dis 21:390, 1995

MAAYAN H et al: Infective endocarditis due to *Moraxella lacunata*: Report of 4 patients and review of published cases of *Moraxella* endocarditis. Scand J Infect Dis 36:878, 2005

MURPHY TF et al: *Moraxella catarrhalis* in chronic obstructive pulmonary disease: Burden of disease and immune response. Am J Respir Crit Care Med 172:195, 2005

SETHI S et al: New strains of bacteria and exacerbations of chronic obstructive pulmonary disease. N Engl J Med 347:465, 2002

TALAN DA et al: Bacteriologic analysis of infected dog and cat bites. N Engl J Med 340:85, 1999

VERDUIN CM et al: *Moraxella catarrhalis*: From emerging to established pathogen. Clin Microbiol Rev 15:125, 2002

139 *Haemophilus* Infections
Timothy F. Murphy

HAEMOPHILUS INFLUENZAE

MICROBIOLOGY

Haemophilus influenzae was first recognized in 1892 by Pfeiffer, who erroneously concluded that the bacterium was the cause of influenza. The bacterium is a small (1- by 0.3-μm) gram-negative organism of variable shape; hence, it is often described as a pleomorphic coccobacillus. In clinical specimens such as cerebrospinal fluid (CSF) and sputum, it frequently stains only faintly with phenosafranin and therefore can easily be overlooked.

H. influenzae grows both aerobically and anaerobically. Its aerobic growth requires two factors: hemin (X factor) and nicotinamide adenine dinucleotide (V factor). These requirements are used in the clinical laboratory to identify the bacterium. Caution must be used to distinguish *H. influenzae* from *H. haemolyticus*, a respiratory tract commensal that has identical growth requirements. *H. haemolyticus* has classically been distinguished from *H. influenzae* by hemolysis on horse blood agar. However, a significant proportion of isolates of *H. haemolyticus* have recently been recognized as nonhemolytic. Analysis of 16S ribosomal sequences is one reliable method to distinguish these two species.

Six major serotypes of *H. influenzae* have been identified; designated *a* through *f*, they are based on antigenically distinct polysaccharide capsules. In addition, some strains lack a polysaccharide capsule and are referred to as *nontypable* strains. Type b and nontypable strains are the most relevant strains clinically (Table 139-1), although encapsulated strains other than type b can cause disease. *H. influenzae* was the first free-living organism to have its entire genome sequenced.

The antigenically distinct type b capsule is a linear polymer composed of ribosyl-ribitol phosphate. Strains of *H. influenzae* type b (Hib) cause disease primarily in infants and children <6 years of age. Nontypable strains are primarily mucosal pathogens but occasionally cause invasive disease.

EPIDEMIOLOGY AND TRANSMISSION

H. influenzae, an exclusively human pathogen, is spread by airborne droplets or by direct contact with secretions or fomites. Nontypable strains colonize the upper respiratory tract of up to three-fourths of healthy adults. Colonization with nontypable *H. influenzae* is a dynamic process; new strains are acquired and other strains are replaced periodically.

The widespread use of Hib conjugate vaccines in many industrialized countries has resulted in striking decreases in the rate of nasopharyngeal colonization by Hib and in the incidence of Hib infection (Fig. 139-1). However, the majority of the world's children remain unimmunized. Worldwide, invasive Hib disease occurs predominantly in unimmunized children and in those who have not completed the primary immunization series.

FIGURE 139-1 Estimated incidence (rate per 100,000) of invasive disease due to *Haemophilus influenzae* type b among children <5 years of age: 1987–2000. (*Data from the Centers for Disease Control and Prevention.*)

Certain groups have a higher incidence of invasive Hib disease than the general population. The incidence of meningitis due to Hib has been three to four times higher among black children than among white children in several studies. In some Native American groups, the incidence of invasive Hib disease is 10 times higher than that in the general population. Although this increased incidence has not yet been accounted for, several factors may be relevant, including age at exposure to the bacterium, socioeconomic conditions, and genetic differences in the ability to mount an immune response.

PATHOGENESIS

Hib strains cause systemic disease by invasion and hematogenous spread from the respiratory tract to distant sites such as the meninges, bones, and joints. The type b polysaccharide capsule is an important virulence factor affecting the bacterium's ability to avoid opsonization and cause systemic disease.

Nontypable strains cause disease by local invasion of mucosal surfaces. Otitis media results when bacteria reach the middle ear by way of the eustachian tube. Adults with chronic bronchitis experience recurrent lower respiratory tract infection due to nontypable strains. In addition, persistent nontypable *H. influenzae* colonization of the lower airways of adults with chronic obstructive pulmonary disease (COPD) contributes to the airway inflammation that is a hallmark of the disease. The incidence of invasive disease caused by nontypable strains is low.

IMMUNE RESPONSE

Antibody to the capsule is important in protection from infection by Hib strains. The level of (maternally acquired) serum antibody to the capsular polysaccharide, which is a polymer of polyribitol ribose phosphate (PRP), declines from birth to 6 months of age and, in the absence of vaccination, remains low until ~2 or 3 years of age. The age at the antibody nadir correlates with that of the peak incidence of type b disease. Antibody to PRP then appears partly as a result of exposure to Hib or cross-reacting antigens. Systemic Hib disease is unusual after the age of 6 years because of the presence of protective antibody. Vaccines in which PRP is conjugated to protein carrier molecules have been developed and are now used widely. These vaccines generate an antibody response to PRP in infants and effectively prevent invasive infections in infants and children.

Since nontypable strains lack a capsule, the immune response to infection is directed at noncapsular antigens. These antigens have generated considerable interest as immune targets and potential vaccine components. The human immune response to nontypable strains appears to be strain-specific, accounting in part for the propensity of these strains to cause recurrent otitis media and recurrent exacerbations of chronic bronchitis in immunocompetent hosts.

CLINICAL MANIFESTATIONS

Hib The most serious manifestation of infection with Hib is *meningitis* (Chap. 376). The age of peak incidence varies somewhat among populations, depending in part on the use of vaccine, but this infec-

TABLE 139-1 CHARACTERISTICS OF TYPE b AND NONTYPABLE STRAINS OF *HAEMOPHILUS INFLUENZAE*

Feature	Type b Strains	Nontypable Strains
Capsule	Ribosyl-ribitol phosphate	Unencapsulated
Pathogenesis	Invasive infections due to hematogenous spread	Mucosal infections due to contiguous spread
Clinical manifestations	Meningitis and invasive infections in incompletely immunized infants and children	Otitis media in infants and children; lower respiratory tract infections in adults with chronic bronchitis
Evolutionary history	Basically clonal	Genetically diverse
Vaccine	Highly effective conjugate vaccines	None available; under development

CHAPTER 139

Haemophilus Infections

tion primarily affects infants <2 years of age. The clinical manifestations of Hib meningitis are similar to those of meningitis caused by other bacterial pathogens. Fever and altered central nervous system function are the most common features at presentation. Nuchal rigidity may or may not be evident. Subdural effusion, the most common complication, is suspected when, despite 2 or 3 days of appropriate antibiotic therapy, the infant has seizures, hemiparesis, or continued obtundation. The overall mortality rate from Hib meningitis is ~5%, and the morbidity rate is high. Of survivors, 6% have permanent sensorineural hearing loss, and about one-fourth have a significant handicap of some type. If more subtle handicaps are sought, up to half of survivors are found to have some neurologic sequelae, such as partial hearing loss and delayed language development.

Epiglottitis (Chap. 31) is a life-threatening Hib infection involving cellulitis of the epiglottis and supraglottic tissues. It can lead to acute upper airway obstruction. Its unique epidemiologic features are its occurrence in an older age group (2–7 years old) than other Hib infections and its absence among Navajo Indians and Alaskan Eskimos. Sore throat and fever rapidly progress to dysphagia, drooling, and airway obstruction. Epiglottitis also occurs in adults.

Cellulitis (Chap. 119) due to Hib occurs in young children. The most common location is on the head or neck, and the involved area sometimes takes on a characteristic bluish-red color. Most patients have bacteremia, and 10% have an additional focus of infection.

Hib causes *pneumonia* in infants. The infection is clinically indistinguishable from other types of bacterial pneumonia (e.g., pneumococcal pneumonia) except that Hib is more likely to involve the pleura.

Several less common invasive conditions can be important clinical manifestations of Hib infection in children. These include osteomyelitis, septic arthritis, pericarditis, orbital cellulitis, endophthalmitis, urinary tract infection, abscesses, and bacteremia without an identifiable focus. As has been mentioned, Hib infections are unusual among patients >6 years old.

Nontypable *H. influenzae* Nontypable *H. influenzae* is a common cause of community-acquired bacterial pneumonia in adults. Nontypable *H. influenzae* pneumonia is especially common among patients with COPD or AIDS. The clinical features of *H. influenzae* pneumonia are similar to those of other types of bacterial pneumonia (including pneumococcal pneumonia). Patients present with fever, cough, and purulent sputum, usually of several days' duration. Chest radiography reveals alveolar infiltrates in a patchy or lobar distribution. Gram-stained sputum contains a predominance of small, pleomorphic, coccobacillary gram-negative bacteria.

Exacerbations of COPD caused by nontypable *H. influenzae* are characterized by increased cough, sputum production, and shortness of breath. Fever is low-grade, and no infiltrates are evident on chest x-ray.

Nontypable *H. influenzae* is one of the three most common causes of childhood otitis media (the other two being *Streptococcus pneumoniae* and *Moraxella catarrhalis*) (Chap. 31). Infants are febrile and irritable, while older children report ear pain. Symptoms of viral upper respiratory infection often precede otitis media. The diagnosis is made by pneumatic otoscopy. An etiologic diagnosis, although not routinely sought, can be established by tympanocentesis and culture of middle-ear fluid. The increasing use of pneumococcal polysaccharide conjugate vaccines in infants is resulting in a relative increase in the proportion of otitis media cases that are caused by *H. influenzae*.

Nontypable *H. influenzae* also causes puerperal sepsis and is an important cause of neonatal bacteremia. These nontypable strains, which are closely related to *H. haemolyticus*, tend to be of biotype IV and cause invasive disease after colonizing the female genital tract.

Nontypable *H. influenzae* causes sinusitis (Chap. 31) in adults and children. In addition, the bacterium is a less common cause of various invasive infections that are reported primarily as small-series descriptions and case reports. These infections include empyema, adult epiglottitis, pericarditis, cellulitis, septic arthritis, osteomyelitis, endocarditis, cholecystitis, intraabdominal infections, urinary tract infections, mastoiditis, aortic graft infection, and bacteremia without a detectable focus.

DIAGNOSIS

The most reliable method for establishing a diagnosis of Hib infection is recovery of the organism in culture. The CSF of a patient in whom meningitis is suspected should be subjected to Gram's staining and culture. The presence of gram-negative coccobacilli in Gram-stained CSF is strong evidence for Hib meningitis. Recovery of the organism from CSF confirms the diagnosis. Cultures of other normally sterile body fluids, such as blood, joint fluid, pleural fluid, pericardial fluid, and subdural effusion, are confirmatory in other infections.

Detection of PRP is an important adjunct to culture in rapid diagnosis of Hib meningitis. Immunoelectrophoresis, latex agglutination, coagglutination, and enzyme-linked immunosorbent assay are effective in detecting PRP. These assays are particularly helpful when patients have received prior antimicrobial therapy and thus are especially likely to have negative cultures.

Before the early 1980s, nontypable strains of *H. influenzae* were frequently misidentified as Hib because of their autoagglutination when serotypes were determined in agglutination assays. Since nontypable *H. influenzae* is primarily a mucosal pathogen, it is a component of a mixed flora; this situation makes etiologic diagnosis challenging. Nontypable *H. influenzae* infection is strongly suggested by the predominance of gram-negative coccobacilli among abundant polymorphonuclear leukocytes in a Gram-stained sputum specimen from a patient in whom pneumonia or tracheobronchitis is suspected. A sputum culture is helpful when interpreted along with the results of Gram's staining. Although bacteremia is detectable in a small proportion of patients with pneumonia due to nontypable *H. influenzae*, most such patients have negative blood cultures.

A diagnosis of otitis media is based on the detection by pneumatic otoscopy of fluid in the middle ear. An etiologic diagnosis requires tympanocentesis but is not routinely sought. An invasive procedure is also required to determine the etiology of sinusitis; thus, treatment is often empirical once the diagnosis is suspected in light of clinical symptoms and sinus radiographs.

℞ HAEMOPHILUS INFLUENZAE

Initial therapy for meningitis due to Hib should consist of a cephalosporin such as ceftriaxone or cefotaxime. For children, the dosage of ceftriaxone is 75–100 mg/kg daily given in two doses 12 h apart. The pediatric dosage of cefotaxime is 200 mg/kg daily given in four doses 6 h apart. Adult dosages are 2 g every 12 h for ceftriaxone and 2 g every 4–6 h for cefotaxime. An alternative regimen for initial therapy is ampicillin (200–300 mg/kg daily in four divided doses) plus chloramphenicol (75–100 mg/kg daily in four divided doses). Therapy should continue for a total of 1–2 weeks.

Administration of glucocorticoids to patients with Hib meningitis reduces the incidence of neurologic sequelae. The presumed mechanism is reduction of the inflammation induced by bacterial cell-wall mediators of inflammation when cells are killed by antimicrobial agents. Dexamethasone (0.6 mg/kg per day intravenously in four divided doses for 2 days) is recommended for the treatment of Hib meningitis in children >2 months of age.

Invasive infections other than meningitis are treated with the same antimicrobial agents. For epiglottitis, the dosage of ceftriaxone is 50 mg/kg daily, and the dosage of cefotaxime is 150 mg/kg daily, given in three divided doses 8 h apart. Epiglottitis constitutes a medical emergency, and maintenance of an airway is critical. The duration of therapy is determined by the clinical response. A course of 1–2 weeks is usually appropriate.

Many infections caused by nontypable strains of *H. influenzae*, such as otitis media, sinusitis, and exacerbations of COPD, can be treated with oral antimicrobial agents. Approximately 20–35% of nontypable strains produce β-lactamase (with the exact proportion depending on geographic location), and these strains are resistant to ampicillin. Several agents have excellent activity against nontypable *H. influenzae*, including amoxicillin/clavulanic acid, various extended-spectrum cephalosporins, the macrolides azithromycin and clarithromycin, and the new ketolide telithromycin. Fluoroquinolones are highly active against *H. influenzae* and are useful in adults with exacerbations of COPD. However, fluoroquinolones are not currently recommended for the treatment of children or pregnant women because of possible effects on articular cartilage.

In addition to β-lactamase production, alteration of penicillin-binding proteins—a second mechanism of ampicillin resistance—has been detected in isolates of *H. influenzae*. Although rare in the United States, these β-lactamase-negative ampicillin-resistant strains are increasing in prevalence in Europe and Japan. Continued monitoring of the evolving antimicrobial susceptibility patterns of *H. influenzae* will be important.

PREVENTION

Vaccination (See also Chap. 116) The development of conjugate vaccines that prevent invasive infections with Hib in infants and children has been a dramatic success. Three such vaccines are licensed in the United States. In addition to eliciting protective antibody, these vaccines prevent disease by reducing rates of pharyngeal colonization with Hib.

The widespread use of conjugate vaccines has dramatically reduced the incidence of Hib disease in developed countries. Even though the manufacture of Hib vaccines is costly, vaccination is cost-effective. The Global Alliance for Vaccines and Immunizations has recognized the underuse of Hib conjugate vaccines. The disease burden has been reduced in developing countries that have implemented routine vaccination (e.g., The Gambia, Chile). An important obstacle to more widespread vaccination is the lack of data on the epidemiology and burden of Hib disease in many developing countries.

All children should be immunized with an Hib conjugate vaccine, receiving the first dose at ~2 months of age, the rest of the primary series at 2–6 months of age, and a booster dose at 12–15 months of age. Specific recommendations vary for the different conjugate vaccines. The reader is referred to the recommendations of the American Academy of Pediatrics (Chap. 116 and *www.cispimmunize.org*). Currently, no vaccines are available for the prevention of disease caused by nontypable *H. influenzae*.

Chemoprophylaxis The risk of secondary disease is greater than normal among household contacts of patients with Hib disease. Therefore, all children and adults (except pregnant women) in households with at least one incompletely immunized contact <4 years of age should receive prophylaxis with oral rifampin. When two or more cases of invasive Hib disease have occurred within 60 days at a child-care facility attended by incompletely vaccinated children, administration of rifampin to all attendees and personnel is indicated, as is recommended for household contacts. Chemoprophylaxis is not indicated in nursery and child-care contacts of a single index case. The reader is referred to the recommendations of the American Academy of Pediatrics.

HAEMOPHILUS INFLUENZAE BIOGROUP AEGYPTIUS

H. influenzae biogroup aegyptius was formerly called *Haemophilus aegyptius* because of phenotypic characteristics distinct from those of *H. influenzae*. However, later studies involving DNA hybridization and DNA transformation demonstrated that *H. aegyptius* and *H. influenzae* are members of the same species.

H. influenzae biogroup aegyptius has long been associated with conjunctivitis. Moreover, this strain is now known to be the cause of Brazilian purpuric fever (BPF), which was first recognized in 1984 in the rural Brazilian town of Promissão. The sharing of many phenotypic and genotypic characteristics by the various strains of *H. influenzae* biogroup aegyptius that cause BPF indicates that these strains represent a clone of *H. influenzae* that has acquired specific virulence factors, several of which are associated with a pathogenicity island. The age of peak incidence of BPF is 1–4 years, with a range of 3 months to 8 years. The illness can occur sporadically or in outbreaks. Typically, after an episode of purulent conjunctivitis, high fever occurs in association with vomiting and abdominal pain. Within 12–48 h after onset, the patient develops petechiae, purpura, and peripheral necrosis and experiences vascular collapse. The characteristic laboratory features are thrombocytopenia, prolonged prothrombin time, uniformly unrevealing CSF findings, and blood cultures positive for *H. influenzae* biogroup aegyptius. Initial reports cited high mortality (70%), but subsequent studies have indicated that milder forms of the illness exist. Most patients have resolved or resolving purulent conjunctivitis, and culture of the conjunctiva is positive in approximately one-third of cases. BPF has been seen in several towns in Brazil and on two occasions in Australia.

HAEMOPHILUS DUCREYI

Haemophilus ducreyi is the etiologic agent of chancroid (Chap. 124), a sexually transmitted disease characterized by genital ulceration and inguinal adenitis. *H. ducreyi* poses a significant health problem in developing countries. Although this infection is less common in the United States, its incidence has increased dramatically in the past several years. In addition to being a cause of morbidity in itself, chancroid is associated with HIV infection because of the role played by genital ulceration in HIV transmission.

MICROBIOLOGY

H. ducreyi is a highly fastidious coccobacillary gram-negative bacterium whose growth requires X factor (hemin). Although, in light of this requirement, the bacterium has been classified in the genus *Haemophilus*, DNA homology and chemotaxonomic studies have established substantial differences between *H. ducreyi* and other *Haemophilus* species. Taxonomic reclassification of the organism is likely in the future but awaits further study.

The histology of the genital ulcer of chancroid is characterized by perivascular and interstitial infiltrates of macrophages and of CD4+ and CD8+ T lymphocytes. The appearance is consistent with a delayed-type hypersensitivity, cell-mediated immune response. The presence of CD4+ T cells and macrophages in the ulcer may explain, in part, the facilitation of HIV transmission in patients with chancroid.

EPIDEMIOLOGY AND PREVALENCE

Chancroid is a common cause of genital ulcers in developing countries. In the United States, chancroid is now endemic in some regions, and several large outbreaks have occurred since 1981. Recurring epidemiologic themes have been apparent in these outbreaks: (1) transmission has been predominantly heterosexual; (2) males have outnumbered females by ratios of 3:1 to 25:1; (3) prostitutes have been important in transmission of the infection; and (4) chancroid has been strongly associated with illicit drug use.

CLINICAL MANIFESTATIONS

Infection is acquired as the result of a break in the epithelium during sexual contact with an infected individual. After an incubation period of 4–7 days, the initial lesion—a papule with surrounding erythema—appears. In 2 or 3 days, the papule evolves into a pustule, which spontaneously ruptures and forms a sharply circumscribed ulcer that is generally not indurated (Fig. 139-2). The ulcers are painful and bleed easily; little or no inflammation of the surrounding skin is evident. Approximately half of patients develop enlarged, tender inguinal lymph nodes, which frequently become fluctuant and spontaneously rupture. Patients usually seek medical care after 1–3 weeks of painful symptoms.

The presentation of chancroid does not usually include all of the typical clinical features and is sometimes atypical. Multiple ulcers can coalesce to form giant ulcers. Ulcers can appear and then resolve, with inguinal adenitis (Fig. 139-2) and suppuration following 1–3 weeks later; this clinical picture can be confused with that of lymphogranuloma venereum (Chap. 169). Multiple small ulcers can resemble folliculitis. Other differential diagnostic considerations include the various infections causing genital ulceration, such as primary syphilis, condyloma latum of secondary syphilis, genital herpes, and donovanosis. In rare cases chancroid lesions become secondarily infected with bacteria; the result is extensive inflammation.

DIAGNOSIS

Clinical diagnosis of chancroid is often inaccurate, and laboratory confirmation should be attempted in suspected cases. Gram's staining

FIGURE 139-2 Chancroid with characteristic penile ulcers and associated left inguinal adenitis (bubo).

of a swab of the lesion may reveal a predominance of characteristic gram-negative coccobacilli, but the presence of other bacteria often makes it difficult to interpret this result. An accurate diagnosis of chancroid relies on culture of *H. ducreyi* from the lesion. In addition, aspiration and culture of suppurative lymph nodes should be considered. Since the organism can be difficult to grow, the use of selective and supplemented media is necessary. A multiplex polymerase chain reaction assay has been developed for simultaneous amplification of DNA targets from *H. ducreyi*, *Treponema pallidum*, and herpes simplex virus types 1 and 2. When this assay becomes commercially available, it will be a useful diagnostic tool with which to identify the etiology of genital ulcers.

R_x *HAEMOPHILUS DUCREYI*

The treatment regimen recommended by the Centers for Disease Control and Prevention is a single 1-g oral dose of azithromycin. Alternative regimens include ceftriaxone (250 mg intramuscularly in a single dose), ciprofloxacin (500 mg orally bid for 3 days), or erythromycin base (500 mg orally

tid for 7 days). Isolates from patients who do not respond promptly to treatment should be tested for antimicrobial susceptibility. In patients with HIV infection, healing may be slow and longer courses of treatment may be necessary. Clinical treatment failure in HIV-seropositive patients may reflect co-infection, especially with herpes simplex virus. Contacts of patients with chancroid should be identified and treated, whether or not symptoms are present, if they had sexual contact with the patient during the 10 days preceding the patient's onset of symptoms.

FURTHER READINGS

BONG CT et al: *Haemophilus ducreyi*: Clinical features, epidemiology, and prospects for disease control. Microbes Infect 4:1141, 2002

CASEY JR, PICHICHERO ME: Changes in frequency and pathogens causing acute otitis media in 1995–2003. Pediatr Infect Dis J 23:824, 2004

COMMITTEE ON INFECTIOUS DISEASES: *Haemophilus influenzae* infections, in *2003 Red Book, Report of the Committee on Infectious Diseases*, 26th ed, LK Pickering et al (eds). Elk Grove Village, IL, American Academy of Pediatrics, 2003

DOMINGUEZ SR, DAUM RS: Toward global *Haemophilus influenzae* type b immunization. Clin Infect Dis 37:1600, 2003

HEILMANN KP et al: Decreasing prevalence of beta-lactamase production among respiratory tract isolates of *Haemophilus influenzae* in the United States. Antimicrob Agents Chemother 49:2561, 2005

KELLY DF et al: *Haemophilus influenzae* type b conjugate vaccines. Immunology 113:163, 2004

LIEBOWITZ E et al: *Haemophilus influenzae*: A significant pathogen in acute otitis media. Pediatr Infect Dis J 23:1142, 2004

MCGILLIVARY G et al: Cloning and sequencing of a genomic island found in the Brazilian purpuric fever clone of *Haemophilus influenzae* biogroup aegyptius. Infect Immun 73:1927, 2005

MURPHY TF: Respiratory infections caused by non-typeable *Haemophilus influenzae*. Curr Opin Infect Dis 16:129, 2003

———— et al: Persistent colonization by *Haemophilus influenzae* in chronic obstructive pulmonary disease. Am J Respir Crit Care Med 170:266, 2004

SETHI S et al: Strain-specific immune response to *Haemophilus influenzae* in chronic obstructive pulmonary disease. Am J Respir Crit Care Med 169:448, 2004

140 Infections Due to the HACEK Group and Miscellaneous Gram-Negative Bacteria
Tamar F. Barlam, Dennis L. Kasper

THE HACEK GROUP

HACEK organisms are a group of fastidious, slow-growing, gram-negative bacteria whose growth requires an atmosphere of carbon dioxide. Species belonging to this group include several *Haemophilus* species, *Actinobacillus actinomycetemcomitans*, *Cardiobacterium hominis*, *Eikenella corrodens*, and *Kingella kingae*. HACEK bacteria normally reside in the oral cavity and have been associated with local infections in the mouth. They are also known to cause severe systemic infections—most often bacterial endocarditis, which can develop on either native or prosthetic valves (Chap. 118).

HACEK ENDOCARDITIS

In large series, up to 3% of cases of infective endocarditis are attributable to HACEK organisms, most often *A. actinomycetemcomitans*, *Haemophilus* species, and *C. hominis*. The clinical course of HACEK

endocarditis tends to be subacute; however, embolization is common. The overall prevalence of major emboli associated with HACEK endocarditis ranges from 28 to 71% in different series. On echocardiography, valvular vegetations are seen in up to 85% of patients. The vegetations are frequently large, although vegetation size has not been directly correlated with the risk of embolization. Cultures of blood from patients with suspected HACEK endocarditis may require up to 30 days to become positive, and the microbiology laboratory should be alerted when a HACEK organism is being considered. However, most cultures that ultimately yield a HACEK organism become positive within the first week, especially with improved culture systems such as BACTEC. In addition, polymerase chain reaction techniques are facilitating the diagnosis of HACEK infections. Because of the organisms' slow growth, antimicrobial testing may be difficult, and β-lactamase production may not be detected. E-test methodology may increase the accuracy of susceptibility testing.

***Haemophilus* Species** *Haemophilus* species are differentiated by their in vitro growth requirements for X factor (hemin) and V factor (nicotinamide adenine dinucleotide). *H. aphrophilus* requires only X factor for growth, while species designated *para-* require only V factor. *H. aphrophilus* and *H. parainfluenzae* are the most common *Haemophilus* species isolated from cases of HACEK endocarditis; *H. paraphrophilus* is less common. Invasive infection typically occurs in patients with a history of cardiac valvular disease, often in the setting of a recent dental procedure. Sixty percent of these patients have been ill for <2 months before presentation, and 19–50% develop congestive heart failure. Mortality rates as high as 30–50% have been reported in older series; however, more recent studies have documented mortality rates of <5%. *H. aphrophilus* also causes invasive bone and joint infections, and *H. parainfluenzae* has been isolated from other infections such as meningitis; brain, dental, and liver abscess; pneumonia; and septicemia.

Actinobacillus actinomycetemcomitans *A. actinomycetemcomitans* can be isolated from soft tissue infections and abscesses in association with *Actinomyces israelii*. Typically, patients who develop endocarditis with *A. actinomycetemcomitans* have severe periodontal disease or have recently undergone dental procedures in the setting of underlying cardiac valvular damage. The disease is insidious; patients may be sick for several months before diagnosis. Frequent complications include embolic phenomena, congestive heart failure, and renal failure. *A. actinomycetemcomitans* has been isolated from patients with brain abscess, meningitis, endophthalmitis, parotitis, osteomyelitis, urinary tract infection, pneumonia, and empyema, among other infections.

Cardiobacterium hominis *C. hominis* primarily causes endocarditis in patients with underlying valvular heart disease or with prosthetic valves. This organism most frequently affects the aortic valve. Many patients have signs and symptoms of long-standing infection before diagnosis, with evidence of arterial embolization, vasculitis, cerebrovascular accidents, immune complex glomerulonephritis, or arthritis at presentation. Embolization, mycotic aneurysms, and congestive heart failure are common complications.

Eikenella corrodens *E. corrodens* is most frequently recovered from sites of infection in conjunction with other bacterial species. Clinical sources of *E. corrodens* include sites of human bite wounds (clenched-fist injuries), endocarditis, soft tissue infections, osteomyelitis, respiratory infections, chorioamnionitis, gynecologic infections associated with intrauterine devices, meningitis and brain abscesses, and visceral abscesses.

Kingella kingae Because of improved microbiologic methodology, isolation of *K. kingae* is increasingly common. Inoculation of clinical specimens (e.g., synovial fluid) into aerobic blood culture bottles enhances recovery of this organism. In recent series, *K. kingae* has been the third most common cause of septic arthritis in children <24 months of age; staphylococcal and streptococcal species remain most prevalent. Invasive *K. kingae* infections with bacteremia are associated with upper respiratory tract infections and stomatitis. Both *K. kingae* colonization and primary herpes—a major cause of stomatitis—peak in children 6–48 months of age. *K. kingae* bacteremia can present with a petechial rash similar to that seen in *Neisseria meningitidis* sepsis.

Infective endocarditis, unlike other infections with *K. kingae*, occurs in older children and adults. The majority of patients have preex-

isting valvular disease. There is a high incidence of complications, including arterial emboli, cerebrovascular accidents, tricuspid insufficiency, and congestive heart failure with cardiovascular collapse.

℞ ENDOCARDITIS CAUSED BY HACEK ORGANISMS

See **Table 140-1**. Native-valve endocarditis should be treated for 4 weeks with antibiotics, whereas prosthetic-valve endocarditis requires 6 weeks of therapy. The cure rates for HACEK prosthetic-valve endocarditis appear to be high. Unlike prosthetic-valve endocarditis caused by other gram-negative organisms, HACEK endocarditis is often cured with antibiotic treatment alone—i.e., without surgical intervention.

OTHER GRAM-NEGATIVE BACTERIA

Achromobacter xylosoxidans *A. xylosoxidans* (previously *Alcaligenes xylosoxidans*) is probably part of the endogenous intestinal flora and has been isolated from water sources. Immunocompromised hosts, including patients with cancer and post-chemotherapy neutropenia, cirrhosis, and chronic renal failure, are at increased risk. Nosocomial outbreaks of *A. xylosoxidans* infection have been attributed to contaminated fluids, and clinical illness has been associated with isolates from many sites, including blood (often in the setting of intravascular devices). Community-acquired bacteremia with *A. xylosoxidans* usually occurs in the setting of pneumonia. Metastatic skin lesions are present in one-fifth of cases. The reported mortality rate is 67%—a figure similar to rates for other bacteremic gram-negative pneumonias.

℞ ACHROMOBACTER XYLOSOXIDANS INFECTIONS

Treatment is based on in vitro susceptibility testing of all clinically relevant isolates.

***Aeromonas* Species** More than 85% of *Aeromonas* infections are caused by *A. hydrophila*, *A. caviae*, and *A. veronii* biovar *sobria*. *Aeromonas* proliferates in potable and fresh water and in soil. It remains controversial whether *Aeromonas* is a cause of bacterial gastroenteritis; asymptomatic colonization of the intestinal tract with *Aeromonas* occurs frequently. However, rare cases of hemolytic-uremic syndrome following bloody diarrhea have been shown to be secondary to the presence of *Aeromonas*.

Aeromonas causes sepsis and bacteremia in infants with multiple medical problems and in immunocompromised hosts, particularly those with cancer or hepatobiliary disease. *Aeromonas* infection and sepsis can occur in patients with trauma (including severe trauma with myonecrosis) and in burn patients exposed to *Aeromonas* by environmental (freshwater or soil) contamination of their wounds. Reported mortality rates range from 25% among immunocompromised adults with sepsis to >90% among patients with myonecrosis. *Aeromonas* can produce ecthyma gangrenosum (hemorrhagic vesicles sur-

TABLE 140-1   TREATMENT OF ENDOCARDITIS CAUSED BY HACEK GROUP ORGANISMS[A]

Organism	Initial Therapy	Alternative Agents	Comments
Haemophilus species, *Actinobacillus actinomycetemcomitans*	Ceftriaxone (2 g/d)	Ampicillin/sulbactam (3 g of ampicillin q6h) **or** fluoroquinolones[b]	Ampicillin ± an aminoglycoside can be used if the organism does not produce β-lactamase.[c]
Cardiobacterium hominis	Penicillin (16–18 mU/d in 6 divided doses) or ampicillin (2 g q4h)	Ceftriaxone (2 g/d) **or** ampicillin/sulbactam (3 g of ampicillin q6h)	An aminoglycoside (gentamicin, 3 mg/kg per day in 3 divided doses) may be added, but its value has not been proven. The organism is usually pansensitive, but high-level penicillin resistance has been reported.
Eikenella corrodens	Ampicillin (2 g q4h)	Ceftriaxone (2 g/d) **or** fluoroquinolones[b]	The organism is typically resistant to clindamycin, metronidazole, and aminoglycosides.
Kingella kingae	Ceftriaxone (2 g/d) or ampicillin (3 g q6h)	Fluoroquinolones[b]	The prevalence of β-lactamase-producing strains is increasing. Efficacy for invasive infections is best demonstrated for first-line treatments.

[a]Susceptibility testing should be performed in all cases to guide therapy.
[b]Fluoroquinolones are not recommended for treatment of children <17 years of age.
[c]European guidelines for endocarditis recommend the addition of gentamicin (3 mg/kg per day in 3 divided doses for 2–4 weeks).

rounded by a rim of erythema with central necrosis and ulceration) resembling the lesions seen in *Pseudomonas aeruginosa* infection. *Aeromonas* causes nosocomial infections related to catheters, surgical incisions, or use of leeches. Other manifestations include meningitis, peritonitis, pneumonia, and ocular infections.

℞ AEROMONAS INFECTIONS

Aeromonas species are generally susceptible to fluoroquinolones (e.g., ciprofloxacin at a dosage of 500 mg every 12 h PO or 400 mg every 12 h IV), trimethoprim-sulfamethoxazole (TMP-SMX; trimethoprim dosage, 10 mg/kg per day in 3 or 4 divided doses), third-generation cephalosporins, and aminoglycosides. Because *Aeromonas* can produce various β-lactamases, including carbapenemases, susceptibility testing must be used to guide therapy.

Capnocytophaga Species This genus of fastidious, fusiform, gram-negative coccobacilli is facultatively anaerobic and requires an atmosphere enriched in carbon dioxide for optimal growth. *C. ochracea, C. gingivalis,* and *C. sputigena* have been associated with sepsis in immunocompromised hosts, particularly neutropenic patients with hematologic malignancy, and probably play a role in localized juvenile periodontitis in the immunocompetent host. These species have been isolated from many other sites as well, usually as part of a polymicrobial infection.

C. canimorsus and *C. cynodegmi* are endogenous to the canine mouth (**Chap. e14**). Patients infected with these species frequently have a history of dog bites or of exposure to dogs without scratches or bites. Asplenia, glucocorticoid therapy, and alcohol abuse are predisposing conditions that can be associated with fulminant infections. *C. canimorsus* causes a wide range of infections, including severe sepsis with shock and disseminated intravascular coagulation, meningitis, endocarditis, cellulitis, and septic arthritis.

℞ CAPNOCYTOPHAGA INFECTIONS

Because of increasing β-lactamase production, clindamycin (600–900 mg every 6–8 h) or drug combinations including a penicillin derivative plus a β-lactamase inhibitor—such as ampicillin/sulbactam (1.5–3.0 g of ampicillin every 6 h)—are currently recommended for empirical treatment of infections caused by *C. ochracea, C. gingivalis,* and *C. sputigena*. Infections with *C. canimorsus* should be treated with penicillin (12–18 million units every 4 h). This regimen or ampicillin/sulbactam should be given prophylactically to asplenic patients sustaining dog-bite injuries. *C. canimorsus* is also susceptible to clindamycin, imipenem, fluoroquinolones, and third-generation cephalosporins.

Chryseobacterium Species (Formerly *Flavobacterium*) *C. meningosepticum* is an important cause of nosocomial infections, including outbreaks due to contaminated fluids (e.g., disinfectants and aerosolized antibiotics) and sporadic infections due to indwelling devices, feeding tubes, and other fluid-associated apparatuses. Patients with nosocomial *C. meningosepticum* infection usually have underlying immunosuppression (e.g., related to malignancy). *C. meningosepticum* has been reported to cause meningitis (primarily in neonates), sepsis, endocarditis, bacteremia, soft tissue infections, and pneumonia. *C. indologenes* has caused bacteremia, sepsis, and pneumonia, typically in immunocompromised patients with indwelling devices.

℞ CHRYSEOBACTERIUM INFECTIONS

Chryseobacteria are often susceptible to fluoroquinolones, TMP-SMX, imipenem, and third- or fourth-generation cephalosporins, but susceptibility testing should be performed.

Pasteurella multocida *P. multocida* is a bipolar-staining, gram-negative coccobacillus that colonizes the respiratory and gastrointestinal tracts of domestic animals; oropharyngeal colonization rates are 70–90% in cats and 50–65% in dogs. *P. multocida* can be transmitted to humans through bites or scratches, via the respiratory tract from contact with contaminated dust or infectious droplets, or via deposition of the organism on injured skin or mucosal surfaces during licking. Most human infections affect skin and soft tissue; almost two-thirds of these infections are caused by cats. Patients at the extremes of age or with serious underlying disorders (e.g., cirrhosis) are at increased risk for systemic manifestations, including meningitis, peritonitis, osteomyelitis, endocarditis, and septic shock, but cases have also occurred in healthy individuals. If inhaled, *P. multocida* can cause acute respiratory tract infection, particularly in patients with underlying sinus and pulmonary disease.

℞ PASTEURELLA MULTOCIDA INFECTIONS

P. multocida is susceptible to penicillin, ampicillin, ampicillin/sulbactam, second- and third-generation cephalosporins, tetracyclines, and fluoroquinolones. β-lactamase-producing strains have been reported.

MISCELLANEOUS ORGANISMS

Agrobacterium radiobacter (tumefaciens) has usually been associated with infection in the presence of medical devices, including intravascular catheter–related infections, prosthetic-joint and prosthetic-valve infections, and peritonitis caused by dialysis catheters. Most cases occur in immunocompromised hosts, especially individuals with malignancy or HIV infection. Strains are usually susceptible to fluoroquinolones, third-generation cephalosporins, imipenem, TMP-SMX, and aminoglycosides.

Chromobacterium violaceum, although rarely a human pathogen, reportedly has been responsible for life-threatening infections with severe sepsis and metastatic abscesses, particularly in children with defective neutrophil function (e.g., those with chronic granulomatous disease). *C. violaceum* is generally susceptible to ciprofloxacin (500 mg every 12 h PO or 400 mg every 12 h IV), TMP-SMX, and gentamicin.

Plesiomonas shigelloides is a freshwater organism that causes acute diarrhea (Chap. 122) and occasionally serious extraintestinal disease, most commonly in immunocompromised hosts. *Ochrobactrum anthropi* causes infections related to central venous catheters in compromised hosts; other invasive infections have been described. Other organisms include *Weeksella* species; various CDC groups, such as EF4 and Ve-2; *Flavimonas* species; *Sphingobacterium* species; *Protomonas* species; *Oligella urethralis;* and *Shewanella putrefaciens*. The reader is advised to consult subspecialty texts and references for further guidance on these organisms.

FURTHER READINGS

BROUQUI P, RAOULT D: Endocarditis due to rare and fastidious bacteria. Clin Microbiol Rev 14:177, 2001

CHOMETON S et al: Specific real-time polymerase chain reaction places *Kingella kingae* as the most common cause of osteoarticular infections in young children. Pediatr Infect Dis J 26:377, 2007

ELLIOTT TSJ et al: Guidelines for the antibiotic treatment of endocarditis in adults: Report of the Working Party of the British Society for Antimicrobial Chemotherapy. J Antimicrob Chemother 54:971, 2004

GOLDBERG MH, KATZ J: Infective endocarditis caused by fastidious oro-pharyngeal HACEK micro-organisms. J Oral Maxillofac Surg 64:969, 2006

JOLIVET-GOUGEON A et al: Antimicrobial treatment of *Capnocytophaga* infections. Int J Antimicrob Agents 29:367, 2007

HUANG ST et al: Clinical characteristics of invasive *Haemophilus aphrophilus* infections. J Microbiol Immunol Infect 38:271, 2005

MARTINO R et al: Bacteremia caused by *Capnocytophaga* species in patients with neutropenia and cancer: Results of a multicenter study. Clin Infect Dis 33:E20, 2001

PATUREL L et al: *Actinobacillus actinomycetemcomitans* endocarditis. Clin Microbiol Infect 10:98, 2004

SHIE SS et al: Characteristics of *Achromobacter xylosoxidans* bacteremia in northern Taiwan. J Microbiol Immunol Infect 38:277, 2005

UDAKA T et al: *Eikenella corrodens* in head and neck infections. J Infect 54:343, 2007

141 *Legionella* Infection
Miguel Sabria, Victor L. Yu

Legionellosis refers to the two clinical syndromes caused by bacteria of the genus *Legionella*. *Pontiac fever* is an acute, febrile, self-limited illness that has been serologically linked to *Legionella* species, whereas *Legionnaires' disease* is the designation for pneumonia caused by these species. Legionnaires' disease was first recognized in 1976, when an outbreak of pneumonia took place at a hotel in Philadelphia during the American Legion Convention. The causative agent proved to be a newly discovered bacterium, *Legionella pneumophila*, that was isolated from lung specimens obtained from the victims at autopsy.

MICROBIOLOGY

The family Legionellaceae comprises more than 49 species with more than 64 serogroups. The species *L. pneumophila* causes 80–90% of human infections and includes at least 16 serogroups; serogroups 1, 4, and 6 are most commonly implicated in human infections. To date, 18 species other than *L. pneumophila* have been associated with human infections, among which *L. micdadei* (Pittsburgh pneumonia agent), *L. bozemanii*, *L. dumoffii*, and *L. longbeachae* are the most common.

Members of the Legionellaceae are aerobic gram-negative bacilli that do not grow on routine microbiologic media. Buffered charcoal yeast extract (BCYE) agar is the medium used to grow *Legionella*. Antibiotics added to the medium suppress the growth of competing flora from non-sterile sites, and dyes color the colonies and assist in identification.

The direct fluorescent antibody (DFA) test can definitively identify a number of individual species. In the case of *L. pneumophila*, the sero-group-specific antigen and antibodies detected by immunofluorescence are directed primarily at the lipopolysaccharide, a prominent outer-membrane component. Both polyclonal and monoclonal DFA reagents are commercially available. The monoclonal reagent is less cross-reactive but is specific for *L. pneumophila*.

ECOLOGY AND TRANSMISSION

The natural habitats for *L. pneumophila* are aquatic bodies, including lakes and streams. *L. longbeachae* has been isolated from soil. Legionellae can survive under a wide range of environmental conditions; for example, the organisms can live for years in refrigerated water samples. Natural bodies of water contain only small numbers of legionellae. However, once the organisms enter human-constructed aquatic reservoirs (such as water-distribution systems), they can grow and proliferate. Factors known to enhance colonization by and amplification of legionellae include warm temperatures (25°–42°C), stagnation, and scale and sediment. *L. pneumophila* can form microcolonies within biofilms; its eradication from water-distribution systems requires disinfectants that can penetrate the biofilm. The presence of symbiotic microorganisms, including algae, amebas, ciliated protozoa, and other water-dwelling bacteria, promotes the growth of *L. pneumophila*. Legionellae can invade and multiply within free-living protozoa.

The source of *Legionella* is water. Community-acquired Legionnaires' disease has been linked to colonization of residential and industrial water supplies. Potable-water distribution systems in hospitals, long-term-care facilities, hotels, and large buildings have been implicated. Sporadic community-acquired cases have been linked to residential water systems.

Cooling towers and evaporative condensers have been overestimated as sources of *Legionella*. Early investigations that implicated cooling towers antedated the discovery that the organism could also exist in potable-water distribution systems. It is now known that, in many outbreaks attributed to cooling towers, cases of Legionnaires' disease continued to occur despite disinfection of the cooling towers; the potable water supply was the actual source. Koch's postulates have never been fulfilled for cooling tower–associated outbreaks as they have been for hospital-acquired Legionnaires' disease. Nevertheless, cooling towers are occasionally identified in community-acquired outbreaks.

L. longbeachae infections have been linked to potting soil.

Multiple modes of transmission of *Legionella* to humans exist, including aerosolization, aspiration, and direct instillation into the lungs during respiratory tract manipulations. Aspiration is now known to be the predominant mode of transmission, but it is unclear whether *Legionella* enters the lungs via oropharyngeal colonization or directly via the drinking of contaminated water. Oropharyngeal colonization has been demonstrated in patients undergoing transplantation. Nasogastric tubes have been linked to hospital-acquired Legionnaires' disease; microaspiration of contaminated water was the hypothesized mode of transmission. Surgery with general anesthesia is a known risk factor that is consistent with aspiration. Especially compelling is the reported 30% incidence of postoperative *Legionella* pneumonia among patients undergoing head and neck surgery at a hospital with a contaminated water supply; aspiration is a recognized sequela in such cases. Studies of patients with hospital-acquired Legionnaires' disease have shown that these individuals underwent endotracheal intubation significantly more often and for a significantly longer duration than patients with hospital-acquired pneumonia of other etiologies.

Aerosolization of *Legionella* by devices filled with tap water, including whirlpools, nebulizers, and humidifiers, has been implicated. An ultrasonic mist machine in the produce section of a grocery store was the source in a community outbreak. Pontiac fever has been linked to *Legionella*-containing aerosols from water-using machinery, a cooling tower, air-conditioners, and whirlpools.

EPIDEMIOLOGY

The incidence of Legionnaires' disease depends on the degree of contamination of the aquatic reservoir, the immune status of the persons exposed to water from that reservoir, the intensity of exposure, and the availability of specialized laboratory tests on which the correct diagnosis can be based.

Numerous prospective studies have ranked *Legionella* among the top four microbial causes of community-acquired pneumonia (with *Streptococcus pneumoniae*, *Haemophilus influenzae*, and *Chlamydophila pneumoniae* usually ranked first, second, and third, respectively), accounting for 2–9% of cases. On the basis of a multihospital study of community-acquired pneumonia in Ohio, the Centers for Disease Control and Prevention (CDC) estimated that as many as 18,000 cases of sporadic community-acquired Legionnaires' disease occur annually in the United States and that only 3% of these cases are correctly diagnosed. *Legionella* is responsible for 10–50% of cases of nosocomial pneumonia when a hospital's water system is colonized with the organisms. The incidence of hospital-acquired Legionnaires' disease depends on the degree of contamination of the water system as defined by the rate of positivity of distal water sites (not as defined quantitatively by the number of colony-forming units per milliliter).

Risk factors for Legionnaires' disease include cigarette smoking; chronic lung disease; advanced age; prior hospitalization, with discharge within 10 days before onset of pneumonia symptoms; and immunosuppression. Immunosuppressive conditions that predispose to Legionnaires' disease include transplantation, HIV infection, and treatment with glucocorticoids or tumor necrosis factor α. However, in a large prospective study of community-acquired pneumonia, 28% of patients with Legionnaires' disease did not have these classic risk factors. Surgery is a prominent predisposing factor in hospital-acquired infection, with transplant recipients at highest risk. Hospital-acquired cases are now being recognized among neonates and immunosuppressed children.

Pontiac fever occurs in epidemics. The high attack rate (>90%) reflects airborne transmission.

PATHOGENESIS AND IMMUNITY

Legionella enters the lungs through aspiration or direct inhalation. Attachment to host cells is mediated by bacterial type IV pili, heat-shock proteins, and the major outer-membrane protein. *Legionella* binds to complement CR1 and CR3 integrin receptors on the surface of the host cell. Because the organisms possess pili that may mediate adherence to respiratory tract epithelial cells, conditions that impair mucociliary clearance, including cigarette smoking, lung disease, or alcoholism, predispose to Legionnaires' disease.

Cell-mediated immunity is the primary mechanism of host defense against *Legionella*, as it is against other intracellular pathogens. Thus Legionnaires' disease is more common and its manifestations are more severe among patients with depressed cell-mediated immunity. The disease also occurs with unusual frequency among patients with hairy cell leukemia, which is characterized by monocyte deficiency and dysfunction.

Alveolar macrophages readily phagocytose *Legionella*. The attachment of the bacteria to phagocytes is mediated via Fc receptors and complement receptors, which attach to the bacterial major outer-membrane protein. Binding to these receptors promotes phagocytosis but fails to trigger an oxidative burst. The *L. pneumophila* phagosome resists acidification and evades fusion with late endocytic compartments and lysosomes. Although many legionellae are killed, some proliferate intracellularly until the cells rupture; the bacteria are then phagocytosed again by newly recruited phagocytes, and the cycle begins anew.

The role of neutrophils in immunity appears to be minimal: neutropenic patients are not predisposed to Legionnaires' disease. Although *L. pneumophila* is susceptible to oxygen-dependent microbiologic systems in vitro, it resists killing by neutrophils.

The humoral immune system is active against *Legionella*. Type-specific IgM and IgG antibodies are measurable within weeks of infection. In vitro, antibodies promote killing of *Legionella* by phagocytes (neutrophils, monocytes, and alveolar macrophages). Immunized animals develop a specific antibody response, with subsequent resistance to *Legionella* challenge. However, antibodies neither enhance lysis by complement nor inhibit intracellular multiplication within phagocytes.

Some *L. pneumophila* strains are clearly more virulent than others, although the precise factors mediating virulence remain uncertain. For example, although multiple strains may colonize water-distribution systems, only a few cause disease in patients exposed to water from these systems. At least one surface epitope of *L. pneumophila* serogroup 1 is associated with virulence. Monoclonal antibody subtype mAb2 has been linked to virulence. *L. pneumophila* serogroup 6 is more commonly involved in hospital-acquired Legionnaires' disease and is more likely to be associated with a poor outcome.

The genome of *L. pneumophila* has been sequenced. A broad range of membrane transporters within the genome are thought to optimize the use of nutrients in water and soil. Genes responsible for establishment of an intracellular growth site in human alveolar macrophages and replication in symbiotic microorganisms have been identified.

CLINICAL AND LABORATORY FEATURES

Pontiac Fever   Pontiac fever is an acute, self-limiting, flu-like illness with an incubation period of 24–48 h. Pneumonia does not develop. Malaise, fatigue, and myalgias are the most common symptoms, occurring in 97% of cases. Fever (usually with chills) develops in 80–90% of cases and headache in 80%. Other symptoms (seen in <50% of cases) include arthralgias, nausea, cough, abdominal pain, and diarrhea. Modest leukocytosis with a neutrophilic predominance is sometimes detected. Without antibiotic therapy, complete recovery takes place in only a few days; a few patients may experience lassitude for many weeks thereafter. The diagnosis is established by antibody seroconversion.

Legionnaires' Disease (Pneumonia)   Legionnaires' disease is often included in the differential diagnosis of "atypical pneumonia," along with infection due to *C. pneumoniae, Chlamydophila psittaci, Mycoplasma pneumoniae, Coxiella burnetii*, and some viruses. The clinical similarities among these types of pneumonia include a relatively nonproductive cough and a low incidence of grossly purulent sputum. However, the clinical manifestations of Legionnaires' disease are usually more severe than those of most "atypical" pneumonias, and the course and prognosis of *Legionella* pneumonia more closely resemble those of bacteremic pneumococcal pneumonia than those of pneumonia due to other "atypical" pathogens. Patients with community-ac-

quired Legionnaires' disease are significantly more likely than patients with pneumonia of other etiologies to be admitted to an intensive care unit on presentation.

The incubation period for Legionnaires' disease is usually 2–10 days, although longer incubation periods have been documented. The symptoms and signs may range from a mild cough and a slight fever to stupor with widespread pulmonary infiltrates and multisystem failure. Nonspecific symptoms—malaise, fatigue, anorexia, and headache—are seen early in the illness. Myalgias and arthralgias are uncommon but are prominent in a few patients. Upper respiratory symptoms, including coryza, are rare.

The mild cough of Legionnaires' disease is only slightly productive. Sometimes the sputum is streaked with blood. Chest pain—either pleuritic or nonpleuritic—can be a prominent feature and, when coupled with hemoptysis, can lead to an incorrect diagnosis of pulmonary embolism. Shortness of breath is reported by one-third to one-half of patients.

Gastrointestinal difficulties are often pronounced; abdominal pain, nausea, and vomiting affect 10–20% of patients. Diarrhea (watery rather than bloody) is reported in 25–50% of cases. The most common neurologic abnormalities are confusion or changes in mental status; however, the multitudinous neurologic symptoms reported range from headache and lethargy to encephalopathy.

Patients with Legionnaires' disease virtually always have fever. Temperatures in excess of 40.5°C (104.9°F) were recorded in 20% of the cases in one series. Relative bradycardia has been overemphasized as a useful diagnostic finding; it occurs primarily in older patients with severe pneumonia. Chest examination reveals rales early in the course and evidence of consolidations as the disease progresses. Abdominal examination may reveal generalized or local tenderness.

Although the clinical manifestations often considered classic for Legionnaires' disease (Table 141-1) may suggest the diagnosis, prospective comparative studies have shown that clinical manifestations are generally nonspecific and that Legionnaires' disease is not readily distinguishable from pneumonia of other etiologies. In a review of 13 studies of community-acquired pneumonia, clinical manifestations that occurred significantly more often in Legionnaires' disease included diarrhea, neurologic findings (including confusion), and a temperature of >39°C. Hyponatremia, elevated values in liver function tests, and hematuria also occurred more frequently in Legionnaires' disease. Other laboratory abnormalities include creatine phosphokinase elevation, hypophosphatemia, serum creatinine elevation, and proteinuria.

Extrapulmonary Legionellosis   Since the portal of entry for *Legionella* is the lung in virtually all cases, extrapulmonary manifestations usually result from bloodborne dissemination from the lung. In a prospective survey of patients with Legionnaires' disease diagnosed by isolation of the organism from sputum, *Legionella* was isolated from the blood by a special culture method in 38% of cases.

Legionella has been identified in lymph nodes, spleen, liver, or kidneys in autopsied cases. The most common extrapulmonary site of legionellosis is the heart; numerous reports have described myocarditis, pericarditis, postcardiotomy syndrome, and prosthetic-valve endocarditis. Most cases have been hospital-acquired. In some patients without overt evidence of pneumonia, the organisms may gain entry through a postoperative sternal wound exposed to contaminated tap water or

---

TABLE 141-1   CLINICAL CLUES SUGGESTIVE OF LEGIONNAIRES' DISEASE

Diarrhea

High fever (>40°C; >104°F)

Numerous neutrophils but no organisms revealed by Gram's staining of respiratory secretions

Hyponatremia (serum sodium level <131 mg/dL)

Failure to respond to β-lactam drugs (penicillins or cephalosporins) and aminoglycoside antibiotics

Occurrence of illness in an environment in which the potable water supply is known to be contaminated with *Legionella*

Onset of symptoms within 10 days after discharge from the hospital

FIGURE 141-1 Chest radiographic findings in a 52-year-old man who presented with pneumonia subsequently diagnosed as Legionnaires' disease. The patient was a cigarette smoker with chronic obstructive pulmonary disease and alcoholic cardiomyopathy; he had received glucocorticoids. *L. pneumophila* was identified by DFA stain-ing and culture of sputum. **Left:** Baseline chest radiograph showing long-standing cardiomegaly. **Center:** Admission chest radiograph showing new rounded opacities. **Right:** Chest radiograph taken 3 days after admission, during treatment with erythromycin.

through a mediastinal-tube insertion site. Sinusitis, peritonitis, pyelonephritis, skin and soft tissue infection, septic arthritis, and pancreatitis have been seen predominantly in immunosuppressed patients.

Chest Radiography Virtually all patients with Legionnaires' disease have abnormal chest radiographs showing pulmonary infiltrates at the time of clinical presentation. In a few cases of hospital-acquired disease, fever and respiratory tract symptoms have preceded the radiographic appearance of the infiltrate. Findings on chest radiography are useful for assessing the severity of illness in that they identify multilobar involvement and permit monitoring of disease progression. However, these findings are nonspecific and do not serve to distinguish Legionnaires' disease from pneumonias of other etiologies. Pleural effusion is evident in 28–63% of patients on hospital admission. In immunosuppressed patients, especially those receiving glucocorticoids, distinctive rounded nodular opacities may be seen; these lesions may expand and cavitate (Fig. 141-1). Likewise, abscesses can occur in immunosuppressed hosts. The progression of infiltrates and pleural effusion on chest radiography despite appropriate antibiotic therapy within the first week is common, and radiographic improvement lags behind clinical improvement by several days. Complete clearing of infiltrates requires 1–4 months.

DIAGNOSIS
Because clinical manifestations are nonspecific, the diagnosis of Legionnaires' disease requires special microbiologic tests (Table 141-2). The sensitivity of bronchoscopy specimens is approximately the same as that of sputum samples for culture on selective media; if sputum is not available, bronchoscopy specimens may yield the organism. Bronchoalveolar lavage fluid gives higher yields than bronchial wash specimens. Thoracentesis should be performed if pleural effusion is found, and the fluid should be evaluated by DFA staining, culture, and the antigen assay designed for use with urine (see "Urinary Antigen," below).

TABLE 141-2 UTILITY OF SPECIAL LABORATORY TESTS FOR THE DIAGNOSIS OF LEGIONNAIRES' DISEASE

Test	Sensitivity, %	Specificity, %
Culture		
Sputum[a]	80	100
Transtracheal aspirate	90	100
Direct fluorescent antibody staining of sputum	50–70	96–99
Urinary antigen testing[b]	70	100
Antibody serology[c]	40–60	96–99

[a]Use of multiple selective media with dyes.
[b]Serogroup 1 only.
[c]IgG and IgM testing of both acute- and convalescent-phase sera. A single titer of ≥1:256 is considered presumptive, while fourfold seroconversion is considered definitive.

Staining Gram's staining of material from normally sterile sites, such as pleural fluid or lung tissue, occasionally suggests the diagnosis; efforts to detect *Legionella* in sputum by Gram's staining typically reveal numerous leukocytes but no organisms. When they are visualized, the organisms appear as small, pleomorphic, faint, gram-negative bacilli. *L. micdadei* organisms can be detected as weakly or partially acid-fast bacilli in clinical specimens. Modified acid-fast staining substitutes 1% sulfuric acid for the traditional 3% hydrochloric acid; the less aggressive decolorizer increases the yield of *L. micdadei*. *Legionella*-infected patients have occasionally been treated empirically with antituberculosis medications because of false-positive acid-fast smears.

The DFA test is rapid and highly specific but is less sensitive than culture because large numbers of organisms are required for microscopic visualization. This test is more likely to be positive in advanced than in early disease.

Culture The definitive method for diagnosis of *Legionella* infection is isolation of the organism from respiratory secretions or other specimens. Multiple selective BCYE media containing dyes are required for maximal sensitivity. Colonies grow slowly, requiring 3–5 days to become grossly visible. When culture plates are overgrown with other microflora, pretreatment of the specimen with acid or heat can markedly improve the yield. *L. pneumophila* is often isolated from sputum that is not grossly or microscopically purulent; sputum containing more than 25 epithelial cells per high-power field (a finding that classically suggests contamination) may still yield *L. pneumophila*.

Antibody Detection Antibody testing of both acute- and convalescent-phase sera is necessary. A fourfold rise in titer is diagnostic; 12 weeks are often required for the detection of an antibody response. A single titer of 1:128 in a patient with pneumonia constitutes circumstantial evidence for Legionnaires' disease. Serology is of use primarily in epidemiologic studies. The specificity of serology for *Legionella* species other than *L. pneumophila* is uncertain; there is cross-reactivity with *Legionella* spp. and some gram-negative bacilli.

Urinary Antigen The assay for *Legionella* soluble antigen in urine is rapid, relatively inexpensive, easy to perform, second only to culture in terms of sensitivity, and highly specific. Several enzyme immunoassays and a rapid immunochromatographic assay are commercially available. Like the urinary antigen assay, the rapid immunochromatographic assay is relatively inexpensive and easy to perform. The use of urinary antigen testing in every clinical laboratory is recommended. The urinary antigen test is available only for *L. pneumophila* serogroup 1, which causes ~80% of *Legionella* infections. Cross-reactivity with other *L. pneumophila* serogroups and other *Legionella* species has been detected in up to 22% of urine samples from patients with culture-proven cases. Antigen in urine is detectable 3 days after the onset of clinical disease and disappears over 2 months; positivity can be prolonged when patients receive glucocorticoids. The test is not affected by antibiotic administration.

Molecular Methods   Polymerase chain reaction (PCR) with DNA probes is theoretically more sensitive and specific than other methods. A molecular probe is undergoing evaluation. PCR has proven somewhat useful in the identification of *Legionella* from environmental water specimens. In PCR (unlike culture), epidemiologic links cannot be made since the infecting pathogen is not available for molecular subtyping.

PATHOLOGY

The consistent pathologic features of Legionnaires' disease are confined to the lungs. Multifocal pneumonia, with patchy lobular inflammation and extensive multilobar consolidation, has been observed. Visible abscesses with central necrosis were seen in 20% of autopsied cases in one study. On histologic examination, fibrinopurulent pneumonia with intensive alveolitis and bronchiolitis is evident. The DFA stain is not only specific but also the most sensitive option for visualization of the organism in tissues. Polyvalent but not monoclonal DFA stain can be used for formalinized specimens. Culture is the preferred method for diagnosis based on clinical specimens.

℞ LEGIONELLA INFECTION

Because *Legionella* is an intracellular pathogen, antibiotics that can reach intracellular concentrations exceeding the minimal inhibitory concentration are most likely to be clinically efficacious. The dosages for various drugs used in the treatment of *Legionella* infection are listed in **Table 141-3**.

The newer macrolides (especially azithromycin) and respiratory tract quinolones are now the antibiotics of choice and are effective as monotherapy. Compared with erythromycin, the newer macrolides have superior in vitro activity, display greater intracellular activity, reach higher concentrations in respiratory secretions and in lung tissue, and have fewer adverse effects. The pharmacokinetics of the newer macrolides and quinolones also allow once- or twice-daily dosing. Quinolones are the preferred antibiotics for transplant recipients because both macrolides and rifampin interact pharmacologically with cyclosporine and tacrolimus. Retrospective uncontrolled studies have shown that complications of pneumonia are fewer and clinical response is more rapid in patients receiving quinolones than in those receiving macrolides. Ketolides (telithromycin) are highly active in vitro and in intracellular models, but clinical experience is less extensive than that with macrolides and quinolones. Alternative agents include tetracycline and its analogues doxycycline and minocycline. Tigecycline is active in vitro but clinical experience is lacking. Anecdotal reports have described both successes and failures with trimethoprim-sulfamethoxazole, imipenem, and clindamycin. For severely ill patients with extensive pulmonary infiltrates, a two-drug combination of a newer macrolide or a quinolone with rifampin can be considered for initial treatment.

Initial therapy should be given by the IV route. A clinical response usually occurs within 3–5 days, after which oral therapy can be substituted. The total duration of therapy in the immunocompetent host is 10–14 days; a longer course (3 weeks) may be appropriate for immunosuppressed patients and those with advanced disease. For azithromycin, with its long half-life, a 5- to 10-day course is sufficient.

Pontiac fever requires only symptom-based treatment, not antimicrobial therapy.

PROGNOSIS

Mortality rates for Legionnaires' disease vary with the patient's underlying disease and its severity, the patient's immune status, the severity of pneumonia, and the timing of administration of appropriate antimicrobial therapy. Mortality rates are highest (80%) among immunosuppressed patients who do not receive appropriate antimicrobial therapy early in the course of illness. With appropriate and timely antibiotic treatment, mortality rates from community-acquired Legionnaires' disease among immunocompetent patients range from 0 to 11%; without treatment, the figure may be as high as 31%. In a study of survivors of an outbreak of community-acquired Legionnaires' disease, sequelae of fatigue, neurologic symptoms, and weakness were found in 63–75% of patients 17 months after receipt of antibiotics.

PREVENTION

 Routine environmental culture of hospital water supplies is recommended as an approach to the prevention of hospital-acquired Legionnaires' disease. Guidelines mandating this proactive approach have been adopted in Denmark, France, Germany, Italy, the Netherlands, and Taiwan. The CDC has thus far avoided this issue, but routine-culture guidelines from U.S. health departments have been adopted in Pittsburgh (PA), New York, and Maryland. Positive cultures from the water supply mandate the use of specialized laboratory tests (especially culture on selective media and the urinary antigen test) for patients with hospital-acquired pneumonia. Studies have shown that neither a high degree of outward cleanliness of the water system nor routine application of maintenance measures decreases the frequency or intensity of *Legionella* contamination. Thus, engineering guidelines and building codes, although routinely advocated as preventive measures, have little impact on the presence of *Legionella*.

Disinfection of the water supply is now feasible. Two methods have proven reliable and cost-effective. The superheat-and-flush method requires heating of the water so that the distal-outlet temperature is 70–80°C and flushing of the distal outlets with hot water for at least 30 min. This method is ideal for emergency situations. A commercial copper and silver ionization method has proved effective in numerous hospitals. Carbon dioxide and monochloramine are undergoing evaluation, and preliminary results are promising. Tap water filters have been effective for high-risk patient areas, such as transplantation units. Hyperchlorination is no longer recommended because of its expense, carcinogenicity, corrosive effects on piping, and unreliable efficacy.

FURTHER READINGS

GREENBERG D et al: Problem pathogens: Paediatric legionellosis—implications for improved diagnosis. Lancet Infect Dis 6:529, 2006

LETTINGA KD et al: Health-related quality of life and posttraumatic stress disorder among survivors of an outbreak of Legionnaires' disease. Clin Infect Dis 35:11, 2002

MODOL J et al: Hospital-acquired Legionnaires' disease in a university hospital: Impact of the copper-silver ionization system. Clin Infect Dis 44:263, 2007

TABLE 141-3   ANTIBIOTIC THERAPY FOR *LEGIONELLA* INFECTION

Antimicrobial Agent	Dosage[a]
Macrolides	
Azithromycin	500 mg[b] PO or IV[c] q24h
Clarithromycin	500 mg PO or IV[c] q12h
Quinolones	
Levofloxacin	750 mg IV q24h
	500 mg[b] PO q24h
Ciprofloxacin	400 mg IV q8h
	750 mg PO q12h
Moxifloxacin	400 mg[b] PO q24h
Ketolide	
Telithromycin	800 mg PO q24h
Tetracyclines	
Doxycycline	100 mg[b] PO or IV q12h
Minocycline	100 mg[b] PO or IV q12h
Tetracycline	500 mg PO or IV q6h
Tigecycline	100-mg IV load, then 50 mg IV q12h[d]
Others	
Trimethoprim-sulfamethoxazole	160/800 mg IV q8h
	160/800 mg PO q12h
Rifampin[e]	100–600 mg PO or IV q12h

[a]Dosages are derived from clinical experience.
[b]The authors recommend doubling the first dose.
[c]The IV formulation is not available in some countries.
[d]Undergoing evaluation.
[e]Rifampin should be used only in combination with a macrolide or a quinolone.

MUDER R, YU VL: Infection due to *Legionella* species other than *L. pneumophila*. Clin Infect Dis 35:990, 2002

MULAZIMOGLU L, YU VL: Can Legionnaires' disease be diagnosed by clinical criteria? A critical review. Chest 120:1049, 2001

PEDRO-BOTET ML et al: Legionnaires' disease contracted from patient homes: The coming of the third plague? Eur J Clin Microbiol Infect Dis 21:699, 2002

ROIG J, PEDRO-BOTET ML: *Legionella* spp: Community acquired and nosocomial infections. Curr Opin Infect Dis 16:45, 2003

SABRIA M et al: Fluoroquinolones vs macrolides in the treatment of Legionnaires' disease. Chest 128:1401, 2005

———, YU VL: Hospital-acquired legionellosis: Solutions for preventable infection. Lancet Infect Dis 2:368, 2002

SQUIER CL et al: A proactive approach to prevention of healthcare-acquired Legionnaires' disease: The Allegheny County (Pittsburgh) experience. Am J Infect Control 33:360, 2005

TUBACH F et al: Emergence of *L. pneumophila* pneumonia in patients receiving tumor necrosis factor-α antagonists. Clin Infect Dis 43:e95, 2006

142 Pertussis and Other *Bordetella* Infections

Scott A. Halperin

Pertussis is an acute infection of the respiratory tract caused by *Bordetella pertussis*. The name *pertussis* means "violent cough," which aptly describes the most consistent and prominent feature of the illness. The inspiratory sound made at the end of an episode of paroxysmal coughing gives rise to the common name for the illness, "whooping cough"; however, this feature is variable: it is uncommon among infants ≤6 months of age and is frequently absent in older children and adults. The Chinese name for pertussis is "the 100-day cough," which accurately describes the clinical course of the illness. The identification of *B. pertussis* was first reported by Bordet and Gengou in 1906, and vaccines were produced over the following two decades.

MICROBIOLOGY

Of the nine identified species in the genus *Bordetella*, only three are of major medical significance. *B. pertussis* infects only humans and is the most important *Bordetella* species causing human disease. *B. parapertussis* causes an illness in humans that is similar to pertussis but is typically milder; co-infections with *B. parapertussis* and *B. pertussis* have been documented. *B. bronchiseptica* is an important pathogen of domestic animals that causes kennel cough in dogs, atrophic rhinitis and pneumonia in pigs, and pneumonia in cats. Both respiratory infection and opportunistic infection are occasionally reported in humans. Two additional species, *B. hinzii* and *B. holmesii*, are unusual causes of bacteremia; both have been isolated from patients with sepsis, most often from those who are immunocompromised.

Bordetella species are gram-negative pleomorphic aerobic bacilli that share common genotypic characteristics. *B. pertussis* and *B. parapertussis* are the most similar of the species, but *B. parapertussis* does not express the gene coding for pertussis toxin. *B. pertussis* is a slow-growing fastidious organism that requires selective medium and forms small glistening bifurcated colonies. Suspicious colonies are presumptively identified as *B. pertussis* by direct fluorescent antibody testing or by agglutination with species-specific antiserum. *B. pertussis* is further differentiated from other *Bordetella* species by biochemical and motility characteristics.

B. pertussis produces a wide array of toxins and biologically active products that are important in its pathogenesis and in immunity. Most of these virulence factors are under the control of a single genetic locus that regulates their production, resulting in antigenic modulation and phase variation. Although these processes occur both in vitro and in vivo, their importance in the pathobiology of the organism is unknown; they may play a role in intracellular persistence and person-to-person spread. The organism's most important virulence factor is *pertussis toxin*, which is composed of a B oligomer–binding subunit and an enzymatically active A protomer that ADP-ribosylates a guanine nucleotide-binding regulatory protein (G protein) in target cells, producing a variety of biologic effects. Pertussis toxin has important mitogenic ac-

tivity, affects the circulation of lymphocytes, and serves as an adhesin for bacterial binding to respiratory ciliated cells. Other important virulence factors and adhesins are *filamentous hemagglutinin*, a component of the cell wall, and *pertactin*, an outer-membrane protein. *Fimbriae*, bacterial appendages that play a role in bacterial attachment, are the major antigens against which agglutinating antibodies are directed. These agglutinating antibodies have historically been the primary means of serotyping *B. pertussis* strains. Other virulence factors include tracheal cytotoxin, which causes respiratory epithelial damage; adenylate cyclase toxin, which impairs host immune-cell function; dermonecrotic toxin, which may contribute to respiratory mucosal damage; and lipooligosaccharide, which has properties similar to those of other gram-negative bacterial endotoxins.

EPIDEMIOLOGY

Pertussis is a highly communicable disease, with attack rates of 80–100% among unimmunized household contacts and 20% within households in well-immunized populations. The infection has a worldwide distribution, with cyclical outbreaks every 3–5 years (a pattern that has persisted despite widespread immunization). Pertussis occurs in all months; however, in North America, its activity peaks in summer and autumn.

In developing countries, pertussis remains an important cause of infant morbidity and death. The reported incidence of pertussis worldwide has decreased as a result of improved vaccine coverage. However, coverage rates are still <50% in many developing nations (**Fig. 142-1**); the World Health Organization (WHO) estimates that 90% of the burden of pertussis is in the developing world. In addition, overreporting of immunization coverage and underreporting of disease result in substantial underestimation of the global burden of pertussis (**Fig. 142-2**). The WHO estimates that more than 17.6 million people worldwide were infected by *B. pertussis* in 2003, with 279,000 deaths from pertussis among children.

Before the institution of widespread immunization programs in the developed world, pertussis was one of the most common infectious causes of morbidity and death. In the United States before the 1940s, between 115,000 and 270,000 cases of pertussis were reported annually, with an average yearly rate of 150 cases per 100,000 population. With universal childhood immunization, the number of reported cases fell by >95%, and mortality rates decreased even more dramatically. Only 1010 cases of pertussis were reported in 1976. Since that time, however, rates have slowly increased. In 2003, more than 11,600 cases of pertussis were reported in the United States.

Although thought of as a disease of childhood, pertussis can affect people of all ages and is increasingly being identified as a cause of prolonged coughing illness in adolescents and adults. In unimmunized populations, pertussis incidence peaks during the preschool years, and well over half of children have the disease before reaching adulthood. In highly immunized populations such as those in North America, the peak incidence is among infants <1 year of age who have not completed the three-dose primary immunization series. Recent trends, however, show an increasing incidence of pertussis among adolescents and adults. In the United States between 2001 and 2003, 23% of patients were <1 year of age, 33% were adolescents, and 23% were adults. The figures for adolescents and adults are probably underestimates because

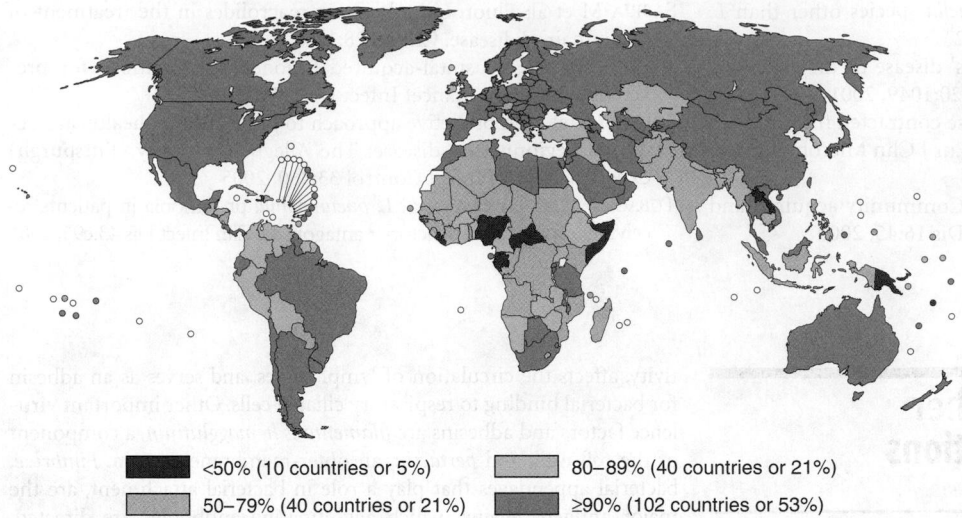

FIGURE 142-1 Immunization coverage with DTP3 vaccines (diphtheria toxoid, tetanus toxoid, and pertussis, 3 doses) in infants, 2004. *(Reprinted with permission of the World Health Organization. Source: WHO/IVB database, 2005. This map does not imply the expression of any opinion whatsoever on the part of the World Health Organization concerning the legal status of any country, territory, city, or area of its authorities or concerning the delimitation of its frontiers or boundaries.)*

Legend:
- <50% (10 countries or 5%)
- 50–79% (40 countries or 21%)
- 80–89% (40 countries or 21%)
- ≥90% (102 countries or 53%)

of a greater degree of underrecognition and underreporting in these age groups. A number of studies of prolonged coughing illness suggest that pertussis may be the etiologic agent in 12–30% of adults with cough that does not improve within 2 weeks. In one study of the efficacy of an acellular pertussis vaccine in adolescents and adults, the incidence of pertussis in the placebo group was 3.7–4.5 cases per 1000 person-years. Although this prospective cohort study yielded a lower estimate than the studies of cough illness, its results still translate to 600,000–800,000 cases of pertussis annually among adults in the United States. Severe morbidity and high mortality rates, however, are restricted almost entirely to infants. In Canada, there were 10 deaths from pertussis between 1991 and 1998; all those who died were infants ≤6 months of age. Although school-age children are the source of infection for most households, adults are the likely source for high-risk infants and may serve as the reservoir of infection between epidemic years.

PATHOGENESIS

Infection with *B. pertussis* is initiated by attachment of the organism to the ciliated epithelial cells of the nasopharynx. Attachment is mediated by surface adhesins (e.g., pertactin and filamentous hemagglutinin), which bind to the integrin family of cell-surface proteins, probably in conjunction with pertussis toxin. The role of fimbriae in adhesion and in maintenance of infection has not been fully delineated. At the site of attachment, the organism multiplies, producing a variety of other toxins that cause local mucosal damage (tracheal cytotoxin, dermonecrotic toxin). Impairment of host defense by *B. pertussis* is mediated by pertussis toxin and adenylate cyclase toxin. There is local cellular invasion, with intracellular bacterial persistence; however, systemic dissemination does not occur. Systemic manifestations (lymphocytosis) result from the effects of the toxins.

The pathogenesis of the clinical manifestations of pertussis is poorly understood. It is not known what causes the hallmark paroxysmal cough. A pivotal role for pertussis toxin has been proposed. Proponents of this position point to the efficacy of preventing clinical symptoms with a vaccine containing only pertussis toxoid. Detractors counter that pertussis toxin is not the critical factor because paroxysmal cough also occurs in patients infected with *B. parapertussis*, which does not produce pertussis toxin. It is thought that neurologic events in pertussis, such as seizures and encephalopathy, are due to hypoxia from coughing paroxysms or apnea rather than to the effects of specific bacterial products. *B. pertussis* pneumonia, which occurs in up to 10% of infants with pertussis, is usually a diffuse bilateral primary infection. In older children and adults with pertussis, pneumonia is often due to secondary bacterial infection with streptococci or staphylococci.

IMMUNITY

Both humoral and cell-mediated immunity are thought to be important in pertussis. Antibodies to pertussis toxin, filamentous hemagglutinin, pertactin, and fimbriae are all protective in animal models. Pertussis agglutinins were correlated with protection in early studies of whole-cell pertussis vaccines. Serologic correlates of protection conferred by acellular pertussis vaccines have not been established, although antibody to pertactin, fimbriae, and (to a lesser degree) pertussis toxin correlated best with protection in two efficacy trials. The duration of immunity after whole-cell pertussis vaccination is short-lived, with little protection remaining after 10–12 years. After a three-dose infant primary series of acellular pertussis vaccine, protection persists for at least 5–6 years; the duration of immunity after a four- or five-dose schedule is not yet known. Although immunity after natural infection has been said to be lifelong, seroepidemiologic evidence suggests that it may not be and that subsequent episodes of clinical pertussis are prevented by intermittent subclinical infection.

CLINICAL MANIFESTATIONS

Pertussis is a prolonged coughing illness with clinical manifestations that vary by age (**Table 142-1**). Although not uncommon among adolescents and adults, classic pertussis is most often seen in preschool and school-age children. After an incubation period averaging 7–10 days, an illness develops that is indistinguishable from the common cold and is characterized by coryza, lacrimation, mild cough, low-grade fever, and malaise. After 1–2 weeks, this *catarrhal phase* evolves into the *paroxysmal phase*: the cough becomes more frequent and spasmodic with repetitive bursts of 5–10 coughs, often within a single expiration. Posttussive vomiting is frequent, with a mucous plug occasionally expelled at the end of an episode. The episode may be terminated by an audible whoop, which occurs upon rapid inspiration against a closed glottis at the end of a paroxysm. During a spasm, there may be impressive neck-vein distension, bulging eyes, tongue protrusion, and cyanosis. Paroxysms may be precipitated by noise, eating, or physical contact. Between

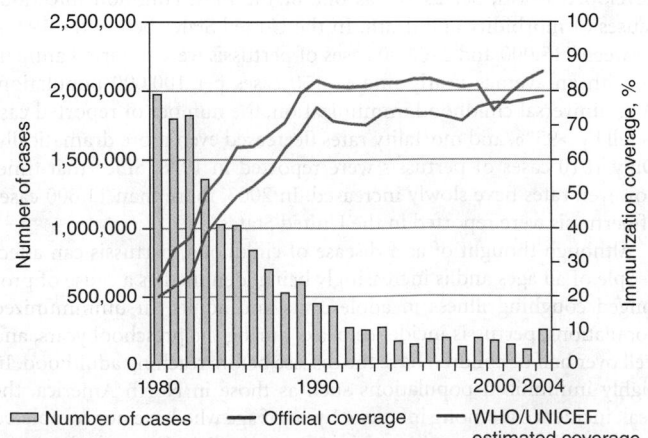

FIGURE 142-2 Global annual reported pertussis incidence and rate of coverage with DTP3 (diphtheria toxoid, tetanus toxoid, and pertussis vaccine, 3 doses), 1980–2004. *(Reprinted with permission of the World Health Organization. Source: WHO/IVB database, 2005.)*

Legend:
- Number of cases
- Official coverage
- WHO/UNICEF estimated coverage

TABLE 142-1 CLINICAL FEATURES OF PERTUSSIS, BY AGE GROUP AND DIAGNOSTIC STATUS

| | Percentage of Patients | | |
| | Adolescents and Adults | | |
Feature	Laboratory Confirmation	No Laboratory Confirmation	Children
Cough	95–100	95–100	95–100
Prolonged	60–80	60–80	60–95
Paroxysmal	60–90	50–90	80–95
Sleep-disturbing	50–80	50–80	90–100
Whoop	10–40	5–30	40–80
Posttussive vomiting	20–50	5–30	80–90

attacks, the patient's appearance is normal but increasing fatigue is evident. The frequency of paroxysmal episodes varies widely, from several per hour to 5–10 per day. Episodes are often worse at night and interfere with sleep. Weight loss is not uncommon as a result of the illness's interference with eating. Most complications occur during the paroxysmal stage. Fever is uncommon and suggests bacterial superinfection.

After 2–4 weeks, the coughing episodes become less frequent and less severe—changes heralding the onset of the *convalescent phase*. This phase can last 1–3 months and is characterized by gradual resolution of coughing episodes. For 6–12 months, intercurrent viral infections may be associated with a recrudescence of paroxysmal cough.

Not all individuals who develop pertussis have classic disease. The clinical manifestations in adolescents and adults are more often atypical. In a German study of pertussis in adults, more than two-thirds had paroxysmal cough and more than one-third had whoop. Adult illness in North America differs from this experience: the cough may be severe and prolonged but is less frequently paroxysmal, and a whoop is uncommon. Vomiting with cough is the best predictor of pertussis as the cause of prolonged cough in adults. Other predictive features are a cough at night and exposure to other individuals with a prolonged coughing illness.

COMPLICATIONS

Complications are frequently associated with pertussis and are more common among infants than among older children or adults. Subconjunctival hemorrhages, abdominal and inguinal hernias, pneumothoraces, and facial and truncal petechiae can result from increased intrathoracic pressure generated by severe fits of coughing. Weight loss can follow decreased caloric intake. In a series of more than 1100 children <2 years of age who were hospitalized with pertussis, 27.1% had apnea, 9.4% had pneumonia, 2.6% had seizures, and 0.4% had encephalopathy; 10 children (0.9%) died. Pneumonia is reported in <5% of adolescents and adults and increases in frequency after 50 years of age. In contrast to the primary *B. pertussis* pneumonia that develops in infants, pneumonia in adolescents and adults with pertussis is usually caused by a secondary infection with encapsulated organisms such as *Streptococcus pneumoniae* or *Haemophilus influenzae*. Pneumothorax, severe weight loss, inguinal hernia, rib fracture, carotid artery aneurysm, and cough syncope have all been reported in adolescents and adults with pertussis.

DIAGNOSIS

If the classic symptoms of pertussis are present, clinical diagnosis is not difficult. However, particularly in older children and adults, it is difficult to differentiate infections caused by *B. pertussis* and *B. parapertussis* from other respiratory tract infections on clinical grounds. Therefore, laboratory confirmation should be attempted in all cases. Lymphocytosis—an absolute lymphocyte count of $>10 \times 10^9/L$—is common among young children (in whom it is unusual with other infections) but not among adolescents and adults. Culture of nasopharyngeal secretions remains the gold standard of diagnosis, although DNA detection by polymerase chain reaction (PCR) is replacing culture in many laboratories because of increased sensitivity and quicker

results. The best specimen is collected by nasopharyngeal aspiration, in which a fine flexible plastic catheter attached to a 10-mL syringe is passed into the nasopharynx and withdrawn while gentle suction is applied. Since *B. pertussis* is highly sensitive to drying, secretions for culture should be inoculated without delay onto appropriate medium (Bordet-Gengou or Regan-Lowe), or the catheter should be flushed with a phosphate-buffered saline solution for culture and/or PCR. An alternative to the aspirate is a Dacron or rayon nasopharyngeal swab; again, inoculation of culture plates should be immediate or an appropriate transport medium (e.g., Regan-Lowe charcoal medium) should be used. Results of PCR can be available within hours; cultures become positive by day 5 of incubation. *B. pertussis* and *B. parapertussis* can be differentiated by agglutination with specific antisera or by direct immunofluorescence.

Nasopharyngeal cultures in untreated pertussis remain positive for a mean of 3 weeks after the onset of illness; these cultures become negative within 5 days of the institution of appropriate antimicrobial therapy. The duration of a positive PCR in untreated pertussis or after therapy is not known but exceeds that of positive cultures. Since much of the period during which the organism can be recovered from the nasopharynx falls into the catarrhal phase, when the etiology of the infection is not suspected, there is only a small window of opportunity for culture-proven diagnosis. Cultures from infants and young children are more frequently positive than those from older children and adults; this difference may reflect earlier presentation of the former age group for medical care. Direct fluorescent antibody tests of nasopharyngeal secretions for direct diagnosis may still be available in some laboratories but should not be used because of poor sensitivity and specificity.

As a result of the difficulties with laboratory diagnosis of pertussis in adolescents, adults, and patients who have been symptomatic for >4 weeks, increasing attention is being given to serologic diagnosis. Enzyme immunoassays detecting IgA and IgG antibodies to pertussis toxin, filamentous hemagglutinin, pertactin, and fimbriae have been developed and assessed for reproducibility. Two- or fourfold increases in antibody titer are suggestive of pertussis, although cross-reactivity of some antigens (such as filamentous hemagglutinin and pertactin) among *Bordetella* species makes it difficult to depend diagnostically on seroconversion involving a single type of antibody. Late presentation for medical care and prior immunization also complicate serologic diagnosis because the first sample obtained may in fact be a convalescent-phase specimen. Criteria for serologic diagnosis based on a single serum specimen compared with established population values are gaining acceptance, and serology will likely become more widely available for the diagnosis of pertussis.

DIFFERENTIAL DIAGNOSIS

A child presenting with paroxysmal cough, posttussive vomiting, and whoop is likely to have an infection caused by *B. pertussis* or *B. parapertussis*; lymphocytosis increases the likelihood of a *B. pertussis* etiology. Viruses such as respiratory syncytial virus and adenovirus have been isolated from patients with clinical pertussis but probably represent co-infection. In adolescents and adults, who often do not have paroxysmal cough or whoop, the differential diagnosis of a prolonged coughing illness is more extensive. Pertussis should be suspected in anyone with a cough that does not improve within 14 days, a paroxysmal cough of any duration, or any respiratory symptoms after contact with a laboratory-confirmed case of pertussis. Other etiologies to consider include infections caused by *Mycoplasma pneumoniae*, *Chlamydia pneumoniae*, adenovirus, influenza virus, and other respiratory viruses. Use of angiotensin-converting enzyme (ACE) inhibitors, reactive airway disease, and gastroesophageal reflux disease are well-described noninfectious causes of prolonged cough in adults.

℞ PERTUSSIS

ANTIBIOTICS The purpose of antibiotic therapy for pertussis is to eradicate the infecting bacteria from the nasopharynx; therapy does not substantially alter the clinical course unless given early in the catarrhal

TABLE 142-2 ANTIMICROBIAL THERAPY FOR PERTUSSIS

Drug	Adult Daily Dose	Frequency	Duration (Days)	Comments
Erythromycin estolate	1–2 g	3 divided doses	7–14	Frequent gastrointestinal side effects
Clarithromycin	500 mg	2 divided doses	7	
Azithromycin	500 mg on day 1, 250 mg subsequently	1 daily dose	5	
Trimethoprim-sulfamethoxazole	160 mg of trimethoprim, 800 mg of sulfamethoxazole	2 divided doses	14	For patients allergic to macrolides; data on effectiveness limited

phase. Macrolide antibiotics are the drugs of choice for treatment of pertussis (Table 142-2); macrolide-resistant *B. pertussis* strains have been reported but are rare. Trimethoprim-sulfamethoxazole is recommended as an alternative for individuals allergic to macrolides.

SUPPORTIVE CARE Young infants have the highest rates of complication and death from pertussis; therefore, most infants (and older children with severe disease) should be hospitalized. A quiet environment may decrease the stimulation that can trigger paroxysmal episodes. Use of β-adrenergic agonists and/or glucocorticoids has been advocated by some authorities but has not been proven to be effective. Cough suppressants are not effective and play no role in the management of pertussis.

INFECTION CONTROL MEASURES Hospitalized patients with pertussis should be placed in respiratory isolation, with the use of precautions appropriate for pathogens spread by large respiratory droplets. Isolation should continue for 5 days after initiation of erythromycin therapy or for 3 weeks (i.e., until nasopharyngeal cultures are consistently negative) when the patient cannot tolerate antimicrobial therapy.

PREVENTION

Chemoprophylaxis Because the risk of transmission of *B. pertussis* within households is high, chemoprophylaxis is widely recommended for household contacts of pertussis cases. The effectiveness of chemoprophylaxis, although unproven, is supported by several epidemiologic studies of institutional and community outbreaks. In the only randomized placebo-controlled study, erythromycin estolate (50 mg/kg per day in three divided doses; maximum dose, 1 g/d) was effective in reducing the incidence of bacteriologically confirmed pertussis by 67%; however, there was no decrease in the incidence of clinical disease. Despite these disappointing results, many authorities continue to recommend chemoprophylaxis, particularly in households with members at high risk of severe disease (children <1 year of age). Data are not available on use of the newer macrolides for chemoprophylaxis, but these drugs are commonly used because of their increased tolerability and their effectiveness.

Immunization (See also Chap. 116) The mainstay of pertussis prevention is active immunization. Pertussis vaccine, now available for >80 years, became widely used in North America after 1940; the reported number of pertussis cases has since fallen by >90%. Whole-cell pertussis vaccines are prepared through the heating, chemical inactivation, and purification of whole *B. pertussis* organisms. Although effective (average efficacy estimate, 85%; range for different products, 30–100%), whole-cell pertussis vaccines are associated with adverse events—both common (fever; injection-site pain, erythema, and swelling; irritability) and uncommon (febrile seizures, hypotonic hyporesponsive episodes). Alleged associations of whole-cell pertussis vaccine with encephalopathy, sudden infant death syndrome, and autism, although not substantiated, have spawned an active anti-immunization lobby. The development of acellular pertussis vaccines, which are effective but less reactogenic, has greatly

alleviated concerns about the inclusion of pertussis vaccine in the combined infant immunization series. Although whole-cell vaccines are still used extensively in the developing world, acellular pertussis vaccines are used exclusively for childhood immunization in much of the developed world. In North America, acellular pertussis vaccines are given as a three-dose primary series at 2, 4, and 6 months of age, with a reinforcing dose at 15–18 months of age and a booster dose at 4–6 years of age.

Although a wide variety of acellular pertussis vaccines were developed, only a few are still widely marketed; all contain pertussis toxoid and filamentous hemagglutinin. One acellular pertussis vaccine also contains pertactin, and another contains pertactin and two types of fimbriae. In light of analyses of phase 3 efficacy studies, most experts have concluded that two-component acellular pertussis vaccines are more effective than monocomponent vaccines and that the addition of pertactin increases efficacy still more. The further addition of fimbriae appears to enhance protective efficacy against milder disease. In two studies, protection conferred by pertussis vaccines correlated best with the production of antibody to pertactin, fimbriae, and pertussis toxin.

The development of acellular pertussis vaccines has sparked interest in the potential for pertussis control in adolescents and adults and in the possibility that pertussis control in those groups will enhance the protection of infants too young to be immunized. Whole-cell pertussis vaccine is contraindicated in individuals ≥7 years of age because of their poor toleration of possible adverse events. However, adult formulations of acellular pertussis vaccines have been shown to be safe, immunogenic, and efficacious in clinical trials in adolescents and adults and are now recommended for routine immunization of these groups in several countries, including the United States.

FURTHER READINGS

DE SERRES G et al: Morbidity of pertussis in adolescents and adults. J Infect Dis 182:174, 2000

HALPERIN SA et al: A randomized, placebo-controlled trial of erythromycin estolate chemoprophylaxis for household contacts of children with culture-positive *Bordetella pertussis* infection. Pediatrics 104:e42, 1999

—— et al: Epidemiological features of pertussis in hospitalized patients in Canada, 1991–1997: Report of the Immunization Monitoring Program—Active (IMPACT). Clin Infect Dis 28:1238, 1999

LEE GM et al: Pertussis in adolescents and adults: Should we vaccinate? Pediatrics 115:1675, 2005

MATTOO S, CHERRY JD: Molecular pathogenesis, epidemiology, and clinical manifestations of respiratory infections due to *Bordetella pertussis* and other *Bordetella* subspecies. Clin Microbiol Rev 18:326, 2005

RIFFELMANN M et al: Pertussis PCR Consensus Group. Nucleic acid amplification tests for diagnosis of *Bordetella* infections. J Clin Microbiol 43:4925, 2005

SKOWRONSKI DM et al: The changing age and seasonal profile of pertussis in Canada. J Infect Dis 185:1448, 2002

TAN T et al: Epidemiology of pertussis. Pediatr Infect Dis J 24(Suppl):S10, 2005

WARD JI et al: APERT Study Group. Efficacy of an acellular pertussis vaccine among adolescents and adults. N Engl J Med 353:1555, 2005

YIH WK et al: The increasing incidence of pertussis in Massachusetts adolescents and adults, 1989–1998. J Infect Dis 182:1409, 2000

143 Diseases Caused by Gram-Negative Enteric Bacilli

Thomas A. Russo, James R. Johnson

GENERAL FEATURES AND PRINCIPLES

EPIDEMIOLOGY

Escherichia coli, Klebsiella, Proteus, Enterobacter, Serratia, Citrobacter, Morganella, Providencia, Edwardsiella, and *Acinetobacter* are components of the normal animal and human colonic flora and/or of the flora of a variety of environmental habitats, including long-term-care facilities (LTCFs) and hospitals. As a result, except for certain pathotypes of intestinal pathogenic *E. coli,* these genera are global pathogens. In healthy humans, *E. coli* is the predominant species of gram-negative bacilli (GNB) in the colonic flora. GNB (primarily *E. coli, Klebsiella,* and *Proteus*) only transiently colonize the oropharynx and skin of healthy individuals. In contrast, in LTCF and hospital settings, a variety of GNB emerge as the dominant flora of both mucosal and skin surfaces, particularly in association with antimicrobial use, severe illness, and extended length of stay. This colonization may lead to subsequent infection; for example, oropharyngeal colonization may lead to pneumonia.

STRUCTURE AND FUNCTION

GNB possess an extracytoplasmic outer membrane, a feature shared generally among gram-negative bacteria. This outer membrane consists of a lipid bilayer with associated proteins, lipoproteins, and polysaccharides [capsule, lipopolysaccharide (LPS)]. The outer membrane interfaces with the bacterial environment, including the human host. A variety of components of the outer membrane are critical determinants in pathogenesis and antimicrobial resistance.

PATHOGENESIS

Multiple bacterial virulence factors are required for the pathogenesis of infections caused by GNB. Possession of specialized virulence genes defines pathogens and enables them to infect the host efficiently. It is becoming clear that hosts and their cognate pathogens have been co-adapting throughout evolutionary history, and it has been speculated that infection is just one point on the spectrum of evolved relationships between microbes and hosts. At one end of this spectrum is a commensal/symbiotic interaction (e.g., mitochondria—formerly bacteria—within eukaryotic cells); at the other end is a lethal outcome, producing a "dead-end relationship" (e.g., Ebola virus). During the host-pathogen "chess match" over time, various and redundant strategies have emerged in both the pathogens and their hosts that enable these partners to maintain their coexistence (Table 143-1).

Extraintestinal pathogenic strains of *E. coli* (ExPEC) and the other genera discussed in this chapter cause infection outside the bowel. All are extracellular pathogens and therefore share certain pathogenic features. Innate immunity (including the activities of complement, antimicrobial peptides, and professional phagocytes) and humoral immunity are the principal host-defense components. Both susceptibility to and severity of infection are increased with dysfunction or deficiencies of these components (Chap. 113). In contrast, the virulence traits of intestinal pathogenic *E. coli*—i.e., the distinctive strains that can cause diarrheal disease—are for the most part different from those of extraintestinal pathogenic *E. coli* and other GNB that cause extraintestinal infections. This difference reflects site-specific differences in host environments and defense mechanisms.

A given extraintestinal pathogen usually possesses multiple adhesins for binding to a variety of host cells (e.g., in *E. coli:* type 1 fimbriae, Sfa/Foc fimbriae, P pili). Nutrient acquisition (e.g., of iron via siderophores) requires many genes that are necessary but not sufficient for pathogenesis. The ability to resist the bactericidal activity of complement and phagocytes in the absence of antibody (e.g., as conferred by capsule or O antigen of LPS) is one of the defining traits of an extracellular pathogen. Tissue damage (e.g., as mediated by hemolysin in the case of *E. coli*) may facilitate spread. Without doubt, many important virulence genes await identification, and our understanding of many aspects of the pathogenesis of infections due to GNB is in its infancy (Chap. 114).

The ability to induce septic shock is another defining feature of these genera. GNB are the most common causes of this potentially lethal syndrome. The lipid A moiety of LPS (via interaction with host Toll-like receptor 4) and probably other bacterial factors as well stimulate a proinflammatory host response that, if overly exuberant, results in shock (Chap. 265).

Many antigenic variants (serotypes) exist in most genera of GNB. For example, there are >150 O-specific antigens and >80 capsular antigens in *E. coli.* This antigenic variability, which permits immune evasion and allows recurrent infection by different strains of the same species, has impeded vaccine development (Chap. 116).

INFECTIOUS SYNDROMES

Although certain strains of *E. coli* have evolved to be strictly intestinal pathogens, causing gastroenteritis by a variety of unique pathogenic mechanisms, extraintestinal infections are the predominant presentation of disease caused by enteric GNB. Depending on both the host and the pathogen, nearly every organ or body cavity can be infected with GNB. *E. coli* and—to a lesser degree—*Klebsiella* and *Proteus* account for most extraintestinal infections due to GNB and are the most virulent pathogens of this group. However, the other genera are becoming increasingly important, particularly among LTCF residents and hospitalized patients. This expanding role is due in large part to the intrinsic or acquired antimicrobial resistance of these organisms and the increasing number of individuals with alterations or disruptions of host defenses. The mortality rate is significant in many GNB infections and correlates with the severity of illness. Especially problematic are pneumonia and bacteremia (arising from any source) when complicated by organ failure (severe sepsis) and/or shock; associated mortality rates are 20–50%.

DIAGNOSIS

Isolation of GNB from ordinarily sterile anatomic sites almost always implies infection, whereas their isolation from nonsterile sites, particularly from open soft-tissue wounds and the respiratory tract, requires clinical correlation to differentiate colonization from infection. Tentative laboratory identification based on lactose fermentation and indole

TABLE 143-1 INTERACTIONS OF EXTRAINTESTINAL PATHOGENIC *E. COLI* WITH THE HUMAN HOST: A PARADIGM FOR EXTRACELLULAR, EXTRAINTESTINAL GRAM-NEGATIVE BACTERIAL PATHOGENS

Bacterial Goal	Host Obstacle	Bacterial Solution
Extraintestinal attachment	Flow of urine, mucociliary blanket	Multiple adhesins (e.g., type 1 fimbriae, Sfa/Foc, P pili)
Nutrient acquisition for growth	Nutrient sequestration (e.g., iron via intracellular storage and extracellular scavenging via lactoferrin and transferrin)	Cellular lysis (e.g., hemolysin); multiple mechanisms for competing for extracellular iron (e.g., siderophores) and other nutrients
Initial avoidance of host bactericidal activity	Complement, phagocytic cells, antimicrobial peptides	Capsular polysaccharide, lipopolysaccharide
Transmission	?	Irritant tissue damage resulting in increased excretion (e.g., toxins such as hemolysin)
Late avoidance of host bactericidal activity	Acquired immunity (e.g., specific antibodies), treatment with antibiotics	? Cell entry, acquisition of antimicrobial resistance

production (described for each genus below), which usually is possible before final identification of the organism and determination of its antimicrobial susceptibilities, may guide empirical antimicrobial therapy.

℞ INFECTIONS CAUSED BY GRAM-NEGATIVE ENTERIC BACILLI

(See also Chap. 127) Accumulating evidence indicates that initiation of appropriate empirical antimicrobial therapy early in the course of GNB infections (particularly serious infections) leads to improved outcomes. Familiarity with evolving patterns of antimicrobial resistance in enteric GNB is necessary in the selection of appropriate empirical therapy. The antimicrobial resistance profiles of GNB vary by species, geographic location, regional antimicrobial use, and hospital site [e.g., intensive care units (ICUs) versus wards]. At present, the most reliably active agents against enteric GNB are the carbapenems (e.g., imipenem), the aminoglycoside amikacin, the fourth-generation cephalosporin cefepime, and piperacillin-tazobactam.

β-Lactamases, which inactivate β-lactam agents, are the most important mediators of resistance to these drugs in GNB. Decreased permeability and/or active efflux of β-lactam agents, although less common, may occur alone or in combination with β-lactamase-mediated resistance. *Broad-spectrum* β-lactamases, which mediate resistance to many penicillins and first-generation cephalosporins, are frequently expressed in enteric GNB. These enzymes are inhibited by agents such as clavulanate. *Extended-spectrum* β-lactamases (ESBLs) confer resistance to the same drugs as broad-spectrum β-lactamases as well as to third-generation cephalosporins, aztreonam, and (in some instances) fourth-generation cephalosporins.

The acquisition of ESBL-encoding genes via transferable plasmids is increasing in GNB worldwide, with rates varying greatly even among hospitals in a given region. To date, ESBLs are most prevalent in *Klebsiella pneumoniae*, *K. oxytoca*, and *E. coli* but also occur (and are probably underrecognized) in *Enterobacter*, *Citrobacter*, *Proteus*, *Serratia*, and other enteric GNB. At present, the regional prevalence of ESBL-producing GNB declines in rank order as follows: Latin America > Western Pacific > Europe > United States and Canada. ESBL-producing GNB are most prevalent in hospitals (ICUs > wards) but recently have emerged in the community. Hospital outbreaks due to ESBL-producing strains have been associated with extensive use of third-generation cephalosporins, particularly ceftazidime. The carbapenems are the most reliably active β-lactam agents against ESBL-expressing strains. GNB that express ESBLs may also possess porin mutations that result in decreased uptake of cephalosporins and β-lactam/β-lactamase inhibitor combinations. Thus, ESBL-producing isolates should be considered resistant to all penicillins, cephalosporins, and aztreonam.

AmpC β-lactamases confer resistance to the same substrates as ESBLs plus the cephamycins, a subset of the second-generation cephalosporins. AmpC enzymes resist inhibition by β-lactamase inhibitors. Constitutive chromosomal AmpC β-lactamases are present in nearly all strains of *Enterobacter*, *Serratia*, *Citrobacter*, *Proteus vulgaris*, *Providencia*, *Morganella*, and *Acinetobacter*, resulting in resistance to aminopenicillins, cefazolin, and cefoxitin. In addition, some strains of *E. coli*, *K. pneumoniae*, and other Enterobacteriaceae have acquired plasmids containing AmpC β-lactamase genes. The fourth-generation cephalosporin cefepime is stable to AmpC β-lactamases and is an appropriate treatment option if the concomitant presence of an ESBL can be excluded.

Carbapenemases confer resistance to the same drugs as ESBLs plus cephamycins and carbapenems. At present, carbapenemase-producing enteric GNB are uncommon. In the United States, strains of *Klebsiella* and *Enterobacter* that possess carbapenemases on transferable plasmids and exhibit resistance to fluoroquinolones and aminoglycosides have been found. Tigecycline (a glycylcycline, a new antimicrobial class) and the polymyxins (agents of last resort, given their potential toxicities) are the most active drugs in vitro, but their clinical efficacy has not been demonstrated.

Resistance to fluoroquinolones usually is due to alterations of the target site (DNA gyrase and/or topoisomerase IV), with or without decreased permeability, active efflux, or protection of the target site. Resistance to fluoroquinolones is increasingly prevalent among GNB; 20–80% of ESBL-producing enteric GNB are also resistant to fluoroquinolones. At present, this drug class should be considered unreliable as empirical therapy for infections due to GNB in critically ill patients.

Not all clinical laboratories screen for ESBLs, screening protocols are limited, and no recommended tests identify AmpC β-lactamases or carbapenemases. For these reasons, these resistance mechanisms are underreported, and it is important to assess the clinical response to treatment in addition to in vitro susceptibility data.

Given the increasing prevalence of multidrug resistance in enteric GNB, it is reasonable—pending susceptibility results—to combine agents for empirical treatment of GNB infections in critically ill patients. Although supporting clinical evidence is limited, combination therapy may increase antimicrobial efficacy and/or diminish the emergence of resistance in some circumstances. In addition, drainage of abscesses and removal of infected foreign bodies are often required for cure.

GNB are commonly involved in polymicrobial infections, in which the role of each specific pathogen is uncertain (Chap. 157). Although some GNB are more pathogenic than others, it is usually prudent, if possible, to design an antimicrobial regimen active against all of the GNB identified, since each is capable of pathogenicity in its own right.

PREVENTION

(See also Chap. 125) Diligent adherence to hand-hygiene protocols by health care personnel and avoidance of inappropriate antimicrobial use are key measures in preventing infection and the further development of antimicrobial resistance. Likewise, avoidance of the use of indwelling devices that predispose to infections due to GNB (e.g., urinary and intravascular catheters, endotracheal tubes) decreases infection risk.

ESCHERICHIA COLI INFECTIONS

COMMENSAL STRAINS

For the most part, commensal *E. coli* variants, which constitute the bulk of the normal facultative intestinal flora in most humans, confer benefits to the host (e.g., resistance to colonization with pathogenic organisms). These strains generally lack the specialized virulence traits that enable extraintestinal and intestinal pathogenic *E. coli* strains to cause disease outside and within the gastrointestinal tract, respectively. However, even commensal *E. coli* strains can be involved in extraintestinal infections in the presence of an aggravating factor, such as a foreign body (e.g., a urinary catheter), host compromise (e.g., local anatomic or functional abnormalities such as urinary or biliary tract obstruction or systemic immunocompromise), or an inoculum that is large or contains a mixture of bacterial species (e.g., fecal contamination of the peritoneal cavity).

EXTRAINTESTINAL PATHOGENIC (ExPEC) STRAINS

The majority of *E. coli* isolates from symptomatic infections of the urinary tract, bloodstream, cerebrospinal fluid, respiratory tract, and peritoneum (spontaneous bacterial peritonitis) can be differentiated from commensal and intestinal pathogenic strains of *E. coli* by virtue of their distinctive virulence factor profiles (Tables 143-1 and **143-2**) and phylogenetic background. ExPEC strains can also cause surgical wound infection, osteomyelitis, and myositis, but the number of cases evaluated to date is too small for a reliable assessment of proportions.

Like commensal *E. coli* (but in contrast to intestinal pathogenic *E. coli*), ExPEC strains are often found in the normal intestinal flora and do not cause gastroenteritis in humans. Although acquisition of an ExPEC strain by the host is a prerequisite for ExPEC infection, it is not the rate-limiting step, which instead is entry of an ExPEC strain from its site of colonization (e.g., the colon, vagina, or oropharynx) into a normally sterile extraintestinal site (e.g., the urinary tract, peritoneal cavity, or lungs). ExPEC strains have acquired genes encoding diverse extraintestinal virulence factors that enable the bacteria to cause infections outside the gastrointestinal tract in both normal and compromised hosts (Table 143-1). These virulence genes are, for the most part, distinct from those that enable intestinal pathogenic strains to cause diarrheal disease. All age groups, all types of hosts, and nearly all organs and anatomic sites are susceptible to infection by ExPEC. Previously healthy hosts infected with ExPEC can become severely ill or die; however, adverse outcomes are more prevalent in the presence of comorbid illnesses and host defense abnormalities. *E. coli* is the most

TABLE 143-2 **INTESTINAL PATHOGENIC _E. COLI_** 939

Pathotype[a]	Epidemiology	Clinical Syndrome[b]	Defining Molecular Trait	Responsible Genetic Element[c]
STEC	Food, water, person-to-person; all ages, industrialized countries	Hemorrhagic colitis, hemolytic-uremic syndrome	Shiga toxin	Lambda-like Stx1- or Stx2-encoding bacteriophage
ETEC	Food, water; young children in and travelers to developing countries	Traveler's diarrhea	Heat-stable and -labile enterotoxins, colonization factors	Virulence plasmid(s)
EPEC	Person-to-person; young children and neonates in developing countries	Watery diarrhea	Localized adherence, attaching and effacing lesion on intestinal epithelium	EPEC adherence factor plasmid pathogenicity island (locus for enterocyte effacement)
EIEC	Food, water; children in and travelers to developing countries	Dysentery	Invasion of colonic epithelial cells, intracellular multiplication, cell-to-cell spread	Multiple genes contained primarily in large virulence plasmid
EAEC	? Food, water; children in and travelers to developing countries; all ages, industrialized countries	Traveler's diarrhea, acute diarrhea, persistent diarrhea	Aggregative/diffuse adherence, virulence factors regulated by AggR	Chromosomal or plasmid-associated adherence and toxin genes

[a]STEC, Shiga toxin–producing _E. coli_; ETEC, enterotoxigenic _E. coli_; EPEC, enteropathogenic _E. coli_; EIEC, enteroinvasive _E. coli_; EAEC, enteroaggregative _E. coli_.

[b]Classic syndromes; see text for details on spectrum of disease.

[c]Pathogenesis is multigenic, including genes in addition to those listed.

common enteric gram-negative species to cause extraintestinal infection in ambulatory, LTCF, and hospital settings. The diversity and the medical and economic impact of ExPEC infections are evident from consideration of the following specific syndromes.

Extraintestinal Infectious Syndromes • _URINARY TRACT INFECTION (UTI)_ The urinary tract is the site most frequently infected by ExPEC. An exceedingly common infection among ambulatory patients, UTI accounts for 1% of ambulatory care visits in the United States and is second only to lower respiratory tract infection among infections responsible for hospitalization. UTIs are best considered by clinical syndrome (e.g., uncomplicated cystitis, pyelonephritis, and catheter-associated UTIs) and within the context of specific hosts (e.g., premenopausal women, compromised hosts; Chap. 282). _E. coli_ is the single most common pathogen for all UTI syndrome/host group combinations. Each year in the United States, _E. coli_ causes 85–95% of an estimated 6–8 million episodes of uncomplicated cystitis in premenopausal women, with an estimated $1 billion in direct health care costs. Furthermore, 20% of women with an initial cystitis episode develop frequent recurrences (from 0.3 to >20 per year).

Uncomplicated cystitis, the most common acute UTI syndrome, is characterized by dysuria, frequency, and suprapubic pain. Fever and/or back pain suggests progression to pyelonephritis. Fever may take 5–7 days to resolve completely in appropriately treated patients with pyelonephritis. Persistently elevated or increasing fever and neutrophil counts should prompt evaluation for intrarenal or perinephric abscess and/or obstruction. Renal parenchymal damage and loss of renal function during pyelonephritis occur primarily with urinary obstruction. Pregnant women are at unusually high risk for developing pyelonephritis, which can adversely affect the outcome of pregnancy. As a result, prenatal screening for and treatment of asymptomatic bacteriuria are standard. Prostatic infection is a potential complication of UTI in men. The diagnosis and treatment of UTI, as detailed in Chap. 282, should be tailored to the individual host, the nature and site of infection, and local patterns of antimicrobial susceptibility.

ABDOMINAL AND PELVIC INFECTION The abdomen/pelvis is the second most common site of extraintestinal infection due to _E. coli_. A wide va-

riety of clinical syndromes occur in this location, including acute peritonitis secondary to fecal contamination, spontaneous bacterial peritonitis, dialysis-associated peritonitis, diverticulitis, appendicitis, intraperitoneal or visceral abscesses (hepatic, pancreatic, splenic), infected pancreatic pseudocysts, and septic cholangitis and/or cholecystitis. In intraabdominal infections, _E. coli_ can be isolated either alone or (as is often the case) along with other facultative and/or anaerobic members of the intestinal flora (Chap. 121).

PNEUMONIA _E. coli_ is not usually considered a cause of pneumonia (Chap. 251). Indeed, enteric GNB account for only 2–5% of cases of community-acquired pneumonia (CAP), in part because these organisms only transiently colonize the oropharynx of a minority of healthy individuals. However, rates of oral colonization with _E. coli_ and other GNB increase with the severity of illness and with antibiotic use. Thus, GNB are a common cause of pneumonia among residents of LTCFs and are the most common cause (60–70% of cases) of hospital-acquired pneumonia (Chap. 125), particularly among postoperative and intensive care patients. Pulmonary infection is usually acquired by small-volume aspiration but occasionally occurs via hematogenous spread, in which case multifocal nodular infiltrates can be seen. Tissue necrosis, probably due to cytotoxins produced by GNB, is common. Despite significant institutional variation, _E. coli_ is generally the third or fourth most commonly isolated gram-negative bacillus in hospital-acquired pneumonia, accounting for 5–8% of episodes in both U.S.-based and European-based studies. Regardless of the host, pneumonia due to enteric GNB is a serious disease, with high crude and attributable mortality rates (20–60% and 10–20%, respectively).

MENINGITIS (See also Chap. 376) _E. coli_ is one of the two leading causes of neonatal meningitis (the other being group B _Streptococcus_). Most of the responsible strains possess the K1 capsular antigen. After the first month of life, _E. coli_ meningitis is uncommon, occurring predominantly in the setting of disruption of the meninges from craniotomy or trauma or in the presence of cirrhosis. In patients with cirrhosis, the meninges are presumably seeded as a result of poor hepatic clearance of portal vein bacteremia.

CELLULITIS/MUSCULOSKELETAL INFECTION _E. coli_ contributes frequently to infection of decubitus ulcers and occasionally to infection of ulcers and wounds of the lower extremity in diabetic patients and other hosts with neurovascular compromise. Osteomyelitis secondary to contiguous spread can occur in these settings. In addition, _E. coli_ occasionally causes cellulitis or infections of burn sites or surgical wounds, particularly when the infection originates close to the perineum. Hematogenously acquired osteomyelitis, particularly of vertebral bodies, is more commonly caused by _E. coli_ than is generally appreciated; this organism accounts for up to 10% of cases in some series (Chap. 120). _E. coli_ occasionally causes orthopedic device–associated infection or septic arthritis and rarely causes hematogenous myositis. Upper-leg myositis or fasciitis due to _E. coli_ should prompt an evaluation for an abdominal source with contiguous spread.

ENDOVASCULAR INFECTION Despite being one of the most common causes of bacteremia, _E. coli_ rarely seeds native or prosthetic heart valves. When the organism does seed native valves, it usually does so in the setting of prior valve disease. *E. coli* infections of aneurysms and vascular grafts are quite uncommon.

MISCELLANEOUS INFECTIONS *E. coli* can cause infection in nearly every organ and anatomic site. It occasionally causes postoperative mediastinitis or complicated sinusitis and uncommonly causes endophthalmitis or brain abscess.

BACTEREMIA *E. coli* bacteremia can arise from primary infection at any extraintestinal site. In addition, primary *E. coli* bacteremia can arise from percutaneous intravascular devices or transrectal prostate biopsy or can result from the increased intestinal mucosal permeability seen in neonates and in the settings of neutropenia and chemotherapy-induced mucositis, trauma, and burns. Roughly equal proportions of *E. coli* bacteremia cases originate in the community and in the hospital. In most studies, *E. coli* and *Staphylococcus aureus* are the two most common blood isolates of clinical significance; *E. coli*, which is isolated in 17–37% of cases, is the gram-negative bacillus most often isolated from the blood in the ambulatory setting and in most LTCF and hospital settings. Isolation of *E. coli* from the blood is almost always clinically significant and typically is accompanied by the sepsis syndrome, severe sepsis (sepsis-induced dysfunction of at least one organ or system), or septic shock (Chap. 265). Calculations based on a conservative estimate for the proportional contribution of *E. coli* to severe sepsis (i.e., 17% of all cases) translate into an estimated 40,000 deaths among the affected patients in the United States in 2001.

The urinary tract is the most common source of *E. coli* bacteremia, accounting for one-half to two-thirds of episodes. Bacteremia from a urinary tract source is particularly common in patients with pyelonephritis, urinary tract obstruction, or instrumentation in the presence of infected urine. The abdomen is the second most common source, accounting for 25% of episodes. Although biliary obstruction (stones, tumor) and overt bowel disruption are responsible for many of these cases, some abdominal sources (e.g., abscesses) are remarkably silent clinically and require identification via imaging studies (e.g., CT). Therefore, the physician should be cautious in designating the urinary tract as the source of *E. coli* bacteremia in the absence of characteristic signs and symptoms of UTI. Soft tissue, bone, pulmonary, and intravascular catheter infections are other sources of *E. coli* bacteremia.

Diagnosis Strains of *E. coli* that cause extraintestinal infections usually grow both aerobically and anaerobically within 24 h on standard diagnostic media and are easily identified by the clinical microbiology laboratory according to routine biochemical criteria. More than 90% of ExPEC strains are rapid lactose fermenters and are indole positive.

℞ EXTRAINTESTINAL *E. COLI* INFECTIONS

In the past, most *E. coli* isolates were highly susceptible to a broad range of antimicrobial agents. Unfortunately, this situation has changed. In general, the frequency of ampicillin resistance precludes its empirical use, even in community-acquired infections. The prevalence of resistance to first-generation cephalosporins and trimethoprim-sulfamethoxazole (TMP-SMX) is increasing among community-acquired strains in the United States (with current rates of 10–40%) and is even higher outside North America. Until recently, TMP-SMX was the drug of choice for the treatment of uncomplicated cystitis in many locales. Although continued empirical use of TMP-SMX will predictably result in ever-diminishing cure rates, a wholesale switch to alternative agents (e.g., fluoroquinolones) will just as predictably accelerate the widespread emergence of resistance to these antimicrobial classes, as is already occurring in some areas. Resistance to fluoroquinolones has increased steadily over the last decade; in 2002–2005, prevalence rates were 5–20% in North America and even higher in other regions. The prevalence of resistance is higher in settings where fluoroquinolone prophylaxis is used extensively (e.g., in patients with leukemia, transplant recipients, and patients with cirrhosis) and among isolates from LTCFs and hospitals. Among quinolone-resistant strains, a significant (30–40%) prevalence of co-resistance to amoxicillin/clavulanic acid and piper-

acillin has been reported. The prevalence of co-resistance to more advanced cephalosporins (second-, third-, and fourth-generation), monobactams (e.g., aztreonam), piperacillin-tazobactam, and the non-amikacin aminoglycosides is increasing but is still generally <10%. Carbapenems (e.g., imipenem) and amikacin are the most predictably active agents. Although relevant clinical experience is limited, tigecycline and polymyxin B (the agent of last resort because of its potential toxicities) are highly active in vitro.

INTESTINAL PATHOGENIC STRAINS

Certain strains of *E. coli* are capable of causing diarrheal disease. Other important intestinal pathogens are discussed in Chaps. 122, 135, and 146–149. At least in the industrialized world, intestinal pathogenic strains of *E. coli* are rarely encountered in the fecal flora of healthy persons and instead appear to be essentially obligate pathogens. These strains have evolved a special ability to cause enteritis, enterocolitis, and colitis when ingested in sufficient quantities by a naive host. At least five distinct pathotypes of intestinal pathogenic *E. coli* exist: (1) Shiga toxin–producing *E. coli* (STEC)/enterohemorrhagic *E. coli* (EHEC), (2) enterotoxigenic *E. coli* (ETEC), (3) enteropathogenic *E. coli* (EPEC), (4) enteroinvasive *E. coli* (EIEC), and (5) enteroaggregative *E. coli* (EAEC). Diffusely adherent *E. coli* (DAEC) and cytodetaching *E. coli* are additional putative pathotypes. Transmission occurs predominantly via contaminated food and water for ETEC, STEC, EIEC, and probably EAEC and by person-to-person spread for EPEC (and occasionally STEC/EHEC). Gastric acidity confers some protection against infection; therefore, persons with decreased stomach acid levels are especially susceptible. Humans are the major reservoir (except for STEC/EHEC); host range appears to be dictated by species-specific attachment factors. Although there is some overlap, each pathotype possesses a unique combination of virulence traits that results in a distinctive intestinal pathogenic mechanism (Table 143-2). These strains are largely incapable of causing disease outside the intestinal tract. Except in the case of STEC/EHEC and perhaps EAEC, disease due to this group of pathogens occurs primarily in developing countries.

Shiga Toxin–Producing and Enterohemorrhagic *E. coli* STEC/EHEC strains constitute an emerging group of pathogens that can cause hemorrhagic colitis and the hemolytic-uremic syndrome (HUS). Several large outbreaks resulting from the consumption of undercooked ground beef and other foods (e.g., fresh spinach) have received significant media attention. O157:H7 is the most prominent serotype, but serogroups O6, O26, O55, O91, O103, O111, O113, and OX3 have also been associated with these syndromes. The ability of STEC/EHEC to produce Shiga toxin (Stx2 and/or Stx1) or related toxins is a critical factor in the expression of clinical disease. *Shigella dysenteriae* strains that produce the closely related Shiga toxin Stx can cause the same syndrome. Stx2 appears to be more important than Stx1 in the development of HUS. All Shiga toxins studied to date are multimers composing one enzymatically active A subunit and five identical B subunits that mediate binding to globoceramides. The A subunit cleaves an adenine from the host cell's 28S rRNA, thereby irreversibly inhibiting ribosomal function. Therefore, Shiga toxins belong to the class of toxins known as *ribosome-inactivating proteins*.

Additional factors, such as acid tolerance and adherence, are necessary for full pathogenicity among STEC strains. Most disease-causing isolates possess the genomic locus for enterocyte effacement (LEE). This pathogenicity island was first described in EPEC strains and contains genes that mediate adherence to intestinal epithelial cells. EHEC strains make up the subgroup of STEC strains that possess stx_1 and/or stx_2 as well as LEE.

Domesticated ruminant animals, particularly cattle and young calves, serve as the major reservoir for STEC/EHEC. Ground beef—the most common food source of STEC/EHEC strains—is often contaminated during processing. Furthermore, manure from cattle or other animals that is used as fertilizer can contaminate produce (potatoes, lettuce, spinach, sprouts, fallen apples), and fecal runoff from this source can contaminate water. It is estimated that <10³ CFU of STEC/

EHEC can cause disease. Therefore, not only can low levels of food or environmental contamination (e.g., in water swallowed while swimming) result in disease, but person-to-person transmission (e.g., at day-care centers and in institutions) is an important route for secondary spread. Laboratory-associated infections also take place. Illness due to this group of pathogens occurs both as outbreaks and as sporadic cases, with a peak incidence in the summer months.

In contrast to other intestinal pathotypes, STEC/EHEC causes infections more frequently in industrialized countries than in developing regions. O157:H7 strains are the fourth most commonly reported cause of bacterial diarrhea in the United States (after *Campylobacter*, *Salmonella*, and *Shigella*). Colonization of the colon and perhaps the ileum results in symptoms after an incubation period of 3 or 4 days. Colonic edema and an initial secretory diarrhea may develop into the STEC/EHEC hallmark syndrome of grossly bloody diarrhea (as detected by history or examination) in >90% of cases. Significant abdominal pain and fecal leukocytes are common (70% of cases), whereas fever is not; a lack of fever often results in diagnostic consideration of noninfectious conditions (e.g., intussusception and inflammatory or ischemic bowel disease). Occasionally, infections caused by *Clostridium difficile*, *Campylobacter*, and *Salmonella* present in a similar fashion. STEC/EHEC disease is usually self-limited, lasting 5–10 days. This infection can be complicated by HUS, which occurs 2–14 days after diarrhea in 2–8% of cases and most often affects very young or elderly patients. It is estimated that >50% of all cases of HUS in the United States are caused by STEC/EHEC. This complication is probably mediated by the systemic translocation of Shiga toxins. Erythrocytes may serve as carriers of Stx to endothelial cells located in the small vessels of the kidney and brain. The subsequent development of thrombotic microangiopathy (perhaps with direct toxin-mediated effects on various nonendothelial cells) commonly produces some combination of fever, thrombocytopenia, renal failure, and encephalopathy. Although the mortality rate with dialysis support is <10%, residual renal and neurologic dysfunction may persist.

Enterotoxigenic *E. coli* In tropical or developing countries, ETEC is a major cause of endemic diarrhea. After weaning, children in these locales commonly experience several episodes of ETEC infection during the first 3 years of life. The incidence of disease diminishes with age, a pattern that correlates with the development of mucosal immunity to colonization factors (i.e., adhesins). In industrialized countries, infection usually follows travel to endemic areas. ETEC is the most common agent of traveler's diarrhea, causing 25–75% of cases. The incidence of infection is decreased by prudent avoidance of potentially contaminated fluids and foods (Chap. 117). ETEC infection is uncommon in the United States, but outbreaks secondary to consumption of food products imported from endemic areas have occurred. A large inoculum (10^6–10^{10} CFU) is needed to produce disease. After ingestion of contaminated water or food (particularly items that are poorly cooked, unpeeled, or unrefrigerated), colonization factor–mediated intestinal adherence occurs over 12–72 h.

Disease is mediated primarily by a heat-labile toxin (LT-1) and/or a heat-stable toxin (STa) that causes net fluid secretion via activation of adenylate cyclase (LT-1) and/or guanylate cyclase (STa) in the jejunum and ileum. The result is watery diarrhea accompanied by cramps. LT-1 consists of an A and a B subunit and is structurally and functionally similar to cholera toxin. Strong binding of the B subunit to the GM_1 ganglioside on intestinal epithelial cells leads to the intracellular translocation of the A subunit, which functions as an ADP-ribosyltransferase. Mature STa is an 18- or 19-amino-acid secreted peptide whose biologic activity is mediated by binding to the guanylate cyclase C found in the brush-border membrane of enterocytes; this binding results in increased intracellular concentrations of cyclic GMP. Characteristically absent are histopathologic changes within the small bowel; mucus, blood, and inflammatory cells in stool; and fever. The disease spectrum ranges from a mild illness to a life-threatening cholera-like syndrome. Although symptoms are usually self-limited (typically lasting for 3 days), infection may result in significant morbidity and mortality when access to health care is limited and when small and/or undernourished children are affected.

Enteropathogenic *E. coli* EPEC causes disease primarily in young children, including neonates. The first *E. coli* pathotype recognized as an agent of diarrheal disease, EPEC was responsible for outbreaks of infantile diarrhea (including some outbreaks in hospital nurseries) in industrialized countries in the 1940s and 1950s. At present, EPEC infection is an uncommon cause of diarrhea in developed countries but is an important cause of diarrhea (both sporadic and epidemic) among infants in developing countries. Breast-feeding diminishes the incidence of EPEC infection. Rapid person-to-person spread may occur. Upon colonization of the small bowel, symptoms develop after a brief incubation period (1 or 2 days). Initial localized adherence leads to a characteristic effacement of microvilli, with the formation of cuplike, actin-rich pedestals. The actual mechanism(s) of diarrhea production are an area of ongoing investigation. Diarrheal stool often contains mucus but not blood. Although usually self-limited (lasting 5–15 days), EPEC diarrhea may persist for weeks.

Enteroinvasive *E. coli* EIEC, a relatively uncommon cause of diarrhea, is rarely identified in the United States, although a few food-related outbreaks have been described. In developing countries, sporadic disease is infrequently recognized in children and travelers. EIEC shares many genetic and clinical features with *Shigella*; however, unlike *Shigella*, EIEC produces disease only at a large inoculum (10^8–10^{10} CFU), with onset generally following an incubation period of 1–3 days. Initially, enterotoxins are believed to induce secretory small-bowel diarrhea. Subsequently, colonization and invasion of the colonic mucosa, followed by replication therein and cell-to-cell spread, result in the development of inflammatory colitis characterized by fever, abdominal pain, tenesmus, and scant stool containing mucus, blood, and inflammatory cells. Symptoms are usually self-limited (7–10 days).

Enteroaggregative and Diffusely Adherent *E. coli* EAEC has been described primarily in developing countries and in young children. However, a recent study indicates that it may be a relatively common cause of diarrhea in all age groups in industrialized countries. EAEC has also been recognized increasingly as an important cause of traveler's diarrhea. A large inoculum is required for infection, which manifests as watery, sometimes prolonged diarrhea. In vitro, the organisms exhibit a diffuse or "stacked-brick" pattern of adherence to epithelial cells. Virulence factors that probably contribute to disease are regulated in part by the transcriptional activator AggR and include the aggregative adherence fimbriae (AAF/I-III) and the enterotoxins Pet, EAST-1, Shet1, and Shet2. Some but not all strains of DAEC are capable of causing diarrheal disease, primarily in children 2–6 years of age in some developing countries. The Afa/Dr adhesins may contribute to the pathogenesis of infection.

Diagnosis A practical approach to the evaluation of diarrhea is to distinguish noninflammatory from inflammatory cases (Chap. 122). ETEC, EPEC, and DAEC are uncommon causes of noninflammatory diarrhea in the United States; EAEC has recently been described as a cause of diarrhea in this country. The diagnosis of these infections requires specialized assays that are not routinely available and whose use is rarely indicated since the diseases are self-limited. ETEC causes the majority and EAEC a minority of cases of noninflammatory traveler's diarrhea. Definitive diagnosis generally is not necessary. Empirical antimicrobial (or symptom-based) treatment, along with rehydration therapy, is a reasonable approach. If diarrhea persists despite treatment, *Giardia* or *Cryptosporidium* (or, in immunocompromised hosts, certain other microbial agents) should be sought. The diagnosis of infection with EIEC, a rare cause of inflammatory diarrhea in the United States, also requires specialized assays. However, evaluation for STEC/EHEC infection, particularly when bloody diarrhea is reported or observed, is appropriate. Although screening for *E. coli* strains that do not ferment sorbitol, with subsequent serotyping for O157, is the most common method currently used to detect STEC/EHEC, testing for Shiga toxins or toxin genes is more sensitive, specific, and rapid. The latter approach offers another advantage as well: it detects both non-O157 STEC/EHEC and sorbitol-fermenting strains of O157:H7, which otherwise are difficult to identify. DNA-based, enzyme-linked immunosorbent, and cytotoxicity assays are in various stages of development and are likely to emerge as the diagnostic standards.

Rx INTESTINAL *E. COLI* INFECTIONS

The mainstay of treatment for all diarrheal syndromes is replacement of water and electrolytes (Chap. 122). The use of prophylactic antibiotics to prevent traveler's diarrhea generally should be discouraged, especially in light of high rates of antimicrobial resistance. However, in selected patients (e.g., those who cannot afford a brief illness or have an increased susceptibility to infection), the use of rifaximin, which is nonabsorbable and well tolerated, is reasonable. When stools are free of mucus and blood, early patient-initiated treatment of traveler's diarrhea with a quinolone or azithromycin decreases the duration of illness, and the use of loperamide may halt symptoms within a few hours (Chap. 122). Although dysentery caused by EIEC is self-limited, treatment hastens the resolution of symptoms, particularly in severe cases. Antimicrobial therapy for STEC/EHEC infection (the presence of which is suggested by bloody diarrhea without fever) should be avoided, since antibiotics may increase the incidence of HUS (possibly via increased production/release of Stx).

KLEBSIELLA INFECTIONS

K. pneumoniae is the most important *Klebsiella* species from a medical standpoint, causing community-acquired, LTCF-acquired, and nosocomial infections. *K. oxytoca* is primarily a pathogen in LTCF and hospital settings. The *K. pneumoniae* subspecies *rhinoscleromatis* and *ozaenae* are usually isolated from patients in tropical climates. *Klebsiella* species are broadly prevalent in the environment and colonize mucosal surfaces of mammals. In healthy humans, *K. pneumoniae* colonization rates are 5–35% in the colon and 1–5% in the oropharynx; the skin is usually colonized only transiently. In LTCFs and hospitals, colonization occurs with *K. oxytoca* as well, and carriage rates are significant among both staff and patients. Person-to-person spread is the predominant mode of acquisition. Classically, *Klebsiella* is associated with CAP, primarily among alcoholics. However, most *Klebsiella* infections now occur in LTCFs and hospitals. *Klebsiella* causes a spectrum of extraintestinal infections similar to that caused by *E. coli*. However, extraintestinal infections due to *Klebsiella* occur at a lower incidence at all sites except the respiratory tract, possibly because of differences in colonization rates and site-specific virulence traits. Antibiotic-resistant strains have been responsible for a number of outbreaks of nosocomial infection in ICUs and neonatal nurseries. The most common clinical syndromes are pneumonia, UTI, abdominal infection, surgical site infection, soft tissue infection, and subsequent bacteremia. *K. pneumoniae* subspecies *rhinoscleromatis* is the causative agent of rhinoscleroma—a granulomatous, slowly progressive (over months to years) infection of the upper respiratory mucosa that causes necrosis and occasional obstruction of the nasal passages. *K. pneumoniae* subspecies *ozaenae* has been implicated in chronic atrophic rhinitis and in rare cases of invasive disease in compromised hosts.

INFECTIOUS SYNDROMES
Pneumonia *K. pneumoniae* causes only a small proportion of cases of CAP (Chap. 251). CAP due to *K. pneumoniae* occurs primarily in hosts with underlying conditions (e.g., alcoholism, diabetes, or chronic lung disease). As in all pneumonias due to enteric GNB, production of purulent sputum and evidence of airspace disease are typically encountered. Presentation with earlier, less extensive infection is more common than the classically described lobar infiltrate with a bulging fissure. Pulmonary necrosis, pleural effusion, and empyema can occur with disease progression. Pulmonary infection is especially common among residents of LTCFs and hospitalized patients because of increased rates of oropharyngeal colonization. Mechanical ventilation is an important risk factor.

UTI *K. pneumoniae* accounts for only 1–2% of UTI episodes among otherwise healthy adults but for 5–17% of episodes of complicated UTI, including infections associated with indwelling bladder catheters.

Abdominal Infection *Klebsiella* causes a spectrum of abdominal infections similar to that caused by *E. coli* but is less frequently isolated from these infections. Recently, however, the incidence of hepatic abscesses caused by *Klebsiella* (the majority due to strains with the K1 capsular serotype) has increased in Taiwan and elsewhere. Diabetes appears to be an important risk factor. Associated bacteremia is common, resulting in metastatic complications (e.g., endophthalmitis and pulmonary, renal, and CNS abscesses).

Other Infections *Klebsiella* cellulitis or soft tissue infection most frequently affects devitalized tissue (e.g., decubitus and diabetic ulcers, burn sites) and immunocompromised hosts. *Klebsiella* causes some cases of surgical site infection, hematogenously derived endophthalmitis (especially that associated with hepatic abscess), and nosocomial sinusitis as well as occasional cases of osteomyelitis contiguous to soft tissue infection, temperate myositis, and meningitis (in the neonatal period or after neurosurgery).

Bacteremia *Klebsiella* infection at any site can produce bacteremia. Infections of the urinary tract, respiratory tract, and abdomen (especially hepatic abscess) each account for 15–30% of *Klebsiella* bacteremias. Intravascular device–related infections account for another 5–15% of episodes and surgical site and miscellaneous infections for the rest. *Klebsiella* is a cause of sepsis in neonates and of bacteremia in neutropenic patients. Like enteric GNB in general, *Klebsiella* rarely causes endocarditis or endovascular infection.

DIAGNOSIS
Klebsiellae are readily isolated and identified in the laboratory. These organisms usually ferment lactose, although the subspecies *rhinoscleromatis* and *ozaenae* are nonfermenters and are indole negative.

Rx KLEBSIELLA INFECTIONS

K. pneumoniae and *K. oxytoca* have antibiotic resistance profiles that are largely similar. These species are intrinsically resistant to ampicillin and ticarcillin. Data from the National Nosocomial Infections Surveillance System (NNIS) indicated that 20.6% of ICU patients were infected with strains resistant to third-generation cephalosporins in 2003—a 47% increase over figures for 1998–2002. Even higher rates have been reported outside North America. This increasing resistance is mediated primarily by plasmid-encoded ESBLs. In addition, these plasmids usually encode resistance to aminoglycosides, tetracyclines, and TMP-SMX. Resistance to β-lactam/β-lactamase inhibitor combinations and second-generation cephalosporins independent of ESBL-containing plasmids has also been described with increasing frequency. The prevalence of quinolone resistance is 15–20% overall and 50% in ESBL-containing strains. Given both the undesirability of treating the latter strains with penicillins or cephalosporins and the quinolone resistance often associated with ESBLs, empirical treatment of serious or health care–associated *Klebsiella* infections with amikacin, carbapenems, or tigecycline (to which resistance rates are generally <10% in North America) is prudent. However, clinical experience with tigecycline is limited, and this approach assumes the continued low prevalence of carbapenemases. Polymyxin B can be considered for use against highly resistant strains but is an agent of last resort because of its potential toxicities.

PROTEUS INFECTIONS

P. mirabilis causes 90% of *Proteus* infections, which occur in the community, LTCFs, and hospitals. *P. vulgaris* and *P. penneri* are associated primarily with infections acquired in LTCFs or hospitals. *Proteus* species are part of the colonic flora of a wide variety of mammals, birds, fish, and reptiles. The ability of these GNB to generate histamine from contaminated fish has implicated them in the pathogenesis of scombroid (fish) poisoning (Chap. 391). *P. mirabilis* colonizes healthy humans (prevalence, 50%), whereas *P. vulgaris* and *P. penneri* are isolated primarily from individuals with underlying disease. The urinary tract is by far the most common site of *Proteus* infection, with adhesins, flagella, IgA protease, and urease representing the principal urovirulence factors. *Proteus* less commonly causes infection at a variety of other extraintestinal sites.

INFECTIOUS SYNDROMES

UTI   Most *Proteus* infections arise from the urinary tract. *P. mirabilis* causes only 1–2% of cases of UTI in healthy women, and *Proteus* species collectively cause only 5% of cases of hospital-acquired UTI. However, *Proteus* is responsible for 10–15% of cases of complicated UTI, primarily those associated with catheterization; in the setting of long-term catheterization, the prevalence of *Proteus* UTI is 20–45%. This high prevalence is due in part to bacterial production of urease, which hydrolyzes urea to ammonia and results in alkalization of the urine. Alkalization of urine, in turn, leads to precipitation of organic and inorganic compounds, with the formation of struvite and carbonate-apatite crystals, the formation of biofilms on catheters, and/or the development of calculi. *Proteus* becomes associated with the stones and biofilms; thereafter, it usually can be eradicated only by the removal of the stones or the catheter. Over time, staghorn calculi may form and lead to obstruction and renal failure. Thus, urine samples with unexplained alkalinity should be cultured for *Proteus*, and identification of a *Proteus* species should prompt an evaluation for urolithiasis.

Other Infections   *Proteus* occasionally causes pneumonia (primarily in LTCF residents or hospitalized patients), nosocomial sinusitis, intraabdominal abscesses, biliary tract infection, surgical site infection, soft tissue infection (especially decubitus and diabetic ulcers), and osteomyelitis (primarily contiguous); in rare cases, it causes temperate myositis. In addition, *Proteus* occasionally causes neonatal meningitis (with the umbilicus often implicated as the source); this disease is often complicated by the development of a cerebral abscess. Otogenic brain abscess also occurs.

Bacteremia   The majority of *Proteus* bacteremias originate from the urinary tract; however, any of the less common sites of infection as well as intravascular devices are also potential sources. Endovascular infection is rare. *Proteus* species are occasional agents of sepsis in neonates and of bacteremia in neutropenic patients.

DIAGNOSIS

Proteus is readily isolated and identified in the laboratory. Most strains are lactose negative, produce H_2S, and demonstrate characteristic swarming motility on agar plates. *P. mirabilis* is indole negative, whereas *P. vulgaris* and *P. penneri* are indole positive.

℞ PROTEUS INFECTIONS

P. mirabilis is usually susceptible to most antimicrobial agents except tetracycline, polymyxin B, and tigecycline. Resistance to ampicillin and first-generation cephalosporins has been acquired by 10–50% of strains. Overall, 10–15% of *P. mirabilis* isolates are resistant to quinolones; 5% of isolates in the United States now produce ESBLs. *P. vulgaris* and *P. penneri* exhibit more extensive drug resistance than does *P. mirabilis*. Resistance to ampicillin and first-generation cephalosporins is the rule, and 30–40% of isolates are resistant to quinolones. Derepression of an inducible chromosomal AmpC β-lactamase (not present in *P. mirabilis*) occurs in up to 30% of isolates. Imipenem, fourth-generation cephalosporins (e.g., cefepime), amikacin, and TMP-SMX display excellent activity against *Proteus* species (90–100% of isolates susceptible).

E. cloacae and *E. aerogenes* are responsible for most *Enterobacter* infections (65–75% and 15–25%, respectively); *E. sakazakii* and *E. gergoviae* are less commonly isolated (1% and <1% of *Enterobacter* isolates, respectively). Enterobacters cause primarily hospital-acquired and other health care–related infections. The organisms are widely prevalent in foods, environmental sources (including equipment at health care facilities), and a wide variety of animals. Few healthy humans are colonized, but the percentage increases significantly in the setting of LTCF residence or hospitalization. Although colonization is an important prelude to infection, direct introduction via IV lines (e.g., contaminated IV fluids or pressure monitors) also occurs. Significant antibiotic resistance has developed in *Enterobacter* species and has contributed to the emergence of the organisms as prominent nosocomial pathogens. Individuals who have previously received antibiotic treatment, have comorbid disease, and are being treated in ICUs are at greatest risk for infection. *Enterobacter* causes a spectrum of extraintestinal infections similar to that described for other GNB.

INFECTIOUS SYNDROMES

Pneumonia, UTI (particularly catheter-related), intravascular device–related infection, surgical site infection, and abdominal infection (primarily postoperative or related to devices such as biliary stents) are the most common syndromes encountered. Nosocomial sinusitis, meningitis related to neurosurgical procedures (including use of pressure monitors), osteomyelitis, and endophthalmitis after eye surgery are less frequent. *E. sakazakii* is associated with neonatal meningitis/sepsis (particularly in premature infants); contaminated formula has been implicated as a source of this infection, which is often complicated by brain abscess or ventriculitis. Bacteremia can result from infection at any of these sites. In *Enterobacter* bacteremia of unclear origin, the contamination of IV fluids or medications, blood components or plasma derivatives, catheter-flushing fluids, pressure monitors, and dialysis equipment should be considered, particularly in an outbreak setting. *Enterobacter* can also cause bacteremia in neutropenic patients. *Enterobacter* endocarditis is rare, occurring primarily in association with illicit IV drug use or prosthetic valves.

DIAGNOSIS

Enterobacter is readily isolated and identified in the laboratory. Most strains are lactose positive and indole negative.

℞ ENTEROBACTER INFECTIONS

Significant antimicrobial resistance exists among *Enterobacter* strains. Ampicillin and the first- and second-generation cephalosporins have little or no activity. The extensive use of third-generation cephalosporins has resulted in the selection of strains that are derepressed for production of AmpC β-lactamase, which confers resistance to third-generation cephalosporins, monobactams (e.g., aztreonam), and (frequently) β-lactam/β-lactamase inhibitor combinations. Resistance may emerge during therapy; in one study, the emergence of resistance was documented in 20% of patients. Resistance should be considered a possibility when clinical deterioration follows initial improvement, and third-generation cephalosporins should be avoided in the treatment of serious *Enterobacter* infections. NNIS data for 2003 identified resistance to third-generation cephalosporins in 31% of ICU isolates. Cefepime is stable, even in the presence of AmpC β-lactamases; thus, it is a suitable option for treatment of *Enterobacter* infections in the absence of a coexistent ESBL. However, the prevalence of ESBL production in *Enterobacter* (particularly in *E. cloacae*) has been increasing and is now 5–30%. Such strains are challenging to treat. Fortunately, in the United States, imipenem, amikacin, and quinolones have generally retained excellent activity (90–99% of isolates susceptible). Although clinical experience is limited, tigecycline is highly active in vitro.

SERRATIA INFECTIONS

S. marcescens causes the majority of *Serratia* infections (>90%), and *S. liquefaciens* is isolated occasionally. Serratiae are found primarily in the environment (including in health care institutions), particularly in moist foci. Although serratiae have been isolated from a variety of animals, healthy humans are rarely colonized. In LTCFs or hospitals, reservoirs for the organisms include health care personnel, food, milk (neonatal units), sinks, respiratory equipment, pressure monitors, IV solutions, multiply accessed medication vials, blood products (e.g., platelets), lotions, irrigation solutions, and even disinfectants. Infection results from either direct inoculation (e.g., via IV fluid) or colonization (primarily of the respiratory tract) and subsequent infection. Sporadic infection is most common, but epidemics and common-source outbreaks occasionally occur. The spectrum of extraintestinal infections caused by *Serratia* is similar to that for other GNB. *Serratia* species account for 1–3% of hospital-acquired infections.

INFECTIOUS SYNDROMES

The respiratory tract, the genitourinary tract, intravascular devices, and surgical wounds are the most common sites of *Serratia* infection and sources of *Serratia* bacteremia. Soft tissue infections (including myositis), osteomyelitis, abdominal and biliary tract infection (postprocedural), contact lens–associated keratitis, endophthalmitis, septic arthritis (primarily from intraarticular injections), and infusion-related bacteremias occur less commonly. Serratiae are uncommon causes of neonatal or postsurgical meningitis and of bacteremia in neutropenic patients. Endocarditis is rare.

DIAGNOSIS

Serratiae are readily cultured and identified by the laboratory and are usually lactose and indole negative. Some *S. marcescens* strains are red-pigmented.

℞ *SERRATIA* INFECTIONS

Most *Serratia* strains (>80%) are resistant to ampicillin, first-generation cephalosporins, and polymyxin B. Derepression of inducible chromosomal AmpC β-lactamases may be preexistent or may develop during therapy. Both in the United States and globally, the prevalence of ESBL-producing isolates is <5%. In general, >90% of *Serratia* isolates are susceptible to other GNB-appropriate antibiotics.

CITROBACTER INFECTIONS

C. freundii and *C. koseri* cause most human *Citrobacter* infections, which are epidemiologically and clinically similar to *Enterobacter* infections. *Citrobacter* species are commonly present in water, food, soil, and certain animals. *Citrobacter* is part of the normal fecal flora in a minority of healthy humans, but colonization rates increase in LTCFs and hospitals—the settings in which nearly all infections occur. *Citrobacter* species account for 1–2% of nosocomial infections. The affected hosts are usually immunocompromised or have comorbid disease. *Citrobacter* causes extraintestinal infections similar to those described for other GNB.

INFECTIOUS SYNDROMES

The urinary tract accounts for 40–50% of *Citrobacter* infections. Less commonly involved sites include the biliary tree (particularly with stones or obstruction), the respiratory tract, surgical sites, soft tissue (e.g., decubitus ulcers), the peritoneum, and intravascular devices. Osteomyelitis (usually from a contiguous focus), neurosurgery-related infection, and myositis occur rarely. *Citrobacter* (particularly *C. koseri*) also uncommonly causes neonatal meningitis, with brain abscess complicating 50–80% of cases. Bacteremia is most often due to UTI, biliary or abdominal infection, or intravascular device infection. *Citrobacter* uncommonly causes bacteremia in neutropenic patients. Endocarditis and endovascular infections are rare.

DIAGNOSIS

Citrobacter species are readily isolated and identified; 35–50% of isolates are lactose positive. *C. freundii* is indole negative, whereas *C. koseri* is indole positive.

℞ *CITROBACTER* INFECTIONS

C. freundii is more resistant to antibiotics than is *C. koseri*. Ampicillin and the first- and second-generation cephalosporins display poor activity. *Citrobacter* species possess inducible AmpC β-lactamases; derepression may be preexistent or may develop during therapy. Resistance to antipseudomonal penicillins, aztreonam, quinolones, gentamicin, and third-generation cephalosporins is variable but increasing. Combination with β-lactamase inhibitors usually does not increase the susceptibility of *Citrobacter* to β-lactam agents. The prevalence of ESBL-producing isolates is <5%. Imipenem, amikacin, cefepime, tigecycline (with which there is limited clinical experience), and polymyxin B (the agent of last resort because of potential toxicities) are most active, with >90% of strains susceptible.

MORGANELLA AND *PROVIDENCIA* INFECTIONS

M. morganii, P. stuartii, and (less frequently) *P. rettgeri* are the members of their respective genera that cause human infections. In terms of epidemiologic associations, pathogenic properties, and clinical manifestations, these organisms are largely similar to *Proteus* species; however, *Morganella* and *Providencia* occur almost exclusively among LTCF residents; to a lesser degree, they affect hospitalized patients.

INFECTIOUS SYNDROMES

These species are primarily urinary tract pathogens, causing UTIs that are most often associated with long-term (>30-day) catheterization. Such infections often lead to biofilm formation and catheter encrustation (sometimes causing catheter obstruction) or to the development of struvite bladder or renal stones (sometimes causing renal obstruction and serving as foci for relapse). Other, less common infectious syndromes include surgical site infection, soft tissue infection (primarily involving decubitus and diabetic ulcers), burn site infection, pneumonia (particularly ventilator-associated), intravascular device infection, and intraabdominal infection. Rarely, the other extraintestinal infections described for GNB also occur. Bacteremia is uncommon; although any infected site can serve as the source, the urinary tract accounts for most cases, and the next most common sources are surgical sites and soft tissues.

DIAGNOSIS

M. morganii and *Providencia* are readily isolated and identified. Nearly all isolates are indole positive but are unable to ferment lactose.

℞ *MORGANELLA* AND *PROVIDENCIA* INFECTIONS

Morganella and *Providencia* may be extensively resistant to antibiotics. Most isolates are resistant to ampicillin, first-generation cephalosporins, tigecycline, and polymyxin B; 40% are resistant to quinolones. *Morganella* and *Providencia* possess inducible AmpC β-lactamases; derepression may be preexistent or may develop during therapy. Resistance to antipseudomonal penicillins, aztreonam, gentamicin, TMP-SMX, and the second- and third-generation cephalosporins is emerging but variable. The β-lactamase inhibitor tazobactam increases susceptibility to β-lactam agents, but sulbactam and clavulanic acid do not. Imipenem, amikacin, and cefepime are the most active agents (>90% of isolates susceptible). Removal of an infected catheter or stone may be critical for eradication of UTI.

EDWARDSIELLA INFECTIONS

 E. tarda is the only member of the genus *Edwardsiella* that is associated with human disease. This organism is found predominantly in freshwater and marine environments and among the animals associated with these settings. Human acquisition occurs primarily during interaction with these reservoirs. *E. tarda* infection is rare in the United States; recently reported cases are mostly from Southeast Asia. This pathogen shares clinical features with both *Salmonella* species and *Vibrio vulnificus*.

INFECTIOUS SYNDROMES

Gastroenteritis is the predominant infectious syndrome (50–80% of infections). Self-limiting watery diarrhea is most common, but severe colitis also occurs. The most common extraintestinal infection is wound infection due to direct inoculation, which is often associated with freshwater-, marine-, or snake-related injuries. Other infectious syndromes result from invasion of the gastrointestinal tract and subsequent bacteremia. Most afflicted hosts have comorbidities (e.g., hepatobiliary disease or iron overload, cancer, or diabetes mellitus). A primary bacteremic syndrome, sometimes complicated by meningitis, has a 40% case-fatality rate. Visceral (primarily hepatic) and intraperitoneal abscesses also occur.

DIAGNOSIS

Although *E. tarda* can readily be isolated and identified, most laboratories do not routinely seek to identify it in stool samples.

℞ *EDWARDSIELLA* INFECTIONS

E. tarda is susceptible to most antimicrobial agents appropriate for use against GNB. Gastroenteritis is generally self-limiting, but treatment with a quinolone may hasten resolution. In the setting of severe sepsis, quinolones, third- or fourth-generation cephalosporins, imipenem, and amikacin—either alone or in combination—are the safest choices pending susceptibility information.

ACINETOBACTER INFECTIONS

The *A. baumannii-calcoaceticus* complex is responsible for most *Acinetobacter* infections. *Acinetobacter* is highly prevalent in the environment, being found in most water and soil samples. Whereas *Acinetobacter* has only occasionally been cultured from the moist skin of healthy humans, colonization of the skin and the respiratory and gastrointestinal tracts is common among residents of LTCFs and hospitalized patients. It is not surprising that the overwhelming majority of *Acinetobacter* infections are acquired in LTCFs and hospitals, where the sources for acquisition include health care personnel, medical equipment, food, and the environment. The spectrum of extraintestinal infections caused by *Acinetobacter* is similar to that caused by other GNB. *Acinetobacter* species account for 1–3% of hospital-acquired infections and primarily affect immunocompromised hosts and patients with comorbid disease, especially patients in ICUs. In some centers, the incidence of *Acinetobacter* infections, particularly those due to antibiotic-resistant strains, is increasing significantly. Both sporadic and epidemic infections occur, usually after the first week of hospitalization. Until recently, *A. baumannii* was best known as an agent of nosocomial infections. However, *A. baumannii* can also cause severe community-acquired pneumonia and diverse infections following battlefield injuries.

INFECTIOUS SYNDROMES

The respiratory tract (particularly in mechanically ventilated patients) and intravascular devices are the favored sites of infection. *A. baumannii* uncommonly causes severe CAP, usually in compromised hosts (e.g., alcoholic patients), with the preponderance of cases reported from warm, humid geographic locales. Infections of the catheterized urinary tract, postoperative sites, burn sites, biliary stents, and sinuses (with tube-related ostial obstruction) are less common, as are neurosurgical infections, which may be associated with devices such as pressure monitors. Infections of soft tissue and bone have been common among soldiers with battlefield injuries. Uncommon infections include ophthalmic infection and peritonitis associated with continuous ambulatory peritoneal dialysis. The respiratory tract and intravascular devices are the most common sources of bacteremia.

DIAGNOSIS

On Gram's stain, *Acinetobacter* organisms usually appear as short GNB or coccobacilli. They are strictly aerobic, nonfermenting, and oxidase negative and are readily isolated and identified.

℞ *ACINETOBACTER* INFECTIONS

Many strains of *Acinetobacter* are extensively resistant to antimicrobial agents. Empirical combination therapy is prudent pending susceptibility studies. Ampicillin, aztreonam, and the first- and second-generation cephalosporins exhibit little or no activity. The prevalences of resistance to antipseudomonal penicillins, quinolones, third-generation cephalosporins, and gentamicin are 20–90%. Ampicillin/sulbactam, rifampin, tetracyclines, imipenem/cilastatin, tigecycline, and amikacin are often active; however, resistance to all of these agents has been reported. Colistin and polymyxin B have been used with some success against extensively resistant isolates but probably should be considered a last resort because of their potential toxicities.

INFECTIONS CAUSED BY MISCELLANEOUS GENERA

Species of *Hafnia, Kluyvera, Cedecea, Pantoea, Ewingella,* and *Photorhabdus* are occasionally isolated from diverse clinical specimens, including blood, sputum, cerebrospinal fluid, joint fluid, bile, and wounds. These organisms are rare and usually opportunistic human pathogens.

FURTHER READINGS

DRUDY D et al: *Enterobacter sakazakii*: An emerging pathogen in powdered infant formula. Clin Infect Dis 42:996, 2006

FANG CT et al: *Klebsiella pneumoniae* genotype K1: An emerging pathogen that causes septic ocular or central nervous system complications from pyogenic liver abscess. Clin Infect Dis 45:284, 2007

FOURNIER PE, RICHET H: The epidemiology and control of *Acinetobacter baumannii* in health care facilities. Clin Infect Dis 44:1577, 2007

HEJAZI A, FALKINER FR: *Serratia marcescens.* J Med Microbiol 46:903, 1997

KAPER J et al: Pathogenic *Escherichia coli.* Nat Rev Microbiol 2:123, 2004

KIM B et al: Bacteraemia due to the tribe Proteeae: A review of 132 cases during a decade (1991-2000). Scand J Infect Dis 35:98, 2003

PATERSON DL: Resistance in gram-negative bacteria: Enterobacteriaceae. Am J Infect Control 34:S20, 2006

RUSSO TA, JOHNSON JR: Medical and economic impact of extraintestinal infections due to *Escherichia coli*: Focus on an increasingly important endemic problem. Microbes Infect 5:449, 2003

SCOTT P et al: An outbreak of multidrug-resistant *Acinetobacter baumannii-calcoaceticus* complex infection in the US military health care system associated with military operations in Iraq. Clin Infect Dis 44:1577, 2007

SHIH CC et al: Bacteremia due to *Citrobacter* species: Significance of primary intraabdominal infection. Clin Infect Dis 23:543, 1996

SLAVEN EM et al: Myonecrosis caused by *Edwardsiella tarda:* A case report and case series of extraintestinal *E. tarda* infections. Clin Infect Dis 32:1430, 2001

CHAPTER 143

Diseases Caused by Gram-Negative Enteric Bacilli

144 *Helicobacter pylori* Infections

John C. Atherton, Martin J. Blaser

DEFINITION

Helicobacter pylori, which persistently colonizes the stomachs of ~50% of the world's human population, is the main risk factor for peptic ulceration (Chap. 287) as well as for gastric adenocarcinoma and gastric MALT (mucosa-associated lymphoid tissue) lymphoma (Chap. 87). Treatment for *H. pylori* has revolutionized the management of peptic ulcer disease, providing a permanent cure in many cases. The prevention of *H. pylori* colonization could potentially represent primary prevention of gastric malignancy and peptic ulceration. However, controversial but increasing evidence indicates that *H. pylori* may in fact offer some protection against recently emergent diseases—most notably gastroesophageal reflux disease (GERD) and its complications (e.g., esophageal adenocarcinoma). Thus, clearance of *H. pylori* from human populations may not be without negative repercussions.

ETIOLOGIC AGENT

H. pylori is a gram-negative bacillus that has naturally colonized humans for at least tens of thousands of years. It is noninvasive and lives in gastric mucus, with a small proportion of the bacteria adherent to the mucosa. Its spiral shape and flagella render *H. pylori* motile in the mucus environment. This organism has several acid-resistance mechanisms, most notably a highly expressed urease that catalyzes urea hydrolysis to produce buffering ammonia. *H. pylori* is microaerophilic (requiring low levels of oxygen), is slow-growing, and requires complex growth media in vitro. Publication of several complete genomic sequences of *H. pylori* since 1997 has led to significant advances in the understanding of the organism's biology.

A very small proportion of gastric *Helicobacter* infections are due to species other than *H. pylori*, which probably are acquired most often as zoonoses. Whether these non-*pylori* gastric helicobacters cause disease remains controversial. In immunocompromised hosts, several nongastric (intestinal) *Helicobacter* species can cause disease with clinical features resembling those of *Campylobacter* infections; these species are covered in Chap. 148.

EPIDEMIOLOGY

The prevalence of *H. pylori* among adults is ~30% in the United States and other developed countries as opposed to >80% in most developing countries. In the United States, prevalence varies with age: ~50% of 60-year-old persons and ~20% of 30-year-old persons are colonized. *H. pylori* is usually acquired in childhood. The age association is due mostly to a birth-cohort effect whereby current 60-year-olds were more commonly colonized as children than current 30-year-olds. Spontaneous acquisition or loss of *H. pylori* in adulthood is uncommon. Other strong risk factors for *H. pylori* colonization are markers of crowding and poor hygiene in childhood. The very low incidence among children in developed countries at present is probably due, at least in part, to improved living standards and increased use of antibiotics.

Humans are the only important reservoir of *H. pylori*. Children may acquire the organism from their parents (more often from the mother) or from other children. Whether transmission usually takes place by the fecal-oral or the oral-oral route is unknown, but *H. pylori* is easily cultured from vomitus and gastroesophageal refluxate and is less easily cultured from stool.

PATHOLOGY AND PATHOGENESIS

H. pylori colonization induces a tissue response in the stomach; termed *chronic superficial gastritis*, this response includes infiltration of the mucosa by both mononuclear and polymorphonuclear cells. (The term *gastritis* should be used specifically to describe histologic features; it has also been used to describe endoscopic appearances and even symptoms, which do not correlate with microscopic findings or

even with the presence of *H. pylori*.) Although *H. pylori* is capable of numerous adaptations that prevent excessive stimulation of the immune system, colonization is accompanied by a considerable persistent immune response, including the production of both local and systemic antibodies as well as cell-mediated responses. However, these responses are ineffective in clearing the bacterium. This inefficient clearing appears to be due in part to *H. pylori*'s downregulation of the immune system, which fosters its own persistence.

Most *H. pylori*–colonized persons do not develop clinical sequelae. That some persons develop overt disease whereas others do not is related to a combination of factors: bacterial strain differences, host susceptibility to disease, and environmental factors. Several *H. pylori* virulence factors are more common among strains that are associated with disease than among those that are not. The *cag* pathogenicity island (PaI) is a group of genes that encodes a secretion system through which a specific protein, CagA, is translocated into epithelial cells. CagA affects host cell signal transduction, inducing proliferative and cytoskeletal changes. The secretion system also induces a proinflammatory cytokine response, which results in enhanced inflammation. Patients with peptic ulcer disease or gastric adenocarcinoma are more likely than persons without these conditions to be colonized by *cag* PaI-positive strains. The secreted *H. pylori* protein VacA occurs in several forms. Strains with the more active forms are more commonly isolated from patients with peptic ulcer disease or gastric carcinoma than from persons without these conditions. BabA and SabA, adhesins expressed by only some strains, are associated with increased gastric inflammation and with increased risk of peptic ulceration and gastric adenocarcinoma. Other *H. pylori* factors that may affect disease risk are still being described.

The best-characterized host determinants of disease are genetic polymorphisms leading to enhanced *H. pylori*–stimulated secretion of proinflammatory cytokines such as interleukin 1β. *H. pylori*–positive individuals with these polymorphisms are at increased risk of hypochlorhydria and gastric adenocarcinoma. In addition, environmental cofactors are important in pathogenesis. Smoking increases the risks of ulcers and cancer in *H. pylori*–positive individuals. Diets high in salt and preserved foods increase cancer risk, whereas diets high in antioxidants and vitamin C are protective.

The pattern of gastric inflammation is associated with disease risk: antral-predominant gastritis is most closely linked with duodenal ulceration, whereas pangastritis is linked with gastric ulceration and adenocarcinoma. This difference probably explains why patients with duodenal ulceration rarely develop gastric adenocarcinoma later in life, despite being colonized by *H. pylori*.

How gastric colonization causes duodenal ulceration is now becoming clearer. *H. pylori*–induced gastritis diminishes the number of somatostatin-producing D cells. Since somatostatin inhibits gastrin release, gastrin levels are higher than in *H. pylori*–negative persons. These increased gastrin levels lead to increased meal-stimulated acid secretion in the gastric corpus, which is only mildly inflamed in antral-predominant gastritis. In turn, increased acid secretion eventually induces protective gastric metaplasia in the duodenum; the duodenum can then become colonized by *H. pylori*, inflamed, and ulcerated.

The pathogenesis of gastric ulceration and that of gastric adenocarcinoma are less well understood, although both conditions arise in association with pan- or corpus-predominant gastritis. The hormonal changes described above still occur, but the inflamed acid-producing gastric corpus produces less acid, with consequent relative hypochlorhydria, despite the hypergastrinemia. Gastric ulcers usually occur at the junction of antral and corpus-type mucosa, and this region is particularly inflamed. Gastric cancer probably stems from progressive DNA damage and the survival of abnormal epithelial cell clones. The DNA damage is thought to be due principally to reactive oxygen and nitrogen species arising from inflammatory cells and perhaps from other bacteria that survive in hypochlorhydric stomachs. Longitudinal analyses of gastric biopsy specimens taken years apart from the same patient show that the common *intestinal* type of gastric adenocarcinoma follows the stepwise changes from simple gastritis to gastric atrophy, intestinal metaplasia,

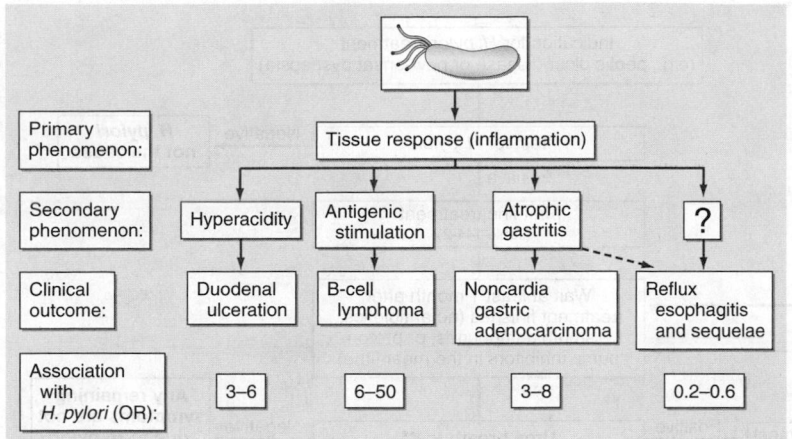

FIGURE 144-1 Schematic of the relationships between colonization with *Helicobacter pylori* and diseases of the upper gastrointestinal tract among persons in developed countries. Essentially all persons colonized with *H. pylori* develop a host response, which is generally termed *chronic gastritis.* The nature of the interaction of the host with the particular bacterial population determines the clinical outcome. *H. pylori* colonization increases the lifetime risk of peptic ulcer disease, noncardia gastric cancer, and B cell non-Hodgkin's gastric lymphoma [odds ratios (ORs) for all, >3]. In contrast, a growing body of evidence indicates that *H. pylori* colonization (especially with *cagA*+ strains) protects against adeno-carcinoma of the esophagus (and the sometimes related gastric cardia) and pre-malignant lesions such as Barrett's esophagus (OR, <1). While the incidences of peptic ulcer disease (cases not due to nonsteroidal anti-inflammatory drugs) and noncardia gastric cancer are declining in developed countries, the incidence of adenocarcinoma of the esophagus is rapidly increasing. [*Adapted from Blaser MJ: Hypothesis: The changing relationships of Helicobacter pylori and humans: Implications for health and disease. J Infect Dis 179:1523, 1999, with permission.*]

and dysplasia. A second, *diffuse* type of gastric adenocarcinoma may arise directly from simple chronic gastritis.

CLINICAL MANIFESTATIONS

Essentially all *H. pylori*–colonized persons have gastric tissue responses, but fewer than 15% develop associated illnesses such as peptic ulceration, gastric adenocarcinoma, or gastric lymphoma (**Fig. 144-1**).

Worldwide, >80% of duodenal ulcers and >60% of gastric ulcers are related to *H. pylori* colonization (Chap. 287), although the proportion of ulcers due to aspirin and nonsteroidal anti-inflammatory drugs (NSAIDs) is increasing, especially in developed countries. The main lines of evidence for an ulcer-promoting role for *H. pylori* are (1) that the presence of the organism is a risk factor for the development of ulcers, (2) that non-NSAID-induced ulcers rarely develop in the absence of *H. pylori*, (3) that eradication of *H. pylori* markedly reduces rates of ulcer relapse, and (4) that experimental *H. pylori* infection of gerbils causes gastric ulceration.

Prospective nested case-control studies have shown that *H. pylori* colonization is a risk factor for adenocarcinomas of the distal (non-cardia) stomach (Chap. 87). Long-term experimental infection of gerbils also may result in gastric adenocarcinoma. Moreover, the presence of *H. pylori* is strongly associated with primary gastric lymphoma, although this condition is less common. Many low-grade gastric B cell lymphomas arising from MALT are driven by T cell stimulation, which in turn is driven by *H. pylori* antigen stimulation; *H. pylori* antigen–driven tumors may regress either fully or partially after *H. pylori* eradication.

Many patients have upper gastrointestinal symptoms but have normal results in upper gastrointestinal endoscopy (so-called functional or nonulcer dyspepsia; Chap. 287). Because *H. pylori* is common, some of these patients will be positive for the organism. *H. pylori* eradication leads to symptom resolution only a little (<10%) more commonly than does placebo treatment. Whether such patients have peptic ulcers in remission at the time of endoscopy or whether a small

subgroup of patients with true functional dyspepsia respond to *H. pylori* treatment is unclear.

Much interest has focused on a possible protective role for *H. pylori* against GERD (Chap. 286) and adenocarcinoma of the esophagus and gastric cardia (Chap. 87). The main lines of evidence for this role are (1) that there is a temporal relationship between a falling prevalence of *H. pylori* colonization and a rising incidence of these conditions, and (2) that, in most studies, the prevalence of *H. pylori* colonization (especially with proinflammatory *cagA*+ strains) is significantly lower among patients with these esophageal diseases than among control subjects. The mechanism underlying this protective effect appears to include *H. pylori*–induced hypochlorhydria. Since, at the individual level, GERD symptoms may decrease, worsen, or remain unchanged after treatment targeting *H. pylori*, concerns about GERD should not affect decisions about *H. pylori* treatment when a definite indication exists.

H. pylori has an increasingly recognized role in other gastric pathologies. It may be one initial precipitant of autoimmune gastritis and pernicious anemia and also may predispose some patients to iron deficiency through hypochlorhydria and reduced iron absorption. In addition, several extragastrointestinal pathologies have been linked with *H. pylori* colonization, although evidence of causality is less strong. Several small studies have documented improvement or resolution of idiopathic thrombocytopenic purpura after treatment for *H. pylori* colonization. A potentially important but even more controversial association is with ischemic heart disease and cerebrovascular disease. However, the strength of these associations is reduced if confounding factors are taken into account, and most authorities consider the associations to be noncausal.

DIAGNOSIS

Tests for *H. pylori* can be divided into two groups: invasive tests, which require upper gastrointestinal endoscopy and are based on the analysis of gastric biopsy specimens, and noninvasive tests (**Table 144-1**). Endoscopy often is not performed in the initial management of young dyspeptic patients without "alarm" symptoms but is commonly used to exclude malignancy in older patients. If endoscopy is performed, the most convenient biopsy-based test is the biopsy urease test, in

TABLE 144-1 TESTS COMMONLY USED TO DETECT *HELICOBACTER PYLORI*

Test	Advantages	Disadvantages
Invasive (Based on Endoscopic Biopsy)		
Biopsy urease test	Quick, simple	Some commercial tests not fully sensitive before 24 h
Histology	May give additional histologic information	Sensitivity dependent on experience and use of special stains
Culture	Permits determination of antibiotic susceptibility	Sensitivity dependent on experience
Noninvasive		
Serology	Inexpensive and convenient	Cannot be used for early follow-up; some commercial kits inaccurate
^{13}C or ^{14}C urea breath test	Inexpensive and simpler than endoscopy; useful for follow-up after treatment	Low-dose irradiation in ^{14}C test (although ^{14}C is rarely used)
Stool antigen test	Inexpensive and convenient; useful for follow-up after treatment; may be useful in children	New test; role not fully established; appears less accurate than urea breath test, particularly when used to assess treatment success

which one large or two small antral biopsy specimens are placed into a gel containing urea and an indicator. The presence of *H. pylori* urease elicits a color change, which often occurs within minutes but can require up to 24 h. Histologic examination of biopsy specimens for *H. pylori* is also accurate, provided that a special stain (e.g., a modified Giemsa or silver stain) permitting optimal visualization of the organism is used. If biopsy specimens are obtained from both antrum and corpus, histologic study yields additional information, including the degree and pattern of inflammation, atrophy, metaplasia, and dysplasia. Microbiologic culture is most specific but may be insensitive because of difficulty with *H. pylori* isolation. Once the organism is cultured, its identity as *H. pylori* can be confirmed by its typical appearance on Gram's stain and its positive reactions in oxidase, catalase, and urease tests. Moreover, the organism's susceptibility to antibiotics can be determined; this information can be clinically useful in difficult cases. The occasional biopsy specimens containing the less common non-*pylori* gastric helicobacters give only weakly positive results in the biopsy urease test. Positive identification of these bacteria requires visualization of the characteristic long, tight spirals in histologic sections.

Noninvasive *H. pylori* testing is the norm if gastric cancer does not need to be excluded by endoscopy. The most consistently accurate test is the urea breath test. In this simple test, the patient drinks a labeled urea solution and then blows into a tube. The urea is labeled with either the nonradioactive isotope ^{13}C or a minute dose of the radioactive isotope ^{14}C. If *H. pylori* urease is present, the urea is hydrolyzed and labeled carbon dioxide is detected in breath samples. The stool antigen test, another simple assay, is more convenient and potentially less expensive than the urea breath test but has been slightly less accurate in some comparative studies. The simplest tests for ascertaining *H. pylori* status are serologic assays measuring specific IgG levels in serum by enzyme-linked immunosorbent assay or immunoblot. The best of these tests are as accurate as other diagnostic methods, but many commercial tests—especially rapid office tests—do not perform well.

The urea breath test, the stool antigen test, and biopsy-based tests can all be used to assess the success of treatment (Fig. 144-2). However, because these tests are dependent on *H. pylori* load, their use <4 weeks after treatment may lead to false-negative results. Furthermore, these tests are unreliable if performed within 4 weeks of intercurrent treatment with antibiotics or bismuth compounds or within 2 weeks of the discontinuation of proton pump inhibitor (PPI) treatment. In the assessment of treatment success, noninvasive tests are normally preferred; however, after gastric ulceration, endoscopy should be repeated to ensure healing and to exclude gastric carcinoma by further histologic sampling. Serologic tests are not used to monitor treatment success, as the gradual drop in titer of *H. pylori*–specific antibodies is too slow to be of practical use.

℞ *H. PYLORI* INFECTIONS

The most clear-cut indications for treatment are *H. pylori*–related duodenal or gastric ulceration or low-grade gastric B cell lymphoma. *H. pylori* should be eradicated in patients with documented ulcer disease, whether or not the ulcers are currently active, to reduce the likelihood of relapse (Fig. 144-2).

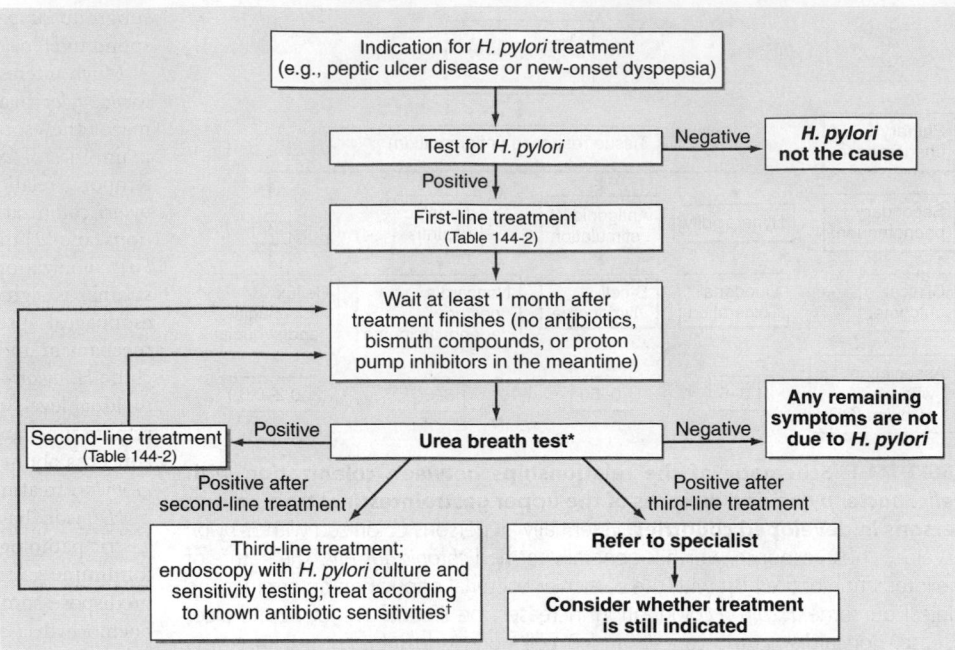

FIGURE 144-2 Algorithm for the management of *Helicobacter pylori* infection. *Occasionally, an endoscopy and a biopsy-based test are used instead of a urea breath test in follow-up after treatment. The main indication for these invasive tests is gastric ulceration; in this condition, as opposed to duodenal ulceration, it is important to check healing and to exclude underlying gastric adenocarcinoma. †Some authorities now use empirical third-line regimens, several of which have been described.

Many guidelines now recommend *H. pylori* treatment in uninvestigated simple dyspepsia following noninvasive diagnosis; others also recommend treatment in functional dyspepsia, in case the patient is one of the perhaps 5–10% to benefit (beyond placebo effects) from such treatment. People with a strong family history of gastric cancer should be treated to eradicate *H. pylori* in the hope that their risk will be reduced. For several reasons, widespread community screening for and treatment of *H. pylori* as primary prophylaxis for gastric cancer and peptic ulcers are not currently recommended. To begin with, it is unclear whether treatment for *H. pylori* reduces the risk of cancer from that in persons who have never acquired the organism. The largest study to date (performed in China) showed no such risk reduction during the 7 years of follow-up. Moreover, treatment has side effects that can be severe in rare cases. Antibiotic resistance may arise in *H. pylori* or other incidentally carried bacteria. Otherwise healthy people may become anxious, especially if treatment is unsuccessful. Finally, it is possible that treatment for *H. pylori* will provoke or exacerbate GERD.

Although *H. pylori* is susceptible to a wide range of antibiotics in vitro, monotherapy has been disappointing in vivo, probably because of inadequate antibiotic delivery to the colonization niche. Failure of monotherapy has prompted the development of multidrug regimens, the most successful of which are triple and quadruple combinations that produce *H. pylori* eradication rates of >90% in many trials and >75% in clinical practice. Current regimens consist of a PPI or ranitidine bismuth citrate and two or three antimicrobial agents given for 7–14 days (Table 144-2).

The two most important factors in successful *H. pylori* treatment are the patient's close compliance with the regimen and the use of drugs to which *H. pylori* has not acquired resistance. Treatment failure following minor lapses in compliance is common and often leads to acquired resistance to metronidazole or clarithromycin. To stress the importance of compliance, written instructions should be given to the patient, and minor side effects of the regimen should be explained. Resistance to metronidazole and clarithromycin is of growing concern. Clarithromycin resistance is less prevalent but, if present, usually results in treatment failure. Metronidazole-resistant strains of *H. pylori* are more common, but these strains still may be cleared by metronidazole-containing regimens. Assessment of antibiotic susceptibilities before treatment would be optimal but is not usually undertaken because endoscopy and mucosal biopsy are necessary to obtain *H. pylori* for culture and because most microbiology laboratories are inexperienced in *H. pylori* culture. In the absence of susceptibility information, a

TABLE 144-2 RECOMMENDED TREATMENT REGIMENS FOR *HELICOBACTER PYLORI*

Regimen, Duration	Drug 1	Drug 2	Drug 3	Drug 4
First-Line Treatment				
Regimen 1: OCA (7–14 days)[a]	Omeprazole[b] (20 mg bid)	Clarithromycin (500 mg bid)	Amoxicillin (1 g bid)	—
Regimen 2: OCM (7–14 days)	Omeprazole[b] (20 mg bid)	Clarithromycin (500 mg bid)	Metronidazole (500 mg bid)	—
Second-Line Treatment[c]				
Regimen 3: OBTM (14 days)[d]	Omeprazole[b] (20 mg bid)	Bismuth subsalicylate (2 tabs qid)	Tetracycline HCl (500 mg qid)	Metronidazole (500 mg tid)

[a]Meta-analyses show that a 14-day course of therapy is slightly superior to a 7-day course. However, the success rate for 7-day therapy is so high in northern Europe (>80%) that 7-day treatment is recommended in most guidelines.

[b]Omeprazole may be replaced with any proton pump inhibitor at an equivalent dosage or, in Regimens 1 and 2, with ranitidine bismuth citrate (400 mg).

[c]An alternative to this second-line therapy is to culture *H. pylori* and to be guided by antibiotic susceptibility data. Patients in whom second-line therapy fails should undergo endoscopy for *H. pylori* culture and antibiotic susceptibility testing.

[d]Data supporting this regimen come mainly from Europe and are based on the use of bismuth subcitrate and metronidazole (400 mg tid).

history of the patient's antibiotic use should be obtained, and, even if only distant exposure is identified (e.g., previous metronidazole consumption for giardiasis or trichomoniasis), use of the agent should be avoided if possible. If initial *H. pylori* treatment fails, two strategies are commonly used (Fig. 144-2). One is re-treatment with a quadruple-drug regimen (Table 144-2). The second is endoscopy, biopsy, and culture plus treatment based on documented antibiotic sensitivities. If re-treatment fails, susceptibility testing should usually be performed, although empirical third-line therapies have been described.

Clearance of non-*pylori* gastric helicobacters can follow the use of bismuth compounds alone or of triple-drug regimens. However, in the absence of trials, it is unclear whether this outcome represents successful treatment or natural clearance of the bacterium.

PREVENTION

Carriage of *H. pylori* has considerable public health significance in developed countries, where it is associated with peptic ulcer disease and gastric adenocarcinoma, and in developing countries, where gastric adenocarcinoma is an even more common cause of cancer death late in life. However, given that *H. pylori* has coevolved with its human host over millennia, preventing or eliminating colonization on a population basis may have distinct disadvantages. For example, absence of *H. pylori* has been reported to increase the risk of diarrheal diseases and of GERD and its complications, including esophageal adenocarcinoma. Recently, we have speculated that the disappearance of *H. pylori* is associated with an increased risk of other emerging diseases reflecting aspects of the current Western lifestyle, such as asthma, obesity, and type 2 diabetes mellitus. If mass prevention were contemplated, vaccination would be the most obvious method, and experimental immunization of animals has given promising results. However, in the United States and other developed countries, rates of *H. pylori* carriage, peptic ulceration, and gastric adenocarcinoma are falling, while rates of esophageal reflux disease and its sequelae are increasing. Thus, prevention of colonization in these countries may be unnecessary or even unwise.

FURTHER READINGS

Blaser MJ: Who are we? Indigenous microbes and the ecology of human diseases. EMBO Rep 7:956, 2006

Blaser MJ, Atherton JC: *Helicobacter pylori* persistence: Biology and disease. J Clin Invest 113:321, 2004

Chen Y, Blaser MJ: Inverse associations of *Helicobacter pylori* with asthma and allergies. Arch Intern Med 167:821, 2007

Franco AT et al: Activation of beta-catenin by carcinogenic *Helicobacter pylori*. Proc Natl Acad Sci USA 102:10646, 2005

Hansson LE et al: The risk of stomach cancer in patients with gastric or duodenal ulcer disease. N Engl J Med 335:242, 1996

Kamangar F et al: Opposing risks of gastric cardia and noncardia gastric adenocarcinomas associated with *Helicobacter pylori* seropositivity. J Natl Cancer Inst 98:1445, 2006

Marshall BJ, Warren JR: Unidentified curved bacilli in the stomach of patients with gastritis and peptic ulceration. Lancet 1:1311, 1984

Odenbreit S et al: Translocation of *Helicobacter pylori* CagA into gastric epithelial cells by type IV secretion. Science 287:1497, 2000

Parsonnet J et al: *Helicobacter pylori* infection and gastric lymphoma. N Engl J Med 330:1267, 1994

Rieder G et al: *Helicobacter pylori* cag-type IV secretion system facilitates corpus colonization to induce precancerous conditions in Mongolian gerbils. Gastroenterology 128:1229, 2005

Tomb JF et al: The complete genome sequence of the gastric pathogen *Helicobacter pylori*. Nature 388:539, 1997

Wong BC et al: *Helicobacter pylori* eradication to prevent gastric cancer in a high-risk region of China: A randomized controlled trial. JAMA 291:187, 2004

145 Infections Due to *Pseudomonas* Species and Related Organisms
Reuben Ramphal

The pseudomonads are a heterogeneous group of gram-negative bacteria that have in common an inability to ferment lactose. Once classified in the genus *Pseudomonas*, the members of this group are now assigned to three medically important genera—*Pseudomonas*, *Burkholderia*, and *Stenotrophomonas*—whose biologic behaviors encompass both similarities and marked differences and whose genetic makeups differ in many respects. The pathogenicity of most pseudomonads is based on opportunism; the exceptions are the organisms that cause melioidosis (*B. pseudomallei*) and glanders (*B. mallei*).

P. aeruginosa, the major pathogen of the group, is mainly associated with infections in hospitalized patients and in patients with cystic fibrosis (CF; Chap. 253). Cytotoxic chemotherapy, mechanical ventilation, and broad-spectrum antibiotic therapy probably paved the way for increasing colonization and infection by *P. aeruginosa*. Since the implementation of these advances in medical therapy, most conditions predisposing to *P. aeruginosa* infections have involved host compromise and/or broad-spectrum antibiotic use. Other members of the genus *Pseudomonas*—*P. putida*, *P. fluorescens*, and *P. stutzeri*—infect humans infrequently.

The genus *Burkholderia* comprises >40 species, of which *B. cepacia* is most frequently encountered in Western countries. Like *P. aeruginosa*, *B. cepacia* is both a nosocomial pathogen and a cause of infection in CF. The other medically important members of this genus are *B. pseudomallei* and *B. mallei*, which, as mentioned above, cause melioidosis and glanders, respectively.

The genus *Stenotrophomonas* contains one species of medical significance, *S. maltophilia* (previously classified in the genera *Pseudomonas* and *Xanthomonas*). This organism is strictly an opportunist that "overgrows" in the setting of potent broad-spectrum antibiotic use.

PSEUDOMONAS AERUGINOSA

EPIDEMIOLOGY

P. aeruginosa is found in most moist environments. Soil, plants, vegetables, tap water, and countertops can all be reservoirs for this microbe, which has simple nutritional needs. Given the ubiquity of *P. aeruginosa*, contact with the organism obviously is not sufficient for colonization or infection. Clinical and experimental observations suggest that *P. aeruginosa* infection often occurs concomitantly with host defense compromise, mucosal trauma, physiologic derangement, and antibiotic-mediated suppression of normal flora. Thus, it comes as no surprise that the majority of *P. aeruginosa* infections occur in intensive care units (ICUs), where these factors frequently converge. It is believed that the organism is initially acquired from environmental sources, but patient-to-patient spread also occurs in clinics and families.

Burn patients once appeared to be unusually susceptible to *P. aeruginosa*. For example, in 1959–1963, *Pseudomonas* burn-wound sepsis was the principal cause of death in 60% of burn patients at the U.S. Army Institute of Surgical Research. For reasons that are unclear, however, *P. aeruginosa* infection in burn patients is no longer the major problem that it was during the 1950s and 1960s. Similarly, in the 1960s, *P. aeruginosa* appeared as a common pathogen in patients receiving cytotoxic chemotherapy at many institutions in the United States, subsequently diminishing in importance. Despite this subsidence, *P. aeruginosa* remains one of the most feared pathogens in this population because of its high mortality rate.

 Moreover, in the Far East and some parts of Latin America, *P. aeruginosa* continues to be the most common cause of gram-negative bacteremia in neutropenic patients.

In contrast to the trends for burn patients and neutropenic patients in the United States, the incidence of *P. aeruginosa* infections among patients with CF has not changed. *P. aeruginosa* remains the most common contributing factor to respiratory failure in CF and is responsible for the majority of deaths among CF patients.

LABORATORY FEATURES

P. aeruginosa is a nonfastidious, motile gram-negative rod that grows on most common laboratory media, including blood and MacConkey agars. It is easily identified in the laboratory on primary-isolation agar plates by pigment production that confers a yellow to dark green or even bluish appearance. Colonies have a shiny "gun-metal" appearance and a characteristic fruity odor. Two of the identifying biochemical characteristics of *P. aeruginosa* are an inability to ferment lactose on MacConkey agar and a positive reaction in the oxidase test. Most strains are identified on the basis of these readily detectable laboratory features even before extensive biochemical testing is done. Some isolates from CF patients are easily identified by their mucoid appearance, which is due to the production of large amounts of the mucoid exopolysaccharide alginate.

PATHOGENESIS

Unraveling the mechanisms underlying disease caused by *P. aeruginosa* has proven challenging. Of the common gram-negative bacteria, no other species produces such a large number of putative virulence factors (Table 145-1). Yet *P. aeruginosa* rarely initiates an infectious process in the absence of host injury or compromise, and few of its putative virulence factors have been shown definitively to be involved in disease in humans. Despite its metabolic versatility and possession of multiple colonizing factors, *P. aeruginosa* exhibits no competitive advantage over enteric bacteria in the human gut; neither is it a normal inhabitant of the human gastrointestinal tract, despite the host's continuous environmental exposure to the organism.

TABLE 145-1 MAIN PUTATIVE VIRULENCE FACTORS OF *PSEUDOMONAS AERUGINOSA*

Substance/ Organelle	Function	Virulence in Animal Disease
Pili	Adhesion to cells	?
Flagella	Adhesion, motility, inflammation	Yes
Lipopolysaccharide	Antiphagocytic activity, inflammation	Yes
Type III secretion system	Cytotoxic activity (ExoU)	Yes
Proteases	Proteolytic activity, cytotoxicity	?
Phospholipases	Cytotoxicity	?
Exotoxin A	Cytotoxicity	?

Acute *P. aeruginosa* Infections • *MOTILITY AND COLONIZATION* A general tenet of bacterial pathogenesis is that most bacteria must adhere to surfaces or colonize a host niche in order to initiate disease. Most pathogens examined thus far possess adherence factors called *adhesins*. *P. aeruginosa* is no exception. Among its many adhesins are its pili, which demonstrate adhesive properties for a variety of cells and adhere best to injured cell surfaces. In the organism's flagellum, the flagellin molecule binds to cells, and the flagellar cap attaches to mucins through the recognition of glycan chains. Nonflagellated *P. aeruginosa* mutants are less virulent or avirulent in some animal models; however, it is unclear whether this decreased virulence is due to the loss of adhesion or to the loss of other flagellar functions. Other *P. aeruginosa* adhesins include the outer core of the lipopolysaccharide (LPS) molecule, which binds to the cystic fibrosis transmembrane conductance regulator (CFTR) and aids in internalization of the organism, and the alginate coat of mucoid strains, which enhances adhesion to cells and mucins. In addition, membrane proteins and lectins have been proposed as colonization factors. It appears that the deletion of any given adhesin is not sufficient to abrogate the ability of *P. aeruginosa* to colonize surfaces.

EVASION OF HOST DEFENSES The transition from bacterial colonization to disease requires the evasion of host defenses by a substantial number of bacteria. *P. aeruginosa* appears to be well equipped for evasion. Attached bacteria inject four known toxins (ExoS, ExoU, ExoT, and ExoY) via a type III secretion system that allows the bacteria to evade phagocytic cells either by cytotoxicity or by inhibition of phagocytosis. Mutants with defects in this system fail to disseminate in some animal models of infection. Secreted toxins such as exotoxin A and leukocidin have the potential to kill phagocytic cells, and multiple secreted elastases may degrade host effector molecules released in response to infection.

TISSUE INJURY Among gram-negative bacteria, *P. aeruginosa* probably produces the largest number of substances that are toxic to cells and thus may injure tissues. The type III toxins are capable of tissue injury. However, their delivery requires the adherence of the organism to cells. Thus, the effects of these toxins are likely to be local or to depend on the presence of vast numbers of bacteria. On the other hand, secreted diffusible toxins can act freely wherever they come into contact with cells. Exotoxin A, four different elastases, at least two phospholipases, rhamnolipids, pyocyanin, and hydrocyanic acid are all produced by this organism and are all capable of inducing host injury.

INFLAMMATORY COMPONENTS The inflammatory response to many products of *P. aeruginosa* is arguably the most important factor in disease causation. For example, injurious inflammatory responses to the lipid A component of the LPSs and to the flagellin are mediated through the Toll-like receptor (TLR) system (principally TLR4 and TLR5). These inflammatory responses are required for successful defense against *P. aeruginosa* (i.e., in their absence, animals are defenseless against *P. aeruginosa* infection), but florid responses are likely to result in disease. When the sepsis syndrome and septic shock develop in *P. aeruginosa* infection, they are probably the result of the host response to one or both of these substances. Another layer of complexity is added by the possibility that injury to cells by many of the described factors may cause cell death and the release of cellular components (e.g., heat-shock proteins) that may activate the TLR system.

Chronic *P. aeruginosa* Infections   Chronic infection due to *P. aeruginosa* occurs mainly in the lungs in the setting of structural pulmonary diseases. The classic example is CF; others include bronchiectasis and chronic relapsing panbronchiolitis, a disease seen in Japan and some Pacific Islands. Hallmarks of these illnesses are altered mucociliary clearance leading to mucus stasis and mucus accumulation in the lungs. There is probably a common factor that selects for *P. aeruginosa* colonization in these lung diseases—perhaps the adhesiveness of *P. aeruginosa* for mucus, a phenomenon that is not noted for most other common gram-negative bacteria, and/or the ability of *P. aeruginosa* to evade host defenses in mucus. Furthermore, *P. aeruginosa* seems to change in ways that allow its prolonged survival in the lung without an early fatal outcome for the host. The strains found in CF patients exhibit minimal production of virulence factors. Some strains even lose the ability to produce pili and flagella, and most become complement-sensitive because of the loss of the O side chain of their LPS molecules. An example of the impact of these changes is found in the organism's discontinuation of the production of flagellin (probably its most strongly proinflammatory molecule) when it encounters purulent mucus. This response probably dampens the host's response, allowing the organism to survive in mucus. *P. aeruginosa* is also believed to lose the ability to secrete many of its injectable toxins during growth in mucus. Although the alginate coat is thought to play a role in the organism's survival, alginate is not essential, since nonmucoid strains are commonly found in chronic lung diseases other than CF. In short, virulence in chronic infections may be mediated mainly by the attenuated host inflammatory response, which slowly injures the lungs over decades.

CLINICAL MANIFESTATIONS

P. aeruginosa causes infections at almost all sites in the body. The infections encountered most commonly in hospitalized patients are described below.

Bacteremia   Crude mortality rates exceeding 50% have been reported among patients with *P. aeruginosa* bacteremia. Consequently, this clinical entity has been much feared, and its management has been attempted with the use of multiple antibiotics. Recent publications report attributable mortality rates of 28–44%, with the precise figure depending on the adequacy of treatment and the seriousness of the underlying disease. In the past, the patient with *P. aeruginosa* bacteremia classically was neutropenic or had a burn injury. Today, however, a minority of patients in these categories have bacteremic *P. aeruginosa* infections. Rather, *P. aeruginosa* bacteremia is seen most often in patients on ICUs.

The clinical presentation of *P. aeruginosa* bacteremia rarely differs from that of sepsis in general (Chap. 264). Patients are usually febrile, but those who are most severely ill may be in shock or even hypothermic. The only point differentiating this entity from gram-negative sepsis of other causes may be the distinctive skin lesions (ecthyma gangrenosum) of *Pseudomonas* infection, which occur almost exclusively in markedly neutropenic patients and patients with AIDS. These small or large, painful, reddish, maculopapular lesions have a geographic margin; they are initially pink, then darken to purple, and finally become black and necrotic (**Fig. 145-1**). Histopathologic studies indicate that the lesions are due to vascular invasion and are teeming with bacteria. Although similar lesions may occur in aspergillosis and mucormycosis, their presence suggests *P. aeruginosa* bacteremia as the most likely diagnosis.

℞ BACTEREMIA

(**Table 145-2**) Antimicrobial treatment of *P. aeruginosa* bacteremia has been controversial. Before 1971, the outcome of *Pseudomonas* bacteremia in febrile neutropenic patients treated with the available agents—gentamicin and the polymyxins—was dismal. Studies published around that time

FIGURE 145-1 Ecthyma gangrenosum in a neutropenic patient 3 days after onset.

indicated that treatment with carbenicillin, with or without an aminoglycoside, significantly improved outcome. Concurrently, several retrospective analyses suggested that the use of two agents that were synergistic against gram-negative pathogens in vitro resulted in better outcomes in neutropenic patients. Thus, combination therapy became the standard of care—first for *P. aeruginosa* bacteremia in febrile neutropenic patients and then for all *P. aeruginosa* infections in neutropenic or nonneutropenic patients.

With the introduction of newer antipseudomonal drugs, a number of studies have revisited the choice between combination treatment and monotherapy for *Pseudomonas* bacteremia. Although the majority of experts still favor combination therapy, most of these observational studies indicate that a single modern antipseudomonal β-lactam agent to which the isolate is sensitive is as efficacious as a combination. Even in patients at greatest risk of early death from *P. aeruginosa* bacteremia (i.e., those with fever and neutropenia), empirical antipseudomonal monotherapy is deemed to be as efficacious as empirical combination therapy by the practice guidelines of the Infectious Diseases Society of America. One firm conclusion is that monotherapy with an aminoglycoside is not optimal.

There are, of course, institutions and countries where rates of susceptibility of *P. aeruginosa* to first-line antibiotics are <80%. When a septic patient with a high probability of *P. aeruginosa* infection is encountered in such settings, empirical combination therapy should be administered until the pathogen is identified and susceptibility data become available. Thereafter, whether one or two agents should be continued remains a matter of individual preference.

Acute Pneumonia   Respiratory infections are the most common of all infections caused by *P. aeruginosa*. This organism appears first or second on most lists of the causes of ventilator-associated pneumonia (VAP). However, much debate centers on the actual role of *P. aeruginosa* in VAP. Many of the relevant data are based on cultures of sputum or endotracheal tube aspirates and may represent nonpathogenic colonization of the tracheobronchial tree, biofilms on the endotracheal tube, or simple tracheobronchitis.

Older reports of *P. aeruginosa* pneumonia described patients with an acute clinical syndrome of fever, chills, cough, and necrotizing pneumonia indistinguishable from other gram-negative bacterial pneumonias. The traditional accounts described a fulminant infection, with cyanosis, tachypnea, copious sputum, and systemic toxicity. Chest radiographs demonstrated bilateral pneumonia, often with nodular densities with or without cavities. This picture is now remarkably rare. Today, the typical patient is using a ventilator, has a slowly progressive infiltrate, and has been colonized with *P. aeruginosa* for days. While some cases may progress rapidly over 48–72 h, they are the exceptions. Nodular densities are not commonly seen. However, infiltrates may go on to necrosis. Necrotizing pneumonia has also been seen in the community (e.g., after inhalation of hot-tub water contaminated with *P. aeruginosa*). The typical patient has fever, leukocytosis, and purulent sputum, and the chest radiograph shows a new infiltrate or the expansion of a preexisting infiltrate. Chest examination generally detects rales or dullness. Of course, such findings are quite common among ventilated patients in the ICU. A sputum Gram's stain showing mainly polymorphonuclear leukocytes (PMNs) in conjunction with a culture positive for *P. aeruginosa* in this setting suggests a diagnosis of acute *P. aeruginosa* pneumonia. The emerging consensus is that an in-

TABLE 145-2 ANTIBIOTIC TREATMENT OF INFECTIONS DUE TO *PSEUDOMONAS AERUGINOSA* AND RELATED SPECIES

Infection	Antibiotics and Dosages	Other Considerations
Bacteremia Nonneutropenic host	Monotherapy: Ceftazidime (2 g q8h IV) or cefepime (2 g q12h IV) Combination therapy: Piperacillin/tazobactam (3.375 g q4h IV) or imipenem (500 mg q6h IV) or meropenem (1 g q8h IV) *plus* Amikacin (7.5 mg/kg q12h or 15 mg/kg q24h IV)	Add an aminoglycoside for patients in shock and in regions or hospitals where rates of resistance to the primary β-lactam agents are high. Tobramycin may be used instead of amikacin (susceptibility permitting).
Neutropenic host	Cefepime (2 g q8h IV) or all other agents in above dosages	
Endocarditis	Antibiotic regimens as for bacteremia for 6–8 weeks	Resistance during therapy is common. Surgery is required for relapse.
Pneumonia	Drugs and dosages as for bacteremia, except that the available carbapenems should not be the primary drugs because of high rates of resistance during therapy	IDSA guidelines recommend the addition of an aminoglycoside or ciprofloxacin. The duration of therapy is 10–14 days.
Bone infection, malignant otitis externa	Cefepime or ceftazidime at the same dosages as for bacteremia; aminoglycosides not a necessary component of therapy; ciprofloxacin (500–750 mg q12h PO) may be used	Duration of therapy varies with the drug used (e.g., 6 weeks for a β-lactam agent; at least 3 months for oral therapy except in puncture-wound osteomyelitis, for which the duration should be 2–4 weeks).
Central nervous system infection	Ceftazidime or cefepime (2 g q8h IV) or meropenem (1 g q8h IV)	Abscesses or other closed-space infections may require drainage. The duration of therapy is ≥2 weeks.
Eye infection Keratitis/ulcer	Topical therapy with tobramycin/ciprofloxacin/levofloxacin eyedrops	Use maximal strengths available or compounded by pharmacy.
Endophthalmitis	Ceftazidime or cefepime as for central nervous system infection *plus* Topical therapy	
Urinary tract infection	Ciprofloxacin (500 mg q12h PO) or levofloxacin (750 mg q24h) or any aminoglycoside (total daily dose given once daily)	Relapse may occur if an obstruction or a foreign body is present.
Multidrug-resistant *P. aeruginosa* infection	Colistin (100 mg q12h IV) for the shortest possible period to obtain a clinical response	Doses used have varied. Dosage adjustment is required in renal failure. Inhaled colistin may be added for pneumonia (100 mg q12h).
Stenotrophomonas maltophilia infection	TMP-SMX (1600/320 mg q12h IV for 14 days) Ticarcillin/clavulanate (3.1 g q4h IV for 14 days)	Resistance to all agents is increasing. Levofloxacin may be an alternative, but there is little published clinical experience with this agent.
Burkholderia cepacia infection	Meropenem (1 g q8h IV for 14 days) TMP-SMX (1600/320 mg q12h IV for 14 days)	Resistance to both agents is increasing. Do not use them in combination because of possible antagonism.
Melioidosis, glanders	Ceftazidime (2 g q6h for 2 weeks) or meropenem (1 g q8h for 2 weeks) or imipenem (500 mg q6h for 2 weeks) *followed by* TMP-SMX (1600/320 mg q12h PO for 3 months)	See "Further Readings" for more details on therapy and alternative agents.

Note: IDSA, Infectious Diseases Society of America; TMP-SMX, trimethoprim-sulfamethoxazole.

vasive procedure (e.g., bronchoalveolar lavage or protected-brush sampling of the distal airways) should be used to obtain samples for quantitative lung cultures in order to substantiate the occurrence of *P. aeruginosa* pneumonia and prevent antibiotic overuse.

℞ ACUTE PNEUMONIA

(Table 145-2) The results of therapy for *P. aeruginosa* pneumonia have been unsatisfactory. Reports suggest mortality rates of 40–80%, but how many of these deaths are attributable to underlying disease remains unknown. The drugs of choice for *P. aeruginosa* pneumonia are similar to those given for bac-

teremia. A potent antipseudomonal β-lactam drug is the mainstay of therapy. Failure rates were high when aminoglycosides were used as single agents, possibly because of binding to airway secretions. Thus a strong case cannot be made for the inclusion of the aminoglycoside component in regimens used against fully susceptible organisms, especially given the evidence that aminoglycosides are not optimally active in the lungs at concentrations normally reached after IV administration. Nonetheless, aminoglycosides are commonly used in clinical practice. Some experts suggest the combination of a β-lactam agent and an antipseudomonal fluoroquinolone instead.

Chronic Respiratory Tract Infections *P. aeruginosa* is responsible for chronic infections of the airways associated with a number of underlying or predisposing conditions—most commonly CF in Caucasian populations (Chap. 253). A state of chronic colonization beginning early in childhood is seen in some Asian populations with chronic or diffuse panbronchiolitis, a disease of unknown etiology. *P. aeruginosa* is one of the organisms that colonizes damaged bronchi in bronchiectasis, a disease secondary to multiple causes in which profound structural abnormalities of the airways result in mucus stasis.

℞ CHRONIC RESPIRATORY TRACT INFECTIONS

Optimal management of chronic *P. aeruginosa* lung infection has not been determined, but it is customary to treat these patients on the basis of bacterial sensitivity. Patients respond clinically to antipseudomonal therapy, but the organism is rarely eradicated. Since eradication is unlikely, the aim of treatment for chronic infection is to quell exacerbations of inflammation. The regimens used are similar to those used for pneumonia, but an aminoglycoside is almost always added because resistance is common in chronic disease. It may be most appropriate to use an inhaled aminoglycoside preparation in order to maximize airway drug levels.

Endovascular Infections Infective endocarditis due to *P. aeruginosa* is seen mainly in IV drug users whose native valves are involved. This organism has also been reported to cause prosthetic valve endocarditis. Sites of prior native-valve injury due to the injection of foreign material such as talc or fibers probably serve as niduses for bacterial attachment to the heart valve. The manifestations of *P. aeruginosa* endocarditis resemble those of other forms of acute endocarditis in IV drug users except that the disease is more indolent than *Staphylococcus aureus* endocarditis. While most disease involves the right side of the heart, left-sided involvement is not rare and multivalvular disease is common. Fever is a common manifestation, as is pulmonary involvement (due to septic emboli to the lungs). Hence, patients may also experience chest pain and hemoptysis. Involvement of the left side of the heart may lead to signs of cardiac failure, systemic emboli, and local cardiac involvement with sinus of Valsalva abscesses and conduction defects. Skin manifestations are rare in this disease, and ecthyma gangrenosum is not seen. The diagnosis is based on positive blood cultures along with clinical signs of endocarditis.

℞ ENDOVASCULAR INFECTIONS

(Table 145-2) It has been customary to use synergistic antibiotic combinations in treating *P. aeruginosa* endocarditis because of the development of resistance during therapy with a single antipseudomonal β-lactam agent. Which combination therapy is preferable is unclear, as all combinations have failed. Cases of *P. aeruginosa* endocarditis that relapse during or fail to respond to therapy are often caused by resistant organisms and may require surgical therapy. Other considerations for valve replacement are similar to those in other forms of endocarditis (Chap. 118).

Bone and Joint Infections Although *P. aeruginosa* is an infrequent cause of bone and joint infections, *Pseudomonas* bacteremia or infective endocarditis caused by the injection of contaminated illicit drugs has been well documented to result in vertebral osteomyelitis and sternoclavicular joint arthritis. The clinical presentation of vertebral *P. aeruginosa* osteomyelitis is more indolent than that of staphylococcal osteomyelitis. The duration of symptoms in IV drug users with vertebral osteomyelitis due to *P. aeruginosa* varies from weeks to months. Fever is not uniformly present; when present, it tends to be low grade. There may be mild tenderness at the site of involvement. Blood cultures are usually negative unless there is concomitant endocarditis. The erythrocyte sedimentation rate (ESR) is generally elevated. Vertebral osteomyelitis due to *P. aeruginosa* has also been reported in the elderly, in whom it originates from urinary tract infections (UTIs). The infection generally involves the lumbosacral area because of a shared venous drainage (Batson's plexus) between the lumbosacral spine and the pelvis. Sternoclavicular septic arthritis due to *P. aeruginosa* is seen almost exclusively in IV drug users. This disease may occur with or without endocarditis, and a primary site of infection often is not found. Plain radiographs show joint or bone involvement. Treatment of these forms of disease is generally successful.

Pseudomonas osteomyelitis of the foot most often follows puncture wounds through sneakers and mostly affects children. The main manifestation is pain in the foot, sometimes with superficial cellulitis around the puncture wound and tenderness on deep palpation of the wound. Multiple joints or bones of the foot may be involved. Systemic symptoms are generally absent, and blood cultures are usually negative. Radiographs may or may not be abnormal, but the bone scan is usually positive, as are MRI studies. Needle aspiration usually yields a diagnosis. Prompt surgery, with exploration of the nail puncture tract and debridement of the involved bones and cartilage, is generally recommended in addition to antibiotic therapy.

Central Nervous System (CNS) Infections CNS infections due to *P. aeruginosa* are relatively rare. Involvement of the CNS is almost always secondary to a surgical procedure or head trauma. The entity seen most often is postoperative or posttraumatic meningitis. Subdural or epidural infection occasionally results from contamination of these areas. Embolic disease arising from endocarditis in IV drug users and leading to brain abscesses has also been described. The cerebrospinal fluid (CSF) profile of *P. aeruginosa* meningitis is no different from that of pyogenic meningitis of any other etiology.

℞ CENTRAL NERVOUS SYSTEM INFECTIONS

(Table 145-2) Treatment of *Pseudomonas* meningitis is difficult; little information has been published, and no controlled trials in humans have been undertaken. However, the general principles involved in the treatment of meningitis apply, including the need for high doses of bactericidal antibiotics to attain high drug levels in the CSF. The agent with which there is the most published experience in *P. aeruginosa* meningitis is ceftazidime, but other antipseudomonal β-lactam drugs that reach high CSF concentrations, such as cefepime and meropenem, have also been used successfully. Other forms of *P. aeruginosa* CNS infection, such as brain abscesses and epidural and subdural empyema, generally require surgical drainage in addition to antibiotic therapy.

Eye Infections Eye infections due to *P. aeruginosa* occur mainly as a result of direct inoculation into the tissue during trauma or surface injury by contact lenses. Keratitis and corneal ulcers are the most common types of eye disease and are often associated with contact lenses (especially the extended-wear variety). Keratitis can be slowly or rapidly progressive, but the classic description is disease progressing over 48 h to involve the entire cornea, with opacification and sometimes perforation. *P. aeruginosa* keratitis should be considered a medical emergency because of the rapidity with which it can progress to loss of sight. *P. aeruginosa* endophthalmitis secondary to bacteremia is the most devastating of *P. aeruginosa* eye infections. The disease is fulminant, with severe pain, chemosis, decreased visual acuity, anterior uveitis, vitreous involvement, and panophthalmitis.

℞ EYE INFECTIONS

(Table 145-2) The usual therapy for keratitis is the administration of topical antibiotics. Therapy for endophthalmitis includes the use of high-dose local and systemic antibiotics (to achieve higher drug concentrations in the eye) and vitrectomy.

Ear Infections *P. aeruginosa* infections of the ears vary from mild swimmer's ear to serious life-threatening infections with neurologic sequelae. Swimmer's ear is common among children and results from infection of moist macerated skin of the external ear canal. Most cases resolve with treatment, but some patients develop chronic drainage. Swimmer's ear is managed with topical antibiotic agents (otic solutions). The most serious form of *Pseudomonas* infection involving the ear has been given various names: two of these designations, malignant otitis externa and necrotizing otitis externa, are now used for the same entity. This disease was originally described in elderly diabetic patients, in whom the majority of cases still occur. However, it has also been described in patients with AIDS and in elderly patients without underlying diabetes or immunocompromise. The usual presenting symptoms are decreased hearing and ear pain, which may be severe and lancinating. The pinna is usually painful, and the external canal may be tender. The ear canal almost always shows signs of inflammation, with granulation tissue and exudate. Tenderness anterior to the tragus may extend as far as the temporomandibular joint and mastoid process. A small minority of patients have systemic symptoms. Patients in whom the diagnosis is made late may present with cranial nerve palsies or even with cavernous venous sinus thrombosis. The ESR is invariably elevated ($\geq$100 mm/h). The diagnosis is made on clinical grounds in severe cases; however, the "gold standard" is a positive technetium-99 bone scan in a patient with otitis externa due to *P. aeruginosa*. In diabetic patients, a positive bone scan constitutes presumptive evidence for this diagnosis and should prompt biopsy or empirical therapy.

℞ EAR INFECTIONS

(Table 145-2) Given the infection of the ear cartilage, sometimes with mastoid or petrous ridge involvement, patients with malignant (necrotizing) otitis externa are treated as for osteomyelitis.

Urinary Tract Infections UTIs due to *P. aeruginosa* generally occur as a complication of a foreign body in the urinary tract, an obstruction in the genitourinary system, or urinary tract instrumentation or surgery.

However, UTIs caused by *P. aeruginosa* have been described in pediatric outpatients without stones or evident obstruction.

℞ URINARY TRACT INFECTIONS

(Table 145-2) Most *P. aeruginosa* UTIs are considered complicated infections that must be treated longer than uncomplicated cystitis. In general, a 7- to 10-day course of treatment suffices, with up to 2 weeks of therapy in cases of pyelonephritis. Urinary catheters, stents, or stones should be removed to prevent relapse, which is common and may be due not to resistance but rather to factors such as a foreign body that has been left in place or an ongoing obstruction.

Skin and Soft Tissue Infections Besides pyoderma gangrenosum in neutropenic patients (an entity described earlier in this chapter), folliculitis and other papular or vesicular lesions due to *P. aeruginosa* have been extensively described and are collectively referred to as *dermatitis*. Multiple outbreaks have been linked to whirlpools, spas, and swimming pools. To prevent such outbreaks, the growth of *P. aeruginosa* in the home and in recreational environments must be controlled by proper chlorination of water. Most cases of hot-tub folliculitis are self-limited, requiring only the avoidance of exposure to the contaminated source of water.

Toe-web infections occur especially often in the tropics, and the "green nail syndrome" is caused by *P. aeruginosa* paronychia, which results from frequent submersion of the hands in water. In the latter entity, the green discoloration results from diffusion of pyocyanin into the nail bed. *P. aeruginosa* remains a prominent cause of burn wound infections in some parts of the world. Its management is best left to specialists in burn wound care.

Infections in Febrile Neutropenic Patients In febrile neutropenia, *P. aeruginosa* has historically been the organism against which empirical coverage is always essential. In the 1960s and early 1970s, *P. aeruginosa* infection occurred commonly in febrile neutropenic patients, with high associated mortality rates. Although in Western countries these infections are now less common, their importance has not diminished because of persistently high mortality rates. In other parts of the world as well, *P. aeruginosa* continues to be a significant problem in febrile neutropenia, causing a larger proportion of infections in febrile neutropenic patients than any other single organism. For example, *P. aeruginosa* was responsible for 28% of documented infections in 499 febrile neutropenic patients in one study from the Indian subcontinent and for 31% of these infections in another. In a large study of infections in leukemia patients from Japan, *P. aeruginosa* was the most frequently documented cause of bacterial infection. In studies performed in North America, northern Europe, and Australia, the incidence of *P. aeruginosa* bacteremia in febrile neutropenia was quite variable. In a review of 97 reports published in 1987–1994, the incidence was reported to be 1–2.5% among febrile neutropenic patients given empirical therapy and 5–12% among microbiologically documented infections. The most common clinical syndromes encountered were bacteremia, pneumonia, and soft tissue infections manifesting mainly as ecthyma gangrenosum.

℞ INFECTIONS IN FEBRILE NEUTROPENIC PATIENTS

(Table 145-2) Compared with rates three decades ago, improved rates of response to antibiotic therapy have been reported in many studies. A study of 127 patients demonstrated a reduction in the mortality rate from 71% to 25% with the introduction of ceftazidime and imipenem. Since neutrophils—the normal host defenses against this organism—are absent in febrile neutropenic patients, maximal doses of antipseudomonal β-lactam antibiotics should be used for the management of *P. aeruginosa* bacteremia in this setting.

Infections in Patients with AIDS Both community- and hospital-acquired *P. aeruginosa* infections were documented in patients with AIDS before the advent of antiretroviral therapy. Since the introduction of protease inhibitors, *P. aeruginosa* infections in AIDS patients have been seen less frequently but still occur, particularly in the form of sinusitis. The clinical presentation of *Pseudomonas* infection (especially pneumonia and bacteremia) in AIDS patients is remarkable in that, although the illness may appear not to be severe, the infection may nonetheless be fatal. Patients with bacteremia may have only a low-grade fever and may present with ecthyma gangrenosum. Bacteremia may herald underlying disease at another site (often pneumonia or sinusitis). Pneumonia, with or without bacteremia, is perhaps the most common type of *P. aeruginosa* infection in AIDS patients. Patients with AIDS and *P. aeruginosa* pneumonia exhibit the classic clinical signs and symptoms of pneumonia, such as fever, productive cough, and chest pain. The infection may be lobar or multilobar and shows no predisposition for any particular location. The most striking feature is the high frequency of cavitary disease.

℞ INFECTIONS IN AIDS PATIENTS

Therapy for any of these conditions in AIDS patients is no different from that in other patients. However, relapse is the rule unless the patient's CD4+ T cell count rises to >50/μL or suppressive antibiotic therapy is given. In attempts to achieve cures and prevent relapses, therapy tends to be more prolonged than that in the immunocompetent patient.

Multidrug-Resistant Infections (Table 145-2) *P. aeruginosa* is notorious for antibiotic resistance. During three decades, the impact of resistance was minimized by the rapid development of potent antipseudomonal agents. However, the situation has recently changed, with the worldwide selection of strains carrying determinants that mediate resistance to β-lactams, fluoroquinolones, and aminoglycosides. This situation has been compounded by the lack of development of new classes of antipseudomonal drugs for nearly two decades. Physicians now resort to drugs such as colistin and polymyxin, which were discarded decades ago. These alternative approaches to the management of multiresistant *P. aeruginosa* infections were first used some time ago in CF patients, who receive colistin (polymyxin E) IV and by aerosol despite its renal toxicity. Colistin is rapidly becoming the last-resort agent of choice, even in non-CF patients infected with multiresistant *P. aeruginosa*.

The clinical outcome of multidrug-resistant *P. aeruginosa* infections treated with colistin is difficult to judge from case reports, especially given the many drugs used in the complicated management of these patients. Although earlier reports described marginal efficacy and serious nephrotoxicity and neurotoxicity, recent reports have been more encouraging. Because colistin shows synergy with other antimicrobial agents in vitro, it may be possible to reduce the dosage—and thus the toxicity—of this drug when it is combined with drugs such as rifampin and β-lactams; however, no studies in humans or animals support this approach at this time.

OTHER PSEUDOMONADS

Stenotrophomonas maltophilia

S. maltophilia is the only potential human pathogen among a genus of ubiquitous organisms found in the rhizosphere (i.e., the soil that surrounds the roots of plants). The organism is an opportunist that is acquired from the environment but is even more limited than *P. aeruginosa* in its ability to colonize patients or cause infections. Immunocompromise is not sufficient to permit these events; rather, major perturbations of the human flora are usually necessary for the establishment of *S. maltophilia*. Accordingly, most cases of human infection occur in the setting of very broad-spectrum antibiotic therapy with agents such as advanced cephalosporins and carbapenems, which eradicate the normal flora and other pathogens. The remarkable ability of *S. maltophilia* to resist virtually all classes of antibiotics is attributable to the possession of antibiotic efflux pumps and of two β-lactamases (L1 and L2) that mediate β-lactam resistance, including that to carbapenems. Fortunately, the virulence of *S. maltophilia* appears to be limited.

Although a serine protease is present in some strains, virulence is probably a result of the host's inflammatory response to components of the organism such as LPS and flagellin. *S. maltophilia* is most commonly found in the respiratory tract of ventilated patients, where the distinction between its roles as a colonizer and as a pathogen is often difficult to make. However, *S. maltophilia* does cause pneumonia and bacteremia in such patients, and these infections have led to septic shock. Also common is central venous line–associated infection (with or without bacteremia), which has been reported most often in patients with cancer. *S. maltophilia* is a rare cause of ecthyma gangrenosum in neutropenic patients. It has been isolated from ~5% of CF patients but is not believed to be a significant pathogen in this setting.

Rx S. MALTOPHILIA

The intrinsic resistance of *S. maltophilia* to most antibiotics renders infection difficult to treat. The antibiotics to which it is most often (although not uniformly) susceptible are trimethoprim-sulfamethoxazole (TMP-SMX), ticarcillin/clavulanate, and levofloxacin (Table 145-2). Consequently, a combination of TMP-SMX and ticarcillin/clavulanate is recommended for initial therapy. Catheters must be removed in the treatment of bacteremia to hasten cure and prevent relapses. The treatment of VAP due to *S. maltophilia* is much more difficult than that of bacteremia, with the frequent development of resistance during therapy.

Burkholderia cepacia

B. cepacia gained notoriety as the cause of a rapidly fatal syndrome of respiratory distress and septicemia (the cepacia syndrome) in CF patients. Previously, it had been recognized as an antibiotic-resistant nosocomial pathogen (then designated *P. cepacia*) in ICU patients. Patients with chronic granulomatous disease are also predisposed to *B. cepacia* lung disease. The organism has been reclassified into nine subgroups, only some of which are common in CF. *B. cepacia* is an environmental organism that inhabits moist environments and is found in the rhizosphere. This organism possesses multiple virulence factors that may play roles in disease as well as colonizing factors that are capable of binding to lung mucus—an ability that may explain the predilection of *B. cepacia* for the lungs in CF. *B. cepacia* secretes elastase and possesses components of an injectable toxin-secretion system like that of *P. aeruginosa*; its LPS is among the most potent of all LPSs in stimulating an inflammatory response in the lungs and may be the cause of the lung disease seen in the cepacia syndrome. The organism can penetrate epithelial surfaces by virtue of motility and inhibition of host innate immune defenses. Besides infecting the lungs in CF, *B. cepacia* appears as an airway colonizer during broad-spectrum antibiotic therapy and is a cause of VAP, catheter-associated infections, and wound infections.

Rx B. CEPACIA

B. cepacia is intrinsically resistant to many antibiotics. Therefore, treatment must be tailored according to sensitivities. TMP-SMX, meropenem, and doxycycline are the most effective agents in vitro and may be started as first-line agents (Table 145-2). Some strains are susceptible to third-generation cephalosporins and fluoroquinolones, and these agents may be used against isolates known to be susceptible. Combination therapy for serious pulmonary infection (e.g., in CF) is suggested for multidrug-resistant strains; the combination of meropenem and TMP-SMX may be antagonistic, however. Resistance to all agents used has been reported during therapy.

Burkholderia pseudomallei

B. pseudomallei is the causative agent of melioidosis, a disease of humans and animals that is geographically restricted to Southeast Asia and northern Australia, with occasional cases in countries such as India and China. This organism may be isolated from individuals returning directly from these endemic regions and from military personnel who have served in endemic regions and then returned home after stops in Europe. Symptoms of this illness may develop only at a later date because of the organism's ability to cause latent infections. *B. pseudomallei* is found in soil and water. Humans and animals are infected by inoculation, inhalation, or ingestion; only rarely is the organism transmitted from person to person. Humans are not colonized without being infected. Among the pseudomonads, *B. pseudomallei* is perhaps the most virulent. Host compromise is not an essential prerequisite for disease, although many patients have common underlying medical diseases (e.g., diabetes or renal failure). *B. pseudomallei* is a facultative intracellular organism whose replication in PMNs and macrophages may be aided by the possession of a polysaccharide capsule. The organism also possesses elements of a type III secretion system that plays a role in its intracellular survival. During infection, there is a florid inflammatory response whose role in disease is unclear.

B. pseudomallei causes a wide spectrum of disease, ranging from asymptomatic infection to abscesses, pneumonia, and disseminated disease. It is a significant cause of fatal community-acquired pneumonia and septicemia in endemic areas, with mortality rates as high as 44% reported in Thailand. Acute pulmonary infections are the most commonly diagnosed form of melioidosis. Pneumonia may be asymptomatic (with routine chest radiographs showing mainly upper-lobe infiltrates) or may present as severe necrotizing disease. *B. pseudomallei* also causes chronic pulmonary infections with systemic manifestations that mimic those of tuberculosis, including chronic cough, fever, hemoptysis, night sweats, and cavitary lung disease. Besides pneumonia, the other principal form of *B. pseudomallei* disease is skin ulceration with associated lymphangitis and regional lymphadenopathy. Spread from the lungs or skin, which is most often documented in debilitated individuals, gives rise to septicemic forms of melioidosis that carry a high mortality rate.

Rx B. PSEUDOMALLEI

B. pseudomallei is susceptible to advanced penicillins and cephalosporins and to carbapenems. Treatment is divided into two stages: an intensive 2-week phase of therapy with ceftazidime or a carbapenem followed by at least 12 weeks of oral TMP-SMX to eradicate the organism and prevent relapse. The recognition of this bacterium as a potential agent of biologic warfare has stimulated interest in the development of a vaccine.

Burkholderia mallei

B. mallei causes the equine disease glanders in Africa, Asia, and South America. The organism was eradicated from Europe and North America decades ago. The last case seen in the United States occurred in 2001 in a laboratory worker; before that, *B. mallei* had last been seen in this country in 1949. In contrast to the other organisms discussed in this chapter, *B. mallei* is not an environmental organism and does not persist outside its equine hosts. Consequently, *B. mallei* infection is an occupational risk for handlers of horses, equine butchers, and veterinarians in areas of the world where it still exists. The polysaccharide capsule is a critical virulence determinant; diabetics are thought to be more susceptible to infection by this organism. The organism is transmitted from animals to humans by inoculation into the skin, where it causes local infection with nodules and lymphadenitis. Regional lymphadenopathy is common. Respiratory secretions from infected horses are extremely infectious. Inhalation results in clinical signs of typical pneumonia but may also cause an acute febrile illness with ulceration of the trachea. The organism may disseminate from the skin or lungs to cause septicemia with signs of sepsis. The septicemic form is frequently associated with shock and a high mortality rate. The infection may also enter a chronic phase and present as disseminated abscesses. *B. mallei* infection may present as early as 1–2 days after inhalation or (in cutaneous disease) may not become evident for months.

Rx B. MALLEI

The antibiotic susceptibility pattern of *B. mallei* is similar to that of *B. pseudomallei*; in addition, the organism is susceptible to the newer macrolides azithromycin and clarithromycin. *B. mallei* infection should be treated with the same drugs and for the same duration as melioidosis.

FURTHER READINGS

CHASTRE J et al: Comparison of 8 vs 15 days of antibiotic therapy for ventilator-associated pneumonia in adults: A randomized trial. JAMA 290:2588, 2003

CURRIE BJ: *Burkholderia pseudomallei* and *Burkholderia mallei*: Melioidosis and glanders, in *Principles and Practice of Infectious Diseases*, 6th ed, GL Mandell et al (eds). Philadelphia, Elsevier Churchill Livingstone, 2005, pp 2622–2632

JOHNSON MP, RAMPHAL R: Malignant external otitis: Report on therapy with ceftazidime and review of therapy and prognosis. Rev Infect Dis 12:173, 1990

KALLEL H et al: Colistin as a salvage therapy for nosocomial infections caused by multidrug-resistant bacteria in the ICU. Int J Antimicrob Agents 28:366, 2006

LODISE TP JR et al: Predictors of 30-day mortality among patients with *Pseudomonas aeruginosa* bloodstream infections: Impact of delayed appropriate antibiotic selection. Antimicrob Agents Chemother 51:3510, 2007

MASCHMEYER G, GÖBEL UB: *Stenotrophomonas maltophilia* and *Burkholderia cepacia*, in *Principles and Practice of Infectious Diseases*, 6th ed, GL Mandell et al (eds). Philadelphia, Elsevier Churchill Livingstone, 2005, pp 2616–2622

MENDELSON MH et al: *Pseudomonas aeruginosa* bacteremia in AIDS. Clin Infect Dis: 886, 1994

MICEK ST et al: *Pseudomonas aeruginosa* bloodstream infection: Importance of appropriate antibiotic therapy. Antimicrob Agents Chemother 49:1306, 2005

OBRITSCH MD et al: Nosocomial infections due to multidrug resistant *Pseudomonas aeruginosa*: Epidemiology and treatment options. Pharmacotherapy 25:1353, 2006

PIER GB, RAMPHAL R et al: *Pseudomonas aeruginosa*, in *Principles and Practice of Infectious Diseases*, 6th ed, GL Mandell et al (eds). Philadelphia, Elsevier Churchill Livingstone, 2005, pp 2587–2615

146 Salmonellosis
David A. Pegues, Samuel I. Miller

Bacteria of the genus *Salmonella* are highly adapted for growth in both humans and animals and cause a wide spectrum of disease. The growth of serotypes *S.* Typhi and *S.* Paratyphi is restricted to human hosts, in whom these organisms cause enteric (typhoid) fever. The remaining serotypes (nontyphoidal *Salmonella*, or NTS) can colonize the gastrointestinal tracts of a broad range of animals, including mammals, reptiles, birds, and insects. More than 200 serotypes are pathogenic to humans, in whom they often cause gastroenteritis and can be associated with localized infections and/or bacteremia.

ETIOLOGY

This large genus of gram-negative bacilli within the family Enterobacteriaceae consists of two species: *S. choleraesuis*, which contains six subspecies, and *S. bongori*. *S. choleraesuis* subspecies I contains almost all the serotypes pathogenic for humans. Because the designation *S. choleraesuis* refers to both a species and a serotype, the species designation *S. enterica* has been recommended and widely adopted. According to the current *Salmonella* nomenclature system, the full taxonomic designation *Salmonella enterica* subspecies *enterica* serotype Typhimurium can be shortened to *Salmonella* serotype Typhimurium or simply *Salmonella* Typhimurium.

Members of the seven *Salmonella* subspecies are classified into >2400 serotypes (serovars) according to the somatic O antigen [lipopolysaccharide (LPS) cell-wall components], the surface Vi antigen (restricted to *S.* Typhi and *S.* Paratyphi C), and the flagellar H antigen. For simplicity, most *Salmonella* serotypes are named for the city where they were identified, and the serotype is often used as the species designation.

Salmonellae are gram-negative, non-spore-forming, facultatively anaerobic bacilli that measure 2–3 by 0.4–0.6 μm. The initial identification of salmonellae in the clinical microbiology laboratory is based on growth characteristics. Salmonellae, like other Enterobacteriaceae, produce acid on glucose fermentation, reduce nitrates, and do not produce cytochrome oxidase. In addition, all salmonellae except *S.* Gallinarum-Pullorum are motile by means of peritrichous flagella, and all but *S.* Typhi produce gas (H_2S) on sugar fermentation. Notably, only 1% of clinical isolates ferment lactose; a high level of suspicion must be maintained to detect these rare clinical lactose-fermenting isolates.

Although serotyping of all surface antigens can be used for formal identification, most laboratories perform a few simple agglutination reactions that define specific O-antigen serogroups, designated A, B, C_1, C_2, D, and E. Strains in these six serogroups cause ~99% of *Salmo-nella* infections in humans and warm-blooded animals. Molecular typing methods, including pulsed-field gel electrophoresis, are used in epidemiologic investigations to differentiate *Salmonella* strains of a common serotype.

PATHOGENESIS

All *Salmonella* infections begin with ingestion of organisms in contaminated food or water. The infectious dose is 10^3–10^6 colony-forming units. Conditions that decrease either stomach acidity (an age of <1 year, antacid ingestion, or achlorhydric disease) or intestinal integrity (inflammatory bowel disease, prior gastrointestinal surgery, or alteration of the intestinal flora by antibiotic administration) increase susceptibility to *Salmonella* infection.

Once salmonellae reach the small intestine, they penetrate the mucous layer of the gut and traverse the intestinal layer through phagocytic microfold (M) cells that reside within Peyer's patches. Salmonellae can trigger the formation of membrane ruffles in normally nonphagocytic epithelial cells. These ruffles reach out and enclose adherent bacteria within large vesicles by a process referred to as *bacteria-mediated endocytosis* (BME). BME is dependent on the direct delivery of *Salmonella* proteins into the cytoplasm of epithelial cells by a specialized bacterial secretion system (*type III secretion*). These bacterial proteins mediate alterations in the actin cytoskeleton that are required for *Salmonella* uptake.

After crossing the epithelial layer of the small intestine, *S.* Typhi and *S.* Paratyphi, which cause enteric (typhoid) fever, are phagocytosed by macrophages. These salmonellae survive the antimicrobial environment of the macrophage by sensing environmental signals that trigger alterations in regulatory systems of the phagocytosed bacteria. For example, PhoP/PhoQ (the best-characterized regulatory system) triggers the expression of outer-membrane proteins and mediates modifications in LPS so that the altered bacterial surface can resist microbicidal activities and potentially alter host cell signaling. In addition, salmonellae encode a second type III secretion system that directly delivers bacterial proteins across the phagosome membrane into the macrophage cytoplasm. This secretion system functions to remodel the *Salmonella*-containing vacuole, promoting bacterial survival and replication.

Once phagocytosed, salmonellae disseminate throughout the body in macrophages via the lymphatics and colonize reticuloendothelial tissues (liver, spleen, lymph nodes, and bone marrow). Patients have relatively few or no signs and symptoms during this initial incubation stage. Signs and symptoms, including fever and abdominal pain, probably result from secretion of cytokines by macrophages and epithelial cells in response to bacterial products that are recognized by innate immune receptors when a critical number of organisms have replicated. Over time, the development of hepatosplenomegaly is likely to be related to the recruitment of mononuclear cells and the development of a specific acquired cell-mediated immune response to *S. typhi* colonization. The recruitment of additional mononuclear cells and lymphocytes to Peyer's patches during the several weeks after initial colonization/infection can result in marked enlargement and necrosis of the Peyer's patches, which may be mediated by bacterial products that promote cell death as well as the inflammatory response.

In contrast to enteric fever, which is characterized by an infiltration of mononuclear cells into the small-bowel mucosa, NTS gastroenteritis is characterized by massive polymorphonuclear leukocyte (PMN) infiltration into both the large- and small-bowel mucosa. This response appears to depend on the induction of interleukin (IL) 8, a strong neutrophil chemotactic factor, which is secreted by intestinal cells as a result of *Salmonella* colonization and translocation of bacterial proteins into host cell cytoplasm. The degranulation and release of toxic substances by neutrophils may result in damage to the intestinal mucosa, causing the inflammatory diarrhea observed with nontyphoidal gastroenteritis.

ENTERIC (TYPHOID) FEVER

Typhoid fever is a systemic disease characterized by fever and abdominal pain and caused by dissemination of *S.* Typhi or *S.* Paratyphi. The disease was initially called *typhoid fever* because of its clinical similarity to typhus. However, in the early 1800s, typhoid fever was clearly defined pathologically as a unique illness on the basis of its association with enlarged Peyer's patches and mesenteric lymph nodes. In 1869, given the anatomic site of infection, the term *enteric fever* was proposed as an alternative designation to distinguish typhoid fever from typhus. However, to this day, the two designations are used interchangeably.

EPIDEMIOLOGY

In contrast to other *Salmonella* serotypes, the etiologic agents of enteric fever—*S.* Typhi and *S.* Paratyphi serotypes A, B, and C—have no known hosts other than humans. Most commonly, food-borne or waterborne transmission results from fecal contamination by ill or asymptomatic chronic carriers. Sexual transmission between male partners has been described. Health care workers occasionally acquire enteric fever after exposure to infected patients or during processing of clinical specimens and cultures.

With improvements in food handling and water/sewage treatment, enteric fever has become rare in developed nations. Worldwide, however, there were an estimated 22 million cases of enteric fever, with 200,000 deaths, in 2002. The incidence is highest (>100 cases per 100,000 population per year) in south-central and Southeast Asia; medium (10–100 cases per 100,000) in the rest of Asia, Africa, Latin America, and Oceania (excluding Australia and New Zealand); and low in other parts of the world. A high incidence of enteric fever correlates with poor sanitation and lack of access to clean drinking water. In endemic regions, enteric fever is more common in urban than rural areas and among young children and adolescents. Risk factors include contaminated water or ice, flooding, food and drinks purchased from street vendors, raw fruits and vegetables grown in fields fertilized with sewage, ill household contacts, lack of hand washing and toilet access, and evidence of prior *Helicobacter pylori* infection (an association probably related to chronically reduced gastric acidity). It is estimated that there is one case of paratyphoid fever for every four cases of typhoid fever, but the incidence of infection associated with *S.* Paratyphi A appears to be increasing, especially in India.

Legend:
- Endemic disease
- Multidrug-resistant strains reported
- Nalidixic acid-resistant strains reported

Multidrug-resistant (MDR) strains of *S.* Typhi emerged in 1989 in China and Southeast Asia and have since disseminated widely (Fig. 146-1). These strains contain plasmids encoding resistance to chloramphenicol, ampicillin, and trimethoprim—antibiotics long used to treat enteric fever. With the increased use of fluoroquinolones to treat MDR enteric fever, strains of *S.* Typhi and *S.* Paratyphi with reduced susceptibility to ciprofloxacin [minimal inhibitory concentration (MIC), 0.125–1.0 µg/mL] have emerged in India and Vietnam and have been associated with clinical treatment failure. Testing of isolates for resistance to the first-generation quinolone nalidixic acid detects most but not all strains with reduced susceptibility to ciprofloxacin.

The incidence of enteric fever among U.S. travelers is estimated at 3–30 cases per 100,000. Of 1393 cases reported to the Centers for Disease Control and Prevention (CDC) in 1994–1999, 74% were associated with recent international travel, most commonly to India (30%), Pakistan (13%), Mexico (12%), Bangladesh (8%), the Philippines (8%), and Haiti (5%). Likewise, of 356 cases reported in the United States in 2003, ~74% occurred in persons who reported international travel during the preceding 6 weeks. Only 4% of travelers diagnosed with enteric fever gave a history of *S.* Typhi vaccination within the previous 5 years. Increased rates of MDR *S.* Typhi and *S.* Paratyphi have been reported among travelers. In 1996–1997, 80% of U.S. travelers with enteric fever acquired in Vietnam were infected with MDR *S.* Typhi strains. Of the 25–30% of reported cases of enteric fever in the United States that are domestically acquired, the majority are sporadic, but 7% have occurred in recognized outbreaks linked to contaminated food products and previously unrecognized chronic carriers. An increasing proportion of cases (currently ~80%) are associated with foreign-born U.S. residents visiting friends and relatives in their native countries.

CLINICAL COURSE

Enteric fever is a misnomer, in that the hallmark features of this disease—fever and abdominal pain—are variable. While fever is documented at presentation in >75% of cases, abdominal pain is reported in only 30–40%. Thus, a high index of suspicion for this potentially fatal systemic illness is necessary when a person presents with fever and a history of recent travel to a developing country.

The incubation period for *S.* Typhi averages 10–14 days but ranges from 3 to 21 days, with the duration likely reflecting the inoculum size and the host's health and immune status. The most prominent symptom is prolonged fever (38.8°–40.5°C; 101.8°–104.9°F), which can continue for up to 4 weeks if untreated. *S.* Paratyphi A is thought to cause milder disease than *S.* Typhi, with predominantly gastrointestinal symptoms. However, a prospective study of 669 consecutive cases of enteric fever in Kathmandu, Nepal, found that the infections were clinically indistinguishable. In this series, symptoms reported on initial medical evaluation included headache (80%), chills (35–45%), cough (30%), sweating (20–25%), myalgias (20%), malaise (10%), and arthralgia (2–4%). Gastrointestinal symptoms included anorexia (55%), abdominal pain (30–40%), nausea (18–24%), vomiting (18%), and diarrhea (22–28%) more commonly than constipation (13–16%). Physical findings included coated tongue (51–56%), splenomegaly (5–6%), and abdominal tenderness (4–5%).

Early physical findings of enteric fever include rash ("rose spots"), hepatosplenomegaly (3–6%), epistaxis, and relative bradycardia at the peak of high fever. Rose spots (Fig. 146-2) make up a faint, salmon-colored, blanching, maculopapular rash located primarily on the trunk and chest. The rash is evident in ~30% of patients at the end of the first week and resolves without a trace after 2–5 days. Patients can have two or three crops of lesions, and *Salmonella* can be cultured from punch biopsies of these lesions. The faintness of the rash makes it difficult to detect in highly pigmented patients.

The development of severe disease (which occurs in ~10–15% of patients) depends on host factors (immunosuppression, antacid therapy, previous exposure, and vaccination), strain virulence and inoculum, and choice of antibiotic therapy. Gastrointestinal bleeding (10–20%) and intestinal perforation (1–3%) most commonly occur in the third and fourth weeks of illness and result from hyperplasia, ulceration, and necrosis of the ileocecal Peyer's patches at the initial site of *Salmonella* infiltration. Both complications are life-threatening and require immediate fluid resuscitation and surgical intervention, with broadened antibiotic coverage for polymicrobial peritonitis (Chap. 121) and treatment of gastrointestinal hemorrhages, including bowel resection. Neurologic manifestations occur in 2–40% of patients and include meningitis, Guillain-Barré syndrome, neuritis, and neuropsychiatric symptoms (described as "muttering delirium" or "coma vigil"), with picking at bedclothes or imaginary objects.

Rare complications whose incidences are reduced by prompt antibiotic treatment include disseminated intravascular coagulation, hematophagocytic syndrome, pancreatitis, hepatic and splenic abscesses and granulomas, endocarditis, pericarditis, myocarditis, orchitis, hepatitis, glomerulonephritis, pyelonephritis and hemolytic uremic syndrome, severe pneumonia, arthritis, osteomyelitis, and parotitis. Up to 10% of patients develop mild relapse, usually within 2–3 weeks of fever resolution and in association with the same strain type and susceptibility profile.

Up to 10% of untreated patients with typhoid fever excrete *S.* Typhi in the feces for up to 3 months, and 1–4% develop chronic asymptomatic carriage, shedding *S.* Typhi in either urine or stool for >1 year. Chronic carriage is more common among women, infants, and persons with biliary abnormalities or concurrent bladder infection with *Schistosoma haematobium*. The anatomic abnormalities associated with the latter conditions presumably allow prolonged colonization.

DIAGNOSIS

Since the clinical presentation of enteric fever is relatively nonspecific, the diagnosis needs to be considered in any febrile traveler returning from a developing country, especially the Indian subcontinent, the Philippines, or Latin America. Other diagnoses that should be considered in these travelers include malaria, hepatitis, bacterial enteritis, dengue fever, rickettsial infections, leptospirosis, amebic liver abscesses, and acute HIV infection (Chap. 117). Other than a positive culture, no specific laboratory test is diagnostic for enteric fever. In 15–25% of cases, leukopenia and neutropenia are detectable. Leukocytosis is more common among children, during the first 10 days of illness, and in cases complicated by intestinal perforation or secondary infection. Other nonspecific laboratory findings include moderately elevated liver function tests and muscle enzyme levels.

The definitive diagnosis of enteric fever requires the isolation of *S.* Typhi or *S.* Paratyphi from blood, bone marrow, other sterile sites, rose spots, stool, or intestinal secretions. The yield of blood cultures is quite variable; sensitivity is as high as 90% during the first week of in-

FIGURE 146-2 "Rose spots," the rash of enteric fever due to *S.* Typhi or *S.* Paratyphi.

fection and decreases to 50% by the third week. A low yield in infected patients is related to low numbers of salmonellae (<15 organisms/mL) and/or to recent antibiotic treatment. Since almost all *S.* Typhi organisms in blood are associated with the mononuclear-cell/platelet fraction, centrifugation of blood and culture of the buffy coat can substantially reduce the time to isolation of the organism but does not increase sensitivity.

Unlike blood culture, bone marrow culture remains highly (90%) sensitive despite ≤5 days of antibiotic therapy. Culture of intestinal secretions (best obtained by a noninvasive duodenal string test) can be positive despite a negative bone marrow culture. If blood, bone marrow, and intestinal secretions are all cultured, the yield is >90%. Stool cultures, while negative in 60–70% of cases during the first week, can become positive during the third week of infection in untreated patients.

Several serologic tests, including the classic Widal test for "febrile agglutinins," are available. None of these tests is sufficiently sensitive or specific to replace culture-based methods for the diagnosis of enteric fever in developed countries. Polymerase chain reaction and DNA probe assays to detect *S.* Typhi in blood are being developed.

℞ ENTERIC (TYPHOID) FEVER

Prompt administration of appropriate antibiotic therapy prevents severe complications of enteric fever and results in a case-fatality rate of <1%. The initial choice of antibiotics depends on the susceptibility of the *S.* Typhi and *S.* Paratyphi strains in the area of residence or travel **(Table 146-1)**. For treatment of drug-susceptible typhoid fever, fluoroquinolones are the most effective class of agents, with cure rates of ~98% and relapse and fecal carriage rates of <2%. Experience is most extensive with ciprofloxacin. Short-course ofloxacin therapy is similarly successful against infection caused by nalidixic acid–susceptible strains. However, the increased incidence of nalidixic acid–resistant (NAR) *S.* Typhi in Asia, which is probably related to the widespread availability of fluoroquinolones over the counter, is now limiting the use of this drug class for empirical therapy. Patients infected with NAR *S.* Typhi strains should be treated with ceftriaxone, azithromycin, or high-dose ciprofloxacin. However, high-dose fluoroquinolone therapy for NAR enteric fever has been associated with delayed resolution of fever and high rates of fecal carriage during convalescence.

Ceftriaxone, cefotaxime, and (oral) cefixime are effective for treatment of MDR enteric fever, including NAR and fluoroquinolone-resistant strains. These agents clear fever in ~1 week, with failure rates of ~5–10%, fecal carriage rates of <3%, and relapse rates of 3–6%. Oral azithromycin results in defervescence in 4–6 days, with rates of relapse and convalescent stool carriage of <3%. Despite efficient in vitro killing of *Salmonella*, first- and second-generation cephalosporins as well as aminoglycosides are ineffective in treating clinical infections.

Patients with persistent vomiting, diarrhea, and/or abdominal distension should be hospitalized and given supportive therapy as well as a pa-

TABLE 146-1 ANTIBIOTIC THERAPY FOR ENTERIC FEVER IN ADULTS

Indication	Agent	Dosage (Route)	Duration, Days
Empirical Treatment			
	Ceftriaxone[a]	1–2 g/d (IV)	7–14
	Azithromycin	1 g/d (PO)	5
Fully Susceptible			
	Ciprofloxacin[b] (first line)	500 mg bid (PO) or 400 mg q12h (IV)	5–7
	Amoxicillin (second line)	1 g tid (PO) or 2 g q6h (IV)	14
	Chloramphenicol	25 mg/kg tid (PO or IV)	14–21
	Trimethoprim-sulfamethoxazole	160/800 mg bid (PO)	14
Multidrug-Resistant			
	Ciprofloxacin	500 mg bid (PO) or 400 mg q12h (IV)	5–7
	Ceftriaxone	2–3 g/d (IV)	7–14
	Azithromycin	1 g/d (PO)[c]	5
Nalidixic Acid–Resistant			
	Ceftriaxone	1–2 g/d (IV)	7–14
	Azithromycin	1 g/d (PO)	5
	High-dose ciprofloxacin	750 mg bid (PO) or 400 mg q8h (IV)	10–14

[a]Or another third-generation cephalosporin [e.g., cefotaxime, 2 g q8h (IV), or cefixime, 400 mg bid (PO)].
[b]Or ofloxacin, 400 mg bid (PO) for 2–5 days.
[c]Or 1 g on day 1 followed by 500 mg/d PO for 6 days.

renteral third-generation cephalosporin or fluoroquinolone, depending on the susceptibility profile. Therapy should be administered for at least 10 days or for 5 days after fever resolution.

In a randomized, prospective, double-blind study of critically ill patients with enteric fever (i.e., those with shock and obtundation) in Indonesia in the early 1980s, the administration of dexamethasone (3-mg initial dose followed by eight doses of 1 mg/kg every 6 h) with chloramphenicol was associated with a substantially lower mortality rate than treatment with chloramphenicol alone (10% vs 55%). Although this study has not been repeated in the "post-chloramphenicol era," severe enteric fever remains one of the few indications for glucocorticoid treatment of an acute bacterial infection.

The 1–5% of patients who develop chronic carriage of *Salmonella* can be treated for 4–6 weeks with an appropriate oral antibiotic. Treatment with oral amoxicillin, trimethoprim-sulfamethoxazole (TMP-SMX), ciprofloxacin, or norfloxacin is ~80% effective in eradicating chronic carriage of susceptible organisms. However, in cases of anatomic abnormality (e.g., biliary or kidney stones), eradication often requires both antibiotic therapy and surgical correction.

PREVENTION AND CONTROL

Theoretically, it is possible to eliminate the salmonellae that cause enteric fever since they survive only in human hosts and are spread by contaminated food and water. However, given the high prevalence of the disease in developing countries that lack adequate sewage disposal and water treatment, this goal is currently unrealistic. Thus, travelers to developing countries should be advised to monitor their food and water intake carefully and to consider vaccination.

Two typhoid vaccines are commercially available: (1) Ty21a, an oral live attenuated *S.* Typhi vaccine (given on days 1, 3, 5, and 7, with a booster every 5 years); and (2) Vi CPS, a parenteral vaccine consisting of purified Vi polysaccharide from the bacterial capsule (given in 1 dose, with a booster every 2 years). The old parenteral whole-cell typhoid/paratyphoid A and B vaccine is no longer licensed, largely because of significant side effects (see below). An acetone-killed whole-cell vaccine is available only for use by the U.S. military. The minimal age for vaccination is 6 years for Ty21a and 2 years for Vi CPS. Currently, there is no licensed vaccine for paratyphoid fever.

A large-scale meta-analysis of vaccine trials comparing whole-cell vaccine, Ty21a, and Vi CPS in populations in endemic areas indicates that, while all three vaccines are similarly effective for the first year, the 3-year cumulative efficacy of the whole-cell vaccine (73%) exceeds that of both Ty21a (51%) and Vi CPS (55%). In addition, the heat-killed whole-cell vaccine maintains its efficacy for 5 years, whereas Ty21a and Vi CPS maintain their efficacy for 4 and 2 years, respectively. However, the whole-cell vaccine is associated with a much higher incidence of side effects (especially fever: 16% vs 1–2%) than the other two vaccines.

Vi CPS typhoid vaccine is poorly immunogenic in children <5 years of age because of T cell–independent properties. In the recently developed Vi-rEPA vaccine, Vi is bound to a nontoxic recombinant protein that is identical to *Pseudomonas aeruginosa* exotoxin A. In 2- to 4-year-olds, two injections of Vi-rEPA induced higher T-cell responses and higher levels of serum IgG antibody to Vi than did Vi CPS in 5- to 14-year-olds. In a two-dose trial in 2- to 5-year-old children in Vietnam, Vi-rEPA provided 91% efficacy at 27 months and 88% efficacy at 43 months and was very well tolerated. Similar results were obtained in a trial in Cambodia. This vaccine is not yet commercially available in the United States. At least three new live vaccines are in clinical development and may prove more efficacious and longer-lasting than previous live vaccines.

Although data on typhoid vaccines in travelers are limited, some evidence suggests that efficacy rates may be substantially lower than those for local populations in endemic areas. Both the CDC and the World Health Organization recommend typhoid vaccination for travelers to typhoid-endemic countries. Recent analyses from the CDC found that 16% of travel-associated cases occurred among persons who stayed at their travel destination for ≤2 weeks. Thus, vaccination should be strongly considered even for persons planning short-term travel to high-risk areas such as the Indian subcontinent. In the United States, persons who have intimate or household contact with a chronic carrier or laboratory workers who frequently deal with *S.* Typhi also should receive typhoid vaccine.

Enteric fever is a notifiable disease in the United States. Individual health departments have their own guidelines for allowing ill or colonized food handlers or health care workers to return to their jobs. The reporting system enables public health departments to identify potential source patients and to treat chronic carriers in order to prevent further outbreaks. In addition, since 1–4% of patients with *S.* Typhi infection become chronic carriers, it is important to monitor patients (especially child-care providers and food handlers) for chronic carriage and to treat this condition if indicated.

NONTYPHOIDAL SALMONELLOSIS

EPIDEMIOLOGY

During 1996–1999, there were an estimated 1.4 million cases of nontyphoidal salmonellosis in the United States, resulting in 168,000 physician office visits, 15,000 hospitalizations, and 400 deaths annually. In 2004, the incidence of NTS infection in this country was 14.7 per 100,000 persons—the highest rate among the nine food-borne enteric pathogens under active surveillance. Five serotypes accounted for 57% of U.S. infections in 2004: Typhimurium (20%), Enteritidis (15%), Newport (10%), Javiana (7%), and Heidelberg (5%).

The incidence of nontyphoidal salmonellosis is highest during the rainy season in tropical climates and during the warmer months in temperate climates, coinciding with the peak in food-borne outbreaks. Rates of morbidity and mortality associated with NTS are highest among the elderly, infants, and immunocompromised individuals, including those with hemoglobinopathies, HIV infection, or infections that cause blockade of the reticuloendothelial system (e.g., bartonellosis, malaria, schistosomiasis, and histoplasmosis).

Unlike *S.* Typhi and *S.* Paratyphi, whose only reservoir is humans, NTS can be acquired from multiple animal reservoirs. Transmission is most commonly associated with animal food products, especially eggs, poultry, undercooked ground meat, and dairy products and fresh produce contaminated with animal waste.

S. Enteritidis infection associated with chicken eggs emerged as a major cause of foodborne disease during the 1980s and 1990s. *S.* Enteritidis infection of the ovaries and upper oviduct tissue of hens results in contamination of egg contents before shell deposition. Infection is spread to egg-laying hens from breeding flocks and through contact with rodents and manure. Of the 360 outbreaks of *S.* Enteritidis with a confirmed source that were reported to the CDC in 1985–1998, 279 (78%) were associated with raw or undercooked eggs. After peaking at 3.9 cases per 100,000 U.S. population in 1995, the incidence of *S.* Enteritidis infection declined dramatically to 1.98 per 100,000 in 1999; this decrease probably reflected improved on-farm control measures, refrigeration, and education of consumers and food-service workers. Transmission via contaminated eggs can be prevented by cooking eggs until the yolk is solidified and through pasteurization of egg products.

Centralization of food processing and widespread food distribution have contributed to the increased incidence of NTS in developing countries. Manufactured foods to which recent *Salmonella* outbreaks have been traced include pasteurized milk, infant formula, powdered milk products, and various processed foods. Large outbreaks have also been linked to fresh produce, including alfalfa sprouts, cantaloupe, fresh-squeezed orange juice, and tomatoes; these items become contaminated by manure or water at a single site and then are widely distributed.

An estimated 6% of sporadic *Salmonella* infections in the United States are attributed to contact with reptiles and amphibians, especially iguanas, snakes, turtles, and lizards. Reptile-associated *Salmonella* infection more commonly leads to hospitalization and more frequently involves infants than do other *Salmonella* infections. Other pets, including African hedgehogs, snakes, birds, rodents, baby chicks, ducklings, dogs, and cats, are also potential sources of NTS.

Increasing antibiotic resistance in NTS species is a global problem and has been linked to the widespread use of antimicrobial agents in food animals and especially in animal feed. In the early 1990s, *S.* Typhimurium definitive phage type 104 (DT104), characterized by resistance to ≥5 antibiotics (ampicillin, chloramphenicol, streptomycin, sulfonamides, and tetracyclines; R-type ACSSuT), emerged worldwide. From 1979–1980 to 2001, the prevalence of *S.* Typhimurium ACSSuT increased in the United States from 0.6% to 7% of all NTS isolates, and most (65%) of these ACSSuT isolates were phage type DT104. Acquisition is associated with exposure to ill farm animals and to various meat products, including uncooked or undercooked ground beef. In an analysis of U.S. surveillance data for 1996–2001, antibiotic-resistant NTS strains, especially *S.* Typhimurium DT104, were associated with an increased risk of bloodstream infection and hospitalization. NAR and trimethoprim-resistant DT104 strains are emerging, especially in the United Kingdom.

Because of increased resistance to conventional antibiotics such as ampicillin and TMP-SMX, extended-spectrum cephalosporins and fluoroquinolones have emerged as the agents of choice for the treatment of MDR NTS infections. With the increased use of these agents, the CDC reported that the prevalence of ceftriaxone-resistant NTS strains rose from 0 in 1995 to 0.5% in 1998. Of the ceftriaxone-resistant isolates, 77% were from children <18 years of age, in whom ceftriaxone is the antibiotic of choice for treatment of invasive infection. These strains contained plasmid-encoded AmpC β-lactamases that were probably acquired by horizontal genetic transfer from *Escherichia coli* strains in food-producing animals—an event linked to the widespread use of the veterinary cephalosporin ceftiofur.

Resistance to nalidixic acid and fluoroquinolones also has begun to emerge and is most commonly associated with point mutations in the DNA gyrase genes *gyr*A and *gyr*B. Nalidixic acid resistance is a good predictor of reduced susceptibility to clinically useful fluoroquinolones. From 1994–1995 to 2000, the rate of NAR NTS isolates in the United States increased fivefold (from 0.5% to 2.5%). In Denmark, infection with NAR *S.* Typhimurium DT104 has been linked to swine and associated with a threefold higher risk of invasive disease or death within 90 days. In Taiwan in 2000, a strain of ciprofloxacin-resistant (MIC, ≥4 μg/mL) *S.* Choleraesuis caused a large outbreak of invasive infections that was linked to the use of enrofloxacin in swine feed.

CLINICAL MANIFESTATIONS

Gastroenteritis Infection with NTS most often results in gastroenteritis indistinguishable from that caused by other enteric pathogens. Nausea, vomiting, and diarrhea occur 6–48 h after the ingestion of contaminated food or water. Patients often experience abdominal cramping and fever (38–39°C; 100.5–102.2°F). Diarrheal stools are usually loose, nonbloody, and of moderate volume. However, large-volume watery stools, bloody stools, or symptoms of dysentery may occur. Rarely, NTS causes pseudoappendicitis or an illness that mimics inflammatory bowel disease.

Gastroenteritis caused by NTS is usually self-limited. Diarrhea resolves within 3–7 days and fever within 72 h. Stool cultures remain positive for 4–5 weeks after infection and—in rare cases of chronic carriage (<1%)—for >1 year. Antibiotic treatment usually is not recommended and in some studies has prolonged fecal carriage. Neonates, the elderly, and immunosuppressed patients (e.g., transplant recipients, HIV-infected persons) with NTS gastroenteritis are especially susceptible to dehydration and dissemination and may require hospitalization and antibiotic therapy. Acute NTS gastroenteritis was associated with a threefold increased risk of dyspepsia and irritable bowel syndrome at 1 year in a recent study from Spain.

Bacteremia and Endovascular Infections Up to 5% of patients with NTS gastroenteritis develop bacteremia; of these, 5–10% develop localized infections. Bacteremia and metastatic infection are most common with *S.* Choleraesuis and *S.* Dublin and among infants, the elderly, and immunocompromised patients. NTS endovascular infection should be suspected in high-grade bacteremia, especially with preexisting valvular heart disease, atherosclerotic vascular disease, prosthetic vascular graft, or aortic aneurysm. Arteritis should be suspected in elderly patients with prolonged fever and back, chest, or abdominal pain developing after an episode of gastroenteritis. Endocarditis and arteritis are rare (<1% of cases) but are associated with potentially fatal complications, including valve perforation, endomyocardial abscess, infected mural thrombus, pericarditis, mycotic aneurysms, aneurysm rupture, aortoenteric fistula, and vertebral osteomyelitis.

Localized Infections • *INTRAABDOMINAL INFECTIONS* Intraabdominal infections due to NTS are rare and usually manifest as hepatic or splenic abscesses or as cholecystitis. Risk factors include hepatobiliary anatomic abnormalities (e.g., gallstones), abdominal malignancy, and sickle cell disease (especially with splenic abscesses). Eradication of the infection often requires surgical correction of abnormalities and percutaneous drainage of abscesses.

CENTRAL NERVOUS SYSTEM INFECTIONS Meningitis most commonly develops in infants 1–4 months of age. It often results in severe sequelae (including seizures, hydrocephalus, brain infarction, and mental retardation) with death in up to 60% of cases. Other rare central nervous system infections include ventriculitis, subdural empyema, and brain abscesses.

PULMONARY INFECTIONS NTS pulmonary infections usually present as lobar pneumonia, and complications include lung abscess, empyema, and bronchopleural fistula formation. The majority of cases occur in patients with lung cancer, structural lung disease, sickle cell disease, or glucocorticoid use.

URINARY AND GENITAL TRACT INFECTIONS Urinary tract infections caused by NTS present as either cystitis or pyelonephritis. Risk factors include malignancy, urolithiasis, structural abnormalities, HIV infection, and renal transplantation. NTS genital infections are rare and include ovarian and testicular abscesses, prostatitis, and epididymitis. Like other focal infections, both genital and urinary tract infections can be complicated by abscess formation.

BONE, JOINT, AND SOFT TISSUE INFECTIONS *Salmonella* osteomyelitis most commonly affects the femur, tibia, humerus, or lumbar vertebrae and is most often seen in association with sickle cell disease, hemoglobinopathies, or preexisting bone disease (e.g., fractures). Prolonged antibiotic treatment is recommended to decrease the risk of relapse and chronic osteomyelitis. Septic arthritis occurs in the same patient population as osteomyelitis and usually involves the knee, hip, or shoulder joints. Reactive arthritis (Reiter's syndrome) can follow NTS gastroenteritis and is seen most frequently in persons with the HLA-B27 histocompatibility antigen. NTS rarely can cause soft tissue infections, usually at sites of local trauma in immunosuppressed patients.

DIAGNOSIS

The diagnosis of NTS infection is based on the isolation of the organism from freshly passed stool or from blood or another ordinarily sterile body fluid. All salmonellae isolated in clinical laboratories should be sent to local public health departments for serotyping. Blood cultures should be done whenever a patient has prolonged or recurrent fever. Endovascular infection should be suspected if there is high-grade bacteremia (>50% of three or more blood cultures positive). Echocardiography, computed tomography, and indium-labeled white cell scanning are used to identify localized infection. When another localized infection is suspected, joint fluid, abscess drainage, or cerebrospinal fluid should be cultured, as clinically indicated.

℞ NONTYPHOIDAL SALMONELLOSIS

Antibiotics should not be used routinely to treat uncomplicated NTS gastroenteritis. The symptoms are usually self-limited, and the duration of fever and diarrhea is not significantly decreased by antibiotic therapy. In addition, antibiotic treatment has been associated with increased rates of relapse and prolonged gastrointestinal carriage. Dehydration secondary to diarrhea should be treated with fluid and electrolyte replacement.

Preemptive antibiotic treatment (Table 146-2) should be considered for patients at increased risk for invasive NTS infection, including neonates (probably up to 3 months of age); persons >50 years of age with suspected atherosclerosis; and patients with immunosuppression, cardiac valvular or endovascular abnormalities, or significant joint disease. Treatment should consist of an oral or IV antibiotic administered for 48–72 h or until the patient becomes afebrile. Immunocompromised persons may require up to 7–14 days of therapy. The <1% of persons who develop chronic carriage of NTS should receive a prolonged antibiotic course, as described above for chronic carriage of S. Typhi.

Because of the increasing prevalence of antibiotic resistance, empirical therapy for life-threatening NTS bacteremia or focal NTS infection should include a third-generation cephalosporin or a fluoroquinolone (Table 146-2). If the bacteremia is low-grade (<50% of blood cultures positive), the patient should be treated for 7–14 days. Patients with AIDS and NTS bacteremia should receive 1–2 weeks of IV antibiotic therapy followed by 4 weeks of oral therapy with a fluoroquinolone. Patients whose infections relapse after this regimen should receive long-term suppressive therapy with a fluoroquinolone or TMP-SMX, as indicated by bacterial sensitivities.

If the patient has endocarditis or arteritis, treatment for 6 weeks with an IV β-lactam antibiotic (such as ceftriaxone or ampicillin) is indicated. IV ciprofloxacin followed by prolonged oral therapy is an option, but published experience is limited. Early surgical resection of infected aneurysms or other infected endovascular sites is recommended. Patients with infected prosthetic vascular grafts that cannot be resected have been maintained successfully on chronic suppressive oral therapy. For extraintestinal nonvascular infections, a 2- to 4-week course of antibiotic therapy (depending on the infection site) is usually recommended. In chronic osteomyelitis, abscess, or urinary or hepatobiliary infection associated with anatomic abnormalities, surgical resection or drainage may be required in addition to prolonged antibiotic therapy for eradication of infection.

PREVENTION AND CONTROL

Despite widespread efforts to prevent or reduce bacterial contamination of animal-derived food products and to improve food-safety education and training, recent declines in the incidence of NTS in the United States have been modest compared with those of other food-borne pathogens. This observation probably reflects the complex epidemiology of NTS. Identifying effective risk-reduction strategies requires monitoring of every step of food production, from handling of raw animal or plant products to preparation of finished foods. Contaminated food can be made safe for consumption by pasteurization, irradiation, or proper cooking. All cases of NTS infection should be reported to local public health departments, since tracking and monitoring of these cases can identify the source(s) of infection and help authorities anticipate large outbreaks. Lastly, the prudent use of antimicrobial agents in both humans and animals is needed to limit the emergence of MDR *Salmonella*.

FURTHER READINGS

COHEN JI et al: Extra-intestinal manifestations of *Salmonella* infections. Medicine 66:349, 1987

GLYNN MK et al: Emergence of multidrug-resistant *Salmonella enterica* serotype *typhimurium* DT104 infections in the United States. N Engl J Med 338:1333, 1998

TABLE 146-2	ANTIBIOTIC THERAPY FOR NONTYPHOIDAL *SALMONELLA* INFECTION IN ADULTS		
Indication	Agent	Dosage (Route)	Duration, Days
Preemptive Treatment[a]			
	Ciprofloxacin[b]	500 mg bid (PO)	2–3
Severe Gastroenteritis[c]			
	Ciprofloxacin	500 mg bid (PO) or 400 mg q12h (IV)	3–7
	Trimethoprim-sulfamethoxazole	160/800 mg bid (PO)	
	Amoxicillin	1 g tid (PO)	
	Ceftriaxone	1–2 g/d (IV)	
Bacteremia			
	Ceftriaxone[d]	2 g/d (IV)	7–14
	Ciprofloxacin	400 mg q12h (IV), then 500 mg bid (PO)	
Endocarditis or Arteritis			
	Ceftriaxone	2 g/d (IV)	42
	Ciprofloxacin	400 mg q8h (IV), then 750 mg bid (PO)	
	Ampicillin	2 g q4h (IV)	
Meningitis			
	Ceftriaxone	2 g q12 h (IV)	14–21
	Ampicillin	2 g q4h (IV)	
Other Localized Infection			
	Ceftriaxone	2 g/d (IV)	14–28
	Ciprofloxacin	500 mg bid (PO) or 400 mg q12h (IV)	
	Ampicillin	2 g q6h (IV)	

[a]Consider for neonates; persons >50 years of age with possible atherosclerotic vascular disease; and patients with immunosuppression, endovascular graft, or joint prosthesis.
[b]Or ofloxacin, 400 mg bid (PO).
[c]Consider on an individualized basis for patients with severe diarrhea and high fever who require hospitalization.
[d]Or cefotaxime, 2 g q8h (IV).

962   Hoffman SL et al: Reduction in mortality in chloramphenicol-treated severe typhoid fever by high-dose dexamethasone. N Engl J Med 310:82, 1984

Lin FY et al: The efficacy of a *Salmonella typhi* Vi conjugate vaccine in two-to-five-year-old children. N Engl J Med 344:1263, 2001

Maskey AP et al: *Salmonella* enteric serovar Paratyphi A and *S. enterica* serovar Typhi cause indistinguishable clinical syndromes in Kathmandu, Nepal. Clin Infect Dis 42:1247, 2006

Ohl ME, Miller SI: *Salmonella*: A model for bacterial pathogenesis. Annu Rev Med 52:259, 2001

Steinberg EB et al: Typhoid fever in travelers: Who should be targeted for prevention. Clin Infect Dis 39:186, 2004

Su LH et al: Antimicrobial resistance in nontyphoid *Salmonella* serotypes: A global challenge. Clin Infect Dis 39:546, 2004

Varma JK et al: Antimicrobial-resistant nontyphoidal *Salmonella* is associated with excess bloodstream infections and hospitalizations. J Infect Dis 191:554, 2005

147 Shigellosis

Philippe Sansonetti, Jean Bergounioux

The discovery of *Shigella* as the etiologic agent of dysentery—a clinical syndrome of fever, intestinal cramps, and frequent passage of small, bloody, mucopurulent stools—is attributed to the Japanese microbiologist Kiyoshi Shiga, who isolated the Shiga bacillus (now known as *Shigella dysenteriae* type 1) from patients' stools in 1897 during a large and devastating dysentery epidemic. *Shigella* cannot be distinguished from *Escherichia coli* by DNA hybridization and remains a separate species only on historical and clinical grounds.

DEFINITION

Shigella is a non-spore-forming, gram-negative bacterium that, unlike *E. coli*, is nonmotile and does not produce gas from sugars, decarboxylate lysine, or hydrolyze arginine. Some serovars produce indole, and occasional strains utilize sodium acetate. *S. dysenteriae*, *S. flexneri*, *S. boydii*, and *S. sonnei* (serogroups A, B, C, and D, respectively) can be differentiated on the basis of biochemical and serologic characteristics. Genome sequencing of *E. coli* K12, *S. flexneri* 2a, *S. sonnei*, *S. dysenteriae* type 1, and *S. boydii* has revealed that these species have ~93% of genes in common. The three major genomic "signatures" of *Shigella* are (1) a 215-kb virulence plasmid that carries most of the genes required for pathogenicity (particularly invasive capacity); (2) the lack or alteration of genetic sequences encoding products (e.g., lysine decarboxylase) that, if expressed, would attenuate pathogenicity; and (3) in *S. dysenteriae* type 1, the presence of genes encoding Shiga toxin, a potent cytotoxin.

EPIDEMIOLOGY

The human intestinal tract represents the major reservoir of *Shigella*, which is also found (albeit rarely) in the higher primates. Because excretion of shigellae is greatest in the acute phase of disease, the bacteria are transmitted most efficiently by the fecal-oral route. Most cases of shigellosis are caused by person-to-person transmission, although some outbreaks reflect contamination of water or food. *Shigella* can also be transmitted by flies and, given its capacity to survive in foodstuffs, can be a significant cause of food-borne infection. The high-level infectivity of *Shigella* is reflected by the very small inoculum required for experimental infection of volunteers [100 colony-forming units (CFU)], by the very high attack rates during outbreaks in day care centers (33–73%), and by the high rates of secondary cases among family members of sick children (26–33%). Shigellosis can also be transmitted sexually.

In a review published under the auspices of the World Health Organization (WHO), the total annual number of cases in 1966–1997 was estimated at 165 million, and 69% of these cases occurred in children <5 years of age. In this review, the annual number of deaths was calculated to range between 500,000 and 1.1 million. More recent data (2000–2004) from six Asian countries (Bangladesh, China, Pakistan, Indonesia, Vietnam, and Thailand) indicate that even though the incidence of shigellosis remains stable, mortality rates associated with this disease may have decreased significantly, possibly as a result of improved nutritional standards. However, extensive and essentially uncontrolled use of antibiotics has increased the risk of emergence of multidrug-resistant *Shigella* strains.

Throughout history, *Shigella* epidemics have often occurred in settings of human crowding under poor hygienic conditions—e.g., among soldiers in campaigning armies, inhabitants of besieged cities, groups on pilgrimages, and refugees in camps. Epidemics follow a cyclic pattern in areas such as the Indian subcontinent and sub-Saharan Africa. These devastating epidemics, which are most often caused by *S. dysenteriae* type 1, are characterized by high attack rates and high mortality rates. In Bangladesh, for instance, an epidemic caused by *S. dysenteriae* type 1 was associated with a 42% increase in mortality rates among children 1–4 years of age. Apart from these epidemics, shigellosis is essentially an endemic disease, with 99% of cases occurring in the developing world and particularly high prevalences in the most impoverished areas, where personal and general hygiene is substandard. *S. flexneri* isolates predominate in less well-developed areas, whereas *S. sonnei* is more prevalent in economically emerging regions and in the industrialized world.

An often-overlooked complication of shigellosis is the short- and long-term impairment of the nutritional status of infected children in endemic areas. Combined with anorexia, the exudative enteropathy resulting from mucosal abrasions contributes to rapid exacerbation of the patient's nutritional status. Shigellosis is thus a major contributor to stunted growth among children in developing countries.

PATHOGENESIS AND PATHOLOGY

Shigella infection occurs through oral contamination. Direct fecal-oral transmission predominates since the organism is not well adapted to survive in the environment. Resistance to low-pH conditions allows shigellae to survive passage through the gastric barrier, an ability that may explain in part why a small inoculum (as few as 100 CFU) is sufficient to cause infection.

The watery diarrhea that usually precedes the dysenteric syndrome is attributable to active secretion and abnormal water reabsorption, a secretory effect at the jejunal level described in experimentally infected rhesus monkeys. This initial purge is probably due to the combined action of an enterotoxin (ShET-1) and mucosal inflammation. The dysenteric syndrome, manifested by bloody and mucopurulent stools, reflects invasion of the mucosa.

The pathogenesis of *Shigella* is essentially determined by a large virulence plasmid of 214 kb comprising ~100 genes, of which 25 encode a type III secretion system that inserts into the membrane of the host cell to allow effectors to transit from the bacterial cytoplasm to the cell cytoplasm (Fig. 147-1). Bacteria are thereby able to invade intestinal epithelial cells by inducing their own uptake after the initial crossing of the epithelial barrier through M cells (the specialized translocating epithelial cells in the follicle-associated epithelium that covers mucosal lymphoid nodules). The organisms induce apoptosis of subepithelial resident macrophages. Once inside the cytoplasm of intestinal epithelial cells, *Shigella* effectors trigger the cytoskeletal rearrangements necessary to direct uptake of the organism into the epithelial cell. The *Shigella*-containing vacuole is then quickly lysed, releasing bacteria into the cytosol.

Intracellular shigellae next use cytoskeletal components to propel themselves inside the infected cell; when the moving organism and the

FIGURE 147-1 Invasive strategy of *Shigella flexneri*. IL, interleukin; NLR, nod-like receptor; PMN, polymorphonuclear leukocyte.

Figure labels:
- *Shigella*
- M cell
- Epithelial cell
- IcsA
- Activation of NF-κB caused by IL-1β and intracellular NLR activation
- Cell-to-cell spread
- IL-8
- Macrophages
- IpaB IpaC IpaA + type III secretion
- IL-1β
- Disruption of epithelial permeability barrier by PMNs
- Macrophage apoptosis Caspase-I activation by IpaB
  -Bacterial survival
  -Initiation of inflammation
- Massive invasion of epithelium
- IL-18

host cell membrane come into contact, cellular protrusions form and are engulfed by neighboring cells. This series of events permits bacterial cell-to-cell spread that is protected from immune effector mechanisms.

Cytokines released by a growing number of infected intestinal epithelial cells attract increased numbers of immune cells [particularly polymorphonuclear leukocytes (PMNs)] to the infected site, thus further destabilizing the epithelial barrier, exacerbating inflammation, and leading to the acute colitis that characterizes shigellosis. Recent evidence indicates that some of the type III secretion system–injected effectors can control the extent of inflammation, thus facilitating bacterial survival.

Shiga toxin produced by *S. dysenteriae* type 1 increases disease severity. Shiga toxin and Shiga-like toxins belong to a group of A1-B5 protein toxins whose B subunit binds to the cell surface and whose catalytic A subunit expresses an RNA N-glycosidase on 28S ribosomal RNA. These events lead to inhibition of binding of the amino-acyl-tRNA to the 60S ribosomal subunit and thus to a general shutoff of cell protein biosynthesis. Shiga toxins are translocated from the bowel into the circulation. After binding to the receptor globotriaosylceramide on target cells in the kidney, toxin is internalized by receptor-mediated endocytosis and interacts with the subcellular machinery to inhibit protein synthesis. The consequent pathophysiologic changes may result in hemolytic-uremic syndrome (HUS; see below).

CLINICAL MANIFESTATIONS

The presentation and severity of shigellosis depend to some extent on the infecting species but even more on the age and the immunologic and nutritional status of the host. Poverty and a poor hygienic environment are strongly related to the number and severity of diarrheal episodes, especially in children <5 years old.

Shigellosis typically evolves through four phases: incubation, watery diarrhea, dysentery, and the postinfectious phase. The incubation period usually lasts 1–4 days but may be as long as 8 days. Typical initial manifestations are transient fever, limited watery diarrhea, malaise, and anorexia. Signs and symptoms may range from mild abdominal discomfort to severe cramps, diarrhea, fever, vomiting, and tenesmus. The manifestations are usually exacerbated in children, with temperatures up to 40°–41°C and more severe anorexia and watery diarrhea. Unlike most diarrheal syndromes, dysenteric syndromes do not have dehydration as a major feature. This initial phase may represent the only clinical manifestation of shigellosis, especially in developed countries. Otherwise, dysentery follows within hours or days and is characterized by small volumes of bloody mucopurulent stools with increased tenesmus and abdominal cramps. At this stage, *Shigella* produces acute colitis involving mainly the dis-

tal colon and the rectum. Endoscopy demonstrates an edematous and hemorrhagic mucosa, with ulcerations and possibly overlying exudates resembling pseudomembranes. The extent of the lesions correlates with the number and frequency of stools and with the degree of protein loss by exudative mechanisms. Most episodes are self-limited and resolve without treatment in 1 week. With appropriate treatment, recovery takes place within a few days to a week, with no sequelae.

Acute life-threatening complications are seen most often in children <5 years of age, particularly affecting malnourished children in developing countries. Risk factors for death include nonbloody diarrhea, moderate to severe dehydration, bacteremia, absence of fever, abdominal tenderness, and rectal prolapse. Major complications are predominantly intestinal (e.g., toxic megacolon, intestinal perforations, rectal prolapse) or metabolic (e.g., hypoglycemia, hyponatremia, dehydration). Bacteremia is rare and is reported most frequently in severely malnourished children, HIV-infected patients, and patients with defects in innate immunity. Alterations of consciousness, including seizures, delirium, and coma, may occur, especially in children <5 years old, and are associated with a poor prognosis; fever and severe metabolic alterations are more often the major causes of altered consciousness than is meningitis or the Ekiri syndrome (toxic encephalopathy associated with bizarre posturing, cerebral edema, and fatty degeneration of viscera), which has been reported in Japanese children. Pneumonia, vaginitis, and keratoconjunctivitis due to *Shigella* are rarely reported. In the absence of serious malnutrition, severe and very unusual clinical manifestations, such as meningitis, may be linked to disorders of immune function and require relevant investigations.

Two complications of particular importance are toxic megacolon and HUS. Toxic megacolon is a consequence of severe inflammation extending to the colonic smooth-muscle layer and causing paralysis and dilatation. The patient presents with abdominal distention and tenderness, with or without signs of localized or generalized peritonitis. The abdominal x-ray characteristically shows marked dilatation of the transverse colon (with the greatest distention in the ascending and descending colons); thumbprinting caused by mucosal inflammatory edema; and loss of the normal haustral pattern associated with pseudopolyps, often extending into the lumen. Pneumatosis coli is an occasional finding. If perforation occurs, radiographic signs of pneumoperitoneum may be apparent. Predisposing factors (e.g., hypokalemia and use of opioids, anticholinergics, loperamide, psyllium seeds, and antidepressants) should be sought.

Shiga toxin produced by *S. dysenteriae* type 1 has been linked to HUS in developing countries but rarely in industrialized countries. HUS is an early complication that most often develops after several days of diarrhea. Clinical examination shows pallor, asthenia, and irritability and, in some cases, bleeding of the nose and gums, oliguria, and increasing edema. HUS is a nonimmune (Coombs test–negative) hemolytic anemia defined by a diagnostic triad: microangiopathic hemolytic anemia [hemoglobin level typically <80 g/L (<8 g/dL)], thrombocytopenia (mild to moderate in severity; typically <60,000 platelets/μL), and acute renal failure due to thrombosis of the glomerular capillaries (with markedly elevated creatinine levels). Anemia is severe, with fragmented red blood cells (schizocytes) in the peripheral smear, high serum concentrations of lactate dehydrogenase and free circulating hemoglobin, and elevated reticulocyte counts. Acute renal failure occurs in 55–70% of cases; however, renal function recovers in most of these cases (up to 70% in various series). Leukemoid reactions, with leukocyte counts of 50,000/μL, are sometimes noted in association with HUS.

The postinfectious immunologic complication known as reactive arthritis (Reiter's syndrome) can develop weeks or months after shigellosis, especially in patients expressing the histocompatibility antigen HLA-B27. About 3% of patients infected with *S. flexneri* later develop Reiter's syndrome, with arthritis, ocular inflammation, and urethritis—a condition that can last for months or years and progress to difficult-to-treat chronic arthritis. Postinfectious arthropathy occurs only after infection with *S. flexneri* and not after infection with the other *Shigella* serotypes.

LABORATORY DIAGNOSIS

 The differential diagnosis in patients with a dysenteric syndrome depends on the clinical and environmental context. In developing areas, infectious diarrhea caused by other invasive pathogenic bacteria (*Salmonella enteritidis, Campylobacter jejuni, Clostridium difficile, Yersinia enterocolitica*) or parasites (*Entamoeba histolytica*) should be considered. Only bacteriologic and parasitologic examinations of stool can truly differentiate among these pathogens. A first flare of inflammatory bowel disease, such as Crohn's disease or ulcerative colitis (Chap. 289), should be considered in patients in industrialized countries. Despite similar symptoms, anamnesis discriminates between shigellosis, which usually follows recent travel in an endemic zone, and these other conditions.

Microscopic examination of stool smears shows the presence of erythrophagocytic trophozoites with very few PMNs in *E. histolytica* infection, whereas bacterial enteroinvasive infections (particularly shigellosis) are characterized by high PMN counts in each microscopic field. However, because shigellosis often manifests only as watery diarrhea, systematic attempts to isolate *Shigella* are necessary.

The "gold standard" for the diagnosis of *Shigella* infection remains the isolation and identification of the pathogen from fecal material. One major difficulty, particularly in endemic areas where laboratory facilities are not immediately available, is the fragility of *Shigella* and its common disappearance during transport, especially with rapid changes in temperature and pH. In the absence of a reliable enrichment medium, buffered glycerol saline or Cary-Blair medium can be used as a holding medium, but prompt inoculation onto isolation medium is essential. The probability of isolation is higher if the portion of stools that contains bloody and/or mucopurulent material is directly sampled. Rectal swabs can be used as they offer the highest rate of successful isolation during the acute phase of disease. Blood cultures are positive in <5% of cases and should be done only when a patient presents with a clinical picture of severe sepsis.

In addition to quick processing, the use of several media increases the likelihood of successful isolation: a nonselective medium such as bromocresol-purple agar lactose; a low-selectivity medium such as MacConkey or eosin-methylene blue; and a high-selectivity medium such as Hektoen, *Salmonella-Shigella*, or xylose-lysine-deoxycholate agar. After incubation on these media for 12–18 h at 37°C, shigellae appear as non-lactose-fermenting colonies that measure 0.5–1 mm in diameter and have a convex, translucent, smooth surface. Suspected colonies on nonselective or low-selectivity medium can be subcultured on a high-selectivity medium before being specifically identified or can be identified directly by standard commercial systems on the basis of four major characteristics: glucose positivity (usually without production of gas), lactose negativity, H₂S negativity, and lack of motility. The four *Shigella* serogroups (A–D) can then be differentiated by additional characteristics. This approach adds time and difficulty to the identification process, however; thus, after presumptive diagnosis, the use of serologic methods—e.g., slide agglutination, with group- and then type-specific antisera—should be considered. Group-specific antisera are widely available; in contrast, because of the large number of serotypes and sub-serotypes that must be considered, type-specific antisera are rare and more expensive and are often restricted to reference laboratories.

Rx SHIGELLOSIS

ANTIBIOTIC SUSCEPTIBILITY OF *SHIGELLA* As an enteroinvasive disease, shigellosis requires antibiotic treatment. Since the mid-1960s, however, increasing resistance to multiple drugs has been a dominant factor in treatment decisions. Resistance rates are highly dependent on the geographic area. Clonal spread of particular strains and horizontal transfer of resistance determinants, particularly via plasmids and transposons, contribute to multidrug resistance. Quinolone resistance is essentially due to chromosomal mutations affecting DNA gyrase and topoisomerase IV. A review of the antibiotic resistance history of *Shigella* in India found that, after their introduction in the late 1980s, the second-generation quinolones norfloxacin, ciprofloxacin, and ofloxacin were highly effective in the treatment of shigellosis, including cases caused by multidrug-resistant strains of *S. dysenteriae* type 1. In contrast, investigations of recent outbreaks in India and Bangladesh have shown high levels of resistance (generally 5%) to norfloxacin, ciprofloxacin, and ofloxacin among certain isolates. The incidence of multidrug resistance parallels widespread uncontrolled use of antibiotics (particularly in developing areas), calls for the rational use of effective drugs, and underscores the need for alternative drugs to treat infections caused by resistant strains.

ANTIBIOTIC TREATMENT OF SHIGELLOSIS (Table 147-1) Because of the ready transmissibility of *Shigella*, current public health recommendations in the United States are that every case be treated with antibiotics. Ciprofloxacin is recommended as first-line treatment. A number of other drugs have been tested and shown to be effective, including ceftriaxone, azithromycin, pivmecillinam, and some fifth-generation quinolones. While infections caused by non-*dysenteriae Shigella* in immunocompetent individuals are routinely treated with a 3-day course of antibiotics, it is recommended that *S. dysenteriae* infections be treated for 5 days and that *Shigella* infections in immunocompromised patients be treated for 7–10 days.

Treatment for shigellosis must be adapted to the clinical context, with the recognition that the most fragile patients are children <5 years old, who represent two-thirds of all cases worldwide. There are few data on the use of quinolones in children. The half-life of ciprofloxacin is longer in infants than in older individuals. The ciprofloxacin dose generally recommended for children is 30 mg/kg per day in two divided doses. Adults living in areas with high hygienic standards are likely to develop milder, shorter-duration disease, whereas infants in endemic areas can develop severe, sometimes fatal dysentery. In the former setting, treatment will remain minimal and bacteriologic proof of infection will often come after symptoms have resolved; in the latter setting, more aggressive measures, possibly including resuscitation, may be required.

REHYDRATION AND NUTRITION *Shigella* infection rarely causes significant dehydration. Cases requiring aggressive rehydration (particularly in industrialized countries) are uncommon. In developing countries, malnu-

TABLE 147-1 RECOMMENDED ANTIMICROBIAL THERAPY FOR SHIGELLOSIS

Antimicrobial Agent	Treatment Schedule		Limitations
	In Children	**In Adults**	
First line			
Ciprofloxacin	15 mg/kg	500 mg	
	2 times per day for 3 days, PO		
Second line			
Pivmecillinam	20 mg/kg	100 mg	Cost
	4 times per day for 5 days, PO		No pediatric formulation
			Frequent administration
			Resistance emerging
Ceftriaxone	50–100 mg/kg	–	Efficacy not validated
	Once a day IM for 2–5 days		Must be injected
Azithromycin	6–20 mg/kg	1–1.5 g	Cost
	Once a day for 1–5 days, PO		Efficacy not validated
			MIC near serum concentration
			Resistance emerges rapidly and spreads to other bacteria

Source: WHO Library Cataloguing-in-Publication Data: Guidelines for the control of shigellosis, including epidemics due to *Shigella dysenteriae* type 1 (www.searo.who.int/LinkFiles/CAH_Publications_shigella.pdf).

trition remains the primary indicator for diarrhea-related death, highlighting the importance of nutrition in early management. Rehydration should be oral unless the patient is comatose or presents in shock. Because of the improved effectiveness of reduced-osmolarity oral rehydration solution (especially for children with acute noncholera diarrhea), the WHO and UNICEF now recommend a standard solution of 245 mOsm/L (sodium, 75 mmol/L; chloride, 65 mmol/L; glucose (anhydrous), 75 mmol/L; potassium, 20 mmol/L; citrate, 10 mmol/L). In shigellosis, as in acute infectious diarrhea of most etiologies (including cholera), the coupled transport of sodium to glucose or other solutes is largely unaffected, and oral rehydration therapy represents the easiest and most efficient form of rehydration, especially in severe cases.

Nutrition should be started as soon as possible after completion of initial rehydration. Early refeeding is safe, well tolerated, and clinically beneficial. Because breast-feeding reduces diarrheal losses and the need for oral rehydration in infants, it should be maintained in the absence of contraindications (e.g., maternal HIV infection).

NONSPECIFIC, SYMPTOM-BASED THERAPY   Antimotility agents have been implicated in prolonged fever in volunteers with shigellosis. These agents are suspected of increasing the risk of toxic megacolon and are thought to have been responsible for HUS in children infected by Shiga toxin–producing strains of *E. coli*. For safety reasons, it is better to avoid antimotility agents in bloody diarrhea.

TREATMENT OF COMPLICATIONS   There is no consensus regarding the best treatment for toxic megacolon. The patient should be assessed frequently by both medical and surgical teams. Anemia, dehydration, and electrolyte deficits (particularly hypokalemia) may aggravate colonic atony and should be actively treated. Nasogastric aspiration helps to deflate the colon. Parenteral nutrition has not been proved to be beneficial. Fever persisting beyond 48–72 h raises the possibility of local perforation or abscess. Most studies recommend colectomy if, after 48–72 h, colonic distention persists. However, some physicians recommend continuation of medical therapy for up to 7 days if the patient seems to be improving clinically despite persistent megacolon without free perforation. Intestinal perforation, either isolated or complicating toxic megacolon, requires surgical treatment and intensive medical support.

Rectal prolapse must be treated as soon as possible. With the health care provider using surgical gloves or a soft warm wet cloth and the patient in the knee-chest position, the prolapsed rectum is gently pushed back into place. If edema of the rectal mucosa is evident (rendering reintegration difficult), it can be osmotically reduced by applying gauze impregnated with a warm solution of saturated magnesium sulfate. Rectal prolapse often relapses but usually resolves along with the resolution of dysentery.

HUS must be treated by water restriction, including discontinuation of oral rehydration solution and potassium-rich alimentation. Hemofiltration is usually required.

PREVENTION
Hand washing after defecation or handling of children's feces and before handling of food is recommended. However, this protocol entails an average of 32 hand washes per day, with consumption of 20 L of water. If soap is too costly, ash or mud can be used, but access to water remains essential. Stool precautions, together with a cleaning protocol for medical staff as well as for patients, have proven useful in limiting the spread of infection during *Shigella* outbreaks. Ideally, patients should have a negative stool culture before their infection is considered cured. Recurrences are rare if treatment and prevention are correctly implemented.

Although several live attenuated oral and subunit parenteral vaccine candidates have been produced and are undergoing clinical trials, no vaccine against shigellosis is currently available. Especially given the rapid progression of antibiotic resistance in *Shigella*, a vaccine is urgently needed.

FURTHER READINGS

BENNISH ML, WOJTYNIAK BJ: Mortality due to shigellosis: Community and hospital data. Rev Infect Dis 13(Suppl 4):S245, 1991

COSSART P, SANSONETTI PJ: Bacterial invasion: The paradigms of enteroinvasive pathogens. Science 304:242, 2004

KOTLOFF KL et al: Overview of live vaccine strategies against *Shigella*, in *New Generation Vaccines*, 3d ed, MM Levine et al (eds). London, Informa Healthcare, 2004, pp 723–735

——— et al: Global burden of *Shigella* infections: Implications for vaccine development and implementation of control strategies. Bull World Health Organ 77:651, 1999

NIYOGI SK: Shigellosis. J Microbiol 43:133, 2005

PHALIPON A, SANSONETTI PJ: Shigella's ways of manipulating the host intestinal innate and adaptive immune system: A tool box for survival? Immunol Cell Biol 85:119, 2007

VON SEIDLEIN L et al: A multicentre study of *Shigella* diarrhoea in six Asian countries: Disease burden, clinical manifestations, and microbiology. PLoS Med 3(9):e353, 2006

WORLD HEALTH ORGANIZATION: Guidelines for the control of shigellosis, including epidemics due to *Shigella dysenteriae* type 1. WHO Library Cataloguing-in-Publication Data (*www.searo.who.int/LinkFiles/CAH_Publications_shigella.pdf*)

148 Infections Due to *Campylobacter* and Related Species
Martin J. Blaser

DEFINITION
Bacteria of the genus *Campylobacter* and of the related genera *Arcobacter* and *Helicobacter* (Chap. 144) cause a variety of inflammatory conditions. Although acute diarrheal illnesses are most common, these organisms may cause infections in virtually all parts of the body, especially in compromised hosts, and these infections may have late nonsuppurative sequelae. The designation *Campylobacter* comes from the Greek for "curved rod" and refers to the organism's vibrio-like morphology.

ETIOLOGY
Campylobacters are motile, non-spore-forming, curved, gram-negative rods. Originally known as *Vibrio fetus*, these bacilli were reclassified as a new genus in 1973, after their dissimilarity to other vibrios was recog-

nized. More than 15 species have since been identified. These species are currently divided into three genera: *Campylobacter*, *Arcobacter*, and *Helicobacter*. Not all of the species are pathogens of humans. The human pathogens fall into two major groups: those that primarily cause diarrheal disease and those that cause extraintestinal infection. The principal diarrheal pathogen is *C. jejuni*, which accounts for 80–90% of all cases of recognized illness due to campylobacters and related genera. Other organisms that cause diarrheal disease include *C. coli, C. upsaliensis, C. lari, C. hyointestinalis, C. fetus, A. butzleri, A. cryaerophilus, H. cinaedi,* and *H. fennelliae*. The two *Helicobacter* species causing diarrheal disease, *H. cinaedi* and *H. fennelliae*, are intestinal rather than gastric organisms; in terms of the clinical features of the illnesses they cause, these species most closely resemble *Campylobacter* rather than *H. pylori* (Chap. 144) and thus are considered in this chapter.

The major species causing extraintestinal illnesses is *C. fetus*. However, any of the diarrheal agents listed above may cause systemic or localized infection as well. Neither aerobes nor strict anaerobes, these microaerophilic organisms are adapted for survival in the gastrointestinal mucous layer. This chapter focuses on *C. jejuni* and *C. fetus* as the major pathogens in and prototypes for their groups. The key features of infection are listed by species (excluding *C. jejuni*, described in detail in the text below) in Table 148-1.

TABLE 148-1 CLINICAL FEATURES ASSOCIATED WITH INFECTION DUE TO "ATYPICAL" *CAMPYLOBACTER* AND RELATED SPECIES IMPLICATED AS CAUSES OF HUMAN ILLNESS

Species	Common Clinical Features	Less Common Clinical Features	Additional Information
Campylobacter coli	Fever, diarrhea, abdominal pain	Bacteremia[a]	Clinically indistinguishable from *C. jejuni*
Campylobacter fetus	Bacteremia,[a] sepsis, meningitis, vascular infections	Diarrhea, relapsing fevers	Not usually isolated from media containing cephalothin or incubated at 42°C
Campylobacter upsaliensis	Watery diarrhea, low-grade fever, abdominal pain	Bacteremia, abscesses	Difficult to isolate because of cephalothin susceptibility
Campylobacter lari	Abdominal pain, diarrhea	Colitis, appendicitis	Seagulls frequently colonized; organism often transmitted to humans via contaminated water
Campylobacter hyointestinalis	Watery or bloody diarrhea, vomiting, abdominal pain	Bacteremia	Causes proliferative enteritis in swine
Helicobacter fennelliae	Chronic mild diarrhea, abdominal cramps, proctitis	Bacteremia[a]	Best treated with fluoroquinolones
Helicobacter cinaedi	Chronic mild diarrhea, abdominal cramps, proctitis	Bacteremia[a]	Best treated with fluoroquinolones; identified in healthy hamsters
Campylobacter jejuni subspecies *doylei*	Diarrhea	Chronic gastritis, bacteremia[b]	Uncertain role as human pathogen
Arcobacter cryaerophilus	Diarrhea	Bacteremia	Cultured under aerobic conditions
Arcobacter butzleri	Fever, diarrhea, abdominal pain, nausea	Bacteremia, appendicitis	Cultured under aerobic conditions; enzootic in nonhuman primates
Campylobacter sputorum	Pulmonary, perianal, groin, and axillary abscesses	Bacteremia	Three clinically relevant biovars: *C. sputorum* subspecies *sputorum*, *C. sputorum* subspecies *bubulus*, and *Campylobacter mucosalis*

[a]In immunocompromised hosts, especially HIV-infected persons.
[b]In children.

Source: Adapted from BM Allos, MJ Blaser: *Campylobacter jejuni* and the expanding spectrum of related infections. Clin Infect Dis 20:1092, 1995.

EPIDEMIOLOGY

Campylobacters are found in the gastrointestinal tract of many animals used for food (including poultry, cattle, sheep, and swine) and many household pets (including birds, dogs, and cats). These microorganisms usually do not cause illness in their animal hosts. In most cases, campylobacters are transmitted to humans in raw or undercooked food products or through direct contact with infected animals. In the United States and other developed countries, ingestion of contaminated poultry that has not been sufficiently cooked is the most common mode of acquisition (30–70% of cases). Other modes include ingestion of raw (unpasteurized) milk or untreated water, contact with infected household pets, travel to developing countries (campylobacters being among the leading causes of traveler's diarrhea; Chaps. 117 and 122), oral-anal sexual contact, and (occasionally) contact with an index case who is incontinent of stool.

Campylobacter infections are common. Several studies indicate that, in the United States, diarrheal disease due to campylobacters is more common than that due to *Salmonella* and *Shigella* combined. Infections occur throughout the year, but their incidence peaks during summer and early autumn. Persons of all ages are affected; however, attack rates for *C. jejuni* are highest among young children and young adults, while those for *C. fetus* are highest at the extremes of age. Systemic infections due to *C. fetus* (and to other *Campylobacter* and related species) are most common among compromised hosts. Persons at increased risk include those with AIDS, hypogammaglobulinemia, neoplasia, liver disease, diabetes mellitus, and generalized atherosclerosis as well as neonates and pregnant women. However, apparently healthy nonpregnant persons occasionally develop transient *Campylobacter* bacteremia as part of a gastrointestinal illness.

In developing countries, *C. jejuni* infections are hyperendemic, with the highest rates among children <2 years old. Infection rates fall with age, as does the illness-to-infection ratio. These observations suggest that frequent exposure to *C. jejuni* leads to the acquisition of immunity.

PATHOLOGY AND PATHOGENESIS

Many *C. jejuni* infections are subclinical, especially in hosts in developing countries who have had multiple prior infections and thus are partially immune. Most illnesses occur within 2–4 days (range, 1–7 days) of exposure to the organism in food or water. The sites of tissue injury include the jejunum, ileum, and colon. Biopsies show an acute nonspecific inflammatory reaction, with neutrophils, monocytes, and eosinophils in the lamina propria, as well as damage to the epithelium, including loss of mucus, glandular degeneration, and crypt abscesses. Biopsy findings may be consistent with Crohn's disease or ulcerative colitis, but these "idiopathic" chronic inflammatory diseases should not be diagnosed unless infectious colitis, *specifically including* that due to infection with *Campylobacter* species and related organisms, has been ruled out.

The high frequency of *C. jejuni* infections and their severity and recurrence among hypogammaglobulinemic patients suggest that antibodies are important in protective immunity. The pathogenesis of infection is uncertain. Both the motility of the strain and its capacity to adhere to host tissues appear to favor disease, but classic enterotoxins and cytotoxins (although described and including cytolethal distending toxin, or CDT) appear not to play substantial roles in tissue injury or disease production. The organisms have been visualized in the epithelium, albeit in low numbers. The documentation of a significant tissue response and occasionally of *C. jejuni* bacteremia further suggests that tissue invasion is clinically significant, and in vitro studies are consistent with this pathogenetic feature.

The pathogenesis of *C. fetus* infections is better defined. Virtually all clinical isolates of *C. fetus* possess a proteinaceous capsule-like structure (an S-layer) that renders the organisms resistant to complement-mediated killing and opsonization. As a result, *C. fetus* can cause bacteremia and can seed sites beyond the intestinal tract. The ability of the organism to switch the S-layer proteins expressed—a phenomenon that results in antigenic variability—may contribute to the chronicity and high rate of recurrence of *C. fetus* infections in compromised hosts.

CLINICAL MANIFESTATIONS

The clinical features of infections due to *Campylobacter* and the related *Arcobacter* and intestinal *Helicobacter* species causing enteric disease appear to be highly similar. *C. jejuni* can be considered the prototype, in part because it is by far the most common enteric pathogen. A prodrome of fever, headache, myalgia, and/or malaise often occurs 12–48 h before the onset of diarrheal symptoms. The most common signs and symptoms of the intestinal phase are diarrhea, abdominal pain, and fever. The degree of diarrhea varies from several loose stools to grossly bloody stools; most patients presenting for medical attention have ≥10 bowel movements on the worst day of illness. Abdominal pain usually consists of cramping and may be the most prominent symptom. Pain is usually generalized but may become localized; *C. jejuni* infection may cause pseudoappendicitis. Fever may be the only initial manifestation of *C. jejuni* infection, a situation mimicking the early stages of typhoid fever. Febrile young children may develop convulsions. *Campylobacter* enteritis is generally self-limited; however, symptoms persist for >1 week in 10–20% of patients seeking medical attention, and clinical relapses occur in 5–10% of untreated patients.

C. fetus may cause a diarrheal illness similar to that due to *C. jejuni*, especially in normal hosts. This organism may also cause either intermittent diarrhea or nonspecific abdominal pain without localizing signs. Sequelae are uncommon, and the outcome is benign. *C. fetus* may also cause a prolonged relapsing systemic illness (with fever, chills, and myalgias) that has no obvious primary source; this manifestation is especially common among compromised hosts. Secondary seeding of an organ (e.g., meninges, brain, bone, urinary tract, or soft tissue) complicates the course, which may be fulminant. *C. fetus* infections have a tropism for vascular sites: endocarditis, mycotic aneurysm, and septic thrombophlebitis may all occur. Infection during pregnancy often leads to fetal death. A variety of *Campylobacter* species and *H. cinaedi* can cause recurrent cellulitis with fever and bacteremia in immunocompromised hosts.

COMPLICATIONS

Except in infection with *C. fetus*, bacteremia is uncommon, developing most often in immunocompromised hosts and at the extremes of age. Three patterns of extraintestinal infection have been noted: (1) transient bacteremia in a normal host with enteritis (benign course, no specific treatment needed); (2) sustained bacteremia or focal infection in a normal host (bacteremia originating from enteritis, with patients responding well to antimicrobial therapy); and (3) sustained bacteremia or focal infection in a compromised host. Enteritis may not be clinically apparent. Antimicrobial therapy, possibly prolonged, is necessary for suppression or cure of the infection.

Campylobacter, *Arcobacter*, and intestinal *Helicobacter* infections in patients with AIDS or hypogammaglobulinemia may be severe, persistent, and extraintestinal; relapse after cessation of therapy is common. Hypogammaglobulinemic patients may also develop osteomyelitis and an erysipelas-like rash or cellulitis.

Local suppurative complications of infection include cholecystitis, pancreatitis, and cystitis; distant complications include meningitis, endocarditis, arthritis, peritonitis, cellulitis, and septic abortion. All these complications are rare, except in immunocompromised hosts. Hepatitis, interstitial nephritis, and the hemolytic-uremic syndrome occasionally complicate acute infection. Reactive arthritis and other rheumatologic complaints may develop several weeks after infection, especially in persons with the HLA-B27 phenotype. Guillain-Barré syndrome (or its Miller Fisher or cranial polyneuropathy variant) follows *Campylobacter* infections uncommonly—i.e., in 1 of every 1000–2000 cases or, for certain *C. jejuni* serotypes (such as O19), in 1 of every 100–200 cases. Despite the low frequency of this complication, it is now estimated that *Campylobacter* infections, because of their high incidence, may trigger 20–40% of all cases of Guillain-Barré syndrome. Immunoproliferative small-intestinal disease (*alpha chain disease*), a form of lymphoma that originates in small-intestinal mucosa-associated lymphoid tissue, has been associated with *C. jejuni*; antimicrobial therapy has led to marked clinical improvement.

DIAGNOSIS

In patients with *Campylobacter* enteritis, peripheral leukocyte counts reflect the severity of the inflammatory process. However, stools from nearly all *Campylobacter*-infected patients presenting for medical attention in the United States contain leukocytes or erythrocytes. Fecal smears should be treated with Gram's or Wright's stain and examined in all suspected cases. When the diagnosis of *Campylobacter* enteritis is suspected on the basis of findings indicating inflammatory diarrhea (fever, fecal leukocytes), clinicians can ask the laboratory to attempt the visualization of organisms with characteristic vibrioid morphology by direct microscopic examination of stools with Gram's staining or to use phase-contrast or dark-field microscopy to identify the organisms' characteristic "darting" motility. Confirmation of the diagnosis of *Campylobacter* infection is based on identification of an isolate from cultures of stool, blood, or another site. *Campylobacter*-specific media

should be used to culture stools from all patients with inflammatory or bloody diarrhea. Since all *Campylobacter* species are fastidious, they will not be isolated unless selective media or other selective techniques are used. Not all media are equally useful for isolation of the broad array of campylobacters; therefore, failure to isolate campylobacters from stool does not entirely rule out their presence. The detection of the organisms in stool almost always implies infection; there is a brief period of postconvalescent fecal carriage and no commensalism in humans. In contrast, *C. sputorum* and related organisms found in the oral cavity are commensals with rare pathogenic significance. Because of low levels of metabolic activity in standard blood culture media, *Campylobacter* bacteremia may be difficult to detect unless laboratorians are looking for low-positive results in quantitative assays.

DIFFERENTIAL DIAGNOSIS

The symptoms of *Campylobacter* enteritis are not sufficiently unusual to distinguish this illness from that due to *Salmonella*, *Shigella*, *Yersinia*, and other pathogens. The combination of fever and fecal leukocytes or erythrocytes is indicative of inflammatory diarrhea, and definitive diagnosis is based on culture or demonstration of the characteristic organisms on stained fecal smears. Similarly, extraintestinal *Campylobacter* illness is diagnosed by culture. Infection due to *Campylobacter* should be suspected in the setting of septic abortion, and that due to *C. fetus* should be suspected specifically in the setting of septic thrombophlebitis. It is important to reiterate that (1) the presentation of *Campylobacter* enteritis may mimic that of ulcerative colitis or Crohn's disease, (2) *Campylobacter* enteritis is much more common than either of the latter (especially among young adults), and (3) biopsy may not distinguish among these entities. Thus a diagnosis of inflammatory bowel disease should not be made until *Campylobacter* infection has been ruled out, especially in persons with a history of foreign travel, significant animal contact, immunodeficiency, or exposure incurring a high risk of transmission.

℞ INFECTIONS DUE TO *CAMPYLOBACTER* AND RELATED SPECIES

Fluid and electrolyte replacement is central to the treatment of diarrheal illnesses (Chap. 122). Even among patients presenting for medical attention with *Campylobacter* enteritis, not all clearly benefit from specific antimicrobial therapy. Indications for therapy include high fever, bloody diarrhea, severe diarrhea, persistence for >1 week, and worsening of symptoms. A 5- to 7-day course of erythromycin (250 mg orally four times daily or—for children—30–50 mg/kg per day, in divided doses) is the regimen of choice. Both clinical trials and in vitro susceptibility testing indicate that other macrolides, including clarithromycin and azithromycin, also are useful therapeutic agents. An alternative regimen for adults is ciprofloxacin (500 mg orally twice daily) or another fluoroquinolone for 5–7 days, but resistance to this class of agents as well as to tetracyclines has been increasing. Patients infected with antibiotic-resistant strains are at increased risk of adverse outcomes. Use of antimotility agents, which may prolong the duration of symptoms and have been associated with toxic megacolon and with death, is not recommended.

For systemic infections, treatment with gentamicin (1.7 mg/kg IV every 8 h after a loading dose of 2 mg/kg), imipenem (500 mg IV every 6 h), or chloramphenicol (50 mg/kg IV each day in three or four divided doses) should be started empirically, but susceptibility testing should then be performed. Ciprofloxacin and amoxicillin/clavulanate are alternative agents for susceptible strains. In the absence of immunocompromise or endovascular infections, therapy should be administered for 14 days. For immunocompromised patients with systemic infections due to *C. fetus* and for patients with endovascular infections, prolonged therapy (for up to 4 weeks) is usually necessary. For recurrent infections in immunocompromised hosts, lifelong therapy/prophylaxis is sometimes necessary.

PROGNOSIS

Nearly all patients recover fully from *Campylobacter* enteritis, either spontaneously or after antimicrobial therapy. Volume depletion probably contributes to the few deaths that are reported. As stated above, occasional patients develop reactive arthritis or Guillain-Barré syndrome or its variants. Systemic infection with *C. fetus* is much more often fatal than that due to related species; this higher mortality rate reflects in part the population affected. Prognosis depends on the rapidity with which appropriate therapy is begun. Otherwise-healthy hosts usually survive *C. fetus* infections without sequelae. Compromised hosts often have recurrent and/or life-threatening infections due to a variety of *Campylobacter* species.

FURTHER READINGS

HELMS M et al: Adverse health events associated with antimicrobial drug resistance in *Campylobacter* species: A registry-based cohort study. J Infect Dis 191:1050, 2005

LANG DR et al (eds): Development of Guillain-Barré syndrome following *Campylobacter* infection. J Infect Dis 176(Suppl 2):S91, 1997

LECUIT M et al: Immunoproliferative small intestinal disease associated with *Campylobacter jejuni*. N Engl J Med 350:239, 2004

MEAD PS et al: Food-related illness and death in the United States. Emerg Infect Dis 5:607, 1999

NACHAMKIN I, BLASER MJ (eds): *Campylobacter jejuni*, 2d ed. Washington, American Society for Microbiology, 2000

SMITH KE et al: Quinolone-resistant *Campylobacter jejuni* infections in Minnesota, 1992–1998. Investigation Team. N Engl J Med 340:1525, 1999

149 Cholera and Other Vibrioses
Matthew K. Waldor, Gerald T. Keusch

Members of the genus *Vibrio* cause a number of important infectious syndromes. Classic among them is cholera, a devastating diarrheal disease caused by *V. cholerae* that has been responsible for seven global pandemics and much suffering over the past two centuries. Epidemic cholera remains a significant public health concern in the developing world today. Other vibrioses caused by other *Vibrio* species include syndromes of diarrhea, soft tissue infection, or primary sepsis. All *Vibrio* species are highly motile, facultatively anaerobic, curved gram-negative rods with one or more flagella. In nature, vibrios most commonly reside in tidal rivers and bays under conditions of moderate salinity. They proliferate in the summer months when water temperatures exceed 20°C. As might be expected, the illnesses they cause also increase in frequency during the warm months.

CHOLERA

DEFINITION

Cholera is an acute diarrheal disease that can, in a matter of hours, result in profound, rapidly progressive dehydration and death. Accordingly, cholera gravis (the severe form of cholera) is a much-feared disease, particularly in its epidemic presentation. Fortunately, prompt aggressive fluid repletion and supportive care can obviate the high mortality that cholera has historically wrought. While the term *cholera* has occasionally been applied to any severely dehydrating secretory diarrheal illness, whether infectious in etiology or not, it has generally referred to disease caused by *V. cholerae* serogroup O1. In 1992, however, a new serogroup (O139) that causes epidemic cholera emerged on the Indian subcontinent and has since killed thousands of people.

MICROBIOLOGY AND EPIDEMIOLOGY

The species *V. cholerae* comprises a host of organisms classified on the basis of the carbohydrate determinants of their lipopolysaccharide (LPS) O antigens. Some 200 serogroups have now been recognized. They are divided into those that agglutinate in antisera to the O1 group antigen (*V. cholerae* O1) and those that do not (non-O1 *V. cholerae*). Although some non-O1 *V. cholerae* serogroups have occasionally caused sporadic outbreaks of diarrhea, serogroup O1 was, until the emergence of serogroup O139, the exclusive cause of epidemic cholera. Two biotypes of *V. cholerae* O1, classical and El Tor, are distinguished. Each biotype is further subdivided into two serotypes, termed *Inaba* and *Ogawa*.

The natural habitat of *V. cholerae* is coastal salt water and brackish estuaries, where the organism lives in close relation to plankton. Humans become infected incidentally but, once infected, can act as vehicles for spread. Ingestion of water contaminated by human feces is the most common means of acquisition of *V. cholerae*. Consumption of contaminated food can also contribute to spread. There is no known animal reservoir. While the infectious dose is relatively high, it is markedly reduced in hypochlorhydric persons, in those using antacids, and when gastric acidity is buffered by a meal. Cholera is predominantly a pediatric disease in endemic areas, but it affects adults and children equally when newly introduced into a population. Children <2 years of age are less likely to develop severe cholera than are older children, perhaps because of passive immunity acquired from breast milk. In endemic areas, the disease is more common in the summer and fall months. For unexplained reasons, susceptibility to cholera is significantly influenced by ABO blood group status; persons with type O blood are at greatest risk, while those with type AB are at least risk.

Cholera is native to the Ganges delta in the Indian subcontinent. Since 1817, seven global pandemics have occurred. The current (seventh) pandemic—the first due to the El Tor biotype—began in Indonesia in 1961 and spread throughout Asia as *V. cholerae* El Tor displaced the endemic classical strain. In the early 1970s, El Tor cholera erupted in Africa, causing major epidemics before becoming a persistent endemic problem. Currently, >90% of cholera cases reported annually to the World Health Organization (WHO) are from Africa (Fig. 149-1). In the period 2000–2004, the annual worldwide number of cholera cases reported to the WHO remained stable at ~100,000. This number is certainly a significant underestimate, as several nations with endemic cholera do not report cholera cases to the WHO.

The recent history of cholera has been punctuated by severe outbreaks. Such outbreaks are often precipitated by war or other circumstances that lead to the breakdown of public health measures. Such was the case in the camps for Rwandan refugees set up in 1994 around Goma, Zaire.

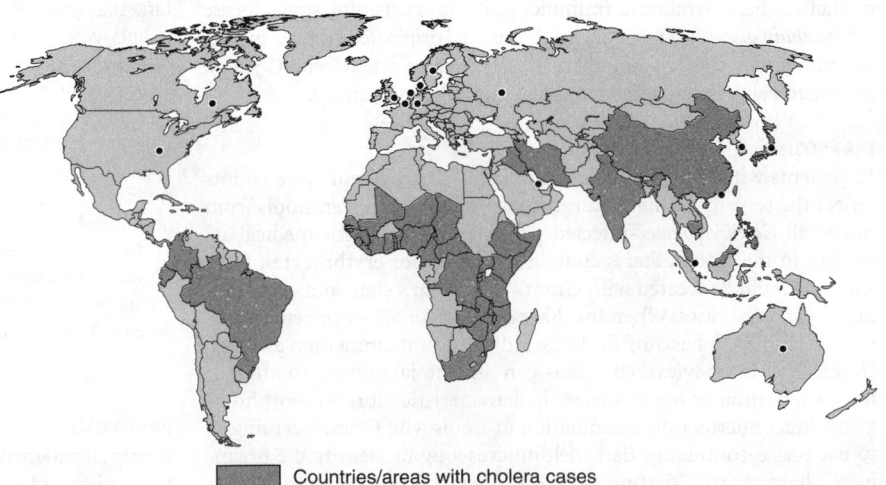

FIGURE 149-1 World distribution of cholera in 2004. *(Adapted from WHO: Cholera, 2004.)*

Countries/areas with cholera cases

● Imported cholera cases

FIGURE 149-2 Spread of *Vibrio cholerae* O1 in the Americas, 1991–1994. *(Courtesy of Dr. Robert V. Tauxe, Centers for Disease Control and Prevention, Atlanta; with permission.)*

FIGURE 149-3 Spread of *Vibrio cholerae* O139 in the Indian subcontinent and elsewhere in Asia, 1992–1994. *(Courtesy of Dr. Robert V. Tauxe, CDC, Atlanta; with permission.)*

Since 1973, sporadic endemic infections due to *V. cholerae* O1 strains related to the seventh-pandemic strain have been recognized along the U.S. Gulf Coast of Louisiana and Texas. These infections are typically associated with the consumption of contaminated, locally harvested shellfish. Occasionally, cases in U.S. locations remote from the Gulf Coast have been linked to shipped-in Gulf Coast seafood.

It was not until 1991 that the current cholera pandemic reached Latin America. Beginning along the Peruvian coast in January 1991, the disease spread in an explosive epidemic to virtually all of South and Central America and to Mexico (Fig. 149-2). About 400,000 cases were reported in the first year of the outbreak, and >1 million had been reported by the end of 1994. While the cumulative mortality rate has been <1%, the mortality rate approached 30% in the communities first affected, where a lack of familiarity with the disease led initially to the deployment of ineffective treatment. Intensive education of health care providers and of the community at large has enhanced awareness of the disease and its appropriate management and has greatly diminished mortality. As it did in Africa two decades earlier, the epidemic El Tor strain proved capable of establishing itself in inland waters rather than in its classic niche of coastal salt waters; the organism has already become endemic in many of the Latin American countries into which it was recently introduced. Cases linked to the Latin American epidemic have occurred (via importation of contaminated seafood) in the United States. Although secondary spread of this strain has not taken place in the United States, these events underscore the need for vigilance among health care professionals, even in locations remote from an epidemic.

In October 1992, a large-scale outbreak of clinical cholera occurred in southeastern India. The etiologic agent proved to be of a novel *V. cholerae* serogroup. This strain spread rapidly up and down the coast of the Bay of Bengal, reaching Bangladesh in December 1992. There alone, it caused more than 100,000 cases of cholera in the first 3 months of 1993. It subsequently spread across the Indian subcontinent and to neighboring countries, affecting Pakistan, Nepal, western China, Thailand, and Malaysia by the end of 1994 (Fig. 149-3). The organism has since been designated *V. cholerae* O139 Bengal in recognition of its novel O antigen and its geographic origin. The clinical manifestations and epidemiologic features of the disease caused by *V. cholerae* O139 Bengal are indistinguishable from those of O1 cholera. Immunity to the latter, however, is not protective against the former. Because naturally acquired immunity to *V. cholerae* O1 does not cross-protect

against *V. cholerae* O139 Bengal, vaccines being developed against the former are unlikely to be effective against the latter.

Some authorities believed that the emergence of *V. cholerae* O139 signaled the beginning of the eighth global cholera pandemic. Indeed, just as O1 El Tor replaced the classical biotype that preceded it, O139 Bengal in 1993 rapidly replaced O1 El Tor as the most common environmental isolate and the predominant cause of clinical cholera in the areas in which it had appeared. However, by the beginning of 1994, O1 El Tor had resumed its dominance in Bangladesh. *V. cholerae* O139 has not spread outside of Asia, and currently, in most regions of Southeast Asia, *V. cholerae* O1 remains dominant.

PATHOGENESIS

In the final analysis, cholera is a toxin-mediated disease. Its characteristic watery diarrhea is due to the action of cholera toxin, a potent protein enterotoxin elaborated by the organism after it colonizes the small intestine. For *V. cholerae* to colonize the small intestine and produce cholera toxin, it must first recognize, contend with, and traverse several hostile environments. The first of these is the acidic milieu of the stomach. To elude the bactericidal effects of gastric acidity, *V. cholerae* relies, at least in part, on a relatively large inoculum size (compared to that needed for colonization by *Shigella*, for instance). The organism must next traverse the mucous layer lining the small bowel. *V. cholerae* chemotaxis and motility and the action of a variety of proteases may allow the organism to traverse this gel covering the intestinal epithelium. The toxin-coregulated pilus (TCP), so named because its synthesis is regulated in parallel with that of cholera toxin, is essential for *V. cholerae* intestinal colonization. Cholera toxin, TCP, and several other virulence factors are coordinately regulated by ToxR. This protein modulates the expression of virulence genes in response to environmental signals via a cascade of regulatory proteins. Additional regulatory processes, including bacterial responses to the density of the bacterial population (in a phenomenon known as *quorum sensing*), control the virulence of *V. cholerae*.

Once established in the human small bowel, the organism produces cholera toxin, which consists of a monomeric enzymatic moiety (the A subunit) and a pentameric binding moiety (the B subunit). The B pentamer binds to G_{M1} ganglioside, a glycolipid on the surface of epithelial cells that serves as the toxin receptor and makes possible the delivery of the A subunit to its cytosolic target. The activated A subunit (A_1) irreversibly transfers ADP-ribose from nicotinamide adenine dinucleotide to its specific target protein, the GTP-binding regulatory component of adenylate cyclase. The ADP-ribosylated G protein upregulates the activity of adenylate cyclase; the result is the intracellular accumulation of high levels of cyclic AMP. In intestinal epithelial cells, cyclic AMP inhibits the absorptive sodium transport system in villus cells and activates the secretory chloride transport system in crypt cells, and these events lead to the accumulation of sodium chloride in the intestinal lumen. Since water moves passively to maintain osmolality, isotonic fluid accumulates in the lumen. When the volume of that fluid exceeds the capacity of the rest of the gut to resorb it, watery diarrhea results. Unless the wasted fluid and electrolytes are adequately replaced, shock (due to profound dehydration) and acidosis (due to loss of bicarbonate) follow. Although perturbation of the adenylate cyclase pathway is the primary mechanism by which cholera toxin causes excess fluid secretion, increasing evidence indicates that cholera toxin also enhances intestinal secretion via prostaglandins and/or neural histamine receptors.

The genes encoding cholera toxin (*ctxAB*) are part of the genome of a bacteriophage designated CTXΦ. The receptor for this phage on the *V. cholerae* surface is the intestinal colonization factor TCP. Since *ctxAB* is part of a mobile genetic element (CTXΦ), horizontal transfer of this bacteriophage may account for the emergence of new toxigenic *V. cholerae* serogroups. Many of the other genes important for *V. cholerae* pathogenicity, including the genes encoding the biosynthesis of TCP, those encoding accessory colonization factors, and those regulating virulence gene expression, are clustered together in the *V. cholerae* pathogenicity island. Similar clustering of virulence genes is found in other bacterial pathogens. It is believed that pathogenicity islands are acquired by horizontal gene transfer.

V. cholerae O139 Bengal is closely related to the O1 El Tor strains of the seventh pandemic and seems to have arisen from them by horizontal gene transfer. It shares the virulence attributes and general pathogenic mechanisms of O1 vibrios. *V. cholerae* O139 Bengal is in fact virtually identical to the seventh-pandemic strains of *V. cholerae* O1 El Tor except for two important differences: production of the novel O139 LPS and of an immunologically related O-antigen polysaccharide capsule. Encapsulation is not a feature of O1 strains and may explain the resistance of O139 strains to human serum in vitro as well as the occasional development of O139 bacteremia.

CLINICAL MANIFESTATIONS

After a 24- to 48-h incubation period, cholera begins with the sudden onset of painless watery diarrhea that may quickly become voluminous and is often followed shortly by vomiting. In severe cases, stool volume can exceed 250 mL/kg in the first 24 h. If fluids and electrolytes are not replaced, hypovolemic shock and death ensue. Fever is usually absent. Muscle cramps due to electrolyte disturbances are common. The stool has a characteristic appearance: a nonbilious, gray, slightly cloudy fluid with flecks of mucus, no blood, and a somewhat sweet, inoffensive odor. It has been called "rice-water" stool because of its resemblance to the water in which rice has been washed. Clinical symptoms parallel volume contraction: At losses of 3–5% of normal body weight, thirst develops; at 5–8%, postural hypotension, weakness, tachycardia, and decreased skin turgor are documented; and at >10%, oliguria, weak or absent pulses, sunken eyes (and, in infants, sunken fontanelles), wrinkled ("washerwoman") skin, somnolence, and coma are characteristic. Complications derive exclusively from the effects of volume and electrolyte depletion and include renal failure due to acute tubular necrosis. Thus, if the patient is adequately treated with fluid and electrolytes, complications are averted and the process is self-limited, resolving in a few days.

Laboratory data usually reveal an elevated hematocrit (due to hemoconcentration) in nonanemic patients; mild neutrophilic leukocytosis; elevated levels of blood urea nitrogen and creatinine consistent with prerenal azotemia; normal sodium, potassium, and chloride levels; a markedly reduced bicarbonate level (<15 mmol/L); and an elevated anion gap (due to increases in serum lactate, protein, and phosphate). Arterial pH is usually low (~7.2).

DIAGNOSIS

The clinical suspicion of cholera can be confirmed by the identification of *V. cholerae* in stool; however, the organism must be specifically sought. With experience, it can be detected directly by dark-field microscopy on a wet mount of fresh stool, and its serotype can be discerned by immobilization with specific antiserum. Laboratory isolation of the organism requires the use of a selective medium. The best of these is thiosulfate–citrate–bile salts–sucrose (TCBS) agar, on which the organism grows as a flat yellow colony. If a delay in sample processing is expected, Carey-Blair transport medium and/or alkaline-peptone water-enrichment medium should be inoculated as well. In endemic areas, there is little need for biochemical confirmation and characterization, although these tasks may be worthwhile in places where *V. cholerae* is an uncommon isolate. Standard microbiologic biochemical testing for Enterobacteriaceae will suffice for identification of *V. cholerae*. All vibrios are oxidase-positive.

The yield of stool cultures for the diagnosis of *V. cholerae* infection declines late in the course of the illness or when effective antibacterial therapy is initiated. Monoclonal antibody–based diagnostic kits and methods based on the polymerase chain reaction and on DNA probes have been developed for detection of *V. cholerae* O1 and O139.

℞ CHOLERA

Cholera is simple to treat; only the rapid and adequate replacement of fluids, electrolytes, and base is required. The mortality rate for appropriately treated disease is usually <1%. However, analysis of a large outbreak of cholera among airline travelers from an endemic country to the United States revealed frequent misdiagnoses by U.S. health professionals and poor appreciation on their part of the principles of management. Fluid replacement may be given orally, but oral rehydration is not always feasible in the presence of significant vomiting. Oral rehydration takes advantage of the hexose-Na⁺ cotransport mechanism to move Na⁺ across the gut mucosa together with an actively transported molecule such as glucose. For the sake of simplicity, the WHO advises routine use of a single solution of oral rehydration salts (ORS) for diarrheal disease rather than encouraging attempts to choose among multiple formulations according to etiology (Table 149-1). If available, rice-based ORS is considered superior to standard ORS in the treatment of cholera.

For initial management of severely dehydrated patients, IV fluid replacement is preferable. Because profound acidosis (pH < 7.2) is common in this group, Ringer's lactate is the best choice among commercial products (Table 149-2). It must be used with additional potassium supplements, preferably given by mouth. The total fluid deficit in severely dehydrated patients (≥10% of body weight) can be replaced safely within the first 4 h of therapy, half within the first hour. Thereafter, oral therapy can usually be initiated, with the goal of maintaining fluid intake equal to fluid output. However, patients with continued large-volume diarrhea may require prolonged IV treatment to keep up with gastrointestinal fluid losses. Severe hypokalemia can develop but will respond to potassium given either IV or orally. In the absence of adequate staff to monitor the patient's progress, the oral route of rehydration and potassium replacement is safer than the IV route.

Although not necessary for cure, the use of an antibiotic to which the organism is susceptible diminishes the duration and volume of fluid loss and

TABLE 149-1	COMPOSITION OF WORLD HEALTH ORGANIZATION ORAL REHYDRATION SOLUTION (ORS)ᵃ,ᵇ

Constituent	Concentration, mmol/L
Na⁺	75
K⁺	20
Cl⁻	65
Citrateᶜ	10
Glucose	75

ᵃContains (per package, to be added to 1 L of drinking water): NaCl, 2.6 g; Na₃C₆H₅O₇·2H₂O, 2.9 g; KCl, 1.5 g; and glucose, 15 g.
ᵇIf prepackaged ORS is unavailable, a simple homemade alternative can be prepared by combining 5 g NaCl (about 1 level teaspoon) with either 50 g precooked rice cereal or 40 g sucrose in 1 L of drinking water. In that case, potassium must be supplied separately (e.g., in orange juice or coconut water).
ᶜ10 mmol citrate per liter, which supplies 30 mmol HCO₃/L.

TABLE 149-2 ELECTROLYTE COMPOSITION OF CHOLERA STOOL AND OF INTRAVENOUS REHYDRATION SOLUTION

	Concentration, mmol/L			
Substance	Na+	K+	Cl−	Base
Stool				
Adult	135	15	90	30
Child	100	25	90	30
Ringer's lactate	130	4[a]	109	28

[a]Potassium supplements, preferably administered by mouth, are required to replace the usual potassium losses from stool.

hastens clearance of the organism from the stool. Single-dose tetracycline (2 g) or doxycycline (300 mg) is effective in adults but is not recommended for children <8 years of age because of possible deposition in bone and developing teeth. Emerging drug resistance is an ever-present concern. For adults with cholera in areas where tetracycline resistance is prevalent, ciprofloxacin [either in a single dose (30 mg/kg, not to exceed a total dose of 1 g) or in a short course (15 mg/kg bid for 3 days, not to exceed a total daily dose of 1 g)], erythromycin (a total of 40 mg/kg daily in three divided doses for 3 days), or a single 1-g dose of azithromycin is a clinically effective substitute. These drugs are highly effective in reducing total stool output and are significantly better than trimethoprim-sulfamethoxazole. For children, furazolidone has been the recommended agent and trimethoprim-sulfamethoxazole the second choice. Because of cost and/or toxicity issues related to the other drugs, erythromycin is a good choice for pediatric cholera.

PREVENTION

Provision of safe water and facilities for sanitary disposal of feces, improved nutrition, and attention to food preparation and storage in the household can significantly reduce the incidence of cholera.

Much effort has been devoted to the development of an effective cholera vaccine over the past two decades, with a particular focus on oral vaccine strains. Traditional killed cholera vaccine given intramuscularly provides little protection to nonimmune subjects and predictably causes adverse effects, including pain at the injection site, malaise, and fever. The vaccine's limited efficacy is due, at least in part, to its failure to induce a local immune response at the intestinal mucosal surface.

Two types of oral cholera vaccines have been developed. The first is a killed whole-cell (WC) vaccine. Two formulations of the killed WC vaccine have been prepared: one that also contains the nontoxic B subunit of cholera toxin (WC/BS) and one composed solely of killed bacteria. In field trials in Bangladesh, both of the killed vaccines offered significant protection from cholera compared with placebo for the first 6 months after vaccination, with protection rates of ~58% for WC and 85% for WC/BS. Protective efficacy rates for both vaccines declined to ~50% by 3 years after vaccine administration. Immunity was relatively sustained in persons vaccinated at an age of >5 years but was not well sustained in younger vaccinees. The WC/BS vaccine proved effective in a trial conducted in a sub-Saharan African population with a high prevalence of HIV infection. Killed oral vaccines also confer herd protection to unvaccinated individuals living in proximity to vaccinated individuals. Serious consideration should be given to the administration of the WC/BS vaccine in high-risk environments such as refugee camps. The WC/BS vaccine is available in Europe but not in the United States.

The second approach is a live attenuated vaccine strain developed, for example, by the isolation or creation of mutants lacking the genes encoding cholera toxin. Strain CVD 103-HgR, an oral live cholera vaccine licensed for immunization of travelers in Europe, is derived from a classical biotype strain of *V. cholerae* and contains a deletion of the cholera toxin A subunit gene. This strain has been extensively tested in volunteers; a single dose yielded a high degree of

protection against experimental challenge with classical *V. cholerae* strains, with almost no side effects. Protective efficacy was not as great against challenge with El Tor *V. cholerae*. Unfortunately, in a large field trial in Indonesian children, this vaccine failed to induce protection against clinical cholera. Other live attenuated vaccine candidate strains have been prepared from El Tor and O139 *V. cholerae* and are now undergoing clinical trials. Because of the minimal efficacy of existing parenteral vaccines, cholera immunization is recommended for U.S. travelers only if it is mandated by the countries they plan to visit.

OTHER *VIBRIO* SPECIES

The genus *Vibrio* includes several human pathogens that do not cause cholera. Abundant in coastal waters throughout the world, noncholera vibrios can reach high concentrations in the tissues of filter-feeding mollusks. As a result, human infection commonly follows the ingestion of seawater or of raw or undercooked shellfish (Table 149-3). Most noncholera vibrios can be cultured on blood or MacConkey agar, which contains enough salt to support the growth of these halophilic species. In the microbiology laboratory, the species of noncholera vibrios are distinguished by standard biochemical tests. The most important of these organisms are *V. parahaemolyticus* and *V. vulnificus*.

The two major types of syndromes for which these species are responsible are gastrointestinal illness (due to *V. parahaemolyticus*, non-O1 *V. cholerae*, *V. mimicus*, *V. fluvialis*, *V. hollisae*, and *V. furnissii*) and soft tissue infections (due to *V. vulnificus*, *V. alginolyticus*, and *V. damselae*). *V. vulnificus* is also a cause of primary sepsis in some compromised individuals. *V. parahaemolyticus* causes rare cases of wound infection and otitis and very rare cases of sepsis.

SPECIES ASSOCIATED PRIMARILY WITH GASTROINTESTINAL ILLNESS

V. parahaemolyticus Widespread in marine environments, *V. parahaemolyticus* grows in saline concentrations up to 8–10%. This species was originally implicated in enteritis in Japan in 1953, accounting for 24% of reported cases in one study—a rate that presumably was due to the common practice of eating raw seafood in that country. *V. parahaemolyticus* has since been identified as a significant intestinal pathogen in many regions of the world. In the United States, common-source outbreaks of diarrhea caused by this organism have been linked to the consumption of undercooked or improperly handled seafood or of other foods contaminated by seawater. Since the mid-1990s, the incidence of *V. parahaemolyticus* infections has increased in several countries, including the United States. Serotypes O3:K6, O4:K68, and O1:K-untypable, which are genetically related to one another, account for this increase. The enteropathogenicity of *V. parahaemolyticus* is closely linked to its ability to cause hemolysis on Wagatsuma agar (i.e., the *Kanagawa phenomenon*). Although the mechanism by which the organism causes diarrhea remains unclear, the genome sequence of *V. parahaemolyticus* contains a pathogenicity island—a cluster of likely virulence-associated genes. *V. parahaemolyticus* should be considered

TABLE 149-3 FEATURES OF SELECTED NONCHOLERA VIBRIOSES

Organism	Vehicle or Activity	Host at Risk	Syndrome
V. parahaemolyticus	Shellfish, seawater	Normal	Gastroenteritis
	Seawater	Normal	Wound infection
Non-O1 *V. cholerae*	Shellfish, travel	Normal	Gastroenteritis
	Seawater	Normal	Wound infection, otitis media
V. vulnificus	Shellfish	Immunosuppressed[a]	Sepsis, secondary cellulitis
	Seawater	Normal	Wound infection, cellulitis
V. alginolyticus	Seawater	Normal	Wound infection, cellulitis, otitis
	Seawater	Burned, other immunosuppressed	Sepsis

[a]Especially with liver disease or hemochromatosis.
Source: Table 161-3 in *Harrison's Principles of Internal Medicine*, 14th edition.

a possible etiologic agent in all cases of diarrhea that can be linked epidemiologically to seafood consumption or to the sea itself.

Infections with *V. parahaemolyticus* can result in two distinct gastrointestinal presentations. The more common of the two presentations (including nearly all cases in North America) is characterized by watery diarrhea, usually occurring in conjunction with abdominal cramps, nausea, and vomiting and accompanied in ~25% of cases by fever and chills. After an incubation period of 4 h to 4 days, symptoms develop and persist for a median of 3 days. Dysentery, the less common presentation, is characterized by severe abdominal cramps, nausea, vomiting, and bloody or mucoid stools.

Most cases of *V. parahaemolyticus*–associated gastrointestinal illness, regardless of the presentation, are self-limited and require neither antimicrobial treatment nor hospitalization. Deaths are extremely rare. Severe infections are associated with underlying diseases, including diabetes, preexisting liver disease, iron-overload states, or immunosuppression. The occasional severe case should be treated with fluid replacement and antibiotics, as described above for cholera.

Non-O1 *V. cholerae* The heterogeneous non-O1 *V. cholerae* organisms cannot be distinguished from *V. cholerae* O1 by routine biochemical tests but do not agglutinate in O1 antiserum. Non-O1 strains have caused several well-studied food-borne outbreaks of gastroenteritis and have also been responsible for sporadic cases of otitis media, wound infection, and bacteremia. Like other vibrios, non-O1 *V. cholerae* organisms are widely distributed in marine environments. In most instances, recognized cases in the United States have been associated with the consumption of raw oysters or with recent travel, typically to Mexico. The broad clinical spectrum of diarrheal illness caused by these organisms is probably due to the group's heterogeneous virulence attributes. *V. cholerae* O139 Bengal, although technically a non-O1 vibrio, is not grouped with these pathogens because it can cause epidemic cholera.

In the United States, about half of all non-O1 *V. cholerae* isolates are from stool samples. The typical incubation period for gastroenteritis due to these organisms is <2 days, and the illness lasts for ~2–7 days. Patients' stools may be copious and watery or may be partly formed, less voluminous, and bloody or mucoid. Diarrhea can result in severe dehydration. Many cases include abdominal cramps, nausea, vomiting, and fever. Like those with cholera, patients who are seriously dehydrated should receive oral or IV fluids; the value of antibiotics is not clear.

Extraintestinal infections due to non-O1 *V. cholerae* commonly follow occupational or recreational exposure to seawater. Around 10% of non-O1 *V. cholerae* isolates come from cases of wound infection, 10% from cases of otitis media, and 20% from cases of bacteremia (which is particularly likely to develop in patients with liver disease). Extraintestinal infections should be treated with antibiotics. Information to guide antibiotic selection and dosing is limited, but most strains are sensitive in vitro to tetracycline, ciprofloxacin, and third-generation cephalosporins.

SPECIES ASSOCIATED PRIMARILY WITH SOFT TISSUE INFECTION OR BACTEREMIA
(See also Chap. 119)

V. vulnificus *V. vulnificus* is the most common cause of severe vibrio infections in the United States. Like most vibrios, this organism proliferates in the warm summer months and requires a saline environment for growth. In this country, infections in humans typically occur in coastal states between May and October and most commonly affect men >40 years of age. *V. vulnificus* has been linked to two distinct syndromes: primary sepsis, which usually occurs in patients with underlying liver disease, and primary wound infection, which generally affects people without underlying disease. Some authors have suggested that *V. vulnificus* also causes gastroenteritis independent of other clinical manifestations. *V. vulnificus* is endowed with a number of virulence attributes, including a capsule that confers resistance to phagocytosis and to the bactericidal activity of human serum as well as a cytolysin. Measured as the 50% lethal dose in mice, the organism's virulence is considerably increased under conditions of iron overload; this obser-

vation is consistent with the propensity of *V. vulnificus* to infect patients who have hemochromatosis.

Primary sepsis most often develops in patients who have cirrhosis or hemochromatosis. However, *V. vulnificus* bacteremia can also affect individuals who have hematopoietic disorders or chronic renal insufficiency, those who are using immunosuppressive medications or alcohol, or (in rare instances) those who have no known underlying disease. After a median incubation period of 16 h, the patient develops malaise, chills, fever, and prostration. One-third of patients develop hypotension, which is often apparent at admission. Cutaneous manifestations develop in most cases (usually within 36 h of onset) and characteristically involve the extremities (the lower more often than the upper). In a common sequence, erythematous patches are followed by ecchymoses, vesicles, and bullae. In fact, sepsis and bullous skin lesions suggest the diagnosis in appropriate settings. Necrosis and sloughing may also be evident. Laboratory studies reveal leukopenia more often than leukocytosis, thrombocytopenia, or elevated levels of fibrin split products. *V. vulnificus* can be cultured from blood or cutaneous lesions. The mortality rate approaches 50%, with most deaths due to uncontrolled sepsis. Accordingly, prompt treatment is critical and should include empirical antibiotic administration, aggressive debridement, and general supportive care. *V. vulnificus* is sensitive in vitro to a number of antibiotics, including tetracycline, fluoroquinolones, and third-generation cephalosporins. Data from animal models suggest that either a fluoroquinolone or the combination of minocycline and cefotaxime should be used in the treatment of *V. vulnificus* septicemia.

V. vulnificus can infect either a fresh or an old wound that comes into contact with seawater; the patient may or may not have underlying disease. After a short incubation period (4 h to 4 days; mean, 12 h), the disease begins with swelling, erythema, and (in many cases) intense pain around the wound. These signs and symptoms are followed by cellulitis, which spreads rapidly and is sometimes accompanied by vesicular, bullous, or necrotic lesions. Metastatic events are uncommon. Most patients have a fever and leukocytosis. *V. vulnificus* can be cultured from skin lesions and occasionally from the blood. Prompt antibiotic therapy and debridement are usually curative.

V. alginolyticus First identified as a pathogen of humans in 1973, *V. alginolyticus* occasionally causes eye, ear, and wound infections. This species is the most salt-tolerant of the vibrios and can grow in salt concentrations of >10%. Most clinical isolates come from superinfected wounds that presumably become contaminated at the beach. Although severity varies, *V. alginolyticus* infection tends not to be serious and generally responds well to antibiotic therapy and drainage. A few cases of otitis externa, otitis media, and conjunctivitis due to this pathogen have been described. Tetracycline treatment usually results in cure. *V. alginolyticus* is a rare cause of bacteremia in immunocompromised hosts.

ACKNOWLEDGMENT
The authors gratefully acknowledge the valuable contributions of Dr. Robert Deresiewicz, a coauthor of this chapter for the 14th edition.

FURTHER READINGS

LUCAS MES et al: Effectiveness of mass oral cholera vaccination in Beira, Mozambique. N Engl J Med 352:757, 2005

SACK DA et al: Cholera. Lancet 363:223, 2004

SAHA D et al: Single-dose azithromycin for the treatment of cholera in adults. N Engl J Med 354:2452, 2006

TANG HJ et al: In vitro and in vivo activities of newer fluoroquinolones against *Vibrio vulnificus*. Antimicrob Agents Chemother 46:3580, 2002

WORLD HEALTH ORGANIZATION: *The Treatment of Diarrhoea: A Manual for Physicians and Other Senior Health Workers.* Geneva, World Health Organization, 2005 (*www.who.int/child-adolescent-health/New_Publications/CHILD_HEALTH/ISBN_92_4_159318_0.pdf*)

———: Cholera, 2004. Wkly Epidemiol Rec 80:261, 2005 (*www.who.int/wer*)

150 Brucellosis
Michael J. Corbel, Nicholas J. Beeching

DEFINITION

Brucellosis is a bacterial zoonosis transmitted directly or indirectly to humans from infected animals, predominantly domesticated ruminants and swine. The disease is known colloquially as *undulant fever* because of its remittent character. Its distribution is worldwide apart from the few countries where it has been eradicated from the animal reservoir. Although brucellosis commonly presents as an acute febrile illness, its clinical manifestations vary widely, and definitive signs indicative of the diagnosis may be lacking. Thus the clinical diagnosis usually must be supported by the results of bacteriologic and/or serologic tests.

ETIOLOGIC AGENTS

Human brucellosis is caused by strains of *Brucella*, a bacterial genus that has been suggested, on genetic grounds, to comprise a single species, *Brucella melitensis*, with a number of biologic variants that exhibit particular host preferences. Recently, this view has been challenged on the basis of detailed differences in chromosomal structure and host preference. The traditional classification into nomen species is now favored both because of these differences and because this classification scheme closely reflects the epidemiologic patterns of the infection. The nomen system recognizes *B. melitensis*, which is the commonest cause of symptomatic disease in humans and for which the main sources are sheep, goats, and camels; *B. abortus*, which is usually acquired from cattle or buffalo: *B. suis*, which generally is acquired from swine but has one variant enzootic in reindeer and caribou and another in rodents; and *B. canis*, which is acquired most often from dogs. *B. ovis*, which causes reproductive disease in sheep, and *B. neotomae*, which is specific for desert rodents, have not been clearly implicated in human disease. Other brucellae have been isolated from marine mammals, and two new nomen species, *B. cetaceae* and *B. pinnipediae*, have been proposed. At least one case of laboratory-acquired human disease due to one of these proposed species has been described, and apparent cases of natural infection have been reported. As infections in marine mammals seem widespread, more cases of zoonotic infection may be identified.

All brucellae are small, gram-negative, unencapsulated, nonsporulating rods or coccobacilli. They grow aerobically on peptone-based medium incubated at 37° C; the growth of some types is improved by supplementary CO_2. In vivo, brucellae behave as facultative intracellular parasites. The organisms are sensitive to sunlight, ionizing radiation, and moderate heat; they are killed by boiling and pasteurization but are resistant to freezing and drying. Their resistance to drying renders brucellae stable in aerosol form, facilitating airborne transmission. The organisms can survive for up to 2 months in soft cheeses made from goat's or sheep's milk; for at least 6 weeks in dry soil contaminated with infected urine, vaginal discharge, or placental or fetal tissues; and for at least 6 months in damp soil or liquid manure kept under cool dark conditions. Brucellae are easily killed by a wide range of common disinfectants used under optimal conditions but are likely to be much more resistant at low temperatures or in the presence of heavy organic contamination.

EPIDEMIOLOGY

Brucellosis is a zoonosis whose occurrence is closely related to its prevalence in domesticated animals. The true global prevalence of human brucellosis is unknown because of the imprecision of diagnosis and the inadequacy of reporting and surveillance systems in many countries. Even in developed countries, the true incidence may be 10–20 times higher than the reported figures. Bovine brucellosis has been the target of control programs in many parts of the world and has been eradicated from the cattle populations of Australia, New Zealand, Bulgaria, Canada, Cyprus, Great Britain (including the Channel Islands), Japan, Luxembourg, Romania, the Scandinavian countries, Switzerland, and the Czech and Slovak Republics. Its incidence has been reduced to a low level in the United States and most Western European countries, with a varied picture in other parts of the world. There is evidence of a resurgence in Eastern Europe following economic changes in recent years, and new outbreaks have also occurred in Ireland. Efforts to eradicate *B. melitensis* infection from sheep and goat populations have been much less successful. These efforts have relied heavily on vaccination programs, which have tended to fluctuate with changing economic and political conditions. In some countries (e.g., Israel), *B. melitensis* has caused serious outbreaks in cattle. Infections with *B. melitensis* still pose a major public health problem in Mediterranean countries; in western, central, and southern Asia; and in parts of Africa and South and Central America.

Human brucellosis is usually associated with occupational or domestic exposure to infected animals or their products. Farmers, shepherds, goatherds, veterinarians, and employees in slaughterhouses and meat-processing plants in endemic areas are occupationally exposed to infection. Family members of individuals involved in animal husbandry may be at risk, although it is often difficult to differentiate food-borne infection from environmental contamination under these circumstances. Laboratory workers who handle cultures or infected samples are also at risk. Travelers and urban dwellers usually acquire the infection through consumption of contaminated foods. In countries that have eradicated the disease, new cases are most commonly acquired abroad. Dairy products, especially soft cheeses, unpasteurized milk, and ice cream, are the most frequently implicated sources of infection; raw meat and bone marrow may be sources under exceptional circumstances. Infections acquired through cosmetic treatments using materials of fetal origin have been reported. Person-to-person transmission is extremely rare, as is transfer of infection by blood or tissue donation. Although brucellosis is a chronic intracellular infection, there is no evidence for increased prevalence or severity among individuals with HIV infection or with immunodeficiency or immunosuppression of other etiologies.

Brucellosis may be acquired by ingestion, inhalation, or mucosal or percutaneous exposure. Accidental injection of the live vaccine strains of *B. abortus* (19 and RB51) and *B. melitensis* (Rev 1) can cause disease. *B. melitensis* and *B. suis* have been developed as biological weapons by several countries and could be exploited for bioterrorism (Chap. 214). This possibility should be borne in mind in the event of sudden unexplained outbreaks.

IMMUNITY AND PATHOGENESIS

Exposure to brucellosis elicits both humoral and cell-mediated immune responses. The mechanisms of protective immunity against human brucellosis are presumed to be similar to those documented in laboratory animals. The response to infection and its outcome are influenced by the virulence, phase, and species of the infecting strain. Differences have been reported between *B. abortus* and *B. suis* in the modes of cellular entry and subsequent compartmentalization and processing. Antibodies promote clearance of extracellular brucellae by bactericidal action and by facilitation of phagocytosis by polymorphonuclear and mononuclear phagocytes; however, antibodies alone cannot eradicate infection. Organisms taken up by macrophages and other cells can establish persistent intracellular infections. The key target cell is the macrophage, and bacterial mechanisms for suppressing intracellular killing and apoptosis result in very large intracellular populations. Opsonized bacteria are actively phagocytosed by neutrophilic granulocytes and by monocytes. In these and other cells, initial attachment takes place via specific receptors, including Fc, C3, fibronectin, and mannose-binding proteins. Opsonized—but not unopsonized—bacteria trigger an oxidative burst inside phagocytes. Unopsonized bacteria are internalized via similar receptors but at much lower efficiency. Smooth strains enter host cells via lipid rafts. Smooth lipopolysaccharide (LPS), β-cyclic glucan, and possibly an invasion-attachment protein (IalB) are involved in this process. Tumor necrosis factor α (TNF-α) produced early in the course of infection stimulates cytotoxic lymphocytes and activates macrophages, which can kill intracellular brucellae (probably mainly through production of reactive oxygen and nitrogen intermediates) and may clear infection. However, virulent *Brucella* cells can suppress the TNF-α response, and control of infection in this situation depends on macrophage activation and interferon γ (IFN-γ) responses. Cytokines such as interleukin (IL) 12 promote production of IFN-γ, which drives T_H1-type responses and stimulates macrophage activation. Inflammatory cytokines, including IL-4, IL-6, and IL-10, downregulate the protective response. As in other types of intracellular infection, it is assumed that initial replication of brucellae takes place within cells of the lymph nodes draining the point of entry. Subsequent hematogenous spread may result in chronic localizing infection at almost any site, although the reticuloendothelial system, musculoskeletal tissues, and genitourinary system are most frequently targeted. Both acute and chronic inflammatory responses develop in brucellosis, and the local tissue response may include granuloma formation with or without necrosis and caseation. Abscesses may also develop, especially in chronic localized infection.

The determinants of pathogenicity of *Brucella* have not been fully characterized, and the mechanisms underlying the manifestations of brucellosis are incompletely understood. The organism's survival strategy is centered on processes that permit survival within monocytic cells. The smooth *Brucella* LPS, which has an unusual O-chain and core-lipid composition, has relatively low endotoxin activity and plays a key role in pyrogenicity and in resistance to phagocytosis and serum killing in the nonimmune host. LPS is believed also to play a key role in suppressing phagosome-lysosome fusion and diverting the internalized bacteria into vacuoles located in endoplasmic reticulum, where intracellular replication takes place. Specific exotoxins have not been isolated, but a type IV secretion system (VirB) that regulates intracellular survival and trafficking has been identified. In *B. abortus* this system can be activated extracellularly, but in *B. suis* it is activated (by low pH) only during intracellular growth. Brucellae then produce acid-stable proteins that facilitate the organisms' survival in phagosomes and may enhance their resistance to reactive oxygen intermediates. Virulent brucellae are resistant to defensins and produce a Cu-Zn superoxide dismutase that increases their resistance to reactive oxygen intermediates.

CLINICAL FEATURES

Brucellosis almost invariably causes fever, which may be associated with profuse sweats, especially at night. In endemic areas, brucellosis may be difficult to distinguish from the many other causes of fever. However, two features recognized in the nineteenth century distinguish brucellosis from other tropical fevers, such as typhoid and malaria. (1) Left untreated, the fever of brucellosis shows an undulating pattern that persists for weeks before the commencement of an afebrile period that may be followed by relapse. (2) The fever of brucellosis is associated with musculoskeletal symptoms and signs in about one-half of all patients.

The clinical syndromes caused by the different nomen species are similar, although *B. melitensis* tends to be associated with a more acute and aggressive presentation and *B. suis* with focal abscess induction. *B. abortus* infections may be more insidious in onset and more likely to become chronic.

The incubation period varies from 1 week to several months, and the onset of fever and other symptoms may be abrupt or insidious. In addition to experiencing fever and sweats, patients become increasingly apathetic and fatigued; lose appetite and weight; and have nonspecific myalgia, headache, and chills. Overall, the presentation of brucellosis often fits one of three patterns: febrile illness that resembles typhoid but is less severe; fever and acute monoarthritis, typically of the hip or knee, in a young child; and long-lasting fever, misery, and low-back or hip pain in an older man. In an endemic area (e.g., much of the Middle East), a patient with fever and difficulty walking into the clinic would be regarded as having brucellosis until it was proved otherwise.

Diagnostic clues in the patient's history include travel to an endemic area, employment in a diagnostic microbiology laboratory, con-

TABLE 150-1	RADIOLOGY OF THE SPINE: DIFFERENTIATION OF BRUCELLOSIS FROM TUBERCULOSIS	
	Brucellosis	**Tuberculosis**
Site	Lumbar and others	Dorsolumbar
Vertebrae	Multiple or contiguous	Contiguous
Diskitis	Late	Early
Body	Intact until late	Morphology lost early
Canal compression	Rare	Common
Epiphysitis	Anterosuperior (Pom's sign)	General: upper and lower disk regions, central, subperiosteal
Osteophyte	Anterolateral (parrot beak)	Unusual
Deformity	Wedging uncommon	Anterior wedge, gibbus
Recovery	Sclerosis, whole body	Variable
Paravertebral abscess	Small, well-localized	Common and discrete loss, transverse process
Psoas abscess	Rare	More likely

sumption of unpasteurized milk products (including soft cheeses), contact with animals, and—in an endemic setting—a history of similar illness in the family (documented in almost 50% of cases).

Focal features are present in the majority of patients. The most common are musculoskeletal pain and physical findings in the peripheral and axial skeleton (~40% of cases). Osteomyelitis more commonly involves the lumbar and low thoracic vertebrae than the cervical and high thoracic spine. Individual joints that are most commonly affected by septic arthritis are the knee, hip, sacroiliac, shoulder, and sternoclavicular joints; the pattern may be one of monoarthritis or polyarthritis. Osteomyelitis may also accompany septic arthritis.

In addition to the usual causes of vertebral osteomyelitis or septic arthritis, the most important differential diagnosis is tuberculosis. This point influences the therapeutic approach as well as the prognosis, given that several antimicrobial agents used to treat brucellosis are also used to treat tuberculosis. Septic arthritis in brucellosis progresses slowly, starting with small pericapsular erosions. In the vertebrae, anterior erosions of the superior end plate are typically the first features to become evident, with eventual involvement and sclerosis of the whole vertebra. Anterior osteophytes eventually develop, but vertebral destruction or impingement on the spinal cord is rare and usually suggests tuberculosis (Table 150-1).

Other systems may be involved in a manner that resembles typhoid. About one-quarter of patients have a dry cough, usually with few changes visible on the chest x-ray, although pneumonia, empyema, intrathoracic adenopathy, or lung abscess can occur. One-quarter of patients have hepatosplenomegaly, and 10–20% have significant lymphadenopathy; the differential diagnosis includes glandular fever–like illness such as that caused by Epstein-Barr virus, *Toxoplasma*, and cytomegalovirus; HIV infection; or tuberculosis. Up to 10% of men have acute epididymoorchitis, which must be distinguished from mumps and from surgical problems such as torsion. Prostatitis, inflammation of the seminal vesicles, salpingitis, and pyelonephritis all occur. There is an increased incidence of fetal loss among infected pregnant women, although teratogenicity has not been described and the tendency to cause abortions is much less pronounced in humans than in farm animals.

Neurologic involvement is common, with depression and lethargy whose severity may not be truly appreciated by either the patient or the physician until after treatment. A small proportion of patients develop lymphocytic meningoencephalitis that mimics neurotuberculosis or noninfectious conditions and that may be complicated by intracerebral abscess, a variety of cranial nerve deficits, or ruptured mycotic aneurysms.

Endocarditis occurs in ~1% of cases, most often affecting the aortic valve (natural or prosthetic). Any site in the body may be involved in metastatic abscess formation or inflammation; the female breast and the thyroid gland are affected particularly often. Nonspecific maculo-

FIGURE 150-1 Liver biopsy specimen from a patient with brucellosis shows a noncaseating granuloma. *[From Mandell's Atlas of Infectious Diseases, Vol II, in DL Stevens (ed): Skin, Soft Tissue, Bone and Joint Infections, Fig. 5-9; with permission.]*

papular rashes and other skin manifestations are uncommon and are rarely noticed by the patient even if they are present.

DIAGNOSIS

Because the clinical picture of brucellosis is not distinctive, the diagnosis must be based on a history of potential exposure, a presentation consistent with the disease, and supporting laboratory findings. Results of routine biochemical assays are usually within normal limits, although serum levels of hepatic enzymes and bilirubin may be elevated. Peripheral leukocyte counts are usually normal or low, with relative lymphocytosis. Mild anemia may be documented. Thrombocytopenia and disseminated intravascular coagulation with raised levels of fibrinogen degradation products can develop. The erythrocyte sedimentation rate and C-reactive protein levels are often normal but may be raised.

In body fluids such as cerebrospinal fluid (CSF) or joint fluid, lymphocytosis and low glucose levels are the norm. Elevated CSF levels of adenosine deaminase cannot be used to distinguish tubercular meningitis, as they may also be found in brucellosis. Biopsied samples of tissues such as lymph node or liver may show noncaseating granulomas (Fig. 150-1) without acid/alcohol-fast bacilli. The radiologic features of bony disease develop late and are much more subtle than those of tuberculosis or septic arthritis of other etiologies, with less bone and joint destruction. Isotope scanning is more sensitive than plain x-ray and continues to give positive results long after successful treatment.

Isolation of brucellae from blood, CSF, bone marrow, or joint fluid or from a tissue aspirate or biopsy sample is definitive, and attempts at isolation are usually successful in 50–70% of cases. Duplicate cultures should be incubated for up to 6 weeks (in air and 10% CO$_2$, respectively). Concentration and lysis of buffy coat cells before culture may increase the isolation rate. Cultures in modern nonradiometric or similar signaling systems (e.g., Bactec) usually become positive within 7–10 days but should be maintained for at least 3 weeks before the results are declared negative. All cultures should be handled under containment conditions appropriate for dangerous pathogens. *Brucella* spp. may be misidentified as *Agrobacterium*, *Ochrobactrum*, or *Psychrobacter (Moraxella) phenylpyruvicus* by the gallery identification strips commonly used in the diagnostic laboratory.

The peripheral blood–based polymerase chain reaction (PCR) has enormous potential to detect bacteremia, to predict relapse, and to exclude "chronic brucellosis." PCR is probably more sensitive and is certainly quicker than blood culture, and it does not carry the attendant biohazard risk posed by culture. Nucleic acid amplification techniques are now quite widely used, although no single standardized procedure has been adopted. Primers for the spacer region between the genes encoding the 16S and 23S ribosomal RNAs (*rrs-rrl*), the outer membrane

protein Omp2, the insertion sequence *IS711*, and protein BCSP31 are sensitive and specific. Blood and other tissues are the most suitable samples for analysis.

Serologic examination often provides the only positive laboratory findings in brucellosis. In acute infection, IgM antibodies appear early and are followed by IgG and IgA. All these antibodies are active in agglutination tests, whether performed by tube, plate, or microagglutination methods. The majority of patients have detectable agglutinins at this stage. As the disease progresses, IgM levels decline, and the avidity and subclass distribution of IgG and IgA change. The result is reduced or undetectable agglutinin titers. However, the antibodies are detectable by alternative tests, including the complement fixation test, Coombs' antiglobulin test, and enzyme-linked immunosorbent assay. There is no clear cutoff value for a diagnostic titer. Rather, serology results must be interpreted in the context of exposure history and clinical presentation. In endemic areas or in settings of potential occupational exposure, agglutinin titers of 1:320–1:640 or higher are considered diagnostic; in nonendemic areas, a titer of ≥1:160 is considered significant. Repetition of tests after 2–4 weeks may demonstrate a rising titer.

In most centers, the standard agglutination test (SAT) is still the mainstay of serologic diagnosis, although some investigators rely on the rose bengal test, which has not been fully validated for human diagnostic use. Dipstick assays for anti-*Brucella* IgM are useful for the diagnosis of acute infection but are less sensitive for infection with symptoms of several months' duration. In an endemic setting, >90% of patients with acute bacteremia have SAT titers of at least 1:320.

Antibody to the *Brucella* LPS O chain—the dominant antigen—is detected by all the conventional tests that employ smooth *B. abortus* cells as antigen. Since *B. abortus* cross-reacts with *B. melitensis* and *B. suis*, there is no advantage in replicating the tests with these antigens. Cross-reactions also occur with the O chains of some other gram-negative bacteria, including *Escherichia coli* O157, *Francisella tularensis*, *Salmonella enterica* group N, *Stenotrophomonas maltophilia*, and *Vibrio cholerae*. Cross-reactions do not occur with the cell-surface antigens of rough *Brucella* strains such as *B. canis* or *B. ovis*; serologic tests for these nomen species must employ an antigen prepared from either one. Most protein antigens are shared by all *Brucella* strains, and some are also common to *Ochrobactrum* species. Immunoblotting against protein extracts has been advocated as a differential test, but no validated procedure is yet available.

℞ BRUCELLOSIS

The broad aims of antimicrobial therapy are to treat current infection and relieve its symptoms and to prevent relapse. Focal disease presentations may require specific intervention in addition to more prolonged and tailored antibiotic therapy. In addition, tuberculosis must always be excluded, or—to prevent the emergence of resistance—therapy must be tailored to specifically exclude drugs active against tuberculosis (e.g., rifampin used alone) or to include a full antituberculous regimen.

Early experience with streptomycin monotherapy showed that relapse was common; thus dual therapy with tetracyclines became the norm. This is still the most effective combination, but alternatives may be used, with the options depending on local or national policy about the use of rifampin for the treatment of nonmycobacterial infection. Antimicrobial efficacy can usually be predicted by in vitro testing; however, the use of fluoroquinolones remains controversial despite the good in vitro activity and white cell penetration of most agents of this class. Low intravacuolar pH is probably a factor in the poor performance of these drugs.

For adults with acute nonfocal brucellosis (duration, <1 month), a 6-week course of therapy incorporating at least two antimicrobial agents is required. Complex or focal disease necessitates ≥3 months of therapy. Adherence to the therapeutic regimen is very important, and poor compliance underlies almost all cases of apparent treatment failure; such failure is rarely due to the emergence of drug resistance, although increasing resistance to trimethoprim-sulfamethoxazole (TMP-SMX) has been reported at one center. There is good retrospective evidence that a 3-week course of two agents is as effective as a 6-week course for treatment and prevention of relapse in children, but this point has not yet been proven in prospective studies.

The "gold standard" for the treatment of brucellosis in adults is IM streptomycin (0.75–1 g daily for 14–21 days) together with doxycycline (100 mg twice daily for 6 weeks). In both clinical trials and observational studies, relapse follows such treatment in 5–10% of patients. The usual alternative regimen (and the current World Health Organization recommendation) is rifampin (600–900 mg/d) plus doxycycline (100 mg twice daily) for 6 weeks. The relapse/failure rate is ~10% in trial conditions but rises to >20% in many nontrial situations, possibly because doxycycline levels are reduced and clearance rates increased by concomitant rifampin administration. Patients who cannot tolerate or receive tetracyclines (children, pregnant women) can be given high-dose TMP-SMX instead (2 or 3 standard-strength tablets twice daily for adults, depending on weight).

Evidence is beginning to accumulate that other aminoglycosides can be substituted for streptomycin—e.g., netilmicin or gentamicin given at a dosage of 5–6 mg/kg per day for at least 2 weeks. (Shorter courses have been associated with high failure rates in adults.) A 5- to 7-day course of therapy with gentamicin (and a 3-week course of TMP-SMX) is probably adequate for children with uncomplicated disease. Early experience with fluoroquinolone monotherapy was disappointing, but high-dose ofloxacin (400 mg twice daily) or ciprofloxacin (500 mg twice daily), given together with rifampin for 6 weeks, may become accepted as an alternative to the other 6-week regimens for adults.

Significant neurologic disease due to *Brucella* requires prolonged treatment (i.e., for 3–6 months), usually with ceftriaxone supplementation of a standard regimen. *Brucella* endocarditis is treated with at least three drugs (an aminoglycoside, a tetracycline, and rifampin), and many experts add ceftriaxone and/or a fluoroquinolone to reduce the need for valve replacement. Treatment is usually given for at least 6 months, and clinical endpoints for its discontinuation are often difficult to define. Surgery is still required for the majority of cases of infection of prosthetic heart valves and prosthetic joints.

There is no evidence base to guide prophylaxis after exposure to brucellae (e.g., in the laboratory), inadvertent immunization with live vaccine intended for use in animals, or deliberately released brucellae. Most authorities recommend the administration of rifampin plus doxycycline for 3 weeks after a low-risk exposure (e.g., a nonspecific laboratory accident) and for 6 weeks after a major exposure to aerosol or injected material. However, such regimens are poorly tolerated, and doxycycline monotherapy of the same duration may be substituted.

PROGNOSIS AND FOLLOW-UP

Relapse occurs in up to 30% of poorly compliant patients. Thus patients should ideally be followed clinically for up to 2 years to detect relapse, which responds to a prolonged course of the same therapy used originally. The general well-being and the body weight of the patient are more useful guides than serology to lack of relapse. IgG antibody levels detected by the SAT and its variants can remain in the diagnostic range for >2 years after successful treatment. Complement fixation titers usually fall to normal within 1 year of cure. Immunity is not solid; patients can be reinfected after repeated exposures. Fewer than 1% of patients die of brucellosis. When the outcome is fatal, death is usually a consequence of cardiac involvement; more rarely, it results from severe neurologic disease. Despite the low mortality rate, recovery from brucellosis is slow, and the illness can cause prolonged inactivity, with consequent domestic and economic losses.

The existence of a prolonged chronic brucellosis state after successful treatment remains controversial. Evaluation of patients in whom this state is considered (often those with work-related exposure to brucellae) includes careful exclusion of malingering, nonspecific chronic fatigue syndromes, and other causes of excessive sweating, such as alcohol abuse and obesity. In the future, the availability of more sensitive assays to detect *Brucella* antigen or DNA may help to identify patients with ongoing infection.

PREVENTION

Vaccines based on live attenuated *Brucella* strains, such as *B. abortus* strain 19BA or 104M, have been used in some countries to protect high-risk populations but have displayed only short-term efficacy and high reactogenicity. Subunit vaccines have been developed but are of uncertain value and cannot be recommended at present. Research in this area has been stimulated by interest in biodefense (Chap. 214) and may eventually yield new products, some of which may be based on the live attenuated WR 201 variant of *B. melitensis* strain 16M. The mainstay of veterinary prevention is a national commitment to testing and slaughter of infected herds/flocks (with compensation for owners), control of animal movement, and active immunization of animals. These measures are usually sufficient to control human disease as well. In their absence, pasteurization of all milk products before consumption is sufficient to prevent nonoccupational animal-to-human transmission. All cases of brucellosis in animals and humans should be reported to the appropriate public health authorities.

FURTHER READINGS

ALMUNEEF M, MEMISH ZA: Prevalence of brucella antibodies after acute brucellosis. J Chemother 15:148, 2003

CORBEL MJ, BANAI M: Genus *Brucella* Meyer and Shaw 1920,173[AL], in *Bergey's Manual of Systematic Bacteriology*, 2d ed, vol 2: *The Proteobacteria*, DJ Bruner et al (eds). New York, Springer, 2006, pp 370–386

HASANJANI ROUSHAN MR et al: Efficacy of gentamicin and doxycycline versus streptomycin plus doxycycline in the treatment of brucellosis in humans. Clin Infect Dis 42:1075, 2006

KHAN MY et al: Brucellosis in pregnant women. Clin Infect Dis 32:1172, 2000

MALEY MW et al: Prevention of laboratory-acquired brucellosis: Significant side effects of prophylaxis. Clin Infect Dis 42:433, 2006

MEMISH Z et al: *Brucella* bacteraemia: Clinical and laboratory observations in 160 patients. J Infect 40:59, 2000

NAVARRO E et al: Use of real time quantitative polymerase chain reaction to monitor the evolution of *Brucella melitensis* DNA load during therapy and post-therapy follow-up in patients with brucellosis. Clin Infect Dis 42:1266, 2006

PAPPAS G et al: New approaches to the antibiotic therapy of brucellosis. Int J Antimicrob Agents 26:101, 2005

——— et al: Brucellosis. N Engl J Med 352:2325, 2005

SALTOGLU N et al: Efficacy of rifampicin plus doxycycline versus rifampicin plus quinolone in the treatment of brucellosis. Saudi Med J 23:921, 2002

151 Tularemia
Richard F. Jacobs, Gordon E. Schutze

DEFINITION

Tularemia is a zoonosis caused by *Francisella tularensis*. Humans of any age, sex, or race are universally susceptible to this systemic infection. Tularemia is primarily a disease of wild animals and persists in contaminated environments, ectoparasites, and animal carriers. Human infection is incidental and usually results from interaction with biting or blood-sucking insects, contact with wild or domestic animals, ingestion of contaminated water or food, or inhalation of infective aerosols.

Tularemia is common in Arkansas, Oklahoma, and Missouri, where >50% of the cases in the United States occur. Increasing numbers of cases have been reported from the Scandinavian countries, eastern Europe, and Siberia. The illness is characterized by various clinical syndromes, the most common of which consists of an ulcerative lesion at the site of inoculation, with regional lymphadenopathy and lymphadenitis. Systemic manifestations, including pneumonia, typhoidal tularemia, and fever without localizing findings, pose a greater diagnostic challenge.

ETIOLOGY AND EPIDEMIOLOGY

With rare exceptions, tularemia is the only disease produced by *F. tularensis*—a small (0.2 μm by 0.2–0.7 μm), gram-negative, pleomorphic, nonmotile, non-spore-forming bacillus. Bipolar staining results in a coccoid appearance. The organism is a thinly encapsulated, nonpiliated strict aerobe that invades host cells. In nature, *F. tularensis* is a hardy organism that persists for weeks or months in mud, water, and decaying animal carcasses. Dozens of biting and blood-sucking insects, especially ticks and tabanid flies, serve as vectors. Ticks and wild rabbits are the source for most of the human cases in the endemic areas of the southeastern and Rocky Mountain states. In Utah, Nevada, and California, tabanid flies are the most common vectors. Animal reservoirs include wild rabbits, squirrels, birds, sheep, beavers, muskrats, and domestic dogs and cats. Person-to-person transmission is rare or nonexistent. Tularemia is more common among men than among women.

The two main biovars of *F. tularensis*—*tularensis* (type A) and *holarctica* (type B)—are both found in the United States. Type A produces more serious disease in humans; without treatment, the associated fatality rate is ~5%. Type B produces a milder, often subclinical infection that is usually contracted from water or marine mammals. Although all strains appear serologically identical, individual strains may possess varying degrees of virulence. Currently, there are four proposed subspecies among which 16S RNA analyses show ≥ 99.8% similarity. *F. tularensis* does not produce an exotoxin, but an endotoxin similar to that of other gram-negative bacilli has been identified. The progression of illness depends on the organism's virulence, the inoculum size, the portal of entry, and the host's immune status.

Ticks pass *F. tularensis* to their offspring transovarially. The organism is found in tick feces but not in large quantities in tick salivary glands. In the United States, the disease is carried by *Dermacentor andersoni* (Rocky Mountain wood tick), *D. variabilis* (American dog tick), *D. occidentalis* (Pacific coast dog tick), and *Amblyomma americanum* (Lone Star tick). *F. tularensis* is transmitted frequently during blood meals taken by embedded ticks after hours of attachment. It is the taking of a blood meal through a fecally contaminated field that transmits the organism. Transmission of the organism by ticks and tabanid flies takes place mainly in the spring and summer. However, continued transmission in the winter by trapped or hunted animals has been documented. The organism is extremely infectious. Biosafety level 2 is recommended for clinical laboratory work with material whose contamination with *F. tularensis* is suspected, and biosafety level 3 is required for culture of the organism in large quantities. Issues related to the intentional spread of tularemia through ingestion or inhalation are discussed in Chap. 214.

PATHOGENESIS AND PATHOLOGY

The most common portal of entry for human infection is through skin or mucous membranes, either directly—through the bite of ticks, other arthropods, or other animals—or via inapparent abrasions. Inhalation or ingestion of *F. tularensis* also can result in infection. Although >10^8 organisms are usually required to produce infection via the oral route (oropharyngeal or gastrointestinal tularemia), fewer than 50 organisms will result in infection when injected into the skin (ulceroglandular/glandular tularemia) or inhaled (tularemia pneumonia). After inoculation into the skin, the organism multiplies locally; within 2–5 days (range, 1–10 days), it produces an erythematous, tender, or pruritic papule. The papule rapidly enlarges and forms an ulcer with a black base (chancriform lesion). The bacteria spread to regional lymph nodes, producing lymphadenopathy (buboes), and, with bacteremia, may spread to distant organs.

Tularemia is characterized by mononuclear cell infiltration with pyogranulomatous pathology. The histopathologic findings can be quite similar to those in tuberculosis, although tularemia develops more rapidly. As a facultatively intracellular bacterium, *F. tularensis* can parasitize both phagocytic and nonphagocytic host cells and can survive intracellularly for prolonged periods. In the acute phase of infection, the primary organs affected (skin, lymph nodes, liver, and spleen) include areas of focal necrosis, initially surrounded by polymorphonuclear leukocytes (PMNs). Subsequently, granulomas form, with epithelioid cells, lymphocytes, and multinucleated giant cells surrounded by areas of necrosis. These areas may resemble caseation necrosis but later coalesce to form abscesses.

Conjunctival inoculation can result in infection of the eye, with regional lymph node enlargement (preauricular lymphadenopathy, Parinaud's complex). Aerosolization and inhalation or hematogenous spread of organisms can result in pneumonia. In the lung, an inflammatory reaction develops, including foci of alveolar necrosis and cell infiltration (initially polymorphonuclear and later mononuclear) with granulomas. Chest roentgenograms usually reveal bilateral patchy infiltrates rather than large areas of consolidation. Pleural effusions are common and may contain blood. Lymphadenopathy occurs in regions draining infected organs. Therefore, in pulmonary infection, mediastinal adenopathy may be evident, whereas patients with oropharyngeal tularemia develop cervical lymphadenopathy. In gastrointestinal or typhoidal tularemia, mesenteric lymphadenopathy may follow the ingestion of large numbers of organisms. (The term *typhoidal tularemia* may be used to describe severe bacteremic disease, irrespective of the mode of transmission or portal of entry.) Meningitis has been reported as a primary or secondary manifestation of bacteremia. Patients may also present with fever and no localizing signs.

IMMUNOLOGY

Infection with *F. tularensis* stimulates the host to produce antibodies. However, this antibody response probably plays only a minor role in the containment of infection. In contrast, cell-mediated immunity, which develops over 2–4 weeks, plays a major role in containment and eradication. Macrophages, once activated, can kill *F. tularensis*. Recovery from infection generally renders the patient resistant to reinfection; this point is not completely understood.

Immunospecific protection against tularemia can be afforded either by natural infection or by vaccination with live attenuated strains of *F. tularensis*. Killed vaccines, on the other hand, induce no protection against virulent *F. tularensis*. After natural infection or vaccination, serum antibodies to surface-exposed carbohydrate antigens predominate, whereas T cell determinants are located on membrane proteins beneath the bacterial capsule. T cell responses are thought to be due to priming by the organism. The anamnestic T cell response to *F. tularensis* seems to involve a multitude of microbial proteins, each with a distinct set of T cell determinants. A predominant role for CD4+ T cells is supported by the results of experiments in mice, which indicated that resistance to infection was restricted at the level of the major histocompatibility complex (MHC) class II determinants. Humans primed to *F. tularensis* (like those primed to *Mycobacterium tuberculosis*) show a T$_H$1-like response. T cell proliferation is associated with the production of interleukin (IL) 2 and interferon γ but with little or no production of IL-4. Recent evidence indicates that the percentage of γδ T cells expressing tumor necrosis factor α is decreased during the first 7–40 days after infection. This decrease may reflect the modulation of an inflammatory response. Investigations of neutrophils in tularemia suggest that PMNs are needed for defense against primary infection. PMNs may restrict the growth of *F. tularensis* before the organism becomes intracellular.

CLINICAL MANIFESTATIONS

Tularemia often starts with a sudden onset of fever, chills, headache, and generalized myalgias and arthralgias (Table 151-1). This onset takes place when the organism penetrates the skin, is ingested, or is inhaled. An incubation period of 2–10 days is followed by the formation of an ulcer at the site of penetration, with local inflammation. The ulcer may persist for several months as organisms are transported via the lymphatics to the re-

TABLE 151-1 CLINICAL PRESENTATION OF TULAREMIA

Sign or Symptom	Rate of Occurrence, %	
	Children	Adults
Lymphadenopathy	96	65
Fever (≥38.3°C or ≥101°F)	87	21
Ulcer/eschar/papule	45	51
Myalgias/arthralgias	39	2
Headache	9	5
Cough	9	5
Pharyngitis	43	—
Diarrhea	43	—

Source: Adapted from RF Jacobs, JP Narain: Tularemia in adults and children: A changing presentation. *Pediatrics* 76:818, 1985; with permission.

FIGURE 151-1   An 8-year-old boy with inguinal lymphadenitis and associated tick-bite site characteristic of ulceroglandular tularemia.

gional lymph nodes. These nodes enlarge and may become necrotic and suppurative. If the organism enters the bloodstream, widespread dissemination as well as signs and symptoms of endotoxemia may result.

In the United States, most patients with tularemia (75–85%) acquire the infection by inoculation of the skin. In adults, the most common localized form is inguinal/femoral lymphadenopathy; in children, it is cervical lymphadenopathy. About 20% of patients develop a generalized maculopapular rash, which occasionally becomes pustular. Erythema nodosum occurs infrequently. The clinical manifestations of tularemia have been divided into various syndromes, which are listed in Table 151-2.

Ulceroglandular/Glandular Tularemia   These two forms of tularemia account for ~75–85% of cases. The predominant form in children involves cervical or posterior auricular lymphadenopathy and is usually related to tick bites on the head and neck. In adults, the most common form is inguinal/femoral lymphadenopathy resulting from insect and tick exposures on the lower limbs. In cases related to wild game, the usual portal of entry for *F. tularensis* is either an injury sustained while skinning or cleaning an animal carcass or a bite (usually on the hand). Epitrochlear lymphadenopathy/lymphadenitis is common in patients with bite-related injuries.

In ulceroglandular tularemia, the ulcer is erythematous, indurated, and nonhealing, with a punched-out appearance that lasts 1–3 weeks. The papule may begin as an erythematous lesion that is tender or pruritic; it evolves over several days into an ulcer with sharply demarcated edges and a yellow exudate. The ulcer gradually develops a black base, and simultaneously the regional lymph nodes become tender and severely enlarged (Fig. 151-1). The affected lymph nodes may become fluctuant and drain spontaneously, but usually the condition resolves with effective treatment. Late suppuration of lymph nodes has been described in up to 25% of patients with ulceroglandular/glandular tularemia. Examination of material taken from these late fluctuant nodes after successful antimicrobial treatment reveals sterile necrotic tissue. In 5–10% of patients, the skin lesion may be inapparent, with lymphadenopathy plus systemic signs and symptoms the only physical findings (*glandular tularemia*). Conversely, a tick or deerfly bite on the trunk may result in an ulcer without evident lymphadenopathy.

TABLE 151-2   CLINICAL SYNDROMES OF TULAREMIA

Syndrome	Rate of Occurrence, %	
	Children	Adults
Ulceroglandular	45	51
Glandular	25	12
Pulmonary (pneumonia)	14	18
Oropharyngeal	4	—
Oculoglandular	2	—
Typhoidal	2	12
Unclassified	6	11

Source: Adapted from RF Jacobs, JP Narain: Tularemia in adults and children: A changing presentation. *Pediatrics* 76:818, 1985; with permission.

Oculoglandular Tularemia   In ~1% of patients, the portal of entry for *F. tularensis* is the conjunctiva. Usually, the organism reaches the conjunctiva through contact with contaminated fingers. The inflamed conjunctiva is painful, with numerous yellowish nodules and pinpoint ulcers. Purulent conjunctivitis with regional lymphadenopathy (preauricular, submandibular, or cervical) is evident. Because of debilitating pain, the patient may seek medical attention before regional lymphadenopathy develops. Painful preauricular lymphadenopathy is unique to tularemia and distinguishes it from cat-scratch disease, tuberculosis, sporotrichosis, and syphilis. Corneal perforation may occur.

Oropharyngeal and Gastrointestinal Tularemia   Rarely, tularemia follows ingestion of contaminated undercooked meat, oral inoculation of *F. tularensis* from the hands in association with the skinning and cleaning of animal carcasses, or consumption of contaminated food or water. Oral inoculation may result in acute, exudative, or membranous pharyngitis associated with cervical lymphadenopathy or in ulcerative intestinal lesions associated with mesenteric lymphadenopathy, diarrhea, abdominal pain, nausea, vomiting, and gastrointestinal bleeding. Infected tonsils become enlarged and develop a yellowish-white pseudomembrane, which can be confused with that of diphtheria. The clinical severity of gastrointestinal tularemia varies from mild, unexplained, persistent diarrhea with no other symptoms to a fulminant, fatal disease. In fatal cases, the extensive intestinal ulceration found at autopsy suggests an enormous inoculum.

Pulmonary Tularemia   Tularemia pneumonia presents as variable parenchymal infiltrates that are unresponsive to treatment with β-lactam antibiotics. Tularemia must be considered in the differential diagnosis of atypical pneumonia in a patient with a history of travel to an endemic area. The disease can result from inhalation of an infectious aerosol or can spread to the lungs and pleura after bloodstream dissemination. Inhalation-related pneumonia has been described in laboratory workers after exposure to contaminated materials and is associated with a relatively high mortality rate. Exposure to *F. tularensis* in aerosols from live domestic animals or dead wildlife (including birds) has been reported to cause pneumonia. Hematogenous dissemination to the lungs occurs in 10–15% of cases of ulceroglandular tularemia and in about half of cases of typhoidal tularemia. Previously, tularemia pneumonia was thought to be a disease of older patients, but as many as 10–15% of children with clinical manifestations of tularemia have parenchymal infiltrates detected by chest roentgenography. Patients with pneumonia usually have a nonproductive cough and may have dyspnea or pleuritic chest pain. Roentgenograms of the chest usually reveal bilateral patchy infiltrates (described as ovoid or lobar densities), lobar parenchymal infiltrates, and cavitary lesions. Pleural effusions may have a predominance of mononuclear leukocytes or PMNs and sometimes red blood cells. Empyema may develop. Blood cultures may be positive for *F. tularensis*.

Typhoidal Tularemia The typhoidal presentation is now considered rare in the United States. The source of infection in typhoidal tularemia is usually associated with pharyngeal and/or gastrointestinal inoculation or bacteremic disease. Fever usually develops without apparent skin lesions or lymphadenopathy. Some patients have cervical and mesenteric lymphadenopathy. In the absence of a history of possible contact with a vector, diagnosis can be extremely difficult. Blood cultures may be positive and patients may present with classic sepsis or septic shock in this acute systemic form of the infection. Typhoidal tularemia is usually associated with a huge inoculum or with a pre-existing compromising condition. High continuous fevers, signs of endotoxemia, and severe headache are common. The patient may be delirious and may develop prostration and shock. If presumptive antibiotic therapy in culture-negative cases does not include an aminoglycoside, the mortality rate can approach 30%.

Other Manifestations *F. tularensis* infection has been associated with meningitis, pericarditis, hepatitis, peritonitis, endocarditis, osteomyelitis, and sepsis and septic shock with rhabdomyolysis and acute renal failure. In the rare cases of tularemia meningitis, a predominantly lymphocytic response is demonstrated in cerebrospinal fluid.

DIFFERENTIAL DIAGNOSIS

When patients in endemic areas present with fever, chronic ulcerative skin lesions, and large tender lymph nodes (Fig. 151-1), a diagnosis of tularemia should be made presumptively, and confirmatory diagnostic testing and appropriate therapy should be undertaken. When the possibility of tularemia is considered in a nonendemic area, an attempt should be made to identify contact with a potential animal vector. The level of suspicion should be especially high in hunters, trappers, game wardens, veterinarians, laboratory workers, and individuals exposed to an insect or another animal vector. However, up to 40% of patients with tularemia have no known history of epidemiologic contact with an animal vector.

The characteristic presentation of ulceroglandular tularemia does not pose a diagnostic problem, but a less classic progression of regional lymphadenopathy or glandular tularemia must be differentiated from other diseases (Table 151-3). The skin lesion of tularemia may resemble those seen in various other diseases but is generally accompanied by more impressive regional lymphadenopathy. In children, the differentiation of tularemia from cat-scratch disease is made more difficult by the chronic papulovesicular lesion associated with *Bartonella henselae* infection (Chap. 153). Oropharyngeal tularemia can resemble and must be differentiated from pharyngitis due to other bacteria or viruses. Tularemia pneumonia may resemble any atypical pneumonia. Typhoidal tularemia may resemble a variety of other infections.

LABORATORY DIAGNOSIS

Direct microscopic examination of polychromatically stained tissue smears or clinical specimens reveals *F. tularensis* organisms, singly and in groups, both intra- and extracellularly. Gram's staining of clinical or biopsy material is of little value, as the small, weakly staining, gram-negative, nonmotile, non-spore-forming bacteria are difficult to distinguish from the background. An indirect fluorescent antibody test with commercially available antisera can be useful, although false-positive results due to *Legionella* spp. have been reported.

The diagnosis of tularemia is most frequently confirmed by agglutination testing. Microagglutination and tube agglutination are the

TABLE 151-3   TULAREMIA: DIFFERENTIAL DIAGNOSIS, BY CLINICAL DISEASE CATEGORY

Glandular	Oropharyngeal	Typhoidal	Pneumonia
Pyogenic bacterial infection[a]	Group A streptococcal pharyngitis	Typhoid fever	*Mycoplasma pneumoniae* pneumonia
Nontuberculous mycobacterial infection	*Arcanobacterium haemolyticum* pharyngitis	Other *Salmonella* bacteremias	*Chlamydophila pneumoniae* pneumonia
Sporotrichosis	Diphtheria	Rocky Mountain spotted fever	Psittacosis
Tuberculosis	Infectious mononucleosis	Human monocytotropic ehrlichiosis	*Legionella pneumophila* pneumonia
Syphilis	Various viral infections[b]	Human granulocytotropic ehrlichiosis	Q fever
Anthrax		Infectious mononucleosis	Histoplasmosis
Rat-bite fever		Brucellosis	Blastomycosis
Scrub typhus		Toxoplasmosis	Coccidioidomycosis
Plague		Tuberculosis	Various viral infections[d]
Lymphogranuloma venereum		Sarcoidosis	
Cat-scratch disease		Malignancy[c]	

[a]*Staphylococcus aureus, Streptococcus pyogenes.*
[b]Adenovirus, enteroviruses, parainfluenza virus, influenza virus A and B, respiratory syncytial virus.
[c]Hematologic and reticuloendothelial malignancies.
[d]Influenza virus A and B, parainfluenza virus, respiratory syncytial virus, adenovirus, enteroviruses, hantavirus.

techniques most commonly used to detect antibody to *F. tularensis*. In the standard tube agglutination test, a single titer of ≥1:160 is interpreted as a presumptive positive result. A fourfold increase in titer between paired serum samples collected 2–3 weeks apart is considered diagnostic. False-negative serologic responses are obtained early in infection; up to 30% of patients infected for 3 weeks have sera that test negative. Late in infection, titers into the thousands are common, and titers of 1:20–1:80 may persist for years. Enzyme-linked immunosorbent assays have proved useful for the detection of both antibodies and antigens. Analysis of urine for *F. tularensis* antigen has yielded promising results in clinical trials, but facilities for this type of analysis are not widely available. A skin test for delayed hypersensitivity to *F. tularensis* turns positive during the first week of illness and remains positive for years. The skin-test antigen, which is not commercially available, can boost titers of agglutinating antibody.

Culture and isolation of *F. tularensis* are difficult. In one study, the organism was isolated in only 10% of more than 1000 human cases, 84% of which were confirmed by serology. The medium of choice is cysteine-glucose-blood agar. *F. tularensis* can be isolated directly from infected ulcer scrapings, lymph-node biopsy specimens, gastric washings, sputum, and blood cultures. Colonies are blue-gray, round, smooth, and slightly mucoid. On media containing blood, a small zone of α hemolysis usually surrounds the colony. Slide agglutination tests or direct fluorescent antibody tests with commercially available antisera can be applied directly to culture suspensions for identification. Most clinical laboratories will not attempt to culture *F. tularensis* because of the infectivity of the organism from the culture media. Although tularemia is not spread from person to person, the organism can be inhaled from culture plates and infect unsuspecting laboratory workers. In most clinical laboratories, biosafety level 2 practices are recommended to handle clinical specimens thought to contain *F. tularensis*.

A variety of polymerase chain reaction (PCR) methods have been used to detect *F. tularensis* DNA in multiple clinical specimens. The majority of these methods target the genes encoding the outer-membrane proteins (e.g., *fopA* or *tul4*). A 16S rDNA sequence identification PCR is helpful when the patient's clinical information does not lead the clinician to suspect a diagnosis of tularemia.

℞ TULAREMIA

F. tularensis cannot be subjected to standardized antimicrobial susceptibility testing because the organism will not grow on the media used. A wide variety of antibiotics, including all β-lactam antibiotics and the newer cephalosporins, are ineffective for the treatment of tularemia. Several studies indicated that third-generation cephalosporins were active against *F. tularensis* in vitro, but clinical case reports suggested a nearly universal failure rate of ceftriaxone in pediatric patients with tularemia. Although in vitro data indicate that imipenem may be active, therapy with imipenem, sulfanilamides, and macrolides is not presently recommended because of the lack of relevant clinical data. Fluoroquinolones have shown promise in terms of their relatively low toxicity and their potential for oral administration. With intracellular activity, fluoroquinolones have been used for successful treatment of tularemia and are candidates for primary or alternative therapy, pending clinical trials. The use of these agents should also be considered when patients are allergic or intolerant to other treatments. When used, ciprofloxacin should be given for a total of 10 days. Chloramphenicol and tetracycline have been used successfully for treatment of the acute stages of tularemia but have been associated with higher relapse rates (up to 20%) than conventionally used agents. Oral chloramphenicol is no longer available in the United States.

Gentamicin is considered the drug of choice for both adults and children. The dosage for adults is 5 mg/kg daily in two divided doses. The dosage for children is 2.5 mg/kg tid or 5 mg/kg bid. Gentamicin therapy is typically continued for 7–10 days; however, in mild to moderate cases of tularemia in which the patient becomes afebrile within the first 48–72 h of gentamicin treatment, a 5- to 7-day course has been successful.

If available (shortages have been reported over the past several years), streptomycin given intramuscularly also is effective. The dosage for adults is 2 g/d in two divided doses. For children, the dosage is 30 mg/kg daily in two divided doses (maximal daily dose, 2 g). After a clinical response is demonstrated at 3–5 days, the dose can be reduced to 10–15 mg/kg daily in two divided doses. The total duration of streptomycin therapy in both adults and children is usually 10 days.

Virtually all strains of *F. tularensis* are susceptible to streptomycin and gentamicin. In successfully treated patients, defervescence usually occurs within 2 days, but skin lesions and lymph nodes may take 1–2 weeks to heal. When therapy is not initiated within the first several days of illness, defervescence may be delayed. Relapses are uncommon with streptomycin or gentamicin therapy. Late lymph-node suppuration, however, occurs in ~40% of children, regardless of the treatment received. These nodes have typically been found to contain sterile necrotic tissue without evidence of active infection. Patients with fluctuant nodes should receive several days of antibiotic therapy before drainage to minimize the risk to hospital personnel. Unlike streptomycin and gentamicin, tobramycin is ineffective in the treatment of tularemia and should not be used.

PROGNOSIS

If tularemia goes untreated, symptoms usually last 1–4 weeks but may continue for months. The mortality rate from severe untreated infection (including all cases of untreated tularemia pneumonia and typhoidal tularemia) can be as high as 30%. However, the overall mortality rate for untreated tularemia is <8%. Mortality is <1% with appropriate treatment. Poor outcomes are often associated with long delays in diagnosis and treatment. Lifelong immunity usually follows tularemia.

PREVENTION

The prevention of tularemia is based on avoidance of exposure to biting and blood-sucking insects, especially ticks and deerflies. A vaccine made from live attenuated *F. tularensis* was developed in the United States and found to be effective. Because of difficulty with standardization, however, the vaccine is not currently licensed in the United States or Europe. A live attenuated vaccine is still available in some parts of the former Soviet Union. Prophylaxis of tularemia has not proved effective in patients with embedded ticks or insect bites. However, in patients who are known to have been exposed to large quantities of organisms (e.g., in the laboratory) and who have incubating infection with *F. tularensis*, early treatment can prevent the development of significant clinical disease.

FURTHER READINGS

BARNS SM et al: Detection of diverse new *Francisella*-like bacteria in environmental samples. Appl Environ Microbiol 71:5494, 2005

CENTERS FOR DISEASE CONTROL AND PREVENTION: Tularemia—United States, 1990–2000. MMWR 51:181, 2002

DE LA PUENTE-REDONDO VA et al: Comparison of different PCR approaches for typing of *Francisella tularensis* strains. J Clin Microbiol 38:1016, 2000

DENNIS DT et al: Tularemia as a biological weapon: Medical and public health management. JAMA 285:2763, 2001

ELIASSON H et al: The 2000 tularemia outbreak: A case-control study of risk factors in disease-endemic and emergent areas, Sweden. Emerg Infect Dis 8:956, 2002

IKÄHEIMO I et al: In vitro antibiotic susceptibility of *Francisella tularensis* isolated from humans and animals. J Antimicrob Chemother 46:287, 2000

JOHANSSON A et al: In vitro susceptibility to quinolones of *Francisella tularensis* subspecies *tularensis*. Scand J Infect Dis 34:327, 2002

PETERSEN JM et al: Methods for the enhanced recovery of *Francisella tularensis* cultures. Appl Environ Microbiol 70:3733, 2004

TARNVIK A et al: Tularemia in Europe: An epidemiological overview. Scand J Infect Dis 36:350, 2004

VERSAGE JL et al: Development of a multitarget real-time TaqMan PCR assay for enhanced detection of *Francisella tularensis* in complex specimens. J Clin Microbiol 41:5492, 2003

152 Plague and Other *Yersinia* Infections
David T. Dennis, Grant L. Campbell

PLAGUE

DEFINITION

Plague is an acute febrile disease caused by infection with *Yersinia pestis*. Human cases are infrequent and are curable with antibiotics. Plague is, however, one of the most virulent and potentially lethal bacterial diseases known, and fatality rates remain high among patients who are not treated in the early stages of infection. Plague occurs in widely scattered foci in Asia, Africa, and the Americas (Fig. 152-1), where its usual hosts are various wild rodents and human-associated rats. Infection is transmitted to humans typically by flea bite and infrequently by direct contact with infected animal tissues or by airborne droplet. The principal clinical forms of plague are bubonic, septicemic, and pneumonic. Although most cases are now sporadic, occurring singly or in small clusters, the potential for outbreaks and epidemic spread remains. Because of its virulence and transmissibility, *Y. pestis* is considered an important potential agent of biological terrorism that requires special countermeasures to protect the public's health (Chap. 214).

ETIOLOGIC AGENT

Y. pestis is a gram-negative coccobacillus in the family Enterobacteriaceae. Genomic analysis suggests that it has only recently evolved from *Y. pseudotuberculosis*. *Y. pestis* is microaerophilic, nonmotile, nonsporulating, oxidase and urease negative, and biochemically unreactive. The organism is nonfastidious and infective for laboratory rodents. It grows well, if slowly, on routinely used microbiologic media (e.g., sheep blood agar, brain-heart infusion broth, and MacConkey agar). *Y. pestis* can multiply within a wide range of temperatures (−2°C to 45°C) and pH values (5.0–9.6), but optimal growth occurs at 28°C and at pH ~7.4. When stained with a polychromatic stain (e.g., Wayson or Giemsa), *Y. pestis* isolated from clinical specimens exhibits a characteristic bipolar appearance, resembling closed safety pins. The bacterium is nonencapsulated but, when grown at ≥30°C, produces a plasmid-expressed envelope glycoprotein, fraction 1 (F1) antigen—a virulence factor that serves as the principal immunodiagnostic marker of infection.

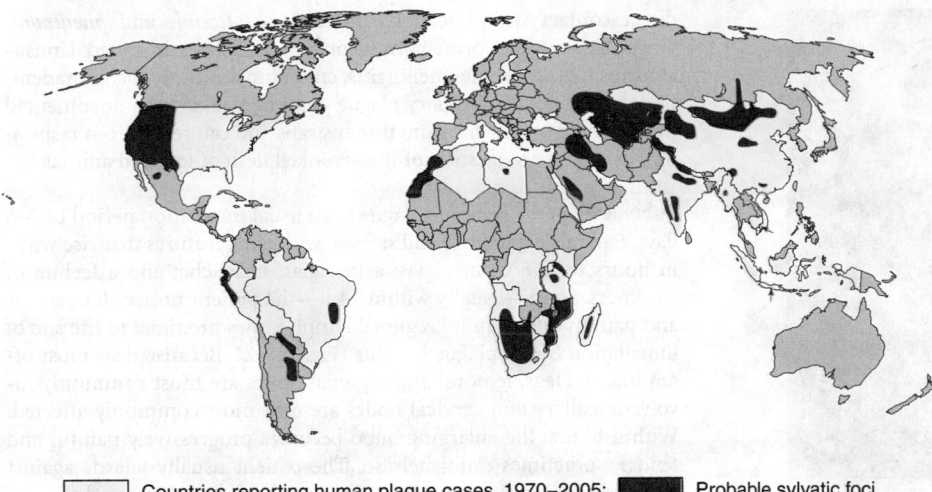

Countries reporting human plague cases, 1970–2005; ▮ Probable sylvatic foci

FIGURE 152-1   Approximate global distribution of *Yersinia pestis*. *(Compiled from WHO, CDC, and country sources.)*

EPIDEMIOLOGY

Y. pestis is maintained in well-established "silent" enzootic cycles involving relatively resistant wild rodents and their fleas in remote, lightly populated areas of Asia, Africa, and the Americas and in limited rural foci in extreme southeastern Europe near the Caspian Sea (Fig. 152-1). Humans and mammals other than rodents are incidental hosts. Outbreaks (epizootics) of plague in susceptible rodent populations may result in widespread rodent die-offs, an avid search by their fleas for new hosts, and an increased risk of spread of infection to humans. In the United States, the principal epizootic hosts are various ground squirrels, prairie dogs, and chipmunks; various burrowing rodents act as reservoir hosts in natural areas elsewhere in the world. *Y. pestis* occasionally spills over from wild rodents to rat species that inhabit cultivated fields and adjacent homes, villages, and towns. The organism can then be transported from towns to cities by these highly adaptable rats and their fleas.

Plague in populated areas is most likely to develop when sanitation is poor and rats are numerous—especially the common black or roof rat (*Rattus rattus*), its close relatives, and the larger brown sewer or Norway rat (*R. norvegicus*). The cosmopolitan oriental rat flea *Xenopsylla cheopis* and (in southern Africa and Brazil) the related species *X. brasiliensis* are efficient vectors of the plague bacillus from rat to rat and from rats to humans. *Y. pestis* multiplies to enormous numbers in the foregut (proventriculus) of these fleas, resulting in a bolus of organisms and clotted blood that blocks the passage of subsequent blood meals. This blockage occurs at temperatures of ≤28°C and depends on a single protease expressed by the plasminogen activator (*pla*) gene of a 9.5-kb plasmid of *Y. pestis*. Regurgitation by a "blocked" flea while it feeds facilitates transmission of the plague bacillus to the new host. Except for large outbreaks of pneumonic plague in Manchuria in the early part of the twentieth century, person-to-person respiratory transmission of plague has since occurred only sporadically and has been limited to clusters of close, direct contacts of pneumonic plague patients, such as household members and caregivers.

International health regulations require that national authorities immediately report plague cases to the World Health Organization (WHO). During 1989–2003, a total of 38,359 human cases of plague were reported to the WHO from 25 countries (a mean of 2557 cases per year). The reported case-fatality rate was 7%. More than 80% (31,273) of the total number of cases were reported from Africa, ~14% (5449) from Asia, and the rest (1637) from the Americas.

In the United States, 5–10 human plague cases typically are reported each year. Most cases occur in New Mexico, Arizona, Colorado, and California (http://www.cdc.gov/ncidod/dvbid/plague/plagwest.htm). The most common modes of transmission are flea bite and direct contact with infected animals, especially exposure to an infected domestic cat. The overall case-fatality rate is ~10%. Most cases of plague occur

in the summer months, when rodents and their fleas are most active. The disease is acquired often in the environs of the patient's residential property and less often during work or recreation in natural areas remote from the patient's place of residence. The arid Native American reservations of New Mexico and Arizona are active plague foci, and Native Americans account for a disproportionately high percentage of plague cases.

Plague can be transmitted during the skinning and handling of carcasses of wild animals such as rabbits and hares, prairie dogs, wildcats, and coyotes. Such direct inoculation of mammal-adapted organisms expressing the F1 antigen is associated with primary septicemia and high mortality rates. Pharyngeal plague can result from the ingestion of undercooked contaminated meat; outbreaks of pharyngeal plague have been reported among persons eating undercooked camel and goat meat. Plague can also be acquired by inhalation of infective respiratory droplets and perhaps by manual transfer of infected fluids to the mouth during the handling of infected animal tissues.

Carnivores, including dogs and cats, can become infected with *Y. pestis* by eating infected rodents and possibly by being bitten by infective fleas. Although clinical plague commonly develops in infected cats, it rarely does so in infected dogs. Both dogs and cats may transport infected fleas from rodent-infested areas to the home environment.

PATHOGENESIS AND PATHOLOGY

Y. pestis is highly invasive and pathogenic. The mechanisms by which the organism causes disease are incompletely understood, but both chromosome- and plasmid-encoded gene products as well as altered cell-mediated immune responses are involved. Three plasmids encode for a variety of known or presumed virulence factors, including the F1 envelope antigen and various *Yersinia* outer-membrane proteins, which confer bacterial resistance to phagocytosis; the V antigen, which is essential for virulence and suppresses the synthesis of various proinflammatory cytokines (e.g., interferon γ and tumor necrosis factor α); pesticin, which interferes with iron uptake; a protease that activates plasminogen and degrades serum complement and is thought to enhance dissemination of *Y. pestis* following inoculation of the skin; a coagulase; and a fibrinolysin. A chromosomally encoded lipopolysaccharide endotoxin is important in sepsis, playing a role in triggering the systemic inflammatory response syndrome and its complications.

Y. pestis organisms inoculated through the skin or mucous membranes are typically carried to regional lymph nodes via lymphatic channels, although direct bloodstream inoculation and dissemination may take place. Mononuclear phagocytes, which can phagocytize *Y. pestis* organisms without destroying them, may play a role in dissemination of the infection to distant sites. Plague can involve almost any organ, and untreated plague generally results in widespread and massive tissue destruction. In the early stages, infected lymph nodes (*buboes*, Fig. 152-2) are characterized by edema and congestion without inflammatory infiltrates or apparent vascular injury. Fully developed buboes contain huge numbers of infectious plague organisms and show distorted or obliterated lymph node architecture with loss of vascular integrity, hemorrhage, necrosis, infiltration of polymorphonuclear neutrophils (PMNs), and extensive serosanguineous effusion. The effusion typically involves perinodal tissues. If several adjacent lymph nodes are involved, a boggy edematous mass can result.

Primary septicemic plague consists of sepsis in the absence of a bubo; secondary septicemic plague is a complication of bubonic or pneumonic plague that occurs when local host defenses are breached. In fatal septicemic plague, multifocal hepatic and splenic necrosis is com-

FIGURE 152-2 Plague patient in the southwestern United States with a left axillary bubo and an unusual plague ulcer and eschar at the site of the infective flea bite.

direct contact with infectious materials. *Septicemic* and *pneumonic* plague can be either primary or secondary to metastatic spread. Unusual forms include plague meningitis, endophthalmitis, and lymphadenitis at multiple sites. Primary plague pharyngitis has been documented by culture of organisms from throat swabs and can result from respiratory exposure or ingestion of undercooked flesh of infected animals.

Bubonic Plague   Bubonic plague has a usual incubation period of 2–6 days. Patients experience chills; fever, with temperatures that rise within hours to ≥38°C; myalgias; arthralgias; headache; and a feeling of weakness. Soon—usually within 24 h—the patient notices tenderness and pain in one or more regional lymph nodes proximal to the site of inoculation of the plague bacillus (Fig. 152-2). Because fleas most often bite the legs, femoral and inguinal nodes are most commonly involved; axillary and cervical nodes are next most commonly affected. Within hours, the enlarging bubo becomes progressively painful and tender, sometimes exquisitely so. The patient usually guards against palpation and limits movement, pressure, and stretch around the bubo. The surrounding tissue often becomes edematous, sometimes markedly so, and the overlying skin may be erythematous, warm, and tense. Inspection of the skin surrounding or distal to the bubo sometimes reveals the site of a flea bite marked by a papule, pustule, or ulcer. The ulcer may be covered by an eschar (Fig. 152-2). A list of lymphadenitic conditions that could be confused with bubonic plague includes *Staphylococcus aureus* and group A β-hemolytic streptococcal infections, cat-scratch disease, tularemia, and—in filariasis-endemic areas—acute filarial lymphadenitis. The bubo of plague is distinguishable from lymphadenitis of most other causes, however, by its rapid onset, its extreme tenderness, the accompanying signs of toxemia, and the absence of cellulitis or obvious ascending lymphangitis. The pain and swelling of bubonic plague can be confused with a strangulated hernia or trauma.

Treated in the uncomplicated state with an appropriate antibiotic, bubonic plague usually responds quickly, with resolution of fever and alleviation of other systemic manifestations over 2–5 days. Buboes often remain enlarged and tender for a week or more after the initiation of treatment and can become fluctuant. Without effective antimicrobial treatment, patients with typical bubonic plague manifest an increasingly toxic state of fever, tachycardia, lethargy leading to prostration, agitation and confusion, and (occasionally) convulsions and delirium. Secondary plague sepsis may result in an alarmingly rapid and refractory cascade of DIC, bleeding, shock, and organ failure.

Septicemic Plague   Primary septicemia, which accounts for ~20% of cases in the United States, develops in the absence of a detectable bubo. The diagnosis often is not suspected until preliminary blood culture results are reported to be positive by the laboratory. *Y. pestis*, however, can also be cultured from the blood of most patients with

mon. Diffuse interstitial myocarditis with cardiac dilatation is sometimes found. If disseminated intravascular coagulation (DIC) ensues, vascular necrosis may lead to widespread cutaneous, mucosal, and serosal ecchymoses and petechiae. Acral ischemia and resulting gangrene sometimes develop.

Primary plague pneumonia generally begins as a lobular process and then extends by confluence, becoming lobar and then multilobar (Fig. 152-3). Plague organisms are typically most numerous in the alveoli. Secondary plague pneumonia begins more diffusely, with organisms at first most numerous in the interstitium. In advanced cases of both primary and secondary plague pneumonia, affected lung tissue is characterized by edema, hemorrhagic necrosis, and infiltration by neutrophilic leukocytes.

CLINICAL MANIFESTATIONS

Plague is characterized by a rapid onset of fever and other systemic manifestations of gram-negative bacterial infection. If it is not quickly and correctly treated, plague can follow a toxic course, resulting in shock, multiple-organ failure, and death. In humans, the three principal forms of plague are bubonic, septicemic, and pneumonic. *Bubonic* plague, accounting in the United States for ~75% of cases, is almost always caused by the bite of an infected flea but occasionally results from

FIGURE 152-3 Sequential chest radiographs of a patient with fatal primary plague pneumonia. *Left:* Upright posteroanterior film taken at admission to hospital emergency department on third day of illness, showing segmental consolidation of right upper lobe. ***Center:*** Portable anteroposterior film taken 8 h after admission, showing extension of pneumonia to right middle and right lower lobes.

Right: Portable anteroposterior film taken 13 h after admission (when patient had clinical adult respiratory distress syndrome), showing diffuse infiltration throughout right lung and patchy infiltration of left lower lung. A cavity later developed at the site of initial right-upper-lobe consolidation.

bubonic plague, and bacteremia must be distinguished from septicemia, in which the patient is desperately ill and requires aggressive care. Septic patients often present with gastrointestinal symptoms of nausea, vomiting, diarrhea, and abdominal pain, which may confound the correct diagnosis. In the United States in 1947–2001, 55 cases of primary septicemic plague with 13 deaths were reported, for a case-fatality rate of 24%. Petechiae, ecchymoses, bleeding from puncture wounds and orifices, and gangrene of acral parts are manifestations of DIC; refractory hypotension, renal shutdown, obtundation, and other signs of shock are preterminal events. Adult respiratory distress syndrome (ARDS) can occur at any stage of septicemic plague. The differential diagnosis of septicemic plague includes sepsis of other gram-negative bacterial etiology, meningococcemia, and acute severe viral infections such as hantavirus illness.

Pneumonic Plague Pneumonic plague is the most life-threatening form of the disease. Primary pneumonic plague accounts for ~5% of plague cases in the United States. The incubation period for primary pneumonic plague is usually 3–5 days (range, 1–7 days). The onset is most often sudden, with chills, fever, headache, myalgias, weakness, and dizziness. Pulmonary signs, including tachypnea and dyspnea, cough, sputum production, and chest pain, typically arise on the second day of illness and may be accompanied by hemoptysis, increasing respiratory distress, cardiopulmonary insufficiency, and circulatory collapse. In primary plague pneumonia, the sputum is most often watery or mucoid, frothy, and blood-tinged, but it may become frankly bloody. Pulmonary signs in primary pneumonic plague may indicate involvement of a single lobe in the early stage, with rapidly developing segmental consolidation before bronchopneumonic spread to other lobes of the same and opposite lungs (Fig. 152-3). Liquefaction necrosis and cavitation may occur early in areas of consolidation and may or may not leave significant residual scarring.

Secondary plague pneumonia, which occurs in 10–15% of bubonic plague cases in the United States, typically manifests first as diffuse interstitial pneumonitis in which sputum production is scant; because the sputum is more likely to be inspissated and tenacious in character than the sputum found in primary pneumonia, it may be less infectious. In the United States in 1947–2001, 46 cases of secondary pneumonic plague and 8 cases of primary pneumonic plague were described, with no known transmission to contacts and an overall case-fatality rate of 41%.

Plague Meningitis Meningitis is an unusual manifestation of plague. In the United States, there were 17 meningitis cases among the 409 evaluable plague cases reported during 1947–2005. All cases of meningitis were complications of bubonic plague, and all but three patients survived. Although meningitis may be a part of the initial presentation of plague, its onset is often delayed and is a manifestation of insufficient treatment. Recent cases in the United States have occurred in association with treatment of bubonic plague with tetracyclines, which are bacteriostatic against *Y. pestis*. Chronic relapsing meningeal plague over periods of weeks or even months was described in the preantibiotic era. The affected patients typically present with fever, headache, meningismus, and neutrophilic pleocytosis.

Plague Pharyngitis Plague pharyngitis presents as fever, sore throat, cervical lymphadenitis, and headache and is often indistinguishable clinically from pharyngitis and tonsillitis of other infectious etiologies, especially streptococcal pharyngitis. Plague pharyngitis can be difficult to distinguish from cervical bubonic plague arising from an infective flea bite on the head and neck region.

LABORATORY FINDINGS AND DIAGNOSIS

A high index of clinical suspicion and a thorough clinical and epidemiologic examination are required for timely diagnosis and treatment. When the diagnosis of plague is delayed or missed, a high case-fatality rate results; infected travelers who seek medical care after they have left endemic areas (peripatetic plague cases) are at especially high risk.

When the diagnosis of plague is being considered, close communication between clinicians and the diagnostic laboratory and between the diagnostic laboratory and a qualified reference laboratory is essential. Tests for plague are highly reliable when conducted by laboratory personnel experienced with *Y. pestis*, but such expertise is usually limited to selected reference laboratories, including state health department laboratories in some plague-endemic states and the CDC plague laboratory (Fort Collins, CO; tel. 970-221-6400).

When plague is suspected, specimens should be collected promptly for laboratory studies, chest roentgenograms should be obtained, and specific antimicrobial therapy should be initiated pending confirmation. Appropriate diagnostic specimens for smear and culture include blood from all patients; lymph node aspirates from those with buboes; sputum samples, pharyngeal swabs, and lower respiratory secretions from those with suspected pneumonic plague; and cerebrospinal fluid (CSF) from those with meningeal signs. Since early buboes are often exquisitely tender and are seldom fluctuant or necrotic, they usually require aspiration under local anesthesia after the injection of 1–2 mL of normal saline (sterile but nonbacteriostatic) into the bubo with a 20- to 22-gauge needle. Typically, aspiration produces a scant amount of serosanguineous fluid.

Patients with plague typically have white blood cell (WBC) counts of 10,000–25,000/μL, with a predominance of PMNs and a left shift. Leukemoid reactions, with WBC counts as high as 100,000/μL, can occur. Modest thrombocytopenia is usually present, and fibrin-fibrinogen split products are often detected, even in patients without frank DIC. In plague pneumonia, stained respiratory secretions usually contain PMNs and characteristic bipolar-staining bacilli. In *Y. pestis* septicemia, visualization of the characteristic bacilli in a routine blood smear or a buffy-coat smear is an uncommon but grave prognostic sign (Fig. 152-4). In patients with plague meningitis, PMN pleocytosis is typical, and the bacilli are usually visible in stained CSF smears.

A variety of appropriate culture media (including brain-heart infusion broth, sheep blood agar, and MacConkey agar) should be inoculated with a portion of each specimen. Moreover, for each specimen, at least one smear should be examined immediately with Wayson or Giemsa stain and at least one with Gram's stain; a smear should also be submitted to a reference laboratory for direct fluorescent antibody testing, antigen-capture enzyme-linked immunosorbent assay (ELISA), polymerase chain reaction (PCR) analysis, or testing by another rapid detection method (e.g., immunochromatographic hand-held assay). An acute-phase serum specimen should be tested for antibody to *Y. pestis*; whenever possible, a convalescent-phase serum specimen collected 3–4 weeks later should also be tested. When a patient dies and plague is suspected, appropriate autopsy tissues for culture, direct fluorescent antibody testing, and immunohistochemical staining include buboes, all solid organs (especially liver, spleen, and lung), and bone marrow. If culture of such specimens is to be attempted, they should be sent to the laboratory either fresh or frozen on dry ice, not in preservatives or fixatives. If necessary, Cary-Blair or a similar medium can be used to transport *Y. pestis*–infected tissues.

FIGURE 152-4 Peripheral blood smear from a patient with fatal plague septicemia and shock, showing characteristic bipolar-staining *Y. pestis* bacilli (Wright's stain, oil immersion).

Laboratory confirmation of plague depends on the isolation of *Y. pestis* from cultures of body fluids or tissues. Cultures of three blood samples taken over a 45-min period before treatment usually result in isolation of the bacterium. *Y. pestis* strains are readily distinguished from those of the closely related species *Y. pseudotuberculosis* by differences in biochemical profile, temperature-dependent susceptibility to lysis by a *Y. pestis*–specific bacteriophage, and motility. Automated bacteriologic test systems can be used to assist in the identification of isolates as *Y. pestis*, but *Y. pestis* can be misidentified (e.g., as *Y. pseudotuberculosis*) or overlooked if these systems are improperly programmed.

In the absence of *Y. pestis* isolation, plague cases can be confirmed either by the demonstration of seroconversion (a fourfold or greater titer rise) to *Y. pestis* F1 antigen in passive hemagglutination tests of acute- and convalescent-phase serum specimens or by detection of an antibody titer of >128 in a single serum sample from a patient with a plague-compatible illness who has not received plague vaccine. The specificity of a positive passive-hemagglutination test requires confirmation with the F1 antigen hemagglutination-inhibition test. A few plague patients seroconvert to F1 antigen as early as 5 days after the onset of illness; most seroconvert 1–2 weeks after onset; a few seroconvert >3 weeks after onset; and a few (<5%) fail to seroconvert at all. Early, specific antibiotic treatment may delay seroconversion by several weeks. After seroconversion, positive serologic titers diminish gradually over months to years. ELISAs for IgM and IgG antibodies to *Y. pestis* are replacing hemagglutination tests in some laboratories. Other new test methods include those mentioned above: antigen-capture ELISAs, PCR, and immunochromatographic hand-held assays for rapid identification of *Y. pestis* in aspirates, sputum, and other infected body fluids or tissues. The hand-held assays can be used at the bedside in the remote rural settings where most plague cases occur and could prove important in responding to bioterrorism (Chap. 214).

℞ PLAGUE

Left untreated, plague is fatal in >50% of bubonic cases and in nearly all septicemic and pneumonic cases. The overall mortality rate for plague cases in the United States since 1950 has been ~14%; deaths are almost always due to delays in seeking treatment, misdiagnosis, delays in the institution of treatment, or incorrect treatment. Rapid diagnosis and appropriate antimicrobial therapy are essential.

Guidelines for the treatment of plague are given in **Table 152-1**. Although streptomycin is the drug of choice, gentamicin is increasingly used for the treatment of plague in the United States because of its ready availability; it is probably as effective as streptomycin and less toxic. Alternative antibiotics include the tetracyclines and chloramphenicol; these agents are usually given orally with initial loading doses but may be given intravenously to critically ill patients and to patients who cannot tolerate oral medication.

Doxycycline is considered the tetracycline of choice. Penicillins, cephalosporins, and macrolides are suboptimal and should not be used. Trimethoprim-sulfamethoxazole (TMP-SMX) has been used successfully to treat bubonic plague but is not considered a first-line agent. Chloramphenicol may be indicated for the treatment of plague meningitis, pleuritis, endophthalmitis, and myocarditis because of its superior tissue penetration; it is used alone or in combination with streptomycin or another first-line agent. In general, antimicrobial treatment should be continued for 7–10 days or for at least 3 days after the patient has become afebrile and has made a clinical recovery. Patients initially given IV antibiotics may be switched to oral regimens upon clinical improvement. Such improvement is usually evident 2–3 days after the start of treatment, even though fever may continue for several days. National bioterrorism-response protocols propose gentamicin, ciprofloxacin, and doxycycline as antimicrobial agents of first choice for treatment and postexposure prophylaxis in the event of an attack using *Y. pestis* (Chap. 214).

Complications of sepsis require intensive monitoring and close physiologic support, as outlined elsewhere (Chaps. 110 and 265). Buboes may require surgical drainage. Abscessed nodes can cause recurrent fever in patients who have apparently recovered; the cause may be occult if intrathoracic or intraabdominal nodes are involved. Although *Y. pestis* is considered to be genetically stable, a multidrug-resistant strain was isolated from a plague patient in Madagascar. This strain exhibited resistance (mediated by a transferable plasmid) to principal first-line antibiotics used for treatment and prophylaxis of plague.

PREVENTION AND CONTROL

Persons at greatest risk for plague in the United States are individuals who live, work, and participate in outdoor recreational activities in areas of those western states in which plague is enzootic. Surveillance, education, and environmental management are the cornerstones of prevention and control. Personal protective measures include the avoidance of areas with known epizootic plague (in which warning signs may be posted) and of sick or dead animals; the use of repellents, insecticides, and protective clothing when at risk of exposure to rodents' fleas; and the wearing of gloves when handling animal carcasses. Short-term antibiotic prophylaxis (**Table 152-2**) is recommended for persons known to have had close contact with a patient with suspected or confirmed pneumonic plague. The recommended duration of postexposure prophylaxis is 5 days. Patients in whom respiratory plague is suspected should be managed under isolation, with use of respiratory-droplet precautions until pneumonia has been ruled out or until 48 h of effective antimicrobial therapy has been administered, after which standard infection-control precautions are adequate. Masks that block droplets are considered to be protective against respiratory transmission of plague and would be expected to be an important tool to prevent secondary plague spread in the event of bioterrorism (Chap. 214).

Rodent food (garbage, pet food) and habitats (brush piles, junk heaps, woodpiles) should be eliminated in residential and occupational environments; buildings and food stores should be rodent-proofed. The con-

TABLE 152-1 GUIDELINES FOR THE TREATMENT OF PLAGUE

Drug	Daily Dosage	Interval, h	Route(s) of Administration
Streptomycin			
Adults	2 g	12	IM
Children	30 mg/kg	12	IM
Gentamicin			
Adults	3–5 mg/kg[a]	8	IM or IV
Children	6.0–7.5 mg/kg	8	IM or IV
Infants/neonates	7.5 mg/kg	8	IM or IV
Tetracycline			
Adults	2 g	6	PO or IV
Children ≥8 y	25–50 mg/kg	6	PO or IV
Doxycycline			
Adults	200 mg	12 or 24	PO or IV
Children ≥8 y	4.4 mg/kg	12 or 24	PO or IV
Chloramphenicol			
Adults	50 mg/kg[b]	6	PO or IV
Children ≥1 y	50 mg/kg[b]	6	PO or IV

[a]Dosage should be reduced to 3 mg/kg daily as soon as clinically indicated.
[b]For meningitis, up to 100 (mg/kg)/d initially.

TABLE 152-2 GUIDELINES FOR PLAGUE PROPHYLAXIS

Drug	Daily Dosage	Interval, h	Route of Administration
Tetracycline			
Adults	1–2 g	6 or 12	PO
Children ≥8 y	25–50 mg/kg	6 or 12	PO
Doxycycline			
Adults	100–200 mg	12 or 24	PO
Children ≥8 y	2–4 mg/kg	12 or 24	PO
Trimethoprim-sulfamethoxazole			
Adults	320 mg[a]	12	PO
Children ≥2 mo	8 mg/kg[a]	12	PO
Ciprofloxacin[b]			
Adults	1 g	12	PO
Children	40 mg/kg	12	PO

[a]Trimethoprim component.
[b]Recommended as an alternative to doxycycline in bioterrorism-response plans.

trol of fleas with insecticides is a key public health measure in situations where epizootic plague activity places humans at high risk; this effort includes dusting and spraying of rodent burrows, rodent runs, and other sites where rodents and their fleas are found. In plague-endemic areas of the western United States, persons should keep their dogs and cats free of fleas and restrained. The decision to control plague by killing rodents should be left to public health authorities, and such a program should be carried out only in conjunction with effective flea control. Killing of rodents has no lasting benefit without environmental sanitation.

The previously used killed, whole-cell plague vaccine is no longer available in the United States. New and improved vaccines that use recombinant F1 and V antigens to induce protective antibodies are undergoing clinical trials. In the United States, the indications for use of these newer vaccines would probably be similar to those for the previously available killed vaccine, which was mostly limited to protecting laboratory personnel who routinely worked with Y. pestis and some persons whose vocations brought them into regular contact with wild rodents and their fleas in areas with enzootic or epizootic plague. In addition, a vaccine might be useful in protecting selected persons at risk from biowarfare or bioterrorism.

OTHER YERSINIA INFECTIONS

DEFINITION

Yersiniosis is an uncommon bacterial zoonosis caused primarily by infection with either of two enteropathogenic Yersinia species: Y. enterocolitica or Y. pseudotuberculosis. Reservoir hosts of these bacteria include swine and other wild and domestic animals, and transmission to humans is predominantly via the oral route. Both sporadic cases and common-source outbreaks occur. The most frequent acute clinical manifestations are (1) enteritis or enterocolitis with self-limited diarrhea (especially with Y. enterocolitica) and (2) mesenteric adenitis and terminal ileitis (especially with Y. pseudotuberculosis), which can be confused with acute appendicitis. Septicemia and metastatic focal infections are less common. Yersiniosis can be complicated by nonsuppurative, extraintestinal, inflammatory sequelae—e.g., reactive arthritis (Chap. 318) and erythema nodosum (Chap. 18). Other nonplague Yersinia species, including Y. intermedia, Y. frederiksenii, and Y. kristensenii, have been associated with enteritis or enterocolitis in humans (particularly immunocompromised adults), but little is known about their pathogenicity, public health importance, or clinical management.

ETIOLOGIC AGENTS

Y. enterocolitica and Y. pseudotuberculosis are pleomorphic gram-negative bacilli in the family Enterobacteriaceae. These organisms can multiply within a wide temperature range (−1°C to 45°C). Pathogenic Y. enterocolitica isolates are most commonly identified by biotyping based on biochemical profiles and serotyping according to somatic O and H antigens. Six biotypes and >60 serotypes of Y. enterocolitica are recognized. A separate serotyping system for Y. pseudotuberculosis (also based on somatic antigens) has distinguished six major serotypes (I–VI) and their subtypes.

EPIDEMIOLOGY

Yersinia enterocolitica Y. enterocolitica is distributed worldwide and has been isolated from soil, fresh water, contaminated foodstuffs (e.g., meat, milk, and vegetables), and a wide variety of wild and domestic animals. Many serotypes isolated from environmental sources, however, evidently are not human pathogens. Most human infections have been caused by Y. enterocolitica serotypes O:3; O:5,27; O:8; and O:9. These serotypes are primarily associated with wild and domestic mammals. The recognized incidence of these infections and their sequelae is highest in Scandinavia and some other northern European countries, but reliable population-based estimates of incidence are unavailable.

All age groups are susceptible to Y. enterocolitica infections, but the majority of cases of enterocolitis are in children 1–4 years old. These infections show a modest predilection for males. Mesenteric adenitis

and terminal ileitis are most common among older children and young adults. Risk factors for Y. enterocolitica septicemia and metastatic focal infections include chronic liver disease, malignancy, diabetes mellitus, immunosuppressive therapy, HIV disease, alcoholism, malnutrition, advanced age, iron overload (see "Pathogenesis and Pathology," below), and hemolytic anemias (including the thalassemias). The nonsuppurative sequelae of yersiniosis are most common among adults. HLA-B27 is expressed in 70–80% of patients who develop reactive arthritis associated with yersiniosis. HLA-B27 is not a risk factor for Yersinia-induced erythema nodosum; females with this condition outnumber males by 2 to 1.

Among Y. enterocolitica strains isolated from patients in recent decades, serotypes O:3 and O:9 have predominated in Europe, while serotype O:3 has predominated in Canada, Japan, and the United States. The apparent incidence of Yersinia-induced nonsuppurative sequelae reportedly is 10–30% in Scandinavia and much lower in most other countries, including the United States.

Common-source outbreaks of Y. enterocolitica enteritis have been traced to such vehicles as raw milk, contaminated pasteurized milk, and foods prepared with contaminated fresh water. Because Y. enterocolitica commonly colonizes the gastrointestinal tracts of swine, sporadic human cases and outbreaks of yersiniosis have also been associated with the preparation or ingestion of raw pork products (e.g., chitterlings). In some cases of yersiniosis, circumstantial evidence suggests transmission via contact with dogs and cats or their feces. Several nosocomial outbreaks of Y. enterocolitica infection have been described; fecal-oral transmission from person to person was suspected. Fecal-oral transmission among family members may also explain occasional secondary cases in households. In a prospective study of 50 children with Y. enterocolitica enteritis, fecal excretion of the organism persisted for an average of 27 days (range, 4–79 days) after the cessation of symptoms. A chronic carrier state, however, has not been demonstrated. Y. enterocolitica is a rare but often lethal cause of transfusion-associated septicemia. The explanation is that blood donors occasionally have transient, occult Y. enterocolitica bacteremia and that this organism can slowly multiply to high concentrations in blood refrigerated for at least 10 days.

Yersinia pseudotuberculosis The ecology of Y. pseudotuberculosis seems to parallel that of Y. enterocolitica closely. Y. pseudotuberculosis is also widespread in wild and domestic animals and is isolated from many environmental sources. Swine appear to be an important reservoir for pathogenic strains. Although human infections appear to be relatively rare, large common-source epidemics can occur.

PATHOGENESIS AND PATHOLOGY

With rare exceptions (e.g., transmission via contaminated blood products or direct cutaneous inoculation), the enteropathogenic yersiniae are thought to enter the host via the oral route. The incubation period averages 5 days (range, 1–11 days). Studies of animals have shown that the organisms initially invade the ileal epithelium, then are translocated via M cells into the lamina propria, and finally enter Peyer's patches, where they replicate. They subsequently drain into the mesenteric lymph nodes, which undergo hyperplasia and from which the bacteria can be disseminated. The mesenteric lymph nodes can become intensely swollen and matted and are occasionally detected on physical examination as a tender right-lower-quadrant mass. Intestinal inflammation (most commonly of the distal ileum and less commonly of the ascending colon) develops and may be accompanied by mucosal ulcerations and by the shedding of PMNs and red blood cells into the intestinal lumen. In relatively severe cases, thrombosis of mesenteric blood vessels, intestinal hemorrhage, and necrosis can occur. In patients with enteropathogenic yersinial infections who undergo exploratory laparotomy, the appendix usually is histologically normal or shows only lymphoid hyperplasia, but frank suppuration is sometimes evident.

A plasmid of ~70 kb is essential for virulence of the enteropathogenic yersiniae because it encodes at least six Yersinia outer-membrane proteins, which confer a variety of pathogenic properties—e.g., cytotoxicity; resistance to phagocytosis by PMNs; and the ability to cause monocyte apoptosis (programmed cell death), to suppress the host's expression of tumor necrosis factor α, and to interfere with platelet aggregation and host complement activation. A chromosomal gene (*inv*) encodes for the surface protein invasin, which is necessary for yersinial invasion of nonphagocytic host cells (e.g., epithelial cells) in vitro and which facilitates the translocation of bacteria across the intestinal epithelium. Both *Y. enterocolitica* and *Y. pseudotuberculosis* can express at least one protein superantigen that selectively stimulates the proliferation of T cells. Many strains of *Y. enterocolitica* produce a heat-stable enterotoxin that is similar to *Escherichia coli* enterotoxin. The cell walls of *Y. enterocolitica* and *Y. pseudotuberculosis* contain a lipopolysaccharide (endotoxin). Some *Yersinia* strains are unable to synthesize bacterial iron chelators called *siderophores*. However, they can exploit host-chelated iron stores and the drug deferoxamine (a siderophore produced by *Streptomyces pilosus*). Therefore, iron overload (e.g., caused by hemodialysis or multiple transfusions) and deferoxamine therapy appear to be independent risk factors for *Y. enterocolitica* bacteremia, especially that involving serotypes O:3 and O:9, and to a lesser degree for *Y. pseudotuberculosis* bacteremia.

Immunogenetic factors and cell-mediated immune responses are clearly involved in the pathogenesis of reactive arthritis following infection with the enteropathogenic yersiniae. As noted above, most patients with *Yersinia*-induced reactive arthritis express HLA-B27. In addition, *Y. pseudotuberculosis* shares at least one cross-reactive epitope with HLA-B27, and *Y. enterocolitica* infection alters the expression of serologic HLA-B27 epitopes on lymphocytes and monocytes. In patients with reactive arthritis following *Y. enterocolitica* infection, yersinial antigens are commonly detectable in synovial fluid cells in the apparent absence of whole organisms. Thus, it is unknown whether the arthritis results from occult bacterial persistence through self-tolerance of HLA-B27 with a failure of cross-reactive immune responses to yersiniae, from an immune response to common antigenic determinants shared by the bacteria and host HLA-B27 (i.e., molecular mimicry), or from other mechanisms. The pathogenesis of *Yersinia*-induced erythema nodosum is obscure.

In some assays, patients with Graves' disease have an increased prevalence of serum antibodies to *Y. enterocolitica*, and the immunoglobulins of patients recovering from *Y. enterocolitica* infections react with the human thyroid-stimulating hormone receptor. However, a link between *Y. enterocolitica* infection and the subsequent development of autoimmune thyroiditis has not been convincingly demonstrated. Similarly, the hypothesis that the nonplague yersinioses can trigger ulcerative colitis or Crohn's disease remains intriguing but unproven.

CLINICAL MANIFESTATIONS

Yersinia enterocolitica The principal clinical manifestations of *Y. enterocolitica* infection are enteritis, enterocolitis, mesenteric adenitis, and terminal ileitis. Less common manifestations include exudative pharyngitis, septicemia, metastatic focal infections, reactive polyarthritis, and erythema nodosum. When age groups are combined, the most common presentation of *Y. enterocolitica* infection is acute diarrhea from enteritis or enterocolitis. Low-grade fever and cramping abdominal pain occur in most cases, nausea and vomiting in 15–40%, hematochezia in up to 30%, and a generalized maculopapular skin rash in a few cases. Diarrhea persists for an average of 2 weeks (range, 1 day to many months), during which the frequency of bowel movements diminishes. Uncommonly, enteritis or enterocolitis can be complicated by severe abdominal pain and high fever. Rare (and sometimes fatal) complications include diffuse inflammation, ulceration, hemorrhage, and necrosis of the small bowel and colon; intestinal perforation; peritonitis; ascending cholangitis; mesenteric vein thrombosis; diverticulitis; toxic megacolon; and ileocecal intussusception.

The syndrome of mesenteric adenitis and terminal ileitis without diarrhea is easily confused with appendicitis. Low-grade fever and right-lower-quadrant pain, tenderness, guarding, and rebound tenderness are common. During six recognized common-source outbreaks in the United States, 10% of 444 patients with symptomatic undiagnosed *Y. enterocolitica* infections underwent laparotomy for suspected appendicitis; surgical incisions became infected with *Y. enterocolitica* in a few of these cases.

Acute pharyngitis and pharyngotonsillitis, with or without cervical adenitis or intestinal illness, are less common but potentially lethal manifestations of *Y. enterocolitica* infection, particularly in adults. *Y. enterocolitica* septicemia generally presents as a severe illness with fever and leukocytosis, often with abdominal pain and jaundice and without localized signs of infection. Metastatic focal *Y. enterocolitica* infections can occur with or without clinically apparent bacteremia and can affect almost any organ system. Examples include abscess formation (e.g., in liver, spleen, kidney, lung, skeletal muscle, lymph node, or cutaneous tissue), osteomyelitis, meningitis, peritonitis, urinary tract infection, pneumonia, empyema, endocarditis, pericarditis, mycotic aneurysm, septic arthritis, suppurative conjunctivitis, panophthalmitis, Parinaud's oculoglandular syndrome, and cutaneous pustules or bullae.

In Scandinavia, the incidence of reactive arthritis following *Y. enterocolitica* infection among adults is estimated to be at least 10%. About 80% of these patients have prior symptoms such as fever, diarrhea, or abdominal pain. Typically, these symptoms precede the arthritis by 1 week and are of short duration. The most commonly affected joints are the knees and ankles, but other joints can be involved. Typically, multiple (two to eight) joints become involved sequentially and asymmetrically over a period of a few days to 2 weeks, after which no additional joints are affected. Monarticular arthritis occurs less commonly. In two-thirds of cases, the acute arthritis remits spontaneously within 1–3 months. Chronic joint disease is documented in a minority of cases. A few HLA-B27-positive patients with *Y. enterocolitica*–induced arthritis have subsequent ankylosing spondylitis, but this development is best explained by the fact that HLA-B27 is a major risk factor for each of these diseases. Mild, self-limited myocarditis accompanies ~10% of cases of *Yersinia*-induced arthritis and can occur independently. Typical manifestations include cardiac murmurs and transient electrocardiographic abnormalities, such as prolongation of the PR interval and nonspecific ST-segment and T-wave changes. The syndrome of *Yersinia*-induced arthritis and carditis can be confused with acute rheumatic fever. In Scandinavia, erythema nodosum occurs in 15–20% of patients with yersiniosis, usually within a few days to 3 weeks after the onset of intestinal illness. Lesions typically are located on the lower extremities and resolve within 1 month. Less commonly reported nonsuppurative sequelae of *Y. enterocolitica* infections include reactive uveitis, iritis, conjunctivitis, urethritis, and glomerulonephritis. The complete triad of Reiter's syndrome (arthritis, conjunctivitis, and urethritis) is seen in 5–10% of patients with *Yersinia*-induced arthritis.

Yersinia pseudotuberculosis The most common clinical presentation of *Y. pseudotuberculosis* infection is fever and abdominal pain caused by mesenteric adenitis; diarrheal illness is less common than in *Y. enterocolitica* infection. Systemic manifestations, including septicemia, focal infections, reactive arthritis, and erythema nodosum, are generally similar to those associated with *Y. enterocolitica* infection. In addition, *Y. pseudotuberculosis* has been associated with a scarlet fever–like syndrome, acute interstitial nephritis, and hemolytic-uremic syndrome.

LABORATORY FINDINGS AND DIAGNOSIS

Results of routine laboratory tests in most patients with yersiniosis are nonspecific. Leukocyte counts are usually normal or slightly elevated, often with a modest left shift. Standard microbiologic methods are sufficient to isolate *Y. enterocolitica* and *Y. pseudotuberculosis* from otherwise-sterile sites, such as blood, CSF, lymph node tissue, and peritoneal fluid, and from abscesses. Isolation of these organisms from feces is impeded by their slow growth and the overgrowth of normal fecal flora on culture media routinely used to select for enteric bacteria. The yield from feces and other grossly contaminated specimens can be increased by the use of *Yersinia*-selective [e.g., cefsulodin-Irgasan-novobiocin (CIN)] agar and by cold enrichment. Because bacteriologic procedures designed to isolate yersiniae from feces are not considered cost-effective, many laboratories undertake them by special request only.

The results of serologic tests can be used to support a diagnosis of yersiniosis. Agglutination tests or ELISAs are used most commonly; immunoblotting has also been used. The existence of multiple serotypes makes routine serologic tests laborious; thus these tests are generally conducted only in research laboratories or large commercial laboratories. Since these tests are experimental and are neither standardized nor well validated, and since some strains of *Yersinia* cross-react with other bacteria (e.g., *Brucella*, *Salmonella*, *Vibrio*, and *Borrelia*) and with serum from some patients with thyroiditis, results should be interpreted with caution. In typical uncomplicated cases of yersiniosis, agglutinin titers begin to rise within the first week of illness, peak in the second week, and then gradually diminish and return to normal within 3–6 months, although agglutinating antibody may remain detectable for several years in some cases. Because an initial serum specimen is often collected ≥1 week after the onset of illness, when agglutinin titers are already high, it is usually impossible to document a fourfold or greater rise in titer between paired specimens (although a fourfold or greater fall in titer may be found). Immunohistochemical techniques and PCR tests to detect yersinial antigens and DNA, respectively, in clinical specimens are experimental at this time.

In patients with *Yersinia*-induced reactive arthritis, synovial fluid is sterile and the leukocyte count ranges from a few hundred to 60,000/μL, with a majority of PMNs. The erythrocyte sedimentation rate is often >100 mm/h. Rheumatoid factor and antinuclear antibodies are usually absent. The diagnosis of *Yersinia*-induced reactive arthritis or other nonsuppurative inflammatory sequelae can be difficult, especially when triggering infections are asymptomatic or clinically mild or occur several weeks before the diagnosis is attempted. Because the isolation of a pathogenic *Yersinia* strain from feces is the most specific diagnostic test in such cases, it should be attempted. Since culture is of limited sensitivity in this clinical setting, a high index of suspicion and positive results of serologic tests for *Y. enterocolitica* or *Y. pseudotuberculosis* are usually required for diagnosis.

℞ OTHER *YERSINIA* INFECTIONS

The effectiveness of antimicrobial agents in the treatment of yersinial enteritis, enterocolitis, mesenteric adenitis, or terminal ileitis has not been established. These conditions are usually self-limited, and their treatment is symptom-based and supportive. In uncomplicated cases, diarrhea should be treated with fluid and electrolyte replacement, with the route of delivery dependent on clinical severity. Enteric precautions are advisable for patients hospitalized with yersinial diarrhea. In general, antimicrobial treatment should be reserved for patients with septicemia, metastatic focal infections, or immunosuppression and enterocolitis. Controlled clinical comparisons of antimicrobial agents in the treatment of severe cases of yersiniosis have not yet been conducted. In such cases, drug selection should ultimately be guided by clinical response and bacterial sensitivity patterns. Clinical isolates of *Y. enterocolitica* and *Y. pseudotuberculosis* are usually susceptible in vitro to aminoglycosides, third-generation cephalosporins, chloramphenicol, quinolones, tetracyclines, and TMP-SMX. In laboratory animals infected with enteropathogenic yersiniae, the fluoro-

quinolones have exerted the strongest bactericidal effects in vivo; clinical experience with these drugs against these pathogens in humans is promising but limited. Because they produce β-lactamases, isolates typically are resistant to penicillin, ampicillin, carbenicillin, and first-generation and most second-generation cephalosporins. Optimal dosages and durations of therapy have not been established. Mortality rates from *Y. enterocolitica* septicemia are ~10% despite treatment. Focal extraintestinal infections may require at least 3 weeks of therapy. No role for antimicrobial agents in the management of the nonsuppurative inflammatory manifestations of yersiniosis has been established. Patients with reactive arthritis may benefit from treatment with nonsteroidal anti-inflammatory drugs, intraarticular steroid injections, and physical therapy.

PREVENTION AND CONTROL

The importance of safe food-handling and food-preparation practices in the prevention of yersiniosis cannot be overemphasized. Caution is particularly warranted in the case of pork and other animal products. The consumption of raw or undercooked meats, especially pork, should be avoided. Increased efforts to prevent the spread of enteric pathogens in household, pet-care, day-care, and hospital settings and in the food industry would be likely to decrease the incidence of yersiniosis. Current regulations of the U.S. Food and Drug Administration require visual inspection of packed red cell units before transfusion, with the discarding of units in which bacterial contamination is suspected on the basis of darkening (reflecting decreased oxygen saturation and hemolysis). Since the risk is minimal, more specific measures to further decrease the likelihood of transfusion of *Y. enterocolitica*–contaminated blood products (e.g., limiting the period for which red cells can be stored before transfusion) have not been widely implemented.

Yersiniosis is not routinely reportable to public health authorities in most jurisdictions. However, clinicians who suspect a common-source outbreak (e.g., because they have documented a familial case cluster) or some other public health threat (e.g., because they have found *Y. enterocolitica* bacteremia in a recent blood donor) should consult promptly with local public health officials.

FURTHER READINGS

ABDEL-HAQ NM et al: Antibiotic susceptibilities of *Yersinia enterocolitica* recovered from children over a 12-year period. Int J Antimicrob Agents 27:449, 2006

DAS R et al: Study of proinflammatory responses induced by *Yersinia pestis* in human monocytes using cDNA arrays. Genes Immun 8:308, 2007

EISEN RJ et al: Human plague in the southwestern United States, 1957–2004: Spatial models of elevated risk of human exposure to *Yersinia pestis*. J Med Entomol 44:530, 2007

GRAHEK-OGDEN D: Outbreak of *Yersinia enterocolitica* serogroup O:9 infection and processed pork, Norway. Emerg Infect Dis 13:754, 2007

PERDIKOGIANNI C et al: *Yersinia enterocolitica* infection mimicking surgical conditions. Pediatr Surg Int 22:589, 2006

PRENTICE MB, RAHALISON L: Plague. Lancet 369:1196, 2007

153 *Bartonella* Infections, Including Cat-Scratch Disease
David H. Spach, Emily Darby

Bartonella species are gram-negative bacteria that can cause an array of infectious diseases, including cat-scratch disease (CSD), bacillary angiomatosis, bacteremia, culture-negative endocarditis, trench fever,

and bartonellosis (Table 153-1). Three *Bartonella* species play a major role in causing human disease: *B. bacilliformis*, *B. quintana*, and *B. henselae*. Recent advances in molecular diagnostics have expanded the list of diseases known to be caused by *Bartonella* species.

CAT-SCRATCH DISEASE

DEFINITION AND ETIOLOGY

CSD is typically a self-limited illness characterized by regional lymphadenopathy lasting weeks to months. *B. henselae* is the primary caus-

TABLE 153-1 MAJOR DISEASES CAUSED BY *BARTONELLA* SPECIES

Disease	Organism	Risk Factor
Cat-scratch disease	*B. henselae*	Cat scratch or bite
Bacillary angiomatosis	*B. quintana, B. henselae*	Cat scratch or bite
Bacillary peliosis	*B. henselae*	Cat scratch or bite
Trench fever	*B. quintana*	Homelessness, body louse infestation, alcoholism
Endocarditis	*B. quintana, B. henselae, B. elizabethae*	As for cat-scratch disease and trench fever
Bartonellosis	*B. bacilliformis*	Sandfly bite

ative agent. Infrequently, patients with CSD develop disseminated *B. henselae* infection.

EPIDEMIOLOGY

CSD has a global distribution. In the United States, the annual incidence is ~4–9 cases per 100,000 persons, with ~40% of cases involving adults. Cats are the primary host for *B. henselae* and transmit the infection to humans via a scratch, bite, or lick. In cats (particularly kittens), the incidence of asymptomatic *B. henselae* bacteremia is high. The cat flea (*Ctenocephalides felis*) serves as the vector for transmission between animals. Rarely, CSD occurs after exposure to dogs.

CLINICAL PRESENTATION

The initial clinical manifestation—the primary inoculation lesion—consists of a 0.5- to 1-cm papule, vesicle, or nodule that appears at the site where *B. henselae* is introduced and persists for ~1–3 weeks. Adenopathy typically develops 2–3 weeks after the initial scratch or bite (range, 3–50 days). Unilateral solitary or regional lymphadenopathy (Fig. 153-1) occurs in more than 90% of patients; its location corresponds with the route of lymphatic drainage. Lymph nodes are tender, firm, and mobile, and ~10% suppurate; overlying erythema is occasionally present. Nonspecific systemic symptoms, such as fever, anorexia, headache, myalgias, malaise, and abdominal pain, are variably present at this stage. Lymphadenopathy usually resolves within 3 months.

Atypical presentations of CSD are described in up to one-quarter of cases. Parinaud's oculoglandular syndrome is a frequently reported atypical presentation that follows inoculation of bacteria onto the conjunctiva or eyelid. Patients develop unilateral manifestations that may include conjunctivitis, granulomatous lesions, and preauricular lymphadenopathy. Systemic spread of *B. henselae* may occur independent of lymphadenopathy or may follow the more typical manifestations of the disease. Disseminated disease most often involves the nervous system, visceral organs, or bone. Patients with neuroretinitis generally present with sudden, painless loss of vision. Most ocular abnormalities caused by CSD usually resolve within several months without residual damage; however, some patients have long-lasting visual deficits. Other rare complications include encephalitis, peripheral nerve abnormalities, myelitis, facial palsy, and granulomatous hepatitis or splenitis.

PATHOLOGY

Early in the course of CSD, histologic examination of lymph nodes reveals follicular hyperplasia and arteriolar proliferation. Cortical granulomas, with occasional multinucleated giant cells, neutrophilic infiltrates, and coalescing microabscesses (stellate microabscesses), appear within weeks; the granulomas are surrounded by histiocytes and peripheral lymphocytes. Warthin-Starry stain may reveal typical clusters of pleomorphic gram-negative organisms within areas of necrosis, blood vessel walls, or erythrocytes.

DIAGNOSIS

A suspected diagnosis of CSD is usually based on a typical clinical presentation in conjunction with a history of recent cat exposure. Results of routine laboratory studies are generally normal. The differential diagnosis most often includes lymphoma, mycobacterial infection, and soft tissue infection caused by methicillin-resistant *Staphylococcus au-*

FIGURE 153-1 Characteristic regional (axillary) lymphadenopathy in a patient with cat-scratch disease.

reus. Not only can CSD overlap clinically with lymphoma and mycobacterial infection; it can also occur in conjunction with these diseases. Serologic tests for antibody to *B. henselae* can support the clinical diagnosis but do not have optimal sensitivity and specificity. Accordingly, in most instances, lymph node biopsy or aspiration is required to rule out other diseases and establish the diagnosis. In this situation, polymerase chain reaction (PCR) analysis of the tissue sample is generally preferred. Cultures of lymph node tissue are rarely positive.

℞ CAT-SCRATCH DISEASE

(Table 153-2) In most cases of typical CSD, illness eventually resolves without therapy. Studies of antimicrobial treatment for CSD in immunocompetent patients have demonstrated only modest benefit. Some experts advocate reassurance and supportive care for management of lymphadenopathy in immunocompetent patients, whereas others recommend treatment with azithromycin to expedite resolution of lymphadenopathy. Antimicrobial therapy is uniformly recommended for immunosuppressed patients with CSD. Most clinicians treat atypical manifestations of CSD, but there are few data to guide the management of atypical disease.

BARTONELLA INFECTIONS IN HIV-INFECTED PERSONS

B. henselae and *B. quintana* can cause a broad spectrum of disease in HIV-infected individuals, including bacillary angiomatosis, peliosis hepatis, osteomyelitis, unexplained fever, bacteremia, and endocarditis. Bacillary angiomatosis is the most common of these manifestations (Chap. 182). Regardless of the manifestations, serologic tests may help support the diagnosis. (See below for a full discussion of all these specific conditions.)

℞ *BARTONELLA* INFECTIONS IN HIV-INFECTED PERSONS

As detailed below, antibiotic therapy (Table 153-2) is strongly recommended for all HIV-infected patients with *Bartonella* infections. Indeed, visceral disease may be progressive and fatal without appropriate antibiotic therapy. Relapses of *Bartonella* infections in HIV-infected persons are common, particularly after relatively short antibiotic courses.

BACILLARY ANGIOMATOSIS AND PELIOSIS HEPATIS

ETIOLOGY AND EPIDEMIOLOGY

Bacillary angiomatosis and peliosis hepatis occur primarily in HIV-infected persons whose CD4+ T cell counts are <100/μL. Earlier studies suggested that ~1 in 1000 HIV-infected persons developed bacillary angiomatosis; however, this incidence has declined in recent years, probably

TABLE 153-2 TREATMENT OF ADULTS WITH DISEASE CAUSED BY BARTONELLA SPECIES[a]

Disease	Treatment
Cat-scratch disease	
Lymphadenopathy	Consider azithromycin (500 mg PO on day 1, then 250 mg PO qd for 4 days)
Retinitis	Doxycycline (100 mg PO bid for 4–6 weeks) *plus*
	Rifampin (300 mg PO bid for 4–6 weeks)
Bacillary angiomatosis	Erythromycin (500 mg PO qid for 3 months) *or*
	Doxycycline (100 mg PO bid for 3 months)
Bacillary peliosis	Erythromycin (500 mg PO qid for 4 months) *or*
	Doxycycline (100 mg PO bid for 4 months)
Bartonella endocarditis	
Suspected	Gentamicin (3 mg/kg qd IV for 14 days) *plus* ceftriaxone (2 g IV qd for 6 weeks) *with or without*
	Doxycycline (100 mg PO bid for 6 weeks)
Confirmed	Gentamicin (3 mg/kg qd IV for 14 days) *plus*
	Doxycycline (100 mg PO bid for 6 weeks)
Trench fever	Doxycycline (200 mg PO qd for 4 weeks) *plus*
	Gentamicin (3 mg/kg qd IV for 14 days)
Bartonellosis	
Oroya fever	Chloramphenicol (500 mg PO or IV qid for 14 days) *plus* a β-lactam agent *or*
	Ciprofloxacin (500 mg bid for 10 days)
Verruga peruana	Rifampin (10 mg/kg qd PO for 14 days) *or*
	Streptomycin (15–20 mg/kg qd IM for 10 days)

[a]Based on recommendations from Rolain et al, 2004.

FIGURE 153-2 Nodular lesion of bacillary angiomatosis with superficial ulceration in an AIDS patient with advanced immunodeficiency.

stroma containing a mixture of inflammatory cells, dilated capillaries, and clumps of granular material. Warthin-Starry stain may reveal bacilli.

DIAGNOSIS

The diagnosis of bacillary angiomatosis is ideally based on histologic findings (see "Pathology," above).

℞ BACILLARY ANGIOMATOSIS AND PELIOSIS HEPATIS

(Table 153-2) As stated above, prolonged therapy with oral erythromycin or doxycycline is recommended for both bacillary angiomatosis and peliosis hepatis.

as a result of effective antiretroviral therapy and the consequent decrease in the number of patients with advanced immunodeficiency. Cutaneous bacillary angiomatosis is caused by *B. henselae* or *B. quintana*, subcutaneous nodules and lytic bone predominantly by *B. quintana*, and bacillary peliosis by *B. henselae*. Risk factors for *B. henselae* infection consist of contact with cats or fleas, whereas *B. quintana* infections are associated with low income, homelessness, and louse infestation.

CLINICAL PRESENTATION

Patients with bacillary angiomatosis most often present with painless cutaneous lesions, but other manifestations include subcutaneous masses or nodules (Fig. 153-2), superficial ulcerated plaques, and verrucous growths. The cutaneous lesions may be single or multiple and may vary in color from tan to red to deep purple. The differential diagnosis of cutaneous bacillary angiomatosis includes Kaposi's sarcoma, pyogenic granuloma, and subcutaneous tumors. Painful osseous lesions may develop beneath the cutaneous lesions. Bacillary angiomatosis may rarely involve the oropharynx, lungs, heart, intestines, lymph nodes, muscle, or brain. Patients with bacillary peliosis usually present with nonspecific systemic symptoms, with or without cutaneous involvement. Radiographic studies of osseous bacillary angiomatosis typically demonstrate lytic bone lesions on plain films and focal uptake of technetium on bone scans. Imaging of patients with peliosis hepatis generally reveals hypodense regions in the liver. In patients with advanced immunodeficiency, *B. henselae* and *B. quintana* can cause unexplained fever. In addition, *B. henselae* or *B. quintana* is occasionally identified as the cause of endocarditis in HIV-infected persons.

PATHOLOGY

Histologic examination of bacillary angiomatosis lesions demonstrates lobular proliferation of blood vessels lined by enlarged endothelial cells with a mixed infiltrate of neutrophils and lymphocytes. Examination of bacillary peliosis tissue reveals small blood-filled cystic lesions partially lined by endothelial cells and generally surrounded by a fibromyxoid

TRENCH FEVER

DEFINITION AND ETIOLOGY

Trench fever, a febrile illness caused by *B. quintana*, was initially described in World War I, during which the disease developed in an estimated 1 million soldiers on the western and eastern European fronts. In modern times, *B. quintana* infection has resurfaced as "urban trench fever."

EPIDEMIOLOGY

Available data suggest that *B. quintana* has a global distribution, and cases of trench fever have now been reported sporadically throughout the world. Risk factors associated with urban trench fever include poverty, homelessness, and alcoholism. Multiple studies have established the body louse as the principal vector for transmitting *B. quintana* to humans. No animal reservoirs have been identified.

CLINICAL PRESENTATION

Reports of classic trench fever in World War I described an incubation period of 5–20 days followed by one of four patterns of illness: (1) a solitary episode of fever; (2) a brief febrile period typically lasting <1 week; (3) febrile episodes lasting ~5 days interspersed with asymptomatic intervals of ~5 days ("quintan fever"); and (4) a persistent and debilitating febrile illness, often lasting >1 month. Despite the seriousness of the illness, mortality rates are low. In modern-day cases, patients have presented with nonspecific and inconsistent clinical symptoms that have included fever, headache, weight loss, and leg pain. Many patients in contemporary case series have been diagnosed with chronic bacteremia (often asymptomatic), and occasional patients have been diagnosed with culture-negative endocarditis (see below).

DIAGNOSIS

The diagnosis of urban trench fever is most often made on the basis of serologic studies or by isolating *B. quintana* from blood cultures. In patients with endocarditis who require valve replacement surgery, PCR testing of valve tissue can establish the diagnosis.

PART 7

Infectious Diseases

℞ TRENCH FEVER

(Table 153-2) Relatively few data exist regarding optimal therapy for urban trench fever. Mild cases can be treated with doxycycline. However, patients with bacteremia should receive both doxycycline and gentamicin, mainly to prevent the development of endocarditis. Patients with documented endocarditis also should receive doxycycline plus gentamicin.

ENDOCARDITIS

DEFINITION AND ETIOLOGY

Bartonella species have now been established as an important cause of "culture-negative" endocarditis. Although reports have identified five *Bartonella* species as causes of infective endocarditis in humans, >95% of cases have involved either *B. quintana* or *B. henselae*.

EPIDEMIOLOGY

Sporadic cases of *Bartonella*-associated endocarditis have been reported in multiple regions of the world. Most cases have involved adults, and most have affected native heart valves. Identified risk factors for *B. quintana* endocarditis consist of homelessness and infestation with body lice, whereas exposure to cats and previous valvular heart disease are associated with *B. henselae* endocarditis.

CLINICAL PRESENTATION

Clinical findings in *Bartonella* endocarditis resemble the typical findings in subacute bacterial endocarditis. Because blood cultures usually have no evident growth in the first 7–10 days, *Bartonella* endocarditis often is initially diagnosed as culture-negative endocarditis.

DIAGNOSIS

The diagnosis of endocarditis is based on clinical, laboratory, and echocardiographic findings. The identification of *Bartonella* as the specific pathogen causing endocarditis can prove challenging, especially since only ~25% of patients with *Bartonella* endocarditis have *Bartonella* isolated from blood cultures. The yield of blood cultures is enhanced by extended incubation (for 4–6 weeks). In patients from whose blood cultures *Bartonella* is not isolated, the diagnosis is usually based on either a strongly positive serologic test or evidence (most often obtained with a PCR-based method) of *Bartonella* in cardiac valve tissue.

℞ ENDOCARDITIS

(Table 153-2) For "culture-negative" endocarditis in which *Bartonella* is the suspected cause, empirical treatment consists of ceftriaxone plus gentamicin, with or without doxycycline. For confirmed *Bartonella* endocarditis, treatment consists of doxycycline plus gentamicin. If gentamicin cannot be used, rifampin should be considered as a substitute.

BARTONELLOSIS (CARRIÓN'S DISEASE)

DEFINITION AND ETIOLOGY

Bartonellosis, or Carrión's disease, is caused by *B. bacilliformis*. The disease is characterized by two distinct phases: (1) an acute febrile hematic phase, known as Oroya fever; and (2) an eruptive phase manifested by cutaneous lesions, known as verruga peruana. In 1885, Daniel Carrión, a Peruvian medical student, established the common source of the two phases of this illness by inoculating himself with material from a verruga peruana lesion and subsequently developing fatal Oroya fever.

EPIDEMIOLOGY

Bartonellosis occurs endemically in certain regions of South America. It has been reported predominantly in river valleys of the Andes Mountains in Peru as well as in some localized regions of Colombia and Ecuador. The sandfly *Lutzomyia verrucarum* serves as the vector for *B. bacilliformis* and transmits the organism to humans via a bite on the skin. Most patients with acute bartonellosis are immunologically naïve, and most cases involve tourists and transient workers. In contrast, the eruptive phase of bartonellosis most often occurs among the native population in the Andes.

CLINICAL PRESENTATION

The clinical manifestations of acute bartonellosis typically begin ~3 weeks after inoculation of *B. bacilliformis* and include fever, malaise, changes in mental status, hepatomegaly, lymphadenopathy, and profound macrocytic anemia. Patients are typically bacteremic with *B. bacilliformis* at this phase. Without antimicrobial therapy, the mortality rate exceeds 40%; infections with other pathogens and noninfectious complications contribute to this high mortality rate. Treatment with chloramphenicol during the acute phase decreases, but does not eliminate, the risk of developing eruptive bartonellosis. Only ~5% of persons with eruptive cutaneous verrugas recall having experienced an acute febrile illness in the preceding 3 months. The cutaneous verrugas typically manifest as reddish-purple pruritic papules or nodules and may resemble the cutaneous lesions of bacillary angiomatosis. Untreated, the lesions can persist for years.

DIAGNOSIS

The diagnosis of acute bartonellosis can reliably be made by detection of intraerythrocytic organisms in a Wright-Giemsa-stained thin blood smear. In addition, most patients have positive blood cultures, but 2–3 weeks are typically required for the organism's isolation. For patients with cutaneous verrugas in the eruptive phase, biopsy should be performed. Histopathologic examination characteristically shows intense proliferation of newly formed capillaries and marked endothelial hyperplasia. The yield of blood smear and blood culture is markedly lower among patients in the eruptive phase. The utility of serologic tests is high for patients in both phases.

℞ BARTONELLOSIS

(Table 153-2) Use of chloramphenicol plus a second antimicrobial agent (generally a β-lactam) is generally recommended to provide effective treatment of *B. bacilliformis* and to cover any likely concomitant secondary bacterial infection. Treatment with ciprofloxacin, streptomycin, tetracycline, and erythromycin is also effective. Rifampin or streptomycin should be used to treat chronic bartonellosis.

FURTHER READINGS

Foucault C et al: *Bartonella quintana* characteristics and clinical management. Emerg Infect Dis 12:217, 2006

Hansmann Y et al: Diagnosis of cat scratch disease with detection of *Bartonella henselae* by PCR: A study of patients with lymph node enlargement. J Clin Microbiol 43:3800, 2005

Houpikian P, Raoult D: Blood culture–negative endocarditis in a reference center: Etiologic diagnosis of 348 cases. Medicine (Baltimore) 84:162, 2005

Maguina C et al: Bartonellosis (Carrión's disease) in the modern era. Clin Infect Dis 33:772, 2001

Mohle-Boetani JC et al: Bacillary angiomatosis and bacillary peliosis in patients infected with human immunodeficiency virus: Clinical characteristics in a case-control study. Clin Infect Dis 22:794, 1996

Ohl ME, Spach DH: *Bartonella quintana* and urban trench fever. Clin Infect Dis 31:131, 2000

Rolain JM et al: Lymph node biopsy specimens and diagnosis of cat scratch disease. Emerg Infect Dis 12:1338, 2006

Rolain JM et al: Recommendations for treatment of human infections caused by *Bartonella* species. Antimicrob Agents Chemother 48:1921, 2004

Spach DH, Koehler JE: *Bartonella*-associated infections. Infect Dis Clin North Am 12:137, 1998

154 Donovanosis
Gavin Hart

Donovanosis is a chronic, progressively destructive bacterial infection of the genital region that is generally regarded as sexually transmitted (see "Epidemiology," below). The disease has been known by many other names, the most common of which are *granuloma inguinale* and *granuloma venereum*.

ETIOLOGY

Donovanosis is caused by *Klebsiella granulomatis* (formerly known as *Calymmatobacterium granulomatis*), an intracellular, gram-negative, pleomorphic, encapsulated (when mature) bacterium measuring 1.5 by 0.7 µm. *K. granulomatis* shares many morphologic and serologic characteristics and >99% homology at the nucleotide level with *Klebsiella* species that are pathogenic to humans. Polymerase chain reaction (PCR) amplification of the *phoE* gene shows it to be closely related to that in *Klebsiella pneumoniae*, *K. rhinoscleromatis*, and *K. ozaenae*. Electron microscopy shows typical gram-negative morphology and a large capsule but no flagella. Filiform or vesicular protrusions occur on a corrugated cell wall.

EPIDEMIOLOGY

Donovanosis is endemic among Aborigines in central Australia as well as in Papua New Guinea, southeastern India, southern Africa, Vietnam, the Caribbean, Brazil, and Argentina. In the first half of the twentieth century, the disease was endemic in parts of the United States (with an estimated 5000–10,000 cases in 1947); small epidemics still occur in this country and in other developed countries. The decline in the United States to fewer than 20 reported cases annually in the past decade has probably resulted from lower transmission rates due to earlier presentation for increasingly effective antibiotic therapy. More than 70% of cases involve persons 20–40 years of age.

The infection is predominantly sexually transmitted, but extragenital skin lesions can follow transmission from concurrent genital lesions via the fingers or through other nonsexual contact, and autoinoculation may produce new lesions from contact with adjacent skin ("kissing" lesions). Infants born to infected mothers have acquired infection at birth.

CLINICAL MANIFESTATIONS

The incubation period is usually 1–4 weeks but may extend to 1 year. Skin lesions have been detected in infants 6 weeks to 6 months after birth. The disease begins as one or more subcutaneous nodules that erode through the skin to produce clean, granulomatous, sharply defined, usually painless lesions (Fig. 154-1). These lesions, which bleed readily on contact, slowly enlarge. The genitalia are involved in 90% of cases, the inguinal region in 10%, and the anal region in 5–10%. Genital swelling, particularly of the labia, is a common feature and occasionally progresses to pseudoelephantiasis. Phimosis and paraphimosis are common local complications, and progressive erosion of affected tissues may completely destroy the penis or other organs. Less common clinical variants include a hypertrophic form (cauliflower- or wartlike lesions), a necrotic form (destructive lesions with foul-smelling exudate, often resembling amebiasis), and a sclerotic or cicatricial form, which has a dry base with extensive scar tissue. Tissue destruction may be greater in patients co-infected with HIV than in those without HIV infection.

Extragenital lesions occur in at least 6% of cases. Oral donovanosis, the most common extragenital manifestation, presents as pain or bleeding in the mouth, lesions on the lips, or extensive swelling of the gums and palate. Donovanosis may affect most bones, and sometimes many bones are affected at the same time; the tibia is involved in >50% of such cases. Bony lesions are associated with constitutional symptoms (weight loss, fever, night sweats, and malaise) and are usually found in women. More than 50% of women with donovanosis have

FIGURE 154-1 Multiple granulomatous lesions of the penis in a patient with donovanosis.

primary lesions on the cervix. Prompt pelvic examinations and early diagnosis are likely to substantially decrease the morbidity and mortality (likely outcomes in misdiagnosed spinal lesions) associated with extragenital donovanosis in women.

DIAGNOSIS

Laboratory Diagnosis The preferred diagnostic method involves demonstration of typical intracellular Donovan bodies within large mononuclear cells visualized in smears prepared from lesions (Fig. 154-2) or biopsy specimens. With typical beefy lesions, a small piece of tissue is removed with forceps and scalpel, and a crush impression of the deep surface is made on a glass slide. The smear is air-dried, heat-fixed, and stained with Giemsa, Leishman's, or Wright's stain. For dry, flat, or necrotic lesions, a punch-biopsy specimen should be obtained from the advancing edge. This specimen can be used to prepare a smear or embedded for histologic examination (with a silver stain). Histologic ex-

FIGURE 154-2 The typical appearance of Donovan bodies is seen in a large mononuclear cell (20–90 µm in diameter; Giemsa stain; original magnification, ×1000). The host cell nucleus is usually oval, eccentric, and vesicular or pyknotic. The causative organisms appear as bipolar-staining (closed safety-pin) forms that measure 1–1.5 µm in length and 0.5–0.7 µm in diameter and are contained in cytoplasmic vacuoles.

TABLE 154-1 DIFFERENTIAL DIAGNOSIS OF DONOVANOSIS	
Disease (Chapter)	**Distinguishing Features**
Secondary syphilis: condylomata lata (162)	White or pale moist plaques in anogenital region (as opposed to bright red donovanosis lesions); lesions subside within 1 week of treatment with benzathine penicillin, 2.4 mU (whereas donovanosis lesions remain unchanged)
Squamous cell carcinoma (83)	Histologic appearance
Penile amebiasis (202)	Microscopic identification of *Entamoeba histolytica*
Chancroid: pseudogranuloma inguinale (139)	Culture of *Haemophilus ducreyi*
Tuberculosis (158)	Histologic features of bony lesions
Actinomycosis (156)	Microscopic identification of sulfur granules
Rhinoscleroma (143)	Histologic features
Leishmaniasis (205)	Histologic features
Histoplasmosis (192)	Histologic features

amination shows epithelial proliferation, often simulating neoplasia, with a heavy inflammatory infiltrate of plasma cells, some neutrophils, and few if any lymphocytes. *K. granulomatis* has never been grown on artificial solid media but has been cultured in chicken embryonic yolk sacs, on human monocytes, and on human epithelial (HEp-2) cells. A diagnostic PCR test has been developed and incorporated into a colorimetric detection system for *K. granulomatis*. A serologic test, based on indirect immunofluorescence, is more useful in confirming the diagnosis in cases with long-standing lesions than in early disease.

Differential Diagnosis The differential diagnosis of donovanosis is summarized in Table 154-1. Syphilis and donovanosis frequently coexist because syphilis is usually highly prevalent in areas where donovanosis is endemic; thus positive syphilis serology does not exclude a diagnosis of donovanosis. Genital ulcers are a risk factor for HIV acquisition in developing countries, and patients with donovanosis should be tested for HIV infection.

℞ DONOVANOSIS

Table 154-2 shows the most effective regimens for treating donovanosis. Doxycycline offers the advantage of convenient administration and has been widely used in developed countries, but azithromycin is increasingly

TABLE 154-2 THE MOST EFFECTIVE ANTIBIOTIC REGIMENS FOR TREATMENT OF DONOVANOSIS[a]	
Antibiotic	**Oral Dosage**
Azithromycin	1 g weekly or 500 mg/d
Erythromycin	500 mg qid
Tetracycline	500 mg qid
Doxycycline	100 mg bid
Trimethoprim-sulfamethoxazole	1 double-strength tablet[b] bid
Chloramphenicol	500 mg tid

[a]Patients should be examined weekly, and therapy should be continued until lesions have healed (3–5 weeks, except in severe cases).
[b]160 mg/800 mg.

being used as first-choice therapy. Extensive lesions have been cured with oral azithromycin at a dosage of 500 mg/d, but the more convenient dose of 1 g weekly is also effective. Although chloramphenicol is the drug of choice in some developing countries, it is unlikely to be acceptable in developed countries because of bone marrow toxicity. Penicillin is not effective for treating donovanosis. Patients should be examined weekly, and therapy should be continued until lesions have healed (3–5 weeks, except in severe cases). If antibiotic therapy is stopped earlier, lesions often continue to heal, but the relapse rate is higher. If the lesions are unchanged after 2 weeks of treatment, an alternative antibiotic regimen should be used.

The treatment regimens listed in Table 154-2—perhaps with increased duration—are usually adequate in HIV-infected patients without immunosuppression, but an increasing failure rate has been reported in immunosuppressed patients, for whom daily administration of azithromycin is recommended if other regimens fail to elicit a response.

FURTHER READINGS

See *www.stdservices.on.net/std/donovanosis/Default.htm* for an illustrated lecture and a comprehensive bibliography on donovanosis.

HART G: Donovanosis (granuloma inguinale), in *Atlas of Infectious Diseases*, vol V: *Sexually Transmitted Diseases*, MF Rein (ed). Philadelphia, Churchill Livingstone, 1996, pp 17.1–17.10

———: Donovanosis. Clin Infect Dis 25:24, 1997

O'FARRELL N: Donovanosis. Sex Transm Infect 78:452, 2002

SARDANA K, SEHGAL V: Genital ulcer disease and human immunodeficiency virus: A focus. Int J Dermatol 44:391, 2005

WU JJ et al: Selected sexually transmitted diseases and their relationship to HIV. Clin Dermatol 22:499, 2004

SECTION 7 MISCELLANEOUS BACTERIAL INFECTIONS

155 Nocardiosis
Gregory A. Filice

Nocardiosis refers to disease caused by bacteria of the genus *Nocardia*. Pneumonia and disseminated disease are most common. Other forms include cellulitis, lymphocutaneous syndrome, actinomycetoma, and keratitis.

MICROBIOLOGY

Nocardiae are saprophytic aerobic actinomycetes and are common worldwide in soil, where they contribute to decay of organic matter. Nocardial taxonomy is complex and incompletely understood. As taxonomy continues to evolve, any nocardiae isolated from a human should be considered potential pathogens.

Nocardia asteroides, which is most commonly isolated from clinical material and associated with invasive disease, is actually a species complex. Six other *Nocardia* species [*N. brasiliensis*, *N. otitidiscaviarum* (formerly *N. caviae*), *N. farcinica*, *N. nova*, *N. transvalensis*, and *N. pseudobrasiliensis*] have been firmly established as human pathogens, and at least 11 additional species have been associated with human disease.

N. farcinica is a less common human pathogen than *N. asteroides* but is more virulent and prone to dissemination. *N. pseudobrasiliensis* is most often associated with invasive disease, and *N. brasiliensis* is usually associated with disease limited to the skin. *N. transvalensis* is generally associated with pulmonary or systemic disease in immunosuppressed patients or with actinomycetoma, an indolent, slowly progressive disease of skin and underlying tissues with nodular swellings and draining sinuses.

EPIDEMIOLOGY

Approximately 1100 cases of nocardial infection are diagnosed annually in the United States, 85% of them pulmonary and/or systemic.

The annual incidence is ~0.375 cases per 100,000 persons. The disease is more common among adults than among children and among males than among females. Nearly all cases are sporadic, but outbreaks have been associated with contamination of the hospital environment, solutions, or drug injection equipment. Person-to-person spread is not well documented. There is no known seasonality.

The risk of pulmonary or disseminated disease is greater than usual among persons with deficient cell-mediated immunity, especially that associated with lymphoma, transplantation, glucocorticoid therapy, or AIDS. The incidence is ~140-fold greater among patients with AIDS and ~340-fold greater among bone marrow transplant recipients than in general populations. In AIDS, nocardiosis usually affects persons with <250 CD4+ T lymphocytes/μL. Nocardiosis has also been associated with pulmonary alveolar proteinosis, tuberculosis and other mycobacterial diseases, chronic granulomatous disease, interleukin 12 deficiency, and treatment with monoclonal antibodies to tumor necrosis factor. Any child with nocardiosis and no known cause of immunosuppression should undergo tests to determine the adequacy of the phagocytic respiratory burst.

Actinomycetoma associated with *N. brasiliensis*, *N. asteroides*, *N. otitidiscaviarum*, and *N. transvalensis* occurs mainly in tropical and subtropical regions, especially those of Mexico, Central and South America, Africa, and India. The most important risk factor is frequent contact with soil or vegetable matter.

PATHOLOGY AND PATHOGENESIS

Pneumonia and disseminated disease are both thought to follow inhalation of fragmented bacterial mycelia. The characteristic histologic feature of nocardiosis is an abscess with extensive neutrophil infiltration and prominent necrosis. Granulation tissue usually surrounds the lesions, but extensive fibrosis or encapsulation is uncommon. Actinomycetoma is characterized by suppurative inflammation with sinus tract formation. Granules—microcolonies composed of dense masses of bacterial filaments extending radially from a central core—are occasionally observed in histologic preparations. They are frequently found in discharges from lesions of actinomycetoma but almost never from lesions in other forms of nocardiosis. Infrequently, nocardiae and other indolent pathogens, including fungi or mycobacteria, are isolated from the same patient.

Nocardiae have evolved a number of properties that enable them to survive within phagocytes, including neutralization of oxidants, prevention of phagosome-lysosome fusion, and prevention of phagosome acidification. Neutrophils phagocytose the organisms and limit their growth but do not kill them efficiently. Cell-mediated immunity is important for definitive control and elimination of nocardiae.

CLINICAL MANIFESTATIONS

Respiratory Tract Disease Pneumonia, the most common form of nocardial disease in the respiratory tract, is typically subacute; symptoms have usually been present for days or weeks at presentation. The onset is occasionally more acute in immunosuppressed patients. Cough is prominent and produces small amounts of thick, purulent sputum that is not malodorous. Fever, anorexia, weight loss, and malaise are common; dyspnea, pleuritic pain, and hemoptysis are less common. Remissions and exacerbations over several weeks are frequent. Roentgenographic patterns vary, but some are highly suggestive of nocardial pneumonia. Infiltrates vary in size and are typically of at least moderate density. Single or multiple nodules are common (Figs. 155-1 and 155-2), sometimes suggesting tumor metastases. Infiltrates and nodules tend to cavitate (Fig. 155-2). Empyema is present in one-third of cases.

Nocardiosis may spread directly from the lungs to adjacent tissues. Pericarditis, mediastinitis, and the superior vena cava syndrome have all been reported. Nocardial laryngitis, tracheitis, and bronchitis are much less common than pneumonia. In the major airways, disease often presents as a nodular or granulomatous mass. A few cases of sinusitis have been reported.

FIGURE 155-1 Nocardial pneumonia. Discrete nodular infiltrates are present in midlung fields on both sides.

Nocardiae are sometimes isolated from respiratory secretions of patients without apparent nocardial disease. These patients usually have chronic pulmonary disease with airway or parenchymal abnormalities and do not necessarily require treatment for nocardiosis (see "Diagnosis," below).

Extrapulmonary Disease In half of all cases of pulmonary nocardiosis, disease appears outside the lungs. In one-fifth of cases of disseminated disease, lung disease is not apparent. The most common site of dissemination is the brain. Other common sites include the skin and supporting structures, kidneys, bone, and muscle, but almost any organ can be involved. Peritonitis and epididymo-orchitis have been reported recently. Nocardiae have been recovered from blood in a few cases of pneumonia, disseminated disease, or central venous catheter

FIGURE 155-2 Nocardial pneumonia. A CT scan shows bilateral nodules, with cavitation in the nodule in the left lung.

FIGURE 155-3 **Nocardial abscesses** in the right occipital lobe.

FIGURE 155-4 **Nocardial actinomycetoma** illustrating common features including swelling, multiple sinus tracts, and involvement of the foot. *(Image provided by Amor Khachemoune and Ronald O. Perelman, New York University School of Medicine.)*

infection. Nocardial endocarditis occurs rarely and can affect either native or prosthetic valves.

The typical manifestation of extrapulmonary dissemination is a subacute abscess. A minority of abscesses outside the lungs or central nervous system (CNS) form fistulae and discharge small amounts of pus. In CNS infections, brain abscesses are usually supratentorial, are often multiloculated, and may be single or multiple (Fig. 155-3). Brain abscesses tend to burrow into the ventricles or extend out into the subarachnoid space. The symptoms and signs are somewhat more indolent than those of other types of bacterial brain abscess. Meningitis is uncommon and is usually due to spread from a nearby brain abscess. Nocardiae are not easily recovered from cerebrospinal fluid (CSF).

Disease following Transcutaneous Inoculation Disease that follows transcutaneous nocardial inoculation usually takes one of three forms: cellulitis, lymphocutaneous syndrome, or actinomycetoma.

Cellulitis generally begins 1–3 weeks after a recognized breach of the skin, often with soil contamination. Subacute cellulitis, with pain, swelling, erythema, and warmth, develops over days to weeks. The lesions are usually firm and not fluctuant. Disease may progress to involve underlying muscles, tendons, bones, or joints. Dissemination is rare. *N. brasiliensis* is the most common isolate, but *N. asteroides* is often isolated from people living in cooler climates.

Lymphocutaneous disease usually begins as a pyodermatous lesion at the site of inoculation, with central ulceration and purulent or honey-colored drainage. Subcutaneous nodules often appear along lymphatics that drain the primary lesion. The lymphangitic form closely resembles lymphocutaneous sporotrichosis (Chap. 199). Most cases of the lymphocutaneous syndrome are associated with *N. brasiliensis*.

Actinomycetoma (Fig. 155-4) usually begins with a nodular swelling, sometimes at a site of local trauma. Lesions typically develop on the feet or hands but may involve the posterior part of the neck, the upper back, the head, and other sites. The nodule eventually breaks down, and a fistula appears. This fistula is typically followed by others. The fistulae tend to come and go, with new ones forming as old ones disappear. The discharge is serous or purulent, may be bloody, and often contains 0.1- to 2-mm white granules consisting of masses of mycelia. The lesions spread slowly along fascial planes to involve adjacent areas of skin, subcutaneous tissue, and bone. Over months or years, there may be extensive deformation of the affected part. Lesions

involving soft tissues are only mildly painful; those affecting bones or joints are more so. Systemic symptoms are absent or minimal. Infection rarely disseminates from actinomycetoma, and lesions on the hands and feet usually cause only local disability. Lesions on the head, neck, and trunk can invade locally to involve deep organs, with consequent severe disability or death.

Eye Infections *Nocardia* species (particularly *N. asteroides*) are uncommon causes of subacute keratitis, usually following eye trauma. Nocardial endophthalmitis can develop after eye surgery. In one series, nocardiae accounted for more than half of culture-proved cases of endophthalmitis after cataract surgery. Endophthalmitis can also occur during disseminated disease. Nocardial infection of lachrymal glands has been reported.

DIAGNOSIS

The first step in diagnosis is examination of sputum or pus for crooked, branching, beaded, gram-positive filaments 1 μm wide and up to 50 μm long (Fig. 155-5). Most nocardiae are acid-fast in direct smears if a weak acid is used for decolorization (e.g., in the modified Kinyoun, Ziehl-Neelsen, and Fite-Faraco methods). The organisms often take up silver stains. Nocardiae grow relatively slowly; colonies may take up to 2 weeks to appear and may not develop their characteristic appearance for up to 4 weeks. Several blood culture systems support nocardial growth. Yield in manual systems is enhanced when blood cultures are incubated aerobically for up to 4 weeks and when blind subcultures are performed. Nocardial growth is so different from that of more common pathogens that the laboratory should be alerted when

FIGURE 155-5 **Gram-stained sputum from a patient with nocardial pneumonia.** *(Image provided by Charles Cartwright and Susan Nelson, Hennepin County Medical Center, Minneapolis, MN.)*

nocardiosis is suspected in order to maximize the likelihood of isolation. Since nocardiae are among the few aerobic microorganisms that use paraffin as a carbon source, paraffin baiting can be used to isolate the organisms from mixed cultures.

In nocardial pneumonia, sputum smears are often negative. Unless the diagnosis can be made in smear-negative cases by sampling lesions in more accessible sites, bronchoscopy or lung aspiration is usually necessary. Transtracheal aspiration should be avoided, as it frequently leads to nocardial cellulitis in tissues around the puncture wound.

To evaluate the possibility of dissemination in patients with nocardial pneumonia, a careful history should be obtained and a thorough physical examination performed. Suggestive symptoms or signs should be pursued with further diagnostic tests. CT or MRI of the head, with and without contrast material, should be undertaken if signs or symptoms suggest brain involvement. Some authorities recommend brain imaging in all cases of pulmonary or disseminated disease.

When clinically indicated, CSF or urine should be concentrated and then cultured. In actinomycetoma, granules should be sought in the discharge. Suspect particles should be washed in saline, examined microscopically, and cultured.

Isolation of nocardiae from sputum or blood occasionally represents colonization, transient infection, or contamination. In typical cases of respiratory tract colonization, Gram-stained specimens are negative and cultures are only intermittently positive. A positive sputum culture in an immunosuppressed patient usually reflects disease. When nocardiae are isolated from an immunocompetent patient without apparent nocardial disease, the patient should be observed carefully without treatment. A patient with a host-defense defect that increases the risk of nocardiosis should usually receive antimicrobial treatment.

Nocardia species are difficult to differentiate from one another with standard biochemical tests. The Clinical and Laboratory Standards Institute has published a broth microdilution method for nocardiae, but experience with nocardiae and quality-control testing are required for reliable results. Isolates from patients with systemic or severe disease should be sent to a reference laboratory for definitive identification and susceptibility testing.

Several presumptive diagnostic tests for nocardial infection have been studied, including tests for antibodies, nocardial metabolites, and nocardial DNA. None is ready for clinical use at this time.

Rx NOCARDIOSIS

Sulfonamides are the drugs of choice for nocardiosis (Table 155-1). The combination of sulfamethoxazole (SMX) and trimethoprim (TMP) is probably equivalent to sulfonamides; some authorities believe that the combination may in fact be more effective, but it also poses a modestly greater risk of hematologic toxicity. At the outset, 10–20 mg of TMP per kg and 50–100 mg of SMX per kg should be given each day in two divided doses. Later, the daily doses can be decreased to as little as 5 mg/kg and 25 mg/kg, respectively. In difficult cases, sulfonamide levels should be measured and dosages adjusted to keep serum concentrations between 100 and 150 μg/mL. In persons with sulfonamide allergies, desensitization usually allows continuation of therapy with these effective and inexpensive drugs.

Minocycline is the best-established alternative oral drug and should be given in doses of 100–200 mg twice a day. Other tetracyclines are usually ineffective. Linezolid appears to be active in vitro and has been effective in a few clinical cases. *N. nova* infections can be treated with erythromycin (500–750 mg four times a day) and/or ampicillin (1 g four times a day), but other *Nocardia* species are often resistant to both drugs. Amoxicillin (500 mg) combined with clavulanic acid (125 mg), given three times a day, has been effective in a few cases but should be avoided in cases due to *N. nova*, in which clavulanate induces β-lactamase production. Ofloxacin (400 mg twice a day) and clarithromycin (500 mg twice a day) have each been successful in a few cases.

Amikacin, the best-established parenteral drug, is given in doses of 5–7.5 mg/kg every 12 h. Serum levels should be monitored during prolonged therapy in patients with diminished renal function and in the elderly. Newer β-lactam antibiotics, including cefotaxime, ceftizoxime, ceftriaxone, and imipenem, are usually effective. These agents may be less effective in some cases caused by *N. farcinica*.

In vitro, *N. farcinica* differs from most nocardiae in that it is resistant to cephalosporins in most cases and to imipenem in one-fifth of cases. *N. pseudobrasiliensis* often exhibits resistance to minocycline or amoxicillin/clavulanic acid and susceptibility to ciprofloxacin or clarithromycin. *N. transvalensis* displays increased resistance to many antimicrobial agents, including amikacin, tobramycin, cefotaxime, ceftriaxone, and amoxicillin/clavulanic acid. *N. nova* isolates appear to be susceptible to ampicillin and erythromycin in vitro but also produce β-lactamase constitutively or in the presence of a β-lactam drug.

Use of SMX and TMP in high-risk populations to prevent *Pneumocystis* disease or urinary tract infections appears to reduce the risk of nocardiosis as well. However, the incidence of nocardiosis is low enough that prophylaxis of this disease is not recommended.

In patients with nocardiosis who need immunosuppressive therapy for an underlying disease or prevention of transplant rejection, such therapy should be continued. In many cases, two or more antimicrobial agents have been used to treat nocardiosis, often in combinations including drugs that are usually effective by themselves, like a sulfonamide or minocycline. Whether such combination therapy is better than monotherapy is not known, and it certainly increases the risk of toxicity. In treating patients with severe disease, some experts begin with a combination including TMP-SMX, amikacin, and ceftriaxone or imipenem. If combination therapy is used initially, a single drug should be used after clinical improvement, which usually occurs within the first week or two of treatment.

Surgical management of nocardial disease is similar to that of other bacterial diseases. Brain abscesses should be aspirated, drained, or excised if the diagnosis is unclear, if an abscess is large and accessible, or if an abscess fails to respond to chemotherapy. Small or inaccessible brain abscesses should be treated medically; clinical improvement should be noticeable within 1–2 weeks. Brain imaging should be repeated to document the resolution of lesions, although abatement on images often lags behind clinical improvement.

Antimicrobial therapy usually suffices for nocardial actinomycetoma. In deep or extensive cases, drainage or excision of heavily involved tissue may facilitate healing, but structure and function should be preserved whenever possible.

Nocardial infections tend to relapse (particularly in patients with chronic gran-

TABLE 155-1 TREATMENT FOR NOCARDIOSIS

Disease	Duration	Drugs (Daily Dose)[a]
Pulmonary or systemic		Systemic therapy
Intact host defenses	6–12 mo	Oral
Deficient host defenses	12 mo[b]	1. Trimethoprim (10–20 mg/kg) and
CNS disease	12 mo[c]	sulfamethoxazole (50–100 mg/kg)
Cellulitis, lymphocutaneous syndrome	2 mo	2. Minocycline (200–400 mg)
Osteomyelitis, arthritis, laryngitis, sinusitis	4 mo	3. Linezolid (1200 mg) Parenteral 1. Amikacin (10–15 mg/kg)
Actinomycetoma	6–12 mo after clinical cure	2. Cefotaxime (6 g), ceftizoxime (6 g), ceftriaxone (1–2 g), imipenem (2 g)
Keratitis	Topical: Until apparent cure	1. Sulfonamide drops 2. Amikacin drops
	Systemic: Until 2–4 mo after apparent cure	Drugs for systemic therapy as listed above

[a]For each category, choices are numbered in order of preference.
[b]In some patients with AIDS or chronic granulomatous disease, therapy for pulmonary or systemic disease must be continued indefinitely.
[c]If all apparent CNS disease has been excised, the duration of therapy may be reduced to 6 months.

ulomatous disease), and long courses of antimicrobial therapy are necessary. If disease is unusually extensive, if the patient is immunosuppressed, or if the response to therapy is slow, the recommendations in Table 155-1 should be exceeded.

The mortality rate for pulmonary or disseminated nocardiosis outside the CNS should be <5%. CNS disease carries a higher mortality rate. Patients should be followed carefully for at least 6 months after therapy has ended.

FURTHER READINGS

BROWN-ELLIOTT BA et al: Clinical and laboratory features of the *Nocardia* spp. based on current molecular taxonomy. Clin Microbiol Rev 19:259, 2006

CHOUCIÑO C et al: Nocardial infections in bone marrow transplant recipients. Clin Infect Dis 23:1012, 1996

FABRE S et al: Primary cutaneous *Nocardia otitidiscaviarum* infection in a patient with rheumatoid arthritis treated with infliximab. J Rheumatol 32:2432, 2005

FILICE GA: Nocardiosis in persons with human immunodeficiency virus infection, transplant recipients, and large, geographically defined populations. J Lab Clin Med 145:156, 2005

LALITHA P et al: Postcataract endophthalmitis in South India incidence and outcome. Ophthalmology 112:1884, 2005

PALMER DL et al: Diagnostic and therapeutic considerations in *Nocardia asteroides* infection. Medicine 53:391, 1974

POONWAN N et al: Characterization of clinical isolates of pathogenic *Nocardia* strains and related actinomycetes in Thailand from 1996 to 2003. Mycopathologia 159:361, 2005

ROUTH JC et al: Epididymo-orchitis and testicular abscess due to *Nocardia asteroides* complex. Urology 65:591, 2005

RUPPRECHT TA, PFISTER HW: Clinical experience with linezolid for the treatment of central nervous system infections. Eur J Neurol 12:536, 2005

UTTAMCHANDANI RB et al: Nocardiosis in 30 patients with advanced human immunodeficiency virus infection: Clinical features and outcome. Clin Infect Dis 18:348, 1994

156 Actinomycosis
Thomas A. Russo

Actinomycosis is an indolent, slowly progressive infection caused by anaerobic or microaerophilic bacteria, primarily of the genus *Actinomyces*, that colonize the mouth, colon, and vagina. Mucosal disruption may lead to infection at virtually any site in the body. In vivo growth of actinomycetes usually results in the formation of characteristic clumps called *grains* or *sulfur granules*. The clinical presentations of actinomycosis are myriad. Common in the preantibiotic era, actinomycosis has diminished in incidence, as has its timely recognition. Actinomycosis has been called the most misdiagnosed disease, and it has been said that no disease is so often missed by experienced clinicians. Thus this entity remains a diagnostic challenge.

Three clinical presentations that should prompt consideration of this unique infection are (1) the combination of chronicity, progression across tissue boundaries, and mass-like features (mimicking malignancy, with which it is often confused); (2) the development of a sinus tract, which may spontaneously resolve and recur; and (3) a refractory or relapsing infection after a short course of therapy, since cure of established actinomycosis requires prolonged treatment. An awareness of the full spectrum of the disease will expedite its diagnosis and treatment and will minimize the unnecessary surgical interventions, morbidity, and mortality that are reported all too often.

ETIOLOGIC AGENTS

Actinomycosis is most commonly caused by *A. israelii. A. naeslundii, A. odontolyticus, A. viscosus, A. meyeri, A. gerencseriae*, and *Propionibacterium propionicum* are established but less common causes. Most if not all actinomycotic infections are polymicrobial. *Actinobacillus actinomycetemcomitans, Eikenella corrodens*, Enterobacteriaceae, and species of *Fusobacterium, Bacteroides, Capnocytophaga, Staphylococcus*, and *Streptococcus* are commonly isolated with actinomycetes in various combinations, depending on the site of infection. The contribution of these other species to the pathogenesis of actinomycosis is uncertain.

Comparative 16S rRNA gene sequencing has led to the identification of an ever-expanding list of *Actinomyces* spp., presently numbered at 92. Increasing data support *A. europaeus, A. neuii, A. radingae, A. graevenitzii, A. turicensis, A. cardiffensis, A. houstonensis, A. hongkongensis*, and *A. funkei* as additional causes of human actinomycosis.

EPIDEMIOLOGY

Actinomycosis has no geographic boundaries and occurs throughout life, with a peak incidence in the middle decades. Males have a threefold higher incidence than females, possibly because of poorer dental hygiene and/or more frequent trauma. Factors that have probably contributed to the decrease in actinomycosis incidence since the advent of antibiotics include improved dental hygiene and the initiation of antimicrobial treatment before the disease develops fully. Individuals who do not seek or have access to health care are undoubtedly at higher risk.

PATHOGENESIS AND PATHOLOGY

The etiologic agents of actinomycosis are members of the normal oral flora and are often cultured from the bronchi, the gastrointestinal tract, and the female genital tract. The critical step in the development of actinomycosis is disruption of the mucosal barrier. Local infection may ensue. Once established, actinomycosis spreads contiguously in a slow progressive manner, ignoring tissue planes. Although acute inflammation may initially develop at the infection site, the hallmark of actinomycosis is the characteristic chronic, indolent phase manifested by lesions that usually appear as single or multiple indurations. Central necrosis consisting of neutrophils and sulfur granules develops and is virtually diagnostic. The fibrotic walls of the mass are typically described as "wooden." The responsible bacterial and/or host factors have not been identified. Over time, sinus tracts to the skin, adjacent organs, or bone may develop. In rare instances, distant hematogenous seeding may occur. As mentioned above, these unique features of actinomycosis mimic malignancy, with which it is often confused.

Foreign bodies appear to facilitate infection. This association most frequently involves intrauterine contraceptive devices (IUCDs). An increasing number of reports have described an association of actinomycosis with HIV infection, transplantation, and radio- or chemotherapy. Ulcerative mucosal infections (e.g., by herpes simplex virus or cytomegalovirus) and abnormalities in host defenses may facilitate the development of actinomycosis in the latter settings.

CLINICAL MANIFESTATIONS

Oral-Cervicofacial Disease Actinomycosis occurs most frequently at an oral, cervical, or facial site, usually as a soft tissue swelling, abscess, or mass lesion that is often mistaken for a neoplasm. The angle of the jaw is generally involved, but a diagnosis of actinomycosis should be considered with any mass lesion or relapsing infection in the head and neck (Chap. 31). Otitis, sinusitis, and canaliculitis also can develop. Pain, fever, and leukocytosis are variably reported. Contiguous extension to the cranium, cervical spine, or thorax is a potential sequela.

Thoracic Disease Thoracic actinomycosis usually follows an indolent progressive course, with involvement of the pulmonary parenchyma and/or the pleural space. Chest pain, fever, and weight loss are common. A cough, when present, is variably productive. The usual radiographic finding is either a mass lesion or pneumonia. On computed

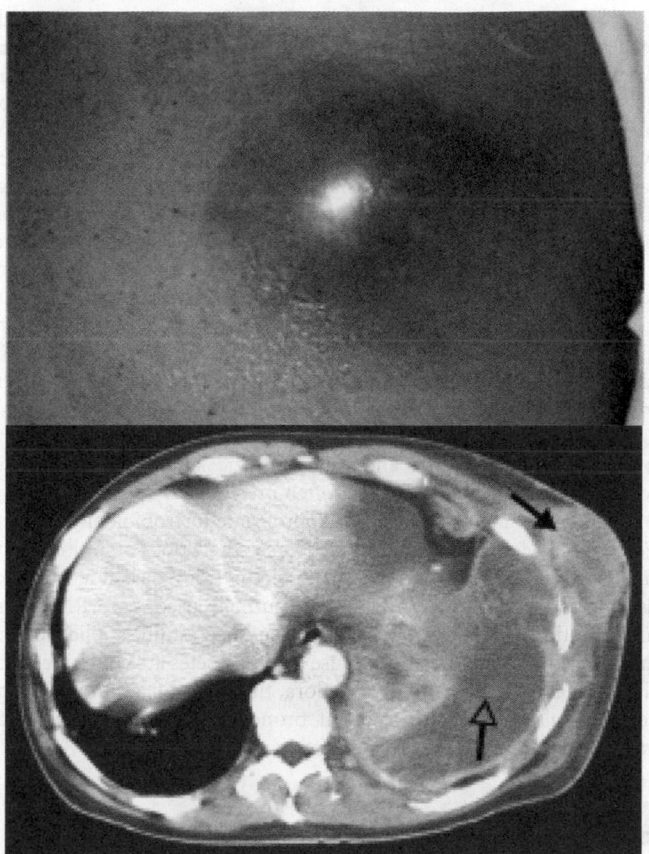

FIGURE 156-1 **Thoracic actinomycosis. *Top:*** A chest wall mass from extension of pulmonary infection. ***Bottom:*** Pulmonary infection is complicated by empyema (*open arrow*) and extension to the chest wall (*closed arrow*). (*Courtesy of Dr. C. B. Hsiao, Division of Infectious Diseases, Department of Medicine, State University of New York at Buffalo; with permission.*)

tomography (CT), central areas of low attenuation and ringlike rim enhancement may be seen. Cavitary disease or hilar adenopathy may develop. More than 50% of cases include pleural thickening, effusion, or empyema (Fig. 156-1). Rarely, pulmonary nodules or endobronchial lesions occur. Pulmonary lesions suggestive of actinomycosis may cross fissures or pleura; may involve the mediastinum, contiguous bone, or chest wall; or may be associated with a sinus tract. In the ab-

sence of these findings, thoracic actinomycosis is usually mistaken for a neoplasm or for pneumonia due to more usual causes.

Mediastinal infection is uncommon, usually arising from thoracic extension but rarely resulting from perforation of the esophagus, from trauma, or from head and neck or abdominal disease. The structures within the mediastinum and the heart can be involved in various combinations; consequently, the possible presentations are diverse. Primary endocarditis and isolated disease of the breast have been described.

Abdominal Disease Abdominal actinomycosis poses a great diagnostic challenge. Months or years usually pass from the inciting event (e.g., appendicitis, diverticulitis, peptic ulcer disease, foreign-body perforation, bowel surgery, or ascension from IUCD-associated pelvic disease) to clinical recognition. Because of the flow of peritoneal fluid and/or the direct extension of primary disease, virtually any abdominal organ, region, or space can be involved. The disease usually presents as an abscess, a mass, or a mixed lesion that is often fixed to underlying tissue and mistaken for a tumor. On CT, enhancement is most often heterogeneous and adjacent bowel is thickened. Sinus tracts to the abdominal wall, to the perianal region, or between the bowel and other organs may develop and mimic inflammatory bowel disease (Chap. 289). Recurrent disease or a wound or fistula that fails to heal suggests actinomycosis.

Hepatic infection usually presents as one or more abscesses or masses (Fig. 156-2). Isolated disease presumably develops via hematogenous seeding from cryptic foci. Imaging and percutaneous techniques have resulted in improved diagnosis and treatment.

All levels of the urogenital tract can be infected. Renal disease usually presents as pyelonephritis and/or renal and perinephric abscess. Bladder involvement, usually due to extension of pelvic disease, may result in ureteral obstruction or fistulas to bowel, skin, or uterus. *Actinomyces* can be detected in urine with appropriate stains and cultures.

Pelvic Disease Actinomycotic involvement of the pelvis occurs most commonly in association with an IUCD. When an IUCD is in place or has recently been removed, pelvic symptoms should prompt consideration of actinomycosis. The risk, although not quantified, appears small. The disease rarely develops when the IUCD has been in place for <1 year, but the risk increases with time. Actinomycosis can also present months after IUCD removal. Symptoms are typically indolent; fever, weight loss, abdominal pain, and abnormal vaginal bleeding or discharge are the most common. The earliest stage of disease—often endometritis—commonly progresses to pelvic masses or a tuboovarian abscess (Fig. 156-3). Unfortunately, because the diagnosis is often

FIGURE 156-2 **Hepatic-splenic actinomycosis. *A.*** Computed tomogram showing multiple hepatic abscesses and a small splenic lesion due to *A. israelii*. Arrow indicates extension outside the liver. ***Inset:*** Gram's stain of abscess fluid demonstrating beaded filamentous gram-positive rods. ***B.*** Subsequent formation of a sinus tract. (*Reprinted with permission from Saad M: Actinomyces hepatic abscess with cutaneous fistula. N Engl J Med 353:e16, 2005. © 2005 Massachusetts Medical Society. All rights reserved.*)

FIGURE 156-3 Computed tomogram showing pelvic actinomycosis associated with an intrauterine contraceptive device. The device is encased by endometrial fibrosis (*solid arrow*); also visible are paraendometrial fibrosis (*open triangular arrowhead*) and an area of suppuration (*open arrow*).

delayed, a "frozen pelvis" mimicking malignancy or endometriosis can develop by the time of recognition.

An unresolved issue is whether screening of cervical or endometrial specimens for *Actinomyces*-like organisms (ALOs) can predict or prevent IUCD-associated disease. Although the risk appears small, the consequences of infection are significant. Therefore, until more quantitative data become available, it seems prudent to remove the IUCD in the presence of symptoms that cannot be accounted for, regardless of whether ALOs or immunofluorescence-positive organisms are detected, and—if advanced disease is excluded—to initiate a 14-day course of empirical treatment for possible early pelvic actinomycosis. The detection of ALOs or immunofluorescence-positive organisms in the absence of symptoms warrants education of the patient and close follow-up but not removal of the IUCD unless a suitable contraceptive alternative is agreed on.

Central Nervous System Disease Actinomycosis of the central nervous system (CNS) is rare. Single or multiple brain abscesses are most common. An abscess usually appears on CT as a ring-enhancing lesion with a thick wall that may be irregular or nodular. Meningitis, epidural or subdural space infection, and cavernous sinus syndrome also have been described.

Musculoskeletal and Soft Tissue Infection Actinomycotic infection of bone is usually due to adjacent soft-tissue infection but may be associated with trauma (e.g., fracture of the mandible) or hematogenous spread. Because of slow disease progression, new bone formation and bone destruction are seen concomitantly. Infection of an extremity is uncommon and is usually a result of trauma. Skin, subcutaneous tissue, muscle, and bone (with periostitis or acute or chronic osteomyelitis) are involved alone or in various combinations. Cutaneous sinus tracts frequently develop.

Disseminated Disease Hematogenous dissemination of disease from any location rarely results in multiple-organ involvement. The lungs and liver are most commonly affected, with the presentation of multiple nodules mimicking disseminated malignancy. The clinical presentation may be surprisingly indolent given the extent of disease.

DIAGNOSIS
The diagnosis of actinomycosis is rarely considered. All too often, the first mention of actinomycosis is by the pathologist after extensive surgery. Since medical therapy alone is often sufficient for cure, the challenge for the clinician is to consider the possibility of actinomycosis, to diagnose it in the least invasive fashion, and to avoid unnecessary surgery. The clinical and radiographic presentations that suggest actinomycosis are discussed above. Aspirations and biopsies (with or without CT or ultrasound guidance) are being used successfully to obtain clinical material for diagnosis, although surgery may be required. The diagnosis is most commonly made by microscopic identification of sulfur granules (an in vivo matrix of bacteria, calcium phosphate, and host material) in pus or tissues. Occasionally, these granules are identified grossly from draining sinus tracts or pus. Although sulfur granules are a defining characteristic of actinomycosis, granules are also found in mycetoma (Chaps. 155 and 199) and botryomycosis (a chronic suppurative bacterial infection of soft tissue or, in rare cases, visceral tissue that produces clumps of bacteria resembling granules). These entities can easily be differentiated from actinomycosis with appropriate histopathologic and microbiologic studies. Microbiologic identification of actinomycetes is often precluded by prior antimicrobial therapy or failure to perform appropriate microbiologic cultures. For optimal yield, the avoidance of even a single dose of antibiotics is mandatory. Primary isolation usually requires 5–7 days but may take as long as 2–4 weeks. Although not routinely used, 16S rRNA gene amplification and sequencing have been successfully applied to increase diagnostic sensitivity. Because actinomycetes are components of the normal oral and genital-tract flora, their identification in the absence of sulfur granules in sputum, bronchial washings, and cervicovaginal secretions is of little significance.

℞ ACTINOMYCOSIS

Decisions about treatment are based on the collective clinical experience of the past 50 years. Actinomycosis requires prolonged treatment with high doses of antimicrobial agents. The need for intensive treatment is presumably due to the drugs' poor penetration of the thick-walled masses common in this infection and/or the sulfur granules themselves. Although therapy must be individualized, the intravenous administration of 18–24 million units of penicillin daily for 2–6 weeks, followed by oral therapy with penicillin or amoxicillin (total duration, 6–12 months), is a reasonable

TABLE 156-1 APPROPRIATE AND INAPPROPRIATE ANTIBIOTIC THERAPY FOR ACTINOMYCOSIS[a]

Category	Agent
Extensive successful clinical experience[b]	Penicillin: 18–24 mU/d IV q4h, 1–2 g/d PO q6h
	Erythromycin: 2–4 g/d IV q6h, 1–2 g/d PO q6h
	Tetracycline: 1–2 g/d PO q6h
	Doxycycline: 200 mg/d IV or PO q12–24h
	Minocycline: 200 mg/d IV or PO q12h
	Clindamycin: 2.7 g/d IV q8h, 1.2–1.8 g/d PO q6–8h
Anecdotal successful clinical experience	Ceftriaxone
	Ceftizoxime
	Imipenem
	Piperacillin-tazobactam
Agents that should be avoided	Metronidazole
	Aminoglycosides
	Oxacillin
	Dicloxacillin
	Cephalexin
Agents predicted to be efficacious on the basis of in vitro activity	Moxifloxacin
	Vancomycin
	Linezolid
	Quinupristin-dalfopristin

[a]Additional coverage for concomitant "companion" bacteria may be required.
[b]Controlled evaluations have not been performed. Dose and duration require individualization depending on the host, site, and extent of infection. As a general rule, a maximal parenteral antimicrobial dose for 2–6 weeks followed by oral therapy, for a total duration of 6–12 months, is required for serious infections and bulky disease, whereas a shorter course may suffice for less extensive disease, particularly in the oral-cervicofacial region.

guideline for serious infections and bulky disease. Less extensive disease, particularly that involving the oral-cervicofacial region, may be cured with a shorter course. If therapy is extended beyond the resolution of measurable disease, the risk of relapse—a clinical hallmark of this infection—will be minimized; CT and magnetic resonance imaging (MRI) are generally the most sensitive and objective techniques by which to accomplish this goal. A similar approach is reasonable for immunocompromised patients, although refractory disease has been described in HIV-infected individuals. Suitable alternative antimicrobial agents and those deemed unreliable are listed in **Table 156-1**. Although the role played by "companion" microbes in actinomycosis is unclear, many isolates are pathogens in their own right, and a regimen covering these organisms during the initial treatment course is reasonable.

Combined medical-surgical therapy is still advocated by some authorities. However, an increasing body of literature now supports an initial attempt at cure with medical therapy alone, even in extensive disease. CT and MRI should be used to monitor the response to therapy. In most cases, either surgery can be avoided or a less extensive procedure can be used. This approach is particularly valuable in sparing critical organs, such as the bladder or the reproductive organs in women of child-bearing age. For a well-defined abscess, percutaneous drainage in combination with medical therapy is a reasonable approach. When a critical location is involved (e.g.,

the epidural space, the CNS) or when suitable medical therapy fails, surgical intervention may be appropriate.

FURTHER READINGS

CLARRIDGE JE III, ZHANG Q: Genotypic diversity of clinical *Actinomyces* species: Phenotype, source, and disease correlation among genospecies. J Clin Microbiol 40:3442, 2002

COLMEGNA I et al: Disseminated *Actinomyces meyeri* infection resembling lung cancer with brain metastases. Am J Med Sci 326:152, 2003

KAYIKCIOGLU F et al: *Actinomyces* infection in the female genital tract. Eur J Obstet Gynecol Reprod Biol 118:77, 2005

LECOUVET F et al: The etiologic diagnosis of infectious discitis is improved by amplification-based DNA analysis. Arthritis Rheum 50:2985, 2004

PULVERER G et al: Human cervicofacial actinomyceses: Microbiologic data for 1997 cases. Clin Infect Dis 37:490, 2003

RUSSO TA: Actinomycosis, in *Principles and Practice of Infectious Diseases*, 6th ed, GL Mandell et al (eds). New York, Churchill Livingstone, 2005, pp 2924–2934

157 Infections Due to Mixed Anaerobic Organisms
Dennis L. Kasper, Ronit Cohen-Poradosu

DEFINITIONS

Anaerobic bacteria are organisms that require reduced oxygen tension for growth, failing to grow on the surface of solid media in 10% CO_2 in air. (In contrast, *microaerophilic bacteria* can grow in an atmosphere of 10% CO_2 in air or under anaerobic or aerobic conditions, although they grow best in the presence of only a small amount of atmospheric oxygen, and *facultative bacteria* can grow in the presence or absence of air.) This chapter describes infections caused by nonsporulating anaerobic bacteria. In general, anaerobes associated with human infections are relatively aerotolerant. They can survive for as long as 72 h in the presence of oxygen, although generally they do not multiply in this environment. A far smaller number of pathogenic anaerobic bacteria (which are also part of the normal flora) die after brief contact with oxygen, even in low concentrations.

The nonsporulating anaerobic bacteria exist as components of the normal flora on the mucosal surfaces of humans and animals. The major reservoirs of these bacteria are the mouth, lower gastrointestinal (GI) tract, skin, and female genital tract (Table 157-1). Among the constituents of the oral flora, anaerobes are the predominant commensal organisms, ranging in concentration from 10^9/mL in saliva to 10^{12}/mL in gingival scrapings. In the oral cavity, the ratio of anaerobic to aerobic bacteria ranges from 1:1 on the surface of a tooth to 1000:1 in the gingival crevices. Anaerobic bacteria are not found in appreciable numbers in the normal upper intestine until the distal ileum. In the colon, the proportion of anaerobes increases significantly, as does the overall bacterial count. In the colon, for example, there are 10^{11}–10^{12} organisms per gram of stool, and >99% of these organisms are anaerobic, with an anaerobe-to-aerobe ratio of ~1000:1. In the female genital tract, there are ~10^9 organisms per milliliter of secretions, with an anaerobe-to-aerobe ratio of ~10:1.

Anaerobes play a key role in maintaining the balance between the host and its colonizing organisms. Hundreds of species of anaerobic bacteria have been identified as part of the normal flora of humans. Identification of as many as 500 anaerobic species in fecal specimens reflects the diversity of the anaerobic flora. Despite the complex array of bacteria in the normal flora, relatively few species are isolated commonly from human infection. Anaerobic infections occur when the harmonious relationship between the host and the bacteria is disrupted. Any site in the body is susceptible to infection with these indigenous organisms when a mucosal barrier or the skin is compromised by surgery, trauma, tumor, ischemia, or necrosis, all of which can reduce local tissue redox potentials. Because the sites that are colonized by anaerobes contain many species of bacteria, disruption of anatomic barriers allows the penetration of many organisms, resulting in mixed infections involving multiple species of anaerobes combined with facultative or microaerophilic organisms. Such mixed infections are seen in the head and neck (chronic sinusitis, chronic otitis media, Ludwig's angina, and periodontal abscesses). Brain abscesses and subdural empyema are the most common anaerobic infections of the central nervous system (CNS). Anaerobes are responsible for pleuropulmonary diseases such as aspiration pneumonia, necrotizing pneumonia, lung abscess, and empyema.

TABLE 157-1	ANAEROBIC HUMAN FLORA: AN OVERVIEW		
Anatomic Site	**Total Bacteria**[a]	**Aerobic/ Anaerobic Ratio**	**Potential Pathogens**
Oral cavity			
Saliva	10^8–10^9	1:1	*Fusobacterium nucleatum, Prevotella melaninogenica, Prevotella oralis* group, *Bacteroides ureolyticus* group, *Peptostreptococcus* spp.
Tooth surface	10^{10}–10^{11}	1:1	
Gingival crevices	10^{11}–10^{12}	10^3:1	
Gastrointestinal tract			
Stomach	0–10^5	1:1	
Jejunum/ileum	10^4–10^7	1:1	
Terminal ileum and colon	10^{11}–10^{12}	10^3:1	*Bacteroides* spp. (principally members of the B. fragilis group), *Prevotella* spp., *Clostridium* spp., *Peptostreptococcus* spp.
Female genital tract	10^7–10^9	10:1	*Peptostreptococcus* spp., *Bacteroides* spp., *Prevotella bivia*

[a]Per gram or milliliter.

These organisms also play an important role in various intraabdominal infections, such as peritonitis and intraabdominal and hepatic abscesses (Chap. 121). They are isolated frequently in female genital tract infections, such as salpingitis, pelvic peritonitis, tuboovarian abscess, vulvovaginal abscess, septic abortion, and endometritis (Chap. 124). Anaerobic bacteria are also found often in infections of the skin, soft tissues, and bones and in bacteremia.

ETIOLOGY

The taxonomic classification of anaerobes is rapidly evolving, with frequent changes in nomenclature based on newly discovered relationships among bacterial species. The major anaerobic gram-positive cocci that produce disease are *Peptostreptococcus* spp. The major species of this genus that are involved in infections are *Peptostreptococcus micros*, *P. magnus*, *P. asaccharolyticus*, *P. anaerobius*, and *P. prevotii*. Clostridia (Chap. 135) are gram-positive rods that are isolated from wounds, abscesses, sites of abdominal infection, and blood. The principal anaerobic gram-negative bacilli found in human infections are the *Bacteroides fragilis* group as well as *Fusobacterium*, *Prevotella*, and *Porphyromonas* spp. Other members of the Bacteroidaceae family include *Bilophila wadsworthia*, an organism that has been isolated from infected sites and has been reported to cause serious infections. Gram-positive anaerobic non-spore-forming bacilli are uncommon as etiologic agents of human infection. *Propionibacterium acnes*, a rare cause of foreign-body infections, is one of the few nonclostridial gram-positive rods associated with infections.

The *B. fragilis* group contains the anaerobic pathogens most frequently isolated from clinical infections. Members of this group are part of the normal bowel flora; they include several distinct species, such as *B. fragilis*, *B. thetaiotaomicron*, *B. vulgatus*, *B. uniformis*, *B. ovatus*, and *Parabacteroides distasonis*. *B. fragilis* is the most important clinical isolate. However, in cultures of commensal fecal flora, *B. fragilis* is isolated in lower numbers than some of the other *Bacteroides* spp.

A second major group of phenotypically similar organisms is part of the indigenous oral flora. Thus these organisms are found at infected sites that can be seeded with oral microflora. Many of these species are pigment-producing bacteria belonging to two distinct genera, *Prevotella* and *Porphyromonas*; these genera comprise several pathogenic species, including *Porphyromonas gingivalis*, *Porphyromonas asaccharolytica*, and *Prevotella oralis*. *Porphyromonas* and *Prevotella* spp. cause localized infections that can spread contiguously.

In female genital tract infections, organisms normally colonizing the vagina (e.g., *Prevotella bivia* and *Prevotella disiens*) are the most frequent isolates, although *B. fragilis* is not uncommon. The *Fusobacterium* species *F. necrophorum*, *F. nucleatum*, and *F. varium*, which reside primarily in the oral cavity and the GI tract, are also isolated from clinical infections, including necrotizing pneumonia and abscesses. The skin flora contains anaerobic bacteria as well: *Propionibacterium* (mainly *P. acnes*) and peptostreptococci.

Infections caused by anaerobic bacteria most frequently are due to more than one organism. These polymicrobial infections may be caused by one or several anaerobic species or by a combination of anaerobic organisms and microaerophilic or facultative bacteria acting synergistically.

APPROACH TO THE PATIENT:
Infections Due to Mixed Anaerobic Organisms

The physician must consider several points when approaching the patient with presumptive infection due to anaerobic bacteria.

1. Most of the organisms colonizing mucosal sites are harmless commensals; very few cause disease. When these organisms do cause disease, it often occurs in proximity to the mucosal site they colonize.
2. For anaerobes to cause tissue infection, they must spread beyond the normal mucosal barriers.

3. Conditions favoring the propagation of these bacteria, particularly a lowered oxidation-reduction potential, are necessary. These conditions exist at sites of trauma, tissue destruction, compromised vascular supply, and complications of preexisting infection, which produce necrosis.
4. There is a complex array of infecting flora. For example, as many as 12 types of organisms can be isolated from a suppurative site.
5. Anaerobic organisms tend to be found in abscess cavities or in necrotic tissue. The failure of an abscess to yield organisms on routine culture is a clue that the abscess is likely to contain anaerobic bacteria. Often smears of this "sterile pus" are found to be teeming with bacteria when Gram's stain is applied. Malodorous pus suggests anaerobic infection. Although some facultative organisms (e.g., *Staphylococcus aureus*) are also capable of causing abscesses, abscesses in organs or deeper body tissues should call to mind anaerobic infection.
6. Gas is found in many anaerobic infections of deep tissues but is not diagnostic because it can be produced by aerobic bacteria as well.
7. Although a putrid-smelling infection site or discharge is considered diagnostic for anaerobic infection, this manifestation usually develops late in the course and is present in only 30–50% of cases.
8. Some species (the best example being the *B. fragilis* group) require specific therapy. However, many synergistic infections can be cured with antibiotics directed at some but not all of the organisms involved. Antibiotic therapy, combined with debridement and drainage, disrupts the interdependent relationship among the bacteria, and some species that are resistant to the antibiotic do not survive without the co-infecting organisms.
9. Manifestations of severe sepsis and disseminated intravascular coagulation (DIC) are unusual in patients with purely anaerobic infection.

EPIDEMIOLOGY

Difficulties in the performance of appropriate cultures, contamination of cultures by aerobic bacteria or components of the normal flora, and the lack of readily available, reliable culture techniques have made it impossible to obtain accurate data on incidence or prevalence. However, anaerobic infections are encountered frequently in hospitals with active surgical, trauma, and obstetric and gynecologic services. Depending on the institution, anaerobic bacteria account for 0.5–12% of all cases of bacteremia.

PATHOGENESIS

Anaerobic bacterial infections usually occur when an anatomic barrier becomes disrupted and constituents of the local flora enter a site that was previously sterile. Because of the specific growth requirements of anaerobic organisms and their presence as commensals on mucosal surfaces, conditions must arise that allow these organisms to penetrate mucosal barriers and enter tissue with a lowered oxidation-reduction potential. Therefore, tissue ischemia, trauma, surgery, perforated viscus, shock, and aspiration provide environments conducive to the proliferation of anaerobes. In the case of a perforated viscus, hundreds of species of anaerobic bacteria are spilled into the peritoneal cavity, but many of these organisms are unable to survive because the highly vascularized tissue provides a sufficiently high redox potential. The entry of oxygen into the environment results in the selection of the more aerotolerant anaerobic organisms.

The ability of an organism to adhere to host tissues is important to the establishment of infection. Some oral species adhere to crevicular epithelium in the oral cavity. *Prevotella melaninogenica* actually attaches to other microorganisms; *P. gingivalis* is a common isolate in periodontal disease. These organisms have fimbriae that facilitate attachment. Some *Bacteroides* strains appear to be piliated, a characteristic that may account for their ability to adhere.

The most extensively studied virulence factor of the nonsporulating anaerobes is the capsular polysaccharide complex of *B. fragilis*. This organism is unique among anaerobes in its potential for virulence during growth at normally sterile sites. Although it constitutes only 0.5–1% of the normal colonic flora, *B. fragilis* is the anaerobe most commonly isolated from intraabdominal infections and bacteremia. One polysaccharide of *B. fragilis* possesses distinct biologic properties, such as the ability (owing to a unique zwitterionic motif of charged sugars) to promote abscess formation. Intraabdominal abscess induction is related to the capacity of the polysaccharide to stimulate the release of cytokines and chemokines—in particular, interleukin (IL) 8, IL-17, and tumor necrosis factor (TNF) α—from resident peritoneal cells. The release of cytokines and chemokines results in the chemotaxis of polymorphonuclear neutrophils (PMNs) into the peritoneum, where they adhere to mesothelial cells induced by TNF-α to upregulate their expression of intercellular adhesion molecule 1 (ICAM-1). PMNs adherent to ICAM-1-expressing cells probably represent the nidus for an abscess. Prophylactic or therapeutic administration of the polysaccharide to experimental animals confers protection against abscess induction after challenge with intestinal microorganisms capable of inducing abscesses. This protection is mediated by T cells controlling cytokine release; IL-10 appears to be the cytokine primarily responsible for downregulating the tissue response of abscess formation. Although abscesses constitute a host response that localizes and contains infecting bacteria, abscess formation in patients with sepsis often results in severe and chronic illness that requires surgical drainage in combination with antimicrobial therapy.

Anaerobic bacteria produce a number of exoproteins that are capable of enhancing the organisms' virulence. The collagenase produced by *P. gingivalis* may enhance tissue destruction. An enterotoxin has been identified in *B. fragilis* strains associated with diarrheal disease in animals and young children. Anaerobic gram-negative bacteria such as *B. fragilis* possess lipopolysaccharides (LPSs, endotoxins) that are 100–1000 times less biologically potent than endotoxins associated with aerobic gram-negative bacteria. This relative biologic inactivity may account for the lower frequency of DIC and purpura in *Bacteroides* bacteremia than in facultative and aerobic gram-negative bacillary bacteremia. An exception is the LPS from *Fusobacterium*, which may account for the severity of Lemierre's syndrome.

CLINICAL MANIFESTATIONS

Anaerobic Infections of the Mouth, Head, and Neck

(See also Chap. 31) Anaerobic bacteria are commonly involved in infections of the mouth, head, and neck. The predominant isolates are components of the normal flora of the upper airways—mainly the *Bacteroides oralis* group, pigmented *Prevotella* spp., *P. asaccharolytica*, *Fusobacterium* spp., peptostreptococci, and microaerophilic streptococci.

Soft tissue infections of the oral-facial area may or may not be odontogenic. Odontogenic infections—primarily dental caries and periodontal disease—are common and have both local consequences (especially tooth loss) and the potential for life-threatening spread to the deep fascial spaces of the head and neck. Infections of the mouth can arise from either the supragingival or the subgingival dental plaque composed of bacteria colonizing the tooth surface. Supragingival plaque formation begins with the adherence of gram-positive bacteria to the tooth surface. This form of plaque is influenced by salivary and dietary components, oral hygiene, and local host factors. Supragingival plaque can lead to dental caries and, with further invasion, to pulpitis (endodontic infection) that can further perforate the alveolar bone, causing periapical abscess. Subgingival plaque is associated with periodontal infections (e.g., gingivitis, periodontitis, and periodontal abscess) that can further disseminate to adjacent structures such as the mandible, causing osteomyelitis of the maxillary sinuses. Periodontitis may also result in spreading infection that can involve adjacent bone or soft tissues.

NECROTIZING ULCERATIVE GINGIVITIS

Gingivitis may become a necrotizing infection (trench mouth, Vincent's stomatitis). The onset of disease is usually sudden and is associated with tender bleeding gums, foul breath, and a bad taste. The gingival mucosa, especially the papillae between the teeth, becomes ulcerated and may be covered by a gray exudate, which is removable with gentle pressure. Patients may become systemically ill, developing fever, cervical lymphadenopathy, and leukocytosis. Occasionally, ulcerative gingivitis can spread to the buccal mucosa, the teeth, and the mandible or maxilla, resulting in widespread destruction of bone and soft tissue. This infection is termed *acute necrotizing ulcerative mucositis* (cancrum oris, noma). It destroys tissue rapidly, causing the teeth to fall out and large areas of bone—or even the whole mandible—to be sloughed. A strong putrid odor is frequently detected, although the lesions are not painful. The gangrenous lesions eventually heal, leaving large disfiguring defects. This infection most commonly follows a debilitating illness or affects severely malnourished children. It has been known to complicate leukemia or to develop in individuals with a genetic deficiency of catalase.

ACUTE NECROTIZING INFECTIONS OF THE PHARYNX

These infections usually occur in association with ulcerative gingivitis. Symptoms include an extremely sore throat, foul breath, and a bad taste accompanied by fever and a sensation of choking. Examination of the pharynx demonstrates that the tonsillar pillars are swollen, red, ulcerated, and covered with a grayish membrane that peels easily. Lymphadenopathy and leukocytosis are common. The disease may last for only a few days or, if not treated, may persist for weeks. Lesions begin unilaterally but may spread to the other side of the pharynx or the larynx. Aspiration of the infected material by the patient can result in lung abscesses.

PERIPHARYNGEAL SPACE INFECTIONS

These infections arise from the spread of organisms from the upper airways to potential spaces formed by the fascial planes of the head and neck. The etiology is typically polymicrobial and represents the normal flora of the mucosa of the originating site.

Peritonsillar abscess (*quinsy*) is a complication of acute tonsillitis caused mainly by a mixed flora containing anaerobes and group A *Streptococcus*. In submandibular space infection (*Ludwig's angina*), 80% of cases are caused by infection of the tissues surrounding the second and third molar teeth. This infection results in marked local swelling of tissues, with pain, trismus, and superior and posterior displacement of the tongue. Submandibular swelling of the neck can impair swallowing and cause respiratory obstruction. In some cases, tracheotomy may be life-saving. *Cervicofacial actinomycosis* (Chap. 156) is caused by a branching, gram-positive, non-spore-forming, strict/facultative anaerobe that is a part of the normal oral flora. This chronic disease is characterized by abscesses, draining sinus tracts, fistula, bone destruction, and fibrosis. It can easily be mistaken for malignancy or granulomatous disease. Actinomycosis less frequently involves the thorax, abdomen, pelvis, and CNS.

SINUSITIS AND OTITIS

Anaerobic bacteria have been implicated in chronic sinusitis but play little role in acute sinusitis. In chronic sinusitis, anaerobic bacteria are found in 0–52% of cases, depending on the method used to collect specimens. In one study, cultures of samples from patients with chronic sinusitis and patients with an acute exacerbation of chronic sinusitis yielded aerobes only in 25% and 27% of cases, respectively; anaerobes only in 34% and 37%; and mixed organisms in 41% and 37%. The predominant aerobic bacteria were Enterobacteriaceae and *S. aureus* in both groups; in addition, *Streptococcus pneumoniae* was commonly isolated from the acute-exacerbation group. The predominant anaerobic bacteria in both groups were *Peptostreptococcus* spp., *Fusobacterium* spp., anaerobic gram-negative bacilli, and *P. acnes*.

Anaerobic bacteria are much more easily implicated in chronic suppurative otitis media than in acute otitis media. Purulent exudate from chronically draining ears has been found to contain anaerobes, particularly *Bacteroides* spp., in up to 50% of cases. *B. fragilis* has been isolated from up to 28% of patients with chronic otitis media.

COMPLICATIONS OF ANAEROBIC HEAD AND NECK INFECTIONS Contiguous craniad spread of these infections may result in osteomyelitis of the skull or mandible or in intracranial infections such as brain abscess and subdural empyema. Caudal spread can produce mediastinitis or pleuropulmonary infection. Hematogenous complications may also result from anaerobic infections of the head and neck. Bacteremia, which occasionally is polymicrobial, can lead to endocarditis or other distant infections. Lemierre's syndrome, which has been uncommon in the antimicrobial era, is an acute oropharyngeal infection with secondary septic thrombophlebitis of the internal jugular vein and frequent metastasis, most commonly to the lung. *F. necrophorum* is the usual cause. This infection typically begins with pharyngitis, which is followed by local invasion in the lateral pharyngeal space with resultant internal jugular vein thrombophlebitis. A typical clinical triad seen in recent series is pharyngitis, a tender/swollen neck, and noncavitating pulmonary infiltrates.

CNS Infections CNS infections associated with anaerobic bacteria are brain abscess (Chap. 376), epidural abscess, and subdural empyema. Anaerobic meningitis is rare and is usually related to parameningeal collection or shunt infection. If optimal bacteriologic techniques are employed, as many as 85% of brain abscesses yield anaerobic bacteria, which usually originate from otolaryngeal infection. Commonly isolated are peptostreptococci, *Fusobacterium* spp., *Bacteroides* spp., and *Prevotella* spp. Facultative or microaerophilic streptococci and coliforms are often part of a mixed infecting flora in brain abscesses.

Pleuropulmonary Infections Anaerobic pleuropulmonary infections result from the aspiration of oropharyngeal contents, often in the context of an altered state of consciousness or an absent gag reflex. Four clinical syndromes are associated with anaerobic pleuropulmonary infection produced by aspiration: simple aspiration pneumonia, necrotizing pneumonia, lung abscess, and empyema.

ASPIRATION PNEUMONITIS Bacterial aspiration pneumonitis must be distinguished from two other clinical syndromes associated with aspiration that are not of bacterial etiology. One syndrome results from aspiration of solids, usually food. Obstruction of major airways typically results in atelectasis and moderate nonspecific inflammation. Therapy consists of removal of the foreign body.

The second aspiration syndrome is more easily confused with bacterial aspiration. *Mendelson's syndrome*, a chemical pneumonitis, results from regurgitation of stomach contents and aspiration of chemical material, usually acidic gastric juices. Pulmonary inflammation—including the destruction of the alveolar lining, with transudation of fluid into the alveolar space—occurs with remarkable rapidity. Typically this syndrome develops within hours, often following anesthesia when the gag reflex is depressed. The patient becomes tachypneic, hypoxic, and febrile. The leukocyte count may rise, and the chest x-ray may evolve suddenly from normal to a complete bilateral "whiteout" within 8–24 h. Sputum production is minimal. The pulmonary signs and symptoms can resolve quickly with symptom-based therapy or can culminate in respiratory failure, with the subsequent development of bacterial superinfection over a period of days. Antibiotic therapy is not indicated unless bacterial infection supervenes.

In contrast to these syndromes, bacterial aspiration pneumonia develops over a period of several days or weeks rather than hours. It is seen in patients who are hospitalized and have a depressed gag reflex, impaired swallowing, or a tracheal or nasogastric tube; elderly patients; and patients with transiently impaired consciousness in the wake of seizures, cerebrovascular accidents, or alcoholic blackouts. Patients who enter the hospital with this syndrome typically have been ill for several days and generally report low-grade fever, malaise, and sputum production. In some patients, weight loss and anemia reflect a more chronic process. Usually the history reveals factors predisposing to aspiration, such as alcohol overdose or residence in a nursing home. Examination sometimes yields evidence of periodontal disease. Sputum characteristically is not malodorous unless the process has been

under way for at least a week. A mixed bacterial flora with many PMNs is evident on Gram's staining of sputum. Expectorated sputum is unreliable for anaerobic cultures because of inevitable contamination by normal oral flora. Reliable specimens for culture can be obtained by transtracheal or transthoracic aspiration—techniques that are rarely used at present. Culture of protected-brush specimens or bronchoalveolar lavage fluid obtained by bronchoscopy is controversial.

Chest x-rays show consolidation in dependent pulmonary segments: in the basilar segments of the lower lobes if the patient has aspirated while upright and in either the posterior segment of the upper lobe (usually on the right side) or the superior segment of the lower lobe if the patient has aspirated while supine. The organisms isolated from the lungs reflect the pharyngeal flora; pigmented and nonpigmented *Prevotella* spp., *Peptostreptococcus* spp., *Bacteroides* spp., *Fusobacterium* spp., and anaerobic cocci are the most common isolates. The patient who aspirates in the hospital may also have a mixed infection involving enteric gram-negative rods. In a study on the microbiology of severe aspiration pneumonia in institutionalized elderly patients, gram-negative bacilli were cultured in 49% of cases (with an anaerobe also recovered in 14% of this group), anaerobes in 16%, and *S. aureus* in 12%.

NECROTIZING PNEUMONITIS This form of anaerobic pneumonitis is characterized by numerous small abscesses that spread to involve several pulmonary segments. The process can be indolent or fulminating. This syndrome is less common than either aspiration pneumonia or lung abscess and includes features of both types of infection.

ANAEROBIC LUNG ABSCESSES These abscesses result from subacute anaerobic pulmonary infection. The clinical syndrome typically involves a history of constitutional signs and symptoms (including malaise, weight loss, fever, night sweats, and foul-smelling sputum), perhaps over a period of weeks (Chap. 251). Patients who develop lung abscesses characteristically have dental infection and periodontitis, but lung abscesses in edentulous patients have been reported. Abscess cavities may be single or multiple and generally occur in dependent pulmonary segments (Fig. 157-1). Anaerobic abscesses must be distinguished from lesions associated with tuberculosis, neoplasia, and other conditions. Oral anaerobes predominate and are found in 60–80% of cases. There is also an important role for microaerophilic streptococci such as *S. milleri*. *S. aureus* and enteric gram-negative bacilli may be found as well. Septic pulmonary emboli may originate from intraabdominal or female genital tract infections and can produce anaerobic pneumonia.

EMPYEMA Empyema is a manifestation of long-standing anaerobic pulmonary infection. The clinical presentation, which includes foul-smelling sputum, resembles that of other anaerobic pulmonary infections. Patients may report pleuritic chest pain and marked chest-wall tenderness.

FIGURE 157-1 Chest radiograph of right-lower-lobe lung abscess in a 60-year-old alcoholic patient. [*From GL Mandell (ed): Atlas of Infectious Diseases, Vol VI. Philadelphia, Current Medicine Inc, Churchill Livingstone, 1996; with permission.*]

PART 7

Infectious Diseases

Empyema may be masked by overlying pneumonitis and should be considered especially in cases of persistent fever despite antibiotic therapy. Diligent physical examination and the use of ultrasound to localize a loculated empyema are important diagnostic tools. The collection of a foul-smelling exudate by thoracentesis is typical. Cultures of infected pleural fluid yield an average of 3.5 anaerobes and 0.6 facultative or aerobic bacterial species. Drainage is required. Defervescence, a return to a feeling of well-being, and resolution of the process may require several months.

Extension from a subdiaphragmatic infection may also result in anaerobic empyema.

Intraabdominal Infections Intraabdominal infections—mainly peritonitis and abscesses—are usually polymicrobial and represent the normal intestinal (especially colonic) flora. These infections usually follow a breach in the mucosal barrier occurring as a result of appendicitis, diverticulitis, neoplasm, inflammatory bowel disease, surgery, or trauma. On average, four to six species are isolated per specimen submitted to the microbiology laboratory, with a predominance of coliforms, anaerobes, and enterococci. The most common isolates are *Escherichia coli* and *B. fragilis*. Disease originating from proximal-bowel perforation reflects the flora of this site, with a predominance of aerobic and anaerobic gram-positive bacteria and *Candida*.

Enterotoxigenic *B. fragilis* has been associated with watery diarrhea in a few young children and adults. In case-control studies of children with undiagnosed diarrheal disease, enterotoxigenic *B. fragilis* was isolated from significantly more children with diarrhea than children in the control group. Neutropenic enterocolitis (typhlitis) has been associated with anaerobic infection of the cecum but—in the setting of neutropenia (Chap. 82)—may involve the entire bowel. Patients usually present with fever; abdominal pain, tenderness, and distention; and watery diarrhea. The bowel wall is edematous with hemorrhage and necrosis. The primary pathogen is thought by some authorities to be *Clostridium septicum*, but other clostridia and mixed anaerobic infections have also been implicated. More than 50% of patients developing early clinical signs can benefit from antibiotic therapy and bowel rest. Surgery is sometimes required to remove gangrenous bowel. See Chap. 121 for a complete discussion of intraabdominal infections.

Pelvic Infections The vagina of a healthy woman is one of the major reservoirs of anaerobic and aerobic bacteria. In the normal flora of the female genital tract, anaerobes outnumber aerobes by a ratio of ~10:1 and include anaerobic gram-positive cocci and *Bacteroides* spp. Anaerobes are isolated from most women with genital tract infections that are not caused by a sexually transmitted pathogen. The major anaerobic pathogens are *B. fragilis*, *P. bivia*, *P. disiens*, *P. melaninogenica*, anaerobic cocci, and *Clostridium* spp. Anaerobes are frequently encountered in tuboovarian abscess, septic abortion, pelvic abscess, endometritis, and postoperative wound infection, particularly following hysterectomy. Although these infections are often of mixed etiology, involving both anaerobes and coliforms, pure anaerobic infections without coliform or other facultative bacterial species occur more often in pelvic than in intraabdominal sites and are characterized by drainage of foul-smelling pus or blood from the uterus, generalized uterine or local pelvic tenderness, and continued fever and chills. Suppurative thrombophlebitis of the pelvic veins may complicate the infections and lead to repeated episodes of septic pulmonary emboli.

Anaerobic bacteria have been thought to be contributing factors in the etiology of bacterial vaginosis. This syndrome of unknown etiology is characterized by a profuse malodorous discharge and a change in the bacterial ecology that results in replacement of the *Lactobacillus*-dominated normal flora with an overgrowth of bacterial species including *Gardnerella vaginalis*, *Prevotella* spp., *Mobiluncus* spp., peptostreptococci, and genital mycoplasmas. A study based on 16S rRNA identification found other anaerobes that were predominant in cases but not in controls: *Atopobium*, *Leptotrichia*, *Megasphaera*, and *Eggerthella*. Anaerobic bacteria are thought to play a role in the etiology of pelvic inflammatory disease (Chap. 124), and several investigations

have shown an association between bacterial vaginosis and the development of pelvic inflammatory disease.

Pelvic infections due to *Actinomyces* spp. have been associated with the use of intrauterine devices (Chap. 156).

Skin and Soft Tissue Infections Injury to skin, bone, or soft tissue by trauma, ischemia, or surgery creates a suitable environment for anaerobic infections. These infections are most frequently found in sites prone to contamination with feces or with upper airway secretions—e.g., wounds associated with intestinal surgery, decubitus ulcers, or human bites. Deep soft-tissue infections associated with anaerobic bacteria are crepitant cellulitis, synergistic cellulitis, gangrene, and necrotizing fasciitis (Chaps. 119 and 135). Moreover, these organisms have been isolated from cutaneous abscesses, rectal abscesses, and axillary sweat gland infections (hidradenitis suppurativa). Anaerobes are frequently cultured from foot ulcers of diabetic patients.

These soft tissue or skin infections are usually polymicrobial. A mean of 4.8 bacterial species are isolated, with an anaerobe-to-aerobe ratio of ~3:2. The most frequently isolated organisms include *Bacteroides* spp., peptostreptococci, enterococci, clostridia, and *Proteus* spp. The involvement of anaerobes in these types of infections is associated with a higher frequency of fever, foul-smelling lesions, gas in the tissues, and visible foot ulcer.

Anaerobic bacterial synergistic gangrene (*Meleney's gangrene*), a rare infection of the superficial fascia, is characterized by exquisite pain, redness, and swelling followed by induration. Erythema surrounds a central zone of necrosis. A granulating ulcer forms at the original center as necrosis and erythema extend outward. Symptoms are limited to pain; fever is not typical. These infections usually involve a combination of *Peptostreptococcus* spp. and *S. aureus*; the usual site of infection is an abdominal surgical wound or the area surrounding an ulcer on an extremity. Treatment includes surgical removal of necrotic tissue and antimicrobial administration.

Necrotizing fasciitis, a rapidly spreading destructive disease of the fascia, is usually attributed to group A streptococci (Chap. 130) but can also be a mixed infection involving anaerobes and aerobes, usually after surgeries and in patients with diabetes or peripheral vascular disease. The most frequently isolated anaerobes in these infections are *Peptostreptococcus* and *Bacteroides* spp. Gas may be found in the tissues. Similarly, myonecrosis can be associated with mixed anaerobic infection. *Fournier's gangrene* consists of cellulitis involving the scrotum, perineum, and anterior abdominal wall, with mixed anaerobic organisms spreading along deep external fascial planes and causing extensive loss of skin.

Bone and Joint Infections Although actinomycosis (Chap. 156) accounts on a worldwide basis for most anaerobic infections in bone, organisms including peptostreptococci or microaerophilic cocci, *Bacteroides* spp., *Fusobacterium* spp., and *Clostridium* spp. can also be involved. These infections frequently arise adjacent to soft tissue infections. Hematogenous seeding of bone is uncommon. *Prevotella* and *Porphyromonas* spp. are detected in infections involving the maxilla and mandible, whereas *Clostridium* spp. have been reported as anaerobic pathogens in cases of osteomyelitis of the long bones following fracture or trauma. Fusobacteria have been isolated in pure culture from sites of osteomyelitis adjacent to the perinasal sinuses. Peptostreptococci and microaerophilic cocci have been reported as significant pathogens in infections involving the skull, mastoid, and prosthetic implants placed in bone. In patients with osteomyelitis (Chap. 120), the most reliable culture specimen is a bone biopsy sample free of normal uninfected skin and subcutaneous tissue. In patients with anaerobic osteomyelitis, a mixed flora is frequently isolated from a bone biopsy specimen.

In cases of anaerobic septic arthritis, the most common isolates are *Fusobacterium* spp. Most of the patients involved have uncontrolled peritonsillar infections progressing to septic cervical venous thrombophlebitis (Lemierre's syndrome) and resulting in hematogenous dissemination with a predilection for the joints. Unlike anaerobic osteomyelitis, anaerobic pyoarthritis in most cases is not polymicrobial and may be acquired hematogenously. Anaerobes are important pathogens in infections involving prosthetic joints; in these infections, the causative organisms (such as *Peptostreptococcus* spp. and *P. acnes*) are part of the normal skin flora.

Bacteremia Transient bacteremia is a well-known event in healthy people whose anatomic mucosal barriers have been injured (e.g., during dental extractions or dental scaling). These bacteremic episodes, which are often due to anaerobes, have no pathologic consequences. However, anaerobic bacteria are found in cultures of blood from clinically ill patients when proper culture techniques are used. Anaerobes have accounted for 0.5–12% of all bacteremias, depending on the institution. *B. fragilis* is the single most common anaerobic isolate from the bloodstream, accounting for 60–80% of anaerobic bacteremias.

In recent years, the rate of isolation of anaerobic bacteria from blood cultures has been decreasing. Studies from the 1970s and early 1980s found that 10–15% of positive blood cultures yielded anaerobes, while more recent surveys have found rates as low as 4%. This change may be related to the administration of antibiotic prophylaxis before intestinal surgery, the earlier recognition of localized infections, and the empirical use of broad-spectrum antibiotics for presumed infection. However, anaerobic bacteremia may be reemerging. Comparing two periods (1993–1996 and 2001–2004), investigators at the Mayo Clinics found a 74% increase in the incidence of anaerobic bacteremias per 100,000 patient-days; this finding contrasts with a 45% decrease in incidence from 1977 to 1988 at the same institution.

Once the organism in the blood has been identified, both the portal of bloodstream entry and the underlying problem that probably led to seeding of the bloodstream can often be deduced from an understanding of the organism's normal site of residence. For example, mixed anaerobic bacteremia including *B. fragilis* usually implies colonic pathology with mucosal disruption from neoplasia, diverticulitis, or some other inflammatory lesion. The initial manifestations are determined by the portal of entry and reflect the localized condition. When bloodstream invasion occurs, patients can become extremely ill, with rigors and hectic fevers. The clinical picture may be quite similar to that seen in sepsis involving aerobic gram-negative bacilli. Although complications of anaerobic bacteremia (e.g., septic thrombophlebitis and septic shock) have been reported, their incidence in association with anaerobic bacteremia is low. Anaerobic bacteremia is potentially fatal and requires rapid diagnosis and appropriate therapy. The mortality rate appears to increase with the age of the patient (with reported rates of >66% among patients >60 years old), with the isolation of multiple species from the bloodstream, and with the failure to surgically remove a focus of infection.

Endocarditis and Pericarditis (See also Chap. 118) Endocarditis due to anaerobes is uncommon. However, anaerobic streptococci, which are often classified incorrectly, are responsible for this disease more frequently than is generally appreciated. Gram-negative anaerobes are unusual causes of endocarditis. Signs and symptoms of anaerobic endocarditis are similar to those of endocarditis due to facultative organisms. Mortality rates of 21–43% have been reported for anaerobic endocarditis.

Anaerobes, particularly *B. fragilis* and *Peptostreptococcus* spp., are uncommonly found in infected pericardial fluids. Anaerobic pericarditis is associated with a mortality rate of >50%.

DIAGNOSIS
There are three critical steps in the diagnosis of anaerobic infection: (1) proper specimen collection; (2) rapid transport of the specimens to the microbiology laboratory, preferably in anaerobic transport media; and (3) proper handling of the specimens by the laboratory. Specimens must be collected by meticulous sampling of infected sites, with avoidance of contamination by the normal flora. When such contamination is likely, the specimen is unacceptable. Examples of specimens unacceptable for anaerobic culture include sputum collected by expectoration or nasal tracheal suction, bronchoscopy specimens, samples collected directly through the vaginal vault, urine collected by voiding, and feces. Specimens appropriate for anaerobic culture include sterile body fluids such as blood, pleural fluid, peritoneal fluid, cerebrospinal fluid, and aspirates or biopsies from normally sterile sites.

Because even brief exposure to oxygen may kill some anaerobic organisms and result in failure to isolate them in the laboratory, air must be expelled from the syringe used to aspirate the abscess cavity, and the needle must be capped with a sterile rubber stopper. It is also important to remember that prior antibiotic therapy reduces cultivability of these bacteria. Specimens can be injected into transport bottles containing a reduced medium or taken immediately in syringes to the laboratory for direct culture on anaerobic media. In general, swabs should not be used. If a swab must be used, it should be placed in a reduced semisolid carrying medium before transport to the laboratory. Delays in transport may lead to a failure to isolate anaerobes due to exposure to oxygen or overgrowth of facultative organisms, which may eliminate or obscure any anaerobes that are present. All clinical specimens from suspected anaerobic infections should be Gram-stained and examined for organisms with characteristic morphology. It is not unusual for organisms to be observed on Gram's staining but not isolated in culture. If purulent materials are found to be sterile or organisms are seen on Gram's staining but do not grow in the culture, the involvement of anaerobes should be suspected.

Because of the time and difficulty involved in the isolation of anaerobic bacteria, diagnosis of anaerobic infections must frequently be based on presumptive evidence. Certain sites with lowered oxidation-reduction potential (e.g., avascular necrotic tissues) favor the diagnosis of an anaerobic infection. When infections occur in proximity to mucosal surfaces normally harboring an anaerobic flora, such as the GI tract, female genital tract, or oropharynx, anaerobes should be considered as potential etiologic agents. A foul odor is often indicative of anaerobes, which produce certain organic acids as they proliferate in necrotic tissue. Although these odors are nearly pathognomonic for anaerobic infection, the absence of odor does not exclude an anaerobic etiology. Because anaerobes often coexist with other bacteria to cause mixed or synergistic infection, Gram's staining of exudate frequently reveals numerous pleomorphic cocci and bacilli suggestive of anaerobes. Sometimes these organisms have morphologic characteristics associated with specific species.

The presence of gas in tissues is highly suggestive, but not diagnostic, of anaerobic infection. When cultures of obviously infected sites yield no growth, streptococci only, or a single aerobic species (such as *E. coli*) and Gram's staining reveals a mixed flora, the implication is that the anaerobic microorganisms failed to grow because of inadequate transport and/or culture techniques. Failure of an infection to respond to antibiotics that are not active against anaerobes (e.g., aminoglycosides and—in some circumstances—penicillin, cephalosporins, or tetracyclines) suggests an anaerobic etiology.

Rx ANAEROBIC INFECTIONS

Successful therapy for anaerobic infections requires the administration of a combination of appropriate antibiotics, surgical resection, debridement of devitalized tissues, and drainage either by surgery or percutaneously (guided by an imaging technique such as CT, MRI, or ultrasound). Perforations must be closed promptly, closed spaces drained, tissue compartments decompressed, and an adequate blood supply established. Abscess cavities should be drained as soon as fluctuation or localization occurs.

ANTIBIOTIC THERAPY AND RESISTANCE Decisions about the treatment of anaerobic infections with antibiotics are usually based on known resistance patterns in certain species, on the likelihood of encountering a given species in the case at hand, and on Gram's stain findings. Antibiotics active against clinically relevant anaerobes can be grouped into four categories on the basis of their predicted activity (**Table 157-2**). (Nearly all the drugs listed have toxic side effects, which are described in detail in Chap. 127.) In many infections, anaerobes are mixed with coliforms and other facultative organisms. The best therapeutic regimens, therefore, are usually those active against both aerobic and anaerobic bac-

TABLE 157-2 ANTIMICROBIAL THERAPY FOR INFECTIONS INVOLVING COMMONLY ENCOUNTERED ANAEROBIC GRAM-NEGATIVE RODS

Category 1 (<2% Resistance)	Category 2 (<15% Resistance)	Category 3 (Variable Resistance)	Category 4 (Resistance)
Carbapenems (imipenem, meropenem)	Cephamycins	Penicillin	Aminoglycosides
Metronidazole[a]	Clindamycin	Cephalosporins	Monobactams
β-Lactam/β-lactamase inhibitor combination (ampicillin/sulbactam, ticarcillin/clavulanic acid, piperacillin/tazobactam)	High-dose antipseudomonal penicillins	Tetracycline	Trimethoprim-sulfamethoxazole
Chloramphenicol[b]		Vancomycin	
		Erythromycin	
		Tigecycline	
		Newer quinolones (moxifloxacin, gatifloxacin)	

[a]Usually needs to be given in combination with aerobic bacterial coverage. For infections originating below the diaphragm, aerobic gram-negative coverage is essential. For infections from an oral source, aerobic gram-positive coverage is added. Metronidazole also is not active against *Actinomyces, Propionibacterium*, or other gram-positive non-spore-forming bacilli (e.g., *Eubacterium, Bifidobacterium*) and is unreliable against peptostreptococci.
[b]Chloramphenicol is probably not as effective as other category 1 antimicrobials in treating anaerobic infections.

teria. The choice of empirical antibiotics for the anaerobes in mixed infections can nearly always be made reliably, since patterns of antimicrobial susceptibility are usually predictable (Chap. 127 and Table 157-2).

Antibiotic susceptibility testing of anaerobic bacteria has been difficult and controversial. Owing to the slow growth rate of many anaerobes, the lack of standardized testing methods and of clinically relevant standards for resistance, and the generally good results obtained with empirical therapy, there has been limited interest in testing these organisms for antibiotic susceptibility. However, a recent study of antibiotic-treated patients with *Bacteroides* isolates from blood found mortality rates of 45% among those whose isolates were deemed resistant to the agent used and 16% among those whose isolates were deemed sensitive. These figures suggest that in vitro susceptibility testing should be performed for *Bacteroides* isolates from hospitalized patients with bacteremia and that the results of this testing should guide treatment. In general, cure rates of >80% can be attained among *Bacteroides*-infected patients with appropriate antimicrobial therapy and drainage. Of the drugs active against most clinically relevant anaerobes, metronidazole, β-lactam/β-lactamase inhibitor combinations, and carbapenems are preferred.

Antibiotic resistance in anaerobic bacteria is an increasing problem. Nearly all organisms in the *B. fragilis* group (>97%) are resistant to penicillin G. The cephamycins (cefoxitin and cefotetan) are more active against this group, but resistance rates between 8% and 14% were observed between 1987 and 2000. Rates of resistance to β-lactam agents among anaerobes other than *Bacteroides* are lower but highly variable. β-Lactam/β-lactamase inhibitor combinations such as ampicillin/sulbactam, ticarcillin/clavulanic acid, and piperacillin/tazobactam are usually a good option. Metronidazole is active against gram-negative anaerobes, including the *B. fragilis* group; resistance is rare but has been reported. Resistance to metronidazole is more common among gram-positive anaerobes, including *P. acnes, Actinomyces* spp., lactobacilli, and anaerobic streptococci. In the United States, rates of clindamycin resistance among isolates of the *B. fragilis* group increased from 3% in 1982 to 16% in 1996 and 26% in 2000, with figures as high as 44% in some series. Rates of resistance to clindamycin among non-*Bacteroides* anaerobes are much lower (<10%).

If a patient fails to respond to one of the category 1 or category 2 drugs (Table 157-2), consideration should be given to alternative therapy and to determination of the resistance patterns among *Bacteroides* isolates. Although in vitro resistance of *Bacteroides* spp. to chloramphenicol has not been reported, this drug may not be as effective as other category 1 drugs. Newer available options include tigecycline, the first glycylcycline to be approved by the U.S. Food and Drug Administration. Tigecycline is active against some anaerobic bacteria, including *Peptostreptococcus* spp., *Propionibacterium* spp., *Prevotella* spp., *Fusobacterium* spp., and most *Bacteroides* spp. Its efficacy for treatment of intraabdominal infections was comparable to that of imipenem in two phase 2 clinical trials. Data from in vitro susceptibility studies and clinical trials suggest that the newer fluoroquinolones (e.g., moxifloxacin, gatifloxacin, and gemifloxacin) will be useful in the treatment of mixed aerobic-anaerobic infections. However, these drugs exhibit relatively weak in vitro activity against many *Bacteroides* spp. other than *B. fragilis*, including *B. thetaiotaomicron, B. vulgatus*, and *B. uniformis*.

TREATMENT OF INFECTIONS AT SPECIFIC SITES In clinical situations, specific regimens must be tailored to the initial site of infection. The duration of therapy also depends on the infection site; the reader is referred to specific chapters on sites of infection for recommendations.

β-Lactamase production has been reported in anaerobic strains that are usually isolated from infections originating above the diaphragm. Up to 60% of clinical isolates classified as *Prevotella* or *Porphyromonas* spp., non–*B. fragilis* species of *Bacteroides*, or *Fusobacterium* spp. reportedly produce β-lactamase. The clinical significance of resistance in these organisms has been suggested by studies showing clindamycin to be superior to penicillin (which for many years was considered the therapeutic "gold standard") for the treatment of lung abscesses. Presumably, the success of clindamycin is attributable to a broader spectrum of activity against oral anaerobes; thus, a combination of penicillin and metronidazole or another antibiotic combination that is active against both oral anaerobes and aerobes is likely to be as effective as clindamycin. Bronchoscopy in lung abscess is indicated only to rule out airway obstruction and does not enhance drainage; in any event, it should be delayed until the antimicrobial regimen has begun to affect the disease process so that the procedure does not spread the infection. Surgery is almost never indicated because of the danger of spilling the abscess contents into the lungs.

Although many oral anaerobic infections and most cases of anaerobic pneumonia still respond to penicillin therapy, some infections due to oral organisms fail to respond to this drug, and in these cases the use of a drug that is effective against penicillin-resistant anaerobes is recommended (Table 157-2). Life-threatening infections involving the anaerobic flora of the mouth, such as space infections of the head and neck, should be treated empirically as if penicillin-resistant anaerobes are involved. Less serious infections involving the oral microflora can be treated with penicillin alone; metronidazole can be added (or clindamycin can be substituted) if the patient responds poorly to penicillin therapy. Combinations of antibiotics used to treat mixed infections of oral origin must include drugs active against the gram-positive aerobic flora of the mouth.

Chloramphenicol has been used successfully against anaerobic CNS infections at doses of 30–60 mg/kg per day, with the exact dose depending on the severity of illness. However, penicillin G and metronidazole also cross the blood-brain barrier and are bactericidal for many anaerobic organisms (Chap. 376).

Anaerobic infections arising below the diaphragm (e.g., colonic and intraabdominal infections) must be treated specifically with agents active against *Bacteroides* spp. (Table 157-2). In intraabdominal sepsis (Chap. 121), the use of antibiotics effective against penicillin-resistant anaerobes has clearly reduced the incidence of postoperative infections and serious infectious complications. Specifically, a drug from category 1 (Table 157-2) must be included for broad-spectrum coverage. Recommended doses for commonly used category 1 drugs are given in **Table 157-3**. Therapy for intraabdominal sepsis must also include drugs active against the gram-neg-

TABLE 157-3 DOSES AND SCHEDULES FOR TREATMENT OF SERIOUS INFECTIONS DUE TO COMMONLY ENCOUNTERED ANAEROBIC GRAM-NEGATIVE RODS

First-Line Therapy	Dose	Schedule[a]
Metronidazole[b]	500 mg	q6h
Ticarcillin/clavulanic acid	3.1 g	q4h
Piperacillin/tazobactam	3.375 g	q6h
Imipenem	0.5 g	q6h
Meropenem	1.0 g	q8h

[a]See disease-specific chapters for recommendations on duration of therapy.
[b]Should generally be used in conjunction with drugs active against aerobic or facultative organisms.
Note: All drugs are given by the IV route.

ative aerobic flora of the bowel. If the involvement of gram-positive bacteria such as enterococci is suspected, either ampicillin or vancomycin should be added. A meta-analysis of 40 randomized or quasi-randomized controlled trials of 16 antibiotic regimens for secondary peritonitis showed equivalent clinical success for all regimens.

Cases of anaerobic osteomyelitis in which a mixed flora is isolated from a bone biopsy specimen should be treated with a regimen that covers all the isolates. When an anaerobic organism is recognized as a major or sole pathogen infecting a joint, the duration of treatment should be similar to that used for arthritis caused by aerobic bacteria (Chap. 328). Therapy includes the management of underlying disease states, the administration of appropriate antimicrobial agents, temporary joint immobilization, percutaneous drainage of effusions, and (usually) the removal of infected prostheses or internal fixation devices. Surgical drainage and debridement procedures such as sequestrectomy are essential for the removal of necrotic tissue that can sustain anaerobic infections.

The outcome of anaerobic bacteremia is significantly better in patients either initially given or switched to appropriate therapy based on known antibiotic susceptibilities.

FAILURE OF THERAPY Anaerobic infections that fail to respond to treatment or that relapse should be reassessed. Consideration should be given to additional surgical drainage or debridement. Superinfections with resistant gram-negative facultative or aerobic bacteria should be ruled out. The possibility of drug resistance must be entertained; if resistance is involved, repeated cultures may yield the pathogenic organism.

SUPPORTIVE MEASURES Other supportive measures in the management of anaerobic infections include careful attention to fluid and electrolyte balance (since extensive local edema may lead to hypoalbuminemia), hemodynamic support for septic shock, immobilization of infected extremities, maintenance of adequate nutrition during chronic infections by parenteral hyperalimentation, relief of pain, and anticoagulation with heparin for thrombophlebitis. For patients with severe anaerobic infections of soft tissues, hyperbaric oxygen therapy is advocated by some experts, but its value has not been proven in controlled trials.

FURTHER READINGS

ALDRIDGE KE et al: Bacteremia due to *Bacteroides fragilis* group: Distribution of species, beta-lactamase production and antimicrobial susceptibility patterns. Antimicrob Agents Chemother 47:148, 2003

KURIYAMA T et al: Antimicrobial susceptibility of 800 anaerobic isolates from patients with dentoalveolar infection to 13 oral antibiotics. Oral Microbiol Immunol 22:285, 2007

LASSMAN B et al: Reemergence of anaerobic bacteremia. Clin Infect Dis 44:895, 2007

MAZMANIAN SK et al: The love-hate relationship between bacterial polysaccharides and the immune system. Nat Rev Immunol 6:849, 2006

SALONEN JH et al: Clinical significance and outcome of anaerobic bacteremia. Clin Infect Dis 26:1413, 1998

SNYDMAN DR et al: National survey on the susceptibility of *Bacteroides fragilis* group: Report and analysis of trends in the United States from 1997 to 2004. Antimicrob Agents Chemother 51:1649, 2007

SOLOMKIN JS et al: Guidelines for the selection of anti-infective agents for complicated intra-abdominal infections. Clin Infect Dis 37:997, 2003

TZIANABOS AO et al: Anaerobic infections: General concepts, in *Principles and Practice of Infectious Diseases*, 6th ed, GL Mandell et al (eds). Philadelphia, Elsevier Churchill Livingstone, 2005, pp 2810–2816

SECTION 8   MYCOBACTERIAL DISEASES

158   Tuberculosis
Mario C. Raviglione, Richard J. O'Brien

Tuberculosis, one of the oldest diseases known to affect humans, is a major cause of death worldwide. This disease, which is caused by bacteria of the *Mycobacterium tuberculosis* complex, usually affects the lungs, although other organs are involved in up to one-third of cases. If properly treated, tuberculosis caused by drug-susceptible strains is curable in virtually all cases. If untreated, the disease may be fatal within 5 years in 50–65% of cases. Transmission usually takes place through the airborne spread of droplet nuclei produced by patients with infectious pulmonary tuberculosis.

ETIOLOGIC AGENT

Mycobacteria belong to the family Mycobacteriaceae and the order Actinomycetales. Of the pathogenic species belonging to the *M. tuberculosis* complex, the most common and important agent of human disease is *M. tuberculosis*. The complex includes *M. bovis* (the bovine tubercle bacillus—characteristically resistant to pyrazinamide, once an important cause of tuberculosis transmitted by unpasteurized milk, and currently the cause of a small percentage of cases worldwide), *M. caprae* (related to *M. bovis*), *M. africanum* (isolated from cases in West, Central, and East Africa), *M. microti* (the "vole" bacillus, a less virulent and rarely encountered organism), *M. pinnipedii* (a bacillus infecting seals and sea lions in the southern hemisphere and recently isolated from humans), and *M. canettii* (a rare isolate from East African cases that produces unusual smooth colonies on solid media and is considered closely related to a supposed progenitor type).

M. tuberculosis is a rod-shaped, non-spore-forming, thin aerobic bacterium measuring 0.5 μm by 3 μm. Mycobacteria, including *M. tuberculosis*, are often neutral on Gram's staining. However, once stained, the bacilli cannot be decolorized by acid alcohol; this characteristic justifies their classification as acid-fast bacilli (AFB; Fig. 158-1). Acid fastness is due mainly to the organisms' high content of mycolic acids, long-chain cross-linked fatty acids, and other cell-wall lipids. Microorganisms other than mycobacteria that display some acid fastness include species of *Nocardia* and *Rhodococcus*, *Legionella micdadei*, and the protozoa *Isospora* and *Cryptosporidium*. In the mycobacterial cell wall, lipids (e.g., mycolic acids) are linked to underlying arabinogalactan and peptidoglycan. This structure confers very low permeability of the cell wall, thus reducing the effectiveness of most antibiotics. Another molecule in the mycobacterial cell wall, lipoarabinomannan, is involved in the pathogen-host interaction and facilitates the survival of *M. tuberculosis* within macrophages. The complete genome sequence of *M. tuberculosis* comprises 4043 genes encoding 3993 proteins and 50 genes encoding RNAs; its high guanine-plus-cytosine content (65.6%) is indicative of an aerobic lifestyle. A large proportion of genes are devoted to the production of enzymes involved in cell wall metabolism.

EPIDEMIOLOGY

More than 5 million new cases of tuberculosis (all forms, both pulmonary and extrapulmonary) were reported to the World Health Organization (WHO) in 2005; >90% of cases were reported from developing countries. However, because of insufficient case detection and incomplete notification, reported cases represent only ~60% of total estimated cases. The WHO estimated that 8.8 million new cases of tuberculosis occurred worldwide in 2005, 95% of them in developing countries of Asia (4.9 million), Africa (2.6 million), the Middle East

FIGURE 158-1 **Acid-fast bacillus smear** showing *M. tuberculosis* bacilli. *(Courtesy of the CDC, Atlanta.)*

(0.6 million), and Latin America (0.4 million). It is further estimated that 1.6 million deaths from tuberculosis occurred in 2005, 95% of them in developing countries. Estimates of tuberculosis incidence rates (per 100,000 population) and numbers of tuberculosis-related deaths in 2005 are depicted in Fig. 158-2 and Fig. 158-3, respectively.

During the late 1980s and early 1990s, numbers of reported cases of tuberculosis increased in industrialized countries. These increases were related largely to immigration from countries with a high prevalence of tuberculosis; infection with HIV; social problems, such as increased urban poverty, homelessness, and drug abuse; and dismantling of tuberculosis services. During the past few years, numbers of reported cases have begun to decline again or stabilized in industrialized nations. In the United States, with the implementation of stronger control programs, the decrease resumed in 1993. In 2005, 14,097 cases of tuberculosis (4.8 cases per 100,000 population) were reported to the Centers for Disease Control and Prevention (CDC).

In the United States, tuberculosis is uncommon among young adults of European descent, who have only rarely been exposed to *M. tuberculosis* infection during recent decades. In contrast, because of a high risk in the past, the prevalence of *M. tuberculosis* infection is relatively high among elderly Caucasians, who remain at increased risk of developing active tuberculosis. Tuberculosis in the United States is also a disease of young adult members of the HIV-infected, immigrant, and disadvantaged/marginalized populations. Similarly, in Europe, tuberculosis has reemerged as an important public health problem, mainly as a result of cases among immigrants from high-prevalence countries.

Recent data on trends indicate that in 2005 tuberculosis incidence was stable or falling in most regions; the result is a small decline globally from figures in previous years. This global reduction is due largely to an apparent peaking in sub-Saharan Africa, where incidence had risen steeply since the 1980s as a result of the HIV epidemic and the paucity of health services. In eastern Europe, incidence increased during the 1990s because of deterioration in socioeconomic conditions and the health care infrastructure; however, after peaking in 2001, incidence has recently stabilized.

FROM EXPOSURE TO INFECTION

M. tuberculosis is most commonly transmitted from a person with infectious pulmonary tuberculosis to others by droplet nuclei, which are aerosolized by coughing, sneezing, or speaking. The tiny droplets dry rapidly; the smallest (<5–10 μm in diameter) may remain suspended in the air for several hours and may reach the terminal air passages when inhaled. There may be as many as 3000 infectious nuclei per cough. Other routes of transmission of tubercle bacilli (e.g., through the skin or the placenta) are uncommon and of no epidemiologic significance.

The probability of contact with a person who has an infectious form of tuberculosis, the intimacy and duration of that contact, the degree of infectiousness of the case, and the shared environment in which the contact takes place are all important determinants of the likelihood of transmission. Several studies of close-contact situations have clearly demonstrated that tuberculosis patients whose sputum contains AFB visible by microscopy are the most likely to transmit the infection. The most infectious patients have cavitary pulmonary disease or, much less commonly, laryngeal tuberculosis and produce sputum containing as many as 10^5–10^7 AFB/mL. Patients with sputum smear–negative/culture-positive tuberculosis are less infectious, and those with culture-negative pulmonary disease and extrapulmonary tuberculosis are essentially noninfectious. Because persons with both HIV infection and tuberculosis are less likely to have cavitations, they may be less infectious than persons without HIV co-infection. Crowding in poorly ventilated rooms is one of the most important factors in the transmission of tubercle bacilli, since it increases the intensity of contact with a case.

In short, the risk of acquiring *M. tuberculosis* infection is determined mainly by exogenous factors. Because of delays in seeking care and in making a diagnosis, it is estimated that, in high-prevalence settings, up to 20 contacts may be infected by each AFB-positive case before the index case is found to have tuberculosis.

FROM INFECTION TO DISEASE

Unlike the risk of acquiring infection with *M. tuberculosis*, the risk of developing disease after being infected depends largely on endogenous fac-

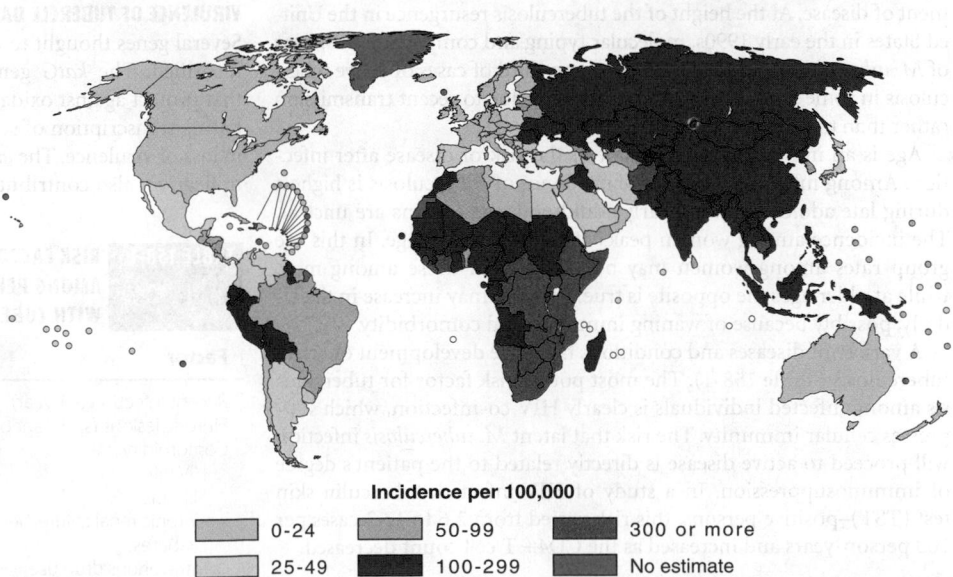

Incidence per 100,000

0-24	50-99	300 or more
25-49	100-299	No estimate

FIGURE 158-2 **Estimated tuberculosis incidence rates (per 100,000 population) in 2005.** The designations employed and the presentation of material on this map do not imply the expression of any opinion whatsoever on the part of the WHO concerning the legal status of any country, territory, city, or area or of its authorities or concerning the delimitation of its frontiers or boundaries. White lines on maps represent approximate border lines for which there may not yet be full agreement. *(Courtesy of the Stop TB Department, WHO; with permission.)*

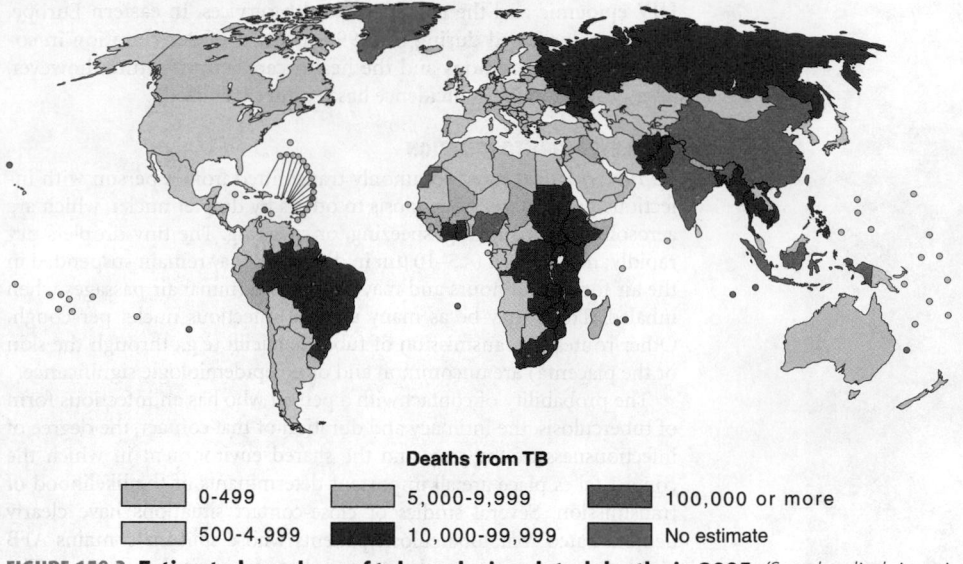

Deaths from TB

0-499	5,000-9,999	100,000 or more
500-4,999	10,000-99,999	No estimate

FIGURE 158-3 Estimated numbers of tuberculosis-related deaths in 2005. *(See also disclaimer in Fig. 158-2. Courtesy of the Stop TB Department, WHO; with permission.)*

tors, such as the individual's innate immunologic and nonimmunologic defenses and level of function of cell-mediated immunity (CMI). Clinical illness directly following infection is classified as *primary tuberculosis* and is common among children up to 4 years of age and among immunocompromised persons. Although primary tuberculosis may be severe and disseminated, it is not generally associated with high-level transmissibility. When infection is acquired later in life, the chance is greater that the mature immune system will contain it at least temporarily. The majority of infected individuals who ultimately develop tuberculosis do so within the first year or two after infection. Dormant bacilli, however, may persist for years before reactivating to produce *secondary* (or *postprimary*) *tuberculosis*, which, because of frequent cavitation, is more often infectious than is primary disease. Overall, it is estimated that up to 10% of infected persons will eventually develop active tuberculosis in their lifetime. The risk is much higher among HIV-infected persons. Reinfection of a previously infected individual, which is common in areas with high rates of tuberculosis transmission, may also favor the development of disease. At the height of the tuberculosis resurgence in the United States in the early 1990s, molecular typing and comparison of strains of *M. tuberculosis* suggested that up to one-third of cases of active tuberculosis in some inner-city communities were due to recent transmission rather than to reactivation of latent infection.

Age is an important determinant of the risk of disease after infection. Among infected persons, the incidence of tuberculosis is highest during late adolescence and early adulthood; the reasons are unclear. The incidence among women peaks at 25–34 years of age. In this age group rates among women may be higher than those among men, while at older ages the opposite is true. The risk may increase in the elderly, possibly because of waning immunity and comorbidity.

A variety of diseases and conditions favor the development of active tuberculosis (Table 158-1). The most potent risk factor for tuberculosis among infected individuals is clearly HIV co-infection, which suppresses cellular immunity. The risk that latent *M. tuberculosis* infection will proceed to active disease is directly related to the patient's degree of immunosuppression. In a study of HIV-infected, tuberculin skin test (TST)–positive persons, this risk varied from 2.6 to 13.3 cases per 100 person-years and increased as the CD4+ T cell count decreased.

NATURAL HISTORY OF DISEASE

Studies conducted in various countries before the advent of chemotherapy showed that untreated tuberculosis is often fatal. About one-third of patients died within 1 year after diagnosis, and one-half died within 5 years. The 5-year mortality rate among sputum smear–positive cases

was 65%. Of the survivors at 5 years, ~60% had undergone spontaneous remission, while the remainder were still excreting tubercle bacilli.

With effective, timely, and proper chemotherapy, patients have a very high chance of being cured. However, improper use of antituberculosis drugs, while reducing mortality rates, may also result in large numbers of chronic infectious cases, often with drug-resistant bacilli.

PATHOGENESIS AND IMMUNITY

INFECTION AND MACROPHAGE INVASION

The interaction of *M. tuberculosis* with the human host begins when droplet nuclei containing microorganisms from infectious patients are inhaled. While the majority of inhaled bacilli are trapped in the upper airways and expelled by ciliated mucosal cells, a fraction (usually <10%) reach the alveoli. There, alveolar macrophages that have not yet been activated phagocytize the bacilli. Invasion of macrophages by mycobacteria results largely from binding of the bacterial cell wall with a variety of macrophage cell-surface molecules, including complement receptors, mannose receptor, immunoglobulin GFcγ receptor, and type A scavenger receptors. Phagocytosis is enhanced by complement activation leading to opsonization of bacilli with C3 activation products such as C3b. After a phagosome forms, the survival of *M. tuberculosis* within it seems to depend on reduced acidification due to lack of accumulation of vesicular proton-adenosine triphosphatase. A complex series of events is probably generated by the bacterial cell-wall glycolipid lipoarabinomannan (LAM). LAM inhibits the intracellular increase of Ca^{2+}. Thus the Ca^{2+}/calmodulin pathway (leading to phagosome-lysosome fusion) is impaired, and the bacilli may survive within the phagosomes. If the bacilli are successful in arresting phagosome maturation, then replication begins and the macrophage eventually ruptures and releases its bacillary contents.

VIRULENCE OF TUBERCLE BACILLI

Several genes thought to confer virulence to *M. tuberculosis* have been identified. The *katG* gene encodes for catalase/peroxidase enzymes that protect against oxidative stress; *rpoV* is the main sigma factor initiating transcription of several genes. Defects in these two genes result in loss of virulence. The *erp* gene, encoding a protein required for multiplication, also contributes to virulence. Strains of the Beijing/W ge-

TABLE 158-1	RISK FACTORS FOR ACTIVE TUBERCULOSIS AMONG PERSONS WHO HAVE BEEN INFECTED WITH TUBERCLE BACILLI
Factor	**Relative Risk/Odds[a]**
Recent infection (<1 year)	12.9
Fibrotic lesions (spontaneously healed)	2–20
Comorbidity	
HIV infection	100
Silicosis	30
Chronic renal failure/hemodialysis	10–25
Diabetes	2–4
Intravenous drug use	10–30
Immunosuppressive treatment	10
Gastrectomy	2–5
Jejunoileal bypass	30–60
Posttransplantation period (renal, cardiac)	20–70
Malnutrition and severe underweight	2

[a]Old infection = 1.

notype family have been identified in outbreak conditions in a variety of settings worldwide and have been associated with higher mortality rates and occasionally with multidrug resistance.

INNATE RESISTANCE TO INFECTION

Several observations suggest that genetic factors play a key role in innate nonimmune resistance to infection with *M. tuberculosis* and the development of disease. The existence of this resistance, which is polygenic in nature, is suggested by the differing degrees of susceptibility to tuberculosis in different populations. In mice, a gene called *Nramp1* (natural resistance–associated macrophage protein 1) plays a regulatory role in resistance/susceptibility to mycobacteria. The human homologue NRAMP1, which maps to chromosome 2q, may play a role in determining susceptibility to tuberculosis, as is suggested by a study among West Africans. Polymorphisms in multiple genes, such as those encoding for histocompatibility leukocyte antigen (HLA), interferon γ (IFN-γ), T cell growth factor β (TGF-β), interleukin (IL) 10, mannose-binding protein, IFN-γ receptor, Toll-like receptor (TLR) 2, vitamin D receptor, and IL-1, have been associated with susceptibility to tuberculosis.

THE HOST RESPONSE

In the initial stage of host-bacterium interaction, either fusion between phagosomes and lysosomes occurs, preventing bacillary survival, or the bacilli begin to multiply, ultimately killing the macrophage. A variety of chemoattractants that are released after cell lysis (e.g., complement components, bacterial molecules, and cytokines) recruit additional immature monocyte-derived macrophages, including dendritic cells, which migrate to the draining lymph nodes and present mycobacterial antigens to T lymphocytes. At this point, the development of CMI and humoral immunity begins. These initial stages of infection are usually asymptomatic.

About 2–4 weeks after infection, two host responses to *M. tuberculosis* develop: a macrophage-activating CMI response and a tissue-damaging response. The *macrophage-activating response* is a T cell–mediated phenomenon resulting in the activation of macrophages that are capable of killing and digesting tubercle bacilli. The *tissue-damaging response* is the result of a delayed-type hypersensitivity (DTH) reaction to various bacillary antigens; it destroys unactivated macrophages that contain multiplying bacilli but also causes caseous necrosis of the involved tissues (see below). Although both of these responses can inhibit mycobacterial growth, it is the balance between the two that determines the form of tuberculosis that will develop subsequently.

GRANULOMA FORMATION

With the development of specific immunity and the accumulation of large numbers of activated macrophages at the site of the primary lesion, granulomatous lesions (tubercles) are formed. These lesions consist of accumulations of lymphocytes and activated macrophages that evolve toward epithelioid and giant cell morphologies. Initially, the tissue-damaging response can limit mycobacterial growth within macrophages. As stated above, this response, mediated by various bacterial products, not only destroys macrophages but also produces early solid necrosis in the center of the tubercle. Although *M. tuberculosis* can survive, its growth is inhibited within this necrotic environment by low oxygen tension and low pH. At this point, some lesions may heal by fibrosis, with subsequent calcification, whereas inflammation and necrosis occur in other lesions.

THE MACROPHAGE-ACTIVATING RESPONSE

CMI is critical at this early stage. In the majority of infected individuals, local macrophages are activated when bacillary antigens processed by macrophages stimulate T lymphocytes to release a variety of lymphokines. These activated macrophages aggregate around the lesion's center and effectively neutralize tubercle bacilli without causing further tissue destruction. In the central part of the lesion, the necrotic material resembles soft cheese (*caseous necrosis*)—a phenomenon that may also be observed in other conditions, such as neoplasms. Even when healing takes place, viable bacilli may remain dormant within macrophages or in the necrotic material for many years. These "healed" lesions in the lung parenchyma and hilar lymph nodes may later undergo calcification.

In a minority of cases, the macrophage-activating response is weak, and mycobacterial growth can be inhibited only by intensified DTH reactions, which lead to lung tissue destruction. The lesion tends to enlarge further, and the surrounding tissue is progressively damaged. At the center of the lesion, the caseous material liquefies. Bronchial walls as well as blood vessels are invaded and destroyed, and cavities are formed. The liquefied caseous material, containing large numbers of bacilli, is drained through bronchi. Within the cavity, tubercle bacilli multiply, spill into the airways, and are discharged into the environment through expiratory maneuvers such as coughing and talking. In the early stages of infection, bacilli are usually transported by macrophages to regional lymph nodes, from which they gain access to the bloodstream and disseminate widely throughout the body. The resulting lesions may undergo the same evolution as those in the lungs, although most tend to heal. In young children with poor natural immunity, hematogenous dissemination may result in fatal miliary tuberculosis or tuberculous meningitis.

ROLE OF MACROPHAGES AND MONOCYTES

While CMI confers partial protection against *M. tuberculosis*, humoral immunity plays a less well-defined role in protection (although evidence is accumulating on the existence of LAM antibodies, which may prevent dissemination of infection in children). In the case of CMI, two types of cells are essential: macrophages, which directly phagocytize tubercle bacilli, and T cells (mainly CD4+ T lymphocytes), which induce protection through the production of cytokines, especially IFN-γ. After infection with *M. tuberculosis*, alveolar macrophages secrete various cytokines responsible for a number of events (e.g., the formation of granulomas) as well as systemic effects (e.g., fever and weight loss). Monocytes and macrophages attracted to the site are key components of the immune response. Their primary mechanism is probably related to production of nitric oxide, which has antimycobacterial activity and increases synthesis of cytokines such as tumor necrosis factor α (TNF-α) and IL-1, which in turn regulate release of reactive nitrogen intermediates. In addition, macrophages can undergo apoptosis—a defensive mechanism to prevent release of cytokines and bacilli via their sequestration in the apoptotic cell.

ROLE OF T LYMPHOCYTES

Alveolar macrophages, monocytes, and dendritic cells are also critical in processing and presenting antigens to T lymphocytes, primarily CD4+ and CD8+ T cells; the result is the activation and proliferation of CD4+ T lymphocytes, which are crucial to the host's defense against *M. tuberculosis*. Qualitative and quantitative defects of CD4+ T cells explain the inability of HIV-infected individuals to contain mycobacterial proliferation. Activated CD4+ T lymphocytes can differentiate into cytokine-producing T_H1 or T_H2 cells. T_H1 cells produce IFN-γ—an activator of macrophages and monocytes—and IL-2. T_H2 cells produce IL-4, IL-5, IL-10, and IL-13 and also may promote humoral immunity. The interplay of these various cytokines and their cross-regulation determine the host's response. The role of cytokines in promoting intracellular killing of mycobacteria, however, has not been entirely elucidated. IFN-γ may induce the generation of reactive nitrogen intermediates and regulate genes involved in bactericidal effects. TNF-α also seems to be important.

Observations made originally in transgenic knockout mice and more recently in humans suggest that other T cell subsets, especially CD8+ T cells, may play an important role. CD8+ T cells have been associated with protective activities via cytotoxic responses and lysis of infected cells as well as with production of IFN-γ and TNF-α. Finally, natural killer cells act as co-regulators of CD8+ T cell lytic activities, and γδ T cells are increasingly thought to be involved in protective responses in humans.

MYCOBACTERIAL LIPIDS AND PROTEINS

Lipids have been involved in mycobacterial recognition by the innate immune system, and lipoproteins (such as 19-kDa lipoprotein) have been proven to trigger potent signals through TLRs present in blood dendritic cells. *M. tuberculosis* possesses various protein antigens. Some are present in the cytoplasm and cell wall; others are secreted. That the latter are more important in eliciting a T lymphocyte response is suggested by experiments documenting the appearance of protective immunity in animals after immunization with live, protein-secreting mycobacteria. Among the antigens that may play a protective role are the 30-kDa (or 85B) and ESAT-6 antigens. Protective immunity is probably the result of reactivity to many different mycobacterial antigens.

SKIN TEST REACTIVITY

Coincident with the appearance of immunity, DTH to *M. tuberculosis* develops. This reactivity is the basis of the TST, which is used primarily for the detection of *M. tuberculosis* infection in persons without symptoms. The cellular mechanisms responsible for TST reactivity are related mainly to previously sensitized CD4+ T lymphocytes, which are attracted to the skin-test site. There, they proliferate and produce cytokines. While DTH is associated with protective immunity (TST-positive persons being less susceptible to a new *M. tuberculosis* infection than TST-negative persons), it by no means guarantees protection against reactivation. In fact, cases of active tuberculosis are often accompanied by strongly positive skin-test reactions. There is also evidence of reinfection with a new strain of *M. tuberculosis* in patients previously treated for active disease. This evidence underscores the fact that previous latent or active tuberculosis may not confer fully protective immunity.

CLINICAL MANIFESTATIONS

Tuberculosis is classified as pulmonary, extrapulmonary, or both. Before the advent of HIV infection, ~80% of all new cases of tuberculosis were limited to the lungs. However, up to two-thirds of HIV-infected patients with tuberculosis may have both pulmonary and extrapulmonary disease or extrapulmonary disease alone.

PULMONARY TUBERCULOSIS

Pulmonary tuberculosis can be categorized as primary or postprimary (secondary).

Primary Disease   Primary pulmonary tuberculosis occurs soon after the initial infection with tubercle bacilli. In areas of high tuberculosis transmission, this form of disease is often seen in children. Because most inspired air is distributed to the middle and lower lung zones, these areas of the lungs are most commonly involved in primary tuberculosis. The lesion forming after infection is usually peripheral and accompanied in more than half of cases by hilar or paratracheal lymphadenopathy, which may not be detectable on chest radiography. In the majority of cases, the lesion heals spontaneously and may later be evident as a small calcified nodule (*Ghon lesion*).

In children and in persons with impaired immunity (e.g., those with malnutrition or HIV infection), primary pulmonary tuberculosis may progress rapidly to clinical illness. The initial lesion increases in size and can evolve in different ways. Pleural effusion, which is found in up to two-thirds of cases, results from the penetration of bacilli into the pleural space from an adjacent subpleural focus. In severe cases, the primary site rapidly enlarges, its central portion undergoes necrosis, and cavitation develops (*progressive primary tuberculosis*). Tuberculosis in young children is almost invariably accompanied by hilar or mediastinal lymphadenopathy due to the spread of bacilli from the lung parenchyma through lymphatic vessels. Enlarged lymph nodes may compress bronchi, causing obstruction and subsequent segmental or lobar collapse. Partial obstruction may cause obstructive emphysema, and bronchiectasis may also develop. Hematogenous dissemination, which is common and often asymptomatic, may result in the most severe manifestations of primary *M. tuberculosis* infection. Bacilli reach the bloodstream from the pulmonary lesion or the lymph nodes and disseminate into various organs, where they may produce granulomatous lesions. Although healing frequently takes place, immunocompromised persons (e.g., patients with HIV infection) may develop miliary tuberculosis and/or tuberculous meningitis.

Postprimary Disease   Also called *adult-type*, *reactivation*, or *secondary tuberculosis*, postprimary disease results from endogenous reactivation of latent infection and is usually localized to the apical and posterior segments of the upper lobes, where the substantially higher mean oxygen tension (compared with that in the lower zones) favors mycobacterial growth. In addition, the superior segments of the lower lobes are frequently involved. The extent of lung parenchymal involvement varies greatly, from small infiltrates to extensive cavitary disease. With cavity formation, liquefied necrotic contents are ultimately discharged into the airways, resulting in satellite lesions within the lungs that may in turn undergo cavitation (Figs. 158-4 and 158-5). Massive involvement of pulmonary segments or lobes, with coalescence of lesions, produces tuberculous pneumonia. While up to one-third of untreated patients reportedly succumb to severe pulmonary tuberculosis within a few weeks or months after onset (the classical "galloping consumption" of the past), others undergo a process of spontaneous remission or proceed along a chronic, progressively debilitating course ("consumption"). Under these circumstances, some pulmonary lesions become fibrotic and may later calcify, but cavities persist in other parts of the lungs. Individuals with such chronic disease continue to discharge tubercle bacilli into the environment. Most patients respond to treatment, with defervescence, decreasing cough, weight gain, and a general improvement in well-being within several weeks.

Early in the course of disease, symptoms and signs are often nonspecific and insidious, consisting mainly of fever and night sweats, weight loss, anorexia, general malaise, and weakness. However, in the majority of cases, cough eventually develops—often initially nonproductive and subsequently accompanied by the production of purulent sputum, sometimes with blood streaking. Massive hemoptysis may ensue as a consequence of the erosion of a blood vessel in the wall of a cavity. Hemoptysis, however, may also result from rupture of a dilated vessel in a cavity (*Rasmussen's aneurysm*) or from aspergilloma formation in an old cavity. Pleuritic chest pain sometimes develops in patients with subpleural parenchymal lesions. Extensive disease may produce dyspnea and, in rare instances, adult respiratory distress syndrome (ARDS).

Physical findings are of limited use in pulmonary tuberculosis. Many patients have no abnormalities detectable by chest examina-

FIGURE 158-4 Chest radiograph showing a right upper-lobe infiltrate and a cavity with an air-fluid level in a patient with active tuberculosis. *(Courtesy of Dr. Andrea Gori, Department of Infectious Diseases, S. Paolo University Hospital, Milan, Italy; with permission.)*

FIGURE 158-5 CT scan showing a large cavity in the right lung of a patient with active tuberculosis. *(Courtesy of Dr. Enrico Girardi, National Institute for Infectious Diseases, Spallanzani Hospital, Rome, Italy; with permission.)*

tion, whereas others have detectable rales in the involved areas during inspiration, especially after coughing. Occasionally, rhonchi due to partial bronchial obstruction and classic amphoric breath sounds in areas with large cavities may be heard. Systemic features include fever (often low-grade and intermittent) in up to 80% of cases and wasting. Absence of fever, however, does not exclude tuberculosis. In some cases, pallor and finger clubbing develop. The most common hematologic findings are mild anemia and leukocytosis. Hyponatremia due to the syndrome of inappropriate secretion of antidiuretic hormone (SIADH) has also been reported.

EXTRAPULMONARY TUBERCULOSIS

In order of frequency, the extrapulmonary sites most commonly involved in tuberculosis are the lymph nodes, pleura, genitourinary tract, bones and joints, meninges, peritoneum, and pericardium. However, virtually all organ systems may be affected. As a result of hematogenous dissemination in HIV-infected individuals, extrapulmonary tuberculosis is seen more commonly today than in the past.

Lymph-Node Tuberculosis (Tuberculous Lymphadenitis) The most common presentation of extrapulmonary tuberculosis (>40% of cases in the United States in recent series), lymph-node disease is particularly frequent among HIV-infected patients. In the United States, children and women (particularly non-Caucasians) also seem to be especially susceptible. Once caused mainly by *M. bovis*, tuberculous lymphadenitis is today due largely to *M. tuberculosis*. Lymph-node tuberculosis presents as painless swelling of the lymph nodes, most commonly at posterior cervical and supraclavicular sites (a condition historically referred to as *scrofula*). Lymph nodes are usually discrete and nontender in early disease but may be inflamed and have a fistulous tract draining caseous material. Associated pulmonary disease is seen in >40% of cases. Systemic symptoms are usually limited to HIV-infected patients. The diagnosis is established only by fine-needle aspiration or surgical biopsy. AFB are seen in up to 50% of cases, cultures are positive in 70–80%, and histologic examination shows granulomatous lesions. Among HIV-infected patients, granulomas usually are not seen. Differential diagnosis includes a variety of infectious conditions, neoplastic diseases such as lymphomas or metastatic carcinomas, and rare disorders like Kikuchi disease (necrotizing histiocytic lymphadenitis), Kimura's disease, and Castleman's disease.

Pleural Tuberculosis Involvement of the pleura, which accounts for ~20% of extrapulmonary cases in the United States, is common in primary tuberculosis and may result from either contiguous spread of pa-

renchymal inflammation or, as in many cases of pleurisy accompanying postprimary disease, actual penetration by tubercle bacilli into the pleural space. Depending on the extent of reactivity, the effusion may be small, remain unnoticed, and resolve spontaneously or may be sufficiently large to cause symptoms such as fever, pleuritic chest pain, and dyspnea. Physical findings are those of pleural effusion: dullness to percussion and absence of breath sounds. A chest radiograph reveals the effusion and, in up to one-third of cases, also shows a parenchymal lesion. Thoracentesis is required to ascertain the nature of the effusion and to differentiate it from manifestations of other etiologies. The fluid is straw-colored and at times hemorrhagic; it is an exudate with a protein concentration >50% of that in serum (usually ~4–6 g/dL), a normal to low glucose concentration, a pH of ~7.3 (occasionally <7.2), and detectable white blood cells (usually 500–6000/μL). Neutrophils may predominate in the early stage, while mononuclear cells are the typical finding later. Mesothelial cells are generally rare or absent. AFB are seen on direct smear in only 10–25% of cases, but cultures may be positive for *M. tuberculosis* in 25–75% of cases; positive cultures are more common among postprimary cases. Determination of the pleural concentration of adenosine deaminase (ADA) is a useful screening test: tuberculosis is virtually excluded if the value is very low. Needle biopsy of the pleura is often required for diagnosis and reveals granulomas and/or yields a positive culture in up to 80% of cases. This form of pleural tuberculosis responds well to chemotherapy and may resolve spontaneously. The usefulness of glucocorticoid administration is doubtful.

Tuberculous empyema is a less common complication of pulmonary tuberculosis. It is usually the result of the rupture of a cavity, with spillage of a large number of organisms into the pleural space. This process may create a bronchopleural fistula with evident air in the pleural space. A chest radiograph shows hydropneumothorax with an air-fluid level. The pleural fluid is purulent and thick and contains large numbers of lymphocytes. Acid-fast smears and mycobacterial cultures are often positive. Surgical drainage is usually required as an adjunct to chemotherapy. Tuberculous empyema may result in severe pleural fibrosis and restrictive lung disease. Removal of the thickened visceral pleura (decortication) is occasionally necessary to improve lung function.

Tuberculosis of the Upper Airways Nearly always a complication of advanced cavitary pulmonary tuberculosis, tuberculosis of the upper airways may involve the larynx, pharynx, and epiglottis. Symptoms include hoarseness, dysphonia, and dysphagia in addition to chronic productive cough. Findings depend on the site of involvement, and ulcerations may be seen on laryngoscopy. Acid-fast smear of the sputum is often positive, but biopsy may be necessary in some cases to establish the diagnosis. Carcinoma of the larynx may have similar features but is usually painless.

Genitourinary Tuberculosis Genitourinary tuberculosis, which accounts for ~15% of all extrapulmonary cases in the United States, may involve any portion of the genitourinary tract. Local symptoms predominate, and up to one-third of patients may concomitantly have pulmonary disease. Urinary frequency, dysuria, nocturia, hematuria, and flank or abdominal pain are common presentations. However, patients may be asymptomatic and the disease discovered only after severe destructive lesions of the kidneys have developed. Urinalysis gives abnormal results in 90% of cases, revealing pyuria and hematuria. The documentation of culture-negative pyuria in acidic urine raises the suspicion of tuberculosis. Intravenous pyelography, abdominal CT, or MRI (Fig. 158-6) may show deformities and obstructions, and calcifications and ureteral strictures are suggestive findings. Culture of three morning urine specimens yields a definitive diagnosis in nearly 90% of cases. Severe ureteral strictures may lead to hydronephrosis and renal damage.

Genital tuberculosis is diagnosed more commonly in female than in male patients. In female patients, it affects the fallopian tubes and the endometrium and may cause infertility, pelvic pain, and menstrual abnormalities. Diagnosis requires biopsy or culture of specimens obtained by dilatation and curettage. In male patients, tuberculosis

FIGURE 158-6 MRI of culture-confirmed renal tuberculosis. T2-weighted coronary plane: coronal sections showing several renal lesions in both the cortical and the medullary tissues of the right kidney. *(Courtesy of Dr. Alberto Matteelli, Department of Infectious Diseases, University of Brescia, Italy; with permission.)*

preferentially affects the epididymis, producing a slightly tender mass that may drain externally through a fistulous tract; orchitis and prostatitis may also develop. In almost half of cases of genitourinary tuberculosis, urinary tract disease is also present. Genitourinary tuberculosis responds well to chemotherapy.

Skeletal Tuberculosis In the United States, tuberculosis of the bones and joints is responsible for ~10% of extrapulmonary cases. In bone and joint disease, pathogenesis is related to reactivation of hematogenous foci or to spread from adjacent paravertebral lymph nodes. Weight-bearing joints (the spine in 40% of cases, the hips in 13%, and the knees in 10%) are most commonly affected. Spinal tuberculosis (Pott's disease or tuberculous spondylitis; Fig. 158-7) often involves two or more adjacent vertebral bodies. While the upper thoracic spine is the most common site of spinal tuberculosis in children, the lower thoracic and upper lumbar vertebrae are usually affected in adults. From the anterior superior or inferior angle of the vertebral body, the lesion slowly reaches the adjacent body, later affecting the intervertebral disk. With advanced disease, collapse of vertebral bodies results in kyphosis (*gibbus*). A paravertebral "cold" abscess may also form. In the

FIGURE 158-7 CT scan demonstrating destruction of the right pedicle of T10 due to Pott's disease. The patient, a 70-year-old Asian woman, presented with back pain and weight loss and had biopsy-proven tuberculosis. *(Courtesy of Charles L. Daley, M.D., University of California, San Francisco; with permission.)*

upper spine, this abscess may track to and penetrate the chest wall, presenting as a soft tissue mass; in the lower spine, it may reach the inguinal ligaments or present as a psoas abscess. CT or MRI reveals the characteristic lesion and suggests its etiology. The differential diagnosis includes tumors and other infections. Pyogenic bacterial osteomyelitis, in particular, involves the disk very early and produces rapid sclerosis. Aspiration of the abscess or bone biopsy confirms the tuberculous etiology, as cultures are usually positive and histologic findings highly typical. A catastrophic complication of Pott's disease is paraplegia, which is usually due to an abscess or a lesion compressing the spinal cord. Paraparesis due to a large abscess is a medical emergency and requires rapid drainage. Tuberculosis of the hip joints, usually involving the head of the femur, causes pain; tuberculosis of the knee produces pain and swelling. If the disease goes unrecognized, the joints may be destroyed. Diagnosis requires examination of the synovial fluid, which is thick in appearance, with a high protein concentration and a variable cell count. Although synovial fluid culture is positive in a high percentage of cases, synovial biopsy and tissue culture may be necessary to establish the diagnosis. Skeletal tuberculosis responds to chemotherapy, but severe cases may require surgery.

Tuberculous Meningitis and Tuberculoma Tuberculosis of the central nervous system (CNS) accounts for ~5% of extrapulmonary cases in the United States. It is seen most often in young children but also develops in adults, especially those infected with HIV. Tuberculous meningitis results from the hematogenous spread of primary or postprimary pulmonary disease or from the rupture of a subependymal tubercle into the subarachnoid space. In more than half of cases, evidence of old pulmonary lesions or a miliary pattern is found on chest radiography. The disease often presents subtly as headache and slight mental changes after a prodrome of weeks of low-grade fever, malaise, anorexia, and irritability. If not recognized, tuberculous meningitis may evolve acutely with severe headache, confusion, lethargy, altered sensorium, and neck rigidity. Typically, the disease evolves over 1–2 weeks, a course longer than that of bacterial meningitis. Paresis of cranial nerves (ocular nerves in particular) is a frequent finding, and the involvement of cerebral arteries may produce focal ischemia. The ultimate evolution is toward coma, with hydrocephalus and intracranial hypertension.

Lumbar puncture is the cornerstone of diagnosis. In general, examination of the cerebrospinal fluid (CSF) reveals a high leukocyte count (up to 1000/μL), usually with a predominance of lymphocytes but sometimes with a predominance of neutrophils in the early stage; a protein content of 1–8 g/L (100–800 mg/dL); and a low glucose concentration. However, any of these three parameters can be within the normal range. AFB are seen on direct smear of CSF sediment in up to one-third of cases, but repeated lumbar punctures increase the yield. Culture of CSF is diagnostic in up to 80% of cases and remains the gold standard. Polymerase chain reaction (PCR) has a sensitivity of up to 80%, but rates of false-positivity reach 10%. The ADA concentration may be a sensitive test but has low specificity. Imaging studies (CT and MRI) may show hydrocephalus and abnormal enhancement of basal cisterns or ependyma.

If unrecognized, tuberculous meningitis is uniformly fatal. This disease responds to chemotherapy; however, neurologic sequelae are documented in 25% of treated cases, in most of which the diagnosis has been delayed. Clinical trials have demonstrated that patients given adjunctive glucocorticoids may experience faster resolution of CSF abnormalities and elevated CSF pressure. In a recent study, adjunctive dexamethasone (0.4 mg/kg per day given IV and tapering by 0.1 mg/kg per week until the fourth week, when 0.1 mg/kg per day was administered; followed by 4 mg/d given by mouth and tapering by 1 mg per week until the fourth week, when 1 mg/d was administered) significantly enhanced the chances of survival among persons >14 years of age but did not reduce the frequency of neurologic sequelae.

Tuberculoma, an uncommon manifestation of CNS tuberculosis, presents as one or more space-occupying lesions and usually causes seizures and focal signs. CT or MRI reveals contrast-enhanced ring lesions, but biopsy is necessary to establish the diagnosis.

Gastrointestinal Tuberculosis Gastrointestinal tuberculosis is uncommon, making up 3.5% of extrapulmonary cases in the United States. Various pathogenetic mechanisms are involved: swallowing of sputum with direct seeding, hematogenous spread, or (largely in developing areas) ingestion of milk from cows affected by bovine tuberculosis. Although any portion of the gastrointestinal tract may be affected, the terminal ileum and the cecum are the sites most commonly involved. Abdominal pain (at times similar to that associated with appendicitis) and swelling, obstruction, hematochezia, and a palpable mass in the abdomen are common findings at presentation. Fever, weight loss, anorexia, and night sweats are also common. With intestinal-wall involvement, ulcerations and fistulae may simulate Crohn's disease; the differential diagnosis with this entity is always difficult. Anal fistulae should prompt an evaluation for rectal tuberculosis. As surgery is required in most cases, the diagnosis can be established by histologic examination and culture of specimens obtained intraoperatively.

Tuberculous peritonitis follows either the direct spread of tubercle bacilli from ruptured lymph nodes and intraabdominal organs (e.g., genital tuberculosis in women) or hematogenous seeding. Nonspecific abdominal pain, fever, and ascites should raise the suspicion of tuberculous peritonitis. The coexistence of cirrhosis (Chap. 301) in patients with tuberculous peritonitis complicates the diagnosis. In tuberculous peritonitis, paracentesis reveals an exudative fluid with a high protein content and leukocytosis that is usually lymphocytic (although neutrophils occasionally predominate). The yield of direct smear and culture is relatively low; culture of a large volume of ascitic fluid can increase the yield, but peritoneal biopsy (with a specimen best obtained by laparoscopy) is often needed to establish the diagnosis.

Pericardial Tuberculosis (Tuberculous Pericarditis) Due to direct progression of a primary focus within the pericardium, to reactivation of a latent focus, or to rupture of an adjacent subcarinal lymph node, pericardial tuberculosis has often been a disease of the elderly in countries with low tuberculosis prevalence but also develops frequently in HIV-infected patients. Case-fatality rates are as high as 40% in some series. The onset may be subacute, although an acute presentation, with dyspnea, fever, dull retrosternal pain, and a pericardial friction rub, is possible. An effusion eventually develops in many cases; cardiovascular symptoms and signs of cardiac tamponade may ultimately appear (Chap. 232). In the presence of effusion, tuberculosis must be suspected if the patient belongs to a high-risk population (HIV-infected, originating in a high-prevalence country); if there is evidence of previous tuberculosis in other organs; or if echocardiography, CT, or MRI shows effusion and thickness across the pericardial space. A definitive diagnosis can be obtained by pericardiocentesis under echocardiographic guidance. The pericardial fluid must be submitted for biochemical, cytologic, and microbiologic study. The effusion is exudative in nature, with a high count of leukocytes (predominantly mononuclear cells). Hemorrhagic effusion is frequent. Direct smear examination is very rarely positive. Culture of pericardial fluid reveals *M. tuberculosis* in up to two-thirds of cases, while pericardial biopsy has a higher yield. High levels of ADA and IFN-γ may also suggest a tuberculous etiology.

Without treatment, pericardial tuberculosis is usually fatal. Even with treatment, complications may develop, including chronic constrictive pericarditis with thickening of the pericardium, fibrosis, and sometimes calcification, which may be visible on a chest radiograph. A course of glucocorticoid treatment (e.g., prednisone, 20–60 mg/d for up to 6 weeks) is useful in the management of acute disease, reducing effusion, facilitating hemodynamic recovery, and thus decreasing mortality rates. Progression to chronic constrictive pericarditis, however, seems unaffected by such therapy.

Miliary or Disseminated Tuberculosis Miliary tuberculosis is due to hematogenous spread of tubercle bacilli. Although in children it is often the consequence of primary infection, in adults it may be due to either recent infection or reactivation of old disseminated foci. The lesions are usually yellowish granulomas 1–2 mm in diameter that resemble millet seeds (thus the term *miliary*, coined by nineteenth-century pathologists).

Clinical manifestations are nonspecific and protean, depending on the predominant site of involvement. Fever, night sweats, anorexia, weakness, and weight loss are presenting symptoms in the majority of cases. At times patients have a cough and other respiratory symptoms due to pulmonary involvement as well as abdominal symptoms. Physical findings include hepatomegaly, splenomegaly, and lymphadenopathy. Eye examination may reveal choroidal tubercles, which are pathognomonic of miliary tuberculosis, in up to 30% of cases. Meningismus occurs in <10% of cases.

A high index of suspicion is required for the diagnosis of miliary tuberculosis. Frequently, chest radiography reveals a miliary reticulonodular pattern (more easily seen on underpenetrated film), although no radiographic abnormality may be evident early in the course and among HIV-infected patients. Other radiologic findings include large infiltrates, interstitial infiltrates (especially in HIV-infected patients), and pleural effusion. Sputum smear microscopy is negative in 80% of cases. Various hematologic abnormalities may be seen, including anemia with leukopenia, lymphopenia, neutrophilic leukocytosis and leukemoid reactions, and polycythemia. Disseminated intravascular coagulation has been reported. Elevation of alkaline phosphatase levels and other abnormal values in liver function tests are detected in patients with severe hepatic involvement. The TST may be negative in up to half of cases, but reactivity may be restored during chemotherapy. Bronchoalveolar lavage and transbronchial biopsy are more likely to provide bacteriologic confirmation, and granulomas are evident in liver or bone-marrow biopsy specimens from many patients. If it goes unrecognized, miliary tuberculosis is lethal; with proper early treatment, however, it is amenable to cure. Glucocorticoid therapy has not proved beneficial.

A rare presentation seen in the elderly is *cryptic miliary tuberculosis*, which has a chronic course characterized by mild intermittent fever, anemia, and—ultimately—meningeal involvement preceding death. An acute septicemic form, *nonreactive miliary tuberculosis*, occurs very rarely and is due to massive hematogenous dissemination of tubercle bacilli. Pancytopenia is common in this form of disease, which is rapidly fatal. At postmortem examination, multiple necrotic but nongranulomatous ("nonreactive") lesions are detected.

Less Common Extrapulmonary Forms Tuberculosis may cause chorioretinitis, uveitis, panophthalmitis, and painful hypersensitivity-related phlyctenular conjunctivitis. Tuberculous otitis is rare and presents as hearing loss, otorrhea, and tympanic membrane perforation. In the nasopharynx, tuberculosis may simulate Wegener's granulomatosis. Cutaneous manifestations of tuberculosis include primary infection due to direct inoculation, abscesses and chronic ulcers, scrofuloderma, lupus vulgaris (a smoldering disease with nodules, plaques, and fissures), miliary lesions, and erythema nodosum. Adrenal tuberculosis is a manifestation of disseminated disease presenting rarely as adrenal insufficiency. Finally, congenital tuberculosis results from transplacental spread of tubercle bacilli to the fetus or from ingestion of contaminated amniotic fluid. This rare disease affects the liver, spleen, lymph nodes, and various other organs.

HIV-ASSOCIATED TUBERCULOSIS

(See also Chap. 182) Tuberculosis is one of the most common diseases among HIV-infected persons worldwide. In some African countries, the rate of HIV infection among tuberculosis patients reaches 70–80% in certain urban settings. A person with a positive TST who acquires HIV infection has a 3–13% annual risk of developing active tuberculosis. A new tuberculosis infection acquired by an HIV-infected individual may evolve to active disease in a matter of weeks rather than months or years.

Tuberculosis can appear at any stage of HIV infection, and its presentation varies with the stage. When CMI is only partially compromised, pulmonary tuberculosis presents in a typical manner (Figs. 158-4 and 158-5), with upper-lobe infiltrates and cavitation and without significant lymphadenopathy or pleural effusion. In late stages of HIV infection, a primary tuberculosis–like pattern, with diffuse interstitial or miliary infiltrates, little or no cavitation, and intrathoracic lymphadenopathy, is more common. Overall, sputum smears may be positive less frequently among tuberculosis patients with HIV infection than among those without; thus, the diagnosis of tuberculosis may be unusually difficult, especially in view of the variety of HIV-related pulmonary conditions mimicking tuberculosis.

Extrapulmonary tuberculosis is common among HIV-infected patients. In various series, extrapulmonary tuberculosis—alone or in association with pulmonary disease—has been documented in 40–60% of all cases in HIV–co-infected individuals. The most common forms are lymphatic, disseminated, pleural, and pericardial. Mycobacteremia and meningitis are also frequent, particularly in advanced HIV disease.

The diagnosis of tuberculosis in HIV-infected patients may be difficult not only because of the increased frequency of sputum-smear negativity (up to 40% in culture-proven pulmonary cases) but also because of atypical radiographic findings, a lack of classic granuloma formation in the late stages, and a negative TST. Delays in treatment may prove fatal. Recommendations for the prevention and treatment of tuberculosis in HIV-infected individuals are provided below.

DIAGNOSIS OF TUBERCULOSIS

The key to the diagnosis of tuberculosis is a high index of suspicion. Diagnosis is not difficult with a high-risk patient—e.g., a homeless alcoholic who presents with typical symptoms and a classic chest radiograph showing upper-lobe infiltrates with cavities (Fig. 158-4). On the other hand, the diagnosis can easily be missed in an elderly nursing home resident or a teenager with a focal infiltrate.

Often, the diagnosis is first entertained when the chest radiograph of a patient being evaluated for respiratory symptoms is abnormal. If the patient has no complicating medical conditions that cause immunosuppression, the chest radiograph may show typical upper-lobe infiltrates with cavitation (Fig. 158-4). The longer the delay between the onset of symptoms and the diagnosis, the more likely is the finding of cavitary disease. In contrast, immunosuppressed patients, including those with HIV infection, may have "atypical" findings on chest radiography—e.g., lower-zone infiltrates without cavity formation.

AFB MICROSCOPY

A presumptive diagnosis is commonly based on the finding of AFB on microscopic examination of a diagnostic specimen, such as a smear of expectorated sputum or of tissue (e.g., a lymph node biopsy). Although rapid and inexpensive, AFB microscopy has relatively low sensitivity (40–60%) in confirmed cases of pulmonary tuberculosis. Most modern laboratories processing large numbers of diagnostic specimens use auramine-rhodamine staining and fluorescence microscopy. The more traditional method—light microscopy of specimens stained with Kinyoun or Ziehl-Neelsen basic fuchsin dyes—is satisfactory, although more time-consuming. For patients with suspected pulmonary tuberculosis, three sputum specimens, preferably collected early in the morning, should be submitted to the laboratory for AFB smear and mycobacterial culture. If tissue is obtained, it is critical that the portion of the specimen intended for culture not be put in formaldehyde. The use of AFB microscopy on urine or gastric lavage fluid is limited by the presence of commensal mycobacteria that can cause false-positive results.

MYCOBACTERIAL CULTURE

Definitive diagnosis depends on the isolation and identification of *M. tuberculosis* from a clinical specimen or the identification of specific sequences of DNA in a nucleic acid amplification test (see below). Specimens may be inoculated onto egg- or agar-based medium (e.g., Löwenstein-Jensen or Middlebrook 7H10) and incubated at 37°C (under 5% CO_2 for Middlebrook medium). Because most species of mycobacteria, including *M. tuberculosis*, grow slowly, 4–8 weeks may be required before growth is detected. Although *M. tuberculosis* may be presumptively identified on the basis of growth time and colony pigmentation and morphology, a variety of biochemical tests have traditionally been used to speciate mycobacterial isolates. In modern, well-equipped laborato-

ries, the use of broth-based culture for isolation and speciation by molecular methods or high-pressure liquid chromatography of mycolic acids has replaced isolation on solid media and identification by biochemical tests. These new methods have decreased the time required for bacteriologic confirmation to 2–3 weeks.

NUCLEIC ACID AMPLIFICATION

Several test systems based on amplification of mycobacterial nucleic acid are available. These systems permit the diagnosis of tuberculosis in as little as several hours, with high specificity and sensitivity approaching that of culture. These tests are most useful for the rapid confirmation of tuberculosis in persons with AFB-positive specimens but also have utility for the diagnosis of AFB-negative pulmonary and extrapulmonary tuberculosis.

DRUG SUSCEPTIBILITY TESTING

In general, the initial isolate of *M. tuberculosis* should be tested for susceptibility to isoniazid, rifampin, and ethambutol. In addition, expanded susceptibility testing is mandatory when resistance to one or more of these drugs is found or the patient either fails to respond to initial therapy or has a relapse after the completion of treatment (see "Treatment Failure and Relapse," below). Susceptibility testing may be conducted directly (with the clinical specimen) or indirectly (with mycobacterial cultures) on solid or liquid medium. Results are obtained most rapidly by direct susceptibility testing on liquid medium, with an average reporting time of 3 weeks. With indirect testing on solid medium, results may be unavailable for ≥8 weeks. Molecular methods for the rapid identification of genetic mutations known to be associated with resistance to rifampin and isoniazid have been developed but are not marketed in the United States.

RADIOGRAPHIC PROCEDURES

As noted above, the initial suspicion of pulmonary tuberculosis is often based on abnormal chest radiographic findings in a patient with respiratory symptoms. Although the "classic" picture is that of upper-lobe disease with infiltrates and cavities (Fig. 158-4), virtually any radiographic pattern—from a normal film or a solitary pulmonary nodule to diffuse alveolar infiltrates in a patient with ARDS—may be seen. In the era of AIDS, no radiographic pattern can be considered pathognomonic. CT (Fig. 158-5) may be useful in interpreting questionable findings on plain chest radiography and may be helpful in diagnosing some forms of extrapulmonary tuberculosis [e.g., Pott's disease (Fig. 158-7)]. MRI is useful in the diagnosis of intracranial tuberculosis.

ADDITIONAL DIAGNOSTIC PROCEDURES

Other diagnostic tests may be used when pulmonary tuberculosis is suspected. Sputum induction by ultrasonic nebulization of hypertonic saline may be useful for patients who cannot produce a sputum specimen spontaneously. Frequently, patients with radiographic abnormalities that are consistent with other diagnoses (e.g., bronchogenic carcinoma) undergo fiberoptic bronchoscopy with bronchial brushings and endobronchial or transbronchial biopsy of the lesion. Bronchoalveolar lavage of a lung segment containing an abnormality may also be performed. In all cases, it is essential that specimens be submitted for AFB smear and mycobacterial culture. For the diagnosis of primary pulmonary tuberculosis in children, who often do not expectorate sputum, specimens from early-morning gastric lavage may yield positive cultures.

Invasive diagnostic procedures are indicated for patients with suspected extrapulmonary tuberculosis. In addition to testing of specimens from involved sites (e.g., CSF for tuberculous meningitis, pleural fluid and biopsy samples for pleural disease), biopsy and culture of bone marrow and liver tissue have a good diagnostic yield in disseminated (miliary) tuberculosis, particularly in HIV-infected patients, who also have a high frequency of positive blood cultures.

In some cases, cultures are negative but a clinical diagnosis of tuberculosis is supported by consistent epidemiologic evidence (e.g., a history of close contact with an infectious patient), a positive TST, and a compatible clinical and radiographic response to treatment. In the United States and other industrialized countries with low rates of tuberculosis, some patients with limited abnormalities on chest radiographs and sputum positive for AFB are infected with nontuberculous mycobacteria, most commonly organisms of the *M. avium* complex (MAC) or *M. kansasii* (Chap. 160). Factors favoring the diagnosis of nontuberculous mycobacterial disease over tuberculosis include an absence of risk factors for tuberculosis, a negative TST, and underlying chronic pulmonary disease.

Patients with HIV-associated tuberculosis pose several diagnostic problems (see "HIV-Associated Tuberculosis," above). Moreover, HIV-infected patients with sputum culture–positive, AFB-positive tuberculosis may present with a normal chest radiograph. With the advent of highly active antiretroviral therapy, the occurrence of disseminated MAC disease that can be confused with tuberculosis has become much less common.

SEROLOGIC AND OTHER DIAGNOSTIC TESTS FOR ACTIVE TUBERCULOSIS

A number of serologic tests based on detection of antibodies to a variety of mycobacterial antigens are marketed in developing countries but not in the United States. Careful independent assessments of these tests suggest that they are not useful as diagnostic aids, especially in persons with a low probability of tuberculosis. Various methods aimed at detection of mycobacterial antigens in diagnostic specimens are being investigated but are limited at present by low sensitivity. Determination of ADA levels in pleural fluid may be useful in the diagnosis of pleural tuberculosis; the utility of this test in the diagnosis of other forms of extrapulmonary tuberculosis (e.g., pericardial, peritoneal, and meningeal) is less clear.

DIAGNOSIS OF LATENT *M. TUBERCULOSIS* INFECTION

Tuberculin Skin Testing In 1891, Robert Koch discovered that components of *M. tuberculosis* in a concentrated liquid culture medium, subsequently named "old tuberculin" (OT), were capable of eliciting a skin reaction when injected subcutaneously into patients with tuberculosis. In 1932, Seibert and Munday purified this product by ammonium sulfate precipitation to produce an active protein fraction known as *tuberculin purified protein derivative (PPD)*. In 1941, PPD-S, developed by Seibert and Glenn, was chosen as the international standard. Later, the WHO and UNICEF sponsored large-scale production of a master batch of PPD (RT23) and made it available for general use. The greatest limitation of PPD is its lack of mycobacterial species specificity, a property due to the large number of proteins in this product that are highly conserved in the various species. In addition, subjectivity of the skin-reaction interpretation, deterioration of the product, and batch-to-batch variations limit the usefulness of PPD.

Skin testing with tuberculin-PPD (TST) is most widely used in screening for latent *M. tuberculosis* infection (LTBI). The test is of limited value in the diagnosis of active tuberculosis because of its relatively low sensitivity and specificity and its inability to discriminate between latent infection and active disease. False-negative reactions are common in immunosuppressed patients and in those with overwhelming tuberculosis. False-positive reactions may be caused by infections with nontuberculous mycobacteria (Chap. 160) and by bacille Calmette-Guérin (BCG) vaccination.

IFN-γ Release Assays (IGRAs) Recently, two in vitro assays that measure T cell release of IFN-γ in response to stimulation with the highly tuberculosis-specific antigens ESAT-6 and CFP-10 have become commercially available. QuantiFERON-TB Gold® (Cellestis Ltd., Carnegie, Australia) is a whole-blood enzyme-linked immunosorbent assay (ELISA) for measurement of IFN-γ, and T-SPOT.TB® (Oxford Immunotec, Oxford, UK) is an enzyme-linked immunospot (ELISpot) assay.

IGRAs are more specific than the TST as a result of less cross-reactivity due to BCG vaccination and sensitization by nontuberculous mycobacteria. IGRAs also appear to be at least as sensitive as the TST for active tuberculosis (used as a surrogate for LTBI). Although diagnostic sensitivity for LTBI cannot be directly estimated because of the

absence of a gold standard, these tests have shown better correlation than the TST with exposure to *M. tuberculosis* in contact investigations in low-incidence settings.

Other potential advantages of IGRAs include logistical convenience, the need for fewer patient visits to complete testing, the avoidance of unreliable and somewhat subjective measurements such as skin induration, and the ability to perform serial testing without inducing the boosting phenomenon (a spurious TST conversion due to boosting of reactivity on subsequent TSTs among BCG-vaccinated persons and those infected with other mycobacteria). Because of the high specificity and other potential advantages, IGRAs are likely to replace the TST for LTBI diagnosis in low-incidence, high-income settings where cross-reactivity due to BCG might adversely impact the interpretation and utility of the TST. Direct comparative studies in routine practice thus far suggest that the ELISpot has a lower rate of indeterminate results and probably a higher degree of diagnostic sensitivity than the whole-blood ELISA. Further studies are under way to assess the performance of these tests in contact investigations and in persons with suspected tuberculosis disease, health care workers, HIV-infected individuals, persons with iatrogenic immunosuppression, and children.

℞ TUBERCULOSIS

The two aims of tuberculosis treatment are to interrupt tuberculosis transmission by rendering patients noninfectious and to prevent morbidity and death by curing patients with tuberculosis. Chemotherapy for tuberculosis became possible with the discovery of streptomycin in the mid-1940s. Randomized clinical trials clearly indicated that the administration of streptomycin to patients with chronic tuberculosis reduced mortality rates and led to cure in the majority of cases. However, monotherapy with streptomycin was frequently associated with the development of resistance to this drug and the attendant failure of treatment. With the discovery of para-aminosalicylic acid (PAS) and isoniazid, it became axiomatic that cure of tuberculosis required the concomitant administration of at least two agents to which the organism was susceptible. Furthermore, early clinical trials demonstrated that a long period of treatment—i.e., 12–24 months— was required to prevent recurrence.

The introduction of rifampin in the early 1970s heralded the era of effective short-course chemotherapy, with a treatment duration of <12 months. The discovery that pyrazinamide, which was first used in the 1950s, augmented the potency of isoniazid/rifampin regimens led to the use of a 6-month course of this triple-drug regimen as standard therapy.

DRUGS Four major drugs are considered the first-line agents for the treatment of tuberculosis: isoniazid, rifampin, pyrazinamide, and ethambutol **(Table 158-2)**. These drugs are well absorbed after oral administration, with peak serum levels at 2–4 h and nearly complete elimination within 24 h. These agents are recommended on the basis of their bactericidal activity (i.e., their ability to rapidly reduce the number of viable organisms and render patients noninfectious), their sterilizing activity (i.e., their ability to kill all bacilli and thus sterilize the affected tissues, measured in terms of the ability to prevent relapses), and their low rate of induction of drug resistance. Rifapentine and rifabutin, two drugs related to rifampin, are also available in the United States and are useful for selected patients. **For a detailed discussion of the drugs used for the treatment of tuberculosis, see Chap. 161.**

Because of a lower degree of efficacy and a higher degree of intolerability and toxicity, six classes of second-line drugs are generally used only for the treatment of patients with tuberculosis resistant to first-line drugs. Included in this group are the injectable aminoglycosides streptomycin (formerly a first-line agent), kanamycin, and amikacin; the injectable polypeptide capreomycin; the oral agents ethionamide, cycloserine, and PAS; and the fluoroquinolone antibiotics. Of the quinolones, third-generation agents are preferred: levofloxacin, gatifloxacin (no longer marketed in the United States), and moxifloxacin. Amithiozone (thiacetazone) is still used in some developing countries but is associated with severe and sometimes even fatal skin reactions among HIV-infected patients. Other drugs of unproven efficacy that have been used in the treatment of patients with resistance to most of the first- and second-line agents include clofazimine, amoxicillin/clavulanic acid, and linezolid.

TABLE 158-2 RECOMMENDED DOSAGE[a] FOR INITIAL TREATMENT OF TUBERCULOSIS IN ADULTS[b]

Drug	Dosage	
	Daily Dose	**Thrice-Weekly Dose[c]**
Isoniazid	5 mg/kg, max 300 mg	15 mg/kg, max 900 mg
Rifampin	10 mg/kg, max 600 mg	10 mg/kg, max 600 mg
Pyrazinamide	20–25 mg/kg, max 2 g	30–40 mg/kg, max 3 g
Ethambutol[d]	15–20 mg/kg	25–30 mg/kg

[a]The duration of treatment for individual drugs varies by regimen, as detailed in Table 158-3.

[b]Dosages for children are similar, except that some authorities recommend higher doses of isoniazid (10–15 mg/kg daily; 20–30 mg/kg intermittent) and rifampin (10–20 mg/kg).

[c]Dosages for twice-weekly administration are the same for isoniazid and rifampin but are higher for pyrazinamide (50 mg/kg, with a maximum of 4 g/d) and ethambutol (40–50 mg/d).

[d]In certain settings, streptomycin (15 mg/kg daily, with a maximum dose of 1 g; or 25–30 mg/kg thrice weekly, with a maximum dose of 1.5 g) can replace ethambutol in the initial phase of treatment. However, streptomycin is no longer considered a first-line drug by the ATS, the IDSA, or the CDC.

Source: Based on recommendations of the American Thoracic Society, the Infectious Diseases Society of America, and the Centers for Disease Control and Prevention.

REGIMENS Standard short-course regimens are divided into an initial, or bactericidal, phase and a continuation, or sterilizing, phase. During the initial phase, the majority of the tubercle bacilli are killed, symptoms resolve, and usually the patient becomes noninfectious. The continuation phase is required to eliminate persisting mycobacteria and prevent relapse.

The treatment regimen of choice for virtually all forms of tuberculosis in both adults and children consists of a 2-month initial phase of isoniazid, rifampin, pyrazinamide, and ethambutol followed by a 4-month continuation phase of isoniazid and rifampin (**Table 158-3**). Treatment may be given daily throughout the course or intermittently (either three times weekly throughout the course or twice weekly after an initial phase of daily therapy, although the twice-weekly option is not recommended by the WHO). A continuation phase of once-weekly rifapentine and isoniazid is equally effective for HIV-seronegative patients with noncavitary pulmonary tuberculosis who have negative sputum cultures at 2 months. Intermittent treatment is especially useful for patients whose therapy is being directly observed (see below). Patients with cavitary pulmonary tuberculosis and delayed sputum-culture conversion (i.e., those who remain culture-positive at 2 months) should have the continuation phase extended by 3 months, for a total course of 9 months. For patients with sputum culture–negative pulmonary tuberculosis, the duration of treatment may be reduced to a total of 4 months. To prevent isoniazid-related neuropathy, pyridoxine (10–25 mg/d) should be added to the regimen given to persons at high risk of vitamin B6 deficiency (e.g., alcoholics; malnourished persons; pregnant and lactating women; and patients with conditions such as chronic renal failure, diabetes, and HIV infection, which are also associated with neuropathy). A full course of therapy (completion of treatment) is defined more accurately by the total number of doses taken than by the duration of treatment.

Specific recommendations on the required numbers of doses for each of the various treatment regimens have been published jointly by the American Thoracic Society, the Infectious Diseases Society of America, and the CDC. In some developing countries where the ability to ensure compliance with treatment is limited, a continuation-phase regimen of daily isoniazid and ethambutol for 6 months is acceptable. However, this regimen is associated with a higher rate of relapse and failure, especially among HIV-infected patients.

Lack of adherence to treatment is recognized worldwide as the most important impediment to cure. Moreover, the tubercle bacilli infecting patients who do not adhere to the prescribed regimen are likely to become drug resistant. Both patient- and provider-related factors may affect compliance. Patient-related factors include a lack of belief that the illness is significant and/or that treatment will have a beneficial effect; the existence of concomitant medical conditions (notably substance abuse); lack of social support; and poverty, with attendant joblessness and homelessness. Provider-related factors that may promote compliance include the education and encouragement of patients, the offering of convenient clinic hours, and the provision of incentives and enablers such as meals and travel vouchers.

In addition to specific measures addressing noncompliance, two other strategic approaches are used: direct observation of treatment and provision of fixed-drug-combination (FDC) products. Because it is difficult to predict which patients will adhere to the recommended treatment, all patients should have their therapy directly supervised, especially during the initial phase. In the United States, personnel to supervise therapy are usually available through tuberculosis control programs of local public health departments. Supervision increases the proportion of patients completing treatment and greatly lessens the chances of relapse and acquired drug resistance. FDC products (e.g., isoniazid/rifampin, isoniazid/rifampin/pyrazinamide, and isoniazid/rifampin/pyrazinamide/ethambutol) are available

TABLE 158-3 RECOMMENDED ANTITUBERCULOSIS TREATMENT REGIMENS

Indication	Initial Phase		Continuation Phase	
	Duration, Months	**Drugs**	**Duration, Months**	**Drugs**
New smear- or culture-positive cases	2	HRZE[a,b]	4	HR[a,c,d]
New culture-negative cases	2	HRZE[a]	2	HR[a]
Pregnancy	2	HRE[e]	7	HR
Failure and relapse[f]	—	—	—	—
Resistance (or intolerance) to H	Throughout (6)	RZE[g]		
Resistance to H + R	Throughout (12–18)	ZEQ + S (or another injectable agent[h])		
Resistance to all first-line drugs	Throughout (24)	1 injectable agent[h] + 3 of these 4: ethionamide, cycloserine, Q, PAS		
Standardized re-treatment (susceptibility testing unavailable)	3	HRZES[i]	5	HRE
Drug intolerance to R	Throughout (12)[j]	HZE		
Drug intolerance to Z	2	HRE	7	HR

[a]All drugs can be given daily or intermittently (three times weekly throughout or twice weekly after 2–8 weeks of daily therapy during the initial phase).

[b]Streptomycin can be used in place of ethambutol but is no longer considered to be a first-line drug by ATS/IDSA/CDC.

[c]The continuation phase should be extended to 7 months for patients with cavitary pulmonary tuberculosis who remain sputum culture–positive after the initial phase of treatment.

[d]HIV-negative patients with noncavitary pulmonary tuberculosis who have negative sputum AFB smears after the initial phase of treatment can be given once-weekly rifapentine/isoniazid in the continuation phase.

[e]The 6-month regimen with pyrazinamide can probably be used safely during pregnancy and is recommended by the WHO and the International Union Against Tuberculosis and Lung Disease. If pyrazinamide is not included in the initial treatment regimen, the minimum duration of therapy is 9 months.

[f]Regimen is tailored according to the results of drug susceptibility tests.

[g]A fluoroquinolone may strengthen the regimen for patients with extensive disease.

[h]Amikacin, kanamycin, or capreomycin. All these agents should be discontinued after 2–6 months, depending upon tolerance and response.

[i]Streptomycin should be discontinued after 2 months. This regimen is less effective for patients in whom treatment has failed, who have an increased probability of rifampin-resistant disease. In such cases, the re-treatment regimen might include second-line drugs chosen in light of the likely pattern of drug resistance.

[j]Streptomycin for the initial 2 months or a fluoroquinolone might strengthen the regimen for patients with extensive disease.

Abbreviations: H, isoniazid; R, rifampin; Z, pyrazinamide; E, ethambutol; S, streptomycin; Q, a quinolone antibiotic; PAS, para-aminosalicylic acid.

(except, in the United States, for the four-drug FDC) and are strongly recommended as a means of minimizing the likelihood of prescription error and of the development of drug resistance as the result of monotherapy. In some formulations of these combination products, the bioavailability of rifampin has been found to be substandard. In North America and Europe, regulatory authorities ensure that combination products are of good quality; however, this type of quality assurance cannot be assumed to take place in less affluent countries. Alternative regimens for patients who exhibit drug intolerance or adverse reactions are listed in Table 158-3. However, severe side effects prompting discontinuation of any of the first-line drugs and use of these alternative regimens are uncommon.

MONITORING TREATMENT RESPONSE AND DRUG TOXICITY

Bacteriologic evaluation is the preferred method of monitoring the response to treatment for tuberculosis. Patients with pulmonary disease should have their sputum examined monthly until cultures become negative. With the recommended regimen, >80% of patients will have negative sputum cultures at the end of the second month of treatment. By the end of the third month, virtually all patients should be culture-negative. In some patients, especially those with extensive cavitary disease and large numbers of organisms, AFB smear conversion may lag behind culture conversion. This phenomenon is presumably due to the expectoration and microscopic visualization of dead bacilli. As noted above, patients with cavitary disease who do not achieve sputum culture conversion by 2 months require extended treatment. When a patient's sputum cultures remain positive at ≥3 months, treatment failure and drug resistance or poor adherence with the regimen should be suspected (see below). A sputum specimen should be collected by the end of treatment to document cure. If mycobacterial cultures are not practical, then monitoring by AFB smear examination should be undertaken at 2, 5, and 6 months. Smears that are positive after 5 months of treatment in a patient known to be adherent are indicative of treatment failure.

Bacteriologic monitoring of patients with extrapulmonary tuberculosis is more difficult and often not feasible. In these cases, the response to treatment must be assessed clinically and radiographically.

Monitoring of the response to treatment during chemotherapy by serial chest radiographs is not recommended, as radiographic changes may lag behind bacteriologic response and are not highly sensitive. After the completion of treatment, neither sputum examination nor chest radiography is recommended for routine follow-up purposes. However, a chest radiograph obtained at the end of treatment may be useful for comparative purposes should the patient develop symptoms of recurrent tuberculosis months or years later. Patients should be instructed to report promptly for medical assessment should they develop any such symptoms.

During treatment, patients should be monitored for drug toxicity (see Table 161-3). The most common adverse reaction of significance is hepatitis. Patients should be carefully educated about the signs and symptoms of drug-induced hepatitis (e.g., dark urine, loss of appetite) and should be instructed to discontinue treatment promptly and see their health care provider should these symptoms occur. Although biochemical monitoring is not routinely recommended, all adult patients should undergo baseline assessment of liver function (e.g., measurement of serum levels of hepatic aminotransferases and serum bilirubin). Older patients, those with concomitant diseases, those with a history of hepatic disease (especially hepatitis C), and those using alcohol daily should be monitored especially closely (i.e., monthly), with repeated measurements of aminotransferases, during the initial phase of treatment. Up to 20% of patients have small increases in aspartate aminotransferase (up to three times the upper limit of normal) that are not accompanied by symptoms and are of no consequence. For patients with symptomatic hepatitis and those with marked (five- to sixfold) elevations in serum levels of aspartate aminotransferase, treatment should be stopped and drugs reintroduced one at a time after liver function has returned to normal.

Hypersensitivity reactions usually require the discontinuation of all drugs and rechallenge to determine which agent is the culprit. Because of the variety of regimens available, it is usually not necessary—although it is possible—to desensitize patients. Hyperuricemia and arthralgia caused by pyrazinamide can usually be managed by the administration of acetylsalicylic acid; however, pyrazinamide treatment should be stopped if the patient develops gouty arthritis. Individuals who develop autoimmune thrombocytopenia secondary to rifampin therapy should not receive the

drug thereafter. Similarly, the occurrence of optic neuritis with ethambutol is an indication for permanent discontinuation of this drug. Other common manifestations of drug intolerance, such as pruritus and gastrointestinal upset, can generally be managed without the interruption of therapy.

TREATMENT FAILURE AND RELAPSE   As stated above, treatment failure should be suspected when a patient's sputum cultures remain positive after 3 months or when AFB smears remain positive after 5 months. In the management of such patients, it is imperative that the current isolate be tested for susceptibility to first- and second-line agents. When the results of susceptibility testing are expected to become available within a few weeks, changes in the regimen can be postponed until that time. However, if the patient's clinical condition is deteriorating, an earlier change in regimen may be indicated. A cardinal rule in the latter situation is always to add more than one drug at a time to a failing regimen: at least two and preferably three drugs that have never been used and to which the bacilli are likely to be susceptible should be added. The patient may continue to take isoniazid and rifampin along with these new agents pending the results of susceptibility tests.

The mycobacterial strains infecting patients who experience a relapse after apparently successful treatment are less likely to have acquired drug resistance (see below) than are strains from patients in whom treatment has failed. However, if the regimen administered initially does not contain rifampin, the probability of isoniazid resistance is high. Acquired resistance is uncommon among strains from patients who relapse after completing a standard short-course regimen. However, it is prudent to begin the treatment of all patients who have relapsed with all four first-line drugs plus streptomycin, pending the results of susceptibility testing. In less affluent countries and other settings where facilities for culture and drug susceptibility testing are not available, a standard regimen should be used in all instances of relapse and treatment failure (Table 158-3).

DRUG-RESISTANT TUBERCULOSIS   Strains of *M. tuberculosis* resistant to individual drugs arise by spontaneous point mutations in the mycobacterial genome, which occur at low but predictable rates. Because there is no cross-resistance among the commonly used drugs, the probability that a strain will be resistant to two drugs is the product of the probabilities of resistance to each drug and thus is low. The development of drug-resistant tuberculosis is invariably the result of monotherapy—i.e., the failure of the health care provider to prescribe at least two drugs to which tubercle bacilli are susceptible or of the patient to take properly prescribed therapy.

Drug-resistant tuberculosis may be either primary or acquired. Primary drug resistance is that in a strain infecting a patient who has not previously been treated. Acquired resistance develops during treatment with an inappropriate regimen. In North America and Europe, rates of primary resistance are generally low, and isoniazid resistance is most common. In the United States, while primary isoniazid resistance was stable at ~7–8% between 1993 and 2002, the rate of primary multidrug-resistant (MDR) tuberculosis (defined as tuberculosis due to a strain resistant at least to isoniazid and rifampin) declined from 2.5% to 1%. Resistance rates are higher among foreign-born and HIV-infected patients. Worldwide, MDR tuberculosis is a serious problem in some regions, especially in the former Soviet Union and parts of Asia **(Fig. 158-8)**. As noted above, drug-resistant tuberculosis can be prevented by adherence to the principles of sound therapy: the inclusion of at least two bactericidal drugs to which the organism is susceptible, the use of FDC products, and the verification that patients complete the prescribed course.

Although the 6-month regimen described in Table 158-3 is generally effective for patients with initial isoniazid-resistant disease, it is prudent to include ethambutol and pyrazinamide for the full 6 months. In such cases, isoniazid probably does not contribute to a successful outcome and should be omitted. MDR tuberculosis is more difficult to manage than is disease caused by a drug-susceptible organism, especially because resistance to other first-line drugs as well as to isoniazid and rifampin is common. For strains resistant to isoniazid and rifampin, combinations of a fluoroquinolone, ethambutol, pyrazinamide, and streptomycin (or, for strains resistant to streptomycin as well, another injectable agent such as amikacin or kanamycin), given for 18–24 months and for at least 9 months after sputum culture conversion, may be effective. For patients with bacilli resistant to all of the first-line agents, cure may be attained with a combi-

PART 7

Infectious Diseases

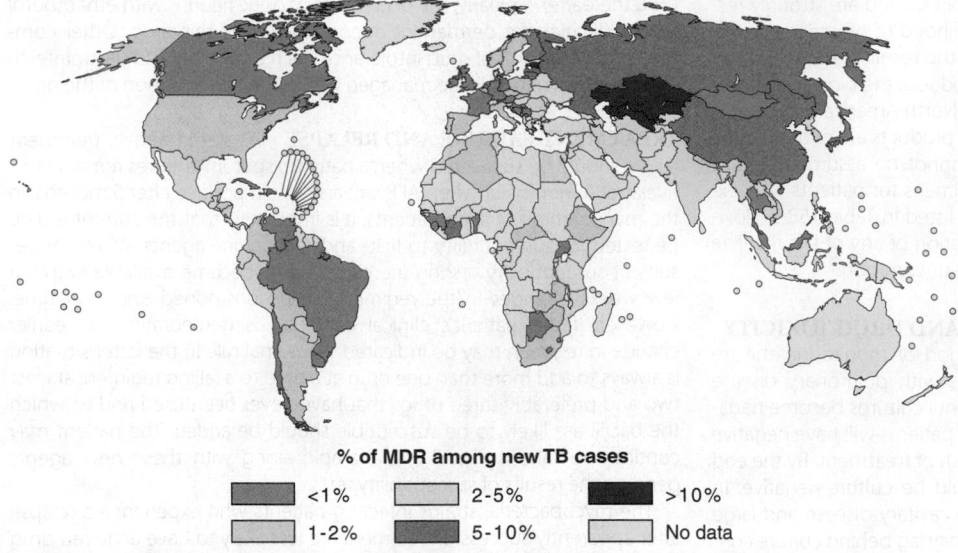

% of MDR among new TB cases

<1%   2-5%   >10%

1-2%   5-10%   No data

FIGURE 158-8 Percentage of new tuberculosis cases exhibiting multidrug resistance in all countries surveyed by the WHO/Union Global Drug Resistance Surveillance Project during 1994–2005. *(See also disclaimer in Fig. 158-2. Courtesy of the Stop TB Department, WHO; with permission.)*

nation of four second-line drugs, including one injectable agent (Table 158-3). The optimal duration of treatment in this situation is not known; however, a duration of 24 months is recommended. MDR strains of *M. tuberculosis* that are also resistant to at least the fluoroquinolones and one or more of the injectable drugs amikacin, kanamycin, or capreomycin [extensive drug-resistant (XDR) strains] have fewer treatment options and a much poorer prognosis. For patients with localized disease and sufficient pulmonary reserve, lobectomy or pneumonectomy may be helpful. Because the management of patients with MDR and XDR tuberculosis is complicated by both social and medical factors, care of these patients should be restricted to those tuberculosis control programs with resources and capacity and to specialized centers.

HIV-ASSOCIATED TUBERCULOSIS In general, the standard treatment regimens are equally efficacious in HIV-negative and HIV-positive patients. However, adverse drug effects may be more pronounced in HIV-infected patients. Since these effects may include serious or even fatal skin reactions to amithiozone (thiacetazone), this drug, which has been used in place of ethambutol in developing countries, is no longer recommended by the WHO.

Three important considerations are relevant to tuberculosis treatment in HIV-infected patients: an increased frequency of paradoxical reactions, drug interactions between antiretroviral therapy and rifamycins, and development of rifampin monoresistance with widely spaced intermittent treatment. Exacerbations in symptoms, signs, and laboratory or radiographic manifestations of tuberculosis—termed the *immune reconstitution inflammatory syndrome* (IRIS)—have been associated with the administration of antiretroviral regimens. IRIS is more common among patients with advanced immunosuppression and extrapulmonary tuberculosis. The presumed pathogenesis of IRIS is an immune response that is elicited by antigens released as bacilli are killed during effective chemotherapy and that is temporally associated with improving immune function. The first priority in the management of a possible case of IRIS is to ensure that the clinical syndrome does not represent a failure of tuberculosis treatment or the development of another infection. Mild paradoxical reactions can be managed with symptom-based treatment. Glucocorticoids have been used for more severe reactions, although their use in this setting has not been formally evaluated in clinical trials.

Most HIV-infected tuberculosis patients are candidates for antiretroviral therapy, although the optimal timing of this treatment is not known. Rifampin, a potent inducer of enzymes of the cytochrome P450 system, lowers serum levels of many HIV protease inhibitors and some nonnucleoside reverse transcriptase inhibitors—essential drugs used in antiretroviral regimens. In such cases, rifabutin, which has much less enzyme-inducing activity, has been recommended in place of rifampin. However, dosage adjustment for rifabutin and/or the antiretroviral drugs may be necessary.

Because recommendations are frequently updated, consultation of the CDC website is advised (*www.cdc.gov/tb/TB_HIV_Drugs/default.htm*).

Several clinical trials of HIV-associated tuberculosis have found that patients with advanced immunosuppression (CD4+ T cell counts of <100/µL) are prone to treatment failure and relapse with rifampin-resistant organisms when treated with "highly intermittent" (i.e., once- or twice-weekly) rifamycin-containing regimens. Consequently, it is recommended that these patients receive daily or thrice-weekly therapy for the entire course.

SPECIAL CLINICAL SITUATIONS
Although comparative clinical trials of treatment for extrapulmonary tuberculosis are limited, the available evidence indicates that most forms of disease can be treated with the 6-month regimen recommended for patients with pulmonary disease. The American Academy of Pediatrics recommends that children with bone and joint tuberculosis, tuberculous meningitis, or miliary tuberculosis receive 9–12 months of treatment.

Treatment for tuberculosis may be complicated by underlying medical problems that require special consideration (see Table 161-1). As a rule, patients with chronic renal failure should not receive aminoglycosides and should receive ethambutol only if serum levels can be monitored. Isoniazid, rifampin, and pyrazinamide may be given in the usual doses in cases of mild to moderate renal failure, but the dosages of isoniazid and pyrazinamide should be reduced for all patients with severe renal failure except those undergoing hemodialysis. Patients with hepatic disease pose a special problem because of the hepatotoxicity of isoniazid, rifampin, and pyrazinamide. Patients with severe hepatic disease may be treated with ethambutol, streptomycin, and possibly another drug (e.g., a fluoroquinolone); if required, isoniazid and rifampin may be administered under close supervision. The use of pyrazinamide by patients with liver failure should be avoided. Silicotuberculosis necessitates the extension of therapy by at least 2 months.

The regimen of choice for pregnant women (Tables 161-1 and 158-3) is 9 months of treatment with isoniazid and rifampin supplemented by ethambutol for the first 2 months. Although the WHO has recommended routine use of pyrazinamide in pregnant women, this drug has not been recommended in the United States because of insufficient data documenting its safety in pregnancy. Streptomycin is contraindicated because it is known to cause eighth-cranial-nerve damage in the fetus. Treatment for tuberculosis is not a contraindication to breast-feeding; most of the drugs administered will be present in small quantities in breast milk, albeit at concentrations far too low to provide any therapeutic or prophylactic benefit to the child.

Medical consultation on difficult-to-manage cases is provided by the CDC Regional Training and Medical Consultation Centers (*http://www.cdc.gov/tb/rtmcc.htm*).

PREVENTION

By far the best way to prevent tuberculosis is to diagnose and isolate infectious cases rapidly and administer appropriate treatment until patients are rendered noninfectious and the disease is cured. Additional strategies include BCG vaccination and treatment of persons with latent tuberculosis infection who are at high risk of developing active disease.

BCG VACCINATION
BCG was derived from an attenuated strain of *M. bovis* and first administered to humans in 1921. Many BCG vaccines are available worldwide; all are derived from the original strain, but the vaccines vary in efficacy, ranging from 80% to nil in randomized, placebo-controlled trials. A similar range of efficacy was found in recent observational studies (case-control, historic cohort, and cross-sectional) in

areas where infants are vaccinated at birth. These studies also found higher rates of efficacy in the protection of infants and young children from relatively serious forms of tuberculosis, such as tuberculous meningitis and miliary tuberculosis.

BCG vaccine is safe and rarely causes serious complications. The local tissue response begins 2–3 weeks after vaccination, with scar formation and healing within 3 months. Side effects—most commonly, ulceration at the vaccination site and regional lymphadenitis—occur in 1–10% of vaccinated persons. Some vaccine strains have caused osteomyelitis in ~1 case per million doses administered. Disseminated BCG infection and death have occurred in 1–10 cases per 10 million doses administered, although this problem is restricted almost exclusively to persons with impaired immunity, such as children with severe combined immunodeficiency syndrome or adults with HIV infection. BCG vaccination induces TST reactivity, which tends to wane with time. The presence or size of TST reactions after vaccination does not predict the degree of protection afforded.

BCG vaccine is recommended for routine use at birth in countries with high tuberculosis prevalence. However, because of the low risk of transmission of tuberculosis in the United States, the unreliable protection afforded by BCG, and its impact on the TST, the vaccine has never been recommended for general use in the United States. The CDC has recommended that HIV-infected adults and children not receive BCG vaccine, although the WHO has recommended that asymptomatic HIV-infected children residing in tuberculosis-endemic areas receive BCG.

Rx LATENT TUBERCULOSIS INFECTION

Treatment of selected persons with LTBI aims at preventing active disease. This intervention (formerly called *preventive chemotherapy* or *chemoprophylaxis*) is based on the results of a large number of randomized, placebo-controlled clinical trials demonstrating that a 6- to 12-month course of isoniazid reduces the risk of active tuberculosis in infected people by up to 90%. Analysis of available data indicates that the optimal duration of treatment is 9–10 months. In the absence of reinfection, the protective effect is believed to be lifelong. Clinical trials have shown that isoniazid reduces rates of tuberculosis among TST-positive persons with HIV infection. Studies in HIV-infected patients have also demonstrated the effectiveness of shorter courses of rifampin-based treatment.

In most cases, candidates for treatment of LTBI (Table 158-4) are identified by the TST of persons in defined high-risk groups. For skin testing, 5 tuberculin units of polysorbate-stabilized PPD should be injected intradermally into the volar surface of the forearm (Mantoux method). Multipuncture tests are not recommended. Reactions are read at 48–72 h as the transverse diameter (in millimeters) of induration; the diameter of erythema is not considered. In some persons, TST reactivity wanes with time but can be recalled by a second skin test administered ≥1 week after the first (i.e., two-step testing). For persons periodically undergoing the TST, such as health care workers and individuals admitted to long-term-care institutions, initial two-step testing may preclude subsequent misclassification of persons with boosted reactions as TST converters.

The cutoff for a positive TST (and thus for treatment) is related both to the probability that the reaction represents true infection and to the likelihood that the individual, if truly infected, will develop tuberculosis (Table 158-4). Thus, positive reactions for close contacts of infectious cases, persons with HIV infection, persons receiving drugs that suppress the immune system, and previously untreated persons whose chest radiograph is consistent with healed tuberculosis are defined as an area of induration ≥5 mm in diameter. A 10-mm cutoff is used to define positive reactions in most other at-risk persons. For persons with a very low risk of developing tuberculosis if infected, a cutoff of 15 mm is used. (Except for employment purposes where longitudinal screening is anticipated, the TST is not indicated for these low-risk persons.) Treatment should be considered for persons from tuberculosis-endemic countries who have a history of BCG vaccination. A positive reaction in an IGRA is not based on the degree of response—i.e., the level of IFN-γ induced.

Some TST-negative individuals are also candidates for treatment. Infants and children who have come into contact with infectious cases should be treated and should have a repeat skin test 2 or 3 months after contact

TABLE 158-4 TUBERCULIN REACTION SIZE AND TREATMENT OF LATENT TUBERCULOSIS INFECTION

Risk Group	Tuberculin Reaction Size, mm
HIV-infected persons or persons receiving immunosuppressive therapy	≥5
Close contacts of tuberculosis patients	≥5[a]
Persons with fibrotic lesions on chest radiography	≥5
Recently infected persons (≤2 years)	≥10
Persons with high-risk medical conditions[b]	≥10
Low-risk persons[c]	≥15

[a]Tuberculin-negative contacts, especially children, should receive prophylaxis for 2–3 months after contact ends and should then undergo repeat TST. Those whose results remain negative should discontinue prophylaxis. HIV-infected contacts should receive a full course of treatment regardless of TST results.

[b]Includes diabetes mellitus, some hematologic and reticuloendothelial diseases, injection drug use (with HIV seronegativity), end-stage renal disease, and clinical situations associated with rapid weight loss.

[c]Except for employment purposes where longitudinal TST screening is anticipated, TST is not indicated for these low-risk persons. A decision to treat should be based on individual risk/benefit considerations.

ment. HIV-infected persons who have been exposed to an infectious tuberculosis patient should receive treatment regardless of the TST result.

Isoniazid is administered at a daily dose of 5 mg/kg (up to 300 mg/d) for 9 months (Table 158-5). On the basis of cost-benefit analyses, a 6-month period of treatment has been recommended in the past and may be considered for HIV-negative adults with normal chest radiographs when financial considerations are important. When supervised treatment is desirable and feasible, isoniazid may be given at a dose of 15 mg/kg (up to 900 mg) twice weekly. An alternative regimen for adults is 4 months of daily rifampin. A 3-month regimen of isoniazid and rifampin is recommended in the United Kingdom for both adults and children. A previously recommended regimen of 2 months of rifampin and pyrazinamide has been associated with serious and fatal hepatotoxicity and now is generally not recommended. The rifampin regimen should be considered for persons who are likely to have been infected with an isoniazid-resistant strain.

Isoniazid should not be given to persons with active liver disease. All persons at increased risk of hepatotoxicity (e.g., those abusing alcohol daily and those with a history of liver disease) should undergo baseline and then monthly assessment of liver function. All patients should be carefully educated about hepatitis and instructed to discontinue use of the drug immediately should any symptoms develop. Moreover, patients should be seen and questioned monthly during therapy about adverse reactions and should be given no more than 1 month's supply of drug at each visit.

It may be more difficult to ensure compliance when treating persons with latent infection than when treating those with active tuberculosis. If family members of active cases are being treated, compliance and monitoring may be easier. When feasible, twice-weekly supervised therapy may increase the likelihood of completion. As in active cases, the provision of incentives may also be helpful.

PRINCIPLES OF TUBERCULOSIS CONTROL

The highest priority in any tuberculosis control program is the prompt detection of cases and the provision of short-course chemotherapy to all tuberculosis patients under proper case-management conditions, including directly observed therapy. In addition, in low-prevalence countries with adequate resources, screening of high-risk groups (such as immigrants from high-prevalence countries, migratory workers, prisoners, the homeless, substance abusers, and HIV-seropositive persons) is recommended. TST-positive high-risk persons should be treated for latent infection. Contact investigation is an important component of efficient tuberculosis control. In the United States, a great deal of attention has been given to the transmission of tuberculosis (particularly in association with HIV infection) in institutional settings such as hospitals, homeless shelters, and prisons. Measures to limit such transmission include respiratory isolation of persons with

CHAPTER 158 Tuberculosis

TABLE 158-5 REVISED DRUG REGIMENS FOR TREATMENT OF LATENT TUBERCULOSIS INFECTION (LTBI) IN ADULTS

Drug	Interval and Duration	Comments[a]	Rating[b] (Evidence[c]) HIV-Negative	Rating[b] (Evidence[c]) HIV-Infected
Isoniazid	Daily for 9 months[d,e]	In HIV-infected persons, isoniazid may be administered concurrently with nucleoside reverse transcriptase inhibitors, protease inhibitors, or nonnucleoside reverse transcriptase inhibitors (NNRTIs).	A (II)	A (II)
	Twice weekly for 9 months[d,e]	Directly observed therapy (DOT) must be used with twice-weekly dosing.	B (II)	B (II)
	Daily for 6 months[e]	Regimen is not indicated for HIV-infected persons, those with fibrotic lesions on chest radiographs, or children.	B (I)	C (I)
	Twice weekly for 6 months[e]	DOT must be used with twice-weekly dosing.	B (II)	C (I)
Rifampin[f]	Daily for 4 months	Regimen is used for contacts of patients with isoniazid-resistant, rifampin-susceptible tuberculosis. In HIV-infected persons, most protease inhibitors and delavirdine should not be administered concurrently with rifampin. Rifabutin, with appropriate dose adjustments, can be used with protease inhibitors (saquinavir should be augmented with ritonavir) and NNRTIs (except delavirdine). Clinicians should consult web-based updates for the latest specific recommendations.	B (II)	B (III)
Rifampin plus pyrazinamide (RZ)	Daily for 2 months	Regimen generally should not be offered for treatment of LTBI in either HIV-infected or HIV-negative persons.	D (II)	D (II)
	Twice weekly for 2–3 months		D (III)	D (III)

[a]Interactions with HIV-related drugs are updated frequently and are available at http://www.aidsinfo.nih.gov/guidelines.
[b]Strength of the recommendation: A. Both strong evidence of efficacy and substantial clinical benefit support recommendation for use. Should always be offered. B. Moderate evidence for efficacy or strong evidence for efficacy but only limited clinical benefit supports recommendation for use. Should generally be offered. C. Evidence for efficacy is insufficient to support a recommendation for or against use, or evidence for efficacy might not outweigh adverse consequences (e.g., drug toxicity, drug interactions) or cost of the treatment or alternative approaches. Optional. D. Moderate evidence for lack of efficacy or for adverse outcome supports a recommendation against use. Should generally not be offered. E. Good evidence for lack of efficacy or for adverse outcome supports a recommendation against use. Should never be offered.
[c]Quality of evidence supporting the recommendation: I. Evidence from at least one properly randomized controlled trial. II. Evidence from at least one well-designed clinical trial without randomization, from cohort or case-controlled analytic studies (preferably from more than one center), from multiple time-series studies, or from dramatic results in uncontrolled experiments. III. Evidence from opinions of respected authorities based on clinical experience, descriptive studies, or reports of expert committees.
[d]Recommended regimen for persons aged <18 years.
[e]Recommended regimen for pregnant women.
[f]The substitution of rifapentine for rifampin is not recommended because rifapentine's safety and effectiveness have not been established for patients with LTBI.
Source: Adapted from CDC: Targeted tuberculin testing and treatment of latent tuberculosis infection. MMWR 49(RR-6), 2000

suspected tuberculosis until they are proven to be noninfectious (i.e., by sputum AFB smear negativity), proper ventilation in rooms of patients with infectious tuberculosis, use of ultraviolet irradiation in areas of increased risk of tuberculosis transmission, and periodic screening of personnel who may come into contact with known or unsuspected cases of tuberculosis. In the past, radiographic surveys, especially those conducted with portable equipment and miniature films, were advocated for case finding. Today, however, the prevalence of tuberculosis in industrialized countries is sufficiently low that "mass miniature radiography" is not cost-effective.

In high-prevalence countries, many tuberculosis control programs have made good progress in reducing morbidity and mortality during the past decade by adopting and implementing the DOTS strategy promoted by the WHO. This strategy consists of: (1) political commitment with increased and sustained financing; (2) case detection through quality-assured bacteriology (starting with microscopic examination of sputum from patients with cough of >2–3 weeks' duration); (3) administration of standardized treatment, with supervision and patient support; (4) an effective drug supply and management system; and (5) a monitoring and evaluation system, with impact measurement (including assessment of treatment outcomes—e.g., cure, completion of treatment without bacteriologic proof of cure, death, treatment failure, and default—in all cases registered and notified). In 2006, the WHO indicated that, while DOTS remains the essential component of any control strategy, additional steps must be undertaken to reach the 2015 tuberculosis control targets set within the United Nations Millennium Development Goals. Thus, a new "Stop TB Strategy" with six components has been promoted: (1) Pursue high-quality DOTS expansion and enhancement. (2) Address HIV-associated tuberculosis, MDR tuberculosis, and other special challenges. (3) Contribute to health system strengthening. (4) Engage all care providers. (5) Empower people with tuberculosis and communities. (6) Enable and promote research. As part of the fourth component, new evidence-based International Standards for Tuberculosis Care, focused on diagnosis, treatment, and public health responsibilities, have recently been introduced for wide adoption by medical and professional societies, academic institutions, and all practitioners worldwide.

FURTHER READINGS

AMERICAN THORACIC SOCIETY, CENTERS FOR DISEASE CONTROL AND PREVENTION: Targeted tuberculin testing and treatment of latent tuberculosis infection. Am J Respir Crit Care Med 161:S221, 2000

AMERICAN THORACIC SOCIETY, INFECTIOUS DISEASES SOCIETY OF AMERICA, CENTERS FOR DISEASE CONTROL AND PREVENTION: Treatment of tuberculosis. Am J Respir Crit Care Med 167:603, 2003

CENTERS FOR DISEASE CONTROL AND PREVENTION: Control of tuberculosis in the United States: Recommendations from the American Thoracic Society, CDC, and the Infectious Diseases Society of America. MMWR 54:RR1, 2005

HOPEWELL PC et al: International standards for tuberculosis care. Lancet Infect Dis 6:710, 2006

PAI M et al: New tools and emerging technologies for the diagnosis of tuberculosis. Part I: Latent tuberculosis. Part II: Active tuberculosis and drug resistance. Expert Rev Mol Diagn 6:413, 2006

RAVIGLIONE MC, SMITH IM: XDR tuberculosis—Implications for global public health. N Engl J Med 356:656, 2007

———, UPLEKAR M: WHO's new Stop TB Strategy. Lancet 367:952, 2006

REID A et al: Towards universal access to HIV prevention, treatment, care and support: The role of tuberculosis/HIV collaboration. Lancet Infect Dis 6:483, 2006

WORLD HEALTH ORGANIZATION: Guidelines for the programmatic management of drug-resistant tuberculosis. Geneva, WHO, 2006

159 Leprosy (Hansen's Disease)
Robert H. Gelber

Leprosy, first described in ancient Indian texts from the sixth century B.C., is a nonfatal, chronic infectious disease caused by *Mycobacterium leprae*, whose clinical manifestations are largely confined to the skin, peripheral nervous system, upper respiratory tract, eyes, and testes. The unique tropism of *M. leprae* for peripheral nerves (from large nerve trunks to microscopic dermal nerves) and certain immunologically mediated reactional states are the major causes of morbidity in leprosy. The propensity of the disease, when untreated, to result in characteristic deformities and the recognition in most cultures that the disease is communicable from person to person have resulted historically in a profound social stigma. Today, with early diagnosis and the institution of appropriate and effective antimicrobial therapy, patients can lead productive lives in the community, and deformities and other visible manifestations can largely be prevented.

ETIOLOGY

M. leprae is an obligate intracellular bacillus (0.3–1 μm wide and 1–8 μm long) that is confined to humans, armadillos in certain locales, and sphagnum moss. The organism is acid-fast, indistinguishable microscopically from other mycobacteria, and ideally detected in tissue sections by a modified Fite stain. Strain variability has been documented in this organism. *M. leprae* produces no known toxins and is well adapted to penetrate and reside within macrophages, yet it may survive outside the body for months. In untreated patients, only ~1% of *M. leprae* organisms are viable. The morphologic index (MI), a measure of the number of acid-fast bacilli (AFB) in skin scrapings that stain uniformly bright, correlates with viability. The bacteriologic index (BI), a logarithmic-scaled measure of the density of *M. leprae* in the dermis, may be as high as 4–6+ in untreated patients, falling by 1 unit per year during effective therapy; the rate of decrease is independent of the relative potency of effective antimicrobial therapy. A rising MI or BI suggests relapse and perhaps—if the patient is being treated—drug resistance. The latter possibility can be confirmed or excluded in the mouse model.

As a result of reductive evolution, almost half of the *M. leprae* genome contains nonfunctional genes; only 1605 genes encode for proteins, and 1439 genes are shared with *Mycobacterium tuberculosis*. In contrast, *M. tuberculosis* uses 91% of its genome to encode for 4000 proteins. Among the lost genes in *M. leprae* are those for catabolic and respiratory pathways; transport systems; purine, methionine, and glutamine synthesis; and nitrogen regulation. The genome of *M. leprae* provides a metabolic rationale for its obligate intracellular existence and reliance on host biochemical support, a template for targets of drug development, and ultimately a pathway to cultivation. The finding of strain variability among *M. leprae* isolates has provided a powerful tool with which to address anew the organism's epidemiology and pathobiology and to determine whether relapse represents reactivation or reinfection. The bacterium's complex cell wall contains large amounts of an *M. leprae*–specific phenolic glycolipid (PGL-1), which is detected in serologic tests. The unique trisaccharide of *M. leprae* binds to the basal lamina of Schwann cells; this interaction is probably relevant to the fact that *M. leprae* is the only bacterium to invade peripheral nerves.

Although it was the first bacterium to be etiologically associated with human disease, *M. leprae* remains one of the few bacterial species that still has not been cultivated on artificial medium or tissue culture. The multiplication of *M. leprae* in mouse footpads (albeit limited, with a doubling time of ~2 weeks) has provided a means to evaluate antimicrobial agents, monitor clinical trials, and screen vaccines. *M. leprae* grows best in cooler tissues (the skin, peripheral nerves, anterior chamber of the eye, upper respiratory tract, and testes), sparing warmer areas of the skin (the axilla, groin, scalp, and midline of the back).

EPIDEMIOLOGY

Demographics Leprosy is almost exclusively a disease of the developing world, affecting areas of Asia, Africa, Latin America, and the Pacific (Fig. 159-1). While Africa has the highest disease prevalence, Asia has the most cases. More than 80% of the world's cases occur in a few countries: India, China, Myanmar, Indonesia, Brazil, Nigeria, Madagascar, and Nepal. Within endemic locales, the distribution of leprosy is quite uneven, with areas of high prevalence bordering on areas with little or no disease. In Brazil the majority of cases occur in the Amazon basin and two western states, while in Mexico leprosy is mostly confined to the Pacific coast. Except as imported cases, leprosy is largely absent from the United States, Canada, and northwestern Europe. In the United States, ~4000 persons have leprosy and 100–200 new cases are reported annually, most of them in California, Texas, New York, and Hawaii among immigrants from Mexico, Southeast Asia, the Philippines, and the Caribbean. The comparative genomics of single-nucleotide polymorphisms support the likelihood that four distinct strains exist, having originated in East Africa or Central Asia. A mutation spread to Europe and subsequently underwent two separate mutations that were then followed by spread to West Africa and the Americas.

The global prevalence of leprosy is difficult to assess, given that many of the locales with high prevalence lack a significant medical or public health infrastructure. Estimates range from 0.6 to 8 million affected individuals. The lower estimate includes only persons who have not completed chemotherapy, excluding those who may be physically or psychologically damaged from leprosy and who may yet relapse or develop immune-mediated reactions. The higher figure includes patients whose infections probably are already cured and many who have no leprosy-related deformity or disability. Although the figures on the worldwide prevalence of leprosy are debatable, it is not falling; there are an estimated 600,000 new cases annually, 60% of them in India.

Leprosy is associated with poverty and rural residence. It appears not to be associated with AIDS, perhaps because of leprosy's long in-

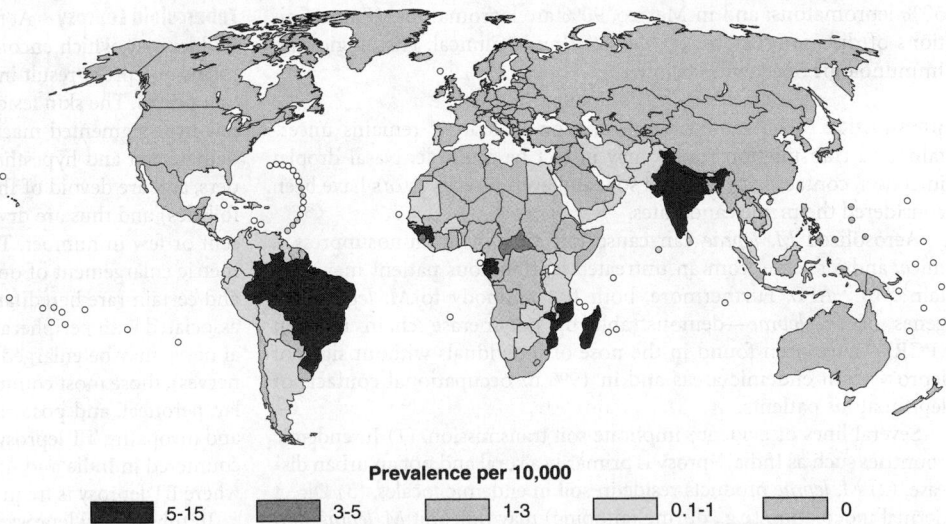

Prevalence per 10,000

| 5-15 | 3-5 | 1-3 | 0.1-1 | 0 |

FIGURE 159-1 Estimated prevalence of leprosy at the turn of the millennium. Because data on leprosy prevalence in many endemic countries are unreliable, global prevalence is difficult to assess with any great degree of accuracy; however, it is not falling (see text). *(Courtesy of Patrick J. Brennan, Ph.D., with permission; www.cvmbs.colostate.edu/microbiology/leprosy/globalleprosy3.html.)*

TABLE 159-1 CLINICAL, BACTERIOLOGIC, PATHOLOGIC, AND IMMUNOLOGIC SPECTRUM OF LEPROSY

Feature	Tuberculoid (TT, BT) Leprosy	Borderline (BB, BL) Leprosy	Lepromatous (LL) Leprosy
Skin lesions	One or a few sharply defined annular asymmetric macules or plaques with a tendency toward central clearing, elevated borders	Intermediate between BT and LL type lesions; ill-defined plaques with an occasional sharp margin; few or many in number	Symmetric, poorly marginated, multiple infiltrated nodules and plaques or diffuse infiltration; xanthoma-like or dermatofibroma papules; leonine facies and eyebrow alopecia
Nerve lesions	Skin lesions anesthetic early; nerve near lesions sometimes enlarged; nerve abscesses most common in BT	Hypesthetic or anesthetic skin lesions; nerve trunk palsies, at times symmetric	Hypesthesia a late sign; nerve palsies variable; acral, distal, symmetric anesthesia common
Acid-fast bacilli (BI^a)	0–1+	3–5+	4–6+
Lymphocytes	2+	1+	0–1+
Macrophage differentiation	Epithelioid	Epithelioid in BB; usually undifferentiated, but may have foamy changes in BL	Foamy change the rule; may be undifferentiated in early lesions
Langhans' giant cells	1–3+	—	—
Lepromin skin test	+++	—	—
Lymphocyte transformation test	Generally positive	1–10%	1–2%
CD4+/CD8+ T-cell ratio in lesions	1.2	BB (NT); BL: 0.48	0.50
M. leprae PGL-1 antibodies	60%	85%	95%

^{a}See text.

Abbreviations: BB, mid-borderline; BL, borderline lepromatous; BT, borderline tuberculoid; TT, polar tuberculoid; LL, polar lepromatous; BI, bacteriologic index; NT, not tested; PGL-1, phenolic glycolipid 1.

cubation period. Most people appear to be naturally immune to leprosy and do not develop disease manifestations after exposure. The time of peak onset is in the second and third decades of life. The most severe lepromatous form of leprosy is twice as common among men as among women and is rarely encountered in children. The frequency of the polar forms of leprosy in different countries varies widely and may in part be genetically determined; certain HLA associations are known for both polar forms of leprosy (see below). In India and Africa, 90% of cases are tuberculoid; in Southeast Asia, 50% are tuberculoid and 50% lepromatous; and in Mexico, 90% are lepromatous. (For definitions of disease types, see Table 159-1 and "Clinical, Histologic, and Immunologic Spectrum," below.)

Transmission The route of transmission of leprosy remains uncertain, and transmission routes may in fact be multiple. Nasal droplet infection, contact with infected soil, and even insect vectors have been considered the prime candidates.

Aerosolized *M. leprae* can cause infection in immunosuppressed mice, and a sneeze from an untreated lepromatous patient may contain >10^{10} AFB. Furthermore, both IgA antibody to *M. leprae* and genes of *M. leprae*—demonstrable by polymerase chain reaction (PCR)—have been found in the nose of individuals without signs of leprosy from endemic areas and in 19% of occupational contacts of lepromatous patients.

Several lines of evidence implicate soil transmission. (1) In endemic countries such as India, leprosy is primarily a rural and not an urban disease. (2) *M. leprae* products reside in soil in endemic locales. (3) Direct dermal inoculation (e.g., during tattooing) may transmit *M. leprae*, and common sites of leprosy in children are the buttocks and thighs, suggesting that microinoculation of infected soil may transmit the disease.

Evidence for insect vectors of leprosy includes the demonstration that bedbugs and mosquitoes in the vicinity of leprosaria regularly harbor

M. leprae and that experimentally infected mosquitoes can transmit infection to mice. Skin-to-skin contact is generally not considered an important route of transmission.

In endemic countries, ~50% of leprosy patients have a history of intimate contact with an infected person (often a household member), while, for unknown reasons, leprosy patients in nonendemic locales can identify such contact only 10% of the time. Moreover, household contact with an infected lepromatous case carries an eventual risk of disease acquisition of ~10% in endemic areas as opposed to only 1% in nonendemic locales. Contact with a tuberculoid case carries a very low risk. Physicians and nurses caring for leprosy patients and the co-workers of these patients are not at risk for leprosy.

M. leprae causes disease primarily in humans. However, in Texas and Louisiana, 15% of nine-banded armadillos are infected, and armadillo contact occasionally results in human disease. Armadillos develop disseminated infection after IV inoculation of live *M. leprae*.

CLINICAL, HISTOLOGIC, AND IMMUNOLOGIC SPECTRUM

The incubation period prior to manifestation of clinical disease can vary between 2 and 40 years, although it is generally 5–7 years in duration. Leprosy presents as a spectrum of clinical manifestations that have bacteriologic, pathologic, and immunologic counterparts. The spectrum from polar tuberculoid (TT) to borderline tuberculoid (BT) to mid-borderline (BB, which is rarely encountered) to borderline lepromatous (BL) to polar lepromatous (LL) disease is associated with an evolution from asymmetric localized macules and plaques to nodular and indurated symmetric generalized skin manifestations, an increasing bacterial load, and loss of *M. leprae*–specific cellular immunity (Table 159-1). Distinguishing dermatopathologic characteristics include the number of lymphocytes, giant cells, and AFB as well as the nature of epithelioid cell differentiation. Where a patient presents on the clinical spectrum largely determines prognosis, complications, reactional states, and the intensity of antimicrobial therapy required.

Tuberculoid Leprosy At the less severe end of the spectrum is tuberculoid leprosy, which encompasses TT and BT disease. In general, these forms of leprosy result in symptoms confined to the skin and peripheral nerves. The skin lesions of tuberculoid leprosy consist of one or a few hypopigmented macules or plaques (Fig. 159-2) that are sharply demarcated and hypesthetic, often have erythematous or raised borders, and are devoid of the normal skin organs (sweat glands and hair follicles) and thus are dry, scaly, and anhidrotic. AFB are generally absent or few in number. Tuberculoid leprosy patients may have asymmetric enlargement of one or a few peripheral nerves. Indeed, leprosy and certain rare hereditary neuropathies are the only human diseases associated with peripheral-nerve enlargement. Although any peripheral nerve may be enlarged (including small digital and supraclavicular nerves), those most commonly affected are the ulnar, posterior auricular, peroneal, and posterior tibial nerves, with associated hypesthesia and myopathy. TT leprosy is the most common form of the disease encountered in India and Africa but is virtually absent in Southeast Asia, where BT leprosy is frequent.

In tuberculoid leprosy, T cells breach the perineurium, and destruction of Schwann cells and axons may be evident, resulting in fibrosis of the epineurium, replacement of the endoneurium with epithelial granulomas, and occasionally caseous necrosis. Such invasion and destruction of nerves in the dermis by T cells are pathognomonic for leprosy.

FIGURE 159-2 Tuberculoid (TT) leprosy: a well-defined, hypopigmented, anesthetic macule with anhidrosis and a raised granular margin *(arrowhead)*.

Circulating lymphocytes from patients with tuberculoid leprosy readily recognize *M. leprae* and its constituent proteins, patients have positive lepromin skin tests (see "Diagnosis," below), and—owing to a type 1 cytokine pattern in tuberculoid tissues—strong T cell and macrophage activation results in a localized infection. In tuberculoid leprosy tissue, there is a 2:1 predominance of helper CD4+ over CD8+ T lymphocytes. Tuberculoid tissues are rich in the mRNAs of the proinflammatory T_H1 family of cytokines: interleukin (IL) 2, interferon γ (IFN-γ), and IL-12; in contrast, IL-4, IL-5, and IL-10 mRNAs are scarce.

Lepromatous Leprosy Lepromatous leprosy patients present with symmetrically distributed skin nodules (Fig. 159-3), raised plaques, or diffuse dermal infiltration, which, when on the face, results in leonine facies. Late manifestations include loss of eyebrows (initially the lateral margins only) and eyelashes, pendulous earlobes, and dry scaling skin, particularly on the feet. In LL leprosy, bacilli are numerous in the skin (as many as 10^9/g), where they are often found in large clumps (*globi*), and in peripheral nerves, where they initially invade Schwann cells, resulting in foamy degenerative myelination and axonal degeneration and later in Wallerian degeneration. In addition, bacilli are plentiful in circulating blood and in all organ systems except the lungs and the central nervous system. Nevertheless, patients are afebrile, and there is no evidence of major organ system

FIGURE 159-3 Lepromatous (LL) leprosy: advanced nodular lesions.

dysfunction. Found almost exclusively in western Mexico and the Caribbean is a form of lepromatous leprosy without visible skin lesions but with diffuse dermal infiltration and a demonstrably thickened dermis, termed *diffuse lepromatosis*. In lepromatous leprosy, nerve enlargement and damage tend to be symmetric, result from actual bacillary invasion, and are more insidious but ultimately more extensive than in tuberculoid leprosy. Patients with LL leprosy have acral, distal, symmetric peripheral neuropathy and a tendency toward symmetric nerve-trunk enlargement. They may also have signs and symptoms related to involvement of the upper respiratory tract, the anterior chamber of the eye, and the testes.

In untreated LL patients, lymphocytes regularly fail to recognize either *M. leprae* or its protein constituents, and lepromin skin tests are negative (see "Diagnosis," below). This loss of protective cellular immunity appears to be antigen-specific, as patients are not unusually susceptible to opportunistic infections, cancer, or AIDS and maintain delayed-type hypersensitivity to *Candida*, *Trichophyton*, mumps, tetanus toxoid, and even purified protein derivative of tuberculin. At times, *M. leprae*–specific anergy is reversible with effective chemotherapy. In LL tissues, there is a 2:1 ratio of CD8+ to CD4+ T lymphocytes. LL patients have a predominant T_H2 response and hyperglobulinemia, and LL tissues demonstrate a T_H2 cytokine profile, being rich in mRNAs for IL-4, IL-5, and IL-10 and poor in those for IL-2, IFN-γ, and IL-12. It appears that cytokines mediate a protective tissue response in leprosy, as injection of IFN-γ or IL-2 into lepromatous lesions causes a loss of AFB and histopathologic conversion toward a tuberculoid pattern. Macrophages of lepromatous leprosy patients appear to be functionally intact; circulating monocytes exhibit normal microbicidal function and responsiveness to IFN-γ.

Reactional States Lepra reactions comprise several common immunologically mediated inflammatory states that cause considerable morbidity. Some of these reactions precede diagnosis and the institution of effective antimicrobial therapy; indeed, these reactions may precipitate presentation for medical attention and diagnosis. Other reactions occur after the initiation of appropriate chemotherapy and may cause patients to perceive that their leprosy is worsening and to lose confidence in conventional therapy. Only by warning patients of the potential for these reactions and describing their manifestations can physicians treating leprosy patients ensure continued credibility.

TYPE 1 LEPRA REACTIONS (DOWNGRADING AND REVERSAL REACTIONS) Type 1 lepra reactions occur in almost half of patients with borderline forms of leprosy but not in patients with pure lepromatous disease. Manifestations include classic signs of inflammation within previously involved macules, papules, and plaques and, on occasion, the appearance of new skin lesions, neuritis, and (less commonly) fever—generally low-grade. The nerve trunk most commonly involved in this process is the ulnar nerve at the elbow, which may be painful and exquisitely tender. If patients with affected nerves are not treated promptly with glucocorticoids (see below), irreversible nerve damage may result in as little as 24 h. The most dramatic manifestation is footdrop, which occurs when the peroneal nerve is involved.

When type 1 lepra reactions precede the initiation of appropriate antimicrobial therapy, they are termed *downgrading reactions*, and the case becomes histologically more lepromatous; when they occur after the initiation of therapy, they are termed *reversal reactions*, and the case becomes more tuberculoid. Reversal reactions often occur in the first months or years after the initiation of therapy but may also develop several years thereafter.

Edema is the most characteristic microscopic feature of type 1 lepra lesions, whose diagnosis is primarily clinical. Reversal reactions are typified by a T_H1 cytokine profile, with an influx of CD4+ helper cells and increased levels of IFN-γ and IL-2. In addition, type 1 reactions are associated with large numbers of T cells bearing γ/δ receptors—a unique feature of leprosy.

TYPE 2 LEPRA REACTIONS: ERYTHEMA NODOSUM LEPROSUM Erythema nodosum leprosum (ENL) (Fig. 159-4) occurs exclusively in patients near

FIGURE 159-4 Moderately severe skin lesions of erythema no-dosum leprosum (ENL), some with postulation and ulceration.

the lepromatous end of the leprosy spectrum (BL-LL), affecting nearly 50% of this group. Although ENL may precede leprosy diagnosis and initiation of therapy (sometimes, in fact, prompting the diagnosis), in 90% of cases it follows the institution of chemotherapy, generally within 2 years. The most common features of ENL are crops of painful erythematous papules that resolve spontaneously in a few days to a week but may recur; malaise; and fever that can be profound. However, patients may also experience symptoms of neuritis, lymphadenitis, uveitis, orchitis, and glomerulonephritis and may develop anemia, leukocytosis, and abnormal liver function tests (particularly increased aminotransferase levels). Individual patients may have either a single bout of ENL or chronic recurrent manifestations. Bouts may be either mild or severe and generalized; in rare instances, ENL results in death.

Skin biopsy of ENL papules reveals vasculitis or panniculitis, sometimes with many lymphocytes but characteristically with polymorphonuclear leukocytes as well.

Elevated levels of circulating tumor necrosis factor (TNF) have been demonstrated in ENL; thus, TNF may play a central role in the pathobiology of this syndrome. ENL is thought to be a consequence of immune complex deposition, given its T_H2 cytokine profile and its high levels of IL-6 and IL-8. However, in ENL tissue, the presence of HLA-DR framework antigen of epidermal cells—considered a marker for a delayed-type hypersensitivity response—and evidence of higher levels of IL-2 and IFN-γ than are usually seen in polar lepromatous disease suggest an alternative mechanism.

LUCIO'S PHENOMENON Lucio's phenomenon is an unusual reaction seen exclusively in patients from the Caribbean and Mexico who have the diffuse lepromatosis form of lepromatous leprosy, most often those who are untreated. Patients with this reaction develop recurrent crops of large, sharply marginated, ulcerative lesions—particularly on the lower extremities—that may be generalized and, when so, are frequently fatal as a result of secondary infection and consequent septic bacteremia. Histologically, the lesions are characterized by ischemic necrosis of the epidermis and superficial dermis, heavy parasitism of endothelial cells with AFB, and endothelial proliferation and thrombus formation in the larger vessels of the deeper dermis. Like ENL, the Lucio phenomenon is probably mediated by immune complexes.

Complications • *THE EXTREMITIES* Complications of the extremities in leprosy patients are primarily a consequence of neuropathy leading to insensitivity and myopathy. Insensitivity affects fine touch, pain, and heat receptors but generally spares position and vibration appreciation. The most commonly affected nerve trunk is the ulnar nerve at the elbow, whose involvement results in clawing of the fourth and fifth fingers, loss of dorsal interosseous musculature in the affected hand, and loss of sensation in these distributions. Median nerve involvement in leprosy impairs thumb opposition and grasp; radial

nerve dysfunction, although rare in leprosy, leads to wristdrop. Tendon transfers can restore hand function but should not be performed until 6 months after the initiation of antimicrobial therapy and the conclusion of episodes of acute neuritis.

Plantar ulceration, particularly at the metatarsal heads, is probably the most frequent complication of leprous neuropathy. Therapy requires careful debridement; administration of appropriate antibiotics; avoidance of weight-bearing until ulcerations are healed, with slowly progressive ambulation thereafter; and wearing of special shoes to prevent recurrence.

Footdrop as a result of peroneal nerve palsy should be treated with a simple nonmetallic brace within the shoe or with surgical correction attained by tendon transfers. Although uncommon, Charcot's joints, particularly of the foot and ankle, may result from leprosy.

The loss of distal digits in leprosy is a consequence of insensitivity, trauma, secondary infection, and—in lepromatous patients—a poorly understood and sometimes profound osteolytic process. Conscientious protection of the extremities during cooking and work and the early institution of therapy have substantially reduced the frequency and severity of distal digit loss in recent times.

THE NOSE In lepromatous leprosy, bacillary invasion of the nasal mucosa can result in chronic nasal congestion and epistaxis. Saline nose drops may relieve these symptoms. Long-untreated LL leprosy may further result in destruction of the nasal cartilage, with consequent saddle-nose deformity or anosmia (more common in the preantibiotic era than at present). Nasal reconstructive procedures can ameliorate significant cosmetic defects.

THE EYE Owing to cranial nerve palsies, lagophthalmos and corneal insensitivity may complicate leprosy, resulting in trauma, secondary infection, and (without treatment) corneal ulcerations and opacities. For patients with these conditions, eyedrops during the day and ointments at night provide some protection from such consequences. Furthermore, in LL leprosy, the anterior chamber of the eye is invaded by bacilli, and ENL may result in uveitis, with consequent cataracts and glaucoma. Thus leprosy is a major cause of blindness in the developing world. Slit-lamp evaluation of LL patients often reveals "corneal beading," representing globi of *M. leprae*.

THE TESTES *M. leprae* invades the testes, while ENL may cause orchitis. Thus males with lepromatous leprosy often manifest mild to severe testicular dysfunction, with an elevation of luteinizing and follicle-stimulating hormones, decreased testosterone, and aspermia or hypospermia in 85% of LL patients but in only 25% of BL patients. LL patients may become impotent and infertile. Impotence is sometimes responsive to testosterone replacement.

AMYLOIDOSIS Secondary amyloidosis is a complication of LL leprosy and ENL that is encountered infrequently in the antibiotic era. This complication may result in abnormalities of hepatic and particularly renal function.

NERVE ABSCESSES Patients with various forms of leprosy, but particularly those with the BT form, may develop abscesses of nerves (most commonly the ulnar) with an adjacent cellulitic appearance of the skin. In such conditions, the affected nerve is swollen and exquisitely tender. Although glucocorticoids may reduce signs of inflammation, rapid surgical decompression is necessary to prevent irreversible sequelae.

DIAGNOSIS

Leprosy most commonly presents with both characteristic skin lesions and skin histopathology. Thus the disease should be suspected when a patient from an endemic area has suggestive skin lesions or peripheral neuropathy. The diagnosis should be confirmed by histopathology. In tuberculoid leprosy, lesional areas—preferably the advancing edge—must be biopsied because normal-appearing skin does not have pathologic features. In lepromatous leprosy, nodules, plaques, and indurated areas are optimal biopsy sites, but biopsies of normal-appearing skin are also generally diagnostic. Lepromatous leprosy is associated with diffuse hyperglobulinemia, which may result in false-positive serologic tests (e.g., VDRL, RA, ANA) and therefore may cause diagnostic confusion. On occasion, tuberculoid lesions may not (1) appear typical, (2) be hypesthetic, and (3) contain granulomas but only nonspecific lymphocytic infiltrates. In such instances, two of these three characteristics are considered sufficient for a diagnosis. It is preferable to overdiagnose leprosy rather than to allow a patient to remain untreated.

IgM antibodies to PGL-1 are found in 95% of untreated lepromatous leprosy patients; the titer decreases with effective therapy. However, in tuberculoid leprosy—the form of disease most often associated with diagnostic uncertainty owing to the absence or paucity of AFB—patients have significant antibodies to PGL-1 only 60% of the time; moreover, in endemic locales, exposed individuals without clinical leprosy may harbor antibodies to PGL-1. Thus PGL-1 serology is of little diagnostic utility in tuberculoid leprosy. Heat-killed *M. leprae* (lepromin) has been used as a skin test reagent. It generally elicits a reaction in tuberculoid leprosy patients, may do so in individuals without leprosy, and gives negative results in lepromatous leprosy patients; consequently, it is likewise of little diagnostic value. Unfortunately, PCR of the skin for *M. leprae*, although positive in LL and BL leprosy, yields negative results in 50% of tuberculoid leprosy cases, again offering little diagnostic assistance.

Included in the differential diagnosis of lesions that resemble leprosy are sarcoidosis, leishmaniasis, lupus vulgaris, dermatofibroma, histiocytoma, lymphoma, syphilis, yaws, granuloma annulare, and various other disorders causing hypopigmentation (notably pityriasis alba, tinea, and vitiligo). Sarcoidosis may result in perineural inflammation, but actual granuloma formation within dermal nerves is pathognomonic for leprosy. In lepromatous leprosy, sputum specimens may be loaded with AFB—a finding that can be inappropriately interpreted as representing pulmonary tuberculosis.

℞ LEPROSY

ANTIMICROBIAL THERAPY   Active Agents   Established agents used to treat leprosy include dapsone (50–100 mg/d), clofazimine (50–100 mg/d, 100 mg three times weekly, or 300 mg monthly), and rifampin (600 mg daily or monthly). Of these drugs, only rifampin is bactericidal. The sulfones (folate antagonists), the foremost of which is dapsone, were the first antimicrobial agents found to be effective for the treatment of leprosy and are still the mainstay of therapy. With sulfone treatment, skin lesions resolve and numbers of viable bacilli in the skin are reduced. Although primarily bacteriostatic, dapsone monotherapy results in only a 2.5% resistance-related relapse rate; after ≥18 years of therapy and subsequent discontinuation, only another 10% of patients relapse, developing new, usually asymptomatic, shiny, "histoid" nodules. Dapsone is generally safe and inexpensive. Individuals with glucose-6-phosphate dehydrogenase deficiency who are treated with dapsone may develop severe hemolysis; those without this deficiency also have reduced red cell survival and a hemoglobin decrease averaging 1 g/dL. Dapsone's usefulness is limited occasionally by allergic dermatitis and rarely by the sulfone syndrome (including high fever, anemia, exfoliative dermatitis, and a mononucleosis-type blood picture). It must be remembered that rifampin induces microsomal enzymes, necessitating increased doses of medications such as glucocorticoids and oral birth control regimens. Clofazimine is often cosmetically unacceptable to light-skinned leprosy patients because it causes a red-black skin discoloration that accumulates, particularly in lesional areas, and makes the patient's diagnosis obvious to members of the community.

Other antimicrobial agents active against *M. leprae* in animal models and at the usual daily doses used in clinical trials include ethionamide/prothionamide; the aminoglycosides streptomycin, kanamycin, and amikacin (but not gentamicin or tobramycin); minocycline; clarithromycin; and several fluoroquinolones, particularly ofloxacin. Next to rifampin, minocycline, clarithromycin, and ofloxacin appear to be most bactericidal for *M. leprae*, but these drugs have not been used extensively in leprosy control programs. Most recently, rifapentine and moxifloxacin have been found to be especially potent against *M. leprae*. In preliminary clinical trials, moxifloxacin has been matched in potency only by rifampin.

Choice of Regimens   Antimicrobial therapy for leprosy must be individualized, depending on the clinical/pathologic form of the disease encountered. Tuberculoid leprosy, which is associated with a low bacterial burden and a protective cellular immune response, is the easiest form to treat and can be reliably cured with a finite course of chemotherapy. In contrast, lepromatous leprosy may have a higher bacillary load than any other human bacterial disease, and the absence of a salutary T cell repertoire requires prolonged or even lifelong chemotherapy. Hence, careful classification of disease prior to therapy is important.

In developed countries, clinical experience with leprosy classification is limited; fortunately, however, the resources needed for skin biopsy are highly accessible and pathologic interpretation is readily available. In developing countries, clinical expertise is greater but is now waning substantially as the care of leprosy patients is integrated into general health services. In addition, access to dermatopathology services is often limited. In such instances, skin smears may prove useful, but in many locales access to the resources needed for their preparation and interpretation may also be unavailable. Use of skin smears is no longer encouraged by the World Health Organization (WHO) and is often replaced by mere counting of lesions, which, together with the lack of histopathology, may negatively affect decisions about chemotherapy, increase the potential for reactions, and worsen the ultimate prognosis.

A reasoned approach to the treatment of leprosy is confounded by these and several other issues:

1. Even without therapy, TT leprosy may heal spontaneously, and prolonged dapsone monotherapy (even for LL leprosy) is generally curative in 80% of cases.
2. In tuberculoid disease, there are often no bacilli found in the skin prior to therapy, and thus there is no objective measure of therapeutic success. Furthermore, despite adequate treatment, TT and particularly BT lesions often resolve little or incompletely, while relapse and late type 1 lepra reactions can be difficult to distinguish.
3. LL leprosy patients commonly harbor viable persistent *M. leprae* organisms after prolonged intensive therapy; the propensity of these organisms to initiate clinical relapse is unclear. Because relapse in LL patients after discontinuation of rifampin-containing regimens usually begins only after 7–10 years, follow-up over the very long term is necessary to assess ultimate clinical outcomes.
4. Even though primary dapsone resistance is exceedingly rare and multidrug therapy is generally recommended (at least for lepromatous leprosy), there is a paucity of information from experimental animals and clinical trials on the optimal combination of antimicrobial agents, dosing schedule, or duration of therapy.

In 1982, the WHO made recommendations for "the chemotherapy of leprosy for control programs." These recommendations came on the heels of the demonstration of the relative success of long-term dapsone monotherapy and in the context of concerns about dapsone resistance. Other complicating considerations included the limited resources available for leprosy care in the very areas where it is most prevalent and the frustration and discouragement of patients and program managers with the previous requirement for lifelong therapy for many leprosy patients. The WHO delineated for the first time a finite duration of therapy for all forms of leprosy and—given the prohibitive cost of daily rifampin treatment in developing countries—encouraged the monthly administration of this agent as part of a multidrug regimen.

Over the ensuing years, these WHO recommendations have been broadly implemented, and the duration of therapy required, particularly for lepromatous leprosy, has been progressively shortened. For treatment purposes, the WHO classifies patients as *paucibacillary* or *multibacillary*. Previously, patients without demonstrable AFB in the dermis were classified as paucibacillary and those with AFB as multibacillary. Currently, owing to the perceived unreliability of skin smears in the field, patients are classified as multibacillary if they have six or more skin lesions and as paucibacillary if they have fewer. The WHO recommends that paucibacillary adults be treated with 100 mg of dapsone daily and 600 mg of rifampin monthly (supervised) for 6 months **(Table 159-2)**. For patients with single-lesion paucibacillary leprosy, the WHO recommends as an alternative a single dose of rifampin (600 mg), ofloxacin (400 mg), and minocycline (100 mg). Multibacillary adults should be treated with 100 mg of dapsone plus 50 mg of clofazimine daily (unsupervised) and with 600 mg of rifampin plus 300 mg of clofazimine monthly (supervised). Originally, the WHO recommended that lepromatous patients be treated for 2 years or until smears became nega-

TABLE 159-2 ANTIMICROBIAL REGIMENS RECOMMENDED FOR THE TREATMENT OF LEPROSY IN ADULTS

Form of Leprosy	More Intensive Regimen	WHO Recommended Regimen (1982)
Tuberculoid (paucibacillary)	Dapsone (100 mg/d) for 5 years	Dapsone (100 mg/d, unsupervised) plus rifampin (600 mg/month, supervised) for 6 months
Lepromatous (multibacillary)	Rifampin (600 mg/d) for 3 years plus dapsone (100 mg/d) indefinitely	Dapsone (100 mg/d) plus clofazimine (50 mg/d), unsupervised; and rifampin (600 mg) plus clofazimine (300 mg) monthly (supervised) for 1–2 years

Note: See text for discussion and comparison of WHO recommendations and more intensive approach as well as alternative WHO regimen for single-lesion paucibacillary leprosy.

tive (generally in ~5 years); subsequently, the acceptable course was reduced to 1 year—a change that remains especially controversial in the absence of supporting clinical trials.

Several factors have caused many authorities to question the WHO recommendations and to favor a more intensive approach. Among these factors are—for multibacillary patients—a high (double-digit) relapse rate in three locales (reaching 20–40% in one locale, with the rate directly related to the initial bacterial burden) and—for paucibacillary patients—demonstrable lesional activity for years in fully half of patients after the completion of therapy. The more intensive approach (Table 159-2) calls for tuberculoid leprosy to be treated with dapsone (100 mg/d) for 5 years and for lepromatous leprosy to be treated with rifampin (600 mg/d) for 3 years and with dapsone (100 mg/d) throughout life.

On effective antimicrobial therapy, new skin lesions and signs and symptoms of peripheral neuropathy cease appearing. Nodules and plaques of lepromatous leprosy noticeably flatten in 1–2 months and resolve in 1 year or a few years, while tuberculoid skin lesions may disappear, improve, or remain relatively unchanged. Although the peripheral neuropathy of leprosy may improve somewhat in the first few months of therapy, rarely is it significantly ameliorated by treatment.

THERAPY FOR REACTIONS   Type 1   Type 1 lepra reactions are best treated with glucocorticoids (e.g., prednisone, initially at doses of 40–60 mg/d). As the inflammation subsides, the glucocorticoid dose can be tapered, but steroid therapy must be continued for at least 3 months lest recurrence supervene. Because of the myriad toxicities of prolonged glucocorticoid therapy, the indications for its initiation are strictly limited to lesions whose intense inflammation poses a threat of ulceration; lesions at cosmetically important sites, such as the face; and cases in which neuritis is present. Mild to moderate lepra reactions that do not meet these criteria should be tolerated and glucocorticoid treatment withheld. Thalidomide is ineffective against type 1 lepra reactions. Clofazimine (200–300 mg/d) is of questionable benefit but in any event is far less efficacious than glucocorticoids.

Type 2   Treatment of ENL must be individualized. If ENL is mild (i.e., without fever or other organ involvement, with occasional crops of only a few skin papules), it may be treated with antipyretics alone. However, in cases with many skin lesions, fever, malaise, and other tissue involvement, brief courses (1–2 weeks) of glucocorticoids (initially 40–60 mg/d) are often effective. With or without therapy, individual inflamed papules last for >1 week. Successful therapy is defined by the cessation of skin lesion development and the disappearance of other systemic signs and symptoms. If, despite two courses of glucocorticoid therapy, ENL appears to be recurring and persisting, treatment with thalidomide (100–300 mg nightly) should be initiated, with the dose depending on the initial severity of the reaction. Because even a single dose of thalidomide administered early in pregnancy may result in severe birth defects, including phocomelia, the use of this drug in the United States for the treatment of fertile female patients is tightly regulated and requires informed consent, prior pregnancy testing, and maintenance of birth control measures. Although the mechanism of thalidomide's dramatic action against ENL is not entirely clear, the drug's efficacy is probably attributable to its reduction of TNF levels and IgM synthesis and its slowing of polymorphonuclear leukocyte migration. After the

reaction is controlled, lower doses of thalidomide (50–200 mg nightly) are effective in preventing relapses of ENL. Clofazimine in high doses (300 mg nightly) has some efficacy against ENL, but its use permits only a modest reduction of the glucocorticoid dose necessary for ENL control.

Lucio's Phenomenon   Neither glucocorticoids nor thalidomide is effective against this syndrome. Optimal wound care and therapy for bacteremia are indicated. Ulcers tend to be chronic and heal poorly. In severe cases, exchange transfusion may prove useful.

PREVENTION AND CONTROL

Vaccination at birth with bacille Calmette-Guérin (BCG) has proved variably effective in preventing leprosy: the results have ranged from total inefficacy to 80% efficacy. The addition of heat-killed *M. leprae* to BCG does not increase vaccine efficacy. Because whole mycobacteria contain large amounts of lipids and carbohydrates that have proven in vitro to be immunosuppressive for lymphocytes and macrophages, *M. leprae* proteins may prove to be superior vaccines. Data from a mouse model support this possibility.

Chemoprophylaxis with dapsone may reduce the number of cases of tuberculoid leprosy but not of lepromatous leprosy and hence is not recommended, even for household contacts. Because leprosy transmission appears to require close prolonged household contact, hospitalized patients need not be isolated.

In 1992, the WHO—on the basis of that organization's treatment recommendations—launched a landmark campaign to eliminate leprosy as a public health problem by the year 2000 (goal, <1 case per 10,000 population). The campaign mobilized and energized nongovernmental organizations and national health services to treat leprosy with multiple drugs and to clean up outdated registries. In these respects, the effort has proven hugely successful, with >6 million patients completing therapy. However, the target of leprosy elimination has not yet been reached. In fact, the success of the WHO campaign in reducing the number of cases worldwide has been largely attributable to the redefinition of what constitutes a case of leprosy. Formerly calculated by disease prevalence, the case count is now limited to those not yet treated with multiple drugs. In each of the 23 countries with the largest number of leprosy cases, the annual incidence of leprosy is stable or actually rising. Furthermore, after the completion of therapy, when a patient is no longer considered to represent a "case," half of all patients continue to manifest disease activity for years; relapse rates (at least for multibacillary patients) are unacceptably high; disabilities and deformities go unchecked; and the social stigma of the disease persists.

During most of the twentieth century, nongovernmental organizations, particularly Christian missionaries, provided a medical infrastructure devoted to the care and treatment of leprosy patients—the envy of those with other medical priorities in the developing world. With the public perception that leprosy is near eradication, resources for patient care are rapidly being diverted, and the burden of patient care is being transferred to nonexistent or overloaded national health services and to health workers who lack the tools and skills needed for disease diagnosis, classification, and nuanced therapy (particularly in cases of reactional neuritis). Thus the prerequisites for a salutary outcome increasingly go unmet.

FURTHER READINGS

COLE ST et al: Massive gene decay in the leprosy bacillus. Nature 409:1007, 2001

GELBER RH: The chemotherapy of leprosy: Lessons learned, some forgotten, current status and future prospects. Malaysian Journal of Dermatology 18:10, 2005

——— et al: The relapse rate in MB leprosy patients treated with 2-years of WHO-MDT is not low. Int J Lepr Other Mycobact Dis 72:493, 2004

LOCKWOOD D: Leprosy elimination—a virtual phenomenon or a reality? BMJ 324:1516, 2002

MODLIN RL, REA TH: Immunology of leprosy granulomas. Springer Semin Immunopathol 10:359, 1998

MONET M et al: On the origin of leprosy. Science 308:1040, 2005

RIDLEY DS: Histological classification and the immunological spectrum of leprosy. Bull World Health Organ 51:451, 1974

SHEPARD CC: The experimental disease that follows injection of human leprosy bacilli into foot pads of mice. J Exp Med 112:445, 1960

WARWICK JB, LOCKWOOD D: Leprosy. Lancet 363:1209, 2004

WHO EXPERT COMMITTEE ON LEPROSY: Seventh Report. WHO Tech Rep Ser No. 874. Geneva, World Health Organization, 1998

160 Nontuberculous Mycobacteria

C. Fordham von Reyn

The designation *nontuberculous mycobacteria* (NTM) encompasses the mycobacterial species other than organisms of the *Mycobacterium tuberculosis* complex and *M. leprae*. The NTM are distributed widely in the environment, are typically acquired from environmental sources, and therefore are also referred to as *environmental mycobacteria*. Most species are less virulent for humans than *M. tuberculosis*. Thus symptomatic infections are often associated with local or generalized defects in host defenses. Because isolation of NTM from a clinical specimen may represent true infection, colonization, or environmental contamination, strict criteria are required to assess the clinical significance of a positive culture. Although the >90 species of NTM have been associated with a wide variety of infections, most infections are due to a relatively limited number of species that cause characteristic patterns of disease (Table 160-1).

MICROBIOLOGY

Like *M. tuberculosis*, NTM organisms are acid-fast bacilli (AFB), resisting decolorization after staining. NTM have conventionally been characterized by the time required for clinical specimens to yield visible growth on solid media. Rapidly growing NTM species, such as *M. abscessus*, *M. fortuitum*, and *M. chelonae*, appear within 7 days. These organisms grow on standard microbiologic media and thus may be reported even when the clinician has not explicitly requested cultures for mycobacteria. Slow-growing species, in contrast, often take 2–3 weeks to grow on solid media and require special mycobacterial media such as Lowenstein-Jensen or Middlebrook. Accordingly, slow-growing NTM species are usually isolated only when the clinician specifically requests cultures for mycobacteria. Representative slow-growing species include *M. avium*, *M. kansasii*, *M. ulcerans*, and *M. marinum*. The automated broth culture systems now used in many laboratories may permit isolation of slow-growing NTM organisms within 10–14 days.

Further classification based on colony pigmentation (Runyon classification) has been replaced by the use of DNA probes for identification of common species such as *M. avium*, *M. intracellulare*, *M. gordonae* (which is rarely pathogenic), and *M. kansasii*. Less common species may be identified rapidly on the basis of fatty acid composition or DNA sequencing. Molecular strain typing ("fingerprinting") based on analysis of polymorphisms among large restriction fragments can be used to determine whether two or more isolates are genotypically and, by implication, epidemiologically related. This technique has been useful for identifying common-source outbreaks of infection or contamination.

Antibiotic susceptibility testing should be performed for rapidly growing NTM species. However, susceptibility testing of slow-growing species is of limited value: testing methods are not well standardized, and the relevance of the results to outcome is uncertain since patients are usually treated with multiple-drug regimens. As discussed later in this chapter, testing of *M. avium* or *M. kansasii* for susceptibility to specific drugs may be useful in certain situations.

DISTRIBUTION

NTM have a waxy, hydrophobic, triple-layered cell wall that renders them unusually resistant to varied physical conditions and chemical agents (including disinfectants such as chlorine at concentrations used in drinking water). These organisms can make use of a wide variety of carbon and nitrogen sources and can survive in nutrient-poor environments. Thus they are widely distributed in water, biofilms, and soil as well as in numerous animal species. Optimal growth temperatures vary and may influence distribution. For example, *M. avium* and *M. intracellulare* are often isolated from potable hot-water sources, whereas *M. marinum* is found in the cooler water of fish tanks. Most species of NTM are obligate aerobes and grow best at acid pH. Soil and natural water samples from most regions of the world contain numerous species of NTM, which are as common in northern regions (e.g., Finland) as they are in more temperate areas (e.g., the southern United States).

EPIDEMIOLOGY

Asymptomatic infections with NTM are common in humans and are probably acquired most often from childhood contact with soil, water, and possibly animals. Studies with skin-test agents derived from NTM indicate that 30–40% of adults in the northern and southern United States have had prior unrecognized or asymptomatic infection with NTM—most often with organisms of the *M. avium* complex (MAC). Since latent infection is not a recognized characteristic of NTM, most symptomatic infections are thought to represent recent exposure. Molecular methods have identified clusters of infections and pseudoinfections associated with potable water as well as nosocomial infections

TABLE 160-1 MAIN SPECIES OF NONTUBERCULOUS MYCOBACTERIA (NTM) AND PATTERNS OF DISEASE

Species	Growth on Solid Media	Environmental Reservoir	Patterns of Disease[a]			
			Cutaneous	Pulmonary	Disseminated	Other
M. avium	Slow	Hot water systems, natural water, soil	−	++	+++	Lymphadenitis
M. intracellulare	Slow	Hot water systems, natural water, soil	−	+++	+	Lymphadenitis
M. kansasii	Slow	Potable and natural water	−	+++	++	−
M. abscessus, M. chelonae, M. fortuitum	Rapid	Potable and natural water, soil	++	+	−	Sporotrichoid spread
M. marinum	Slow	Fish tanks, salt water	++	−	−	Sporotrichoid spread
M. ulcerans	Slow	Natural water	++	−	−	"Buruli ulcer," osteomyelitis

[a]Symbols indicate relative prevalence among NTM infections of the indicated species and pattern of disease: +++, most common; ++, common; +, reported but uncommon; −, rare or not reported.

related to clinical procedures such as endoscopy and surgery. Environmental exposures are assumed to cause most symptomatic infections; however, this point has been difficult to document by molecular methods, presumably because there are many potential exposures (some of which are sporadic) and because a specific NTM species may be present only transiently or in low numbers in any given source.

PATHOGENESIS

NTM may be acquired through cutaneous, respiratory, gastrointestinal, or (rarely) parenteral exposure. Organisms are ingested by host macrophages and may survive within these cells to replicate and cause symptomatic infection. Disease manifestations in immunocompetent hosts are due to host cellular immune responses and the formation of granulomas. Intracellular killing of mycobacteria, with ultimate control of infection, requires the action of cellular immune mechanisms including proliferation of CD4+ T lymphocytes and elaboration of interferon γ (IFN-γ) and interleukin 12. Deficiencies in CD4+ T cell function due to HIV infection, anti–tumor necrosis factor (TNF) therapy, and inherited deficiencies in the production of or response to IFN-γ are associated with disseminated NTM infection (Chap. 182).

The cellular immune response to NTM may be evident in tuberculin skin testing or newer interferon-γ release assays (IGRAs). Tuberculin skin testing with *M. tuberculosis* purified protein derivative may elicit small reactions with some NTM and larger reactions (comparable to those in tuberculosis) among immunocompetent individuals infected with *M. marinum* or *M. kansasii*. IGRAs that employ *M. tuberculosis*–specific antigens (ESAT-6, CFP-10) are negative in most NTM infections but may be positive with *M. marinum* or *M. kansasii*.

There is no convincing evidence that NTM can establish latent infection with subsequent clinical reactivation—a pattern characteristic of *M. tuberculosis*. Asymptomatic infection with NTM in a healthy host may induce beneficial immunity; persons with skin-test reactivity to NTM antigens (e.g., *M. intracellulare*) are at decreased risk for the subsequent development of tuberculosis. Likewise, immunization with bacille Calmette-Guérin (BCG) from *M. bovis* provides protection against childhood cervical adenitis due to NTM.

CLINICAL SYNDROMES

Cutaneous Disease   NTM can cause a variety of cutaneous disease syndromes when inoculated directly from an environmental source into an area of open or diseased skin or into a surgical wound. These organisms are also associated with localized or disseminated cutaneous disease in immunosuppressed patients. *M. abscessus*, *M. fortuitum*, *M. chelonae*, *M. marinum*, and *M. ulcerans* are the most commonly involved species. Cutaneous disease may be nodular or ulcerating, sometimes with reddish-blue discoloration and typically with minimal drainage. Lesions may be single, or the infection may spread proximally up the lymphatics, producing additional nodules (sporotrichoid spread). In compromised hosts, disseminated lesions may appear as a result of bacteremic spread. Clinical suspicion of NTM infection is based on chronicity, the absence of bacterial growth on routine culture, and the failure to respond to standard antibacterial therapy. Biopsies often reveal granuloma formation, and acid-fast stains may be positive.

Pulmonary Disease   NTM species cause chronic progressive pulmonary infection both in normal hosts and in those with underlying pulmonary disease or immunosuppression. The clinical features may resemble slowly progressive pulmonary tuberculosis, which is often the initial diagnosis in patients with positive AFB smears. Among patients born in the United States, pulmonary disease due to AFB is more likely to be due to NTM than to *M. tuberculosis*.

The diagnosis of pulmonary infection with NTM is complicated by the variability in clinical and radiologic manifestations, the frequent presence of significant prior pulmonary disease, and the fact that isolation of NTM from the sputum may represent harmless colonization of the lower respiratory tract. The diagnosis should be based on specific, validated criteria that emphasize a compatible clinical syndrome, char-

TABLE 160-2	ATS/IDSA CRITERIA FOR THE DIAGNOSIS OF PULMONARY DISEASE DUE TO NONTUBERCULOUS MYCOBACTERIA[a]
Category	**Requirement**
Clinical	Pulmonary symptoms (e.g., chronic cough) and appropriate exclusion of other diagnoses
Radiologic	Chest x-ray: nodular or cavitary opacities *or* High-resolution CT: multifocal bronchiectasis with multiple small nodules
Bacteriologic	Sputum: ≥2 positive cultures *or* Bronchial wash or lavage: ≥1 positive culture *or* Lung biopsy: granulomatous inflammation or positive stain for acid-fast bacilli plus ≥1 positive culture (of biopsy, sputum, or bronchial wash sample)

[a]Diagnosis requires the fulfillment of clinical criteria plus one radiologic criterion and one bacteriologic criterion. ATS, American Thoracic Society; IDSA, Infectious Diseases Society of America.
Source: Griffith et al, 2007.

acteristic findings on chest x-ray or CT, and repeated isolation of NTM from the sputum or growth of NTM from a lung biopsy (Table 160-2).

In immunocompetent hosts, infection may result in the onset of chronic cough, dyspnea, and fatigue; fever is unusual. Pathologic and radiologic manifestations of pulmonary infection due to NTM include the formation of solitary or multiple nodules, chronic pneumonitis, bronchiectasis, cavity formation, or a combination of these features. In some patients with NTM pulmonary disease, CT shows a characteristic pattern of small cylindrical bronchiectasis and multiple small (<5-mm) nodules and fibrosis. Compared with patients who have tuberculosis, those who have lung disease caused by NTM are more likely to have bilateral and midzone infiltrates and less likely to have pleural effusions. Patients with characteristic radiologic findings and negative results of routine sputum cultures for mycobacteria should have bronchoscopy and transbronchial biopsy performed in an attempt to identify granulomas and AFB. In patients with chronic pulmonary disease, the superimposition of infection with NTM may not be associated with easily recognizable changes in symptoms or radiologic features.

Together, MAC organisms (especially *M. intracellulare*) are the most common cause of pulmonary disease due to NTM in developed countries; next in frequency are *M. kansasii* (United States, Europe, South Africa), *M. abscessus* (United States), *M. xenopi* (Europe, Canada), and *M. malmoense* (United Kingdom, northern Europe). However, isolation of NTM from the sputum must be considered in the context of clinical manifestations. For example, NTM (most prominently, MAC organisms; less commonly, *M. abscessus*) can be cultured from 13% of cystic fibrosis patients in the United States (Chap. 253); however, not all of these patients appear to have invasive NTM disease. Although invasive disease should be strongly suspected when the same NTM species is isolated on multiple occasions from a patient with lung disease, even persistent organisms may represent colonization or slowly progressive disease apparent only on long-term follow-up. Additional laboratory tests (e.g., immunologic assessments) are of no value in the diagnosis.

Although treatment should be considered in patients who meet the clinical, radiologic, and microbiologic criteria for NTM disease (Table 160-2), several other factors require consideration. For example, whereas species such as *M. kansasii* are usually pathogenic and a single isolate may be significant, species such as *M. gordonae* are rarely pathogenic, even when isolated repeatedly. In addition, in some patients with true invasive disease, infection may progress so slowly that it is unlikely to have much impact on longevity determined by age or comorbid illness. Since therapy for NTM requires prolonged administration of multiple drugs and is associated with significant side effects, the decision to institute treatment in patients with noncavitary disease who do not have clearly progressive pulmonary disease should be made with careful deliberation after a period of clinical and radiologic follow-up.

Disseminated Disease   Patients with impaired cellular immunity—most notably, patients with advanced HIV disease (Chap. 182), immunosuppressed recipients of solid-organ or hematopoietic stem-cell transplants (Chap. 126), and patients receiving anti-TNF therapy—are susceptible to disseminated disease due to NTM. Other predisposing conditions include treatment with glucocorticoids, lymphoma and leukemia (especially hairy cell leukemia), and heritable disorders of IFN-γ production and function. *M. avium* and *M. kansasii* are the species most commonly isolated in disseminated disease, but numerous other organisms (e.g., *M. genavense*, *M. haemophilum*) have also been recovered.

Patients with disseminated infection present with fever, weight loss, and fatigue and sometimes with hepatosplenomegaly or lymphadenopathy. Chest radiographs are typically normal in infection with *M. avium* (although they may show a miliary pattern) but are usually abnormal with *M. kansasii*. Laboratory studies may demonstrate anemia and an elevated level of alkaline phosphatase in serum. Disseminated disease is characterized by the widespread presence of foamy macrophages with AFB, which may be demonstrated in biopsy samples of bone marrow, intestine, or liver. Granulomas are typically absent in patients with impaired cellular immunity. In most cases, the diagnosis can be established by one or two sets of mycobacterial blood cultures, which will be positive for the etiologic mycobacteria in 2–3 weeks. Treatment requires long-term administration of a multiple-drug antimycobacterial regimen and attempts to ameliorate the defect in cellular immunity [e.g., institution of antiretroviral therapy (ART) and discontinuation of glucocorticoid administration].

Other Disease NTM have been associated with disease at numerous other anatomic locations, including ocular infections, mastoiditis, sinusitis, mastitis, catheter site infections, endocarditis, meningitis, peritonitis, appendicitis, pericarditis, pyelonephritis, prostatitis, tenosynovitis, bursitis, septic arthritis, osteomyelitis, and lymphadenitis (especially in children). Accumulating data support an association between infection with *M. avium* subspecies *paratuberculosis* and Crohn's disease.

ORGANISMS

M. AVIUM COMPLEX

Pulmonary Disease MAC organisms (*M. avium*, *M. intracellulare*, and genetically related unnamed species) are more common than *M. tuberculosis* as a cause of mycobacterial pulmonary disease among persons born in the United States. Epidemiologic data support a marked increase in the incidence of MAC infection over the past two to three decades. Two patterns of MAC disease are recognized: one form is typically the primary basis for a diagnosis of pulmonary disease and is often nodular/bronchiectatic, whereas the other form develops as a secondary complication of underlying pulmonary disease and is sometimes fibrocavitary (Table 160-3). The description of subtle defects in cellular immune responses and body morphotype in patients with primary disease raises the possibility of an as-yet-undefined immune defect predisposing to MAC infection. Patients with secondary disease include those with chronic obstructive pulmonary disease, prior tuberculosis, cystic fibrosis, or pulmonary alveolar proteinosis. The sources of infection have not been identified.

CLINICAL FEATURES AND DIAGNOSIS Symptoms and diagnostic studies are described above (see "Clinical Syndromes"). CT identifies characteristic cylindrical bronchiectasis with nodule formation, documents the extent of disease, and establishes a baseline for possible treatment. Standard diagnostic criteria should be applied (Table 160-2). Isolates from patients with prolonged prior macrolide exposure or prior treatment failure should be tested for susceptibility to clarithromycin.

TABLE 160-3	TYPICAL FEATURES OF PRIMARY AND SECONDARY PULMONARY DISEASE DUE TO THE *M. AVIUM* COMPLEX	
Feature	**Primary**	**Secondary**
Age	>50 years	30–70 (mean, 60) years
Sex	F > M	M > F
Underlying disease	None definitively identified; subtle defect in cellular immunity postulated	Chronic obstructive pulmonary disease, cystic fibrosis, prior tuberculosis, alveolar proteinosis
Radiologic features	Typically nodular (<5 mm)/ bronchiectatic (cylindrical) with midzone involvement	Sometimes fibrocavitary; infiltrates or nodules in some cases

℞ MAC PULMONARY DISEASE

Treatment should be initiated in most patients with secondary MAC pulmonary disease. For patients with primary MAC pulmonary disease, decisions about treatment must be made on an individual basis. A period of observation before consideration of treatment may be useful when there is no evidence of a progressive pulmonary process and when the patient's age or underlying disease is likely to be the critical determinant of survival over the next few years.

Recommended treatment for MAC pulmonary disease includes two drugs: daily clarithromycin (or thrice-weekly azithromycin) and ethambutol. Some authorities recommend a three-drug regimen including these two agents plus rifampin, although there are no comparative data for two- versus three-drug regimens and concomitant administration of rifampin lowers serum levels of clarithromycin (Table 160-4). For seriously ill patients with advanced disease, a four-drug regimen including the three drugs listed above as well as streptomycin or amikacin for the first 2 months should be considered. In many cases, treatment may serve only to halt the progression of radiologic findings; in some cases, symptoms and radiologic findings improve. The response to treatment is best in patients whose isolates have the lowest minimum inhibitory concentrations of clarithromycin. As many as 30% of patients treated with standard drugs at standard doses cannot tolerate therapy, generally because of gastrointestinal side effects. Rifabutin appears to have the highest rate of side effects. Stepwise introduction of drugs at 1-week intervals, starting with half the usual dose, may improve tolerance. In many cases, final doses need to be reduced or drugs eliminated or replaced with alternatives. Gatifloxacin and

TABLE 160-4	REGIMENS FOR PREVENTION AND TREATMENT OF DISEASE DUE TO THE *M. AVIUM* COMPLEX	
Category	**Regimen**	**Indication and Duration**
Pulmonary Disease		
Treatment	Clarithromycin (250–500 mg bid[a]) or azithromycin (250 mg/d[b]) **plus** Ethambutol (15 mg/kg qd)[c]	Treat when patient meets ATS/IDSA criteria (Table 160-2) and has secondary MAC disease or has primary MAC disease plus indication for treatment (see text). Treat for 18 months or until 12 months after conversion of sputum culture.
Disseminated Disease		
Treatment	Clarithromycin (500 mg PO bid) or azithromycin (500 mg daily[b]) **plus** Ethambutol (15 mg/kg qd[d])	Treat when MAC blood culture is positive or MAC is isolated from ordinarily sterile site. Continue with secondary prevention.
Prevention	Azithromycin (1200 mg PO weekly[b]) or clarithromycin (500 mg PO bid)	Treat when CD4+ T cell count is <50/μL. Discontinue if CD4+ T cell count exceeds 100/μL for >3 months during antiretroviral therapy.

[a]Give 250 mg of clarithromycin bid if the patient weighs <50 kg.
[b]Azithromycin is preferred to clarithromycin in pregnancy.
[c]An intermittent three-drug regimen with concomitant rifampin, rather than a daily two-drug regimen, is recommended in the current ATS/IDSA guidelines (Griffith et al, 2007) but not by this author; a four-drug regimen including streptomycin may be indicated in severe cases.
[d]Concomitant rifabutin (150–300 mg/d) may protect against the development of clarithromycin resistance and be associated with a modest clinical benefit but can cause interactions with antiretroviral therapy.

CHAPTER 160

Nontuberculous Mycobacteria

moxifloxacin exhibit in vitro activity against many strains but have not been studied for the treatment of pulmonary disease due to MAC.

For patients with positive sputum cultures who receive a macrolide-containing regimen, treatment should be continued for at least 12 months after cultures revert to negative; the typical duration is 18 months. The duration of therapy with other regimens may need to be extended to 24 months. Approximately 20% of patients experience treatment failure or relapse; some apparent treatment failures may actually represent reinfection. Surgical resection is an option for patients with localized disease who are intolerant of or unresponsive to multiple-drug therapy; however, this approach is associated with postoperative complications in as many as 20% of patients and should be undertaken only by surgeons who have considerable experience with this intervention.

Hot-Tub Lung Hot-tub lung is a form of hypersensitivity pneumonitis due to NTM, most commonly MAC organisms. Affected individuals present with cough, fever, and dyspnea after repeated exposure to indoor hot tubs contaminated with MAC. Some patients are hypoxemic. The chest x-ray shows diffuse nodular infiltrates, and high-resolution CT may also demonstrate ground-glass infiltrates. MAC organisms can be isolated from expectorated sputum or lung tissue, and biopsy specimens display centrilobular and bronchocentric granuloma formation. Resolution typically follows avoidance of exposure and/or treatment with glucocorticoids. Most patients do not appear to require specific antimicrobial therapy.

Disseminated Disease Disseminated MAC disease occurs principally among patients with immunosuppression (including those with advanced HIV disease) who live in developed countries but are not receiving ART. Almost all cases occur at CD4+ T cell counts of <100/μL, and the risk is ~20% per year for untreated patients with CD4+ T cell counts of <50/μL. The risk of disease is essentially eliminated for recipients of ART who have an increase in CD4+ T cell count to >100/μL that is maintained for 3 months. Most cases are due to *M. avium*, and molecular studies indicate that as many as 25% of disseminated infections involve more than one strain. Strains causing bacteremia differ genetically from those typically isolated from respiratory sources or the environment. Molecular techniques have documented nosocomial acquisition from potable hot water and have demonstrated common genotypes among isolates from humans and those from peat used in potting soil. Epidemiologic studies have demonstrated an increased risk associated with consumption of untreated spring water and of raw or partially cooked fish or shellfish and a decreased risk associated with showering. Overall, sources of acquisition appear to be diverse and exposure is probably unavoidable; at this time, no specific behavioral changes can be recommended for at-risk patients.

CLINICAL FEATURES AND DIAGNOSIS Disseminated MAC infection in AIDS is associated with fever, weakness, and weight loss and usually presents as a wasting syndrome in patients who are not receiving ART or chemoprophylaxis for *M. avium* (Chap. 182). Untreated disease shortens the survival period of patients with advanced AIDS by 4–5 months. Laboratory findings may include anemia, hypoalbuminemia, and elevated serum levels of alkaline phosphatase and lactate dehydrogenase. HIV-infected patients with prior disseminated MAC infection or unrecognized or subclinical MAC infection may experience an immune reconstitution syndrome when they start to receive ART (Chap. 182). This syndrome presents 1–12 weeks after the institution of ART and often manifests as localized (or generalized) culture-positive lymphadenitis with blood cultures negative for *M. avium*.

℞ DISSEMINATED MAC DISEASE

Disseminated MAC disease requires treatment with the combination of clarithromycin and ethambutol, with or without rifabutin (Table 160-4), along with ART for HIV. Antimycobacterial treatment should be continued for at least 12 months and until the CD4+ T cell count has been >100/μL for

at least 6 months. The immune reconstitution syndrome should be treated with initiation or continuation of the same antimycobacterial regimen.

PREVENTION Chemoprophylaxis is highly effective for the prevention of disseminated MAC infection in AIDS (Table 160-4). Weekly azithromycin administration should be instituted when the CD4+ T cell count is <50/μL or when a patient with HIV infection has had an AIDS-defining opportunistic infection (e.g., *Pneumocystis* infection). Chemoprophylaxis may be discontinued when the CD4+ T cell count has been >100/μL for >3 months.

M. KANSASII

Pulmonary Disease Pulmonary disease due to *M. kansasii* has been reported from many areas of the world, including North America, Europe, and South Africa. In the United States, *M. kansasii* is the second most common cause of lung disease due to NTM and is distributed largely in central and southern states and California. The average age of onset is 60 years, and most patients have predisposing factors, such as chronic obstructive pulmonary disease, carcinoma of the lung, silicosis, or prior tuberculosis. However, pulmonary infection sometimes occurs in persons without predisposing disease and has also been associated with poverty. Disease may sometimes wax and wane over many years; this pattern is assumed to represent chronic infection rather than reactivation. Localized pulmonary infection has been described in South African miners with early HIV infection and preserved CD4+ T cell counts. The source of infection has not been identified, although *M. kansasii* has been isolated from both potable and natural water sources.

CLINICAL FEATURES AND DIAGNOSIS *M. kansasii* is the most pathogenic nontuberculous mycobacterial species affecting the lung, and the clinical features of *M. kansasii* disease resemble those of tuberculosis. Most cases include cough and sputum production; 30% include frank hemoptysis. Systemic signs and symptoms, including fever, night sweats, and weight loss, are reported by as many as 50% of patients. However, symptoms may be subtle or absent in patients with underlying malignancy. Chest radiographs show cavitation in 50% of patients, pleural scarring in 40%, and infiltrates in 30%; abnormalities are most prominent in the apices. Clinical and radiographic effects progress in the absence of treatment.

Sputum samples should be obtained for AFB staining and mycobacterial culture. The isolation of *M. kansasii* sometimes represents colonization; the diagnostic criteria in Table 160-2 are useful when multiple sputum samples can be obtained. However, the growth of *M. kansasii* from even a single sputum culture should be considered to have potential clinical significance, especially in HIV-positive patients. Testing of *M. kansasii* isolates for susceptibility to rifampin is recommended.

℞ M. KANSASII PULMONARY DISEASE

For rifampin-susceptible strains of *M. kansasii*, the recommended regimen is daily rifampin (600 mg), isoniazid (300 mg), and ethambutol (15 mg/kg). Sputum cultures almost always become negative by 4 months; patients should be treated for at least 12 months after the last positive culture. Resistance to rifampin may develop, in which case clarithromycin or azithromycin may be substituted.

Disseminated Disease Disseminated *M. kansasii* disease occurs principally among patients with advanced AIDS and CD4+ T cell counts of <100/μL. It has also been reported in patients with leukemia, lymphoma, or solid-organ transplantation.

CLINICAL FEATURES AND DIAGNOSIS Symptoms are similar to those reported for disseminated MAC infection, although in disseminated *M. kansasii* infection cough is more common and chest radiographs more often demonstrate alveolar or interstitial infiltrates or cavities. An immune reconstitution syndrome may follow the institution of ART in HIV-infected patients, manifesting as cervical or mediastinal lymphadenitis (Chap. 182).

The diagnosis is established by the isolation of *M. kansasii* from a normally sterile parenchymal site or from blood. In one series of cases, concurrent disseminated infection with a second NTM species (most often *M. avium*) was found in one-third of patients. The isolation of *M. kansasii* from sputum from a patient with advanced HIV disease suggests disseminated infection and is an indication for mycobacterial blood culture.

℞ *M. KANSASII* DISSEMINATED DISEASE

Treatment of disseminated *M. kansasii* disease is the same as that for pulmonary disease due to this organism. Patients with AIDS should receive an ART regimen that is compatible with a rifamycin (rifampin or rifabutin). Untreated disease is associated with shortened survival, and the response to treatment is good in patients who do not have rapidly progressive HIV infection. HIV-positive patients who experience clearing of systemic symptoms and have positive cultures with sustained recovery of the CD4+ T cell count can probably have treatment discontinued (as described above for *M. avium* infection). There is no recommended prophylactic regimen, although the azithromycin regimen given to prevent disseminated *M. avium* infection may also be effective in preventing disseminated *M. kansasii* infection.

M. ABSCESSUS, *M. CHELONAE*, AND *M. FORTUITUM*

Three rapidly growing NTM species are prominent in reports of human infection and colonization: *M. abscessus*, *M. chelonae*, and *M. fortuitum*. These organisms are acquired from water, soil, or nosocomial sources. The most common clinical manifestation of infection is disseminated cutaneous disease in patients who have defects in cellular immunity or are receiving glucocorticoid therapy. Immunocompetent hosts can develop localized cutaneous infection in surgical or traumatic wounds, from contaminated injections, or after body piercing. Cutaneous lesions are cellulitic or nodular; are typically erythematous, indurated, and tender; and may progress to ulceration and purulent drainage. Proximal sporotrichoid spread has also been reported. Pulmonary infection (usually due to *M. abscessus*) is the next most common manifestation and occurs principally in patients with underlying lung disease, such as cystic fibrosis.

The rapidly growing NTM species may be isolated from clinical specimens submitted for routine microbiologic testing. However, reliable evaluation requires inoculation onto special mycobacterial media and an extended incubation period. Because rapidly growing NTM species are also common laboratory contaminants, numerous false alarms in the form of pseudoepidemics have been reported.

℞ *M. ABSCESSUS*, *M. CHELONAE*, AND *M. FORTUITUM* INFECTIONS

Treatment varies with the patient group and with the species of rapidly growing NTM. Susceptibility tests should be performed and used to guide antibiotic selection. All three species are usually susceptible to clarithromycin and amikacin; *M. abscessus* and *M. fortuitum* are also susceptible to cefoxitin and imipenem. Other agents that may be active include doxycycline and fluoroquinolones. Patients with localized cutaneous disease may respond to a single active agent (e.g., clarithromycin at a dosage of 500 mg twice daily by mouth for ≥2 weeks). Up to 6 months of therapy may be optimal for bacteremic or disseminated cutaneous disease, and a second agent should be added on the basis of susceptibility tests. Pulmonary disease due to *M. fortuitum* or *M. chelonae* should be treated with two active agents (usually including clarithromycin) until sputum cultures have been negative for 12 months. Pulmonary disease due to *M. abscessus* is especially difficult to treat since prolonged therapy is necessary and the most active drugs require parenteral administration and carry a significant risk of toxicity with prolonged use. The most potent regimen is typically IV amikacin (10–15 mg/kg daily) and IV cefoxitin (3 g every 6 h) or imipenem (500 mg every 6–12 h) with oral clarithromycin (500 mg twice daily). Expert consultation should be sought for management of this chronic, often incurable pulmonary infection.

M. MARINUM

M. marinum is widely distributed in water and causes chronic cutaneous infection when an open cutaneous lesion is exposed to a colonized water source. Most infections are due to hand or upper-extremity exposure to fish tanks, and some are due to shellfish or marine exposures. Swimming pools are no longer a common source of infection because of current chlorination standards. *M. marinum* grows optimally at 30°C—a lower temperature than is optimal for most pathogenic mycobacteria. After a median incubation period of 21 days (≥30 days in 35% of cases), a granulomatous or ulcerating skin lesion develops at the site of entry, with subsequent sporotrichoid spread in many cases. In some patients, especially those with serious underlying disease and those receiving immunosuppressive therapy, infection may extend to deeper structures, producing tenosynovitis or osteomyelitis. The diagnosis is established by mycobacterial culture of a biopsied lesion or by demonstration of granulomas or AFB in a biopsy sample from a patient with a compatible exposure history.

℞ *M. MARINUM* INFECTIONS

Treatment consists of the combination of clarithromycin and ethambutol; the regimen is given for 1–2 months after resolution of lesions—typically 3–4 months in total. Surgical debridement may be necessary in extensive or deep disease; however, routine incision and drainage are not helpful. Rifampin should be added in cases of osteomyelitis. Persons with occupational or avocational exposure to fish tanks or salt water should wear waterproof gloves to prevent infection of open cutaneous lesions.

M. ULCERANS

M. ulcerans causes cutaneous infection (Buruli ulcer) in endemic regions of Central and West Africa, Central and South America, Malaysia, Indonesia, Papua New Guinea, and Australia. The organism is closely related to *M. marinum*, has a similar temperature for optimal growth, and has been isolated from natural bodies of water. Most cases of human infection occur on the bare arms or legs of children or young adults living near rivers, lakes, or swamps. Transmission is thought to result from minor trauma or the bite of an aquatic insect. The initial lesion is a small painless nodule that progresses to a deep ulcer. The ulcer expands, resulting in sloughing of skin and subcutaneous tissue; osteomyelitis may also occur. Stellate scarring and deforming contractures may result from extensive necrosis.

Biopsy analyses demonstrate extracellular AFB in early lesions, with a limited inflammatory reaction. Tissue destruction extends beyond the area of demonstrable bacterial infection and has been attributed to a unique mycobacterial toxin, mycolactone.

℞ *M. ULCERANS* INFECTIONS

Antimicrobial therapy has not yet been shown to be beneficial, although rifampin, dapsone, clarithromycin, streptomycin, and amikacin display in vitro activity against *M. ulcerans*. Surgical treatment is of primary importance, and skin grafting may be required. Immunization with BCG reduces the risk of disease by ~50%.

OTHER NTM SPECIES

Numerous other NTM species have been associated with human disease, although they may represent contaminants in clinical specimens. Species and sites of possible infection include *M. celatum* (lung, lymph nodes), *M. genavense* (disseminated), *M. gordonae* (skin, contaminant), *M. haemophilum* (skin, disseminated), *M. malmoense* (lung), *M. simiae* (lung, disseminated), *M. scrofulaceum* (lymphadenitis), *M. szulgai* (skin, lung), and *M. xenopi* (lung, disseminated).

FURTHER READINGS

DOUCETTE K, FISHMAN JA: Nontuberculous mycobacterial infection in hematopoietic stem cell and solid organ transplant recipients. Clin Infect Dis 38:1428, 2004

GRIFFITH DE et al: An official ATS/IDSA statement: Diagnosis, treatment and prevention of nontuberculous mycobacterial diseases. Am J Respir Crit Care Med 175:367, 2007

HANAK V et al: Hot tub lung: Presenting features and clinical course of 21 patients. Respir Med 100:610, 2006

KOBASHI Y et al: Relationship between clinical efficacy of treatment of pulmonary *Mycobacterium avium* complex disease and drug-sensitivity testing of *M. avium* complex isolates. J Infect Chemother 12:195, 2006

PHILLIPS M, VON REYN CF: Nosocomial infections due to nontuberculous mycobacteria. Clin Infect Dis 33:1363, 2001

REED C et al: Environmental risk factors for infection with *Mycobacterium avium* complex. Am J Epidemiol 164:32, 2006

VON REYN CF et al: Skin test reactions to *Mycobacterium tuberculosis* purified protein derivative and *Mycobacterium avium* sensitin among health care workers and medical students in the United States. Int J Tuberc Lung Dis 5:1122, 2001

161 Antimycobacterial Agents
Richard J. Wallace, Jr., David E. Griffith

The physician is greatly challenged to provide optimal therapy for mycobacterial illnesses because of the increase in both drug-susceptible and multidrug-resistant tuberculosis; the increasing number of pathogenic nontuberculous mycobacteria (NTM); drug-related toxicities and drug-drug interactions (especially in patients who have AIDS, with their complex antiretroviral drug regimens); and the plethora of new antibiotics with antimycobacterial potential. This chapter reviews the therapeutic agents used for treatment of tuberculosis, leprosy (Hansen's disease), and diseases caused by NTM, including the *Mycobacterium avium* complex (MAC), *M. kansasii*, the rapidly growing mycobacteria, and *M. marinum*. The use of first-line antimycobacterial agents in patients with renal or hepatic disease and in pregnant women is summarized in Table 161-1. The effects of antimycobacterial agents on the levels, activity, and toxicity of other commonly used drugs are summarized in Table 161-2. The reader is referred to the other chapters in this section for a more complete discussion of therapy for specific mycobacterial diseases.

TUBERCULOSIS

Drugs used to treat tuberculosis have been classified into first-line and second-line agents. *First-line essential* antituberculous agents are the most effective and are a necessary component of any short-course therapeutic regimen. The four drugs in this category are rifampin, isoniazid, ethambutol, and pyrazinamide. The *first-line supplemental* agents, which are highly effective with acceptable toxicity, include rifabutin, rifapentine, and streptomycin. *Second-line* antituberculous drugs are clinically much less effective than first-line agents and elicit severe reactions much more frequently. These drugs are rarely used in therapy and then only by caregivers experienced with their use. The older agents include para-aminosalicylic acid (PAS), ethionamide, cycloserine, amikacin, and capreomycin. Favorable experience in patients with tuberculosis resistant to or intolerant of first-line drugs suggests that the fluoroquinolones levofloxacin and moxifloxacin are important additions to multidrug antituberculous regimens; thus these agents have now been added to the list of second-line drugs.

FIRST-LINE ESSENTIAL ANTITUBERCULOUS DRUGS

Rifampin Rifampin, a semisynthetic derivative of *Streptomyces mediterranei*, is considered the most important and potent antituberculous agent. It is also active against a wide spectrum of other organisms, including some gram-positive and gram-negative bacteria, *Legionella* spp., *M. kansasii*, and *M. marinum*.

MECHANISM OF ACTION Rifampin has both intracellular and extracellular bactericidal activity. It blocks RNA synthesis by specifically binding and inhibiting DNA-dependent RNA polymerase. Susceptible strains of *M. tuberculosis* as well as *M. kansasii* and *M. marinum* are inhibited by ≤1 µg/mL.

PHARMACOLOGY Rifampin is a fat-soluble complex macrocyclic antibiotic that is absorbed readily after either PO or IV administration. Serum levels of 10–20 µg/mL follow a standard adult oral dose of 600 mg. Rifampin distributes well throughout most body tissues, including inflamed meninges. The fact that rifampin turns body fluids (urine, saliva, sputum, tears) a red-orange color makes it simple and inexpensive to check on patients' compliance with therapy. Rifampin is excreted primarily through the bile and the enterohepatic circulation, while 30–40% of a dose is excreted via the kidneys. The drug is administered three times weekly, twice weekly, or daily at a dose of 600 mg for adults (10 mg/kg) and 10–20 mg/kg for children. As mentioned above, rifampin is also available for IV administration.

ADVERSE EFFECTS (Table 161-3) Rifampin is generally well tolerated; the most common adverse event is gastrointestinal upset. This drug rarely causes hepatocellular injury when given alone; however, hepatitis is more common when rifampin is given in combination with isoniazid or pyrazinamide. Other adverse effects of rifampin include rash (0.8%), hemolytic anemia (<1%), thrombocytopenia, and immunosuppression of unknown clinical importance. Rifampin is a potent inducer of the hepatic microsomal enzymes and thereby decreases the half-life of a number of drugs, including digoxin, warfarin, prednisone, cyclosporine, methadone, oral contraceptives, clarithromycin, the HIV protease inhibitors, the HIV nonnucleoside reverse transcriptase inhibitors, and quinidine (Table 161-2). The dose of rifampin generally does not require reduction in patients with

TABLE 161-1 USE OF FIRST-LINE ANTIMYCOBACTERIAL AGENTS IN PATIENTS WITH RENAL OR HEPATIC DISEASE AND IN PREGNANT WOMEN

| | | Use in Indicated Circumstances | | |
| | | Renal Disease: Creatinine Clearance Rate | | |
Agent	Severe Hepatic Disease	<60 but >30 mL/min	≤30 mL/min	Pregnancy[a]
Azithromycin	No change	No change	?Decrease dose	No evidence of risk (B)
Clarithromycin	No change	No change	Decrease dose	Risk cannot be ruled out (C)
Ethambutol	No change	No change	No change	Risk cannot be ruled out (C)
Isoniazid	Avoid use or monitor carefully	No change	No change	Risk cannot be ruled out (C)
Pyrazinamide	Avoid use or monitor carefully	No change	Decrease dose[b]	Risk cannot be ruled out (C)[c]
Rifabutin	No change	No change	No change	No evidence of risk (B)
Rifampin	Avoid use or monitor carefully	No change	No change	Risk cannot be ruled out (C)
Rifapentine	Avoid use or monitor carefully	No change	No change	Risk cannot be ruled out (C)
Streptomycin	No change	Decrease dose	Decrease dose and frequency	Definite evidence of risk (D)

[a]Based on Food and Drug Administration pregnancy categories of A–D, X.
[b]Prudent but not absolutely necessary.
[c]Use in pregnancy is recommended by international organizations outside the United States.

PART 7 Infectious Diseases

TABLE 161-2 EFFECTS OF MAJOR ANTIMYCOBACTERIAL AGENTS ON LEVELS/ACTIVITY/TOXICITY OF OTHER COMMONLY USED DRUGS[a]

Rifampin/rifabutin[b]	Isoniazid
Acetaminophen ($\downarrow$)	Alcohol ($\uparrow$ in risk of hepatitis)
Antiarrhythmics ($\downarrow$)	Carbamazepine ($\uparrow$)
Anticonvulsants ($\downarrow$)	Diphenylhydantoin ($\uparrow$)
Azole antifungals ($\downarrow$)	Enflurane ($\uparrow$ in risk of renal failure)
Barbiturates ($\downarrow$)	Warfarin ($\uparrow$)
β Blockers ($\downarrow$)	**Clarithromycin**
Calcium channel blockers ($\downarrow$)	Astemizole ($\uparrow$)
Chloramphenicol ($\downarrow$)	Carbamazepine ($\uparrow$)
Clarithromycin ($\downarrow$)	Digoxin ($\uparrow$)
Cyclosporine ($\downarrow$)	Rifabutin ($\uparrow$)
Dapsone ($\downarrow$)	Ritonavir ($\downarrow$)
Delavirdine ($\downarrow$)	Terfenadine ($\uparrow$)
Diazepam ($\downarrow$)	Zidovudine ($\downarrow$)
Digoxin ($\downarrow$)	
Doxycycline ($\downarrow$)	
Fluoroquinolones ($\downarrow$)	
Glucocorticoids ($\downarrow$)	
Halothane ($\downarrow$)	
Hormonal contraceptives ($\downarrow$)	
Narcotics ($\downarrow$)	
NNRTIs[c] ($\downarrow$)	
Oral hypoglycemics ($\downarrow$)	
Probenecid ($\downarrow$)	
Protease inhibitors ($\downarrow$)	
Quinidine ($\downarrow$)	
Theophylline ($\downarrow$)	
Tricyclic antidepressants ($\downarrow$)	
Warfarin ($\downarrow$)	
Zidovudine ($\downarrow$)	

[a] The following antimycobacterial agents have no or minimal effects on other drugs: amikacin, azithromycin, capreomycin, ethambutol, streptomycin, pyrazinamide.
[b] Rifabutin, which induces the cytochrome P450 system, has the same effects ($\downarrow$) as rifampin but to a lesser degree. All drugs whose half-life is decreased by rifampin induction of hepatic microsomal enzymes may be subject to the same effect when coadministered with rifabutin; however, this point has not yet been studied.
[c] NNRTIs, nonnucleoside reverse transcriptase inhibitors.

renal failure, especially those receiving intermittent rifampin treatment (Table 161-1).

RESISTANCE Acquired resistance to rifampin results from spontaneous point mutations that alter the β subunit of the RNA polymerase

(*rpoB*) gene. Studies have shown that 96% of rifampin-resistant strains have a missense mutation within a 91-bp central core region of the gene. Rifampin-resistant strains of *M. leprae* have similar mutations that alter a single serine residue (Ser-425) in the same core region of the *rpoB* gene. Intrinsic resistance to rifampin is relatively common among most species of rapidly growing and slowly growing NTM; the mechanisms underlying this resistance have yet to be determined.

Isoniazid After rifampin, isoniazid is considered the best antituberculous drug available. Isoniazid should be included in all tuberculosis treatment regimens unless the organism is resistant. This agent is inexpensive, readily synthesized, available worldwide, highly selective for mycobacteria, and well tolerated, with only 5% of patients exhibiting adverse effects.

MECHANISM OF ACTION Isoniazid is the hydrazide of isonicotinic acid, a small, water-soluble molecule that easily penetrates the cell. Its mechanism of action involves inhibition of mycolic acid cell-wall synthesis via oxygen-dependent pathways such as the catalase-peroxidase reaction. Isoniazid is bacteriostatic against resting bacilli and bactericidal against rapidly multiplying organisms, both extracellularly and intracellularly. The minimal inhibitory concentrations (MICs) of isoniazid for wild-type (untreated) strains of *M. tuberculosis* are <0.1 µg/mL, while those for *M. kansasii* are usually 0.5–2.0 µg/mL. The MICs of this drug for other NTM are often higher.

PHARMACOLOGY Both oral and IM preparations of isoniazid are readily absorbed. The standard adult daily oral dose of 300 mg produces peak serum levels of 3–5 µg/mL. Isoniazid diffuses well throughout the body and reaches therapeutic concentrations in serum, cerebrospinal fluid (CSF), and infected tissue, including caseous granulomas. Isoniazid is metabolized in the liver via acetylation and hydrolysis; its metabolites are excreted into the urine. The rate of acetylation is genetically controlled. The recommended daily dose for the treatment of tuberculosis in the United States is 5 mg/kg for adults and 10–20 mg/kg for children, with a maximal daily dose of 300 mg for both groups. (Tuberculosis organizations outside the United States have recommended 5 mg/kg daily for both groups.) For intermittent therapy (usually directly observed), a maximal dose of 900 mg twice or thrice weekly is used. Isoniazid does not require dosage adjustment in patients with renal insufficiency or with end-stage renal disease requiring chronic hemodialysis. Although not approved by the U.S. Food and Drug Administration (FDA), IV isoniazid can be given in an urgent situation.

TABLE 161-3 MONITORING SIDE EFFECTS OF COMMON ANTITUBERCULOUS DRUGS

Drug	Side Effect	Management
Rifampin	Rash	Observe patient/stop drug if significant
	Liver dysfunction	Monitor AST/limit alcohol consumption/monitor for hepatitis symptoms
	Flulike syndrome	Administer at least twice weekly/limit dose to 10 mg/kg (adults)
	Red-orange urine	Reassure patient
	Drug interactions	Consider monitoring levels of other drugs affected by rifampin, especially with contraceptives, anticoagulants, and digoxin/avoid use with protease inhibitors
	Fever, chills	Stop drug
Isoniazid	Hepatitis	Monitor AST/limit alcohol consumption/monitor for hepatitis symptoms/educate patient/stop drug at first symptoms of hepatitis (nausea, vomiting, anorexia, flulike syndrome)
	Peripheral neuritis	Administer vitamin B_6
	Optic neuritis	Administer vitamin B_6/stop drug
	Seizures	Administer vitamin B_6
Pyrazinamide	Hepatitis	Monitor AST/limit daily dosage to 15–30 mg/kg/discontinue with signs or symptoms of hepatitis
	Hyperuricemia	Monitor uric acid level only in cases of gout or renal failure
Ethambutol	Optic neuritis	Use 25 mg/kg daily only for first 2 months (except in drug-resistant tuberculosis), then use lower daily dose (15 mg/kg) when possible/monitor visual acuity (eye chart) and red-green color vision (Ishihara Color Book) at baseline and with any visual complaint/educate patient/stop drug at first change in vision, get ophthalmologic evaluation
Streptomycin, amikacin, capreomycin	Ototoxicity, renal toxicity	Limit dose and duration of therapy as much as possible/avoid daily therapy in patients >50 years old/monitor BUN and serum creatinine levels and possibly conduct audiometry before and as needed during therapy/question patient regularly about tinnitus, dizziness, vertigo, and decreased hearing/measure serum drug levels if possible/educate patient/stop drug at first development of adverse effect (usually tinnitus)

Note: AST, aspartate aminotransferase; BUN, blood urea nitrogen.

ADVERSE EFFECTS (Table 161-3) The two most important adverse effects of isoniazid therapy are hepatotoxicity and peripheral neuropathy. Other adverse reactions are either rare or less significant and include rash (2%), fever (1.2%), anemia, acne, arthritic symptoms, a systemic lupus erythematosus–like syndrome, optic atrophy, seizures, and psychiatric symptoms. Isoniazid-associated hepatotoxicity includes asymptomatic transient elevation in aminotransferase levels (20%), symptomatic hepatitis (<1%), and fulminant hepatitis with hepatic failure (<<0.01%). Isoniazid-associated hepatitis is idiosyncratic and increases in incidence with age, daily alcohol consumption, concomitant rifampin administration, and active hepatitis B infection as well as in women who are pregnant or in the immediate postpartum period (up to 3 months after delivery). Appropriate clinical monitoring of patients receiving isoniazid includes at least monthly questioning about hepatitis-related symptoms and filling of prescriptions for no more than 1 month's worth of medication. Clinical monitoring is essential for all patients since discontinuation of the drug at the onset of hepatitis symptoms reduces the risk of progression to fatal hepatitis. The Centers for Disease Control and Prevention (CDC) and the American Thoracic Society (ATS) recommend that serum concentrations of alanine aminotransferase (ALT) be determined at baseline in patients with liver disorders or HIV infection, in women who are pregnant or in the immediate postpartum period (3 months), in persons with a history of liver disease (e.g., hepatitis B or C, alcoholic hepatitis, or cirrhosis), in persons who use alcohol regularly, and in other individuals at risk for chronic liver disease who are receiving isoniazid for treatment of latent tuberculosis. Baseline testing is no longer routinely indicated in persons >35 years of age. Routine laboratory monitoring during isoniazid treatment is indicated for patients whose baseline liver function tests yield abnormal results and for persons at risk for hepatic disease, including the groups just mentioned. Measurement of the ALT level is mandatory whenever a patient notices the onset of symptoms suggestive of isoniazid-associated hepatitis (e.g., fever, anorexia, nausea, vomiting, and/or a flulike syndrome including fever and myalgias), and treatment should be discontinued until the relationship between therapy and symptoms is ascertained. The CDC and the ATS recommend that isoniazid should be discontinued whenever (1) an asymptomatic elevation of the ALT level exceeds five times the upper limit of normal or (2) the ALT is three times the upper limit of normal in conjunction with hepatitis symptoms or jaundice. Peripheral neuritis associated with isoniazid is uncommon and probably relates to interference with pyridoxine (vitamin B$_6$) metabolism. The risk of isoniazid-related neurotoxicity is greatest for patients with preexisting disorders that also pose a risk of neuropathy, such as diabetes, alcohol abuse, or malnutrition. In these patients, the prophylactic administration of 25–50 mg of pyridoxine daily should be considered.

RESISTANCE The molecular sites of isoniazid resistance have been detailed. Most isoniazid-resistant strains have amino acid changes in either the catalase-peroxidase gene (*katG*) or the promoter of a two-gene locus known as *inhA*. Missense mutations or deletion of *katG* is also associated with reduced catalase and peroxidase activity. Rates of primary isoniazid resistance in untreated patients are much higher in many foreign-born populations than in populations born in the United States.

Ethambutol A derivative of ethylenediamine, ethambutol is a water-soluble compound that is active only against mycobacteria. Susceptible species include *M. tuberculosis*, *M. marinum*, *M. kansasii*, and MAC organisms. Among first-line drugs, ethambutol is the least potent against *M. tuberculosis*. It is used most often with rifampin for treatment of tuberculosis in patients who cannot tolerate isoniazid or who are thought or known to be infected with isoniazid-resistant organisms.

MECHANISM OF ACTION Ethambutol at standard doses is bacteriostatic against *M. tuberculosis*. Its primary mechanism of action appears to be inhibition of an arabinosyltransferase that mediates the polymerization of arabinose into arabinogalactan within the cell wall.

PHARMACOLOGY After oral administration, 75–80% of a dose of ethambutol is absorbed from the gastrointestinal tract. Peak serum levels of 2–4 µg/mL are achieved 2–4 h after the standard adult daily dose of 15 mg/kg. The drug's distribution throughout the body is adequate except in the CSF, where it reaches only low levels. However, ethambutol can reach CSF levels up to 50% as high as peak plasma levels when administered at a daily dosage of 25 mg/kg (which may be given in one daily dose) for the first 2 months, with subsequent reduction to 15 mg/kg. In cases of drug-resistant tuberculosis or where retreatment is necessary, the higher dose may be given for the duration. For intermittent therapy, the dosage is 50 mg/kg twice weekly or 30 mg/kg thrice weekly. The dosage must be lowered for patients with renal insufficiency (a creatinine clearance rate of <50 mL/min) to prevent drug accumulation and toxicity.

ADVERSE EFFECTS (Table 161-3) Ethambutol is usually well tolerated. Retrobulbar optic neuritis is the most serious adverse effect; axial or central neuritis—the only form reported in patients taking doses of <30 mg/kg—involves the papillomacular bundle of fibers and results in reduced visual acuity, central scotoma, and loss of ability to see green. Symptoms of ocular toxicity typically develop several months after initiation of therapy, but rapid-onset optic neuritis has been reported. The risk of optic neuritis depends on the dose and duration of therapy: this reaction develops in 5% of patients receiving a daily dose of 25 mg/kg but in fewer than 1% of patients given a daily dose of 15 mg/kg. Patients taking the lower dose should be tested for visual acuity and red-green color discrimination at baseline and whenever there is a subjective change in vision. Patients taking the higher dose should be tested at baseline, monthly thereafter, and whenever there is a subjective change in vision. Intermittent (three times weekly) administration of ethambutol at 25 mg/kg per dose appears to be better tolerated than daily administration of 15 mg/kg, especially in elderly populations being treated for MAC infection. Optic neuritis with associated visual loss is usually reversible, but recovery may take >6 months.

Other adverse effects of ethambutol are infrequent. Hyperuricemia occurs but is usually asymptomatic. Peripheral sensory neuropathy occurs in rare instances. Optic neuritis is rare at the low dose in children; however, the use of ethambutol in very young children is problematic because visual complications are difficult to monitor.

RESISTANCE Ethambutol resistance in *M. tuberculosis* most commonly relates to missense mutations in the *embB* gene that encodes for arabinosyltransferase. Such mutations have been found in 70% of resistant strains and involve amino acid replacements at position 306 or 406 in ~90% of cases. Species of NTM that are intrinsically resistant to ethambutol have variant amino acids in this region of the gene, while susceptible species have the same amino acid sequences as *M. tuberculosis*.

Pyrazinamide A derivative of nicotinic acid, pyrazinamide is an important bactericidal drug used in short-course therapy for tuberculosis.

MECHANISM OF ACTION Pyrazinamide is similar to isoniazid in its narrow spectrum of antibacterial activity, which essentially includes only *M. tuberculosis*. The drug is bactericidal to slowly metabolizing organisms located within the acidic environment of the phagocyte or caseous granuloma; it is active only at a pH of <6.0. Pyrazinamide is considered a prodrug and is converted by the tubercle bacillus to the active form pyrazinoic acid. The target for this compound is thought to be a fatty acid synthase gene (*fasI*). Susceptible strains of *M. tuberculosis* are inhibited by 20 µg/mL.

PHARMACOLOGY Pyrazinamide is well absorbed after oral administration, with a plasma concentration range of 20–60 µg/mL 1–2 h after oral ingestion of the currently recommended adult daily dose of 15–30 mg/kg (maximum, 2 g/d). The drug is well distributed throughout the body. Levels in CSF are excellent, reaching 50–100% of levels in serum. The serum half-life of the drug is 9–11 h. Pyrazinamide is metabolized by at least two major pathways and one minor pathway in the liver; its several metabolites include pyrazinoic acid, 5-hydroxypyrazinamide, and 5-hydroxypyrazinoic acid. Pyrazinamide is not available in a parenteral formulation.

ADVERSE EFFECTS (Table 161-3) At the high dosages used in the past, hepatotoxicity was a prominent complication of pyrazinamide therapy. However, at the currently recommended dosages, the frequency of hepatotoxicity is no higher than that for concomitant isoniazid and rifampin therapy. Although pyrazinamide is recommended by international tuberculosis organizations for routine use in pregnancy, it is not recommended in the United States because of inadequate teratogenicity data (Table 161-1). The combination of rifampin/pyrazinamide once recommended for treatment of latent tuberculosis has recently been shown to be associated with an unacceptably high rate of hepatitis. Hyperuricemia is a common adverse effect of pyrazinamide therapy; the incidence is probably reduced by concurrent rifampin therapy. Clinical gout is seen only rarely. Polyarthralgias are encountered fairly commonly but are not related to the hyperuricemia.

RESISTANCE Resistance to pyrazinamide is associated with loss of pyrazinamidase activity such that pyrazinamide is no longer converted to pyrazinoic acid. More than 90% of isolates with MICs of >100 µg/mL have mutations in the *pncA* gene, which encodes for pyrazinamidase. All strains of *M. bovis* are naturally resistant to pyrazinamide and have a point substitution within the *pncA* gene.

FIRST-LINE SUPPLEMENTAL DRUGS

Streptomycin An aminoglycoside isolated from *Streptomyces griseus*, streptomycin is available for IM and IV administration only. In the United States, it is the least-used first-line supplemental drug for tuberculosis because of its toxicity, the difficulty in obtaining adequate CSF levels, and the inconvenience of parenteral administration. In developing countries, however, streptomycin is frequently used because of its low cost. The drug is active against untreated strains of *M. tuberculosis*, *M. kansasii*, and *M. marinum* and against some strains of MAC organisms at achievable serum levels.

MECHANISM OF ACTION Streptomycin inhibits protein synthesis by disruption of ribosomal function.

PHARMACOLOGY Serum levels of streptomycin peak at 25–40 µg/mL after a 1.0-g dose. Streptomycin is bactericidal for rapidly dividing extracellular mycobacteria but is ineffective in the acidic environment within the macrophage. It diffuses poorly into the meninges and, in patients with meningitis, reaches CSF levels that are only 20% of serum levels.

The usual adult dose of streptomycin for a 70-kg patient under age 50 is 0.5–1.0 g (10–15 mg/kg) given IM daily or five times per week; the pediatric dose is 20–40 mg/kg daily, with a maximum of 1 g/d. Because streptomycin is eliminated almost exclusively by the kidneys, the dosage must be lowered and the frequency of administration reduced (to only two or three times per week) in most patients >50 years of age and in any patient with renal impairment (Table 161-1) or reduced body weight. Streptomycin can be given IV, although this approach is not approved by the FDA.

ADVERSE EFFECTS (Table 161-3) Adverse reactions to streptomycin therapy occur in 10–20% of recipients. Ototoxicity and renal toxicity are the most common and the most serious. Renal toxicity, usually manifested as nonoliguric renal failure, is less common with streptomycin than with other frequently used aminoglycosides, such as gentamicin. Ototoxicity involves both hearing loss and vestibular dysfunction. The latter is more common and includes loss of balance, vertigo, and tinnitus. Patients receiving streptomycin must be monitored carefully for these adverse effects. Less serious reactions include perioral paresthesia, eosinophilia, rash, and drug fever.

RESISTANCE In two-thirds of streptomycin-resistant strains of *M. tuberculosis*, mutations have been identified in one of two targets: a 16S rRNA gene (*rrs*) or the gene encoding ribosomal protein S12 (*rpsL*). Both targets are believed to be involved in streptomycin ribosomal binding. No mutational change has been identified in the other one-third of resistant isolates. Strains of *M. tuberculosis* resistant to streptomycin are not cross-resistant to capreomycin or amikacin.

Rifabutin Rifabutin, a semisynthetic rifamycin spiropiperidyl derivative, shares many characteristics with rifampin, including activity against *M. tuberculosis*. Rifabutin is also active against some strains of rifampin-resistant *M. tuberculosis* and is more active than rifampin against the *M. avium* complex and other NTM. To date, rifabutin has been most useful in the prophylaxis of disseminated MAC infection and in the treatment of drug-resistant tuberculosis. Rifabutin is recommended in place of rifampin for the treatment of HIV-positive individuals who are also taking protease inhibitors because its effect on these agents is less pronounced (Table 161-2).

MECHANISM OF ACTION In *Escherichia coli* and *Bacillus subtilis*, rifabutin inhibits DNA-dependent RNA polymerase in the same manner as rifampin. Its mode of action against mycobacteria is believed to be the same.

PHARMACOLOGY The pharmacology of rifabutin is dramatically different from that of rifampin. Rifabutin is readily absorbed after a single oral dose of 300 mg and reaches peak serum levels (0.35 µg/mL) in 2–4 h. This lipophilic drug distributes best to tissues: tissue levels are 5–10 times higher than plasma levels. CSF concentrations are 30–70% of plasma levels in HIV-infected patients who have meningitis. The drug's slow clearance via hepatic metabolism and renal excretion results in a mean serum half-life of 45 h, which is much longer than the 3- to 5-h half-life of rifampin. Clarithromycin (but not azithromycin) and fluconazole appear to block the hepatic metabolism of rifabutin, with consequent increases in serum levels. Adjustment of dosage is usually unnecessary in elderly patients and in patients with reduced hepatic or renal function (Table 161-1).

ADVERSE EFFECTS The majority of rifabutin's adverse effects are dose related. These events occur most frequently in patients receiving >300 mg/d. The most common symptoms are gastrointestinal; other reactions include rash, headache, asthenia, chest pain, myalgia, and insomnia. Like those taking rifampin, most patients taking rifabutin have discolored (orange to tan) urine and other body fluids. Less common adverse reactions include fever, chills, a flulike syndrome, anterior uveitis, hepatitis, *Clostridium difficile*–associated diarrhea, a diffuse polymyalgia syndrome, and a yellow skin discoloration ("pseudojaundice"). Laboratory abnormalities include neutropenia, leukopenia, thrombocytopenia, and increased levels of liver enzymes. Rifabutin induces hepatic cytochrome P450 enzymes but does so much less strongly than rifampin.

RESISTANCE Resistance to rifabutin is attributable to the same mechanism as that to rifampin—i.e., mutations involving the *rpoB* gene. However, of the 14 mutant *rpoB* alleles that confer resistance to rifampin, only 9 confer high-level resistance to rifabutin; the remaining 5 result in only small changes in rifabutin MICs, which remain at ≤0.5 µg/mL. Thus rifabutin inhibits about one-quarter of rifampin-resistant strains of *M. tuberculosis*.

Rifapentine A semisynthetic cyclopentyl rifamycin antibiotic, rifapentine received accelerated approval from the FDA for the treatment of tuberculosis. It is the first new drug approved for tuberculosis in the United States in 30 years. While similar to rifampin, rifapentine is lipophilic and longer acting—characteristics that enhance patient compliance; the drug can be administered at a dose of 600 mg once or twice weekly. Rifapentine has not yet been approved for the treatment of patients with HIV disease because rifapentine/rifampin monoresistance frequently develops in HIV-positive patients receiving isoniazid plus once-weekly rifapentine.

MECHANISM OF ACTION Rifapentine exerts its bactericidal effect by inhibiting DNA-dependent RNA polymerase in susceptible bacteria. The MICs of rifapentine for rifampin-susceptible strains of *M. tuberculosis* range from 0.03 to 0.12 μg/mL.

PHARMACOLOGY After oral administration, rifapentine reaches peak serum concentrations in 5–6 h and achieves a steady state in 10 days. The half-life of rifapentine and its active metabolite 25-desacetyl rifapentine is ~13 h. The administered dose is excreted via the liver (70%).

ADVERSE EFFECTS Rifapentine's adverse-event pattern is similar to that of rifampin. Rifapentine induces the hepatic cytochrome P450 enzymes CYP3A4 and 2C8/9. Current induction studies suggest that its potential for drug-drug interaction may be lower than that of rifampin but greater than that of rifabutin. Drugs potentially affected by concomitant administration of rifapentine are listed under "Rifampin/rifabutin" in Table 161-2. Rifapentine is in category C for use in pregnancy (Table 161-1) because of its teratogenesis in rats and rabbits.

RESISTANCE Strains of *M. tuberculosis* resistant to rifapentine, rifampin, and rifabutin all involve spontaneous point mutations in the *rpoB* gene. All strains resistant to rifampin are also resistant to rifapentine.

SECOND-LINE ANTITUBERCULOUS DRUGS

Second-line and/or newer antituberculosis agents are used either when tuberculosis is drug resistant or when first-line supplemental drugs are not available. The more important second-line drugs are discussed below in their general (descending) order of usefulness.

Quinolones The mode of action of the fluorinated quinolones presumably is the prevention of DNA synthesis through the inhibition of DNA gyrase. Ofloxacin, levofloxacin, ciprofloxacin, and moxifloxacin are active against many mycobacteria, including *M. tuberculosis, M. leprae, M. marinum, M. kansasii,* and *M. fortuitum.* Levofloxacin and moxifloxacin are the most active quinolones against *M. tuberculosis.* Recent studies suggest that use of moxifloxacin may reduce the duration of therapy for drug-susceptible tuberculosis. These drugs are well absorbed orally, reach high serum levels, and distribute well to body tissues and fluids. While not approved for antituberculous therapy in the United States, ofloxacin—used in combination with isoniazid and rifampin for the treatment of pulmonary tuberculosis—has been as active and safe as ethambutol in initial trials. Adverse effects are relatively uncommon, occurring in 0.5–10% of cases and consisting mostly of benign reactions such as gastrointestinal intolerance, rashes, dizziness, and headache. The quinolones are rapidly becoming some of the most important and effective drugs for the treatment of patients who have resistant tuberculosis or are intolerant to first-line essential drugs. Some experts would classify the quinolones, especially moxifloxacin, as first-line supplemental agents. The quinolones can also be administered IV.

Mycobacterial resistance to the fluoroquinolones develops rapidly. Its molecular basis is complex; only some strains exhibit missense mutations in the A subunit (*gyrA* gene) of DNA gyrase. Fluoroquinolone-resistant tuberculosis is a source of growing concern. Because of their broad spectrum and the ease with which mutational resistance develops, antituberculous therapy with quinolones should be reserved (pending the results of ongoing studies) for patients with multidrug-resistant disease and for those who cannot tolerate first-line drugs.

Capreomycin Capreomycin, a complex cyclic polypeptide antibiotic derived from *Streptomyces capreolus,* is similar to streptomycin in terms of dosing, mechanism of action, pharmacology, and toxicity. It is administered only by the IM route in doses of 10–15 mg/kg daily or five times per week (maximal daily dose, 1 g), with peak blood levels of 20–40 μg/mL. After 2–4 months, the dosage should be reduced to 1 g two or three times a week. Cross-resistance to kanamycin and amikacin—but not to streptomycin—is common. After streptomycin, capreomycin is the injectable drug of choice for tuberculosis.

Amikacin This well-known aminoglycoside is bactericidal to extracellular organisms. Amikacin is active against *M. tuberculosis* and several of the nontuberculous species, including the rapidly growing mycobacteria, *M. kansasii, M. leprae,* and the *M. avium* complex. The usual adult dosage is 7–10 mg/kg IM or IV three to five times per week (generally no more than 500–750 mg/d). Resistance relates to a single A → G base-pair change at position 1408 in the 16S ribosomal RNA gene.

Ethionamide Like isoniazid and pyrazinamide, ethionamide is a derivative of isonicotinic acid. This agent is bacteriostatic against metabolizing *M. tuberculosis* and some NTM. It is most useful in the treatment of multidrug-resistant tuberculosis. However, its use is severely limited by its toxicity and frequent side effects, which include intense gastrointestinal intolerance (anorexia, vomiting, and dysgeusia), serious neurologic reactions, reversible hepatitis (5% of cases), hypersensitivity reactions, and hypothyroidism.

Para-Aminosalicylic Acid PAS as a calcium or sodium salt inhibits the growth of *M. tuberculosis* by impairing folate synthesis. It is rarely indicated for the treatment of tuberculosis because of its low level of antituberculous activity and its high level of gastrointestinal toxicity (manifesting as nausea, vomiting, and diarrhea). Enteric-coated PAS granules (4 g every 8 h) may be better tolerated than other formulations and produce higher therapeutic blood levels. The drug has a short half-life (1 h), and 80% of the dose is excreted in the urine.

Cycloserine Cycloserine (D-4-amino-3-isoxazolidinone) is produced by *Streptomyces orchidaceus* and is active against a broad spectrum of bacteria, including *M. tuberculosis.* Cycloserine is well absorbed after oral administration and is widely distributed throughout body fluids, including the CSF. Serious side effects limit the use of this drug and include psychosis (with suicide in some cases), seizures, peripheral neuropathy, headaches, somnolence, and allergic reactions. Cycloserine should not be given to patients with epilepsy, active alcohol abuse, severe renal insufficiency, or a history of depression or psychosis.

NEWER ANTITUBERCULOUS DRUGS

A number of drugs are being evaluated for their antituberculous activity. This group includes newer rifamycins, fluoroquinolones, oxazolidinones (linezolid; see below), nitroimidazopyrans, and diarylquinolines. Although it is not clear how many of the new agents will prove to be clinically useful, there are currently more antituberculosis drugs in development than at any previous time.

Linezolid Linezolid is one of a new class of gram-positive-active antimicrobial agents called oxazolidinones that inhibit protein synthesis by binding to the 70S ribosomal initiation complex. Linezolid has very low MICs against both drug-susceptible and drug-resistant *M. tuberculosis* in vitro and has been used successfully as a component of multidrug regimens in a small number of patients with drug-resistant tuberculosis. This agent is available in IV and oral forms. Linezolid is associated with frequent, severe adverse events, including bone marrow suppression (which appears to be dose dependent and reversible) and peripheral neuropathy (which appears to be neither dose dependent nor reversible).

LEPROSY (HANSEN'S DISEASE)

Therapy for leprosy remains difficult, especially in developing countries. Obstacles include the long courses of drug therapy required, the high cost and limited availability of most drugs, the frequency of adverse drug reactions, the difficulty of determining a treatment endpoint, and (given that *M. leprae* still cannot be grown in vitro) the difficulty of conducting susceptibility testing. While many drugs are active against *M. leprae,* efficacy in the treatment of leprosy has been established only for dapsone, rifampin, clofazimine, and ethionamide; because of its potentially severe side effects, the WHO no longer recommends ethionamide for the treatment of leprosy. Initiation of multidrug treatment has reduced the problem of acquired drug resistance seen previously with dapsone monotherapy.

Rifampin Rifampin is considered the most active agent for the treatment of leprosy. Its worldwide use is limited only by its cost. This drug is highly bactericidal against *M. leprae* and reduces the number of viable bacilli in patients' tissues faster than any other available agent. Rifampin must be combined with other antileprosy drugs to forestall resistance. For cost reasons, the drug dose of 600 mg is given once a month (supervised) outside the United States, but this dose is given daily in the United States. For details on pharmacology, adverse events, and resistance, see relevant sections under "Tuberculosis."

Dapsone Dapsone (4,4′-diaminodiphenylsulfone) inhibits bacterial folic acid synthesis. It is now considered the second most active drug (after rifampin) in the treatment of leprosy because of its ready availability, low cost, and low toxicity and the susceptibility of untreated strains of *M. leprae* to low concentrations.

PHARMACOLOGY Dapsone is well absorbed orally and distributes well throughout the body. The usual daily dosage is 100 mg for adults and 0.9–1.4 mg/kg for children. Plasma concentrations peak within 1–3 h. The median elimination half-life is 22 h. Dapsone is cleared by acetylation in the liver. The drug is 70% bound to plasma protein. Usual daily doses produce serum concentrations of 10–15 μg/mL, which far exceed the MIC for *M. leprae* (0.01–0.001 μg/mL).

ADVERSE EFFECTS Hemolysis and methemoglobinemia are common untoward reactions to dapsone. Patients should be screened for glucose-6-phosphate dehydrogenase deficiency to prevent serious drug-induced hemolysis. However, most patients tolerate dapsone therapy well with adequate clinical and laboratory supervision. Other side effects include gastrointestinal intolerance, headache, pruritus, peripheral neuropathies, nephrotic syndrome, fever, and rash.

Clofazimine A phenazine iminoquinone dye, clofazimine is weakly bactericidal against *M. leprae*. It is useful in treating dapsone-resistant leprosy and may lessen the severity of erythema nodosum leprosum (ENL). Clofazimine's mode of action is not well understood. Its serum half-life is ~60–70 days; only a small proportion of the dose is excreted daily into the urine or bile. Bactericidal activity is very slow and is evident for ~50 days after administration. The usual adult dosage is 50–100 mg/d, 100 mg three times a week, or (for treatment of ENL) 300 mg/d. Untoward effects include skin discoloration and, less commonly, gastrointestinal intolerance.

Other Agents A number of other drugs exhibit significant activity against *M. leprae*, but clinical experience with these agents is lacking. Thalidomide is now approved by the FDA for treatment of ENL. This drug is sedating and extremely teratogenic and should *never* be taken by anyone who is or may become pregnant. Physicians wishing to prescribe thalidomide must register with the System for Thalidomide Education and Prescribing Safety (S.T.E.P.S.) at 1-888-423-5436 (Celgene Corporation). The newer macrolide antibiotics (particularly clarithromycin), minocycline (a long-acting tetracycline), and a number of fluoroquinolones (including ofloxacin, sparfloxacin, and pefloxacin) have shown promising bactericidal activity against *M. leprae*. For the most minor form of leprosy, the WHO now suggests the use of single-dose rifampin/ofloxacin/minocycline (ROM).

NONTUBERCULOUS MYCOBACTERIA

Although less pathogenic than *M. tuberculosis*, NTM can cause pulmonary, skin, bone, joint, lymph node, and soft tissue infection as well as disseminated disease in immunocompromised hosts, including patients with AIDS. MAC organisms and *M. kansasii* are the two most common causes of NTM pulmonary infection. Up to 40% of AIDS patients with CD4+ T cell counts of <50/μL develop disseminated disease due to *M. avium* unless they are receiving specific *M. avium* prophylaxis.

Clarithromycin Clarithromycin (6-0-methylerythromycin) is a newer macrolide that is similar to erythromycin in its mechanism of action. It is well absorbed with or without meals but may elicit gastrointestinal intolerance. Clarithromycin distributes well into body tissues and fluids and is highly concentrated in macrophages. The drug is metabolized in the liver, with ~30% of a given dose excreted in the urine. The dosage should be reduced if the creatinine clearance rate is ≤30 mL/min. Like erythromycin, clarithromycin binds with plasma proteins (65–70%) and can raise the levels of drugs such as theophylline and carbamazepine. Serum levels of clarithromycin are reduced by rifampin and, to a lesser degree, by rifabutin; clarithromycin increases serum levels of rifabutin and some antihistamines (e.g., terfenadine), thus potentially increasing their toxicity. The drug is also highly active not only against MAC organisms but also against almost all other NTM, including *M. marinum, M. kansasii, M. haemophilum, M. genavense, M. xenopi, M. abscessus,* and *M. chelonae*. Recent studies have shown that most members of the *M. fortuitum* group are resistant to macrolides on the basis of chromosomal *erm* genes. Standard antimycobacterial doses have been 500 mg twice daily or, in the case of MAC pulmonary disease, three times weekly. The more common side effects of high doses include nausea, vomiting, and (occasionally) abnormal liver function tests. A bitter taste is common even with routine doses. Most gastrointestinal side effects can be minimized by reducing the dose or using slow-release formulations. Clarithromycin is teratogenic in laboratory animals and is in category C for use in pregnancy (Table 161-1). Resistance results from point mutations involving adenine at position 2058 or 2059 in the 23S ribosomal RNA gene macrolide binding site and is a major concern for all slowly growing species and the rapid growers *M. chelonae* and *M. abscessus*, which have only a single copy of the ribosomal genes.

Azithromycin Azithromycin is a macrolide that belongs to the family of azalides. This drug reaches much lower serum levels than clarithromycin (usually ≤0.5 μg/mL), but its high tissue and macrophage concentrations and longer half-life suggest the feasibility of intermittent therapy. Azithromycin is involved in few drug interactions since it does not affect the cytochrome P450 system. The usual doses are 250–500 mg three times weekly (MAC therapy) or 1200 mg once a week (prophylaxis for disseminated *M. avium*). No alteration in dose is required in renal failure. The most common side effects are gastrointestinal symptoms and reversible hearing loss. Resistance to azithromycin develops by the same mechanism as that to clarithromycin, with cross-resistance between the two macrolides.

Therapy for Specific NTM Infections • *MAC ORGANISMS* The treatment of MAC lung disease involves the use of two or three drugs administered either daily or three times per week. Given the potential for drug-related toxicity and the remaining uncertainties about the optimal regimen and schedule, treatment frequently needs to be individualized.

Therapy for MAC lung disease in the adult patient with nodular disease and bronchiectasis usually involves the administration of clarithromycin (500 mg morning and night), ethambutol (25 mg/kg), and rifampin (600 mg) on a Monday–Wednesday–Friday schedule. For patients with upper-lobe cavitary disease, daily therapy is usually recommended. Therapy is generally continued until cultures have been negative for 12 months.

For disseminated disease in AIDS, daily administration of one of the newer macrolides (clarithromycin or azithromycin) and ethambutol (15 mg/kg) is considered an essential component of any treatment regimen, with rifabutin (300 mg) a commonly used third drug. Other alternative drugs include streptomycin and amikacin. Clofazimine appears to increase mortality risk and should be avoided. For prophylaxis of disseminated MAC disease, rifabutin (300 mg/d), clarithromycin (500 mg twice daily), and azithromycin (1200 mg once weekly) have all been effective in controlled or comparative clinical trials. Once-weekly azithromycin is the drug most often used.

M. KANSASII *M. kansasii* is usually susceptible to most antituberculous drugs except for pyrazinamide. Current ATS recommendations for the treatment of *M. kansasii* pulmonary disease are daily isoniazid (300 mg), rifampin (600 mg), and ethambutol (15 mg/kg); this regimen is continued until 12 months after the last positive sputum culture. In patients taking protease inhibitors, rifabutin (150 mg/d) or clarithromycin

(500 mg twice daily) should be substituted for rifampin. The potential advantages of the highly active rifabutin and the newer macrolides in immunocompetent patients have not been studied.

RAPIDLY GROWING MYCOBACTERIA The *M. fortuitum* group, *M. abscessus*, and *M. chelonae* account for >80% of cases of clinical disease due to rapidly growing mycobacteria. These organisms are resistant to antituberculous agents other than amikacin but are variably susceptible to several traditional antibiotics. Clarithromycin has dramatically changed the approach to therapy for infections with rapidly growing mycobacteria, since it inhibits most species. Other drugs with good activity include amikacin, cefoxitin, doxycycline, imipenem, the fluorinated quinolones, sulfonamides, and linezolid.

M. MARINUM *M. marinum*, a cause of posttraumatic localized skin infection, is typically susceptible to minocycline, rifampin, ethambutol, clarithromycin, and trimethoprim-sulfamethoxazole and is resistant to isoniazid.

FURTHER READINGS

AMERICAN THORACIC SOCIETY: Targeted tuberculin testing and treatment of latent tuberculosis infection. Am J Respir Crit Care Med 161:S221, 2000

———/CENTERS FOR DISEASE CONTROL AND PREVENTION/INFECTIOUS DISEASES SOCIETY OF AMERICA: Treatment of tuberculosis. Am J Respir Crit Care Med 167:603, 2003

BOCK NN et al: A prospective, randomized, double-blind study of the tolerability of rifapentine 600, 900, and 1,200 mg plus isoniazid in the continuation phase of tuberculosis treatment. Am J Respir Crit Care Med 165:1526, 2002

BURMAN WJ et al: Moxifloxacin versus ethambutol in the first 2 months of treatment for pulmonary tuberculosis. Am J Respir Crit Care Med 174:331, 2006

GRIFFITH DE et al: An official ATS/IDSA statement: Diagnosis, treatment, and prevention of nontuberculous mycobacterial diseases. Am J Respir Crit Care Med 175:367, 2007

JASMER RM et al: Short-course rifampin and pyrazinamide compared with isoniazid for latent tuberculosis infection: A multicenter clinical trial. Ann Intern Med 137:640, 2002

MUSSER JM: Antimicrobial agent resistance in mycobacteria: Molecular genetic insights. Clin Microbiol Rev 8:496, 1995

SAUKKONEN JJ et al: An official ATS statement: Hepatotoxicity of antituberculosis therapy. Am J Respir Crit Care Med 174:935, 2006

WHO EXPERT COMMITTEE ON LEPROSY: Seventh Report. Geneva, World Health Organization, 1998, Technical Report Series, No. 874

SECTION 9 SPIROCHETAL DISEASES

162 Syphilis
Sheila A. Lukehart

DEFINITION

Syphilis, a chronic systemic infection caused by *Treponema pallidum* subspecies *pallidum*, is usually sexually transmitted and is characterized by episodes of active disease interrupted by periods of latency. After an incubation period averaging 2–6 weeks, a primary lesion appears, often associated with regional lymphadenopathy. The secondary stage, associated with generalized mucocutaneous lesions and generalized lymphadenopathy, is followed by a latent period of subclinical infection lasting years or decades. In about one-third of untreated cases, the tertiary stage appears, characterized by progressive destructive mucocutaneous, musculoskeletal, or parenchymal lesions; aortitis; or symptomatic central nervous system (CNS) disease.

ETIOLOGY

The Spirochaetales include three genera that are pathogenic for humans and for a variety of other animals: *Leptospira*, which causes human leptospirosis (Chap. 164); *Borrelia*, which causes relapsing fever and Lyme disease (Chaps. 165 and 166); and *Treponema*, which causes the diseases known as treponematoses (see also Chap. 163). The genus *Treponema* includes *T. pallidum* subspecies *pallidum*, which causes venereal syphilis; *T. pallidum* subspecies *pertenue*, which causes yaws; *T. pallidum* subspecies *endemicum*, which causes endemic syphilis or bejel; and *T. carateum*, which causes pinta. Until recently, the subspecies were distinguished primarily by the clinical syndromes they produce. Researchers have now identified molecular signatures that can differentiate the three subspecies of *T. pallidum* by culture-independent, polymerase chain reaction (PCR)–based methods. Other *Treponema* species found in the human mouth, genital mucosa, and gastrointestinal tract have been associated with disease (e.g., periodontitis), but their role as primary etiologic agents is unclear.

T. pallidum subspecies *pallidum* (referred to hereafter simply as *T. pallidum*), a thin spiral organism, has a cell body surrounded by a trilaminar cytoplasmic membrane, a delicate peptidoglycan layer providing some structural rigidity, and a lipid-rich outer membrane containing relatively few integral membrane proteins. Endoflagella wind around the cell body in the periplasmic space and are responsible for motility.

T. pallidum cannot be cultured in vitro, and little was known about its metabolism until the genome was sequenced in 1998. This spirochete possesses severely limited metabolic capabilities, lacking the genes required for de novo synthesis of most amino acids, nucleotides, and lipids. In addition, *T. pallidum* lacks genes encoding the enzymes of the Krebs cycle and oxidative phosphorylation. To compensate, the organism contains numerous genes predicted to code for transporters of amino acids, carbohydrates, and cations. In addition, genome analyses and other studies have revealed the existence of a 12-member gene family (called *tpr*) that bears similarities to variable outer-membrane antigens of other spirochetes. One member, TprK, has discrete variable (V) regions that are targets of the humoral immune response. Data suggest that sequence variation occurs in TprK during infection and that this variation is a mechanism for immune invasion.

The only known natural host for *T. pallidum* is the human host. *T. pallidum* can infect many mammals, but only humans, higher apes, and a few laboratory animals regularly develop syphilitic lesions. Virulent strains of *T. pallidum* are grown in rabbits.

EPIDEMIOLOGY

Nearly all cases of syphilis are acquired by sexual contact with infectious lesions (i.e., the chancre, mucous patch, skin rash, or condylomata lata). Less common modes of transmission include nonsexual personal contact, infection in utero, blood transfusion, and organ transplantation.

SYPHILIS IN THE UNITED STATES

With the advent of penicillin therapy, the total number of cases of syphilis reported annually in the United States declined significantly to a low of 31,575 in 2000—a 95% decrease from 1943. In 2005, 33,278 cases were reported. Surveillance of the number of new cases of primary and secondary (infectious) syphilis, which is a better indicator of disease activity, has revealed multiple cycles of 7–10 years, each with a rapid rise and fall in incidence. The current increase in infectious syphilis (to 8724 cases in 2005) began in the western United States in 1997 and has particularly affected men who have sex with men (MSM), many of whom are co-infected with HIV. This outbreak has spread to large cities on the west coast of North America and to major cities elsewhere in the United States. It has been suggested that the regular fluctuation in syphilis rates is due to herd immunity in susceptible populations. Although there are no data to suggest that persons treated for syphilis possess significant resistance to reinfection, it has been recognized for many years that persons with untreated syphilis are refractory to symptomatic reinfection.

The populations at highest risk for acquiring syphilis have changed over time, with outbreaks among MSM in the late 1970s and early 1980s as well as at present. The epidemic that peaked in 1990 predominantly involved African-American heterosexual men and women and occurred largely in urban areas, where infectious syphilis was correlated significantly with the exchange of sex for crack cocaine. Since 1996, syphilis rates have declined among African Americans but remain higher than those for other racial/ethnic groups. Foci of syphilis still exist in a small number of counties in the southern United States.

The incidence of congenital syphilis roughly parallels that of infectious syphilis in females. The number of reported cases of congenital syphilis among infants ≤1 year of age fell to a low of 107 cases in 1978, when infectious syphilis was most prevalent among homosexual and bisexual men, and then rose dramatically from 1986 to 1991 during the epidemic in African-American women. In 2005, 329 cases were reported. It is important to note that the case definition for congenital syphilis was broadened in 1989 and now includes all live or stillborn infants delivered to women with untreated or inadequately treated syphilis.

One-third to one-half of individuals named as sexual contacts of persons with infectious syphilis become infected. Many sexual contacts will already have developed manifestations of syphilis when they are first seen, and ~30% of apparently uninfected contacts who are examined within 30 days of exposure actually have incubating infection and will later develop infectious syphilis if not treated. Thus, identification and treatment of all recently exposed sexual contacts are important aspects of syphilis control. Also important is the identification of infected persons by serologic testing of pregnant women, persons admitted to hospitals, and military inductees. Routine premarital serologic testing for syphilis is controversial because of low yield.

GLOBAL SYPHILIS

Syphilis remains a significant health problem globally, with an estimated 12 million new infections per year. The regions that are most affected include sub-Saharan Africa, South America, and Southeast Asia (Fig. 162-1). Some African studies have shown antenatal syphilis seropositivity rates as high as 30%, and congenital syphilis has been reported to account for up to 50% of stillbirths. Large increases in syphilis have occurred in the independent states of the former Soviet Union, and higher numbers of cases have recently been reported in European countries.

NATURAL COURSE AND PATHOGENESIS OF UNTREATED SYPHILIS

T. pallidum rapidly penetrates intact mucous membranes or microscopic abrasions in skin and within a few hours enters the lymphatics and blood to produce systemic infection and metastatic foci long before the appearance of a primary lesion. Blood from a patient with in-

cubating or early syphilis is infectious. The generation time of *T. pallidum* during early active disease in vivo is estimated to be ~30 h, and the incubation period of syphilis is inversely proportional to the number of organisms inoculated. The 50% infectious dose for intradermal inoculation in humans has been calculated to be 57 organisms, and the treponeme concentration generally reaches 10^7/g of tissue before a clinical lesion appears. The median incubation period in humans (~21 days) suggests an average inoculum of 500–1000 infectious organisms for naturally acquired disease; the incubation period rarely exceeds 6 weeks.

The primary lesion appears at the site of inoculation, usually persists for 4–6 weeks, and then heals spontaneously. Histopathologic examination shows perivascular infiltration, chiefly by CD4+ and CD8+ T lymphocytes, plasma cells, and macrophages, with capillary endothelial proliferation and subsequent obliteration of small blood vessels. The cellular infiltration displays a T_H1-type cytokine profile consistent with the activation of macrophages. Phagocytosis of opsonized organisms by activated macrophages ultimately causes their destruction, resulting in spontaneous resolution of the chancre.

The generalized parenchymal, constitutional, and mucocutaneous manifestations of secondary syphilis usually appear ~6–8 weeks after the chancre heals. Approximately 15% of patients with secondary syphilis still have persisting or healing chancres, and the stages may overlap more frequently in persons with concurrent HIV infection. In other patients, secondary lesions may appear several months after the chancre has healed, and some patients may enter the latent stage without ever recognizing secondary lesions. The histopathologic features of secondary maculopapular skin lesions are hyperkeratosis of the epidermis; capillary proliferation with endothelial swelling in the superficial corium; and dermal papillae with transmigration of polymorphonuclear leukocytes and, in the deeper corium, perivascular infiltration by CD8+ T lymphocytes, CD4+ T lymphocytes, macrophages, and plasma cells. Treponemes are found in many tissues, including the aqueous humor of the eye and the cerebrospinal fluid (CSF). Invasion of the CNS by *T. pallidum* occurs during the first weeks or months of infection, and CSF abnormalities are detected in as many as 40% of patients during the secondary stage. Clinical hepatitis and immune complex–induced membranous glomerulonephritis are relatively rare but recognized manifestations of secondary syphilis; liver function tests may yield abnormal results in up to one-quarter of patients with early syphilis. Generalized nontender lymphadenopathy is noted in 85% of patients with secondary syphilis. The paradoxical appearance of secondary manifestations despite high titers of antibody (including immobilizing antibody) to *T. pallidum* is unexplained but may result from antigenic variation or changes in expression of surface antigens. Secondary lesions subside within 2–6 weeks, and the infection enters the latent stage, which is detectable only by serologic testing. In the preantibiotic era, up to 25% of untreated patients experienced at least one generalized or localized mucocutaneous relapse, usually during the first

FIGURE 162-1   Estimated annual new cases of syphilis among adults, 1999. *(Courtesy of the World Health Organization.)*

year. Therefore, identification and examination of sexual contacts are most important for patients with syphilis of <1 year's duration. Recurrent generalized rash is now rare.

About one-third of patients with untreated latent syphilis developed clinically apparent tertiary disease in the preantibiotic era. In industrialized countries today, specific treatment for early and latent syphilis and coincidental therapy have nearly eliminated tertiary disease except for cases of neurosyphilis in HIV-infected persons. In the past, the most common types of tertiary disease were the gumma (a usually benign granulomatous lesion), cardiovascular syphilis (usually involving the vasa vasorum of the ascending aorta and resulting in aneurysm), and symptomatic neurosyphilis (tabes dorsalis and paresis). Asymptomatic CNS involvement, however, is still demonstrable in up to 25% of patients with late latent syphilis. The factors that contribute to the development and progression of tertiary disease are unknown.

The course of untreated syphilis was studied retrospectively in a group of nearly 2000 patients with primary or secondary disease diagnosed clinically (the Oslo Study, 1891–1951) and was assessed prospectively in 431 African-American men with seropositive latent syphilis of ≥3 years' duration (the notorious Tuskegee Study, 1932–1972). In the Oslo Study, 24% of patients developed relapsing secondary lesions within 4 years, and 28% eventually developed one or more manifestations of tertiary syphilis. Cardiovascular syphilis, including aortitis, was detected in 10% of patients, none of whom had been infected before age 15; 7% of patients developed symptomatic neurosyphilis, and 16% developed benign tertiary syphilis (gummas of the skin, mucous membranes, and skeleton). Syphilis was the primary cause of death in 15% of men and 8% of women. Cardiovascular syphilis was documented in 35% of men and 22% of women who eventually came to autopsy. In general, serious late complications were nearly twice as common among men as among women.

The Tuskegee Study showed that the death rate among untreated African-American men with syphilis (25–50 years old) was 17% higher than that among uninfected subjects and that 30% of all deaths were attributable to cardiovascular or CNS syphilis. By far the most important factor in increased mortality was cardiovascular syphilis. Anatomic evidence of aortitis was found in 40–60% of autopsied subjects with syphilis (vs. 15% of control subjects), whereas CNS syphilis was found in only 4%. Rates of hypertension were also higher among the infected subjects. The ethical issues eventually raised by this study, begun in the preantibiotic era but continuing into the early 1970s, had a major influence on the development of current guidelines for human medical experimentation, and the history of the study may still contribute to a reluctance of some African Americans to participate as subjects in clinical research.

These two studies both showed that about one-third of patients with untreated syphilis develop clinical or pathologic evidence of tertiary syphilis, that about one-fourth die as a direct result of tertiary syphilis, and that there is additional excess mortality not directly attributable to tertiary syphilis.

CLINICAL MANIFESTATIONS

Primary Syphilis The typical primary chancre usually begins as a single painless papule that rapidly becomes eroded and usually becomes indurated, with a characteristic cartilaginous consistency on palpation of the edge and base of the ulcer. In heterosexual men the chancre is usually located on the penis (Fig. 162-2), whereas in homosexual men it is often found in the anal canal or rectum, in the mouth, or on the external genitalia. In women, common primary sites are the cervix and labia. Consequently, primary syphilis goes unrecognized in women and homosexual men more often than in heterosexual men. Multiple primary lesions may be more common among men with concurrent HIV infection.

Atypical primary lesions are common. The clinical appearance depends on the number of treponemes inoculated and on the immunologic status of the patient. A large inoculum produces a dark-field-positive ulcerative lesion in nonimmune volunteers but may produce a small dark-field-negative papule, an asymptomatic but seropositive latent infection, or no response at all in some individuals with a history of syphilis. A small

FIGURE 162-2 Primary syphilis with a firm, nontender chancre.

inoculum may produce only a papular lesion, even in nonimmune individuals. Therefore, syphilis should be considered even in the evaluation of trivial or atypical dark-field-negative genital lesions. The genital lesions that most commonly must be differentiated from those of primary syphilis include those caused by herpes simplex virus infection (Chap. 172), chancroid (Chap. 139), traumatic injury, and donovanosis (Chap. 154). *Primary genital herpes* may produce inguinal adenopathy, but the nodes are tender and the lesions consist of multiple painful vesicles, which later ulcerate and are often accompanied by systemic symptoms, including fever. *Recurrent genital herpes* typically begins with a unilateral cluster of painful vesicles, usually without associated adenopathy. *Chancroid* produces painful, superficial, exudative, nonindurated ulcers, more often multiple than in syphilis (see Fig. 139-2); adenopathy is common, can be either unilateral or bilateral, is tender, and may be suppurative. *Donovanosis*, which is rare in the United States and Europe, is usually seen as a granulomatous ulcer that, although painless, is friable.

Regional (usually inguinal) lymphadenopathy accompanies the primary syphilitic lesion, appearing within 1 week of lesion onset. The nodes are firm, nonsuppurative, and painless. Inguinal lymphadenopathy is bilateral and may occur with anal as well as with external genital chancres. The chancre generally heals within 4–6 weeks (range, 2–12 weeks), but lymphadenopathy may persist for months.

Secondary Syphilis The protean manifestations of the secondary stage usually include localized or diffuse mucocutaneous lesions and generalized nontender lymphadenopathy. As stated above, the healing primary chancre is still present in 15% of cases, and the stages may overlap more frequently in persons with concurrent HIV infection than in those without this co-infection. The skin rash consists of macular, papular, papulosquamous, and occasionally pustular syphilides; often more than one form is present simultaneously. The eruption may be very subtle, and 25% of patients with a discernible rash may be unaware that they have dermatologic manifestations. Initial lesions are pale red or pink, nonpruritic, discrete macules distributed on the trunk and proximal extremities; these macules progress to papular lesions (Fig. 162-3) that are distributed widely and that frequently involve the palms and soles (Fig. 162-4, left). Rarely, severe necrotic lesions (*lues maligna*) may appear. Involvement of the hair follicles may result in patchy alopecia of the scalp hair, eyebrows, or beard in up to 5% of cases.

In warm, moist, intertriginous areas (commonly the perianal region, vulva, and scrotum), papules can enlarge to produce broad, moist, pink or gray-white, highly infectious lesions (*condylomata lata*) in 10% of patients with secondary syphilis. Superficial mucosal erosions (*mucous patches*) occur in 10–15% of patients and commonly involve the oral or genital mucosa (Fig. 162-4, right). The typical mucous patch is a painless silver-gray erosion surrounded by a red periphery.

Constitutional symptoms that may accompany or precede secondary syphilis include sore throat (15–30%), fever (5–8%), weight loss (2–20%), malaise (25%), anorexia (2–10%), headache (10%), and

FIGURE 162-3 Secondary syphilis: the papulosquamous truncal eruption.

meningismus (5%). *Acute meningitis* occurs in only 1–2% of cases, but cell and protein concentrations in CSF are increased in ≥30% of cases. *T. pallidum* has been recovered from CSF during primary and secondary syphilis in 30% of cases; this finding is often but not always associated with other CSF abnormalities.

Less common complications of secondary syphilis include hepatitis, nephropathy, gastrointestinal involvement (hypertrophic gastritis, patchy proctitis, or a rectosigmoid mass), arthritis, and periostitis. Ocular findings that suggest secondary syphilis include pupillary abnormalities and optic neuritis as well as the classic iritis or uveitis. The diagnosis of secondary syphilis is often considered in the affected patients only after they fail to respond to steroid therapy. Anterior uveitis has been reported in 5–10% of patients with secondary syphilis, and *T. pallidum* has been demonstrated in the aqueous humor from such patients. Hepatic involvement is common in syphilis; although it is usually asymptomatic, up to 25% of patients may have abnormal liver function tests. Frank *syphilitic hepatitis* is distinguished by an unusually high serum level of alkaline phosphatase and by a nonspecific histologic appearance that is unlike that of viral hepatitis and includes moderate inflammation with polymorphonuclear leukocytes and lymphocytes, some hepatocellular damage, and no cholestasis. *Renal involvement* usually results from immune complex deposition and produces proteinuria associated with an acute nephrotic syndrome (or rarely with hemorrhagic glomerulonephritis). Like those of primary syphilis, the manifestations of the secondary stage resolve spontaneously, usually within 1–6 months.

Latent Syphilis Positive serologic tests for syphilis, together with a normal CSF examination and the absence of clinical manifestations of syphilis, indicate a diagnosis of latent syphilis. The diagnosis is often suspected on the basis of a history of primary or secondary lesions, a history of exposure to syphilis, or the delivery of an infant with congenital syphilis. A previous negative serologic test or a history of lesions or exposure may help establish the duration of latent infection, which is an important factor in the selection of appropriate therapy. *Early latent* syphilis is limited to the first year after infection, whereas *late latent* syphilis is defined as that of ≥1 year's (or unknown) duration. *T. pallidum* may still seed the bloodstream intermittently during the latent stage, and pregnant women with latent syphilis may infect the fetus in utero. Moreover, syphilis has been transmitted through blood transfusion or organ donation from patients with latent syphilis. It was previously thought that untreated late latent syphilis had three possible outcomes: (1) persistent lifelong infection; (2) development of late syphilis; or (3) spontaneous cure, with reversion of serologic tests to negative. It is now apparent, however, that the more sensitive treponemal antibody tests rarely, if ever, become negative without treatment. Although progression to clinically evident late syphilis is very rare today, the occurrence of spontaneous cure is in doubt.

Involvement of the CNS Traditionally, neurosyphilis has been considered a late manifestation of syphilis, but this view is inaccurate. CNS syphilis represents a continuum encompassing early invasion (usually within the first weeks or months of infection), months to years of asymptomatic involvement, and, in some cases, development of early or late neurologic manifestations.

ASYMPTOMATIC NEUROSYPHILIS The diagnosis of asymptomatic neurosyphilis is made in patients who lack neurologic symptoms and signs but who have CSF abnormalities including mononuclear pleocytosis, increased protein concentrations, or a reactive Venereal Disease Research Laboratory (VDRL) slide test. Such abnormalities are found in up to one-quarter of patients with untreated latent syphilis, and these patients are at risk for development of neurologic complications. In primary and secondary syphilis, such abnormalities may be found in up to 40% of untreated patients, and *T. pallidum* can be isolated from CSF of 30% of patients even in the absence of other CSF abnormalities. Although the therapeutic implications of these findings in early syphilis are uncertain, it seems appropriate to conclude that even patients with early syphilis who have such findings do indeed have asymptomatic neurosyphilis and should be treated for neurosyphilis. In patients with untreated asymptomatic neurosyphilis, the overall cumulative probability of progression to clinical neurosyphilis is ~20% in the first 10 years but increases with time; the likelihood is highest among patients with the greatest degree of pleocytosis or protein elevation. Patients with untreated latent syphilis and normal CSF probably run no risk of subsequent neurosyphilis. In one study, neurosyphilis was associated with a rapid plasma reagin (RPR) titer of ≥1:32, regardless of clinical stage or HIV infection status.

SYMPTOMATIC NEUROSYPHILIS
Although mixed features are common, the major clinical categories of symptomatic neurosyphilis include meningeal, meningovascular, and parenchymatous syphilis. The last category includes general paresis and tabes dorsalis. The onset of symptoms usually comes <1 year after infection for meningeal syphilis, at 5–10 years for meningovascular syphilis, at 20 years for general paresis, and at 25–30 years for tabes dorsalis. However, symptomatic neurosyphilis, particularly

FIGURE 162-4 Secondary syphilis. *Left:* Papules on the palms. ***Right:*** Mucous patches on the tongue. *(Courtesy of Ron Roddy; with permission.)*

in the antibiotic era, often presents not as a classic picture but rather as mixed and subtle or incomplete syndromes.

Meningeal syphilis may involve either the brain or the spinal cord, and patients may present with headache, nausea, vomiting, neck stiffness, cranial nerve involvement, seizures, and changes in mental status. This condition may be concurrent with or may follow the secondary stage. Patients presenting with uveitis or iritis frequently have meningeal syphilis.

Meningovascular syphilis reflects diffuse inflammation of the pia and arachnoid together with evidence of focal or widespread arterial involvement of small, medium, or large vessels. The most common presentation is a stroke syndrome involving the middle cerebral artery of a relatively young adult. However, unlike the usual thrombotic or embolic stroke syndrome of sudden onset, meningovascular syphilis often becomes manifest after a subacute encephalitic prodrome (with headaches, vertigo, insomnia, and psychological abnormalities), which is followed by a gradually progressive vascular syndrome.

The manifestations of *general paresis* reflect widespread late parenchymal damage and include abnormalities corresponding to the mnemonic *paresis*: *p*ersonality, *a*ffect, *r*eflexes (hyperactive), *e*ye (e.g., Argyll Robertson pupils), *s*ensorium (illusions, delusions, hallucinations), *i*ntellect (a decrease in recent memory and in the capacity for orientation, calculations, judgment, and insight), and *s*peech. *Tabes dorsalis* is a late manifestation of syphilis that presents as symptoms and signs of demyelination of the posterior columns, dorsal roots, and dorsal root ganglia. Symptoms include ataxic wide-based gait and footslap; paresthesia; bladder disturbances; impotence; areflexia; and loss of position, deep pain, and temperature sensations. Trophic joint degeneration (Charcot's joints) and perforating ulceration of the feet can result from loss of pain sensation. The small, irregular Argyll Robertson pupil, a feature of both tabes dorsalis and paresis, reacts to accommodation but not to light. *Optic atrophy* also occurs frequently in association with tabes.

Other Manifestations of Late Syphilis The slowly progressive inflammatory disease leading to tertiary manifestations begins early during the pathogenesis of syphilis, although these manifestations may not become clinically apparent for years. Early syphilitic aortitis becomes evident soon after secondary lesions subside, and treponemes that trigger the development of gummas may have seeded the tissue years earlier.

CARDIOVASCULAR SYPHILIS Cardiovascular manifestations, usually appearing 10–40 years after infection, are attributable to endarteritis obliterans of the vasa vasorum, which provide the blood supply to large vessels. This condition results in uncomplicated aortitis, aortic regurgitation, saccular aneurysm (usually of the ascending aorta), or coronary ostial stenosis. In the preantibiotic era, symptomatic cardiovascular complications developed in ~10% of persons with late untreated syphilis, although syphilitic aortitis was demonstrated at autopsy in about one-half of African-American men with untreated syphilis. Today, this form of late syphilis is rarely seen in the developed world.

Linear calcification of the ascending aorta on chest x-ray films suggests asymptomatic syphilitic aortitis, as arteriosclerosis seldom produces this sign. Syphilitic aneurysms—usually saccular, occasionally fusiform—do not lead to dissection. Only 1 in 10 aortic aneurysms of syphilitic origin involves the abdominal aorta.

LATE BENIGN SYPHILIS (GUMMA) Gummas are usually solitary lesions ranging from microscopic to several centimeters in diameter. Histologic examination shows a granulomatous inflammation, with a central area of necrosis due to endarteritis obliterans. Although rarely demonstrated microscopically, *T. pallidum* has reportedly been recovered from these lesions, and penicillin treatment results in rapid resolution, confirming the treponemal stimulus for the inflammation. Common sites include the skin and skeletal system; however, any organ may be involved. Gummas of the skin produce indolent, painless, indurated nodular or ulcerative lesions that may resemble other chronic granulomatous conditions, including tuberculosis, sarcoido-

sis, leprosy, and deep fungal infections. Skeletal gummas most frequently involve the long bones, although any bone may be affected. Radiographic abnormalities with advanced gummas of bone include periostitis or destructive or sclerosing osteitis. Upper respiratory gummas can lead to perforation of the nasal septum or palate.

Congenital Syphilis Transmission of *T. pallidum* from a syphilitic woman to her fetus across the placenta may occur at any stage of pregnancy, but fetal damage generally does not occur until after the fourth month of gestation, when fetal immunologic competence begins to develop. This timing suggests that the pathogenesis of congenital syphilis depends on the host immune response rather than on a direct toxic effect of *T. pallidum*. The risk of fetal infection during untreated early maternal syphilis is ~75–95%, decreasing to ~35% for maternal syphilis of >2 years' duration. Adequate treatment of the mother before the 16th week of pregnancy should prevent fetal damage, and treatment of the mother before the third trimester should adequately treat the infected fetus. Untreated maternal infection may result in a rate of fetal loss of up to 40% (with stillbirth more common than abortion because of the late onset of fetal pathology), prematurity, neonatal death, or nonfatal congenital syphilis. Among infants born alive, only fulminant congenital syphilis is clinically apparent at birth, and these babies have a very poor prognosis. The most common clinical problem is the healthy-appearing baby born to a mother with a positive serologic test. Routine serologic testing in early pregnancy is considered cost-effective in virtually all populations, even in areas with a low prenatal prevalence of syphilis. Where the prevalence of syphilis is high or when the patient is at high risk of reinfection, serologic testing should be repeated in the third trimester and at delivery. Neonatal congenital syphilis must be differentiated from other generalized congenital infections, including rubella, cytomegalovirus or herpes simplex virus infection, and toxoplasmosis, as well as from erythroblastosis fetalis.

The manifestations of congenital syphilis can be divided into three types according to their timing: (1) early manifestations, which appear within the first 2 years of life (often at 2–10 weeks of age), are infectious, and resemble the manifestations of severe secondary syphilis in the adult; (2) late manifestations, which appear after 2 years and are noninfectious; and (3) residual stigmata. The earliest sign of congenital syphilis (appearing 2–6 weeks after birth) is usually rhinitis, or "snuffles" (23%), which is soon followed by other mucocutaneous lesions (35–41%). These may include bullae (syphilitic pemphigus), vesicles, superficial desquamation, petechiae, and (later) papulosquamous lesions, mucous patches, and condylomata lata. The most common early manifestations are bone changes (61%), including osteochondritis, osteitis, and periostitis detectable by x-ray examination of long bones; hepatosplenomegaly (50%); lymphadenopathy (32%); anemia (34%); jaundice (30%); thrombocytopenia; and leukocytosis. CNS invasion by *T. pallidum* is detectable in 22% of infected neonates. Neonatal death is usually due to pulmonary hemorrhage, secondary bacterial infection, or severe hepatitis.

Late congenital syphilis (untreated after 2 years of age) is subclinical in 60% of cases; the clinical spectrum in the remainder of cases differs in certain respects from that of acquired late syphilis in the adult. For example, cardiovascular manifestations rarely develop in late congenital syphilis, whereas interstitial keratitis is much more common and occurs between the ages of 5 and 25. Other manifestations include eighth-nerve deafness and recurrent arthropathy. Bilateral knee effusions are known as *Clutton's joints*. Asymptomatic neurosyphilis is present in about one-third of untreated patients, and clinical neurosyphilis occurs in one-quarter of untreated individuals >6 years old. Gummatous periostitis occurs between the ages of 5 and 20 and, as in nonvenereal endemic syphilis, tends to cause destructive lesions of the palate and nasal septum.

Classic stigmata include *Hutchinson's teeth* (centrally notched, widely spaced, peg-shaped upper central incisors), "mulberry" molars (sixth-year molars with multiple, poorly developed cusps), saddle nose, and saber shins.

LABORATORY EXAMINATIONS

Demonstration of the Organism *T. pallidum* cannot be detected by culture. Historically, dark-field microscopy and immunofluorescence antibody staining have been used to identify this spirochete in samples from moist lesions such as chancres or condylomata lata, but these tests are rarely available today outside of research laboratories. More sensitive PCR tests have been developed but are not commercially available.

T. pallidum can be found in tissue with appropriate silver stains, but these results should be interpreted with caution because artifacts resembling *T. pallidum* are often seen. Tissue treponemes can be demonstrated more reliably in research laboratories by PCR or by immunofluorescence or immunohistochemical methods using specific monoclonal or polyclonal antibodies to *T. pallidum*.

Serologic Tests for Syphilis There are two types of serologic test for syphilis: nontreponemal and treponemal. Both are reactive in persons with any treponemal infection, including yaws, pinta, and endemic syphilis.

The most widely used nontreponemal antibody tests for syphilis are the RPR and VDRL tests, which measure IgG and IgM directed against a cardiolipin-lecithin-cholesterol antigen complex. The RPR test is easier to perform and uses unheated serum; it is the test of choice for rapid serologic diagnosis in a clinical setting and can be automated. The VDRL test remains the standard for examining CSF.

The RPR and VDRL tests are used for screening or for quantitation of serum antibody. The titer reflects disease activity, rising during the evolution of early syphilis and often exceeding 1:32 in secondary syphilis. A persistent fall by two dilutions (fourfold) or more after treatment of early syphilis is considered an adequate response to therapy. VDRL titers do not correspond directly to RPR titers, and sequential quantitative testing (as for response to therapy) must employ a single test.

The treponemal tests measure antibodies to native or recombinant *T. pallidum* antigens. These include the fluorescent treponemal antibody–absorbed (FTA-ABS) test and several agglutination assays. The microhemagglutination assay for *T. pallidum* (MHA-TP) has been replaced by the Serodia TP-PA test (Fujirebio, Tokyo), which is more sensitive for primary syphilis. The *T. pallidum* hemagglutination test (TPHA) is widely used in Europe but is not available in the United States. When used to confirm positive nontreponemal test results, treponemal tests have a very high positive predictive value for diagnosis of syphilis. In a screening setting, however, these tests give false-positive results at rates as high as 1–2%. New enzyme-linked immunosorbent assays have also been approved as confirmatory tests.

 Considerable interest has recently been focused on point-of-care immunochromatographic strip tests that can be used in the field or in resource-poor settings.

The relative sensitivities of the standard tests for untreated syphilis are shown in Table 162-1. All tests may be nonreactive in early primary syphilis, although the treponemal tests have slightly higher sensitivity during this stage. All tests are reactive during secondary syphilis. (Fewer than 1% of patients with secondary syphilis have a VDRL test that is nonreactive or weakly reactive with undiluted serum but is positive at higher serum

dilutions—the *prozone phenomenon*.) Whereas nontreponemal test titers will decline or the tests will become nonreactive after therapy for early syphilis, treponemal tests often remain reactive after therapy and are not helpful in determining infection status of persons with past syphilis.

For practical purposes, most clinicians need to be familiar with the three uses of serologic tests for syphilis: (1) screening or diagnostic purposes (RPR or VDRL), (2) quantitative measurement of antibody to assess clinical syphilis activity or to monitor response to therapy (RPR or VDRL), and (3) confirmation of a syphilis diagnosis in a patient with a reactive RPR or VDRL test (FTA-ABS or Serodia TP-PA).

IgM testing is not useful for adult syphilis. Moreover, no commercially available IgM test is recommended for evaluation of infants with suspected congenital syphilis.

False-Positive Serologic Tests for Syphilis The lipid antigens of nontreponemal tests are found in human tissues, and the tests may be reactive (usually with titers ≤1:8) in persons without treponemal infection. Among patients selected on the basis of risk factors, clinical suspicion, or history of exposure, <1% of reactive tests are falsely positive. Modern VDRL and RPR tests are 97–99% specific, and false-positive reactions are largely limited to persons with autoimmune conditions or injection drug use. The prevalence of false-positive results increases with advancing age, approaching 10% among persons >70 years old. In a patient with a false-positive nontreponemal test, syphilis is excluded by a nonreactive treponemal test.

Evaluation for Neurosyphilis Involvement of the CNS is detected by examination of CSF for pleocytosis (>5 white blood cells/mm³), increased protein concentration (>45 mg/dL), or VDRL reactivity. CSF abnormalities can be demonstrated in up to 40% of cases of primary or secondary syphilis and in 25% of cases of latent syphilis. In older asymptomatic seropositive individuals, the yield of lumbar puncture is relatively low. *T. pallidum* has been recovered by CSF inoculation into rabbits from up to 30% of patients with primary or secondary syphilis but rarely from those with latent syphilis. The presence of *T. pallidum* in CSF is often associated with other CSF abnormalities; however, organisms can be recovered from patients with otherwise-normal CSF. Before the advent of penicillin, the risk of developing clinical neurosyphilis was roughly proportional to the intensity of CSF changes. CSF examination is recommended by the Centers for Disease Control and Prevention (CDC) in the evaluation of any seropositive patient with neurologic or ophthalmic signs and symptoms, patients with other late syphilis, cases of suspected treatment failure, and HIV-infected patients with untreated late latent syphilis or syphilis of unknown duration. The possibility of asymptomatic neurosyphilis in some patients with early disease is not addressed by these recommendations. Because standard therapy with penicillin G benzathine fails to result in treponemicidal drug levels in the CSF, some experts also advise lumbar puncture in early syphilis, particularly in patients with HIV infection or with nontreponemal test titers of ≥1:32.

The CSF VDRL test is highly specific but is insensitive and may be nonreactive even in cases of symptomatic neurosyphilis. The degree of sensitivity is highest in meningovascular syphilis and paresis and is lower in asymptomatic neurosyphilis and tabes dorsalis. The unabsorbed FTA test on CSF is reactive far more often than the CSF VDRL test in all stages of syphilis, but FTA reactivity may reflect passive transfer of serum antibody into the CSF. A nonreactive CSF FTA test, however, may be used to rule out neurosyphilis.

Evaluation for Syphilis in HIV-Infected Patients Because persons at highest risk for syphilis are also at increased risk for HIV infection, these two infections frequently coexist. There is evidence that syphilis and other genital-ulcer diseases may be important risk factors for the acquisition and transmission of HIV infection.

The manifestations of syphilis may be altered in patients with concurrent HIV infection, and multiple cases of neurologic relapse after standard therapy have been reported in HIV-infected patients. *T. pallidum* has been isolated from the CSF of several patients after penicillin G benzathine therapy for early syphilis. A multicenter U.S. study of early syphilis found simi-

	Mean Percentage Positive (Range) at Indicated Stage of Disease[b]			
Test[a]	Primary	Secondary	Latent	Tertiary
VDRL, RPR	78 (74–87)	100	95 (88–100)	71 (37–94)
FTA-ABS	84 (70–100)	100	100	96
TP-PA[c]	89	100	100	NA

TABLE 162-1 SENSITIVITY OF SERODIAGNOSTIC TESTS IN UNTREATED SYPHILIS

[a]The specificity for each of these tests is 94–99%.
[b]In CDC studies.
[c]Limited numbers of sera have been evaluated by TP-PA.
Source: Modified from SA Larsen et al: Clin Microbiol Rev 8:1, 1995; and V Pope et al: J Clin Microbiol 38:2543, 2000.

lar clinical responses to therapy in persons with and without concurrent HIV infection, although the study lacked sufficient statistical power to exclude an effect of HIV and 41% of subjects were lost to follow-up. Serologically defined treatment failure was more common among HIV-infected patients than among those without this co-infection. This investigation confirmed the high rate of CNS invasion in early syphilis and the persistence of *T. pallidum* after standard therapy: 11 of 43 HIV-infected patients and 21 of 88 HIV-uninfected patients had *T. pallidum* detectable in CSF before therapy; 7 of the 35 patients who underwent lumbar puncture after therapy (some HIV-infected and others uninfected) still had *T. pallidum* detectable in CSF.

There is no clear evidence that the sensitivity of serologic tests for syphilis differs in HIV-infected versus HIV-uninfected patients. Rates of decline of serologic titers appear to be slower in HIV-infected individuals. The clinical significance of this observation is unclear.

Persons with newly diagnosed HIV infection should be tested for syphilis; conversely, all patients with newly diagnosed syphilis should be tested for HIV infection. Some authorities, persuaded by reports of persistent *T. pallidum* in CSF of HIV-infected persons after standard therapy for early syphilis, recommend CSF examination for evidence of neurosyphilis for all co-infected patients, regardless of the stage of syphilis, with treatment for neurosyphilis if CSF abnormalities are found. Others believe that standard therapy is sufficient for all cases of early syphilis, without CSF examination. Serologic testing after treatment is important for all patients with syphilis, particularly for those also infected with HIV.

℞ SYPHILIS

TREATMENT OF ACQUIRED SYPHILIS The CDC's 2006 guidelines for the treatment of syphilis are summarized in **Table 162-2** and are discussed below. Penicillin G is the drug of choice for all stages of syphilis. *T. pallidum* is killed by very low concentrations of penicillin G, although a long period of exposure to penicillin is required because of the unusually slow rate of multiplication of the organism. The efficacy of penicillin against syphilis remains undiminished after 60 years of use. Other antibiotics effective in syphilis include the tetracyclines, erythromycin, and the cephalosporins. Aminoglycosides and spectinomycin inhibit *T. pallidum* only in very large doses, and the sulfonamides and the quinolones are inactive. Azithromycin has shown significant promise as an effective oral agent against *T. pallidum*; however, recent studies have documented clinical failures associated with a mutation in the 23S rRNA gene known to confer macrolide resistance. Strains harboring this mutation are present in >50% of recent isolates from Seattle and San Francisco. In contrast, an ongoing trial of single-dose azithromycin for early syphilis in Madagascar and several eastern U.S. sites has not documented clinical failures. Thus, the prevalence of resistant strains varies by geographic location. In all cases, careful follow-up should be assured for any patient treated for syphilis with azithromycin.

Early Syphilis Patients and Their Contacts Penicillin G benzathine is the most widely used agent for the treatment of early syphilis; a single dose of 2.4 million units is recommended. Preventive treatment is also recommended for individuals who have been exposed to infectious syphilis within the previous 3 months. *The regimens recommended for prevention are the same as those recommended for early syphilis.*

Penicillin G benzathine cures >95% of cases of early syphilis. Clinical relapse can follow treatment with penicillin G benzathine in patients with both HIV infection and early syphilis. Because the risk of neurologic relapse may be higher in HIV-infected patients, some experts recommend exami-

Stage of Syphilis	Patients without Penicillin Allergy	Patients with Confirmed Penicillin Allergy
Primary, secondary, or early latent	Penicillin G benzathine (single dose of 2.4 mU IM)	Tetracycline hydrochloride (500 mg PO qid) or doxycycline (100 mg PO bid) for 2 weeks
Late latent (or latent of uncertain duration), cardiovascular, or benign tertiary	Lumbar puncture CSF normal: Penicillin G benzathine (2.4 mU IM weekly for 3 weeks) CSF abnormal: Treat as neurosyphilis	Lumbar puncture CSF normal and patient not infected with HIV: Tetracycline hydrochloride (500 mg PO qid) or doxycycline (100 mg PO bid) for 4 weeks CSF normal and patient infected with HIV: Desensitization and treatment with penicillin if compliance cannot be ensured CSF abnormal: Treat as neurosyphilis
Neurosyphilis (asymptomatic or symptomatic)	Aqueous penicillin G (18–24 mU/d IV, given as 3–4 mU q4h or continuous infusion) for 10–14 days *or* Aqueous penicillin G procaine (2.4 mU/d IM) plus oral probenecid (500 mg qid), both for 10–14 days	Desensitization and treatment with penicillin
Syphilis in pregnancy	According to stage	Desensitization and treatment with penicillin

aSee text for full discussion of indications for lumbar puncture and syphilis therapy in HIV-infected individuals.
Abbreviations: mU, million units; CSF, cerebrospinal fluid.
Source: These recommendations are based on those issued by the Centers for Disease Control and Prevention in 2006.

nation of CSF from HIV-seropositive individuals with syphilis at any stage, particularly if the RPR or VDRL titer is ≥1:32. Therapy appropriate for neurosyphilis should be given if there is any evidence of CNS syphilis.

Late Latent and Late Syphilis If CSF abnormalities are found, the patient should be treated for neurosyphilis. If CSF is normal, the recommended treatment is penicillin G benzathine (7.2 million units total; Table 162-2). The clinical response to treatment for benign tertiary syphilis is usually impressive. However, responses to therapy for cardiovascular syphilis are not dramatic because aortic aneurysm and aortic regurgitation cannot be reversed by antibiotic treatment.

Penicillin-Allergic Patients For penicillin-allergic patients with syphilis, a 2-week (early syphilis) or 4-week (late or late latent syphilis) course of therapy with doxycycline or tetracycline is recommended. These regimens appear to be effective in early syphilis but have not been tested for late or late latent syphilis, and compliance may be problematic. Limited studies suggest that ceftriaxone (1 g/d, given IM or IV, for 8–10 days) is effective for early syphilis. These nonpenicillin regimens have not been carefully evaluated in HIV-infected individuals and should be used with caution. If compliance and follow-up cannot be ensured, penicillin-allergic HIV-infected persons with late latent or late syphilis should be desensitized and treated with penicillin.

Neurosyphilis Penicillin G benzathine, given in total doses of up to 7.2 million units, does not produce detectable concentrations of penicillin G in CSF and should not be used for treatment of neurosyphilis. Asymptomatic neurosyphilis may relapse following treatment with benzathine penicillin, and the risk of relapse may be higher in HIV-infected patients. Administration of IV aqueous crystalline penicillin G in recommended doses is thought to ensure treponemicidal concentrations of penicillin G in CSF. The clinical response to penicillin therapy for meningeal syphilis is dramatic, but treatment of neurosyphilis with existing parenchymal damage may only arrest disease progression.

Some recent publications have reported neurologic relapse even after high-dose IV penicillin therapy for neurosyphilis in HIV-infected patients. No alternative therapies have been explored, but careful follow-up is essential, and re-treatment is warranted in such patients.

No data support the use of antibiotics other than penicillin G for the treatment of neurosyphilis. In patients with penicillin allergy demonstrated by skin testing, desensitization and treatment with penicillin is the recommended course.

Management of Syphilis in Pregnancy Every pregnant woman should undergo a nontreponemal test at her first prenatal visit and, if at high risk

Stage of Syphilis	Tests to Perform	When to Perform	Re-Treatment[a] Considered If:
Primary or secondary	Quantitative RPR or VDRL[b]	HIV-uninfected: 6 and 12 months HIV-infected: 3, 6, 9, 12, and 24 months	1. Titer increases by fourfold *or* 2. Titer fails to decline by fourfold or test fails to become nonreactive by 6 months *or* 3. Clinical signs persist or recur
Latent or late	Quantitative RPR or VDRL[b]	HIV-uninfected: 6, 12, and 24 months HIV-infected: 6, 12, 18, and 24 months	1. Titer increases by fourfold *or* 2. Initial titer of ≥1:32 fails to decline by fourfold by 6 months *or* 3. New clinical signs develop
Neurosyphilis (asymptomatic or symptomatic)	1. If CSF pleocytosis was documented initially, repeat CSF exam. 2. Monitor decline in CSF protein and CSF-VDRL. (Note: Rate of decline may be slow.) 3. Quantitative serum RPR or VDRL.[b]	1. Every 6 months until CSF cell count is normal 2. Until normal 3. 6, 12, 18, and 24 months	1. CSF cell count has not decreased at 6 months *or* 2. CSF is not normal after 2 years

[a]Try to distinguish between reinfection and treatment failure. If no clear evidence of re-infection exists, perform CSF examination. If CSF is normal, treat as for late latent syphilis (Table 162-2). If CSF is abnormal, treat as for neurosyphilis (Table 162-2) .

[b]VDRL and RPR titers cannot be compared; use the same test for each follow-up sample.

of exposure, again in the third trimester and at delivery. In the untreated pregnant patient with presumed syphilis, expeditious treatment appropriate to the stage of the disease is essential. Patients should be warned of the risk of a Jarisch-Herxheimer reaction, which may be associated with mild premature contractions but rarely results in premature delivery.

Penicillin is the only recommended agent for the treatment of syphilis in pregnancy. If the patient has a documented penicillin allergy, desensitization and penicillin therapy should be undertaken according to the CDC's 2006 treatment guidelines. After treatment, a quantitative nontreponemal test should be repeated monthly throughout pregnancy to assess therapeutic efficacy. Treated women whose antibody titers rise by fourfold or who do not show a fourfold decrease in titer over a 3-month period should be re-treated.

EVALUATION AND MANAGEMENT OF CONGENITAL
SYPHILIS Whether or not they are infected, newborn infants of mothers with reactive serologic tests may themselves have reactive tests because of transplacental transfer of maternal IgG antibody. For asymptomatic infants born to women treated adequately with penicillin during the first or second trimester of pregnancy, monthly quantitative nontreponemal tests may be performed to monitor for appropriate reduction in antibody titers. Rising or persistent titers indicate infection, and the infant should be treated. Detection of neonatal IgM antibody may be useful, but no commercially available test is currently recommended.

An infant should be treated at birth if the treatment status of the seropositive mother is unknown; if the mother has received inadequate or nonpenicillin therapy or has received penicillin therapy in the third trimester; or if the infant may be difficult to follow. The CSF should be examined to obtain baseline values before treatment. Penicillin is the only recommended drug for the treatment of syphilis in infants. Specific recommendations for the treatment of infants and older children are included in the CDC's 2006 guidelines.

JARISCH-HERXHEIMER REACTION A dramatic though usually
mild reaction consisting of fever, chills, myalgias, headache, tachycardia, increased respiratory rate, increased circulating neutrophil count, and vasodilation with mild hypotension may follow the initiation of treatment for syphilis. This reaction is thought to be a response to lipoproteins released by dying *T. pallidum* organisms. The Jarisch-Herxheimer reaction occurs in ~50% of patients with primary syphilis, 90% of those with secondary syphilis, and a lower proportion of persons with later-stage disease. Defervescence takes place within 12–24 h. In patients with secondary syphilis, erythema and edema of the mucocutaneous lesions may increase. Patients should be warned to expect such symptoms, which can be managed with symptom-based treatment. Steroid and other anti-inflammatory therapy is not required for this mild transient reaction.

FOLLOW-UP EVALUATION OF RESPONSES TO THERAPY Efficacy of treatment should be assessed by monitoring of the quantitative VDRL or RPR titer (**Table 162-3**). More frequent serologic examination is recommended for patients concurrently infected with HIV. Because the FTA-ABS and agglutination tests remain positive in most patients treated

for seropositive syphilis, these tests are not useful in following the response to therapy. After successful treatment of seropositive first-episode primary or secondary syphilis, the VDRL or RPR titer progressively declines, becoming negative by 12 months in 40–75% of seropositive primary cases and in 20–40% of secondary cases. Patients with a history of syphilis have less rapid declines in titer and are less likely to become VDRL- or RPR-negative. Re-treatment should be considered if serologic responses are not adequate or if clinical signs persist or recur. Because it is difficult to differentiate treatment failure from reinfection, the CSF should be examined, with treatment for neurosyphilis if CSF is abnormal and treatment for late latent syphilis if CSF is normal.

Patients treated for late latent syphilis frequently have low initial VDRL or RPR titers and may not have a fourfold decline after therapy with penicillin. Re-treatment is not warranted unless the titer rises or signs and symptoms of syphilis appear. Because treponemal tests may remain positive despite treatment for seropositive syphilis, these tests are not useful in following the response to therapy.

The activity of neurosyphilis correlates best with CSF pleocytosis, and this measure provides the most sensitive index of response to treatment. An elevated CSF cell count falls to normal in 3–12 months in adequately treated HIV-uninfected patients. The persistence of mild pleocytosis in HIV-infected patients may be due to the presence of HIV in CSF; this scenario may be difficult to distinguish from treatment failure. Elevated levels of CSF protein fall more slowly, and the CSF VDRL titer declines gradually over a period of several years.

IMMUNITY TO SYPHILIS

The rate of development of acquired resistance to *T. pallidum* after natural or experimental infection is related to the size of the antigenic stimulus, which depends on both the size of the infecting inoculum and the duration of infection before treatment. The role of serum antibody in conferring immunity to syphilis remains undefined, although antibodies have been implicated in strain-specific immunity. Cellular immunity is considered to be of major importance in immunity and in the healing of early lesions. The cellular infiltration, predominantly T lymphocytes and macrophages, produces a T_H1 cytokine milieu consistent with the clearance of organisms by activated macrophages. Specific antibody enhances phagocytosis and is required for macrophage-mediated killing of *T. pallidum*. Recent studies indicate that sequence variation of TprK occurs during *T. pallidum* infection. This observation suggests a role for antigenic variation in the persistence of infection and in susceptibility to reinfection with another strain. No likely vaccine candidate antigens have been identified to date.

FURTHER READINGS

CENTERS FOR DISEASE CONTROL AND PREVENTION: 2006 Sexually transmitted diseases treatment guidelines. MMWR 55:22, 2006

CENTURION-LARA A et al: Gene conversion: A mechanism for generation of heterogeneity in the *tprK* gene of *Treponema pallidum* during infection. Mol Microbiol 52:1579, 2004

GRASSLY NC et al: Host immunity and synchronized epidemics of syphilis across the United States. Nature 433:417, 2005

LUKEHART SA et al: Macrolide resistance in *Treponema pallidum* in the United States and Ireland. N Engl J Med 351:154, 2004

MARRA CM et al: Cerebrospinal fluid abnormalities in patients with syphilis: Association with clinical and laboratory features. J Infect Dis 189:369, 2004

———— et al: Normalization of cerebrospinal fluid abnormalities after neurosyphilis therapy: Does HIV status matter? Clin Infect Dis 38:1001, 2004

MICHELOW IC et al: Central nervous system infection in congenital syphilis. N Engl J Med 346:1792, 2002

PEELING R et al: Avoiding HIV and dying of syphilis. Lancet 364:1561, 2004

ROLFS RT et al: A randomized trial of enhanced therapy for early syphilis in patients with and without human immunodeficiency virus infection. N Engl J Med 337:307, 1997

163 Endemic Treponematoses
Sheila A. Lukehart

The endemic, or nonvenereal, treponematoses are bacterial infections caused by close relatives of *Treponema pallidum* subspecies *pallidum*, the etiologic agent of venereal syphilis (Chap. 162). Yaws, pinta, and endemic syphilis are distinguished from venereal syphilis by mode of transmission, age of acquisition, geographic distribution, and clinical features. These infections are limited to rural areas of developing nations and are seen in developed countries only in recent immigrants from endemic regions. Our "knowledge" about the endemic treponematoses is based on observations of health care workers who have visited endemic areas; virtually no well-designed studies of the natural history, diagnosis, or treatment of these infections have been conducted. The treponemal infections are compared and contrasted in Table 163-1.

EPIDEMIOLOGY

The endemic treponematoses are chronic diseases transmitted by direct contact during childhood and, like syphilis, can cause severe late manifestations years after initial infection. In a World Health Organization (WHO)–sponsored mass eradication campaign from 1952 to 1969, more than 160 million people in Africa, Asia, and South America were examined for treponemal infections, and more than 50 million cases, contacts, and latent infections were treated. This campaign reduced the prevalence of active yaws from >20% to <1% in many areas. In recent decades, lack of focused surveillance and diversion of resources have resulted in a resurgence of these infections in some regions. The estimated geographic distribution of the endemic treponematoses in the 1990s is shown in Fig. 163-1. The most recent WHO estimate (1997) suggested that there are 460,000 new cases per year and a prevalence of 3 million infected persons. Areas of resurgent yaws morbidity include West Africa (Ivory Coast, Ghana, Togo, Benin), the Central African Republic, Nigeria, and rural Democratic Republic of Congo (formerly Zaire). The prevalence of endemic syphilis is estimated to be >10% in some regions of Mali, Niger, Burkina Faso, and Senegal. In Asia and the Pacific Islands, recent reports suggest active outbreaks of yaws in Papua New Guinea, East Timor, Vanuatu, Laos, Kampuchea, and Indonesia. India renewed its focus on yaws eradication in 1996 and reported no cases in 2004. In the Americas, foci of yaws persist in Haiti and other Caribbean islands, Peru, Colombia, Ecuador, Brazil, Guyana, and Surinam. Pinta is limited to Central America and northern South America, where it is found rarely and only in remote villages.

MICROBIOLOGY

The etiologic agents of the endemic treponematoses are *T. pallidum* subspecies *pertenue* (yaws), *T. pallidum* subspecies *endemicum* (endemic syphilis), and *T. carateum* (pinta). These little-studied organisms are morphologically identical to *T. pallidum* subspecies *pallidum*, and no antigenic differences among them have been identified to date. A controversy has existed about whether the pathogenic treponemes are truly different organisms. Three of the four organisms are classified as subspecies of *T. pallidum*; the fourth (*T. carateum*) remains a separate species simply because no organisms have been available for genetic studies. Molecular signatures that can differentiate the causative agents of venereal syphilis, yaws, and bejel have been identified by polymerase chain reaction amplification of *tpr* genes and restriction digestion. Whether these genetic differences are related to the distinct clinical courses of these diseases has not been determined.

CLINICAL FEATURES

All of the treponemal infections are chronic and are characterized by defined disease stages, with a localized primary lesion, disseminated secondary lesions, periods of latency, and possible late lesions. Primary and secondary stages are more frequently overlapping in yaws and endemic syphilis, and the late manifestations of pinta are very mild relative to the destructive lesions of the other treponematoses. The current preference is to divide the clinical course of the endemic treponematoses into "early" and "late" stages.

TABLE 163-1 COMPARISON OF THE TREPONEMES AND ASSOCIATED DISEASES

Feature	Venereal Syphilis	Yaws	Endemic Syphilis	Pinta
Organism	*T. pallidum* subsp. *pallidum*	*T. pallidum* subsp. *pertenue*	*T. pallidum* subsp. *endemicum*	*T. carateum*
Mode of transmission	Sexual, transplacental	Skin-to-skin	Household contacts: mouth-to-mouth or via shared drinking/eating utensils	Skin-to-skin
Usual age of acquisition	Adulthood	Early childhood	Early childhood	Late childhood
Primary lesion	Cutaneous ulcer (chancre)	Papilloma, often ulcerative	Rarely seen	Nonulcerating papule with satellites, pruritic
Location	Genital, oral, anal	Extremities	Oral	Extremities, face
Secondary lesions	Mucocutaneous lesions; condylomata lata	Cutaneous papulosquamous lesions; osteoperiostitis	Florid mucocutaneous lesions (mucous patch, split papule, condyloma latum); osteoperiostitis	Pintides, pigmented, pruritic
Infectious relapses	~25%	Common	Unknown	None
Late complications	Gummas, cardiovascular and CNS involvement[a]	Destructive gummas of skin, bone, cartilage	Destructive gummas of skin, bone, cartilage	Nondestructive, dyschromic, achromic macules

[a]CNS involvement in the endemic treponematoses has been postulated by some investigators (see text).

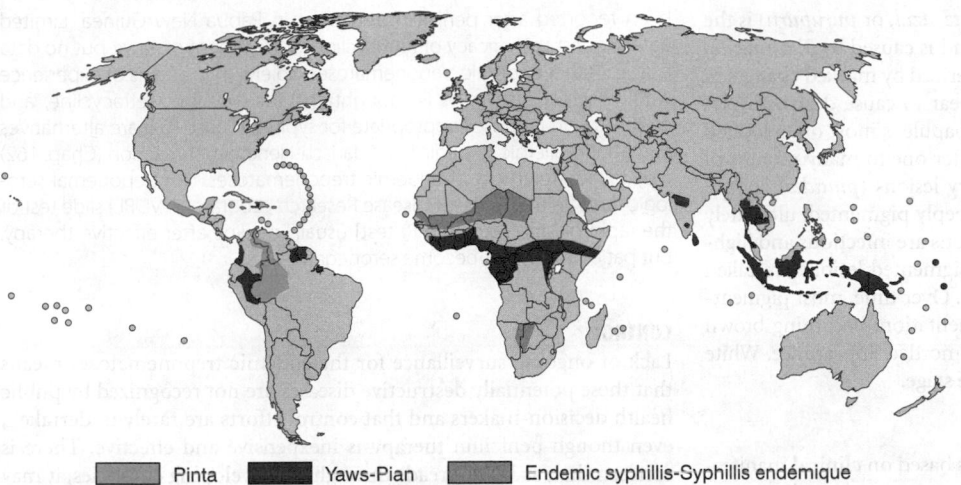

FIGURE 163-1 Geographic distribution of endemic treponematoses in the 1990s.

Legend: Pinta | Yaws-Pian | Endemic syphillis-Syphillis endémique

The major clinical features differing between venereal syphilis and the nonvenereal infections are the apparent lack of congenital transmission and of central nervous system (CNS) involvement in the nonvenereal infections. It is not known whether these distinctions are entirely accurate. Because of the high degree of genetic relatedness among the organisms, there is little biologic reason to think that *T. pallidum* subspecies *endemicum* and *T. pallidum* subspecies *pertenue* would be unable to cross the blood-brain barrier or to invade the placenta. These organisms are like *T. pallidum* subspecies *pallidum* in that they can disseminate from the site of primary infection and can persist for decades. The lack of recognized congenital infection may be due to the fact that childhood infections are in the latent stage (low bacterial load) before girls reach sexual maturity. Neurologic involvement may go unrecognized because of the lack of trained medical personnel in endemic regions, the delay of many years between infection and possible CNS manifestations, or a low rate of symptomatic CNS disease. Some published evidence supports congenital transmission as well as cardiovascular, ophthalmologic, and CNS involvement in yaws. Although the reported studies have been small, have failed to control for other causes of CNS abnormalities, have not included specific treponemal serologic tests, and have not analyzed the response to therapy, it may be erroneous to accept unquestioningly the frequently repeated belief that these organisms fail to cause such manifestations.

Yaws Also known as *pian*, *framboesia*, or *bouba*, yaws is caused by *T. pallidum* subspecies *pertenue* and is characterized by the development of one or several primary lesions ("mother yaw"), which is followed by the appearance of multiple disseminated skin lesions. All early skin lesions are infectious and may persist for many months; cutaneous relapses are common during the first 5 years. Late manifestations, affecting 10% of untreated persons, are destructive and can involve skin, bone, and joints.

The infection is transmitted by direct contact with infectious lesions, often during play or group sleeping, and may be enhanced by disruption of the skin by insect bites or abrasions. After an average of 3–4 weeks, the first lesion begins as a papule—usually on an extremity—and then enlarges (particularly during moist warm weather) to become papillomatous or "raspberry-like" (thus the name "framboesia") (Fig. 163-2). Regional lymphadenopathy develops, and the lesion usually heals within 6 months; dissemination is thought to occur during the early weeks of infection. A generalized secondary eruption, accompanied by generalized lymphadenopathy, appears either concurrent with or following the primary lesion, may take several forms (macular, papular, or papillomatous), and may become secondarily infected with other bacteria. Painful papillomatous lesions on the soles of the feet result in a painful crablike gait ("crab yaws"), and periostitis may result in nocturnal bone pain and polydactylitis. Late yaws is manifested by gummas of the skin and long bone, hyperkeratoses of the palms and soles, osteitis and periostitis, and hydrarthrosis. The late gummatous lesions are characteristically extensive. Destruction of the nose, maxilla, palate, and pharynx is termed *gangosa* and is similar to the destructive lesions seen in leprosy and leishmaniasis.

Endemic Syphilis Endemic syphilis, also called *bejel*, *siti*, *dichuchwa*, *njovera*, or *skerljevo*, is caused by *T. pallidum* subspecies *endemicum*. The early lesions are localized primarily to the mucocutaneous and mucosal surfaces, and the infection may be transmitted by direct contact, by kissing, or by sharing drinking and eating utensils. A role for insects in transmission has been suggested but is unproven. The initial lesion, usually an intraoral papule (Fig. 163-2), often goes unrecognized and is followed by mucous patches on the oral mucosa and mucocutaneous lesions resembling the condylomata lata of secondary syphilis. This eruption may last for months or even years, and treponemes can readily be demonstrated in early lesions. Periostitis and regional lymphadenopathy are common. After a variable period of latency, late manifestations may appear, including osseous and cutaneous gummas. Destructive gummas, osteitis, and gangosa are more common in endemic syphilis than in late yaws.

CHAPTER 163

Endemic Treponematoses

  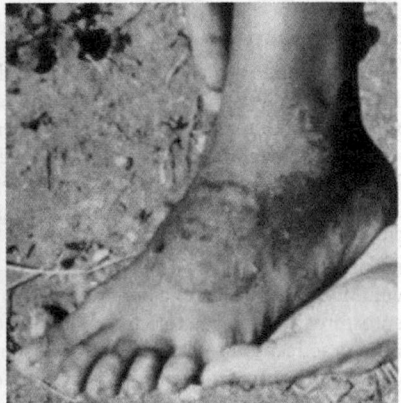

FIGURE 163-2 Clinical manifestations of endemic treponematoses. *Left:* Papillomatous primary lesion of yaws. *Center:* Split papules of early endemic syphilis. *Right:* Pigmented macules of pinta. (From PL Perine et al. Handbook of Endemic Treponematoses, Geneva,

Pinta Pinta (also called *mal del pinto, carate, azul,* or *purupuru*) is the most benign of the treponemal infections and is caused by *T. carateum*. This disease has three stages that are characterized by marked changes in skin color (Fig. 163-2), but it does not appear to cause destructive lesions or to involve other tissues. The initial papule is most often located on the extremities or face and is pruritic. After one to many months of infection, numerous disseminated secondary lesions (*pintides*) appear. These lesions are initially red but become deeply pigmented, ultimately turning a dark slate blue. The secondary lesions are infectious and highly pruritic and may persist for years. Late pigmented lesions are called *dyschromic macules* and contain treponemes. Over time, most pigmented lesions show varying degrees of depigmentation, becoming brown and eventually white and giving the skin a mottled appearance. White achromic lesions are characteristic of the late stage.

DIAGNOSIS

Diagnosis of the endemic treponematoses is based on clinical manifestations and, when available, dark-field microscopy and serologic testing. The same tests that are used for venereal syphilis (Chap. 162) become reactive during all treponemal infections, and there is no serologic test that can discriminate among the different infections. The nonvenereal treponemal infections should be considered in the evaluation of a reactive syphilis serology in any person who has emigrated from an endemic area.

℞ ENDEMIC TREPONEMATOSES

The recommended therapy for patients and their contacts is benzathine penicillin (1.2 million units IM for adults; 600,000 units for children <10 years old). This dose is half of that recommended for early venereal syphilis, and no controlled efficacy studies have been conducted. Definitive evidence of resistance to penicillin is lacking, although relapsing lesions have

been reported after penicillin treatment in Papua New Guinea. Limited data suggest the efficacy of tetracycline for treatment of yaws, but no data exist for other endemic treponematoses. Solely on the basis of experience with venereal syphilis, it is thought that doxycycline, tetracycline, and erythromycin (at doses appropriate for syphilis; Chap. 162) are alternatives for patients allergic to penicillin. A Jarisch-Herxheimer reaction (Chap. 162) may follow treatment of endemic treponematoses. Nontreponemal serologic titers [in the Venereal Disease Research Laboratory (VDRL) slide test or the rapid plasma reagin (RPR) test] usually decline after effective therapy, but patients may not become seronegative.

CONTROL

Lack of ongoing surveillance for the endemic treponematoses means that these potentially destructive diseases are not recognized by public health decision-makers and that control efforts are rarely undertaken, even though penicillin therapy is inexpensive and effective. There is concern that, as HIV spreads throughout developing countries, it may markedly affect the manifestations and transmission of the endemic treponematoses.

FURTHER READINGS

ANTAL GM et al: The endemic treponematoses. Microbes Infect 4:83, 2002

BORA D et al: Yaws and its eradication in India—a brief review. J Commun Dis 37:1, 2005

CENTURION-LARA A et al: Molecular differentiation of *Treponema pallidum* subspecies. J Clin Microbiol 44:3377, 2006

ENGELKENS HJH et al: Nonvenereal treponematoses in tropical countries. Clin Dermatol 17:143, 1999

WALKER SL et al: Yaws—a review of the last 50 years. Int J Dermatol 39:258, 2000

164 Leptospirosis
Peter Speelman, Rudy Hartskeerl

Leptospirosis is an emerging infectious disease of global importance, as illustrated by recent large outbreaks in Asia, Central and South America, and the United States. The disease is caused by pathogenic leptospires and is characterized by a broad spectrum of clinical manifestations, varying from inapparent infection to fulminant, fatal disease. In its mild form, leptospirosis may present as an influenza-like illness with headache and myalgias. Severe leptospirosis, characterized by jaundice, renal dysfunction, and hemorrhagic diathesis, is referred to as *Weil's syndrome*.

ETIOLOGIC AGENTS

Leptospires are spirochetes belonging to the order Spirochaetales and the family Leptospiraceae. Traditionally, the genus *Leptospira* comprised two species: the pathogenic *L. interrogans* and the free-living *L. biflexa*; the current designations are *L. interrogans sensu lato* and *L. biflexa sensu lato*, respectively. Seventeen genomospecies of pathogenic leptospires are now recognized on the basis of their DNA relatedness. The genome sequences of two strains have been published, and reporting of the genomes of other strains is in progress. This information will undoubtedly lead to a better understanding of the pathogenesis of leptospirosis. However, for clinical and epidemiologic reasons, it is still more practical to use a classification system based on serologic differences. The pathogenic leptospires are divided into serovars according to their antigenic composition. More than 250 serovars make up the 26 serogroups.

Leptospires are coiled, thin, highly motile organisms with hooked ends and two periplasmic flagella that permit burrowing into tissue

(Fig. 164-1). These organisms are 6–20 μm long and ~0.1 μm wide. They stain poorly but can be seen microscopically by dark-field examination and after silver impregnation staining. Leptospires require special media and conditions for growth; it may take weeks for cultures to become positive.

EPIDEMIOLOGY

Leptospirosis is an important zoonosis with a worldwide distribution, affecting at least 160 mammalian species. Rodents, especially rats, are the most important reservoir, although other wild mammals as well as domestic and farm animals may also harbor leptospires. These microorganisms establish a symbiotic relationship

FIGURE 164-1 Scanning electron micrograph of leptospires.

with their host and can persist in the renal tubules for years. Some serovars are generally associated with particular animals (e.g., Icterohaemorrhagiae and Copenhageni with rats, Grippotyphosa with voles, Hardjo with cattle, Canicola with dogs, and Pomona with pigs) but may occur in other animals as well.

In most countries, leptospirosis in humans is an underestimated problem. This infection occurs most commonly in the tropics because the climate as well as the sometimes-poor hygienic conditions favor the pathogen's survival and distribution. Most cases occur in men, with a peak incidence during the summer and fall in Western countries and during the rainy season in the tropics. Transmission of leptospires to humans may follow direct contact with urine, blood, or tissue from an infected animal or exposure to a contaminated environment; human-to-human transmission is rare. Since leptospires are excreted in the urine and can survive in water for many months, water is an important vehicle in their transmission. Epidemics of leptospirosis may result from exposure to flood waters contaminated by urine from infected animals, as has been reported from Nicaragua.

Reliable data on morbidity and mortality from leptospirosis have gradually started to appear. In 1999, more than 500,000 cases were reported from China, with case-fatality rates ranging from 0.9 to 7.9%. In Brazil, more than 28,000 cases were reported in the same year. Although humans are commonly infected with leptospires, only a minority become symptomatic or develop severe leptospirosis. In an ongoing cohort study in Brazil, 5% of the persons studied have been infected, whereas the incidence of severe leptospirosis is 9.5 per 100,000 cases.

In the United States, the 40–120 cases reported annually to the Centers for Disease Control and Prevention (CDC) surely represent a significant underestimation of the total number. Certain occupational groups are at especially high risk; included are veterinarians, agricultural workers, sewage workers, slaughterhouse employees, and workers in the fishing industry. Such individuals may acquire leptospirosis through direct exposure to or contact with contaminated water and soil. Leptospirosis has also been recognized in deteriorating inner cities and suburbs where rat populations are expanding. One report described leptospirosis in urban residents of Baltimore who were sporadically exposed to rat urine.

Recreational exposure and domestic-animal contact are also prominent sources of leptospirosis. Recreational water activities, such as canoeing, windsurfing, swimming, and waterskiing, place persons at risk. Several outbreaks have followed sporting events. For example, a large outbreak occurred in 1998 among athletes after a triathlon in Illinois. Ingestion of one or more swallows of lake water was a prominent risk factor for illness. Heavy rains that preceded the triathlon, with consequent agricultural runoff, are likely to have increased the level of leptospiral contamination in the lake water. In 2000, 80 participants contracted leptospirosis during an Eco-Challenge multisport endurance race in Malaysian Borneo. Swimming in the Segama River was an independent risk factor for infection.

In a study in the Netherlands, 14% of patients with confirmed leptospirosis had acquired the infection while traveling in tropical countries, most often in Southeast Asia. Transmission via laboratory accidents has been reported but is rare. Leptospirosis develops occasionally after unanticipated immersion in contaminated water (e.g., in an automobile accident) and rarely after an animal bite.

PATHOGENESIS

The pathogenesis of leptospirosis is incompletely understood. Leptospires enter the host through abrasions in the skin or through intact mucous membranes, especially the conjunctiva and the lining of the oro- and nasopharynx. Drinking of contaminated water may introduce leptospires through the mouth, throat, or esophagus. After entry of the organisms, leptospiremia develops, with subsequent spread to all organs. Multiplication takes place in blood and in tissues, and leptospires can be isolated from blood and cerebrospinal fluid (CSF) during the first 4–10 days of illness. CSF examination during this period documents pleocytosis in the majority of instances, but only a minority of patients develop symptoms and signs of meningitis at this point.

All forms of leptospires can damage the wall of small blood vessels; this damage leads to vasculitis with leakage and extravasation of cells, including hemorrhages. The most important known pathogenic properties of leptospires are adhesion to cell surfaces and cellular toxicity.

Vasculitis is responsible for the most important manifestations of the disease. Although leptospires mainly infect the kidneys and liver, any organ may be affected. In the kidney, leptospires migrate to the interstitium, renal tubules, and tubular lumen, causing interstitial nephritis and tubular necrosis. Hypovolemia due to dehydration or altered capillary permeability may contribute to the development of renal failure. In the liver, centrilobular necrosis with proliferation of Kupffer cells may be found. However, severe hepatocellular necrosis is not a feature of leptospirosis. Pulmonary involvement is the result of hemorrhage and not of inflammation. Invasion of skeletal muscle by leptospires results in swelling, vacuolation of the myofibrils, and focal necrosis. In severe leptospirosis, vasculitis may ultimately impair the microcirculation and increase capillary permeability, resulting in fluid leakage and hypovolemia.

When antibodies are formed, leptospires are eliminated from all sites in the host except the eye, the proximal renal tubules, and perhaps the brain, where they may persist for weeks or months. The persistence of leptospires in the aqueous humor occasionally causes chronic or recurrent uveitis. The systemic immune response is effective in eliminating the organism but may also produce symptomatic inflammatory reactions. A rise in antibody titer coincides with the development of meningitis; this association suggests that an immunologic mechanism is responsible.

After the start of antimicrobial treatment for leptospirosis, a Jarisch-Herxheimer reaction similar to that seen in other spirochetal diseases may develop. Although frequently described in older publications, this reaction seems to be a rare event in leptospirosis and is certainly less frequent in this infection than in other spirochetal diseases.

CLINICAL MANIFESTATIONS

(Fig. 164-2) Many *Leptospira*-infected persons remain asymptomatic. Serologic evidence of past inapparent infection is frequently found in persons who have been exposed to leptospires but have not become ill. In symptomatic cases of leptospirosis, clinical manifestations vary from mild to serious or even fatal. More than 90% of symptomatic persons have the relatively mild and usually anicteric form of leptospirosis, with or without meningitis. Severe leptospirosis with profound jaundice (Weil's syndrome) develops in 5–10% of infected individuals. The idea that distinct clinical syndromes are associated with specific serogroups has been refuted, although some serovars tend to cause more severe disease than others.

The incubation period is usually 1–2 weeks but ranges from 2 to 20 days (Fig. 164-2). Typically, an acute leptospiremic phase is followed by an immune leptospiruric phase. The distinction between the first and second phases is not always clear, and milder cases do not always include the second phase.

Anicteric Leptospirosis Leptospirosis may present as an acute influenza-like illness, with fever, chills, severe headache, nausea, vomiting, and myalgias. Muscle pain, which especially affects the calves, back, and abdomen, is an important feature of leptospiral infection. Less common features include sore throat and rash. The patient usually has an intense headache (frontal or retroorbital) and sometimes develops photophobia. Mental confusion may be evident. Pulmonary involvement, manifested in most cases by cough and chest pain and in a few cases by hemoptysis, is not uncommon.

The most common finding on physical examination is fever with conjunctival suffusion. Less common findings include muscle tenderness, lymphadenopathy, pharyngeal injection, rash, hepatomegaly, and splenomegaly. The rash may be macular, maculopapular, erythematous, urticarial, or hemorrhagic. Mild jaundice may be present.

Most patients become asymptomatic within 1 week. After an interval of 1–3 days, the illness recurs in a number of cases. The start of this second (immune) phase coincides with the development of antibodies. Symptoms are more variable than during the first (leptospiremic) phase. Usually the symptoms last for only a few days, but occasionally they per-

FIGURE 164-2 Biphasic nature of leptospirosis and relevant investigations at different stages of disease. Specimens 1 and 2 for serology are acute-phase serum samples; specimen 3 is a convalescent-phase serum sample that may facilitate detection of a delayed immune response; and specimens 4 and 5 are follow-up serum samples that can provide epidemiologic information, such as the presumptive infecting serogroup. [*Reprinted as adapted by Levett (from Turner LH: Leptospirosis. BMJ 1:231, 1969) with permission from the American Society for Microbiology and the BMJ Publishing Group.*]

sist for weeks. Often the fever is less pronounced and the myalgias are less severe than in the leptospiremic phase. An important event during the immune phase is the development of aseptic meningitis. Although no more than 15% of all patients have symptoms and signs of meningitis, many patients have CSF pleocytosis. Meningeal symptoms usually disappear within a few days but may persist for weeks. Similarly, pleocytosis generally disappears within 2 weeks but occasionally persists for months. Aseptic meningitis is more common among children than among adults. Iritis, iridocyclitis, and chorioretinitis—late complications that may persist for years—can become apparent as early as the third week but often present several months after the initial illness. One epidemic of uveitis among patients with leptospirosis has been reported. Mortality rates in anicteric leptospirosis are low, although death as a result of pulmonary hemorrhage occurred in 2.4% of cases in a Chinese outbreak.

Severe Leptospirosis (Weil's Syndrome) Weil's syndrome, the most severe form of leptospirosis, is characterized by jaundice, renal dysfunction, and hemorrhagic diathesis; by pulmonary involvement in many cases; and by mortality rates of 5–15%. In Europe, this syndrome is frequently but not exclusively associated with infection due to serovar Icterohaemorrhagiae/Copenhageni. The onset of illness is no different from that of less severe leptospirosis; however, after 4–9 days, jaundice as well as renal and vascular dysfunction generally develop. Although some degree of defervescence may be noted after the first week of illness, a biphasic disease pattern like that seen in anicteric leptospirosis is lacking. The jaundice of Weil's syndrome, which can be profound and give an orange cast to the skin, is usually not associated with severe hepatic necrosis. Death is rarely due to liver failure. Hepatomegaly and tenderness in the right upper quadrant are usually detected. Splenomegaly is found in 20% of cases.

Renal failure may develop, often during the second week of illness. Hypovolemia and decreased renal perfusion contribute to the development of acute tubular necrosis with oliguria or anuria. Dialysis is sometimes required, although a fair number of cases can be managed without dialysis. Renal function may be completely regained.

Pulmonary involvement occurs frequently; in some clusters of cases, it is a major manifestation, resulting in cough, dyspnea, chest pain, and blood-stained sputum and sometimes in hemoptysis or even respiratory failure. Hemorrhagic manifestations are seen in Weil's syndrome: epistaxis, petechiae, purpura, and ecchymoses are found commonly, while severe gastrointestinal bleeding and adrenal or subarachnoid hemorrhage are detected rarely.

Rhabdomyolysis, hemolysis, myocarditis, pericarditis, congestive heart failure, cardiogenic shock, adult respiratory distress syndrome, necrotizing pancreatitis, and multiorgan failure have all been described during severe leptospirosis.

LABORATORY AND RADIOLOGIC FINDINGS

(Fig. 164-2) The kidneys are invariably involved in leptospirosis. Related findings range from urinary sediment changes (leukocytes, erythrocytes, and hyaline or granular casts) and mild proteinuria in anicteric leptospirosis to renal failure and azotemia in severe disease.

The erythrocyte sedimentation rate is usually elevated. In anicteric leptospirosis, peripheral leukocyte counts range from 3000 to 26,000/μL, with a left shift; in Weil's syndrome, leukocytosis is often marked. Mild thrombocytopenia occurs in up to 50% of patients and is associated with renal failure.

In contrast to patients with acute viral hepatitis, those with leptospirosis typically have elevated serum levels of bilirubin and alkaline phosphatase as well as mild increases (up to 200 U/L) in serum levels of aminotransferases. In Weil's syndrome, the prothrombin time may be prolonged but can be corrected with vitamin K. Levels of creatine phosphokinase, which are elevated in up to 50% of patients with leptospirosis during the first week of illness, may help to differentiate this infection from viral hepatitis.

When a meningeal reaction develops, polymorphonuclear leukocytes predominate initially and the number of mononuclear cells increases later. The protein concentration in the CSF may be elevated; CSF glucose levels are normal.

In severe leptospirosis, pulmonary radiographic abnormalities are more common than would be expected on the basis of physical examination. These abnormalities most frequently develop 3–9 days after the onset of illness. The most common radiographic finding is a patchy alveolar pattern that corresponds to scattered alveolar hemorrhage. Radiographic abnormalities most often affect the lower lobes in the periphery of the lung fields.

DIAGNOSIS

(Fig. 164-2) A definite diagnosis of leptospirosis is based either on isolation of the organism from the patient or on seroconversion or a rise in antibody titer in the microscopic agglutination test (MAT). In the United States, the MAT is performed only at the CDC. In cases with strong clinical evidence of infection, a single antibody titer of 1:200–1:800 (depending on whether the case occurs in a low- or high-endemic area) in the MAT is required. Preferably, a fourfold or greater rise in titer is detected between acute- and convalescent-phase serum specimens. Antibodies generally do not reach detectable levels until the second week of illness. The antibody response can be affected by early treatment.

The MAT, which uses a battery of live leptospiral strains, and the enzyme-linked immunosorbent assay (ELISA), which uses a broadly reacting antigen, are the standard serologic procedures. These tests usually are available only in specialized laboratories and are used for determination of the antibody titer and for tentative identification of the serogroup—and in some cases the serovar—involved (thus the importance of using antigens representative of the serovars prevalent in the particular geographic area). Since cross-reactions occur frequently, however, it is often impossible to identify the infecting serogroup or serovar. Serologic testing cannot be used as the basis for a decision about whether to start treatment.

In addition to the MAT and the ELISA, various rapid tests with diagnostic value (some of them commercially available) have been developed. These rapid tests, which mainly apply lateral flow, (latex) agglutination, or ELISA methodology, have reasonable sensitivity and specificity; variation in reported data probably reflects differences in test interpretation, (re)exposure risks, and serovar distribution and the use of biased serum panels. These methods do not require culture or MAT facilities. However, in endemic areas, pooled serum samples from the local population are required as positive and negative controls. Polymerase chain reaction techniques have been developed but so far have not found widespread use outside research and reference laboratories.

Leptospires can be isolated from blood and/or CSF during the first 10 days of illness and from urine for several weeks beginning at ~1 week. Cultures most often become positive after 2–4 weeks, with a range of 1 week to 6 months. Sometimes urine cultures remain positive for months or years after the start of illness. For isolation of leptospires from body fluids or tissues, Ellinghausen-McCullough-Johnson-Harris (EMJH) medium is useful; other possibilities are Fletcher medium and Korthof medium. Specimens can be mailed to a reference laboratory for culture, since leptospires remain viable in anticoagulated blood (heparin, EDTA, or citrate) for up to 11 days at room temperature. Isolation of leptospires is important since it is the only way the infecting serovar can be correctly identified. Dark-field examination of blood or urine frequently results in misdiagnosis and should not be used.

DIFFERENTIAL DIAGNOSIS

Leptospirosis should be differentiated from other febrile illnesses associated with headache and muscle pain, such as dengue, malaria, enteric fever, viral hepatitis, *Hantavirus* infections, and rickettsial diseases. In light of the strong similarity in epidemiology and clinical presentation between leptospirosis and *Hantavirus* infections and given the reported occurrence of dual infections, it is advisable to conduct serologic testing for *Hantavirus* in cases of suspected leptospirosis. When patients have a flulike disease with disproportionately severe myalgia or aseptic meningitis, a diagnosis of leptospirosis should be considered.

℞ LEPTOSPIROSIS

Although a review of antibiotics for the treatment of leptospirosis concluded that there is insufficient evidence to provide clear guidelines for practice, the outcomes of the randomized clinical trials included in this review suggest that penicillin and doxycycline may be useful agents. Accordingly, these are the most commonly used antibiotics. Treatment should be initiated as early as possible; nevertheless, contrary to previous reports, treatment started after the first 4 days of illness is still effective. In milder cases, oral treatment with tetracycline, doxycycline, ampicillin, or amoxicillin should be considered. For severe cases of leptospirosis, intravenous administration of penicillin G, amoxicillin, ampicillin, or erythromycin is recommended **(Table 164-1)**. One comparative trial of the efficacy of ceftriaxone and penicillin for the treatment of severe leptospirosis found no significant differences between the two drugs in terms of complications or mortality rates. Another open-label randomized study compared parenteral cefotaxime, penicillin G, and doxycycline for the treatment of suspected severe leptospirosis. Among 264 patients with leptospirosis confirmed by serologic testing or culture, the mortality rate was 5%. There were no significant differences between antibiotics with regard to associated mortality, defervescence, or time to resolution of abnormal laboratory findings. Thus doxycycline, cefotaxime, or ceftriaxone is a satisfactory alternative to penicillin G for the treatment of severe leptospirosis.

In rare cases, a Jarisch-Herxheimer reaction develops within hours after the start of antimicrobial therapy (see "Pathogenesis" above). Although so far the only effective mode of management is supportive, the role of antibodies to tumor necrosis factor in the treatment of this reaction deserves further study. A beneficial effect of the use of such antibodies for the modulation of the reaction has been demonstrated in patients with louseborne relapsing fever. Patients with severe leptospirosis and renal failure may require dialysis. Those with Weil's syndrome may need transfusions of whole blood and/or platelets. Intensive care may be necessary.

TABLE 164-1 TREATMENT AND CHEMOPROPHYLAXIS OF LEPTOSPIROSIS

Purpose of Drug Administration	Regimen
Treatment	
Mild leptospirosis	Doxycycline, 100 mg orally bid *or* Ampicillin, 500–750 mg orally qid *or* Amoxicillin, 500 mg orally qid
Moderate/severe leptospirosis	Penicillin G, 1.5 million units IV qid *or* Ampicillin, 1 g IV qid *or* Amoxicillin, 1 g IV qid *or* Ceftriaxone, 1 g IV once daily *or* Cefotaxime, 1 g IV qid *or* Erythromycin, 500 mg IV qid
Chemoprophylaxis	Doxycycline, 200 mg orally once a week

Note: All regimens used for treatment are administered for 7 days.

PROGNOSIS

Most patients with leptospirosis recover. Mortality rates are highest among patients who are elderly and those who have Weil's syndrome. Leptospirosis during pregnancy is associated with high rates of fetal mortality. Long-term follow-up of patients with renal failure and hepatic dysfunction has documented good recovery of renal and hepatic function.

PREVENTION

Individuals who may be exposed to leptospires through their occupations or their involvement in recreational water activities should be informed about the risks. Measures for controlling leptospirosis include avoidance of exposure to urine and tissues from infected animals, vaccination of animals, and rodent control. The animal vaccine used in a given area should contain the serovars known to be present in that area. Unfortunately, some vaccinated animals still excrete leptospires in their urine. Vaccination of humans against a specific serovar prevalent in an area has been undertaken in some European and Asian countries and has proved effective. Although a large-scale trial of vaccine in humans has been reported from Cuba, no conclusions can be drawn about efficacy and adverse reactions because of insufficient details on study design. Chemoprophylaxis with doxycycline (200 mg once a week) has appeared to be efficacious to some extent but is indicated only in rare instances of sustained short-term exposure (Table 164-1).

FURTHER READINGS

BHARTI AR et al: Leptospirosis: A zoonotic disease of global importance. Lancet Infect Dis 3:757, 2003

GUIDUGLI F et al: Antibiotics for leptospirosis. Cochrane Database Syst Rev 2:CD001306, 2000

LEVETT PN: Leptospirosis. Clin Microbiol Rev 14:296, 2001

MORGAN J et al: Outbreak of leptospirosis among triathlon participants and community residents in Springfield, Illinois, 1998. Clin Infect Dis 34:1593, 2002

PANAPHUT T et al: Ceftriaxone compared with sodium penicillin G for treatment of severe leptospirosis. Clin Infect Dis 36:1507, 2003

SEHGAL SC et al: Randomized controlled trial of doxycycline prophylaxis against leptospirosis in an endemic area. Int J Antimicrob Agents 13:249, 2000

SEJVAR J et al: Leptospirosis in "Eco-Challenge" athletes, Malaysian Borneo, 2000. Emerg Infect Dis 9:702, 2003

SUPPUTAMONGKOL Y et al: An open, randomized, controlled trial of penicillin, doxycycline, and cefotaxime for patients with severe leptospirosis. Clin Infect Dis 39:1417, 2004

VINETZ JM: Leptospirosis. Curr Opin Infect Dis 14:527, 2001

WORLD HEALTH ORGANIZATION/INTERNATIONAL LEPTOSPIROSIS SOCIETY: *Human Leptospirosis: Guidance for Diagnosis, Surveillance and Control.* Geneva, World Health Organization, 2003, 109 pp

165 Relapsing Fever
David T. Dennis

DEFINITION

The term *relapsing fever* describes two distinct diseases. *Tick-borne (endemic) relapsing fever* (TBRF) is a zoonosis that is transmitted principally from rodents to humans by the bite of various soft ticks. *Louse-borne (epidemic) relapsing fever* (LBRF) is a disease of humans that is transmitted from one person to another by the body louse. Both diseases are characterized by recurrent acute episodes of spirochetemia and fever alternating with variable periods of remission.

ETIOLOGY

Relapsing fever is caused by infection with spirochetal gram-negative bacteria of the genus *Borrelia* (family Spirochaetaceae). The borreliae are helical in shape and average 0.2–0.5 μm in width and 5–20 μm in length. They comprise an outer membrane, an intermediate peptidoglycan layer, and an inner cytoplasmic membrane, which encloses the protoplasmic cylinder. A variable number of periplasmic flagella are situated beneath the outer membrane. Relapsing-fever borreliae are slow-growing and microaerophilic; they grow best at 30°–35°C in Barbour-Stoenner-Kelly (BSK II) medium.

B. recurrentis is the only species that causes LBRF. Most of the various species of *Borrelia* that cause TBRF are named after the species of *Ornithodoros* tick responsible for their transmission. In North America, TBRF is caused mostly by *B. hermsii* and only occasionally by *B. turicatae*; *B. duttoni* is the most common cause of TBRF in sub-Saharan Africa, an area of high endemicity. Borreliae are unique among bacteria in having a genome composed of a linear chromosome and a series of linear and circular plasmids. The sequences of both the flagellin and the 16S ribosomal RNA genes are homogeneous among LBRF strains; in contrast, there is considerable heterogeneity of these genes between Old World and New World TBRF strains. A unique process of DNA rearrangement within *vmp* genes located on linear plasmids results in extensive variation in the expression of the surface antigens in relapsing fever borreliae. These *vmp* genes encode variable major proteins (VMPs) found on the spirochete's outer-membrane surface. The antigenic variation generated by sequential expression of previously silent *vmp* genes allows the borreliae to intermittently escape the immune response of the host and results in the febrile spirochetemic relapses that are characteristic of infection with these organisms.

EPIDEMIOLOGY

Louse-Borne Relapsing Fever Body lice (*Pediculus humanus* var. *corporis*) become infected with *B. recurrentis* by feeding on spirochetemic humans, the only reservoirs of infection. In lice, *B. recurrentis* spirochetes are found almost exclusively in the hemolymph; humans acquire infection when body lice are crushed and their infective fluids enter breaks in the skin, typically abrasions caused by scratching of pruritic louse bites. Spirochetes are *not* transmitted directly by the bite of a louse (anterior station transmission) but may possibly be transmitted in a manner similar to epidemic typhus by percutaneous inoculation of louse feces (posterior station transmission). Lice have a life span of only a few weeks, feed at frequent intervals, and survive only a few days off the human host. Typically, body lice reside in seams of clothing and bedclothes, where they deposit their eggs (nits). Head lice have not been shown to be vectors of LBRF.

LBRF has severely affected military and civilian populations disrupted by war and other disasters. Historically, the disease has been most common among slum dwellers, prisoners, and others living in impoverished, overcrowded, and unhygienic conditions. In the first half of the twentieth century, during periods of war and famine, both LBRF and louse-borne typhus were epidemic in Eastern Europe, the Balkans, and the former Soviet Union. The global distribution and incidence of LBRF have been substantially reduced by improvements in standards of living, sanitation, and hygiene; LBRF is now an important disease only in northeastern Africa, especially the highlands of Ethiopia, where an estimated 10,000 cases occur annually. LBRF has repeatedly spilled out of Ethiopia into populations of displaced persons in neighboring Somalia and Sudan.

Short-term visitors to endemic areas are at almost no risk of LBRF. Persons who have close contact with LBRF-affected populations (such as relief workers) can acquire the disease from lice or by direct contact with contaminated blood.

Tick-Borne Relapsing Fever Argasid ticks of the genus *Ornithodoros* transmit TBRF through their saliva and excreta when they take blood meals. Ticks typically become infected with TBRF borreliae as part of a zoonotic cycle when they feed on spirochetemic rodents and lagomorphs; the exception is *O. moubata*, a tick species that is thought to acquire *B. duttoni* only by feeding on infected humans. Ticks transmit TBRF borreliae vertically from one stage to the next; in some species, infection is transmitted transovarially over several generations. Soft ticks are hardy and can survive for as long as 10 years with only an occasional blood meal. These ticks feed painlessly, relatively quickly (for 20–45 min), and usually at night while hosts are sleeping. Thus patients with TBRF are often unaware of tick exposures.

TBRF borreliae are widely distributed throughout the world. Human infection with these organisms is generally underrecognized and underreported. TBRF is most highly endemic in sub-Saharan Africa but is also found in countries of the Mediterranean littoral, Middle Eastern states, southern Russia, the Indian subcontinent, Central Asia, and China and rarely in North, Central, and South America. The disease typically occurs sporadically or in small—often familial—clusters. Infected soft ticks may cause repeated infections among persons living or sleeping in the same dwelling. In sub-Saharan Africa, *O. moubata*, the vector of *B. duttoni*, infests native huts and rest houses, hiding in crevices of floors and walls during the day and emerging at night to feed on sleeping inhabitants.

In the United States, TBRF occurs west of the Mississippi River, especially in forested mountainous areas of far western states, where *B. hermsii* is the causative agent. Less commonly, persons become infected with *B. turicatae* after exposures in tick-infested caves in semidesert areas of the Southwest. On average, ~35 cases of TBRF are reported annually in the United States. *B. hermsii* infections most often occur during spring and summer months among persons sleeping in rustic mountain cabins and vacation homes and occasionally in permanent residences and in outdoor settings. The vertebrate reservoirs of infection are chipmunks and other rodents that nest in foundations, wall spaces, and attics of these dwellings. Outbreaks caused by *B. hermsii* have taken place among persons staying in cabins along the north rim of the Grand Canyon and in the mountains of California, Idaho, and Colorado. In North America, most recent cases have been reported from Washington, California, Colorado, Idaho, Oregon, and British Columbia.

PATHOGENESIS AND PATHOLOGY

In humans, relapsing-fever borreliae pass through the skin or mucous membranes, multiply in the blood, and circulate in great numbers during febrile periods. The organisms have also been found in the liver, spleen, bone marrow, and central nervous system (CNS) and may be sequestered at these sites during periods of remission. The severity of disease is positively correlated with spirochete density in the blood. Even though the pathophysiologic manifestations of the disease resemble responses to endotoxin, and although plasma from some patients with relapsing fever coagulates *Limulus* amebocyte lysates, borreliae and other spirochetes have not been shown to express a true lipopolysaccharide (endotoxin) molecule. Infection with *B. recurrentis* has been shown, however, to activate protein mediators of inflammation, such as Hageman factor (factor XII), prekallikrein, and proteins of the complement system; furthermore, a spirochetal heat-stable pyrogenic factor stimulates mononuclear phagocytes to express increased amounts of leukocyte pyrogen and thromboplastin.

The treatment of relapsing fever with antibiotics may provoke a Jarisch-Herxheimer reaction (see "Rx: Relapsing Fever," below). In patients with LBRF, this reaction has been associated with a release of various cytokines into the plasma, including interleukin 6, interleukin 8, C-reactive protein, and large amounts of tumor necrosis factor α (TNF-α). Pretreatment of LBRF patients with antibody to TNF-α suppresses Jarisch-Herxheimer reactions and reduces plasma concentrations of certain cytokines.

Death due to TBRF is rare. In contrast, fatality rates of 20% have been recorded during outbreaks of LBRF in malnourished and stressed populations. Relapsing fever in pregnancy can result in abortion, stillbirth, and fatal neonatal infections. Autopsies of patients with relapsing fever most often reveal hepatosplenomegaly and variable edema and swelling of other organs, including brain, lungs, and kidneys. On microscopic examination, the spleen is congested and contains multiple microabscesses composed of mononuclear cells that replace the white pulp, the myocardium displays diffuse histiocytic inflammation and interstitial edema, and the liver has areas of midzonal necrosis. Petechial hemorrhages are commonly evident over the surfaces of the meninges, pleura, heart, spleen, liver, kidneys, and mesentery. Subcapsular and parenchymal hemorrhagic infarcts of the spleen, heart, liver, and brain are sometimes grossly visible.

CLINICAL MANIFESTATIONS

The clinical manifestations of LBRF and TBRF are similar. The common signs and symptoms of TBRF, as documented in North America, are listed in Table 165-1. The mean incubation period is 7 days (range, 2–18 days), and the onset of illness is sudden, with fever, headache, shaking chills, sweats, myalgias, and arthralgias. The arthralgia of relapsing fever can be severe, involving small and large joints, but there is no evidence of arthritis. Dizziness, nausea, and vomiting are common. Sleep may be difficult and is sometimes accompanied by disturbing dreams. The patient is coherent but withdrawn, thirsty, and uninterested in food and other outside stimuli. The fever is high from the first, with the temperature usually reaching ≥40°C (≥104°F) and then becoming irregular in pattern. High fever is sometimes accompanied by delirium. Patients are usually tachycardic and mildly tachypneic and become prostrate as the disease progresses. Some patients have meningismus. The conjunctivae are often injected, and photophobia is common. The sclerae may become icteric, particularly in the later stages of illness. The mucous membranes may be dry, and patients are often dehydrated. Scattered petechiae develop on the trunk, extremities, and mucous membranes in one-third or more of patients with LBRF but in a smaller proportion of patients with TBRF. A nonproductive cough is common, but chest sounds are usually normal; pleuritic pain and an accompanying pleuritic rub are sometimes noted. Cardiac findings are compatible with a high-output state; tachycardia and summation gallop are common. Tender enlargement of the spleen and liver frequently occurs in the acute phase of illness.

TABLE 165-1 MANIFESTATIONS OF TICK-BORNE RELAPSING FEVER ACQUIRED IN THE NORTHWESTERN UNITED STATES AND SOUTHWESTERN BRITISH COLUMBIA

Sign or Symptom	%	Sign or Symptom	%
Headache	94	Photophobia	25
Myalgia	92	Neck pain	24
Chills	88	Rash	18
Nausea	76	Dysuria	13
Arthralgia	73	Jaundice	10
Vomiting	71	Hepatomegaly	10
Abdominal pain	44	Splenomegaly	6
Confusion	38	Conjunctival injection	5
Dry cough	27	Eschar	2
Eye pain	26	Meningitis	2
Diarrhea	25	Nuchal rigidity	2
Dizziness	25		

Source: From a review of 182 cases reported in the period 1980–1995 (Dworkin et al.).

Epistaxis and blood-tinged sputum are common complications, and gastrointestinal and CNS hemorrhage can occur. Because of bleeding, outbreaks of LBRF have been initially confused with viral hemorrhagic fever. Other complications of variable incidence include iridocyclitis, optic neuritis, lymphocytic meningitis, coma, isolated cranial-nerve palsy, pneumonitis, myocarditis, and splenic rupture. Acute respiratory distress syndrome is becoming increasingly recognized as a complication of TBRF in the United States. However, life-threatening complications are unusual in otherwise healthy persons given supportive care, especially if the illness is diagnosed and treated early. Children generally have a milder course of illness than adults.

Without treatment, symptoms intensify over 2–7 days (average, 5 days in LBRF and 3 days in TBRF), ending in a spontaneous crisis that coincides with the disappearance of spirochetes from the circulation. The crisis comprises two phases over several hours: a *chill phase*, characterized by rigors, rising temperature, and hypermetabolism, and a *flush phase* of falling temperature, diaphoresis, and a decreased effective circulating blood volume. The pathophysiologic events associated with this crisis are magnified when precipitated by antibiotic treatment and are indistinguishable from the Jarisch-Herxheimer reaction of treated syphilis (see "Rx: Relapsing Fever," below). The crisis is followed by a period of exhaustion, sleep, and an uneventful recovery. Orthostatic hypotension is typical in the early recovery phase. Not uncommonly, in the first week of convalescence, the patient experiences 1 or 2 days of mild fever unassociated with detectable spirochetemia. In untreated patients, spirochetemia and symptoms may recur after a period of several days or weeks (average interval to first relapse, 9 days in LBRF and 7 days in TBRF). Only one or two relapses characteristically occur in untreated patients with LBRF, whereas as many as 10 (average, three) can occur in untreated patients with TBRF. In most cases, the illness becomes shorter and milder and the afebrile intervals longer with each relapse. Because of the great antigenic variation among *Borrelia* strains, infection confers only partial immunity, and repeated infections of the same individual have been recorded.

DIFFERENTIAL DIAGNOSIS AND LABORATORY FINDINGS

Diseases that should be considered in the differential diagnosis of relapsing fever or that may complicate relapsing fever include typhus fever, typhoid fever, nontyphoidal salmonellosis, malaria, dengue and other arboviral illnesses, tuberculosis, leptospirosis, and viral hemorrhagic fevers. In the United States, the geographic distribution of Colorado tick fever (Chap. 189) overlaps that of TBRF, and the two diseases have similar manifestations early in their courses.

The diagnosis of relapsing fever is confirmed most easily by the detection of spirochetes in blood, bone marrow aspirates, or cerebrospinal fluid. Motile spirochetes can be seen when specimens are examined by dark-field microscopy. Fixed organisms are clearly visible in Wright-, Giemsa-, or acridine orange–stained preparations of thin or dehemoglobinized thick smears of peripheral blood or buffy-coat preparations (Fig. 165-1). Organisms are most numerous in specimens taken during periods of high temperature preceding the crisis; smears of peripheral blood are positive in ≥70% of patients with LBRF and in a lower percentage of patients with TBRF. In reference laboratories, relapsing-fever spirochetes are cultured from blood by the inoculation of BSK II medium or by the intraperitoneal inoculation of immature laboratory mice. Serum antibodies to *Borrelia* can be detected by enzyme immunoassays, indirect fluorescent antibody (IFA) assay, and Western immunoblotting using whole-cell sonicates as antigen; however, these tests are unstandardized and are subject to insensitivity and cross-reactivity with other spirochetal agents, including *B. burgdorferi* (the agent of Lyme disease) and *Treponema pallidum*. The Western immunoblot test employing species-specific recombinant glycerophosphodiester phosphodiesterase (GlpQ) as antigen is more sensitive and specific than the whole-cell sonicate IFA test or the enzyme-linked immunosorbent assay.

Other laboratory findings in relapsing fever are nonspecific. The leukocyte count is normal or moderately elevated, with an unremarkable cell differential. Serum bilirubin levels are generally only slightly

FIGURE 165-1 Photomicrograph of tick-borne relapsing fever spirochete (*B. hermsii*) in a Wright-Giemsa-stained peripheral blood film.

elevated. Thrombocytopenia commonly occurs in relapsing-fever patients during the acute phase of the illness; platelet counts rebound during early convalescence. Prothrombin and partial thromboplastin times are often moderately prolonged during acute illness, as are standardized bleeding times. Fibrinogen concentrations in the blood are normal, and fibrinolysis is mild or absent. Results of the Rumpel-Leede tourniquet test for capillary fragility are negative, despite the presence of petechiae.

℞ RELAPSING FEVER

Relapsing-fever borreliae are exquisitely sensitive to antibiotics. Treatment with doxycycline (or another tetracycline), erythromycin, or chloramphenicol produces rapid clearance of spirochetes and a remission of symptoms **(Table 165-2)**. The response to a single dose of penicillin may be delayed and incomplete. Although a single dose of doxycycline (or another tetracycline), erythromycin, or chloramphenicol is highly effective in the treatment of LBRF, less is known about the efficacy of single-dose treatment of TBRF. Empirical treatment of TBRF for 7 days is therefore recommended to reduce the risk of persisting or relapsing borreliosis. For children <8 years of age and for pregnant women, erythromycin or penicillin may be preferred, given the potential adverse effects of tetracyclines.

Treatment of LBRF with a rapidly acting antibiotic regularly precipitates a Jarisch-Herxheimer-like reaction within 1–4 h of the first dose. This reac-

TABLE 165-2 ANTIBIOTIC TREATMENT OF LOUSE-BORNE AND TICK-BORNE RELAPSING FEVER IN ADULTS

Medication	Louse-Borne Relapsing Fever (Single Dose)	Tick-Borne Relapsing Fever (7-Day Schedule)
Oral		
Erythromycin	500 mg	500 mg q6h
Tetracycline	500 mg	500 mg q6h
Doxycycline	100 mg	100 mg q12h
Chloramphenicol	500 mg	500 mg q6h
Parenteral[a]		
Erythromycin	500 mg	500 mg q6h
Tetracycline	250 mg	250 mg q6h
Doxycycline	100 mg	100 mg q12h
Chloramphenicol	500 mg	500 mg q6h
Penicillin G (procaine)	600,000 IU	600,000 IU daily

[a]For tick-borne relapsing fever, parenteral therapy is used only until oral treatment is tolerated.

tion, which occurs in >50% of treated TBRF patients in North America, tends to be more severe when the patient has LBRF rather than TBRF and when high numbers of spirochetes are circulating in the bloodstream. In the chill phase of the reaction, rigors and rising fever are accompanied by an increasing metabolic rate, alveolar hyperventilation, high cardiac output, increasing peripheral vascular resistance, and decreased pulmonary arterial pressure. The body temperature commonly rises to ≥41°C (≥105.8°F). This high fever is accompanied often by agitation and confusion and sometimes by delirium. Fever can be partially controlled by the use of a cooling blanket and ice packs and by sponging of the patient with tepid water and alcohol. The chill phase terminates after 10–30 min, giving way to a flush phase characterized by a fall in body temperature, drenching sweats, and sometimes (more commonly in LBRF) a potentially dangerous fall in systemic arterial pressure and rise in pulmonary arterial pressure. Although cardiac output is maintained at high levels, the effective circulating blood volume decreases as peripheral vascular resistance falls. Vital signs must be monitored carefully during this period of the reaction, which usually lasts ≤8 h. Clinical and electrocardiographic evidence of myocarditis and myocardial dysfunction includes a prolonged QT_c interval, a third heart sound (S_3), elevated central venous pressure, arterial hypotension, and rare pulmonary congestion. The use of delayed-release IM penicillin may prolong or delay the clearance of spirochetes and thereby attenuate the accompanying Jarisch-Herxheimer reaction, but this response is not predictable; furthermore, single-dose penicillin treatment sometimes results in relapse of spirochetemia and symptoms. Glucocorticoids and nonsteroidal anti-inflammatory agents do not prevent or significantly modify the cardiopulmonary disturbances of the Jarisch-Herxheimer reaction, although hydrocortisone and acetaminophen given at the same time as antibiotics reduce peak body temperature. Although pretreatment with antibody to TNF-α may moderate the Jarisch-Herxheimer reaction in treated patients with LBRF, its use in LBRF is impractical and its use in TBRF (whose treatment is typically associated with a relatively mild Jarisch-Herxheimer reaction) is not warranted. Close monitoring of fluid balance, arterial and venous pressures, and myocardial function is advised in supportive management of the Jarisch-Herxheimer reaction in patients with LBRF.

The management of patients with relapsing fever–induced myocardial dysfunction requires caution in the administration of IV fluids and, in some cases, use of short-term inotropic therapy. The inability of heparin to control bleeding in LBRF suggests that disseminated intravascular coagulation is not important in its causation. Vitamin K and other soluble vitamins are sometimes given to counter dietary deficiencies in patients with LBRF. Because postural hypotension is often pronounced during the acute phase of relapsing fever and in the early stage of recovery, patients should be assisted when arising from bed.

Untreated LBRF has a high case-fatality rate, especially among persons in otherwise poor health, such as those in famine-affected populations. The fatality rate among treated persons is usually <5%. In general, TBRF is a milder disease than LBRF: the spontaneous crisis and the Jarisch-Herxheimer reactions are less pronounced and the case-fatality rates are lower for TBRF than for LBRF.

PREVENTION AND CONTROL

LBRF is best prevented by addressing socioeconomic circumstances that promote louse infestation (crowding, poverty, homelessness), by applying hygienic practices that reduce numbers of body lice (washing clothes, drying clothes in direct sunlight, changing clothes at frequent intervals), and by delousing. In infested situations like those in refugee camps, individuals, their clothes, and their bedding should be deloused with appropriate acaricides, such as 0.5% permethrin dust. Impregnation of clothing with liquid permethrin, a residual acaricide, can provide long-term protection against infestation. Spread of infection can be controlled by early case detection and treatment of infected persons and close contacts. In outbreaks of fever that involve louse-infested populations, empirical single-dose treatment with doxycycline will be effective against typhus as well as LBRF. *B. recurrentis* has a fragile life cycle and is eradicable.

In TBRF-endemic areas, risk of exposure can be reduced by avoiding rodent- and tick-infested dwellings and infested natural sites and by applying control measures. Access of rodents to foundation spaces, attics, and other harborages in dwellings, outbuildings, and their surroundings should be eliminated. Rodents and rodent nests should be removed from infested buildings. Tick harborages can be chemically treated by pest-control specialists using various acaricides, such as carbaryl, diazinon, chlorpyrifos, pyrethrins, and malathion. Persons who enter tick-infested sites can protect themselves by wearing clothing that denies ticks access to the skin, by applying repellents to exposed skin and to clothing, and by applying an acaricide containing permethrin to clothing. Reporting of suspected cases of relapsing fever to public health authorities is important so that an epidemiologic investigation and control measures can be initiated promptly. Prompt diagnosis and treatment of relapsing fever in pregnant women is important in avoiding the potentially severe consequences of fetal or neonatal infection.

FURTHER READINGS

CUTLER SJ et al: *Borrelia recurrentis* characterization and comparison with relapsing fever, Lyme-associated, and other *Borrelia* spp. Int J Syst Bacteriol 47:958, 1997

DAI Q et al: Antigenic variation by *Borrelia hermsii* occurs through recombination between extragenic repetitive elements on linear plasmids. Mol Microbiol 60:1329, 2006

DWORKIN MS et al: Tick-borne relapsing fever in North America. Med Clin North Am 86:417, 2002

GOODMAN JL et al (eds): *Tick-Borne Diseases of Humans.* Washington, DC, ASM Press, 2005

LONDONO D et al: Cardiac apoptosis in severe relapsing fever borreliosis. Infect Immun 73:7669, 2005

PAROLA P, RAOULT D: Ticks and tickborne bacterial diseases in humans: An emerging infectious threat. Clin Infect Dis 32:897, 2001

PAUL WS et al: Outbreak of tick-borne relapsing fever at the north rim of the Grand Canyon: Evidence for effectiveness of preventive measures. Am J Trop Med Hyg 66:71, 2002

PORCELLA SF et al: Serodiagnosis of louse-borne relapsing fever with glycerophosphodiester phosphodiesterase (GlpQ) from *Borrelia recurrentis*. J Clin Microbiol 38:3561, 2000

TAL H et al: Postexposure treatment with doxycycline for the prevention of tick-borne relapsing fever. N Engl J Med 355:148, 2006

VIAL L et al: Incidence of tick-borne relapsing fever in west Africa: Longitudinal study. Lancet 368:37, 2006

166 Lyme Borreliosis
Allen C. Steere

DEFINITION

Lyme borreliosis is caused by a spirochete, *Borrelia burgdorferi sensu lato*, that is transmitted by ticks of the *Ixodes ricinus* complex. The infection usually begins with a characteristic expanding skin lesion, erythema migrans (EM; stage 1, localized infection). After several days or weeks, the spirochete may spread to many different sites (stage 2, disseminated infection). Possible manifestations of disseminated infection include secondary annular skin lesions, meningitis, cranial neuritis, radiculoneuritis, peripheral neuritis, carditis, atrioventricular nodal block, or migratory musculoskeletal pain. Months or years later (usually after periods of latent infection), intermittent or chronic arthritis, chronic encephalopathy or polyneuropathy, or acrodermatitis may develop (stage 3, persistent infection). Most patients experience early symptoms of the illness during the summer, but the infection may not become symptomatic until it progresses to stage 2 or 3.

Lyme disease was recognized as a separate entity in 1976 because of geographic clustering of children in Lyme, Connecticut, who were thought to have juvenile rheumatoid arthritis. It became apparent that Lyme disease was a multisystem illness that affected primarily the skin, nervous system, heart, and joints. Epidemiologic studies of patients with EM implicated certain *Ixodes* ticks as vectors of the disease. Early in the twentieth century, EM had been described in Europe and attributed to *I. ricinus* tick bites. In 1982, a previously unrecognized spirochete, now called *Borrelia burgdorferi*, was recovered from *Ixodes scapularis* ticks and then from patients with Lyme disease. The entity is now called Lyme disease or Lyme borreliosis.

ETIOLOGIC AGENT

B. burgdorferi, the causative agent of Lyme disease, is a fastidious, microaerophilic bacterium. The spirochete's genome is quite small (~1.5 Mb) and consists of a highly unusual linear chromosome of 950 kb as well as 9 circular and 12 linear plasmids. The most remarkable aspect of the *B. burgdorferi* genome is that there are sequences for more than 100 known or predicted lipoproteins—a larger number than in any other organism. The spirochete has few proteins with biosynthetic activity and depends on its host for most of its nutritional requirements. It has no sequences for recognizable toxins.

 Currently, 13 closely related borrelial species are collectively referred to as *Borrelia burgdorferi sensu lato* (*B. burgdorferi* in the general sense). The human infection Lyme borreliosis is caused primarily by three pathogenic genospecies: *B. burgdorferi sensu stricto* (*B. burgdorferi* in the strict sense, hereafter referred to as *B. burgdorferi*), *Borrelia garinii*, and *Borrelia afzelii*. *B. burgdorferi* is the sole cause of the infection in the United States; all three genospecies are found in Europe, and the latter two species occur in Asia.

EPIDEMIOLOGY

The 13 known genospecies of *B. burgdorferi sensu lato* live in nature in enzootic cycles involving 14 different species of ticks that are part of the *I. ricinus* complex. *I. scapularis* (Fig. 392-1) is the principal vector in the northeastern United States from Maine to Virginia and in the midwestern states of Wisconsin and Minnesota. *I. pacificus* is the vector in the western states of California and Oregon. The disease is acquired throughout Europe (from Great Britain to Scandinavia to European Russia), where *I. ricinus* is the vector, and in Asian Russia, China, and Japan, where *I. persulcatus* is the vector. These ticks may transmit other diseases as well. In the United States, *I. scapularis* also transmits babesiosis and human anaplasmosis; in Europe and Asia, *I. ricinus* and *I. persulcatus* also transmit tick-borne encephalitis.

Ticks of the *I. ricinus* complex have larval, nymphal, and adult stages. They require a blood meal at each stage. The risk of infection in a given area depends largely on the density of these ticks as well as their feeding habits and animal hosts, which have evolved differently in different locations. For *I. scapularis* in the northeastern United States, the white-footed mouse and certain other rodents are the preferred hosts of the immature larvae and nymphs. It is critical that both of the tick's immature stages feed on the same host, because the life cycle of the spirochete depends on horizontal transmission: in early summer from infected nymphs to mice and in late summer from infected mice to larvae, which then molt to become the infected nymphs that will begin the cycle again the following year. It is the tiny nymphal tick that is primarily responsible for transmission of the disease to humans during the early summer months. White-tailed deer, which are not involved in the life cycle of the spirochete, are the preferred host for the adult stage of *I. scapularis* and seem to be critical to the tick's survival.

Lyme disease is now the most common vector-borne infection in the United States and Europe. Since surveillance was begun by the Centers for Disease Control and Prevention (CDC) in 1982, the number of cases in the United States has increased dramatically. More than 20,000 new cases are now reported each summer. In Europe, the highest reported frequencies of the disease are in the middle of the continent and in Scandinavia.

PATHOGENESIS AND IMMUNITY

To maintain its complex enzootic cycle, *B. burgdorferi* must adapt to two markedly different environments: the tick and the mammalian host. The spirochete expresses outer-surface protein A (OspA) in the midgut of the tick, whereas OspC is upregulated as the organism travels to the tick's salivary gland. There, OspC binds a tick salivary-gland protein (Salp15), which is required for infection of the mammalian host. The tick must usually be attached for at least 24 h for transmission of *B. burgdorferi*.

After injection into the human skin, *B. burgdorferi* may migrate outward, producing EM, and may spread hematogenously or in the lymph to other organs. The only known virulence factors of *B. burgdorferi* are surface proteins that allow the spirochete to attach to mammalian proteins, integrins, glycosaminoglycans, or glycoproteins. For example, spread through the skin and other tissue matrices may be facilitated by the binding of human plasminogen and its activators to the surface of the spirochete. Some *Borrelia* strains bind complement regulator–acquiring surface proteins (FHL-1/reconectin, or factor H), which help to protect spirochetes from complement-mediated lysis. Dissemination of the organism in the blood is facilitated by binding to the fibrinogen receptor on activated platelets ($\alpha_{IIb}\beta_3$) and the vitronectin receptor ($\alpha_v\beta_3$) on endothelial cells. Spirochetal decorin-binding proteins A and B bind decorin, a glycosaminoglycan on collagen fibrils; this binding may explain why the organism is commonly aligned with collagen fibrils in the extracellular matrix in the heart, nervous system, or joints.

To control and eradicate *B. burgdorferi*, the host mounts both innate and adaptive immune responses, resulting in macrophage- and antibody-mediated killing of the spirochete. As part of the innate immune response, complement may lyse the spirochete in the skin. Chemokines released by constituent cells in the skin lead to the recruitment of neutrophils and macrophages; the latter release potent proinflammatory cytokines. The purpose of the adaptive immune response appears to be the production of specific antibodies, which opsonize the organism—a step necessary for optimal spirochetal killing. Histologic examination of all affected tissues reveals an infiltration of lymphocytes, macrophages, and plasma cells with some degree of vascular damage (including mild vasculitis or hypervascular occlusion). These findings suggest that the spirochete may have been present in or around blood vessels.

Despite the innate and adaptive immune responses, *B. burgdorferi* may sometimes survive in certain sites, such as collagen bundles in synovial tissue. The ability of the spirochete to downregulate the expression of surface-exposed protein antigens and, in the case of the VlsE lipoprotein, the ability to change amino acid sequences in the protein are important mechanisms of immune evasion. However, in the battle between *B. burgdorferi* survival factors and host immune responses, spirochetes do not seem to be able to survive indefinitely against the immune responses of normal human patients. Moreover, the organisms do not have mechanisms that help to protect them from antibiotic therapy. For example, *B. burgdorferi* has only been seen extracellularly in affected tissues; it has not been shown to "hide out" in intracellular locations, thereby evading antibiotic exposure.

CLINICAL MANIFESTATIONS

Early Infection: Stage 1 (Localized Infection)   Because of the small size of nymphal ixodid ticks, most patients do not remember the preceding tick bite. After an incubation period of 3–32 days, EM, which occurs at the site of the tick bite, usually begins as a red macule or papule that expands slowly to form a large annular lesion (Fig. 166-1). As the lesion increases in size, it often develops a bright red outer border and partial central clearing. The center of the lesion sometimes becomes intensely erythematous and indurated, vesicular, or necrotic. In other instances, the expanding lesion remains an even, intense red; several red rings are found within an outside ring; or the central area turns

FIGURE 166-1   A classic erythema migrans lesion (9 cm in diameter) is shown near the right axilla. The lesion has partial central clearing, a bright red outer border, and a target center. *(Courtesy of Vijay K. Sikand, MD; with permission.)*

blue before the lesion clears. Although EM can be located anywhere, the thigh, groin, and axilla are particularly common sites. The lesion is warm but not often painful. Approximately 20% of patients do not exhibit this characteristic skin manifestation.

Early Infection: Stage 2 (Disseminated Infection)   In cases in the United States, *B. burgdorferi* often spreads hematogenously to many sites within days or weeks after the onset of EM. In these cases, patients may develop secondary annular skin lesions similar in appearance to the initial lesion. Skin involvement is commonly accompanied by severe headache, mild stiffness of the neck, fever, chills, migratory musculoskeletal pain, arthralgias, and profound malaise and fatigue. Less common manifestations include generalized lymphadenopathy or splenomegaly, hepatitis, sore throat, nonproductive cough, conjunctivitis, iritis, or testicular swelling. Except for fatigue and lethargy, which are often constant, the early signs and symptoms of Lyme disease are typically intermittent and changing. Even in untreated patients, the early symptoms usually become less severe or disappear within several weeks. In ~15% of patients, the infection presents with these nonspecific systemic symptoms.

Symptoms suggestive of meningeal irritation may develop early in Lyme disease when EM is present but usually are not associated with cerebrospinal fluid (CSF) pleocytosis or an objective neurologic deficit. After several weeks or months, ~15% of untreated patients develop frank neurologic abnormalities, including meningitis, subtle encephalitic signs, cranial neuritis (including bilateral facial palsy), motor or sensory radiculoneuropathy, peripheral neuropathy, mononeuritis multiplex, cerebellar ataxia, or myelitis—alone or in various combinations. In the United States, the usual pattern consists of fluctuating symptoms of meningitis accompanied by facial palsy and peripheral radiculoneuropathy. Lymphocytic pleocytosis (~100 cells/μL) is found in CSF, often along with elevated protein levels and normal or slightly low glucose concentrations. In Europe and Asia, the first neurologic sign is characteristically radicular pain, which is followed by the development of CSF pleocytosis (called meningopolyneuritis, or *Bannwarth's syndrome*); meningeal or encephalitic signs are frequently absent. In children, the optic nerve may be affected because of inflammation or increased intracranial pressure, which may lead to blindness. These early neurologic abnormalities usually resolve completely within months, but in rare cases chronic neurologic disease may occur later.

Within several weeks after the onset of illness, ~8% of patients develop cardiac involvement. The most common abnormality is a fluctuating degree of atrioventricular block (first-degree, Wenckebach, or complete heart block). Some patients have more diffuse cardiac involvement, including electrocardiographic changes indicative of acute myopericarditis, left ventricular dysfunction evident on radionuclide scans, or (in rare cases) cardiomegaly or pancarditis. Cardiac involvement usually lasts for only a few weeks but may recur. Chronic cardiomyopathy caused by *B. burgdorferi* has been reported in Europe.

During this stage, musculoskeletal pain is common. The typical pattern consists of migratory pain in joints, tendons, bursae, muscles, or bones (usually without joint swelling) lasting for hours or days and affecting one or two locations at a time.

Late Infection: Stage 3 (Persistent Infection) Months after the onset of infection, ~60% of patients in the United States who have received no antibiotic treatment develop frank arthritis. The typical pattern comprises intermittent attacks of oligoarticular arthritis in large joints (especially the knees), lasting for weeks or months in a given joint. A few small joints or periarticular sites may also be affected, primarily during early attacks. The number of patients who continue to have recurrent attacks decreases each year. However, in a small percentage of cases, involvement of large joints—usually one or both knees—becomes chronic and may lead to erosion of cartilage and bone.

White cell counts in joint fluid range from 500–110,000/μL (average, 25,000/μL); most of these cells are polymorphonuclear leukocytes. Tests for rheumatoid factor or antinuclear antibodies usually give negative results. Examination of synovial biopsy samples reveals fibrin deposits, villous hypertrophy, vascular proliferation, microangiopathic lesions, and a heavy infiltration of lymphocytes and plasma cells.

Although most patients with Lyme arthritis respond well to antibiotic therapy, a small percentage have persistent arthritis for months or even for several years after the apparent eradication of spirochetes from the joints by antibiotic therapy. Compared with antibiotic-responsive patients, those with antibiotic-refractory arthritis have a higher frequency of certain class II major histocompatibility complex molecules (particularly HLA-DRBI*0401 or -*0101 molecules) that bind an epitope of OspA (OspA$_{163-175}$), and they often exhibit T cell recognition of this epitope. In addition, these patients have significantly higher levels of proinflammatory chemokines and cytokines in joint fluid (especially CXCL9 and interferon γ) than do antibiotic-responsive patients; these higher levels persist during the postantibiotic period, when polymerase chain reaction (PCR) results for *B. burgdorferi* DNA are uniformly negative. It has been postulated that, in these genetically susceptible individuals, *B. burgdorferi* may trigger autoimmunity within the proinflammatory milieu of the joints.

Although less common, chronic neurologic involvement may also become apparent months to several years after the onset of infection, sometimes following long periods of latent infection. The most common form of chronic central nervous system involvement is subtle encephalopathy affecting memory, mood, or sleep, and the most common form of peripheral neuropathy is an axonal polyneuropathy manifested as either distal paresthesia or spinal radicular pain. Patients with encephalopathy frequently have evidence of memory impairment in neuropsychological tests and abnormal results in CSF analyses. In cases of polyneuropathy, electromyography generally shows extensive abnormalities of proximal and distal nerve segments. Encephalomyelitis or leukoencephalitis, a rare manifestation of Lyme borreliosis associated primarily with *B. garinii* infection in Europe, is a severe neurologic disorder that may include spastic paraparesis, upper motor-neuron bladder dysfunction, and, rarely, lesions in the periventricular white matter.

Acrodermatitis chronica atrophicans, the late skin manifestation of the disorder, has been associated primarily with *B. afzelii* infection in Europe and Asia. It has been observed especially often in elderly women. The skin lesions, which are usually found on the acral surface of an arm or leg, begin insidiously with reddish-violaceous discoloration; they become sclerotic or atrophic over a period of years.

The basic patterns of Lyme borreliosis are similar worldwide, but there are regional variations, primarily between the illness found in America, which is caused exclusively by *B. burgdorferi*, and that found in Europe, which is caused primarily by *B. afzelii* and *B. garinii*. With each of the *Borrelia* spp., the infection usually begins with EM. However, *B. burgdorferi* often disseminates widely; it is particularly arthritogenic, and it may cause antibiotic-refractory arthritis. *B. garinii* typically disseminates less widely, but it is especially neurotropic and

may cause borrelial encephalomyelitis. *B. afzelii* often infects only the skin but may persist in that site, where it may cause several different dermatoborrelioses, including acrodermatitis chronica atrophicans.

DIAGNOSIS

The culture of *B. burgdorferi* in Barbour-Stoenner-Kelly (BSK) medium permits definitive diagnosis, but this method has been used primarily in research studies. Moreover, with a few exceptions, positive cultures have been obtained only early in the illness—particularly from biopsy samples of EM skin lesions, less often from plasma samples, and occasionally from CSF samples. Later in the infection, PCR is greatly superior to culture for the detection of *B. burgdorferi* DNA in joint fluid—the major use for PCR testing in Lyme disease. However, the sensitivity of PCR determinations in CSF from patients with neuroborreliosis has been much lower. There seems to be little if any role for PCR in the detection of *B. burgdorferi* DNA in blood or urine samples. Moreover, this procedure, which must be carefully controlled to prevent contamination, is not routinely available.

Because of the problems associated with direct detection of *B. burgdorferi*, Lyme disease is usually diagnosed by the recognition of a characteristic clinical picture with serologic confirmation. Although serologic testing may yield negative results during the first several weeks of infection, most patients have a positive antibody response to *B. burgdorferi* after that time. The limitation of serologic tests is that they do not clearly distinguish between active and inactive infection. Patients with previous Lyme disease—particularly in cases progressing to late stages—often remain seropositive for years, even after adequate antibiotic treatment. In addition, ~10% of patients are seropositive because of asymptomatic infection. If these individuals subsequently develop another illness, the positive serologic test for Lyme disease may cause diagnostic confusion. According to an algorithm published by the American College of Physicians (Table 166-1), serologic testing for Lyme disease is recommended only for patients with at least an intermediate pretest probability of Lyme disease, such as those with oligoarticular arthritis. It should not be used as a screening procedure in patients with pain or fatigue syndromes. In such patients, the probability of a false-positive serologic result is higher than that of a true-positive result.

For serologic analysis of Lyme disease in the United States, the CDC recommends a two-step approach in which samples are first tested by enzyme-linked immunosorbent assay (ELISA) and equivocal or positive results are then tested by Western blotting. During the first month of infection, both IgM and IgG responses to the spirochete should be determined, preferably in both acute- and convalescent-phase serum samples. Approximately 20–30% of patients have a positive response detectable in acute-phase samples, whereas ~70–80% have a positive response during convalescence (2–4 weeks later). After 1 month of infection (by which time most patients with active Lyme disease have disseminated infection), the sensitivity and specificity of the IgG response to the spirochete are both very high—in the range of 95–99%—as determined by the two-test approach of ELISA and Western blot. At this point and thereafter, a single test (that for IgG) is usually sufficient. In persons with illness of >1

TABLE 166-1	**ALGORITHM FOR TESTING FOR AND TREATING LYME DISEASE**

Pretest Probability	Example	Recommendation
High	Patients with erythema migrans	Empirical antibiotic treatment without serologic testing
Intermediate	Patients with oligoarticular arthritis	Serologic testing and antibiotic treatment if test results are positive
Low	Patients with nonspecific symptoms (myalgias, arthralgias, fatigue)	Neither serologic testing nor antibiotic treatment

Source: Adapted from the recommendations of the American College of Physicians (G Nichol et al: Ann Intern Med 128:37, 1998, with permission).

month's duration, a positive IgM test result alone is likely to be false-positive and therefore should not be used to support the diagnosis.

According to current criteria adopted by the CDC, an IgM Western blot is considered positive if two of the following three bands are present: 23, 39, and 41 kDa. However, the combination of the 23- and 41-kDa bands may still represent a false-positive result. An IgG blot is considered positive if 5 of the following 10 bands are present: 18, 23, 28, 30, 39, 41, 45, 58, 66, and 93 kDa. In European cases, there is less expansion of the antibody response, and no single set of criteria for the interpretation of immunoblots results in high levels of sensitivity and specificity in all countries.

Several second-generation tests that use recombinant spirochetal proteins or synthetic peptides have shown promising results. For example, an IgG ELISA employing a 26-mer peptide from invariant region 6 (IR$_6$) of the VlsE lipoprotein has a sensitivity and a specificity similar to those achieved with the IgM and IgG two-test approach using sonicated whole spirochetes. However, the IR$_6$ ELISA has a limitation similar to that affecting standard serology, in that a positive test result does not distinguish clearly between active and past infection. The IR$_6$ ELISA may be of value with regard to European as well as American strains of the spirochete.

DIFFERENTIAL DIAGNOSIS

Classic EM is a slowly expanding erythema, often with partial central clearing. If the lesion expands little, it may represent the red papule of an uninfected tick bite. If the lesion expands rapidly, it may represent cellulitis (e.g., streptococcal cellulitis) or an allergic reaction, perhaps to tick saliva. Patients with secondary annular lesions may be thought to have erythema multiforme, but neither the development of blistering mucosal lesions nor the involvement of the palms or soles is a feature of *B. burgdorferi* infection. In the southeastern United States, an EM-like skin lesion, sometimes with mild systemic symptoms, may be associated with *Amblyomma americanum* tick bites, but the cause of this illness has not yet been identified.

In the United States, *I. scapularis* ticks may transmit not only *B. burgdorferi* but also *Babesia microti*, a red blood cell parasite (Chap. 204), or *Anaplasma phagocytophilum*, the agent of human granulocytotropic anaplasmosis (formerly human granulocytotropic ehrlichiosis; Chap. 167). Although babesiosis and anaplasmosis are most often asymptomatic, infection with any of these three agents may cause nonspecific systemic symptoms, and co-infected patients may have more severe or persistent symptoms than patients infected with a single agent. Standard blood counts may yield clues regarding the presence of co-infection. Anaplasmosis may cause leukopenia or thrombocytopenia, and babesiosis may cause thrombocytopenia or (in severe cases) hemolytic anemia. IgM serologic responses may confuse the diagnosis. For example, *A. phagocytophilum* may elicit a positive IgM response to *B. burgdorferi*. The frequency of co-infection in different studies has been variable. In one prospective study, 4% of patients with EM had evidence of co-infection.

Facial palsy caused by *B. burgdorferi*, which occurs in the early disseminated phase of the infection (often in July, August, or September), is usually recognized by its association with EM. However, in rare cases, facial palsy without EM may be the presenting manifestation of Lyme disease. In such cases, both the IgM and the IgG responses to the spirochete are usually positive. The most common infectious agents that cause facial palsy are herpes simplex virus type 1 (Bell's palsy; Chap. 172) and varicella-zoster virus (Ramsay Hunt syndrome; Chap. 173).

Later in the infection, oligoarticular Lyme arthritis most resembles reactive arthritis in an adult or the pauciarticular form of juvenile rheumatoid arthritis in a child. Patients with Lyme arthritis usually have the highest IgG antibody responses seen in the infection, with reactivity to many spirochetal proteins.

The most common problem in diagnosis is to mistake Lyme disease for chronic fatigue syndrome (Chap. 384) or fibromyalgia (Chap. 329). This difficulty is compounded by the fact that a small percentage of patients do in fact develop these chronic pain or fatigue syndromes in association with or soon after Lyme disease. Compared with Lyme disease, chronic fatigue syndrome or fibromyalgia tends to produce more generalized and disabling symptoms, including marked fatigue, severe headache, diffuse musculoskeletal pain, multiple symmetric tender points in characteristic locations, pain and stiffness in many joints, diffuse dysesthesia, difficulty with concentration, and sleep disturbances. Patients with chronic fatigue syndrome or fibromyalgia lack evidence of joint inflammation; they have normal results in neurologic tests; and they usually have a greater degree of anxiety and depression than patients with chronic neuroborreliosis.

℞ LYME BORRELIOSIS

As outlined in the algorithm in **Fig. 166-2**, the various manifestations of Lyme disease can usually be treated successfully with orally administered antibiotics; the exceptions are objective neurologic abnormalities and third-degree atrioventricular heart block, which are generally treated with IV antibiotics. For early Lyme disease, doxycycline is effective in men and in nonpregnant women. An advantage of this regimen is that it is also effective against *A. phagocytophilum*, which is transmitted by the same tick that transmits the Lyme disease agent. Amoxicillin, cefuroxime axetil, and erythromycin or its congeners are second-, third-, and fourth-choice alternatives, respectively. In children, amoxicillin is effective (not more than 2 g/d); in cases of penicillin allergy, cefuroxime axetil or erythromycin may be used. In contrast to second- or third-generation cephalosporin antibiotics, first-generation cephalosporins, such as cephalexin, are not effective. For patients with infection localized to the skin, a 14-day course of therapy is generally sufficient; in contrast, for patients with disseminated infection, a 21-day course is recommended. Approximately 15% of patients experience a Jarisch-Herxheimer-like reaction during the first 24 h of therapy. In multicenter studies, >90% of patients whose early Lyme disease was treated with these regimens had satisfactory outcomes. Although some pa-

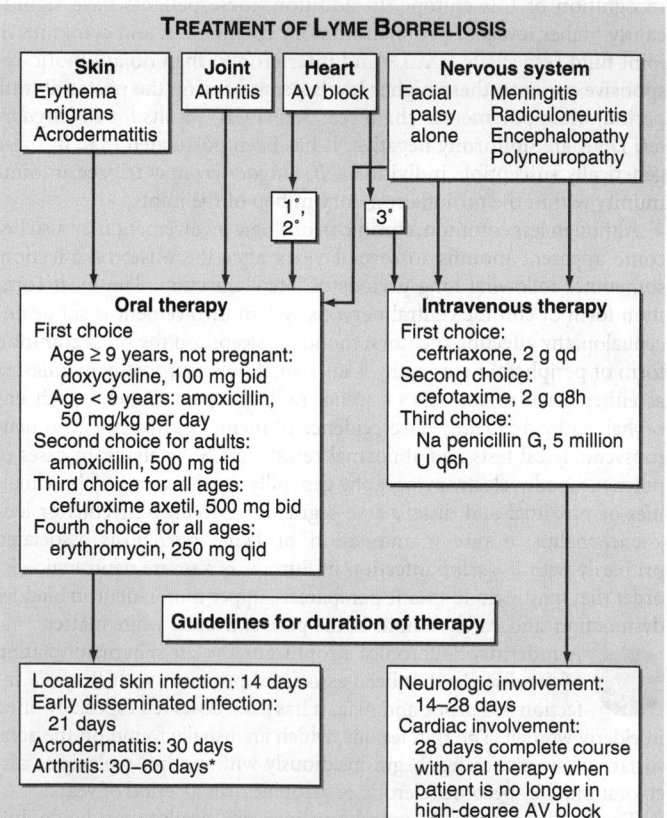

TREATMENT OF LYME BORRELIOSIS

Skin	Joint	Heart	Nervous system	
Erythema migrans Acrodermatitis	Arthritis	AV block	Facial palsy alone	Meningitis Radiculoneuritis Encephalopathy Polyneuropathy

1°, 2°   3°

Oral therapy
First choice
  Age ≥ 9 years, not pregnant: doxycycline, 100 mg bid
  Age < 9 years: amoxicillin, 50 mg/kg per day
Second choice for adults: amoxicillin, 500 mg tid
Third choice for all ages: cefuroxime axetil, 500 mg bid
Fourth choice for all ages: erythromycin, 250 mg qid

Intravenous therapy
First choice: ceftriaxone, 2 g qd
Second choice: cefotaxime, 2 g q8h
Third choice: Na penicillin G, 5 million U q6h

Guidelines for duration of therapy

Localized skin infection: 14 days
Early disseminated infection: 21 days
Acrodermatitis: 30 days
Arthritis: 30–60 days*

Neurologic involvement: 14–28 days
Cardiac involvement: 28 days complete course with oral therapy when patient is no longer in high-degree AV block

FIGURE 166-2 Algorithm for the treatment of the various acute or chronic manifestations of Lyme borreliosis. AV, atrioventricular. *For Lyme arthritis, IV ceftriaxone (2 g given once a day for 14–28 days) is also effective and is necessary for a small percentage of patients; however, compared with oral treatment, this regimen is less convenient to administer, has more side effects, and is more expensive.

tients reported symptoms after treatment, objective evidence of persistent infection or relapse was rare, and re-treatment was usually unnecessary.

Oral administration of doxycycline or amoxicillin for 30 days is recommended for the initial treatment of Lyme arthritis in patients who do not have concomitant neurologic involvement. Among patients with arthritis who do not respond to oral antibiotics, re-treatment with IV ceftriaxone for 28 days is appropriate. In patients with arthritis in whom joint inflammation persists for months or even several years after both oral and IV antibiotics, despite a negative PCR result for *B. burgdorferi* DNA in joint fluid, treatment with anti-inflammatory agents or synovectomy may be successful.

For objective neurologic abnormalities (with the possible exception of facial palsy alone), parenteral antibiotic therapy is indicated. IV ceftriaxone, given for 14–28 days, is most commonly used for this purpose, but IV cefotaxime or IV penicillin G for the same duration may also be effective. In patients with high-degree atrioventricular block or a PR interval > 0.3 s, IV therapy for at least part of the course and cardiac monitoring are recommended, but the insertion of a permanent pacemaker is not necessary.

It is unclear how and whether asymptomatic infection should be treated, but patients with such infection are often given a course of oral antibiotics. Because maternal-fetal transmission of *B. burgdorferi* seems to occur rarely (if at all), standard therapy for the manifestations of the illness is recommended for pregnant women. Long-term persistence of *B. burgdorferi* has not been documented in any large series of patients after treatment with currently recommended regimens. Therefore, there is no indication for multiple, repeated antibiotic courses in the treatment of Lyme disease.

After appropriately treated Lyme disease, a small percentage of patients continue to have subjective symptoms, primarily musculoskeletal pain, neurocognitive difficulties, or fatigue. This *chronic Lyme disease* or *post–Lyme syndrome* is a disabling condition that is similar to chronic fatigue syndrome or fibromyalgia. In a large study, one group of patients with post–Lyme syndrome received IV ceftriaxone for 30 days followed by oral doxycycline for 60 days, while another group received IV and oral placebo preparations for the same durations. No significant differences were found between groups in the numbers of patients reporting that their symptoms had improved, become worse, or stayed the same. Such patients are best treated for the relief of symptoms rather than with prolonged courses of antibiotics.

The risk of infection with *B. burgdorferi* after a recognized tick bite is so low that antibiotic prophylaxis is not routinely indicated. However, if an attached, engorged *I. scapularis* nymph is found or if follow-up is anticipated to be difficult, a single 200-mg dose of doxycycline, which usually prevents Lyme disease when given within 72 h after the tick bite, may be administered.

PROGNOSIS

The response to treatment is best early in the disease. Later treatment of Lyme borreliosis is still effective, but the period of convalescence may be longer. Eventually, most patients recover with minimal or no residual deficits.

REINFECTION

Reinfection may occur after EM when patients are treated with antimicrobial agents. In such cases, the immune response is not adequate to provide protection from subsequent infection. However, patients who develop an expanded immune response to the spirochete over a period of months (such as those with Lyme arthritis) have protective immunity for a period of years and do not acquire the infection again.

PREVENTION

Protective measures for the prevention of Lyme disease may include the avoidance of tick-infested areas, the use of repellents and acaricides, tick checks, and modification of landscapes in or near residential areas. Although a vaccine for Lyme disease used to be available, the manufacturer has discontinued its production. Therefore, no vaccine is now commercially available for the prevention of this infection.

FURTHER READINGS

BACON RM et al: Serodiagnosis of Lyme disease by kinetic immunosorbent assay using recombinant VlsE1 or peptide antigens of *Borrelia burgdorferi* compared with 2-tiered testing using whole-cell lysates. J Infect Dis 187:1187, 2003

KLEMPNER MS et al: Two controlled trials of antibiotic treatment in patients with persistent symptoms and a history of Lyme disease. N Engl J Med 345:85, 2001

NADELMAN RB et al: Prophylaxis with single-dose doxycycline for the prevention of Lyme disease after *Ixodes scapularis* tick bite. N Engl J Med 345:79, 2001

STEERE AC: Lyme disease. N Engl J Med 345:115, 2001

———, ANGELIS SM: Therapy for Lyme arthritis: Strategies for the treatment of antibiotic-refractory arthritis. Arthritis Rheum 54:3079, 2006

——— et al: Antibiotic-refractory Lyme arthritis is associated with HLA-DR molecules that bind a *Borrelia burgdorferi* peptide. J Exp Med 203:961, 2006

——— et al: The emergence of Lyme disease. J Clin Invest 113:1093, 2004

WORMSER GP et al: The clinical assessment, treatment and prevention of Lyme disease, anaplasmosis, and babesiosis: Clinical practice guidelines of the Infectious Diseases Society of America. Clin Infect Dis 43:1089, 2006

SECTION 10 DISEASES CAUSED BY RICKETTSIAE, MYCOPLASMAS, AND CHLAMYDIAE

167 Rickettsial Diseases

David H. Walker, J. Stephen Dumler, Thomas Marrie

The rickettsiae are a heterogeneous group of small, obligately intracellular, gram-negative coccobacilli and short bacilli, most of which are transmitted by a tick, mite, flea, or louse vector. Except for louse-borne typhus, humans are incidental hosts. Among rickettsiae, *Coxiella burnetii*, *Rickettsia prowazekii*, and *R. typhi* have the well-documented ability to survive for an extended period outside the reservoir or vector and to be extremely infectious: inhalation of a single *Coxiella* microorganism can cause pneumonia. High infectivity and severe illness after inhalation make *R. prowazekii*, *R. rickettsii*, *R. typhi*, *R. conorii*, and *C. burnetii* bioterrorism threats.

 Clinical infections with rickettsiae can be classified according to (1) the taxonomy and diverse microbial characteristics of the agents, which belong to six genera (*Rickettsia*, *Orientia*, *Ehrlichia*, *Anaplasma*, *Neorickettsia*, and *Coxiella*); (2) epidemiology; or (3) clinical manifestations. The clinical manifestations of all the acute presentations are similar during the first 5 days: fever, headache, and myalgias with or without nausea, vomiting, and cough. As the course progresses, clinical manifestations—including occurrence of a macular, maculopapular, or vesicular rash; eschar; pneumonitis; and meningoencephalitis—vary from one disease to another. Given the 12 etiologic agents with varied mechanisms of transmission, geographic distribu-

TABLE 167-1 FEATURES OF SELECTED RICKETTSIAL INFECTIONS

Disease	Organism	Transmission	Geographic Range	Incubation Period (Days)	Duration (Days)	Rash (%)	Eschar (%)	Lymphade-nopathy[a]
Rocky Mountain spotted fever	Rickettsia rickettsii	Tick bite: Dermacentor andersoni	United States	2–14	10–20	90	<1	+
		D. variabilis	United States					
		Amblyomma cajennense, A. aureolatum	Central/South America					
		Rhipicephalus sanguineus	Mexico, United States					
Mediterranean spotted fever[b]	R. conorii	Tick bite: R. sanguineus, R. pumilio	Southern Europe, Africa, Middle East, Central Asia	5–7	7–14	97	50	+
African tick-bite fever	R. africae	Tick bite: A. hebraeum, A. variegatum	Sub-Saharan Africa, West Indies	4–10	?	50	90	++++
Rickettsialpox	R. akari	Mite bite: Liponyssoides sanguineus	United States, Ukraine, Croatia	10–17	3–11	100	90	+++
Flea-borne spotted fever	R. felis	Flea (mechanism undetermined): Ctenocephalides felis	North and South America, Europe	8–16	8–16	80	15	—
Epidemic typhus	R. prowazekii	Louse feces: Pediculus humanus corporis, fleas and lice of flying squirrels, or recrudescence	Worldwide	7–14	10–18	80	None	—
Tick-borne lymphadenopathy	R. slovaca	Tick bite: Dermacentor marginatus, D. reticularis	Europe	7–9	17–180	5	100	++++
Murine typhus	R. typhi	Flea feces: Xenopsylla cheopis, C. felis, others	Worldwide	8–16	8–16	80	None	—
Human monocytotropic ehrlichiosis	Ehrlichia chaffeensis	Tick bite: Amblyomma americanum, D. variabilis	United States	1–21	3–21	36	None	++
Human granulocytotropic anaplasmosis	Anaplasma phagocytophilum	Tick bite: Ixodes scapularis, I. ricinus, I. pacificus	United States, Europe, Asia	1–21	3–14	Rare	None	—
Scrub typhus	Orientia tsutsugamushi	Mite bite: Leptotrombidium deliense, others	Asia, Australia, New Guinea, Pacific Islands	9–18	6–21	50	35	+++
Q fever	Coxiella burnetii	Inhalation of aerosols of infected parturition material (sheep, dogs, others), ingestion of infected milk or milk products	Worldwide	3–30	5–57	<1	None	—

[a]++++, severe; +++, marked; ++, moderate; +, present in a small portion of cases; —, not a noted feature.
[b]Eschar is usually present at the bite site.

tions, and associated disease manifestations, the consideration of rickettsial diseases as a single entity poses complex challenges (Table 167-1).

Establishing the etiologic diagnosis of rickettsioses is very difficult during the acute stage of illness, and definitive diagnosis usually requires the examination of paired serum samples after convalescence. Heightened clinical suspicion is based on epidemiologic data, history of exposure to vectors or reservoir animals, travel to endemic locations, clinical manifestations (sometimes including rash or eschar), and characteristic laboratory findings [including thrombocytopenia, normal or low white blood cell (WBC) counts, elevated hepatic enzyme levels, and hyponatremia]. Such suspicion should prompt empirical treatment. Doxycycline is the drug of choice for most of these infections. Only one agent, C. burnetii, has been documented to cause chronic illness. One other, R. prowazekii, causes recrudescent illness (Brill-Zinsser disease) when latent infection is reactivated years after resolution of the acute illness.

Rickettsial infections dominated by fever may resolve without further clinical evolution. However, after nonspecific early manifestations, the illnesses can also evolve along one or more of several principal clinical lines: (1) development of a macular or maculopapular rash; (2) development of an eschar at the site of tick or mite feeding; (3) development of a vesicular rash (often in rickettsialpox and African tick-bite fever); (4) development of pneumonitis with chest radiographic opacities and/or rales [Q fever and severe cases of Rocky Mountain spotted fever (RMSF), Mediterranean spotted fever (MSF), louse-borne typhus, human monocytotropic ehrlichiosis (HME), human granulocytotropic anaplasmosis (HGA), scrub typhus, and murine typhus]; (5) development of meningoencephalitis [louse-borne typhus and severe cases of RMSF, scrub typhus, HME, murine typhus, MSF, and (rarely) Q fever]; and (6) progressive hypotension and multiorgan failure as seen with sepsis or toxic shock syndrome (RMSF, MSF, louse-borne typhus, murine typhus, scrub typhus, HME, and HGA).

Epidemiologic clues to the transmission of a particular pathogen include (1) environmental exposure to ticks, fleas, or mites during the season of activity of the vector species for the disease in the appropriate geographic region (spotted fever and typhus group rickettsioses, scrub typhus, ehrlichioses, anaplasmosis); (2) travel to or residence in an endemic geographic region during the incubation period (Table 167-1); (3) exposure to parturient ruminants, cats, and dogs (Q fever); (4) exposure to flying squirrels (R. prowazekii infection); and (5) history of previous louse-borne typhus (recrudescent typhus).

Clinical laboratory findings, such as thrombocytopenia (particularly in spotted fever and typhus rickettsioses, ehrlichioses, anaplasmosis, and scrub typhus), normal or low WBC counts, mild to moderate serum elevations of hepatic aminotransferases, and hyponatremia suggest some common pathophysiologic mechanisms.

Application of these clinical, epidemiologic, and laboratory principles requires a consideration of the possibility of a rickettsial diagnosis and a knowledge of the individual diseases.

TICK-, MITE-, LOUSE-, AND FLEA-BORNE RICKETTSIOSES

These diseases, caused by organisms of the genera *Rickettsia* and *Orientia* in the family Rickettsiaceae, result from endothelial infection and increased vascular permeability. Pathogenic rickettsial species are very closely related, have small genomes (as a result of reductive evolution, which eliminated genes for biosynthesis of intracellularly available molecules), and are traditionally separated into typhus and spotted fever groups on the basis of lipopolysaccharide antigens. Some diseases and their agents (e.g., *R. africae*, *R. parkeri*, and *R. sibirica*) are too similar to require separate descriptions. Indeed, the similarities among MSF (*R. conorii*, all strains), North Asian tick typhus (*R. sibirica*), Japanese spotted fever (*R. japonica*), and Flinders Island spotted fever (*R. honei*) far outweigh the minor variations. The Rickettsiaceae that cause life-threatening infections are, in order of decreasing case-fatality rate, *R. rickettsii* (RMSF); *R. prowazekii* (louse-borne typhus); *Orientia tsutsugamushi* (scrub typhus); *R. conorii* (MSF); *R. typhi* (murine typhus); and, in rare cases, other spotted fever group organisms. Some agents (e.g., *R. africae*, *R. akari*, *R. slovaca*, *R. honei*, *R. felis*, *R. aeschlimannii*, and *R. parkeri*) have never been documented to cause a fatal illness.

ROCKY MOUNTAIN SPOTTED FEVER

RMSF occurs in 48 states (with the highest prevalence in the south-central and southeastern states) as well as in Canada, Mexico, and Central and South America. The infection is transmitted by *Dermacentor variabilis*, the American dog tick, in the eastern two-thirds of the United States and California; by *D. andersoni*, the Rocky Mountain wood tick, in the western United States; by *Rhipicephalus sanguineus* in Mexico and Arizona; and by *Amblyomma cajennense* in Central and South America. Maintained principally by transovarial transmission from one generation of ticks to the next, *R. rickettsii* can be acquired by uninfected ticks through the ingestion of a blood meal from rickettsemic small mammals.

Humans become infected during tick season (in the Northern Hemisphere, from May to September), although some cases occur in winter. The mortality rate was 20–25% in the preantibiotic era and remains at ~3–5% principally because of delayed diagnosis and treatment. The case-fatality ratio increases with each decade of life above age 20.

Pathogenesis   *R. rickettsii* organisms are inoculated into the dermis along with secretions of the tick's salivary glands after ≥6 h of feeding. The rickettsiae spread lymphohematogenously throughout the body and infect numerous foci of contiguous endothelial cells. The dose-dependent incubation period is ~1 week (range, 2–14 days). Occlusive thrombosis and ischemic necrosis are not the fundamental pathologic basis for tissue and organ injury. Instead, increased vascular permeability, with resulting edema, hypovolemia, and ischemia, is responsible. Consumption of platelets results in thrombocytopenia in 32–52% of patients, but disseminated intravascular coagulation with hypofibrinogenemia is rare. Activation of platelets, generation of thrombin, and activation of the fibrinolytic system all appear to be homeostatic physiologic responses to endothelial injury.

Clinical Manifestations   Early in the illness, when medical attention usually is first sought, RMSF is difficult to distinguish from many self-limiting viral illnesses. Fever, headache, malaise, myalgia, nausea, vomiting, and anorexia are the most common symptoms during the first 3 days. The patient becomes progressively more ill as vascular infection and injury advance. In one large series, only one-third of patients were diagnosed with presumptive RMSF early in the clinical course and treated appropriately as outpatients. In the tertiary care setting, RMSF is all too often recognized only when late severe manifestations, developing at the end of the first week or during the second week of illness in patients without appropriate treatment, prompt return to a physician or hospital and admission to an intensive care unit.

The progressive nature of the infection is clearly manifested in the skin. Rash is evident in only 14% of patients on the first day of illness and in only 49% during the first 3 days. Macules (1–5 mm) appear first on the wrists and ankles and then on the remainder of the extremities

FIGURE 167-1   *Top*: Petechial lesions of Rocky Mountain spotted fever on the lower legs and soles of a young, previously healthy patient. ***Bottom*: Close-up of lesions** from the same patient. *(Photos courtesy of Dr. Lindsey Baden; with permission.)*

and the trunk. Later, more severe vascular damage results in frank hemorrhage at the center of the maculopapule, producing a petechia that does not disappear upon compression (Fig. 167-1). This sequence of events is sometimes delayed or aborted by effective treatment. However, the rash is a variable manifestation, appearing on day 6 or later in 20% of cases and not appearing at all in 9–16% of cases. Petechiae occur in 41–59% of cases, appearing on or after day 6 in 74% of cases that include a rash. Involvement of the palms and soles, often considered diagnostically important, usually develops relatively late in the course (after day 5 in 43% of cases) and does not develop at all in 18–64% of cases.

Hypovolemia leads to prerenal azotemia and (in 17% of cases) hypotension. Infection of the pulmonary microcirculation leads to noncardiogenic pulmonary edema; 12% of patients have severe respiratory disease, and 8% require mechanical ventilation. Cardiac involvement manifests as dysrhythmia in 7–16% of cases.

Besides the preceding respiratory failure, central nervous system (CNS) involvement is the other important determinant of the outcome of RMSF. Encephalitis, presenting as confusion or lethargy, is apparent in 26–28% of cases. Progressively severe encephalitis manifests as stupor or delirium in 21–26% of cases, as ataxia in 18%, as coma in 10%, and as seizures in 8%. Numerous focal neurologic deficits have been reported. Meningoencephalitis results in cerebrospinal fluid (CSF) pleocytosis in 34–38% of cases; usually there are 10–100 cells/μL and a mononuclear predominance, but occasionally there are >100 cells/μL and a polymorphonuclear predominance. The CSF protein concentration is increased in 30–35% of cases, but the CSF glucose concentration is usually normal.

Renal failure, often reversible with rehydration, is caused by acute tubular necrosis in severe cases with shock. Hepatic injury with increased serum aminotransferase concentrations (38% of cases) is due to focal death of individual hepatocytes without hepatic failure. Jaundice is recognized in 9% of cases and an elevated serum bilirubin concentration in 18–30%.

Life-threatening bleeding is rare. Anemia develops in 30% of cases and is severe enough to require transfusions in 11%. Blood is detected in the stools or vomitus of 10% of patients, and death has followed massive upper gastrointestinal hemorrhage.

Other characteristic clinical laboratory findings include increased plasma levels of proteins of the acute-phase response (C-reactive protein, fibrinogen, ferritin, and others), hypoalbuminemia, and hyponatremia (in 56% of cases) due to the appropriate secretion of antidiuretic hormone in response to the hypovolemic state. Myositis occurs occasionally, with marked elevations in serum creatine kinase levels and multifocal rhabdomyonecrosis. Ocular involvement includes conjunctivitis in 30% of cases and retinal vein engorgement, flame hemorrhages, arterial occlusion, and papilledema with normal CSF pressure in some instances.

In untreated cases, the patient usually dies 8–15 days after onset. A rare presentation, fulminant RMSF, is fatal within 5 days after onset. This fulminant presentation is seen most often in black males with glucose-6-phosphate dehydrogenase (G6PD) deficiency and may be related to an undefined effect of hemolysis on the rickettsial infection. Although survivors of RMSF usually return to their previous state of health, permanent sequelae, including neurologic deficits and gangrene necessitating amputation of extremities, may follow severe illness.

Diagnosis   The diagnosis of RMSF during the acute stage is more difficult than is generally appreciated. The most important epidemiologic factor is a history of exposure to a potentially tick-infested environment within the 12 days preceding disease onset during a season of possible tick activity. However, only 60% of patients actually recall being bitten by a tick during the incubation period.

The differential diagnosis for early clinical manifestations of RMSF (fever, headache, and myalgia without a rash) includes influenza, enteroviral infection, infectious mononucleosis, viral hepatitis, leptospirosis, typhoid fever, gram-negative or gram-positive bacterial sepsis, HME, HGA, murine typhus, sylvatic flying-squirrel typhus, and rickettsialpox. Enterocolitis may be suggested by nausea, vomiting, and abdominal pain; prominence of abdominal tenderness has resulted in exploratory laparotomy. CNS involvement may masquerade as bacterial or viral meningoencephalitis. Cough, pulmonary signs, and chest radiographic opacities may lead to a diagnostic consideration of bronchitis or pneumonia.

At presentation during the first 3 days of illness, only 3% of patients exhibit the classic triad of fever, rash, and history of tick exposure. When a rash appears, a diagnosis of RMSF should certainly be considered. However, many illnesses considered in the differential diagnosis may also be associated with a rash, including rubeola, rubella, meningococcemia, disseminated gonococcal infection, secondary syphilis, toxic shock syndrome, drug hypersensitivity, idiopathic thrombocytopenic purpura, thrombotic thrombocytopenic purpura, Kawasaki syndrome, and immune complex vasculitis. Conversely, any person in an endemic area with a provisional diagnosis of one of the above illnesses may have RMSF. Thus, if a viral infection is suspected during RMSF season in an endemic area, it should always be kept in mind that RMSF can mimic viral infection early in the course; if the illness worsens over the next couple of days after initial presentation, the patient should return for reevaluation.

The most common serologic test for confirmation of the diagnosis is the indirect immunofluorescence assay. Not until 7–10 days after onset is a diagnostic titer of ≥1:64 usually detectable. The sensitivity and specificity of the indirect immunofluorescence assay are 94–100% and 100%, respectively. It is important to understand that serologic tests for RMSF are usually negative at the time of presentation for medical care and that treatment should not be delayed while a positive serologic result is awaited.

The only diagnostic test that is useful during the acute illness is immunohistologic examination of a cutaneous biopsy sample from a rash lesion for *R. rickettsii*. Examination of a 3-mm punch biopsy from such a lesion is 70% sensitive and 100% specific. Polymerase chain reaction

(PCR) amplification and detection of *R. rickettsii* DNA in peripheral blood is a relatively insensitive approach except when the patient is already in the preterminal state. Rickettsiae are present in large quantities in heavily infected foci of endothelial cells but in relatively low quantities in the circulation. Cultivation of rickettsiae in cell culture is feasible but is seldom undertaken because of biohazard concerns.

℞ ROCKY MOUNTAIN SPOTTED FEVER

The drug of choice for the treatment of both children and adults with RMSF is doxycycline, except when the patient is pregnant or allergic to this drug (see below). Because of the severity of RMSF, immediate empirical administration of doxycycline should be strongly considered for any patient with a consistent clinical presentation in the appropriate epidemiologic setting. Doxycycline is administered orally (or, in the presence of coma or vomiting, intravenously) at 200 mg/d in two divided doses. For children with suspected RMSF, up to five courses of doxycycline may be administered with minimal risk of dental staining. Other regimens include oral tetracycline (25–50 mg/kg per day) in four divided doses. Treatment with chloramphenicol is advised only for patients who are pregnant or allergic to doxycycline. The antirickettsial drug should be administered until the patient has been afebrile and improving clinically for 2–3 days. β-Lactam antibiotics, erythromycin, and aminoglycosides have no role in the treatment of RMSF, and sulfa-containing drugs are likely to exacerbate this infection. There is little clinical experience with fluoroquinolones, clarithromycin, and azithromycin, which are not recommended. The most seriously ill patients are managed in intensive care units, with careful administration of fluids to achieve optimal tissue perfusion without precipitating noncardiogenic pulmonary edema. In some severely ill patients, hypoxemia requires intubation and mechanical ventilation; oliguric or anuric acute renal failure requires hemodialysis; seizures necessitate the use of antiseizure medication; anemia or severe hemorrhage necessitates transfusions of packed red blood cells; or bleeding with severe thrombocytopenia requires platelet transfusions. Heparin is not a useful component of treatment, and there is no evidence that glucocorticoids affect outcome.

Prevention   Avoidance of tick bites is the only available preventive approach. Use of protective clothing and tick repellents, inspection of the body once or twice a day, and removal of ticks before they inoculate rickettsiae reduce the risk of infection.

MEDITERRANEAN SPOTTED FEVER (BOUTONNEUSE FEVER), AFRICAN TICK-BITE FEVER, AND OTHER TICK-BORNE SPOTTED FEVERS

R. conorii is prevalent in southern Europe, Africa, and southwestern and south-central Asia. Regional names for the disease caused by this organism include Mediterranean spotted fever, Kenya tick typhus, Indian tick typhus, Israeli spotted fever, and Astrakhan spotted fever. The disease is characterized by high fever, rash, and—in most geographic locales—an inoculation eschar (*tâche noire*) at the site of the tick bite. A severe form of the disease (mortality rate, 50%) occurs in patients with diabetes, alcoholism, or heart failure.

African tick-bite fever, caused by *R. africae*, occurs in rural areas of sub-Saharan Africa and in the Caribbean islands and is transmitted by *Amblyomma hebraeum* and *A. variegatum* ticks. The average incubation period is 7 days. The mild illness consists of headache, fever, eschar, and regional lymphadenopathy. *Amblyomma* ticks often feed in groups, with the consequent development of multiple eschars. Rash may be vesicular, sparse, or absent altogether. Because of tourism in sub-Saharan Africa, African tick-bite fever is the most frequently imported rickettsiosis in Europe and North America. A similar disease caused by the very closely related *R. parkeri* is transmitted by *A. maculatum* in the United States and *A. triste* in South America.

R. japonica causes *Japanese spotted fever*, which also occurs in Korea. A similar disease in northern Asia is caused by *R. sibirica*. *Queensland tick typhus* due to *R. australis* is transmitted by *Ixodes holocyclus*. *Flinders Island spotted fever*, found on the island for which it is named as well as in other parts of Tasmania, in mainland Australia, and in southeastern Asia, is caused by *R. honei*. In Europe, patients infected with *R. slovaca* after a wintertime *Dermacentor* tick bite manifest an afebrile illness with an eschar (usually on the scalp) and regional lymphadenopathy.

Diagnosis Diagnosis of these tick-borne spotted fevers is based on clinical and epidemiologic findings and is confirmed by serology, immunohistochemical demonstration of rickettsiae in skin biopsy specimens, cell-culture isolation of rickettsiae, or PCR of skin biopsy or blood samples. The serologic identification of the etiologic species requires knowledge of all the potential agents as well as expensive, laborious cross-adsorption of the patient's serum. In an endemic area, patients presenting with fever, rash, and/or a skin lesion consisting of a black necrotic area or a crust surrounded by erythema should be considered to have one of these rickettsial spotted fevers.

℞ TICK-BORNE SPOTTED FEVERS

Successful therapeutic agents include doxycycline (100 mg bid orally for 1–5 days), ciprofloxacin (750 mg bid orally for 5 days), and chloramphenicol (500 mg qid orally for 7–10 days). Pregnant patients may be treated with josamycin (3 g/d orally for 5 days). Data on the efficacy of treatment of mildly ill children with clarithromycin or azithromycin should not be extrapolated to adults or to patients with moderate or severe illness.

RICKETTSIALPOX

R. akari infects mice and their mites (*Liponyssoides sanguineus*), which maintain the organisms by transovarian transmission.

Epidemiology Rickettsialpox is recognized principally in New York City, but cases have also been reported in other urban and rural locations in the United States and in Ukraine, Croatia, and Turkey. Investigation of eschars suspected of representing bioterrorism-associated cutaneous anthrax has revealed that rickettsialpox occurs more frequently than previously realized.

Clinical Manifestations A papule forms at the site of the mite's feeding, develops a central vesicle, and becomes a 1- to 2.5-cm painless black crusted eschar surrounded by an erythematous halo (**Fig. 167-2**). Enlargement of the regional lymph nodes draining the eschar suggests initial lymphogenous spread. After an incubation period of 10–17 days, during which the eschar and regional lymphadenopathy frequently go unnoticed, onset is marked by malaise, chills, fever, headache, and myalgia. A macular rash appears 2–6 days after onset and evolves sequentially into papules, vesicles, and crusts that heal without scarring (**Fig. 167-3**). The rash may remain macular or maculopapular. Some patients develop nausea, vomiting, abdominal pain, cough, conjunctivitis, or photophobia. If untreated, fever lasts 6–10 days.

FIGURE 167-2 Eschar at the site of the mite bite in a patient with rickettsialpox. *(Reprinted from A Krusell et al: Emerg Infect Dis 8:727, 2002. Photo obtained by Dr. Kenneth Kaye.)*

FIGURE 167-3 *Top:* Papulovesicular lesions on the trunk of the patient with rickettsialpox shown in Fig. 167-2. ***Bottom:* Close-up of lesions** from the same patient. *(Reprinted from A Krusell et al: Emerg Infect Dis 8:727, 2002. Photos obtained by Dr. Kenneth Kaye.)*

Diagnosis and Treatment Clinical, epidemiologic, and convalescent serologic data establish the diagnosis of a spotted fever group rickettsiosis that is seldom pursued further. Doxycycline is the drug of choice for treatment.

FLEA-BORNE SPOTTED FEVER

An emerging rickettsiosis caused by *R. felis* probably occurs worldwide. Maintained transovarially in the geographically widespread cat flea *Ctenocephalides felis*, the infection has been described as moderately severe, with fever, rash, headache, and CNS and gastrointestinal symptoms.

ENDEMIC MURINE TYPHUS

Epidemiology *R. typhi* is maintained in mammalian host/flea cycles, with rats (*Rattus rattus* and *R. norvegicus*) and the Oriental rat flea (*Xenopsylla cheopis*) as the classic zoonotic niche. Fleas acquire *R. typhi* from rickettsemic rats and carry the organism throughout their life span. Nonimmune rats and humans are infected when rickettsia-laden flea feces contaminate pruritic bite lesions; less frequently, the flea bite transmits the organisms. Transmission also may occur via inhalation of aerosolized rickettsiae from flea feces. Infected rats appear healthy, although they are rickettsemic for ~2 weeks.

Murine typhus occurs mainly in southern Texas and southern California, where the classic rat/flea cycle is absent and an opossum/cat flea (*C. felis*) cycle is prominent. Globally, endemic typhus occurs year-round, mainly in warm (often coastal) areas throughout the tropics and subtropics, where it is highly prevalent though often unrecognized. The incidence peaks from April through June in southern Texas and during the warm months of summer and early fall in other geographic locations. Patients seldom recall exposure to fleas, although exposure to animals such as cats, opossums, and rats is reported in nearly 40% of cases.

Clinical Manifestations   The incubation period of experimental murine typhus averages 11 days (range, 8–16 days). Headache, myalgia, arthralgia, nausea, and malaise develop 1–3 days before onset of chills and fever. Nearly all patients experience nausea and vomiting early in the illness.

The duration of untreated illness averages 12 days (range, 9–18 days). Rash is present in only 13% of patients at presentation for medical care (usually ~4 days after onset of fever), appearing an average of 2 days later in half of the remaining patients and never appearing in the others. The initial macular rash is often detected by careful inspection of the axilla or the inner surface of the arm. Subsequently, the rash becomes maculopapular, involving the trunk more often than the extremities; it is seldom petechial and rarely involves the face, palms, or soles. A rash is detected in only 20% of patients with darkly pigmented skin.

Pulmonary involvement is frequently prominent; 35% of patients have a hacking, nonproductive cough, and 23% of patients who undergo chest radiography have pulmonary densities due to interstitial pneumonia, pulmonary edema, and pleural effusions. Bibasilar rales are the most common pulmonary sign. Less common clinical manifestations include abdominal pain, confusion, stupor, seizures, ataxia, coma, and jaundice. Clinical laboratory studies frequently reveal anemia and leukopenia early in the course, leukocytosis late in the course, thrombocytopenia, hyponatremia, hypoalbuminemia, mildly increased serum hepatic aminotransferases, and prerenal azotemia. Complications may include respiratory failure, hematemesis, cerebral hemorrhage, and hemolysis. Severe illness necessitates the admission of 10% of hospitalized patients to an intensive care unit. Greater severity is generally associated with old age, underlying disease, and treatment with a sulfonamide; the case-fatality rate is 1%. In a study of children with murine typhus, 50% suffered only nocturnal fevers, feeling well enough for active daytime play.

Diagnosis and Treatment   Cultivation, PCR, or cross-adsorption serologic studies of acute- and convalescent-phase sera can provide a specific diagnosis, and an immunohistochemical method for identification of typhus group-specific antigens has been developed. Nevertheless, most patients are treated empirically with doxycycline (100 mg bid orally for 7–15 days) on the basis of clinical suspicion. Serologic methods are usually used when laboratory confirmation of the diagnosis is sought.

EPIDEMIC (LOUSE-BORNE) TYPHUS

The human body louse (*Pediculus humanus corporis*) lives in clothing under poor hygienic conditions and usually in impoverished cold areas. Lice acquire *R. prowazekii* when they ingest blood from a rickettsemic patient. The rickettsiae multiply in the midgut epithelial cells of the louse and are shed in the louse's feces. The infected louse leaves a febrile person and deposits infected feces on its subsequent host during its blood meal; the patient autoinoculates the organisms by scratching. The louse is killed by the rickettsiae and does not pass *R. prowazekii* to its offspring.

Epidemic typhus haunts regions afflicted by wars and disasters. An outbreak involved 100,000 people in refugee camps in Burundi in 1997. A small focus occurred in Russia in 1998; sporadic cases have been reported from Algeria, and frequent outbreaks have occurred in Peru. Eastern flying-squirrels (*Glaucomys volans*) and their lice and fleas maintain *R. prowazekii* in a zoonotic cycle. The fleas transmit the infection sporadically to humans.

Brill-Zinsser disease is a recrudescent illness occurring years after acute epidemic typhus, probably as a result of waning immunity. Typhus infection remains latent for years; its reactivation results in sporadic cases of disease in louse-free populations or in epidemics in louse-infested populations.

Rickettsiae are potential agents of bioterrorism (Chap. 214). Infections with *R. prowazekii* and *R. rickettsii* have high case-fatality ratios.

These organisms cause difficult-to-diagnose diseases, are highly infectious when inhaled as aerosols, and have been selected for resistance to tetracycline or chloramphenicol in the laboratory.

Clinical Manifestations   After an incubation period of ~1 week, the onset of illness is abrupt, with prostration, severe headache, and fever rising rapidly to 38.8°–40.0°C (102°–104°F). Cough is prominent, occurring in 70% of patients. Myalgias are usually severe. In the outbreak in Burundi, the disease was referred to as sutama ("crouching"), a designation reflecting the posture of patients attempting to alleviate the pain. A rash begins on the upper trunk, usually on the fifth day, and then becomes generalized, involving the entire body except the face, palms, and soles. Initially, this rash is macular; without treatment, it becomes maculopapular, petechial, and confluent. The rash often is not detected on black skin; 60% of African patients have spotless epidemic typhus. Photophobia, with considerable conjunctival injection and eye pain, is frequent. The tongue may be dry, brown, and furred. Confusion and coma are common. Skin necrosis and gangrene of the digits as well as interstitial pneumonia may occur in severe cases. Untreated disease is fatal in 7–40% of cases, with outcome depending primarily on the condition of the host. Patients with untreated infections develop renal insufficiency and multiorgan involvement in which neurologic manifestations are frequently prominent. Overall, 12% of patients with epidemic typhus have neurologic involvement. Infection associated with North American flying squirrels is a milder illness; whether this milder disease is due to host factors (e.g., better health status) or attenuated virulence is unknown.

Diagnosis and Treatment   Epidemic typhus is sometimes misdiagnosed as typhoid fever in tropical countries (Chap. 146). The means even for serologic studies are often unavailable in settings of louse-borne typhus. Epidemics may be recognized by the serologic or immunohistochemical diagnosis of a single case or by detection of *R. prowazekii* in a louse found on a patient. Cross-adsorption indirect fluorescent antibody (IFA) studies can distinguish *R. prowazekii* and *R. typhi* infections. Doxycycline (200 mg/d, given in two divided doses) is administered orally or—if the patient is comatose or vomiting—intravenously. Although under epidemic conditions a single 200-mg dose has proved effective, treatment is generally continued until 2–3 days after defervescence. Pregnant patients should be evaluated individually and treated with either chloramphenicol early in pregnancy or, if necessary, doxycycline late in pregnancy.

Prevention   Prevention of epidemic typhus involves control of body lice. Clothes should be changed regularly, and insecticides should be used every 6 weeks to control the louse population.

SCRUB TYPHUS

O. tsutsugamushi differs substantially from *Rickettsia* species both genetically and in terms of cell wall composition (i.e., it lacks lipopolysaccharide and peptidoglycan). *O. tsutsugamushi* is maintained by transovarian transmission in trombiculid mites. After hatching, infected larval mites (chiggers, the only stage that feeds on a host) inoculate organisms into the skin. Infected chiggers are found particularly in areas of heavy scrub vegetation during the wet season, when mites lay eggs.

Scrub typhus is endemic in eastern and southern Asia, northern Australia, and islands of the western Pacific and Indian Oceans. Infections are prevalent in these regions; in some areas, >3% of the population is infected or reinfected each month. Immunity wanes over 1–3 years, and the organism exhibits remarkable antigenic diversity.

Clinical Manifestations   Illness varies from mild and self-limiting to fatal. After an incubation period of 6–21 days, onset is characterized by fever, headache, myalgia, cough, and gastrointestinal symptoms. Some patients recover spontaneously after a few days. The classic case description includes an eschar where the chigger feeds, regional lymphadenopathy, and a maculopapular rash—signs that are seldom seen in indigenous patients. Fewer than 50% of Westerners develop an eschar, and fewer than 40% develop a rash (on day 4–6 of illness). Severe cases typically include encephalitis and interstitial pneumonia due to vascular injury. The case-fatality rate for untreated classic cases is 7% but would probably be lower if all mild cases were diagnosed.

Diagnosis and Treatment Serologic assays (IFA, indirect immunoperoxidase, and enzyme immunoassays) are the mainstays of laboratory diagnosis. Patients are treated with doxycycline (100 mg bid orally for 7–15 days) or chloramphenicol (500 mg qid orally for 7–15 days). Some cases of scrub typhus in Thailand are caused by doxycycline- or chloramphenicol-resistant strains that are susceptible to rifampin. Azithromycin and clarithromycin have been used successfully in a few patients.

EHRLICHIOSES AND ANAPLASMOSIS

Ehrlichioses are acute febrile infections caused by members of the family Anaplasmataceae, which is made up of obligately intracellular organisms transmitted by ticks and contains four genera: *Ehrlichia*, *Anaplasma*, *Wolbachia*, and *Neorickettsia*. The bacteria reside in vertebrate reservoirs and target vacuoles of hematopoietic cells (Fig. 167-4). Two *Ehrlichia* species and one *Anaplasma* species cause human infections that can be severe and frequent. *E. chaffeensis*, the agent of HME, infects predominantly mononuclear phagocytic cells. *E. ewingii* and *A. phagocytophilum* infect neutrophils.

Ehrlichia and *Anaplasma* are maintained by horizontal tick-mammal-tick transmission, and humans are only inadvertently infected. Wolbachiae are associated with human diseases caused by filariae, since they are important for filarial viability and pathogenicity; antibiotic treatment targeting wolbachiae is a strategy for the control of filariasis. Neorickettsiae parasitize flukes that in turn parasitize aquatic snails, fish, and insects. Only a single human neorickettsiosis has been described: sennetsu fever, an infectious mononucleosis–like illness that was first identified in 1953. Transmission is probably due to the ingestion of raw fish containing *N. sennetsu*–infected flukes.

HUMAN MONOCYTOTROPIC EHRLICHIOSIS
Epidemiology More than 2657 cases of *E. chaffeensis* infection had been reported to the Centers for Disease Control and Prevention (CDC) as of September 2006. However, active prospective surveillance has demonstrated an incidence as high as 414 cases per 100,000 population in some regions of the United States. Most *E. chaffeensis* infections are

FIGURE 167-4 Peripheral blood smear from a patient with human granulocytotropic anaplasmosis. A neutrophil contains two morulae (vacuoles filled with *A. phagocytophilum*). (*Photo courtesy of Dr. J. Stephen Dumler.*)

identified in the south-central, southeastern, and mid-Atlantic states, but cases have also been recognized in California. All life stages of the Lone Star tick (*A. americanum*) vector feed on white-tailed deer—a major reservoir host. Subclinically infected dogs and coyotes also serve as reservoirs. Tick bites and exposures are reported by patients, frequently in rural areas and especially in May through July. The median age of HME patients is 53 years; however, severe and fatal infections in children are also well recognized. Of patients with HME, 61% are male.

Clinical Manifestations *E. chaffeensis* disseminates hematogenously from the dermal blood pool created by the feeding tick. After a median incubation period of 8 days, illness develops. Clinical manifestations are undifferentiated and include fever (97% of cases), headache (80%), myalgia (57%), and malaise (82%). Less frequently observed are nausea, vomiting, and diarrhea (23–64%); cough (26%); rash (31% overall, 6% at presentation); and confusion (19%). HME can be severe: 62% of patients with documented cases are hospitalized, and ~3% die. Severe complications include toxic shock–like or septic shock–like syndromes, adult respiratory distress syndrome, cardiac failure, hepatitis, meningoencephalitis, hemorrhage, and—in immunocompromised patients—overwhelming infection. Laboratory findings are valuable in the differential diagnosis of HME; 62% of patients have leukopenia (initially lymphopenia, later neutropenia), 71% have thrombocytopenia, and 83% have elevated serum levels of hepatic aminotransferases. Despite low blood cell counts, the bone marrow is hypercellular, and noncaseating granulomas may be present. Vasculitis is not a component of HME.

Diagnosis Because HME can be fatal, empirical antibiotic therapy based on clinical diagnosis is required. This diagnosis is suggested by fever with a known tick exposure during the preceding 3 weeks, thrombocytopenia and/or leukopenia, and increased serum aminotransferase activities. Morulae are infrequently demonstrated on peripheral blood smears. Active HME can be confirmed by PCR amplification of *E. chaffeensis* nucleic acids in blood obtained before the start of doxycycline therapy. Retrospective serodiagnosis requires a consistent clinical picture and a fourfold increase in *E. chaffeensis* antibody titer (to ≥1:64 in paired sera obtained ~3 weeks apart). Separate specific diagnostic tests are necessary for HME and HGA.

EHRLICHIOSIS EWINGII
Ehrlichia ewingii, originally a neutrophil pathogen causing febrile lameness in dogs, resembles *E. chaffeensis* in its tick vector (*A. americanum*) and vertebrate reservoirs (white-tailed deer and dogs). *E. ewingii* illness is similar to but less severe than HME. The majority of cases have occurred in immunocompromised patients. No specific diagnostic test for ehrlichiosis ewingii is readily available.

℞ EHRLICHIOSES

Doxycycline is effective for HME and ehrlichiosis ewingii. Therapy with doxycycline (100 mg given orally or intravenously twice daily) or tetracycline (250–500 mg given orally every 6 h) lowers hospitalization rates and shortens fever duration. *E. chaffeensis* is not susceptible to chloramphenicol in vitro, and the use of this drug is controversial. While a few reports document *E. chaffeensis* persistence in humans, this finding is rare; most infections are cured by short courses of doxycycline (continuing for 3–5 days after defervescence). Although poorly studied, rifampin may be suitable when doxycycline is contraindicated.

Prevention HME and ehrlichiosis ewingii are prevented by the avoidance of ticks in endemic areas. The use of protective clothing and tick repellents, careful postexposure tick searches, and prompt removal of attached ticks markedly diminish infection risk.

HUMAN GRANULOCYTOTROPIC ANAPLASMOSIS
Epidemiology As of September 2006, 3257 cases of HGA had been reported to the CDC, most in the upper midwestern and northeastern

United States; the case distribution is similar to that for Lyme disease because of the shared *I. scapularis* tick vector. White-footed mice and white-tailed deer in the United States and red deer in Europe are natural reservoirs for *A. phagocytophilum*. HGA incidence peaks in May through July, but the disease can occur throughout the year with exposure to *Ixodes* ticks. HGA often affects males (57%) and older persons (median age, 51 years).

Clinical Manifestations Seroprevalence rates are high in endemic regions; thus it seems likely that most individuals develop subclinical infections. The incubation period for HGA is 4–8 days, after which the disease manifests as fever (93% of cases), myalgia (77%), headache (76%), and malaise (94%). A minority of patients develop nausea, vomiting, or diarrhea (16–38%); cough (19%); or confusion (17%). Rash (6%) is almost invariably concurrent erythema migrans attributable to Lyme disease. Most patients develop thrombocytopenia (71%) and/or leukopenia (49%) with increased serum hepatic aminotransferase activities (71%).

Severe complications occur most often in the elderly and include adult respiratory distress syndrome, a toxic shock–like syndrome, and life-threatening opportunistic infections. Meningoencephalitis has not been conclusively documented with HGA, but brachial plexopathy and demyelinating polyneuropathy are reported. For HGA, 7% of patients require intensive care, and the case-fatality rate is 0.5%. Neither vasculitis nor granulomas are components of HGA. While co-infections with *Borrelia burgdorferi* and *Babesia microti* [transmitted by the same tick vector(s)] occur, there is little evidence of comorbidity or persistence.

Diagnosis HGA should be included in the differential diagnosis of influenza-like illnesses during seasons with *Ixodes* tick activity (May through December), especially with tick bite or exposure. Concurrent thrombocytopenia, leukopenia, or elevation in serum alanine or aspartate aminotransferase further increases the likelihood of HGA. Many HGA patients develop Lyme disease antibodies in the absence of clinical findings consistent with that diagnosis. Thus, HGA should be considered in the differential diagnosis of atypical severe Lyme disease presentations. Peripheral blood film examination for neutrophil morulae can yield a diagnosis in 20–75% of infections. PCR testing of blood from patients with active disease before doxycycline therapy is sensitive and specific. Serodiagnosis is retrospective, requiring a four-fold increase in *A. phagocytophilum* antibody titer (to ≥1:80) in paired serum samples obtained 1 month apart. In regions where seroprevalence is high, a single acute-phase titer may be misleading.

℞ **HUMAN GRANULOCYTOTROPIC ANAPLASMOSIS**

No prospective studies of therapy for HGA have been conducted. However, doxycycline (100 mg by mouth twice daily) is effective. Rifampin therapy is associated with improvement of HGA in pregnant women and children. Most treated patients defervesce within 24–48 h.

Prevention HGA prevention requires tick avoidance. Transmission can be documented as few as 4 h after a tick bite.

Q FEVER

Q fever results from infection with *C. burnetii*. This organism forms spores that allow its survival in harsh environments. *Coxiella* escapes intracellular killing in macrophages by inhibiting the final phagosome maturation step (cathepsin fusion) and adapts to the acidic phagolysosome.

Q fever encompasses two broad clinical syndromes: acute and chronic infection. The host's immune response (rather than the infecting strain) most likely determines whether chronic Q fever develops. *C. burnetii* survives in monocytes from patients with chronic Q fever but not in those from patients with acute Q fever or from uninfected persons. Impairment of the bactericidal activity of the *C. burnetii*–infected monocyte seems to be due to overproduction of interleukin 10.

The CD4+/CD8+ ratio is decreased in Q fever endocarditis. Very few organisms and a strong cellular response are observed in patients with acute Q fever, while many organisms and a moderate cellular response are seen in chronic Q fever. Immunologic control of *C. burnetii* is T cell–dependent, but 80–90% of bone marrow aspirates obtained after recovery from Q fever contain *C. burnetii* DNA.

Epidemiology Q fever is a zoonosis. The primary sources of human infection are infected cattle, sheep, and goats. However, cats, rabbits, pigeons, and dogs have also transmitted *C. burnetii* to humans. The wildlife reservoir includes ticks. In the infected female mammal, *C. burnetii* localizes to the uterus and the mammary glands. Infection is reactivated during pregnancy. High concentrations of *C. burnetii* are found in the placenta. At the time of parturition, *C. burnetii* organisms are released into the air, and infection follows inhalation of aerosolized organisms by a susceptible host. Soil is contaminated during parturition, and *C. burnetii* aerosols can be generated months later during windstorms. Individuals up to 18 km from the source have been infected. *C. burnetii* is a potential agent of bioterrorism.

Persons at risk for Q fever include abattoir workers, veterinarians, and other individuals who have contact with infected animals, particularly newborn animals or products of conception. The organism is shed in milk for weeks to months after parturition. The ingestion of contaminated milk in some geographic areas probably represents a major route of transmission to humans, although the experimental evidence on this point is contradictory. In rare instances, human-to-human transmission has followed labor and childbirth in an infected woman, autopsy of an infected individual, or blood transfusion. Some evidence suggests that *C. burnetii* can be sexually transmitted among humans. Nevertheless, the vast majority of Q fever cases result from inhalation of contaminated aerosols.

Infections due to *C. burnetii* occur in most geographic locations except New Zealand and Antarctica. The primary manifestations of acute Q fever vary with the area. For example, the primary manifestation is pneumonia in Nova Scotia (Canada) but is granulomatous hepatitis in Marseille (France). These differences may reflect the route of infection—i.e., the ingestion of contaminated milk for hepatitis and inhalation of contaminated aerosols for pneumonia.

Young age seems to be protective against infection with *C. burnetii*. In a large outbreak in Switzerland, symptomatic infection occurred five times more often among persons >15 years of age than among those <15 years old. In many outbreaks, men are affected more commonly than women. In France, despite similar occupational exposure of the sexes, the male-to-female ratio is 2.45:1; this difference reflects the fact that female sex hormones are partially protective against infection.

Clinical Manifestations • ***ACUTE Q FEVER*** The incubation period for acute Q fever is 3–30 days. The symptoms are nonspecific; common among them are fever, extreme fatigue, and severe headache. Other symptoms include chills, sweats, nausea, vomiting, and diarrhea, which occur in 5–20% of patients. Cough develops in about half of patients with Q fever pneumonia. Neurologic manifestations of acute Q fever are uncommon; however, in one outbreak in the United Kingdom, 23% of 102 patients had neurologic signs and symptoms as the major manifestation. A nonspecific rash may be evident in 4–18% of patients. The WBC count is usually normal. Thrombocytopenia occurs in ~25% of patients, and reactive thrombocytosis (with platelet counts sometimes exceeding $10^6/\mu L$) frequently develops during recovery. Chest radiography may show an opacity that is indistinguishable from that seen in pneumonia of other etiologies. Multiple rounded opacities are common. In one study of 1070 patients with acute Q fever in southern France, 40% of patients presented with hepatitis, 17% with pneumonia, 20% with both pneumonia and hepatitis, 14% with isolated fever, 2% with CNS disease, and 1% with pericarditis and myocarditis.

Acute Q fever occasionally complicates pregnancy. In one series, Q fever in pregnancy resulted in premature birth in 35% of cases, and 43% of pregnancies ended in abortion or neonatal death. In Halifax, Nova Scotia, a current or previous neonatal death was three times more likely among women seropositive for *C. burnetii* than among seronegative women. Up to 70% of cases of Q fever in children are asymptomatic. Only a few cases of Q fever endocarditis have been reported in children.

In Australia and the United Kingdom, a fatigue state lasting 5–10 years has followed Q fever in 8–15% of cases. Low levels of *C. burnetii* DNA have been detected in the affected patients 0.75–5 years after infection. Patients who develop Q fever fatigue syndrome have a higher frequency of carriage of HLA-DRB1*11 and of the 2/2 genotype of the interferon γ intron 1 microsatellite.

Patients with acute Q fever and lesions of native heart valves, prosthetic heart valves, or prosthetic intravascular material should undergo serologic monitoring every 4 months for 2 years. If the phase I IgG titer is >1:800, further investigation is warranted. Some authorities recommend that patients with valvulopathy and acute Q fever receive doxycycline and hydroxychloroquine for 12 months to prevent chronic Q fever.

CHRONIC Q FEVER Chronic Q fever, which almost always implies endocarditis, usually occurs in patients with previous valvular heart disease, immunosuppression, or chronic renal insufficiency. Fever is usually absent or low grade. Patients may have nonspecific symptoms for up to 1 year before diagnosis. Valvular vegetations are detected in only 12% of patients by transthoracic echocardiography, but the rate of detection may be higher with transesophageal echocardiography. The vegetations in chronic Q fever endocarditis differ from those in bacterial endocarditis, manifesting as endothelialized nodules on the valves. A high index of suspicion is necessary for a correct diagnosis. The disease should be suspected in all patients with culture-negative endocarditis. In addition, all patients with valvular heart disease and an unexplained purpuric eruption, renal insufficiency, stroke, and/or progressive heart failure should be tested for *C. burnetii* infection. Patients with chronic Q fever have hepatomegaly and/or splenomegaly, which, in combination with rheumatoid factor, elevated erythrocyte sedimentation rate, high C-reactive protein level, and/or increased γ-globulin concentrations (up to 60–70 g/L), suggests this diagnosis. Other manifestations of chronic Q fever include infection of vascular prostheses, aneurysms, and bone as well as chronic sternal wound infection. Unusual manifestations include chronic thrombocytopenia, mixed cryoglobulinemia, and livedo reticularis.

Diagnosis Isolation of *C. burnetii* from buffy-coat blood samples or tissue specimens by a shell-vial technique is seldom attempted because of biohazard concerns. PCR detects *C. burnetii* DNA in tissues, including paraffin-embedded tissues. Serology is the most commonly used diagnostic tool. Indirect immunofluorescence is sensitive and specific and is the method of choice. Rheumatoid factor should be adsorbed from the specimen before testing. An IgG titer of ≥1:800 to phase I antigen is suggestive of chronic Q fever. In chronic infection, the antibody titer to phase I antigen is usually much higher than that to phase II antigen; the reverse is true in acute infection, in which a fourfold rise in titer may be demonstrated between acute- and convalescent-phase serum samples.

℞ Q FEVER

Treatment of acute Q fever with doxycycline (100 mg twice daily for 14 days) is usually successful. Quinolones are also effective. When Q fever is diagnosed in a pregnant woman, treatment with trimethoprim-sulfamethoxazole is recommended for the duration of the pregnancy.

The treatment of chronic Q fever is difficult and requires careful follow-up. Addition of hydroxychloroquine (to alkalinize the phagolysosome) renders doxycycline bactericidal against *C. burnetii*, and this combination is currently the favored regimen. Treatment with doxycycline (100 mg bid) and hydroxychloroquine (200 mg tid; plasma concentration maintained at

0.8–1.2 μg/mL) for 18 months is superior to a regimen of doxycycline and ofloxacin. Optimal management of Q fever endocarditis entails determination of the minimal inhibitory concentration (MIC) of doxycycline for the patient's isolate and measurement of serum doxycycline levels. A serum level–to–doxycycline MIC ratio of ≥1 is associated with a rapid decline in phase I antibodies. Patients treated with this regimen must be advised about photosensitivity and retinal toxicity risks. The doxycycline-hydroxychloroquine regimen was successful in one patient with HIV infection and Q fever endocarditis. The Jarisch-Herxheimer reaction occasionally complicates the treatment of chronic Q fever.

Treatment of *C. burnetii*–infected aortic aneurysms is the same as that for Q fever endocarditis. Surgical intervention is often required.

If doxycycline-hydroxychloroquine cannot be used, the regimen should include at least two antibiotics active against *C. burnetii*. Rifampin (300 mg once daily) combined with doxycycline (100 mg twice daily) or ciprofloxacin (750 mg twice daily) has been used successfully. The optimal duration of antibiotic therapy for chronic Q fever remains undetermined. The authors recommend at least 3 years of treatment, with discontinuation only if the phase I IgA antibody titer is ≤1:50 and the IgG phase I titer is ≤1:200.

THERAPY WITH BIOLOGIC MODIFYING AGENTS Interferon γ was successful in the treatment of a 3-year-old boy with prolonged fever, abdominal pain, and thrombocytopenia due to *C. burnetii* that was not eradicated with conventional antibiotic therapy. Many patients with granulomatous hepatitis due to Q fever have a prolonged febrile illness that is unresponsive to antibiotics. For these individuals, treatment with prednisone (0.5 mg/kg) has resulted in defervescence within 2–15 days. After defervescence, the glucocorticoid dose is tapered over the next month.

Prevention A whole-cell vaccine (Q-Vax) licensed in Australia effectively prevents Q fever in abattoir workers. Before administration of the vaccine, skin testing with intradermal diluted *C. burnetii* vaccine is performed, serologic testing is undertaken, and a history of possible Q fever is sought. Vaccine is given only to patients with no history of Q fever and negative results in serologic and skin tests.

Good animal-husbandry practices are important in preventing widespread contamination of the environment by *C. burnetii*. These practices include isolating aborting animals for up to 14 days, raising feed bunks to prevent contamination of feed by excreta, destroying aborted materials (i.e., burning and burying fetal membranes and stillborn animals), and wearing masks and gloves when handling aborted materials. Only seronegative pregnant animals should be used in research settings, and only seronegative animals should be permitted in petting zoos.

ACKNOWLEDGMENT
The contributions of Didier Raoult, MD, to this chapter in previous editions are gratefully acknowledged.

FURTHER READINGS

BLANCO JR et al (eds): *Century of Rickettsiology: Emerging, Reemerging Rickettsioses, Molecular Diagnostics, and Emerging Veterinary Rickettsioses.* Malden, MA, Blackwell Scientific, 2006

CHAPMAN AS et al: Diagnosis and management of tickborne rickettsial diseases: Rocky Mountain spotted fever, ehrlichioses, and anaplasmosis—United States. MMWR 55:1, 2006

DUMLER JS: *Anaplasma* and *Ehrlichia* infection. Ann NY Acad Sci 1063:361, 2005

MCQUISTON JH et al: National surveillance and the epidemiology of Q fever in the United States, 1978–2004. Am J Trop Med Hyg 75:36, 2006

RAOULT D et al: Q fever 1985–1998. Clinical and epidemiologic features of 1,383 infections. Medicine (Baltimore) 79:109, 2000

WALKER DH: Rickettsiae and rickettsial infections: The current state of knowledge. Clin Infect Dis 45(Suppl1):539, 2007

168 Infections Due to Mycoplasmas
William M. McCormack

Mycoplasmas, the smallest free-living organisms known, are prokaryotes that are bounded only by a plasma membrane. Their lack of a cell wall is associated with cellular pleomorphism and resistance to cell wall–active antimicrobial agents, such as penicillins and cephalosporins. The organisms' small genome limits biosynthesis and explains the difficulties encountered with in vitro cultivation. Mycoplasmas typically colonize mucosal surfaces of the respiratory and urogenital tracts of many animal species. Of the 17 species of mycoplasmas recovered from humans, most are commensals. *Mycoplasma pneumoniae* causes upper and lower respiratory tract infections. *M. genitalium* and ureaplasmas are established causes of urethritis and have been implicated in other genital conditions. *M. hominis* and ureaplasmas are part of the complex microbial flora of bacterial vaginosis (Chap. 124). The two biovars of *Ureaplasma*, previously classified together as *U. urealyticum*, have recently been separated into two species: *U. parvum* and *U. urealyticum*.

MECHANISMS OF PATHOGENICITY
Adherence of mycoplasmas to the surface of the host cell is necessary for colonization and infection. Some pathogenic mycoplasmas are flask-shaped, with specialized tips that enhance adherence. *M. pneumoniae* adheres via a network of interactive adhesins and accessory proteins and produces hydrogen peroxide, which may cause injury to host cells. *M. hominis* metabolizes arginine, with the production of potentially cytotoxic amounts of ammonia. Ureaplasmas have been placed in a separate genus because of their unique urease activity; the metabolism of urea also produces ammonia. *M. pneumoniae* may evoke IgM autoantibodies that agglutinate human erythrocytes at 4°C. These cold agglutinins can cause anemia and other complications.

MYCOPLASMA PNEUMONIAE
Epidemiology   *M. pneumoniae* causes upper and lower respiratory tract symptoms in all age groups, with the highest attack rates in 5- to 20-year-olds. Infection with *M. pneumoniae* is acquired by inhalation of aerosols. The incubation period is 2–3 weeks, considerably longer than that of most other respiratory infections. Although epidemics have taken place in closed populations, such as those at schools and military installations, most cases occur sporadically or in families. Cases in families typically occur serially and are separated by 2- to 3-week intervals. Infections in adults are often the result of contact with children.

Infection with *M. pneumoniae* occurs worldwide and year round, with epidemics every few years. Some studies have noted an increase in the number of cases during the autumn months in temperate climates. Although pneumonia is the classic presentation, nonpneumonic infection is considerably more common. In very young children, most infections result only in upper respiratory symptoms, whereas children >5 years of age and adults may have bronchitis and pneumonia.

Clinical Presentation   After the prolonged incubation period, fever and constitutional symptoms develop along with headache and cough, both of which can be prominent and distressing. Symptoms typically progress less rapidly than those of viral respiratory tract infections. In the minority (perhaps 5–10%) of infected individuals who develop tracheobronchitis or pneumonia, cough becomes more prominent. Sputum, if produced at all, is usually white and may be tinged with blood. The temperature seldom rises above 38.9°–39.4°C (102°–103°F). Shaking chills, myalgias, and gastrointestinal symptoms (e.g., nausea, vomiting, and diarrhea) are unusual. Chest muscle soreness may result from frequent and prolonged coughing, but true pleuritic pain is uncommon.

Pharyngeal injection is often noted. Cervical lymph node enlargement is unusual. Ear pain due to bullous myringitis (blisters on the tympanic membrane) is a unique but uncommon manifestation. As in other "atypical" pneumonias, findings on auscultation of the lung may be normal or nearly normal despite striking radiographic abnormalities. Pleural effusions develop in <20% of patients.

M. pneumoniae infection may be particularly severe in patients who have sickle cell disease and other hemoglobin S–related hemoglobinopathies. The functional asplenia seen in sickle cell disease may contribute to severe disease as it does in pneumococcal infection. Severe respiratory distress and large pleural effusions may occur.

Extrapulmonary Manifestations   A broad array of extrapulmonary abnormalities have been associated with *M. pneumoniae* infection (Table 168-1). Although these events are unusual, they complicate other respiratory diseases even more rarely and often provide the only clue that an otherwise-unremarkable respiratory infection may be mycoplasmal. Erythema multiforme (Stevens-Johnson syndrome; see Fig. 52-9) typically occurs in young male patients with *M. pneumoniae* infection. Digital necrosis has been seen in patients with sickle cell disease who develop very high titers of cold agglutinins. Arthralgias are not unusual in patients who have mycoplasmal pneumonia; mycoplasmal arthritis is rare except in patients who have hypogammaglobulinemia.

The pathogenesis of the extrapulmonary manifestations of *M. pneumoniae* infection is controversial. Occasional reports have described the identification of *M. pneumoniae* or its nucleic acids in involved tissues. The fact that most attempts at detection have yielded negative results, however, suggests that these extrapulmonary complications have an immunologic basis.

Diagnosis   Most infections with *M. pneumoniae* are not diagnosed, as they are indistinguishable from upper and lower respiratory tract infections caused by myriad other viral and bacterial pathogens. When the diagnosis is suspected, it is usually because illness is prolonged or extrapulmonary manifestations develop. The white blood cell count is generally somewhat elevated, with few immature cells. Gram's staining of sputum shows leukocytes without a predominance of any bacterial morphologic type. Since *M. pneumoniae* lacks a cell wall, it cannot be detected on Gram's stain. In patients who have pneumonia, the chest radiograph may show reticulonodular or interstitial infiltration, primarily in the lower lobes. As in other "atypical" pneumonias, radiographic abnormalities may be more prominent than would be predicted by auscultation of the chest.

M. pneumoniae can be grown on artificial media, but the process is exacting, requires special media, and takes upwards of 2 weeks. Thus, mycoplasmal cultures do not provide timely information to aid in patient management. The same, unfortunately, is true of serologic diagnosis. Specific antibodies can be detected by enzyme-linked immunoassays, indirect immunofluorescence, or complement fixation but do not develop early enough to guide decisions regarding treatment. As with most serologic tests, examination of paired acute- and convalescent-phase serum specimens is required for good sensitivity and specificity.

TABLE 168-1   EXTRAPULMONARY MANIFESTATIONS OF *MYCOPLASMA PNEUMONIAE* INFECTION

System	Manifestations
Dermatologic	Erythema multiforme
	Maculopapular exanthems
	Vesicular exanthems
	Erythema nodosum
	Urticaria
Cardiovascular	Myocarditis
	Pericarditis
Neurologic	Encephalitis
	Aseptic meningitis
	Cerebellar ataxia
	Guillain-Barré syndrome
	Transverse myelitis
	Polyradiculopathy
Rheumatologic	Arthralgias
	Arthritis
	Juvenile-onset spondyloarthropathy
Hematologic	Hemolytic anemia
	Coagulopathies

Cold agglutinins are nonspecific but develop within the first 7–10 days in more than half of patients with *M. pneumoniae* pneumonia and may be detectable when the patient presents to a health care provider. In a patient with a compatible clinical picture, a cold agglutinin titer of ≥1:32 supports the diagnosis of mycoplasmal pneumonia. Cold agglutinin determinations are readily available from diagnostic laboratories. The test can also be performed at the bedside by the addition of 1 mL of the patient's blood to a tube containing anticoagulant (e.g., a tube used to collect blood for determination of prothrombin activity). Before cooling, the nonaggregated red blood cells coat the sides of the inverted tube. The blood is cooled to 4°C when the tube is placed in an ice bath for 3–5 min or in a standard refrigerator. In a positive test, clumps of red blood cells can be observed when the tube is inverted. Rewarming of the sample to 37°C in an incubator or by exposure to body heat should reverse the agglutination. A positive "bedside" cold agglutinin test is equivalent to a laboratory titer of ≥1:64.

The lack of sensitive, specific, and timely diagnostic tests has prompted the development of a variety of antigen detection tests (e.g., nucleic acid amplification) that do not involve serology or the cultivation of live organisms. Since many viral and bacterial infections result in clinical presentations similar to that caused by *M. pneumoniae*, examination of specimens for single antigens is unlikely to be useful. Multiplex nucleic acid amplification tests that examine a single throat swab or sputum sample for the most likely causative microorganisms have been developed. Such tests may provide more precise etiologic diagnosis of upper and lower respiratory tract infections.

℞ PNEUMONIA CAUSED BY *M. PNEUMONIAE*

Pneumonia due to *M. pneumoniae* is usually self-limited and is seldom life-threatening. Effective antimicrobial agents do shorten the duration of illness and, by reducing coughing, may conceivably render the patient less infectious. Although symptoms are alleviated by antimicrobial treatment, the organism usually is not eradicated. Cultures positive for *M. pneumoniae* may persist for months despite clinically effective antimicrobial therapy. The beneficial effects, if any, of such treatment on extrapulmonary manifestations of *M. pneumoniae* infection are unknown.

Because most mycoplasmal infections are not specifically diagnosed, management is directed at one of two syndromes: upper respiratory tract infection or community-acquired pneumonia. Upper respiratory infections, whether caused by viruses or by *M. pneumoniae*, do not require antimicrobial treatment. Community-acquired pneumonia (Chap. 251) may be caused by bacteria such as *Streptococcus pneumoniae* and *Haemophilus influenzae* or by "atypical" agents such as *Chlamydophila pneumoniae*, *Legionella pneumophila*, and *M. pneumoniae*. Recommended treatment regimens are detailed in **Tables 168-2** and **168-3**. Treatment of documented *M. pneumoniae* pneumonia is usually continued for 14–21 days.

GENITAL MYCOPLASMAS   (See also Chap. 124)

Epidemiology   *M. hominis*, *U. urealyticum*, and *U. parvum* are the most prevalent genital mycoplasmas. Infants may become colonized with these organisms during passage through a colonized birth canal.

TABLE 168-2	ORAL ANTIMICROBIAL AGENTS FOR THE TREATMENT OF AMBULATORY PATIENTS WITH COMMUNITY-ACQUIRED PNEUMONIA

Agent	Dose and Schedule
Doxycycline	100 mg bid
Erythromycin	500 mg qid
Clarithromycin	500 mg bid
Azithromycin	500 mg qd
Levofloxacin	500 mg qd
Moxifloxacin	400 mg qd
Gemifloxacin	320 mg qd

Note: Treatment of documented *M. pneumoniae* pneumonia is usually continued for 14–21 days.

TABLE 168-3	ANTIMICROBIAL AGENTS FOR THE TREATMENT OF HOSPITALIZED PATIENTS WITH COMMUNITY-ACQUIRED PNEUMONIA

1. Intravenous ceftriaxone (1.0 g/d) *or*
   Intravenous cefotaxime (1.0 g q8h) *or*
   Intravenous ampicillin/sulbactam (1.5–3.0 g q6h)
   plus
   Intravenous or oral erythromycin (500 mg qid) *or*
   Intravenous or oral azithromycin (500 mg qd) *or*
   Oral clarithromycin (500 mg bid)
2. Intravenous or oral levofloxacin (500 mg qd)
3. Intravenous or oral moxifloxacin (400 mg qd)

Note: Treatment of documented *M. pneumoniae* pneumonia is usually continued for 14–21 days.

Neonatal colonization tends not to persist. Only ~10% of prepubertal girls and even fewer prepubertal boys are colonized with ureaplasmas. After puberty, colonization occurs mainly as a result of sexual activity. Among adults, disadvantaged populations have higher colonization rates. Ureaplasmas can be cultured from the vaginas of ~80% of women cared for in public clinics and about half of women cared for by private obstetricians and gynecologists. Similarly, vaginal *M. hominis* is found in ~50% of women attending public clinics and in ~20% of private patients. Men have somewhat lower rates of genital colonization than women. In short, *U. urealyticum*, *U. parvum*, and *M. hominis* are frequently detected in genital specimens from healthy, sexually experienced adults. Evaluation of the role of these organisms in human disease must take into account their high prevalence among healthy people.

M. fermentans colonizes both the respiratory and genital tracts in >20% of adults. There is no convincing evidence that *M. fermentans* causes human disease. *M. genitalium* is a fastidious organism that is difficult to cultivate. Polymerase chain reaction (PCR) studies have identified the organism more successfully.

Association with Human Disease • *NONGONOCOCCAL URETHRITIS (NGU)*
Although *Chlamydia trachomatis* is the organism most firmly implicated in the etiology of NGU, there is no doubt that sexually transmitted ureaplasmas and *M. genitalium* also cause some cases. The ubiquity of ureaplasmas among men who do not have urethritis and the difficulty of identifying *M. genitalium* do not allow precise estimation of the proportion of cases of NGU caused by each of these mycoplasmas.

EPIDIDYMITIS AND PROSTATITIS   Ureaplasmas may be an occasional cause of epididymitis. *M. hominis* has not been implicated in this disease. Neither organism has been convincingly associated with prostatitis.

PELVIC INFLAMMATORY DISEASE (PID)   *M. hominis* and ureaplasmas are prominent components of the complex microbial flora of bacterial vaginosis. Since bacterial vaginosis is associated with PID, it is difficult to determine whether these organisms play an independent role in this condition. Although *M. genitalium* is not associated with bacterial vaginosis, preliminary studies have linked it to cervicitis, PID, and tubal factor infertility in women who are not infected with either *Neisseria gonorrhoeae* or *C. trachomatis*.

DISORDERS OF REPRODUCTION   Ureaplasmas have been considered as causes of involuntary infertility in both men and women, but there is no convincing evidence for such an association. These organisms have been associated with chorioamnionitis and preterm birth. Given the close association of ureaplasmas with bacterial vaginosis, a condition that is strongly associated with chorioamnionitis and preterm birth, it is difficult to define an independent role for ureaplasmas in these conditions. In infants of very low birth weight, ureaplasmas have been shown to cause pneumonia and long-term respiratory dysfunction. *M. hominis* can cause postpartum fever, which has been associated with isolation of this organism from blood and its occasional dissemination to joints, resulting in septic arthritis.

EXTRAGENITAL INFECTIONS   Sexually acquired reactive arthritis and Reiter's syndrome may be triggered by ureaplasmas, although *C. trachomatis* is the usual triggering agent. Patients who have hypogammaglobulinemia may develop chronic arthritis due to ureaplasmas and some other mycoplasmal species. *M. hominis* has been identified in patients with post-thoracotomy sternal wound infection and in rare instances of prosthetic heart valve and prosthetic joint infection.

Diagnosis   There is seldom any reason to examine specimens from the lower genital tract (vagina, male urethra) for mycoplasmas. The ubiquity of the organisms among healthy individuals makes a positive result uninterpretable. The organisms should be sought only in specimens from normally sterile areas, such as joint fluid with evidence of inflammation and cultures negative for conventional microorganisms.

M. hominis can replicate in many routine blood culture media without changing the appearance of the media. Although the organism forms nonhemolytic pinpoint colonies on blood agar, it cannot be visualized in gram-stained smears of these colonies. Neither ureaplasmas nor *M. genitalium* will grow in ordinary microbiologic media.

Microbiologic diagnosis of genital mycoplasmal infection requires specially prepared media and is beyond the capability of all but reference and research laboratories. Nucleic acid amplification tests such as PCR have been developed.

℞ GENITAL MYCOPLASMAS

Ureaplasmas, *M. genitalium*, and *M. hominis* are usually susceptible to tetracyclines (e.g., doxycycline). Infections caused by tetracycline-resistant ureaplasmas can be treated with erythromycin, while those due to tetracycline-resistant strains of *M. hominis* respond to treatment with clindamycin. As noted above, a specific microbiologic diagnosis of mycoplasmal infection is seldom made. Appropriate treatment provides antimicrobial coverage for the organisms that cause the particular syndrome. Accordingly, NGU is treated with doxycycline (100 mg orally twice a day for 7 days) or azithromycin (1.0 g as a single oral dose) to provide activity against *C. trachomatis, U. urealyticum, U. parvum,* and *M. genitalium.* Recommended regimens for the treatment of PID provide antimicrobial activity against gonococci, chlamydiae, and anaerobes as well as genital mycoplasmas.

FURTHER READINGS

ALEXANDER ER et al: Pneumonia due to *Mycoplasma pneumoniae.* N Engl J Med 275:131, 1966

MANDELL LA et al: Update of practice guidelines for the management of community-acquired pneumonia in immunocompetent adults. Clin Infect Dis 37:1405, 2003

MOROZUMI M et al: Simultaneous detection of pathogens in clinical samples from patients with community-acquired pneumonia by real-time PCR with pathogen-specific molecular beacon probes. J Clin Microbiol 44:1440, 2006

MURRAY HW et al: The protean manifestations of *Mycoplasma pneumoniae* in adults. Am J Med 58:229, 1975

TAYLOR SN: *Mycoplasma genitalium.* Curr Infect Dis Rep 7:453, 2005

WAITES KB et al: Mycoplasmas and ureaplasmas as neonatal pathogens. Clin Microbiol Rev 18:757, 2005

169 Chlamydial Infections
Walter E. Stamm

Three chlamydial species cause human infections: *Chlamydia trachomatis, Chlamydophila psittaci,* and *Chlamydophila pneumoniae. C. psittaci* is widely distributed in nature, producing genital, conjunctival, intestinal, or respiratory infections in many mammalian and avian species. Genital infections with *C. psittaci* have been well characterized in several species and cause abortion and infertility. Although mammalian strains of *C. psittaci* are not known to infect humans, avian strains occasionally do so, causing pneumonia and the systemic illness known as *psittacosis. C. pneumoniae* is a fastidious chlamydial species that appears to be a common cause of upper respiratory tract infection and pneumonia, primarily in children and young adults, and is a cause of recurrent respiratory infections in older adults. Studies have also linked *C. pneumoniae* infection to atherosclerotic cardiovascular disease and perhaps to asthma. No animal reservoir has been identified for *C. pneumoniae*; it appears to be an exclusively human pathogen spread via the respiratory route through close personal contact. *C. trachomatis* is also an exclusively human pathogen and was identified as the cause of trachoma in the 1940s. Since then, *C. trachomatis* has been recognized as a major cause of sexually transmitted and perinatal infection.

Chlamydiae are obligate intracellular bacteria that are classified in their own order, Chlamydiales (Fig. 169-1). They possess both DNA and RNA, have a cell wall and ribosomes similar to those of gram-negative bacteria, and are inhibited by antibiotics such as tetracycline. A unique feature of all chlamydiae is their complex reproductive cycle (Fig. 169-2). Two forms of the microorganism—the extracellular elementary body (EB) and the intracellular reticulate body (RB)—participate in this cycle. The EB is adapted for extracellular survival and is the infective form transmitted from one person to another. EBs attach to susceptible target cells (usually columnar or transitional epithelial cells) and enter the cells inside a phagosome. Within 8 h of cell entry, the EBs reorganize into RBs, which are adapted to intracellular survival and multiplication. They undergo binary fission, eventually producing

FIGURE 169-1 Chlamydial intracellular inclusions filled with smaller dense elementary bodies and larger reticulate bodies.

numerous replicates contained within the intracellular membrane-bound "inclusion body," which occupies much of the infected host cell. Chlamydial inclusions resist lysosomal fusion until late in the developmental cycle. After 24 h, the RBs condense and form EBs still

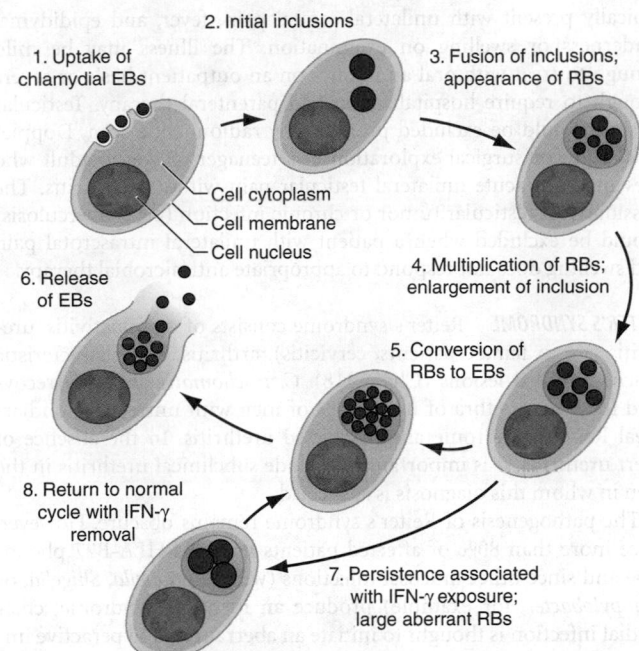

1. Uptake of chlamydial EBs

2. Initial inclusions

3. Fusion of inclusions; appearance of RBs

Cell cytoplasm
Cell membrane
Cell nucleus

6. Release of EBs

4. Multiplication of RBs; enlargement of inclusion

5. Conversion of RBs to EBs

8. Return to normal cycle with IFN-γ removal

7. Persistence associated with IFN-γ exposure; large aberrant RBs

FIGURE 169-2 Chlamydial life cycle. EBs, elementary bodies; RBs, reticulate bodies; IFN-γ, interferon γ.

contained within the inclusion. The inclusion then lyses, releasing EBs from the cell to initiate infection of adjacent cells or transmission to another person. Under some conditions [e.g., exposure to interferon γ (IFN-γ) or antibiotics], an altered life cycle is induced in which large, metabolically inactive RBs persist but do not replicate. Removal of the IFN-γ or antibiotics is followed by restoration of the normal life cycle.

Studies with monoclonal antibodies and nucleotide sequencing of the major outer-membrane protein have delineated at least 20 serotypes of *C. trachomatis*. According to the classification of Wang and Grayston, strains associated with trachoma are generally of the A, B, Ba, and C serovars, while serovars D through K are largely associated with sexually transmitted and perinatally acquired infections. Serovars L₁, L₂, and L₃ produce lymphogranuloma venereum (LGV) and hemorrhagic proctocolitis. The LGV strains exhibit unique biologic behavior in that they are more invasive than the other serovars, produce disease in lymphatic tissue, grow readily in cell culture systems and macrophages, and are lethal when inoculated intracerebrally into mice and monkeys. Non-LGV strains of *C. trachomatis* characteristically produce infections involving the superficial columnar epithelium of the eye, genitalia, and respiratory tract.

C. trachomatis is an infrequent cause of endocarditis, peritonitis, pleuritis, and possibly periappendicitis and occasionally causes respiratory infections in older children and adults. Some immunosuppressed patients with pneumonia have had either serologic or cultural evidence of *C. trachomatis* infection, but more data are necessary to define a pathogenic role for this organism in these patients.

C. TRACHOMATIS INFECTIONS

GENITAL INFECTIONS

Genital infections caused by *C. trachomatis* represent the most common bacterial sexually transmitted infections (STIs) in the United States (Chap. 124). An estimated 4 million cases occur each year. In adults, the clinical spectrum of sexually transmitted *C. trachomatis* infections parallels that of gonococcal infections. Both infections have been associated with urethritis, proctitis, and conjunctivitis in both sexes; with epididymitis in men; and with mucopurulent cervicitis (MPC), acute salpingitis, bartholinitis, and the Fitz-Hugh–Curtis syndrome (perihepatitis) in women. Moreover, both infections can be associated with septic arthritis. In general, however, chlamydial infections produce fewer symptoms and signs than gonococcal infections at the

same anatomic site; in fact, chlamydial infections are often totally asymptomatic. Increasing evidence suggests that many chlamydial infections of the genital tract, especially in women, persist for months without producing symptoms. Simultaneous infection with *C. trachomatis* often occurs in women with cervical gonococcal infection and in heterosexual men with gonococcal urethritis.

Epidemiology Infections due to *C. trachomatis* have been reportable in the United States since 1985, and national incidence data show steadily rising numbers of reported infections, probably reflecting both increased testing and increased reporting more than increasing incidence. Most testing to date has focused on women, and thus the reported incidence is severalfold greater among women than among men; this difference likely represents a surveillance artifact.

The age of peak incidence of genital *C. trachomatis* infections, as of other STIs, is the late teens and early twenties. The prevalence of chlamydial urethral infection among young men is at least 3–5% for those seen in general medical settings or in urban high schools and is >10% for asymptomatic soldiers undergoing routine physical examination; 15–20% of heterosexual men seen in sexually transmitted disease (STD) clinics may be positive for *C. trachomatis*. In areas where chlamydial control programs have been implemented, the overall prevalence may be markedly reduced. In short, the prevalence among men varies widely with the population group studied and with the geographic locale. With the newer, more sensitive nucleic acid amplification tests (NAATs), such as polymerase chain reaction (PCR) and transcription-mediated amplification (TMA), prevalences in most populations have been 10–30% higher than those measured with older, less sensitive tests.

The prevalence of cervical infection among women is ~5% for asymptomatic college students and prenatal patients in the United States, >10% for women seen in family planning clinics, and >20% for women seen in STD clinics. As in men, the prevalence of genital *C. trachomatis* infections varies substantially by geographic locale, with the highest rates in the southeastern United States. However, substantial prevalences (~8%) of asymptomatic chlamydial infection have been demonstrated among young female military recruits from all parts of the United States. In this country, the prevalence of *C. trachomatis* in the cervix of pregnant women is 5–10 times higher than that of *Neisseria gonorrhoeae*. The prevalence of genital infection with either agent is highest among individuals who are between the ages of 18 and 24, single, and non-Caucasian (e.g., African-American or Latino). Recurrent chlamydial infections occur frequently in these same risk groups and are often acquired from untreated sexual partners. Use of oral contraceptive pills and the presence of cervical ectopy also confer an increased risk of chlamydial infection. The proportion of infections that are asymptomatic appears to be higher for *C. trachomatis* than for *N. gonorrhoeae*, and symptomatic *C. trachomatis* infections are clinically less severe. Mild or asymptomatic chlamydial infections of the fallopian tubes nonetheless cause ongoing tubal damage and infertility. Furthermore, because the total number of *C. trachomatis* infections exceeds the total number of *N. gonorrhoeae* infections in industrialized countries, the total morbidity caused by *C. trachomatis* genital infections in these countries exceeds that caused by *N. gonorrhoeae*. The prevalence of *C. trachomatis* is higher than that of *N. gonorrhoeae* in industrialized countries, in part because measures such as treatment of sex partners and routine cultures for case detection in asymptomatic individuals have been applied much longer and more effectively to the control of gonorrhea than to the control of *C. trachomatis* infection.

Pathogenesis *C. trachomatis* preferentially infects the columnar epithelium of the eye and the respiratory and genital tracts. The infection induces an immune response but often persists for months or years in the absence of antimicrobial therapy. Serious sequelae often occur in association with repeated or persistent infections. The precise mechanism through which repeated or persistent infection elicits an inflammatory response that leads to tubal scarring and damage in the female upper genital tract is not yet clear. One antigen, the chlamydial 60-kDa heat-shock protein, may be involved in inducing a pathologic immune response or may elicit antibodies that cross-react with human heat-shock proteins. Several complete chlamydial genomes have been sequenced, and genetic studies may soon offer further insights into the pathogenic mechanisms of *C. trachomatis*.

Clinical Manifestations · *NONGONOCOCCAL AND POSTGONOCOCCAL URETHRITIS* Nongonococcal urethritis (NGU) is a diagnosis of exclusion that is applied to men with symptoms and/or signs of urethritis who do not have gonorrhea. Postgonococcal urethritis (PGU) refers to NGU developing in men 2–3 weeks after treatment of gonococcal urethritis with single doses of agents such as penicillins or cephalosporins that lack antimicrobial activity against chlamydiae. Since current treatment regimens for gonorrhea include tetracycline, doxycycline, or azithromycin for possible concomitant chlamydial infection, both the incidence of PGU and the causative role of chlamydiae in this syndrome have declined. *C. trachomatis* causes 20–40% of cases of NGU in heterosexual men but is less commonly isolated from homosexual men with this syndrome. The cause of most of the remaining cases of NGU is uncertain; considerable evidence suggests that *Ureaplasma urealyticum* and *Mycoplasma genitalium* cause many cases of NGU, while *Trichomonas vaginalis* and herpes simplex virus (HSV) cause some cases.

NGU is diagnosed by documentation of a leukocytic urethral exudate and by exclusion of gonorrhea by Gram's staining or culture. *C. trachomatis* urethritis is generally less severe than gonococcal urethritis, although in an individual patient these two forms of urethritis cannot be reliably differentiated solely on clinical grounds. Symptoms include urethral discharge (often whitish and mucoid rather than frankly purulent), dysuria, and urethral itching. Physical examination may reveal meatal erythema and tenderness and a urethral exudate that is often demonstrable only by stripping of the urethra.

At least one-third of males with *C. trachomatis* urethral infection have no demonstrable signs or symptoms of urethritis. Use of NAATs on first-void urine specimens to diagnose chlamydial infections in men has facilitated broader-based testing for asymptomatic infection in males. As a result, asymptomatic chlamydial urethritis has been demonstrated in 5–10% of sexually active adolescent males screened in school-based clinics or community centers. Such patients generally have first-glass pyuria (≥15 leukocytes per 400× microscopic field in the sediment of first-void urine), a positive leukocyte esterase test, or an increased number of leukocytes on a Gram-stained smear prepared from a urogenital swab inserted 1–2 cm into the anterior urethra. For the enumeration of leukocytes, the smear is first scanned at low power to identify areas of the slide containing the highest concentration of leukocytes. These areas are then examined under oil immersion (1000×). An average of four or more leukocytes in at least three of five 1000× oil-immersion fields is indicative of urethritis and correlates with the recovery of *C. trachomatis*. To differentiate between true urethritis and functional symptoms among symptomatic patients or to make a presumptive diagnosis of *C. trachomatis* infection in "high-risk" but asymptomatic men (e.g., male patients in STD clinics, sex partners of women with nongonococcal salpingitis or MPC, fathers of children with inclusion conjunctivitis), the examination of an endourethral specimen for increased leukocytes is useful if specific diagnostic tests for chlamydiae are not available. Alternatively, urethritis can be assayed noninvasively by examination of a first-void urine sample for pyuria, either by microscopy or by the leukocyte esterase test. Urine (or a urethral swab) can also be directly tested for chlamydiae or gonococci by DNA amplification methods, as described below.

EPIDIDYMITIS *C. trachomatis* is the foremost cause of epididymitis in sexually active heterosexual men <35 years of age, accounting for ~70% of cases. *N. gonorrhoeae* causes most of the remaining cases, and some men have simultaneous infections with both pathogens, usually accompanied by asymptomatic urethritis as defined above. In homosexual men, sexually transmitted coliform infection acquired via insertive rectal intercourse may cause epididymitis. Coliform bacteria and *Pseudomonas aeruginosa*, usually detected in association with preceding urologic instrumentation or surgery, are the most common causes of epididymitis in men over 35. Men with chlamydial epididymitis

typically present with unilateral scrotal pain, fever, and epididymal tenderness or swelling on examination. The illness may be mild enough to treat with oral antibiotics on an outpatient basis or severe enough to require hospitalization and parenteral therapy. Testicular torsion should be excluded promptly by radionuclide scan, Doppler flow study, or surgical exploration in a teenager or young adult who presents with acute unilateral testicular pain without urethritis. The possibility of testicular tumor or chronic infection (e.g., tuberculosis) should be excluded when a patient with unilateral intrascrotal pain and swelling does not respond to appropriate antimicrobial therapy.

REITER'S SYNDROME Reiter's syndrome consists of conjunctivitis, urethritis (or, in female patients, cervicitis), arthritis, and characteristic mucocutaneous lesions (Chap. 318). *C. trachomatis* has been recovered from the urethra of up to 70% of men with untreated nondiarrheal Reiter's syndrome and associated urethritis. In the absence of overt urethritis, it is important to exclude subclinical urethritis in the men in whom this diagnosis is suspected.

The pathogenesis of Reiter's syndrome remains obscure. However, since more than 80% of affected patients have the HLA-B27 phenotype and since other mucosal infections (with *Salmonella*, *Shigella*, or *Campylobacter*, for example) produce an identical syndrome, chlamydial infection is thought to initiate an aberrant and hyperactive immune response that produces inflammation at the involved target organs in these genetically predisposed individuals. Evidence of exaggerated cell-mediated and humoral immune responses to chlamydial antigens in Reiter's syndrome supports this hypothesis. The presumptive demonstration of chlamydial EBs and chlamydial DNA in the joint fluid and synovial tissue of patients with Reiter's syndrome suggests that chlamydiae may actually spread from genital to joint tissues in these patients, perhaps in macrophages.

PROCTITIS *C. trachomatis* strains of either the genital immunotypes D through K or the LGV immunotypes cause proctitis in homosexual men who practice receptive anorectal intercourse. In the United States, the vast majority of cases are due to immunotypes D through K and present either as asymptomatic infection or as mild proctitis not unlike gonococcal proctitis. These infections may develop in heterosexual women as well. Patients present with mild rectal pain, mucous discharge, tenesmus, and (occasionally) bleeding. Nearly all have neutrophils in Gram-stained rectal samples. Anoscopy in these non-LGV cases of chlamydial proctitis reveals mild, patchy mucosal friability and mucopurulent discharge, and the disease process is limited to the distal rectum. LGV strains produce more severe ulcerative proctitis or proctocolitis that can be confused clinically with HSV proctitis (severe rectal pain, rectal bleeding, discharge, and tenesmus) and that histologically resembles Crohn's disease in that giant cell formation and granulomas can be seen (Chap. 289). In the United States, these cases of LGV proctitis occur almost exclusively in homosexual men, many of whom are positive for HIV.

MUCOPURULENT CERVICITIS Although many women with *C. trachomatis* infection of the cervix have no symptoms or signs, a careful speculum examination reveals evidence of MPC in 30–50% of cases. As is discussed more fully in Chap. 124, MPC is associated with yellow mucopurulent endocervical discharge and with ≥20 neutrophils per 1000× microscopic field within strands of cervical mucus on a thinly smeared, Gram-stained preparation of endocervical exudate. Other characteristic findings include edema of the zone of cervical ectopy and a propensity of the mucosa to bleed on minor trauma—e.g., when specimens are collected with a swab. A Pap smear shows increased numbers of neutrophils as well as a characteristic pattern of mononuclear inflammatory cells, including plasma cells, transformed lymphocytes, and histiocytes. Cervical biopsy shows a predominantly mononuclear cell infiltrate of the subepithelial stroma, often with follicular cervicitis.

PELVIC INFLAMMATORY DISEASE (See also Chap. 124) In the United States, *C. trachomatis* has been identified in the fallopian tubes or endometrium of up to 50% of women with pelvic inflammatory disease

(PID), and its role as an important etiologic agent in this syndrome is well accepted. PID occurs via ascending intraluminal spread of *C. trachomatis* from the lower genital tract. MPC is thus followed by endometritis, endosalpingitis, and finally pelvic peritonitis. Evidence of MPC is usually found in women with laparoscopically verified salpingitis. Similarly, endometritis, demonstrated by endometrial biopsy showing plasma cell infiltration of the endometrial epithelium, is documented in most women with laparoscopically verified chlamydial (or gonococcal) salpingitis. Chlamydial endometritis can also occur in the absence of clinical evidence of salpingitis: ~40–50% of women with MPC have plasma cell endometritis. Histologic evidence of endometritis has been correlated with an "endometritis syndrome" consisting of vaginal bleeding, lower abdominal pain, and uterine tenderness in the absence of adnexal tenderness. Chlamydial salpingitis produces milder symptoms than does gonococcal salpingitis and may be associated with less marked adnexal tenderness. Thus mild adnexal or uterine tenderness in sexually active women with cervicitis suggests PID.

Infertility associated with fallopian-tube scarring has been strongly linked to antecedent *C. trachomatis* infection in serologic studies. Since many infertile women with tubal scarring and antichlamydial antibody have no history of PID, it appears that subclinical tubal infection ("silent salpingitis") may produce scarring. Studies in animals and humans with salpingitis and tubal scarring suggest the continuing presence of persistent, slowly replicating chlamydial infection in tubal tissue. While the pathogenesis of *C. trachomatis*–induced tubal scarring remains poorly understood, antibodies to the chlamydial 60-kDa heat-shock protein have been correlated with tubal infertility, ectopic pregnancy, and Fitz-Hugh–Curtis syndrome (see below). Thus this antigen may initiate an immune-mediated process that ultimately damages the fallopian tube. Host genetic susceptibility, as defined by HLA type, may also play an important role.

Perihepatitis, or the Fitz-Hugh–Curtis syndrome, was originally described as a complication of gonococcal PID. The syndrome should be suspected whenever a young, sexually active woman presents with an illness resembling cholecystitis (fever and right-upper-quadrant pain of subacute or acute onset). Symptoms and signs of salpingitis may be minimal. Cultural and/or serologic evidence of *C. trachomatis* infection is found in three-quarters of women with this syndrome.

URETHRAL SYNDROME IN WOMEN In the absence of infection with uropathogens such as coliforms or *Staphylococcus saprophyticus*, *C. trachomatis* is the pathogen most commonly isolated from college women with dysuria, frequency, and pyuria (Chap. 282). This organism can also be isolated from the urethra of women without symptoms of urethritis, and up to 25% of female STD clinic patients with chlamydial urogenital infection have cultures positive for *C. trachomatis* from the urethra only.

INFECTION IN PREGNANCY AND THE NEONATAL PERIOD Studies in the United States have demonstrated that 5–25% of pregnant women have *C. trachomatis* infections of the cervix. In these studies, approximately one-half to two-thirds of children exposed during birth have acquired *C. trachomatis* infection. Roughly half of the infected infants (25% of the group exposed) have developed clinical evidence of inclusion conjunctivitis. In addition to infecting the eye, *C. trachomatis* has been isolated frequently and persistently from the nasopharynx, rectum, and vagina of such infants, occasionally for >1 year in the absence of treatment. Pneumonia develops in 10% of children infected perinatally, and otitis media may in some cases result from perinatally acquired chlamydial infection.

Neonatal chlamydial conjunctivitis has an acute onset 5–14 days after birth and often produces a profuse mucopurulent discharge. However, it is impossible to differentiate chlamydial conjunctivitis from other forms of neonatal conjunctivitis (such as that due to *N. gonorrhoeae*, *Haemophilus influenzae*, *Streptococcus pneumoniae*, or HSV) on clinical grounds; thus laboratory diagnosis is required. Inclusions within epithelial cells are often detected in Giemsa-stained conjunctival smears, but these smears are considerably less sensitive than cultures, antigen detection tests, or NAATs for chlamydiae. Gram-stained smears may show gonococci or occasional small gram-negative coccobacilli in *Haemophilus* conjunctivitis, but smears should be accompanied by cultures for these agents.

C. trachomatis causes a distinctive pneumonia syndrome in infants. Epidemiologic studies have linked chlamydial pulmonary infection in infants with increased occurrence of subacute lung disease (bronchitis, asthma, wheezing) in later childhood.

Lymphogranuloma Venereum • *DEFINITION* LGV is an STI caused by *C. trachomatis* strains of the L_1, L_2, and L_3 serovars. In the United States, most cases are caused by L_2 organisms. Classically, acute LGV is characterized by a transient primary genital lesion followed by multilocular suppurative regional lymphadenopathy. However, patients exposed via insertive rectal intercourse usually develop hemorrhagic proctitis with regional lymphadenitis. Acute LGV is almost always associated with systemic symptoms such as fever and leukocytosis but is rarely associated with systemic complications such as meningoencephalitis. Without treatment, late complications that develop after a period of years include genital elephantiasis due to lymphatic involvement; strictures; and fistulas of the penis, urethra, and rectum.

EPIDEMIOLOGY LGV is usually sexually transmitted, but occasional transmission by nonsexual personal contact, fomites, or laboratory accidents has been documented. Laboratory work involving the creation of aerosols of LGV organisms (e.g., sonication, homogenization) must be conducted only with appropriate measures for biologic containment.

The peak incidence of LGV corresponds to the age of greatest sexual activity: the second and third decades of life. The worldwide incidence of LGV is falling, but the disease is still endemic and a major cause of morbidity in Asia, Africa, South America, and parts of the Caribbean. In the Bahamas, an apparent outbreak of LGV was described in association with a concurrent increase in heterosexual infection with HIV. For more than a decade, however, the reported incidence of LGV in the United States has been only 0.1 case per 100,000 persons. Recently, clusters of LGV cases have been described in the United States and in Western Europe, largely among men having sex with men. These cases have usually presented as hemorrhagic proctocolitis in HIV-positive men. More widespread use of NAATs for identification of rectal infections may have enhanced case recognition.

The frequency of infection following exposure is believed to be much lower for LGV than for gonorrhea and syphilis. Early manifestations are recognized more often in men than in women, who usually present with late complications. In the United States, where the reported male-to-female ratio of cases is 3.4:1, most cases involve homosexually active men and persons returning from abroad (travelers, sailors, and military personnel). The main reservoir of infection, although it has not been directly demonstrated, is presumed to be asymptomatically infected individuals.

CLINICAL MANIFESTATIONS A *primary genital lesion* develops 3 days to 3 weeks after exposure. It is a small, painless vesicle or nonindurated ulcer or papule located on the penis in men and on the labia, posterior vagina, or fourchette in women. The primary lesion is noticed by fewer than one-third of men with LGV and only rarely by women. It heals in a few days without scarring and, even when noticed, is usually recognized as LGV only in retrospect. LGV strains of *C. trachomatis* have occasionally been recovered from genital ulcers and from the urethra of men and the endocervix of women who present with inguinal adenopathy; these areas may be the primary site of infection in some cases.

Primary anal or *rectal infection* develops after receptive anorectal intercourse. In women, rectal infection with LGV (or non-LGV) strains of *C. trachomatis* presumably can also arise by the contiguous spread of infected secretions along the perineum (as in rectal gonococcal infections in women) or perhaps by spread to the rectum via the pelvic lymphatics.

From the site of the primary urethral, genital, anal, or rectal infection, the organism spreads via the regional lymphatics. Penile, vulvar, or anal infection can lead to inguinal and femoral lymphadenitis. Rectal infection produces hypogastric and deep iliac lymphadenitis. Upper vaginal or cervical infection results in enlargement of the obturator and iliac nodes.

The most common presenting picture in heterosexual men is the *inguinal syndrome*, which is characterized by painful inguinal lymphadenopathy beginning 2–6 weeks after presumed exposure; in rare instances, the onset comes after a few months. The inguinal adenopathy is unilateral in two-thirds of cases, and palpable enlargement of the iliac and femoral nodes is often evident on the same side as the enlarged inguinal nodes. The nodes are initially discrete, but progressive periadenitis results in a matted mass of nodes that becomes fluctuant and suppurative. The overlying skin becomes fixed, inflamed, and thin and finally develops multiple draining fistulas. Extensive enlargement of chains of inguinal nodes above and below the inguinal ligament ("the sign of the groove") is not specific and, although not uncommon, is documented in only a minority of cases. On histologic examination, infected nodes are initially found to have characteristic small stellate abscesses surrounded by histiocytes. These abscesses coalesce to form large, necrotic, suppurative foci. Spontaneous healing usually takes place after several months; inguinal scars or granulomatous masses of various sizes persist for life. Massive pelvic lymphadenopathy may lead to exploratory laparotomy.

As NAATs for *C. trachomatis* are being used more often, increasing numbers of cases of LGV proctitis are being recognized in homosexual men. Such patients present with anorectal pain and mucopurulent, bloody rectal discharge. Although these patients may report diarrhea, they are often referring not to diarrhea but rather to frequent, painful, unsuccessful attempts at defecation (tenesmus). Sigmoidoscopy reveals ulcerative proctitis or proctocolitis, with purulent exudate and mucosal bleeding. The histopathologic findings in the rectal mucosa include granulomas with giant cells, crypt abscesses, and extensive inflammation. These clinical, sigmoidoscopic, and histopathologic findings may closely resemble those of Crohn's disease of the rectum.

Constitutional symptoms are common during the stage of regional lymphadenopathy and, in cases of proctitis, may include fever, chills, headache, meningismus, anorexia, myalgias, and arthralgias. These findings in the presence of lymphadenopathy are sometimes mistakenly interpreted as malignant lymphoma. Other systemic complications are infrequent but include arthritis with sterile effusion, aseptic meningitis, meningoencephalitis, conjunctivitis, hepatitis, and erythema nodosum. Chlamydiae have been recovered from the cerebrospinal fluid and in one case were isolated from the blood of a patient with severe constitutional symptoms—a result indicating the dissemination of infection. Laboratory-acquired infections suspected of being due to the inhalation of aerosols have been associated with mediastinal lymphadenitis, pneumonitis, and pleural effusion.

Complications of untreated anorectal infection include perirectal abscess; fistula in ano; and rectovaginal, rectovesical, and ischiorectal fistulas. Secondary bacterial infection probably contributes to these complications. Rectal stricture is a late complication of anorectal infection and usually develops 2–6 cm from the anal orifice—i.e., at a site within reach on digital rectal examination. Proximal extension of the stricture for several centimeters may lead to a mistaken clinical and radiographic diagnosis of carcinoma.

A small percentage of cases of LGV in men present as chronic progressive infiltrative, ulcerative, or fistular lesions of the penis, urethra, or scrotum. Associated lymphatic obstruction may produce elephantiasis. When urethral stricture occurs, it usually involves the posterior urethra and causes incontinence or difficulty with urination.

Approach to the Diagnosis and Treatment of *C. trachomatis* Genital Infections

Four types of laboratory procedure are available to confirm *C. trachomatis* infection: direct microscopic examination of tissue scrapings for typical intracytoplasmic inclusions or EBs; isolation of the organism in cell culture; demonstration of chlamydial antigens by immunologic detection or demonstration of chlamydial genes in NAATs; and detection of antibody in serum or in local secretions.

Except in conjunctivitis, direct microscopic examination of Giemsa-stained cell scrapings for typical inclusions has an unacceptably low degree of sensitivity, and false-positive interpretations by inexperienced observers are also common. Even for conjunctivitis, this approach has been replaced by direct fluorescent antibody staining of conjunctival smears to identify chlamydial EBs with specific monoclonal antibodies (see below) or, where available, NAATs.

Cell culture techniques for isolation of *C. trachomatis* are available only in large medical centers. In addition to limited availability, other disadvantages of cell culture include its low and variable level of sensitivity (40–80%), its requirement for rigorous transport conditions, and its high cost and technically demanding nature. Therefore, nonculture alternatives involving antigen detection or nucleic acid amplification have been developed. In the direct immunofluorescent antibody (DFA) slide test, potentially infected genital or ocular secretions are smeared onto a slide, fixed, and stained with fluorescein-conjugated monoclonal antibody specific for chlamydial antigens. The observation of fluorescing EBs confirms the diagnosis. Enzyme-linked immunosorbent assay (ELISA) techniques for the detection of chlamydial antigens provide another alternative to culture. The reported sensitivity and specificity of these tests for genital infections (as compared with culture) have been 60–80% and 97–99%, respectively, in high-risk populations. More recently, NAATs have been developed for chlamydial diagnosis using PCR, ligase chain reaction (LCR), TMA, and other techniques. These tests are quite clearly the most sensitive and specific chlamydial diagnostic methods available; they are also the most expensive. Because of their very high analytic sensitivity, NAATs allow the use of novel specimens: these tests can detect chlamydial genes in first-void urine samples or patient-collected vaginal swabs with a high degree of sensitivity and specificity. The use of urine specimens and patient-collected vaginal swabs rather than conventional urethral and cervical swabs is particularly appealing for public-health chlamydial screening programs because of the ease of sample collection and transport, even in community-based settings. These tests have also facilitated population-based studies of chlamydial infections.

Serologic tests are of limited usefulness in the diagnosis of most chlamydial oculogenital infections. The complement fixation test with heat-stable, genus-specific antigen has been used with some success to diagnose LGV but is insensitive in infections due to non-LGV strains of *C. trachomatis*. The microimmunofluorescence (micro-IF) test with *C. trachomatis* antigens is more sensitive but is generally available only in research laboratories. The test measures antibodies by serovar specificity and by immunoglobulin class (IgM, IgG, IgA, secretory IgA) in both serum and local secretions. Cross-reacting antibodies to *C. pneumoniae* may sometimes be problematic. Serologic diagnosis by the micro-IF test may be useful in infant pneumonia (in which high-titer IgM antibody and/or fourfold rises in titer are often demonstrated), in chlamydial salpingitis (especially Fitz-Hugh–Curtis syndrome), and in LGV. In all of these more invasive syndromes, high antibody levels are present.

Table 169-1 summarizes the diagnostic tests of choice for patients with suspected *C. trachomatis* infection. It is clear that, in most settings and for most purposes, sensitivity and specificity will be greatest with NAATs. For patients to whom medicolegal considerations may apply (victims of sexual or child abuse), cultures or NAATs should always be used. In men with suspected urethritis, application of NAATs to a first-void urine specimen offers a sensitive and noninvasive diagnostic method other than the use of urethral swabs. For the diagnosis of urogenital (cervical or urethral) infections in women, testing of a first-void urine specimen by nucleic acid amplification methods is about as sensitive as testing of a cervical swab. Patient-collected vaginal swabs analyzed by NAAT have also been used successfully and with equal sensitivity and specificity. Since chlamydial diagnostic testing has become more widely available and is now more sensitive and specific than in the past, its use for specific diagnosis in patients with suspected chlamydial syndromes (e.g., MPC, NGU, and PID) and their partners should be promoted. High priority should also be given to the screening of asymptomatic high-risk women who would not otherwise receive treatment for presumptive chlamydial infection, especially those seen in high-risk settings (e.g., STD clinics or abortion clinics) and those with a high-risk profile (e.g., sexually active and ≤ 21 years of age, new sex partner within the preceding 2 months, or more than one current sex partner). Similar screening programs should be used to detect and treat asymptomatic urethritis in high-risk adolescent males. Where implemented, screening programs of this type have generally been associated with reductions in the prevalence of chlamydial infection and of its complications, such as PID, ectopic pregnancy, and infertility.

TABLE 169-1 DIAGNOSTIC TESTS FOR SEXUALLY TRANSMITTED AND PERINATAL *CHLAMYDIA TRACHOMATIS* INFECTION

Infection	Suggestive Signs/Symptoms	Presumptive Diagnosis[a]	Confirmatory Test of Choice
Men			
NGU, PGU	Discharge, dysuria	Gram's stain with >4 neutrophils per oil-immersion field; no gonococci	Urine or urethral NAAT for *C. trachomatis*
Epididymitis	Unilateral intrascrotal swelling, pain, tenderness; fever; NGU	Gram's stain with >4 neutrophils per oil-immersion field; no gonococci; urinalysis with pyuria	Urine or urethral NAAT for *C. trachomatis*
Women			
Cervicitis	Mucopurulent cervical discharge, bleeding and edema of the zone of cervical ectopy	Cervical Gram's stain with ≥20 neutrophils per oil-immersion field in cervical mucus	Urine, cervical, or vaginal NAAT for *C. trachomatis*
Salpingitis	Lower abdominal pain, cervical motion tenderness, adnexal tenderness or masses	*C. trachomatis* always potentially present in salpingitis	Urine, cervical, or vaginal NAAT for *C. trachomatis*
Urethritis	Dysuria and frequency without hematuria	MPC; sterile pyuria; negative routine urine culture	Urine or urethral NAAT for *C. trachomatis*
Adults of Either Sex			
Proctitis	Rectal pain, discharge, tenesmus, bleeding; history of receptive anorectal intercourse	Negative gonococcal culture and Gram's stain; at least 1 neutrophil per oil-immersion field in rectal Gram's stain	Rectal NAAT for *C. trachomatis* or culture
Reiter's syndrome	NGU, arthritis, conjunctivitis, typical skin lesions	Gram's stain with >4 neutrophils per oil-immersion field; lack of gonococci indicative of NGU	Urine or urethral NAAT for *C. trachomatis*
LGV	Regional adenopathy, primary lesion, proctitis, systemic symptoms	None	Culture of LGV strain from node or rectum, occasionally from urethra or cervix; NAAT for *C. trachomatis* from these sites; LGV CF titer, ≥1:64; micro-IF titer, ≥1:512
Neonates			
Conjunctivitis	Purulent conjunctival discharge 6–18 days after delivery	Negative culture and Gram's stain for gonococci, *Haemophilus* spp., pneumococci, staphylococci	Conjunctival NAAT for *C. trachomatis*; FA-stained scraping of conjunctival material
Infant pneumonia	Afebrile, staccato cough, diffuse rales, bilateral hyperinflation, interstitial infiltrates	None	Chlamydial culture or NAAT of sputum, pharynx, eye, rectum; micro-IF antibody to *C. trachomatis*—fourfold change in IgG or IgM antibody titer

[a]A presumptive diagnosis of chlamydial infection is often made in the syndromes listed when gonococci are not found. A positive test for *Neisseria gonorrhoeae* does not exclude the involvement of *C. trachomatis*, which often is present in patients with gonorrhea.

Note: CF, complement-fixing; FA, fluorescent antibody; LGV, lymphogranuloma venereum; micro-IF, microimmunofluorescence; MPC, mucopurulent cervicitis; NAAT, nucleic acid amplification test; NGU, nongonococcal urethritis; PGU, postgonococcal urethritis.

℞ *C. TRACHOMATIS* GENITAL AND PERINATAL INFECTIONS

Until the introduction of azithromycin, chlamydial infections could not be eradicated by single-dose or short-term antimicrobial regimens, and most uncomplicated genital infections in adults were treated with a 7-day course of doxycycline or tetracycline. A 2-week course is recommended for complicated chlamydial infections (e.g., PID, epididymitis) and at least a 3-week course of doxycycline (100 mg orally bid) or erythromycin base (500 mg orally qid) for LGV. Failure of treatment with a tetracycline in genital infections usually indicates poor compliance or reinfection rather than the involvement of a drug-resistant strain. To date, clinically significant drug resistance has not been observed in *C. trachomatis* infection.

Therapy for *C. trachomatis* urethritis is more efficacious than therapy for nonchlamydial NGU. *C. trachomatis* is eradicated from the urethra in nearly all cases by treatment with tetracycline hydrochloride (500 mg qid for 7 days) or doxycycline (100 mg by mouth bid for 7 days).

Eradication of *C. trachomatis* from the cervix by tetracycline and doxycycline, with doses and durations similar to those specified above for urethritis, has been demonstrated. Azithromycin (a single oral 1-g dose) is the regimen of choice for pregnant women with *C. trachomatis* infection. However, amoxicillin (500 mg tid for 7 days) can also be given to pregnant women. Tetracycline hydrochloride (500 mg qid) or doxycycline (100 mg bid) for 14 days produces clinical and microbiologic cure of epididymitis and PID associated with *C. trachomatis* infection, but in this situation a tetracycline should always be used together with a drug that is highly effective against gonorrhea.

Azithromycin is highly active against *C. trachomatis*; exhibits prolonged bioavailability; is concentrated intracellularly; and has, for the first time, made it possible to use single-dose therapy for chlamydial infection. In comparative trials, a 1-g single dose of azithromycin has been as effective as 7 days of doxycycline therapy for uncomplicated chlamydial infection. Azithromycin causes fewer adverse gastrointestinal reactions than do older macrolides such as erythromycin. The single-dose regimen of azithromycin has great appeal for the treatment of patients with uncomplicated chlamydial infection (especially those without symptoms and those with a likelihood of poor compliance) and of sexual partners of infected patients. These advantages must be weighed against the considerably greater cost of azithromycin. Whenever possible, the single 1-g dose should be given as directly observed therapy. Although not approved by the U.S. Food and Drug Administration for the treatment of pregnant women, the 1-g single-dose regimen of azithromycin appears to be safe and effective for this purpose.

Of the fluoroquinolones, ofloxacin (300 mg by mouth bid for 7 days) and levofloxacin (500 mg/d by mouth for 7 days) are as effective as doxycycline for the treatment of chlamydial infection and appear to be safe and well tolerated. These drugs cannot be used in pregnancy.

TREATMENT OF SEX PARTNERS The continued high prevalence of chlamydial infections in most parts of the United States is due primarily to the failure to diagnose—and therefore treat—patients with symptomatic or asymptomatic infection and their sex partners. *C. trachomatis* urethral or cervical infection has been well documented in a high proportion of the sex partners of patients with NGU, epididymitis, Reiter's syndrome, salpingitis, or endocervicitis. If possible, confirmatory laboratory tests for *Chlamydia* should be undertaken in these individuals, but even those without positive tests or evidence of clinical disease who have recently been exposed to proven or possible chlamydial infection (e.g., NGU) should be offered therapy. A novel approach is the use of partner-delivered therapy, in which the infected patient receives treatment and is also provided with single-dose azithromycin to give to his or her sex partner(s).

CHAPTER 169 Chlamydial Infections

TREATMENT OF NEONATES AND INFANTS In neonates with conjunctivitis or infants with pneumonia, erythromycin ethylsuccinate or estolate can be given orally at a dosage of 50 mg/kg per day, preferably in four divided doses, for 2 weeks. Careful attention must be given to compliance with therapy—a frequent problem. Relapses of eye infection are common after treatment with topical erythromycin or tetracycline ophthalmic ointment and may also follow oral erythromycin therapy. Thus follow-up cultures should be performed after treatment. Both parents should be examined for *C. trachomatis* infection and, if diagnostic testing is not readily available, should be treated with doxycycline or azithromycin.

Prevention Efforts to develop a vaccine for chlamydial infection have not yet been successful. Early diagnosis and treatment shorten the duration of the infectious period and therefore constitute primary prevention of chlamydial infection. By the early 1990s, one of the 10 regions of the United States (Region X, the Pacific Northwest) had formally undertaken a chlamydial control program involving widespread screening of women attending family planning clinics. In women meeting the criteria for high risk, ~500,000 tests per year were conducted at 150 such clinics throughout the region. Within 5 years, the prevalence of chlamydial infection had been reduced by >30% in this population. However, the chlamydial prevalence in Region X has since leveled off and even begun to increase once again. Thus, further study of chlamydial screening programs and their impact on *Chlamydia*-associated reproductive sequelae is needed. While most regions of the United States have now initiated screening programs, some family planning and STD clinics still do not offer chlamydial testing. The availability of highly sensitive and specific diagnostic tests that can be done with urine specimens and of single-dose therapy makes it feasible to mount an effective chlamydial control program nationwide, with screening of high-risk persons both in traditional health care settings and in novel community- and school-based settings.

TRACHOMA AND ADULT INCLUSION CONJUNCTIVITIS

Definition *Trachoma* is a chronic conjunctivitis associated with infection by *C. trachomatis* serovar A, B, Ba, or C. It has been responsible for an estimated 20 million cases of blindness throughout the world and remains an important cause of preventable blindness. *Inclusion conjunctivitis* is an acute ocular infection caused by sexually transmitted *C. trachomatis* strains (usually serovars D through K) in adults exposed to infected genital secretions and in their newborn offspring.

Epidemiology In trachoma-endemic areas where the classic eye disease is seen, *C. trachomatis* is transmitted from eye to eye via hands, flies, towels, and other fomites; serovar A, B, Ba, or C is usually involved. The worldwide incidence and severity of trachoma have decreased dramatically during the past 35 years, mainly as a result of improving hygienic and economic conditions. However, endemic trachoma is still the major cause of preventable blindness in northern Africa, sub-Saharan Africa, the Middle East, and parts of Asia. Transmission occurs primarily through close personal contact, particularly among young children in rural communities with limited water supplies. In endemic areas, trachoma is associated with repeated exposure and reinfection, but the infection can also become chronic and persistent. Acute relapse of old trachoma occasionally follows treatment with cortisone eye ointment or develops in very old persons who were exposed in their youth.

Clinical Manifestations Both endemic trachoma and adult inclusion conjunctivitis present initially as a conjunctivitis characterized by small lymphoid follicles in the conjunctiva. In regions with hyperendemic classic blinding trachoma, the disease usually starts insidiously before the age of 2 years. Reinfection is common and probably contributes to the pathogenesis of trachoma. Studies using PCR techniques indicate that chlamydial DNA is often present in the ocular secretions of patients with trachoma, even in the absence of positive cultures. Thus persistent infection may be more common than was previously thought.

The cornea becomes involved, with inflammatory leukocytic infiltrations and superficial vascularization (pannus formation). As the inflammation continues, conjunctival scarring eventually distorts the eyelids, causing them to turn inward so that the inturned lashes constantly abrade the eyeball (trichiasis and entropion); eventually the corneal epithelium is abraded and may ulcerate, with subsequent corneal scarring and blindness. Destruction of the conjunctival goblet cells, lacrimal ducts, and lacrimal gland may produce a "dry-eye" syndrome, with resultant corneal opacity due to drying (xerosis) or secondary bacterial corneal ulcers.

Communities with blinding trachoma often experience seasonal epidemics of conjunctivitis due to *H. influenzae* that contribute to the intensity of the inflammatory process. In such areas the active infectious process usually resolves spontaneously in affected persons at 10–15 years of age, but the conjunctival scars continue to shrink, producing trichiasis and entropion and subsequent corneal scarring in adults. In areas with milder and less prevalent disease, the process may be much slower, with active disease continuing into adulthood; blindness is rare in these cases.

Eye infection with genital *C. trachomatis* strains in sexually active young adults presents as the acute onset of unilateral follicular conjunctivitis and preauricular lymphadenopathy similar to that seen in acute adenovirus or herpesvirus conjunctivitis. If untreated, the disease may persist for 6 weeks to 2 years. It is frequently associated with corneal inflammation in the form of discrete opacities ("infiltrates"), punctate epithelial erosions, and minor degrees of superficial corneal vascularization. Very rarely, conjunctival scarring and eyelid distortion occur, particularly in patients treated for many months with topical glucocorticoids. Recurrent eye infections develop most often in patients whose sexual consorts are not treated with antimicrobial agents.

Diagnosis The clinical diagnosis of classic trachoma can be made if two of the following signs are present: (1) lymphoid follicles on the upper tarsal conjunctiva; (2) typical conjunctival scarring; (3) vascular pannus; or (4) limbal follicles or their sequelae, Herbert's pits. The clinical diagnosis of endemic trachoma should be confirmed by laboratory tests in children with more marked degrees of inflammation. Intracytoplasmic chlamydial inclusions are found in 10–60% of Giemsa-stained conjunctival smears in such populations, but chlamydial NAATs are more sensitive and are often positive when smears or cultures are negative. Follicular conjunctivitis in adult Europeans or Americans living in trachomatous regions is rarely due to trachoma.

℞ ADULT INCLUSION CONJUNCTIVITIS

Adult inclusion conjunctivitis responds well to treatment with the same regimens used for treatment of uncomplicated genital infections—namely, azithromycin (a 1-g single oral dose) or doxycycline (100 mg bid for 7 days). Simultaneous treatment of all sexual consorts of the patient is also necessary to prevent ocular reinfection and to avoid chlamydial genital disease. Topical antibiotic treatment is not required for patients who receive systemic antibiotics.

Prevention Efforts to develop a trachoma vaccine have not yet been successful. General hygienic measures associated with improved living standards are effective in the elimination of endemic trachoma. An adequate water supply for personal cleanliness may be a critical factor. In some areas the reduction of numbers of flies in the household is important. The key elements of the World Health Organization's Global Campaign to Eliminate Trachoma are encompassed in the S-A-F-E strategy: surgery for deformed eyelids; periodic mass treatment with azithromycin; face washing; and environmental improvements. Mass treatment of entire villages with single-dose azithromycin has been associated with marked declines in chlamydial infection and eye disease.

C. PSITTACI INFECTIONS

Definition Psittacosis is primarily an infectious disease of birds and mammals that is caused by *C. psittaci*. Transmission of infection from birds to humans results in a febrile illness characterized by pneumonitis and systemic manifestations. Inapparent infections or mild influenza-like illnesses may also occur. The term *ornithosis* is sometimes applied to infections contracted from birds other than parrots or parakeets, but *psittacosis* is the preferred generic term for all forms of the disease.

Epidemiology Almost any avian species can harbor *C. psittaci*. Psittacine birds (parrots, parakeets, budgerigars) are most commonly infected, but human cases have been traced to contact with pigeons, ducks, turkeys, chickens, and many other birds. Psittacosis may be considered an occupational disease of pet-shop owners, poultry workers, pigeon fanciers, taxidermists, veterinarians, and zoo attendants. Incidence has increased during the past 25 years, with cases and outbreaks occurring primarily among employees of poultry-processing plants. It is suspected that many cases go undiagnosed and unreported.

C. psittaci is present in nasal secretions, excreta, tissues, and feathers of infected birds. Although the disease can be fatal, infected birds frequently show only minor evidence of illness, such as ruffled feathers, lethargy, and anorexia. Asymptomatic avian carriers are common, and complete recovery may be followed by continued shedding of the organism for many months.

Psittacosis is almost always transmitted to humans by the respiratory route. On rare occasions the disease may be acquired from the bite of a pet bird. Prolonged contact is not essential for transmission of the disease; spending a few minutes in an environment previously occupied by an infected bird has resulted in human infection. In one outbreak, gardening rather than direct exposure to birds was associated with infection. A psittacosis-like agent has been transmitted among hospital personnel, with severe and sometimes fatal infections. There is evidence that these "human" strains are more virulent than avian organisms. There is no record of infection acquired by the ingestion of poultry products.

Pathogenesis The psittacosis agent gains entrance to the body through the upper respiratory tract, spreads via the bloodstream, and eventually localizes in the pulmonary alveoli and in the reticuloendothelial cells of the spleen and liver. Invasion of the lung probably takes place by way of the bloodstream rather than by direct extension from the upper air passages. A lymphocytic inflammatory response occurs on both the interstitial and the respiratory surfaces of the alveoli as well as in the perivascular spaces. The alveolar walls and interstitial tissues of the lung are thickened, edematous, necrotic, and occasionally hemorrhagic. Histologic examination of the affected areas reveals alveolar spaces filled with fluid, erythrocytes, and lymphocytes. The picture is not pathognomonic for psittacosis unless macrophages containing characteristic cytoplasmic inclusion bodies (Levinthal-Coles-Lillie bodies) are identified. The respiratory epithelium of the bronchi and bronchioles usually remains intact.

Clinical Manifestations The clinical manifestations and course of psittacosis are extremely variable. After an incubation period of 7–14 days or longer, the disease may start abruptly with shaking chills and fever, with temperatures ranging as high as 40.5°C (105°F); however, the onset is often gradual, with fever increasing over 3–4 days. Headache is almost always prominent, is usually diffuse and excruciating, and is often the chief complaint.

Many patients present with a dry hacking cough that is usually nonproductive, but small amounts of mucoid or bloody sputum may be raised as the disease progresses. Cough may begin early in the course of the disease or as late as 5 days after the onset of fever. Chest pain, pleurisy with effusion, or a friction rub may all occur but are rare. Pericarditis and myocarditis have been reported. Most patients have a normal or slightly increased respiratory rate; marked dyspnea with cyanosis occurs only in severe psittacosis with extensive pulmonary involvement. In psittacosis, as in mycoplasmal pneumonias, the physical signs of pneumonitis tend to be less prominent than symptoms and x-ray findings would suggest. The initial examination may reveal fine sibilant rales, or clinical evidence of pneumonia may be completely lacking. Rales usually become audible and more numerous as the illness progresses. Signs of frank pulmonary consolidation are usually absent. Symptoms of upper respiratory tract infection are not prominent, although mild sore throat, pharyngitis, and cervical adenopathy are often documented; on occasion, the last may be the only manifestation of illness. Epistaxis is encountered early in the course of nearly one-fourth of cases. Photophobia is also common.

Patients often report generalized myalgia, and spasm and stiffness of the muscles of the back and neck may lead to an erroneous diagnosis of meningitis. Lethargy, mental depression, agitation, insomnia, and disorientation have been prominent features of the illness in some epidemics but not in others; delirium and stupor develop near the end of the first week in severe cases. Occasional patients are comatose when first seen; the diagnosis of psittacosis may be elusive in these cases. Gastrointestinal manifestations such as abdominal pain, nausea, vomiting, or diarrhea are noted in some cases; constipation and abdominal distention sometimes occur as late complications. Icterus, the result of severe hepatic involvement, is a rare and ominous finding. A faint macular rash (Horder's spots) resembling the rose spots of typhoid fever has been described.

Patients without cough or other clinical evidence of respiratory involvement present with fever of unknown origin (Chap. 19). The pulse rate is slow in relation to the fever. When splenomegaly is noted in a patient with acute pneumonitis, psittacosis should be considered; the reported incidence of splenomegaly in this disease ranges from 10 to 70%. Nontender hepatic enlargement also occurs, but jaundice is rare. Thrombophlebitis is not unusual during convalescence; indeed, pulmonary infarction is sometimes a late complication and may be fatal.

In untreated cases of psittacosis, sustained or mildly remittent fever persists for 10 days to 3 weeks or occasionally for as long as 3 months. Over this period, the respiratory manifestations gradually abate. Psittacosis contracted from parrots or parakeets is more likely to be a severe, prolonged illness than infection acquired from pigeons or barnyard fowl. Relapses occur but are rare. Occasional patients develop endocarditis, and *C. psittaci* infection should be considered in cases of culture-negative endocarditis. Secondary bacterial infections are uncommon. Immunity to reinfection is probably permanent.

Laboratory Findings The chest x-ray in psittacosis is nonspecific and may show pneumonic lesions that are usually patchy in appearance but can be hazy, diffuse, homogeneous, lobar, atelectatic, wedge-shaped, nodular, or miliary. The white blood cell count is normal or moderately decreased in the acute phase of the disease but may rise in convalescence. The erythrocyte sedimentation rate frequently is not elevated. Transient proteinuria is common. The cerebrospinal fluid sometimes contains a few mononuclear cells but is otherwise normal. Despite hepatomegaly, the results of liver function tests are generally normal or only mildly elevated.

The diagnosis can be confirmed only by isolation of the causative microorganism or by serologic studies. The agent is present in the blood during the acute phase of the disease and in the bronchial secretions for weeks or sometimes years after infection, but it is difficult to isolate. Further, the organism is hazardous to work with in the laboratory, and most clinical laboratories do not offer culture for *C. psittaci*. Thus psittacosis is most readily diagnosed by the demonstration of a rising titer of complement fixation antibody in the serum of a patient with a compatible clinical syndrome. Both an acute-phase and a convalescent-phase specimen should always be tested. *C. trachomatis*, *C. psittaci*, and *C. pneumoniae* all share a genus-specific "group" antigen, which is the basis of the complement fixation test. Thus acute infections with *C. trachomatis* or *C. pneumoniae* can also produce titer rises in this test. However, these three species have different major outer-membrane proteins that are the principal antigens in the micro-IF test. If there is doubt as to the interpretation of the complement fixation test, the micro-IF test can be used to differentiate among these antigens. The prompt initiation of treatment with tetracycline has been shown to delay an antibody rise in convalescence for several weeks or months.

Differential Diagnosis A history of exposure to birds may be the only clinical basis for differentiating psittacosis from a variety of infectious and noninfectious febrile disorders. The list of pulmonary diseases that may be confused with psittacosis includes *Mycoplasma* pneumonia, *C. pneumoniae* pneumonia, legionellosis, viral pneumonia, Q fever, coccidioidomycosis, tuberculosis, enterovirus infection, carcinoma of the lung with bronchial obstruction, and common bacterial pneumonias. In the early stages, before pneumonitis appears, psittacosis may be mistaken for influenza, typhoid fever, miliary tuberculosis, or infectious mononucleosis.

Rx C. PSITTACI INFECTIONS

The tetracyclines are consistently effective in the treatment of psittacosis. Defervescence and alleviation of symptoms usually take place within 24–48 h after the institution of therapy with 2 g daily in four divided doses. To avoid relapse, treatment should probably be continued for at least 7–14 days after defervescence. Doxycycline (100 mg by mouth bid) can also be used. In severe cases, hospitalization and pulmonary intensive care may be indicated. Sulfonamides are not active against *C. psittaci*. Erythromycin can be used in patients allergic to or intolerant of tetracyclines. Limited data from studies in vitro and in animal models suggest that azithromycin and some fluoroquinolones are active against *C. psittaci*.

C. PNEUMONIAE INFECTIONS

Definition *C. pneumoniae* can be distinguished from the other two chlamydial species causing human infections on the basis of DNA hybridization and EB morphology. Although *C. pneumoniae* can be grown in a variety of cell cultures, it is considerably more difficult to culture than other chlamydiae, especially from clinical specimens. HL cells appear to be the most effective cell line for isolation of *C. pneumoniae*.

Epidemiology Knowledge of the epidemiology of *C. pneumoniae* infections comes primarily from serologic studies. Infections begin to occur in late childhood, achieve peak incidence in early adulthood, and continue throughout adult life.

Seroprevalence in the many adult populations that have been tested throughout the world exceeds 40%—a figure suggesting that *C. pneumoniae* infections are ubiquitous. Secondary episodes (reinfections) appear to occur commonly in older adults throughout life. *C. pneumoniae* also produces epidemics of pneumonia and respiratory illness, especially in close residential quarters such as military barracks. The incidence of infections outside of epidemics remains poorly defined. The organism appears to be transmitted from person to person, probably primarily in schools and family units.

Pathogenesis Little is known about the pathogenesis of *C. pneumoniae* infection. The infection begins in the upper respiratory tract and in many persons is a long-lived asymptomatic condition of the upper respiratory mucosal surfaces. However, evidence of replication within vascular endothelium and synovial membranes of joints shows that, in at least some individuals, the organism is transported to distant sites, perhaps within macrophages. A *C. pneumoniae* outer-membrane protein may induce host immune responses whose cross-reaction with human proteins results in an autoimmune reaction.

Clinical Manifestations The clinical spectrum of *C. pneumoniae* infection includes acute pharyngitis, sinusitis, bronchitis, and pneumonitis, primarily in young adults. The clinical manifestations of primary infection appear to be more severe and prolonged than those of reinfection. The pneumonitis resembles that of *Mycoplasma* pneumonia in that leukocytosis is frequently lacking and patients often have prominent antecedent upper respiratory tract symptoms, fever, nonproductive cough, mild to moderate illness, minimal findings on chest auscultation, and small segmental infiltrates on chest x-ray. In elderly patients, pneumonia due to *C. pneumoniae* can be especially severe and may necessitate hospitalization and respiratory support.

Epidemiologic studies have demonstrated an association between serologic evidence of *C. pneumoniae* infection and atherosclerotic disease of the coronary and other arteries. In addition, *C. pneumoniae* has been identified in atherosclerotic plaques by electron microscopy, DNA hybridization, and immunocytochemistry. The organism has also been recovered in culture from atheromatous plaque—a result indicating the presence of viable replicating bacteria in vessels. Evidence from animal models supports the hypothesis that *C. pneumoniae* infection of the upper respiratory tract is followed by recovery of the organism from atheromatous lesions in the aorta and that the infection accelerates the process of atherosclerosis, especially in hypercholesterolemic animals. Antimicrobial treatment of the infected animals reverses the increased risk of atherosclerosis. In humans, two small trials in patients with unstable angina or recent myocardial infarction suggested that antibiotics reduce subsequent untoward cardiac events. However, larger trials have not demonstrated that various antibiotic regimens affect the risk of these events.

Diagnosis Diagnosis of *C. pneumoniae* infection is difficult because cell culture techniques are not available for routine clinical use and non-culture tests using antigen detection methods or DNA probes have not been developed for commercial use. Acute- and convalescent-phase sera can be tested for chlamydial complement fixation antibody to make a retrospective diagnosis. However, this test does not distinguish *C. pneumoniae* infection from infection due to *C. trachomatis* or *C. psittaci*.

Rx C. PNEUMONIAE INFECTIONS

Although few controlled trials of treatment have been reported, *C. pneumoniae* is inhibited in vitro by erythromycin, tetracycline, azithromycin, clarithromycin, gatifloxacin, and gemifloxacin. Recommended therapy consists of 2 g/d of either tetracycline or erythromycin for 10–14 days. Other macrolides (e.g., azithromycin) and some fluoroquinolones (e.g., levofloxacin and gatifloxacin) also appear to be effective.

FURTHER READINGS

ADIMORA AA: Treatment of uncomplicated genital *Chlamydia trachomatis* infections in adults. Clin Infect Dis 35(Suppl 2):S183, 2002

CASSELL JA et al: Trends in sexually transmitted infections in general practice 1990–2000: Population based study using data from the UK general practice research database. BMJ 332:332, 2006

CHIDAMBARAN JD et al: Effect of a single mass antibiotic distribution on the prevalence of infectious trachoma. JAMA 295:1142, 2006

GOLDEN MR et al: Effect of expedited treatment of sex partners on recurrent or persistent gonorrhea or chlamydial infection. N Engl J Med 352:676, 2005

GRAYSTON JT et al: Azithromycin for the secondary prevention of coronary events. N Engl J Med 352:1637, 2005

———: Infections caused by *Chlamydia pneumoniae*, strain TWAR. Clin Infect Dis 15:757, 1992

HOLMES KK, STAMM WE: Lower genital tract infections in women: Cystitis, urethritis, vulvovaginitis, and cervicitis, in *Sexually Transmitted Diseases*, 4th ed, KK Holmes et al (eds). New York, McGraw-Hill, 2008

SOLOMON AW et al: Mass treatment with single-dose azithromycin for trachoma. N Engl J Med 351:1962, 2004

STAMM WE: *Chlamydia* screening: Expanding the scope. Ann Intern Med 141:570, 2004

———: *Chlamydia trachomatis*: The persistent pathogen. Sex Transm Dis 13:684, 2001

———: *Chlamydia trachomatis* infections in adults, in *Sexually Transmitted Diseases*, 4th ed, KK Holmes et al (eds). New York, McGraw-Hill, 2008

SECTION 11 VIRAL DISEASES: GENERAL CONSIDERATIONS

170 Medical Virology
Fred Wang, Elliott Kieff

DEFINING A VIRUS

Viruses consist of a nucleic acid surrounded by one or more proteins. Some viruses also have an outer-membrane envelope. Viruses are obligate intracellular parasites: they can replicate only within cells since their nucleic acids do not encode the many enzymes necessary for protein, carbohydrate, or lipid metabolism and for the generation of high-energy phosphates. Typically, viral nucleic acids encode proteins necessary for replicating and packaging their nucleic acids within the biochemical milieu of host cells.

Viruses differ from viroids, prions, and virusoids. *Virusoids* are nucleic acids that depend on helper viruses to package their nucleic acids into virus-like particles. *Viroids* are naked, cyclical, mostly double-stranded, small RNAs. Viroids appear to be restricted to plants, spread from cell to cell, and are replicated by cellular RNA polymerase II. *Prions* (Chap. 378) are abnormal protein molecules that can spread. These molecules reproduce by changing the structure of their normal cellular protein counterparts. Prions have been implicated in neurodegenerative conditions such as Creutzfeldt-Jakob disease, Gerstmann-Sträussler disease, kuru, and human bovine spongiform encephalopathy ("mad cow disease").

VIRAL STRUCTURE

Viruses have from a few to several hundred genes. These genes may be in a single-strand or double-strand DNA genome or in a single-strand sense, a single-strand or segmented antisense, or a double-strand segmented RNA genome. Sense-strand RNA genomes can be translated directly into protein. Sense and antisense genomes are also referred to as *positive-strand* and *negative-strand genomes*, respectively. The viral nucleic acid is usually associated with one or more virus-encoded nucleoproteins in the core of the viral particle. The viral nucleic acid and nucleoproteins are almost always enclosed in a protein shell called a *capsid*. Because of the limited genetic complexity of viruses, their capsids are usually composed of multimers of identical capsomeres. Capsomeres are in turn composed of one or a few proteins. Capsids have icosahedral or helical symmetry. Icosahedral structures approximate spheres but have two-, three-, and fivefold axes of symmetry, while helical structures have only a twofold axis of symmetry. The entire structural unit of nucleic acid, nucleoprotein(s), and capsid is called a *nucleocapsid*.

Many human viruses are simply composed of a core and a capsid. For these viruses, the outer surface of the capsid mediates contact with uninfected cells. Other viruses are more complex and have an outer lipid-containing envelope derived from virus-modified membranes of the infected cell. The piece of infected-cell membrane that becomes the viral envelope has usually been modified during infection by the insertion of virus-encoded glycoproteins, which usually mediate contact of enveloped viruses with uninfected cells. Matrix or tegument proteins fill the space between the nucleocapsid and the envelope in many enveloped viruses. In general, enveloped viruses are sensitive to lipid solvents and nonionic detergents that can dissolve the envelope, while viruses that consist only of nucleocapsids are somewhat resistant. A schematic diagram for large and complex herpesviruses is shown in **Fig. 170-1**. Prototypical pathogenic human viruses are listed in **Table 170-1**. The relative sizes and structures of typical pathogenic human viruses are shown in **Fig. 170-2**.

TAXONOMY OF PATHOGENIC HUMAN VIRUSES

As is apparent from Table 170-1 and Fig. 170-2, the classification of viruses into orders and families is based on nucleic acid composition, nucleocapsid size and symmetry, and presence or absence of an envelope. Viruses of a single family have similar types of genomes and are often morphologically indistinguishable in electron micrographs. Further subclassification into genera depends on similarities in epidemiology and biologic effects and on the degree of colinear nucleic acid sequence homology.

Most human viruses have a common name related to their pathologic effects or the circumstances of their discovery. Formal species names have been assigned by the International Committee on Taxonomy of Viruses. The formal designation consists of the name of the host followed by the family or genus of the virus and a number. This dual terminology has created a confusing situation in which viruses are referred to and referenced by either name—e.g., varicella-zoster virus (VZV) or human herpesvirus (HHV) 3.

VIRAL INFECTION IN VITRO

STAGES OF VIRAL INFECTION AT THE CELLULAR LEVEL
Viral Interactions with the Cell Surface and Cell Entry Viral infection is initiated by adsorption of the virus to the cell surface. Adsorption results from the molecular interaction of viral surface proteins with receptors on the cell's plasma membrane (see Table 114-1). For example, a poliovirus capsid protein binds to a cell plasma-membrane protein of the immunoglobulin superfamily type. A rhinovirus capsid protein binds to intercellular adhesion molecule 1. An echovirus capsid protein binds to an integrin. The influenza A virus envelope hemagglutinin protein binds to sialic acid. The HIV envelope glycoprotein binds to CD4 and then engages one of several chemokine receptors that function as coreceptors for the virus. Herpes simplex virus (HSV) envelope glycoproteins bind to heparan sulfate on cell surfaces and then engage one of several immunoglobulin superfamily or tumor necrosis factor (TNF) receptors. Epstein-Barr virus (EBV) glycoprotein gp350 binds to the B lymphocyte complement receptor CD21 and then engages major histocompatibility complex (MHC) class II molecules as a coreceptor. Adsorption characteristically proceeds almost as well at 4°C as at 37°C. Adsorbed virus can still be neutralized by antibody. Adsorption frequently initiates changes in virion surface proteins that

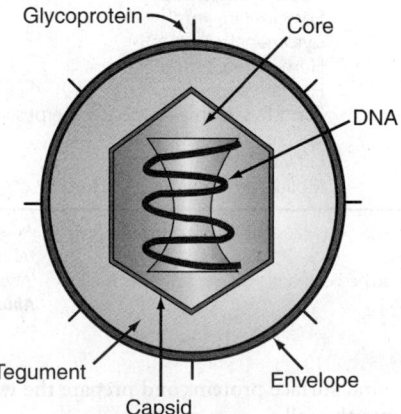

FIGURE 170-1 Schematic diagram of an enveloped herpesvirus with an icosahedral nucleocapsid. The approximate respective dimensions of the nucleocapsid and the enveloped particles are 110 and 180 nm. The capsid is composed of 162 capsomeres: 150 with sixfold and 12 with fivefold axes of symmetry.

TABLE 170-1 VIRUS FAMILIES PATHOGENIC FOR HUMANS

Family	Representative Viruses	Type of RNA/DNA	Lipid Envelope
RNA Viruses			
Picornaviridae	Poliovirus	(+) RNA	No
	Coxsackievirus		
	Echovirus		
	Enterovirus		
	Rhinovirus		
	Hepatitis A virus		
Caliciviridae	Norwalk agent	(+) RNA	No
	Hepatitis E virus		
Togaviridae	Rubella virus	(+) RNA	Yes
	Eastern equine encephalitis virus		
	Western equine encephalitis virus		
Flaviviridae	Yellow fever virus	(+) RNA	Yes
	Dengue virus		
	St. Louis encephalitis virus		
	West Nile virus		
	Hepatitis C virus		
	Hepatitis G virus		
Coronaviridae	Coronaviruses[a]	(+) RNA	Yes
Rhabdoviridae	Rabies virus	(–) RNA	Yes
	Vesicular stomatitis virus		
Filoviridae	Marburg virus	(–) RNA	Yes
	Ebola virus		
Paramyxoviridae	Parainfluenza virus	(–) RNA	Yes
	Respiratory syncytial virus		
	Newcastle disease virus		
	Mumps virus		
	Rubeola (measles) virus		
Orthomyxoviridae	Influenza A, B, and C viruses	(–) RNA, 8 segments	Yes
Bunyaviridae	Hantavirus	(–) RNA, 3 circular segments	Yes
	California encephalitis virus		
	Sandfly fever virus		
Arenaviridae	Lymphocytic choriomeningitis virus	(–) RNA, 2 circular segments	Yes
	Lassa fever virus		
	South American hemorrhagic fever virus		
Reoviridae	Rotavirus	ds RNA, 10–12 segments	No
	Reovirus		
	Colorado tick fever virus		
Retroviridae	Human T-lymphotropic virus types I and II	(+) RNA, 2 identical segments	Yes
	Human immunodeficiency virus types 1 and 2		
DNA Viruses			
Hepadnaviridae	Hepatitis B virus	ds DNA with ss portions	Yes
Parvoviridae	Parvovirus B19	ss DNA	No
Papovaviridae	Human papillomaviruses	ds DNA	No
	JC virus		
	BK virus		
Adenoviridae	Human adenoviruses	ds DNA	No
Herpesviridae	Herpes simplex virus types 1 and 2[b]	ds DNA	Yes
	Varicella-zoster virus[c]		
	Epstein-Barr virus[d]		
	Cytomegalovirus[e]		
	Human herpesvirus 6		
	Human herpesvirus 7		
	Kaposi's sarcoma–associated herpesvirus[f]		
Poxviridae	Variola (smallpox) virus	ds DNA	Yes
	Orf virus		
	Molluscum contagiosum virus		

[a]Including the coronavirus causing severe acute respiratory syndrome (SARS).
[b]Also called human herpesvirus (HHV) 1 and 2, respectively.
[c]Also called HHV-3.
[d]Also called HHV-4.
[e]Also called HHV-5.
[f]Also called HHV-8.
Abbreviations: ds, double-strand; ss, single-strand.

destabilize the viral surface proteins and prepare the way for the next stage of entry into the cell.

After adsorption, viruses penetrate the cell membrane by fusing with it. The fusion reaction results in the virus's partial decomposition. The virus becomes insensitive to neutralizing antibody as it penetrates, becomes uncoated, and enters the cytoplasm. Penetration and uncoating result in viral nucleocapsid or nucleoprotein entry into the cytoplasm.

Penetration and uncoating as well as subsequent steps in viral replication depend on the cell's energy metabolism and on biochemical changes in the cell's plasma membrane and cytoskeleton. Therefore, penetration proceeds slowly at temperatures <37°C. Interaction of viral surface proteins with cell receptors can induce receptor aggregation at the site of adsorption. Receptor aggregation can trigger signaling events within the cytoplasm and changes in the plasma membrane. The cell frequently misperceives that the receptor has encountered its "normal ligand." Aggregated receptor may be internalized with the attached virus in an endocytic process. Viral endocytosis may proceed through clathrin-coated pits. Endocytosis is important in the entry of viruses as diverse as picornaviruses, influenza viruses, HIV, adenoviruses, and herpesviruses. In many cases, entry of the virus into the cytoplasm depends on acidification of the viral endosome.

Influenza virus provides a well-studied example of the effect of low pH on viral penetration. Influenza hemagglutinin mediates adsorption, receptor aggregation, and endocytosis. In low-pH endosomes, changes in the conformation of the hemagglutinin expose amphipathic domains that interact chemically with the cell membrane and initiate fusion of the viral and cellular membranes. (The HIV envelope glycoprotein undergoes similar conformational changes after interaction with CD4 and chemokine receptors.) For influenza virus, the M2 membrane protein also plays a key role in the uncoating of the viral envelope by providing an ion channel in the envelope. The fusion of viral proteins with cell membranes is a crucial step in viral infection, resulting in the mixture of viral envelope lipids and proteins with cell membrane lipids and proteins and (in this case) in the penetration of the influenza nucleocapsid into the cytoplasm. Viral glycoproteins other than the protein that mediates initial adsorption may be critical in mediating envelope fusion with cell membranes, which involves hydrophobic interactions. The hydrophobic interactions required for fusion can be susceptible to chemical inhibition or blockade.

Viral Gene Expression and Replication

After uncoating and release of viral nucleoprotein into the cytoplasm, the viral genome is transported to a site for expression and replication. In order to produce infectious progeny, viruses must (1) produce proteins necessary to replicate their nucleic acid, (2) produce structural proteins, and (3) assemble the nucleic acid and proteins into progeny virions. Different viruses use different strategies and gene repertoires to accomplish these goals. DNA viruses, except for poxviruses, replicate their nucleic acid and assemble into nucleocapsid complexes in the cell

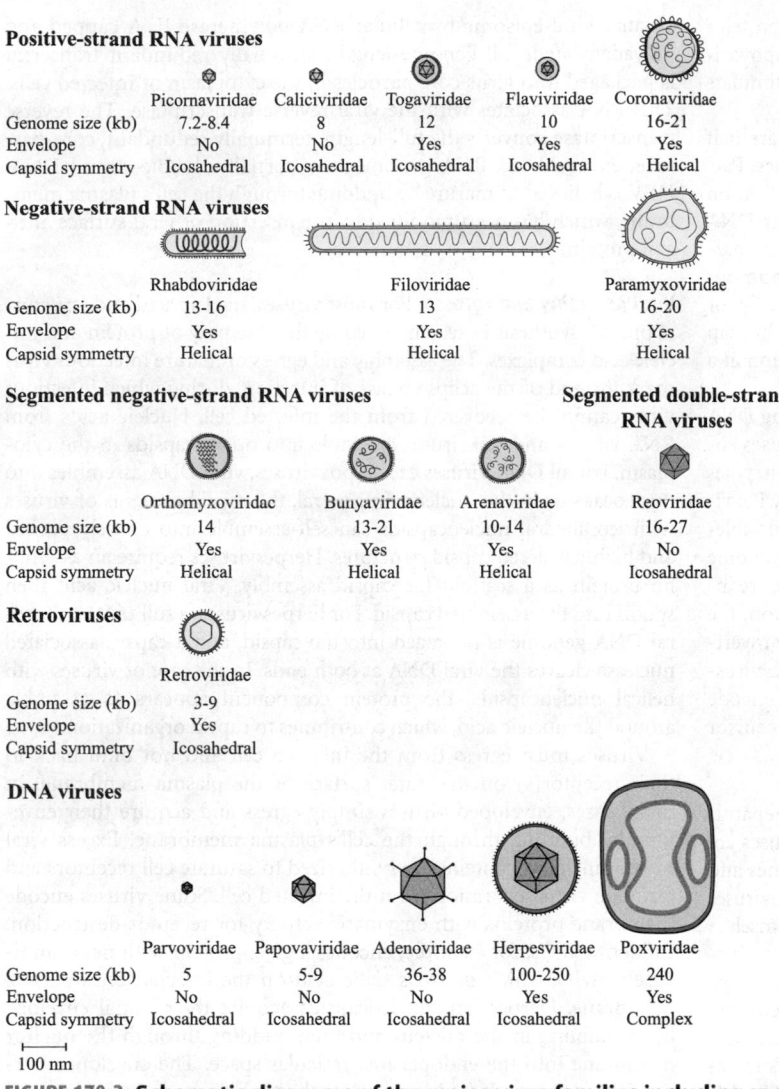

Positive-strand RNA viruses

	Picornaviridae	Caliciviridae	Togaviridae	Flaviviridae	Coronaviridae
Genome size (kb)	7.2-8.4	8	12	10	16-21
Envelope	No	No	Yes	Yes	Yes
Capsid symmetry	Icosahedral	Icosahedral	Icosahedral	Icosahedral	Helical

Negative-strand RNA viruses

	Rhabdoviridae	Filoviridae	Paramyxoviridae
Genome size (kb)	13-16	13	16-20
Envelope	Yes	Yes	Yes
Capsid symmetry	Helical	Helical	Helical

Segmented negative-strand RNA viruses   **Segmented double-strand RNA viruses**

	Orthomyxoviridae	Bunyaviridae	Arenaviridae	Reoviridae
Genome size (kb)	14	13-21	10-14	16-27
Envelope	Yes	Yes	Yes	No
Capsid symmetry	Helical	Helical	Helical	Icosahedral

Retroviruses

	Retroviridae
Genome size (kb)	3-9
Envelope	Yes
Capsid symmetry	Icosahedral

DNA viruses

	Parvoviridae	Papovaviridae	Adenoviridae	Herpesviridae	Poxviridae
Genome size (kb)	5	5-9	36-38	100-250	240
Envelope	No	No	No	Yes	Yes
Capsid symmetry	Icosahedral	Icosahedral	Icosahedral	Icosahedral	Complex

├── 100 nm

FIGURE 170-2 Schematic diagrams of the major virus families including species that infect humans. The viruses are grouped by genome type and are drawn approximately to scale. Prototype viruses of each family that cause human disease are listed in Table 170-1.

nucleus. RNA viruses, except for influenza viruses, transcribe and replicate their nucleic acid and assemble entirely in the cytoplasm. Thus, the replication strategies of DNA and RNA viruses are presented separately below. Positive-strand and negative-strand RNA viruses are discussed separately. Medically important viruses of each group are used for illustrative purposes.

POSITIVE-STRAND RNA VIRUSES

Medically important positive-strand RNA viruses include picornaviruses, flaviviruses, togaviruses, caliciviruses, and coronaviruses. Genomic RNA from positive-strand RNA viruses is released into the cytoplasm without associated enzymes. Cell ribosomes recognize and associate with an internal ribosome entry sequence in the viral genomic RNA and translate a polyprotein that is a fusion of many or all of the viral proteins. The viral RNA polymerase and other viral proteins are cleaved from the polyprotein by protease components of the polyprotein. Antigenomic RNA is then transcribed from the genomic RNA template. Positive-strand genomes and mRNAs are next transcribed from the antigenomic RNA by the viral RNA polymerase. Positive-strand genomic RNA is encapsidated in the cytoplasm.

NEGATIVE-STRAND RNA VIRUSES

Medically important negative-strand RNA viruses include rhabdoviruses, filoviruses, paramyxoviruses, myxoviruses, and bunyaviruses. Negative-strand RNA virus genomes are released into the cytoplasm with an associated RNA polymerase and one or more accessory proteins. Some of these genomes are seg-

mented. Except for influenza viruses, negative-strand RNA viruses replicate entirely in the cytoplasm. The viral RNA polymerase transcribes messenger RNAs (mRNAs) as well as full-length antigenomic RNA, which is the template for replication of genomic RNA. These mRNAs encode for the viral RNA polymerase and accessory factors as well as for viral structural proteins. Influenza virus is an unusual negative-strand RNA virus that transcribes its mRNAs and antigenomic RNAs in the cell's nucleus. All negative-strand RNA viruses, including influenza viruses, assemble in the cytoplasm.

DOUBLE-STRAND SEGMENTED RNA VIRUSES

These viruses, which are taxonomically grouped in the reovirus family, have 10–12 RNA segments that make up their genome. The medically important viruses in this group are rotaviruses and Colorado tick fever virus. Reovirus virions include an RNA polymerase complex. Reoviruses replicate and assemble in the cytoplasm.

DNA VIRUSES

Medically important DNA viruses include parvoviruses, papovaviruses [e.g., human papillomaviruses (HPVs) and polyomaviruses], adenoviruses, herpesviruses, and poxviruses. Other than poxviruses, most DNA virus genomes must get to the cell's nucleus for transcription by cellular RNA polymerase II. For example, after receptor binding and fusion, herpesvirus nucleocapsids are released into the cytoplasm along with tegument proteins. The complex is then transported along microtubules to nuclear pores, and the DNA is released into the nucleus.

Transcriptional regulation and mRNA processing for nuclear DNA viruses depend on both viral and cellular proteins. For HSVs, a virus tegument protein activates transcription of viral immediate-early genes, a class of genes expressed immediately after infection. Transcription of immediate-early genes requires the viral tegument protein and preexisting cellular transcription factors. One of the key preexisting cellular factors for HSV-1 immediate-early gene transcription is docked in the cytoplasm in neurons. Nuclear absence of this cell factor important for viral gene transcription may explain why HSV-1 goes into a latent state in neurons and how lytic infection is activated by signaling in a latently infected cell.

DNA virus gene transcription is usually regulated and proceeds in an organized cascade. Transcription and expression of adenovirus and herpesvirus immediate-early genes turn on the promoters for early genes, whereas poxvirus virions carry all the factors necessary for early-gene transcription. Smaller DNA viruses are not as dependent on transactivators encoded from the viral genome for early-gene transcription. Most early genes encode proteins that are necessary for viral DNA synthesis and for the turn-on of late-gene transcription. Late genes encode mostly viral structural proteins or viral proteins necessary for the assembly and egress of the virus from the infected cell. Late-gene transcription is continuously dependent on DNA replication. Therefore, inhibitors of DNA replication also stop late-gene transcription.

Each DNA virus family uses unique mechanisms for replicating its DNA. Herpesvirus DNAs are linear in the virion but circularize in the infected cell. In lytic virus infection, circular herpesvirus genomes are replicated into linear concatemers through a "rolling-circle" mechanism. Herpesviruses encode a DNA polymerase and at least six other viral proteins necessary for viral DNA replication; these viruses also encode several enzymes that increase the pool of precursor deoxynucleotide triphosphates. Adenovirus genomes are linear in the virion and are replicated into complementary linear copies by a virus-encoded DNA polymerase and an initiator protein complex. The double-strand circular papovavirus genomes are replicated into progeny circular DNA molecules by cellular DNA replication enzymes. Two viral early proteins contribute to viral DNA replication and to the persistence of papovavirus DNA in latently infected cells. Early papovavirus proteins stimulate cells to remain in cycle, thus facilitating viral DNA replication.

Parvoviruses are the smallest DNA viruses: their genomes are half the size of the papovavirus genomes and include only two genes. Parvoviruses have negative single-strand DNA genomes. The replication of autonomous parvoviruses, such as B19, depends on cellular DNA replication and requires the virus-encoded Rep protein. Other parvoviruses, such as adeno-associated virus (AAV), are not autonomous and require helper viruses of the adenovirus or herpesvirus family for their replication. AAV has been touted as a potentially safe human gene therapy vector because its Rep protein causes its integration at a single chromosomal site.

Poxviruses are the largest DNA viruses and are unique among DNA viruses in replicating and assembling in the cytoplasm. Poxviruses encode transcription factors and an RNA polymerase as well as enzymes for RNA capping and polyadenylation and for DNA synthesis. Poxvirus DNA also has a unique structure. The two strands of the double-strand linear DNA are covalently linked at the ends so that the genome is also a covalently closed single-strand circle. In addition, there are inverted repeats at the ends of the DNA. During DNA replication, the genome is cleaved within the terminal inverted repeat, and the inverted repeats self-prime complementary-strand synthesis by the virus-encoded DNA polymerase. Like herpesviruses, poxviruses encode several enzymes that increase deoxynucleotide triphosphate precursor levels and thus facilitate viral DNA synthesis.

VIRUSES WITH BOTH RNA AND DNA GENOMES Retroviruses and hepatitis B virus (HBV) are not purely RNA or DNA viruses. Retroviruses are enveloped RNA viruses with two identical sense-strand genomes and associated reverse transcriptase and integrase enzymes. Retroviruses differ from all other viruses in that they reverse-transcribe themselves into partially duplicated double-strand DNA copies and then routinely integrate into the host genome as part of their replication strategy. Cellular RNA polymerase II and transcription factors regulate transcription from the integrated provirus genome. Some retroviruses also encode for regulators of transcription and RNA processing, such as Tax and Rex in human T-lymphotropic virus (HTLV) types I and II and Tat and Rev in HIV-1 and HIV-2. HIV genomes also encode for the additional accessory proteins Vpr, Vpu, and Vif, which are important for efficient infection and immune escape. Full-length proviral transcripts are made from a promoter in the viral terminal repeat and serve as both genomic RNAs that will be packaged in the nucleocapsids and mRNAs that encode for the viral Gag protein, polymerase/integrase protein, and envelope glycoprotein. The Gag protein includes a protease that cleaves it into several components, including a viral matrix protein that coats the viral RNA. Viral RNA polymerase/integrase, matrix protein, and cellular tRNA are key components of the viral nucleocapsid. The HIV Gag protease has been an important target for inhibition of HIV replication. Remnants and even complete copies of simple retroviral DNA in the human genome indicate that there may be replication-competent simple human retroviruses. However, replication has not been documented or associated with any disease. Integrated retroviral DNAs are also present in other animal species, such as pigs. These porcine retroviruses are a potential cause for concern in xenotransplantation because retroviral replication could cause disease in humans. Since the retroviral DNA is integrated into the porcine genome, special pathogen-free breeding practices cannot cleanse the donor herd of retroviral infection.

HBV is unique because virion DNA expression in infected cells results in the packaging of reverse transcriptase and genomic RNA in the virion. The genomic RNA is then copied into an incomplete double-strand circular DNA genome before the virion matures and is released from the infected cell. On entry of HBV into the cytoplasm of an infected cell, the virion reverse transcriptase/DNA polymerase completes DNA synthesis, and the covalently closed circular genome resides in the nucleus. Viral mRNAs are transcribed from the closed circular viral episome by cellular RNA polymerase II. A capped and polyadenylated, full-genome-length, terminally redundant transcript is packaged into virus core particles in the cytoplasm of infected cells. This RNA associates with the viral reverse transcriptase. The reverse transcriptase converts the full-length, terminally redundant, core-particle, encapsidated RNA genome into partially double-strand DNA. HBV is believed to mature by budding through the cell's plasma membrane, which has been modified by the insertion of viral surface antigen protein.

Viral Assembly and Egress For most viruses, nucleic acid and structural protein synthesis is accompanied by the assembly of protein and nucleic acid complexes. The assembly and egress of mature infectious virus mark the end of the eclipse phase of infection, during which infectious virus cannot be recovered from the infected cell. Nucleic acids from RNA viruses and poxviruses assemble into nucleocapsids in the cytoplasm. For all DNA viruses except poxviruses, viral DNA assembles into nucleocapsids in the nucleus. In general, the capsid proteins of viruses with icosahedral nucleocapsids can self-assemble into densely packed and highly ordered capsid structures. Herpesviruses require an assemblin protein as a scaffold for capsid assembly. Viral nucleic acid then spools into the assembled capsid. For herpesviruses, a full unit of the viral DNA genome is packaged into the capsid, and a capsid-associated nuclease cleaves the viral DNA at both ends. In the case of viruses with helical nucleocapsids, the protein component appears to assemble around the nucleic acid, which contributes to capsid organization.

Viruses must egress from the infected cell and not bind back to their receptor(s) on the outer surface of the plasma membrane. In many cases, enveloped viruses simply egress and acquire their envelope by budding through the cell's plasma membrane. Excess viral membrane glycoproteins are synthesized to saturate cell receptors and facilitate virus separation from the infected cell. Some viruses encode membrane proteins with enzymatic activity for receptor destruction. Influenza virus, for example, encodes a glycoprotein with neuraminidase activity, which destroys sialic acid on the infected cell's plasma membrane. Herpesvirus nucleocapsids acquire their initial envelope by assembling in the nucleus and then budding through the nuclear membrane into the endoplasmic reticular space. The enveloped herpesvirus is then released from the cell either by maturation in cytoplasmic vesicles, which fuse with the plasma membrane and release the virus by exocytosis, or by "de-envelopment" into the cytoplasm and "re-envelopment" at the Golgi or plasma membrane. In most instances, nonenveloped viruses appear to depend on the death and dissolution of the infected cell for their release.

FIDELITY OF VIRAL REPLICATION

Hundreds or thousands of progeny may be produced from a single virus-infected cell. Many particles partially assemble and never mature into virions. Many mature-appearing virions are imperfect and have only incomplete or nonfunctional genomes. Despite the inefficiency of assembly, a typical virus-infected cell releases 10–1000 infectious progeny. Some of these progeny may contain genomes that differ from those of the virus that infected the cell. Smaller, "defective" virus genomes have been noted with the replication of many RNA and DNA viruses. Virions with defective genomes can be produced in large numbers through packaging of incompletely synthesized nucleic acid. Adenovirus packaging is notoriously inefficient, and a high ratio of particle to infectious virus may limit the amount of recombinant adenovirus that can be administered for gene therapy. Mutant viral genomes are also produced and can be of medical significance. In general, viral nucleic acid replication is more error-prone than cellular nucleic acid replication. RNA polymerases and reverse transcriptases are significantly more error-prone than DNA polymerases. Mutant viruses can be virulent and may preferentially cause disease through evasion of the host immune response or through resistance to antiviral drugs. Persistent hepatitis C virus (HCV) infection is due in part to genome mutation and persistent immune escape. Viral nucleic acids can also mutate by recombination or reassortment between two related viruses in a single infected cell. While this occurrence is unusual under most circumstances of natural infection, the changes can be substantial and can significantly alter virulence or epidemiology. Reassortment of an avian or mammalian influenza A hemagglutinin gene into a human influenza background is believed to play a role in the emergence of new epidemic influenza A strains.

VIRAL GENES NOT REQUIRED FOR VIRAL REPLICATION

Viruses frequently have genes encoding proteins that are not directly involved in replication or packaging of the viral nucleic acid, in virion assembly, or in regulation of the transcription of viral genes involved in those processes. Most of these proteins fall into five classes: (1) proteins that directly or indirectly alter cell growth; (2) proteins that inhibit cellular RNA or protein synthesis so that viral mRNA can be efficiently transcribed or translated; (3) proteins that promote cell survival or inhibit apoptosis so that progeny virus can mature and escape from the infected cell; (4) proteins that inhibit the host interferon response; and (5) proteins that downregulate host inflammatory or immune responses so that virus infection can proceed in an infected person to the extent consistent with the survival of the virus and its efficient transmission to a new host. More complex viruses of the poxvirus or herpesvirus family encode many proteins that serve these functions. Some of these viral proteins have motifs similar to those of cell proteins, while others are quite novel. Virology has increasingly focused on these more sophisticated strategies evolved by viruses to permit the establishment of long-term infection in humans and other animals. These strategies often provide unique insights into the control of cell growth, cell survival, macromolecular synthesis, proteolytic processing, immune or inflammatory suppression, immune resistance, cytokine mimicry, or cytokine blockade.

HOST RANGE

The concept of host range was originally based on the cell types in which a virus replicated in tissue culture. For the most part, the host range is limited by specific cell-surface proteins required for viral adsorption or penetration—i.e., to the cell types that express receptors or coreceptors for a specific virus. Another common basis for host-range limitation is the degree of transcriptional activity from viral promoters in different cell types. Most DNA viruses depend not only on cellular RNA polymerase II and the basal components of the cellular transcription complex but also on activated components and transcriptional accessory factors, both of which differ among differentiated tissues, among cells at various phases of the cell cycle, and between resting and cycling cells.

The importance of host range factors is illustrated by the identification of determinants that prevent certain animal viruses from infecting humans. The SARS coronavirus and the influenza virus strain from the 1918 pandemic are believed to have originated from animal viruses in which minor genetic mutations resulted in more efficient human infection or enhanced transmission among humans.

VIRAL CYTOPATHIC EFFECTS AND INHIBITORS OF APOPTOSIS

The replication of almost all viruses has adverse effects on the infected cell, inhibiting cellular synthesis of DNA, RNA, or proteins. This inhibitory effect probably stems from the viruses' need to prevent or limit nonspecific, innate host resistance factors, including interferon (IFN). Most commonly, viruses specifically inhibit host protein synthesis by attacking a component of the translational initiation complex—frequently, a component that is not required for efficient translation of viral RNAs. Poliovirus protease 2A, for example, cleaves a cellular component of the complex that ordinarily facilitates translation of cell mRNAs by interacting with their cap structure. Poliovirus RNA is efficiently translated without a cap since it has an internal ribosome entry sequence. Influenza virus inhibits the processing of mRNA by snatching cap structures from nascent cell RNAs and using them as primers in the synthesis of viral mRNA. HSV has a virion tegument protein that inhibits cellular mRNA translation.

Apoptosis is the expected consequence of virus-induced inhibition of cellular macromolecular synthesis and viral nucleic acid replication.

While the induction of apoptosis may be important for the release of some viruses (particularly nonenveloped viruses), many viruses have acquired genes or parts of genes that enable them to forestall infected-cell apoptosis. This delay may be advantageous in allowing the completion of viral replication. Adenoviruses and herpesviruses encode analogues of the cellular Bc12 protein, which blocks mitochondrial enhancement of proapoptotic stimuli. Poxviruses and some herpesviruses encode caspase inhibitors. Many viruses, including HPVs and adenoviruses, encode proteins that inhibit p53 or its downstream proapoptotic effects.

VIRAL INFECTION IN VIVO

TRANSMISSION

The capsid and envelope of a virus protect its genome and permit its efficient transmission from cell to cell and to prospective hosts. Most common viral infections are spread by direct contact, by ingestion of contaminated water or food, or by inhalation of aerosolized particles. In all these situations, infection begins on an epithelial or mucosal surface and spreads along it or from it to deeper tissues. Infection may then spread through the body via the bloodstream, lymphatics, or neural circuits. Parenteral inoculation can also transmit some viral infections among humans or from animals (including insects) to humans.

Some viruses are transmitted only between humans. The dependence of smallpox and poliovirus infections on interhuman transmission makes it feasible to eliminate these viruses from human circulation by mass vaccination. In contrast, herpesviruses survive over time by establishing persistent infection in humans for decades, with eventual reactivation and infection of new and naïve generations.

Animals are important reservoirs and vectors for transmission of viruses causing human disease. Herpes B, monkeypox, and viral hemorrhagic fevers are examples of zoonotic infections caused by direct contact with animals or transmission from animals through other vectors. These infections may not be sustainable among humans alone because of the lack of efficient interhuman transmission. SARS resulted when an animal coronavirus apparently gained access to the human population concomitant with a mutation that enhanced its pathogenicity and spread in humans. Avian influenza viruses have drawn increased public attention because of their potential to undergo genetic changes and contribute to human disease.

PRIMARY INFECTION

The first (primary) episode of viral infection usually lasts from several days to several weeks. During this period, the concentration of virus at sites of infection rises and then falls, usually to unmeasurable levels. The rate at which the intensity of viral infection rises and falls at a given site depends on the accessibility of that organ or tissue to both the virus and systemic immune effectors, the intrinsic ability of the virus to replicate at that site, and endogenous nonspecific and specific resistance. Typically, infections with enterovirus, mumps virus, measles virus, rubella virus, rotavirus, influenza virus, AAV, adenovirus, HSV, and VZV are cleared from almost all sites within 3–4 weeks. Some of these viruses are especially proficient in altering or evading the innate and acquired immune responses; thus primary infection with AAV, EBV, or cytomegalovirus (CMV) can last for several months. Characteristically, primary infections due to HBV, HCV, hepatitis D virus (HDV), HIV, HPV, and molluscum contagiosum virus extend beyond several weeks. For some of these viruses (e.g., HPV, HBV, HCV, HDV, and molluscum contagiosum virus), the primary phase of infection is almost indistinguishable from the persistent phase.

Disease manifestations usually arise as a consequence of viral replication and the resultant inflammatory response at a specific site but do not necessarily correlate with levels of replication at that site. For example, the clinical manifestations of limited infection with poliovirus, enterovirus, rabies virus, measles virus, mumps virus, or HSV in neural cells are severe relative to the level of viral replication at mucosal surfaces. Similarly, significant morbidity may accompany in utero fetal infection with rubella virus or CMV.

Primary infections are cleared by nonspecific innate and specific adaptive immune responses. Thereafter, an immunocompetent host is usually immune to the disease manifestations of reinfection by the same virus. Immunity frequently does not prevent transient surface colonization on reexposure, persistent colonization, or even limited deep infection.

PERSISTENT AND LATENT INFECTIONS

Relatively few viruses cause persistent or latent infections. HBV, HCV, rabies virus, measles virus, HIV, HTLV, HPV, HHV, and some poxviruses are notable exceptions. The mechanisms for persistent infection vary widely. HCV RNA polymerase and HIV reverse transcriptase have high mutation rates, and the generation of variant genomes that evade the host immune response facilitates persistent infection. HIV is also directly immunosuppressive, depleting CD4+ T lymphocytes and compromising CD8+ cytotoxic T cell immune responsiveness. Moreover, HIV encodes a Nef protein that downmodulates MHC class I expression, rendering HIV-infected cells partially resistant to immune CD8+ cytolysis.

In contrast, DNA viruses have much lower mutation rates. Their persistence in human populations can be due to their ability to establish latent infection and to reactivate from latency. In this instance, *latency* is defined as a state of infection in which the virus is not replicating. Viral genes associated with lytic infection are not expressed, and infectious virus is not made. The complete viral genome is present and may be replicated by cellular DNA polymerase in conjunction with the cell genome replication. HPVs establish latent infection in basal epithelial cells, which replicate. Some of the progeny cells provide a stable supply of latently infected basal cells, while others go on to squamous differentiation and, in the process, become permissive for lytic viral infection. For herpesviruses, latent infection is established in nonreplicating neural cells (HSV and VZV) or in replicating cells of hematopoietic lineages [EBV and probably CMV, HHV-6, HHV-7, and Kaposi's sarcoma–associated herpesvirus (KSHV, also known as HHV-8)]. In their latent stage, HPV and herpesvirus genomes are largely hidden from the normal immune response. It is still not fully understood how partially latent and reactivated HPV and herpesvirus infections escape immediate and effective immune responses in highly immune hosts. HPV, HSV, and VZV may be somewhat protected because they replicate in middle and upper layers of the squamous epithelium—sites not routinely visited by immune and inflammatory cells. HSV and CMV are also known to encode proteins that downregulate MHC class I expression and antigenic peptide presentation on infected cells, thereby enabling these cells to escape CD8+ T lymphocyte cytotoxicity.

Like other poxviruses, molluscum contagiosum virus cannot establish latent infection but rather causes persistent infection in hypertrophic lesions that last for months or years. This virus encodes a chemokine homologue that probably blocks inflammatory responses and an MHC class I analogue that may block cytotoxic T lymphocyte attack.

PERSISTENT VIRAL INFECTIONS AND CANCER

Persistent viral infection is estimated to be the root cause of as many as 20% of human malignancies. For the most part, cancer is an accidental and highly unusual or long-term effect of infection with oncogenic human viruses. In these malignancies, viral infection is a critical and ultimately determinative early step, forcing infected cells to enter the cell cycle and enhancing their survival. An unusual virus-infected cell undergoes the subsequent genetic changes that permit the enhanced autonomous growth and survival characteristic of a malignant cell.

Most hepatocellular carcinoma is now believed to be caused by chronic inflammatory, immune, and regenerative responses to HBV or HCV infection. Epidemiologic data firmly link HBV and HCV infections to hepatocellular carcinoma. These infections elicit repetitive cycles of virus-induced liver injury followed by tissue repair and regeneration. Over decades, chronic virus infection, repetitive tissue regeneration, and acquired chromosomal changes can result in enhanced cell proliferation and survival and eventually in hepatocellular carcinoma. In rare instances, HBV DNA integrates into cellular DNA—an event that probably contributes to the development of some tumors.

Almost all cervical carcinoma is caused by persistent infection with "high-risk" genital HPV strains. Whereas HBV and HCV infections stimulate cell growth indirectly in response to virus-induced injury, proteins E6 and E7 of HPV type 16 or 18 can directly affect cell growth by causing the loss of p53 and RB, two cell proteins with tumor-suppressive function. These viral proteins can also increase genomic instability. However, like HBV and HCV infections, HPV infection alone is not sufficient for carcinogenesis. Cervical carcinoma is inevitably associated with persistent HPV infection and integration of the HPV genome into chromosomal DNA. Integrations that result in overexpression of E6 and E7 from HPV type 16 or 18 can cause profound changes in cell growth and survival, and subsequent chromosomal changes accumulating over ensuing cycles of cell growth can lead to malignant conversion and cervical carcinoma.

EBV infection and expression of the latent-infection viral proteins can immortalize B lymphocyte growth in tissue culture. In most humans, the immune response to the strongly antigenic EBV latent-infection proteins prevents uncontrolled B cell lymphoproliferation. However, when humans are immunosuppressed by posttransplantation medications, HIV infection, or genetic immunodeficiencies, EBV-induced B cell malignancies can emerge.

EBV infection also plays a role in the long-term development of certain B lymphocyte and epithelial cell malignancies. Persistent EBV infection and expression of the EBV oncogene LMP1 in latently infected epithelial cells appear to be critical early steps in the evolution of anaplastic nasopharyngeal carcinoma, a common malignancy in Chinese and North African populations. As in other virus-associated malignancies, genomic instability and chromosomal abnormalities contribute to the development of EBV-associated nasopharyngeal carcinomas. High-level LMP1 expression in Reed-Sternberg cells is also a hallmark of many cases of Hodgkin's disease. LMP1-induced nuclear factor κB (NF-κB) activity may rescue and prolong the survival of defective B cells that are normally eliminated by apoptosis, thereby allowing the acquisition of other genetic changes leading to malignant Reed-Sternberg cells.

The HTLV-I Tax and Rex proteins appear to be critical to the initiation of cutaneous adult T cell lymphoma/leukemias that may occur long after primary HTLV-I infection. Tax-induced NF-κB activation may contribute to cytokine production, infected cell survival, and eventual outgrowth of malignant cells.

Molecular data confirm the presence of KSHV DNA in all Kaposi's tumors, including those associated with HIV infection, transplantation, and familial transmission. KSHV infection is also etiologically implicated in pleural-effusion lymphomas and multicentric Castleman's disease, which are more common among HIV-infected than among HIV-uninfected people. Several KSHV proteins that can be expressed in latently infected cells, such as v-cyclin, v-interferon regulatory factor (v-IRF), and latency-associated nuclear antigen (LANA), are implicated in increased cell proliferation and survival.

Evidence supporting a causal role of viral infection in these malignancies includes (1) epidemiologic data, (2) the presence of viral DNA in all tumor cells, (3) the ability of the viruses to transform human cells in culture, (4) the results of in vitro assays for transforming effects of specific viral genes on cell growth or survival, and (5) pathologic data indicating the expression of transforming viral genes in premalignant or malignant cells in vivo. Virus-related malignancies provide an opportunity to expand our understanding of the biologic mechanisms important in the development of cancer; they also offer unique opportunities for the development of vaccines and therapeutics that could prevent or specifically treat cancers associated with virus infection. Widespread immunization against hepatitis B has resulted in a decreased prevalence of HBV-associated hepatitis and will likely prevent most HBV-related liver cancers. Studies of an HPV vaccine have shown reduced rates of colonization with high-risk HPV strains and a decreased risk of cervical cancer. The successful use of in vitro–expanded EBV-specific T cell populations to treat or prevent EBV-associated posttransplantation lymphoproliferative disease demonstrates the potential of immunotherapy against virus-associated cancers.

RESISTANCE TO VIRAL INFECTIONS

Resistance to viral infections is initially provided by factors that are not virus-specific. Physical protection is afforded by the cornified layers of the skin and by mucous secretions that continuously sweep over mucosal surfaces. Once the first cell is infected, IFNs are induced and confer resistance to virus replication. Viral infection may also trigger the release of other cytokines from infected cells; these cytokines may be chemotactic to inflammatory and immune cells. Viral protein epitopes expressed on the cell surface in the context of MHC class I and II proteins stimulate the expansion of T cell populations with T cell receptors that can recognize the virus-encoded peptides. Cytokines, inflammatory agents, and antigens released by virus-induced cell death further attract inflammatory cells, dendritic cells, granulocytes, natural killer (NK) cells, and B lymphocytes to the sites of initial infection and to draining lymph nodes. IFNs and NK cells are particularly important in containing viral infection for the first several days. Granulocytes and macrophages are also important in the phagocytosis and degradation of viruses, especially after an initial antibody response.

By 7–10 days after infection, virus-specific antibody responses, virus-specific HLA class II–restricted CD4+ helper T lymphocyte responses, and virus-specific HLA class I–restricted CD8+ cytotoxic T lymphocyte responses have developed. These responses, whose magnitude typically increases over the second and third weeks of infection, are important in rapid recovery. Also between the second and third weeks, the antibody type usually changes from IgM to IgG; IgG or IgA antibody can then be detected at infected mucosal surfaces. Antibody may directly neutralize virus by binding to its surface and preventing its adsorption or penetration. Complement usually enhances antibody-mediated virus neutralization. Antibody and complement can also lyse virus-infected cells that express viral proteins on their surface. A cell infected with a replicating enveloped virus usually expresses the virus-envelope glycoproteins on the cell plasma membrane. Specific antibodies can bind to the glycoproteins, fix complement, and lyse the infected cell.

Antibody and CD4+/CD8+ T lymphocyte responses tend to persist for several months after primary infection. Antibody-producing lymphocytes persist in small numbers as memory cells and begin to proliferate rapidly in response to a second infection, providing an early barrier to reinfection with the same virus. Immunologic memory for T cell responses appears to be shorter-lived. Redevelopment of T cell immunity may take longer than secondary antibody responses, particularly when many years have elapsed between primary infection and reexposure. However, persistent infections or frequent reactivations from latency can result in sustained high-level T cell responses. For example, EBV and CMV typically induce high-level CD4+ and CD8+ T cell responses that are sustained for decades after primary infection.

Some viruses have genes that alter innate and acquired host defenses. Adenoviruses encode small RNAs that inhibit IFN-induced, PKR-mediated shutoff of infected-cell protein synthesis. Furthermore, adenovirus E1A can directly inhibit IFN-mediated changes in cell gene transcription. Moreover, adenovirus E3 proteins prevent TNF-induced cytolysis and block HLA class I antigen synthesis by the infected cell. HSV ICP47 and CMV US11 block class I antigen presentation. EBV encodes an interleukin (IL) 10 homologue that inhibits NK and T cell responses. Vaccinia virus encodes a soluble receptor for IFN-α and binding proteins for IFN-γ, IL-1, IL-18, and TNF, which inhibit host innate and adaptive immune responses. Vaccinia virus also encodes a caspase inhibitor that inhibits the ability of CD8+ cytotoxic cells to kill virus-infected cells. Some poxviruses and herpesviruses also encode chemokine-binding proteins that inhibit cellular inflammatory responses. The adoption of these strategies by viruses highlights the importance of the corresponding host resistance factors in containing viral infection and the importance of redundancy in host resistance.

The host inflammatory and immune response to viral infection does not come without a price. This response contributes to the symptoms, signs, and other pathophysiologic manifestations of viral infection. Inflammation at sites of viral infection can subvert an effective immune response and induce tissue death and dysfunction. Moreover, immune responses to viral infection could, in principle, result in immune attack upon cross-reactive epitopes on normal cells, with consequent autoimmunity. While such effects have been demonstrated in experimental models, their role in the autoimmune manifestations of primary or recurrent human viral infections is uncertain.

INTERFERONS

All human cells can synthesize IFN-α or -β in response to viral infection. These IFN responses are usually induced by the presence of double-strand viral RNA, which can be made by both RNA and DNA viruses and sensed by double-strand RNA binding proteins in the cell cytoplasm, such as PKR and RIG-I. IFN-γ is not highly related to IFN-α or -β and is produced mainly by NK cells and by immune T lymphocytes responding to IL-12. IFN-α and -β bind to the IFN-α receptor, while IFN-γ binds to a different but related receptor. Both receptors signal through receptor-associated JAK kinases and other cytoplasmic proteins, including "STAT" proteins. STAT proteins are tyrosine-phosphorylated by JAK kinases, translocate to the nucleus, and activate promoters for specific cell genes. Three types of antiviral effects are induced by IFN at the transcriptional level. The first effect is attributable to the induction of 2′-5′ oligo(A) synthetases, which require double-strand RNA for their activation. Activated synthetase polymerizes oligo(A) and thereby activates RNAse L, which in turn degrades single-strand RNA. The second effect takes place through the induction of PKR, a serine and threonine kinase that is also activated by double-strand RNA. PKR phosphorylates and negatively regulates the translational initiation factor eIF2-α, shutting down protein synthesis in the infected cell. A third effect is initiated through the induction of Mx proteins, a family of GTPases that is particularly important in inhibiting the replication of influenza virus and vesicular stomatitis virus (VSV). These IFN effects are mostly directed against the infected cell, causing both viral and cellular dysfunction and thereby limiting viral replication.

DIAGNOSTIC VIROLOGY

A wide variety of methods are now used to diagnose viral infection. Serology and viral isolation in tissue culture remain important standards. Acute- and convalescent-phase sera with rising titers of antibody to virus-specific antigens and a shift from IgM to IgG antibodies are generally accepted as diagnostic of acute viral infection. Serologic diagnosis is based on a >4-fold rise in IgG antibody concentration when acute- and convalescent-phase serum samples are analyzed at the same time.

Immunofluorescence, hemadsorption, and hemagglutination assays for antiviral antibodies are labor-intensive and are being replaced by enzyme-linked immunosorbent assays (ELISAs). ELISAs generally use specific viral proteins that are most frequently targeted by the antibody response. The proteins are purified from virus-infected cells or produced by recombinant DNA technology and are attached to a solid phase, where they can be incubated with serum, washed to eliminate nonspecific antibodies, and allowed to react with an enzyme-linked reagent to detect human IgG or IgM antibody specifically adhering to the viral antigen. The amount of antibody can then be quantitated by the intensity of a color reaction mediated by the linked enzyme. ELISAs can be sensitive and automated. Western blots can confirm the presence of antibody to multiple specific viral proteins simultaneously. The proteins are separated by size and transferred to an inert membrane, where they are incubated with serum antibodies. Western blots have an internal specificity control, since the level of reactivity for viral proteins can be compared with that for cellular proteins in the same sample. Western blots require individual evaluation and are inherently difficult to quantitate or automate.

Virus isolation in tissue culture depends on infection of susceptible cells and amplification by replication in infected cells. Virus growth in cell cultures can frequently be identified by its effects on cell morphology under light microscopy. For example, HSV produces a typical cytopathic effect in rabbit kidney cells within 3 days. Other viral cytopathic effects may not be as diagnostically useful. Identification usually requires confirmation by staining with virus-specific monoclonal antibodies. The efficiency and speed of virus identification can be enhanced by combining short-term culture with immune detection. In assays with "shell vials" of tissue culture cells growing on a coverslip, viral infection can be detected by staining of the culture with a monoclonal antibody to a specific viral protein expressed early in viral replication. Thus, virus-infected cells can be detected within hours or days of inoculation; several rounds of infection would be required to produce a visible cytopathic effect.

Virus isolation in tissue culture also depends on the collection of specimens from the appropriate site and the rapid transport of these specimens in the appropriate medium to the virology laboratory. Rapid transport maintains viral viability and limits bacterial and fungal overgrowth. Enveloped viruses are generally much more sensitive to freezing and thawing than nonenveloped viruses. The most appropriate site for culture depends on the pathogenesis of the virus in question. Nasopharyngeal, tracheal, or endobronchial aspirates are most appropriate for the identification of respiratory viruses. Sputum cultures generally are less appropriate because bacterial contamination and viscosity threaten tissue-culture cell viability. Aspirates of vesicular fluid are useful for isolation of HSV and VZV. Nasopharyngeal aspirates and stool specimens may be useful when the patient has fever and a rash and an enteroviral infection is suspected. Adenoviruses can be cultured from the urine of patients with hemorrhagic cystitis. CMV can frequently be isolated from cultures of urine or buffy coat. Biopsy material can be effectively cultured when viruses infect major organs, as in HSV encephalitis or adenovirus pneumonia.

Virus isolation does not necessarily establish disease causality. Viruses can persistently or intermittently colonize normal human mucosal surfaces. Saliva can be positive for herpesviruses, and normal urine samples can be positive for CMV. Isolations from blood, cerebrospinal fluid (CSF), or tissue are more often diagnostic of significant viral infection.

Another method aimed at increasing the speed of viral diagnosis is direct testing for antigen or cytopathic effects. Virus-infected cells from the patient may be detected by staining with virus-specific monoclonal antibodies; e.g., epithelial cells obtained by nasopharyngeal aspiration can be stained with a variety of monoclonal antibodies to respiratory viruses.

Nucleic acid amplification techniques bring speed, sensitivity, and specificity to diagnostic virology. The ability to directly amplify minute amounts of viral nucleic acids present in specimens means that detection no longer depends on viable virus and its replication. For example, amplification and detection of HSV nucleic acids in the CSF of patients with HSV encephalitis is a more sensitive detection method than culture of virus from CSF. The extreme sensitivity of these tests can be a problem, since subclinical infection or contamination can lead to false-positive results. Detection of viral nucleic acids does not necessarily indicate virus-induced disease.

Measurement of the amount of viral RNA or DNA in peripheral blood is an important means of determining which patients are at increased risk for virus-induced disease and of evaluating clinical responses to antiviral chemotherapy. Nucleic acid technologies for RNA quantification are routinely used in AIDS patients to evaluate responses to antiviral agents and to detect virus resistance or noncompliance with therapy. Viral-load measurements are also useful for evaluating the treatment of patients with HBV and HCV infections. Nucleic acid testing or direct staining with CMV-specific monoclonal antibodies to quantitate virus-infected cells in the peripheral blood (CMV antigenemia) is useful for identifying immunosuppressed patients who may be at risk for CMV-induced disease.

DRUG TREATMENT FOR VIRAL INFECTIONS

Multiple steps in the viral life cycle can be effectively targeted by antiviral drugs. Nucleoside and nonnucleoside reverse transcriptase inhibitors prevent synthesis of the HIV provirus, while protease inhibitors block maturation of the HIV polyprotein after infection of the cell. Enfuvirtide is a small peptide derived from HIV gp41 that acts before infection by preventing a conformational change required for virus fusion. Integrase inhibitors are now in clinical testing. Amantadine and rimantadine inhibit the influenza M2 protein, preventing release of viral RNA early during infection, whereas zanamivir and oseltamivir inhibit the influenza neuraminidase, which is necessary for the efficient release of mature virions from infected cells.

Virus genomes can evolve resistance to drugs by mutation and selection, by recombination with a drug-resistant virus, or (in the case of influenza virus and other multicomponent RNA virus genomes) by reassortment. The emergence of drug-resistant strains can limit therapeutic efficacy. As with antibacterial therapy, excessive and inappropriate use of antiviral therapy can select for the emergence of drug-resistant strains. HIV genotyping is a rapid method for identifying drug-resistant viruses. Resistance to reverse transcriptase or protease inhibitors has been associated with specific mutations in the reverse transcriptase or protease genes. Identification of these mutations by polymerase chain reaction amplification and nucleic acid sequencing can be clinically useful for determining which antiviral agents may still be effective. Drug resistance in herpesviruses is a more unusual problem.

IMMUNIZATION FOR THE PREVENTION OF VIRAL INFECTIONS

Viral vaccines are among the outstanding accomplishments of medical science. Smallpox has been eradicated except as a potential weapon of biological warfare or bioterrorism (Chap. 214). Poliovirus eradication may soon follow. Measles can be contained or eliminated. Excess mortality due to influenza virus epidemics can be prevented, and the threat of influenza pandemics can be decreased by contemporary killed or live attenuated influenza vaccines. Mumps, rubella, and chickenpox are well controlled by childhood vaccination in the developed world. Reimmunization of mature adults can be used to control herpes zoster. New rotavirus vaccines are entering the market. Widespread HBV vaccination has dramatically lowered the frequency of acute and chronic hepatitis and is expected to lead to a dramatic decrease in the incidence of hepatocellular carcinoma. Use of purified proteins, genetically engineered live-virus vaccines, and recombinant DNA–based strategies will make it possible to immunize against severe infections with other viruses. The development of effective vaccines against HIV and HCV is complicated by the high mutation rate of RNA polymerase and reverse transcriptase, the evolutionary and individual divergence of HIV and HCV genomes, and repeated high-level exposure in some populations. Concerns about the use of smallpox and other viruses as weapons necessitate maintenance of immunity to agents that are not naturally encountered.

VIRUSES AS NOVEL THERAPEUTIC TOOLS OR AGENTS

Viruses are being experimentally developed for the delivery of biotherapeutics or novel vaccines. Foreign genes can be inserted into viral nucleic acids, and the recombinant virus vectors can be used to infect the patient or the patient's cells ex vivo. Retroviruses integrate into the cell genome and have been used to functionally replace the abnormal gene in T cells of patients with severe combined immunodeficiency, thereby restoring immune function. Recombinant adenovirus, AAV, and retroviruses are being explored for use in diseases due to single-gene defects, such as cystic fibrosis and hemophilia. Recombinant poxviruses and adenoviruses are also being used experimentally as vaccine vectors. Viral vectors are being tested experimentally for expressing cytokines that can enhance immunity against tumor cells or for expressing proteins that can increase the sensitivity of tumor cells to chemotherapy. Live HSV is now being used experimentally to kill glioblastoma cells after injections into tumors.

For improved safety, nonreplicating viruses are frequently employed in clinical trial settings. Potential adverse events associated with virus-mediated gene transfer include the induction of inflammatory and antiviral immune responses. Integration is useful for permanent gene therapy, but integrations can induce disease by enhancing or interrupting the expression of important cellular genes.

FURTHER READINGS

FINLAY BB, MCFADDEN G: Anti-immunology: Evasion of the host immune system by bacterial and viral pathogens. Cell 124:767, 2006

HILLEMAN MR: Strategies and mechanisms for host and pathogen survival in acute and persistent viral infections. Proc Natl Acad Sci USA 101(Suppl 2):14560, 2004

KNIPE DM et al (eds): *Fields Virology*, 6th ed. New York, Lippincott Williams & Wilkins, 2006

MUNGER K et al: Viral carcinogenesis and genomic instability. EXS 96:179, 2006

171 Antiviral Chemotherapy, Excluding Antiretroviral Drugs

Lindsey R. Baden, Raphael Dolin

The field of antiviral therapy—both the number of antiviral drugs and our understanding of their optimal use—continues to lag behind the field of antibacterial drug treatment, in which >70 years of experience have now been accumulated, but significant progress has been made in recent years on new drugs for several viral infections.

The development of antiviral drugs poses several challenges. Viruses replicate intracellularly and often employ host cell enzymes, macromolecules, and organelles for synthesis of viral particles. Therefore, useful antiviral compounds must discriminate between host and viral functions with a high degree of specificity; agents without such selectivity are likely to be too toxic for clinical use.

The development of laboratory assays to assist clinicians in the appropriate use of antiviral drugs is also in its early stages. Phenotypic and genotypic assays for resistance to antiviral drugs are becoming more widely available, and correlations of laboratory results with clinical outcomes in various settings are beginning to be defined. Of particular note has been the development of highly sensitive and specific methods that measure the concentration of virus in blood (*virus load*) and permit direct assessment of the antiviral effect of a given drug regimen in that compartment in the host. Virus load measurements have been useful in recognizing the risk of disease progression in patients with certain viral infections and in identifying patients to whom antiviral chemotherapy might be of greatest benefit. Like any in vitro laboratory test, these tests yield results that are highly dependent on (and likely to vary with) the laboratory techniques employed.

Information regarding the pharmacokinetics of some antiviral drugs, particularly in diverse clinical settings, is limited. Assays to measure the concentrations of these drugs, especially of their active moieties within cells, are primarily research procedures and are not widely available to clinicians. Thus, there are relatively few guidelines for adjusting dosages of antiviral agents to maximize antiviral activity and minimize toxicity. Consequently, clinical use of antiviral drugs must be accompanied by particular vigilance with regard to unanticipated adverse effects.

Like that of other infections, the course of viral infections is profoundly affected by an interplay of the pathogen with a complex set of host defenses. The presence or absence of preexisting immunity, the ability to mount humoral and/or cell-mediated immune responses, and the stimulation of innate immunity are important determinants of the outcome of viral infections. The state of the host's defenses needs to be considered when antiviral agents are used or evaluated.

As with any therapy, the optimal use of antiviral compounds requires a specific and timely diagnosis. For some viral infections, such as herpes zoster, the clinical manifestations are so characteristic that a diagnosis can be made on clinical grounds alone. For other viral infections, such as influenza A, epidemiologic information (e.g., the documentation of a community-wide outbreak) can be used to make a presumptive diagnosis with a high degree of accuracy. However, for most other viral infections, including herpes simplex encephalitis, cytomegaloviral infections other than retinitis, and enteroviral infections, diagnosis on clinical grounds alone cannot be accomplished with certainty. For such infections, rapid viral diagnostic techniques are of great importance. Considerable progress has been made in recent years in the development of such tests, which are now widely available for a number of viral infections.

Despite these complexities, the efficacy of a number of antiviral compounds has been clearly established in rigorously conducted and controlled studies. As summarized in Table 171-1, this chapter reviews the antiviral drugs that are currently approved or are likely to be considered for approval in the near future for use against viral infections other than those caused by HIV. Antiretroviral drugs are reviewed in Chap. 182.

TABLE 171-1	ANTIVIRAL CHEMOTHERAPY AND CHEMOPROPHYLAXIS			
Infection	**Drug**	**Route**	**Dosage**	**Comment**
Influenza A and B				
Prophylaxis	Oseltamivir	Oral	Adults: 75 mg/d Children ≥1 yr: 30–75 mg/d, depending on weight	Prophylaxis must continue for the duration of the outbreak and can be administered simultaneously with inactivated vaccine. Unless the sensitivity of isolates is known, neither amantadine nor rimantadine is currently recommended for prophylaxis or therapy because of the high rate of resistance in influenza A/H3N2 viruses since the 2005–2006 season.
	Zanamivir	Inhaled orally	Adults and children ≥5 yrs: 10 mg/d	
	Amantadine[a] or rimantadine[a]	Oral	Adults: 200 mg/d Children 1–9 yrs: 5 mg/kg per day (maximum, 150 mg/d)	
Treatment	Oseltamivir	Oral	Adults: 75 mg bid for 5 days Children 1–12 yrs: 30–75 mg bid for 5 days	When started within 2 days of onset, zanamivir and oseltamivir reduce symptoms by 1.0–1.5 and 1.3 days, respectively, in uncomplicated disease. Zanamivir may exacerbate bronchospasm in patients with asthma. Oseltamivir's side effects of nausea and vomiting can be reduced in frequency by drug administration with food. Amantadine and rimantadine are similarly effective in uncomplicated influenza caused by sensitive viruses. None of the listed drugs has been thoroughly studied in complicated cases (e.g., pneumonia).
	Zanamivir	Inhaled orally	Adults and children ≥7 yrs: 10 mg bid for 5 days	
	Amantadine[a]	Oral	Adults: 100 qd or bid Children 1–9 yrs: 5 mg/kg per day (maximum, 150 mg/d) for 5–7 days	
	Rimantadine[a]	Oral	100 qd or bid for 5–7 days in adults	
RSV infection	Ribavirin	Small-particle aerosol	Administered continuously from reservoir containing 20 mg/mL for 3–6 days	Ribavirin is used for treatment of infants and young children hospitalized with RSV pneumonia and bronchiolitis.
CMV retinitis in immunocompromised host (AIDS)	Ganciclovir	IV	5 mg/kg bid for 14–21 days; then 5 mg/kg per day as maintenance dose	Ganciclovir, valganciclovir, foscarnet, and cidofovir are approved for treatment of CMV retinitis in patients with AIDS. They are also used for colitis, pneumonia, or "wasting" syndrome associated with CMV and for prevention of CMV disease in transplant recipients. Valganciclovir has largely supplanted oral ganciclovir and is frequently used in place of IV ganciclovir.
		Oral	1 g tid as maintenance dose	
	Valganciclovir	Oral	900 mg bid for 21 days; then 900 mg/d as maintenance dose	

(continued)

TABLE 171-1 ANTIVIRAL CHEMOTHERAPY AND CHEMOPROPHYLAXIS (CONTINUED)

Infection	Drug	Route	Dosage	Comment
CMV retinitis (continued)	Foscarnet	IV	60 mg/kg q8h for 14–21 days; then 90–120 mg/kg per day as maintenance dose	Foscarnet is not myelosuppressive and is active against acyclovir- and ganciclovir-resistant herpesviruses.
	Cidofovir	IV	5 mg/kg once weekly for 2 weeks, then once every other week; given with probenecid and hydration	
	Fomivirsen	Intravitreal	330 mg on day 1 and day 15, followed by 330 mg monthly as maintenance	Fomivirsen has reduced the rate of progression of CMV retinitis in patients in whom other regimens have failed or have not been well tolerated. The major form of toxicity is ocular inflammation.
Varicella				
Immunocompetent host	Acyclovir	Oral	20 mg/kg (maximum, 800 mg) 4 or 5 times daily for 5 days	Treatment confers modest clinical benefit when administered within 24 h of rash onset.
Immunocompromised host	Acyclovir	IV	10 mg/kg q8h for 7 days	A change to oral valacyclovir can be considered once fever has subsided if there is no evidence of visceral involvement.
Herpes simplex encephalitis	Acyclovir	IV	10 mg/kg q8h for 14–21 days	Results are optimal when therapy is initiated early. Some authorities recommend treatment for 21 days to prevent relapses.
Neonatal herpes simplex	Acyclovir	IV	10 mg/kg q8h for 14–21 days	Serious morbidity is common despite therapy. Prolonged oral administration of acyclovir after initial IV therapy has been suggested because of long-term sequelae associated with cutaneous recurrences of HSV infection.
Genital herpes simplex				
Primary (treatment)	Acyclovir	IV	5 mg/kg q8h for 5–10 days	The IV route is preferred for infections severe enough to warrant hospitalization or with neurologic complications.
		Oral	200 mg 5 times daily for 10 days	The oral route is preferred for patients whose condition does not warrant hospitalization. Adequate hydration must be maintained.
	Acyclovir	Topical	5% ointment; 4–6 applications daily for 7–10 days	Topical use—largely supplemented by oral therapy—may obviate systemic administration to pregnant women. Systemic symptoms and untreated areas are not affected.
	Valacyclovir	Oral	1 g bid for 10 days	Valacyclovir appears to be as effective as acyclovir but can be administered less frequently.
	Famciclovir	Oral	250 mg tid for 5–10 days[b]	Famciclovir appears to be similar in effectiveness to acyclovir.
Recurrent (treatment)	Acyclovir	Oral	200 mg 5 times daily for 5 days	Clinical effect is modest and is enhanced if therapy is initiated early. Treatment does not affect recurrence rates.
	Famciclovir	Oral	1000 mg bid for 1 day	
	Valacyclovir	Oral	500 mg bid for 3 days	
Recurrent (suppression)	Acyclovir	Oral	400 mg bid for ≥12 months	Suppressive therapy is recommended only for patients with at least 6–10 recurrences per year. "Breakthrough" occasionally takes place, and asymptomatic shedding of virus occurs. The need for suppressive therapy should be reevaluated after 1 year. Suppression with valacyclovir reduces transmission of genital HSV among discordant couples.
	Valacyclovir	Oral	500–1000 mg/d	
	Famciclovir	Oral	125–250 mg bid	
Mucocutaneous herpes simplex in immuno-compromised host				
Treatment	Acyclovir	IV	5 mg/kg q8h for 7 days	The choice of the IV or oral route depends on the severity of infection and the patient's ability to take oral medication. Oral or IV treatment has supplanted topical therapy except for small, easily accessible lesions. Foscarnet is used for acyclovir-resistant viruses.
		Oral	400 mg 5 times daily for 10 days	
		Topical	5% ointment; 4–6 applications daily for 7 days or until healed	
	Valacyclovir	Oral	1 g tid for 7 days[b]	
	Famciclovir	Oral	500 mg bid for 4 days[c]	
Prevention of recurrence during intense immunosuppression	Acyclovir	Oral	200 mg bid	Treatment is administered during periods when intense immunosuppression is expected—e.g., during antitumor chemotherapy or after transplantation—and is usually continued for 2–3 months.
		IV	5 mg/kg q12h	
	Valacyclovir	Oral	1 g tid[b]	
	Famciclovir	Oral	500 mg bid[b]	
Herpes simplex orolabialis (recurrent)	Penciclovir	Topical	1.0% cream applied q2h during waking hours for 4 days	Treatment shortens healing time and symptoms by 0.5–1.0 day (compared with placebo).
	Valacyclovir	Oral	2 g q12h for 1 day	Therapy begun at the earliest symptom reduces disease duration by 1 day.
	Famciclovir[b]	Oral	500 mg tid for 5 days	Therapy begun 48 h after UV light exposure decreases time to healing by 2 days.
	Docosonal[d]	Topical	10% cream 5 times daily until healed	Application at initial symptoms reduces healing time by 1 day.
Herpes simplex keratitis	Trifluridine	Topical	1 drop of 1% ophthalmic solution q2h while awake (maximum, 9 drops daily)	Therapy should be undertaken in consultation with an ophthalmologist.
	Vidarabine	Topical	0.5-in. ribbon of 3% ophthalmic ointment 5 times daily	

(continued)

TABLE 171-1 ANTIVIRAL CHEMOTHERAPY AND CHEMOPROPHYLAXIS (CONTINUED)

Infection	Drug	Route	Dosage	Comment
Herpes zoster				
Immunocompetent host	Valacyclovir	Oral	1 g tid for 7 days	Valacyclovir may be more effective than acyclovir for pain relief; otherwise, it has a similar effect on cutaneous lesions and should be given within 72 h of rash onset.
	Famciclovir	Oral	500 mg q8h for 7 days	The duration of postherpetic neuralgia is shorter than with placebo. Famciclovir showed overall efficacy similar to that of acyclovir in a comparative trial. It should be given ≤72 h after rash onset.
	Acyclovir	Oral	800 mg 5 times daily for 7–10 days	Acyclovir causes faster resolution of skin lesions than placebo and provides some relief of acute symptoms if given within 72 h of rash onset. Combined with tapering doses of prednisone, acyclovir improves quality-of-life outcomes.
Immunocompromised host	Acyclovir	IV	10 mg/kg q8h for 7 days	Effectiveness in localized zoster is most marked when treatment is given early. Foscarnet may be used for VZV infections that are resistant to acyclovir.
		Oral	800 mg 5 times daily for 7 days	
	Famciclovir	Oral	500 mg tid for 10 days[b]	
Herpes zoster ophthalmicus	Acyclovir	Oral	600 mg 5 times daily for 10 days	Treatment reduces ocular complications, including ocular keratitis and uveitis.
Condyloma acuminatum	IFN-α2b	Intralesional	1 million units per wart (maximum of 5) thrice weekly for 3 weeks	Intralesional treatment frequently results in regression of warts, but lesions often recur. Parenteral administration may be useful if lesions are numerous.
	IFN-αn3	Intralesional	250,000 units per wart (maximum of 10) twice weekly for up to 8 weeks	
Chronic hepatitis B	IFN-α2b	SC	5 million units daily or 10 million units thrice weekly for 16–24 weeks	HBeAg and DNA are eliminated in 33–37% of cases. Histopathologic improvement is also seen.
	Pegylated IFN-α2a	SC	180 μg weekly for 48 weeks	HBeAg and DNA are eliminated in 32–43% of recipients.
	Lamivudine	Oral	100 mg/d for 12–18 months; 150 mg bid as part of therapy for HIV infection	The efficacy of lamivudine is similar to that of IFN, but lamivudine is better tolerated. Resistance develops in 24% of recipients when lamivudine is used as monotherapy for 1 year.
	Adefovir dipivoxil	Oral	10 mg/d for 48 months	A return of ALT levels to normal is documented in 48–72% of recipients and improved liver histopathology in 53–64%. Adefovir is effective in lamivudine-resistant hepatitis B. Renal function should be monitored.
	Entecavir	Oral	0.5 mg/d for 48 weeks (1 mg/d if HBV is resistant to lamivudine)	Normalization of ALT is seen in 68–78% of recipients and loss of HBeAg in 21%. Entecavir is active against lamivudine-resistant HBV.
	Telbivudine	Oral	600 mg/d for 52 weeks	Reduction of HBV DNA by >5 $\log_{10}$ copies/mL along with either normalization of ALT or loss of serum HBeAg is seen in 75% of recipients. Myopathy may occur.
Chronic hepatitis C	IFN-α2a or IFN-α2b	SC	3 million units thrice weekly for 12–18 months	A return of ALT levels to normal is documented in 54% of recipients but is sustained in only 28%. Improvement in liver histopathology is seen.
	IFN-α2b/ ribavirin	SC (IFN)/oral (ribavirin)	3 million units thrice weekly (IFN)/1000–1200 mg daily (ribavirin) for 6–12 months	Combination therapy results in sustained responses in up to 40–50% of all recipients.
	Pegylated IFN-α2b	SC	1 μg/kg weekly for 12–24 months	The slower clearance of pegylated IFNs than of standard IFNs permits once-weekly administration. The pegylated formulations appear to be superior to standard IFNs in tolerability and efficacy, both as monotherapy and in combination with ribavirin. Sustained virologic responses were seen in 42–46% of genotype 1 patients and in 76–82% of those infected with genotype 2 or 3.
	Pegylated IFN-α2a	SC	180 μg weekly for 12–24 months	
	Pegylated IFN-α2b/ ribavirin	SC (IFN)/oral (ribavirin)	1.5 μg/kg weekly (IFN)/800–1200 mg daily (ribavirin)[d] for 24–48 weeks	
	Pegylated IFN-α2a/ ribavirin	SC (IFN)/oral (ribavirin)	180 μg weekly (IFN)/800–1200 mg daily (ribavirin) for 24–48 weeks	
	IFN-alfacon	SC	9–15 μg thrice weekly for 6–12 months	Doses of 9 and 15 μg are equivalent to IFN-α2a and IFN-α2b doses of 3 million and 5 million units, respectively.
Chronic hepatitis D	IFN-α2a or IFN-α2b	SC	9 million units thrice weekly for 12 months	The overall efficacy and the optimal regimen and duration of therapy have not been established. Responses usually are not sustained when therapy is stopped.

[a]Influenza A only. Unless isolate sensitivity is known, not recommended for prophylaxis or therapy since 2005–2006 because of high rates of resistance in influenza A/H3N2 viruses.

[b]Not approved for this indication by the U.S. Food and Drug Administration (FDA).

[c]Approved by the FDA for treatment of HIV-infected individuals.

[d]Active ingredient: benzyl alcohol. Available without prescription.

Abbreviations: ALT, alanine aminotransferase; CMV, cytomegalovirus; HBeAg, hepatitis B e antigen; HBV, hepatitis B virus; HSV, herpes simplex virus; IFN, interferon; RSV, respiratory syncytial virus; UV, ultraviolet; VZV, varicella-zoster virus.

ZANAMIVIR AND OSELTAMIVIR

Zanamivir and oseltamivir are inhibitors of the influenza viral neuraminidase enzyme, which is essential for release of the virus from infected cells and for its subsequent spread throughout the respiratory tract of the infected host. The enzyme cleaves terminal sialic acid residues and thus destroys the cellular receptors to which the viral hemagglutinin attaches. Zanamivir and oseltamivir are sialic acid transition-state analogues and are highly active and specific inhibitors of the neuraminidases of both influenza A and B viruses. The antineuraminidase activity of the two drugs is similar, although zanamivir has somewhat greater in vitro activity against influenza B. Both zanamivir and oseltamivir act through competitive and reversible inhibition of the active site of influenza A and B viral neuraminidases and have relatively little effect on mammalian cell enzymes.

Oseltamivir phosphate is an ethyl ester prodrug that is converted to oseltamivir carboxylate by esterases in the liver. Orally administered oseltamivir has a bioavailability of >60% and a plasma half-life of 7–9 h. The drug is excreted unmetabolized, primarily by the kidneys. Zanamivir has low oral bioavailability and is administered orally via a hand-held inhaler. By this route, ~15% of the dose is deposited in the lower respiratory tract, and low plasma levels of the drug are detected.

Orally inhaled zanamivir is generally well tolerated, although exacerbations of asthma may occur. The toxicities most frequently encountered with orally administered oseltamivir are nausea, gastrointestinal discomfort, and (less commonly) vomiting. Gastrointestinal discomfort is usually transient and is less likely if the drug is administered with food. Recently, neuropsychiatric events (delirium, self-injury) have been reported in children who have been taking oseltamivir, primarily in Japan.

Inhaled zanamivir and orally administered oseltamivir have been effective in the treatment of naturally occurring influenza A or B in otherwise-healthy adults. In placebo-controlled studies, illness has been shortened by 1.0–1.5 days of therapy with either of these drugs when treatment is administered within 2 days of onset. A recent meta-analysis of clinical studies of oseltamivir suggests that treatment may reduce the likelihood of certain respiratory tract complications of influenza. Once-daily inhaled zanamivir or once-daily orally administered oseltamivir provides effective prophylaxis against laboratory-documented influenza A– and influenza B–associated illness.

The emergence of viruses resistant to zanamivir or oseltamivir occurs but appears to be less frequent than the emergence of resistance to the adamantanes in clinical studies carried out thus far. In one pediatric study, 5.5% of patients treated with oseltamivir developed resistant isolates. A somewhat higher rate of resistance was noted in a recent pediatric study of oseltamivir from Japan. Resistance to the neuraminidase inhibitors may develop by changes in the viral neuraminidase enzyme, by changes in the hemagglutinin that make it more resistant to the actions of the neuraminidase, or by both mechanisms. Some isolates that are resistant to oseltamivir may remain sensitive to zanamivir. Since the mechanisms of action of the neuraminidase inhibitors differ from those of the adamantanes (see below), zanamivir and oseltamivir are active against strains of influenza A virus that are resistant to amantadine and rimantadine.

Zanamivir and oseltamivir have been approved by the U.S. Food and Drug Administration (FDA) for treatment of influenza in adults and in children (those ≥7 years old for zanamivir and those ≥1 year old for oseltamivir) who have been symptomatic for ≤2 days. Oseltamivir is approved for prophylaxis of influenza in individuals ≥1 year of age and zanamivir for those ≥5 years of age (Table 171-1).

AMANTADINE AND RIMANTADINE

Amantadine and the closely related compound rimantadine are primary symmetric amines that display antiviral activity limited to influenza A viruses. Amantadine and rimantadine have been shown to be efficacious in the prophylaxis and treatment of influenza A infections in humans for >40 years. High frequencies of resistance to these drugs

were noted among influenza A/H3N2 viruses in the 2005–2006 influenza season and continue to be seen up to the present (2006–2007). Therefore, these agents are no longer recommended unless the sensitivity of the individual influenza A isolate is known, in which case their use may be considered. Amantadine and rimantadine act through inhibition of the ion channel function of the influenza A M2 matrix protein, on which appropriate uncoating of the virus depends. A substitution of a single amino acid at critical sites in the M2 protein can result in a virus that is resistant to amantadine and rimantadine.

Amantadine and rimantadine have been shown to be effective in the prophylaxis of influenza A in large-scale studies of young adults and in less extensive studies of children and elderly persons. In such studies, efficacy rates of 55–80% in the prevention of influenza-like illness were noted, and even higher rates were reported when virus-specific attack rates were calculated. Amantadine and rimantadine have also been found to be effective in the treatment of influenza A infection in studies involving predominantly young adults and, to a lesser extent, children. Administration of these compounds within 24–72 h after the onset of illness has resulted in a reduction of the duration of signs and symptoms by ~50% from that in placebo recipients. The effect on signs and symptoms of illness is superior to that of commonly used antipyretic-analgesic agents. Only anecdotal reports are available concerning the efficacy of amantadine or rimantadine in the prevention or treatment of complications of influenza (e.g., pneumonia).

Amantadine and rimantadine are available only in oral formulations and are ordinarily administered to adults once or twice daily, with a dosage of 100–200 mg/d. Despite their structural similarities, the two compounds have different pharmacokinetics. Amantadine is not metabolized and is excreted almost entirely by the kidney, with a half-life of 12–17 h and peak plasma concentrations of 0.4 μg/mL. In contrast, rimantadine is extensively metabolized to hydroxylated derivatives and has a half-life of 30 h. Only 30–40% of an orally administered dose of rimantadine is recovered in the urine. The peak plasma levels of rimantadine are approximately half those of amantadine, but rimantadine is concentrated in respiratory secretions to a greater extent than amantadine. For prophylaxis, the compounds must be administered daily for the period at risk (i.e., the peak duration of the outbreak). For therapy, amantadine or rimantadine is generally administered for 5–7 days.

Although these compounds are generally well tolerated, 5–10% of amantadine recipients experience mild central nervous system side effects consisting primarily of dizziness, anxiety, insomnia, and difficulty in concentrating. These effects are rapidly reversible upon cessation of the drug's administration. At a dose of 200 mg/d, rimantadine is better tolerated than amantadine; in a large-scale study of young adults, adverse effects were no more frequent among rimantadine recipients than among placebo recipients. Seizures and worsening of congestive heart failure have also been reported in patients treated with amantadine, although a causal relationship has not been established. The dosage of amantadine should be reduced to 100 mg/d in patients with renal insufficiency [i.e., a creatinine clearance rate (Cr_{Cl}) of <50 mL/min] and in the elderly. A rimantadine dose of 100 mg/d should be used for patients with a Cr_{Cl} of <10 mL/min and in the elderly.

RIBAVIRIN

Ribavirin is a synthetic nucleoside analogue that inhibits a wide range of RNA and DNA viruses. The mechanism of action of ribavirin is not completely defined and may be different for different groups of viruses. Ribavirin-5′-monophosphate blocks the conversion of inosine-5′-monophosphate to xanthosine-5′-monophosphate and interferes with the synthesis of guanine nucleotides as well as that of both RNA and DNA. Ribavirin-5′-monophosphate also inhibits capping of virus-specific messenger RNA in certain viral systems. In studies demonstrating the effectiveness of ribavirin in the treatment of respiratory syncytial virus (RSV) infection in infants, the compound was administered as a small-particle aerosol. In infants with RSV infection who were given ribavirin by continuous aerosol for 3–6 days, illness and lower respiratory tract signs resolved more rapidly and arterial oxygen desaturation was less pronounced than in placebo-treated groups. In addition, ribavirin has had a beneficial clinical effect in infants with RSV infection who require mechanical ventilation. Aerosolized ribavirin has also been administered to older children and adults with severe RSV and parainfluenza virus infections (including immunosuppressed patients) and to older children and adults with influenza A or B infection, but the benefit of this treatment, if any, is unclear. In RSV infections in immunosuppressed patients, ribavirin is often given in combination with immunoglobulins.

Orally administered ribavirin has not been effective in the treatment of influenza A virus infections. IV or oral ribavirin has reduced mortality rates among patients with Lassa fever; it has been particularly effective in this regard when given within the first 6 days of illness. IV ribavirin has been reported to be of clinical benefit in the treatment of hemorrhagic fever with renal syndrome caused by Hantaan virus and as therapy for Argentinian hemorrhagic fever. Moreover, oral ribavirin has been recommended for the treatment and prophylaxis of Congo-Crimean hemorrhagic fever. An open-label trial suggested that oral ribavirin may be beneficial in the treatment of Nipah virus encephalitis. Use of IV ribavirin in patients with hantavirus pulmonary syndrome in the United States has not been associated with clear-cut benefits. Oral administration of ribavirin reduces serum aminotransferase levels in patients with chronic hepatitis C virus (HCV) infection; since it appears not to reduce serum HCV RNA levels, the mechanism of this effect is unclear. The drug provides added benefit when given by mouth in doses of 800–1200 mg/d in combination with interferon (IFN) α2b or α2a (see below), and the ribavirin/IFN combination has been approved for the treatment of patients with chronic HCV infection.

Large doses of ribavirin (800–1000 mg/d PO) have been associated with reversible hematopoietic toxicity. This effect has not been observed with aerosolized ribavirin, apparently because little drug is absorbed systemically. Aerosolized administration of ribavirin is generally well tolerated but occasionally is associated with bronchospasm, rash, or conjunctival irritation. Aerosolized ribavirin has been approved for treatment of RSV infection in infants and should be administered under close supervision—particularly in the setting of mechanical ventilation, where precipitation of the drug is possible. Health care workers exposed to the drug have experienced minor toxicity, including eye and respiratory tract irritation. Because ribavirin is mutagenic, teratogenic, and embryotoxic, its use is generally contraindicated in pregnancy. Its administration as an aerosol poses a risk to pregnant health care workers.

ANTIVIRAL DRUGS ACTIVE AGAINST HERPESVIRUS INFECTIONS

ACYCLOVIR AND VALACYCLOVIR

Acyclovir is a highly potent and selective inhibitor of the replication of certain herpesviruses, including herpes simplex virus (HSV) types 1 and 2, varicella-zoster virus (VZV), and Epstein-Barr virus (EBV). It is relatively ineffective in the treatment of human cytomegalovirus (CMV) infections; however, some studies have indicated its effectiveness in the prevention of CMV-associated disease in immunosuppressed patients. Valacyclovir, the L-valyl ester of acyclovir, is converted almost entirely to acyclovir by intestinal and hepatic hydrolysis after oral administration. Valacyclovir has pharmacokinetic advantages over orally administered acyclovir: it exhibits significantly greater oral bioavailability, results in higher blood levels, and can be given less frequently than acyclovir (two or three rather than five times daily).

The high degree of selectivity of acyclovir is related to its mechanism of action, which requires that the compound first be phosphorylated to acyclovir monophosphate. This phosphorylation occurs efficiently in herpesvirus-infected cells by means of a virus-coded thymidine kinase. In uninfected mammalian cells, little phosphorylation of acyclovir occurs, and the drug is therefore concentrated in herpesvirus-infected cells. Acyclovir monophosphate is subsequently converted by host cell kinases to a triphosphate that is a potent inhibitor of virus-induced DNA polymerase but has relatively little effect on host-cell DNA

polymerase. Acyclovir triphosphate can also be incorporated into viral DNA, with early chain termination.

Acyclovir is available in IV, oral, and topical forms, while valacyclovir is available in an oral formulation. IV acyclovir is markedly effective in the treatment of mucocutaneous HSV infections in immunocompromised hosts, in whom it reduces time to healing, duration of pain, and virus shedding. When administered prophylactically during periods of intense immunosuppression (e.g., related to chemotherapy for leukemia or transplantation) and before the development of lesions, IV acyclovir reduces the frequency of HSV-associated disease. After prophylaxis is discontinued, HSV lesions recur. IV acyclovir is also effective in the treatment of HSV encephalitis; two comparative trials have indicated that acyclovir is more effective than vidarabine for this indication (see below).

Because VZV is generally less sensitive to acyclovir than is HSV, higher doses of acyclovir must be used to treat VZV infections. In immunocompromised patients with herpes zoster, IV acyclovir reduces the frequency of cutaneous dissemination and visceral complications and—in one comparative trial—was more effective than vidarabine. Acyclovir, administered at doses of 800 mg PO five times a day, had a modest beneficial effect on localized herpes zoster lesions in both immunocompromised and immunocompetent patients. Combination of acyclovir with a tapering regimen of prednisone appeared to be more effective than acyclovir alone in terms of quality-of-life outcomes in immunocompetent patients over age 50 with herpes zoster. A comparative study of acyclovir (800 mg PO five times daily) and valacyclovir (1 g PO tid) in immunocompetent patients with herpes zoster indicated that the latter drug may be more effective in eliciting the resolution of zoster-associated pain. Orally administered acyclovir (600 mg five times a day) reduced complications of herpes zoster ophthalmicus in a placebo-controlled trial.

In chickenpox, a modest overall clinical benefit is attained when oral acyclovir therapy is begun within 24 h of the onset of rash in otherwise-healthy children (20 mg/kg, up to a maximum of 800 mg, four times a day) or adults (800 mg five times a day). IV acyclovir has also been reported to be effective in the treatment of immunocompromised children with chickenpox.

The most widespread use of acyclovir is in the treatment of genital HSV infections. IV or oral acyclovir or oral valacyclovir has shortened the duration of symptoms, reduced virus shedding, and accelerated healing when employed for the treatment of primary genital HSV infections. Oral acyclovir and valacyclovir have also had a modest effect in treatment of recurrent genital HSV infections. However, the failure of treatment of either primary or recurrent disease to reduce the frequency of subsequent recurrences has indicated that acyclovir is ineffective in eliminating latent infection. Chronic oral administration of acyclovir for ≥1–6 years or of valacyclovir for ≥1 year has reduced the frequency of recurrences markedly during therapy; once the drug is discontinued, lesions recur. In one study, suppressive therapy with valacyclovir (500 mg once daily for 8 months) reduced transmission of HSV-2 genital infections among discordant couples by 50%. A modest effect on herpes labialis (i.e., a reduction of disease duration by 1 day) was seen when valacyclovir was administered upon detection of the first symptom of a lesion at a dose of 2 g every 12 h for 1 day. In AIDS patients, chronic or intermittent administration of acyclovir has been associated with the development of HSV and VZV strains resistant to the action of the drug and with clinical failures. The most common mechanism of resistance is a deficiency of the virus-induced thymidine kinase. Patients with HSV or VZV infections resistant to acyclovir have frequently responded to foscarnet.

With the availability of the oral and IV forms, there are few indications for topical acyclovir, although treatment with this formulation has been modestly beneficial in primary genital HSV infections and in mucocutaneous HSV infections in immunocompromised hosts.

Overall, acyclovir is remarkably well tolerated and is generally free of toxicity. The most frequently encountered form of toxicity is renal dysfunction because of drug crystallization, particularly after rapid IV administration or with inadequate hydration. Central nervous system changes, including lethargy and tremors, are occasionally reported, primarily in immunosuppressed patients. However, whether these changes are related to acyclovir, to concurrent administration of other therapy, or to underlying infection remains unclear. Acyclovir is excreted primarily unmetabolized by the kidney via both glomerular filtration and tubular secretion. Approximately 15% of a dose of acyclovir is metabolized to 9-[(carboxymethoxy)methyl]guanine or other minor metabolites. Reduction in dosage is indicated in patients with a Cr_{Cl} of <50 mL/min. The half-life of acyclovir is ~3 h in normal adults, and the peak plasma concentration after a 1-h infusion of a dose of 5 mg/kg is 9.8 μg/mL. Approximately 22% of an orally administered acyclovir dose is absorbed, and peak plasma concentrations of 0.3–0.9 μg/mL are attained after administration of a 200-mg dose. Acyclovir penetrates relatively well into the cerebrospinal fluid (CSF), with concentrations approaching half of those found in plasma.

Acyclovir causes chromosomal breakage at high doses, but its administration to pregnant women has not been associated with fetal abnormalities. Nonetheless, the potential risks and benefits of acyclovir should be carefully assessed before the drug is used in pregnancy.

Valacyclovir exhibits three to five times greater bioavailability than acyclovir. The concentration-time curve for valacyclovir, given as 1 g PO three times daily, is similar to that for acyclovir, given as 5 mg/kg IV every 8 h. The safety profiles of valacyclovir and acyclovir are similar, although thrombotic thrombocytopenic purpura/hemolytic-uremic syndrome has been reported in immunocompromised patients who have received high doses of valacyclovir (8 g/d). Valacyclovir is approved for the treatment of herpes zoster, of initial and recurrent episodes of genital HSV infections in immunocompetent adults, and of herpes labialis as well as for suppressive treatment of genital herpes. Although it has not been extensively studied in other clinical settings involving HSV or VZV infections, many consultants use valacyclovir rather than oral acyclovir in settings where the latter has been approved because of valacyclovir's superior pharmacokinetics and more convenient dosing schedule.

CIDOFOVIR

Cidofovir is a phosphonate nucleotide analogue of cytosine. Its major use is in CMV infections, particularly retinitis, but it is active against a broad range of herpesviruses, including HSV, human herpesvirus (HHV) type 6, HHV-8, and certain other DNA viruses such as polyomaviruses, papillomaviruses, adenoviruses, and poxviruses, including variola (smallpox) and vaccinia. Cidofovir does not require initial phosphorylation by virus-induced kinases; the drug is phosphorylated by host cell enzymes to cidofovir diphosphate, which is a competitive inhibitor of viral DNA polymerases and, to a lesser extent, of host cell DNA polymerases. Incorporation of cidofovir diphosphate slows or terminates nascent DNA chain elongation. Cidofovir is active against HSV isolates that are resistant to acyclovir because of absent or altered thymidine kinase and against CMV isolates that are resistant to ganciclovir because of UL97 phosphotransferase mutations. Cidofovir is usually active against foscarnet-resistant CMV, although cross-resistance to foscarnet as well as to ganciclovir has been described.

Cidofovir has poor oral availability and is administered IV. It is excreted primarily by the kidney and has a plasma half-life of 2.6 h. Cidofovir diphosphate's intracellular half-life of >48 h is the basis for the recommended dosing regimen of 5 mg/kg once a week for the initial 2 weeks and then 5 mg/kg every other week. The major toxic effect of cidofovir is proximal renal tubular injury, as manifested by elevated serum creatinine levels and proteinuria. The risk of nephrotoxicity can be reduced by vigorous saline hydration and by concomitant oral administration of probenecid. Neutropenia, rashes, and gastrointestinal tolerance may also occur.

IV cidofovir has been approved for the treatment of CMV retinitis in AIDS patients who are intolerant of ganciclovir or foscarnet or in whom those drugs have failed. In a controlled study, a maintenance dosage of 5 mg/kg per week administered to AIDS patients reduced the progression of CMV retinitis from that seen at 3 mg/kg. IV cidofovir has been reported anecdotally to be effective for treatment of acyclo-

vir-resistant mucocutaneous HSV infections. Likewise, topically administered cidofovir is reportedly beneficial against these infections in HIV-infected patients; it is also being studied for the treatment of anogenital warts. Anecdotal use of IV cidofovir has been described in disseminated adenoviral infections in immunosuppressed patients, but its efficacy, if any, is not known. An ophthalmic formulation is being studied as treatment for adenoviral keratoconjunctivitis. Intravitreal cidofovir has been used to treat CMV retinitis but has been associated with significant toxicity.

FOMIVIRSEN

Fomivirsen is the first antisense oligonucleotide approved by the FDA for therapy in humans. This phosphorothioate oligonucleotide, 21 nucleotides in length, inhibits CMV replication through interaction with CMV messenger RNA. Fomivirsen is complementary to messenger transcripts of the major immediate early region 2 (IE2) of CMV, which codes for proteins regulating viral gene expression. In addition to its antisense mechanism of action, fomivirsen may exert activity against CMV through inhibition of viral adsorption to cells as well as direct inhibition of viral replication. Because of its different mechanism of action, fomivirsen is active against CMV isolates that are resistant to nucleoside or nucleotide analogues, such as ganciclovir, foscarnet, or cidofovir.

Fomivirsen has been approved for intravitreal administration in the treatment of CMV retinitis in AIDS patients who have failed to respond to other treatments or cannot tolerate them. Injections of 330 mg for two doses 2 weeks apart, followed by maintenance doses of 330 mg monthly, significantly reduce the rate of progression of CMV retinitis. The major toxicity is ocular inflammation, including vitritis and iritis, which usually responds to topically administered glucocorticoids.

GANCICLOVIR AND VALGANCICLOVIR

An analogue of acyclovir, ganciclovir is active against HSV and VZV and is markedly more active than acyclovir against CMV. Ganciclovir triphosphate inhibits CMV DNA polymerase and can be incorporated into CMV DNA, whose elongation it eventually terminates. In HSV- and VZV-infected cells, ganciclovir is phosphorylated by virus-encoded thymidine kinases; in CMV-infected cells, it is phosphorylated by a viral kinase encoded by the UL97 gene. Ganciclovir triphosphate is present in tenfold higher concentrations in CMV-infected cells than in uninfected cells. Ganciclovir is approved for the treatment of CMV retinitis in immunosuppressed patients and for the prevention of CMV disease in transplant recipients. It is widely used for the treatment of other CMV-associated syndromes, including pneumonia, esophagogastrointestinal infections, hepatitis, and "wasting" illness.

Ganciclovir is available for IV or oral administration. Because its oral bioavailability is low (5–9%), relatively large doses (1 g three times daily) must be administered by this route. Oral ganciclovir has largely been supplanted by valganciclovir, which is the L-valyl ester of ganciclovir. Valganciclovir is well absorbed orally, with a bioavailability of 60%, and is rapidly hydrolyzed to ganciclovir in the intestine and liver. The area under the curve for a 900-mg dose of valganciclovir is equivalent to that for 5 mg/kg of ganciclovir given IV, although peak serum concentrations are ~40% lower for valganciclovir. The serum half-life is 3.5 h after IV administration of ganciclovir and 4.0 h after PO administration of valganciclovir. Ganciclovir is excreted primarily by the kidneys in an unmetabolized form, and its dosage should be reduced in cases of renal failure. The most commonly employed dosage for initial IV therapy is 5 mg/kg every 12 h for 14–21 days; this regimen is followed by an IV maintenance dose of 5 mg/kg per day or five times per week. For oral therapy with valganciclovir, the dose is 900 mg twice daily for 21 days followed by 900 mg once a day for maintenance, with dose adjustment in patients with renal dysfunction. Intraocular ganciclovir, given by either intravitreal injection or intraocular implantation, has also been used to treat CMV retinitis.

Ganciclovir is effective as prophylaxis against CMV-associated disease in organ and bone marrow transplant recipients. Oral ganciclovir administered prophylactically to AIDS patients with CD4+ T cell counts of <100/μL has provided protection against the development of CMV retinitis. However, the long-term benefits of this approach to prophylaxis in AIDS patients have not been established, and most experts do not recommend the use of oral ganciclovir for this purpose. As already mentioned, valganciclovir has supplanted oral ganciclovir in settings where oral prophylaxis or therapy is considered.

The administration of ganciclovir has been associated with profound bone marrow suppression, particularly neutropenia, which significantly limits the drug's use in many patients. Bone marrow toxicity is potentiated in the setting of renal dysfunction and when other bone marrow suppressants, such as zidovudine, are used concomitantly.

Resistance has been noted in CMV isolates obtained after therapy with ganciclovir, especially in patients with AIDS. Such resistance may develop through a mutation in either the viral UL97 gene or the viral DNA polymerase. Ganciclovir-resistant isolates are usually sensitive to foscarnet (see below) or cidofovir (see above).

FAMCICLOVIR AND PENCICLOVIR

Famciclovir is the diacetyl 6-deoxyester of the guanosine analogue penciclovir. Famciclovir is well absorbed orally, has a bioavailability of 77%, and is rapidly converted to penciclovir by deacetylation and oxidation in the intestine and liver. Penciclovir's spectrum of activity and mechanism of action are similar to those of acyclovir. Thus, penciclovir is usually not active against acyclovir-resistant viruses. However, some acyclovir-resistant viruses with altered thymidine kinase or DNA polymerase substrate specificity may be sensitive to penciclovir. This drug is phosphorylated initially by a virus-encoded thymidine kinase and subsequently by cellular kinases to penciclovir triphosphate, which inhibits HSV-1, HSV-2, VZV, and EBV as well as hepatitis B virus (HBV). The serum half-life of penciclovir is 2 h, but the intracellular half-life of penciclovir triphosphate is 7–20 h—markedly longer than that of acyclovir triphosphate. The latter is the basis for the less frequent (twice-daily) dosing schedule for famciclovir than for acyclovir. Penciclovir is eliminated primarily in the urine by both glomerular filtration and tubular secretion. The usually recommended dosage interval should be adjusted for renal insufficiency.

Clinical trials involving immunocompetent adults with herpes zoster showed that famciclovir was superior to placebo in eliciting the resolution of skin lesions and virus shedding and in shortening the duration of postherpetic neuralgia; moreover, administered at 500 mg every 8 h, famciclovir was at least as effective as acyclovir administered at a dose of 800 mg PO five times daily. Famciclovir was also effective in the treatment of herpes zoster in immunosuppressed patients. Clinical trials have demonstrated its effectiveness in the suppression of genital HSV infections for up to 1 year and in the treatment of initial and recurrent episodes of genital herpes. Famciclovir is effective as therapy for mucocutaneous HSV infections in HIV-infected patients. Application of a 1% penciclovir cream reduces the duration of signs and symptoms of herpes labialis in immunocompetent patients (by 0.5–1.0 day) and has been approved for that purpose by the FDA. Famciclovir is generally well tolerated, with occasional headache, nausea, and diarrhea reported in frequencies similar to those among placebo recipients. The administration of high doses of famciclovir for 2 years was associated with an increased incidence of mammary adenocarcinomas in female rats, but the clinical significance of this effect is unknown.

FOSCARNET

Foscarnet (phosphonoformic acid) is a pyrophosphate-containing compound that potently inhibits herpesviruses, including CMV. This drug inhibits DNA polymerases at the pyrophosphate binding site at concentrations that have relatively little effect on cellular polymerases. Foscarnet does not require phosphorylation to exert its antiviral activity and is therefore active against HSV and VZV isolates that are resistant to acyclovir because of deficiencies in thymidine kinase as well as against most ganciclovir-resistant strains of CMV. Foscarnet also inhibits the reverse transcriptase of HIV and is active against HIV in vivo.

Foscarnet is poorly soluble and must be administered IV via an infusion pump in a dilute solution over 1–2 h. The plasma half-life of foscarnet is 3–5 h and increases with decreasing renal function, since the drug is eliminated primarily by the kidneys. It has been estimated that 10–28% of a dose may be deposited in bone, where it can persist for months. The most common initial dosage of foscarnet—60 mg/kg every 8 h for 14–21 days—is followed by a maintenance dose of 90–120 mg/kg once a day.

Foscarnet is approved for the treatment of CMV retinitis in patients with AIDS and of acyclovir-resistant mucocutaneous HSV infections. In a comparative clinical trial, the drug appeared to be about as efficacious as ganciclovir against CMV retinitis but was associated with a longer survival period, possibly because of its activity against HIV. Intraocular foscarnet has been used to treat CMV retinitis. Foscarnet has also been employed to treat acyclovir-resistant HSV and VZV infections as well as ganciclovir-resistant CMV infections, although resistance to foscarnet has been reported in CMV isolates obtained during therapy. Foscarnet has also been used to treat HHV-6 infections in immunosuppressed patients.

The major form of toxicity associated with foscarnet is renal impairment. Thus renal function should be monitored closely, particularly during the initial phase of therapy. Since foscarnet binds divalent metal ions, hypocalcemia, hypomagnesemia, hypokalemia, and hypo- or hyperphosphatemia can develop. Saline hydration and slow infusion appear to protect the patient against nephrotoxicity and electrolyte disturbances. Although hematologic abnormalities have been documented (most commonly anemia), foscarnet is not generally myelosuppressive and may be administered concomitantly with myelosuppressive medications such as zidovudine.

TRIFLURIDINE

Trifluridine is a pyrimidine nucleoside active against HSV-1, HSV-2, and CMV. Trifluridine monophosphate irreversibly inhibits thymidylate synthetase, and trifluridine triphosphate inhibits viral and, to a lesser extent, cellular DNA polymerases. Because of systemic toxicity, its use is limited to topical therapy. Trifluridine is approved for treatment of HSV keratitis, for which trials have shown that it is more effective than topical idoxuridine but similar in efficacy to topical vidarabine. The drug has benefited some patients with HSV keratitis who have failed to respond to idoxuridine or vidarabine. Topical application of trifluridine to sites of acyclovir-resistant HSV mucocutaneous infections has also been beneficial in some cases.

VIDARABINE

Vidarabine is a purine nucleoside analogue with activity against HSV-1, HSV-2, VZV, and EBV. Vidarabine inhibits viral DNA synthesis through its 5′-triphosphorylated metabolite, although its precise molecular mechanisms of action are not completely understood. IV-administered vidarabine has been shown to be effective in the treatment of herpes simplex encephalitis, mucocutaneous HSV infections, herpes zoster in immunocompromised patients, and neonatal HSV infections. Its use has been supplanted by that of IV acyclovir, which is more effective and easier to administer. Production of the IV preparation has been discontinued by the manufacturer, but vidarabine is available as an ophthalmic ointment, which is effective in the treatment of HSV keratitis.

ANTIVIRAL DRUGS ACTIVE AGAINST HEPATITIS VIRUSES

LAMIVUDINE

Lamivudine is a pyrimidine nucleoside analogue that is used primarily in combination therapy against HIV infection (Chap. 182). It is also active against HBV through inhibition of the viral DNA polymerase and has been approved for the treatment of chronic HBV infection. At doses of 100 mg/d for 1 year, lamivudine is well tolerated and results in suppression of HBV DNA levels, normalization of serum aminotransferase levels in 50–70% of patients, and reduction of hepatic inflammation and fibrosis in 50–60% of patients. Loss of hepatitis B e antigen (HBeAg) occurs in 30% of patients. Resistance to lamivudine develops in 24% of patients treated for 1 year and is associated with changes in the YMDD motif of HBV DNA polymerase. This is an important limitation of monotherapy with the drug. Lamivudine is being evaluated as a component of combination regimens (with IFNs and other nucleoside or nucleotide analogues listed below) for the treatment of hepatitis B. Lamivudine appears to be useful in the prevention or suppression of HBV infection associated with liver transplantation.

ADEFOVIR

Adefovir dipivoxil is an acyclic nucleotide analogue of adenosine monophosphate that has activity against HBV, HIV, HSV, and CMV. It is phosphorylated by cellular kinases to the active triphosphate moiety, which is a competitive inhibitor of HBV DNA polymerase and results in chain termination after incorporation into nascent viral DNA. Adefovir is administered orally and is eliminated primarily by the kidneys, with a plasma half-life of 7.5 h. In clinical studies, therapy with adefovir at a dose of 10 mg/d for 48 weeks resulted in normalization of alanine aminotransferase (ALT) levels in 48–72% of patients and improved liver histology in 53–64%; it also resulted in a 3.6-log$_{10}$ reduction in the number of HBV DNA copies per milliliter of plasma. Adefovir was effective in treatment-naive patients as well as in those infected with lamivudine-resistant HBV. Resistance to adefovir appears to develop less readily than that to lamivudine, but adefovir resistance rates of 15–18% have been reported after 192 weeks of treatment. This agent is generally well tolerated. Significant nephrotoxicity attributable to adefovir is uncommon at the dose employed in the treatment of HBV infections (10 mg/d) but is a treatment-limiting adverse effect at the higher doses used in therapy for HIV infections (30–120 mg/d). In any case, renal function should be monitored in patients taking adefovir, even at the lower dose. Adefovir is approved only for treatment of chronic HBV infection.

TENOFOVIR

Tenofovir disoproxil fumarate is a nucleotide analogue of adenosine monophosphate with activity against both retroviruses and hepadnaviruses. In patients co-infected with HIV and HBV, tenofovir reduces HBV loads by 3–4 log$_{10}$ copies/mL at 24 weeks and is effective against lamivudine-resistant HBV. The drug is approved only for treatment of HIV infection, but its use should be considered in patients co-infected with HIV and HBV. **For a more detailed discussion of tenofovir, see Chap. 182.**

ENTECAVIR

Entecavir is a cyclopentyl guanosine analogue that inhibits HBV through inhibition of HBV DNA polymerase by entecavir triphosphate and is also active against HIV. In vitro, entecavir is more potent than lamivudine or adefovir against HBV and is also effective against lamivudine-resistant HBV. Administration of entecavir at a dose of 0.5 mg/d PO for 48 weeks results in a reduction of HBV DNA by 5.0–6.9 log$_{10}$ copies/mL, normalization of ALT values in 68–78% of recipients, and loss of HBeAg in 21%. Entecavir is highly bioavailable but should be taken on an empty stomach since food interferes with its absorption. The drug is eliminated primarily in unchanged form by the kidneys, and its dosage should be adjusted for patients with Cr$_{Cl}$ values of <50 mg/min. Overall, entecavir is well tolerated. Resistance to entecavir has not been observed during the treatment of naïve patients; however, resistance was noted in 7–10% of lamivudine-refractory patients at 48 weeks of treatment with entecavir. Entecavir-resistant strains appear to be sensitive to adefovir. As with other anti-HBV treatments, exacerbation of hepatitis may occur when entecavir therapy is stopped. Entecavir is approved for treatment of chronic hepatitis B in adults.

TELBIVUDINE

Telbivudine is the β-L enantiomer of thymidine and is a potent inhibitor of HBV. Its active form is telbivudine triphosphate, which inhibits HBV DNA polymerase but has little or no activity against human DNA polymerase. Administration of telbivudine at a dose of 600 mg/d PO for 52 weeks to patients with chronic hepatitis B resulted in reduction of HBV DNA by >5 log$_{10}$ copies/mL along with either loss of serum HBeAg or normalization of ALT in 75% of recipients. After 2 years of therapy, resistance to telbivudine was noted in isolates from 8.6–21.6% of patients. Telbivudine-resistant HBV is usually resistant to lamivudine as well but is generally susceptible to adefovir.

Telbivudine is eliminated primarily by the kidneys, and the dosage should be reduced in patients with a Cl$_{Cr}$ value of <50 mL/min. Telbivudine is generally well tolerated, but increases in serum creatinine kinases and clinically evident myopathy have been observed. As with other anti-HBV drugs, hepatitis may be exacerbated in patients who have discontinued telbivudine therapy. Telbivudine has been approved for treatment of adults with chronic hepatitis B who have evidence of viral replication and either persistent elevation in serum aminotransferases or histologically active disease.

INTERFERONS

IFNs are cytokines that exhibit a broad spectrum of antiviral activities as well as immunomodulating and antiproliferative properties. IFNs are not available for oral administration but must be given IM, SC, or IV. Early studies with human leukocyte IFN demonstrated an effect in the prophylaxis of experimentally induced rhinovirus infections in humans and in the treatment of VZV infections in immunosuppressed patients. DNA recombinant technology has made available highly purified α, β, and γ IFNs that have been evaluated in a variety of viral infections. Results of such trials have confirmed the effectiveness of intranasally administered IFN in the prophylaxis of rhinovirus infections, although its use has been associated with nasal mucosal irritation. Studies have also demonstrated a beneficial effect of intralesionally or systemically administered IFNs on genital warts. The effect of systemic administration consists primarily of a reduction in the size of the warts, and this mode of therapy may be useful in persons who have numerous warts that cannot easily be treated by individual intralesional injections. However, lesions frequently recur after either intralesional or systemic IFN therapy is discontinued.

IFNs have undergone extensive study in the treatment of chronic HBV infection. The administration of IFN-α2b (5 million units daily or 10 million units three times a week for 16–24 weeks) to patients with stable chronic HBV infection resulted in loss of markers of HBV replication, such as HBeAg and HBV DNA, in 33–37% of cases; 8% of patients also became negative for hepatitis B surface antigen. In >80% of patients who lose HBeAg and HBV DNA markers, serum aminotransferases return to normal levels, and both short- and long-term improvements in liver histopathology have been described. Predictors of a favorable response to therapy include low pretherapy levels of HBV DNA, high pretherapy serum levels of ALT, a short duration of chronic HBV infection, and active inflammation in liver histopathology. Poor responses are seen in immunosuppressed patients, including those with HIV infection. A longer duration of therapy (12–24 months) is recommended for HBeAg-negative chronic hepatitis B. Adverse effects of the above doses of IFN are common and include fever, chills, myalgia, fatigue, neurotoxicity (primarily manifested as somnolence, depression, anxiety, and confusion), and leukopenia. Approximately 25% of patients receiving a daily dose of 5 million units require dose reduction, but <5% require discontinuation of therapy. Pegylated IFNs, which are covalently linked with monomethoxy polyethylene glycol, have a markedly reduced clearance rate. Therefore, they can be administered less frequently, are better tolerated, and may be more effective in some settings than standard IFNs (see discussion of hepatitis C below). Pegylated IFN-α2a is approved for the treatment of patients with chronic hepatitis B who are either positive or negative for HBeAg (Table 171-1).

Several IFN preparations, including IFN-α2a, IFN-α2b, IFN-alfacon-1, and IFN-αm1 (lymphoblastoid), have been studied as therapy for chronic HCV infections. A variety of monotherapy regimens have been employed, of which the most common is IFN-α2b or -α2a at 3 million units three times per week for 12–18 months. The addition of oral ribavirin to IFN-α2b—either as initial therapy or after failure of IFN therapy alone—results in significantly higher rates of sustained virologic and/or serum ALT responses (40–50%) than are obtained with monotherapy. Comparative studies indicate that pegylated IFN-α2b or -α2a therapy is more effective than standard IFN treatment against chronic HCV infection. The combination of SC pegylated IFN and oral ribavirin is more convenient and appears to be the most effective regimen for treatment of chronic hepatitis C. With this combination regimen, sustained virologic responses were seen in 42–46% of patients with genotype 1 infection and in 76–82% of patients with genotype 2 or 3 infection. Ribavirin appears to have a small antiviral effect in HCV infection but may also be working through an immuno-modulatory effect in combination with IFN. Optimal results with ribavirin appear to be associated with weight-based dosing. Prognostic factors for a favorable response include an age of <45 years, a short duration of infection, low levels of HCV RNA, and infection with HCV genotypes other than 1. IFN-alfacon, a synthetic "consensus" α interferon, appears to produce response rates similar to those elicited by IFN-α2a or -α2b alone and is also approved in the United States for the treatment of chronic hepatitis C.

The efficacy of IFN-α treatment for chronic hepatitis D remains unestablished. Anecdotal reports suggested that doses ranging from 5 million units daily to 9 million units three times per week for 12 months elicit biochemical and virologic responses. Results from small controlled trials have been inconsistent, and observed responses have not generally been sustained. Limited experience has been published with the use of pegylated IFN-α2b for treatment of hepatitis D, but some consultants prefer this agent for this indication because of its pharmacologic advantages over standard IFN.

FURTHER READINGS

Beutner KR et al: Valaciclovir compared with acyclovir for improved therapy for herpes zoster in immunocompetent adults. Antimicrob Agents Chemother 39:1546, 1995

Couch RB: Drug therapy: Prevention and treatment of influenza. N Engl J Med 343:1778, 2000

Crumpacker CS: Ganciclovir. N Engl J Med 335:721, 1996

Dolin R et al: A controlled trial of amantadine and rimantadine in the prophylaxis of influenza A infection. N Engl J Med 307:580, 1982

Field JJ, Hoofnagle JH: Mechanism of action of interferon and ribavirin in treatment of hepatitis C. Nature 436:967, 2005

Gish RG et al: Safety and antiviral activity of emtricitabine (FTC) for the treatment of chronic hepatitis B infection: A two-year study. J Hepatol 43:60, 2005

Hall CB et al: Aerosolized ribavirin treatment of infants with respiratory syncytial viral infection: A randomized double-blind study. N Engl J Med 308:1443, 1983

Hayden FG: Antiviral drugs (other than antiretrovirals), in *Principles and Practice of Infectious Diseases*, 6th ed, JE Bennett et al (eds). Philadelphia, Elsevier Churchill Livingstone, 2005, pp 514–551

Lai CL et al: Entecavir versus lamivudine for patients with HBeAg-negative chronic hepatitis B. N Engl J Med 354:186, 2006

Lalezari JP et al: Randomized controlled study of the safety and efficacy of IV cidofovir for the treatment of relapsing cytomegalovirus retinitis in patients with AIDS. J AIDS 17:339, 1998

Lok AS et al: Management of hepatitis B: 2000—summary of a workshop. Gastroenterology 120:1828, 2001

Martin DF et al: A controlled trial of valganciclovir as induction therapy for cytomegalovirus retinitis. N Engl J Med 346:1119, 2002

National Institutes of Health Consensus Development Conference Statement: Management of hepatitis C. September 12, 2002 (available at *www.niaid.nih.gov*)

Treanor JJ et al: Efficacy and safety in treating acute influenza: A randomized controlled trial. U.S. Oral Neuraminidase Study Group. JAMA 283:1016, 2000

SECTION 12   INFECTIONS DUE TO DNA VIRUSES

172   Herpes Simplex Viruses
Lawrence Corey

DEFINITION

Herpes simplex viruses (HSV-1, HSV-2; *Herpesvirus hominis*) produce a variety of infections involving mucocutaneous surfaces, the central nervous system (CNS), and—on occasion—visceral organs. Prompt recognition and treatment reduce the morbidity and mortality associated with HSV infections.

ETIOLOGIC AGENT

The genome of HSV is a linear, double-strand DNA molecule (molecular weight, $\sim100 \times 10^6$ units) that encodes >90 transcription units with 84 identified proteins. The genomic structures of the two HSV subtypes are similar. The overall genomic sequence homology between HSV-1 and HSV-2 is ~50%, while the proteome homology is >80%. The homologous sequences are distributed over the entire genome map, and most of the polypeptides specified by one viral type are antigenically related to polypeptides of the other viral type. Many type-specific regions unique to HSV-1 and HSV-2 proteins do exist, however, and a number of them appear to be important in host immunity. These type-specific regions have been used to develop serologic assays that distinguish between the two viral subtypes. Either restriction endonuclease analysis of viral DNA or DNA sequencing can be used to distinguish between the two subtypes and among strains of each subtype. The variability of nucleotide sequences from clinical strains of HSV-1 and HSV-2 is such that HSV isolates obtained from two individuals can be differentiated by restriction enzyme patterns or genomic sequences. Moreover, epidemiologically related sources, such as sexual partners, mother-infant pairs, or persons involved in a common-source outbreak, can be inferred from such patterns.

The viral genome is packaged in a regular icosahedral protein shell (capsid) composed of 162 capsomeres (see Fig. 170-1). The outer covering of the virus is a lipid-containing membrane (envelope) acquired as the DNA-containing capsid buds through the inner nuclear membrane of the host cell. Between the capsid and lipid bilayer of the envelope is the tegument. Viral replication has both nuclear and cytoplasmic phases. Attachment and fusion of the viral envelope and the cell membrane involve several ubiquitous heparin-like surface receptors. Replication is highly regulated. After fusion and entry, the nucleocapsid enters the cytoplasm and several viral proteins are released from the virion. Some of these viral proteins shut off host protein synthesis (by increasing cellular RNA degradation), while others "turn on" the transcription of early genes of HSV replication. These early gene products, designated α *genes*, are required for synthesis of the subsequent polypeptide group, the β polypeptides, many of which are regulatory proteins and enzymes required for DNA replication. Most current antiviral drugs interfere with β proteins, such as the viral DNA polymerase enzyme. The third (γ) class of HSV genes requires viral DNA replication for expression and constitutes most of the structural proteins specified by the virus.

After replication of the viral genome and synthesis of structural proteins, nucleocapsids are assembled in the nucleus of the cell. Envelopment occurs as the nucleocapsids bud through the inner nuclear membrane into the perinuclear space. In some cells, viral replication in the nucleus forms two types of inclusion bodies: type A basophilic Feulgen-positive bodies that contain viral DNA and eosinophilic inclusion bodies that are devoid of viral nucleic acid or protein and represent a "scar" of viral infection. Enveloped virions are then transported via the endoplasmic reticulum and the Golgi apparatus to the cell surface.

HSV infection of some neuronal cells does not result in cell death. Instead, viral genomes are maintained by the cell in a repressed state compatible with survival and normal activities of the cell, a condition called *latency*. Latency is associated with transcription of only a limited number of virus-encoded proteins. Subsequently, the viral genome may become activated; its activation results in the normal pattern of regulated viral gene expression, viral replication, and viral release. The release of HSV from the neuron and its subsequent entry into epithelial cells result in viral replication in these cells, destruction of the cells, and the subsequent reappearance of virus on mucosal surfaces. This process is termed *reactivation*. Whereas infectious virus is rarely recovered from sensory or autonomic nervous system ganglia dissected from cadavers, maintenance and growth of the neural cells (as "explants") in tissue culture result in production of infectious virions and in subsequent permissive infection of susceptible cells (*cocultivation*). The mechanisms by which latency is established, maintained, or broken are incompletely understood. Two RNA "latency-associated" transcripts that overlap the immediate early (α) gene products, called *ICP-O*, are found in abundance in the nuclei of latently infected neurons. Deletion mutants of this region that can become latent have been made. However, the efficiency of their later reactivation is reduced; thus, these latency-associated transcripts may play a role in maintaining rather than in establishing latency. Recent studies suggest that HSV-specific micro-RNAs in these and other regions of the viral genome may play an important role in virus maintenance in and release from neurons. CD8+ T cells have been found in ganglia of experimental animals and humans and appear to influence the process of reactivation, possibly by inducing antiviral factors such as interferon (IFN) γ. At present, strategies to interrupt latency or to maintain molecular latency in neurons are not available. In experimental animals, ultraviolet light, systemic and local immunosuppression, and trauma to the skin or ganglia are associated with reactivation.

PATHOGENESIS

Exposure to HSV at mucosal surfaces or abraded skin sites permits entry of the virus and initiation of its replication in cells of the epidermis and dermis. HSV infections are usually acquired subclinically. Whether clinical or subclinical, HSV acquisition is associated with sufficient viral replication to permit infection of either sensory or autonomic nerve endings. On entry into the neuronal cell, the virus—or, more likely, the nucleocapsid—is transported intra-axonally to the nerve cell bodies in ganglia. In humans, the transit interval from inoculation of virus in peripheral tissue to spread to the ganglia is unknown. During the initial phase of infection, viral replication occurs in ganglia and contiguous neural tissue. Virus then spreads to other mucocutaneous surfaces through centrifugal migration of infectious virions via peripheral sensory nerves. This mode of spread helps explain the large surface area involved, the high frequency of new lesions distant from the initial crop of vesicles that is characteristic in patients with primary genital or oral-labial HSV infection, and the ability to recover virus from neural tissue distant from neurons innervating the inoculation site. Contiguous spread of locally inoculated virus also may take place and allow further mucosal extension of disease. Recent studies have demonstrated HSV viremia—another mechanism for extension of infection throughout the body—in ~30–40% of persons with primary HSV-2 infection. Latent infection with both viral subtypes in both sensory and autonomic ganglia has been demonstrated.

Analysis of the DNA from sequential isolates of HSV or from isolates from multiple infected ganglia in any one individual has revealed similar, if not identical, restriction endonuclease or DNA sequence patterns in most persons. Occasionally (most frequently in immunocompromised persons), multiple strains of the same viral subtype are detected in one individual. As exposure to mucosal shedding is relatively common during a person's lifetime, these data suggest that exogenous infection with different strains of the same subtype is possible.

IMMUNITY

Host responses influence the acquisition of HSV disease, the severity of infection, resistance to the development of latency, the maintenance of latency, and the frequency of recurrences. Both antibody-mediated and cell-mediated reactions are clinically important. Immunocompromised patients with defects in cell-mediated immunity experience more severe and more extensive HSV infections than those with deficits in humoral immunity, such as agammaglobulinemia. Experimental ablation of lymphocytes indicates that T cells play a major role in preventing lethal disseminated disease, although antibodies help reduce virus titers in neural tissue. Some of the clinical manifestations of HSV appear to be related to the host immune response (e.g., stromal opacities associated with recurrent herpetic keratitis). The surface viral glycoproteins have been shown to be targets of antibodies that mediate neutralization and immune-mediated cytolysis (antibody-dependent cell-mediated cytotoxicity). Monoclonal antibodies specific for each of the known viral glycoproteins have, in experimental infections, conferred protection against subsequent neurologic disease or ganglionic latency. In humans, however, subunit glycoprotein vaccines have been only partially successful in reducing acquisition of infection. Multiple cell populations, including natural killer cells, macrophages, and a variety of T lymphocytes, play a role in host defenses against HSV infections, as do lymphokines generated by T lymphocytes. In animals, passive transfer of primed lymphocytes confers protection from subsequent challenge. Maximal protection usually requires the activation of multiple T cell subpopulations, including cytotoxic T cells and T cells responsible for delayed hypersensitivity. The latter cells may confer protection by the antigen-stimulated release of lymphokines (e.g., IFNs), which in turn have a direct antiviral effect and both activate and enhance a variety of specific and nonspecific effector cells. Increasing evidence suggests that HSV-specific CD8+ T cell responses are critical for clearance of virus from lesions. In addition, immunosuppressed patients with frequent and prolonged HSV lesions have fewer functional CD8+ T cells directed at HSV. The HSV virion contains a variety of genes that are directed at the inhibition of host responses. These include gene no. 12 (*US-12*), which can bind to the cellular transporter-activating protein TAP-1 and reduce the ability of this protein to bind HSV peptides to human leukocyte antigen (HLA) class I, thereby reducing recognition of viral proteins by cytotoxic T cells of the host. This effect can be overcome by the addition of IFN-γ, but this reversal requires 24–48 h; thus, the virus has time to replicate and invade other host cells. To date, the immunodominant T cell responses appear to be type-specific. Entry of infectious HSV-1 and HSV-2 inhibits several signaling pathways of both CD4+ and CD8+ T cells, leading to their functional impairment in killing and influencing the spectrum of their cytokine secretion.

EPIDEMIOLOGY

Seroepidemiologic studies have documented HSV infections worldwide. Serologic assays with whole-virus antigen preparations, such as complement fixation, neutralization, indirect immunofluorescence, passive hemagglutination, radioimmunoassay, and enzyme-linked immunosorbent assay, are useful for differentiating uninfected (seronegative) persons from those with past HSV-1 or HSV-2 infection, but they do not reliably distinguish between the two viral subtypes. Serologic assays that identify antibodies to type-specific surface proteins (epitopes) of the two viral subtypes have been developed and can distinguish reliably between the human antibody responses to HSV-1 and HSV-2. The most commonly used assays are those that measure antibodies to glycoprotein G of HSV-1 (gG1) and HSV-2 (gG2). A Western blot assay that can detect several HSV type-specific proteins can also be used.

Infection with HSV-1 is acquired more frequently and earlier than infection with HSV-2. More than 90% of adults have antibodies to

HSV-1 by the fifth decade of life. In populations of low socioeconomic status, most persons acquire HSV-1 infection before the third decade of life.

Antibodies to HSV-2 are not detected routinely until puberty. Antibody prevalence rates correlate with past sexual activity and vary greatly among different population groups. There is some evidence that the prevalence of HSV-2 has decreased slightly over the past 5 years in the United States. Serosurveys indicate that 15–20% of the U.S. population has antibodies to HSV-2. In most routine obstetric and family planning clinics, 25% of women have HSV-2 antibodies, although only 10% of those who are seropositive for HSV-2 report a history of genital lesions. As many as 50% of heterosexual adults attending sexually transmitted disease clinics have antibodies to HSV-2.

A wide variety of serologic surveys have indicated a similar or even higher seroprevalence of HSV-2 in most parts of Central America, South America, and Africa. There is an epidemiologic synergy between HSV-2 and HIV-1. HSV-2 infection is associated with a two- to fourfold increase in HIV-1 acquisition. In addition, HSV-2 is reactivated and transmitted more frequently in persons co-infected with HIV-1 and HSV-2 than in persons not infected with HIV-1. Thus, most areas of the world with a high HIV-1 prevalence also have a high HSV-2 prevalence. In Africa, HSV-2 seroprevalence has ranged from 40% to 70% in obstetric and other sexually experienced populations. Antibody prevalence rates average ~5–10% higher among women than among men.

Several studies suggest that many cases of "asymptomatic" genital HSV-2 infection are, in fact, simply unrecognized: when "asymptomatic" seropositive persons are shown pictures of genital lesions, >60% subsequently identify episodes of symptomatic reactivation. Most important, these asymptomatic seropositive persons with reactivation shed virus on mucosal surfaces almost as frequently as those with symptomatic disease. The large reservoir of unidentified carriers of HSV-2 and the frequent asymptomatic reactivation of the virus from the genital tract have fostered the continued spread of genital herpes throughout the world. HSV-2 infection is an independent risk factor for the acquisition and transmission of infection with HIV-1. Among co-infected persons, HIV-1 virions can be shed from herpetic lesions of the genital region. This shedding may facilitate the spread of HIV through sexual contact.

HSV infections occur throughout the year. Transmission can result from contact with persons who have active ulcerative lesions or with persons who have no clinical manifestations of infection but who are shedding HSV from mucocutaneous surfaces. Studies using the polymerase chain reaction (PCR) have shown that HSV reactivation on genital skin and mucosal surfaces is much more common than previously recognized. Among immunocompetent adults, HSV-2 can be cultured from the genital tract on 2–10% of days tested, and HSV DNA can be detected on 20–30% of days by PCR. Corresponding figures for HSV-1 in oral secretions are similar. Rates of shedding are highest during the initial years after acquisition, with viral shedding occurring on as many as 30–50% of days during this period. Immunosuppressed patients shed HSV from mucosal sites at an even higher frequency (20–80% of days). Reactivation rates vary widely among individuals. Among HIV-positive patients, a low CD4+ T cell count and a heavy viral load are associated with increased rates of HSV reactivation. (Daily antiviral chemotherapy for HSV-2 can markedly reduce shedding rates, as measured by PCR.) These high rates of mucocutaneous reactivation suggest that exposure to HSV from sexual or other close contact (kissing, sharing of glasses or silverware) is common and help explain the continuing spread and high seroprevalence of HSV infections worldwide.

CLINICAL SPECTRUM

HSV has been isolated from nearly all visceral and mucocutaneous sites. The clinical manifestations and course of HSV infection depend on the anatomic site involved, the age and immune status of the host, and the antigenic type of the virus. Primary HSV infections (i.e., first infections with either HSV-1 or HSV-2 in which the host lacks HSV

antibodies in acute-phase serum) are frequently accompanied by systemic signs and symptoms. Compared with recurrent episodes, primary infections, which involve both mucosal and extramucosal sites, are characterized by a longer duration of symptoms and virus isolation from lesions. The incubation period ranges from 1 to 26 days (median, 6–8 days). Both viral subtypes can cause genital and oral-facial infections, and the infections caused by the two subtypes are clinically indistinguishable. However, the frequency of reactivation of infection is influenced by anatomic site and virus type. Genital HSV-2 infection is twice as likely to reactivate and recurs 8–10 times more frequently than genital HSV-1 infection. Conversely, oral-labial HSV-1 infection recurs more frequently than oral-labial HSV-2 infection. Asymptomatic shedding rates follow the same pattern.

Oral-Facial Infections Gingivostomatitis and pharyngitis are the most common clinical manifestations of first-episode HSV-1 infection, while recurrent herpes labialis is the most common clinical manifestation of reactivation HSV-1 infection. HSV pharyngitis and gingivostomatitis usually result from primary infection and are most commonly seen among children and young adults. Clinical symptoms and signs, which include fever, malaise, myalgias, inability to eat, irritability, and cervical adenopathy, may last 3–14 days. Lesions may involve the hard and soft palate, gingiva, tongue, lip, and facial area. HSV-1 or HSV-2 infection of the pharynx usually results in exudative or ulcerative lesions of the posterior pharynx and/or tonsillar pillars. Lesions of the tongue, buccal mucosa, or gingiva may occur later in the course in one-third of cases. Fever lasting 2–7 days and cervical adenopathy are common. It can be difficult to differentiate HSV pharyngitis clinically from bacterial pharyngitis, *Mycoplasma pneumoniae* infections, and pharyngeal ulcerations of noninfectious etiologies (e.g., Stevens-Johnson syndrome). No substantial evidence suggests that reactivation of oral-labial HSV infection is associated with symptomatic recurrent pharyngitis.

Reactivation of HSV from the trigeminal ganglia may be associated with asymptomatic virus excretion in the saliva, development of intraoral mucosal ulcerations, or herpetic ulcerations on the vermilion border of the lip or external facial skin. About 50–70% of seropositive patients undergoing trigeminal nerve-root decompression and 10–15% of those undergoing dental extraction develop oral-labial HSV infection a median of 3 days after these procedures. Clinical differentiation of intraoral mucosal ulcerations due to HSV from aphthous, traumatic, or drug-induced ulcerations is difficult.

In immunosuppressed patients, HSV infection may extend into mucosal and deep cutaneous layers. Friability, necrosis, bleeding, severe pain, and inability to eat or drink may result. The lesions of HSV mucositis are clinically similar to mucosal lesions caused by cytotoxic drug therapy, trauma, or fungal or bacterial infections. Persistent ulcerative HSV infections are among the most common infections in patients with AIDS. HSV and *Candida* infections often occur concurrently. Systemic antiviral therapy speeds the rate of healing and relieves the pain of mucosal HSV infections in immunosuppressed patients. The frequency of HSV reactivation during the early phases of transplantation or induction chemotherapy is high (50–90%), and prophylactic systemic antiviral agents such as IV acyclovir, penciclovir, or the oral congeners of these drugs are used to reduce reactivation rates. Patients with atopic eczema may also develop severe oral-facial HSV infections (*eczema herpeticum*), which may rapidly involve extensive areas of skin and occasionally disseminate to visceral organs. Extensive eczema herpeticum has resolved promptly with the administration of IV acyclovir. Erythema multiforme may also be associated with HSV infections (see Fig. 52-9); some evidence suggests that HSV infection is the precipitating event in ~75% of cases of cutaneous erythema multiforme. HSV antigen has been demonstrated both in circulatory immune complexes and in skin lesion biopsy samples from these cases. Patients with severe HSV-associated erythema multiforme are candidates for chronic suppressive oral antiviral therapy.

HSV-1 and varicella-zoster virus (VZV) have been implicated in the etiology of Bell's palsy (flaccid paralysis of the mandibular portion of

FIGURE 172-1 Genital herpes: primary vulvar infection. Multiple, extremely painful, punched-out, confluent, shallow ulcers on the edematous vulva and perineum. Micturition is often very painful. Associated inguinal lymphadenopathy is common. *(Reprinted with permission from K Wolff, RA Johnson, D Summond: Fitzpatrick's Color Atlas and Synopsis of Clinical Dermatology, 5th ed.)*

the facial nerve). Although uniform recommendations for treatment of this entity are not available, recent evidence suggests that antiviral chemotherapy in conjunction with a short course of glucocorticoids may result in improved outcomes.

Genital Infections First-episode primary genital herpes is characterized by fever, headache, malaise, and myalgias. Pain, itching, dysuria, vaginal and urethral discharge, and tender inguinal lymphadenopathy are the predominant local symptoms. Widely spaced bilateral lesions of the external genitalia are characteristic (Fig. 172-1). Lesions may be present in varying stages, including vesicles, pustules, or painful erythematous ulcers. The cervix and urethra are involved in >80% of women with first-episode infections. First episodes of genital herpes in patients who have had prior HSV-1 infection are associated with systemic symptoms in a few patients and with faster healing than primary genital herpes. The clinical courses of acute first-episode genital herpes are similar for HSV-1 and HSV-2 infection. However, the recurrence rates of genital disease differ with the viral subtype: the 12-month recurrence rates among patients with first-episode HSV-2 and HSV-1 infections are ~90% and ~55%, respectively (median number of recurrences, 4 and <1, respectively). Recurrence rates for genital HSV-2 infections vary greatly among individuals and over time within the same individual. HSV has been isolated from the urethra and urine of men and women without external genital lesions. A clear mucoid discharge and dysuria are characteristics of symptomatic HSV urethritis. HSV has been isolated from the urethra of 5% of women with the dysuria-frequency syndrome. Occasionally, HSV genital tract disease is manifested by endometritis and salpingitis in women and by prostatitis in men. About 15% of cases of HSV-2 acquisition are associated with nonlesional clinical syndromes, such as aseptic meningitis, cervicitis, or urethritis. A more complete discussion of the differential diagnosis of genital herpes is presented in Chap. 124.

Both HSV-1 and HSV-2 can cause symptomatic or asymptomatic rectal and perianal infections. HSV proctitis is usually associated with rectal intercourse. However, subclinical perianal shedding of HSV is detected in women and men who report no rectal intercourse. This phenomenon is due to the establishment of latency in the sacral dermatome from prior genital tract infection, with subsequent reactivation in epithelial cells in the perianal region. Such reactivations are often subclinical. Symptoms of HSV proctitis include anorectal pain, anorectal discharge, tenesmus, and constipation. Sigmoidoscopy reveals ulcerative lesions of the distal 10 cm of the rectal mucosa. Rectal biopsies show mucosal ulceration, necrosis, polymorphonuclear and lymphocytic infiltration of the lamina propria, and (in occasional cases) multinucleated intranuclear inclusion–bearing cells. Perianal herpetic lesions are also found in immunosuppressed patients receiving cytotoxic therapy. Extensive perianal herpetic lesions and/or HSV proctitis is common among patients with HIV infection.

Herpetic Whitlow Herpetic whitlow—HSV infection of the finger—may occur as a complication of primary oral or genital herpes by inoculation of virus through a break in the epidermal surface or by direct introduction of virus into the hand through occupational or some other type of exposure. Clinical signs and symptoms include abrupt-onset edema, erythema, and localized tenderness of the infected finger. Vesicular or pustular lesions of the fingertip that are indistinguishable from lesions of pyogenic bacterial infection are seen. Fever, lymphadenitis, and epitrochlear and axillary lymphadenopathy are common. The infection may recur. Prompt diagnosis (to avoid unnecessary and potentially exacerbating surgical therapy and/or transmission) is essential. Antiviral chemotherapy is usually recommended (see below).

Herpes Gladiatorum HSV may infect almost any area of skin. Mucocutaneous HSV infections of the thorax, ears, face, and hands have been described among wrestlers. Transmission of these infections is facilitated by trauma to the skin sustained during wrestling. Several recent outbreaks have illustrated the importance of prompt diagnosis and therapy to contain the spread of this infection.

Eye Infections HSV infection of the eye is the most common cause of corneal blindness in the United States. HSV keratitis presents as an acute onset of pain, blurred vision, chemosis, conjunctivitis, and characteristic dendritic lesions of the cornea. Use of topical glucocorticoids may exacerbate symptoms and lead to involvement of deep structures of the eye. Debridement, topical antiviral treatment, and/or IFN therapy hastens healing. However, recurrences are common, and the deeper structures of the eye may sustain immunopathologic injury. Stromal keratitis due to HSV appears to be related to T cell–dependent destruction of deep corneal tissue. An HSV-1 epitope that is autoreactive with T cell–targeting corneal antigens has been postulated to be a factor in this infection. Chorioretinitis, usually a manifestation of disseminated HSV infection, may occur in neonates or in patients with HIV infection. HSV and VZV can cause acute necrotizing retinitis as an uncommon but severe manifestation.

Central and Peripheral Nervous System Infections HSV accounts for 10–20% of all cases of sporadic viral encephalitis in the United States. The estimated incidence is ~2.3 cases per 1 million persons per year. Cases are distributed throughout the year, and the age distribution appears to be biphasic, with peaks at 5–30 and >50 years of age. HSV-1 causes >95% of cases.

The pathogenesis of HSV encephalitis varies. In children and young adults, primary HSV infection may result in encephalitis; presumably, exogenously acquired virus enters the CNS by neurotropic spread from the periphery via the olfactory bulb. However, most adults with HSV encephalitis have clinical or serologic evidence of mucocutaneous HSV-1 infection before the onset of CNS symptoms. In ~25% of the cases examined, the HSV-1 strains from the oropharynx and brain tissue of the same patient differ; thus some cases may result from reinfection with another strain of HSV-1 that reaches the CNS. Two theories have been proposed to explain the development of actively replicating HSV in localized areas of the CNS in persons whose ganglionic and CNS isolates are similar. Reactivation of latent HSV-1 infection in trigeminal or autonomic nerve roots may be associated with extension of virus into the CNS via nerves innervating the middle cranial fossa. HSV DNA has been demonstrated by DNA hybridization in brain tissue obtained at autopsy—even from healthy adults. Thus, reactivation of long-standing latent CNS infection may be another mechanism for the development of HSV encephalitis.

Recent studies have identified genetic polymorphisms in two separate genes among children with HSV encephalitis. Peripheral-blood mononuclear cells from these children appear to secrete reduced levels of IFN in response to HSV; if confirmed, this observation suggests that sporadic HSV encephalitis may be related to a variety of host genetic determinants.

The clinical hallmark of HSV encephalitis has been the acute onset of fever and focal neurologic symptoms and signs, especially in the temporal lobe (Fig. 172-2). Clinical differentiation of HSV encephalitis from other viral encephalitides, focal infections, or noninfectious processes is difficult. Elevated cerebrospinal fluid (CSF) protein levels, leukocytosis (predominantly lymphocytes), and red blood cell counts due to hemorrhagic necrosis are common. While brain biopsy has been the gold standard for defining HSV encephalitis, the high sensitivity and specificity of HSV DNA detection by PCR in CSF has largely replaced biopsy for defining HSV CNS infection. Although titers of antibody to HSV in CSF and serum increase in most cases of HSV encephalitis, they rarely do so earlier than 10 days into the illness and therefore, while useful retrospectively, are generally not helpful in establishing an early clinical diagnosis. Demonstration of HSV antigen, HSV DNA, or HSV replication in brain tissue obtained by biopsy is highly sensitive and has a low complication rate; examination of such tissue also provides the best opportunity to identify alternative, potentially treatable causes of encephalitis. Antiviral chemotherapy with acyclovir reduces the rate of death from HSV encephalitis. Even with therapy, however, neurologic sequelae are common, especially in persons >50 years of age. Most authorities recommend the administration of IV acyclovir to patients with presumed HSV encephalitis until the diagnosis is confirmed or an alternative diagnosis is made. Among proven cases of HSV encephalitis, IV therapy is usually recommended until HSV DNA levels in CSF are substantially reduced or nearly undetectable.

HSV DNA has been detected in CSF from 3–15% of persons presenting to the hospital with aseptic meningitis. HSV meningitis, which is usually seen in association with primary genital HSV infection, is an acute, self-limited disease manifested by headache, fever, and mild photophobia and lasting 2–7 days. Lymphocytic pleocytosis in the CSF is characteristic. Neurologic sequelae of HSV meningitis are rare. HSV is the most commonly identified cause of recurrent lymphocytic meningitis (Mollaret's meningitis). Demonstration of HSV antibodies in CSF or persistence of HSV DNA in CSF can establish the diagnosis. For persons with frequent recurrences of HSV meningitis, antiviral therapy has reduced the occurrence of such episodes.

Autonomic nervous system dysfunction, especially of the sacral region, has been reported in association with both HSV and VZV infections. Numbness, tingling of the buttocks or perineal areas, urinary retention, constipation, CSF pleocytosis, and (in males) impotence may occur. Symptoms appear to resolve slowly over days or weeks. Occasionally, hypoesthesia and/or weakness of the lower extremities persists for many months. Rarely, transverse myelitis, manifested by a rapidly progressive symmetric paralysis of the lower extremities or Guillain-Barré syndrome, follows HSV infection. Similarly, peripheral nervous system involvement (Bell's palsy) or cranial polyneuritis may be related to reactivation of HSV-1 infection. Transitory hypoesthesia of the area of skin innervated by the trigeminal nerve and vestibular system dysfunction as

FIGURE 172-2 **CT and diffusion-weighted MRI scans** of the brain of a patient with left-temporal-lobe HSV encephalitis.

measured by electronystagmography are the predominant signs of disease. Whether antiviral chemotherapy can abort these signs or reduce their frequency and severity is not yet known.

Visceral Infections HSV infection of visceral organs usually results from viremia, and multiple-organ involvement is common. Occasionally, however, the clinical manifestations of HSV infection involve only the esophagus, lung, or liver. HSV esophagitis may result from direct extension of oral-pharyngeal HSV infection into the esophagus or may occur de novo by reactivation and spread of HSV to the esophageal mucosa via the vagus nerve. The predominant symptoms of HSV esophagitis are odynophagia, dysphagia, substernal pain, and weight loss. Multiple oval ulcerations appear on an erythematous base with or without a patchy white pseudomembrane. The distal esophagus is most commonly involved. With extensive disease, diffuse friability may spread to the entire esophagus. Neither endoscopic nor barium examination can reliably differentiate HSV esophagitis from *Candida* esophagitis or from esophageal ulcerations due to thermal injury, radiation, or corrosives. Endoscopically obtained secretions for cytologic examination and culture or DNA detection by PCR provide the most useful material for diagnosis. Systemic antiviral chemotherapy usually reduces symptoms and heals esophageal ulcerations.

HSV pneumonitis is uncommon except in severely immunosuppressed patients and may result from extension of herpetic tracheobronchitis into lung parenchyma. Focal necrotizing pneumonitis usually ensues. Hematogenous dissemination of virus from sites of oral or genital mucocutaneous disease may also occur, producing bilateral interstitial pneumonitis. Bacterial, fungal, and parasitic pathogens are commonly present in HSV pneumonitis. The mortality rate from untreated HSV pneumonia in immunosuppressed patients is high (>80%). HSV has also been isolated from the lower respiratory tract of persons with adult respiratory distress syndrome and prolonged intubation. The role of lower respiratory tract HSV infection in overall rates of morbidity and mortality associated with these conditions is unclear.

HSV is an uncommon cause of hepatitis in immunocompetent patients. HSV infection of the liver is associated with fever, abrupt elevations of bilirubin and serum aminotransferase levels, and leukopenia (<4000 white blood cells/μL). Disseminated intravascular coagulation may also develop.

Other reported complications of HSV infection include monarticular arthritis, adrenal necrosis, idiopathic thrombocytopenia, and glomerulonephritis. Disseminated HSV infection in immunocompetent patients is rare. In immunocompromised, burned, or malnourished patients, HSV occasionally disseminates to other visceral organs, such as the adrenal glands, pancreas, small and large intestines, and bone marrow. Rarely, primary HSV infection in pregnancy disseminates and may be associated with the death of both mother and fetus. This uncommon event is usually related to the acquisition of primary infection in the third trimester. Disseminated HSV infection is best detected by the presence of HSV DNA in plasma or blood.

Neonatal HSV Infections Of all HSV-infected populations, neonates (infants younger than 6 weeks) have the highest frequency of visceral and/or CNS infection. Without therapy, the overall rate of death from neonatal herpes is 65%; <10% of neonates with CNS infection develop normally. Although skin lesions are the most commonly recognized features of disease, many infants do not develop lesions at all or do so only well into the course of disease. Neonatal infection is usually acquired perinatally from contact with infected genital secretions at delivery. Congenitally infected infants have been reported. In most series, 30% of neonatal HSV infections are due to HSV-1 and 70% to HSV-2. The risk of developing neonatal HSV infection is 10 times higher for an infant born to a mother who has recently acquired HSV than for other infants. Neonatal HSV-1 infections may also be acquired through postnatal contact with immediate family members who have symptomatic or asymptomatic oral-labial HSV-1 infection or through nosocomial transmission within the hospital. All neonates with presumed neonatal herpes should be treated with IV acyclovir. Antiviral chemotherapy with high-dose IV acyclovir (60 mg/kg per day) has reduced the mortality rate from neonatal herpes to ~15%. However, morbidity, especially among infants with HSV-2 infection involving the CNS, is still very high.

DIAGNOSIS

Both clinical and laboratory criteria are useful for diagnosing HSV infections. A clinical diagnosis can be made accurately when characteristic multiple vesicular lesions on an erythematous base are present. However, herpetic ulcerations may resemble skin ulcerations of other etiologies. Mucosal HSV infections may also present as urethritis or pharyngitis without cutaneous lesions. Thus, laboratory studies to confirm the diagnosis and to guide therapy are recommended. While staining of scrapings from the base of the lesions with Wright's, Giemsa's (Tzanck preparation), or Papanicolaou's stain to detect giant cells or intranuclear inclusions of *Herpesvirus* infection is a well-described procedure, few clinicians are skilled in these techniques, the sensitivity of staining is low (<30% for mucosal swabs), and these cytologic methods do not differentiate between HSV and VZV infections.

HSV infection is best confirmed in the laboratory by detection of virus, viral antigen, or viral DNA in scrapings from lesions. HSV DNA detection by PCR, when available, is the most sensitive laboratory technique. HSV causes a discernible cytopathic effect in a variety of cell culture systems, and this effect can be identified within 48–96 h after inoculation. Spin-amplified culture with subsequent staining for HSV antigen has shortened the time needed to identify HSV to <24 h. The sensitivity of all detection methods depends on the stage of the lesions (with higher sensitivity in vesicular than in ulcerative lesions), on whether the patient has a first or a recurrent episode of the disease (with higher sensitivity in first than in recurrent episodes), and on whether the sample is from an immunosuppressed or an immunocompetent patient (with more antigen or DNA in immunosuppressed patients). Laboratory confirmation permits subtyping of the virus; information on subtype may be useful epidemiologically and may help to predict the frequency of reactivation after first-episode oral-labial or genital HSV infection.

Acute- and convalescent-phase serum can be useful in demonstrating seroconversion during primary HSV-1 or HSV-2 infection. However, few available tests report titers, and increases in index values do not reflect first episodes in all patients. Serologic assays based on type-specific proteins should be used to identify asymptomatic carriers of HSV-1 or HSV-2 infection. No reliable IgM method for defining acute HSV infection is available.

Several studies have shown that persons with previously unrecognized HSV-2 infection can be taught to identify symptomatic reactivations. Individuals seropositive for HSV-2 should be told about the high frequency of subclinical reactivation in mucosal surfaces that are not visible to the eye (e.g., cervix, urethra, perianal skin) or in microscopic ulcerations that may not be clinically symptomatic. Transmission of infection during such episodes is well established. HSV-2-seropositive persons should be educated about the high likelihood of subclinical shedding and the role condoms (male or female) may play in reducing transmission. Antiviral therapy with valacyclovir (500 mg once daily) has been shown to reduce the transmission of HSV-2 between sexual partners.

℞ HERPES SIMPLEX VIRUS INFECTIONS

Many aspects of mucocutaneous and visceral HSV infections are amenable to antiviral chemotherapy. For mucocutaneous infections, acyclovir and its congeners famciclovir and valacyclovir have been the mainstays of therapy. Several antiviral agents are available for topical use in HSV eye infections: idoxuridine, trifluorothymidine, topical vidarabine, and cidofovir. For HSV encephalitis and neonatal herpes, IV acyclovir is the treatment of choice.

All licensed antiviral agents for use against HSV inhibit the viral DNA polymerase. One class of drugs, typified by the drug acyclovir, is made up of substrates for the HSV enzyme thymidine kinase (TK). Acyclovir, ganciclovir, famciclovir, and valacyclovir are all selectively phosphorylated to the monophosphate form in virus-infected cells. Cellular enzymes convert the monophosphate form of the drug to the triphosphate, which is then incorporated into the viral DNA chain.

Acyclovir is the agent most frequently used for the treatment of HSV infections and is available in IV, oral, and topical formulations. Valacyclovir, the valyl ester of acyclovir, offers greater bioavailability than acyclovir and thus can be administered less frequently. Famciclovir, the oral formulation of penciclovir, is clinically effective in the treatment of a variety of HSV-1 and HSV-2 infections. Ganciclovir is active against both HSV-1 and HSV-2; however, it is more toxic than acyclovir, valacyclovir, and famciclovir and generally is not recommended for the treatment of HSV infections. Anecdotal case reports suggest that ganciclovir may also be less effective than acyclovir for treatment of HSV infections.

All three recommended compounds—acyclovir, valacyclovir, and famciclovir—have proved effective in shortening the duration of symptoms and lesions of mucocutaneous HSV infections in both immunocompromised and immunocompetent patients (**Table 172-1**). IV and oral formulations prevent reactivation of HSV in seropositive immunocompromised patients during induction chemotherapy or in the period immediately after bone marrow or solid organ transplantation. Chronic daily suppressive therapy reduces the frequency of reactivation disease among patients with frequent genital or oral-labial herpes. Only valacyclovir has been subjected to clinical trials that demonstrated reduced transmission of HSV-2 infection between sexual partners.

IV acyclovir (30 mg/kg per day, given as a 10-mg/kg infusion over 1 h at 8-h intervals) is effective in reducing rates of death and morbidity from HSV encephalitis. Early initiation of therapy is a critical factor in outcome. The major side effect associated with IV acyclovir is transient renal insufficiency, usually due to crystallization of the compound in the renal parenchyma. This adverse reaction can be avoided if the medication is given slowly over 1 h and the patient is well hydrated. Because CSF levels of acyclovir average only 30–50% of plasma levels, the dosage of acyclovir used for treatment of CNS infection (30 mg/kg per day) is double that used for treatment of mucocutaneous or visceral disease (15 mg/kg per day). Even higher doses of IV acyclovir are used for neonatal HSV infection (60 mg/kg per day in three divided doses).

Among immunocompetent patients, recent studies have shown the effectiveness of short-course, high-dose oral therapy to reduce the signs and symptoms of oral and genital HSV infection. These regimens include valacyclovir (for 1–3 days) for oral-labial HSV and acyclovir (2 days), valacyclovir (3 days), or famciclovir (1 or 2 days) for recurrent-episode genital herpes (Table 172-1). These short-course regimens are less expensive and more convenient but should be reserved for immunocompetent hosts.

SUPPRESSION OF MUCOCUTANEOUS HERPES Recognition of the high frequency of subclinical reactivation provides a well-accepted rationale for the use of daily antiviral therapy to suppress reactivations of HSV, especially in persons with frequent clinical reactivations (e.g., those with recently acquired genital HSV infection). Immunosuppressed persons, including those with HIV infection, may also benefit from daily antiviral therapy. Recent studies have shown the efficacy of daily acyclovir and valacyclovir in reducing the frequency of HSV reactivations among HIV-positive persons. Regimens used include acyclovir (400 mg three times daily), famciclovir (500 mg twice daily), and valacyclovir (1 g twice daily); valacyclovir at a dose of 4 g daily was associated with thrombotic thrombocytopenic purpura in one study of HIV-infected persons. In addition, daily treatment of HSV-2 reduces the titer of HIV RNA in plasma (0.5-log reduction) and in genital mucosa (0.33-log reduction).

REDUCED HSV TRANSMISSION TO SEXUAL PARTNERS
Once-daily valacyclovir (500 mg) has been shown to reduce transmission of HSV-2 between sexual partners. Transmission rates are higher from males to females and among persons with frequent HSV-2 reactivation. Serologic screening can be used to identify at-risk couples. Daily valacyclovir appears more effective at reducing subclinical shedding than daily famciclovir.

ACYCLOVIR RESISTANCE
Acyclovir-resistant strains of HSV have been identified. Most of these strains have an altered substrate specificity for phosphorylating acyclovir. Thus, cross-resistance to famciclovir and valacyclovir is usually found. Occasionally, an isolate with altered TK specificity arises and is sensitive to famciclovir but not to acyclovir. In some patients infected with TK-deficient virus, higher doses of acyclovir are associated with clearing of lesions. In others, clinical disease progresses despite high-dose therapy. Almost all clinically significant acyclovir resistance has been seen in immunocompromised patients, and HSV-2 isolates are more often resistant than HSV-1 strains. A study by the Centers for Disease Control and Prevention indicated that ~5% of HSV-2 isolates from HIV-positive persons exhibit some degree of in vitro resistance to acyclovir. Of HSV-2 isolates from immunocompetent patients attending sexually transmitted disease clinics, <0.5% show reduced in vitro sensitivity to acyclovir. The lack of appreciable change in the frequency of detection of such isolates in the past 20 years probably reflects the reduced transmission of TK-deficient mutants. Isolation of HSV from lesions persisting despite adequate dosages and blood levels of acyclovir should raise the suspicion of acyclovir resistance. Therapy with the antiviral drug foscarnet is useful in acyclovir-resistant cases (Chap. 171). Because of its toxicity and cost, this drug is usually reserved for patients with extensive mucocutaneous infections. Cidofovir is a nucleotide analogue and exists as a phosphonate or monophosphate form. Most TK-deficient strains of HSV are sensitive to cidofovir. Cidofovir ointment speeds healing of acyclovir-resistant lesions. No well-controlled trials of systemic cidofovir have been reported. True TK-negative variants of HSV appear to have a reduced capacity to spread because of altered neurovirulence—a feature important in the relatively infrequent presence of such strains in immunocompetent populations, even with increasing use of antiviral drugs.

TABLE 172-1 ANTIVIRAL CHEMOTHERAPY FOR HSV INFECTION **1101**

I. Mucocutaneous HSV infections

  A. Infections in immunosuppressed patients

    1. Acute symptomatic first or recurrent episodes: IV acyclovir (5 mg/kg q8h) or oral acyclovir (400 mg qid), famciclovir (500 mg bid or tid), or valacyclovir (500 mg bid) is effective. Treatment duration may vary from 7 to 14 days.

    2. Suppression of reactivation disease (genital or oral-labial): IV acyclovir (5 mg/kg q8h) or oral valacyclovir (500 mg bid) or acyclovir (400–800 mg 3–5 times per day) prevents recurrences during the 30-day period immediately after transplantation. Longer-term HSV suppression is often used for persons with continued immunosuppression. In bone marrow and renal transplant recipients, oral valacyclovir (2 g/d) is also effective in reducing cytomegalovirus infection. Oral valacyclovir at a dose of 4 g/d has been associated with thrombotic thrombocytopenic purpura after extended use in HIV-positive persons. In HIV-infected persons, oral acyclovir (400–800 mg bid), valacyclovir (500 mg bid), or famciclovir (500 mg bid) is effective in reducing clinical and subclinical reactivations of HSV-1 and HSV-2.

  B. Infections in immunocompetent patients

    1. Genital herpes

      a. First episodes: Oral acyclovir (200 mg 5 times per day or 400 mg tid), valacyclovir (1 g bid), or famciclovir (250 mg bid) for 7–14 days is effective. IV acyclovir (5 mg/kg q8h for 5 days) is given for severe disease or neurologic complications such as aseptic meningitis.

      b. Symptomatic recurrent genital herpes: Short-course (1- to 3-day) regimens are preferred because of low cost and convenience. Oral acyclovir (800 mg tid for 2 days), valacyclovir (500 mg bid for 3 days), or famciclovir (750 or 1000 mg bid for 1 day, a 1500-mg single dose, or 500 mg stat followed by 250 mg q12h for 3 days) effectively shortens lesion duration. Other options include oral acyclovir (200 mg 5 times per day), valacyclovir (500 mg bid), and famciclovir (125 mg bid for 5 days).

      c. Suppression of recurrent genital herpes: Oral acyclovir (200-mg capsules tid or qid, 400 mg bid, or 800 mg qd), famciclovir (250 mg bid), or valacyclovir (500 mg daily) is effective. Patients with >9 episodes per year should take oral valacyclovir at a dosage of 1 g daily or 500 mg bid.

    2. Oral-labial HSV infections

      a. First episode: Oral acyclovir (200 mg) is given 4 or 5 times per day; an oral acyclovir suspension can be used (600 mg/m² qid). Oral famciclovir (250 mg bid) or valacyclovir (1 g bid) has been used clinically.

      b. Recurrent episodes: If initiated at the onset of the prodrome, single-dose or 1-day therapy effectively reduces pain and speeds healing. Regimens include oral famciclovir (a 1500-mg single dose or 750 mg bid for 1 day) or valacyclovir (a 2-g single dose or 2 g bid for 1 day). Self-initiated therapy with 6-times-daily topical penciclovir cream effectively speeds healing of oral-labial HSV. Topical acyclovir cream has also been shown to speed healing.

      c. Suppression of reactivation of oral-labial HSV: If started before exposure and continued for the duration of exposure (usually 5–10 days), oral acyclovir (400 mg bid) prevents reactivation of recurrent oral-labial HSV infection associated with severe sun exposure.

    3. Surgical prophylaxis of oral or genital HSV infection: Several surgical procedures, such as laser skin resurfacing, trigeminal nerve-root decompression, and lumbar disk surgery, have been associated with HSV reactivation. IV acyclovir (5 mg/kg q8h) or oral acyclovir (800 mg bid), valacyclovir (500 mg bid), or famciclovir (250 mg bid) effectively reduces reactivation. Therapy should be initiated 48 h before surgery and continued for 3–7 days.

    4. Herpetic whitlow: Oral acyclovir (200 mg) is given 5 times daily for 7–10 days.

    5. HSV proctitis: Oral acyclovir (400 mg 5 times per day) is useful in shortening the course of infection. In immunosuppressed patients or in patients with severe infection, IV acyclovir (5 mg/kg q8h) may be useful.

    6. Herpetic eye infections: In acute keratitis, topical trifluorothymidine, vidarabine, idoxuridine, acyclovir, penciclovir, and interferon are all beneficial. Debridement may be required. Topical steroids may worsen disease.

II. CNS HSV infections

  A. HSV encephalitis: IV acyclovir (10 mg/kg q8h; 30 mg/kg per day) is given for 10 days or until HSV DNA is no longer detected in CSF.

  B. HSV aseptic meningitis: No studies of systemic antiviral chemotherapy exist. If therapy is to be given, IV acyclovir (15–30 mg/kg per day) should be used.

  C. Autonomic radiculopathy: No studies are available. Most authorities recommend a trial of IV acyclovir.

III. Neonatal HSV infections: Oral acyclovir (60 mg/kg per day, divided into 3 doses) is given. The recommended duration of treatment is 21 days. Monitoring for relapse should be undertaken, and some authorities recommend continued suppression with oral acyclovir suspension for 3–4 months.

IV. Visceral HSV infections

  A. HSV esophagitis: IV acyclovir (15 mg/kg per day). In some patients with milder forms of immunosuppression, oral therapy with valacyclovir or famciclovir is effective.

  B. HSV pneumonitis: No controlled studies exist. IV acyclovir (15 mg/kg per day) should be considered.

V. Disseminated HSV infections: No controlled studies exist. IV acyclovir (5 mg/kg q8h) should be tried. Adjustments for renal insufficiency may be needed. No definite evidence indicates that therapy will decrease the risk of death.

VI. Erythema multiforme associated with HSV: Anecdotal observations suggest that oral acyclovir (400 mg bid or tid) or valacyclovir (500 mg bid) will suppress erythema multiforme.

VII. Infections due to acyclovir-resistant HSV: IV foscarnet (40 mg/kg IV q8h) should be given until lesions heal. The optimal duration of therapy and the usefulness of its continuation to suppress lesions are unclear. Some patients may benefit from cutaneous application of trifluorothymidine or 5% cidofovir gel.

The success of efforts to control HSV disease on a population basis through suppressive antiviral chemotherapy and/or educational programs will be limited.

Barrier forms of contraception (especially condoms) decrease the likelihood of transmission of HSV infection, particularly during periods of asymptomatic viral excretion. When lesions are present, HSV infection may be transmitted by skin-to-skin contact despite the use of a condom. Nevertheless, the available data suggest that consistent condom use is an effective means of reducing the risk of genital HSV-2 transmission. Chronic daily antiviral therapy with valacyclovir can also be partially effective in reducing acquisition of HSV-2, especially among susceptible women. There are no comparative efficacy studies of valacyclovir versus condom use. Most authorities suggest both approaches. The need for a vaccine to prevent acquisition of HSV infection is great, especially in light of the role HSV-2 plays in enhancing the acquisition and transmission of HIV-1.

A substantial portion of neonatal HSV cases could be prevented by reducing the acquisition of HSV by women in the third trimester of pregnancy. Identification of women susceptible to HSV acquisition in pregnancy through serologic screening, with a focus on counseling against unprotected oral or genital sex, is receiving increasing attention. Neonatal HSV infection can result from either the acquisition of maternal infection near term or the reactivation of infection at delivery in the already-infected mother. Thus strategies for reducing neonatal HSV are complex. Some authorities have recommended that antiviral therapy with acyclovir or valacyclovir be given to HSV-2-infected women in late pregnancy as a means of reducing reactivation of HSV-2 at term. Data are not available to support the efficacy of this approach. Moreover, the high treatment-to-prevention ratio makes this a dubious public health approach, even though it can reduce the frequency of HSV-associated cesarean delivery.

FURTHER READINGS

BROWN ZA et al: Effect of serologic status and cesarean delivery on transmission rates of herpes simplex virus from mother to infant. JAMA 289:203, 2003

CHILUKURI S, ROSEN T: Management of acyclovir-resistant herpes simplex virus. Dermatol Clin 21:311, 2003

COREY L et al: The effects of herpes simplex virus-2 on HIV-1 acquisition and transmission: A review of two overlapping epidemics. J AIDS 35:435, 2004

KIMBERLIN DW et al: Safety and efficacy of high-dose intravenous acyclovir in the management of neonatal herpes simplex virus infections. Pediatrics 108:230, 2001

WALD A et al: The relationship between condom use and herpes simplex virus acquisition. Ann Intern Med 143:707, 2005

WHITLEY RJ et al: Herpes simplex encephalitis: Adolescents and adults. Antiviral Res 71:141, 2006

173 Varicella-Zoster Virus Infections
Richard J. Whitley

DEFINITION

Varicella-zoster virus (VZV) causes two distinct clinical entities: varicella (chickenpox) and herpes zoster (shingles). Chickenpox, a ubiquitous and extremely contagious infection, is usually a benign illness of childhood characterized by an exanthematous vesicular rash. With reactivation of latent VZV (which is most common after the sixth decade of life), herpes zoster presents as a dermatomal vesicular rash, usually associated with severe pain.

ETIOLOGY

A clinical association between varicella and herpes zoster has been recognized for nearly 100 years. Early in the twentieth century, similarities in the histopathologic features of skin lesions resulting from varicella and herpes zoster were demonstrated. Viral isolates from patients with chickenpox and herpes zoster produced similar alterations in tissue culture—specifically, the appearance of eosinophilic intranuclear inclusions and multinucleated giant cells. These results suggested that the viruses were biologically similar. Restriction endonuclease analyses of viral DNA from a patient with chickenpox who subsequently developed herpes zoster verified the molecular identity of the two viruses responsible for these different clinical presentations.

VZV is a member of the family Herpesviridae, sharing with other members such structural characteristics as a lipid envelope surrounding a nucleocapsid with icosahedral symmetry, a total diameter of ~180–200 nm, and centrally located double-stranded DNA that is ~125,000 bp in length.

PATHOGENESIS AND PATHOLOGY

Primary Infection Transmission occurs readily by the respiratory route; the subsequent localized replication of the virus at an undefined site (presumably the nasopharynx) leads to seeding of the reticuloendothelial system and ultimately to the development of viremia. Viremia in patients with chickenpox is reflected in the diffuse and scattered nature of the skin lesions and can be verified in selected cases by the recovery of VZV from the blood or routinely by the detection of viral DNA in either blood or lesions by polymerase chain reaction (PCR). Vesicles involve the corium and dermis, with degenerative changes characterized by ballooning, the presence of multinucleated giant cells, and eosinophilic intranuclear inclusions. Infection may involve localized blood vessels of the skin, resulting in necrosis and epidermal hemorrhage. With the evolution of disease, the vesicular fluid becomes cloudy because of the recruitment of polymorphonuclear leukocytes and the presence of degenerated cells and fibrin. Ultimately, the vesicles either rupture and release their fluid (which includes infectious virus) or are gradually reabsorbed.

Recurrent Infection The mechanism of reactivation of VZV that results in herpes zoster is unknown. Presumably, the virus infects dorsal root ganglia during chickenpox, where it remains latent until reactivated. Histopathologic examination of representative dorsal root ganglia during active herpes zoster demonstrates hemorrhage, edema, and lymphocytic infiltration.

Active replication of VZV in other organs, such as the lung or the brain, can occur during either chickenpox or herpes zoster but is uncommon in the immunocompetent host. Pulmonary involvement is characterized by interstitial pneumonitis, multinucleated giant cell formation, intranuclear inclusions, and pulmonary hemorrhage. Central nervous system (CNS) infection leads to histopathologic evidence of perivascular cuffing similar to that encountered in measles and other viral encephalitides. Focal hemorrhagic necrosis of the brain, characteristic of herpes simplex virus (HSV) encephalitis, is uncommon in VZV infection.

EPIDEMIOLOGY AND CLINICAL MANIFESTATIONS

Chickenpox Humans are the only known reservoir for VZV. Chickenpox is highly contagious, with an attack rate of at least 90% among susceptible (seronegative) individuals. Persons of both sexes and all races are infected equally often. The virus is endemic in the population at large; however, it becomes epidemic among susceptible individuals during seasonal peaks—namely, late winter and early spring in the temperate zone. Historically, children 5–9 years old are most commonly affected and account for 50% of all cases. Most other cases involve children 1–4 and 10–14 years old. Approximately 10% of the population of the United States over the age of 15 is susceptible to infection. VZV vaccination during the second year of life is dramatically changing the epidemiology of infection. As a consequence, the annualized incidence of chickenpox is decreasing significantly.

The incubation period of chickenpox ranges from 10 to 21 days but is usually 14–17 days. Secondary attack rates in susceptible siblings within a household are 70–90%. Patients are infectious ~48 h before onset of the vesicular rash, during the period of vesicle formation (which generally lasts 4–5 days), and until all vesicles are crusted.

Clinically, chickenpox presents as a rash, low-grade fever, and malaise, although a few patients develop a prodrome 1–2 days before onset of the exanthem. In the immunocompetent patient, chickenpox is usually a benign illness associated with lassitude and with body temperatures of 37.8°–39.4°C (100°–103°F) of 3–5 days' duration. The skin lesions—the hallmark of the infection—include maculopapules, vesicles, and scabs in various stages of evolution (Fig. 173-1). These lesions, which evolve from maculopapules to vesicles over hours to days, appear on the trunk and face and rapidly spread to involve other areas of the body. Most are small and have an erythematous base with a diameter of 5–10 mm. Successive crops appear over a 2- to 4-day period. Lesions can also be found on the mucosa of the pharynx and/or the vagina. Their severity varies from one person to another. Some individuals have very few lesions, while others have as many as 2000. Younger children tend to have fewer vesicles than older individuals. Secondary and tertiary cases within families are associated with a relatively large number of vesicles. Immunocompromised patients—both children and adults, particularly those with leukemia—have lesions (often with a hemorrhagic base) that are more numerous and take longer to heal than those of immunocompetent patients. Immunocompromised individuals are also at greater risk for visceral complications, which occur in 30–50% of cases and are fatal 15% of the time in the absence of antiviral therapy.

The most common infectious complication of varicella is secondary bacterial superinfection of the skin, which is usually caused by *Streptococcus pyogenes* or *Staphylococcus aureus,* including strains that are methicillin resistant. Skin infection results from excoriation of lesions after scratching. Gram's staining of skin lesions should help clarify the etiology of unusually erythematous and pustulated lesions.

The most common extracutaneous site of involvement in children is the CNS. The syndrome of acute cerebellar ataxia and meningeal inflammation generally appears ~21 days after onset of the rash and rarely develops in the preeruptive phase. The cerebrospinal fluid (CSF) contains lymphocytes and elevated levels of protein. CNS involvement

is a benign complication of VZV infection in children and generally does not require hospitalization. Aseptic meningitis, encephalitis, transverse myelitis, Guillain-Barré syndrome, and Reye's syndrome can also occur. Encephalitis is reported in 0.1–0.2% of children with chickenpox. Other than supportive care, no specific therapy is available for patients with CNS involvement.

Varicella pneumonia, the most serious complication following chickenpox, develops more commonly in adults (up to 20% of cases) than in children and is particularly severe in pregnant women. Pneumonia due to VZV usually has its onset 3–5 days into the illness and is associated with tachypnea, cough, dyspnea, and fever. Cyanosis, pleuritic chest pain, and hemoptysis are common. Roentgenographic evidence of disease consists of nodular infiltrates and interstitial pneumonitis. Resolution of pneumonitis parallels improvement of the skin rash; however, patients may have persistent fever and compromised pulmonary function for weeks.

Other complications of chickenpox include myocarditis, corneal lesions, nephritis, arthritis, bleeding diatheses, acute glomerulonephritis, and hepatitis. Hepatic involvement, distinct from Reye's syndrome and usually asymptomatic, is common in chickenpox and is generally characterized by elevated levels of liver enzymes, particularly aspartate and alanine aminotransferases.

Perinatal varicella is associated with a high mortality rate when maternal disease develops within 5 days before delivery or within 48 h thereafter. Because the newborn does not receive protective transplacental antibodies and has an immature immune system, the illness may be unusually severe. The reported mortality rate is as high as 30% in this group. *Congenital varicella,* with clinical manifestations of limb hypoplasia, cicatricial skin lesions, and microcephaly at birth, is extremely uncommon.

Herpes Zoster Herpes zoster (also called shingles) is a sporadic disease that results from reactivation of latent VZV from dorsal root ganglia. Most patients have no history of recent exposure to other individuals with VZV infection. Herpes zoster occurs at all ages, but its incidence is highest (5–10 cases per 1000 persons) among individuals in the sixth decade of life and beyond. Recent data suggest that 1.2 million cases occur annually in the United States. Recurrent herpes zoster is exceedingly rare except in immunocompromised hosts, especially those with AIDS.

Herpes zoster is characterized by a unilateral vesicular eruption within a dermatome, often associated with severe pain. The dermatomes from T3 to L3 are most frequently involved. If the ophthalmic branch of the trigeminal nerve is involved, *zoster ophthalmicus* results. The factors responsible for the reactivation of VZV are not known. In children, reactivation is usually benign; in adults, it can be debilitating. The continuum of pain from onset to resolution is known as *zoster-associated pain.* The onset of disease is heralded by pain within the dermatome, which may precede lesions by 48–72 h; an erythematous maculopapular rash evolves rapidly into vesicular lesions (Fig. 173-2). In the normal host, these lesions may remain few in number and continue to form for only 3–5 days. The total duration of disease is generally 7–10 days; however, it may take as long as 2–4 weeks for the skin to return to normal. Patients with herpes zoster can transmit infection to seronegative individuals, with consequent chickenpox. In a few patients, characteristic localization of pain to a dermatome with serologic evidence of herpes zoster has been reported in the absence of skin lesions. When branches of the trigeminal nerve are involved, lesions may appear on the face, in the mouth, in the eye, or on the tongue. Zoster ophthalmicus is usually a debilitating condition that can result in blindness in the absence of antiviral therapy. In the *Ramsay Hunt syndrome,* pain and vesicles appear in the external auditory canal, and patients lose their sense of taste in the anterior two-thirds of the tongue while developing ipsilateral facial palsy. The geniculate ganglion of the sensory branch of the facial nerve is involved.

In both normal and immunocompromised hosts, the most debilitating complication of herpes zoster is pain associated with acute neuritis and postherpetic neuralgia. Postherpetic neuralgia is uncommon in young individuals; however, at least 50% of zoster patients over age

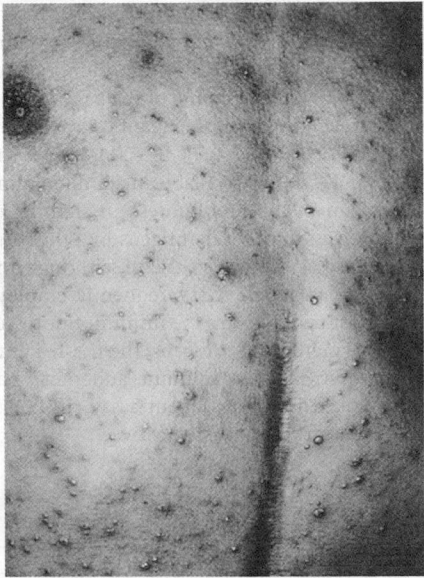

FIGURE 173-1 Numerous varicella lesions at various stages of evolution: vesicles on an erythematous base, umbilical vesicles, and crusts.

FIGURE 173-2 Close-up of lesions of disseminated zoster. Note lesions at different stages of evolution, including pustules and crusting. (*Photo courtesy of Lindsey Baden; with permission.*)

FIGURE 173-3 Herpes zoster is seen in this HIV-infected patient as hemorrhagic vesicles and pustules on an erythematous base grouped in a dermatomal distribution.

50 report some degree of pain in the involved dermatome months after the resolution of cutaneous disease. Changes in sensation in the dermatome, resulting in either hypo- or hyperesthesia, are common.

CNS involvement may follow localized herpes zoster. Many patients without signs of meningeal irritation have CSF pleocytosis and moderately elevated levels of CSF protein. Symptomatic meningoencephalitis is characterized by headache, fever, photophobia, meningitis, and vomiting. A rare manifestation of CNS involvement is granulomatous angiitis with contralateral hemiplegia, which can be diagnosed by cerebral arteriography. Other neurologic manifestations include transverse myelitis with or without motor paralysis.

Like chickenpox, herpes zoster is more severe in immunocompromised than immunocompetent individuals. Lesions continue to form for >1 week, and scabbing is not complete in most cases until 3 weeks into the illness. Patients with Hodgkin's disease and non-Hodgkin's lymphoma are at greatest risk for progressive herpes zoster. Cutaneous dissemination (Fig. 173-3) develops in ~40% of these patients. Among patients with cutaneous dissemination, the risk of pneumonitis, meningoencephalitis, hepatitis, and other serious complications is increased by 5–10%. However, even in immunocompromised patients, disseminated zoster is rarely fatal.

Recipients of hematopoietic stem cell transplants are at particularly high risk of VZV infection. Of all cases of posttransplantation VZV infection, 30% occur within 1 year (50% of these within 9 months); 45% of the patients involved have cutaneous or visceral dissemination. The mortality rate in this situation is 10%. Postherpetic neuralgia, scarring, and bacterial superinfection are especially common in VZV infections occurring within 9 months of transplantation. Among infected patients, concomitant graft-versus-host disease increases the chance of dissemination and/or death.

DIFFERENTIAL DIAGNOSIS

The diagnosis of chickenpox is not difficult. The characteristic rash and a history of recent exposure should lead to a prompt diagnosis. Other viral infections that can mimic chickenpox include disseminated HSV infection in patients with atopic dermatitis and the disseminated vesiculopapular lesions sometimes associated with coxsackievirus infection, echovirus infection, or atypical measles. However, these rashes are more commonly morbilliform with a hemorrhagic component rather than vesicular or vesiculopustular. Rickettsialpox (Chap. 167) can be confused with chickenpox; however, rickettsialpox can be distinguished easily by detection of the "herald spot" at the site of the mite bite and the development of a more pronounced headache. Serologic testing is also useful in differentiating rickettsialpox from varicella and can confirm susceptibility in adults unsure of their chickenpox history. Concern about smallpox has recently increased because of the threat of bioterrorism (Chap. 214). The lesions of smallpox are larger than those of chickenpox and are all at the same stage of evolution at any given time.

Unilateral vesicular lesions in a dermatomal pattern should lead rapidly to the diagnosis of herpes zoster, although the occurrence of shingles without a rash has been reported. Both HSV infections and coxsackievirus infections can cause dermatomal vesicular lesions. Supportive diagnostic virology and fluorescent staining of skin scrapings with monoclonal antibodies are helpful in ensuring the proper diagnosis. In the prodromal stage of herpes zoster, the diagnosis can be exceedingly difficult and may be made only after lesions have appeared or by retrospective serologic assessment.

LABORATORY FINDINGS

Unequivocal confirmation of the diagnosis is possible only through the isolation of VZV in susceptible tissue-culture cell lines, the demonstration of either seroconversion or a fourfold or greater rise in antibody titer between convalescent- and acute-phase serum specimens, or the detection of VZV DNA by PCR. A rapid impression can be obtained by a Tzanck smear, with scraping of the base of the lesions in an attempt to demonstrate multinucleated giant cells, although the sensitivity of this method is low (~60%). PCR technology for the detection of viral DNA in vesicular fluid is available in a limited number of diagnostic laboratories. Direct immunofluorescent staining of cells from the lesion base or detection of viral antigens by other assays (such as the immunoperoxidase assay) is also useful, although these tests are not commercially available. The most frequently employed serologic tools for assessing host response are the immunofluorescent detection of antibodies to VZV membrane antigens, the fluorescent antibody to membrane antigen (FAMA) test, immune adherence hemagglutination, and enzyme-linked immunosorbent assay (ELISA). The FAMA test and the ELISA appear to be most sensitive.

℞ VARICELLA-ZOSTER VIRUS INFECTION

Medical management of chickenpox in the immunologically normal host is directed toward the prevention of avoidable complications. Obviously, good hygiene includes daily bathing and soaks. Secondary bacterial infection of the skin can be avoided by meticulous skin care, particularly with close cropping of fingernails. Pruritus can be decreased with topical dressings or the administration of antipruritic drugs. Tepid water baths and wet compresses are better than drying lotions for the relief of itching. Administration of aspirin to children with chickenpox should be avoided because of the association of aspirin derivatives with the development of Reye's syndrome. Acyclovir therapy (800 mg by mouth five times daily for 5–7 days) is recommended for adolescents and adults with chickenpox of ≤24 h duration. Likewise, acyclovir therapy may be of benefit to children <12 years of age if initiated early in the disease (<24 h) at a dose of 20 mg/kg every 6 h. The second-generation antiherpetic drugs valacyclovir and famciclovir are probably as efficacious or more so; however, no controlled clinical trials comparing these drugs have been reported. The advantages (i.e., pharmacokinetics) of the second-generation agents are described in Chap. 171.

Aluminum acetate soaks for the management of herpes zoster can be both soothing and cleansing. Patients with herpes zoster benefit from oral antiviral therapy, as evidenced by accelerated healing of lesions and resolution of zoster-associated pain with acyclovir, valacyclovir, or famciclovir. Acyclovir, now off patent, is administered at a dosage of 800 mg five times daily for 7–10 days. Famciclovir, the prodrug of penciclovir, is at least as effective as acyclovir and perhaps more so. One study showed twofold faster resolution of postherpetic neuralgia in famciclovir-treated patients with zoster than in recipients of placebo. The dose is 500 mg by mouth three times daily for 7 days. Valacyclovir, the prodrug of acyclovir, accelerates healing and resolution of zoster-associated pain more promptly than acyclovir. The dose is 1 g by mouth three times daily for 5–7 days. Compared with acyclovir, both famciclovir and valacyclovir offer the advantage of less frequent administration.

In severely immunocompromised hosts (e.g., transplant recipients, patients with lymphoproliferative malignancies), both chickenpox and herpes zoster (including disseminated disease) should be treated, at least at the outset, with intravenous acyclovir, which reduces the occurrence of visceral complications but has no effect on healing of skin lesions or pain. The dose is 10–12.5 mg/kg every 8 h for 7 days. For low-risk immunocompromised hosts, oral therapy with valacyclovir or famciclovir appears beneficial. Concomitant with the administration of intravenous acyclovir, it is desirable to wean these patients from immunosuppressive treatment.

Patients with varicella pneumonia may require removal of bronchial secretions and ventilatory support. Persons with zoster ophthalmicus should be referred immediately to an ophthalmologist. Therapy for this condition consists of the administration of analgesics for severe pain and the use of atropine. Acyclovir, valacyclovir, and famciclovir all accelerate healing.

The management of acute neuritis and/or postherpetic neuralgia can be particularly difficult. In addition to the judicious use of analgesics, ranging from nonnarcotics to narcotic derivatives, drugs such as gabapentin, pregabalin, amitriptyline hydrochloride, lidocaine patches, and fluphenazine hydrochloride are reportedly beneficial for pain relief. In one study, glucocorticoid therapy administered early in the course of localized herpes zoster significantly accelerated such quality-of-life improvements as a return to usual activity and termination of analgesia. The dose of prednisone administered orally was 60 mg/d on days 1–7, 30 mg/d on days 8–14, and 15 mg/d on days 15–21. This regimen is appropriate only for relatively healthy elderly persons with moderate or severe pain at presentation. Patients with osteoporosis, diabetes mellitus, glycosuria, or hypertension may not be appropriate candidates. Glucocorticoids should not be used without concomitant antiviral therapy.

PREVENTION

Three methods are used for the prevention of VZV infections. First, a live attenuated varicella vaccine (Oka) is recommended for all children >1 year of age (up to 12 years of age) who have not had chickenpox and for adults known to be seronegative for VZV. A single dose of vaccine is administered to children, whereas adults require two doses. The vaccine is both safe and efficacious. Breakthrough cases are mild and may result in spread of the vaccine virus to susceptible contacts. The universal vaccination of children is resulting in a decreased incidence of chickenpox in sentinel communities. Furthermore, inactivation of the vaccine virus significantly decreases the occurrence of herpes zoster after hematopoietic stem-cell transplantation. After administration of a vaccine with 18 times the viral content of the Oka vaccine to indi-

TABLE 173-1 RECOMMENDATIONS FOR VZIG ADMINISTRATION   1105

Exposure Criteria

1. Exposure to person with chickenpox or zoster
   a. Household: residence in the same household
   b. Playmate: face-to-face indoor play
   c. Hospital
      Varicella: same 2- to 4-bed room or adjacent beds in large ward, face-to-face contact with infectious staff member or patient, visit by a person deemed contagious
      Zoster: intimate contact (e.g., touching or hugging) with a person deemed contagious
   d. Newborn infant: onset of varicella in the mother ≤5 days before delivery or ≤48 h after delivery; VZIG not indicated if the mother has zoster
2. Patient should receive VZIG as soon as possible but not >96 h after exposure

Candidates (Provided They Have Significant Exposure) Include:

1. Immunocompromised susceptible children without a history of varicella or varicella immunization
2. Susceptible pregnant women
3. Newborn infants whose mother had onset of chickenpox within 5 days before or within 48 h after delivery
4. Hospitalized premature infant (≥28 weeks of gestation) whose mother lacks a reliable history of chickenpox or serologic evidence of protection against varicella
5. Hospitalized premature infant (<28 weeks of gestation or ≤1000-g birth weight), regardless of maternal history of varicella or varicella-zoster virus serologic status

viduals >60 years of age, the incidence of shingles was found to decrease by 51%, the burden of illness by 61%, and the incidence of postherpetic neuralgia by 66%. The Advisory Committee on Immunization Practices has therefore recommended that persons in this age group be offered this vaccine in order to reduce the frequency of shingles and the severity of postherpetic neuralgia.

A second approach is to administer varicella-zoster immune globulin (VZIG) to individuals who are susceptible, are at high risk for developing complications of varicella, and have had a significant exposure. This product should be given within 96 h (preferably within 72 h) of the exposure. Indications for administration of VZIG appear in Table 173-1. Unfortunately, the availability of this product in the future will be limited at best.

Lastly, antiviral therapy can be given as prophylaxis to individuals at high risk who are ineligible for vaccine or who are beyond the 96-h window after direct contact. While the initial studies have used acyclovir, similar benefit can be anticipated with either valacyclovir or famciclovir. Therapy is instituted 7 days after intense exposure. At this time, the host is midway into the incubation period. This approach significantly decreases disease severity, if not totally preventing disease.

FURTHER READINGS

ARVIN A: Aging, immunity, and the varicella-zoster virus. N Engl J Med 352:2266, 2005

GNANN JW, WHITLEY RJ: Herpes zoster. N Engl J Med 347:340, 2002

IZURIETA HS et al: Postlicensure effectiveness of varicella vaccine during an outbreak in a child care center. JAMA 278:1495, 1997

NGUYEN HQ et al: Decline in mortality due to varicella after implementation of varicella vaccination in the United States. N Engl J Med 352:450, 2005

OXMAN MN et al: A vaccine to prevent herpes zoster and postherpetic neuralgia in older adults. N Engl J Med 352:2271, 2005

ROWBOTHAM M et al: Gabapentin for the treatment of postherpetic neuralgia. A randomized controlled trial. JAMA 280:1837, 1998

SEWARD JF et al: Contagiousness of varicella in vaccinated cases: A household contact study. JAMA 292:704, 2004

——— et al: Varicella disease after introduction of varicella vaccine in the United States, 1995-2000. JAMA 28:606, 2002

174 Epstein-Barr Virus Infections, Including Infectious Mononucleosis

Jeffrey I. Cohen

DEFINITION

Epstein-Barr virus (EBV) is the cause of heterophile-positive infectious mononucleosis (IM), which is characterized by fever, sore throat, lymphadenopathy, and atypical lymphocytosis. EBV is also associated with several human tumors, including nasopharyngeal carcinoma, Burkitt's lymphoma, Hodgkin's disease, and (in patients with immunodeficiencies) B cell lymphoma. The virus, a member of the family Herpesviridae, consists of a linear DNA core surrounded by a nucleocapsid and an envelope that contains glycoproteins. The two types of EBV that are widely prevalent in nature are not distinguishable by conventional serologic tests.

EPIDEMIOLOGY

EBV infections occur worldwide. These infections are most common in early childhood, with a second peak during late adolescence. By adulthood, more than 90% of individuals have been infected and have antibodies to the virus. IM is usually a disease of young adults. In lower socioeconomic groups and in areas of the world with lower standards of hygiene (e.g., developing countries), EBV tends to infect children at an early age, and symptomatic IM is uncommon. In areas with higher standards of hygiene, infection with EBV is often delayed until adulthood, and IM is more prevalent.

EBV is spread by contact with oral secretions. The virus is frequently transmitted from asymptomatic adults to infants and among young adults by transfer of saliva during kissing. Transmission by less intimate contact is rare. EBV has been transmitted by blood transfusion and by bone marrow transplantation. More than 90% of asymptomatic seropositive individuals shed the virus in oropharyngeal secretions. Shedding is increased in immunocompromised patients and those with IM.

PATHOGENESIS

EBV is transmitted by salivary secretions. The virus infects the epithelium of the oropharynx and the salivary glands and is shed from these cells. While B cells may become infected after contact with epithelial cells, studies suggest that lymphocytes in the tonsillar crypts can be infected directly. The virus then spreads through the bloodstream. The proliferation and expansion of EBV-infected B cells along with reactive T cells during IM result in enlargement of lymphoid tissue. Polyclonal activation of B cells leads to the production of antibodies to host-cell and viral proteins. During the acute phase of IM, up to 1 in every 100 B cells in the peripheral blood is infected by EBV; after recovery, 1–50 in every 1 million B cells is infected. During IM, there is an inverted CD4+/CD8+ T cell ratio. The percentage of CD4+ T cells decreases, while there are large clonal expansions of CD8+ T cells; up to 40% of CD8+ T cells are directed against EBV antigens during acute infection. Data suggest that memory B cells, not epithelial cells, are the reservoir for EBV in the body. When patients are treated with acyclovir, shedding of EBV from the oropharynx stops but the virus persists in B cells.

The EBV receptor (CD21) on the surface of B cells is also the receptor for the C3d component of complement. EBV infection of epithelial cells results in viral replication and production of virions. When B cells are infected by EBV in vitro, they become transformed and can proliferate indefinitely. During latent infection of B cells, only the EBV nuclear antigens (EBNAs), latent membrane proteins (LMPs), and small EBV RNAs are expressed in vitro. EBV-transformed B cells secrete immunoglobulin; only a small fraction of cells produce virus.

Cellular immunity is more important than humoral immunity in controlling EBV infection. In the initial phase of infection, suppressor T cells, natural killer cells, and nonspecific cytotoxic T cells are impor-

tant in controlling the proliferation of EBV-infected B cells. Levels of markers of T cell activation and serum interferon (IFN) γ are elevated. Later in infection, HLA-restricted cytotoxic T cells that recognize EBNAs and LMPs and destroy EBV-infected cells are generated. Studies have shown that one of the late genes expressed during EBV replication, *BCRF1*, is a homologue of interleukin 10 and can inhibit the production of IFN-γ by mononuclear cells in vitro.

If T cell immunity is compromised, EBV-infected B cells may begin to proliferate. When EBV is associated with lymphoma, virus-induced proliferation is but one step in a multistep process of neoplastic transformation. In many EBV-containing tumors, LMP-1 mimics members of the tumor necrosis factor receptor family (e.g., CD40), transmitting growth-proliferating signals.

CLINICAL MANIFESTATIONS

Signs and Symptoms Most EBV infections in infants and young children either are asymptomatic or present as mild pharyngitis with or without tonsillitis. In contrast, up to 75% of infections in adolescents present as IM. IM in the elderly presents relatively often as nonspecific symptoms, including prolonged fever, fatigue, myalgia, and malaise. In contrast, pharyngitis, lymphadenopathy, splenomegaly, and atypical lymphocytes are relatively rare in elderly patients.

The incubation period for IM in young adults is ~4–6 weeks. A prodrome of fatigue, malaise, and myalgia may last for 1–2 weeks before the onset of fever, sore throat, and lymphadenopathy. Fever is usually low-grade and is most common in the first 2 weeks of the illness; however, it may persist for >1 month. Common signs and symptoms are listed along with their frequencies in Table 174-1. Lymphadenopathy and pharyngitis are most prominent during the first 2 weeks of the illness, while splenomegaly is more prominent during the second and third weeks. Lymphadenopathy most often affects the posterior cervical nodes but may be generalized. Enlarged lymph nodes are frequently tender and symmetric but are not fixed in place. Pharyngitis, often the most prominent sign, can be accompanied by enlargement of the tonsils with an exudate resembling that of streptococcal pharyngitis. A morbilliform or papular rash, usually on the arms or trunk, develops in ~5% of cases (Fig. 174-1). Most patients treated with ampicillin develop a macular rash; this rash is not predictive of future adverse reactions to penicillins. Erythema nodosum and erythema multiforme have also been described (Chap. 54). Most patients have symptoms for 2–4 weeks, but malaise and difficulty concentrating can persist for months.

Laboratory Findings The white blood cell count is usually elevated and peaks at 10,000–20,000/μL during the second or third week of illness. Lymphocytosis is usually demonstrable, with >10% atypical lymphocytes. The latter cells are enlarged lymphocytes that have abundant cytoplasm, vacuoles, and indentations of the cell membrane (Fig. 174-2). CD8+ cells predominate among the atypical lympho-

TABLE 174-1 SIGNS AND SYMPTOMS OF INFECTIOUS MONONUCLEOSIS	
Manifestation	**Median Percentage of Patients (Range)**
Symptoms	
Sore throat	75 (50–87)
Malaise	47 (42–76)
Headache	38 (22–67)
Abdominal pain, nausea, or vomiting	17 (5–25)
Chills	10 (9–11)
Signs	
Lymphadenopathy	95 (83–100)
Fever	93 (60–100)
Pharyngitis or tonsillitis	82 (68–90)
Splenomegaly	51 (43–64)
Hepatomegaly	11 (6–15)
Rash	10 (0–25)
Periorbital edema	13 (2–34)
Palatal enanthem	7 (3–13)
Jaundice	5 (2–10)

FIGURE 174-1 Rash in a patient with infectious mononucleosis due to Epstein-Barr virus. *(Courtesy of Maria Turner, MD; with permission.)*

cytes. Low-grade neutropenia and thrombocytopenia are common during the first month of illness. Liver function is abnormal in >90% of cases. Serum levels of aminotransferases and alkaline phosphatase are usually mildly elevated. The serum concentration of bilirubin is elevated in ~40% of cases.

Complications Most cases of IM are self-limited. Deaths are very rare and most often are due to central nervous system (CNS) complications, splenic rupture, upper airway obstruction, or bacterial superinfection.

When CNS complications develop, they usually do so during the first 2 weeks of EBV infection; in some patients, especially children, they are the only clinical manifestations of IM. Heterophile antibodies and atypical lymphocytes may be absent. Meningitis and encephalitis are the most common neurologic abnormalities, and patients may present with headache, meningismus, or cerebellar ataxia. Acute hemiplegia and psychosis have also been described. The cerebrospinal fluid (CSF) contains mainly lymphocytes, with occasional atypical lymphocytes. Most cases resolve without neurologic sequelae. Acute EBV infection has also been associated with cranial nerve palsies (especially those involving cranial nerve VII), Guillain-Barré syndrome, acute transverse myelitis, and peripheral neuritis.

Autoimmune hemolytic anemia occurs in ~2% of cases during the first 2 weeks. In most cases, the anemia is Coombs-positive, with cold agglutinins directed against the i red blood cell antigen. Most patients with hemolysis have mild anemia that lasts for 1–2 months, but some

patients have severe disease with hemoglobinuria and jaundice. Nonspecific antibody responses may also include rheumatoid factor, antinuclear antibodies, anti–smooth muscle antibodies, antiplatelet antibodies, and cryoglobulins. IM has been associated with red-cell aplasia, severe granulocytopenia, thrombocytopenia, pancytopenia, and hemophagocytic syndrome. The spleen ruptures in <0.5% of cases. Splenic rupture is more common among male than female patients and may manifest as abdominal pain, referred shoulder pain, or hemodynamic compromise.

Hypertrophy of lymphoid tissue in the tonsils or adenoids can result in upper airway obstruction, as can inflammation and edema of the epiglottis, pharynx, or uvula. About 10% of patients with IM develop streptococcal pharyngitis after their initial sore throat resolves.

Other rare complications associated with acute EBV infection include hepatitis (which can be fulminant), myocarditis or pericarditis with electrocardiographic changes, pneumonia with pleural effusion, interstitial nephritis, genital ulcerations, and vasculitis.

EBV-Associated Diseases Other Than IM EBV-associated lymphoproliferative disease has been described in patients with congenital or acquired immunodeficiency, including those with severe combined immunodeficiency, patients with AIDS, and recipients of bone marrow or organ transplants who are receiving immunosuppressive drugs (especially cyclosporine). Proliferating EBV-infected B cells infiltrate lymph nodes and multiple organs, and patients present with fever and lymphadenopathy or gastrointestinal symptoms. Pathologic studies show B cell hyperplasia or poly- or monoclonal lymphoma. The X-linked lymphoproliferative syndrome (Duncan's disease) is a recessive disorder of young boys who have a normal response to childhood infections but develop fatal lymphoproliferative disorders after infection with EBV. The protein associated with this syndrome (SAP) binds to a protein that mediates interactions of B and T cells. Most patients with this syndrome die of acute IM. Others develop hypogammaglobulinemia, malignant B cell lymphomas, aplastic anemia, or agranulocytosis. IM has also proved fatal to some patients with no obvious preexisting immune abnormality.

Oral hairy leukoplakia (Fig. 174-3) is an early manifestation of infection with HIV in adults (Chap. 182). Most patients present with raised, white corrugated lesions on the tongue (and occasionally on the buccal mucosa) that contain EBV DNA. Children infected with HIV can develop lymphoid interstitial pneumonitis; EBV DNA is often found in lung tissue from these patients.

Patients with chronic fatigue syndrome may have titers of antibody to EBV that are elevated but are not significantly different from those in healthy EBV-seropositive adults. While some patients have malaise and fatigue that persist for weeks or months after IM, persistent EBV infection is not a cause of chronic fatigue syndrome. Chronic active EBV infection is very rare and is distinct from chronic fatigue syndrome. The affected patients have an illness lasting >6 months, with elevated levels of EBV DNA in the blood, very high titers of antibody to EBV, and evidence of organ involvement, including hepatospleno-

FIGURE 174-2 Atypical lymphocytes from a patient with infectious mononucleosis due to Epstein-Barr virus.

FIGURE 174-3 Oral hairy leukoplakia often presents as white plaques on the lateral surface of the tongue and is associated with Epstein-Barr virus infection.

megaly, lymphadenopathy, and pneumonitis, uveitis, or neurologic disease.

EBV is associated with several malignancies. About 15% of cases of Burkitt's lymphoma in the United States and ~90% of those in Africa are associated with EBV (Chap. 105). African patients with Burkitt's lymphoma have high levels of antibody to EBV, and their tumor tissue usually contains viral DNA. Malaria infection in Africa may impair cellular immunity to EBV and induce polyclonal B cell activation with an expansion of EBV-infected B cells. These changes may enhance the proliferation of B cells, increasing the likelihood of a *c-myc* translocation—the hallmark of Burkitt's lymphoma. EBV-containing Burkitt's lymphoma also occurs in patients with AIDS.

Anaplastic nasopharyngeal carcinoma is uniformly associated with EBV; the affected tissues contain viral DNA and antigens. Patients with nasopharyngeal carcinoma often have elevated titers of antibody to EBV (Chap. 84). High levels of EBV plasma DNA before treatment or detectable levels of EBV DNA after radiation therapy correlate with lower rates of overall survival and relapse-free survival among patients with nasopharyngeal carcinoma.

EBV has been associated with Hodgkin's disease, especially the mixed-cellularity type (Chap. 105). Patients with Hodgkin's disease often have elevated titers of antibody to EBV. In about half of cases, viral DNA and antigens are found in Reed-Sternberg cells. The risk of EBV-positive Hodgkin's disease is significantly increased in young adults after EBV-seropositive IM. About 50% of non-Hodgkin's lymphomas in patients with AIDS are EBV-positive.

In some cases, EBV DNA has been detected in tumors from immunocompetent patients with tonsillar carcinoma, angioimmunoblastic lymphadenopathy, angiocentric nasal NK/T cell immunoproliferative lesions, T cell lymphoma, thymoma, gastric carcinoma, and CNS lymphoma. Studies have demonstrated viral DNA in leiomyosarcomas from AIDS patients and in smooth-muscle tumors from organ transplant recipients. Virtually all CNS lymphomas in AIDS patients are associated with EBV. While serologic studies have found higher levels of antibodies to EBV before the onset of multiple sclerosis in persons ≥25 years old, other studies (including measurement of EBV antibody titers in the CSF) are needed to ascertain a possible causal relationship.

DIAGNOSIS
Serologic Testing The heterophile test is used for the diagnosis of IM in children and adults (Table 174-2). In the test for this antibody, human serum is absorbed with guinea pig kidney, and the heterophile titer is defined as the greatest serum dilution that agglutinates sheep, horse, or cow erythrocytes. Although heterophile antibody binds to certain animal erythrocytes, it does not interact with EBV proteins. A titer of ≥40-fold is diagnostic of acute EBV infection in a patient who has symptoms compatible with IM and atypical lymphocytes. Tests for heterophile antibodies are positive in 40% of patients with IM during the first week of illness and in 80–90% during the third week. Therefore, repeated testing may be necessary, especially if the initial test is performed early. Tests usually remain positive for 3 months after the onset of illness, but heterophile antibodies can persist for up to 1 year. These antibodies usually are not detectable in children <5 years of age, in the elderly, or in patients presenting with symptoms not typical of IM. The commercially available monospot test for heterophile antibodies is somewhat more sensitive than the classic heterophile test. The monospot test is ~75% sensitive and ~90% specific compared with EBV-specific serologies. False-positive monospot results are more common among persons with connective tissue disease, lymphoma, viral hepatitis, and malaria.

EBV-specific antibody testing is used for patients with suspected acute EBV infection who lack heterophile antibodies and for patients with

TABLE 174-2	SEROLOGIC FEATURES OF EBV-ASSOCIATED DISEASES						
		Result in Indicated Test[a]					
			Anti-VCA		Anti-EA		
Condition	**Heterophile**	**IgM**	**IgG**	**EA-D**	**EA-R**	**Anti-EBNA**
Acute infectious mononucleosis	+	+	++	+	−	−
Convalescence	±	−	+	−	±	+
Past infection	−	−	+	−	−	+
Reactivation with immunodeficiency	−	−	++	+	+	±
Burkitt's lymphoma	−	−	+++	±	++	+
Nasopharyngeal carcinoma	−	−	+++	++	±	+

[a]VCA, viral capsid antigen; EA, early antigen; EA-D antibody, antibody to early antigen in diffuse pattern in nucleus and cytoplasm of infected cells; EA-R antibody, antibody to early antigen restricted to the cytoplasm; and EBNA, Epstein-Barr nuclear antigen.
Source: Adapted from Okano, 1988.

atypical infections (Table 174-2). Titers of IgM and IgG antibodies to viral capsid antigen (VCA) are elevated in the serum of more than 90% of patients at the onset of disease. IgM antibody to VCA is most useful for the diagnosis of acute IM because it is present at elevated titers only during the first 2–3 months of the disease; in contrast, IgG antibody to VCA is usually not useful for diagnosis of IM but is often used to assess past exposure to EBV because it persists for life. Seroconversion to EBNA positivity is also useful for the diagnosis of acute infection with EBV. Antibodies to EBNA become detectable relatively late (3–6 weeks after the onset of symptoms) in nearly all cases of acute EBV infection and persist for the lifetime of the patient. These antibodies may be lacking in immunodeficient patients and in those with chronic active EBV infection.

Titers of other antibodies may also be elevated in IM; however, these elevations are less useful for diagnosis. Antibodies to early antigens (EAs) are found either in a diffuse pattern in the nucleus and cytoplasm of infected cells (EA-D antibody) or restricted to the cytoplasm (EA-R antibody). These antibodies are detectable 3–4 weeks after the onset of symptoms in patients with IM. About 70% of individuals with IM have EA-D antibodies during the illness; the presence of EA-D antibodies is especially likely in patients with relatively severe disease. These antibodies usually persist for only 3–6 months. Levels of EA-D antibodies are also elevated in patients with nasopharyngeal carcinoma or chronic active EBV infection. EA-R antibodies are only occasionally detected in patients with IM but are often found at elevated titers in patients with African Burkitt's lymphoma or chronic active EBV infection. IgA antibodies to EBV antigens have proved useful for the identification of patients with nasopharyngeal carcinoma and of persons at high risk for the disease.

Other Studies Detection of EBV DNA, RNA, or proteins has been valuable in demonstrating the association of the virus with various malignancies. The polymerase chain reaction has been used to detect EBV DNA in the CSF of some AIDS patients with lymphomas and to monitor the amount of EBV DNA in the blood of patients with lymphoproliferative disease. Detection of high levels of EBV DNA in blood during the first few weeks of IM may be useful if serologic studies yield equivocal results. Culture of EBV from throat washings or blood is not helpful in the diagnosis of acute infection, since EBV commonly persists in the oropharynx and in B cells for the lifetime of the infected individual.

Differential Diagnosis Whereas ~90% of cases of IM are due to EBV, 5–10% of cases are due to cytomegalovirus (CMV). CMV is the most common cause of heterophile-negative mononucleosis, usually presenting in older patients. IM caused by CMV is associated with a lower frequency of sore throat, splenomegaly, and lymphadenopathy than IM due to EBV. Less common causes of IM include acute infection with *Toxoplasma*, HIV, human herpesvirus 6, and hepatitis viruses as well as drug hypersensitivity reactions. Other diseases that share some of the features of IM include rubella, acute infectious lymphocytosis in children, and lymphoma or leukemia.

TABLE 174-3 TREATMENT OPTIONS FOR POSTTRANSPLANTATION EBV LYMPHOPROLIFERATIVE DISEASE

1. Reduction of immunosuppression, when possible
2. Excision of localized lesions
3. Interferon α
4. Monoclonal antibody to CD20 (rituximab)
5. Radiation therapy (especially for CNS lesions)
6. For stem cell transplant recipients: donor lymphocyte infusions or donor EBV-specific cytotoxic T cell infusions[a]
7. For solid organ transplant recipients: autologous or HLA-matched, EBV-specific, cytotoxic T cell infusions[a]
8. Cytotoxic chemotherapy

[a]Infused T cells must be HLA matched; lymphoproliferative lesions are usually of donor origin for stem cell transplant recipients and of recipient origin for solid organ transplant recipients.

℞ EBV-ASSOCIATED DISEASE

Therapy for IM consists of supportive measures, with rest and analgesia. Excessive physical activity during the first month should be avoided to reduce the possibility of splenic rupture, which necessitates splenectomy. Glucocorticoid therapy is not indicated for uncomplicated IM and in fact may predispose to bacterial superinfection. Prednisone (40–60 mg/d for 2–3 days, with subsequent tapering of the dose over 1–2 weeks) has been used for the prevention of airway obstruction in patients with severe tonsillar hypertrophy, for autoimmune hemolytic anemia, and for severe thrombocytopenia. Glucocorticoids have also been administered to a few selected patients with severe malaise and fever and to patients with severe CNS or cardiac disease. Acyclovir has had no significant clinical impact on IM in controlled trials. In one study, the combination of acyclovir and prednisolone had no significant effect on the duration of symptoms of IM.

Acyclovir, at a dosage of 400–800 mg five times daily, has been effective for the treatment of oral hairy leukoplakia (despite common relapses). The posttransplantation EBV lymphoproliferative syndrome (Chap. 126) generally does not respond to antiviral therapy. When possible, therapy should be directed toward reduction of immunosuppression (Table 174-3). IFN α or antibody to CD20 has been effective in some cases. Infusions of donor lymphocytes are often effective for stem cell transplant recipients, although graft-versus-host disease can occur. Infusions of EBV-specific cytotoxic T cells have been used to prevent EBV lymphoproliferative disease in high-risk settings as well as to treat the disease. Infusion of autologous EBV-specific cytotoxic T lymphocytes has shown promise in small studies of patients with nasopharyngeal carcinoma and Hodgkin's disease. Treatment of two cases of X-linked lymphoproliferative syndrome with antibody to CD20 resulted in a successful outcome of what otherwise would probably have been fatal acute EBV infection.

PREVENTION

The isolation of patients with IM is unnecessary. Vaccines directed against the major EBV glycoprotein have been effective in animal studies and are undergoing clinical trials.

FURTHER READINGS

AUWAERTER PG: Infectious mononucleosis in middle age. JAMA 281:454, 1999

BOLLARD CM et al: Cytotoxic T lymphocyte therapy for Epstein-Barr virus positive Hodgkin's disease. J Exp Med 200:1623, 2004

CHOQUET S et al: Efficacy and safety of rituximab in B-cell post-transplant lymphoproliferative disorders: Results of a prospective multicenter phase 2 study. Blood 107:3053, 2006

COHEN JI: Epstein-Barr virus infection. N Engl J Med 343:481, 2000

FAFI-KREMER S et al: Long term shedding of infectious Epstein-Barr virus after infectious mononucleosis. J Infect Dis 191:985, 2005

HAQUE T et al: Allogeneic cytotoxic T-cell therapy for EBV-positive posttransplantation lymphoproliferative disease: results of a phase 2 multicenter clinical trial. Blood 110:1123, 2007

MILNONE MC et al: Treatment of primary Epstein-Barr virus infection in patients with X-linked lymphoproliferative disease using B-cell-directed therapy. Blood 105:994, 2005

TORRE D, TAMBINI R: Acyclovir for treatment of infectious mononucleosis: A meta-analysis. Scand J Infect Dis 31:543, 1999

WILLIAMS H, CRAWFORD DH: Epstein-Barr virus: The impact of scientific advances on clinical practice. Blood 107:862, 2006

175 Cytomegalovirus and Human Herpesvirus Types 6, 7, and 8

Martin S. Hirsch

CYTOMEGALOVIRUS

DEFINITION

Cytomegalovirus (CMV), which was initially isolated from patients with congenital cytomegalic inclusion disease, is now recognized as an important pathogen in all age groups. In addition to inducing severe birth defects, CMV causes a wide spectrum of disorders in older children and adults, ranging from an asymptomatic, subclinical infection to a mononucleosis syndrome in healthy individuals to disseminated disease in immunocompromised patients. Human CMV is one of several related species-specific viruses that cause similar diseases in various animals. All are associated with the production of characteristic enlarged cells—hence the name *cytomegalovirus*.

CMV, a β-herpesvirus, has double-strand DNA, four species of mRNA, a protein capsid, and a lipoprotein envelope. Like other herpesviruses, CMV demonstrates icosahedral symmetry, replicates in the cell nucleus, and can cause either a lytic and productive or a latent infection. CMV can be distinguished from other herpesviruses by certain biologic properties, such as host range and type of cytopathology. Viral replication is associated with production of large intranuclear inclusions and smaller cytoplasmic inclusions. CMV appears to replicate in a variety of cell types in vivo; in tissue culture it grows preferentially in fibroblasts. Although there is little evidence that CMV is oncogenic in vivo, it does transform fibroblasts in rare instances, and genomic transforming fragments have been identified.

EPIDEMIOLOGY

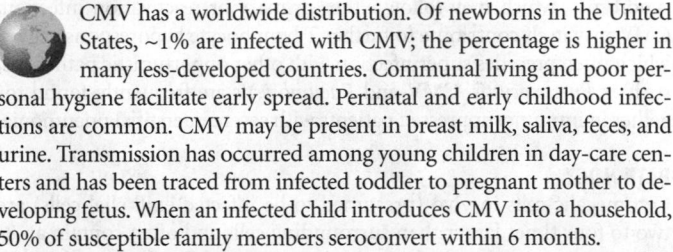 CMV has a worldwide distribution. Of newborns in the United States, ~1% are infected with CMV; the percentage is higher in many less-developed countries. Communal living and poor personal hygiene facilitate early spread. Perinatal and early childhood infections are common. CMV may be present in breast milk, saliva, feces, and urine. Transmission has occurred among young children in day-care centers and has been traced from infected toddler to pregnant mother to developing fetus. When an infected child introduces CMV into a household, 50% of susceptible family members seroconvert within 6 months.

CMV is not readily spread by casual contact but rather requires repeated or prolonged intimate exposure for transmission. In late adolescence and young adulthood, CMV is often transmitted sexually, and asymptomatic carriage in semen or cervical secretions is common. Antibody to CMV is present at detectable levels in a high proportion of sexually active men and women, who may harbor several strains simultaneously. Transfusion of whole blood or certain blood products containing viable leukocytes may transmit CMV, with a frequency of 0.14–10% per unit transfused.

Once infected, an individual generally carries CMV for life. The infection usually remains silent. However, CMV reactivation syndromes develop frequently when T lymphocyte–mediated immunity is compromised—for example, after organ transplantation or in association with lymphoid neoplasms and certain acquired immunodeficiencies (in particular, HIV infection; Chap. 182). Most primary CMV infections in organ transplant recipients (Chap. 126) result from transmission in the graft itself. In CMV-seropositive transplant recipients, infection results from reactivation of latent virus or, less commonly, from reinfection by a new strain. CMV infection may be associated with coronary artery stenosis following heart transplantation or coronary angioplasty, but this association requires further validation.

PATHOGENESIS

Congenital CMV infection can result from either primary or reactivation infection of the mother. However, clinical disease in the fetus or newborn is almost exclusively related to primary maternal infection (Table 175-1). The factors determining the severity of congenital infection are unknown; a deficient capacity to produce precipitating antibodies and to mount T cell responses to CMV is associated with relatively severe disease.

Primary infection in late childhood or adulthood is often associated with a vigorous T lymphocyte response that may contribute to the development of a mononucleosis syndrome similar to that observed after Epstein-Barr virus (EBV) infection (Chap. 174). The hallmark of such infection is the appearance of atypical lymphocytes in the peripheral blood; these cells are predominantly activated CD8+ T lymphocytes. Polyclonal activation of B cells by CMV contributes to the development of rheumatoid factors and other autoantibodies during mononucleosis.

Once acquired, CMV persists indefinitely in host tissues. The sites of persistent infection probably include multiple cell types and various organs. Transmission via blood transfusion or organ transplantation is due to silent infections in these tissues. Autopsy studies suggest that salivary glands and bowel may be sites of latent infection.

If the host's T cell responses become compromised by disease or by iatrogenic immunosuppression, latent virus can be reactivated to cause a variety of syndromes. Chronic antigenic stimulation in the presence of immunosuppression (for example, after tissue transplantation) appears to be an ideal setting for CMV activation and CMV-induced disease. Certain particularly potent suppressants of T cell immunity (e.g., antithymocyte globulin) are associated with a high rate of clinical CMV syndromes, which may follow either primary or reactivation infection. CMV may itself contribute to further T lymphocyte hyporesponsiveness, which often precedes superinfection with other opportunistic pathogens, such as *Pneumocystis*. CMV and *Pneumocystis* are frequently found together in immunosuppressed patients with severe interstitial pneumonia.

PATHOLOGY

Cytomegalic cells in vivo (presumed to be infected epithelial cells) are two to four times larger than surrounding cells and often contain an 8- to 10-μm intranuclear inclusion that is eccentrically placed and is surrounded by a clear halo, producing an "owl's eye" appearance. Smaller granular cytoplasmic inclusions are demonstrated occasionally. Cytomegalic cells are found in a wide variety of organs, including the salivary gland, lung, liver, kidney, intestine, pancreas, adrenal gland, and central nervous system.

The cellular inflammatory response to infection consists of plasma cells, lymphocytes, and monocyte-macrophages. Granulomatous reactions occasionally develop, particularly in the liver. Immunopathologic reactions may contribute to CMV disease. Immune complexes have been detected in infected infants, sometimes in association with CMV-related glomerulopathies. Immune-complex glomerulopathy has also been observed in some CMV-infected patients after renal transplantation.

Population	Risk Factors	Principal Syndromes	Treatment	Prevention
Fetus	Primary maternal infection/early pregnancy	Cytomegalic inclusion disease	None (?ganciclovir)	Avoidance of exposure or maternal treatment with CMV immunoglobulin during pregnancy
Organ transplant recipient	Serostatus of donor and recipient; immunosuppressive regimen; degree of rejection	Febrile leukopenia; pneumonia; gastrointestinal disease	Ganciclovir or valganciclovir	Donor matching; prophylaxis or preemptive therapy with ganciclovir or valganciclovir
Bone marrow transplant recipient	Graft-vs.-host disease; older age; seropositive recipient; viremia	Pneumonia; gastrointestinal disease	Ganciclovir plus CMV immunoglobulin	Donor matching; prophylaxis or preemptive therapy with ganciclovir or valganciclovir
Person with AIDS	<100 CD4+ T cells per microliter; CMV seropositivity	Retinitis; gastrointestinal disease; neurologic disease	Ganciclovir, valganciclovir, foscarnet, or cidofovir	Oral valganciclovir

TABLE 175-1 CMV DISEASE IN THE IMMUNOCOMPROMISED HOST

CLINICAL MANIFESTATIONS

Congenital CMV Infection Fetal infections range from inapparent to severe and disseminated. Cytomegalic inclusion disease develops in ~5% of infected fetuses and is seen almost exclusively in infants born to mothers who develop primary infections during pregnancy. Petechiae, hepatosplenomegaly, and jaundice are the most common presenting features (60–80% of cases). Microcephaly with or without cerebral calcifications, intrauterine growth retardation, and prematurity are reported in 30–50% of cases. Inguinal hernias and chorioretinitis are less common. Laboratory abnormalities include elevated alanine aminotransferase levels, thrombocytopenia, conjugated hyperbilirubinemia, hemolysis, and elevated cerebrospinal fluid protein levels. The prognosis for severely infected infants is poor; the mortality rate is 20–30%, and few survivors escape intellectual or hearing difficulties later in childhood. The differential diagnosis of cytomegalic inclusion disease in infants includes syphilis, rubella, toxoplasmosis, infection with herpes simplex virus or enterovirus, and bacterial sepsis.

Most congenital CMV infections are clinically inapparent at birth. Of asymptomatically infected infants, 5–25% develop significant psychomotor, hearing, ocular, or dental abnormalities over the next several years.

Perinatal CMV Infection The newborn may acquire CMV at delivery by passage through an infected birth canal or by postnatal contact with infected breast milk or other maternal secretions. Of infants who are breast-fed for >1 month by seropositive mothers, 40–60% become infected. Iatrogenic transmission can result from neonatal blood transfusion; screening of blood products before transfusion into low-birth-weight seronegative infants or seronegative pregnant women decreases risk.

The great majority of infants infected at or after delivery remain asymptomatic. However, protracted interstitial pneumonitis has been associated with perinatally acquired CMV infection, particularly in premature infants, and occasionally has been accompanied by infection with *Chlamydia trachomatis*, *Pneumocystis*, or *Ureaplasma urealyticum*. Poor weight gain, adenopathy, rash, hepatitis, anemia, and atypical lymphocytosis may also be found, and CMV excretion often persists for months or years.

CMV Mononucleosis The most common clinical manifestation of CMV infection in normal hosts beyond the neonatal period is a heterophile antibody–negative mononucleosis syndrome, which may develop spontaneously or follow transfusion of leukocyte-containing blood products. Although the syndrome occurs at all ages, it most often involves sexually active young adults. With incubation periods of 20–60 days, the illness generally lasts for 2–6 weeks. Prolonged high fevers, sometimes with chills, profound fatigue, and malaise, characterize this disorder. Myalgias, headache, and splenomegaly are common, but in CMV (as opposed to EBV) mononucleosis, exudative pharyngitis and cervical lymphadenopathy are rare. Occasional patients develop rubelliform rashes, often after exposure to ampicillin or certain other antibiotics. Less common are interstitial or segmental pneumonia, myocarditis, pleuritis, arthritis, and encephalitis. In rare cases, Guillain-Barré syndrome complicates CMV mononucleosis. The characteristic laboratory abnormality is relative lymphocytosis in peripheral blood, with >10% atypical lymphocytes. Total leukocyte counts may be low, normal, or markedly elevated. Although significant jaundice is uncommon, serum aminotransferase and alkaline phosphatase levels are often moderately elevated. Heterophile antibodies are absent; however, transient immunologic abnormalities are common and may include the presence of cryoglobulins, rheumatoid factors, cold agglutinins, and antinuclear antibodies. Hemolytic anemia, thrombocytopenia, and granulocytopenia complicate recovery in rare instances.

Most patients recover without sequelae, although postviral asthenia may persist for months. The excretion of CMV in urine, genital secretions, and/or saliva often continues for months or years. Rarely, CMV infection is fatal in immunocompetent hosts; survivors can have recurrent episodes of fever and malaise, sometimes associated with autonomic nervous system dysfunction (e.g., attacks of sweating or flushing).

CMV Infection in the Immunocompromised Host (Table 175-1) CMV appears to be the most common and important viral pathogen complicating organ transplantation (Chap. 126). In recipients of kidney, heart, lung, and liver transplants, CMV induces a variety of syndromes, including fever and leukopenia, hepatitis, pneumonitis, esophagitis, gastritis, colitis, and retinitis. CMV disease may be an independent risk factor for both graft loss and death. The period of maximal risk is between 1 and 4 months after transplantation, although retinitis may be a later complication. Disease likelihood and viral replication levels generally are greater after primary infection than after reactivation. In addition, molecular studies indicate that seropositive transplant recipients are susceptible to reinfection with donor-derived, genotypically variant CMV, and such infection often results in disease. Reactivation infection, although common, is less likely than primary infection to be important clinically. The risk of clinical disease is related to various factors, such as the degree of immunosuppression; the use of antibodies to T cell receptors; and co-infection with other pathogens. The transplanted organ is particularly vulnerable as a target for CMV infection; thus, there is a tendency for CMV hepatitis to follow liver transplantation and for CMV pneumonitis to follow lung transplantation.

CMV pneumonia occurs in 15–20% of bone marrow transplant recipients; the case-fatality rate is 84–88%, although the risk of severe disease may be reduced by prophylaxis or preemptive therapy with antiviral drugs. The risk is greatest 5–13 weeks after transplantation, and identified risk factors include certain types of immunosuppressive therapy, acute graft-versus-host disease, older age, viremia, and pretransplantation seropositivity.

CMV is an important pathogen in patients with advanced HIV infection (Chap. 182), in whom it often causes retinitis or disseminated disease, particularly when peripheral-blood CD4+ T cell counts fall below 50–100/μL. As treatment for underlying HIV infection has improved, the incidence of serious CMV infections (e.g., retinitis) has decreased. However, during the first few weeks after institution of highly active antiretroviral therapy, acute flare-ups of CMV retinitis may occur secondary to an immune reconstitution inflammatory syndrome.

Syndromes produced by CMV in immunocompromised hosts often begin with prolonged fever, malaise, anorexia, fatigue, night sweats, and arthralgias or myalgias. Liver function abnormalities, leukopenia, thrombocytopenia, and atypical lymphocytosis may be observed during these episodes. The development of tachypnea, hypoxia, and unproductive cough signals respiratory involvement. Radiologic examination of the lung often shows bilateral interstitial or reticulonodular infiltrates that begin in the periphery of the lower lobes and spread centrally and superiorly; localized segmental, nodular, or alveolar patterns are less common. The differential diagnosis includes *Pneumocystis* infection; other viral, bacterial, or fungal infections; pulmonary hemorrhage; and injury secondary to irradiation or to treatment with cytotoxic drugs.

Gastrointestinal CMV involvement may be localized or extensive and almost exclusively affects compromised hosts. Ulcers of the esophagus, stomach, small intestine, or colon may result in bleeding or perforation. CMV infection may lead to exacerbations of underlying ulcerative colitis. Hepatitis occurs frequently, particularly after liver transplantation, and acalculous cholecystitis and adrenalitis have been described.

CMV rarely causes meningoencephalitis in otherwise-healthy individuals. Two forms of CMV encephalitis are seen in patients with AIDS. One resembles HIV encephalitis and presents as progressive dementia; the other is a ventriculoencephalitis characterized by cranial-nerve deficits, nystagmus, disorientation, lethargy, and ventriculomegaly. In immunocompromised patients, CMV can also cause subacute progressive polyradiculopathy, which is often reversible if recognized and treated promptly.

CMV retinitis is an important cause of blindness in immunocompromised patients, particularly patients with advanced AIDS (Chap. 182). Early lesions consist of small, opaque, white areas of granular retinal necrosis that spread in a centrifugal manner and are later accompanied by hemorrhages, vessel sheathing, and retinal edema (Fig. 175-1). CMV retinopathy must be distinguished from that due to other conditions, including toxoplasmosis, candidiasis, and herpes simplex virus infection.

Fatal CMV infections are often associated with persistent viremia and the involvement of multiple organ systems. Progressive pulmonary infiltrates, pancytopenia, hyperamylasemia, and hypotension are characteristic features that are frequently found in conjunction with a terminal bacterial, fungal, or protozoan superinfection. Extensive adrenal necrosis with CMV inclusions is often documented at autopsy, as is CMV involvement of many other organs.

DIAGNOSIS

The diagnosis of CMV infection usually cannot be made reliably on clinical grounds alone. Isolation of CMV or detection of its antigens or DNA in appropriate clinical specimens is the preferred approach. Virus excretion or viremia is readily detected by culture of appropriate specimens on human fibroblast monolayers. If CMV titers are high, as is common in congenital disseminated infection and in patients with AIDS, characteristic cytopathic effects may be detected within a few days. However, in some situations (e.g., CMV mononucleosis), viral titers are low, and cytopathic effects may take several weeks to appear. Many laboratories expedite diagnosis with an overnight tissue-culture

FIGURE 175-1 Cytomegalovirus infection in a patient with AIDS may appear as an arcuate zone of retinitis with hemorrhages and optic disk swelling. Often CMV is confined to the retinal periphery, beyond view of the direct ophthalmoscope.

method (shell vial assay) involving centrifugation and an immunocytochemical detection technique employing monoclonal antibodies to an immediate-early CMV antigen. Isolation of virus from urine or saliva does not, by itself, constitute proof of acute infection, since excretion from these sites may continue for months or years after illness. Detection of viremia is a better predictor of acute infection.

Detection of CMV antigens (pp65) in peripheral-blood leukocytes or of CMV DNA in blood or tissues may hasten diagnosis. Such assays may yield a positive result several days earlier than culture methods. The most sensitive way to detect CMV in blood or other fluids may be by amplifying CMV DNA by polymerase chain reaction (PCR). PCR detection of CMV DNA in blood may predict the risk for disease progression, and PCR detection of CMV DNA in cerebrospinal fluid is useful in the diagnosis of CMV encephalitis or polyradiculopathy.

A variety of serologic assays detect increases in titers of antibody to CMV antigens. An increased antibody level may not be detectable for up to 4 weeks after primary infection, and titers often remain high for years after infection. For this reason, single-sample antibody determinations are of no value in assessing the acuteness of infection. Detection of CMV-specific IgM is sometimes useful in the diagnosis of recent or active infection; circulating rheumatoid factors may result in occasional false-positive IgM tests.

Rx CYTOMEGALOVIRUS INFECTION

Several measures are useful for the prevention of CMV infection in high-risk patients. The use of blood from seronegative donors or of blood that has been frozen, thawed, and deglycerolized greatly decreases the rate of transfusion-associated transmission. Matching of organ or bone marrow transplants by CMV serology, with exclusive use of organs from seronegative donors in seronegative recipients, reduces rates of primary infection after transplantation. Both live attenuated and CMV subunit vaccines have been evaluated, but neither is close to approval for general use.

CMV immune or hyperimmune globulin has been reported (1) to reduce rates of CMV-associated syndromes and of fungal or parasitic superinfections among seronegative renal transplant recipients and (2) to prevent congenital CMV infection in infants of women with primary infection during pregnancy. Studies in bone marrow transplant recipients have produced conflicting results. Prophylactic acyclovir or valacyclovir may reduce rates of CMV infection and disease in certain seronegative renal transplant recipients, although neither drug is effective in the treatment of active CMV disease.

Ganciclovir is a guanosine derivative that has considerably more activity against CMV than its congener acyclovir. After intracellular conversion by a viral phosphotransferase encoded by CMV gene region UL97, ganciclovir triphosphate is a selective inhibitor of CMV DNA polymerase. Several clinical studies have indicated response rates of 70–90% among patients with AIDS who are given ganciclovir for the treatment of CMV retinitis or colitis. In bone marrow transplant recipients with CMV pneumonia, ganciclovir is less effective when given alone, but it elicits a favorable clinical response 50–70% of the time when combined with CMV immune globulin. Prophylactic or suppressive ganciclovir may be useful in high-risk bone marrow or organ transplant recipients (e.g., those who are CMV-seropositive before transplantation or who are CMV culture–positive afterward). In many patients with AIDS, persistently low CD4+ T cell counts, and CMV disease, clinical and virologic relapses occur promptly if treatment with ganciclovir is discontinued. Therefore, prolonged maintenance regimens are recommended for such patients. Resistance to ganciclovir is common among patients treated for >3 months and is usually related to mutations in the CMV UL97 gene.

Valganciclovir is an orally bioavailable prodrug that is rapidly metabolized to ganciclovir in intestinal tissues and the liver. Approximately 60% of an oral dose of valganciclovir is absorbed. An oral valganciclovir dose of 900 mg results in ganciclovir blood levels similar to those obtained with an IV ganciclovir dose of 5 mg/kg. Oral valganciclovir appears to be as effective as IV ganciclovir for both CMV retinitis induction and maintenance regimens. Furthermore, the adverse-event profiles and rates of resistance development for the two drugs are similar.

Ganciclovir or valganciclovir therapy for CMV retinitis consists of a 14- to 21-day induction course (5 mg/kg IV twice daily for ganciclovir or 900 mg twice daily for valganciclovir) followed by prolonged maintenance therapy.

For parenteral maintenance, the ganciclovir dose is 5 mg/kg daily or 6 mg/kg 5 days per week; for oral maintenance, 900 mg of valganciclovir once daily is recommended. Peripheral-blood neutropenia develops in 16–29% of treated patients but may be ameliorated by granulocyte colony-stimulating factor or granulocyte-macrophage colony-stimulating factor. Discontinuation of maintenance therapy should be considered in patients with AIDS who, while receiving antiretroviral therapy, have a sustained (>6-month) increase in CD4+ T cell counts to >100–150/μL.

Ganciclovir may also be administered via a slow-release pellet sutured into the eye. Although this intraocular device provides good local protection, contralateral eye disease and disseminated disease are not affected, and early retinal detachment is possible. A combination of intraocular and systemic therapy may be better than the intraocular implant alone.

Foscarnet (sodium phosphonoformate) inhibits CMV DNA polymerase. Because this agent does not require phosphorylation to be active, it is also effective against most ganciclovir-resistant isolates. Foscarnet is less well tolerated than ganciclovir and causes considerable toxicity, including renal dysfunction, hypomagnesemia, hypokalemia, hypocalcemia, genital ulcers, dysuria, nausea, and paresthesia. Moreover, foscarnet administration requires the use of an infusion pump and close clinical monitoring. With aggressive hydration and dose adjustments for renal dysfunction, the toxicity of foscarnet can be reduced. The use of foscarnet should be avoided when a saline load cannot be tolerated (e.g., in cardiomyopathy). The approved induction regimen is 60 mg/kg every 8 h for 2 weeks, although 90 mg/kg every 12 h is equally effective and no more toxic. Maintenance infusions should deliver 90–120 mg/kg once daily. No oral preparation is available. Foscarnet-resistant virus may emerge during extended therapy.

Cidofovir is a nucleotide analogue with a long intracellular half-life that allows intermittent IV administration. Induction regimens of 5 mg/kg weekly for 2 weeks are followed by maintenance regimens of 3–5 mg/kg every 2 weeks. Cidofovir can cause severe nephrotoxicity through dose-dependent proximal tubular cell injury; however, this adverse effect can be tempered somewhat by saline hydration and probenecid.

It is not clear whether universal prophylaxis or preemptive therapy is the preferable approach in CMV-seropositive immunocompromised hosts. Both ganciclovir and valganciclovir have been used successfully for prophylaxis and preemptive therapy in transplant recipients. For patients with advanced HIV infection (CD4+ T cell counts of <50/μL), some authorities have advocated prophylaxis with oral ganciclovir or valganciclovir. However, side effects, lack of proven benefit, possible induction of viral resistance, and high cost have precluded the wide acceptance of this practice. Preemptive ganciclovir or valganciclovir therapy based on detection of CMV viremia by either antigenemia or PCR techniques is under study.

HUMAN HERPESVIRUS TYPES 6, 7, AND 8

Human herpesvirus (HHV) type 6 was first isolated in 1986 from peripheral-blood leukocytes of six persons with various lymphoproliferative disorders. The virus has a worldwide distribution, and two genetically distinct variants (HHV-6A and HHV-6B) are now recognized. HHV-6 appears to be transmitted by saliva and possibly by genital secretions.

Infection with HHV-6 frequently occurs during infancy as maternal antibody wanes. The peak age of acquisition is 9–21 months; by 24 months, seropositivity rates approach 80%. Older siblings appear to serve as a source of transmission. Congenital infection may also occur. Most infected children develop symptoms (fever, fussiness, and diarrhea). A minority develop exanthem subitum (roseola infantum), a common illness characterized by fever with subsequent rash. Approximately 10–20% of febrile seizures without rash during infancy are caused by HHV-6.

In older age groups, HHV-6 has been associated with mononucleosis syndromes, focal encephalitis, and (in immunocompromised hosts) pneumonitis and disseminated disease. In transplant recipients, HHV-6 infection may be associated with similar syndromes and with graft dysfunction. High plasma loads of HHV-6 DNA in stem cell transplant recipients are associated with allelic-mismatched donors, use of steroids, delayed monocyte and platelet engraftment, development of limbic encephalitis, and increased all-cause mortality. Like many other viruses, HHV-6 has been implicated in the pathogenesis of multiple sclerosis, although further study is needed to distinguish between association and etiology.

HHV-7 was isolated in 1990 from T lymphocytes from the peripheral blood of a healthy 26-year-old man. The virus is frequently acquired during childhood, albeit at a later age than HHV-6. HHV-7 is commonly present in saliva, which is presumed to be the principal source of infection; breast milk can also carry the virus. Viremia can be associated with either primary or reactivation infection. The most common clinical manifestations of childhood HHV-7 infections are fever and seizures. Some children present with respiratory or gastrointestinal signs and symptoms. An association has been made between HHV-7 and pityriasis rosea, but evidence is insufficient to indicate a causal relationship.

HHV-6, HHV-7, and CMV infections may cluster in transplant recipients, making it difficult to sort out the roles of the various agents in individual clinical syndromes. HHV-6 and HHV-7 appear to be susceptible to ganciclovir and foscarnet, although definitive evidence of clinical responses is lacking.

Unique herpesvirus-like DNA sequences were reported during 1994 and 1995 in tissues derived from Kaposi's sarcoma (KS) and body cavity-based lymphoma occurring in patients with AIDS. The virus from which these sequences were derived is designated HHV-8 or Kaposi's sarcoma-associated herpesvirus (KSHV). HHV-8, which infects certain B lymphocytes and endothelium-derived spindle cells, appears to be causally related not only to KS but also to a subgroup of AIDS-related B cell body cavity-based lymphomas (primary effusion lymphomas) and to multicentric Castleman's disease, a lymphoproliferative disorder of B cells. Initial suggestions that HHV-8 is associated with primary pulmonary hypertension have not been confirmed by subsequent studies.

Unlike other herpesvirus infections, HHV-8 infection is much more common in some geographic areas (e.g., central and southern Africa) than in others (North America, Asia, northern Europe). In high-prevalence areas, infection occurs in childhood, seropositivity is associated with having a seropositive mother or (to a lesser extent) older sibling, and HHV-8 may be transmitted in saliva. In low-prevalence areas, infections typically occur in adults, probably with sexual transmission. Concurrent epidemics of HIV-1 and HHV-8 infections among certain populations (e.g., homosexual and bisexual men) in the late 1970s and early 1980s appear to have resulted in the frequent association of AIDS and KS. Transmission of HHV-8 may also be associated with organ transplantation and injection drug use.

Primary HHV-8 infection in immunocompetent children may manifest as fever and maculopapular rash. Among individuals with intact immunity, chronic asymptomatic infection is the rule, and neoplastic disorders generally develop only after subsequent immunocompromise. Immunocompromised persons with primary infection may present with fever, splenomegaly, lymphoid hyperplasia, pancytopenia, or rapid-onset KS. Quantitative analysis of HHV-8 DNA suggests a predominance of latently infected cells in KS lesions and frequent lytic replication in multicentric Castleman's disease.

Effective antiretroviral therapy for HIV-infected individuals has led to a marked reduction in rates of KS among persons dually infected with HHV-8 and HIV in resource-rich areas. HHV-8 itself is susceptible in vitro to ganciclovir, foscarnet, and cidofovir, although clinical evidence for benefit of these agents is lacking.

FURTHER READINGS

ASAHI-OZAKI Y et al: Quantitative analysis of Kaposi sarcoma–associated herpesvirus (KSHV) in KSHV-associated diseases. J Infect Dis 193:773, 2006

CANNON MJ et al: Blood-borne and sexual transmission of human herpesvirus 8 in women with or at risk for human immunodeficiency virus infection. N Engl J Med 344:637, 2001

HALL CB et al: Characteristics and acquisition of human herpesvirus (HHV)-7 infections in relation to infection with HHV-6. J Infect Dis 193:1063, 2006

HEINEMAN TC et al: A phase 1 study of 4 live, recombinant human cytomegalovirus Towne/Toledo chimeric vaccines. J Infect Dis 193:1350, 2006

KALIL AC et al: Meta-analysis: The efficacy of strategies to prevent organ disease by cytomegalovirus in solid organ transplant recipients. Ann Intern Med 143:870, 2005

MARTIN DF et al: A controlled trial of valganciclovir as induction therapy for cytomegalovirus retinitis. N Engl J Med 346:1119, 2002

MBULAITEYE S et al: Molecular evidence for mother-to-child transmission of Kaposi sarcoma–associated herpesvirus in Uganda and K1 gene evolution within the host. J Infect Dis 193:1250, 2006

NIGRO G et al: Passive immunization during pregnancy for congenital cytomegalovirus infection. N Engl J Med 353:1350, 2005

OGATA M et al: Human herpesvirus 6 DNA in plasma after allogeneic stem cell transplantation: Incidence and clinical significance. J Infect Dis 193:68, 2006

ZERR DM et al: A population-based study of primary human herpesvirus 6 infection. N Engl J Med 352:768, 2005

176 Molluscum Contagiosum, Monkeypox, and Other Poxviruses, Excluding Smallpox Virus

Fred Wang

The poxvirus family includes a large number of related DNA viruses that infect various vertebrate hosts. The poxviruses responsible for infections in humans, along with the main manifestations of these infections, are listed in Table 176-1. Infections with orthopoxviruses—e.g., smallpox (variola major) virus (Chap. 214) or the zoonotic monkeypox virus—can result in systemic, potentially lethal human disease. Other poxvirus infections cause primarily localized skin disease in humans.

MOLLUSCUM CONTAGIOSUM

Molluscum contagiosum virus is an obligate human pathogen that causes distinctive proliferative skin lesions. These lesions measure 2–5 mm in diameter and are pearly, flesh-colored, and umbilicated, with a characteristic dimple at the center (Fig. 176-1). A relative lack of inflammation and necrosis distinguishes these proliferative lesions from other poxvirus lesions. Lesions may be found—singly or in clusters—anywhere on the body except on the palms and soles and may be associated with an eczematous rash.

Molluscum contagiosum is the most common human disease resulting from poxvirus infection and is transmitted by close contact, including sexual intercourse. Swimming pools are a common vector for transmission. Atopy and compromise of skin integrity increase the risk of

TABLE 176-1   POXVIRUSES AND HUMAN INFECTIONS

Genus	Species	Human Disease
Orthopoxvirus	Variola[a]	Smallpox, systemic
	Monkeypox	Smallpox-like, systemic
	Vaccinia	Local pox lesion, occasionally systemic
	Cowpox	Local pox lesions
Molluscipoxvirus	Molluscum contagiosum	Molluscum contagiosum, multiple cutaneous lesions
Parapoxvirus	Orf	Contagious pustular dermatitis, local pox lesions
	Pseudocowpox	Milker's nodule, local pox lesions
Yatapoxvirus	Tanapox	Local pox lesions

[a]See Chap. 214.

FIGURE 176-1 Molluscum contagiosum is a cutaneous poxvirus infection characterized by multiple umbilicated flesh-colored or hypopigmented papules.

infection. The incubation period ranges from 2 weeks to 6 months, with an average of 2–7 weeks. In most cases, the disease is self-limited and regresses spontaneously after 3–4 months in immunocompetent hosts. There are no systemic complications, but skin lesions may persist for 3–5 years. Molluscum contagiosum develops especially often in association with advanced HIV infection; the prevalence is 5–18% among HIV-infected patients (Chap. 182). The disease is often more generalized, severe, and persistent in AIDS patients than in other groups, frequently involving the face and upper body. Paradoxically, rates of molluscum contagiosum are reportedly elevated among patients receiving antiretroviral therapy. Moreover, the disease can be exacerbated in the immune reconstitution inflammatory syndrome (IRIS) associated with the initiation of antiretroviral therapy. Extensive molluscum contagiosum has also been reported in conjunction with other types of immunodeficiency.

The diagnosis of molluscum contagiosum is typically made by its clinical presentation and can be confirmed by histologic demonstration of the cytoplasmic eosinophilic inclusions, or *molluscum bodies*, that are characteristic of poxvirus replication. Molluscum contagiosum virus cannot be propagated in vitro, but electron microscopy and molecular studies can be used for its identification.

There is no specific systemic treatment for molluscum contagiosum, but a variety of techniques for physical ablation have been used. Cidofovir displays in vitro activity against many poxviruses, including smallpox virus and molluscum contagiosum virus, and case reports suggest that parenteral or topical cidofovir may have some efficacy in the treatment of recalcitrant molluscum contagiosum in immunosuppressed hosts.

MONKEYPOX

Although monkeypox virus was named after the animal from which it was originally isolated, rodents are the primary viral reservoir. Human infections with monkeypox virus typically occur in Africa when humans come into direct contact with infected animals. Human disease is rare and is characterized by a systemic illness and a vesicular rash similar to those of variola. The clinical presentation of monkeypox can be confused with that of the more

common varicella-zoster virus infection (Chap. 173). Compared with the lesions of this herpesvirus infection, monkeypox lesions tend to be more uniform (i.e., in the same stage of development), diffuse, and peripheral in distribution. Lymphadenopathy is a prominent feature of monkeypox infection.

The first outbreak of human monkeypox infection in the Western Hemisphere occurred in the midwestern United States during May and June 2003, when more than 70 cases were reported, of which 35 were laboratory confirmed. The outbreak was linked to contact with pet prairie dogs that had become infected while being housed with rodents imported from Ghana. Patients presented most frequently with fever, rash, and lymphadenopathy ~12 days after exposure. The median durations of fever and rash were 8 and 12 days, respectively. Of the nine patients who were hospitalized, five were judged to be severely ill, but there were no deaths. Smallpox vaccination can provide cross-reactive immunity to monkeypox infection; nevertheless, there were no significant clinical differences between vaccinated and unvaccinated individuals in this outbreak. Additional studies of people exposed in the outbreak detected subclinical infection in a few vaccinated individuals—an observation suggesting the possibility of long-term vaccine protection. The risk of human disease from animal orthopoxvirus infections may increase as smallpox immunity wanes in the general population and the popularity of exotic animals as household pets grows.

OTHER ZOONOTIC POXVIRUS INFECTIONS

Orf virus and *pseudocowpox* virus are parapoxviruses that naturally infect sheep and cattle. Direct contact with infected animals can result in human infections, typically on the hands, with the development of a nodular, highly vascular proliferative lesion that may ulcerate. Human orf virus infection is also called *ecthyma contagiosum*, and human pseudocowpox virus infection causes "milker's nodules."

Zoonotic infection with *cowpox* virus causes painful hemorrhagic lesions, mostly on the hands or face, with fever or flulike symptoms and lymphadenitis. Lesions generally resolve in 6–8 weeks. Human infection with *tanapox* virus occurs after contact with infected monkeys. In most cases, a febrile prodrome is followed by eruption of a single nodular lesion on the exposed area, but multiple lesions have also been reported. The lesions are relatively large, often break down to form an ulcer, and resolve in 5–6 weeks.

FURTHER READINGS

CENTERS FOR DISEASE CONTROL AND PREVENTION: Update: Multistate outbreak of monkeypox—Illinois, Indiana, Kansas, Missouri, Ohio, and Wisconsin, 2003. MMWR 52:642, 2003

DHAR AD et al: Tanapox infection in a college student. N Engl J Med 350:361, 2004

HAMMARLUND E et al: Multiple diagnostic techniques identify previously vaccinated individuals with protective immunity against monkeypox. Nat Med 11:1005, 2005

HUHN GD et al: Clinical characteristics of human monkeypox, and risk factors for severe disease. Clin Infect Dis 41:1742, 2005

REED KD et al: The detection of monkeypox in humans in the Western Hemisphere. N Engl J Med 350:342, 2004

177 Parvovirus Infections
Kevin E. Brown

Parvoviruses, members of the family Parvoviridae, are small (diameter, ~22 nm), nonenveloped, icosahedral-shaped viruses with a linear single-stranded DNA genome of ~5000 nucleotides. These viruses are dependent on either rapidly dividing host cells or helper viruses for

replication. At least four types of parvovirus infect humans: parvovirus B19, adeno-associated viruses (AAVs), the recently described PARV4/5 virus, and human bocavirus (HBoV). To date, only B19 has been shown definitively to be a human pathogen.

PARVOVIRUS B19

DEFINITION

B19 is the type member of the genus *Erythrovirus*. On the basis of viral sequence, B19 is divided into three genotypes (designated 1, 2, and 3), but only a single B19 antigenic type has been described. Genotypes 2 and 3 are detected relatively infrequently in Europe and the United States.

EPIDEMIOLOGY

B19 exclusively infects humans, and infection is endemic in virtually all parts of the world. Transmission occurs predominantly via the respiratory route and is followed by the onset of rash and arthralgia. By the age of 15 years, ~ 50% of children have detectable IgG; this figure rises to >90% among the elderly. In pregnant women, the estimated annual seroconversion rate is ~1%. Within households, secondary infection rates approach 50%.

Detection of high-titer B19 in blood is not unusual (see "Pathogenesis," below). Transmission can occur as a result of transfusion, most commonly of pooled components. To reduce the risk of transmission, plasma pools are screened by nucleic acid amplification technology, and high-titer pools are discarded. B19 is resistant to both heat and solvent-detergent inactivation.

PATHOGENESIS

B19 replicates primarily in erythroid progenitors. This specificity is due in part to the limited tissue distribution of the B19 receptor, blood group P antigen (globoside). Infection leads to high-titer viremia, with >10^12 virus particles/mL detectable in the blood at the apex (Fig. 177-1), and virus-induced cytotoxicity results in cessation of red cell production. In immunocompetent individuals, viremia and arrest of erythropoiesis are transient and resolve as the IgM and IgG antibody response is mounted. In individuals with normal erythropoiesis, there is only a minimal drop in hemoglobin levels; however, in those with increased erythropoiesis (especially with hemolytic anemia), this cessation of red cell production can induce a transient crisis with severe anemia

(Fig. 177-1). Similarly, if an individual (or, after maternal infection, a fetus) does not mount a neutralizing antibody response and halt the lytic infection, erythroid production is compromised and chronic anemia develops (Fig. 177-1).

The immune-mediated phase of illness, which begins 2–3 weeks after infection as the IgM response peaks, manifests as the rash of fifth disease together with arthralgia and/or frank arthritis. Low-level B19 DNA can be detected by polymerase chain reaction (PCR) in blood and tissues for months to years after acute infection.

The B19 receptor is found in a variety of other cells and tissues, including megakaryocytes, endothelial cells, placenta, myocardium, and liver. Infection of these tissues by B19 may be responsible for some of the more unusual presentations of the infection. Rare individuals who lack P antigen are naturally resistant to B19 infection.

CLINICAL MANIFESTATIONS

Erythema Infectiosum Most B19 infections are asymptomatic. The main manifestation of symptomatic B19 infection is erythema infectiosum, also known as *fifth disease* or *slapped-cheek disease* (Fig. 177-2). Infection begins with a minor febrile prodrome ~7–10 days after exposure, and the classic facial rash develops several days later. The rash may spread to the extremities in a lacy reticular pattern. However, its intensity and distribution vary, and the B19-induced rash is difficult to distinguish from other viral exanthems. Adults may not exhibit the "slapped-cheek" phenomenon.

Polyarthropathy Syndrome Although uncommon among children, arthropathy occurs in ~50% of adults and is more common among women than among men. The distribution of the affected joints is often symmetrical, with arthralgia affecting the small joints of the hands

FIGURE 177-1 Schematic of the time course of B19 infection in (**A**) normals (erythema infectiosum), (**B**) transient aplastic crisis (TAC), and (**C**) chronic anemia/pure red-cell aplasia (PRCA). (*Reprinted with* *permission from Young and Brown, 2004.*)

FIGURE 177-2 Child with erythema infectiosum, or fifth disease, showing typical "slapped-cheek" appearance. *(Courtesy of Bernard Cohen, Virus Reference Department, Health Protection Agency, London; with permission.)*

and occasionally the ankles, knees, and wrists. Resolution usually occurs within a few weeks, but recurring symptoms can continue for months.

Transient Aplastic Crisis Asymptomatic transient reticulocytopenia occurs in most individuals with B19 infection. However, in patients who depend on continual rapid production of red cells, infection can cause transient aplastic crisis (TAC). Affected individuals include those with hemolytic disorders, hemoglobinopathies, red cell enzymopathies, and autoimmune hemolytic anemias. Patients present with symptoms of severe anemia, and bone marrow examination reveals an absence of erythroid precursors and characteristic giant pronormoblasts.

Pure Red-Cell Aplasia/Chronic Anemia
Chronic B19 infection has been reported in a wide range of immunosuppressed patients, including those with congenital immunodeficiency, AIDS (Chap. 182), lymphoproliferative disorders (especially acute lymphocytic leukemia), and transplantation (Chap. 126). Patients have persistent anemia with reticulocytopenia, absent or low levels of B19 IgG, high levels of B19 DNA in serum, and—in many cases—scattered giant pronormoblasts in bone marrow. Rarely, nonerythroid hematologic lineages are also affected. Transient neutropenia, lymphopenia, and thrombocytopenia (including idiopathic thrombocytopenic purpura) have been observed. B19 occasionally causes a hemophagocytic syndrome.

A recent study in Papua New Guinea, where malaria is endemic, suggested that B19 infection plays a major role in the development of severe anemia. Further studies must determine whether B19 infection contributes to severe anemia in other malarial regions.

Hydrops Fetalis B19 infection during pregnancy can lead to hydrops fetalis and/or fetal loss. The risk of transplacental fetal infection is ~30%, and the risk of fetal loss (predominantly early in the second trimester) is ~9%. The risk of congenital infection is <1%. Although B19 does not appear to be teratogenic, anecdotal cases of eye damage and CNS abnormalities have been reported. Cases of congenital anemia have also been described. B19 probably causes 10–20% of all cases of nonimmune hydrops.

Unusual Manifestations Hepatitis, vasculitis, myocarditis, glomerulosclerosis, and central nervous system (CNS) disease have all been reported. However, B19 DNA can be detected by PCR for years in many tissues; this finding is of no known clinical significance, but its interpretation may cause confusion regarding B19 disease association.

DIAGNOSIS
Diagnosis of B19 infection in immunocompetent individuals is generally based on detection of B19 IgM antibodies (Table 177-1). IgM can be detected at the time of rash in erythema infectiosum and by the third day of TAC in patients with hematologic disorders; these antibodies remain detectable for ~3 months. B19 IgG is detectable by the seventh day of illness and persists throughout life. Detection of B19 DNA should be used for the diagnosis of early TAC or chronic anemia. Although B19 levels fall rapidly with the development of the immune response, DNA can be detectable by PCR for months or even years after infection, even in healthy individuals; therefore, quantitative PCR should be used. In acute infection at the height of viremia, >10^{12} B19 DNA genome equivalents (ge)/mL of serum can be detected; however, titers fall rapidly within 2 days. Patients with aplastic crisis or B19-induced chronic anemia generally have >10^5 B19 DNA ge/mL.

℞ PARVOVIRUS INFECTION

No antiviral drug effective against B19 is available, and treatment of B19 infection often targets symptoms only. TAC precipitated by B19 infection frequently necessitates symptom-based treatment with blood transfusions. In patients receiving chemotherapy, temporary cessation of treatment may result in an immune response and resolution. If this approach is unsuccessful or not applicable, commercial immune globulin (IVIg; Gammagard, Sandoglobulin) from healthy blood donors can cure or ameliorate

TABLE 177-1	DISEASES ASSOCIATED WITH HUMAN PARVOVIRUS B19 INFECTION AND METHODS OF DIAGNOSIS				
Disease	**Host(s)**	**IgM**	**IgG**	**PCR**	**Quantitative PCR**
Fifth disease Polyarthropathy syndrome	Healthy children Healthy adults (especially women)	Positive Positive within 3 months of onset	Positive Positive	Positive Positive	
Transient aplastic crisis	Patients with increased erythropoiesis			Positive	Often > 10^{12} ge/mL, but rapidly decreases
Persistent anemia/pure red-cell aplasia	Immunodeficient or immunocompetent patients	Negative/weakly positive	Negative/weakly positive	Positive	Often > 10^{12} ge/mL, but should be >10^6 in the absence of treatment
Hydrops fetalis/congenital anemia	Fetus (<20 weeks)			Positive amniotic fluid or tissue	

Note: ge, genome equivalents; PCR, polymerase chain reaction.

persistent B19 infection in immunosuppressed patients. Generally, the dose used is 400 mg/kg daily for 5–10 days. Like patients with TAC, immunosuppressed patients with persistent B19 infection should be considered infectious. Administration of IVIg is not beneficial for erythema infectiosum or B19-associated polyarthropathy. Intrauterine blood transfusion can prevent fetal loss in some cases of fetal hydrops.

PREVENTION

No vaccine has been approved for the prevention of B19 infection. A vaccine based on virus-like particles expressed in insect cells is under development; the results of phase 1 trials were promising.

OTHER PARVOVIRUSES

ADENO-ASSOCIATED VIRUSES

Antibody studies indicate that AAV infections are common in childhood, but AAVs have not been associated with any disease and are considered nonpathogenic. Most of the interest in AAVs is related to their potential use as vectors for gene therapy.

PARV4/5

The PARV4 viral sequence was initially detected in a patient with an acute viral syndrome. Similar sequences, including the related PARV5 sequence, have been detected in pooled plasma collections. The DNA sequence of PARV4/5 is distinctly different from that of all other parvoviruses, and this virus cannot be classified within the current *Parvovirus* genus. Preliminary serologic studies indicate that PARV4/5 infection is common in childhood, but no association with disease has been shown.

HUMAN BOCAVIRUS

Animal bocaviruses are associated with mild respiratory symptoms and enteritis in young animals. HBoV was recently identified in the respiratory tract of young children with lower respiratory tract infections. However, its contribution to pathogenesis is unknown, and HBoV sequences are often found in the presence of other pathogens. The relation of HBoV and PARV4/5 viruses to the commonly observed fecal parvoviruses also remains to be established.

FURTHER READINGS

ALLANDER T et al: Cloning of a human parvovirus by molecular screening of respiratory tract samples. Proc Natl Acad Sci USA 102:12891, 2005

BROWN KE, YOUNG NS: Parvovirus B19, in NS Young et al (eds). *Clinical Hematology*. Philadelphia, Mosby Elsevier, 2006, pp 981–991

———— et al: Resistance to parvovirus B19 infection due to lack of virus receptor (erythrocyte P antigen). N Engl J Med 330:1192, 1994

———— et al: Erythrocyte P antigen: Cellular receptor for B19 parvovirus. Science 262:114, 1993

FRYER JF et al: Novel parvovirus and related variant in human plasma. Emerg Infect Dis 12:151, 2006

KERR JR et al: *Parvoviruses*. London, Hodder Arnold, 2006

KURTZMAN GJ et al: Chronic bone marrow failure due to persistent B19 parvovirus infection. N Engl J Med 317:287, 1987

WILDIG J et al: Parvovirus B19 infection contributes to severe anemia in young children in Papua New Guinea. J Infect Dis 194:146, 2006

YOUNG NS, BROWN KE: Parvovirus B19. N Engl J Med 350:586, 2004

178 Human Papillomavirus Infections

Richard C. Reichman

DEFINITION

Human papillomaviruses (HPVs) selectively infect the epithelium of skin and mucous membranes. These infections may be asymptomatic, produce warts, or be associated with a variety of both benign and malignant neoplasias.

ETIOLOGIC AGENT

Papillomaviruses are members of the family Papillomaviridae. They are nonenveloped, measure 50–55 nm in diameter, have icosahedral capsids composed of 72 capsomeres, and contain a double-strand circular DNA genome of ~7900 base pairs. The genomic organization of all papillomaviruses is similar and consists of an early (E) region, a late (L) region, and a noncoding upstream regulatory region (URR). Oncogenic HPV types can immortalize human keratinocytes, and this activity has been mapped to products of early genes E6 and E7. E6 protein facilitates the degradation of the p53 tumor-suppressor protein, and E7 protein binds the retinoblastoma gene product and related proteins. The E1 and E2 proteins modulate viral DNA replication and regulate gene expression. The L1 gene codes for the major capsid protein, which makes up 80% of the virion mass. L2 codes for a minor capsid protein. Type-specific conformational antigenic determinants are located on the virion surface. Papillomavirus types are distinguished from one another by the degree of nucleic acid sequence homology. Distinct types share <90% of their DNA sequences in L1. More than 100 HPV types are recognized, and individual types are associated with specific clinical manifestations. For example, HPV-1 causes plantar warts, HPV-6 causes anogenital warts, and HPV-16 infection can produce cervical dysplasia and invasive cervical cancer. HPVs are species-specific and have not been propagated in tissue culture or in common experimental animals. However, some HPV types have been produced in human tissues implanted in immunodeficient mice.

EPIDEMIOLOGY

There are few good studies of the incidence or prevalence of human warts in well-defined populations. Common warts (*verruca vulgaris*) are found in as many as 25% of some groups and are most prevalent among young children. Plantar warts (*verruca plantaris*) are also widely prevalent; they occur most often among adolescents and young adults. Anogenital warts (*condyloma acuminatum*) represent one of the most common sexually transmitted diseases in the United States. HPV infection of the uterine cervix produces the squamous cell abnormalities most frequently detected on Papanicolaou smears.

Most anogenital HPV infections are transmitted through direct contact with infectious lesions. However, lesion characteristics that are associated with transmission, including appearance, have not been defined, and individuals without obvious disease may transmit infection. Close personal contact is also assumed to play a role in the transmission of most cutaneous warts; the importance of fomites in this setting is not clear. Minor trauma at the site of inoculation may facilitate transmission. Recurrent respiratory papillomatosis in young children is an uncommon disease that is acquired from the infected maternal genital tract. In adults, orogenital sexual contact may transmit the disease.

According to a consensus panel gathered by the World Health Organization, a large body of epidemiologic and biologic data has established that some HPV infections cause cervical cancer. For example, >95% of cervical cancers contain HPV DNA of oncogenic (high-risk) types, such as 16, 18, 31, 33, and 45. HPV DNA is also present in the precursor lesions of cervical cancer (cervical intraepithelial neoplasias). Such lesions containing DNA of oncogenic types are more likely to progress than those associated with low-risk HPV types, such as 6 and 11. HPV DNA is transcribed in tumor tissues, and many epidemiologic studies have confirmed a strong relationship between HPV infection (with or without cofactors) and the development of cervical cancer. Definitive proof of the causative role of high-risk HPV types in the pathogenesis of high-grade cervical dysplasia has been provided by the results of recently conducted trials of HPV vaccines. However, it is important to realize that most cervical HPV infections, including those caused by high-risk types, are self-limited. Infection with high-risk HPV types has also been associated with squamous cell carcinomas and dysplasias of the penis, anus, vagina, and vulva. In patients with *epidermodysplasia verruciformis* (see "Clinical Manifestations," below), squamous cell cancers develop frequently at sites infected with specific HPV types, including 5 and 8.

CLINICAL MANIFESTATIONS

The clinical manifestations of HPV infection depend on the location of lesions and the type of virus. Common warts usually occur on the hands as flesh-colored to brown, exophytic, and hyperkeratotic papules. Plantar warts may be quite painful; they can be differentiated from calluses by paring of the surface to reveal thrombosed capillaries. Flat warts (*verruca plana*) are most common among children and occur on the face, neck, chest, and flexor surfaces of the forearms and legs.

Anogenital warts develop on the skin and mucosal surfaces of external genitalia and perianal areas (Fig. 178-1). Among circumcised men, warts are most commonly found on the penile shaft. Lesions frequently occur at the urethral meatus and may extend proximally. Receptive anal intercourse predisposes both men and women to the development of perianal warts, but such lesions occasionally develop without such a history. In women, warts appear first at the posterior introitus and adjacent labia. They then spread to other parts of the vulva and commonly involve the vagina and cervix. In both sexes, external warts suggest the presence of internal lesions; however, internal lesions may be present without external warts, particularly in women. The differential diagnosis of anogenital warts includes condylomata lata of secondary syphilis, molluscum contagiosum, hirsutoid papillomatosis (pearly penile papules), fibroepitheliomas, and a variety of benign and malignant mucocutaneous neoplasms. Respiratory papillomatosis in young children, which may be life-threatening, presents as hoarseness, stridor, or respiratory distress. The disease in adults is usually milder.

Immunosuppressed patients, particularly those undergoing organ transplantation, often develop pityriasis versicolor–like lesions, from which DNA of several HPV types has been extracted. Occasionally, such lesions appear to undergo malignant transformation. Patients infected with HIV are often infected with uncommon HPV types, frequently have severe clinical manifestations of HPV infection, and are at high risk for cervical and anal dysplasia as well as for invasive cancer. HPV disease in patients with HIV infection may be associated with multiple HPV types, is difficult to treat, and often recurs (Chap. 182).

FIGURE 178-1 Anogenital warts are lesions produced by human papillomavirus and in this patient are seen as multiple verrucous papules coalescing into plaques.

Epidermodysplasia verruciformis is a rare autosomal recessive disease characterized by an inability to control HPV infection. Patients are often infected with unique HPV types (i.e., types that affect only this group) and frequently develop cutaneous squamous cell malignancies, particularly in sun-exposed areas. The lesions resemble flat warts or macules similar to those of pityriasis versicolor.

The complications of warts include itching and occasionally bleeding. In rare cases, warts become secondarily infected with bacteria or fungi. Large masses of warts may cause mechanical problems, such as obstruction of the birth canal or the urinary tract. Dysplasias of the uterine cervix are generally asymptomatic until frank carcinoma develops. Patients with anogenital HPV disease may develop serious psychological symptoms due to anxiety and depression over this condition.

PATHOGENESIS

The incubation period of HPV disease is usually 3–4 months (range, 1 month to 2 years). All types of squamous epithelium can be infected by HPV, and the gross and histologic appearances of individual lesions vary with the site of infection and the type of virus. The replication of HPV begins with the infection of basal cells. As cellular differentiation proceeds, HPV DNA replicates and is transcribed. Ultimately, virions are assembled in the nucleus and released when keratinocytes are shed. This process is associated with proliferation of all epidermal layers except the basal layer and produces acanthosis, parakeratosis, and hyperkeratosis. Koilocytes—large round cells with pyknotic nuclei—appear in the granular layer. Histologically normal epithelium may contain HPV DNA, and residual DNA after treatment can be associated with recurrent disease.

Episomal HPV DNA is present in the nuclei of infected cells in benign lesions caused by HPV. However, in severe dysplasias and cancers, HPV DNA is generally integrated, with disruption of the E1/E2 open reading frames. This disruption leads to upregulation of E6 and E7 and subsequent interference with cellular tumor-suppressor proteins. Expression of E6 and E7 proteins of oncogenic HPV types is necessary for the development and maintenance of the transformed state in both cervical cancers and cell lines derived from these tumors.

Host defense responses to HPV infection remain incompletely understood. However, several studies of recently developed HPV vaccines have demonstrated that production of high titers of type-specific neutralizing antibodies by vaccinated individuals is associated with type-specific protection from HPV infection and disease. Because patients with defects in cell-mediated immune responses (including transplant recipients and patients with HIV infection) frequently develop severe HPV disease, such responses are probably important for the control of established virus replication and disease. Histologic studies demonstrating an epidermal lymphomonocytic infiltrate in resolving warts suggest that local immunity may be of particular importance in the resolution of disease. HPV infection also elicits a detectable serologic response in many patients. Using HPV virus-like particles (VLPs) as antigens, type-specific antibodies can be found in sera of about two-thirds of patients with anogenital infection. Antibodies to E-region proteins, most notably E7, have been detected among patients with cervical carcinoma.

DIAGNOSIS

Most warts that are visible to the naked eye can be diagnosed correctly by history and physical examination alone. The use of a colposcope is invaluable in assessing vaginal and cervical lesions and is helpful in the diagnosis of oral and cutaneous HPV disease as well. Application of 3–5% solutions of acetic acid may aid in the visualization of lesions, although the sensitivity and specificity of this procedure are unknown. Papanicolaou smears prepared from cervical or anal scrapings often show cytologic evidence of HPV infection. Persistent or atypical lesions should be biopsied and examined by routine histologic methods. The most sensitive and specific methods of virologic diagnosis use techniques such as the polymerase chain reaction or the hybrid capture assay to detect HPV nucleic acids and to identify specific virus types. Such tests may be useful in the diagnosis and management of cervical HPV disease, although their utility may vary according to the preva-

TABLE 178-1	TREATMENT OF EXTERNAL, EXOPHYTIC ANOGENITAL WARTS

I. Administered by provider
  A. Cryotherapy with liquid nitrogen or cryoprobe weekly
  B. Podophyllin resin, 10–25% weekly for up to 4 weeks
  C. Trichloroacetic acid or bichloroacetic acid, 80–90% weekly
  D. Surgical excision
  E. Other regimens
    1. Intralesionally administered interferon
    2. Laser surgery
II. Administered by patient
  A. Podofilox, 0.5% solution or gel twice daily for 3 days, followed by 4
    days without therapy. This cycle may be repeated four times.
  B. Imiquimod, 5% cream 3 times per week for up to 16 weeks

Source: Modified from Centers for Disease Control and Prevention: MMWR 55(RR-11):1, 2006 (www.cdc.gov/mmwr/preview/mmwrhtml/rr5511a1/htm).

lence of disease and the availability of traditional cytologic and histologic testing. Serologic techniques to diagnose HPV infection are not helpful in individual cases and are not widely available.

℞ HUMAN PAPILLOMAVIRUS INFECTIONS

(Table 178-1) Decisions regarding the initiation of therapy should be made with the recognition that currently available modes of treatment are not completely effective and some have significant side effects. In addition, treatment may be expensive, and many HPV lesions resolve spontaneously. Frequently used therapies include cryosurgery, application of caustic agents, electrodesiccation, surgical excision, and ablation with a laser. Topical antimetabolites such as 5-fluorouracil have also been used. Both failure and recurrence have been well documented with all of these methods of treatment. Cryosurgery is the initial treatment of choice for condyloma acuminatum. Topically applied podophyllum preparations as well as podofilox may also be used. Various interferon preparations have been employed with modest success in the treatment of respiratory papillomatosis and condyloma acuminatum. A topically applied interferon inducer, imiquimod, is also of benefit in the treatment of condyloma acuminatum. The diagnosis and management of anogenital dysplasias and of internal anogenital warts require special skills and resources, and patients with such lesions should be referred to a qualified specialist.

PREVENTION

Recently developed HPV VLP vaccines dramatically reduce rates of infection and disease produced by the HPV types in the vaccines. These products are directed against virus types that cause anogenital tract disease and are derived from expression of the major capsid protein (L1) gene in tissue culture. When expressed using appropriate vectors and tissue culture systems, L1 self-assembles into a VLP that cannot be distinguished morphologically or antigenically from its wild-type counterpart (Fig. 178-2) but that contains no viral nucleic acid. Currently, one quadrivalent product (Gardasil, Merck) containing HPV types 6, 11, 16, and 18 has been licensed in the United States and recommended by the Centers for Disease Control and Prevention for administration to girls and young women 9–26 years of age. Another product (Cervarix, GlaxoSmithKline) contains HPV types 16 and 18 and is likely to be available in the near future. HPV types 6 and 11 cause 90% of anogenital warts, whereas types 16 and 18 are responsible for 70% of cervical cancers. Because 30% of cervical cancers are caused by HPV types not contained in the vaccines, no changes in cervical cancer screening programs are currently recommended. Barrier methods of contraception may also be helpful in preventing transmission of condyloma acuminatum and other anogenital HPV-associated diseases.

FURTHER READINGS

BONNEZ W, REICHMAN RC: Papillomaviruses, in *Principles and Practice of Infectious Diseases*, 6th ed, GL Mandell et al (eds). Churchill Livingstone, New York, 2005, pp 1841–1856

CENTERS FOR DISEASE CONTROL AND PREVENTION: Sexually transmitted diseases treatment guidelines, 2006. MMWR 55(RR-11):1, 2006 (*www.cdc.gov/mmwr/preview/mmwrhtml/rr5511a1.htm*)

HARPER DM et al: Sustained efficacy up to 4.5 years of a bivalent L1 virus-like particle vaccine against human papillomavirus types 16 and 18: Follow-up from a randomised control trial. Lancet 367:1247, 2006

LUQUE AE et al: Prevalence of human papillomavirus (HPV) genotypes and relation to cervical cytology among HIV-1 infected women in Rochester, New York. J Infect Dis 194:428, 2006

VILLA LL et al: High sustained efficacy of a prophylactic quadrivalent human papillomavirus types 6/11/16/18 L1 virus-like particle vaccine through 5 years of follow-up. Br J Cancer 11:1459, 2006

HPV-11 virus particles

HPV-11 virus-like particles

FIGURE 178-2 HPV-11 virus-like particles produced in insect cells (**right**) are morphologically and antigenically indistinguishable from wild-type HPV-11 particles (**left**). *(Images courtesy of Drs. William Bonnez and Robert C. Rose; with permission.)*

179 Common Viral Respiratory Infections and Severe Acute Respiratory Syndrome (SARS)

Raphael Dolin

GENERAL CONSIDERATIONS

Acute viral respiratory illnesses are among the most common of human diseases, accounting for one-half or more of all acute illnesses. The incidence of acute respiratory disease in the United States is 3–5.6 cases per person per year. The rates are highest among children <1 year old (6.1–8.3 cases per year) and remain high until age 6, when a progressive decrease begins. Adults have 3–4 cases per person per year. Morbidity from acute respiratory illnesses accounts for 30–50% of time lost from work by adults and for 60–80% of time lost from school by children. The use of antibacterial agents to treat viral respiratory infections represents a major source of abuse of that category of drugs.

It has been estimated that two-thirds to three-fourths of cases of acute respiratory illnesses are caused by viruses. More than 200 antigenically distinct viruses from 10 genera have been reported to cause acute respiratory illness, and it is likely that additional agents will be described in the future. The vast majority of these viral infections involve the upper respiratory tract, but lower respiratory tract disease can also develop, particularly in younger age groups, in the elderly, and in certain epidemiologic settings.

The illnesses caused by respiratory viruses traditionally have been divided into multiple distinct syndromes, such as the "common cold," pharyngitis, croup (laryngotracheobronchitis), tracheitis, bronchiolitis, bronchitis, and pneumonia. Each of these general categories of illness has a certain epidemiologic and clinical profile; for example, croup occurs exclusively in very young children and has a characteristic clinical course. Some types of respiratory illness are more likely to be associated with certain viruses (e.g., the common cold with rhinoviruses), while others occupy characteristic epidemiologic niches (e.g., adenovirus infections in military recruits). The syndromes most commonly associated with infections with the major respiratory virus groups are summarized in Table 179-1. Most respiratory viruses clearly have the potential to cause more than one type of respiratory illness, and features of several types of illness may be found in the same patient. Moreover, the clinical illnesses induced by these viruses are rarely sufficiently distinctive to permit an etiologic diagnosis on clinical grounds alone, although the epidemiologic setting increases the likelihood that one group of viruses rather than another is involved. In general, laboratory methods must be relied on to establish a specific viral diagnosis.

This chapter reviews viral infections caused by six of the major groups of respiratory viruses: rhinoviruses, coronaviruses, respiratory syncytial viruses, metapneumoviruses, parainfluenza viruses, and adenoviruses. The extraordinary outbreaks of lower respiratory tract disease associated with coronaviruses (severe acute respiratory syndrome, or SARS) in 2002–2003 are also discussed. Influenza viruses, which are a major cause of death as well as morbidity, are reviewed in Chap. 180. Herpesviruses, which occasionally cause pharyngitis and which also cause lower respiratory tract disease in immunosuppressed patients, are reviewed in Chap. 172. Enteroviruses, which account for occasional respiratory illnesses during the summer months, are reviewed in Chap. 184.

RHINOVIRUS INFECTIONS

ETIOLOGIC AGENT

Rhinoviruses are members of the Picornaviridae family, small (15–30 nm) nonenveloped viruses that contain a single-stranded RNA genome. In contrast to other members of the picornavirus family, such as enteroviruses, rhinoviruses are acid-labile and are almost completely inactivated at pH ≤ 3. Rhinoviruses grow preferentially at 33°–34°C (the temperature of the human nasal passages) rather than at 37°C (the temperature of the lower respiratory tract). Of the 102 recognized serotypes of rhinovirus, 91 use intercellular adhesion molecule 1 (ICAM-1) as a cellular receptor and constitute the "major" receptor group, 10 use the low-density lipoprotein receptor and constitute the "minor" receptor group, and 1 uses decay-accelerating factor.

EPIDEMIOLOGY

Rhinoviruses are a prominent cause of the common cold and have been detected in up to 50% of common cold–like illnesses by tissue culture and polymerase chain reaction (PCR) techniques. Overall rates of rhinovirus infection are higher among infants and young children

TABLE 179-1	ILLNESSES ASSOCIATED WITH RESPIRATORY VIRUSES		
	Frequency of Respiratory Syndromes		
Virus	**Most Frequent**	**Occasional**	**Infrequent**
Rhinoviruses	Common cold	Exacerbation of chronic bronchitis and asthma	Pneumonia in children
Coronaviruses[a]	Common cold	Exacerbation of chronic bronchitis and asthma	Pneumonia and bronchiolitis
Human respiratory syncytial virus	Pneumonia and bronchiolitis in young children	Common cold in adults	Pneumonia in elderly and immunosuppressed patients
Parainfluenza viruses	Croup and lower respiratory tract disease in young children	Pharyngitis and common cold	Tracheobronchitis in adults; lower respiratory tract disease in immunosuppressed patients
Adenoviruses	Common cold and pharyngitis in children	Outbreaks of acute respiratory disease in military recruits[b]	Pneumonia in children; lower respiratory tract and disseminated disease in immunosuppressed patients
Influenza A viruses	Influenza[c]	Pneumonia and excess mortality in high-risk patients	Pneumonia in healthy individuals
Influenza B viruses	Influenza[c]	Rhinitis or pharyngitis alone	Pneumonia
Enteroviruses	Acute undifferentiated febrile illnesses[d]	Rhinitis or pharyngitis alone	Pneumonia
Herpes simplex viruses	Gingivostomatitis in children; pharyngotonsillitis in adults	Tracheitis and pneumonia in immunocompromised patients	Disseminated infection in immunocompromised patients
Human metapneumoviruses[e]	Lower respiratory tract disease in children	Upper respiratory tract illness in adults	Pneumonia in elderly and immunosuppressed patients

[a]SARS-associated coronavirus (SARS-CoV) caused epidemics of pneumonia from November 2002 to July 2003 (see text).
[b]Serotypes 4 and 7.
[c]Fever, cough, myalgia, malaise.
[d]May or may not have a respiratory component.
[e]Newly recognized human metapneumoviruses cause upper and lower respiratory tract illnesses; their relative frequency is under investigation.

and decrease with increasing age. Rhinovirus infections occur throughout the year, with seasonal peaks in early fall and spring in temperate climates. These infections are most often introduced into families by preschool or grade-school children <6 years old. Of initial illnesses in family settings, 25–70% are followed by secondary cases, with the highest attack rates among the youngest siblings at home. Attack rates also increase with family size.

Rhinoviruses appear to spread through direct contact with infected secretions, usually respiratory droplets. In some studies of volunteers, transmission was most efficient by hand-to-hand contact, with subsequent self-inoculation of the conjunctival or nasal mucosa. Other studies demonstrated transmission by large- or small-particle aerosol. Virus can be recovered from plastic surfaces inoculated 1–3 h previously; this observation suggests that environmental surfaces contribute to transmission. In studies of married couples in which neither partner had detectable serum antibody, transmission was associated with prolonged contact (≥122 h) during a 7-day period. Transmission was infrequent unless (1) virus was recoverable from the donor's hands and nasal mucosa, (2) at least 1000 $TCID_{50}$ of virus was present in nasal washes from the donor, and (3) the donor was at least moderately symptomatic with the "cold." Despite anecdotal observations, exposure to cold temperatures, fatigue, and sleep deprivation have not been associated with increased rates of rhinovirus-induced illness in volunteers, although some studies have suggested that psychologically defined "stress" may contribute to development of symptoms.

Infection with rhinoviruses is worldwide in distribution. By adulthood, nearly all individuals have neutralizing antibodies to multiple serotypes, although the prevalence of antibody to any one serotype varies widely. Multiple serotypes circulate simultaneously, and generally no single serotype or group of serotypes has been more prevalent than the others.

PATHOGENESIS

Rhinoviruses infect cells through attachment to specific cellular receptors; as mentioned above, most serotypes attach to ICAM-1, while a few use the low-density lipoprotein receptor. Relatively limited information is available on the histopathology and pathogenesis of acute rhinovirus infections in humans. Examination of biopsy specimens obtained during experimentally induced and naturally occurring illness indicates that the nasal mucosa is edematous, is often hyperemic, and—during acute illness—is covered by a mucoid discharge. There is a mild infiltrate with inflammatory cells, including neutrophils, lymphocytes, plasma cells, and eosinophils. Mucus-secreting glands in the submucosa appear hyperactive; the nasal turbinates are engorged, a condition that may lead to obstruction of nearby openings of sinus cavities. Several mediators—e.g., bradykinin; lysylbradykinin; prostaglandins; histamine; interleukins 1β, 6, and 8; and tumor necrosis factor α—have been linked to the development of signs and symptoms in rhinovirus-induced colds.

The incubation period for rhinovirus illness is short, generally 1–2 days. Virus shedding coincides with the onset of illness or may begin shortly before symptoms develop. The mechanisms of immunity to rhinovirus are not well worked out. In some studies, the presence of homotypic antibody has been associated with significantly reduced rates of subsequent infection and illness, but data conflict regarding the relative importance of serum and local antibody in protection from rhinovirus infection.

CLINICAL MANIFESTATIONS

The most common clinical manifestations of rhinovirus infections are those of the common cold. Illness usually begins with rhinorrhea and sneezing accompanied by nasal congestion. The throat is frequently sore, and in some cases sore throat is the initial complaint. Systemic signs and symptoms, such as malaise and headache, are mild or absent, and fever is unusual. Illness generally lasts for 4–9 days and resolves spontaneously without sequelae. In children, bronchitis, bronchiolitis, and bronchopneumonia have been reported; nevertheless, it appears that rhinoviruses are not major causes of lower respiratory tract disease in children. Rhinoviruses may cause exacerbations of asthma and chronic pulmonary disease in adults. The vast majority of rhinovirus infections resolve without sequelae, but complications related to obstruction of the eustachian tubes or sinus ostia, including otitis media or acute sinusitis, can develop. In immunosuppressed patients, particularly bone marrow transplant recipients, severe and even fatal pneumonias have been associated with rhinovirus infections.

DIAGNOSIS

Although rhinoviruses are the most frequently recognized cause of the common cold, similar illnesses are caused by a variety of other viruses, and a specific viral etiologic diagnosis cannot be made on clinical grounds alone. Rather, rhinovirus infection is diagnosed by isolation of the virus from nasal washes or nasal secretions in tissue culture. In practice, this procedure is rarely undertaken because of the benign, self-limited nature of the illness. In most settings, detection of rhinovirus RNA by PCR is more sensitive than that by tissue culture; however, PCR for rhinoviruses is largely a research procedure. Given the many serotypes of rhinovirus, diagnosis by serum antibody tests is currently impractical. Likewise, common laboratory tests, such as white blood cell count and erythrocyte sedimentation rate, are not helpful.

℞ RHINOVIRUS INFECTIONS

Because rhinovirus infections are generally mild and self-limited, treatment is not usually necessary. Therapy in the form of first-generation antihistamines and nonsteroidal anti-inflammatory drugs may be beneficial in patients with particularly pronounced symptoms, and an oral decongestant may be added if nasal obstruction is particularly troublesome. Reduction of activity is prudent in instances of significant discomfort or fatigability. Antibacterial agents should be used only if bacterial complications such as otitis media or sinusitis develop. Specific antiviral therapy is not available.

PREVENTION

Intranasal application of interferon sprays has been effective in the prophylaxis of rhinovirus infections but is also associated with local irritation of the nasal mucosa. Studies of the prevention of rhinovirus infection by administration of antibodies to ICAM-1 or by the soluble purified receptors themselves have yielded disappointing results. Experimental vaccines to certain rhinovirus serotypes have been generated, but their usefulness is questionable because of the myriad serotypes and the uncertainty about mechanisms of immunity. Thorough hand washing, environmental decontamination, and protection against autoinoculation may help to reduce rates of transmission of infection.

CORONAVIRUS INFECTIONS, INCLUDING SARS

ETIOLOGIC AGENT

Coronaviruses are pleomorphic, single-stranded RNA viruses that measure 100–160 nm in diameter. The name derives from the crownlike appearance produced by the club-shaped projections that stud the viral envelope. Coronaviruses infect a wide variety of animal species and have been divided into three antigenic groups. Previously recognized coronaviruses that infect humans fell into two of these groups (serogroups I and II), which include human isolates HCoV-229E and HCoV-OC43, respectively. The coronavirus associated with SARS (SARS-CoV) was first believed to represent a novel group but now is considered to be a distantly related member of group II (Fig. 179-1). To date, the SARS-CoV strains that have been fully sequenced have shown only minimal variation.

In general, human coronaviruses have been difficult to cultivate in vitro, and some strains grow only in human tracheal organ cultures rather than in tissue culture. SARS-CoV is an exception whose ready growth in African green monkey kidney (Vero E6) cells greatly facilitates its study.

EPIDEMIOLOGY

 Generally, human coronavirus infections are present throughout the world. Seroprevalence studies of strains HCoV-229E and HCoV-OC43 have demonstrated that serum antibodies are acquired early in life and increase in prevalence with advancing age, so that >80% of adult populations have antibodies as measured by enzyme-linked immunosorbent assay (ELISA). Overall, coronaviruses account for

FIGURE 179-1 Electron micrograph of SARS-associated coronavirus (SARS-CoV) isolated in fetal rhesus kidney tissue culture from a lung biopsy sample from a patient with SARS. Viral particles are 55–90 mm in diameter. [*Reprinted with permission from Elsevier (JSM Peiris et al., Lancet 361:1319, 2003).*]

10–35% of common colds, depending on the season. Coronavirus infections appear to be particularly prevalent in late fall, winter, and early spring—times when rhinovirus infections are less common.

An extraordinary outbreak of the coronavirus-associated illness known as SARS occurred in 2002–2003. The outbreak apparently began in southern China and eventually resulted in 8096 recognized cases in 28 countries in Asia, Europe, and North and South America; ~90% of cases occurred in China and Hong Kong. The natural reservoir of SARS-CoV appears to be the horseshoe bat, and the outbreak may have originated from human contact with infected semidomesticated animals such as the palm civet. In most cases, however, the infection was transmitted from human to human. Case-fatality rates varied among the outbreaks, with an overall figure of ~9.5%. The disease appeared to be somewhat milder in cases in the United States and was clearly less severe among children. The outbreak ceased in 2003; 17 cases were detected in 2004, mostly in laboratory-associated settings, and no cases were reported in 2005–2006.

The mechanisms of transmission of SARS are incompletely understood. Clusters of cases suggest that spread may occur by both large and small aerosols and perhaps by the fecal-oral route as well. The outbreak of illness in a large apartment complex in Hong Kong suggested that environmental sources, such as sewage or water, may also play a role in transmission. Some ill individuals ("super-spreaders") appeared to be hyperinfectious and were capable of transmitting infection to 10–40 contacts, although most infections resulted in spread either to no one or to three or fewer individuals.

PATHOGENESIS

Coronaviruses that cause the common cold (e.g., strains HCoV-229E and HCoV-OC43) infect ciliated epithelial cells in the nasopharynx via the aminopeptidase N receptor (group I) or a sialic acid receptor (group II). Viral replication leads to damage of ciliated cells and induction of chemokines and interleukins, with consequent common-cold symptoms similar to those induced by rhinoviruses.

SARS-CoV infects cells of the respiratory tract via the angiotensin-converting enzyme 2 receptor. The result is a systemic illness in which virus is also found in the bloodstream, in the urine, and (for up to 2 months) in the stool. Virus persists in the respiratory tract for 2–3 weeks, and titers peak ~10 days after the onset of systemic illness. Pulmonary pathology consists of hyaline membrane formation, desquamation of pneumocytes in alveolar spaces, and an interstitial infiltrate made up of lymphocytes and mononuclear cells. Giant cells are frequently seen, and coronavirus particles have been detected in type II pneumocytes. Elevated levels of proinflammatory cytokines and chemokines have been detected in sera from patients with SARS.

CLINICAL MANIFESTATIONS

After an incubation period that generally lasts 2–7 days (range, 1–14 days), SARS usually begins as a systemic illness marked by the onset of fever, which is often accompanied by malaise, headache, and myalgias and is followed in 1–2 days by a nonproductive cough and dyspnea. Approximately 25% of patients have diarrhea. Chest x-rays can show a variety of infiltrates, including patchy areas of consolidation—most frequently in peripheral and lower lung fields—or interstitial infiltrates, which can progress to diffuse involvement (Fig. 179-2).

In severe cases, respiratory function may worsen during the second week of illness and progress to frank adult respiratory distress syndrome (ARDS) accompanied by multiorgan dysfunction. Risk factors for severe disease include an age of >50 years and comorbidities such as cardiovascular disease, diabetes, or hepatitis. Illness in pregnant women may be particularly severe, but SARS-CoV infection appears to be milder in children than in adults.

The clinical features of common colds caused by human coronaviruses are similar to those of illness caused by rhinoviruses. In studies of volunteers, the mean incubation period of colds induced by coronaviruses (3 days) is somewhat longer than that of illness caused by rhinoviruses, and the duration of illness is somewhat shorter (mean, 6–7 days). In some studies, the amount of nasal discharge was greater in colds induced by coronaviruses than in those induced by rhinoviruses. Coronaviruses other than SARS-CoV have been recovered occasionally from infants with pneumonia and from military recruits with lower respiratory tract disease and have been associated with worsening of chronic bronchitis. Two novel coronaviruses, HCoV-NL63 (group I) and HCoV-HKU1 (group II), have recently been isolated from patients hospitalized with acute respiratory illness. Their role as causes of human respiratory disease remains to be determined.

LABORATORY FINDINGS AND DIAGNOSIS

Laboratory abnormalities in SARS include lymphopenia, which is present in ~50% of cases and which mostly affects CD4+ T cells but also involves CD8+ T cells and NK cells. Total white blood cell counts

FIGURE 179-2 Chest x-rays of a 46-year-old man with SARS. The left lower lung infiltrate seen initially (**A**) progressed to multiple bilateral opacities (**B**). (*Reprinted with permission from N Lee et al. © 2003 Massachusetts Medical Society.*)

are normal or slightly low, and thrombocytopenia may develop as the illness progresses. Elevated serum levels of aminotransferases, creatine kinase, and lactate dehydrogenase have been reported.

A rapid diagnosis of SARS-CoV infection can be made by reverse-transcriptase PCR (RT-PCR) of respiratory tract samples and plasma early in illness and of urine and stool later on. SARS-CoV can also be grown from respiratory tract samples by inoculation into Vero E6 tissue culture cells, in which a cytopathic effect is seen within days. RT-PCR appears to be more sensitive than tissue culture, but only around one-third of cases are positive by PCR at initial presentation. Serum antibodies can be detected by ELISA or immunofluorescence, and nearly all patients develop detectable serum antibodies within 28 days after the onset of illness.

Laboratory diagnosis of coronavirus-induced colds is rarely required. Coronaviruses that cause those illnesses are frequently difficult to cultivate in vitro but can be detected in clinical samples by ELISA or immunofluorescence assays or by RT-PCR for viral RNA. These research procedures can be used to detect coronaviruses in unusual clinical settings.

℞ CORONAVIRUS INFECTIONS

There is no specific therapy of established efficacy for SARS. Although ribavirin has frequently been used, it has little if any activity against SARS-CoV in vitro, and no beneficial effect on the course of illness has been demonstrated. Because of suggestions that immunopathology may contribute to the disease, glucocorticoids have also been widely used, but their benefit, if any, is likewise unestablished. Supportive care to maintain pulmonary and other organ system functions remains the mainstay of therapy.

The approach to the treatment of common colds caused by coronaviruses is similar to that discussed above for rhinovirus-induced illnesses.

PREVENTION

The recognition of SARS led to a worldwide mobilization of public health resources to apply infection-control practices to contain the disease. Case definitions were established, travel advisories were proposed, and quarantines were imposed in certain locales. As of this writing, no additional cases of SARS have been reported since 2004. However, it remains unknown whether the disappearance of cases is a result of control measures, whether it is part of a seasonal or otherwise unexplained epidemiologic pattern of SARS, or when or whether SARS might reemerge. The U.S. Centers for Disease Control and Prevention and the World Health Organization maintain recommendations for surveillance and assessment of potential cases of SARS (*www.cdc.gov/ncidod/sars/*). The frequent transmission of the disease to health care workers makes it mandatory that strict infection-control practices be employed by health care facilities to prevent airborne, droplet, and contact transmission from any suspected cases of SARS. Health care workers who enter areas in which patients with SARS may be present should don gowns, gloves, and eye and respiratory protective equipment (e.g., an N95 filtering facepiece respirator certified by the National Institute for Occupational Safety and Health).

Vaccines have been developed against several animal coronaviruses but not against known human coronaviruses. The emergence of SARS-CoV has stimulated interest in the development of vaccines against such agents.

HUMAN RESPIRATORY SYNCYTIAL VIRUS INFECTIONS

ETIOLOGIC AGENT

Human respiratory syncytial virus, previously referred to as RSV and now designated HRSV, is a member of the Paramyxoviridae family (genus *Pneumovirus*). HRSV, an enveloped virus ~150–350 nm in diameter, is so named because its replication in vitro leads to the fusion of neighboring cells into large multinucleated syncytia. The single-stranded RNA genome codes for 11 virus-specific proteins. Viral RNA is contained in a helical nucleocapsid surrounded by a lipid envelope bearing two glycoproteins: the G protein, by which the virus attaches to cells, and the F (fusion) protein, which facilitates entry of the virus into the cell by fusing

host and viral membranes. HRSV was once considered to be of a single antigenic type, but two distinct subgroups (A and B) and multiple subtypes within each subgroup have now been described. Antigenic diversity is reflected by differences in the G protein, while the F protein is highly conserved. Both antigenic groups can circulate simultaneously in outbreaks, although there are typically alternating patterns in which one subgroup predominates over 1- to 2-year periods. Infections with group B viruses may be somewhat milder than those with group A viruses.

EPIDEMIOLOGY

HRSV is a major respiratory pathogen of young children and the foremost cause of lower respiratory disease in infants. Infection with HRSV is seen throughout the world in annual epidemics that occur in late fall, winter, or spring and last up to 5 months. The virus is rarely encountered during the summer. Rates of illness are highest among infants 1–6 months of age, peaking at 2–3 months of age. The attack rates among susceptible infants and children are extraordinarily high, approaching 100% in settings such as day-care centers where large numbers of susceptible infants are present. By age 2, virtually all children will have been infected with HRSV. HRSV accounts for 20–25% of hospital admissions of young infants and children for pneumonia and for up to 75% of cases of bronchiolitis in this age group. It has been estimated that more than half of infants who are at risk will become infected during an HRSV epidemic.

In older children and adults, reinfection with HRSV is frequent but disease is milder than in infancy. A common cold–like syndrome is the illness most commonly associated with HRSV infection in adults. Severe lower respiratory tract disease with pneumonitis can occur in elderly (often institutionalized) adults and in patients with immunocompromising disorders or treatment, including recipients of stem cell and solid-organ transplants. HRSV is also an important nosocomial pathogen; during an outbreak, it can infect pediatric patients and up to 25–50% of the staff on pediatric wards. The spread of HRSV among families is efficient: up to 40% of siblings may become infected when the virus is introduced into the family setting.

HRSV is transmitted primarily by close contact with contaminated fingers or fomites and by self-inoculation of the conjunctiva or anterior nares. Virus may also be spread by coarse aerosols produced by coughing or sneezing, but it is inefficiently spread by fine-particle aerosols. The incubation period is ~4–6 days, and virus shedding may last for ≥2 weeks in children and for shorter periods in adults. In immunosuppressed patients, shedding can continue for weeks.

PATHOGENESIS

Little is known about the histopathology of minor HRSV infection. Severe bronchiolitis or pneumonia is characterized by necrosis of the bronchiolar epithelium and a peribronchiolar infiltrate of lymphocytes and mononuclear cells. Interalveolar thickening and filling of alveolar spaces with fluid can also be found. The correlates of protective immunity to HRSV are incompletely understood. Because reinfection occurs frequently and is often associated with illness, the immunity that develops after single episodes of infection clearly is not complete or long-lasting. However, the cumulative effect of multiple reinfections is to temper subsequent disease and to provide some temporary measure of protection against infection. Studies of experimentally induced disease in healthy volunteers indicate that the presence of nasal IgA neutralizing antibody correlates more closely with protection than does the presence of serum antibody. Studies in infants, however, suggest that maternally acquired antibody provides some protection from lower respiratory tract disease, although illness can be severe even in infants who have moderate levels of maternally derived serum antibody. The relatively severe disease observed in immunosuppressed patients and experimental animal models indicates that cell-mediated immunity is an important mechanism of host defense against HRSV. Evidence suggests that class I MHC-restricted cytotoxic T cells may be particularly important in this regard.

CLINICAL MANIFESTATIONS

HRSV infection leads to a wide spectrum of respiratory illnesses. In infants, 25–40% of infections result in lower respiratory tract involvement, including pneumonia, bronchiolitis, and tracheobronchitis. In this age group, illness begins most frequently with rhinorrhea, low-grade fever, and mild systemic symptoms, often accompanied by cough and wheezing. Most patients recover gradually over 1–2 weeks. In more severe illness, tachypnea and dyspnea develop, and eventually frank hypoxia, cyanosis, and apnea can ensue. Physical examination may reveal diffuse wheezing, rhonchi, and rales. Chest radiography shows hyperexpansion, peribronchial thickening, and variable infiltrates ranging from diffuse interstitial infiltrates to segmental or lobar consolidation. Illness may be particularly severe in children born prematurely and in those with congenital cardiac disease, bronchopulmonary dysplasia, nephrotic syndrome, or immunosuppression. One study documented a 37% mortality rate among infants with HRSV pneumonia and congenital cardiac disease.

In adults, the most common symptoms of HRSV infection are those of the common cold, with rhinorrhea, sore throat, and cough. Illness is occasionally associated with moderate systemic symptoms such as malaise, headache, and fever. HRSV has also been reported to cause lower respiratory tract disease with fever in adults, including severe pneumonia in the elderly—particularly in nursing-home residents, among whom its impact can rival that of influenza. HRSV pneumonia can be a significant cause of morbidity and death among patients undergoing stem cell and solid-organ transplantation, where case-fatality rates of 20–80% have been reported. Sinusitis, otitis media, and worsening of chronic obstructive and reactive airway disease have also been associated with HRSV infection.

LABORATORY FINDINGS AND DIAGNOSIS

The diagnosis of HRSV infection can be suspected on the basis of a suggestive epidemiologic setting—that is, severe illness among infants during an outbreak of HRSV in the community. Infections in older children and adults cannot be differentiated with certainty from those caused by other respiratory viruses. The specific diagnosis is established by detection of HRSV in respiratory secretions, such as sputum, throat swabs, or nasopharyngeal washes. Virus can be isolated in tissue culture and is identified specifically by immunofluorescence, ELISA, or other immunologic techniques. Rapid viral diagnosis is available by immunofluorescence techniques or ELISA of nasopharyngeal washes, aspirates, and (less satisfactorily) nasopharyngeal swabs. With specimens from children, these techniques have sensitivities and specificities of 80–95%; they are somewhat less sensitive with specimens from adults. Serologic diagnosis may be made by comparison of acute- and convalescent-phase serum specimens by ELISA or by neutralization or complement-fixation tests. These tests may be useful in older children and adults but are less sensitive in children <4 months of age.

℞ HUMAN RESPIRATORY SYNCYTIAL VIRUS INFECTIONS

Treatment of upper respiratory tract HRSV infection is aimed primarily at the alleviation of symptoms and is similar to that for other viral infections of the upper respiratory tract. For lower respiratory tract infections, respiratory therapy, including hydration, suctioning of secretions, and administration of humidified oxygen and antibronchospastic agents, is given as needed. In severe hypoxia, intubation and ventilatory assistance may be required. Studies of infants with HRSV infection who were given aerosolized ribavirin, a nucleoside analogue active in vitro against HRSV, demonstrated a modest beneficial effect on the resolution of lower respiratory tract illness, including alleviation of blood-gas abnormalities. The American Academy of Pediatrics recommends that treatment with aerosolized ribavirin "may be considered" for infants who are severely ill or who are at high risk for complications of HRSV infection; included are premature infants and those with bronchopulmonary dysplasia, congenital heart disease, or immunosuppression. The efficacy of ribavirin against HRSV pneumonia in older children and adults, including those with immunosuppression, has not been established. Administration of standard immunoglobulin, immunoglobulin with high titers of antibody to HRSV (RSVIg), or chimeric mouse-human monoclonal IgG antibody to HRSV (palivizumab) has not been found to be beneficial in the treatment of HRSV pneumonia. Combined therapy with aerosolized ribavirin and palivizumab is being evaluated in immunosuppressed patients with HRSV pneumonia.

PREVENTION

Monthly administration of RSVIg or palivizumab has been approved as prophylaxis against HRSV for children <2 years of age who have bronchopulmonary dysplasia or cyanotic heart disease or who were born prematurely. Considerable interest exists in the development of vaccines against HRSV. Inactivated whole-virus vaccines have been ineffective; in one study, they actually potentiated disease in infants. Other approaches include immunization with purified F and G surface glycoproteins of HRSV or generation of stable, live attenuated virus vaccines. In settings such as pediatric wards where rates of transmission are high, barrier methods for the protection of hands and conjunctivae may be useful in reducing the spread of virus.

HUMAN METAPNEUMOVIRUS INFECTIONS

ETIOLOGIC AGENT

Human metapneumovirus (HMPV) is a recently described viral respiratory pathogen that has been assigned to the Paramyxoviridae family (genus *Metapneumovirus*). Its morphology and genomic organization are similar to those of avian metapneumoviruses, which are recognized respiratory pathogens of turkeys. HMPV particles may be spherical, filamentous, or pleomorphic in shape and measure 150–600 nm in diameter. Particles contain 15-nm projections from the surface that are similar in appearance to those of other Paramyxoviridae. The single-stranded RNA genome codes for nine proteins that, except for the absence of nonstructural proteins, generally correspond to those of HRSV. There is only one antigenic type; two closely related genetic subgroups (A and B) have been described.

EPIDEMIOLOGY

HMPV infections are worldwide in distribution, are most frequent during the winter, and occur early in life, so that serum antibodies to the virus are present in nearly all children by the age of 5. HMPV infections have been detected in older age groups, including elderly adults, and in both immunocompetent and immunosuppressed hosts. To date, studies indicate that HMPV infections account for 4% of respiratory tract illnesses requiring hospitalization of children, 12% of outpatient lower respiratory illnesses, and 2–4% of acute respiratory illnesses in ambulatory adults and elderly patients. HMPV has been detected in a few cases of SARS, but its role (if any) in these illnesses has not been established. Assessment of the overall significance of HMPV infections awaits the conduct of large-scale epidemiologic studies.

CLINICAL MANIFESTATIONS

The spectrum of clinical illnesses associated with HMPV is similar to that associated with HRSV and includes both upper and lower respiratory tract illnesses, such as bronchiolitis, croup, and pneumonia. Reinfection with HMPV is common in older children and adults and has manifestations ranging from subclinical infections to common cold syndromes and occasionally pneumonia, which is seen primarily in elderly patients and those with cardiopulmonary diseases. Serious HMPV infections occur in immunocompromised patients, including those with neoplasia and stem cell transplants.

DIAGNOSIS

HMPV can be detected in nasal aspirates and respiratory secretions by PCR or by growth in rhesus monkey kidney (LLC-MK2) tissue cultures. Rapid immunodetection methods are under development. A serologic diagnosis can be made by ELISA, which uses HMPV-infected tissue culture lysates as sources of antigens.

℞ HUMAN METAPNEUMOVIRUS INFECTIONS

Treatment for HMPV infections is primarily supportive and symptom-based. Ribavirin and RSVIg are both active against HMPV in vitro, but their efficacy in vivo is unknown.

PREVENTION

Vaccines against HMPV are in the early stages of development.

PARAINFLUENZA VIRUS INFECTIONS

ETIOLOGIC AGENT

Parainfluenza viruses belong to the Paramyxoviridae family (genera *Respirovirus* and *Rubulavirus*). They are 150–200 nm in diameter, are enveloped, and contain a single-stranded RNA genome. The envelope is studded with two glycoproteins: one possesses both hemagglutinin and neuraminidase activity, and the other contains fusion activity. The viral RNA genome is enclosed in a helical nucleocapsid and codes for six structural and several accessory proteins. There are four distinct serotypes of parainfluenza virus, all of which share certain antigens with other members of the Paramyxoviridae family, including mumps and Newcastle disease viruses.

EPIDEMIOLOGY

Parainfluenza viruses are distributed throughout the world; infection with type 4 (subtypes 4A and 4B) has been reported less widely, probably because type 4 is more difficult to grow in tissue culture. Infection is acquired in early childhood, so that by 5 years of age most children have antibodies to serotypes 1, 2, and 3. Types 1 and 2 cause epidemics during the fall, often occurring in an alternate-year pattern. Type 3 infection has been detected during all seasons of the year, but epidemics have occurred annually in the spring.

The contribution of parainfluenza infections to respiratory disease varies with both the location and the year. In studies conducted in the United States, parainfluenza virus infections have accounted for 4.3–22% of respiratory illnesses in children. In adults, parainfluenza infections are generally mild and account for <10% of respiratory illnesses. The major importance of parainfluenza viruses is as a cause of respiratory illness in young children, in whom they rank second only to HRSV as causes of lower respiratory tract illness. Parainfluenza virus type 1 is the most frequent cause of croup (laryngotracheobronchitis) in children, while serotype 2 causes similar, although generally less severe, disease. Type 3 is an important cause of bronchiolitis and pneumonia in infants, while illnesses associated with type 4 have generally been mild. Unlike types 1 and 2, type 3 frequently causes illness during the first month of life, when passively acquired maternal antibody is still present. Parainfluenza viruses are spread through infected respiratory secretions, primarily by person-to-person contact and/or by large droplets. The incubation period has varied from 3 to 6 days in experimental infections but may be somewhat shorter for naturally occurring disease in children.

PATHOGENESIS

Immunity to parainfluenza viruses is incompletely understood, but evidence suggests that immunity to infections with serotypes 1 and 2 is mediated by local IgA antibodies in the respiratory tract. Passively acquired serum neutralizing antibodies also confer some protection against infection with types 1, 2, and (to a lesser degree) 3. Studies in experimental animal models and in immunosuppressed patients suggest that T cell–mediated immunity may also be important in parainfluenza virus infections.

CLINICAL MANIFESTATIONS

Parainfluenza virus infections occur most frequently among children, in whom initial infection with serotype 1, 2, or 3 is associated with an acute febrile illness 50–80% of the time. Children may present with coryza, sore throat, hoarseness, and cough that may or may not be croupy. In severe croup, fever persists, with worsening coryza and sore throat. A brassy or barking cough may progress to frank stridor. Most children recover over the next 1 or 2 days, although progressive airway obstruction and hypoxia ensue occasionally. If bronchiolitis or pneumonia develops, progressive cough accompanied by wheezing, tachypnea, and intercostal retractions may occur. In this setting, sputum production increases modestly. Physical examination shows nasopha-ryngeal discharge and oropharyngeal injection, along with rhonchi, wheezes, or coarse breath sounds. Chest x-rays can show air trapping and occasionally interstitial infiltrates.

In older children and adults, parainfluenza infections tend to be milder, presenting most frequently as a common cold or as hoarseness, with or without cough. Lower respiratory tract involvement in older children and adults is uncommon, but tracheobronchitis in adults has been reported. Severe, prolonged, and even fatal parainfluenza infection has been reported in children and adults with severe immunosuppression, including stem cell and solid-organ transplant recipients.

LABORATORY FINDINGS AND DIAGNOSIS

The clinical syndromes caused by parainfluenza viruses (with the possible exception of croup in young children) are not sufficiently distinctive to be diagnosed on clinical grounds alone. A specific diagnosis is established by detection of virus in respiratory tract secretions, throat swabs, or nasopharyngeal washings. Viral growth in tissue culture is detected either by hemagglutination or by a cytopathic effect. Rapid viral diagnosis may be made by identification of parainfluenza antigens in exfoliated cells from the respiratory tract with immunofluorescence or ELISA, although these techniques appear to be less sensitive than tissue culture. Highly specific and sensitive PCR assays have also been developed. Serologic diagnosis can be established by hemagglutination inhibition, complement-fixation, or neutralization tests of acute- and convalescent-phase specimens. However, since frequent heterotypic responses occur among the parainfluenza serotypes, the serotype causing illness often cannot be identified by serologic techniques alone.

Acute epiglottitis caused by *Haemophilus influenzae* type b must be differentiated from viral croup. Influenza A virus is also a common cause of croup during epidemic periods.

℞ PARAINFLUENZA VIRUS INFECTIONS

For upper respiratory tract illness, symptoms can be treated as discussed for other viral respiratory tract illnesses. If complications such as sinusitis, otitis, or superimposed bacterial bronchitis develop, appropriate antibacterial antibiotics should be administered. Mild cases of croup should be treated with bed rest and moist air generated by vaporizers. More severe cases require hospitalization and close observation for the development of respiratory distress. If acute respiratory distress develops, humidified oxygen and intermittent racemic epinephrine are usually administered. Aerosolized or systemically administered glucocorticoids are beneficial; the latter have a more profound effect. No specific antiviral therapy is available, although ribavirin is active against parainfluenza viruses in vitro and anecdotal reports describe its use clinically, particularly in immunosuppressed patients.

PREVENTION

Vaccines against parainfluenza viruses are under development.

ADENOVIRUS INFECTIONS

ETIOLOGIC AGENT

Adenoviruses are complex DNA viruses that measure 70–80 nm in diameter. Human adenoviruses belong to the genus *Mastadenovirus*, which includes 51 serotypes. Adenoviruses have a characteristic morphology consisting of an icosahedral shell composed of 20 equilateral triangular faces and 12 vertices. The protein coat (capsid) consists of hexon subunits with group-specific and type-specific antigenic determinants and penton subunits at each vertex primarily containing group-specific antigens. A fiber with a knob at the end projects from each penton; this fiber contains type-specific and some group-specific antigens. Human adenoviruses have been divided into six subgenera (A through F) on the basis of the homology of DNA genomes and other properties. The adenovirus genome is a linear double-stranded DNA that codes for structural and nonstructural polypeptides. The replicative cycle of adenovirus may result either in lytic infection of cells or in the establishment of a latent infection (primarily involving lymphoid cells). Some adenovirus types can induce oncogenic transformation, and tumor formation has been observed in rodents; however, despite intensive investigation, adenoviruses have not been associated with tumors in humans.

EPIDEMIOLOGY

Adenovirus infections most frequently affect infants and children. Infections occur throughout the year but are most common from fall to spring. Adenoviruses account for ~10% of acute respiratory infections in children but for <2% of respiratory illnesses in civilian adults. Nearly 100% of adults have serum antibody to multiple serotypes—a finding indicating that infection is common in childhood. Types 1, 2, 3, and 5 are the most frequent isolates from children. Certain adenovirus serotypes—particularly 4 and 7 but also 3, 14, and 21—are associated with outbreaks of acute respiratory disease in military recruits in winter and spring. Adenovirus infection can be transmitted by inhalation of aerosolized virus, by inoculation of virus into conjunctival sacs, and probably by the fecal-oral route as well. Type-specific antibody generally develops after infection and is associated with protection, albeit incomplete, against infection with the same serotype.

CLINICAL MANIFESTATIONS

In children, adenoviruses cause a variety of clinical syndromes. The most common is an acute upper respiratory tract infection, with prominent rhinitis. On occasion, lower respiratory tract disease, including bronchiolitis and pneumonia, also develops. Adenoviruses, particularly types 3 and 7, cause pharyngoconjunctival fever, a characteristic acute febrile illness of children that occurs in outbreaks, most often in summer camps. The syndrome is marked by bilateral conjunctivitis in which the bulbar and palpebral conjunctivae have a granular appearance. Low-grade fever is frequently present for the first 3 to 5 days, and rhinitis, sore throat, and cervical adenopathy develop. The illness generally lasts for 1–2 weeks and resolves spontaneously. Febrile pharyngitis without conjunctivitis has also been associated with adenovirus infection. Adenoviruses have been isolated from cases of whooping cough with or without *Bordetella pertussis*; the significance of adenovirus in that disease is unknown.

In adults, the most frequently reported illness has been acute respiratory disease caused by adenovirus types 4 and 7 in military recruits. This illness is marked by a prominent sore throat and the gradual onset of fever, which often reaches 39°C (102.2°F) on the second or third day of illness. Cough is almost always present, and coryza and regional lymphadenopathy are frequently seen. Physical examination may show pharyngeal edema, injection, and tonsillar enlargement with little or no exudate. If pneumonia has developed, auscultation and x-ray of the chest may indicate areas of patchy infiltration.

Adenoviruses have been associated with a number of non–respiratory tract diseases, including acute diarrheal illness caused by types 40 and 41 in young children and hemorrhagic cystitis caused by types 11 and 21. Epidemic keratoconjunctivitis, caused most frequently by types 8, 19, and 37, has been associated with contaminated common sources such as ophthalmic solutions and roller towels. Adenoviruses have also been implicated in disseminated disease and pneumonia in immunosuppressed patients, including recipients of solid-organ or stem cell transplants. In stem cell transplant recipients, adenovirus infections have manifested as pneumonia, hepatitis, nephritis, colitis, encephalitis, and hemorrhagic cystitis. In solid-organ transplant recipients, adenovirus infection may involve the organ transplanted (e.g., hepatitis in liver transplants, nephritis in renal transplants) but can disseminate to other organs as well. In patients with AIDS, high-numbered and intermediate adenovirus serotypes have been isolated, usually in the setting of low CD4+ T cell counts, but their isolation often has not been clearly linked to disease manifestations. Adenovirus nucleic acids have been detected in myocardial cells from patients with "idiopathic" myocardiopathies, and adenoviruses have been suggested as causative agents in some cases.

LABORATORY FINDINGS AND DIAGNOSIS

Adenovirus infection should be suspected in the epidemiologic setting of acute respiratory disease in military recruits and in certain of the clinical syndromes (such as pharyngoconjunctival fever or epidemic keratoconjunctivitis) in which outbreaks of characteristic illnesses occur. In most cases, however, illnesses caused by adenovirus infection cannot be differentiated from those caused by a number of other viral respiratory agents and *Mycoplasma pneumoniae*. A definitive diagnosis of adenovirus infection is established by detection of the virus in tissue culture (as evidenced by cytopathic changes) and by specific identification with immunofluorescence or other immunologic techniques. Rapid viral diagnosis can be established by immunofluorescence or ELISA of nasopharyngeal aspirates, conjunctival or respiratory secretions, urine, or stool. Highly sensitive and specific PCR assays and nucleic acid hybridization are also available. Adenovirus types 40 and 41, which have been associated with diarrheal disease in children, require special tissue-culture cells for isolation, and these serotypes are most commonly detected by direct ELISA of stool. Serum antibody rises can be demonstrated by complement-fixation or neutralization tests, ELISA, radioimmunoassay, or (for those adenoviruses that hemagglutinate red cells) hemagglutination inhibition tests.

℞ ADENOVIRUS INFECTIONS

Only symptom-based treatment and supportive therapy are available for adenovirus infections, and clinically useful antiviral therapy has not been established. Ribavirin and cidofovir have activity in vitro against certain adenoviruses. Retrospective studies and anecdotes describe the use of these agents in disseminated adenovirus infections, but definitive efficacy data from controlled studies are not available.

PREVENTION

Live vaccines have been developed against adenovirus types 4 and 7 and have been used to control illness among military recruits. These vaccines consist of live, unattenuated virus administered in enteric-coated capsules. Infection of the gastrointestinal tract with types 4 and 7 does not cause disease but stimulates local and systemic antibodies that are protective against subsequent acute respiratory disease due to those serotypes. This vaccine has not been produced since 1999, and outbreaks of acute respiratory illness caused by adenovirus types 4 and 7 have emerged again among military recruits. Therefore, a program to redevelop type 4 and 7 vaccines is under way. Adenoviruses are also being studied as live-virus vectors for the delivery of vaccine antigens and for gene therapy.

FURTHER READINGS

AMERICAN ACADEMY OF PEDIATRICS: Diagnosis and management of bronchiolitis. Pediatrics 118:1774, 2006

CHANOCK RM et al: Serious respiratory tract disease caused by respiratory syncytial virus: Prospects for improved therapy and effective immunization. Pediatrics 90:137, 1992

CHRISTIAN MD et al: Severe acute respiratory syndrome. Clin Infect Dis 38:1420, 2004

GRAHAM BS et al: Respiratory syncytial virus immunobiology and pathogenesis. Virology 297:1, 2002

GWALTNEY JM: Rhinoviruses, in *Principles and Practice of Infectious Diseases*, 6th ed, GF Mandell et al (eds). Philadelphia, Elsevier, 2005, pp 2185–2193

LEE N et al: A major outbreak of severe acute respiratory syndrome in Hong Kong. N Engl J Med 348:1986, 2003

PEIRIS JS et al: Severe acute respiratory syndrome. Nat Med 10:S88, 2004

PERET T et al: Characterization of human metapneumoviruses isolated from patients in North America. J Infect Dis 185:1660, 2002

STOCKTON J et al: Human metapneumovirus as a cause of community-acquired respiratory illness. Emerg Infect Dis 8:897, 2002

WRIGHT PF: Parainfluenza viruses, in *Viral Infections of the Respiratory Tract*, R Dolin, PF Wright (eds). New York, Marcel Dekker, 1999

180 Influenza
Raphael Dolin

DEFINITION

Influenza is an acute respiratory illness caused by infection with influenza viruses. The illness affects the upper and/or lower respiratory tract and is often accompanied by systemic signs and symptoms such as fever, headache, myalgia, and weakness. Outbreaks of illness of variable extent and severity occur nearly every winter. Such outbreaks result in significant morbidity in the general population and in increased mortality rates among certain high-risk patients, mainly as a result of pulmonary complications.

ETIOLOGIC AGENT

Influenza viruses are members of the Orthomyxoviridae family, of which influenza A, B, and C viruses constitute three separate genera. The designation of influenza viruses as type A, B, or C is based on antigenic characteristics of the nucleoprotein (NP) and matrix (M) protein antigens. Influenza A viruses are further subdivided (subtyped) on the basis of the surface hemagglutinin (H) and neuraminidase (N) antigens (see below); individual strains are designated according to the site of origin, isolate number, year of isolation, and subtype—for example, influenza A/Hiroshima/52/2005 (H3N2). Influenza A has 16 distinct H subtypes and 9 distinct N subtypes, of which only H1, H2, H3, N1, and N2 have been associated with epidemics of disease in humans. Influenza B and C viruses are similarly designated, but H and N antigens from these viruses do not receive subtype designations, since intratypic variations in influenza B antigens are less extensive than those in influenza A viruses and may not occur with influenza C virus.

Influenza A and B viruses are major human pathogens and the most extensively studied of the Orthomyxoviridae. Type A and type B viruses are morphologically similar. The virions are irregularly shaped spherical particles, measure 80–120 nm in diameter, and have a lipid envelope from the surface of which the H and N glycoproteins project (Fig. 180-1). The hemagglutinin is the site by which the virus binds to sialic acid cell receptors, whereas the neuraminidase degrades the receptor and plays a role in the release of the virus from infected cells after replication has taken place. Influenza viruses enter cells by receptor-mediated endocytosis, forming a virus-containing endosome. The viral hemagglutinin mediates fusion of the endosomal membrane with the virus envelope, and viral nucleocapsids are subsequently released into the cytoplasm. Immune responses to the H antigen are the major determinants of protection against infection with influenza virus, while those to the N antigen limit viral spread and contribute to reduction of the infection. The lipid envelope of influenza A virus also contains the M proteins M1 and M2, which are involved in stabilization of the lipid envelope and in virus assembly. The virion also contains the NP antigen, which is associated with the viral genome, as well as three polymerase (P) proteins that are essential for transcription and synthesis of viral RNA. Two nonstructural proteins function as an interferon antagonist and posttranscriptional regulator (NS1) and a nuclear export factor (NS2 or NEP).

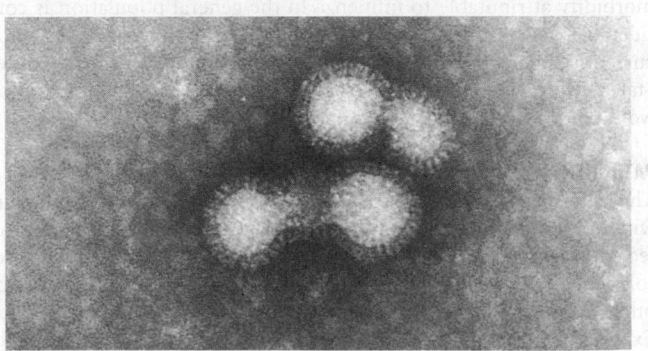

FIGURE 180-1 An electron micrograph of influenza A virus (× 40,000).

TABLE 180-1	EMERGENCE OF ANTIGENIC SUBTYPES OF INFLUENZA A VIRUS ASSOCIATED WITH PANDEMIC OR EPIDEMIC DISEASE	
Years	**Subtype**	**Extent of Outbreak**
1889–90	H2N8[a]	Severe pandemic
1900–03	H3N8[b]	?Moderate epidemic
1918–19	H1N1[b] (formerly HswN1)	Severe pandemic
1933–35	H1N1[b] (formerly H0N1)	Mild epidemic
1946–47	H1N1	Mild epidemic
1957–58	H2N2	Severe pandemic
1968–69	H3N2	Moderate pandemic
1977–78[c]	H1N1	Mild pandemic

[a]As determined by retrospective serologic survey of individuals alive during those years ("seroarcheology").
[b]Hemagglutinins formerly designated as Hsw and H0 are now classified as variants of H1.
[c]From this time until the present (2006–2007), viruses of the H1N1 and H3N2 subtypes have circulated either in alternating years or concurrently.

The genomes of influenza A and B viruses consist of eight single-stranded RNA segments, which code for the structural and nonstructural proteins. Because the genome is segmented, the opportunity for gene reassortment during infection is high; reassortment often occurs during infection of cells with more than one influenza A virus.

EPIDEMIOLOGY

Influenza outbreaks are recorded virtually every year, although their extent and severity vary widely. Localized outbreaks take place at variable intervals, usually every 1–3 years. Global pandemics have occurred at variable intervals, but much less frequently than interpandemic outbreaks (Table 180-1). The most recent pandemic occurred in 1977—some 30 years ago as of this writing; because of this relatively long interval, concern exists that the next pandemic may be imminent.

Influenza A Virus · *ANTIGENIC VARIATION AND INFLUENZA OUTBREAKS* The most extensive and severe outbreaks are caused by influenza A viruses, in part because of the remarkable propensity of the H and N antigens of these viruses to undergo periodic antigenic variation. Major antigenic variations, called *antigenic shifts*, may be associated with pandemics and are restricted to influenza A viruses. Minor variations are called *antigenic drifts*. These types of antigenic variation may involve the hemagglutinin alone or both the hemagglutinin and the neuraminidase. An example of an antigenic shift involving both the hemagglutinin and the neuraminidase is that of 1957, when the predominant influenza A virus subtype shifted from H1N1 to H2N2; this shift resulted in a severe pandemic, with an estimated 70,000 excess deaths (i.e., deaths in excess of the number expected without an influenza epidemic) in the United States alone. In 1968, an antigenic shift involving only the hemagglutinin occurred (H2N2 to H3N2); the subsequent pandemic was less severe than that of 1957. In 1977, an H1N1 virus emerged and caused a pandemic that primarily affected younger individuals (i.e., those born after 1957). As can be seen in Table 180-1, H1N1 viruses circulated from 1918 to 1956; thus, individuals born prior to 1957 would be expected to have some degree of immunity to H1N1 viruses. During most outbreaks of influenza A, a single subtype has circulated at a time. However, since 1977, H1N1 and H3N2 viruses have circulated simultaneously, resulting in outbreaks of varying severity. In some outbreaks, influenza B viruses have also circulated simultaneously with influenza A viruses.

AVIAN INFLUENZA In 1997, human cases of influenza caused by avian influenza viruses (A/H5N1) were detected in Hong Kong during an extensive outbreak of influenza in poultry. Between that time and January 2007, 261 cases of avian influenza in humans were reported in 10 countries in Asia and the Middle East. Nearly all of these cases were associated with contact with infected poultry. Efficient person-to-person transmission has not been observed to date. Mortality rates have been high (60%), and clinical manifestations have differed somewhat from those associated with "typical" outbreaks of influenza (see below). Transmission of avian influenza A/H7N7 viruses from infected poultry to humans has been observed in The Netherlands, resulting predominantly in cases of conjunctivitis and some respiratory illnesses. Infection with avian A/H9N2 viruses along with mild respiratory illness has been reported in children in Hong Kong. Because of the absence of widespread immunity to the H5, H7, and H9 viruses, concern has been raised that avian-to-human transmission may be the basis for the emergence of pandemic strains.

The origin of actual pandemic influenza A virus strains has now been partially elucidated with molecular virologic techniques. It appears that the pandemic strains of 1957 and 1968 resulted from a genetic reassortment between human viruses and avian viruses with novel surface glycoproteins (H2N2, H3). The influenza virus responsible for the most severe pandemic of modern times (1918–1919) appears to have represented an adaptation of an avian virus to efficient infection of humans. Close molecular surveillance of the avian viruses currently infecting humans is being conducted to provide early detection of possible pandemic strains.

FEATURES OF PANDEMIC AND INTERPANDEMIC INFLUENZA A   Pandemics provide the most dramatic evidence of the impact of influenza A. However, illnesses occurring between pandemics (interpandemic disease) account for extensive mortality and morbidity, albeit over a longer period. In the United States, influenza was associated with at least 19,000 excess deaths per season in 1976–1990 and with 36,000 excess deaths per season in 1990–1999. On average, there were 226,000 influenza-associated hospitalizations per year in this country in 1979–2001.

Influenza A viruses that circulate between pandemics demonstrate antigenic drifts in the H antigen. These antigenic drifts result from point mutations involving the RNA segment that codes for the hemagglutinin, which occur most frequently in five hypervariable regions. Epidemiologically significant strains—that is, those with the potential to cause widespread outbreaks—exhibit changes in amino acids in at least two of the major antigenic sites in the hemagglutinin molecule. Since two point mutations are unlikely to occur simultaneously, it is believed that antigenic drifts result from point mutations occurring sequentially during the spread of virus from person to person. Antigenic drifts have been reported nearly annually since 1977 for H1N1 viruses and since 1968 for H3N2 viruses.

Influenza A epidemics begin abruptly, peak over a 2- to 3-week period, generally last for 2–3 months, and often subside almost as rapidly as they began. The first indication of influenza activity in a community is an increase in the number of children with febrile respiratory illnesses who present for medical attention. This increase is followed by increases in rates of influenza-like illnesses among adults and eventually by an increase in hospital admissions for patients with pneumonia, worsening of congestive heart failure, and exacerbations of chronic pulmonary disease. Rates of absence from work and school also rise at this time. An increase in the number of deaths caused by pneumonia and influenza is generally a late observation in an outbreak. Attack rates have been highly variable from outbreak to outbreak but most commonly are in the range of 10–20% of the general population. During the pandemic of 1957, it was estimated that the attack rate of clinical influenza exceeded 50% in urban populations and that an additional 25% or more of individuals in these populations may have been subclinically infected with influenza A virus. Among institutionalized populations and in semiclosed settings with many susceptible individuals, even higher attack rates have been reported.

Epidemics of influenza A occur almost exclusively during the winter months in the temperate zones of the northern and southern hemispheres. In those locations, it is highly unusual to detect influenza A virus at other times, although rises in serum antibody titer or even outbreaks have been noted rarely during warm-weather months. In contrast, influenza virus infections occur throughout the year in the tropics. Where or how influenza A virus persists between outbreaks in temperate zones is unknown. It is possible that influenza A viruses are maintained in the human population on a worldwide basis by person-to-person transmission and that large population clusters support a low level of interepidemic transmission. Alternatively, human strains may persist in animal reservoirs. Convincing evidence to support either explanation is not available. In the modern era, rapid transportation may contribute to the transmission of viruses among widespread geographic locales.

The factors that result in the inception and termination of outbreaks of influenza A are incompletely understood. A major determinant of the extent and severity of an outbreak is the level of immunity in the population at risk. With the emergence of an antigenically novel influenza virus to which little or no immunity is present in a community, extensive outbreaks may occur. When the absence of immunity is worldwide, epidemic disease may spread around the globe, resulting in a pandemic. Such pandemic waves can continue for several years, until immunity in the population reaches a high level. In the years following pandemic influenza, antigenic drifts among influenza viruses result in outbreaks of variable severity in populations with high levels of immunity to the pandemic strain that circulated earlier. This situation persists until another antigenically novel pandemic strain emerges. On the other hand, outbreaks sometimes end despite the persistence of a large pool of susceptible individuals in the population. It has been suggested that certain influenza A viruses, such as recently circulating A/H1N1 strains, may be intrinsically less virulent and cause less severe disease than other variants, even in immunologically virgin subjects. If so, then other (undefined) factors besides the level of preexisting immunity must play a role in the epidemiology of influenza.

Influenza B and C Viruses   Influenza B virus causes outbreaks that are generally less extensive and are associated with less severe disease than those caused by influenza A virus. The hemagglutinin and neuraminidase of influenza B virus undergo less frequent and less extensive variation than those of influenza A viruses; this characteristic may account, in part, for the lesser extent of disease. Influenza B outbreaks are seen most frequently in schools and military camps, although outbreaks in institutions in which elderly individuals reside have also been noted on occasion. The most serious complication of influenza B virus infection is Reye's syndrome (Chap. 303).

In contrast to influenza A and B viruses, influenza C virus appears to be a relatively minor cause of disease in humans. It has been associated with common cold–like symptoms and occasionally with lower respiratory tract illness. Serum antibody to this virus is widely prevalent and indicates that asymptomatic infection may be common.

Influenza-Associated Morbidity and Mortality   The morbidity and mortality caused by influenza outbreaks continue to be substantial. Most individuals who die in this setting have underlying diseases that place them at high risk for complications of influenza. Excess hospitalizations for groups of adults and children with high-risk medical conditions ranged from 56 to 1900 per 100,000 during outbreaks of influenza in 1973–1993. The most prominent high-risk conditions are chronic cardiac and pulmonary diseases and old age. Mortality rates among individuals with chronic metabolic or renal disease or certain immunosuppressive diseases have also been elevated, albeit lower than those among patients with chronic cardiopulmonary diseases. The morbidity attributable to influenza in the general population is considerable. It is estimated that interpandemic outbreaks of influenza currently incur annual costs of more than $12 billion in the United States. If a pandemic were to occur, it is estimated that annual costs would range from $71 to $167 billion for attack rates of 15–35%.

PATHOGENESIS AND IMMUNITY

The initial event in influenza is infection of the respiratory epithelium with influenza virus acquired from respiratory secretions of acutely infected individuals. In all likelihood, the virus is transmitted via aerosols generated by coughs and sneezes, although hand-to-hand contact, other personal contact, and even fomite transmission may take place. Experimental evidence suggests that infection by a small-particle aerosol (particle diameter, <10 μm) is more efficient than that by larger droplets. Initially, viral infection involves the ciliated columnar epithelial cells, but it may also involve other respiratory tract cells, including alveolar cells, mucous gland cells, and macrophages. In infected cells, virus replicates within 4–6 h, after which infectious virus is released to infect adjacent or nearby cells. In this way, infection spreads from a few foci to a large number of respiratory cells over several hours. In experimentally induced infection, the incubation period of illness has ranged from 18 to 72 h, depending on the size of the viral inoculum. Histopathologic study reveals degenerative changes, including granulation, vacuolization, swelling, and pyknotic nuclei, in infected ciliated cells. The cells eventually become necrotic and desquamate; in some areas, previously columnar epithelium is replaced by flattened and metaplastic epithelial cells. The severity of illness is correlated with the quantity of virus shed in secretions; thus, the degree of viral replication itself may be an important factor in pathogenesis. Despite the frequent development of systemic signs and symptoms such as fever, headache, and myalgias, influenza virus has only rarely been detected in extrapulmonary sites (including the bloodstream). Evidence suggests that the pathogenesis of systemic symptoms in influenza may be related to the induction of certain cytokines, particularly tumor necrosis factor α, interferon α, interleukin 6, and interleukin 8, in respiratory secretions and in the bloodstream.

The host response to influenza infections involves a complex interplay of humoral antibody, local antibody, cell-mediated immunity, interferon, and other host defenses. Serum antibody responses, which can be detected by the second week after primary infection, are measured by a variety of techniques: hemagglutination inhibition (HI), complement fixation (CF), neutralization, enzyme-linked immunosorbent assay (ELISA), and antineuraminidase antibody assay. Antibodies to the hemagglutinin appear to be the most important mediators of immunity; in several studies, HI titers of ≥40 have been associated with protection from infection. Secretory antibodies produced in the respiratory tract are predominantly of the IgA class and also play a major role in protection against infection. Secretory antibody neutralization titers of ≥ 4 have also been associated with protection. A variety of cell-mediated immune responses, both antigen-specific and antigen-nonspecific, can be detected early after infection and depend on the prior immune status of the host. These responses include T cell proliferative, T cell cytotoxic, and natural killer cell activity. In humans, CD8+ HLA class I–restricted cytotoxic T lymphocytes (CTLs) are directed at conserved regions of internal proteins (NP, M, and polymerases) as well as against the surface proteins (H and N). Interferons can be detected in respiratory secretions shortly after the shedding of virus has begun, and rises in interferon titers coincide with decreases in virus shedding.

The host defense factors responsible for cessation of virus shedding and resolution of illness have not been defined specifically. Virus shedding generally stops within 2–5 days after symptoms first appear, at a time when serum and local antibody responses often are not detectable by conventional techniques (although antibody rises may be detected earlier by use of highly sensitive techniques, particularly in individuals with previous immunity to the virus). It has been suggested that interferon, cell-mediated immune responses, and/or nonspecific inflammatory responses all contribute to the resolution of illness. CTL responses may be particularly important in this regard.

CLINICAL MANIFESTATIONS
Influenza has most frequently been described as an illness characterized by the abrupt onset of systemic symptoms, such as headache, feverishness, chills, myalgia, or malaise, and accompanying respiratory tract signs, particularly cough and sore throat. In many cases, the onset is so abrupt that patients can recall the precise time they became ill. However, the spectrum of clinical presentations is wide, ranging from a mild, afebrile respiratory illness similar to the common cold (with either a gradual or an abrupt onset) to severe prostration with relatively few respiratory signs and symptoms. In most of the cases that come to a physician's attention, the patient has a fever, with temperatures of 38°–41°C (100.4°–105.8°F). A rapid temperature rise within the first 24 h of illness is generally followed by gradual defervescence over 2–3 days, although, on occasion, fever may last as long as 1 week. Patients report a feverish feeling and chilliness, but true rigors are rare. Headache, either generalized or frontal, is often particularly troublesome. Myalgias may involve any part of the body but are most common in the legs and lumbosacral area. Arthralgias may also develop.

Respiratory symptoms often become more prominent as systemic symptoms subside. Many patients have a sore throat or persistent cough, which may last for ≥ 1 week and which is often accompanied by substernal discomfort. Ocular signs and symptoms include pain on motion of the eyes, photophobia, and burning of the eyes.

Physical findings are usually minimal in uncomplicated influenza. Early in the illness, the patient appears flushed, and the skin is hot and dry, although diaphoresis and mottled extremities are sometimes evident, particularly in older patients. Examination of the pharynx may yield surprisingly unremarkable results despite a severe sore throat, but injection of the mucous membranes and postnasal discharge are apparent in some cases. Mild cervical lymphadenopathy may be noted, especially in younger individuals. The results of chest examination are largely negative in uncomplicated influenza, although rhonchi, wheezes, and scattered rales have been reported with variable frequency in different outbreaks. Frank dyspnea, hyperpnea, cyanosis, diffuse rales, and signs of consolidation are indicative of pulmonary complications. Patients with apparently uncomplicated influenza have been reported to have a variety of mild ventilatory defects and increased alveolar-capillary diffusion gradients; thus, subclinical pulmonary involvement may be more common than is appreciated.

In uncomplicated influenza, the acute illness generally resolves over 2–5 days, and most patients have largely recovered in 1 week, although cough may persist 1–2 weeks longer. In a significant minority (particularly the elderly), however, symptoms of weakness or lassitude (postinfluenzal asthenia) may persist for several weeks and may prove troublesome for persons who wish to resume their full level of activity promptly. The pathogenetic basis for this asthenia is unknown, although pulmonary function abnormalities may persist for several weeks after uncomplicated influenza.

COMPLICATIONS
Complications of influenza occur most frequently in patients >64 years old and in those with certain chronic disorders, including cardiac or pulmonary diseases, diabetes mellitus, hemoglobinopathies, renal dysfunction, and immunosuppression. Pregnancy in the second or third trimester also predisposes to complications with influenza. Children <2 years old (especially infants) are also at high risk for complications.

Pulmonary Complications · *PNEUMONIA* The most significant complication of influenza is pneumonia: "primary" influenza viral pneumonia, secondary bacterial pneumonia, or mixed viral and bacterial pneumonia.

PRIMARY INFLUENZA VIRAL PNEUMONIA Primary influenza viral pneumonia is the least common but most severe of the pneumonic complications. It presents as acute influenza that does not resolve but instead progresses relentlessly, with persistent fever, dyspnea, and eventual cyanosis. Sputum production is generally scanty, but the sputum can contain blood. Few physical signs may be evident early in the illness. In more advanced cases, diffuse rales may be noted, and chest x-ray findings consistent with diffuse interstitial infiltrates and/or acute respiratory distress syndrome may be present. In such cases, arterial blood-gas determinations show marked hypoxia. Viral cultures of respiratory secretions and lung parenchyma, especially if samples are taken early in illness, yield high titers of virus. In fatal cases of primary viral pneumonia, histopathologic examination reveals a marked inflammatory reaction in the alveolar septa, with edema and infiltration by lymphocytes, macrophages, occasional plasma cells, and variable numbers of neutrophils. Fibrin thrombi in alveolar capillaries, along with necrosis and hemorrhage, have also been noted. Eosinophilic hyaline membranes can be found lining alveoli and alveolar ducts.

Primary influenza viral pneumonia has a predilection for individuals with cardiac disease, particularly those with mitral stenosis, but has also been reported in otherwise-healthy young adults as well as in older individuals with chronic pulmonary disorders. In some epidemics of influenza (notably those of 1918 and 1957), pregnancy increased the risk of primary influenza pneumonia. Subsequent epidemics of influenza have been associated with increased rates of hospitalization among pregnant women.

SECONDARY BACTERIAL PNEUMONIA Secondary bacterial pneumonia follows acute influenza. Improvement of the patient's condition over 2–3 days is followed by a reappearance of fever along with clinical signs and symptoms of bacterial pneumonia, including cough, production of purulent sputum, and physical and x-ray signs of consolidation. The most common bacterial pathogens in this setting are *Streptococcus pneumoniae*, *Staphylococcus aureus*, and *Haemophilus influenzae*—organisms that can colonize the nasopharynx and that cause infection in the wake of changes in bronchopulmonary defenses. The etiology can often be determined by Gram's staining and culture of an appropriately obtained sputum specimen. Secondary bacterial pneumonia occurs most frequently in high-risk individuals with chronic pulmonary and cardiac disease and in elderly individuals. Patients with secondary bacterial pneumonia often respond to antibiotic therapy when it is instituted promptly.

MIXED VIRAL AND BACTERIAL PNEUMONIA Perhaps the most common pneumonic complications during outbreaks of influenza have mixed features of viral and bacterial pneumonia. Patients may experience a gradual progression of their acute illness or may show transient improvement followed by clinical exacerbation, with eventual manifestation of the clinical features of bacterial pneumonia. Sputum cultures may contain both influenza A virus and one of the bacterial pathogens described above. Patchy infiltrates or areas of consolidation may be detected by physical examination and chest x-ray. Patients with mixed viral and bacterial pneumonia generally have less widespread involvement of the lung than those with primary viral pneumonia, and their bacterial infections may respond to appropriate antibacterial drugs. Mixed viral and bacterial pneumonia occurs primarily in patients with chronic cardiovascular and pulmonary diseases.

OTHER PULMONARY COMPLICATIONS Other pulmonary complications associated with influenza include worsening of chronic obstructive pulmonary disease and exacerbation of chronic bronchitis and asthma. In children, influenza infection may present as croup. Sinusitis as well as otitis media (the latter occurring particularly often in children) may also be associated with influenza.

Extrapulmonary Complications In addition to the pulmonary complications of influenza, a number of extrapulmonary complications may occur. These include *Reye's syndrome* (Chap. 303), a serious complication in children that is associated with influenza B and to a lesser extent with influenza A virus infection as well as with varicella-zoster virus infection. An epidemiologic association between Reye's syndrome and aspirin therapy for the antecedent viral infection has been noted, and the syndrome's incidence has decreased markedly with widespread warnings regarding aspirin use by children with acute viral respiratory infections.

Myositis, rhabdomyolysis, and myoglobinuria are occasional complications of influenza infection. Although myalgias are exceedingly common in influenza, true myositis is rare. Patients with acute myositis have exquisite tenderness of the affected muscles, most commonly in the legs, and may not be able to tolerate even the slightest pressure, such as the touch of bedsheets. In the most severe cases, there is frank swelling and bogginess of muscles. Serum levels of creatine phosphokinase and aldolase are markedly elevated, and an occasional patient develops renal failure from myoglobinuria. The pathogenesis of influenza-associated myositis is also unclear, although the presence of influenza virus in affected muscles has been reported.

Myocarditis and pericarditis were reported in association with influenza virus infection during the 1918–1919 pandemic; these reports were based largely on histopathologic findings, and these complications have been reported only infrequently since that time. Electrocardiographic changes during acute influenza are common among patients who have cardiac disease but have been ascribed most often to exacerbations of the underlying cardiac disease rather than to direct involvement of the myocardium with influenza virus.

Central nervous system (CNS) diseases, including encephalitis, transverse myelitis, and Guillain-Barré syndrome, have been reported during influenza. The etiologic relationship of influenza virus to such CNS illnesses remains uncertain. Toxic shock syndrome associated with *S. aureus* or group A streptococcal infection following acute influenza infection has also been reported (Chaps. 129 and 130).

In addition to complications involving the specific organ systems described above, influenza outbreaks include a number of cases in which elderly and other high-risk individuals develop influenza and subsequently experience a gradual deterioration of underlying cardiovascular, pulmonary, or renal function—changes that occasionally are irreversible and lead to death. These deaths contribute to the overall excess mortality associated with influenza A outbreaks.

Complications of Avian Influenza Cases of influenza caused by avian A/H5N1 virus are reportedly associated with high rates of pneumonia (>50%) and extrapulmonary manifestations such as diarrhea and CNS involvement. Deaths have been associated with multisystem dysfunction, including cardiac and renal failure.

LABORATORY FINDINGS AND DIAGNOSIS

During acute influenza, virus may be detected in throat swabs, nasopharyngeal washes, or sputum. The virus can be isolated by use of tissue culture—or, less commonly, chick embryos—within 48–72 h after inoculation. Most commonly, the laboratory diagnosis is established with rapid viral tests that detect viral nucleoprotein or neuraminidase by means of immunologic or enzymatic techniques that are highly sensitive and 60–90% as specific as tissue culture. Viral nucleic acids can also be detected in clinical samples by reverse transcriptase polymerase chain reaction. The type of the infecting influenza virus (A or B) may be determined by either immunofluorescence or HI techniques, and the hemagglutinin subtype of influenza A virus (H1, H2, or H3) may be identified by HI with use of subtype-specific antisera. Serologic methods for diagnosis require comparison of antibody titers in sera obtained during the acute illness with those in sera obtained 10–14 days after the onset of illness and are useful primarily in retrospect. Fourfold or greater titer rises as detected by HI or CF or significant rises as measured by ELISA are diagnostic of acute infection. CF tests are generally less sensitive than other serologic techniques, but, as they detect type-specific antigens, they may be particularly useful when subtype-specific reagents are not available.

Other laboratory tests generally are not helpful in the specific diagnosis of influenza virus infection. Leukocyte counts are variable, frequently being low early in illness and normal or slightly elevated later. Severe leukopenia has been described in overwhelming viral or bacterial infection, while leukocytosis with >15,000 cells/μL raises the suspicion of secondary bacterial infection.

DIFFERENTIAL DIAGNOSIS

During a community-wide outbreak, a clinical diagnosis of influenza can be made with a high degree of certainty in patients who present to a physician's office with the typical febrile respiratory illness described above. In the absence of an outbreak (i.e., in sporadic or isolated cases), influenza may be difficult to differentiate on clinical grounds alone from an acute respiratory illness caused by any of a variety of respiratory viruses or by *Mycoplasma pneumoniae*. Severe streptococcal pharyngitis or early bacterial pneumonia may mimic acute influenza, although bacterial pneumonias generally do not run a self-limited course. Purulent sputum in which a bacterial pathogen can be detected by Gram's staining is an important diagnostic feature in bacterial pneumonia.

TABLE 180-2 ANTIVIRAL MEDICATIONS FOR TREATMENT AND PROPHYLAXIS OF INFLUENZA

	Age Group (years)		
Antiviral Drug	**Children (≤12)**	**13–64**	**≥65**
Oseltamivir			
Treatment, influenza A and B	Age 1–12, dose varies by weight[a]	75 mg PO bid	75 mg PO bid
Prophylaxis, influenza A and B	Age 1–12, dose varies by weight[b]	75 PO qd	75 mg PO qd
Zanamivir			
Treatment, influenza A and B	Age 7–12, 10 mg bid by inhalation	10 mg bid by inhalation	10 mg bid by inhalation
Prophylaxis, influenza A and B	Age 5–12, 10 mg qd by inhalation	10 mg qd by inhalation	10 mg qd by inhalation
Amantadine[c]			
Treatment, influenza A	Age 1–9, 5 mg/kg in 2 divided doses, up to 150 mg/d	Age ≥10, 100 mg PO bid	≤100 mg/d
Prophylaxis, influenza A	Age 1–9, 5 mg/kg in 2 divided doses, up to 150 mg/d	Age ≥10, 100 mg PO bid	≤100 mg/d
Rimantadine[c]			
Treatment, influenza A	Not approved	100 mg PO bid	100–200 mg/d
Prophylaxis, influenza A	Age 1–9, 5 mg/kg in 2 divided doses, up to 150 mg/d	Age ≥10, 100 mg PO bid	100–200 mg/d

[a]<15 kg: 30 mg bid; >15–23 kg: 45 mg bid; >23–40 kg: 60 mg bid; >40 kg: 75 mg bid.
[b]<15 kg: 30 mg qd; >15–23 kg: 45 mg qd; >23–40 kg: 60 mg qd; >40 kg: 75 mg qd.
[c]Amantadine and rimantadine are not currently recommended (2006–2007) because of widespread resistance in influenza A/H3N2 viruses. Their use may be reconsidered if viral susceptibility is reestablished.

℞ **INFLUENZA**

In uncomplicated cases of influenza, symptom-based therapy with acetaminophen for the relief of headache, myalgia, and fever may be considered, but the use of salicylates should be avoided in children <18 years of age because of the possible association of salicylates with Reye's syndrome. Since cough is ordinarily self-limited, treatment with cough suppressants generally is not indicated, although codeine-containing compounds may be employed if the cough is particularly troublesome. Patients should be advised to rest and maintain hydration during acute illness and to return to full activity only gradually after illness has resolved, especially if it has been severe.

Specific antiviral therapy is available for influenza **(Table 180-2)**: the neuraminidase inhibitors zanamivir and oseltamivir for both influenza A and influenza B and the adamantane agents amantadine and rimantadine for influenza A (Chap. 171) In 2005–2006, resistance to amantadine was reported in >90% of A/H3N2 viral isolates; thus amantadine and rimantadine are no longer recommended, but their use may be reconsidered if sensitivity becomes reestablished.

Oseltamivir (administered orally at a dose of 75 mg twice a day for 5 days) or zanamivir (which must be given by an oral inhalation device; 10 mg twice a day for 5 days) reduces the duration of signs and symptoms of influenza by 1–1.5 days if treatment is started within 2 days of the onset of illness. Zanamivir may exacerbate bronchospasm in asthmatic patients, and oseltamivir has been associated with nausea and vomiting, whose frequency can be reduced by administration of the drug with food. Oseltamivir has also been associated with neuropsychiatric side effects in children.

If begun within 48 h of the onset of illness due to sensitive influenza A virus strains, treatment with amantadine or rimantadine reduces the duration of systemic and respiratory symptoms of influenza by ~50%. Of individuals who receive amantadine, 5–10% experience mild CNS side effects, primarily jitteriness, anxiety, insomnia, or difficulty concentrating. These side effects disappear promptly upon cessation of therapy. Rimantadine appears to be equally efficacious and is associated with less frequent CNS side effects than is amantadine. In adults, the usual dose of amantadine or rimantadine is 200 mg/d for 3–7 days. Since both drugs are excreted via the kidney, the dose should be reduced to ≤100 mg/d in elderly patients and in patients with renal insufficiency. Resistant viruses emerge frequently during treatment with amantadine or rimantadine and can be transmitted among family members. Development of resistance to zanamivir or oseltamivir appears to be less common but can occur. Ribavirin is a nucleoside analogue with activity against influenza A and B viruses in vitro. It has been reported to be variably effective against influenza when administered as an aerosol but ineffective when administered orally. Its efficacy in the treatment of influenza A or B is unestablished.

Studies demonstrating the therapeutic efficacy of antiviral compounds in influenza have primarily involved young adults with uncomplicated disease. A meta-analysis of studies with oseltamivir suggests that treatment may reduce the likelihood of some lower respiratory tract complications of influenza. However, it is not known whether antiviral agents are themselves effective in the treatment of influenza pneumonia or of other complications of influenza. Therapy for primary influenza pneumonia is directed at maintaining oxygenation and is most appropriately undertaken in an intensive care unit, with aggressive respiratory and hemodynamic support as needed. Bypass membrane oxygenators have been employed in this setting with variable results. When an acute respiratory distress syndrome develops, fluids must be administered cautiously, with close monitoring of blood gases and hemodynamic function.

Antibacterial drugs should be reserved for the treatment of bacterial complications of acute influenza, such as secondary bacterial pneumonia. The choice of antibiotics should be guided by Gram's staining and culture of appropriate specimens of respiratory secretions, such as sputum or transtracheal aspirates. If the etiology of a case of bacterial pneumonia is unclear from an examination of respiratory secretions, empirical antibiotics effective against the most common bacterial pathogens in this setting (*S. pneumoniae, S. aureus,* and *H. influenzae*) should be selected (Chaps. 128, 129, and 139).

PROPHYLAXIS

Inactivated and live attenuated vaccines against influenza are available, and their use represents the major public health measure for prevention of influenza. The vast majority of currently used vaccines are inactivated ("killed") preparations derived from influenza A and B viruses that circulated during the previous influenza season. If the vaccine virus and the currently circulating viruses are closely related, 50–80% protection against influenza would be expected from inactivated vaccines. The available inactivated vaccines have been highly purified and are associated with few reactions. Up to 5% of individuals experience low-grade fever and mild systemic symptoms 8–24 h after vaccination, and up to one-third develop mild redness or tenderness at the vaccination site. Since the vaccine is produced in eggs, individuals with true hypersensitivity to egg products either should be desensitized or should not be vaccinated. Although the 1976 swine influenza vaccine appears to have been associated with an increased frequency of Guillain-Barré syndrome, influenza vaccines administered since 1976 generally have not been. Possible exceptions were noted during the 1992–1993 and 1993–1994 influenza seasons, when there may have been an excess risk of Guillain-Barré syndrome of slightly more than 1 case per million vaccine recipients. However, the overall health risk following influenza outweighs the potential risk associated with vaccination.

The U.S. Public Health Service recommends the administration of inactivated influenza vaccine to individuals who, because of age or underlying disease, are at increased risk for complications of influenza and to the contacts of these individuals (Table 180-3). Inactivated vaccines may be administered safely to immunocompromised patients. Influenza vaccination is not associated with exacerbations of chronic nervous-system diseases such as multiple sclerosis. Vaccine should be administered early in the autumn before influenza outbreaks occur and should then be given annually to maintain immunity against the most current influenza virus strains.

TABLE 180-3   PERSONS FOR WHOM ANNUAL INFLUENZA VACCINATION IS RECOMMENDED

Children 6–59 months old
Women who will be pregnant during the influenza season
Persons ≥50 years old
Children and adolescents (6 months to 18 years old) who are receiving long-term aspirin therapy and therefore may be at risk for developing Reye's syndrome after influenza
Adults and children who have chronic disorders of the pulmonary or cardiovascular systems, including asthma[a]
Adults and children who have required regular medical follow-up or hospitalization during the preceding year because of chronic metabolic diseases (including diabetes mellitus), renal dysfunction, hemoglobinopathies, or immunodeficiency (including immunodeficiency caused by medications or by HIV)
Adults and children who have any condition (e.g., cognitive dysfunction, spinal cord injuries, seizure disorders, or other neuromuscular disorders) that can compromise respiratory function or the handling of respiratory secretions or can increase the risk of aspiration
Residents of nursing homes and other chronic-care facilities that house persons of any age who have chronic medical conditions
Persons who live with or care for persons at high risk for influenza-related complications, including healthy household contacts of and caregivers for children from birth through 59 months of age
Health care workers

[a]Hypertension itself is not considered a chronic disorder for which influenza vaccination is recommended.
Source: Centers for Disease Control and Prevention: Prevention and control of influenza: Recommendations of the Advisory Committee on Immunization Practices (ACIP). MMWR 55(RR-11):1, 2006.

A live attenuated influenza vaccine that is administered by intranasal spray is also available. The vaccine is generated by reassortment between currently circulating strains of influenza A and B virus and a cold-adapted, attenuated master strain. The cold-adapted vaccine is well tolerated and highly efficacious (92% protective) in young children; in one study, it provided protection against a circulating influenza virus that had drifted antigenically away from the vaccine strain. Live attenuated vaccine is approved for use in healthy persons 5–49 years of age.

Antiviral drugs may also be used as chemoprophylaxis against influenza (Table 180-2). Chemoprophylaxis with oseltamivir (75 mg/d by mouth) or zanamivir (10 mg/d inhaled) has been 84–89% efficacious against influenza A and B. Chemoprophylaxis with amantadine or rimantadine is no longer recommended because of reports of widespread resistance to these drugs. In earlier studies with sensitive viruses, prophylaxis with amantadine or rimantadine (100–200 mg/d) was 70–100% effective against illness associated with influenza A. Chemo-

prophylaxis is most likely to be used for high-risk individuals who have not received influenza vaccine or in a situation where the vaccines previously administered are relatively ineffective because of antigenic changes in the circulating virus. During an outbreak, antiviral chemoprophylaxis can be administered simultaneously with inactivated vaccine, since the drugs do not interfere with an immune response to the vaccine. In fact, there is evidence that the protective effects of chemoprophylaxis and inactivated vaccine may be additive. However, concurrent administration of chemoprophylaxis and the live attenuated vaccine may interfere with the immune response to the latter. Antiviral drugs should not be administered until at least 2 weeks after administration of live vaccine, and vaccination with live vaccine should not begin until at least 48 h after antiviral drug administration has been stopped. Chemoprophylaxis may also be employed to control nosocomial outbreaks of influenza. For that purpose, prophylaxis should be instituted promptly when influenza activity is detected and must be continued daily for the duration of the outbreak.

FURTHER READINGS

BEIGEL JH et al: Avian influenza A (H5N1) infection in humans. N Engl J Med 353:1374, 2005

BELSHE RB et al: The efficacy of live attenuated, cold adapted trivalent, intranasal influenza vaccine in children. N Engl J Med 38:1405, 1998

CENTERS FOR DISEASE CONTROL AND PREVENTION: Prevention and control of influenza. MMWR 55(RR–11):1, 2006

COOPER NJ et al: Effectiveness of neuraminidase inhibitors in treatment and prevention of influenza A and B: Systematic review and meta-analysis of randomized controlled trials. BMJ 326:1235, 2003

DOLIN R: Interpandemic as well as pandemic disease. N Engl J Med 353:2535, 2005

HAYDEN FG et al: Use of the selective oral neuraminidase inhibitor oseltamivir to prevent influenza. N Engl J Med 341:1336, 1999

MELTZER MI et al: The economic impact of pandemic influenza in the United States: Priorities for intervention. Emerg Infect Dis 5:659, 1999

MIST [MANAGEMENT OF INFLUENZA IN THE SOUTHERN HEMISPHERE TRIALISTS] STUDY GROUP: Randomized trial of efficacy and safety of inhaled zanamivir in treatment of influenza A and B infections. Lancet 352:1871, 1998

NEUZIL KM et al: Influenza-associated morbidity and mortality in young and middle-aged women. JAMA 281:901, 1999

SIMONSEN L et al: Pandemic vs epidemic mortality: A pattern of changing age distribution. J Infect Dis 178:53, 1998

TREANOR JJ: Influenza virus, in *Principles and Practice of Infectious Diseases*, 6th ed, GL Mandell et al (eds). Philadelphia, Elsevier, 2005, pp 2201–2203

SECTION 14   INFECTIONS DUE TO HUMAN IMMUNODEFICIENCY VIRUS AND OTHER HUMAN RETROVIRUSES

181   The Human Retroviruses
Dan L. Longo, Anthony S. Fauci

The retroviruses, which make up a large family (Retroviridae), infect mainly vertebrates. These viruses have a unique replication cycle whereby their genetic information is encoded by RNA rather than DNA. Retroviruses contain an RNA-dependent DNA polymerase (a reverse transcriptase) that directs the synthesis of a DNA form of the viral genome after infection of a host cell. The designation *retrovirus*

denotes that information in the form of RNA is transcribed into DNA in the host cell—a sequence that overturned a central dogma of molecular biology: that information passes unidirectionally from DNA to RNA to protein. The observation that RNA was the source of genetic information in the causative agents of certain animal tumors led to a number of paradigm-shifting biologic insights regarding not only the direction of genetic information passage but also the viral etiology of certain cancers and the concept of oncogenes as normal host genes scavenged and altered by a viral vector.

The family Retroviridae includes three subfamilies (Table 181-1): Oncovirinae, of which human T cell lymphotropic virus (HTLV) type I is the most important in humans; Lentivirinae, of which HIV is the

TABLE 181-1   CLASSIFICATION OF RETROVIRUSES: THE FAMILY RETROVIRIDAE

Subfamily, Group[a]	Example(s)	Feature
Oncovirinae (oncogenic viruses)		
Avian leukosis	Rous sarcoma virus	Contains *src* oncogene
Mammalian C-type	Abelson leukemia virus	Contains *abl* oncogene
B-type	Murine mammary tumor virus	Can be endogenous or exogenous
D-type	Mason-Pfizer monkey virus	—
HTLV-BLV	HTLV-I	Causes T-cell lymphoma and neurologic disease
Lentivirinae (slow viruses)	HIV-1, HIV-2	Cause AIDS
	Visna virus	Causes lung and brain diseases in sheep
	Feline immunodeficiency virus	Causes immunodeficiency in cats
Spumavirinae (foamy viruses)	Simian foamy virus, human foamy virus	Cause no known disease

[a]The Oncovirinae were originally grouped into types A–D on the basis of morphologic features (size, core location, budding) under electron microscopy; however, this system has been replaced by groupings based on relationships of genome structure and sequence.

Note: HTLV, human T cell lymphotropic virus; BLV, bovine leukemia virus.

most important in humans; and Spumavirinae, the "foamy" viruses, named for the pathologic appearance of infected cells. A number of spumaviruses have been isolated from humans; however, they are not associated with any known disease and therefore are not discussed further in this chapter.

The wide variety of interactions of a retrovirus with its host range from completely benign events (e.g., silent carriage of endogenous retroviral sequences in the germ-line genome of many animal species) to rapidly fatal infections (e.g., exogenous infection with an oncogenic virus such as Rous sarcoma virus in chickens). The ability of retroviruses to acquire and alter the structure and function of host cell sequences has revolutionized our understanding of molecular carcinogenesis. The viruses can insert into the germ-line genome of the host cell and behave as a transposable or movable genetic element. They can activate or inactivate genes near the site of integration into the genome. They can rapidly alter their own genome by recombination and mutation under selective environmental stimuli.

Most human viral diseases occur as a consequence of either tissue destruction by the virus itself or the host's response to the virus. Although these mechanisms are operative in retroviral infections, retroviruses have additional mechanisms of inducing disease, including the malignant transformation of an infected cell and the induction of an immunodeficiency state that leads to opportunistic diseases (infections and neoplasms; Chap. 182).

STRUCTURE AND LIFE CYCLE

Despite the wide range of biologic consequences of retroviral infection, all retroviruses are similar in structure, genome organization, and mode of replication. Retroviruses are 70–130 nm in diameter and have a lipid-containing envelope surrounding an icosahedral capsid with a dense inner core. The core contains two identical copies of the single-strand RNA genome. The RNA molecules are 8–10 kb long and are complexed with reverse transcriptase and tRNA. Other viral proteins, such as integrase, are also components of the virion particle. The RNA has features usually found in mRNA: a cap site at the 5′ end of the molecule, which is important in the initiation of mRNA translation, and a polyadenylation site at the 3′ end, which influences mRNA turnover (i.e., messages with shorter polyA tails turn over faster than messages with longer polyA tails). However, the retroviral RNA is not translated; instead it is transcribed into DNA. The DNA form of the retroviral genome is called a *provirus*.

The replication cycle of retroviruses proceeds in two phases (**Fig. 181-1**). In the first phase, the virus enters the cytoplasm after binding to a specific cell-surface receptor; the viral RNA and reverse transcriptase synthesize a double-strand DNA version of the RNA template; and the provirus moves into the nucleus and integrates into the host

cell genome. This proviral integration is permanent. Although some animal retroviruses integrate into a single specific site of the host genome in every infected cell, the four known human retroviruses (HTLV-I, HTLV-II, HIV-1, and HIV-2) integrate randomly. This first phase of replication depends entirely on gene products in the virus. The second phase includes the synthesis and processing of viral genomes, mRNAs, and proteins using host cell machinery, often under the influence of viral gene products. Virions are assembled and released from the cell by budding from the membrane; host cell membrane proteins are frequently incorporated into the envelope of the virus. Proviral integration occurs during the S-phase of the cell cycle; thus, in general, nondividing cells are resistant to retroviral infection. Only the lentiviruses are able to infect nondividing cells. Once a host cell is infected, it is infected for the life of the cell.

Retroviral genomes include both coding and noncoding sequences (**Fig. 181-2**). In general, noncoding sequences are important recognition signals for DNA or RNA synthesis or processing events and are located in the 5′ and 3′ terminal regions of the genome. All retroviral genomes are terminally redundant, containing identical sequences called *long terminal repeats* (LTRs). The ends of the retroviral RNA genome differ slightly in sequence from the integrated retroviral DNA. In the latter, the LTR sequences are repeated in both the 5′ and the 3′ terminus of the virus. The LTRs contain sequences involved in initiating the expression of the viral proteins, the integration of the provirus, and the polyadenylation of viral RNAs. The primer binding site, which is critical for the initiation of reverse transcription, and the viral packaging sequences are located outside the LTR sequences. The coding regions include the *gag* (group-specific antigen, core protein), *pol* (RNA-dependent DNA polymerase), and *env* (envelope) genes. The *gag* gene encodes a precursor polyprotein that is cleaved to form three to five capsid proteins; a fraction of the Gag precursor proteins also contain a protease responsible for cleaving the Gag and Pol polyproteins. A Gag-Pol polyprotein gives rise to the protease that is responsible for cleaving the Gag-Pol polyprotein. The *pol* gene encodes three proteins: the reverse transcriptase, the integrase, and the protease. The reverse transcriptase functions to copy the viral RNA into the double-strand DNA provirus, which inserts itself into the host cell DNA via the action of integrase. The protease functions to cleave the Gag-Pol polyprotein into smaller protein products. The *env* gene encodes the envelope glycoproteins: one protein that binds to specific surface receptors and determines what cell types can be infected and a smaller transmembrane protein that anchors the complex to the envelope. **Figure 181-3** shows how the retroviral gene products make up the virus structure.

HTLVs have a region between *env* and the 3′ LTR that encodes at least two proteins in overlapping reading frames: Tax, a 40-kDa protein that does not bind to DNA but induces the expression of host cell transcription factors that alter host cell gene expression; and Rex, a 27-kDa protein that regulates the expression of viral mRNAs. These two proteins are produced from messages that are similar but that are spliced differently from overlapping but distinct exons.

The lentiviruses in general, and HIV-1 and -2 in particular, contain a larger genome than other pathogenic retroviruses. They contain an untranslated region between *pol* and *env* that encodes portions of several proteins, varying with the reading frame into which the mRNA is spliced. Tat is a 14-kDa protein that augments the expression of virus from the LTR. The Rev protein of HIV-1, similar to the Rex protein of HTLV, regulates RNA splicing and/or RNA transport. The Nef protein downregulates CD4, the cellular receptor for HIV; alters host T cell activation pathways; and enhances viral infectivity. The Vif protein is necessary for the proper assembly of the HIV nucleoprotein core in

FIGURE 181-1 The life cycle of retroviruses. A. Overview of virus replication. The retrovirus enters a target cell by binding to a specific cell-surface receptor; once the virus is internalized, its RNA is released from the nucleocapsid and is reverse-transcribed into proviral DNA. The provirus is inserted into the genome and then transcribed into RNA; the RNA is translated; and virions assemble and are extruded from the cell membrane by budding. **B.** Overview of retroviral gene expression. The provirus is transcribed, capped, and polyadenylated. Viral RNA molecules then have one of three fates: they are exported to the cytoplasm, where they are packaged as the viral RNA in infectious viral particles; they are spliced to form the message for the envelope polyprotein; or they are translated into Gag and Pol proteins. Most of the messages for the Pol protein fail to initiate Pol translation because of a stop codon before its initiation; however, in a fraction of the messages, the stop codon is missed and the Pol proteins are translated. [*Modified from JM Coffin, in BN Fields, DM Knipe (eds): Fields Virology. New York, Raven, 1990; with permission.*]

many types of cells; without Vif, proviral DNA is not efficiently produced in these infected cells. In addition, the Vif protein targets APOBEC (apolipoprotein B mRNA-editing enzyme catalytic polypeptide, a cytidine deaminase that mutates the viral sequence) for proteasomal degradation, thus blocking its virus-suppressing effect. Vpr, Vpu (HIV-1 only), and Vpx (HIV-2 only) are viral proteins encoded by translation of the same message in different reading frames. As noted above, oncogenic retroviruses depend on cell proliferation for their replication; lentiviruses can infect nondividing cells, largely through effects mediated by Vpr. Vpr facilitates transport of the provirus into the nucleus and can induce other cellular changes, such as G_2 growth arrest and differentiation of some target cells. Vpx is structurally related to Vpr, but its functions are not fully defined. Vpu promotes the degradation of CD4 in the endoplasmic reticulum and stimulates the release of virions from infected cells.

Retroviruses can be either exogenously acquired by infection with a virion capable of replication or transmitted in the germ line as endoge-

nous virus. Endogenous retroviruses are often replication-defective. The human genome contains endogenous retroviral sequences, but there are no known replication-competent endogenous retroviruses in humans.

In general, viruses that contain only the *gag*, *pol*, and *env* genes either are not pathogenic or take a long time to induce disease; these observations indicate the importance of the other regulatory genes in viral disease pathogenesis. The pathogenesis of neoplastic transformation by retroviruses relies on the chance integration of the provirus at a spot in the genome that will result in the expression of a cellular gene (proto-oncogene) that becomes transforming by virtue of its unregulated expression. For example, avian leukosis virus causes B cell leukemia by inducing the expression of *myc*. Some retroviruses possess captured and altered cellular genes near their integration site, and these viral oncogenes are capable of transforming the infected host cell. Viruses that have oncogenes often have lost a portion of their genome that is required for replication. Such viruses need helper viruses to reproduce, a feature that may explain why these acute transforming retroviruses are rare in nature. All human retroviruses identified to date are exogenous and are not acutely transforming (i.e., they lack a transforming oncogene).

These remarkable properties of retroviruses have led to experimental efforts to use them as vectors to insert specific genes into particular cell types, a process known as *gene therapy* or *gene transfer*. The process could be used to repair a genetic defect or to introduce a new property that could be used therapeutically; for example, a gene (e.g., thymidine kinase) that would make a tumor cell susceptible to killing by a drug (e.g., ganciclovir) could be inserted. One source of concern about the use of retroviral vectors in humans is that replication-competent viruses might rescue endogenous retroviral replication, with unpredictable results. This concern is not merely hypothetical: the detection of proteins encoded by endogenous retroviral sequences on the surface of cancer cells implies that the genetic events leading to the cancer were able to activate the synthesis of these usually silent genes.

HUMAN T CELL LYMPHOTROPIC VIRUS

HTLV-I was isolated in 1980 from a T cell lymphoma cell line from a patient originally thought to have cutaneous T cell lymphoma. Later it became clear that the patient had a distinct form of lymphoma (originally reported in Japan) called *adult T cell leukemia/lymphoma* (ATL). Serologic data have determined that HTLV-I is the cause of at least two important diseases: ATL and tropical spastic paraparesis, also called *HTLV-I-associated myelopathy* (HAM). HTLV-I may also play a role in infective dermatitis and uveitis syndromes.

Two years after the isolation of HTLV-I, HTLV-II was isolated from a patient with an unusual form of hairy cell leukemia that affected T cells. Although early epidemiologic studies of HTLV-II failed to reveal a consistent disease association, more recent studies suggest an association of HTLV-II with human disease (see "Associated Diseases" under "Features of HTLV-II Infection," below), particularly among injection drug users.

BIOLOGY AND MOLECULAR BIOLOGY

Because the biology of HTLV-I and that of HTLV-II are similar, the following discussion will focus on HTLV-I.

The human glucose transporter protein 1 (GLUT-1) functions as a receptor for HTLV-I, probably acting together with neuropilin-1 (NRP1). Generally, only T cells are productively infected, but infection of B cells and other cell types is occasionally detected. The most common outcome of HTLV-I infection is latent carriage of randomly integrated provirus in CD4+ T cells. HTLV-I does not contain an oncogene and does not insert into a unique site in the genome. Indeed, most infected cells express no viral gene products. The only viral gene product that is routinely expressed in tumor cells transformed by HTLV-I in vivo is *tax*, and even *tax* is not expressed in the tumor cells of many ATL patients. Cells transformed in vitro, by contrast, actively transcribe HTLV-I RNA and produce infectious virions. Most HTLV-I-transformed cell lines are the result of the infection of a normal host T cell in vitro. It is difficult to establish cell lines derived from authentic ATL cells.

FIGURE 181-2 Genomic structure of retroviruses. The murine leukemia virus MuLV has the typical three structural genes: *gag*, *pol*, and *env*. The *gag* region gives rise to three proteins: matrix (MA), capsid (CA), and nucleic acid–binding (NC) proteins. The *pol* region encodes both a protease (PR) responsible for cleaving the viral polyproteins and a reverse transcriptase (RT). In addition, HIV *pol* encodes an integrase (IN). The *env* region encodes a surface protein (SU) and a small transmembrane protein (TM). The human retroviruses have additional gene products translated in each of the three possible reading frames. HTLV-I and HTLV-II have *tax* and *rex* genes with exons on either side of the *env* gene. HIV-1 and HIV-2 have six accessory gene products: *tat, rev, vif, nef, vpr*, and either *vpu* (in HIV-1) or *vpx* (in HIV-2). The genes for these proteins are located mainly between the *pol* and *env* genes. LTR, long terminal repeat.

Although *tax* does not itself bind to DNA, it does induce the expression of a wide range of host cell gene products, including transcription factors (especially c-rel/NF-κB, ets-1 and -2, and members of the fos/jun family), cytokines [e.g., interleukin (IL) 2, granulocyte-macrophage colony-stimulating factor, and tumor necrosis factor (TNF)], and membrane proteins and receptors [major histocompatibility (MHC) molecules and IL-2 receptor α]. The genes activated by *tax* are generally controlled by transcription factors of the c-rel/NF-κB and cyclic AMP response element binding (CREB) protein families. It is unclear how this induction of host gene expression leads to neoplastic transformation; *tax* can interfere with G_1 and mitotic cell-cycle checkpoints, block apoptosis, inhibit DNA repair, and promote antigen-independent T cell proliferation. Induction of a cytokine-autocrine loop has been proposed; however, IL-2 is not the crucial cytokine. The involvement of IL-4, IL-7, and IL-15 has been proposed.

In light of the irregular expression of *tax* in ATL cells, it has been suggested that *tax* is important in the early phases of transformation but is not essential for the maintenance of the transformed state. As is clear from the epidemiology of HTLV-I infection, transformation of an infected cell is a rare event and may depend on heterogeneous second, third, or fourth genetic hits. No consistent chromosomal abnormalities have been described in ATL; however, individual cases with p53 mutations and translocations involving the T cell receptor genes on chromosome 14 have been reported. *Tax* may repress certain DNA repair enzymes, permitting the accumulation of genetic damage that would normally be repaired. However, the molecular pathogenesis of HTLV-I–induced neoplasia is not fully understood.

FEATURES OF HTLV-I INFECTION

Epidemiology HTLV-I infection is transmitted in at least three ways: from mother to child, especially via breast milk; through sexual activity, more commonly from men to women; and through the blood—via contaminated transfusions or contaminated needles. The virus is most commonly transmitted perinatally. Compared with HIV, which can be transmitted in cell-free form, HTLV-I is less infectious, and its transmission usually requires cell-to-cell contact.

HTLV-I is endemic in southwestern Japan and Okinawa, where >1 million persons are infected. Antibodies to HTLV-I are present in the serum of up to 35% of Okinawans, 10% of residents of the Japanese island of Kyushu, and <1% of persons in nonendemic regions of Japan. Despite this high prevalence of infection, only ~500 cases of ATL are diagnosed in this area each year. Clusters of infection have been noted in other areas of the Orient, such as Taiwan; in the Caribbean basin, including northeastern South America; in northwestern South America; in central and southern Africa; in Italy, Israel, Iran, and Papua New Guinea; in the Arctic; and in the southeastern part of the United States (Fig. 181-4). An estimated 15–20 million persons have HTLV-I infection worldwide.

A progressive spastic or ataxic myelopathy developing in an individual who is HTLV-I positive (i.e., who has serum antibodies to HTLV-I) is likely to be due to direct infection of the nervous system with the virus; a similar disorder may result from infection with HIV or HTLV-II. In rare instances, patients with HAM are seronegative but have detectable antibody to HTLV-I in the cerebrospinal fluid (CSF).

The cumulative lifetime risk of developing ATL is 3% among HTLV-I–infected patients, with a threefold greater risk among men than among women; a similar cumulative risk is projected for HAM (4%), but with women more commonly affected than men. The distribution of the two diseases overlaps the distribution of HTLV-I, with >95% of affected patients showing serologic evidence of HTLV-I infection. The latency period between infection and the emergence of disease is 20–30 years for ATL. For HAM, the median latency period is ~3.3 years (range, 4 months to 30 years). The development of ATL is rare among persons

	HTLV-I	HIV-1
SU	gp46	gp120
TM	p21	gp41
NC	p15	p7
PR	p14	p10
RT	p95	p66
IN	—	p32
MA	p19	p17
CA	p24	p24
RNA	9kb	10kb

FIGURE 181-3 Schematic structure of human retroviruses. The surface glycoprotein (SU) is responsible for binding to receptors of host cells. The transmembrane protein (TM) anchors SU to the virus. NC is a nucleic acid–binding protein found in association with the viral RNA. A protease (PR) cleaves the polyproteins encoded by the *gag, pol*, and *env* genes into their functional components. RT is reverse transcriptase, and IN is an integrase present in some retroviruses (e.g., HIV-1) that facilitates insertion of the provirus into the host genome. The matrix protein (MA) is a Gag protein closely associated with the lipid of the envelope. The capsid protein (CA) forms the major internal structure of the virus, the core shell.

FIGURE 181-4 Global distribution of HTLV-I infection. Countries with a prevalence of HTLV-I infection of 1–5% are shaded darkly. Note that the distribution of infected patients is not uniform in endemic countries. For example, the people of southwestern Japan and northeastern Brazil are more commonly affected than those in other regions of those countries.

infected by blood products; however, ~20% of patients with HAM acquire HTLV-I from contaminated blood. ATL is more common among perinatally infected individuals, whereas HAM is more common among persons infected via sexual transmission.

Associated Diseases • ATL Four clinical types of HTLV-I-induced neoplasia have been described: acute, lymphomatous, chronic, and smoldering. All of these tumors are monoclonal proliferations of CD4+ post-thymic T cells with clonal proviral integrations and clonal T cell receptor gene rearrangements.

Acute ATL About 60% of patients who develop malignancy have classic acute ATL, which is characterized by a short clinical prodrome (~2 weeks between the first symptoms and the diagnosis) and an aggressive natural history (median survival period, 6 months). The clinical picture is dominated by rapidly progressive skin lesions, pulmonary involvement, hypercalcemia, and lymphocytosis with cells containing lobulated or "flower-shaped" nuclei (see Fig. 105-10). The malignant cells have monoclonal proviral integrations and express CD4, CD3, and CD25 (low-affinity IL-2 receptors) on their surface. Serum levels of CD25 can be used as a tumor marker. Anemia and thrombocytopenia are rare. The skin lesions may be difficult to distinguish from those in mycosis fungoides. Lytic bone lesions, which are common, do not contain tumor cells but rather are composed of osteolytic cells, usually without osteoblastic activity. Despite the leukemic picture, bone marrow involvement is patchy in most cases.

The hypercalcemia of ATL is multifactorial; the tumor cells produce osteoclast-activating factors (TNF-α, IL-1, lymphotoxin) and can also produce a parathyroid hormone–like molecule. Affected patients have an underlying immunodeficiency that makes them susceptible to opportunistic infections similar to those seen in patients with AIDS (Chap. 182). The pathogenesis of the immunodeficiency is unclear. Pulmonary infiltrates in ATL patients reflect leukemic infiltration half the time and opportunistic infections with organisms such as *Pneumocystis* and other fungi the other half. Gastrointestinal symptoms are nearly always related to opportunistic infection. *Strongyloides stercoralis* is a gastrointestinal parasite that has a pattern of endemic distribution similar to that of HTLV-I. HTLV-I-infected persons also infected with this parasite may develop ATL more often or more rapidly than those without *Strongyloides* infections. Serum concentrations of lactate dehydrogenase (LDH) and alkaline phosphatase are often elevated in ATL. About 10% of patients have leptomeningeal involvement leading to weakness, altered mental status, paresthesia, and/or headache. Unlike other forms of central nervous system (CNS) lymphoma, ATL may be accompanied by normal CSF protein levels. The diagnosis depends on finding ATL cells in the CSF (Chap. 105).

Lymphomatous ATL The lymphomatous type of ATL occurs in ~20% of patients and is similar to the acute form in its natural history and clinical course, except that circulating abnormal cells are rare and lymphadenopathy is evident. The histology of the lymphoma is variable but does not influence the natural history. In general, the diagnosis is suspected on the basis of the patient's birthplace (see "Epidemiology," above) and the presence of skin lesions and hypercalcemia. The diagnosis is confirmed by the detection of antibodies to HTLV-I in serum.

Chronic ATL Patients with the chronic form of ATL generally have normal serum levels of calcium and LDH and no involvement of the CNS, bone, or gastrointestinal tract. The median duration of survival for these patients is 2 years. In some cases, chronic ATL progresses to the acute form of the disease.

Smoldering ATL Fewer than 5% of patients have the smoldering form of ATL. In this form, the malignant cells have monoclonal proviral integration; <5% of peripheral blood cells exhibit typical morphologic abnormalities; hypercalcemia, adenopathy, and hepatosplenomegaly do not develop; the CNS, the bones, and the gastrointestinal tract are not involved; and skin lesions and pulmonary lesions may be present. The median survival period of this small subset of patients appears to be ≥5 years.

HAM (TROPICAL SPASTIC PARAPARESIS) In contrast to ATL, in which there is a slight predominance of male patients, HAM affects females disproportionately. HAM resembles multiple sclerosis in certain ways (Chap. 375). The onset is insidious. Symptoms include weakness or stiffness in one or both legs, back pain, and urinary incontinence. Sensory changes are usually mild, but peripheral neuropathy may develop. The disease generally takes the form of slowly progressive and unremitting thoracic myelopathy; one-third of patients are bedridden within 10 years of diagnosis, and one-half are unable to walk unassisted by this point. Patients display spastic paraparesis or paraplegia with hyperreflexia, ankle clonus, and extensor plantar responses. Cognitive function is usually spared; cranial nerve abnormalities are unusual.

MRI reveals lesions in both the white matter and the paraventricular regions of the brain as well as in the spinal cord. Pathologic examination of the spinal cord shows symmetric degeneration of the lateral columns, including the corticospinal tracts; some cases involve the posterior columns as well. The spinal meninges and cord parenchyma contain an inflammatory infiltrate with myelin destruction.

HTLV-I is not usually found in cells of the CNS but may be detected in a small population of lymphocytes present in the CSF. In general, HTLV-I replication is greater in HAM than in ATL, and patients with HAM have a stronger immune response to the virus. Antibodies to HTLV-I are present in the serum and appear to be produced in the CSF of HAM patients, where titers are often higher than in the serum. The pathophysiology of HAM may involve the induction of autoimmune destruction of neural cells by T cells with specificity for viral components such as Tax or Env proteins. One theory is that susceptibility to HAM may be related to the presence of human leukocyte antigen (HLA) alleles capable of presenting viral antigens in a fashion that leads to autoimmunity. Insufficient data are available to confirm an HLA association. However, antibodies in the sera of HAM patients have been shown to bind a neuron-specific antigen [heteronuclear ribonuclear protein A1 (hnRNP A1)] and to interfere with neurotransmission in vitro.

It is unclear what factors influence whether HTLV-I infection will cause disease and, if it does, whether it will induce a neoplasm (ATL) or an autoimmune disorder (HAM). Differences in viral strains, the susceptibility of particular MHC haplotypes, the route of HTLV-I infection, the viral load, and the nature of the HTLV-I-related immune response are putative factors, but few definitive data are available.

OTHER PUTATIVE HTLV-I-RELATED DISEASES In areas where HTLV-I is endemic, diverse inflammatory and autoimmune diseases have been attributed to the virus, including uveitis, dermatitis, pneumonitis, rheumatoid arthritis, and polymyositis. However, a causal relationship between HTLV-I and these illnesses has not been established.

Prevention Women in endemic areas should not breast-feed their children, and blood donors should be screened for serum antibodies to HTLV-I. As in the prevention of HIV infection, the practice of safe sex and the avoidance of needle sharing are important.

℞ HTLV-I INFECTION

For the small number of patients who develop HTLV-I-related disease, therapies are not curative. In patients with the acute and lymphomatous types of ATL, the disease progresses rapidly. Hypercalcemia is generally controlled by glucocorticoid administration and cytotoxic therapy directed against the neoplasm. The tumor is highly responsive to combination chemotherapy that is employed against other forms of lymphoma; however, patients are susceptible to overwhelming bacterial and opportunistic infections, and ATL relapses within 4–10 months after remission in most cases. The combination of interferon α and zidovudine may extend survival. Because viral replication is not clearly associated with ATL progression, zidovudine is probably effective through its cytotoxic effects (as a chain-terminating thymidine analogue) rather than its antiviral effects. An experimental approach using an yttrium 90–labeled or toxin-conjugated antibody to the IL-2 receptor appears promising but is not widely available. Patients with the chronic or smoldering form of ATL may be managed with an expectant approach: treat any infections, and watch and wait for signs of progression to acute disease.

Patients with HAM may obtain some benefit from the use of glucocorticoids to reduce inflammation. Antiretroviral regimens have not been effective. In one study, danazol (200 mg three times daily) produced significant neurologic improvement in five of six treated patients, with resolution of urinary incontinence in two cases, decreased spasticity in three, and restoration of the ability to walk after confinement to a wheelchair in two. Physical therapy and rehabilitation are important components of management.

FEATURES OF HTLV-II INFECTION

Epidemiology HTLV-II is endemic in certain Native American tribes and in Africa. It is generally considered to be a New World virus that was brought from Asia to the Americas 10,000–40,000 years ago during the migration of infected populations across the Bering land bridge. The mode of transmission of HTLV-II is probably the same as that of HTLV-I (see above). HTLV-II may be less readily transmitted sexually than HTLV-I.

Studies of large cohorts of injection drug users with serologic assays that reliably distinguish HTLV-I from HTLV-II indicated that the vast majority of HTLV-positive cohort members were infected with HTLV-II. The seroprevalence of HTLV in a cohort of 7841 injection drug users from drug treatment centers in Baltimore, Chicago, Los Angeles, New Jersey (Asbury Park and Trenton), New York City (Brooklyn and Har-

lem), Philadelphia, and San Antonio was 20.9%, with >97% of cases due to HTLV-II. The seroprevalence of HTLV-II was higher in the Southwest and the Midwest than in the Northeast. In contrast, the seroprevalence of HIV-1 was higher in the Northeast than in the Southwest or the Midwest. Approximately 3% of the cohort members were infected with both HTLV-II and HIV-1. The seroprevalence of HTLV-II increased linearly with age. Women were significantly more likely to be infected with HTLV-II than were men; the virus is thought to be more efficiently transmitted from male to female than from female to male.

Associated Diseases Although HTLV-II was isolated from a patient with a T cell variant of hairy cell leukemia, this virus has not been consistently associated with a particular disease and in fact has been thought of as "a virus searching for a disease." However, evidence is accumulating that HTLV-II may play a role in certain neurologic, hematologic, and dermatologic diseases. These data require confirmation, particularly in light of the previous confusion regarding the relative prevalences of HTLV-I and HTLV-II among injection drug users.

Prevention Avoidance of needle sharing, adherence to safe-sex practices, screening of blood (by assays for HTLV-I, which also detect HTLV-II), and avoidance of breast-feeding by infected women are important principles in the prevention of spread of HTLV-II.

HUMAN IMMUNODEFICIENCY VIRUS

HIV-1 and HIV-2 are members of the lentivirus subfamily of Retroviridae and are the only lentiviruses known to infect humans. The lentiviruses are slow-acting by comparison with viruses that cause acute infection (e.g., influenza virus) but not by comparison with other retroviruses. The features of acute primary infection with HIV resemble those of more classic acute infections. The characteristic chronicity of HIV disease is consistent with the designation *lentivirus*. For a detailed discussion of HIV, see Chap. 182.

FURTHER READINGS

GHEZ D et al: Neuropilin-1 is involved in human T-cell lymphotropic virus type 1 entry. J Virol 80:6844, 2006

KASHANCHI F, BRADY JN: Transcriptional and post-transcriptional gene regulation of HTLV-1. Oncogene 24:5938, 2005

LEE SM et al: HTLV-1 induced molecular mimicry in neurological disease. Curr Top Microbiol Immunol 296:125, 2005

MANEL N et al: HTLV-I tropism and envelope receptor. Oncogene 24:6016, 2005

MATSUOKA M, JEANG KT: Human T-cell leukaemia virus type 1 (HTLV-1) infectivity and cellular transformation. Nat Rev Cancer 7:270, 2007

PELOPONESE JM et al: Modulation of nuclear factor-κB by human T cell leukemia virus type 1 Tax protein. Immunol Res 34:1, 2006

PROIETTI FA et al: Global epidemiology of HTLV-I infection and associated diseases. Oncogene 24:6058, 2005

TAYLOR GP, MATSUOKA M: Natural history of adult T-cell leukemia/lymphoma and approaches to therapy. Oncogene 24:6047, 2005

182 Human Immunodeficiency Virus Disease: AIDS and Related Disorders
Anthony S. Fauci, H. Clifford Lane

AIDS was first recognized in the United States in the summer of 1981, when the U.S. Centers for Disease Control and Prevention (CDC) re-

ported the unexplained occurrence of *Pneumocystis jiroveci* (formerly *P. carinii*) pneumonia in five previously healthy homosexual men in Los Angeles and of Kaposi's sarcoma (KS) with or without *P. jiroveci* pneumonia in 26 previously healthy homosexual men in New York and Los Angeles. Within months, the disease became recognized in male and female injection drug users (IDUs) and soon thereafter in recipients of blood transfusions and in hemophiliacs. As the epidemiologic pattern of the disease unfolded, it became clear that an infectious agent transmissible by sexual (homosexual and heterosexual) contact and blood or blood products was the most likely etiologic cause of the epidemic.

In 1983, human immunodeficiency virus (HIV) was isolated from a patient with lymphadenopathy, and by 1984 it was demonstrated clearly to be the causative agent of AIDS. In 1985, a sensitive enzyme-linked immunosorbent assay (ELISA) was developed, which led to an appreciation of the scope and evolution of the HIV epidemic at first in the United States and other developed nations and ultimately among developing nations throughout the world (see below). The staggering worldwide evolution of the HIV pandemic has been matched by an explosion of information in the areas of HIV virology, pathogenesis (both immunologic and virologic), treatment of HIV disease, treatment and prophylaxis of the opportunistic diseases associated with HIV infection, prevention of infection, and vaccine development. The information flow related to HIV disease is enormous and continues to expand, and it has become almost impossible for the health care generalist to stay abreast of the literature. The purpose of this chapter is to present the most current information available on the scope of the epidemic; on its pathogenesis, treatment, and prevention; and on prospects for vaccine development. Above all, the aim is to provide a solid scientific basis and practical clinical guidelines for a state-of-the-art approach to the HIV-infected patient.

DEFINITION

The current CDC classification system for HIV-infected adolescents and adults categorizes persons on the basis of clinical conditions associated with HIV infection and CD4+ T lymphocyte counts. The system is based on three ranges of CD4+ T lymphocyte counts and three clinical categories and is represented by a matrix of nine mutually exclusive categories (Tables 182-1 and 182-2). Using this system, any HIV-infected individual with a CD4+ T cell count of <200/μL has AIDS by definition, regardless of the presence of symptoms or opportunistic diseases (Table 182-1). Once individuals have had a clinical condition in category B, their disease classification cannot be reverted back to category A, even if the condition resolves; the same holds true for category C in relation to category B.

The definition of AIDS is indeed complex and comprehensive and was established not for the practical care of patients, but for surveillance purposes. Thus, the clinician should not focus on whether or not the patient fulfills the strict definition of AIDS, but should view HIV disease as a spectrum ranging from primary infection, with or without the acute syndrome, to the asymptomatic stage, to advanced disease (see below).

ETIOLOGIC AGENT

The etiologic agent of AIDS is HIV, which belongs to the family of human retroviruses (Retroviridae) and the subfamily of lentiviruses (Chap. 181). Nononcogenic lentiviruses cause disease in other animal species, including sheep, horses, goats, cattle, cats, and monkeys. The four recognized human retroviruses belong to two distinct groups: the human T lymphotropic viruses (HTLV)-I and HTLV-II, which are transforming retroviruses; and the human immunodeficiency viruses, HIV-1 and HIV-2, which cause cytopathic effects either directly or indirectly (see

| TABLE 182-1 | 1993 REVISED CLASSIFICATION SYSTEM FOR HIV INFECTION AND EXPANDED AIDS SURVEILLANCE CASE DEFINITION FOR ADOLESCENTS AND ADULTS[a] |

CD4+ T Cell Categories	Clinical Categories		
	A Asymptomatic, Acute (Primary) HIV or PGL[b]	B Symptomatic, Not A or C Conditions	C AIDS-Indicator Conditions
>500/μL	A1	B1	C1
200–499/μL	A2	B2	C2
<200/μL	A3	B3	C3

[a]The shaded areas indicate the expanded AIDS surveillance case definition.
[b]PGL, progressive generalized lymphadenopathy.
Source: MMWR 42(No. RR-17), December 18, 1992.

| TABLE 182-2 | CLINICAL CATEGORIES OF HIV INFECTION |

Category A: Consists of one or more of the conditions listed below in an adolescent or adult (>13 years) with documented HIV infection. Conditions listed in categories B and C must not have occurred.
  Asymptomatic HIV infection
  Persistent generalized lymphadenopathy
  Acute (primary) HIV infection with accompanying illness or history of acute HIV infection
Category B: Consists of symptomatic conditions in an HIV-infected adolescent or adult that are not included among conditions listed in clinical category C and that meet at least one of the following criteria: (1) The conditions are attributed to HIV infection or are indicative of a defect in cell-mediated immunity; or (2) the conditions are considered by physicians to have a clinical course or to require management that is complicated by HIV infection. Examples include, but are not limited to, the following:
  Bacillary angiomatosis
  Candidiasis, oropharyngeal (thrush)
  Candidiasis, vulvovaginal; persistent, frequent, or poorly responsive to therapy
  Cervical dysplasia (moderate or severe)/cervical carcinoma in situ
  Constitutional symptoms, such as fever (38.5°C) or diarrhea lasting >1 month
  Hairy leukoplakia, oral
  Herpes zoster (shingles), involving at least two distinct episodes or more than one dermatome
  Idiopathic thrombocytopenic purpura
  Listeriosis
  Pelvic inflammatory disease, particularly if complicated by tuboovarian abscess
  Peripheral neuropathy
Category C: Conditions listed in the AIDS surveillance case definition.
  Candidiasis of bronchi, trachea, or lungs
  Candidiasis, esophageal
  Cervical cancer, invasive[a]
  Coccidioidomycosis, disseminated or extrapulmonary
  Cryptococcosis, extrapulmonary
  Cryptosporidiosis, chronic intestinal (>1 month's duration)
  Cytomegalovirus disease (other than liver, spleen, or nodes)
  Cytomegalovirus retinitis (with loss of vision)
  Encephalopathy, HIV-related
  Herpes simplex: chronic ulcer(s) (>1 month's duration); or bronchitis, pneumonia, or esophagitis
  Histoplasmosis, disseminated or extrapulmonary
  Isosporiasis, chronic intestinal (>1 month's duration)
  Kaposi's sarcoma
  Lymphoma, Burkitt's (or equivalent term)
  Lymphoma, primary, of brain
  Mycobacterium avium complex or *M. kansasii*, disseminated or extrapulmonary
  Mycobacterium tuberculosis, any site (pulmonary[a] or extrapulmonary)
  Mycobacterium, other species or unidentified species, disseminated or extrapulmonary
  Pneumocystis jiroveci pneumonia
  Pneumonia, recurrent[a]
  Progressive multifocal leukoencephalopathy
  Salmonella septicemia, recurrent
  Toxoplasmosis of brain
  Wasting syndrome due to HIV

[a]Added in the 1993 expansion of the AIDS surveillance case definition.
Source: MMWR 42(No. RR-17), December 18, 1992.

below and Chap. 181). The most common cause of HIV disease throughout the world, and certainly in the United States, is HIV-1, which comprises several subtypes with different geographic distributions (see below). HIV-2 was first identified in 1986 in West African patients and was originally confined to West Africa. However, a number of cases that can be traced to West Africa or to sexual contacts with West Africans have been identified throughout the world. Both HIV-1 and HIV-2 are zoonotic infections. The *Pan troglodytes troglodytes* species of chimpanzees has been established as the natural reservoir of HIV-1 and the most likely source of original human infection. HIV-2 is more closely related phylogenetically to the simian immunodeficiency virus (SIV) found in sooty mangabeys than it is to HIV-1. The taxonomic relationship among primate lentiviruses is shown in Fig. 182-1.

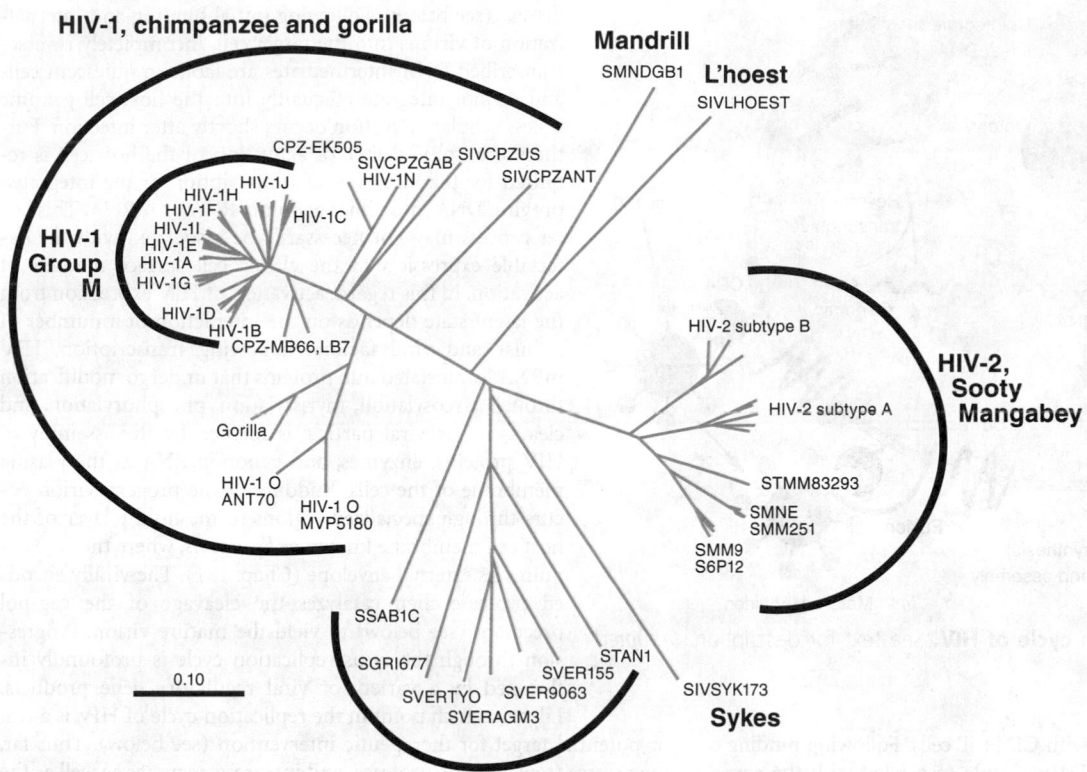

FIGURE 182-1 **A phylogenetic tree, based on the complete genomes of primate immunodeficiency viruses.** The scale at the bottom (0.10) indicates a 10% difference at the nucleotide level. (*Prepared by Brian Foley, PhD, of the HIV Sequence Database, Theoretical Biology and Biophysics Group, Los Alamos National Laboratory.*)

MORPHOLOGY OF HIV

Electron microscopy shows that the HIV virion is an icosahedral structure (Fig. 182-2A) containing numerous external spikes formed by the two major envelope proteins, the external gp120 and the transmembrane gp41. The virion buds from the surface of the infected cell and incorporates a variety of host proteins, including major histocompatibility complex (MHC) class I and II antigens (Chap. 309), into its lipid bilayer. The structure of HIV-1 is schematically diagrammed in Fig. 182-2B (Chap. 181).

REPLICATION CYCLE OF HIV

HIV is an RNA virus whose hallmark is the reverse transcription of its genomic RNA to DNA by the enzyme *reverse transcriptase*. The replication cycle of HIV begins with the high-affinity binding of the gp120 protein via a portion of its V1 region near the N terminus to its receptor on

the host cell surface, the CD4 molecule (Fig. 182-3). The CD4 molecule is a 55-kDa protein found predominantly on a subset of T lymphocytes that are responsible for helper function in the immune system (Chap. 308). It is also expressed on the surface of monocytes/macrophages and dendritic/Langerhans cells. Once gp120 binds to CD4, the gp120 undergoes a conformational change that facilitates binding to one of a group of co-receptors. The two major co-receptors for HIV-1 are CCR5 and CXCR4. Both receptors belong to the family of seven-transmembrane-domain G protein–coupled cellular receptors, and the use of one or the other or both receptors by the virus for entry into the cell is an important determinant of the cellular tropism of the virus (see below for details). Certain dendritic cells express a diversity of C-type lectin receptors on their surface, one of which is called *DC-SIGN*, that also bind with high affinity to the HIV gp120 envelope protein, allowing the dendritic cell to facilitate the binding of virus to the CD4+ T cell upon

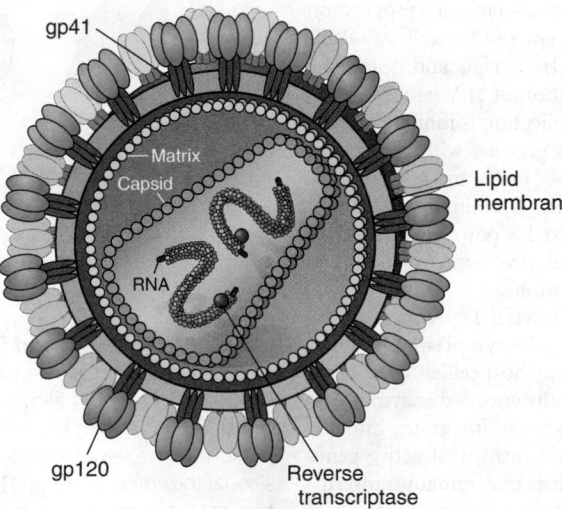

FIGURE 182-2 *A.* **Electron micrograph of HIV.** Figure illustrates a typical virion following budding from the surface of a CD4+ T lymphocyte, together with two additional incomplete virions in the process of budding from the cell membrane. *B.* Structure of HIV-1, including the gp120 outer membrane, gp41 transmembrane components of the envelope, genomic RNA, enzyme reverse transcriptase, p18(17) inner membrane (matrix), and p24 core protein (capsid) (copyright by George V. Kelvin). (*Adapted from RC Gallo: Sci Am 256:46, 1987.*)

A   *B*

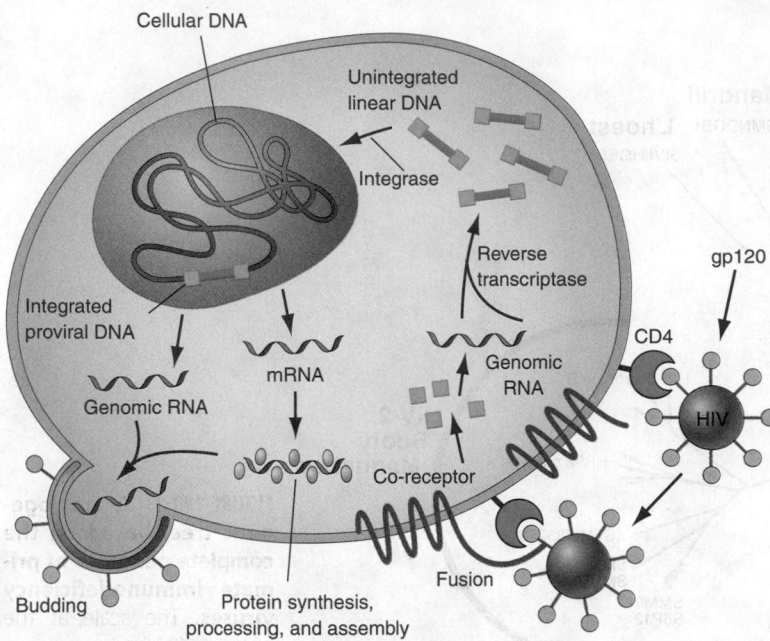

FIGURE 182-3 The replication cycle of HIV. See text for description. *(Adapted from Fauci, 1996.)*

PART 7

Infectious Diseases

engagement of dendritic cells with CD4+ T cells. Following binding of the envelope protein to the CD4 molecule associated with the above-mentioned conformational change in the viral envelope gp120, fusion with the host cell membrane occurs via the newly exposed gp41 molecule penetrating the plasma membrane of the target cell and then coiling upon itself to bring the virion and target cell together. Following fusion, the preintegration complex, composed of viral RNA and viral enzymes and surrounded by a capsid protein coat, is released into the cytoplasm of the target cell **(Fig. 182-4)**. As the preintegration complex traverses the cytoplasm to reach the nucleus (Fig. 182-3), the viral reverse transcriptase enzyme catalyzes the reverse transcription of the genomic RNA into DNA, and the protein coat opens to release the resulting double-stranded HIV-DNA. At this point in the replication cycle, the viral genome is vulnerable to cellular factors that can block the progression of infection. In particular, the cytoplasmic TRIM5-α protein in rhesus macaque cells blocks SIV replication at a point shortly after the virus fuses with the host cell. Although the exact mechanisms of action of TRIM5-α remain unclear, the human form is inhibited by cyclophilin A and is not effective in restricting HIV replication in human cells. The recently described APOBEC family of cellular proteins also inhibits progression of virus infection after virus has entered the cell. APOBEC proteins bind to nascent reverse transcripts and deaminate viral cytidine, causing hypermutation of HIV genomes. It is still not clear whether (1) viral replication is inhibited by the binding of APOBEC to the virus genome with subsequent accumulation of reverse transcripts, or (2) by the hypermutations caused by the enzymatic deaminase activity of APOBEC proteins. HIV has evolved a powerful strategy to protect itself from APOBEC. The viral protein Vif targets APOBEC for proteasomal degradation.

With activation of the cell, the viral DNA accesses the nuclear pore and is exported from the cytoplasm to the nucleus, where it is integrated into the host cell chromosomes through the action of another virally encoded enzyme, *integrase*. HIV provirus (DNA) selectively integrates into the nuclear DNA preferentially within introns of active genes and regional hotspots. This provirus may remain transcriptionally inactive (latent) or it may manifest varying levels of gene expression, up to active production of virus.

Cellular activation plays an important role in the replication cycle of HIV and is critical to the pathogenesis of HIV disease (see below). Following initial binding and internalization of virions into the target cell, incompletely reverse-transcribed DNA intermediates are labile in quiescent cells and do not integrate efficiently into the host cell genome unless cellular activation occurs shortly after infection. Furthermore, some degree of activation of the host cell is required for the initiation of transcription of the integrated proviral DNA into either genomic RNA or mRNA. This latter process may not necessarily be associated with the detectable expression of the classic cell surface markers of activation. In this regard, activation of HIV expression from the latent state depends on the interaction of a number of cellular and viral factors. Following transcription, HIV mRNA is translated into proteins that undergo modification through glycosylation, myristylation, phosphorylation, and cleavage. The viral particle is formed by the assembly of HIV proteins, enzymes, and genomic RNA at the plasma membrane of the cells. Budding of the progeny virion occurs through specialized regions in the lipid bilayer of the host cell membrane known as *lipid rafts*, where the core acquires its external envelope (Chap. 181). The virally encoded protease then catalyzes the cleavage of the gag-pol precursor (see below) to yield the mature virion. Progression through the virus replication cycle is profoundly influenced by a variety of viral regulatory gene products. Likewise, each point in the replication cycle of HIV is a real or potential target for therapeutic intervention (see below). Thus far, the reverse transcriptase, protease, and integrase enzymes as well as the process of virus–target cell binding and fusion have proven clinically to be susceptible to pharmacologic disruption (see below). Inhibitors of the maturation process of virions during the latter phase of the replication cycle are currently being evaluated in clinical trials.

HIV GENOME

Figure 182-5 illustrates schematically the arrangement of the HIV genome. Like other retroviruses, HIV-1 has genes that encode the structural proteins of the virus: *gag* encodes the proteins that form the core of the virion (including p24 antigen); *pol* encodes the enzymes responsible for protease processing of viral proteins, reverse transcription, and integration; and *env* encodes the envelope glycoproteins. However, HIV-1 is more complex than other retroviruses, particularly those of the nonprimate group, in that it also contains at least six other genes

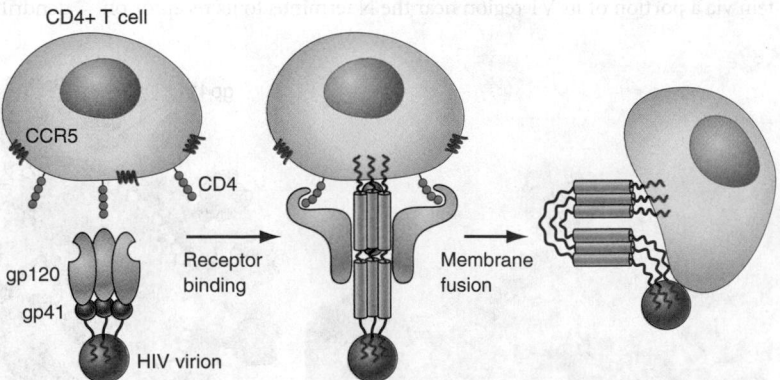

FIGURE 182-4 Binding and fusion of HIV-1 with its target cell. HIV-1 binds to its target cell via the CD4 molecule, leading to a conformational change in the gp120 molecule that allows it to bind to the co-receptor CCR5 (for R5-using viruses). The virus then firmly attaches to the host cell membrane in a coiled-spring fashion via the newly exposed gp41 molecule. Virus-cell fusion occurs as the transitional intermediate of gp41 undergoes further changes to form a hairpin structure that draws the two membranes into close proximity (see text for details). *(Adapted from D Montefiori, JP Moore: Science 283:336, 1999; with permission.)*

LTR: Long terminal repeat
Contains control regions that bind host transcription factors (NF-κB, NFAT, Sp.1, TBP)
Required for the initiation of transcription
Contains RNA trans-acting response element (TAR) that binds Tat

vif: Viral infectivity factor (p23)
Overcomes inhibitory effects of APOBEC, preventing hypermutation and viral DNA degradation

vpu: Viral protein U
Promotes CD4 degradation and influences virion release

env: gp 160 envelope protein
Cleaved in endoplasmic reticulum to gp 120 (SU) and gp41 (TM)
gp 120 mediates CD4 and chemokine receptor binding, while gp41 mediates fusion
Contains RNA response element (RRE) that binds Rev

nef: Negative effector (p27)
Promotes down-regulation of surface CD4 and MHC 1 expression
Blocks apoptosis
Enhance virion infectivity
Alters state of cellular activation
Progression to disease slowed significantly in absence of NEF

gag: Pr55^gag
Polyprotein processed by PR
MA, matrix (p17)
Undergoes myristylation that helps target gag polyprotein to lipid rafts;
CA, capsid (p24) Binds cyclophilin A
NC, nucleocapsid (p7) Zn finger, RNA-binding protein
p6
Interacts with Vpr; contains late domain (PTAP) that binds TSG101 and participates in terminal stops of virion budding

pol: Polymerase
Encodes a variety of viral enzymes, including PR (p10), RT, and RNAase H (p66/51), and IN (p32) all processed by PR

vpr: Viral protein R (p15)
Promotes G2 cell-cycle arrest
Facilitates HIV infection of macrophages

rev: Regulator of viral gene expression (p19)
Binds RRE
Inhibits viral RNA splicing and promotes nuclear export of incompletely spliced viral RNAs

tat: Transcriptional activator (p14)
Binds TAR
In presence of host cyclin T1 and CDK9 enhances RNA Pol II elongation on the viral DNA template

FIGURE 182-5 Organization of the genome of the HIV provirus together with a summary description of its nine genes encoding 15 proteins. *(Adapted from Greene and Peterlin.)*

(*tat, rev, nef, vif, vpr,* and *vpu*), which code for proteins involved in the modification of the host cell to enhance virus growth and the regulation of viral gene expression (Chap. 181). Several of these proteins are thought to play a role in the pathogenesis of HIV disease; their various functions are listed in Fig. 182-5. Flanking these genes are the long terminal repeats (LTRs), which contain regulatory elements involved in gene expression (Fig. 182-5). The major difference between the genomes of HIV-1 and HIV-2 is the fact that HIV-2 lacks the *vpu* gene and has a *vpx* gene not contained in HIV-1.

MOLECULAR HETEROGENEITY OF HIV-1

Molecular analyses of HIV isolates reveal varying levels of sequence diversity over all regions of the viral genome. For example, the degree of difference in the coding sequences of the viral envelope protein ranges from a few percent (very close, between isolates from the same infected individual) to 50% (extreme diversity, between isolates from the different groups of HIV-1, M, N, and O; see below). The changes tend to cluster in hypervariable regions. HIV can evolve by several means, including simple base substitution, insertions and deletions, recombination, and gain and loss of glycosylation sites. HIV sequence diversity arises directly from the limited fidelity of the reverse transcriptase. The balance of immune pressure and functional constraints on proteins influences the regional level of variation within proteins. For example, Envelope, which is exposed on the surface of the virion and is under immune selective pressure from both antibodies and cytolytic T lymphocytes, is extremely variable, with clusters of mutations in hypervariable domains. In contrast, Reverse Transcriptase, with important enzymatic functions, is relatively conserved, particularly around the active site. The extraordinary variability of HIV-1 is in marked contrast to the relative stability of HTLV-I and -II.

There are three groups of HIV-1: group M (major), which is responsible for most of the infections in the world; group O (outlier), a relatively rare viral form found originally in Cameroon, Gabon, and France; and group N, first identified in a Cameroonian woman with AIDS; only a few cases of the latter have been identified. Among primate lentiviruses, HIV-1 is most closely related to viruses isolated from chimpanzees and gorillas. The chimpanzee subspecies *Pan troglodytes troglodytes* has been established to be the natural reservoir of the HIV-1 M and N groups. The HIV-1 O group is most closely related to viruses found in Cameroonian gorillas. The M group comprises nine subtypes, or *clades*, designated A, B, C, D, F, G, H, J, and K, as well as a growing number of major and minor circulating recombinant forms (CRFs). CRFs are generated by infection of an individual with two subtypes that then recombine and create a virus with a selective advantage. These CRFs range from highly prevalent forms such as the AE virus, CRF01_AE, which is predominant in southeast Asia and often referred to simply as E, despite the fact that the parental E virus has never been found, and CRF02_AG from west and central Africa, to a large number of CRFs that are relatively rare. The subtypes and CRFs create the major lineages of the M group of HIV-1. The picture has been complicated somewhat when it was found that some subtypes are not equidistant from one another, while others contained sequences so diverse that they could not properly be considered to be the same subtype. Thus, the term *sub-subtype* was introduced, and subtypes A and F are now subdivided into A1 and A2, F1 and F2. It has also been argued that subtypes B and D are really too close to be separate subtypes and should be considered sub-subtypes; it was decided, however, not to increase the confusion by renaming the clades (Fig. 182-6).

The global patterns of HIV-1 variation likely result from accidents of viral trafficking. Subtype B viruses, which now differ by up to 17% in their *env* coding sequences, are the overwhelmingly predominant viruses seen in the United States, Canada, certain countries in South America, western Europe, and Australia. Other subtypes are also present in these countries to varying degrees. It is thought that, purely by chance, subtype B was seeded into the United States in the late 1970s, thereby establishing an overwhelming founder effect. Subtype C viruses (of the M group) are the most common form worldwide; many countries have co-circulating viral subtypes that are giving rise to new CRFs. **Figure 182-7** schematically diagrams the worldwide distribution of HIV-1 subtypes by region. Seven strains account for the

FIGURE 182-6 Phylogenetic tree constructed from representative viral envelope sequences of the subtypes and CRF01 in HIV-1 group M, some isolates from groups N and O (also HIV-1 human), CPZ (chimpanzee), and gorilla (GOR). The scale bar at the bottom indicates the genetic distances between the sequences. A1 and A2, F1 and F2 are subtypes; CRF01_AE is unique in the envelope gene but similar to subtype A in the rest of the genome. *(Courtesy of Brian Foley, PhD, Bette Korber, PhD, and Thomas Leitner, PhD, HIV Database, Los Alamos National Laboratory; with permission.)*

majority of HIV infections globally: HIV-1 subtypes A, B, C, D, G and two of the CRFs, CRF01_AE and CRF02_AG. The predominant subtype in Europe, Australia, and the Americas is subtype B. In sub-Saharan Africa, home to approximately two-thirds of all individuals living with HIV/AIDS, >50% of infections are caused by subtype C, with smaller proportions of infections caused by subtype A, subtype G, CRF02_AG, and other subtypes and recombinants. In Asia, HIV-1 isolates of the CRF01_AE lineage and subtypes C and B predominate. CRF01_AE accounts for most infections in south and southeast Asia, while subtype C is prevalent in India (see "HIV Infection and AIDS Worldwide," below). Sequence analyses of HIV-1 isolates from infected individuals indicate that recombination among viruses of different clades likely occurs as a result of infection of an individual with viruses

of more than one subtype, particularly in geographic areas where subtypes overlap.

TRANSMISSION

HIV is transmitted by both homosexual and heterosexual contact; by blood and blood products; and by infected mothers to infants either intrapartum, perinatally, or via breast milk. After >25 years of scrutiny, there is no evidence that HIV is transmitted by casual contact or that the virus can be spread by insects, such as by a mosquito bite.

SEXUAL TRANSMISSION

HIV infection is predominantly a sexually transmitted disease (STD) worldwide. In the United States, ~49% of the HIV/AIDS cases diagnosed in 2005 among adults and adolescents were attributed to male-to-male sexual contact. Heterosexual contact accounted for another 32%.

Worldwide, the most common mode of infection, particularly in developing countries, is clearly heterosexual transmission. Furthermore, the yearly incidence of new cases of AIDS attributed to heterosexual transmission of HIV is steadily increasing in the United States, mainly among minorities, particularly women in minority groups **(Fig. 182-8)**.

HIV has been demonstrated in seminal fluid both within infected mononuclear cells and in cell-free material. The virus appears to concentrate in the seminal fluid, particularly in situations where there are increased numbers of lymphocytes and monocytes in the fluid, as in genital inflammatory states such as urethritis and epididymitis, conditions closely associated with other STDs (see below). The virus has also been demonstrated in cervical smears and vaginal fluid. There is a strong association of HIV transmission with receptive anal intercourse, probably because only a thin, fragile rectal mucosal membrane separates the deposited semen from potentially susceptible cells in and beneath the mucosa and trauma may be associated with anal intercourse. Anal douching and sexual practices that traumatize the rectal mucosa also increase the likelihood of infection. It is likely that anal intercourse provides at least two modalities of infection: (1) direct inoculation into blood in cases of traumatic tears in the mucosa; and (2) infection of susceptible target cells, such as Langerhans cells, in the mucosal layer in the absence of trauma (see below). Although the vaginal mucosa is sev-

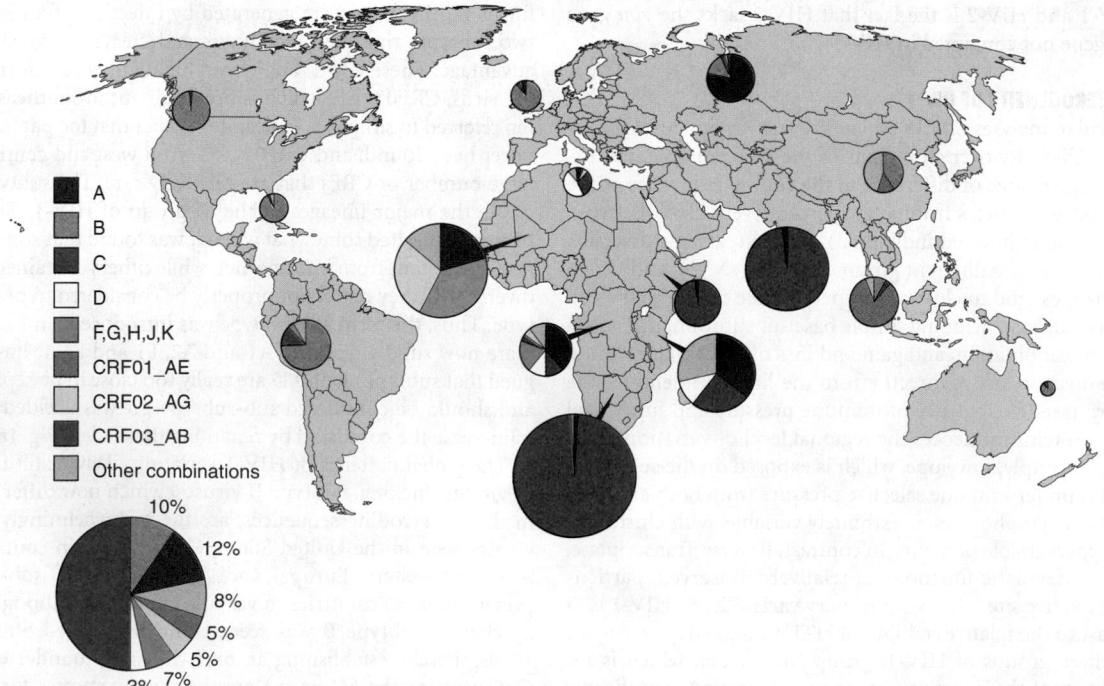

FIGURE 182-7 Geographic distribution of HIV-1 subtypes and recombinants. The prevalence of HIV-1 genetic subtypes varies by geographic region. The proportions of subtypes in different regions are indicated by pie charts. *(From J Hemelaar et al: AIDS 20:W13, 2006.)*

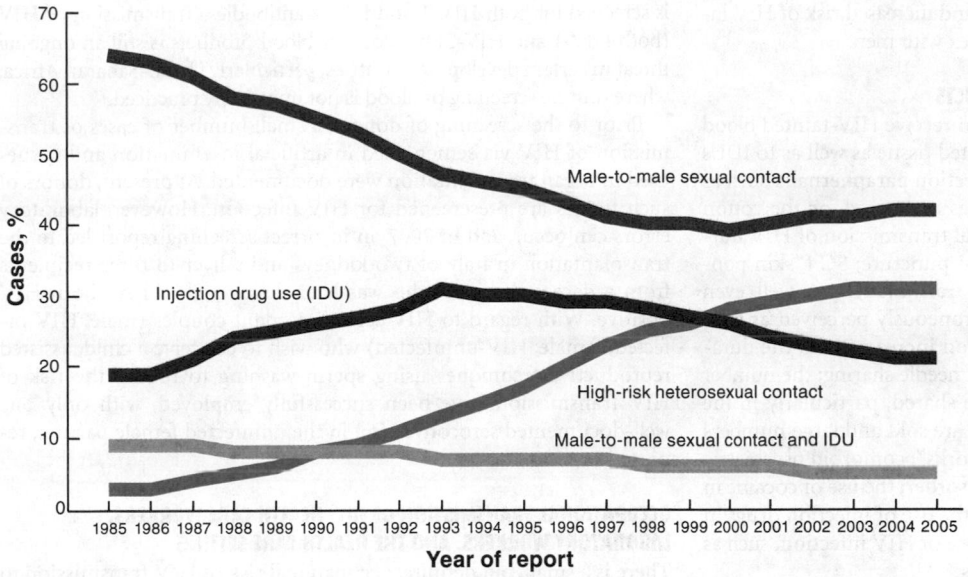

FIGURE 182-8 AIDS cases among U.S. adults and adolescents by exposure category and year of diagnosis. The proportion of AIDS cases attributed to heterosexual contact with a person known to have or at high risk for HIV infection (high-risk heterosexual) increased from 3% in 1985 to 31% in 2005. *[From The Centers for Disease Control and Prevention (CDC).]*

early stage of HIV infection when plasma HIV RNA levels are highest and in advanced disease as the viral set point increases (Fig. 182-9).

A number of studies have indicated that male *circumcision* is associated with a lower risk of HIV infection among men. This difference may be due to increased susceptibility of uncircumcised men to ulcerative STDs, as well as other factors such as microtrauma to the foreskin and glans penis. In addition, the highly vascularized inner foreskin tissue contains a high density of Langerhans cells as well as increased numbers of CD4+ T cells, macrophages, and other cellular targets for HIV. Finally, the moist environment under the foreskin may promote the presence or persistence of microbial flora that, via inflammatory changes, may lead to even higher concentrations of target cells for HIV in the foreskin. In some studies the use of oral contraceptives was associated with an increase in incidence of HIV infection over and above that which might be expected by not using a condom for birth control. This phenomenon may be due to drug-induced changes in the cervical mucosa, rendering it more vulnerable to penetration by the virus. Adolescent girls might also be more susceptible to infection upon exposure due to the properties of an immature genital tract with increased cervical ectopy or exposed columnar epithelium.

Oral sex is a much less efficient mode of transmission of HIV than is receptive anal intercourse. A number of studies have reported that the incidence of transmission of infection by oral sex among couples discordant for HIV was extremely low. However, there have been reports of documented HIV transmission resulting solely from receptive fellatio and insertive cunnilingus. Therefore, the assumption that receptive oral sex is completely safe is not warranted. The association of alcohol consumption and illicit drug use with unsafe sexual behavior, both homosexual and heterosexual, leads to an increased risk of sexual transmission of HIV. Methamphetamine ("crystal meth," "tina") and other so-called club drugs (e.g., ecstasy, ketamine, and gamma hydroxybutyrate), sometimes taken in conjunction with sildenafil (Viagra) or related drugs have

eral layers thicker than the rectal mucosa and less likely to be traumatized during intercourse, it is clear that the virus can be transmitted to either partner through vaginal intercourse. Studies in the United States and Europe have found that male-to-female HIV transmission is usually more efficient than female-to-male transmission, but small numbers of HIV-positive female index partners limit conclusive sex-specific estimates of transmission probabilities per sex act. The differences in reported transmission rates between men and women may be due in part to the prolonged exposure to infected seminal fluid of the vaginal and cervical mucosa, as well as the endometrium (when semen enters through the cervical os). By comparison, the penis and urethral orifice are exposed relatively briefly to infected vaginal fluid. Among various cofactors examined in studies of heterosexual HIV transmission, the presence of other sexually transmitted diseases (STDs; see below) has been strongly associated with HIV transmission. In this regard, there is a close association between genital ulcerations and transmission, from the standpoints of both susceptibility to infection and infectivity. Infections with microorganisms such as *Treponema pallidum* (Chap. 162), *Haemophilus ducreyi* (Chap. 139), and herpes simplex virus (HSV; Chap. 172) are important causes of genital ulcerations linked to transmission of HIV. In addition, pathogens responsible for nonulcerative inflammatory STDs such as those caused by *Chlamydia trachomatis* (Chap. 169), *Neisseria gonorrhoeae* (Chap. 137), and *Trichomonas vaginalis* (Chap. 208) are also associated with an increased risk of transmission of HIV infection. Bacterial vaginosis, an infection related to sexual behavior, but not strictly an STD, may also be linked to an increased risk of transmission of HIV infection. Several studies suggest that treating other STDs and genital tract syndromes may help prevent transmission of HIV. This effect is most prominent in populations in which the prevalence of HIV infection is relatively low. In studies conducted in Uganda, the chief predictor of heterosexual transmission of HIV was the level of plasma viremia. In a cohort of couples in which one partner was HIV-infected and one was initially uninfected, the mean serum HIV RNA level was significantly higher among HIV-infected subjects whose partners seroconverted than among those whose partners did not seroconvert. In fact, transmission was rare when the infected partner had a plasma level of <1500 copies of HIV RNA per milliliter. The rate of HIV transmission per coital act was highest during the

FIGURE 182-9 HIV transmission rate per coital act among 235 HIV serodiscordant couples in Uganda, and 95% confidence intervals, by follow-up interval. The risk of HIV transmission was highest during early-stage and late-stage infection. *(From Wawer et al.)*

been associated with risky sexual practices and increased risk of HIV infection, particularly among men who have sex with men.

TRANSMISSION BY BLOOD AND BLOOD PRODUCTS

HIV can be transmitted to individuals who receive HIV-tainted blood transfusions, blood products, or transplanted tissue as well as to IDUs who are exposed to HIV while sharing injection paraphernalia such as needles, syringes, the water in which drugs are mixed, or the cotton through which drugs are filtered. Parenteral transmission of HIV during injection drug use does not require IV puncture; SC ("skin popping") or IM ("muscling") injections can transmit HIV as well, even though these behaviors are sometimes erroneously perceived as low-risk. Among IDUs, the risk of HIV infection increases with the duration of injection drug use; the frequency of needle sharing; the number of partners with whom paraphernalia are shared, particularly in the setting of "shooting galleries" where drugs are sold and large numbers of IDUs may share a limited number of "works"; comorbid psychiatric conditions such as antisocial personality disorder; the use of cocaine in injectable form or smoked as "crack"; and the use of injection drugs in a geographic location with a high prevalence of HIV infection, such as certain inner-city areas in the United States.

The first transfusion-associated cases of AIDS were reported in 1982, and by the end of 2005, >9300 individuals in the United States who survived the illness for which they received HIV-contaminated blood transfusions, blood components, or transplanted tissue had developed AIDS. Virtually all these cases were due to HIV infection prior to the spring of 1985, when mandatory testing of donated blood for HIV-1 was initiated. It is estimated that 90–100% of individuals who were exposed to HIV-contaminated products became infected. Transfusions of whole blood, packed red blood cells, platelets, leukocytes, and plasma are all capable of transmitting HIV infection. In contrast, hyperimmune γ globulin, hepatitis B immune globulin, plasma-derived hepatitis B vaccine, and Rh$_0$ immune globulin have not been associated with transmission of HIV infection. The procedures involved in processing these products either inactivate or remove the virus.

In addition to the above, an estimated 8000–10,000 individuals in the United States with hemophilia or other clotting disorders were infected with HIV by receipt of HIV-contaminated fresh-frozen plasma or concentrates of clotting factors; by the end of 2005, >5400 of these individuals had developed AIDS. Currently, in the United States and in most developed countries, the following measures have made the risk of transmission of HIV infection by transfused blood or blood products extremely small: (1) the screening of all blood for HIV nucleic acid, p24 antigen, and/or anti-HIV antibodies; (2) the self-deferral of donors on the basis of risk behavior; (3) the screening out of HIV-negative individuals with positive surrogate laboratory parameters of HIV infection, such as hepatitis B and C; and (4) serologic testing for syphilis. The chance of infection of a hemophiliac via clotting factor concentrates has essentially been eliminated because of the added layer of safety resulting from heat treatment of the concentrates.

It is currently estimated that the risk of infection with HIV in the United States via transfused screened blood is approximately 1 in 1.5 million donations. Therefore, among the ~15 million donations collected in the United States each year, about 10 infectious donations are available for transfusion. Thus, despite the best efforts of science, one cannot completely eliminate the risk of transfusion-related transmission of HIV since current technology cannot detect HIV RNA for the first 1–2 weeks following infection due to the low levels of viremia. There have been several reports of sporadic breakdowns in routinely available screening procedures in certain countries, where contaminated blood was allowed to be transfused, resulting in small clusters of patients becoming infected. In China, a disturbingly large number of persons have become infected by selling blood in situations where the collectors reused needles that were contaminated and, in some instances, mixed blood products from a number of individuals, separated the plasma, and reinfused red blood cells back into individual donors.

There have been no reported cases of transmission of HIV-2 in the United States via donated blood or tissues, and, currently, donated blood is screened for both HIV-1 and HIV-2 antibodies. Transmission of HIV (both HIV-1 and HIV-2) by blood or blood products is still an ongoing threat in certain developing countries, particularly in sub-Saharan Africa, where routine screening of blood is not universally practiced.

Prior to the screening of donors, a small number of cases of transmission of HIV via semen used in artificial insemination and tissues used in organ transplantation were documented. At present, donors of such tissues are prescreened for HIV infection. However, laboratory errors can occur, and in 2007 an incorrect screening report led to the transplantation in Italy of two kidneys and a liver to three recipients from a deceased donor who was later discovered to have been HIV positive. With regard to HIV sero-discordant couples (male, HIV infected; female, HIV-uninfected) who wish to conceive a child, assisted reproductive techniques using sperm-washing to reduce the risk of HIV transmission have been successfully employed, with only one well-documented seroconversion in the uninfected female partner, reported in 1990.

OCCUPATIONAL TRANSMISSION OF HIV: HEALTH CARE WORKERS, LABORATORY WORKERS, AND THE HEALTH CARE SETTING

There is a small, but definite, occupational risk of HIV transmission to health care workers and laboratory personnel and potentially others who work with HIV-containing materials, particularly when sharp objects are used. An estimated 600,000–800,000 health care workers are stuck with needles or other sharp medical instruments in the United States each year.

Exposures that place a health care worker at potential risk of HIV infection are percutaneous injuries (e.g., a needle stick or cut with a sharp object) or contact of mucous membrane or nonintact skin (e.g., exposed skin that is chapped, abraded, or afflicted with dermatitis) with blood, tissue, or other potentially infectious body fluids. Large, multi-institutional studies have indicated that the risk of HIV transmission following skin puncture from a needle or a sharp object that was contaminated with blood from a person with documented HIV infection is ~0.3% and after a mucous membrane exposure it is 0.09% (see "HIV and the Health Care Worker," below). HIV transmission after non-intact skin exposure has been documented, but the average risk for transmission by this route has not been precisely determined; however, it is estimated to be less than the risk for mucous membrane exposure. Transmission of HIV through intact skin has not been documented.

In addition to blood and visibly bloody body fluids, semen and vaginal secretions are also considered potentially infectious but have not been implicated in occupational transmission from patients to health care workers. The following fluids are also considered potentially infectious: cerebrospinal fluid, synovial fluid, pleural fluid, peritoneal fluid, pericardial fluid, and amniotic fluid. The risk for transmission after exposure to fluids or tissues other than HIV-infected blood also has not been quantified but is probably considerably lower than for blood exposures. Feces, nasal secretions, saliva, sputum, sweat, tears, urine, and vomitus are not considered potentially infectious unless they are visibly bloody. Rare cases of HIV transmission via human bites have been reported, but not after an occupational exposure.

An increased risk for HIV infection following percutaneous exposures to HIV-infected blood is associated with exposures involving a relatively large quantity of blood, as in the case of a device visibly contaminated with the patient's blood, a procedure that involves a needle placed directly in a vein or artery, or a deep injury. Factors that might be associated with mucocutaneous transmission of HIV include exposure to an unusually large volume of blood, prolonged contact, and a potential portal of entry. In addition, the risk increases for exposures to blood from patients with advanced-stage disease, owing to the higher titer of HIV in the blood as well as to other factors, such as the presence of more virulent strains of virus. The use of antiretroviral drugs as postexposure prophylaxis decreases the risk of infection compared to historic controls in occupationally exposed health care workers (see "HIV and the Health Care Worker," below). The risk of hepatitis B virus (HBV) infection following a similar type of exposure is ~6–30% in nonimmune individuals; if a susceptible worker is exposed to HBV, postexposure prophylaxis with hepatitis B immune globulin and initiation of HBV vaccine is >90% effective in preventing HBV infection. The risk of hepatitis C virus (HCV) infection following percutaneous injury is ~1.8% (Chap. 298).

Since the beginning of the HIV epidemic, there have been at least three reported instances in which transmission of infection from a health care worker to patients seemed highly probable. One cluster of infections involved an HIV-infected dentist in Florida who apparently infected as many as six of his patients, most likely through contaminated instruments. Another case involved an HIV-infected orthopedic surgeon in France who apparently infected a patient during placement of a total hip prosthesis. A third case involved the apparent transmission of HIV from an HIV-infected nurse to a surgical patient in France. Breaches in infection control and the reuse of contaminated syringes have also resulted in the transmission of HIV from patient to patient in hospitals, nursing homes, and outpatient settings. For example, in the only report of HIV transmission from patient to patient during a surgical procedure, four patients in Australia were apparently infected by an HIV-negative general surgeon during routine outpatient surgery. Although the mechanism of transmission was not definitively identified, a failure on the part of the surgeon to sterilize instruments properly following prior surgery on an HIV-infected patient was considered a likely explanation for this outbreak. Three patients (two in hospitals in the United States and one in the Netherlands) undergoing nuclear medicine procedures were reported to have inadvertently received IV injections of blood or other material from patients infected with HIV. Hemodialysis centers have also been implicated in several reported HIV transmission incidents.

The most dramatic reports involved transmission of HIV to 8000–10,000 children in Romanian orphanages in the 1980s. Other large incidents occurred in hospitals in Russia and Libya in the late 1980s and late 1990s, respectively. Each of these incidents received considerable attention and likely was related to reuse of contaminated needles and/or administration of contaminated blood products. Despite the small number of documented cases, the risk of HIV transmission involving health care workers (infected or not) to patients is extremely low in developed countries; in fact, too low to be measured accurately. In this regard, several epidemiologic studies have been performed tracing thousands of patients of HIV-infected dentists, physicians, surgeons, obstetricians, and gynecologists, and no other cases of HIV infection that could be linked to the health care providers were identified. The very rare occurrence of transmission of HIV as well as HBV and HCV to and from health care workers in the workplace underscores the importance of the use of universal precautions when caring for all patients (see below and Chap. 125).

MATERNAL-FETAL/INFANT TRANSMISSION

HIV infection can be transmitted from an infected mother to her fetus during pregnancy, during delivery, or by breast-feeding. This is an extremely important form of transmission of HIV infection in certain developing countries, where the proportion of infected women to infected men is ~1:1. Virologic analysis of aborted fetuses indicate that HIV can be transmitted to the fetus as early as the first and second trimester of pregnancy. However, maternal transmission to the fetus occurs most commonly in the perinatal period. Two studies performed in Rwanda and the former Zaire indicated that the relative proportions of mother-to-child transmissions were 23–30% before birth, 50–65% during birth, and 12–20% via breast-feeding.

In the absence of prophylactic antiretroviral therapy to the mother during pregnancy, labor, and delivery, and to the fetus following birth (see below), the probability of transmission of HIV from mother to infant/fetus ranges from 15–25% in industrialized countries and from 25–35% in developing countries. These differences may relate to the adequacy of prenatal care as well as to the stage of HIV disease and the general health of the mother during pregnancy. Higher rates of transmission have been reported to be associated with many factors, the best documented of which is the presence of high maternal levels of plasma viremia. In one study of 552 singleton pregnancies in the United States,

the rate of mother-to-baby transmission was 0% among women with <1000 copies of HIV RNA per milliliter of blood, 16.6% among women with 1000–10,000 copies/mL, 21.3% among women with 10,001–50,000 copies/mL, 30.9% among women with 50,001–100,000 copies/mL, and 40.6% among women with >100,000 copies/mL. However, there may not be a lower "threshold" below which transmission never occurs, since other studies have reported transmission by women with viral RNA levels <50 copies/mL. Low maternal CD4+ T cell counts have also been associated with higher rates of transmission; however, since low CD4+ T cell counts are often associated with high levels of plasma viremia, in one study using multivariate analysis including plasma viral load and CD4+ T cell count, only the level of plasma HIV RNA was significant. Increased mother-to-child transmission is also correlated with closer HLA match between mother and child. A prolonged interval between membrane rupture and delivery is another well-documented risk factor for transmission. Other conditions that are potential risk factors, but which have not been consistently demonstrated, are the presence of chorioamnionitis at delivery; STDs during pregnancy; hard drug use during pregnancy; cigarette smoking; preterm delivery; and obstetrical procedures such as amniocentesis, amnioscopy, fetal scalp electrodes, and episiotomy. In a study conducted in the United States and France, zidovudine treatment of HIV-infected pregnant women from the beginning of the second trimester through delivery and of the infant for 6 weeks following birth dramatically decreased the rate of intrapartum and perinatal transmission of HIV infection from 22.6% in the untreated group to <5%. The rate of mother-to-child transmission is approaching 1% or less in pregnant women who are receiving combination antiretroviral therapy for their HIV infection. Such treatment, combined with cesarean section delivery, has rendered mother-to-child transmission of HIV an unusual event in the United States and other developed nations. In developed countries, current recommendations to reduce perinatal transmission of HIV include universal voluntary HIV testing and counseling of pregnant women, antiretroviral prophylaxis with one or more drugs in cases in which the mother does not require therapy for her HIV infection, combination therapy for women who do require therapy, obstetric management that attempts to minimize exposure of the infant to maternal blood and genital secretions, and avoidance of breast-feeding. It is recommended that the choice of antiretroviral therapy for pregnant women should be based on the same considerations used for women who are not pregnant, with discussion of the recognized and unknown risks and benefits of such therapy during pregnancy (see below under "Treatment"). This approach has led to a remarkable decrease in the number of infants infected with HIV through mother-to-child transmission in the United States, from an estimated peak of 1750 HIV-infected infants born each year during the early to mid-1990s to 280–370 infants in 2000, and a dramatic decrease in reported AIDS cases among children (Fig. 182-10). Certain studies have demonstrated that truncated regimens of zidovudine alone or in combination with lamivudine given to the mother during the last few weeks of pregnancy or even only during labor and delivery, and to the infant for a week or less, significantly reduced transmission to the infant compared to placebo. Short-course prophylactic antiretroviral (ARV) regimens, such as a single dose of nevirapine given to the mother at the onset of labor and a single dose to the infant within 72 h of birth, are of particular relevance to low- to mid-income nations because of the low cost and the fact that in these regions perinatal care is often not available and pregnant women are often seen by a health care provider for the first time at or near the time of delivery. Indeed, short-course ARV regimens have now been used for several years in developing nations for the prevention of mother-to-child transmission. It is estimated that the successful implementation of such regimens has saved as many as 1000 babies per day from becoming infected with HIV, the vast majority of whom are in sub-Saharan Africa. Given that combination ARV therapy is now increasingly available to individuals in developing countries due to the lower cost of drugs and programs that are making drugs available to these regions of the world, combinations of drugs are being used more frequently, where available, to treat HIV-infected pregnant women who require therapy notwithstanding their pregnancy. This has had the

FIGURE 182-10 Estimated numbers of AIDS cases in children <13 years of age, by year of diagnosis, 1992–2005, 50 states and the District of Columbia. *(From CDC.)*

effect of benefitting the women, blocking HIV transmission to the fetus, and protecting against subsequent transmission by breast-feeding (see below).

Breast-feeding is an important modality of transmission of HIV infection in developing countries, particularly where mothers continue to breast-feed for prolonged periods. The risk factors for mother-to-child transmission of HIV via breast-feeding are not fully understood; factors that increase the likelihood of transmission include detectable levels of HIV in breast milk, the presence of mastitis, low maternal CD4+ T cell counts, and maternal vitamin A deficiency. The risk of HIV infection via breast-feeding is highest in the early months of breast-feeding. In addition, exclusive breast-feeding has been reported to carry a lower risk of HIV transmission than mixed feeding. Certainly in developed countries, breast-feeding by an infected mother should be avoided. However, there is disagreement regarding recommendations for breast-feeding in certain developing countries, where breast milk is the only source of adequate nutrition as well as immunity against potentially serious infections for the infant. The optimal approach to prevent transmission by infected mothers who choose to breast-feed would be to provide continual treatment to the infected mother. This approach has become more feasible as ARV therapy becomes more widely available in developing countries. Despite progress in this regard, ARV therapy is currently available to only ~25% of persons in developing nations who require it. Therefore, alternative approaches to block transmission by breast-feeding are being tested. In this regard, studies are being conducted to determine whether intermittent administration of nevirapine, which has a relatively long half-life, to uninfected babies born of infected mothers decreases the incidence of infection via breast-feeding.

TRANSMISSION BY OTHER BODY FLUIDS

Although HIV can be isolated typically in low titers from saliva of a small proportion of infected individuals, there is no convincing evidence that saliva can transmit HIV infection, either through kissing or through other exposures, such as occupationally to health care workers. Saliva contains endogenous antiviral factors; among these factors, HIV-specific immunoglobulins of IgA, IgG, and IgM isotypes are detected readily in salivary secretions of infected individuals. It has been suggested that large glycoproteins such as mucins and thrombospondin-1 sequester HIV into aggregates for clearance by the host. In addition, a number of soluble salivary factors inhibit HIV to various degrees in vitro, probably by targeting host cell receptors rather than the virus itself. Perhaps the best-studied of these, secretory leukocyte protease inhibitor (SLPI), blocks HIV infection in several cell culture systems, and it is found in saliva at levels that approximate those required for inhibition of HIV in vitro. In this regard, higher salivary levels of SLPI in breast-fed infants were associated with a decreased risk of HIV transmission through breast milk. It has also been suggested that submandibular sa-

liva reduces HIV infectivity by stripping gp120 from the surface of virions, and that saliva-mediated disruption and lysis of HIV-infected cells occurs because of the hypotonicity of oral secretions. There have been outlier cases of suspected transmission by saliva, but these have probably been blood-to-blood transmissions. Transmission of HIV by a human bite can occur but is a rare event; at least four cases of such transmission have been reported. In addition, a most unusual form of HIV transmission from infected children to mothers in the former Soviet Union has been identified. In those cases, the children (infected through transfusion) were said to have bleeding sores in the mouth, and the mothers were said to have lacerations and abrasions on and around the nipples of the breast resulting from trauma from the children's teeth. Breast-feeding had been continued until the children were older than is usual in other developed countries.

Although virus can be identified, if not isolated, from virtually any body fluid, there is no evidence that HIV transmission can occur as a result of exposure to tears, sweat, and urine. However, there have been isolated cases of transmission of HIV infection by body fluids that may or may not have been contaminated with blood. Most of these situations occurred in the setting of a close relative providing intensive nursing care for an HIV-infected person without observing universal precautions, underscoring the importance of observing such precautions in the handling of body fluids and wastes from HIV-infected individuals (see below).

EPIDEMIOLOGY

HIV INFECTION AND AIDS WORLDWIDE

HIV infection/AIDS is a global pandemic, with cases reported from virtually every country. At the end of 2007, 33.2 million individuals were living with HIV infection (range: 30.6–36.1 million) according to the Joint United Nations Programme on HIV/AIDS (UNAIDS). More than 95% of people living with HIV/AIDS reside in low- and middle-income countries; ~50% are female, and 2.5 million are children <15 years. The global distribution of these cases is illustrated in **Fig. 182-11**.

In 2007, there were an estimated 2.5 million new cases of HIV infection worldwide, including 420,000 in children <15 years. In 2007, global AIDS deaths totaled 2.1 million (including 330,000 children <15 years). UNAIDS estimates that global HIV prevalence has been level since 2001. HIV incidence likely peaked in the late 1990s at >3 million new infections per year (**Fig. 182-12**). Recent reductions in global HIV incidence likely reflect natural trends in the pandemic as well as the results of prevention programs resulting in behavior change.

The HIV epidemic has occurred in "waves" in different regions of the world, each wave having somewhat different characteristics depending on the demographics of the country and region in question and the timing of the introduction of HIV into the population. Although the AIDS epidemic was first recognized in the United States and shortly thereafter in Western Europe, it very likely began in sub-Saharan Africa (see above), which has been particularly devastated by the epidemic. More than two-thirds of all people with HIV infection (~22.5 million) live in that region, even though sub-Saharan Africa is home to just 10–11% of the world's population (Fig. 182-11). Within the region, southern Africa is worst-affected. In eight southern African countries, available seroprevalence data indicate that >15% of the adult population aged 15–49 is HIV-infected. In addition, among high-risk individuals (e.g., commercial sex workers, patients attending STD clinics) who live in urban areas of sub-Saharan Africa, seroprevalence is now >50% in some countries. According to projections of the

FIGURE 182-11 Estimated number of adults and children living with HIV infection as of December, 2007. Total: 33.2 (30.6–36.1) million. *[From United Nations AIDS Program (UNAIDS).]*

United Nations Population Division, life expectancies in several highly affected countries could drop to <40 years, well below what they would have been without HIV/AIDS and below levels reached in the pre-AIDS era (Fig. 182-13).

In Asia, an estimated 4.9 million people were living with HIV at the end of 2007. National HIV prevalence is highest in southeast Asia, with wide variation in trends between different countries. The epidemic in Asia lagged temporally behind that in Africa; however, the populations of many Asian nations are so large (especially India and China) that even low national HIV prevalence rates result in large numbers of people living with HIV. Encouragingly, HIV prevalence has declined in Myanmar, Cambodia and in Thailand; however, HIV prevalence continues to increase in other countries such as Indonesia and Vietnam.

The epidemic is expanding in Eastern Europe and Central Asia, where ~1.6 million people were living with HIV at the end of 2007. Ninety percent of new HIV infections reported in 2007 occurred in two countries, the Russian Federation and Ukraine. Driven initially by injection drug use and increasingly by heterosexual transmission, the number of new infections in this region has increased dramatically over the past decade.

Approximately 1.8 million people are living with HIV/AIDS in Latin America and the Caribbean. Brazil is home to the largest number of HIV-infected people in the region. However, the epidemic has been slowed in that country due to successful treatment and prevention efforts. The Caribbean region has the highest regional adult seroprevalence rate after Africa, due in large part to the huge case load in Haiti. Approximately 2.1 million people are living with HIV/AIDS in North America and in Western and Central Europe.

The major mode of HIV transmission worldwide is unquestionably heterosexual sex; this is particularly true, and has been so since the beginning of the epidemic, in developing countries, where the numbers of infected men and women are approximately equal. The epidemic in most developed countries was first introduced among men who have sex with men and, to a greater or lesser degree (depending on the individual country), among IDUs. In this regard, the total numbers of AIDS cases in those countries still reflect a high proportion of cases among these high-risk groups. However, in most developed countries, including the United States (see above and below), there has been a gradual shift toward heterosexual transmission (Fig. 182-8).

AIDS IN THE UNITED STATES

AIDS has had—and will continue to have—an extraordinary public health impact in the United States. As of January 1, 2006, an estimated 984,155 cases of AIDS had been diagnosed in the United States and dependent areas, and ~550,394 AIDS-related deaths had occurred. AIDS cases have been reported in all 50 states, the District of Columbia; and in U.S. dependencies, possessions, and associated nations. An estimated 1.1 million individuals in the United States are living with HIV infection, one-quarter of whom are unaware of their infection. The estimated

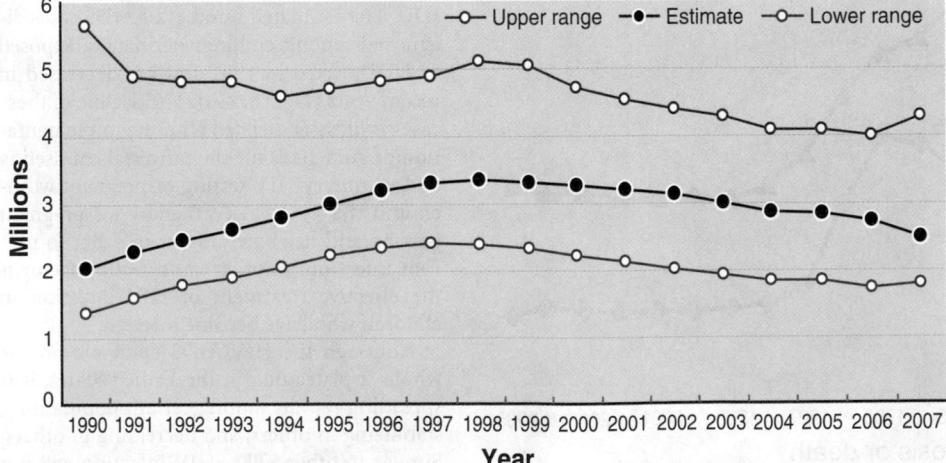

ESTIMATED NUMBER OF PEOPLE NEWLY INFECTED WITH HIV GLOBALLY, 1990–2007

FIGURE 182-12 Estimated number of people newly infected with HIV globally, 1990–2007. *[From United Nations AIDS Program (UNAIDS).]*

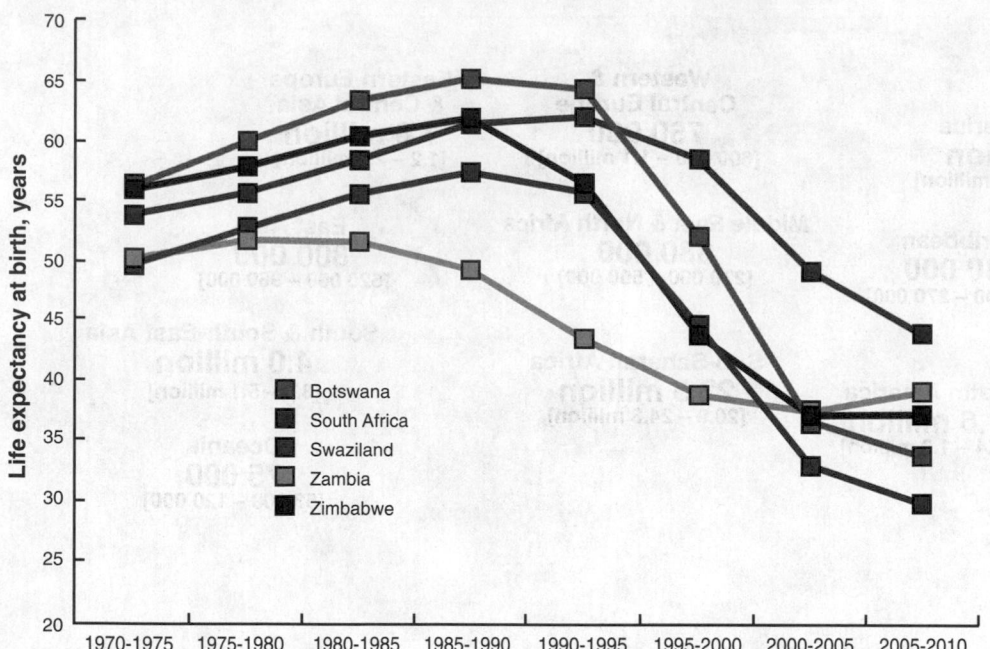

FIGURE 182-13 The impact of HIV/AIDS on life expectancy in five Sub-Saharan African countries, 1970–2010. *[From United Nations AIDS Program (UNAIDS).]*

HIV seroprevalence rate among adults aged 15–49 years in the United States is ~0.6%. Prevalence is highest among young adults in their late twenties and thirties and among minorities.

The number of AIDS cases and deaths rose steadily through the 1980s; AIDS cases peaked in 1993 and deaths in 1995 **(Fig. 182-14)**. Since then, the annual numbers of AIDS-related deaths in the United States have fallen ~70%. This trend is due to several factors, including the improved prophylaxis and treatment of opportunistic infections, the growing experience among the health professions in caring for HIV-infected individuals, improved access to health care, and a decrease in new infections due to saturational effects and prevention efforts. However, the most influential factor clearly has been the increased use of potent ARV drugs, generally administered in a combination of three or four agents (see below).

Approximately 40,000 individuals are newly infected each year in the United States, a figure that has remained stable for at least 15

years. Among adults and adolescents newly diagnosed with HIV infection (regardless of AIDS status) in the United States in 2005, ~74% are men and ~26% are women **(Fig. 182-15)**. Of new HIV/AIDS diagnoses among men, ~67% were due to male-to-male sexual contact, ~15% to heterosexual contact, ~13% to injection drug use, and ~5% to a combination of male-to-male sexual contact and injection drug use. Of new HIV/AIDS diagnoses among women, ~80% were due to heterosexual contact and ~20% to injection drug use.

HIV transmission patterns in the United States have shifted over time. When one looks at the totality of data collected from the beginning of the epidemic, ~46% of all AIDS cases are among men who have had sex with men. However, since the mid-1980s the proportion of newly reported cases of AIDS in this population has declined from ~64% of cases diagnosed in 1985 to ~42% of cases diagnosed in 2005 (Fig. 182-8). Meanwhile, the proportion of new AIDS cases attributed to heterosexual contact has increased dramatically, from 3% in 1985 to 31% in 2005. The share of AIDS diagnoses due to injection drug use was 19% in 1985, peaked at 31% in 1993, and was 21% in 2005. Women are increasingly affected: the proportion of AIDS cases among female adults and adolescents (age >13 years) increased from 7% in 1985 to 27% in 2005.

HIV infection and AIDS have disproportionately affected minority populations in the United States. Among those diagnosed with HIV (regardless of AIDS status) in 2005, 49% percent were African Americans, a group that comprises only 13% of the U.S. population **(Fig. 182-16)**. An estimated 3% of black men and 1% of black women in their thirties are living with HIV infection. HIV/AIDS ranked ninth among all causes of mortality in the United States in 2004 among those aged 35–64 years, but among African Americans it ranked third.

As of January 1, 2006, an estimated 9112 cases of AIDS in children <13 years old had been diagnosed, and ~54% of these children have died. Approximately 93% of these children were born to mothers who were HIV-infected or who were at risk for HIV infection and, in the majority of those cases, the mother was either an IDU or the heterosexual partner of an IDU. The estimated number of AIDS cases diagnosed among children perinatally exposed to HIV peaked in 1992 and has decreased in recent years (Fig. 182-10). The decline of these cases is likely associated with the implementation of guidelines for the universal counseling and voluntary HIV testing of pregnant women and the use of ARV therapy for pregnant women and newborn infants in order to prevent infection. Another contributing factor is the effective treatment of HIV infection in children who have become infected.

Although the HIV/AIDS epidemic on the whole is plateauing in the United States, it is spreading rapidly among certain populations, stabilizing in others, and decreasing in others. Similar to other STDs, HIV infection will not spread homogeneously throughout the population of the United States. However, it is clear

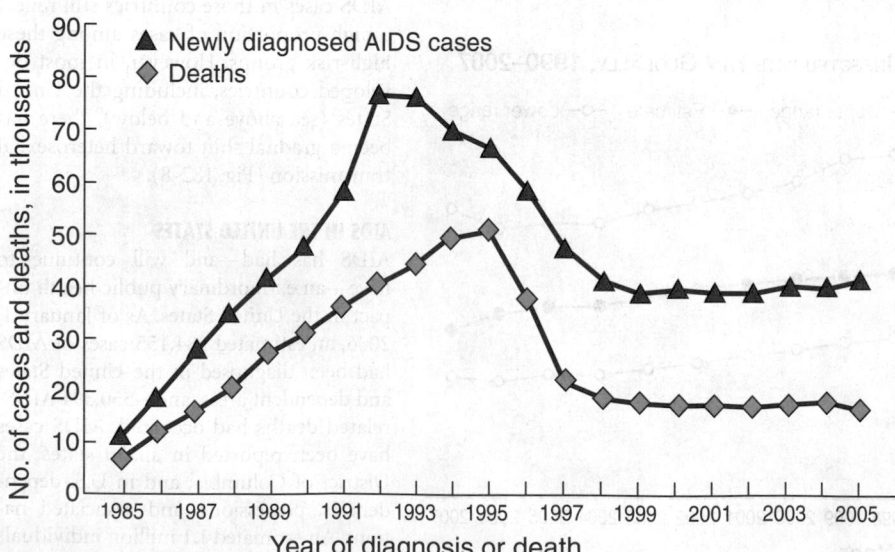

FIGURE 182-14 Estimated number of AIDS cases and AIDS deaths, United States, 1985–2005. *(From CDC.)*

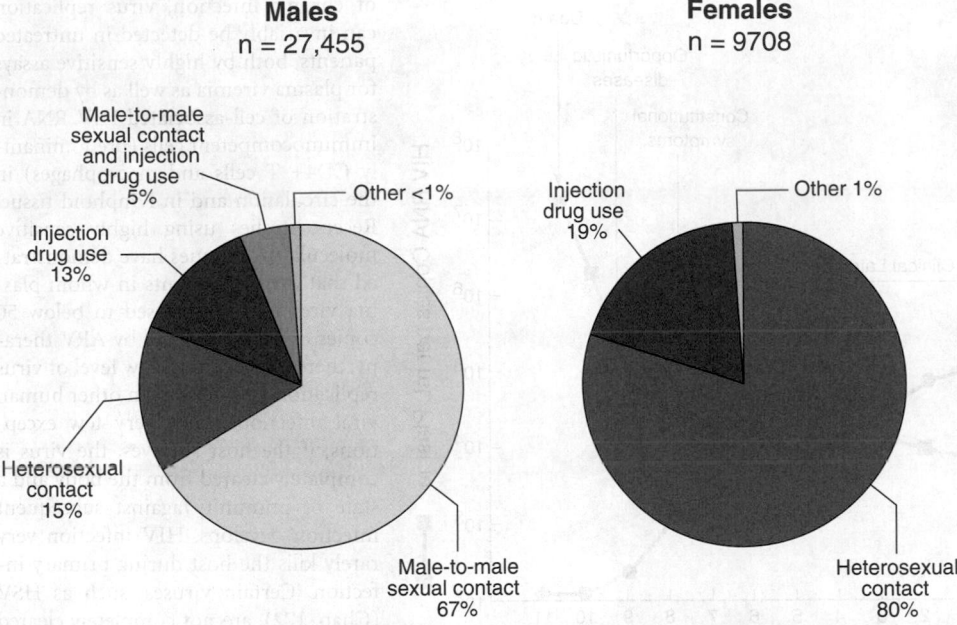

Males
n = 27,455

Females
n = 9708

Male-to-male sexual contact and injection drug use 5%

Injection drug use 13%

Other <1%

Injection drug use 19%

Other 1%

Heterosexual contact 15%

Male-to-male sexual contact 67%

Heterosexual contact 80%

FIGURE 182-15 Transmission categories of adults and adolescents with HIV/AIDS diagnosed during 2005 in the United States. Estimates based on data from 33 states with long-term, confidential, name-based HIV infection reporting. Data include persons with a diagnosis of HIV infection regardless of AIDS status at diagnosis. *(From CDC.)*

that anyone who practices high-risk behavior is at risk for HIV infection. In addition, recent increases in infections and AIDS cases among young men who have sex with men and among heterosexuals (particularly sexual partners of IDUs, women, and adolescents) as well as the spread in pockets of poverty in both urban and rural regions (particularly among underserved minority populations in the southern United States with inadequate access to health care) testify to the fact that the epidemic of HIV infection in the United States remains a public health problem of major proportions.

PATHOPHYSIOLOGY AND PATHOGENESIS

The hallmark of HIV disease is a profound immunodeficiency resulting primarily from a progressive quantitative and qualitative deficien-

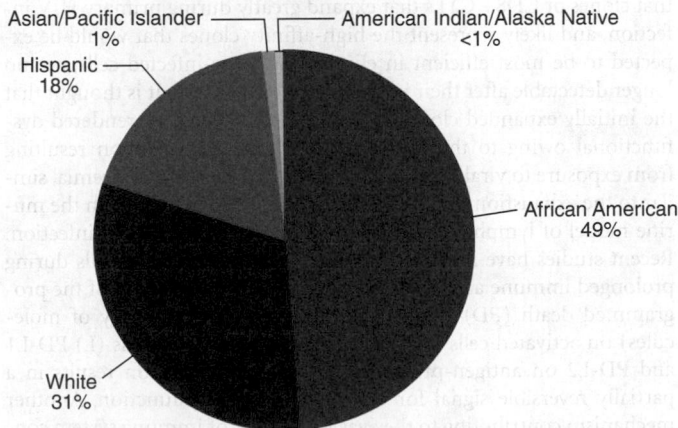

n = 37,331

Asian/Pacific Islander 1%

American Indian/Alaska Native <1%

Hispanic 18%

African American 49%

White 31%

FIGURE 182-16 Race/ethnicity of persons (including children) with HIV/AIDS diagnosed during 2005 in the United States. Estimates based on data from 33 states with long-term, confidential, name-based HIV infection reporting. Data include persons with a diagnosis of HIV infection regardless of AIDS status at diagnosis. *(From CDC.)*

cy of the subset of T lymphocytes referred to as *helper T cells*. This subset of T cells is defined phenotypically by the presence on its surface of the CD4 molecule (Chap. 308), which serves as the primary cellular receptor for HIV. A co-receptor must also be present together with CD4 for efficient fusion and entry of HIV-1 into its target cells (Figs. 182-3 and 182-4). HIV uses two major co-receptors for fusion and entry; these co-receptors are also the primary receptors for certain chemoattractive cytokines termed *chemokines* and belong to the seven-transmembrane-domain G protein–coupled family of receptors. CCR5 and CXCR4 are the major co-receptors used by HIV (see above and below). A number of mechanisms responsible for cellular depletion and/or immune dysfunction of CD4+ T cells have been demonstrated in vitro; these include direct infection and destruction of these cells by HIV and immune clearance of infected cells, as well as indirect effects such as immune exhaustion due to aberrant cellular activation and activation-induced cell death (see below). Patients with CD4+ T cell levels below certain thresholds (see below) are at high risk of developing a variety of opportunistic diseases, particularly the infections and neoplasms that are AIDS-defining illnesses. Some features of AIDS, such as Kaposi's sarcoma and neurologic abnormalities (see below), cannot be explained completely by the immunodeficiency caused by HIV infection, since these complications may occur prior to the development of severe immunologic impairment.

The combination of viral pathogenic and immunopathogenic events that occurs during the course of HIV disease from the moment of initial (primary) infection through the development of advanced-stage disease is complex and varied. It is important to appreciate that the pathogenic mechanisms of HIV disease are multifactorial and multiphasic and are different at different stages of the disease. Therefore, it is essential to consider the typical clinical course of an untreated HIV-infected individual in order to more fully appreciate these pathogenic events (Fig. 182-17).

PRIMARY HIV INFECTION, INITIAL VIREMIA, AND DISSEMINATION OF VIRUS
The events associated with primary HIV infection are likely critical determinants of the subsequent course of HIV disease. In particular, the early dissemination of virus to lymphoid organs, particularly the gut-associated lymphoid tissue (GALT), is a major factor in the establishment of a chronic and persistent infection (see below). The initial infection of susceptible cells may vary somewhat with the route of infection. Virus that enters directly into the bloodstream via infected blood or blood products (i.e., transfusions, use of contaminated needles for injecting drugs, sharp-object injuries, maternal-to-fetal transmission either intrapartum or perinatally, or sexual intercourse where there is enough trauma to cause bleeding) is likely cleared from the circulation to the spleen and other lymphoid organs, where primary focal infections begin, followed by wider dissemination throughout other lymphoid tissues, particularly the GALT, leading to a burst of viremia. Dendritic cells play an important role in the initiation of HIV infection. These cells express a diversity of C-type lectin receptors on their surface, one of which is called *DC-SIGN* (see above). DC-SIGN binds with high affinity to the HIV envelope gp120 and can retain infectious particles for days in vitro. In this regard, dendritic cells can trap HIV and mediate the efficient transinfection of CD4+ T cells. In addition, DC-SIGN may also facilitate CD4-mediated infection of dendritic cells. These mechanisms likely op-

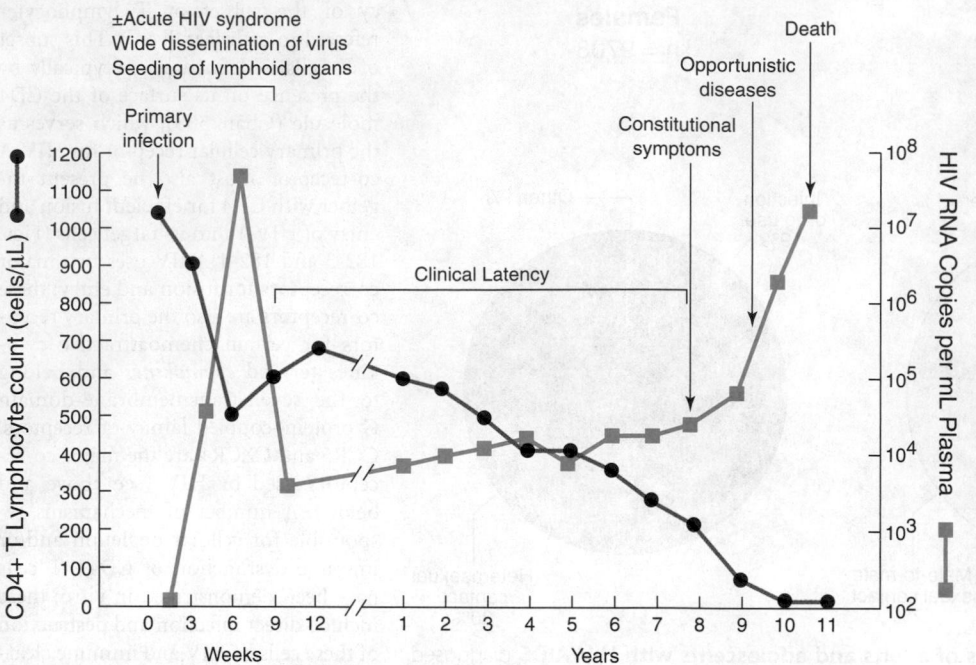

FIGURE 182-17 Typical course of an untreated HIV-infected individual. See text for detailed description. [From G Pantaleo et al: N Engl J Med 328(5):327, 1993. Copyright 1993 Massachusetts Medical Society. All rights reserved.]

erate in humans when HIV enters "locally" (as opposed to directly into the blood) and encounters mucosal dendritic cells via the vagina, rectum, or urethra during intercourse or via the upper gastrointestinal tract from swallowed infected breast milk or rarely semen or vaginal fluid. In primary HIV infection, virus replication in CD4+ T cells intensifies prior to the initiation of an HIV-specific immune response (see below, Fig.182-17), with a burst of viremia resulting from the rapid replication of virus in susceptible cells in lymphoid organs (particularly the GALT), with subsequent dissemination of virus to the brain and other tissues. Of note, animal studies have demonstrated that a significant percentage of CD4+ T cells (particularly memory cells) in the GALT is depleted early after SIV infection, via either direct infection of cells or bystander cell killing. The repopulation of such cells may be extremely problematic, even after initiation of ARV therapy. Individuals who experience the "acute HIV syndrome," which occurs to varying degrees in ~50% of individuals with primary infection, have high levels of viremia measured in millions of copies of HIV RNA per milliliter that last for several weeks (see below). Acute mononucleosis-like symptoms are well correlated with the presence of viremia. Virtually all patients develop some degree of viremia during primary infection, which contributes to virus dissemination throughout the lymphoid tissue (see above), even though they may remain asymptomatic or not recall experiencing symptoms. It appears that the initial level of plasma viremia in primary HIV infection does not necessarily determine the rate of disease progression; however, the set point of the level of steady-state plasma viremia after ~1 year does seem to correlate with the slope of disease progression (see below).

ESTABLISHMENT OF CHRONIC AND PERSISTENT INFECTION

Persistent Virus Replication   HIV infection is unique among human viral infections. Despite the robust cellular and humoral immune responses that are mounted following primary infection (see below), once infection has been established the virus succeeds in escaping immune-mediated clearance (see below), paradoxically seems to thrive on immune activation, and is never eliminated completely from the body. Rather, a chronic infection develops that persists with varying degrees of continual virus replication in the untreated patient for a median of ~10 years before the patient becomes clinically ill (see below). It is this establishment of a chronic, persistent infection that is the hallmark of HIV disease. Throughout the often protracted course

of chronic infection, virus replication can invariably be detected in untreated patients, both by highly sensitive assays for plasma viremia as well as by demonstration of cell-associated HIV RNA in immunocompetent cells (predominantly CD4+ T cells and macrophages) in the circulation and in lymphoid tissue. Recent studies using highly sensitive molecular techniques have demonstrated that even in patients in whom plasma viremia is suppressed to below 50 copies of HIV RNA/mL by ARV therapy, there is a continual low level of virus replication (see below). In other human viral infections, with very few exceptions, if the host survives, the virus is completely cleared from the body and a state of immunity against subsequent infection develops. HIV infection very rarely kills the host during primary infection. Certain viruses, such as HSV (Chap. 172), are not completely cleared from the body after infection but instead enter a latent state; in these cases, clinical latency is accompanied by microbiologic latency. This is not the case with HIV infection as described above. Chronicity associated with persistent virus replication can also be seen in certain cases of HBV and HCV infections (Chap. 300); however, in these infections the immune system is not a target of the virus.

Evasion of Immune System Control   Inherent to the establishment of chronicity of HIV infection is the ability of the virus to evade elimination and control by the immune system. There are a number of mechanisms whereby the virus accomplishes this evasion. Paramount among these is the establishment of a sustained level of replication associated with the generation of viral diversity via mutation and recombination, thus providing a means to evade control and elimination by the immune system. The selection of mutants that escape control by CD8+ cytolytic T lymphocytes (CTLs) is critical to the propagation and progression of HIV infection. The high rate of virus replication and the continual mutation of virus also contribute to the inability of neutralizing antibody to contain the virus quasispecies present in an individual at any given time. Molecular analysis of clonotypes has demonstrated that clones of CD8+ CTLs that expand greatly during primary HIV infection, and likely represent the high-affinity clones that would be expected to be most efficient in eliminating virus-infected cells, are no longer detectable after their initial burst of expansion. It is thought that the initially expanded clones may have been deleted or rendered dysfunctional owing to the overwhelming immune activation resulting from exposure to viral antigens during the initial burst of viremia, similar to the exhaustion of CD8+ CTLs that has been reported in the murine model of lymphocytic choriomeningitis virus (LCMV) infection. Recent studies have indicated that exhaustion of effector cells during prolonged immune activation is associated with expression of the programmed death (PD)-1 molecule (of the B7-CD28 family of molecules) on activated cells and its interaction with its ligands (L) PD-L1 and PD-L2 on antigen-presenting cells. This interaction results in a partially reversible signal for cell death and/or dysfunction. Another mechanism contributing to the evasion by HIV of immune system control is the downregulation of HLA class I molecules on the surface of HIV-infected cells by the Nef protein of HIV, resulting in the lack of ability of the CD8+ CTL to recognize and kill the infected target cell. Although this downregulation of HLA class I molecules would favor elimination of HIV-infected cells by natural killer (NK) cells, this latter mechanism does not seem to remove HIV-infected cells effectively (see below). The principal targets of neutralizing antibodies against HIV are the envelope proteins gp120 and gp41. HIV employs three mechanisms to evade neutralizing responses: hypervariability in the primary sequence of the envelope, extensive glycosylation of the envelope, and conformational masking of neutralizing epitopes.

CD4+ T cell help is essential for the integrity of antigen-specific immune responses, both humoral and cell-mediated. HIV preferentially infects activated CD4+ T cells including HIV-specific CD4+ T cells, and so this loss of viral-specific helper T cell responses has profound negative consequences for the immunologic control of HIV replication. Furthermore, this loss occurs early in the course of infection, and animal studies indicate that 40–70% of all memory CD4+ T cells in the GALT are eliminated during acute infection. Another means of escape of HIV-infected cells from elimination by CD8+ CTLs is the sequestration of infected cells in immunologically privileged sites such as the central nervous system (CNS).

Finally, the escape of HIV from elimination during primary infection allows the formation of a pool of latently infected cells that cannot be eliminated by virus-specific CTLs (see below). Thus, despite a potent immune response and the marked downregulation of virus replication following primary HIV infection, HIV succeeds in establishing a state of chronic infection with a variable degree of persistent virus replication. In most cases, during this period patients make the clinical transition from acute primary infection to variable periods of clinical latency or smoldering disease activity(see below).

Reservoirs of HIV-Infected Cells: Obstacle to the Eradication of Virus

There exists in virtually all HIV-infected individuals a pool of latently infected, resting CD4+ T cells that serves as at least one component of the persistent reservoir of virus. Such cells manifest postintegration latency in that the HIV provirus integrates into the genome of the cell and can remain in this state until an activation signal drives the expression of HIV transcripts and ultimately replication-competent virus. This form of latency is to be distinguished from preintegration latency, in which HIV enters a resting CD4+ T cell and, in the absence of an activation signal, only a limited degree of reverse transcription of the HIV genome occurs. This period of preintegration latency may last hours to days, and if no activation signal is delivered to the cell, the proviral DNA loses its capacity to initiate a productive infection. If these cells do become activated, reverse transcription proceeds to completion and the virus continues along its replication cycle (see above and Fig. 182-18). The pool of cells that are in the postintegration state of latency is established early during the course of primary HIV infection. Despite the suppression of plasma viremia to <50 copies of HIV RNA per milliliter by potent combinations of several ARV drugs administered over several years, this pool of latently infected cells persists and can give rise to replication-competent virus. Modeling studies built on projections of decay curves (see below) have estimated that in such a setting of prolonged suppression, it would require from 7–70 years for the pool of latently infected cells to be completely eliminated. Furthermore, the reservoir of latently infected cells is replenished during minor detectable rebounds of virus replication that may occur intermittently, during the low levels of persistent virus replication that goes undetectable (see below) (Fig. 182-18), even in patients who for the most part are treated successfully, and certainly during major rebounds of viremia in patients whose therapy is interrupted for a period of weeks or longer. Over the past several years attempts have been made to eliminate HIV in the latent viral reservoir using agents that stimulate resting CD4+ T cells during the course of antiretroviral therapy; however, such attempts have been unsuccessful. As more sophisticated techniques become available for measuring extremely low levels of virus replication, it is becoming clear that virus replication continually occurs at very low levels in a substantial proportion of individuals whose viral load is "undetectable" by the standard assays of plasma viremia (see above and below). Thus, although a small pool of truly resting, latently infected cells exists at any given point in time, this pool is continually being activated and replenished by ongoing low levels of virus replication. Reservoirs of HIV infected

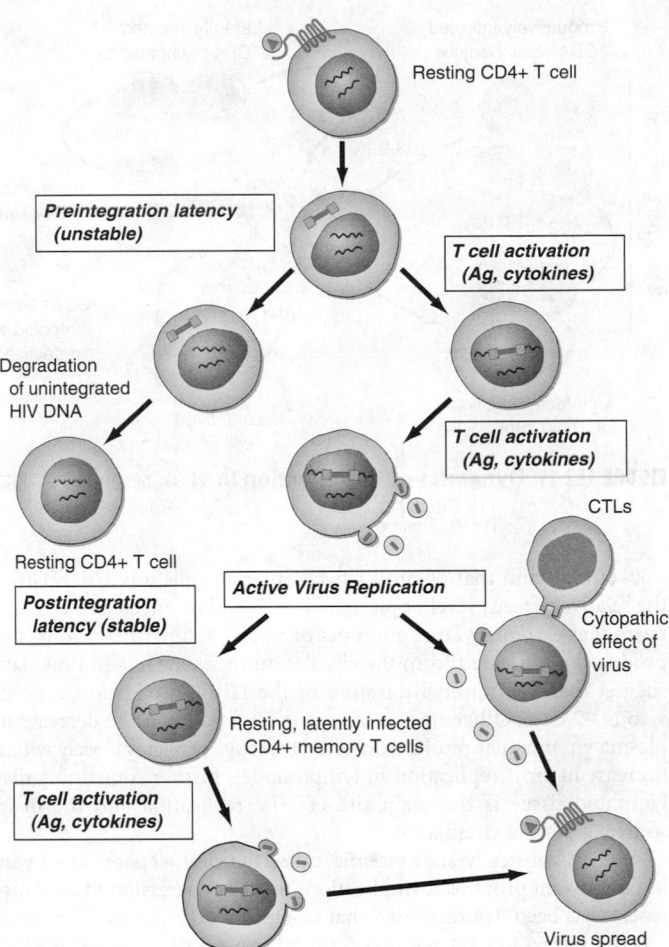

FIGURE 182-18 Generation of latently infected, resting CD4+ T cells in HIV-infected individuals. See text for details. Ag, antigen; CTLs, cytolytic T lymphocytes. *(Courtesy of TW Chun; with permission.)*

cells, latent or otherwise, can exist in a number of compartments including the lymphoid tissue, peripheral blood, and the CNS (likely in cells of the monocyte/macrophage lineage) as well as in other unidentified locations. Thus, this persistent reservoir of infected cells at various stages of latency and/or low levels of persistent virus replication are major obstacles to any goal of eradication of virus from infected individuals, despite the favorable clinical outcomes that have resulted from ARV therapy (see below).

Viral Dynamics   The dynamics of viral production and turnover have been quantified using mathematical modeling in the setting of the administration of reverse transcriptase and protease inhibitors to HIV-infected individuals in clinical studies. Treatment with these drugs resulted in a precipitous decline in the level of plasma viremia, which typically fell by well over 90% within 2 weeks. The number of CD4+ T cells in the blood increased concurrently, which suggested that the killing of CD4+ T cells was linked directly to the levels of replicating virus. However, a significant component of the early rise in CD4+ T cell numbers following the initiation of therapy may be due to the redistribution of cells into the peripheral blood from other body compartments as a consequence of therapy-related diminution in viremia-associated immune system activation. It was determined on the basis of modeling the kinetics of viral decline and the emergence of resistant mutants during therapy that 93–99% of the circulating virus originated from recently infected, rapidly turning over CD4+ T cells and that ~1–7% of circulating virus originated from longer-lived cells, likely monocytes/macrophages. A negligible amount of circulating virus originated from the pool of latently infected cells (see above) (Fig. 182-19). It was also determined that the half-life of a circulating virion was

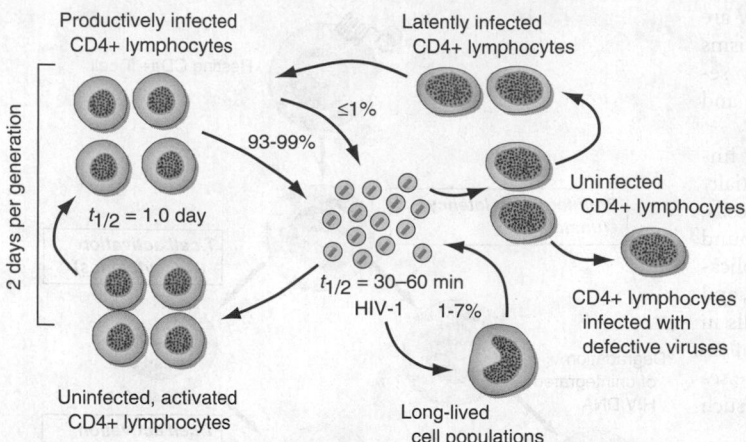

FIGURE 182-19 Dynamics of HIV infection in vivo. See text for detailed description. *(From AS Perelson et al: Science 271:1582, 1996.)*

~30–60 min and that of productively infected cells was 1 day. Given the relatively steady level of plasma viremia and of infected cells, it appears that extremely large amounts of virus ($\sim 10^{10}$–10^{11} virions) are produced and cleared from the circulation each day. In addition, data suggest that the minimal duration of the HIV-1 replication cycle in vivo is ~2 days. Other studies have demonstrated that the decrease in plasma viremia that results from ARV therapy correlates closely with a decrease in virus replication in lymph nodes, further confirming that lymphoid tissue is the main site of HIV replication and the main source of plasma viremia.

The level of steady-state viremia, called the viral *set point*, at ~1 year has important prognostic implications for the progression of HIV disease. It has been demonstrated that as a group HIV-infected individuals who have a low set point at 6 months to 1 year progress to AIDS much more slowly than individuals whose set point is very high at that time (Fig. 182-20). Levels of viremia generally increase as disease progresses. Measurement of the level of viremia is critical in guiding therapeutic decisions in HIV-infected individuals (see below).

Clinical Latency versus Microbiologic Latency With the exception of long-term nonprogressors (see below), the level of CD4+ T cells in the blood decreases progressively in HIV-infected individuals. The decline in CD4+ T cells may be gradual or abrupt, the latter usually reflecting a significant spike in the level of plasma viremia. Most patients are relatively asymptomatic while this progressive decline is taking place (see below) and are often described as being in a state of *clinical latency*. However, this term is misleading; it does not mean disease latency, since progression, although slow in many cases, is generally relentless during this period. Furthermore, clinical latency should not be confused with microbiologic latency, since some level of virus replication invariably occurs during this period of clinical latency. Even in those rare patients who have <50 copies of HIV RNA per milliliter in the absence of therapy, there is virtually always some degree of ongoing virus replication.

ADVANCED HIV DISEASE

In untreated patients or in patients in whom therapy has not adequately controlled virus replication (see below), after a variable period, usually measured in years, the CD4+ T cell count falls below a critical level (<200/μL) and the patient becomes highly susceptible to opportunistic disease (Fig. 182-17). For this reason, the CDC case definition of AIDS includes all HIV-infected individuals with CD4+ T cell counts below this level (Table 182-1). Patients may experience constitutional signs and symptoms or may develop an opportunistic disease abruptly without any prior symptoms, although the latter scenario is unusual. The depletion

of CD4+ T cells continues to be progressive and unrelenting in this phase. It is not uncommon for CD4+ T cell counts in the untreated patient to drop as low as 10/μL or even to zero. In countries where ARV therapy and prophylaxis and treatment for opportunistic infections are readily accessible to such patients, survival is increased dramatically even with this level of advanced disease. In contrast, untreated patients who progress to this severest form of immunodeficiency usually succumb to opportunistic infections or neoplasms (see below).

LONG-TERM SURVIVORS AND LONG-TERM NONPROGRESSORS

The prognosis for HIV-infected individuals who have access to health care and ARV therapy has improved greatly since the beginning of the epidemic. The median time from primary HIV infection to the development of AIDS in untreated individuals in the developed world is ~10 years. This period has been markedly extended by the wide availability of combinations of ARV drugs in the developed world, and increasingly in low- to mid-income countries; the full extent of this benefit is yet to be realized (see below). It is important to distinguish between the terms *long-term survivor* and *long-term nonprogressor*. Long-term nonprogressors are by definition long-term survivors; however, the reverse is not always true. The definitions of these categories are empirical and continue to change as more data are collected from prospective cohort studies. Predictions from one study that antedated the availability of effective ARV therapy estimated that ~13% of homosexual/bisexual men who were infected at an early age may remain free of clinical AIDS for >20 years. Originally, individuals were considered to be long-term survivors if they remained alive for 10–15 years after initial infection. Currently, individuals are considered to be long-term survivors if they remain alive for ≥20 years after initial infection. In most such individuals the disease has progressed, in that they have significant immunodeficiency, and many have experienced opportunistic diseases. Some of these individuals have CD4+ T cell counts that have decreased to ≤200/μL but have remained stable at that level for years. The mechanisms of this stabilization are not entirely clear but may relate to the beneficial effects of ARV therapy and prophylaxis against opportunistic infections. In addition, a number of viral and/or host determinants likely contribute to the long-term survival of these individuals. Quantitative and qualitative aspects of the HIV-specific immune response, as well as recognized and unrecognized genetic factors (see below), may also contribute to the long-term survival of these individuals.

Definitions of long-term nonprogressors have varied considerably over the years, and so such individuals constitute a heterogeneous

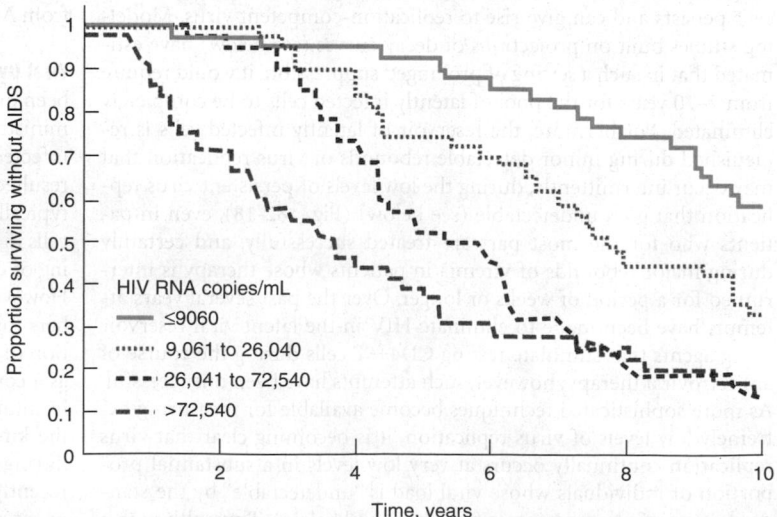

FIGURE 182-20 Relationship between levels of virus and rates of disease progression. Kaplan-Meier curves for AIDS-free survival stratified by baseline HIV-1 RNA categories (copies per milliliter). *(From Mellors et al.)*

group. Originally, individuals considered to be long-term nonprogressors were those who had been infected with HIV for a long period (≥10 years), whose CD4+ T cell counts were in the normal range and remained stable over years, and who had not received ARV therapy. Such patients had relatively low, but usually detectable, levels of plasma viremia, generally normal immune function according to commonly measured parameters (skin tests, in vitro lymphocyte responses to various mitogens and antigens), and normal-appearing lymphoid tissue architecture as determined on lymph node biopsy. In general, long-term nonprogressors manifested robust HIV-specific immune responses, both humoral (neutralizing antibodies) and cell-mediated (HIV-specific CTLs). However, this may also be true of some individuals early in the course of disease who ultimately progress to advanced disease. No qualitative abnormalities in the virus were detected in most of these patients. However, a small subset of patients did have defective virus; in particular, in one cohort of five long-term nonprogressors, the virus had a defect in the *nef* gene. In another report, a blood donor in Australia who was HIV-infected and a group of seven individuals who were infected by blood or blood products from that donor remained free of HIV-related disease and maintained normal and stable CD4+ T cell counts for several years after infection. Sequence analysis of viruses isolated from the donor and recipients revealed similar deletions in the *nef* gene and the region of overlap of *nef* and the U3 region of the HIV LTR (Fig. 182-5). The vast majority of these originally reported long-term nonprogressors have now gone on to progressive disease. More recently, cohorts of rare long-term nonprogressors have been described who have been infected for 20 years with normal CD4+ T cell counts and who typically maintain plasma viral RNA <50 copies per milliliter without ARV therapy. When these more stringent definitions based predominantly on levels of plasma viremia are applied, very strong associations with HLA B*5701 or HLA B*2705 alleles have been found. In addition, the HIV-specific CD8+ T cell response in these patients is highly focused on B5701-restricted peptides, suggesting that the B5701 molecule plays a direct role in restriction of virus replication in these individuals, although the precise mechanisms of this effect remain unclear.

A number of other host genetic factors exert more modest effects on restriction of HIV replication, yet they also may be associated with slower progression of disease (see "Genetic Factors in HIV Pathogenesis," below). The precise role of host factors in long-term nonprogression remains unclear. There is no single genetic determinant for nonprogression. However, several genetic variants and mutations have been demonstrated to result in a delay in the progression of HIV disease. These include heterozygosity for the *CCR5-Δ32* deletion, heterozygosity for the *CCR2-64I* mutation, homozygosity for the *SDF1-3′A* mutation, and heterozygosity for the *RANTES-28G* mutation (see "Genetic Factors in HIV Pathogenesis," below). Since CCR5 is the major co-receptor for R5 or macrophage-tropic strains of HIV and since individuals who are homozygous for the *CCR5-Δ32* deletion are, with rare exceptions, protected against HIV infection, the potential mechanism for slow progression in heterozygotes is clear. In addition, certain single nucleotide polymorphisms in the *CCR5* promoter have been shown to be associated with slower progression of disease. The reason for the slowing of progression of HIV disease in individuals who are heterozygous for the *CCR2-64I* mutation is less clear; however, it has been demonstrated that CXCR4 can dimerize with the CCR2-64I mutant but not with wild-type CCR2. This dimerization may reduce the amount of CXCR4 on the cell surface and as a result inhibit infection with X4 viruses. Homozygosity for the *SDF1-3′* A mutation may upregulate the *SDF1* gene enabling SDF-1, which is the natural ligand for CXCR4, to compete more effectively with X4 virus for the CXCR4 co-receptor. The *RANTES-28G* mutation increases RANTES (CCL5) expression, which is the natural ligand for CCR5 and may thus inhibit infection with R5 viruses. The gene *CCL3L1* codes for MIP1αP and has an influence on both susceptibility to infection and disease progression based upon the gene copy number in the individual. Finally, maximal HLA heterozygosity of class I loci (A, B, and C) has been shown to be associated with delayed progression of HIV disease. Al-though most long-term nonprogressors have robust HIV-specific immune responses as well as competent CD8+ T cell suppressors of HIV replication, it is unclear whether these factors are directly responsible for the state of nonprogression. A substantial proportion of HIV-infected individuals manifest comparable immune responses early in the course of their disease and still experience disease progression. As noted above, long-term nonprogressors likely represent a heterogeneous group. It has recently been reported in some cohorts that individuals co-infected with HIV and *GB virus C* (GBV-C) have lower mortality than HIV-infected individuals without GBV-C infection. The precise mechanisms of this apparent beneficial effect are unclear at present.

LYMPHOID ORGANS AND HIV PATHOGENESIS

Regardless of the portal of entry of HIV, lymphoid tissues are the major anatomic sites for the establishment and propagation of HIV infection (see above). Despite the use of measurements of plasma viremia to determine the level of disease activity, virus replication occurs mainly in lymphoid tissue and not in blood; indeed, the level of plasma viremia directly reflects virus production in lymphoid tissue.

Some patients experience progressive generalized lymphadenopathy (see below) early in the course of the infection; others experience varying degrees of transient lymphadenopathy. Lymphadenopathy reflects the cellular activation and immune response to the virus in the lymphoid tissue, which is generally characterized by follicular or germinal center hyperplasia. Lymphoid tissue involvement is a common denominator of virtually all patients with HIV infection, even those without easily detectable lymphadenopathy.

Simultaneous examinations of lymph tissue and peripheral blood in patients and monkeys during various stages of HIV and SIV infection, respectively, have led to substantial insight into the pathogenesis of HIV disease. In most of the original human studies, peripheral lymph nodes have been used predominantly as the source of lymphoid tissue. More recent studies in monkeys and humans have focused on the GALT, where the earliest burst of virus replication occurs associated with marked depletion of CD4+ T cells (see below). In detailed studies in peripheral lymph node tissue, using a combination of polymerase chain reaction (PCR) techniques for HIV DNA and HIV RNA in tissue and HIV RNA in plasma, in situ hybridization for HIV RNA, and light and electron microscopy, the following picture has emerged. During acute HIV infection high levels of plasma viremia at first originating from virus replication in the GALT occurs with dissemination of virus to peripheral lymphoid tissue where extensive viral replication in individual cells is demonstrated. A profound degree of cellular activation occurs (see below) and is reflected in follicular or germinal center hyperplasia. At this time copious amounts of extracellular virions (both infectious and defective) are trapped on the processes of the follicular dendritic cells (FDCs) in the germinal centers of the lymph nodes. Virions that have bound complement components on their surfaces attach to the surface of FDCs via interactions with complement receptors and likely via Fc receptors that bind to antibodies that are attached to the virions. In situ hybridization reveals expression of virus in individual cells of the paracortical area and, to a lesser extent, the germinal center (Fig. 182-21). The persistence of trapped virus after the transition from acute to chronic infection likely reflects a steady state whereby trapped virus turns over and is replaced by fresh virions, which are continually produced to a greater or lesser degree in individual patients. The trapped virus, either as whole virion or shed envelope, serves as a continual activator of CD4+ T cells, thus driving further virus replication.

During early-stage HIV disease, the architecture of the germinal centers is generally preserved and may even be hyperplastic owing to in situ proliferation of cells (mostly B lymphocytes) and recruitment to the lymph nodes of a number of cell types (B cells, CD4+ and CD8+ T cells). Electron-microscopic studies have demonstrated a fine network of FDCs with many long, fingerlike processes that envelop virtually every lymphocyte in the germinal center. Extracellular virions can be seen attached to the processes, yet the FDCs appear to be relatively healthy. The trapping of antigen is a physiologically normal function

FIGURE 182-21 HIV in the lymph node of an HIV-infected individual. An individual cell infected with HIV shown expressing HIV RNA by in situ hybridization using a radiolabeled molecular probe. Original ×500. *(Adapted from G Pantaleo et al: Nature 362:355, 1993.)*

for the FDCs, which present antigen to B cells and contribute to the generation of B cell memory. However, in the case of HIV, the trapped virions serve as a persistent source of cellular activation, resulting in the secretion of proinflammatory cytokines such as interleukin (IL)-1β, tumor necrosis factor (TNF)-α, and IL-6, which can upregulate virus replication in infected cells (see below). Furthermore, although trapped virus is coated by neutralizing antibodies, it has been demonstrated that certain of these virions remain infectious for CD4+ T cells while attached to the processes of the FDCs. CD4+ T cells that migrate into the germinal center to provide help to B cells in the generation of an HIV-specific immune response are susceptible to infection by these trapped virions. Thus, in HIV infection, a normal physiologic function of the immune system, which contributes to the clearance of virus as well as to the generation of a specific immune response, can also have deleterious consequences.

As the disease progresses, the architecture of the germinal centers begins to show disruption, and the trapping efficiency of the lymphoid tissue diminishes. Electron microscopy reveals swollen organelles, and the FDCs begin to undergo cell death. The mechanisms of FDC death remain unclear; there is no indication by electron microscopy of copious virus replication or budding of virions off the cell in great quantities. This process of FDC death is accompanied by the deposition of collagen, leading to irreparable damage to the germinal centers. As the disease progresses to an advanced stage, there is complete disruption of the architecture of the germinal centers, accompanied by dissolution of the FDC network and massive dropout of FDCs. At this point, the lymph nodes are "burnt out." This destruction of lymphoid tissue compounds the immunodeficiency of HIV disease and contributes both to the inability to control HIV replication (leading usually to high levels of plasma viremia in the untreated or inadequately treated patient) and to the inability to mount adequate immune responses against opportunistic pathogens. The events from primary infection to the ultimate destruction of the immune system are illustrated in **Fig. 182-22**. Recently, nonhuman primate studies and some human studies have examined GALT at various stages of HIV disease. It is noteworthy that prior to infection approximately half of all CD4+ T cells in the jejunum express the HIV cellular co-receptor CCR5, rendering them highly susceptible to infection. Within the GALT, the basal level of activation combined with virus-mediated cellular activation results in the infection and elimination of an estimated 50–90% of CD4+ T cells in the gut. The extent of this early damage to GALT, which comprises a major component of lymphoid tissue in the body, plays a role in determining the potential for immunologic recovery of the memory cell subset.

CELLULAR ACTIVATION AND HIV PATHOGENESIS

Activation of the immune system is an essential component of an appropriate immune response to a foreign antigen. The immune system is normally in a state of homeostasis, awaiting perturbation by foreign antigenic stimuli. Once the immune response deals with and clears the antigen, the system returns to relative quiescence (Chap. 308). In HIV infection, however, the immune system is chronically activated, providing the cell substrates necessary for persistent virus replication throughout the course of HIV disease, particularly in the untreated patient (see above) and to variable degrees even in certain patients receiving ARV

FIGURE 182-22 Events that transpire from primary HIV infection through the establishment of chronic persistent infection to the ultimate destruction of the immune system. See text for details. CTLs, cytolytic T lymphocytes; GALT, gut-associated lymphoid tissue.

therapy whose level of plasma viremia is suppressed to below the level of detection by standard assays (see below). Aberrant immune activation is the hallmark of HIV infection and is a critical component of the pathogenesis of HIV disease. This activated state is reflected by hyperactivation of B cells leading to hypergammaglobulinemia; spontaneous lymphocyte proliferation; activation of monocytes; expression of activation markers on CD4+ and CD8+ T cells; increased activation-associated cellular apoptosis; lymph node hyperplasia, particularly early in the course of disease (see above); increased secretion of proinflammatory cytokines (see below); elevated levels of neopterin, β_2-microglobulin, acid-labile interferon, and soluble IL-2 receptors; and autoimmune phenomena (see below). Even in the absence of direct infection of a target cell, HIV envelope proteins can interact with cellular receptors (CD4 molecules and chemokine receptors) to deliver potent activation signals resulting in calcium flux, the phosphorylation of certain proteins involved in signal transduction, co-localization of cytoplasmic proteins including those involved in cell trafficking, immune dysfunction, and, under certain circumstances, apoptosis (see below). The secretion of certain proinflammatory and immunoregulatory cytokines is both a consequence of the aberrant immune activation associated with HIV infection and a mechanism of propagation of the process of aberrant cellular activation (see below).

In addition to endogenous factors such as cytokines, a number of exogenous factors such as other microbes that are associated with heightened cellular activation can enhance HIV replication and thus may have important effects on HIV pathogenesis. Co-infection in vivo or in vitro with a range of viruses, such as HSV types 1 and 2, cytomegalovirus (CMV), human herpesvirus (HHV) 6, Epstein-Barr virus (EBV), HBV, adenovirus, and HTLV-I have been shown to upregulate HIV expression. Other microbes, such as *Mycoplasma*, have been reported to contribute to the induction of HIV expression. In addition, infestation with nematodes has been shown to be associated with a heightened state of immune activation that facilitates HIV replication; in certain studies deworming of the infected host has resulted in a decrease in plasma viremia. Two diseases of extraordinary global health significance, malaria and tuberculosis (TB), have been shown to increase HIV viral load in dually infected individuals. Globally, *Mycobacterium tuberculosis* is probably the most common opportunistic infection in HIV-infected individuals (see below and Chap. 158). In addition to the fact that HIV-infected individuals are more likely to develop active TB after exposure, it has been demonstrated that active TB can accelerate the course of HIV infection. It has also been shown that levels of plasma viremia are greatly elevated in HIV-infected individuals with active TB, compared to pre-TB levels and levels of viremia after successful treatment of the active TB. In vitro studies demonstrated that virus replication was markedly enhanced in lymphocytes of HIV-infected individuals who were skin test–positive for purified protein derivative (PPD) when PPD antigen was added to culture, resulting in cellular activation. Confirmatory evidence that antigen-induced activation was a major contributor to the accelerated viremia in HIV-infected individuals with active TB was provided by studies in which HIV-infected individuals were immunized with common recall antigens such as tetanus toxoid, influenza, or pneumococcal polysaccharide. Under these circumstances, a transient elevation of plasma viremia accompanied the cellular activation induced by the immunization. A greater degree of induction of virus was seen in those individuals with early-stage as opposed to advanced stage HIV disease (i.e., in those with more competent immune systems), and the degree of virus induction correlated with the level of immune system activation. The situation is similar in the interaction between HIV and malaria parasites (Chap. 203). Acute infection of HIV-infected individuals with *Plasmodium falciparum* increases HIV viral load and the increased viral load is reversed by effective malaria treatment

Persistent immune activation may have several deleterious consequences. From a virologic standpoint, although quiescent CD4+ T cells can be infected with HIV, reverse transcription, integration, and virus spread are much more efficient in activated cells. Furthermore, cellular activation induces expression of virus in cells latently infected with HIV (see above). From an immunologic standpoint, chronic exposure of the immune system to a particular antigen over an extended period may ultimately lead to an inability to sustain an adequate immune response to the antigen in question. In many chronic viral infections, including HIV infection, persistent viremia is associated with "functional exhaustion" and apoptosis of virus-specific T cells. It has been demonstrated that this phenomenon may be mediated, at least in part, by the engagement of PD-1, which is highly expressed on the majority of HIV-specific T cells, with its ligands (PD-L1 and PD-L2) on antigen-presenting cells and epithelial cells, resulting in either T cell death or anergy (see above). Furthermore, the ability of the immune system to respond to a broad spectrum of antigens may be compromised if immunocompetent cells are maintained in a state of chronic activation. In addition, activation of the immune system may favor the elimination of cells via programmed cell death (apoptosis) (see below) as well as the secretion of certain cytokines that can induce HIV expression (see below).

The deleterious effects of chronic immune activation on the progression of HIV disease are well established. As in most conditions of persistent antigen exposure, the host must maintain sufficient activation of antigen (HIV)-specific responses but must also prevent excessive activation and potential immune-mediated damage to tissues. Certain studies suggest that normal immunosuppressive mechanisms that act to keep hyperimmune activation in check, particularly CD4+, FoxP3+, CD25+ regulatory T cells (T-regs), may be dysfunctional or depleted in the context of advanced HIV disease.

Apoptosis *Apoptosis* is a form of programmed cell death that is a normal mechanism for the elimination of effete cells in organogenesis as well as in the cellular proliferation that occurs during a normal immune response (Chap. 308). Apoptosis is strictly dependent on cellular activation, and the aberrant cellular activation associated with HIV disease (see above) is correlated with a heightened state of apoptosis. It has been hypothesized that, in HIV infection, sequential activation signals delivered to CD4+ T cells induce apoptosis. Cross-linking of the CD4 molecule by gp120 or gp120/anti-gp120 complexes delivers the first of two signals required for apoptosis. The second signal supposedly leading to cell death is delivered via the T cell receptor by antigen. According to this hypothesis, direct infection of CD4+ T cells is not required for apoptosis to occur, although it has been demonstrated that alterations in tyrosine kinase activity of HIV-infected cells may induce the cell to undergo apoptosis. HIV can trigger both Fas-dependent and Fas-independent pathways of apoptosis. Mechanisms involved in this process include upregulation of Fas and Fas ligand, upregulation of caspase-1 and caspase-6, downregulation of the antiapoptotic Bcl-2 protein, and activation of cyclin-dependent kinases. Certain viral gene products have been associated with enhanced susceptibility to apoptosis including Env, Tat, and Vpr. In contrast, Nef has been shown to possess antiapoptotic properties. A number of studies, including those examining lymphoid tissue, have demonstrated that the rate of apoptosis is elevated in HIV infection and that apoptosis is seen in "bystander" cells such as CD8+ T cells and B cells as well as in CD4+ T cells. The intensity of apoptosis correlates with the general state of activation of the immune system and not with the stage of disease or with viral burden. It is likely that apoptosis of immunocompetent cells contributes to the immune abnormalities in HIV disease; however, this is probably a nonspecific mechanism that merely reflects the aberrant state of immune activation.

Autoimmune Phenomena The autoimmune phenomena that are common in HIV-infected individuals reflect, at least in part, chronic immune system activation as well as molecular mimicry by viral components. Although these phenomena usually occur in the absence of autoimmune disease, a wide spectrum of clinical manifestations that may be associated with autoimmunity have been described (see below). Autoimmune phenomena include antibodies to lymphocytes and, less commonly, to platelets and neutrophils. Antiplatelet antibodies have some clinical relevance, in that they may contribute to the thrombocytopenia of HIV disease (see below). Antibodies to nuclear and cytoplasmic components of cells have been reported, as have antibodies to cardiolipin; CD4 molecules; CD43 molecules, C1q-A; variable regions of the T cell receptor α, β, and γ chains; Fas; denatured collagen; and IL-2. In addition, autoantibodies to a range of serum proteins, including albumin, immunoglobulin, and thyroglobulin, have been reported. There is antigenic cross-reactivity between HIV viral proteins (gp120 and gp41) and MHC class II determinants, and anti-MHC class II antibodies have been reported in HIV infection. These antibodies could potentially lead to the elimination of MHC class II–bearing cells via antibody-dependent cellular cytotoxicity (ADCC), although this has not been clearly demonstrated to occur (Chap. 308). In addition, regions of homology exist between HIV envelope glycoproteins and IL-2 as well as MHC class I molecules. With the widespread use of effective antiretroviral therapy, an *immune reconstitution inflammatory syndrome* (IRIS) has become increasingly more common. IRIS is an autoimmune-like phenomenon characterized by a paradoxical deterioration of clinical condition, which is usually compartmentalized to a particular organ system, in individuals in whom ARV therapy has recently been initiated. It is associated with a decrease in viral load and at least partial recovery of immune competence, usually associated with increases in CD4+ T cell counts. The immunopathogenesis is felt to be related to an increase in immune response against the presence of residual antigens that are usually microbial and is commonly seen with underlying *Mycobacterium tuberculosis* and cryptococcosis. This syndrome is discussed in more detail below.

THE CYTOKINE NETWORK IN HIV PATHOGENESIS

The immune system is homeostatically regulated by a complex network of immunoregulatory cytokines, which are pleiotropic and redundant and operate in an autocrine and paracrine manner. They are expressed continuously, even during periods of apparent quiescence of the immune system. On perturbation of the immune system by antigenic challenge, the expression of cytokines increases to varying degrees (Chap. 308). Cytokines that are important components of this immunoregulatory network have been demonstrated to play a major role in the regulation of HIV expression in vitro. Potent modulation of HIV expression has been demonstrated either by manipulating endogenous cytokines or by adding exogenous cytokines to culture. Cytokines that induce HIV expression in one or more of these systems include IL-1, IL-2, IL-3, IL-6, IL-12, TNF-α, TNF-β, macrophage colony-stimulating factor (M-CSF), and granulocyte-macrophage colony-stimulating factor (GM-CSF). Among these cytokines, the most consistent and potent inducers of HIV expression are the *proinflammatory cytokines* TNF-α, IL-1β, and IL-6. Interferon (IFN)-α and -β suppress HIV replication, whereas transforming growth factor (TGF) β, IL-4, IL-10, and IFN-γ can either induce or suppress HIV expression, depending on the system involved. The *CC-chemokines* RANTES (CCL5), macrophage inflammatory protein (MIP)-1α (CCL3), and MIP-1β (CCL4) (Chap. 308) inhibit infection by and spread of R5 HIV-1 strains, while *stromal cell–derived factor* (SDF) 1 inhibits infection by and spread of X4 strains (see below). The alpha defensin family of cytokines has been shown to inhibit both R5 and X4 viruses, and other soluble factors that have not yet been fully characterized have also been shown to suppress HIV replication.

The molecular mechanisms of HIV regulation are best understood for TNF-α, which activates NF-κB proteins that function as transcriptional activators of HIV expression. The HIV-inducing effect of IL-1β is thought to occur at the level of viral transcription in an NF-κB-independent manner. IL-6, GM-CSF, and IFN-γ regulate HIV expression mainly by posttranscriptional mechanisms. Elevated levels of TNF-α and IL-6 have been demonstrated in plasma and cerebrospinal fluid (CSF), and increased expression of TNF-α, IL-1β, IFN-γ, and IL-6 has been demonstrated in the lymph nodes of HIV-infected individuals. The mechanisms whereby the CC-chemokines RANTES (CCL5), MIP-1α (CCL3), and MIP-1β (CCL4) inhibit infection of R5 strains of HIV or SDF-1 blocks X4 strains of HIV involve blocking of the binding of the virus to its co-receptors, the CC-chemokine receptor CCR5 and the CXC-chemokine receptor CXCR4, respectively (see above and below). However, several CC-chemokines, including but not limited

to CCL3, -4, and -5, induce intracellular signals that actually enhance infection by X4 strains of virus at both the entry and postentry levels. The mechanisms whereby other less well characterized factors (see above) inhibit HIV replication are not completely understood.

Blocking of endogenous HIV-inducing cytokines or addition of inhibitors of HIV-suppressor cytokines in cultures of peripheral blood and lymph node mononuclear cells from HIV-infected individuals has demonstrated that HIV replication is controlled tightly by endogenous cytokines that act synergistically and in an autocrine and paracrine manner, similar to their physiologic function in the regulation of the immune system. Indeed, the net level of virus replication in an HIV-infected individual reflects at least in part a balance between inductive and suppressive host factors, mediated mainly by cytokines.

LYMPHOCYTE TURNOVER IN HIV INFECTION

The immune systems of patients with HIV infection are characterized by a profound increase in lymphocyte turnover that is immediately reduced with effective ARV therapy. Studies utilizing in vivo or in vitro labelling of lymphocytes in the S-phase of the cell cycle have demonstrated a tight correlation between the degree of lymphocyte turnover and plasma levels of HIV RNA. This increase in turnover is seen in CD4+ and CD8+ T lymphocytes as well as B lymphocytes and can be observed in peripheral blood and lymphoid tissue. Mathematical models derived from these data suggest that one can view the lymphoid pool as consisting of dynamically distinct subpopulations of cells that are differentially affected by HIV infection. A major consequence of HIV infection appears to be a shift in cells from a more quiescent pool to a pool with a higher turnover rate. It is likely that a consequence of a higher rate of turnover is a higher rate of cell death. The role of the thymus in adult human T cell homeostasis and HIV pathogenesis is an area of controversy. While some data point to an important role for the thymus in maintaining T cell numbers and suggest that impairment of thymic function may be responsible for the declines in CD4+ T cells seen in the setting of HIV infection, other studies have concluded that the thymus plays a minor role in HIV pathogenesis. Among the data supporting an important role for the thymus are those that demonstrate an increase in the levels of T cell receptor excision circles (TRECs) following initiation of ARV therapy. TRECs are a byproduct of T cell development and represent episomal fragments of DNA that are excised during T cell receptor gene rearrangement (Chap. 308). Levels of TRECs will be the net result of changes in thymic output together with changes in T cell turnover. An increase in thymic output and/or a decrease in T cell turnover will lead to an increase in levels of TRECs. While it is clear that levels of TRECs increase following initiation of ARV therapy, it is not clear whether this is a consequence of increased thymic output or decreased T cell turnover.

THE ROLE OF CO-RECEPTORS IN HIV PATHOGENESIS

As mentioned above, HIV-1 utilizes two major co-receptors along with CD4 to bind to, fuse with, and enter target cells; these co-receptors are CCR5 and CXCR4, which are also receptors for certain endogenous chemokines. Strains of HIV that utilize CCR5 as a co-receptor are referred to as *R5 viruses*. Strains of HIV that utilize CXCR4 are referred to as *X4 viruses*. Many virus strains are *dual tropic* in that they utilize both CCR5 and CXCR4; these are referred to as *R5X4 viruses*.

The natural chemokine ligands for the major HIV co-receptors can readily block entry of HIV. For example, the CC-chemokines RANTES (CCL5), MIP-1α (CCL3), and MIP-1β (CCL4), which are the natural ligands for CCR5, block entry of R5 viruses, whereas SDF-1, the natural ligand for CXCR4, blocks entry of X4 viruses. The mechanism of inhibition of viral entry is a steric inhibition of binding that is not dependent on signal transduction (**Fig. 182-23**).

The transmitting virus is almost invariably an R5 virus that predominates during the early stages of HIV disease. In ~40% of HIV-infected individuals, there is a transition to a predominantly X4 virus that is associated with a relatively rapid progression of disease. However, at least 60% of infected individuals progress in their disease while maintaining predominance of an R5 virus. It should be pointed out

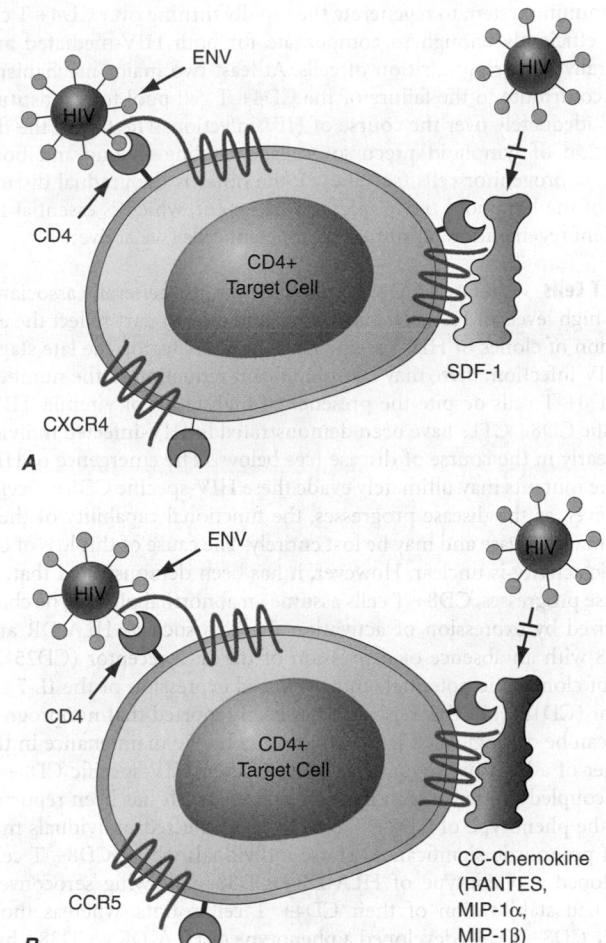

FIGURE 182-23 Model for the role of co-receptors CXCR4 and CCR5 in the efficient binding and entry of X4 (*A*) and R5 (*B*) strains of HIV-1, respectively, into CD4+ target cells. Blocking of this initial event in the virus life cycle can be accomplished by inhibition of binding to the co-receptor by the normal ligand for the receptor in question. The ligand for CXCR4 is stromal cell–derived factor (SDF-1); the ligands for CCR5 are RANTES, MIP-1α, and MIP-1β.

that clade C viruses, unlike other subgroups, almost never switch from CCR5 tropism to CXCR4 tropism; the reason for this difference is unclear. Other chemokine receptor family members may function as co-receptors for HIV and SIV entry, but to a much lesser extent than do CCR5 and CXCR4; these include CCR3, BOB/GPR15, CXCR6 (Bonzo/STRL33/TYMSTR), CCR2, CCR8, CX3CR1(V28), and GPR1.

The basis for the tropism of different envelope glycoproteins for either CCR5 or CXCR4 relates to the ability of the HIV envelope, including the third variable region (V3 loop) of gp120, to interact with these co-receptors. In this regard, binding of gp120 to CD4 induces a conformational change in gp120 that increases its affinity for CCR5 (see above). Finally, R5 viruses are more efficient in infecting monocytes/macrophages and microglial cells of the brain (see "Neuropathogenesis," below).

CELLULAR TARGETS OF HIV

Although the CD4+ T lymphocytes and CD4+ cells of monocyte lineage are the principal targets of HIV, virtually any cell that expresses the CD4 molecule together with co-receptor molecules (see above and below) can potentially be infected with HIV. Circulating dendritic cells have been reported to express low levels of CD4 and, depending on their stage of maturation, these cells can be infected with HIV (see below). Epidermal Langerhans cells express CD4 and have been infected by HIV in vivo. In vitro, HIV has been reported also to infect a wide range of cells and cell lines that express low levels of CD4, no detect-

able CD4, or only CD4 mRNA; among these are FDCs, megakaryocytes, eosinophils, astrocytes, oligodendrocytes, microglial cells, CD8+ T cells, B cells, and NK cells as well as a variety of organ-specific cells. Since the only cells that have been shown unequivocally to be infected with HIV and to support replication of the virus are CD4+ T lymphocytes and cells of monocyte/macrophage lineage, the relevance of the in vitro infection of these other cell types is questionable.

Of potentially important clinical relevance is the demonstration that thymic precursor cells, which were assumed to be negative for CD3, CD4, and CD8 molecules, actually do express low levels of CD4 and can be infected with HIV in vitro. In addition, human thymic epithelial cells transplanted into an immunodeficient mouse can be infected with HIV by direct inoculation of virus into the thymus. Since these cells may play a role in the normal regeneration of CD4+ T cells, it is possible that their infection and depletion contribute, at least in part, to the impaired ability of the CD4+ T cell pool to completely reconstitute itself in certain infected individuals in whom ARV therapy has suppressed viral replication to <50 copies of HIV RNA per milliliter (see below). In addition, CD34+ monocyte precursor cells have been shown to be infected in vivo in patients with advanced HIV disease. It is likely that these cells express low levels of CD4, and therefore it is not essential to invoke CD4-independent mechanisms to explain the infection.

ABNORMALITIES OF MONONUCLEAR CELLS

CD4+ T Cells The range of T cell abnormalities in advanced HIV infection is broad. The defects are both quantitative and qualitative and affect virtually every limb of the immune system (see below), indicating the critical dependence of the integrity of the immune system on the inducer/helper function of CD4+ T cells. In advanced HIV disease, most of the observed immune defects can ultimately be explained by the quantitative depletion of CD4+ T cells. However, T cell dysfunction (see below) can be demonstrated in patients early in the course of infection, even when the CD4+ T cell count is in the low-normal range. The degree and spectrum of dysfunctions increase as the disease progresses. One of the first abnormalities to be detected is a defect in response to remote recall antigens, such as tetanus toxoid and influenza, at a time when mononuclear cells can still respond normally to mitogenic stimulation. Indeed, defects of central memory cells are a critical component of HIV immunopathogenesis. The progressive loss of antigen-specific CD4+ T cells has important implications for the control of HIV infection. In this regard, there is a correlation between the maintenance of HIV-specific CD4+ T cell proliferative responses and improved control of infection. Essentially every T cell function has been reported to be abnormal at some stage of HIV infection. These abnormalities include defective T cell cloning and colony-forming efficiencies, impaired expression of IL-2 receptors, defective IL-2 production, reduced expression of the IL-7 receptor (CD127), and decreased IFN-γ production in response to antigens. The proportion of CD4+ T cells that express CD28, which is a major co-stimulatory molecule necessary for the normal activation of T cells, is reduced during HIV infection. Cells lacking expression of CD28 do not respond normally to activation signals and may express markers of terminal activation including HLA-DR, CD38, and CD45RO. CD4+ T cells from HIV-infected individuals express abnormally low levels of CD40 ligand, which may contribute to the dysregulation of B cell function observed in HIV disease. As mentioned above (see "Cellular Activation and HIV Pathogenesis"), a subset of CD4+ T cells referred to as *T regulatory cells*, or T-regs, may be involved in dampening aberrant immune activation that propagates HIV replication. The presence of these T-reg cells correlates with lower viral loads and higher CD4+/CD8+ T cell ratios. A loss of this T-reg capability with advanced disease may be detrimental to the control of virus replication.

It is difficult to explain completely the profound immunodeficiency noted in HIV-infected individuals solely on the basis of direct infection and quantitative depletion of CD4+ T cells. This is particularly apparent during the early stages of HIV disease, when CD4+ T cell numbers may be only marginally decreased. In this regard, it is likely that CD4+ T cell dysfunction results from a combination of depletion

TABLE 182-3	MECHANISMS OF CD4+ T CELL DYSFUNCTION AND DEPLETION

Direct Mechanisms	Indirect Mechanisms
Loss of plasma membrane integrity due to viral budding	Aberrant intracellular signaling events
Accumulation of unintegrated viral DNA	Autoimmunity
Interference with cellular RNA processing	Innocent bystander killing of viral antigen–coated cells
Intracellular gp120-CD4 autofusion events	Apoptosis
	Inhibition of lymphopoiesis
	Activation-induced cell death
Syncytia formation	Elimination of HIV-infected cells by virus-specific immune responses

of cells due to direct infection of the cell and a number of virus-related but indirect effects on the cell (Table 182-3). Indeed, it has been demonstrated that patients with high levels of plasma viremia have a variety of subtle abnormalities of CD4+ T cell function, particularly involving aberrancies in signal transduction pathways. These abnormalities could be due either to aberrant activation induced by the cascade of cytokines that are expressed in viremic patients or by the direct effect of virus on the cell. In this regard, certain of these abnormalities can be reproduced by exposing CD4+ T cells of normal individuals to oligomeric HIV envelope proteins in vitro (see below).

Single-cell killing and the formation of syncytia between infected and uninfected cells have been demonstrated clearly in vitro, although there is little evidence that this process occurs in vivo. Cytopathicity in an infected cell in vitro may result from a number of mechanisms, including copious budding of virions from the cell surface with resulting disruption of the integrity of the cell membrane; interference with cellular RNA processing or the accumulation of high levels of heterodisperse RNA molecules; disruption of cellular protein synthesis owing to high levels of viral RNA; accumulation of high levels of unintegrated viral DNA in the cell cytoplasm; induction of aberrant patterns of protein tyrosine phosphorylation; and the interaction between HIV gp120 and CD4 intracellularly. Strain differences in single-cell killing are determined largely by gp120 sequences, which supports the importance of the viral envelope in this process. Humoral and cellular immune responses to HIV may contribute to protective immunity by eliminating virus and virus-infected cells (see below). However, since the main targets of HIV infection are immunocompetent cells, these responses may contribute to immune cell depletion and immunologic dysfunction by eliminating both infected cells and "innocent bystander" cells. Soluble viral proteins, particularly gp120, can bind with high affinity to the CD4 molecules on uninfected T cells and monocytes; in addition, virus and/or viral proteins can bind to dendritic cells or FDCs. HIV-specific antibody can recognize these bound molecules and potentially collaborate in the elimination of the cells by ADCC.

Nonpolymorphic determinants of MHC class I products share a degree of homology with gp120 and gp41 proteins of HIV. Such similarities may lead to the generation of autoantibodies to self-MHC determinants. Anti-HLA-DR antibodies have been demonstrated in the sera of HIV-infected individuals (see "Autoimmune Phenomena," above). These antibodies could contribute to the elimination of HLA-DR–expressing cells by ADCC; in addition, it has been suggested that these antibodies may inhibit certain T cell functions that involve HLA-DR molecules.

HIV envelope glycoproteins gp120 and gp160 manifest high-affinity binding to CD4 as well as to various chemokine receptors (see above). Intracellular signals transduced by gp120 through both CD4 and CCR5/CXCR4 have been associated with a number of immunopathogenic processes including anergy, apoptosis, and abnormalities of cell trafficking. The molecular mechanisms responsible for these abnormalities include dysregulation of the T cell receptor–phosphoinositide pathway, p56lck activation, phosphorylation of focal adhesion kinase, activation of the MAP kinase and ras signaling pathways, and downregulation of the co-stimulatory molecules CD40 ligand and CD80.

Finally, the inexorable decline in CD4+ T cell counts that occurs in most HIV-infected individuals may result in part from the inability of the immune system to regenerate the rapidly turning over CD4+ T cell pool efficiently enough to compensate for both HIV-mediated and naturally occurring attrition of cells. At least two major mechanisms may contribute to the failure of the CD4+ T cell pool to reconstitute itself adequately over the course of HIV infection. The first is the destruction of lymphoid precursor cells, including thymic and bone marrow progenitor cells (see above); the other is the gradual disruption of the lymphoid tissue microenvironment, which is essential for efficient regeneration of immunocompetent cells (see above).

CD8+ T Cells A relative CD8+ T lymphocytosis is generally associated with high levels of HIV plasma viremia and may in part reflect the expansion of clones of HIV-specific CD8+ CTLs. During the late stages of HIV infection, there may be a significant reduction in the numbers of CD8+ T cells despite the presence of high levels of viremia. HIV-specific CD8+ CTLs have been demonstrated in HIV-infected individuals early in the course of disease (see below). The emergence of HIV escape mutants may ultimately evade these HIV-specific CD8+ T cells. However, as the disease progresses, the functional capability of these cells may decrease and may be lost entirely. The cause of this loss of cytolytic activity is unclear. However, it has been demonstrated that, as disease progresses, CD8+ T cells assume an abnormal phenotype characterized by expression of activation markers such as HLA-DR and CD38 with an absence of expression of the IL-2 receptor (CD25), a loss of clonogenic potential, and a reduced expression of the IL-7 receptor (CD127). In this regard, it has been reported that nonprogressors can be distinguished from progressors by the maintenance in the former of a high proliferative capacity of their HIV-specific CD8+ T cells coupled to increases in perforin expression. It has been reported that the phenotype of CD8+ T cells in HIV-infected individuals may be of prognostic significance. Those individuals whose CD8+ T cells developed a phenotype of HLA-DR+/CD38– following seroconversion had stabilization of their CD4+ T cell counts, whereas those whose CD8+ T cells developed a phenotype of HLA-DR+/CD38+ had a more aggressive course and a poorer prognosis. In addition to the defects in HIV-specific CTLs, functional defects in other MHC-restricted CTLs, such as those directed against influenza and CMV, have been demonstrated. CD8+ T cells secrete a variety of soluble factors that inhibit HIV replication including the CC-chemokines RANTES (CCL5), MIP-1α (CCL3), and MIP-1β (CCL4) as well as one or more as yet poorly identified factors (see above). The presence of high levels of HIV viremia in vivo as well as exposure of CD8+ T cells in vitro to HIV envelope, both of which are associated with aberrant immune activation, has been shown to be associated with a variety of cellular functional abnormalities. Furthermore, since the integrity of CD8+ T cell function depends in part on adequate inductive signals from CD4+ T cells, the defect in CD8+ CTLs is likely compounded by the quantitative loss and qualitative dysfunction of CD4+ T cells. Finally, as mentioned above, certain cell surface negative regulatory molecules such as CTLA-4 and PD-1 are upregulated on activated T cells, and engagement of these molecules with their ligands may play a role in the exhaustion and death of CD8+, HIV-specific T cells.

B Cells The predominant defect in B cells from HIV-infected individuals is one of aberrant cellular activation, which is reflected by spontaneous proliferation and immunoglobulin secretion and by increased spontaneous secretion of TNF-α and IL-6. In addition, B cells from HIV viremic patients manifest a decreased capacity to mount a proliferative response to ligation of the B cell antigen receptor (surface IgM) at the same time as they are capable of robust differentiation in response to a variety of stimuli. B cells from HIV-infected individuals manifest enhanced spontaneous in vitro transformation with EBV, a process that is likely due to defective T cell immune surveillance. The in vivo counterpart of this phenomenon is an increase in the incidence of EBV-related B cell lymphomas in HIV-infected individuals. Untransformed B cells cannot be infected with HIV. However, HIV or its products can activate B cells directly; portions of the HIV gp41 envelope protein have been reported to induce polyclonal B cell activation. In addition, it has been reported that products of the VH₃ genes on the surface of B cells can serve as a receptor for HIV. B cells from patients with high levels of viremia bind virions to their surface via the CD21 complement receptor. It is likely that in vivo activation of B cells by replication-competent or -defective virus as well as viral products during the viremic state account at least in part for the spontaneous activation of these cells noted ex vivo. B cell subpopulations from HIV-infected individuals undergo a number of changes over the course of HIV disease, including the attrition of memory B cells; the appearance of mature, activated B cells defined by reduced expression of CD21, increased expression of activation markers, increased secretion of immunoglobulins, and increased susceptibility to Fas-mediated apoptosis; and the appearance of immature B cells associated with CD4+ T cell lymphopenia. Cognate B cell–CD4+ T cell interactions are abnormal in viremic HIV-infected individuals in that B cells respond poorly to CD4+ T cell help and CD4+ T cells receive inadequate co-stimulatory signals from activated B cells. In vivo, the aberrant activated state of B cells manifests itself by hypergammaglobulinemia and by the presence of circulating immune complexes and autoantibodies (see above). HIV-infected individuals respond poorly to primary and secondary immunizations with protein and polysaccharide antigens. Using immunization with influenza vaccine it has been demonstrated that there is a memory B cell defect in HIV-infected individuals, particularly those with high levels of HIV viremia. Taken together, these B cell defects are likely responsible in part for the increase in certain bacterial infections seen in advanced HIV disease in adults, as well as for the important role of bacterial infections in the morbidity and mortality of HIV-infected children, who cannot mount an adequate humoral response to common bacterial pathogens. The absolute number of circulating B cells may be depressed in HIV infection; this phenomenon likely reflects increased activation-induced apoptosis as well as a redistribution of cells out of the circulation and into the lymphoid tissue—phenomena that are associated with ongoing viral replication.

Monocytes/Macrophages   Circulating monocytes are generally normal in number in HIV-infected individuals. Monocytes express the CD4 molecule and several co-receptors for HIV on their surface, including CCR5, CXCR4, and CCR3, and thus are targets of HIV infection. The degree of cytopathicity of HIV for cells of the monocyte lineage is low, and HIV can replicate extensively in cells of the monocyte lineage with relatively little cytopathic effect. Hence, monocyte-lineage cells may play a role in the dissemination of HIV in the body and can serve as reservoirs of HIV infection, thus representing an obstacle to the eradication of HIV by ARV drugs. In vivo infection of circulating monocytes is difficult to demonstrate; however, infection of tissue macrophages and macrophage-lineage cells in the brain (infiltrating macrophages or resident microglial cells) and lung (pulmonary alveolar macrophages) can be demonstrated easily. Tissue macrophages are an important source of HIV during the inflammatory response associated with opportunistic infections. Infection of monocyte precursors in the bone marrow may directly or indirectly be responsible for certain of the hematologic abnormalities in HIV-infected individuals. A number of abnormalities of circulating monocytes have been reported in HIV-infected individuals, including decreased secretion of IL-1 and IL-12; increased secretion of IL-10; defects in antigen presentation and induction of T cell responses due to decreased MHC class II expression; and abnormalities of Fc receptor function, C3 receptor–mediated clearance, oxidative burst responses, and certain cytotoxic functions such as ADCC, possibly related to low levels of expression of Fc and complement receptors. Exposure of monocytes to viral proteins such as gp120 and Tat, as well as to certain cytokines, can cause abnormal activation, and this may play a role in cellular dysfunction (see above).

Dendritic and Langerhans Cells   Dendritic cells may play an important role in the initiation of HIV infection by virtue of the ability of HIV to bind to cell surface C-type lectin receptors, particularly DC-SIGN (see above). This allows efficient presentation of virus to CD4+ T cell tar-

gets that become infected; complexes of infected CD4+ T cells and dendritic cells provide an optimal microenvironment for virus replication. There has been considerable disagreement regarding the HIV infectibility and hence the depletion as well as the dysfunction of dendritic cells themselves. Depending on their state of maturation, dendritic cells express varying levels of CD4 as well as several chemokine receptors. In this regard, it appears that the ability of a dendritic cell to become infected depends in part on its state of maturation. Mature dendritic cells have been demonstrated to be infectable by both R5 and X4 isolates of HIV-1. Immature tissue dendritic cells have been less well studied in their native state. Even in those dendritic cells in which infection occurs, the efficiency of infection and level of productivity of infection is quite low compared to CD4+ T cells.

Natural Killer Cells   The role of NK cells is to provide immunosurveillance against virus-infected cells, certain tumor cells, and allogeneic cells (Chap. 308). Functional abnormalities in NK cells have been observed throughout the course of HIV disease, and the severity of these abnormalities increases as disease progresses. HIV infection of target cells downregulates HLA-A and -B, but not HLA-C and -D molecules; this may explain in part the relative inability of NK cells to kill HIV-infected target cells. Most studies report that NK cells are normal in number; however, patients with high levels of virus replication manifest an abnormal representation of a functionally defective CD56–/CD16+ NK cell subset. This abnormal subset of NK cells manifests an increased expression of inhibitory NK cell receptors (iNKRs) and a substantial decrease in expression of natural cytotoxicity receptors (NCRs) and shows a markedly impaired lytic activity. The overrepresentation of this abnormal subset of NK cells may explain in part the observed defects in NK cell function in HIV-infected individuals. NK cells also serve as important sources of HIV-inhibitory CC-chemokines. NK cells isolated from HIV-infected individuals constitutively produce high levels of MIP-1α (CCL3), MIP-1β (CCL4), and RANTES (CCL5). In addition, high levels of these chemokines are seen when NK cells are stimulated with IL-2 or IL-15 or when CD16 is cross-linked or during the process of lytic killing of target cells. HIV-infected patients with high levels of plasma viremia manifest a decreased ability, compared to HIV-infected individuals who are aviremic, of their NK cells to block HIV replication in vitro in assays of both cell contact and supernatant-mediated suppression of virus. Finally, NK cell–dendritic cell interactions are important for normal immune function. NK cells and dendritic cells reciprocally modulate each other's activation and maturation. These interactions are markedly impaired in HIV-infected individuals with high levels of plasma viremia.

GENETIC FACTORS IN HIV PATHOGENESIS

MHC Genes   Several reports have described MHC alleles and other host factors that may influence the pathogenesis and course of HIV disease. These include associations with transmission and with the type of clinical course, such as slow or rapid rates of progression to AIDS (Table 182-4). For example, researchers recently employed a whole-genome association strategy to identify two independently acting groups of polymorphisms associated with HLA loci B and C, which explained 15% of the variation in viral load among individuals during the asymptomatic period of infection. A number of mechanisms have been proposed whereby MHC-encoded molecules might predispose an individual either to rapid progression or to nonprogression to AIDS. These proposed mechanisms include the ability to present certain immunodominant HIV T helper or CTL epitopes, leading to a relatively protective immune response against HIV and hence to a slower rate of disease progression. In contrast, certain MHC class I or class II alleles might predispose an individual to an immunopathogenic response against viral epitopes in certain tissues, such as the CNS or lungs, or against certain HIV-infected cell types, such as macrophages or dendritic cells/Langerhans cells. In addition, certain rare MHC class I and class II alleles might facilitate rapid recognition of HIV-infected cells from the infecting partner in primary HIV infection and promote rejection of these cells by alloreactive responses.

Similarly, common MHC alleles could lead to less effective removal of HIV-infected allogeneic cells. In this regard, it has been demonstrated that allele sharing at HLA-B loci is associated with increased risk of transmission of HIV infection between heterosexual Zambian couples discordant for HIV. It has been clearly demonstrated that maximal *HLA* heterozygosity for class I loci (A, B, and C) is associated with a delayed onset of AIDS among HIV-infected individuals, whereas homozygosity for these loci was associated with a more rapid progression to AIDS and death. This observation is likely due to the fact that individuals who are heterozygous at *HLA* loci are able to present a greater variety of antigenic peptides to cytotoxic T lymphocytes than are homozygotes, resulting in a more effective immune response against a number of pathogens including HIV. Of particular note is the fact that the HLA class I alleles B*35 and Cw*04 were consistently associated with rapid development of AIDS. Other data have indicated that transporter associated with antigen-processing (TAP) genes play a role in determining the outcome of HIV infection. HLA profiles that reflect certain combinations of MHC-encoded TAP and class I and class II genes are strongly associated with different rates of progression to AIDS. A recent finding of genetic association with HIV disease progression has highlighted the role for NK cells in HIV disease. A single nucleotide polymorphism (SNP) in the killer immunoglobulin-like receptor (KIR) gene was shown to be strongly associated with rapid progression to AIDS. However, when the KIR3 DS1 SNP was present with HLA-B Bw4-80I, the resultant phenotype was delayed progression to AIDS, even though this HLA-B allele alone has no effect on HIV disease progression. Furthermore, the KIR3 DS1/HLA-B Bw4-80I-carrying individuals had a significantly reduced viral load, beginning early in the course of infection, and protection against opportunistic infections during the later stages of the disease. This observation points to the potential role of NK cells in the maintenance of the viral set point, and strongly suggests that HLA-B Bw4-80I serves

TABLE 182-4 HOST GENETIC FACTORS THAT INFLUENCE RISK OF TRANSMISSION AND RATES OF DISEASE PROGRESSION TO AIDS

	MHC Genes	
	HLA Class I[a]	**HLA Class II**[a]
Disease progression		
Rapid	**A23, A24,** A26, A28, A29, A31, B7 supertype, **B*08,** B14, B21, **B22,** B25, **B35,** B37, B38, **B53,** B44, B49, **C4, C7,** C8, C16, **homozygosity for class I alleles**	**DRB1*01, DRB1*03,** DRB1*05, DRB1*11
Slow	A10, A19, A*30, **A32,** B14, B16, B17, B18, **B27,** B*39, B51, **B57,** B58, C8, **heterozygosity for class I alleles**	DRB1*03, DRB1*13
Transmission		
Increased risk	A2, B21, B35, Cw4, **allele sharing between HIV donor and recipient**	DRB1*05, DRB1*06, DRB1*13
Reduced risk	A2/A6802 supertype, A11, B18, B52, B57, B58, C2	

Factor	Association
Chemokine and Chemokine Receptor Genes	
CCR5	Homozygous defect involving a 32-bp deletion corresponding to the second extracellular loop of the receptor results in loss of surface expression, and consequently, resistance to infection; heterozygous defect appears to result in partial protection against transmission and disease progression. Several single nucleotide polymorphisms (SNPs) in the CCR5 promoter have been identified that along with the CCR2-64I polymorphism define nine human haplogroups (HHA to HHE, HHF*1, HHF*2, HHG*1 and HHG*2). Homozygosity for the HHE haplotype is associated with an increased risk of transmission and an accelerated rate of disease progression.
CCR2	Heterozygosity for the CCR2-64I polymorphism is associated with a slower rate of disease progression, and in one study this effect was found to be more prominent in African Americans.
CX3CR1	Mutations 249I and 280M are associated with a rapid rate of disease progression to AIDS in a French-Caucasian cohort. Inconsistent effects were detected in other cohorts.
CCL3L1 (MIP-1αP)	The copy number of CCL3L1 varies within and among populations (range 0–10 copies per diploid genome). A copy number lower than the average gene dose found in a population is associated with an increased risk of acquiring HIV and a more rapid rate of disease progression to AIDS.
CCL5 (RANTES)	SNPs in the promoter, intron, and 3'-untranslated region can influence transcription and protein production, and consequently, affect risk of acquiring HIV and rates of disease progression. For example, a haplotype defined by two promoter SNPs (-471A/-96C) is associated with a faster rate of disease progression in European Americans. However, the -471A/-96G haplotype is found mostly in populations from East Asia, and this haplotype was associated with a slow rate of disease progression in a Japanese cohort.
CCL2 (MCP-1)	The MCP-1 -2578G allele results in increased transcription, protein production, and monocyte recruitment. Homozygosity for the MCP-1 -2578G allele is associated with an enhanced risk of developing HIV-1-associated dementia and a rapid disease course.
CXCL12 (SDF-1)	The SDF-1 3'A SNP in the 3' untranslated region was initially reported to be associated with a slower disease rate of progression in a large U.S.-based cohort, but the results in other cohorts suggest an opposite effect.
Cytokine Genes	
IL-10	Individuals carrying the IL-10-592A promoter allele were at increased risk for HIV infection and, once infected, progressed more rapidly than did homozygotes for the alternative IL-10-5'-592 C/C genotype.
IL-4	The IL-4-589T results in higher levels of IL-4 production in vivo, resulting in downregulation of CCR5. However, the effects of this polymorphism on disease progression are inconsistent.
IL-6	A single report showed that possession of the IL-6 promoter polymorphism (-174G) is associated with an increased risk of developing Kaposi sarcoma in HIV-1-positive individuals.
TNF-α	A single report showed that the SNP TNF-α-238A, but not the -308A allele correlates with a higher frequency of lipodystrophy.
Other Genes	
APOBEC3G	The 186R allele is associated with a decline in CD4 T cells and an accelerated rate of progression to AIDS in African Americans.
VDR	Homozygosity for the vitamin D receptor gene polymorphism B (VDR-BB) correlates with a rapid progression to AIDS.
MBL2	Conflicting effects have been reported for MBL variants.
Gene-Gene Interactions	
KIR gene with HLA-B	In the absence of HLA-B Bw4-80I, KIR3DS1 is strongly associated with rapid progression to AIDS. This effect is reversed by the presence of HLA-B Bw4-80I. Individuals carrying both genes have a delayed progression to AIDS; in the absence of KIR3DS1, HLA-B Bw4-80I has no effect on disease progression.
CCL3L1 and CCR5	Based on possession of a low or high copy number of CCL3L1 (CCL3L1^{low} or CCL3L1^{high}) and a detrimental or nondetrimental (CCR5^{det} or CCR5^{nondet}) CCR5 genotype, variations in these two genes segregate into four genetic risk groups (GRGs). In HIV-infected adults followed in a U.S.-based cohort, an association for a low, moderate, and high risk of acquiring HIV or progressing rapidly to AIDS and death was detected in those possessing a CCL3L1^{high}/CCR5^{nondet}, CCL3L1^{high}/CCR5^{det} or CCL3L1^{low}/CCR5^{nondet}, and CCL3L1^{low}/CCR5^{det} GRG, respectively.

[a]For MHC genes, bold denotes alleles that in multiple reports have been shown to have consistent effects in different cohorts, whereas italic denotes alleles that have been show to have effects in a few cohorts. HH, human haplogroup.

Sources: Sunil K. Ahuja, MD, and adapted from HA Stephens: Trends Immunol 26(1):41, 2005; M Carrington, SJ O'Brien: Annu Rev Med 54:535 2003; Epub 2001 Dec 3; RA Kaslow et al: J Infect Dis. 191 [Suppl 1]:S68, 2005; A Telenti, G Bleiber: Future Virol 1:55, 2006.

as the ligand activating the KIR, resulting in the death of the target cell. These gene-gene interactions between KIR and MHC genes are illustrated in Table 182-4.

Chemokine Receptors   The most dramatic example of a genetic factor influencing HIV infection and/or pathogenesis relates to the gene that codes for the HIV cellular co-receptor CCR5. Rare individuals have been reported who had repetitive sexual exposure to HIV in high-risk situations but remained uninfected. The peripheral blood mononuclear cells of two such individuals were found to be highly resistant to infection in vitro with R5 strains of HIV-1 but were readily infected with X4 strains. Genetic analysis revealed that these two individuals inherited a homozygous defect in the gene that codes for CCR5, the cellular co-receptor for R5 strains of HIV-1. The defective *CCR5* allele contained a 32-bp deletion corresponding to the second extracellular loop of the receptor (*Δ32* allele). The encoded protein was severely truncated and the receptor was nonfunctional, explaining the refractoriness to infection with R5 strains of HIV-1. Population studies revealed that ~1% of the Caucasian population of western European ancestry possessed the homozygous defect. Up to 20% of individuals of European descent were found to be heterozygous for the *CCR5 Δ32* allele. Of note, cohort studies of hundreds of DNA samples originating from western and central Africa and Far East Asia indicate that the *CCR5 Δ32* allele is either absent or extremely rare in these populations. A number of studies found that the frequency of *CCR5 Δ32* allele was enriched in exposed, uninfected individuals. Furthermore, in a cohort of 1400 HIV-1–infected Caucasian individuals, no subject homozygous for the mutation was found, strongly supporting the concept that the homozygous defect confers protection against infection. This finding is particularly compelling in light of the fact that transmitting viruses are strongly biased toward R5 strains of HIV-1 (see above). Of note, several individuals have been identified who were homozygous for the *CCR5 Δ32* defect who in fact did become infected with HIV. These individuals were found to have an X4 strain of HIV that was associated in some cases with an accelerated course of disease. In some studies, HIV-infected individuals who are heterozygous for the *CCR5 Δ32* allele had a slower rate of disease progression. Slow progression of HIV disease is also seen in individuals who are heterozygous for the *CCR2-64I* polymorphism. This *CCR2-64I* allele–associated effect could be due to its linkage with SNPs in the *CCR5* promoter that are known to influence disease progression rates and/or due to dimerization of CXCR4 with the mutated *CCR2-64I* resulting in a decreased expression of CXCR4 on the cell surface.

A number of SNPs in the *CCR5* promoter have been associated with varied rates of disease progression. The promoter SNPs along the *CCR5 Δ32* and CCR2-V64I alleles define nine *CCR5* human haplogroups (HH)designated as HHA through HHE, and HHG*1, HHG*2, HHF*1 and HHF*2 (Table 182-4). Studies have shown that homozygosity for the HHE haplotype is associated with an increased risk of acquiring HIV and progressing rapidly to AIDS. Pairing of the HHC and the *CCR5 Δ32*-containing HHG*2 haplotype is associated with a slower rate of disease progression and reduced risk of acquiring HIV.

Chemokines   The varied distribution of the copy number of *CCL3L1* and *RANTES* polymorphisms provides some striking examples of the effect of chemokine genes on HIV pathogenesis. The *CCL3L1* gene encodes MIP-1αP, the most potent agonist of CCR5 and HIV-suppressive chemokine for R5 strains of HIV-1. This gene is present in a range of copy numbers in and among different racial groups. Individuals with fewer than average copy numbers for their racial group showed both an increased susceptibility to infection with HIV and a faster rate of progression to AIDS. When the interaction of this gene with the different *CCR5* alleles was examined, individuals with a low *CCL3L1* gene dose and certain *CCR5* alleles, which have a detrimental effect on disease progression, were shown to have a significantly greater risk of transmission and faster disease progression rates. SNPs have been identified in the gene that encodes for CCL5 (*RANTES*), another potent agonist of CCR5 and an R5 HIV-suppressive chemokine. Some of

these SNPs correlate with either an increased or decreased *CCL5* gene transcription and this is thought to underlie the disease associations detected. For example, the *CCL5* -96G SNP upregulates *CCL5* gene transcription and is associated with delayed progression to AIDS in a Japanese cohort; the prevalence of this allele is very low in other populations. The opposite effects are observed for an intronic *CCL5* SNP designated as In1.1C. This SNP is associated with decreased *CCL5* gene transcription and correlates strongly with a rapid progression rate to AIDS. Other SNPs that decrease *CCL5* gene transcription are associated with a higher rate of HIV infection. The results of these genotype-phenotype studies with *CCL3L1* and *CCL5* genes reinforce the central role for R5 viruses in the establishment of HIV infection.

Additional associations for other chemokines have been noted. CCL2 is a one of the most potent chemokines that attracts and activates mononuclear phagocytes (MP). In a U.S. population-based study, homozygosity for the *CCL2* (*MCP-1*) -2578G allele was associated with a 50% reduction in the risk of acquiring HIV-1. However, once HIV-1 infection was established, this same *CCL2* genotype was associated with accelerated disease progression and a 4.5-fold increased risk of HIV-associated dementia. Possession of the *CCL2* -2578G allele is associated with increased CCL2 serum levels and recruitment of MPs to inflamed tissues. Since recruitment of MPs to the CNS and the activation status of MPs in the CNS is thought to be a key determinant of HIV-associated dementia, these association studies implicate a central role for CCL2 in the pathogenesis of HIV-related CNS disease.

Cytokines   In addition to the chemokine receptors and chemokines, polymorphisms in cytokine genes have also been found to influence intersubject differences in susceptibility to HIV/AIDS. Individuals who carry a certain allele (-592A) of the IL-10 promoter are at increased risk of infection and, once infected, progress more rapidly than homozygotes for the alternative genotype. The mechanism of this effect is felt to be a downregulation of the inhibitory cytokine IL-10 resulting in facilitation of HIV replication. The SNP, IL-4 -589T, increases IL-4 production. This allele associates with a slower progression to AIDS, presumably through the downregulation of CCR5 by higher and more sustained levels of IL-4. However, the effects of this IL-4 polymorphism on disease progression are inconsistent in different studies.

Other Genes   Additional genes such as those involved in innate immunity, lipid metabolism, and cell cycle have also been found to be associated with altered HIV/AIDS susceptibility. For example, a histidine-arginine change at position 186 in the gene that encodes APOBEC3G is found at a higher frequency in individuals of African descent and is associated with more rapid disease progression rates. Homozygosity for the vitamin D receptor form B correlates with rapid progression to AIDS. The mechanism is thought to relate to the known effects of vitamin D on immune modulation.

The effects of some genes [e.g., *CX3CR1, CXCL12 (SDF-1), IL-4, IL-6, TNF-α,* and *MBL2*] on HIV pathogenesis are either from a single cohort or the findings are inconsistent in different cohorts. Nevertheless, there is growing appreciation that the evolutionary histories of human populations have had a significant impact on the distribution of variation of some genes that are thought to play a key role in HIV-1/AIDS pathogenesis, and that this might be responsible, in part, for the heterogeneous nature of the epidemiology of the HIV-1 pandemic.

NEUROPATHOGENESIS

While there has been a remarkable decrease in the incidence of HIV encephalopathy among those with access to treatment in the era of effective ARV therapy, HIV-infected individuals can still experience a variety of neurologic abnormalities due either to opportunistic infections and neoplasms or to direct effects of HIV or its products (see below). With regard to the latter, HIV has been demonstrated in the brain and CSF of infected individuals with and without neuropsychiatric abnormalities. The main cell types that are infected in the brain in vivo are the perivascular macrophages and the microglial cells; monocytes that have already been infected in the blood can migrate into the brain, where they then reside as macrophages, or macrophages can be directly infected within the brain. The precise mechanisms whereby HIV enters the brain are unclear; however, they are thought to relate, at least in part, to the ability of virus-infected and immune-activated macrophages to induce adhesion molecules such as E-selectin and vascular cell adhesion molecule-1 (VCAM-1) on brain endothelium. Other studies have demonstrated that HIV gp120 enhances the expression of intercellular adhesion molecule-1 (ICAM-1) in glial cells; this effect may facilitate entry of HIV-infected cells into the CNS and may promote syncytia formation. Virus isolates from the brain are preferentially R5 strains as opposed to X4 strains (see above); in this regard, HIV-infected individuals who are heterozygous for *CCR5-Δ32* appear to be relatively protected against the development of HIV encephalopathy compared to wild-type individuals. Distinct HIV envelope sequences are associated with the clinical expression of the AIDS dementia complex (see below). There is no convincing evidence that brain cells other than those of monocyte/macrophage lineage can be productively infected in vivo. Astrocytes have been reported to be susceptible to HIV infection in vitro despite the fact that they do not express detectable levels of cell-surface CD4 or the main HIV co-receptors. Nonetheless, they do not support active virus replication. There is no convincing evidence that oligodendrocytes or neurons can be infected with HIV (see below).

HIV-infected individuals may manifest white matter lesions as well as neuronal loss. Given the absence of evidence of HIV infection of neurons either in vivo or in vitro, it is highly unlikely that direct infection of these cells accounts for their loss. Rather, the HIV-mediated effects on neurons and oligodendrocytes are thought to involve indirect pathways whereby viral proteins, particularly gp120 and Tat, trigger the release of endogenous neurotoxins from macrophages and to a lesser extent from astrocytes. In addition, it has been demonstrated that both HIV-1 Nef and Tat can induce chemotaxis of leukocytes, including monocytes, into the CNS. Neurotoxins can be released from monocytes as a consequence of infection and/or immune activation. Monocyte-derived neurotoxic factors have been reported to kill neurons via the *N*-methyl-D-aspartate (NMDA) receptor. In addition, HIV gp120 shed by virus-infected monocytes could cause neurotoxicity by antagonizing the function of vasoactive intestinal peptide (VIP), by elevating intracellular calcium levels, and by decreasing nerve growth factor levels in the cerebral cortex. A variety of monocyte-derived cytokines can contribute directly or indirectly to the neurotoxic effects in HIV infection; these include TNF-α, IL-1, IL-6, TGF-β, IFN-γ, platelet-activating factor, and endothelin. Furthermore, among the CC-chemokines, elevated levels of monocyte chemotactic protein (MCP)1 in the brain and CSF have been shown to correlate best with the presence and degree of HIV encephalopathy. In addition, infection and/or activation of monocyte-lineage cells can result in increased production of eicosanoids, nitric oxide, and quinolinic acid, which may contribute to neurotoxicity. Astrocytes may play diverse roles in HIV neuropathogenesis. Reactive gliosis or astrocytosis has been demonstrated in the brains of HIV-infected individuals, and TNF-α and IL-6 have been shown to induce astrocyte proliferation. In addition, astrocyte-derived IL-6 can induce HIV expression in infected cells in vitro. Furthermore, it has been suggested that astrocytes may downregulate macrophage-produced neurotoxins. It has been reported that HIV-infected individuals with the E4 allele for apolipoprotein E (apo E) are at increased risk for AIDS encephalopathy and peripheral neuropathy. The likelihood that HIV or its products are involved in neuropathogenesis is supported by the observation that neuropsychiatric abnormalities may undergo remarkable and rapid improvement upon the initiation of ARV therapy.

It has also been suggested that the CNS may serve as a relatively sequestered site for a reservoir of latently infected cells and for the slow, continual replication of HIV that might be a barrier for the eradication of virus by ARV therapy (see "Reservoirs of HIV-Infected Cells: Obstacle to the Eradication of Virus," above).

PATHOGENESIS OF KAPOSI'S SARCOMA

There are at least four distinct epidemiologic forms of KS: (1) the classic form that occurs in older men of predominantly Mediterranean or eastern European Jewish backgrounds with no recognized contributing factors; (2) the equatorial African form that occurs in all ages, also without any recognized precipitating factors; (3) the form associated with organ transplantation and its attendant iatrogenic immunosuppressed state; and (4) the form associated with HIV-1 infection. In the latter two forms, KS is an opportunistic disease; in HIV-infected individuals, unlike typical opportunistic infections, its occurrence is not strictly related to the level of depression of CD4+ T cell counts (see below). The pathogenesis of KS is complex; fundamentally, it is an angioproliferative disease that is not a true neoplastic sarcoma, at least not in its early stages. It is a manifestation of excessive proliferation of spindle cells that are believed to be of vascular origin and have features in common with endothelial and smooth-muscle cells. In HIV disease the development of KS is dependent on the interplay of a variety of factors including HIV-1 itself, human herpes virus 8 (HHV-8), immune activation, and cytokine secretion. A number of epidemiologic and virologic studies have clearly linked HHV-8, which is also referred to as *Kaposi's sarcoma–associated herpesvirus* (KSHV), to KS not only in HIV-infected individuals but also in individuals with the other forms of KS. HHV-8 is a γ-herpesvirus related to EBV and herpesvirus saimiri. It encodes a homologue to human IL-6 and in addition to KS has been implicated in the pathogenesis of body cavity lymphoma, multiple myeloma, and monoclonal gammopathy of undetermined significance. Sequences of HHV-8 are found universally in the lesions of KS, and patients with KS are virtually all seropositive for HHV-8. HHV-8 DNA sequences can be found in the B cells of 30–50% of patients with KS and 7% of patients with AIDS without clinically apparent KS.

Between 1 and 2% of eligible blood donors are positive for antibodies to HHV-8, while the prevalence of HHV-8 seropositivity in HIV-infected men is 30–35%. The prevalence in HIV-infected women is ~4%. This finding is reflective of the lower incidence of KS in women. It has been debated whether HHV-8 is actually the transforming agent in KS; the bulk of the cells in the tumor lesions of KS are not neoplastic cells. However, it has been demonstrated that endothelial cells can be transformed in vitro by HHV-8. In this regard, HHV-8 possesses a number of genes including homologues of the IL-8 receptor, Bcl-2, and cyclin D, which can potentially transform the host cell. Despite the complexity of the pathogenic events associated with the development of KS in HIV-infected individuals, HHV-8 is the etiologic agent of this disease. The initiation and/or propagation of KS requires an activated state and is mediated, at least in part, by cytokines. A number of factors, including TNF-α, IL-1β, IL-6, GM-CSF, basic fibroblast growth factor, and oncostatin M, function in an autocrine and paracrine manner to sustain the growth and chemotaxis of the KS spindle cells. In this regard, KSHV-derived IL-6 has been demonstrated to induce proliferation of lymphoma cells and to inhibit the cytostatic effects of INF-α on KSHV-infected lymphoma cells.

IMMUNE RESPONSE TO HIV

As detailed above and below, following the initial burst of viremia during primary infection, HIV-infected individuals mount robust immune responses that in most cases substantially curtail the levels of plasma viremia and likely contribute to delaying the ultimate development of clinically apparent disease for a median of 10 years in untreated individuals. This immune response contains elements of both humoral and cell-mediated immunity involving both innate and adaptive immune responses (Table 182-5; Fig. 182-24). It is directed against multiple antigenic determinants of the HIV virion as well as against viral proteins expressed on the surface of infected cells. Ironically, those CD4+ T cells with T cell receptors specific for HIV are theoretically those CD4+ T cells most likely to be activated and thus to serve as early targets for productive HIV infection and the cell death or dysfunction associated with infection. Thus, an early consequence of HIV infection is interference with and decrease of the helper cell population needed to generate an effective immune response.

Although a great deal of investigation has been directed toward delineating and better understanding the components of this immune

TABLE 182-5 ELEMENTS OF THE IMMUNE RESPONSE TO HIV

Humoral immunity
  Binding antibodies
  Neutralizing antibodies
    Type specific
    Group specific
  Antibodies participating in antibody-dependent cellular cytotoxicity (ADCC)
    Protective
    Pathogenic (bystander killing)
  Enhancing antibodies
  Complement
Cell-mediated immunity
  Helper CD4+ T lymphocytes
  Class I MHC–restricted cytotoxic CD8+ T lymphocytes
  CD8+ T cell–mediated inhibition (noncytolytic)
  ADCC
  Natural killer cells

response, it remains unclear which immunologic effector mechanisms are most important in delaying progression of infection and which, if any, play a role in the pathogenesis of HIV disease. This lack of knowl-

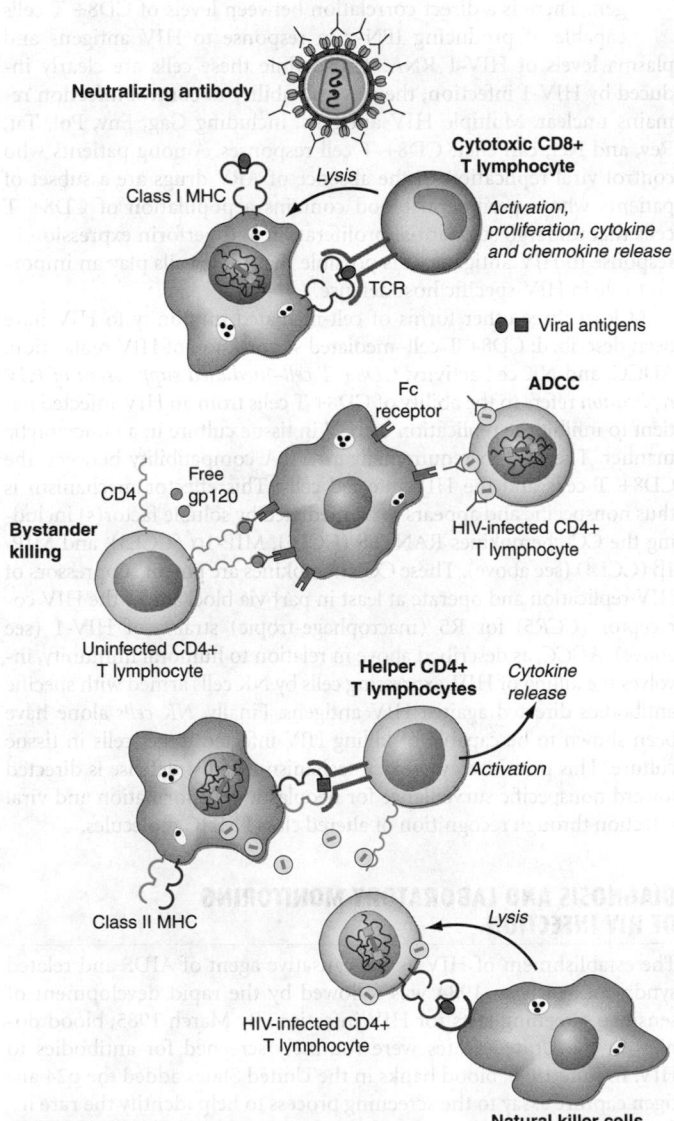

FIGURE 182-24 Schematic representation of the different immunologic effector mechanisms thought to be active in the setting of HIV infection. Detailed descriptions are given in the text. TCR, T cell receptor; ADCC, antibody-dependent cellular cytotoxicity; MHC, major histocompatibility complex.

edge has also hampered the ability to develop an effective vaccine for HIV disease.

HUMORAL IMMUNE RESPONSE

Antibodies to HIV usually appear within 6 weeks and almost invariably within 12 weeks of primary infection (Fig. 182-25); rare exceptions are individuals who have defects in the ability to produce HIV-specific antibodies. Detection of these antibodies forms the basis of most diagnostic screening tests for HIV infection. The appearance of HIV-binding antibodies detected by ELISA and Western blot assays occurs prior to the appearance of neutralizing antibodies; the latter generally appear following the initial decreases in plasma viremia, which is more closely related to the appearance of HIV-specific CD8+ T lymphocytes. The first antibodies detected are those directed against the structural or gag proteins of HIV, p24 and p17, and the gag precursor p55. The development of antibodies to p24 is associated with a decrease in the serum levels of free p24 antigen. Antibodies to the gag proteins are followed by the appearance of antibodies to the envelope proteins (gp160, gp120, p88, and gp41) and to the products of the *pol* gene (p31, p51, and p66). In addition, one may see antibodies to the low-molecular-weight regulatory proteins encoded by the HIV genes *vpr*, *vpu*, *vif*, *rev*, *tat*, and *nef*. On rare occasion, levels of HIV-specific antibodies may decline during treatment of acute HIV infection.

While antibodies to multiple antigens of HIV are produced, the precise functional significance of these different antibodies is unclear. The only viral proteins that elicit neutralizing antibodies are the envelope proteins gp120 and gp41. As noted above, the envelope of HIV consists of an outer envelope glycoprotein with a molecular mass of 120 kDa and a transmembrane glycoprotein with a molecular mass of 41 kDa. These are initially synthesized as a 160-kDa precursor that is cleaved by cellular proteases. Most of the antienvelope antibodies are directed either toward an epitope in the gp41 region comprising amino acids 579–613 or toward a hypervariable region in the gp120 molecule, known as the *V3 loop region*, comprising amino acids 303–338. This V3 region is a major site for the development of mutations that lead to variants of HIV that are not well recognized by the immune system.

Antibodies directed toward the envelope proteins of HIV have been characterized both as being protective and as possibly contributing to the pathogenesis of HIV disease. Among the protective antibodies are those that function to neutralize HIV directly and prevent the spread of infection to additional cells, as well as those that participate in ADCC. Within the first 6 months of infection neutralizing antibodies appear; however, the virus quickly escapes these neutralizing antibodies. One of the principal mechanisms of immune escape is the addition of N-linked glycosylation sites. The added carbohydrate moieties interfere with envelope recognition by these initial antibodies. The hyperglycosylation of the envelope protein has been termed the *glycan shield*. Neutralizing antibodies appear to be of two forms, type-specific and group-specific. *Type-specific neutralizing antibodies* are generally directed to the V3 loop region. These antibodies neutralize only viruses of a given strain and are present in low titer in most infected individuals. *Group-specific neutralizing antibodies* are capable of neutralizing a wide variety of HIV isolates. At least two forms of group-specific antibodies have been identified: those binding to amino acids 423–437 of gp120, which lie close to the CD4 binding site, and those binding to amino acids 728–745 of gp41, which lie proximal to the viral membrane. The other major class of protective antibodies are those that participate in ADCC, which is actually a form of cell-mediated immunity (Chap. 308) in which NK cells that bear Fc receptors are armed with specific anti-HIV antibodies that bind to the NK cells via their Fc portion. These armed NK cells then bind to and destroy cells expressing HIV antigens. Antibodies to both gp120 and gp41 have been shown to participate in ADCC-mediated killing of HIV-infected cells. The levels of antienvelope antibodies capable of mediating ADCC are highest in the earlier stages of HIV infection. In vitro, IL-2 can augment ADCC-mediated killing.

In addition to playing a role in host defense, HIV-specific antibodies have also been implicated in disease pathogenesis. Antibodies di-

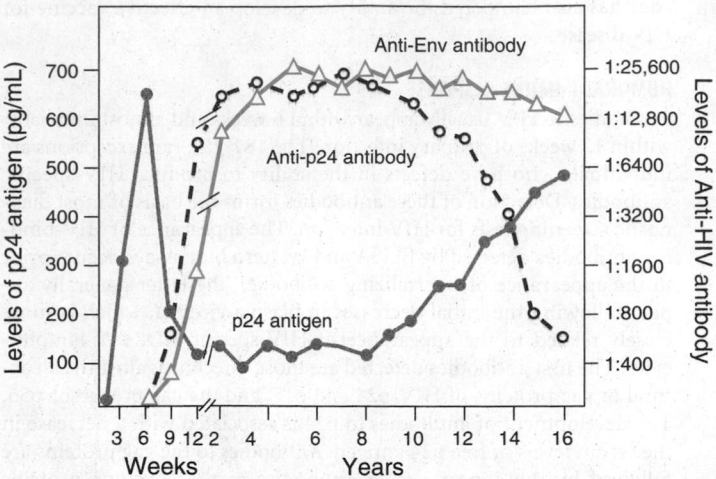

FIGURE 182-25 Relationship between antigenemia and the development of antibodies to HIV. Antibodies to HIV proteins are generally seen 6–12 weeks following infection and 3–6 weeks after the development of plasma viremia. Late in the course of illness, antibody levels to p24 decline, generally in association with a rising titer of p24 antigen.

rected to gp41, when present in low titer, have been shown in vitro to be capable of facilitating infection of cells through an Fc receptor–mediated mechanism known as *antibody enhancement*. Thus, the same regions of the envelope protein of HIV that give rise to antibodies capable of mediating ADCC also elicit the production of antibodies that can facilitate infection of cells in vitro. In addition, it has been postulated that anti-gp120 antibodies that participate in the ADCC killing of HIV-infected cells might also kill uninfected CD4+ T cells if the uninfected cells had bound free gp120, a phenomenon referred to as *bystander killing*. One of the most primitive components of the humoral immune system is the complement system (Chap. 308). This element of innate immunity consists of ~30 proteins that are found circulating in blood or associated with cell membranes. While HIV alone is capable of directly activating the complement cascade, the resulting lysis is weak due to the presence of host cell regulatory proteins captured in the virion envelope during budding. It is possible that complement-opsonized HIV virions have increased infectivity in a manner analogous to antibody-mediated enhancement.

CELLULAR IMMUNE RESPONSE

Given the fact that T cell–mediated immunity is known to play a major role in host defense against most viral infections (Chap. 308), it is generally thought to be an important component of the host immune response to HIV. T cell immunity can be divided into two major categories, mediated respectively by the *helper/inducer CD4+ T cells* and the *cytotoxic/immunoregulatory CD8+ T cells*.

HIV-specific CD4+ T cells can be detected in the majority of HIV-infected patients through the use of flow cytometry to measure intracellular cytokine production in response to MHC class II tetramers pulsed with HIV peptides or through lymphocyte proliferation assays utilizing HIV antigens such as p24. HIV-specific CD4+ T cells may be preferential targets of HIV infection by HIV-infected antigen-presenting cells during the generation of an immune response to HIV (see above). However, they also are likely to undergo clonal expansions in response to HIV antigens and thus survive as a population of cells. No clear correlations exist between levels of HIV-specific CD4+ T lymphocytes and plasma HIV RNA levels; however, in the setting of high viral loads, CD4+ T cell responses to HIV antigens appear to shift from one of proliferation and IL-2 production to one of IFN-γ production. Thus, while a reverse correlation exists between the level of p24-specific proliferation and levels of plasma HIV viremia, the nature of the causal relationship between these parameters is unclear.

MHC class I–restricted, HIV-specific CD8+ T cells have been identified in the peripheral blood of patients with HIV-1 infection. These cells include CTLs that produce perforins and T cells that can be induced by HIV antigens to express an array of cytokines such as IFN-γ. CTLs have been identified in the peripheral blood of patients within weeks of HIV infection. These CD8+ T lymphocytes, through their HIV-specific antigen receptors, bind to and cause the lytic destruction of target cells bearing autologous MHC class I molecules associated with HIV antigens. Two types of CTL activity can be demonstrated in the peripheral blood or lymph node mononuclear cells of HIV-infected individuals. The first type directly lyses appropriate target cells in culture without prior in vitro stimulation (*spontaneous CTL activity*). The other type of CTL activity reflects the *precursor frequency of CTLs* (CTLp); this type of CTL activity can be demonstrated by stimulation of CD8+ T cells in vitro with a mitogen such as phytohemagglutinin or anti-CD3 antibody.

In addition to CTLs, CD8+ T cells capable of being induced by HIV antigens to express cytokines such as IFN-γ also appear in the setting of HIV-1 infection. It is not clear whether these are the same or different effector pools compared to those cells mediating cytotoxicity; in addition, the relative roles of each in host defense against HIV are not fully understood. It does appear that these CD8+ T cells are driven to in vivo expansion by HIV antigen. There is a direct correlation between levels of CD8+ T cells capable of producing IFN-γ in response to HIV antigens and plasma levels of HIV-1 RNA. Thus, while these cells are clearly induced by HIV-1 infection, their overall ability to control infection remains unclear. Multiple HIV antigens, including Gag, Env, Pol, Tat, Rev, and Nef, can elicit CD8+ T cell responses. Among patients who control viral replication in the absence of ARV drugs are a subset of patients whose peripheral blood contains a population of CD8+ T cells that undergo substantial proliferation and perforin expression in response to HIV antigens. It is possible that these cells play an important role in HIV-specific host defense.

At least three other forms of cell-mediated immunity to HIV have been described: CD8+ T cell–mediated suppression of HIV replication, ADCC, and NK cell activity. *CD8+ T cell–mediated suppression of HIV replication* refers to the ability of CD8+ T cells from an HIV-infected patient to inhibit the replication of HIV in tissue culture in a noncytolytic manner. There is no requirement for HLA compatibility between the CD8+ T cells and the HIV-infected cells. This effector mechanism is thus nonspecific and appears to be mediated by soluble factor(s) including the CC-chemokines RANTES (CCL5), MIP-1α (CCL3), and MIP-1β (CCL4) (see above). These CC-chemokines are potent suppressors of HIV replication and operate at least in part via blockade of the HIV coreceptor (*CCR5*) for R5 (macrophage-tropic) strains of HIV-1 (see above). *ADCC*, as described above in relation to humoral immunity, involves the killing of HIV-expressing cells by NK cells armed with specific antibodies directed against HIV antigens. Finally, *NK cells* alone have been shown to be capable of killing HIV-infected target cells in tissue culture. This primitive cytotoxic mechanism of host defense is directed toward nonspecific surveillance for neoplastic transformation and viral infection through recognition of altered class I MHC molecules.

DIAGNOSIS AND LABORATORY MONITORING OF HIV INFECTION

The establishment of HIV as the causative agent of AIDS and related syndromes early in 1984 was followed by the rapid development of sensitive screening tests for HIV infection. By March 1985, blood donors in the United States were routinely screened for antibodies to HIV. In June 1996, blood banks in the United States added the p24 antigen capture assay to the screening process to help identify the rare infected individuals who were donating blood in the time (up to 3 months) between infection and the development of antibodies. In 2002 the ability to detect early infection with HIV was further enhanced by the licensure of nucleic acid testing (NAT) as a routine part of blood donor screening. These refinements decreased the interval between infection and detection (window period) from 22 days for

A
1. Virus digested: digest separated into components by molecular weight
2. Proteins transferred to filter paper: reaction with test serum
3. Enzyme-conjugated antihuman antibody added
4. Substrate added and color noted

B
1. Positive HIV-1 infection
2. gp 160 immunization
3. Indeterminate (HIV-2 infection)
4. Indeterminate (cross-reacting antibody to p24)
5. Negative

FIGURE 182-26 Western blot assay for detection of antibodies to HIV. A. Schematic representation of how a Western blot is performed. **B.** Examples of patterns of Western blot reactivity. In each instance the Western blot strip contains antigens to HIV-1. The sera from the patient immunized to the HIV-1 envelope contains only antibodies to the HIV-1 envelope proteins. The sera from the patient with HIV-2 infection cross-reacts with both *reverse transcriptase* and *gag* gene products of HIV-1.

antibody testing to 16 days with p24 antigen testing and subsequently to 12 days with nucleic acid testing. The development of sensitive assays for monitoring levels of plasma viremia ushered in a new era of being able to monitor the progression of HIV disease more closely. Utilization of these tests, coupled with the measurement of levels of CD4+ T lymphocytes in peripheral blood, is essential in the management of patients with HIV infection.

DIAGNOSIS OF HIV INFECTION
The CDC has recommended that screening for HIV infection be performed as a matter of routine health care. The diagnosis of HIV infection depends upon the demonstration of antibodies to HIV and/or the direct detection of HIV or one of its components. As noted above, antibodies to HIV generally appear in the circulation 2–12 weeks following infection.

The standard blood screening test for HIV infection is the ELISA, also referred to as an *enzyme immunoassay* (EIA). This solid-phase assay is an extremely good screening test with a sensitivity of >99.5%. Most diagnostic laboratories use a commercial EIA kit that contains antigens from both HIV-1 and HIV-2 and thus are able to detect either. These kits use both natural and recombinant antigens and are continuously updated to increase their sensitivity to newly discovered species, such as group O viruses (Fig. 182-6). The fourth generation EIA tests combine detection of antibodies to HIV with detection of the p24 antigen of HIV. EIA tests are generally scored as positive (highly reactive), negative (nonreactive), or indeterminate (partially reactive). While the EIA is an extremely sensitive test, it is not optimal with regard to specificity. This is particularly true in studies of low-risk individuals, such as volunteer blood donors. In this latter population, only 10% of EIA-positive individuals are subsequently confirmed to have HIV infection. Among the factors associated with false-positive EIA tests are antibodies to class II antigens, autoantibodies, hepatic disease, recent influenza vaccination, and acute viral infections. For these reasons, anyone suspected of having HIV infection based upon a positive or inconclusive EIA result must have the result confirmed with a more specific assay such as the Western blot. One can estimate whether or not an individual has a recent infection with HIV-1 by comparing the results on a standard assay that will score positive for all infected individuals to the results on an assay modified to be less sensitive ("de-

tuned assay") that will score positive only for individuals with established HIV infection. In rare instances, an HIV-infected individual treated early in the course of infection may revert to a negative EIA. This does *not* indicate clearing of infection; rather, it signifies levels of ongoing exposure to virus insufficient to maintain a measurable antibody response. When these individuals have discontinued therapy, viruses and antibodies have reappeared.

The most commonly used confirmatory test is the Western blot (Fig. 182-26). This assay takes advantage of the fact that multiple HIV antigens of different, well-characterized molecular weights elicit the production of specific antibodies. These antigens can be separated on the basis of molecular weight, and antibodies to each component can be detected as discrete bands on the Western blot. A negative Western blot is one in which no bands are present at molecular weights corresponding to HIV gene products. In a patient with a positive or indeterminate EIA and a negative Western blot, one can conclude with certainty that the EIA reactivity was a false positive. On the other hand, a Western blot demonstrating antibodies to products of all three of the major genes of HIV (*gag*, *pol*, and *env*) is conclusive evidence of infection with HIV. Criteria established by the U.S. Food & Drug Administration (FDA) in 1993 for a positive Western blot state that a result is considered positive if antibodies exist to two of the three HIV proteins: p24, gp41, and gp120/160. Using these criteria, ~10% of all blood donors deemed positive for HIV-1 infection lacked an antibody band to the *pol* gene product p31. Some 50% of these blood donors were subsequently found to be false positives. Thus, the absence of the p31 band should increase the suspicion that one may be dealing with a false-positive test result. In this setting it is prudent to obtain additional confirmation with an RNA-based test and/or a follow-up Western blot. By definition, Western blot patterns of reactivity that do not fall into the positive or negative categories are considered "indeterminate." There are two possible explanations for an indeterminate Western blot result. The most likely explanation in a low-risk individual is that the patient being tested has antibodies that cross-react with one of the proteins of HIV. The most common patterns of cross-reactivity are antibodies that react with p24 and/or p55. The least likely explanation in this setting is that the individual is infected with HIV and is in the process of mounting a classic antibody response. In either instance, the Western blot should be repeated in 1 month to determine whether or not the indeterminate pattern is a pattern in evolution.

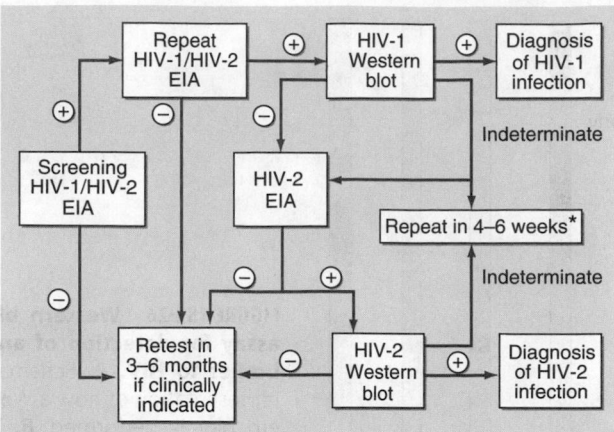

FIGURE 182-27 Algorithm for the use of serologic tests in the diagnosis of HIV-1 or HIV-2 infection. *Stable indeterminate Western blot 4–6 weeks later makes HIV infection unlikely. However, it should be repeated twice at 3-month intervals to rule out HIV infection. Alternatively, one may test for HIV-1 p24 antigen or HIV RNA.

In addition, one may attempt to confirm a diagnosis of HIV infection with the p24 antigen capture assay or one of the tests for HIV RNA (discussed below). While the Western blot is an excellent confirmatory test for HIV infection in patients with a positive or indeterminate EIA, it is a poor screening test. Among individuals with a negative EIA and PCR for HIV, 20–30% may show one or more bands on Western blot. While these bands are usually faint and represent cross-reactivity, their presence creates a situation in which other diagnostic modalities (such as DNA PCR, RNA PCR, the bDNA assay, or p24 antigen capture) must be employed to ensure that the bands do not indicate early HIV infection.

A guideline for the use of these serologic tests in attempting to make a diagnosis of HIV infection is depicted in Fig. 182-27. In patients in whom HIV infection is suspected, the appropriate initial test is the EIA. If the result is negative, unless there is strong reason to suspect early HIV infection (as in a patient exposed within the previous 3 months), the diagnosis is ruled out and retesting should be performed only as clinically indicated. If the EIA is indeterminate or positive, the test should be repeated. If the repeat is negative on two occasions, one can assume that the initial positive reading was due to a technical error in the performance of the assay and that the patient is negative. If the repeat is indeterminate or positive, one should proceed to the HIV-1 Western blot. If the Western blot is positive, the diagnosis is HIV-1 infection. If the Western blot is negative, the EIA can be assumed to have been a false positive for HIV-1 and the diagnosis of HIV-1 infection is ruled out. It would be prudent at this point to perform specific serologic testing for HIV-2 following the same type of algorithm. If the Western blot for HIV-1 is indeterminate, it should be repeated in 4–6 weeks; in addition, one may proceed to a p24 antigen capture assay, HIV-1 RNA assay, or HIV-1 DNA PCR and specific serologic testing for HIV-2. If the p24 and HIV RNA assays are negative and there is no progression in the Western blot, a diagnosis of HIV-1 is ruled out. If either the p24 or HIV-1 RNA assay is positive and/or the HIV-1 Western blot shows progression, a tentative diagnosis of HIV-1 infection can be made and later confirmed with a follow-up Western blot demonstrating a positive pattern. In addition to these standard laboratory-based assays for detecting antibodies to HIV, a series of point-of-care tests are also available. Among the most popular of these is the OraQuick Rapid HIV-1 antibody test that can be run on blood, plasma, or saliva. The sensitivity and specificity of this

test are each ~99%. While negative results from this test are adequate to rule out a diagnosis of HIV infection, a positive finding should be considered preliminary and confirmed with standard serologic testing, as described above.

As mentioned above, a variety of laboratory tests are available for the direct detection of HIV or its components (Table 182-6; Fig. 182-28). These tests may be of considerable help in making a diagnosis of HIV infection when the Western blot results are indeterminate. In addition, the tests detecting levels of HIV RNA can be used to determine prognosis and to assess the response to ARV therapies. The simplest of the direct detection tests is the *p24 antigen capture assay*. This is an EIA-type assay in which the solid phase consists of antibodies to the p24 antigen of HIV. It detects the viral protein p24 in the blood of HIV-infected individuals where it exists either as free antigen or complexed to anti-p24 antibodies. Overall, ~30% of individuals with untreated HIV infection have detectable levels of free p24 antigen. This increases to ~50% when samples are treated with a weak acid to dissociate antigen-antibody complexes. Throughout the course of HIV infection, an equilibrium exists between p24 antigen and anti-p24 antibodies. During the first few weeks of infection, before an immune response develops, there is a brisk rise in p24 antigen levels (Fig. 182-25). After the development of anti-p24 antibodies, these levels decline. Late in the course of infection, when circulating levels of virus are high, p24 antigen levels also increase, particularly when detected by techniques involving dissociation of antigen-antibody complexes. The p24 antigen capture assay has its greatest use as a screening test for HIV infection in patients suspected of having the acute HIV syndrome, as high levels of p24 antigen are present prior to the development of antibodies. Its use for routine blood donor screening for HIV infection has been replaced by use of nucleic acid testing. The ability to measure and monitor levels of HIV RNA in the plasma of patients with HIV infection has been of extraordinary value in furthering our understanding of the pathogenesis of HIV infection and in providing a diagnostic tool in settings where measurements of anti-HIV antibodies may be misleading, such as in acute infection and neonatal infection. Three assays are predominantly used for this purpose. They are reverse transcriptase PCR (*RT-PCR*; Amplicor); branched DNA (*bDNA*; VERSANT); and nucleic acid sequence–based amplification (*NASBA*; NucliSens). These tests are of value in making a diagnosis of HIV infection, in establishing initial prognosis, in determining the need for therapy, and for monitoring the effects of therapy. In addition to these three commercially available tests, the *DNA PCR* is also employed by research laboratories for making a diagnosis of HIV infection by amplifying HIV proviral DNA from peripheral blood mononuclear cells. The commercially available RNA detection tests have a sensitivity of 40–80 copies of HIV RNA per milliliter of plasma. Research laboratory–based RNA assays can detect as few as one HIV RNA copy per milliliter, while the DNA PCR tests can detect proviral DNA at a frequency of one copy per 10,000–100,000 cells. Thus, these tests are ex-

TABLE 182-6	CHARACTERISTICS OF TESTS FOR DIRECT DETECTION OF HIV		
Test	**Technique**	**Sensitivity**[a]	**Cost/ Test**[b]
Immune complex–dissociated p24 antigen capture assay	Measurement of levels of HIV-1 core protein in an EIA-based format following dissociation of antigen-antibody complexes by weak acid treatment	Positive in 50% of patients; detects down to 15 pg/mL of p24 protein	$1–2
HIV RNA by PCR	PCR amplification of cDNA generated from viral RNA (target amplification)	Reliable to 40 copies/mL of HIV RNA	$75–150
HIV RNA by bDNA	Measurement of levels of particle-associated HIV RNA in a nucleic acid capture assay employing signal amplification	Reliable to 50 copies/mL of HIV RNA	$75–150
HIV RNA by NucliSens	Isothermic nucleic acid amplification with internal controls	Reliable to 80 copies/mL of HIV RNA	$75–150

[a]Sensitivity figures refer to those approved by the US FDA.
[b]Prices may be lower in large volume settings.
Note: EIA, enzyme immunoassay; PCR, polymerase chain reaction.

FIGURE 182-28 Comparison of RT-PCR and bDNA assays. A. Schematic representation of reverse transcriptase–polymerase chain reaction (RT-PCR) and bDNA assays. See text for detailed description. **B.** Scatter plot of $\log_{10}$ v3-bDNA versus $\log_{10}$ RT-PCR with the line of equity (solid) and the fitted regression line (hatched). The equation for the fitted regression line is given in the lower-right-hand corner. There is good agreement between the two assays. v3, version 3 of the bDNA assay. *(Adapted from HC Highbarger et al: J Clin Microbiol 37:3612, 1999.)*

tremely sensitive. One frequent consequence of a high degree of sensitivity is some loss of specificity, and false-positive results have been reported with each of these techniques. For this reason, a positive EIA with a confirmatory Western blot remains the "gold standard" for a diagnosis of HIV infection, and the interpretation of other test results must be done with this in mind.

In the RT-PCR technique, following DNase treatment, a cDNA copy is made of all RNA species present in plasma. Insofar as HIV is an RNA virus, this will result in the production of DNA copies of the HIV genome in amounts proportional to the amount of HIV RNA present in plasma. This cDNA is then amplified and characterized using standard PCR techniques, employing primer pairs that can distinguish genomic cDNA from messenger cDNA. The bDNA assay involves the use of a solid-phase nucleic acid capture system and signal amplification through successive nucleic acid hybridizations to detect small quantities of HIV RNA. Both tests can achieve a tenfold increase in sensitivity to 40–50 copies of HIV RNA per milliliter with a preconcentration step in which plasma undergoes ultracentrifugation to pellet the viral particles. The NASBA technique involves the isothermal amplification of a sequence within the gag region of HIV in the presence of internal standards and employs the production of multiple RNA copies through the action of T7-RNA polymerase. The resulting RNA species are quantitated through hybridization with a molecular beacon DNA probe that is quenched in the absence of hybridization. The lower limit of detection for the NucliSens assay is 80 copies/mL.

In addition to being a diagnostic and prognostic tool, RT-PCR is also useful for amplifying defined areas of the HIV genome for sequence analysis and has become an important technique for studies of sequence diversity and microbial resistance to ARV agents. In patients with a positive or indeterminate EIA test and an indeterminate Western blot, and in patients in whom serologic testing may be unreliable (such as patients with hypogammaglobulinemia or advanced HIV disease), these tests for quantitating HIV RNA in plasma provide valuable tools for making a diagnosis of HIV infection; however, they should be used for diagnosis only when standard serologic testing has failed to provide a definitive result.

LABORATORY MONITORING OF PATIENTS WITH HIV INFECTION

The epidemic of HIV infection and AIDS has provided the clinician with new challenges for integrating clinical and laboratory data to effect optimal patient management. The close relationship between clinical manifestations of HIV infection and CD4+ T cell count has made measurement of the latter a routine part of the evaluation of HIV-infected individuals. Determinations of CD4+ T cell counts and measurements of the levels of HIV RNA in serum or plasma provide a powerful set of tools for determining prognosis and monitoring response to therapy.

CD4+ T Cell Counts The CD4+ T cell count is the laboratory test generally accepted as the best indicator of the immediate state of immunologic competence of the patient with HIV infection. This measurement, which can be made directly or calculated as the product of the percent of CD4+ T cells (determined by flow cytometry) and the total lymphocyte count [determined by the white blood cell count (WBC) and the differential percent], has been shown to correlate very well with the level of immunologic competence. Patients with CD4+ T cell counts <200/µL are at high risk of disease from *P. jiroveci*, while patients with CD4+ T cell counts <50/µL are at high risk of disease from CMV, mycobacteria of the *M. avium* complex (MAC) and/or *T. gondii* (Fig. 182-29). Patients with HIV infection should have CD4+ T cell measurements performed at the time of diagnosis and every 3–6 months thereafter. More frequent measurements should be made if a declining trend is noted. According to most guidelines, a CD4 T cell count <350/µL is an indication for consideration of initiating ARV therapy, and a decline in CD4+ T cell count of >25% is an indication for considering a change in therapy. Once the CD4+ T cell count is <200/µL, patients should be placed on a regimen for *P. jiroveci* prophylaxis, and once the count is <50/µL, primary prophylaxis for MAC infection is indicated. As with any laboratory measurement, one may wish to obtain two determinations prior to any significant changes in patient management based upon CD4+ T cell count alone. In patients with hypersplenism or who have undergone splenectomy the CD4+ T cell percentage may be a more reliable indication of immune function than the CD4+ T cell count. A CD4+ T cell percent of 15 is comparable to a CD4+ T cell count of 200/µL.

HIV RNA Determinations Facilitated by highly sensitive techniques for the precise quantitation of small amounts of nucleic acids, the measurement of serum or plasma levels of HIV RNA has become an essential component in the monitoring of patients with HIV infection. As discussed under diagnosis of HIV infection, the two most commonly used techniques are the RT-PCR assay and the bDNA assay. Both assays generate data in the form of number of copies of HIV RNA per milliliter of serum or plasma. Standard assays can detect as few as 40–50 copies of HIV RNA per milliliter of plasma, while research-based assays can detect down to one copy per milliliter. Although earlier versions of the bDNA assay generated values that were ~50% of those of the RT-PCR assay, the more recent versions (version 3 or higher) provide numbers essentially identical to those of the RT-PCR test (Fig. 182-28). While it is common practice to describe levels of HIV RNA

FIGURE 182-29 Relationship between CD4+ T cell counts and the development of opportunistic diseases. Boxplot of the median (line inside the box), first quartile (bottom of the box), third quartile (top of the box), and mean (asterisk) CD4+ lymphocyte count at the time of the development of opportunistic disease. Can, candidal esophagitis; CMV, cytomegalovirus infection; Crp, cryptosporidiosis; Cry, cryptococcal meningitis; DEM, AIDS dementia complex; HSV, herpes simplex virus infection; HZos, herpes zoster; KS, Kaposi's sarcoma; MAC, *Mycobacterium avium* complex bacteremia; NHL, non-Hodgkin's lymphoma; PCP, primary *Pneumocystis jiroveci* pneumonia; PCP2, secondary *P. jiroveci* pneumonia; PML, progressive multifocal leukoencephalopathy; Tox, *Toxoplasma gondii* encephalitis; WS, wasting syndrome. *(From RD Moore, RE Chaisson: Ann Intern Med 124:633, 1996.)*

below these cut-offs as "undetectable," this is a term that should be avoided as it is imprecise and leaves the false impression that the level of virus is 0. By utilizing more sensitive, nested PCR techniques and by studying tissue levels of virus as well as plasma levels, HIV RNA can be detected in virtually every patient with HIV infection. Measurements of changes in HIV RNA levels over time have been of great value in delineating the relationship between levels of virus and rates of disease progression (Fig. 182-20), the rates of viral turnover, the relationship between immune system activation and viral replication, and the time to development of drug resistance. HIV RNA measurements are greatly influenced by the state of activation of the immune system and may fluctuate greatly in the setting of secondary infections or immunization. For these reasons, decisions based upon HIV RNA levels should never be made on a single determination. Measurements of plasma HIV RNA levels should be made at the time of HIV diagnosis and every 3–6 months thereafter in the untreated patient. In general, most guidelines suggest that therapy be considered in patients with >100,000 copies of HIV RNA per milliliter (see below). Following the initiation of therapy or any change in therapy, plasma HIV RNA levels should be monitored approximately every 4 weeks until the effectiveness of the therapeutic regimen is determined by the development of a new steady-state level of HIV RNA. In most instances of effective therapy this will be <50 copies per milliliter. This level of virus is generally achieved within 6 months of the initiation of effective treatment. During therapy, levels of HIV RNA should be monitored every 3–4 months to evaluate the continuing effectiveness of therapy.

HIV Resistance Testing The availability of multiple ARV drugs as treatment options has generated a great deal of interest in the potential for measuring the sensitivity of an individual's HIV virus(es) to different ARV agents. HIV resistance testing can be done through either genotypic or phenotypic measurements. In the genotypic assays, sequence analyses of the HIV genomes obtained from patients are compared to sequences of viruses with known ARV resistance profiles. In the phenotypic assays, the in vivo growth of viral isolates obtained from the patient are compared to the growth of reference strains of the virus in the presence or absence of different ARV drugs. A modification of this phenotypic approach utilizes a comparison of the enzymatic activities of the reverse transcriptase or protease genes obtained by molecular cloning of patients' isolates to the enzymatic activities of genes obtained from ref-

erence strains of HIV in the presence or absence of different drugs targeted to these genes. These tests are quite good in identifying those ARV agents that have been utilized in the past and suggesting agents that may be of future value in a given patient. Drug resistance testing in the setting of virologic failure should be performed while the patient is still on the failing regimen because of the propensity for the pool of HIV quasispecies to rapidly revert to wild-type in the absence of the selective pressure of ARV therapy. In the hands of experts, resistance testing enhances the short-term ability to decrease viral load by ~0.5 log compared to changing drugs merely on the basis of drug history. In addition to the use of resistance testing to help in the selection of new drugs in patients with virologic failure, it may also be of value in selecting an initial regimen for treatment of therapy-naïve individuals. This is particularly true in geographic areas with a high level of background resistance.

Co-Receptor Tropism Assays Following the licensure of maraviroc as the first CCR5 antagonist for the treatment of HIV infection (see below), it became necessary to be able to determine whether or not a patient's virus was likely to respond to this treatment. Patients tend to have CCR5-tropic virus (see above) early in the course of infection with a trend toward CXCR4 viruses later in disease. Maraviroc is only effective against CCR5-tropic viruses. Due to the fact that the genotypic determinants of cellular tropism are poorly defined, a phenotypic assay is necessary to determine this property of HIV. Two commercial assays; the Trofile assay (Monogram Biosciences) and the Phenoscript assay (VIRalliance), are available to make this determination. These assays clone the envelope regions of the patient's virus into an indicator virus that is then used to infect target cells expressing either CCR5 or CXCR4 as their co-receptor. These assays take weeks to perform and are expensive.

Other Tests A variety of other laboratory tests have been studied as potential markers of HIV disease activity. Among these are quantitative culture of replication-competent HIV from plasma, peripheral blood mononuclear cells, or resting CD4+ T cells; circulating levels of β_2-microglobulin, soluble IL-2 receptor, IgA, acid-labile endogenous interferon, or TNF-α; and the presence or absence of activation markers such as CD38, HLA-DR, or PD-1 on CD8+ T cells. While these measurements have value as markers of disease activity and help to increase our understanding of the pathogenesis of HIV disease, they do not currently play a major role in the monitoring of patients with HIV infection.

CLINICAL MANIFESTATIONS

The clinical consequences of HIV infection encompass a spectrum ranging from an acute syndrome associated with primary infection to a prolonged asymptomatic state to advanced disease. It is best to regard HIV disease as beginning at the time of primary infection and progressing through various stages. As mentioned above, active virus replication and progressive immunologic impairment occur throughout the course of HIV infection in most patients. With the exception of the rare true long-term nonprogressors (see above), HIV disease in untreated patients inexorably progresses even during the clinically latent stage. However, ARV therapy has had a major impact on blocking or slowing the progression of disease over extended periods of time in a substantial proportion of adequately treated patients (see below).

FIGURE 182-30 The acute HIV syndrome. See text for detailed description. *(Adapted from G Pantaleo et al: N Engl J Med 328:327, 1993. Copyright 1993 Massachusetts Medical Society. All rights reserved.)*

THE ACUTE HIV SYNDROME

It is estimated that 50–70% of individuals with HIV infection experience an acute clinical syndrome ~3–6 weeks after primary infection (Fig. 182-30). Varying degrees of clinical severity have been reported, and although it has been suggested that symptomatic seroconversion leading to the seeking of medical attention indicates an increased risk for an accelerated course of disease, there does not appear to be a correlation between the level of the initial burst of viremia in acute HIV infection and the subsequent course of disease. The typical clinical findings in the acute HIV syndrome are listed in Table 182-7; they occur along with a burst of plasma viremia. It has been reported that several symptoms of the acute HIV syndrome (fever, skin rash, pharyngitis, and myalgia) occur less frequently in those infected by injection drug use versus those infected by sexual contact. The syndrome is typical of an acute viral syndrome and has been likened to acute infectious mononucleosis. Symptoms usually persist for one to several weeks and gradually subside as an immune response to HIV develops and the levels of plasma viremia decrease. Opportunistic infections have been reported during this stage of infection, reflecting the immunodeficiency that results from reduced numbers of CD4+ T cells and likely also from the dysfunction of CD4+ T cells owing to viral protein and endogenous cytokine-induced perturbations of cells (see "Mechanisms of CD4+ T Lymphocyte Depletion and Dysfunction," above) associated with the extremely high levels of plasma viremia. A number of immunologic abnormalities accompany the acute HIV syndrome, including multiphasic perturbations of the numbers of circulating lymphocyte subsets. The number of total lymphocytes and T cell subsets (CD4+ and CD8+) are initially reduced. An inversion of the CD4+/CD8+ T cell ratio occurs later because of a rise in the number of CD8+ T cells. In fact, there may be a selective and transient expansion of CD8+ T cell subsets, as determined by T cell receptor analysis (see above). The total circulating CD8+ T cell count may remain elevated or return to normal; however, CD4+ T cell levels usually remain somewhat depressed, although there may be a slight rebound toward normal. Lymphadenopathy occurs in ~70% of individuals with primary HIV infection. Most patients recover spontaneously from this syndrome and many are left with only a mildly depressed CD4+ T cell count that remains stable for a variable period before beginning its progressive decline (see below); in some individuals, the CD4+ T cell count returns to the normal range. Approximately 10% of patients manifest a fulminant course of immunologic and clinical deterioration after primary infection, even after the disappearance of initial symptoms. In most patients, primary infection with or without the acute syndrome is followed by a prolonged period of clinical latency or smoldering low disease activity. A small percentage of HIV-infected individuals treated with ARV drugs during acute infection may revert to a negative EIA test during the time they remain on therapy. They rapidly re-seroconvert with the discontinuation of treatment.

TABLE 182-7 CLINICAL FINDINGS IN THE ACUTE HIV SYNDROME 1169

General	Neurologic
Fever	Meningitis
Pharyngitis	Encephalitis
Lymphadenopathy	Peripheral neuropathy
Headache/retroorbital pain	Myelopathy
Arthralgias/myalgias	Dermatologic
Lethargy/malaise	Erythematous maculopapular
Anorexia/weight loss	rash
Nausea/vomiting/diarrhea	Mucocutaneous ulceration

Source: From B Tindall, DA Cooper: AIDS 5:1, 1991.

THE ASYMPTOMATIC STAGE—CLINICAL LATENCY

Although the length of time from initial infection to the development of clinical disease varies greatly, the median time for untreated patients is ~10 years. As emphasized above, HIV disease with active virus replication is ongoing and progressive during this asymptomatic period. The rate of disease progression is directly correlated with HIV RNA levels. Patients with high levels of HIV RNA in plasma progress to symptomatic disease faster than do patients with low levels of HIV RNA (Fig. 182-20). Some patients referred to as *long-term nonprogressors* show little if any decline in CD4+ T cell counts over extended periods of time. These patients generally have extremely low levels of HIV RNA with a subset, referred to as *elite nonprogressors*, exhibiting HIV RNA levels <50 copies per milliliter. Certain other patients remain entirely asymptomatic despite the fact that their CD4+ T cell counts show a steady progressive decline to extremely low levels. In these patients, the appearance of an opportunistic disease may be the first manifestation of HIV infection. During the asymptomatic period of HIV infection, the average rate of CD4+ T cell decline is ~50/μL per year. When the CD4+ T cell count falls to <200/μL, the resulting state of immunodeficiency is severe enough to place the patient at high risk for opportunistic infection and neoplasms, and hence for clinically apparent disease.

SYMPTOMATIC DISEASE

Symptoms of HIV disease can appear at any time during the course of HIV infection. Generally speaking, the spectrum of illnesses that one observes changes as the CD4+ T cell count declines. The more severe and life-threatening complications of HIV infection occur in patients with CD4+ T cell counts <200/μL. A diagnosis of AIDS is made in anyone with HIV infection and a CD4+ T cell count <200/μL and in anyone with HIV infection who develops one of the HIV-associated diseases considered to be indicative of a severe defect in cell-mediated immunity (category C, Table 182-2). While the causative agents of the secondary infections are characteristically opportunistic organisms such as *P. jiroveci*, atypical mycobacteria, CMV, and other organisms that do not ordinarily cause disease in the absence of a compromised immune system, they also include common bacterial and mycobacterial pathogens. Fewer than 50% of deaths among AIDS patients are as a direct result of an AIDS-defining illness, and the average CD4+ T cell count of an HIV-infected patient at the time of death is just over 300 cells/μL. Similarly, following the widespread use of combination ARV therapy and implementation of guidelines for the prevention of opportunistic infections (Table 182-8), the incidence of secondary infections has decreased dramatically (Fig. 182-31). Overall, the clinical spectrum of HIV disease is constantly changing as patients live longer and new and better approaches to treatment and prophylaxis are developed. In addition to the classic AIDS-defining illnesses, patients with HIV infection also have an increase in serious non-AIDS illnesses, including cardiovascular, renal, and hepatic disease. The physician providing care to a patient with HIV infection must be well versed in general internal medicine as well as HIV-related infectious diseases and new clinical syndromes related to chronic illness and long-term ARV therapy. In general, it should be stressed that a key element of treatment of symptomatic complications of HIV disease, whether they are primary or secondary, is achieving good control of HIV replication through the use of combination ARV therapy and instituting primary and secondary prophylaxis for opportunistic infections as indicated.

TABLE 182-8 NIH/CDC/IDSA 2008 GUIDELINES FOR THE PREVENTION OF OPPORTUNISTIC INFECTIONS IN PERSONS INFECTED WITH HIV

Pathogen	Indications	First Choice(s)	Alternatives
Recommended as Standard of Care for Primary and Secondary Prophylaxis			
Pneumocystis jiroveci	CD4+ T cell count <200/μL or Oropharyngeal candidiasis or Prior bout of PCP	Trimethoprim/sulfamethoxazole (TMP/SMZ), 1 DS tablet qd PO	Dapsone 50 mg bid PO or 100 mg/d PO Dapsone 50 mg/d PO + Pyrimethamine 50 mg/wk PO + Leucovorin 25 mg/wk PO
	May stop prophylaxis if CD4+ T cell count > 200/μL for ≥3 mo	TMP/SMZ, 1 SS tablet qd PO	Dapsone 200 mg PO + Pyrimethamine 75 mg PO + Leucovorin 25 mg PO weekly Aerosolized pentamidine, 300 mg qm via Respirgard II nebulizer Atovaquone 1500 mg/d PO TMP/SMZ 1 DS tablet PO 3×/wk
Mycobacterium tuberculosis			
Isoniazid sensitive	Skin test >5 mm or Prior positive test without treatment or Close contact with case of active pulmonary TB	Isoniazid 300 mg PO + Pyridoxine 50 mg PO qd ×9 mo Isoniazid 900 mg PO + Pyridoxine 100 mg PO 2 ×/wk ×9 mo	Isoniazid 900 mg PO + pyridoxine 50 mg PO 2×/wk × 9 mo Isoniazid 300 mg + rifampin 600 mg (or rifabutin 300 mg) + pyridoxine 50 mg/d ×4 mo
Isoniazid resistant	Same with high probability of exposure to isoniazid-resistant TB	Rifabutin 300 mg or Rifampin 600 mg PO qd ×4 mo	
Multidrug resistant	Same with high probability of exposure to multidrug resistant TB	Consult local public health authorities	
Mycobacterium-avium complex	CD4+ T cell count <50/μL	Azithromycin 1200 mg weekly PO or Clarithromycin 500 mg bid PO	Rifabutin 300 mg/d PO Azithromycin 1200 mg weekly PO + Rifabutin 300 mg/d PO
	Prior documented disseminated disease May stop prophylaxis if CD4+ T cell count > 100/μL for ≥3 mo	Clarithromycin 500 mg bid PO + Ethambutol 15 (mg/kg)/d PO +/– Rifabutin 300 mg/d PO	Azithromycin 500 mg/d PO + Ethambutol 15 (mg/kg)/d PO +/– Rifabutin 300 mg/d PO
Toxoplasma gondii	TOXO IgG antibody and CD4+ T cell count <100/μL	TMP/SMZ 1 DS tablet PO qd	TMP/SMZ 1 DS 3× weekly Dapsone 50 mg/d PO + Pyrimethamine 50 mg weekly PO + Leucovorin 25 mg weekly PO Dapsone 200 mg PO + Pyrimethamine 75 mg PO + Leucovorin 25 mg PO weekly Atovaquone 1500 mg PO +/– Pyrimethamine 25 mg PO + Leucovorin 10 mg PO daily
	Prior toxoplasmic encephalitis and CD4+ T cell count <200	Sulfadiazine 500–1000 mg qid PO + pyrimethamine 25–50 mg/d PO + leucovorin 10–25 mg/d PO	Clindamycin 600 mg q8h PO + Pyrimethamine 25–50 mg/d PO + Leucovorin 10–25 mg/d PO
	May stop prophylaxis if CD4+ T cell count >200/μL for ≥3 months		Atovaquone 750 mg PO q6–12 h +/– Pyrimethamine 25 mg/d + Leucovorin 10 mg/d PO
Varicella zoster virus	Significant exposure to chickenpox or shingles in a patient with no history of immunization or prior exposure to either	Varicella zoster immune globulin 6.25 mL, IM, within 96 h of exposure	
Cryptococcus neoformans	Prior documented disease May stop prophylaxis if CD4+ T cell count >200 for 6 mo and no evidence of active infection	Fluconazole 200 mg/d PO	Itraconazole 200 mg/d PO
Histoplasma capsulatum	Prior documented disease May stop prophylaxis after 1 year if CD4+ T cell count >150 and patient on ARV therapy for ≥6 mo	Itraconazole 200 mg bid PO	Fluconazole 800 mg/d PO
Coccidioides immitis	Prior documented disease or Positive serology and CD4+ T cell count <250 [For this indication prophylaxis can be stopped if CD4+ T cell count ≥250 for 6 mo.]	Fluconazole 400 mg/d PO	Itraconazole 200 mg bid PO
Penicillium marneffei	Prior documented disease May stop secondary prophylaxis in patients on ARVs with CD4+ T cell count >100 for ≥6 mo	Itraconazole 200 mg/d PO	
Salmonella species	Prior bacteremia	Ciprofloxacin 500 mg bid PO for 6 mo or more	
Bartonella	Prior infection May stop if CD4+ T cell count >200 for >3 mo	Doxycycline 200 mg/d Azithromycin 1200 mg weekly PO Clarithromycin 500 mg bid PO	
Cytomegalovirus	Prior end-organ disease May stop prophylaxis if CD4+ T cell count > 100/μL for 6 mo and no evidence of active CMV disease Restart if prior retinitis and CD4+ T cells <100/μL	Ganciclovir, 5–6 mg/kg 5–7 d/wk IV Valganciclovir 900 mg bid PO Foscarnet 90–120 (mg/kg)/d IV Ganciclovir sustained-release implant q6–9mo + Valganciclovir 900 mg bid PO	Cidofovir 5 mg/kg every other week IV + Probenecid Formivirsen 330 μg intravitreal q2–4 wk Valganciclovir 900 mg PO daily Formivirsen, 1 vial injected into the vitreous q2–4wk

(continued)

Pathogen	Indications	First Choice(s)	Alternatives
Immunizations Generally Recommended			
Hepatitis B virus	All susceptible (anti-HBc and anti-HBs negative) patients	Hepatitis B vaccine: 3 doses	
Hepatitis A virus	All susceptible (anti-HAV negative) patients	Hepatitis A vaccine: 2 doses	
Influenza virus	All patients annually	Inactivated trivalent influenza virus vaccine 1 dose yearly	Oseltamivir 75 mg PO qd Rimantadine or amantadine 100 mg PO bid (influenza A only)
Streptococcus pneumoniae	All patients, preferably before CD4+ T cell count ≥200/μL	Pneumoccal vaccine 0.5 mL IM ×1 if CD4+ T cell count >200/μL Reimmunize patients initially immunized at a CD4+ T cell count <100/μL whose CD4+ T cell count then increases to >200/μL	
Human papilloma virus	Girls and women 9–26 years of age	HPV vaccine; 3 doses	
Recommended for Prevention of Severe or Frequent Recurrences			
Herpes simplex	Frequent/severe recurrences	Acyclovir 200 mg tid PO Acyclovir 400 mg bid PO Famciclovir 250 mg bid PO	Valacyclovir 500 mg PO bid
Candida	Frequent/severe recurrences	Fluconazole 100–200 mg/d PO	Itraconazole solution 200 mg/d PO

Note: DS, double strength; SS, single strength; PCP, *Pneumocystis carinii* pneumonia; TB, tuberculosis.

Disease of the Respiratory System Acute bronchitis and sinusitis are prevalent during all stages of HIV infection. The most severe cases tend to occur in patients with lower CD4+ T cell counts. Sinusitis presents as

FIGURE 182-31 A. Decrease in the incidence of opportunistic infections and Kaposi's sarcoma in HIV-infected individuals with CD4+ T cell counts <100/μL from 1992 through 1998. [*Adapted and updated from FJ Palella et al: N Engl J Med 338:853, 1998, and JE Kaplan et al: Clin Infect Dis 30(S1):S5, 2000, with permission.*] **B.** Quarterly incidence rates of cytomegalovirus (CMV), *Pneumocystis jiroveci* pneumonia (PCP), and *Mycobacterium avium* complex (MAC) from 1995–2001. (*From FJ Palella et al: AIDS 16:1617, 2002.*)

fever, nasal congestion, and headache. The diagnosis is made by CT or MRI. The maxillary sinuses are most commonly involved; however, disease is also frequently seen in the ethmoid, sphenoid, and frontal sinuses. While some patients may improve without antibiotic therapy, radiographic improvement is quicker and more pronounced in patients who have received antimicrobial therapy. It is postulated that this high incidence of sinusitis results from an increased frequency of infection with encapsulated organisms such as *H. influenzae* and *Streptococcus pneumoniae*. In patients with low CD4+ T cell counts one may see mucormycosis infections of the sinuses. In contrast to the course of this infection in other patient populations, mucormycosis of the sinuses in patients with HIV infection may progress more slowly. In this setting aggressive, frequent local debridement in addition to local and systemic amphotericin B may be needed for effective treatment.

Pulmonary disease is one of the most frequent complications of HIV infection. The most common manifestation of pulmonary disease is pneumonia. The two most common causes of pneumonia are bacterial infections and the unicellular fungus *P. jiroveci* infection. Other major causes of pulmonary infiltrates include mycobacterial infections, other fungal infections, nonspecific interstitial pneumonitis, KS, and lymphoma.

Pneumonia is seen with an increased frequency in patients with HIV infection; they appear to be particularly prone to infections with encapsulated organisms. *S. pneumoniae* (Chap. 128) and *H. influenzae* (Chap. 139) are responsible for most cases of bacterial pneumonia in patients with AIDS. This may be a consequence of altered B cell function and/or defects in neutrophil function that may be secondary to HIV disease (see above). *S. pneumoniae* (pneumococcal) infection may be the earliest serious infection to occur in patients with HIV disease. This can present as pneumonia, sinusitis, and/or bacteremia. Patients with untreated HIV infection have a sixfold increase in the incidence of pneumococcal pneumonia and a 100-fold increase in the incidence of pneumococcal bacteremia. Pneumococcal disease may be seen in patients with relatively intact immune systems. In one study, the baseline CD4+ T cell count at the time of a first episode of pneumococcal pneumonia was ~300/μL. Of interest is the fact that the inflammatory response to pneumococcal infection appears proportional to the CD4+ T cell count. Due to this high risk of pneumococcal disease, immunization with pneumococcal polysaccharide is one of the generally recommended prophylactic measures for patients with HIV infection. This is likely most effective if given while the CD4+ T cell count is >200/μL. It is less clear whether this intervention is effective when given to patients with more advanced disease and high viral loads.

CHAPTER 182

Human Immunodeficiency Virus Disease: AIDS and Related Disorders

Pneumocystis pneumonia (PCP), once the hallmark of AIDS, has dramatically declined in incidence following the development of effective prophylactic regimens and the widespread use of combination ARV therapy. It is, however, the single most common cause of pneumonia in patients with HIV infection in the United States and can be identified as a likely etiologic agent in 25% of cases of pneumonia in patients with HIV infection. Approximately 25% of cases of HIV-associated PCP occur in patients who are unaware of their HIV status. The risk of PCP is greatest among those who have experienced a previous bout of PCP and those who have CD4+ T cell counts of <200/μL. Overall, 79% of patients with PCP have CD4+ T cell counts <100/μL and 95% of patients have CD4+ T cell counts <200/μL. Recurrent fever, night sweats, thrush, and unexplained weight loss are also associated with an increased incidence of PCP. For these reasons, it is strongly recommended that all patients with CD4+ T cell counts <200/μL (or a CD4 percentage <15) receive some form of PCP prophylaxis. The incidence of PCP is approaching zero in patients with known HIV infection receiving appropriate ARV therapy and prophylaxis. In the United States, primary PCP is now occurring at a median CD4+ T cell count of 36/μL, while secondary PCP is occurring at a median CD4+ T cell count of 10/μL. Patients with PCP generally present with fever and a cough that is usually nonproductive or productive of only scant amounts of white sputum. They may complain of a characteristic retrosternal chest pain that is worse on inspiration and is described as sharp or burning. HIV-associated PCP may have an indolent course characterized by weeks of vague symptoms and should be included in the differential diagnosis of fever, pulmonary complaints, or unexplained weight loss in any patient with HIV infection and <200 CD4+ T cells/μL. The most common finding on chest x-ray is either a normal film, if the disease is suspected early, or a faint bilateral interstitial infiltrate. The classic finding of a dense perihilar infiltrate is unusual in patients with AIDS. In patients with PCP who have been receiving aerosolized pentamidine for prophylaxis, one may see an x-ray picture of upper lobe cavitary disease, reminiscent of TB. Other less common findings on chest x-ray include lobar infiltrates and pleural effusions. Routine laboratory evaluation is usually of little help in the differential diagnosis of PCP. A mild leukocytosis is common, although this may not be obvious in patients with prior neutropenia. Arterial blood gases may indicate hypoxemia with a decline in Pa_{O_2} and an increase in the arterial-alveolar (a − A) gradient. Arterial blood gas measurements not only aid in making the diagnosis of PCP but also provide important information for staging the severity of the disease and directing treatment (see below). A definitive diagnosis of PCP requires demonstration of the organism in samples obtained from induced sputum, bronchoalveolar lavage, transbronchial biopsy, or open lung biopsy. PCR has been used to detect specific DNA sequences for *P. jiroveci* in clinical specimens where histologic examinations have failed to make a diagnosis.

In addition to pneumonia, a number of other clinical problems have been reported in HIV-infected patients as a result of infection with *P. jiroveci*. Otic involvement may be seen as a primary infection, presenting as a polypoid mass involving the external auditory canal. In patients receiving aerosolized pentamidine for prophylaxis against PCP one may see a variety of extrapulmonary manifestations of *P. jiroveci*. These include ophthalmic lesions of the choroid, a necrotizing vasculitis that resembles Burger's disease, bone marrow hypoplasia, and intestinal obstruction. Other organs that have been involved include lymph nodes, spleen, liver, kidney, pancreas, pericardium, heart, thyroid, and adrenals. Organ infection may be associated with cystic lesions that may appear calcified on CT or ultrasound.

The standard treatment for PCP or disseminated pneumocystosis is trimethoprim/sulfamethoxazole (TMP/SMX). A high incidence of side effects, particularly skin rash and bone marrow suppression, is seen with TMP/SMX in patients with HIV infection. Alternative treatments for mild to moderate PCP include dapsone/trimethoprim and clindamycin/primaquine. Intravenous pentamidine is the treatment of choice for severe disease in the patient unable to tolerate TMP/SMX. For patients with a Pa_{O_2} < 70 mmHg or with an a − A gradient >35 mmHg,

adjunct glucocorticoid therapy should be used in addition to specific antimicrobials. Overall, treatment should be for 21 days and followed by secondary prophylaxis. Prophylaxis for PCP is indicated for any HIV-infected individual who has experienced a prior bout of PCP, any patient with a CD4+ T cell count of <200/μL or a CD4 percentage <15, any patient with unexplained fever for >2 weeks, and any patient with a history of oropharyngeal candidiasis. The preferred regimen for prophylaxis is TMP/SMX, one double-strength tablet daily. This regimen also provides protection against toxoplasmosis and some bacterial respiratory pathogens. For patients who cannot tolerate TMP/SMX, alternatives for prophylaxis include dapsone plus pyrimethamine plus leucovorin, aerosolized pentamidine administered by the Respirgard II nebulizer, and atovaquone. Primary or secondary prophylaxis for PCP can be discontinued in those patients treated with combination ARV therapy who maintain good suppression of HIV (<50 copies per milliliter) and CD4+ T cell counts >200/μL for 3–6 months.

M. tuberculosis, once thought to be on its way to extinction in the United States, experienced a resurgence associated with the HIV epidemic (Chap. 158). Worldwide, approximately one-third of all AIDS-related deaths are associated with TB. In the United States ~5% of AIDS patients have active TB. HIV infection increases the risk of developing active TB by a factor of 100. For the patient with untreated HIV infection and a positive PPD skin test, the rate of reactivation TB is 7–10% per year. Untreated TB can accelerate the course of HIV infection. Levels of plasma HIV RNA increase in the setting of active TB and decline in the setting of successful TB treatment. Active TB is most common in patients 25–44 years of age, in African Americans and Hispanics, in patients in New York City and Miami, and in patients in developing countries. In these demographic groups, 20–70% of the new cases of active TB are in patients with HIV infection. The epidemic of TB embedded in the epidemic of HIV infection probably represents the greatest health risk to the general public and the health care profession associated with the HIV epidemic. In contrast to infection with atypical mycobacteria such as MAC, active TB often develops relatively early in the course of HIV infection and may be an early clinical sign of HIV disease. In one study, the median CD4+ T cell count at presentation of TB was 326/μL. The clinical manifestations of TB in HIV-infected patients are quite varied and generally show different patterns as a function of the CD4+ T cell count. In patients with relatively high CD4+ T cell counts, the typical pattern of pulmonary reactivation occurs in which patients present with fever, cough, dyspnea on exertion, weight loss, night sweats, and a chest x-ray revealing cavitary apical disease of the upper lobes. In patients with lower CD4+ T cell counts, disseminated disease is more common. In these patients the chest x-ray may reveal diffuse or lower lobe bilateral reticulonodular infiltrates consistent with miliary spread, pleural effusions, and hilar and/or mediastinal adenopathy. Infection may be present in bone, brain, meninges, gastrointestinal tract, lymph nodes (particularly cervical lymph nodes), and viscera. Approximately 60–80% of patients have pulmonary disease, and 30–40% have extrapulmonary disease. Respiratory isolation and a negative-pressure room should be used for patients in whom a diagnosis of pulmonary TB is being considered. This approach is critical to limit nosocomial and community spread of infection. Culture of the organism from an involved site provides a definitive diagnosis. Blood cultures are positive in 15% of patients. This figure is higher in patients with lower CD4 +T cell counts. In the setting of fulminant disease one cannot rely upon the accuracy of a negative PPD skin test to rule out a diagnosis of TB. TB is one of the conditions associated with HIV infection for which cure is possible with appropriate therapy. Therapy for TB is generally the same in the HIV-infected patient as in the HIV-negative patient (Chap. 158). Due to the possibility of multidrug resistant or extensively drug-resistant TB, drug susceptibility testing should be performed to guide therapy. Due to pharmacokinetic interactions, adjusted doses of rifabutin should be substituted for rifampin in patients receiving the HIV protease inhibitors or nonnucleoside reverse transcriptase inhibitors. Treatment is most effective in programs that involve directly observed therapy. Initiation of ARV therapy and/or anti-TB therapy may be associated with clinical deterioration due to immune reconstitution inflammatory syndrome (IRIS) reactions. These are most common in patients initiating both treatments at the same time, occur several weeks following initiation of therapy, and are seen more frequently in patients with advanced HIV disease. Effective prevention of active TB can be a reality if the health care professional is aggressive in looking for evidence of latent TB by making sure that all patients with HIV infection receive a PPD skin test or evaluation with an interferon-γ release assay. Anergy testing is not of value in this setting. HIV-infected individuals with a skin test reaction of >5 mm, a positive interferon-γ release assay or those who are close household contacts of persons with active TB should receive treatment with 9 months of isoniazid.

Atypical mycobacterial infections are also seen with an increased frequency in patients with HIV infection. Infections with at least 12 different mycobacteria have been reported, including *M. bovis* and representatives of all four Runyon groups. The most common atypical mycobacterial infection is with *M. avium* or *M. intracellulare* species—MAC. Infections with MAC are seen mainly in patients in the United States and are rare in Africa. It has been suggested that prior infection with *M. tuberculosis* decreases the risk of MAC infection. MAC infections probably arise from organisms that are ubiquitous in the environment, including both soil and water. The presumed portals of entry are the respiratory and gastrointestinal tract. MAC infection is a late complication of HIV infection, predominantly occurring in patients with CD4+ T cell counts of <50/μL. The average CD4+ T cell count at the time of diagnosis is 10/μL. The most common presentation is disseminated disease with fever, weight loss, and night sweats. At least 85% of patients with MAC infection are mycobacteremic, and large numbers of organisms can often be demonstrated on bone marrow biopsy. The chest x-ray is abnormal in ~25% of patients, with the most common pattern being that of a bilateral, lower lobe infiltrate suggestive of miliary spread. Alveolar or nodular infiltrates and hilar and/or mediastinal adenopathy can also occur. Other clinical findings include endobronchial lesions, abdominal pain, diarrhea, and lymphadenopathy. The diagnosis is made by the culture of blood or involved tissue. The finding of two consecutive sputum samples positive for MAC is highly suggestive of pulmonary infection. Cultures may take 2 weeks to turn positive. Therapy consists of a macrolide, usually clarithromycin, with ethambutol. Some physicians elect to add a third drug from among rifabutin, ciprofloxacin, or amikacin in patients with extensive disease. Therapy is generally for life; however, with the use of highly active antiretroviral therapy (HAART), it is possible to discontinue therapy in patients with sustained suppression of HIV replication and CD4+ T cell counts >100/μL for 3–6 months. Primary prophylaxis for MAC is indicated in patients with HIV infection and CD4+ T cell counts <50/μL. This may be discontinued in patients in whom HAART induces a sustained suppression of viral replication and increases in CD4+ T cell counts to >100/μL for 3–6 months.

Rhodococcus equi is a gram-positive pleomorphic acid-fast nonspore-forming bacillus that can cause pulmonary and/or disseminated infection in patients with HIV infection. Fever and cough are the most common presenting signs. Radiographically one may see cavitary lesions and consolidation. Blood cultures are often positive. Treatment is based upon antimicrobial sensitivity testing.

Fungal infections of the lung, in addition to PCP, can be seen in patients with AIDS. Patients with pulmonary cryptococcal disease present with fever, cough, dyspnea, and in some cases, hemoptysis. A focal or diffuse interstitial infiltrate is seen on chest x-ray in >90% of patients. In addition, one may see lobar disease, cavitary disease, pleural effusions, and hilar or mediastinal adenopathy. Over half of patients are fungemic, and 90% of patients have concomitant CNS infection. *Coccidioides immitis* is a mold that is endemic in the southwest United States. It can cause a reactivation pulmonary syndrome in patients with HIV infection. Most patients with this condition will have CD4+ T cell counts <250/μL. Patients present with fever, weight loss, cough, and extensive, diffuse reticulonodular infiltrates on chest x-ray. One may also see nodules, cavities, pleural effusions, and hilar adenopathy. While serologic testing is of value in the immunocompe-

tent host, serologies are negative in 25% of HIV-infected patients with coccidioidal infection. Invasive aspergillosis is not an AIDS-defining illness and is generally not seen in patients with AIDS in the absence of neutropenia or administration of glucocorticoids. *Aspergillus* infection may have an unusual presentation in the respiratory tract of patients with AIDS where it gives the appearance of a pseudomembranous tracheobronchitis. Primary pulmonary infection of the lung may be seen with *histoplasmosis*. The most common pulmonary manifestation of histoplasmosis, however, is in the setting of disseminated disease, presumably due to reactivation. In this setting respiratory symptoms are usually minimal, with cough and dyspnea occurring in 10–30% of patients. The chest x-ray is abnormal in ~50% of patients, showing either a diffuse interstitial infiltrate or diffuse small nodules.

Two forms of *idiopathic interstitial pneumonia* have been identified in patients with HIV infection: lymphoid interstitial pneumonitis (LIP) and nonspecific interstitial pneumonitis (NIP). LIP, a common finding in children, is seen in about 1% of adult patients with untreated HIV infection. This disorder is characterized by a benign infiltrate of the lung and is thought to be part of the polyclonal activation of lymphocytes seen in the context of HIV and EBV infections. Transbronchial biopsy is diagnostic in 50% of the cases, with an open-lung biopsy required for diagnosis in the remainder of cases. This condition is generally self-limited and no specific treatment is necessary. Severe cases have been managed with brief courses of glucocorticoids. Although rarely a clinical problem since the use of HAART, evidence of NIP may be seen in up to half of all patients with untreated HIV infection. Histologically, interstitial infiltrates of lymphocytes and plasma cells in a perivascular and peribronchial distribution are present. When symptomatic, patients present with fever and nonproductive cough occasionally accompanied by mild chest discomfort. Chest x-ray is usually normal or may reveal a faint interstitial pattern. Similar to LIP, NIP is a self-limited process for which no therapy is indicated other than appropriate management of the underlying HIV infection. HIV-related pulmonary arterial hypertension (HIV-PAH) is seen in ~0.5% of HIV-infected individuals. Patients may present with an array of symptoms including shortness of breath, fatigue, syncope, chest pain, and signs of right-sided heart failure. Chest x-ray reveals dilated pulmonary vessels and right-sided cardiomegaly with right ventricular hypertrophy seen on electrocardiogram. ARV therapy does not appear to be of clear benefit, and the prognosis is quite poor with a median survival in the range of 2 years.

Neoplastic diseases of the lung including KS and lymphoma are discussed below in the section on malignancies.

Diseases of the Cardiovascular System   Heart disease is a relatively common postmortem finding in HIV-infected patients (25–75% in autopsy series). Cardiovascular disease may be seen as a direct consequence of HIV infection or as a consequence of ARV therapy as part of the lipodystrophy syndrome. As a primary consequence of HIV infection, the most common clinically significant finding is a dilated cardiomyopathy associated with congestive heart failure (CHF), referred to as *HIV-associated cardiomyopathy*. This generally occurs as a late complication of HIV infection and, histologically, displays elements of myocarditis. For this reason some have advocated treatment with intravenous immunoglobulin (IVIg). HIV can be directly demonstrated in cardiac tissue in this setting, and there is debate over whether or not it plays a direct role in this condition. Patients present with typical findings of CHF, namely edema and shortness of breath. Patients with HIV infection may also develop cardiomyopathy as side effects of IFN-α or nucleoside analogue therapy. These are reversible once therapy is stopped. KS, cryptococcosis, Chagas' disease, and toxoplasmosis can involve the myocardium, leading to cardiomyopathy. In one series, most patients with HIV infection and a treatable myocarditis were found to have myocarditis associated with toxoplasmosis. Most of these patients also had evidence of CNS toxoplasmosis. Thus, MRI or double-dose contrast CT scan of the brain should be included in the workup of any patient with advanced HIV infection and cardiomyopathy.

A variety of other cardiovascular problems are found in patients with HIV infection. Pericardial effusions may be seen in the setting of advanced HIV infection. Predisposing factors include TB, CHF, mycobacterial infection, cryptococcal infection, pulmonary infection, lymphoma, and KS. While pericarditis is quite rare, in one series 5% of patients with HIV disease had pericardial effusions that were considered to be moderate or severe. Tamponade and death have occurred in association with pericardial KS, presumably owing to acute hemorrhage. Nonbacterial thrombotic endocarditis has been reported and should be considered in patients with unexplained embolic phenomena. Intravenous pentamidine, when given rapidly, can result in hypotension as a consequence of cardiovascular collapse. A high percentage of patients have hypertriglyceridemia and elevations in serum cholesterol, and coronary artery disease has been a relatively frequent finding at autopsy. This problem appears to becoming even more prevalent as a side effect of HAART and in particular in patients with co-infection with HCV. While the clinical significance of these findings has not been precisely defined, recent data suggest a linear relationship between time on HAART and development of ischemic heart disease. In one large series the overall rate of myocardial infarction (MI) was 3.5/1000 years, 28% of these events were fatal, and MI was responsible for 7% of all deaths in the cohort. The risk of MI increased by 26% per year of HAART. This small increase in the risk of death from MI in the setting of HAART has to be balanced against the marked increase in overall survival brought about by HAART. Efforts to decrease the risk of cardiovascular diseases by minimizing the time on HAART were associated with a paradoxical increase in the rate of cardiovascular disease suggesting that the pathogenesis of cardiovascular diseases in the setting of HIV infection is multifactorial, with HIV infection and the resulting immune activation and coagulopathy likely playing a significant role.

Diseases of the Oropharynx and Gastrointestinal System   Oropharyngeal and gastrointestinal diseases are common features of HIV infection. They are most frequently due to secondary infections. In addition, oral and gastrointestinal lesions may occur with KS and lymphoma.

Oral lesions, including *thrush*, *hairy leukoplakia*, and *aphthous ulcers* (Fig. 182-32), are particularly common in patients with untreated HIV infection. Thrush, due to *Candida* infection, and oral hairy leukoplakia, presumed due to EBV, are usually indicative of fairly advanced immunologic decline; they generally occur in patients with CD4+ T cell counts of <300/μL. In one study, 59% of patients with oral candidiasis went on to develop AIDS in the next year. Thrush appears as a white, cheesy exudate, often on an erythematous mucosa in the posterior oropharynx. While most commonly seen on the soft palate, early lesions are often found along the gingival border. The diagnosis is made by direct examination of a scraping for pseudohyphal elements. Culturing is of no diagnostic value, as most patients with HIV infection will have a positive throat culture for *Candida* even in the absence of thrush. Oral hairy leukoplakia presents as white, frondlike lesions, generally along the lateral borders of the tongue and sometimes on the adjacent buccal mucosa (Fig. 182-32). Despite its name, oral hairy leukoplakia is not considered a premalignant condition. Lesions are associated with florid replication of EBV. While usually more disconcerting

FIGURE 182-32 Various oral lesions in HIV-infected individuals. A. Thrush. **B.** Hairy leukoplakia. **C.** Aphthous ulcer. **D.** Kaposi's sarcoma.

FIGURE 182-33 Barium swallow of a patient with *Candida* esophagitis. The flow of barium along the mucosal surface is grossly irregular.

as a sign of HIV-associated immunodeficiency than a clinical problem in need of treatment, severe cases have been reported to respond to topical podophyllin or systemic therapy with anti-herpesvirus agents. Aphthous ulcers of the posterior oropharynx are also seen with regularity in patients with HIV infection (Fig. 182-32). These lesions are of unknown etiology and can be quite painful and interfere with swallowing. Topical anesthetics provide immediate symptomatic relief of short duration. The fact that thalidomide is an effective treatment for this condition suggests that the pathogenesis may involve the action of tissue-destructive cytokines. Palatal, glossal, or gingival ulcers may also result from cryptococcal disease or histoplasmosis.

Esophagitis (Fig. 182-33) may present with odynophagia and retrosternal pain. Upper endoscopy is generally required to make an accurate diagnosis. Esophagitis may be due to *Candida*, CMV, or HSV. While CMV tends to be associated with a single large ulcer, HSV infection is more often associated with multiple small ulcers. The esophagus may also be the site of KS and lymphoma. Like the oral mucosa, the esophageal mucosa may have large, painful ulcers of unclear etiology that may respond to thalidomide. While achlorhydria is a common problem in patients with HIV infection, other gastric problems are generally rare. Among the conditions involving the stomach are KS and lymphoma. Infections of the small and large intestine leading to diarrhea, abdominal pain, and occasionally fever are among the most significant gastrointestinal problems in HIV-infected patients. They include infections with bacteria, protozoa, and viruses.

Bacteria may be responsible for secondary infections of the gastrointestinal tract. Infections with enteric pathogens such as *Salmonella*, *Shigella*, and *Campylobacter* are more common in homosexual men and are often more severe and more apt to relapse in patients with HIV infection. Patients with untreated HIV have approximately a 20-fold increased risk of infection with *S. typhimurium*. They may present with a variety of nonspecific symptoms including fever, anorexia, fatigue, and malaise of several weeks' duration. Diarrhea is common but may be absent. Diagnosis is made by culture of blood and stool. Long-term therapy with ciprofloxacin is the recommended treatment. HIV-infected patients also have an increased incidence of *S. typhi* infection in areas of the world where typhoid is a problem. *Shigella* spp., particularly *S. flexneri*, can cause severe intestinal disease in HIV-infected individuals. Up to 50% of patients will develop bacteremia. *Campylobacter* in-

fections occur with an increased frequency in patients with HIV infection. While *C. jejuni* is the strain most frequently isolated, infections with many other strains have been reported. Patients usually present with crampy abdominal pain, fever, and bloody diarrhea. Infection may present as proctitis. Stool examination reveals the presence of fecal leukocytes. Systemic infection can occur, with up to 10% of infected patients exhibiting bacteremia. Most strains are sensitive to erythromycin. Abdominal pain and diarrhea may be seen with MAC infection.

Fungal infections may also be a cause of diarrhea in patients with HIV infection. Histoplasmosis, coccidioidomycosis, and penicilliosis have all been identified as a cause of fever and diarrhea in patients with HIV infection. Peritonitis has been seen with *C. immitis*.

Cryptosporidia, microsporidia, and *Isospora belli* (Chap. 208) are the most common opportunistic protozoa that infect the gastrointestinal tract and cause diarrhea in HIV-infected patients. Cryptosporidial infection may present in a variety of ways, ranging from a self-limited or intermittent diarrheal illness in patients in the early stages of HIV infection to a severe, life-threatening diarrhea in severely immunodeficient individuals. In patients with untreated HIV infection and CD4+ T cell counts of <300/μL, the incidence of cryptosporidiosis is ~1% per year. In 75% of cases the diarrhea is accompanied by crampy abdominal pain, and 25% of patients have nausea and/or vomiting. Cryptosporidia may also cause biliary tract disease in the HIV-infected patient, leading to cholecystitis with or without accompanying cholangitis. The diagnosis of cryptosporidial diarrhea is made by stool examination. The diarrhea is noninflammatory, and the characteristic finding is the presence of oocysts that stain with acid-fast dyes. Therapy is predominantly supportive, and marked improvements have been reported in the setting of effective ARV therapy. Treatment with up to 2000 mg/d of nitazoxanide (NTZ) is associated with improvement in symptoms or a decrease in shedding of organisms in about half of patients. Its overall role in the management of this condition remains unclear. Patients can minimize their risk of developing cryptosporidiosis by avoiding contact with human and animal feces and by not drinking untreated water from lakes or rivers.

Microsporidia are small, unicellular, obligate intracellular parasites that reside in the cytoplasm of enteric cells (Chap. 208). The main species causing disease in humans is *Enterocytozoon bieneusi*. The clinical manifestations are similar to those described for cryptosporidia and include abdominal pain and diarrhea. The small size of the organism may make it difficult to detect; however, with the use of chromotrope-based stains, organisms can be identified in stool samples by light microscopy. Definitive diagnosis generally depends on electron-microscopic examination of a stool specimen, intestinal aspirate, or intestinal biopsy specimen. In contrast to cryptosporidia, microsporidia have been noted in a variety of extraintestinal locations, including the eye, muscle, and liver, and have been associated with conjunctivitis and hepatitis. Albendazole, 400 mg bid, has been reported to be of benefit in some patients.

I. belli is a coccidian parasite (Chap. 208) most commonly found as a cause of diarrhea in patients from the Caribbean and Africa. Its cysts appear in the stool as large, acid-fast structures that can be differentiated from those of cryptosporidia on the basis of size, shape, and number of sporocysts. The clinical syndromes of *Isospora* infection are identical to those caused by cryptosporidia. The important distinction is that infection with *Isospora* is generally relatively easy to treat with TMP/SMX. While relapses are common, a thrice-weekly regimen of TMP/SMX appears adequate to prevent recurrence.

CMV colitis was once seen as a consequence of advanced immunodeficiency in 5–10% of patients with AIDS. It is much less common with the advent of HAART. CMV colitis presents as diarrhea, abdominal pain, weight loss, and anorexia. The diarrhea is usually nonbloody, and the diagnosis is achieved through endoscopy and biopsy. Multiple mucosal ulcerations are seen at endoscopy, and biopsies reveal characteristic intranuclear inclusion bodies. Secondary bacteremias may result as a consequence of thinning of the bowel wall. Treatment is with either ganciclovir or foscarnet for 3–6 weeks. Relapses are common, and maintenance therapy is typically necessary in patients whose HIV infection is poorly controlled. Patients with CMV disease of the gastrointestinal tract should be carefully monitored for evidence of CMV retinitis.

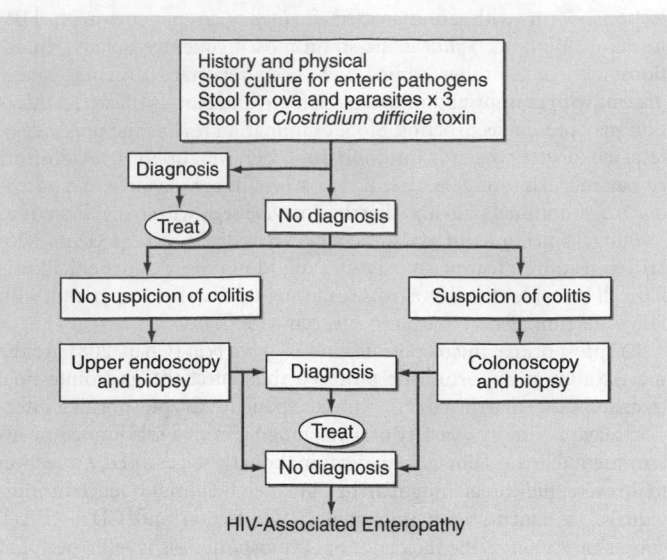

FIGURE 182-34 Algorithm for the evaluation of diarrhea in a patient with HIV infection. HIV-associated enteropathy is a diagnosis of exclusion and can be made only after other, generally treatable, forms of diarrheal illness have been ruled out.

FIGURE 182-35 Severe, erosive perirectal herpes simplex in a patient with AIDS.

In addition to disease caused by specific secondary infections, patients with HIV infection may also experience a chronic diarrheal syndrome for which no etiologic agent other than HIV can be identified. This entity is referred to as *AIDS enteropathy* or *HIV enteropathy*. It is most likely a direct result of HIV infection in the gastrointestinal tract. Histologic examination of the small bowel in these patients reveals low-grade mucosal atrophy with a decrease in mitotic figures, suggesting a hyporegenerative state. Patients often have decreased or absent small-bowel lactase and malabsorption with accompanying weight loss.

The initial evaluation of a patient with HIV infection and diarrhea should include a set of stool examinations, including culture, examination for ova and parasites, and examination for *Clostridium difficile* toxin. Approximately 50% of the time this workup will demonstrate infection with pathogenic bacteria, mycobacteria, or protozoa. If the initial stool examinations are negative, additional evaluation, including upper and/or lower endoscopy with biopsy, will yield a diagnosis of microsporidial or mycobacterial infection of the small intestine ~30% of the time. In patients for whom this diagnostic evaluation is nonrevealing, a presumptive diagnosis of HIV enteropathy can be made if the diarrhea has persisted for >1 month. An algorithm for the evaluation of diarrhea in patients with HIV infection is given in Fig. 182-34.

Rectal lesions are common in HIV-infected patients, particularly the perirectal ulcers and erosions due to the reactivation of HSV (Fig. 182-35). These may appear quite atypical, as denuded skin without vesicles, and they respond well to treatment with acyclovir, famciclovir, or foscarnet. Other rectal lesions encountered in patients with HIV infection include condylomata acuminata, KS, and intraepithelial neoplasia (see below).

Hepatobiliary Disease Diseases of the hepatobiliary system are a major problem in patients with HIV infection. It has been estimated that approximately one-third of the deaths of patients with HIV infection are in some way related to liver disease. While this is predominantly a reflection of the problems encountered in the setting of co-infection with hepatitis B or C, it is also a reflection of the hepatic injury, ranging from hepatic steatosis to hypersensitivity reactions to immune reconstitution, that can be seen in the context of ARV therapy.

The prevalence of co-infection with HIV and hepatitis viruses varies by geographic region. In the United States, ~90% of HIV-infected individuals have evidence of infection with HBV; 6–14% have chronic HBV infection; 5–50% of patients are co-infected with HCV; and co-infection with hepatitis D, E, and/or G viruses is common. Among IV

drug users with HIV infection, rates of HCV infection range from 70–95%. HIV infection has a significant impact on the course of hepatitis virus infection. It is associated with approximately a threefold increase in the development of persistent hepatitis B surface antigenemia. Patients infected with both HBV and HIV have decreased evidence of inflammatory liver disease. The presumption that this is due to the immunosuppressive effects of HIV infection is supported by the observations that this situation can be reversed, and one may see the development of more severe hepatitis following the initiation of effective ARV therapy. In studies of the impact of HIV on HBV infection four- to tenfold increases in liver-related mortality have been noted in patients with HIV and active HBV infection compared to rates in patients with either infection alone. There is a slight increase in overall mortality in HIV-infected individuals who are also hepatitis B surface antigen (HBsAg) positive. IFN-α is less successful as a treatment of HBV in patients with HIV co-infection, and lamivudine, emtricitabine, or adefovir/tenofovir and entecavir alone or in combination are useful in the treatment of hepatitis B in patients with HIV infection. It is important to remember that all the above-mentioned drugs also have activity against HIV and should not be used as single agents in patients with HIV infection, in order to avoid the rapid development of resistant quasispecies of HIV. HCV infection is more severe in the patient with HIV infection; it does not appear to affect overall mortality in HIV-infected individuals when other variables such as age, baseline CD4+ T cell count, and use of HAART are taken into account. In the setting of HIV and HCV co-infection, levels of HCV are approximately tenfold higher than in the HIV-negative patient with HCV infection and there is a tenfold increased risk of death due to liver disease in co-infected patients. Treatment for HCV infection consists of pegylated IFN-α and ribavirin. If a 2-log drop in levels of HCV RNA is not seen within 12 weeks, it is unlikely that therapy will be of value. Hepatitis A virus infection is not seen with an increased frequency in patients with HIV infection. It is recommended that all patients with HIV infection who have not experienced natural infection be immunized with hepatitis A and/or hepatitis B vaccines. Infection with hepatitis G virus, also known as GB virus C, is seen in ~50% of patients with HIV infection. For reasons that are currently unclear there are data to suggest that patients with HIV infection co-infected with this virus have a decreased rate of progression to AIDS.

A variety of other infections may also involve the liver. Granulomatous hepatitis may be seen as a consequence of mycobacterial or fungal infections, particularly MAC infection. Hepatic masses may be seen in the context of TB, peliosis hepatis, or fungal infection. Among the fungal opportunistic infections *C. immitis* and *Histoplasma capsulatum* are those most likely to involve the liver. Biliary tract disease in the form of papillary stenosis or sclerosing cholangitis has been reported in the context of cryptosporidiosis, CMV infection, and KS.

Many of the drugs used to treat HIV infection are metabolized by the liver and can cause liver injury. Fatal hepatic reactions have been reported with a wide array of ARVs including nucleoside analogues, nonnucleoside analogues, and protease inhibitors. Nucleoside analogues work by inhibiting DNA synthesis. This can result in toxicity to mitochondria, which can lead to disturbances in oxidative metabolism. This may manifest as hepatic steatosis and, in severe cases, lactic acidosis and fulminant liver failure. It is important to be aware of this condition and to watch for it in patients with HIV infection receiving nucleoside analogues. It is reversible if diagnosed early and the offending agent(s) discontinued. Nevirapine has been associated with at times fatal fulminant and cholestatic hepatitis, hepatic necrosis, and hepatic failure. Indinavir may cause mild to moderate elevations in serum bilirubin in 10–15% of patients in a syndrome similar to Gilbert's syndrome. A similar pattern of hepatic injury may be seen with atazanavir. In the patient receiving HAART with an unexplained increase in hepatic transaminases, strong consideration should be given to drug toxicity. *Pancreatic injury* is most commonly a consequence of drug toxicity, notably that secondary to pentamidine or dideoxynucleosides. While up to half of patients in some series have biochemical evidence of pancreatic injury, <5% of patients show any clinical evidence of pancreatitis that is not linked to a drug toxicity.

Diseases of the Kidney and Genitourinary Tract Diseases of the kidney or genitourinary tract may be a direct consequence of HIV infection, due to an opportunistic infection or neoplasm, or related to drug toxicity. *HIV-associated nephropathy* was first described in IDUs and was initially thought to be IDU nephropathy in patients with HIV infection; it is now recognized as a true direct complication of HIV infection. Although the majority of patients have CD4+ T cell counts <200/μL, HIV-associated nephropathy can be an early manifestation of HIV infection and is also seen in children. Over 90% of reported cases have been in African-American or Hispanic individuals; the disease is not only more prevalent in these populations but also more severe and is the third leading cause of end-stage renal failure among African Americans aged 20–64 in the United States. Proteinuria is the hallmark of this disorder. Overall, microalbuminuria is seen in ~20% of untreated HIV-infected patients; significant proteinuria is seen in closer to 2%. Edema and hypertension are rare. Ultrasound examination reveals enlarged, hyperechogenic kidneys. A definitive diagnosis is obtained through renal biopsy. Histologically, focal segmental glomerulosclerosis is present in 80%, and mesangial proliferation in 10–15% of cases. Prior to effective antiretroviral therapy, this disease was characterized by relatively rapid progression to end-stage renal disease and patients with HIV-associated nephropathy should be treated for their HIV infection regardless of CD4+ T cell count. Treatment with angiotensin-converting enzyme (ACE) inhibitors and/or prednisone, 60 mg/d, has also been reported to be of benefit in some cases. The incidence of this disease in patients receiving adequate ARV therapy has not been well defined; however, the impression is that it has decreased in frequency and severity. It is the leading cause of end-stage renal disease in patients with HIV infection.

Among the drugs commonly associated with renal damage in patients with HIV disease are pentamidine, amphotericin, adefovir, cidofovir, tenofovir, and foscarnet. TMP/SMX may compete for tubular secretion with creatinine and cause an increase in the serum creatinine level. Sulfadiazine may crystallize in the kidney and result in an easily reversible form of renal shutdown. One of the most common drug-induced renal complications is indinavir-associated renal calculi. This condition is seen in ~10% of patients receiving this HIV protease inhibitor. It may present with a variety of manifestations, ranging from asymptomatic hematuria to renal colic. Adequate hydration is the mainstay of treatment and prevention for this condition.

Genitourinary tract infections are seen with a high frequency in patients with HIV infection; they present with skin lesions, dysuria, he-

maturia, and/or pyuria and are managed in the same fashion as in patients without HIV infection. Infections with HSV are covered below under dermatologic disorders. Infections with *T. pallidum*, the etiologic agent of *syphilis*, play an important role in the HIV epidemic (Chap. 181). In HIV-negative individuals, genital syphilitic ulcers as well as the ulcers of chancroid are major predisposing factors for heterosexual transmission of HIV infection. While most HIV-infected individuals with syphilis have a typical presentation, a variety of formerly rare clinical problems may be encountered in the setting of dual infection. Among them are *lues maligna*, an ulcerating lesion of the skin due to a necrotizing vasculitis; unexplained fever; nephrotic syndrome; and neurosyphilis. The most common presentation of syphilis in the HIV-infected patient is that of *condylomata lata*, a form of secondary syphilis. Neurosyphilis may be asymptomatic or may present as acute meningitis, neuroretinitis, deafness, or stroke. The rate of neurosyphilis may be as high as 1% in patients with HIV infection. As a consequence of the immunologic abnormalities seen in the setting of HIV infection, diagnosis of syphilis through standard serologic testing may be challenging. On the one hand, a significant number of patients have false-positive Venereal Disease Research Laboratory (VDRL) tests due to polyclonal B cell activation. On the other hand, the development of a new positive VDRL may be delayed in patients with new infections, and the anti-fluorescent treponema antibody (anti-FTA) test may be negative due to immunodeficiency. Thus, dark-field examination of appropriate specimens should be performed in any patient in whom syphilis is suspected, even if the patient has a negative VDRL. Similarly, any patient with a positive serum VDRL test, neurologic findings, and an abnormal spinal fluid examination should be considered to have neurosyphilis, regardless of the CSF VDRL result. In any setting, patients treated for syphilis need to be carefully monitored to ensure adequate therapy.

Vulvovaginal candidiasis is a common problem in women with HIV infection. Symptoms include pruritus, discomfort, dyspareunia, and dysuria. Vulvar infection may present as a morbilliform rash that may extend to the thighs. Vaginal infection is usually associated with a white discharge, and plaques may be seen along an erythematous vaginal wall. Diagnosis is made by microscopic examination of the discharge for pseudohyphal elements in a 10% potassium hydroxide solution. Mild disease can be treated with topical therapy. More serious disease can be treated with fluconazole. Other causes of vaginitis include *Trichomonas* and mixed bacteria.

Diseases of the Endocrine System and Metabolic Disorders A variety of endocrine and metabolic disorders are seen in the context of HIV infection. Between 33 and 75% of patients with HIV infection receiving HAART develop a syndrome often referred to as *lipodystrophy*, consisting of elevations in plasma triglycerides, total cholesterol, and apolipoprotein B, as well as hyperinsulinemia and hyperglycemia. Many of the patients have been noted to have a characteristic set of body habitus changes associated with fat redistribution, consisting of truncal obesity coupled with peripheral wasting (Fig. 182-36). Truncal obesity is apparent as an increase in abdominal girth related to increases in mesenteric fat, a dorsocervical fat pad ("buffalo hump") reminiscent of patients with Cushing's syndrome, and enlargement of the breasts. The peripheral wasting or lipoatrophy is particularly noticeable in the face and buttocks and by the prominence of the veins in the legs. These changes may develop at any time ranging from ~6 weeks to several years following the initiation of HAART. Approximately 20% of the patients with HIV-associated lipodystrophy meet the criteria for the *metabolic syndrome* as defined by The International Diabetes Federation or The U.S. National Cholesterol Education Program Adult Treatment Panel III. The lipodystrophy syndrome has been reported in association with regimens containing a variety of different drugs, and while initially reported in the setting of protease inhibitor therapy, it appears similar changes can also be induced by potent protease-sparing regimens. It has been suggested that the lipoatrophy changes are particularly severe in patients receiving thymidine analogues. National Cholesterol Education Program (NCEP) guidelines should be followed in the management of these lipid abnor-

FIGURE 182-36 Characteristics of lipodystrophy. A. Truncal obesity and buffalo hump. **B.** Facial wasting. **C.** Accumulation of intraabdominal fat on CT scan.

malities (Chap. 235). Due to concerns regarding drug interactions, the most commonly utilized agents in this setting are gemfibrozil and atorvastatin. In addition to these abnormalities, patients with HIV infection treated with HAART have been found to have an increased incidence of osteonecrosis or avascular necrosis of the hip and shoulders. In a study of asymptomatic patients, 4.4% were found to have evidence of osteonecrosis on MRI. This complication has been associated with the use of lipid-lowering agents, systemic glucocorticoids, or testosterone; body-building exercise; alcohol consumption; and the presence of anticardiolipin antibodies. Osteoporosis has been reported in 7% of women with HIV infection, with 41% of women demonstrating some degree of osteopenia. In addition, lactic acidosis is associated with ARV therapy. This is most commonly seen with nucleoside analogue reverse transcriptase inhibitors and can be fatal (see below).

Patients with advanced HIV disease may develop hyponatremia due to the syndrome of inappropriate antidiuretic hormone (vasopressin) secretion (SIADH) as a consequence of increased free water intake and decreased free water excretion. SIADH is usually seen in conjunction with pulmonary or CNS disease. Low serum sodium may also be due to adrenal insufficiency; concomitant high serum potassium should alert one to this possibility. Adrenal gland disease may be due to mycobacterial infections, CMV disease, cryptococcal disease, histoplasmosis, or ketoconazole toxicity.

Thyroid function may be altered in 10–15% of patients with HIV infection. Both hypo- and hyperthyroidism may be seen. The predominant abnormality is subclinical hypothyroidism. In the setting of HAART up to 10% of patients have been noted to have elevated thyroid-stimulating hormone levels, suggesting that this may be a manifestation of immune reconstitution. Immune-reconstitution Graves' disease may occur as a late (9–48 months) complication of HAART. In advanced HIV disease, infection of the thyroid gland may occur with opportunistic pathogens,

including *P. jiroveci*, CMV, mycobacteria, *Toxoplasma gondii*, and *Cryptococcus neoformans*. These infections are generally associated with a nontender, diffuse enlargement of the thyroid gland. Thyroid function is usually normal. Diagnosis is made by fine-needle aspirate or open biopsy.

Advanced HIV disease is associated with *hypogonadism* in ~50% of men. While this is generally a complication of underlying illness, testicular dysfunction may also be a side effect of ganciclovir therapy. In some surveys, up to two-thirds of patients report decreased libido and one-third complain of impotence. Androgen-replacement therapy should be considered in patients with symptomatic hypogonadism. HIV infection does not seem to have a significant effect on the menstrual cycle outside the setting of advanced disease.

Rheumatologic Diseases Immunologic and rheumatologic disorders are common in patients with HIV infection and range from excessive immediate-type hypersensitivity reactions (Chap. 311) to an increase in the incidence of reactive arthritis (Chap. 318) to conditions characterized by a diffuse infiltrative lymphocytosis. The occurrence of these phenomena is an apparent paradox in the setting of the profound immunodeficiency and immunosuppression that characterizes HIV infection.

Drug allergies are the most significant allergic reactions occurring in HIV-infected patients and appear to become more common as the disease progresses. They occur in up to 65% of patients who receive therapy with TMP/SMX for PCP. In general, these drug reactions are characterized by erythematous, morbilliform eruptions that are pruritic, tend to coalesce, and are often associated with fever. Nonetheless, ~33% of patients can be maintained on the offending therapy, and thus these reactions are not an immediate indication to stop the drug. Anaphylaxis is extremely rare in patients with HIV infection, and patients who have a cutaneous reaction during a single course of therapy can still be considered candidates for future treatment or prophylaxis with the same agent. The one exception to this is the nucleoside analogue abacavir, where fatal hypersensitivity reactions have been reported with rechallenge. This hypersensitivity is strongly associated with the HLA-B57 haplotype and a hypersensitivity reaction to abacavir is an absolute contraindication to future therapy. For other agents, including TMP/SMX, desensitization regimens are moderately successful. While the mechanisms underlying these allergic-type reactions remain unknown, patients with HIV infection have been noted to have elevated IgE levels that increase as the CD4+ T cell count declines. The numerous examples of patients with multiple drug reactions suggest that a common pathway is involved.

HIV infection shares many similarities with a variety of autoimmune diseases, including a substantial polyclonal B cell activation that is associated with a high incidence of antiphospholipid antibodies, such as anticardiolipin antibodies, VDRL antibodies, and lupus-like anticoagulants. In addition, HIV-infected individuals have an increased incidence of antinuclear antibodies. Despite these serologic findings, there is no evidence that HIV-infected individuals have an increase in two of the more common autoimmune diseases, i.e., systemic lupus erythematosus and rheumatoid arthritis. In fact, it has been observed that these diseases may be somewhat ameliorated by the concomitant presence of HIV infection, suggesting that an intact CD4+ T cell limb of the immune response plays an integral role in the pathogenesis of these conditions. Similarly, there are anecdotal reports of patients with common variable immunodeficiency (Chap. 310), characterized by hypogammaglobulinemia, who have had a normalization of Ig levels following the development of HIV infection, suggesting a possible role for overactive CD4+ T cell immunity in certain forms of that syndrome. The one autoimmune disease that may occur with an increased frequency in patients with HIV infection is a variant of primary Sjögren's syndrome (Chap. 317). Patients with HIV infection may develop a syndrome consisting of parotid gland enlargement, dry eyes, and dry mouth that is associated with lymphocytic infiltrates of the salivary gland and lung. In contrast to Sjögren's syndrome, in which these infiltrates are composed predominantly of CD4+ T cells, in patients with HIV infection the infiltrates are composed predominantly of CD8+ T cells. In addition, while patients with Sjögren's syndrome are mainly women who have autoantibodies to Ro and La and who frequently have HLA-DR3 or -B8 MHC haplotypes, HIV-infected individuals with this syndrome are usually African-American men who do not have anti-Ro or anti-La and who most often are HLA-DR5. This syndrome appears to be less common with the increased use of effective ARV therapy. The term *diffuse infiltrative lymphocytosis syndrome* (DILS) has been proposed to describe this entity and to distinguish it from Sjögren's syndrome.

Approximately one-third of HIV-infected individuals experience arthralgias; furthermore, 5–10% are diagnosed as having some form of reactive arthritis, such as Reiter's syndrome or psoriatic arthritis (Chap. 318). These syndromes occur with increasing frequency as the competency of the immune system declines. This association may be related to an increase in the number of infections with organisms that may trigger a reactive arthritis with progressive immunodeficiency or to a loss of important regulatory T cells. Reactive arthritides in HIV-infected individuals generally respond well to standard treatment; however, therapy with methotrexate has been associated with an increase in the incidence of opportunistic infections and should be used with caution and only in severe cases.

HIV-infected individuals also experience a variety of joint problems without obvious cause that are referred to generically as *HIV- or AIDS-associated arthropathy*. This syndrome is characterized by subacute oligoarticular arthritis developing over a period of 1–6 weeks and lasting 6 weeks to 6 months. It generally involves the large joints, predominantly the knees and ankles, and is nonerosive with only a mild inflammatory response. X-rays of the joint are nonrevealing. Nonsteroidal anti-inflammatory drugs are only marginally helpful; however, relief has been noted with the use of intraarticular glucocorticoids. A second form of arthritis also thought to be secondary to HIV infection is called *painful articular syndrome*. This condition, reported as occurring in as many as 10% of AIDS patients, presents as an acute, severe, sharp pain in the affected joint. It affects primarily the knees, elbows, and shoulders; lasts 2–24 h; and may be severe enough to require narcotic analgesics. The cause of this arthropathy is unclear; however, it is thought to result from a direct effect of HIV on the joint. This condition is reminiscent of the fact that other lentiviruses, in particular the caprine arthritis-encephalitis virus, are capable of directly causing arthritis.

A variety of other immunologic or rheumatologic diseases have been reported in HIV-infected individuals, either de novo or in association with opportunistic infections or drugs. Using the criteria of widespread musculoskeletal pain of at least 3 months' duration and the presence of at least 11 of 18 possible tender points by digital palpation, 11% of an HIV-infected cohort containing 55% IDUs were diagnosed as having *fibromyalgia* (Chap. 329). While the incidence of frank arthritis was less in this population than in other studied populations that consisted predominantly of homosexual men, these data support the concept that there are musculoskeletal problems that occur as a direct result of HIV infection. In addition there have been reports of leukocytoclastic vasculitis in the setting of zidovudine therapy. CNS angiitis and polymyositis have also been reported in HIV-infected individuals. Septic arthritis is surprisingly rare, especially given the increased incidence of staphylococcal bacteremias seen in this population. When septic arthritis has been reported, it has usually been due to *Staphylococcus aureus*, systemic fungal infections with *C. neoformans*, *Sporothrix schenckii*, or *H. capsulatum* or to systemic mycobac-

terial infection with *M. tuberculosis*, *M. haemophilum*, *M. avium*, or *M. kansasii*.

As noted above, 4.4% of patients with HIV infection were found to have some evidence of osteonecrosis by MRI during systematic screening of asymptomatic patients. The percentage of patients with symptomatic osteonecrosis has been estimated to be as high as 1%. While this problem was first recognized in the setting of HAART, it has been difficult to establish a cause-and-effect relationship. Alcohol consumption and a history of glucocorticoid use have been particularly associated with this condition in patients with HIV infection.

Immune Reconstitution Inflammatory Syndrome Following the initiation of effective ARV therapy, a paradoxical worsening of preexisting, untreated, or partially treated opportunistic infections may be noted (Table 182-9). These IRISs are particularly common in patients with underlying untreated mycobacterial infections. They are seen in anywhere from 10–50% of patients, depending upon the clinical setting, and are most common in patients starting therapy with CD4+ T cell counts <50 cells/μL who have a precipitous drop in HIV RNA levels following the initiation of HAART. Signs and symptoms may appear anywhere from 2 weeks to 2 years after the initiation of HAART and can include localized lymphadenitis, prolonged fever, pulmonary infiltrates, increased intracranial pressure, uveitis, and Graves' disease. The clinical course can be protracted and severe cases can be fatal. The underlying mechanism appears to be related to a phenomenon similar to type IV hypersensitivity reactions and reflects the immediate improvements in immune function that occur as levels of HIV RNA drop and the immunosuppressive effects of HIV infection are controlled. In severe cases, the use of immunosuppressive drugs such as glucocorticoids may be required to blunt the inflammatory component of these reactions while specific antimicrobial therapy takes effect.

Diseases of the Hematopoietic System Disorders of the hematopoietic system including lymphadenopathy, anemia, leukopenia, and/or thrombocytopenia are common throughout the course of HIV infection and may be the direct result of HIV, manifestations of secondary infections and neoplasms, or side effects of therapy (Table 182-10). Direct histologic examination and culture of lymph node or bone marrow tissue are often diagnostic. A significant percentage of bone marrow aspirates from patients with HIV infection have been reported to contain lymphoid aggregates, the precise significance of which is unknown. Initiation of HAART will lead to reversal of most hematologic complications that are the direct result of HIV infection.

Some patients, otherwise asymptomatic, may develop *persistent generalized lymphadenopathy* as an early clinical manifestation of HIV

TABLE 182-9 CHARACTERISTICS OF IMMUNE RECONSTITUTION INFLAMMATORY SYNDROME (IRIS)

- Paradoxical worsening of clinical condition following the initiation of antiretroviral therapy
- Occurs weeks to months following the initiation of antiretroviral therapy
- Most common in patients starting therapy with a CD4+ T cell count under 50/μL who experience a precipitous drop in viral load
- Frequently seen in the setting of tuberculosis
- Can be fatal

TABLE 182-10 CAUSES OF BONE MARROW SUPPRESSION IN PATIENTS WITH HIV INFECTION

HIV infection	Medications
Mycobacterial infections	Zidovudine
Fungal infections	Dapsone
B19 parvovirus infection	Trimethoprim/sulfamethoxazole
Lymphoma	Pyrimethamine
	5-Flucytosine
	Ganciclovir
	Interferon-α
	Trimetrexate
	Foscarnet

infection. This condition is defined as the presence of enlarged lymph nodes (>1 cm) in two or more extrainguinal sites for >3 months without an obvious cause. The lymphadenopathy is due to marked follicular hyperplasia in the node in response to HIV infection. The nodes are generally discrete and freely movable. This feature of HIV disease may be seen at any point in the spectrum of immune dysfunction and is not associated with an increased likelihood of developing AIDS. Paradoxically, a loss in lymphadenopathy or a decrease in lymph node size outside the setting of ARV therapy may be a prognostic marker of disease progression. In patients with CD4+ T cell counts >200/μL, the differential diagnosis of lymphadenopathy includes KS, TB, Castleman's disease, and lymphoma. In patients with more advanced disease, lymphadenopathy may also be due to atypical mycobacterial infection, toxoplasmosis, systemic fungal infection, or bacillary angiomatosis. While indicated in patients with CD4+ T cell counts <200/μL, lymph node biopsy is not indicated in patients with early-stage disease unless there are signs and symptoms of systemic illness, such as fever and weight loss, or unless the nodes begin to enlarge, become fixed, or coalesce. Monoclonal gammopathy of unknown significance (MGUS; Chap. 106), defined as the presence of a serum monoclonal IgG, IgA, or IgM in the absence of a clear cause, has been reported in 3% of patients with HIV infection. The overall clinical significance of this finding in patients with HIV infection is unclear, although it has been associated with other viral infections, non-Hodgkin's lymphoma, and plasma cell malignancy.

Anemia is the most common hematologic abnormality in HIV-infected patients and in the absence of a specific treatable cause is independently associated with a poor prognosis. While generally mild, anemia can be quite severe and require chronic blood transfusions. Among the specific reversible causes of anemia in the setting of HIV infection are drug toxicity, systemic fungal and mycobacterial infections, nutritional deficiencies, and parvovirus B19 infections. Zidovudine may block erythroid maturation, prior to its effects on other marrow elements. A characteristic feature of zidovudine therapy is an elevated mean corpuscular volume (MCV). Another drug used in patients with HIV infection that has a selective effect on the erythroid series is dapsone. This drug can cause a serious hemolytic anemia in patients who are deficient in glucose-6-phosphate dehydrogenase and can create a functional anemia in others through induction of methemoglobinemia. Folate levels are usually normal in HIV-infected individuals; however, vitamin B$_{12}$ levels may be depressed as a consequence of achlorhydria or malabsorption. True autoimmune hemolytic anemia is rare, although ~20% of patients with HIV infection may have a positive direct antiglobulin test as a consequence of polyclonal B cell activation. Infection with parvovirus B19 may also cause anemia. It is important to recognize this possibility given the fact that it responds well to treatment with IVIg. Erythropoietin levels in patients with HIV infection and anemia are generally less than expected given the degree of anemia. Treatment with erythropoietin at doses of 100 μg/kg three times a week may result in an increase in hemoglobulin levels. An exception to this is a subset of patients with zidovudine-associated anemia in whom erythropoietin levels may be quite high.

During the course of HIV infection, neutropenia may be seen in approximately half of patients. In most instances it is mild; however, it can be severe and can put patients at risk of spontaneous bacterial infections. This is most frequently seen in patients with severely advanced HIV disease and in patients receiving any of a number of potentially myelosuppressive therapies. In the setting of neutropenia, diseases that are not commonly seen in HIV-infected patients, such as aspergillosis or mucormycosis, may occur. The potential role of colony-stimulating factors in the management of patients with HIV infection has undergone extensive evaluation. Both granulocyte colony-stimulating factor (G-CSF) and GM-CSF increase neutrophil counts in patients with HIV infection regardless of the cause of the neutropenia. Earlier concerns about the potential of these agents to also increase levels of HIV were not confirmed in controlled clinical trials.

Thrombocytopenia may be an early consequence of HIV infection. Approximately 3% of patients with untreated HIV infection and CD4+ T cell counts ≥400/μL have platelet counts <150,000/μL. For untreated patients with CD4+ T cell counts <400/μL, this incidence increases to 10%. Thrombocytopenia is rarely a serious clinical problem in patients with HIV infection and generally responds well to ARV therapy. Clinically, it resembles the thrombocytopenia seen in patients with idiopathic thrombocytopenic purpura (Chap. 109). Immune complexes containing anti-gp120 antibodies and anti-anti-gp120 antibodies have been noted in the circulation and on the surface of platelets in patients with HIV infection. Patients with HIV infection have also been noted to have a platelet-specific antibody directed toward a 25-kDa component of the surface of the platelet. Other data suggest that the thrombocytopenia in patients with HIV infection may be due to a direct effect of HIV on megakaryocytes. Whatever the cause, it is very clear that the most effective medical approach to this problem has been the use of HAART. For patients with platelet counts <20,000/μL a more aggressive approach combining IVIg or anti-Rh Ig for an immediate response with ARV therapy for a more lasting response is appropriate. Rituximab has been used with some success in otherwise refractory cases. Splenectomy is a rarely needed option and is reserved for patients refractory to medical management. Because of the risk of serious infection with encapsulated organisms, all patients with HIV infection about to undergo splenectomy should be immunized with pneumococcal polysaccharide. It should be noted that, in addition to causing an increase in the platelet count, removal of the spleen will result in an increase in the peripheral blood lymphocyte count, making CD4+ T cell counts unreliable. In this setting, the clinician should rely on the CD4+ T cell percent for making diagnostic decisions with respect to the likelihood of opportunistic infections. A CD4+ T cell percent of 15 is approximately equivalent to a CD4+ T cell count of 200/μL. In patients with early HIV infection, thrombocytopenia has also been reported as a consequence of classic thrombotic thrombocytopenic purpura (Chap. 109). This clinical syndrome, consisting of fever, thrombocytopenia, hemolytic anemia, and neurologic and renal dysfunction, is a rare complication of early HIV infection. As in other settings, the appropriate management is the use of salicylates and plasma exchange. Other causes of thrombocytopenia include lymphoma, mycobacterial infections, and fungal infections.

Approximately 4% of patients with HIV infection experience venous thrombotic events such as deep vein thrombosis or pulmonary embolism. Among the factors associated with clinical thrombosis are age over 45, history of an opportunistic infection, and estrogen use.

Abnormalities of the coagulation cascade including decreased protein S activity, increases in factor VIII, and the presence of anticardiolipin antibodies have been reported in patients with HIV infection. Elevations in D-dimer appear predictive of a poor clinical outcome.

Dermatologic Diseases Dermatologic problems occur in >90% of patients with HIV infection. From the macular, roseola-like rash seen with the acute seroconversion syndrome to extensive end-stage KS, cutaneous manifestations of HIV disease can be seen throughout the course of HIV infection. Among the more common nonneoplastic problems are seborrheic dermatitis, folliculitis, and opportunistic infections. Extrapulmonary pneumocystosis may cause a necrotizing vasculitis. Neoplastic conditions are covered below in the section on malignant diseases.

Seborrheic dermatitis occurs in 3% of the general population and in up to 50% of patients with HIV infection. Seborrheic dermatitis increases in prevalence and severity as the CD4+ T cell count declines. In HIV-infected patients, seborrheic dermatitis may be aggravated by concomitant infection with *Pityrosporum*, a yeastlike fungus; use of topical antifungal agents has been recommended in cases refractory to standard topical treatment.

Folliculitis is among the most prevalent dermatologic disorders in patients with HIV infection and is seen in ~20% of patients. It is more common in patients with CD4+ T cell counts <200 cells/μL. One form of folliculitis, *eosinophilic pustular folliculitis,* is a rare dermatologic condition that is seen with increased frequency in patients with HIV infection. It presents as multiple, urticarial perifollicular papules that may coalesce into plaquelike lesions. Skin biopsy reveals an eosinophilic infiltrate of the hair follicle, which in certain cases has been associated with the presence of a mite. Patients typically have an elevated serum IgE level and may respond to treatment with topical antihelminthics. Pruritus is a common symptom in patients with HIV infection and can lead to prurigo nodularis. Patients with HIV infection have also been reported to develop a severe form of *Norwegian scabies* with hyperkeratotic psoriasiform lesions.

Both *psoriasis* and *ichthyosis*, although they are not reported to be increased in frequency, may be particularly severe when they occur in patients with HIV infection. Preexisting psoriasis may become guttate in appearance and more refractory to treatment in the setting of HIV infection.

Reactivation herpes zoster (*shingles*) is seen in 10–20% of patients with HIV infection. This reactivation syndrome of varicella-zoster virus indicates a modest decline in immune function and may be the first indication of clinical immunodeficiency. In one series, patients who developed shingles did so an average of 5 years after HIV infection. In a cohort of patients with HIV infection and localized zoster, the subsequent rate of the development of AIDS was 1% per month. In that study, AIDS was more likely to develop if the outbreak of zoster was associated with severe pain, extensive skin involvement, or involvement of cranial or cervical dermatomes. The clinical manifestations of reactivation zoster in HIV-infected patients, although indicative of immunologic compromise, are not as severe as those seen in other immunodeficient conditions. Thus, while lesions may extend over several dermatomes and frank cutaneous dissemination may be seen, visceral involvement has not been reported. In contrast to patients without a known underlying immunodeficiency state, patients with HIV infection tend to have recurrences of zoster with a relapse rate of ~20%. Acyclovir or famciclovir is the treatment of choice. Foscarnet may be of value in patients with acyclovir-resistant virus.

Infection with *herpes simplex virus* in HIV-infected individuals is associated with recurrent orolabial, genital, and perianal lesions as part of recurrent reactivation syndromes (Chap. 172). As HIV disease progresses and the CD4+ T cell count declines, these infections become more frequent and severe. Lesions often appear as beefy red, are exquisitely painful, and have a tendency to occur high in the gluteal cleft (Fig. 182-35). Perirectal HSV may be associated with proctitis and anal fissures. HSV should be high in the differential diagnosis of any HIV-infected patient with a poorly healing, painful perirectal lesion. In addition to recurrent mucosal ulcers, recurrent HSV infection in the form of *herpetic whitlow* can be a problem in patients with HIV infection, presenting with painful vesicles or extensive cutaneous erosion. Acyclovir or famciclovir is the treatment of choice in these settings. Of note is the fact that even subclinical reactivation of herpes simplex may be associated with increases in plasma HIV RNA levels. In a cohort of patients from Burkina Faso seropositive for HIV-1 and HSV-2 with CD4+ T cell counts >200 cells/μL, chronic use of valacyclovir was associated with a 0.5 log decrease in HIV viral load. Thus, consideration should be given to chronic suppressive therapy in patients with recurrent outbreaks of herpesvirus.

Diffuse skin eruptions due to *Molluscum contagiosum* may be seen in patients with advanced HIV infection. These flesh-colored, umbilicated lesions may be treated with local therapy. They tend to regress with effective ARV therapy. Similarly, *condyloma acuminatum* lesions may be more severe and more widely distributed in patients with low CD4+ T cell counts. Atypical mycobacterial infections may present as erythematous cutaneous nodules as may fungal infections, *Bartonella*, *Acanthamoeba*, and KS.

The skin of patients with HIV infection is often a target organ for drug reactions (Chap. 56). Although most skin reactions are mild and not necessarily an indication to discontinue therapy, patients may have particularly severe cutaneous reactions, including erythroderma and *Stevens-Johnson syndrome*, as a reaction to drugs, particularly sulfa drugs, the nonnucleoside reverse transcriptase inhibitors, abacavir, amprenavir, darunavir, fosamprenavir, and tipranavir. Similarly, patients with HIV infection are often quite photosensitive and burn easi-

TABLE 182-11 **NEUROLOGIC DISEASES IN PATIENTS WITH HIV INFECTION** **1181**

Opportunistic infections	Myelopathy
Toxoplasmosis	Vacuolar myelopathy
Cryptococcosis	Pure sensory ataxia
Progressive multifocal	Paresthesia/dysesthesia
leukoencephalopathy	Peripheral neuropathy
Cytomegalovirus	Acute inflammatory demyelinat-
Syphilis	ing polyneuropathy (Guillain-
Mycobacterium tuberculosis	Barré syndrome)
HTLV-I infection	Chronic inflammatory demyelin-
Neoplasms	ating polyneuropathy (CIDP)
Primary CNS lymphoma	Mononeuritis multiplex
Kaposi's sarcoma	Distal symmetric polyneuropathy
Result of HIV-1 infection	Myopathy
Aseptic meningitis	
HIV-associated neurocognitive	
impairment, including HIV	
encephalopathy/AIDS	
dementia complex	

ly following exposure to sunlight or as a side effect of radiation therapy (Chap. 57).

HIV infection and its treatment may be accompanied by cosmetic changes of the skin that are not of great clinical importance but may be troubling to patients. Yellowing of the nails and straightening of the hair, particularly in African-American patients, have been reported as a consequence of HIV infection. Zidovudine therapy has been associated with elongation of the eyelashes and the development of a bluish discoloration to the nails, again more common in African-American patients. Therapy with clofazimine may cause a yellow-orange discoloration of the skin and urine.

Neurologic Diseases Clinical disease of the nervous system accounts for a significant degree of morbidity in a high percentage of patients with HIV infection (Table 182-11). The neurologic problems that occur in HIV-infected individuals may be either primary to the pathogenic processes of HIV infection or secondary to opportunistic infections or neoplasms (see above). Among the more frequent opportunistic diseases that involve the CNS are toxoplasmosis, cryptococcosis, progressive multifocal leukoencephalopathy, and primary CNS lymphoma. Other less common problems include mycobacterial infections; syphilis; and infection with CMV, HTLV-I, *T. cruzi*, or *Acanthamoeba*. Overall, secondary diseases of the CNS occur in approximately one-third of patients with AIDS. These data antedate the widespread use of combination ARV therapy, and this frequency is considerably less in patients receiving effective ARV drugs. Primary processes related to HIV infection of the nervous system are reminiscent of those seen with other lentiviruses, such as the Visna-Maedi virus of sheep.

Neurologic problems directly attributable to HIV occur throughout the course of infection and may be inflammatory, demyelinating, or degenerative in nature. The term *HIV-associated neurocognitive impairment* (HNCI) is used to describe a spectrum of disorders that range from asymptomatic to apparent only through extensive neuropsychiatric testing to clinically severe. The most severe form, the *AIDS dementia complex*, or *HIV encephalopathy*, is considered an AIDS-defining illness. Most HIV-infected patients have some neurologic problem during the course of their disease. As noted in the section on pathogenesis, damage to the CNS may be a direct result of viral infection of the CNS macrophages or glial cells or may be secondary to the release of neurotoxins and potentially toxic cytokines such as IL-1β, TNF-α, IL-6, and TGF-β. It has been reported that HIV-infected individuals with the E4 allele for apo E are at increased risk for AIDS encephalopathy and peripheral neuropathy. Virtually all patients with HIV infection have some degree of nervous system involvement with the virus. This is evidenced by the fact that CSF findings are abnormal in ~90% of patients, even during the asymptomatic phase of HIV infection. CSF abnormalities include pleocytosis (50–65% of patients), detection of viral RNA (~75%), elevated CSF protein (35%), and evidence of intrathecal synthesis of anti-HIV antibodies (90%). It is important to point out that evidence of infection of the CNS with HIV does not imply impairment of cognitive function. The neurologic function of an HIV-infected individual should be considered normal unless clinical signs and symptoms suggest otherwise.

Aseptic meningitis may be seen in any but the very late stages of HIV infection. In the setting of acute primary infection patients may experience a syndrome of headache, photophobia, and meningismus. Rarely, an acute encephalopathy due to encephalitis may occur. Cranial nerve involvement may be seen, predominantly cranial nerve VII but occasionally V and/or VIII. CSF findings include a lymphocytic pleocytosis, elevated protein level, and normal glucose level. This syndrome, which cannot be clinically differentiated from other viral meningitides (Chap. 377), usually resolves spontaneously within 2–4 weeks; however, in some patients, signs and symptoms may become chronic. Aseptic meningitis may occur any time in the course of HIV infection; however, it is rare following the development of AIDS. This fact suggests that clinical aseptic meningitis in the context of HIV infection is an immune-mediated disease.

C. neoformans is the leading infectious cause of meningitis in patients with AIDS (Chap. 195). It is the initial AIDS-defining illness in ~2% of patients and generally occurs in patients with CD4+ T cell counts <100/μL. Cryptococcal meningitis is particularly common in patients with AIDS in Africa, occurring in ~20% of patients. Most patients present with a picture of subacute meningoencephalitis with fever, nausea, vomiting, altered mental status, headache, and meningeal signs. The incidence of seizures and focal neurologic deficits is low. The CSF profile may be normal or may show only modest elevations in WBC or protein levels and decreases in glucose. In addition to meningitis, patients may develop cryptococcomas and cranial nerve involvement. Approximately one-third of patients also have pulmonary disease. Uncommon manifestations of cryptococcal infection include skin lesions that resemble *molluscum contagiosum*, lymphadenopathy, palatal and glossal ulcers, arthritis, gastroenteritis, myocarditis, and prostatitis. The prostate gland may serve as a reservoir for smoldering cryptococcal infection. The diagnosis of cryptococcal meningitis is made by identification of organisms in spinal fluid with India ink examination or by the detection of cryptococcal antigen. A biopsy may be needed to make a diagnosis of CNS cryptococcoma. Treatment is with IV amphotericin B, at a dose of 0.7 mg/kg daily, with flucytosine, 25 mg/kg qid for 2 weeks, followed by fluconazole, 400 mg/d PO for 10 weeks, and then fluconazole, 200 mg/d until the CD4+ T cell count has increased to >200 cells/μL for 6 months in response to HAART. Repeated lumbar puncture may be required to manage increased intracranial pressure. Symptoms may recur with initiation of HAART as an immune reconstitution syndrome (see above). Other fungi that may cause meningitis in patients with HIV infection are *C. immitis* and *H. capsulatum*. Meningoencephalitis has also been reported due to *Acanthamoeba* or *Naegleria*.

HIV encephalopathy, also called HIV-associated dementia or AIDS dementia complex, consists of a constellation of signs and symptoms of CNS disease. While this is generally a late complication of HIV infection that progresses slowly over months, it can be seen in patients with CD4+ T cell counts >350 cells/μL. A major feature of this entity is the development of dementia, defined as a decline in cognitive ability from a previous level. It may present as impaired ability to concentrate, increased forgetfulness, difficulty reading, or increased difficulty performing complex tasks. Initially these symptoms may be indistinguishable from findings of situational depression or fatigue. In contrast to "cortical" dementia (such as Alzheimer's disease), aphasia,

TABLE 182-12	CLINICAL STAGING OF HIV ENCEPHALOPATHY (AIDS DEMENTIA COMPLEX)
Stage	**Definition**
Stage 0 (normal)	Normal mental and motor function
Stage 0.5 (equivocal/ subclinical)	Absent, minimal, or equivocal symptoms without impairment of work or capacity to perform activities of daily living. Mild signs (snout response, slowed ocular or extremity movements) may be present. Gait and strength are normal.
Stage 1 (mild)	Able to perform all but the more demanding aspects of work or activities of daily living but with unequivocal evidence (signs or symptoms that may include performance on neuropsychological testing) of functional, intellectual, or motor impairment. Can walk without assistance.
Stage 2 (moderate)	Able to perform basic activities of self-care but cannot work or maintain the more demanding aspects of daily life. Ambulatory, but may require a single prop.
Stage 3 (severe)	Major intellectual incapacity (cannot follow news or personal events, cannot sustain complex conversation, considerable slowing of all output) or motor disability (cannot walk unassisted, usually with slowing and clumsiness of arms as well).
Stage 4 (end-stage)	Nearly vegetative. Intellectual and social comprehension and output are at a rudimentary level. Nearly or absolutely mute. Paraparetic or paraplegic with urinary and fecal incontinence.

Source: Adapted from JJ Sidtis, RW Price, Neurology 40:197, 1990.

apraxia, and agnosia are uncommon, leading some investigators to classify HIV encephalopathy as a "subcortical dementia" (see below). In addition to dementia, patients with HIV encephalopathy may also have motor and behavioral abnormalities. Among the motor problems are unsteady gait, poor balance, tremor, and difficulty with rapid alternating movements. Increased tone and deep tendon reflexes may be found in patients with spinal cord involvement. Late stages may be complicated by bowel and/or bladder incontinence. Behavioral problems include apathy and lack of initiative, with progression to a vegetative state in some instances. Some patients develop a state of agitation or mild mania. These changes usually occur without significant changes in level of alertness. This is in contrast to the finding of somnolence in patients with dementia due to toxic/metabolic encephalopathies.

HIV encephalopathy is the initial AIDS-defining illness in ~3% of patients with HIV infection and thus only rarely precedes clinical evidence of immunodeficiency. Clinically significant encephalopathy eventually develops in ~25% of patients with AIDS. As immunologic function declines, the risk and severity of HIV encephalopathy increase. Autopsy series suggest that 80–90% of patients with HIV infection have histologic evidence of CNS involvement. Several classification schemes have been developed for grading HIV encephalopathy; a commonly used clinical staging system is outlined in Table 182-12.

The precise cause of HIV encephalopathy remains unclear, although the condition is thought to be a result of a combination of direct effects of HIV on the CNS and associated immune activation. HIV has been found in the brains of patients with HIV encephalopathy by Southern blot, in situ hybridization, PCR, and electron microscopy. Multinucleated giant cells, macrophages, and microglial cells appear to be the main cell types harboring virus in the CNS. Histologically, the major changes are seen in the subcortical areas of the brain and include pallor and gliosis, multinucleated giant cell encephalitis, and vacuolar myelopathy. Less commonly, diffuse or focal spongiform changes occur in the white matter. Areas of the brain involved in motor, language, and judgment are most severely affected.

There are no specific criteria for a diagnosis of HIV encephalopathy, and this syndrome must be differentiated from a number of other diseases that affect the CNS of HIV-infected patients (Table 182-11). The diagnosis of dementia depends upon demonstrating a decline in cognitive function. This can be accomplished objectively with the use of a Mini-Mental Status Examination (MMSE) in patients for whom prior scores are available. For this reason, it is advisable for all patients with a diagnosis of HIV infection to have a baseline MMSE. However, changes in MMSE scores may be absent in patients with mild HIV encephalopathy. Imaging studies of the CNS, by either MRI or CT, often demonstrate evidence of cerebral atrophy (Fig. 182-37). MRI may also reveal small areas of increased density on T2-weighted images. Lumbar puncture is an important element of the evaluation of patients with HIV infection and neurologic abnormalities. It is generally most

FIGURE 182-37 AIDS dementia complex. Postcontrast CT scan through the lateral ventricles of a 47-year-old man with AIDS, altered mental status, and dementia. The lateral and third ventricles and the cerebral sulci are abnormally prominent. Mild white matter hypodensity is also seen adjacent to the frontal horns of the lateral ventricles.

helpful in ruling out or making a diagnosis of opportunistic infections. In HIV encephalopathy, patients may have the nonspecific findings of an increase in CSF cells and protein level. While HIV RNA can often be detected in the spinal fluid and HIV can be cultured from the CSF, this finding is not specific for HIV encephalopathy. There appears to be no correlation between the presence of HIV in the CSF and the presence of HIV encephalopathy. Elevated levels of macrophage chemoattractant protein (MCP-1), β_2-microglobulin, neopterin, and quinolinic acid (a metabolite of tryptophan reported to cause CNS injury) have been noted in the CSF of patients with HIV encephalopathy. These findings suggest that these factors as well as inflammatory cytokines may be involved in the pathogenesis of this syndrome.

Combination ARV therapy is of benefit in patients with HIV encephalopathy. Improvement in neuropsychiatric test scores has been noted for both adult and pediatric patients treated with ARVs. The rapid improvement in cognitive function noted with the initiation of ARV therapy suggests that at least some component of this problem is quickly reversible, again supporting at least a partial role of soluble mediators in the pathogenesis. It should also be noted that these patients have an increased sensitivity to the side effects of neuroleptic drugs. The use of these drugs for symptomatic treatment is associated with an increased risk of extrapyramidal side effects; therefore, patients with HIV encephalopathy who receive these agents must be monitored carefully.

Seizures may be a consequence of opportunistic infections, neoplasms, or HIV encephalopathy (Table 182-13). The seizure threshold is often lower than normal in patients with advanced HIV infection due to the frequent presence of electrolyte abnormalities. Seizures are

TABLE 182-13	CAUSES OF SEIZURES IN PATIENTS WITH HIV INFECTION	
Disease	**Overall Contribution to First Seizure, %**	**Fraction of Patients Who Have Seizures, %**
HIV encephalopathy	24–47	7–50
Cerebral toxoplasmosis	28	15–40
Cryptococcal meningitis	13	8
Primary central nervous system lymphoma	4	15–30
Progressive multifocal leukoencephalopathy	1	

Source: From DM Holtzman et al: Am J Med 87:173, 1989.

seen in 15–40% of patients with cerebral toxoplasmosis, 15–35% of patients with primary CNS lymphoma, 8% of patients with cryptococcal meningitis, and 7–50% of patients with HIV encephalopathy. Seizures may also be seen in patients with CNS tuberculosis, aseptic meningitis, and progressive multifocal leukoencephalopathy. Seizures may be the presenting clinical symptom of HIV disease. In one study of 100 patients with HIV infection presenting with a first seizure, cerebral mass lesions were the most common cause, responsible for 32 of the 100 new-onset seizures. Of these 32 cases, 28 were due to toxoplasmosis and 4 to lymphoma. HIV encephalopathy accounted for an additional 24 new-onset seizures. Cryptococcal meningitis was the third most common diagnosis, responsible for 13 of the 100 seizures. In 23 cases, no cause could be found, and it is possible that these cases represent a subcategory of HIV encephalopathy. Of these 23 cases, 16 (70%) had two or more seizures, suggesting that anticonvulsant therapy is indicated in all patients with HIV infection and seizures unless a rapidly correctable cause is found. While phenytoin remains the initial treatment of choice, hypersensitivity reactions to this drug have been reported in >10% of patients with AIDS, and therefore the use of phenobarbital or valproic acid must be considered as alternatives.

Patients with HIV infection may present with *focal neurologic deficits* from a variety of causes. The most common causes are toxoplasmosis, progressive multifocal leukoencephalopathy, and CNS lymphoma. Other causes include cryptococcal infections (discussed above; also Chap. 195), stroke, and reactivation Chagas' disease.

Toxoplasmosis has been one of the most common causes of secondary CNS infections in patients with AIDS, but its incidence is decreasing in the era of HAART. It is most common in patients from the Caribbean and from France. Toxoplasmosis is generally a late complication of HIV infection and usually occurs in patients with CD4+ T cell counts <200/μL. Cerebral toxoplasmosis is thought to represent a reactivation syndrome. It is 10 times more common in patients with antibodies to the organism than in patients who are seronegative. Patients diagnosed with HIV infection should be screened for IgG antibodies to *T. gondii* during the time of their initial workup. Those who are seronegative should be counseled about ways to minimize the risk of primary infection including avoiding the consumption of undercooked meat and careful hand washing after contact with soil or changing the cat litter box. The most common clinical presentation of cerebral toxoplasmosis in patients with HIV infection is fever, headache, and focal neurologic deficits. Patients may present with seizure, hemiparesis, or aphasia as a manifestation of these focal deficits or with a picture more influenced by the accompanying cerebral edema and characterized by confusion, dementia, and lethargy, which can progress to coma. The diagnosis is usually suspected on the basis of MRI findings of multiple lesions in multiple locations, although in some cases only a single lesion is seen. Pathologically, these lesions generally exhibit inflammation and central necrosis and, as a result, demonstrate ring enhancement on contrast MRI (Fig. 182-38) or, if MRI is unavailable or contraindicated, on double-dose contrast CT. There is usually evidence of surrounding edema. In addition to toxoplasmosis, the differential diagnosis of single or multiple enhancing mass lesions in the HIV-infected patient includes primary CNS lymphoma (see below) and, less commonly, TB or fungal or bacterial abscesses. The definitive diagnostic procedure is brain biopsy. However, given the morbidity than can accompany this procedure, it is usually reserved for the patient who has failed 2–4 weeks of empirical therapy. If the patient is seronegative for *T. gondii*, the likelihood that a mass lesion is due to toxoplasmosis is <10%. In that setting, one may choose to be more aggressive and perform a brain biopsy sooner. Standard treatment is sulfadiazine and pyrimethamine with leucovorin as needed for a minimum of 4–6 weeks. Alternative therapeutic regimens include clindamycin in combination with pyrimethamine; atovaquone plus pyrimethamine; and azithromycin plus pyrimethamine plus rifabutin. Relapses are common, and it is recommended that patients with a history of prior toxoplasmic encephalitis receive maintenance therapy with sulfadiazine, pyrimethamine, and leucovorin as long as their CD4+ T cell counts remain <200 cells/μL. Patients with CD4+ T

FIGURE 182-38 Central nervous system toxoplasmosis. A coronal postcontrast T1-weighted MR scan demonstrates a peripheral enhancing lesion in the left frontal lobe, associated with an eccentric nodular area of enhancement (*arrow*); this so-called eccentric target sign is typical of toxoplasmosis.

cell counts <100/μL and IgG antibody to *Toxoplasma* should receive primary prophylaxis for toxoplasmosis. Fortunately, the same daily regimen of a single double-strength tablet of TMP/SMX used for *P. jiroveci* prophylaxis provides adequate primary protection against toxoplasmosis. Secondary prophylaxis/maintenance therapy for toxoplasmosis may be discontinued in the setting of effective ARV therapy and increases in CD4+ T cell counts to >200/μL for 6 months.

JC virus, a human polyomavirus that is the etiologic agent of *progressive multifocal leukoencephalopathy* (PML), is an important opportunistic pathogen in patients with AIDS (Chap. 377). While ~70% of the general adult population have antibodies to JC virus, indicative of prior infection, <10% of healthy adults show any evidence of ongoing viral replication. PML is the only known clinical manifestation of JC virus infection. It is a late manifestation of AIDS and is seen in ~4% of patients with AIDS. The lesions of PML begin as small foci of demyelination in subcortical white matter that eventually coalesce. The cerebral hemispheres, cerebellum, and brainstem may all be involved. Patients typically have a protracted course with multifocal neurologic deficits, with or without changes in mental status. Approximately 20% of patients experience seizures. Ataxia, hemiparesis, visual field defects, aphasia, and sensory defects may occur. MRI typically reveals multiple, nonenhancing white matter lesions that may coalesce and have a predilection for the occipital and parietal lobes. The lesions show signal hyperintensity on T2-weighted images and diminished signal on T1-weighted images. The measurement of JC virus DNA levels in CSF has a diagnostic sensitivity of 76% and a specificity of close to 100%. Prior to the availability of potent ARV combination therapy, the majority of patients with PML died within 3–6 months of the onset of symptoms. Paradoxical worsening of PML has been seen with initiation of HAART as an immune reconstitution syndrome. There is no specific treatment for PML; however, a minimal median survival of 18 months and survival of >7 years have been reported in patients with PML treated with HAART for their HIV disease. Unfortunately only ~50% of patients with HIV infection and PML show neurologic improvement with HAART. Studies with other antiviral agents such as cidofovir have failed to show clear benefit. Factors influencing a favorable prognosis for PML in the setting of HIV infection include a CD4+ T cell count >100/μL at baseline and the ability to maintain an HIV viral load of <500 copies per milliliter. Baseline HIV-1 viral load does not have independent predictive value of survival. PML is one of the few opportunistic infections that continues to occur with some frequency despite the widespread use of HAART.

Reactivation American trypanosomiasis may present as acute meningoencephalitis with focal neurologic signs, fever, headache, vomiting, and seizures. In South America, reactivation of *Chagas' disease* is considered to be an AIDS-defining condition and may be the initial AIDS-defining condition. Lesions appear radiographically as single or multiple hypodense areas, typically with ring enhancement and edema. They are found predominantly in the subcortical areas, a feature that differentiates them from the deeper lesions of toxoplasmosis. *Trypanosoma cruzi* amastigotes, or trypanosomes, can be identified from biopsy specimens or CSF. Other CSF findings include elevated protein and a mild (<100 cells/μL) lymphocytic pleocytosis. Organisms can also be identified by direct examination of the blood. Treatment consists of benzimidazole (2.5 mg/kg bid) or nifurtimox (2 mg/kg qid) for at least 60 days, followed by maintenance therapy for the duration of immunodeficiency with either drug at a dose of 5 mg/kg three times a week. As is the case with cerebral toxoplasmosis, successful therapy with ARVs may allow discontinuation of therapy for Chagas' disease.

Stroke may occur in patients with HIV infection. In contrast to the other causes of focal neurologic deficits in patients with HIV infection, the symptoms of a stroke are sudden in onset. Among the secondary infectious diseases in patients with HIV infection that may be associated with stroke are vasculitis due to cerebral varicella zoster or neurosyphilis and septic embolism in association with fungal infection. Other elements of the differential diagnosis of stroke in the patient with HIV infection include atherosclerotic cerebral vascular disease, thrombotic thrombocytopenic purpura, and cocaine or amphetamine use.

Primary CNS lymphoma is discussed below in the section on neoplastic diseases.

Spinal cord disease, or myelopathy, is present in ~20% of patients with AIDS, often as part of HIV encephalopathy. In fact, 90% of the patients with HIV-associated myelopathy have some evidence of dementia, suggesting that similar pathologic processes may be responsible for both conditions. Three main types of spinal cord disease are seen in patients with AIDS. The first of these is a vacuolar myelopathy, as discussed above under HIV encephalopathy. This condition is pathologically similar to subacute combined degeneration of the cord such as occurs with pernicious anemia. Although vitamin B$_{12}$ deficiency can be seen in patients with AIDS as a primary complication of HIV infection, it does not appear to be responsible for the myelopathy seen in the majority of patients. Vacuolar myelopathy is characterized by a subacute onset and often presents with gait disturbances, predominantly ataxia and spasticity; it may progress to include bladder and bowel dysfunction. Physical findings include evidence of increased deep tendon reflexes and extensor plantar responses. The second form of spinal cord disease involves the dorsal columns and presents as a pure sensory ataxia. The third form is also sensory in nature and presents with paresthesias and dysesthesias of the lower extremities. In contrast to the cognitive problems seen in patients with HIV encephalopathy, these spinal cord syndromes do not respond well to ARV drugs, and therapy is mainly supportive.

One important disease of the spinal cord that also involves the peripheral nerves is a *myelopathy* and *polyradiculopathy* seen in association with CMV infection. This entity is generally seen late in the course of HIV infection and is fulminant in onset, with lower extremity and sacral paresthesias, difficulty in walking, areflexia, ascending sensory loss, and urinary retention. The clinical course is rapidly progressive over a period of weeks. CSF examination reveals a predominantly neutrophilic pleocytosis, and CMV DNA can be detected by CSF PCR. Therapy with ganciclovir or foscarnet can lead to rapid improvement, and prompt initiation of foscarnet or ganciclovir therapy is important in minimizing the degree of permanent neurologic damage. Combination therapy with both drugs should be considered in patients who have been previously treated for CMV disease. Other diseases involving the spinal cord in patients with HIV infection include HTLV-I-associated myelopathy (HAM) (Chap. 181), neurosyphilis (Chap. 162), infection with herpes simplex (Chap. 172) or varicellazoster (Chap. 173), TB (Chap. 158), and lymphoma (Chap. 105).

Peripheral neuropathies are common in patients with HIV infection. They occur at all stages of illness and take a variety of forms. Early in the course of HIV infection, an acute inflammatory demyelinating polyneuropathy resembling Guillain-Barré syndrome may occur (Chap. 381). In other patients, a progressive or relapsing-remitting inflammatory neuropathy resembling chronic inflammatory demyelinating polyneuropathy (CIDP) has been noted. Patients commonly present with progressive weakness, areflexia, and minimal sensory changes. CSF examination often reveals a mononuclear pleocytosis, and peripheral nerve biopsy demonstrates a perivascular infiltrate suggesting an autoimmune etiology. Plasma exchange or IVIg has been tried with variable success. Because of the immunosuppressive effects of glucocorticoids, they should be reserved for severe cases of CIDP refractory to other measures. Another autoimmune peripheral neuropathy seen in patients with AIDS is mononeuritis multiplex (Chaps. 381 and 319) due to a necrotizing arteritis of peripheral nerves. The most common peripheral neuropathy in patients with HIV infection is a *distal sensory polyneuropathy* that may be a direct consequence of HIV infection or a side effect of dideoxynucleoside therapy. Two-thirds of patients with AIDS may be shown by electrophysiologic studies to have some evidence of peripheral nerve disease. Presenting symptoms are usually painful burning sensations in the feet and lower extremities. Findings on examination include a stocking-type sensory loss to pinprick, temperature, and touch sensation and a loss of ankle reflexes. Motor changes are mild and are usually limited to weakness of the intrinsic foot muscles. Response of this condition to ARVs has been variable, perhaps because ARVs are responsible for the problem in some instances. When due to dideoxynucleoside therapy, patients with lower extremity peripheral neuropathy may complain of a sensation that they are walking on ice. Other entities in the differential diagnosis of peripheral neuropathy include diabetes mellitus, vitamin B_{12} deficiency, and side effects from metronidazole or dapsone. For distal symmetric polyneuropathy that fails to resolve following the discontinuation of dideoxynucleosides, therapy is symptomatic; gabapentin, carbamazepine, tricyclics, or analgesics may be effective for dysesthesias. Treatment-naive patients may respond to combination ARV therapy.

Myopathy may complicate the course of HIV infection; causes include HIV infection itself, zidovudine, and the generalized wasting syndrome. HIV-associated myopathy may range in severity from an asymptomatic elevation in creatine kinase levels to a subacute syndrome characterized by proximal muscle weakness and myalgias. Quite pronounced elevations in creatine kinase may occur in asymptomatic patients, particularly after exercise. The clinical significance of this as an isolated laboratory finding is unclear. A variety of both inflammatory and noninflammatory pathologic processes have been noted in patients with more severe myopathy, including myofiber necrosis with inflammatory cells, nemaline rod bodies, cytoplasmic bodies, and mitochondrial abnormalities. Profound muscle wasting, often with muscle pain, may be seen after prolonged zidovudine therapy. This toxic side effect of the drug is dose-dependent and is related to its ability to interfere with the function of mitochondrial polymerases. It is reversible following discontinuation of the drug. Red ragged fibers are a histologic hallmark of zidovudine-induced myopathy.

Ophthalmologic Disease Ophthalmologic problems occur in ~50% of patients with advanced HIV infection. The most common abnormal findings on funduscopic examination are cotton-wool spots. These are hard white spots that appear on the surface of the retina and often have an irregular edge. They represent areas of retinal ischemia secondary to microvascular disease. At times they are associated with small areas of hemorrhage and thus can be difficult to distinguish from CMV retinitis. In contrast to CMV retinitis, however, these lesions are not associated with visual loss and tend to remain stable or improve over time.

One of the most devastating consequences of HIV infection is CMV retinitis. Patients at high risk of CMV retinitis (CD4+ T cell count <100/μL) should undergo an ophthalmologic examination every 3–6 months. The majority of cases of CMV retinitis occur in patients with a CD4+ T cell count <50/μL. Prior to the availability of HAART, this CMV reactivation syndrome was seen in 25–30% of patients with AIDS. CMV retinitis usually presents as a painless, progressive loss of vision. Patients may also complain of blurred vision, "floaters," and scintillations. The disease is usually bilateral, although typically it affects one eye more than

the other. The diagnosis is made on clinical grounds by an experienced ophthalmologist. The characteristic retinal appearance is that of perivascular hemorrhage and exudate. In situations where the diagnosis is in doubt due to an atypical presentation or an unexpected lack of response to therapy, vitreous or aqueous humor sampling with molecular diagnostic techniques may be of value. CMV infection of the retina results in a necrotic inflammatory process, and the visual loss that develops is irreversible. CMV retinitis may be complicated by rhegmatogenous retinal detachment as a consequence of retinal atrophy in areas of prior inflammation. Therapy for CMV retinitis consists of oral valganciclovir, IV ganciclovir, or IV foscarnet, with cidofovir as an alternative. Combination therapy with ganciclovir and foscarnet has been shown to be slightly more effective than either ganciclovir or foscarnet alone in the patient with relapsed CMV retinitis. A 3-week induction course is followed by maintenance therapy with oral valganciclovir. If CMV disease is limited to the eye, a ganciclovir-releasing intraocular implant, periodic injections of the antisense nucleic acid preparation fomivirsen, or intravitreal injections of ganciclovir or foscarnet may be considered; some choose to combine intraocular implants with oral valganciclovir. Intravitreal injections of cidofovir are generally avoided due to the increased risk of uveitis and hypotony. Maintenance therapy is continued until the CD4+ T cell count remains >100–150/μL for >6 months. The majority of patients with HIV infection and CMV disease develop some degree of uveitis with the initiation of ARV therapy. The etiology of this is unknown; however, it has been suggested that this may be due to the generation of an enhanced immune response to CMV as an IRIS (see above). In some instances this has required the use of topical glucocorticoids.

Both HSV and varicella zoster virus can cause a rapidly progressing, bilateral necrotizing retinitis referred to as the *acute retinal necrosis syndrome*, or *progressive outer retinal necrosis* (PORN). This syndrome, in contrast to CMV retinitis, is associated with pain, keratitis, and iritis. It is often associated with orolabial HSV or trigeminal zoster. Ophthalmologic examination reveals widespread pale gray peripheral lesions. This condition is often complicated by retinal detachment. It is important to recognize and treat this condition with IV acyclovir as quickly as possible to minimize the loss of vision.

Several other secondary infections may cause ocular problems in HIV-infected patients. *P. jiroveci* can cause a lesion of the choroid that may be detected as an incidental finding on ophthalmologic examination. These lesions are typically bilateral, are from half to twice the disc diameter in size, and appear as slightly elevated yellow-white plaques. They are usually asymptomatic and may be confused with cotton-wool spots. Chorioretinitis due to toxoplasmosis can be seen alone or, more commonly, in association with CNS toxoplasmosis. KS may involve the eyelid or conjunctiva while lymphoma may involve the retina.

Additional Disseminated Infections and Wasting Syndrome Infections with species of the small, gram-negative rickettsia-like organism *Bartonella* (Chap. 153) are seen with increased frequency in patients with HIV infection. While not considered an AIDS-defining illness by the CDC, many experts view infection with *Bartonella* as indicative of a severe defect in cell-mediated immunity. It is usually seen in patients with CD4+ T cell counts <100/μL. Among the clinical manifestations of *Bartonella* infection are bacillary angiomatosis, cat-scratch disease, and trench fever. *Bacillary angiomatosis* is usually due to infection with *B. henselae*. It is characterized by a vascular proliferation that leads to a variety of skin lesions that have been confused with the skin lesions of KS. In contrast to the lesions of KS, the lesions of bacillary angiomatosis generally blanch, are painful, and typically occur in the setting of systemic symptoms. Infection can extend to the lymph nodes, liver (peliosis hepatis), spleen, bone, heart, CNS, respiratory tract, and gastrointestinal tract. *Cat-scratch disease* generally begins with a papule at the site of inoculation. This is followed several weeks later by the development of regional adenopathy and malaise. Infection with *B. quintana* is transmitted by lice and has been associated with case reports of trench fever, endocarditis, adenopathy, and bacillary angiomatosis. The organism is quite difficult to culture, and diagnosis often relies upon identifying the organism in biopsy specimens using the Warthin-Starry or similar stains. Treatment is with either erythromycin or doxycycline for at least 3 months.

Histoplasmosis is an opportunistic infection that is seen most frequently in patients in the Mississippi and Ohio River valleys, Puerto Rico, the Dominican Republic, and South America. These are all areas in which infection with *H. capsulatum* is endemic (Chap. 192). Because of this limited geographic distribution, the percentage of AIDS cases in the United States with histoplasmosis is only ~0.5. Histoplasmosis is generally a late manifestation of HIV infection; however, it may be the initial AIDS-defining condition. In one study, the median CD4+ T cell count for patients with histoplasmosis and AIDS was 33/μL. While disease due to *H. capsulatum* may present as a primary infection of the lung, disseminated disease, presumably due to reactivation, is the most common presentation in HIV-infected patients. Patients usually present with a 4- to 8-week history of fever and weight loss. Hepatosplenomegaly and lymphadenopathy are each seen in about 25% of patients. CNS disease, either meningitis or a mass lesion, is seen in 15% of patients. Bone marrow involvement is common, with thrombocytopenia, neutropenia, and anemia occurring in 33% of patients. Approximately 7% of patients have mucocutaneous lesions consisting of a maculopapular rash and skin or oral ulcers. Respiratory symptoms are usually mild, with chest x-ray showing a diffuse infiltrate or diffuse small nodules in ~50% of cases. Diagnosis is made by culturing the organisms from blood, bone marrow, or tissue. Treatment is typically with amphotericin B, 0.7–1.0 mg/kg daily to a total dose of 1 g followed by maintenance therapy with itraconazole. In the setting of mild infection, it may be appropriate to treat with itraconazole alone.

Following the spread of HIV infection to southeast Asia, disseminated infection with the fungus *Penicillium marneffei* was recognized as a complication of HIV infection and is considered an AIDS-defining condition in those parts of the world where it occurs. *P. marneffei* is the third most common AIDS-defining illness in Thailand, following TB and cryptococcosis. It is more frequently diagnosed in the rainy than the dry season. Clinical features include fever, generalized lymphadenopathy, hepatosplenomegaly, anemia, thrombocytopenia, and papular skin lesions with central umbilication. Treatment is with amphotericin B followed by itraconazole.

Visceral leishmaniasis (Chap. 205) is recognized with increasing frequency in patients with HIV infection who live in or travel to areas endemic for this protozoal infection transmitted by sandflies. The clinical presentation is one of hepatosplenomegaly, fever, and hematologic abnormalities. Lymphadenopathy and other constitutional symptoms may be present. A chronic, relapsing course is seen in two-thirds of co-infected patients. Organisms can be isolated from cultures of bone marrow aspirates. Histologic stains may be negative, and antibody titers are of little help. Patients with HIV infection usually respond well initially to standard therapy with amphotericin B or pentavalent antimony compounds. Eradication of the organism is difficult, however, and relapses are common.

Patients with HIV infection are at increased risk of clinical malaria. This is particularly true for patients from nonendemic areas with presumed primary infection and in patients with lower CD4+ T cell counts. HIV-positive individuals with CD4+ T cell counts <300 cells/μL have a poorer response to malaria treatment than others. Co-infection with malaria is associated with a modest increase in HIV viral load. The risk of malaria may be decreased with TMP/SMX prophylaxis.

Generalized wasting is an AIDS-defining condition; it is defined as involuntary weight loss of >10% associated with intermittent or constant fever and chronic diarrhea or fatigue lasting >30 days in the absence of a defined cause other than HIV infection. It is the initial AIDS-defining condition in ~10% of patients with AIDS in the United States and is an indication for initiation of HAART. A constant feature of this syndrome is severe muscle wasting with scattered myofiber degeneration and occasional evidence of myositis. Glucocorticoids may be of some benefit; however, this approach must be carefully weighed against the risk of compounding the immunodeficiency of HIV infection. Androgenic steroids, growth hormone, and total parenteral nutrition have been used as therapeutic interventions with variable success.

Neoplastic Diseases   The neoplastic diseases clearly seen with an increased frequency in patients with HIV infection are KS and non-Hodgkin's lymphoma. In addition, there also appears to be an increased incidence of Hodgkin's disease; multiple myeloma; leukemia; melanoma; and cervical, brain, testicular, oral, lung, and anal cancers. Recent years have witnessed a marked reduction in the incidence of KS (Fig. 182-31) and improvements in the outcomes of HIV-infected patients with non-AIDS-defining malignancies. These changes are primarily due to the use of potent ARV therapy. Rates of non-Hodgkin's lymphoma have declined as well; however, this decline has not been as dramatic as the decline in rates of KS. In contrast, HAART has had little effect on human papilloma virus (HPV)-associated malignancies. As patients with HIV infection live longer, a wider array of cancers are being seen in this population of patients. While some may only reflect known risk factors (i.e., smoking) that are increased in patients with HIV infection, some may be a direct consequence of HIV.

Kaposi's sarcoma is a multicentric neoplasm consisting of multiple vascular nodules appearing in the skin, mucous membranes, and viscera. The course ranges from indolent, with only minor skin or lymph node involvement, to fulminant, with extensive cutaneous and visceral involvement. In the initial period of the AIDS epidemic, KS was a prominent clinical feature of the first cases of AIDS, occurring in 79% of the patients diagnosed in 1981. By 1989 it was seen in only 25% of cases, by 1992 the number had decreased to 9%, and by 1997 the number was <1%. HHV-8 or KSHV has been strongly implicated as a viral cofactor in the pathogenesis of KS (see above).

Clinically, KS has varied presentations and may be seen at any stage of HIV infection, even in the presence of a normal CD4+ T cell count. The initial lesion may be a small, raised reddish-purple nodule on the skin (Fig. 182-39), a discoloration on the oral mucosa (Fig. 182-32D), or a swollen lymph node. Lesions often appear in sun-exposed areas, particularly the tip of the nose, and have a propensity to occur in areas of trauma (Koebner phenomenon). Because of the vascular nature of the tumors and the presence of extravasated red blood cells in the lesions, their colors range from reddish to purple to brown and often take the appearance of a bruise, with yellowish discoloration and tattooing. Lesions range in size from a few millimeters to several centimeters in diameter and may be either discrete or confluent. KS lesions most commonly appear as raised macules; however, they can also be papular, particularly in patients with higher CD4+ T cell counts. Confluent lesions may give rise to surrounding lymphedema and may be disfiguring when they involve the face and disabling when they involve the lower extremities or the surfaces of joints. Apart from skin, lymph nodes, gastrointestinal tract, and lung are the organ systems most commonly affected by KS. Lesions have been reported in virtually every organ, including the heart and the CNS. In contrast to most malignancies, in which lymph node involvement implies metastatic spread and a poor prognosis, lymph node involvement may be seen very early in KS and is of no special clinical significance. In fact, some patients

FIGURE 182-39 Kaposi's sarcoma in a patient with AIDS demonstrating patch, plaque, and tumor stages.

FIGURE 182-40 Chest x-ray of a patient with AIDS and pulmonary Kaposi's sarcoma. The characteristic findings include dense bilateral lower lobe infiltrates obscuring the heart borders and a pleural effusion.

may present with disease limited to the lymph nodes. These are generally patients with relatively intact immune function and thus the patients with the best prognosis. Pulmonary involvement with KS generally presents with shortness of breath. Some 80% of patients with pulmonary KS also have cutaneous lesions. The chest x-ray characteristically shows bilateral lower lobe infiltrates that obscure the margins of the mediastinum and diaphragm (Fig. 182-40). Pleural effusions are seen in 70% of cases of pulmonary KS, a fact that is often helpful in the differential diagnosis. Gastrointestinal involvement is seen in 50% of patients and usually takes one of two forms: (1) mucosal involvement, which may lead to bleeding that can be severe; these patients sometimes also develop symptoms of gastrointestinal obstruction if lesions become large; and (2) biliary tract involvement. KS lesions may infiltrate the gallbladder and biliary tree, leading to a clinical picture of obstructive jaundice similar to that seen with sclerosing cholangitis. Several staging systems have been proposed for KS. One in common use was developed by the National Institute of Allergy and Infectious Diseases AIDS Clinical Trials Group; it distinguishes patients on the basis of tumor extent, immunologic function, and presence or absence of systemic disease (Table 182-14).

A diagnosis of KS is based upon biopsy of a suspicious lesion. Histologically one sees a proliferation of spindle cells and endothelial cells, extravasation of red blood cells, hemosiderin-laden macrophages, and, in early cases, an inflammatory cell infiltrate. Included in the differential diagnosis are lymphoma (particularly for oral lesions), bacillary angiomatosis, and cutaneous mycobacterial infections.

Management of KS (Table 182-15) should be carried out in consultation with an expert since definitive treatment guidelines do not exist.

TABLE 182-15 **MANAGEMENT OF AIDS-ASSOCIATED KAPOSI'S SARCOMA** **1187**

Observation and optimization of antiretroviral therapy
Single or limited number of lesions
Radiation
Intralesional vinblastine
Cryotherapy
Extensive disease
Initial therapy
Interferon-α (if CD4+ T cells >150/μL)
Liposomal daunorubicin
Subsequent therapy
Liposomal doxorubicin
Paclitaxel
Combination chemotherapy with low-dose doxorubicin, bleomycin, and vinblastine (ABV)
Radiation treatment

In the majority of cases, effective ARV therapy will go a long way in achieving control. Indeed, spontaneous regressions have been reported in the setting of HAART. For patients in whom tumor persists or in whom control of HIV replication is not possible, a variety of options exist. In some cases, lesions remain quite indolent, and many of these patients can be managed with no specific treatment. Fewer than 10% of AIDS patients with KS die as a consequence of their malignancy, and death from secondary infections is considerably more common. Thus, whenever possible one should avoid treatment regimens that may further suppress the immune system and increase susceptibility to opportunistic infections. Treatment is indicated under two main circumstances. The first is when a single lesion or a limited number of lesions are causing significant discomfort or cosmetic problems, such as with prominent facial lesions, lesions overlying a joint, or lesions in the oropharynx that interfere with swallowing or breathing. Under these circumstances, treatment with localized radiation, intralesional vinblastine, or cryotherapy may be helpful. It should be noted that patients with HIV infection are particularly sensitive to the side effects of radiation therapy. This is especially true with respect to the development of radiation-induced mucositis; doses of radiation directed at mucosal surfaces, particularly in the head and neck region, should be adjusted accordingly. The use of systemic therapy, either IFN-α or chemotherapy, should be considered in patients with a large number of lesions or in patients with visceral involvement. The single most important determinant of response appears to be the CD4+ T cell count. This relationship between response rate and baseline CD4+ T cell count is particularly true for IFN-α. The response rate for patients with CD4+ T cell counts >600/μL is ~80%, while the response rate for patients with counts <150/μL is <10%. In contrast to the other systemic therapies, IFN-α provides an added advantage of having ARV activity; thus, it may be the appropriate first choice for single-agent systemic therapy for early patients with disseminated disease. A variety of chemotherapeutic agents have also been shown to have activity against KS. Three of them, liposomal daunorubicin, liposomal doxorubicin, and paclitaxel, have been approved by the FDA for this indication. Liposomal daunorubicin is approved as first-line therapy for patients with advanced KS. It has fewer side effects than conventional chemotherapy. In contrast, liposomal doxorubicin and paclitaxel are approved only for KS patients who have failed standard chemotherapy. Response rates vary from 23–88%, appear to be comparable to what had been achieved earlier with combination chemotherapy regimens, and are greatly influenced by CD4+ T cell count.

Lymphomas occur with an increased frequency in patients with congenital or acquired T cell immunodeficiencies (Chap. 310). AIDS is no exception; at least 6% of all patients with AIDS develop lymphoma at some time during the course of their illness. This is a 120-fold

TABLE 182-14 **NATIONAL INSTITUTE OF ALLERGY AND INFECTIOUS DISEASES AIDS CLINICAL TRIALS GROUP TIS STAGING SYSTEM FOR KAPOSI'S SARCOMA**

Parameter	Good Risk (Stage 0): All of the Following	Poor Risk (Stage 1): Any of the Following
Tumor (T)	Confined to skin and/or lymph nodes and/or minimal oral disease	Tumor-associated edema or ulceration Extensive oral lesions Gastrointestinal lesions Nonnodal visceral lesions
Immune system (I)	CD4+ T cell count ≥200/μL	CD4+ T cell count <200/μL
Systemic illness (S)	No B symptoms[a] Karnofsky performance status ≥70 No history of opportunistic infection, neurologic disease, lymphoma, or thrush	B symptoms[a] present Karnofsky performance status <70 History of opportunistic infection, neurologic disease, lymphoma, or thrush

[a]Defined as unexplained fever, night sweats, >10% involuntary weight loss, or diarrhea persisting for more than 2 weeks.

increase in incidence compared to the general population. In contrast to the situation with KS, primary CNS lymphoma, and most opportunistic infections, the incidence of AIDS-associated systemic lymphomas has not experienced as dramatic a decrease as a consequence of the widespread use of effective ARV therapy. Lymphoma occurs in all risk groups, with the highest incidence in patients with hemophilia and the lowest incidence in patients from the Caribbean or Africa with heterosexually acquired infection. Lymphoma is a late manifestation of HIV infection, generally occurring in patients with CD4+ T cell counts <200/μL. As HIV disease progresses, the risk of lymphoma increases. In contrast to KS, which occurs at a relatively constant rate throughout the course of HIV disease, the attack rate for lymphoma increases exponentially with increasing duration of HIV infection and decreasing level of immunologic function. At 3 years following a diagnosis of HIV infection, the risk of lymphoma is 0.8% per year; by 8 years after infection, it is 2.6% per year. As individuals with HIV infection live longer as a consequence of improved ARV therapy and better treatment and prophylaxis of opportunistic infections, it is anticipated that the incidence of lymphomas may increase.

Three main categories of lymphoma are seen in patients with HIV infection: grade III or IV immunoblastic lymphoma, Burkitt's lymphoma, and primary CNS lymphoma. Approximately 90% of these lymphomas are B cell in phenotype, and half contain EBV DNA. These tumors may be either monoclonal or oligoclonal in nature and are probably in some way related to the pronounced polyclonal B cell activation seen in patients with AIDS.

Immunoblastic lymphomas account for ~60% of the cases of lymphoma in patients with AIDS. These are generally high grade and would have been classified as diffuse histiocytic lymphomas in earlier classification schemes. This tumor is more common in older patients, increasing in incidence from 0% in HIV-infected individuals <1 year old to >3% in those >50. One variant of immunoblastic lymphoma is body cavity lymphoma. This malignancy presents with lymphomatous pleural, pericardial, and/or peritoneal effusions in the absence of discrete nodal or extranodal masses. The tumor cells do not express surface markers for B cells or T cells. HHV-8 DNA sequences have been found in the genomes of the malignant cells from patients with body cavity lymphomas (see above).

Small noncleaved cell lymphoma (*Burkitt's lymphoma*) accounts for ~20% of the cases of lymphoma in patients with AIDS. It is most frequent in patients 10–19 years old and usually demonstrates characteristic c-*myc* translocations from chromosome 8 to chromosomes 14 or 22. Burkitt's lymphoma is not commonly seen in the setting of immunodeficiency other than HIV-associated immunodeficiency, and the incidence of this particular tumor is over 1000-fold higher in the setting of HIV infection than in the general population. In contrast to African Burkitt's lymphoma, where 97% of the cases contain EBV genome, only 50% of HIV-associated Burkitt's lymphomas are EBV-positive.

Primary CNS lymphoma accounts for ~20% of the cases of lymphoma in patients with HIV infection. In contrast to HIV-associated Burkitt's lymphoma, primary CNS lymphomas are usually positive for EBV. In one study, the incidence of Epstein-Barr positivity was 100%. This malignancy does not have a predilection for any particular age group. The median CD4+ T cell count at the time of diagnosis is ~50/μL. Thus, CNS lymphoma generally presents at a later stage of HIV infection than systemic lymphoma. This fact may at least in part explain the poorer prognosis for this subset of patients.

The clinical presentation of lymphoma in patients with HIV infection is quite varied, ranging from focal seizures to rapidly growing mass lesions in the oral mucosa (Fig. 182-41) to persistent unexplained fever. At least 80% of patients present with extranodal disease, and a similar percentage have B-type symptoms of fever, night sweats, or weight loss. Virtually any site in the body may be involved. The most common extranodal site is the CNS, which is involved in approximately one-third of all patients with lymphoma. Approximately 60% of these cases are primary CNS lymphoma. Primary CNS lymphoma generally presents with focal neurologic deficits, including cranial nerve findings, headaches, and/or seizures. MRI or CT generally re-

FIGURE 182-41 Diffuse histiocytic lymphoma involving the hard palate of a patient with AIDS.

veals a limited number (one to three) of 3- to 5-cm lesions (Fig. 182-42). The lesions often show ring enhancement on contrast administration and may occur in any location. Locations that are most commonly involved with CNS lymphoma are deep in the white matter. Contrast enhancement is usually less pronounced than that seen with toxoplasmosis. The main diseases in the differential diagnosis are cerebral toxoplasmosis and cerebral Chagas' disease. In addition to the 20% of lymphomas in HIV-infected individuals that are primary CNS lymphomas, CNS disease is also seen in HIV-infected patients with systemic lymphoma. Approximately 20% of patients with systemic lymphoma have CNS disease in the form of leptomeningeal involvement. This fact underscores the importance of lumbar puncture in the staging evaluation of patients with systemic lymphoma.

Systemic lymphoma is seen at earlier stages of HIV infection than primary CNS lymphoma. In one series the mean CD4+ T cell count was 189/μL. In addition to lymph node involvement, systemic lymphoma may commonly involve the gastrointestinal tract, bone marrow, liver, and lung. Gastrointestinal tract involvement is seen in ~25% of patients. Any site in the gastrointestinal tract may be involved, and patients may complain of difficulty swallowing or abdominal pain. The diagnosis is usually suspected on the basis of CT or MRI of the abdomen. Bone marrow involvement is seen in ~20% of patients and may lead to pancytopenia. Liver and lung involvement are each seen in ~10% of patients. Pulmonary disease may present as either a mass lesion, multiple nodules, or an interstitial infiltrate.

FIGURE 182-42 Central nervous system lymphoma. Postcontrast T1-weighted MR scan in a patient with AIDS, an altered mental status, and hemiparesis. Multiple enhancing lesions, some ring-enhancing, are present. The left Sylvian lesion shows gyral and subcortical enhancement, and the lesions in the caudate and splenium (*arrowheads*) show enhancement of adjacent ependymal surfaces.

Both conventional and unconventional approaches have been employed in an attempt to treat HIV-related lymphomas. Systemic lymphoma is generally treated by the oncologist with combination chemotherapy. Earlier disappointing figures are being replaced with more optimistic results for the treatment of systemic lymphoma following the availability of more effective combination ARV therapy. As in most situations in patients with HIV disease, those with the higher CD4+ T cell counts tend to do better. Response rates as high as 72% with a median survival of 33 months and disease-free intervals up to 9 years have been reported. Treatment of primary CNS lymphoma remains a significant challenge. Treatment is complicated by the fact that this illness usually occurs in patients with advanced HIV disease. Palliative measures such as radiation therapy provide some relief. The prognosis remains poor in this group, with a 2-year survival of 29%.

Multicentric Castleman's disease is an HHV-8 associated lymphoproliferative disorder that is seen with an increased frequency in patients with HIV infection. While not a true malignancy, it shares many features with lymphoma including generalized lymphadenopathy, hepatosplenomegaly, and systemic symptoms of fever, fatigue, and weight loss. Pulmonary symptoms may be seen in ~50% of patients. Kaposi's sarcoma is present in 75–82% of cases. Lymph node biopsies reveal a predominance of interfollicular plasma cells and/or germinal centers with vascularization and an "onion skin" appearance (hyaline vascular). Prior to the availability of HAART, HIV-infected patients with multicentric Castleman's disease had a 15-fold increased risk of developing non-Hodgkin's lymphoma compared to HIV-infected patients in general. Treatment typically involves chemotherapy. Anecdotal reports of success with rituximab suggest that more specific treatment may be successful, although in one series treatment with rituximab was associated with worsening of coexisting KS. The median survival of patients with treated multicentric Castleman's disease pre-HAART was 14 months. This has increased to 4 years in the era of HAART.

Evidence of infection with *human papilloma virus* (HPV), associated with *intraepithelial dysplasia of the cervix* or *anus*, is approximately twice as common in HIV-infected individuals as in the general population and can lead to intraepithelial neoplasia and eventually invasive cancer. In separate studies, HIV-infected men were examined for evidence of anal dysplasia, and Papanicolaou (Pap) smears were found to be abnormal in 20–80%. These changes tend to persist and are generally not affected by HAART, raising the possibility of a subsequent transition to a more malignant condition. While the incidence of an abnormal Pap smear of the cervix is ~5% in otherwise healthy women, the incidence of abnormal cervical smears in women with HIV infection is 30–60%, and *invasive cervical cancer* is included as an AIDS-defining condition. Thus far, however, only small increases in the incidence of cervical or anal cancer have been seen as a consequence of HIV infection. However, given this high rate of dysplasia, a comprehensive gynecologic and rectal examination, including Pap smear, is indicated at the initial evaluation and 6 months later for all patients with HIV infection. If these examinations are negative at both time points, the patient should be followed with yearly evaluations. If an initial or repeat Pap smear shows evidence of severe inflammation with reactive squamous changes, the next Pap smear should be performed at 3 months. If, at any time, a Pap smear shows evidence of squamous intraepithelial lesions, colposcopic examination with biopsies as indicated should be performed. The 2-year survival rate for HIV infected patients with invasive cervical cancer is 64% compared to 79% in non-HIV-infected patients. The most common HPV genotypes in the general population and the genotypes upon which current HPV vaccines are based are 16 and 18. This is not the case in the HIV-infected population where other genotypes such as 56 and 53 predominate. This raises concerns as to the potential effectiveness of the current HPV vaccines for HIV-infected patients.

IDIOPATHIC CD4+ T LYMPHOCYTOPENIA

A syndrome was recognized in 1992 that was characterized by an absolute CD4+ T cell count of <300/μL or <20% of total T cells on a mini-mum of two occasions at least 6 weeks apart; no evidence of HIV-1, HIV-2, HTLV-I, or HTLV-II on testing; and the absence of any defined immunodeficiency or therapy associated with decreased levels of CD4+ T cells. By mid-1993, ~100 patients had been described. After extensive multicenter investigations, a series of reports were published in early 1993, which together allowed a number of conclusions. Idiopathic CD4+ lymphocytopenia (ICL) is a very rare syndrome, as determined by studies of blood donors and cohorts of HIV-seronegative men who have sex with men. Cases were clearly identified as early as 1983, and cases remarkably similar to ICL had been identified decades ago. The definition of ICL based on CD4+ T cell counts coincided with the ready availability of testing for CD4+ T cells in patients suspected of being immunosuppressed. Although, as a result of immune deficiency, certain patients with ICL develop some of the opportunistic diseases (particularly cryptococcosis) seen in HIV-infected patients, the syndrome is demographically, clinically, and immunologically unlike HIV infection and AIDS. Fewer than half of the reported ICL patients had risk factors for HIV infection, and there were wide geographic and age distributions. The fact that a significant proportion of patients did have risk factors probably reflects a selection bias, in that physicians who take care of HIV-infected patients are more likely to monitor CD4+ T cells. Approximately one-third of the patients are women, compared to 16% of women among HIV-infected individuals in the United States. Many patients with ICL remained clinically stable, and their condition did not deteriorate progressively as is common with seriously immunodeficient HIV-infected patients. Certain patients with ICL even experienced spontaneous reversal of the CD4+ T lymphocytopenia. Immunologic abnormalities in ICL are somewhat different from those of HIV infection. ICL patients often also have decreases in CD8+ T cells and in B cells. Furthermore, immunoglobulin levels were either normal or, more commonly, decreased in patients with ICL, compared to the usual hypergammaglobulinemia of HIV-infected individuals. Finally, virologic studies revealed no evidence of HIV-1, HIV-2, HTLV-I, or HTLV-II or of any other mononuclear cell–tropic virus. Furthermore, there was no epidemiologic evidence to suggest that a transmissible microbe was involved. The cases of ICL were widely dispersed, with no clustering. Close contacts and sexual partners who were studied were clinically well and were serologically, immunologically, and virologically negative for HIV. ICL is a heterogeneous syndrome, and it is highly likely that there is no common cause; however, there may be common causes among subgroups of patients that are currently unrecognized.

Patients who present with laboratory data consistent with ICL should be worked up for underlying diseases that could be responsible for the immune deficiency. If no underlying cause is detected, no specific therapy should be initiated. However, if opportunistic diseases occur, they should be treated appropriately (see above). Depending on the level of the CD4+ T cell count, patients should receive prophylaxis for the commonly encountered opportunistic infections.

℞ AIDS AND RELATED DISORDERS

GENERAL PRINCIPLES OF PATIENT MANAGEMENT   The CDC guidelines call for the testing for HIV infection to be a part of routine medical care. It is recommended that the patient be informed of the intention to test as is the case with other routine laboratory determinations and be given the opportunity to "opt out." Such an approach is critical to the goal of identifying as many infected individuals as possible since ~25% of the >1 million individuals in the United States who are HIV-infected are not aware of their status. Under these circumstances of routine testing, although desirable, pretest counseling may not always be built into the testing process. However, no matter how well prepared a patient is for adversity, the discovery of a diagnosis of HIV infection is a devastating event. Thus, physicians should be sensitive to this fact and, where possible, execute some degree of pretest counseling to at least partially prepare the patient should the results demonstrate the presence of HIV infection. Following a diagnosis of HIV infection, the health care provider should be prepared to activate support systems immediately for the newly diagnosed patient. These should include an experienced social worker or nurse who can spend time talking to the person and ensuring that he or she is emotionally stable. Most communities have HIV support centers that can be of great help in these difficult situations.

The treatment of patients with HIV infection requires not only a comprehensive knowledge of the possible disease processes that may occur and up-to-date knowledge of and experience with ARV therapy, but also the ability to deal with the problems of a chronic, potentially life-threatening illness. A comprehensive knowledge of internal medicine is required to deal with the changing spectrum of illness associated with HIV infection. Great advances have been made in the treatment of patients with HIV infection. The appropriate use of potent combination ARV therapy and other treatment and prophylactic interventions is of critical importance in providing each patient with the best opportunity to live a long and healthy life despite the presence of HIV infection. In contrast to the earlier days of this epidemic, a diagnosis of HIV infection need no longer be equated with an inevitably fatal disease. In addition to medical interventions, the health care provider has a responsibility to provide each patient with appropriate counseling and education concerning their disease as part of a comprehensive care plan. Patients must be educated about the potential transmissibility of their infection and about the fact that while health care providers may refer to levels of the virus as "undetectable," this is more a reflection of the sensitivity of the assay being used to measure the virus than a comment on the presence or absence of the virus. It is important for patients to be aware that the virus is still present and capable of being transmitted at all stages of HIV disease. Thus, there need to be frank discussions concerning sexual practices and the sharing of needles. The treating physician must not only be aware of the latest medications available for patients with HIV infection but must also educate patients concerning the natural history of their illness and listen and be sensitive to their fears and concerns. As with other diseases, therapeutic decisions should be made in consultation with the patient, when possible, and with the patient's proxy if the patient is incapable of making decisions. In this regard, it is recommended that all patients with HIV infection, and in particular those with CD4+ T cell counts <200/μL, designate a trusted individual with durable power of attorney to make medical decisions on their behalf, if necessary.

Following a diagnosis of HIV infection, there are several examinations and laboratory studies that should be performed to help determine the extent of disease and provide baseline standards for future reference (**Table 182-16**). In addition to routine chemistry, fasting lipid profile, fasting glucose and hematology screening panels, Pap smear, and chest x-ray, one should also obtain a CD4+ T cell count, two separate plasma HIV RNA levels, an HIV resistance test, an RPR or VDRL test, an anti-*Toxoplasma* antibody titer, and serologies for hepatitis A, B, and C. A PPD test should be done, and a MMSE performed and recorded. Patients should be immunized with pneumococcal polysaccharide and, if seronegative for these viruses, with hepatitis A and hepatitis B vaccines. The status of hepatitis C infection should be determined. In addition, patients should be counseled with regard to sexual practices and needle sharing, and counseling should be offered to those whom the patient knows or suspects may also be infected. Once these baseline activities are performed, short- and long-term medical management strategies should be developed based upon the most recent information available and modified as new information becomes available. The field of HIV medicine is changing rapidly, and it is difficult to

TABLE 182-16 INITIAL EVALUATION OF THE PATIENT WITH HIV INFECTION

History and physical examination
Routine chemistry and hematology
Lipid profile and fasting glucose
CD4+ T lymphocyte count
Two plasma HIV RNA levels
HIV resistance testing
RPR test
Anti-*Toxoplasma* antibody titer
PPD skin test
Mini-mental status examination
Serologies for hepatitis A, hepatitis B, and hepatitis C
Immunization with pneumococcal polysaccharide; influenza as indicated
Immunization with hepatitis A and hepatitis B if seronegative
Counseling regarding natural history and transmission
Help contacting others who might be infected

Note: VDRL, Venereal Disease Research Laboratory; PPD, purified protein derivative.

TABLE 182-17 RESOURCES AVAILABLE ON THE WORLD WIDE WEB ON HIV DISEASE

http://www.aidsinfo.nih.gov	AIDS info, a service of the U.S. Department of Health and Human Services, posts federally approved treatment guidelines for HIV and AIDS; provides information on federally funded and privately funded clinical trials and CDC publications and data
http://www.cdcnpin.org	Updates on epidemiologic data from the CDC

Note: CDC, Centers for Disease Control and Prevention.

remain fully up to date. Fortunately there are a series of excellent sites on the internet that are frequently updated, and they provide the most recent information on a variety of topics, including consensus panel reports on treatment (**Table 182-17**).

ANTIRETROVIRAL THERAPY Combination antiretroviral therapy (ART), or highly active antiretroviral therapy (HAART), is the cornerstone of management of patients with HIV infection. Following the initiation of widespread use of HAART in the United States in 1995–1996, marked declines have been noted in the incidence of most AIDS-defining conditions (Fig. 182-31). Suppression of HIV replication is an important component in prolonging life as well as in improving the quality of life in patients with HIV infection. Adequate suppression requires strict adherence to prescribed regimens of ARV drugs. This has been facilitated by the coformulations of ARVs and the development of once-daily regimens. Unfortunately, many of the most important questions related to the treatment of HIV disease currently lack definitive answers. Among them are the questions of when should therapy be started, what is the best initial regimen, when should a given regimen be changed, and what should it be changed to when a change is made. Notwithstanding these uncertainties, the physician and patient must come to a mutually agreeable plan based upon the best available data. In an effort to facilitate this process, the U.S. Department of Health and Human Services has published a series of frequently updated guidelines including the "*Principles of Therapy of HIV Infection,*" "*Guidelines for the Use of Antiretroviral Agents in HIV-Infected Adults and Adolescents,*" and "*Guidelines for the Prevention of Opportunistic Infections in Persons Infected with Human Immunodeficiency Virus.*" At present, an extensive clinical trials network, involving both clinical investigators and patient advocates, is in place attempting to develop improved approaches to therapy. Consortia comprising representatives of academia, industry, independent foundations, and the federal government are involved in the process of drug development, including a wide-ranging series of clinical trials. As a result, new therapies and new therapeutic strategies are continually emerging. New drugs are often available through expanded access programs prior to official licensure. Given the complexity of this field, decisions regarding ARV therapy are best made in consultation with experts. Currently available drugs for the treatment of HIV infection fall into four categories: those that inhibit the viral reverse transcriptase enzyme, those that inhibit the viral protease enzyme, those that inhibit the viral integrase enzyme, and those that interfere with viral entry (**Table 182-18, Fig. 182-43**).

The FDA-approved reverse transcriptase inhibitors include the *nucleoside analogues* zidovudine, didanosine, zalcitabine, stavudine, lamivudine, abacavir, and emtricitabine; the *nucleotide analogue* tenofovir; and the *nonnucleoside reverse transcriptase inhibitors* nevirapine, delavirdine, and efavirenz (Fig. 182-43; Table 182-18). These were the first class of drugs that were licensed for the treatment of HIV infection. They are indicated for this use as part of combination regimens. It should be stressed that none of these drugs should be used as monotherapy for HIV infection due to the relative ease with which drug resistance may develop under such circumstances. Thus, when lamivudine or tenofovir are used to treat hepatitis B infection in the setting of HIV infection, one should ensure that the patient is also on additional ARV medication. The reverse transcriptase inhibitors block the HIV replication cycle at the point of RNA-dependent DNA synthesis, the reverse transcription step. While the nonnucleoside reverse transcriptase inhibitors are quite selective for the HIV-1 reverse transcriptase, the nucleoside and nucleotide analogues inhibit a variety of DNA polymerization reactions in addition to those of the HIV-1 reverse transcriptase. For this reason, serious side effects are more varied with the nucleoside analogues and include mitochondrial damage that can lead to hepatic steatosis and lactic acidosis as

Drug	Status	Indication	Dose in Combination	Supporting Data	Toxicity
Reverse Transcriptase Inhibitors					
Zidovudine (AZT, azidothymidine, Retrovir, 3′azido-3′-deoxythymidine)	Licensed	Treatment of HIV infection in combination with other antiretroviral agents Prevention of maternal-fetal HIV transmission	200 mg q8h or 300 mg bid	19 vs 1 death in original placebo-controlled trial in 281 patients with AIDS or ARC. Decreased progression to AIDS in patients with CD4+ T cell counts <500/μL, n = 2051 In pregnant women with CD4+ T cell count ≥200/μL, AZT PO beginning at weeks 14–34 of gestation plus IV drug during labor and delivery plus PO AZT to infant for 6 wk decreased transmission of HIV by 67.5% (from 25.5% to 8.3%), n = 363	Anemia, granulocytopenia, myopathy, lactic acidosis, hepatomegaly with steatosis, headache, nausea
Didanosine (Videx, Videx EC, ddI, dideoxyinosine, 2′,3′-dideoxy-inosine)	Licensed	For treatment of HIV infection in combination with other antiretroviral agents	Buffered: Requires 2 tablets to achieve adequate buffering of stomach acid; should be administered on an empty stomach ≥60 kg: 200 mg bid <60 kg: 125 mg bid Enteric coated: ≥60 kg: 400 mg qd < 60 kg: 250 mg qd	Clinically superior to AZT as monotherapy in 913 patients with prior AZT therapy. Clinically superior to AZT and comparable to AZT + ddI and AZT + ddC in 1067 AZT-naive patients with CD4+ T cell counts of 200–500/μL	Pancreatitis, peripheral neuropathy, abnormalities on liver function tests, lactic acidosis, hepatomegaly with steatosis
Zalcitabine (ddC, HIVID, 2′3′-dideoxy-cytidine)	Licensed Discontinued in 2006	In combination with other antiretroviral agents for the treatment of HIV infection	0.75 mg tid	Clinically inferior to AZT monotherapy as initial treatment. Clinically as good as ddI in advanced patients intolerant to AZT. In combination with AZT, was clinically superior to AZT alone in patients with AIDS or CD4+ T cell count <350/μL	Peripheral neuropathy, pancreatitis, lactic acidosis, hepatomegaly with steatosis, oral ulcers
Stavudine (d4T, Zerit, 2′3′-didehydro-3′-dideoxythymidine)	Licensed	Treatment of HIV-infected patients in combination with other antiretroviral agents	≥60 kg: 40 mg bid <60 kg: 30 mg bid	Superior to AZT with respect to changes in CD4+ T cell counts in 359 patients who had received ≥24 wk of AZT. Following 12 wk of randomization, the CD4+ T cell count had decreased in AZT-treated controls by a mean of 22/μL, while in stavudine-treated patients, it had increased by a mean of 22/μL	Peripheral neuropathy, pancreatitis, lactic acidosis, hepatomegaly with steatosis, ascending neuromuscular weakness, lipodystrophy
Lamivudine (Epivir, 2′3′-dideoxy-3′-thiacytidine, 3TC)	Licensed	In combination with other antiretroviral agents for the treatment of HIV infection	150 mg bid 300 mg qd	Superior to AZT alone with respect to changes in CD4 counts in 495 patients who were zidovudine-naive and 477 patients who were zidovudine-experienced. Overall CD4+ T cell counts for the zidovudine group were at baseline by 24 wk, while in the group treated with zidovudine plus lamivudine, they were 10–50 cells/μL above baseline. 54% decrease in progression to AIDS/death compared to AZT alone	Hepatotoxicity
Emtricitabine (FTC, Emtriva)	Licensed	In combination with other antiretroviral agents for the treatment of HIV infection	200 mg qd	Comparable to d4T in combination with ddI and efavirenz in 571 treatment-naive patients. Similar to 3TC in combination with AZT or d4T + NNRT1 or PI in 440 patients doing well for at least 12 weeks on a 3TC regimen	Hepatotoxicity
Abacavir (Ziagen)	Licensed	For treatment of HIV infection in combination with other antiretroviral agents	300 mg bid	Abacavir + AZT + 3TC equivalent to indinavir + AZT + 3TC with regard to viral load suppression (~60% in each group with <400 HIV RNA copies/mL plasma) and CD4 cell increase (~100/μL in each group) at 24 weeks	Hypersensitivity reaction (can be fatal); fever, rash, nausea, vomiting, malaise or fatigue, and loss of appetite
Tenofovir (Viread)	Licensed	For use in combination with other antiretroviral agents when treatment is indicated	300 mg qd	Reduction of ~0.6 log in HIV-1 RNA levels when added to background regimen in treatment-experienced patients	Potential for renal toxicity

(continued)

Drug	Status	Indication	Dose in Combination	Supporting Data	Toxicity
Delavirdine (Rescriptor)	Licensed	For use in combination with appropriate antiretrovirals when treatment is warranted	400 mg tid	Delavirdine + AZT superior to AZT alone with regard to viral load suppression at 52 weeks	Skin rash, abnormalities in liver function tests
Nevirapine (Viramune)	Licensed	In combination with other antiretroviral agents for treatment of progressive HIV infection	200 mg/d × 14 days then 200 mg bid	Increases in CD4+ T cell count, decrease in HIV RNA when used in combination with nucleosides	Skin rash, hepatotoxicity
Efavirenz (Sustiva)	Licensed	For treatment of HIV infection in combination with other antiretroviral agents	600 mg qhs	Efavirenz + AZT + 3TC comparable to indinavir + AZT + 3TC with regard to viral load suppression (a higher percentage of the efavirenz group achieved viral load <50 copies/mL; however, the discontinuation rate in the indinavir group was unexpectedly high, accounting for most treatment "failures"); CD4 cell increase (~140/μL in each group) at 24 weeks	Rash, dysphoria, elevated liver function tests, drowsiness, abnormal dreams, depression
Etravirine	Expanded access 1-866-889-2074	Pending	Pending	Pending	Rash, headache, dizziness, nausea, diarrhea

Protease Inhibitors

Drug	Status	Indication	Dose in Combination	Supporting Data	Toxicity
Saquinavir mesylate (Invirase—hard gel capsule)	Licensed	In combination with other antiretroviral agents when therapy is warranted	1000 mg + 100 mg ritonavir bid	Increases in CD4+ T cell counts, reduction in HIV RNA most pronounced in combination therapy with ddC. 50% reduction in first AIDS-defining event or death in combination with ddC compared to either agent alone	Diarrhea, nausea, headaches, hyperglycemia, fat redistribution, lipid abnormalities
(Fortovase—soft gel capsule)	Licensed Discontinued 2006	For use in combination with other antiretroviral agents when treatment is warranted	1200 mg tid	Reduction in the mortality rate and AIDS-defining events for patients who received hard-gel formulation in combination with ddC	Diarrhea, nausea, abdominal pain, headaches, hyperglycemia, fat redistribution, lipid abnormalities
Ritonavir (Norvir)	Licensed	In combination with other antiretroviral agents for treatment of HIV infection when treatment is warranted	600 mg bid	Reduction in the cumulative incidence of clinical progression or death from 34 to 17% in patients with CD4+ T cell count <100/μL treated for a median of 6 months	Nausea, abdominal pain, hyperglycemia, fat redistribution, lipid abnormalities, may alter levels of many other drugs, including saquinavir
Indinavir sulfate (Crixivan)	Licensed	For treatment of HIV infection in combination with other antiretroviral agents when antiretroviral treatment is warranted	800 mg q8h or 800 mg + 100 mg ritonavir bid or 1000 mg q8h when used with efavirenz or nevirapine	Increase in CD4+ T cell count by 100/μL and 2-log decrease in HIV RNA levels when given in combination with zidovudine and lamivudine. Decrease of 50% in risk of progression to AIDS or death when given with zidovudine and lamivudine compared with zidovudine and lamivudine alone	Nephrolithiasis, indirect hyperbilirubinemia, hyperglycemia, fat redistribution, lipid abnormalities
Nelfinavir mesylate (Viracept)	Licensed	For treatment of HIV infection in combination with other antiretroviral agents when antiretroviral therapy is warranted	750 mg tid or 1250 mg bid	2.0-log decline in HIV RNA when given in combination with stavudine	Diarrhea, loose stools, hyperglycemia, fat redistribution, lipid abnormalities. May contain traces of the potential carcinogen/teratogen ethyl methane sulfonate
Amprenavir (Agenerase)	Licensed	In combination with other antiretroviral agents for treatment of HIV infection	1200 mg bid or 600 mg + 100 mg ritonavir bid or 1200 mg + 200 mg ritonavir qd	In treatment-naïve patients, amprenavir + AZT + 3TC superior to AZT + 3TC with regard to viral load suppression (53% vs 11% with <400 HIV RNA copies/mL plasma at 24 weeks). CD4+ T cell responses similar between treatment groups. In treatment-experienced patients, amprenavir + NRTIs similar to indinavir + NRTIs with regard to viral load suppression (43% vs 53% with <400 HIV RNA copies/mL plasma at 24 weeks). CD4+ T cell responses superior in the indinavir + NRTIs group	Nausea, vomiting, diarrhea, rash, oral paresthesias, elevated liver function tests, hyperglycemia, fat redistribution, lipid abnormalities
Fosamprenavir (Lexiva)	Licensed		1400 mg bid or 700 mg + 100 mg ritonavir bid		

(continued)

Drug	Status	Indication	Dose in Combination	Supporting Data	Toxicity
Lopinavir/ritonavir (Kaletra)	Licensed	For treatment of HIV infection in combination with other antiretroviral agents	400 mg/100 mg bid	In treatment-naïve patients, lopinavir/ritonavir + d4T + 3TC superior to nelfinavir+ d4T + 3TC with regard to viral load suppression (79% vs 64% with <400 HIV RNA copies/mL at 40 weeks). CD4+ T cell increases similar in both groups.	Diarrhea, hyperglycemia, fat redistribution, lipid abnormalities
Atazanavir (Reyataz)	Licensed	For treatment of HIV infection in combination with other antiretroviral agents	400 mg qd or 300 mg qd +Ritonavir 100 mg qd when given with efavirenz	Comparable to efavirenz when given in combination with AZT + 3TC in a study of 810 treatment-naive patients. Comparable to nelfinavir when given in combination with d4T + 3TC in a study of 467 treatment-naive patients.	Hyperbilirubinemia, PR prolongation, nausea, vomiting, hyperglycemia, fat maldistribution
Tipranavir (Aptlvus)	Licensed	In combination with 200 mg ritonavir for combination therapy in treatment-experienced adults	500 mg + 200 mg ritonavir twice daily	At 24 weeks, patients with prior extensive exposure to ARVs showed a −0.8 log change in HIV RNA levels and a 34 cell increase in CD4+ T cells compound to −0.25 log and 4 cells in the control arm. Inferior to lopinavir/ritonavir in a randomized, controlled trial in naïve patients.	Diarrhea, nausea, fatigue, headache, skin rash, hepatotoxicity, intracranial hemorrhage
Darunavir (Prezista)	Licensed	In combination with 100 mg ritonavir for combination therapy in treatment-experienced adults	600 mg + 100 mg ritonavir twice daily with food	At 24 weeks, patients with prior extensive exposure to antiretrovirals treated with a new combination including darunavir showed a −1.89 log change in HIV RNA levels and a 92 cell increase in CD4+ T cells compared to −0.48 log and 17 cells in the control arm.	Diarrhea, nausea, headache

Entry Inhibitors

Drug	Status	Indication	Dose in Combination	Supporting Data	Toxicity
Enfuvirtide (Fuzeon)	Licensed	In combination with other agents in treatment-experienced patients with evidence of HIV-1 replication despite ongoing antiretroviral therapy	90 mg SC bid	In treatment of experienced patients, superior to placebo when added to new optimized background (37% vs 16% with <400 HIV RNA copies/mL at 24 weeks; + 71 vs + 35 CD4+ T cells at 24 weeks)	Local injection reactions, hypersensitivity reactions, increased rate of bacterial pneumonia
Maraviroc (Selzentry)	Licensed	In combination with other antiretroviral agents in treatment experienced adults infected with only CCR5-tropic HIV-1 that is resistant to multiple antiretroviral agents	150–600 mg bid depending upon concomitant medications (see text)	At 24 weeks, among 635 patients with CCR5-tropic virus and HIV-1 RNA >5000 copies/mL despite at least 6 months of prior therapy with at least one agent from 3 of the 4 antiretroviral drug classes, 61% of patients randomized to maraviroc achieved HIV RNA levels <400 copies/mL compared to 28% of patients randomized to placebo	Hepatotoxicity, nasopharyngitis, fever, cough, rash, abdominal pain, dizziness, fever, musculoskeletal symptoms

Integrase Inhibitor

Drug	Status	Indication	Dose in Combination	Supporting Data	Toxicity
Raltegravir (Isentress)	Licensed	In combination with other antiretroviral agents in treatment experienced patients with evidence of ongoing HIV-1 replication	400 mg bid	At 24 weeks, among 436 patients with three-class drug resistance, 76% of patients randomized to receive raltegravir achieved HIV RNA levels <400 copies/mL compared to 41% of patients randomized to receive placebo	Nausea, rash

Note: ARC, AIDS-related complex; NRTIs, nonnucleoside reverse transcriptase inhibitors.

CHAPTER 182

Human Immunodeficiency Virus Disease: AIDS and Related Disorders

well as peripheral neuropathy and pancreatitis. One of the more recently recognized problems that has been encountered with the widespread use of HAART therapy has been a syndrome of hyperlipidemia, glucose intolerance/insulin resistance, and fat redistribution often referred to as *lipodystrophy syndrome* (discussed above under metabolic abnormalities).

Zidovudine (AZT; 3'-azido-2',3'-dideoxythymidine) was the first drug approved for the treatment of HIV infection and is the prototype nucleoside analogue. These compounds, in which the hydroxyl group in the 3' position of the ribose moiety is substituted with a hydrogen or other chemical group, act as DNA chain terminators owing to their inability to form a 3'-5' phosphodiester linkage with another nucleoside. They bind much more avidly to the active site of the RNA-dependent DNA polymerase of HIV (reverse transcriptase) than to the active site of mammalian cell DNA polymerases; this explains their selective effect on HIV replication. Zidovudine also has a relatively high avidity for the DNA polymerase-γ of human mitochondria. This may contribute to the development of the fatty liver and the myopathy sometimes observed in patients taking zidovudine. As with all the nucleoside analogues, the active form of zidovudine is the triphosphate, and the rate of phosphorylation, a thymidine kinase–dependent pathway, may be different in different cells. This may explain why zidovudine is more effective at inhibiting HIV replication in some cells than others. The clinical benefit of zidovudine was clearly established in 1986 in a phase II, randomized, placebo-controlled trial in patients with advanced HIV disease. However, while treatment of patients with early stages of HIV infection with zidovudine monotherapy was associated with increases in CD4+ T cell count, it was not associated with a better overall outcome than waiting until later to treat. Subsequent trials established the ability of this drug to dramatically decrease the incidence of perinatal transmission of HIV from infected mother to infant. Eventually a series of studies demonstrated the superiority of combination ARV regimens over zidovudine alone, and combination therapy (discussed below) remains the standard of treatment today. Among the side effects of zidovudine at the initiation of therapy are fatigue, malaise, nausea, and headache. These side effects often subside over time. Patients on zidovudine may develop a macrocytic anemia, neutropenia, myopathy, cardiomyopathy, and lactic acidosis associated with fatty infiltration of the liver. As with every ARV drug, HIV has the ability to develop resistance to zidovudine. Zidovudine resistance has been reported to occur ~6 months following the initiation of zidovudine monotherapy. More recently, zidovudine-resistant viruses have been noted in patients with acute infection prior to the initiation of therapy,

implying that zidovudine-resistant viruses can be transmitted from person to person. Resistance emerges more rapidly in late-stage patients, presumably as a consequence of a greater degree of viral replication and thus a greater opportunity for mutation. A variety of amino acid changes including substitutions, insertions, and deletions have been reported to confer zidovudine resistance **(Fig. 182-44)**. One combination preparation, Combivir, consists of zidovudine and lamivudine, while another, Trizivir, consists of zidovudine, lamivudine, and abacavir.

Didanosine (ddI; 2',3'-dideoxyinosine) was the second drug licensed for the treatment of HIV infection, followed shortly thereafter by zalcitabine. Didanosine is metabolized to dideoxyadenosine in vivo. It is best absorbed on an empty stomach at a high pH. The toxicity profile of didanosine is quite different from that of zidovudine. The most common toxicity is a painful sensory peripheral neuropathy that occurs in ~30% of patients receiving >400 mg/d. It generally resolves with discontinuation of the drug and may not recur if the drug is resumed at a reduced dose. At higher doses than are currently used one may see pancreatitis in ~10% of patients. Pancreatitis associated with didanosine therapy can be fatal. Didanosine should be discontinued if a patient experiences abdominal pain consistent with pancreatitis or if an elevated serum amylase or lipase level is found in association with an edematous pancreas on ultrasound. Didanosine is contraindicated in patients with a prior history of pancreatitis, regardless of etiology. A higher incidence of didanosine-associated toxicities has been seen when it is used in combination with stavudine, hydroxyurea, ribavirin, or tenofovir.

Zalcitabine (ddC; 2',3'-dideoxycytidine) is rarely used today in the management of patients with HIV infection and was discontinued from the US market in 2006. Among the nucleoside analogues licensed for the treatment of HIV infection, it is probably the weakest. The main toxicities of ddC are peripheral neuropathy and pancreatitis.

Stavudine (d4T; 2',3'-didehydro-3'-deoxythymidine) was the fourth drug licensed for the treatment of HIV infection and was discontinued from the US market in 2006. Like zidovudine, stavudine is a thymidine analogue. These two drugs are antagonistic in vitro and in vivo and should not be given together. Stavudine has been associated with a higher incidence of mitochondrial toxicity than the other licensed nucleoside analogues. Peripheral neuropathy, lipoatrophy, lactic acidosis, and hepatic steatosis are the main toxicities of stavudine.

Lamivudine (3TC; 2',3'-dideoxy-3'-thiacytidine) is the fifth of the nucleoside analogues to be licensed in the United States. In actual practice, lami-

FIGURE 182-43 Molecular structures of antiretroviral agents.

Protease Inhibitors

Ritonavir

Nelfinavir mesylate

Lopinavir

Saquinavir mesylate

Indinavir sulfate

Amprenavir

Atazanavir

Tipranavir

Darunavir

Entry Inhibitors

Enfuvirtide

Maraviroc

Integrase Inhibitor

Raltegravir

FIGURE 182-43 (*Continued*)

MUTATIONS IN THE REVERSE TRANSCRIPTASE GENE ASSOCIATED WITH RESISTANCE TO REVERSE TRANSCRIPTASE INHIBITORS

Nucleoside and Nucleotide Reverse Transcriptase Inhibitors (nRTIs)[1]

Multi-nRTI Resistance: 69 Insertion Complex[2] (affects all nRTIs currently approved by the US FDA)

	M	A		K			L	T	K
	41	62	69	70			210	215	219
	L	V	Insert	R			W	Y	Q
								F	E

Multi-nRTI Resistance: 151 Complex[3] (affects all nRTIs currently approved by the US FDA except tenofovir)

	A		V	F		F	Q
	62		75	77		116	151
	V		I	L		Y	M

Multi-nRTI Resistance: Thymidine Analogue-associated Mutations[4,5] (TAMs; affects all nRTIs currently approved by the US FDA)

	M		D	K			L	T	K
	41		67	70			210	215	219
	L		N	R			W	Y	Q
								F	E

Abacavir[6]

	K		L		Y		M
	65		74		115		184
	R		V		F		V

Didanosine[7,8]

	K		L
	65		74
	R		V

Emtricitabine

	K		M
	65		184
	R		V
			I

Lamivudine

	K		M
	65		184
	R		V
			I

Stavudine[4,5,9,10]

	M		D	K			L	T	K
	41		67	70			210	215	219
	L		N	R			W	Y	Q
								F	E

Tenofovir[11]

	K	K
	65	70
	R	R

Zidovudine[4,5,9,10]

	M		D	K			L	T	K
	41		67	70			210	215	219
	L		N	R			W	Y	Q
								F	E

Nonnucleoside Reverse Transcriptase Inhibitors (NNRTIs)[1,12]

Efavirenz

	L	K	V	V		Y		Y	G		P
	100	103	106	108		181		188	190		225
	I	N	M	I		C		L	S		H
						I			A		

Etravirine[13] (expanded access)

	V	A	L	K	V		V	Y		G
	90	98	100	101	106		179	181		190
	I	G	I	E	I		D	C		S
				P			F	I		A
								V		

Nevirapine

	L	K	V	V		Y		Y	G
	100	103	106	108		181		188	190
	I	N	A	I		C		C	A
			M			I		L	
								H	

FIGURE 182-44 Amino acid substitutions conferring resistance to antiretroviral drugs. For each amino acid residue, the letter above the bar indicates the amino acid associated with wild-type virus and the letter(s) below indicate the substitution(s) that confer viral resistance. The number shows the position of the mutation in the protein. Mutations selected by protease inhibitors in Gag cleavage sites are not listed. HR1 indicates first heptad repeat; NAMs indicates nRTI-associated mutations; nRTI indicates nucleoside reverse transcriptase inhibitor; NNRTI indicates nonnucleoside reverse transcriptase inhibitor; PI indicates protease inhibitor. Amino acid abbreviations: A, alanine; C, cysteine; D, aspartate; E, glutamine; F, phenylalanine; G, glycine; H, histidine; I, isoleucine; K, lysine; L, leucine; M, methionine; N, asparagine; P, proline; Q, glutamine; R, arginine; S, serine; T, threonine; V, valine; W, tryptophan; Y, tyrosine. [*Reprinted with permission from the International AIDS Society—USA. Johnson VA, Brun-Vézinet F, Clotet B, Günthard HF, Kuritzkes DR, Pillay D, Schapiro JM, and Richman DD. Update of the Drug Resistance Mutations in HIV-1: 2007. Topics in HIV Medicine. 2007; 15(4):119–125. Updated information (and thorough explanatory notes) is available at www.iasusa.org.*]

MUTATIONS IN THE PROTEASE GENE ASSOCIATED WITH RESISTANCE TO PROTEASE INHIBITORS[14,15,16,17]

Atazanavir +/– ritonavir[18]

Pos	10	16	20	24	32	33	34	36	46	48	**50**	53	54	60	62	64	71	73	82	**84**	85	**88**	90	93
WT	L	G	K	L	V	L	E	M	M	G	I	F	I	D	I	I	A	G	V	I	I	N	L	I
Mut	I,F,V,C	E	R,M,I,T,V	I		I,F,V	Q	I,L,V	I,L	V	L,Y		L,V,M,T,A	E	V	L,M,V	V,I,T,L	C,S,T,A	A,T,F,I	V	V	S	M	L,M

Fosamprenavir/ritonavir

Pos	10	32	46	47	**50**	54	73	76	82	**84**	90
WT	L	V	M	I	I	I	G	L	V	I	L
Mut	I,F,R,V	I	I,L	V	V,L	L,V,M	S	V	A,F,S,T	V	M

Darunavir/ritonavir[19]

Pos	11	32	33	47	**50**	54	73	**76**	**84**	89
WT	V	V	L	I	I	I	G	L	I	L
Mut	I	I	F	V	V	M,L	S	V	V	V

Indinavir/ritonavir[20]

Pos	10	20	24	32	36	**46**	54	71	73	76	77	82	84	90
WT	L	K	L	V	M	M	I	A	G	L	L	V	I	L
Mut	I,R,V	M,R	I	I	I	I,L	V	V,T	S,A	V	I	A,F,T	V	M

Lopinavir/ritonavir[21]

Pos	10	20	24	**32**	33	46	**47**	50	53	54	63	71	73	76	**82**	84	90
WT	L	K	L	V	L	M	I	I	F	I	L	A	G	L	V	I	L
Mut	F,I,R,V	M,R	I	I	F	I,L	V,A	V	L	V,L,A,M,T,S	P	V,T	S	V	A,F,T,S	V	M

Nelfinavir[20,22]

Pos	10	**30**	36	46	71	77	82	84	88	**90**
WT	L	D	M	M	A	V	V	I	N	L
Mut	F,I	N	I	I,L	V,T	I	A,F,T,S	V	D,S	M

Saquinavir/ritonavir

Pos	10	24	**48**	54	62	71	73	77	82	84	**90**
WT	L	L	G	I	I	A	G	V	V	I	L
Mut	I,R,V	I	V	V,L	V	V,T	S		A,F,T,S	V	M

Tipranavir/ritonavir[23]

Pos	10	13	20	**33**	35	36	43	46	47	54	58	69	74	**82**	83	**84**	90
WT	L	I	K	L	E	M	K	M	I	I	Q	H	T	V	N	I	L
Mut	V	V	M,R	F	G	I	T	L	V	A,M,V	E	K	P	L,T	D	V	M

MUTATIONS IN THE ENVELOPE GENE ASSOCIATED WITH RESISTANCE TO ENTRY INHIBITORS

Enfuvirtide[24]

Pos	36	37	38	39	40	42	43
WT	G	I	V	Q	Q	N	N
Mut	D,S	V	A,M,E	R	H	T	D

Maraviroc[25] See User Note

MUTATIONS IN THE INTEGRASE GENE ASSOCIATED WITH RESISTANCE TO INTEGRASE INHIBITORS

Raltegravir[26] (expanded access)

Pos	148	155
WT	Q	N
Mut	H,K,R	H

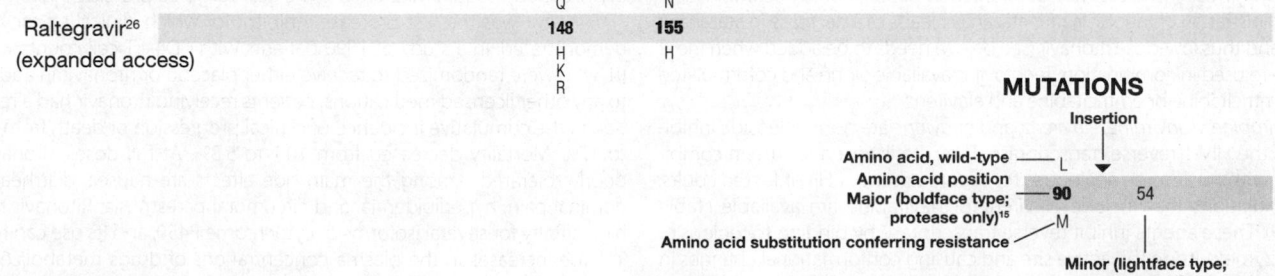

MUTATIONS

- Insertion
- Amino acid, wild-type — L
- Amino acid position — **90** · 54
- Major (boldface type; protease only)[15]
- Amino acid substitution conferring resistance — M
- Minor (lightface type; protease only)[15]

FIGURE 182-44 (*Continued*)

vudine or the closely related drug emtricitabine is a frequent element of many different combination regimens currently in use. These two drugs and the nucleotide reverse transcriptase inhibitor tenofovir (see below) also have activity against hepatitis B virus. For this reason flares of hepatitis may be seen in co-infected patients starting and or stopping these agents due to the confounding issues of direct effects of treatment and the potential for the IRIS (see above). To prevent the development of resistant strains of HIV, these drugs should never be used on their own for the treatment of hepatitis B in the patient with HIV infection. Lamivudine is available either alone or in coformulations including zidovudine and/or abacavir **(Table 182-19)**. One reason behind the excellent synergy seen between lamivudine and the other nucleoside analogues may be that strains of HIV resistant to lamivudine (M184V substitution) appear to have enhanced sensitivity to other nucleosides, and thus development of dual resistance is more difficult. In addition, there is a suggestion that 3TC-resistant strains of HIV may be less virulent and are less able to generate new mutants than are strains of HIV that are 3TC-sensitive. Lamivudine is among the best tolerated and least toxic nucleoside analogues.

Emtricitabine (FTC; 5-fluoro-1-(2R,5S)-[2-(hydroxymethyl)-1,3-oxathiolan-5-y]cytosine) is the negative enantiomer of a thio analogue of cytidine with a fluorine in the 5 position. It is licensed for use in combination with other ARV agents for treatment of HIV-1 infection in adults. Compared to lamivudine, it is similar in activity and has a longer half-life. It is available either alone or co-formulated with tenofovir or tenofovir and efavirenz (Table 182-19). Resistance to emtricitabine is associated with the M184V mutation in reverse transcriptase. Viruses showing the K65R mutation in reverse transcriptase may have reduced susceptibility to emtricitabine.

Abacavir {(1S,cis)-4-[2-amino-6-(cyclopropylamino)-9H-purin-9-yl]-2-cyclopentene-1-methanol sulfate (salt)(2:1)} is a synthetic carbocyclic analogue of the nucleoside guanosine. It is licensed to be used in combination with other ARV agents for the treatment of HIV-1 infection. Hypersensitivity reactions that may occur with initial therapy or rechallenge have been reported in ~4% of patients treated with this drug, and patients developing signs or symptoms of hypersensitivity such as fever, skin rash, fatigue, and gastrointestinal symptoms should discontinue the drug and not restart it. Fatal hypersensitivity reactions have been reported with rechallenge. Abacavir hypersensitivity appears to occur with a higher frequency in patients who are HLA-B57. It has been recommended that patients be screened for HLA-B57 prior to initiation of abacavir and that abacavir only be used as a last resort in patients who are HLA-B57 postive. Abacavir-resistant strains of HIV are typically also resistant to lamivudine, didanosine, and zalcitabine. Abacavir is formulated alone as well as in combination with lamivudine or zidovudine and lamivudine.

Tenofovir disoproxil fumarate (9-[(R)-2-[[bis[[(isopropoxycarbonyl)oxy]methoxy]phosphinyl]methoxy]propyl]adenine fumarate (1:1)) is an acyclic nucleoside phosphonate diester analogue of adenosine monophosphate. It undergoes diester hydrolysis to form the nucleoside monophosphate tenofovir and is the first nucleotide analogue to be licensed for treatment of HIV infection. It is indicated in combination with other ARV agents for the treatment of HIV-1 infection. HIV isolates with increased resistance typically express a K65R mutation in reverse transcriptase and a three- to fourfold reduction in sensitivity to tenofovir. Tenofovir is primarily eliminated by the kidneys, and renal impairment including a Fanconi-like syndrome with hypophosphatemia may occur. Tenofovir is contraindicated in patients with renal impairment. Coadministration with didanosine leads to a 60% increase in didanosine levels, and thus doses of didanosine need to be adjusted and patients monitored carefully if these two drugs are used in combination. In addition CD4+ T cell increases may be blunted in patients on this combination. Coadministration of tenofovir with atazanavir leads to a decrease in atazanavir levels and thus low-dose ritonavir (see below) needs to be added when these drugs are used in combination. Tenofovir is available alone and coformulated with emtricitabine or emtricitabine and efavirenz.

Nevirapine, delavirdine, efavirenz, and *etravirine* are nonnucleoside inhibitors of the HIV-1 reverse transcriptase. They are licensed for use in combination with nucleoside analogues for the treatment of HIV-infected adults. Coformulations that include efavirenz or nevirapine are available (Table 182-19). These agents inhibit reverse transcriptase by binding to regions of the enzyme outside the active site and causing conformational changes in the enzyme that render it inactive. Although these agents are active in the nanomolar range, they are also very selective for the reverse transcriptase of HIV-1, have no activity against HIV-2, and, when used as monotherapy,

TABLE 182-19 COMBINATION FORMULATIONS OF ANTIRETROVIRAL DRUGS

Name	Combination
Combivir	Zidovudine + lamivudine
Epzicom	Zidovudine + abacavir
Trizivir	Zidovudine + lamivudine + abacavir
Truvada	Tenofovir + emtricitabine
Atripla	Tenofovir + emtricitabine + efavirenz
Triomune*a*	Stavudine + lamivudine + nevirapine

*a*Not licensed in the United States.

are associated with the rapid emergence of drug-resistant mutants (Table 182-18; Fig. 182-44). Efavirenz is administered once a day, nevirapine and etravirine twice a day, and delavirdine three times a day. All four drugs are associated with the development of a maculopapular rash, generally seen within the first few weeks of therapy. While it is possible to treat through this rash, it is important to be sure that one is not dealing with a more severe eruption such as Stevens-Johnson syndrome by looking carefully for signs of mucosal involvement, significant fever, or painful lesions with desquamation. Severe, life-threatening, and in some cases fatal hepatotoxicity, including fulminant and cholestatic hepatitis, hepatic necrosis, and hepatic failure, have been reported in patients treated with nevirapine. There is a suggestion that this is more common in women with higher CD4+ T cell counts. Many patients treated with efavirenz note a feeling of light-headedness, dizziness, or out of sorts following the initiation of therapy. Some complain of vivid dreams. These symptoms tend to disappear after several weeks of therapy. Aside from difficulties with dreams, taking efavirenz at bedtime may minimize the side effects. Efavirenz may cause fetal harm when administered during the first trimester to a pregnant woman. Women of childbearing potential should undergo pregnancy testing prior to initiation of efavirenz. Efavirenz is commonly used in combination with two nucleoside analogues as part of initial treatment regimens. Etravirine is a diarylpyrimidine derivative that is currently available on expanded access for treatment of HIV infection in combination with other agents. In contrast to the other nonnucleoside reverse transcriptase inhibitors, which all exhibit cross-resistance, etravirine may be active against strains of HIV that are resistant to other nonnucleoside reverse transcriptase inhibitors. Among its side effects are rash, headache, nausea, and diarrhea.

The HIV-1 protease inhibitors (saquinavir, indinavir, ritonavir, nelfinavir, amprenavir, fosamprenavir, lopinavir/ritonavir, atazanavir, tipranavir, and darunavir) are a major part of the therapeutic armamentarium of ARVs. When used as part of initial regimens in combination with reverse transcriptase inhibitors, these agents have been shown to be capable of suppressing levels of HIV replication to under 50 copies per milliliter in the majority of patients for a minimum of 5 years. As in the case of reverse transcriptase inhibitors, resistance to protease inhibitors can develop rapidly in the setting of monotherapy, and thus these agents should be used only as part of combination therapeutic regimens. A summary of known resistance mutations for protease inhibitors is shown in Fig. 182-44.

Saquinavir was the first of the HIV-1 protease inhibitors to be licensed. It is typically given with low doses of ritonavir to obtain therapeutic levels. Saquinavir is metabolized by the cytochrome P450 system in both the gastrointestinal tract and the liver. Low-dose ritonavir results in inhibition of cytochrome P450 action. Thus, when both drugs are administered together there is an increase in saquinavir levels. This use of low doses of ritonavir to provide pharmacodynamic boosting of other agents is a common strategy in HIV therapy. Saquinavir is among the best-tolerated protease inhibitors.

Ritonavir was the first protease inhibitor for which clinical efficacy was demonstrated. In a study of 1090 patients with CD4+ T cell counts <100/μL who were randomized to receive either placebo or ritonavir in addition to any other licensed medications, patients receiving ritonavir had a reduction in the cumulative incidence of clinical progression or death from 34% to 17%. Mortality decreased from 10.1 to 5.8%. At full doses, ritonavir is poorly tolerated. Among the main side effects are nausea, diarrhea, abdominal pain, hyperlipidemia, and circumoral paresthesia. Ritonavir has a high affinity for several isoforms of cytochrome P450, and its use can result in large increases in the plasma concentrations of drugs metabolized by this pathway. Among the agents affected in this manner are most other protease inhibitors, macrolide antibiotics, R-warfarin, ondansetron, rifabutin, most calcium channel blockers, glucocorticoids, and some of the chemotherapeutic agents used to treat KS and/or lymphomas. In addition, ritonavir may increase the activity of glucuronyltransferases, thus decreasing the levels of drugs metabolized by this pathway. Overall, great care must be taken when prescribing additional drugs to patients taking protease inhibitors in general and ritonavir in particular. As mentioned above, the pharmacodynamic boosting property of ritonavir, seen with doses as low as 100–200 mg once or twice a day, is often used in the setting of combination ARV therapy for HIV infection to derive more convenient regimens. For example, when given with low-dose ritonavir, saquinavir and indinavir can both be given on twice-a-day schedules and taken with food.

Indinavir was the first protease inhibitor used in combination with dual nucleoside therapy. The combination of zidovudine, lamivudine, and indinavir was the first "triple combination" shown to have a profound effect on HIV replication. The main side effects of indinavir are nephrolithiasis (seen in 4% of patients) and asymptomatic indirect hyperbilirubinemia (seen in 10%). Indinavir is predominantly metabolized by the liver. The dose should be lowered in patients with cirrhosis. Levels of indinavir are decreased during concurrent therapy with rifabutin, efavirenz, or nevirapine and increased during concurrent therapy with ketoconazole, delavirdine, or ritonavir. Dosages should be modified appropriately in these circumstances (Table 182-18).

Nelfinavir was approved in 1997 and *amprenavir* was approved in 1999 for the treatment of adult or pediatric HIV infection when ARV therapy is warranted. As with most of the newer ARV agents, these approvals were based on randomized, controlled trials that demonstrated decreases in plasma HIV RNA levels and increases in CD4+ T cell counts. The presence of the potential carcinogen and teratogen ethyl methanesulfonate in nelfinavir preparations makes it a drug to be avoided in pregnant women. Both nelfinavir and amprenavir have unique resistance profiles. Nelfinavir resistance is associated with a D30N substitution in the protease gene. Viruses harboring this single mutation retain sensitivity to other protease inhibitors. While it has been suggested that for this reason nelfinavir is a good initial protease inhibitor, enthusiasm for its use has waned following the 48-week clinical trials data demonstrating the virologic inferiority of nelfinavir to lopinavir/ritonavir, to fosamprenavir, and to efavirenz. Protease inhibitor resistance typically involves multiple amino acid substitutions and reduced susceptibility across the class. Amprenavir resistance is associated with a unique substitution at amino acid 50 (I50V). Nelfinavir and amprenavir are both associated with gastrointestinal side effects. About 1% of patients receiving amprenavir have experienced severe and life-threatening skin reactions. An additional disadvantage of amprenavir is that the original formulation requires the patient to take 8 large capsules twice a day. Amprenavir has largely been replaced by fosamprenavir (see below).

Fosamprenavir was licensed in 2003 for the treatment of HIV infection in combination with other ARV agents in adults. It is a prodrug of amprenavir that is rapidly converted to amprenavir by cellular phosphatases. It is supplied as a 700-mg tablet. The recommended dosage is 1400 mg bid or 700 mg bid with ritonavir, 100 mg bid, or 1400 mg once a day with ritonavir, 200 mg once a day. As noted above, ritonavir-boosted fosamprenavir has been shown to be comparable to lopinavir/ritonavir and efavirenz in combination regimens.

Lopinavir/ritonavir (Kaletra) is a fixed-dose combination of the protease inhibitors lopinavir (200 mg) and ritonavir (50 mg). It was licensed in 2000 for treatment of HIV-1 infection in adults and children in combination with other agents. A main advantage of this pill is that it combines the pharmacologic enhancement of low-dose ritonavir with a second protease inhibitor in a single capsule. In a randomized, controlled trial, this combination capsule was found to be superior to nelfinavir. Its main complications are gastrointestinal upset and hyperlipidemia.

Atazanavir is an azapeptide inhibitor of the HIV-1 protease that was licensed in 2003. An advantage of atazanavir is that total cholesterol and triglyceride levels do not increase as much with atazanavir as with other protease inhibitors. This coupled with the fact that it can be given on a once-daily schedule has made atazanavir a popular component of initial treatment regimens. Atazanavir is associated with increases in serum bilirubin and prolongations of the ECG PR interval. Atazanavir-resistant isolates emerging in previously treatment-naïve individuals frequently harbor an I50L substitution. This mutation in some instances is associated with increased sensitivity to other protease inhibitors. Atazanavir requires an acidic gastric pH for absorption, and its use in combination with a proton pump inhibitor is contraindicated due to concerns about absorption. Ata-

zanavir is an inhibitor of cytochrome P3A and its use may be associated with increased levels of calcium channel blockers, macrolide antibiotics, HMB-CoA reductase inhibitors, and sildenafil. Levels of atazanavir are lower in the presence of tenofovir or efavirenz. In these settings, levels of atazanavir should be boosted with the use of low-dose ritonavir.

Tipranavir is a non-peptidic HIV protease inhibitor licensed in 2005. It is licensed for use in combination with 200 mg ritonavir and is indicated for combination ARV therapy of HIV-1 infection in treatment-experienced adults or in adults with evidence of HIV-1 strains resistant to multiple protease inhibitors. Tipranavir was found to be inferior to lopinavir/ritonavir in a randomized controlled trial in naïve patients. In that study, at lower doses it was virologically inferior while at higher doses it exhibited a greater degree of hepatotoxicity. The main side effects of tipranavir are gastrointestinal intolerance and skin rash; the latter is seen in ~10% of patients and may be related to the sulfonamide moiety in the molecule. Tipranavir coadministered with ritonavir has also been associated with reports of intracranial hemorrhage as well as reports of clinical hepatitis and hepatic decompensation, including some fatalities in both settings. The risk of hepatotoxicity is increased in patients with hepatitis B or C co-infection.

Darunavir is a non-peptidic HIV protease inhibitor licensed in 2006 to be coadministered with 100 mg of ritonavir and other ARV agents for the treatment of HIV infection in ARV treatment–experienced adults. This indication is based on the fact that the trials leading to licensure of darunavir were carried out in treatment-experienced patients. In these studies 46% of patients achieved a reduction in HIV RNA viral loads to <50 copies per milliliter. Studies are underway in treatment-naïve patients. Skin rash, which may be severe, is seen in 7% of patients and may be related to the sulfonamide moiety contained in the molecule. Gastrointestinal intolerance and headache are the other most frequent side effects.

Entry inhibitors act by interfering with the binding of HIV to its receptor or co-receptor or by interfering with the process of fusion (see above). The first drug in this class to be licensed was the fusion inhibitor *enfuvirtide*, or T-20, followed by the CCR5 antagonist *maraviroc*. A variety of additional small molecules that bind to HIV-1 co-receptors are currently in clinical trials.

Enfuvirtide is a linear 36-amino-acid synthetic peptide with the *N*-terminus acetylated and the *C*-terminus a carboxamide. It is composed of naturally occurring L-amino acid residues and interferes with the fusion of the viral and cellular membranes by binding to the HR1 region in the gp41 subunit of the HIV-1 envelope. This binding interferes with the coil-coil interaction required to approximate the two membranes. Resistant isolates of HIV exhibit amino acid changes in positions 36–45 of gp41. In two independent studies, patients who had persistent viremia despite prior treatment with agents from all three available classes of drugs were randomized to receive an individualized regimen (based upon prior treatment history and resistance profile) with or without enfuvirtide. The change in plasma HIV-1 RNA from baseline was ~1 log greater (–1.53 vs. –0.68) in patients randomized to receive enfuvirtide. Among the drawbacks of this agent are the requirement for twice-a-day injection, the occurrence of injection site reactions in close to 100% of patients, and an increase in bacterial pneumonia in the enfuvirtide-treated patients compared to the patients in the control arm (4.68 vs. 0.61 events per 100 patient years) in the phase III studies.

Maraviroc is a CCR5 antagonist that interferes with HIV binding at the stage of co-receptor engagement. It was licensed in 2007 for treatment of HIV infection in combination with other agents in treatment-experienced patients infected with only CCR5-tropic virus resistant to multiple agents. A co-receptor tropism assay should be performed if one is considering the use of maraviroc to ensure that the potential patient is harboring R5 virus. In phase III trials of treatment-experienced patients randomized to receive optimal therapy plus maraviroc or placebo, 61% of patients randomized to maraviroc achieved HIV RNA levels <400 copies/mL compared to 28% of patients randomized to placebo. An allergic reaction-associated hepatotoxicity has been reported with maraviroc. Among the most common side effects of maraviroc are dizziness due to postural hypotension, cough, fever, colds, rash, muscle and joint pain, and stomach pain. Maraviroc is a substrate of CYP3A and Pgp and the recommend dose varies depending upon concomitant medications. In combination with nucleoside analogues, tipranavir/ritonavir, enfuvirtide and/or nevirapine the dose is 300 mg twice daily. In the presence of CYP3A inhibitors such as most protease inhibitors the dose is 150 mg twice daily and in presence of CYP3A inducers such as efavirenz the dose is 600 mg twice daily.

The newest class of ARV compounds are the *integrase inhibitors*. *Raltegravir* is an inhibitor of the viral enzyme integrase and the first of this class to be approved. It was approved in 2007 for treatment of HIV infection in combination with other agents in treatment experienced patients. Raltegravir exhibits a wide range of activity against HIV-1 and HIV-2 including viruses with multiple resistance mutations to other classes of drugs. As with several other compounds, resistance to raltegravir comes at the expense of replicative fitness. In two phase III studies in which 436 patients with 3-class ARV drug resistance were randomized to an optimized background regimen with raltegravir or placebo, 76% of patients receiving raltegravir achieved HIV RNA levels <400 copies/mL compared to 41% of patients randomized to the placebo arm. In contrast to many other antiretroviral drugs the side effect profile of raltegravir is minimal with similar side effect profiles noted for the raltegravir and placebo groups.

PRINCIPLES OF THERAPY The principles of therapy for HIV infection have been articulated by a panel sponsored by the U.S. Department of Health and Human Services as a working group of the NIH Office of AIDS Research Advisory Council These principles are summarized in **Table 182-20**. As noted in these guidelines, eradication of HIV infection has not yet been possible. Treatment decisions must take into account the fact that one is dealing with a chronic infection. While early therapy is generally the rule in infectious diseases, immediate treatment of every HIV-infected individual upon diagnosis may not be prudent, and therapeutic decisions must take into account the balance between risks and benefits. While it seems reasonable to assume that the complications associated with ARV therapy could be minimized by regimens designed to minimize exposure to the drugs in question, all efforts to do so have paradoxically been associated with an increase in serious adverse events in the patients randomized to intermittent therapy suggesting that some "non-AIDS" associated serious adverse events such as heart attack and stroke may be linked to HIV replication. Thus, unless contraindicated for reasons of toxicity, patients started on ARV therapy should remain on ARV therapy.

At present, a reasonable course of action is to initiate ARV therapy in anyone with the acute HIV syndrome; all pregnant women; patients with symptomatic disease; and patients with asymptomatic disease with CD4+ T cell counts <350/μL **(Table 182-21)**. In addition, one may wish to administer a 6-week course of therapy to uninfected individuals immediately following a high-risk exposure to HIV.

Once the decision has been made to initiate therapy, the health care provider must decide which drugs to use as the first regimen. The decision regarding choice of drugs not only will affect the immediate response to

therapy but also will have implications regarding options for future therapeutic regimens. The initial regimen is usually the most effective insofar as the virus has yet to develop significant resistance. The two options for initial therapy most commonly in use today are two different three-drug regimens. The first regimen utilizes two nucleoside analogues (one of which is usually lamivudine or emtricitabine) and a nonnucleoside reverse transcriptase inhibitor. The second regimen utilizes two nucleoside analogues and a protease inhibitor. Unfortunately there are no clear data at present on which to base distinctions between these two approaches. Following the initiation of therapy one should expect a 1 log (tenfold) reduction in plasma HIV RNA levels within 1–2 months and eventually a decline in plasma HIV RNA levels to <50 copies per milliliter. During this same time there should be a rise in the CD4+ T cell count of 100–150/μL that is particularly brisk during the first month of therapy. Many clinicians feel that failure to achieve this endpoint is an indication for a change in therapy. Other reasons for a change in therapy include a persistently declining CD4+ T cell count, clinical deterioration, or drug toxicity **(Table 182-22)**. As in the case of initiating therapy, changing therapy may have a lasting impact on future therapeutic options. When changing therapy because of treatment failure (clinical progression or worsening laboratory parameters), it is important to attempt to provide a regimen with at least two new active drugs. This decision can be guided by resistance testing (see below). In the patient in whom a change is made for reasons of drug toxicity, a simple replacement of one drug is reasonable. It should be stressed that in attempting to sort out a drug toxicity it may be advisable to hold all therapy for a period of time to distinguish between drug toxicity and disease progression. Drug toxicity will usually begin to show signs of reversal within 1–2 weeks. Prior to changing a treatment regimen because of drug failure, it is important to ensure that the patient has been adherent to the prescribed regimen. As in the case of initial therapy, the simpler the new therapeutic regimen, the easier it is for the patient to be compliant. Plasma HIV RNA levels and CD4+ T lymphocyte counts should be monitored every 3–4 months during therapy and more frequently if one is contemplating a change in regimen or immediately following a change in regimen.

In an attempt to determine an optimal therapeutic regimen, one may attempt to measure ARV drug susceptibility through genotyping or phenotyping of HIV quasispecies and determine adequacy of dosing through measurement of drug levels. Genotyping may be done through dideoxynucleotide sequencing, DNA chip hybridization, or line probe assays. Phe-

---

TABLE 182-21 INDICATIONS FOR THE INITIATION OF ANTIRETROVIRAL THERAPY IN PATIENTS WITH HIV INFECTION

I. Acute infection syndrome
II. Chronic infection
  A. Symptomatic disease (including HIV-associated nephropathy)
  B. Asymptomatic diseases
    1. CD4+ T cell count <350/μL[a]
    2. Pregnancy
III. Postexposure prophylaxis

[a]This is an area of controversy. Some experts would wait until the CD4 cell count declines to 200/μL, some would treat everyone with a viral load >100,000 copies/mL, whereas others would treat everyone regardless of CD4+ T cell count.
Source: *Guidelines for the Use of Antiretroviral Agents in HIV-Infected Adults and Adolescents,* USPH.

TABLE 182-20 PRINCIPLES OF THERAPY OF HIV INFECTION

1. Ongoing HIV replication leads to immune system damage and progression to AIDS.
2. Plasma HIV RNA levels indicate the magnitude of HIV replication and the rate of CD4+ T cell destruction. CD4+ T cell counts indicate the current level of competence of the immune system.
3. Rates of disease progression differ among individuals, and treatment decisions should be individualized based upon plasma HIV RNA levels and CD4+ T cell counts.
4. Maximal suppression of viral replication is a goal of therapy; the greater the suppression the less likely the appearance of drug-resistant quasispecies.
5. The most effective therapeutic strategies involve the simultaneous initiation of combinations of effective anti-HIV drugs with which the patient has not been previously treated and that are not cross-resistant with antiretroviral agents that the patient has already received.
6. The antiretroviral drugs used in combination regimens should be used according to optimum schedules and dosages.
7. The number of available drugs is limited. Any decisions on antiretroviral therapy have a long-term impact on future options for the patient.
8. Women should receive optimal antiretroviral therapy regardless of pregnancy status.
9. The same principles apply to children and adults. The treatment of HIV-infected children involves unique pharmacologic, virologic, and immunologic considerations.
10. Compliance is an important part of ensuring maximal effect from a given regimen. The simpler the regimen, the easier it is for the patient to be compliant.

Source: Modified from *Principles of Therapy of HIV Infection,* USPHS, and the Henry J. Kaiser Family Foundation.

TABLE 182-22 INDICATIONS FOR CHANGING ANTIRETROVIRAL THERAPY IN PATIENTS WITH HIV INFECTION[a]

Less than a 1-log drop in plasma HIV RNA by 4 weeks following the initiation of therapy
A reproducible significant increase (defined as 3-fold or greater) from the nadir of plasma HIV RNA level not attributable to intercurrent infection, vaccination, or test methodology
Persistently declining CD4+ T cell numbers
Clinical deterioration
Side effects

[a]Generally speaking, a change should involve the initiation of at least 2 drugs felt to be effective in the given patient. The exception to this is when change is being made to manage toxicity, in which case a single substitution is reasonable.
Source: *Guidelines for the Use of Antiretroviral Agents in HIV-Infected Adults and Adolescents,* USPHS.

notypic assays typically measure the enzymatic activity of viral enzymes in the presence or absence of different concentrations of different drugs and have also been used to determine co-receptor tropism. These assays will generally detect quasispecies present at a frequency of ≥10%. The precise role of resistance testing in the management of patients with HIV infection is not yet clear. It is generally recommended that resistance testing be used in selecting initial therapy in settings where the risk of transmission of resistant virus is high (such as the United States and Europe) and in determining new regimens for patients experiencing virologic failure while on therapy. Resistance testing may be of particular value in distinguishing drug-resistant virus from poor patient compliance. Due to the rapid rate at which drug-resistant viruses revert to wild-type, it is recommended that resistant testing performed in the setting of drug failure be carried out while the patient is still on the failing regimen. Measurement of plasma drug levels can also be used to tailor an individual treatment. The inhibitory quotient, defined as the trough blood level/IC50 of the patient's virus, is used by some to determine the adequacy of dosing of a given treatment regimen.

In addition to the licensed medications discussed above, a large number of experimental agents are being evaluated as possible therapies for HIV infection. Therapeutic strategies are being developed that interfere with virtually every step of the replication cycle of the virus (Fig. 182-3). In addition, as more is discovered about the role of the immune system in controlling viral replication, additional strategies, generically referred to as "immune-based therapies," are being developed as a complement to antiviral therapy. Among the antiviral agents in early clinical trials are additional nucleoside and nucleotide analogues, protease inhibitors, fusion inhibitors, receptor and co-receptor antagonists, and integrase inhibitors as well as new anti-viral strategies including antisense nucleic acids and maturation inhibitors. Among the immune-based therapies being evaluated are IFN-α, bone marrow transplantation, adoptive transfer of lymphocytes genetically modified to resist infection or enhance HIV-specific immunity, active immunotherapy with inactivated HIV or its components, IL-2, and IL-7.

HIV AND THE HEALTH CARE WORKER

Health care workers, especially those who deal with large numbers of HIV-infected patients, have a small but definite risk of becoming infected with HIV as a result of professional activities (see "Occupational Transmission of HIV: Health Care Workers, Laboratory Workers, and the Health Care Setting," above). The first case of HIV transmission from a patient to health care worker was reported in 1984. By the end of 2002, 106 health care workers worldwide were documented as having seroconverted to HIV following occupational HIV exposure; another 238 possible occupational seroconversions had been reported. Only three of these cases were reported from sub-Saharan Africa, where HIV is most prevalent. Hence it is likely that the global prevalence of occupationally acquired HIV infection is much higher than has been reported.

In the United States 57 health care workers have become infected with HIV by occupational exposure; 26 have developed AIDS. The individuals who seroconverted include 19 laboratory workers (16 of whom were clinical laboratory workers), 24 nurses, 6 physicians, 2 surgical technicians, 1 dialysis technician, 1 respiratory therapist, 1 health aide, 1 embalmer/morgue technician, and 2 housekeeper/maintenance workers. The exposures included 48 percutaneous (puncture/cut injury), 5 mucocutaneous (mucous membrane and/or skin), 2 both percutaneous and mucocutaneous, and 2 unknown route of exposure. Forty-nine exposures were to HIV-infected blood, three to concentrated virus in a laboratory, one to visibly bloody fluid, and four to an unspecified fluid. As of January 1, 2003, there had been 139 other cases of HIV infection or AIDS among health care workers who have not reported other risk factors for HIV infection and who report a history of exposure to blood, body fluids, or HIV-infected laboratory material, but for whom seroconversion after exposure was not documented. The number of these workers who actually acquired their infection through occupational exposures is not known. Taken together, the data from several large studies suggest that the risk of HIV infection following a percutaneous exposure to HIV-contaminated blood is ~0.3%, and after a mucous membrane exposure, ~0.09%. Although episodes of HIV transmission after nonin-

tact skin exposure have been documented, the average risk for transmission by this route has not been precisely quantified but is estimated to be less than the risk for mucous membrane exposures. The risk for transmission after exposure to fluids or tissues other than HIV-infected blood also has not been quantified but is probably considerably lower than for blood exposures. A seroprevalence survey of 3420 orthopedic surgeons, 75% of whom practiced in an area with a relatively high prevalence of HIV infection and 39% of whom reported percutaneous exposure to patient blood, usually through an accident involving a suture needle, failed to reveal any cases of possible occupational infection, suggesting that the risk of infection with a suture needle may be considerably less than that with a blood-drawing needle.

Most cases of health care worker seroconversion occur as a result of needle-stick injuries. When one considers the circumstances that result in needle-stick injuries, it is immediately obvious that adhering to the standard guidelines for dealing with sharp objects would result in a significant decrease in this type of accident. In one study, 27% of needle-stick injuries resulted from improper disposal of the needle (over half of these were due to recapping the needle), 23% occurred during attempts to start an IV line, 22% occurred during blood drawing, 16% were associated with an IM or SC injection, and 12% were associated with giving an IV infusion.

Clinicians should consider potential occupational exposures to HIV as urgent medical concerns to ensure timely postexposure management and possible administration of postexposure ARV prophylaxis (PEP). Recommendations regarding PEP must take into account that several circumstances determine the risk of transmission of HIV following occupational exposure. In this regard, several factors have been associated with an increased risk for occupational transmission of HIV infection, including deep injury, the presence of visible blood on the instrument causing the exposure, injury with a device that had been placed in the vein or artery of the source patient, terminal illness in the source patient, and lack of postexposure ARV therapy in the exposed health care worker. Other important considerations when considering PEP in the health care worker include known or suspected pregnancy or breast-feeding, the possibility of exposure to drug-resistant virus, and toxicities of PEP regimens. Regardless of the decision to use PEP, the wound should be cleansed immediately and antiseptic applied. If a decision is made to offer PEP, U.S. Public Health Service guidelines recommend (1) a combination of two nucleoside analogue reverse transcriptase inhibitors given for 4 weeks for less severe exposures, or (2) a combination of two nucleoside analogue reverse transcriptase inhibitors plus a third drug given for 4 weeks for more severe exposures. Most clinicians administer the latter regimen in all cases in which a decision is made to treat. Detailed guidelines are available from the *Updated U.S. Public Health Service Guidelines for the Management of Occupational Exposures to HIV and Recommendations for Postexposure Prophylaxis* (CDC, 2005). The report emphasizes the importance of adherence to PEP when it is indicated; follow-up of exposed workers to improve PEP adherences, monitoring for adverse events (including seroconversion), and expert consultation in the management of exposures.

For consultation on the treatment of occupational exposures to HIV and other bloodborne pathogens, the clinician managing the exposed patient can call the National Clinicians' Post-Exposure Prophylaxis Hotline (Pepsine) at 888-HIV-4911 (888-448-4911). This service is available 24 h a day, at no charge (additional information on the Internet is available at *http://www.ucsf.edu/hivcntr*). Pepsine support may be especially useful in challenging situations, such as when drug-resistant HIV strains are suspected or the health care worker is pregnant.

Health care workers can minimize their risk of occupational HIV infection by following the CDC guidelines of July 1991, which include adherence to universal precautions, refraining from direct patient care if one has exudative lesions or weeping dermatitis, and disinfecting and sterilizing reusable devices employed in invasive procedures. The premise of universal precautions is that every specimen should be handled as if it came from someone infected with a bloodborne pathogen. All samples should be double-bagged, gloves should be worn when drawing blood, and spills should be immediately disinfected with bleach.

In attempting to put this small but definite risk to the health care worker in perspective, it is important to point out that ~200 health care workers die each year as a result of occupationally acquired hepatitis B infection. The tragedy in this instance is that these infections and deaths due to HBV could be greatly decreased by more extended use of the HBV vaccine. The risk of HBV infection following a needle-stick injury from a hepatitis antigen–positive patient is much higher than the risk of HIV infection (see "Transmission," above). There are multiple examples of needle-stick injuries where the patient was positive for both HBV and HIV and the health care worker became infected only with HBV. For these reasons, it is advisable, given the high prevalence of HBV infection in HIV-infected individuals, that all health care workers dealing with HIV-infected patients be immunized with the HBV vaccine.

TB is another infection common to HIV-infected patients that can be transmitted to the health care worker. For this reason, all health care workers should know their PPD status, have it checked yearly, and receive 6 months of isoniazid treatment if their skin test converts to positive. In addition, all patients in whom a diagnosis of TB is being entertained should be placed immediately in respiratory isolation, pending results of the diagnostic evaluation. The emergence of drug-resistant organisms, including the extensively drug resistant TB strains that have been identified in Africa, has made TB an increasing problem for health care workers. This is particularly true for the health care worker with preexisting HIV infection.

One of the most charged issues ever to come between health care workers and patients is that of transmission of infection from HIV-infected health care workers to their patients. This is discussed under "Occupational Transmission of HIV: Health Care Workers, Laboratory Workers, and the Health Care Setting," above. Theoretically, the same universal precautions that are used to protect the health care worker from the HIV-infected patient will also protect the patient from the HIV-infected health care worker.

VACCINES

Given that human behavior, especially human sexual behavior, is extremely difficult to change, a critical modality for preventing the spread of HIV infection is the development of a safe and effective vaccine. Historically, vaccines have provided a safe, cost-effective, and efficient means of preventing illness, disability, and death from infectious diseases. Successful vaccines for the most part are predicated on the assumption that the body can mount an adequate immune response to the microbe or virus in question during natural infection, and that the vaccine will mimic the natural response to infection. Even with serious diseases such as smallpox, poliomyelitis, measles, and influenza among others, the body in the vast majority of cases clears the infectious agent and provides protection against future exposure. Unfortunately, this is not the case with HIV infection since the natural immune response to HIV infection is unable to clear the virus from the body and cases of superinfection have been reported. Some of the factors that contribute to the problematic nature of development of a preventive HIV vaccine are the high mutability of the virus, the fact that the infection can be transmitted by cell-free or cell-associated virus, the likely need for the development of effective mucosal immunity, and the fact that it has been difficult to establish the precise correlates of protective immunity to HIV infection. Some HIV-infected individuals are long-term non-progressors (see above), and a number of individuals have been exposed to HIV multiple times but remain uninfected; these facts suggest that there are elements of an HIV-specific immune response that have the potential to be protective. Early attempts to develop a vaccine with the envelope protein gp120 aimed at inducing neutralizing antibodies in humans were performed based on the induction of neutralizing antibodies in non-human primates. The significance of the laboratory assays were unknown at the time, and the elicited antisera failed to neutralize primary isolates of HIV cultured and tested in fresh peripheral blood mononuclear cells. In this regard, two phase 3 trials were undertaken in the United States and Thailand using soluble gp120, and the vaccines failed to protect human volunteers from HIV infection. It should be pointed out that while the ideal goal of an HIV vaccine is to prevent infection, a vaccine given to an uninfected individual that significantly alters the course of disease or the infectivity of the individual, should that person become infected, could have an impact not only on the individual in question but also on the spread of infection in the community. In this regard, a number of studies in monkeys using vaccines that induce predominantly cellular (T cell) immune responses have not protected the animals against infection but have lowered the initial burst of viremia following acute infection as well as decreased temporarily the viral set point. Since most sexually transmitted HIV infections occur when the transmitting partner is experiencing high levels of viremia such as during the acute phase of HIV infection or during the advanced stage of disease when the viral load is high, such a vaccine, which might limit the initial burst of viremia in primary infection and decrease the established viral set point, could have benefits for the individual as well as for their sexual partners. It is clear that it will take several years of clinical trials to establish the efficacy or lack thereof of a candidate vaccine for HIV.

PREVENTION

Education, counseling, and behavior modification are the cornerstones of an HIV prevention strategy. A major problem in the United States and elsewhere is that many infections are passed on by those who do not know that they are infected. Of the >1 million persons in the United States who are HIV-infected, it is estimated that ~25% do not know their HIV status and thus may be putting others at risk by their own behavior. In this regard, the CDC has recently recommended that HIV testing become part of routine medical care and that all individuals between the ages of 13 and 64 years be informed of the testing and be tested without the need for written informed consent. The individual could "opt out" of testing, but if not, testing would be routinely administered. In addition to identifying individuals who might benefit from ARV therapy, information gathered from such an approach should serve as the basis for behavior-modification programs, both for infected individuals who may be unaware of their HIV status and who could infect others and for uninfected individuals practicing high-risk behavior. The practice of "safer sex" is the most effective way for sexually active uninfected individuals to avoid contracting HIV infection and for infected individuals to avoid spreading infection. Abstinence from sexual relations is the only absolute way to prevent sexual transmission of HIV infection. However, for many individuals this may not be feasible, and there are a number of relatively safe practices that can markedly decrease the chances of transmission of HIV infection. Partners engaged in monogamous sexual relationships who wish to be assured of safety should both be tested for HIV antibody. If both are negative, it must be understood that any divergence from monogamy puts both partners at risk; open discussion of the importance of honesty in such relationships should be encouraged. When the HIV status of either partner is not known, or when one partner is positive, there are a number of options. Use of condoms can markedly decrease the chance of HIV transmission. It should be remembered that condoms are not 100% effective in preventing transmission of HIV infection, and there is an ~10% failure rate of condoms used for contraceptive purposes. Most condom failures result from breakage or improper usage, such as not wearing the condom for the entire period of intercourse. Latex condoms are preferable, since virus has been shown to leak through natural skin condoms. Petroleum-based gels should never be used for lubrication of the condom, since they increase the likelihood of condom rupture. Some men who have sex with men practice fellatio as a "minimal risk" activity compared to anal intercourse. It should be emphasized that receptive fellatio is definitely not safe sex, and although the incidence of transmission via fellatio is considerably less than that of rectal or vaginal intercourse, there has been documentation of transmission of HIV where receptive fellatio was the only sexual act performed (see "Transmission," above). Topical microbicides for vaginal and anal use are being pursued actively as a means by which individuals could avoid infection when the insertive partner cannot be relied on to use a condom. Three clinical trials in South Africa, Uganda, and Kenya have shown that adult male circumcision results in an ~50% reduction in HIV acquisition in the circumcised subject. Clearly, this approach has considerable potential as a preventive strategy for HIV infection and is currently being pursued, particularly in developing nations, as a component of HIV prevention. Kissing is considered safe, although there is a theoretical possibility of transmission via virus in saliva. The low concentration of virus in saliva of infected individuals, as well as the presence in saliva of HIV-inhibitory proteins (see above), lessens any risk of transmission by kissing.

The most effective way to prevent transmission of HIV infection among IDUs is to stop the use of injectable drugs. Unfortunately, that is extremely difficult to accomplish unless the individual enters a treatment program. For those who will not or cannot participate in a drug treatment program and who will continue to inject drugs, the avoidance of sharing of needles and other paraphernalia ("works") is the next best way to avoid transmission of infection. However, the cultural and social factors that contribute to the sharing of paraphernalia are complex and difficult to overcome. In addition, needles and syringes may be in short supply. Under these circumstances, paraphernalia should be cleaned after each usage with a virucidal solution, such as undiluted sodium hypochlorite (household bleach). Data from a number of studies have indicated that programs that provide sterile needles to addicts in exchange for used needles have resulted in a decrease in HIV transmission without increasing the use of injection drugs. It is important for IDUs to be tested for HIV infection and counseled, to avoid transmission to their sexual partners. Secondary and tertiary spread of HIV infection by the heterosexual route within settings of a high level of injection drug use has increased greatly in the United States, particularly among African Americans (see above). Studies are underway to determine the safety and efficacy of preexposure as well as postexposure administration of ARV drugs for the prevention of HIV infection.

Transmission of HIV via transfused blood or blood products has been decreased dramatically by a combination of screening of all blood donors for HIV infection by assays for both HIV antibody and nucleic acid and self-deferral of individuals at risk for HIV infection. In addition, clotting factor concentrates are heat-treated, essentially eliminating the risk to hemophiliacs who require these products. Autologous transfusions are preferable to transfusions from another individual. However, logistic constraints as well as the unpredictability of the need for most transfusions limit the feasibility of this approach. At present the risk of becoming HIV-infected from a contaminated blood transfusion is approximately 1 in 1.5 million donations.

Treatment of an HIV-infected mother with ARV therapy during pregnancy and the infant during the first weeks following birth has proved very effective in dramatically decreasing mother-to-child transmission of HIV. In situations such as that seen in certain developing countries where pregnant women frequently present to a health care system during labor, administration of a short course (as little as a single dose of one drug) of ARV therapy to the mother during labor and to the infant within 48 h of birth has also been successful in decreasing the incidence of mother-to-child transmission of HIV.

HIV can be transmitted via breast milk and colostrum. The avoidance of breast-feeding may not be practical in developing countries, where nutritional concerns override the risk of HIV transmission. However, it is becoming appreciated that 5–15% of infants who were born of HIV-infected mothers and who were fortunate enough not to have been infected intrapartum or peripartum become infected via breast-feeding. Therefore, in developing countries, breast-feeding from an infected mother should be avoided if at all possible. Unfortunately, this is rarely the case, and given the disadvantages of withholding breast-feeding in developing countries (see above), health authorities in most developing countries continue to recommend breast-feeding despite the potential for HIV transmission. Treatment of the infected mother with ARV therapy, in addition to decreasing perinatal mother-to-child transmission, can also decrease transmission by breast-feeding. In developed countries such as the United States, where bottled formula and milk are readily accessible, breast-feeding is absolutely contraindicated when a mother is HIV positive.

FURTHER READINGS

BAILEY RC et al: Male circumcision for HIV prevention in young men in Casuum, Kenya: A randomised controlled trial. Lancet 369:643, 2007

BENSON CA et al: Treating opportunistic infections among HIV-infected adults and adolescents. Recommendations from CDC, the National Institutes of Health, and the HIV Medicine Association/Infectious Diseases Society of America. MMWR 53(RR-15):1, 2004. Updates available at http://www.aidsinfo.nih.gov

BRENNER BG et al: High rates of forward transmission events after acute/early HIV-1 infection. J Infect Dis 195:951, 2007

CENTERS FOR DISEASE CONTROL AND PREVENTION: Revised guidelines for HIV counseling, testing, and referral. MMWR Recomm Rep 50(RR-19):1, 2001

———: Updated U.S. Public Health Service guidelines for the management of occupational exposures to HIV and recommendations for postexposure prophylaxis. MMWR Recomm Rep 54(RR-9): 1, 2005

———: HIV/AIDS Surveillance Report, 2005;17 (Revised ed), 2007. Available at http://www.cdc.gov/hiv/

———: Revised recommendations for HIV testing of adults, adolescents, and pregnant women in health-care settings. MMWR Recomm Rep 55(RR-14):1, 2006

———: Essential Components of a Comprehensive Strategy to Prevent Domestic HIV, 2006. Available at http://www.cdc.gov/Hiv/resources/reports/comp_hiv_prev/index.htm

———; HEALTH RESOURCES AND SERVICES ADMINISTRATION; NATIONAL INSTITUTES OF HEALTH; HIV MEDICINE ASSOCIATION OF THE INFECTIOUS DISEASES SOCIETY OF AMERICA: Incorporating HIV prevention into the medical care of persons living with HIV. MMWR Recomm Rep 52(RR-12):1, 2003

CENTLIVRE M et al: In HIV-1 pathogenesis the die is cast during primary infection. AIDS 21:1, 2007

COHEN MS, PILCHER CD: Amplified HIV transmission and new approaches to HIV prevention. J Infect Dis 191:1391, 2005

COLLINS LS et al: Multicentric Castleman's disease in HIV infection. Int J STD AIDS 17:19, 2006

COREY L: Synergistic copathogens—HIV-1 and HSV-2. N Engl J Med 356:854, 2007

DEEKS SG, WALKER BD: Human immunodeficiency virus controllers: Mechanisms of durable virus control in the absence of antiretroviral therapy. Immunity 27:406, 2007

DEPARTMENT OF HEALTH AND HUMAN SERVICES PANEL ON ANTIRETROVIRAL GUIDELINES FOR ADULTS AND ADOLESCENTS: Guidelines for the Use of Antiretroviral Agents in HIV-1-Infected Adults and Adolescents, October 10, 2006. Updates available at http://www.aidsinfo.nih.gov

DORAK MT et al: Transmission of HIV-1 and HLA-B allele-sharing within serodiscordant heterosexual Zambian couples. Lancet 363:2137, 2004

DRUMRIGHT L et al: Unprotected anal intercourse and substance use among men who have sex with men with recent HIV infection. J AIDS 43:344, 2006

ESTE JA, TELENTI A: HIV entry inhibitors. Lancet 370:81, 2007

FAUCI AS: Host factors and the pathogenesis of HIV-induced disease. Nature 384:529, 1996

———: The AIDS epidemic—considerations for the 21st century. N Engl J Med 341:1046, 1999

FELLAY J et al: A whole-genome association study of major determinants for host control of HIV-1. Science 317:944, 2007

FREEMAN GJ et al: Reinvigorating exhausted HIV-specific T cells via PD-1–PD-1 ligand blockade. J Exp Med 203:2223, 2006

FREIBERG M et al: The association between hepatitis C infection and prevalent cardiovascular disease among HIV-infected individuals. AIDS 21:193, 2007

GERETTI AM: Epidemiology of antiretroviral drug resistance in drug-naive persons. Curr Opin Infect Dis 20:22, 2007

Gonzalez-Scarano F, Martin-Garcia J: The neuropathogenesis of AIDS. Nat Rev Immunol 5:69, 2005

Gray RH et al: Male circumcision for HIV prevention in men in Rakai, Uganda: A randomised trial. Lancet 369:657, 2007

Greene WC, Peterlin BM: Charting HIV's remarkable voyage through the cell: Basic science as a passport to future therapy. Nat Med 8:673, 2002

Gutierrez F et al: Osteonecrosis in patients infected with HIV: clinical epidemiology and natural history in a large case series from Spain. J AIDS 42(3):286, 2006

Hammer SM et al: Treatment for adult HIV infection: 2006 recommendations of the International AIDS Society-USA panel. JAMA 296:827, 2006

Han Y et al: Experimental approaches to the study of HIV-1 latency. Nat Rev Microbiol 5:95, 2007

Ho DD et al: Rapid turnover of plasma virions and CD4 lymphocytes in HIV infection. Nature 373:123, 1995

Hoffman RM, Currier JS: Management of antiretroviral treatment-related complications. Infect Clin Dis North Am 21:103, 2007

Huang L et al: Current concepts: Intensive care of patients with HIV Infection. N Engl J Med 355:173, 2006

Izzedine H, Deray G: The nephrologist in the HAART era. AIDS 21:409, 2007

Johnston MI, Fauci AS: An HIV vaccine: Evolving concepts. N Engl J Med 356:2073, 2007

Joint United Nations Programme on HIV/AIDS (UNAIDS): Report on the global AIDS epidemic, 2006

———: AIDS epidemic update, 2007

Kaplan JE et al: Guidelines for preventing opportunistic infections among HIV-infected persons—2002. Recommendations of the U.S. Public Health Service and the Infectious Diseases Society of America. MMWR Recomm Rep 51(RR-8):1, 2002. Updates available at *http://www.aidsinfo.nih.gov*

Keele BF et al: Chimpanzee reservoirs of pandemic and nonpandemic HIV-1. Science 313:523, 2006

Keruly JC, Moore RD: Immune status at presentation to care did not improve among antiretroviral-naive persons from 1990 to 2006. Clin Infect Dis 45:1369, 2007

Koziel MJ, Peters MG: Current concepts: Viral hepatitis in HIV infection. N Engl J Med 356:1445, 2007

Lipman M, Breen R: Immune reconstitution inflammatory syndrome in HIV. Curr Opin Infect Dis 19:20, 2006

Lyles CM et al: Best-evidence interventions: Findings from a systematic review of HIV behavioral interventions for US populations at high risk, 2000–2004. Am J Public Health 97:133, 2007

Mangili A et al: Risk of cardiovascular disease in a cohort of HIV-infected adults: A study using carotid intima-media thickness and coronary artery calcium score. Clin Infect Dis 43:1482, 2006

May MT et al: HIV treatment response and prognosis in Europe and North America in the first decade of highly active antiretroviral therapy: A collaborative analysis. Lancet 368:451, 2006

Mellors JW et al: Prognosis in HIV-1 infection predicted by the quantity of virus in plasma. Science 272:1167, 1996

Morse CG, Kovacs JA: Metabolic and skeletal complications of HIV infection: The price of success. JAMA 296:844, 2006

Pantaleo G, Fauci AS: HIV infection is active and progressive in lymphoid tissue during the clinically latent stage of disease. Nature 362:355, 1993

Palefsky JM et al: Anal intraepithelial neoplasia in the highly active antiretroviral therapy era among HIV-positive men who have sex with men. AIDS 19:1407, 2005

Palella FJ Jr et al: Mortality in the highly active antiretroviral therapy era: Changing causes of death and disease in the HIV Outpatient Study. J AIDS 43(1):27, 2006

Perinatal HIV Guidelines Working Group: U.S. Public Health Service Task Force recommendations for use of antiretroviral drugs in pregnant HIV-1-infected women for maternal health and interventions to reduce perinatal HIV-1 transmission in the United States, November 2, 2007. Updates available at *http://www.aidsinfo.nih.gov*

Shelburne SA et al: Incidence and risk factors for immune reconstitution inflammatory syndrome during highly active antiretroviral therapy. AIDS 19:399, 2005

Silvestri G et al: Understanding the benign nature of SIV infection in natural hosts. J Clin Invest 11:3148, 2007

Simon V et al: HIV/AIDS epidemiology, pathogenesis, prevention, and treatment. Lancet 368:489, 2006

Stephens HA: HIV-1 diversity versus HLA class I polymorphism. Trends Immunol 26:41, 2005

U.S. Public Health Service: Updated U.S. Public Health Service Guidelines for the Management of Occupational Exposures to HBV, HCV, and HIV and Recommendations for Postexposure Prophylaxis. MMWR Recomm Rep 50(RR-11):1, 2001. Updates available at *http://www.aidsinfo.nih.gov*

The Strategies for Management of Antiretroviral Therapy (SMART) Study Group: CD4+ count-guided interruption of antiretroviral treatment. N Engl J Med 355(22):2283, 2006

Volmink J et al: Antiretrovirals for reducing the risk of mother-to-child transmission of HIV infection. Cochrane Database Syst Rev 1:CD003510, 2007

Walensky RP et al: The survival benefits of AIDS treatment in the United States. J Infect Dis 194:11, 2006

Wawer MJ et al: Rates of HIV-1 transmission per coital act, by stage of HIV-1 infection, in Rakai, Uganda. J Infect Dis 191:1403, 2005

Wei X et al: Viral dynamics in human immunodeficiency virus type 1 infection. Nature 373:117, 1995

Wells CD et al: HIV infection and multidrug-resistant tuberculosis: The perfect storm. J Infect Dis 196(Suppl 1):S86, 2007

Zancanaro PCQ et al: Cutaneous manifestations of HIV in the era of highly active antiretroviral therapy: An institutional urban clinic experience. J Am Acad Dermatol 54(4):581, 2006

SECTION 15 — INFECTIONS DUE TO RNA VIRUSES

183 Viral Gastroenteritis

Umesh D. Parashar, Roger I. Glass

Acute infectious gastroenteritis is a common illness that affects persons of all ages worldwide. It is a leading cause of mortality among children in developing countries, accounting for an estimated 2 million deaths each year, and is responsible for up to 10–12% of all hospitalizations among children in industrialized countries, including the United States. Elderly persons, especially those with debilitating health conditions, are also at risk of severe complications and death from acute gastroenteritis. Among healthy young adults, acute gastroenteritis is rarely fatal but incurs substantial medical and social costs, including those of time lost from work.

Several enteric viruses have been recognized as important etiologic agents of acute infectious gastroenteritis (Table 183-1, Fig. 183-1). Illness caused by these viruses is characterized by the acute onset of vomiting and/or diarrhea, which may be accompanied by fever, nausea, abdominal cramps, anorexia, and malaise. As shown in Table 183-2,

TABLE 183-1 **VIRAL CAUSES OF GASTROENTERITIS AMONG HUMANS**

Virus	Family	Genome	Primary Age Group at Risk	Clinical Severity	Detection Assays[a]
Group A rotavirus	Reoviridae	Double-strand segmented RNA	Children <5 years	+++	EM, EIA (commercial), PAGE, RT-PCR
Norovirus	Caliciviridae	Positive-sense single-strand RNA	All ages	++	EM, EIA, RT-PCR
Sapovirus	Caliciviridae	Positive-sense single-strand RNA	Children <5 years	+	EM, EIA, RT-PCR
Astrovirus	Astroviridae	Positive-sense single-strand RNA	Children <5 years	+	EM, EIA, RT-PCR
Adenovirus (types 40 and 41)	Adenoviridae	Double-strand DNA	Children <5 years	+/++	EM, EIA (commercial), PCR

[a]EIA, enzyme immunoassay; EM, electron microscopy; PAGE, polyacrylamide gel electrophoresis; PCR, polymerase chain reaction; RT-PCR, reverse-transcriptase PCR.

several features can help distinguish gastroenteritis caused by viruses from that caused by bacterial agents. However, the distinction based on clinical and epidemiologic parameters alone is often difficult, and laboratory tests may be required to confirm the diagnosis.

HUMAN CALICIVIRUSES

Etiologic Agent The Norwalk virus is the prototype strain of a group of nonenveloped, small (27–40 nm), round, icosahedral viruses with relatively amorphous surface features on visualization by electron microscopy. These viruses have been difficult to classify because they have not been adapted to cell culture, they often are shed in low titers for only a few days, and no animal models are available. Molecular cloning and characterization have demonstrated that these viruses have a single, positive-strand RNA genome ~7.5 kb in length and that they possess a single virion-associated protein—similar to that of typical caliciviruses—with a molecular mass of 60 kDa. On the basis of these molecular characteristics, these viruses are presently classified in two genera belonging to the family Caliciviridae: the *noroviruses* and the *sapoviruses* (previously called Norwalk-like viruses and Sapporo-like viruses, respectively).

Epidemiology Infections with the Norwalk and related human caliciviruses are common worldwide, and most adults have antibodies to these viruses. Antibody is acquired at an earlier age in developing countries—a pattern consistent with the presumed fecal-oral mode of transmission. Infections occur year-round, although, in temperate climates, a distinct increase has been noted in cold-weather months. Noroviruses may be the most common infectious agents of mild gastroenteritis in the community and affect all age groups, whereas sapoviruses primarily cause gastroenteritis in children. Noroviruses also cause traveler's diarrhea, and outbreaks have occurred among military personnel deployed to various parts of the world. The etiologic role of noroviruses in moderate and severe gastroenteritis requiring a visit to a physician or hospitalization is still being studied. However, the limited data available indicate that norovirus may be the second most common viral agent (after rotavirus) among young children and the most common agent among older children and adults. Noroviruses are also recognized as the major cause of epidemics of gastroenteritis worldwide. In the United States, >90% of outbreaks of nonbacterial gastroenteritis are caused by noroviruses. Epidemics occur throughout the year, in all age groups, and in a variety of settings.

Virus is transmitted predominantly by the fecal-oral route but is also present in vomitus. Because an inoculum with very few viruses can be infectious, transmission can occur by aerosolization, by contact with contaminated fomites, and by person-to-person contact. Viral shedding and infectivity are greatest during the acute illness, but challenge studies with Norwalk virus in volunteers indicate that viral antigen may be shed by asymptomatically infected persons and also by symptomatic persons before the onset of symptoms and for up to 2 weeks after the resolution of illness. In one study, 11 of 15 norovirus-infected children <2 years of age shed the virus for >2 weeks after onset; this group included 3 infants <6 months of age who shed virus for 42–47 days or even longer.

Pathogenesis The exact sites and cellular receptors for attachment of viral particles have not been determined. Data suggest that carbohydrates that are similar to human histo-blood group antigens and are present on the gastroduodenal epithelium of individuals with the secretor phenotype may serve as ligands for the attachment of Norwalk virus. Additional studies must more fully elucidate norovirus-carbohydrate interactions, including potential strain-specific variations. After the infection of volunteers, reversible lesions are noted in the upper jejunum, with broadening and blunting of the villi, shortening of the microvilli, vacuolization of the lining epithelium, crypt hyperplasia, and infiltration of the lamina propria by polymorphonuclear neutrophils and lymphocytes. The lesions persist for at least 4 days after the resolution of symptoms and are associated with malabsorption of carbohydrates and fats and a decreased level of brush-border enzymes. Adenylate cyclase activity is not altered. No histopathologic changes are seen in the stomach or colon, but gastric motor function is delayed, and this alteration is believed to contribute to the nausea and vomiting that are typical of this illness.

Clinical Manifestations Gastroenteritis caused by Norwalk and related human caliciviruses has a sudden onset, following an average incubation period of 24 h (range, 12–72 h). The illness generally lasts 12–60 h and is characterized by one or more of the following symptoms:

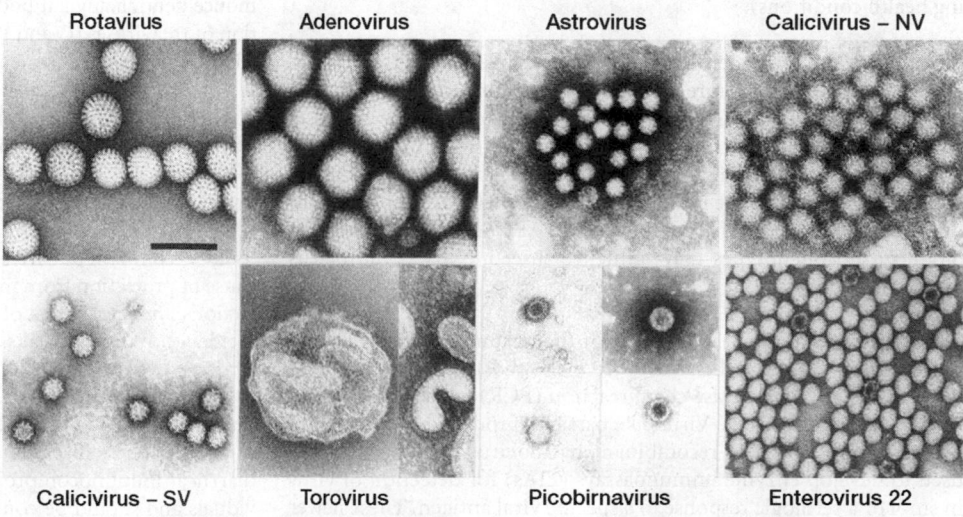

FIGURE 183-1 **Viral agents of gastroenteritis.** NV, Norwalk-like virus; SV, Sapporo-like virus.

TABLE 183-2 CHARACTERISTICS OF GASTROENTERITIS CAUSED BY VIRAL AND BACTERIAL AGENTS

Feature	Viral Gastroenteritis	Bacterial Gastroenteritis
Setting	Incidence similar in developing and developed countries	More common in settings with poor hygiene and sanitation
Infectious dose	Low (10–100 viral particles) for most agents	High (>10^5 bacteria) for *Escherichia coli*, *Salmonella*, *Vibrio*; medium (10^2–10^5 bacteria) for *Campylobacter jejuni*; low (10–100 bacteria) for *Shigella*
Seasonality	In temperate climates, winter seasonality for most agents; year-round occurrence in tropical areas	More common in summer or rainy months, particularly in developing countries with a high disease burden
Incubation period	1–3 days for most agents; can be shorter for norovirus	1–7 days for common agents (e.g., *Campylobacter*, *E. coli*, *Shigella*, *Salmonella*); a few hours for bacteria producing preformed toxins (e.g., *Staphylococcus aureus*, *Bacillus cereus*)
Reservoir	Primarily humans	Depending on species, human (e.g., *Shigella*, *Salmonella*), animal (e.g., *Campylobacter*, *Salmonella*, *E. coli*), and water (e.g., *Vibrio*) reservoirs exist.
Fever	Common with rotavirus and norovirus; uncommon with other agents	Common with agents causing inflammatory diarrhea (e.g., *Salmonella*, *Shigella*)
Vomiting	Prominent and can be the only presenting feature, especially in children	Common with bacteria producing preformed toxins; less prominent in diarrhea due to other agents
Diarrhea	Common; nonbloody in almost all cases	Prominent and frequently bloody with agents causing inflammatory diarrhea
Duration	1–3 days for norovirus and sapovirus; 2–8 days for other viruses	1–2 days for bacteria producing preformed toxins; 2–8 days for most other bacteria
Diagnosis	This is often a diagnosis of exclusion in clinical practice. Commercial enzyme immunoassays are available for detection of rotavirus and adenovirus, but identification of other agents is limited to research and public health laboratories.	Fecal examination for leukocytes and blood is helpful in differential diagnosis. Culture of stool specimens, sometimes on special media, can identify several pathogens. Molecular techniques are useful epidemiologic tools but are not routinely used in most laboratories.
Treatment	Supportive therapy to maintain adequate hydration and nutrition should be given. Antibiotics and antimotility agents are contraindicated.	Supportive hydration therapy is adequate for most patients. Antibiotics are recommended for patients with dysentery caused by *Shigella* or *Vibrio cholerae* and for some patients with *Clostridium difficile* colitis.

nausea, vomiting, abdominal cramps, and diarrhea. Vomiting is more prevalent among children, whereas a greater proportion of adults develop diarrhea. Constitutional symptoms are common, including headache, fever, chills, and myalgias. Noroviruses appear to cause more severe illness than sapoviruses, although both illnesses are less severe than that due to rotavirus. The stools are characteristically loose and watery, without blood, mucus, or leukocytes. White cell counts are generally normal; rarely, leukocytosis with relative lymphopenia may be observed. Death is a rare outcome and usually results from severe dehydration in vulnerable persons (e.g., elderly patients with debilitating health conditions).

Immunity Approximately 50% of persons challenged with Norwalk virus become ill and acquire short-term immunity against the infecting strain. Immunity to Norwalk virus appears to correlate inversely with level of antibody; i.e., persons with higher levels of preexisting antibody to Norwalk virus are more susceptible to illness. This observation suggests that some individuals have a genetic predisposition to illness. Recent data indicate that specific ABO, Lewis, and secretor blood group phenotypes may influence susceptibility to norovirus infection.

Diagnosis Cloning and sequencing of the genomes of Norwalk and several other human caliciviruses have allowed the development of assays based on polymerase chain reaction (PCR) for detection of virus in stool and vomitus. Virus-like particles produced by expression of capsid proteins in a recombinant baculovirus vector have been used to develop enzyme immunoassays (EIAs) for detection of virus in stool or a serologic response to a specific viral antigen. These newer diagnostic techniques are considerably more sensitive than previous

detection methods, such as electron microscopy, immune electron microscopy, and EIAs based on reagents derived from humans. However, no currently available single assay can detect all human caliciviruses because of their great genetic and antigenic diversity. In addition, the assays are still cumbersome and are available primarily in research laboratories, although they are increasingly being adopted by public health laboratories for routine screening of fecal specimens from patients affected by outbreaks of gastroenteritis. Commercial EIA kits have been developed but are still being evaluated to determine their optimal use for both outbreak-related and sporadic acute gastroenteritis cases.

℞ INFECTIONS WITH NORWALK AND RELATED HUMAN CALICIVIRUSES

The disease is self-limited, and oral rehydration therapy is generally adequate. If severe dehydration develops, IV fluid therapy is indicated. No specific antiviral therapy is available.

Prevention Epidemic prevention relies on situation-specific measures, such as control of contamination of food and water, exclusion of ill food handlers, and reduction of person-to-person spread through good personal hygiene and disinfection of contaminated fomites. The role of immunoprophylaxis is not clear, given the lack of long-term immunity from natural disease and the paradoxical inverse association between the level of immune response and protection from disease.

ROTAVIRUS

Etiologic Agent Rotaviruses are members of the family Reoviridae. The viral genome consists of 11 segments of double-strand RNA that are enclosed in a triple-layered, nonenveloped, icosahedral capsid 75 nm in diameter. Viral protein 6 (VP6), the major structural protein, is the target of commercial immunoassays and determines the group specificity of rotaviruses. There are seven major groups of rotavirus (A through G); human illness is caused primarily by group A and, to a much lesser extent, by groups B and C. Two outer-capsid proteins, VP7 (G-protein) and VP4 (P-protein), determine serotype specificity, induce neutralizing antibodies, and form the basis for binary classification of rotaviruses (G and P types). The segmented genome of rotavirus allows genetic reassortment (i.e., exchange of genome segments between viruses) during co-infection—a property that may play a role in viral evolution and has been utilized in the development of reassortant animal-human rotavirus–based vaccines.

 Epidemiology Worldwide, nearly all children are infected with rotavirus by 3–5 years of age. Neonatal infections are common but are often asymptomatic or mild, presumably because of protection from maternal antibody or breast-feeding. First infections after 3 months of age are likely to be symptomatic, and the incidence of disease peaks among children 4–23 months of age. Reinfections are common, but the severity of disease decreases with each repeat infection. Therefore, severe rotavirus infections are relatively uncommon among older children and adults. Nevertheless, rotavirus can cause illness in parents and caretakers of children with rotavirus diarrhea, immunocompromised persons, travelers, and elderly individuals and should be considered in the differential diagnosis of gastroenteritis among adults. In temperate climates, rotavirus disease

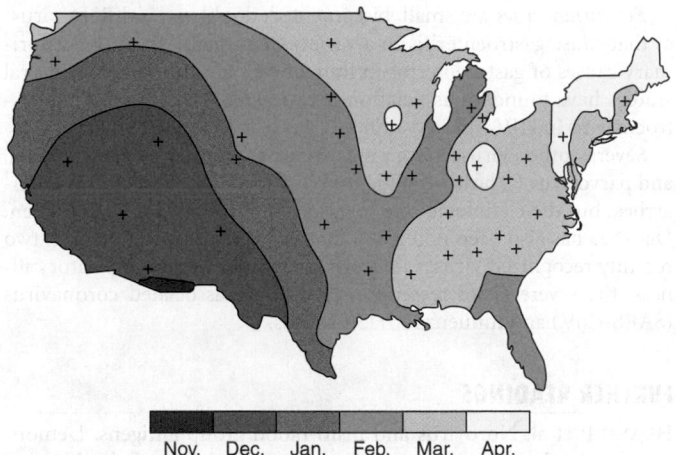

FIGURE 183-2 Time of peak rotavirus activity in the contiguous 48 states: United States, July 1991 to June 1997. Data are from ~90 U.S. laboratories. *(Adapted from TJ Torok et al: Visualizing geographic and temporal trends in rotavirus activity in the United States, 1991 to 1996. National Respiratory and Enteric Virus Surveillance System Collaborating Laboratories. Pediatr Infect Dis J 16:941, 1997.)*

occurs predominantly during the cooler fall and winter months. In the United States, the rotavirus season each year begins in the Southwest during the autumn (October through December) and migrates across the continent, peaking in the Northeast during the spring (March through May) (Fig. 183-2); the reasons for this characteristic pattern are not clear. In tropical settings, rotavirus disease occurs year-round, with less pronounced seasonal peaks.

Rotavirus gastroenteritis is more frequently associated with dehydration than is gastroenteritis caused by other pathogens. Therefore, the proportion of gastroenteritis cases that are attributable to rotavirus increases with increasing severity of illness, ranging from a median of 8% in the community to 18% among outpatients and 40% among hospitalized patients. Each year, rotavirus is estimated to cause ~500,000 childhood deaths worldwide.

During episodes of rotavirus-associated diarrhea, virus is shed in large quantities in stool (10^7–10^{12}/g). Viral shedding detectable by EIA usually subsides within 1 week but may persist for >30 days in immunocompromised individuals. Viral shedding may be detected for longer periods by sensitive molecular assays, such as PCR. The virus is transmitted predominantly through the fecal-oral route. Spread through respiratory secretions, person-to-person contact, or contaminated environmental surfaces has also been postulated to explain the rapid acquisition of antibody in the first 3 years of life, regardless of sanitary conditions.

At least 10 different G serotypes of group A rotavirus have been identified in humans, but only five types (G1 through G4 and G9) are common. While human rotavirus strains that possess a high degree of genetic homology with animal strains have been identified, animal-to-human transmission appears to be uncommon.

Group B rotaviruses have been associated with several large epidemics of severe gastroenteritis among adults in China since 1982 and have recently been identified in India but not in other parts of the world. Group C rotaviruses have been associated with a small proportion of pediatric gastroenteritis cases in several countries worldwide.

Pathogenesis Rotaviruses infect and ultimately destroy mature enterocytes in the villous epithelium of the proximal small intestine. The loss of absorptive villous epithelium, coupled with the proliferation of secretory crypt cells, results in secretory diarrhea. Brush-border enzymes characteristic of differentiated cells are reduced, and this change leads to the accumulation of unmetabolized disaccharides and consequent osmotic diarrhea. Studies in mice indicate that a nonstructural rotavirus protein, NSP4, functions as an enterotoxin and contributes to secretory diarrhea by altering epithelial cell function and perme-

ability. In addition, rotavirus may evoke fluid secretion through activation of the enteric nervous system in the intestinal wall. Recent data indicate that rotavirus antigenemia and viremia are common among children with acute rotavirus infection, although the antigen and RNA levels in serum are substantially lower than those in stool.

Clinical Manifestations The clinical spectrum of rotavirus infection ranges from subclinical infection to severe gastroenteritis leading to life-threatening dehydration. After an incubation period of 1–3 days, the illness has an abrupt onset, with vomiting frequently preceding the onset of diarrhea. Up to one-third of patients may have a temperature of >39°C. The stools are characteristically loose and watery and only infrequently contain red or white cells. Gastrointestinal symptoms generally resolve in 3–7 days.

Respiratory and neurologic features in children with rotavirus infection have been reported, but causal associations have not been proven. Moreover, rotavirus infection has been associated with a variety of other clinical conditions (e.g., sudden infant death syndrome, necrotizing enterocolitis, intussusception, Kawasaki disease, and type 1 diabetes), but no causal relationship has been confirmed with any of these syndromes.

Rotavirus does not appear to be a major opportunistic pathogen in children with HIV infection. In severely immunodeficient children, rotavirus can cause protracted diarrhea with prolonged viral excretion and, in rare instances, can disseminate systemically. Persons who are immunosuppressed for bone marrow transplantation are also at risk for severe or even fatal rotavirus disease.

Immunity Protection against rotavirus disease is correlated with the presence of virus-specific secretory IgA antibodies in the intestine and, to some extent, the serum. Because virus-specific IgA production at the intestinal surface is short-lived, complete protection against disease is only temporary. However, each infection and subsequent reinfection confers progressively greater immunity; thus severe disease is most common among young children with first or second infections. Immunologic memory is believed to be important in the attenuation of disease severity upon reinfection.

Diagnosis Illness caused by rotavirus is difficult to distinguish clinically from that caused by other enteric viruses. Because large quantities of virus are shed in feces, the diagnosis can usually be confirmed by a wide variety of commercially available EIAs or by techniques for detecting viral RNA, such as gel electrophoresis, probe hybridization, or PCR.

℞ ROTAVIRUS INFECTIONS

Rotavirus gastroenteritis can lead to severe dehydration. Thus appropriate treatment should be instituted early. Standard oral rehydration therapy is successful in most children who can take oral fluids, but IV fluid replacement may be required for patients who are severely dehydrated or are unable to tolerate oral therapy because of frequent vomiting. The therapeutic role of probiotics, bismuth subsalicylate, enkephalinase inhibitors, and nitazoxanide has been evaluated in clinical studies but is not clearly defined. Antibiotics and antimotility agents should be avoided. In immunocompromised children with chronic symptomatic rotavirus disease, orally administered immunoglobulins or colostrum may resolve symptoms, but the choice of agents and their doses have not been well studied and are often empirical.

Prevention Efforts to develop rotavirus vaccines were pursued because it was apparent—given the similar rates in less developed and industrialized nations—that improvements in hygiene and sanitation were unlikely to reduce disease incidence. The first rotavirus vaccine licensed in the United States in 1998 was withdrawn from the market within 1 year because it was linked with intussusception, a severe bowel obstruction.

 In 2006, promising safety and efficacy results for two new rotavirus vaccines were reported from large clinical trials conducted in North America, Europe, and Latin America. One of these vaccines, a multivalent bovine-human reassortant rotavirus-based preparation, was recommended for routine immunization of all U.S. infants in early 2006. The second vaccine, based on a single attenuated human rotavirus strain, is not licensed in the United States but has been introduced in immunization programs in several countries in Latin America and Europe.

Global Considerations Rotavirus is ubiquitous and infects nearly all children worldwide by 5 years of age. However, compared with rotavirus disease in industrialized countries, that in developing countries occurs at a younger age, is less seasonal, is more often associated with severe outcomes (including death), and is more frequently caused by uncommon rotavirus strains. The different epidemiology of rotavirus disease and the greater prevalence of co-infection with other enteric pathogens, of comorbidities, and of malnutrition in developing countries may adversely affect the performance of rotavirus vaccines. Therefore, before global recommendations for vaccine use can be issued, it is vital to evaluate the efficacy of rotavirus vaccines in resource-poor settings of Africa and Asia. Trials in these areas are under way.

OTHER VIRAL AGENTS OF GASTROENTERITIS

Enteric *adenoviruses* of serotypes 40 and 41 belonging to subgroup F are 70- to 80-nm viruses with double-strand DNA that cause ~2–12% of all diarrhea episodes in young children. Unlike adenoviruses that cause respiratory illness, enteric adenoviruses are difficult to cultivate in cell lines, but they can be detected with commercially available EIAs.

Astroviruses, 28- to 30-nm viruses with a characteristic icosahedral structure, contain a positive-sense, single-strand RNA. At least seven serotypes have been identified, of which serotype 1 is most common. Astroviruses are primarily pediatric pathogens, causing ~2–10% of cases of mild to moderate gastroenteritis in children. The availability of simple immunoassays to detect virus in fecal specimens and of molecular methods to confirm and characterize strains will permit more comprehensive assessment of the etiologic role of these agents.

Toroviruses are 100- to 140-nm, enveloped, positive-strand RNA viruses that are recognized as causes of gastroenteritis in horses (Berne virus) and cattle (Breda virus). Their role as a cause of diarrhea in humans is still unclear, but studies from Canada have demonstrated associations between torovirus excretion and both nosocomial gastroenteritis and necrotizing enterocolitis in neonates. These associations require further evaluation.

Picobirnaviruses are small, bisegmented, double-strand RNA viruses that cause gastroenteritis in a variety of animals. Their role as primary causes of gastroenteritis in humans remains unclear, but several studies have found an association between picobirnaviruses and gastroenteritis in HIV-infected adults.

Several other viruses (e.g., enteroviruses, reoviruses, pestiviruses, and parvovirus B) have been identified in the feces of patients with diarrhea, but their etiologic role in gastroenteritis has not been proven. Diarrhea has also been noted as a manifestation of infection with two recently recognized viruses that primarily cause severe respiratory illness: the severe acute respiratory syndrome–associated coronavirus (SARS-CoV) and influenza A/H5N1 virus.

FURTHER READINGS

HUANG P et al: Norovirus and histo-blood group antigens: Demonstration of a wide spectrum of strain specificities and classification of two major binding groups among multiple binding patterns. J Virol 79:6714, 2005

KO G et al: Noroviruses as a cause of traveler's diarrhea among students from the United States visiting Mexico. J Clin Microbiol 43:6126, 2005

LEUNG WK et al: Enteric involvement of severe acute respiratory syndrome–associated coronavirus infection. Gastroenterology 125:1011, 2003

LODHA A et al: Human torovirus: A new virus associated with neonatal necrotizing enterocolitis. Acta Paediatr 94:1085, 2005

MURATA T et al: Prolonged norovirus shedding in infants <or=6 months of age with gastroenteritis. Pediatr Infect Dis J 26:46, 2007

RAY P et al: Quantitative evaluation of rotaviral antigenemia in children with acute rotaviral diarrhea. J Infect Dis 194:588, 2006

ROSSIGNOL JF et al: Effect of nitazoxanide for treatment of severe rotavirus diarrhoea: Randomised double-blind placebo-controlled trial. Lancet 368:124, 2006

RUIZ-PALACIOS G et al: Safety and efficacy of an attenuated vaccine against severe rotavirus gastroenteritis. N Engl J Med 354:11, 2006

TRAN TH et al: Avian influenza A (H5N1) in 10 patients in Vietnam. N Engl J Med 350:1179, 2004

VESIKARI T et al: Safety and efficacy of a pentavalent human-bovine (WC3) reassortant rotavirus vaccine. N Engl J Med 354:23, 2006

184 Enteroviruses and Reoviruses
Jeffrey I. Cohen

ENTEROVIRUSES

CLASSIFICATION AND CHARACTERIZATION

Enteroviruses are so named because of their ability to multiply in the gastrointestinal tract. Despite their name, these viruses are not a prominent cause of gastroenteritis. Enteroviruses encompass 65 human serotypes: 3 serotypes of poliovirus, 23 serotypes of coxsackievirus A, 6 serotypes of coxsackievirus B, 29 serotypes of echovirus, and enteroviruses 68–71. Enteroviruses 73–102 have recently been identified in humans by molecular techniques, but their clinical features have not been described. Enterovirus surveillance conducted in the United States by the Centers for Disease Control and Prevention (CDC) in 2002–2004 showed that two enteroviruses—echoviruses 9 and 30—accounted for 59% of all enterovirus isolates.

Human enteroviruses contain a single-stranded RNA genome surrounded by an icosahedral capsid comprising four viral proteins. These viruses have no lipid envelope and are stable in acidic environments, including the stomach. They are resistant to inactivation by standard disinfectants (e.g., alcohol, detergents) and can persist for days at room temperature.

PATHOGENESIS AND IMMUNITY

Much of what is known about the pathogenesis of enteroviruses has been derived from studies of poliovirus infection. After ingestion, poliovirus is thought to infect epithelial cells in the mucosa of the gastrointestinal tract and then to spread to and replicate in the submucosal lymphoid tissue of the tonsils and Peyer's patches. The virus next spreads to the regional lymph nodes, a viremic phase ensues, and the virus replicates in organs of the reticuloendothelial system. In some cases, a second viremia occurs and the virus replicates further in various tissues, sometimes causing symptomatic disease.

It is uncertain whether poliovirus reaches the central nervous system (CNS) during viremia or whether it also spreads via peripheral nerves. Since viremia precedes the onset of neurologic disease in humans and in experimentally infected chimpanzees, it has been assumed that the virus enters the CNS via the bloodstream. The poliovirus receptor is a member of the immunoglobulin superfamily. Poliovirus infection is limited to primates, largely because their cells express the viral receptor. Studies demonstrating the poliovirus receptor in the end-plate region of muscle at the neuromuscular junction suggest that, if the virus enters the muscle during viremia, it could travel across the neuromuscular junction up the axon to the anterior horn cells. Studies of monkeys and of transgenic mice expressing the poliovirus receptor show that, after IM injection, poliovirus does not reach the spinal cord if the sciatic nerve is cut. Taken together, these findings suggest that poliovirus can spread directly from muscle to the CNS by neural pathways. Intercellular adhesion molecule 1 (ICAM-1) is a receptor for coxsackieviruses A13, A18, and A21; CAR for coxsackievirus B; VLA-2 integrin for echovirus types 1 and 8; and CD55 for enterovirus 70 and some serotypes of coxsackievirus A and B and echovirus.

Poliovirus can usually be cultured from the blood 3–5 days after infection, before the development of neutralizing antibodies. While viral replication at secondary sites begins to slow 1 week after infection, it continues in the gastrointestinal tract. Poliovirus is shed from the oropharynx for up to 3 weeks after infection and from the gastrointestinal tract for as long as 12 weeks; immunodeficient patients can shed poliovirus for up to 20 years. During replication in the gastrointestinal tract, attenuated oral poliovirus can mutate, reverting to a more neurovirulent phenotype within a few days. The clinical significance of this increased neurovirulence is unknown.

Humoral and secretory immunity in the gastrointestinal tract is important for the control of enterovirus infections. Enteroviruses induce specific IgM, which usually persists for <6 months, and specific IgG, which persists for life. Capsid protein VP1 is the predominant target of neutralizing antibody, which generally confers lifelong protection against subsequent disease caused by the same serotype but does not prevent infection or virus shedding. Enteroviruses also induce cellular immunity, but the significance of this mechanism in limiting infection is uncertain. Patients with impaired cellular immunity are not known to develop unusually severe disease when infected with enteroviruses. In contrast, the severe infections in patients with agammaglobulinemia emphasize the importance of humoral immunity in controlling enterovirus infections. Disseminated enterovirus infections have occurred in stem cell transplant recipients. IgA antibodies are instrumental in reducing poliovirus replication in and shedding from the gastrointestinal tract. Breast milk contains IgA specific for enteroviruses and can protect humans from infection.

EPIDEMIOLOGY

Enteroviruses have a worldwide distribution. More than 50% of nonpoliovirus enterovirus infections and more than 90% of poliovirus infections are subclinical. When symptoms do develop, they are usually nonspecific and occur in conjunction with fever; only a minority of infections are associated with specific clinical syndromes. The incubation period for most enterovirus infections ranges from 2 to 14 days but usually is <1 week.

Enterovirus infection is more common in socioeconomically disadvantaged areas, especially in those where conditions are crowded and in tropical areas where hygiene is poor. Infection is most common among infants and young children; serious illness develops most often during the first few days of life and in older children and adults. In developing countries, where children are infected at an early age, poliovirus infection has less often been associated with paralysis; in countries with better hygiene, older children and adults are more likely to be seronegative, become infected, and develop paralysis. Passively acquired maternal antibody reduces the risk of symptomatic infection in neonates. Young children are the most frequent shedders of enteroviruses and are usually the index cases in family outbreaks. In temperate climates, enterovirus infections occur most often in the summer and fall; no seasonal pattern is apparent in the tropics.

Most enteroviruses are transmitted primarily by the fecal-oral route from fecally contaminated fingers or inanimate objects. Patients are most infectious shortly before and after the onset of symptomatic disease, when virus is present in the stool and throat. The ingestion of virus-contaminated food or water can also cause disease. Certain enteroviruses (such as enterovirus 70, which causes acute hemorrhagic conjunctivitis) can be transmitted by direct inoculation from the fingers to the eye. Airborne transmission is important for some viruses that cause respiratory tract disease, such as coxsackievirus A21. Enteroviruses can be transmitted across the placenta from mother to fetus, causing severe disease in the newborn. The transmission of enteroviruses through blood transfusions or insect bites has not been documented. Nosocomial spread of coxsackievirus and echovirus has taken place in hospital nurseries.

CLINICAL FEATURES

Poliovirus Infection Most infections with poliovirus are asymptomatic. After an incubation period of 3–6 days, ~5% of patients present with a minor illness (abortive poliomyelitis) manifested by fever, malaise, sore throat, anorexia, myalgias, and headache. This condition usually resolves in 3 days. About 1% of patients present with aseptic meningitis (nonparalytic poliomyelitis). Examination of cerebrospinal fluid (CSF) reveals lymphocytic pleocytosis, a normal glucose level, and a normal or slightly elevated protein level; CSF polymorphonuclear leukocytes may be present early. In some patients, especially children, malaise and fever precede the onset of aseptic meningitis.

PARALYTIC POLIOMYELITIS The least common presentation is that of paralytic disease. After one or several days, signs of aseptic meningitis are followed by severe back, neck, and muscle pain and by the rapid or gradual development of motor weakness. In some cases the disease appears to be biphasic, with aseptic meningitis followed first by apparent recovery but then (1–2 days later) by the return of fever and the development of paralysis; this form is more common among children than among adults. Weakness is generally asymmetric, is proximal more than distal, and may involve the legs (most commonly); the arms; or the abdominal, thoracic, or bulbar muscles. Paralysis develops during the febrile phase of the illness and usually does not progress after defervescence. Urinary retention may also occur. Examination reveals weakness, fasciculations, decreased muscle tone, and reduced or absent reflexes in affected areas. Transient hyperreflexia sometimes precedes the loss of reflexes. Patients frequently report sensory symptoms, but objective sensory testing usually yields normal results. Bulbar paralysis may lead to dysphagia, difficulty in handling secretions, or dysphonia. Respiratory insufficiency due to aspiration, involvement of the respiratory center in the medulla, or paralysis of the phrenic or intercostal nerves may develop, and severe medullary involvement may lead to circulatory collapse. Most patients with paralysis recover some function weeks to months after infection. About two-thirds of patients have residual neurologic sequelae.

Paralytic disease is more common among older individuals, pregnant women, and persons exercising strenuously or undergoing trauma at the time of CNS symptoms. Tonsillectomy predisposes to bulbar poliomyelitis, and IM injections increase the risk of paralysis in the involved limb(s).

VACCINE-ASSOCIATED POLIOMYELITIS Until recently, poliomyelitis due to live poliovirus vaccine occurred in the United States. The risk of developing poliomyelitis after oral vaccination is estimated at 1 case per 2.5 million doses. The risk is ~2000 times higher among immunodeficient persons, especially in persons with hypo- or agammaglobulinemia. Before 1997, an average of eight cases of vaccine-associated poliomyelitis occurred—in both vaccinees and their contacts—in the United States each year. With the change in recommendations first to a sequential regimen of inactivated poliovirus vaccine (IPV) and oral poliovirus vaccine (OPV) in 1997 and then to an all-IPV regimen in 2000, the number of cases of vaccine-associated polio declined. From 1997 to 1999, six such cases were reported in the United States; no cases have been reported since 1999.

POSTPOLIO SYNDROME The *postpolio syndrome* presents as a new onset of weakness, fatigue, fasciculations, and pain with additional atrophy of the muscle group involved during the initial paralytic disease 20–40 years earlier. The syndrome is more common among women and with increasing time after acute disease. The onset is usually insidious, and weakness occasionally extends to muscles that were not involved during the initial illness. The prognosis is generally good; progression to further

TABLE 184-1 MANIFESTATIONS COMMONLY ASSOCIATED WITH ENTEROVIRUS SEROTYPES

Manifestation	Serotype(s) of Indicated Virus	
	Coxsackievirus	Echovirus (E) and Enterovirus (Ent)
Acute hemorrhagic conjunctivitis	A24	E70
Aseptic meningitis	A2, 4, 7, 9, 10; B1-5	E4, 6, 7, 9, 11, 13, 16, 18, 19, 30, 33; Ent70, 71
Encephalitis	A9; B1-5	E3, 4, 6, 9, 11, 25, 30; Ent71
Exanthem	A4, 5, 9, 10, 16; B1, 3-5	E4-7, 9, 11, 16-19, 25, 30; Ent71
Generalized disease of the newborn	B1-5	E4-6, 7, 9, 11, 14, 16, 18, 19
Hand-foot-and-mouth disease	A5, 7, 9, 10, 16; B1, 2, 5	Ent71
Herpangina	A1-10, 16, 22; B1-5	E6, 9, 11, 16, 17, 25; Ent71
Myocarditis, pericarditis	A4, 9, 16; B1-5	E6, 9, 11, 22
Paralysis	A4, 7, 9; B1-5	E2, 4, 6, 9, 11, 30; Ent70, 71
Pleurodynia	A1, 2, 4, 6, 9, 10, 16; B1-6	E1-3, 6, 7, 9, 11, 12, 14, 16, 19, 24, 25, 30
Pneumonia	A9, 16; B1-5	E6, 7, 9, 11, 12, 19, 20, 30; Ent68, 71

weakness is usually slow, with plateau periods of 1–10 years. The postpolio syndrome is thought to be due to progressive dysfunction and loss of motor neurons that compensated for the neurons lost during the original infection and not to persistent or reactivated poliovirus infection.

Other Enteroviruses An estimated 5–10 million cases of symptomatic disease due to enteroviruses other than poliovirus occur in the United States each year. Among neonates, enteroviruses are the most common cause of aseptic meningitis and nonspecific febrile illnesses. Certain clinical syndromes are more likely to be caused by certain serotypes (Table 184-1), but there is much overlap. In 2002–2004, 85% of enterovirus infections were caused by only 9 human serotypes. Echoviruses 9 and 30 accounted for 60% of recognized enterovirus infections.

NONSPECIFIC FEBRILE ILLNESS (SUMMER GRIPPE) The most common clinical manifestation of enterovirus infection is a nonspecific febrile illness. After an incubation period of 3–6 days, patients present with an acute onset of fever, malaise, and headache. Occasional cases are associated with upper respiratory symptoms, and some cases include nausea and vomiting. Symptoms often last for 3–4 days, and most cases resolve in a week. While infections with other respiratory viruses occur more often from late fall to early spring, enterovirus febrile illness frequently occurs in the summer and early fall.

GENERALIZED DISEASE OF THE NEWBORN Most serious enterovirus infections in infants develop during the first week of life, although severe disease can occur up to 3 months of age. Neonates often present with an illness resembling bacterial sepsis, with fever, irritability, and lethargy. Laboratory abnormalities include leukocytosis with a left shift, thrombocytopenia, elevated values in liver function tests, and CSF pleocytosis. The illness can be complicated by myocarditis and hypotension, fulminant hepatitis and disseminated intravascular coagulation, meningitis or meningoencephalitis, or pneumonia. It may be difficult to distinguish neonatal enterovirus infection from bacterial sepsis, although a history of a recent virus-like illness in the mother provides a clue.

ASEPTIC MENINGITIS AND ENCEPHALITIS Enteroviruses are the cause of up to 90% of cases of aseptic meningitis in children and young adults in which an etiologic agent can be identified. Patients with aseptic meningitis typically present with an acute onset of fever, chills, headache, photophobia, and pain on eye movement. Nausea and vomiting are also common. Examination reveals meningismus without localizing neurologic signs; drowsiness or irritability may also be apparent. In some cas-

es, a febrile illness may be reported that remits but returns several days later in conjunction with signs of meningitis. Other systemic manifestations may provide clues to an enteroviral cause, including diarrhea, myalgias, rash, pleurodynia, myocarditis, and herpangina. Examination of the CSF invariably reveals pleocytosis; early in the course, polymorphonuclear leukocytes may be present or even predominant—a finding that raises the possibility of bacterial or other nonviral causes of meningitis. Partially treated bacterial meningitis may be particularly difficult to exclude in some instances. A useful rule is that the CSF cell count in enteroviral meningitis shows a shift to lymphocytic predominance within 24 h of presentation, and the total count generally does not exceed 1000 cells/μL. Additional CSF findings consist of a normal glucose content and a normal or only slightly elevated (by ≤100 mg/dL) level of protein. Enteroviruses and mumps virus may produce a similar picture of meningitis; a low CSF glucose level suggests mumps, whereas a normal CSF glucose level and transient CSF polymorphonuclear pleocytosis suggest enterovirus infection. Enteroviral meningitis is more frequent in summer and fall in temperate climates, while viral meningitis of other etiologies (e.g., mumps) is more common in winter and spring. Symptoms ordinarily resolve within a week, although CSF abnormalities can persist for several weeks. Enteroviral meningitis is often more severe in adults than in children. Neurologic sequelae are rare, and most patients have an excellent prognosis.

Enteroviral encephalitis is much less common than enteroviral aseptic meningitis. Occasional highly inflammatory cases of enteroviral meningitis may be complicated by a mild form of encephalitis that is recognized on the basis of progressive lethargy, disorientation, and sometimes seizures. Less commonly, severe primary encephalitis may develop. An estimated 10–20% of cases of viral encephalitis are due to enteroviruses. Immunocompetent patients generally have a good prognosis.

Patients with hypogammaglobulinemia or agammaglobulinemia or severe combined immunodeficiency may develop chronic meningitis or encephalitis; about half of these patients have a dermatomyositis-like syndrome, with peripheral edema, rash, and myositis. They may also have chronic hepatitis. Patients may develop neurologic disease while receiving gamma globulin replacement therapy. Echoviruses (especially echovirus 11) are the most common pathogens in this situation.

Paralytic disease due to enteroviruses other than poliovirus occurs sporadically and is usually less severe than poliomyelitis. Most cases are due to enterovirus 70 or 71 or to coxsackievirus A7 or A9. Guillain-Barré syndrome is also associated with enterovirus infection. While some studies have suggested a link between enteroviruses and the chronic fatigue syndrome, most recent studies have not demonstrated such an association.

PLEURODYNIA (BORNHOLM DISEASE) Patients with pleurodynia present with an acute onset of fever and spasms of pleuritic chest or upper abdominal pain. Chest pain is more common in adults, and abdominal pain is more common in children. Paroxysms of severe, knifelike pain usually last 15–30 min and are associated with diaphoresis and tachypnea. Fever peaks within an hour after the onset of paroxysms and subsides when pain resolves. The involved muscles are tender to palpation, and a pleural rub may be detected. The white blood cell count and chest x-ray are usually normal. Most cases are due to coxsackievirus B and occur during epidemics. Symptoms resolve in a few days, and recurrences are rare. Treatment includes the administration of nonsteroidal anti-inflammatory agents or the application of heat to the affected muscles.

MYOCARDITIS AND PERICARDITIS Enteroviruses are estimated to cause up to one-third of cases of acute myocarditis. Coxsackievirus B and its RNA have been detected in pericardial fluid and myocardial tissue in some cases of acute myocarditis and pericarditis. Most cases of enteroviral myocarditis or pericarditis occur in newborns, adolescents, or young adults. More than two-thirds of patients are male. Patients often present with an upper respiratory tract infection that is followed by fever, chest pain, dyspnea, arrhythmias, and occasionally heart failure. A pericardial friction rub is documented in half of cases, and the electrocardiogram shows ST-segment elevations or ST- and T-wave abnormalities. Serum levels of myocardial enzymes are often elevated. Neonates commonly have severe disease, while most older children and adults recover completely. Up to 10% of cases progress to chronic dilated cardiomyopathy. Chronic constrictive pericarditis may also be a sequela.

EXANTHEMS Enterovirus infection is the leading cause of exanthems in children in the summer and fall. While exanthems are associated with many enteroviruses, certain types have been linked to specific syndromes. Echoviruses 9 and 16 have frequently been associated with exanthem and fever. Rashes may be discrete (rubelliform) or confluent (morbilliform), beginning on the face and spreading to the trunk and extremities. Echovirus 9 is the most common cause of rubelliform rash. Unlike the rash of rubella, the enteroviral rash occurs in the summer and is not associated with lymphadenopathy. Roseola-like rashes develop after defervescence, with macules and papules on the face and trunk. The Boston exanthem, caused by echovirus 16, is a roseola-like rash that often affects multiple members of a family. A variety of other rashes have been associated with enteroviruses, including erythema multiforme and vesicular, urticarial, petechial, or purpuric lesions. Enanthems also occur, including lesions that resemble the Koplik's spots seen with measles.

HAND-FOOT-AND-MOUTH DISEASE After an incubation period of 4–6 days, patients with hand-foot-and-mouth disease present with fever, anorexia, and malaise; these manifestations are followed by the development of sore throat and vesicles (Fig. 184-1A) on the buccal mucosa and often on the tongue and then by the appearance of tender vesicular lesions on the dorsum of the hands, sometimes with involvement of the palms. The vesicles may form bullae and quickly ulcerate. About one-third of patients also have lesions on the palate, uvula, or tonsillar pillars, and one-third have a rash on the feet (including the soles) or on the buttocks. The disease is highly infectious, with attack rates of close to 100% among young children. The lesions usually resolve in 1 week. Most cases are due to coxsackievirus A16 or enterovirus 71.

An epidemic of enterovirus 71 infection in Taiwan in 1998 resulted in thousands of cases of hand-foot-and-mouth disease or herpangina. Severe complications included CNS disease, myocarditis, and pulmonary hemorrhage. About 90% of those who died were children ≤5 years old, and these deaths were associated with pulmonary edema or pulmonary hemorrhage. CNS disease included aseptic meningitis, flaccid paralysis (similar to poliomyelitis), or rhombencephalitis with myoclonus and tremor or ataxia. The mean age of patients with CNS complications was 2.5 years, and MRI in cases with encephalitis usually showed brain-stem lesions. Follow-up of children at 6 months showed persistent dysphagia, cranial nerve palsies, hypoventilation, limb weakness, and atrophy.

HERPANGINA Herpangina is usually caused by coxsackievirus A and presents as acute-onset fever, sore throat, dysphagia, and grayish-white papulovesicular lesions on an erythematous base that ulcerate (Fig. 184-1B). The lesions can persist for weeks; are present on the soft palate, anterior pillars of the tonsils, and uvula; and are concentrated in the posterior portion of the mouth. In contrast to herpes stomatitis, enteroviral herpangina is not associated with gingivitis. Acute lymphonodular pharyngitis associated with coxsackievirus A10 presents as white or yellow nodules surrounded by erythema in the posterior oropharynx. The lesions do not ulcerate.

ACUTE HEMORRHAGIC CONJUNCTIVITIS Patients with acute hemorrhagic conjunctivitis present with an acute onset of severe eye pain, blurred vision, photophobia, and watery discharge from the eye. Examination reveals edema, chemosis, and subconjunctival hemorrhage and often shows punctate keratitis and conjunctival follicles as well (Fig. 184-1C). Preauricular adenopathy is often found. Epidemics and

FIGURE 184-1 A. Tender vesicles and erosions in the mouth of a patient with hand-foot-and-mouth disease. **B.** Soft-palate lesions of herpangina due to coxsackievirus. **C.** Acute hemorrhagic conjunctivitis due to enterovirus 71. (*Images B and C are reprinted with permission from Redbook 2006: Committee on Infectious Diseases, 27th ed. Elk Grove Village, IL: American Academy of Pediatrics.*)

nosocomial spread have been associated with enterovirus 70 and cox-sackievirus A24. Systemic symptoms, including headache and fever, develop in 20% of cases, and recovery is usually complete in 10 days. The sudden onset and short duration of the illness help to distinguish acute hemorrhagic conjunctivitis from other ocular infections such as those due to adenovirus and *Chlamydia*. Paralysis has been associated with some cases of acute hemorrhagic conjunctivitis due to enterovirus 70 during epidemics.

OTHER MANIFESTATIONS Enteroviruses are an infrequent cause of childhood pneumonia and the common cold. Coxsackievirus B has been isolated at autopsy from the pancreas of a few children presenting with type 1 diabetes mellitus; however, most attempts to isolate the virus have been unsuccessful. Other diseases that have been associated with enterovirus infection include parotitis, bronchitis, bronchiolitis, croup, infectious lymphocytosis, polymyositis, acute arthritis, and acute nephritis.

DIAGNOSIS

Isolation of enterovirus in cell culture is the traditional diagnostic procedure. While cultures of stool, nasopharyngeal, or throat samples from patients with enterovirus diseases are often positive, isolation of the virus from these sites does not prove that it is directly associated with disease because these sites are frequently colonized for weeks in patients with subclinical infections. Isolation of virus from the throat is more likely to be associated with disease than isolation from the stool since virus is shed for shorter periods from the throat. Cultures of CSF, serum, fluid from body cavities, or tissues are positive less frequently, but a positive result is indicative of disease caused by enterovirus. In some cases, the virus is isolated only from the blood or only from the CSF; therefore, it is important to culture multiple sites. Cultures are more likely to be positive earlier than later in the course of infection. Most human enteroviruses can be detected within a week after inoculation of cell cultures. Cultures may be negative because of the presence of neutralizing antibody, lack of susceptibility of the cells used, or inappropriate handling of the specimen. Coxsackievirus A may require inoculation into special cell-culture lines or into suckling mice.

Identification of the enterovirus serotype is useful primarily for epidemiologic studies and, with a few exceptions, has little clinical utility. It is important to identify serious infections with enterovirus during epidemics and to distinguish the vaccine strain of poliovirus from the other enteroviruses in the throat or in the feces. Stool and throat samples for culture as well as acute- and convalescent-phase serum specimens should be obtained from all patients with suspected poliomyelitis. In the absence of a positive CSF culture, a positive culture of stool obtained within the first 2 weeks after the onset of symptoms is most often used to confirm the diagnosis of poliomyelitis. If poliovirus infection is suspected, two or more fecal and throat swab samples should be obtained at least 1 day apart and cultured for enterovirus as soon as possible. If poliovirus is isolated, it should be sent to the CDC for identification as either wild-type or vaccine virus.

The polymerase chain reaction (PCR) has been used to amplify viral nucleic acid from CSF, serum, urine, throat swabs, and tissues. A single pair of PCR primers can detect >92% of the serotypes that infect humans. With the proper controls, PCR of the CSF is highly sensitive (≥95%) and specific (>80%) and is more rapid than culture. PCR of the CSF is less likely to be positive when patients present ≥3 days after the onset of meningitis rather than earlier; in these cases, PCR of fecal specimens should be considered, although the test is less specific than PCR of CSF. PCR of serum is also highly sensitive and specific in the diagnosis of disseminated disease. PCR may be particularly helpful for the diagnosis and follow-up of enterovirus disease in immunodeficient patients receiving immunoglobulin therapy, whose viral cultures may be negative. Antigen detection and hybridization of enterovirus sequences in human tissues with a specific probe are additional options, but these techniques are generally less sensitive than PCR.

Serologic diagnosis of enterovirus infection is limited by the large number of serotypes and the lack of a common antigen. Demonstration of seroconversion may be useful in rare cases for confirmation of culture results, but serologic testing is usually limited to epidemiologic studies. Serum should be collected and frozen soon after the onset of disease and again ~4 weeks later. Measurement of neutralizing titers is the most accurate method for antibody determination; measurement of complement-fixation titers is usually less sensitive. Titers of virus-specific IgM are elevated in both acute and chronic infection.

℞ ENTEROVIRUS INFECTIONS

Most enterovirus infections are mild and resolve spontaneously; however, intensive supportive care may be needed for cardiac, hepatic, or CNS disease. IV, intrathecal, or intraventricular immunoglobulin has been used with apparent success for the treatment of chronic enterovirus meningoencephalitis and dermatomyositis in patients with hypogammaglobulinemia or agammaglobulinemia. The disease may stabilize or resolve during therapy; however, some patients decline inexorably despite therapy. IV administration of immunoglobulin with high titers of antibody to the infecting virus has been used in some cases of life-threatening infection in neonates, who may not have maternally acquired antibody. In one trial involving neonates with enterovirus infections, immunoglobulin containing very high titers of antibody to the infecting virus reduced rates of viremia; however, the study was too small to show a substantial clinical benefit. The level of enteroviral antibodies varies with the immunoglobulin preparation. For a time, pleconaril was given to patients with severe enterovirus infections on a compassionate-use basis, but this drug is no longer available for this use. Glucocorticoids are contraindicated.

Good hand-washing practices and the use of gowns and gloves are important in limiting nosocomial transmission of enteroviruses during epidemics. Enteric precautions are indicated for 7 days after the onset of enterovirus infections.

PREVENTION AND ERADICATION OF POLIOVIRUS

(See also Chap. 116) After a peak of 57,879 cases of poliomyelitis in the United States in 1952, the introduction of inactivated vaccine in 1955 and of oral vaccine in 1961 ultimately eradicated disease due to wild-type poliovirus in the Western Hemisphere. Such disease has not been documented in the United States since 1979, when cases occurred among religious groups who had declined immunization. In the Western Hemisphere, paralysis due to wild-type poliovirus was last documented in 1991.

In 1988, the World Health Organization adopted a resolution to eradicate poliomyelitis by the year 2000. From 1988 to 2001, the number of cases worldwide decreased by >99%, with fewer than 1000 confirmed cases reported in 2001. In 2002, however, there were ~1900 cases of polio, with ~1500 reported in India. Wild-type poliovirus type 2 has not been detected in the world since 1999. The Americas were certified free of indigenous wild-type poliovirus transmission in 1994, the Western Pacific Region in 2000, and the European Region in 2002. The total number of cases worldwide fell to a nadir of 498 in 2001. However, from 2002 to 2005, 21 countries previously free of polio reported cases imported from 6 polio-endemic countries. By 2006, polio transmission had been reduced or interrupted in most of these 21 countries, and polio was endemic in only 4 countries, with a total of 2000 cases (Table 184-2). Preliminary data indicate a total of 1959 cases in 2006, with ~90% of cases from Nigeria and India. Polio is a source of concern for unimmunized or partially immunized travelers to these regions. Outbreaks of polio in Europe and North America have been traced to cases imported from the Indian subcontinent. Clearly, global eradication of polio is necessary to eliminate the risk of importation of wild-type virus. Outbreaks are thought to have been facilitated by suboptimal rates of vaccination, isolated pockets of unvaccinated children, poor sanitation and crowding, improper vaccine-storage conditions, and a reduced level of response to one of the serotypes in the vaccine. While the global eradication campaign has markedly reduced the number of cases of polio, doubts have been raised as to whether eradication is a realistic goal given the large number of asymptomatic cases and the political instability in developing countries.

Outbreaks of poliomyelitis due to circulating vaccine-derived poliovirus have recently occurred. In Egypt, 30 cases of vaccine-derived polio oc-

TABLE 184-2	LABORATORY-CONFIRMED CASES OF POLIOMYELITIS IN 2006	

Country	Type of Transmission	Number of Cases
Nigeria	Endemic	1123[a]
India	Endemic	676
Pakistan	Endemic	40
Afghanistan	Endemic	31
Somalia	Imported	35
Others[b]	Imported	93
Others[c]	Vaccine-derived	2
Total		**2000**

[a]Of these cases, 1 was vaccine-derived.
[b]Imported cases: Namibia, 19; Bangladesh, 18; Ethiopia, 17; Democratic Republic of the Congo, 13; Niger, 11; Nepal, 5; Angola, 2; Cameroon, 2; Kenya, 2; Indonesia, 2; Chad, 1; Yemen, 1.
[c]Vaccine-derived cases: Myanmar, 1; Cambodia, 1.
Source: World Health Organization.

TABLE 184-3	RECOMMENDATIONS FOR POLIOVIRUS VACCINATION OF ADULTS

1. Most adults in the United States have been vaccinated during childhood and have little risk of exposure to wild-type virus in the United States. Immunization is recommended for those with a higher risk of exposure than the general population, including:
   a. travelers to areas where poliovirus is or may be epidemic or endemic;
   b. members of communities or population groups with disease caused by wild-type polioviruses;
   c. laboratory workers handling specimens that may contain wild-type polioviruses; and
   d. health care workers in close contact with patients who may be excreting wild-type polioviruses.
2. Three doses of IPV are recommended for adults who need to be immunized. The second dose should be given 1–2 months after the first dose; the third dose should be given 6–12 months after the second dose.
3. Adults who are at increased risk of exposure to wild-type poliovirus and who have previously completed primary immunization should receive a single dose of IPV. Adults who did not complete primary immunization should receive the remaining vaccinations with IPV.

Note: IPV, inactivated poliovirus vaccine.
Source: Modified from Pickering LK, ed. Redbook 2006: Committee on Infectious Diseases, 27th ed. Elk Grove Village, IL: American Academy of Pediatrics.

curred in 1988–1993; in the Dominican Republic and Haiti, 21 cases occurred in 2000–2001; and fewer than 5 cases each occurred in the Philippines (2001), Madagascar (2002), and China (2004). These OPV-derived viruses reverted to a more neurovirulent phenotype after undetected circulation (probably for >2 years). The epidemic in Hispaniola was rapidly terminated after intensive vaccination with OPV. In 2005, a case of vaccine-derived polio occurred in an unvaccinated U.S. woman returning from a visit to Central and South America. In the same year, an unvaccinated immunocompromised infant in Minnesota was found to be shedding vaccine-derived poliovirus; further investigation identified 3 other infants in the same community who were shedding the virus. All 4 infants were asymptomatic. These outbreaks emphasize the need for maintaining high levels of vaccine coverage and continued surveillance for circulating virus.

IPV is used in most industrialized countries and OPV in most developing countries, including those in which polio still is or recently was endemic. After several doses of OPV alone, the seropositivity rate for individual poliovirus serotypes may still be suboptimal for children in developing countries; one or more supplemental doses of IPV can increase the rate of seropositivity for these serotypes. While IM injections of other vaccines (live or attenuated) can be given concurrently with OPV, unnecessary IM injections should be avoided during the first month after vaccination because they increase the risk of vaccine-associated paralysis. Since 1988, an enhanced-potency inactivated poliovirus vaccine has been available in the United States.

OPV and IPV induce antibodies that persist for at least 5 years. Both vaccines induce IgG and IgA antibodies. Compared with recipients of IPV, recipients of OPV shed less virus and less frequently develop reinfection with wild-type virus after exposure to poliovirus. Although IPV is safe and efficacious, OPV offers the advantages of ease of administration, lower cost, and induction of intestinal immunity resulting in a reduction in the risk of community transmission of wild-type virus. Because of progress toward global eradication of polio (with a reduced risk of imported cases) and the continued occurrence of cases of vaccine-associated polio, an all-IPV regimen was recommended in 2000 for childhood poliovirus vaccination in the United States, with vaccine administration at 2, 4, and 6–18 months and 4–6 years of age. The risk of vaccine-associated polio should be discussed before OPV is administered. Recommendations for vaccination of adults are listed in Table 184-3.

There are concerns about discontinuing vaccination in the event that endemic spread of poliovirus is eliminated. Among the reasons for these concerns are that poliovirus is shed from some immunocompromised persons for several years, that vaccine-derived poliovirus can circulate and cause disease, and that wild-type poliovirus is present in a large number of laboratories. A national survey began in October 2002 to encourage laboratories to dispose of all unneeded wild-type poliovirus materials and to identify laboratories that have wild-type poliovirus or specimens that may contain virus.

REOVIRUSES

Reoviruses are double-stranded RNA viruses encompassing three serotypes. Serologic studies indicate that most humans are infected with reoviruses during childhood. Most infections either are asymptomatic or cause very mild disease. One outbreak of reovirus infection in children resulted in minor upper respiratory tract symptoms. Reovirus is considered a rare cause of mild gastroenteritis in infants and children. Speculation regarding an association of reovirus type 3 with idiopathic neonatal hepatitis and extrahepatic biliary atresia is based on an elevated prevalence of antibody to reovirus among some of these patients and the detection of viral RNA by PCR in hepatobiliary tissues in some studies.

FURTHER READINGS

ALEXANDER LN et al: Vaccine policy changes and epidemiology of poliomyelitis in the United States. JAMA 292:1696, 2004

ARITA I et al: Is polio eradication realistic? Science 312:852, 2006

CENTERS FOR DISEASE CONTROL AND PREVENTION: Enterovirus surveillance—United States, 2002–2004. MMWR 55:153, 2006

————: Resurgence of wild poliovirus type 1 transmission and consequences of importation—21 countries, 2002–2005. MMWR 55:145, 2006

CHANG L-Y et al: Transmission and clinical features of enterovirus 71 infections in household contacts in Taiwan. JAMA 291:222, 2004

JUBELT B, AAGRE JC: Characteristics and management of postpolio syndrome. JAMA 284:412, 2000

KEW O et al: Vaccine-derived polioviruses and the endgame strategy for global polio eradication. Annu Rev Microbiol 59:587, 2005

KUPILIA L et al: Diagnosis of enteroviral meningitis by use of polymerase chain reaction of cerebrospinal fluid, stool, and serum specimens. Clin Infect Dis 40:982, 2005

MACLENNAN C et al: Failure to clear persistent vaccine-derived neurovirulent poliovirus infection in an immunocompromised man. Lancet 363:1509, 2004

PEREZ-VELEZ CM et al: Outbreak of neurologic enterovirus type 71 disease: A diagnostic challenge. Clin Infect Dis 45:950, 2007

THOMPSON KM, TEBBENS RJ: Eradication versus control for poliomyelitis: An economic analysis. Lancet 369:1363, 2007

185 Measles (Rubeola)
Anne Gershon

DEFINITION

Measles (rubeola) is a highly contagious, acute, exanthematous respiratory disease with a characteristic clinical picture and a pathognomonic enanthem: Koplik's spots, an eruption on the buccal mucous membranes (Fig. 185-1).

A successful live attenuated measles vaccine became available in 1963 in the United States and elsewhere, and measles is now an unusual disease in most developed countries where this vaccine is widely used. However, measles continues to occur sporadically in miniepidemics in the United States, and major epidemics in developing nations make this disease a persistent cause of childhood morbidity and mortality.

In 2000, measles was the fifth leading cause of childhood mortality worldwide, with an estimated 777,000 deaths. The incidence of global measles in 2004 is shown in Fig. 185-2.

ETIOLOGIC AGENT

Measles virus is the only member of the genus *Morbillivirus* that infects humans. Part of the family Paramyxoviridae, it is related to viruses causing similar infections in other mammals: distemper, rinderpest, morbilli, and *peste des petits ruminants*. There is only one antigenic type. Virions—pleomorphic spheres with a diameter of 100–250 nm—consist of six proteins. The inner capsid is composed of RNA and three proteins. The outer envelope consists of a matrix protein bearing short surface-glycoprotein projections or peplomers, one a hemagglutinin (H) and the other a fusion (F) protein. Sequencing of the single-stranded genome makes it possible to distinguish vaccine-type from wild-type virus. The genetic variability of wild-type virus (23 genotypes identified) permits identification of strains endemic within a given locale where measles cases have occurred. The cellular receptors for measles virus are the CD46 and CD150 molecules expressed on many human cells.

EPIDEMIOLOGY

Measles has a worldwide distribution; humans are the only natural hosts, although other primates can be experimentally infected. During the prevaccination era in the United States, measles epidemics took place every 2–5 years. In epidemic years, roughly half a million measles cases occurred; 99% of adults had serologic evidence of previous measles infection. After the live attenuated vaccine became available, the number of cases reported to the Centers for Disease Control and Prevention fell, with a nadir of 1497 cases in 1983. In 1990, after an upsurge to more than 27,000 cases (with 89 deaths), the disease was once more brought under control, mainly through the routine administration of two doses of vaccine. Reasons for the resurgence included failure to immunize young children, especially in inner-city areas; primary vaccine failure (rate, ~5%); and (rarely) waning immunity.

Between 1993 and 1996, fewer than 1000 cases per year were reported in the United States; 309 cases were reported in 1995, 116 in 2001, and only 37 in 2004. Molecular studies indicated interruption of transmission of indigenous measles in 1993. Most cases since have resulted from international importations of the virus by immigrants or U.S. citizens returning from travel abroad. Mortality rates are highest among children <2 years of age and among

FIGURE 185-1 Koplik's spots, which manifest as white or bluish lesions with an erythematous halo on the buccal mucosa, usually occur in the first 2 days of measles symptoms and may briefly overlap the measles exanthem. The presence of the erythematous halo differentiates Koplik's spots from Fordyce's spots (ectopic sebaceous glands), which occur in the mouths of healthy individuals. *(Source: Centers for Disease Control and Prevention. Photo selected by Dr. Kenneth Kaye.)*

adults. Patients with impaired cell-mediated immunity are at especially high risk for severe or even fatal measles. The measles-associated mortality rate in the United States is ~0.3%; in developing countries, it frequently exceeds 1% and sometimes approaches 10% because of malnutrition and associated immunodeficiency and HIV infection.

Measles virus is transmitted by respiratory secretions, predominantly through exposure to aerosols but also through direct contact with larger droplets. Patients are contagious from 1 or 2 days before symptom onset until 4 days after the rash appears. Infectivity peaks during the prodromal phase. The mean intervals from infection to symptom onset and rash appearance are 10 and 14 days, respectively.

PATHOGENESIS, IMMUNITY, AND PATHOLOGY

Measles virus invades the respiratory epithelium and spreads via the bloodstream to the reticuloendothelial system, from which it infects

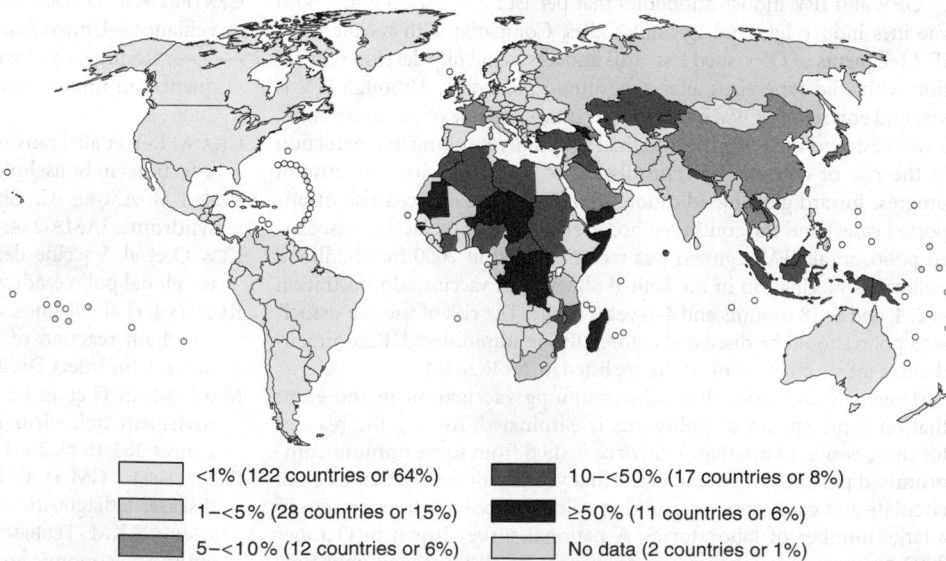

<1% (122 countries or 64%)	10–<50% (17 countries or 8%)
1–<5% (28 countries or 15%)	≥50% (11 countries or 6%)
5–<10% (12 countries or 6%)	No data (2 countries or 1%)

FIGURE 185-2 Worldwide reported measles incidence rate per 100,000 population, 2004. *(Source: WHO/IBV database, 2005. This map does not imply the expression of any opinion whatsoever on the part of the World Health Organization concerning the legal status of any country, territory, city, or area of its authorities or concerning the delimitation of its frontiers or boundaries.)*

white blood cells, thereby establishing infection of the skin, respiratory tract, and other organs. Both viremia and viruria develop. Multinucleated giant cells with inclusion bodies in the nucleus and cytoplasm (Warthin-Finkeldey cells) are found in respiratory and lymphoid tissues and are pathognomonic for measles. Direct invasion of T lymphocytes and increased levels of suppressive cytokines (e.g., interleukin 4) may play a role in the temporary depression of cellular immunity that accompanies and transiently follows measles. The major infected cell in the blood is the monocyte. Infection of the entire respiratory tract accounts for the characteristic cough and coryza of measles and for the less frequent manifestations of croup, bronchiolitis, and pneumonia. Generalized damage to the respiratory tract, with loss of cilia, predisposes to secondary bacterial infections such as pneumonia and otitis media.

Specific antibodies are not detectable before the onset of rash. Cellular immunity (consisting of cytotoxic T cells and possibly natural killer cells) plays a prominent role in host defense, and patients who are deficient in cellular immunity are at high risk for severe measles. Children with isolated agammaglobulinemia are not at increased risk. Immune reactions to the virus in the endothelial cells of dermal capillaries play a substantial role in the development of Koplik's spots (the pathognomonic enanthem) and rash; in immunodeficient hosts, measles may be severe despite the absence of these manifestations. Measles antigens have been demonstrated in involved skin during early stages of the illness.

Pathologic changes in measles encephalitis include focal hemorrhage, congestion, and perivascular demyelination. Measles virus is rarely isolated from cerebrospinal fluid (CSF) in cases of encephalitis, which are thought to be due to the interaction of virus-infected cells with local cellular immune factors.

CLINICAL MANIFESTATIONS

Measles begins with a 2- to 4-day respiratory prodrome of malaise, cough, coryza, conjunctivitis with lacrimation, nasal discharge, and increasing fever [with temperatures as high as 40.6°C (105°F), probably reflecting secondary viremia]. At this stage of the illness, in which the rash has not yet developed, influenza may be suspected. Just before rash onset, Koplik's spots appear as 1- to 2-mm blue-white spots on a bright red background (Fig. 185-1). Without adequate illumination for examination, they may be overlooked. Koplik's spots are typically located on the buccal mucosa, alongside the second molars, and may be extensive; they are not associated with any other infectious disease. The spots wane after the onset of rash and soon disappear. The entire buccal and inner labial mucosa may be inflamed, and the lips may be reddened.

The characteristic erythematous, nonpruritic, maculopapular rash of measles begins at the hairline and behind the ears, spreads down the trunk and limbs to include the palms and soles, and often becomes confluent (Fig. 185-3). At this time, the patient is at the most severe point of the illness. By the fourth day, the rash begins to fade in the order in which it appeared. Brownish discoloration of the skin and desquamation may occur later. Fever usually resolves by the fourth or fifth day after the onset of rash; prolonged fever suggests a complication of measles. Lymphadenopathy, diarrhea, vomiting, and splenomegaly are common features. The chest x-ray may be abnormal, even in uncomplicated measles, because of the propensity of measles virus to invade the respiratory tract. The entire illness, which usually lasts ~10 days, tends to be more severe in adults than in children, with higher fever, more prominent rash, and a higher incidence of complications.

Milder forms of the illness with less intense symptoms and a milder rash, termed *modified measles*, may occur in individuals with preexisting partial immunity induced by active or passive vaccination. These patients include infants <1 year of age who retain some proportion of passively acquired maternal antibodies. On occasion, individuals with a history of immunization may develop modified measles.

COMPLICATIONS

The complications of measles (Table 185-1) can be divided into three groups, according to the site involved: the respiratory tract, the central nervous system (CNS), and the gastrointestinal tract. Respiratory tract

FIGURE 185-3 In measles, discrete erythematous lesions become confluent as the rash spreads downward. *(Reprinted with permission from Fitzpatrick TB et al: Color Atlas & Synopsis of Clinical Dermatology, 4th ed. New York, McGraw-Hill, 2001, p 775.)*

involvement, manifested as laryngitis, croup, or bronchitis, occurs in the majority of cases of uncomplicated measles. In young children, otitis media is the most common complication. Pneumonia is a frequent reason for hospitalization, especially of adults. The pneumonia is of viral origin in the majority of cases, but secondary bacterial infection (most commonly caused by streptococci, pneumococci, or staphylococci) also develops with some frequency. Primary giant-cell (Hecht's) pneumonia is most often documented in immunocompromised and/or malnourished patients.

Encephalographic abnormalities in the absence of symptoms of CNS disease are extremely common in measles. Symptomatic CNS disease may present with fever, headache, drowsiness, coma, and/or seizures. Symptoms usually begin within days after the onset of rash but occasionally appear for the first time several weeks later. About 10% of patients do not survive acute measles encephalitis; a significant percentage of survivors have permanent sequelae (e.g., mental retardation or epilepsy). Most cases appear to result from an immune-mediated response to myelin proteins (postinfectious encephalomyelitis) and not directly from viral infection of the CNS (Chap. 375). Rarely, transverse myelitis follows measles. Immunocompromised patients are at risk for progressive fatal encephalitis 1–6 months after measles; in some cases, even though prior measles has not been recognized, the virus is identified at autopsy. Sub-

TABLE 185-1 COMPLICATIONS OF MEASLES

Complication	Comments
Otitis media	Very common in infants with measles
Pneumonia	May be primary viral pneumonia or bacterial superinfection; frequent reason for hospitalization of adults; measles rash sometimes lacking in immunocompromised patients with measles pneumonia
Croup	Occasionally severe, requiring intubation in infants
Gastroenteritis	Diarrhea can be life threatening in infants
Cervical adenitis	Due to lymphoid hyperplasia as host response to virus; common
Acute encephalitis	May be mild to severe/fatal; occurs in 1 in 1000 cases of measles; cerebral and cerebellar forms; immune-mediated pathogenesis
Subacute sclerosing panencephalitis (SSPE)	In 1 in 100,000 cases of measles, usually when measles occurs in infancy; seen 5–10 years later. In the United States, most children with SSPE were born in another country where measles vaccine is not routinely used.

acute sclerosing panencephalitis (SSPE)—a protracted, chronic, extremely rare form of measles encephalitis—sometimes follows measles and is particularly common among children who have measles before the age of 2 years (Chap. 376). As a result of widespread vaccination, SSPE has virtually disappeared in the United States. Typically, progressive dementia evolves over several months. SSPE is thought to be due to a complex interaction of the host with defective measles virus.

Gastrointestinal complications of measles include gastroenteritis, hepatitis, appendicitis, ileocolitis, and mesenteric adenitis. It is not uncommon to detect high levels of alanine and aspartate aminotransferases in the absence of gastrointestinal signs such as jaundice.

Rare complications include myocarditis, glomerulonephritis, and postinfectious thrombocytopenic purpura. Measles can exacerbate preexisting tuberculosis, presumably through virus-induced depression of cellular immunity. Natural measles and immunization against measles can result in tuberculin skin-test anergy lasting for ~1 month.

ATYPICAL MEASLES

An atypical form of measles has been reported in individuals who received formalin-inactivated measles vaccine (used in the United States in 1963–1967 and in Canada until 1970) and subsequently were exposed to measles virus. After a several-day prodrome of fever, myalgia, and headache, the rash appears (Fig. 185-4); it begins peripherally and can be urticarial, maculopapular, hemorrhagic, and/or vesicular. Fever is high and accompanied by edema of the extremities, interstitial pulmonary infiltrates, hepatitis, and (on occasion) pleural effusion. The differential diagnosis includes Rocky Mountain spotted fever, Henoch-Schönlein purpura, meningococcemia, drug allergy, toxic shock syndrome, and varicella. Despite its severity, the illness is self-limited. Measles virus cannot be isolated from these patients. This disease is believed to be due to hypersensitivity to measles virus induced by the inactivated vaccine. To prevent it, adults who received formalin-inactivated measles vaccine should be immunized with live attenuated measles vaccine. Because inactivated measles vaccine has not been available for >35 years, atypical measles has virtually disappeared.

MEASLES IN THE IMMUNOCOMPROMISED HOST

Patients with defects in cell-mediated immunity are at risk for severe protracted and fatal measles. Included in this category are patients with congenital cellular immune defects or malignancy, recipients of immunosuppressive therapy, or persons infected with HIV. In these patients, measles may not be accompanied by a rash. Complications are primary measles (giant-cell) pneumonia, progressive encephalitis beginning weeks or months after initial infection, and (in HIV-infected patients) progression to AIDS.

FIGURE 185-4 Petechial lesions in a patient with atypical measles. *(Photo courtesy of Stephen E. Gellis, MD; with permission.)*

MEASLES IN ADULTS

Measles is naturally a disease of childhood and, like many other viral infections, is more severe in adults than in children. About 3% of young adults with measles develop primary viral pneumonia and require hospitalization. Hepatitis and bronchospasm are more common among adults with measles than among children, and the rash is more severe and more confluent in adults. Bacterial superinfection is more common among adults, more than one-third of whom develop respiratory complications such as otitis media, sinusitis, and pneumonia. Adults may develop measles because they were never immunized or (more rarely) because their vaccine-induced immunity has waned. Very low titers of antibody to measles virus have been associated with lack of protection.

LABORATORY FINDINGS

Lymphopenia and neutropenia are common in measles and may be due to invasion of leukocytes by the virus, with subsequent cell death. Leukocytosis may herald a bacterial superinfection. Patients with measles encephalitis usually have an elevated protein concentration in CSF as well as lymphocytosis.

DIAGNOSIS

A specific diagnosis of measles can be made quickly by immunofluorescent staining of a smear of respiratory secretions for measles antigen; monoclonal antibodies conjugated to fluorescein are commercially available. Secretions can be examined microscopically for multinucleated giant cells. Measles virus can be demonstrated by culture or polymerase chain reaction in respiratory secretions or urine. A number of serologic tests are available. A serologic diagnosis by enzyme immunoassay (EIA) cannot necessarily be made rapidly if acute- and convalescent-phase serum specimens are examined. However, EIA measurement of specific IgM permits diagnosis on the basis of an acute-phase serum sample. Specific IgM antibodies are detectable within 1–2 days after rash onset, and the IgG titer rises significantly after 10 days. Atypical measles and SSPE are associated with extremely high levels of measles antibodies in blood and/or CSF.

DIFFERENTIAL DIAGNOSIS

Classic measles—with Koplik's spots, cough, coryza, conjunctivitis, and a rash beginning on the head—is easily diagnosed on clinical grounds. Modified measles is more difficult to diagnose because one or more characteristic signs or symptoms may be lacking. The differential diagnosis of measles includes Kawasaki disease, scarlet fever, infectious mononucleosis, toxoplasmosis, drug eruption, and *Mycoplasma pneumoniae* infection. In the differential diagnosis of measles, attention should be paid to the current epidemiology of the disease in the community and to the patient's history of measles vaccination and foreign travel.

PREVENTION

The development of live attenuated measles vaccine by Enders and colleagues was a milestone in American medicine. This vaccine, used in the United States for the routine immunization of children since 1963, induces seroconversion in ~95% of recipients and probably confers lifelong protection. Waning immunity to measles after immunization is rare. For the past three decades, measles vaccine has been available as the combination vaccine measles-mumps-rubella (MMR); this vaccine should be administered to children at 12–15 months of age. (Vaccination at 12 months is preferred for infants whose mothers were immunized against measles in childhood.) A second dose of MMR vaccine is recommended for school-age children. This two-dose policy was developed in the late 1980s in response to measles outbreaks in the United States. MMR vaccine is likely to be supplanted by MMRV vaccine, which also covers varicella and was licensed by the U.S. Food and Drug Administration in 2005. MMRV vaccine is licensed only for children 1–13 years of age.

Older susceptible persons should be immunized. Individuals should be considered susceptible to measles unless they have documentation of physician-diagnosed measles or of the receipt of two doses of vaccine, have laboratory evidence of measles immunity, or were born before 1957. Rarely, individuals born before 1957 develop measles, and those who are at risk of exposure to measles (e.g., health care workers, teachers, and international travelers) should be tested for measles antibody and immunized if necessary. Approximately 10% of healthy vaccinees develop a fever, with temperatures up to 39.4°C (103°F), 5–7 days after vaccination; this fever lasts 1–5 days and is accompanied by a transient rash. Individuals previously immunized only with killed vaccine are considered susceptible and should receive at least one dose—preferably two doses—of MMR vaccine. Transient adverse reactions in these individuals include fever, malaise, and redness and swelling at the injection site.

Because of the severity of measles in this group and the lack of reported problems following vaccination, children with asymptomatic HIV infection should receive MMR vaccine; those with severe immunosuppression (<15% CD4+ T lymphocytes) should not. A case of fatal measles due to vaccine-type virus was reported in a college student with AIDS in 1998. Measles vaccine is contraindicated for persons with impaired cell-mediated immunity, for pregnant women, and for persons with a history of anaphylaxis due to egg protein or neomycin. Minor illnesses, with or without fever and a history of convulsions, are not contraindications to vaccination. Vaccination should be deferred for 6–11 months after the receipt of immune globulin or of blood products containing antibodies and for at least 3 months after the discontinuation of immunosuppressive treatment. Vaccine failures have been ascribed to faulty vaccine storage, the presence of maternally derived antibodies in infants, and simultaneous administration of measles vaccine and immune globulin.

The only temporally related causal complications of measles vaccination are febrile seizures, which rarely have long-term sequelae; self-limited thrombocytopenia; and rare anaphylaxis. An exhaustive analysis conducted in 2000 by a number of official committees, including those of the American Academy of Pediatrics and the Institute of Medicine, found no causal relationship between MMR vaccination and subsequent development of autism.

Children and adults who are susceptible to measles and are exposed to the disease should receive postexposure prophylaxis. Standard immune globulin, given intramuscularly within 6 days of exposure, can exert a protective or modifying effect. The dose is 0.25 mL/kg for healthy persons and 0.5 mL/kg for immunocompromised persons, with a maximum dose of 15 mL. Immune globulin is particularly strongly indicated for susceptible household contacts, especially those <1 year of age, and for immunocompromised persons. HIV-infected individuals, particularly those with severe immunosuppression, should be given immune globulin after exposure, regardless of their measles immune status and whether or not they are receiving intravenous immune globulin. Vaccination within 72 h of exposure may also provide

protection against clinical measles but is contraindicated in immuno-compromised patients. Vaccine and immune globulin should not be given concurrently.

Rx MEASLES

Therapy for measles is largely supportive and symptom based. Patients with otitis media and pneumonia should be given standard antibiotics. Patients with encephalitis need supportive care, including observation for increased intracranial pressure. Controlled trials suggest clinical benefit from high doses of vitamin A in severe or potentially severe measles, especially in children <2 years old who are or may be malnourished. On the basis of limited data, a dose of 50,000 IU is used for infants 1–6 months old; 100,000 IU is recommended for infants 7–12 months old and 200,000 IU for children >1 year old. A single dose is administered on two consecutive days. In the United States, vitamin A treatment is recommended for young children hospitalized for measles and for pediatric measles patients with immunodeficiency, clinical evidence of vitamin A deficiency, impaired intestinal absorption, moderate to severe malnutrition, or recent immigration from an area where there is high mortality from measles. Transient vomiting and headache may be associated with the administration of vitamin A. Ribavirin is effective against measles virus in vitro and may be considered for use in immunocompromised individuals.

FURTHER READINGS

CENTERS FOR DISEASE CONTROL AND PREVENTION: Measles, mumps, and rubella—vaccine use and strategies for elimination of measles, rubella, and congenital rubella syndrome and control of mumps. MMWR Morb Mortal Wkly Rep 47:1, 1998

———: Measles—United States, 2004. MMWR Morb Mortal Wkly Rep 54:1229, 2005

D'SOUZA RM, D'SOUZA R: Vitamin A for preventing secondary infections in children with measles—a systematic review. J Trop Pediatr 48:72, 2002

FORNI AL et al: Severe measles pneumonitis in adults: Evaluation of clinical characteristics and therapy with intravenous ribavirin. Clin Infect Dis 19:454, 1994

IMMUNIZATION SAFETY REVIEW COMMITTEE, INSTITUTE OF MEDICINE: Immunization Safety Review: Measles-Mumps-Rubella Vaccine and Autism, K Stratton et al (eds). Washington, DC, National Academy of Sciences, 2001 (www.nap.edu/catalog/10101.html)

KAPLAN LJ et al: Severe measles in immunocompromised patients. JAMA 267:1237, 1992

STALKUP JR: A review of measles virus. Dermatol Clin 20:209, 2002

YEUNG LF et al: A limited measles outbreak in a highly vaccinated US boarding school. Pediatrics 116:1287, 2005

186 Rubella (German Measles)
Anne Gershon

DEFINITION

Rubella is an acute viral infection of children and adults that characteristically includes rash, fever, and lymphadenopathy and has a broad spectrum of other possible manifestations. However, a high percentage of rubella infections in both children and adults are subclinical. In addition, the illness can resemble a mild attack of measles (rubeola) and can cause arthritis, especially in adults. Rubella was formerly known as *German measles* because it was first distinguished clinically from rubeola in Germany, where it generated much medical interest in the mid-eighteenth and early nineteenth centuries. Rubella during pregnancy can lead to fetal infection, with the production of a significant

constellation of malformations (*congenital rubella syndrome*) in a high proportion of infected fetuses. Rubella virus was first isolated in cell culture just before the last pandemic of the disease began in 1962. Since the licensing of rubella vaccine in the United States in 1969, there have been no further epidemics in this country.

ETIOLOGIC AGENT

Rubella virus, a togavirus, is the only member of the *Rubivirus* genus and is closely related to the alphaviruses. Unlike these agents, however, it does not require a vector for transmission. Moreover, there is no RNA sequence homology between rubella virus and the alphaviruses.

The rubella virion is composed of an inner icosahedral capsid of RNA and protein that is surrounded by a lipid-containing envelope with glycoprotein spikes and a diameter of ~60 nm. The structural proteins associated with rubella virus are E1 and E2 (transmembrane envelope glycoproteins) and C (the capsid protein that surrounds the viral RNA). Only one serotype has been identified.

EPIDEMIOLOGY

In the United States during the prevaccine era, rubella was most common in the spring and most often affected school-age children; only 80–90% of adults were immune; and major epidemics occurred every 6–9 years. The most recent epidemic in the United States occurred in 1964–1965, when more than 12 million cases of postnatal rubella and more than 20,000 cases of the congenital rubella syndrome were reported. Although there have been no epidemics since the introduction of live attenuated rubella vaccine in 1969, limited outbreaks have been reported in settings where susceptible individuals come into close contact with one another (e.g., schools and workplaces). Since 2001, the annual incidences of rubella have been the lowest ever recorded in the United States. In 2001–2004, an average of only 14 cases of postnatally acquired rubella were reported annually to the Centers for Disease Control and Prevention (CDC). During these 4 years, only 4 confirmed cases of congenital rubella syndrome were reported. Three of the affected infants were born to women who had immigrated to the United States. Currently, 91% of U.S. residents are estimated to be immune to rubella, and at least 95% of schoolchildren have been immunized. When rubella is reported in the United States, the genotype of the virus is consistent with an imported agent.

 Although rubella is no longer considered endemic in the United States, global challenges remain. According to the World Health Organization, 57% of countries included rubella vaccine in their national programs in 2003, but rubella continues to be endemic in many areas of the world.

Whether symptomatic or subclinical, rubella is contagious, albeit less so than measles. Its incubation period is 18 days on average, with a range of 12–23 days. The virus, which is spread in droplets shed in respiratory secretions, infects the respiratory tract and then the bloodstream. In postnatally acquired infections, rubella virus is shed during the prodromal phase of the illness, and shedding from the pharynx can continue for ~1 week after onset. Despite high titers of specific neutralizing antibodies, infants with congenital rubella may excrete rubella virus from the respiratory tract and in the urine until the age of 2 years. This excretion raises important issues related to infection control in hospital and day-care settings. Persons recently immunized with live attenuated rubella vaccine do not transmit the vaccine virus to others, although low titers of rubella virus may be detected transiently in the pharynx.

After an attack of rubella, specific antibodies and cell-mediated immunity develop and probably play a significant role in protection against future disease. Asymptomatic reinfection at the level of the respiratory tract is common upon re-exposure to the virus but is rarely, if ever, associated with viremia.

Rubella virus has been cultured from respiratory secretions during reinfection. Fetal infection may occur during maternal reinfection but is acknowledged to be extremely rare because of the absence of maternal viremia under these circumstances. Viremia following reinfection of individuals immunized against rubella also is rare.

Although the current level of congenital rubella in the United States is exceedingly low, it has been observed that young immigrants to the United States from countries in Latin America and the Caribbean, where rubella vaccine is not routinely given to children, are at increased risk for rubella susceptibility. Because infants with the congenital rubella syndrome have been born to immigrant Hispanic women, increasing efforts have been made to identify and vaccinate such women before they become pregnant.

PATHOGENESIS AND PATHOLOGY

Little is known about the microscopic pathology of postnatally acquired rubella because the disease is invariably self-limited. Like that of measles, the rash of rubella is immunologically mediated; its onset coincides with the development of specific antibodies. Viremia can be demonstrated for ~1 week before and ends within a few days after the onset of rash.

The cause of the damage to cells and organs in congenital rubella is not well understood. Proposed mechanisms of fetal damage include mitotic arrest of cells, tissue necrosis without inflammation, and chromo-

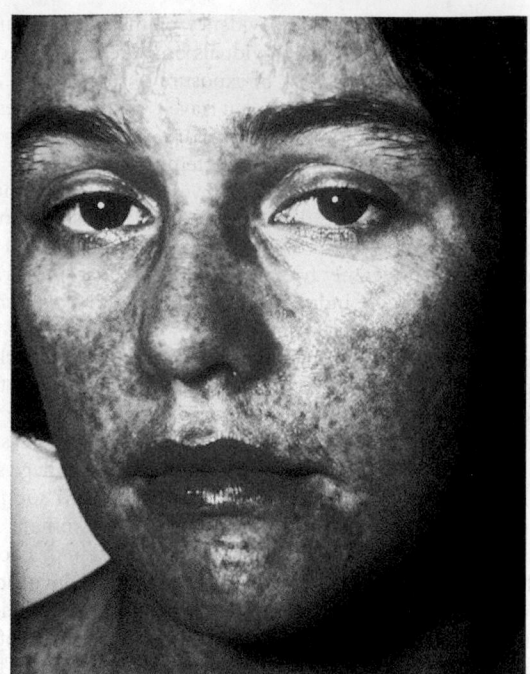

FIGURE 186-1 In rubella, an erythematous exanthem spreads from the hairline downward and clears as it spreads. *(Photo courtesy of Stephen E. Gellis, MD; with permission.)*

somal damage. The growth of the fetus may be retarded. Other findings may include decreased numbers of megakaryocytes in the bone marrow, extramedullary hematopoiesis, and interstitial pneumonia.

CLINICAL MANIFESTATIONS

Postnatally Acquired Rubella   Infection acquired after birth usually results in an extremely mild or subclinical illness. A prodromal phase is uncommon in children; adults may have more severe disease, with a brief prodrome of malaise, fever, and anorexia. The foremost symptoms of postnatally acquired rubella include posterior auricular, cervical, and suboccipital lymphadenopathy; fever; and rash. The rash often begins on the face (Fig. 186-1) and spreads down the body. It is maculopapular but not confluent, is sometimes accompanied by mild coryza and conjunctivitis, and generally lasts for 3–5 days. A petechial enanthem on the soft palate, designated *Forschheimer spots*, may occur but is not specific for rubella. Fever may be absent entirely or may be present for only several days in the early phase of the illness.

Complications of postnatally acquired rubella are uncommon; bacterial superinfection is rare. One particularly troublesome complication is seen almost exclusively in women: arthritis, most frequently involving the fingers, wrists, and/or knees. Arthritis develops as the rash is appearing and may take several weeks to resolve. Chronic arthritis resulting from rubella is extremely rare. Rubella virus has been isolated from joint fluid during acute rubella arthritis and from peripheral blood in chronic rubella arthritis.

Another complication of postnatally acquired rubella is hemorrhage due to both thrombocytopenia and vascular damage; this complication occurs in 1 of every 3000 patients. Thrombocytopenia may last for weeks or months; it can have long-term consequences if there is bleeding into organs such as the eye or the brain.

Both children and adults may develop encephalitis after rubella; the incidence is about five times lower than that of encephalitis following measles. Adults are more likely than children to develop encephalitis; the mortality rate from this complication is 20–50%. Mild hepatitis is an unusual complication. Immunosuppressed patients are not at increased risk for rubella as they are for measles.

Congenital Rubella   Maternal infection in early pregnancy can lead to fetal infection, with resultant congenital rubella. The classic signs of

TABLE 186-1	CLINICAL PROBLEMS ASSOCIATED WITH THE CONGENITAL RUBELLA SYNDROME	
Transient Signs/Symptoms (at Birth Only)	**Permanent Signs/Symptoms (Developmental)**
Bony abnormalities	Autism
Cloudy cornea	Behavioral disorders
Hemolytic anemia	Congenital heart disease (patent ductus
Hepatitis	arteriosus, pulmonic stenosis)
Hepatosplenomegaly	Cryptorchidism
Jaundice	Deafness
Low birth weight	Degenerative brain disease
Lymphadenopathy	Diabetes mellitus
Meningoencephalitis	Glaucoma
Rubella viral pneumonia	Inguinal hernia
Thrombocytopenic purpura	Mental retardation
	Microcephaly
	Myopia
	Precocious puberty
	Retinopathy
	Seizures
	Spastic diplegia
	Thyroid disorders

congenital rubella are cataract, heart disease, deafness, and myriad other defects (Table 186-1). The most important factor in the pathogenicity of rubella virus for the fetus is gestational age at the time of infection. Maternal infection during the first trimester leads to fetal infection in ~50% of cases; maternal infection early in the second trimester leads to fetal infection in about one-third of cases. Fetal malformations not only are more common after maternal infection in the first trimester but also tend to be more severe and to involve more organ systems. Whereas a fetus infected in the fourth week of gestation may develop many problems, one infected later (e.g., in the twentieth week) may have isolated deafness as the only symptom.

DIAGNOSIS

Because postnatally acquired rubella is often a mild disease and because many cases are subclinical, diagnosis on clinical grounds can be difficult. Other diseases that may mimic rubella include toxoplasmosis, scarlet fever, modified measles, roseola, fifth disease (erythema infectiosum due to parvovirus B19), and enteroviral infection. Routine laboratory tests usually reveal leukopenia and atypical lymphocytes.

The isolation of rubella virus in cell cultures of throat samples, urine, or other secretions is difficult and expensive but is sometimes undertaken. Polymerase chain reaction (PCR) is also useful for diagnosis. These techniques are particularly useful when congenital rubella is suspected. A laboratory diagnosis may also be made serologically. The most commonly used test is an enzyme-linked immunosorbent assay (ELISA) for IgG and IgM antibodies. Acute rubella is diagnosed by the documentation of a fourfold or greater rise in the titer of IgG antibodies in paired acute- and convalescent-phase serum specimens or by the detection of rubella-specific IgM antibodies in one serum specimen. However, false-negative and false-positive IgM reactions are sometimes obtained. Moreover, true-positive IgM reactions can occur in both primary infection and reinfection. Congenital rubella is diagnosed by the isolation of rubella virus, a positive PCR assay, the detection of IgM antibodies in a single serum sample, and/or the documentation of either the persistence of rubella antibodies in serum beyond 1 year of age or a rising antibody titer anytime during infancy in an unvaccinated child. Biopsied tissues and/or blood and cerebrospinal fluid have also been used for the demonstration of rubella antigens with monoclonal antibodies and for the detection of rubella RNA by in situ hybridization and PCR.

Cases of suspected postnatal or congenital rubella should be reported to the CDC.

PREVENTION

Live attenuated rubella vaccine was licensed in 1969, 7 years after rubella virus was first isolated in culture. This vaccine was developed as a strategy to prevent congenital rubella by ensuring that very few pregnant women would be susceptible and that there would be little circulating wild-type virus. Rubella vaccine induces seroconversion in >95% of recipients. Since its licensure, there have been no major epidemics in the United States, and the number of cases has declined by 98%. The vaccine currently licensed in the United States, RA 27/3, is propagated in human diploid cells and is more immunogenic (particularly with regard to the stimulation of secretory immunity) than previously licensed vaccines. The present vaccination strategy, developed in part when measles was not being adequately controlled, is to immunize all infants at 12–15 months of age with measles-mumps-rubella (MMR) vaccine and to administer a second dose in early childhood. Rubella vaccine may also be administered to anyone who is thought to be susceptible to the infection and is not pregnant; it is particularly important that hospital workers of either sex be immune to rubella so that nosocomial transmission is avoided. Although there has been little change in the prevalence of immunity to rubella among women of childbearing age (~80%), the incidence of congenital rubella is extremely low, with fewer than 10 cases annually. It is likely that, although antibody may be undetectable years after immunization, protection against infection—possibly due to cell-mediated immunity—is the rule. At present, there is little if any evidence of significant waning of clinically important immunity to rubella with time.

On occasion, rubella vaccine may cause arthralgia or arthritis, especially in young women. Very rarely, rubella vaccination results in chronic arthritis; however, even cases of frank arthritis in vaccinees are generally self-limited, lasting only ~1 week.

After investigation of a series of more than 400 women who were inadvertently immunized during pregnancy and who carried their infants to term, the CDC has concluded that vaccine-type rubella virus either does not cause the congenital rubella syndrome at all or does so at an incidence too low to be detected. Nonetheless, rubella vaccine is contraindicated for use in pregnant women, and it is recommended that pregnancy be avoided for at least 3 months after rubella vaccination. It is acceptable for rubella-susceptible children whose mothers also are susceptible to be immunized, as vaccine recipients do not shed rubella virus or transmit it to susceptible individuals. Although it is recommended that rubella vaccine not be given to immunosuppressed persons, the vaccine is given to children infected with HIV. No adverse effects of rubella vaccine have been reported in immunocompromised patients.

℞ RUBELLA

There is no specific therapy for rubella. At one time, immune globulin was used in an effort to prevent congenital rubella when pregnant women became infected. However, because administration of immune globulin did not prevent maternal viremia, this approach was discarded. Symptom-based treatment is given for manifestations such as fever, arthralgia, and arthritis.

FURTHER READINGS

ANDRADE JQ et al: Rubella in pregnancy: Intrauterine transmission and perinatal outcome during a Brazilian epidemic. J Clin Virol 35:285, 2005

BANATVALA JE, BROWN DWG: Rubella. Lancet 363:1127, 2004

CENTERS FOR DISEASE CONTROL AND PREVENTION: Measles, mumps, and rubella—vaccine use and strategies for elimination of measles, rubella, and congenital rubella syndrome and control of mumps. MMWR Morb Mortal Wkly Rep 47:1, 1998

———: Control and prevention of rubella: Evaluation and management of suspected outbreaks, rubella in pregnant women, and surveillance for congenital rubella syndrome. MMWR Morb Mortal Wkly Rep 50:1, 2001

———: Elimination of rubella and congenital rubella syndrome—United States, 1969–2004. MMWR Morb Mortal Wkly Rep 54:279, 2005

———: Imported case of congenital rubella syndrome—New Hampshire, 2005. MMWR Morb Mortal Wkly Rep 54:1160, 2005

DANAVARO-HOLLIDAY MC et al: A large rubella outbreak with spread from the workplace to the community. JAMA 284:2733, 2000

PLOTKIN SA, REEF S: Rubella vaccine, in *Vaccines*, SA Plotkin and WA Orenstein (eds). Philadelphia, Saunders, 2004, pp 389–440

REEF SE et al: The changing epidemiology of rubella in the 1990s: On the verge of elimination and new challenges for control and prevention. JAMA 287:464, 2002

SHERIDAN E: Congenital rubella syndrome: A risk in immigrant populations. Lancet 359:674, 2002

187 Mumps
Anne Gershon

DEFINITION

Mumps is an acute, systemic, communicable viral infection whose most distinctive feature is swelling of one or both parotid glands. Involvement of other salivary glands, the meninges, the pancreas, and the gonads also is common.

ETIOLOGIC AGENT

Mumps virus, a paramyxovirus, is pleomorphic and has a diameter ranging from 100 to 300 nm. The virion is composed of RNA and seven proteins. The RNA is surrounded by an envelope composed of glycoproteins, including a hemagglutinin-neuraminidase (HN), a hemolysis cell fusion antigen (F), and a matrix envelope protein (M). A fourth protein (SH) may also be membrane-associated. There are three internal components: a nucleocapsid protein (NP), a phosphoprotein (P), and a large protein (L). There is only one antigenic type of mumps virus. Polymerase chain reaction (PCR) has detected geographic differences among mumps viruses from different locales.

EPIDEMIOLOGY

After the introduction of mumps vaccine in 1967, the incidence of clinical mumps declined significantly in the United States. In 1968 (before widespread immunization), 185,691 cases of mumps were reported in this country. The 231–277 cases reported annually in 2001–2005 represent a >99% reduction from prevaccine levels. Before widespread vaccination, the incidence of mumps was highest in the winter and spring, with epidemics every 2–5 years. At that time, mumps was principally a disease of childhood, although today >50% of cases occur in young adults. Epidemics tended to occur in confined populations (e.g., in schools and the military services).

The incubation period of mumps generally ranges from 14 to 18 days, with extremes of 7 and 23 days. However, because a contact may be shedding virus before the onset of clinical disease or (like one-third of patients) may have subclinical infection, the incubation period in individual cases is often uncertain. One attack of mumps usually confers lifelong immunity. Long-term immunity is also associated with immunization.

PATHOGENESIS

Mumps virus is transmitted by droplet nuclei, saliva, and fomites. Replication of the virus in the epithelium of the upper respiratory tract leads to viremia, which is followed by infection of glandular tissues and/or the central nervous system (CNS).

Little is known of the pathology of mumps since the disease is rarely fatal. The affected glands contain perivascular and interstitial mononuclear cell infiltrates with prominent edema. Necrosis of acinar and epithelial duct cells is evident in the salivary glands and in the germinal epithelium of the seminiferous tubules.

CLINICAL MANIFESTATIONS

The prodrome of mumps consists of fever, malaise, myalgia, and anorexia. Parotitis, if it develops, usually does so within the next 24 h but may be delayed for as long as a week; it is generally bilateral, although the onset on the two sides may not be synchronous and at times only one side is affected. The submaxillary and sublingual glands are in-volved less often than the parotid and are almost never involved alone. Swelling of the parotid is accompanied by tenderness and obliteration of the space between the ear lobe and the angle of the mandible (Fig. 187-1). The patient frequently reports an earache and finds it difficult to eat, swallow, or talk. Glandular swelling increases for a few days and then gradually subsides, disappearing within a week. The orifice of Stensen's duct is commonly red and swollen. Presternal pitting edema has been described in ~5% of mumps cases, often in association with submandibular adenitis.

Other than parotitis, orchitis is the most common manifestation of mumps among postpubertal males, developing in ~20% of cases. The testis is painful, tender, and enlarged to several times its normal size; accompanying fever is common. Later, testicular atrophy develops in half of the affected men. Since orchitis is bilateral in <15% of cases, sterility after mumps is rare. Oophoritis in women—far less common than orchitis in men—may cause lower abdominal pain but does not lead to sterility.

Aseptic meningitis, which may develop before, during, after, or in the absence of parotitis, is common in both children and adults. Symptoms include stiff neck, headache, and drowsiness. Pleocytosis of the cerebrospinal fluid (CSF), with up to 1000 cells/µL, may develop in up to 50% of cases of clinical mumps, but clinical signs of meningeal irritation are documented in only 5–25% of cases. Within the first 24 h, polymorphonuclear leukocytes may predominate in CSF, but by the second day nearly all the cells are lymphocytes. The glucose level in CSF may be abnormally low, and this finding may arouse suspicion of bacterial meningitis. Aseptic meningitis due to mumps without parotitis is indistinguishable clinically from that caused by other viruses. Mumps meningitis is almost invariably self-limited, although cranial nerve palsies have occasionally led to permanent sequelae, particularly deafness. More rarely, mumps virus may cause encephalitis, which presents as high fever with marked changes in the level of consciousness and frequently results in permanent sequelae in survivors. Other CNS problems occasionally associated with mumps include cerebellar ataxia, facial palsy, transverse myelitis, Guillain-Barré syndrome, and aqueductal stenosis leading to hydrocephalus.

Mumps pancreatitis, which may present as abdominal pain, is difficult to diagnose because an elevated serum amylase level can be associated with either parotitis or pancreatitis. Other unusual complications of mumps include myocarditis, mastitis, thyroiditis, nephritis, arthritis, and thrombocytopenic purpura. An excessive number of sponta-

FIGURE 187-1 Schematic drawing of parotid gland infected with mumps virus (*right*) compared with normal gland (*left*). An enlarged cervical lymph node is usually posterior to the imaginary line. (*Reprinted with permission from Gershon A et al: Mumps, in Krugman's Infectious Diseases of Children, 11th ed. Philadelphia, Elsevier, 2004, p 392.*)

TABLE 187-1 DIFFERENTIAL DIAGNOSIS OF PAROTITIS

Etiology	Comments
Systemic Infections	
Mumps	Rare in countries with vaccination programs
Coxsackievirus infection	Particularly likely in children
HIV infection	In HIV-positive children receiving no antiretroviral therapy; additional disease manifestations likely
Parainfluenza virus type 3 infection	Particularly likely in children; associated with acute respiratory tract symptoms
Influenza A virus infection	Seasonal (winter, spring); associated with acute respiratory tract symptoms
Cat-scratch disease	Unusual but described
Epstein-Barr virus infection	Unusual but described
Systemic Noninfectious Causes	
Sarcoidosis	Additional manifestations of disease likely
Sjögren's syndrome	Additional manifestations of disease likely
Uremia	Additional manifestations of disease likely
Diabetes mellitus	Additional manifestations of disease likely
Drugs	Phenylbutazone, thiouracil
Unilateral Parotitis	
Ductal obstruction due to stones or strictures	Unilateral, gradual onset, suppurative
Parotid cyst	Unilateral, gradual onset
Parotid tumor	Unilateral, gradual onset
Acute Suppurative Parotitis	
Staphylococcus aureus, *Streptococcus* species, and (rarely) gram-negative bacteria, anaerobes	

neous abortions are associated with gestational mumps when the disease occurs during the first trimester. Mumps in pregnancy does not lead to premature birth or fetal malformations.

DIFFERENTIAL DIAGNOSIS

Because of widespread vaccination, mumps is currently a rare disease in the United States. The diagnosis is made easily in patients with acute bilateral parotitis and a history of recent exposure. When parotitis is unilateral or absent or when sites other than the parotid gland are involved, laboratory diagnosis may be required.

The differential diagnosis of parotitis is presented in Table 187-1. Other entities should be considered when manifestations consistent with mumps appear in organs other than the parotid. Testicular torsion may produce a painful scrotal mass resembling that seen in mumps orchitis. Other viruses (e.g., enteroviruses) may cause aseptic meningitis that is clinically indistinguishable from that due to mumps virus.

Myocarditis as a severe but usually self-limited complication of mumps has been described. Molecular diagnostic assays have implicated mumps virus in some cases of endocardial fibroelastosis following myocarditis.

LABORATORY DIAGNOSIS

Mumps virus is readily isolated after inoculation of appropriate clinical specimens into cell cultures. The virus can be identified rapidly in shell vial cultures by immunofluorescence. Mumps virus may be recovered from saliva, throat, and urine during the first few days of illness and from the CSF of patients with mumps meningitis. Shedding of virus in the urine may persist for as long as 2 weeks. PCR also is used to detect mumps virus in clinical specimens. No particular peripheral blood cell count is characteristic of mumps.

Highly sensitive enzyme-linked immunosorbent assays are useful for serologic diagnosis of mumps and for determination of susceptibility to the disease. Acute mumps can be diagnosed either by the examination of acute- and convalescent-phase sera for a significant increase in IgG antibody levels or by the demonstration of specific IgM in one serum specimen. The mumps skin test is no longer used.

PREVENTION

Live attenuated mumps vaccine (Jeryl Lynn strain) induces antibodies that protect the recipient against infection in >95% of cases. Mumps vaccine is usually administered as part of the measles-mumps-rubella (MMR) vaccine at the age of 12–15 months and again at 4–12 years of age. MMR vaccine will probably be supplanted by MMRV vaccine, which also covers varicella. Licensed by the U.S. Food and Drug Administration in 2005, MMRV is licensed for use only in children 1–13 years of age. Vaccination is also recommended for susceptible older children, adolescents, and adults, particularly male adolescents who have not had mumps. For these patients, either MMR or monovalent mumps vaccine may be given; two doses are preferred. Inadvertent immunization of individuals who are already immune is not associated with significant adverse reactions. Mumps vaccine is not recommended for pregnant women, for patients receiving glucocorticoids, or for other immunocompromised hosts. However, children with HIV infection who are not severely immunocompromised can safely be immunized against mumps; MMR vaccine is usually used for this purpose (Chap. 116). Occasionally, febrile reactions and parotitis have been reported soon after mumps vaccination. Allergic reactions after vaccination, such as rash and pruritus, occur uncommonly and are usually mild and self-limited. In the United States, the incidence of encephalitis during the month after mumps vaccination is no greater than the background incidence rate of encephalitis in the population.

℞ MUMPS

Therapy for parotitis and other manifestations of mumps is symptom-based. The administration of analgesics and the application of warm or cold compresses to the parotid area may be helpful. Mumps immune globulin is of no value. Testicular pain may be minimized by the local application of cold compresses and gentle support for the scrotum. Anesthetic blocks also may be used. Neither the administration of glucocorticoids nor incision of the tunica albuginea is of proven value for the treatment of severe orchitis. Anecdotal information on a small number of patients with orchitis suggests that administration of interferon α may be helpful.

FURTHER READINGS

BRISS PA et al: Sustained transmission of mumps in a highly vaccinated population: Assessment of primary vaccine failure and waning vaccine-induced immunity. J Infect Dis 169:77, 1994

CENTERS FOR DISEASE CONTROL AND PREVENTION: Mumps epidemic—United Kingdom, 2004–2005. MMWR Morb Mortal Wkly Rep 55:173, 2006

———: Mumps outbreak at a summer camp—New York, 2005. MMWR Morb Mortal Wkly Rep 55:175, 2006

———: Update: Multistate outbreak of mumps—United States, January 1–May 2, 2006. MMWR Morb Mortal Wkly Rep 55:559, 2006

———: Measles, mumps, and rubella—vaccine use and strategies for elimination of measles, rubella, and congenital rubella syndrome and control of mumps. MMWR Morb Mortal Wkly Rep 47:1, 1998

CHAUDARY S et al: Fulminant mumps myocarditis. Ann Intern Med 110:569, 1989

DAVIDKIN I et al: Etiology of mumps-like illnesses in children and adolescents vaccinated for measles, mumps, and rubella. J Infect Dis 191:719, 2005

GUT JP et al: Symptomatic mumps reinfections. J Med Virol 45:17, 1995

MCDONALD JC et al: Clinical and epidemiologic features of mumps encephalitis and possible causes of vaccine-related disease. Pediatr Infect Dis J 8:751, 1989

UCHIDA K et al: Rapid and sensitive detection of mumps virus RNA directly from clinical samples by real-time PCR. J Med Virol 75:470, 2005

188 Rabies and Other Rhabdovirus Infections

Alan C. Jackson, Eric C. Johannsen

RABIES

Rabies is an acute viral disease of the central nervous system (CNS) that is transmitted to humans by infected animals. After a prodromal phase, rabies manifests most often as encephalitis—or less frequently as a paralytic form of the disease—and then progresses to coma and death.

ETIOLOGIC AGENT

Rabies virus is a member of the genus *Lyssavirus* in the family Rhabdoviridae, which includes vesicular stomatitis virus (VSV), a bovine pathogen of significant economic importance that can infect humans (see "Other Rhabdoviruses," below). *Rhabdos*, meaning "rodlike," refers to the distinctive elongated shape of these viruses. Their enveloped virions contain a single-strand, nonsegmented, negative-sense RNA. The rabies virus genome consists of 11,932 nucleotides and encodes five proteins: nucleocapsid, matrix, phosphoprotein, glycoprotein, and an RNA polymerase. Each animal reservoir harbors one or more distinct rabies virus variants that can be distinguished by the sequence of the nucleocapsid gene.

EPIDEMIOLOGY

Rabies is a zoonosis that is generally transmitted to humans by the bite of a rabid animal. Understanding the epizootiology of rabies is essential in evaluating the need for rabies postexposure prophylaxis (PEP; see "Prevention," below). Rabies virus can infect most mammals and is worldwide in distribution.

Historically, dogs were the primary reservoir and vector for rabies, and they remain the major source of transmission to humans in Asia and Africa (see "Global Considerations," below). Coordinated vaccination and surveillance programs have essentially eliminated the rabies reservoir in dogs in North America and Europe and have uncovered previously unsuspected reservoirs in wildlife species. Surveillance data from 2006 identified 6940 confirmed animal cases of rabies in the United States. Only 8% of these cases were in domestic animals, including 318 cases in cats, 82 in cattle, and 79 in dogs. Essentially all infections of domestic animals were the result of "spillover" from wildlife reservoirs, not of transmission from one domestic animal to another. In North America, bats, raccoons, skunks, and foxes have endemic rabies virus infection. The importance of each reservoir varies geographically: rabies in raccoons is endemic on the east coast; rabies in skunks occurs predominantly in the Midwest, with another focus in California; and rabies in foxes is found in parts of Texas, Arizona, and Alaska. Rabies in bats is not geographically restricted.

Because each species harbors one or more specific rabies virus variants (or strains), it is possible to trace the source of a human infection even when there is no known exposure. Since 1990, bats have accounted for most cases of human rabies in the United States, with the majority of the remaining cases due to dog exposures occurring in other countries. The majority of human rabies cases acquired from bats have been associated with a single variant (Ln/Ps) harbored by silver-haired and eastern pipistrelle bats. The implication is that the Ln/Ps variant may have particular attributes that render it capable of readily establishing human infections—e.g., an affinity for specific cell receptors or more efficient initial replication in nonneuronal tissues. A contributing factor may be that rabies virus can be transmitted by minor, seemingly unimportant or unrecognized bat bites. In contrast, bites of terrestrial mammals are more likely to receive medical attention. Fatal cases of rabies have resulted when the significance of a known bat exposure was not appreciated. In circumstances where a bat bite or bat salivary contact with broken skin or mucous membranes cannot be excluded (e.g., when a bat is found in a room with an infant or a sleeping adult), the bat should be tested for rabies and expert consultation sought.

Nonbite exposures only rarely transmit rabies virus infection. Exposures to aerosols in the laboratory or in caves containing millions of bats have resulted in human rabies. Transplanted corneal tissue has been the source of eight cases of human rabies, and strict guidelines for donor screening have been adopted in an effort to eliminate this risk. In 2004, three deaths resulted from transplantation of solid organs and another death from transplantation of a vascular conduit from a donor who was initially thought to have died from an intracranial hemorrhage but was retrospectively diagnosed with rabies. Although all organ donors are screened and tested for infectious risks, routine testing of donors for rabies in the absence of epidemiologic risk has not been recommended. There are no known instances in which health care workers have acquired rabies from infected patients. However, standard universal and respiratory precautions should be observed by care givers because contact of the patients' saliva or neuronal tissue with mucous membranes or nonintact skin could result in transmission.

PATHOGENESIS

The incubation period of rabies (defined as the interval between virus exposure and onset of clinical disease) is usually 1–3 months but in rare cases is as short as 2 weeks or >1 year. During most of the incubation period, rabies virus is thought to be present at or close to the site of inoculation (Fig. 188-1), predominantly in muscle cells. Administration of rabies PEP during this incubation period is critical; the benefit of PEP in preventing disease progression once rabies virus has entered peripheral nerves is limited. Several receptors probably account for the ability of rabies virus to infect both sensory and motor neurons. The virus is known to bind to nicotinic acetylcholine receptors, and acetylcholine receptor blockade inhibits rabies virus attachment. Experimental evidence also supports a role for the neural cell adhesion molecule and the p75^{NTR} neurotrophin receptor as receptors for rabies virus. After entering sensory and motor neurons, rabies virus spreads centripetally at a rate of 100–400 mm/d via fast axonal transport to the spinal cord or brainstem. Once the virus enters the CNS, it spreads rapidly throughout the gray matter via established neuroanatomic connections. There are inflammatory changes, but there are few degenerative changes involving neurons and little evidence of neuronal death. These observations have led to the concept that neuronal dysfunction—rather than neuronal death—is responsible for clinical disease in rabies. The basis for the behavioral changes, including aggression, is not well understood. After CNS infection is established, there is centrifugal spread along peripheral nerves to other tissues, including the salivary glands, liver, muscle, skin, adrenal glands, and heart. Rabies virus replication in acinar cells of the salivary glands results in viral excretion in the saliva of rabid animals.

Pathology studies show mild inflammatory changes in the CNS in rabies, with mononuclear inflammatory infiltration in the leptomeninges, perivascular regions, and parenchyma, including microglial nodules called *Babes nodules*. Degenerative neuronal changes are usually not prominent, and neuronophagia is observed occasionally. The most characteristic pathologic finding in rabies is the *Negri body* (Fig. 188-2). Negri bodies are eosinophilic cytoplasmic inclusions in brain neurons and are composed of randomly oriented rabies virus nucleocapsids embedded in an amorphous substance or matrix. These inclusions occur in a minority of infected cells, are most commonly present in Purkinje cells of the cerebellum and in pyramidal cells in the hippocampus, and are less frequently seen in cortical neurons and in the brainstem. For obscure reasons, Negri bodies are rarely produced in infections caused by laboratory variants of rabies virus, whereas wild, or "street," rabies infection results in Negri bodies in ~80% of cases. Thus, the absence of Negri bodies does not exclude the diagnosis.

CLINICAL MANIFESTATIONS

Rabies has the highest case-fatality rate of any infectious disease. Although the diagnosis of rabies should be considered in any case of unexplained encephalitis or flaccid paralysis accompanied by fever, efforts to prevent the disease are appropriately focused on early identification of draft of air (aerophobia). These symptoms are probably due to dysfunction of infected brainstem neurons that normally inhibit inspiratory neurons near the nucleus ambiguus, resulting in exaggerated defense reflexes that protect the respiratory tract. The combination of hypersalivation and pharyngeal dysfunction is also responsible for the classic appearance of "foaming at the mouth" (Fig. 188-3). Brainstem dysfunction progresses rapidly, and coma followed within days by death is the rule unless the course is prolonged by supportive measures. With such measures, late complications can include disturbances of water balance (syndrome of inappropriate antidiuretic hormone secretion or diabetes insipidus), noncardiogenic pulmonary edema, and cardiac arrhythmias due to brainstem dysfunction and/or myocarditis.

Paralytic Rabies For unknown reasons, muscle weakness predominates and cardinal features of encephalitic rabies (hydrophobia, aerophobia, fluctuating consciousness) are lacking in ~20% of rabies cases. Paralytic rabies is characterized by early and prominent muscle weakness, often beginning in the bitten extremity and spreading to produce quadriparesis and facial weakness. Sphincter involvement is common, but sensory involvement is usually mild. Guillain-Barré syndrome is a common misdiagnosis. Transplantation of corneal tissue from donors in whom paralytic rabies was misdiagnosed as Guillain-Barré syndrome has resulted in clinical rabies and death in recipients. Patients with paralytic rabies generally survive a few days longer than is typical in encephalitic rabies, but multiple-organ failure ensues even with aggressive supportive care.

LABORATORY INVESTIGATIONS

During the early clinical stages of rabies, laboratory findings are nonspecific. Complete blood counts are usually normal. Examination of cerebrospinal fluid (CSF) often reveals mild mononuclear cell pleocytosis with a mildly elevated protein level. Severe pleocytosis (>1000 cells/μL) is unusual and should prompt a search for an alternative diagnosis. CT head scans are usually normal in rabies. MRI brain scans sometimes show signal abnormalities in the brainstem or other areas, but these findings are variable and nonspecific. Electroencephalograms show only nonspecific abnormalities. The most important tests in suspected cases of rabies are those that may identify an alternative, potentially treatable diagnosis (see "Differential Diagnosis," below).

DIAGNOSIS

In North America, a diagnosis of rabies often is not considered until relatively late in the clinical course, even with a typical clinical presentation. This diagnosis should be considered in patients presenting with acute encephalitis or with unexplained ascending paralysis, including

FIGURE 188-1 Schematic representation of the pathogenetic events following peripheral inoculation of rabies virus. *(Adapted from Jackson AC: Human disease, in Rabies, edited by AC Jackson and WH Wunner, 2002, Academic Press, San Diego, pp 219-244; with permission.)*

Labels in figure:
Brain
6. Infection of brain neurons with neuronal dysfunction
Eye
7. Centrifugal spread along nerves to salivary glands, skin, cornea, and other organs
Salivary glands
3. Virus binds to nicotinic acetylcholine receptors at neuromuscular junction
5. Replication in motor neurons of the spinal cord and local dorsal root ganglia and rapid ascent to brain
Dorsal root ganglion
Sensory nerves to skin
Skeletal muscle
4. Virus travels within axons in peripheral nerves via retrograde fast axonal transport
2. Viral replication in muscle
Spinal cord
1. Virus inoculated

rabies exposure and administration of PEP. After an asymptomatic incubation period, clinical rabies progresses through three general phases: a prodrome, an acute neurologic phase, and coma/death (Table 188-1).

Prodromal Features Clinically apparent rabies infection begins with nonspecific prodromal symptoms, including fever, malaise, headache, nausea, and vomiting. Anxiety or agitation may also occur. Paresthesias, pain, or pruritus near the site of the exposure occurs in 50–80% of patients and suggests rabies. The wound has usually healed by this point, and these symptoms may reflect infection of local dorsal root or cranial sensory ganglia.

Encephalitic Rabies Two acute neurologic forms of rabies are seen in humans: encephalitic (furious) in 80% and paralytic in 20%. Manifestations of encephalitic rabies may be seen in many other viral encephalitides as well. These features include fever, confusion, hallucinations, combativeness, muscle spasms, hyperactivity, and seizures. Autonomic dysfunction is common and may result in hypersalivation, excessive perspiration, gooseflesh, pupillary dilation, and/or priapism. In encephalitic rabies, episodes of hyperexcitability are typically followed by periods of complete lucidity that become shorter as the disease progresses. Rabies encephalitis is most distinguished by early brainstem involvement, which results in the classic symptoms of hydrophobia and aerophobia: involuntary, painful contraction of the diaphragm and accessory respiratory, laryngeal, and pharyngeal muscles in response to swallowing liquids (hydrophobia) or a

TABLE 188-1   PROGRESSION OF RABIES VIRUS INFECTION

Phase	Duration	Signs/Symptoms
Incubation period	1–3 months[a]	None
Prodrome	1–7 days	Fever, malaise, headache, nausea, vomiting, agitation, focal paresthesias, pain
Acute neurologic phase		
Encephalitic (80%)	1–7 days	Fever, confusion, hallucinations, hyperactivity, pharyngeal spasms (hydrophobia/aerophobia), seizures
Paralytic (20%)	2–10 days	Ascending flaccid paralysis
Coma/death	1–14 days	...

[a]Typical duration, with a possible range of 2 weeks to >1 year.

FIGURE 188-2 Three large Negri bodies in the cytoplasm of a cerebellar Purkinje cell from an 8-year-old boy who died of rabies after being bitten by a rabid dog in Mexico. *(From AC Jackson, E Lopez-Corella, N Engl J Med 335:568, 1996. © Massachusetts Medical Society.)*

those in whom Guillain-Barré syndrome is suspected. A lack of animal-bite history or a lack of hydrophobia is not unusual in rabies. Once rabies is suspected, rabies-specific tests should be employed to confirm the diagnosis. Diagnostically useful specimens include serum, CSF, fresh saliva, brain tissue (when available), and skin biopsy samples from the neck. Because skin biopsy relies on the demonstration of rabies virus in cutaneous nerves at the base of hair follicles, samples from the neck should include at least 10 hair follicles. Multiple testing modalities are required to ensure a high negative predictive value. For example, because rabies virus infects immunologically privileged neuronal tissues, serum antibodies often do not develop until very late in the disease.

FIGURE 188-3 Hydrophobic spasm of inspiratory muscles associated with terror in a patient with encephalitic (furious) rabies who is attempting to swallow water. *(Copyright DA Warrell, Oxford, UK; with permission.)*

Rabies Virus–Specific Antibodies In a previously unimmunized patient, serum neutralizing antibodies to rabies virus are diagnostic. Antibodies may be detected within a few days after the onset of symptoms, but some patients die without detectable antibodies. The presence of rabies virus–specific antibodies in the CSF suggests rabies, regardless of immunization status.

Reverse Transcription Polymerase Chain Reaction (RT-PCR) Detection of rabies virus RNA by RT-PCR is highly sensitive and specific. This technique can detect virus in fresh saliva samples, CSF, and tissue. In addition, RT-PCR can distinguish between rabies virus variants, permitting the investigator to infer the likely source of an infection.

Direct Fluorescent Antibody (DFA) Testing DFA testing with rabies antibodies conjugated to fluorescent dyes is highly sensitive and specific and can be applied to brain tissue or skin biopsies from the nape of the neck. In the latter samples, rabies virus can be detected in cutaneous nerves at the base of hair follicles.

DIFFERENTIAL DIAGNOSIS

Early in the course of illness, rabies is frequently indistinguishable from other causes of encephalitis. Herpes simplex virus type 1 and rarely other herpesviruses cause sporadic cases of encephalitis and are important considerations because they require specific treatment. During summer months, enteroviruses and arthropod-borne viruses are an important diagnostic consideration. PCR testing of CSF for specific viruses should be guided by local epidemiologic patterns. Immune-mediated postviral encephalitis may follow infection with influenza, measles, mumps, varicella-zoster, and other viruses. It is important to recognize that immune-mediated encephalitis may occur as a sequela of immunization with rabies vaccine derived from neural tissues (e.g., Semple vaccine). Drug reactions and vasculitis are other important noninfectious causes of encephalitis that must be considered. A conversion disorder due to an exaggerated fear of rabies ("rabies hysteria") can produce symptoms that closely resemble those of rabies (e.g., aggressive behavior, inability to swallow or communicate); an unusually short "incubation period" can be an important clue to the correct diagnosis.

As previously mentioned, paralytic rabies may mimic Guillain-Barré syndrome. In these cases, the documentation of fever or bladder dysfunction can suggest the diagnosis of rabies. Conversely, Guillain-Barré syndrome may rarely occur as a complication of rabies vaccination and may be mistaken for paralytic rabies (i.e., vaccine failure).

℞ RABIES

There is no established treatment for rabies. There have been several recent treatment failures of antiviral therapy, ketamine, and therapeutic coma—measures that were used in a healthy survivor who had rabies virus antibodies present at the time of presentation. Expert opinion should be sought before any course of experimental therapy is embarked upon. A palliative approach may be appropriate for some patients.

PROGNOSIS

Rabies is an almost uniformly fatal disease but is almost always preventable with appropriate postexposure therapy during the incubation period (see below). There are only six well-documented cases of survival after symptomatic rabies infection. All but one of the patients involved had received rabies vaccine before disease onset; these patients represented failures of postexposure rabies prophylaxis. Most patients with rabies die within several days, even with aggressive care in a critical care unit.

PREVENTION

Postexposure Prophylaxis Since there is no effective therapy for rabies, it is extremely important to prevent the disease after an animal exposure. Figure 188-4 shows the steps involved in making decisions about rabies PEP. On the basis of the history of the exposure and local epidemiologic information, the physician must decide whether initia-

FIGURE 188-4 Algorithm for rabies postexposure prophylaxis.
RIG, rabies immune globulin. *[From L Corey, in Harrison's Principles of Internal Medicine, 15th ed. E Braunwald et al (eds): New York, McGraw-Hill, 2001, adapted with permission.]*

Rabies prophylaxis

Did the animal bite the patient or did saliva contaminate a scratch, abrasion, open wound, or mucous membrane? — No → None

Yes ↓

Is rabies known or suspected to be present in the species and the geographic area? — No → None

Yes ↓

Was the animal captured? — No → RIG and vaccine

Yes ↓

Was the animal a normally behaving dog, cat, or ferret? — Yes → Does the animal become ill under observation over the next 10 days? — No → None

No ↓ ← Yes

Does laboratory examination of the brain by fluorescent antibody staining confirm rabies? — No → None

Yes ↓

RIG and vaccine

---

tion of PEP is warranted. Healthy dogs, cats, or ferrets may be confined and observed for 10 days. PEP is not necessary if the animal remains healthy. If the animal develops signs of rabies during the observation period, it should be euthanized immediately, and the head should be transported to the laboratory under refrigeration and examined for the presence of rabies virus by DFA testing and viral isolation using cell culture or mouse inoculation. Any animal other than a dog, cat, or ferret should be euthanized immediately and the head submitted for examination. In high-risk exposures and in areas where canine rabies is endemic, rabies prophylaxis should be initiated without waiting for laboratory results. If the laboratory results prove to be negative, it may safely be concluded that the animal's saliva did not contain rabies virus, and immunization should be discontinued. If an animal escapes after an exposure, it must be considered rabid, and PEP must be initiated unless information from public health officials indicates otherwise (i.e., there is no endemic rabies in the area). PEP may be warranted when a person present in the same space as a bat (e.g., a small child or a sleeping adult) cannot reliably rule out contact with an unrecognized bite.

PEP includes local wound care and both active and passive immunization. Local wound care is essential and may decrease the risk of rabies virus infection by as much as 90%. Wound care should not be delayed, even if the initiation of immunization is postponed pending the results of the 10-day observation period. All bite wounds and scratches should be washed thoroughly with soap and water. Devitalized tissues should be debrided, tetanus prophylaxis given, and antibiotic treatment initiated whenever indicated.

All previously unvaccinated persons should be passively immunized with rabies immune globulin (RIG). If RIG is not immediately available, it should be administered no later than 7 days after the first vaccine dose. After day 7, endogenous antibodies are being produced, and passive immunization may actually be counterproductive. If anatomically feasible,

the entire dose of RIG (20 IU/kg) should be infused at the site of the bite; otherwise, any RIG remaining after infiltration of the bite site should be administered IM at a distant site. With multiple or large wounds, the RIG preparation may be diluted in order to obtain a sufficient volume for adequate infiltration of all wound sites. If the exposure involves a mucous membrane, the entire dose should be administered IM. Rabies vaccine and RIG should never be administered at the same site or with the same syringe. Commercially available RIG in the United States is purified from the serum of hyperimmunized human donors. These human RIG preparations are much better tolerated than are the equine-derived preparations still in use in some countries (see "Global Considerations," below). Serious adverse effects of human RIG are uncommon. Local pain and low-grade fever may occur.

Two purified inactivated rabies vaccines are available for rabies PEP in the United States. They are highly immunogenic and remarkably safe compared with earlier vaccines. Five 1-mL doses of rabies vaccine should be given IM in the deltoid area. (The anterolateral aspect of the thigh is also acceptable in children.) Gluteal injections, which may not always reach muscle, should not be given and have been associated with rare vaccine failures. Ideally, the first dose should be given as soon as possible after exposure; failing that, it should be given without further delay. The four additional doses should be given on days 3, 7, 14, and 28. Pregnancy is not a contraindication for immunization. Glucocorticoids and other immunosuppressive medications may interfere with the development of active immunity and should not be administered during PEP unless they are essential. In several studies, all persons vaccinated with the above schedule developed a serologic response within 2–4 weeks. Routine measurement of serum neutralizing antibody titers is not required, but titers should be measured 2–4 weeks after immunization in immunocompromised persons. Local reactions (pain, erythema, edema, and pruritus) and mild systemic reactions (fever, myalgias, headache, and nausea) are common; anti-inflammatory and antipyretic medications may be used, but immunization should not be discontinued. Systemic allergic reactions are uncommon, but anaphylaxis does occur rarely and can be treated with epinephrine and antihistamines. The risk of rabies development should be carefully considered before the decision is made to discontinue vaccination because of an adverse reaction. Advice and assistance from state health officials or the Centers for Disease Control and Prevention may be helpful in managing adverse reactions to vaccine.

Preexposure Rabies Vaccination Preexposure rabies prophylaxis should be considered for people with an occupational or recreational risk of rabies exposures, including certain travelers to rabies-endemic areas. This primary schedule consists of three doses of rabies vaccine given on days 0, 7, and 21 or 28. Serum neutralizing antibody tests help determine the need for subsequent booster doses. When a previously immunized individual is exposed to rabies, two booster doses of vaccine should be administered on days 0 and 3. Wound care remains critical. RIG should not be administered to previously vaccinated persons.

GLOBAL CONSIDERATIONS

Worldwide, endemic canine rabies is estimated to cause 55,000 human deaths annually. Most of these deaths occur in Asia and Africa, with rural populations and children most frequently affected. Because of this distribution, most of the burden of rabies PEP is borne by those least able to pay. In Latin America, rabies control efforts in dogs have been quite successful in recent years. In Europe and Canada, an epizootic of rabies in red foxes has been partly controlled by widespread use of baits containing rabies vaccine.

In addition to the rabies vaccines discussed above, vaccines grown in either primary cell lines (hamster or dog kidney) or continuous cell lines (Vero cells) are satisfactory and are available in many countries outside the United States. Less expensive vaccines derived from neural tissues have been used in developing countries; however, these vaccines are associated with serious neuroparalytic complications, and their use should be discontinued as soon as possible. Worldwide, >10 million individuals receive postexposure vaccination against rabies each year.

If human RIG is unavailable, purified equine RIG can be used in the same manner at a dose of 40 IU/kg. Before the administration of equine RIG, hypersensitivity should be assessed by intradermal testing with a 1:10 dilution. The incidence of anaphylactic reactions and serum sickness has been low with recent equine RIG products.

OTHER RHABDOVIRUSES

OTHER LYSSAVIRUSES

A growing number of lyssaviruses other than rabies virus have been discovered to infect bat populations throughout the world. Four of these viruses have produced at least one case of human illness indistinguishable from rabies: European bat lyssaviruses 1 and 2, Australian bat lyssavirus, and the Duvenhage virus (in Africa). Mokola virus, a lyssavirus that has been isolated from shrews with an unknown reservoir species, has also produced human illness in Africa.

VESICULAR STOMATITIS VIRUS

Vesicular stomatitis is a viral disease of cattle, horses, pigs, and some wild mammals. VSV is a member of the genus *Vesiculovirus* in the family Rhabdoviridae. Outbreaks of vesicular stomatitis in animals occur sporadically in the southwestern United States. The infection is associated with severe vesiculation and ulceration of oral tissues, teats, and feet and may be clinically indistinguishable from the more dangerous foot-and-mouth disease. Epidemics are usually seasonal and are probably due to arthropod vectors. Direct animal-to-animal spread can also occur, although the virus cannot penetrate intact skin. Transmission to humans usually results from direct contact with infected animals

(particularly cattle) and occasionally follows laboratory exposure. In human disease, early conjunctivitis is followed by an acute influenza-like illness with fever, chills, nausea, vomiting, headache, retrobulbar pain, myalgias, substernal pain, malaise, pharyngitis, and lymphadenitis. Small vesicular lesions may be present on the buccal mucosa or on the fingers. The illness usually lasts 3–6 days, with a subsequent full recovery. Subclinical infections are common. A serologic diagnosis can be made on the basis of a rise in titer of complement-fixing or neutralizing antibodies. Therapy is symptom-based.

FURTHER READINGS

BAER GM (ed): *The Natural History of Rabies*, 2d ed. Boca Raton, CRC Press, 1991

CENTERS FOR DISEASE CONTROL AND PREVENTION: Human rabies prevention—United States, 1999: Recommendations of the Advisory Committee on Immunization Practices (ACIP). MMWR 48(RR-1):1, 1999

JACKSON AC: Rabies: New insights into pathogenesis and treatment. Curr Opin Neurol 19:267, 2006

———, WUNNER WH (eds): *Rabies*, 2d ed. London, Elsevier, 2007

LETCHWORTH GJ et al: Vesicular stomatitis. Vet J 157:239, 1999

WARRELL MJ, WARRELL DA: Rabies and other lyssavirus diseases. Lancet 363:959, 2004

WILLOUGHBY RE JR et al: Survival after treatment of rabies with induction of coma. N Engl J Med 352:2508, 2005

WORLD HEALTH ORGANIZATION: *WHO Expert Consultation on Rabies: First Report*. First Report ed. Geneva, WHO, 2005

189 Infections Caused by Arthropod- and Rodent-Borne Viruses
Clarence J. Peters

Some zoonotic viruses are transmitted in nature without regard to humans and only incidentally infect and produce disease in humans; in addition, a few agents are regularly spread among humans by arthropods. Most of these viruses either are maintained by arthropods or chronically infect rodents. Obviously, the mode of transmission is not a rational basis for taxonomic classification. Indeed, zoonotic viruses from at least seven families act as significant human pathogens (Table 189-1). The virus families differ fundamentally from one another in terms of morphology, replication mechanisms, and genetics. Information on a virus's membership in a family or genus is enlightening with regard to maintenance strategies, sensitivity to antiviral agents, and some aspects of pathogenesis but does not necessarily predict which clinical syndromes (if any) the virus will cause in humans.

FAMILIES OF ARTHROPOD- AND RODENT-BORNE VIRUSES (TABLE 189-1)

The Arenaviridae The Arenaviridae are spherical, 110- to 130-nm particles that bud from the cell's plasma membrane and utilize ambisense RNA genomes with two segments for replication. There are two main phylogenetic branches of Arenaviridae: the Old World viruses, such as Lassa fever and lymphocytic choriomeningitis (LCM) viruses, and the New World viruses, including those causing the South American hemorrhagic fevers (HFs). Arenaviruses persist in nature by chronically infecting rodents with a striking one-virus–one-rodent species relationship. These rodent infections result in long-term virus excretion and perhaps in lifelong viremia; vertical infection is common with some arenaviruses. Humans become infected through the inhalation of aerosols containing arenaviruses, which are then deposit-

ed in the terminal air passages, and probably also through close contact with rodents and their excreta, which results in the contamination of mucous membranes or breaks in the skin.

The Bunyaviridae The family Bunyaviridae includes four medically significant genera. All of these spherical viruses have three negative-sense RNA segments maturing into 90- to 120-nm particles in the Golgi complex and exiting the cell by exocytosis. Viruses of the genus *Bunyavirus* are largely mosquito-borne and have a viremic vertebrate intermediate host; many are also transovarially transmitted in their specific mosquito host. One serologic group also uses biting midges as vectors. Sandflies or mosquitoes are the vectors for the genus *Phlebovirus* (named after phlebotomus fever or sandfly fever, the best-known disease associated with the genus), while ticks serve as vectors for the genus *Nairovirus*. Viruses of both of these genera are also associated with vertical transmission in the arthropod host and with horizontal spread through viremic vertebrate hosts. The genus *Hantavirus* is unique among the Bunyaviridae in that it is not transmitted by arthropods but is maintained in nature by rodent hosts that chronically shed virus. Like the arenaviruses, the hantaviruses usually display striking virus–rodent species specificity. Hantaviruses do not cause chronic viremia in their rodent hosts and are transmitted only horizontally from rodent to rodent.

Other Families The Flaviviridae are positive-sense, single-strand RNA viruses that form particles of 40–50 nm in the endoplasmic reticulum. The flaviviruses discussed here are from the genus *Flavivirus* and make up two phylogenetically and antigenically distinct divisions transmitted among vertebrates by mosquitoes and ticks, respectively. The mosquito-borne viruses fall into phylogenetic groups that include yellow fever virus, the four dengue viruses, and encephalitis viruses, while the tick-borne group encompasses a geographically varied spectrum of species, some of which are responsible for encephalitis or for hemorrhagic disease with encephalitis. The Reoviridae are double-strand RNA viruses with multisegmented genomes. These 80-nm particles are the only viruses discussed in this chapter that do not have a lipid envelope and thus are insensitive to detergents. The Togaviridae

TABLE 189-1 MAJOR ZOONOTIC VIRUS FAMILIES AND SOME CHARACTERISTICS OF TYPICAL MEMBERS

Family	Genus or Group	Syndrome(s): Typical Viruses	Maintenance Strategy
Arenaviridae	Old World complex	FM, E: Lymphocytic choriomeningitis virus	Chronic infection of rodents, often with persistent viremia; vertical transmission common
		HF: Lassa fever virus	
	New World or Tacaribe complex	HF: South American HF viruses (Machupo, Junin, Guanarito, Sabia)	Chronic infection of rodents, sometimes with persistent viremia; vertical infection may occur
Bunyaviridae	*Bunyavirus*	E: California serogroup viruses (La Crosse, Jamestown Canyon, California encephalitis)	Mosquito-vertebrate cycle; transovarial transmission in mosquito common
		FM: Bunyamwera, group C, Tahyna viruses	
		FM: Oropouche virus	Transmitted by *Culicoides*
	Phlebovirus	FM: Sandfly fever, Toscana viruses	Sandfly transmission between vertebrates, with prominent transovarial component in sandfly
		FM: Punta Toro virus	
		HF, FM, E: Rift Valley fever virus	Mosquito-vertebrate transmission, with transovarial component in mosquito
	Nairovirus	HF: Crimean-Congo HF virus	Tick-vertebrate, with transovarial transmission in tick
	Hantavirus	HF: Hantaan, Dobrava, Puumala viruses	Rodent reservoir; chronic virus shedding, but chronic viremia unknown
		HF: Sin Nombre and related hantaviruses	Sigmodontine rodent reservoir
Filoviridae[a]	*Ebolavirus, Marburgvirus*	HF: Marburg viruses, Ebola viruses (4 species)	Unknown
Flaviviridae	*Flavivirus* (mosquito-borne)	HF: Yellow fever virus	Mosquito-vertebrate; transovarial rare
		FM, HF: Dengue viruses (4 serotypes)	
		E: St. Louis, Japanese, West Nile, and Murray Valley encephalitis viruses; Rocio viruses	
	Flavivirus (tick-borne)	E: Central European tick-borne encephalitis, Russian spring-summer encephalitis, Powassan viruses	Tick-vertebrate
		HF: Omsk HF, Kyasanur Forest disease viruses	
Reoviridae	*Coltivirus*	FM, E: Colorado tick fever virus	Tick-vertebrate
	Orbivirus	FM, E: Orungo, Kemerovo viruses	Arthropod-vertebrate
Rhabdoviridae[b]	*Vesiculovirus*	FM: Vesicular stomatitis virus (Indiana, New Jersey); Chandipura, Piry viruses	Sandfly-vertebrate, with prominent transovarial component in sandfly
Togaviridae	*Alphavirus*	AR: Sindbis, chikungunya, Mayaro, Ross River, Barmah Forest viruses	Mosquito-vertebrate
		E: Eastern, western, and Venezuelan equine encephalitis viruses	

[a]The Filoviridae are discussed in Chap. 190.
[b]The Rhabdoviridae are discussed in Chap. 188.

Note: Abbreviations refer to the disease syndrome most commonly associated with the virus: FM, fever, myalgia; AR, arthritis, rash; E, encephalitis; HF, hemorrhagic fever.

have a single positive-strand RNA genome and bud particles of ~60–70 nm from the plasma membrane. The togaviruses discussed here are all members of the genus *Alphavirus* and are transmitted among vertebrates by mosquitoes in their natural cycle. The Filoviridae and the Rhabdoviridae are discussed in Chaps. 190 and 188, respectively.

PROMINENT FEATURES OF ARTHROPOD- AND RODENT-BORNE VIRUSES
Although this chapter discusses the major features of selected arthropod- and rodent-borne viruses, it does not deal with >500 other distinct recognized zoonotic viruses, about one-fourth of which infect humans. Zoonotic viruses are undergoing genetic evolution, "new" zoonotic viruses are being discovered, and the epidemiology of zoonotic viruses is continuing to evolve through environmental changes affecting vectors, reservoirs, and humans. These zoonotic viruses are most numerous in the tropics but are also found in temperate and frigid climates. Their distribution and seasonal activity may be variable and often depend largely on ecologic conditions such as rainfall and temperature, which in turn affect the density of vectors and reservoirs and the development of infection therein.

Maintenance and Transmission Arthropod-borne viruses infect their vectors after the ingestion of a blood meal from a viremic vertebrate. The vectors then develop chronic, systemic infection as the viruses penetrate the gut and spread throughout the body. The viruses eventually reach the salivary glands during a period that is referred to as *extrinsic incubation* and that typically lasts 1–3 weeks in mosquitoes. At this point, an arthropod is competent to continue the chain of transmission by infecting another vertebrate when a subsequent blood meal is taken. The arthropod generally is unharmed by the infection, and the natural vertebrate partner usually has only transient viremia with no overt disease. An alternative mechanism for virus maintenance in its arthropod host is transovarial transmission, which is common among members of the family Bunyaviridae.

Rodent-borne viruses such as the hantaviruses and arenaviruses are maintained in nature by chronic infection transmitted between rodents. As in arthropod-borne virus cycles, there is usually a high degree of rodent-virus specificity, and there is no overt disease in the reservoir/vector.

Epidemiology The distribution of arthropod- and rodent-borne viruses is restricted by the areas inhabited by their reservoir/vectors and provides an important clue in the differential diagnosis. Table 189-2 shows the approximate geographic distribution of the most important of these viruses. Members of each family, each genus, and even each serologically related group usually occur in each area but may not be pathogenic in all areas or may not be a commonly recognized cause of disease in all areas and so may not be included in the table.

Most of these diseases are acquired in a rural setting; a few have urban vectors. Seoul, sandfly fever, and Oropouche viruses are examples of urban viruses, but the most notable are yellow fever, dengue, and chikungunya viruses. A history of mosquito bite has little diagnostic significance in the individual; a history of tick bite is more diagnostically specific. Rodent exposure is often reported by persons infected with an arenavirus or a hantavirus but again has little specificity. Indeed, aerosols may infect persons who have no recollection of having even seen rodents.

Syndromes Human disease caused by arthropod- and rodent-borne viruses is often subclinical. The spectrum of possible responses to infection is wide, and our knowledge of the outcome of most of these infections is limited. The usual disease syndromes associated with these viruses have been grouped into four categories: fever and myalgia, arthritis and rash, encephalitis, and hemorrhagic fever. Although for the purposes of this discussion most viruses have been placed in a single group, the categories often overlap. For example, West Nile and Venezuelan equine encephalitis viruses are discussed as encephalitis viruses,

TABLE 189-2 GEOGRAPHIC DISTRIBUTION OF SOME IMPORTANT AND COMMONLY ENCOUNTERED HUMAN ZOONOTIC VIRAL DISEASES

Area	Arenaviridae	Bunyaviridae	Flaviviridae	Rhabdoviridae	Togaviridae
North America	Lymphocytic choriomeningitis	La Crosse, Jamestown Canyon, California encephalitis; hantavirus pulmonary syndrome	St. Louis, Powassan, West Nile encephalitis; dengue	Vesicular stomatitis	Eastern, western equine encephalitis
South America	Bolivian, Argentine, Venezuelan, and Brazilian HF; lymphocytic choriomeningitis	Oropouche, group C, Punta Toro infection; hantavirus pulmonary syndrome	Yellow fever, dengue, Rocio virus infection	Vesicular stomatitis, Piry virus infection	Mayaro virus infection, Venezuelan equine encephalitis
Europe	Lymphocytic choriomeningitis	Tahyna, Toscana, sandfly fever; HF with renal syndrome	West Nile, Central European tick-borne, Russian spring-summer encephalitis	—	Sindbis virus infection
Middle East	—	Sandfly fever, Crimean-Congo HF	West Nile encephalitis, dengue	—	—
Eastern Asia	—	Sandfly fever; Hantaan, Seoul virus infection	Dengue; Japanese, Russian spring-summer encephalitis; Omsk HF	Chandipura virus infection	—
Southwestern Asia	—	Sandfly fever, Crimean-Congo HF	West Nile, Japanese encephalitis; dengue; Kyasanur Forest disease	—	Chikungunya virus infection
Southeast Asia	—	Seoul virus infection	Japanese encephalitis, dengue	—	Chikungunya virus infection
Africa	Lassa fever	Bunyamwera virus infection, Rift Valley fever	Yellow fever, dengue	—	Sindbis, chikungunya virus infection
Australia	—	—	Murray Valley encephalitis, dengue	—	Ross River, Barmah Forest virus infection

Note: HF, hemorrhagic fever.

but during epidemics they may cause many cases of milder febrile syndromes and relatively uncommon cases of encephalitis. Similarly, Rift Valley fever virus is best known as a cause of HF, but the attack rates for febrile disease are far higher, and encephalitis is occasionally seen as well. LCM virus is classified as a cause of fever and myalgia because this syndrome is its most common disease manifestation and because, even when central nervous system (CNS) disease occurs, it is usually mild and is preceded by fever and myalgia. Dengue virus infection is considered as a cause of fever and myalgia (dengue fever) because this is by far the most common manifestation worldwide and is the syndrome most likely to be seen in the United States; however, dengue HF is also discussed in the HF section because of its complicated pathogenesis and importance in pediatric practice in certain areas of the world.

Diagnosis Laboratory diagnosis is required in any given case, although epidemics occasionally provide clinical and epidemiologic clues on which an educated guess as to etiology can be based. For most arthropod- and rodent-borne viruses, acute-phase serum samples (collected within 3 or 4 days of onset) have yielded isolates, and paired sera have been used to demonstrate rising antibody titers by a variety of tests. Intensive efforts to develop rapid tests for HF have resulted in an antigen-detection enzyme-linked immunosorbent assay (ELISA) and an IgM-capture ELISA that can provide a diagnosis based on a single serum sample within a few hours and are particularly useful in severe cases. More sensitive reverse-transcription polymerase chain reaction (RT-PCR) tests may yield diagnoses based on samples without detectable antigen and may also provide useful genetic information about the virus. Hantavirus infections differ from others discussed here in that severe acute disease is immunopathologic; patients present with serum IgM that serves as the basis for a sensitive and specific test.

At diagnosis, patients with encephalitis are generally no longer viremic or antigenemic and usually do not have virus in cerebrospinal fluid (CSF). In this situation, the value of serologic methods and RT-PCR is being validated. IgM capture is increasingly being used for the simultaneous testing of serum and CSF. IgG ELISA or classic serology is useful in the evaluation of past exposure to the viruses, many of which circulate in areas with a minimal medical infrastructure and sometimes cause mild or subclinical infection.

The remainder of this chapter offers general descriptions of the broad syndromes caused by arthropod- and rodent-borne viruses. Most of the diseases under consideration have not been studied in detail with modern medical approaches; thus available data may be incomplete or biased.

FEVER AND MYALGIA

Fever and myalgia constitute the syndrome most commonly associated with zoonotic virus infection. Many of the numerous viruses belonging to the families listed in Table 189-1 probably cause this syndrome, but several viruses have been selected for inclusion in the table because of their prominent associations with the syndrome and their biomedical importance.

The syndrome typically begins with the abrupt onset of fever, chills, intense myalgia, and malaise. Patients may also report joint pains, but no true arthritis is detectable. Anorexia is characteristic and may be accompanied by nausea or even vomiting. Headache is common and may be severe, with photophobia and retroorbital pain. Physical findings are minimal and are usually confined to conjunctival injection with pain on palpation of muscles or the epigastrium. The duration of symptoms is quite variable but generally is 2–5 days, with a biphasic course in some instances. The spectrum of disease varies from subclinical to temporarily incapacitating.

Less constant findings include a maculopapular rash. Epistaxis may occur but does not necessarily indicate a bleeding diathesis. A minority of the cases caused by some viruses are known or suspected to include aseptic meningitis, but this diagnosis is difficult to make in remote areas, given the patients' photophobia and myalgia as well as the lack of opportunity to examine the CSF. Although pharyngitis may be noted or radiographic evidence of pulmonary infiltrates found in some cases, these viruses are not primary respiratory pathogens. The differential diagnosis includes anicteric leptospirosis, rickettsial diseases, and the early stages of other syndromes discussed in this chapter. These diseases are often described as "flulike," but the usual absence of cough and coryza makes influenza an unlikely confounder except at the earliest stages.

Complete recovery is generally the outcome in this syndrome, although prolonged asthenia and nonspecific symptoms have been described in some cases, particularly after infection with LCM or dengue virus. Treatment is supportive, with aspirin avoided because of the potential for exacerbated bleeding and Reye's syndrome. Efforts at prevention are best based on vector control, which, however, may be expensive or impossible. For mosquito control, destruction of breeding sites is generally the most economically and environmentally sound approach. Measures taken by the individual to avoid the vector can be valuable. Avoiding the vector's habitat and times of peak activity, using screens or other barriers (e.g., permethrin-impregnated bed nets) to prevent the vector from entering dwellings, judiciously applying arthropod repellents such as diethyltoluamide (DEET) to the skin, and wearing permethrin-impregnated clothing are all possible approaches, depending on the vector and its habits.

LYMPHOCYTIC CHORIOMENINGITIS

LCM is transmitted from the common house mouse (*Mus musculus*) to humans by aerosols of excreta and secreta. LCM virus, an arenavirus, is maintained in the mouse mainly by vertical transmission from infected dams. The vertically infected mouse remains viremic for life, with high concentrations of virus in all tissues. Infected colonies of pet hamsters have also served as a link to humans. LCM virus is widely used in immunology laboratories as a model of T cell function and can silently infect cell cultures and passaged tumor lines, resulting in infections among scientists and animal caretakers. Patients with LCM may have a history of residence in rodent-infested housing or other exposure to rodents. An antibody prevalence of ~5–10% has been reported among adults from the United States, Argentina, and endemic areas of Germany.

LCM differs from the general syndrome of fever and myalgia in that its onset is gradual. Among the conditions occasionally associated with LCM are orchitis, transient alopecia, arthritis, pharyngitis, cough, and maculopapular rash. An estimated one-fourth of patients or fewer experience a febrile phase of 3–6 days and then, after a brief remission, develop renewed fever accompanied by severe headache, nausea and vomiting, and meningeal signs lasting for ~1 week. These patients virtually always recover fully, as do the uncommon patients with clear-cut signs of encephalitis. Recovery may be delayed by transient hydrocephalus.

During the initial febrile phase, leukopenia and thrombocytopenia are common and virus can usually be isolated from blood. During the CNS phase, virus may be found in the CSF, but antibodies are present in blood. The pathogenesis of LCM is thought to resemble that following direct intracranial inoculation of the virus into adult mice; the onset of the immune response leads to T cell–mediated immunopathologic meningitis. During the meningeal phase, CSF mononuclear-cell counts range from the hundreds to the low thousands per microliter, and hypoglycorrhachia is found in one-third of cases. The IgM-capture ELISA of serum and CSF is usually positive; RT-PCR assays have been developed for application to CSF. Recent infections transmitted by organ transplantation did not include evidence of an immune response, followed a fulminant course (not unlike that of Lassa fever), and required immunohistochemistry or RT-PCR for diagnosis.

Infection with LCM virus should be suspected in acutely ill febrile patients with marked leukopenia and thrombocytopenia. In cases of aseptic meningitis, any of the following should suggest LCM: well-marked febrile prodrome, adult age, autumn seasonality, low CSF glucose levels, or CSF mononuclear cell counts of >1000/μL.

In pregnant women, LCM virus infection may lead to fetal invasion with consequent congenital hydrocephalus and chorioretinitis. Since the maternal infection may be mild, consisting of only a short febrile illness, antibodies to the virus should be sought in both the mother and the fetus in suspicious circumstances, particularly TORCH-negative neonatal hydrocephalus. [TORCH is a battery of tests encompassing *t*oxoplasmosis, *o*ther conditions (congenital syphilis and viral infection), *r*ubella, *c*ytomegalovirus infection, and *h*erpes simplex virus infection.]

BUNYAMWERA VIRUS INFECTION

The mosquito-transmitted Bunyamwera serogroup viruses are found on every continent except Australia and Antarctica. Bunyamwera virus and its close relative Ilesha virus commonly cause febrile disease in Africa. Nigari virus, a reassortant of Bunyamwera virus, has recently been identified as an important human pathogen in Africa. Other related viruses are implicated in such disease in Southeast Asia (Batai virus), Europe (Calovo virus), and South America (Wyeomyia virus). In North America, Cache Valley virus has been implicated in febrile hu-

man disease and in rare instances of more serious systemic illness; the presence of serum antibodies to this virus may be associated with congenital malformations. In Central America, the closely related Fort Sherman virus causes the fever-myalgia syndrome.

GROUP C VIRUS INFECTION

The group C viruses include at least 11 agents transmitted by mosquitoes in neotropical forests. These agents are among the most common causes of arboviral infection in humans entering American jungles and cause acute febrile disease.

TAHYNA VIRUS INFECTION

This California serogroup virus (see discussion of California encephalitis, below) occurs in central and western Europe, and related viruses are emerging in Russia. The significance of Tahyna virus in human health has been well studied only in the Czech and Slovak Republics; there, the virus was found to be a prominent cause of febrile disease, in some cases causing pharyngitis, pulmonary syndromes, and aseptic meningitis. The potential for arboviruses to be unexpectedly involved in such cases in areas of high mosquito prevalence needs to be kept in mind.

OROPOUCHE FEVER

Oropouche virus is transmitted in Central and South America by a biting midge, *Culicoides paraensis*, which often breeds to high density in cacao husks and other vegetable detritus found in towns and cities. Explosive epidemics involving thousands of cases have been reported from several towns in Brazil and Peru. Rash and aseptic meningitis have been detected in a number of cases.

SANDFLY FEVER

The sandfly *Phlebotomus papatasi* transmits sandfly fever. Female sandflies may be infected by the oral route as they take a blood meal and may transmit the virus to offspring when they lay their eggs after a second blood meal. This prominent transovarial pattern was the first to be recognized among dipterans and complicates virus control. A previous designation for sandfly fever, "3-day fever," instructively describes the brief, debilitating course associated with this essentially benign infection. There is neither a rash nor CNS involvement, and complete recovery is the rule.

Sandfly fever is found in the circum-Mediterranean area, extending to the east through the Balkans into China as well as into the Middle East and southwestern Asia. The vector is found in both rural and urban settings and is known for its small size, which enables it to penetrate standard mosquito screens and netting, and for its short flight range. Epidemics have been described in the wake of natural disasters and wars. In parts of Europe, sandfly populations and virus transmission were greatly reduced by the extensive residual spraying conducted after World War II to control malaria, and the incidence continues to be low. A common pattern of disease in endemic areas consists of high attack rates among travelers and military personnel with little or no disease in the local population, who are protected after childhood infection. More than 30 related phleboviruses are transmitted by sandflies and mosquitoes, but most are of unknown significance in terms of human health.

TOSCANA VIRUS DISEASE

Toscana virus is a *Phlebovirus* (family Bunyaviridae) transmitted primarily by the circum-Mediterranean sandfly *P. perniciosus*. The vertebrate amplifying host, if one exists, is unknown. Toscana virus infection is common during the summer among rural residents and vacationers, particularly in Italy, Spain, and Portugal; a number of cases have been identified in travelers returning to Germany and Scandinavia. The disease may manifest as an uncomplicated febrile illness but is often associated with aseptic meningitis, with virus isolated from the CSF.

PUNTA TORO VIRUS DISEASE

Of the several phleboviruses that are associated with New World sandflies and infect humans, Punta Toro virus is the best known. The disease caused by this virus is clinically similar to but epidemiologically different from that caused by the Naples or Sicilian sandfly fever viruses. Punta Toro virus infections are sporadic and are acquired in the tropical forest, where the vectors rest on tree buttresses. Epidemics have not been reported, but antibody prevalences among inhabitants of villages in the endemic areas indicate a cumulative lifetime exposure rate of >50%.

DENGUE FEVER

All four distinct dengue viruses (dengue 1–4) have *Aedes aegypti* as their principal vector, and all cause a similar clinical syndrome. In rare cases, second infection with a serotype of dengue virus different from that involved in the primary infection leads to dengue HF with severe shock (see below). Sporadic cases are seen in the settings of endemic transmission and epidemic disease. Year-round transmission between latitudes 25°N and 25°S has been established, and seasonal forays of the viruses to points as far north as Philadelphia are thought to have taken place in the United States. Dengue fever is seen in the Caribbean region, including Puerto Rico. With increasing spread of the vector mosquito throughout the tropics and subtropics, large areas of the world have become vulnerable to the introduction of dengue viruses, particularly through air travel by infected humans, and both dengue fever and the related dengue HF are becoming increasingly common. Conditions favorable to dengue transmission exist in the southern United States, and bursts of dengue fever activity are to be expected in this region, particularly along the Mexican border, where water may be stored in containers and *A. aegypti* numbers may therefore be greatest. This mosquito, which is also an efficient vector of the yellow fever and chikungunya viruses, typically breeds near human habitation, using relatively fresh water from sources such as water jars, vases, discarded containers, coconut husks, and old tires. *A. aegypti* usually inhabits dwellings and bites during the day.

After an incubation period of 2–7 days, the typical patient experiences the sudden onset of fever, headache, retroorbital pain, and back pain along with the severe myalgia that gave rise to the colloquial designation "break-bone fever." There is often a macular rash on the first day as well as adenopathy, palatal vesicles, and scleral injection. The illness may last a week, with additional symptoms usually including anorexia, nausea or vomiting, marked cutaneous hypersensitivity, and—near the time of defervescence—a maculopapular rash beginning on the trunk and spreading to the extremities and the face. Epistaxis and scattered petechiae are often noted in uncomplicated dengue, and preexisting gastrointestinal lesions may bleed during the acute illness.

Laboratory findings include leukopenia, thrombocytopenia, and, in many cases, serum aminotransferase elevations. The diagnosis is made by IgM ELISA or paired serology during recovery or by antigen-detection ELISA or RT-PCR during the acute phase. Virus is readily isolated from blood in the acute phase if mosquito inoculation or mosquito cell culture is used.

COLORADO TICK FEVER

Several hundred cases of Colorado tick fever are reported annually in the United States. The infection is acquired between March and November through the bite of an infected *Dermacentor andersoni* tick in mountainous western regions at altitudes of 1200–3000 m (4000–10,000 ft). Small mammals serve as the amplifying host. The most common presentation consists of fever and myalgia; meningoencephalitis is not uncommon, and hemorrhagic disease, pericarditis, myocarditis, orchitis, and pulmonary presentations are also reported. Rash develops in a substantial minority of cases. The disease usually lasts 7–10 days and is often biphasic. The most important differential diagnostic considerations since the beginning of the twentieth century have been Rocky Mountain spotted fever and tularemia. In Colorado, Colorado tick fever is much more common than Rocky Mountain spotted fever.

Infection of erythroblasts and other marrow cells by Colorado tick fever virus results in the appearance and persistence (for several weeks) of erythrocytes containing the virus. This feature, detected in smears stained by immunofluorescence, can be diagnostically helpful. The clinical laboratory detects leukopenia and thrombocytopenia.

ORBIVIRUS INFECTION

The orbiviruses encompass many human and veterinary pathogens. For example, Orungo virus is widely transmitted by mosquitoes in tropical Africa and causes febrile disease in humans. The Kemerovo complex includes the Kemerovo, Lipovnik, and Tribec viruses of Russia and central Europe; these viruses are transmitted by ticks and are associated with febrile and neurologic disease.

ENCEPHALITIS

Arboviral encephalitis is a seasonal disease, commonly occurring in the warmer months. Its incidence varies markedly with time and place, depending on ecologic factors. The causative viruses differ substantially in terms of case-infection ratio (i.e., the ratio of clinical to subclinical infections), mortality rate, and residua (Table 189-3). Humans are not an important amplifier of these viruses.

All the viral encephalitides discussed in this section have a similar pathogenesis as far as is known. An infected arthropod ingests a blood meal from a human and infects the host. The initial period of viremia is thought to originate most commonly from the lymphoid system. Viremia leads to CNS invasion, presumably through infection of olfactory neuroepithelium with passage through the cribriform plate or through infection of brain capillaries and multifocal entry into the CNS. During the viremic phase, there may be little or no recognized disease except in the case of tick-borne flaviviral encephalitis, in which there may be a clearly delineated phase of fever and systemic illness. The disease process in the CNS arises partly from direct neuronal infection and subsequent damage and partly from edema, inflammation, and other indirect effects. The usual pathologic picture is one of focal necrosis of neurons, inflammatory glial nodules, and perivascular lymphoid cuffing; the severity and distribution of these abnormalities vary with the infecting virus. Involved areas display the "luxury perfusion" phenomenon, with normal or increased total blood flow and low oxygen extraction.

The typical patient presents with a prodrome of nonspecific constitutional symptoms, including fever, abdominal pain, vertigo, sore throat, and respiratory symptoms. Headache, meningeal signs, photophobia, and vomiting follow quickly. Involvement of deeper structures may be signaled by lethargy, somnolence, and intellectual deficit (as disclosed by the mental status examination or failure at serial 7 subtraction); more severely affected patients are obviously disoriented and may be comatose. Tremors, loss of abdominal reflexes, cranial nerve palsies, hemiparesis, monoparesis, difficulty in swallowing, and frontal lobe signs are all common. Spinal and motor neuron diseases are documented with West Nile and Japanese encephalitis viruses. Convulsions and focal signs may be evident early or may appear during the course of the disease. Some patients present with an abrupt onset of fever, convulsions, and other signs of CNS involvement. The results of human infection range from no significant symptoms through febrile headache to aseptic meningitis and finally to full-blown encephalitis; the proportions and severity of these manifestations vary with the infecting virus.

The acute encephalitis usually lasts from a few days to as long as 2–3 weeks, but recovery may be slow, with weeks or months required for the return of maximal recoupable function. Difficulty concentrating, fatigability, tremors, and personality changes are common during recovery. The acute illness requires management of a comatose patient who may have intracranial pressure elevations, inappropriate secretion of antidiuretic hormone, respiratory failure, and convulsions. There is no specific therapy for these viral encephalitides. The only practical preventive measures are vector management and personal protection against the arthropod transmitting the virus; for Japanese encephalitis or tick-borne encephalitis, vaccination should be considered in certain circumstances (see relevant sections below).

TABLE 189-3 PROMINENT FEATURES OF ARBOVIRAL ENCEPHALITIS

Virus	Natural Cycle	Incubation Period, Days	Annual No. of Cases	Case-to-Infection Ratio	Age of Cases	Case-Fatality Rate, %	Residua
La Crosse	*Aedes triseriatus*–chipmunk (transovarial component in mosquito also important)	~3–7	70 (U.S.)	<1:1000	<15 years	<0.5	Recurrent seizures in ~10%; severe deficits in rare cases; decreased school performance and behavioral change suspected in small proportion
St. Louis	*Culex tarsalis, C. pipiens, C. quinquefasciatus*–birds	4–21	85, with hundreds to thousands in epidemic years (U.S.)	<1:200	Milder cases in the young; more severe cases in adults >40 years old, particularly the elderly	7	Common in the elderly
Japanese	*Culex tritaeniorhynchus*–birds	5–15	>25,000	1:200–300	All ages; children in highly endemic areas	20–50	Common (approximately half of cases); may be severe
West Nile	*Culex* mosquitoes–birds	3–6	?	Very low	Mainly the elderly	5–10	Uncommon
Central European	*Ixodes ricinus*–rodents, insectivores	7–14	Thousands	1:12	All ages; milder in children	1–5	20%
Russian spring-summer	*I. persulcatus*–rodents, insectivores	7–14	Hundreds	—	All ages; milder in children	20	Approximately half of cases; often severe; limb-girdle paralysis
Powassan	*I. cookei*–wild mammals	~10	~1 (U.S.)	—	All ages; some predilection for children	~10	Common (approximately half of cases)
Eastern equine	*Culiseta melanura*–birds	~5–10	5 (U.S.)	1:40 adult 1:17 child	All ages; predilection for children	50–75	Common
Western equine	*Culex tarsalis*–birds	~5–10	~20 (U.S.)	1:1000 adult 1:50 child 1:1 infant	All ages; predilection for children <2 years old (increased mortality in elderly)	3–7	Common only among infants <1 year old
Venezuelan equine (epidemic)	Unknown (multiple mosquito species and horses in epidemics)	1–5	?	1:250 adult 1:25 child (approximate)	All ages; predilection for children	~10	

The diagnosis of arboviral encephalitis depends on the careful evaluation of a febrile patient with CNS disease, with rapid identification of treatable herpes simplex encephalitis, ruling out of brain abscess, exclusion of bacterial meningitis by serial CSF examination, and performance of laboratory studies to define the viral etiology. Leptospirosis, neurosyphilis, Lyme disease, cat-scratch fever, and newer viral encephalitides such as Nipah virus infection from Malaysia should be considered. The CSF examination usually shows a modest cell count—in the tens or hundreds or perhaps a few thousand. Early in the process, a significant proportion of these cells may be polymorphonuclear leukocytes, but usually there is a mononuclear cell predominance. CSF glucose levels are usually normal. There are exceptions to this pattern of findings. In eastern equine encephalitis, for example, polymorphonuclear leukocytes may predominate during the first 72 h of disease and hypoglycorrhachia may be detected. In LCM, lymphocyte counts may be in the thousands, and the glucose concentration may be diminished. Experience with imaging studies is still evolving; clearly, however, both CT and MRI may be normal, except for evidence of preexisting conditions, or sometimes may suggest diffuse edema. Several patients with eastern equine encephalitis have had focal abnormalities, and individuals with severe Japanese encephalitis have presented with bilateral thalamic lesions that have often been hemorrhagic. Electroencephalography usually shows diffuse abnormalities and is not directly helpful.

A humoral immune response is usually detectable at or near the onset of disease. Both serum and CSF should be examined for IgM antibodies. Virus generally cannot be isolated from blood or CSF, although Japanese encephalitis virus has been recovered from CSF in severe cases. RT-PCR analysis of CSF may yield positive results. Virus can be obtained from and viral antigen is present in brain tissue, although its distribution may be focal.

CALIFORNIA, LA CROSSE, AND JAMESTOWN CANYON VIRUS ENCEPHALITIS

The isolation of California encephalitis virus established the California serogroup of viruses as a cause of encephalitis, and its use as a diagnostic antigen led to the description of many cases of "California encephalitis." In fact, however, this virus has been implicated in only a few cases of encephalitis, and the serologically related La Crosse virus is the major cause of encephalitis among viruses in the California serogroup. "California encephalitis" due to La Crosse virus infection is most commonly reported from the upper Midwest but is also found in other areas of the central and eastern United States, most often in West Virginia, Tennessee, North Carolina, and Georgia. The serogroup includes 13 other viruses, some of which may also be involved in human disease that is misattributed because of the complexity of the group's serology; these viruses include the Jamestown Canyon, snowshoe hare, Inkoo, and Trivittatus viruses, all of which have *Aedes* mosquitoes as their vector and all of which have a strong element of transovarial transmission in their natural cycles.

The mosquito vector of La Crosse virus is *A. triseriatus*. In addition to a prominent transovarial component of transmission, a mosquito can become infected through feeding on viremic chipmunks and other mammals as well as through venereal transmission from another mosquito. The mosquito breeds in sites such as tree holes and abandoned tires and bites during daylight hours. These habits correlate with the risk factors for human cases: recreation in forested areas, residence at the forest's edge, and the presence of abandoned tires around the home. Intensive environmental modification based on these findings has reduced the incidence of disease in a highly endemic area in the

Midwest. Most cases occur from July through September. The Asian tiger mosquito, *A. albopictus*, efficiently transmits the virus to mice and also transmits the agent transovarially in the laboratory; this aggressive anthropophilic mosquito has the capacity to urbanize, and its possible impact on transmission to humans is of concern.

An antibody prevalence of ≥20% in endemic areas indicates that infection is common, but CNS disease has been recognized primarily in children <15 years of age. The illness varies from a picture of aseptic meningitis accompanied by confusion to severe and occasionally fatal encephalitis. Although there may be prodromal symptoms, the onset of CNS disease is sudden, with fever, headache, and lethargy often joined by nausea and vomiting, convulsions (in one-half of patients), and coma (in one-third of patients). Focal seizures, hemiparesis, tremor, aphasia, chorea, Babinski signs, and other evidence of significant neurologic dysfunction are common, but residua are not. Perhaps 10% of patients have recurrent seizures in the succeeding months. Other serious sequelae are rare, although a decrease in scholastic standing has been reported and mild personality change has occasionally been suggested. Treatment is supportive over a 1- to 2-week acute phase during which status epilepticus, cerebral edema, and inappropriate secretion of antidiuretic hormone are important concerns. Ribavirin has been used in severe cases, and a clinical trial of this drug is under way.

The blood leukocyte count is commonly elevated, sometimes reaching levels of 20,000/μL, and there is usually a left shift. CSF cell counts are typically 30–500/μL with a mononuclear cell predominance (although 25–90% of cells are polymorphonuclear in some cases). The protein level is normal or slightly increased, and the glucose level is normal. Specific virologic diagnosis based on IgM-capture assays of serum and CSF is efficient. The only human anatomic site from which virus has been isolated is the brain.

Jamestown Canyon virus has been implicated in several cases of encephalitis in adults; in these cases, the disease was usually associated with a significant respiratory illness at onset. Human infection with this virus has been documented in New York, Wisconsin, Ohio, Michigan, Ontario, and other areas of North America where the vector mosquito, *A. stimulans*, feeds on its main host, the white-tailed deer.

ST. LOUIS ENCEPHALITIS

St. Louis encephalitis virus is transmitted between *Culex* mosquitoes and birds. This virus causes low-level endemic infection among rural residents of the western and central United States, where *C. tarsalis* is the vector (see "Western Equine Encephalitis," below), but the more urbanized mosquito species *C. pipiens* and *C. quinquefasciatus* have been responsible for epidemics resulting in hundreds or even thousands of cases in cities of the central and eastern United States. Most cases occur in June through October. The urban mosquitoes breed in accumulations of stagnant water and sewage with high organic content and readily bite humans in and around houses at dusk. The elimination of open sewers and trash-filled drainage systems is expensive and may not be possible, but screening of houses and implementation of personal protective measures may be an effective approach for individuals. The rural vector is most active at dusk and outdoors; its bites can be avoided by modification of activities and use of repellents.

Disease severity increases with age: infections that result in aseptic meningitis or mild encephalitis are concentrated in children and young adults, while severe and fatal cases primarily affect the elderly. Infection rates are similar in all age groups; thus the greater susceptibility of older persons to disease is a biologic consequence of aging. The disease has an abrupt onset, sometimes following a prodrome, and begins with fever, lethargy, confusion, and headache. In addition, nuchal rigidity, hypotonia, hyperreflexia, myoclonus, and tremor are common. Severe cases can include cranial nerve palsies, hemiparesis, and convulsions. Patients often report dysuria and may have viral antigen in urine as well as pyuria. The overall mortality rate is generally ~7% but may reach 20% among patients over the age of 60. Recovery is slow. Emotional lability, difficulties in concentration and memory, asthenia, and tremor are commonly prolonged in older patients.

The CSF of patients with St. Louis encephalitis usually contains tens to hundreds of cells, with a lymphocytic predominance and a normal glucose level. Leukocytosis with a left shift is often documented.

JAPANESE ENCEPHALITIS

Japanese encephalitis virus is found throughout Asia, including far eastern Russia, Japan, China, India, Pakistan, and Southeast Asia, and causes occasional epidemics on western Pacific islands. The virus has been detected in the Torres Strait islands, and a human encephalitis case has been identified on the nearby Australian mainland. This flavivirus is particularly common in areas where irrigated rice fields attract the natural avian vertebrate hosts and provide abundant breeding sites for mosquitoes such as *C. tritaeniorhynchus*, which transmit the virus to humans. Additional amplification by pigs, which suffer abortion, and horses, which develop encephalitis, may be significant as well. Vaccination of these additional amplifying hosts may reduce the transmission of the virus. An effective, formalin-inactivated vaccine purified from mouse brain is produced in Japan and licensed for human use in the United States. It is given on days 0, 7, and 30 or—with some sacrifice in serum neutralizing titer—on days 0, 7, and 14. Vaccination is indicated for summer travelers to rural Asia, where the risk of clinical disease may be 0.05–2.1/10,000 per week (Table 116-2). The severe and often fatal disease reported in expatriates must be balanced against the 0.1–1% chance of a late systemic or cutaneous allergic reaction. These reactions are rarely fatal but may be severe and have been known to begin 1–9 days after vaccination, with associated pruritus, urticaria, and angioedema. Live attenuated vaccines are being used in China but are not recommended in the United States at this time.

WEST NILE VIRUS INFECTION

West Nile virus is transmitted among wild birds by *Culex* mosquitoes in Africa, the Middle East, southern Europe, and Asia. It is a common cause of febrile disease without CNS involvement, but it occasionally causes aseptic meningitis and severe encephalitis; these serious infections are particularly common among the elderly. The febrile-myalgic syndrome caused by West Nile virus differs from many others by the frequent appearance of a maculopapular rash concentrated on the trunk and lymphadenopathy. Headache, ocular pain, sore throat, nausea and vomiting, and arthralgia (but not arthritis) are common accompaniments. In addition, the virus has been implicated in severe and fatal hepatic necrosis in Africa.

West Nile virus was introduced into New York City in 1999 and subsequently spread to other areas of the northeastern United States, causing >60 cases of aseptic meningitis or encephalitis among humans as well as die-offs among crows, exotic zoo birds, and other birds. The virus has continued to spread and is now found in almost all states, Canada, and Mexico. *C. pipiens* remains the major vector in the northeastern United States, but several other *Culex* species are also involved, and blue jays compete with crows as amplifiers and lethal targets in other areas of the country. Annually, ~1000–3000 cases of encephalitis with ~100–300 deaths are reported in the United States. The ratio of CNS involvement to infection is thought to be ~1:100; the remainder of patients have subclinical infection or West Nile fever. Encephalitis, sequelae, and death are all more common among the elderly, diabetics, and patients with previous CNS insults. In addition to the more severe motor and cognitive sequelae, milder findings may include tremor, slight abnormalities in motor skills, and loss of executive functions. Intense clinical interest and the availability of laboratory diagnostic methods have made it possible to define a number of unusual clinical features, including chorioretinitis, flaccid paralysis with histologic lesions resembling poliomyelitis, and initial presentation with fever and focal neurologic deficits in the absence of diffuse encephalitis. Immunosuppressed patients may have fulminant courses or develop persistent CNS infection. Virus transmission through both transplantation and blood transfusion has necessitated screening of blood and organ donors by nucleic acid–based tests.

West Nile virus falls into the same phylogenetic group of flaviviruses as St. Louis and Japanese encephalitis viruses, as do Murray Valley and

Rocio viruses. The latter two viruses are both maintained in mosquitoes and birds and produce a clinical picture resembling that of Japanese encephalitis. Murray Valley virus has caused occasional epidemics and sporadic cases in Australia. Rocio virus caused recurrent epidemics in a focal area of Brazil in 1975–1977 and then virtually disappeared.

CENTRAL EUROPEAN TICK-BORNE ENCEPHALITIS AND RUSSIAN SPRING-SUMMER ENCEPHALITIS

A spectrum of tick-borne flaviviruses has been identified across the Eurasian land mass. Many are known mainly as agricultural pathogens (e.g., louping ill virus in the United Kingdom). From Scandinavia to the Urals, central European tick-borne encephalitis is transmitted by *Ixodes ricinus*. Human cases occur between April and October, with a peak in June and July. A related and more virulent virus is that of Russian spring-summer encephalitis, which is associated with *I. persulcatus* and is distributed from Europe across the Urals to the Pacific Ocean. The ticks transmit the disease primarily in the spring and early summer, with a lower rate of transmission later in summer. Small mammals are the vertebrate amplifiers for both viruses. The risk varies by geographic area and can be highly localized within a given area; human cases usually follow outdoor activities or consumption of raw milk from infected goats or other infected animals.

After an incubation period of 7–14 days or perhaps longer, the central European viruses classically result in a febrile-myalgic phase that lasts for 2–4 days and is thought to correlate with viremia. A subsequent remission for several days is followed by the recurrence of fever and the onset of meningeal signs. The CNS phase varies from mild aseptic meningitis, which is more common among younger patients, to severe encephalitis with coma, convulsions, tremors, and motor signs lasting for 7–10 days before improvement begins. Spinal and medullary involvement can lead to typical limb-girdle paralysis and to respiratory paralysis. Most patients recover, only a minority with significant deficits. Infections with the Far Eastern viruses generally run a more abrupt course. The encephalitic syndrome caused by these viruses sometimes begins without a remission and has more severe manifestations than the European syndrome. Mortality is high, and major sequelae—most notably, lower motor neuron paralyses of the proximal muscles of the extremities, trunk, and neck—are common.

In the early stage of the illness, virus may be isolated from the blood. In the CNS phase, IgM antibodies are detectable in serum and/or CSF. Thrombocytopenia sometimes develops during the initial febrile illness, which resembles the early hemorrhagic phase of some other tick-borne flaviviral infections, such as Kyasanur Forest disease. Other tick-borne flaviviruses are less common causes of encephalitis, including louping ill virus in the United Kingdom and Powassan virus.

There is no specific therapy for infection with these viruses. However, effective alum-adjuvanted, formalin-inactivated vaccines are produced in Austria, Germany, and Russia. Two doses of the Austrian vaccine separated by an interval of 1–3 months appear to be effective in the field, and antibody responses are similar when vaccine is given on days 0 and 14. Other vaccines have elicited similar neutralizing antibody titers. Since rare cases of postvaccination Guillain-Barré syndrome have been reported, vaccination should be reserved for persons likely to experience rural exposure in an endemic area during the season of transmission. Cross-neutralization for the central European and Far Eastern strains has been established, but there are no published field studies on cross-protection of formalin-inactivated vaccines. Because 0.2–4% of ticks in endemic areas may be infected, tick bites raise the issue of immunoglobulin prophylaxis. Prompt administration of high-titered specific preparations should probably be undertaken, although no controlled data are available to prove the efficacy of this measure. Immunoglobulin should not be administered late because of the risk of antibody-mediated enhancement.

POWASSAN ENCEPHALITIS

Powassan virus is a member of the tick-borne encephalitis virus complex and is transmitted by *I. cookei* among small mammals in eastern Canada and the United States, where it has been responsible for 20 recognized cases of human disease. Other ticks may transmit the virus in a wider geographic area, and there is some concern that *I. scapularis* (also called *I. dammini*), a competent vector in the laboratory, may become involved as it becomes more prominent in the United States. Patients with Powassan encephalitis (many of whom are children) present in May through December after outdoor exposure and an incubation period thought to be ~1 week. Powassan encephalitis is severe, and sequelae are common.

EASTERN EQUINE ENCEPHALITIS

Eastern equine encephalitis is found primarily within endemic swampy foci along the eastern coast of the United States, with a few inland foci as far removed as Michigan. Human cases present from June through October, when the bird–*Culiseta* mosquito cycle spills over into other mosquito species such as *A. sollicitans* or *A. vexans*, which are more likely to bite mammals. There is concern over the potential role of the introduced anthropophilic mosquito species *A. albopictus*, which has been found to be naturally infected and is an effective vector in the laboratory. Horses are a common target for the virus; contact with unvaccinated horses may be associated with human disease, but horses probably do not play a significant role in amplification of the virus.

Eastern equine encephalitis is one of the most destructive of the arboviral conditions, with a brusque onset, rapid progression, high mortality, and frequent residua. This severity is reflected in the extensive necrotic lesions and polymorphonuclear infiltrates found at postmortem examination of the brain and the acute polymorphonuclear CSF pleocytosis often occurring during the first 1–3 days of disease. In addition, leukocytosis with a left shift is a common feature. A formalin-inactivated vaccine has been used to protect laboratory workers but is not generally available or applicable.

WESTERN EQUINE ENCEPHALITIS

The primary maintenance cycle for western equine encephalitis virus in the United States is between *C. tarsalis* and birds, principally sparrows and finches. Equines and humans become infected, and both species suffer encephalitis without amplifying the virus in nature. St. Louis encephalitis is transmitted in a similar cycle in the same region but causes human disease about a month earlier than the period (July through October) in which western equine encephalitis virus is active. Large epidemics of western equine encephalitis took place in the western and central United States and Canada during the 1930s to 1950s, but in recent years the disease has been uncommon. There were 41 reported cases in the United States in 1987 but only 5 reported cases from 1988 to 2001. This decline in incidence may reflect in part the integrated approach to mosquito management that has been employed in irrigation projects and the increasing use of agricultural pesticides; it almost certainly reflects the increased tendency for humans to be indoors behind closed windows at dusk—the peak period of biting by the major vector.

Western equine encephalitis virus causes a typical diffuse viral encephalitis with an increased attack rate and increased morbidity among the young, particularly children <2 years old. In addition, mortality rates are high among the young and the very elderly. One-third of individuals who have convulsions during the acute illness have subsequent seizure activity. Infants <1 year old—particularly those in the first months of life—are at serious risk of motor and intellectual damage. Twice as many males as females develop clinical encephalitis after 5–9 years of age; this difference may be related to greater outdoor exposure of boys to the vector but is also likely to be due in part to biologic differences. A formalin-inactivated vaccine has been used to protect laboratory workers but is not generally available or applicable.

VENEZUELAN EQUINE ENCEPHALITIS

There are six known types of virus in the Venezuelan equine encephalitis complex. An important distinction is between the *epizootic* viruses (subtypes IAB and IC) and the *enzootic* viruses (subtypes ID to IF and types II to VI). The epizootic viruses have an unknown natural cycle but periodically cause extensive epidemics in equines and humans in the Americas. These epidemics rely on the high-level viremia in horses and mules that results in the infection of several species of mosquitoes, which in turn infect humans and perpetuate virus transmission. Humans also have high-level viremia but probably are not important in virus transmission. Enzootic viruses are found primarily in humid tropical forest habitats and are maintained between *Culex* mosquitoes and rodents; these viruses cause human disease but are not pathogenic for horses and do not cause epizootics.

Epizootics of Venezuelan equine encephalitis occurred repeatedly in Venezuela, Colombia, Ecuador, Peru, and other South American countries at intervals of ≤10 years from the 1930s until 1969, when a massive epizootic spread throughout Central America and Mexico, reaching southern Texas in 1972. Genetic sequencing of the virus from the 1969–1972 outbreak suggested that it originated from residual "un-inactivated" virus in veterinary vaccines. The outbreak was terminated in Texas with the use of a live attenuated vaccine (TC-83) originally developed for human use by the U.S. Army; the epizootic virus was then used for further production of inactivated veterinary vaccines. No further epizootic disease was identified until 1995 and subsequently, when additional epizootics took place in Colombia, Venezuela, and Mexico. The viruses involved in these epizootics as well as previously epizootic subtype IC viruses have been shown to be close phylogenetic relatives of known enzootic subtype ID viruses. This finding suggests that active evolution and selection of epizootic viruses are under way in northern South America.

During epizootics, extensive human infection is the rule, with clinical disease in 10–60% of infected individuals. Most infections result in notable acute febrile disease, while relatively few result in encephalitis. A low rate of CNS invasion is supported by the absence of encephalitis among the many infections resulting from exposure to aerosols in the laboratory or from vaccine accidents. The most recent large epizootic of Venezuelan equine encephalitis occurred in Colombia and Venezuela in 1995; of the >85,000 clinical cases, 4% (with a higher proportion among children than adults) included neurologic symptoms and 300 ended in death.

Enzootic strains of Venezuelan equine encephalitis virus are common causes of acute febrile disease, particularly in areas such as the Florida Everglades and the humid Atlantic coast of Central America. Encephalitis has been documented only in the Florida infections; the three cases were caused by type II enzootic virus, also called *Everglades virus*. All three patients had preexisting cerebral disease. Extrapolation from the rate of genetic change suggests that Everglades virus may have been introduced into Florida <200 years ago and that it is most closely related to the ID subtypes that appear to have given evolutionary rise to the epizootic strains active in South America.

The prevention of epizootic Venezuelan equine encephalitis depends on vaccination of horses with the attenuated TC-83 vaccine or with an inactivated vaccine prepared from that strain. Humans can be protected with similar vaccines, but the use of such products is restricted to laboratory personnel because of reactogenicity and limited availability. In addition, wild-type virus and perhaps TC-83 vaccine may have some degree of fetal pathogenicity. Enzootic viruses are genetically and antigenically different from epizootic viruses, and protection against the former with vaccines prepared from the latter is relatively ineffective.

ARTHRITIS AND RASH

True arthritis is a common accompaniment of several viral diseases, such as rubella (caused by a non-alphavirus togavirus), parvovirus B19 infection, and hepatitis B; it is an occasional accompaniment of infection due to mumps virus, enteroviruses, herpesviruses, and adenoviruses. It is not generally appreciated that the alphaviruses are also common causes of arthritis. In fact, the alphaviruses discussed below all cause acute febrile diseases accompanied by the development of true arthritis and a maculopapular rash. Rheumatic involvement includes arthralgia alone, periarticular swelling, and (less commonly) joint effusions. Most of these diseases are less severe and have fewer articular manifestations

in children than in adults. In temperate climates, these are summer diseases. No specific therapy or licensed vaccines exist.

SINDBIS VIRUS INFECTION

Sindbis virus is transmitted among birds by mosquitoes. Infections with the northern European strains of this virus (which cause, for example, Pogosta disease in Finland, Karelian fever in the independent states of the former Soviet Union, and Okelbo disease in Sweden) and with the genetically related southern African strains are particularly likely to result in the arthritis-rash syndrome. Exposure to a rural environment is commonly associated with this infection, which has an incubation period of <1 week.

The disease begins with rash and arthralgia. Constitutional symptoms are not marked, and fever is modest or lacking altogether. The rash, which lasts ~1 week, begins on the trunk, spreads to the extremities, and evolves from macules to papules that often vesiculate. The arthritis of this condition is multiarticular, migratory, and incapacitating, with resolution of the acute phase in a few days. Wrists, ankles, phalangeal joints, knees, elbows, and—to a much lesser extent—proximal and axial joints are involved. Persistence of joint pains and occasionally of arthritis is a major problem and may go on for months or even years despite a lack of deformity.

CHIKUNGUNYA VIRUS INFECTION

It is likely that chikungunya virus ("that which bends up") is of African origin and is maintained among nonhuman primates on that continent by *Aedes* mosquitoes of the subgenus *Stegomyia* in a fashion similar to yellow fever virus. Like yellow fever virus, chikungunya virus is readily transmitted among humans in urban areas by *A. aegypti*. The *A. aegypti*–chikungunya virus transmission cycle has also been introduced into Asia, where it poses a prominent health problem. The disease is endemic in rural areas of Africa, and intermittent epidemics take place in towns and cities of Africa and Asia. In 2004, a massive epidemic in the Indian Ocean region began; it now appears to have been spread totally by travelers. *A. albopictus* was identified as the major vector, and there were multiple exportations to temperate zones and to areas where *A. aegypti* is present. Chikungunya is one more reason (in addition to dengue and yellow fever) that *A. aegypti* must be controlled.

Full-blown disease is most common among adults, in whom the clinical picture may be dramatic. The abrupt onset follows an incubation period of 2–3 days. Fever and severe arthralgia are accompanied by chills and constitutional symptoms such as headache, photophobia, conjunctival injection, anorexia, nausea, and abdominal pain. Migratory polyarthritis mainly affects the small joints of the hands, wrists, ankles, and feet, with lesser involvement of the larger joints. Rash may appear at the outset or several days into the illness; its development often coincides with defervescence, which takes place around day 2 or 3 of disease. The rash is most intense on the trunk and limbs and may desquamate. Petechiae are occasionally seen, and epistaxis is not uncommon, but this virus is not a regular cause of the HF syndrome, even in children. A few patients develop leukopenia. Elevated levels of aspartate aminotransferase (AST) and C-reactive protein have been described, as have mildly decreased platelet counts. Recovery may require weeks. Some older patients continue to experience stiffness, joint pain, and recurrent effusions for several years; this persistence may be especially common in HLA-B27 patients. An investigational live attenuated vaccine has been developed but requires additional testing. It appears to be headed for further development and commercial manufacture stimulated by the Indian Ocean outbreak.

A related virus, O'nyong-nyong, caused a major epidemic of arthritis and rash involving at least 2 million people as it moved across eastern and central Africa in the 1960s. After its mysterious emergence, the virus virtually disappeared, leaving only occasional evidence of its persistence in Kenya until a transient resurgence of epidemic activity in 1997.

MAYARO FEVER

Mayaro virus is maintained in the forests of the Americas by *Haemagogus* mosquitoes and nonhuman primates. It causes a frequently endemic and sometimes epidemic infection of humans and appears to produce a syndrome resembling chikungunya virus infection.

EPIDEMIC POLYARTHRITIS (ROSS RIVER VIRUS INFECTION)

Ross River virus has caused epidemics of distinctive clinical disease in Australia since the beginning of the twentieth century and continues to be responsible for thousands of cases in rural and suburban areas annually. The virus is transmitted by *A. vigilax* and other mosquitoes, and its persistence is thought to involve transovarial transmission. No definitive vertebrate host has been identified, but several mammalian species, including wallabies, have been suggested. Endemic transmission has also been documented in New Guinea, and in 1979 the virus swept through the eastern Pacific Islands, causing hundreds of thousands of illnesses. The virus was carried from island to island by infected humans and was believed to have been transmitted among humans by *A. polynesiensis* and *A. aegypti*.

The incubation period is 7–11 days long, and the onset of illness is sudden, with joint pain usually ushering in the disease. The rash generally develops coincidentally or follows shortly but in some cases precedes joint pains by several days. Constitutional symptoms such as low-grade fever, asthenia, myalgia, headache, and nausea are not prominent and indeed are absent in many cases. Most patients are incapacitated for considerable periods by joint involvement, which interferes with sleeping, walking, and grasping. Wrist, ankle, metacarpophalangeal, interphalangeal, and knee joints are the most commonly involved, although toes, shoulders, and elbows may be affected with some frequency. Periarticular swelling and tenosynovitis are common, and one-third of patients have true arthritis. Only half of all arthritis patients can resume normal activities within 4 weeks, and 10% still must limit their activity at 3 months. Occasional patients are symptomatic for 1–3 years but without progressive arthropathy. Aspirin and nonsteroidal anti-inflammatory drugs are effective for the treatment of symptoms.

Clinical laboratory values are normal or variable in Ross River virus infection. Tests for rheumatoid factor and antinuclear antibodies are negative, and the erythrocyte sedimentation rate is acutely elevated. Joint fluid contains 1000–60,000 mononuclear cells/μL, and Ross River virus antigen is demonstrable in macrophages. IgM antibodies are valuable in the diagnosis of this infection, although they occasionally persist for years. The isolation of the virus from blood by mosquito inoculation or mosquito cell culture is possible early in the illness. Because of the great economic impact of annual epidemics in Australia, an inactivated vaccine is being developed and has been found to be protective in mice.

Perhaps because of the local interest in arboviruses in general and in Ross River virus in particular, other arthritogenic arboviruses have been identified in Australia, including Gan Gan virus, a member of the family Bunyaviridae; Kokobera virus, a flavivirus; and Barmah Forest virus, an alphavirus. The last virus is a common cause of infection and must be differentiated from Ross River virus by specific testing.

HEMORRHAGIC FEVERS

The viral HF syndrome is a constellation of findings based on vascular instability and decreased vascular integrity. An assault, direct or indirect, on the microvasculature leads to increased permeability and (particularly when platelet function is decreased) to actual disruption and local hemorrhage. Blood pressure is decreased, and in severe cases shock supervenes. Cutaneous flushing and conjunctival suffusion are examples of common, observable abnormalities in the control of local circulation. The hemorrhage is inconstant and is in most cases an indication of widespread vascular damage rather than a life-threatening loss of blood volume. Disseminated intravascular coagulation (DIC) is occasionally found in any severely ill patient with HF but is thought to occur regularly only in the early phases of HF with renal syndrome, Crimean-Congo HF, and perhaps some cases of filovirus HF. In some viral HF syndromes, specific organs may be particularly impaired, such as the kidney in HF with renal syndrome, the lung in hantavirus pulmonary syndrome, or the liver in yellow fever, but in all these diseases the generalized circulatory disturbance is critically important.

The pathogenesis of HF is poorly understood and varies among the viruses regularly implicated in the syndrome, which number more than a dozen. In some cases direct damage to the vascular system or even to parenchymal cells of target organs is important, whereas in others soluble mediators are thought to play the major role. The acute phase in most cases of HF is associated with ongoing virus replication and viremia. Exceptions are the hantavirus diseases and dengue HF/dengue shock syndrome (DHF/DSS), in which the immune response plays a major pathogenic role.

The HF syndromes all begin with fever and myalgia, usually of abrupt onset. Within a few days the patient presents for medical attention because of increasing prostration that is often accompanied by severe headache, dizziness, photophobia, hyperesthesia, abdominal or chest pain, anorexia, nausea or vomiting, and other gastrointestinal disturbances. Initial examination often reveals only an acutely ill patient with conjunctival suffusion, tenderness to palpation of muscles or abdomen, and borderline hypotension or postural hypotension, perhaps with tachycardia. Petechiae (often best visualized in the axillae), flushing of the head and thorax, periorbital edema, and proteinuria are common. Levels of AST are usually elevated at presentation or within a day or two thereafter. Hemoconcentration from vascular leakage, which is usually evident, is most marked in hantavirus diseases and in DHF/DSS. The seriously ill patient progresses to more severe symptoms and develops shock and other findings typical of the causative virus. Shock, multifocal bleeding, and CNS involvement (encephalopathy, coma, convulsions) are all poor prognostic signs.

One of the major diagnostic clues is travel to an endemic area within the incubation period for a given syndrome (Table 189-4). Except for Seoul, dengue, and yellow fever virus infections, which have urban vectors, travel to a rural setting is especially suggestive of a diagnosis of HF.

Early recognition is important because of the need for virus-specific therapy and supportive measures, including prompt, atraumatic hospitalization; judicious fluid therapy that takes into account the patient's increased capillary permeability; administration of cardiotonic drugs; use of pressors to maintain blood pressure at levels that will support renal perfusion; treatment of the relatively common secondary bacterial infections; replacement of clotting factors and platelets as indicated; and the usual precautionary measures used in the treatment of patients with hemorrhagic diatheses. DIC should be treated only if clear laboratory evidence of its existence is found and if laboratory monitoring of therapy is feasible; there is no proven benefit of such therapy. The available evidence suggests that HF patients have a decreased cardiac output and will respond poorly to fluid loading as it is often practiced in the treatment of shock associated with bacterial sepsis. Specific therapy is available for several of the HF syndromes. In addition, several diseases considered in the differential diagnosis—malaria, shigellosis, typhoid, leptospirosis, relapsing fever, and rickettsial disease—are treatable and potentially lethal. Strict barrier nursing and other precautions against infection of medical staff and visitors are indicated in HF except that due to hantaviruses, yellow fever, Rift Valley fever, and dengue.

LASSA FEVER

Lassa virus is known to cause endemic and epidemic disease in Nigeria, Sierra Leone, Guinea, and Liberia, although it is probably more widely distributed in West Africa. This virus and its relatives exist elsewhere in Africa, but their health significance is unknown. Like other arenaviruses, Lassa virus is spread to humans by small-particle aerosols from chronically infected rodents and may also be acquired during the capture or eating of these animals. It can be transmitted by close person-to-person contact. The virus is often present in urine during convalescence and is suspected to be present in seminal fluid early in recovery. Nosocomial spread has occurred but is uncommon if proper sterile parenteral techniques are used. Individuals of all ages and both sexes are affected; the incidence of disease is highest in the dry season, but transmission takes place year-round. In countries where Lassa virus is endemic, Lassa fever can be a prominent cause of febrile disease. For example, in one hospital in Sierra Leone, laboratory-confirmed Lassa fever is consistently responsible for one-fifth of ad-

TABLE 189-4   VIRAL HEMORRHAGIC FEVER (HF) SYNDROMES AND THEIR DISTRIBUTION

Disease	Incubation Period, Days	Case-Infection Ratio	Case-Fatality Rate, %	Geographic Range	Target Population
Lassa fever	5–16	Mild infections probably common	15	West Africa	All ages, both sexes
South American HF	7–14	Most infections (more than half) result in disease	15–30	Selected rural areas of Bolivia, Argentina, Venezuela, and Brazil	Bolivia: Men in countryside; all ages, both sexes in villages Argentina: All ages, both sexes; excess exposure and disease in men Venezuela: All ages, both sexes
Rift Valley fever	2–5	~1:100^a	~50	Sub-Saharan Africa, Madagascar, Egypt	All ages, both sexes; more often diagnosed in men; preexisting liver disease may predispose
Crimean-Congo HF	3–12	≥1:5	15–30	Africa, Middle East, Turkey, Balkans, southern region of former Soviet Union, western China	All ages, both sexes; men more exposed in some settings
HF with renal syndrome	9–35	Hantaan, >1:1.25; Puumala, 1:20	Hantaan, 5–15; Puumala, <1	Worldwide, depending on rodent reservoir	Excess of male patients (partly due to greater exposure); mainly adults
Hantavirus pulmonary syndrome	~7–28	Very high	40–50	Americas	Excess of male patients due to some occupational exposure; mainly adults
Marburg or Ebola HF	3–16	High	25–90	Sub-Saharan Africa	All ages, both sexes; children less exposed
Yellow fever	3–6	1:2–1:20	20	Africa, South America	All ages, both sexes; adults more exposed in jungle setting; preexisting flavivirus immunity may cross-protect
Dengue HF/dengue shock syndrome	2–7	Nonimmune, 1:10,000; heterologous immune, 1:100	<1 with supportive treatment	Tropics and subtropics worldwide	Predominantly children; previous heterologous dengue infection predisposes to HF
Kyasanur Forest/Omsk HF	3–8	Variable	0.5–10	Mysore State, India/western Siberia	Variable

^{a}Figure is for HF cases only. Most infections with Rift Valley fever virus result in fever and myalgia rather than HF.

missions to the medical wards. There are probably tens of thousands of Lassa fever cases annually in West Africa alone.

Among the HF agents, only the arenaviruses are typically associated with a gradual onset of illness. The average case of Lassa fever has a gradual onset that gives way to more severe constitutional symptoms and prostration. Bleeding is seen in only ~15–30% of cases. A maculopapular rash is often noted in light-skinned Lassa patients. Effusions are common, and male-dominant pericarditis may develop late. The fetal death rate is 92% in the last trimester, when the maternal mortality rate is also increased from the usual 15–30%; these figures suggest that interruption of the pregnancy of infected women should be considered. White blood cell counts are normal or slightly elevated, and platelet counts are normal or somewhat low. Deafness coincides with clinical improvement in ~20% of cases and is permanent and bilateral in some. Reinfection may occur but has not been associated with severe disease.

High-level viremia or a high serum concentration of AST statistically predicts a fatal outcome. Thus patients with an AST level of >150 IU/mL should be treated with IV ribavirin. This antiviral nucleoside analogue appears to be effective in reducing mortality rates from the levels documented among retrospective controls, and its only major side effect is reversible anemia that usually does not require transfusion. The drug should be given by slow IV infusion in a dose of 32 mg/kg; this dose should be followed by 16 mg/kg every 6 h for 4 days and then by 8 mg/kg every 8 h for 6 days.

SOUTH AMERICAN HF SYNDROMES (ARGENTINE, BOLIVIAN, VENEZUELAN, AND BRAZILIAN)

These diseases are similar to one another clinically, but their epidemiology differs with the habits of their rodent reservoirs and the interactions of these animals with humans. Person-to-person or nosocomial transmission is rare but has occurred.

The basic disease resembles Lassa fever, with two marked differences. First, thrombocytopenia—often marked—is the rule, and bleeding is quite common. Second, CNS dysfunction is much more common

than in Lassa fever and is often manifested by marked confusion, tremors of the upper extremities and tongue, and cerebellar signs. Some cases follow a predominantly neurologic course, with a poor prognosis. The clinical laboratory is helpful in diagnosis since thrombocytopenia, leukopenia, and proteinuria are typical findings.

Argentine HF is readily treated with convalescent-phase plasma given within the first 8 days of illness. In the absence of passive antibody therapy, IV ribavirin in the dose recommended for Lassa fever is likely to be effective in all the South American HF syndromes. The transmission of the disease from men convalescing from Argentine HF to their wives suggests the need for counseling of arenavirus HF patients concerning the avoidance of intimate contacts for several weeks after recovery. A safe, effective, live attenuated vaccine exists for Argentine HF. In experimental animals, this vaccine is cross-protective against the Bolivian HF virus.

RIFT VALLEY FEVER

The mosquito-borne Rift Valley fever virus is also a pathogen of domestic animals such as sheep, cattle, and goats. It is maintained in nature by transovarial transmission in floodwater *Aedes* mosquitoes and presumably also has a vertebrate amplifier. Epizootics and epidemics occur when sheep or cattle become infected during particularly heavy rains; developing high-level viremia, these animals infect many species of mosquitoes. Remote sensing via satellite can detect the ecologic changes associated with high rainfall that predict the likelihood of Rift Valley fever transmission; it can also detect the special depressions from which the floodwater *Aedes* mosquito vectors emerge. In addition, the virus is infectious when transmitted by contact with blood or aerosols from domestic animals or their abortuses. The slaughtered meat is not infectious; anaerobic glycolysis in postmortem tissues results in an acidic environment that rapidly inactivates Bunyaviridae such as Rift Valley fever virus and Crimean-Congo HF virus. The natural range of Rift Valley fever virus is confined to sub-Saharan Africa, where its circulation is markedly enhanced by substantial rainfall such as that which occurred during the El Niño phenomenon of 1997; subsequent spread to the Arabian Peninsula caused epidemic disease in 2000. The virus has also been found in Madagascar and has been introduced into Egypt, where it caused major epidemics in 1977–1979, 1993, and subsequently. Neither person-to-person nor nosocomial transmission has been documented.

Rift Valley fever virus is unusual in that it causes several clinical syndromes. Most infections are manifested as the febrile-myalgic syndrome. A small proportion of infections result in HF with especially prominent liver involvement. Renal failure and DIC are also common features. Perhaps 10% of otherwise mild infections lead to retinal vasculitis; funduscopic examination reveals edema, hemorrhages, and infarction, and some patients have permanently impaired vision. A small proportion of cases (<1 in 200) are followed by typical viral encephalitis. One of the complicated syndromes does not appear to predispose to another.

There is no proven therapy for any of the syndromes described above. Both retinal disease and encephalitis occur after the acute febrile syndrome has ended and serum neutralizing antibody has developed—events suggesting that only supportive care need be given. Epidemic disease is best prevented by vaccination of livestock. The established ability of this virus to propagate after an introduction into Egypt suggests that other potentially receptive areas, including the United States, should have a response ready for such an eventuality. It seems likely that this disease, like Venezuelan equine encephalitis, can be controlled only with adequate stocks of an effective live attenuated vaccine, and there are no such global stocks. A formalin-inactivated vaccine confers immunity to humans, but quantities are limited and three injections are required; this vaccine is recommended for exposed laboratory workers and for veterinarians working in sub-Saharan Africa.

CRIMEAN-CONGO HF

This severe HF syndrome has a wide geographic distribution, potentially being found wherever ticks of the genus *Hyalomma* occur. The propensity of these ticks to feed on domestic livestock and certain wild mammals means that veterinary serosurveys are the most effective mechanism for the surveillance of virus circulation in a region. Human infection is acquired via a tick bite or during the crushing of infected ticks. Domestic animals do not become ill but do develop viremia; thus there is danger of infection at the time of slaughter and for a brief interval thereafter (through contact with hides or carcasses). Cases have followed sheep shearing. An epidemic in South Africa was associated with slaughter of tick-infested ostriches. Nosocomial epidemics are common and are usually related to extensive blood exposure or needle sticks.

Although generally similar to other HF syndromes, Crimean-Congo HF causes extensive liver damage, resulting in jaundice in some cases. Clinical laboratory values indicate DIC and show elevations in AST, creatine phosphokinase, and bilirubin. Patients with fatal cases generally have more marked changes, even in the early days of illness, and also develop leukocytosis rather than leukopenia. In addition, thrombocytopenia is more marked and develops earlier in cases with a fatal outcome.

No controlled trials have been performed with IV ribavirin, but clinical experience and retrospective comparison of patients with ominous clinical laboratory values suggest that ribavirin is efficacious and should be given. No human or veterinary vaccines are recommended.

HF WITH RENAL SYNDROME

This disease, the first to be identified as an HF, is widely distributed over Europe and Asia; the major causative viruses and their rodent reservoirs on these two continents are Puumala virus (bank vole, *Clethrionomys glareolus*) and Hantaan virus (striped field mouse, *Apodemus agrarius*), respectively. Other potential causative viruses exist, including Dobrava virus (yellow-necked field mouse, *A. flavicollis*), which causes severe HF with renal syndrome in the Balkans. Seoul virus is associated with the Norway or sewer rat, *Rattus norvegicus*, and has a worldwide distribution through the migration of the rodent; it is associated with mild or moderate HF with renal syndrome in Asia, but in

many areas of the world the human disease has been difficult to identify. Most cases occur in rural residents or vacationers; the exception is Seoul virus disease, which may be acquired in an urban or rural setting or from contaminated laboratory rat colonies. Classic Hantaan disease in Korea (Korean HF) and in rural China (epidemic HF) is most common in spring and fall and is related to rodent density and agricultural practices. Human infection is acquired primarily through aerosols of rodent urine, although virus is also present in saliva and feces. Patients with hantavirus diseases are not infectious. HF with renal syndrome is the most important form of HF today, with >100,000 cases of severe disease in Asia annually and milder Puumala infections numbering in the thousands as well.

Severe cases of HF with renal syndrome caused by Hantaan virus evolve in identifiable stages: the febrile stage with myalgia, lasting 3 or 4 days; the hypotensive stage, often associated with shock and lasting from a few hours to 48 h; the oliguric stage with renal failure, lasting 3–10 days; and the polyuric stage with diuresis and hyposthenuria.

The *febrile stage* is initiated by the abrupt onset of fever, headache, severe myalgia, thirst, anorexia, and often nausea and vomiting. Photophobia, retroorbital pain, and pain on ocular movement are common, and the vision may become blurred with ciliary body inflammation. Flushing over the face, the V area of the neck, and the back is characteristic, as are pharyngeal injection, periorbital edema, and conjunctival suffusion. Petechiae often develop in areas of pressure, the conjunctivae, and the axillae. Back pain and tenderness to percussion at the costovertebral angle reflect massive retroperitoneal edema. Laboratory evidence of mild to moderate DIC is present. Other laboratory findings include proteinuria and an active urinary sediment.

The *hypotensive stage* is ushered in by falling blood pressure and sometimes by shock. The relative bradycardia typical of the febrile phase is replaced by tachycardia. Kinin activation is marked. The rising hematocrit reflects increasing vascular leakage. Leukocytosis with a left shift develops, and thrombocytopenia continues. Atypical lymphocytes—which in fact are activated CD8+ (and, to a lesser extent, CD4+) T cells—circulate. Proteinuria is marked, and the urine's specific gravity falls to 1.010. The renal circulation is congested and compromised from local and systemic circulatory changes resulting in necrosis of tubules, particularly at the corticomedullary junction, and oliguria.

During the *oliguric stage*, hemorrhagic tendencies continue, probably in large part because of uremic bleeding defects. The oliguria persists for 3–10 days before the return of renal function marks the onset of the *polyuric stage*, which carries the danger of dehydration and electrolyte abnormalities.

Mild cases of HF with renal syndrome may be much less stereotypical. The presentation may include only fever, gastrointestinal abnormalities, and transient oliguria followed by hyposthenuria.

HF with renal syndrome should be suspected in patients with rural exposure in an endemic area. Prompt recognition of the disease permits rapid hospitalization and expectant management of shock and renal failure. Useful clinical laboratory parameters include leukocytosis, which may be leukemoid and is associated with a left shift; thrombocytopenia; and proteinuria. Mainstays of therapy are the management of shock, reliance on pressors, modest crystalloid infusion, IV use of human serum albumin, and treatment of renal failure with prompt dialysis for the usual indications. Hydration may result in pulmonary edema, and hypertension should be avoided because of the possibility of intracranial hemorrhage. Use of IV ribavirin has reduced mortality and morbidity in severe cases provided treatment is begun within the first 4 days of illness. The case-fatality ratio may be as high as 15% but with proper therapy should be <5%. Sequelae have not been definitively established, but there is a correlation in the United States between chronic hypertensive renal failure and the presence of antibodies to Seoul virus.

Infections with Puumala virus, the most common cause of HF with renal syndrome in Europe, result in a much attenuated picture but the same general presentation. The syndrome may be referred to by its former name, *nephropathia epidemica*. Bleeding manifestations are found in only 10% of cases, hypotension rather than shock is usually seen, and oliguria is present in only about half of patients. The dominant features may be fever, abdominal pain, proteinuria, mild oliguria, and sometimes blurred vision or glaucoma followed by polyuria and hyposthenuria in recovery. The mortality rate is <1%.

The diagnosis is readily made by IgM-capture ELISA, which should be positive at admission or within 24–48 h thereafter. The isolation of virus is difficult, but RT-PCR of a blood clot collected early in the clinical course or of tissues obtained postmortem will give positive results. Such testing is usually undertaken only if definitive identification of the infecting viral species is required or if molecular epidemiologic questions exist.

HANTAVIRUS PULMONARY SYNDROME

Hantavirus pulmonary syndrome was discovered in 1993, but retrospective identification of cases by immunohistochemistry (1978) and serology (1959) support the idea that it is a recently discovered rather than a truly new disease. The causative agents are hantaviruses of a distinct phylogenetic lineage that is associated with the rodent subfamily Sigmodontinae. Sin Nombre virus, which chronically infects the deer mouse (*Peromyscus maniculatus*), is the most important agent of hantavirus pulmonary syndrome in the United States. The disease is also caused by a Sin Nombre virus variant from the white-footed mouse (*P. leucopus*), by Black Creek Canal virus (*Sigmodon hispidus*, the cotton rat), and by Bayou virus (*Oryzomys palustris*, the rice rat). Several other related viruses cause the disease in South America, but Andes virus is unusual in that it, alone among hantaviruses, has been implicated in human-to-human transmission. The disease is linked to rodent exposure and particularly affects rural residents living in dwellings permeable to rodent entry or working at occupations that pose a risk of rodent exposure. Each rodent species has its own particular habits; in the case of the deer mouse, these behaviors include living in and around human habitation.

The disease begins with a prodrome of ~3–4 days (range, 1–11 days) comprising fever, myalgia, malaise, and often gastrointestinal disturbances such as nausea, vomiting, and abdominal pain. Dizziness is common and vertigo occasional. Severe prodromal symptoms bring some individuals to medical attention, but patients are usually recognized as the cardiopulmonary phase begins. Typically, there is slightly lowered blood pressure, tachycardia, tachypnea, mild hypoxemia, and early radiographic signs of pulmonary edema. Physical findings in the chest are often surprisingly scant. The conjunctival and cutaneous signs of vascular involvement seen in other types of HF are absent. During the next few hours, decompensation may progress rapidly to severe hypoxemia and respiratory failure. Most patients surviving the first 48 h of hospitalization are extubated and discharged within a few days, with no apparent residua.

Management during the first few hours after presentation is critical. The goal is to prevent severe hypoxemia by oxygen therapy, with intubation and intensive respiratory management if needed. During this period, hypotension and shock with increasing hematocrit invite aggressive fluid administration, but this intervention should be undertaken with great caution. Because of low cardiac output with myocardial depression and increased pulmonary vascular permeability, shock should be managed expectantly with pressors and modest infusion of fluid guided by the pulmonary capillary wedge pressure. Mild cases can be managed by frequent monitoring and oxygen administration without intubation. Many patients require intubation to manage hypoxemia and also develop shock. Mortality rates remain at ~30–40% even with good management. The antiviral drug ribavirin inhibits the virus in vitro but did not have a marked effect on patients treated in an open-label study.

During the prodrome, the differential diagnosis of hantavirus pulmonary syndrome is difficult, but by the time of presentation or within 24 h thereafter, a number of diagnostically helpful clinical features become apparent. Cough is not usually present at the outset but may develop later. Interstitial edema is evident on the chest x-ray. Later, bilateral alveolar edema with a central distribution develops in the setting of a normal-sized heart; occasionally, the edema is initially unilateral. Pleural effusions are often seen. Thrombocytopenia, circu-

lating atypical lymphocytes, and a left shift (often with leukocytosis) are almost always evident; thrombocytopenia is a particularly important early clue. Hemoconcentration, proteinuria, and hypoalbuminemia should also be sought. Although thrombocytopenia virtually always develops and prolongation of the partial thromboplastin time is the rule, clinical evidence for coagulopathy or laboratory indications of DIC are found in only a minority of cases, usually in severely ill patients. Patients with severe illness also have acidosis and elevated serum levels of lactate. Mildly increased values in renal function tests are common, but patients with severe cases often have markedly elevated concentrations of serum creatinine; some of the viruses other than Sin Nombre virus have been associated with more kidney involvement, but few such cases have been studied. The differential diagnosis includes abdominal surgical conditions and pyelonephritis as well as rickettsial disease, sepsis, meningococcemia, plague, tularemia, influenza, and relapsing fever.

A specific diagnosis is best made by IgM testing of acute-phase serum, which has yielded positive results even in the prodrome. Tests using a Sin Nombre virus antigen detect the related hantaviruses causing the pulmonary syndrome in the Americas. Occasionally, heterologous viruses will react only in the IgG ELISA, but this finding is highly suspicious given the very low seroprevalence of these viruses in normal populations. RT-PCR is usually positive when used to test blood clots obtained in the first 7–9 days of illness as well as tissues; this test is useful in identifying the infecting virus in areas outside the home range of the deer mouse and in atypical cases.

YELLOW FEVER

Yellow fever virus caused major epidemics in the Americas, Africa, and Europe before the discovery of mosquito transmission in 1900 led to its control through attacks on its urban vector, *A. aegypti*. Only then was it found that a jungle cycle also existed in Africa, involving other *Aedes* mosquitoes and monkeys, and that colonization of the New World with *A. aegypti*, originally an African species, had established urban yellow fever as well as an independent sylvatic yellow fever cycle involving *Haemagogus* mosquitoes and New World monkeys in American jungles. Today, urban yellow fever transmission occurs only in some African cities, but the threat exists in the great cities of South America, where reinfestation by *A. aegypti* has taken place and dengue transmission by the same mosquito is common. As late as 1905, New Orleans suffered >3000 cases with 452 deaths from "yellow jack." Despite the existence of a highly effective and safe vaccine, several hundred jungle yellow fever cases occur annually in South America, and thousands of jungle and urban cases occur each year in Africa.

Yellow fever is a typical HF accompanied by prominent hepatic necrosis. A period of viremia, typically lasting 3 or 4 days, is followed by a period of "intoxication." During the latter phase in severe cases, the characteristic jaundice, hemorrhages, black vomit, anuria, and terminal delirium occur, perhaps related in part to extensive hepatic involvement. Blood leukocyte counts may be normal or reduced and are often high in terminal stages. Albuminuria is usually noted and may be marked; as renal function fails in terminal or severe cases, the level of blood urea nitrogen rises proportionally. Abnormalities detected in liver function tests range from modest elevations of AST levels in mild cases to severe derangement.

Urban yellow fever can be prevented by the control of *A. aegypti*. The continuing sylvatic cycle requires vaccination of all visitors to areas of potential transmission. With few exceptions, reactions to vaccine are minimal; immunity is provided within 10 days and lasts for at least 10 years. An egg allergy dictates caution in vaccine administration. Although there are no documented harmful effects of the vaccine on the fetus, pregnant women should be immunized only if they are definitely at risk of yellow fever exposure. Since vaccination has been associated with several cases of encephalitis in children <6 months of age, it should be delayed until after 12 months of age unless the risk of exposure is very high. Rare, serious, multisystemic adverse reactions (occasionally fatal) have been reported, particularly affecting the elderly; nevertheless, the number of deaths of unvaccinated travelers with yellow fever exceeds the number of deaths from vaccination, and a liberal vaccination policy for travelers to involved areas should be pursued. Timely information on changes in yellow fever distribution and yellow fever vaccine requirements can be obtained from Health Information for Travelers, Centers for Disease Control and Prevention, Atlanta, GA 30333; by fax request (404-332-4565; document number 220022); by phone (404-332-4559); or via the Internet (*www.cdc.gov*).

DENGUE HEMORRHAGIC FEVER/DENGUE SHOCK SYNDROME

A syndrome of HF noted in the 1950s among children in the Philippines and Southeast Asia was soon associated with dengue virus infections, particularly those occurring against a background of previous exposure to another dengue-virus serotype. The transient heterotypic protection after dengue virus infection is replaced within several weeks by the potential for heterotypic infection resulting in typical dengue fever (see above) or—uncommonly—in enhanced disease (secondary DHF/DSS). In rare instances, primary dengue infections lead to an HF syndrome, but much less is known about pathogenesis in this situation. In the past 20 years, *A. aegypti* has progressively reinvaded Latin America and other areas, and frequent travel by infected individuals has introduced multiple strains of dengue virus from many geographic areas. Thus the pattern of hyperendemic transmission of multiple dengue serotypes has now been established in the Americas and the Caribbean and has led to the emergence of DHF/DSS as a major problem there as well. Millions of dengue infections, including many thousands of cases of DHF/DSS, occur annually. The severe syndrome is unlikely to be seen in U.S. citizens since few children have the dengue antibodies that can trigger the pathogenetic cascade when a second infection is acquired.

Macrophage/monocyte infection is central to the pathogenesis of dengue fever and to the origin of DHF/DSS. Previous infection with a heterologous dengue-virus serotype may result in the production of nonprotective antiviral antibodies that nevertheless bind to the virion's surface and through interaction with the Fc receptor focus secondary dengue viruses on the target cell, the result being enhanced infection. The host is also primed for a secondary antibody response when viral antigens are released and immune complexes lead to activation of the classic complement pathway, with consequent phlogistic effects. Cross-reactivity at the T cell level results in the release of physiologically active cytokines, including interferon γ and tumor necrosis factor α. The induction of vascular permeability and shock depends on multiple factors, including the following:

1. *Presence of enhancing and nonneutralizing antibodies*—Transplacental maternal antibody may be present in infants <9 months old, or antibody elicited by previous heterologous dengue infection may be present in older individuals. T cell reactivity is also intimately involved.
2. *Age*—Susceptibility to DHF/DSS drops considerably after 12 years of age.
3. *Sex*—Females are more often affected than males.
4. *Race*—Caucasians are more often affected than blacks.
5. *Nutritional status*—Malnutrition is protective.
6. *Sequence of infection*—For example, serotype 1 followed by serotype 2 seems to be more dangerous than serotype 4 followed by serotype 2.
7. *Infecting serotype*—Type 2 is apparently more dangerous than other serotypes.

In addition, there is considerable variation among strains of a given serotype, with Southeast Asian serotype 2 strains having more potential to cause DHF/DSS than others.

Dengue HF is identified by the detection of bleeding tendencies (tourniquet test, petechiae) or overt bleeding in the absence of underlying causes such as preexisting gastrointestinal lesions. Dengue shock syndrome, usually accompanied by hemorrhagic signs, is much more serious and results from increased vascular permeability leading to shock. In mild DHF/DSS, restlessness, lethargy, thrombocytopenia (<100,000/μL), and hemoconcentration are detected 2–5 days after the onset of typical dengue fever, usually at the time of defervescence. The maculopapular rash that often develops in dengue fever may also appear in DHF/DSS. In more severe cases, frank shock is apparent, with low pulse pressure, cyanosis, hepatomegaly, pleural effusions, ascites, and in some cases severe ecchymoses and gastrointestinal bleeding. The period of shock lasts only 1 or 2 days, and most patients respond promptly to close monitoring, oxygen administration, and infusion of crystalloid or—in severe cases—colloid. The case-fatality rates reported vary greatly with case ascertainment and the quality of treatment; however, most DHF/DSS patients respond well to supportive therapy, and the overall mortality rate at an experienced center in the tropics is probably as low as 1%.

A virologic diagnosis can be made by the usual means, although multiple flavivirus infections lead to a broad immune response to several members of the group, and this situation may result in a lack of virus specificity of the IgM and IgG immune responses. A secondary antibody response can be sought with tests against several flavivirus antigens to demonstrate the characteristic wide spectrum of reactivity.

The key to control of both dengue fever and DHF/DSS is the control of *A. aegypti*, which also reduces the risk of urban yellow fever and chikungunya virus circulation. Control efforts have been handicapped by the presence of nondegradable tires and long-lived plastic containers in trash repositories, insecticide resistance, urban poverty, and an inability of the public health community to mobilize the populace to respond to the need to eliminate mosquito breeding sites. Live attenuated dengue vaccines are in the late stages of development and have produced promising results in early tests. Whether vaccines can provide safe, durable immunity to an immunopathologic disease such as DHF/DSS in endemic areas is an issue that will have to be tested, but it is hoped that vaccination will reduce transmission to negligible levels.

KYASANUR FOREST DISEASE AND OMSK HEMORRHAGIC FEVER

See Chap. 189 in *Harrison's Online* (*www.harrisonsonline.com*).

FILOVIRUS HEMORRHAGIC FEVER

See Chap. 190.

FURTHER READINGS

BRUNO P et al: The protean manifestations of hemorrhagic fever with renal syndrome. A retrospective review of 26 cases from Korea. Ann Intern Med 113:385, 1990

CALISHER CH: Medically important arboviruses of the United States and Canada. Clin Microbiol Rev 7:89, 1994

CENTERS FOR DISEASE CONTROL AND PREVENTION: Update: Management of patients with suspected viral hemorrhagic fever—United States. MMWR 44:475, 1995 (*http://www.cdc.gov/mmwr/preview/mmwrhtml/00038033.htm*)

DERESIEWICZ RL et al: Clinical and neuroradiographic manifestations of eastern equine encephalitis. N Engl J Med 336:1867, 1997

ENRIA D et al: Arenaviruses, in *Tropical Infectious Diseases: Principles, Pathogens, & Practice*, RL Guerrant et al (eds). New York, Saunders, 1999, pp 1189–1212

PETERS CJ, KHAN AS: Hantavirus pulmonary syndrome: The new American hemorrhagic fever. Clin Infect Dis 34:1224, 2002

RIVAS F et al: Epidemic Venezuelan equine encephalitis in La Guajira, Colombia, 1995. J Infect Dis 175:828, 1997

SOLOMON SR, VAUGHN DW: Pathogenesis and clinical features of Japanese encephalitis and West Nile virus infections. Curr Top Microbiol Immunol 267:171, 2002

SOLOMON T et al: West Nile encephalitis. BMJ 326:865, 2003

WURTZ R, PALEOLOGOS N: La Crosse encephalitis presenting like herpes simplex encephalitis in an immunocompromised adult. Clin Infect Dis 31:1113, 2000

CHAPTER 189

Infections Caused by Arthropod- and Rodent-Borne Viruses

190 Ebola and Marburg Viruses
Clarence J. Peters

DEFINITION

Both Marburg virus and Ebola virus cause an acute febrile illness associated with high mortality. This illness is characterized by multisystem involvement that begins with the abrupt onset of headache, myalgias, and fever and proceeds to prostration, rash, and shock and often to bleeding manifestations. Epidemics usually begin with a single case acquired from an unknown reservoir in nature and spread mainly through close contact with sick persons or their body fluids, either at home or in the hospital.

ETIOLOGY

The family Filoviridae (Fig. 190-1) comprises two antigenically and genetically distinct genera: *Marburgvirus* and *Ebolavirus*. *Ebolavirus* has four readily distinguishable species named for their original sites of recognition: Zaire, Sudan, Côte d'Ivoire, and Reston. Except for the Reston virus, all the Filoviridae are African viruses that cause severe and often fatal disease in humans. The Reston virus, which has been exported from the Philippines on several occasions, has caused fatal infections in monkeys but only subclinical infections in humans. Different strains of the four Ebola species, isolated over time and space, exhibit remarkable sequence conservation, indicating marked genetic stability in their selective niche.

Typical filovirus particles contain a single linear, negative-sense, single-stranded RNA arranged in a helical nucleocapsid. The virions are 790–970 nm in length; they may also appear in elongated, contorted forms. The lipid envelope confers sensitivity to lipid solvents and common detergents. The viruses are largely destroyed by heat (60°C, 30 min) and by acidity but may persist for weeks in blood at room temperature. The surface glycoprotein self-associates to form the virion surface spikes, which presumably mediate attachment to cells and fusion. The glycoprotein's high sugar content may contribute to its low capacity to elicit neutralizing antibodies. A smaller form of the glycoprotein, bearing many of its antigenic determinants, is produced by in vitro–infected cells and is found in the circulation in human disease; it has been speculated that this circulating soluble protein may suppress the immune response to the virion surface protein or block antiviral effector mechanisms. Both Marburg virus and Ebola virus are biosafety level 4 pathogens because of their high associated mortality rate and aerosol infectivity.

FIGURE 190-1 Ebola virions: diagnostic specimen from the first passage in Vero cells of a blood sample from a patient. Some of the filamentous (negatively stained) virions were fused together, end-to-end, giving the appearance of a "bowl of spaghetti." This image was from the first isolation and visualization of Ebola virus in 1970. *(Courtesy of Fredrick A. Murphy, MD, University of Texas Medical Branch, Galveston, Texas; with permission.)*

EPIDEMIOLOGY

Marburg virus was first identified in Germany in 1967, when infected African green monkeys (*Cercopithecus aethiops*) imported from Uganda transmitted the agent to workers in a vaccine laboratory. Of the 25 human cases acquired from monkeys, seven ended in death. The six secondary cases were associated with close contact or parenteral exposure. Secondary spread to the wife of one patient was documented, and virus was isolated from the husband's semen despite the presence of circulating antibodies. Subsequently, isolated cases of Marburg virus infection have been reported from eastern and southern Africa, with limited spread.

In 1999, repeated transmission of Marburg virus to workers in a gold mine in eastern Democratic Republic of the Congo was documented. The secondary spread of the virus among patients' families was more extensive than previously noted, resembling that of Ebola virus and emphasizing the importance of hygiene and proper barrier nursing in the epidemiology of these viruses in Africa.

In 2004–2005, an alarming, massive Marburg virus epidemic, with >250 cases, occurred in Angola. The epidemiologic features resembled those of the Ebola virus epidemics described below, and the case-fatality rate was 90%. This high figure may have been due in part to poor conditions in African hospitals; however, the virus isolated in this epidemic was slightly different phylogenetically from other known strains and exhibited increased virulence in nonhuman primates.

In 1976, epidemics of severe hemorrhagic fever (550 human cases) occurred simultaneously in Zaire and Sudan, and Ebola virus was found to be the etiologic agent. Later, it was shown that different species of virus (with associated mortality rates of 90% and 50%, respectively) had caused the two epidemics. Both epidemics were associated with interhuman spread (particularly in the hospital setting) and the use of unsterilized needles and syringes—a common practice in developing-country hospitals. The epidemics dwindled as the clinics were closed and as people in the endemic area increasingly shunned affected persons and avoided traditional burial practices.

The Zaire Ebola virus recurred in a major epidemic (317 cases, 88% mortality rate) in the Democratic Republic of the Congo in 1995 and in smaller epidemics in Gabon in 1994–1996. Mortality rates were high, transmission to caregivers and others who had direct contact with body fluids was common, and poor hygiene in hospitals exacerbated spread. In the Congo epidemic, an index case was infected in Kikwit in January 1995. The epidemic smoldered until April, when intense nosocomial transmission forced closure of the hospitals; samples were finally sent to the laboratory for Ebola testing, which yielded positive results within a few hours. International assistance, with barrier nursing instruction and materials, was provided; nosocomial transmission ceased, hospitals reopened, and patients were segregated to prevent intrafamilial spread. The last case was reported in June 1995.

Separate emergences of Ebola virus (Zaire) were detected in Gabon in 1994–2003, usually in association with deep-forest exposure and subsequent familial and nosocomial transmission. Die-offs of nonhuman primates were sometimes documented, and Ebola infection was confirmed in at least some animals. In a 1996 episode, a physician exposed to Ebola-infected patients traveled to South Africa with a fever; a nurse who assisted in a cutdown on the physician developed Ebola hemorrhagic fever and died despite intensive care. The index patient was identified retrospectively on the basis of serum antibodies and virus isolation from semen. No additional cases were detected from care of the primary or secondary case, nor were there any secondary cases following care of an unsuspected Côte d'Ivoire Ebola case in Switzerland. Thus, distant transport of Ebola virus is an established risk, but limited nosocomial spread occurs under proper hygienic conditions.

In 2000–2001, an indolent outbreak of Sudan Ebola virus claimed the lives of 224 (53%) of 425 patients with presumptive cases in Uganda.

Reston Ebola virus was first seen in the United States in 1989, when it caused a fatal, highly transmissible disease among cynomolgus macaques imported from the Philippines and quarantined in Reston, Virginia, pending distribution to biomedical researchers. This and other appearances of the Reston virus have been traced to a single export facility in the Philippines, but no source in nature has been established.

Epidemiologic studies (including a specific search in the Kikwit epidemic) have failed to yield evidence for an important role of airborne particles in human disease. This lack of epidemiologic evidence is surprising and seems to conflict with the viruses' classification as biosafety level 4 pathogens (which is based in part on their aerosol infectivity) and with formal laboratory assessments showing a high degree of aerosol infectivity for monkeys. Sick humans apparently do not usually generate sufficient amounts of infectious aerosols to pose a significant hazard to those around them.

Although numerous die-offs have recently been reported among chimpanzees and gorillas (some even threatening the viability of these endangered species), these animals (like humans) appear to be sentinels for virus activity. Speculation about the true reservoirs has centered on bats, and preliminary evidence indicates that bats may indeed be the reservoirs of filoviruses. This evidence includes the detection of antibodies and reverse-transcriptase polymerase chain reaction (RT-PCR) products in bats, the epidemiologic findings in subterranean gold mines in Durba (Democratic Republic of the Congo) where Marburg transmission has occurred, and reported associations of human antibody production with the handling of bats.

PATHOLOGY AND PATHOGENESIS

In humans and in animal models, Ebola and Marburg viruses replicate well in virtually all cell types, including endothelial cells, macrophages, and parenchymal cells of multiple organs. The earliest involvement—that of the mononuclear phagocyte system—is responsible for initiation of the disease process. Viral replication is associated with cellular necrosis both in vivo and in vitro. Significant findings at the light-microscopic level include liver necrosis with Councilman bodies, intracellular inclusions that correlate with extensive collections of viral nucleocapsids, interstitial pneumonitis, cerebral glial nodules, and small infarcts. Antigen and virions are abundant in fibroblasts, interstitium, and (to a lesser extent) the appendages of the subcutaneous tissues in fatal cases; escape through small breaks in the skin or possibly through sweat glands may occur and, if so, may be correlated with the established epidemiologic risk of close contact with patients and the touching of the deceased. Inflammatory cells are not prominent, even in necrotic areas.

In addition to sustaining direct damage from viral infection, patients infected with Ebola virus (Zaire) have high circulating levels of proinflammatory cytokines, which presumably contribute to the severity of the illness. In fact, the virus interacts intimately with the cellular cytokine system. It is resistant to the antiviral effects of interferon α, although this mediator is amply induced. Viral infection of endothelial cells selectively inhibits the expression of major histocompatibility complex class I molecules and blocks the induction of several genes by the interferons. In addition, glycoprotein expression inhibits αV integrin expression, an effect that has been shown to lead to detachment and subsequent death of endothelial cells in vitro.

Acute infection is associated with high levels of circulating virus and viral antigen. Clinical improvement takes place when viral titers decrease concomitantly with the onset of a virus-specific immune response, as detected by enzyme-linked immunosorbent assay (ELISA) or fluorescent antibody testing. In fatal cases, there is usually little evidence of an antibody response, and there is extensive depletion of spleen and lymph nodes. Recovery is apparently mediated by the cellular immune response: convalescent-phase plasma has little in vitro virus-neutralizing capacity and is not protective in passive transfer experiments in monkey and guinea pig models.

CLINICAL MANIFESTATIONS

After an incubation period of ~7–10 days (range, 3–16 days), the patient abruptly develops fever, severe headache, malaise, myalgia, nausea, and vomiting. Continued fever is joined by diarrhea (often severe), chest pain (accompanied by cough), prostration, and depressed mentation. In light-skinned patients (and less often in dark-skinned individuals), a maculopapular rash appears around day 5–7 and is followed by desquamation. Bleeding may begin about this time and is apparent from any mucosal site and into the skin. In some epidemics, fewer than half of patients have had overt bleeding, and this manifestation has been absent even in some fatal cases. Additional findings include edema of the face, neck, and/or scrotum; hepatomegaly; flushing; conjunctival injection; and pharyngitis. Around 10–12 days after the onset of disease, the sustained fever may break, with improvement and eventual recovery of the patient. Recrudescence of fever may be associated with secondary bacterial infections or possibly with localized virus persistence. Late hepatitis, uveitis, and orchitis have been reported, with isolation of virus from semen or detection of PCR products in vaginal secretions for several weeks.

LABORATORY FINDINGS

Leukopenia is common early on; neutrophilia has its onset later. Platelet counts fall below (sometimes much below) 50,000/μL. Laboratory evidence of disseminated intravascular coagulation is found, but its clinical significance and the need for therapy are controversial. Serum levels of alanine and aspartate aminotransferases (particularly the latter) rise progressively, and jaundice develops in some cases. The serum amylase level may be elevated, and this elevation may be associated with abdominal pain, suggesting pancreatitis. Proteinuria is usual; decreased kidney function is proportional to shock.

DIAGNOSIS

Most patients acutely ill as a result of infection with Ebola or Marburg virus have high concentrations of virus in blood. Antigen-detection ELISA is a sensitive, robust diagnostic modality. Virus isolation and RT-PCR are also effective and provide additional sensitivity in some cases. Patients who are recovering develop IgM and IgG antibodies that are best detected by ELISA but are also reactive in the less specific fluorescent antibody test. Skin biopsies are an extremely useful adjunct in postmortem diagnosis of infection with Ebola virus (and, to a lesser extent, Marburg virus) because of the presence of large amounts of viral antigen, the relatively low risk posed by sample collection, and the lack of cold-chain requirements for formalin-fixed tissues.

℞ EBOLA AND MARBURG VIRUS INFECTIONS

No virus-specific therapy is available, and—given the extensive viral involvement in fatal cases—supportive treatment may not be as useful as was once hoped. However, recent studies in rhesus monkeys have shown improved survival among animals treated with an inhibitor of factor VIIa/tissue factor or with activated protein C. Vigorous treatment of shock should take into account the likelihood of vascular leak in the pulmonary and systemic circulation and of myocardial functional compromise. The membrane fusion mechanism of Ebola virus resembles that of retroviruses, and the identification of "fusogenic" sequences suggests that inhibitors of cell entry may be developed. Despite the poor neutralizing capacity of polyclonal convalescent-phase sera, phage display of immunoglobulin mRNA from convalescent-phase bone marrow has yielded monoclonal antibodies that have in vitro neutralizing capacity and mediate protection in guinea pig models (but, unfortunately, not in monkey models).

PREVENTION

No vaccine or antiviral drug is currently available, but barrier nursing precautions in African hospitals can greatly decrease the spread of the virus beyond the index case and thus prevent epidemics of infection with filoviruses and with other agents as well. An adenovirus-vectored Ebola glycoprotein gene has proved protective in nonhuman primates and is undergoing phase 1 trials in humans.

FURTHER READINGS

FELDMANN H et al: Proceedings of an international symposium on filoviruses. J Infect Dis Suppl, 2007

GEISBERT TW et al: Treatment of Ebola virus infection with a recombinant inhibitor of factor VIIa/tissue factor: A study in rhesus monkeys. Lancet 362:1953, 2003

PETERS CJ, LeDUC JW: An introduction to Ebola: The virus and

1242

the disease. J Infect Dis 179(Suppl 1):ix, 1999 (Also available at *www.journals.uchicago.edu/JID/*)

SANCHEZ A et al: Analysis of human peripheral blood samples from fatal and nonfatal cases of Ebola (Sudan) hemorrhagic fever: Cellular responses, virus load, and nitric oxide levels. J Virol 78:10370, 2004

SULLIVAN NT: Accelerated vaccination for Ebola virus haemorrhagic fever in non-human primates. Nature 424:681, 2003

TOWNER JS et al: *Marburgvirus* genomics and association with a large hemorrhagic fever outbreak in Angola. J Virol 80:6497, 2006

SECTION 16 — FUNGAL AND ALGAL INFECTIONS

191 Diagnosis and Treatment of Fungal Infections
John E. Edwards, Jr.

TERMINOLOGY AND MICROBIOLOGY

Traditionally, fungal infections have been classified into specific categories based on both anatomic location and epidemiology. The most common general anatomic categories are mucocutaneous and deep organ infection; the most common general epidemiologic categories are endemic and opportunistic. Although *mucocutaneous infections* can cause serious morbidity, they are rarely fatal. *Deep organ infections* also cause severe illness in many cases but, in contrast to mucocutaneous infections, are often fatal. The *endemic mycoses* (e.g., coccidioidomycosis) are infections caused by fungal organisms that are not part of the normal human microbial flora and are acquired from environmental sources. In contrast, *opportunistic mycoses* are caused by organisms (e.g., *Candida* and *Aspergillus*) that frequently are components of the normal human flora and whose ubiquity in nature renders them easily acquired by the immunocompromised host. Opportunistic fungi cause serious infections when the immunologic response of the host becomes ineffective, allowing the organisms to transition from harmless commensals to invasive pathogens. Frequently, the diminished effectiveness of the immune system is a result of advanced modern therapies that coincidentally either unbalance the host's microflora or directly interfere with immunologic responses. Endemic mycoses cause more severe illness in immunocompromised patients than in immunocompetent individuals.

Patients acquire infection with endemic fungi almost exclusively by inhalation. The soil is the natural reservoir for the vast majority of endemic mycoses. The dermatophytic fungi may be acquired by human-to-human transmission, but the majority of infections result from environmental contact. In contrast, the opportunistic fungus *Candida* invades the host from normal sites of colonization, usually the mucous membranes of the gastrointestinal tract. In general, innate immunity is the primary defense mechanism against fungi. Although antibodies are formed during many fungal infections (and even during commensalism), they generally do not constitute the primary mode of defense. Nevertheless, in selected infections, as discussed below, measurement of antibody titers may be a useful diagnostic test.

Three other terms frequently used in clinical discussions of fungal infections are *yeast*, *mold*, and *dimorphic fungus*. *Yeasts* are seen as rounded single cells or as budding organisms. *Candida* and *Cryptococcus* are traditionally classified as yeasts. Molds grow as filamentous forms called *hyphae* both at room temperature and when they invade tissue. *Aspergillus*, *Rhizopus* [the species that causes mucormycosis (zygomycosis)], and fungi commonly infecting the skin to cause ringworm and related cutaneous conditions are classified as molds. Variations occur within this classification of yeasts and molds. For instance, when *Candida* infects tissue, both yeasts and filamentous forms may occur (except with *C. glabrata*, which forms only yeasts in tissue); in contrast, *Cryptococcus* exists only in yeast form. *Dimorphic* is the term used to describe fungi that grow as yeasts or large spherical structures in tissue but as filamentous forms at room temperature in the environment. Classified in this group are the organisms causing blastomycosis, paracoccidioidomycosis, coccidioidomycosis, histoplasmosis, blastomycosis, and sporotrichosis.

The incidence of fungal infections has risen substantially over the past several decades. Opportunistic infections have increased in frequency as a consequence of intentional immunosuppression in organ and stem cell transplantation and many other diseases, the administration of cytotoxic chemotherapy for cancers, and the liberal use of antibacterial agents. The incidence of endemic mycoses has increased in geographic locations where there has been substantial population growth.

DIAGNOSIS

The definitive diagnosis of any fungal infection requires histopathologic identification of the fungus invading tissue, accompanied by evidence of an inflammatory response. The identification of an inflammatory response has been especially important with regard to *Aspergillus* infection. *Aspergillus* is ubiquitous and can float from the air onto biopsy material. Therefore, in rare but important instances, this fungus is an ex vivo contaminant during processing of a specimen for microscopy, with a consequent incorrect diagnosis. The stains most commonly used to identify fungi are periodic acid–Schiff and Gomori methenamine silver. *Candida*, unlike other fungi, is visible on gram-stained tissue smears. Hematoxylin and eosin stain is not sufficient to identify *Candida* in tissue specimens. When positive, an India ink preparation of cerebrospinal fluid (CSF) is diagnostic for cryptococcosis. Most laboratories now use calcofluor white staining coupled with fluorescent microscopy to identify fungi in fluid specimens.

Extensive investigations of the diagnosis of deep organ fungal infections have yielded a variety of tests with different degrees of specificity and sensitivity. The most reliable tests are the detection of antibody to *Coccidioides immitis* and *Histoplasma capsulatum* in serum and CSF, the detection of cryptococcal polysaccharide antigen in serum and CSF, and the detection of *Histoplasma* antigen in urine or serum. The test for galactomannan has been used extensively in Europe and is now approved in the United States for diagnosis of aspergillosis. This test requires additional validation before its true usefulness can be determined. Sources of concern are the incidence of false-negative results and the need for multiple serial tests to reduce this incidence. The β-glucan test for *Candida* is also under evaluation but, like the galactomannan test, requires additional validation. Numerous polymerase chain reaction assays to detect antigens are in the developmental stages, as are nucleic acid hybridization techniques; however, these methods are not currently used on a widespread basis in major medical centers.

Of the fungal organisms, *Candida* is by far most frequently recovered from blood. Although *Candida* species can be detected with any of the automated blood culture systems widely used at present, the lysis-centrifugation technique increases the sensitivity of blood cultures for less common organisms (e.g., *H. capsulatum*) and should be used when disseminated fungal infection is suspected.

Except in the cases of coccidioidomycosis, cryptococcosis, and histoplasmosis, there are no fully validated and widely used tests for serodiagnosis of disseminated fungal infection. Skin tests for the endemic mycoses are no longer available.

This discussion is intended as a brief overview of general strategies for the use of antifungal agents in the treatment of fungal infections. Details on regimens, schedules, and strategies are discussed in the chapters on specific mycoses that follow in this section.

Since fungal organisms are eukaryotic cells that contain most of the same organelles (with many of the same physiologic functions) as human cells, the identification of drugs that selectively kill or inhibit fungi but are not toxic to human cells has been highly problematic. Far fewer antifungal than antibacterial agents have been introduced into clinical medicine.

AMPHOTERICIN B (AmB)   The introduction of AmB in the late 1950s revolutionized the treatment of fungal infections in deep organs. Before AmB became available, cryptococcal meningitis and other disseminated fungal infections were nearly always fatal. For nearly a decade after AmB was introduced, it was the only effective agent for the treatment of life-threatening fungal infections. AmB remains the broadest-spectrum antifungal agent but carries several disadvantages, including significant nephrotoxicity, lack of an oral preparation, and unpleasant side effects (fever, chills, and nausea) during treatment. To circumvent nephrotoxicity and infusion side effects, lipid formulations of AmB were developed and have virtually replaced the original colloidal deoxycholate formulation in clinical use (although the older formulation is still available). The lipid formulations include liposomal AmB (L-AB; 435 mg/kg per day) and AmB lipid complex (ABLC; 5 mg/kg per day). A third preparation, AmB colloidal dispersion (ABCD; 3–4 mg/kg per day), is rarely used because of the high incidence of side effects associated with infusion. (The doses listed are standard doses for adults with invasive infection.)

The lipid formulations of AmB have the disadvantage of being considerably more expensive than the deoxycholate formulation. Experience is still accumulating on the comparative efficacy, toxicity, and advantages of the different formulations for specific clinical fungal infections [e.g., central nervous system (CNS) infection]. Whether there is a clinically significant difference in these drugs with respect to CNS penetration or nephrotoxicity remains controversial. Despite these issues and despite the expense, the lipid formulations are now much more commonly used than AmB deoxycholate in the United States.

AZOLES   This class of antifungal drugs offers important advantages over AmB: the azoles cause little or no nephrotoxicity and are available in oral preparations. Early azoles included ketoconazole and miconazole, which have been replaced by newer agents for the treatment of deep organ fungal infections. The azoles' mechanism of action is inhibition of ergosterol synthesis in the fungal cell wall. Unlike AmB, these drugs are considered fungistatic, not -cidal.

Fluconazole   Since its introduction, fluconazole has played an extremely important role in the treatment of a wide variety of serious fungal infections. Its major advantages are the availability of both oral and IV formulations, a long half-life, satisfactory penetration of most body fluids (including ocular fluid and CSF), and minimal toxicity (especially relative to AmB). Its disadvantages include (usually reversible) hepatotoxicity and—at high doses—alopecia, muscle weakness, and dry mouth with a metallic taste. Fluconazole is not effective for the treatment of aspergillosis, mucormycosis, or *Scedosporium apiospermum* infections. It is less effective than the newer azoles against *C. glabrata* and *C. krusei*.

Fluconazole has become the agent of choice for the treatment of coccidioidal meningitis, although relapses have followed therapy with this drug. In addition, fluconazole is useful for both consolidation and maintenance therapy for cryptococcal meningitis. This agent has been shown to be as efficacious as AmB in the treatment of candidemia. The effectiveness of fluconazole in candidemia and the drug's relatively minimal toxicity, in conjunction with the inadequacy of diagnostic tests for widespread hematogenously disseminated candidiasis, have led to a change in the paradigm for candidemia management. The standard of care is now to treat all candidemic patients with an antifungal agent and to change all their intravascular lines, if feasible, rather than merely to remove a singular suspect intravascular line and then observe the patient. The usual fluconazole regimen for treatment of candidemia is 400 mg/d given until 2 weeks after the last positive blood culture.

Fluconazole is considered effective as fungal prophylaxis in bone marrow transplant recipients and high-risk liver transplant patients. Its use for pro-phylaxis in patients with leukemia, in AIDS patients with low CD4+ T cell counts, and in patients on surgical intensive care units remains controversial.

Voriconazole   Like fluconazole, voriconazole is available in both oral and IV formulations. Voriconazole has a broader spectrum than fluconazole against *Candida* species (including *C. glabrata* and *C. krusei*) and is active against *Aspergillus*, *Scedosporium*, and *Fusarium*. It is generally considered the first-line drug of choice for treatment of aspergillosis. A few case reports have shown voriconazole to be effective in individual patients with coccidioidomycosis, blastomycosis, and histoplasmosis, but (because of limited data) this agent is not recommended for treatment of the endemic mycoses. Among the disadvantages of voriconazole (compared with fluconazole) are its more numerous interactions with many of the drugs used in patients predisposed to fungal infections. Hepatotoxicity, skin rashes (including photosensitivity), and visual disturbances are relatively common. Voriconazole is also considerably more expensive than fluconazole. Moreover, it is advisable to monitor voriconazole levels in certain patients since (1) this drug is completely metabolized in the liver by CYP2C9, CYP3A4, and CYP2C19; and (2) human genetic variability in CYP2C19 activity exists. Dosages should be reduced accordingly in those patients with liver failure. Dose adjustments for renal insufficiency are not necessary; however, because the IV formulation is prepared in cyclodextrin, it should not be given to patients with severe renal insufficiency.

Itraconazole   Itraconazole is available in IV and oral (capsule and suspension) formulations. Varying blood levels among patients taking oral itraconazole reflect a disadvantage compared with the other azoles. Itraconazole is the drug of choice for mild to moderate histoplasmosis and blastomycosis and has often been used for chronic mucocutaneous candidiasis. It has been approved by the U.S. Food and Drug Administration (FDA) for use in febrile neutropenic patients. Itraconazole has also proven useful for the treatment of chronic coccidioidomycosis, sporotrichosis, and *S. apiospermum* infection. The mucocutaneous and cutaneous fungal infections that have been treated successfully with itraconazole include oropharyngeal candidiasis (especially in AIDS patients), tinea versicolor, tinea capitis, and onychomycosis. Disadvantages of itraconazole include its poor penetration into the CSF, the use of cyclodextrin in both the oral suspension and the IV preparation, the variable absorption of the capsules, and the need for monitoring of blood levels in patients taking capsules for disseminated mycoses. In recent years, reported cases of severe congestive heart failure in patients taking itraconazole have been a source of concern. Like the other azoles, itraconazole can cause hepatic toxicity.

Posaconazole   Posaconazole is approved by the FDA for prophylaxis of aspergillosis and candidiasis in patients at high risk for developing these infections because of severe immunocompromise. This drug has also been evaluated for the treatment of zygomycosis, fusariosis, aspergillosis, and oropharyngeal candidiasis. The relevant studies of posaconazole in zygomycosis, fusariosis, and aspergillosis have examined salvage therapy. A study of >90 patients whose zygomycosis was refractory to other therapy yielded encouraging results. No trials of posaconazole for the treatment of candidemia have yet been reported. Case reports have described the drug's efficacy in coccidioidomycosis and histoplasmosis. Controlled trials have shown its effectiveness as a prophylactic agent in patients with acute leukemia and in bone marrow transplant recipients. In addition, posaconazole has been found to be effective against fluconazole-resistant *Candida* species. The results of a large-scale study of the use of posaconazole as salvage therapy for aspergillosis have been promising but, as of this writing, have not been published in a peer-reviewed format.

ECHINOCANDINS   The echinocandins, including the approved drugs caspofungin, anidulafungin, and micafungin, have added considerably to the antifungal armamentarium. All three of these agents inhibit β-1,3-glucan synthase, which is necessary for cell wall synthesis in fungi and is not a component of human cells. None of these agents is available in an oral formulation. The echinocandins are considered fungicidal for *Candida* and fungistatic for *Aspergillus*. Their greatest use to date is against candidal infections. They offer two advantages: broad-spectrum activity against all *Candida* species and relatively low toxicity. The minimum inhibitory concentrations (MICs) of all the echinocandins are highest against *C. parapsilosis*; it is not clear whether these higher MIC values represent less clinical effectiveness against this species. The echinocandins are among the safest antifungal agents.

In controlled trials, *caspofungin* has been at least as efficacious as AmB for the treatment of candidemia and invasive candidiasis and as efficacious as fluconazole for the treatment of candidal esophagitis. In addition, caspofungin has been efficacious as salvage therapy for aspergillosis. At present, it is used most extensively for the treatment of candidemic patients, especially before the infecting species is precisely identified.

Anidulafungin has been approved by the FDA as therapy for candidemia in nonneutropenic patients and for *Candida* esophagitis, intraabdominal infection, and peritonitis. In controlled trials, anidulafungin has been more efficacious than fluconazole against candidemia and invasive candidiasis and as efficacious as fluconazole against candidal esophagitis. When anidulafungin is used with cyclosporine, tacrolimus, or voriconazole, no dosage adjustment is required for either drug in the combination.

Micafungin has been approved for the treatment of esophageal candidiasis and for prophylaxis in patients receiving stem cell transplants. Studies thus far have shown that coadministration of micafungin and cyclosporine does not require dose adjustments for either drug. When micafungin is given with sirolimus, the AUC rises for sirolimus, usually necessitating a reduction in its dose. In open-label trials, favorable results have been obtained with micafungin for the treatment of deep-seated *Aspergillus* and *Candida* infections.

FLUCYTOSINE (5-FLUOROCYTOSINE)   The use of flucytosine has diminished in recent years as newer antifungal drugs have been developed. Flucytosine has a unique mechanism of action based on intrafungal conversion to 5-fluorouracil, which is toxic to the cell. Development of resistance to the compound has limited its use as a single agent. Flucytosine is nearly always used in combination with AmB. Its good penetration into the CSF makes it attractive for use with AmB for treatment of cryptococcal meningitis. Flucytosine has also been recommended for the treatment of candidal meningitis in combination with AmB; comparative trials with AmB alone have not been done. Significant and frequent bone marrow depression is seen with flucytosine when this drug is used with AmB.

GRISEOFULVIN AND TERBINAFINE   Historically, griseofulvin has been useful primarily for ringworm infection. This agent is usually given for relatively long periods. Terbinafine has been used primarily for onychomycosis but also for ringworm. In comparative studies, terbinafine has been as effective as itraconazole and more effective than griseofulvin for both conditions.

TOPICAL ANTIFUNGAL AGENTS   A detailed discussion of the agents used for the treatment of cutaneous fungal infections and onychomycosis is beyond the scope of this chapter; the reader is referred to the dermatology literature. Many classes of compounds have been used to treat the common fungal infections of the skin. Among the azoles used are clotrimazole, econazole, miconazole, oxiconazole, sulconazole, ketoconazole, tioconazole, butaconazole, and terconazole. In general, topical treatment of vaginal candidiasis has been successful. Since there is considered to be little difference in the efficacy of the various vaginal preparations, the choice of agent is made by the physician and/or the patient on the basis of preference and availability. Fluconazole given orally at 150 mg has the advantage of not requiring repeated intravaginal application. Nystatin is a polyene that has been used for both oropharyngeal thrush and vaginal candidiasis. Useful agents in other classes include ciclopirox olamine, halprogin, terbinafine, naftifine, tolnaftate, and undecylenic acid.

FURTHER READINGS

BATTI Z et al: Review of epidemiology, diagnosis, and treatment of invasive mould infections in allogeneic hematopoietic stem cell transplant recipients. Mycopathologia 162:1, 2006

CHU JH et al: Hospitalizations for endemic mycoses: A population-based national study. Clin Infect Dis 42:822, 2006

DEPAUW BE: Increasing fungal infections in the intensive care unit. Surg Infect (Larchmt) 7(Suppl 2):S93, 2006

DISMUKES WE: Antifungal therapy: Lessons learned over the past 27 years. Clin Infect Dis 42:1289, 2006

ENOCH DA et al: Invasive fungal infections: A review of epidemiology and management options. J Med Microbiol 55:809, 2006

KAUFFMAN CA: Clinical efficacy of new antifungal agents. Curr Opin Microbiol 9:1, 2006

LIPSETT PA: Surgical critical care: Fungal infections in surgical patients. Crit Care Med 34(9 Suppl):S215, 2006

MANDELL GL et al (eds): Mycoses, in *Principles and Practice of Infectious Diseases*, 6th ed. Elsevier Churchill Livingstone, Philadelphia, 2005, pp 2935–3094

WHEAT LJ: Antigen detection, serology, and molecular diagnosis of invasive mycoses in the immunocompromised host. Transpl Infect Dis 8:128, 2006

192   Histoplasmosis
Chadi A. Hage, L. Joseph Wheat

ETIOLOGY

Histoplasma capsulatum, a thermal dimorphic fungus, is the etiologic agent of histoplasmosis. In most endemic areas, *H. capsulatum* var. *capsulatum* is the causative agent; in Africa, *H. capsulatum* var. *duboisii* is also found. Mycelia—the naturally infectious form of *Histoplasma*—have a characteristic appearance, with microconidial and macroconidial forms. Microconidia are oval and are small enough (2–5 μm) to reach the terminal bronchioles and alveoli. Shortly after infecting the host, mycelia transform into the yeasts that are found inside macrophages and other phagocytes. The yeast forms are characteristically small (2–5 μm), with occasional narrow budding. In the laboratory, mycelia are best grown at room temperature, whereas yeasts are grown at 37°C on enriched media.

EPIDEMIOLOGY

Histoplasmosis is the most prevalent endemic mycosis in North America. Although this fungal disease has been reported throughout the world, its endemicity is particularly notable in certain parts of North, Central, and South America; Africa; and Asia. In the United States, the endemic areas spread over the Ohio and Mississippi river valleys. This pattern is related to the humid and acidic nature of the soil in these areas. Soil enriched with bird or bat droppings promotes the growth and sporulation of *Histoplasma*. Disruption of soil containing the organism leads to aerosolization of the microconidia and exposure of humans nearby. Activities associated with high-level exposure include spelunking, excavation, cleaning of chicken coops, demolition and remodeling of old buildings, and cutting of dead trees. Most cases seen outside of highly endemic areas represent imported disease—e.g., cases reported in Europe after travel to the Americas, Africa, or Asia.

PATHOGENESIS AND PATHOLOGY

Infection follows inhalation of microconidia (Fig. 192-1). Once they reach the alveolar spaces, microconidia are rapidly recognized and engulfed by alveolar macrophages. At this point, the microconidia transform into budding yeasts (Fig. 192-2), a process that is integral to the pathogenesis of histoplasmosis and is dependent on the availability of calcium and iron inside the phagocytes. The yeasts are capable of growing and multiplying inside resting macrophages. Neutrophils and then lymphocytes are attracted to the site of infection. Before the development of cellular immunity, yeasts use the phagosomes as a vehicle for translocation to local draining lymph nodes, whence they spread hematogenously throughout the reticuloendothelial system. Adequate cellular immunity develops ~2 weeks after infection. T cells produce interferon γ to assist the macrophages in killing the organism and controlling the progression of disease. Interleukin 12 and tumor necrosis factor α (TNF-α) play an essential role in cellular immunity to *H. capsulatum*. In the immunocompetent host, macrophages, lymphocytes, and epithelial cells eventually organize and form granulo-

FIGURE 192-1 Spiked spherical conidia of *H. capsulatum* (lactolphenol cotton blue stain).

FIGURE 192-3 Intracellular yeasts (*arrows*) of *H. capsulatum* in a liver biopsy specimen (hematoxylin and eosin stain).

mas that contain the organisms. These granulomas typically fibrose and calcify; calcified mediastinal lymph nodes and hepatosplenic calcifications are frequently found in healthy individuals from endemic areas. In immunocompetent hosts, infection with *H. capsulatum* confers some immunity to reinfection. In patients with impaired cellular immunity, the infection is not contained and can disseminate. Progressive disseminated histoplasmosis (PDH) can involve multiple organs, most commonly the bone marrow, spleen, liver (Fig. 192-3), adrenal glands, and mucocutaneous membranes. Unlike latent tuberculosis, latent histoplasmosis is rarely reactivated.

Structural lung disease (e.g., emphysema) impairs the clearance of pulmonary histoplasmosis, and chronic pulmonary disease can result. This chronic process is characterized by progressive inflammation, tissue necrosis, and fibrosis mimicking cavitary tuberculosis.

CLINICAL MANIFESTATIONS

The clinical spectrum of histoplasmosis ranges from asymptomatic infection to life-threatening illness. The attack rate and the extent and severity of the disease depend on the intensity of exposure, the im-

FIGURE 192-2 Small (2–5 μm) narrow budding yeasts of *H. capsulatum* from bronchoalveolar lavage fluid (Grocott's methenamine silver stain).

mune status of the exposed individual, and the underlying lung architecture of the host.

In immunocompetent individuals with low-level exposure, most *Histoplasma* infections are either asymptomatic or mild and self-limited. Of adults residing in endemic areas, 50–80% have skin-test and/or radiographic evidence of previous infection without clinical manifestations. When symptoms do develop, they usually appear 2–4 weeks after exposure. Heavy exposure leads to a flulike illness with fever, chills, sweats, headache, myalgia, anorexia, cough, dyspnea, and chest pain. Chest radiographs usually show signs of pneumonitis with hilar or mediastinal adenopathy. Pulmonary infiltrates may be focal with light exposure or diffuse with heavy exposure. Rheumatologic symptoms of arthralgia or arthritis, often associated with erythema nodosum, occur in 5–10% of patients with acute histoplasmosis. Pericarditis may also develop. These manifestations represent inflammatory responses to the acute infection rather than its direct effects. Hilar or mediastinal lymph nodes may undergo necrosis and coalesce to form large mediastinal masses that can cause compression of great vessels, proximal airways, and the esophagus. These necrotic lymph nodes also may rupture and create fistulas between mediastinal structures (e.g., bronchoesophageal fistulas).

PDH is typically seen in immunocompromised individuals, who account for ~70% of cases. Common risk factors include AIDS (CD4+ T cell count, <200/μL), extremes of age, and the use of immunosuppressive medications such as prednisone, methotrexate, and anti-TNF-α agents. The spectrum of PDH ranges from an acute, rapidly fatal course—with diffuse interstitial or reticulonodular lung infiltrates causing respiratory failure, shock, coagulopathy, and multiorgan failure—to a more subacute course with a focal organ distribution. Common manifestations include fever and weight loss. Hepatosplenomegaly is also common. Other findings may include meningitis or focal brain lesions, ulcerations of the oral mucosa, gastrointestinal ulcerations, and adrenal insufficiency. Prompt recognition of this devastating illness is of paramount importance in patients with more severe manifestations or with underlying immunosuppression, especially AIDS (Chap. 182).

Chronic cavitary histoplasmosis is seen in smokers who have structural lung disease (e.g., bullous emphysema). This chronic illness is characterized by productive cough, dyspnea, low-grade fever, night sweats, and weight loss. Chest radiographs usually show upper-lobe infiltrates, cavitation, and pleural thickening—findings resembling those of tuberculosis. Without treatment, the course is slowly progressive.

Fibrosing mediastinitis is an uncommon and serious complication of histoplasmosis. In certain patients, acute infection is followed for unknown reasons by progressive fibrosis around the hilar and mediastinal lymph nodes. Involvement may be unilateral or bilateral; bilateral involvement carries a worse prognosis. Major manifestations include superior vena cava syndrome, obstruction of pulmonary vessels, and

TABLE 192-1 RECOMMENDATIONS FOR THE TREATMENT OF HISTOPLASMOSIS

Type of Histoplasmosis	Treatment Recommendations	Comments
Acute pulmonary, moderate to severe illness with diffuse infiltrates and/or hypoxemia	Lipid amphotericin B (3–5 mg/kg per day) ± glucocorticoids for 1–2 weeks; then itraconazole (200 mg twice daily) for 12 weeks. Monitor renal and hepatic function.	Patients with mild cases usually recover without therapy, but itraconazole should be considered if the patient's condition has not improved after 1 month.
Chronic/cavitary pulmonary	Itraconazole (200 mg once or twice daily) for at least 12 months. Monitor hepatic function.	Continue treatment until radiographic findings show no further improvement. Monitor for relapse after treatment is stopped.
Progressive disseminated	Lipid amphotericin B (3–5 mg/kg per day) for 1–2 weeks; then itraconazole (200 mg twice daily) for at least 12 months. Monitor renal and hepatic function.	Liposomal amphotericin B is preferred, but the amphotericin B lipid complex may be used because of cost. Chronic maintenance therapy may be necessary if the degree of immunosuppression cannot be reduced.
Central nervous system	Liposomal amphotericin B (5 mg/kg per day) for 4–6 weeks; then itraconazole (200 mg 2 or 3 times daily) for at least 12 months. Monitor renal and hepatic function.	A longer course of lipid amphotericin B is recommended because of the high risk of relapse. Itraconazole should be continued until cerebrospinal fluid or CT abnormalities clear.

recurrent airway obstruction. Patients may experience recurrent pneumonia, hemoptysis, or respiratory failure. Fibrosing mediastinitis is fatal in up to one-third of cases.

In healed histoplasmosis, calcified mediastinal nodes or lung parenchyma may erode through the walls of the airways and cause hemoptysis. This condition is called *broncholithiasis*.

 African histoplasmosis caused by *H. capsulatum* var. *duboisii* is clinically distinct and is characterized by frequent skin and bone involvement.

DIAGNOSIS

Fungal culture remains the gold standard diagnostic test for histoplasmosis. However, culture results may not be known for up to 1 month, and cultures are often negative in less severe cases. Cultures are positive in ~75% of cases of PDH and chronic pulmonary histoplasmosis. Cultures of bronchoalveolar lavage (BAL) fluid are positive in about half of patients with acute pulmonary histoplasmosis causing diffuse infiltrates with hypoxemia. In PDH, the culture yield is highest for BAL fluid, bone marrow aspirate, and blood. Cultures of sputum or bronchial washings are usually positive in chronic pulmonary histoplasmosis. Cultures are typically negative, however, in other forms of histoplasmosis.

Fungal stains of cytopathology or biopsy materials showing structures resembling *Histoplasma* yeasts are helpful in the diagnosis of PDH, yielding positive results in about half of cases. Yeasts can be seen in BAL fluid (Fig. 192-2) from patients with diffuse pulmonary infiltrates, in bone marrow biopsy samples, and in biopsy specimens of other involved organs (e.g., the adrenal glands). Occasionally, yeasts are seen in blood smears from patients with severe PDH. However, staining artifacts and other fungal elements may be misidentified as *Histoplasma* yeasts.

The detection of *Histoplasma* antigen in body fluids is extremely useful in the diagnosis of PDH and acute diffuse pulmonary histoplasmosis. The sensitivity of this technique is >90% for urine and 80% for serum from patients with PDH and ~75% for urine from patients with acute pulmonary histoplasmosis. Antigen can be detected in cerebrospinal fluid from patients with meningitis and in BAL fluid from those with pneumonia. Cross-reactivity occurs with African histoplasmosis, blastomycosis, coccidioidomycosis, paracoccidioidomycosis, and *Penicillium marneffei* infection.

Serologic tests, including immunodiffusion and complement fixation, are especially useful for the diagnosis of self-limited acute pulmonary histoplasmosis; however, at least 1 month is required for the production of antibodies after acute infection. A fourfold rise in antibody titer may be seen in patients with acute pulmonary histoplasmosis. Serologic tests are also useful for the diagnosis of chronic pulmonary histoplasmosis. Limitations of serology, however, include insensitivity early in the course of infection in immunosuppressed patients and the persistence of detectable antibody for several years after infection. Pos-

itive results from past infection may lead to a misdiagnosis of active histoplasmosis in a patient with another disease process.

℞ HISTOPLASMOSIS

Treatment recommendations for histoplasmosis are summarized in **Table 192-1**. Treatment is indicated for all patients with PDH or chronic pulmonary histoplasmosis as well as for symptomatic patients with acute pulmonary histoplasmosis causing diffuse infiltrates, especially with hypoxemia. In the vast majority of cases, however, acute pulmonary histoplasmosis resolves without therapy, and treatment is not recommended.

The preferred treatments for histoplasmosis include the lipid formulations of amphotericin B in more severe cases and itraconazole in others. Liposomal amphotericin B has been more effective than the deoxycholate formulation for treatment of PDH in patients with AIDS. The deoxycholate formulation of amphotericin B is an alternative to a lipid formulation in patients who are at a low risk for nephrotoxicity. Posaconazole, voriconazole, and fluconazole are alternatives for patients who cannot take itraconazole.

In severe cases requiring hospitalization, a lipid formulation of amphotericin B is followed by itraconazole. In patients with meningitis, a lipid formulation of amphotericin B should be given for 4–6 weeks before the switch to itraconazole. In immunosuppressed patients, the degree of immunosuppression should be reduced if possible. Antiretroviral treatment improves the outcome of PDH in patients with AIDS and is recommended.

Blood levels of itraconazole should be monitored to ensure adequate drug exposure, and drug interactions should be carefully assessed: itraconazole not only is cleared by cytochrome P450 metabolism but also inhibits cytochrome P450. This profile causes interactions with many other medications.

The duration of treatment for acute pulmonary histoplasmosis is 6–12 weeks, while that for PDH and chronic pulmonary histoplasmosis is ≥1 year. Antigen levels in urine and serum should be monitored during and for at least 1 year after therapy for PDH. Stable or rising antigen levels suggest treatment failure or relapse.

Previously, lifelong itraconazole maintenance therapy was recommended for patients with AIDS once histoplasmosis was diagnosed. Today, however, maintenance therapy is not required for patients who respond well to antiretroviral therapy, with CD4+ T cell counts of at least 150/μL (preferably >250/μL); who complete at least 1 year of itraconazole therapy; and who exhibit neither clinical evidence of active histoplasmosis nor an antigenuria level of >4 ng/mL.

Fibrosing mediastinitis, which represents a chronic fibrotic reaction to past mediastinal histoplasmosis rather than an active infection, does not respond to antifungal therapy. While treatment is often prescribed for patients with acute pulmonary histoplasmosis who have not recovered within 1 month and for those with persistent mediastinal lymphadenopathy, the effectiveness of antifungal therapy in these situations is unknown.

FURTHER READINGS

GOLDMAN M et al: Safety of discontinuation of maintenance therapy for disseminated histoplasmosis after immunologic response to antiretroviral therapy. Clin Infect Dis 38:1485, 2004

GOODWIN R et al: Histoplasmosis in normal hosts. Medicine (Baltimore) 60:231, 1981

JOHNSON PC et al: Safety and efficacy of liposomal amphotericin B compared with conventional amphotericin B for induction therapy of histoplasmosis in patients with AIDS. Ann Intern Med 137:105, 2002

KAUFFMAN CA: Histoplasmosis: A clinical and laboratory update. Clin Microb Rev 20:115, 2007

NEWMAN SL: Cell-mediated immunity to *Histoplasma capsulatum*. Semin Respir Infect 16:102, 2001

VAIL GM et al: Incidence of histoplasmosis following allogeneic bone marrow transplant or solid organ transplant in a hyperendemic area. Transpl Infect Dis 4:148, 2002

WHEAT LJ: Current diagnosis of histoplasmosis. Trends Microbiol 11:488, 2003

———: Histoplasmosis. Experience during outbreaks in Indianapolis and review of the literature. Medicine (Baltimore) 76:339, 1997

———: Improvements in diagnosis of histoplasmosis. Expert Opin Biol Ther 6:1207, 2006

——— et al: Clinical practice guidelines for the management of patients with histoplasmosis: 2007 update by the Infectious Diseases Society of America. Clin Infect Dis 45:807, 2007

——— et al: Pulmonary histoplasmosis syndromes: Recognition, diagnosis, and management. Semin Respir Crit Care Med 25:129, 2004

193 Coccidioidomycosis
Neil M. Ampel

DEFINITION AND ETIOLOGY

Coccidioidomycosis, commonly known as valley fever, is caused by the dimorphic soil-dwelling fungus *Coccidioides*. Genetic analysis has demonstrated the existence of two species, *C. immitis* and *C. posadasii*. These species are indistinguishable with regard to the clinical disease they cause as well as in routine laboratory tests. Thus, the organism will be referred to simply as *Coccidioides* for the remainder of this chapter.

EPIDEMIOLOGY

Coccidioidomycosis is confined to the Western Hemisphere between the latitudes of 40°N and 40°S. In the United States, areas of high endemicity include the southern portion of the San Joaquin Valley of California, the south-central region of Arizona, and the southwestern Rio Grande Valley. However, infection may be acquired in other areas of the southwestern United States, including the southern coastal counties in California, southern Nevada, and southwestern Utah. Outside the United States, coccidioidomycosis is endemic to northern Mexico as well as to localized regions of Central America. In South America, there are endemic foci in Colombia, Venezuela, northeastern Brazil, Paraguay, Bolivia, and north-central Argentina.

The risk of infection is increased by direct exposure to soil harboring *Coccidioides*. Because of difficulty in isolating *Coccidioides* from the soil, the precise characteristics of potentially infectious soil are not known. In general, *Coccidioides* appears to be supported in previously uncultivated desert soil, such as that found in the Lower Sonoran Life Zone. However, several outbreaks have been associated with soil from archaeologic excavations of Amerindian sites both within and outside of the recognized endemic region.

In endemic areas, many cases of *Coccidioides* infection occur without obvious soil or dust exposure. Climatic factors appear to increase the infection rate in these regions. In particular, periods of dryness after rainy seasons have been associated with marked increases in the number of cases.

Recently, the number of cases of symptomatic coccidioidomycosis has increased dramatically in south-central Arizona, where most of the state's population resides. The factors causing this increase have not been fully elucidated; however, an influx of older, susceptible individuals into the region as well as increased construction in previously undeveloped desert appear to be involved.

PATHOGENESIS, PATHOLOGY, AND IMMUNE RESPONSE

On agar media and in the soil, *Coccidioides* exists as a filamentous mold. Within this mycelial structure, individual filaments (*hyphae*) elongate and branch, some growing upward. Cells within the hyphae degenerate, leaving alternating barrel-shaped viable cells called *arthroconidia*. Measuring only ~2 × 5 μm, arthroconidia may become airborne for extended periods. The small size of the arthroconidia also allows them to evade initial mechanical mucosal defenses and reach the alveolus, where infection is initiated in the nonimmune host.

Once in a susceptible host, the arthroconidia enlarge, become rounded, and develop internal septations. The resulting structures, called *spherules* (Fig. 193-1), may attain sizes of 80 μm and are unique to *Coccidioides*. The septations encompass uninuclear elements called *endospores*. Spherules may rupture and release packets of endospores that can themselves develop into spherules, thus propagating infection locally. If returned to artificial media or the soil, the fungus reverts to its mycelial stage.

Clinical observations and data from studies of animals strongly support the critical role of a robust cellular immune response in the host's control of coccidioidomycosis. Necrotizing granulomas containing spherules are typically identified in patients with resolved pulmonary infection. In disseminated disease, granulomas are generally

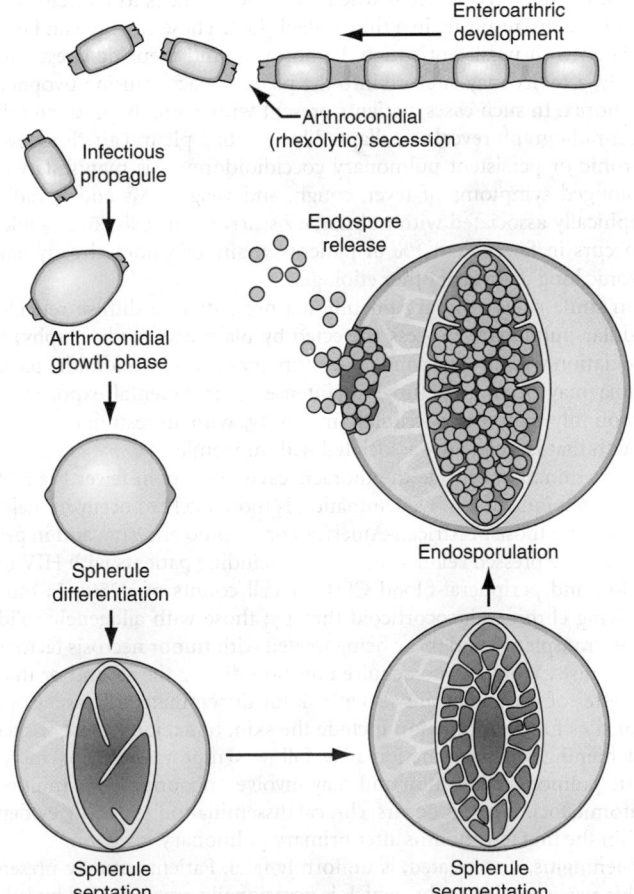

FIGURE 193-1 Life cycle of *Coccidioides*. *(From Kirkland TN, Fierer J: Coccidioidomycosis: A reemerging infectious disease. Emerg Infect Dis 2:192, 1996.)*

poorly formed or do not develop at all, and a polymorphonuclear leukocyte response occurs frequently. In patients who are asymptomatic or in whom the initial pulmonary infection resolves, delayed-type hypersensitivity to coccidioidal antigens is routinely documented.

CLINICAL AND LABORATORY MANIFESTATIONS

Coccidioidomycosis is protean in its manifestations. Of infected individuals, 60% are completely asymptomatic, and the remaining 40% have symptoms that are related principally to pulmonary infection, including fever, cough, and pleuritic chest pain. The risk of symptomatic illness increases with age. Coccidioidomycosis is commonly misdiagnosed as community-acquired bacterial pneumonia.

There are several cutaneous manifestations of primary pulmonary coccidioidomycosis. Toxic erythema consisting of a maculopapular rash has been noted in some cases. Erythema nodosum (typically over the lower extremities) or erythema multiforme (usually in a necklace distribution) may occur; these manifestations are seen particularly often in women. Arthralgias and arthritis may develop. The diagnosis of primary pulmonary coccidioidomycosis is suggested by a history of night sweats or profound fatigue as well as by peripheral-blood eosinophilia or hilar or mediastinal lymphadenopathy on chest radiography. While pleuritic chest pain is common, pleural effusion is less so, occurring in fewer than 10% of cases. Such effusions are invariably associated with a pulmonary infiltrate on the same side. The cellular content of these effusions is mononuclear in nature; *Coccidioides* is rarely grown from effusions.

Although primary pulmonary coccidioidomycosis usually resolves without sequelae, several complications may ensue. Pulmonary nodules are residua of primary pneumonia. Generally single, located in the upper lobes, and ≤4 cm in diameter, nodules are often discovered on a routine chest radiograph in an asymptomatic patient. Calcification is uncommon.

Pulmonary cavities occur when a nodule extrudes its contents into the bronchus, resulting in a thin-walled shell. These cavities can be associated with persistent cough, hemoptysis, and pleuritic chest pain. Rarely, a cavity may rupture into the pleural space, causing pyopneumothorax. In such cases, patients present with acute dyspnea, and the chest radiograph reveals a collapsed lung with a pleural air-fluid level. Chronic or persistent pulmonary coccidioidomycosis manifests with prolonged symptoms of fever, cough, and weight loss and is radiographically associated with pulmonary scarring, fibrosis, and cavities. It occurs in fewer than 1% of patients, many of whom already have chronic lung disease of other etiologies.

In some cases, primary pneumonia presents as a diffuse reticulonodular pulmonary process (detected by plain chest radiography) in association with dyspnea and fever. Primary diffuse coccidioidal pneumonia may occur in settings of intense environmental exposure or profoundly suppressed cellular immunity, with unrestrained fungal growth that is frequently associated with fungemia.

Dissemination outside the thoracic cavity occurs in fewer than 1% of infected individuals. Dissemination is more likely to occur in males, particularly those of African-American or Filipino ancestry, and in persons with depressed cellular immunity, including patients with HIV infection and peripheral-blood CD4+ T cell counts of <250/μL; those receiving chronic glucocorticoid therapy; those with allogeneic solid-organ transplants; and those being treated with tumor necrosis factor α antagonists. Women who acquire infection during the second or third trimester of pregnancy are also at risk for disseminated disease. Common sites for dissemination include the skin, bone, joints, soft tissues, and meninges. Dissemination may follow symptomatic or asymptomatic pulmonary infection and may involve only one site or multiple anatomic foci. When it occurs, clinical dissemination is usually evident within the first few months after primary pulmonary infection.

Meningitis, if untreated, is uniformly fatal. Patients usually present with a persistent headache, which is occasionally accompanied by lethargy and confusion. Nuchal rigidity, if present, is not severe. Examination of cerebrospinal fluid (CSF) demonstrates lymphocytic pleocytosis with profound hypoglycorrhachia and elevated protein levels. CSF eo-sinophilia is occasionally documented. With or without appropriate therapy, patients may develop hydrocephalus, which presents clinically as a marked decline in mental status, often with gait disturbances.

DIAGNOSIS

As mentioned above, coccidioidomycosis is often misdiagnosed as community-acquired bacterial pneumonia. Serology plays an important role in establishing the diagnosis of coccidioidomycosis. Several techniques are available, including the traditional tube-precipitin (TP) and complement-fixation (CF) assays, immunodiffusion (IDTP and IDCF), and enzyme immunoassay (EIA) to detect IgM and IgG antibodies. TP antibody is found in serum soon after infection and persists for weeks. TP titers are not useful for gauging disease progression, and this antibody is not found in the CSF. Titers of CF antibody generally rise later than do those of TP antibody, and CF antibody usually persists longer. Rising CF titers are associated with clinical progression, and the presence of CF antibody in CSF is an indicator for coccidioidal meningitis.

Because of its commercial availability, the coccidioidal EIA is frequently used as a screening tool for coccidioidal serology. However, the frequent false-positive results obtained with the IgM EIA make this test unreliable. Instead, the traditional TP or IDTP should be used. In addition, while the sensitivity and specificity of the IgG EIA appear to be high when compared with those of the CF and IDCF assays, the optical density obtained in the EIA does not correlate with the serologic titer of either of the latter tests.

Coccidioides grows within 3–7 days at 37°C on a variety of artificial media, including blood agar. Therefore, it is always useful to obtain samples of sputum or other respiratory fluids and tissues for culture in suspected cases of coccidioidomycosis. The clinical laboratory should be alerted to the possibility of this diagnosis, since *Coccidioides* can pose a significant hazard to laboratory workers if it is inadvertently inhaled. *Coccidioides* can also be identified directly. While treatment of samples with potassium hydroxide is rarely fruitful in establishing the diagnosis, examination of sputum or other respiratory fluids after Papanicolaou or Gomori methenamine silver staining reveals spherules in a significant proportion of patients with pulmonary coccidioidomycosis. For fixed tissues (e.g., those obtained from biopsy specimens), spherules with surrounding inflammation can be demonstrated with hematoxylin-eosin or Gomori methenamine silver staining.

Rx COCCIDIOIDOMYCOSIS

(Table 193-1) Currently, there are two main classes of antifungals useful for the treatment of coccidioidomycosis. While once routinely prescribed, amphotericin B in all its formulations is now reserved for only the most severe cases of dissemination and for intrathecal or intraventricular administration to patients with coccidioidal meningitis in whom triazole therapy has failed. The original formulation of amphotericin B, which is dispersed with deoxycholate, is usually administered intravenously in doses of 0.7–1.0 mg/kg either daily or three times per week. The newer lipid-based formulations—amphotericin B lipid complex (ABLC), amphotericin B colloidal dispersion (ABCD), and amphotericin B liposomal complex—appear to offer no therapeutic advantage over the deoxycholate formulation but are associated with less renal toxicity. The lipid dispersions are administered intravenously at doses of 5 mg/kg daily or three times per week.

Triazole antifungals are the principal drugs now used to treat most cases of coccidioidomycosis. Clinical trials have demonstrated the usefulness of both fluconazole and itraconazole, and evidence indicates that itraconazole may be more efficacious against bone and joint disease. Because of its demonstrated penetration into CSF, fluconazole is the azole of choice for the treatment of coccidioidal meningitis. For both drugs, a minimal oral adult dosage of 400 mg/d should be used. The maximal dose of itraconazole is 200 mg three times daily, but higher doses of fluconazole may be given. Two newer triazole antifungals, posaconazole and voriconazole, are now available. However, given the paucity of clinical data, the high cost, and (particularly for voriconazole) the potential toxicity, these agents should be reserved for cases that remain recalcitrant when treated with fluconazole or itraconazole. High-dose triazole therapy may be teratogen-

TABLE 193-1	CLINICAL PRESENTATIONS OF COCCIDIOIDOMYCOSIS, THEIR FREQUENCY, AND RECOMMENDED INITIAL THERAPY FOR THE IMMUNOCOMPETENT HOST

Clinical Presentation	Frequency, %	Recommended Therapy
Asymptomatic	60	None
Primary pneumonia (focal)	40	In most cases, none[a]
Diffuse pneumonia	<1	Amphotericin B followed by prolonged oral triazole therapy
Pulmonary sequelae	5	
Nodule	—	None
Cavity	—	In most cases, none[b]
Chronic pneumonia	—	Prolonged triazole therapy
Disseminated disease	≤1	
Skin, bone, joint, soft tissue	—	Prolonged triazole therapy[c]
Meningitis	—	Life-long triazole therapy[d]

[a]Treatment is indicated for hosts with depressed cellular immunity as well as for those with prolonged symptoms and signs of increased severity, including night sweats for >3 weeks, weight loss of >10%, a complement-fixation titer of >16, and extensive pulmonary involvement on chest radiography.
[b]Treatment (usually the oral triazoles fluconazole and itraconazole) is recommended for persistent symptoms.
[c]In severe cases, some clinicians would use amphotericin B as initial therapy.
[d]Intraventricular or intrathecal amphotericin B is recommended in cases of triazole failure. Hydrocephalus may occur, requiring a CSF shunt.

ic; thus, amphotericin B should be considered as therapy for coccidioidomycosis in pregnant women.

Most patients with focal primary pulmonary coccidioidomycosis require no therapy. Patients for whom antifungal therapy should be considered include those with underlying cellular immunodeficiencies and those with prolonged symptoms and signs of extensive disease. Specific criteria include symptoms persisting for ≥2 months, night sweats occurring for >3 weeks, weight loss of >10%, a serum CF antibody titer of >1:16, and extensive pulmonary involvement apparent on chest radiograph.

Diffuse pulmonary coccidioidomycosis represents a special situation. Because most patients with this form of disease are profoundly hypoxemic and critically ill, many clinicians favor beginning therapy with amphotericin B and switching to an oral triazole once clinical improvement occurs.

The nodules that may follow primary pulmonary coccidioidomycosis do not require treatment. However, nodules are not easily distinguished from pulmonary malignancies by means of radiographic imaging (including positron emission tomography scans). Close clinical follow-up and biopsy may be required to distinguish these two entities. Most pulmonary cavities do not require therapy. Antifungal treatment should be considered in patients with persistent cough, pleuritic chest pain, and hemoptysis. Occasionally, pulmonary coccidioidal cavities become secondarily infected. This development is usually manifested by an air-fluid level within the cavity. Bacterial flora or *Aspergillus* species are commonly involved, and therapy directed at these organisms should be considered. Surgery is rarely required except in cases of persistent hemoptysis or pyopneumothorax. For chronic pulmonary coccidioidomycosis, prolonged antifungal thera-

py—lasting for at least 1 year—is usually required, with monitoring of symptoms, radiographic changes, sputum cultures, and serologic titers.

Most cases of disseminated coccidioidomycosis require prolonged antifungal therapy. Duration of treatment is based on resolution of the signs and symptoms of the lesion in conjunction with a significant decline in serum CF antibody titer. Such therapy routinely is continued for at least several years. Relapse occurs in 15–30% of individuals once therapy is discontinued.

Coccidioidal meningitis poses a special challenge. While most patients with this form of disease respond to treatment with oral triazoles, 80% experience relapse when therapy is stopped. Thus, life-long therapy is recommended. In cases of triazole failure, intrathecal or intraventricular amphotericin B may be used. Installation requires considerable expertise and should be performed only by an experienced health care provider. Shunting of CSF in addition to appropriate antifungal therapy is required in cases of meningitis complicated by hydrocephalus. It is prudent to obtain expert consultation in all cases of coccidioidal meningitis.

PREVENTION

There are no proven methods to reduce the risk of acquiring coccidioidomycosis among residents of an endemic region. Avoidance of direct contact with uncultivated soil or with visible dust containing soil presumably reduces the risk. Prophylactic antifungal therapy may be useful in patients who have evidence of active or recent coccidioidomycosis and are about to undergo allogeneic solid-organ transplantation. Data on the use of antifungal agents for prophylaxis in other situations are scanty and do not suggest efficacy.

FURTHER READINGS

BERGSTROM L et al: Increased risk of coccidioidomycosis in patients treated with tumor necrosis factor alpha antagonists. Arthritis Rheum 50:1959, 2004

BLAIR JE et al: The prevention of recrudescent coccidioidomycosis after solid organ transplantation. Transplantation 83:1182, 2007

DiCAUDO DJ et al: The exanthem of acute pulmonary coccidioidomycosis: Clinical and histopathologic features of 3 cases and review of the literature. Arch Dermatol 142:744, 2006

DRUTZ DJ, CATANZARO A: Coccidioidomycosis (parts I and II). Am Rev Respir Dis 117:559 and 727, 1978

FISHER MC et al: Molecular and phenotypic description of *Coccidioides posadasii* sp. nov., previously recognized as the non-California population of *Coccidioides immitis*. Mycologia 94:73, 2002

GALGIANI JN et al: Coccidioidomycosis. Clin Infect Dis 41:1217, 2005

——— et al: Comparison of oral fluconazole and itraconazole for progressive, nonmeningeal coccidioidomycosis. A randomized, double-blind trial. Mycoses Study Group. Ann Intern Med 133:676, 2000

PARK BJ et al: An epidemic of coccidioidomycosis in Arizona associated with climatic changes, 1998–2001. J Infect Dis 191:1981, 2005

VALDIVIA L et al: Coccidioidomycosis as a common cause of community-acquired pneumonia. Emerg Infect Dis 12:958, 2006

194 Blastomycosis

Stanley W. Chapman, Donna C. Sullivan

Blastomycosis is a systemic pyogranulomatous infection, primarily involving the lungs, that arises after inhalation of the conidia of *Blastomyces dermatitidis*. Pulmonary blastomycosis varies from an asymptomatic infection to acute or chronic pneumonia. Hematogenous dissemination occurs frequently. Extrapulmonary disease of the skin, bones, and genitourinary system is common, but almost any organ can be infected.

ETIOLOGIC AGENT

B. dermatitidis is the asexual state of *Ajellomyces dermatitidis*. Two serotypes have been identified on the basis of the presence or absence of the A antigen. *B. dermatitidis* exhibits thermal dimorphism, growing as the mycelial phase at room temperature and as the yeast phase at 37°C. Primary isolation is most dependable for the mycelial phase incubated at 30°C. Definitive identification usually requires conversion to the yeast phase at 37°C or, more commonly, the use of nucleic acid amplification techniques (e.g., AccuProbe, Gen-Probe, San Diego, CA) that detect mycelial-phase growth. Yeast cells are usually 8–15 μm in diameter, have thick refractile cell walls, are multinucleate, and reproduce by a single, large, broad-based bud.

EPIDEMIOLOGY

Most cases of blastomycosis have been reported in North America. Endemic areas include the southeastern and south-central states bordering the Mississippi and Ohio river basins, the midwestern states and Canadian provinces bordering the Great Lakes, and a small area in New York and Canada along the St. Lawrence River. Outside North America, blastomycosis has been reported most frequently in Africa.

Early studies of endemic cases indicated that middle-aged men with outdoor occupations were at greatest risk. Reported outbreaks, however, do not suggest a predilection according to sex, age, race, occupation, or season. *B. dermatitidis* probably grows as microfoci in the warm, moist soil of wooded areas rich in organic debris. Exposure to soil, whether related to work or recreation, appears to be the common factor associated with infection.

PATHOGENESIS

After inhalation, the conidia of *B. dermatitidis* are susceptible to phagocytosis and killing in the lungs by polymorphonuclear leukocytes, monocytes, and alveolar macrophages. This phagocytic response represents innate immunity and probably explains the high frequency of asymptomatic infections in outbreaks. Conidia that escape phagocytosis rapidly convert to the yeast phase in tissue. The greater resistance of the thick-walled yeast form to phagocytosis and killing probably contributes to infection. This yeast-phase conversion also induces the expression of the 120-kDa glycoprotein BAD-1, which is an adhesin, an essential virulence factor, and the major epitope for humoral and cellular immunity. The primary acquired host defense against *B. dermatitidis* is cellular immunity mediated by antigen-specific T cells and lymphokine-activated macrophages.

APPROACH TO THE PATIENT:
Blastomycosis

Whether acute or chronic, blastomycosis mimics many other disease processes. For example, acute pulmonary blastomycosis may present with signs and symptoms indistinguishable from those of bacterial pneumonia or influenza. Chronic pulmonary blastomycosis most commonly mimics malignancy or tuberculosis. Skin lesions are often misdiagnosed as basal cell or squamous cell carcinoma, pyoderma gangrenosum, or keratoacanthoma. Laryngeal lesions are frequently mistaken for squamous cell carcinoma. Thus, the clinician must maintain a high index of suspicion and perform a careful histologic evaluation of secretions or biopsy material from patients who live in or have visited regions endemic for blastomycosis.

CLINICAL MANIFESTATIONS

Acute pulmonary infection is usually diagnosed in association with point-source outbreaks and is accompanied by the abrupt onset of fever, chills, pleuritic chest pain, arthralgias, and myalgias. Cough is initially nonproductive but frequently becomes purulent as disease progresses. Chest radiographs usually reveal alveolar infiltrates with consolidation. Pleural effusions and hilar adenopathy are uncommon. Most patients diagnosed with pulmonary blastomycosis have chronic indolent pneumonia with signs and symptoms of fever, weight loss, productive cough, and hemoptysis. The most common radiologic findings are alveolar infiltrates with or without cavitation, mass lesions that mimic bronchogenic carcinoma, and fibronodular infiltrates. Respiratory failure (adult respiratory distress syndrome) associated with miliary disease or diffuse pulmonary infiltrates is more common among immunocompromised patients, especially those in the late

TABLE 194-1 TREATMENT OF BLASTOMYCOSIS

Disease	Primary Therapy	Alternative Therapy
Immunocompetent Patient/Life-Threatening Disease		
Pulmonary	AmB,[a] 0.7–1.0 mg/kg qd (total dose: 1.5–2.5 g)	Itraconazole, 200–400 mg/d (once patient's condition has stabilized)
Disseminated CNS	AmB, 0.7–1.0 mg/kg qd (total dose: at least 2 g)	Fluconazole, 800 mg/d (if patient is intolerant to full course of AmB)
Non-CNS	AmB, 0.7–1.0 mg/kg qd (total dose: 1.5–2.5 g)	Itraconazole, 200–400 mg/d (once patient's condition has stabilized)
Immunocompetent Patient/Non-Life-Threatening Disease		
Pulmonary or disseminated (non-CNS)	Itraconazole, 200–400 mg/d or AmB, 0.5–0.7 mg/kg qd (in patients intolerant to itraconazole or whose disease progresses despite therapy)	Fluconazole, 400–800 mg/d or Ketoconazole, 400–800 mg/d
Immunocompromised Patient[b]		
All infections	AmB, 0.7–1.0 mg/kg qd (total dose: 1.5–2.5 g)	Itraconazole, 200–400 mg/d (non-CNS disease, once clinically improved)

[a] In all regimens listed, an AmB lipid formulation (3.0–5.0 mg/kg qd) can be substituted for AmB deoxycholate.
[b] Suppressive therapy with itraconazole may be considered for patients whose immunocompromised state continues. Fluconazole (800 mg/d) may be useful for patients who have CNS disease or are intolerant to itraconazole.
Note: AmB, amphotericin B; CNS, central nervous system.

stages of AIDS (Chap. 182). Mortality rates are ≥50% among these patients, and most deaths occur within the first few days of therapy.

Skin disease is the most common extrapulmonary manifestation of blastomycosis. Two types of skin lesions occur: verrucous (more common) and ulcerative. Osteomyelitis is associated with as many as one-fourth of *B. dermatitidis* infections. The vertebrae, pelvis, sacrum, skull, ribs, or long bones are most frequently involved. Patients with *B. dermatitidis* osteomyelitis often present with contiguous soft-tissue abscesses or chronic draining sinuses. In men, blastomycosis may involve the prostate and epididymis. Central nervous system (CNS) disease occurs in <5% of immunocompetent patients with blastomycosis. In AIDS patients, however, CNS disease has been reported in ~40% of cases, usually presenting as a brain abscess. Less common forms of CNS disease are cranial or spinal epidural abscess and meningitis.

DIAGNOSIS

Definitive diagnosis of blastomycosis requires growth of the organism from sputum, pus, or biopsy material. A presumptive diagnosis is made by visualization of the characteristic broad-based budding yeast in clinical specimens. Serologic diagnosis of blastomycosis is of limited usefulness because of cross-reactivity with other fungal antigens.

A *Blastomyces* antigen assay that detects antigen in urine and serum is commercially available (Mira Vista Diagnostics, Indianapolis, IN). Antigen detection in urine appears to be more sensitive than serum antigen detection. This antigen test may be useful for monitoring of patients during therapy or for early detection of relapse.

℞ BLASTOMYCOSIS

The Infectious Diseases Society of America has published guidelines for the treatment of blastomycosis. Selection of an appropriate therapeutic regimen must be based on the clinical form and severity of the disease, the immune status of the patient, and the toxicity of the antifungal agent (Table 194-1). Although spontaneous cures of acute pulmonary infection have been well documented, there are no criteria by which to distinguish patients whose disease will progress or disseminate. Thus, almost all patients with blastomycosis should be treated.

Itraconazole is the agent of choice for immunocompetent patients with mild to moderate pulmonary or non-CNS extrapulmonary disease.

Therapy is continued for 6–12 months. Amphotericin B is the preferred initial treatment for patients who are severely immunocompromised, who have life-threatening disease or CNS disease, or whose disease progresses during treatment with itraconazole. Although not rigorously studied, lipid formulations of amphotericin B can provide an alternative for patients who cannot tolerate amphotericin B deoxycholate. Most patients with non-CNS disease whose clinical condition improves after an initial course of amphotericin B (usually 2 weeks in duration) can be switched to itraconazole to complete 6–12 months of therapy. Fluconazole, because of its excellent penetration of the CNS, may have a role in the treatment of patients with brain abscess or meningitis after an initial course of amphotericin B.

The newer triazoles voriconazole and posaconazole have not been studied extensively in human cases of blastomycosis. The echinocandins have variable activity against *B. dermatitidis* and have no place in the treatment of blastomycosis.

PROGNOSIS

Clinical and mycologic response rates are 90–95% among compliant immunocompetent patients given itraconazole for mild to moderate pulmonary and extrapulmonary disease without CNS involvement.

195 Cryptococcosis
Arturo Casadevall

DEFINITION AND ETIOLOGY

Cryptococcus neoformans, a yeast-like fungus, is the etiologic agent of cryptococcosis. Cryptococcal strains are antigenically and genetically diverse. Both *C. neoformans* and *C. gattii* are pathogenic for humans and can cause cryptococcosis. *C. neoformans* consists of serotypes A and D, and *C. gattii* consists of serotypes B and C. Currently, most authorities further subdivide *C. neoformans* into two varieties: *grubii* (serotype A) and *neoformans* (serotype D). Most clinical microbiology laboratories do not routinely distinguish among cryptococcal species and varieties but rather identify all isolates simply as *C. neoformans*.

EPIDEMIOLOGY

Cryptococcosis was first described in the 1890s but remained relatively rare until the mid-twentieth century, when advances in diagnosis and increases in the number of immunosuppressed individuals markedly raised its reported prevalence. The spectrum of disease caused by *C. neoformans* consists predominantly of meningoencephalitis and pneumonia, but skin and soft tissue infections also occur. Serologic studies have shown that, although cryptococcal *infection* is common among immunocompetent individuals, cryptococcal *disease* (cryptococcosis) is relatively rare in the absence of impaired immunity. Individuals at high risk for cryptococcosis include patients with hematologic malignancies, recipients of solid organ transplants who require ongoing immunosuppressive therapy, persons whose medical conditions necessitate glucocorticoid therapy, and patients with advanced HIV infection and CD4+ T lymphocyte counts of <200/μL. Since the onset of the HIV pandemic in the early 1980s, the overwhelming majority of cryptococcosis cases have occurred in patients with AIDS (Chap. 182). To understand the impact of HIV infection on the epidemiology of cryptococcosis, it is instructive to note that in the early 1990s there were >1000 cases of cryptococcal meningitis each year in New York City—a figure far exceeding that for all cases of bacterial meningitis. With the advent of effective antiretroviral therapy, the incidence of AIDS-related cryptococcosis has been sharply reduced among treated individuals; however, the disease remains distressingly common in regions where antiretroviral therapy is not readily available, such as Africa and Asia, where up to one-third of patients with AIDS have cryptococcosis.

Bone and joint disease usually requires 12 months of therapy. The <5% of infections that relapse after an initial course of itraconazole usually respond well to a second treatment course.

FURTHER READINGS

BRADSHER RW: Blastomycosis, in *Clinical Mycology*, WE Dismukes et al (eds). New York, Oxford University Press, 2003, pp 299–310

—— et al: Blastomycosis. Infect Dis Clin North Am 17:21, 2003

CHAPMAN SW: *Blastomyces dermatitidis*, in *Principles and Practice of Infectious Diseases*, 6th ed, GL Mandell et al (eds). New York, Churchill Livingstone, 2005, pp 3026–3040

——, SULLIVAN DC: Diagnosis and treatment of blastomycosis, in *Diagnosis and Treatment of Human Mycoses*, D Hospental, M Rinaldi (eds). Totowa, NJ, Humana Press, 2007

—— et al: Practice guidelines for the management of patients with blastomycosis. Clin Infect Dis 30:679, 2000 (updates: *www.idsociety.org*)

DEEPE GS et al: Progress in vaccination for histoplasmosis and blastomycosis: Coping with cellular immunity. Med Mycol 43:381, 2005

Cryptococcal infection is acquired from the environment. *C. neoformans* and *C. gattii* inhabit different ecologic niches. *C. neoformans* is frequently found in soils contaminated with avian excreta and can easily be recovered from shaded and humid soils contaminated with pigeon droppings. In contrast, *C. gattii* is not found in bird feces. Instead, it inhabits a variety of arboreal species, including several types of eucalyptus tree. *C. neoformans* strains are found throughout the world; however, var. *grubii* (serotype A) strains are far more common than var. *neoformans* (serotype D) strains among both clinical and environmental isolates. The geographic distribution of *C. gattii* was thought to be largely limited to tropical regions until an outbreak of cryptococcosis caused by a new serotype B strain began in Vancouver in 1999. In addition to the different geographic distributions of the two cryptococcal species, individual susceptibility to these species affects epidemiology. Cryptococcosis caused by the *C. neoformans* varieties occurs mostly in individuals with AIDS (Chap. 182) and other forms of impaired immunity. In contrast, *C. gattii*–related disease is not associated with specific immune deficits and often occurs in immunocompetent individuals.

PATHOGENESIS

Cryptococcal infection is acquired by inhalation of aerosolized infectious particles. The exact nature of these particles is not known; the two leading candidate forms are small desiccated yeast cells and basidiospores. Little is known about the pathogenesis of initial infection. Serologic studies have shown that cryptococcal infection is acquired in childhood, but it is not known whether the initial infection is symptomatic. Given serologic documentation that cryptococcal infection is common yet cryptococcal disease is rare, the consensus is that pulmonary defense mechanisms in immunologically intact individuals are highly effective at containing *C. neoformans*. It is not clear whether initial infection leads to a state of immunity or whether most individuals are subject throughout life to frequent and recurrent infections that resolve without clinical disease. However, evidence indicates that some human cryptococcal infections lead to a state of latency in which viable organisms are harbored for prolonged periods, possibly in granulomas. Thus the inhalation of *C. neoformans* can be followed by clearance of the organism or establishment of the latent state. The consequences of prolonged harboring of *C. neoformans* in the lung are not known, but evidence from animal studies indicates that the organism's prolonged presence could alter the immunologic milieu in the lung and predispose to allergic airway disease.

Cryptococcosis usually presents clinically as chronic meningoencephalitis. The mechanisms by which *C. neoformans* undergoes extrapulmonary

FIGURE 195-1 Cryptococcal antigen in human brain tissue, as revealed by immunohistochemical staining. Brown areas show polysaccharide deposits in the midbrain of a patient who died of cryptococcal meningitis. *(Reprinted with permission from SC Lee et al: Hum Pathol 27:839, 1996.)*

dissemination and enters the central nervous system (CNS) remain poorly understood. There is evidence that yeast cells can migrate directly across the endothelium by a mechanism that may be associated with changes in polysaccharide structure. *C. neoformans* has well-defined virulence factors that include the polysaccharide capsule, the ability to make melanin, and the elaboration of enzymes (e.g., phospholipase and urease) that enhance the survival of fungal cells in tissue. Among these virulence factors, the capsule and melanin production have been most extensively studied. The *C. neoformans* capsule is antiphagocytic, and the capsular polysaccharide has been associated with numerous deleterious effects on host immune function. Cryptococcal infections elicit little or no tissue inflammatory response. The immune dysfunction seen in cryptococcosis has been attributed to the release of copious amounts of capsular polysaccharide into tissues, where it probably interferes with local immune responses (Fig. 195-1). In clinical practice, the cryptococcal polysaccharide is the antigen that is measured as a diagnostic marker of *C. neoformans* infection.

APPROACH TO THE PATIENT:
Cryptococcosis

Cryptococcosis should be included in the differential diagnosis when any patient presents with findings suggestive of chronic meningitis. Concern about cryptococcosis is heightened by a history of headache and neurologic symptoms in a patient with an underlying immunosuppressive disorder or state that is associated with an increased incidence of cryptococcosis, such as advanced HIV infection or solid organ transplantation.

CLINICAL MANIFESTATIONS
The clinical manifestations of cryptococcosis reflect the site of fungal infection. *C. neoformans* infection can affect any tissue or organ, but the majority of cases that come to clinical attention involve the CNS and/or the lungs. CNS involvement usually presents as signs and symptoms of chronic meningitis, such as headache, fever, lethargy, sensorium deficits, memory deficits, cranial nerve paresis, vision deficits, and meningismus. Cryptococcal meningitis differs from bacterial meningitis in that many *Cryptococcus*-infected patients present with symptoms of several weeks' duration. In addition, classic characteristics of meningeal irritation, such as meningismus, may be absent in cryptococcal meningitis. Indolent cases can present as subacute dementia. Meningeal cryptococcosis can lead to sudden catastrophic vision loss.

Pulmonary cryptococcosis usually presents as cough, increased sputum production, and chest pain. Patients infected with *C. gattii* can present with granulomatous pulmonary masses known as *cryptococco-*

mas. Fever develops in a minority of cases. Like CNS disease, pulmonary cryptococcosis can follow an indolent course, and the majority of cases probably do not come to clinical attention. In fact, many cases are discovered incidentally during the workup of an abnormal chest radiograph obtained for other diagnostic purposes. Pulmonary cryptococcosis is often associated with antecedent diseases such as malignancy, diabetes, and tuberculosis.

Skin lesions are common in patients with disseminated cryptococcosis and can be highly variable, including papules, plaques, purpura, vesicles, tumor-like lesions, and rashes. The spectrum of cryptococcosis in HIV-infected patients is so varied and has changed so much since the advent of antiretroviral therapy that a distinction between HIV-related and HIV-unrelated cryptococcosis is no longer pertinent. In patients with AIDS and solid organ transplant recipients, the lesions of cutaneous cryptococcosis often resemble those of molluscum contagiosum (Fig. 195-2; Chap. 182).

DIAGNOSIS
A diagnosis of cryptococcosis requires the demonstration of *C. neoformans* in normally sterile tissues. Visualization of the capsule of fungal cells in cerebrospinal fluid (CSF) mixed with India ink is a useful rapid diagnostic technique. *C. neoformans* cells in India ink have a distinctive appearance because their capsules exclude ink particles. However, the CSF India ink examination may yield negative results in patients with a low fungal burden. This examination should be performed by a trained individual, since leukocytes and fat globules can sometimes be mistaken for fungal cells. Cultures of CSF and blood that are positive for *C. neoformans* are diagnostic for cryptococcosis. In cryptococcal meningitis, CSF examination usually reveals evidence of chronic meningitis with mononuclear cell pleocytosis and increased protein levels. A particularly useful test is cryptococcal antigen (CRAg) detection in CSF and blood. The assay is based on serologic detection of cryptococcal polysaccharide and is both sensitive and specific. A positive cryptococcal antigen test provides strong presumptive evidence for cryptococcosis; however, because the result is often negative in pulmonary cryptococcosis, the test is less useful in the diagnosis of pulmonary disease.

℞ CRYPTOCOCCOSIS

Both the site of infection and the immune status of the host must be considered in the selection of therapy for cryptococcosis. The disease has two

FIGURE 195-2 Disseminated fungal infection. A liver transplant recipient developed six cutaneous lesions similar to the one shown. Biopsy and serum antigen testing demonstrated *Cryptococcus*. Important features of the lesion include a benign-appearing fleshy papule with central umbilication resembling molluscum contagiosum. *(Photo courtesy of Dr. Lindsey Baden; with permission.)*

general patterns of manifestation: (1) pulmonary cryptococcosis, with no evidence of extrapulmonary dissemination; and (2) extrapulmonary (systemic) cryptococcosis, with or without meningoencephalitis. Pulmonary cryptococcosis in an immunocompetent host sometimes resolves without therapy. However, given the propensity of *C. neoformans* to disseminate from the lung, the inability to gauge the host's immune status precisely, and the availability of low-toxicity therapy in the form of fluconazole, the current recommendation is for pulmonary cryptococcosis in an immunocompetent individual to be treated with fluconazole (200–400 mg/d for 3–6 months). Extrapulmonary cryptococcosis without CNS involvement in an immunocompetent host can be treated with the same regimen, although amphotericin B (AmB; 0.5–1.0 mg/kg daily for 4–6 weeks) may be required for more severe cases. In general, extrapulmonary cryptococcosis without CNS involvement requires less intensive therapy—with the caveat that morbidity and death in cryptococcosis are associated with meningeal involvement. Thus the decision to categorize cryptococcosis as "extrapulmonary without CNS involvement" should be made only after careful evaluation of the CSF reveals no evidence of *C. neoformans* infection. For CNS involvement in a host without AIDS or obvious immune impairment, most authorities recommend initial therapy with AmB (0.5–1.0 mg/kg daily) during an induction phase, which is followed by prolonged therapy with fluconazole (400 mg/d) during a consolidation phase. For cryptococcal meningoencephalitis without a concomitant immunosuppressive condition, the recommended regimen is AmB (0.5–1.0 mg/kg) plus flucytosine (100 mg/kg) daily for 6–10 weeks. Alternatively, patients can be treated with AmB (0.5–1.0 mg/kg) plus flucytosine (100 mg/kg) daily for 2 weeks and then with fluconazole (400 mg/d) for at least 10 weeks. Patients with immunosuppression are treated with the same initial regimens except that consolidation therapy with fluconazole is given for a prolonged period to prevent relapse.

Cryptococcosis in patients with HIV infection always requires aggressive therapy and is considered incurable unless immune function improves. Consequently, therapy for cryptococcosis in the setting of AIDS has two phases: induction therapy (intended to reduce the fungal burden and alleviate symptoms) and lifelong maintenance therapy (to prevent a symptomatic clinical relapse). Pulmonary and extrapulmonary cryptococcosis without evidence of CNS involvement can be treated with fluconazole (200–400 mg/d). In patients who have more extensive disease, flucytosine (100 mg/d) may be added to the fluconazole regimen for 10 weeks, with lifelong fluconazole maintenance therapy thereafter. For HIV-infected patients with evidence of CNS involvement, most authorities recommend induction therapy with AmB. An acceptable regimen is AmB (0.7–1.0 mg/kg) plus flucytosine (100 mg) daily for 2 weeks followed by fluconazole (400 mg/d) for at least 10 weeks and then by lifelong maintenance therapy with fluconazole (200 mg/d). Fluconazole (400–800 mg/d) plus flucytosine (150–100 mg/d) for 6–10 weeks followed by fluconazole (200 mg/d) as maintenance therapy can be used as an alternative. Lipid formulations of AmB can be substituted for AmB deoxycholate in patients with renal impairment. Neither caspofungin nor mycofungin is effective against *C. neoformans*, and neither drug has a role in the treatment of cryptococcosis. Cryptococcal meningoencephalitis is often associated with increased intracranial pressure, which is believed to be responsible for damage to the brain and cranial nerves. Appropriate management of CNS cryptococcosis requires careful attention to the management of intracranial pressure, including the reduction of pressure by repeated therapeutic lumbar puncture and the placement of shunts.

In HIV-infected patients with previously treated cryptococcosis who are receiving fluconazole maintenance therapy, it may be possible to discontinue antifungal drug treatment if antiretroviral therapy results in immunologic improvement. However, certain recipients of maintenance therapy who have a history of successfully treated cryptococcosis can develop a troublesome immune reconstitution syndrome when antiretroviral therapy produces a rebound in immunologic function.

PROGNOSIS AND COMPLICATIONS

Even with antifungal therapy, cryptococcosis is associated with high rates of morbidity and death. For the majority of patients with cryptococcosis, the most important prognostic factor is the extent and the duration of the underlying immunologic deficits that predisposed them to develop the disease. Therefore, cryptococcosis is often curable with antifungal therapy in individuals with no apparent immunologic dysfunction, but, in patients with severe immunosuppression (e.g., those with AIDS), the best that can be hoped for is that antifungal therapy will induce remission, which can then be maintained with lifelong suppressive therapy. Before the advent of antiretroviral therapy, the median overall survival period for AIDS patients with cryptococcosis was <1 year. Cryptococcosis in patients with underlying neoplastic disease has a particularly poor prognosis. For CNS cryptococcosis, poor prognostic markers are a positive CSF assay for yeast cells by initial India ink examination (evidence of a heavy fungal burden), high CSF pressure, low CSF glucose levels, low CSF pleocytosis (<2/µL), recovery of yeast cells from extraneural sites, the absence of antibody to *C. neoformans*, a CSF or serum cryptococcal antigen level of ≥1:32, and concomitant glucocorticoid therapy or hematologic malignancy. A response to treatment does not guarantee cure since relapse of cryptococcosis is common even among patients with relatively intact immune systems. Complications of CNS cryptococcosis include cranial nerve deficits, vision loss, and cognitive impairment.

PREVENTION

No vaccine is available for cryptococcosis. In patients at high risk (e.g., those with advanced HIV infection and CD4+ T lymphocyte counts of <200/µL), primary prophylaxis with fluconazole (200 mg/d) is effective in reducing the prevalence of disease. Since antiretroviral therapy raises the CD4+ T lymphocyte count, it constitutes an immunologic form of prophylaxis. However, cryptococcosis in the setting of immune reconstitution has been reported in patients with HIV infection and recipients of solid organ transplants.

FURTHER READINGS

ABERT J et al: A pilot study of the discontinuation of antifungal therapy for disseminated cryptococcal disease in patients with acquired immunodeficiency syndrome, following immunologic response to antiretroviral therapy. J Infect Dis 185:1179, 2002

CHAYAKULKEEREE M, PERFECT JP: Cryptococcosis. Infect Dis Clin North Am 20:507, 2006

LILIANG P et al: Use of ventriculoperitoneal shunts to treat uncontrollable intracranial hypertension in patients who have cryptococcal meningitis without hydrocephalus. Clin Infect Dis 34:E64, 2002

LORTHOLARY O et al: Incidence and risk factors of immune reconstitution inflammatory syndrome complicating HIV-associated cryptococcosis in France. AIDS 19:1043, 2005

MASUR H et al: Guidelines for preventing opportunistic infections among HIV-infected persons—2002. Ann Intern Med 137:435, 2002

SAAG MS et al: Practice guidelines for the management of cryptococcal disease. Clin Infect Dis 30:710, 2000

196 Candidiasis
John E. Edwards, Jr.

The genus *Candida* encompasses more than 150 species, only a few of which cause disease in humans. With rare exceptions, the human pathogens are *C. albicans, C. guilliermondii, C. krusei, C. parapsilosis, C. tropicalis, C. kefyr, C. lusitaniae, C. dubliniensis,* and *C. glabrata.* Ubiquitous in nature, these organisms are found on inanimate objects, in foods, and on animals and are normal commensals of humans. They inhabit the gastrointestinal tract (including the mouth and oropharynx), the female genital tract, and the skin. Although cases of candidiasis have been described since antiquity in debilitated patients, the advent of *Candida* species as common human pathogens dates to the introduction of modern therapeutic approaches that suppress normal host defense mechanisms. Of these relatively recent advances, the most important is the use of antibacterial agents that alter the normal human microbial flora and allow nonbacterial species to become more prevalent in the commensal flora. With the introduction of antifungal agents, the causes of *Candida* infections shifted from an almost complete dominance of *C. albicans* to the common involvement of *C. glabrata* and the other species listed above. The non-*albicans* species now account for approximately half of all cases of candidemia and hematogenously disseminated candidiasis. Recognition of this change is clinically important, since the various species differ in susceptibility to the newer antifungal agents. In developed countries, where medical therapeutics are commonly used, *Candida* species are now among the most common nosocomial pathogens. In the United States, these species are the fourth most common isolates from the blood of hospitalized patients.

Candida is a small, thin-walled, ovoid yeast that measures 4–6 μm in diameter and reproduces by budding. Organisms of this genus occur in three forms in tissue: blastospores, pseudohyphae, and hyphae. *Candida* grows readily on simple medium; lysis centrifugation enhances its recovery from blood. Species are identified by biochemical testing (currently with automated devices) or on special agar.

PATHOGENESIS

In the most serious form of *Candida* infection, the organisms disseminate hematogenously and form microabscesses and small macroabscesses in major organs. Although the exact mechanism is not known, *Candida* probably enters the bloodstream from mucosal surfaces after growing to large numbers as a consequence of bacterial suppression by antibacterial drugs; alternatively, in some instances, the organism may enter from the skin. A change from the blastospore stage to the pseudohyphal and hyphal stages is generally considered integral to the organism's penetration into tissue. However, *C. glabrata* can cause extensive infection even though it does not transform into pseudohyphae or hyphae. Numerous reviews of cases of hematogenously disseminated candidiasis have identified the following predisposing factors or conditions: antibacterial agents, indwelling intravascular catheters, hyperalimentation fluids, indwelling urinary catheters, parenteral glucocorticoids, respirators, neutropenia, abdominal and thoracic surgery, cytotoxic chemotherapy, and immunosuppressive agents for organ transplantation. Patients with severe burns, low-birth-weight neonates, and persons using illicit IV drugs are also susceptible. HIV-infected patients with low CD4+ T cell counts and patients with diabetes are susceptible to mucocutaneous infection, which may eventually develop into the disseminated form when other predisposing factors are encountered. Women who receive antibacterial agents may develop vaginal candidiasis.

Innate immunity is the most important defense mechanism against hematogenously disseminated candidiasis, and the neutrophil is the most important component of this defense. Although many immunocompetent individuals have antibodies to *Candida*, the role of these antibodies in defense against the organism is not clear.

CLINICAL MANIFESTATIONS

Mucocutaneous Candidiasis   *Thrush* is characterized by white, adherent, painless, discrete or confluent patches in the mouth, tongue, or esophagus, occasionally with fissuring at the corners of the mouth. This form of *Candida* disease may also occur at points of contact with dentures. Organisms are identifiable in gram-stained scrapings from lesions. The occurrence of thrush in a young, otherwise healthy-appearing person should prompt an investigation for underlying HIV infection. More commonly, thrush is seen as a nonspecific manifestation of severe debilitating illness. Vulvovaginal candidiasis is accompanied by pruritus, pain, and vaginal discharge that is usually thin but may contain whitish "curds" in severe cases.

Other Candida *skin infections* include paronychia, a painful swelling at the nail-skin interface; onychomycosis, a fungal nail infection rarely caused by this genus; intertrigo, an erythematous irritation with redness and pustules in the skin folds; balanitis, an erythematous-pustular infection of the glans penis; erosio interdigitalis blastomycetica, an infection between the digits of the hands or toes; folliculitis, with pustules developing most frequently in the area of the beard; perianal candidiasis, a pruritic, erythematous, pustular infection surrounding the anus; and diaper rash, a common erythematous-pustular perineal infection in infants. Generalized disseminated cutaneous candidiasis, another form of infection that occurs primarily in infants, is characterized by widespread eruptions over the trunk, thorax, and extremities. The diagnostic macronodular lesions of hematogenously disseminated candidiasis (Fig. 196-1) indicate a high probability for dissemination to multiple organs as well as the skin. While the lesions are seen predominantly in immunocompromised patients treated with cytotoxic drugs, they may also develop in patients without neutropenia.

Chronic mucocutaneous candidiasis is a heterogeneous infection of the hair, nails, skin, and mucous membranes that persists despite intermittent therapy. The onset of disease usually comes in infancy or within the first two decades of life but in rare cases can come in later life. The condition may be mild and limited to a specific area of the skin or nails, or it may take a severely disfiguring form (*Candida* granuloma) characterized by exophytic outgrowths on the skin. The condition is usually associated with specific immunologic dysfunction; most frequently reported is a failure of T lymphocytes to proliferate or to stimulate cytokines in response to stimulation by *Candida* antigens in vitro. Approximately half of patients have associated endocrine abnormalities that together are designated the *autoimmune polyendocri-*

FIGURE 196-1 Macronodular skin lesions associated with hematogenously disseminated candidiasis. *Candida* organisms are usually but not always visible on histopathologic examination. The fungi grow when a portion of the biopsied specimen is cultured. Therefore, for optimal identification, both histopathology and culture should be performed. (*Image courtesy of Dr. Noah Craft and the Victor Newcomer collection at UCLA, archived by Logical Images, Inc.; with permission.*)

nopathy–candidiasis–ectodermal dystrophy (APECED) syndrome. This syndrome is due to mutations in the autoimmune regulator (*AIRE*) gene and is most prevalent among Finns, Iranian Jews, Sardinians, northern Italians, and Swedes. Conditions that usually follow the onset of the disease include hypoparathyroidism, adrenal insufficiency, autoimmune thyroiditis, Graves' disease, chronic active hepatitis, alopecia, juvenile-onset pernicious anemia, malabsorption, and primary hypogonadism. In addition, dental enamel dysplasia, vitiligo, pitted nail dystrophy, and calcification of the tympanic membranes may occur. Patients with chronic mucocutaneous candidiasis rarely develop hematogenously disseminated candidiasis, probably because their neutrophil function remains intact.

Deeply Invasive Candidiasis   Deeply invasive *Candida* infections may or may not be due to hematogenous seeding. Deep esophageal infection may result from penetration by organisms from superficial esophageal erosions; joint or deep wound infection from contiguous spread of organisms from the skin; kidney infection from catheter-initiated spread of organisms through the urinary tract; infection of intraabdominal organs and the peritoneum from perforation of the gastrointestinal tract; and gallbladder infection from retrograde migration of organisms from the gastrointestinal tract into the biliary drainage system.

However, far more commonly, deeply invasive candidiasis is a result of hematogenous seeding of various organs as a complication of candidemia. Once the organism gains access to the intravascular compartment (either from the gastrointestinal tract or, less often, from the skin through the site of an indwelling intravascular catheter), it may spread hematogenously to a variety of deep organs. The brain, chorioretina (Fig. 196-2), heart, and kidneys are most commonly infected and the liver and spleen less commonly so (most often in neutropenic patients). In fact, nearly any organ can become involved, including the endocrine glands, pancreas, heart valves (native or prosthetic), skeletal muscle, joints (native or prosthetic), bone, and meninges. *Candida* organisms may also spread hematogenously to the skin and cause classic macronodular lesions (Fig. 196-1). Frequently, painful muscular involvement is also evident beneath the area of affected skin. Chorioretinal involvement and skin involvement are highly significant, since both findings are associated with a very high probability of abscess formation in multiple deep organs as a result of generalized hematogenous seeding. Ocular involvement (Fig. 196-2) may require specific treatment, such as partial vitrectomy to prevent permanent blindness.

FIGURE 196-2 Hematogenous *Candida* endophthalmitis. A classic off-white lesion projecting from the chorioretina into the vitreous causes the surrounding haze. The lesion is composed primarily of inflammatory cells rather than organisms. Lesions of this type may progress to cause extensive vitreal inflammation and eventual loss of the eye. Partial vitrectomy, combined with IV and possibly intravitreal antifungal therapy, may be helpful in controlling the lesions. (*Image courtesy of Dr. Gary Holland; with permission.*)

Disease	Preferred Treatment	Alternatives
Cutaneous	Topical azole	Topical nystatin
Vulvovaginal	Oral fluconazole (150 mg) or azole cream or suppository	Nystatin suppository
Thrush	Clotrimazole troches	Nystatin
Esophageal	Fluconazole tablets (100–200 mg/d) or itraconazole solution (200 mg/d)	Caspofungin, micafungin, or amphotericin B

TABLE 196-1   TREATMENT OF MUCOCUTANEOUS CANDIDAL INFECTIONS

An ocular examination is indicated for all patients with candidemia, whether or not they have ocular manifestations.

DIAGNOSIS

The diagnosis of *Candida* infection is established by visualization of pseudohyphae or hyphae on wet mount (saline and 10% KOH), tissue Gram's stain, periodic acid–Schiff stain, or methenamine silver stain in the presence of inflammation. Absence of organisms on hematoxylin-eosin staining does not reliably exclude *Candida* infection. The most challenging aspect of diagnosis is determining which patients with *Candida* isolates have hematogenously disseminated candidiasis. For instance, recovery of *Candida* from sputum, urine, or peritoneal catheters may indicate mere colonization rather than deep-seated infection, and *Candida* isolation from the blood of patients with indwelling intravascular catheters may reflect inconsequential seeding of the blood from or growth of the organisms on the catheter. Despite extensive research into both antigen and antibody detection systems, there is currently no widely available and validated diagnostic test to distinguish patients with inconsequential seeding of the blood from those whose positive blood cultures represent hematogenous dissemination to multiple organs. Many studies are under way to establish the utility of the β-glucan test. Meanwhile, the presence of ocular or macronodular skin lesions is highly suggestive of widespread infection of multiple deep organs.

℞ CANDIDA INFECTIONS

MUCOCUTANEOUS *CANDIDA* INFECTION   The treatment of mucocutaneous candidiasis is summarized in **Table 196-1**.

CANDIDEMIA AND SUSPECTED HEMATOGENOUSLY DISSEMINATED CANDIDIASIS   All patients with candidemia are now treated with a systemic antifungal agent. A certain percentage of patients, including many of those who have candidemia associated with an indwelling intravascular catheter, probably have "benign" candidemia rather than deep-organ seeding. However, because there is no reliable way to distinguish benign candidemia from deep-organ infection, and because antifungal drugs less toxic than amphotericin B are available, it has become the standard of practice to treat all patients with candidemia, whether or not there is clinical evidence of deep-organ involvement. In addition, if an indwelling intravascular catheter may be involved, it is best to remove or replace the device whenever possible.

The drugs used for the treatment of candidemia and suspected disseminated candidiasis are listed in **Table 196-2**. Various lipid formulations of amphotericin B, three echinocandins, and the azoles fluconazole and voriconazole are used; no agent within a given class has been clearly identified as superior to the others. Most institutions choose an agent from each class on the basis of their own specific microbial epidemiology, strategies to minimize toxicities, and cost considerations. Unless azole resistance is considered likely, fluconazole is the agent of choice for the treatment of candidemia and suspected disseminated candidiasis in nonneutropenic, hemodynamically stable patients. Initial treatment in the context of likely azole resistance depends, as mentioned above, on the epidemiology of the individual hospital. For example, certain hospitals have a high rate of recovery of *C. glabrata*, while others do not. For hemodynamically unstable or neutropenic patients, initial treatment with broader-spectrum agents is desirable; these drugs include polyenes, echinocandins, or later-generation azoles such as voriconazole. Once the clinical response has been assessed and the pathogen specifically identified, the regimen can be altered

TABLE 196-2 AVAILABLE AGENTS FOR THE TREATMENT OF DISSEMINATED CANDIDIASIS

Agent	Route of Administration	Comment
Amphotericin B deoxycholate	IV only	Being replaced by lipid formulations
Amphotericin B lipid formulations		Not FDA approved as primary therapy, but used commonly because less toxic than amphotericin B deoxycholate; ABCD associated with frequent infusion reactions
Liposomal (AmBisome, Abelcet)	IV only	
Lipid complex (ABLC)	IV only	
Colloidal dispersion (ABCD)	IV only	
Azoles		
Fluconazole	IV and oral	Most commonly used
Voriconazole	IV and oral	Multiple drug interactions
Echinocandins		Broad spectrum against *Candida* species
Caspofungin	IV only	Approved for disseminated candidiasis
Anidulafungin	IV only	Approved for disseminated candidiasis
Micafungin	IV only	Under evaluation for disseminated candidiasis

Note: Although ketoconazole is approved for the treatment of disseminated candidiasis, it has been replaced by the newer agents listed in this table.
Abbreviation: FDA, U.S. Food and Drug Administration.

accordingly. At present, the vast majority of *C. albicans* isolates are sensitive to fluconazole. Isolates of *C. glabrata* and *C. krusei* are less sensitive to fluconazole and more sensitive to polyenes and echinocandins. *C. parapsilosis* is less sensitive to echinocandins in vitro, although the clinical significance of this finding is not known.

Some generalizations about the management of specific *Candida* infections are possible. Recovery of *Candida* from sputum is almost never indicative of underlying pulmonary candidiasis and does not by itself warrant antifungal treatment. Similarly, *Candida* in the urine of a patient with an indwelling bladder catheter may represent colonization only rather than bladder or kidney infection; however, the threshold for systemic treatment is lower in severely ill patients in this category since it is not possible to distinguish colonization from lower or upper urinary tract infection. If the isolate is *C. albicans*, most clinicians use oral fluconazole rather than a bladder washout with amphotericin, which was more commonly used in the past. The significance of the recovery of *Candida* from abdominal drains in postoperative patients is also unclear, but again, the threshold for treatment is generally low because most of the affected patients have been subjected to factors predisposing to disseminated candidiasis.

Removal of the infected valve and long-term antifungal therapy constitute appropriate treatment for *Candida* endocarditis. Although definitive studies are not available, patients usually are treated for weeks with a systemic antifungal agent and then given chronic suppressive therapy for months or years (and sometimes indefinitely) with an oral azole.

Hematogenous *Candida* endophthalmitis is a special problem requiring ophthalmologic consultation. In lesions that are expanding or that threaten the macula, an IV polyene combined with flucytosine has been the regimen of choice. However, as more data on the azoles and echinocandins become available, new strategies may evolve. Of paramount importance is the decision to perform a partial vitrectomy. This procedure debulks the infection and can preserve sight, which may otherwise be lost as a result of vitreal scarring. All patients with candidemia should undergo ophthalmologic examination because of the relatively high frequency of this ocular complication. Not only can this examination detect a developing eye lesion early in its course; in addition, identification of a lesion signifies a probability of ~90% of deep-organ abscesses and may prompt prolongation of therapy for candidemia beyond the recommended 2 weeks after the last positive blood culture.

Although the basis for the consensus is a very small data set, the recommended treatment for *Candida* meningitis is a polyene plus flucytosine. Successful treatment of *Candida*-infected prosthetic material (e.g., an artificial joint) nearly always requires removal of the infected material followed by long-term administration of an antifungal agent selected on the basis of the isolate's sensitivity and the logistics of administration.

PROPHYLAXIS

The use of antifungal agents to prevent *Candida* infections has been controversial, but some general principles have emerged. Most centers administer prophylactic fluconazole (400 mg/d) to recipients of allogeneic stem cell transplants. High-risk liver transplant recipients are also given fluconazole prophylaxis in most centers. The use of prophylaxis for neutropenic patients has varied considerably from center to center; most centers that elect to give prophylaxis to this population use either fluconazole or a comparatively low dose of an IV polyene—either amphotericin B deoxycholate or a lipid formulation of this agent. Some centers have used itraconazole suspension.

Prophylaxis is sometimes given to surgical patients at very high risk. The widespread use of prophylaxis in general surgical or medical intensive care units is not—and should not be—a common practice for three reasons: (1) the incidence of disseminated candidiasis is relatively low, (2) the cost-benefit ratio is suboptimal, and (3) increased resistance with widespread prophylaxis is a valid concern.

Prophylaxis for oropharyngeal or esophageal candidiasis in HIV-infected patients is not recommended unless there are frequent recurrences.

FURTHER READINGS

EDWARDS JE JR: Candidiasis, in *Principles and Practice of Infectious Diseases*, 6th ed, GL Mandell et al (eds). Philadelphia, Elsevier Churchill Livingstone, 2005, pp 2938–2973

KAUFFMAN CA: Clinical efficacy of new antifungal agents. Curr Opin Microbiol 9:1, 2006

MASCHMEYER G: The changing epidemiology of invasive fungal infections: New threats. Int J Antimicrob Agents 27(Suppl 1):3, 2006

OSTROSKY-ZEICHNER L et al: Multicenter clinical evaluation of the $(1\rightarrow3)$ beta-D-glucan assay as an aid to diagnosis of fungal infections in humans. Clin Infect Dis 41:654, 2005

PAPPAS PG et al: Guidelines for treatment of candidiasis. Clin Infect Dis 38:161, 2004

RUHNKE M: Epidemiology of *Candida albicans* infections and role of non-*Candida-albicans* yeasts. Curr Drug Targets 7:495, 2006

SOBEL JD: Current trends and challenges in candidiasis. Oncology (Williston Park) 18(Suppl 13):7, 2004

SPELLBERG BJ et al: Current treatment strategies for disseminated candidiasis. Clin Infect Dis 42:244, 2006

TORTORANO AM et al: Candidaemia in Europe: Epidemiology and resistance. Int J Antimicrob Agents 27:359, 2006

197 Aspergillosis
David W. Denning

Aspergillosis is the collective term used to describe all disease entities caused by any one of ~35 pathogenic and allergenic species of *Aspergillus*. Only those species that grow at 37°C can cause invasive infection, al-

though some species without this capability can cause allergic syndromes. *A. fumigatus* is responsible for most cases of invasive aspergillosis, almost all cases of chronic aspergillosis, and most allergic syndromes. *A. flavus* is more prevalent in some hospitals and causes a higher proportion of cases of sinus and cutaneous infection and keratitis than *A. fumigatus*. *A. niger* can cause invasive infection but more commonly colonizes the respiratory tract and causes external otitis. *A. terreus* causes only invasive disease, usually with a poor prognosis. *A. nidulans* occasionally causes invasive infection, primarily in patients with chronic granulomatous disease.

EPIDEMIOLOGY AND ECOLOGY

Aspergillus has a worldwide distribution, most commonly growing in decomposing plant materials (i.e., compost) and in bedding. This hyaline (nonpigmented), septate, branching mold produces vast numbers of conidia (spores) on stalks above the surface of mycelial growth. Aspergilli are found in indoor and outdoor air, on surfaces, and in water from surface reservoirs. Daily exposures vary from a few to many millions of conidia; the latter high numbers of conidia are encountered in hay barns and other very dusty environments. The required size of the infecting inoculum is uncertain; however, only intense exposures (e.g., during construction work, handling of moldy bark or hay, or composting) are sufficient to cause disease in healthy immunocompetent individuals. Allergic syndromes may be exacerbated by continuous antigenic exposure arising from sinus or airway colonization or from nail infection. High-efficiency particulate air (HEPA) filtration is often protective against infection; thus HEPA filters should be installed and monitored for efficiency in operating rooms and in hospital environments that house very high-risk patients.

The incubation period of invasive aspergillosis after exposure is highly variable, extending in documented cases from 2 to 90 days. Thus community-acquired acquisition of an infecting strain frequently manifests as invasive infection during hospitalization, although nosocomial acquisition is also common. Outbreaks usually are directly related to a contaminated air source in the hospital.

RISK FACTORS AND PATHOGENESIS

The primary risk factors for invasive aspergillosis are profound neutropenia and glucocorticoid use; risk increases with longer duration of these conditions. Higher doses of glucocorticoids increase the risk of both acquisition of invasive aspergillosis and death from the infection. Neutrophil and/or phagocyte dysfunction is also an important risk factor, as evidenced by aspergillosis in chronic granulomatous disease, advanced HIV infection, and relapsed leukemia. An increasing incidence of invasive aspergillosis in medical intensive care units suggests that, in patients who are not immunocompromised, temporary abrogation of protective responses as a result of glucocorticoid use or a general anti-inflammatory state is a significant risk factor. Many patients have some evidence of prior pulmonary disease—typically, a history of pneumonia or chronic obstructive pulmonary disease. Glucocorticoid use does not appear to predispose to invasive *Aspergillus* sinusitis but probably increases the risk of dissemination after pulmonary infection.

Patients with chronic pulmonary aspergillosis have a wide spectrum of underlying pulmonary disease, often tuberculosis or sarcoidosis. Patients are immunocompetent except that a genetic defect in mannose-binding protein is common, as are some cytokine regulation defects, most of which are consistent with an inability to mount an inflammatory immune (T_H1-like) response. Glucocorticoids accelerate disease progression.

Allergic bronchopulmonary aspergillosis (ABPA) is associated with certain HLA class II types; polymorphisms of interleukin (IL) 4Ra, IL-10, and SPA2 genes; and heterozygosity of the cystic fibrosis transmembrane conductance regulator (*CFTR*) gene. These associations suggest a strong genetic basis for the development of a T_H2-like and "allergic" response to *A. fumigatus*; this response probably is also protective against invasive disease, since high-dose glucocorticoid treatment for exacerbations of ABPA almost never leads to invasive aspergillosis.

CLINICAL FEATURES AND APPROACH TO THE PATIENT

(Table 197-1)

TABLE 197-1 MAJOR MANIFESTATIONS OF ASPERGILLOSIS

Organ	Major Manifestations in Indicated Type of Disease			
	Invasive (Acute and Subacute)	Chronic	Saprophytic	Allergic
Lung	Angioinvasive in neutropenia, non-angioinvasive, granulomatous	Chronic cavitary, chronic fibrosing	Aspergilloma (single), airway colonization	Allergic bronchopulmonary, severe asthma with fungal sensitization, extrinsic allergic alveolitis
Sinus	Acute invasive	Chronic invasive, chronic granulomatous	Maxillary fungal ball	Allergic fungal sinusitis, eosinophilic fungal rhinosinusitis
Brain	Abscess, hemorrhagic infarction, meningitis, mycotic cerebral aneurysm	Granulomatous, meningitis	None	None
Skin	Acute disseminated, locally invasive (trauma, burns, IV access)	External otitis, onychomycosis	None	None
Heart	Endocarditis (native or prosthetic), pericarditis	None	None	None
Eye	Keratitis, endophthalmitis (postoperative and disseminated)	None	None	None described

Invasive Pulmonary Aspergillosis Both the frequency of invasive disease and the pace of its progression increase with greater degrees of immunocompromise (Fig. 197-1). Invasive aspergillosis is arbitrarily divided into acute and subacute forms that have courses of ≤1 month and 1–3 months, respectively. More than 80% of cases of invasive aspergillosis involve the lungs. The most common clinical features are no symptoms at all, fever, cough (sometimes productive), nondescript chest discomfort, trivial hemoptysis, and shortness of breath. Although the fever often responds to glucocorticoids, the disease progresses. The keys to early diagnosis in at-risk patients are a high index of suspicion, screening for circulating antigen, and urgent CT of the thorax.

Invasive Sinusitis The sinuses are involved in 5–10% of cases of invasive aspergillosis, especially in patients with leukemia and recipients of hematopoietic stem cell transplants. In addition to fever, the most common features are nasal or facial discomfort, blocked nose, and nasal discharge (sometimes bloody). Direct examination of the interior of the nose reveals dusky or necrotic-looking tissue in any location. CT or MRI of the sinuses is essential but does not distinguish invasive *Aspergillus* sinusitis from pre-existing allergic sinusitis, bacterial sinusitis, or other fungal sinusitis early in the disease process.

Disseminated Aspergillosis In the most severely immunocompromised patients, *Aspergillus* disseminates from the lungs to multiple organs—most often to the brain but also to the skin, thyroid, bone, kidney, liver, gastrointestinal tract, eye, and heart valve. Aside from cutaneous lesions, the most common features are gradual clinical deterioration over 1–3 days, with low-grade fever and features of mild sepsis, and multiple nonspecific abnormalities in laboratory tests. In most cases, at least one localization becomes apparent. Blood cultures are not helpful since they are almost always negative.

Cerebral Aspergillosis Hematogenous dissemination to the brain is a devastating complication of invasive aspergillosis. Single or multiple lesions may develop. In acute disease, hemorrhagic infarction is most typical, and cerebral abscess is common. Rarer manifestations include meningitis, mycotic aneurysm, and cerebral granuloma. Local spread also occurs, resulting in a single abscess. Postoperative infection from cranial sinuses is occasionally recorded and is exacerbated by glucocorticoid use after neurosurgery. The presentation can be either acute or subacute, with mood changes, focal signs, seizures, and decline in mental status. Cerebral granuloma can mimic a primary or secondary tumor. MRI is the most useful immediate investigation; unenhanced CT of the brain is usually nonspecific, and contrast is often contraindicated in the affected patients because of poor renal function.

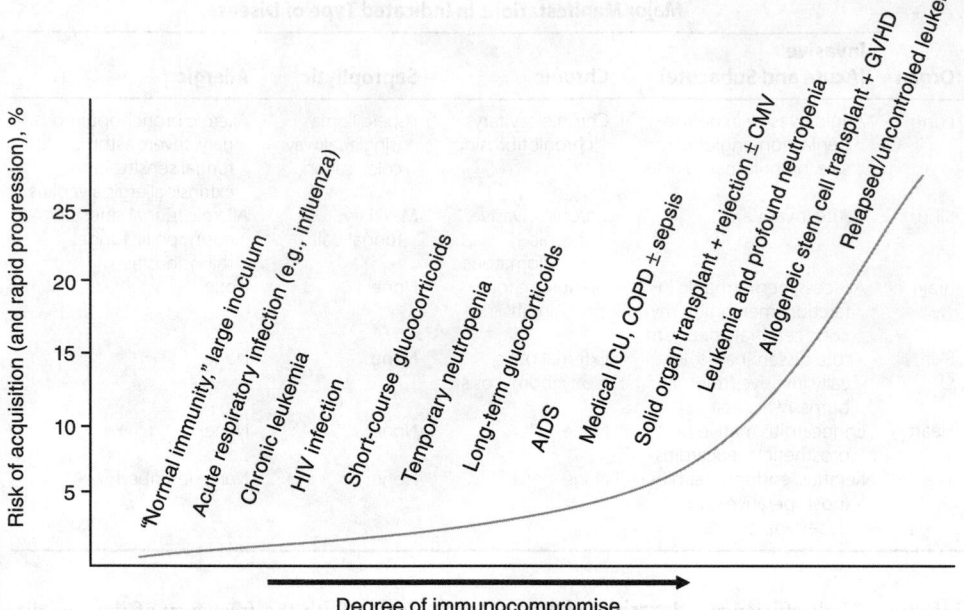

FIGURE 197-1 Invasive aspergillosis: conditions placing patients at elevated risk of acquisition and relatively rapid progression. ICU, intensive care unit; COPD, chronic obstructive pulmonary disease; CMV, cytomegalovirus; GVHD, graft-vs-host disease.

Endocarditis Most cases of *Aspergillus* endocarditis are prosthetic valve infections resulting from contamination during surgery. Native valve disease is reported, especially as a feature of disseminated infection and in persons using illicit IV drugs. Culture-negative endocarditis with large vegetations is the most common presentation, but embolectomy reveals the diagnosis in a few cases.

Cutaneous Aspergillosis Dissemination of *Aspergillus* occasionally results in cutaneous features, usually an erythematous or purplish nontender area that progresses to a necrotic eschar. Direct invasion of the skin occurs in neutropenic patients at the site of IV catheter insertion and in burn patients. Rapidly progressive local aspergillosis of the skin and underlying tissue may follow trauma, and wounds may become infected with *Aspergillus* after surgery.

Chronic Pulmonary Aspergillosis The hallmark of chronic cavitary pulmonary aspergillosis (also called semi-invasive aspergillosis, chronic necrotizing aspergillosis, or complex aspergilloma) (Fig. 197-2) is one or more pulmonary cavities expanding over a period of months or years in association with pulmonary symptoms and systemic manifestations such as fatigue and weight loss. (Pulmonary aspergillosis developing over <3 months is better classified as subacute invasive aspergillosis.) Often mistaken initially for tuberculosis, almost all cases occur in patients with prior pulmonary disease (e.g., tuberculosis, atypical mycobacterial infection, sarcoidosis, ankylosing spondylitis, rheumatoid lung disease, pneumothorax, bullae) or prior lung surgery. The onset is insidious, and systemic features are sometimes more prominent than pulmonary symptoms. Cavities may have a fluid level or a well-formed fungal ball, but pericavitary infiltrates and multiple cavities—with or without pleural thickening—are typical. Antibodies to *Aspergillus* are almost always detectable in blood, usually as precipitating antibody and sometimes at high titers. Some patients have concurrent infections—even without a fungal ball—with atypical mycobacteria and/or other bacterial pathogens, such as *Staphylococcus aureus* or *Pseudomonas aeruginosa*. If untreated, chronic pulmonary aspergillosis typically progresses (sometimes relatively rapidly) to unilateral or upper-lobe fibrosis. This end-stage entity is termed *chronic fibrosing pulmonary aspergillosis*.

Aspergilloma Aspergilloma (fungal ball) occurs in up to 20% of residual chest cavities ≥2 cm in diameter. Some fungal balls remain stable in a single cavity for many years, and 10% resolve spontaneously. However, aspergillomas are often a feature of chronic pulmonary aspergillosis with its associated features. Signs and symptoms associated with single (simple) aspergillomas are minor, including a cough (sometimes productive), hemoptysis, wheezing, and mild fatigue. More significant signs and symptoms are associated with chronic cavitary pulmonary aspergillosis. The vast majority of fungal balls are caused by *A. fumigatus*, but *A. niger* has been implicated, particularly in diabetic patients; aspergillomas due to *A. niger* can lead to oxalosis with renal dysfunction. The most significant complication of aspergilloma is life-threatening hemoptysis, which may be the presenting manifestation.

Chronic Sinusitis Three entities are subsumed under this broad label: sinus aspergilloma, chronic invasive sinusitis, and chronic granulomatous sinusitis. *Sinus aspergilloma* is limited to the maxillary sinus and consists of a chronic saprophytic entity in which the sinus cavity is filled with a fungal ball. This form of disease is associated with prior upper-jaw root canal work and chronic (bacterial) sinusitis. About 90% of CT scans show focal hyperattenuation related to concretions; on MRI scans, the T2-weighted signal is decreased, whereas that of bacterial sinusitis is increased. Removal of the fungal ball is curative. No tissue invasion is demonstrable histologically or radiologically.

In contrast, *chronic invasive sinusitis* is a slowly destructive process that most commonly affects the ethmoid and sphenoid sinuses but can involve any sinus. Patients are usually but not always immunocompro-

FIGURE 197-2 CT scan image of the chest in a patient with longstanding bilateral chronic cavitary pulmonary aspergillosis. He had a prior history of several bilateral pneumothoraces and required bilateral pleurodesis (1990). CT scan then demonstrated multiple bullae, and sputum cultures grew *A. fumigatus*. The patient had initially weakly and later strongly positive serum *Aspergillus* antibody tests (precipitins). This scan (2003) shows a mixture of thick- and thin-walled cavities in both lungs, with a large cavity containing a probable fungal ball protruding into the large cavity on the right. There is also considerable pleural thickening bilaterally.

mised to some degree (e.g., as a result of diabetes or HIV infection). Imaging of the cranial sinuses shows opacification of one or more sinuses, local bone destruction, and invasion of local structures. The differential diagnosis is wide, as numerous other fungi may cause a similar disease and sphenoid sinusitis is often caused by bacteria. Apart from a history of chronic nasal discharge and blockage, loss of the sense of smell, and persistent headache, the usual presenting features are related to local involvement of critical structures. The orbital apex syndrome (blindness and proptosis) is characteristic. Facial swelling, cavernous sinus thrombosis, carotid artery occlusion, pituitary fossa, and brain and skull base invasion have been described.

Chronic granulomatous sinusitis due to *Aspergillus* is most commonly seen in the Middle East and India and is often caused by *A. flavus*. It typically presents late, with facial swelling and unilateral proptosis. The prominent granulomatous reaction histologically distinguishes this disease from chronic invasive sinusitis, in which tissue necrosis with a low-grade mixed-cell infiltrate is typical.

Allergic Bronchopulmonary Aspergillosis   In almost all cases, ABPA represents a hypersensitivity reaction to *A. fumigatus*; rare cases are due to other aspergilli and other fungi. ABPA occurs in ~1% of patients with asthma and in up to 15% of adults with cystic fibrosis, and occasional cases are reported in patients without either of these diseases. Episodes of bronchial obstruction with mucous plugs leading to coughing fits, "pneumonia," consolidation, and breathlessness are typical. Many patients report coughing up thick sputum casts, usually brown or clear. Eosinophilia commonly develops before systemic glucocorticoids are given. The cardinal diagnostic tests include an elevated serum level of total IgE (usually >1000 IU/mL), a positive skin-prick test to *A. fumigatus* extract, or detection of *Aspergillus*-specific IgE and IgG (precipitating) antibodies. Central bronchiectasis is characteristic, but patients may present before it becomes apparent.

Severe Asthma with Fungal Sensitization (SAFS)   Many adults with severe asthma do not fulfill the criteria for ABPA and yet are allergic to fungi. Although *A. fumigatus* is a common allergen, numerous other fungi (e.g., *Cladosporium* and *Alternaria* spp.) are implicated by skin-prick testing and/or specific IgE radioallergosorbent (RAST) testing.

Allergic Sinusitis   Like the lungs, the sinuses manifest allergic responses to *Aspergillus* and other fungi. The affected patients present with chronic (i.e., perennial) sinusitis typically requiring multiple course of antibiotics that are of only limited benefit. Many of these patients have nasal polyps, and all have congested nasal mucosa and sinuses full of mucoid material. The histologic hallmark of allergic fungal sinusitis is local eosinophilia and the breakdown products of eosinophils, Charcot-Leyden crystals. Removal of abnormal mucus and polyps, with local and occasionally systemic administration of glucocorticoids, usually leads to resolution. Persistent or recurrent signs and symptoms may require more extensive surgery (ethmoidectomy) and possibly local antifungal therapy.

Superficial Aspergillosis   *Aspergillus* can cause keratitis and otitis externa. The former may be difficult to diagnose early enough to save the patient's sight. Treatment requires local surgical debridement as well as both systemic and topical antifungal therapy. Otitis externa is a common problem for which local debridement and local application of antifungal agents constitute the most common approach to treatment.

DIAGNOSIS

Several techniques are required to establish the diagnosis of any form of aspergillosis with confidence. Patients with acute invasive aspergillosis have a relatively heavy load of fungus in the affected organ; thus culture, molecular diagnosis, antigen detection, and histopathology usually confirm the diagnosis. However, the pace of progression leaves only a narrow window for making the diagnosis without losing the patient, and some invasive procedures are not possible because of coagulopathy, respiratory compromise, and other factors. Currently,

~40% of cases of invasive aspergillosis are missed clinically and are diagnosed only at autopsy. Histologic examination of affected tissue reveals either infarction, with invasion of blood vessels by many fungal hyphae, or acute necrosis, with limited inflammation and hyphae. *Aspergillus* hyphae are hyaline, narrow, and septate, with branching at 45°; no yeast forms are present in infected tissue. Hyphae can be seen in cytology or microscopy preparations, which therefore provide a rapid means of presumptive diagnosis.

Culture is important in confirming the diagnosis, given that multiple other (rarer) fungi can mimic *Aspergillus* spp. histologically. Bacterial agar is less sensitive than fungal media for culture. Thus, if physicians do not request fungal culture, the diagnosis may be missed. Culture may be falsely positive (e.g., in patients whose airways are colonized by *Aspergillus*) or falsely negative. Only 10–30% of patients with invasive aspergillosis have a positive culture at any time. Molecular diagnostic techniques promise to be both faster and more sensitive than culture.

The *Aspergillus* antigen test relies on detection of galactomannan release from *Aspergillus* spp. during growth. Antigen testing in high-risk patients is best done prospectively, as positive results usually precede clinical or radiologic features by several days. Antigen testing may be falsely positive in patients receiving certain β-lactam/β-lactamase inhibitor antibiotic combinations, such as tazocillin/sulbactam and amoxicillin/clavulanic acid; in these cases, a second test is required for confirmation. Antigen testing and molecular testing on bronchoalveolar lavage fluid and cerebrospinal fluid are useful if performed before antifungal therapy has been given for more than a few days. The sensitivity of antigen detection is reduced by antifungal prophylaxis.

Definitive confirmation of the diagnosis requires (1) a positive culture of a sample taken directly from an ordinarily sterile site (e.g., a brain abscess) or (2) positive results of both histologic testing and culture of a sample taken from an affected organ (e.g., sinuses or skin). Most diagnoses of invasive aspergillosis are inferred from fewer data, including the presence of the *halo sign* on a high-resolution thoracic CT scan, in which a localized ground-glass appearance representing hemorrhagic infarction surrounds a nodule. While a halo sign may be produced by other fungi, *Aspergillus* spp. are by far the most common cause. Halo signs are present for ~7 days early in the course of infection in neutropenic patients and are a good prognostic feature. Thick CT sections can give the false appearance of a halo sign, as can other technical factors. Other common radiologic features of invasive pulmonary aspergillosis include pleural-based infarction or cavitation.

For chronic invasive aspergillosis, *Aspergillus* antibody testing is invaluable although relatively imprecise. Titers fall with successful therapy. Cultures are infrequently positive. Some patients with chronic pulmonary aspergillosis also have elevated titers of total serum IgE and *Aspergillus*-specific IgE.

ABPA and SAFS are diagnosed serologically or with skin-prick tests. Allergic *Aspergillus* sinusitis is usually diagnosed histologically, although precipitating antibodies in blood may also be useful.

℞ ASPERGILLOSIS

Antifungal drugs active against *Aspergillus* include voriconazole, itraconazole, posaconazole, caspofungin, micafungin, and amphotericin B. Initial IV administration is preferred for acute invasive aspergillosis and oral administration for all other disease that requires antifungal therapy. Current recommendations are shown in **Table 197-2**. Voriconazole is the preferred agent for invasive aspergillosis; caspofungin, posaconazole, and lipid-associated amphotericin B are second-line agents. Amphotericin B is not active against *A. terreus* or *A. nidulans*. An infectious disease consultation is advised for patients with invasive disease, given the complexity of management. It is not clear whether combination therapy for acute invasive aspergillosis is beneficial, but it is widely used for very ill patients and for those with a poor prognosis. Commonly used combinations include an azole with either caspofungin or micafungin. The interactions of voriconazole and itraconazole with many drugs must be considered before these agents are prescribed. In addition, the effects of both drugs vary substantially from one patient to another, and many authorities recommend monitoring to ensure that drug concentrations are adequate but not excessive. The duration of therapy for invasive aspergillosis

TABLE 197-2 TREATMENT OF ASPERGILLOSIS

Indication	Primary Treatment	Evidence Level[a]	Precautions	Secondary Treatment	Comments
Invasive[a]	Voriconazole	AI	Drug interactions (especially with rifampin), renal failure (IV only)	Amphotericin B, caspofungin, posaconazole, micafungin	As primary therapy, voriconazole carries 20% more responses than amphotericin B. If azole prophylaxis fails, it is unclear whether a class change is required for therapy.
Prophylaxis	Itraconazole solution, posaconazole	AI	Diarrhea and vomiting with itraconazole, vincristine interaction	Micafungin, aerosolized amphotericin B	Some centers monitor plasma levels of itraconazole.
ABPA	Itraconazole	AI	Some glucocorticoid interactions, including with inhaled formulations	Voriconazole	Long-term therapy is helpful in most patients. Others can discontinue treatment. No evidence indicates whether or not therapy modifies progression to bronchiectasis/fibrosis.
Single aspergilloma	Surgery	BII	Multicavity disease: poor outcome of surgery; medical therapy preferable	Itraconazole, voriconazole, intracavity amphotericin B	Single large cavities with an aspergilloma are best resected.
Chronic pulmonary[b]	Itraconazole	BII	Poor absorption of capsules with proton pump inhibitors or H_2 blockers	Voriconazole, IV amphotericin B	Resistance may emerge during treatment, especially if plasma drug levels are subtherapeutic.

Note: The oral dose is usually 200 mg bid for voriconazole and itraconazole and 400 mg bid for posaconazole. The IV dose of voriconazole is 6 mg/kg twice at 12-h intervals (loading doses) followed by 4 mg/kg q12h. Plasma monitoring is helpful in optimizing the dosage. Caspofungin is given as a single loading dose of 70 mg, followed by 50 mg/d; some authorities use 70 mg/d for patients weighing >80 kg, and lower doses are required with hepatic dysfunction. Micafungin is given as 50 mg/d for prophylaxis and as at least 150 mg/d for treatment; this drug is not yet approved by the U.S. Food and Drug Administration (FDA) for this indication. Amphotericin B deoxycholate is given at a daily dose of 1 mg/kg if tolerated. Several strategies are available for minimizing renal dysfunction. Lipid-associated amphotericin B is given at 3 mg/kg (AmBisome) or 5 mg/kg (Abelcet). Different regimens are available for aerosolized amphotericin B, but none is FDA approved. Other considerations that may alter dose selection or route include age; concomitant medications; renal, hepatic, or intestinal dysfunction; and drug tolerability.
[a]Evidence levels are those used in treatment guidelines (Stevens DA et al: Practice guidelines for diseases caused by *Aspergillus*. Clin Infect Dis 30:696, 2000).
[b]An infectious disease consultation is appropriate for these patients.

varies from ~3 months to several years, depending on the patient's immune status and response to therapy. Relapse occurs if the response is suboptimal and immune reconstitution is not complete.

Itraconazole is the preferred oral agent for chronic and allergic forms of aspergillosis. Voriconazole and posaconazole can be substituted when failure, emergence of resistance, or adverse events occur. An itraconazole dose of 200 mg twice daily is recommended, with monitoring of drug concentrations in the blood. Chronic cavitary pulmonary aspergillosis probably requires life-long therapy, whereas the duration of treatment for other forms of chronic and allergic aspergillosis requires case-by-case evaluation.

Resistance to one or more azoles, although uncommon, may develop during long-term treatment, and a positive culture during antifungal therapy is an indication for susceptibility testing. Glucocorticoids should be used with caution in chronic cavitary pulmonary aspergillosis.

Surgical treatment is important in several forms of aspergillosis, including maxillary fungal ball and single aspergillomas, in which surgery is curative; invasive aspergillosis involving bone, heart valve, sinuses, proximal areas of the lung, and areas impinging on the great vessels; brain abscess; keratitis; and endophthalmitis. In allergic fungal sinusitis, removal of abnormal mucus and polyps, with local and occasionally systemic glucocorticoid treatment, usually leads to resolution. Persistent or recurrent signs and symptoms may require more extensive surgery (ethmoidectomy) and possibly local antifungal therapy. Surgery is problematic in chronic pulmonary aspergillosis, usually resulting in serious complications. Bronchial artery embolization is preferred for problematic hemoptysis.

PROPHYLAXIS

In situations in which moderate or high risk is predicted (e.g., after induction therapy for acute myeloid leukemia), the need for antifungal prophylaxis for superficial and systemic candidiasis and for invasive aspergillosis is generally accepted. Fluconazole is commonly used in these situations but has no activity against *Aspergillus* spp. Itraconazole capsules are ineffective, and itraconazole solution offers only modest efficacy. Posaconazole solution is probably more effective. Some data support the use of IV low-dose micafungin. No prophylactic regimen is completely successful.

OUTCOME

Invasive aspergillosis is curable if immune reconstitution occurs, whereas allergic and chronic forms are not. The mortality rate for invasive aspergillosis is ~50% if the infection is diagnosed and treated but is 100% if the diagnosis is missed. Cerebral aspergillosis, *Aspergillus* endocarditis, and bilateral extensive invasive pulmonary aspergillosis have very poor outcomes, as does invasive infection in patients with late-stage AIDS, patients with relapsed uncontrolled leukemia, and recipients of allogeneic hematopoietic stem cell transplants.

FURTHER READINGS

CLANCY CJ et al: Bronchoalveolar lavage galactomannan in diagnosis of invasive aspergillosis among solid-organ transplant recipients. J Clin Microbiol 45:1759, 2007

CAMUSET J et al: Treatment of chronic pulmonary aspergillosis by voriconazole in nonimmunocompromised patients. Chest 131:1435, 2007

DENNING DW et al: The link between fungi and asthma—a summary of the evidence. Eur Respir J 27:615, 2006

HERBRECHT R et al: Voriconazole versus amphotericin B for primary therapy of invasive aspergillosis. N Engl J Med 347:408, 2002

HOPE WW et al: Laboratory diagnosis of invasive aspergillosis. Lancet Infect Dis 9:609, 2005

——— et al: The invasive and saprophytic syndromes due to *Aspergillus* spp. Med Mycol 43(Suppl 1):S207, 2005

MEERSSEMAN W et al: Invasive aspergillosis in the intensive care unit. Clin Infect Dis 45:205, 2007

MOSS RB: Pathophysiology and immunology of allergic bronchopulmonary aspergillosis. Med Mycol 43(Suppl1):S203, 2005

PASQUALOTTO AC, DENNING DW: Post-operative aspergillosis. Clin Microbiol Rev 12:1060, 2006

TEKAIA F, LATGE JP: *Aspergillus fumigatus*: Saprophyte or pathogen? Curr Opin Microbiol 8:385, 2005

198 Mucormycosis
Alan M. Sugar

Mucormycosis (also called *zygomycosis*) is a serious, relatively uncommon invasive fungal infection and one of the most aggressive and lethal invasive mycoses. Physicians caring for patients with diabetes mellitus, immunocompromise (including that following organ transplantation), or iron overload syndromes (particularly those associated with hemodialysis) should be acutely aware of the enhanced susceptibility of these individuals to infection with the Mucorales. Timely diagnosis is critical to survival and minimization of morbidity. Institution of aggressive surgical and medical therapy is critical in maximizing the likelihood of a good outcome. Delay in considering the diagnosis and instituting appropriate therapeutic measures results in increasingly severe disfigurement at best and in death at worst.

ETIOLOGY
Fungi from the order Mucorales are the etiologic agents of mucormycosis. Despite the name of this infection, *Mucor* is not the most common genus recovered from patients. Rather, *Rhizopus* and *Rhizomucor* are the genera usually cultured from tissue samples. Other, less common fungi, including *Absidia*, *Cunninghamella*, *Apophysomyces*, and *Saksenaea*, are increasingly being isolated and, for the most part, cause similar clinical syndromes. Thus, there is no specific clinical feature that permits identification of the precise fungus involved. Submission of appropriate biopsy material to the microbiology laboratory is mandatory to ensure a pathogen's identification.

PATHOGENESIS
Mucorales are found commonly in the environment, and spores of these usually nonpathogenic fungi are likely to be inhaled daily. In the normal human lung, spores are inhibited from germinating into hyphae by alveolar macrophages. However, in diabetic patients, especially those with elevated blood sugar levels and acidemia, the spores germinate, hyphae develop (Fig. 198-1), and the fungi begin an inexorable march throughout the lung tissue, invading blood vessels and surrounding tissues. As blood vessels become involved, thrombosis occurs, tissue necrosis results, and the fungi continue to grow in this devitalized tissue. The use of deferoxamine to treat iron overload is a risk factor for mucormycosis; the siderophore supplies the fungi with iron that enhances their growth.

Spores settle in the upper airways, lower airways, or gastrointestinal tract and can spread beyond the initial site of infection, causing disseminated mucormycosis. Increasingly, patients are presenting with extensive cutaneous involvement after direct implantation of spores into the skin as a result of trauma (e.g., that sustained in a motor vehicle accident). The pathology in all these sites is the same, with blood vessel invasion and tissue necrosis as hallmarks and specific organ dysfunction depending on the location of the infection.

CLINICAL MANIFESTATIONS
The manifestations of mucormycosis depend on the site of infection. Patients with *rhinocerebral mucormycosis* may present with symptoms typical of sinusitis. However, progression of symptoms over several days indicates a more serious process than the more common bacterial or viral sinusitis. As the infection spreads, hypesthesia or numbness of the face overlying the infection may develop. Concomitant symptoms include headache, bloody nasal discharge, and changes in mental status. The black eschar of the palate is widely described as a hallmark of rhinocerebral mucormycosis, but the astute clinician will recognize earlier manifestations of this end-stage lesion reflecting invasion of the palate. These subtler lesions, which may consist of discolored, often hyperemic areas on the palate, will, if untreated, progress rapidly to the commonly recognized black eschar, which indicates angioinvasion and tissue necrosis. Involvement of the orbit (Fig. 198-2) compromises proper ocular-muscle function and normal movement of the eye within the skull, resulting in double vision. If the blood supply to the eye is affected by invasion of the retinal artery, blindness develops, often quite rapidly. Proptosis and ptosis are late findings reflecting a mass lesion within the orbit and cranial nerve involvement, respectively. Progression of the infection into the brain results in the formation of brain abscesses and phlegmon; symptoms and signs depend on the location of these lesions. Cavernous sinus thrombosis is an ominous sign. CT and MRI reveal sinus opacification and destruction of contiguous bone, and brain involvement can be readily appreciated.

Pulmonary mucormycosis presents as severe, progressive, tissue-destructive pneumonia. Neutropenia is a common predisposing factor. A high fever and a critical clinical condition are typical. Cavitation of involved lung develops rapidly, and hematogenous spread beyond the lungs to the brain and other organs may occur.

Gastrointestinal mucormycosis occurs primarily in those patients with protein-calorie malnutrition and usually presents as a perforated viscus. Premortem diagnosis is rare, and most patients with this form of mucormycosis do not survive.

Cutaneous mucormycosis is more common than disease at other sites and develops after traumatic injuries in which wounds are contaminated with dirt. Areas of tissue necrosis enlarge rapidly, involving all layers of the skin and underlying structures.

A

B

FIGURE 198-1 **A.** Hematoxylin and eosin–stained section of lung tissue showing the broad, infrequently septate, thin-walled hyphae of *Absidia corymbifera*. **B.** Grocott's methenamine silver–stained section of lung tissue showing typical zygomycete hyphae of *A. corymbifera*. (*Courtesy of David Ellis, PhD, Mycology Unit, Women's and Children's Hospital, Adelaide, Australia; with permission.*)

FIGURE 198-2 **A.** Rhinocerebral zygomycosis caused by *Rhizopus oryzae*, with extensive involvement of the orbit. **B.** Associated MRI scan. *(Courtesy of David Ellis, PhD, Mycology Unit, Women's and Children's Hospital, Adelaide, Australia; with permission.)*

DIAGNOSIS

Laboratory Features There are no pathognomonic hematologic changes. The abnormalities that are found reflect underlying predisposing conditions (e.g., diabetic ketoacidosis) and general indications of infection, such as elevated white blood cell counts and acute-phase reactant levels. Blood cultures are virtually always negative.

Microscopic examination and culture of biopsy samples from the involved area are critical in making an accurate diagnosis. As much tissue as possible should be submitted to the microbiology and histopathology laboratories. Swabs are insufficient. These fungi grow rapidly and are usually visible on culture plates within a day or two. Their identification is based on traditional morphologic features. Fixed tissue samples are treated with special stains for fungi; for example, Gomori methenamine silver stains the fungi black against a green background, and periodic acid–Schiff stains the hyphae red. Mucorales appear as broad (diameter, 6–50 μm), usually nonseptate hyphae with branches at right angles; the organisms are often described as ribbon-like. Hyphae cut and viewed on end can deceptively appear yeast-like. The microscopic appearance of the Mucorales is sufficiently different from that of *Aspergillus*, *Fusarium*, and other pathogenic molds (which characteristically appear as narrow, septate hyphae with narrow-angle branching) that a pathologist can readily make a preliminary diagnosis of mucormycosis. Identification of the specific organism requires culture. In the laboratory, each species of Mucorales exhibits characteristic morphologic features that permit specific identification. Molecular methods of speciation are still used only as research tools.

Differential Diagnosis Other fungal infections, including aspergillosis, fusariosis, and scedosporiosis, must be ruled out by culture and histopathologic analysis. Microscopic examination easily distinguishes the etiologic agents of these infections from the Mucorales. Aggressive pyogenic bacterial infections—e.g., those caused by *Pseudomonas*, *Aeromonas*, or *Vibrio* species; *Staphylococcus aureus*; and a variety of anaerobes—occasionally produce similar clinical presentations but can be ruled out by Gram's staining, culture, and microscopic analysis of tissue samples.

℞ MUCORMYCOSIS

Three factors are key to a successful outcome of therapy for mucormycosis: (1) reversal of the underlying predisposition; (2) aggressive surgical debridement; and (3) aggressive antifungal therapy, with early initiation and high drug doses. Failure to undertake all three of these interventions simultaneously has a significant and negative impact on outcome.

Reversal of underlying disease is relatively easy in patients with diabetic ketoacidosis but is more difficult in patients who require continued immunosuppression for control of an underlying disease or after organ transplantation. In all cases, minimization of immunosuppressive medications enhances overall control of the fungal infection.

Aggressive surgical debridement requires the removal of all dead tissue and of tissue that appears to be so severely compromised that its continued viability is in question. Extensive reconstructive surgery may be required once the infection has been cured.

Traditionally, high-dose conventional amphotericin B has been used for the treatment of mucormycosis, but doses have been limited to <1.5 mg/kg per day because of the nearly universal development of nephrotoxicity. Use of lipid formulations at doses of 15–20 mg/kg per day (AmBisome) or 15 mg/kg per day (Abelcet) maximizes the amount of amphotericin B delivered to the tissues as well as the speed of its delivery. At these doses, nephrotoxicity occurs in <50% of patients.

Posaconazole, an experimental triazole antifungal agent, has been shown to be active against mucormycosis in mouse models of infection and in patients who cannot tolerate or do not respond to other antifungal drugs. The precise clinical role for posaconazole in the treatment of mucormycosis is not clear, but this drug may prove to be a valuable alternative to amphotericin B in selected cases. Given the relative rarity of mucormycosis, it is not likely that a randomized study will rigorously compare the roles of the various antifungal agents.

The optimal duration of therapy for mucormycosis is not known precisely. If possible, antifungal administration should be continued for at least 3 months after (1) all clinical abnormalities resolve or stabilize, leaving no clinical evidence of infection at the involved site(s); and (2) scans, x-rays, and laboratory studies yield normal or stable results. Careful follow-up should continue for at least 1 year to confirm that there is no evidence of recurrent infection. With this approach, recurrences should be rare.

FURTHER READINGS

CHAYAKULKEEREE M et al: Zygomycosis: The re-emerging fungal infection. Eur J Clin Microbiol Infect Dis 25:215, 2006

DAVARI HR et al: Outcome of mucormycosis in liver transplantation: Four cases and a review of literature. Exp Clin Transplant 1:147, 2003

GONZALEZ CE et al: Zygomycosis. Infect Dis Clin North Am 16:895, 2002

GREENBERG RN et al: Posaconazole as salvage therapy for zygomycosis. Antimicrob Agents Chemother 50:126, 2006

GREENBERG RN et al: Zygomycosis (mucormycosis): Emerging clinical importance and new treatments. Curr Opin Infect Dis 17:517, 2004

LIANG KP et al: Rhino-orbitocerebral mucormycosis caused by *Apophysomyces elegans*. J Clin Microbiol 44:892, 2006

O'NEILL BM et al: Disseminated rhinocerebral mucormycosis: A case report and review of the literature. J Oral Maxillofac Surg 64:326, 2006

PRABHU RM et al: Mucormycosis and entomophthoramycosis: A review of the clinical manifestations, diagnosis and treatment. Clin Microbiol Infect 10(Suppl 1):31, 2004

RODEN MM et al: Epidemiology and outcome of zygomycosis: A review of 929 reported cases. Clin Infect Dis 41:634, 2005

SPELLBERG B et al: Novel perspectives on mucormycosis: Pathophysiology, presentation, and management. Clin Microbiol Rev 18:556, 2005

199 Miscellaneous Mycoses and Algal Infections
Stanley W. Chapman, Donna C. Sullivan

MYCOSES

The clinical spectrum of fungal disease varies from superficial infections of the skin, hair, and nails to life-threatening systemic infections. Superficial infections involve the outermost layers of skin and hair and are associated with little or no inflammation. Cutaneous infections involve deeper layers of the skin, hair follicles, and nails and are accompanied by inflammation. Subcutaneous infections involve the dermis and subcutaneous tissues. Systemic disease involves deep tissue invasion of one or more internal organs and usually follows inhalation of the fungus. In immunocompromised patients, disseminated disease may result from superficial, cutaneous, or subcutaneous fungal infections.

SUPERFICIAL INFECTIONS

Malasseziasis Tinea (pityriasis) versicolor, caused by lipophilic yeasts of the genus *Malassezia,* is the most common superficial skin infection. The clinical presentation usually consists of scaly hypo- or hyperpigmented macular lesions on the chest, back, neck, and arms.

ETIOLOGIC AGENTS *Malassezia* species are components of the human cutaneous flora that are dimorphic, existing in both yeast and mycelial phases. Each phase was originally classified as a separate genus: *Pityrosporum* for the yeast form and *Malassezia* for the mycelial form. The two genera were reclassified in 1986 as a single genus, *Malassezia.* Initially, only one species, *M. furfur,* was recognized, but seven distinct species have since been identified: *M. furfur, M. sympodialis, M. obtusa, M. globosa, M. restricta, M. slooffiae,* and *M. pachydermatis.*

EPIDEMIOLOGY *Malassezia* species can be isolated from sebaceous-rich areas of the skin, most frequently from the chest and the midline of the back. The prevalence of tinea versicolor in susceptible age groups (primarily adolescents and young adults) is low in temperate climates but may reach 40–60% in tropical climates.

PATHOGENESIS The pathogenesis of tinea versicolor is unclear but may involve the conversion of colonizing yeasts into the mycelial form, which then invades the stratum corneum.

CLINICAL MANIFESTATIONS The lesions of tinea versicolor are usually asymptomatic. Most patients seek medical advice for cosmetic reasons. Lesions typically appear as patches of pink or coppery-brown skin but may appear paler than the surrounding skin, especially in dark-skinned individuals. Although some patients report mild pruritus, the lesions do not usually elicit an immune response. Other cutaneous manifestations associated with *Malassezia* species include seborrheic dermatitis, folliculitis, atopic dermatitis, and dandruff.

DIAGNOSIS Tinea versicolor is diagnosed on clinical grounds by the characteristic distribution and appearance of skin lesions. Lesions may fluoresce yellow-green under long-wave UVA (Wood's light). Treatment of skin scrapings with potassium hydroxide (KOH) reveals yeasts and hyphal elements with a "spaghetti and meatballs" appearance.

℞ MALASSEZIASIS

Malassezia species are susceptible to a variety of topical antifungal agents, including 2.5% selenium sulfide shampoo (a 10- to 15-min application followed by rinsing); topical azoles such as clotrimazole, miconazole, econazole, and ketoconazole; terbinafine gel; and ciclopirox cream/solution. The typical treatment duration is 2 weeks. In patients with extensive or persistent lesions, short-course or pulse therapy with oral ketoconazole (a single 400-mg dose), fluconazole (a single 400-mg dose or 150 mg every week for 4 weeks), or itraconazole (200 mg every other day for 7 days) has proved effective.

COMPLICATIONS *M. furfur* is lipophilic and causes catheter-related fungemia in premature neonates and immunocompromised adults receiving IV lipids by central venous catheter. Infection of the lungs is pronounced and frequently results in respiratory failure. *M. pachydermatis,* although not lipophilic, is an increasingly important pathogen in neonatal intensive care units. When its presence is suspected, the microbiology laboratory should be notified because its isolation requires special culture conditions. Catheter-related *Malassezia* infections should be managed with prompt catheter removal and systemic antifungal therapy with amphotericin B or an azole (Table 199-1). Because transmission of both *M. furfur* and *M. pachydermatis* on the hands of health care workers has been documented, a strict handwashing protocol should be enforced when outbreaks are identified.

PROGNOSIS In general, the prognosis in tinea versicolor is excellent, but the disease recurs in up to 80% of patients within 2 years after cessation of treatment. Early diagnosis and treatment in patients with disseminated infection improve outcome.

Other Superficial Mycoses Tinea nigra is a rare infection of the palms caused by the dematiaceous fungus *Hortaea* (formerly *Exophiala*) *werneckii.* Two types of piedra characterized by nodules of fungal elements on the hair shaft have been reported: black piedra caused by *Piedraia hortae* and white piedra caused by *Trichosporon* species (which may also be associated with other superficial infections as well as with invasive trichosporonosis). *T. beigelii* has historically been the most significant pathogen in the genus *Trichosporon.* Recently proposed revisions in classification and nomenclature are based on analysis of 26S rRNA sequences and use of nonmolecular techniques to differentiate 17 species—only 6 of which cause human disease—and 5 varieties of *Trichosporon.* Under this system, *T. beigelii* will be designated *T. cutaneum.* The other five human pathogens included in this revised classification are *T. asteroides, T. ovoides, T. inkin, T. asahii,* and *T. mucoides.* In addition, four serotypes of *Trichosporon* (serotypes I, II, III, and I-III) have been recognized, of which only serotypes I (*T. cutaneum* and *T. mucoides*) and II (*T. asahii, T. asteroides, T. inkin,* and *T. ovoides*) are pathogenic. Given that this revised nomenclature has not been universally adopted, the previous classification system may remain in use for some time and may be a source of confusion.

T. ovoides is usually associated with white piedra of the scalp, whereas *T. inkin* is primarily associated with white piedra of the groin. *T. ovoides* has also been implicated in summer-type hypersensitivity pneumonitis. The treatment of white piedra requires shaving off all the hair in the affected areas and applying a topical azole for 1–4 months.

CUTANEOUS INFECTIONS

The cutaneous mycoses are caused by *dermatophytes,* which infect keratinized tissues, including skin, hair follicles, and nails. These der-

TABLE 199-1 SYSTEMIC THERAPY FOR MISCELLANEOUS INVASIVE MYCOSES AND THE ALGAL INFECTION PROTOTHECOSIS

Type of Infection	First-Line Therapy	Alternative Therapy
Malasseziasis		
Central venous catheter–related infections	Removal of central venous catheter AmB[a]	In vitro susceptibility studies indicate that azoles may offer a therapeutic alternative.
Trichosporonosis	AmB in combination with voriconazole[b] (300 mg bid)	GM-CSF or IFN-γ may be a useful therapeutic adjunct.
Sporotrichosis		
Cutaneous/ lympho-cutaneous	Itraconazole[c] (100–200 mg/d for 3–6 months)	Terbinafine, 500–1000 mg/d
Non-life-threatening pulmonary, osteoarticular, or disseminated disease	Itraconazole (200 mg bid for 12 months)	AmB (lipid formulation) *or* fluconazole (800 mg/d for 12 months) in patients who cannot tolerate AmB or itraconazole
Life-threatening pulmonary or disseminated disease	AmB	Selected patients may be switched to oral itraconazole (200 mg bid for 12 months)
Eumycetoma	Surgery in combination with: Ketoconazole (200–400 mg/d) *or* Voriconazole (600 mg/d) *or* Terbinafine (500 mg/d)	Posaconazole is currently being evaluated.
Dematiaceous fungal infections	Surgical excision or cryosurgery combined with:	...
Chromoblastomycosis	Itraconazole (200–600 mg/d), alone or with 5-fluorocytosine (50–100 mg/kg qd in 3 or 4 divided doses)	
Phaeohyphomycosis		
Cutaneous or subcutaneous disease	Itraconazole (200 mg once or twice daily before surgery and to prevent relapse)	
Systemic/CNS	AmB in combination with itraconazole (200 mg bid) or voriconazole (200 mg bid)	
Paracoccidioidomycosis		
Mild to moderate disease	Itraconazole (200–400 mg/d)	...
Severe disease	AmB	Selected patients may be switched to itraconazole after an initial course of AmB.
Penicilliosis		
Mild to moderate disease	Itraconazole (200 mg bid for 2 months)	...
Severe disease	AmB	Selected patients may be switched to itraconazole (200 mg bid) after an initial course of AmB. The duration of primary treatment is 2 months.
Suppressive therapy for patients with HIV infection or AIDS	Itraconazole (200 mg/d)	
Fusariosis and pseudallescheriasis/scedosporiosis	IV voriconazole (6 mg/kg q12h for first 24 h, then 4 mg/kg q12h until neutropenia resolves and clinical response is documented)	Selected patients may be switched to oral voriconazole (200 mg bid) after a clinical response and reversal of neutropenia.
Protothecosis	Itraconazole (200 mg/d for 2 months or until lesions resolve)	Disseminated infections should be treated with IV AmB.

[a]Unless otherwise noted, AmB dosages are 0.6–1.0 mg/kg per day of the deoxycholate formulation or 3–5 mg/kg per day of a lipid formulation.

[b]An initial loading dose of voriconazole is recommended on day 1 for both IV therapy (6 mg/kg q12h) and oral therapy (400 mg q12h).

[c]An initial loading dose of itraconazole is recommended for both IV therapy (200 mg bid for 2 days) and oral therapy (200 mg bid for 2 days).

Note: AmB, amphotericin B; CNS, central nervous system; GM-CSF, granulocyte-macrophage colony-stimulating factor; IFN-γ, interferon γ.

matophytic fungi invade the epidermis and elicit an inflammatory reaction, including redness and pruritus. Dermatophytic infections are designated according to the anatomic location of the lesions—e.g., tinea corporis (the trunk, shoulders, or limbs), *tinea cruris* (the warm moist areas of the groin, perianal, and perineal areas), *tinea faciei* (the nonhairy areas of the face), *tinea pedis* (the feet), *tinea unguium* (the nails), and *tinea capitis* (the scalp).

ETIOLOGIC AGENTS Three genera of dermatophytes—*Microsporum, Trichophyton,* and *Epidermophyton*—are associated with human infec-

tions. Members of these genera can be divided into three groups according to their natural reservoir and potential for infection: anthropophilic, zoophilic, and geophilic organisms.

EPIDEMIOLOGY Tinea is common worldwide. It is estimated that more than 8 million office visits to primary care physicians are made annually for tinea-related symptoms.

PATHOGENESIS Dermatophytic fungi release proteolytic enzymes and keratinases into the skin. These exocellular enzymes release nutrients and facilitate dissemination through the stratum corneum. A specific host immune response is directed against the organisms.

CLINICAL MANIFESTATIONS Any dermatophyte can cause tinea corporis, which is commonly called "ringworm" because of the typical appearance of lesions: annular scaly patches with raised, erythematous vesicular borders and central clearing. Tinea faciei, like tinea corporis, can be caused by any dermatophyte. *T. rubrum* and *E. floccosum* are common causes of tinea cruris; similar lesions can be caused by *Candida* infection.

Tinea pedis, the most common clinical dermatophytic infection, usually presents with interdigital cracking, scaling, and maceration. Hyperkeratosis and peeling of the soles of the feet are common, with a scaly red "moccasin-like" appearance in chronic cases. The most common cause of tinea pedis is *T. rubrum*. Clinical lesions similar to those of tinea pedis can be caused by nondermatophytic fungi, yeasts, and bacteria.

Tinea unguium is caused by *T. rubrum, T. mentagrophytes,* and *E. floccosum*. The term *onychomycosis* encompasses nail infections due to either dermatophytes or nondermatophytic fungi. Dermatophytes cause 80–90% of cases of onychomycosis. The prevalence of these infections is ~2% among young adults and increases to 20% among individuals 40–60 years of age. Onychomycosis occurs in diabetic patients at the same rate as in the general population but poses a greater risk of bacterial superinfection in diabetes.

Tinea capitis is a common dermatophytic disease of children but is relatively rare among adults. The clinical presentation may vary from a diffuse scaly scalp to scattered areas of scale with or without alopecia. Hair may break off at the scalp ("black-dot ringworm"). Pruritus is not a constant symptom. Inflammatory responses may be minimal or severe, with the formation of a kerion characterized by alopecia, a tender or painful boggy scalp, purulent drainage, and localized lymphadenopathy. *T. tonsurans* is the most common dermatophyte associated with tinea capitis.

DIAGNOSIS Some skin lesions have distinctive characteristics that allow a presumptive diagnosis, and topical therapy is often initiated solely on the basis of the lesions' appearance. However, the ease of obtaining specimens for microscopic examination and culture should encourage definitive diagnosis. Scrapings of skin lesions can be examined as a wet preparation, with a drop of 10% KOH used to dissolve cells and debris. Samples for fungal cultures should be obtained from patients whose history, physical examination, and KOH-treated specimens are inconclusive with regard to the diagnosis of dermatophytic infection. It is recommended that a definitive diagnosis be established in patients before systemic antifungal agents are administered.

Rx CUTANEOUS INFECTIONS

Most tinea infections can be treated with topical agents alone. Many such antifungal agents are widely available as both prescription and over-the-counter products. Topical imidazoles (e.g., clotrimazole, miconazole, econazole, and ketoconazole) are generally well tolerated and efficacious when used twice daily for at least 2 weeks. The allylamines, including terbinafine and naftifine (available in 1% creams or 1% solutions), provide cure rates of ≥75% and require only once-daily application for shorter periods. Tolnaftate powder is best suited for prevention of tinea pedis.

Systemic therapy is indicated for patients who are unresponsive to topical therapy; for those who have infections involving the scalp or bearded areas, who have hyperkeratotic areas on the palms or soles, or who have widespread disease; and for immunocompromised individuals. Once-daily itraconazole (200 mg), terbinafine (250 mg), and griseofulvin (500 mg of the microcrystalline formulation or 375 mg of the ultramicrocrystalline formulation) has proved effective. Treatment should be administered until lesions resolve. For patients with nail disease, itraconazole (200 mg/d) or terbinafine (250 mg/d) is preferred. The duration of therapy is 2–3 months for fingernails and 4–6 months for toenails. Pulse therapy with itraconazole and terbinafine is an option. Relapse of nail disease is common.

COMPLICATIONS Sites of tinea pedis frequently become superinfected with bacteria. Sometimes these infections are serious, especially in diabetic patients, patients who have undergone saphenous-vein harvest for coronary artery bypass grafts, and patients with any significant venous incompetence.

SUBCUTANEOUS INFECTIONS
Fungal infections that primarily involve the dermis and subcutaneous tissue result from implantation of the organism in the skin through trauma. The major subcutaneous mycoses are sporotrichosis, mycetoma, chromoblastomycosis, and phaeohyphomycosis.

Sporotrichosis Sporotrichosis most commonly presents as chronic cutaneous, lymphocutaneous, and/or subcutaneous disease. This infection may also be extracutaneous, occurring at pulmonary, osteoarticular, or disseminated sites.

ETIOLOGIC AGENT Sporotrichosis is caused by the thermally dimorphic fungus *Sporothrix schenckii*, which is found in soil, plants, and moss and on animals. *S. schenckii* exists worldwide but is most common in tropical and warmer temperate regions, such as Mexico and Central and South America.

EPIDEMIOLOGY Sporotrichosis is usually an occupational disease of gardeners, farmers, forestry workers, florists, and horticulturists. There have been well-documented epidemics (e.g., among South African gold miners) as well as scattered outbreaks (e.g., among workers handling sphagnum, hay, and wood). Recent reports indicate that infection can be related to zoonotic spread from cats and armadillos.

PATHOGENESIS Sporotrichosis most often follows inoculation of the organism into the skin.

CLINICAL MANIFESTATIONS The majority of infections with *S. schenckii* present either as fixed cutaneous sporotrichosis or as lymphangitic or lymphocutaneous disease. Fixed cutaneous disease (plaque sporotrichosis) is limited to the site of inoculation. The primary lesion enlarges and may ulcerate and become verrucous. In lymphocutaneous disease, which accounts for ~80% of cases, secondary lesions ascend along the lymphatics that drain the area, producing small painless nodules that erupt, drain, and ulcerate. Other organisms (e.g., nontuberculous mycobacteria, *Nocardia*, *Leishmania*, and chromoblastomycotic agents) may cause similar lesions. Osteoarticular sporotrichosis is an uncommon complication but may cause granulomatous tenosynovitis and bursitis, particularly in alcoholic patients. Pulmonary sporotrichosis following inhalation of *S. schenckii* conidia has been reported in alcoholic patients with chronic obstructive pulmonary disease. Disseminated disease, including that involving the central nervous system, is most likely to occur in patients who have AIDS or are otherwise immunocompromised.

DIAGNOSIS A definitive diagnosis is made by culture of *S. schenckii* on any of a variety of media. Histopathologic examination of biopsy material may also contribute to the diagnosis, with detection of the characteristic ovoid or cigar-shaped yeast forms.

Rx SPOROTRICHOSIS

Sporotrichosis requires systemic therapy (Table 199-1). Historically, oral therapy with a saturated solution of potassium iodide (SSKI; 5 drops 3 times daily, increasing to 40–50 drops 3 times daily as tolerated) has been successful, but the use of this intervention is often limited by its toxicity. Because it has fewer side effects and is better tolerated, oral itraconazole has replaced SSKI as the treatment of choice for cutaneous and lymphocutaneous sporotrichosis. Terbinafine has also been effective against lymphocutaneous disease, although it has not been approved for this indication by the U.S. Food and Drug Administration. Patients with non-life-threatening pulmonary disease and those with osteoarticular disease should be treated with itraconazole for at least 12 months. Amphotericin B is the preferred agent for patients with life-threatening pulmonary disease or disseminated infection, for patients who cannot tolerate itraconazole, and for patients in whom itraconazole treatment has failed.

COMPLICATIONS Hematogenous dissemination of *S. schenckii* is most common among immunocompromised patients, including those with HIV infection or AIDS. These patients may develop widespread cutaneous ulcers, granulomas, and systemic disease with pulmonary, meningeal, articular, or generalized infection.

PROGNOSIS Success rates of 90–100% have been reported for itraconazole treatment of lymphocutaneous sporotrichosis. A clinical response usually occurs within 4–6 weeks of the start of therapy. Patients who relapse usually respond to a second course of itraconazole.

Mycetoma Mycetoma is a chronic suppurative infection that begins in the subcutaneous tissue and spreads to fascia and bone. Mycetoma due to fungi is called *eumycetoma*, while that caused by actinomycetes is referred to as *actinomycetoma*. Both diseases are characterized by abscesses containing grains composed of large aggregates of filaments (fungal or actinomycete). Traumatic inoculation is responsible for initial infection.

ETIOLOGY AND EPIDEMIOLOGY Mycetomas are common in Mexico, Central America, Venezuela, Brazil, Africa, the Middle East, India, Pakistan, and Bangladesh. The most common cause of eumycetoma worldwide is *Madurella mycetomatis*, while the rare cases that occur in the United States are associated with *Pseudallescheria boydii*. Actinomycetoma, the usual form of mycetoma in Mexico and Central America, is associated with *Nocardia brasiliensis*, *Streptomyces somaliensis*, *Actinomadura madurae*, and *Actinomadura pelletieri*.

CLINICAL MANIFESTATIONS Clinically, eumycetoma and actinomycetoma are similar, beginning as small, firm, painless subcutaneous plaques or nodules on the foot or leg and, less frequently, on the arms, torso, and scalp. Patients usually present with draining sinus tracts, subcutaneous abscesses, fibrosis with woody induration, and extension to fascia and bone.

DIAGNOSIS Diagnosis is based on visualization of grains in pus, sinus exudate, or tissue biopsy. Fungal hyphae must be distinguished from the filamentous forms seen in actinomycetoma. Organisms associated with mycetoma, whether fungi or actinomycetes, can be grown on a variety of culture media.

℞ MYCETOMA

The treatment of mycetoma is problematic. A combined medical/surgical approach is the option of choice (Table 199-1). Because actinomycetoma does not respond to antifungal agents, the differentiation between eumycetoma and actinomycetoma is crucial. (For the treatment of actinomycetoma, see Chaps. 155 and 156.) Amphotericin B has not generally been effective for the treatment of eumycetoma. A limited number of patients have responded to long-term azole therapy. Posaconazole, an investigational agent, may have a role in the treatment of eumycetoma in the future.

Dematiaceous Fungal Infections Of the many names applied to infections caused by brown- or black-pigmented soil fungi, *phaeohyphomycosis* and *chromoblastomycosis* are the most widely accepted. Phaeohyphomycosis refers to infections in which the organisms in tissue occur as pigmented yeast-like forms and/or hyphae. Chromoblastomycosis is distinguished by the presence of pigmented sclerotic bodies in tissue.

Chromoblastomycosis is characterized by slow-growing verrucous plaques or nodules, usually on the lower extremities. The most common etiologic agents are *Fonsecaea pedrosoi, F. compacta, Phialophora verrucosa, Rhinocladiella aquaspersa,* and *Cladosporium (Cladophialophora) carrionii.* Most cases affect rural workers living in tropical and subtropical regions, and infection is acquired by traumatic inoculation. Small verrucous papules enlarge slowly but remain painless. Lesions seen in late stages may be superficial or raised purplish irregular plaques; less commonly, they may be nodular, tumorous, verrucous, or cicatricial. In advanced cases, secondary lymphedema, bacterial infections, and keratin necrosis can develop. Although histologic examination of scrapings or biopsy material for characteristic sclerotic bodies can lead to the diagnosis of chromoblastomycosis, culture is required for identification of the causative agent. Treatment is difficult, although many therapeutic interventions have been described (Table 199-1). Results are best when early surgical excision or cryosurgery is used in combination with antifungal therapy. Treatment with itraconazole—either alone or with 5-fluorocytosine—has had some success.

Phaeohyphomycosis presents in four clinical forms: superficial, cutaneous-corneal, subcutaneous, and systemic. *Exophiala jeanselmei, Wangiella dermatitidis,* and *Bipolaris* species are the most common etiologic agents. The route of infection is most likely implantation, with the subsequent formation of an inflammatory cyst. A single inflammatory nondraining cyst located on a proximal limb is the most typical presentation. The diagnosis is usually made by histopathologic detection (in biopsy material) of a fibrous capsule with a granulomatous reaction and a necrotic center. Culture is required to identify specific organisms. Surgical excision of the lesion is essential. Itraconazole treatment reduces the size of large lesions before excision and prevents relapse afterward (Table 199-1). Cerebral phaeohyphomycosis is thought to be due to direct extension from adjacent paranasal sinuses or from a penetrating trauma to the head. Most cases present as a brain abscess with focal neurologic deficits and/or generalized seizures. A review of 101 cases revealed that one-half of patients had no apparent immunocompromising condition. Infections in immunocompromised patients are more likely to disseminate; disseminated infections have been reported in patients with HIV infection, solid-

organ transplant recipients, patients with malignancies, and one pregnant woman. Rhinocerebral disease requires surgical drainage along with antifungal therapy. A combination of amphotericin B and itraconazole or voriconazole is recommended.

SYSTEMIC MYCOSES

Paracoccidioidomycosis Often referred to as South American blastomycosis, paracoccidioidomycosis is a systemic disease caused by the dimorphic fungus *Paracoccidioides brasiliensis.* Pulmonary infection follows inhalation of conidia and may disseminate to other organs, producing secondary lesions in the skin, lymph nodes, and adrenal glands. Subclinical infections have been documented in healthy residents of endemic regions. Paracoccidioidomycosis is most common in Venezuela, Colombia, Ecuador, Argentina, and Brazil. Histopathologic examination of clinical specimens may reveal globose yeast cells with multiple buds. Definitive diagnosis relies on culture of the organism. Itraconazole treatment has been effective (Table 199-1). An initial course of amphotericin B may be required in seriously ill patients.

Penicilliosis Caused by the thermally dimorphic fungus *Penicillium marneffei,* penicilliosis is a disease of immunocompromised individuals living in or traveling to Southeast Asia. The primary portal of entry is the lungs, and hematologic dissemination follows. Clinical manifestations are similar to those of disseminated histoplasmosis and include fever, chills, weight loss, anemia, generalized lymphadenopathy, and hepatomegaly. Diffuse papular lesions similar to those of molluscum contagiosum are common in patients with HIV infection or AIDS. Small yeast cells may be seen on histopathologic examination of tissue, but definitive diagnosis depends on culture. Amphotericin B is the treatment of choice for severely ill patients (Table 199-1). Patients who have less severe disease or who have responded to an initial course of amphotericin B may be treated with itraconazole. Primary therapy is usually given for 2 months; in patients with HIV infection or AIDS, suppressive therapy with itraconazole may be useful in preventing relapse.

Fusariosis Fusariosis is an invasive mold infection associated with *Fusarium* species, most commonly *F. solani.* The skin and respiratory tract are the primary portals of entry. Localized skin infections may occur at sites of trauma in immunocompetent hosts. Disease may disseminate from the skin or respiratory tract in immunocompromised patients; 90% of such cases are reported in neutropenic patients with leukemia or recipients of allogeneic bone marrow transplants. The clinical presentation is generally nonspecific, with fever and skin lesions that eventually become necrotic and resemble ecthyma gangrenosum. Clinical, radiographic, and pathologic findings are similar to those in invasive aspergillosis or zygomycosis. Blood cultures are positive in up to 50% of cases, and the presence of a mold in cultured blood from neutropenic patients suggests fusariosis. *Fusarium* species are often resistant to antifungal therapy. High-dose amphotericin B has met with limited success. Therapy with voriconazole (Table 199-1) has been successful in a few patients. Therapy is continued until neutropenia resolves and a clinical response is documented. The prognosis of disseminated infection is related to the reversal of neutropenia and other immunodeficiencies.

Pseudallescheriasis and Scedosporiosis The emerging pathogens, *P. boydii, Scedosporium apiospermum* (the asexual form of *P. boydii*), and *S. prolificans* are molds that cause rare sinopulmonary infections in immunocompetent hosts and that may present as fungus balls in the lungs or paranasal sinuses. Severe pneumonia, invasive sinusitis, and hematogenous dissemination (including brain abscess) occur in immunosuppressed hosts, especially bone marrow transplant recipients. The hyphal elements seen in the tissues of patients with *Pseudallescheria* and *Scedosporium* infections resemble those seen in intravascular invasion by *Aspergillus.* The outcome of treatment is poor, and most patients with disseminated disease die. Amphotericin B is not effective in the treatment of pseudallescheriasis or scedosporiosis. A small number of patients have been cured with voriconazole in the same doses listed for fusariosis (Table 199-1). Surgical debridement and drainage of abscesses may also be necessary.

Trichosporonosis *Trichosporon* species, predominantly *T. asahii* and to a lesser extent *T. mucoides*, can cause disseminated trichosporonosis in immunocompromised patients, especially those with profound neutropenia. Unpublished studies describe isolation of *Trichosporon* from pubic sites of white piedra, sputum, skin lesions, and blood. *T. pullulans* (formerly *Monilia pullulans*) is a rare cause of systemic infection. Portals of entry include the skin, gastrointestinal tract, and lungs. The clinical presentation mimics candidiasis. Cultures of blood, skin lesions, or biopsy specimens confirm the diagnosis. *Trichosporon* shares antigens with *Cryptococcus neoformans* and produces positive results in the latex agglutination test. Treatment of *Trichosporon* infections is complicated by resistance to amphotericin B. Mortality rates of >80% have been reported. The azoles, especially voriconazole, have been effective alone or in combination with amphotericin B (Table 199-1). Adjunctive therapy with granulocyte-macrophage colony-stimulating factor or interferon γ may be beneficial. The prognosis, however, is related to the resolution of neutropenia.

ALGAL INFECTIONS

Prototheca, an achlorophyllic alga common in nature, has been associated with rare human infections in Europe, Asia, Oceania, and the United States (particularly the southeastern states). This organism has been isolated from slime flux of trees, industrial ponds, tap water, sewage systems, swimming pools, and soil. Infections with *P. wickerhamii* and *P. zopfii* occur primarily in immunocompromised patients. Protothecosis may present as a cutaneous disease with erythematous nodules, plaques, or superficial ulcers on exposed skin; as olecranon

bursitis; or as a systemic infection. Histologic examination of biopsy material may reveal multinucleated giant cells and extra- and intracellular, basophilic to amphiphilic organisms containing endospores. *Prototheca* can be cultured on Sabouraud's agar. The most frequently used therapeutic agent is amphotericin B, which has proved effective even in patients with disseminated protothecosis. Azole antifungal agents such as itraconazole, ketoconazole, and fluconazole have also been used successfully. Surgical excision may play a role in the treatment of localized cutaneous lesions.

FURTHER READINGS

ALY R: Skin, hair, and nail fungal infections. Infect Dis Clin Pract 10:117, 1998

CHAPMAN SW, DANIEL CR III: Cutaneous manifestations of fungal infection. Infect Dis Clin North Am 4:879, 1994

DIGNANI MC ct al: Immunomodulation with interferon-gamma and colony-stimulating factors for refractory fungal infections in patients with leukemia. Cancer 104:199, 2005

FLEMING RV, ANAISSIE EJ: Emerging fungal infections, in *Fungal Infections in the Immunocompromised Patient*, JR Wingard, EJ Anaissie (eds). Boca Raton, Taylor & Francis Group, 2005, pp 311–340

——— et al: Emerging and less common fungal pathogens. Infect Dis Clin North Am 16:915, 2002

QUEIROZ-TELLES F et al: Subcutaneous mycoses. Infect Dis Clin North Am 17:59, 2003

SEGAL BH et al: Fungal infections in nontransplant patients with hematologic malignancies. Infect Dis Clin North Am 16:935, 2002

SILVEIRA F, NUCCI M: Emergence of black moulds in fungal disease: Epidemiology and therapy. Curr Opin Infect Dis 14:679, 2001

www.doctorfungus.org

200 *Pneumocystis* Infection
A. George Smulian, Peter D. Walzer

DEFINITION AND DESCRIPTION

Pneumocystis is an opportunistic fungal pulmonary pathogen that is an important cause of pneumonia in the immunocompromised host. Although organisms within the *Pneumocystis* genus are morphologically very similar, they are genetically diverse and host-specific. *P. jirovecii* infects humans, whereas *P. carinii*—the original species described in 1909—infects rats. For clarity, only the genus designation *Pneumocystis* will be used in this chapter.

Developmental stages of the organism include the trophic form, the cyst, and the precyst (an intermediate stage). The life cycle of *Pneumocystis* probably involves sexual and asexual reproduction, although definitive proof awaits the development of a reliable culture system. *Pneumocystis* contains several different antigen groups, the most prominent of which is the 95- to 140-kDa major surface glycoprotein (MSG). MSG plays a central role in the interaction of *Pneumocystis* with its host.

EPIDEMIOLOGY

Serologic surveys have demonstrated that *Pneumocystis* has a worldwide distribution and that most healthy children have been exposed to the organism by 3–4 years of age. Airborne transmission of *Pneumocystis* has been documented in animal studies; person-to-person transmission has been suggested by hospital outbreaks of *Pneumocystis* pneumonia (PcP) and by molecular epidemiologic analysis of isolates. *Pneumocystis* colonization of immunocompetent individuals has been detected by polymerase chain reaction (PCR) techniques.

PATHOGENESIS AND PATHOLOGY

The host factors that predispose to the development of PcP include defects in cellular and humoral immunity. The risk of PcP among HIV-infected patients rises markedly when circulating CD4+ T cell counts fall below 200/μL. Other persons at risk for PcP are patients receiving immunosuppressive agents (particularly glucocorticoids) for cancer and organ transplantation; those receiving biologic agents such as infliximab and etanercept for rheumatoid arthritis and inflammatory bowel disease; children with primary immunodeficiency diseases; and premature malnourished infants.

The principal host effector cells against *Pneumocystis* are alveolar macrophages, which ingest and kill the organism, releasing a variety of inflammatory mediators. Proliferating organisms remain extracellular within the alveolus, attaching tightly to type I cells. Alveolar damage results in increased alveolar-capillary permeability and surfactant abnormalities, including a fall in phospholipids and an increase in surfactant proteins A and D. The host inflammatory response to lung injury leads to increases in levels of interleukin 8 and in neutrophil counts in bronchoalveolar lavage (BAL) fluid. These changes correlate with disease severity.

On lung sections stained with hematoxylin and eosin, the alveoli are filled with a typical foamy, vacuolated exudate. Severe disease may include interstitial edema, fibrosis, and hyaline membrane formation. The host inflammatory changes usually consist of hypertrophy of alveolar type II cells, a typical reparative response, and a mild mononuclear cell interstitial infiltrate. Malnourished infants display an intense plasma cell infiltrate that gave the disease its early name: interstitial plasma cell pneumonia.

CLINICAL FEATURES

Patients with PcP develop dyspnea, fever, and nonproductive cough. HIV-infected patients are usually ill for several weeks and may have relatively subtle manifestations. Symptoms in non-HIV-infected pa-

FIGURE 200-1 **A.** Chest radiograph depicting diffuse infiltrates in an HIV-infected patient with PcP. **B.** High-resolution CT of the lung show-ing ground-glass opacification in an HIV-infected patient with PcP. *(Courtesy of Dr. Cristopher Meyer, with permission.)*

tients are of shorter duration and often begin after the glucocorticoid dose has been tapered. A high index of suspicion and a thorough history are key factors in early detection.

Physical findings include tachypnea, tachycardia, and cyanosis, but lung auscultation reveals few abnormalities. Reduced arterial oxygen pressure (Pa_{O_2}), increased alveolar-arterial oxygen gradient ($PA_{O_2} - Pa_{O_2}$), and respiratory alkalosis are evident. Diffusion capacity is reduced, and heightened uptake with nonspecific nuclear imaging techniques (gallium scan) may be noted. Elevated serum concentrations of lactate dehydrogenase, reflecting lung parenchymal damage, have been reported; however, the increase is not specific for PcP.

The classic findings on chest radiography consist of bilateral diffuse infiltrates beginning in the perihilar regions (Fig. 200-1*A*), but various atypical manifestations (nodular densities, cavitary lesions) have also been reported. Pneumothorax occurs, and its management is often difficult. Early in the course of PcP, the chest radiograph may be normal, although high-resolution CT of the lung may reveal ground-glass opacities at this stage (Fig. 200-1*B*).

While *Pneumocystis* usually remains confined to the lungs, cases of disseminated infection have occurred in both HIV-infected and non-HIV-infected patients. Common sites of involvement include the lymph nodes, spleen, liver, and bone marrow.

DIAGNOSIS

Because of the nonspecific nature of the clinical picture, the diagnosis must be based on specific identification of the organism. A definitive diagnosis is made by histopathologic staining. Traditional cell wall stains such as methenamine silver selectively stain the wall of *Pneumocystis* cysts, while reagents such as Wright-Giemsa stain the nuclei of all developmental stages. Immunofluorescence with monoclonal antibodies is more sensitive and specific than histologic staining. DNA amplification by PCR may become part of routine diagnostics but may not distinguish colonization from infection.

The successful diagnosis of PcP depends on the collection of proper specimens. In general, the yield from different diagnostic procedures is higher in HIV-infected patients than in non-HIV-infected patients because of the higher organism burden in the former group. Sputum induction and oral washes have gained popularity as simple, noninvasive techniques; however, these procedures require trained and dedicated personnel. Fiberoptic bronchoscopy with BAL, which provides information about the organism burden, the host inflammatory response, and the presence of other opportunistic infections, continues to be the mainstay of *Pneumocystis* diagnosis. Transbronchial biopsy and open lung biopsy, the most invasive procedures, are used only when a diagnosis cannot be made by BAL.

COURSE AND PROGNOSIS

In the typical case of untreated PcP, progressive respiratory embarrassment leads to death. Therapy is most effective when instituted early, before there is extensive alveolar damage. If examination of induced sputum is nondiagnostic and BAL cannot be performed in a timely manner, empirical therapy for PcP is reasonable. However, this practice does not eliminate the need for a specific etiologic diagnosis. With improved management of HIV and its complications, mortality from PcP is 15–20% at 1 month and 50–55% at 1 year. Rates of early death remain high among patients who require mechanical ventilation (60%) and among non-HIV-infected patients (40%).

℞ *PNEUMOCYSTIS* INFECTION

Trimethoprim-sulfamethoxazole (TMP-SMX), which acts by inhibiting folic acid synthesis, is considered the drug of choice for all forms of PcP (**Table 200-1**). Therapy is continued for 14 days in non-HIV-infected patients and for 21 days in persons infected with HIV. Since HIV-infected patients respond more slowly than non-HIV-infected patients, it is prudent to wait at least 7 days after the initiation of treatment before concluding that therapy has failed. TMP-SMX is well tolerated by non-HIV-infected patients, whereas more than half of HIV-infected patients experience serious adverse reactions.

Several alternative regimens are available for the treatment of mild to moderate cases of PcP (a Pa_{O_2} of >70 mmHg or a $PA_{O_2} - Pa_{O_2}$ of <35 mmHg on breathing room air). TMP plus dapsone and clindamycin plus primaquine are about as effective as TMP-SMX. Dapsone and primaquine should not be administered to patients with glucose-6-phosphate dehydrogenase (G6PD) deficiency. Atovaquone is less effective than TMP-SMX but is better tolerated. Since *Pneumocystis* lacks ergosterol, it is not susceptible to antifungal agents that inhibit ergosterol synthesis.

Alternative regimens that are recommended for the treatment of moderate to severe PcP (a Pa_{O_2} of ≤70 mmHg or a $PA_{O_2} - Pa_{O_2}$ of ≥35 mmHg) are parenteral pentamidine, parenteral clindamycin plus primaquine, or trimetrexate plus leucovorin. Parenteral clindamycin plus primaquine may be more efficacious than pentamidine.

Molecular evidence of resistance to sulfonamides and to atovaquone has emerged among human *Pneumocystis* isolates. Although prior sulfonamide exposure is a risk factor, this resistance has also occurred in HIV-infected patients who have never received sulfonamides. The outcome of therapy appears to be linked more strongly to traditional measures—e.g., high Acute Physiology, Age, and Chronic Health Evaluation III (APACHE III) scores, need for positive-pressure ventilation, delayed intubation, and development of pneumothorax—than to the presence of molecular markers of sulfonamide resistance. HIV-infected patients frequently experience deterioration of respiratory function shortly after receiving anti-*Pneumocystis* drugs. The adjunctive administration of tapering doses of glucocorticoids to HIV-infected patients with moderate to severe PcP can prevent this

TABLE 200-1	TREATMENT OF PNEUMOCYSTOSIS
Drug(s), Dose, Route	**Adverse Effects**
First Choice[a]	
TMP-SMX (5 mg/kg TMP, 25 mg/kg SMX[b]) q6–8 h PO or IV	Fever, rash, cytopenias, hepatitis, hyperkalemia, GI disturbances
Other Agents[a]	
TMP, 5 mg/kg q6–8h, plus dapsone, 100 mg qd PO	Hemolysis (G6PD deficiency), methemoglobinemia, fever, rash, GI disturbances
Atovaquone, 750 mg bid PO	Rash, fever, GI and hepatic disturbances
Clindamycin, 300–450 mg q6h PO or 600 mg q6–8h IV, plus primaquine, 15–30 mg qd PO	Hemolysis (G6PD deficiency), methemoglobinemia, rash, colitis, neutropenia
Pentamidine, 3–4 mg/kg qd IV	Hypotension, azotemia, cardiac arrhythmias, pancreatitis, dysglycemias, hypocalcemia, neutropenia, hepatitis
Trimetrexate, 45 mg/m^2 qd IV, plus leucovorin,[c] 20 mg/kg q6h PO or IV	Cytopenias, peripheral neuropathy, hepatic disturbances
Adjunctive Agent	
Prednisone, 40 mg bid × 5 d, 40 mg qd × 5 d, 20 mg qd × 11 d; PO or IV	Immunosuppression, peptic ulcer, hyperglycemia, mood changes, hypertension

[a]Therapy is administered for 14 days to non-HIV-infected patients and for 21 days to HIV-infected patients.
[b]Equivalent of 2 double-strength (DS) tablets. (One DS tablet contains 160 mg of TMP and 800 mg of SMX.)
[c]Leucovorin prevents bone marrow toxicity from trimetrexate.
Note: GI, gastrointestinal; G6PD, glucose-6-phosphate dehydrogenase; TMP-SMX, trimethoprim-sulfamethoxazole.

TABLE 200-2	PROPHYLAXIS OF PNEUMOCYSTOSIS[a]
Drug(s), Dose, Route	**Comments**
First Choice	
TMP-SMX, 1 DS tablet or 1 SS tablet qd PO[b]	TMP-SMX can be safely reintroduced in some patients who have experienced mild to moderate side effects.
Other Agents	
Dapsone, 50 mg bid or 100 mg qd PO	—
Dapsone, 50 mg qd PO, plus pyrimethamine, 50 mg weekly PO, plus leucovorin, 25 mg weekly PO	Leucovorin prevents bone marrow toxicity from pyrimethamine.
Dapsone, 200 mg weekly PO, plus pyrimethamine, 75 mg weekly PO, plus leucovorin, 25 mg weekly PO	Leucovorin prevents bone marrow toxicity from pyrimethamine.
Pentamidine, 300 mg monthly via Respirgard II nebulizer	Adverse reactions include cough and bronchospasm.
Atovaquone, 1500 mg qd PO	—
TMP-SMX, 1 DS tablet three times weekly PO	TMP-SMX can be safely reintroduced in some patients who have experienced mild to moderate side effects.

[a]For list of adverse effects, see Table 200-1.
[b]One DS tablet contains 160 mg of TMP and 800 mg of SMX.
Note: DS, double-strength; SS, single-strength; TMP-SMX, trimethoprim-sulfamethoxazole.

problem and improve the rate of survival (Table 200-1). For maximal benefit, this adjunctive therapy should be started early in the course of the illness. The use of steroids as adjunctive therapy in HIV-infected patients with mild PcP or in non-HIV-infected patients remains to be evaluated.

PREVENTION

Prophylaxis is indicated for HIV-infected patients with CD4+ T cell counts of <200/µL or a history of oropharyngeal candidiasis and for both HIV-infected and non-HIV-infected patients who have recovered from PcP. Prophylaxis may be discontinued in HIV-infected patients once CD4+ T cell counts have risen to >200/µL and remained at that level for ≥3 months. Primary prophylaxis guidelines for immunocompromised hosts not infected with HIV are less clear.

TMP-SMX is the drug of choice for primary and secondary prophylaxis (Table 200-2). This agent also provides protection against toxoplasmosis and some bacterial infections. Alternative regimens are available for individuals intolerant of TMP-SMX (Table 200-2). Although there are no specific recommendations for preventing the spread of *Pneumocystis* in health care facilities, it seems prudent to prevent direct contact between patients with PcP and other susceptible hosts.

FURTHER READINGS

CENTERS FOR DISEASE CONTROL AND PREVENTION: Treating opportunistic infections among HIV-infected adults and adolescents: Recommendations from the CDC, the National Institutes of Health and the HIV Medicine Association/Infectious Diseases Society of America. MMWR 53(RR-15):1, 2004

DALY KR et al: Antibody responses to the *Pneumocystis jirovecii* major surface glycoprotein. Emerg Infect Dis 12:1231, 2006

FESTIC E et al: Acute respiratory failure due to *Pneumocystis* pneumonia in patients without human immunodeficiency virus infection: Outcome and associated features. Chest 128:573, 2005

MEDRANO FJ et al: *Pneumocystis jirovecii* in general population. Emerg Infect Dis 11:245, 2005

MILLER RF et al: Improved survival for HIV infected patients with severe *Pneumocystis jirovecii* pneumonia is independent of highly active antiretroviral therapy. Thorax 61:716, 2006

REDHEAD SA et al: *Pneumocystis* and *Trypanosoma cruzi*: Nomenclature and typifications. J Eukaryot Microbiol 53:1, 2006

THOMAS CF JR, LIMPER AH: *Pneumocystis* pneumonia. N Engl J Med 350:2487, 2004

ZAR HJ: Pneumonia in HIV-infected and HIV-uninfected children in developing countries: Epidemiology, clinical features, and management. Curr Opin Pulm Med 10:176, 2004

Pneumocystis Infection

SECTION 17 PROTOZOAL AND HELMINTHIC INFECTIONS: GENERAL CONSIDERATIONS

201 Agents Used to Treat Parasitic Infections

Thomas A. Moore

Parasitic infections afflict more than half of the world's population and impose a substantial health burden, particularly in underdeveloped nations, where they are most prevalent. The remarkable success of global campaigns aimed at controlling or eliminating ancient scourges such as dracunculiasis and onchocerciasis has been offset by the spread of other diseases such as trypanosomiasis due to crumbling infrastructures in settings of HIV infection, civil war, and unstable government. The reach of some parasitic diseases, including malaria, has expanded over the past few decades as a result of factors such as deforestation, population shifts, global warming, and other climatic events. Despite major efforts at vaccine development and vector control, chemotherapy remains the single most effective means of controlling parasitic infections. However, efforts to combat the spread of some diseases are hindered by the development and spread of drug re-

sistance, the limited introduction of new antiparasitic agents, and the proliferation of counterfeit medications. Significant advances toward the reduction of the burden of parasitic disease have nevertheless been made, and the significant increase in funding of global health initiatives offers promise for the future.

This chapter deals exclusively with the agents used to treat infections due to parasites. Specific treatment recommendations for the parasitic diseases of humans are listed in subsequent chapters. The pharmacology of the antiparasitic agents is discussed in great detail in Chap. e17.

Table 201-1 presents a brief overview of each agent (including some drugs that are covered in other chapters), along with its major toxicities, spectrum of activity, and safety for use during pregnancy and lactation. Many of the agents are approved by the U.S. Food and Drug Administration but are considered investigational for the treatment of certain infections; these drugs are marked accordingly in the table. In addition, drugs available only through the Centers for Disease Control and Prevention (CDC) Drug Service (telephone: 404-639-3670 or 404-639-2888; www.cdc.gov/ncidod/dpd/professional/drug_service.htm) or only through their manufacturers (whose contact information may be available from the CDC) are specified by footnotes in the table.

TABLE 201-1 OVERVIEW OF AGENTS USED FOR THE TREATMENT OF PARASITIC INFECTIONS

Drugs by Class	Parasitic Infection(s)	Adverse Effects	Major Drug-Drug Interactions	Pregnancy Class[a]	Breast Milk
4-Aminoquinolines					
Amodiaquine	Malaria[b]	Agranulocytosis, hepatotoxicity	No information	Not assigned	No information
Chloroquine	Malaria[b]	*Occasional:* pruritus, nausea, vomiting, headache, hair depigmentation, exfoliative dermatitis, reversible corneal opacity. *Rare:* irreversible retinal injury, nail discoloration, blood dyscrasias	Antacids and kaolin: reduced absorption of chloroquine Ampicillin: bioavailability reduced by chloroquine Cimetidine: increased serum levels of chloroquine Cyclosporine: serum levels increased by chloroquine	Not assigned[c]	Yes
8-Aminoquinolines					
Primaquine	Malaria[b]	*Frequent:* hemolysis in patients with G6PD deficiency. *Occasional:* methemoglobinemia, GI disturbances. *Rare:* CNS symptoms	Quinacrine: potentiated toxicity of primaquine	Contraindicated	No information
Tafenoquine	Malaria[b]	*Frequent:* hemolysis in patients with G6PD deficiency, mild GI upset. *Occasional:* methemoglobinemia, headaches	No information	Not assigned	No information
Aminoalcohols					
Halofantrine	Malaria[b]	*Frequent:* abdominal pain, diarrhea. *Occasional:* ECG disturbances (dose-related prolongation of QTc and PR interval), nausea, pruritus. Contraindicated in persons who have cardiac disease or who have taken mefloquine in the preceding 3 weeks	Concomitant use of agents that prolong QTc interval contraindicated	C	No information
Lumefantrine	Malaria	*Occasional:* nausea, vomiting, diarrhea, abdominal pain, anorexia, headache, dizziness	No major interactions	Not assigned	No information
Aminoglycosides					
Paromomycin	Amebiasis,[b] infection with *Dientamoeba fragilis*, giardiasis, cryptosporidiosis, leishmaniasis	*Frequent:* GI disturbances (oral dosing only). *Occasional:* nephrotoxicity, ototoxicity, vestibular toxicity (parenteral dosing only)	No major interactions	Not assigned[c]	No information

(continued)

TABLE 201-1 OVERVIEW OF AGENTS USED FOR THE TREATMENT OF PARASITIC INFECTIONS (CONTINUED)

Drugs by Class	Parasitic Infection(s)	Adverse Effects	Major Drug-Drug Interactions	Pregnancy Class[a]	Breast Milk

Amphotericin B
  Amphotericin B deoxycholate
  Amphotec (InterMune)
  Amphotericin B lipid complex, ABLC (Abelcet)
  Amphotericin B, liposomal (AmBisome)
	Leishmaniasis,[d] amebic meningoencephalitis	*Frequent:* fever, chills, hypokalemia, hypomagnesemia, nephrotoxicity. *Occasional:* vomiting, dyspnea, hypotension	Antineoplastic agents: renal toxicity, bronchospasm, hypotension
			Glucocorticoids, ACTH, digitalis: hypokalemia
			Zidovudine: increased myelo- and nephrotoxicity
				B	No information

Antimonials Pentavalent antimony[e]	Leishmaniasis	*Frequent:* arthralgias/myalgias, pancreatitis, ECG changes (QT prolongation, T wave flattening or inversion)	No major interactions	Not assigned	Yes
Meglumine antimonate		*Frequent:* arthralgias/myalgias, pancreatitis, ECG changes (QT prolongation, T wave flattening or inversion)	Antiarrhythmics and tricyclic antidepressants: increased risk of cardiotoxicity	Not assigned	No information
Artemisinin and derivatives	Malaria	*Occasional:* neurotoxicity (ataxia, convulsions), nausea, vomiting, anorexia, contact dermatitis		Not assigned	No information
Arteether Artemether			No information No clinically significant interactions		
Artesunate			Mefloquine: levels decreased and clearance accelerated by artesunate		
Dihydroartemisinin			Mefloquine: increased absorption		
Atovaquone	Malaria,[a] babesiosis	*Frequent:* nausea, vomiting. *Occasional:* abdominal pain, headache	Plasma levels decreased by rifampin, tetracycline; bioavailability decreased by metoclopramide	C	No information

Azoles
  Fluconazole
  Itraconazole
  Ketoconazole
	Leishmaniasis	*Serious:* hepatotoxicity. *Rare:* exfoliative skin disorders, anaphylaxis	Warfarin, oral hypoglycemics, phenytoin, cyclosporine, theophylline, digoxin, dofetilide, quinidine, carbamazepine, rifabutin, busulfan, docetaxel, vinca alkaloids, pimozide, alprazolam, diazepam, midazolam, triazolam, verapamil, atorvastatin, cerivastatin, lovastatin, simvastatin, tacrolimus, sirolimus, indinavir, ritonavir, saquinavir, alfentanil, buspirone, methylprednisolone, trimetrexate: plasma levels increased by azoles
			Carbamazepine, phenobarbital, phenytoin, isoniazid, rifabutin, rifampin, antacids, H2-receptor antagonists, proton pump inhibitors, nevirapine: decreased plasma levels of azoles
			Clarithromycin, erythromycin, indinavir, ritonavir: increased plasma levels of azoles
				C	Yes

Benzimidazoles Albendazole	Ascariasis, capillariasis, clonorchiasis, cutaneous larva migrans, cysticercosis,[b] echinococcosis,[b] enterobiasis, eosinophilic enterocolitis, gnathostomiasis, hookworm, lymphatic filariasis, microsporidiosis, strongyloidiasis, trichinellosis, trichostrongyliasis, trichuriasis, visceral larva migrans	*Occasional:* nausea, vomiting, abdominal pain, headache, reversible alopecia, elevated aminotransferases. *Rare:* leukopenia, rash	Dexamethasone, praziquantel: plasma level of albendazole sulfoxide increased by ~50%	C	Yes[f]

(continued)

TABLE 201-1 **OVERVIEW OF AGENTS USED FOR THE TREATMENT OF PARASITIC INFECTIONS (CONTINUED)**

Drugs by Class	Parasitic Infection(s)	Adverse Effects	Major Drug-Drug Interactions	Pregnancy Class[a]	Breast Milk
Mebendazole	Ascariasis,[b] capillariasis, eosinophilic enterocolitis, enterobiasis,[b] hookworm,[b] trichinellosis, trichostrongyliasis, trichuriasis,[b] visceral larva migrans	*Occasional:* diarrhea, abdominal pain, elevated aminotransferases. *Rare:* agranulocytosis, thrombocytopenia, alopecia	Cimetidine: inhibited mebendazole metabolism	C	No information
Thiabendazole	Strongyloidiasis,[b] cutaneous larva migrans,[b] visceral larva migrans[b]	*Frequent:* anorexia, nausea, vomiting, diarrhea, headache, dizziness, asparagus-like urine odor. *Occasional:* drowsiness, giddiness, crystalluria, elevated aminotransferases, psychosis. *Rare:* hepatitis, seizures, angioneurotic edema, Stevens-Johnson syndrome, tinnitus	Theophylline: serum levels increased by thiabendazole	C	No information
Triclabendazole	Fascioliasis, paragonimiasis	*Occasional:* abdominal cramps, diarrhea, biliary colic, transient headache	No information	Not assigned	Yes
Benznidazole	Chagas' disease	*Frequent:* rash, pruritus, nausea, leukopenia, paresthesias	No major interactions	Not assigned	No information
Bithionol[e]	Fascioliasis, paragonimiasis	Diarrhea, abdominal cramps (usually mild and transient)			
Clindamycin	Babesiosis, malaria, toxoplasmosis	*Occasional:* pseudomembranous colitis, abdominal pain, diarrhea, nausea/vomiting. *Rare:* pruritus, skin rashes	No major interactions	B	Yes[f]
Diloxanide furoate	Amebiasis	*Frequent:* flatulence. *Occasional:* nausea, vomiting, diarrhea. *Rare:* pruritus	None reported	Contraindicated	No information
Eflornithine[g] (difluoromethylornithine, DFMO)	Trypanosomiasis	*Frequent:* pancytopenia. *Occasional:* diarrhea, seizures. *Rare:* transient hearing loss	No major interactions	Contraindicated	No information
Emetine and dehydroemetine[e]	Amebiasis, fascioliasis	*Severe:* cardiotoxicity. *Frequent:* pain at injection site. *Occasional:* dizziness, headache, GI symptoms	None reported	X	No information
Folate antagonists Dihydrofolate reductase inhibitors Pyrimethamine	Malaria,[b] isosporiasis, toxoplasmosis[b]	*Occasional:* folate deficiency. *Rare:* rash, seizures, severe skin reactions (toxic epidermal necrolysis, erythema multiforme, Stevens-Johnson syndrome)	Sulfonamides, proguanil, zidovudine: increased risk of bone marrow suppression when used concomitantly	C	Yes
Proguanil and chlorproguanil	Malaria	*Occasional:* urticaria. *Rare:* hematuria, GI disturbances	No major interactions	C	Yes
Trimethoprim	Cyclosporiasis, isosporiasis	Hyperkalemia, GI upset, mild stomatitis	Methotrexate: reduced clearance Warfarin: effect prolonged Phenytoin: hepatic metabolism increased	C	Yes
Dihydropteroate synthetase inhibitors: sulfonamides Sulfadiazine Sulfamethoxazole Sulfadoxine	Malaria,[b] toxoplasmosis[b]	*Frequent:* GI disturbances, allergic skin reactions, crystalluria. *Rare:* severe skin reactions (toxic epidermal necrolysis, erythema multiforme, Stevens-Johnson syndrome), agranulocytosis, aplastic anemia, hypersensitivity of the respiratory tract, hepatitis, interstitial nephritis, hypoglycemia, aseptic meningitis	Thiazide diuretics: increased risk of thrombocytopenia in elderly patients Warfarin: effect prolonged by sulfonamides Methotrexate: levels increased by sulfonamides Phenytoin: metabolism impaired by sulfonamides Sulfonylureas: effect prolonged by sulfonamides	B	Yes
Dihydropteroate synthetase inhibitors: sulfones Dapsone	Leishmaniasis, malaria, toxoplasmosis	*Frequent:* rash, anorexia. *Occasional:* hemolysis, methemoglobinemia, neuropathy, allergic dermatitis, anorexia, nausea, vomiting, tachycardia, headache, insomnia, psychosis, hepatitis. *Rare:* agranulocytosis	Rifampin: lowered plasma levels of dapsone	C	Yes
Fumagillin	Microsporidiosis	*Rare:* neutropenia, thrombocytopenia	None reported	No information	No information

(continued)

Drugs by Class	Parasitic Infection(s)	Adverse Effects	Major Drug-Drug Interactions	Pregnancy Class[a]	Breast Milk
Furazolidone	Giardiasis	*Frequent:* nausea/vomiting, brown urine. *Occasional:* rectal itching, headache. *Rare:* hemolytic anemia, disulfiram-like reactions, MAO-inhibitor interactions	Risk of hypertensive crisis when administered for >5 days with MAO inhibitors	C	No information
Iodoquinol	Amebiasis,[b] balantidiasis, *D. fragilis* infection	*Occasional:* headache, rash, pruritus, thyrotoxicosis, nausea, vomiting, abdominal pain, diarrhea. *Rare:* optic neuritis, peripheral neuropathy, seizures, encephalopathy	No major interactions	C	No information
Ivermectin	Ascariasis, cutaneous larva migrans, gnathostomiasis, loiasis, lymphatic filariases, onchocerciasis,[b] scabies, strongyloidiasis,[b] trichuriasis	*Occasional:* fever, pruritus, headache, myalgias. *Rare:* hypotension	No major interactions	C	Yes[f]
Levamisole	Ascariasis, hookworm	*Frequent:* GI disturbances, dizziness, headache. *Rare:* agranulocytosis, peripheral neuropathy	Alcohol: disulfiram-like effect Warfarin: prolonged prothrombin time	C	No information
Macrolides Azithromycin	Babesiosis	*Occasional:* nausea, vomiting, diarrhea, abdominal pain. *Rare:* angioedema, cholestatic jaundice	Cyclosporine and digoxin: levels increased by azithromycin Nelfinavir: increased levels of azithromycin	B	Yes
Spiramycin[g]	Toxoplasmosis	*Occasional:* GI disturbances, transient skin eruptions. *Rare:* thrombocytopenia, QT prolongation in an infant, cholestatic hepatitis	No major interactions	Not assigned[c]	Yes[f]
Mefloquine	Malaria[b]	*Frequent:* lightheadedness, nausea, headache. *Occasional:* confusion; nightmares; insomnia; visual disturbance; transient and clinically silent ECG abnormalities, including sinus bradycardia, sinus arrhythmia, first-degree AV block, prolongation of QTc interval, and abnormal T waves. *Rare:* psychosis, convulsions, hypotension	Administration of halofantrine <3 weeks after mefloquine use may produce fatal QTc prolongation. Mefloquine may lower plasma levels of anticonvulsants. Levels decreased and clearance accelerated by artesunate	C	Yes
Melarsoprol[e]	Trypanosomiasis	*Frequent:* myocardial injury, encephalopathy, peripheral neuropathy, hypertension. *Occasional:* G6PD-induced hemolysis, erythema nodosum leprosum. *Rare:* hypotension	No major interactions	Not assigned	No information
Metrifonate	Schistosomiasis	*Frequent:* abdominal pain, nausea, vomiting, diarrhea, headache, vertigo, bronchospasm. *Rare:* cholinergic symptoms	No major interactions	B	No
Miltefosine	Leishmaniasis	*Frequent:* mild and transient (1–2 days) GI disturbances within first 2 weeks of therapy (resolve after treatment completion); motion sickness. *Occasional:* reversible elevations of creatinine and aminotransferases	No major interactions	Not assigned	No information
Niclosamide	Intestinal cestodes[b]	*Occasional:* nausea, vomiting, dizziness, pruritus	No major interactions	B	No information
Nifurtimox[e]	Chagas' disease	*Frequent:* nausea, vomiting, abdominal pain, insomnia, paresthesias, weakness, tremors. *Rare:* seizures (all are reversible and dose-related)	No major interactions	Not assigned	No information
Nitazoxanide	Cryptosporidiosis,[b] giardiasis[b]	*Occasional:* abdominal pain, diarrhea. *Rare:* vomiting, headache	No major interactions	B	No information
Nitroimidazoles Metronidazole	Amebiasis,[b] balantidiasis, dracunculiasis, giardiasis, trichomoniasis,[b] *D. fragilis* infection	*Frequent:* nausea, headache, anorexia, metallic aftertaste. *Occasional:* vomiting, insomnia, vertigo, paresthesias, disulfiram-like effects. *Rare:* seizures, peripheral neuropathy	Warfarin: effect enhanced by metronidazole Disulfiram: psychotic reaction Phenobarbital, phenytoin: accelerate elimination of metronidazole Lithium: serum levels elevated by metronidazole Cimetidine: prolonged half-life of metronidazole	B	Yes

(continued)

TABLE 201-1 **OVERVIEW OF AGENTS USED FOR THE TREATMENT OF PARASITIC INFECTIONS (CONTINUED)**

Drugs by Class	Parasitic Infection(s)	Adverse Effects	Major Drug-Drug Interactions	Pregnancy Class[a]	Breast Milk
Tinidazole	Amebiasis,[b] giardiasis, trichomoniasis	*Occasional:* nausea, vomiting, metallic taste	See metronidazole	C	Yes
Oxamniquine	Schistosomiasis	*Occasional:* dizziness, drowsiness, headache, orange urine, elevated aminotransferases. *Rare:* seizures	No major interactions	C	No information
Paromomycin	Amebiasis,[b] *D. fragilis* infection, giardiasis, cryptosporidiosis, leishmaniasis	*Frequent:* GI disturbances (oral dosing only). *Occasional:* nephrotoxicity, ototoxicity, vestibular toxicity (parenteral dosing only)	No major interactions	Oral: B Parenteral: not assigned[c]	No information
Pentamidine isethionate	Leishmaniasis, trypanosomiasis	*Frequent:* hypotension, hypoglycemia, pancreatitis, sterile abscesses at IM injection sites, GI disturbances, reversible renal failure. *Occasional:* hepatotoxicity, cardiotoxicity, delirium. *Rare:* anaphylaxis	No major interactions	C	No information
Piperazine and derivatives					
Piperazine	Ascariasis, enterobiasis	*Occasional:* nausea, vomiting, diarrhea, abdominal pain, headache. *Rare:* neurotoxicity, seizures	None reported	C	No information
Diethylcarbamazine[e]	Lymphatic filariasis, loiasis, tropical pulmonary eosinophilia	*Frequent:* dose-related nausea, vomiting. *Rare:* fever, chills, arthralgias, headaches	None reported	Not assigned[c]	No information
Praziquantel	Clonorchiasis,[b] cysticercosis, diphyllobothriasis, hymenolepiasis, taeniasis, opisthorchiasis, intestinal trematodes, paragonimiasis, schistosomiasis[b]	*Frequent:* abdominal pain, diarrhea, dizziness, headache, malaise. *Occasional:* fever, nausea. *Rare:* pruritus, singultus	No major interactions	B	Yes
Pyrantel pamoate	Ascariasis, eosinophilic enterocolitis, enterobiasis,[b] hookworm, trichostrongyliasis	*Occasional:* GI disturbances, headache, dizziness, elevated aminotransferases	No major interactions	C	No information
Quinacrine[g]	Giardiasis[b]	*Frequent:* headache, nausea, vomiting, bitter taste. *Occasional:* yellow-orange discoloration of skin, sclerae, urine; begins after 1 week of treatment and lasts up to 4 months after drug discontinuation. *Rare:* psychosis, exfoliative dermatitis, retinopathy, G6PD-induced hemolysis, exacerbation of psoriasis, disulfiram-like effects	Primaquine: toxicity potentiated by quinacrine	C	No information
Quinine and quinidine	Malaria, babesiosis	*Frequent:* cinchonism (tinnitus, high-tone deafness, headache, dysphoria, nausea, vomiting, abdominal pain, visual disturbances, postural hypotension), hyperinsulinemia resulting in life-threatening hypoglycemia. *Occasional:* deafness, hemolytic anemia, arrhythmias, hypotension due to rapid IV infusion	Carbonic-anhydrase inhibitors, thiazide diuretics: reduced renal elimination of quinidine Amiodarone, cimetidine: increased quinidine levels Nifedipine: decreased quinidine levels; quinidine slows metabolism of nifedipine Phenobarbital, phenytoin, rifampin: accelerated hepatic elimination of quinidine Verapamil: reduced hepatic clearance of quinidine Diltiazem: decreased clearance of quinidine	X	Yes[f]
Quinolones					
Ciprofloxacin	Cyclosporiasis, isosporiasis	*Occasional:* nausea, diarrhea, vomiting, abdominal pain/discomfort, headache, restlessness, rash. *Rare:* myalgias/arthralgias, tendon rupture, CNS symptoms (nervousness, agitation, insomnia, anxiety, nightmares or paranoia); convulsions	Probenecid: increased serum levels of ciprofloxacin Theophylline, warfarin: serum levels increased by ciprofloxacin	C	Yes

(continued)

Drugs by Class	**Parasitic Infection(s)**	**Adverse Effects**	**Major Drug-Drug Interactions**	**Pregnancy Class[a]**	**Breast Milk**
Suramin[e]	Trypanosomiasis	*Frequent:* immediate: fever, urticaria, nausea, vomiting, hypotension; delayed (up to 24 h): exfoliative dermatitis, stomatitis, paresthesias, photophobia, renal dysfunction. *Occasional:* nephrotoxicity, adrenal toxicity, optic atrophy, anaphylaxis	No major interactions	Not assigned	No information
Tetracyclines	Balantidiasis, *D. fragilis* infection, malaria; lymphatic filariasis (doxycycline)	*Frequent:* GI disturbances. *Occasional:* photosensitivity dermatitis. *Rare:* exfoliative dermatitis, esophagitis, hepatotoxicity	Warfarin: effect prolonged by tetracyclines	D	Yes

[a]Based on U.S. Food and Drug Administration (FDA) pregnancy categories of A–D, X.
[b]Approved by the FDA for this indication.
[c]Use in pregnancy is recommended by international organizations outside the United States.
[d]Only AmBisome has been approved for this indication.
[e]Available through the Centers for Disease Control and Prevention (CDC).
[f]Not believed to be harmful.
[g]Available through the manufacturer.

Note: ACTH, adrenocorticotropic hormone; AV, atrioventricular; CNS, central nervous system; ECG, electrocardiogram; G6PD, glucose 6-phosphate dehydrogenase; MAO, monoamine oxidase.

FURTHER READINGS

ABRAMOWICZ M (ed): Drugs for parasitic infections. Med Lett Drugs Ther 46:1, 2004

MOORE TA, MCCARTHY JS: Benzimidazoles (albendazole, mebendazole, thiabendazole, triclabendazole), in *Antimicrobial Therapy and Vaccines*, 2d ed, VL Yu et al (eds). Pittsburgh, ESun Technologies, 2005, pp 1021–1036

SHAPIRO TA, GOLDBERG DE: Drugs used in the chemotherapy of protozoal infections: Malaria, in *Goodman and Gilman's The Pharmacological Basis of Therapeutics*, 11th ed, L Brunton et al (eds). New York, McGraw-Hill, 2005, pp 1021–1048

WINSTANLEY P, WARD S: Malaria chemotherapy. Adv Parasitol 61:47, 2006

WORLD HEALTH ORGANIZATION: *Model Prescribing Information: Drugs Used in Parasitic Diseases*, 2d ed. Geneva, WHO, 1995

SECTION 18 PROTOZOAL INFECTIONS

202 Amebiasis and Infection with Free-Living Amebas
Sharon L. Reed

AMEBIASIS

DEFINITION

Amebiasis is an infection with the intestinal protozoan *Entamoeba histolytica*. About 90% of infections are asymptomatic, and the remaining 10% produce a spectrum of clinical syndromes ranging from dysentery to abscesses of the liver or other organs.

LIFE CYCLE AND TRANSMISSION

E. histolytica is acquired by ingestion of viable cysts from fecally contaminated water, food, or hands. Food-borne exposure is most prevalent and is particularly likely when food handlers are shedding cysts or food is being grown with feces-contaminated soil, fertilizer, or water. Besides the drinking of contaminated water, less common means of transmission include oral and anal sexual practices and—in rare instances—direct rectal inoculation through colonic irrigation devices. Motile trophozoites are released from cysts in the small intestine and, in most patients, remain as harmless commensals in the large bowel. After encystation, infectious cysts are shed in the stool and can survive for several weeks in a moist environment. In some patients, the trophozoites invade either the bowel mucosa, causing symptomatic colitis, or the bloodstream, causing distant abscesses of the liver, lungs, or brain. The trophozoites may not encyst in patients with active dysentery, and motile hematophagous trophozoites are frequently present in fresh stools. Trophozoites are rapidly killed by exposure to air or stomach acid, however, and therefore cannot transmit infection.

EPIDEMIOLOGY

About 10% of the world's population is infected with *Entamoeba*, the majority with noninvasive *Entamoeba dispar*. Amebiasis results from infection with *E. histolytica* and is the third most common cause of death from parasitic disease (after schistosomiasis and malaria). The wide spectrum of clinical disease caused by *Entamoeba* is due in part to the differences between these two infecting species. Cysts of *E. histolytica* and *E. dispar* are morphologically identical, but *E. histolytica* has unique isoenzymes, surface antigens, DNA markers, and virulence properties (Table 202-1). Most asymptomatic carriers, including homosexual men and patients with AIDS, harbor *E. dispar* and have self-limited infections. These observations indicate that *E. dispar* is incapable of causing invasive disease, since *Cryptosporidium* and *Isospora belli*, which also cause only self-limited illnesses in immunocompetent people, cause devastating diarrhea in

TABLE 202-1 *E. HISTOLYTICA* AND *E. DISPAR*, COMPARED AND CONTRASTED

Similarities

1. Both species are spread through ingestion of infectious cysts.
2. Cysts of the two species are morphologically identical.
3. Both species colonize the large intestine.

Differences

1. Only *E. histolytica* causes invasive disease.
2. Only *E. histolytica* infections elicit a positive amebic serology.
3. The two species have distinct rRNA sequences.
4. The two species have distinct surface antigens and isoenzyme markers.
5. Gal/GalNAc lectin can be used to differentiate the two species in stool ELISA.

Note: ELISA, enzyme-linked immunosorbent assay; Gal/GalNAc, galactose *N*-acetylgalactosamine. See text.

FIGURE 202-1 Trophozoite of *E. histolytica* demonstrating a single nucleus with a central, dot-like nucleolus (trichrome stain).

patients with AIDS. However, host factors play a role as well. In one study, 10% of asymptomatic patients who were colonized with *E. histolytica* went on to develop amebic colitis, while the rest remained asymptomatic and cleared the infection within 1 year.

Areas of highest incidence (due to inadequate sanitation and crowding) include most developing countries in the tropics, particularly Mexico, India, and nations of Central and South America, tropical Asia, and Africa. In a 4-year follow-up study of preschool children in a highly endemic area of Bangladesh, 80% of children had at least one episode of infection with *E. histolytica* and 53% had more than one episode. Naturally acquired immunity did develop but was usually short-lived and correlated with the presence in the stool of secretory IgA antibody to the major adherence lectin galactose *N*-acetylgalactosamine (Gal/GalNAc). The main groups at risk for amebiasis in developed countries are returned travelers, recent immigrants, homosexual men, and inmates of institutions.

PATHOGENESIS AND PATHOLOGY

Both trophozoites (Fig. 202-1) and cysts (Fig. 202-2) are found in the intestinal lumen, but only trophozoites of *E. histolytica* invade tissue. The trophozoite is 20–60 μm in diameter and contains vacuoles and a nucleus with a characteristic central nucleolus. In animals, depletion of intestinal mucus, diffuse inflammation, and disruption of the epithelial barrier occur before trophozoites actually come into contact with the colonic mucosa. Trophozoites attach to colonic mucus and epithelial cells by Gal/GalNAc. The earliest intestinal lesions are microulcerations of the mucosa of the cecum, sigmoid colon, or rectum that release erythrocytes, inflammatory cells, and epithelial cells. Proctoscopy reveals small ulcers with heaped-up margins and normal in-

tervening mucosa. Submucosal extension of ulcerations under viable-appearing surface mucosa causes the classic "flask-shaped" ulcer containing trophozoites at the margins of dead and viable tissues. Although neutrophilic infiltrates may accompany the early lesions in animals, human intestinal infection is marked by a paucity of inflammatory cells, probably in part because of the killing of neutrophils by trophozoites (Fig. 202-3). Treated ulcers characteristically heal with little or no scarring. Occasionally, however, full-thickness necrosis and perforation occur.

Rarely, intestinal infection results in the formation of a mass lesion, or *ameboma*, in the bowel lumen. The overlying mucosa is usually thin and ulcerated, while other layers of the wall are thickened, edematous, and hemorrhagic; this condition results in exuberant formation of granulation tissue with little fibrous-tissue response.

A number of virulence factors have been linked to the ability of *E. histolytica* to invade through the interglandular epithelium. One consists of the extracellular cysteine proteinases that degrade collagen, elastin, IgA, IgG, and the anaphylatoxins C3a and C5a. Other enzymes may disrupt glycoprotein bonds between mucosal epithelial cells in the gut. Amebas can lyse neutrophils, monocytes, lymphocytes, and cells of colonic and hepatic lines. The cytolytic effect of amebas appears to require direct contact with target cells and may be linked to the release of phospholipase A and pore-forming peptides. *E. histolytica* trophozoites also cause apoptosis of human cells.

Liver abscesses are always preceded by intestinal colonization, which may be asymptomatic. Blood vessels may be compromised early by wall lysis and thrombus formation. Trophozoites invade veins to reach the liver through the portal venous system. *E. histolytica* is resistant to complement-mediated lysis—a property critical to survival in the bloodstream. In contrast, *E. dispar* is rapidly lysed by complement and is thus restricted to the bowel lumen. Inoculation of amebas into the portal system of hamsters results in an acute cellular infiltrate consisting predominantly of neutrophils. Later, the neutrophils are lysed by contact with amebas, and the release of neutrophil toxins may contribute to necrosis of hepatocytes. The liver parenchyma is replaced by necrotic material that is surrounded by a thin rim of congested liver tissue. The necrotic contents of a liver abscess are classically described as "anchovy paste," although the fluid is variable in color and is composed of bacteriologically sterile granular debris with few or no cells. Amebas, if seen, tend to be found near the capsule of the abscess.

A study in Bangladeshi schoolchildren revealed that an intestinal IgA response to Gal/GalNAc reduced the risk of new *E. histolytica* infection by 64%. Serum IgG antibody is not protective; titers correlate with the duration of illness rather than with the severity of disease. Indeed, Bangladeshi children with a serum IgG response were more likely than those without such a response to develop new *E. histolytica* infection. Studies of animals suggest that cell-mediated immunity may

FIGURE 202-2 Cyst of *E. histolytica* showing three of the four nuclei (trichrome stain).

FIGURE 202-3 Pathology of amebic ulcer with colonic invasion. Arrow points to trophozoites (hematoxylin and eosin, 400X).

be important for protection, although patients with AIDS appear not to be predisposed to more severe disease.

CLINICAL SYNDROMES

Intestinal Amebiasis   The most common type of amebic infection is asymptomatic cyst passage. Even in highly endemic areas, most patients harbor *E. dispar*.

Symptomatic amebic colitis develops 2–6 weeks after the ingestion of infectious cysts. A gradual onset of lower abdominal pain and mild diarrhea is followed by malaise, weight loss, and diffuse lower abdominal or back pain. Cecal involvement may mimic acute appendicitis. Patients with full-blown dysentery may pass 10–12 stools per day. The stools contain little fecal material and consist mainly of blood and mucus. In contrast to those with bacterial diarrhea, fewer than 40% of patients with amebic dysentery are febrile. Virtually all patients have heme-positive stools.

More fulminant intestinal infection, with severe abdominal pain, high fever, and profuse diarrhea, is rare and occurs predominantly in children. Patients may develop toxic megacolon, in which there is severe bowel dilation with intramural air. Patients receiving glucocorticoids are at risk for severe amebiasis. Uncommonly, patients develop a chronic form of amebic colitis, which can be confused with inflammatory bowel disease. The association between severe amebiasis complications and glucocorticoid therapy emphasizes the importance of excluding amebiasis when inflammatory bowel disease is suspected. An occasional patient presents with only an asymptomatic or tender abdominal mass caused by an ameboma, which is easily confused with cancer on barium studies. A positive serologic test or biopsy can prevent unnecessary surgery in this setting. The syndrome of postamebic colitis—persistent diarrhea following documented cure of amebic colitis—is controversial; no evidence of recurrent amebic infection can be found, and re-treatment usually has no effect.

Amebic Liver Abscess   Extraintestinal infection by *E. histolytica* most often involves the liver. Of travelers who develop an amebic liver abscess after leaving an endemic area, 95% do so within 5 months. Young patients with an amebic liver abscess are more likely than older patients to present in the acute phase with prominent symptoms of <10 days' duration. Most patients are febrile and have right-upper-quadrant pain, which may be dull or pleuritic in nature and may radiate to the shoulder. Point tenderness over the liver and right-sided pleural effusion are common. Jaundice is rare. Although the initial site of infection is the colon, fewer than one-third of patients with an amebic abscess have active diarrhea. Older patients from endemic areas are more likely to have a subacute course lasting 6 months, with weight loss and hepatomegaly. About one-third of patients with chronic presentations are febrile. Thus, the clinical diagnosis of an amebic liver abscess may be difficult to establish because the symptoms and signs are often nonspecific. Since 10–15% of patients present only with fever, amebic liver abscess must be considered in the differential diagnosis of fever of unknown origin (Chap. 19).

Complications of Amebic Liver Abscess   Pleuropulmonary involvement, which is reported in 20–30% of patients, is the most frequent complication of amebic liver abscess. Manifestations include sterile effusions, contiguous spread from the liver, and rupture into the pleural space. Sterile effusions and contiguous spread usually resolve with medical therapy, but frank rupture into the pleural space requires drainage. A hepatobronchial fistula may cause cough productive of large amounts of necrotic material that may contain amebas. This dramatic complication carries a good prognosis. Abscesses that rupture into the peritoneum may present as an indolent leak or an acute abdomen and require both percutaneous catheter drainage and medical therapy. Rupture into the pericardium, usually from abscesses of the left lobe of the liver, carries the gravest prognosis; it can occur during medical therapy and requires surgical drainage.

Other Extraintestinal Sites   The genitourinary tract may become involved by direct extension of amebiasis from the colon or by hematogenous spread of the infection. Painful genital ulcers, characterized by a punched-out appearance and profuse discharge, may develop secondary to extension from either the intestine or the liver. Both these conditions respond well to medical therapy. Cerebral involvement has been reported in fewer than 0.1% of patients in large clinical series. Symptoms and prognosis depend on the size and location of the lesion.

DIAGNOSTIC TESTS

Laboratory Diagnosis   Stool examinations, serologic tests, and noninvasive imaging of the liver are the most important procedures in the diagnosis of amebiasis. Fecal findings suggestive of amebic colitis include a positive test for heme, a paucity of neutrophils, and amebic cysts or trophozoites. The definitive diagnosis of amebic colitis is made by the demonstration of hematophagous trophozoites of *E. histolytica* (Fig. 202-1). Because trophozoites are killed rapidly by water, drying, or barium, it is important to examine at least three fresh stool specimens. Examination of a combination of wet mounts, iodine-stained concentrates, and trichrome-stained preparations of fresh stool and concentrates for cysts (Fig. 202-2) or trophozoites (Fig. 202-1) confirms the diagnosis in 75–95% of cases. Cultures of amebas are more sensitive but are not routinely available. If stool examinations are negative, sigmoidoscopy with biopsy of the edge of ulcers may increase the yield, but this procedure is dangerous during fulminant colitis because of the risk of perforation. Trophozoites in a biopsy specimen from a colonic mass confirm the diagnosis of ameboma, but trophozoites are rare in liver aspirates because they are found in the abscess capsule and not in the readily aspirated necrotic center. Accurate diagnosis requires experience, since the trophozoites may be confused with neutrophils and the cysts must be differentiated morphologically from *Entamoeba hartmanni*, *Entamoeba coli*, and *Endolimax nana*, which do not cause clinical disease and do not warrant therapy. Unfortunately, the cysts of *E. histolytica* cannot be distinguished microscopically from those of *E. dispar*. Therefore, the microscopic diagnosis of *E. histolytica* can be made only by the detection of *Entamoeba* trophozoites that have ingested erythrocytes. In terms of sensitivity, stool diagnostic tests based on the detection of the Gal/GalNAc lectin of *E. histolytica* compare favorably with the polymerase chain reaction and with isolation in culture followed by isoenzyme analysis.

Serology is an important addition to the methods used for parasitologic diagnosis of invasive amebiasis. Enzyme-linked immunosorbent assays (ELISAs) and agar gel diffusion assays are positive in more than 90% of patients with colitis, amebomas, or liver abscess. Positive results in conjunction with the appropriate clinical syndrome suggest active disease because serologic findings usually revert to negative within 6–12 months. Even in highly endemic areas such as South Africa, fewer than 10% of asymptomatic individuals have a positive amebic serology. The interpretation of the indirect hemagglutination test is more difficult because titers may remain positive for as long as 10 years.

Up to 10% of patients with acute amebic liver abscess may have negative serologic findings; in suspected cases with an initially negative result, testing should be repeated in a week. In contrast to carriers of *E. dispar*, most asymptomatic carriers of *E. histolytica* develop antibodies. Thus, serologic tests are helpful in assessing the risk of invasive amebiasis in asymptomatic, cyst-passing individuals in nonendemic areas. Serologic tests also should be performed in patients with ulcerative colitis before the institution of glucocorticoid therapy to prevent the development of severe colitis or toxic megacolon owing to unsuspected amebiasis.

Routine hematology and chemistry tests usually are not very helpful in the diagnosis of invasive amebiasis. About three-fourths of patients with an amebic liver abscess have leukocytosis (>10,000 cells/μL); this condition is particularly likely if symptoms are acute or complications have developed. Invasive amebiasis does not elicit eosinophilia. Anemia, if present, is usually multifactorial. Even with large liver abscesses, liver enzyme levels are normal or minimally elevated. The alkaline phosphatase level is most often elevated and may remain so for months. Aminotransferase elevations suggest acute disease or a complication.

FIGURE 202-4 Abdominal CT scan of a large amebic abscess of the right lobe of the liver. *(Courtesy of the Department of Radiology, UCSD Medical Center, San Diego; with permission.)*

Radiographic Studies Radiographic barium studies are potentially dangerous in acute amebic colitis. Amebomas are usually identified first by a barium enema, but biopsy is necessary for differentiation from carcinoma.

Radiographic techniques such as ultrasonography, CT, and MRI are all useful for detection of the round or oval hypoechoic cyst. More than 80% of patients who have had symptoms for >10 days have a single abscess of the right lobe of the liver (Fig. 202-4). Approximately 50% of patients who have had symptoms for <10 days have multiple abscesses. Findings associated with complications include large abscesses (>10 cm) in the superior part of the right lobe, which may rupture into the pleural space; multiple lesions, which must be differentiated from pyogenic abscesses; and lesions of the left lobe, which may rupture into the pericardium. Because abscesses resolve slowly and may increase in size in patients who are responding clinically to therapy, frequent follow-up ultrasonography may prove confusing. Complete resolution of a liver abscess within 6 months can be anticipated in two-thirds of patients, but 10% may have persistent abnormalities for a year.

DIFFERENTIAL DIAGNOSIS

The differential diagnosis of intestinal amebiasis includes bacterial diarrheas (Chap. 122) caused by *Campylobacter* (Chap. 148); enteroinvasive *Escherichia coli* (Chap. 143); and species of *Shigella* (Chap. 147), *Salmonella* (Chap. 146), and *Vibrio* (Chap. 149). Although the typical patient with amebic colitis has less prominent fever than in these other conditions as well as heme-positive stools with few neutrophils, correct diagnosis requires bacterial cultures, microscopic examination of stools, and amebic serologic testing. As has already been mentioned, amebiasis must be ruled out in any patient thought to have inflammatory bowel disease.

Because of the variety of presenting signs and symptoms, amebic liver abscess can easily be confused with pulmonary or gallbladder disease or with any febrile illness with few localizing signs, such as malaria (Chap. 203) or typhoid fever (Chap. 146). The diagnosis should be considered in members of high-risk groups who have recently traveled outside the United States (Chap. 117) and in inmates of institutions. Once radiographic studies have identified an abscess in the liver, the most important differential diagnosis is between amebic and pyogenic abscess. Patients with pyogenic abscess typically are older and have a history of underlying bowel disease or recent surgery. Amebic serology is helpful, but aspiration of the abscess, with Gram's staining and culture of the material, may be required for differentiation of the two diseases.

℞ AMEBIASIS

INTESTINAL DISEASE (Table 202-2) The drugs used to treat amebiasis can be classified according to their primary site of action. Luminal amebi-

TABLE 202-2	DRUG THERAPY FOR AMEBIASIS
Indication	**Therapy**
Asymptomatic carriage	Luminal agent: iodoquinol (650-mg tablets), 650 mg tid for 20 days; *or* paromomycin (250-mg tablets), 500 mg tid for 10 days
Acute colitis	Metronidazole (250- or 500-mg tablets), 750 mg PO or IV tid for 5–10 days, *plus* Luminal agent as above
Amebic liver abscess	Metronidazole, 750 mg PO or IV for 5–10 days, *or* Tinidazole, 2 g PO once, *or* Ornidazole,[a] 2 g PO once, *plus* Luminal agent as above

[a]Not available in the United States.

cides are poorly absorbed and reach high concentrations in the bowel, but their activity is limited to cysts and trophozoites close to the mucosa. Only two luminal drugs are available in the United States: iodoquinol and paromomycin. Indications for the use of luminal agents include eradication of cysts in patients with colitis or a liver abscess and treatment of asymptomatic carriers. The majority of asymptomatic individuals who pass cysts are colonized with *E. dispar*, which does not warrant specific therapy. However, it is prudent to treat asymptomatic individuals who pass cysts unless *E. dispar* colonization can be definitively demonstrated by specific antigen-detection tests.

Tissue amebicides reach high concentrations in the blood and tissue after oral or parenteral administration. The development of nitroimidazole compounds, especially metronidazole, was a major advance in the treatment of invasive amebiasis. Patients with amebic colitis should be treated with intravenous or oral metronidazole. Side effects include nausea, vomiting, abdominal discomfort, and a disulfiram-like reaction. Another longer-acting imidazole compound, tinidazole, is also effective and was recently approved in the United States. All patients should also receive a full course of therapy with a luminal agent, since metronidazole does not eradicate cysts. Resistance to metronidazole has been selected in the laboratory but has not been found in clinical isolates. Relapses are not uncommon and probably represent reinfection or failure to eradicate amebas from the bowel because of an inadequate dosage or duration of therapy.

AMEBIC LIVER ABSCESS Metronidazole is the drug of choice for amebic liver abscess. Longer-acting nitroimidazoles (tinidazole and ornidazole) have been effective as single-dose therapy in developing countries. With early diagnosis and therapy, mortality rates from uncomplicated amebic liver abscess are <1%. The second-line therapeutic agents emetine and chloroquine should be avoided if possible because of the potential cardiovascular and gastrointestinal side effects of the former and the higher relapse rates with the latter. There is no evidence that combined therapy with two drugs is more effective than the single-drug regimen. Studies of South Africans with liver abscesses demonstrated that 72% of patients without intestinal symptoms had bowel infection with *E. histolytica*; thus, all treatment regimens should include a luminal agent to eradicate cysts and prevent further transmission. Amebic liver abscess recurs rarely.

ASPIRATION OF LIVER ABSCESSES More than 90% of patients respond dramatically to metronidazole therapy with decreases in both pain and fever within 72 h. Indications for aspiration of liver abscesses are (1) the need to rule out a pyogenic abscess, particularly in patients with multiple lesions; (2) the lack of a clinical response in 3–5 days; (3) the threat of imminent rupture; and (4) the need to prevent rupture of left-lobe abscesses into the pericardium. There is no evidence that aspiration, even of large abscesses (up to 10 cm), accelerates healing. Percutaneous drainage may be successful even if the liver abscess has already ruptured. Surgery should be reserved for instances of bowel perforation and rupture into the pericardium.

PREVENTION

Amebic infection is spread by ingestion of food or water contaminated with cysts. Since an asymptomatic carrier may excrete up to 15 million cysts per day, prevention of infection requires adequate sanitation and eradication of cyst carriage. In high-risk areas, infection can be minimized by the avoidance of unpeeled fruits and vegetables and the use of bottled water. Because cysts are resistant to readily attainable levels of chlorine, disinfection by iodination (tetraglycine hydroperiodide) is recommended. There is no effective prophylaxis.

INFECTION WITH FREE-LIVING AMEBAS

EPIDEMIOLOGY

Free-living amebas of the genera *Acanthamoeba* and *Naegleria* are distributed throughout the world and have been isolated from a wide variety of fresh and brackish water, including that from lakes, taps, hot springs, swimming pools, and heating and air-conditioning units, and even from the nasal passages of healthy children. Encystation may protect the protozoa from desiccation and food deprivation. The persistence of *Legionella pneumophila* in water supplies may be attributable in part to chronic infection of free-living amebas, particularly *Naegleria*. Free-living amebas of the genus *Balamuthia* have only recently been isolated from soil samples, including a sample from a flowerpot linked to a fatal infection in a child.

NAEGLERIA INFECTIONS

Primary amebic meningoencephalitis caused by *Naegleria fowleri* follows the aspiration of water contaminated with trophozoites or cysts or the inhalation of contaminated dust, leading to invasion of the olfactory neuroepithelium. After an incubation period of 2–15 days, severe headache, high fever, nausea, vomiting, and meningismus develop. Photophobia and palsies of the third, fourth, and sixth cranial nerves are common. Rapid progression to seizures and coma may follow. The prognosis is uniformly poor: most patients die within a week. Only a few survivors, treated with high-dose amphotericin B and rifampin, have been reported. Infection is most common in otherwise-healthy children or young adults, who often report recent swimming in lakes or heated swimming pools.

The diagnosis of *Naegleria* infection should be considered in any patient who has purulent meningitis without evidence of bacteria on Gram's staining, antigen detection assay, and culture. Other laboratory findings resemble those for fulminant bacterial meningitis, with elevated intracranial pressure, high white blood cell counts (up to 20,000/μL), and elevated protein concentrations and low glucose levels in cerebrospinal fluid (CSF). Diagnosis depends on the detection of motile trophozoites in wet mounts of fresh spinal fluid. Antibodies to *Naegleria* spp. have been detected in normal adults; serologic testing is not useful in the diagnosis of acute infection.

ACANTHAMOEBA INFECTIONS

Granulomatous Amebic Encephalitis   Infection with *Acanthamoeba* species follows a more indolent course and typically occurs in chronically ill or debilitated patients. Risk factors include lymphoproliferative disorders, chemotherapy, glucocorticoid therapy, lupus erythematosus, and AIDS. Infection usually reaches the central nervous system (CNS) hematogenously from a primary focus in the sinuses, skin, or lungs. In the CNS, the onset is insidious, and the syndrome often mimics a space-occupying lesion. Altered mental status, headache, and stiff neck may be accompanied by focal findings such as cranial nerve palsies, ataxia, and hemiparesis. Cutaneous ulcers or hard nodules containing amebas are frequently detected in AIDS patients with disseminated *Acanthamoeba* infection.

Examination of the CSF for trophozoites may be diagnostically helpful, but lumbar puncture may be contraindicated because of increased intracerebral pressure. CT frequently reveals cortical and subcortical lesions of decreased density consistent with embolic infarcts. In other patients, multiple enhancing lesions with edema may mimic the computed tomographic appearance of toxoplasmosis (Chap. 207). Demonstration of the trophozoites and cysts of *Acanthamoeba* on wet mounts or in biopsy specimens establishes the diagnosis. Culture on nonnutrient agar plates seeded with *E. coli* may also be helpful. Fluorescein-labeled antiserum is available from the Centers for Disease

FIGURE 202-5 Double-walled cyst of *Acanthamoeba castellani*, as seen by phase-contrast microscopy. *[From DJ Krogstad et al, in A Balows et al (eds): Manual of Clinical Microbiology, 5th ed. Washington, DC, American Society for Microbiology, 1991.]*

Control and Prevention (CDC) for the detection of protozoa in biopsy specimens. Granulomatous amebic encephalitis in patients with AIDS may have an accelerated course (with survival for only 3–40 days) because of the difficulty these individuals have in forming granulomas. Various antimicrobial agents have been used to treat *Acanthamoeba* infection, including pentamidine, trimethoprim-sulfamethoxazole, and fluconazole, but the infection is almost uniformly fatal.

Keratitis   The incidence of keratitis caused by *Acanthamoeba* has increased in the past 20 years, in part as a result of improved diagnosis. Earlier infections were associated with trauma to the eye and exposure to contaminated water. At present, most infections are linked to extended-wear contact lenses, and rare cases are associated with laser-assisted in situ keratomileusis (LASIK). Risk factors include the use of homemade saline, the wearing of lenses while swimming, and inadequate disinfection. Since contact lenses presumably cause microscopic trauma, the early corneal findings may be nonspecific. The first symptoms usually include tearing and the painful sensation of a foreign body. Once infection is established, progression is rapid; the characteristic clinical sign is an annular, paracentral corneal ring representing a corneal abscess. Deeper corneal invasion and loss of vision may follow.

The differential diagnosis includes bacterial, mycobacterial, and herpetic infection. The irregular polygonal cysts of *Acanthamoeba* (Fig. 202-5) may be identified in corneal scrapings or biopsy material, and trophozoites can be grown on special media. Cysts are resistant to available drugs, and the results of medical therapy have been disappointing. Some reports have suggested partial responses to propamidine isethionate eyedrops. Severe infections usually require keratoplasty.

BALAMUTHIA INFECTIONS

Balamuthia mandrillaris, a free-living ameba previously referred to as a leptomyxid ameba, is an important etiologic agent of amebic meningoencephalitis in immunocompetent hosts. The course is typically subacute, with focal neurologic signs, fever, seizures, and headaches leading to death within 1 week to several months after onset. Examination of CSF reveals mononuclear or neutrophilic pleocytosis, elevated protein levels, and normal to low glucose concentrations. Multiple hypodense lesions are usually detected with imaging studies. This mixed picture of space-occupying lesions with CSF pleocytosis is suggestive of *Balamuthia*. Detection of an indirect fluorescent antibody response may be helpful in noninvasive diagnosis, but usually a definitive diagnosis is made post-mortem. Fluorescent antibody is available from the CDC. The variety of drugs used to treat the few surviving patients (numbering fewer than five in the United States) include pentamidine, flucytosine, sulfadiazine, and macrolides. The differential diagnosis includes tuberculomas (Chap. 158) and neurocysticercosis (Chap. 213).

FURTHER READINGS

DEETZ TR et al: Successful treatment of *Balamuthia* amoebic encephalitis: Presentation of two cases. Clin Infect Dis 37:1304, 2003

HAQUE R et al: *Entamoeba histolytica* infection in children and protection from subsequent amebiasis. Infect Immun 37:1304, 2003

HUSTON CD et al: Caspase-3-dependent killing of host cells by the parasite *Entamoeba histolytica*. Cell Microbiol 2:617, 2000

KUMAR R, LLOYD D: Recent advances in the treatment of *Acanthamoeba* keratitis. Clin Infect Dis 35:434, 2002

PETRI WA et al: The bittersweet interface of parasite and host lectin-carbohydrate interactions during human invasion by the parasite *Entamoeba histolytica*. Annu Rev Microbiol 56:39, 2002

QUE X, REED SL: Cysteine proteinases and the pathogenesis of amebiasis. Clin Microbiol Rev 13:196, 2002

SCHUSTER FL, VISVESVARA GS: Free-living amoebae as opportunistic and non-opportunistic pathogens of humans and animals. Int J Parasitol 345:1001, 2004

SOLAYMANI-MOHAMMADI S et al: Comparison of a stool antigen detection kit and PCR for diagnosis of *Entamoeba histolytica* and *Entamoeba dispar* infections in asymptomatic cyst passers in Iran. J Clin Microbiol 44:2258, 2006

STANLEY SL: Amoebiasis. Lancet 361:1025, 2006

———, REED SL: Microbes and microbial toxins: Paradigms for microbial-mucosal interactions. VI. *Entamoeba histolytica*: Parasite-host interactions. Am J Physiol Gastrointest Liver Physiol 280:G1049, 2001

203 Malaria
Nicholas J. White, Joel G. Breman

Humanity has but three great enemies: Fever, famine and war; of these by far the greatest, by far the most terrible, is fever.

William Osler

Malaria is a protozoan disease transmitted by the bite of infected *Anopheles* mosquitoes. It is the most important of the parasitic diseases of humans, with transmission in 107 countries containing 3 billion people and causing 1–3 million deaths each year. Malaria has now been eliminated from the United States, Canada, Europe, and Russia but, despite enormous control efforts, has resurged in many parts of the tropics. Added to this resurgence are the increasing problems of drug resistance of the parasite and insecticide resistance of the vectors. Occasional local transmission after importation of malaria has occurred recently in several southern and eastern areas of the United States and in Europe, indicating the continual danger to nonmalarious countries. Although there are promising new control and research initiatives, malaria remains today, as it has been for centuries, a heavy burden on tropical communities, a threat to nonendemic countries, and a danger to travelers.

ETIOLOGY AND PATHOGENESIS

Four species of the genus *Plasmodium* cause nearly all malarial infections in humans (although rare infections involve species normally affecting other primates). These are *P. falciparum*, *P. vivax*, *P. ovale*, and *P. malariae* (Table 203-1). Almost all deaths are caused by falciparum malaria. Human infection begins when a female anopheline mosquito inoculates plasmodial *sporozoites* from its salivary gland during a blood meal (Fig. 203-1). These microscopic motile forms of the malarial parasite are carried rapidly via the bloodstream to the liver, where they invade hepatic parenchymal cells and begin a period of asexual reproduction. By this amplification process (known as *intrahepatic* or *preerythrocytic schizogony* or *merogony*), a single sporozoite eventually may produce from 10,000 to >30,000 daughter merozoites. The swollen infected liver cell eventually bursts, discharging motile *merozoites* into the bloodstream. These then invade the red blood cells (RBCs) and multiply six- to twentyfold every 48–72 h. When the parasites reach densities of ~50/μL of blood, the symptomatic stage of the infection begins. In *P. vivax* and *P. ovale* infections, a proportion of the intrahepatic forms do not divide immediately but remain dormant for a period ranging from 3 weeks to a year or longer before reproduction begins. These dormant forms, or *hypnozoites*, are the cause of the relapses that characterize infection with these two species.

After entry into the bloodstream, merozoites rapidly invade erythrocytes and become *trophozoites*. Attachment is mediated via a specific erythrocyte surface receptor. In the case of *P. vivax*, this receptor is related to the Duffy blood-group antigen Fy^a or Fy^b. Most West Africans and people with origins in that region carry the Duffy-negative FyFy phenotype and are therefore resistant to *P. vivax* malaria. During the early stage of intraerythrocytic development, the small "ring forms" of the four parasitic species appear similar under light microscopy. As the trophozoites enlarge, species-specific characteristics become evident, pigment becomes visible, and the parasite assumes an irregular or ameboid shape. By the end of the 48-h intraerythrocytic life cycle (72 h for *P. malariae*), the parasite has consumed nearly all the hemoglobin and grown to occupy most of the RBC. It is now called a *schizont*. Multiple nuclear divisions have taken place (*schizogony* or *merogony*), and the RBC then ruptures to release 6–30 daughter merozoites, each potentially capable of invading a new RBC and repeating the cycle. The disease in human beings is caused by the direct effects of RBC invasion and destruction by the asexual parasite and the host's reaction. After a series of asexual cycles (*P. falciparum*) or immediately after release from the liver (*P. vivax*, *P. ovale*, *P. malariae*), some of the para-

TABLE 203-1 **CHARACTERISTICS OF *PLASMODIUM* SPECIES INFECTING HUMANS**

Characteristic	Finding for Indicated Species			
	P. falciparum	*P. vivax*	*P. ovale*	*P. malariae*
Duration of intrahepatic phase (days)	5.5	8	9	15
Number of merozoites released per infected hepatocyte	30,000	10,000	15,000	15,000
Duration of erythrocytic cycle (hours)	48	48	50	72
Red cell preference	Younger cells (but can invade cells of all ages)	Reticulocytes and cells up to 2 weeks old	Reticulocytes	Older cells
Morphology	Usually only ring forms^a; banana-shaped gametocytes	Irregularly shaped large rings and trophozoites; enlarged erythrocytes; Schüffner's dots	Infected erythrocytes, enlarged and oval with tufted ends; Schüffner's dots	Band or rectangular forms of trophozoites common
Pigment color	Black	Yellow-brown	Dark brown	Brown-black
Ability to cause relapses	No	Yes	Yes	No

^{a}Parasitemias of >2% are suggestive of *P. falciparum* infection.

sites develop into morphologically distinct, longer-lived sexual forms (*gametocytes*) that can transmit malaria.

After being ingested in the blood meal of a biting female anopheline mosquito, the male and female gametocytes form a zygote in the insect's midgut. This zygote matures into an ookinete, which penetrates and encysts in the mosquito's gut wall. The resulting oocyst expands by asexual division until it bursts to liberate myriad motile sporozoites, which then migrate in the hemolymph to the salivary gland of the mosquito to await inoculation into another human at the next feeding.

EPIDEMIOLOGY

Malaria occurs throughout most of the tropical regions of the world (Fig. 203-2). *P. falciparum* predominates in Africa, New Guinea, and Haiti; *P. vivax* is more common in Central America. The prevalence of these two species is approximately equal in South America, the Indian subcontinent, eastern Asia, and Oceania. *P. malariae* is found in most endemic areas, especially throughout sub-Saharan Africa, but is much less common. *P. ovale* is relatively unusual outside of Africa and, where it is found, comprises <1% of isolates.

The epidemiology of malaria is complex and may vary considerably even within relatively small geographic areas. Endemicity traditionally has been defined in terms of parasitemia rates or palpable-spleen rates in children 2–9 years of age as hypoendemic (<10%), mesoendemic (11–50%), hyperendemic (51–75%), and holoendemic (>75%); however, it is uncommon to use these indices for planning control programs. In holo- and hyperendemic areas (e.g., certain regions of tropical Africa or coastal New Guinea) where there is intense *P. falciparum* transmission, people may sustain more than one infectious mosquito bite per day and are infected repeatedly throughout their lives. In such settings, rates of morbidity and mortality due to malaria are considerable during childhood. Immunity against disease is hard won in these areas, and the burden of disease in young children is high; by adulthood, however, most malarial infections are asymptomatic. Constant, frequent, year-round infection is termed *stable transmission*. In areas where transmission is low, erratic, or focal, full protective immunity is not acquired, and symptomatic disease may occur at all ages. This situation usually exists in hypoendemic areas and is termed *unstable transmission*. Even in stable transmission areas, there is often an increased incidence of symptomatic malaria coinciding with increased mosquito breeding and transmission during the rainy season. Malaria behaves like an epidemic disease in some areas, particularly those with unstable malaria, such as northern India, Sri Lanka, Southeast Asia, Ethiopia, Eritrea, Rwanda, Burundi, southern Africa, and Madagascar. An epidemic can develop when there are changes in environmental, economic, or social conditions, such as heavy rains following drought or migrations (usually of refugees or workers) from a nonmalarious region to an area of high transmission; a breakdown in malaria control and prevention services can intensify epidemic conditions. This situation usually results in considerable mortality among all age groups.

The principal determinants of the epidemiology of malaria are the number (density), the human-biting habits, and the longevity of the anopheline mosquito vectors. Not all of the >400 anophelines can transmit malaria, and those that do vary considerably in their efficiency as malaria vectors. More specifically, the transmission of malaria is directly proportional to the density of the vector, the square of the number of human bites per day per mosquito, and the tenth power of the probability of the mosquito's surviving for 1 day. Mosquito longevity is particularly important, because the portion of the parasite's life cycle that takes place within the mosquito—from gametocyte ingestion to

FIGURE 203-1 The malaria transmission cycle from mosquito to human. RBC, red blood cell.

subsequent inoculation (*sporogony*)—lasts 8–30 days, depending on ambient temperature; thus, to transmit malaria, the mosquito must survive for >7 days. In general, at temperatures below 16°–18°C, sporogony is not completed and transmission does not occur, although malaria outbreaks and transmission have recently occurred in the highlands of east Africa—areas (>1500 m) previously free of vectors. The most effective mosquito vectors of malaria are those, such as *Anopheles gambiae* in Africa, which are long-lived, occur in high densities in tropical climates, breed readily, and bite humans in preference to other animals. The entomologic inoculation rate (the number of sporozoite-positive mosquito bites per person per year) is the most common measure of malaria transmission and varies from <1 in some parts of Latin America and Southeast Asia to >300 in parts of tropical Africa.

ERYTHROCYTE CHANGES IN MALARIA

After invading an erythrocyte, the growing malarial parasite progressively consumes and degrades intracellular proteins, principally hemoglobin. The potentially toxic heme is detoxified by polymerization to biologically inert hemozoin (malaria pigment). The parasite also alters the RBC membrane by changing its transport properties, exposing cryptic surface antigens, and inserting new parasite-derived proteins. The RBC becomes more irregular in shape, more antigenic, and less deformable.

In *P. falciparum* infections, membrane protuberances appear on the erythrocyte's surface 12–15 h after the cell's invasion. These "knobs" extrude a high-molecular-weight, antigenically variant, strain-specific erythrocyte membrane adhesive protein (PfEMP1) that mediates attachment to receptors on venular and capillary endothelium—an event termed *cytoadherence*. Several vascular receptors have been identified, of which intercellular adhesion molecule 1 (ICAM-1) is probably the most important in the brain, chondroitin sulfate B in the placenta, and CD36 in most other organs. Thus, the infected erythrocytes stick inside and eventually block capillaries and venules. At the same stage, these *P. falciparum*–infected RBCs may also adhere to uninfected RBCs (to form rosettes) and to other parasitized erythrocytes (agglutination). The processes of cytoadherence, rosetting, and agglutination are central to the pathogenesis of falciparum malaria. They result in the sequestration of RBCs containing mature forms of the parasite in vital organs (particularly the brain), where they interfere with microcirculatory flow and metabolism. Sequestered parasites continue to develop out of reach of the principal host defense mechanism: splenic processing and filtration. As a consequence, only the younger ring forms of the asexual parasites are seen circulating in the peripheral blood in falciparum malaria, and the level of peripheral parasitemia underestimates the true number of par-

FIGURE 203-2 Malaria-endemic countries in the Americas (***bottom***) and in Africa, the Middle East, Asia, and the South Pacific (***top***), 2007. CAR, Central African Republic; DCOR, Democratic Republic of the Congo; UAE, United Arab Emirates.

Malaria-Endemic Areas
- ⬤ Chloroquine-resistant
- ⬤ Chloroquine-sensitive
- ◯ None

asites within the body. Severe malaria is also associated with reduced deformability of the uninfected erythrocytes, which compromises their passage through the partially obstructed capillaries and venules and shortens RBC survival.

In the other three ("benign") malarias, sequestration does not occur, and all stages of the parasite's development are evident on peripheral blood smears. Whereas *P. vivax*, *P. ovale*, and *P. malariae* show a marked predilection for either young RBCs (*P. vivax*, *P. ovale*) or old cells (*P. malariae*) and produce a level of parasitemia that is seldom >2%, *P. falciparum* can invade erythrocytes of all ages and may be associated with very high levels of parasitemia.

HOST RESPONSE

Initially, the host responds to plasmodial infection by activating nonspecific defense mechanisms. Splenic immunologic and filtrative clearance

functions are augmented in malaria, and the removal of both parasitized and uninfected erythrocytes is accelerated. The parasitized cells escaping splenic removal are destroyed when the schizont ruptures. The material released induces the activation of macrophages and the release of proinflammatory mononuclear cell–derived cytokines, which cause fever and exert other pathologic effects. Temperatures of ≥40°C damage mature parasites; in untreated infections, the effect of such temperatures is to further synchronize the parasitic cycle, with eventual production of the regular fever spikes and rigors that originally served to characterize the different malarias. These regular fever patterns (tertian, every 2 days; quartan, every 3 days) are seldom seen today in patients who receive prompt and effective antimalarial treatment.

The geographic distributions of sickle cell disease, ovalocytosis, thalassemia, and glucose-6-phosphate dehydrogenase (G6PD) deficiency closely resemble that of malaria before the introduction of control measures. This similarity suggests that these genetic disorders confer protection against death from falciparum malaria. For example, HbA/S heterozygotes (sickle cell trait) have a sixfold reduction in the risk of dying from severe falciparum malaria. This decrease in risk appears to be related to impaired parasite growth at low oxygen tensions. Parasite multiplication in HbA/E heterozygotes is reduced at high parasite densities. In Melanesia, children with α-thalassemia appear to have more frequent malaria (both vivax and falciparum) in the early years of life, and this pattern of infection appears to protect against severe disease. In Melanesian ovalocytosis, rigid erythrocytes resist merozoite invasion, and the intraerythrocytic milieu is hostile.

Nonspecific host defense mechanisms stop the infection's expansion, and the subsequent specific immune response controls the infection. Eventually, exposure to sufficient strains confers protection from high-level parasitemia and disease but not from infection. As a result of this state of infection without illness (*premunition*), asymptomatic parasitemia is common among adults and older children living in regions with stable and intense transmission (i.e., holo- or hyperendemic areas). Immunity is mainly specific for both the species and the strain of infecting malarial parasite. Both humoral immunity and cellular immunity are necessary for protection, but the mechanisms of each are incompletely understood (Fig. 203-1). Immune individuals have a polyclonal increase in serum levels of IgM, IgG, and IgA, although much of this antibody is unrelated to protection. Antibodies to a variety of parasitic antigens presumably act in concert to limit in vivo replication of the parasite. In the case of falciparum malaria, the most important of these antigens is the surface adhesin—the variant protein PfEMP1 mentioned above. Passively transferred IgG from immune adults has been shown to reduce levels of parasitemia in children; although parasitemia in very young infants can occur, passive transfer of maternal antibody contributes to the relative (but not complete) protection of infants from severe malaria in the first months of life. This complex immunity to disease declines when a person lives outside an endemic area for several months or longer.

Several factors retard the development of cellular immunity to malaria. These factors include the absence of major histocompatibility antigens on the surface of infected RBCs, which precludes direct T cell recognition; malaria antigen–specific immune unresponsiveness; and the enormous strain diversity of malarial parasites, along with the ability of the parasites to express variant immunodominant antigens on the erythrocyte surface that change during the period of infection. Parasites may persist in the blood for months (or, in the case of *P. malariae*, for many years) if treatment is not given. The complexity of the immune response in malaria, the sophistication of the parasites' evasion mechanisms, and the lack of a good in vitro correlate with clinical immunity have all slowed progress toward an effective vaccine.

CLINICAL FEATURES

Malaria is a very common cause of fever in tropical countries. The first symptoms of malaria are nonspecific; the lack of a sense of well-being, headache, fatigue, abdominal discomfort, and muscle aches followed by fever are all similar to the symptoms of a minor viral illness. In some instances, a prominence of headache, chest pain, abdominal pain, arthralgia, myalgia, or diarrhea may suggest another diagnosis. Although headache may be severe in malaria, there is no neck stiffness or photophobia resembling that in meningitis. While myalgia may be prominent, it is not usually as severe as in dengue fever, and the muscles are not tender as in leptospirosis or typhus. Nausea, vomiting, and orthostatic hypotension are common. The classic malarial paroxysms, in which fever spikes, chills, and rigors occur at regular intervals, are relatively unusual and suggest infection with *P. vivax* or *P. ovale*. The fever is irregular at first (that of falciparum malaria may never become regular); the temperature of nonimmune individuals and children often rises above 40°C in conjunction with tachycardia and sometimes delirium. Although childhood febrile convulsions may occur with any of the malarias, generalized seizures are specifically associated with falciparum malaria and may herald the de-

velopment of cerebral disease. Many clinical abnormalities have been described in acute malaria, but most patients with uncomplicated infections have few abnormal physical findings other than fever, malaise, mild anemia, and (in some cases) a palpable spleen. Anemia is common among young children living in areas with stable transmission, particularly where resistance has compromised the efficacy of antimalarial drugs. In nonimmune individuals with acute malaria, the spleen takes several days to become palpable, but splenic enlargement is found in a high proportion of otherwise healthy individuals in malaria-endemic areas and reflects repeated infections. Slight enlargement of the liver is also common, particularly among young children. Mild jaundice is common among adults; it may develop in patients with otherwise uncomplicated falciparum malaria and usually resolves over 1–3 weeks. Malaria is not associated with a rash like those seen in meningococcal septicemia, typhus, enteric fever, viral exanthems, and drug reactions. Petechial hemorrhages in the skin or mucous membranes—features of viral hemorrhagic fevers and leptospirosis—develop only rarely in severe falciparum malaria.

SEVERE FALCIPARUM MALARIA
Appropriately and promptly treated, uncomplicated falciparum malaria (i.e., the patient can swallow medicines and food) carries a mortality rate of ~0.1%. However, once vital-organ dysfunction occurs or the total proportion of erythrocytes infected increases to >2% (a level corresponding to >10^{12} parasites in an adult), mortality risk rises steeply. The major manifestations of severe falciparum malaria are shown in Table 203-2, and features indicating a poor prognosis are listed in Table 203-3.

Cerebral Malaria Coma is a characteristic and ominous feature of falciparum malaria and, despite treatment, is associated with death rates of ~20% among adults and 15% among children. Any obtundation, delirium, or abnormal behavior should be taken very seriously. The onset may be gradual or sudden following a convulsion.

Cerebral malaria manifests as diffuse symmetric encephalopathy; focal neurologic signs are unusual. Although some passive resistance to head flexion may be detected, signs of meningeal irritation are lacking. The eyes may be divergent and a pout reflex is common, but other primitive reflexes are usually absent. The corneal reflexes are preserved, except in deep coma. Muscle tone may be either increased or decreased. The tendon reflexes are variable, and the plantar reflexes may be flexor or extensor; the abdominal and cremasteric reflexes are absent. Flexor or extensor posturing may be seen. Approximately 15% of patients have retinal hemorrhages; with pupillary dilatation and indirect ophthalmoscopy, this figure increases to 30–40%. Other funduscopic abnormalities (Fig. 203-3) include discrete spots of retinal opacification (30–60%), papilledema (8% among children, rare among adults), cotton wool spots (<5%), and decolorization of a retinal vessel or segment of vessel (occasional cases). Convulsions, usually generalized and often repeated, occur in up to 50% of children with cerebral malaria. More covert seizure activity is also common, particularly among children, and may manifest as repetitive tonic-clonic eye movements or even hypersalivation. Whereas adults rarely (i.e., in <3% of cases) suffer neurologic sequelae, ~15% of children surviving cerebral malaria—especially those with hypoglycemia, severe anemia, repeated seizures, and deep coma—have some residual neurologic deficit when they regain consciousness; hemiplegia, cerebral palsy, cortical blindness, deafness, and impaired cognition and learning (all of varying duration) have been reported. Approximately 10% of children surviving cerebral malaria have a persistent language deficit. The incidence of epilepsy is increased and the life expectancy decreased among these children.

Hypoglycemia Hypoglycemia, an important and common complication of severe malaria, is associated with a poor prognosis and is particularly problematic in children and pregnant women. Hypoglycemia in malaria results from a failure of hepatic gluconeogenesis and an increase in the consumption of glucose by both host and, to a much less-

TABLE 203-2 MANIFESTATIONS OF SEVERE FALCIPARUM MALARIA

Signs	Manifestations
Major	
Unarousable coma/ cerebral malaria	Failure to localize or respond appropriately to noxious stimuli; coma persisting for >30 min after generalized convulsion
Acidemia/acidosis	Arterial pH <7.25 or plasma bicarbonate level of <15 mmol/L; venous lactate level of >5 mmol/L; manifests as labored deep breathing, often termed "respiratory distress"
Severe normochro- mic, normocytic anemia	Hematocrit of <15% or hemoglobin level of <50 g/L (<5 g/dL) with parasitemia level of >100,000/μL
Renal failure	Urine output (24 h) of <400 mL in adults or <12 mL/kg in children; no improvement with rehy- dration; serum creatinine level of >265 μmol/L (>3.0 mg/dL)
Pulmonary edema/ adult respiratory distress syndrome	Noncardiogenic pulmonary edema, often aggravated by overhydration
Hypoglycemia	Plasma glucose level of <2.2 mmol/L (<40 mg/dL)
Hypotension/shock	Systolic blood pressure of <50 mmHg in children 1–5 years or <80 mmHg in adults; core/skin tem- perature difference of >10°C; capillary refill >2 s
Bleeding/dissemi- nated intravascu- lar coagulation	Significant bleeding and hemorrhage from the gums, nose, and gastrointestinal tract and/or evi- dence of disseminated intravascular coagulation
Convulsions	More than two generalized seizures in 24 h; signs of continued seizure activity sometimes subtle (e.g., tonic-clonic eye movements without limb or face movement)
Hemoglobinuria[a]	Macroscopic black, brown, or red urine; not associ- ated with effects of oxidant drugs and red blood cell enzyme defects (such as G6PD deficiency)
Other	
Impaired conscious- ness/arousable	Unable to sit or stand without support
Extreme weakness	Prostration; inability to sit unaided[b]
Hyperparasitemia	Parasitemia level of >5% in nonimmune patients (>20% in any patient)
Jaundice	Serum bilirubin level of >50 mmol/L (>3.0 mg/dL) if combined with other evidence of vital-organ dysfunction

[a]Hemoglobinuria may occur in uncomplicated malaria.
[b]In a child who is normally able to sit.
Note: G6PD, glucose-6-phosphate dehydrogenase.

TABLE 203-3 FEATURES INDICATING A POOR PROGNOSIS IN SEVERE FALCIPARUM MALARIA

Clinical
  Marked agitation
  Hyperventilation (respiratory distress)
  Hypothermia (<36.5°C)
  Bleeding
  Deep coma
  Repeated convulsions
  Anuria
  Shock
Laboratory
  Biochemistry
    Hypoglycemia (<2.2 mmol/L)
    Hyperlactatemia (>5 mmol/L)
    Acidosis (arterial pH <7.3, serum HCO3 <15 mmol/L)
    Elevated serum creatinine (>265 μmol/L)
    Elevated total bilirubin (>50 μmol/L)
    Elevated liver enzymes (AST/ALT 3 times upper limit of normal, 5-nucleotidase ↑)
    Elevated muscle enzymes (CPK ↑, myoglobin ↑)
    Elevated urate (>600 μmol/L)
  Hematology
    Leukocytosis (>12,000/μL)
    Severe anemia (PCV <15%)
    Coagulopathy
      Decreased platelet count (<50,000/μL)
      Prolonged prothrombin time (>3 s)
      Prolonged partial thromboplastin time
      Decreased fibrinogen (<200 mg/dL)
  Parasitology
    Hyperparasitemia
      Increased mortality at >100,000/μL
      High mortality at >500,000/μL
      >20% of parasites identified as pigment-containing trophozoites and schizonts
      >5% of neutrophils with visible pigment

Note: ALT, alanine aminotransferase; AST, aspartate aminotransferase; CPK, creatine phosphokinase; PCV, packed cell volume.

Noncardiogenic Pulmonary Edema Adults with severe falciparum ma- laria may develop noncardiogenic pulmonary edema even after several days of antimalarial therapy. The pathogenesis of this variant of the

er extent, the malaria parasites. To compound the situation, quinine and quinidine—drugs used for the treatment of severe chloroquine-resistant malaria—are powerful stimulants of pancreatic insulin secre- tion. Hyperinsulinemic hypoglycemia is especially troublesome in pregnant women receiving quinine treatment. In severe disease, the clinical diagnosis of hypoglycemia is difficult: the usual physical signs (sweating, gooseflesh, tachycardia) are absent, and the neurologic im- pairment caused by hypoglycemia cannot be distinguished from that caused by malaria.

Acidosis Acidosis, an important cause of death from severe malaria, results from accumulation of organic acids. Hyperlactatemia com- monly coexists with hypoglycemia. In adults, coexisting renal impair- ment often compounds the acidosis; in children, ketoacidosis may also contribute. Other still-unidentified organic acids are major contribu- tors to acidosis. Acidotic breathing, sometimes called respiratory dis- tress, is a sign of poor prognosis. It is often followed by circulatory failure refractory to volume expansion or inotropic drugs and ulti- mately by respiratory arrest. The plasma concentrations of bicarbon- ate or lactate are the best biochemical prognosticators in severe malaria. Lactic acidosis is caused by the combination of anaerobic gly- colysis in tissues where sequestered parasites interfere with microcir- culatory flow, hypovolemia, lactate production by the parasites, and a failure of hepatic and renal lactate clearance. The prognosis of severe acidosis is poor.

FIGURE 203-3 The eye in cerebral malaria: perimacular whitening and pale-centered retinal hemorrhages. *(Courtesy of N. Beare, T. Taylor, S. Harding, S. Lewallen, and M. Molyneux; with permission.)*

adult respiratory distress syndrome is unclear. The mortality rate is >80%. This condition can be aggravated by overly vigorous administration of IV fluid. Noncardiogenic pulmonary edema can also develop in otherwise uncomplicated vivax malaria, where recovery is usual.

Renal Impairment   Renal impairment is common among adults with severe falciparum malaria but rare among children. The pathogenesis of renal failure is unclear but may be related to erythrocyte sequestration interfering with renal microcirculatory flow and metabolism. Clinically and pathologically, this syndrome manifests as acute tubular necrosis, although renal cortical necrosis never develops. Acute renal failure may occur simultaneously with other vital-organ dysfunction (in which case the mortality risk is high) or may progress as other disease manifestations resolve. In survivors, urine flow resumes in a median of 4 days, and serum creatinine levels return to normal in a mean of 17 days (Chap. 273). Early dialysis or hemofiltration considerably enhances the likelihood of a patient's survival, particularly in acute hypercatabolic renal failure.

Hematologic Abnormalities   Anemia results from accelerated RBC removal by the spleen, obligatory RBC destruction at parasite schizogony, and ineffective erythropoiesis. In severe malaria, both infected and uninfected RBCs show reduced deformability, which correlates with prognosis and development of anemia. Splenic clearance of all RBCs is increased. In nonimmune individuals and in areas with unstable transmission, anemia can develop rapidly and transfusion is often required. As a consequence of repeated malarial infections, children in many areas of Africa may develop severe anemia resulting from both shortened RBC survival and marked dyserythropoiesis. Anemia is a common consequence of antimalarial drug resistance, which results in repeated or continued infection.

Slight coagulation abnormalities are common in falciparum malaria, and mild thrombocytopenia is usual. Of patients with severe malaria, <5% have significant bleeding with evidence of disseminated intravascular coagulation. Hematemesis from stress ulceration or acute gastric erosions may also occur.

Liver Dysfunction   Mild hemolytic jaundice is common in malaria. Severe jaundice is associated with *P. falciparum* infections; is more common among adults than among children; and results from hemolysis, hepatocyte injury, and cholestasis. When accompanied by other vital-organ dysfunction (often renal impairment), liver dysfunction carries a poor prognosis. Hepatic dysfunction contributes to hypoglycemia, lactic acidosis, and impaired drug metabolism. Occasional patients with falciparum malaria may develop deep jaundice (with hemolytic, hepatitic, and cholestatic components) without evidence of other vital-organ dysfunction.

Other Complications   Septicemia may complicate severe malaria, particularly in children. In endemic areas, *Salmonella* bacteremia has been associated specifically with *P. falciparum* infections. Chest infections and catheter-induced urinary tract infections are common among patients who are unconscious for >3 days. Aspiration pneumonia may follow generalized convulsions. The frequency of complications of severe falciparum malaria is summarized in Table 203-4.

MALARIA IN PREGNANCY

In heavily endemic (hyper- and holoendemic) areas, falciparum malaria in primi- and secundigravid women is associated with low birth weight (average reduction, ~170 g) and consequently increased infant and childhood mortality. In general, infected mothers in areas of stable transmission remain asymptomatic despite intense accumulation of parasitized erythrocytes in the placental microcirculation. Maternal HIV infection predisposes pregnant women to malaria, predisposes their newborns to congenital malarial infection, and exacerbates the reduction in birth weight associated with malaria.

In areas with unstable transmission of malaria, pregnant women are prone to severe infections and are particularly vulnerable to high-

Complication	Nonpregnant Adults	Pregnant Women	Children
Anemia	+	++	+++
Convulsions	+	+	+++
Hypoglycemia	+	+++	+++
Jaundice	+++	+++	+
Renal failure	+++	+++	−
Pulmonary edema	++	+++	+

Key: −, rare; +, infrequent; ++, frequent; +++, very frequent.

edema. Fetal distress, premature labor, and stillbirth or low birth weight are common results. Fetal death is usual in severe malaria. Congenital malaria occurs in <5% of newborns whose mothers are infected; its frequency and the level of parasitemia are related directly to the parasite density in maternal blood and in the placenta. *P. vivax* malaria in pregnancy is also associated with a reduction in birth weight (average, 110 g), but, in contrast to the situation in falciparum malaria, this effect is more pronounced in multigravid than in primigravid women.

MALARIA IN CHILDREN

Most of the estimated 1–3 million persons who die of falciparum malaria each year are young African children. Convulsions, coma, hypoglycemia, metabolic acidosis, and severe anemia are relatively common among children with severe malaria, whereas deep jaundice, acute renal failure, and acute pulmonary edema are unusual. Severely anemic children may present with labored deep breathing, which in the past has been attributed incorrectly to "anemic congestive cardiac failure" but in fact is usually caused by metabolic acidosis, often compounded by hypovolemia. Evidence is accruing that severe malaria can result in long-term neurocognitive and developmental deficits. In general, children tolerate antimalarial drugs well and respond rapidly to treatment.

TRANSFUSION MALARIA

Malaria can be transmitted by blood transfusion, needle-stick injury, sharing of needles by infected injection drug users, or organ transplantation. The incubation period in these settings is often short because there is no preerythrocytic stage of development. The clinical features and management of these cases are the same as for naturally acquired infections. Radical chemotherapy with primaquine is unnecessary for transfusion-transmitted *P. vivax* and *P. ovale* infections.

CHRONIC COMPLICATIONS OF MALARIA

TROPICAL SPLENOMEGALY (HYPERREACTIVE MALARIAL SPLENOMEGALY)

Chronic or repeated malarial infections produce hypergammaglobulinemia; normochromic, normocytic anemia; and, in certain situations, splenomegaly. Some residents of malaria-endemic areas in tropical Africa and Asia exhibit an abnormal immunologic response to repeated infections that is characterized by massive splenomegaly, hepatomegaly, marked elevations in serum titers of IgM and malarial antibody, hepatic sinusoidal lymphocytosis, and (in Africa) peripheral B cell lymphocytosis. This syndrome has been associated with the production of cytotoxic IgM antibodies to CD8+ T lymphocytes, antibodies to CD5+ T lymphocytes, and an increase in the ratio of CD4+ T cells to CD8+ T cells. These events may lead to uninhibited B cell production of IgM and the formation of cryoglobulins (IgM aggregates and immune complexes). This immunologic process stimulates reticuloendothelial hyperplasia and clearance activity and eventually produces splenomegaly. Patients with hyperreactive malarial splenomegaly (HMS) present with an abdominal mass or a dragging sensation in the abdomen and occasional sharp abdominal pains suggesting perisplenitis. Anemia and some degree of pancytopenia are usually evident, and in some cases malarial parasites cannot be found in peripheral-blood smears. Vulnerability to respira-

FIGURE 203-4 Thin blood films of *Plasmodium falciparum*. A. Young trophozoites. **B.** Old trophozoites. **C.** Pigment in polymorphonuclear cells and trophozoites. **D.** Mature schizonts. **E.** Female gametocytes. **F.** Male gametocytes. (*Reproduced from Bench Aids for the Diagnosis of Malaria Infections, 2d ed, with the permission of the World Health Organization.*)

pattern with nonselective proteinuria. Quartan nephropathy usually responds poorly to treatment with either antimalarial agents or glucocorticoids and cytotoxic drugs.

BURKITT'S LYMPHOMA AND EPSTEIN-BARR VIRUS INFECTION

It is possible that malaria-related immunosuppression provokes infection with lymphoma viruses. Burkitt's lymphoma is strongly associated with Epstein-Barr virus. The prevalence of this childhood tumor is high in malarious areas of Africa.

DIAGNOSIS

DEMONSTRATION OF THE PARASITE

The diagnosis of malaria rests on the demonstration of asexual forms of the parasite in stained peripheral-blood smears. After a negative blood smear, repeat smears should be made if there is a high degree of suspicion. Of the Romanowsky stains, Giemsa at pH 7.2 is preferred; Wright's, Field's, or Leishman's stain can also be used. Both thin (**Figs. 203-4** and **203-5**; see also **Figs. e18-1** and **e18-2**) and thick (**Figs. 203-6, 203-7, 203-8,** and **203-9**) blood smears should be examined. The thin blood smear should be rapidly air-dried, fixed in anhydrous methanol, and stained; the RBCs in the tail of the film should then be examined under oil immersion (×1000 magnification). The level

tory and skin infections is increased; many patients die of overwhelming sepsis. Persons with HMS who are living in endemic areas should receive antimalarial chemoprophylaxis; the results are usually good. In nonendemic areas, antimalarial treatment is advised. In some cases refractory to therapy, clonal lymphoproliferation may develop and then evolve into a malignant lymphoproliferative disorder.

QUARTAN MALARIAL NEPHROPATHY

Chronic or repeated infections with *P. malariae* (and possibly with other malarial species) may cause soluble immune-complex injury to the renal glomeruli, resulting in the nephrotic syndrome. Other unidentified factors must contribute to this process since only a very small proportion of infected patients develop renal disease. The histologic appearance is that of focal or segmental glomerulonephritis with splitting of the capillary basement membrane. Subendothelial dense deposits are seen on electron microscopy, and immunofluorescence reveals deposits of complement and immunoglobulins; in samples of renal tissue from children, *P. malariae* antigens are often visible. A coarse-granular pattern of basement membrane immunofluorescent deposits (predominantly IgG3) with selective proteinuria carries a better prognosis than a fine-granular, predominantly IgG2

FIGURE 203-5 Thin blood films of *Plasmodium vivax*. A. Young trophozoites. **B.** Old trophozoites. **C.** Mature schizonts. **D.** Female gametocytes. **E.** Male gametocytes. (*Reproduced from Bench Aids for the Diagnosis of Malaria Infections, 2d ed, with the permission of the World Health Organization.*)

FIGURE 203-6 Thick blood films of *Plasmodium falciparum*. A. Trophozoites. **B.** Gametocytes. *(Reproduced from Bench Aids for the Diagnosis of Malaria Infections, 2d ed, with the permission of the World Health Organization.)*

of parasitemia is expressed as the number of parasitized erythrocytes per 1000 RBCs. The thick blood film should be of uneven thickness. The smear should be dried thoroughly and stained without fixing. As many layers of erythrocytes overlie one another and are lysed during the staining procedure, the thick film has the advantage of concentrating the parasites (by 40- to 100-fold compared with a thin blood film) and thus

increasing diagnostic sensitivity. Both parasites and white blood cells (WBCs) are counted, and the number of parasites per unit volume is calculated from the total leukocyte count. Alternatively, a WBC count of 8000/μL is assumed. This figure is converted to the number of parasitized erythrocytes per microliter. A minimum of 200 WBCs should be counted under oil immersion. Interpretation of blood smear films requires some experience because artifacts are common. Before a thick smear is judged to be negative, 100–200 fields should be examined under oil immersion. In high-transmission areas, the presence of up to 10,000 parasites/μL of blood may be tolerated without symptoms or signs in partially immune individuals. Thus the detection of malaria parasites is sensitive but only poorly specific in identifying malaria as the cause of illness.

Rapid, simple, sensitive, and specific antibody-based diagnostic stick or card tests that detect *P. falciparum*–specific, histidine-rich protein 2 (PfHRP2) or lactate dehydrogenase antigens in finger-prick blood samples have been introduced (Table 203-5). Some of these tests carry a second antibody, which allows falciparum malaria to be distinguished from the less dangerous malarias. PfHRP2-based tests may remain positive for several weeks after acute infection. This feature is a disadvantage in high-transmission areas where infections are frequent but is of value in the diagnosis of severe malaria in patients who have taken antimalarial drugs and cleared peripheral parasitemia (but in whom the PfHRP2 test remains strongly positive).

FIGURE 203-7 Thick blood films of *Plasmodium vivax*. A. Trophozoites. **B.** Schizonts. **C.** Gametocytes. *(Reproduced from Bench Aids for the Diagnosis of Malaria Infections, 2d ed, with the permission of the World Health Organization.)*

FIGURE 203-8 Thick blood films of *Plasmodium ovale*. A. Trophozoites. **B.** Schizonts. **C.** Gametocytes. *(Reproduced from Bench Aids for the Diagnosis of Malaria Infections, 2d ed, with the permission of the World Health Organization.)*

The relationship between parasitemia and prognosis is complex; in general, patients with $>10^5$ parasites/μL are at increased risk of dying, but nonimmune patients may die with much lower counts, and partially immune persons may tolerate parasitemia levels many times higher with only minor symptoms. In severe malaria, a poor prognosis is indicated by a predominance of more mature *P. falciparum* parasites (i.e., >20% of parasites with visible pigment) in the peripheral blood film or by the presence of phagocytosed malarial pigment in >5% of neutrophils. In *P. falciparum* infections, gametocytemia peaks 1 week after the peak of asexual parasites. Because the mature gametocytes of *P. falciparum* are not affected by most antimalarial drugs, their persistence does not constitute evidence of drug resistance. Phagocytosed malarial pigment is sometimes seen inside peripheral-blood monocytes or polymorphonuclear leukocytes and may provide a clue to recent infection if malaria parasites are not detectable. After the clearance of the parasites, this intraphagocytic malarial pigment is often evident for several days in the peripheral blood or for longer in bone marrow aspirates or smears of fluid expressed after intradermal puncture. Staining of parasites with the fluorescent dye acridine orange allows more rapid diagnosis of malaria (but not speciation of the infection) in patients with low-level parasitemia.

LABORATORY FINDINGS

Normochromic, normocytic anemia is usual. The leukocyte count is generally normal, although it may be raised in very severe infections. There is slight monocytosis, lymphopenia, and eosinopenia, with reactive lymphocytosis and eosinophilia in the weeks after the acute infection. The erythrocyte

FIGURE 203-9 Thick blood films of *Plasmodium malariae*. A. Trophozoites. **B.** Schizonts. **C.** Gametocytes. *(Reproduced from Bench Aids for the Diagnosis of Malaria Infections, 2d ed, with the permission of the World Health Organization.)*

CHAPTER 203 Malaria

TABLE 203-5 METHODS FOR THE DIAGNOSIS OF MALARIA[a]

Method	Procedure	Advantages	Disadvantages
Thick blood film[b]	Blood should be uneven in thickness but sufficiently thin to read watch hands through part of the spot. Stain dried, unfixed blood spot with Giemsa, Field's, or other Romanowsky stain. Count number of asexual parasites per 200 WBCs (or per 500 at low densities). Count gametocytes separately.[c]	Sensitive (0.001% parasitemia); species specific; inexpensive	Requires experience (artifacts may be misinterpreted as low-level parasitemia); underestimates true count
Thin blood film[d]	Stain fixed smear with Giemsa, Field's, or other Romanowsky stain. Count number of RBCs containing asexual parasites per 1000 RBCs. In severe malaria, assess stage of parasite development and count neutrophils containing malaria pigment.[e] Count gametocytes separately.[c]	Rapid; species specific; inexpensive; in severe malaria, provides prognostic information[e]	Insensitive (<0.05% parasitemia); uneven distribution of *P. vivax*, as enlarged infected red cells concentrate at leading edge
PfHRP2 dipstick or card test	A drop of blood is placed on the stick or card, which is then immersed in washing solutions. Monoclonal antibody captures the parasite antigen and reads out as a colored band.	Robust and relatively inexpensive; rapid; sensitivity similar to or slightly lower than that of thick films (~0.001% parasitemia)	Detects only *Plasmodium falciparum*; remains positive for weeks after infection[f]; does not quantitate *P. falciparum* parasitemia
Plasmodium LDH dipstick or card test	A drop of blood is placed on the stick or card, which is then immersed in washing solutions. Monoclonal antibodies capture the parasite antigens and read out as colored bands. One band is genus specific (all malarias), and the other is specific for *P. falciparum*.	Rapid; sensitivity similar to or slightly lower than that of thick films for *P. falciparum* (~0.001% parasitemia)	Slightly more difficult preparation than PfHRP2 tests; may miss low-level parasitemia with *P. vivax*, *P. ovale*, and *P. malariae* and does not speciate these organisms; does not quantitate *P. falciparum* parasitemia
Microtube concentration methods with acridine orange staining	Blood is collected in a specialized tube containing acridine orange, anticoagulant, and a float. After centrifugation, which concentrates the parasitized cells around the float, fluorescence microscopy is performed.	Sensitivity similar or superior to that of thick films (~0.001% parasitemia); ideal for processing large numbers of samples rapidly	Does not speciate or quantitate; requires fluorescence microscopy

[a]Malaria cannot be diagnosed clinically with accuracy, but treatment should be started on clinical grounds if the laboratory confirmation is likely to be delayed. In areas of the world where malaria is endemic and transmission is high, low-level asymptomatic parasitemia is common in otherwise-healthy people. Thus malaria may not be the cause of a fever, although in this context the presence of >10,000 parasites/μL (~0.2% parasitemia) *does* indicate that malaria is the cause. Antibody and polymerase chain reaction tests have no role in the diagnosis of malaria.
[b]Asexual parasites/200 WBCs × 40 = parasite count/μL (assumes a WBC count of 8000/μL). See Figs. 203-6 through 203-9.
[c]Gametocytemia may persist for days or weeks after clearance of asexual parasites. Gametocytemia without asexual parasitemia does not indicate active infection.
[d]Parasitized RBCs (%) × hematocrit × 1256 = parasite count/μL. See Figs. 203-3 and 203-4.
[e]The presence of >100,000 parasites/μL (~2% parasitemia) is associated with an increased risk of severe malaria, but some patients have severe malaria with lower counts. At any level of parasitemia, the finding that >50% of parasites are tiny rings (cytoplasm width less than half of nucleus width) carries a relatively good prognosis. The presence of visible pigment in >20% of parasites or of phagocytosed pigment in >5% of polymorphonuclear leukocytes (indicating massive recent schizogony) carries a worse prognosis.
[f]Persistence of PfHRP2 is a disadvantage in high-transmission settings, where many asymptomatic people have positive tests, but can be used to diagnostic advantage in low-transmission settings when a sick patient has received previous unknown treatment (which, in endemic areas, often consists of antimalarial drugs). A positive PfHRP2 test indicates that the illness is falciparum malaria, even if the blood smear is negative.
Note: LDH, lactate dehydrogenase; PfHRP2, *P. falciparum* histidine-rich protein 2; RBCs, red blood cells; WBCs, white blood cells.

sedimentation rate, plasma viscosity, and levels of C-reactive protein and other acute-phase proteins are high. The platelet count is usually reduced to ~10^5/μL. Severe infections may be accompanied by prolonged prothrombin and partial thromboplastin times and by more severe thrombocytopenia. Levels of antithrombin III are reduced even in mild infection. In uncomplicated malaria, plasma concentrations of electrolytes, blood urea nitrogen (BUN), and creatinine are usually normal. Findings in severe malaria may include metabolic acidosis, with low plasma concentrations of glucose, sodium, bicarbonate, calcium, phosphate, and albumin together with elevations in lactate, BUN, creatinine, urate, muscle and liver enzymes, and conjugated and unconjugated bilirubin. Hypergammaglobulinemia is usual in immune and semi-immune subjects. Urinalysis generally gives normal results. In adults and children with cerebral malaria, the mean opening pressure at lumbar puncture is ~160 mm of cerebrospinal fluid (CSF); usually the CSF is normal or has a slightly elevated total protein level [<1.0 g/L (<100 mg/dL)] and cell count (<20/μL).

℞ MALARIA

(Table 203-6) When a patient in or from a malarious area presents with fever, thick and thin blood smears should be prepared and examined immediately to confirm the diagnosis and identify the species of infecting parasite (Figs. 203-4 through 203-9). Repeat blood smears should be performed at least every 12–24 h for 2 days if the first smears are negative and malaria is strongly suspected. Alternatively, a rapid antigen detection card or stick test should be performed. Patients with severe malaria or those unable to take oral drugs should receive parenteral antimalarial therapy. If there is any doubt about the resistance status of the infecting organism, it should be considered resistant. Antimalarial susceptibility testing can be performed but is not generally available and yields results too slowly to influence the choice of treatment. Several drugs are available for oral treatment, and the choice of drug depends on the likely sensitivity of the infecting parasites. Despite recent evidence of chloroquine resistance in *P. vivax* (from parts of Indonesia, Oceania, eastern and southern Asia, and Central and South America), chloroquine remains the treatment of choice for the "benign" human malarias (*P. vivax, P. ovale, P. malariae*) except in Indonesia and Papua New Guinea, where high levels of resistance are prevalent.

The treatment of falciparum malaria has changed radically in recent years. In endemic areas, the World Health Organization now recommends artemisinin-based combinations as first-line treatment for uncomplicated falciparum malaria everywhere. These rapidly and reliably effective drugs are often unavailable in temperate countries (including the United States), where treatment recommendations are limited by the registered available drugs. Fake or substandard drugs, including antimalarial agents, are being sold in many low-income countries; thus, careful attention is required at purchase, especially when the patient fails to respond as expected. Characteristics of antimalarial drugs are shown in **Table 203-7**.

SEVERE MALARIA In large studies conducted in Asia, parenteral artesunate, a water-soluble artemisinin derivative, has been shown to reduce mortality rates in severe falciparum malaria by 35% from rates obtained with quinine. Artesunate has therefore become the drug of choice. Artesunate is given by the IV route but can also be given by IM injection. Artemether and

TABLE 203-6 REGIMENS FOR THE TREATMENT OF MALARIA

Type of Disease or Treatment	Regimen(s)
Uncomplicated Malaria	
Known chloroquine-sensitive strains of *Plasmodium vivax, P. malariae, P. ovale, P. falciparum*[a]	Chloroquine (10 mg of base/kg stat followed by 5 mg/kg at 12, 24, and 36 h or by 10 mg/kg at 24 h and 5 mg/kg at 48 h) *or* Amodiaquine (10–12 mg of base/kg qd for 3 days)
Radical treatment for *P. vivax* or *P. ovale* infection	In addition to chloroquine or amodiaquine as detailed above, primaquine (0.25 mg of base/kg qd; 0.375–0.5 mg of base/kg qd in Southeast Asia and Oceania) should be given for 14 days to prevent relapse. In mild G6PD deficiency, 0.75 mg of base/kg should be given once weekly for 6 weeks. Primaquine should not be given in severe G6PD deficiency.
Sensitive *P. falciparum* malaria[b]	Artesunate[c] (4 mg/kg qd for 3 days) plus sulfadoxine (25 mg/kg)/pyrimethamine (1.25 mg/kg) as a single dose *or* Artesunate[c] (4 mg/kg qd for 3 days) plus amodiaquine (10 mg of base/kg qd for 3 days)[d]
Multidrug-resistant *P. falciparum* malaria	Either artemether-lumefantrine[c] (1.5/9 mg/kg bid for 3 days with food) or artesunate[c] (4 mg/kg qd for 3 days) *plus* Mefloquine (25 mg of base/kg—either 8 mg/kg qd for 3 days or 15 mg/kg on day 2 and then 10 mg/kg on day 3)[d]
Second-line treatment/treatment of imported malaria	Either artesunate[c] (2 mg/kg qd for 7 days) or quinine (10 mg of salt/kg tid for 7 days) *plus 1 of the following 3:* 1. Tetracycline[e] (4 mg/kg qid for 7 days) 2. Doxycycline[e] (3 mg/kg qd for 7 days) 3. Clindamycin (10 mg/kg bid for 7 days) *or* Atovaquone-proguanil (20/8 mg/kg qd for 3 days with food)
Severe Falciparum Malaria[f]	
	Artesunate[c] (2.4 mg/kg stat IV followed by 2.4 mg/kg at 12 and 24 h and then daily if necessary)[g] *or* Artemether[c] (3.2 mg/kg stat IM followed by 1.6 mg/kg qd) *or* Quinine dihydrochloride (20 mg of salt/kg[h] infused over 4 h, followed by 10 mg of salt/kg infused over 2–8 h q8h[i]) *or* Quinidine (10 mg of base/kg[h] infused over 1–2 h, followed by 1.2 mg of base/kg per hour[i] with electrocardiographic monitoring)

[a]Very few areas now have chloroquine-sensitive malaria (Fig. 203-2).

[b]In areas where the partner drug to artesunate is known to be effective.

[c]Artemisinin derivatives are not registered in the United States and some other temperate countries.

[d]Fixed-dose coformulated combinations are available.

[e]Tetracycline and doxycycline should not be given to pregnant women or to children <8 years of age.

[f]Oral treatment should be substituted as soon as the patient recovers sufficiently to take fluids by mouth.

[g]Artesunate is the drug of choice when available. The data from large studies in Southeast Asia showed a 35% reduction in mortality rate from that with quinine. Severe malaria in children in high-transmission settings has different characteristics; thus trials are ongoing in Africa comparing artesunate with quinine to determine whether there is a survival benefit in African children.

[h]A loading dose should not be given if therapeutic doses of quinine or quinidine have definitely been administered in the previous 24 h. Some authorities recommend a lower dose of quinidine.

[i]Infusions can be given in 0.9% saline and 5% or 10% dextrose in water. Infusion rates for quinine and quinidine should be carefully controlled.

Note: G6PD, glucose-6-phosphate dehydrogenase.

the closely related drug artemotil (arteether) are oil-based formulations given by IM injection; they are erratically absorbed and do not confer the same survival benefit as artesunate. A rectal formulation of artesunate has been developed as a community-based prereferral treatment for patients in the rural tropics who cannot take oral medications. Although the artemisinin compounds are safer than quinine and considerably safer than quinidine, only one formulation is available in the United States. IV artesunate has recently been approved by the FDA for emergency use for severe malaria through the Centers for Disease Control and Prevention (CDC) Drug Service (see end of chapter for contact information). The antiarrhythmic quinidine gluconate is as effective as quinine and, as it is more readily available, has replaced quinine for the treatment of malaria in the United States. The administration of quinidine must be closely monitored if dysrhythmias and hypotension are to be avoided. Total plasma levels >8 µg/mL, a QT_c interval >0.6 s, or QRS widening beyond 25% of baseline are indications for slowing infusion rates. If arrhythmia or saline-unresponsive hypotension develops, treatment with this drug should be discontinued. Quinine is safer than quinidine; cardiovascular monitoring is not required except when the recipient has cardiac disease.

Severe falciparum malaria constitutes a medical emergency requiring intensive nursing care and careful management. The patient should be weighed and, if comatose, placed on his or her side or prone. Frequent evaluation of the patient's condition is essential. Ancillary drugs such as high-dose glucocorticoids, urea, heparin, dextran, desferrioxamine, antibody to tumor necrosis factor α, and high-dose phenobarbital (20 mg/kg) have proved either ineffective or harmful in clinical trials and should not be used. In acute renal failure or severe metabolic acidosis, hemofiltration or hemodialysis should be started as early as possible.

Parenteral antimalarial treatment should be started as soon as possible. If artemether, quinine, or quinidine is used, an initial loading dose must be given so that therapeutic concentrations are reached as soon as possible. Both quinine and quinidine will cause dangerous hypotension if injected rapidly; when given IV, they must be administered carefully by rate-controlled infusion only. If this approach is not possible, quinine may be given by deep IM injections into the anterior thigh. The optimal therapeutic range for quinine and quinidine in severe malaria is not known with certainty, but total plasma concentrations of 8–15 mg/L for quinine and 3.5–8.0 mg/L for quinidine are effective and do not cause serious toxicity. The systemic clearance and apparent volume of distribution of these alkaloids are markedly reduced and plasma protein binding is increased in severe malaria, so that the blood concentrations attained with a given dose are higher. If the patient remains seriously ill or in acute renal failure for >2 days, maintenance doses of quinine or quinidine should be reduced by 30–50% to prevent toxic accumulation of the drug. The initial doses should never be reduced. If one of the artemisinin derivatives is given, dose reductions are unnecessary, even in renal failure. Exchange transfusion should be considered for severely ill patients, although the precise indications for this procedure have not been agreed upon. It has been recommended that—if safe and feasible—exchange should be considered for patients with severe malaria, but there is no clear evidence that this measure is beneficial. The role of prophylactic anticonvulsants is uncertain. If respiratory support is not available, then a full loading dose of phenobarbital (20 mg/kg) to prevent convulsions should not be given as it may cause respiratory arrest.

When the patient is unconscious, the blood glucose level should be measured every 4–6 h, and values <2.2 mmol/L (40 mg/dL) should mandate treatment with IV dextrose. All patients treated with IV quinine or quinidine should receive a continuous infusion of 5–10% dextrose. The parasite count and hematocrit level should be measured every 6–12 h. Anemia develops rapidly; if the hematocrit falls to <20%, then whole blood (preferably fresh) or packed cells should be transfused slowly, with careful attention to circulatory status. Renal function should be checked daily. Children presenting with severe anemia and acidotic breathing are often

TABLE 203-7 **PROPERTIES OF ANTIMALARIAL DRUGS**

Drug(s)	Pharmacokinetic Properties	Antimalarial Activity	Minor Toxicity	Major Toxicity
Quinine, quinidine	Good oral and IM absorption (quinine); Cl and V_d reduced, but plasma protein binding (principally to $\propto_1$ acid glycoprotein) increased (90%) in malaria; quinine $t_{1/2}$: 16 h in malaria, 11 h in healthy persons; quinidine $t_{1/2}$: 13 h in malaria, 8 h in healthy persons	Acts mainly on trophozoite blood stage; kills gametocytes of *P. vivax*, *P. ovale*, and *P. malariae* (but not *P. falciparum*); no action on liver stages	*Common:* "Cinchonism": tinnitus, high-tone hearing loss, nausea, vomiting, dysphoria, postural hypotension; ECG QT_c interval prolongation (quinine usually by <10% but quinidine by up to 25%) *Rare:* Diarrhea, visual disturbance, rashes *Note:* Very bitter taste	*Common:* Hypoglycemia *Rare:* Hypotension, blindness, deafness, cardiac arrhythmias, thrombocytopenia, hemolysis, hemolytic-uremic syndrome, vasculitis, cholestatic hepatitis, neuromuscular paralysis *Note:* Quinidine more cardiotoxic
Chloroquine	Good oral absorption, very rapid IM and SC absorption; complex pharmacokinetics; enormous Cl and V_d (unaffected by malaria); blood concentration profile determined by distribution processes in malaria; $t_{1/2}$: 1–2 months	As for quinine but acts slightly earlier in asexual cycle	*Common:* Nausea, dysphoria, pruritus in dark-skinned patients, postural hypotension *Rare:* Accommodation difficulties, keratopathy, rash *Note:* Bitter taste, well tolerated	*Acute:* Hypotensive shock (parenteral), cardiac arrhythmias, neuropsychiatric reactions *Chronic:* Retinopathy (cumulative dose, >100 g), skeletal and cardiac myopathy
Amodiaquine	Good oral absorption; largely converted to active metabolite desethylamodiaquine	As for chloroquine	Nausea (tastes better than chloroquine)	Agranulocytosis; hepatitis, mainly with prophylactic use
Mefloquine	Adequate oral absorption; no parenteral preparation; $t_{1/2}$: 14–20 days (shorter in malaria)	As for quinine	Nausea, giddiness, dysphoria, fuzzy thinking, sleeplessness, nightmares, sense of dissociation	Neuropsychiatric reactions, convulsions, encephalopathy
Tetracycline, doxycycline[a]	Excellent absorption; $t_{1/2}$: 8 h for tetracycline, 18 h for doxycycline	Weak antimalarial activity; should not be used alone for treatment	Gastrointestinal intolerance, deposition in growing bones and teeth, photosensitivity, moniliasis, benign intracranial hypertension	Renal failure in patients with impaired renal function (tetracycline)
Halofantrine[b]	Highly variable absorption related to fat intake; $t_{1/2}$: 1–3 days (active desbutyl metabolite $t_{1/2}$: 3–7 days)	As for quinine	Diarrhea	Cardiac conduction disturbances; atrioventricular block; ECG QT_c interval prolongation; potentially lethal ventricular tachyarrhythmias
Artemisinin and derivatives (artemether, artesunate)	Good oral absorption, slow and variable absorption of IM artemether; artesunate and artemether biotransformed to active metabolite dihydroartemisinin; all drugs eliminated very rapidly; $t_{1/2}$: <1 h	Broader stage specificity and more rapid than other drugs; no action on liver stages; kills all but fully mature gametocytes of *P. falciparum*	Reduction in reticulocyte count (but not anemia)	Anaphylaxis, urticaria, fever
Pyrimethamine	Good oral absorption, variable IM absorption; $t_{1/2}$: 4 days	For blood stages, acts mainly on mature forms; causal prophylactic	Well tolerated	Megaloblastic anemia, pancytopenia, pulmonary infiltration
Proguanil (chloroguanide)	Good oral absorption; biotransformed to active metabolite cycloguanil; $t_{1/2}$: 16 h; biotransformation reduced by oral contraceptive use and in pregnancy	Causal prophylactic; not used alone for treatment	Well tolerated; mouth ulcers and rare alopecia	Megaloblastic anemia in renal failure
Primaquine	Complete oral absorption; active compound not known; $t_{1/2}$: 7 h	Radical cure; eradicates hepatic forms of *P. vivax* and *P. ovale*; kills all stages of gametocyte development of *P. falciparum*	Nausea, vomiting, diarrhea, abdominal pain, hemolysis, methemoglobinemia	Massive hemolysis in subjects with severe G6PD deficiency
Atovaquone	Highly variable absorption related to fat intake; $t_{1/2}$: 30–70 h	Acts mainly on trophozoite blood stage	None identified	None identified
Lumefantrine	Highly variable absorption related to fat intake; $t_{1/2}$: 3–4 days	As for quinine	None identified	None identified

[a]Tetracycline and doxycycline should not be given to pregnant women or to children <8 years of age.
[b]Halofantrine should not be used by patients with long ECG QT_c intervals or known conduction disturbances or by those taking drugs that may affect ventricular repolarization, e.g., quinidine, quinine, mefloquine, chloroquine, neuroleptics, antiarrhythmics, tricyclic antidepressants, terfenadine, or astemizole.

Abbreviations: Cl, systemic clearance; V_d, total apparent volume of distribution; IM, intramuscular; SC, subcutaneous; ECG, electrocardiogram; G6PD, glucose-6-phosphate dehydrogenase.

hypovolemic; in this situation, resuscitation with crystalloids or blood is indicated. Accurate assessment is vital. Management of fluid balance is difficult in severe malaria, particularly in adults, because of the thin dividing line between overhydration (leading to pulmonary edema) and underhydration (contributing to renal impairment). If necessary, central venous pressures should be measured and maintained in the low-normal range. As soon as the patient can take fluids, oral therapy should be substituted for parenteral treatment.

UNCOMPLICATED MALARIA   Infections due to *P. vivax*, *P. malariae*, and *P. ovale* should be treated with oral chloroquine (total dose, 25 mg of base/kg). In much of the tropics, drug-resistant *P. falciparum* has been increasing in distribution, frequency, and intensity. Chloroquine-resistant *P. falciparum* is now present throughout most of the tropical world, and resistance to sulfadoxine/pyrimethamine is widespread and increasing. It is now accepted that, to prevent resistance, falciparum malaria should be treated with drug combinations and not with single drugs in endemic areas; the same rationale has been applied successfully to the treatment of tuberculosis and HIV/AIDS. This combination strategy is based on simultaneous use of two or more drugs with different modes of action: one is usually an artemisinin derivative (artesunate, artemether, or dihydroartemisinin) given for 3 days, and the other is usually a slower-acting antimalarial to which *P. falciparum* is sensitive. Artemisinin combination regimens now constitute first-line recommended treatment for falciparum malaria. In areas with multidrug-resistant falciparum malaria (parts of Asia and South America), either artemether-lumefantrine or artesunate-mefloquine should be used. Although significant resistance to mefloquine has been documented in Thailand, Myanmar, Vietnam, Laos, and Cambodia **(Fig. 203-10)**, mefloquine is usually effective against multidrug-resistant strains of *P. falciparum* outside these areas and, in combination with artesunate, achieves cure rates exceeding 90% nearly everywhere. Atovaquone-proguanil is also highly effective. In areas with more drug-sensitive isolates, atovaquone-proguanil, mefloquine, artesunate-amodiaquine, or artesunate-sulfadoxine/pyrimethamine can be used, depending on the prevailing drug susceptibility pattern. These 3-day regimens are all well tolerated, although mefloquine is associated with increased rates of vomiting and dizziness. As second-line treatment for recrudescence following first-line therapy, a 7-day course of either artesunate or quinine plus tetracycline, doxycycline, or clindamycin is effective. Tetracycline and doxycycline cannot be given to pregnant women or to children <8 years of age. Oral quinine is extremely bitter and regularly produces cinchonism comprising tinnitus, high-tone deafness, nausea, vomiting, and dysphoria. Adherence is poor with the required 7-day regimens of quinine.

Patients should be monitored for vomiting for 1 h after the administration of any oral antimalarial drug. If there is vomiting, the dose should be repeated. Symptom-based treatment, with tepid sponging and acetaminophen administration, lowers fever and thereby reduces the patient's propensity to vomit these drugs. Minor central nervous system reactions (nausea, dizziness, sleep disturbances) are common. The incidence of serious adverse neuropsychiatric reactions to mefloquine treatment is ~1 in 1000 in Asia but may be as high as 1 in 200 among Africans and Caucasians. All the antimalarial quinolines (chloroquine, mefloquine, and quinine) exacerbate the orthostatic hypotension associated with malaria, and all are tolerated better by children than by adults. Pregnant women, young children, patients unable to tolerate oral therapy, and nonimmune subjects (e.g., travelers) with suspected malaria should be evaluated carefully and hospitalization considered. If there is any doubt as to the identity of the infecting malarial species, treatment for falciparum malaria should be given. A negative blood smear does not rule out malaria; thick blood films should be checked 1 and 2 days later to exclude the diagnosis. Nonimmune patients receiving treatment for malaria should have daily parasite counts performed until negative thick films indicate clearance of the parasite. If the level of parasitemia does not fall below 25% of the admission value in 48 h or if parasitemia has not cleared by 7 days (and adherence is assured), drug resistance is likely and the regimen should be changed. If treatment failures occur with commonly used antimalarial agents, alternative drugs should be used.

To eradicate persistent liver stages and prevent relapse (radical treatment), primaquine (0.25–0.5 mg of base/kg, adult dose) should be given daily for 14 days to patients with *P. vivax* or *P. ovale* infections after laboratory tests for G6PD deficiency have proved negative. A total dose of 22.5–30 mg for an adult is recommended for infections acquired in Southeast Asia and Oceania. If the patient has a mild variant of G6PD deficiency, primaquine can be given in a dose of 0.75 mg of base/kg (45 mg maximum) once weekly for 6 weeks.

COMPLICATIONS   **Acute Renal Failure**   If the level of BUN or creatinine rises despite adequate rehydration, fluid administration should be restricted to prevent volume overload. As in other forms of hypercatabolic acute renal failure, renal replacement is best performed early (Chap. 273). Hemofiltration and hemodialysis are more effective than peritoneal dialysis and are associated with lower mortality. Some patients with renal impairment pass small volumes of urine sufficient to allow control of fluid balance; these cases can be managed conservatively if other indications for

FIGURE 203-10 Mefloquine resistance in *Plasmodium falciparum* in Southeast Asia: high-level mefloquine resistance (*brown*), low-level mefloquine resistance (*red*), and mefloquine sensitivity (failure rate, <20%; *green*). There is insufficient information for the other areas.

dialysis do not arise. Renal function usually improves within days, but full recovery may take weeks.

Acute Pulmonary Edema   Patients should be positioned with the head of the bed at a 45° elevation and given oxygen and IV diuretics. Pulmonary artery occlusion pressures may be normal, indicating increased pulmonary capillary permeability. Positive-pressure ventilation should be started early if the immediate measures fail (Chap. 228).

Hypoglycemia   An initial slow injection of 50% dextrose (0.5 g/kg) should be followed by an infusion of 10% dextrose (0.10 g/kg per hour). The blood glucose level should be checked regularly thereafter as recurrent hypoglycemia is common, particularly among patients receiving quinine or quinidine. In severely ill patients, hypoglycemia commonly occurs together with metabolic (lactic) acidosis and carries a poor prognosis.

Other Complications   Patients who develop spontaneous bleeding should be given fresh blood and IV vitamin K. Convulsions should be treated with IV or rectal benzodiazepines and, if necessary, respiratory support. Aspiration pneumonia should be suspected in any unconscious patient with convulsions, particularly with persistent hyperventilation; IV antimicrobial agents and oxygen should be administered, and pulmonary toilet should be undertaken. Hypoglycemia or gram-negative septicemia should be suspected when the condition of any patient suddenly deteriorates for no obvious reason during antimalarial treatment. Systemic *Salmonella* infections are common complications among African children with falciparum malaria. Antibiotics should be considered for severely ill patients not responding to antimalarial treatment.

PREVENTION

These are halcyon days for malaria prevention and control. New drugs have been discovered and developed; highly effective drugs, insecticide-treated nets, and insecticides for spraying dwellings are being purchased for endemic countries by the Global Fund to Fight HIV/AIDS, Tuberculosis, and Malaria and the President's Malaria Initiative; and even stronger support is being advocated by the Roll Back Malaria Partnership, the Global Health Council, and other supporters of malaria control and research. Still, the eradication of malaria is not yet feasible because of the widespread distribution of *Anopheles* breeding

TABLE 203-8 DRUGS USED IN THE PROPHYLAXIS OF MALARIA

Drug	Usage	Adult Dose	Pediatric Dose	Comments
Atovaquone/ proguanil (Malarone)	Prophylaxis in areas with chloroquine- or mefloquine-resistant *Plasmodium falciparum*	1 adult tablet PO[a]	5–8 kg: ¹/₂ pediatric tablet[b] daily ≥8–10 kg: ³/₄ pediatric tablet daily ≥10–20 kg: 1 pediatric tablet daily ≥20–30 kg: 2 pediatric tablets daily ≥30–40 kg: 3 pediatric tablets daily ≥40 kg: 1 adult tablet daily	Begin 1–2 days before travel to malarious areas. Take daily at the same time each day while in the malarious area and for 7 days after leaving such areas. Atovaquone-proguanil is contraindicated in persons with severe renal impairment (creatinine clearance rate <30 mL/min). It is not recommended for children weighing <5 kg, pregnant women, or women breast-feeding infants weighing <5 kg. Atovaquone/proguanil should be taken with food or a milky drink.
Chloroquine phosphate (Aralen and generic)	Prophylaxis only in areas with chloroquine-sensitive *P. falciparum*[c]	300 mg of base (500 mg of salt) PO once weekly	5 mg/kg of base (8.3 mg of salt/kg) PO once weekly, up to a maximum adult dose of 300 mg of base	Begin 1–2 weeks before travel to malarious areas. Take weekly on the same day of the week while in the malarious areas and for 4 weeks after leaving such areas. Chloroquine phosphate may exacerbate psoriasis.
Doxycycline (many brand names and generic)	Prophylaxis in areas with chloroquine- or mefloquine-resistant *P. falciparum*[c]	100 mg PO qd	≥8 years of age: 2 mg/kg, up to adult dose	Begin 1–2 days before travel to malarious areas. Take daily at the same time each day while in the malarious areas and for 4 weeks after leaving such areas. Doxycycline is contraindicated in children <8 years of age and in pregnant women.
Hydroxychloroquine sulfate (Plaquenil)	An alternative to chloroquine for primary prophylaxis only in areas with chloroquine-sensitive *P. falciparum*[c]	310 mg of base (400 mg of salt) PO once weekly	5 mg of base/kg (6.5 mg of salt/kg) PO once weekly, up to maximum adult dose of 310 mg of base	Begin 1–2 weeks before travel to malarious areas. Take weekly on the same day of the week while in the malarious areas and for 4 weeks after leaving such areas. Hydroxychloroquine may exacerbate psoriasis.
Mefloquine (Lariam and generic)	Prophylaxis in areas with chloroquine-resistant *P. falciparum*	228 mg of base (250 mg of salt) PO once weekly	≤9 kg: 4.6 mg of base/kg (5 mg of salt/kg) PO once weekly 10–19 kg: ¹/₄ tablet once weekly 20–30 kg: ¹/₂ tablet once weekly 31–45 kg: ³/₄ tablet once weekly ≥46 kg: 1 tablet once weekly	Begin 1–2 weeks before travel to malarious areas. Take weekly on the same day of the week while in the malarious areas and for 4 weeks after leaving such areas. Mefloquine is contraindicated in persons allergic to this drug or related compounds (e.g., quinine and quinidine) and in persons with active or recent depression, generalized anxiety disorder, psychosis, schizophrenia, other major psychiatric disorders, or seizures. Use with caution in persons with psychiatric disturbances or a history of depression. Mefloquine is not recommended for persons with cardiac conduction abnormalities.
Primaquine	An option for prophylaxis in special circumstances	30 mg of base (52.6 mg of salt) PO qd	0.5 mg of base/kg (0.8 mg of salt/kg) PO qd, up to adult dose; should be taken with food	Begin 1–2 days before travel to malarious areas. Take daily at the same time each day while in the malarious areas and for 7 days after leaving such areas. Primaquine is contraindicated in persons with G6PD1 deficiency. It is also contraindicated during pregnancy and in lactation unless the infant being breast-fed has a documented normal G6PD level. Use in consultation with malaria experts.
Primaquine	Used for presumptive antirelapse therapy (terminal prophylaxis) to decrease risk of relapses of *P. vivax* and *P. ovale*.	30 mg of base (52.6 mg of salt) PO qd for 14 days after departure from the malarious area	0.5 mg of base/kg (0.8 mg of salt/kg), up to adult dose, PO qd for 14 days after departure from the malarious area	This therapy is indicated for persons who have had prolonged exposure to *P. vivax* and/or *P. ovale*. It is contraindicated in persons with G6PD1 deficiency as well as during pregnancy and in lactation unless the infant being breast-fed has a documented normal G6PD level.

[a]An adult tablet contains 250 mg of atovaquone and 100 mg of proguanil hydrochloride.
[b]A pediatric tablet contains 62.5 mg of atovaquone and 25 mg of proguanil hydrochloride.
[c]Very few areas now have chloroquine-sensitive malaria (Fig. 203-2).

Source: CDC: *http://wwwn.cdc.gov/travel/contentMalariaDrugsHC.aspx*, accessed September 13, 2007.

sites; the great number of infected persons; the continued use of ineffective antimalarial drugs; and inadequacies in human and material resources, infrastructure, and control programs. Malaria may be contained by judicious use of insecticides to kill the mosquito vector, rapid diagnosis, appropriate patient management, and—where effective and feasible—administration of intermittent presumptive treatment or chemoprophylaxis to high-risk groups. Malaria researchers are intensifying their efforts to gain a better understanding of parasite-human-mosquito interactions and to develop more effective control and prevention interventions. Despite the enormous investment in efforts to develop a malaria vaccine, no safe, effective, long-lasting vaccine is likely to be available for general use in the near future (Chap. 116). While there is promise for one or more malaria vaccines on the more distant horizon, prevention and control measures continue to rely on antivector and drug-use strategies.

PERSONAL PROTECTION AGAINST MALARIA

Simple measures to reduce the frequency of mosquito bites in malarious areas are very important. These measures include the avoidance of exposure to mosquitoes at their peak feeding times (usually dusk and dawn) and throughout the night as well as the use of insect repellents containing DEET (10–35%) or picaridin (7%; if DEET is unacceptable), suitable clothing, and insecticide-impregnated bed nets or other materials. Widespread use of bed nets treated with residual pyrethroids reduces the incidence of malaria in areas where vectors bite indoors at night and has been shown to reduce mortality rates in western and eastern Africa.

CHEMOPROPHYLAXIS

(Table 203-8; *http://wwwn.cdc.gov/travel/contentMalariaDrugsHC. aspx*; accessed September 13, 2007) Recommendations for prophylaxis depend on knowledge of local patterns of plasmodial drug sensitivity and

PART 7
Infectious Diseases

the likelihood of acquiring malarial infection. When there is uncertainty, drugs effective against resistant *P. falciparum* should be used [atovaquone-proguanil (Malarone), doxycycline, mefloquine, or primaquine]. Chemoprophylaxis is never entirely reliable, and malaria should always be considered in the differential diagnosis of fever in patients who have traveled to endemic areas, even if they are taking prophylactic antimalarial drugs.

Pregnant women traveling to malarious areas should be warned about the potential risks. All pregnant women at risk in endemic areas should be encouraged to attend regular antenatal clinics. Mefloquine is the only drug advised for pregnant women traveling to areas with drug-resistant malaria; this drug is generally considered safe in the second and third trimesters of pregnancy, and the limited data on first-trimester exposure are reassuring. The safety of other prophylactic antimalarial agents in pregnancy has not been established. Antimalarial prophylaxis has been shown to reduce mortality rates among children between the ages of 3 months and 4 years in malaria-endemic areas; however, it is not a logistically or economically feasible option in many countries. The alternative—to give intermittent treatment doses [intermittent preventive treatment (IPT)]—shows promise for more widespread use in infants, young children, and pregnant women. Children born to nonimmune mothers in endemic areas (usually expatriates moving to malaria-endemic areas) should receive prophylaxis from birth.

Travelers should start taking antimalarial drugs 2 days to 1–2 weeks before departure so that any untoward reactions can be detected and so that therapeutic antimalarial blood concentrations will be present when needed (Table 203-8). Antimalarial prophylaxis should continue for 4 weeks after the traveler has left the endemic area, except if atovaquone-proguanil or primaquine has been taken; these drugs have significant activities against the liver stage of the infection (causal prophylaxis) and can be discontinued 1 week after departure from the endemic area. Presumptive self-treatment for malaria with atovaquone-proguanil (for 3 consecutive days) or another drug can be considered under special circumstances; medical advice on self-treatment should be sought before departure for malarious areas and as soon as possible after illness begins.

Atovaquone-proguanil (Malarone; 3.75/1.5 mg/kg or 250/100 mg, daily adult dose) is a fixed-combination, once-daily prophylactic agent that is very well tolerated by adults and children, with fewer adverse gastrointestinal effects than chloroquine-proguanil and fewer adverse central nervous system effects than mefloquine. It is proguanil itself, rather than the antifolate metabolite cycloguanil, that acts synergistically with atovaquone. This combination is effective against all types of malaria, including multidrug-resistant falciparum malaria. Atovaquone-proguanil is best taken with food or a milky drink to optimize absorption. There are insufficient data on the safety of this regimen in pregnancy.

Mefloquine (250 mg of salt weekly, adult dose) has been widely used for malarial prophylaxis because it is usually effective against multidrug-resistant falciparum malaria and is reasonably well tolerated. Mild nausea, dizziness, fuzzy thinking, disturbed sleep patterns, vivid dreams, and malaise are relatively common. Approximately 1 in every 10,000 recipients develops an acute reversible neuropsychiatric reaction manifested by confusion, psychosis, convulsions, or encephalopathy. The role of mefloquine prophylaxis during pregnancy remains uncertain; in studies in Africa, mefloquine prophylaxis was found to be effective and safe during pregnancy. However, in one study from Thailand, treatment of malaria with mefloquine was associated with an increased risk of stillbirth.

Daily administration of doxycycline (100 mg daily, adult dose) is an effective alternative to atovaquone-proguanil or mefloquine. Doxycycline is generally well tolerated but may cause vulvovaginal thrush, diarrhea, and photosensitivity and cannot be used by children <8 years old or by pregnant women.

Chloroquine remains the drug of choice for the prevention of infection with drug-sensitive *P. falciparum* (now found in very few areas of the world) and with the other human malarial species (although chloroquine-resistant *P. vivax* has been reported from parts of eastern Asia, Oceania, and Central and South America). Chloroquine is generally well tolerated, although some patients cannot take the drug because of malaise, headache, visual symptoms (from reversible keratopathy), gastrointestinal in-

tolerance, or (in dark-skinned patients) pruritus. A concomitant filarial infection may provoke or aggravate chloroquine-induced pruritus. Chloroquine is considered safe in pregnancy. With chronic administration for >5 years, a characteristic dose-related retinopathy may develop, but this condition is rare at the doses used for antimalarial prophylaxis. Idiosyncratic or allergic reactions are also rare. Skeletal and cardiac myopathy are potential problems with protracted prophylactic use; they are more likely to occur with the high doses used in the treatment of rheumatoid arthritis. Neuropsychiatric reactions and skin rashes are unusual. When used continuously, amodiaquine, a related aminoquinoline, is associated with a high risk of agranulocytosis (~1 person in 2000) and hepatotoxicity (~1 person in 16,000) and should not be used for prophylaxis.

Primaquine (0.5 mg of base/kg or 30 mg, daily adult dose taken with food) has proved safe and effective in the prevention of drug-resistant falciparum and vivax malaria in adults. This drug can be considered for persons who are traveling to areas with or without drug-resistant *P. falciparum* and who are intolerant to other recommended drugs. Abdominal pain and oxidant hemolysis—the principal adverse effects—are not common as long as the drug is taken with food and is not given to G6PD-deficient persons. Primaquine should not be given to pregnant women or neonates. Travelers must be tested for G6PD deficiency and be shown to have a level in the normal range before receiving primaquine. In G6PD deficiency, primaquine can cause hemolysis that is sometimes fatal.

In the past, the dihydrofolate reductase inhibitors pyrimethamine and proguanil (chloroguanide) have been administered widely, but the rapid selection of resistance in both *P. falciparum* and *P. vivax* has limited their use. Whereas antimalarial quinolines such as chloroquine act on the erythrocyte stage of parasitic development, the dihydrofolate reductase inhibitors also inhibit preerythrocytic growth in the liver (causal prophylaxis) and development in the mosquito (sporontocidal activity). Proguanil is safe and well tolerated, although mouth ulceration occurs in ~8% of persons using this drug; it is considered safe for antimalarial prophylaxis in pregnancy. The prophylactic use of the combination of pyrimethamine and sulfadoxine is not recommended because of an unacceptable incidence of severe toxicity, principally exfoliative dermatitis and other skin rashes, agranulocytosis, hepatitis, and pulmonary eosinophilia (incidence, 1:7000; fatal reactions, 1:18,000). The combination of pyrimethamine with dapsone (0.2/1.5 mg/kg weekly; 12.5/100 mg, adult dose) is a third-line alternative available in some countries. Dapsone may cause methemoglobinemia and allergic reactions and (at higher doses) may pose a significant risk of agranulocytosis. Proguanil and the pyrimethamine-dapsone combination are not available in the United States.

Because of the increasing spread and intensity of antimalarial drug resistance (Figs. 203-2 and 203-10), the Centers for Disease Control and Prevention (CDC; *http://www.cdc.gov/malaria/index.htm*), which recommends a daily dose of atovaquone-proguanil for all travelers, maintains an updated 24-h travel and malaria information audiotape that can be accessed by touch-tone telephone (877-FYI-TRIP). Regional and disease-specific documents may be requested from the CDC Fax Information Service (888-232-3299). Consultation for the evaluation of prophylaxis failures or treatment of malaria can be obtained from state and local health departments and the CDC Malaria Hotline (770-488-7788) or the CDC Emergency Operations Center (770-488-7100).

FURTHER READINGS

BAIRD JK et al: Prevention and treatment of vivax malaria. Curr Infect Dis Rep 9:39, 2007

CENTERS FOR DISEASE CONTROL AND PREVENTION: Treatment of malaria (guidelines for clinicians). Atlanta, Department of Health and Human Services, 2000; available online at *http://www.cdc.gov/malaria/diagnosis_treatment/tx_clinicians.htm*

DONDORP A et al: Artesunate versus quinine for treatment of severe falciparum malaria: A randomised trial. Lancet 366:717, 2005

PHU NH et al: Hemofiltration and peritoneal dialysis in infection-associated acute renal failure in Vietnam. N Engl J Med 347:895, 2002

WHITE NJ: The assessment of antimalarial drug efficacy. Trends Parasitol 18:865, 2002

1294 WORLD HEALTH ORGANIZATION: Severe falciparum malaria. Trans R Soc Trop Med Hyg 94(Suppl 1):51, 2000

———: Guidelines for the treatment of malaria. Geneva, World Health Organization, 2006

———: Assessment and monitoring of antimalarial drug efficacy for the treatment of uncomplicated falciparum malaria. WHO/HTM/RBM/2003.50; available online at *http://www.who.int/malaria/docs/ProtocolWHO.pdf*

204 Babesiosis

Jeffrey A. Gelfand, Edouard Vannier

Babesiosis is an emerging infection transmitted by ticks and caused by intraerythrocytic protozoa of the genus *Babesia*. Wild and domestic animals are natural reservoirs of *Babesia* species. Only in the past 50 years has *Babesia* been appreciated to be a pathogen in humans. Usually a mild flulike illness in young and healthy people, babesiosis may develop into a life-threatening malaria-like syndrome in asplenic, immunocompromised, or elderly patients.

ETIOLOGY AND NATURAL CYCLE

In the northeastern United States, *Babesia microti* is transmitted to humans by the hard-bodied tick *Ixodes scapularis* (*I. dammini*). In the fall, adult ticks feed primarily on white-tailed deer. Deer are incompetent reservoirs for *B. microti* but are essential for the maintenance of *I. scapularis*. Adult ticks overwinter and lay eggs in the spring. The eggs hatch into larvae in late July. In August and September, larvae become infected as they feed on *B. microti*–infected white-footed mice. In the spring of the following year, larvae molt into nymphs that remain infected with *B. microti* (transstadial transmission). Early in the summer, these nymphs feed on white-footed mice that become reservoirs of *B. microti*. Transmission of *B. microti* to humans is incidental and occurs primarily at the nymphal stage.

In Europe, *I. ricinus* is regarded as the main vector for infection of humans with *B. divergens*, a pathogen of cattle. *B. divergens* is maintained in the life cycle of the tick by transstadial and transovarial transmission. Nymphs and adults are considered the primary vectors in bovine and human babesiosis.

As ticks feed, *Babesia*-infected red blood cells (RBCs) accumulate in their gut. Gametes fuse into zygotes that translocate across the epithelium, enter the hemolymph, and become kinetes. Some kinetes reach salivary acini and undergo hypertrophy to become dormant sporoblasts. Upon attachment of the tick to the host, sporogony is initiated. In the last hours of feeding, sporozoites are deposited in the host dermis. Once in the blood, sporozoites invade erythrocytes to become trophozoites. Trophozoites undergo asynchronous schizogony, resulting in the budding of two or four merozoites. Tetrads ("Maltese crosses") are pathognomonic of *B. microti* and other small *Babesia* species (e.g., *B. duncani*) but are seen only rarely in blood smears during infection.

EPIDEMIOLOGY

United States Babesiosis due to *B. microti* is an emerging infection in the United States. Most of the >300 documented cases have occurred in coastal southern New England (from eastern Connecticut to Cape Cod, MA) and the chain of islands off the coast, particularly Nantucket Island and Martha's Vineyard (MA); Block Island (RI); and eastern Long Island, Shelter Island, and Fire Island (NY). Several cases have been reported from upstate New York, New Jersey, and Pennsylvania and from the upper Midwest (Wisconsin, Minnesota). Because babesiosis is not a notifiable disease in every state and asymptomatic infection is common, the incidence of *B. microti* infection is greatly underestimated. In New York state alone, >800 cases have been reported in the past decade. In Washington state and northern California, nine cases have been attributed to *B. duncani* (isolates WA1 and CA5), *B. duncani*–type parasites (WA2 and CA6), and other closely related babesial parasites (CA1–4). These organisms are antigenically distinct from *B. microti* and belong to the clade of piroplasms found in dogs (*B. conradae*) and wild animals in the western United States. As asymptomatic infection may persist for

months without detectable parasitemia, babesiosis may be transmitted by blood transfusion, especially in endemic areas. More than 50 transfusion-transmitted cases have been attributed to *B. microti* and two to *B. duncani* (WA1 and WA2). Neonatal babesiosis is rare and has been acquired by vertical transmission, blood transfusion, or tick bite. Lastly, *B. divergens*–like parasites have been implicated in three cases of acute babesiosis (one each in Missouri, Kentucky, and Washington state).

Other Countries Babesiosis is rare in Europe, with half of the >35 cases documented in France and the British Isles. In addition to the original case from Croatia, cases have been reported from the central Alpine region (Austria, Italy, Switzerland) and from southern Europe (Spain, Portugal). Most cases have involved asplenic patients and have been attributed to *B. divergens*. *B. microti* has been implicated in only a handful of cases, although serologic evidence of *B. microti* infection has emerged from Switzerland and midwestern Germany. A study of two patients from Austria and Italy has identified *Babesia* EU1 as a novel pathogen that belongs to the *B. divergens* clade and is closely related to *B. odocoilei*, a parasite of white-tailed deer.

Sporadic cases of human babesiosis have been described in Mexico, Colombia, the Canary Islands, Ivory Coast, Egypt, Mozambique, South Africa, and India. Cases due to *B. microti*–like piroplasms have been reported from Taiwan and Japan.

CLINICAL PRESENTATION

Infections with *B. microti* vary in severity. Asymptomatic infection or self-limiting flulike illness occurs in ~25% of adults and ~50% of children. The incubation period lasts 1–6 weeks. Onset is gradual. The most common manifestations are fever (intermittent or sustained, with temperatures sometimes reaching 40°C), fatigue, malaise, shaking chills, sweats, myalgias, and arthralgias. Less frequent symptoms include shortness of breath, headache, anorexia, and nausea. Malaise, myalgias, arthralgias, and shortness of breath may help differentiate babesiosis from other febrile illnesses. Fever is the salient feature on physical examination. Mild splenomegaly and hepatomegaly may be noted. Jaundice is rare.

Low hematocrit, low hemoglobin, and hemoglobinuria are consistent with hemolytic anemia. The parasitemia level is usually 1–10% in immunocompetent hosts but can reach 85% in asplenic patients. Reticulocyte counts are elevated, white blood cell (WBC) counts are normal or slightly low, and thrombocytopenia is common. Levels of liver enzymes (including alkaline phosphatase, lactate dehydrogenase, aspartate and alanine aminotransferases, and bilirubin) are elevated. With hemolysis, the serum haptoglobin concentration is low, and urinalysis may show hemoglobinuria and proteinuria.

Complications of babesiosis include acute respiratory failure, disseminated intravascular coagulation, congestive heart failure, and renal failure. *B. microti* infection may be fatal in 5–10% of cases in hospitalized patients. Severe anemia (hemoglobin concentration, <10 g/dL) and high-level parasitemia (>10%) are risk factors for complications. Alkaline phosphatase levels of >125 U/L, WBC counts of >5 × 10^9/L, and male gender are strong predictors of severe disease, as defined by death, hospitalization for >2 weeks, or admission to an intensive care unit for >2 days. Severe babesiosis is common among asplenic patients, patients co-infected with *Borrelia burgdorferi* (i.e., those with Lyme disease), persons >50 years of age, and individuals with comorbidities, including HIV infection, cancer, and other diseases associated with immunosuppression. Infection may recrudesce after splenectomy or immunosuppressive therapy.

Babesiosis due to *B. divergens* occurs most often in asplenic patients. After an incubation period of 1–3 weeks, disease suddenly appears. Hemoglobinuria—the presenting symptom—is followed by jaundice, persistent high fever (40°–41°C), myalgias, shaking chills, and drenching sweats. Babesiosis may evolve into a shocklike syndrome, with renal failure and pulmonary edema. The parasitemia level can reach 80%. Hemoglobin levels may plunge to 4–8 g/dL. The mortality rate remains high (42%).

Infections with *B. duncani* and related parasites range from asymptomatic to severe and are sometimes fatal.

DIAGNOSIS

A diagnosis of babesiosis should be considered for any symptomatic patient who resides or travels in endemic areas. The tick bite often goes unnoticed. Because symptoms are nonspecific, the diagnosis requires laboratory testing. Babesiosis is diagnosed by microscopic examination of Giemsa-stained thin blood smears. *Babesia* spp. appear annular, oval, or piriform. Ring forms are most common and do not contain the central brownish deposits (hemozoin) typical of *Plasmodium falciparum*. Tetrads are indicative of small babesial parasites, such as *B. microti* and *B. duncani*. An indirect immunofluorescent antibody test (IFAT) for *B. microti* is available from the Centers for Disease Control and Prevention. A serum IgG titer of ≥1:64 is diagnostic. The latter test has good predictive value for infection but must be interpreted in the clinical context; antibodies do not develop until at least 1 week into the illness, and serologic testing does not distinguish prior infection from active infection. Thus, IFAT is ideal for detection of past or persistent infection but not of fulminant acute infection. Antibodies to *B. microti* do not react with *B. divergens* or *B. duncani*. The persistence of low-grade infection is best diagnosed by polymerase chain reaction (PCR)–based amplification of the babesial 18S rRNA gene in blood samples. As primers are species-specific, this assay is a valuable adjunct in the diagnosis of babesiosis.

℞ BABESIOSIS

(See **Table 204-1**) Whether *B. microti* infection should be treated depends on the clinical context. Asymptomatic infections need not be treated, but if *Babesia* organisms continue to be seen on blood smear or by PCR for >3 months, treatment should be considered. Symptomatic infections should not be treated if blood smear and PCR are both negative for *Babesia*. If *Babesia* is detected in blood samples from symptomatic patients, treatment should be initiated.

A combination of atovaquone and azithromycin, given for 7–10 days, constitutes initial therapy for non-life-threatening (mild) babesiosis due to *B. microti*. For immunocompromised patients, higher doses of azithromycin (600–1000 mg/d) than those listed in the table are used. A combination of clindamycin and quinine is given for 7–10 days to patients with severe *B. microti* babesiosis; whenever possible, clindamycin should be given IV rather than PO. Partial or complete RBC exchange transfusion is advised in severe babesiosis, which is defined as a parasitemia level of >10%; significant hemolysis; or renal, hepatic, or pulmonary compromise. Treatment failures have been described with the recommended medical regimens. Other combination therapies may be used. A combination of azithromycin and quinine was effective in two patients with infection refractory to clindamycin plus quinine. One patient with AIDS and chronic babesiosis was treated successfully with a combination of clindamycin, doxycycline, and azithromycin after becoming allergic to quinine.

In patients with mild *B. microti* babesiosis, symptoms should improve within the first 48 h of therapy and should resolve within 3 months. In patients with severe babesiosis, hematocrit and parasitemia should be monitored each day or every other day until symptoms recede and the parasitemia level is <5%. Re-treatment may be required if the babesial parasite or amplifiable babesial DNA is detected for >3 months after initial

TABLE 204-1 ANTIBIOTIC REGIMENS FOR THE TREATMENT OF BABESIOSIS			
Organism	**Severity**	**Adults**	**Children**
B. microti	Mild[a]	Atovaquone (750 mg q12h PO) *plus* Azithromycin (500–1000 mg/d PO on day 1, 250 mg/d PO thereafter)	Atovaquone (20 mg/kg q12h PO; maximum, 750 mg/dose) *plus* Azithromycin [10 mg/kg qd PO on day 1 (maximum, 500 mg/dose), 5 mg/kg qd PO thereafter (maximum, 250 mg/dose)]
	Severe[a]	Clindamycin (300–600 mg q6h IV or 600 mg q8h PO) *plus* Quinine (650 mg q6–8h PO) *plus* Consider RBC exchange transfusion	Clindamycin (7–10 mg/kg q6–8h IV or 7–10 mg/kg q6–8h PO; maximum, 600 mg/dose) *plus* Quinine (8 mg/kg q8h PO; maximum, 650 mg/dose) *plus* Consider RBC exchange transfusion
B. divergens	Mild or severe[b]	Immediate complete RBC exchange transfusion *plus* Clindamycin (600 mg q6–8h IV) *plus* Quinine (650 mg q8h PO)	Immediate complete RBC exchange transfusion *plus* Clindamycin (7–10 mg/kg q6–8h IV; maximum, 600 mg/dose) *plus* Quinine (8 mg/kg q8h PO; maximum, 650 mg/dose)

[a]Treatment duration: 7–10 days.
[b]Treatment duration: generally 7–10 days, but may vary.
Note: RBC, red blood cell.

therapy, but routine testing is not needed for immunocompetent patients who are asymptomatic. Underlying immunodeficiency (such as malignancy or HIV infection) should be considered in patients with severe or prolonged episodes of babesiosis. There is increasing evidence that immunosuppressed patients may need treatment for considerably longer periods.

Patients with babesiosis should be evaluated for Lyme disease (Chap. 166) and human granulocytotropic anaplasmosis (Chap. 167), as all three infections may be acquired from the same tick vector. In endemic areas for these infections, relevant antimicrobial therapy should be considered when an intercurrent infection is strongly suspected.

B. divergens infection is often severe and progresses rapidly. The recommended treatment is immediate complete blood exchange transfusion and medical therapy with IV clindamycin plus oral quinine. Exchange transfusion ensures a complete and rapid removal of parasitized RBCs, RBC debris, and inflammatory mediators. Although uninfected RBCs are introduced by exchange transfusion, anemia may persist for >1 month. If so, additional transfusion is needed.

PREVENTION

Individuals who live or travel in endemic areas, especially those at increased risk for severe babesiosis, should be advised to avoid tick exposure by wearing protective clothing (long sleeves/long pants, with pants tucked into socks); applying tick repellents (such as DEET) to clothing; and limiting outdoor activities, especially between May and September, when infection risk is highest. Thorough skin examination after outdoor exposure allows removal of ticks within 24 h of attachment—i.e., before transmission can occur.

FURTHER READINGS

AGUILAR-DELFIN I et al: Resistance to acute babesiosis is associated with interleukin-12 and gamma interferon–mediated responses and requires macrophages and natural killer cells. Infect Immun 71:2002, 2003

HOLMAN PJ: Phylogenetic and biologic evidence that *Babesia divergens* is not endemic in the United States. Ann NY Acad Sci 1081:518, 2006

THOMPSON C et al: Coinfecting deer-associated zoonoses: Lyme disease, babesiosis, and ehrlichiosis. Clin Infect Dis 33:676, 2001

YOKOYAMA N et al: Erythrocyte invasion by *Babesia* parasites: Current advances in the elucidation of the molecular interactions between the protozoan ligands and host receptors in the invasion stage. Vet Parasitol 138:22, 2006

205 Leishmaniasis
Barbara L. Herwaldt

The term *leishmaniasis* encompasses multiple clinical syndromes. Most notable are visceral, cutaneous, and mucosal leishmaniasis, which result from infection of macrophages throughout the reticuloendothelial system, in the dermis, and in the naso-oropharyngeal mucosa, respectively.

Leishmaniasis, a vector-borne disease caused by obligate intracellular protozoa, is characterized by vast diversity and by specificity within that diversity. The disease is endemic in focal areas of ~90 countries in the tropics, subtropics, and southern Europe, in settings that range from deserts to rain forests and from rural to urban areas. Infection in humans is caused by ~20 *Leishmania* species (*Leishmania* and *Viannia* subgenera) (Table 205-1), which are transmitted by ~30 species of phlebotomine sandflies [*Phlebotomus* (Old World) and *Lutzomyia* (New World)]. Amid this diversity, particular parasite, vector, and host species maintain the transmission cycle in a given setting.

Both the diversity and the specificity of the disease confound attempts to generalize about any aspect of leishmaniasis, including control measures and clinical management. The multitudinous possible combinations of *Leishmania* species/strains, syndromes, and geographic areas—modified by host factors and immunoinflammatory responses—may be associated with clinically relevant differences, such as diverse manifestations of infection and diverse responses to particular therapies. It is essential that clinicians understand the dangers associated with extrapolating data from one setting to another and the importance of individualizing patient care, with expert consultation.

LIFE CYCLE AND IMMUNOREGULATION

Leishmania parasites, which target and persist in tissue macrophages, are transmitted by the bite of female phlebotomine sandflies. While probing for a blood meal, sandflies regurgitate the parasite's flagellated promastigote stage into the host's skin; sandfly salivary components with immunomodulating effects have been shown to promote experimental infection. Promastigotes bind to receptors on macrophages, are phagocytized, and transform within phagolysosomes into nonflagellated amastigotes (Fig. 205-1), which replicate and infect additional macrophages. Amastigotes ingested by sandflies transform back into infective promastigotes. Other modes of transmission include congenital and parenteral (e.g., by blood transfusion or needle sharing).

Leishmaniasis is viewed as a model system for exploring immunoregulatory responses to intracellular pathogens. Murine models of *L. major* infection exemplify the T_H1/T_H2 paradigm, in which polarized T_H1 and T_H2 responses govern resistance and susceptibility, respectively. Production of interferon γ (IFN-γ) by T_H1 and natural killer cells confers resistance; interleukin (IL) 12 induces naïve T cells to differentiate into T_H1 cells and induces T cells and natural killer cells to produce IFN-γ. In contrast, expansion of IL-4-producing T_H2 cells and IL-10 mediate susceptibility.

Although the immunoregulatory responses are more complex and less polarized in humans than in inbred mice, key principles are evident. The immunoinflammatory response is central to pathogenesis, healing is associated with activation of macrophages to kill intracellular amastigotes, and persistent infection is characteristic. Although the correlates of immunity are not fully defined and may differ between treated and untreated persons, nonsterile cure is a mixed blessing: quiescent parasites may help the host maintain a protective T cell–mediated immune response but may also serve as a source for activation of latent or clinically cured infection if the protective mechanisms fail.

EPIDEMIOLOGY, PREVENTION, AND CONTROL

 Leishmaniasis is endemic or emerging in focal areas of ~90 countries in Asia, the Middle East, southern Europe, and Africa (Old World disease) and the Americas (New World disease) (Table 205-1). Upwards of several hundred thousand cases of visceral leishmaniasis and 1–1.5 million cases of cutaneous leishmaniasis occur annually. Leishmaniasis is associated with the loss of ~2.4 million disability-adjusted life-years.

More than 90% of the world's cases of visceral leishmaniasis occur in three regions: (1) southern Asia or the Indian subcontinent, particularly in Bihar State in northeastern India and in foci in Bangladesh and Nepal; (2) eastern Africa (Sudan and neighboring countries); and (3) the Americas, particularly in periurban areas of northeastern Brazil.

TABLE 205-1 *LEISHMANIA* SPECIES THAT CAUSE DISEASE IN HUMANS

Species[a]	Clinical Syndrome[b]	Geographic Distribution[c]
Subgenus *Leishmania*		
L. donovani complex		
L. donovani sensu stricto	VL (PKDL, OWCL)	China, Indian subcontinent (southern Asia), southwestern Asia, Ethiopia,[d] Kenya, Somalia, Sudan, Uganda; possibly sporadic elsewhere in sub-Saharan Africa
L. infantum sensu stricto[e]	VL (OWCL)	China, central and southwestern Asia, Middle East, southern Europe, northern Africa, Ethiopia,[d] Sudan; sporadic elsewhere in sub-Saharan Africa
L. chagasi[e]	VL (NWCL)	Central and South America
L. mexicana complex		
L. mexicana	NWCL (DCL)	Mexico, Central and South America; sporadic in Texas and Oklahoma
L. amazonensis	NWCL (ML, DCL, VL)	Panama and South America
L. tropica	OWCL (VL)[f]	Central Asia, India, Pakistan, southwestern Asia, Middle East, Turkey, Greece, northern Africa, Ethiopia,[d] Kenya, Namibia
L. major	OWCL	Central Asia, India, Pakistan, southwestern Asia, Middle East, Turkey, northern Africa, Sahel region of north-central Africa, Ethiopia,[d] Sudan, Kenya
L. aethiopica	OWCL (DCL)	Ethiopia,[d] Kenya, Uganda
Subgenus *Viannia*		
L. (V.) braziliensis	NWCL (ML)	Central and South America
L. (V.) guyanensis	NWCL (ML)	South America
L. (V.) panamensis	NWCL (ML)	Central America, Venezuela, Colombia, Ecuador, Peru
L. (V.) peruviana	NWCL[g]	Peru (western slopes of Andes)

[a]Species other than those listed here have been reported to infect humans.

[b]DCL, diffuse cutaneous leishmaniasis; ML, mucosal leishmaniasis; NWCL, New World (American) cutaneous leishmaniasis; OWCL, Old World cutaneous leishmaniasis; PKDL, post–kala-azar dermal leishmaniasis; VL, visceral leishmaniasis. Clinical syndromes less frequently associated with the various species are shown in parentheses.

[c]The geographic distribution is highly focal within countries/regions, and the order in which areas are listed does not reflect the level of endemicity. (See text for further information.) The geographic distribution of cases evaluated in countries such as the United States reflects travel and immigration patterns.

[d]Cutaneous and visceral leishmaniasis also are endemic in parts of Eritrea, but the causative species have not been well established.

[e]"*L. infantum*" and "*L. chagasi*" are considered synonymous.

[f]*L. tropica* also causes leishmaniasis recidivans and viscerotropic leishmaniasis.

[g]The cutaneous leishmaniasis syndrome caused by this species is called *uta*.

FIGURE 205-1 Amastigotes (the tissue stage of *Leishmania* parasites) in a Giemsa-stained impression smear of tissue from a patient with cutaneous leishmaniasis. Amastigotes are oval or egg shaped and ~2–4 µm in length. Their internal organelles include a nucleus (*larger arrow*) and rod-shaped kinetoplast (*smaller arrow*). In particular, the kinetoplast, a specialized mitochondrial structure that contains extranuclear DNA, should be visualized. The extracellular amastigotes probably were released from macrophages during manipulation of the specimen. Magnification: ×1000, obtained using a ×100 oil-immersion objective. (*Photograph courtesy of H. Bishop; with permission.*)

The predominant etiologic agents are *L. donovani* in southern Asia and eastern Africa and *L. infantum/L. chagasi* elsewhere in the Old and New Worlds. These organisms can also cause cutaneous leishmaniasis.

More than 90% of the world's cases of cutaneous leishmaniasis occur in Afghanistan (Fig. 205-2), Algeria, Iran, Iraq, Pakistan, Saudi Arabia, and Syria (Old World) and in Brazil and Peru (New World). The predominant etiologic agents are *L. tropica*, *L. major*, and *L. aethiopica* (Old World) and species of the *L. mexicana* complex and the *Viannia* subgenus (New World).

In general, prevention and control measures are difficult to sustain and must be tailored to the setting. Vaccine strategies are being explored. Vector characteristics contribute to the focality of transmission in time and place and have implications for preventive measures. Sandflies are nocturnal (i.e., most active from dusk to dawn), have a limited flight range (usually remaining within a few hundred meters of their breeding site), and are small (about one-third the size of mosquitoes). Personal protective measures include minimizing nocturnal outdoor activities, wearing protective clothing, and applying insect repellent to exposed skin. In settings with domiciliary transmission, spraying dwellings with residual-action insecticides and using bed nets treated with long-lasting insecticides may be protective.

Most transmission cycles traditionally have been classified as zoonotic, except for the anthroponotic cycles of *L. donovani* (in southern Asia and potentially in eastern Africa) and *L. tropica*. However, some zoonotic cycles may be partially anthroponotic (and vice versa), and transmission patterns can evolve (e.g., from predominantly sylvatic to include domiciliary transmission) in the context of environmental and epidemiologic changes.

If transmission is exclusively or partially anthroponotic, treatment of infected persons can serve as a control measure, and suboptimal treatment can lead to dissemination of drug resistance. In southern Asia, which arguably carries ~70% of the global burden of visceral leishmaniasis, transmission of *L. donovani* is anthroponotic and largely intra- or peridomiciliary. In 2005, India, Nepal, and Bangladesh resolved to collaborate to reduce the annual incidence of visceral leishmaniasis to <1 case per 10,000 persons by the year 2015. For areas where canids are reservoir hosts (*L. infantum/L. chagasi*–endemic regions), various control strategies are being explored (e.g., insecticide-impregnated dog collars and vaccine candidates).

VISCERAL LEISHMANIASIS

The general term *visceral leishmaniasis* encompasses a broad spectrum of severity and manifestations, with a chronic, subacute, or acute onset and an incubation period of weeks, months, or sometimes years. In contrast, the term *kala-azar* typically is reserved for advanced, life-threatening disease. Although *kala-azar* means black [*kala*] fever [*azar*] in Hindi, darkening of the skin is uncommon. The classic manifestations of advanced disease include prolonged fever; cachexia (malnutrition being both a risk factor for and a sequela of visceral leishmaniasis); hepatosplenomegaly (with splenomegaly usually predominant and the spleen sometimes massive); anemia; leukopenia (neutropenia, marked eosinopenia, and relative lymphocytosis and monocytosis); thrombocytopenia, sometimes associated with bleeding; hypergammaglobulinemia (chiefly IgG, from polyclonal B cell activation); and hypoalbuminemia. The differential diagnosis includes tropical and infectious diseases that cause fever or organomegaly (e.g., typhoid fever, subacute bacterial endocarditis, miliary tuberculosis, brucellosis, histoplasmosis, tropical splenomegaly syndrome, and schistosomiasis) and myeloproliferative diseases (e.g., leukemia and lymphoma).

Post–kala-azar dermal leishmaniasis (PKDL) is a syndrome characterized by skin lesions (including macules, papules, nodules, and patches) that are typically most prominent on the face and that develop during or after therapy for visceral leishmaniasis. In Sudan, PKDL is noted in ~50% of patients from 0 to 6 months after therapy and usually heals spontaneously. In contrast, in India, PKDL is noted in ~5–10% of patients, occurring several years after treatment and usually requiring further therapy. PKDL can be confused with miliaria rubra, syphilis, yaws, and leprosy.

The diagnosis of visceral leishmaniasis should be considered for HIV-infected patients who have ever been in leishmaniasis-endemic areas and have manifestations consistent with visceral infection. The leishmanial infection may have been acquired recently (e.g., from a contaminated syringe) or may represent activation of latent infection acquired in

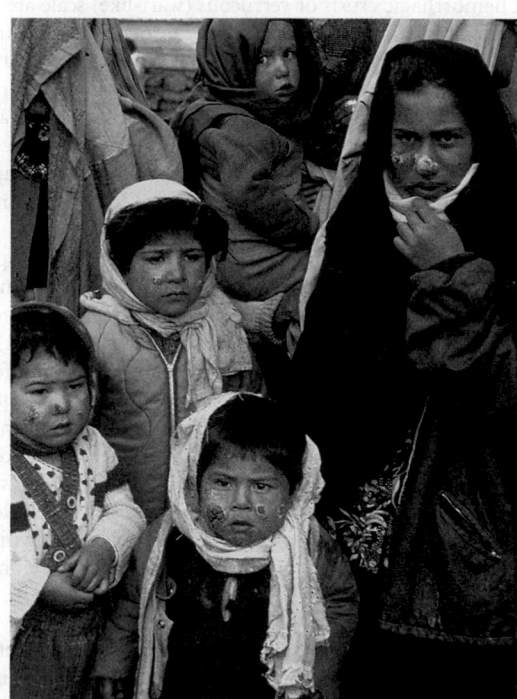

FIGURE 205-2 People in Kabul, Afghanistan, standing in line for hours on a bitterly cold day in February 1997 at a treatment center for cutaneous leishmaniasis. Kabul is experiencing a prolonged epidemic of anthroponotic cutaneous leishmaniasis caused by *Leishmania tropica*. [*Photograph courtesy of Dr. R. Ashford and reprinted with permission from Elsevier Science (Lancet 354:1193, 1999).*]

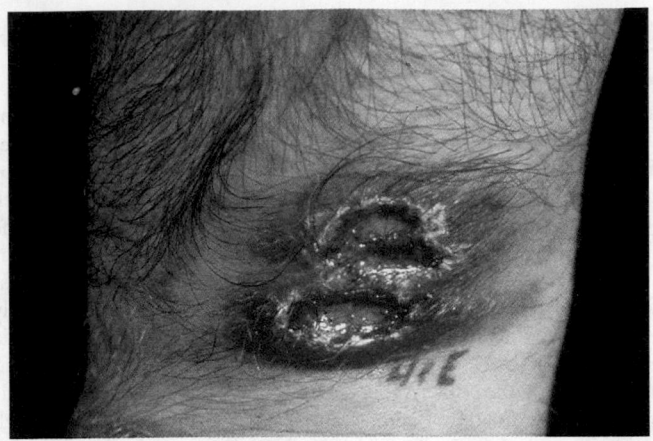

FIGURE 205-3 Ulcerative skin lesions with raised outer borders on the arm of a patient with New World (American) cutaneous leishmaniasis acquired in Costa Rica. *(Photograph courtesy of Dr. A. Wright, with permission.)*

the distant past; most co-infected patients with clinically evident visceral infection have CD4+ T lymphocyte counts of <200/μL.

Most cases of *Leishmania*-HIV co-infection have been reported from southern Europe (particularly Spain, France, Italy, and Portugal). Whereas antiretroviral therapy has decreased the incidence of clinically manifest leishmanial infection in Europe, increasing numbers of co-infected cases are being reported in resource-poor countries.

CUTANEOUS LEISHMANIASIS

Typically, the incubation period of cutaneous leishmaniasis ranges from weeks to months. Lesions progress from papules to plaques (which can be smooth or scaly and develop central ulceration; Fig. 205-3) to atrophic scars. The spectrum includes papulonodular, nodular, and noduloulcerative lesions. Multiple primary lesions, satellite lesions, regional adenopathy, nodular lymphangitis, secondary bacterial infection, and thick hemorrhagic crusts or verrucous (wart-like) scale are variably present. Both active and healed lesions can cause considerable morbidity. Spontaneous resolution does not preclude reactivation of infection, dissemination to mucous membranes (see below), or reinfection.

Cutaneous leishmaniasis can be confused with tropical, traumatic, and venous-stasis ulcers; foreign-body reactions; myiasis; infected insect bites; impetigo, ecthyma, and pyoderma gangrenosum; superficial and deep fungal, mycobacterial, and spirochetal infections; and cutaneous sarcoidosis and neoplasms.

The polyparasitic and oligoparasitic ends of the disease spectrum are represented by diffuse cutaneous leishmaniasis (DCL) and leishmaniasis recidivans, respectively. DCL, which typically is caused by *L. aethiopica* (Old World) and *L. mexicana* species (New World), develops in the context of *Leishmania*-specific anergy and is manifested by chronic, disseminated, nonulcerative lesions, with abundant parasites but few lymphocytes. DCL should be differentiated from benign disseminated cutaneous leishmaniasis, lepromatous leprosy, and PKDL. Leishmaniasis recidivans, which most characteristically is caused by *L. tropica*, is a hyperergic variant with scarce parasites. It resembles lupus vulgaris and is characterized by a chronic, solitary plaque (typically on the cheek) that heals centrally but slowly expands at the periphery.

MUCOSAL LEISHMANIASIS

Traditionally, the term *mucosal leishmaniasis* (or *espundia*) refers to a potentially disfiguring sequela of New World cutaneous leishmaniasis that results from dissemination of parasites from the skin to the naso-oropharyngeal mucosa. Mucosal leishmaniasis is caused by species in the *Viannia* subgenus [especially *L. (V.) braziliensis* and *L. (V.) panamensis* but also *L. (V.) guyanensis*] and by *L. amazonensis* (Table 205-1).

The magnitudes and the determinants (both parasite- and host-related) of the risks for mucosal dissemination and mucosal disease are poorly defined. Overall risk estimates for mucosal disease typically are ≤5%

(~1–10%). The risk appears to be higher in South America and southern Central America than in *L. Viannia*–endemic regions further north (e.g., in Guatemala and Mexico). Mucosal and cutaneous lesions can be noted concomitantly or appear decades apart. Mucosal disease typically is noted within several years after the resolution of the original cutaneous lesions, which usually were not treated or were treated suboptimally.

The initial manifestations of mucosal disease typically are persistent, unusual nasal symptoms (e.g., epistaxis and stuffiness), with erythema and edema of the nasal mucosa, which can be followed by progressive, ulcerative destruction of the naso-oropharyngeal mucosa and surrounding tissues in the context of a hyperactive immune response. The differential diagnosis includes other infectious diseases (e.g., rhinoscleroma, paracoccidioidomycosis, histoplasmosis, leprosy, syphilis, and tertiary yaws), sarcoidosis, neoplasms, and mucosal ulceration from cocaine use.

DIAGNOSIS

PRINCIPLES AND PERSPECTIVE

Leishmaniasis often is diagnosed presumptively by clinical and epidemiologic criteria. Definitive diagnosis requires demonstration of the parasite in specimens from infected sites, which typically relies on classic microbiologic methods—i.e., detection of amastigotes by light microscopic examination of stained slides or detection of promastigotes by in vitro culture. In general, amastigotes, including their characteristic internal organelles (Fig. 205-1), are more easily recognizable on Giemsa-stained smears (e.g., thin smears of dermal scrapings or bone marrow aspirates and impression smears of biopsy specimens) than in tissue sections, particularly if organisms are rare.

Leishmania species can be distinguished by isoenzyme analysis of cultured promastigotes or determination of monoclonal antibody specificity. Molecular techniques of assorted types, with diverse genetic markers, are at various stages of development and validation for diagnosis of leishmaniasis and identification of species. Analyses of the genomes and the proteome profiles of *Leishmania* species may lead to novel diagnostic approaches.

Immunologic diagnostic methods include serologic assays and tests for *Leishmania*-specific cell-mediated immunity (e.g., skin testing for delayed-type hypersensitivity reactions). The utility of such methods depends in part on the syndrome. Most serologic assays do not reliably distinguish active from quiescent infection. No leishmanin skin-test preparation has been approved for use in the United States.

VISCERAL LEISHMANIASIS

Patients with advanced visceral leishmaniasis commonly have relatively heavy parasite burdens and high-level antibody responses that are not protective but are useful diagnostically; skin-test reactivity develops after recovery. Aspirates and biopsy specimens (e.g., of spleen, bone marrow, liver, or lymph node) are useful for parasitologic confirmation by traditional and molecular methods. Although the diagnostic yield is highest for splenic aspirates (>95%), bone marrow aspiration is safer.

In the appropriate setting, seropositivity is often the diagnostic standard. Although test performance can vary by region, approaches that offer the potential for improved field applicability include direct agglutination testing with freeze-dried antigen and immunochromatographic dipstick testing of fingerstick blood for antibody to recombinant antigens or synthetic peptides (e.g., rK39). In addition, assays for detection of leishmanial antigen in urine are being evaluated.

The sensitivity of serologic methods is lower in HIV-infected patients than in persons not infected with HIV (~50% vs. >90%). In contrast, the parasites may be abundant in typical sites (e.g., bone marrow), in atypical sites (e.g., gastrointestinal tissue), and in circulating monocytes—a circumstance that facilitates parasitologic diagnosis. The sensitivities of peripheral-blood smear and buffy-coat culture are ~50% and ~70%, respectively. PCR may be even more sensitive.

CUTANEOUS AND MUCOSAL LEISHMANIASIS

Aspirates and biopsy specimens of skin lesions and lymph nodes are useful for parasitologic confirmation of cutaneous and mucosal leishmaniasis by traditional and molecular methods. Parasitologic confirmation of mucosal leishmaniasis—a pauciparasitic syndrome—by traditional methods can be difficult. Serologic testing usually is not helpful for patients with cutaneous leishmaniasis; except in patients with DCL and some patients with mucosal leishmaniasis, antibody is either undetectable or present at low levels. In contrast, skin-test reactivity usually develops during active infection except in patients with DCL.

Rx LEISHMANIASIS

PRINCIPLES AND PERSPECTIVE   **(Table 205-2)** Decisions about whether and how to treat leishmaniasis should be individualized. For cases in which systemic treatment is indicated, the parenterally administered pentavalent antimonial (Sb^V) compounds sodium stibogluconate and meglumine antimonate have been the mainstays of therapy for more than half a century. Manifestations of toxicity (e.g., body aches, malaise, elevated aminotransferase levels, chemical pancreatitis, and electrocardiographic abnormalities) are commonly noted but usually do not limit therapy and are reversible.

Conventional amphotericin B deoxycholate and pentamidine isethionate, the traditional parenteral alternatives to Sb^V, were previously relegated to second-line status, largely because of less experience with their use for the treatment of leishmaniasis and greater concern about their induction of potentially serious or irreversible toxicities (e.g., renal impairment). Amphotericin B, which has high-level, broad-spectrum antileishmanial activity, has been upgraded to first-line status in settings in which its benefits outweigh its risks (e.g., for Sb^V-resistant visceral leishmaniasis).

Lipid formulations of amphotericin B passively target the agent to macrophage-rich organs, resulting in less renal and other toxicity and permitting the use of higher daily doses and shorter courses of therapy. Targeting of drug to the reticuloendothelial system is ideal for visceral leishmaniasis but may not be advantageous for other syndromes. For amphotericin B and other antileishmanial agents, various delivery/targeting mechanisms and formulations are being explored.

Although some alternative therapies may have utility in particular settings, even data from well-conducted clinical trials cannot necessarily be generalized to other contexts. Of particular note, data from the many clinical trials of therapy for visceral leishmaniasis in foci in northeastern India are not necessarily directly applicable to visceral leishmaniasis caused by *L. donovani* in other foci in southern Asia or elsewhere (e.g., eastern Africa) or to visceral infection caused by *L. infantum/chagasi*—let alone to other leishmanial syndromes.

Except for the development of resistance to Sb^V and pentamidine, Indian kalaazar typically is easier to treat than visceral leishmaniasis elsewhere: i.e., it is more responsive to therapy, even with lower total doses. Counterintuitively, visceral leishmaniasis often is easier to treat than cutaneous or mucosal leishmaniasis. Achieving

adequate drug levels in the phagolysosomes of dermal and mucosal macrophages can be challenging, and the difficulty can be compounded by the fact that some dermotropic species are intrinsically less sensitive than *L. donovani* to particular drugs.

Some of these issues are exemplified by miltefosine, the first highly active oral agent for visceral leishmaniasis. Both experimental (in vitro) and clinical data indicate that *L. donovani* (the agent of Indian visceral leishmaniasis) is highly sensitive to miltefosine, whereas other species are variably responsive. In addition, the long half-life of the drug and suboptimal treatment predispose to the development of resistance. The most common side effects of therapy include gastrointestinal symptoms and reversible elevations in creatinine and aminotransferase levels. Miltefosine's teratogenicity in animals has implications for its use in women of child-bearing age (Table 205-2).

TABLE 205-2	PARENTERAL AND ORAL DRUG REGIMENS FOR TREATMENT OF LEISHMANIASIS^a	
Clinical Syndrome, Drug	**Route of Administration**	**Regimen**
Visceral Leishmaniasis		
Parenteral therapy		
Pentavalent antimony^b	IV, IM	20 mg Sb^V/kg qd for 28 days
Amphotericin B, lipid formulation^c	IV	2–5 mg/kg qd (total: usually ~15–21 mg/kg)
Amphotericin B (deoxycholate)	IV	0.5–1 mg/kg qod or qd (total: usually ~15–20 mg/kg)
Paromomycin sulfate^d	IV, IM	15–20 mg/kg qd for ~21 days
Pentamidine isethionate	IV, IM	4 mg/kg qod or thrice weekly for ~15–30 doses
Oral therapy		
Miltefosine^{d,e}	PO	2.5 mg/kg qd for 28 days
Cutaneous Leishmaniasis		
Parenteral therapy		
Pentavalent antimony^b	IV, IM	20 mg Sb^V/kg qd for 10–20 days (standard recommendation: 20 days)
Pentamidine isethionate	IV, IM	2 mg/kg qod for 7 doses
Amphotericin B (deoxycholate)	IV	0.5–1 mg/kg qod or qd (total: up to ~20 mg/kg)
Oral therapy		
Fluconazole	PO	200 mg qd for 6 weeks^f
Ketoconazole	PO	600 mg qd for 28 days^f
Itraconazole	PO	200 mg bid for 28 days^f
Miltefosine^{d,e}	PO	2.5 mg/kg qd for 28 days
Mucosal Leishmaniasis		
Pentavalent antimony^b	IV, IM	20 mg Sb^V/kg qd for 28 days
Amphotericin B (deoxycholate)	IV	1 mg/kg qod or qd (total: usually ~20–40 mg/kg)
Pentamidine isethionate	IV, IM	2–4 mg/kg qod or thrice weekly for ≥15 doses

^{a}See text for additional details and perspective about the drugs and regimens in this table and about treatment of leishmaniasis in general. Some of the listed drugs are effective only against certain *Leishmania* species/strains and only in certain areas of the world. Classification of drugs/regimens in such categories as first-line, alternative, (in)effective, investigational, (un)available, and cost-prohibitive is highly dependent on the setting. Ranges shown for doses and durations of therapy reflect variability both in dosage regimens among clinical trials and in responsiveness in different settings. To maximize effectiveness and minimize toxicity, the listed regimens should be individualized according to the particularities of the case and in consultation with an expert. Children may need different dosage regimens. Except for liposomal amphotericin B (see footnote c), as of this writing, none of the drugs listed is licensed by the U.S. Food and Drug Administration (FDA) for the treatment of leishmaniasis per se.
^{b}The Centers for Disease Control and Prevention (CDC) provides the pentavalent antimonial (Sb^V) compound sodium stibogluconate (Pentostam; Glaxo Operations UK Limited, Barnard Castle, United Kingdom; 100 mg Sb^V/mL) to U.S.-licensed physicians through the CDC Drug Service (404-639-3670) under an IND mechanism with the FDA. The other widely used Sb^V compound, meglumine antimonate (Glucantime; typically, ~85 mg Sb^V/mL), is available primarily in Spanish- and French-speaking areas of the world. Locally made (generic) Sb^V preparations may have different Sb^V concentrations and may vary in quality and safety.
^{c}The lipid formulations of amphotericin B include liposomal amphotericin B and amphotericin B lipid complex. In 1997, the FDA approved the following regimen of liposomal amphotericin B for immunocompetent patients with visceral leishmaniasis: 3 mg/kg qd on days 1–5, 14, and 21, for a total of 21 mg/kg. For immunosuppressed patients, the approved regimen is 4 mg/kg qd on days 1–5, 10, 17, 24, 31, and 38, for a total of 40 mg/kg. Many alternative regimens have been proposed for immunocompetent patients in various regions of the world; the regimens vary with respect to total and daily doses, number of doses, and intervals between doses. See text for perspective on the use of lipid formulations of amphotericin B for treatment of cutaneous and mucosal leishmaniasis.
^{d}Not commercially available in the United States as of this writing.
^{e}Miltefosine, which is teratogenic in animals, should not be used to treat pregnant women. Women of child-bearing age should use effective birth control during treatment and for 2 months thereafter. See text regarding the treatment of mucosal leishmaniasis.
^{f}Adult dosage.

VISCERAL LEISHMANIASIS The primary goal of treatment for visceral leishmaniasis is to prevent death. Highly effective antileishmanial therapy is essential, as is supportive care (e.g., therapy for malnutrition, anemia, bleeding, and intercurrent infections). In most regions, Sb^V therapy remains highly effective. However, use of an alternative agent should be considered if high-level Sb^V resistance is prevalent or if non-Sb^V therapy is advantageous for other reasons (e.g., duration, cost, or tolerability). In general, most patients feel better and become afebrile during the first week of therapy; resolution of splenomegaly and hematologic abnormalities may require weeks or months.

In northeastern India, districts of Bihar State north of the Ganges River constitute the epicenter of the epidemic of Sb^V resistance, which is spreading—to varying degrees—to contiguous areas of India and southern Nepal. Conventional amphotericin B has become first-line therapy where Sb^V and pentamidine are no longer effective. Lipid formulations of amphotericin B, which are cost-prohibitive where they are most needed, are increasingly being used in southern Europe.

The anthroponotic transmission of *L. donovani* in southern Asia is both a blessing and a curse: a blessing because treatment can serve as a control measure, and a curse because suboptimal treatment can and does lead to the development and dissemination of drug resistance and thereby to the elimination of drugs from the limited armamentarium and to the demise of patients who cannot afford or access the few alternatives. In this context, the oral agent miltefosine, which is registered for commercial use in India and some other countries, has great potential but also is highly vulnerable. The advent of oral therapy translates into unsupervised outpatient treatment, in which patients buy the quantity of drug they can afford and prematurely stop therapy when their supply is depleted or their symptoms are alleviated. Unless protective measures are implemented (e.g., with directly observed or multidrug therapy), drug resistance almost assuredly will develop and spread. The oral agent sitamaquine, an 8-amino-quinoline, is being field-tested in various regions but appears to have a narrow therapeutic window and can cause nephrotoxicity.

The aminoglycoside paromomycin (the chemical equivalent of aminosidine) is a candidate parenteral agent for use alone or in drug combinations. To date, the rates of response in field tests have been variable; response rates may be higher in India than in eastern Africa.

Patients who are co-infected with HIV may initially respond well to standard therapy but typically experience more toxicity. Antiretroviral therapy delays but does not prevent relapses. Consensus approaches to treatment and secondary prophylaxis have not been established.

CUTANEOUS LEISHMANIASIS Decisions about clinical management of cutaneous leishmaniasis should be based on consideration of goals (e.g., accelerating the healing of skin lesions, decreasing morbidity, decreasing risks for local and mucosal dissemination and relapse), parasite factors (e.g., tissue tropisms and drug sensitivities), and the extent to which the lesions are of concern or are bothersome because of their location (e.g., on the face or near joints), number, size, persistence, or other features (e.g., nodular lymphangitis). When optimal effectiveness is important, parenteral Sb^V therapy is generally recommended. The first sign of a clinical response typically is decreasing induration, and relapses usually are noted first at the margins of healed lesions.

Although clinical trials of conventional amphotericin B for cutaneous leishmaniasis have not been conducted and standard dosage regimens have not been established, this agent almost assuredly is highly and broadly effective, albeit potentially toxic. Conflicting, limited data are available for lipid formulations. Pentamidine was effective in Colombia [predominantly against *L. (V.) panamensis*] but not in Peru [against *L. (V.) braziliensis*].

The effectiveness of the oral agent miltefosine is species and strain dependent. For example, this drug has been effective against *L. (V.) panamensis* in Colombia but ineffective against *L. (V.) braziliensis* in Guatemala. At best, azoles have shown modest activity against particular species in isolated studies—e.g., ketoconazole and itraconazole against *L. mexicana* in Guatemala, ketoconazole against *L. (V.) panamensis* in Panama, and fluconazole against *L. major* in Saudi Arabia. Itraconazole has been ineffective against *L. (V.) panamensis* in Colombia.

Local therapy can be considered for some cases without demonstrable local dissemination or risk of mucosal dissemination (e.g., for relatively benign lesions caused by *L. mexicana* or *L. major*). Examples of approaches being used or evaluated in some settings include intralesional Sb^V, various formulations of paromomycin ointments, topical immunomodulators, thermotherapy, and cryotherapy.

MUCOSAL LEISHMANIASIS The traditional treatment options for mucosal leishmaniasis include Sb^V and conventional amphotericin B; conflicting, limited data are available for lipid formulations of the latter drug. The response rates approach those for cutaneous leishmaniasis if mucosal disease is detected and treated at early stages, whereas advanced disease may be unresponsive or relapse repeatedly. Oral miltefosine therapy shows promise, on the basis of a clinical trial in Bolivia. Adjunctive immunotherapy is being evaluated. Concomitant glucocorticoid therapy is indicated if respiratory compromise develops after initiation of therapy.

FURTHER READINGS

ALVAR J et al: Chemotherapy in the treatment and control of leishmaniasis. Adv Parasitol 61:223, 2006

COLER RN, REED SG: Second-generation vaccines against leishmaniasis. Trends Parasitol 21:244, 2005

CROFT SL et al: Drug resistance in leishmaniasis. Clin Microbiol Rev 19:111, 2006

CRUZ I et al: *Leishmania*/HIV co-infections in the second decade. Indian J Med Res 123:357, 2006

HERWALDT BL: Leishmaniasis. Lancet 354:1191, 1999

MURRAY HW et al: Advances in leishmaniasis. Lancet 366:1561, 2005

SMITH DF et al: Comparative genomics: From genotype to disease phenotype in the leishmaniases. Int J Parasitol 37:1173, 2007

206 Trypanosomiasis
Louis V. Kirchhoff

The genus *Trypanosoma* contains many species of protozoans. *Trypanosoma cruzi*, the cause of Chagas' disease in the Americas, and the two trypanosome subspecies that cause human African trypanosomiasis, *Trypanosoma brucei gambiense* and *T. brucei rhodesiense*, are the only members of the genus that cause disease in humans.

CHAGAS' DISEASE

DEFINITION

Chagas' disease, or American trypanosomiasis, is a zoonosis caused by the protozoan parasite *T. cruzi*. Acute Chagas' disease is usually a mild febrile illness that results from initial infection with the organism. After spontaneous resolution of the acute illness, most infected persons remain for life in the indeterminate phase of chronic Chagas' disease, which is characterized by subpatent parasitemia, easily detectable antibodies to *T. cruzi*, and an absence of symptoms. In a minority of chronically infected patients, cardiac and gastrointestinal lesions develop that can result in serious morbidity and even death.

LIFE CYCLE AND TRANSMISSION

T. cruzi is transmitted among its mammalian hosts by hematophagous triatomine insects, often called *reduviid bugs*. The insects become infected by sucking blood from animals or humans who have circulating parasites. Ingested organisms multiply in the gut of the triatomines, and infective forms are discharged with the feces at the time of subsequent blood meals. Transmission to a second vertebrate host occurs when breaks in the skin, mucous membranes, or conjunctivae become contaminated with bug feces that contain infective parasites. *T. cruzi* can also be transmitted by the transfusion of blood donated by infected persons, by organ transplantation, from mother to fetus, and in laboratory accidents.

PART 7 Infectious Diseases

PATHOLOGY

An indurated inflammatory lesion called a *chagoma* often appears at the parasites' portal of entry. Local histologic changes include the presence of parasites within leukocytes and cells of subcutaneous tissues and the development of interstitial edema, lymphocytic infiltration, and reactive hyperplasia of adjacent lymph nodes. After dissemination of the organisms through the lymphatics and the bloodstream, muscles (including the myocardium) may become heavily parasitized (Fig. 206-1). The characteristic pseudocysts present in sections of infected tissues are intracellular aggregates of multiplying parasites.

In the minority of persons with chronic *T. cruzi* infections who develop related clinical manifestations, the heart is the organ most commonly affected. Changes include thinning of the ventricular walls, biventricular enlargement, apical aneurysms, and mural thrombi. Widespread lymphocytic infiltration, diffuse interstitial fibrosis, and atrophy of myocardial cells are often apparent, but parasites are difficult to find in myocardial tissue. Conduction-system involvement often affects the right branch and the left anterior branch of the bundle of His. In chronic Chagas' disease of the gastrointestinal tract (megadisease), the esophagus and colon may exhibit varying degrees of dilatation. On microscopic examination, focal inflammatory lesions with lymphocytic infiltration are seen, and the number of neurons in the myenteric plexus may be markedly reduced. Accumulating experimental evidence implicates the persistence of parasites and the accompanying chronic inflammation—rather than autoimmune mechanisms—as the basis for the pathology in patients with chronic *T. cruzi* infection.

EPIDEMIOLOGY

T. cruzi is found only in the Americas. Wild and domestic mammals harboring *T. cruzi* and infected triatomines are found in spotty distributions from the southern United States to southern Argentina. Humans become involved in the cycle of transmission when infected vectors take up residence in the primitive wood, adobe, and stone houses common in much of Latin America. Thus human *T. cruzi* infection is a health problem primarily among the poor in rural areas of Mexico and Central and South America. Most new *T. cruzi* infections in rural settings occur in children, but the incidence is unknown because most cases go undiagnosed. Historically, transfusion-associated transmission of *T. cruzi* has been a serious public health problem in many endemic countries. However, with some notable exceptions, transmission by this route has been markedly reduced as effective programs for the screening of donated blood have been implemented. Several dozen patients with HIV and chronic *T. cruzi* infections who underwent acute recrudescence of the latter have been described. These patients generally presented with *T. cruzi* brain abscesses, a manifestation of the illness that does not occur in immunocompetent persons. Currently, it is estimated that 12 million people are chronically infected with *T. cruzi* and that 25,000 deaths due to the illness occur each year. Of chronically infected persons, 10–30% eventually develop symptomatic cardiac lesions or gastrointestinal disease. The resulting morbidity and mortality make Chagas' disease the most important parasitic disease burden in Latin America.

In recent years, the rate of *T. cruzi* transmission has decreased markedly in several endemic countries as a result of successful programs involving vector control, blood-bank screening, and education of at-risk populations. A major program begun in 1991 in the "southern cone" nations of South America (Uruguay, Paraguay, Bolivia, Brazil, Chile, and Argentina) has provided the framework for much of this progress. Uruguay and Chile were certified transmission-free in the late 1990s, and Brazil was declared free of transmission in 2006. Transmission has been reduced markedly in Argentina as well. Similar control programs have been initiated in the countries of northern South America and in the Central American nations.

Acute Chagas' disease is rare in the United States. Five cases of autochthonous transmission and five instances of transmission by blood transfusion have been reported. Moreover, *T. cruzi* was transmitted to five recipients of organs from three *T. cruzi*–infected donors. Two of these recipients became infected through cardiac transplants. Acute Chagas' disease has not been reported in tourists returning to the United States from Latin America, although two such instances have been reported in Europe. In contrast, the prevalence of chronic *T. cruzi* infections in the United States has increased considerably in recent years. Data from the 2000 census indicate that >12 million immigrants from Chagas'-endemic countries currently live in the United States, ~8 million of whom are Mexicans. The prevalence of *T. cruzi* infection in Mexico is 0.5–1.0%, and most of the 4 million immigrants from Chagas'-endemic nations who are not Mexicans come from countries in which the prevalence of *T. cruzi* infection is greater than it is in Mexico. The total number of *T. cruzi*–infected persons living in the United States can be estimated reasonably to be 80,000–120,000. The number of instances of transfusion-associated transmission in this country is likely to be considerably greater than the number reported. Screening of the U.S. blood supply for evidence of *T. cruzi* infection has recently begun (see "Diagnosis," below).

CLINICAL COURSE

The first signs of acute Chagas' disease develop at least 1 week after invasion by the parasites. When the organisms enter through a break in the skin, an indurated area of erythema and swelling (the chagoma), accompanied by local lymphadenopathy, may appear. *Romaña's sign*—the classic finding in acute Chagas' disease, which consists of unilateral painless edema of the palpebrae and periocular tissues—can result when the conjunctiva is the portal of entry (Fig. 206-2). These initial local signs may be followed by malaise, fever, anorexia, and edema of the face and lower extremities. A morbilliform rash may also appear. Generalized lymphadenopathy and hepatosplenomegaly may develop. Severe myocarditis develops rarely; most deaths in acute Chagas' disease are due to heart failure. Neurologic signs are not common, but meningoencephalitis occurs occasionally. The acute symptoms resolve spontaneously in virtually all patients, who then enter the asymptomatic or indeterminate phase of chronic *T. cruzi* infection.

Symptomatic chronic Chagas' disease becomes apparent years or even decades after the initial infection. The heart is commonly involved, and symptoms are caused by rhythm disturbances, dilated cardiomyopathy, and thromboembolism. Right bundle-branch block is a common electrocardiographic abnormality, but other types of atrioventricular block, premature ventricular contractions, and tachy- and bradyarrhythmias occur frequently. Cardiomyopathy often results in right-sided or biventricular heart failure. Embolization of mural thrombi to the brain or other areas may take place. Patients with megaesophagus suffer from dysphagia, odynophagia, chest pain, and regurgitation. Aspiration can occur (especially during sleep) in patients with severe esophageal dysfunction, and repeated episodes of aspiration pneumonitis are common. Weight loss, cachexia, and pulmonary infection can result in death. Patients with megacolon are

FIGURE 206-1 *Trypanosoma cruzi* in the heart muscle of a child who died of acute Chagas' myocarditis. An infected myocyte containing several dozen *T. cruzi* amastigotes is in the center of the field (hematoxylin and eosin, ×900).

FIGURE 206-2 Romaña's sign in an Argentinean patient with acute *T. cruzi* infection. *(Courtesy of Dr. Humberto Lugones, Centro de Chagas, Santiago del Estero, Argentina; with permission.)*

plagued by abdominal pain and chronic constipation, and advanced megacolon can cause obstruction, volvulus, septicemia, and death.

DIAGNOSIS

The diagnosis of acute Chagas' disease requires the detection of parasites. Microscopic examination of fresh anticoagulated blood or of the buffy coat is the simplest way to see the motile organisms. Parasites also can be seen in Giemsa-stained thin and thick blood smears. Microhematocrit tubes containing acridine orange as a stain can be used for the same purpose. When repeated attempts to visualize the organisms are unsuccessful, polymerase chain reaction (PCR) or hemoculture in special media can be performed. When used by experienced personnel, all of these methods yield positive results in a high proportion of cases of acute Chagas' disease. Hemoculture has the disadvantage of taking several weeks to give positive results. Serologic testing plays no role in diagnosing acute Chagas' disease.

Chronic Chagas' disease is diagnosed by the detection of specific antibodies that bind to *T. cruzi* antigens. Demonstration of the parasite is not of primary importance. In Latin America, ~20 assays are commercially available, including several based on recombinant antigens. Unfortunately, these tests have varying levels of sensitivity and specificity, and false-positive reactions are a particular problem—typically with samples from patients who have other infectious and parasitic diseases or autoimmune disorders. In addition, confirmatory testing has presented a persistent challenge. For these reasons, it is generally recommended that specimens be tested in at least two assays and that well-characterized positive and negative comparison samples be included in each run. The radioimmune precipitation assay (Chagas' RIPA) is a highly sensitive and specific confirmatory method for detecting antibodies to *T. cruzi* [approved under the Clinical Laboratory Improvement Amendment (CLIA) and available in the author's laboratory]. In December 2006, the U.S. Food and Drug Administration (FDA) approved a test to screen blood and organ donors for *T. cruzi* infection (Ortho *T. cruzi* ELISA Test System, Ortho-Clinical Diagnostics, Raritan, NJ). In late January 2007, the American Red Cross and Blood Systems, Inc.—blood-collection agencies that together account for ~65% of the U.S. blood supply—initiated screening of all the donations they process for *T. cruzi*. The Chagas' RIPA is being used as the confirmatory assay. Data generated during the first 2 months of screening suggest that if 65% of the blood supply continues to be tested, ~1500 Ortho-reactive donors will be identified annually, ~350 of

whom will be RIPA-positive; these figures reflect an overall prevalence of ~1 in 30,000 donors. The use of PCR assays to detect *T. cruzi* DNA in chronically infected persons has been studied extensively. The sensitivity of this approach has not been shown to be reliably greater than that of serology, and no PCR assays are commercially available.

℞ CHAGAS' DISEASE

Therapy for Chagas' disease is unsatisfactory. For many years, only two drugs—nifurtimox and benznidazole—have been available for this purpose. Unfortunately, both drugs lack efficacy and often cause severe side effects.

In acute Chagas' disease, nifurtimox markedly reduces the duration of symptoms and parasitemia and decreases the mortality rate. Nevertheless, limited studies have shown that only ~70% of acute infections are cured parasitologically by a full course of treatment. Despite its limitations, treatment with nifurtimox should be initiated as early as possible in acute Chagas' disease. Common adverse effects of nifurtimox include abdominal pain, anorexia, nausea, vomiting, and weight loss. Neurologic reactions to the drug may include restlessness, disorientation, insomnia, twitching, paresthesia, polyneuritis, and seizures. These symptoms usually disappear when the dosage is reduced or treatment is discontinued. The recommended daily dosage is 8–10 mg/kg for adults, 12.5–15 mg/kg for adolescents, and 15–20 mg/kg for children 1–10 years of age. The drug should be given orally in four divided doses each day, and therapy should be continued for 90–120 days. Nifurtimox is available from the Drug Service of the Centers for Disease Control and Prevention (CDC) in Atlanta (telephone number, 770-639-3670).

The efficacy of benznidazole is similar to that of nifurtimox; a cure rate of 90% among congenitally infected infants treated before their first birthday has been reported. Adverse effects include peripheral neuropathy, rash, and granulocytopenia. The recommended oral dosage is 5 mg/kg per day for 60 days. Benznidazole is generally considered the drug of choice in Latin America.

The question of whether patients in the indeterminate or chronic symptomatic phase of Chagas' disease should be treated with nifurtimox or benznidazole has been debated for years. The fact that parasitologic cure rates in chronically infected persons may be <10% is central to this controversy. There is no convincing evidence from properly controlled trials that treatment of adults with long-standing *T. cruzi* infections with either of the drugs is beneficial. The current consensus of Latin American authorities is that all *T. cruzi*–infected persons up to 18 years old should be given benznidazole or nifurtimox.

The usefulness of allopurinol, fluconazole, and itraconazole for the treatment of acute Chagas' disease has been studied in laboratory animals and to a lesser extent in humans. None of these drugs has exhibited a level of anti–*T. cruzi* activity that warrants its use in patients. Several newer antifungal azoles have shown promise in animal studies but have not yet been tested in humans.

Patients who develop cardiac and/or gastrointestinal disease in association with *T. cruzi* infection should be referred to appropriate subspecialists for further evaluation and treatment. Cardiac transplantation is an option for patients with end-stage chagasic cardiopathies, and >100 such transplantations have been done in Brazil and the United States. The survival rate among Chagas' disease cardiac transplant recipients is higher than that among persons receiving cardiac transplants for other reasons. This better outcome may be due to the fact that lesions are limited to the heart in most patients with symptomatic chronic Chagas' disease.

PREVENTION

Since drug therapy is unsatisfactory and vaccines are not available, the control of *T. cruzi* transmission in endemic countries must depend on reduction of domiciliary vector populations by spraying of insecticides, improvements in housing, and education of at-risk persons. As noted above, these measures, coupled with serologic screening of blood donors, have markedly reduced transmission of the parasite in many endemic countries. Tourists would be wise to avoid sleeping in dilapidated houses in rural areas of endemic countries. Mosquito nets and insect repellent provide additional protection.

In view of the possibly serious consequences of chronic *T. cruzi* infection, it would be prudent for all immigrants from endemic regions living in the United States to be tested for evidence of infection. Identification of persons harboring the parasite would permit periodic electrocardiographic monitoring, which can be important because pacemakers benefit some patients who develop ominous rhythm disturbances. The possibility of congenital transmission is yet another justification for screening. Guidance for the evaluation and long-term monitoring of *T. cruzi*–infected persons is being developed by staff at the CDC.

Laboratory personnel should wear gloves and eye protection when working with *T. cruzi* and infected vectors.

SLEEPING SICKNESS

DEFINITION

Sleeping sickness, or human African trypanosomiasis (HAT), is caused by flagellated protozoan parasites that belong to the *T. brucei* complex and are transmitted to humans by tsetse flies. In untreated patients, the trypanosomes first cause a febrile illness that is followed months or years later by progressive neurologic impairment and death.

THE PARASITES AND THEIR TRANSMISSION

The East African (*rhodesiense*) and the West African (*gambiense*) forms of sleeping sickness are caused, respectively, by two trypanosome subspecies: *T. brucei rhodesiense* and *T. brucei gambiense*. These subspecies are morphologically indistinguishable but cause illnesses that are epidemiologically and clinically distinct (Table 206-1). The parasites are transmitted by blood-sucking tsetse flies of the genus *Glossina*. The insects acquire the infection when they ingest blood from infected mammalian hosts. After many cycles of multiplication in the midgut of the vector, the parasites migrate to the salivary glands. Their transmission takes place when they are inoculated into a mammalian host during a subsequent blood meal. The injected trypanosomes multiply in the blood (Fig. 206-3) and other extracellular spaces and evade immune destruction for long periods by undergoing antigenic variation, a process driven by gene switching in which the antigenic structure of the organisms' surface coat of glycoproteins changes periodically.

PATHOGENESIS AND PATHOLOGY

A self-limited inflammatory lesion (trypanosomal chancre) may appear a week or so after the bite of an infected tsetse fly. A systemic febrile illness then evolves as the parasites are disseminated through the lymphatics and bloodstream. Systemic HAT without central nervous system (CNS) involvement is generally referred to as *stage I disease*. In this stage, widespread lymphadenopathy and splenomegaly reflect marked lymphocytic and histiocytic proliferation and invasion of morular cells, which are plasmacytes that may be involved in the pro-

FIGURE 206-3 *Trypanosoma brucei rhodesiense* forms in rat blood. The slender parasite is thought to be the form that multiplies in mammalian hosts, while the stumpy forms are nondividing and are capable of infecting insect vectors (Giemsa, ×1200). *(Courtesy of Dr. G. A. Cook, Madison, WI; with permission.)*

duction of IgM. Endarteritis, with perivascular infiltration of both parasites and lymphocytes, may develop in lymph nodes and the spleen. Myocarditis develops frequently in patients with stage I disease and is especially common in *T. b. rhodesiense* infections.

Hematologic manifestations that accompany stage I HAT include moderate leukocytosis, thrombocytopenia, and anemia. High levels of immunoglobulins, consisting primarily of polyclonal IgM, are a constant feature, and heterophile antibodies, antibodies to DNA, and rheumatoid factor are often detected. High levels of antigen-antibody complexes may play a role in the tissue damage and increased vascular permeability that facilitate dissemination of the parasites.

Stage II disease involves invasion of the CNS. The presence of trypanosomes in perivascular areas is accompanied by intense infiltration of mononuclear cells. Abnormalities in cerebrospinal fluid (CSF) include increased pressure, elevated total protein concentration, and pleocytosis. In addition, trypanosomes are frequently found in CSF.

EPIDEMIOLOGY

The trypanosomes that cause sleeping sickness are found only in Africa. Approximately 50 million persons are at risk of acquiring HAT, and tens of thousands of new cases occur every year. Precise data are not available because health statistics are often incomplete in the developing countries where HAT is endemic. Sleeping sickness has undergone a resurgence in recent years, with major epidemics in the Sudan, Ivory Coast, Chad, the Central African Republic, and several other endemic countries.

Humans are the only reservoir of *T. b. gambiense*, which occurs in widely distributed foci in tropical rain forests of Central and West Africa. *Gambiense* trypanosomiasis is primarily a problem in rural populations; tourists rarely become infected. Trypanotolerant antelope species in savanna and woodland areas of Central and East Africa are the principal reservoir of *T. b. rhodesiense*. Cattle can also be infected with this and other trypanosome species but generally succumb to the infection. Since risk results for the most part from contact with tsetse flies that feed on wild animals, humans acquire *T. b. rhodesiense* infection only incidentally, usually while visiting or working in areas where infected game and vectors are present. Roughly one or two patients with HAT acquired in East African game parks (and typically caused by *T. b. rhodesiense*) are reported to the CDC each year.

CLINICAL COURSE

A painful trypanosomal chancre appears in some patients at the site of inoculation of the parasite. Hematogenous and lymphatic dissemination (stage I disease) is marked by the onset of fever. Typically, bouts of

TABLE 206-1	COMPARISON OF WEST AFRICAN AND EAST AFRICAN TRYPANOSOMIASES	
Point of Comparison	**West African (*Gambiense*)**	**East African (*Rhodesiense*)**
Organism	*T. b. gambiense*	*T. b. rhodesiense*
Vectors	Tsetse flies (palpalis group)	Tsetse flies (morsitans group)
Primary reservoir	Humans	Antelope and cattle
Human illness	Chronic (late CNS disease)	Acute (early CNS disease)
Duration of illness	Months to years	<9 months
Lymphadenopathy	Prominent	Minimal
Parasitemia	Low	High
Diagnosis by rodent inoculation	No	Yes
Epidemiology	Rural populations	Workers in wild areas, rural populations, tourists in game parks

Abbreviation: CNS, central nervous system.
Source: Reprinted with permission from LV Kirchhoff in GL Mandell et al (eds): *Principles and Practice of Infectious Diseases*, 6th ed. Philadelphia, Elsevier Churchill Livingstone, 2005.

high temperatures lasting several days are separated by afebrile periods. Lymphadenopathy is prominent in *T. b. gambiense* trypanosomiasis. The nodes are discrete, movable, rubbery, and nontender. Cervical nodes are often visible, and enlargement of the nodes of the posterior cervical triangle, or *Winterbottom's sign*, is a classic finding. Pruritus and maculopapular rashes are common. Inconstant findings include malaise, headache, arthralgias, weight loss, edema, hepatosplenomegaly, and tachycardia. The differential diagnosis of stage I HAT includes many diseases that are common in the tropics and are associated with fevers. HIV infection, malaria, and typhoid fever are common in populations at risk for HAT and need to be considered.

CNS invasion (stage II disease) is characterized by the insidious development of protean neurologic manifestations that are accompanied by progressive abnormalities in the CSF. A picture of progressive indifference and daytime somnolence develops (hence the designation "sleeping sickness"), sometimes alternating with restlessness and insomnia at night. A listless gaze accompanies a loss of spontaneity, and speech may become halting and indistinct. Extrapyramidal signs may include choreiform movements, tremors, and fasciculations. Ataxia is frequent, and the patient may appear to have Parkinson's disease, with a shuffling gait, hypertonia, and tremors. In the final phase, progressive neurologic impairment ends in coma and death.

The most striking difference between the West African and East African trypanosomiases is that the latter illness tends to follow a more acute course. Typically, in tourists with *T. b. rhodesiense* disease, systemic signs of infection, such as fever, malaise, and headache, appear before the end of the trip or shortly after the return home. Persistent tachycardia unrelated to fever is common early in the course of *T. b. rhodesiense* trypanosomiasis, and death may result from arrhythmias and congestive heart failure before CNS disease develops. In general, untreated *T. b. rhodesiense* trypanosomiasis leads to death in a matter of weeks to months, often without a clear distinction between the hemolymphatic and CNS stages. In contrast, *T. b. gambiense* disease can smolder for many months or even for years.

DIAGNOSIS

A definitive diagnosis of HAT requires detection of the parasite. If a chancre is present, fluid should be expressed and examined directly by light microscopy for the highly motile trypanosomes. The fluid also should be fixed and stained with Giemsa. Material obtained by needle aspiration of lymph nodes early in the illness should be examined similarly. Examination of wet preparations and Giemsa-stained thin and thick films of serial blood samples is also useful. If parasites are not seen initially in blood, efforts should be made to concentrate the organisms; the simplest method involves the use of microhematocrit tubes containing acridine orange. In these tubes the parasites are separated from blood cells by centrifugation and are easily seen under light microscopy because of the stain. Alternatively, the buffy coat from 10–15 mL of anticoagulated blood can be examined directly under a microscope. The likelihood of finding parasites in blood is higher in stage I than in stage II disease and in patients infected with *T. b. rhodesiense* rather than *T. b. gambiense*. Trypanosomes may also be seen in material aspirated from the bone marrow; the aspirate can be inoculated into liquid culture medium, as can blood, buffy coat, lymph node aspirates, and CSF. Finally, *T. b. rhodesiense* infection can be detected by inoculation of these specimens into mice or rats, which—when positive—results in patent parasitemias in a week or two. Although this method is highly sensitive for the detection of *T. b. rhodesiense*, it does not detect *T. b. gambiense* because of host specificity.

It is essential to examine CSF from all patients in whom HAT is suspected. Abnormalities in the CSF that may be associated with stage II disease include an increase in the CSF mononuclear cell count as well as increases in opening pressure and in levels of total protein and IgM. Trypanosomes may be seen in the sediment of centrifuged CSF. Any CSF abnormality in a patient in whom trypanosomes have been found at other sites must be viewed as pathognomonic for CNS involvement and thus must prompt specific treatment for CNS disease. In patients with CSF pleocytosis in whom parasites are not found, tuberculous

TABLE 206-2	TREATMENT OF HUMAN AFRICAN TRYPANOSOMIASES[a]	
	Clinical Stage	
Causative Organism	**I (Normal CSF)**	**II (Abnormal CSF)**
T. brucei gambiense (West African)	Pentamidine Alternative: Suramin	Eflornithine Alternative: Melarsoprol
T. brucei rhodesiense (East African)	Suramin	Melarsoprol

[a]For doses and duration, see text.
Note: CSF, cerebrospinal fluid.

meningitis and HIV-associated CNS infections such as cryptococcosis should be considered in the differential diagnosis.

A number of serologic assays are available to aid in the diagnosis of HAT, but their variable sensitivity and specificity mandate that decisions about treatment be based on demonstration of the parasite. These tests are of value for epidemiologic surveys. PCR assays for detecting African trypanosomes in humans have been developed, but none is commercially available.

℞ SLEEPING SICKNESS

The drugs used for treatment of HAT are suramin, pentamidine, eflornithine, and the organic arsenical melarsoprol. In the United States these drugs can be obtained from the CDC. Therapy for HAT must be individualized on the basis of the infecting subspecies, the presence or absence of CNS disease, adverse reactions, and occasionally drug resistance. The choices of drugs for the treatment of HAT are summarized in **Table 206-2**.

Suramin is highly effective against stage I East African disease. However, it can cause serious adverse effects and must be administered under the close supervision of a physician. A 100- to 200-mg IV test dose should be given to detect hypersensitivity. The dosage for adults is 20 mg/kg on days 1, 5, 12, 18, and 26. The drug is given by slow IV infusion of a freshly prepared 10% aqueous solution. Approximately 1 patient in 20,000 has an immediate, severe, and potentially fatal reaction to the drug, developing nausea, vomiting, shock, and seizures. Less severe reactions include fever, photophobia, pruritus, arthralgias, and skin eruptions. Renal damage is the most common important adverse effect of suramin. Transient proteinuria often appears during treatment. A urinalysis should be done before each dose, and treatment should be discontinued if proteinuria increases or if casts and red cells appear in the sediment. Suramin should not be given to patients with renal insufficiency.

Eflornithine is highly effective for treatment of both stages of West African trypanosomiasis. In the trials on which the FDA based its approval, this agent cured >90% of 600 patients with stage II disease. The recommended treatment schedule is 400 mg/kg per day, given intravenously in four divided doses, for 2 weeks. Adverse reactions include diarrhea, anemia, thrombocytopenia, seizures, and hearing loss. The high dosage and duration of therapy required are disadvantages that make widespread use of eflornithine difficult.

Pentamidine is the first-line drug for patients with stage I West African HAT. The dose for both adults and children is 4 mg/kg per day, given intramuscularly or intravenously, for 10 days. Frequent, immediate adverse reactions include nausea, vomiting, tachycardia, and hypotension. These reactions are usually transient and do not warrant cessation of therapy. Other adverse reactions include nephrotoxicity, abnormal liver function tests, neutropenia, rashes, hypoglycemia, and sterile abscesses.

The arsenical melarsoprol is the drug of choice for the treatment of East African trypanosomiasis with CNS involvement and is an alternative agent for stage II West African disease. Melarsoprol cures both stages of the disease and therefore is also indicated for the treatment of stage I disease in patients who fail to respond to or cannot tolerate suramin or pentamidine. However, because of its relatively high toxicity, melarsoprol is never the first choice for the treatment of stage I disease. For East African disease, the drug should be given to adults in three courses of 3 days each. The dosage is 2–3.6 mg/kg per day, given intravenously in three divided doses for 3 days, followed 1 week later by 3.6 mg/kg per day, also in three divided doses and for 3 days. The latter course is repeated 7 days later. In debilitated patients, suramin is administered for 2–4 days before therapy with melarsoprol is initiated; an 18-mg initial dose of the latter drug, followed by progressive increases to the standard dose, has been recommended. For children, a total of 18–25 mg/kg should be given over 1 month. An IV starting dose of 0.36 mg/kg should be increased gradually to a maximum of 3.6 mg/kg at 1- to 5-day intervals, for a total of 9 or 10 doses. The regimen for West African disease is 2.2 mg/kg per day, given intravenously for 10 days.

Melarsoprol is highly toxic and should be administered with great care. To reduce the likelihood of drug-induced encephalopathy, all patients receiving melarsoprol should be given prednisolone at a dose of 1 mg/kg (up to 40 mg) per day, beginning 1–2 days before the first dose of melarsoprol and continuing through the last dose. Without prednisolone prophylaxis, the incidence of reactive encephalopathy has been reported to be as high as 18% in some series. Clinical manifestations of reactive encephalopathy include high fever, headache, tremor, impaired speech, seizures, and even coma and death. Treatment with melarsoprol should be discontinued at the first sign of encephalopathy but may be restarted cautiously at lower doses a few days after signs have resolved. Extravasation of the drug results in intense local reactions. Vomiting, abdominal pain, nephrotoxicity, and myocardial damage can occur.

PREVENTION

HAT poses complex public-health and epizootic problems in Africa. Considerable progress has been made in some areas through control programs that focus on eradication of vectors and drug treatment of infected humans; however, there is no consensus on the best approach to solving the overall problem, and major epidemics continue to occur. Individuals can reduce their risk of acquiring trypanosomiasis by avoiding areas known to harbor infected insects, by wearing protective clothing, and by using insect repellent. Chemoprophylaxis is not recommended, and no vaccine is available to prevent transmission of the parasites.

FURTHER READINGS

CHANG CD et al: Evaluation of a prototype *Trypanosoma cruzi* antibody assay with recombinant antigens on a fully automated chemiluminescence analyzer for blood donor screening. Transfusion 46:1737, 2006

FIORELLI AI et al: Later evolution after cardiac transplantation in Chagas' disease. Transplant Proc 37:2793, 2005

KIRCHHOFF LV et al: Transfusion-associated Chagas' disease (American trypanosomiasis) in Mexico: Implications for transfusion medicine in the United States. Transfusion 46:298, 2006

LAMBERT N et al: Chagasic encephalitis as the initial manifestation of AIDS. Ann Intern Med 144:941, 2006

MASCOLA L et al: Chagas disease after organ transplantation—Los Angeles, California, 2006. MMWR 55:798, 2006

RASSI A JR et al: Development and validation of a risk score for predicting death in Chagas' heart disease. N Engl J Med 355:799, 2006

SARTORI AM et al: Exacerbation of HIV viral load simultaneously with asymptomatic reactivation of chronic Chagas' disease. Am J Trop Med Hyg 67:521, 2002

SCHMUNIS GA, CRUZ JR: Safety of the blood supply in Latin America. Clin Microbiol Rev 18:12, 2005

WELBURN SC et al: Crisis, what crisis? Control of Rhodesian sleeping sickness. Trends Parasitol 22:123, 2006

207 *Toxoplasma* Infections
Lloyd H. Kasper

DEFINITION

Toxoplasmosis is caused by infection with the obligate intracellular parasite *Toxoplasma gondii*. Acute infection acquired after birth may be asymptomatic but frequently results in the chronic persistence of cysts in the host's tissues. In both acute and chronic toxoplasmosis, the parasite is responsible for clinically evident disease, including lymphadenopathy, encephalitis, myocarditis, and pneumonitis. Congenital toxoplasmosis is an infection of newborns that results from the transplacental passage of parasites from an infected mother to the fetus. These infants usually are asymptomatic at birth but later manifest a wide range of signs and symptoms, including chorioretinitis, strabismus, epilepsy, and psychomotor retardation.

ETIOLOGY

T. gondii is an intracellular coccidian that infects both birds and mammals. There are two distinct stages in the life cycle of *T. gondii* (Fig. 207-1). In the *nonfeline* stage, tissue cysts that contain bradyzoites or sporulated oocysts are ingested by an intermediate host (e.g., a human, mouse, sheep, pig, or bird). The cyst is rapidly digested by the acidic-pH gastric secretions. Bradyzoites or sporozoites are released, enter the small-intestinal epithelium, and transform into rapidly dividing tachyzoites. The tachyzoites can infect and replicate in all mammalian cells except red blood cells. Once attached to the host cell, the parasite penetrates the cell and forms a parasitophorous vacuole within which it divides. Parasite replication continues until the number of parasites within the cell approaches a critical mass and the cell ruptures, releasing parasites that infect adjoining cells.

As a result of this process, an infected organ soon shows evidence of cytopathology. Most tachyzoites are eliminated by the host's humoral and cell-mediated immune responses. Tissue cysts containing many bradyzoites develop 7–10 days after systemic tachyzoite infection. These tissue cysts occur in various host organs but persist principally within the central nervous system (CNS) and muscle. The development of this chronic stage completes the nonfeline portion of the life cycle. Active infection in the immunocompromised host is most likely to be due to the spontaneous release of encysted parasites that undergo rapid transformation into tachyzoites within the CNS.

The principal (*feline*) stage in the life cycle takes place in the cat (the definitive host) and its prey. The parasite's sexual phase is defined by the formation of oocysts within the feline host. This enteroepithelial cycle begins with the ingestion of the bradyzoite tissue cysts and culminates (after several intermediate stages) in the production of gametes. Gamete fusion produces a zygote, which envelops itself in a rigid wall and is secreted in the feces as an unsporulated oocyst. After 2–3 days of exposure to air at ambient temperature, the noninfectious oocyst sporulates to produce eight sporozoite progeny. The sporulated oocyst can be ingested by an intermediate host, such as a person emptying a cat's litter box or a pig rummaging in a barnyard. It is in the intermediate host that *T. gondii* completes its life cycle.

EPIDEMIOLOGY

T. gondii infects a wide range of mammals and birds. Its seroprevalence depends on the locale and the age of the population. Generally, hot arid climatic conditions are associated with a low prevalence of infection. In the United States and most European countries, the seroprevalence increases with age and exposure. For example, in the United States, 5–30% of individuals 10–19 years old and 10–67% of those >50 years old have serologic evidence of exposure; seroprevalence increases by ~1% per year. In Central America, France, Turkey, and Brazil, the seroprevalence is higher. There may be as many as 2100 cases of toxoplasmic encephalitis (TE) each year in the United States.

TRANSMISSION

Oral Transmission The principal source of human *Toxoplasma* infection remains uncertain. Transmission usually takes place by the oral route and can be attributable to ingestion of either sporulated oocysts from contaminated soil or bradyzoites from undercooked meat. During

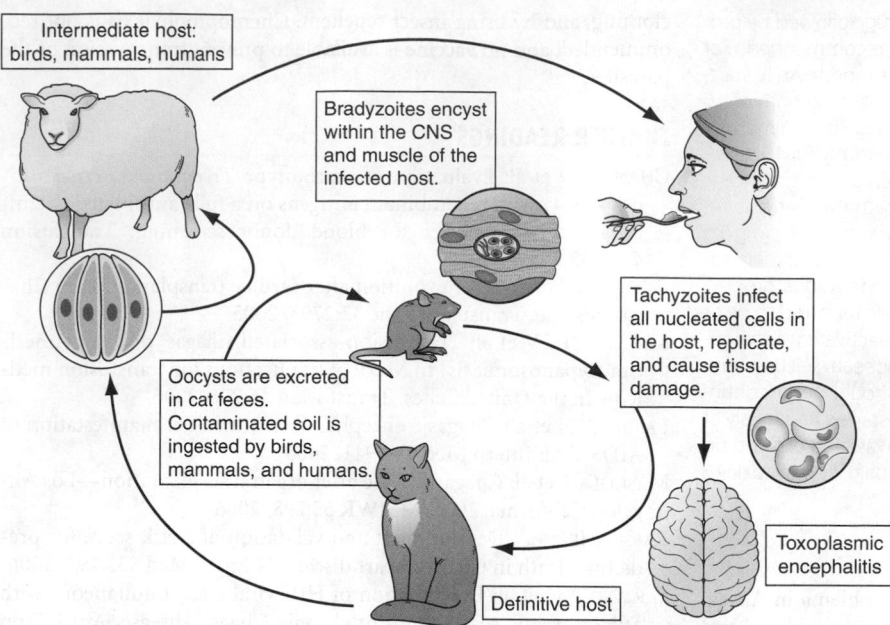

Intermediate host:
birds, mammals, humans

Bradyzoites encyst
within the CNS
and muscle of the
infected host.

Tachyzoites infect
all nucleated cells in
the host, replicate,
and cause tissue
damage.

Oocysts are excreted
in cat feces.
Contaminated soil is
ingested by birds,
mammals, and humans.

Toxoplasmic
encephalitis

Definitive host

FIGURE 207-1 Life cycle of *Toxoplasma gondii*. The cat is the definitive host in which the sexual phase of the cycle is completed. Oocysts shed in cat feces can infect a wide range of animals, including birds, rodents, grazing domestic animals, and humans. The bradyzoites found in the muscle of food animals may infect humans who eat insufficiently cooked meat products, particularly lamb and pork. Although human disease can take many forms, congenital infection and encephalitis from reactivation of latent infection in the brains of immunosuppressed persons are the most important manifestations. CNS, central nervous system. *(Courtesy of Dominique Buzoni-Gatel, Institut Pasteur, Paris; with permission.)*

acute feline infection, a cat may excrete as many as 100 million parasites per day. These very stable sporozoite-containing oocysts are highly infectious and may remain viable for many years in the soil. Humans infected during a well-documented outbreak of oocyst-transmitted infection develop stage-specific antibodies to the oocyst/sporozoite.

Children and adults also can acquire infection from tissue cysts containing bradyzoites. The ingestion of a single cyst is all that is required for human infection. Undercooking or insufficient freezing of meat is an important source of infection in the developed world. In the United States, 10–20% of lamb products and 25–35% of pork products show evidence of cysts that contain bradyzoites. The incidence in beef is much lower—perhaps as low as 1%. Direct ingestion of bradyzoite cysts in these various meat products leads to acute infection.

Transmission via Blood or Organs In addition to oral transmission, direct transmission of the parasite by blood or organ products during transplantation takes place at a low rate. Viable parasites can be cultured from refrigerated anticoagulated blood, which may be a source of infection in individuals receiving blood transfusions. *T. gondii* infection also has been reported in kidney and heart transplant recipients who were uninfected before transplantation.

Transplacental Transmission About one-third of all women who acquire infection with *T. gondii* during pregnancy transmit the parasite to the fetus; the remainder give birth to normal, uninfected babies. Of the various factors that influence fetal outcome, gestational age at the time of infection is the most critical (see below). Few data support a role for recrudescent maternal infection as the source of congenital disease. Thus, women who are seropositive before pregnancy usually are protected against acute infection and do not give birth to congenitally infected neonates.

The following general guidelines can be used to evaluate congenital infection. There is essentially no risk if the mother becomes infected ≥6 months before conception. If infection is acquired <6 months before conception, the likelihood of transplacental infection increases as the interval between infection and conception decreases. In pregnancy, if

the mother becomes infected during the first trimester, the incidence of transplacental infection is lowest (~15%), but the disease in the neonate is most severe. If maternal infection occurs during the third trimester, the incidence of transplacental infection is greatest (65%), but the infant is usually asymptomatic at birth. Infected infants who are normal at birth may have a higher incidence of learning disabilities and chronic neurologic sequelae than uninfected children. Only a small proportion (20%) of women infected with *T. gondii* develop clinical signs of infection. Often the diagnosis is first appreciated when routine postconception serologic tests show evidence of specific antibody.

PATHOGENESIS

Upon the host's ingestion of either tissue cysts containing bradyzoites or oocysts containing sporozoites, the parasites are released from the cysts by a digestive process. Bradyzoites are resistant to the effect of pepsin and invade the host's gastrointestinal tract. Within enterocytes (or other gut-associated cells), the parasites undergo morphologic transformation, giving rise to invasive tachyzoites. These tachyzoites induce a parasite-specific secretory IgA response. From the gastrointestinal tract, parasites are disseminated to a variety of organs, particularly lymphatic tissue, skeletal muscle, myocardium, retina, placenta, and the CNS. At these sites, the parasite infects host cells, replicates, and invades the adjoining cells. In this fashion, the hallmarks of the infection develop: cell death and focal necrosis surrounded by an acute inflammatory response.

In the immunocompetent host, both the humoral and the cellular immune responses control infection; parasite virulence and tissue tropism may be strain specific. Tachyzoites are sequestered by a variety of immune mechanisms, including induction of parasiticidal antibody, activation of macrophages with radical intermediates, production of interferon γ (IFN-γ), and stimulation of cytotoxic T lymphocytes of the CD8+ phenotype. These antigen-specific lymphocytes are capable of killing both extracellular parasites and target cells infected with parasites. As tachyzoites are cleared from the acutely infected host, tissue cysts containing bradyzoites begin to appear, usually within the CNS and the retina. In the immunocompromised or fetal host, the immune factors necessary to control the spread of tachyzoite infection are lacking. This altered immune state allows the persistence of tachyzoites and gives rise to progressive focal destruction that results in organ failure (i.e., necrotizing encephalitis, pneumonia, and myocarditis).

Persistence of infection with cysts containing bradyzoites is common in the immunocompetent host. This lifelong infection usually remains subclinical. Although bradyzoites are in a slow metabolic phase, cysts do degenerate and rupture within the CNS. This degenerative process, with the development of new bradyzoite-containing cysts, is the most probable source of recrudescent infection in immunocompromised individuals and the most likely stimulus for the persistence of antibody titers in the immunocompetent host.

PATHOLOGY

Cell death and focal necrosis due to replicating tachyzoites induce an intense mononuclear inflammatory response in any tissue or cell type infected. Tachyzoites rarely can be visualized by routine histopathologic staining of these inflammatory lesions. However, immunofluorescent staining with parasitic antigen–specific antibodies can reveal either the organism itself or evidence of antigen. In contrast to this inflammatory process caused by tachyzoites, bradyzoite-containing cysts cause inflammation only at the early stages of development, and even this inflammation may be a response to the presence of tachyzoite antigens. Once the cysts reach maturity, the inflammatory process can no longer be detected, and the cysts remain immunologically quiescent within the brain matrix until they rupture.

Lymph Nodes During acute infection, lymph node biopsy demonstrates characteristic findings, including follicular hyperplasia and irregular clusters of tissue macrophages with eosinophilic cytoplasm. Granulomas rarely are evident in these specimens. Although tachyzoites are not usually visible, they can be sought either by subinoculation of infected tissue into mice, with resultant disease, or by polymerase chain reaction (PCR). PCR amplification of DNA fragments representing either p30 (SAG-1) or p22 (SAG-2) surface antigen or B1 antigen is an effective and sensitive assay for establishing lymph node infection by tachyzoites.

Eyes In the eye, infiltrates of monocytes, lymphocytes, and plasma cells may produce uni- or multifocal lesions. Granulomatous lesions and chorioretinitis can be observed in the posterior chamber after acute necrotizing retinitis. Other ocular complications include iridocyclitis, cataracts, and glaucoma.

Central Nervous System During CNS involvement, both focal and diffuse meningoencephalitis can be documented, with evidence of necrosis and microglial nodules. Necrotizing encephalitis in patients without AIDS is characterized by small diffuse lesions with perivascular cuffing in contiguous areas. In the AIDS population, polymorphonuclear leukocytes may be present in addition to monocytes, lymphocytes, and plasma cells. Cysts containing bradyzoites frequently are found contiguous with the necrotic tissue border. As stated previously, it is estimated that there are as many as 2100 cases of TE in the United States each year.

Lungs and Heart Among patients with AIDS who die of toxoplasmosis, 40–70% have involvement of the lungs and heart. Interstitial pneumonitis can develop in neonates and immunocompromised patients. Thickened and edematous alveolar septa infiltrated with mononuclear and plasma cells are apparent. This inflammation may extend to the endothelial walls. Tachyzoites and bradyzoite-containing cysts have been observed within the alveolar membrane. Superimposed bronchopneumonia can be caused by other microbial agents. Cysts and aggregates of parasites in cardiac muscle tissue are evident in patients with AIDS who die of toxoplasmosis. Focal necrosis surrounded by inflammatory cells is associated with hyaline necrosis and disrupted myocardial cells. Pericarditis is associated with toxoplasmosis in some patients.

Gastrointestinal Tract Acute infection in certain strains of inbred mice (B6) results in lethal ileitis within 7–9 days. This inflammatory bowel disease has been recognized in several mammalian species, including pigs and nonhuman primates. The association between human inflammatory bowel disease and either acute or recurrent *Toxoplasma* infection has not been established.

Other Sites Pathologic changes during disseminated infection are similar to those described for the lymph nodes, eyes, and CNS. In patients with AIDS, the skeletal muscle, pancreas, stomach, and kidneys can be involved, with necrosis, invasion by inflammatory cells, and (rarely) tachyzoites detectable by routine staining. Large necrotic lesions may cause direct tissue destruction. In addition, secondary effects from acute infection of these various organs, including pancreatitis, myositis, and glomerulonephritis, have been reported.

HOST IMMUNE RESPONSE

Acute *Toxoplasma* infection evokes a cascade of protective immune responses in the immunocompetent host. *Toxoplasma* enters the host at the gut mucosal level and evokes a mucosal immune response that includes the production of antigen-specific secretory IgA. Titers of serum IgA antibody directed at p30 (SAG-1) are a useful marker for congenital and acute toxoplasmosis. Milk-whey IgA from acutely in-

fected mothers contains a high titer of antibody to *T. gondii* and can block infection of enterocytes in vitro. In mice, IgA intestinal secretions directed at the parasite are abundant and are associated with the induction of mucosal T cells.

Within the host, *T. gondii* rapidly induces detectable levels of both IgM and IgG serum antibodies. Monoclonal gammopathy of the IgG class can occur in congenitally infected infants. IgM levels may be increased in newborns with congenital infection. The polyclonal IgG antibodies evoked by infection are parasiticidal in vitro in the presence of serum complement and are the basis for the Sabin-Feldman dye test. However, cell-mediated immunity is the major protective response evoked by the parasite during host infection. Macrophages are activated after phagocytosis of antibody-opsonized parasites. This activation can lead to death of the parasite by either an oxygen-dependent or an oxygen-independent process. If the parasite is not phagocytosed and enters the macrophage by active penetration, it continues to replicate, and this replication may represent the mechanism for transport and dissemination to distant organs. *Toxoplasma* stimulates a robust interleukin (IL) 12 response by human dendritic cells. The requirement for costimulation via CD40/154 has been established. The CD4+ and CD8+ T cell responses are antigen-specific and further stimulate the production of a variety of important lymphokines that expand the T cell and natural killer cell repertoire. *T. gondii* is a potent inducer of a T_H1 phenotype, with IL-12 and IFN-γ playing an essential role in the control of the parasites' growth in the host. Regulation of the inflammatory response is at least partially under the control of a T_H2 response that includes the production of IL-4 and IL-10 in seropositive individuals. Both asymptomatic patients and those with active infection may have a depressed CD4+ to CD8+ ratio. This shift may be correlated with a disease syndrome but is not necessarily correlated with disease outcome. Human T cell clones of both the CD4+ and the CD8+ phenotypes are cytolytic against parasite-infected macrophages. These T cell clones produce cytokines that are "microbistatic." IL-18, IL-7, and IL-15 upregulate the production of IFN-γ and may be important during acute and chronic infection. The effect of IFN-γ may be paradoxical, with stimulation of a host downregulatory response as well.

Although in patients with AIDS *T. gondii* infection is believed to be recrudescent, determination of antibody titers is not helpful in establishing reactivation. Because of the severe depletion in CD4+ T cells, quite frequently there is no observed increase in antibody titer during exacerbation of infection. T cells from AIDS patients with reactivation of toxoplasmosis fail to secrete both IFN-γ and IL-2. This alteration in the production of these critical immune cytokines contributes to the persistence of infection. *Toxoplasma* infection frequently develops late in the course of AIDS, when the loss of T cell–dependent protective mechanisms, particularly CD8+ T cells, becomes most pronounced.

CLINICAL MANIFESTATIONS

In persons whose immune systems are intact, acute toxoplasmosis is usually asymptomatic and self-limited. This condition can go unrecognized in 80–90% of adults and children with acquired infection. The asymptomatic nature of this infection makes diagnosis difficult in mothers infected during pregnancy. In contrast, the wide range of clinical manifestations in congenitally infected children includes severe neurologic complications such as hydrocephalus, microcephaly, mental retardation, and chorioretinitis. If prenatal infection is severe, multiorgan failure and subsequent intrauterine fetal death can occur. In children and adults, chronic infection can persist throughout life, with little consequence to the immunocompetent host.

Toxoplasmosis in Immunocompetent Patients The most common manifestation of acute toxoplasmosis is cervical lymphadenopathy. The nodes may be single or multiple, are usually nontender, are discrete, and vary in firmness. Lymphadenopathy also may be found in suboccipital, supraclavicular, inguinal, and mediastinal areas. Generalized lymphadenopathy occurs in 20–30% of symptomatic patients. Between 20 and 40% of patients with lymphadenopathy also have headache, malaise, fatigue, and fever [usually with a temperature of <40°C (<104°F)]. A smaller proportion of symptomatic individuals have myalgia, sore throat, abdominal pain, maculopapular rash, meningoencephalitis, and confusion. Rare complications associated with infection in the normal immune host include pneumonia, myocarditis, encephalopathy, pericarditis, and polymyositis. Symptoms associated with acute infection usually resolve within several weeks, although the lymphadenopathy may persist for some months. In one epidemic, toxoplasmosis was diagnosed correctly in only 3 of the 25 patients who consulted physicians. If toxoplasmosis is considered in the differential diagnosis, routine laboratory and serologic screening should precede node biopsy.

The results of routine laboratory studies are usually unremarkable except for minimal lymphocytosis, an elevated erythrocyte sedimentation rate, and a nominal increase in liver aminotransferases. Evaluation of cerebrospinal fluid (CSF) in cases with evidence of encephalopathy or meningoencephalitis shows an elevation of intracranial pressure, mononuclear pleocytosis (10–50 cells/mL), a slight increase in protein concentration, and (occasionally) an increase in the gamma globulin level. PCR amplification of the *Toxoplasma* DNA target sequence in CSF may be beneficial. The CSF of chronically infected individuals is normal.

Infection of Immunocompromised Patients Patients with AIDS and those receiving immunosuppressive therapy for lymphoproliferative disorders are at greatest risk for developing acute toxoplasmosis. This predilection may be due either to reactivation of latent infection or to acquisition of parasites from exogenous sources such as blood or transplanted organs. In individuals with AIDS, >95% of cases of TE are believed to be due to recrudescent infection. In most of these cases, encephalitis develops when the CD4+ T cell count falls below 100/μL. In immunocompromised hosts, the disease may be rapidly fatal if untreated. Thus accurate diagnosis and initiation of appropriate therapy are necessary to prevent fulminant infection.

Toxoplasmosis is a principal opportunistic infection of the CNS in persons with AIDS. Although geographic origin may be related to frequency of infection, it has no correlation with the severity of disease in immunocompromised hosts. Individuals with AIDS who are seropositive for *T. gondii* are at very high risk for encephalitis. In the United States, about one-third of the 15–40% of adult AIDS patients who are latently infected with *T. gondii* develop TE.

The signs and symptoms of acute toxoplasmosis in immunocompromised patients principally involve the CNS (**Fig. 207-2**). More than 50% of patients with clinical manifestations have intracerebral involvement. Clinical findings at presentation range from nonfocal to focal dysfunction. CNS findings include encephalopathy, meningoencephalitis, and mass lesions. Patients may present with altered mental status (75%), fever (10–72%), seizures (33%), headaches (56%), and focal neurologic findings (60%), including motor deficits, cranial nerve palsies, movement disorders, dysmetria, visual-field loss, and aphasia. Patients who present with evidence of diffuse cortical dysfunction develop evidence of focal neurologic disease as infection progresses. This altered condition is due not only to the necrotizing encephalitis caused by direct invasion by the parasite but also to secondary effects, including vasculitis, edema, and hemorrhage. The onset of infection can range from an insidious process over several weeks to an acute confusional state with fulminant focal deficits, including hemiparesis, hemiplegia, visual-field defects, localized headache, and focal seizures.

Although lesions can occur anywhere in the CNS, the areas most often involved appear to be the brainstem, basal ganglia, pituitary gland, and corticomedullary junction. Brainstem involvement gives rise to a variety of neurologic dysfunctions, including cranial nerve palsy, dysmetria, and ataxia. With basal ganglionic infection, patients may develop hydrocephalus, choreiform movements, and choreoathetosis. Because *Toxoplasma*

FIGURE 207-2 Toxoplasmic encephalitis in a 36-year-old patient with AIDS. The multiple lesions are demonstrated by magnetic resonance scanning (T1 weighted with gadolinium enhancement). *(Courtesy of Clifford Eskey, Dartmouth Hitchcock Medical Center, Hanover, NH; with permission.)*

usually causes encephalitis, meningeal involvement is uncommon, and thus CSF findings may be unremarkable or may include a modest increase in cell count and in protein—but not glucose—concentration.

Cerebral toxoplasmosis must be differentiated from other opportunistic infections or tumors in the CNS of AIDS patients. The differential diagnosis includes herpes simplex encephalitis, cryptococcal meningitis, progressive multifocal leukoencephalopathy, and primary CNS lymphoma. Involvement of the pituitary gland can give rise to panhypopituitarism and hyponatremia from inappropriate secretion of vasopressin (antidiuretic hormone). AIDS-dementia complex may present as cognitive impairment, attention loss, and altered memory. Brain biopsy in patients who have been treated for TE but who continue to exhibit neurologic dysfunction often fails to identify organisms.

Autopsies of *Toxoplasma*-infected patients have demonstrated the involvement of multiple organs, including the lungs, gastrointestinal tract, pancreas, skin, eyes, heart, and liver. *Toxoplasma* pneumonia can be confused with *Pneumocystis* pneumonia (PcP). Respiratory involvement usually presents as dyspnea, fever, and a nonproductive cough and may rapidly progress to acute respiratory failure with hemoptysis, metabolic acidosis, hypotension, and (occasionally) disseminated intravascular coagulation. Histopathologic studies demonstrate necrosis and a mixed cellular infiltrate. The presence of organisms is a helpful diagnostic indicator, but organisms can also be found in healthy tissue. Infection of the heart is usually asymptomatic but can be associated with cardiac tamponade or biventricular failure. Infections of the gastrointestinal tract and the liver have been documented.

Congenital Toxoplasmosis Between 400 and 4000 infants born each year in the United States are affected by congenital toxoplasmosis. Infection of the placenta leads to hematogenous infection of the fetus. As stated earlier, the proportion of fetuses that become infected increases but the clinical severity of the infection declines as gestation proceeds. Persistence of *T. gondii* can ultimately result in reactivation and further damage decades later. Factors associated with relatively severe disabilities include delays in diagnosis and in initiation of therapy, neonatal hypoxia and hypoglycemia, profound visual impairment (see "Ocular Infection," below), uncorrected hydrocephalus, and increased intracranial pressure. If treated appropriately, upwards of 70% of children have normal developmental, neurologic, and ophthalmologic findings at follow-up evaluations. Treatment for 1 year with pyrimethamine and a sulfonamide is tolerated with minimal toxicity (see "Treatment," below).

Ocular Infection Infection with *T. gondii* is estimated to cause 35% of all cases of chorioretinitis in the United States and Europe. Most ocular involvement is believed to be due to congenital infection, with a very low incidence following acquired infection. Between 1 and 3% of all patients with AIDS develop debilitating chorioretinitis due to *T. gondii*. A variety of ocular manifestations are documented, including blurred vision, scotoma, photophobia, and eye pain. Macular involvement occurs with loss of central vision, and nystagmus is secondary to poor fixation. Involvement of the extraocular muscles may lead to disorders of convergence and to strabismus. Ophthalmologic examination should be undertaken in newborns with suspected congenital infection. As the inflammation resolves, vision improves, but episodic flare-ups of chorioretinitis, which progressively destroy retinal tissue and lead to glaucoma, are common.

The ophthalmologic examination reveals yellow-white, cotton-like patches with indistinct margins of hyperemia. As the lesions age, white plaques with distinct borders and black spots within the retinal pigment become more apparent. Lesions usually are located near the posterior pole of the retina; they may be single but are more commonly multiple. Congenital lesions may be unilateral or bilateral and show evidence of massive chorioretinal degeneration with extensive fibrosis. Surrounding these areas of involvement are a normal retina and vasculature. In patients with AIDS, retinal lesions are often large, with diffuse retinal necrosis, and include both free tachyzoites and cysts containing bradyzoites. Toxoplasmic chorioretinitis may be a prodrome to the development of encephalitis.

DIAGNOSIS

Tissue and Body Fluids
The differential diagnosis of acute toxoplasmosis can be made by appropriate culture, serologic testing, and PCR (Table 207-1). Although difficult, the isolation of *T. gondii* from blood or other body fluids can be accomplished after subinoculation of the sample into the peritoneal cavity of mice. Mice should be tested for organisms in the peritoneal fluid 6–10 days after inoculation. If no parasites are found in the mouse's peritoneal fluid, its anti-*Toxoplasma* serum titer can be evaluated 4–6 weeks after inoculation. Isolation of *T. gondii* from the patient's body fluids reflects acute infection, whereas isolation from biopsied tissue is an indication only of the presence of tissue cysts and should not be misinterpreted as evidence of acute toxoplasmosis. Persistent parasitemia in patients with latent, asymptomatic infection is rare. Histologic examination of lymph nodes may suggest the characteristic changes described above. Demonstration of tachyzoites in lymph nodes establishes the diagnosis of acute toxoplasmosis. Like subinoculation into mice, histologic demonstration of cysts containing bradyzoites confirms prior infection with *T. gondii* but is nondiagnostic for acute infection.

TABLE 207-1 DIFFERENTIAL LABORATORY DIAGNOSIS OF TOXOPLASMOSIS

Clinical Setting	Alternative Diagnosis	Distinguishing Characteristics
Mononucleosis syndrome	Epstein-Barr virus	Serologic test
	Cytomegalovirus	Serologic test
	HIV	Serologic test
Congenital infection	Cytomegalovirus	Viral culture
	Herpes simplex virus	Viral culture
	Rubella virus	Viral culture/serologic test
	Syphilis	Serologic test
	Listeriosis	Bacterial culture
Retinochoroiditis in immunocompetent individual	Tuberculosis	Bacterial culture
	Syphilis	Serologic test
	Histoplasmosis	Serologic test/culture
Retinochoroiditis in AIDS	Cytomegalovirus	Viral culture/PCR
	Syphilis	Serologic test
	Herpes simplex virus	Viral culture/PCR
	Varicella-zoster virus	Viral culture/PCR
	Fungal infection	Culture
CNS lesions in AIDS	Lymphoma or metastatic tumor	Tissue biopsy
	Brain abscess	Bacterial culture
	Progressive multifocal leukoencephalopathy	PCR
	Fungal/mycobacterial infection	Biopsy and culture

Source: Adapted from Schwartzman JD: Toxoplasmosis, in *Principles and Practice of Clinical Parasitology.* Hoboken, Wiley, 2001.

Serology
The procedures just described have great diagnostic value but are limited by difficulties encountered either in the growth of parasites in vivo or in the identification of tachyzoites by histochemical methods. Serologic testing has become the routine method of diagnosis. A wide range of serologic tests that can be used to measure antibody to *T. gondii* are available commercially.

Diagnosis of acute infection with *T. gondii* can be established by detection of the simultaneous presence of IgG and IgM antibodies to *Toxoplasma* in serum. The presence of circulating IgA favors the diagnosis of an acute infection. The Sabin-Feldman dye test, the indirect fluorescent antibody test, and the enzyme-linked immunosorbent assay (ELISA) all satisfactorily measure circulating IgG antibody to *Toxoplasma*. Positive IgG titers (>1:10) can be detected as early as 2–3 weeks after infection. These titers usually peak at 6–8 weeks and decline slowly to a new baseline level that persists for life. It is necessary to measure the serum IgM titer in concert with the IgG titer to better establish the time of infection. The methods currently available for this determination are the double-sandwich IgM-ELISA and the IgM-immunosorbent assay (IgM-ISAGA). Both of these assays are specific and sensitive, and their use precludes the false-positive results associated with tests for rheumatoid factor and antinuclear antibody. The double-sandwich IgA-ELISA is more sensitive than the IgM-ELISA for detecting congenital infection in the fetus and newborn.

 Recently, the results obtained with PCR have suggested high sensitivity, specificity, and clinical utility in the diagnosis of TE in resource-poor settings.

Molecular Diagnostics
Molecular approaches can directly detect *T. gondii* in biologic samples independent of the serologic response. Specific molecular analysis for either the B1 gene or the 529-bp sequence is useful. Real-time PCR is a promising technique that can provide quantitative results. Isolates can be genotyped and polymorphic sequences can be obtained, with the consequent identification of the precise strain. Knowledge of the correct sequence is important in studies on the correlation of clinical signs and symptoms of disease with the *T. gondii* genotype.

The Immunocompetent Adult or Child
For the patient who presents with lymphadenopathy only, a positive IgM titer is an indication of acute infection—and an indication for therapy, if that is clinically warranted (see "Treatment," below). The serum IgM titer should be determined again in 3 weeks. An elevation in the IgG titer without an increase in the IgM titer suggests that infection is present but is not acute. If there is a borderline increase in either IgG or IgM, the titers should be reassessed in 3–4 weeks.

The Immunocompromised Host
A presumptive clinical diagnosis of TE in patients with AIDS is based on clinical presentation, history of exposure (as evidenced by positive serology), and radiologic evaluation. To detect latent infection with *T. gondii*, HIV-infected persons should be tested for IgG antibody to *Toxoplasma* soon after HIV infection is diagnosed. When these criteria are used, the predictive value is as high as 80%. More than 97% of patients with AIDS and toxoplasmosis have IgG antibody to *T. gondii* in serum. IgM serum antibody usually is not detectable. Attempts to evaluate rising IgG titers or to determine whether IgM is present are not productive. Serologic evidence of infection virtually always precedes the development of TE. It is therefore important to determine the *Toxoplasma* antibody status of all patients infected with HIV. Antibody titers may range from negative to 1:1024 in patients with AIDS and TE. Fewer than 3% of patients have no demonstrable antibody to *Toxoplasma* at diagnosis. Intrathecal antibody to *T. gondii* may be present; determination of the titer may help identify prior infection.

Patients with TE have focal or multifocal abnormalities demonstrable by CT or MRI. Neuroradiologic evaluation should include double-dose contrast CT of the head. By this test, single and frequently multiple contrast-enhancing lesions (<2 cm) may be identified. MRI usually demonstrates multiple lesions located in both hemispheres, with the basal ganglia and corticomedullary junction most commonly involved; MRI provides a more sensitive evaluation of the efficacy of therapy than does CT (Fig. 207-2). These findings are not pathognomonic of *Toxoplasma* infection, since 40% of CNS lymphomas are multifocal and 50% are ring-enhancing. For both MRI and CT scans, the rate of false-negative results is ~10%. The finding of a single lesion on an MRI scan increases the likelihood of primary CNS lymphoma (in which solitary lesions are four times more likely than in TE) and strengthens the argument for the performance of a brain biopsy. A therapeutic trial of anti-*Toxoplasma* medications is frequently used to assess the diagnosis. Treatment of presumptive TE with pyrimethamine plus clindamycin results in quantifiable clinical improvement in >50% of patients by day 3. By day 7, >90% of treated patients show evidence of improvement. In contrast, if patients fail to respond or have lymphoma, clinical signs and symptoms worsen by day 7. Patients in this category require brain biopsy with or without a change in therapy. This procedure can now be performed by a stereotactic CT-guided method that reduces the potential for complications. Brain biopsy for *T. gondii* identifies organisms in 50–75% of cases. PCR amplification of genetic material of the parasite found in the CSF may prove diagnostically beneficial in the future.

Now used in some centers, single-photon emission CT (SPECT) has been touted as a definitive means of detecting or ruling out *Toxoplasma* infection when a CNS lesion is suspected. In the future, SPECT may well be widely used for this purpose.

As in other conditions, the radiologic response may lag behind the clinical response. Resolution of lesions may take from 3 weeks to 6 months. Some patients show clinical improvement despite worsening radiographic findings.

Congenital Infection The issue of concern when a pregnant woman has evidence of recent *T. gondii* infection is obviously whether the fetus is infected. PCR analysis of the amniotic fluid for the B1 gene of *T. gondii* has replaced fetal blood sampling. Serologic diagnosis is based on the persistence of IgG antibody or a positive IgM titer after the first week of life (a time frame that excludes placental leak). The IgG determination should be repeated every 2 months. An increase in IgM beyond the first week of life is indicative of acute infection. However, up to 25% of infected newborns may be seronegative and have normal routine physical examinations. Thus assessment of the eye and the brain, with ophthalmologic testing, CSF evaluation, and radiologic studies, is important in establishing the diagnosis.

Ocular Toxoplasmosis Because of the congenital nature of ocular toxoplasmosis, the serum antibody titer may not correlate with the presence of active lesions in the fundus. In general, a positive IgG titer (measured in undiluted serum if necessary) in conjunction with typical lesions establishes the diagnosis. Antibody production is expressed in terms of the Goldmann-Witmer coefficient (C), in which $C =$ [anti-*Toxoplasma* IgG (aqueous humor/serum)]/[total IgG (serum/aqueous humor)]. The positive cutoff of 3 is the generally accepted discrimination level. The sensitivity of this index as a diagnostic tool lies between 60 and 85%, with a specificity close to 90% in persons of European or North American origin. Confirmation of local specific antibody production in the eye indicates that the site of inflammatory activity is localized to this organ. However, two-thirds of patients without evidence of specific antibody production at initial clinical presentation later develop a detectable titer. If lesions are atypical and the titer is in the low-positive range, the diagnosis is presumptive. The parasitic antigen–specific polyclonal IgG assay as well as parasitic antigen–specific PCR may facilitate the diagnosis. Accordingly, the clinical diagnosis of ocular toxoplasmosis can be supported in 60–90% of cases by laboratory tests, depending on the time of anterior chamber puncture and the panel of antibody analyses used. In the remaining cases, the possibility of a falsely negative laboratory diagnosis or of an incorrect clinical diagnosis cannot be clarified further.

℞ TOXOPLASMOSIS

CONGENITAL INFECTION Congenitally infected neonates are treated with daily oral pyrimethamine (0.5–1 mg/kg) and sulfadiazine (100 mg/kg)

for 1 year. In addition, therapy with spiramycin (100 mg/kg per day) plus prednisone (1 mg/kg per day) is efficacious for congenital infection.

INFECTION IN IMMUNOCOMPETENT PATIENTS Immunologically competent adults and older children who have only lymphadenopathy do not require specific therapy unless they have persistent, severe symptoms. Patients with ocular toxoplasmosis should be treated for 1 month with pyrimethamine plus either sulfadiazine or clindamycin. Prenatal antibiotic therapy can reduce the number of infants severely affected by *Toxoplasma* infection.

INFECTION IN IMMUNOCOMPROMISED PATIENTS **Primary Prophylaxis** Patients with AIDS should be treated for acute toxoplasmosis; in immunocompromised patients, toxoplasmosis is rapidly fatal if untreated. Before the introduction of antiretroviral therapy (ART), the median survival time was >1 year for patients who could tolerate treatment for TE. Despite their toxicity, the drugs used to treat TE were required for survival prior to ART. The incidence of TE has declined as survival of patients with HIV infection has increased as a result of ART.

In Africa, many patients are diagnosed with HIV infection only after developing opportunistic infections such as TE. Hence, the optimal management of these opportunistic infections is important if the benefits of subsequent ART are to be realized. AIDS patients who are seropositive for *T. gondii* and who have a CD4+ T lymphocyte count of <100/μL should receive prophylaxis against TE. A recent Cochrane analysis of clinical trials of TE treatment failed to document the superiority of any one regimen. Of the currently available agents, trimethoprim-sulfamethoxazole (TMP-SMX) appears to be an effective alternative for TE in resource-poor settings where the preferred combination of pyrimethamine plus sulfadiazine is not available. The daily dose of TMP-SMX recommended as the preferred regimen for PcP prophylaxis (one double-strength tablet) is effective against TE. If patients cannot tolerate TMP-SMX, the recommended alternative is dapsone-pyrimethamine, which is also effective against PcP. Atovaquone with or without pyrimethamine also can be considered. Prophylactic monotherapy with dapsone, pyrimethamine, azithromycin, clarithromycin, or aerosolized pentamidine is probably insufficient. AIDS patients who are seronegative for *Toxoplasma* and are not receiving prophylaxis for PcP should be retested for IgG antibody to *Toxoplasma* if their CD4+ T cell count drops to <100/μL. If seroconversion has taken place, then the patient should be given prophylaxis as described above.

Discontinuing Primary Prophylaxis Some current studies indicate that prophylaxis against TE can be discontinued in patients who have responded to ART and whose CD4+ T lymphocyte count has been >200/μL for 3 months. Although patients with CD4+ T lymphocyte counts of <100/μL are at greatest risk for developing TE, the risk that this condition will develop when the count has increased to 100–200/μL has not been established. Thus, prophylaxis should indeed be discontinued only when the count has increased to >200/μL. Continued prophylaxis at a CD4+ count of >200/μL has only a limited preventive effect against TE. Discontinuation of therapy reduces the pill burden; the potential for drug toxicity, drug interaction, or selection of drug-resistant pathogens; and cost. Prophylaxis should be recommenced if the CD4+ T lymphocyte count again decreases to <100–200/μL.

Individuals who have completed initial therapy for TE should receive treatment indefinitely unless immune reconstitution, with a CD4+ T cell count of >200/μL, occurs as a consequence of ART. Combination therapy with pyrimethamine plus sulfadiazine plus leucovorin is effective for this purpose. An alternative to sulfadiazine in this regimen is clindamycin. Unfortunately, only the combination of pyrimethamine plus sulfadiazine provides protection against PcP as well.

Discontinuing Secondary Prophylaxis (Chronic Maintenance Therapy) Patients receiving secondary prophylaxis for TE are at low risk for recurrence when they have completed initial therapy for TE, remain asymptomatic, and have a CD4+ T lymphocyte count of >200/μL for at least 6 months after ART. This recommendation is based on recent observations in a large cohort (381 patients) and is consistent with more extensive data indicating the safety of discontinuing secondary prophylaxis for other opportunistic infections during advanced HIV disease. Discontinuation of chronic maintenance therapy among these patients appears reasonable. A repeat MRI brain scan is recommended. Secondary prophylaxis should be reintroduced if the CD4+ T lymphocyte count decreases to <200/μL.

PREVENTION

All HIV-infected persons, including those who lack IgG antibody to *Toxoplasma*, should be counseled regarding sources of *Toxoplasma* infection. The chances of primary infection with *Toxoplasma* can be reduced by not eating undercooked meat and by avoiding oocyst-contaminated material (i.e., a cat's litter box). Specifically, lamb, beef, and pork should be cooked to an internal temperature of 165°–170°F; from a more practical perspective, meat cooked until it is no longer pink inside usually satisfies this requirement. Hands should be washed thoroughly after work in the garden, and all fruits and vegetables should be washed. If the patient owns a cat, the litter box should be cleaned or changed daily, preferably by an HIV-negative, nonpregnant person; alternatively, patients should wash their hands thoroughly after changing the litter box. Patients should be encouraged to keep their cats inside and not to adopt or handle stray cats. Cats should be fed only canned or dried commercial food or well-cooked table food, not raw or undercooked meats. Patients need not be advised to part with their cats or to have their cats tested for toxoplasmosis. Blood intended for transfusion into *Toxoplasma*-seronegative immunocompromised individuals should be screened for antibody to *T. gondii*. Although such serologic screening is not routinely performed, seronegative women should be screened for evidence of infection several times during pregnancy if they are exposed to environmental conditions that put them at risk for infection with *T. gondii*. HIV-positive individuals should adhere closely to these preventive measures.

FURTHER READINGS

DEDICOAT M: Management of toxoplasmic encephalitis in HIV-infected adults (with an emphasis on resource-poor settings). Cochrane Database Syst Rev 3:CD005420, 2006

GARWEG JG: Determinants of immunodiagnostic success in human ocular toxoplasmosis. Parasite Immunol 27:61, 2005

LEHMANN T et al: Globalization and the population structure of *Toxoplasma gondii*. Proc Natl Acad Sci USA 103:11423, 2006

MASUR H et al: Guidelines for preventing opportunistic infections among HIV-infected persons—2002. Ann Intern Med 137:435, 2002

MCLEOD R et al: Outcome of treatment for congenital toxoplasmosis, 1981–2004: The National Collaborative Chicago-Based, Congenital Toxoplasmosis Study. Clin Infect Dis 42:1383, 2006

MIRO JM et al: Discontinuation of primary and secondary *Toxoplasma gondii* prophylaxis is safe in HIV-infected patients after immunological restoration with highly active antiretroviral therapy: Results of an open, randomized, multicenter clinical trial. Clin Infect Dis 43:79, 2006

MOCROFT A et al: Decline in the AIDS and death rates in the EuroSIDA study: An observational study. Lancet 362:22, 2003

SCHMIDT DR et al: The national neonatal screening programme for congenital toxoplasmosis in Denmark: Results from the initial four years, 1999–2002. Arch Dis Child 91:661, 2006

SWITAJ K et al: Recent trends in molecular diagnostics for *Toxoplasma gondii* infections. Clin Microbiol Infect 11:170, 2005

208 Protozoal Intestinal Infections and Trichomoniasis

Peter F. Weller

PROTOZOAL INFECTIONS

GIARDIASIS

Giardia lamblia (also known as *G. intestinalis*) is a cosmopolitan protozoal parasite that inhabits the small intestines of humans and other mammals.

Giardiasis is one of the most common parasitic diseases in both developed and developing countries worldwide, causing both endemic and epidemic intestinal disease and diarrhea.

Life Cycle and Epidemiology (Fig. 208-1) Infection follows the ingestion of environmentally hardy cysts, which excyst in the small intestine, releasing flagellated trophozoites (Fig. 208-2) that multiply by binary fission. *Giardia* remains a pathogen of the proximal small bowel and does not disseminate hematogenously. Trophozoites remain free in the lumen or attach to the mucosal epithelium by means of a ventral sucking disk. As a trophozoite encounters altered conditions, it forms a morphologically distinct cyst, which is the stage of the parasite usually found in the feces. Trophozoites may be present and even predominate in loose or watery stools, but it is the resistant cyst that survives outside the body and is responsible for transmission. Cysts do not tolerate heating, desiccation, or continued exposure to feces but do remain viable for months in cold fresh water. The number of cysts excreted varies widely but can approach 10^7 per gram of stool.

Ingestion of as few as 10 cysts is sufficient to cause infection in humans. Because cysts are infectious when excreted, person-to-person transmission occurs where fecal hygiene is poor. Giardiasis, as symptomatic or asymptomatic infections, is especially prevalent in day-care centers; person-to-person spread also takes place in other institutional settings with poor fecal hygiene and during anal-oral contact. If food is contaminated with *Giardia* cysts after cooking or preparation, foodborne transmission can occur. Waterborne transmission accounts for episodic infections (e.g., in campers and travelers) and for major epidemics in metropolitan areas. Surface water, ranging from mountain streams to large municipal reservoirs, can become contaminated with fecally derived *Giardia* cysts; outmoded water systems are subject to cross-contamination from leaking sewer lines. The efficacy of water as a means of transmission is enhanced by the small infectious inoculum of *Giardia*, the prolonged survival of cysts in cold water, and the resistance of cysts to killing by routine chlorination methods that are adequate for controlling bacteria. Viable cysts can be eradicated from water by either boiling or filtration. In the United States, *Giardia* (like *Cryptosporidium*; see below) is a common cause of waterborne epidemics of gastroenteritis. *Giardia* is common in developing countries, and infections may be acquired by travelers.

The importance of animal reservoirs as sources of infection for humans is unclear. *Giardia* parasites morphologically similar to those in humans are found in many mammals, including beavers from reservoirs implicated in epidemics, dogs, and cats.

Giardiasis, like cryptosporidiosis, creates a significant economic burden because of the costs incurred in the installation of water filtration systems required to prevent waterborne epidemics, in the management of epidemics that involve large communities, and in the evaluation and treatment of endemic infections.

Pathophysiology The reasons that some, but not all, infected patients develop clinical manifestations and the mechanisms by which *Giardia* causes alterations in small-bowel function are largely unknown. Although trophozoites adhere to the epithelium, they do not cause invasive or locally destructive alterations. The lactose intolerance and, in a minority of infected adults and children, significant malabsorption that develop are clinical signs of the loss of brush-border enzyme activities. In most infections, the morphology of the bowel is unaltered; however, in a few cases (usually in chronically infected, symptomatic patients), the histopathologic findings (including flattened villi) and the clinical manifestations resemble those of tropical sprue and gluten-sensitive enteropathy. The pathogenesis of diarrhea in giardiasis is not known.

The natural history of *Giardia* infection varies markedly. Infections may be aborted, transient, recurrent, or chronic. Parasite as well as host factors may be important in determining the course of infection and disease. Both cellular and humoral responses develop in human infections, but their precise roles in the control of infection and/or dis-

Excystation follows exposure to stomach acid and intestinal proteases, releasing trophozoite forms that multiply by binary fission and reside in the upper small bowel adherent to enterocytes.

Causes: Asymptomatic infection, acute diarrhea, or chronic diarrhea and malabsorption. Small bowel may demonstrate villous blunting, crypt hypertrophy, and mucosal inflammation.

Encystation occurs under conditions of bile salt concentration changes and alkaline pH. Smooth-walled cysts can contain two trophozoites.

Cyst are ingested (10-25 cysts) in contaminated water or food or by direct fecal-oral transmission (as in day care centers).

Cysts can survive in the environment (up to several weeks in cold water). They may also infect nonhuman mammalian species.

Cysts and trophozoites are passed in the stool into the environment.

FIGURE 208-1 Life cycle of *Giardia*. (*Reprinted from RL Guerrant et al: Tropical Infectious Disease: Principles, Pathogens and Practice, 2d ed, 2006, p 987, with permission from Elsevier Science.*)

FIGURE 208-2 Flagellated, binucleate ***Giardia*** trophozoite.

ease are unknown. Because patients with hypogammaglobulinemia suffer from prolonged, severe infections that are poorly responsive to treatment, humoral immune responses appear to be important. The greater susceptibility of the young than of the old and of newly exposed persons than of chronically exposed populations suggests that at least partial protective immunity may develop. *Giardia* isolates vary genotypically, biochemically, and biologically, and variations among isolates may contribute to different courses of infection.

Clinical Manifestations Disease manifestations of giardiasis range from asymptomatic carriage to fulminant diarrhea and malabsorption. Most infected persons are asymptomatic, but in epidemics the proportion of symptomatic cases may be higher. Symptoms may develop suddenly or gradually. In persons with acute giardiasis, symptoms develop after an incubation period that lasts at least 5–6 days and usually 1–3 weeks. Prominent early symptoms include diarrhea, abdominal pain, bloating, belching, flatus, nausea, and vomiting. Although diarrhea is common, upper intestinal manifestations such as nausea, vomiting, bloating, and abdominal pain may predominate. The duration of acute giardiasis is usually >1 week, although diarrhea often subsides. Individuals with chronic giardiasis may present with or without having experienced an antecedent acute symptomatic episode. Diarrhea is not necessarily prominent, but increased flatus, loose stools, sulfurous belching, and (in

some instances) weight loss occur. Symptoms may be continual or episodic and can persist for years. Some persons who have relatively mild symptoms for long periods recognize the extent of their discomfort only in retrospect. Fever, the presence of blood and/or mucus in the stools, and other signs and symptoms of colitis are uncommon and suggest a different diagnosis or a concomitant illness. Symptoms tend to be intermittent yet recurring and gradually debilitating, in contrast with the acute disabling symptoms associated with many enteric bacterial infections. Because of the less severe illness and the propensity for chronic infections, patients may seek medical advice late in the course of the illness; however, disease can be severe, resulting in malabsorption, weight loss, growth retardation, and dehydration. A number of extraintestinal manifestations have been described, such as urticaria, anterior uveitis, and arthritis; whether these are caused by giardiasis or concomitant processes is unclear.

Giardiasis can be severe in patients with hypogammaglobulinemia and can complicate other preexisting intestinal diseases, such as that occurring in cystic fibrosis. In patients with AIDS, *Giardia* can cause enteric illness that is refractory to treatment.

Diagnosis (Table 208-1) Giardiasis is diagnosed by detection of parasite antigens in the feces or by identification of cysts in the feces or of trophozoites in the feces or small intestines. Cysts are oval, measure 8–12 μm × 7–10 μm, and characteristically contain four nuclei. Trophozoites are pear-shaped, dorsally convex, flattened parasites with two nuclei and four pairs of flagella (Fig. 208-2). The diagnosis is sometimes difficult to establish. Direct examination of fresh or properly preserved stools as well as concentration methods should be used. Because cyst excretion is variable and may be undetectable at times, repeated examination of stool, sampling of duodenal fluid, and biopsy of the small intestine may be required to detect the parasite. Tests for parasitic antigens in stool are at least as sensitive and specific as good microscopic examinations and are easier to perform. All of these methods occasionally yield false-negative results.

TABLE 208-1	DIAGNOSIS OF INTESTINAL PROTOZOAL INFECTIONS			
Parasite	Stool O+P[a]	Fecal Acid-Fast Stain	Stool Antigen Immunoassays	Other
Giardia	+		+	
Cryptosporidium	–	+	+	
Isospora	–	+		
Cyclospora	–	+		
Microsporidia	–			Special fecal stains, tissue biopsies

[a]O+P, ova and parasites.

℞ GIARDIASIS

Cure rates with metronidazole (250 mg thrice daily for 5 days) are usually >90%. Tinidazole (2 g once by mouth) is reportedly more effective than metronidazole. Nitazoxanide (500 mg twice daily for 3 days) is an alternative agent for treatment of giardiasis. Paromomycin, an oral aminoglycoside that is not well absorbed, can be given to symptomatic pregnant patients, although information is limited on how effectively this agent eradicates infection.

Almost all patients respond to therapy and are cured, although some with chronic giardiasis experience delayed resolution of symptoms after eradication of *Giardia*. For many of the latter patients, residual symptoms probably reflect delayed regeneration of intestinal brush-border enzymes. Continued infection should be documented by stool examinations before treatment is repeated. Patients who remain infected after repeated treatments should be evaluated for reinfection through family members, close personal contacts, and environmental sources as well as for hypogammaglobulinemia. In cases refractory to multiple treatment courses, prolonged therapy with metronidazole (750 mg thrice daily for 21 days) has been successful.

Prevention   Although *Giardia* is extremely infectious, disease can be prevented by consumption of noncontaminated food and water and by personal hygiene when caring for infected children. Boiling or filtering potentially contaminated water prevents infection.

CRYPTOSPORIDIOSIS

The coccidian parasite *Cryptosporidium* causes diarrheal disease that is self-limited in immunocompetent human hosts but can be severe in persons with AIDS or other forms of immunodeficiency. Two species of *Cryptosporidium*, *C. hominis* and *C. parvum*, cause most human infections.

Life Cycle and Epidemiology   *Cryptosporidium* species are widely distributed in the world. Cryptosporidiosis is acquired by the consumption of oocysts (50% infectious dose: ~132 oocysts in nonimmune individuals), which excyst to liberate sporozoites that in turn enter and infect intestinal epithelial cells. The parasite's further development involves both asexual and sexual cycles, which produce forms capable of infecting other epithelial cells and of generating oocysts that are passed in the feces. *Cryptosporidium* species infect a number of animals, and *C. parvum* can spread from infected animals to humans. Since oocysts are immediately infectious when passed in feces, person-to-person transmission takes place in day-care centers and among household contacts and medical providers. Waterborne transmission (especially that of *C. hominis*) accounts for infections in travelers and for common-source epidemics. Oocysts are quite hardy and resist killing by routine chlorination. Both drinking water and recreational water (e.g., pools, waterslides) have been increasingly recognized as sources of infection.

Pathophysiology   Although intestinal epithelial cells harbor cryptosporidia in an intracellular vacuole, the means by which secretory diarrhea is elicited remain uncertain. No characteristic pathologic changes are found by biopsy. The distribution of infection can be spotty within the principal site of infection, the small bowel. Cryptosporidia are found in the pharynx, stomach, and large bowel of some patients and at times in the respiratory tract. Especially in patients with AIDS, involvement of the biliary tract can cause papillary stenosis, sclerosing cholangitis, or cholecystitis.

Clinical Manifestations   Asymptomatic infections can occur in both immunocompetent and immunocompromised hosts. In immunocompetent persons, symptoms develop after an incubation period of ~1 week and consist principally of watery nonbloody diarrhea, sometimes in conjunction with abdominal pain, nausea, anorexia, fever, and/or weight loss. In these hosts, the illness usually subsides after 1–2 weeks. In contrast, in immunocompromised hosts (especially those with AIDS and CD4+ T cell counts <100/μL), diarrhea can be chronic, persistent, and remarkably profuse, causing clinically significant fluid and electro-lyte depletion. Stool volumes may range from 1 to 25 L/d. Weight loss, wasting, and abdominal pain may be severe. Biliary tract involvement can manifest as midepigastric or right upper quadrant pain.

Diagnosis   (Table 208-1) Evaluation starts with fecal examination for small oocysts, which are smaller (4–5 μm in diameter) than the fecal stages of most other parasites. Because conventional stool examination for ova and parasites does not detect *Cryptosporidium*, specific testing must be requested. Detection is enhanced by evaluation of stools (obtained on multiple days) by several techniques, including modified acid-fast and direct immunofluorescent stains and enzyme immunoassays. Cryptosporidia can also be identified by light and electron microscopy at the apical surfaces of intestinal epithelium from biopsy specimens of the small bowel and, less frequently, the large bowel.

℞ CRYPTOSPORIDIOSIS

Nitazoxanide is approved by the U.S. Food and Drug Administration for the treatment of cryptosporidiosis and is available in tablet form for adults (500 mg twice daily for 3 days) and as an elixir for children. To date, however, this agent has not been effective for the treatment of HIV-infected patients, in whom improved immune status due to antiretroviral therapy can lead to amelioration of cryptosporidiosis. Otherwise, treatment includes supportive care with replacement of fluids and electrolytes and administration of antidiarrheal agents. Biliary tract obstruction may require papillotomy or T-tube placement. Prevention requires minimizing exposure to infectious oocysts in human or animal feces. Use of submicron water filters may minimize acquisition of infection from drinking water.

ISOSPORIASIS

The coccidian parasite *Isospora belli* causes human intestinal disease. Infection is acquired by the consumption of oocysts, after which the parasite invades intestinal epithelial cells and undergoes both sexual and asexual cycles of development. Oocysts excreted in stool are not immediately infectious but must undergo further maturation.

Although *I. belli* infects many animals, little is known about the epidemiology or prevalence of this parasite in humans. It appears to be most common in tropical and subtropical countries. Acute infections can begin abruptly with fever, abdominal pain, and watery nonbloody diarrhea and can last for weeks or months. In patients who have AIDS or are immunocompromised for other reasons, infections often are not self-limited but rather resemble cryptosporidiosis, with chronic, profuse watery diarrhea. Eosinophilia, which is not found in other enteric protozoan infections, may be detectable. The diagnosis (Table 208-1) is usually made by detection of the large (~25-μm) oocysts in stool by modified acid-fast staining. Oocyst excretion may be low-level and intermittent; if repeated stool examinations are unrevealing, sampling of duodenal contents by aspiration or small-bowel biopsy (often with electron-microscopic examination) may be necessary.

℞ ISOSPORIASIS

Trimethoprim-sulfamethoxazole (TMP-SMX; 160/800 mg four times daily for 10 days, and for HIV-infected patients, then three times daily for 3 weeks) is effective. For patients intolerant of sulfonamides, pyrimethamine (50–75 mg/d) can be used. Relapses can occur in persons with AIDS and necessitate maintenance therapy with TMP-SMX (160/800 mg three times per week).

CYCLOSPORIASIS

Cyclospora cayetanensis, a cause of diarrheal illness, is globally distributed: illness due to *C. cayetanensis* has been reported in the United States, Asia, Africa, Latin America, and Europe. The epidemiology of this parasite has not yet been fully defined, but waterborne transmission and food-borne transmission by basil and imported raspberries have been recognized. The full spectrum of illness attributable to *Cyclospora* has not been delineated. Some patients may harbor the infection without symptoms, but many have diarrhea, flulike symptoms, and flatulence and belching. The illness can be self-limited, can wax and wane, or in many cases can involve prolonged diarrhea, anorexia, and upper gastrointestinal symptoms, with sustained fatigue and weight loss in some instances. Diarrheal illness may persist for >1 month. *Cyclospora* can cause enteric illness in patients infected with HIV.

The parasite is detectable in epithelial cells of small-bowel biopsy samples and elicits secretory diarrhea by unknown means. The absence of fecal blood and leukocytes indicates that disease due to *Cyclospora* is not caused by destruction of the small-bowel mucosa. The diagnosis (Table 208-1) can be made by detection of spherical 8- to 10-μm oocysts in the stool, although routine stool O and P examinations are not sufficient. Specific fecal examinations must be requested to detect the oocysts, which are variably acid-fast and are fluorescent when viewed with ultraviolet light microscopy. Cyclosporiasis should be considered in the differential diagnosis of prolonged diarrhea, with or without a history of travel by the patient to other countries.

℞ CYCLOSPORIASIS

Cyclosporiasis is treated with TMP-SMX (160/800 mg twice daily for 7 days). HIV-infected patients may experience relapses after such treatment and thus may require longer-term suppressive maintenance therapy.

MICROSPORIDIOSIS

Microsporidia are obligate intracellular spore-forming protozoa that infect many animals and cause disease in humans, especially as opportunistic pathogens in AIDS. Microsporidia are members of a distinct phylum, Microspora, which contains dozens of genera and hundreds of species. The various microsporidia are differentiated by their developmental life cycles, ultrastructural features, and molecular taxonomy based on ribosomal RNA. The complex life cycles of the organisms result in the production of infectious spores (Fig. 208-3). Currently, eight genera of microsporidia—*Encephalitozoon, Pleistophora, Nosema, Vittaforma, Trachipleistophora, Brachiola, Microsporidium,* and *Enterocytozoon*—are recognized as causes of human disease. Although some microsporidia are probably prevalent causes of self-limited or asymptomatic infections in immunocompetent patients, little is known about how microsporidiosis is acquired.

Microsporidiosis is most common among patients with AIDS, less common among patients with other types of immunocompromise, and rare among immunocompetent hosts. In patients with AIDS, intestinal infections with *Enterocytozoon bieneusi* and *Encephalitozoon* (formerly *Septata*) *intestinalis* are recognized to contribute to chronic diarrhea and wasting; these infections are found in 10–40% of patients with chronic diarrhea. Both organisms have been found in the biliary tracts of patients with cholecystitis. *E. intestinalis* may also disseminate to cause fever, diarrhea, sinusitis, cholangitis, and bronchiolitis. In patients with AIDS, *Encephalitozoon hellem* has caused superficial keratoconjunctivitis as well as sinusitis, respiratory tract disease, and disseminated infection. Myositis due to *Pleistophora* has been documented. *Nosema, Vittaforma,* and *Microspo-*

ridium have caused stromal keratitis associated with trauma in immunocompetent patients.

Microsporidia are small gram-positive organisms with mature spores measuring 0.5–2 μm × 1–4 μm. Diagnosis of microsporidial infections in tissue often requires electron microscopy, although intracellular spores can be visualized by light microscopy with hematoxylin and eosin, Giemsa, or tissue Gram's stain. For the diagnosis of intestinal microsporidiosis, modified trichrome or chromotrope 2R-based staining and Uvitex 2B or calcofluor fluorescent staining reveal spores in smears of feces or duodenal aspirates. Definitive therapies for microsporidial infections remain to be established. For superficial keratoconjunctivitis due to *E. hellem*, topical therapy with fumagillin suspension has shown promise (Chap. 201). For enteric infections with *E. bieneusi* and *E. intestinalis* in HIV-infected patients, therapy with albendazole may be efficacious (Chap. 201).

OTHER INTESTINAL PROTOZOA

Balantidiasis   *Balantidium coli* is a large ciliated protozoal parasite that can produce a spectrum of large-intestinal disease analogous to amebiasis.

 The parasite is widely distributed in the world. Since it infects pigs, cases in humans are more common where pigs are raised. Infective cysts can be transmitted from person to person and

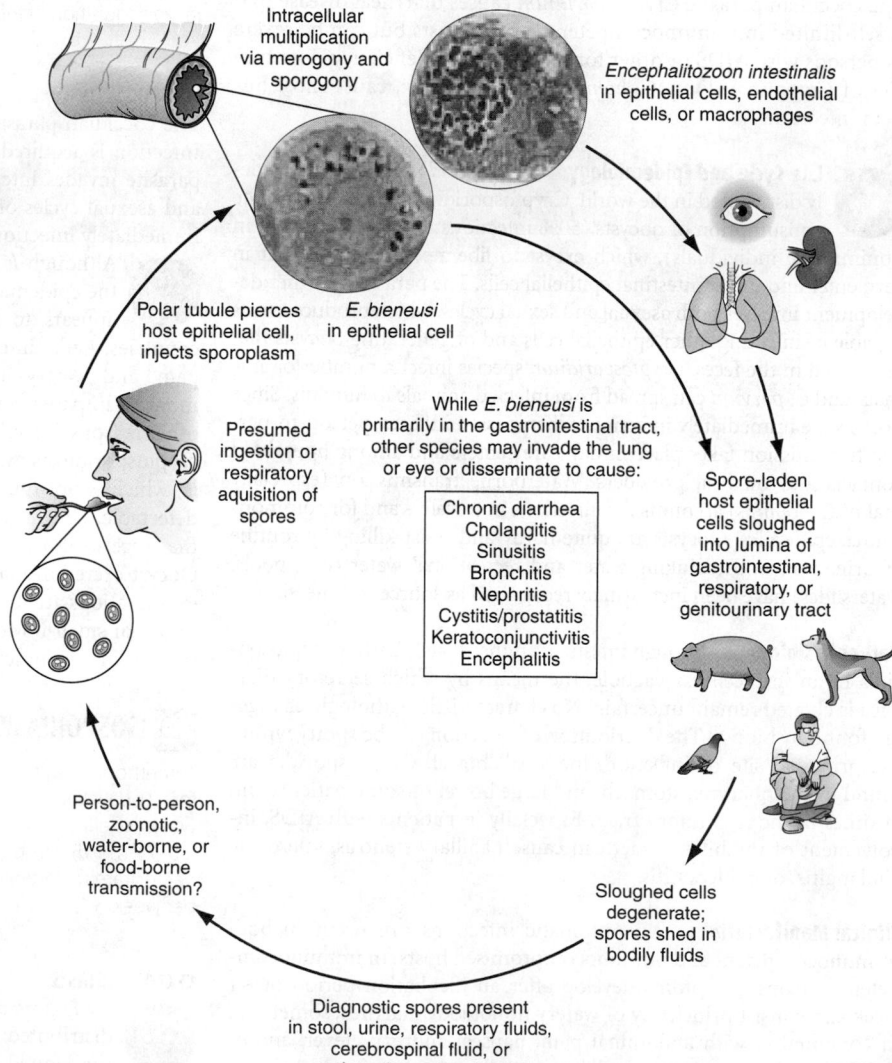

FIGURE 208-3   Life cycle of microsporidia. (*Reprinted from RL Guerrant et al: Tropical Infectious Disease: Principles, Pathogens and Practice, 2d ed, 2006, p 1128, with permission from Elsevier Science.*)

Figure labels:
Microsporidia
Enterocytozoon bieneusi, Encephalitozoon spp., et al.

Intracellular multiplication via merogony and sporogony

Encephalitozoon intestinalis in epithelial cells, endothelial cells, or macrophages

Polar tubule pierces host epithelial cell, injects sporoplasm

E. bieneusi in epithelial cell

Presumed ingestion or respiratory aquisition of spores

While *E. bieneusi* is primarily in the gastrointestinal tract, other species may invade the lung or eye or disseminate to cause:

Chronic diarrhea
Cholangitis
Sinusitis
Bronchitis
Nephritis
Cystitis/prostatitis
Keratoconjunctivitis
Encephalitis

Spore-laden host epithelial cells sloughed into lumina of gastrointestinal, respiratory, or genitourinary tract

Person-to-person, zoonotic, water-borne, or food-borne transmission?

Sloughed cells degenerate; spores shed in bodily fluids

Diagnostic spores present in stool, urine, respiratory fluids, cerebrospinal fluid, or various tissue specimens through water, but many cases are due to the ingestion of cysts derived from porcine feces in association with slaughtering, with use of pig feces for fertilizer, or with contamination of water supplies by pig feces.

Ingested cysts liberate trophozoites, which reside and replicate in the large bowel. Many patients remain asymptomatic, but some have persisting intermittent diarrhea, and a few develop more fulminant dysentery. In symptomatic individuals, the pathology in the bowel—both gross and microscopic—is similar to that seen in amebiasis, with varying degrees of mucosal invasion, focal necrosis, and ulceration. Balantidiasis, unlike amebiasis, does not spread hematogenously to other organs. The diagnosis is made by detection of the trophozoite stage in stool or sampled colonic tissue. Tetracycline (500 mg four times daily for 10 days) is an effective therapeutic agent.

Blastocystis hominis Infection *B. hominis*, while believed by some to be a protozoan capable of causing intestinal disease, remains an organism of uncertain pathogenicity. Some patients who pass *B. hominis* in their stools are asymptomatic, whereas others have diarrhea and associated intestinal symptoms. Diligent evaluation reveals other potential bacterial, viral, or protozoal causes of diarrhea in some but not all patients with symptoms. Because the pathogenicity of *B. hominis* is uncertain and because therapy for *Blastocystis* infection is neither specific nor uniformly effective, patients with prominent intestinal symptoms should be fully evaluated for other infectious causes of diarrhea. If diarrheal symptoms associated with *Blastocystis* are prominent, either metronidazole (750 mg thrice daily for 10 days) or TMP-SMX (160 mg/800 mg twice daily for 7 days) can be used.

Dientamoeba fragilis Infection *D. fragilis* is unique among intestinal protozoa in that it has a trophozoite stage but not a cyst stage. How trophozoites survive to transmit infection is not known. When symptoms develop in patients with *D. fragilis* infection, they are generally mild and include intermittent diarrhea, abdominal pain, and anorexia. The diagnosis is made by the detection of trophozoites in stool; the lability of these forms accounts for the greater yield when fecal samples are preserved immediately after collection. Since fecal excretion rates vary, examination of several samples obtained on alternate days increases the rate of detection. Iodoquinol (650 mg three times daily for 20 days), paromomycin (25–35 mg/kg per day in three doses for 7 days), metronidazole (500–750 mg three times daily for 10 days), or tetracycline (500 mg four times daily for 10 days) is appropriate for treatment.

TRICHOMONIASIS

Various species of trichomonads can be found in the mouth (in association with periodontitis) and occasionally in the gastrointestinal tract. *Trichomonas vaginalis*—one of the most prevalent protozoal parasites in the United States—is a pathogen of the genitourinary tract and a major cause of symptomatic vaginitis.

LIFE CYCLE AND EPIDEMIOLOGY

T. vaginalis is a pear-shaped, actively motile organism that measures about 10×7 μm, replicates by binary fission, and inhabits the lower genital tract of females and the urethra and prostate of males. In the United States, it accounts for ~3 million infections per year in women. While the organism can survive for a few hours in moist environments and could be acquired by direct contact, person-to-person venereal transmission accounts for virtually all cases of trichomoniasis. Its prevalence is greatest among persons with multiple sexual partners and among those with other sexually transmitted diseases (Chap. 124).

CLINICAL MANIFESTATIONS

Many men infected with *T. vaginalis* are asymptomatic, although some develop urethritis and a few have epididymitis or prostatitis. In con-

trast, infection in women, which has an incubation period of 5–28 days, is usually symptomatic and manifests with malodorous vaginal discharge (often yellow), vulvar erythema and itching, dysuria or urinary frequency (in 30–50% of patients), and dyspareunia. These manifestations, however, do not clearly distinguish trichomoniasis from other types of infectious vaginitis.

DIAGNOSIS

Detection of motile trichomonads by microscopic examination of wet mounts of vaginal or prostatic secretions has been the conventional means of diagnosis. Although this approach provides an immediate diagnosis, its sensitivity for the detection of *T. vaginalis* is only ~50–60% in routine evaluations of vaginal secretions. Direct immunofluorescent antibody staining is more sensitive (70–90%) than wet-mount examinations. *T. vaginalis* can be recovered from the urethra of both males and females and is detectable in males after prostatic massage. Culture of the parasite is the most sensitive means of detection; however, the facilities for culture are not generally available, and detection of the organism takes 3–7 days.

℞ TRICHOMONIASIS

Metronidazole, given either as a single 2-g dose or in 500-mg doses twice daily for 7 days, is usually effective. Tinidazole (a single 2-g dose) is also effective. All sexual partners must be treated concurrently to prevent reinfection, especially from asymptomatic males. In males with persistent symptomatic urethritis after therapy for nongonococcal urethritis, metronidazole therapy should be considered for possible trichomoniasis. Alternatives to metronidazole for treatment during pregnancy are not readily available, although use of 100-mg clotrimazole vaginal suppositories nightly for 2 weeks may cure some infections in pregnant women. Reinfection often accounts for apparent treatment failures, but strains of *T. vaginalis* exhibiting high-level resistance to metronidazole have been encountered. Treatment of these resistant infections with higher oral doses, parenteral doses, or concurrent oral and vaginal doses of metronidazole or with tinidazole has been successful.

FURTHER READINGS

CHEX XM et al: Cryptosporidiosis. N Engl J Med 346:1723, 2002

CDC DIVISION OF PARASITIC DISEASES. *http://www.cdc.gov/ncidod/dpd/default.htm*

DIDIER ES: Microsporidiosis: An emerging and opportunistic infection in humans and animals. Acta Trop 94:61, 2005

LEDER K et al: No correlation between clinical symptoms and *Blastocystis hominis* in immunocompetent individuals. J Gastroenterol Hepatol 20:1390, 2005

ROXSTROM-LINDQUIST K et al: Giardia immunity—an update. Trends Parasitol 22:26, 2006

VANDENBERG O et al: Clinical and microbiological features of dientamoebiasis in patients suspected of suffering from a parasitic gastrointestinal illness: A comparison of *Dientamoeba fragilis* and *Giardia lamblia* infections. Int J Infect Dis 10:255, 2006

VAN DER POL B et al: Prevalence, incidence, natural history, and response to treatment of *Trichomonas vaginalis* infection among adolescent women. J Infect Dis 192:2039, 2005

WEISS LM, SCHWARTZ DA: Microsporidiosis, in *Tropical Infectious Diseases: Principles, Pathogens and Practice*, 2d ed, RL Guerrant et al (eds). Elsevier, Philadelphia, 2006, pp 1126–1140

WEITZEL T et al: Epidemiological and clinical features of travel-associated cryptosporidiosis. Clin Microbiol Infect 12:921, 2006

YODER JS, BEACH MJ: Cryptosporidiosis surveillance—United States, 2003–2005. MMWR Surveill Summ 56:1, 2007

——— et al: Giardiasis surveillance—United States, 2003–2005. MMWR Surveill Summ 56:11, 2007

209 | Trichinella and Other Tissue Nematodes

Peter F. Weller

Nematodes are elongated, symmetric roundworms. Parasitic nematodes of medical significance may be broadly classified as either predominantly intestinal or tissue nematodes. This chapter covers trichinellosis, visceral and ocular larva migrans, cutaneous larva migrans, cerebral angiostrongyliasis, and gnathostomiasis. All are zoonotic infections caused by incidental exposure to infectious nematodes. The clinical symptoms of these infections are due largely to invasive larval stages that (except in the case of *Trichinella*) do not reach maturity in humans.

TRICHINELLOSIS

Trichinellosis develops after the ingestion of meat containing cysts of *Trichinella*—for example, pork or other meat from a carnivore. Although most infections are mild and asymptomatic, heavy infections can cause severe enteritis, periorbital edema, myositis, and (infrequently) death.

Life Cycle and Epidemiology   Eight species of *Trichinella* are recognized as causes of infection in humans. Two species are distributed worldwide: *T. spiralis*, which is found in a great variety of carnivorous and omnivorous animals, and *T. pseudospiralis*, which is found in mammals and birds.

T. nativa is present in Arctic regions and infects bears; *T. nelsoni* is found in equatorial eastern Africa, where it is common among felid predators and scavengers such as hyenas and bush pigs; and *T. britovi* is found in Europe, western Africa, and western Asia among carnivores but not among domestic swine. *T. murrelli* is present in North American game animals.

After human consumption of trichinous meat, encysted larvae are liberated by digestive acid and pepsin (Fig. 209-1). The larvae invade the small-bowel mucosa and mature into adult worms. After ~1 week, female worms release newborn larvae that migrate via the circulation to striated muscle. The larvae of all species except *T. pseudospiralis*, *T. papuae*, and *T. zimbabwensis* then encyst by inducing a radical transformation in the muscle cell architecture. Although host immune responses may help to expel intestinal adult worms, they have little effect on muscle-dwelling larvae.

Human trichinellosis is often caused by the ingestion of infected pork products and thus can occur in almost any location where the meat of domestic or wild swine is eaten. Human trichinellosis also may be acquired from the meat of other animals, including dogs (in parts of Asia and Africa), horses (in Italy and France), and bears and walruses (in northern regions). Although cattle (being herbivores) are not natural hosts of *Trichinella*, beef has been implicated in outbreaks when contaminated or adulterated with trichinous pork.

Laws that prohibit the feeding of uncooked garbage to pigs have greatly reduced the transmission of trichinellosis in the United States. About 12 cases of trichinellosis are reported annually in this country, but most mild cases probably remain undiagnosed. Recent U.S. and Canadian outbreaks have been attributable to consumption of wild game (especially bear meat) and, less frequently, of pork.

Pathogenesis and Clinical Features   Clinical symptoms of trichinellosis arise from the successive phases of parasite enteric invasion, larval migration, and muscle encystment (Fig. 209-1). Most light infections (those with <10 larvae per gram of muscle) are asymptomatic, whereas heavy infections (which can involve >50 larvae per gram of muscle) can be life-threatening. Invasion of the gut by large numbers of parasites occasionally provokes diarrhea during the first week after infection. Abdominal pain, constipation, nausea, or vomiting also may be prominent.

Symptoms due to larval migration and muscle invasion begin to appear in the second week after infection. The migrating *Trichinella* larvae provoke a marked local and systemic hypersensitivity reaction, with fever and hypereosinophilia. Periorbital and facial edema is common, as are hemorrhages in the subconjunctivae, retina, and nail beds ("splinter" hemorrhages). A maculopapular rash, headache, cough, dyspnea, or dysphagia sometimes develops. Myocarditis with tachyarrhythmias or heart failure—and, less commonly, encephalitis or pneumonitis—may develop and accounts for most deaths of patients with trichinellosis.

Upon onset of larval encystment in muscle 2–3 weeks after infection, symptoms of myositis with myalgias, muscle edema, and weakness develop, usually overlapping with the inflammatory reactions to

Larvae migrate, penetrate striated muscle, reside in "nurse-cells," and encyst,* causing:

Muscle pain, fever, periorbital edema, eosinophilia, occasional CNS or cardiac damage

Larvae are released in the stomach and mature into adults over 1–2 wks in the small bowel, causing:

Irritation and mild abdominal cramping or even diarrhea

Encysted larvae ingested in undercooked pork, boar, horse, or bear

Similar cycle (as humans) in swine or other carnivores (rats, bears, foxes, dogs, or horses)

*T. papuae, T. zimbabwensis, and T. pseudospiralis do not encyst.

FIGURE 209-1   Life cycle of Trichinella spiralis (cosmopolitan); *nelsoni* (equatorial Africa); *britovi* (Europe, western Africa, western Asia); *nativa* (Arctic); *murrelli* (North America); *papuae* (Papua New Guinea); *zimbabwensis* (Tanzania); and *pseudospiralis* (cosmopolitan). *[Reprinted from Guerrant RL et al (eds): Tropical Infectious Diseases: Principles, Pathogens and Practice, 2d ed, p 1218. © 2006, with permission from Elsevier Science.]*

migrating larvae. The most commonly involved muscle groups include the extraocular muscles; the biceps; and the muscles of the jaw, neck, lower back, and diaphragm. Peaking ~3 weeks after infection, symptoms subside only gradually during a prolonged convalescence. Uncommon infections with *T. pseudospiralis*, whose larvae do not encapsulate in muscles, elicit prolonged polymyositis-like illness.

Laboratory Findings and Diagnosis   Blood eosinophilia develops in >90% of patients with symptomatic trichinellosis and may peak at a level of >50% between 2 and 4 weeks after infection. Serum levels of muscle enzymes, including creatine phosphokinase, are elevated in most symptomatic patients. Patients should be questioned thoroughly about their consumption of pork or wild-animal meat and about illness in other individuals who ate the same meat. A presumptive clinical diagnosis can be based on fevers, eosinophilia, periorbital edema, and myalgias after a suspect meal. A rise in the titer of parasite-specific antibody, which usually does not occur until after the third week of infection, confirms the diagnosis. Alternatively, a definitive diagnosis requires surgical biopsy of at least 1 g of involved muscle; the yields are highest near tendon insertions. The fresh muscle tissue should be compressed between glass slides and examined microscopically (Fig. 209-2), because larvae may be overlooked by examination of routine histopathologic sections alone.

℞ TRICHINELLOSIS

Most lightly infected patients recover uneventfully with bed rest, antipyretics, and analgesics. Glucocorticoids like prednisone **(Table 209-1)** are beneficial for severe myositis and myocarditis. Mebendazole and albendazole are active against enteric stages of the parasite, but their efficacy against encysted larvae has not been conclusively demonstrated.

Prevention   Larvae may be killed by cooking pork until it is no longer pink or by freezing it at −15°C for 3 weeks. However, Arctic *T. nativa* larvae in walrus or bear meat are relatively resistant and may remain viable despite freezing.

VISCERAL AND OCULAR LARVA MIGRANS

Visceral larva migrans is a syndrome caused by nematodes that are normally parasitic for nonhuman host species. In humans, the nematode larvae do not develop into adult worms but instead migrate through host tissues and elicit eosinophilic inflammation. The more common form of visceral larva migrans is toxocariasis due to larvae of the canine ascarid *Toxocara canis*, less commonly to the feline ascarid *T. cati*, and even less commonly to the pig ascarid *Ascaris suum*. Rare cases with eosinophilic meningoencephalitis have been caused by the raccoon ascarid *Baylisascaris procyonis*.

Life Cycle and Epidemiology   The canine roundworm *T. canis* is distributed among dogs worldwide. Ingestion of infective eggs by dogs is followed by liberation of *Toxocara* larvae, which penetrate the gut wall and migrate intravascularly into canine tissues, where most remain in a developmentally arrested state. During pregnancy, some larvae resume migration in bitches and infect puppies prenatally (through transplacental transmission) or after birth (through suckling). Thus, in lactating bitches and puppies, larvae return to the intestinal tract and develop into adult worms, which produce eggs that are released in the feces. Humans acquire toxocariasis mainly by eating soil contaminated by puppy feces that contains infective *T. canis* eggs. Visceral larva migrans is most common among children who habitually eat dirt.

FIGURE 209-2   ***Trichinella* larva** encysted in a characteristic hyalinized capsule in striated muscle tissue. *(Photo/Wadsworth Center, New York State Department of Health. Reprinted from CDC MMWR 53:606, 2004; public domain.)*

Pathogenesis and Clinical Features   Clinical disease most commonly afflicts preschool children. After humans ingest *Toxocara* eggs, the larvae hatch and penetrate the intestinal mucosa, from which they are carried by the circulation to a wide variety of organs and tissues. The larvae invade the liver, lungs, central nervous system (CNS), and other sites, provoking intense local eosinophilic granulomatous responses. The degree of clinical illness depends on larval number and tissue distribution, reinfection, and host immune responses. Most light infections are asymptomatic and may be manifest only by blood eosinophilia. Characteristic symptoms of visceral larva migrans include fever, malaise, anorexia and weight loss, cough, wheezing, and rashes. Hepatosplenomegaly is common. These features are often accompanied by extraordinary peripheral eosinophilia, which may approach 90%. Uncommonly, seizures or behavioral disorders develop. Rare deaths are due to severe neurologic, pneumonic, or myocardial involvement.

The ocular form of the larva migrans syndrome occurs when *Toxocara* larvae invade the eye. An eosinophilic granulomatous mass, most commonly in the posterior pole of the retina, develops around the entrapped larva. The retinal lesion can mimic retinoblastoma in appearance, and mistaken diagnosis of the latter condition can lead to unnecessary enucleation. The spectrum of eye involvement also in-

TABLE 209-1	THERAPY FOR TISSUE NEMATODE INFECTIONS	
Infection	**Severity**	**Treatment**
Trichinellosis	Mild	Supportive
	Moderate	Albendazole (400 mg bid × 8–14 days)
		or
		Mebendazole (200–400 mg tid × 3 days, then 400 mg tid × 8–14 days)
	Severe	Add glucocorticoids (e.g., prednisone, 1 mg/kg qd × 5 days)
Visceral larva migrans	Mild to moderate	Supportive
	Severe	Glucocorticoids (as above)
	Ocular	Not fully defined; albendazole (800 mg bid for adults, 400 mg bid for children) with glucocorticoids × 5–20 days has been effective
Cutaneous larva migrans		Ivermectin (single dose, 200 μg/kg)
		or
		Albendazole (200 mg bid × 3 days)
Angiostrongyliasis	Mild to moderate	Supportive
	Severe	Glucocorticoids (as above)
Gnathostomiasis		Ivermectin (200 μg/kg per day × 2 days)
		or
		Albendazole (400 mg bid × 21 days)

1318 cludes endophthalmitis, uveitis, and chorioretinitis. Unilateral visual disturbances, strabismus, and eye pain are the most common presenting symptoms. In contrast to visceral larva migrans, ocular toxocariasis usually develops in older children or young adults with no history of pica; these patients seldom have eosinophilia or visceral manifestations.

Diagnosis   In addition to eosinophilia, leukocytosis and hypergammaglobulinemia may be evident. Transient pulmonary infiltrates are apparent on chest x-rays of about half of patients with symptoms of pneumonitis. The clinical diagnosis can be confirmed by an enzyme-linked immunosorbent assay for toxocaral antibodies. Stool examination for parasite eggs, while important in the evaluation of unexplained eosinophilia, is worthless for toxocariasis, since the larvae do not develop into egg-producing adults in humans.

℞ VISCERAL AND OCULAR LARVA MIGRANS

The vast majority of *Toxocara* infections are self-limited and resolve without specific therapy. In patients with severe myocardial, CNS, or pulmonary involvement, glucocorticoids may be employed to reduce inflammatory complications. Available anthelmintic drugs, including mebendazole and albendazole, have not been shown conclusively to alter the course of larva migrans. Control measures include prohibiting dog excreta in public parks and playgrounds, deworming dogs, and preventing pica in children. Treatment of ocular disease is not fully defined, but the administration of albendazole in conjunction with glucocorticoids has been effective (Table 209-1).

CUTANEOUS LARVA MIGRANS

Cutaneous larva migrans ("creeping eruption") is a serpiginous skin eruption caused by burrowing larvae of animal hookworms, usually the dog and cat hookworm *Ancylostoma braziliense*. The larvae hatch from eggs passed in dog and cat feces and mature in the soil. Humans become infected after skin contact with soil in areas frequented by dogs and cats, such as areas underneath house porches. Cutaneous larva migrans is prevalent among children and travelers in regions with warm humid climates, including the southeastern United States.

After larvae penetrate the skin, erythematous lesions form along the tortuous tracks of their migration through the dermal-epidermal junction; the larvae advance several centimeters in a day. The intensely pruritic lesions may occur anywhere on the body and can be numerous if the patient has lain on the ground. Vesicles and bullae may form later. The animal hookworm larvae do not mature in humans and, without treatment, will die after an interval ranging from weeks to a couple of months, with resolution of skin lesions. The diagnosis is made on clinical grounds. Skin biopsies only rarely detect diagnostic larvae. Symptoms can be alleviated by ivermectin or albendazole (Table 209-1).

ANGIOSTRONGYLIASIS

Angiostrongylus cantonensis, the rat lungworm, is the most common cause of human eosinophilic meningitis (**Fig. 209-3**).

Life Cycle and Epidemiology   This infection occurs principally in Southeast Asia and the Pacific Basin but has spread to other areas of the world. *A. cantonensis* larvae produced by adult worms in the rat lung migrate to the gastrointestinal tract and are expelled with the feces. They develop into infective larvae in land snails and slugs. Humans acquire the infection by ingesting raw infected mollusks; vegetables contaminated by mollusk slime; or crabs, freshwater shrimp, and certain marine fish that have themselves eaten infected mollusks. The larvae then migrate to the brain.

Pathogenesis and Clinical Features   The parasites eventually die in the CNS, but not before initiating pathologic conse-

quences that, in heavy infections, can result in permanent neurologic sequelae or death. Migrating larvae cause marked local eosinophilic inflammation and hemorrhage, with subsequent necrosis and granuloma formation around dying worms. Clinical symptoms develop 2–35 days after the ingestion of larvae. Patients usually present with an insidious or abrupt excruciating frontal, occipital, or bitemporal headache. Neck stiffness, nausea and vomiting, and paresthesias are also common. Fever, cranial and extraocular nerve palsies, seizures, paralysis, and lethargy are uncommon.

Laboratory Findings   Examination of cerebrospinal fluid (CSF) is mandatory in suspected cases and usually reveals an elevated opening pressure, a white blood cell count of 150–2000/μL, and an eosinophilic pleocytosis of >20%. The protein concentration is usually elevated and the glucose level normal. The larvae of *A. cantonensis* are only rarely seen in CSF. Peripheral-blood eosinophilia may be mild. The diagnosis is generally based on the clinical presentation of eosinophilic meningitis together with a compatible epidemiologic history.

℞ ANGIOSTRONGYLIASIS

Specific chemotherapy is not of benefit in angiostrongyliasis; larvicidal agents may exacerbate inflammatory brain lesions. Management consists of supportive measures, including the administration of analgesics, sedatives, and—in severe cases—glucocorticoids (Table 209-1). Repeated lumbar punctures with removal of CSF can relieve symptoms. In most patients, cerebral angiostrongyliasis has a self-limited course, and recovery is complete. The infection may be prevented by adequately cooking snails, crabs, and prawns and inspecting vegetables for mollusk infestation. Other parasitic or fungal causes of eosinophilic meningitis in endemic areas may include gnathostomiasis (see below), paragonimiasis (Chap. 212), schistosomiasis (Chap. 212), neurocysticercosis (Chap. 213), and coccidioidomycosis (Chap. 193).

GNATHOSTOMIASIS

Infection of human tissues with larvae of *Gnathostoma spinigerum* can cause eosinophilic meningoencephalitis, migratory cutaneous swellings, or invasive masses of the eye and visceral organs.

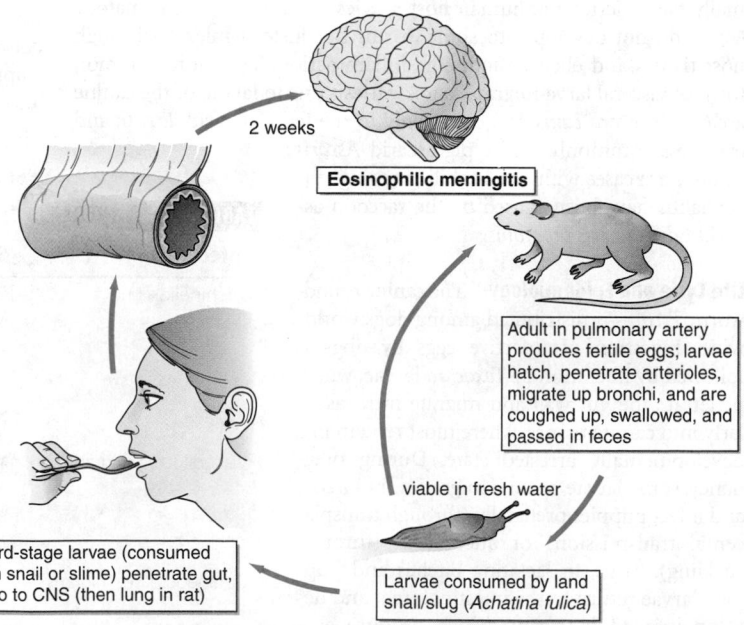

2 weeks

Eosinophilic meningitis

Adult in pulmonary artery produces fertile eggs; larvae hatch, penetrate arterioles, migrate up bronchi, and are coughed up, swallowed, and passed in feces

viable in fresh water

Larvae consumed by land snail/slug (*Achatina fulica*)

3rd-stage larvae (consumed in snail or slime) penetrate gut, go to CNS (then lung in rat)

FIGURE 209-3   Life cycle of *Angiostrongylus cantonensis* (rat lung worm). Also found in Southeast Asia, Pacific Islands, Cuba, Australia, Japan, China, Mauritius, and U.S. ports. [*Reprinted from Guerrant RL et al (eds): Tropical Infectious Diseases: Principles, Pathogens and Practice, 2d ed, p 1225. © 2006, with permission from Elsevier Science.*]

PART 7

Infectious Diseases

Life Cycle and Epidemiology Human gnathostomiasis occurs in many countries and is notably endemic in Southeast Asia and parts of China and Japan. In nature, the mature adult worms parasitize the gastrointestinal tract of dogs and cats. First-stage larvae hatch from eggs passed into water and are ingested by *Cyclops* species (water fleas). Infective third-stage larvae develop in the flesh of many animal species (including fish, frogs, eels, snakes, chickens, and ducks) that have eaten either infected *Cyclops* or another infected second intermediate host. Humans typically acquire the infection by eating raw or undercooked fish or poultry. Raw fish dishes, such as *som fak* in Thailand and *sashimi* in Japan, account for many cases of human gnathostomiasis. Some cases in Thailand result from the local practice of applying frog or snake flesh as a poultice.

Pathogenesis and Clinical Features Clinical symptoms are due to the aberrant migration of a single larva into cutaneous, visceral, neural, or ocular tissues. After invasion, larval migration may cause local inflammation, with pain, cough, or hematuria accompanied by fever and eosinophilia. Painful, itchy, migratory swellings may develop in the skin, particularly in the distal extremities or periorbital area. Cutaneous swellings usually last ~1 week but often recur intermittently over many years. Larval invasion of the eye can provoke a sight-threatening inflammatory response. Invasion of the CNS results in eosinophilic meningitis with myeloencephalitis, a serious complication due to ascending larval migration along a large nerve track. Patients characteristically present with agonizing radicular pain and paresthesias in the trunk or a limb, which are followed shortly by paraplegia. Cerebral involvement, with focal hemorrhages and tissue destruction, is often fatal.

Diagnosis and Treatment Cutaneous migratory swellings with marked peripheral eosinophilia, supported by an appropriate geographic and dietary history, generally constitute an adequate basis for a clinical diagnosis of gnathostomiasis. However, patients may present with ocular or cerebrospinal involvement without antecedent cutaneous swellings. In the latter case, eosinophilic pleocytosis is demonstrable (usually along with hemorrhagic or xanthochromic CSF), but worms are almost never recovered from CSF. Surgical removal of the parasite from subcutaneous or ocular tissue, though rarely feasible, is both diagnostic and therapeutic. Albendazole or ivermectin may be helpful (Table 209-1). At present, cerebrospinal involvement is managed with supportive measures and generally with a course of glucocorticoids. Gnathostomiasis can be prevented by adequate cooking of fish and poultry in endemic areas.

FURTHER READINGS

BARISANI-ASENBAUER T et al: Treatment of ocular toxocariasis with albendazole. J Ocul Pharmacol Ther 17:287, 2001

BOUCHARD O et al: Cutaneous larva migrans in travelers: A prospective study, with assessment of therapy with ivermectin. Clin Infect Dis 31:493, 2000

CDC DIVISION OF PARASITIC DISEASES. *www.cdc.gov/ncidod/dpd/default.htm*

CIANFERONI A et al: Visceral larva migrans associated with earthworm ingestion: Clinical evolution in an adolescent patient. Pediatrics 117:e336, 2006

LIGON BL: Gnathostomiasis: A review of a previously localized zoonosis now crossing numerous geographical boundaries. Semin Pediatr Infect Dis 16:137, 2005

MAGANA M et al: Gnathostomiasis: Clinicopathologic study. Am J Dermatopathol 26:91, 2004

MENARD A et al: Imported cutaneous gnathostomiasis: Report of five cases. Trans R Soc Trop Med Hyg 97:200, 2003

PULJIZ I et al: Electrocardiographic changes in trichinellosis: A retrospective study of 154 patients. Ann Trop Med Parasitol 99:403, 2005

SAKAI S et al: Pulmonary lesions associated with visceral larva migrans due to *Ascaris suum* or *Toxocara canis*: Imaging of six cases. AJR Am J Roentgenol 186:1697, 2006

SLOM TJ et al: An outbreak of eosinophilic meningitis caused by *Angiostrongylus cantonensis* in travelers returning from the Caribbean. N Engl J Med 346:668, 2002

TSAI HC et al: Outbreak of eosinophilic meningitis associated with drinking raw vegetable juice in southern Taiwan. Am J Trop Med Hyg 71:222, 2004

210 Intestinal Nematodes
Peter F. Weller, Thomas B. Nutman

More than a billion persons worldwide are infected with one or more species of intestinal nematodes. Table 210-1 summarizes biologic and clinical features of infections due to the major intestinal parasitic nematodes. These parasites are most common in regions with poor fecal sanitation, particularly in resource-poor countries in the tropics and subtropics, but they have also been seen with increasing frequency among immigrants and refugees to resource-rich countries. Although nematode infections are not usually fatal, they contribute to malnutrition and diminished work capacity. It is interesting that these helminth infections may protect some individuals from allergic disease. Humans may on occasion be infected with nematode parasites that ordinarily infect animals; these zoonotic infections produce diseases such as trichostrongyliasis, anisakiasis, capillariasis, and abdominal angiostrongyliasis.

Intestinal nematodes are roundworms; they range in length from 1 mm to many centimeters when mature (Table 210-1). Their life cycles are complex and highly varied; some species, including *Strongyloides stercoralis* and *Enterobius vermicularis*, can be transmitted directly from person to person, while others, such as *Ascaris lumbricoides*, *Necator americanus*, and *Ancylostoma duodenale*, require a soil phase for development. Because most helminth parasites do not self-replicate, the acquisition of a heavy burden of adult worms requires repeated exposure to the parasite in its infectious stage, whether larva or egg. Hence, clinical disease, as opposed to asymptomatic infection, generally develops only with prolonged residence in an endemic area. In persons with marginal nutrition, intestinal helminth infections may impair growth and development. Eosinophilia and elevated serum IgE levels are features of many helminthic infections and, when unexplained, should always prompt a search for occult helminthiasis. Significant protective immunity to intestinal nematodes appears not to develop in humans, although mechanisms of parasite immune evasion and host immune responses to these infections have not been elucidated in detail.

ASCARIASIS

A. lumbricoides is the largest intestinal nematode parasite of humans, reaching up to 40 cm in length. Most infected individuals have low worm burdens and are asymptomatic. Clinical disease arises from larval migration in the lungs or effects of the adult worms in the intestines.

Life Cycle Adult worms live in the lumen of the small intestine. Mature female *Ascaris* worms are extraordinarily fecund, each producing up to 240,000 eggs a day, which pass with the feces. Ascarid eggs, which are remarkably resistant to environmental stresses, become infective after several weeks of maturation in the soil and can remain infective for years. After infective eggs are swallowed, larvae hatched in the intestine invade the mucosa, migrate through the circulation to the lungs, break into the alveoli, ascend the bronchial tree, and return via

TABLE 210-1 MAJOR HUMAN INTESTINAL PARASITIC NEMATODES

Feature	Ascaris lumbricoides (Roundworm)	Necator americanus, Ancylostoma duodenale (Hookworm)	Strongyloides stercoralis	Trichuris trichiura (Whipworm)	Enterobius vermicularis (Pinworm)
			Parasitic Nematode		
Global prevalence in humans (millions)	1221	740	50	795	300
Endemic areas	Worldwide	Hot, humid regions	Hot, humid regions	Worldwide	Worldwide
Infective stage	Egg	Filariform larva	Filariform larva	Egg	Egg
Route of infection	Oral	Percutaneous	Percutaneous or autoinfection	Oral	Oral
Gastrointestinal location of worms	Jejunal lumen	Jejunal mucosa	Small-bowel mucosa	Cecum, colonic mucosa	Cecum, appendix
Adult worm size	15–40 cm	7–12 mm	2 mm	30–50 mm	8–13 mm (female)
Pulmonary passage of larvae	Yes	Yes	Yes	No	No
Incubation period^a (days)	60–75	40–100	17–28	70–90	35–45
Longevity	1 y	N. americanus: 2–5 y A. duodenale: 6–8 y	Decades (owing to autoinfection)	5 y	2 months
Fecundity (eggs/day/worm)	240,000	N. americanus: 4000–10,000 A. duodenale: 10,000–25,000	5000–10,000	3000–7000	2000
Principal symptoms	Rarely gastrointestinal or biliary obstruction	Iron-deficiency anemia in heavy infection	Gastrointestinal symptoms; malabsorption or sepsis in hyperinfection	Gastrointestinal symptoms, anemia	Perianal pruritus
Diagnostic stage	Eggs in stool	Eggs in fresh stool, larvae in old stool	Larvae in stool or duodenal aspirate; sputum in hyperinfection	Eggs in stool	Eggs from perianal skin on cellulose acetate tape
Treatment	Mebendazole Albendazole Pyrantel pamoate Ivermectin	Mebendazole Pyrantel pamoate Albendazole	1. Ivermectin 2. Albendazole	Mebendazole Albendazole Ivermectin	Mebendazole Pyrantel pamoate Albendazole

^{a}Time from infection to egg production by mature female worm.

swallowing to the small intestine, where they develop into adult worms. Between 2 and 3 months elapse between initial infection and egg production. Adult worms live for 1–2 years.

Epidemiology *Ascaris* is widely distributed in tropical and subtropical regions as well as in other humid areas, including the rural southeastern United States. Transmission typically occurs through fecally contaminated soil and is due either to a lack of sanitary facilities or to the use of human feces as fertilizer. With their propensity for hand-to-mouth fecal carriage, younger children are most affected. Infection outside endemic areas, though uncommon, can occur when eggs on transported vegetables are ingested.

Clinical Features During the lung phase of larval migration, ~9–12 days after egg ingestion, patients may develop an irritating nonproductive cough and burning substernal discomfort that is aggravated by coughing or deep inspiration. Dyspnea and blood-tinged sputum are less common. Fever is usually reported. Eosinophilia develops during this symptomatic phase and subsides slowly over weeks. Chest x-rays may reveal evidence of eosinophilic pneumonitis (Löffler's syndrome), with rounded infiltrates a few millimeters to several centimeters in size. These infiltrates may be transient and intermittent, clearing after several weeks. Where there is seasonal transmission of the parasite, seasonal pneumonitis with eosinophilia may develop in previously infected and sensitized hosts.

In established infections, adult worms in the small intestine usually cause no symptoms. In heavy infections, particularly in children, a large bolus of entangled worms can cause pain and small-bowel obstruction, sometimes complicated by perforation, intussusception, or volvulus. Single worms may cause disease when they migrate into aberrant sites. A large worm can enter and occlude the biliary tree, causing biliary colic, cholecystitis, cholangitis, pancreatitis, or (rarely) intrahepatic abscesses. Migration of an adult worm up the esophagus can provoke coughing and oral expulsion of the worm. In highly endemic areas, intestinal and biliary ascariasis can rival acute appendicitis and gallstones as causes of surgical acute abdomen.

Laboratory Findings Most cases of ascariasis can be diagnosed by microscopic detection of characteristic *Ascaris* eggs (65 by 45 μm) in fecal samples. Occasionally, patients present after passing an adult worm—identifiable by its large size and smooth cream-colored surface—in the stool or through the mouth or nose. During the early transpulmonary migratory phase, when eosinophilic pneumonitis occurs, larvae can be found in sputum or gastric aspirates before diagnostic eggs appear in the stool. The eosinophilia that is prominent during this early stage usually decreases to minimal levels in established infection. Adult worms may be visualized, occasionally serendipitously, on contrast studies of the gastrointestinal tract. A plain abdominal film may reveal masses of worms in gas-filled loops of bowel in patients with intestinal obstruction. Pancreaticobiliary worms can be detected by ultrasound and endoscopic retrograde cholangiopancreatography; the latter method also has been used to extract biliary *Ascaris* worms.

℞ **ASCARIASIS**

Ascariasis should always be treated to prevent potentially serious complications. Albendazole (400 mg once), mebendazole (500 mg once), or ivermectin (150–200 μg/kg once) is effective. These medications are contraindicated in pregnancy, however. Pyrantel pamoate (11 mg/kg once; maximum, 1 g) is safe in pregnancy. Mild diarrhea and abdominal pain are uncommon side effects of these agents. Partial intestinal obstruction should be managed with nasogastric suction, IV fluid administration, and instillation of piperazine through the nasogastric tube, but complete obstruction and its severe complications require immediate surgical intervention.

HOOKWORM

Two hookworm species (*A. duodenale* and *N. americanus*) are responsible for human infections. Most infected individuals are asymptomatic. Hookworm disease develops from a combination of factors—a heavy worm burden, a prolonged duration of infection, and an inadequate iron intake—and results in iron-deficiency anemia and, on occasion, hypoproteinemia.

Life Cycle Adult hookworms, which are ~1 cm long, use buccal teeth (*Ancylostoma*) or cutting plates (*Necator*) to attach to the small-bowel mucosa and suck blood (0.2 mL/d per *Ancylostoma* adult) and interstitial fluid. The adult hookworms produce thousands of eggs daily. The eggs are deposited with feces in soil, where rhabditiform larvae hatch and develop over a 1-week period into infectious filariform larvae. Infective larvae penetrate the skin and reach the lungs by way of the bloodstream. There they invade alveoli and ascend the airways before being swallowed and reaching the small intestine. The prepatent period from skin invasion to appearance of eggs in the feces is ~6–8 weeks, but it may be longer with *A. duodenale*. Larvae of *A. duodenale*, if swallowed, can survive and develop directly in the intestinal mucosa. Adult hookworms may survive over a decade but usually live ~6–8 years for *A. duodenale* and 2–5 years for *N. americanus*.

Epidemiology *A. duodenale* is prevalent in southern Europe, North Africa, and northern Asia, and *N. americanus* is the predominant species in the western hemisphere and equatorial Africa. The two species overlap in many tropical regions, particularly Southeast Asia. In most areas, older children have the highest incidence and greatest intensity of hookworm infection. In rural areas where fields are fertilized with human feces, older working adults also may be heavily affected.

Clinical Features Most hookworm infections are asymptomatic. Infective larvae may provoke pruritic maculopapular dermatitis ("ground itch") at the site of skin penetration as well as serpiginous tracks of subcutaneous migration (similar to those of cutaneous larva migrans; Chap. 209) in previously sensitized hosts. Larvae migrating through the lungs occasionally cause mild transient pneumonitis, but this condition develops less frequently in hookworm infection than in ascariasis. In the early intestinal phase, infected persons may develop epigastric pain (often with postprandial accentuation), inflammatory diarrhea, or other abdominal symptoms accompanied by eosinophilia. The major consequence of chronic hookworm infection is iron deficiency. Symptoms are minimal if iron intake is adequate, but marginally nourished individuals develop symptoms of progressive iron-deficiency anemia and hypoproteinemia, including weakness and shortness of breath.

Laboratory Findings The diagnosis is established by the finding of characteristic 40- by 60-μm oval hookworm eggs in the feces. Stool-concentration procedures may be required to detect light infections. Eggs of the two species are indistinguishable by light microscopy. In a stool sample that is not fresh, the eggs may have hatched to release rhabditiform larvae, which need to be differentiated from those of *S. stercoralis*. Hypochromic microcytic anemia, occasionally with eosinophilia or hypoalbuminemia, is characteristic of hookworm disease.

℞ HOOKWORM INFECTION

Hookworm infection can be eradicated with several safe and highly effective anthelmintic drugs, including albendazole (400 mg once), mebendazole (500 mg once), and pyrantel pamoate (11 mg/kg for 3 days). Mild iron-deficiency anemia can often be treated with oral iron alone. Severe hookworm

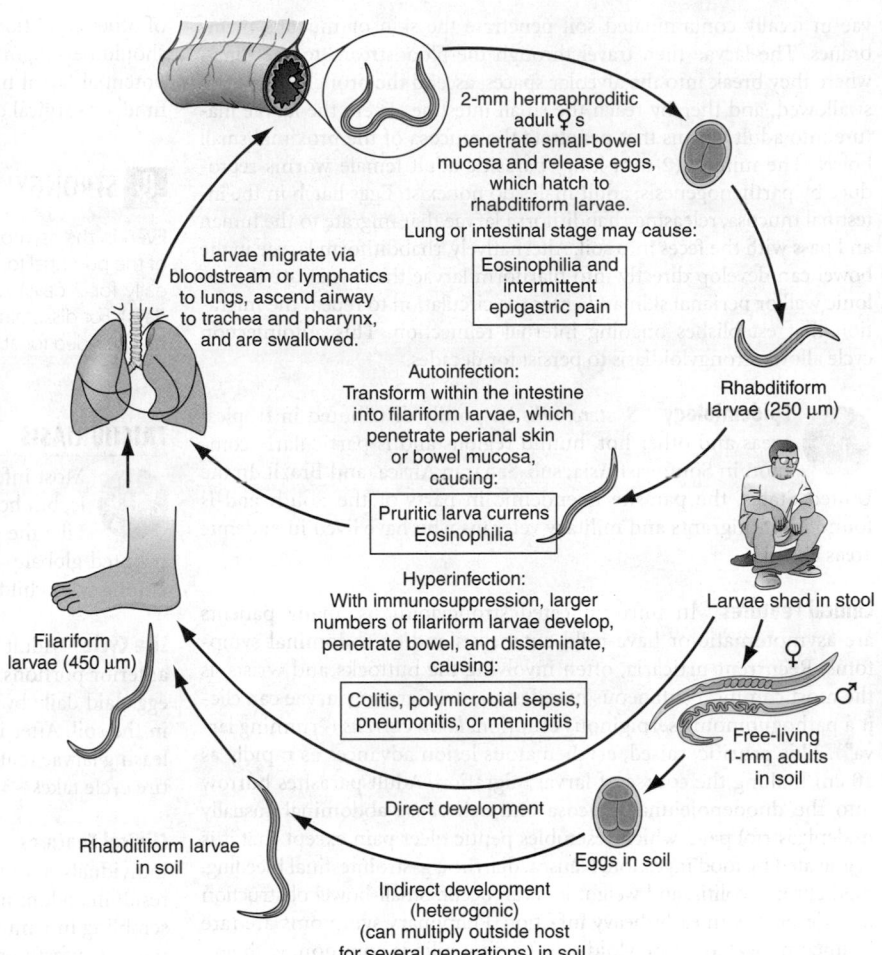

FIGURE 210-1 Life cycle of *Strongyloides stercoralis*. [*Adapted from Guerrant RL et al (eds): Tropical Infectious Diseases: Principles, Pathogens and Practice, 2d ed, p 1276. © 2006, with permission from Elsevier Science.*]

disease with protein loss and malabsorption necessitates nutritional support and oral iron replacement along with deworming.

Ancylostoma caninum and Ancylostoma braziliense *A. caninum*, the canine hookworm, has been identified as a cause of human eosinophilic enteritis, especially in northeastern Australia. In this zoonotic infection, adult hookworms attach to the small intestine (where they may be visualized by endoscopy) and elicit abdominal pain and intense local eosinophilia. Treatment with mebendazole (100 mg twice daily for 3 days) or albendazole (400 mg once) or endoscopic removal is effective. Both of these animal hookworm species can cause cutaneous larva migrans ("creeping eruption"; Chap. 209).

STRONGYLOIDIASIS

S. stercoralis is distinguished by its ability—unusual among helminths—to replicate in the human host. This capacity permits ongoing cycles of autoinfection as infective larvae are internally produced. Strongyloidiasis can thus persist for decades without further exposure of the host to exogenous infective larvae. In immunocompromised hosts, large numbers of invasive *Strongyloides* larvae can disseminate widely and can be fatal.

Life Cycle In addition to a parasitic cycle of development, *Strongyloides* can undergo a free-living cycle of development in the soil (Fig. 210-1). This adaptability facilitates the parasite's survival in the absence of mammalian hosts. Rhabditiform larvae passed in feces can transform into infectious filariform larvae either directly or after a free-living phase of development. Humans acquire strongyloidiasis when filariform larvae in fecally contaminated soil penetrate the skin or mucous membranes. The larvae then travel through the bloodstream to the lungs, where they break into the alveolar spaces, ascend the bronchial tree, are swallowed, and thereby reach the small intestine. There the larvae mature into adult worms that penetrate the mucosa of the proximal small bowel. The minute (2-mm-long) parasitic adult female worms reproduce by parthenogenesis; adult males do not exist. Eggs hatch in the intestinal mucosa, releasing rhabditiform larvae that migrate to the lumen and pass with the feces into soil. Alternatively, rhabditiform larvae in the bowel can develop directly into filariform larvae that penetrate the colonic wall or perianal skin and enter the circulation to repeat the migration that establishes ongoing internal reinfection. This autoinfection cycle allows strongyloidiasis to persist for decades.

 Epidemiology *S. stercoralis* is spottily distributed in tropical areas and other hot, humid regions and is particularly common in Southeast Asia, sub-Saharan Africa, and Brazil. In the United States, the parasite is endemic in parts of the South and is found in immigrants and military veterans who have lived in endemic areas abroad.

Clinical Features In uncomplicated strongyloidiasis, many patients are asymptomatic or have mild cutaneous and/or abdominal symptoms. Recurrent urticaria, often involving the buttocks and wrists, is the most common cutaneous manifestation. Migrating larvae can elicit a pathognomonic serpiginous eruption, *larva currens* ("running larva"). This pruritic, raised, erythematous lesion advances as rapidly as 10 cm/h along the course of larval migration. Adult parasites burrow into the duodenojejunal mucosa and can cause abdominal (usually midepigastric) pain, which resembles peptic ulcer pain except that it is aggravated by food ingestion. Nausea, diarrhea, gastrointestinal bleeding, mild chronic colitis, and weight loss can occur. Small-bowel obstruction may develop with early, heavy infection. Pulmonary symptoms are rare in uncomplicated strongyloidiasis. Eosinophilia is common, with levels fluctuating over time.

The ongoing autoinfection cycle of strongyloidiasis is normally contained by unknown factors of the host's immune system. Abrogation of host immunity, especially with glucocorticoid therapy and much less commonly with other immunosuppressive medications, leads to hyperinfection, with the generation of large numbers of filariform larvae. Colitis, enteritis, or malabsorption may develop. In disseminated strongyloidiasis, larvae may invade not only gastrointestinal tissues and the lungs but also the central nervous system, peritoneum, liver, and kidneys. Moreover, bacteremia may develop because of the passage of enteric flora through disrupted mucosal barriers. Gram-negative sepsis, pneumonia, or meningitis may complicate or dominate the clinical course. Eosinophilia is often absent in severely infected patients. Disseminated strongyloidiasis, particularly in patients with unsuspected infection who are given glucocorticoids, can be fatal. Strongyloidiasis is a frequent complication of infection with human T cell lymphotropic virus type I, but disseminated strongyloidiasis is not common among patients infected with HIV.

Diagnosis In uncomplicated strongyloidiasis, the finding of rhabditiform larvae in feces is diagnostic. Rhabditiform larvae are ~250 μm long, with a short buccal cavity that distinguishes them from hookworm larvae. In uncomplicated infections, few larvae are passed and single stool examinations detect only about one-third of cases. Serial examinations and the use of the agar plate detection method improve the sensitivity of stool diagnosis. In uncomplicated strongyloidiasis (but not in hyperinfection), stool examinations may be repeatedly negative. *Strongyloides* larvae may also be found by sampling of the duodenojejunal contents by aspiration or biopsy. An enzyme-linked immunosorbent assay for serum antibodies to antigens of *Strongyloides* is a sensitive method of diagnosing uncomplicated infections. Such serologic testing should be performed for patients whose geographic histories indicate potential exposure, especially those who exhibit eosinophilia and/or are candidates for glucocorticoid treatment

of other conditions. In disseminated strongyloidiasis, filariform larvae should be sought in stool as well as in samples obtained from sites of potential larval migration, including sputum, bronchoalveolar lavage fluid, or surgical drainage fluid.

 ## STRONGYLOIDIASIS

Even in the asymptomatic state, strongyloidiasis must be treated because of the potential for subsequent fatal hyperinfection. Ivermectin (200 μg/kg daily for 2 days) is more effective than albendazole (400 mg daily for 3 days). For disseminated strongyloidiasis, treatment with ivermectin should be extended for at least 5–7 days or until the parasites are eradicated.

TRICHURIASIS

Most infections with the *Trichuris trichiura* are asymptomatic, but heavy infections may cause gastrointestinal symptoms. Like the other soil-transmitted helminths, whipworm is distributed globally in the tropics and subtropics and is most common among poor children from resource-poor regions of the world.

Life Cycle Adult *Trichuris* worms reside in the colon and cecum, the anterior portions threaded into the superficial mucosa. Thousands of eggs laid daily by adult female worms pass with the feces and mature in the soil. After ingestion, infective eggs hatch in the duodenum, releasing larvae that mature before migrating to the large bowel. The entire cycle takes ~3 months, and adult worms may live for several years.

Clinical Features Tissue reactions to *Trichuris* are mild. Most infected individuals have no symptoms or eosinophilia. Heavy infections may result in abdominal pain, anorexia, and bloody or mucoid diarrhea resembling inflammatory bowel disease. Rectal prolapse can result from massive infections in children, who often suffer from malnourishment and other diarrheal illnesses. Moderately heavy *Trichuris* burdens also contribute to growth retardation.

Diagnosis and Treatment The characteristic 50- by 20-μm lemon-shaped *Trichuris* eggs are readily detected on stool examination. Adult worms, which are 3–5 cm long, are occasionally seen on proctoscopy. Mebendazole (500 mg once) or albendazole (400 mg daily for 3 doses) is safe and effective for treatment. Ivermectin (200 μg/kg daily for 3 doses) is also safe but is not quite as efficacious as the benzimidazoles.

ENTEROBIASIS (PINWORM)

E. vermicularis is more common in temperate countries than in the tropics. In the United States, ~40 million persons are infected with pinworms, with a disproportionate number of cases among children.

Life Cycle and Epidemiology *Enterobius* adult worms are ~1 cm long and dwell in the cecum. Gravid female worms migrate nocturnally into the perianal region and release up to 10,000 immature eggs each. The eggs become infective within hours and are transmitted by hand-to-mouth passage. From ingested eggs, larvae hatch and mature into adults. This life cycle takes ~1 month, and adult worms survive for ~2 months. Self-infection results from perianal scratching and transport of infective eggs on the hands or under the nails to the mouth. Because of the ease of person-to-person spread, pinworm infections are common among family members.

Clinical Features Most pinworm infections are asymptomatic. Perianal pruritus is the cardinal symptom. The itching, which is often worse at night as a result of the nocturnal migration of the female worms, may lead to excoriation and bacterial superinfection. Heavy infections have been claimed to cause abdominal pain and weight loss. On rare occasions, pinworms invade the female genital tract, causing vulvovaginitis and pelvic or peritoneal granulomas. Eosinophilia is uncommon.

Diagnosis   Since pinworm eggs are not released in feces, the diagnosis cannot be made by conventional fecal ova and parasites tests. Instead, eggs are detected by the application of clear cellulose acetate tape to the perianal region in the morning. After the tape is transferred to a slide, microscopic examination will detect pinworm eggs, which are oval, measure 55 by 25 μm, and are flattened along one side.

℞ ENTEROBIASIS

Infected children and adults should be treated with mebendazole (100 mg once), albendazole (400 mg once), or pyrantel pamoate (11 mg/kg once; maximum, 1 g), with the same treatment repeated after 2 weeks. Treatment of household members is advocated to eliminate asymptomatic reservoirs of potential reinfection.

TRICHOSTRONGYLIASIS

Trichostrongylus species, which are normally parasites of herbivorous animals, occasionally infect humans, particularly in Asia and Africa. Humans acquire the infection by accidentally ingesting *Trichostrongylus* larvae on contaminated leafy vegetables. The larvae do not migrate in humans but mature directly into adult worms in the small bowel. These worms ingest far less blood than hookworms; most infected persons are asymptomatic, but heavy infections may give rise to mild anemia and eosinophilia. *Trichostrongylus* eggs in stool examinations resemble those of hookworms but are larger (85 by 115 μm). Treatment consists of mebendazole or albendazole (Chap. 201).

ANISAKIASIS

Anisakiasis is a gastrointestinal infection caused by the accidental ingestion in uncooked saltwater fish of nematode larvae belonging to the family Anisakidae. The incidence of anisakiasis in the United States has increased as a result of the growing popularity of raw fish dishes. Most cases occur in Japan, the Netherlands, and Chile, where raw fish—sashimi, pickled green herring, and ceviche, respectively—are national culinary staples. Anisakid nematodes parasitize large sea mammals such as whales, dolphins, and seals. As part of a complex parasitic life cycle involving marine food chains, infectious larvae migrate to the musculature of a variety of fish. Both *Anisakis simplex* and *Pseudoterranova decipiens* have been implicated in human anisakiasis, but an identical gastric syndrome may be caused by the red larvae of eustrongylid parasites of fish-eating birds.

When humans consume infected raw fish, live larvae may be coughed up within 48 h. Alternatively, larvae may immediately penetrate the mucosa of the stomach. Within hours, violent upper abdominal pain accompanied by nausea and occasionally vomiting ensues, mimicking an acute abdomen. The diagnosis can be established by direct visualization on upper endoscopy, outlining of the worm by contrast radiographic studies, or histopathologic examination of extracted tissue. Extraction of the burrowing larvae during endoscopy is curative. In addition, larvae may pass to the small bowel, where they penetrate the mucosa and provoke a vigorous eosinophilic granulomatous response. Symptoms may appear 1–2 weeks after the infective meal, with intermittent abdominal pain, diarrhea, nausea, and fever resembling the manifestations of Crohn's disease. The diagnosis may be suggested by barium studies and confirmed by curative surgical resection of a granuloma in which the worm is embedded. Anisakid eggs are not found in the stool, since the larvae do not mature in humans. Anisakid larvae in saltwater fish are killed by cooking to 60°C, freezing at –20°C

for 3 days, or commercial blast freezing, but not usually by salting, marinating, or cold smoking. No medical treatment is available; surgical or endoscopic removal should be undertaken.

CAPILLARIASIS

Intestinal capillariasis is caused by ingestion of raw fish infected with *Capillaria philippinensis*. Subsequent autoinfection can lead to a severe wasting syndrome. The disease occurs in the Philippines and Thailand and, on occasion, elsewhere in Asia. The natural cycle of *C. philippinensis* involves fish from fresh and brackish water. When humans eat infected raw fish, the larvae mature in the intestine into adult worms, which produce invasive larvae that cause intestinal inflammation and villus loss. Capillariasis has an insidious onset with nonspecific abdominal pain and watery diarrhea. If untreated, progressive autoinfection can lead to protein-losing enteropathy and severe malabsorption and ultimately to death from cachexia, cardiac failure, or superinfection. The diagnosis is established by identification of the characteristic peanut-shaped (20- by 40-μm) eggs on stool examination. Severely ill patients require hospitalization and supportive therapy in addition to prolonged anthelmintic treatment with mebendazole or albendazole (Chap. 201).

ABDOMINAL ANGIOSTRONGYLIASIS

Abdominal angiostrongyliasis is found in Latin America and Africa. The zoonotic parasite *Angiostrongylus costaricensis* causes eosinophilic ileocolitis after the ingestion of contaminated vegetation. *A. costaricensis* normally parasitizes the cotton rat and other rodents, with slugs and snails serving as intermediate hosts. Humans become infected by accidentally ingesting infective larvae in mollusk slime deposited on fruits and vegetables; children are at highest risk. The larvae penetrate the gut wall and migrate to the mesenteric artery, where they develop into adult worms. Eggs deposited in the gut wall provoke an intense eosinophilic granulomatous reaction, and adult worms may cause mesenteric arteritis, thrombosis, or frank bowel infarction. Symptoms may mimic those of appendicitis, including abdominal pain and tenderness, fever, vomiting, and a palpable mass in the right iliac fossa. Leukocytosis and eosinophilia are prominent. A barium enema may reveal ileocecal-filling defects, but a definitive diagnosis is usually made surgically with partial bowel resection. Pathologic study reveals a thickened bowel wall with eosinophilic granulomas surrounding the *Angiostrongylus* eggs. In nonsurgical cases, the diagnosis rests solely on clinical grounds because larvae and eggs cannot be detected in the stool. Medical therapy for abdominal angiostrongyliasis (mebendazole, thiabendazole; Chap. 201) is of uncertain efficacy. Careful observation and surgical resection for severe symptoms are the mainstays of treatment.

FURTHER READINGS

BETHONY J et al: Soil-transmitted helminth infections: Ascariasis, trichuriasis, and hookworm. Lancet 367:1521, 2006

HOTEZ PJ et al: Hookworm infection. N Engl J Med 351:799, 2004

KEISER PB et al: *Strongyloides stercoralis* in the immunocompromised population. Clin Microbiol Rev 17:208, 2004

LAM CS et al: Disseminated strongyloidiasis: A retrospective study of clinical course and outcome. Eur J Clin Microbiol Infect Dis 25:14, 2006

LIM S et al: Complicated and fatal *Strongyloides* infection in Canadians: Risk factors, diagnosis and management. CMAJ 171:479, 2004

LU LH et al: Human intestinal capillariasis (*Capillaria philippinensis*) in Taiwan. Am J Trop Med Hyg 74:810, 2006

SHAH OJ et al: Biliary ascariasis: A review. World J Surg 30:1500, 2006

211 Filarial and Related Infections
Thomas B. Nutman, Peter F. Weller

Filarial worms are nematodes that dwell in the subcutaneous tissues and the lymphatics. Eight filarial species infect humans (Table 211-1); of these, four—*Wuchereria bancrofti, Brugia malayi, Onchocerca volvulus,* and *Loa loa*—are responsible for most serious filarial infections. Filarial parasites, which infect an estimated 170 million persons worldwide, are transmitted by specific species of mosquitoes or other arthropods and have a complex life cycle including infective larval stages carried by insects and adult worms that reside in either lymphatic or subcutaneous tissues of humans. The offspring of adults are microfilariae, which, depending on their species, are 200–250 μm long and 5–7 μm wide, may or may not be enveloped in a loose sheath, and either circulate in the blood or migrate through the skin (Table 211-1). To complete the life cycle, microfilariae are ingested by the arthropod vector and develop over 1–2 weeks into new infective larvae. Adult worms live for many years, whereas microfilariae survive for 3–36 months. The *Rickettsia*-like endosymbiont *Wolbachia* has been found intracellularly in all stages of *Brugia, Wuchereria, Mansonella,* and *Onchocerca* and is viewed as a possible target for antifilarial chemotherapy.

Usually, infection is established only with repeated, prolonged exposures to infective larvae. Since the clinical manifestations of filarial diseases develop relatively slowly, these infections should be considered to induce chronic diseases with possible long-term debilitating effects. In terms of the nature, severity, and timing of clinical manifestations, patients with filarial infections who are native to endemic areas and undergo lifelong exposure may differ significantly from those who are travelers or who have recently moved to these areas. Characteristically, filarial disease is more acute and intense in newly exposed individuals than in natives of endemic areas.

LYMPHATIC FILARIASIS

Lymphatic filariasis is caused by *W. bancrofti, B. malayi,* or *B. timori.* The threadlike adult parasites reside in lymphatic channels or lymph nodes, where they may remain viable for more than two decades.

EPIDEMIOLOGY

 W. bancrofti, the most widely distributed human filarial parasite, affects an estimated 115 million people and is found throughout the tropics and subtropics, including Asia and the Pacific Islands, Africa, areas of South America, and the Caribbean basin. Humans are the only definitive host for the parasite. Generally, the subperiodic form is found only in the Pacific Islands; elsewhere, *W. bancrofti* is nocturnally periodic. (Nocturnally periodic forms of microfilariae are scarce in peripheral blood by day and increase at night, whereas subperiodic forms are present in peripheral blood at all times and reach maximal levels in the afternoon.) Natural vectors for *W. bancrofti* are *Culex fatigans* mosquitoes in urban settings and anopheline or aedean mosquitoes in rural areas.

Brugian filariasis due to *B. malayi* occurs primarily in China, India, Indonesia, Korea, Japan, Malaysia, and the Philippines. *B. malayi* also has two forms distinguished by the periodicity of microfilaremia. The more common nocturnal form is transmitted in areas of coastal rice fields, while the subperiodic form is found in forests. *B. malayi* naturally infects cats as well as humans. *B. timori* exists only on islands of the Indonesian archipelago.

PATHOLOGY

The principal pathologic changes result from inflammatory damage to the lymphatics, which is typically caused by adult worms and not by microfilariae. Adult worms live in afferent lymphatics or sinuses of lymph nodes and cause lymphatic dilatation and thickening of the vessel walls. The infiltration of plasma cells, eosinophils, and macrophages in and around the infected vessels, along with endothelial and connective tissue proliferation, leads to tortuosity of the lymphatics and damaged or incompetent lymph valves. Lymphedema and chronic-stasis changes with hard or brawny edema develop in the overlying skin. These consequences of filariasis are due both to direct effects of the worms and to the inflammatory response of the host to the parasite. Inflammatory responses are believed to cause the granulomatous and proliferative processes that precede total lymphatic obstruction. It is thought that the lymphatic vessel remains patent as long as the worm remains viable and that the death of the worm leads to enhanced granulomatous reaction and fibrosis. Lymphatic obstruction results, and, despite collateralization of the lymphatics, lymphatic function is compromised.

CLINICAL FEATURES

The most common presentations of the lymphatic filariases are asymptomatic (or subclinical) microfilaremia, hydrocele (Fig. 211-1), acute adenolymphangitis (ADL), and chronic lymphatic disease. In areas where *W. bancrofti* or *B. malayi* is endemic, the overwhelming majority of infected individuals have few overt clinical manifestations of filarial infection despite large numbers of circulating microfilariae in the peripheral blood. Although they may be clinically asymptomatic, virtually all persons with *W. bancrofti* or *B. malayi* microfilaremia have some degree of subclinical disease that includes microscopic hematuria and/or proteinuria, dilated (and tortuous) lymphatics (visualized

TABLE 211-1 CHARACTERISTICS OF THE FILARIAE

Organism	Periodicity	Distribution	Vector	Location of Adult	Microfilarial Location	Sheath
Wuchereria bancrofti	Nocturnal	Cosmopolitan areas worldwide, including South America and Africa	*Culex* (mosquitoes)	Lymphatic tissue	Blood	+
		Mainly India	*Anopheles* (mosquitoes)			
		China, Indonesia	*Aedes* (mosquitoes)			
	Subperiodic	Eastern Pacific	*Aedes* (mosquitoes)	Lymphatic tissue	Blood	+
Brugia malayi	Nocturnal	Southeast Asia, Indonesia, India	*Mansonia, Anopheles* (mosquitoes)	Lymphatic tissue	Blood	+
	Subperiodic	Indonesia, Southeast Asia	*Coquillettidia, Mansonia* (mosquitoes)	Lymphatic tissue	Blood	+
B. timori	Nocturnal	Indonesia	*Anopheles* (mosquitoes)	Lymphatic tissue	Blood	+
Loa loa	Diurnal	West and Central Africa	*Chrysops* (deerflies)	Subcutaneous tissue	Blood	+
Onchocerca volvulus	None	South and Central America, Africa	*Simulium* (blackflies)	Subcutaneous tissue	Skin, eye	–
Mansonella ozzardi	None	South and Central America Caribbean	*Culicoides* (midges) *Simulium* (blackflies)	Undetermined site	Blood	–
M. perstans	None	South and Central America, Africa	*Culicoides* (midges)	Body cavities, mesentery, perirenal tissue	Blood	–
M. streptocerca	None	West and Central Africa	*Culicoides* (midges)	Subcutaneous tissue	Skin	–

FIGURE 211-1 Hydrocele associated with _Wuchereria bancrofti_ infection.

by imaging), and—in men—scrotal lymphangiectasia (detectable by ultrasound). In spite of these findings, the majority of individuals appear to remain clinically asymptomatic for years; relatively few progress to either acute or chronic disease.

ADL is characterized by high fever, lymphatic inflammation (lymphangitis and lymphadenitis), and transient local edema. The lymphangitis is retrograde, extending peripherally from the lymph node draining the area where the adult parasites reside. Regional lymph nodes are often enlarged, and the entire lymphatic channel can become indurated and inflamed. Concomitant local thrombophlebitis can occur as well. In brugian filariasis, a single local abscess may form along the involved lymphatic tract and subsequently rupture to the surface. The lymphadenitis and lymphangitis can involve both the upper and lower extremities in both bancroftian and brugian filariasis, but involvement of the genital lymphatics occurs almost exclusively with _W. bancrofti_ infection. This genital involvement can be manifested by funiculitis, epididymitis, and scrotal pain and tenderness. In endemic areas, another type of acute disease—dermatolymphangioadenitis (DLA)—is recognized as a syndrome that includes high fever, chills, myalgias, and headache. Edematous inflammatory plaques clearly demarcated from normal skin are seen. Vesicles, ulcers, and hyperpigmentation may also be noted. There is often a history of trauma, burns, radiation, insect bites, punctiform lesions, or chemical injury. Entry lesions, especially in the interdigital area, are common. DLA is often diagnosed as cellulitis.

If lymphatic damage progresses, transient lymphedema can develop into lymphatic obstruction and the permanent changes associated with elephantiasis (Fig. 211-2). Brawny edema follows early pitting edema, and thickening of the subcutaneous tissues and hyperkeratosis occur. Fissuring of the skin develops, as do hyperplastic changes. Superinfection of these poorly vascularized tissues becomes a problem. In bancroftian filariasis, in which genital involvement is common, hydroceles may develop (Fig. 211-1); in advanced stages, this condition may evolve into scrotal lymphedema and scrotal elephantiasis. Furthermore, if there is obstruction of the retroperitoneal lymphatics, the increased renal lymphatic pressure leads to rupture of the renal lymphatics and the development of chyluria, which is usually intermittent and most prominent in the morning.

The clinical manifestations of filarial infections in travelers or transmigrants who have recently entered an endemic region are distinctive. Given a sufficient number of bites by infected vectors, usually over a 3- to 6-month period, recently exposed patients can develop acute lymphatic or scrotal inflammation with or without urticaria and localized angioedema. Lymphadenitis of epitrochlear, axillary, femo-

ral, or inguinal lymph nodes is often followed by retrogradely evolving lymphangitis. Acute attacks are short-lived and are not usually accompanied by fever. With prolonged exposure to infected mosquitoes, these attacks, if untreated, become more severe and lead to permanent lymphatic inflammation and obstruction.

DIAGNOSIS

A definitive diagnosis can be made only by detection of the parasites and hence can be difficult. Adult worms localized in lymphatic vessels or nodes are largely inaccessible. Microfilariae can be found in blood, in hydrocele fluid, or (occasionally) in other body fluids. Such fluids can be examined microscopically, either directly or—for greater sensitivity—after concentration of the parasites by the passage of fluid through a polycarbonate cylindrical pore filter (pore size, 3 μm) or by the centrifugation of fluid fixed in 2% formalin (Knott's concentration technique). The timing of blood collection is critical and should be based on the periodicity of the microfilariae in the endemic region involved. Many infected individuals do not have microfilaremia, and definitive diagnosis in such cases can be difficult. Assays for circulating antigens of _W. bancrofti_ permit the diagnosis of microfilaremic and cryptic (amicrofilaremic) infection. Two tests are commercially available: an enzyme-linked immunosorbent assay (ELISA) and a rapid-format immunochromatographic card test. Both assays have sensitivities of 96–100% and specificities approaching 100%. There are currently no tests for circulating antigens in brugian filariasis.

Polymerase chain reaction (PCR)–based assays for DNA of _W. bancrofti_ and _B. malayi_ in blood have been developed. A number of studies indicate that this diagnostic method is of equivalent or greater sensitivity compared with parasitologic methods, detecting patent infection in almost all infected individuals.

In cases of suspected lymphatic filariasis, examination of the scrotum or the female breast by means of high-frequency ultrasound in conjunction with Doppler techniques may result in the identification of motile adult worms within dilated lymphatics. Worms may be visualized in the lymphatics of the spermatic cord in up to 80% of infected men. Live adult worms have a distinctive pattern of movement within the lymphatic vessels (termed the _filaria dance sign_). Radionuclide lymphoscintigraphic imaging of the limbs reliably demonstrates widespread lymphatic abnormalities in both asymptomatic microfilaremic persons and those with clinical manifestations of lymphatic pathology. While of potential utility in the delineation of anatomic changes associated with

FIGURE 211-2 Elephantiasis of the lower extremity associated with _Wuchereria bancrofti_ infection.

infection, lymphoscintigraphy is unlikely to assume primacy in the diagnostic evaluation of individuals with suspected infection; it is principally a research tool, although it has been used more widely for assessment of lymphedema of any cause. Eosinophilia and elevated serum concentrations of IgE and antifilarial antibody support the diagnosis of lymphatic filariasis. There is, however, extensive cross-reactivity between filarial antigens and antigens of other helminths, including the common intestinal roundworms; thus, interpretations of serologic findings can be difficult. In addition, residents of endemic areas can become sensitized to filarial antigens (and thus be serologically positive) through exposure to infected mosquitoes without having patent filarial infections.

The ADL associated with lymphatic filariasis must be distinguished from thrombophlebitis, infection, and trauma. Retrogradely evolving lymphangitis is a characteristic feature that helps distinguish filarial lymphangitis from ascending bacterial lymphangitis. Chronic filarial lymphedema must also be distinguished from the lymphedema of malignancy, postoperative scarring, trauma, chronic edematous states, and congenital lymphatic system abnormalities.

℞ LYMPHATIC FILARIASIS

With newer definitions of clinical syndromes in lymphatic filariasis and new tools to assess clinical status (e.g., ultrasound, lymphoscintigraphy, circulating filarial antigen assays, PCR), approaches to treatment based on infection status can be considered. Diethylcarbamazine (DEC, 6 mg/kg daily for 12 days), which has both macro- and microfilaricidal properties, remains the treatment of choice for the individual with active lymphatic filariasis (microfilaremia, antigen positivity, or adult worms on ultrasound). An alternative treatment is albendazole (400 mg bid for 21 days), although this drug's macrofilaricidal efficacy may be less than that of DEC. An 8-week course of daily doxycycline (targeting the intracellular *Wolbachia* endosymbiont) has significant macrofilaricidal activity, as does a 7-day course of daily DEC/albendazole.

As has already been mentioned, a growing body of evidence indicates that, although they may be asymptomatic, virtually all persons with *W. bancrofti* or *B. malayi* microfilaremia have some degree of subclinical disease (hematuria, proteinuria, abnormalities on lymphoscintigraphy). Thus, early treatment of asymptomatic persons is recommended to prevent further lymphatic damage. For ADL, supportive treatment (including the administration of antipyretics and analgesics) is recommended, as is antibiotic therapy if secondary bacterial infection is likely. Similarly, because lymphatic disease is associated with the presence of adult worms, treatment with DEC is recommended for microfilaria-negative adult-worm carriers.

In persons with chronic manifestations of lymphatic filariasis, treatment regimens that emphasize hygiene, prevention of secondary bacterial infections, and physiotherapy have gained wide acceptance for morbidity control. These regimens are similar to those recommended for lymphedema of most nonfilarial causes and known by a variety of names, including *complex decongestive physiotherapy* and *complex lymphedema therapy*. Hydroceles (Fig. 211-1) can be drained repeatedly or managed surgically. With chronic manifestations of lymphatic filariasis, drug treatment should be reserved for individuals with evidence of active infection; therapy has been associated with clinical improvement and, in some cases, reversal of lymphedema.

The recommended course of DEC treatment (12 days; total dose, 72 mg/kg) has remained standard for many years. However, data indicate that single-dose DEC treatment with 6 mg/kg may be equally efficacious. The 12-day course provides more rapid short-term microfilarial suppression. Regimens that use combinations of single doses of albendazole and either DEC or ivermectin all have a sustained microfilaricidal effect. As mentioned above, an 8-week course of daily doxycycline (200 mg/d) or a 7-day course of daily DEC/albendazole has both significant macrofilaricidal activity and sustained microfilaricidal activity.

Side effects of DEC treatment include fever, chills, arthralgias, headaches, nausea, and vomiting. Both the development and the severity of these reactions are directly related to the number of microfilariae circulating in the bloodstream. The adverse reactions may represent either an acute hypersensitivity reaction to the antigens being released by dead and dying parasites or an inflammatory reaction induced by lipopolysaccharides from the intracellular *Wolbachia* endosymbionts freed from their intracellular niche. Ivermectin has a side effect profile similar to that of DEC when used in lymphatic filariasis. In patients infected with *L. loa*, who have

high levels of *Loa* microfilaremia, DEC—like ivermectin (see "Loiasis," below)—can elicit severe encephalopathic complications. When used in single-dose regimens for the treatment of lymphatic filariasis, albendazole is associated with relatively few side effects.

PREVENTION AND CONTROL

Avoidance of mosquito bites usually is not feasible for residents of endemic areas, but visitors should make use of insect repellent and mosquito nets. Impregnated bednets have a salutary effect. DEC can kill developing forms of filarial parasites and is useful as a prophylactic agent in humans.

Community-based intervention is the current approach to elimination of lymphatic filariasis as a public health problem. The underlying tenet of this approach is that mass annual distribution of antimicrofilarial chemotherapy—albendazole with either DEC (for all areas except those where onchocerciasis is coendemic) or ivermectin—will profoundly suppress microfilaremia. If the suppression is sustained, then transmission can be interrupted. As an added benefit, these combinations have secondary effects on gastrointestinal helminths. An alternative approach to the control of lymphatic filariasis is the use of salt fortified with DEC. Community use of DEC-fortified salt dramatically reduces microfilarial density with no apparent adverse reactions. Community education and clinical care for persons already suffering from the chronic sequelae of lymphatic filariasis are important components of filariasis control and elimination programs.

TROPICAL PULMONARY EOSINOPHILIA

Tropical pulmonary eosinophilia (TPE) is a distinct syndrome that develops in some individuals infected with lymphatic filarial species. This syndrome affects males and females in a ratio of 4:1, often during the third decade of life. The majority of cases have been reported from India, Pakistan, Sri Lanka, Brazil, Guyana, and Southeast Asia.

CLINICAL FEATURES

The main features include a history of residence in filarial-endemic regions, paroxysmal cough and wheezing (usually nocturnal and probably related to the nocturnal periodicity of microfilariae), weight loss, low-grade fever, adenopathy, and pronounced blood eosinophilia (>3000 eosinophils/μL). Chest x-rays or CT scans may be normal but generally show increased bronchovascular markings. Diffuse miliary lesions or mottled opacities may be present in the middle and lower lung fields. Tests of pulmonary function show restrictive abnormalities in most cases and obstructive defects in half. Characteristically, total serum IgE levels (10,000–100,000 ng/mL) and antifilarial antibody titers are markedly elevated.

PATHOLOGY

In TPE, microfilariae and parasite antigens are rapidly cleared from the bloodstream by the lungs. The clinical symptoms result from allergic and inflammatory reactions elicited by the cleared parasites. In some patients, trapping of microfilariae in other reticuloendothelial organs can cause hepatomegaly, splenomegaly, or lymphadenopathy. A prominent, eosinophil-enriched, intraalveolar infiltrate is often reported, and with it comes the release of cytotoxic proinflammatory granular proteins that may mediate some of the pathology seen in TPE. In the absence of successful treatment, interstitial fibrosis can lead to progressive pulmonary damage.

DIFFERENTIAL DIAGNOSIS

TPE must be distinguished from asthma, Löffler's syndrome, allergic bronchopulmonary aspergillosis, allergic granulomatosis with angiitis (Churg-Strauss syndrome), the systemic vasculitides (most notably periarteritis nodosa and Wegener's granulomatosis), chronic eosinophilic pneumonia, and the idiopathic hypereosinophilic syndrome. In addition to a geographic history of filarial exposure, useful features for distinguishing TPE include wheezing that is solely nocturnal, very high levels of antifilarial antibodies, and a rapid initial response to treatment with DEC.

Rx TROPICAL PULMONARY EOSINOPHILIA

ONCHOCERCIASIS

 Onchocerciasis ("river blindness") is caused by the filarial nematode *O. volvulus*, which infects an estimated 13 million individuals. The majority of individuals infected with *O. volvulus* live in the equatorial region of Africa extending from the Atlantic coast to the Red Sea. About 70,000 persons are infected in Guatemala and Mexico, with smaller foci in Venezuela, Colombia, Brazil, Ecuador, Yemen, and Saudi Arabia. Onchocerciasis is the second leading cause of infectious blindness worldwide.

ETIOLOGY AND EPIDEMIOLOGY

Infection in humans begins with the deposition of infective larvae on the skin by the bite of an infected blackfly. The larvae develop into adults, which are typically found in subcutaneous nodules. About 7 months to 3 years after infection, the gravid female releases microfilariae that migrate out of the nodule and throughout the tissues, concentrating in the dermis. Infection is transmitted to other persons when a female fly ingests microfilariae from the host's skin and these microfilariae then develop into infective larvae. Adult *O. volvulus* females and males are ~40–60 cm and ~3–6 cm in length, respectively. The life span of adults can be as long as 18 years, with an average of ~9 years. Because the blackfly vector breeds along free-flowing rivers and streams (particularly in rapids) and generally restricts its flight to an area within several kilometers of these breeding sites, both biting and disease transmission are most intense in these locations.

PATHOLOGY

Onchocerciasis primarily affects the skin, eyes, and lymph nodes. In contrast to the pathology in lymphatic filariasis, the damage in onchocerciasis is elicited by microfilariae and not by adult parasites. In the skin, there are mild but chronic inflammatory changes that can result in loss of elastic fibers, atrophy, and fibrosis. The subcutaneous nodules, or onchocercomata, consist primarily of fibrous tissues surrounding the adult worm, often with a peripheral ring of inflammatory cells. In the eye, neovascularization and corneal scarring lead to corneal opacities and blindness. Inflammation in the anterior and posterior chambers frequently results in anterior uveitis, chorioretinitis, and optic atrophy. Although punctate opacities are due to an inflammatory reaction surrounding dead or dying microfilariae, the pathogenesis of most manifestations of onchocerciasis is still unclear.

CLINICAL FEATURES

Skin Pruritus and rash are the most frequent manifestations of onchocerciasis. The pruritus can be incapacitating; the rash is typically a papular eruption (Fig. 211-3) that is generalized rather than localized to a particular region of the body. Long-term infection results in exaggerated and premature wrinkling of the skin, loss of elastic fibers, and epidermal atrophy that can lead to loose, redundant skin and hypo- or hyperpigmentation. Localized eczematoid dermatitis can cause hyperkeratosis, scaling, and pigmentary changes. In an immunologically hyperreactive form of onchodermatitis (commonly termed *sowdah*, from the Yemeni word meaning "black"), the affected skin darkens as a consequence of the profound inflammation that occurs as microfilariae in the skin are cleared.

 Onchocercomata These subcutaneous nodules, which can be palpable and/or visible, contain the adult worm. In African patients, they are common over the coccyx and sacrum, the trochanter of the femur, the lateral anterior crest, and other bony

FIGURE 211-3 Papular eruption as a consequence of onchocerciasis.

prominences; in patients from South and Central America, nodules tend to develop preferentially in the upper part of the body, particularly on the head, neck, and shoulders.

Nodules vary in size and characteristically are firm and not tender. It has been estimated that, for every palpable nodule, there are four deeper nonpalpable ones.

Ocular Tissue Visual impairment is the most serious complication of onchocerciasis and usually affects only those persons with moderate or heavy infections. Lesions may develop in all parts of the eye. The most common early finding is conjunctivitis with photophobia. Punctate keratitis—acute inflammatory reactions surrounding dying microfilariae and manifested as "snowflake" opacities—is common among younger patients and resolves without apparent complications.

 Sclerosing keratitis occurs in 1–5% of infected persons and is the leading cause of onchocercal blindness in Africa. Anterior uveitis and iridocyclitis develop in ~5% of infected persons in Africa. In Latin America, complications of the anterior uveal tract (pupillary deformity) may cause secondary glaucoma. Characteristic chorioretinal lesions develop as a result of atrophy and hyperpigmentation of the retinal pigment epithelium. Constriction of the visual fields and frank optic atrophy may occur.

Lymph Nodes Mild to moderate lymphadenopathy is common, particularly in the inguinal and femoral areas, where the enlarged nodes may hang down in response to gravity ("hanging groin"), sometimes predisposing to inguinal and femoral hernias.

Systemic Manifestations Some heavily infected individuals develop cachexia with loss of adipose tissue and muscle mass. Among adults who become blind, there is a three- to fourfold increase in the mortality rate.

DIAGNOSIS

Definitive diagnosis depends on the detection of an adult worm in an excised nodule or, more commonly, of microfilariae in a skin snip. Skin snips are obtained with a corneal-scleral punch, which collects a blood-free skin biopsy sample extending to just below the epidermis, or by lifting of the skin with the tip of a needle and excision of a small (1- to 3-mm) piece with a sterile scalpel blade. The biopsy tissue is incubated in tissue culture medium or in saline on a glass slide or flat-bottomed microtiter plate. After incubation for 2–4 h (or occasionally overnight in light infections), microfilariae emergent from the skin can be seen by low-power microscopy.

Eosinophilia and elevated serum IgE levels are common but, because they occur in many parasitic infections, are not diagnostic in

1328 themselves. Assays to detect specific antibodies to *Onchocerca* and PCR to detect onchocercal DNA in skin snips are used in specialized laboratories and are highly sensitive and specific.

The *Mazzotti test* is a provocative technique that can be used in cases where the diagnosis of onchocerciasis is still in doubt (i.e., when skin snips and ocular examination reveal no microfilariae). A small dose of DEC (0.5–1.0 mg/kg) is given orally; the ensuing death of any dermal microfilariae elicits the development or exacerbation of pruritus or dermatitis within hours—an event that strongly suggests onchocerciasis.

℞ ONCHOCERCIASIS

The main goals of therapy are to prevent the development of irreversible lesions and to alleviate symptoms. Surgical excision is recommended when nodules are located on the head (because of the proximity of microfilaria-producing adult worms to the eye), but chemotherapy is the mainstay of management. Ivermectin, a semisynthetic macrocyclic lactone active against microfilariae, is the first-line agent for the treatment of onchocerciasis. It is given orally in a single dose of 150 μg/kg, either yearly or semiannually. Recently, more frequent ivermectin administration (every 3 months) has been suggested to ameliorate pruritus and skin disease. Moreover, quadrennial administration of ivermectin has some macrofilaricidal activity.

After treatment, most individuals have few or no reactions. Pruritus, cutaneous edema, and/or maculopapular rash occurs in ~1–10% of treated individuals.

🌍 In areas of Africa co-endemic for *O. volvulus* and *L. loa*, however, ivermectin is contraindicated (as it is for pregnant or breast-feeding women) because of severe posttreatment encephalopathy seen in patients, especially children, who are heavily microfilaremic for *L. loa* (2000–5000 microfilariae/mL). Although ivermectin treatment results in a marked drop in microfilarial density, its effect can be short-lived (<3 months in some cases). Thus, it is occasionally necessary to give ivermectin more frequently for persistent symptoms. A 6-week course of doxycycline is macrofilaristatic, rendering female adult worms sterile for long periods. Because this agent targets the *Wolbachia* endosymbiont of the filarial parasite, new approaches for definitive treatment (i.e., cure) may become available.

PREVENTION

Vector control has been beneficial in highly endemic areas in which breeding sites are vulnerable to insecticide spraying, but most areas endemic for onchocerciasis are not suited to this type of control. Community-based administration of ivermectin every 6–12 months is being used to interrupt transmission in endemic areas. This measure, in conjunction with vector control, has already helped reduce the prevalence of disease in endemic foci in Africa and Latin America. No drug has proved useful for prophylaxis of *O. volvulus* infection.

LOIASIS

ETIOLOGY AND EPIDEMIOLOGY

🌍 Loiasis is caused by *L. loa* (the African eye worm), which is present in the rain forests of West and Central Africa. Adult parasites (females, 50–70 mm long and 0.5 mm wide; males, 25–35 mm long and 0.25 mm wide) live in subcutaneous tissues. Microfilariae circulate in the blood with a diurnal periodicity that peaks between 12:00 noon and 2:00 P.M.

CLINICAL FEATURES

Manifestations of loiasis in natives of endemic areas may differ from those in temporary residents or visitors. Among the indigenous population, loiasis is often an asymptomatic infection with microfilaremia. Infection may be recognized only after subconjunctival migration of an adult worm (Fig. 211-4) or may be manifested by episodic Calabar swellings—evanescent localized areas of angioedema and erythema developing on the extremities and less frequently at other sites. Nephropathy, encephalopathy, and cardiomyopathy are rare. In patients who are not residents of endemic areas, allergic symptoms predomi-

FIGURE 211-4 Adult *Loa loa* being surgically removed after its subconjunctival migration.

nate, episodes of Calabar swelling tend to be more frequent and debilitating, microfilaremia is rare, and eosinophilia and increased levels of antifilarial antibodies are characteristic.

PATHOLOGY

The pathogenesis of the manifestations of loiasis is poorly understood. Calabar swellings are thought to result from a hypersensitivity reaction to adult worm antigens.

DIAGNOSIS

Definitive diagnosis of loiasis requires the detection of microfilariae in the peripheral blood or the isolation of the adult worm from the eye (Fig. 211-4) or from a subcutaneous biopsy specimen from a site of swelling developing after treatment. PCR-based assays for the detection of *L. loa* DNA in blood are available in specialized laboratories and are highly sensitive and specific. In practice, the diagnosis must often be based on a characteristic history and clinical presentation, blood eosinophilia, and elevated levels of antifilarial antibodies, particularly in travelers to an endemic region, who are usually amicrofilaremic. Other clinical findings in the latter individuals include hypergammaglobulinemia, elevated levels of serum IgE, and elevated leukocyte and eosinophil counts.

℞ LOIASIS

DEC (8–10 mg/kg per day for 21 days) is effective against both the adult and the microfilarial forms of *L. loa*, but multiple courses are frequently necessary before loiasis resolves completely. In cases of heavy microfilaremia, allergic or other inflammatory reactions can take place during treatment, including central nervous system involvement with coma and encephalitis. Heavy infections can be treated initially with apheresis to remove the microfilariae and with glucocorticoids (40–60 mg of prednisone per day) followed by doses of DEC (0.5 mg/kg per day). If antifilarial treatment has no adverse effects, the prednisone dose can be rapidly tapered and the dose of DEC gradually increased to 8–10 mg/kg per day.

Albendazole or ivermectin is effective in reducing microfilarial loads, although neither is approved for this purpose by the U.S. Food and Drug Administration. DEC (300 mg weekly) is an effective prophylactic regimen for loiasis.

STREPTOCERCIASIS

🌍 *Mansonella streptocerca*, found mainly in the tropical forest belt of Africa from Ghana to the Democratic Republic of the Congo, is transmitted by biting midges. The major clinical manifestations involve the skin and include pruritus, papular rashes, and pigmentation changes. Many infected individuals have inguinal adenopathy, although most are asymptomatic. The diagnosis is made by detection of the characteristic microfilariae in skin snips. DEC (6 mg/kg per day in divided doses for 14–21 days) effectively kills both microfilariae and adult worms. As in onchocerciasis, treatment is sometimes accompanied by urticaria, arthralgias, myalgias, headaches, and abdominal discomfort. Ivermectin at a single dose of 150 μg/kg leads to sustained suppression of microfilariae in the skin and is likely to assume primacy in the treatment of streptocerciasis.

MANSONELLA PERSTANS INFECTION

Mansonella perstans, distributed across the center of Africa and in northeastern South America, is transmitted by midges. Adult worms reside in serous cavities—pericardial, pleural, and peritoneal—as well as in the mesentery and the perirenal and retroperitoneal tissues. Microfilariae circulate in the blood without periodicity. The clinical and pathologic features of the infection are poorly defined. Most patients appear to be asymptomatic, but manifestations may include transient angioedema and pruritus of the arms, face, or other parts of the body (analogous to the Calabar swellings of loiasis); fever; headache; arthralgias; and right-upper-quadrant pain. Occasionally, pericarditis and hepatitis occur. The diagnosis is based on the demonstration of microfilariae in blood or serosal effusions. Perstans filariasis is often associated with peripheral-blood eosinophilia and antifilarial antibody elevations. Although DEC (8–10 mg/kg per day for 21 days) is the standard therapeutic agent, there is little evidence that it is effective. Cure is indicated by the disappearance of symptoms and eosinophilia; multiple courses of therapy are usually required. Ivermectin, used in frequent repeated doses, can reduce blood microfilarial levels. Both mebendazole (100 mg bid for 30 days) and albendazole (400 mg bid for 10 days) have occasionally been reported to be effective.

MANSONELLA OZZARDI INFECTION

The distribution of *Mansonella ozzardi* is restricted to Central and South America and certain Caribbean islands. Adult worms are rarely recovered from humans. Microfilariae circulate in the blood without periodicity. Although this organism has often been considered nonpathogenic, headache, articular pain, fever, pulmonary symptoms, adenopathy, hepatomegaly, pruritus, and eosinophilia have been ascribed to *M. ozzardi* infection. The diagnosis is made by detection of microfilariae in peripheral blood. Ivermectin (a single dose of 6 mg) is effective in treating this infection.

DRACUNCULIASIS (GUINEA WORM INFECTION)

ETIOLOGY AND EPIDEMIOLOGY

The incidence of dracunculiasis, caused by *Dracunculus medinensis*, has declined dramatically because of global eradication efforts. Current estimates suggest that there are slightly more than 10,000 cases worldwide, the majority in Sudan, Ghana, and Mali. Asia has now been deemed dracunculiasis-free.

Humans acquire *D. medinensis* when they ingest water containing infective larvae derived from *Cyclops*, a crustacean that is the intermediate host. Larvae penetrate the stomach or intestinal wall, mate, and mature. The adult male probably dies; the female worm develops over a year and migrates to subcutaneous tissues, usually in the lower extremity. As the thin female worm, ranging in length from 30 cm to 1 m, approaches the skin, a blister forms that, over days, breaks down and forms an ulcer. When the blister opens, large numbers of motile, rhabditiform larvae can be released into stagnant water; ingestion by *Cyclops* completes the life cycle.

CLINICAL FEATURES

Few or no clinical manifestations of dracunculiasis are evident until just before the blister forms, when there is an onset of fever and generalized allergic symptoms, including periorbital edema, wheezing, and urticaria. The emergence of the worm is associated with local pain and swelling. When the blister ruptures (usually as a result of immersion in water) and the adult worm releases larva-rich fluid, symptoms are relieved. The shallow ulcer surrounding the emerging adult worm heals over weeks to months. Such ulcers, however, can become secondarily infected, the result being cellulitis, local inflammation, abscess formation, or (uncommonly) tetanus. Occasionally, the adult worm does not emerge but becomes encapsulated and calcified.

DIAGNOSIS

The diagnosis is based on the findings developing with the emergence of the adult worm, as described above.

Rx DRACUNCULIASIS

Gradual extraction of the worm by winding of a few centimeters on a stick each day remains the common and effective practice. Worms may be excised surgically. The administration of metronidazole (250 mg tid for 10 days) may relieve symptoms but has no proven activity against the worm.

PREVENTION

Prevention, which remains the only real control measure, depends on the provision of safe drinking water.

ZOONOTIC FILARIAL INFECTIONS

Dirofilariae that affect primarily dogs, cats, and raccoons occasionally infect humans incidentally, as do *Brugia* and *Onchocerca* parasites that affect small mammals. Because humans are an abnormal host, the parasites never develop fully. Pulmonary dirofilarial infection caused by the canine heartworm *Dirofilaria immitis* generally presents in humans as a solitary pulmonary nodule. Chest pain, hemoptysis, and cough are uncommon. Infections with *D. repens* (from dogs) or *D. tenuis* (from raccoons) can cause local subcutaneous nodules in humans. Zoonotic *Brugia* infection can produce isolated lymph node enlargement, whereas zoonotic *Onchocerca* can cause subconjunctival masses. Eosinophilia levels and antifilarial antibody titers are not commonly elevated. Excisional biopsy is both diagnostic and curative. These infections usually do not respond to chemotherapy.

FURTHER READINGS

BOCKARIE MJ et al: Mass treatment to eliminate filariasis in Papua New Guinea. N Engl J Med 347:1841, 2002

BOUSSINESQ M et al: Clinical picture, epidemiology and outcome of *Loa*-associated serious adverse events related to mass ivermectin treatment of onchocerciasis in Cameroon. Filaria J 2(Suppl 1):S4, 2003

DREYER G et al: Acute attacks in the extremities of persons living in an area endemic for bancroftian filariasis: Differentiation of two syndromes. Trans R Soc Trop Med Hyg 93:413, 1999

GARDON J et al: Serious reactions after mass treatment of onchocerciasis with ivermectin in an area endemic for *Loa loa* infection. Lancet 350:18, 1997

HOERAUF A et al: Onchocerciasis. BMJ 326:207, 2003

——— et al: Depletion of *Wolbachia* endobacteria in *Onchocerca volvulus* by doxycycline and microfilaridermia after ivermectin treatment. Lancet 357:1415, 2001

MCPHERSON T et al: Interdigital lesions and frequency of acute dermatolymphangioadenitis in lymphoedema in a filariasis-endemic area. Br J Dermatol 154:933, 2006

OTTESEN EA: Lymphatic filariasis: Treatment, control and elimination. Adv Parasitol 61:395, 2006

WALTHER M, MULLER R: Diagnosis of human filariases (except onchocerciasis). Adv Parasitol 53:149, 2003

WHO EXPERT COMMITTEE ON ONCHOCERCIASIS: Onchocerciasis and its control: Fourth report. Tech Rep Ser No 852. Geneva, World Health Organization, 1995

212 Schistosomiasis and Other Trematode Infections

Adel A.F. Mahmoud

Trematodes, or flatworms, are a group of morphologically and biologically heterogeneous organisms that belong to the phylum Platyhelminthes. Human infection with trematodes occurs in many geographic areas and can cause considerable morbidity and mortality. For clinical purposes, significant trematode infections of humans may be divided according to tissues invaded by adult flukes: blood, biliary tree, intestines, and lungs (Table 212-1).

Trematodes share some common morphologic features, including macroscopic size (from 1 cm to several cm); dorsoventral, flattened, bilaterally symmetric bodies (adult worms); and the prominence of two suckers. Except for schistosomes, all human parasitic trematodes are hermaphroditic. Their life cycle involves a definitive host (mammalian/human), in which adult worms initiate sexual reproduction, and an intermediate host (snails), in which asexual multiplication of larvae occurs. More than one intermediate host may be necessary for some species of trematodes. Human infection is initiated either by direct penetration of intact skin or by ingestion. Upon maturation within humans, adult flukes initiate sexual reproduction and egg production. Helminth ova leave the definitive host in excreta or sputum and, upon reaching suitable environmental conditions, they hatch, releasing free-living miracidia that seek specific snail intermediate hosts. After asexual reproduction, cercariae are released from infected snails. In certain species, these organisms infect humans; in others, they find a second intermediate host to allow encystment into metacercariae—the infective stage.

The host-parasite relationship in trematode infections is a product of certain biologic features of these organisms: they are multicellular, undergo several developmental changes within the host, and usually result in chronic infections. In general, the distribution of worm infections in human populations is *overdispersed*; i.e., it follows a negative binomial mathematical relationship in which most infected individuals harbor low worm burdens while a small percentage are heavily infected. It is the heavily infected minority who are particularly prone to disease sequelae and who constitute an epidemiologically significant reservoir of infection in endemic areas. Equally important is an appreciation that worms do not multiply within the definitive host and that they have a relatively long life span, ranging from a few months to a few years. Morbidity and death due to trematode infections reflect a multifactorial process that results from the tipping of a delicate balance between intensity of infection and host reactions, which initiate and modulate immunologic and pathologic outcome. Furthermore, the genetics of the parasite and of the human host contribute to the outcome of infection and disease. Infections with trematodes that migrate through or reside in host tissues are associated with a moderate to high degree of peripheral blood eosinophilia; this association is of significance in protective and immunopathologic sequelae and is a useful clinical indicator of infection.

APPROACH TO THE PATIENT: Trematode Infection

The approach to individuals with suspected trematode infection begins with a question: Where have you been? Details of geographic history, exposure to freshwater bodies, and indulgence in local eating habits without ensuring safety of food and drink are all essential elements in the history. The workup plan must include a detailed physical examination and tests appropriate for the suspected infection. Diagnosis is based either on detection of the relevant stage of the parasite in excreta, sputum, or (rarely) tissue samples or on sensitive and specific serologic tests. Consultation with physicians familiar with these infections or with the U.S. Centers for Disease Control and Prevention (CDC) is helpful in guiding diagnosis and selecting therapy.

BLOOD FLUKES: SCHISTOSOMIASIS

Human schistosomiasis is caused by five species of the parasitic trematode genus *Schistosoma*: the intestinal species *S. mansoni*, *S. japonicum*, *S. mekongi*, and *S. intercalatum* and the urinary species *S. haematobium*. Infection may cause considerable morbidity in the intestines, liver, and urinary tract, and a proportion of affected individuals die. Other schistosomes (e.g., avian species) may invade human skin but then die in subcutaneous tissue, producing only self-limiting cutaneous manifestations.

ETIOLOGY

Human infection is initiated by penetration of intact skin with infective cercariae. These organisms, which are released from infected snails in freshwater bodies, measure ~2 mm in length and possess an anterior and a ventral sucker that attach to the skin and facilitate penetration. Once in subcutaneous tissue, cercariae transform into schistosomula, with morphologic, membrane, and immunologic changes. The cercarial outer membrane changes from a trilaminar to a heptalaminar structure that is then maintained throughout the organism's life span in humans. This transformation is thought to be the schistosome's main adaptive mechanism for survival in humans. Schistosomula begin their migration within 2–4 days via venous or lymphatic vessels, reaching the lungs and finally the liver parenchyma. Sexually mature worms descend into the

TABLE 212-1	MAJOR HUMAN TREMATODE INFECTIONS	
Trematode	**Transmission**	**Endemic Area(s)**
Blood Flukes		
Schistosoma mansoni	Skin penetration by cercariae released from snails	Africa, South America, Middle East
S. japonicum	Skin penetration by cercariae released from snails	China, Philippines, Indonesia
S. intercalatum	Skin penetration by cercariae released from snails	West Africa
S. mekongi	Skin penetration by cercariae released from snails	Southeast Asia
S. haematobium	Skin penetration by cercariae released from snails	Africa, Middle East
Biliary (Hepatic) Flukes		
Clonorchis sinensis	Ingestion of metacercariae in freshwater fish	Far East
Opisthorchis viverrini	Ingestion of metacercariae in freshwater fish	Far East, Thailand
O. felineus	Ingestion of metacercariae in freshwater fish	Far East, Europe
Fasciola hepatica	Ingestion of metacercariae on aquatic plants or in water	Worldwide
F. gigantica	Ingestion of metacercariae on aquatic plants or in water	Sporadic, Africa
Intestinal Flukes		
Fasciolopsis buski	Ingestion of metacercariae on aquatic plants	Southeast Asia
Heterophyes heterophyes	Ingestion of metacercariae in freshwater or brackish-water fish	Far East, North Africa
Lung Flukes		
Paragonimus westermani	Ingestion of metacercariae in crayfish or crabs	Global except North America and Europe

worms inhibit the coagulation cascade and evade the effector arms of the host immune responses by still-undetermined mechanisms. The genome of schistosomes is relatively large (~270 Mb) and is arrayed on seven pairs of autosomes and one pair of sex chromosomes. For *S. mansoni*, a total of ~14,000 genes have been estimated; some are species-conserved. The complete sequence of the schistosome genome should be available soon.

EPIDEMIOLOGY

The global distribution of schistosome infection in human populations (Fig. 212-2) is dependent on both parasite and host factors. Information on prevalence and global distribution is inexact. The five *Schistosoma* species are estimated to infect 200–300 million individuals in South America, the Caribbean, Africa, the Middle East, and Southeast Asia. The total population living under conditions favoring transmission approximates double or triple that number—a fact reflecting the public health significance of schistosomiasis.

In endemic areas, the rate of yearly onset of new infection, or incidence, is generally low. Prevalence, on the other hand, starts to be appreciable by the age of 3–4 years and builds to a maximum that varies by endemic region (up to 100%) in the 15- to 20-year age group. Prevalence then stabilizes or decreases slightly in older age groups (>40 years). Intensity of infection (as measured by fecal or urinary egg counts, which correlate with adult worm burdens in most circumstances) follows the increase in prevalence up to the age of 15–20 years and then declines markedly in older age groups. This decline may reflect acquisition of resistance or may be due to changes in water contact patterns, since older people have less exposure. Furthermore, the overdispersed distribution of schistosomes in human populations may be due to the heterogeneity of worm populations, with some more invasive than others; alternatively, it may be due to the demonstrated differences in genetic susceptibility of host populations.

Disease due to schistosome infection is the outcome of parasitologic, host, and additional infectious, nutritional, and environmental factors. Most disease syndromes relate to the presence of one or more of the parasite stages in humans. Disease manifestations in the populations of endemic areas correlate, in general, with the intensity and duration of infection as well as with the age and genetic susceptibility of the host. Overall, disease manifestations are clinically relevant in only a small proportion of persons infected with any of the intestinal schistosomes. In contrast, urinary schistosomiasis manifests clinically in most infected individuals. Recent estimates of total morbidity due to chronic schistosomiasis indicate a significantly greater burden than was previously appreciated.

Patients with both HIV infection and schistosomiasis excrete far fewer eggs in their stools than those infected with *S. mansoni* alone; the mechanism underlying this difference is unknown. Treatment with praziquantel may result in reduced HIV replication and increased CD4+ T lymphocyte counts.

FIGURE 212-1 Morphology of schistosome eggs, the diagnostic stage of the parasite's life cycle. **A.** *S. haematobium* egg found in urine sample. Egg is large (~140 μm long), with a terminal spine. **B.** *S. mansoni* egg found in feces. Egg is large (~150 μm long), with a thin shell and lateral spine. **C.** *S. japonicum* egg found in feces. Egg is smaller than that of *S. mansoni* (~90 μm long), with a small spine or hooklike structure. **D.** *S. mekongi* egg found in feces. Egg is similar to that of *S. japonicum* but smaller (~65 μm long). **E.** *S. intercalatum* egg found in feces. Egg is larger than that of *S. haematobium* (~190 μm long), with a longer, sharply pointed spine. (*From LR Ash, TC Orihel: Atlas of Human Parasitology, 3d ed. Chicago, ASCP Press, 1990; with permission.*)

venous system at specific anatomic locations: intestinal veins (*S. mansoni, S. japonicum, S. mekongi,* and *S. intercalatum*) and vesical veins (*S. haematobium*). After mating, adult gravid females travel against venous blood flow to small tributaries, where they deposit their ova intravascularly. Schistosome ova (Fig. 212-1) have specific morphologic features that vary with the species. Aided by enzymatic secretions through minipores in eggshells, ova move through the venous wall, traversing host tissues to reach the lumen of the intestinal or urinary tract, and are voided with stools or urine. Approximately 50% of ova are retained in host tissues locally (intestines or urinary tract) or are carried by venous blood flow to the liver and other organs. Schistosome ova that reach freshwater bodies hatch, releasing free-living miracidia that seek the snail intermediate host and undergo several asexual multiplication cycles. Finally, infective cercariae are shed from snails.

Adult schistosomes are ~1–2 cm long. Males are slightly shorter than females, with flattened bodies and anteriorly curved edges forming the gynecophoral canal, in which mature adult females are usually held. Females are longer, slender, and rounded in cross-section. The precise nature of biochemical and reproductive exchanges between the two sexes is unknown, as are the regulatory mechanisms for pairing. Adult schistosomes parasitize specific sites in the host venous system. What guides adult intestinal schistosomes to branches of the superior or inferior mesenteric veins or adult *S. haematobium* worms to the vesical plexus is unknown. In addition, adult

PATHOGENESIS AND IMMUNITY

Cercarial invasion is associated with dermatitis arising from dermal and subdermal inflammatory responses, both humoral and cell-me-

FIGURE 212-2 Global distribution of schistosomiasis. A. *S. mansoni* infection (*dark blue*) is endemic in Africa, the Middle East, South America, and a few Caribbean countries. *S. intercalatum* infection (*green*) is endemic in sporadic foci in West and Central Africa. **B.** *S. haematobium* infection (*purple*) is endemic in Africa and the Middle East. The major endemic countries for *S. japonicum* infection (*green*) are China, the Philippines, and Indonesia. *S. mekongi* infection (*red*) is endemic in sporadic foci in Southeast Asia.

diated. As the parasites approach sexual maturity and with the commencement of oviposition, acute schistosomiasis or Katayama fever (a serum sickness–like illness; see "Clinical Features," below) may occur. The associated antigen excess results in formation of soluble immune complexes, which may be deposited in several tissues, initiating multiple pathologic events. In chronic schistosomiasis, most disease manifestations are due to eggs retained in host tissues. The granulomatous response around these ova is cell-mediated and is regulated both positively and negatively by a cascade of cytokine, cellular, and humoral responses. Granuloma formation begins with recruitment of a host of inflammatory cells in response to antigens secreted by the living organism within the ova. Cells recruited initially include phagocytes, antigen-specific T cells, and eosinophils. Fibroblasts, giant cells, and B lymphocytes predominate later. These lesions reach a size many times that of parasite eggs, thus inducing organomegaly and obstruction. Immunomodulation or downregulation of host responses to schistosome eggs plays a significant role in limiting the extent of the granulomatous lesions—and consequently disease—in chronically infected experimental animals or humans. The underlying mechanisms involve another cascade of regulatory cytokines and idiotypic antibodies. Subsequent to the granulomatous response, fibrosis sets in, resulting in more permanent disease sequelae. Because schistosomiasis is also a chronic infection, the accumulation of antigen-antibody complexes results in deposits in renal glomeruli and may cause significant kidney disease.

The better-studied pathologic sequelae in schistosomiasis are those observed in liver disease. Ova that are carried by portal blood embolize to the liver. Because of their size (~150 × 60 μm in the case of *S. mansoni*), they lodge at presinusoidal sites, where granulomas are formed. These granulomas contribute to the hepatomegaly observed in infected individuals. Schistosomal liver enlargement is also associated with certain class I and class II human leukocyte antigen (HLA) haplotypes and markers; its genetic basis appears to be multigenic. Presinusoidal portal blockage causes several hemodynamic changes, including portal hypertension and associated development of portosystemic collaterals at the esophagogastric junction and other sites. Esophageal varices are most likely to break and cause repeated episodes of hematemesis. Because changes in hepatic portal blood flow occur slowly, compensatory arterialization of the blood flow through the liver is established. While this compensatory mechanism may be associated with certain metabolic side effects, retention of hepatocyte perfusion permits maintenance of normal liver function for several years.

The second most significant pathologic change in the liver relates to fibrosis. It is characteristically periportal (Symmers' clay pipe–stem fibrosis) but may be diffuse. Fibrosis, when diffuse, may be seen in areas of egg deposition and granuloma formation but is also seen in distant locations such as portal tracts. Schistosomiasis results in pure fibrotic lesions in the liver; cirrhosis occurs when other nutritional factors or infectious agents (e.g., hepatitis B or C virus) are involved. In recent years, it has been recognized that deposition of fibrotic tissue in the extracellular matrix results from the interaction of T lymphocytes with cells of the fibroblast series; several cytokines, such as interleukin (IL) 2, IL-4, IL-1, and transforming growth factor β (TGF-β), are known to stimulate fibrogenesis. The process may be dependent on the genetic constitution of the host. Furthermore, regulatory cytokines that can suppress fibrogenesis, such as interferon γ (IFN-γ) or IL-12, may play a role in modulating the response.

While the above description focuses on granuloma formation and fibrosis of the liver, similar processes occur in urinary schistosomiasis. Granuloma formation at the lower end of the ureters obstructs urinary flow, with subsequent development of hydroureter and hydronephrosis. Similar lesions in the urinary bladder cause the protrusion of papillomatous structures into its cavity; these may ulcerate and/or bleed. The chronic stage of infection is associated with scarring and deposition of calcium in bladder wall.

Studies on immunity to schistosomiasis, whether innate or adaptive, have expanded our knowledge of the components of these responses and target antigens. The critical question, however, is whether humans acquire immunity to schistosomes. Epidemiologic data suggest the onset of acquired immunity during the course of infection in young adults. Curative treatment of infection divides populations in endemic areas into those who acquire reinfection rapidly (susceptible) and those who follow a protracted course (resistant). This difference may be explained by differences in transmission, immunologic response, or genetic susceptibility. The mechanism of acquired immunity involves antibodies, complement, and several effector cells, particularly eosinophils. Furthermore, the intensity of schistosome infection has been correlated with a region in chromosome 5. In several studies, a few protective schistosome antigens have been identified as vaccine candidates, but none has been evaluated in human populations to date.

CLINICAL FEATURES

In general, disease manifestations of schistosomiasis occur in three stages, which vary not only by species but also by intensity of infection and other host factors, such as age and genetics. During the phase of cercarial invasion, a form of dermatitis may be observed. This so-called swimmers' itch occurs most often with *S. mansoni* and *S. japonicum* infections, manifesting 2 or 3 days after invasion as an itchy maculopapular rash on the affected areas of the skin. The condition is particularly severe when humans are exposed to avian schistosomes. This form of cercarial dermatitis is also seen around freshwater lakes in the northern United States, particularly in the spring. Cercarial dermatitis is a self-limiting clinical entity. During worm maturation and at the beginning of oviposition (i.e., 4–8 weeks after skin invasion), acute schistosomiasis or Katayama fever—a serum sickness–like syndrome with fever, generalized lymphadenopathy, and hepatosplenomegaly—may develop. Individuals with acute schistosomiasis show a high degree of peripheral blood eosinophilia. Parasite-specific antibodies may be detected before schistosome eggs are identified in excreta. Acute schistosomiasis has become an important clinical entity worldwide because of increased travel to endemic areas. Travelers are exposed to parasites while swimming or wading in freshwater bodies and upon their return present with the acute manifestations. The course of acute schistosomiasis is generally benign, but deaths are occasionally reported in association with heavy exposure to schistosomes.

The main clinical manifestations of chronic schistosomiasis are species-dependent. Intestinal species (*S. mansoni, S. japonicum, S. mekongi,* and *S. intercalatum*) cause intestinal and hepatosplenic disease as well as several manifestations associated with portal hypertension. During the intestinal phase, which may begin a few months after infection and may last for years, symptomatic patients characteristically have colicky abdominal pain, bloody diarrhea, and anemia. Patients may also report fatigue and an inability to perform daily routine functions and may show evidence of growth retardation. It has been demonstrated that schistosomiasis morbidity is generally underappreciated. The severity of intestinal schistosomiasis is often related to the intensity of the worm burden. The disease runs a chronic course and may result in colonic polyposis, which has been reported from some endemic areas, such as Egypt.

The hepatosplenic phase of disease manifests early (during the first year of infection, particularly in children) with liver enlargement due to parasite-induced granulomatous lesions. Hepatomegaly is seen in ~15–20% of infected individuals; it correlates roughly with intensity of infection, occurs more often in children, and may be related to specific HLA haplotypes. In subsequent phases of infection, presinusoidal blockage of blood flow leads to portal hypertension and splenomegaly. Moreover, portal hypertension may lead to varices at the lower end of the esophagus and at other sites. Patients with schistosomal liver disease may have right-upper-quadrant "dragging" pain during the hepatomegaly phase, and this pain may move to the left upper quadrant as splenomegaly progresses. Bleeding from esophageal varices may, however, be the first clinical manifestation of this phase. Patients may experience repeated bleeding but seem to tolerate its impact, since an adequate total hepatic blood flow permits normal liver function for a considerable duration. In late-stage disease, typical fibrotic changes occur along with liver function deterioration and the onset of ascites, hypoalbuminemia, and defects in coagulation. Intercurrent viral infections of the liver (especially hepatitis B and C) or nutritional deficiencies may well accelerate or exacerbate the deterioration of hepatic function.

The extent and severity of intestinal and hepatic disease in schistosomiasis mansoni and japonica have been well described. While it was originally thought that *S. japonicum* might induce more severe disease manifestations because the adult worms can produce 10 times more eggs than *S. mansoni,* subsequent field studies have not supported this claim. Clinical observations of individuals infected with *S. mekongi* or *S. intercalatum* have been less detailed, partly because of the limited geographic distribution of these organisms.

The clinical manifestations of *S. haematobium* infection occur relatively early and involve a high percentage of infected individuals. Up to 80% of children infected with *S. haematobium* have dysuria, frequency, and hematuria, which may be terminal. Urine examination reveals blood and albumin as well as an unusually high frequency of bacterial urinary tract infection and urinary sediment cellular metaplasia. These manifestations correlate with intensity of infection, the presence of urinary bladder granulomas, and subsequent ulceration. Along with local effects of granuloma formation in the urinary bladder, obstruction of the lower end of the ureters results in hydroureter and hydronephrosis, which may be seen in 25–50% of infected children. As infection progresses, bladder granulomas undergo fibrosis, which results in typical sandy patches visible on cystoscopy. In many endemic areas, an association between squamous cell carcinoma of the bladder and *S. haematobium* infection has been observed. Such malignancy is detected in a younger age group than is transitional cell carcinoma. In fact, *S. haematobium* has now been classified as a human carcinogen.

Significant disease may occur in other organs during chronic schistosomiasis. Most important are the lungs and central nervous system (CNS); other locations, such as the skin and the genital organs, are far less frequently affected. In pulmonary schistosomiasis, embolized eggs lodge in small arterioles, producing acute necrotizing arteriolitis and granuloma formation. During *S. mansoni* and *S. japonicum* infection, schistosome eggs reach the lungs after the development of portosystemic collateral circulation; in *S. haematobium* infection, ova may reach the lungs directly via connections between the vesical and systemic circulation. Subsequent fibrous tissue deposition leads to endarteritis obliterans, pulmonary hypertension, and cor pulmonale. The most common symptoms are cough, fever, and dyspnea. Cor pulmonale may be diagnosed radiologically on the basis of prominent right side of the heart and dilation of the pulmonary artery. Frank evidence of right-sided heart failure may be seen in late cases.

CNS schistosomiasis is important but less common than pulmonary schistosomiasis. It characteristically occurs as cerebral disease due to *S. japonicum* infection. Migratory worms deposit eggs in the brain and induce a granulomatous response. The frequency of this manifestation among infected individuals in some endemic areas (e.g., the Philippines) is calculated at 2–4%. Jacksonian epilepsy due to *S. japonicum* infection is the second most common cause of epilepsy in these areas. *S. mansoni* and *S. haematobium* infections have been associated with transverse myelitis. This syndrome is thought to be due to eggs traveling to the venous plexus around the spinal cord. In schistosomiasis mansoni, transverse myelitis is usually seen in the chronic stage after the development of portal hypertension and portosystemic shunts, which allow ova to travel to the spinal cord veins. This proposed sequence of events has been challenged because of a few reports of transverse myelitis occurring early in the course of *S. mansoni* infection. More information is needed to confirm these observations. During schistosomiasis haematobia, ova may travel through communication between vesical and systemic veins, resulting in spinal cord disease that may be detected at any stage of infection. Pathologic study of lesions in schistosomal transverse myelitis may reveal eggs along with necrotic or granulomatous lesions. Patients usually present with acute or rapidly progressing lower-leg weakness accompanied by sphincter dysfunction.

DIAGNOSIS

Physicians in areas not endemic for schistosomiasis face considerable diagnostic challenges. In the most common clinical presentation, a traveler returns with symptoms and signs of acute syndromes of schistosomiasis—namely, cercarial dermatitis or Katayama fever. Central to correct diagnosis is a thorough inquiry into travel history and exposure to freshwater bodies, whether slow or fast running. Differential diagnosis of fever in returned travelers includes a spectrum of infections whose etiologies are viral (e.g., Dengue fever), bacterial (e.g., enteric fever, leptospirosis), rickettsial, or protozoal (e.g., malaria). In cases of

Katayama fever, prompt diagnosis is essential and is based on clinical presentation, high-level peripheral blood eosinophilia, and a positive serologic assay for schistosomal antibodies. Two tests are available at the CDC: the Falcon assay screening test/enzyme-linked immunosorbent assay (FAST-ELISA) and the confirmatory enzyme-linked immunoelectrotransfer blot (EITB). Both tests are highly sensitive and ~96% specific. In some instances, examination of stool or urine for ova may yield positive results.

Individuals with established infection are diagnosed by a combination of geographic history, characteristic clinical presentation, and presence of schistosome ova in excreta. The diagnosis may also be established with the serologic assays mentioned above or with those that detect circulating schistosome antigens. These assays can be applied either to blood or to other body fluids (e.g., cerebrospinal fluid). For suspected schistosome infection, stool examination by the Kato thick smear or any other concentration method generally identifies all but the most lightly infected individuals. For *S. haematobium*, urine may be examined by microscopy of sediment or by filtration of a known volume through Nuclepore filters. Kato thick smear and Nuclepore filtration provide quantitative data on the intensity of infection, which is of value in assessing the degree of tissue damage and in monitoring the effect of chemotherapy. Schistosome infection may also be diagnosed by examination of tissue samples, typically rectal biopsies; other biopsy procedures (e.g., liver biopsy) are not needed, except in rare circumstances.

Differential diagnosis of schistosomal hepatomegaly must include viral hepatitis of all etiologies, miliary tuberculosis, malaria, visceral leishmaniasis, ethanol abuse, and causes of hepatic and portal vein obstruction. Differential diagnosis of hematuria in *S. haematobium* infection includes bacterial cystitis, tuberculosis, urinary stones, and malignancy.

℞ SCHISTOSOMIASIS

Treatment of schistosomiasis depends on stage of infection and clinical presentation. Other than topical dermatologic applications for relief of itching, no specific treatment is indicated for cercarial dermatitis caused by avian schistosomes. Therapy for acute schistosomiasis or Katayama fever needs to be adjusted appropriately for each case. While antischistosomal chemotherapy may be used, it does not have a significant impact on maturing worms. In severe acute schistosomiasis, management in an acute-care setting is necessary, with supportive measures and consideration of glucocorticoid treatment. Once the acute critical phase is over, specific chemotherapy is indicated for parasite elimination. For all individuals with established infection, treatment to eradicate the parasite should be administered. The drug of choice is praziquantel, which—depending on the infecting species (Table 212-2)—is administered PO as a total of 40 or 60 mg/kg in two or three doses over a single day. Praziquantel treatment results in parasitologic cure in ~85% of cases and reduces egg counts by >90%. Few side effects have been encountered, and those that do develop usually do not interfere with completion of treatment. Dependence on a single chemotherapeutic agent has raised the possibility of development of resistance in schistosomes; to date, such resistance does not seem to be clinically significant. The effect of antischistosomal treatment on disease manifestations varies by stage. Early hepatomegaly and bladder lesions are known to resolve after chemotherapy, but the late established manifestations, such as fibrosis, do not recede. Additional management modalities are needed for individuals with other manifestations, such as hepatocellular failure or recurrent hematemesis. The use of these interventions is guided by general medical and surgical principles.

PREVENTION AND CONTROL

Transmission of schistosomiasis is dependent on human behavior. Since the geographic distribution of infections in endemic regions of the world is not clearly demarcated, it is prudent for travelers to avoid contact with all freshwater bodies, irrespective of the speed of water flow or unsubstantiated claims of safety. Some topical agents, when applied to skin, may inhibit cercarial penetration, but none is currently available. If exposure occurs, a follow-up

TABLE 212-2 DRUG THERAPY FOR HUMAN TREMATODE INFECTIONS

Infection	Drug of Choice	Adult Dose and Duration
Blood Flukes		
S. mansoni, S. intercalatum, S. haematobium	Praziquantel	20 mg/kg, 2 doses in 1 day
S. japonicum, S. mekongi	Praziquantel	20 mg/kg, 3 doses in 1 day
Biliary (Hepatic) Flukes		
C. sinensis, O. viverrini, O. felineus	Praziquantel	25 mg/kg, 3 doses in 1 day
F. hepatica, F. gigantica	Triclabendazole	10 mg/kg once
Intestinal Flukes		
F. buski, H. heterophyes	Praziquantel	25 mg/kg, 3 doses in 1 day
Lung Flukes		
P. westermani	Praziquantel	25 mg/kg, 3 doses per day for 2 days

visit with a health care provider is strongly recommended. Prevention of infection in inhabitants of endemic areas is a significant challenge. Residents of these regions use freshwater bodies for sanitary, domestic, recreational, and agricultural purposes. Several control measures have been used, including application of molluscicides, provision of sanitary water and sewage disposal, chemotherapy, and health education. Current recommendations to countries endemic for schistosomiasis emphasize the use of multiple approaches. With the advent of an oral, safe, and effective antischistosomal agent, chemotherapy has been most successful in reducing intensity of infection and reversing disease. The duration of this positive impact depends on transmission dynamics of the parasite in any specific endemic region. The ultimate goal of research on prevention and control is development of a vaccine. Although there are a few promising leads, this goal is probably not within reach during the next decade or so.

LIVER (BILIARY) FLUKES

Several species of biliary fluke infecting humans are particularly common in Southeast Asia and Russia. Other species are transmitted in Europe, Africa, and the Americas. On the basis of their migratory pathway in humans, these infections may be divided into the *Clonorchis* and *Fasciola* groups (Table 212-1).

CLONORCHIASIS AND OPISTHORCHIASIS

Infection with *Clonorchis sinensis*, the Chinese or oriental fluke, is endemic among fish-eating mammals in Southeast Asia. Humans are an incidental host; the prevalence of human infection is highest in China, Vietnam, and Korea. Infection with *Opisthorchis viverrini* and *O. felineus* is zoonotic in cats and dogs. Transmission to humans occurs occasionally, particularly in Thailand (*O. viverrini*) and in Southeast Asia and eastern Europe (*O. felineus*). Data on the exact geographic distribution of these infectious agents in human populations are rudimentary.

Infection with any of these three species is established by ingestion of raw or inadequately cooked freshwater fish harboring metacercariae. These organisms excyst in the duodenum, releasing larvae that travel through the ampulla of Vater and mature into adult worms in bile canaliculi. Mature flukes are flat and elongated, measuring 1–2 cm in length. The hermaphroditic worms reproduce by releasing small operculated eggs, which pass with bile into the intestines and are voided with stools. The life cycle is completed in the environment in specific freshwater snails (the first intermediate host) and encystment of metacercariae in freshwater fish.

Except for late sequelae, the exact clinical syndromes caused by clonorchiasis and opisthorchiasis are not well defined. Since most infected individuals harbor a low worm burden, many are asymptomatic. Moderate to heavy infection may be associated with vague right-upper-quadrant pain. In contrast, chronic or repeated infection is associated with manifestations such as cholangitis, cholangiohepatitis, and biliary obstruction. Cholangiocarcinoma is epidemiologically related to *C. sinensis* infection in China and to *O. viverrini* infection in northeastern Thailand. This association has resulted in classification of these infectious agents as human carcinogens.

FASCIOLIASIS

Infections with *Fasciola hepatica* and *F. gigantica* are worldwide zoonoses that are particularly endemic in sheep-raising countries. Human cases have been reported in South America, Europe, Africa, Australia, and the Far East. Recent estimates indicate a worldwide prevalence of 17 million cases. High endemicity has been reported in certain areas of Peru and Bolivia. In most endemic areas the predominant species is *F. hepatica*, but in Asia and Africa a varying degree of overlap with *F. gigantica* has been observed.

Humans acquire fascioliasis by ingestion of metacercariae attached to certain aquatic plants, such as watercress. Infection may also be acquired by consumption of contaminated water or ingestion of food items washed with such water. Acquisition of human infection through consumption of freshly prepared raw liver containing immature flukes has been reported. Infection is initiated when metacercariae excyst, penetrate the gut wall, and travel through the peritoneal cavity to invade the liver capsule. Adult worms finally reach bile ducts, where they produce large operculated eggs, which are voided in bile through the gastrointestinal tract to the outside environment. The flukes' life cycle is completed in specific snails (the first intermediate host) and encystment on aquatic plants.

Clinical features of fascioliasis relate to the stage and intensity of infection. Acute disease develops during parasite migration (1–2 weeks after infection) and includes fever, right-upper-quadrant pain, hepatomegaly, and eosinophilia. CT of the liver may show migratory tracks. Symptoms and signs usually subside as the parasites reach their final habitat. In individuals with chronic infection, bile duct obstruction and biliary cirrhosis are infrequently demonstrated. No relation to hepatic malignancy has been ascribed to fascioliasis.

DIAGNOSIS

Diagnosis of infection with any of the biliary flukes depends on a high degree of suspicion, elicitation of an appropriate geographic history, and stool examination for characteristically shaped parasite ova. Additional evidence may be obtained by documenting peripheral blood eosinophilia or imaging the liver. Serologic testing is helpful, particularly in lightly infected individuals.

℞ BILIARY FLUKES

Drug therapy (praziquantel or triclabendazole) is summarized in Table 212-2. Patients with anatomic lesions in the biliary tract or malignancy are managed according to general medical guidelines.

INTESTINAL FLUKES

Two species of intestinal flukes cause human infection in defined geographic areas worldwide (Table 212-1). The large *Fasciolopsis buski* (adults measure 2 × 7 cm) is endemic in Southeast Asia, while the smaller *Heterophyes heterophyes* is found in the Nile Delta of Egypt and in the Far East. Infection is initiated by ingestion of metacercariae attached to aquatic plants (*F. buski*) or encysted in freshwater or brackish-water fish (*H. heterophyes*). Flukes mature in human intestines, and eggs are passed with stools. Most individuals infected with intestinal flukes are asymptomatic. In heavy *F. buski* infection, diarrhea, abdominal pain, and malabsorption may be encountered. Heavy infection with *H. heterophyes* may be associated with abdominal pain and mucous diarrhea. Diagnosis is established by detection of characteristically shaped ova in stool samples. The drug of choice for treatment is praziquantel (Table 212-2).

LUNG FLUKES

Infection with the lung fluke *Paragonimus westermani* (Table 212-1) and related species (e.g., *P. africanus*) is endemic in many parts of the world, excluding North America and Europe. Endemicity is particularly noticeable in West Africa, Central and South America, and Asia. In nature, the reservoir hosts of *P. westermani* are wild and domestic felines. In Africa, *P. africanus* has been found in other species, such as dogs. Adult lung flukes, which are 7–12 mm in length, are found encapsulated in the lungs of infected persons. In rare circumstances, flukes are found encysted in the CNS (cerebral paragonimiasis) or abdominal cavity. Humans acquire lung fluke infection by ingesting infective metacercariae encysted in the muscles and viscera of crayfish and freshwater crabs. In endemic areas, these crustaceans are consumed either raw or pickled. Once the organisms reach the duodenum, they excyst, penetrate the gut wall, and travel through the peritoneal cavity, diaphragm, and pleural space to reach the lungs. Mature flukes are found in the bronchioles surrounded by cystic lesions. Parasite eggs are either expectorated with sputum or swallowed and passed to the outside environment with feces. The life cycle is completed in snails and freshwater crustacea.

When maturing flukes lodge in lung tissues, they cause hemorrhage and necrosis, resulting in cyst formation. The adjacent lung parenchyma shows evidence of inflammatory infiltration, predominantly by eosinophils. Cysts usually measure 1–2 cm in diameter and may contain one or two worms each. With the onset of oviposition, cysts usually rupture in adjacent bronchioles—an event allowing ova to exit the human host. Older cysts develop thickened walls, which may undergo calcification. During the active phase of paragonimiasis, lung tissues surrounding parasite cysts may contain evidence of pneumonia, bronchitis, bronchiectasis, and fibrosis.

Pulmonary paragonimiasis is particularly symptomatic in persons with moderate to heavy infection. Productive cough with brownish sputum or frank hemoptysis associated with peripheral blood eosinophilia is usually the presenting feature. Chest examination may reveal signs of pleurisy. In chronic cases, bronchitis or bronchiectasis may predominate, but these conditions rarely proceed to lung abscess. Imaging of the lungs demonstrates characteristic features, including patchy densities, cavities, pleural effusion, and ring shadows. Cerebral paragonimiasis presents as either space-occupying lesions or epilepsy.

DIAGNOSIS

Pulmonary paragonimiasis is diagnosed by detection of parasite ova in sputum and/or stools. Serology is of considerable help in egg-negative cases and in cerebral paragonimiasis.

℞ LUNG FLUKES

The drug of choice for treatment is praziquantel (Table 212-2). Other medical or surgical management may be needed for pulmonary or cerebral lesions.

CONTROL AND PREVENTION OF TISSUE FLUKES

For residents of nonendemic areas who are visiting an endemic region, the only effective preventive measure is to avoid ingestion of local plants, fish, or crustaceans; if their ingestion is necessary, these items should be washed or cooked thoroughly. Instruction on water and food preparation and consumption should be included in physicians' advice to travelers (Chap. 117). Interruption of transmission among residents of endemic areas depends on avoiding ingestion of infective stages and disposing of feces and sputum appropriately to prevent hatching of eggs in the environment. These two approaches rely greatly on socioeconomic development and health education. In countries where economic progress has resulted in financial and social improvements, transmission has decreased. The third approach to control in endemic communities entails selective use of chemotherapy for individuals posing the highest risk of transmission—i.e., those with heavy infections. The availability of praziquantel—a broad-spectrum, safe, and effective anthelmintic agent—provides a means for reducing the reservoirs of infection in human populations. However, the existence of most of these helminths as zoonoses in several animal species complicates control efforts.

FURTHER READINGS

ALVES OLIVEIRA LF et al: Cytokine production associated with peripheral fibrosis during chronic schistosomiasis mansoni in humans. Infect Immun 74:1215, 2006

CAFFREY CR: Chemotherapy of schistosomiasis: Present and future. Curr Opin Chem Biol 11:433, 2007

CENTERS FOR DISEASE CONTROL AND PREVENTION: *http://www.cdc.gov/ncidod/dpd*

Drugs for Parasitic Infections. Med Lett Drugs Ther, August 1, 2004

JIA TW et al: Assessment of the age-specific disability weight of chronic schistosomiasis japonica. Bull World Health Organ 85:458, 2007

KALLESTRUP P et al: Schistosomiasis and HIV-1 infection in rural Zimbabwe: Effect of treatment of schistosomiasis on CD4 cell count and plasma HIV-1 RNA load. J Infect Dis 192:1956, 2005

KING CH: Lifting the burden of schistosomiasis—defining elements of infection-associated disease and the benefits of antiparasite treatment. J Infect Dis 196:653, 2007

LIM JH et al: Parasitic diseases of the biliary tract. AJR Am J Roentgenol 188:1596, 2007

LUN ZR et al: Clonorchiasis: A key foodborne zoonosis in China. Lancet Infect Dis 5:31, 2005

MAHMOUD AAFM (ed): Schistosomiasis, in *Tropical Medicine: Science and Practice*, G Pasvol, S Hoffman (eds). London, Imperial College Press, 2001, pp 1–510

STAUFFER WM et al: Biliary liver flukes (opisthorchiasis and clonorchiasis) in immigrants in the United States: Often subtle and diagnosed years after arrival. J Travel Med 11:157, 2004

213 Cestodes
A. Clinton White, Jr., Peter F. Weller

Cestodes, or tapeworms, are segmented worms. The adults reside in the gastrointestinal tract, but the larvae can be found in almost any organ. Human tapeworm infections can be divided into two major clinical groups. In one group, humans are the definitive hosts, with the adult tapeworms living in the gastrointestinal tract (*Taenia saginata, Diphyllobothrium, Hymenolepis,* and *Dipylidium caninum*). In the other, humans are intermediate hosts, with larval-stage parasites present in the tissues; diseases in this category include echinococcosis, sparganosis, and coenurosis. For *Taenia solium,* the human may be either the definitive or the intermediate host.

The ribbon-shaped tapeworm attaches to the intestinal mucosa by means of sucking cups or hooks located on the scolex. Behind the scolex is a short, narrow neck from which proglottids (segments) form. As each proglottid matures, it is displaced further back from the neck by the formation of new, less mature segments. The progressively elongating chain of attached proglottids, called the *strobila,* constitutes the bulk of the tapeworm. The length varies among species. In some, the tapeworm may consist of more than 1000 proglottids and may be several meters long. The mature proglottids are hermaphroditic and produce eggs, which are subsequently released. Since eggs of the different *Taenia* species are morphologically identical, differences in the morphology of the scolex or proglottids provide the basis for diagnostic identification to the species level.

Most human tapeworms require at least one intermediate host for complete larval development. After ingestion of the eggs or proglottids by an intermediate host, the larval oncospheres are activated, escape the egg, and penetrate the intestinal mucosa. The oncosphere migrates to tissues and develops into an encysted form known as a *cysticercus* (single scolex), a *coenurus* (multiple scolices), or a *hydatid* (cyst with daughter cysts, each containing several protoscolices). Ingestion by the definitive host of tissues containing a cyst enables a scolex to develop into a tapeworm.

TAENIASIS SAGINATA

The beef tapeworm *T. saginata* occurs in all countries where raw or undercooked beef is eaten. It is most prevalent in sub-Saharan African and Middle Eastern countries. *T. saginata asiatica* is a variant of *T. saginata* that is found in Asia and for which pigs are the intermediate host.

Etiology and Pathogenesis Humans are the only definitive host for the adult stage of *T. saginata.* This tapeworm, which can reach 8 m in length, inhabits the upper jejunum and has a scolex with four promi-

nent suckers and 1000–2000 proglottids. Each gravid segment has 15–30 uterine branches (in contrast to 8–12 for *T. solium*). The eggs are indistinguishable from those of *T. solium;* they measure 30–40 μm, contain the oncosphere, and have a thick brown striated shell. Eggs deposited on vegetation can live for months or years until they are ingested by cattle or other herbivores. The embryo released after ingestion invades the intestinal wall and is carried to striated muscle, where it transforms into a cysticercus. When ingested in raw or undercooked beef, this form can infect humans. After the cysticercus is ingested, it takes ~2 months for the mature adult worm to develop.

Clinical Manifestations Patients become aware of the infection most commonly by noting passage of proglottids in their feces. The proglottids are often motile, and patients may experience perianal discomfort when proglottids are discharged. Mild abdominal pain or discomfort, nausea, change in appetite, weakness, and weight loss can occur with *T. saginata* infection.

Diagnosis The diagnosis is made by the detection of eggs or proglottids in the stool. Eggs may also be present in the perianal area; thus, if proglottids or eggs are not found in the stool, the perianal region should be examined with use of a cellophane-tape swab (as in pinworm infection; Chap. 210). Distinguishing *T. saginata* from *T. solium* requires examination of mature proglottids or the scolex. Serologic tests are not helpful diagnostically. Eosinophilia and elevated levels of serum IgE may be detected.

℞ TAENIASIS SAGINATA

A single dose of praziquantel (10 mg/kg) is highly effective.

Prevention The major method of preventing infection is the adequate cooking of beef; exposure to temperatures as low as 56°C for 5 min will destroy cysticerci. Refrigeration or salting for long periods or freezing at −10°C for 9 days also kills cysticerci in beef. General preventive measures include inspection of beef and proper disposal of human feces.

TAENIASIS SOLIUM AND CYSTICERCOSIS

The pork tapeworm *T. solium* can cause two distinct forms of infection in humans: adult tapeworms in the intestine or larval forms in the tissues (cysticercosis). Humans are the only definitive hosts for *T. solium;* pigs are the usual intermediate hosts, although other animals may harbor the larval forms.

T. solium exists worldwide but is most prevalent in Latin America, sub-Saharan Africa, China, southern and Southeast Asia, and eastern Europe. Cysticercosis occurs in industrialized nations largely as a result of the immigration of infected persons from endemic areas.

FIGURE 213-1 Neurocysticercosis is caused by *Taenia solium*. Neurologic infection can be classified on the basis of the location and viability of the parasites. When the parasites are in the ventricles, they often cause obstructive hydrocephalus. **Left:** MRI showing a cysticercus in the lateral ventricle, with resultant hydrocephalus. The arrow points to the scolex within the cystic parasite. **Center:** CT showing a parenchymal cysticercus, with enhancement of the cyst wall and an internal scolex (*arrow*). **Right:** Multiple cysticerci, including calcified lesions from prior infection (*arrowheads*), viable cysticerci in the basilar cisterns (*white arrow*), and a large degenerating cysticercus in the Sylvian fissure (*black arrow*). (*Modified with permission from JC Bandres et al: Clin Infect Dis 15:799, 1992. © The University of Chicago Press.*)

Etiology and Pathogenesis The adult tapeworm generally resides in the upper jejunum. The scolex attaches by both sucking disks and two rows of hooklets. Often only one adult worm is present, but that worm may live for years. The tapeworm, usually ~3 m in length, may have as many as 1000 proglottids, each of which produces up to 50,000 eggs. Groups of 3–5 proglottids are generally released and excreted into the feces, and the eggs in these proglottids are infective for both humans and animals. The eggs may survive in the environment for several months. After ingestion of eggs by the pig intermediate host, the larvae are activated, escape the egg, penetrate the intestinal wall, and are carried to many tissues, with a predilection for striated muscle of the neck, tongue, and trunk. Within 60–90 days, the encysted larval stage develops. These cysticerci can survive for months to years. By ingesting undercooked pork containing cysticerci, humans acquire infections that lead to intestinal tapeworms. Infections that cause human cysticercosis follow the ingestion of *T. solium* eggs, usually from close contact with a tapeworm carrier. Autoinfection may occur if an individual with an egg-producing tapeworm ingests eggs derived from his or her own feces.

Clinical Manifestations Intestinal infections with *T. solium* may be asymptomatic. Fecal passage of proglottids may be noted by patients. Other symptoms are infrequent.

In cysticercosis, the clinical manifestations are variable. Cysticerci can be found anywhere in the body but are most commonly detected in the brain, cerebrospinal fluid (CSF), skeletal muscle, subcutaneous tissue, or eye. The clinical presentation of cysticercosis depends on the number and location of cysticerci as well as the extent of associated inflammatory responses or scarring. Neurologic manifestations are the most common (Fig. 213-1). Seizures are associated with inflammation surrounding cysticerci in the brain parenchyma. These seizures may be generalized, focal, or Jacksonian. Hydrocephalus results from obstruction of CSF flow by cysticerci and accompanying inflammation or by CSF outflow obstruction from arachnoiditis. Signs of increased intracranial pressure, including headache, nausea, vomiting, changes in vision, dizziness, ataxia, or confusion, are often evident. Patients with hydrocephalus may develop papilledema or display altered mental status. When cysticerci develop at the base of the brain or in the subarachnoid space, they may cause chronic meningitis or arachnoiditis, communicating hydrocephalus, or strokes.

Diagnosis The diagnosis of intestinal *T. solium* infection is made by the detection of eggs or proglottids, as described for *T. saginata*. In cysticercosis, diagnosis can be difficult. A consensus conference has delineated absolute, major, minor, and epidemiologic criteria for diagnosis (Table 213-1). Diagnostic certainty is possible only with definite demonstration of the parasite (absolute criteria). This task can be accomplished by histologic observation of the parasite in excised tissue, by funduscopic visualization of the parasite in the eye (in the anterior chamber, vitreous, or subretinal spaces), or by neuroimaging studies demonstrating cystic lesions containing a characteristic scolex. In most cases, diagnostic certainty is not possible. Instead, a clinical diagnosis is made on the basis of a combination of clinical presentation, radiographic studies, serologic tests, and exposure history.

Neuroimaging findings suggestive of neurocysticercosis constitute the primary major diagnostic criterion. These findings include cystic lesions with or without enhancement (e.g., ring enhancement), one or more nodular calcifications (which may also have associated enhancement), or focal enhancing lesions. Cysticerci in the brain parenchyma are usually 5–20 mm in diameter and rounded. Cystic lesions in the subarachnoid space or fissures may enlarge up to 6 cm in diameter and may be lobulated. For cysticerci within the subarachnoid space or ventricles, the walls may be very thin and the cyst fluid is often isodense with CSF. Thus, obstructive hydrocephalus or enhancement of the basilar meninges may be the only finding on CT in extraparenchymal neurocysticercosis. Cysticerci in the ventricles or subarachnoid space are usually visible to an experienced neuroradiologist on MRI or on CT with intraventricular contrast injection. CT is more sensitive than MRI in identifying calcified lesions, whereas MRI is better for identifying cystic lesions and enhancement.

The second major diagnostic criterion is detection of specific antibodies to cysticerci. While most tests employing unfractionated antigen have high rates of false-positive and false-negative results, this problem

TABLE 213-1 DIAGNOSTIC CRITERIA FOR HUMAN CYSTICERCOSIS[a]

1. Absolute criteria
   a. Demonstration of cysticerci by histologic or microscopic examination of biopsy material
   b. Visualization of the parasite in the eye by funduscopy
   c. Neuroradiologic demonstration of cystic lesions containing a characteristic scolex
2. Major criteria
   a. Neuroradiologic lesions suggestive of neurocysticercosis
   b. Demonstration of antibodies to cysticerci in serum by enzyme-linked immunoelectrotransfer blot
   c. Resolution of intracranial cystic lesions spontaneously or after therapy with albendazole or praziquantel alone
3. Minor criteria
   a. Lesions compatible with neurocysticercosis detected by neuroimaging studies
   b. Clinical manifestations suggestive of neurocysticercosis
   c. Demonstration of antibodies to cysticerci or cysticercal antigen in cerebrospinal fluid by ELISA
   d. Evidence of cysticercosis outside the central nervous system (e.g., cigar-shaped soft tissue calcifications)
4. Epidemiologic criteria
   a. Residence in a cysticercosis-endemic area
   b. Frequent travel to a cysticercosis-endemic area
   c. Household contact with an individual infected with *Taenia solium*

[a]Diagnosis is confirmed by either one absolute criterion or a combination of two major criteria, one minor criterion, and one epidemiologic criterion. A probable diagnosis is supported by the fulfillment of (1) one major criterion plus two minor criteria; (2) one major criterion plus one minor criterion and one epidemiologic criterion; or (3) three minor criteria plus one epidemiologic criterion.

Note: ELISA, enzyme-linked immunosorbent assay.

Source: Modified from Del Brutto et al.

can be overcome by using the more specific immunoblot assay. An immunoblot assay using lentil-lectin purified glycoproteins has >99% specificity and is highly sensitive. However, patients with single intracranial lesions or with calcifications may be seronegative. With this assay, serum samples provide greater diagnostic sensitivity than CSF. All of the diagnostic antigens have been cloned, and enzyme-linked immunosorbent assays (ELISAs) using recombinant antigens are being developed. Antigen detection assays employing monoclonal antibodies to detect parasite antigen in the blood or spinal fluid may also facilitate diagnosis. However, these assays are not widely available.

Studies have demonstrated that clinical criteria can aid in the diagnosis in selected cases. In patients from endemic areas who had single enhancing lesions presenting with seizures, a normal physical examination, and no evidence of systemic disease (e.g., no fever, adenopathy, or abnormal chest radiograph), the constellation of rounded CT lesions 5–20 mm in diameter with no midline shift was almost always caused by neurocysticercosis. Finally, spontaneous resolution or resolution after therapy with albendazole alone is consistent with neurocysticercosis.

Minor diagnostic criteria include neuroimaging findings consistent with but less characteristic of cysticercosis, clinical manifestations suggestive of neurocysticercosis (e.g., seizures, hydrocephalus, or altered mental status), evidence of cysticercosis outside the central nervous system (CNS; e.g., cigar-shaped soft tissue calcifications), or detection of antibody in CSF by ELISA. Epidemiologic criteria include exposure to a tapeworm carrier or household member infected with *T. solium*, current or prior residence in an endemic area, and frequent travel to an endemic area.

Diagnosis is confirmed in patients with either one absolute criterion or a combination of two major criteria, one minor criterion, and one epidemiologic criterion (Table 213-1). A probable diagnosis is supported by the fulfillment of (1) one major criterion plus two minor criteria; (2) one major criterion plus one minor criterion and one epidemiologic criterion; or (3) three minor criteria plus one epidemiologic criterion. While the CSF is usually abnormal in neurocysticercosis, CSF abnormalities are not pathognomonic. Patients may have CSF pleocytosis with a predominance of lymphocytes, neutrophils, or eosinophils. The protein level in CSF may be elevated; the glucose concentration is usually normal but may be depressed.

℞ TAENIASIS SOLIUM AND CYSTICERCOSIS

Intestinal *T. solium* infection is treated with a single dose of praziquantel (10 mg/kg). However, praziquantel occasionally evokes an inflammatory response in the CNS if concomitant cryptic cysticercosis is present. Niclosamide (2 g) is also effective but is not widely available.

The initial management of neurocysticercosis should focus on symptom-based treatment of seizures or hydrocephalus. Seizures can usually be controlled with antiepileptic treatment. If parenchymal lesions resolve without development of calcifications and patients remain free of seizures, antiepileptic therapy can usually be discontinued after 1–2 years. Placebo-controlled trials are beginning to clarify the clinical advantage of antiparasitic drugs for parenchymal neurocysticercosis. Trends toward faster resolution of neuroradiologic abnormalities have been observed in most studies. The clinical benefits are less dramatic and consist mainly of shortening the period during which recurrent seizures occur and decreasing the number of patients who have many recurrent seizures. For the treatment of patients with brain parenchymal cysticerci, most authorities favor antiparasitic drugs, including praziquantel (50–60 mg/kg daily in three divided doses for 15–30 days) or albendazole (15 mg/kg per day for 8–28 days). Both agents may exacerbate the inflammatory response around the dying parasite, thereby exacerbating seizures or hydrocephalus as well. Thus, patients receiving these drugs should be carefully monitored, and high-dose glucocorticoids should be used during treatment. Since glucocorticoids induce first-pass metabolism of praziquantel and may decrease its antiparasitic effect, cimetidine should be coadministered to inhibit praziquantel metabolism.

For patients with hydrocephalus, the emergent reduction of intracranial pressure is the mainstay of therapy. In the case of obstructive hydrocephalus, the preferred approach is removal of the cysticercus via endoscopic surgery.

However, this intervention is not always possible. An alternative approach is initially to perform a diverting procedure, such as ventriculoperitoneal shunting. Historically, shunts have usually failed, but low failure rates have been attained with administration of antiparasitic drugs and glucocorticoids. Open craniotomy to remove cysticerci is now required only infrequently. For patients with subarachnoid cysts or giant cysticerci, glucocorticoids are needed to reduce arachnoiditis and accompanying vasculitis. Most authorities recommend prolonged courses of antiparasitic drugs and shunting when hydrocephalus is present. In patients with diffuse cerebral edema and elevated intracranial pressure due to multiple inflamed lesions, glucocorticoids are the mainstay of therapy, and antiparasitic drugs should be avoided. For ocular and spinal medullary lesions, drug-induced inflammation may cause irreversible damage. Most patients should be managed surgically, although case reports have described cures with medical therapy.

Prevention Measures for the prevention of intestinal *T. solium* infection consist of the application to pork of precautions similar to those described above for beef with regard to *T. saginata* infection. The prevention of cysticercosis involves minimizing the opportunities for ingestion of fecally derived eggs by means of good personal hygiene, effective fecal disposal, and treatment and prevention of human intestinal infections. Mass chemotherapy has been administered to human and porcine populations in efforts at disease eradication.

ECHINOCOCCOSIS

Echinococcosis is an infection caused in humans by the larval stage of the *Echinococcus granulosus* complex, *E. multilocularis*, or *E. vogeli*. *E. granulosus* complex parasites, which produce unilocular cystic lesions, are prevalent in areas where livestock is raised in association with dogs.

 These parasites are found on all continents, with areas of high prevalence in China, central Asia, the Middle East, the Mediterranean region, eastern Africa, and parts of South America. Molecular evidence suggests that *E. granulosus* strains may actually belong to more than one species; specifically, strains from sheep, cattle, pigs, horses, and camels probably represent separate species. *E. multilocularis*, which causes multilocular alveolar lesions that are locally invasive, is found in Alpine, sub-Arctic, or Arctic regions, including Canada, the United States, and central and northern Europe; China; and central Asia. *E. vogeli* causes polycystic hydatid disease and is found only in Central and South America.

Like other cestodes, echinococcal species have both intermediate and definitive hosts. The definitive hosts are canines that pass eggs in their feces. After the ingestion of eggs, cysts develop in the intermediate hosts—sheep, cattle, humans, goats, camels, and horses for the *E. granulosus* complex and mice and other rodents for *E. multilocularis*. When a dog (*E. granulosus*) or fox (*E. multilocularis*) ingests infected meat containing cysts, the life cycle is completed.

Etiology The small (5-mm-long) adult *E. granulosus* worm, which lives for 5–20 months in the jejunum of dogs, has only three proglottids: one immature, one mature, and one gravid. The gravid segment splits to release eggs that are morphologically similar to *Taenia* eggs and are extremely hardy. After humans ingest the eggs, embryos escape from the eggs, penetrate the intestinal mucosa, enter the portal circulation, and are carried to various organs, most commonly the liver and lungs. Larvae develop into fluid-filled unilocular hydatid cysts that consist of an external membrane and an inner germinal layer. Daughter cysts develop from the inner aspect of the germinal layer, as do germinating cystic structures called *brood capsules*. New larvae, called *protoscolices*, develop in large numbers within the brood capsule. The cysts expand slowly over a period of years.

The life cycle of *E. multilocularis* is similar except that wild canines, such as foxes, serve as the definitive hosts and small rodents serve as the intermediate hosts. The larval form of *E. multilocularis*, however, is quite different in that it remains in the proliferative phase, the parasite is always multilocular, and vesicles without brood capsule or protoscolices progressively invade the host tissue by peripheral extension of processes from the germinal layer.

Clinical Manifestations Slowly enlarging echinococcal cysts generally remain asymptomatic until their expanding size or their space-occupying effect in an involved organ elicits symptoms. The liver and the lungs are the most common sites of these cysts. The liver is involved in about two-thirds of *E. granulosus* infections and in nearly all *E. multilocularis* infections. Since a period of years elapses before cysts enlarge sufficiently to cause symptoms, they may be discovered incidentally on a routine x-ray or ultrasound study.

Patients with hepatic echinococcosis who are symptomatic most often present with abdominal pain or a palpable mass in the right upper quadrant. Compression of a bile duct or leakage of cyst fluid into the biliary tree may mimic recurrent cholelithiasis, and biliary obstruction can result in jaundice. Rupture of or episodic leakage from a hydatid cyst may produce fever, pruritus, urticaria, eosinophilia, or anaphylaxis. Pulmonary hydatid cysts may rupture into the bronchial tree or peritoneal cavity and produce cough, dyspnea, chest pain, or hemoptysis. Rupture of hydatid cysts, which can occur spontaneously or at surgery, may lead to multifocal dissemination of protoscolices, which can form additional cysts. Other presentations are due to the involvement of bone (invasion of the medullary cavity with slow bone erosion producing pathologic fractures), the CNS (space-occupying lesions), the heart (conduction defects, pericarditis), and the pelvis (pelvic mass).

The larval forms of *E. multilocularis* characteristically present as a slowly growing hepatic tumor, with progressive destruction of the liver and extension into vital structures. Patients commonly report upper quadrant and epigastric pain. Liver enlargement and obstructive jaundice may be apparent. The lesions may infiltrate adjoining organs (e.g., diaphragm, kidneys, or lungs) or may metastasize to the spleen, lungs, or brain.

Diagnosis Radiographic and related imaging studies are important in detecting and evaluating echinococcal cysts. Plain films will define pulmonary cysts of *E. granulosus*—usually as rounded masses of uniform density—but may miss cysts in other organs unless there is cyst wall calcification (as occurs in the liver). MRI, CT, and ultrasound reveal well-defined cysts with thick or thin walls. When older cysts contain a layer of hydatid sand that is rich in accumulated protoscolices, these imaging methods may detect this fluid layer of different density. However, the most pathognomonic finding, if demonstrable, is that of daughter cysts within the larger cyst. This finding, like eggshell or mural calcification on CT, is indicative of *E. granulosus* infection and helps to distinguish the cyst from carcinomas, bacterial or amebic liver abscesses, or hemangiomas. In contrast, ultrasound or CT of alveolar hydatid cysts reveals indistinct solid masses with central necrosis and plaquelike calcifications.

A specific diagnosis of *E. granulosus* infection can be made by the examination of aspirated fluids for protoscolices or hooklets, but diagnostic aspiration is not usually recommended because of the risk of fluid leakage resulting in either dissemination of infection or anaphylactic reactions. Serodiagnostic assays can be useful, although a negative test does not exclude the diagnosis of echinococcosis. Cysts in the liver elicit positive antibody responses in ~90% of cases, whereas up to 50% of individuals with cysts in the lungs are seronegative. Detection of antibody to specific echinococcal antigens by immunoblotting has the highest degree of specificity.

℞ ECHINOCOCCOSIS

Therapy for cystic echinococcosis is based on considerations of the size, location, and manifestations of cysts and the overall health of the patient. Surgery has traditionally been the principal definitive method of treatment. Currently, ultrasound staging is recommended for *E. granulosus* infections **(Fig. 213-2)**. For CE1 lesions, uncomplicated CE3 lesions, and some CE2 lesions, PAIR (percutaneous aspiration, infusion of scolicidal agents, and reaspiration) is now recommended instead of surgery. PAIR is contraindicated for superficially located cysts (because of the risk of rupture), for cysts with multiple thick internal septal divisions (honeycombing pattern), and for cysts communicating with the biliary tree. For prophylaxis of secondary peritoneal echinococcosis due to inadvertent spillage of fluid during PAIR, the administration of albendazole (15 mg/kg daily in two divided doses) should be initiated at least 4 days before the procedure and continued for at least 4 weeks afterward. Ultrasound- or CT-guided aspiration allows confirmation of the diagnosis by demonstration of protoscolices in the aspirate. After aspiration, contrast material should be injected to detect occult communications with the biliary tract. Alternatively, the fluid should be checked for bile staining by dipstick. If no bile is found and no communication visualized, the contrast material is reaspirated, with subsequent infusion of scolicidal agents (usually 95% ethanol; alternatively, hypertonic saline). Daughter cysts within the primary cyst may need to be

Echinococcosis cysts

| CL | CE1 | CE2 | CE3 | CE4 | CE5 |

Cystic lesion — Active — Transitional — Inactive

FIGURE 213-2 Management of cystic hydatid disease caused by *Echinococcus granulosus* should be based on viability of the parasite, which can be estimated from radiographic appearance. The ultrasound appearance includes lesions classified as active, transitional, and inactive. *Active* cysts include types CL (with a cystic lesion and no visible cyst wall), CE1 [with a visible cyst wall and internal echoes (snowflake sign)], and CE2 (with a visible cyst wall and internal septation). *Transitional cysts* (CE3) may have detached laminar membranes or may be partially collapsed. *Inactive cysts* include types CE4 (a nonhomogeneous mass) and CE5 (a cyst with a thick calcified wall). [*Adapted from RL Guerrant et al (eds): Tropical Infectious Diseases: Principles, Pathogens and Practice, 2d ed, p 1312. © 2005, with permission from Elsevier Science.*]

punctured separately. In experienced hands, this approach yields rates of cure and relapse equivalent to those following surgery, with less perioperative morbidity and shorter hospitalization.

Surgery remains the treatment of choice for complicated *E. granulosus* cysts (e.g., those communicating with the biliary tract) or for areas where PAIR is not possible. For *E. granulosus*, the preferred surgical approach is pericystectomy, in which the entire cyst and the surrounding fibrous tissue are removed. The risks posed by leakage of fluid during surgery or PAIR include anaphylaxis and dissemination of infectious protoscolices. The latter complication has been minimized by careful attention to the prevention of spillage of the cyst and by soaking of the drapes with hypertonic saline. Infusion of scolicidal agents is no longer recommended because of problems with hypernatremia, intoxication, or sclerosing cholangitis. Albendazole, which is active against *Echinococcus*, should be administered adjunctively, beginning several days before resection and continuing for several weeks for *E. granulosus*. Praziquantel (50 mg/kg daily for 2 weeks) may hasten the death of the protoscolices. Medical therapy with albendazole alone for 12 weeks to 6 months results in cure in ~30% of cases and in improvement in another 50%. In many instances of treatment failure, *E. granulosus* infections are subsequently treated successfully with PAIR or additional courses of medical therapy. Response to treatment is best assessed by serial imaging studies, with attention to cyst size and consistency. Some cysts may not demonstrate complete radiologic resolution even though no viable protoscolices are present. Some of these cysts with partial radiologic resolution (e.g., CE4) can be managed with observation only.

Surgical resection remains the treatment of choice for *E. multilocularis* infection. Complete removal of the parasite continues to offer the best chance for cure. Ongoing therapy with albendazole for at least 2 years after presumptively curative surgery is recommended. Most cases are diagnosed at a stage at which complete resection is not possible; in these cases, albendazole treatment should be continued indefinitely, with careful monitoring. In some cases, liver transplantation has been used because of the size of the necessary liver resection. However, continuous immunosuppression favors the proliferation of *E. multilocularis* larvae and reinfection of the transplant. Thus, indefinite treatment with albendazole is required.

Prevention   In endemic areas, echinococcosis can be prevented by administering praziquantel to infected dogs, by denying dogs access to infected animals, or by vaccinating sheep. Limitation of the number of stray dogs is helpful in reducing the prevalence of infection among humans.

HYMENOLEPIASIS NANA

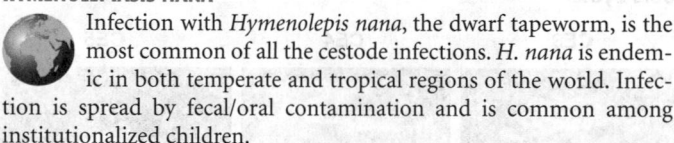 Infection with *Hymenolepis nana*, the dwarf tapeworm, is the most common of all the cestode infections. *H. nana* is endemic in both temperate and tropical regions of the world. Infection is spread by fecal/oral contamination and is common among institutionalized children.

Etiology and Pathogenesis   *H. nana* is the only cestode of humans that does not require an intermediate host. Both the larval and adult phases of the life cycle take place in the human. The adult—the smallest tapeworm parasitizing humans—is ~2 cm long and dwells in the proximal ileum. Proglottids, which are quite small and are rarely seen in the stool, release spherical eggs 30–44 μm in diameter, each of which contains an oncosphere with six hooklets. The eggs are immediately infective and are unable to survive for >10 days in the external environment. *H. nana* can also be acquired by the ingestion of infected insects (especially larval meal-worms and larval fleas). When the egg is ingested by a new host, the oncosphere is freed and penetrates the intestinal villi, becoming a cysticercoid larva. Larvae migrate back into the intestinal lumen, attach to the mucosa, and mature into adult worms over 10–12 days. Eggs may also hatch before passing into the stool, causing internal autoinfection with increasing numbers of intestinal worms. Although the life span of adult *H. nana* worms is only ~4–10 weeks, the autoinfection cycle perpetuates the infection.

Clinical Manifestations   *H. nana* infection, even with many intestinal worms, is usually asymptomatic. When infection is intense, anorexia, abdominal pain, and diarrhea develop.

Diagnosis   Infection is diagnosed by the finding of eggs in the stool.

℞ HYMENOLEPIASIS NANA

Praziquantel (25 mg/kg once) is the treatment of choice, since it acts against both the adult worms and the cysticercoids in the intestinal villi. Nitazoxanide (500 mg bid for 3 days) may be used as an alternative.

Prevention   Good personal hygiene and improved sanitation can eradicate the disease. Epidemics have been controlled by mass chemotherapy coupled with improved hygiene.

HYMENOLEPIASIS DIMINUTA
Hymenolepis diminuta, a cestode of rodents, occasionally infects small children, who ingest the larvae in uncooked cereal foods contaminated by fleas and other insects in which larvae develop. Infection is usually asymptomatic and is diagnosed by the detection of eggs in the stool. Treatment with praziquantel results in cure in most cases.

DIPHYLLOBOTHRIASIS
 Diphyllobothrium latum and other *Diphyllobothrium* species are found in the lakes, rivers, and deltas of the northern hemisphere, Central Africa, and Chile.

Etiology and Pathogenesis   The adult worm—the longest tapeworm (up to 25 m)—attaches to the ileal and occasionally to the jejunal mucosa by its suckers, which are located on its elongated scolex. The adult worm has 3000–4000 proglottids, which release ~1 million eggs daily into the feces. If an egg reaches water, it hatches and releases a free-swimming embryo that can be eaten by small freshwater crustaceans (*Cyclops* or *Diaptomus* species). After an infected crustacean containing a developed procercoid is swallowed by a fish, the larva migrates into the fish's flesh and grows into a plerocercoid, or sparganum larva. Humans acquire the infection by ingesting infected raw or smoked fish. Within 3–5 weeks, the tapeworm matures into an adult in the human intestine.

Clinical Manifestations   Most *D. latum* infections are asymptomatic, although manifestations may include transient abdominal discomfort, diarrhea, vomiting, weakness, and weight loss. Occasionally, infection can cause acute abdominal pain and intestinal obstruction; in rare cases, cholangitis or cholecystitis may be produced by migrating proglottids. Because the tapeworm absorbs large quantities of vitamin B_{12} and interferes with ileal B_{12} absorption, vitamin B_{12} deficiency can develop. Up to 2% of infected patients, especially the elderly, have megaloblastic anemia resembling pernicious anemia and may exhibit neurologic sequelae of B_{12} deficiency.

Diagnosis   The diagnosis is made readily by the detection of the characteristic eggs in the stool. The eggs possess a single shell with an operculum at one end and a knob at the other. Mild to moderate eosinophilia may be detected.

℞ DIPHYLLOBOTHRIASIS

Praziquantel (5–10 mg/kg once) is highly effective. Parenteral vitamin B_{12} should be given if B_{12} deficiency is manifest.

Prevention   Infection can be prevented by heating fish to 54°C for 5 min or by freezing it at −18°C for 24 h. Placing fish in brine with a high salt concentration for long periods kills the eggs.

DIPYLIDIASIS
Dipylidium caninum, a common tapeworm of dogs and cats, may accidentally infect humans. Dogs, cats, and occasionally humans become infected by ingesting fleas harboring cysticercoids. Children are more likely to become infected than adults. Most infections are asymptomatic, but abdominal pain, diarrhea, anal pruritus, urticaria, eosinophilia, or passage of segments in the stool may occur. The diagnosis is made by the

detection of proglottids or ova in the stool. As in *D. latum* infection, therapy consists of praziquantel. Prevention requires anthelmintic treatment and flea control for pet dogs or cats.

SPARGANOSIS

Humans can be infected by the sparganum, or plerocercoid larva, of a diphyllobothrid tapeworm of the genus *Spirometra*. Infection can be acquired by the consumption of water containing infected *Cyclops*; by the ingestion of infected snakes, birds, or mammals; or by the application of infected flesh as poultices. The worm migrates slowly in tissues, and infection commonly presents as a subcutaneous swelling. Periorbital tissues can be involved, and ocular sparganosis may destroy the eye. Surgical excision is used to treat localized sparganosis.

COENUROSIS

This rare infection of humans by the larval stage (coenurus) of the dog tapeworm *Taenia multiceps* or *T. serialis* results in a space-occupying cystic lesion. As in cysticercosis, involvement of the CNS and subcutaneous tissue is most common. Both definitive diagnosis and treatment require surgical excision of the lesion. Chemotherapeutic agents generally are not effective.

WEBSITE OF INTEREST: *CDC Division of Parasitic Diseases. www.cdc.gov/ncidod/dpd/default.htm*

FURTHER READINGS

DEL BRUTTO OH et al: Proposed diagnostic criteria for neurocysticercosis. Neurology 57:177, 2001

ECKERT J, DEPLAZES P: Biological, epidemiological, and clinical aspects of echinococcosis, a zoonosis of increasing concern. Clin Microbiol Rev 17:107, 2004

GARCIA HH et al: A trial of antiparasitic treatment to reduce the rate of seizures due to cerebral cysticercosis. N Engl J Med 350:249, 2004

———— et al: Current consensus guidelines for treatment of neurocysticercosis. Clin Microbiol Rev 15:747, 2002

NASH TE et al: Treatment of neurocysticercosis: Current status and future research needs. Neurology 67:1120, 2006

PAWLOWSKI ZS et al: Echinococcosis in humans: Clinical aspects, diagnosis, and treatment, in *WHO/OIE Manual on Echinococcosis in Humans and Animals: A Public Health Problem of Global Concern*, J Eckert et al (eds). Paris, World Organization for Animal Health, 2001

SCHANTZ PM et al: Echinococcosis, in *Tropical Infectious Diseases: Principles, Pathogens and Practice*, 2d ed, RL Guerrant et al (eds). Philadelphia, Churchill Livingstone, 2005, p 1304

SINGH G, PRABHAKAR S: *Taenia solium Cysticercosis: From Basic Science to Clinical Science.* Wallingford, UK, CABI Publishing, 2002

WORLD HEALTH ORGANIZATION INFORMAL WORKING GROUP ON ECHINOCOCCOSIS: International classification of ultrasound images in cystic echinococcosis for application in clinical and field epidemiological settings. Acta Tropica 85:253, 2003

————: PAIR puncture, aspiration, injection, re-aspiration: An option for the treatment of cystic echinococcosis. WHO/CDS/CSR/APH/2001.6. Geneva, WHO, 2001

214 Microbial Bioterrorism
H. Clifford Lane, Anthony S. Fauci

Descriptions of the use of microbial pathogens as potential weapons of war or terrorism date from ancient times. Among the most frequently cited of such episodes are the poisoning of water supplies in the sixth century B.C. with the fungus *Claviceps purpurea* (rye ergot) by the Assyrians, the hurling of the dead bodies of plague victims over the walls of the city of Kaffa by the Tartar army in 1346, and the efforts by the British to spread smallpox via contaminated blankets to the native American population loyal to the French in 1767. Although the use of chemical weapons in wartime took place in the not-too-distant past (Chap. 215), the tragic events of September 11, 2001, followed closely by the anthrax attacks through the U.S. Postal System, dramatically changed the mindset of the American public regarding both our vulnerability to microbial bioterrorist attacks and the seriousness and intent of the Federal government to protect its citizens against future attacks. Modern science has revealed methods of deliberately spreading or enhancing disease in ways not appreciated by our ancestors. The combination of basic research, good medical practice, and constant vigilance will be needed to defend against such attacks.

Although the potential impact of a bioterrorist attack could be enormous, leading to thousands of deaths and extensive morbidity, acts of bioterrorism would be expected to produce their greatest impact through the fear and terror they generate. In contrast to biowarfare, where the primary goal is destruction of the enemy through mass casualties, an important goal of bioterrorism is to destroy the morale of a society through fear and uncertainty. While the actual biologic impact of a single act may be small, the degree of disruption created by the realization that such an attack is possible may be enormous. This was readily apparent with the impact on the U.S. Postal System and the functional interruption of the activities of the legislative branch of government following the anthrax attacks noted above. Thus, the key to the defense against these attacks is a highly functioning system of public health surveillance and education so that attacks can be quickly recognized and effectively contained. This is complemented by the availability of appropriate countermeasures in the form of diagnostics, therapeutics, and vaccines, both in response to and in anticipation of bioterrorist attacks.

The Working Group for Civilian Biodefense has put together a list of key features that characterize the elements of biologic agents that make them particularly effective as weapons (Table 214-1). Included among these are the ease of spread and transmission of the agent as well as the presence of an adequate database to allow newcomers to the field to quickly apply the good science of others to bad intentions of their own. Agents of bioterrorism may be used in their naturally occurring forms or they can be deliberately modified to provide maximal impact. Among the approaches to maximizing the deleterious effects of biologic agents are the genetic modification of microbes for the

purposes of antimicrobial resistance or evasion by the immune system, creation of fine-particle aerosols, chemical treatment to stabilize and prolong infectivity, and alteration of host range through changes in surface proteins. Certain of these approaches fall under the category of *weaponization*, which is a term generally used to describe the processing of microbes or toxins in a manner that would ensure a devastating effect of a release. For example, weaponization of anthrax by the Soviets comprised the production of vast amounts of spores in a form that maintained aerosolization for prolonged periods of time; the spores were of appropriate size to reach the lower respiratory tract easily and could be delivered in a massive release, such as via widely dispersed bomblets.

The U.S. Centers for Disease Control and Prevention (CDC) classifies potential biologic threats into three categories, A, B, and C (Table 214-2). Category A agents are the highest-priority pathogens. They pose the greatest risk to national security because they (1) can be easily disseminated or transmitted from person to person, (2) result in high mortality rates and have the potential for major public health impact, (3) might cause public panic and social disruption, and (4) require special action for public health preparedness. Category B agents are the second highest priority pathogens and include those that are moderately easy to disseminate, result in moderate morbidity rates and low mortality rates, and require specifically enhanced diagnostic capacity. Category C agents are the third highest priority. These include certain emerging pathogens, to which the general population lacks immunity, that could be engineered for mass dissemination in the future because of availability, ease of production, ease of dissemination, potential for high morbidity and mortality, and major public health impact. A potential pandemic strain of influenza, such as avian influenza, is one such example. It should be pointed out, however, that these designations are empirical, and, depending on evolving circumstances such as intelligence-based threat assessments, the priority rating of any given microbe or toxin could change. The CDC classification system also largely reflects the severity of illness produced by a given agent, rather than its accessibility to potential terrorists.

TABLE 214-2 CDC CATEGORY A, B, AND C AGENTS

Category A
- Anthrax (*Bacillus anthracis*)
- Botulism (*Clostridium botulinum* toxin)
- Plague (*Yersinia pestis*)
- Smallpox (*Variola major*)
- Tularemia (*Francisella tularensis*)
- Viral hemorrhagic fevers
  - Arenaviruses: Lassa, New World (Machupo, Junin, Guanarito, and Sabia)
  - Bunyaviridae: Crimean Congo, Rift Valley
  - Filoviridae: Ebola, Marburg

Category B
- Brucellosis (*Brucella* spp.)
- Epsilon toxin of *Clostridium perfringens*
- Food safety threats (e.g., *Salmonella* spp., *Escherichia coli* 0157:H7, *Shigella*)
- Glanders (*Burkholderia mallei*)
- Melioidosis (*B. pseudomallei*)
- Psittacosis (*Chlamydophila psittaci*)
- Q fever (*Coxiella burnetii*)
- Ricin toxin from *Ricinus communis* (castor beans)
- Staphylococcal enterotoxin B
- Typhus fever (*Rickettsia prowazekii*)
- Viral encephalitis [alphaviruses (e.g., Venezuelan, eastern, and western equine encephalitis)]
- Water safety threats (e.g., *Vibrio cholerae*, *Cryptosporidium parvum*)

Category C
- Emerging infectious diseases threats such as Nipah, hantavirus, SARS coronavirus, and pandemic influenza.

Centers for Disease Control and Prevention and the National Institute of Allergy and Infectious Diseases.

TABLE 214-1 KEY FEATURES OF BIOLOGIC AGENTS USED AS BIOWEAPONS

1. High morbidity and mortality
2. Potential for person-to-person spread
3. Low infective dose and highly infectious by aerosol
4. Lack of rapid diagnostic capability
5. Lack of universally available effective vaccine
6. Potential to cause anxiety
7. Availability of pathogen and feasibility of production
8. Environmental stability
9. Database of prior research and development
10. Potential to be "weaponized"

Source: From L Borio et al: JAMA 287:2391, 2002; with permission.

ANTHRAX

See also Chap. 131.

***Bacillus anthracis* as a Bioweapon**   Anthrax may be the prototypic disease of bioterrorism. Although rarely, if ever, spread from person to person, the illness embodies the other major features of a disease introduced through terrorism, as outlined in Table 214-1. U.S. and British government scientists studied anthrax as a potential biologic weapon beginning approximately at the time of World War II (WWII). Offensive bioweapons activity including bioweapons research on microbes and toxins in the United States ceased in 1969 as a result of two executive orders by President Richard M. Nixon. The 1972 Biological and Toxin Weapons Convention Treaty outlawed research of this type worldwide. Clearly, the Soviet Union was in direct violation of this treaty until at least the Union dissolved in the late 1980s. It is well documented that during this post-treaty period, the Soviets produced and stored tons of anthrax spores for potential use as a bioweapon. At present there is suspicion that research on anthrax as an agent of bioterrorism is ongoing by several nations and extremist groups. One example of this is the release of anthrax spores by the Aum Shrinrikyo cult in Tokyo in 1993. Fortunately, there were no casualties associated with this episode because of the inadvertent use of a nonpathogenic strain of anthrax by the terrorists.

The potential impact of anthrax spores as a bioweapon was clearly demonstrated in 1979 following the accidental release of spores into the atmosphere from a Soviet Union bioweapons facility in Sverdlosk, Russia. While actual figures are not known, at least 77 cases of anthrax were diagnosed with certainty, of which 66 were fatal. These victims were exposed in an area within 4 km downwind of the facility, and deaths due to anthrax were also noted in livestock up to 50 km further downwind. Based on recorded wind patterns, the interval between the time of exposure and development of clinical illness ranged from 2–43 days. The majority of cases were within the first 2 weeks. Death typically occurred within 1–4 days following the onset of symptoms. It is likely that the widespread use of postexposure penicillin prophylaxis limited the total number of cases. The extended period of time between exposure and disease in some individuals supports the data from nonhuman primate studies suggesting the anthrax spores can lie dormant in the respiratory tract for at least 4–6 weeks without evoking an immune response. This extended period of microbiologic latency following exposure poses a significant challenge for management of victims in the postexposure period.

In September 2001, the American public was exposed to anthrax spores as a bioweapon delivered through the U.S. Postal System. The CDC identified 22 confirmed or suspected cases of anthrax as a consequence of this attack. These included 11 patients with inhalational anthrax, of whom 5 died, and 11 patients with cutaneous anthrax (7 confirmed), all of whom survived (Fig. 214-1). Cases occurred in individuals who opened contaminated letters as well as in postal workers involved in the processing of mail. A minimum of five letters mailed from Trenton, NJ, served as the vehicles for these attacks. One of these letters was reported to contain 2 g of material, equivalent to 100 billion to 1 trillion weapon-grade spores. Since studies performed in the 1950s using monkeys exposed to aerosolized anthrax suggested that ~10,000 spores were required to produce lethal disease in 50% of animals exposed to this dose (the LD_{50}), the contents of one letter had the theoretical potential, under optimal conditions, of causing illness or death in up to 50 million individuals when one considers an LD_{50} of 10,000 spores. The strain used in this attack was the Ames strain. Although it was noted to have an inducible beta-lactamase and to constitutively express a cephalosporinase, it was susceptible to all antibiotics standard for *B. anthracis*.

Microbiology and Clinical Features   Anthrax is caused by *B. anthracis*, a gram-positive, nonmotile, spore-forming rod that is found in soil and predominantly causes disease in herbivores such as cattle, goats, and sheep. Anthrax spores can remain viable for decades. The remarkable stability of these spores makes them an ideal bioweapon, and their destruction in decontamination activities can be a challenge. Naturally occurring human infection is generally the result of contact with anthrax-infected animals or animal products such as goat hair. While an LD_{50} of 10,000 spores is a generally accepted number it has also been suggested that as few as one to three spores may be adequate to cause disease in some settings. Advanced technology is likely to be necessary to generate spores of the optimal size (1–5 μm) to travel to the alveolar spaces as a bioweapon.

The three major clinical forms of anthrax are gastrointestinal, cutaneous, and inhalational. *Gastrointestinal anthrax* typically results from the ingestion of contaminated meat; the condition is rarely seen and is unlikely to be the result of a bioterrorism event. The lesion of *cutaneous an-*

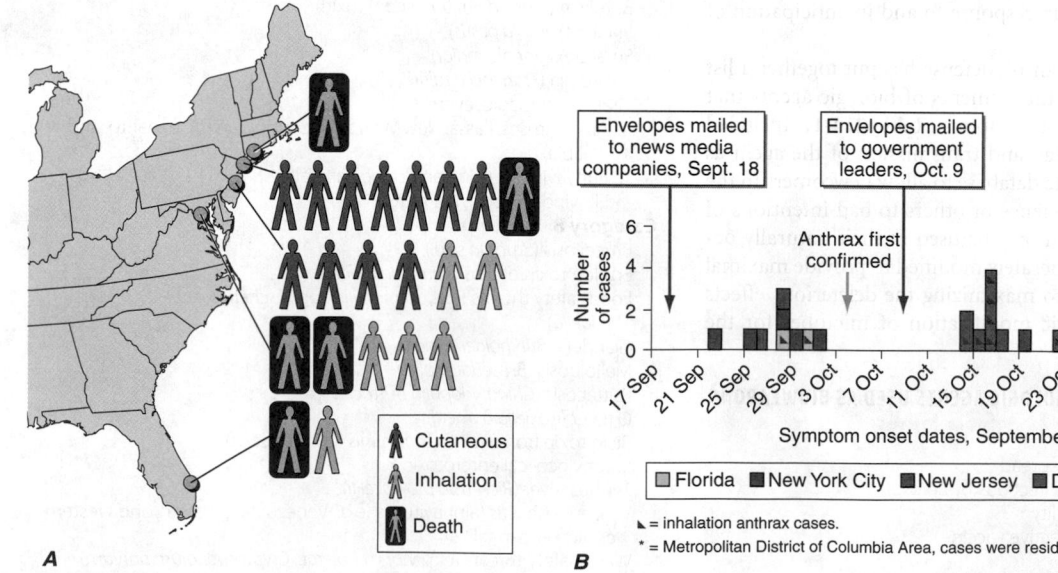

**FIGURE 214-1 Confirmed anthrax cases associated with bioterrorism: United States, 2001. *A.* Geographic location, clinical manifestation, and outcome of the 11 cases of confirmed inhalational and 11 cases of confirmed cutaneous anthrax. *B.* Epidemic curve for 18 confirmed cases of inhalational and cutaneous anthrax and additional 4 cases of suspected cutaneous anthrax. (*From DB Jernigan et al: Investigation of bioterrorism-related anthrax, US 2001: Epidemiologic findings. Emerg Infect Dis 8:1019, 2002; with permission.*)

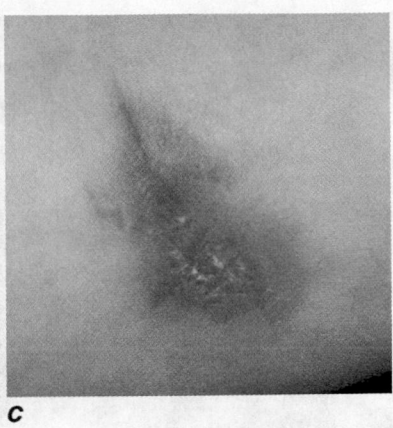

A   **B**   **C**

FIGURE 214-2 Clinical manifestations of a pediatric case of cutaneous anthrax associated with the bioterrorism attack of 2001. The lesion progresses from vesicular on day 5 **(A)** to necrotic with the classic black escar on day 12 **(B)** to a healed scar 2 months later **(C)**. *(Photographs provided by Dr. Mary Wu Chang and (A) reprinted with permission of the New England Journal of Medicine.)*

thrax typically begins as a papule following the introduction of spores through an opening in the skin. This papule then evolves to a painless vesicle followed by the development of a coal-black, necrotic eschar (Fig. 214-2). It is the Greek word for coal (*anthrax*) that gives the organism and the disease its name. Cutaneous anthrax was ~20% fatal prior to the availability of antibiotics. *Inhalational anthrax* is the form most likely to be responsible for death in the setting of a bioterrorist attack. It occurs following the inhalation of spores that become deposited in the alveolar spaces. These spores are phagocytosed by macrophages and transported to the mediastinal and peribronchial lymph nodes where they germinate, leading to active bacterial growth and elaboration of the bacterial products edema toxin and lethal toxin. Subsequent hematogenous spread of bacteria is accompanied by cardiovascular collapse and death. The earliest symptoms are typically a viral-like prodrome with fever, malaise, and abdominal and/or chest symptoms that progress over the course of a few days to a moribund state. A characteristic finding is mediastinal widening and pleural effusions on chest x-ray (Fig. 214-3). While initially thought to be 100% fatal, the experiences at Sverdlosk in 1979 and in the United States in 2001 (see below) indicate that with prompt initiation of antibiotic therapy survival is possible. The characteristics of the 11 cases of inhalational anthrax diagnosed in the United States in 2001 following exposure to contaminated letters postmarked September 18 or October 9, 2001, followed the classic pattern established for this illness, with patients presenting with a rapidly progressive course characterized by fever, fatigue or malaise, nausea or vomiting, cough, and shortness of breath. At presentation, the total white blood cell counts were ~10,000 cells/μL; transaminases tended to be elevated, and all 11 had abnormal findings on chest x-ray and CT. Radiologic findings included infiltrates, mediastinal widening, and hemorrhagic pleural effusions. For cases in which the dates of exposure were known, symptoms appeared within 4–6 days. Death occurred within 7 days of diagnosis in the five fatal cases (overall mortality rate 55%). Rapid diagnosis and prompt initiation of antibiotic therapy were key to survival.

℞ ANTHRAX

Anthrax can be successfully treated if the disease is promptly recognized and appropriate therapy is initiated early. While penicillin, ciprofloxacin, and doxycycline are the currently licensed antibiotics for this indication, clindamycin and rifampin also have in vitro activity against the organism and have been used as part of treatment regimens. Until sensitivity results are known, suspected cases are best managed with a combination of broadly active agents **(Table 214-3)**. Patients with inhalational anthrax are not contagious and do not require special isolation procedures.

Vaccination and Prevention The first successful vaccine for anthrax was developed for animals by Louis Pasteur in 1881. At present, the single vaccine licensed for human use is a product produced from the cell-free culture supernatant of an attenuated, nonencapsulated strain of *B. anthracis* (Stern strain), referred to as *anthrax vaccine adsorbed* (AVA). Clinical trials for safety in humans and efficacy in animals are currently under way to evaluate the role of recombinant protective antigen (one of the major components, along with lethal factor and edema factor, of *B. anthracis* toxins) as an alternative to AVA. In a postexposure setting in non-human primates a 2-week course of AVA + ciprofloxacin was found to be superior to ciprofloxacin alone in preventing the development of clinical disease and death. While the current recommendation for postexposure prophylaxis is 60 days of antibiotics, it would seem prudent to include immunization with anthrax vaccine if available. Given the potential for *B. anthracis* to be engineered to express penicillin resistance, the empirical regimen of choice in this setting is either ciprofloxacin or doxycycline.

PLAGUE
See also Chap. 152.

***Yersinia pestis* as a Bioweapon** Although it lacks the environmental stability of anthrax, the highly contagious nature and high mortality of plague make it a close to ideal agent of bioterrorism, particularly if delivered in a weaponized form. Occupying a unique place in history, plague has been alleged to have been used as a biologic weapon for centuries. The catapulting of plague-infected corpses into besieged fortresses is a practice that was first noted in 1346 during the assault of the city of Kaffa by the Tartars. Although unlikely to have resulted in disease transmission, some believe that this event may have played a role in the start of the Black Death pandemic of the fourteenth and fifteenth centuries in Europe. Given that plague was already moving across Asia toward Europe at this time, it is unclear whether such an allegation is accurate. During WWII, the infamous Unit 731 of the Japanese army was reported to have repeatedly dropped plague-infested fleas over parts of China, including Manchuria. These drops were associated with subsequent outbreaks of plague in the targeted areas. Following WWII, the United States and the Soviet Union conducted programs of research on how to create aerosolized *Y. pestis* that could be used as a bioweapon to cause primary pneumonic plague. As mentioned above, plague was thought to be an excellent bioweapon due to the fact that in addition to causing infection in those inhaling the aerosol, significant numbers of secondary cases of primary pneumonic plague would likely occur due to the contagious nature of the disease and person-to-person transmission via respiratory aerosol. Secondary reports of research conducted during that time suggest that organisms remain viable for up to 1 h and can be dispersed for distances up to 10 km. While the offensive bioweapons program in the United States was terminated prior to production of sufficient quantities of plague organisms for use as a weapon, it is believed that Soviet scientists did manufacture quantities sufficient for such a purpose. It has also been

FIGURE 214-3 Progression of chest x-ray findings in a patient with inhalational anthrax. Findings evolved from subtle hilar prominence and right perihilar infiltrate to a progressively widened medi-astinum, marked perihilar infiltrates, peribronchial cuffing, and air bronchograms. (*From L Borio et al: Death due to bioterrorism-related inhalational anthrax. JAMA 286:2554, 2001; with permission.*)

reported that more than 10 Soviet Institutes and >1000 scientists were working with plague as a biologic weapon. Of concern is the fact that in 1995 a microbiologist in Ohio was arrested for having obtained *Y. pestis* in the mail from the American Type Culture Collection, using a credit card and a false letterhead. In the wake of this incident, the U.S. Congress passed a law in 1997 requiring that anyone intending to send or receive any of 42 different agents that could potentially be used as bioweapons first register with the CDC.

Microbiology and Clinical Features Plague is caused by *Y. pestis*, a nonmotile, gram-negative bacillus that exhibits bipolar, or "safety pin," staining with Wright, Giemsa, or Wayson stains. It has had a major impact on the course of history, thus adding to the element of fear evoked by its mention. The earliest reported plague epidemic was in 224 B.C. in China. The most infamous pandemic began in Europe in the fourteenth century, during which time one-third to one-half of the entire population of Europe was killed. During a plague outbreak in India in 1994, even though the number of confirmed cases was relatively small, it is estimated that 500,000 individuals fled their homes in fear of this disease.

The clinical syndromes of plague generally reflect the mode of infection. *Bubonic plague* is the consequence of an insect bite; primary *pneumonic plague* arises through the inhalation of bacteria. Most of the plague seen in the world today is bubonic plague and is the result of a bite by a plague-infected flea. In part as a consequence of past pandem-

ics, plague infection of rodents exists widely in nature, including in the southwestern United States, and each year thousands of cases of plague occur worldwide through contact with infected animals or fleas. Following inoculation of regurgitated bacteria into the skin by a flea bite, organisms travel through the lymphatics to regional lymph nodes, where they are phagocytized but not destroyed. Inside the cell, they multiply rapidly leading to inflammation, painful lymphadenopathy with necrosis, fever, bacteremia, septicemia, and death. The characteristic enlarged, inflamed lymph nodes, or *buboes*, give this form of plague its name. In some instances, patients may develop bacteremia without lymphadenopathy following infection, a condition referred to as *primary septicemic plague*. Extensive ecchymoses may develop due to disseminated intravascular coagulation, and gangrene of the digits and/or nose may develop in patients with advanced septicemic plague. It is thought that this appearance of some patients gave rise to the term *Black Death* in reference to the plague epidemic of the fourteenth and fifteenth centuries. Some patients may develop pneumonia (secondary pneumonic plague) as a complication of bubonic or septicemic plague. These patients may then transmit the agent to others via the respiratory route, causing cases of primary pneumonic plague. Primary pneumonic plague is the manifestation most likely to occur as the result of a bioterrorist attack, with an aerosol of bacteria spread over a wide area or a particular environment that is densely populated. In this setting patients would be expected to develop fever, cough with hemoptysis, dyspnea, and gastrointestinal

TABLE 214-3 CLINICAL SYNDROMES, PREVENTION, AND TREATMENT STRATEGIES FOR DISEASES CAUSES BY CATEGORY A AGENTS

Agent	Clinical Syndrome	Incubation Period	Diagnosis	Treatment	Prophylaxis
Bacillus anthracis (anthrax)	Cutaneous lesion: Papule to eschar Inhalational disease: Fever, malaise, chest and abdominal discomfort Pleural effusion, widened mediastinum on chest x-ray	1–12 days 1–60 days	Culture, Gram stain, PCR, Wright stain of peripheral smear	Postexposure: Ciprofloxacin, 500 mg, PO bid × 60 d *or* Doxycycline, 100 mg PO bid × 60 d also (Amoxicillin, 500 mg PO q8h, likely to be effective if strain penicillin sensitive) *Active disease:* Ciprofloxacin, 400 mg IV q12h *or* Doxycycline, 100 mg IV q12 *plus* Clindamycin, 900 mg IV q8h and/or rifampin, 300 mg IV q12h; switch to PO when stable ×60 d total *Antitoxin strategies:* Neutralizing monoclonal and polyclonal antibodies are under study	Anthrax vaccine adsorbed Recombinant protective antigen vaccines are under study
Yersinia pestis (pneumonic plague)	Fever, cough, dyspnea, hemoptysis Infiltrates and consolidation on chest x-ray	1–6 days	Culture, Gram stain, direct fluorescent antibody, PCR	Gentamicin, 2.0 mg/kg IV loading then 1.7 mg/kg q8h IV or Streptomycin, 1.0 g q12h IM or IV Alternatives include doxycycline, 100 mg bid PO or IV; chloramphenicol 500 mg qid PO or IV	Doxycycline, 100 mg PO bid (ciprofloxacin may also be active) Formalin-fixed vaccine (FDA licensed; not available) .
Variola major (smallpox)	Fever, malaise, headache, backache, emesis Maculopapular to vesicular to pustular skin lesions	7–17 days	Culture, PCR, electron microscopy	Supportive measures; consideration for cidofovir, anti-vaccinia immunoglobulin	Vaccinia immunization
Francisella tularensis (tularemia)	Fever, chills, malaise, myalgia, chest discomfort, dyspnea, headache, skin rash, pharyngitis, conjunctivitis Hilar adenopathy on chest x-ray	1–14 days	Gram stain, culture, immunohistochemistry, PCR	Streptomycin, 1 g IM bid or Gentamicin, 5 mg/kg per day div q8h IV for 14 days or Doxycycline, 100 mg IV bid or Chloramphenicol, 15 mg/kg IV qid or Ciprofloxacin, 400 mg IV bid	Doxycycline, 100 mg PO bid × 14 days or Ciprofloxacin, 500 mg PO bid × 14 days
Viral hemorrhagic fevers	Fever, myalgia, rash, encephalitis, prostration	2–21 days	RT-PCR, serologic testing for antigen or antibody Viral isolation by CDC or U.S. Army Medical Institute of Infectious Diseases (USAMRIID)	Supportive measures Ribavirin 30 mg/kg up to 2 g × 1, followed by 16 mg/kg IV up to 1 g q6h for 4 days, followed by 8 mg/kg IV up to 0.5 g q8h × 6 days	No known chemoprophylaxis Consideration for ribavirin in high-risk situations Vaccine exists for yellow fever
Botulinum toxin (*Clostridium botulinum*)	Dry mouth, blurred vision, ptosis, weakness, dysarthria, dysphagia, dizziness, respiratory failure, progressive paralysis, dilated pupils	12–72 h	Mouse bioassay, toxin immunoassay	Supportive measures including ventilation 5000–9000 IU equine antitoxin	Administration of antitoxin

Note: CDC, U.S. Centers for Disease Control and Prevention; FDA, U.S. Food and Drug Administration; PCR, polymerase chain reaction; RT-PCR, reverse transcriptase PCR.

symptoms 1–6 days following exposure. Clinical features of pneumonia would be accompanied by pulmonary infiltrates and consolidation on chest x-ray. In the absence of antibiotics, the mortality of this disease is on the order of 85%, and death usually occurs within 2–6 days.

℞ PLAGUE

Streptomycin, tetracycline, and doxycycline are licensed by the U.S. Food and Drug Administration (FDA) for the treatment of plague. Multiple additional antibiotics licensed for other infections are commonly used and are likely effective. Among these are aminoglycosides such as gentamicin, ceph-

alosporins, trimethoprim/sulfamethoxazole, chloramphenicol, and ciprofloxacin (Table 214-3). A multidrug-resistant strain of *Y. pestis* was identified in 1995 from a patient with bubonic plague in Madagascar. While this organism was resistant to streptomycin, ampicillin, chloramphenicol, sulfonamides, and tetracycline, it retained its susceptibility to other aminoglycosides and cephalosporins. Given the subsequent identification of a similar organism in 1997 coupled with the fact that this resistance is plasmid-mediated, it seems likely that genetically modifying *Y. pestis* to a multidrug resistant form is possible. Unlike patients with inhalational anthrax (see above), patients with pulmonary plague should be cared for under conditions of strict respiratory isolation comparable to that used for multidrug-resistant tuberculosis.

Vaccination and Prevention A formalin-fixed, whole-organism vaccine was licensed by the FDA for the prevention of plague. That vaccine is no longer being manufactured, but its potential value as a current countermeasure against bioterrorism would likely have been modest at best as it was ineffective against animal models of primary pneumonic plague. Efforts are under way to develop a second generation of vaccines that will protect against aerosol challenge. Among the candidates being tested are recombinant forms of the F1 and V antigens of *Y. pestis*. It is likely that doxycycline or ciprofloxacin would provide coverage in a chemoprophylaxis setting. Unlike the case with anthrax, in which one has to be concerned about the persistence of ungerminated spores in the respiratory tract, the duration of prophylaxis against plague need only extend to 7 days following exposure.

SMALLPOX

See also Chap. 176.

Variola Virus as a Bioweapon Given that most of the world's population was vaccinated against smallpox, variola virus would not have been considered a good candidate as a bioweapon 30 years ago. However, with the cessation of immunization programs in the United States in 1972 and throughout the world in 1980 due to the successful global eradication of smallpox, close to 50% of the U.S. population is fully susceptible to smallpox today. Given its infectious nature and the 10–30% mortality in unimmunized individuals, the deliberate spread of this virus could have a devastating effect on our society and unleash a previously conquered deadly disease. It is estimated that an initial infection of 50–100 persons in a first-generation of cases could expand by a factor of 10–20 with each succeeding generation in the absence of any effective containment measures. While the likely implementation of an effective public health response makes this scenario unlikely, it does illustrate the potential damage and disruption that can result from a smallpox outbreak.

In 1980, the World Health Organization (WHO) recommended that all immunization programs be terminated; that representative samples of variola virus be transferred to two locations: one at the CDC in Atlanta, GA, in the United States and the other at the Institute of Virus Preparations in the Soviet Union; and that all other stocks of smallpox be destroyed. Several years later, it was recommended that these two authorized collections be destroyed. However, these latter recommendations were placed on hold in the wake of increased concerns on the use of *variola virus* as a biologic weapon and thus the need to maintain an active program of defensive research. Many of these concerns were based upon allegations made by former Soviet officials that extensive programs had been in place in that country for the production and weaponization of large quantities of smallpox virus. The dismantling of these programs with the fall of the Soviet Union and the subsequent weakening of security measures led to fears that stocks of *V. major* may have made their way to other countries or terrorist organizations. In addition, accounts that efforts had been taken to produce recombinant strains of *Variola* that would be more virulent and more contagious than the wild-type virus have led to an increase in the need to be vigilant for the reemergence of this often fatal infectious disease.

Microbiology and Clinical Features Smallpox is caused by one of two variants of variola virus, *V. major* and *V. minor*. Variola is a double-strand DNA virus and member of the Orthopoxvirus genus of the Poxviridae family. Infections with *V. minor* are generally less severe than those of *V. major*, with milder constitutional symptoms and lower mortality rates; thus *V. major* is the only one considered to be a viable bioweapon. Infection with *V. major* typically occurs following contact with an infected person from the time that a maculopapular rash appears on the skin and oropharynx, through the resolution and scabbing of the pustular lesions. Infection occurs principally during close contact, through the inhalation of saliva droplets containing virus from the oropharyngeal exanthem. Aerosolized material from contaminated clothing or linen can also spread infection. Several days after exposure, a primary viremia is believed to occur that results in

dissemination of virus to lymphoid tissues. A secondary viremia occurs ~4 days later that leads to localization of infection in the dermis. Approximately 12–14 days following the initial exposure the patient develops high fever, malaise, vomiting, headache, backache, and a maculopapular rash that begins on the face and extremities and spreads to the trunk (centripetal) with lesions in the same developmental stage in any given location. This is in contrast to the rash of varicella (chickenpox) that begins on the trunk and face and spreads to the extremities (centrifugal) with lesions at all stages of development. The lesions are initially maculopapular and evolve to vesicles that eventually become pustules and then scabs. The oral mucosa also develops maculopapular lesions that evolve to ulcers. The lesions appear over a period of 1–2 days and evolve at the same rate. Although virus can be isolated from the scabs on the skin, the conventional thinking is that once the scabs have formed the patient is no longer contagious. Smallpox is associated with a 10–30% mortality, with patients typically dying of severe systemic illness during the second week of symptoms. Historically, ~5–10% of naturally occurring smallpox cases take either of two highly virulent atypical forms, classified as *hemorrhagic* and *malignant*. These are difficult to recognize because of their atypical presentations. The hemorrhagic form is uniformly fatal and begins with the relatively abrupt onset of a severely prostrating illness characterized by high fevers and severe headache and back and abdominal pain. This form of the illness resembles a severe systemic inflammatory syndrome, in which patients have a high viremia, but die without developing the characteristic rash. Cutaneous erythema develops accompanied by petechiae and hemorrhages into the skin and mucous membranes. Death usually occurs within 5–6 days. The malignant, or "flat," form of smallpox is frequently fatal and has an onset similar to the hemorrhagic form, but with confluent skin lesions developing more slowly and never progressing to the pustular stage.

℞ SMALLPOX

Given the infectious nature of smallpox and the extreme vulnerability of contemporary society, patients who are suspected cases should be handled with strict isolation procedures. While laboratory confirmation of a suspected case by culture and electron microscopy is essential, it is equally important that appropriate precautions be employed when obtaining samples for culture and laboratory testing. All health care and laboratory workers caring for patients should have been recently immunized with vaccinia, and all samples should be transported in doubly sealed containers. Patients should be cared for in negative-pressure rooms with strict isolation precautions.

There is no licensed specific therapy for smallpox, and historic treatments have focused solely on supportive care. While several antiviral agents, including cidofovir, that are licensed for other diseases have in vitro activity against *V. major*, they have never been tested in the setting of human disease. For this reason it is difficult to predict whether or not they would be effective in cases of smallpox and, if effective, whether or not they would be of value in patients with advanced disease. Research programs studying the efficacy of new antiviral compounds against *V. major* are currently under way.

Vaccination and Prevention In 1796 Edward Jenner demonstrated that deliberate infection with cowpox virus could prevent illness on subsequent exposure to smallpox. Today, smallpox is a preventable disease following immunization with vaccinia. The current dilemma facing our society regarding assessment of the risk and/or benefit of smallpox vaccination is that the degree of risk that someone will deliberately and effectively release smallpox into our society is unknown. As a prudent first step in preparedness for a smallpox attack, virtually all members of the U.S. armed services have received primary or booster immunizations with vaccinia. In addition, tens of thousands of civilian health care workers who comprise smallpox-response teams at the state and local public health level have been vaccinated.

Initial fears regarding the immunization of a segment of the American population with vaccinia when there are more individuals receiving

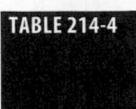

Complication	Number of Cases	DoD Rate per Million Vaccinees (95% Confidence Interval)	Historic Rate Per Million Vaccinees
Mild or temporary:			
Generalized vaccinia, mild	35	67 (52, 85)	45 to 212[a]
Inadvertent inoculation, self	62	119 (98, 142)	606[a]
Vaccinia transfer to contact	28	53 (40, 69)	8 to 27[a]
Moderate or serious:			
Encephalitis	1	2.2 (0.6, 7.2)	2.6 to 8.7[a]
Acute myopericarditis	69	131 (110, 155)	100[b]
Eczema vaccinatum	0	0 (0, 3.7)	2 to 35[a]
Progressive vaccinia	0	0 (0, 3.7)	1 to 7[a]
Death[c]	1	1.9 (0.2, 5.6)	1 to 2[a]

TABLE 214-4 COMPLICATIONS FROM 438,134 ADMINISTRATIONS OF VACCINIA DURING THE UNITED STATES DEPARTMENT OF DEFENSE (DOD) SMALLPOX IMMUNIZATION CAMPAIGN INITIATED IN DECEMBER 2002

[a]Based on adolescent and adult smallpox vaccinations from 1968 studies, both primary and revaccinations.

[b]Based on case series in Finnish military recruits given the Finnish strain of smallpox vaccine.

[c]Potentially attributable to vaccination; after lupus-like illness.

Source: From JD Grabenstein and W Winkenwerder: *http://www.smallpox.mil/event/SPSafetySum.asp*

immunosuppressive drugs and other immunocompromised patients than ever before have largely been dispelled as data are generated from the current military and civilian immunization campaigns. Adverse event rates for the first 450,000 immunizations are similar to and, in certain categories of adverse events, even lower than those from historic data, in which most severe sequelae of vaccination occurred in young infants (Table 214-4). In addition, 11 patients with early stage HIV infection have been inadvertently immunized without problem. One significant concern during the recent immunization campaign, however, has been the description of a syndrome of myopericarditis, which was not appreciated during prior immunization campaigns with vaccinia.

TULAREMIA
See also Chap. 151.

***Francisella tularensis* as a Bioweapon** Tularemia has been studied as an agent of bioterrorism since the mid-twentieth century. It has been speculated by some that the outbreak of tularemia among German and Soviet soldiers during fighting on the Eastern Front during WWII was the consequence of a deliberate release. Unit 731 of the Japanese Army studied the use of tularemia as a bioweapon during WWII. Large preparations were made for mass productive of *F. tularensis* by the United States, but no stockpiling of any agent took place. Stocks of *F. tularensis* were reportedly generated by the Soviet Union in the mid-1950s. It has also been suggested that the Soviet program extended into the era of molecular biology and that some strains were engineered to be resistant to common antibiotics. *F. tularensis* is an extremely infectious organism, and human infections have occurred from merely examining an uncovered petri dish streaked with colonies. Given these facts, it is reasonable to conclude that this organism might be utilized as a bioweapon through either an aerosol or contamination of food or drinking water.

Microbiology and Clinical Features While similar in many ways to anthrax and plague, tularemia, also referred to as rabbit fever or deer fly fever, is neither as lethal nor as fulminant as either of these other two category A bacterial infections. It is, however, extremely infectious, and as few as 10 organisms can lead to establishment of infection. Despite this fact, it is not spread from person to person. Tularemia is

caused by *F. tularensis*, a small, nonmotile, gram-negative coccobacillus. Although it is not a spore-forming organism, it is a hardy bacterium that can survive for weeks in the environment. Infection typically comes from insect bites or contact with organisms in the environment. Large waterborne outbreaks have been recorded. It is most likely that the outbreak among German and Russian soldiers and Russian civilians noted above during WWII represented a large waterborne tularemia outbreak in a *Tularensis*-enzootic area devastated by warfare.

Humans can become infected through a variety of environmental sources. Infection is most common in rural areas where a variety of small mammals may serve as reservoirs. Human infections in the summer are often the result of insect bites from ticks, flies, or mosquitoes that have bitten infected animals. In colder months infections are most likely the result of direct contact with infected mammals and are most common in hunters. In these settings infection typically presents as a systemic illness with an area of inflammation and necrosis at the site of tissue entry. Drinking of contaminated water may lead to an oropharyngeal form of tularemia characterized by pharyngitis with cervical and/or retropharyngeal lymphadenopathy (Chap. 151). The most likely mode of dissemination of tularemia as a biologic weapon would be as an aerosol, as has occurred in a number of natural outbreaks in rural areas, including Martha's Vineyard in the United States. Approximately 1–14 days following exposure by this route one would expect to see inflammation of the airways with pharyngitis, pleuritis, and bronchopneumonia. Typical symptoms would include the abrupt onset of fever, fatigue, chills, headache, and malaise (Table 214-3). Some patients might experience conjunctivitis with ulceration, pharyngitis, and/or cutaneous exanthems. A pulse-temperature dissociation might be present. Approximately 50% of patients would show a pulmonary infiltrate on chest x-ray. Hilar adenopathy might also be present, and a small percent of patients could have adenopathy without infiltrates. The highly variable presentation makes acute recognition of aerosol-disseminated tularemia very difficult. The diagnosis would likely be made by immunohistochemistry or culture of infected tissues or blood. Untreated, mortality rates range from 5–15% for cutaneous routes of infection and 30–60% for infection by inhalation. Since the advent of antibiotic therapy, these rates have dropped to <2%.

℞ TULAREMIA

Both streptomycin and doxycycline are licensed for treatment of tularemia. Other agents likely to be effective include gentamicin, chloramphenicol, and ciprofloxacin (Table 214-3). Given the potential for genetic modification of this organism to yield antibiotic-resistant strains, broad-spectrum coverage should be the rule until sensitivities have been determined. As mentioned above, special isolation procedures are not required.

Vaccination and Prevention There are no vaccines currently licensed for the prevention of tularemia. While a live, attenuated strain of the organism has been used in the past with some reported success, there are inadequate data to support its widespread use at this time. Development of a vaccine for this agent is an important part of the current biodefense research agenda. In the absence of an effective vaccine, post-exposure chemoprophylaxis with either doxycycline or ciprofloxacin appears to be a reasonable approach (Table 214-3).

VIRAL HEMORRHAGIC FEVERS
See also Chaps. 189 and 190.

Hemorrhagic Fever Viruses as Bioweapons Several of the hemorrhagic fever viruses have been reported to have been weaponized by the Soviet Union and the United States. Nonhuman primate studies indicate that infection can be established with very few virions and that infectious aerosol preparations can be produced. Under the guise of wanting to aid victims of an Ebola outbreak, members of the Aum Shrinrikyo cult in Japan were reported to have traveled to central Africa in 1992 in an attempt to obtain Ebola virus for use in a bioterrorist attack. Thus, while there has been no evidence that these agents have ever been used in a biologic attack, there is clear interest in their potential for this purpose.

Microbiology and Clinical Features The viral hemorrhagic fevers are a group of illnesses caused by any one of a number of similar viruses (Table 214-2). These viruses are all enveloped, single-strand RNA viruses that are thought to depend upon a rodent or insect host reservoir for long-term survival. They tend to be geographically restricted according to the migration patterns of their hosts. Great apes are not a natural reservoir for Ebola virus, but large numbers of these animals in sub-Saharan Africa have died from Ebola infection over the past decade. Humans can become infected with hemorrhagic fever viruses if they come into contact with an infected host or other infected animals. Person-to-person transmission, largely through direct contact with virus-containing body fluids, has been documented for Ebola, Marburg and Lassa virus and rarely for the New World arenaviruses. While there is no clear evidence of respiratory spread among humans, these viruses have been shown in animal models to be highly infectious by the aerosol route. This, coupled with mortality rates as high as 90%, makes them excellent candidate agents of bioterrorism.

The clinical features of the viral hemorrhagic fevers vary depending upon the particular agent (Table 214-3). Initial signs and symptoms typically include fever, myalgia, prostration, and disseminated intravascular coagulation with thrombocytopenia and capillary hemorrhage. These findings are consistent with a cytokine-mediated systemic inflammatory syndrome. A variety of different maculopapular or erythematous rashes may be seen. Leukopenia, temperature-pulse dissociation, renal failure, and seizures may also be part of the clinical presentation. Outbreaks of most of these diseases are sporadic and unpredictable. As a consequence, most studies of pathogenesis have been performed using laboratory animals. The diagnosis should be suspected in anyone with temperature >38.3°C for <3 weeks who also exhibits at least two of the following: hemorrhagic or purpuric rash, epistaxis, hematemesis, hemoptysis, or hematochezia in the absence of any other identifiable cause. In this setting, samples of blood should be sent after consultation to the CDC or the U.S. Army Medical Research Institute of Infectious Diseases (USAMRIID) for serologic testing for antigen and antibody as well as reverse transcriptase polymerase chain reaction (RT-PCR) testing for hemorrhagic fever viruses. All samples should be handled with double-bagging. Given how little is known regarding the human-to-human transmission of these viruses, appropriate isolation measures would include full barrier precautions with negative-pressure rooms and use of N95 masks or powered air-purifying respirators (PAPRs). Unprotected skin contact with cadavers has been implicated in the transmission of certain hemorrhagic fever viruses such as Ebola, so it is recommended that autopsies be performed using the strictest measures for protection and that burial or cremation be performed promptly without embalming.

℞ VIRAL HEMORRHAGIC FEVERS

There are no approved and effective antiviral therapies for this class of viruses (Table 214-3). While there are anecdotal reports of the efficacy of ribavirin, interferon-α, or hyperimmune immunoglobulin, definitive data are lacking. The best data for ribavirin are in arenavirus (Lassa and New World) infections. In some in vitro systems specific immunoglobulin has been reported to enhance infectivity, and thus these potential treatments must be approached with caution.

Vaccination and Prevention A live attenuated virus vaccine is available in limited quantities for prevention of yellow fever. There are no other licensed and effective vaccines for these agents. Studies are currently underway examining the potential role of DNA, recombinant viruses, and attenuated viruses as vaccines for several of these infections. Among the most promising at present are vaccines for Argentine, Ebola, Rift Valley, and Kayasanur Forest viruses.

BOTULISM TOXIN (*CLOSTRIDIUM BOTULINUM*)
See also Chap. 135.

Botulinum Toxin as a Bioweapon In a bioterrorist attack, botulinum toxin would likely be dispersed as an aerosol or as contamination of a food supply. While contamination of a water supply is possible, it is likely that any toxin would be rapidly inactivated by the chlorine used to purify drinking water. Similarly, toxin can be inactivated by heating any food to >85°C for >5 min. Without external facilitation, the environmental decay rate is estimated at 1% per minute, and thus the time interval between weapon release and ingestion or inhalation needs to be rather short. The Japanese biologic warfare group, Unit 731, is reported to have conducted experiments on botulism poisoning in prisoners in the 1930s. The United States and the Soviet Union both acknowledged producing botulinum toxin, and there is some evidence that the Soviet Union attempted to create recombinant bacteria containing the gene for botulinum toxin. In records submitted to the United Nations, Iraq admitted to having produced 19,000 L of concentrated toxin—enough toxin to kill the entire population of the world three times over. By many accounts, botulinum toxin was the primary focus of the pre-1991 Iraqi bioweapons program. In addition to these examples of state-supported research into the use of botulinum toxin as a bioweapon, the Aum Shrinrikyo cult unsuccessfully attempted on a least three occasions to disperse botulism toxin into the civilian population of Tokyo.

Microbiology and Clinical Features Unique among the category A agents for not being a live microorganism, botulinum toxin is one of the most potent toxins ever described and is thought by some to be the most poisonous substance in existence. It is estimated that 1 g of botulinum toxin would be sufficient to kill 1 million individuals if adequately dispersed. Botulinum toxin is produced by the gram-positive, spore-forming anaerobe *C. botulinum* (Chap. 135). Its natural habitat is soil. There are seven antigenically distinct forms of botulinum toxin, designated A–G. The majority of naturally occurring human cases are of types A, B, and E. Antitoxin directed toward one of these will have little to no activity against the others. The toxin is a 150-kDa zinc-containing protease that prevents the intracellular fusion of acetylcholine vesicles with the motor neuron membrane, thus preventing the release of acetylcholine. In the absence of acetylcholine-dependent triggering of muscle fibers, a flaccid paralysis develops. Although botulism does not spread from person to person, the ease of production of the toxin coupled with its high morbidity and 60–100% mortality make it a close to ideal bioweapon.

Botulism can result from the presence of *C. botulinum* infection in a wound or the intestine, the ingestion of contaminated food, or the inhalation of aerosolized toxin. The latter two forms are the most likely modes of transmission for bioterrorism. Once toxin is absorbed into the bloodstream it binds to the neuronal cell membrane, enters the cell, and cleaves one of the proteins required for the intracellular binding of the synaptic vesicle to the cell membrane, thus preventing release of the neurotransmitter to the membrane of the adjacent muscle cell. Patients initially develop multiple cranial nerve palsies that are followed by a descending flaccid paralysis. The extent of the neuromuscular compromise is dependent upon the level of toxemia. The majority of patients experience diplopia, dysphagia, dysarthria, dry mouth, ptosis, dilated pupils, fatigue, and extremity weakness. There are minimal true central nervous system effects, and patients rarely show significant alterations in mental status. Severe cases can involve complete muscular collapse, loss of the gag reflex, and respiratory failure, requiring weeks or months of ventilator support. Recovery requires the regeneration of new motor neuron synapses with the muscle cell, a process that can take weeks to months. In the absence of secondary infections, which may be common during the protracted recovery phase of this illness, patients remain afebrile. The diagnosis is suspected on clinical grounds and confirmed by a mouse bioassay or toxin immunoassay.

℞ BOTULISM

Treatment for botulism is mainly supportive and may require intubation, mechanical ventilation, and parenteral nutrition (Table 214-3). If diagnosed early enough, administration of equine antitoxin may reduce the extent of nerve injury and decrease the severity of disease. At present antitoxins are available on a limited basis as a licensed bivalent product with activity against toxin types A and B and as an experimental product with activity against toxin type E. In the event of attack with another toxin type, an investigational antitoxin with activity against all seven toxin types is also available through the U.S. Army. A single dose of antitoxin is usually adequate to neutralize any circulating toxin. Given that these preparations are all derived from horse serum, one needs to be vigilant for hypersensitivity reactions, including serum sickness and anaphylaxis following their administration. Once the damage to the nerve axon has been done, however, there is little possible in the way of specific therapy. At this point vigilance for secondary complications such as infections during the protracted recovery phase is of the utmost importance. Due to their ability to worsen neuromuscular blockade, aminoglycosides and clindamycin should be avoided in the treatment of these infections.

Vaccination and Prevention   A botulinum toxoid preparation has been used as a vaccine for laboratory workers at high risk of exposure and in certain military situations; however, it is not currently available in quantities that could be used for the general population. At present, early recognition of the clinical syndrome and use of appropriate equine antitoxin is the mainstay of prevention of full-blown disease in exposed individuals. The development of human monoclonal antibodies as a replacement for equine antitoxin antibodies is an area of active research interest.

CATEGORY B AND C AGENTS

The category B agents include those that are easy or moderately easy to disseminate and result in moderate morbidity and low mortality rates. A listing of the current category B agents is provided in Table 214-2. As can be seen, it includes a wide array of microorganisms and products of microorganisms. Several of these agents have been used in bioterrorist attacks, although never with the impact of the agents described above. Among the more notorious of these was the contamination of salad bars in Oregon in 1984 with *Salmonella typhimurium* by the religious cult Rajneeshee. In this outbreak, which many consider to be the first bioterrorist attack against U.S. citizens, >750 individuals were poisoned and 40 were hospitalized in an effort to influence a local election. The intentional nature of this outbreak went unrecognized for more than a decade.

Category C agents are the third highest priority agents in the biodefense agenda. These agents include emerging pathogens to which little or no immunity exists in the general population, such as the severe acute respiratory syndrome (SARS) coronavirus or pandemic-potential strains of influenza that could be obtained from nature and deliberately disseminated. These agents are characterized as being relatively easy to produce and disseminate and as having high morbidity and mortality rates as well as a significant public health impact. There is no running list of category C agents at the present time.

PREVENTION AND PREPAREDNESS

As noted above, a large and diverse array of agents has the potential to be used in a bioterrorist attack. In contrast to the military situation with biowarfare, where the primary objective is to inflict mass casualties on a healthy and prepared militia, the objectives of bioterrorism are to harm civilians as well as to create fear and disruption among the civilian population. While the military needs only to prepare their troops to deal with the limited number of agents that pose a legitimate threat of biowarfare, the public health system needs to prepare the entire civilian population to deal with the multitude of agents and settings that could be utilized in a bioterrorism attack. This includes anticipating issues specific to the very young and the very old, the pregnant patient, and the immunocompromised individual. The challenges in this regard are enormous and immediate. While military preparedness emphasizes vaccines toward a limited number of agents, civilian preparedness needs to rely upon rapid diagnosis and treatment of a wide array of conditions.

The medical profession must maintain a high index of suspicion that unusual clinical presentations or the clustering of cases of a rare disease may not be a chance occurrence but rather the first sign of a bioterrorist event. This is particularly true when such diseases occur in traditionally healthy populations, when surprisingly large numbers of rare conditions occur, and when diseases commonly seen in rural settings appear in urban populations. Given the importance of rapid diagnosis and early treatment for many of these conditions, it is essential that the medical care team report any suspected cases of bioterrorism immediately to local and state health authorities and/or to the CDC (888-246-2675). Recent enhancements have been made to the public health surveillance network to facilitate the rapid sharing of information among public health agencies.

At present a series of efforts are taking place to ensure the biomedical security of the civilian population of the United States. The Public Health Service is moving toward a larger, more highly trained, fully deployable force. A Strategic National Stockpile (SNS) has been created by the CDC to provide rapid access to quantities of pharmaceuticals, antidotes, vaccines, and other medical supplies that may be of value in the event of biologic or chemical terrorism. The SNS has two basic components. The first of these consists of "push packages" that can be deployed anywhere in the United States within 12 h. These push packages are a preassembled set of supplies, pharmaceuticals, and medical equipment ready for immediate delivery to the field. They provide treatment for a variety of conditions given the fact that an actual threat may not have been precisely identified at the time of stockpile deployment. The contents of the push packs are constantly updated to ensure that they reflect current needs as determined by national security threat assessments; they include antibiotics for treatment of anthrax, plague, and tularemia as well as a cache of vaccine to deal with a smallpox threat. The second component of the SNS comprises inventories managed by specific vendors and consists of the provision of additional pharmaceuticals, supplies, and/or products tailored to the specific attack.

The number of FDA-approved and -licensed drugs and vaccines for category A and B agents is currently limited and not reflective of the pharmacy of today. In an effort to speed the licensure of additional drugs and vaccines for these diseases, the FDA has proposed a new rule for the licensure of such countermeasures against agents of bioterrorism when adequate and well-controlled clinical efficacy studies cannot be ethically conducted in humans. Thus, for indications in which field trials of prophylaxis or therapy for naturally occurring disease are not feasible, the FDA is proposing to rely on evidence solely from laboratory animal studies. For this rule to apply it must be shown that (1) there are reasonably well-understood pathophysiologic mechanisms for the condition and its treatment; (2) the effect of the intervention is independently substantiated in at least two animal species, including species expected to react with a response predictive for humans; (3) the animal study endpoint is clearly related to the desired benefit in humans; and (4) the data in animals allow selection of an effective dose in humans.

Finally, an initiative referred to as Project BioShield has been established to facilitate biodefense research within the federal government, create a stable source of funding for the purchase of countermeasures against agents of bioterrorism, and create a category of "emergency use authorization" to allow the FDA to approve the use of unlicensed treatments during times of extraordinary unmet needs, as might be present in the context of a bioterrorist attack.

While the prospect of a deliberate attack on civilians with disease-producing agents may seem to be an act of incomprehensible evil, history shows us that it is something that has been done in the past and will likely be done again in the future. It is the responsibility of health care providers to be aware of this possibility, to be able to recognize early signs of a potential bioterrorist attack and alert the public health system, and to respond quickly to provide care to the individual patient. Among the web sites with current information on microbial bioterrorism are *www.bt.cdc.gov, www.niaid.nih.gov, www.jhsph.edu/preparedness,* and *www.cns.miis.edu/research/cbw/index.htm.*

ALIBEK K, HANDELMAN S: *Biohazard: The Chilling True Story of the Largest Covert Biological Weapons in the World, Told from the Inside by the Man Who Ran It*. New York, Random House, 1999

BEIGEL JH et al: Avian influenza A (H5N1) infection in humans. N Engl J Med 353:1375, 2005

CRODDY E (WITH C PEREY-ARMENDARIZ AND J HART): *Chemical and Biological Warfare: A Comprehensive Survey for the Concerned Citizen*. New York, Copernicus Books, 2001

HENDERSON DA et al (eds): *Bioterrorism: Guidelines for Medical and Public Health Management*. JAMA and Archives Journals, AMA Press, 2002

JERNIGAN JA et al: Bioterrorism-related inhalational anthrax: The first 10 cases reported in the United States. Emerg Infect Dis 7:933, 2001

WILKENING DA: Sverdlovsk revisited: Modeling human inhalation anthrax. Proc Natl Acad Sci USA 103:20, 2006

215 Chemical Bioterrorism
Charles G. Hurst, Jonathan Newmark, James A. Romano, Jr.

The use of chemical warfare agents (CWAs) in modern warfare dates back to World War I (WWI). Most recently, sulfur mustard and nerve agents were used by Iraq against the Iranian military and Kurdish civilians. Since the Japanese sarin attacks in 1994–1995 and the terrorist strikes of September 11, 2001, the all too real possibility of chemical or biological terrorism against civilian populations anywhere in the world has attracted increased attention.

Military planners consider the WWI blistering agent, sulfur mustard, and the organophosphorus nerve agents as the most likely agents to be used on the battlefield. In a civilian or terrorist scenario, the choice widens considerably. Cyanide, a common chemical, causes symptoms within seconds and death in 5–10 min if not treated rapidly. Chlorine and phosgene have no specific antidotes but can require intensive care for weeks to months. These agents or one of the industrial HAZMATs will be the likely choice of terrorists. Table 215-1 gives antidote recommendations following exposure to cyanide.

Many mistakenly believe that chemical attacks will always be so severe that little can be done except to bury the dead. History proves the opposite. Even in WWI, when IV fluids, endotracheal tubes, and antibiotics were unavailable, the mortality rate in U.S. forces on the battlefield from chemical warfare agents, chiefly sulfur mustard and the pulmonary intoxicants, was only 1.9%. This was far less than the 7% mortality rate from conventional wounds. In the 1995 Tokyo subway sarin incident, of the 5500 patients who sought medical attention at hospitals, 80% of whom were not actually symptomatic, only 12 died. Recent events should produce not a fatalistic attitude but a realistic wish to understand the pathophysiology of the syndromes these agents cause, with a view to treating expeditiously all patients who present for care and an expectation of saving the vast majority. As we prepare to defend our civilian population from the effects of chemical terrorism, we must also consider the fact that terrorism itself can produce sequelae such as physiologic or neurologic effects that may resemble the effects of nonlethal exposures to CWAs. These effects are due to a general fear of chemicals, fear of decontamination, fear of protective ensemble, or other phobic reactions.

Many writers have pointed out the increased difficulty in differentiating between stress reactions and nerve agent–induced organic brain syndromes. Knowledge of the behavioral effects of CWAs and their medical countermeasures is imperative to ensure that military and civilian medical and mental health organizations can deal with possible incidents involving weapons of mass destruction.

The chemical warfare agents, their NATO codes, and initial effects are listed in Table 215-2.

VESICANTS

Sulfur Mustard Sulfur mustard has been a military threat since it first appeared on the battlefield in Belgium during WWI. In modern times it remains a threat on the battlefield as well as a potential terrorist threat for bioterrorism because of simplicity of manufacture and extreme effectiveness. Sulfur mustard accounted for 70% of the 1.3 million chemical casualties in WWI.

MECHANISM Sulfur mustard constitutes both a vapor and a liquid threat to all exposed epithelial surfaces. Mustard's effects are delayed, appearing hours after exposure. Organs most commonly affected are the skin (with erythema and vesicles), eyes (ranging from mild conjunctivitis to severe eye damage), and airways (ranging from mild upper airway irritation, to severe bronchiolar damage). Following exposure to large quantities of mustard, precursor cells of the bone marrow are damaged, leading to pancytopenia and secondary infection. The gastrointestinal mucosa may be damaged, and there are sometimes central nervous system (CNS) signs of unknown mechanism. No specific antidotes exist; management is entirely supportive. Immediate decontamination of the liquid is the only way to reduce damage. Complete decontamination in 2 min stops clinical injury; decontamination at 5 min will reduce skin injury by ~50%. Table 215-3

TABLE 215-1 ANTIDOTE RECOMMENDATIONS FOLLOWING EXPOSURE TO CYANIDE

Patient	Mild (Conscious)	Severe (Unconscious)	Other Treatment
Child	If patient is conscious and has no other signs or symptoms, antidotes may not be necessary.	Sodium nitrite[a]: 0.12–0.33 mL/kg, not to exceed 10 mL of 3% solution[b] slow IV over no less than 5 min, or slower if hypotension develops *and* Sodium thiosulfate: 1.65 mL/kg of 25% solution IV over 10–20 min	For sodium nitrite–induced orthostatic hypotension, normal saline infusion and supine position are recommended. If still apneic after antidote administration, consider sodium bicarbonate for severe acidosis.
Adult	If patient is conscious and has no other signs or symptoms, antidotes may not be necessary.	Sodium nitrite[a]: 10–20 mL of 3% solution[b] slow IV over no less than 5 min, or slower if hypotension develops *and* Sodium thiosulfate: 50 mL of 25% solution IV over 10–20 min	

[a]If sodium nitrite is unavailable, administer amyl nitrite by inhalation from crushable ampules.
[b]Available in Pasadena Cyanide Antidote Kit, formerly Lilly Cyanide Kit.
Note: Victims whose clothing or skin is contaminated with hydrogen cyanide liquid or solution can secondarily contaminate response personnel by direct contact or through off-gassing vapors. Avoid dermal contact with cyanide-contaminated victims or with gastric contents of victims who may have ingested cyanide-containing materials. Victims exposed only to hydrogen cyanide gas do not pose contamination risks to rescuers. If the patient is a victim of recent smoke inhalation (may have high carboxyhemoglobin levels), administer only sodium thiosulfate.
Source: State of New York, Department of Health.

TABLE 215-2 RECOGNIZING AND DIAGNOSING HEALTH EFFECTS OF CHEMICAL TERRORISM

Agent	Agent Name	Unique Characteristics	Initial Effects
Nerve	Cyclohexyl sarin (GF) Sarin (GB) Soman (GD) Tabun (GA) VX	Miosis (pinpoint pupils) Copious secretions Muscle twitching/fasciculations	Miosis (pinpoint pupils) Blurred/dim vision Headache Nausea, vomiting, diarrhea Copious secretions/sweating Muscle twitching/fasciculations Breathing difficulty Seizures
Asphyxiant/blood	Arsine Cyanogen chloride Hydrogen cyanide	Possible cherry red skin Possible cyanosis Possible frostbite[a]	Confusion Nausea Patients may gasp for air, similar to asphyxiation but more abrupt onset Seizures prior to death
Choking/pulmonary-damaging	Chlorine Hydrogen chloride Nitrogen oxides Phosgene	Chlorine is a greenish-yellow gas with pungent odor Phosgene gas smells like newly mown hay or grass Possible frostbite[a]	Eye and skin irritation Airway irritation Dyspnea, cough Sore throat Chest tightness
Blistering/vesicant	Mustard/Sulfur mustard (HD, H) Mustard gas (H) Nitrogen mustard (HN-1, HN-2, HN-3) Lewisite (L) Phosgene oxime (CX)	Mustard (HD) has an odor like burning garlic or horseradish Lewisite (L) has an odor like penetrating geranium Phosgene oxime (CX) has a pepperish or pungent odor	Severe irritation Redness and blisters of the skin Tearing, conjunctivitis, corneal damage Mild respiratory distress to marked airway damage May cause death
Incapacitating/behavior-altering	Agent 15/BZ	May appear as mass drug intoxication with erratic behaviors, shared realistic and distinct hallucinations, disrobing and confusion Hyperthermia Mydriasis (dilated pupils)	Dry mouth and skin Initial tachycardia Altered consciousness, delusions, denial of illness, belligerence Hyperthermia Ataxia (lack of coordination) Hallucinations Mydriasis (dilated pupils)

[a]Frostbite may occur from skin contact with liquid arsine, cyanogen chloride, or phosgene. **Source:** State of New York, Department of Health.

TABLE 215-3 DECONTAMINATION AND TREATMENT OF CHEMICAL TERRORISM

Agent	Decontamination	First Aid	Other Patient Considerations
Nerve	Remove clothing immediately Gently wash skin with soap and water Do not abrade skin For eyes, flush with plenty of water or normal saline	Atropine before other measures Pralidoxime (2-PAM) chloride	Onset of symptoms from dermal contact with liquid forms may be delayed Repeated antidote administration may be necessary
Asphyxiant/blood	Remove clothing immediately if no frostbite[a] Gently wash skin with soap and water Do not abrade skin For eyes, flush with plenty of water or normal saline	Rapid treatment with oxygen For cyanide, use antidotes (sodium nitrite and then sodium thiosulfate)	Arsine and cyanogen chloride may cause delayed pulmonary edema
Choking/pulmonary-damaging	Remove clothing immediately if no frostbite[a] Gently wash skin with soap and water Do not abrade skin For eyes, flush with plenty of water or normal saline	Fresh air, forced rest Semi-upright position If signs of respiratory distress are present, oxygen with or without positive airway pressure may be needed Other supportive therapy, as needed	May cause delayed pulmonary edema, even following a symptom-free period that varies in duration with the amount inhaled
Blistering/vesicant	Immediate decontamination is essential to minimize damage Remove clothing immediately Gently wash skin with soap and water Do not abrade skin For eyes, flush with plenty of water or normal saline	Immediately decontaminate skin Flush eyes with water or normal saline for 10–15 min If breathing difficulty, give oxygen Supportive care	Mustard has an asymptomatic latent period There is no antidote or treatment for mustard Lewisite has immediate burning pain, blisters later Specific antidote British Anti-Lewisite (BAL) may decrease systemic effects of Lewisite Phosgene oxime causes immediate pain Possible pulmonary edema
Incapacitating/behavior-altering	Remove clothing immediately Gently wash skin with water or soap and water Do not abrade skin	Remove heavy clothing Evaluate mental status Use restraints as needed Monitor core temperature carefully Supportive care	Hyperthermia and self-injury are largest risks Hard to detect because it is an odorless and non-irritating substance Possible serious arrhythmias Specific antidote (physostigmine) may be available

[a]For frostbite areas, do NOT remove any adhering clothing. Wash area with plenty of warm water to release clothing. **Source:** State of New York, Department of Health.

lists approaches to decontamination of mustard and other CWAs.

Mustard dissolves slowly in aqueous media, such as sweat, but once dissolved, it rapidly forms extremely reactive cyclic ethylene sulfonium ions, which react with cell proteins, cell membranes, and especially DNA in rapidly dividing cells. The ability of mustard to react with and alkylate DNA gives rise to the effects by which it has been characterized as "radiomimetic," similar to radiation injury. Mustard has many biologic actions, but its actual mechanism of action is largely unknown. Much of the biologic damage from mustard results from DNA alkylation and crosslinking in rapidly dividing cells: corneal epithelium, basal keratinocytes, bronchial mucosal epithelium, gastrointestinal mucosal epithelium, and bone marrow precursor cells. This may lead to cellular death and inflammatory reactions. In the skin, proteolytic digestion of anchoring filaments at the epidermal-dermal junction may be the major mechanism of action resulting in blister formation. Mustard also possesses mild cholinergic activity, which may be responsible for effects such as early gastrointestinal and CNS symptoms.

Mustard reacts with tissue within minutes of entering the body. Its circulating half-life in unaltered form is extremely brief.

CLINICAL FEATURES   Topical effects of mustard occur in the skin, airways, and eyes, with the eyes being most sensitive, followed by the airways. Absorbed mustard may produce effects in the bone marrow, gastrointestinal tract, and CNS. Direct injury to the gastrointestinal tract may also occur following ingestion of the compound through contamination of water or food.

Erythema is the mildest and earliest form of mustard skin injury. It resembles sunburn and is associated with pruritus, burning, or stinging pain. Erythema begins to appear within 2 h to 2 d after vapor exposure. Time of onset depends on severity of exposure, ambient temperature and humidity, and type of skin. The most sensitive sites are the warm moist locations and thin delicate skin, such as the perineum, external genitalia, axillae, antecubital fossae, and neck.

Within the erythematous areas, small vesicles can develop, which may later coalesce to form bullae (**Fig. 215-1**). The typical bulla is large, dome-shaped, flaccid, thin-walled, translucent, and surrounded by erythema. The blister fluid, a transudate, is clear to straw-colored, which becomes yellow tending to coagulate. The fluid does not contain mustard and is not itself a vesicant. Lesions from high-dose liquid exposure may develop a central zone of coagulation necrosis with blister formation at the periphery. These lesions take longer to heal and are more prone to secondary infection than the uncomplicated lesions seen at lower exposure levels. Severe lesions might require skin grafting.

The primary airway lesion is necrosis of the mucosa with possible damage to underlying smooth muscle. The damage begins in the upper airways and descends to the lower airways in a dose-dependent

FIGURE 215-2 Schematic diagram of pseudomembrane formation as is seen in high-dose sulfur mustard vapor inhalation exposure. In World War I, severe inhalation exposure often caused death via large airways obstruction.

manner. Usually the terminal airways and alveoli are affected only as a terminal event. Pulmonary edema is not usually present unless the damage is very severe, and then it becomes hemorrhagic.

The earliest effects from mustard and perhaps the only effects from a low concentration involve the nose, sinuses, and pharynx. There may be irritation or burning of the nares, epistaxis, sinus pain, and pharyngeal pain. As the concentration increases, laryngitis, voice changes, and nonproductive cough develop. Damage to the trachea and upper bronchi leads to a productive cough. Lower airway involvement causes dyspnea, severe cough, and increasing quantities of sputum. Terminally, there may be necrosis of the smaller airways with hemorrhagic edema into surrounding alveoli. Hemorrhagic pulmonary edema is rare.

Necrosis of airway mucosa causes "pseudomembrane" formation. These membranes may cause obstruction of the bronchi. During WWI, high dose mustard exposure caused acute death via this mechanism in a small minority of cases (**Fig. 215-2**).

The eyes are the organs most sensitive to mustard vapor injury. The latent period is shorter for eye injury than for skin injury and is also exposure concentration–dependent. After low-dose vapor exposure, irritation evidenced by reddening of the eyes may be the only effect. As the dose increases, the injury includes progressively more severe conjunctivitis, photophobia, blepharospasm, pain, and corneal damage (**Fig. 215-3**).

FIGURE 215-1 Large bulla formation from mustard burn in Iranian patient. Although the blisters on this patient's hand involve only 7% of the body surface area, this patient still required hospitalization in a burn intensive care unit.

FIGURE 215-3 World War I photograph of troops exposed to sulfur mustard vapor. The vast majority of these troops survived with no long-term damage to the eyes; however, they were effectively rendered blind for days to weeks.

About 90% of eye injuries related to mustard heal in 2 weeks to 2 months without sequelae. Scarring between the iris and lens may follow severe effects; this scarring may restrict pupillary movements and may predispose victims to glaucoma. The most severe damage is caused by liquid mustard. After extensive eye exposure, severe corneal damage with possible perforation of the cornea and loss of the eye can occur. In some individuals, a latent chronic keratitis sometimes associated with corneal ulcerations has been described as early as 8 months and as late as 20 years after initial exposure.

The mucosa of the gastrointestinal tract is susceptible to mustard damage, either from systemic absorption or ingestion of the agent. Mustard exposure in small amounts will cause nausea and vomiting lasting up to 24 h. The mechanism of the nausea and vomiting is not understood, but mustard does have a cholinergic-like effect. The CNS effects of mustard, likewise, remain poorly defined. Large exposures can cause seizures in animals. Reports from WWI, and again from the Iran-Iraq war, described people exposed to small amounts of mustard acting sluggish, apathetic, and lethargic. These reports suggest that minor psychological problems could linger for a year or longer.

The cause of death in the majority of mustard poisoning cases is sepsis and respiratory failure. Mechanical obstruction via pseudomembrane formation and agent-induced laryngospasm is important in the first 24 h, but only in cases of severe exposure. From the third through the fifth day after exposure, expect a secondary pneumonia due to bacterial invasion of denuded necrotic mucosa. The third wave of death is caused by agent-induced bone marrow suppression, which peaks 7–21 days after exposure and causes death via sepsis.

Rx SULFUR MUSTARD

A patient severely ill from mustard poisoning requires the general supportive care provided for any severely ill patient, as well as the specific care given to a burn patient. Liberal use of systemic analgesics, maintenance of fluid and electrolyte balance, nutrition, appropriate antibiotics, and other supportive measures are necessary (Table 215-3).

The management of a patient exposed to mustard may range from simple, as in the provision of symptomatic care for a sunburn-like erythema, to complex, as in providing total management for a severely ill patient with burns, immunosuppression, and multi-system involvement. Before raw denuded areas of skin develop, especially with less severe exposures, topical cortisone creams or lotions may be of benefit. Some very basic research data point to the early use of anti-inflammatory preparations. Small blisters (<1–2 cm) should be left intact. Because larger bullae will eventually break, they should be carefully unroofed. Denuded areas should be irrigated three to four times daily with saline, other sterile solutions, or soapy water and then liberally covered with the topical antibiotic of choice, such as silver sulfadiazine or mafenide acetate to a thickness of 1–2 mm. Some physicians advocate sterile needle drainage of large blisters, collapsing the blister roof to form a sterile dressing. Mustard blister fluid does not contain sulfur mustard, only sterile tissue fluid. Health care staff should not fear possible contamination. If an antibiotic cream is not available, sterile petrolatum will be useful. Modified Dakins solution (sodium hypochlorite 0.5%) was used both in WWI and in Iranian casualties (1984–1987) for field-expedient irrigation and antisepsis. Large areas of vesication require hospitalization, IV therapy, and whirlpool bath irrigation.

Systemic analgesics should be used liberally, particularly before manipulation of the patient. Monitoring of fluids and electrolytes is important in any sick patient, but it must be recognized that fluid loss is not of the magnitude seen with thermal burns. Overly rigorous hydration seems to have precipitated pulmonary edema in a few Iranian casualties sent to European hospitals.

Conjunctival irritation from a low vapor exposure will respond to any of a number of available ophthalmic solutions after the eyes are thoroughly irrigated. A topical antibiotic applied several times a day will reduce the incidence and severity of infection. Animal laboratory data have shown remarkable results with commercially available topical antibiotic/glucocorticoid ophthalmologic ointments applied early. An ophthalmologist should be consulted. Topical glucocorticoids are not of proven value, but their use during the first few hours or days might significantly reduce inflammation and subsequent damage. Further use should be relegated to an ophthalmologist.

Vaseline or a similar substance should be applied regularly to the edges of the lids to prevent them from sticking together. Topical analgesics may be useful initially if blepharospasm is too severe to permit an adequate examination; however, topical analgesics have limited value.

A productive cough and dyspnea accompanied by fever and leukocytosis occurring within 12–24 h is indicative of a chemical pneumonitis. The clinician must resist the urge to use prophylactic antibiotics for this process. Infection often occurs on the third to fifth day and is signaled by an increased fever, pulmonary infiltrate, and an increase in sputum production with a change in color. Appropriate antibiotic therapy should await confirmation by Gram stain, and later, positive culture and sensitivity.

Intubation may be necessary if laryngeal spasm or edema makes it difficult or becomes life-threatening. Intubation permits better ventilation and facilitates suction of the necrotic and inflammatory debris. Early use of positive end-expiratory pressure (PEEP) or continuous positive airway pressure (CPAP) may be beneficial. Pseudomembrane formation may require fiberoptic bronchoscopy for suctioning of the necrotic debris.

Bronchodilators are of benefit for bronchospasm. If additional relief of bronchospasm is needed, glucocorticoids should be used. There is little evidence that the routine use of glucocorticoids is beneficial, except for additional relief of bronchospasm.

Leukopenia begins around day 3 with major systemic absorption. Marrow suppression peaks at 7–14 days. In the Iran/Iraq war, a white blood count of $\leq 200/\mu L$ usually resulted in death of the patient. Sterilization of the gut by nonabsorbable antibiotics should be considered to reduce the possibility of sepsis from enteric organisms. Cellular replacement (bone marrow transplants or transfusions) may be successful. Granulocyte colony-stimulating factor (G-CSF) produced a 50% reduction in the time for the bone marrow to recover in non-human primates exposed to sulfur mustard. Medication for nausea and vomiting may be necessary for gastrointestinal side effects.

Excellent assessments of the contributions of DNA alkylation, inflammation, activation of proteolytic enzymes, or lipid peroxidation to the mustard injury have been developed in the past 15–20 years. Some examples include (1) the demonstration of up to 75% reduction of inflammation and tissue damage in the mouse ear swelling test by vanilloid compounds, and (2) the demonstration of 50–60% protection by N-acetylcysteine in the generation of free radicals within guinea pig lung exposed to mustard. In many cases, the demonstration of protection is dependent on the availability of sufficient amounts of drug with adequate half-lives. Strategies to enhance bioavailability include attachment of polyethylene glycol to the antioxidant drug/enzyme or delivery of the drug/enzyme in a liposome (or both).

NERVE AGENTS

The organophosphorus nerve agents are the deadliest of the CWAs. They work by inhibition of tissue synaptic acetylcholinesterase, creating an acute cholinergic crisis. Death ensues because of respiratory depression, and can occur within seconds to minutes.

The nerve agents tabun and sarin were first used on the battlefield by Iraq against Iran during the first Persian Gulf War (1984–1987). Estimates of casualties from these agents range from 20,000–100,000. In 1994 and 1995, the Japanese cult Aum Shinrikyo used sarin in two terrorist attacks in Matsumoto and Tokyo.

The "classic" nerve agents include tabun (GA), sarin (GB), soman (GD), cyclosarin (GF), and VX. VR, similar to VX, was manufactured in the former Soviet Union (Table 215-2). The two-letter codes were established by a North Atlantic Treaty Organization (NATO) international convention and convey no clinical implications. All of the nerve agents are organophosphorus compounds, which are liquid at standard temperature and pressure. The "G" agents evaporate at about the rate of water, except for GF, which is oily, and thus will probably have evaporated within 24 h after deposition on the ground. Their high volatility thus makes a spill of any amount a serious vapor hazard. In the Tokyo subway attack where sarin was used, 100% of the symptomatic patients inhaled sarin vapor that spilled out on the floor of the subway cars. VX, an oily liquid, is the exception. Its low vapor pressure makes it much less of a vapor hazard but potentially a greater environmental hazard because it persists in the environment far longer.

MECHANISM   Acetylcholinesterase inhibition accounts for the major life-threatening effects of nerve agent poisoning. Reversal of this inhibition by antidotal therapy is effective, proving that this is the primary toxic action of these poisons. At cholinergic synapses, acetylcholinesterase, bound to the postsynaptic membrane, functions as a turn-off switch to regulate cholinergic transmission. Inhibition of acetylcholinesterases causes the released neurotransmitter, acetylcholine, to accumulate abnormally. End-organ overstimulation, recognized by clinicians as cholinergic crisis, ensues (Fig. 215-4).

CLINICAL FEATURES   Clinical effects of nerve agent exposure are identical for vapor and liquid exposure routes if the dose is sufficiently large. The speed and order of symptom onset will differ (Table 215-2).

Exposure of a patient to nerve agent vapor, overwhelmingly the more likely route of exposure in both battlefield and terrorist scenarios, will cause cholinergic symptoms in the order that the toxin encounters cholinergic synapses. The most exposed synapses on the integument of the human are in the pupillary muscles. Nerve agent vapor easily crosses the cornea, interacts with these synapses, and produces miosis, described by Tokyo subway victims as "the world going black." Rarely this can also cause eye pain and nausea. Exocrine glands located in the nose, mouth, and pharynx next become exposed to the vapor, and cholinergic overload here causes increased secretions, rhinorrhea, excess salivation, and drooling. Next, toxin interacts with exocrine glands in the upper airway, causing bronchorrhea, and with bronchial smooth muscle, causing bronchospasm. This combination of events can cause hypoxia.

Once the victim has inhaled, vapor can passively cross the alveolar-capillary membrane, enter the bloodstream, and, incidentally and asymptomatically, inhibit circulating cholinesterases, particularly free butyrylcholinesterase and erythrocyte acetylcholinesterase, both of which can be assayed. Unfortunately, the assay may not be easily interpreted without a baseline, since cholinesterase levels vary enormously between subjects and over time in an individual healthy patient.

Usually the first organ system to become symptomatic from bloodborne nerve agent exposure is the gastrointestinal tract, where cholinergic overload causes abdominal cramping and pain, nausea, vomiting, and diarrhea. After the gastrointestinal tract is involved, nerve agents will affect the heart, distant exocrine glands, muscles, and brain. Because there are cholinergic synapses on both the vagal (parasympathetic) and sympathetic sides of the autonomic input to the heart, one cannot predict how heart rate and blood pressure will change once intoxicated. Remote exocrine activity will include oversecretion in the salivary, nasal, respiratory, and sweat glands—the patient will be "wet all over." Bloodborne nerve agents will overstimulate neuromuscular junctions in skeletal muscles, causing fasciculations followed by frank twitching. If the process goes on long enough, eventually ATP in muscle will be depleted and flaccid paralysis will ensue.

In the brain, since the cholinergic system is so widely distributed, bloodborne nerve agents will, in sufficient doses, cause rapid loss of consciousness, seizures, and central apnea leading to death within minutes. If respiration is supported, status epilepticus, which does not respond to usual anticonvulsants, may ensue (Chap. 363). If status epilepticus persists, neuronal death and permanent brain dysfunction may occur. Even in mild nerve agent intoxication, patients may recover but may experience weeks of irritability, sleep disturbance, and nonspecific neurobehavioral symptoms.

The time from exposure to development of the full-blown cholinergic crisis from nerve agent vapor inhalation can be minutes or even seconds, yet there is no depot effect. Since nerve agents have a short circulating half-life, if the patient is supported and, ideally, treated with antidotes, improvement should be rapid without subsequent deterioration.

Liquid exposure to nerve agents differs in speed and order of symptom onset. A nerve agent on intact skin will partially evaporate and partially begin to travel through the skin, causing localized sweating

FIGURE 215-4 Schematic diagram of the pathophysiology of nerve agent exposure. Nerve agent (◆) binds to the active site of acetylcholinesterase (AChE), which is shown as floating free in space but is in reality a postsynaptic membrane-bound enzyme. As a result, acetylcholine (●), which is normally released from presynaptic membrane but normally degraded, accumulates, and this leads (↯) to organ overstimulation and cholinergic crisis.

and then localized fasciculations when it encounters neuromuscular junctions. Once in muscle, it will cross into the circulation and cause gastrointestinal discomfort, respiratory distress, heart rate changes, generalized fasciculations and twitching, loss of consciousness, seizures, and central apnea. The time course will be much longer than with vapor inhalation; even a large, lethal droplet can take up to 30 min to have an effect, and a small, sublethal dose could continue to take effect over 18 h. Clinical worsening that occurs hours after treatment has started is far more likely with liquid than with vapor exposure. Additionally, miosis, practically unavoidable with vapor exposure, is not always present with liquid exposure and may be the last symptom to present in this situation. This is due to the relative insulation of the pupillary muscle from the systemic circulation.

Unless removed by specific therapy (oximes), binding of a nerve agent to cholinesterase is essentially irreversible. Erythrocyte acetylcholinesterase activity recovers at about 1% per day. Plasma butyrylcholinesterase recovers more quickly and is a better guide to recovery of tissue enzyme activity.

℞ NERVE AGENTS

Acute nerve agent poisoning is treated by decontamination, respiratory support, and three antidotes—an anticholinergic, an oxime, and an anticonvulsant (Tables 215-3 and 215-4). In acute cases, all of these forms of therapy may be given simultaneously.

DECONTAMINATION   Decontamination of a vapor is formally not necessary, but in the Tokyo subway attack, sarin vapor trapped in the patients' clothing caused miosis in 10% of emergency personnel. Removal of clothing would have obviated most of this problem. Decontamination of liquid is accomplished in the military using the M291 skin decontamination kit, containing an Ambergard resin capable of absorbing liquid off the skin. Civilian agencies now stockpile this product approved by the U.S. Food and Drug Administration (FDA). At hospitals, soap and copious amounts of water should suffice. Physical removal of the agent is superior to all known decontamination solutions and lotions. In any event, decontamination must be accomplished before the patient enters the hospital facility to avoid contaminating the facility and its staff. In patients with contaminated wounds, extract potentially contaminated clothing and other foreign material that may serve as a depot for the liquid agent.

RESPIRATORY SUPPORT   Death from nerve agent poisoning is almost always from respiratory causes. Ventilation will be complicated by increased resistance and secretions. Atropine should be given before ventilation or as ventilation begins, since it will make ventilation far easier.

ANTIDOTAL THERAPY   Atropine   In theory, any anticholinergic could be used to treat nerve agent poisoning, but worldwide the choice is invariably atropine due to its wide temperature stability, rapid effectiveness either IM or IV, and because inadvertent administration of this drug usually causes little CNS dysfunction (Table 215-4). Atropine rapidly reverses cholinergic overload at muscarinic synapses but has little effect at nicotinic synapses. Practically, this implies that atropine can quickly treat the life-threatening respiratory effects of nerve agents but will probably not help neuromuscular and possibly sympathetic effects. In the field, military personnel are given MARK I kits (Fig. 215-5A) containing 2 mg atro-

TABLE 215-4 ANTIDOTE RECOMMENDATIONS FOLLOWING EXPOSURE TO NERVE AGENTS

| Patient Age | Antidotes | | Other Treatment |
	Mild/Moderate Effects[a]	Severe Effects[b]	
Infants (0–2 yrs)	Atropine: 0.05 mg/kg IM, or 0.02 mg/kg IV; and 2-PAM chloride: 15 mg/kg IM or IV slowly	Atropine: 0.1 mg/kg IM, or 0.02 mg/kg IV; and 2-PAM chloride: 25 mg/kg IM, or 15 mg/kg IV slowly	Assisted ventilation after antidotes for severe exposure.
Child (2–10 yrs)	Atropine: 1 mg IM, or 0.02 mg/kg IV; and 2-PAM chloride[c]: 15 mg/kg IM or IV slowly	Atropine: 2 mg IM, or 0.02 mg/kg IV; and 2-PAM chloride[c]: 25 mg/kg IM, or 15 mg/kg IV slowly	Repeat atropine (2 mg IM, or 1 mg IM for infants) at 5- to 10-min intervals until secretions have diminished and breathing is comfortable or airway re-sistance has returned to near normal.
Adolescent (>10 yrs)	Atropine: 2 mg IM, or 0.02 mg/kg IV; and 2-PAM chloride[c]: 15 mg/kg IM or IV slowly	Atropine: 4 mg IM, or 0.02 mg/kg IV; and 2-PAM chloride[c]: 25 mg/kg IM, or 15 mg/kg IV slowly	
Adult	Atropine: 2 to 4 mg IM or IV; and 2-PAM chloride: 600 mg IM, or 15 mg/kg IV slowly	Atropine: 6 mg IM; and 2-PAM chloride: 1800 mg IM, or 15 mg/kg IV slowly	Phentolamine for 2-PAM-induced hy-pertension: (5 mg IV for adults; 1 mg IV for children). Diazepam for convulsions: (0.2 to 0.5 mg IV for infants <5 years: 1 mg IV for children >5 years; 5 mg IV for adults).
Elderly, frail	Atropine: 1 mg IM; and 2-PAM chloride: 10 mg/kg IM, or 5 to 10 mg/kg IV slowly	Atropine: 2 to 4 mg IM; and 2-PAM chloride: 25 mg/kg IM, or 5 to 10 mg/kg IV slowly	

[a]Mild/moderate effects include localized sweating, muscle fasciculations, nausea, vomit-ing, weakness, dyspnea.
[b]Severe effects include unconsciousness, convulsions, apnea, flaccid paralysis.

[c]If calculated dose exceeds the adult IM dose, adjust accordingly.
Note: 2-PAM chloride is pralidoxime chloride or protopam chloride.
Source: State of New York, Department of Health.

pine in autoinjector form for IM use. Civilian agencies are now stockpiling this FDA-approved product as well. One can only give full autoinjector doses and not divide them. The field-loading dose is 2, 4, or 6 mg, with re-treatment every 5–10 min until the patient's breathing and secretions im-prove. The Iranians used larger doses initially during the Iran-Iraq war where oximes were in short supply. When the patient reaches a level of medical care where drugs can be given IV, this is the preferred route; in small children this may be the initial form of atropine therapy. However, pediatric autoinjectors of 0.5 mg and 1.0 mg are now manufactured. There is no upper limit to atropine therapy in a patient either IM or IV; however, a total average adult dose for a severely afflicted patient would usually be 20–30 mg.

In a mildly afflicted patient with miosis and no other systemic symp-toms, atropine or homatropine eye drops may suffice for therapy. This will produce ~24 h of mydriasis. Frank miosis or imperfect accommodation may persist for weeks or even months after all other signs and symptoms have resolved.

Oxime Therapy   Oximes are nucleophiles that reactivate the cholines-terase whose active site has been occupied and bound to nerve agent (Ta-ble 215-4). Therapy with oximes therefore restores normal enzyme function. Oxime therapy is limited by a second side reaction, called "aging," in which a side chain on nerve agents falls off the complex at a characteris-tic rate. "Aged" complexes are negatively charged, and oximes cannot reac-tivate negatively charged complexes. The practical effect of this differs from one nerve agent to another since each ages at a characteristic rate. VX, for practical purposes, never ages, sarin ages in 3–5 h, and tabun ages over a longer period. All of these are so much longer than the patient's ex-pected lifespan after acute nerve agent toxicity that they may be ignored. Soman, on the other hand, ages in 2 min. Thus, after only a few minutes fol-lowing exposure, oximes are useless in treating soman poisoning. The oxime used varies by country; the United States has approved and fielded 2-pralidoxime chloride (2-PAM Cl). MARK I kits (Fig. 215-5A) contain autoin-jectors of 600 mg 2-PAM Cl. Initial field loading doses are 600, 1200, or 1800 mg. Since blood pressure elevation may occur after administration of 45 mg/kg in adults, field use of 2-PAM Cl is restricted to 1800 mg, IM, per hour. During the time when more oxime cannot be given, atropine alone is rec-ommended. In the hospital setting, 2.5–25 mg/kg IV 2-PAM Cl has been found to reactivate 50% of inhibited cholinesterase. The usual recommen-dation is 1000 mg through slow IV drip over 20–30 min, with ≤2500 mg over a period of 1–1.5 h.

Anticonvulsants   Nerve agent–induced seizures do not respond to the usual anticonvulsants used for status epilepticus, including phenytoin, phenobarbital, carbamazepine, valproic acid, and lamotrigine (Chap. 363). The only class of anticonvulsants that has been shown to stop this form of

status are the benzodiazepines. Diazepam is the only benzodiazepine ap-proved for seizures in humans, although other FDA-approved benzodiaze-pines work well against nerve agent–induced seizures in animal models. Diazepam, therefore, is manufactured in 10-mg injectors for IM use and given to U.S. forces for this purpose (**Fig. 215-5B**). Civilian agencies are stockpiling this field product (convulsive antidote for nerve agent, "CANA"), which is not generally used in hospital practice. Extrapolation from animal studies indicates that adults will probably require 30–40 mg diazepam, IM, to stop nerve agent–induced status epilepticus. In the hospital, or in a small child unable to receive the autoinjector, IV diazepam may be used at similar doses. The clinician may confuse seizures with the neuromuscular signs of nerve agent poisoning. In the hospital, early electroencephalogra-phy is advised to distinguish between nonconvulsive status epilepticus, actual seizures, and postictal paralysis. Recent animal studies have shown that the most effective benzodiazepine in this situation is midazolam, which is not FDA-approved for seizures.

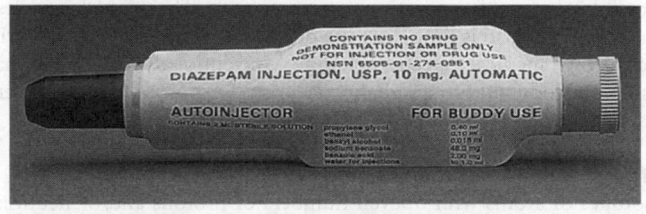

FIGURE 215-5 Antidotes to nerve agents. A. MARK I autoinjector set containing one 600-mg dose of 2-pralidoxime chloride and one 2-mg dose of atropine. Such sets are carried by all U.S. military forces in a po-tentially chemical battlefield and are now being stockpiled by civilian first responders. **B.** Diazepam 10-mg autoinjector. These are carried by all U.S. military forces in a potential chemical battlefield and are being stockpiled by civilian first responders.

Peripheral neuropathy and the so-called intermediate syndrome, prominent long-term effects of insecticide poisoning, are not described in nerve agent survivors.

Recent research has explored approaches leading to a transient "immunity," or drugs that would provide protection against lethal nerve agents yet be devoid of side effects. A novel approach is to use enzymes to scavenge these highly toxic nerve agents before they attack their intended targets. The accumulated work has shown that if a scavenger is present at the time of nerve agent exposure, rapid reduction of toxicant levels is observed. This reduction is so rapid and profound that the need to administer a host of pharmacologically active drugs as antidotes is, in theory, eliminated.

INDUSTRIAL CHEMICALS IN TERRORISM

Many of the chemical warfare agents of WWI, including chlorine, phosgene, and cyanide, are used today in large amounts in industry. They are produced in chemical plants, stockpiled in large tanks, and travel up and down highways and railways in large tanker cars. The rupture of any of these by accident or purposefully could cause many injuries and deaths. Hazardous materials (HAZMATs), not used on the battlefield, can also be used as terrorist weapons. Some of these, including insecticides and ammonia, could wreak as much damage and injury as the weaponized chemical agents.

Recently, insurgents in Iraq used chlorine gas, released from tankers following explosions, as a crude form of chemical weaponry. Using this gas, they killed 12 people and intoxicated more than 140 others in three attacks in February 2007. The clinical course and pathophysiology of the noncardiogenic pulmonary edema induced by chlorine (or phosgene) toxic inhalational injury are described in Chap. 262. Table 215-2 describes the physical appearance and initial physiologic effects of chlorine.

FURTHER READINGS

BROOMFIELD CA et al: Progress on the road to new nerve agent treatments. J Appl Toxicol 21:S43, 2001

GUNDERSON CH et al: Nerve agents: A review. Neurology 42:946, 1992

KARALLIEDDE L et al: Possible immediate and long-term health effects following exposure to chemical warfare agents. Public Health 114:238, 2000

McDONOUGH JH et al: Anticonvulsant treatment of nerve agent seizures: Anticholinergics versus diazepam in soman-intoxicated guinea pigs. Epilepsy Res 38:1, 2000

OKUMURA T et al: Report on 640 victims of the Tokyo subway sarin attack. Ann Emerg Med 28:129, 1996

SIDELL FR: Clinical considerations in nerve agent intoxication, in *Chemical Warfare Agents*, SM Somani (ed). San Diego, California, Academic Press, 1992, pp 156–194

———— et al (eds.): *Medical Aspects of Chemical and Biological Warfare, Volume I of Textbook of Military Medicine*, Walter Reed Army Medical Center, Washington, DC, Borden Institute, 1997. [Available on the website: *http://ccc.apgea.army.mil*]

SMITH WJ: Vesicant agents and antivesicant medical countermeasures: Clinical toxicology and psychological implications. Mil Psychol 14:145, 2002

US ARMY MEDICAL RESEARCH INSTITUTE OF CHEMICAL DEFENSE, CHEMICAL CASUALTY CARE DIVISION: *Medical Management of Chemical Casualties Handbook*, 3d ed. Aberdeen Proving Ground, Maryland, 1999. [Available on the website: *http://ccc.apgea.army.mil*]

WILLEMS JL: Clinical management of mustard gas casualties. Ann Med Milit Belg 3S:1, 1989

216 Radiation Bioterrorism
Zelig A. Tochner, Eli Glatstein

Terror attacks using nuclear or radiation-related devices are an unequivocal threat in the twenty-first century and are capable of unique medical and psychological effects. In this chapter we will focus on the most probable scenarios of possible attacks and the medical principles of handling such threats.

There are two major categories of potential terrorist incidents with widespread radiologic consequences. The first is the use of radiologic dispersal devices. This could cause a purposeful dissemination of radioactive material without nuclear detonation by using conventional explosives with radionuclides, attacking fixed nuclear facilities, or attacking nuclear-powered surface vessels or submarines. Malfunctioning nuclear weapons that are detonated with no nuclear yield (nuclear "duds") and/or installation of radionuclides in food or water are also a possible means of generating a terror attack. The second, and less probable, scenario is the actual use of nuclear weapons. Each scenario has its own medical aspects, including "conventional" blast or thermal injury, introduction to a radiation field, and exposure to either external or internal contamination from a radioactive explosion.

TYPES OF RADIOISOTOPIC RADIATION

Isotopes of atoms with uneven numbers of protons and/or neutrons are typically unstable; such isotopes discharge particles or energy to matter, a process that we define as *radiation*. The main radiation types are alpha, beta, gamma, and neutrons.

Alpha (α) radiation consists of heavy, positively charged particles containing two protons and two neutrons. Alpha particles are usually emitted from isotopes with an atomic number of ≥82, such as uranium or plutonium. Due to their large size, alpha particles have limited penetrating power. Fine obstacles such as cloth or human skin can usually stop them from penetrating into the body, and they represent a small risk to external exposure due to their limited penetration. If they somehow are internalized, then alpha particles can cause significant cellular damage within their immediate proximity.

Beta (β) radiation consists of electrons, which are small, light, negatively charged particles (about 1/2000 the mass of a neutron or proton). They can travel only a short finite distance in tissue, depending on their energy. Exposure to beta particles is common in many radiation accidents. Radioactive iodine, released in nuclear plant accidents, is the best known member of this group. Plastic layers and clothing can stop most beta particles, and their penetration is measured to be a few millimeters. A large quantum of energy to the basal stratum of the skin can cause a burn that is similar to a thermal burn and is treated as such.

Gamma (γ) rays and *x-rays* (both photons) are similar. Gamma rays are uncharged electromagnetic radiation discharged from a nucleus as a wave or photons of energy. X-rays are the product of abrupt mechanical deceleration of electrons striking a heavy target such as tungsten. Gamma and x-rays have similar properties, i.e., no charge and no mass, just energy. Both travel easily through matter, sometimes called *penetrating radiation*, and are the principal type of radiation to cause total-body exposure. If the energy of gamma rays and x-rays is the same, then their biological effects will be the same.

Neutron (η) particles are heavy and uncharged, often emitted during nuclear detonation. They possess a wide energy range; their ability to penetrate tissues is variable, depending upon their energy. They are less likely to be present in most scenarios of radiation bioterrorism.

The ionization resulting from protons, electrons, and gamma rays is either a direct or indirect (i.e., mediated through water) effect of particles or photons on DNA. Ionization of DNA resulting from neutrons is secondary to the neutrons knocking electrons out of their atomic orbit and the formation of free radicals, which can also damage DNA directly.

The commonly used units of radiation are the rad and the gray (Gy). The rad (radiation absorbed dose) is energy deposited within living matter and is equal to 100 ergs/g of tissue.

The traditional rad has been replaced by the Système Internationale (SI) unit of the gray; 100 rad = 1 Gy.

TYPES OF EXPOSURE

Whole-body exposure represents deposition of radiation energy over the entire body. Alpha and beta particles have limited penetration and do not cause significant noncutaneous injury unless emission results from an internalized source. Whole-body exposure from gamma rays, x-rays, or neutrons, which can penetrate through the body (depending on their energy), can result in damage to multiple tissues and organs. The tissue damage is proportional to the radiation exposure of that organ or tissue.

External contamination is a result of fallout of radioactive particles that land on the body surface, clothing, skin, and hair. This is the dominant element to consider in the mass casualty situation resulting from a radioactive terrorist strike. The common contaminants will primarily emit alpha and beta radiation. Alpha particles do not penetrate beyond the skin and thus have minimal systemic effects. Beta emitters can cause significant cutaneous burns and scarring. Gamma emitters may not only cause local damage but can also cause whole-body radiation exposures and injury. The medical treatment is primarily decontamination of the body, including wounds and burns, to prevent the contamination from becoming internalized. Removing the contaminated clothing reduces the contamination significantly and is a first step in the decontamination process. Generally patients will not constitute a significant radiation hazard to health care providers, and life-saving treatment should not be delayed for fear of secondary contamination of the medical team. Any damage to health care personnel will depend directly on the duration of exposure and will be inversely proportional to the square of the distance from any radioactive source. Gowns that can be easily removed are essential to protect health care personnel.

Internal contamination will occur when radioactive material is inhaled, ingested, or able to enter the body through open wounds or burns or via skin absorption. In principle, any externally contaminated casualty should be evaluated for internal contamination. Some isotopes may have toxic effects on specific target organs due to their chemical properties, in addition to radiologic injury. The respiratory system is the main portal of entrance for internal contamination, and the lung is the organ at greatest risk. Aerosol particles <5 μm can reach the alveoli, whereas larger particles will remain in proximal airways. The tiny particles can be absorbed by the lymphatic system or the bloodstream, continuing to irradiate (depending on their biologically active half-life) until being exhaled. Bronchial lavage is often helpful treatment in this situation. Radioactive material entering the gastrointestinal (GI) tract will be absorbed according to its chemical structure and solubility. The insoluble radionuclides may affect the lower GI tract. Intact skin is normally a good barrier to most radionuclides. Penetration through the skin usually takes place when wounds or burns have altered the skin barriers. Therefore, any skin erosion should be cleaned and decontaminated promptly.

Absorbed radioactive materials will travel throughout the body. Liver, kidney, adipose tissue, and bone tend to bind and retain the radioactive material more than other tissues. The medical treatment includes preventing absorption, reducing incorporation, and enhancing elimination (see below).

Localized exposure means close contact between a highly radioactive source and a part of the body, causing discrete damage to the skin and deeper tissues, similar to a thermal burn. Later signs include epilation, erythema, moist desquamation, ulceration, blistering, or necrosis in proportion to exposure. Alopecia, transient or permanent, is dose-related and starts at cutaneous doses >3 Gy. Overt tissue damage can take weeks and even months to develop; the healing process can also be very slow and last for months. Long-term cutaneous changes, including keratosis, fibrosis, and telangiectasias, may appear years after the exposure. Treatment is based on analgesia and infection prophylaxis. Nevertheless, severe burns can often require grafting or even amputation. Long-term radiation effects are characterized by cell loss and cell death.

RADIOLOGIC DISPERSAL EVENTS

Radiologic dispersal incidents are generally of two types resulting from: (1) small, usually localized sources; or (2) wide dispersals over large areas. The radioactive materials can take the form of solid state, aerosol, gas, or liquid. They can be put into food or water, released from vehicles, or be spread by explosion. The principal route of exposure is usually by direct contact between the victim's skin and the radioactive particles, although internal contamination could occur if the material were inhaled or ingested. The radiation field is also a potential source of whole-body exposure. The psychosocial effects that accompany such an event are significant and are beyond the scope of this chapter. A list of radioactive materials, including information on their major properties and medical treatment, is shown in Table 216-1.

In a localized event, the amount and spread of the radioactive materials are usually limited and can be treated like a spill of hazardous material. Protective clothing prevents or minimizes the contamination of emergency responders.

The use of explosives coupled with a large amount of radioactive materials can result in wide dispersion of radiation, which is of far greater concern. Other potential sources of radiation are nuclear reactors, spent nuclear fuel, and transport vehicles. Less probable but still possible is the use of a large source of penetrating radiation without explosion. It is expected that most exposures would be low, and the principal health and psychosocial effects would be similar to the former scenario but on a larger scale.

Whenever an explosion is involved, conventional life-saving treatment should be given first priority. Only then should decontamination and specific treatment be given for the radiation exposure.

Silent exposure represents a scenario in which a powerful radiologic source could be hidden in a crowded place or radiologic materials spread without any awareness or announcement. It might take a long time to recognize the event and the source of exposure. One of the major clues to this situation is the appearance of unusual clinical manifestations in many individuals; such manifestations are often nonspecific and include symptoms of acute radiation sickness (see below) such as headache, fatigue, malaise, and opportunistic infections. GI phenomena such as diarrhea, nausea, vomiting, and anorexia may occur. Dermatologic symptoms (burns, ulceration, and epilation) and hematopoietic manifestations such as bleeding tendency, thrombocytopenia, purpura, lymphopenia, or neutropenia are also possible and dose-related. Careful epidemiologic studies may be necessary to identify the source of such exposure.

NUCLEAR WEAPONS

The most likely scenario of nuclear terror would be the detonation of a single low-yield device. The estimated yield of such device is anywhere between 0.01 and 10 kiloton of TNT, although the probability would more likely be toward the lower yield. Coping with such an event is certainly possible. The effects of such an explosion are a combination of several components: ground shock, air blast, thermal radiation, initial nuclear radiation, residual nuclear radiation, crater formation, and radioactive fallout.

The nuclear detonation, like a conventional explosion, will produce a shock wave that can further damage structures and cause many casualties. In addition, the detonation can produce an extremely hot fireball that can ignite materials and cause severe burns. The detonation also releases an intense pulse of ionizing radiation, mainly gamma rays and neutrons. The radiation produced in the first minute is termed *initial radiation*, while the ongoing radiation due to fallout is termed *residual radiation*. Both types of radiation can cause acute radiation sickness (ARS; see below). The $LD_{50/30}$ (i.e., a dose that causes 50% mortality at 30 days) is ~4 Gy for whole-body exposure without medical support; with medical support, the $LD_{50/30}$ ranges between 8 and 10 Gy. Winds can carry fallout and contaminate large areas.

On top of its effects, a massive blast forms a crater in the soil and usually produces a ground shock compounding the damage and number of casualties. Inhalation of large amounts of radioactive dust causes pneu-

TABLE 216-1 INTERNAL CONTAMINANT RADIONUCLIDES: PROPERTIES AND TREATMENT

Isotope Name	Symbol	Common Usage	Radiation Type $t_{1/2}$ Radiologic $t_{1/2}$ Biologic, days	Exposure Type	Mode of Contamination	Focal Accumulation in Body	Treatment
Manganese	Mn-56	Reactors, research laboratories	β, γ 2.6 h 5.7	External, internal	N/A	Liver	N/A
Cobalt	Co-60	Medical radiotherapy devices, commercial food irradiators	β, γ 5.26 y 9.5	External, internal	Lungs	Liver	Gastric lavage, purgatives; penicillamine in severe cases
Strontium	Sr-90	Fission product of uranium	β 28 y 18,000	Internal	Moderate GI tract	Bones—similar to calcium	Strontium, calcium, ammonium chloride
Molybdenum	Mo-99	Hospitals—scans	β, γ 66.7 h 3	External, internal	N/A	Kidneys	N/A
Technetium	Tc-99m	Hospitals—scans	β, γ 6.049 h 1	External, internal	IV administration	Kidneys, total body	Potassium perchlorate to reduce thyroid dose
Cesium	Cs-137	Medical radiotherapy devices	β, γ 30 y 70	External, internal	Lungs, GI tract, wounds, follows potassium	Renal excretion	Ion-exchange resins, Prussian blue
Gadolinium	Gd-153	Hospitals	β, γ 242 d 1000	External, internal	N/A	N/A	N/A
Iridium	Ir-192	Commercial radiography	β, γ 74 d 50	External, internal	N/A	Spleen	N/A
Radium	Ra-226	Instrument illumination, industrial applications, old medical equipment, former Soviet Union military equipment	α, β, γ 1602 y 16,400	External, internal	GI tract	Bones	MgSO$_4$ lavage, ammonium chloride, calcium alginates
Tritium	H-3	Luminescent gun sights, muzzle-velocity detectors, nuclear weapons	β 12.5 y 12	Internal	Inhalation, GI tract, wounds	Total body	Dilution with controlled water intake, diuretics
Iodine	I-131	Reactor accidents, thyroid ablators	β, γ 8.1 d 138	Internal	Inhalation, GI tract, wounds	Thyroid	Potassium/sodium iodide, propylthiouracil, methimazole
Uranium	U-235	Depleted uranium, natural uranium, fuel rods, weapons-grade material	α, (α, β, γ) 7.1×10^8 y 15	Internal	GI tract	Kidneys, bones	NaHCO$_3$, chelation with EDTA
Plutonium	Pu-239	Produced from uranium in reactors, nuclear weapons	α 2.2×10^4 y 73,000	Internal	Limited lung absorption, high retention	Lungs, bones, bone marrow, liver, gonads	Chelating with DTPA or EDTA
Americium	Am-241	Smoke detectors, nuclear weapon detonation fallout	α 458 y 73,000	Internal	Inhalation, skin wounds	Lungs, liver, bones, bone marrow	Chelating with DTPA or EDTA
Polonium	Po-210	Calibration source	α 138.4 d 60	Internal	Inhalation, wounds	Spleen, kidneys	Lavage, dimercaprol
Thallium	Th-232	Calibration source	α 1.41×10^{10} y 73,000	Internal	N/A	N/A	N/A
Phosphorus	P-32	Research laboratories, medical facilities	β 14.3 d 1155	Internal	Inhalation, GI tract, wounds	Bones, bone marrow, rapidly replicating cells	Lavage, aluminum hydroxide, phosphate

Note: N/A, not available; h, hours; y, years; GI, gastrointestinal.

monitis that can lead to pulmonary fibrosis. Use of a mask covering the mouth and nose can be very helpful. The intense flash of infrared and visible light can cause either temporary or permanent blindness. Cataracts can develop months to years later among those who survive.

ACUTE RADIATION SICKNESS

Radiation interactions with atoms can result in ionization and the formation of free radicals that damage tissue by disrupting chemical bonds and molecular structures in the cell, including DNA. Radiation damage can lead to cell death; those cells that recover may be mutated and at higher risk for subsequent cancer. Cell sensitivity increases as the replication rate increases and the cell differentiation decreases. Bone marrow and mucosal surfaces of the GI tract, which have vast mitotic activity, are significantly more sensitive to radiation than slowly dividing tissues such as bones and muscles. Following exposure of either all or most of the human body to ionizing radiation, ARS can develop. The clinical manifestations of ARS reflect the dose and type of radiation as well as the part of the body exposed.

Clinical Manifestations ARS manifests as three major groups of signs and symptoms: hematopoietic, gastrointestinal, and neurovascular. There are four major stages in ARS: prodrome, latent phase, illness, and either recovery or death. The higher the radiation doses, the shorter and more severe each stage. The prodrome appears within minutes to 4 days postexposure; lasts between a few hours to a few days; and can include nausea, vomiting, anorexia, and diarrhea. At the end of the prodrome, ARS progresses to the latent phase. Minimal or no symptoms are present during the latent phase, which commonly lasts up to 2.5 weeks, but can last up to 6 weeks. The duration depends on the radiation dose, the health of the patient, and the coexisting illness or injury. Following the latent phase, the exposed person manifests illness that may eventuate in recovery or lead to death.

With exposure to doses <1 Gy, ARS is generally mild. At this dose symptoms can be minimal or nonexistent, even if the entire body is exposed to penetrating radiation. The clinical picture will mainly be transient depression of bone marrow (lymphopenia) that lasts up to 2 to 3 weeks and then recovers.

ARS is significantly more acute and severe with exposure to very high doses—>30 Gy. At this dose the prodrome appears in minutes and is followed by 5 to 6 h of latency before a cardiovascular collapse occurs secondary to irreversible damage to the microcirculation.

The type and dose of radiation and the part of the body exposed will determine not only the timing of the different stages of ARS but also the dominant clinical picture. At low radiation doses of 0.7 to 4 Gy, hematopoietic depression due to bone marrow suppression takes place and constitutes the main illness. The patient may develop infections and bleeding secondary to low leukocyte and platelet counts, respectively. The bone marrow will eventually recover in almost all patients if they are supported with transfusions and fluids; antibiotics are often needed in addition. With exposure to 6 to 8 Gy, the clinical picture is significantly more complicated. At these doses the bone marrow will not always recover and death may ensue. A GI syndrome may also accompany the hematopoietic manifestations and further worsen the patient's condition. Compromise of the absorptive layer of the gut alters absorption of fluids, electrolytes, and nutrients. GI injury can lead to vomiting, diarrhea, GI bleeding, sepsis, and electrolyte and fluid imbalance in a patient whose blood counts are compromised for a period of weeks, often leading to death. Whole-body exposure to doses >9–10 Gy is almost always fatal. Crucial elements of the bone marrow simply will not recover. In addition to the GI syndrome associated with very large exposures, patients may develop a neurovascular syndrome; the latter dominates with whole-body doses >20 Gy. Vascular collapse, seizures, confusion, and death usually occur within days. In this variant the prodrome and latent phase both shorten to a few hours.

℞ ACUTE RADIATION SICKNESS

The treatment of ARS is focused on maintaining homeostasis, giving damaged organs the chance to recover. Aggressive support is given to every damaged system. Treatment for the hematopoietic system includes mainly therapy for neutropenia and infection, transfusion and blood products as needed, and hematopoietic growth factors. The value of bone marrow transplantation in this situation is questionable. None of the transplants that were performed among the victims of the nuclear reactor accident in Chernobyl proved successful. Another major component of the treatment of ARS is partial or total parenteral nutrition, to bypass the damaged GI system. For blast and thermal injuries, standard therapy for trauma is given. Psychological support is essential in many cases.

FIGURE 216-1 Algorithm for evacuation in a multicasualties radiologic event.

MEDICAL MANAGEMENT OF RADIATION BIOTERRORISM

Victims of radiation bioterrorism can suffer from conventional thermal or blast injuries, exposure to radiation, and contamination by radioactive materials. Many will have combinations of the above, which can be synergistic and cause higher morbidity and mortality than when they occur alone. The number of casualties will be a major factor in determining the response of the medical system to an act of radiation bioterrorism. If only a few persons are affected, then no significant changes and adaptation of the system are needed to treat the victims. However, if a terror attack results in a large number (dozens, or more) of casualties, then an organized disaster plan at the local and state levels must be invoked to deal with the crisis properly. Medical personnel should have a prior assignment and training and be prepared to function in a scenario with which they are familiar. Stockpiles of specific equipment and medications have to be preplanned (see the Centers for Disease Control and Prevention website—*http://www.bt.cdc.gov*). One of the terrorists' goals is to overwhelm medical facilities and to minimize the salvage of casualties.

Initial management consists of *primary triage and transportation* of the wounded to emergency rooms for treatment. The rationale behind the triage is to sort patients into classes according to the severity of injury, for the purpose of expediting clinical care and maximizing the use of the available clinical services and facilities. Triage requires determination of the level of emergency care needed. The higher the number and range of casualties, the more complex and difficult triage becomes. The mildly wounded and victims of contamination only can be sent to evacuation, registration with disaster response teams, and decontamination and treatment centers. Figure 216-1 illustrates evacuation in a multicasualties radiologic event. In this way, the hospitals themselves can avoid being directly overwhelmed, and those who are severely wounded can receive better treatment. Emergency treatment will be administered initially according to the presence of conventional injuries such as wounds, trauma, and thermal or chemical burns. Individuals with such injuries should be stabilized, if possible, and immediately transported to a medical facility. Removing the victim's clothes and wrapping him or her in clean blankets or nylon sheets reduces both the exposure of the patient and the contamination risk to the staff. However, the possibility of contamination needs to be determined. Less severely injured victims should receive a preliminary decontamination before or during evacuation to a hospital.

One must remember that radionuclide contamination of the skin is commonly not an acute life-threatening situation to the patient or the personnel who care for the patient. Only powerful gamma emitters are likely to cause real damage from contamination. It is important to emphasize that exposure to a radiation field alone does not necessarily create any contamination. The exposed person, if not contaminated, is not radioactive and does not directly emit any radiation.

In order to protect the staff, protective gear (gowns, gloves, masks, and caps) should be used. Protective masks with filters and chemically protective overgarments provide excellent protection from contamination. Waterproof shoe covers are also important. Remaining in the contaminated area and dealing with life-saving procedures should take place according to the "ALARA" principle: as low as reasonably achievable. It is better to send many people for short exposure times than to send a few people for longer periods of time to do the same job.

Decontamination of victims should take place in the field prior to their arrival at medical facilities, but radiologic decontamination should never interfere with medical care. Removal of outer clothing and shoes will usually reduce the patient's contamination by 80–90%. Contaminated clothes should be carefully removed by rolling them over themselves, placing them in marked plastic bags, and removing them to a predefined area for contaminated clothes and equipment. A radiation detector should then be used to check for the presence of any residual radiologic contamination on the patient's body. In order to prevent internalization of the radioactive materials, one should cover open wounds prior to decontamination. Showering or washing of the entire skin and hair is very important. The skin is dried and reassessed for residual contamination until no radiation is found. Contamination-removing chemical agents are more than sufficient to remove radiologic contamination.

Wound decontamination should be as conservative as possible. The main goal is to prevent both extensive local damage and internal contamination through lacerated skin. The bandages should be removed and the wounds flushed. The wound should then be dried and assessed for radiation. This procedure can be repeated again and again until contamination is undetectable. Excision of contaminated wounds should be attempted only when surgically necessary.

In the hospital, staff can wear normal hospital barrier clothing, including two pairs of gloves, a gown, shoe covers, a head cover, and a face mask. Eye protection is recommended. Decontamination of medical personnel is obligatory following emergency treatment and decontamination of the patient. All protective clothing should be placed after use in a designated container for contaminated clothing.

Radiation intensity decays rapidly with the square of the distance from the source, and increasing the distance from the source and decreasing the time spent near it are basic principles of radiation safety. Shielding with lead can be used as protection from small radioactive gamma sources. Geiger counters can detect gamma and beta radiation. Pocket chamber (pencil) dosimeters, film badges, and thermoluminescent dosimeters can measure accumulated exposure to gamma radiation. All of these detectors are in common use in medical facilities and should be used to help and define the level of contamination. Alpha radiation is harder to detect due to its poor penetration. An alpha scintillation counter, which is capable of detecting alpha radiation, is not commonly used in medical facilities.

GUIDELINES FOR HOSPITAL MANAGEMENT

Figure 216-2 illustrates a model for hospital arrangement for triage. Persons contaminated either externally or internally should be identified, externally decontaminated, and, if needed, treated immediately and specifically for internal contamination. In all other cases, the need for treatment of radiation injuries does not constitute a medical emergency. Early actions, such as blood sampling both for assessing the de-

FIGURE 216-2 Flow chart of hospital triage. O.R., operating room.

gree of severity of the exposure and for blood type and cross-matching for possible transfusion, need to be promptly taken if ARS is evident or if exposure is suspected.

In the hospital entrance, a distinct decontamination area should be set up promptly. Separation between clean and contaminated areas is essential. Medical personnel in this area should wear protective gear as noted above. They also should be rotated in their assignments every 1 to 2 h to ensure minimal exposure to radiation. If patients are critically wounded and require either surgery or resuscitation, they need to pass directly to "contaminated" operating rooms or resuscitation sites for life-saving procedures. Once such patients are stable, they should then be decontaminated. It is important to obtain details concerning the exposure, to look for prodromal signs of radiation sickness, and to do a physical examination. One of the best ways to estimate exposure clinically is to measure the time of prodromal appearance. The earlier the prodromal signs and symptoms appear, the higher the dose of radiation exposure. A few laboratory tests need to be routinely taken, such as complete blood count and urinalysis. If internal contamination is suspected, specific treatment should be given, as outlined below.

℞ RADIONUCLIDE CONTAMINATION

Treatment for internal radionuclide contamination should be started as soon as possible after suspected or known exposure. The goal is to leave the smallest amount of radionuclides as possible in the body. Treatment is given in order to reduce absorption and to enhance elimination and excretion.

Clearance of the GI tract may be achieved by stomach lavage; emetics (such as apomorphine, 5 to 10 mg, or ipecac, 1- to 2-g capsules or 15 mL in syrup); or by using purgatives, laxatives, ion exchangers, and aluminum antacids. Prussian blue, 1 g tid for a minimum of 3 weeks, is an ion exchanger used to treat cesium 137 internal contamination. Aluminum antacids (such as aluminum phosphate gel) may reduce strontium uptake in the gut if given immediately after exposure. Aluminum hydroxide is less effective.

Prevention or reversal of radionuclide interaction with tissues can be done by blocking, diluting, mobilizing, and chelating agents. *Blocking agents* prevent entrance of radioactive materials. A good example is potassium iodide (KI), which blocks the uptake of radioactive iodine (^{131}I) by the thyroid. KI is most effective if taken within the first hour after exposure and is still effective 6 h after exposure. The effectiveness subsequently declines until 24 h after exposure; however, it is recommended that KI be taken up to 48 h postexposure. The KI dose is based on age, predicted thyroid exposure, and pregnancy and lactation status. Adults between the ages of 18–40 should receive 130 mg/d for 7–14 days if exposed to ≥10 cGy of radioactive iodine. Other thyroid-blocking agents include prophylthiouracil, 100 mg tid for 8 days, or methimazole, 10 mg tid for 2 days followed by 5 mg tid for 6 days, but they are somewhat less effective.

Diluting agents decrease the absorption of the radionuclide; for example, water may be used as a diluting agent in the treatment for tritium (^{3}H) contamination. The recommended amount is 3–4 L/d for at least 3 weeks.

Mobilizing agents are most effective when given immediately; however, they may be effective for up to 2 weeks after exposure. These include antithyroid drugs, parathyroid extract, glucocorticoids, ammonium chloride, diuretics, expectorants, and inhalants. All of them should induce the release of radionuclides from tissues.

Chelating agents can bind many radioactive materials, after which the complexes are excreted from the human body. In this regard, diethylenetriaminepentaacetic acid (DTPA) either as Ca-DTPA or Zn-DTPA is superior to ethylenediamine tetraacetic acid (EDTA); it was approved by the U.S. Food and Drug Administration (FDA) to treat internal contamination with plutonium, americium and curium, but it also chelates berkelium, californium, or any material with an atomic number >92. Ca-DTPA is more effective than Zn-DTPA during the first 24 h after internal contamination, and both drugs are equally effective after the initial 24 h. If both drugs are available, then Ca-DTPA should be given as the first dose. If additional treatment is needed, treatment should be switched to Zn-DTPA. The dose is 1 g Ca-DTPA or Zn-DTPA, dissolved in 250 mL of normal saline or 5% glucose, given IV over 1 h daily. The duration of chelation treatment depends on the amount of internal contamination and individual response to treatment. DTPA can also be administrated by nebulized inhalation; 1 g is given in 1:1 dilution with water or saline over 15–20 min. Nebulized Zn-DTPA is recommended if the internal contamination is only by inhalation. The IV route is recommended and should be used if the route of internal contamination

TABLE 216-2 COMMON DRUGS^a FOR TREATMENT OF INTERNAL CONTAMINATION

Medication	Administered for Radionuclides	Route of Administration	Dosage	Duration	Mechanism of Action
KI	Iodine-131	PO	130 mg/d for adults >40 with thyroid exposure >500 cGy 130 mg/d for adults 18–40 with thyroid exposure >10 cGy 130 mg/d for pregnant or lactating women with thyroid exposure >5 cGy 65 mg/d for children and adolescents 3–18 with thyroid exposure >5 cGy 32.5 mg/d for infants 1 month to 3 years with thyroid exposure >5 cGy 16 mg/d for neonates from birth to 1 month with thyroid exposure >5 cGy	7–14 days	Blocking agent
Zn-DTPA	Plutonium, trans-plutonium, yttrium, americium, curium	IV	1 g in 250 mL NS or 5% glucose, given in 1–2 h, *or* bolus over 3–4 min	Up to 5 days	Chelating agent
		Inhalation	1 g in 1:1 dilution with water or NS over 15–20 min		
		IM	1 g; not recommended because of pain		
Ca-DTPA	Plutonium, *trans*-plutonium, yttrium, americium, curium	IV	1 g in 250 mL NS or 5% glucose, given in 1–2 h, *or* bolus over 3–4 min	Up to 5 days	Chelating agent
		Inhalation	1 g in 1:1 dilution with water or NS over 15–20 min		
		IM	1 g; not recommended because of pain		
Bicarbonate	Uranium	IV	2 ampules sodium bicarbonate (44.3 meq each, 7.5%) in 1000 mL NS, 125 mL/L, *or* 1 ampule of sodium bicarbonate (44.3 meq, 7.5%) in 500 mL NS, 500 mL/h	Usually IV for the first 24 h, PO for additional 2 days; continuation of treatment for >3 days is rare and can be done according to titration of uranium amounts in the body	Increased excretion via the kidneys
		PO	2 tablets every 4 h until urine pH = 7–8, *or* 4 g (8 tablets) 3 tid		
Prussian blue	Cesium-137	PO	1 g tid with 100–200 mL water, up to 10 g/d	≥3 weeks titrated by urine and fecal bioassay and whole-body counting	Ion exchanger
Water	Tritium (H-3)	PO	>3–4 L per day	3 weeks	Excretion of water
Aluminum phosphate gel	Strontium	PO	100 mL immediately after exposure	Once	Decreased gut absorption
Aluminum hydroxide		PO	60–100 mL	Once	Decreased gut absorption

^{a}Excluding KI, these drugs have not been approved for this purpose by the U.S. Food and Drug Administration at the time of publication.

Note: NS, normal saline.

is not known or if multiple routes of internal contamination are likely. Treating uranium contamination with DTPA is contraindicated, due to its synergistic damage to the kidneys.

Lung lavage can reduce radiation-induced pneumonitis and is indicated only when a large amount of radionuclide enters the lungs and has the potential for acute radiation injury. The procedure requires anesthesia. **Table 216-2** summarizes the common treatment regimens for internal radionuclide contamination.

MEDICAL ASSAY OF THE RADIATION-EXPOSED PATIENT

One of the major difficulties in treating victims exposed to radiation is the determination of the amount of exposure. Clinical assessment of the patient is the best approach. Appearance of an early prodrome indicates high exposure to radiation. Victims who arrive at the hospital complaining of severe weakness, nausea, vomiting, diarrhea, or seizures probably will not survive despite support measures. Decontamination and the use of radiation-detection equipment are both very important. Few tests can be performed in order to estimate the radiation exposure and the contamination. Baseline laboratory tests should include a complete blood count with differential and platelet count, renal evaluation, and determination of electrolytes. Urine and stool samples should be obtained if internal contamination is suspected. Nasal swabs should be taken from each nostril for determination of inhalation of radionuclides. After exhalation, each swab is labeled and sealed in a plastic bag and sent for analysis to appropriate laboratories. Patients exposed to 0.7–4 Gy will develop pancytopenia from as early as 10 days to as long 8 weeks postexposure. Lymphocytes show the most rapid decline, while other leukocytes and platelets decline less rapidly. Erythrocytes are the least vulnerable blood elements.

Absolute lymphocyte counts should be taken every 4–6 h for 5–6 days; they are the most valuable early indicator because they are recognized to be a sensitive marker for radiation damage and correlate with both the exposure and prognosis. A 50% drop in absolute lymphocyte count within the first 24 h indicates a signficant injury. HLA typing is necessary whenever there is suspicion of irreversible bone marrow damage. Lymphocyte chromosomal analysis can detect radiation exposure as low as 0.03–0.06 Gy, and 15 mL of blood should be drawn as early as possible in a heparinized collection tube and kept cool. Radiation-induced chromosomal aberrations in peripheral blood lymphocytes include dicentric chromosomes and ring forms that last for a few weeks. By calibrating a dose-response curve, the radiation dose can be assessed.

Another method for estimating exposure is the micronucleus (MN/Mni) scoring, which is simple and fast but still empirical. An algorithm for the treatment of radiation casualties is shown in **Fig. 216-3**.

FOLLOW-UP

It is desirable to continue follow-up in some circumstances. In general, only persons who are exposed to <8–10 Gy whole-body irradiation have a chance to survive long term, and they are at risk of developing cataracts; sterility; and lung, kidney, and bone marrow problems. Based on their age, gender, and amount and type of exposure, they should be followed for many years. A major public health issue is the risk of secondary malignancy in individuals and populations who were exposed to low doses of radiation. Leukemia, breast, brain, thyroid, and lung cancer are the most common, but the ex-

posed population is at increased risk for many other cancers as well. Appropriate follow-up protocols should be developed based on the type of exposure and the exposed population. In cases of internal contamination, the long-term follow-up should be focused on the organ at risk. Such is the case with uranium contamination, with its nephrotoxic properties.

FURTHER READINGS

DAINIAK N: Hematologic consequences of exposure to ionizing radiation. Exp Hematol 30:513, 2002

GUIDANCE FOR RADIATION ACCIDENT MANAGEMENT, OAK RIDGE–ASSOCIATED UNIVERSITIES: *http://www.orau.gov/reacts/guidance.htm*, updated 03/22/2002

JARRETT D et al (eds): *Medical Management of Radiation Casualties: Handbook.* AFRRI special publication 99-2. Bethesda, MD, Armed Forces Radiobiology Research Institute, 1999 (also available at *http://www.afrri.usuhs.mil.*)

Management of Terrorist Events Involving Radioactive Material. NCRP report no. 138. Bethesda, MD, National Council on Radiation Protection, 2001

METTLER FA JR, VOELZ GL: Major radiation exposure—what to expect and how to respond. N Engl J Med 346:1554, 2002

MOULDER JE: Report on an interagency workshop on the radiobiology of nuclear terrorism. Molecular and Cellular Biology of Moderate Dose (1–10 Sv) Radiation and Potential Mechanisms of Radiation Protection (Bethesda, MD, December 17–18, 2001). Radiat Res 158: 118, 2002

FIGURE 216-3 General guidelines for treatment of radiation casualties. CBC, complete blood count.

217   Basic Biology of the Cardiovascular System

Joseph Loscalzo, Peter Libby, Eugene Braunwald

THE BLOOD VESSEL

VASCULAR ULTRASTRUCTURE

Blood vessels participate in homeostasis on a moment-to-moment basis and contribute to the pathophysiology of diseases of virtually every organ system. Hence, an understanding of the fundamentals of vascular biology furnishes a foundation for understanding normal function of all organ systems and many diseases. The smallest blood vessels, capillaries, consist of a monolayer of endothelial cells in close juxtaposition with occasional smooth-muscle–like cells known as *pericytes* (Fig. 217-1A). Unlike larger vessels, pericytes do not invest the entire microvessel to form a continuous sheath. Veins and arteries typically have a trilaminar structure (Fig. 217-1B–E). The *intima* consists of a monolayer of endothelial cells continuous with those of the capillary trees. The middle layer, or *tunica media*, consists of layers of smooth-muscle cells; in veins, this layer can contain just a few layers of smooth-muscle cells (Fig. 217-1B). The outer layer, the *adventitia*, consists of looser extracellular matrix with occasional fibroblasts, mast cells, and nerve terminals. Larger arteries have their own vasculature, the *vasa vasorum*, which nourish the outer aspects of the tunica media. The adventitia of many veins surpasses the intima in thickness.

The tone of muscular arterioles regulates blood pressure and flow through various arterial beds. These smaller arteries have relatively thick tunica media in relation to the adventitia (Fig. 217-1C). Medium-size muscular arteries likewise contain a prominent tunica media (Fig. 217-1D). Atherosclerosis commonly affects this type of muscular artery. The larger elastic arteries have a much more structured tunica media consisting of concentric bands of smooth-muscle cells interspersed with strata of elastin-rich extracellular matrix sandwiched between continuous layers of smooth-muscle cells (Fig. 217-1E). Larger arteries have a clearly demarcated internal elastic lamina that forms the barrier between the intima and media. An external elastic lamina demarcates the media of arteries from the surrounding adventitia.

ORIGIN OF VASCULAR CELLS

The intima in human arteries often contains occasional resident smooth-muscle cells beneath the monolayer of vascular endothelial cells. The embryonic origin of smooth-muscle cells in various types of artery differs. Some upper-body arterial smooth-muscle cells derive from the neural crest, whereas lower body arteries generally recruit smooth-muscle cells during development from neighboring mesodermal structures, such as the somites. Recent evidence suggests that the bone marrow may give rise to both vascular endothelial cells and smooth-muscle cells, particularly under conditions of repair of injury or vascular lesion formation. Indeed, the ability of bone marrow to repair an injured endothelial monolayer may contribute to maintenance of vascular health and may promote arterial disease when this reparative mechanism fails due to injurious stimuli or age. The precise sources of endothelial and mesenchymal progenitor cells or their stem cell precursors remain the subject of active investigation (Chaps. 66–68).

VASCULAR CELL BIOLOGY

Endothelial Cell   The key cell of the vascular intima, the endothelial cell, has manifold functions in health and disease. Most obviously, the endothelium forms the interface between tissues and the blood compartment. It must, therefore, regulate the entry of molecules and cells into tissues in a selective manner. The ability of endothelial cells to serve as a permselective barrier fails in many vascular disorders, including atherosclerosis and hypertension. This dysregulation of permselectivity also occurs in pulmonary edema and other situations of "capillary leak."

The endothelium also participates in the local regulation of blood flow and vascular caliber. Endogenous substances produced by endothelial cells, such as prostacyclin, endothelium-derived hyperpolarizing factor, and nitric oxide (NO), provide tonic vasodilatory stimuli under physiologic conditions in vivo (Table 217-1). Impaired production or excess catabolism of NO impairs this endothelium-dependent vasodilator function and may contribute to excessive vasoconstriction under various pathologic situations. By contrast, endothelial cells also produce potent vasoconstrictor substances such as endothelin in a regulated fashion. Excessive production of reactive oxygen species, such as superoxide anion (O_2^-), by endothelial or smooth-muscle cells under pathologic conditions (e.g., excessive exposure to angiotensin II) can promote local oxidative stress and inactivate NO.

The endothelial monolayer contributes critically to inflammatory processes involved in normal host defenses and pathologic states. The normal endothelium resists prolonged contact with blood leukocytes; however, when activated by bacterial products, such as endotoxin or proinflammatory cytokines released during infection or injury, endothelial cells express an array of leukocyte adhesion molecules that bind various classes of leukocytes. The endothelial cells appear to recruit selectively different classes of leukocytes under different pathologic conditions. The gamut of adhesion molecules and chemokines generated during acute bacterial processes tends to recruit granulocytes. In chronic inflammatory diseases, such as tuberculosis or atherosclerosis, endothelial cells express adhesion molecules that favor the recruitment of mononuclear leukocytes that characteristically accumulate in these conditions.

The endothelial monolayer also dynamically regulates thrombosis and hemostasis. NO, in addition to its vasodilatory properties, can limit platelet activation and aggregation. Like NO, prostacyclin produced by endothelial cells under normal conditions not only provides a vasodilatory stimulus but also antagonizes platelet activation and aggregation. Thrombomodulin expressed on the surface of endothelial cells binds thrombin at low concentrations and inhibits coagulation through activation of the protein C pathway, leading to enhanced catabolism of clotting factors Va and VIIIa, thereby combating thrombus formation. The surface of endothelial cells contains heparan sulfate glycosaminoglycans that furnish an endogenous antithrombin coating to the vasculature. Endothelial cells also participate actively in fibrinolysis and its regulation. They express receptors for plasminogen activators and produce tissue-type plasminogen activator. Through local generation of plasmin, the normal endothelial monolayer can promote the lysis of nascent thrombi.

When activated by inflammatory cytokines—bacterial endotoxin, or angiotensin II, for example—endothelial cells can produce substantial quantities of the major inhibitor of fibrinolysis, plasminogen activator inhibitor 1 (PAI-1). Thus, under pathologic circumstances, the endothelial cell may promote local thrombus accumulation rather than combat it. Inflammatory stimuli also induce the expression of the potent procoagulant tissue factor, a contributor to disseminated intravascular coagulation in sepsis.

Endothelial cells also participate in the pathophysiology of a number of immune-mediated diseases. Lysis of endothelial cells mediated by complement provides an example of immunologically mediated tissue

FIGURE 217-1 Schematics of the structures of various types of blood vessels. A. Capillaries consist of an endothelial tube in contact with a discontinuous population of pericytes. **B.** Veins typically have thin medias and thicker adventitias. **C.** A small muscular artery consists of a prominent tunica media. **D.** Larger muscular arteries have a prominent media with smooth-muscle cells embedded in a complex extracellular matrix. **E.** Larger elastic arteries have circular layers of elastic tissue alternating with concentric rings of smooth-muscle cells.

injury. Presentation of foreign histocompatibility complex antigens by endothelial cells in solid organ allografts can trigger immunologic rejection. In addition, immune-mediated endothelial injury may contribute in some patients with thrombotic thrombocytopenic purpura and in patients with hemolytic uremic syndrome. Thus, in addition to contributing to innate immune responses, endothelial cells participate actively in both humoral and cellular limbs of the immune response.

Endothelial cells can also regulate growth of the subjacent smooth-muscle cells. Heparan sulfate glycosaminoglycans elaborated by endothelial cells can hold smooth-muscle proliferation in check. In contrast, when exposed to various injurious stimuli, endothelial cells can elaborate growth factors and chemoattractants, such as platelet-derived growth factor, that can promote the migration and proliferation of vascular smooth-muscle cells. Dysregulated elaboration of these growth-stimulatory molecules may promote smooth-muscle accumulation in arterial hyperplastic diseases, including atherosclerosis and in-stent stenosis.

Clinical Assessment of Endothelial Function Endothelial function can be assessed noninvasively and invasively, and typically involves evaluating one measure of endothelial behavior in vivo, viz., endothelium-dependent vasodilation. Using either pharmacologic or mechanical agonists, the endothelium is stimulated to release acutely molecular effectors that alter underlying smooth-muscle cell tone. Invasively, endothelial function can be assessed with the use of agonists that

stimulate release of endothelial NO, such as the cholinergic agonists acetylcholine and methacholine. The typical approach involves measuring quantitatively the change in coronary diameter in response to an intracoronary infusion of these short-lived, rapidly acting agents. Noninvasively, endothelial function can be assessed in the forearm circulation by performing occlusion of brachial artery blood flow with a blood pressure cuff, after which the cuff is deflated and the change in brachial artery blood flow and diameter are measured ultrasonographically (Fig. 217-2). This approach depends upon shear stress-dependent changes in endothelial release of NO following restoration of blood flow, as well as the effect of adenosine released (transiently) from ischemic tissue in the forearm.

Typically, the change in vessel diameter detected by these invasive and noninvasive approaches is ~10%. In individuals with frank atherosclerosis or risk factors for atherosclerosis (especially hypertension, hypercholesterolemia, diabetes mellitus, and smoking), such studies can detect endothelial dysfunction as defined by a smaller change in diameter and, in the extreme case, a so-called paradoxical vasoconstrictor response owing to the direct effect of cholinergic agonists on vascular smooth-muscle cell tone.

VASCULAR SMOOTH-MUSCLE CELL

The vascular smooth-muscle cell, the major cell type of the media layer of blood vessels, also actively contributes to vascular pathobiology. Contraction and relaxation of smooth-muscle cells at the level of the muscular arteries controls blood pressure and, hence, regional blood flow and the afterload experienced by the left ventricle (see below). The vasomotor tone of veins, governed by smooth-muscle cell tone, regulates the capacitance of the venous tree and influences the preload experienced by both ventricles. Smooth-muscle cells in the adult vessel seldom replicate. This homeostatic quiescence of smooth-muscle cells changes under conditions of arterial injury or inflammatory activation. Proliferation and migration of arterial smooth-muscle cells can contribute to the development of arterial stenoses in atherosclerosis, of arteriolar remodeling that can sustain and propagate hypertension, and of the hyperplastic response of arteries injured by angioplasty or stent deployment. In the pulmonary circulation, smooth-muscle migration and proliferation contribute decisively to the pulmonary vascular disease that gradually occurs in response to sustained high-flow states, such as left-to-right shunts. Such pulmonary vascular disease provides a major obstacle to the management of many patients with adult congenital heart disease.

Smooth-muscle cells also secrete the bulk of vascular extracellular matrix. Excessive production of collagen and glycosaminoglycans contributes to the remodeling and altered biology and biomechanics of arteries affected by hypertension or atherosclerosis. In larger elastic arteries, the elastin synthesized by smooth-muscle cells serves to maintain not only normal arterial structure but also hemodynamic function. The ability of the larger arteries, such as the aorta, to store the kinetic energy of systole promotes tissue perfusion during diastole. Arterial stiffness associated with aging or disease, as manifested by a widening pulse pressure, increases left ventricular afterload and portends a poor prognosis.

Like endothelial cells, vascular smooth-muscle cells do not merely respond to vasomotor or inflammatory stimuli elaborated by other

TABLE 217-1 ENDOTHELIAL FUNCTIONS IN HEALTH AND DISEASE	
Homeostatic Phenotype	**Dysfunctional Phenotype**
Vasodilatation	Impaired dilatation, vasoconstriction
Antithrombotic, profibrinolytic	Prothrombotic, antifibrinolytic
Anti-inflammatory	Pro-inflammatory
Antiproliferative	Proproliferative
Antioxidant	Prooxidant

FIGURE 217-2 Assessment of endothelial function in vivo using blood pressure cuff-occlusion and release. Upon deflation of the cuff, changes in diameter (**A**) and blood flow (**B**) of the brachial artery are monitored with an ultrasound probe (**C**). *(Reproduced with permission of J. Vita, MD.)*

cell types but can themselves serve as a source of such stimuli. For example, when stimulated by bacterial endotoxin, smooth-muscle cells can elaborate large quantities of proinflammatory cytokines, such as interleukin 6, as well as lesser quantities of many other proinflammatory mediators. Like endothelial cells, upon inflammatory activation, arterial smooth-muscle cells can produce prothrombotic mediators, such as tissue factor, the antifibrinolytic protein PAI-1, and other molecules that modulate thrombosis and fibrinolysis. Smooth-muscle

cells may also elaborate autocrine growth factors that can amplify hyperplastic responses to arterial injury.

Vascular Smooth-Muscle Cell Function A principal function of vascular smooth-muscle cells is to maintain vessel tone. Vascular smooth-muscle cells contract when stimulated by a rise in intracellular calcium concentration by calcium influx through the plasma membrane and by calcium release from intracellular stores (Fig. 217-3). In vascular smooth-muscle cells, voltage-dependent L-type calcium channels open with membrane depolarization, which is regulated by energy-dependent ion pumps such as the Na^+,K^+-ATPase and ion channels such as the Ca^{2+}-sensitive K^+ channel. Local changes in intracellular calcium concentration, termed *calcium sparks*, result from the influx of calcium through the voltage-dependent calcium channel and are caused by the coordinated activation of a cluster of ryanodine-sensitive calcium release channels in the sarcoplasmic reticulum (see below). Calcium sparks lead to a further direct increase in intracellular calcium concentration and indirectly increase intracellular calcium concentration by activating chloride channels. In addition, calcium sparks reduce contractility by activating large-conductance calcium-sensitive K^+ channels, hyperpolarizing the cell membrane and thereby limiting further voltage-dependent increases in intracellular calcium.

Biochemical agonists also increase intracellular calcium concentration, doing so by receptor-dependent activation of phospholipase C with hydrolysis of phosphatidylinositol 4,5-bisphosphate with generation of diacylglycerol (DAG) and inositol 1,4,5-trisphosphate (IP_3). These membrane lipid derivatives, in turn, activate protein kinase C and increase intracellular calcium concentration. In addition, IP_3 binds to its specific receptor found in the sarcoplasmic reticulum membrane to increase calcium efflux from this calcium storage pool into the cytoplasm.

Vascular smooth-muscle cell contraction is principally controlled by the phosphorylation of myosin light chain, which, in the steady state, depends on the balance between the actions of myosin light chain kinase and myosin light chain phosphatase. Myosin light chain kinase is activated by calcium through the formation of a calcium-calmodulin complex; with phosphorylation of myosin light chain by this kinase, the myosin ATPase activity is increased and contraction sustained. Myosin light chain phosphatase dephosphorylates myosin light chain, reducing myosin ATPase activity and contractile force. Phosphorylation of the myosin binding subunit (thr695) of myosin light chain phosphatase by Rho kinase inhibits phosphatase activity and induces calcium sensitization of the contractile apparatus. Rho kinase is itself activated by the small GTPase RhoA, which is stimulated by guanosine exchange factors and inhibited by GTPase-activating proteins.

Both cyclic AMP and cyclic GMP relax vascular smooth-muscle cells, doing so by complex mechanisms. β-Agonists acting through their G-protein-coupled receptors activate adenylyl cyclase to convert ATP to cyclic AMP; NO and atrial natriuretic peptide acting directly and via a G-protein-coupled receptor, respectively, activate guanylyl cyclase to convert GTP to cyclic GMP. These agents, in turn, activate protein kinase A and protein kinase G, respectively, which inactivates myosin light chain kinase and decreases vascular smooth-muscle cell tone. In addition, protein kinase G can directly interact with the myosin-binding substrate subunit of myosin light chain phosphatase, increasing phosphatase activity and decreasing vascular tone. Lastly, several mechanisms drive NO-dependent, protein kinase G–mediated reductions in vascular smooth-muscle cell calcium concentration, including phosphorylation-dependent inactivation of RhoA; decreased IP_3 formation; phosphorylation of the IP_3 receptor–associated cyclic GMP kinase substrate, with subsequent inhibition of IP_3 receptor function; phosphorylation of phospholamban, which increases calcium ATPase activity and sequestration of calcium in the sarcoplasmic reticulum; and protein kinase G–dependent stimulation of plasma membrane calcium ATPase activity, perhaps by activation of the Na^+,K^+-ATPase or hyperpolarization of the cell membrane by activation of calcium-dependent K^+ channels.

FIGURE 217-3 Regulation of vascular smooth-muscle cell calcium concentration and actomyosin ATPase-dependent contraction. NE, norepinephrine; ET-1, endothelin-1; AngII, angiotensin II; PIP$_2$, phosphatidylinositol 4,5-biphosphate; PLC, phospholipase C; DAG, diacylglycerol; G, G-protein; VDCC, voltage-dependent calcium channel; IP$_3$, inositol 1,4,5-trisphosphate; PKC, protein kinase C; SR, sarcoplasmic reticulum; NO, nitric oxide; ANP, antrial natriuretic peptide; pGC, particular guanylyl cyclase; AC, adenylyl cyclase; sGC, soluble guanylyl cyclase; PKG, protein kinase G; PKA, protein kinase A; MLCK, myosin light chain kinase; MLCP, myosin light chain phosphatase. (Modified from B Berk, in Vascular Medicine, 3d ed, p 23. Philadelphia, Saunders, Elsevier, 2006; with permission.)

Control of Vascular Smooth-Muscle Cell Tone Vascular smooth-muscle cell tone is governed by the autonomic nervous system and by the endothelium in tightly regulated control networks. Autonomic neurons enter the blood vessel media from the adventitia and modulate vascular smooth-muscle cell tone in response to baroreceptors and chemoreceptors within the aortic arch and carotid bodies, and in response to thermoreceptors in the skin. These regulatory components comprise rapidly acting reflex arcs modulated by central inputs that respond to sensory inputs (olfactory, visual, auditory, and tactile) as well as emotional stimuli. Autonomic regulation of vascular tone is mediated by three classes of nerves: *sympathetic*, whose principal neurotransmitters are epinephrine and norepinephrine; *parasympathetic*, whose principal neurotransmitter is acetylcholine; and *nonadrenergic/noncholinergic*, which include two subgroups—nitrergic, whose principal neurotransmitter is NO; and peptidergic, whose principal neurotransmitters are substance P, vasoactive intestinal peptide, calcitonin gene-related peptide, and ATP.

Each of these neurotransmitters acts through specific receptors on the vascular smooth-muscle cell to modulate intracellular calcium and, consequently, contractile tone. Norepinephrine activates α receptors and epinephrine activates α and β receptors (adrenergic receptors); in most blood vessels, norepinephrine activates postjunctional α_1 receptors in large arteries, and α_2 receptors in small arteries and arterioles, leading to vasoconstriction. Most blood vessels express β_2 adrenergic receptors on their vascular smooth-muscle cells and respond to β agonists by cyclic AMP–dependent relaxation. Acetylcholine released from parasympathetic neurons binds to muscarinic receptors (of which there are five subtypes, M_{1-5}) on vascular smooth-muscle cells to yield vasorelaxation. In addition, NO stimulates presynaptic neurons to release acetylcholine, which can stimulate release of NO from the endothelium. Nitrergic neurons release NO produced by neuronal NO synthase,

which causes vascular smooth-muscle cell relaxation via the cyclic GMP–dependent and –independent mechanisms described above. The peptidergic neurotransmitters all potently vasodilate, acting either directly or through endothelium-dependent NO release to decrease vascular smooth-muscle cell tone. The detailed molecular physiology of the autonomic nervous system is provided in Chap. 370.

The endothelium modulates vascular smooth-muscle tone by the direct release of several effectors, including NO, prostacyclin, and endothelium-derived hyperpolarizing factor, all of which cause vasorelaxation; and endothelin, which causes vasoconstriction. The release of these endothelial effectors of vascular smooth-muscle cell tone is stimulated by mechanical (shear stress, cyclic strain, etc.) and biochemical mediators (purinergic agonists, muscarinic agonists, peptidergic agonists), with the biochemical mediators acting through endothelial receptors specific to each class.

In addition to these local, paracrine modulators of vascular smooth-muscle cell tone, circulating mediators can also affect tone, including norepinephrine and epinephrine, vasopressin, angiotensin II, bradykinin, and the natriuretic peptides (ANP, BNP, CNP, and DNP), as discussed above.

VASCULAR REGENERATION

Growing new blood vessels can occur in response to such conditions as chronic hypoxia or tissue ischemia. Growth factors, including vascular endothelial growth factor, activate a signaling cascade that stimulates endothelial proliferation and tube formation, defined as *angiogenesis*. The development of collateral vascular networks in the ischemic myocardium reflects this process and can result from selective activation of endothelial progenitor cells, which may reside in the blood vessel wall or home to the ischemic tissue subtended by an occluded or severely stenotic vessel from the bone marrow. True arterio-

TABLE 217-2 GENETIC POLYMORPHISMS IN VASCULAR FUNCTION AND DISEASE RISK

Gene	Polymorphic Allele	Clinical Implications
α-adrenergic receptors		
α-1A	Arg492Cys	None
α-2B	Glu9/G1712	Increased CHD events
α-2C	A2cDcl3232-325	Ethnic differences in risk of hypertension or heart failure
Angiotensin-converting enzyme (ACE)	Insertion/deletion polymorphism in intron 16	D allele or DD genotype–increased response to ACE inhibitors; inconsistent data for increased risk of atherosclerotic heart disease, and hypertension
Ang II type I receptor	1166A → C Ala-Cys	Increased response to Ang II and increased risk of pregnancy-associated hypertension
β-Adrenergic receptors		
β-1		
	Ser49Gly	Increased HR and DCM risk
	Arg389Gly	Increased heart failure in blacks
β-2		
	Arg16Gly	Familial hypertension, increased obesity risk
	Glu27Gln	Hypertension in white type II diabetics
	Thr164Ile	Decreased agonist affinity and worse HF outcome
B2-Bradykinin receptor	Cys58Thr, Cys412Gly, Thr21Met	Increased risk of hypertension in some ethnic groups
Endothelial nitric oxide synthase (eNOS)	Nucleotide repeats in introns 4 and 13, Glu298Asp	Increased MI and venous thrombosis
	Thr785Cys	Early coronary artery disease

Note: CHD, coronary heart disease; HR, heart rate; DCM, dilated cardiomyopathy; HF, heart failure; MI, myocardial infarction.
Source: Derived from B Schaefer et al: Heart Dis 5:129, 2003.

genesis, or the development of a new blood vessel comprising all three cell layers, does not normally occur in the cardiovascular system of mammals. Recent insights into the molecular determinants and progenitor cells that can recapitulate blood vessel development de novo is the subject of ongoing and rapidly advancing study (Chaps. 66–68).

VASCULAR PHARMACOGENOMICS

The past decade has witnessed considerable progress in efforts to define genetic differences underlying individual differences in vascular pharmacologic responses. Many investigators have focused on receptors and enzymes associated with neurohumoral modulation of vascular function, as well as hepatic enzymes that metabolize drugs affecting vascular tone. The genetic polymorphisms thus far associated with differences in vascular response often (but not invariably) relate to functional differences in the activity or expression of the receptor or enzyme of interest. Some of these polymorphisms appear to be differentially expressed in specific ethnic groups or by sex. A summary of recently identified polymorphisms defining these vascular pharmacogenomic differences is provided in Table 217-2.

CELLULAR BASIS OF CARDIAC CONTRACTION

THE CARDIAC ULTRASTRUCTURE

About three-fourths of the ventricle is composed of individual striated muscle cells (myocytes), normally 60–140 μm in length and 17–25 μm in diameter (Fig. 217-4A). Each cell contains multiple, rodlike cross-banded strands (myofibrils) that run the length of the cell and are, in turn, composed of serially repeating structures, the sarcomeres. The cytoplasm between the myofibrils contains other cell constituents, including the single centrally located nucleus, numerous mitochondria, and the intracellular membrane system, the sarcoplasmic reticulum.

The *sarcomere*, the structural and functional unit of contraction, lies between two adjacent dark lines, the Z lines. The distance between Z lines varies with the degree of contraction or stretch of the muscle

and ranges between 1.6 and 2.2 μm. Within the confines of the sarcomere are alternating light and dark bands, giving the myocardial fibers their striated appearance under the light microscope. At the center of the sarcomere is a dark band of constant length (1.5 μm), the A band, which is flanked by two lighter bands, the I bands, which are of variable length. The sarcomere of heart muscle, like that of skeletal muscle, consists of two sets of interdigitating myofilaments. Thicker filaments, composed principally of the protein myosin, traverse the A band. They are about 10 nm (100 Å) in diameter, with tapered ends. Thinner filaments, composed primarily of actin, course from the Z line through the I band into the A band. They arc approximately 5 nm (50 Å) in diameter and 1.0 μm in length. Thus, thick and thin filaments overlap only within the (dark) A band, while the (light) I band contains only thin filaments. On electron-microscopic examination, bridges may be seen to extend between the thick and thin filaments within the A band; these comprise myosin heads (see below) bound to actin filaments.

THE CONTRACTILE PROCESS

The sliding filament model for muscle contraction rests on the fundamental observation that both the thick and thin filaments are constant in overall length during both contraction and relaxation. With activation, the actin filaments are propelled further into the A band. In the process, the A band remains constant in length, whereas the I band shortens and the Z lines move toward one another.

The *myosin* molecule is a complex, asymmetric fibrous protein with a molecular mass of about 500,000 Da; it has a rodlike portion that is about 150 nm (1500 Å) in length with a globular portion (head) at its end. These globular portions of myosin form the bridges between the myosin and actin molecules and are the site of ATPase activity. In forming the thick myofilament, which is composed of ~300 longitudinally stacked myosin molecules, the rodlike segments of the myosin molecules are laid down in an orderly, polarized manner, leaving the globular portions projecting outward so that they can interact with actin to generate force and shortening (Fig. 217-4B).

Actin has a molecular mass of about 47,000 Da. The thin filament consists of a double helix of two chains of actin molecules wound about each other on a larger molecule, tropomyosin. A group of regulatory proteins—troponins C, I, and T—are spaced at regular intervals on this filament (Fig. 217-5). In contrast to myosin, actin lacks intrinsic enzymatic activity but does combine reversibly with myosin in the presence of ATP and Ca^{2+}. The calcium ion activates the myosin ATPase, which in turn breaks down ATP, the energy source for contraction (Fig. 217-5). The activity of myosin ATPase determines the rate of forming and breaking of the actomyosin cross-bridges and, ultimately, the velocity of muscle contraction. In relaxed muscle, tropomyosin inhibits this interaction. *Titin* (Fig. 217-4D) is a large, flexible, myofibrillar protein that connects myosin to the Z line. Its stretching contributes to the elasticity of the heart.

During activation of the cardiac myocyte, Ca^{2+} becomes attached to troponin C, which results in a conformational change in the regulatory protein tropomyosin; the latter, in turn, exposes the actin cross-bridge interaction sites (Fig. 217-5). Repetitive interaction between myosin heads and actin filaments is termed *cross-bridge cycling*, which results in sliding of the actin along the myosin filaments, ultimately causing muscle shortening and/or the development of tension. The splitting of ATP then dissociates the myosin cross-bridge from actin. In the presence of

FIGURE 217-4 **A** shows the branching myocytes making up the cardiac myofibers. **B** illustrates the critical role played by the changing [Ca²⁺] in the myocardial cytosol. Ca²⁺ ions are schematically shown as entering through the calcium channel that opens in response to the wave of depolarization that travels along the sarcolemma. These Ca²⁺ ions "trigger" the release of more calcium from the sarcoplasmic reticulum (SR) and thereby initiate a contraction-relaxation cycle. Eventually the small quantity of Ca²⁺ that has entered the cell leaves predominantly through an Na⁺/Ca²⁺ exchanger, with a lesser role for the sarcolemmal Ca²⁺ pump. The varying actin-myosin overlap is shown for (**B**) systole, when [Ca²⁺] is maximal, and (**C**) diastole, when [Ca²⁺] is minimal. **D.** The myosin heads, attached to the thick filaments, interact with the thin actin filaments. *(From LH Opie, Heart Physiology, reprinted with permission. Copyright LH Opie, 2004.)*

ATP (Fig. 217-5), linkages between actin and myosin filaments are made and broken cyclically as long as sufficient Ca²⁺ is present; these linkages cease when [Ca²⁺] falls below a critical level, and the troponin-tropomyosin complex once more prevents interactions between the myosin cross-bridges and actin filaments (Fig. 217-6).

Intracytoplasmic Ca²⁺ is a principal mediator of the inotropic state of the heart. The fundamental action of most agents that stimulate myocardial contractility (positive inotropic stimuli), including the digitalis glycosides and β-adrenergic agonists, is to raise the [Ca²⁺] in the vicinity of the myofilaments, which, in turn, triggers cross-bridge cycling. Increased impulse traffic in the cardiac adrenergic nerves stimulates myocardial contractility as a consequence of the release of norepinephrine from cardiac adrenergic nerve endings. Norepineph-

rine activates myocardial β receptors and, through the G$_s$-stimulated guanine nucleotide binding protein, activates the enzyme adenylyl cyclase, which leads to the formation of the intracellular second messenger cyclic AMP from ATP (Fig. 217-6). Cyclic AMP, in turn, activates protein kinase A (PKA), which phosphorylates the Ca²⁺ channel in the myocardial sarcolemma, thereby enhancing the influx of Ca²⁺ into the myocyte. Other functions of PKA are discussed below.

The *sarcoplasmic reticulum* (SR) (Fig. 217-7) is a complex network of anastomosing intracellular channels that invests the myofibrils. Its longitudinally disposed membrane-lined tubules closely invest the surfaces of individual sarcomeres but have no direct continuity with the outside of the cell. However, closely related to the SR, both structurally and functionally, are the transverse tubules, or T system, formed by tubelike invaginations of the sarcolemma that extend into the myocardial fiber along the Z lines, i.e., the ends of the sarcomeres.

CARDIAC ACTIVATION

In the inactive state, the cardiac cell is electrically polarized, i.e., the interior has a negative charge relative to the outside of the cell, with a transmembrane potential of −80 to −100 mV (Chap. 224). The sarcolemma, which in the resting state is largely impermeable to Na⁺, has a Na⁺- and K⁺-stimulating pump energized by ATP that extrudes Na⁺ from the cell; this pump plays a critical role in establishing the resting potential. Thus, intracellular [K⁺] is relatively high and [Na⁺] is far lower, while, conversely, extracellular [Na⁺] is high and [K⁺] is low. At the same time, in the resting state, extracellular [Ca²⁺] greatly exceeds free intracellular [Ca²⁺].

The four phases of the action potential are illustrated in Fig. 224-1B. During the plateau of the action potential (phase 2), there is a slow inward current through L-type Ca²⁺ channels in the sarcolemma (Fig. 217-7). The depolarizing current not only extends across the surface of the cell but penetrates deeply into the cell by way of the ramifying T tubular system. The absolute quantity of Ca²⁺ that crosses the sarcolemma and T system is relatively small and itself appears to be insufficient to bring about full activation of the contractile apparatus. However, this Ca²⁺ current triggers the release of much larger quantities of Ca²⁺ from the SR, a process termed *Ca²⁺-induced Ca²⁺ release*. The latter is a major determinant of intracytoplasmic [Ca²⁺] and therefore of myocardial contractility.

Ca²⁺ is released from the SR through a Ca²⁺ release channel, a cardiac isoform of the ryanodine receptor (RyR2), which controls intracytoplasmic [Ca²⁺] and, as in vascular smooth-muscle cells, leads to the local changes in intracellular [Ca²⁺] called calcium sparks. A number of regulatory proteins, including *calstabin 2*, inhibit RyR2 and, thereby, the release of Ca²⁺ from the SR. PKA dissociates calstabin from the RyR2, enhancing Ca²⁺ release and, thereby, myocardial contractility. Excessive plasma catecholamine levels and cardiac sympathetic neuronal release of norepinephrine cause hyperphosphorylation of PKA, leading to calstabin 2–depleted RyR2. The latter depletes SR Ca²⁺ stores and, thereby, impairs cardiac contraction, leading to heart failure, and also triggers ventricular arrhythmias.

The Ca²⁺ released from the SR then diffuses toward the myofibrils, where, as already described, it combines with troponin C (Fig. 217-6). By repressing this inhibitor of contraction, Ca²⁺ activates the myofilaments to shorten. During repolarization, the activity of the Ca²⁺ pump in the SR, the SR Ca²⁺ ATPase (SERCA$_{2A}$), reaccumulates Ca²⁺ against a concentration gradient, and the Ca²⁺ is stored in the SR by its attachment to a protein, *calsequestrin*. This reaccumulation of Ca²⁺ is

FIGURE 217-5 Four steps in cardiac muscle contraction and relaxation. In relaxed muscle (**upper left**), ATP bound to the myosin cross-bridge dissociates the thick and thin filaments. **Step 1:** Hydrolysis of myosin-bound ATP by the ATPase site on the myosin head transfers the chemical energy of the nucleotide to the activated cross-bridge (**upper right**). When cytosolic Ca^{2+} concentration is low, as in relaxed muscle, the reaction cannot proceed because tropomyosin and the troponin complex on the thin filament do not allow the active sites on actin to interact with the cross-bridges. Therefore, even though the cross-bridges are energized, they cannot interact with actin. **Step 2:** When Ca^{2+} binding to troponin C has exposed active sites on the thin filament, actin interacts with the myosin cross-bridges to form an active complex (**lower right**) in which the energy derived from ATP is retained in the actin-bound cross-bridge, whose orientation has not yet shifted. **Step 3:** The muscle contracts when ADP dissociates from the cross-bridge. This step leads to the formation of the low-energy rigor complex (**lower left**) in which the chemical energy derived from ATP hydrolysis has been expended to perform mechanical work (the "rowing" motion of the cross-bridge). **Step 4:** The muscle returns to its resting state, and the cycle ends when a new molecule of ATP binds to the rigor complex and dissociates the cross-bridge from the thin filament. This cycle continues until calcium is dissociated from troponin C in the thin filament, which causes the contractile proteins to return to the resting state with the cross-bridge in the energized state. ATP, adenosine triphosphate; ATPase, adenosine triphosphatase; ADP, adenosine disphosphate. [From AM Katz: Heart failure: Cardiac function and dysfunction, in Atlas of Heart Diseases, 3d ed, WS Colucci (ed). Philadelphia, Current Medicine, 2002. Reprinted with permission.]

an energy (ATP) requiring process that lowers the cytoplasmic $[Ca^{2+}]$ to a level that inhibits the actomyosin interaction responsible for contraction and in this manner leads to myocardial relaxation. Also, there is an exchange of Ca^{2+} for Na^+ at the sarcolemma (Fig. 217-7), reducing the cytoplasmic $[Ca^{2+}]$. Cyclic AMP–dependent PKA phosphorylates the SR protein *phospholamban*; the latter, in turn, permits activation of the Ca^{2+} pump, thereby increasing the uptake of Ca^{2+} by the SR, accelerating the rate of relaxation and providing larger quantities of Ca^{2+} in the SR for release by subsequent depolarization, thereby stimulating contraction.

Thus, the combination of the cell membrane, transverse tubules, and SR, with their ability to transmit the action potential and to release and then reaccumulate Ca^{2+}, play a fundamental role in the rhythmic contraction and relaxation of heart muscle. Genetic or pharmacologic alterations of any component, whatever its etiology, can disturb these functions.

CONTROL OF CARDIAC PERFORMANCE AND OUTPUT

The extent of shortening of heart muscle and, therefore, the stroke volume of the ventricle in the intact heart depend on three major influences: (1) the length of the muscle at the onset of contraction, i.e., the preload; (2) the tension that the muscle is called upon to develop during contraction, i.e., the afterload; and (3) the contractili-

ty of the muscle, i.e., the extent and velocity of shortening at any given preload and afterload. The major determinants of preload, afterload, and contractility are shown in Table 217-3.

The Role of Muscle Length (Preload) The preload determines the length of the sarcomeres at the onset of contraction. The length of the sarcomeres associated with the most forceful contraction is ~2.2 μm. At this length, the two sets of myofilaments are configured so as to provide the greatest area for their interaction. The length of the sarcomere also regulates the extent of activation of the contractile system, i.e., its sensitivity to Ca^{2+}. According to this concept, termed *length-dependent activation*, the myofilament sensitivity to Ca^{2+} is also maximal at the optimal sarcomere length.

The relation between the initial length of the muscle fibers and the developed force has prime importance for the function of heart muscle. This relationship forms the basis of Starling's law of the heart, which states that, within limits, the force of ventricular contraction depends on the end-diastolic length of the cardiac muscle; in the intact heart the latter relates closely to the ventricular end-diastolic volume.

Cardiac Performance The ventricular end-diastolic or "filling" pressure is sometimes used as a surrogate for the end-diastolic volume. In isolated heart and heart-lung preparations, the stroke volume varies directly with the end-diastolic fiber length (preload) and inversely with the arterial resistance (afterload), and as the heart fails—i.e., as its contractility declines—it delivers a progressively smaller stroke volume from a normal or even elevated end-diastolic volume. The relation between the ventricular end-diastolic pressure and the stroke work of the ventricle (the ventricular function curve) provides a useful definition of the level of contractility of the heart in the intact organism. An increase in contractility is accompanied by a shift of the ventricular function curve upward and to the left (greater stroke work at any level of ventricular end-diastolic pressure, or lower end-diastolic volume at any level of stroke work), while a shift downward and to the right characterizes depression of contractility (Fig. 217-8).

Ventricular Afterload In the intact heart, as in isolated cardiac muscle, the extent (and velocity) of shortening of ventricular muscle fibers at any level of preload and of myocardial contractility relate inversely to the afterload, i.e., the load that opposes shortening. In the intact heart, the afterload may be defined as the tension developed in the ventricular wall during ejection. Afterload is determined by the aortic pressure as well as by the volume and thickness of the ventricular cavity. Laplace's law indicates that the tension of the myocardial fiber is a function of the product of the intracavitary ventricular pressure and ventricular radius divided by the wall thickness. Therefore, at any given level of aortic pressure, the afterload on a dilated left ventricle is higher than that on a normal-sized ventricle. Conversely, at the same aortic pressure and ventricular diastolic volume, the afterload on a hypertrophied ventricle is lower than of a normal chamber. The aortic pressure, in turn, depends on the peripheral vascular resistance, the physical characteristics of the arterial tree, and the volume of blood it contains at the onset of ejection.

FIGURE 217-6 Signal systems involved in positive intropic and lusitropic (enhanced relaxation) effects of β-adrenergic stimulation. When the β-adrenergic agonist interacts with the β receptor, a series of G protein–mediated changes leads to activation of adenylyl cyclase and formation of cyclic adenosine monophosphate (cAMP). The latter acts via protein kinase A to stimulate metabolism (**left**) and to phosphorylate the Ca^{2+} channel protein (**right**). The result is an enhanced opening probability of the Ca^{2+} channel, thereby increasing the inward movement of Ca^{2+} ions through the sarcolemma (SL) of the T tubule. These Ca^{2+} ions release more calcium from the sarcoplasmic reticulum (SR) to increase cytosolic Ca^{2+} and to activate troponin C. Ca^{2+} ions also increase the rate of breakdown of adenosine triphosphate (ATP) to adenosine diphosphate (ADP) and inorganic phosphate (Pi). Enhanced myosin ATPase activity explains the increased rate of contraction, with increased activation of troponin C explaining increased peak force development. An increased rate of relaxation is explained because cAMP also activates the protein phospholamban, situated on the membrane of the SR, that controls the rate of uptake of calcium into the SR. The latter effect explains enhanced relaxation (lusitropic effect). P, phosphorylation; PL, phospholamban; TnI, troponin I. (*Modified from LH Opie, Heart Physiology, reprinted with permission. Copyright LH Opie, 2004.*)

Ventricular afterload critically regulates cardiovascular performance (**Fig. 217-9**). As already noted, elevations of both preload and contractility increase myocardial fiber shortening, while increases in afterload reduce it. The extent of myocardial fiber shortening and left ventricular size determine stroke volume. An increase in arterial pressure induced by vasoconstriction, for example, augments afterload, which opposes myocardial fiber shortening, reducing stroke volume.

When myocardial contractility becomes impaired and the ventricle dilates, afterload rises (Laplace's law) and limits cardiac output. Increased afterload may also result from neural and humoral stimuli that occur in response to a fall in cardiac output. This increased afterload may reduce

FIGURE 217-7 The Ca^{2+} fluxes and key structures involved in cardiac excitation-contraction coupling. The arrows denote the direction of Ca^{2+} fluxes. The thickness of each arrow indicates the magnitude of the calcium flux. Two Ca^{2+} cycles regulate excitation-contraction coupling and relaxation. The larger cycle is entirely intracellular and involves Ca^{2+} fluxes into and out of the sarcoplasmic reticulum, as well as Ca^{2+} binding to and release from troponin C. The smaller extracellular Ca^{2+} cycle occurs when this cation moves into and out of the cell. The action potential opens plasma membrane Ca^{2+} channels to allow passive entry of Ca^{2+} into the cell from the extracellular fluid (**arrow A**). Only a small portion of the Ca^{2+} that enters the cell directly activates the contractile proteins (**arrow A1**). The extracellular cycle is completed when Ca^{2+} is actively transported back out to the extracellular fluid by way of two plasma membrane fluxes mediated by the sodium-calcium exchanger (**arrow B1**) and the plasma membrane calcium pump (**arrow B2**). In the intracellular Ca^{2+} cycle, passive Ca^{2+} release occurs through channels in the cisternae (**arrow C**) and initiates contraction; active Ca^{2+} uptake by the Ca^{2+} pump of the sarcotubular network (**arrow D**) relaxes the heart. Diffusion of Ca^{2+} within the sarcoplasmic reticulum (**arrow G**) returns this activator cation to the cisternae, where it is stored in a complex with calsequestrin and other calcium-binding proteins. Ca^{2+} released from the sarcoplasmic reticulum initiates systole when it binds to troponin C (**arrow E**). Lowering of cytosolic [Ca^{2+}] by the sarcoplasmic reticulum (SR) cause this ion to dissociate from troponin (**arrow F**) and relaxes the heart. Ca^{2+} may also move between mitochondria and cytoplasm (H). (*Adapted from Katz, with permission.*)

cardiac output further, thereby increasing ventricular volume and initiating a vicious circle, especially in patients with ischemic heart disease and limited myocardial O_2 supply. Treatment with vasodilators has the opposite effect; by reducing afterload, cardiac output rises (Chap. 227).

Under normal circumstances, the various influences acting on cardiac performance enumerated above interact in a complex fashion to maintain cardiac output at a level appropriate to the requirements of the metabolizing tissues (Fig. 217-9); interference with a single mechanism may not influence the cardiac output. For example, a moderate reduction of blood volume or the loss of the atrial contribution to ventricular contraction can ordinarily be sustained without a reduction in the cardiac output at rest. Under these circumstances, other factors, such as increases in the frequency of adrenergic nerve impulses to the

TABLE 217-3 DETERMINANTS OF STROKE VOLUME

I. Ventricular Preload
A. Blood volume
B. Distribution of blood volume
  1. Body position
  2. Intrathoracic pressure
  3. Intrapericardial pressure
  4. Venous tone
  5. Pumping action of skeletal muscles
C. Atrial contraction

II. Ventricular Afterload
A. Systemic vascular resistance
B. Elasticity of arterial tree
C. Arterial blood volume
D. Ventricular wall tension
  1. Ventricular radius
  2. Ventricular wall thickness

III. Myocardial Contractility[a]
A. Intramyocardial $[Ca^{2+}]$ ↑↓
B. Cardiac adrenergic nerve activity ↑↓[b]
C. Circulating catecholamines ↑↓[b]
D. Cardiac rate ↑↓[b]
E. Exogenous inotropic agents ↑
F. Myocardial ischemia ↓
G. Myocardial cell death (necrosis, apoptosis, autophagy) ↓
H. Alterations of sarcomeric and cytoskeletal proteins ↓
  1. Genetic
  2. Hemodynamic overload
I. Myocardial fibrosis ↓
J. Chronic overexpression of neurohormones ↓
K. Ventricular remodeling ↓
L. Chronic and/or excessive myocardial hypertrophy ↓

[a]Arrows indicate directional effects of determinants of contractility.
[b]Contractility rises initially but later becomes depressed.

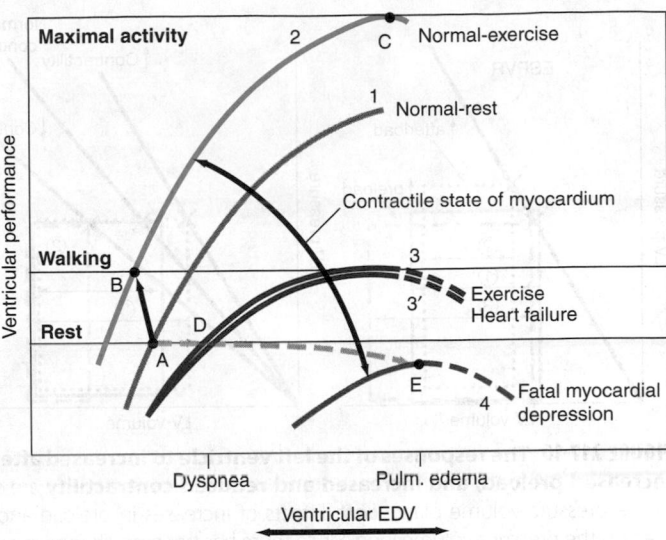

FIGURE 217-8 The interrelations among influences on ventricular end-diastolic volume (EDV) through stretching of the myocardium and the contractile state of the myocardium. Levels of ventricular EDV associated with filling pressures that result in dyspnea and pulmonary edema are shown on the abscissa. Levels of ventricular performance required when the subject is at rest, while walking, and during maximal activity are designated on the ordinate. The broken lines are the descending limbs of the ventricular-performance curves, which are rarely seen during life but show the level of ventricular performance if end-diastolic volume could be elevated to very high levels. For further explanation, see text. [*Modified from WS Colucci and E Braunwald: Pathophysiology of Heart Failure, in Braunwald's Heart Disease, 7th ed, DP Zipes et al (eds). Philadelphia: Elsevier, 2005, pp 509–538.*]

heart, in heart rate, and in venous tone, will serve as compensatory mechanisms and sustain cardiac output in a normal individual.

Exercise The integrated response to exercise illustrates the interactions among the three determinants of stroke volume, i.e., preload, afterload, and contractility (Fig. 217-8). Hyperventilation, the pumping action of the exercising muscles, and venoconstriction during exercise all augment venous return and, hence, ventricular filling and preload (Table 217-3). Simultaneously, the increase in the adrenergic nerve impulse traffic to the myocardium, the increased concentration of circulating catecholamines, and the tachycardia that occur during exercise combine to augment the contractility of the myocardium (Fig. 217-8, curves 1 and 2) and together elevate stroke volume and stroke work, without a change or even a reduction of end-diastolic pressure and volume (Fig. 217-8, points A and B). Vasodilatation occurs in the exercising muscles, thus tending to limit the increase in arterial pressure that would otherwise occur as cardiac output rises to levels as high as five times greater than basal levels during maximal exercise. This vasodilatation ultimately allows the achievement of a greatly elevated cardiac output during exercise, at an arterial pressure only moderately higher than in the resting state.

ASSESSMENT OF CARDIAC FUNCTION

Several techniques can define impaired cardiac function in clinical practice. The cardiac output and stroke volume may be depressed in the presence of heart failure, but, not uncommonly, these variables are within normal limits in this condition. A somewhat more sensitive index of cardiac function is the ejection fraction, i.e., the ratio of stroke volume to end-diastolic volume (normal value = 67 ± 8%), which is frequently depressed in systolic heart failure, even when the stroke volume itself is normal. Alternatively, abnormally elevated ventricular end-diastolic volume (normal value = 75 ± 20 mL/m²) or end-systolic volume (normal value = 25 ± 7 mL/m²) signify impairment of left ventricular systolic function.

Noninvasive techniques, particularly echocardiography as well as radionuclide scintigraphy and cardiac MRI (Chap. 222), have great value in the clinical assessment of myocardial function. They provide mea-

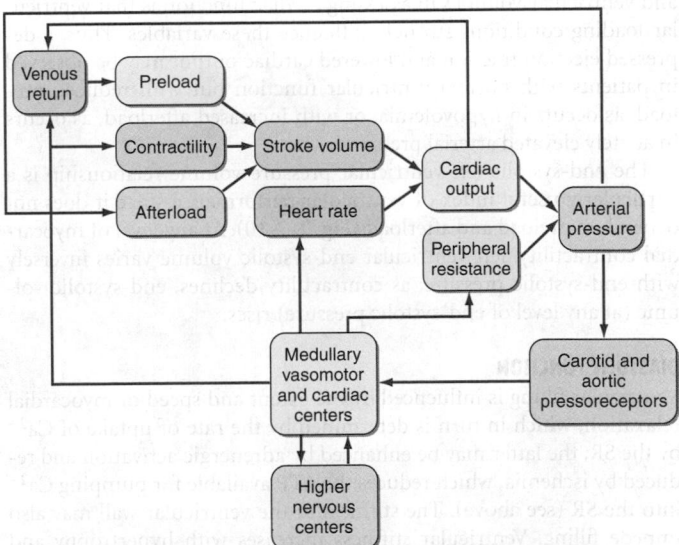

FIGURE 217-9 Interactions in the intact circulation of preload, contractility, and afterload in producing stroke volume. Stroke volume combined with heart rate determines cardiac output, which, when combined with peripheral vascular resistance, determines arterial pressure for tissue perfusion. The characteristics of the arterial system also contribute to afterload, an increase of which reduces stroke volume. The interaction of these components with carotid and aortic arch baroreceptors provides a feedback mechanism to higher medullary and vasomotor cardiac centers and to higher levels in the central nervous system to affect a modulating influence on heart rate, peripheral vascular resistance, venous return, and contractility. [*From MR Starling: Physiology of myocardial contraction, in Atlas of Heart Failure: Cardiac Function and Dysfunction, 3d ed, WS Colucci and E Braunwald (eds). Philadelphia: Current Medicine, 2002, pp 19–35.*]

FIGURE 217-10 The responses of the left ventricle to increased afterload, increased preload, and increased and reduced contractility are shown in the pressure-volume plane. **Left.** Effects of increases in preload and afterload on the pressure-volume loop. Since there has been no change in contractility, ESPVR (the end-systolic pressure volume relation) is unchanged. With an increase in afterload, stroke volume falls (1 → 2); with an increase in preload, stroke volume rises (1 → 3). **Right.** With increased myocardial contractility and constant LV end-diastolic volume, the ESPVR moves to the left of the normal line (lower end-systolic volume at any end-systolic pressure) and stroke volume rises (1 → 3). With reduced myocardial contractility, the ESPVR moves to the right; end-systolic volume is increased and stroke volume falls (1 → 2).

surements of end-diastolic and end-systolic volumes, ejection fraction, and systolic shortening rate, and they allow assessment of ventricular filling (see below) as well as regional contraction and relaxation. The latter measurements are particularly important in ischemic heart disease, as myocardial infarction causes regional myocardial damage.

A limitation of measurements of cardiac output, ejection fraction, and ventricular volumes in assessing cardiac function is that ventricular loading conditions strongly influence these variables. Thus, a depressed ejection fraction and lowered cardiac output may be observed in patients with normal ventricular function but with reduced preload, as occurs in hypovolemia, or with increased afterload, as occurs in acutely elevated arterial pressure.

The end-systolic left ventricular pressure-volume relationship is a particularly useful index of ventricular performance since it does not depend on preload and afterload (Fig. 217-10). At any level of myocardial contractility, left ventricular end-systolic volume varies inversely with end-systolic pressure; as contractility declines, end-systolic volume (at any level of end-systolic pressure) rises.

DIASTOLIC FUNCTION

Ventricular filling is influenced by the extent and speed of myocardial relaxation, which in turn is determined by the rate of uptake of Ca²⁺ by the SR; the latter may be enhanced by adrenergic activation and reduced by ischemia, which reduces the ATP available for pumping Ca²⁺ into the SR (see above). The stiffness of the ventricular wall may also impede filling. Ventricular stiffness increases with hypertrophy and conditions that infiltrate the ventricle, such as amyloid, or by an extrinsic constraint (e.g., pericardial compression) (Fig. 217-11).

Ventricular filling can be assessed by continuously measuring the velocity of flow across the mitral valve using Doppler ultrasound. Normally, the velocity of inflow is more rapid in early diastole than during atrial systole; with mild to moderately impaired relaxation, the rate of early diastolic filling declines, while the rate of presystolic filling rises. With further impairment of filling, the pattern is "pseudo-normalized," and early ventricular filling becomes more rapid as left atrial pressure upstream to the stiff left ventricle rises.

CARDIAC METABOLISM

The heart requires a continuous supply of energy (in the form of ATP) to perform not only its mechanical pumping functions but also to reg-

ulate intracellular and transsarcolemmal ionic movements and concentration gradients. Among its pumping functions, the development of tension, the frequency of contraction, and the level of myocardial contractility are the principal determinants of the heart's substantial energy needs, making its O₂ requirements approximately 15% of that of the entire organism.

Most ATP production depends on the oxidation of substrate [glucose and free fatty acids (FFAs)]. Myocardial FFAs are derived from circulating FFAs, which result principally from lipolysis of adipose tissue, while the myocyte's glucose is obtained from plasma as well as from the cell's breakdown of its glycogen stores (glycogenolysis). There is a reciprocal relation between the utilization of these two principal sources of acetyl CoA in cardiac muscle. Glucose is broken down in the cytoplasm into a three-carbon product, pyruvate, which passes into the mitochondria, where it is metabolized to the two-carbon fragment, acetyl coenzyme A, and undergoes oxidation. FFAs are converted to acyl-CoA in the cytoplasm and acetyl coenzyme A (Co-A) in the mitochondria. Acetyl Co-A enters the citric acid (Krebs) cycle to produce ATP by oxidative phosphorylation within the mitochondria; ATP then enters the cytoplasm from the mitochondrial compartment. Intracellular ADP, resulting from the breakdown of ATP, enhances mitochondrial ATP production.

In the fasted, resting state, circulating FFA concentrations and their myocardial uptake are high, and they are the principal source of acetyl CoA (~70%). In the fed state, with elevations of blood glucose and insulin, glucose oxidation increases and FFA oxidation subsides. Increased cardiac work, the administration of inotropic agents, hypoxia, and mild ischemia all enhance myocardial glucose uptake, glucose production resulting from glycogenolysis, and glucose metabolism to pyruvate (glycolysis). By contrast, β-adrenergic stimulation, as occurs during stress, raises the circulating levels and metabolism of FFAs in favor of glucose. Severe ischemia inhibits the cytoplasmic enzyme pyruvate dehydrogenase, and despite both glycogen and glucose breakdown, glucose is metabolized only to lactic acid (anaerobic glycolysis), which does not enter the citric acid cycle. Anaerobic glycolysis produces much less ATP than aerobic glucose metabolism, in which glucose is metabolized to pyruvate and subsequently

FIGURE 217-11 Mechanisms that cause diastolic dysfunction reflected in the pressure-volume relation. The bottom half of the pressure-volume loop is depicted. Solid lines represent normal subjects; broken lines represent patients with diastolic dysfunction. *(From JD Carroll et al: The differential effects of positive inotropic and vasodilator therapy on diastolic properties in patients with congestive cardiomyopathy. Circulation 74:815, 1986; with permission.)*

oxidized to CO_2. High concentrations of circulating FFAs, which can occur when adrenergic stimulation is superimposed on severe ischemia, reduce oxidative phosphorylation and also cause ATP wastage; the myocardial content of ATP declines, and myocardial contraction becomes impaired. In addition, products of FFA breakdown can exert toxic effects on cardiac cell membranes and may be arrhythmogenic.

Myocardial energy is stored as creatine phosphate (CP), which is in equilibrium with ATP, the immediate source of energy. In states of reduced energy availability, the CP stores decline first. Cardiac hypertrophy, fibrosis, tachycardia, increased wall tension resulting from ventricular dilatation, and increased intracytoplasmic [Ca^{2+}] all contribute to increased myocardial energy needs. When coupled with reduced coronary flow reserve, as occurs with obstruction of coronary arteries or abnormalities of the coronary microcirculation, an imbalance in myocardial ATP production relative to demand may occur, and the resulting ischemia can worsen or cause heart failure.

REGENERATING CARDIAC TISSUE

Until very recently, the mammalian myocardium was viewed as an end-differentiated organ without regeneration potential. Resident and bone marrow–derived stem cells have now been identified, are currently being evaluated as sources of regenerative potential for the heart, and offer the exciting possibility of reconstructing an infarcted or failing ventricle (Chaps. 66, 67).

FURTHER READINGS

COLUCCI WS, BRAUNWALD E (eds): *Atlas of Heart Failure: Cardiac Function and Dysfunction*, 4th ed. Philadelphia, Current Medicine, 2004

DEANFIELD JE et al: Endothelial function and dysfunction: Testing and clinical relevance. Circulation 115:1285, 2007

KATZ AM: *Physiology of the Heart*, 4th ed. Philadelphia, Lippincott Williams and Wilkins, 2005

LIBBY P et al: The vascular endothelium and atherosclerosis, in *The Handbook of Experimental Pharmacology*, S Moncada and EA Higgs (eds). Berlin-Heidelberg, Springer-Verlag, 2006

MAHONEY WM, SCHWARTZ SM: Defining smooth muscle cells and smooth muscle cell injury. J Clin Invest 15:221, 2005

OPIE LH: *Heart Physiology: From Cell to Circulation*, 4th ed. Philadelphia, Lippincott, Williams and Wilkins, 2004

———: Mechanisms of cardiac contraction and relaxation, in *Braunwald's Heart Disease*, 8th ed, P Libby et al (eds). Philadelphia, Elsevier, 2008

WEHRENS XH et al: Intracellular calcium release and cardiac disease. Annu Rev Physiol 67:69, 2005

218 Epidemiology of Cardiovascular Disease

Thomas A. Gaziano, J. Michael Gaziano

Cardiovascular disease (CVD) is now the most common cause of death worldwide. Before 1900, infectious diseases and malnutrition were the most common causes of death throughout the world, and CVD was responsible for <10% of all deaths. Today CVD accounts for ~30% of deaths worldwide, including nearly 40% in high-income countries and about 28% in low- and middle-income countries.

THE EPIDEMIOLOGIC TRANSITION

The global rise in CVD is the result of an unprecedented transformation in the causes of morbidity and mortality during the 20th century. Known as the *epidemiologic transition*, this shift is driven by industrialization, urbanization, and associated lifestyle changes, and it is taking place in every part of the world among all races, ethnic groups, and cultures. The transition is divided into four basic stages: pestilence and famine, receding pandemics, degenerative and human-made diseases, and delayed degenerative diseases. A fifth stage, characterized by an epidemic of inactivity and obesity, may be emerging in some countries (Table 218-1).

Malnutrition, infectious diseases, and high infant and child mortality that are offset by high fertility mark the *age of pestilence and famine*. Tuberculosis, dysentery, cholera, and influenza are often fatal, resulting in a mean life expectancy of about 30 years. Cardiovascular disease, which accounts for <10% of deaths, takes the form of rheumatic heart disease and cardiomyopathies due to infection and malnutrition. Approximately 10% of the world's population remains in the age of pestilence and famine.

Per capita income and life expectancy increase during the *age of receding pandemics* as the emergence of public health systems, cleaner water supplies, and improved nutrition combine to drive down deaths from infectious disease and malnutrition. Infant and childhood mortal-

TABLE 218-1 FIVE STAGES OF EPIDEMIOLOGIC TRANSITION

Stage	Description	Deaths Related to CVD	Predominant CVD Type
Pestilence and famine	Predominance of malnutrition and infectious diseases as causes of death; high rates of infant and child mortality; low mean life expectancy	<10%	Rheumatic heart disease, cardiomyopathies caused by infection and malnutrition
Receding pandemics	Improvements in nutrition and public health, leading to decrease in rates of deaths related to malnutrition and infection; precipitous decline in infant and child mortality rates	10–35%	Rheumatic valvular disease, hypertension, CHD, and stroke (predominantly hemorrhagic)
Degenerative and human-made diseases	Increased fat and caloric intake and decrease in physical activity, leading to emergence of hypertension and atherosclerosis; with increase in life expectancy, mortality from chronic, noncommunicable diseases exceeds mortality from malnutrition and infectious disease	35–65%	CHD and stroke (ischemic and hemorrhagic)
Delayed degenerative diseases	CVD and cancer the major causes of morbidity and mortality; fewer deaths among those with disease and primary events delayed due to better treatment and prevention efforts; decline of age-adjusted CVD mortality; CVD affecting older and older individuals	40–50%	CHD, stroke, and congestive heart failure
Inactivity and obesity	Overweight and obesity increase at alarming rate; diabetes and hypertension increase; leveling off of decline in smoking-rate; physical activity recommendations met by a minority of the population	Possible reversal of age-adjusted declines in mortality	CHD, stroke, and congestive heart failure, peripheral vascular disease

Note: CHD, coronary heart disease; CVD, cardiovascular disease.
Source: Adapted from AR Omran: Milbank Mem Fund Q 49:509, 1971; and SJ Olshansky, AB Ault: Milbank Q 64:355, 1986.

ity also decline, but deaths due to CVD increase to between 10 and 35% of all deaths. Rheumatic valvular disease, hypertension, coronary heart disease, and stroke are the predominant forms of CVD. Almost 40% of the world's population is currently in this stage.

The *age of degenerative and human-made diseases* is distinguished by mortality from noncommunicable diseases—primarily CVD—surpassing mortality from malnutrition and infectious diseases. Caloric intake, particularly from animal fat, increases. Coronary heart disease and stroke are prevalent, and between 35 and 65% of all deaths can be traced to CVD. Typically, the rate of death from coronary heart disease (CHD) exceeds that of stroke by a ratio of 2:1–3:1. During this period, average life expectancy surpasses 50. Roughly 35% of the world's population falls into this category.

In the *age of delayed degenerative diseases*, CVD and cancer remain the major causes of morbidity and mortality, with CVD accounting for 40–50% of all deaths. However, age-adjusted CVD mortality declines, aided by preventive strategies, such as smoking cessation programs and effective blood pressure control; by acute hospital management; and by technological advances, such as the availability of bypass surgery. CHD, stroke, and congestive heart failure are the primary forms of CVD. About 15% of the world's population is now in the age of delayed degenerative diseases or is exiting this age and moving into the fifth stage of the epidemiologic transition.

In the industrialized world, physical activity continues to decline while total caloric intake increases. The resulting epidemic of overweight and obesity may signal the start of the *age of inactivity and obesity*. Rates of type 2 diabetes mellitus, hypertension, and lipid abnormalities are on the rise, trends that are particularly evident in children. If these risk factor trends continue, age-adjusted CVD mortality rates could increase in the coming years.

THE EPIDEMIOLOGIC TRANSITION IN THE UNITED STATES

The United States, like other high-income countries, has proceeded through four stages of the epidemiologic transition. Recent trends, however, suggest that the rates of decline of some chronic and degenerative diseases have slowed. Given the large amount of available data, the United States serves as a useful reference point for comparisons.

The Age of Pestilence and Famine (Before 1900) The American colonies were born into pestilence and famine, with half of the original Pilgrims who arrived in 1620 dying of infection and malnutrition by the following spring. At the end of the 1800s, the U.S. economy was still largely agrarian, with >60% of the population living in rural settings. By 1900, average life expectancy had increased to about 50 years. However, tuberculosis, pneumonia, and other infectious diseases still accounted for more deaths than any other cause. CVD accounted for <10% of all deaths.

The Age of Receding Pandemics (1900–1930) By 1900, a public health infrastructure was in place: 40 states had health departments, many larger towns had major public works efforts to improve the water supply and sewage systems, municipal use of chlorine to disinfect water was widespread, pasteurization and other improvements in food handling were introduced, and the educational quality of health care personnel improved. These changes led to dramatic declines in infectious disease mortality rates. However, the continued shift from a rural, agriculture-based economy to an urban, industrial economy had a number of consequences for risk behaviors and factors for CVD. In particular, consumption of fresh fruits and vegetables declined and consumption of meat and grains increased, resulting in diets that were higher in animal fat and processed carbohydrates. In addition, the availability of factory-rolled cigarettes made them more accessible and affordable for the mass population. Age-adjusted CVD mortality rates rose from 300 per 100,000 people in 1900 to approximately 390 per 100,000 people during this period, driven by rapidly rising CHD rates.

The Age of Degenerative and Human-Made Diseases (1930–1965) During this period, deaths from infectious diseases fell to fewer than 50 per 100,000 population per year, and life expectancy increased to al-

most 70 years. At the same time, the country became increasingly urbanized and industrialized, precipitating a number of important lifestyle changes. By 1955, 55% of adult men were smoking, and fat consumption represented approximately 40% of total calories. Lower activity levels, high-fat diets, and increased smoking pushed CVD death rates to their peak levels.

The Age of Delayed Degenerative Diseases (1965–) Substantial declines in age-adjusted CVD mortality rates began in the mid-1960s. In the 1970s and 1980s, age-adjusted CHD mortality rates fell approximately 2% per year, and stroke rates fell 3% per year. A main characteristic of this phase is the steadily rising age at which a first CVD event occurs. Two significant advances have been attributed to the decline in CVD mortality rates: new therapeutic approaches and the implementation of prevention measures. Treatments once considered advanced, such as angioplasty, bypass surgery, and implantation of defibrillators, are now considered the standard of care. Treatment for hypertension and elevated cholesterol along with the widespread use of aspirin has also made major contributions to reducing deaths from CVD. In addition, Americans were exposed to public health campaigns promoting lifestyle modifications effective at reducing the prevalence of smoking, hypertension, and dyslipidemia.

Is the United States Entering a Fifth Age? Starting in the 1990s, the age-standardized death rate had decreased to an average of about 2% per year for CHD and 1% for stroke. In 2003, the age-standardized death rate for total CVD was 306 per 100,000. The slowing of the decline may be due, in part, to a slowing of the rate of decline in risk factors, such as smoking, and alarming increases in other risk factors, such as obesity and physical inactivity.

CURRENT WORLDWIDE VARIATIONS

An epidemiologic transition much like that which occurred in the United States is occurring throughout the world, but unique regional features have modified aspects of the transition in various parts of the world. In terms of economic development, the world can be divided into two broad categories: (1) high-income countries; and (2) low- and middle-income countries, which can be further subdivided into six distinct economic/geographic regions. Currently, 85% of the world's population lives in low- and middle-income countries, and it is these countries that are driving the rates of change in the global burden of CVD (Fig. 218-1). Three million CVD deaths occurred in high-income countries in 2001, compared to 13 million in the rest of the world.

High-Income Countries Approximately 940 million people live in the high-income countries, where CHD is the dominant form of CVD, with rates that tend to be twofold to fivefold higher than stroke rates. The rates of CVD in Canada, New Zealand, Australia, and Western Europe tend to be similar to those in the United States; however, among the countries of Western Europe, the absolute rates vary threefold with a clear north/south gradient. The highest CVD death rates are in the northern countries, such as Finland, Ireland, and Scotland, with the lowest CVD rates in the Mediterranean countries of France, Spain, and Italy. Japan is unique among the high-income countries: stroke rates increased dramatically over the last century, but CHD rates did not rise as sharply. This difference may stem in part from genetic factors, but it is more likely that the fish- and plant-based, low-fat diet and resulting low cholesterol levels have played a larger role. Importantly, Japanese dietary habits are undergoing substantial changes, reflected in an increase in cholesterol levels.

Low- and Middle-Income Countries The World Bank groups the low- and middle-income countries (gross national income per capita lower than U.S. $9200) into six geographic regions: East Asia and the Pacific, (Eastern) Europe and Central Asia, Latin America and the Caribbean, Middle East and North Africa, South Asia, and Sub-Saharan Africa. Although communicable diseases continue to be a major cause of death, CVD has emerged as a significant health concern in the low- and middle-income countries (Fig. 218-2). In most of these countries, there is an urban/rural gradient for CHD, stroke, and hypertension, with higher rates in urban centers.

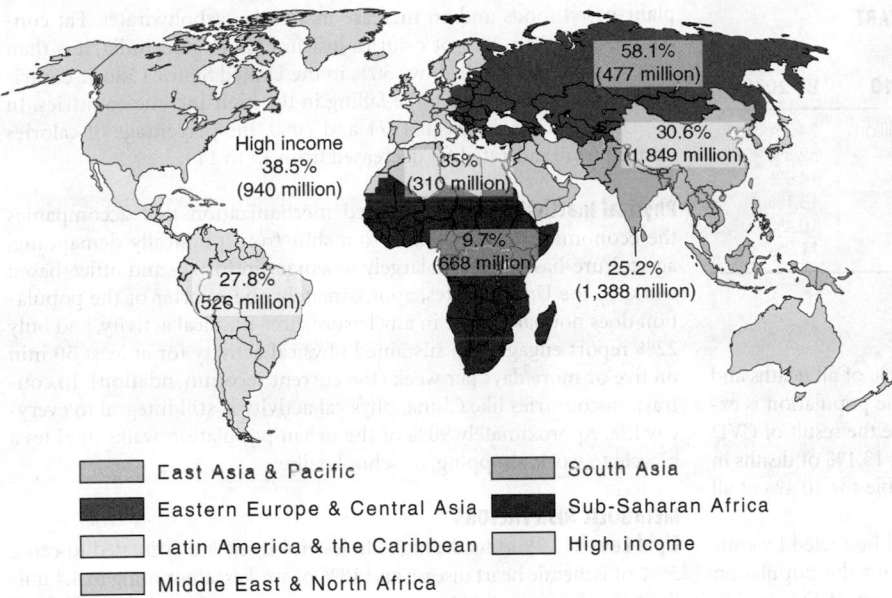

FIGURE 218-1 CVD death as a percentage of total deaths, and total population, in seven economic regions of the world defined by the World Bank. *(Based on data from CD Mathers et al: Deaths and Disease Burden by Cause: Global Burden of Disease Estimates for 2001 by World Bank Country Groups. Disease Control Priorities Working Paper 18. April 2004, revised January 2005.)*

While CVD rates are rapidly rising, there are vast differences among the regions and countries, and even within the countries themselves. Many factors contribute to the heterogeneity. First, the regions are at various stages of the epidemiologic transition. Second, vast differences in lifestyle and behavioral risk factors exist. Third, racial and ethnic differences may lead to altered susceptibilities to various forms of CVD. In addition, it should be noted that for most countries in these regions, accurate country-wide data on cause-specific mortality are not precise, as death certificate completion is not routine, and most countries do not have a centralized registry for deaths.

The *East Asia and Pacific* region appears to be straddling the second and third phases of the epidemiologic transition, with China, Indonesia, and Sri Lanka's large combined population driving most of the trends. Overall, CVD is a major cause of death in China, but like Japan, stroke (particularly hemorrhagic) causes more deaths than CHD. China also appears to have a geographic gradient like that of Western Europe, with higher CVD rates in northern China than in southern China. Other countries, such as Vietnam and Cambodia, are just emerging from the pestilence and famine stage.

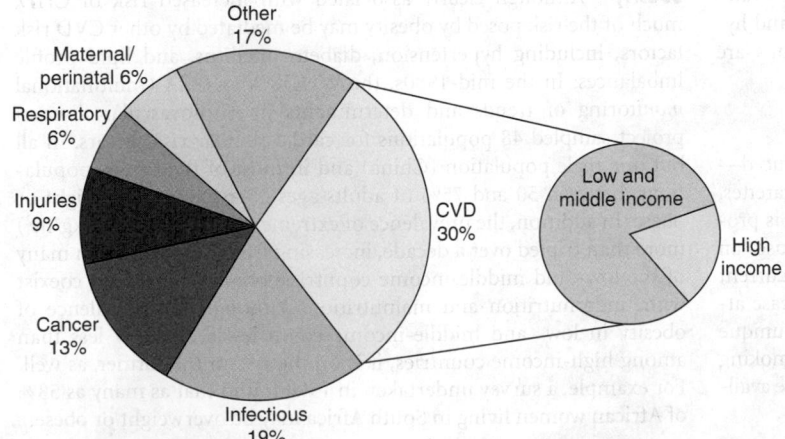

FIGURE 218-2 CVD compared to other causes of death. CVD: cardiovascular disease. *(Based on data from CD Mathers et al: Deaths and Disease Burden by Cause: Global Burden of Disease Estimates for 2001 by World Bank Country Groups. Disease Control Priorities Working Paper 18. April 2004, revised January 2005.)*

The *Eastern Europe and Central Asia* region is firmly in the peak of the third phase, with the highest death rates (58%) due to CVD in the world, nearly double the rate of high-income countries. There is, however, also regional variability. In Russia, increased CVD rates have contributed to falling life expectancy, particularly for men, whose life expectancy has dropped from 71.6 in 1986 to 59 years today. In Poland, by contrast, the age-adjusted mortality rate decreased by approximately 30% for men during the 1990s, and slightly more among women.

In general, the *Latin America and Caribbean* region appears to be in the third phase of the epidemiologic transition, although as in other low- and middle-income regions, there is vast regional heterogeneity, with some areas in the second phase of the transition and some in the fourth. Today, approximately 28% of all deaths in this region are attributable to CVD, with CHD rates higher than stroke rates. Approximately one-quarter of the citizens live in poverty, and many are still dealing with infectious diseases and malnutrition as major problems.

The *Middle East and North Africa* region appears to be entering the third phase of the epidemiologic transition, with rates just below high-income nations. In this region, increasing economic wealth has been accompanied characteristically by urbanization but uncharacteristically by increasing fertility rates as infant and childhood mortality rates have declined. The traditional high-fiber diet, low in fat and cholesterol, has changed rapidly. Over the past few decades, daily fat consumption has increased in most of these countries, ranging from a 13.6% increase in Sudan to a 143.3% increase in Saudi Arabia.

Most people in *South Asia* live in rural India, a country that is experiencing an alarming increase in heart disease. CVD accounted for 32% of all deaths in 2000, and the World Health Organization (WHO) estimates that 60% of the world's cardiac patients will be Indian by 2010. The transition appears to be in the Western style, with CHD as the dominant form of CVD. In 1960, CHD represented 4% of all CVD deaths in India, whereas in 1990 the proportion was >50%. This is somewhat unexpected because stroke tends to be a more dominant factor early in the epidemiologic transition. This finding may reflect inaccuracies in cause-specific mortality estimates or possibly an underlying genetic component. It has been suggested that Indians have exaggerated insulin insensitivity in response to the Western lifestyle pattern that may differentially increase rates of CHD over stroke. Certain remote areas, however, are still emerging from the age of pestilence and famine, with CVD accounting for <10% of total deaths. Rheumatic heart disease continues to be a major cause of morbidity and mortality.

Sub-Saharan Africa remains largely in the first phase of the epidemiologic transition, with CVD rates half of those in high-income nations. Life expectancy has decreased by an average of five years since the early 1990s largely because of HIV/AIDS and other chronic diseases, according to the World Bank; life expectancies are the lowest in the world. While HIV/AIDS is the leading overall cause of death in this region, CVD is the third leading killer and is first among those over the age of 30. Hypertension is now a major public health concern and has resulted in stroke being the dominant form of CVD. Rheumatic heart disease remains an important cause of CVD mortality and morbidity.

GLOBAL TRENDS IN CARDIOVASCULAR DISEASE

In 1990, CVD accounted for 28% of the world's 50.4 million deaths and 9.7% of the 1.4 billion lost disability-adjusted life

TABLE 218-2 ESTIMATED MORBIDITY RELATED TO HEART DISEASE: 2010–2030

Deaths	By 2010	By 2030
CVD deaths: annual number of all deaths	18.1 million	24.2 million
CVD deaths: percentage of all deaths	30.8%	32.5%
CHD deaths: percentage of all male deaths	13.1%	14.9%
CHD deaths: percentage of all female deaths	13.6%	13.1%
Stroke deaths: percentage of all male deaths	9.2%	10.4%
Stroke deaths: percentage of all female deaths	11.5%	11.8%

Note: CVD, cardiovascular disease; CHD, coronary heart disease.
Source: Adapted from Mackay and Mensah.

years (DALYs). By 2001, CVD was responsible for 29% of all deaths and 14% of the 1.5 billion lost DALYs. By 2030, when the population is expected to reach 8.2 billion, 32.5% of all deaths will be the result of CVD (Table 218-2). Of these, 14.9% of deaths in men and 13.1% of deaths in women will be due to CHD. Stroke will be responsible for 10.4% of all male deaths and 11.8% of all female deaths.

In *high-income countries*, population growth will be fueled by emigration from low- and middle-income countries, but the population of high-income countries will shrink as a proportion of the world's population. In high-income countries, the modest decline in CVD death rates begun in the latter third of the 20th century will continue, but the rate of decline appears to be slowing. However, these countries are expected to see an increase in the prevalence of CVD as well as the absolute number of deaths as the population ages.

Significant portions of the population living in *low- and middle-income countries* have entered the third phase of the epidemiologic transition, and some are entering the fourth stage. Changing demographics play a significant role in future predictions for CVD throughout the world. For example, between 1990 and 2001, the population of Eastern Europe and Central Asia grew by 1 million people per year, whereas South Asia added 25 million people each year.

Higher CVD rates will also have an economic impact. Even assuming no increase in CVD risk factors, most countries, but especially India and South Africa, will see a large number of people between 35 and 64 die of CVD over the next 30 years, as well as an increasing level of morbidity among middle-aged people related to heart disease and stroke. In China, it is estimated that there will be 9 million deaths from CVD in 2030—up from 2.4 million in 2002—with half occurring in individuals between 35 and 64 years old.

REGIONAL TRENDS IN RISK FACTORS

As indicated earlier, the global variation in CVD rates is related to temporal and regional variations in known risk behaviors and factors. Ecologic analyses of major CVD risk factors and mortality demonstrate high correlations between expected and observed mortality rates for the three main risk factors—smoking, serum cholesterol, and hypertension—and suggest that many of the regional variations are based on differences in conventional risk factors.

BEHAVIORAL RISK FACTORS

Tobacco Every year, more than 5.5 trillion cigarettes are produced—enough to provide every person on the planet with 1,000 cigarettes. Worldwide, 1.2 billion people smoked in 2000, a number that is projected to increase to 1.6 billion by 2030. Tobacco currently causes an estimated 5 million deaths annually (9% of all deaths). If current smoking patterns continue, by 2030 the global burden of disease attributable to tobacco will reach 10 million deaths annually. A unique feature of low- and middle-income countries is easy access to smoking during the early stages of the epidemiologic transition due to the availability of relatively inexpensive tobacco products.

Diet Total caloric intake per capita increases as countries develop. With regard to CVD, a key element of dietary change is an increase in intake of saturated animal fats and hydrogenated vegetable fats, which contain atherogenic *trans* fatty acids, along with a decrease in intake of

plant-based foods and an increase in simple carbohydrates. Fat contributes less than 20% of calories in rural China and India, less than 30% in Japan, and well above 30% in the United States. Caloric contributions from fat appear to be falling in the high-income countries. In the United States, between 1971 and 2000, the percentage of calories derived from saturated fat decreased from 13 to 11%.

Physical Inactivity The increased mechanization that accompanies the economic transition leads to a shift from physically demanding, agriculture-based work to largely sedentary industry- and office-based work. In the United States, approximately one-quarter of the population does not participate in any leisure-time physical activity, and only 22% report engaging in sustained physical activity for at least 30 min on five or more days per week (the current recommendation). In contrast, in countries like China, physical activity is still integral to everyday life. Approximately 90% of the urban population walks or rides a bicycle to work, shopping, or school daily.

METABOLIC RISK FACTORS

Lipid Levels Worldwide, high cholesterol levels are estimated to cause 56% of ischemic heart disease and 18% of strokes, amounting to 4.4 millions deaths annually. As countries move through the epidemiologic transition, mean population plasma cholesterol levels tend to rise. Social and individual changes that accompany urbanization clearly play a role because plasma cholesterol levels tend to be higher among urban residents than among rural residents. This shift is largely driven by greater consumption of dietary fats—primarily from animal products and processed vegetable oils—and decreased physical activity. In high-income countries, mean population cholesterol levels are generally falling, but in low- and middle-income countries, there is wide variation in these levels.

Hypertension Elevated blood pressure is an early indicator of the epidemiologic transition. Worldwide, approximately 62% of strokes and 49% of cases of ischemic heart disease are attributable to suboptimal (>115 mmHg systolic) blood pressure, which is believed to account for more than 7 million deaths annually. Rising mean blood pressure is apparent as populations industrialize and move from rural to urban settings. Among urban-dwelling men and women in India, for example, the prevalence of hypertension is 25.5% and 29.0%, respectively, whereas it is 14.0% and 10.8%, respectively, in rural communities. One major concern in low- and middle-income countries is the high rate of undetected, and therefore untreated, hypertension. This may explain, at least in part, the higher stroke rates in these countries in relation to CHD rates during the early stages of the transition. The high rates of hypertension, especially undiagnosed hypertension, throughout Asia probably contribute to the high prevalence of hemorrhagic stroke in the region.

Obesity Although clearly associated with increased risk of CHD, much of the risk posed by obesity may be mediated by other CVD risk factors, including hypertension, diabetes mellitus, and lipid profile imbalances. In the mid-1980s, the WHO's MONICA (multinational *moni*toring of trends and determinants in *ca*rdiovascular disease) project sampled 48 populations for cardiovascular risk factors. In all but one male population (China) and in most of the female populations, between 50 and 75% of adults ages 35–64 were overweight or obese. In addition, the prevalence of extreme obesity (BMI ≥40 kg/m^2) more than tripled over a decade, increasing from 1.3 to 4.9%. In many of the low- and middle-income countries, obesity appears to coexist with undernutrition and malnutrition. Although the prevalence of obesity in low- and middle-income countries is certainly less than among high-income countries, it is on the rise in the former, as well. For example, a survey undertaken in 1998 found that as many as 58% of African women living in South Africa may be overweight or obese.

Diabetes Mellitus As a consequence of, or in addition to, increasing body mass index and decreasing levels of physical activity, worldwide rates of diabetes—predominantly type 2 diabetes—are on the rise. In 2003, 194 million adults, or 5% of the world's population, had diabetes, with nearly three-quarters living in high-income countries. By 2025, this number is predicted to increase 72% to 333 million. By 2025, the number of people with type 2 diabetes is projected to double in three of the six low- and middle-income regions: Middle East and North Africa, South Asia, and Sub-Saharan Africa. There appear to be clear genetic susceptibilities to diabetes mellitus in various racial and ethnic groups. For example, migration studies suggest that South Asians and Indians tend to be at higher risk than those of European extraction.

SUMMARY

Although CVD rates are declining in high-income countries, they are increasing in virtually every other region of the world. The consequences of this preventable epidemic will be substantial on many levels—individual mortality and morbidity, family suffering, and staggering economic costs.

Three complementary strategies can be used to lessen the impact. First, the overall burden of CVD risk factors can be lowered through population-wide public health measures, such as national campaigns against cigarette smoking, unhealthy diets, and physical inactivity. Second, it is important to identify higher-risk subgroups of the population who stand to benefit the most from specific, low-cost prevention interventions, including screening for and treatment of hypertension and elevated cholesterol. Simple, low-cost interventions, such as the "polypill," a regimen of aspirin, a statin, and an antihypertensive agent, also need to be explored. Third, resources should be allocated to

acute as well as secondary prevention interventions. For countries with limited resources, a critical first step in developing a comprehensive plan is better assessment of cause-specific mortality and morbidity, as well as the prevalence of the major preventable risk factors.

In the meantime, the high-income countries must continue to bear the burden of research and development aimed at prevention and treatment, being mindful of the economic limitations of many countries. The concept of the epidemiologic transition provides insight into how to alter the course of the CVD epidemic. The efficient transfer of low-cost preventive and therapeutic strategies could alter the natural course of this epidemic and thereby reduce the excess global burden of preventable CVD.

FURTHER READINGS

GAZIANO JM: Global burden of cardiovascular disease, in *Braunwald's Heart Disease: A Textbook of Cardiovascular Medicine*, 8th ed. Philadelphia, Elsevier Saunders, 2008

LOPEZ AD et al (eds): *Global Burden of Disease and Risk Factors*. Washington, D.C.: Oxford University Press, 2006

JAMISON DT et al (eds): *Disease Control Priorities in Developing Countries*, 2nd ed. Washington, D.C., Oxford University Press, 2006

LEEDER S et al: *A Race against Time: The Challenge of Cardiovascular Disease in Developing Economies*. New York: Columbia University, 2004

MACKAY J, MENSAH G: *Atlas of Heart Disease and Stroke*. Geneva: World Health Organization, 2004

---

219 Approach to the Patient with Possible Cardiovascular Disease
Eugene Braunwald

THE MAGNITUDE OF THE PROBLEM

Cardiovascular diseases comprise the most prevalent serious disorders in industrialized nations and are a rapidly growing problem in developing nations (Chap. 218). Although age-adjusted death rates for coronary heart disease have declined by two-thirds in the past four decades in the United States, cardiovascular diseases remain the most common causes of death, responsible for 40% of all deaths, almost 1 million deaths each year. Approximately one-fourth of these deaths are sudden. The growing prevalence of obesity (Chap. 74), type 2 diabetes mellitus (Chap. 338), and metabolic syndrome (Chap. 236), which are important risk factors for atherosclerosis, now threatens to reverse the progress that has been made in the age-adjusted reduction of mortality of coronary heart disease.

For many years cardiovascular disease was considered to be more frequent in men than in women. In fact, the percentage of all deaths secondary to cardiovascular disease is higher among women (43%) than among men (37%). In addition, while the absolute number of deaths secondary to cardiovascular disease has declined over the past decades in men, this number has actually risen in women. Inflammation and the above-mentioned risk factors, i.e., obesity, type 2 diabetes mellitus, and the metabolic syndrome, appear to play a more prominent role in the development of coronary atherosclerosis in women than in men. Coronary artery disease (CAD) is more frequently associated with dysfunction of the coronary microcirculation in women than in men. Exercise electrocardiography has a lower diagnostic accuracy in the prediction of epicardial obstruction in women.

CARDIAC SYMPTOMS

The symptoms caused by heart disease result most commonly from myocardial ischemia, from disturbance of the contraction and/or re-

laxation of the myocardium, from obstruction to blood flow, or from an abnormal cardiac rhythm or rate.

Ischemia, which is caused by an imbalance between the heart's oxygen supply and demand, is manifest most frequently as chest discomfort (Chap. 13), while reduction of the pumping ability of the heart commonly leads to fatigue and elevated intravascular pressure upstream to the failing ventricle. The latter results in abnormal fluid accumulation, with peripheral edema (Chap. 36) or pulmonary congestion and dyspnea (Chap. 33). Obstruction to blood flow, as occurs in valvular stenosis, can cause symptoms resembling those resulting from myocardial failure (Chap. 227). Cardiac arrhythmias often develop suddenly, and the resulting symptoms and signs—palpitations (Chap. 37), dyspnea, hypotension, and syncope (Chap. 21)—generally occur abruptly and may disappear as rapidly as they develop.

Although dyspnea, chest discomfort, edema, and syncope are cardinal manifestations of cardiac disease, they occur in other conditions as well. Thus, dyspnea is observed in disorders as diverse as pulmonary disease, marked obesity, and anxiety (Chap. 33). Similarly, chest discomfort may result from a variety of noncardiac and cardiac causes other than myocardial ischemia (Chap. 13). Edema, an important finding in untreated or inadequately treated heart failure, may also occur with primary renal disease and in hepatic cirrhosis (Chap. 36). Syncope occurs not only with serious cardiac arrhythmias but in a number of neurologic conditions, as well (Chap. 21). Whether or not heart disease is responsible for these symptoms can frequently be determined by carrying out a careful clinical examination (Chap. 220), supplemented by noninvasive testing using electrocardiography at rest and during exercise (Chap. 221), echocardiography, roentgenography, and other forms of myocardial imaging (Chap. 222).

Myocardial or coronary function that may be adequate at rest may be insufficient during exertion. Thus, dyspnea and/or chest discomfort that appear during activity are characteristic of patients with heart disease, while the opposite pattern, i.e., the appearance of these symptoms at rest and their remission during exertion, is rarely observed in such patients. It is important, therefore, to question the patient carefully about the relation of symptoms to exertion.

Many patients with cardiovascular disease may be asymptomatic, both at rest and during exertion, but may present an abnormal physical finding, such as a heart murmur, elevated arterial pressure, or an abnormality of the electrocardiogram (ECG) or of the cardiac silhou-

TABLE 219-1 NEW YORK HEART ASSOCIATION FUNCTIONAL CLASSIFICATION

Class I	Class III
No limitation of physical activity	Marked limitation of physical activity
No symptoms with ordinary exertion	Less than ordinary activity causes symptoms
Class II	Asymptomatic at rest
Slight limitation of physical activity	Class IV
Ordinary activity causes symptoms	Inability to carry out any physical activity without discomfort
	Symptoms at rest

Modified from The Criteria Committee of the New York Heart Association.

ette on the chest roentgenogram or other imaging test. It is important to assess the global risk of CAD in asymptomatic individuals, using a combination of clinical assessment and measurement of cholesterol and its fractions, as well as other biomarkers such as C-reactive protein in some patients (Chap. 235). Since the first clinical manifestation of CAD may be catastrophic—sudden cardiac death, acute myocardial infarction, or stroke in previous asymptomatic persons—it is mandatory to identify those at high risk of such events and institute further testing and preventive measures.

DIAGNOSIS

As outlined by the New York Heart Association, the elements of a complete cardiac diagnosis include the systematic consideration of the following:

1. *The underlying etiology.* Is the disease congenital, hypertensive, ischemic, or inflammatory in origin?
2. *The anatomic abnormalities.* Which chambers are involved? Are they hypertrophied, dilated, or both? Which valves are affected? Are they regurgitant and/or stenotic? Is there pericardial involvement? Has there been a myocardial infarction?
3. *The physiologic disturbances.* Is an arrhythmia present? Is there evidence of congestive heart failure or of myocardial ischemia?
4. *Functional disability.* How strenuous is the physical activity required to elicit symptoms? The classification provided by the New York Heart Association has been found to be useful in describing functional disability (Table 219-1).

One example may serve to illustrate the importance of establishing a complete diagnosis. In a patient who presents with exertional chest discomfort, the identification of myocardial ischemia as the etiology is of great clinical importance. However, the simple recognition of ischemia is insufficient to formulate a therapeutic strategy or prognosis until the underlying anatomic abnormalities responsible for the myocardial ischemia, e.g., coronary atherosclerosis or aortic stenosis, are identified and a judgment is made as to whether other physiologic disturbances that cause an imbalance between myocardial oxygen supply and demand, such as severe anemia, thyrotoxicosis, or supraventricular tachycardia, play a contributory role. Finally, the severity of the disability should govern the extent and tempo of the workup and strongly influence the therapeutic strategy that is selected.

The establishment of a correct and complete cardiac diagnosis usually commences with the history and physical examination (Chap. 220). Indeed, the clinical examination remains the basis for the diagnosis of a wide variety of disorders. The clinical examination may then be supplemented by five types of laboratory tests: (1) ECG (Chap. 221); (2) noninvasive imaging examinations (chest roentgenogram, echocardiogram, radionuclide, computer tomographic and magnetic resonance imaging; Chap. 222); (3) blood tests to assess risk [e.g., lipid determinations, C-reactive protein (Chap. 235)], or cardiac function [e.g., brain natriuretic peptide (BNP); Chap. 227]; (4) occasionally specialized invasive examinations, i.e., cardiac catheterization and coronary arteriography (Chap. 223); and (5) genetic tests to identify monogenic cardiac diseases [e.g., hypertrophic cardiomyopathy (Chap. 231), Marfan syndrome (Chap. 357), and abnormalities of cardiac ion channels that lead to prolongation of the QT interval and an

increase in risk of sudden death (Chap. 226)]. These tests are becoming more widely available.

FAMILY HISTORY

In eliciting the history of a patient with known or suspected cardiovascular disease, particular attention should be directed to the family history. Familial clustering is common in many forms of heart disease. Mendelian transmission of single-gene defects may occur, as in hypertrophic cardiomyopathy (Chap. 231), the Marfan syndrome (Chap. 357), and sudden death associated with a prolonged QT syndrome (Chap. 226). Premature coronary disease and essential hypertension, type 2 diabetes mellitus, and hyperlipidemia (the most important risk factors for coronary artery disease) are usually polygenic disorders. While familial transmission may be less obvious than in the single-gene disorders, it is also helpful in assessing risk and prognosis in polygenic disorders. Familial clustering of cardiovascular diseases may occur not only on a genetic basis but may also be related to familial dietary or behavior patterns, such as excessive ingestion of salt or calories or cigarette smoking.

ASSESSMENT OF FUNCTIONAL IMPAIRMENT

When an attempt is made to determine the severity of functional impairment in a patient with heart disease, it is helpful to ascertain the level of activity and the rate at which it is performed before symptoms develop. Thus, it is not sufficient to state that the patient complains of dyspnea. The breathlessness that occurs after running up two long flights of stairs denotes far less functional impairment than similar symptoms occurring after taking a few steps on level ground. Also, the degree of customary physical activity at work and during recreation should be considered. The development of two-flight dyspnea in a well-conditioned marathon runner may be far more significant than the development of one-flight dyspnea in a previously sedentary person. The history should include a detailed consideration of the patient's therapeutic regimen. For example, the persistence or development of edema, breathlessness, and other manifestations of heart failure in a patient whose diet is rigidly restricted in sodium content and who is receiving optimal doses of diuretics and other therapies for heart failure (Chap. 227) is far graver than are similar manifestations in the absence of these measures. Similarly, the presence of angina pectoris despite treatment with optimal doses of multiple antianginal drugs (Chap. 237) is more serious than it is in a patient on no therapy. In an effort to determine the progression of symptoms, and thereby the severity of the underlying illness, it may be useful to ascertain what, if any, specific tasks the patient could have carried out 6 months or 1 year earlier that he or she cannot carry out at present.

ELECTROCARDIOGRAM

(See also Chap. 221) Although an ECG should usually be recorded in patients with known or suspected heart disease, with the exception of the identification of arrhythmias, of ventricular hypertrophy, and of acute myocardial infarction, it rarely permits establishment of a specific diagnosis. The range of normal electrocardiographic findings is wide, and the tracing can be affected significantly by many noncardiac factors, such as age, body habitus, and serum electrolyte concentrations. In the absence of other abnormal findings, electrocardiographic changes must not be overinterpreted.

ASSESSMENT OF THE PATIENT WITH A HEART MURMUR

(Fig. 219-1) The cause of a heart murmur can often be readily elucidated from a systematic evaluation of its major attributes: timing, duration, intensity, quality, frequency, configuration, location, and radiation when considered in the light of the history, general physical examination, and other features of the cardiac examination, as described in Chap. 220.

The majority of heart murmurs are midsystolic and soft (grades I to II/VI). When such a murmur occurs in an asymptomatic child or young adult *without* other evidence of heart disease on clinical examination, it is usually benign and echocardiography is not generally required. On

EVALUATION OF HEART MURMUR

FIGURE 219-1 An alternative "echocardiography first" approach to the evaluation of a heart murmur that also uses the results of the electrocardiogram (ECG) and chest x-ray in asymptomatic patients with soft midsystolic murmurs and no other physical findings. This algorithm is useful for patients over age 40 years in whom the prevalence of coronary artery disease and aortic stenosis increases as the cause of systolic murmur. [From RA O'Rourke, in Primary Cardiology, 2d ed, E Braunwald, L Goldman (eds). Philadelphia, Saunders, 2003.]

the other hand, two-dimensional and Doppler echocardiography (Chap. 222) are indicated in patients with loud systolic murmurs (grades ≥III/VI), especially those that are holosystolic or late systolic, and in most patients with diastolic or continuous murmurs.

NATURAL HISTORY

Cardiovascular disorders often present acutely, as in a previously asymptomatic person who develops an acute myocardial infarction (Chap. 239) or the previously asymptomatic patient with hypertrophic cardiomyopathy (Chap. 231) or with a prolonged QT interval (Chap. 226) whose first clinical manifestation is syncope or even sudden death. However, the alert physician may recognize the patient at risk of these complications long before they occur and can often take measures to prevent their occurrence. For example, the patient with acute myocardial infarction will often have had risk factors for atherosclerosis for many years. Had these been recognized, their elimination or reduction might have delayed or even prevented the infarction. Similarly, the patient with hypertrophic cardiomyopathy may have had a heart murmur for years, and a family history of this disorder. These findings could have led to an echocardiographic examination and the recognition of the condition and appropriate therapy long before the occurrence of a serious acute manifestation.

Patients with valvular heart disease or idiopathic dilated cardiomyopathy, on the other hand, may have a prolonged course of gradually increasing dyspnea and other manifestations of chronic heart failure that is punctuated by episodes of acute deterioration only late in the course of the disease. It is of great importance to understand the natural history of various cardiac disorders so as to apply diagnostic and therapeutic measures that are appropriate to each stage of the condition as well as to provide the patient and family with an estimate of the prognosis.

PITFALLS IN CARDIOVASCULAR MEDICINE

Increasing subspecialization in internal medicine and the perfection of advanced diagnostic techniques in cardiology can lead to several undesirable consequences. Examples include:

1. Failure by the *noncardiologist* to recognize important cardiac manifestations of systemic illnesses, e.g., the presence of mitral stenosis, patent foramen ovale, and/or transient atrial arrhythmia in a patient with stroke or the presence of pulmonary hypertension and cor pulmonale in a patient with scleroderma or Raynaud's syndrome. A cardiovascular examination should be carried out to identify and estimate the severity of cardiovascular involvement that accompanies many noncardiac disorders.

2. Failure by the *cardiologist* to recognize underlying systemic disorders in patients with heart disease. For example, hyperthyroidism should be tested for in an elderly patient with atrial fibrillation and unexplained heart failure. Similarly, Lyme disease should be considered in a patient with unexplained fluctuating atrioventricular block. A cardiovascular abnormality may provide the clue critical to the recognition of some systemic disorders. For instance, an unexplained pericardial effusion may provide an early clue to the diagnosis of tuberculosis or neoplasm.

3. Overreliance on and overutilization of laboratory tests, particularly invasive techniques for the examination of the cardiovascular system. Cardiac catheterization and coronary arteriography (Chap. 223) provide precise diagnostic information that is critical to clinical evaluation which may be crucial in developing a therapeutic plan in patients with known or suspected CAD. Although a great deal of attention has been directed to these examinations, it is important to recognize that they serve to *supplement*, not *supplant*, a careful examination carried out by clinical and noninvasive techniques. A coronary arteriogram should not be carried out in lieu of a careful history in patients with chest pain suspected of having ischemic heart disease. Although coronary arteriography may establish whether the coronary arteries are obstructed, and if so the severity of the obstruction, the results of the procedure by themselves often do not provide a definite answer to the question of whether a patient's complaint of chest discomfort is attributable to coronary arteriosclerosis and whether or not revascularization is indicated.

Despite the value of invasive tests in certain circumstances, they entail some small risk to the patient, involve discomfort and substantial cost, and place a strain on medical facilities. Therefore, they should be carried out only if, after the results of clinical examination and assessment by noninvasive tests have been considered, the results (of the invasive examination) can be expected to modify the patient's management.

DISEASE PREVENTION AND MANAGEMENT

The prevention of heart disease, especially of CAD, is one of the most important tasks of primary care health givers as well as cardiologists. Prevention begins with risk assessment, followed by attention to lifestyle, such as achieving optimal weight and discontinuing smoking, and aggressive treatment of all abnormal risk factors, such as hypertension, hyperlipidemia, and diabetes mellitus (Chap. 338).

After a complete diagnosis has been established in patients with known heart disease, a number of management options are usually available. Several examples may be used to demonstrate some of the principles of cardiovascular therapeutics:

1. In the absence of evidence of heart disease, a clear, definitive statement to that effect should be made and the patient should *not* be asked to return at intervals for repeated examinations. If there is no evidence for disease, such continued attention may lead to the patient developing inappropriate anxiety and fixation on the heart.

2. If there is no evidence of cardiovascular disease but the patient has one or more risk factors for the development of ischemic heart disease (Chap. 237), a plan for their reduction should be developed and the patient should be retested at intervals to assess compliance and that these risk factors are in fact being reduced.

3. Asymptomatic or mildly symptomatic patients with valvular heart disease that is anatomically severe should be evaluated periodically, every 6 to 12 months, by clinical and noninvasive examinations. Early signs of deterioration of ventricular function may signify the need for surgical treatment before the development of disabling symptoms, irreversible myocardial damage, and excessive risk of surgical treatment (Chap. 230).

4. In patients with CAD (Chap. 237), available practice guidelines should be considered in the decision on the form of treatment (medical, percutaneous coronary intervention, or surgical revascularization). Mechanical revascularization, i.e., the latter two modalities, may be employed too frequently in the United States and perhaps too infrequently in Eastern Europe and developing nations. The mere presence of angina pectoris and/or the demonstration of critical coronary arterial narrowing at angiography should not reflexly evoke a decision to treat the patient by revascularization. Instead, these procedures should be limited to patients with CAD whose angina has not responded adequately to medical treatment or in whom revascularization has been shown to improve the natural history (e.g., acute coronary syndrome, or multivessel CAD with left ventricular dysfunction).

FURTHER READINGS

ABRAMS J: *Synopsis of Cardiac Physical Diagnosis*, 2d ed. Oxford, Butterworth Heinemann, 2001

AMERICAN HEART ASSOCIATION: *Heart Disease and Stroke Statistics, 2006 Update*. Dallas, TX, American Heart Association, *www.americanheart.org*

MORROW DA et al: Chronic coronary artery disease, in *Braunwald's Heart Disease*, 8th ed, P Libby et al (eds). Philadelphia, Saunders, 2008

NATIONAL HEART, LUNG AND BLOOD INSTITUTE: *FY 2005 Fact Book*. Bethesda, MD, National Heart, Lung and Blood Institute, 2006

THE CRITERIA COMMITTEE OF THE NEW YORK HEART ASSOCIATION: *Nomenclature and Criteria for Diagnosis*, 9th ed. Boston, Little, Brown, 1994

THE NHLBI-SPONSORED WOMEN'S ISCHEMIA SYNDROME EVALUATION (WISE): Challenging existing paradigms in ischemic heart disease. J Am Coll Cardiol 47(Suppl S):1, 2006

VANDEN BELT J: The history, in *Classic Teachings in Clinical Cardiology: A Tribute to W. Proctor Harvey*, M Chizner (ed). Cedar Grove, NJ, Laennec, 1996, pp 41–54

SECTION 2 ▸ DIAGNOSIS OF CARDIOVASCULAR DISORDERS

---

220 Physical Examination of the Cardiovascular System
Robert A. O'Rourke, Eugene Braunwald

A precise and detailed physical examination is an often underutilized low-cost method for assessing the cardiovascular system. It frequently provides important information for the appropriate selection of additional noninvasive or invasive tests. First, the general physical appearance should be evaluated. The patient may appear tired because of a chronic low cardiac output; the respiratory rate may be rapid in cases of pulmonary venous congestion. Central cyanosis, often associated with clubbing of the fingers and toes, indicates right-to-left cardiac or extracardiac shunting or inadequate oxygenation of blood by the lungs. Cyanosis in the distal extremities, cool skin, and increased sweating result from vasoconstriction in patients with severe heart failure (Chap. 35). Noncardiovascular details can be equally important. For example, infective endocarditis is the likely diagnosis in patients with petechiae, Osler's nodes, and Janeway lesions (Chap. 118).

The blood pressure should be taken in both arms and with the patient supine and upright; the heart rate should be timed for 30 s. Orthostatic hypotension and tachycardia may indicate a reduced blood volume, while resting tachycardia may be due to heart failure or hypovolemia.

EXAMINATION OF THE RETINA

Visualization of the smaller vessels of the body is possible in the retina. The optic disc should be observed first, with a search for evidence of edema and blurred margins and for cupping with sharp contours. Neovascularization or the pallor of optic atrophy should be excluded. Next, the examiner should scan along the superior temporal arcade, inspecting the arteries for embolic plaques at each bifurcation and noting the arteriovenous crossings for evidence of obscuration of the vein and for marked nicking and narrowing of the vessels, as occurs in hypertension (Chap. 241).

Early diabetic microaneurysms, a manifestation of diabetic microvascular disease, are found just temporal to the fovea, along the horizontal raphe, and cotton-wool infarcts are found circularly around the disc (see Fig. 338-9). Thus, the retina can be searched efficiently for evidence of cardiovascular disease.

Variations in the caliber of a single vessel are more important than arteriovenous ratios. These occur in the form of focal narrowing, or *beading*, and are seen in hypercholesterolemia or spasm. In severe hypertension, hypertensive retinopathy with scattered flame-shaped hemorrhages, very constricted arterioles, and cotton-wool spots are evident (see Fig. 29-7).

Retinal emboli have particular cardiovascular importance. Of these, platelet emboli are both the most common and the most evanescent. Hollenhorst cholesterol plaques may be detected at the same bifurcations for months to years after the embolic shower. Platelet emboli, Hollenhorst plaques, and calcium emboli are usually seen along the course of a retinal artery, and their presence indicates that a patient is shedding from the heart, aorta, great vessels, or carotid arteries (see Fig. 29-5).

EXAMINATION OF THE ABDOMEN

The diameter of the *abdominal* aorta should be estimated. A pulsatile, expansible mass is indicative of an abdominal aortic aneurysm (Chap. 242). An abdominal aortic aneurysm may be missed if the examiner does not assess the area above the umbilicus.

Specific abnormalities of the abdomen may be secondary to heart disease. A large, tender liver is common in patients with heart failure or constrictive pericarditis. Systolic hepatic pulsations are frequent in patients with tricuspid regurgitation. A palpable spleen is a late sign in patients with severe heart failure and is also often evident in patients with infective endocarditis. Ascites may occur with heart failure alone, but it is less common with the use of diuretic therapy. Constrictive pericarditis should be considered when the ascites is out of proportion to peripheral edema. When there is an arteriovenous fistula, a continuous murmur may be heard over the abdomen. A systolic bruit heard over the kidney areas may signify renal artery stenosis in patients with systemic hypertension.

EXAMINATION OF THE EXTREMITIES

Examination of the upper and lower extremities may provide important diagnostic information. Palpation of the peripheral arterial pulses in the upper and lower extremities is necessary to define the adequacy of systemic blood flow and to detect the presence of occlusive arterial lesions. Atherosclerosis of the peripheral arteries may produce intermittent claudication of the buttock, calf, thigh, or foot, with severe disease resulting in tissue damage of the toes. Peripheral atherosclerosis is an important risk factor for coincident ischemic heart disease.

The ankle-brachial index (ABI) is useful in cardiovascular risk assessment. The ABI is the ratio of the systolic blood pressure at the ankle di-

FIGURE 220-1 A. Schematic representation of electrocardiogram, aortic pressure pulse (AOP), phonocardiogram recorded at the apex, and apex cardiogram (ACG). On the phonocardiogram, S₁, S₂, S₃, and S₄ represent the first through fourth heart sounds; OS represents the opening snap of the mitral valve, which occurs coincident with the O point of the apex cardiogram. S₃ occurs coincident with the termination of the rapid-filling wave (RFW) of the ACG, while S₄ occurs coincident with the a wave of the ACG. **B.** Simultaneous recording of electrocardiogram, indirect carotid pulse (CP), phonocardiogram along the left sternal border (LSB), and indirect jugular venous pulse (JVP). ES, ejection sound; SC, systolic click.

vided by the higher of the two arm systolic blood pressures. It reflects the degree of lower-extremity arterial occlusive disease, which is manifest by reduced blood pressure distal to stenotic lesions. Either posterior tibial or dorsalis pedis artery pressures can be used. It is important to note that each equally reflects the status of the aortoiliac and femoropopliteal segments but different tibial arteries; therefore, the resulting ABIs may differ. An arm systolic pressure of 120 mmHg and an ankle systolic pressure of 60 mmHg yields an ABI of 0.5 (60/120). The ABI is inversely related to disease severity. A resting ABI <0.9 is considered abnormal. Lower values correspond to progressively more severe occlusive peripheral arterial disease (PAD) and disabling claudication. An ABI <0.3 is consistent with critical ischemia, rest pain, and tissue loss.

Thrombophlebitis often causes pain (in the calf or thigh) or edema, and when present, pulmonary emboli should be considered as well. Edema of the lower extremities is a sign of heart failure but may also be secondary to local factors, such a varicose veins or thrombophlebitis, or to the removal of veins at coronary artery bypass surgery. Under such circumstances, the edema is often unilateral.

ARTERIAL PRESSURE PULSE

The normal central aortic pulse wave is characterized by a fairly rapid rise to a somewhat rounded peak (Fig. 220-1). The anacrotic shoulder, present on the ascending limb, occurs at the time of peak rate of aortic flow just before maximum pressure is reached. The less-steep descending limb is interrupted by a sharp downward deflection, coincident with aortic valve closure, called the *incisura*. As the pulse wave is transmitted distally, the initial upstroke becomes steeper, the anacrotic shoulder becomes less apparent, and the smoother dicrotic notch replaces the incisure. Accordingly, palpation of a peripheral arterial pulse (e.g., the radial pulse) frequently gives less information than examination of a more central pulse (e.g., the carotid pulse) regarding alterations in left ventricular ejection or aortic valve function. However, certain findings, such as the bisferiens pulse of aortic regurgitation or pulsus alternans, are more evident in peripheral arteries (Fig. 220-2).

The carotid pulse is best examined with the sternocleidomastoid muscle relaxed and with the patient's head rotated slightly toward the examiner. In palpating the brachial arterial pulse, the examiner can support the patient's relaxed elbow with the right arm while compressing the brachial pulse with the thumb. The usual technique is to compress the artery with the thumb or forefinger until the maximum pulse is sensed. Varying degrees of pressure should then be applied while concentrating on the separate phases of the pulse wave. This method,

known as *trisection*, is useful for assessing the sharpness of the upstroke, systolic peak, and diastolic slope of the arterial pulse. In most normal persons, a dicrotic wave is not palpable.

A small weak pulse, *pulsus parvus*, is common in conditions with a diminished left ventricular stroke volume, a narrow pulse pressure, and increased peripheral vascular resistance. A *hypokinetic* pulse may be due to hypovolemia, to left ventricular failure, to restrictive pericardial disease, or to mitral valve stenosis. In aortic valve stenosis, the delayed systolic peak, *pulsus tardus*, results from obstruction to left ventricular ejection (Fig. 220-2B). In contrast, a large, bounding (hyperkinetic) pulse is usually associated with an increased left ventricular stroke volume, a wide pulse pressure, and a decrease in peripheral vascular resistance. This pattern occurs characteristically in patients with an elevated stroke volume, as in complete heart block; with hyperkinetic circulation due to anxiety, anemia, exercise, or fever; or with a rapid runoff of blood from the arterial system (due to a patent ductus arteriosus or peripheral arteriovenous fistula). Patients with mitral regurgitation or a ventricular septal defect may also have a bounding pulse, since vigorous left ventricular ejection produces a rapid upstroke in the arterial pulse, even though the duration of systole and the forward stroke volume may be reduced. In aortic regurgitation, the rapidly rising, bounding arterial pulse results from an increased left ventricular stroke volume and an increased rate of ventricular ejection.

The *bisferiens pulse*, which has two systolic peaks (Fig. 220-2C), is characteristic of aortic regurgitation (with or without accompanying

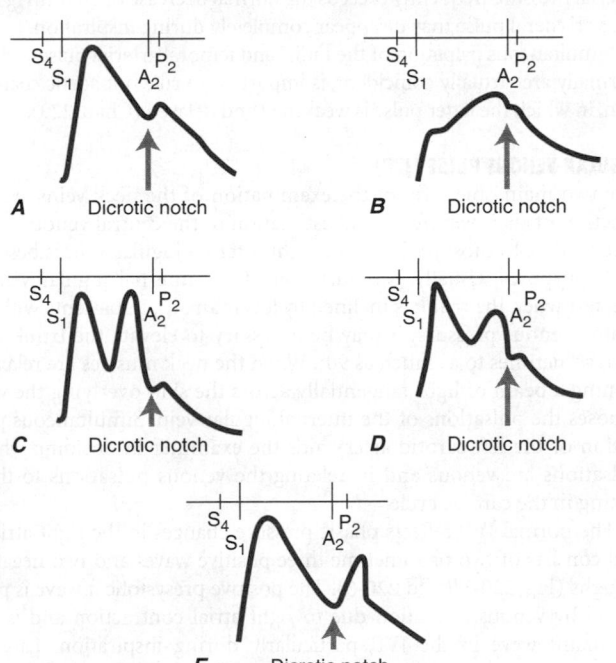

FIGURE 220-2 Schematic diagrams of the configurational changes in carotid pulse and their differential diagnoses. Heart sounds are also illustrated. **A.** Normal. A₂, aortic component of the second heart sound; S₁, first heart sound; S₄, atrial sound. **B.** Anacrotic pulse with a slow initial upstroke. The peak is close to S₂. These features suggest fixed left ventricular outflow obstruction, such as occurs with valvular aortic stenosis. **C.** Pulsus bisferiens with both percussion and tidal waves occurring during systole. This type of carotid pulse contour is most frequently observed in patients with hemodynamically significant aortic regurgitation or combined aortic stenosis and regurgitation with dominant regurgitation. It is rarely appreciated at the bedside by palpation. **D.** In hypertrophic obstructive cardiomyopathy, the pulse wave upstroke rises rapidly and the trough is followed by a smaller slowly rising positive pulse. **E.** A dicrotic pulse results from an accentuated dicrotic wave and tends to occur in patients with sepsis, severe heart failure, hypovolemic shock, cardiac tamponade, and aortic valve replacement. *[From K Chatterjee: Bedside evaluation of the heart: The physical examination, in Cardiology: An Illustrated Text/Reference, K Chatterjee, W Parmley (eds). Philadelphia, JB Lippincott, 1991.]*

stenosis) and of hypertrophic cardiomyopathy (Chap. 231). In the latter condition, the pulse wave upstroke rises rapidly and forcefully, producing the first systolic peak ("percussion wave") (Fig. 220-2*D*). A brief decline in pressure follows because of the sudden midsystolic decrease in the rate of left ventricular ejection, when severe obstruction often develops. This pressure trough is followed by a smaller and more slowly rising positive pulse wave ("tidal wave") produced by continued ventricular ejection and by reflected waves from the periphery. The dicrotic pulse has two palpable waves, one in the systole and one in diastole (Fig. 220-2*E*). It usually denotes a very low stroke volume, particularly in patients with dilated cardiomyopathy.

Pulsus alternans is a pattern in which there is regular alteration of the pressure pulse amplitude, despite a regular rhythm. It is due to alternating left ventricular contractile force, usually indicates severe impairment of left ventricular function, and commonly occurs in patients who also have a loud third heart sound. Pulsus alternans may also occur during or following paroxysmal tachycardia or for several beats following a premature beat in patients without heart disease. In *pulsus bigeminus*, there is also a regular alteration of pressure pulse amplitude, but it is caused by a premature ventricular contraction that follows each regular beat. In *pulsus paradoxus*, the decrease in systolic arterial pressure that normally accompanies the reduction in arterial pulse amplitude during inspiration is accentuated. In patients with pericardial tamponade (Chap. 232), airway obstruction, or superior vena cava obstruction, the decrease in systolic arterial pressure frequently exceeds the normal decrease of 10 mmHg and the peripheral pulse may disappear completely during inspiration.

Simultaneous palpation of the radial and femoral arterial pulses, which normally are virtually coincident, is important to rule out aortic coarctation, in which the latter pulse is weakened and delayed (Chap. 229).

JUGULAR VENOUS PULSE (JVP)

The two main objectives of the examination of the neck veins are inspection of their waveform and estimation of the central venous pressure (CVP). In most patients, the right internal jugular vein is best for both purposes. Usually, the pulsation of the internal jugular vein is greatest when the trunk is inclined by less than 30°. In patients with elevated venous pressure, it may be necessary to elevate the trunk further, sometimes to as much as 90°. When the neck muscles are relaxed, shining a beam of light tangentially across the skin overlying the vein exposes the pulsations of the internal jugular vein. Simultaneous palpation of the left carotid artery aids the examiner in deciding which pulsations are venous and in relating the venous pulsations to their timing in the cardiac cycle.

The normal JVP reflects phasic pressure changes in the right atrium and consists of two or sometime three positive waves and two negative troughs (Fig. 220-1*B* and 220-3). The positive presystolic *a* wave is produced by venous distention due to right atrial contraction and is the dominant wave in the JVP, particularly during inspiration. Large *a* waves indicate that the right atrium is contracting against an increased resistance, such as occurs with tricuspid stenosis (Fig. 220-3) or more commonly with increased resistance to right ventricular filling (pulmonary hypertension or pulmonic stenosis). Large *a* waves also occur during arrhythmias whenever the right atrium contracts while the tricuspid valve is closed by right ventricular systole. Such "cannon" *a* waves may occur regularly (as during junctional rhythm) or irregularly (as in atrioventricular dissociation with ventricular tachycardia or complete heart block). The *a* wave is absent in patients with atrial fibrillation, and there is an increased delay between the *a* wave and the carotid arterial pulse in patients with first-degree atrioventricular block.

The *c* wave, often observed in the JVP (Fig. 220-1), is a positive wave produced by the bulging of the tricuspid valve into the right atrium during right ventricular isovolumetric systole and by the impact of the carotid artery adjacent to the jugular vein. The *x* descent is due both to atrial relaxation and to the downward displacement of the tricuspid valve during ventricular systole. The *x* descent wave during systole is often accentuated in patients with constrictive pericarditis (Fig. 220-3), but the nadir of this wave is reduced with right ventricular dilation and is often reversed in tricuspid regurgitation. The positive,

FIGURE 220-3 Jugular venous pulse. The normal contour is shown by the solid red line. The A-wave (*a*) is absent in atrial fibrillation (dashed green line). The A-wave becomes large when the right atrium contracts against a greater than normal volume of blood, a noncompliant or hypertrophied right ventricle, or a closing or closed tricuspid valve (dashed blue line). Arrows indicate the beginning and the peak of the A-wave. The numbers represent the heart sounds. The fourth heart sound coincides with the peak of the large or giant A-wave. [*From TC Evans et al: Physical examination, in Cardiology: Fundamentals and Practice, 2d ed, ER Giuliani (ed). St. Louis, Mosby-Year Book, 1991, by permission of the Mayo Foundation.*]

late systolic *v* wave results from the increasing volume of blood in the right atrium during ventricular systole when the tricuspid valve is closed. Tricuspid regurgitation causes the *v* wave to be more prominent; when tricuspid regurgitation becomes severe, the combination of a prominent *v* wave and obliteration of the *x* descent results in a single large positive systolic wave. After the *v* wave peaks, the right atrial pressure falls because of the decreased bulging of the tricuspid valve into the right atrium as right ventricular pressure declines and tricuspid valve opens (Fig. 220-3).

This negative descending limb—the *y* descent of the JVP—is produced mainly by the opening of the tricuspid valve and the subsequent rapid inflow of blood into the right ventricle. A rapid, deep *y* descent in early diastole occurs with severe tricuspid regurgitation. A venous pulse characterized by a sharp *y* descent, a deep *y* trough, and a rapid ascent to the baseline is seen in patients with constrictive pericarditis or with severe right-sided heart failure and a high venous pressure. A slow *y* descent in the JVP suggests an obstruction to right ventricular filling, as occurs with tricuspid stenosis or right atrial myxoma.

The right internal jugular is the best vein to use for accurate estimation of the CVP. The sternal angle is used as the reference point because the center of the right atrium lies approximately 5 cm below the sternal angle in the average patient, regardless of body position. The patient is examined at the optimal degree of trunk elevation for visualization of venous pulsations. The vertical distance between the top of the oscillating venous column and the level of the sternal angle is determined; generally it is less than 3 cm (3 cm + 5 cm = 8 cm blood). The most common cause of a high venous pressure is an elevated right ventricular diastolic pressure.

In patients suspected of having right ventricular failure who have a normal CVP at rest, the *abdominojugular reflux test* may be helpful. The palm of the examiner's hand is placed over the abdomen, and firm pressure is applied for 10 s or more. In normal persons, this maneuver does not alter the jugular venous pressure significantly, but when right heart function is impaired, the upper level of venous pulsation usually increases. A positive abdominojugular test is best defined as an increase in JVP during 10 s of firm midabdominal compression followed by a rapid drop in pressure of 4 cm blood on release of the compression. The most common cause of a positive test is right-sided heart failure secondary to elevated left heart filling pressures. Also, abdominal compression may elicit the JVP pattern typical of tricuspid regurgitation when the resting pulse wave is normal. *Kussmaul's sign*—an increase rather than the normal decrease in the CVP during inspiration—is most often caused by severe right-sided heart failure; it is a frequent finding in patients with constrictive pericarditis or right ventricular infarction.

PRECORDIAL PALPATION

The location, amplitude, duration, and direction of the cardiac impulse usually can be best appreciated with the fingertips. The normal left ventricular apex impulse is located at or medial to the left midclavicular line in the fourth or fifth intercostal space. Left ventricular hypertrophy results in exaggeration of the amplitude, duration, and often size of the normal left ventricular thrust. The impulse may be displaced laterally and downward into the sixth or seventh intercostal space, particularly in patients with a left ventricular volume load such as occurs in cases of aortic regurgitation or dilated cardiomyopathy. Right ventricular hypertrophy often results in a sustained systolic lift at the lower left parasternal area, which starts in early systole and is synchronous with the left ventricular apical impulse.

Abnormal precordial pulsations occur during systole in patients with left ventricular dyssynergy due to ischemic heart disease or to diffuse myocardial disease from some other cause. They are most commonly felt in the left midprecordium one or two interspaces above the left ventricular apex.

A left parasternal lift is frequently present in patients with severe mitral regurgitation and is due to anterior displacement of the right ventricle by an enlarged, expanding left atrium. Pulmonary artery pulsation is often visible and palpable in the second left intercostal space. This pulsation usually denotes pulmonary hypertension or increased pulmonary blood flow.

Thrills are palpable, low frequency vibrations associated with heart murmurs. The systolic murmur of mitral regurgitation may be palpated at the cardiac apex. When the palm of the hand is placed over the precordium, the thrill of aortic stenosis crosses the palm toward the right side of the neck, while the thrill of pulmonic stenosis radiates more often to the left side of the neck. The thrill due to a ventricular septal defect is usually located in the third or fourth intercostal spaces near the left sternal border.

Percussion should be performed to identify normal or abnormal position of the heart, stomach, and liver.

CARDIAC AUSCULTATION

To obtain the most information from cardiac auscultation, the observer should keep in mind several principles: (1) Auscultation should be performed in a quiet room to avoid the distracting noises of normal activity. (2) For optimal auscultation, attention must be focused on the phase of the cardiac cycle during which the auscultatory event is expected to occur. (3) The timing of a heart sound or murmur can be determined accurately from its relation to other observable events in the cardiac cycle—the carotid arterial pulse, the apical impulse, or the JVP.

HEART SOUNDS

The major components of heart sounds are vibrations associated with the abrupt acceleration or deceleration of blood in the cardiovascular system. Studies using simultaneous echocardiographic-phonocardiographic recordings indicate that the first and second heart sounds are produced primarily by the closure of the atrioventricular (AV) and semilunar valves and the events that accompany these closures. The intensity of the *first heart sound* (S_1) is influenced by (1) the position of the mitral leaflets at the onset of ventricular systole; (2) the rate of rise of the left ventricular pressure pulse; (3) the presence or absence of structural disease of the mitral valve; and (4) the amount of tissue, air, or fluid between the heart and the stethoscope. S_1 is louder if diastole is shortened because of tachycardia, if AV flow is increased because of high cardiac output or prolonged because of mitral stenosis, or if atrial contraction precedes ventricular contraction by an unusually short interval, reflected in a short PR interval. The loud S_1 in mitral stenosis usually signifies that the valve is pliable and that it remains open at the onset of isovolumetric contraction because of the elevated left atrial pressure. A soft S_1 may be due to poor conduction of sound through the chest wall, a slow rise of the left ventricular pressure pulse, a long PR interval, or imperfect closure due to reduced valve substance, as in mitral regurgitation. S_1 is also soft when the anterior mitral leaflet is immobile because of rigidity and calcification, even in the presence of predominant mitral stenosis.

Splitting of the two high-pitched components of S_1 by 10–30 ms is a normal phenomenon (Fig. 220-1A). The first component of S_1 is usually attributed to mitral valve closure, and the second to tricuspid valve closure. Widening of the S_1 is due most often to complete right bundle branch block and the resulting delay in onset of the right ventricular pressure pulse.

Splitting of the Second Heart Sound This sound (S_2) normally splits into audibly distinct aortic (A_2) and pulmonic (P_2) components during inspiration, when the augmented inflow into the right ventricle increases its stroke volume and ejection period and thus delays closure of the pulmonic valve. P_2 is coincident with the incisura of the pulmonary artery pressure curve, which is separated from the right ventricular pressure tracing by an interval termed the *hangout time*. The absolute value of this interval reflects the resistance to pulmonary vascular bed. This interval is prolonged, and physiologic splitting of S_2 is accentuated, in conditions associated with right ventricular volume overload and a distensible pulmonary vascular bed. However, in patients with an increase in pulmonary vascular resistance, the hangout time is markedly reduced, and narrow splitting of S_2 is present. Splitting that persists with expiration (heard best at the pulmonic area or left sternal border) is usually abnormal when the patient is in the upright position. Such splitting may be due to many causes: delayed activation of the right ventricle (right bundle branch block); left ventricular ectopic beats; a left ventricular pacemaker; prolongation of right ventricular contraction with an increased right ventricular pressure load (pulmonary embolism or pulmonic stenosis); or delayed pulmonic valve closure because of right ventricular volume overload associated with right ventricular failure or diminished impedance of the pulmonary vascular bed and a prolonged hangout time (atrial septal defect).

In pulmonary hypertension, P_2 is loud, and splitting of S_2 may be diminished, normal, or accentuated, depending on the cause of the pulmonary hypertension, the pulmonary vascular resistance, and the presence or absence of right ventricular decompensation. Early aortic valve closure, occurring with mitral regurgitation or a ventricular septal defect, may also produce splitting that persists during expiration. In patients with an atrial septal defect, the proportion of right atrial filling contributed by the left atrium and the venae cavae varies reciprocally during the respiratory cycle, so that right atrial inflow remains relatively constant. Therefore, the volume and duration of right ventricular ejection are not significantly increased by inspiration, and there is little inspiratory exaggeration of the splitting of S_2. This phenomenon, termed *fixed splitting* of the second heart sound, is of considerable diagnostic value.

A delay in aortic valve closure causing P_2 to precede A_2 results in so-called reversed (paradoxic) splitting of S_2. Splitting is then maximal in expiration and decreases during inspiration with the normal delay of pulmonic valve closure. The most common causes of reversed splitting of S_2 are left bundle branch block and delayed excitation of the left ventricle from a right ventricular ectopic beat. Mechanical prolongation of left ventricular systole, resulting in reversed splitting of S_2, may also be caused by severe aortic outflow obstruction, a large aorta-to-pulmonary artery shunt, systolic hypertension, and ischemic heart disease or cardiomyopathy with left ventricular failure. P_2 is normally softer than A_2 in the second left intercostal space; a P_2 that is greater than A_2 in this area suggests pulmonary hypertension (except in patients with atrial septal defect).

Systolic Sounds The *ejection sound* is a sharp, high-pitched event occurring in early systole and closely following the first heart sound (Fig. 220-1B, ES). Ejection sounds occur in the presence of semilunar valve stenosis and in conditions associated with dilation of the aorta or pulmonary artery. *Nonejection clicks*, or *midsystolic clicks*, occurring with or without a late systolic murmur, often denote prolapse of one or both leaflets of the mitral valve (Chap. 230). They probably result from chordae tendineae that are functionally unequal in length and are best heard along the lower left sternal border and at the left ventricular apex. Systolic clicks usually occur later than the systolic ejection sound.

Diastolic Sounds   The *opening snap* (OS) (Fig. 220-1*A*) is a brief, high-pitched, early diastolic sound, which is usually due to stenosis of an AV valve, most often the mitral valve. It is generally heard best at the lower left sternal border and radiates well to the base of the heart. The A$_2$-OS interval is inversely related to the height of the mean left atrial pressure and ranges from 0.04 to 0.12 s. The OS of tricuspid stenosis occurs later in diastole than the mitral OS and is often overlooked. A tumor plop in patients with left atrial myxoma may have the timing of an opening snap, but it is usually lower-pitched.

The *third heart sound* (S$_3$) (Fig. 220-1*A*) is a low-pitched sound produced in the ventricle 0.14–0.16 s after A$_2$, at the termination of rapid filling. This sound is frequent in normal children and in patients with high cardiac output. However, in patients over 40 years, an S$_3$ usually indicates impairment of ventricular function, AV valve regurgitation, or other conditions that increase the rate or volume of ventricular filling. The left-sided S$_3$ is best heard with the bell piece of the stethoscope at the left ventricular apex during expiration and with the patient in the left lateral position. The right-sided S$_3$ is best heard at the left sternal border or just beneath the xiphoid and is usually louder with inspiration. Third heart sounds often disappear with treatment of heart failure. An S$_3$ that is earlier (0.10–0.12 s after A$_2$) and higher-pitched than normal (a pericardial knock) often occurs in patients with constrictive pericarditis (Chap. 232); its presence depends on the restrictive effect of the adherent pericardium, which abruptly halts diastolic filling.

The *fourth heart sound* (S$_4$) is a low-pitched, presystolic sound produced in the ventricle during ventricular filling; it is associated with an effective atrial contraction and is best heard with the bell piece of the stethoscope. The sound is absent in patients with atrial fibrillation. The S$_4$ occurs when diminished ventricular compliance increases the resistance to ventricular filling; it is frequently present in patients with systemic hypertension, aortic stenosis, hypertrophic cardiomyopathy, ischemic heart disease, and acute mitral regurgitation. Most patients with an acute myocardial infarction and sinus rhythm have an audible S$_4$. The S$_4$ is loudest at the left ventricular apex when the patient is in the left lateral position and is accentuated by mild isotonic or isometric exercise in the supine position. The right-sided S$_4$ is present in patients with right ventricular hypertrophy secondary to either pulmonic stenosis or pulmonary hypertension and frequently accompanies a prominent presystolic *a* wave in the JVP. An S$_4$ frequently accompanies delayed AV conduction, even in the absence of clinically detectable heart disease. The incidence of an audible S$_4$ increases with increasing age. Whether an audible S$_4$ in adults without other evidence of cardiac disease is abnormal remains controversial.

HEART MURMURS

(See also **Chap. e8**) The evaluation of the patient with a heart murmur may vary greatly depending on its intensity, timing, location and radiation, and response to various physiologic maneuvers. The intensity (loudness) of murmurs may be graded from I to VI. A grade I murmur is so faint that it can be heard only with special effort; a grade IV murmur is commonly accompanied by a thrill; and a grade VI murmur is audible with the stethoscope removed from contact with the chest. The configuration of a murmur may be crescendo, decrescendo, crescendo-decrescendo (diamond-shaped), or plateau (Fig. 220-4). The precise time of onset and time of cessation of a murmur depend on the instant in the cardiac cycle at which an adequate pressure difference between two chambers arises and disappears.

The location on the chest wall where the murmur is best heard and the areas to which it radiates can aid in identifying the cardiac structure from which the murmur originates. For example, the murmur of aortic valve stenosis is usually loudest in the second right intercostal space and radiates to the carotid arteries. By contrast, the murmur of mitral regurgitation is most often loudest at the cardiac apex, but it may radiate to the left sternal border and base of the heart when the posterior mitral leaflet is predominantly involved or to the axilla and back when the anterior leaflet is more severely affected.

FIGURE 220-4 A. Schematic representation of ECG, aortic pressure (AOP), left ventricular pressure (LVP), and left atrial pressure (LAP). The shaded areas indicate a transvalvular pressure difference during systole. HSM, holosystolic murmur; MSM, midsystolic murmur. **B.** Graphic representation of ECG, aortic pressure (AOP), left ventricular pressure (LVP), and left atrial pressure (LAP) with shaded areas indicating transvalvular diastolic pressure difference. EDM, early diastolic murmur; PSM, presystolic murmur; MDM, middiastolic murmur.

Effects of Physiologic Interventions   By noting changes in the characteristics of the murmur during maneuvers that alter cardiac hemodynamics, its correct origin and significance can usually be identified (Table 220-1).

Systolic Murmurs   •   *HOLOSYSTOLIC (PANSYSTOLIC) MURMURS*   These are generated when there is flow between two chambers that have widely different pressures throughout systole, such as the left ventricle and either the left atrium or the right ventricle. The pressure gradient occurs early in contraction and lasts until relaxation is almost complete. Therefore, holosystolic murmurs begin before aortic ejection, and at the area of maximal intensity they begin with S$_1$ and end after S$_2$. Holosystolic murmurs accompany mitral or tricuspid regurgitation and ventricular septal defect.

The murmur of tricuspid regurgitation associated with pulmonary hypertension is holosystolic and frequently increases during inspiration. Not all patients with mitral or tricuspid regurgitation or ventricular septal defect have holosystolic murmurs. Often, a mild valvular regurgitant jet, detected by color-flow Doppler techniques (Chap. 222), is not associated with an audible murmur.

MIDSYSTOLIC MURMURS   These are also called *systolic ejection murmurs*, which are often crescendo-decrescendo in shape and occur when blood is ejected across the aortic or pulmonic outflow tracts (Fig. 220-4). The murmur starts shortly after S$_1$, when the ventricular pressure becomes high enough to open the semilunar valve. As the velocity of ejection increases, the murmur gets louder; as ejection declines, it diminishes. The murmur ends before the ventricular pressure falls enough to permit closure of the aortic or pulmonic leaflets. When the semilunar valves are normal, an increased flow rate (as occurs in states of elevated cardiac output), ejection into a dilated vessel beyond the valve, or increased transmission of sound through a thin chest wall may be responsible for this murmur. Most benign, functional murmurs are midsystolic and originate from the pulmonary outflow tract. Valvular or subvalvular obstruction of either ventricle may also cause such a midsystolic murmur, the intensity being related to the flow rate.

The murmur of aortic stenosis is the prototype of the left-sided midsystolic murmur. The location and radiation of this murmur are

TABLE 220-1 EFFECTS OF PHYSIOLOGIC AND PHARMACOLOGIC INTERVENTIONS ON THE INTENSITY OF HEART MURMURS AND SOUNDS

Respiration Systolic murmurs due to TR or pulmonic blood flow through a normal or stenotic valve and diastolic murmurs of TS or PR generally increase with inspiration, as do right-sided S_3 and S_4. Left-sided murmurs and sounds usually are louder during expiration, as is the PES.

Valsalva maneuver Most murmurs decrease in length and intensity. Two exceptions are the systolic murmur of HCM, which usually becomes much louder, and that of MVP, which becomes longer and often louder. Following release of the Valsalva maneuver, right-sided murmurs tend to return to control intensity earlier than left-sided murmurs.

After VPB or AF Murmurs originating at normal or stenotic semilunar valves increase in the cardiac cycle following a VPB or in the cycle after a long cycle length in AF. By contrast, systolic murmurs due to AV valve regurgitation either do not change, diminish (papillary muscle dysfunction), or become shorter (MVP).

Positional changes With *standing,* most murmurs diminish, two exceptions being the murmur of HCM, which becomes louder, and that of MVP, which lengthens and often is intensified. With *squatting,* most murmurs become louder, but those of HCM and MVP usually soften and may disappear. Passive leg raising usually produces the same results.

Exercise Murmurs due to blood flow across normal or obstructed valves (e.g., PS, MS) become louder with both isotonic and submaximal isometric (handgrip) exercise. Murmurs of MR, VSD, and AR also increase with handgrip exercise. However, the murmur of HCM often decreases with near maximum handgrip exercise. Left-sided S_4 and S_3 are often accentuated by exercise, particularly when due to ischemic heart disease.

Note: TR, tricuspid regurgitation; TS, tricuspid stenosis; PR, pulmonic regurgitation; HCM, hypertrophic cardiomyopathy; MVP, mitral valve prolapse; PS, pulmonic stenosis; MS, mitral stenosis; MR, mitral regurgitation; PES, pulmonic ejection sound; VSD, ventricular septal defect; AR, aortic regurgitation; VPB, ventricular premature beat; AF, atrial fibrillation.

influenced by the direction of the high-velocity jet within the aortic root. In *valvular aortic stenosis,* the murmur is usually maximal in the second right intercostal space, with radiation into the neck. The murmur may disappear over the sternum and reappear at the apex, leaving a false impression that mitral regurgitation is present (Gallavardin Phenomenon). In hypertrophic cardiomyopathy, the midsystolic murmur originates in the left ventricular cavity and is usually maximal at the lower left sternal edge and apex, with relatively little radiation to the carotids. When the aortic valve is immobile (calcified), the aortic closure sound (A_2) may be soft and inaudible so that the length and configuration of the murmur are difficult to determine.

The patient's age and the area of maximal intensity aid in determining the significance of midsystolic murmurs. Thus, in a young adult with a thin chest and a high velocity of blood flow, a faint or moderate midsystolic murmur heard only in the pulmonic area is usually without clinical significance, while a somewhat louder murmur in the aortic area may indicate congenital aortic stenosis. In elderly patients, pulmonic flow murmurs are rare, while aortic systolic murmurs are common and may be due to aortic dilation, a significant degree of valvular aortic stenosis, or nonstenotic thickening of the aortic valve leaflets. Midsystolic aortic and pulmonic murmurs are intensified during the cardiac cycle following a premature ventricular beat, while those due to mitral regurgitation are unchanged or softer. Echocardiography may be necessary to separate a prominent and exaggerated functional murmur from one due to congenital or acquired semilunar valve stenosis.

EARLY SYSTOLIC MURMURS These murmurs begin with the first heart sound and end in midsystole. In *large ventricular septal defects with pulmonary hypertension,* the shunting at the end of systole may be small or absent, resulting in an early systolic murmur. A similar murmur may occur with very small *muscular ventricular septal defects.* An early systolic murmur is a feature of *tricuspid regurgitation occurring in the absence of pulmonary hypertension,* a lesion that is common in narcotics abusers

with infective endocarditis. Patients with acute mitral regurgitation into a noncompliant left atrium and a large *v* wave often have a loud early systolic murmur that diminishes as the pressure gradient between the left ventricle and left atrium decreases the late systole (Chap. 230).

LATE SYSTOLIC MURMURS These murmurs are faint or moderately loud, high-pitched apical murmurs that start well after ejection and do not mask either heart sound. They are probably related to papillary muscle dysfunction caused by infarction or ischemia of these muscles or to their distortion by left ventricular dilation. They may appear only during angina but are common in patients with myocardial infarction or diffuse myocardial disease. Late systolic murmurs following midsystolic clicks are due to late systolic mitral regurgitation caused by prolapse of the mitral valve into the left atrium (Chap. 230).

Diastolic Murmurs • *EARLY DIASTOLIC MURMURS* These murmurs begin with or shortly after S_2, as soon as the corresponding ventricular pressure falls enough below that in the aorta or pulmonary artery. The high-pitched murmurs of aortic regurgitation or of pulmonic regurgitation due to pulmonary hypertension are generally decrescendo, since there is a progressive decline in the volume or rate of regurgitation during diastole. Faint, high-pitched murmurs of aortic regurgitation are difficult to hear unless they are specifically sought by applying firm pressure with the diaphragm over the left midsternal border while the patient sits leaning forward and holds a breath in full expiration. The diastolic murmur of aortic regurgitation is enhanced by an acute elevation of the arterial pressure, such as occurs with handgrip.

MIDDIASTOLIC MURMURS These usually arise from the mitral or tricuspid valves, occur during early ventricular filling, and are due to disproportion between valve orifice sizes and flow rate. Such murmurs may be quite loud (grade III/VI), despite only slight AV valve stenosis, when there is normal or increased blood flow. Conversely, the murmurs may be soft or even absent despite severe obstruction if the cardiac output is markedly reduced. When stenosis is marked, the diastolic murmur is prolonged, and the duration of the murmur is more reliable than its intensity as an index of the severity of valve obstruction.

The low-pitched, middiastolic murmur of mitral stenosis characteristically follows the OS. It should be specifically sought by placing the bell of the stethoscope at the site of the left ventricular impulse, which is best localized with the patient on the left side. Frequently, the murmur of mitral stenosis is present only at the left ventricular apex, and it may be increased in intensity by mild supine exercise. In tricuspid stenosis, the middiastolic murmur is localized to a relatively limited area along the left sternal edge and may be louder during inspiration.

Middiastolic murmurs may be generated across the mitral valve in cases of mitral regurgitation, patent ductus arteriosus, or ventricular septal defect, and across the tricuspid valve in cases of tricuspid regurgitation or atrial septal defect. These murmurs are related to the very rapid flow across an AV valve, usually follow an S_3, and tend to occur with large left-to-right shunts or severe AV valve regurgitation.

In acute, severe aortic regurgitation, the left ventricular diastolic pressure may exceed the left atrial pressure, resulting in a middiastolic murmur due to "diastolic mitral regurgitation." In severe, chronic aortic regurgitation, a murmur is frequently present that may be either middiastolic or presystolic (Austin-Flint murmur). This murmur appears to originate at the anterior mitral valve leaflet when blood enters the left ventricle simultaneously from both the aortic root and the left atrium.

PRESYSTOLIC MURMURS These murmurs begin during the period of ventricular filling that follows atrial contraction and therefore occur in sinus rhythm. They are usually due to AV valve stenosis and have the same quality as the middiastolic-filling rumble, but they are usually crescendo, reaching peak intensity at the time of a loud S_1. The presystolic murmur corresponds to the AV valve gradient, which may be minimal until the moment of right or left atrial contraction. It is the presystolic murmur that is most characteristic of tricuspid stenosis and sinus rhythm. A right or left *atrial myxoma* may occasionally cause either middiastolic or presystolic murmurs that resemble the murmurs of mitral or tricuspid stenosis.

CONTINUOUS MURMURS These begin in systole, peak near S_2, and continue into all or part of diastole. These murmurs result from continuous flow due to a communication between high- and low-pressure areas that persists through the end of systole and the beginning of diastole. A *patent ductus arteriosus* causes a continuous murmur as long as the pressure in the pulmonary artery is much below that in the aorta. When pulmonary hypertension is present, the diastolic portion may disappear, leaving the murmur confined to systole. Surgically produced connections and the subclavian-pulmonary artery anastomosis result in murmurs similar to that of a patent ductus.

Continuous murmurs may result from congenital or acquired *systemic arteriovenous fistula*, *coronary arteriovenous fistula*, anomalous origin of the left coronary artery from the pulmonary artery, and *communications between the sinus of Valsalva and the right side of the heart.* Murmurs associated with *pulmonary arteriovenous fistulas* may be continuous but are usually only systolic. Continuous murmurs may also be due to disturbances of flow pattern in constricted systemic (e.g., renal) or pulmonary arteries when marked pressure differences between the two sides of the narrow segment persist; a continuous murmur in the back may be present in *coarctation of the aorta*; *pulmonary embolism* may cause continuous murmurs in partially occluded vessels.

The "mammary souffle," an innocent murmur heard over the breasts during late pregnancy and in the early postpartum period, may be systolic or continuous. The innocent cervical venous hum is a continuous murmur usually audible over the medial aspect of the right supraclavicular fossa with the patient upright. The hum is usually louder during diastole and can be abolished instantaneously by digital compression of the ipsilateral internal jugular vein. Transmission of a loud venous hum to the area below the clavicles may result in a mistaken diagnosis of patent ductus arteriosus.

Pericardial Friction Rub (See also Chap. 232) These adventitious sounds may have presystolic, systolic, and early diastolic scratchy components and may be confused with a murmur or extracardiac sound when heard only in systole. A pericardial friction rub is best appreciated with the patient upright and leaning forward and may be accentuated during expiration.

FURTHER READINGS

BRAUNWALD E, PERLOFF JK: Physical examination of the heart and circulation, in *Braunwald's Heart Disease*, 7th ed, D Zipes et al (eds). Philadelphia, Saunders, 2005

GOSWAMI MJ et al: The history, physical examination and cardiac auscultation, in *Hurst's The Heart Manual of Cardiology*, 11th ed, RA O'Rourke et al (eds). New York, McGraw Hill Medical Publishers, 2006

JAVHAR S: The demise of the physical exam. N Engl J Med 354:548, 2006

MARKEL H: The stethoscope and the art of listening. N Engl J Med 354:551, 2006

O'ROURKE RA: Approach to a patient with a heart murmur, in *Primary Cardiology*, 2d ed, E Braunwald, L Goldman (eds). Philadelphia, Saunders, 2003

PERLOFF JK (ed): *Physical Examination of the Heart and Circulation*, 3d ed. Philadelphia, Saunders, 2000

VLACHOPOULOUS C, O'ROURKE MF: Genesis of the normal and abnormal arterial pulse. Curr Probl Cardiol 25:297, 2000

221 Electrocardiography
Ary L. Goldberger

The electrocardiogram (ECG or EKG) is a graphic recording of electric potentials generated by the heart. The signals are detected by means of metal electrodes attached to the extremities and chest wall and are then amplified and recorded by the electrocardiograph. ECG *leads* actually display the instantaneous *differences* in potential between these electrodes.

The clinical utility of the ECG derives from its immediate availability as a noninvasive, inexpensive, and highly versatile test. In addition to its use in detecting arrhythmias, conduction disturbances, and myocardial ischemia, electrocardiography may reveal other findings related to life-threatening metabolic disturbances (e.g., hyperkalemia) or increased susceptibility to sudden cardiac death (e.g., QT prolongation syndromes). The widespread use of coronary fibrinolysis and acute percutaneous coronary interventions in the early therapy of acute myocardial infarction (Chap. 239) has refocused attention on the sensitivity and specificity of ECG signs of myocardial ischemia.

ELECTROPHYSIOLOGY

(See also Chaps. 225 and 226) Depolarization of the heart is the initiating event for cardiac contraction. The electric currents that spread through the heart are produced by three components: cardiac pacemaker cells, specialized conduction tissue, and the heart muscle itself. The ECG, however, records only the depolarization (stimulation) and repolarization (recovery) potentials generated by the atrial and ventricular myocardium.

The depolarization stimulus for the normal heartbeat originates in the *sinoatrial* (SA) *node* (Fig. 221-1), or *sinus node*, a collection of *pacemaker cells*. These cells fire spontaneously; that is, they exhibit *automaticity*. The first phase of cardiac electrical activation is the spread of the depolarization wave through the right and left atria, followed by atrial contraction. Next, the impulse stimulates pacemaker and specialized conduction tissues in the atrioventricular (AV) nodal and His-bundle areas; together, these two regions constitute the AV junction. The bundle of His bifurcates into two main branches, the right and left bundles, which rapidly transmit depolarization wavefronts to the right and left ventricular myocardium by way of Purkinje fibers. The main left bundle bifurcates into two primary subdivisions, a left anterior fascicle and a left posterior fascicle. The depolarization wavefronts then spread through the ventricular wall, from endocardium to epicardium, triggering ventricular contraction.

Since the cardiac depolarization and repolarization waves have direction and magnitude, they can be represented by vectors. *Vectorcardiograms* that measure and display these instantaneous potentials are no longer used much in clinical practice. However, the general princi-

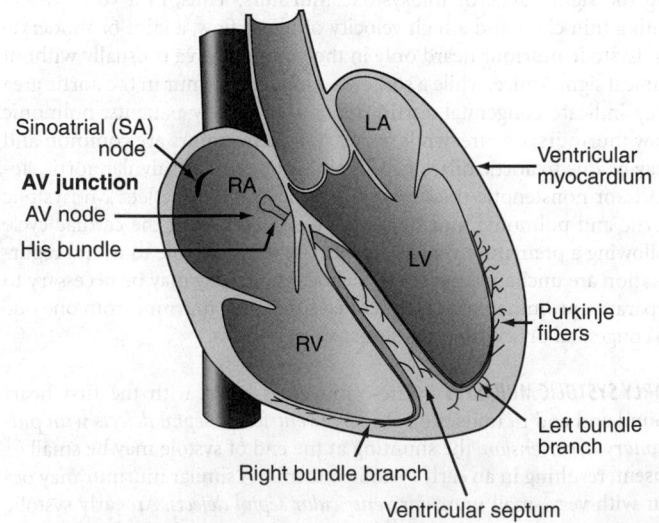

FIGURE 221-1 Schematic of the cardiac conduction system.

FIGURE 221-2 Basic ECG waveforms and intervals. Not shown is the R-R interval, the time between consecutive QRS complexes.

ples of vector analysis remain fundamental to understanding the genesis of normal and pathologic ECG waveforms. Vector analysis illustrates a central concept of electrocardiography—that the ECG records the complex spatial and temporal summation of electrical potentials from multiple myocardial fibers conducted to the surface of the body. This principle accounts for inherent limitations in both ECG *sensitivity* (activity from certain cardiac regions may be canceled out or may be too weak to be recorded) and *specificity* (the same vectorial sum can result from either a selective gain or a loss of forces in opposite directions).

ECG WAVEFORMS AND INTERVALS

The ECG waveforms are labeled alphabetically, beginning with the P wave, which represents atrial depolarization (Fig. 221-2). The QRS complex represents ventricular depolarization, and the ST-T-U complex (ST segment, T wave, and U wave) represents ventricular repolarization. The J point is the junction between the end of the QRS complex and the beginning of the ST segment. Atrial repolarization is usually too low in amplitude to be detected, but it may become apparent in such conditions as acute pericarditis or atrial infarction.

The QRS-T waveforms of the surface ECG correspond in a general way with the different phases of simultaneously obtained ventricular *action potentials*, the intracellular recordings from single myocardial fibers (Chap. 225). The rapid upstroke (phase 0) of the action potential corresponds to the onset of QRS. The plateau (phase 2) corresponds to the isoelectric ST segment, and active repolarization (phase 3) to the inscription of the T wave. Factors that decrease the slope of phase 0 by impairing the influx of Na^+ (e.g., hyperkalemia, or drugs such as flecainide) tend to increase QRS duration. Conditions that prolong phase 2 (use of amiodarone, hypocalcemia) increase the QT interval. In contrast, shortening of ventricular repolarization (phase 2), as by digitalis administration or hypercalcemia, abbreviates the ST segment.

The electrocardiogram is ordinarily recorded on special graph paper which is divided into 1-mm² gridlike boxes. Since the ECG paper speed is generally 25 mm/s, the smallest (1 mm) horizontal divisions correspond to 0.04 (40 ms), with heavier lines at intervals of 0.20 s (200 ms). Vertically, the ECG graph measures the amplitude of a given wave or deflection (1 mV = 10 mm with standard calibration; the voltage criteria for hypertrophy mentioned below are given in millimeters). There are four major ECG intervals: R-R, PR, QRS, and QT (Fig. 221-2). The heart rate (beats per minute) can be readily computed from the interbeat (R-R) interval by dividing the number of large (0.20 s) time units between consecutive R waves into 300 or the number of small (0.04 s) units into 1500. The PR interval measures

the time (normally 120–200 ms) between atrial and ventricular depolarization, which includes the physiologic delay imposed by stimulation of cells in the AV junction area. The QRS interval (normally 100-110 ms or less) reflects the duration of ventricular depolarization. The QT interval includes both ventricular depolarization and repolarization times and varies inversely with the heart rate. A rate-related ("corrected") QT interval, QT_c, can be calculated as $QT/\sqrt{RR}$ and normally is ≤0.44 s. (Some references give QT_c upper normal limits as 0.43 s in men and 0.45 s in women.)

The QRS complex is subdivided into specific deflections or waves. If the initial QRS deflection in a given lead is negative, it is termed a *Q wave*; the first positive deflection is termed an *R wave*. A negative deflection after an R wave is an *S wave*. Subsequent positive or negative waves are labeled R′ and S′, respectively. Lowercase letters (qrs) are used for waves of relatively small amplitude. An entirely negative QRS complex is termed a *QS wave*.

ECG LEADS

The 12 conventional ECG leads record the difference in potential between electrodes placed on the surface of the body. These leads are divided into two groups: six limb (extremity) leads and six chest (precordial) leads. The limb leads record potentials transmitted onto the *frontal plane* (Fig. 221-3A), and the chest leads record potentials transmitted onto the *horizontal plane* (Fig. 221-3B). The six limb leads are further subdivided into three standard "bipolar" leads (I, II, and III) and three augmented "unipolar" leads (aVR, aVL, and aVF). Each standard lead measures the difference in potential between electrodes at two extremities: lead I = left arm – right arm voltages, lead II = left leg – right arm, and lead III = left leg – left arm. The unipolar leads measure the voltage (V) at one locus relative to an electrode (called the *central terminal* or *indifferent electrode*) that has approximately zero potential. Thus, aVR = right arm, aVL = left arm, and aVF = left leg (foot). The lowercase *a* indicates that these unipolar potentials are electrically augmented by 50%. The right leg electrode functions as a ground. The spatial orientation and polarity of the six frontal plane leads is represented on the hexaxial diagram (Fig. 221-4).

The six chest leads (Fig. 221-5) are unipolar recordings obtained by electrodes in the following positions: lead V_1, fourth intercostal space, just to the right of the sternum; lead V_2, fourth intercostal space, just to the left of the sternum; lead V_3, midway between V_2 and V_4; lead V_4, midclavicular line, fifth intercostal space; lead V_5, anterior axillary line, same level as V_4; and lead V_6, midaxillary line, same level as V_4 and V_5.

Together, the frontal and horizontal plane electrodes provide a three-dimensional representation of cardiac electrical activity. Each lead can be likened to a different camera angle "looking" at the same events—atrial and ventricular depolarization and repolarization—from different spatial orientations. The conventional 12-lead ECG can be supplemented with additional leads under special circumstances. For example, right precordial leads V_3R, V_4R, etc., are useful in detect-

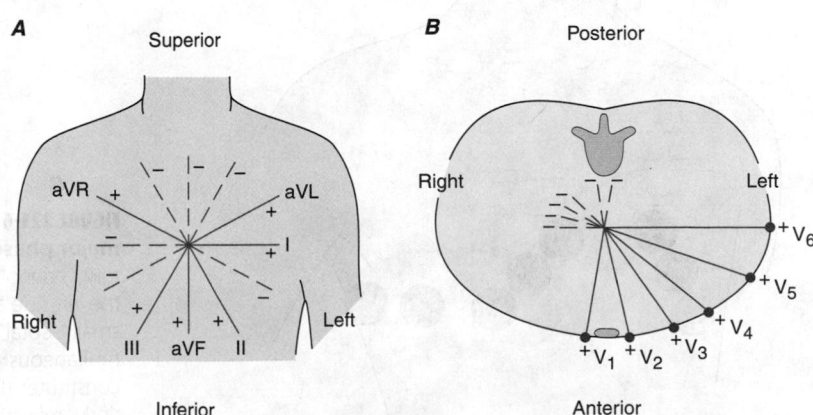

FIGURE 221-3 The six frontal plane (A) and six horizontal plane (B) leads provide a three-dimensional representation of cardiac electrical activity.

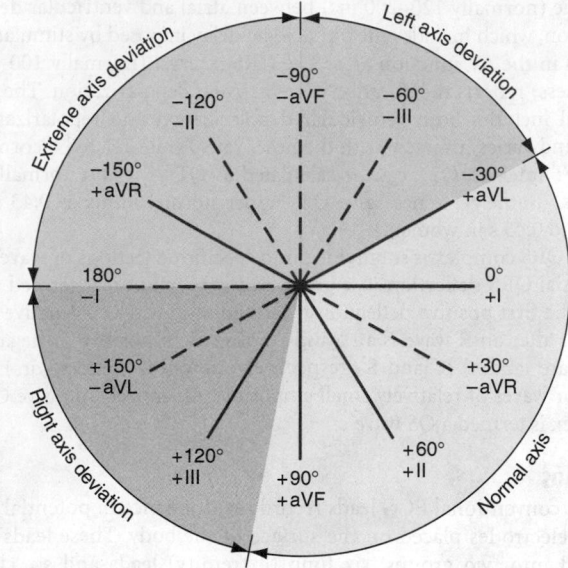

FIGURE 221-4 The frontal plane (limb or extremity) leads are represented on a hexaxial diagram. Each ECG lead has a specific spatial orientation and polarity. The positive pole of each lead axis (*solid line*) and negative pole (*hatched line*) are designated by their angular position relative to the positive pole of lead I (0°). The mean electrical axis of the QRS complex is measured with respect to this display.

ing evidence of acute right ventricular ischemia. Bedside monitors and ambulatory ECG (Holter) recordings usually employ only one or two modified leads. **Intracardiac electrocardiography and electrophysiologic testing are discussed in Chaps. 225 and 226.**

The ECG leads are configured so that a positive (upright) deflection is recorded in a lead if a wave of depolarization spreads toward the positive pole of that lead, and a negative deflection if the wave spreads toward the negative pole. If the mean orientation of the depolarization vector is at right angles to a given lead axis, a biphasic (equally positive and negative) deflection will be recorded.

GENESIS OF THE NORMAL ECG

P WAVE

The normal atrial depolarization vector is oriented downward and toward the subject's left, reflecting the spread of depolarization from the sinus node to the right and then the left atrial myocardium. Since this vector points toward the positive pole of lead II and toward the negative pole of lead aVR, the normal P wave will be positive in lead II and negative in lead aVR. By contrast, activation of the atria from an ectopic pacemaker in the

FIGURE 221-5 The horizontal plane (chest or precordial) leads are obtained with electrodes in the locations shown.

lower part of either atrium or in the AV junction region may produce retrograde P waves (negative in lead II, positive in lead aVR). The normal P wave in lead V_1 may be biphasic with a positive component reflecting right atrial depolarization, followed by a small (<1 mm²) negative component reflecting left atrial depolarization.

QRS COMPLEX

Normal ventricular depolarization proceeds as a rapid, continuous spread of activation wavefronts. This complex process can be divided into two major, sequential phases, and each phase can be represented by a mean vector (Fig. 221-6). The first phase is depolarization of the interventricular septum from the left to the right and anteriorly (vector 1). The second results from the simultaneous depolarization of the right and left ventricles; it is normally dominated by the more massive left ventricle, so that vector 2 points leftward and posteriorly. Therefore, a right precordial lead (V_1) will record this biphasic depolarization process with a small positive deflection (septal r wave) followed by a larger negative deflection (S wave). A left precordial lead, e.g. V_6, will record the same sequence with a small negative deflection (septal q wave) followed by a relatively tall positive deflection (R wave). Intermediate leads show a relative increase in R-wave amplitude (normal R-wave progression) and a decrease in S-wave amplitude progressing across the chest from the right to left. The precordial lead where the R and S waves are of approximately equal amplitude is referred to as the *transition zone* (usually V_3 or V_4) (Fig. 221-7).

The QRS pattern in the extremity leads may vary considerably from one normal subject to another depending on the *electrical axis* of the

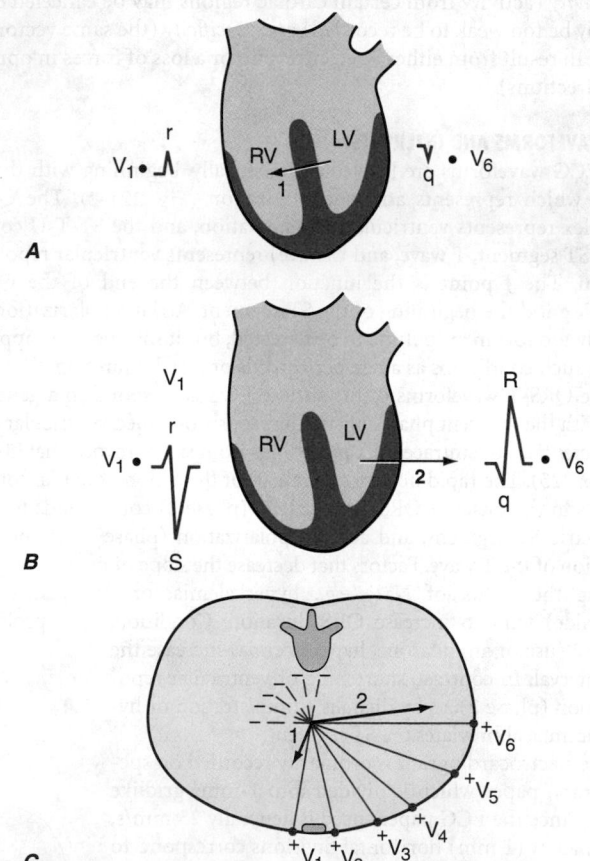

FIGURE 221-6 Ventricular depolarization can be divided into two major phases, each represented by a vector. *A.* The first phase (*arrow 1*) denotes depolarization of the ventricular septum, beginning on the left side and spreading to the right. This process is represented by a small "septal" r wave in lead V_1 and a small septal q wave in lead V_6. ***B.*** Simultaneous depolarization of the left and right ventricles (LV and RV) constitutes the second phase. Vector 2 is oriented to the left and posteriorly, reflecting the electrical predominance of the LV. ***C.*** Vectors (*arrows*) representing these two phases are shown in reference to the horizontal plane leads. (*After Goldberger, 2006.*)

FIGURE 221-7 Normal electrocardiogram from a healthy subject. Sinus rhythm is present with a heart rate of 75 beats per minute. PR interval is 0.16 s; QRS interval (duration) is 0.08 s; QT interval is 0.36 s; QT$_c$ is 0.40 s; the mean QRS axis is about +70°. The precordial leads show normal R-wave progression with the transition zone (R wave = S wave) in lead V$_3$.

QRS, which describes the mean orientation of the QRS vector with reference to the six frontal plane leads. Normally, the QRS axis ranges from −30° to +100° (Fig. 221-4). An axis more negative than −30° is referred to as *left axis deviation*, while an axis more positive than +100° is referred to as *right axis deviation*. Left axis deviation may occur as a normal variant but is more commonly associated with left ventricular hypertrophy, a block in the anterior fascicle of the left bundle system (left anterior fascicular block or hemiblock), or inferior myocardial infarction. Right axis deviation may also occur as a normal variant (particularly in children and young adults); as a spurious finding due to reversal of the left and right arm electrodes; or in conditions such as right ventricular overload (acute or chronic), infarction of the lateral wall of the left ventricle, dextrocardia, left pneumothorax, or left posterior fascicular block.

T WAVE AND U WAVE

Normally, the mean T-wave vector is oriented roughly concordant with the mean QRS vector (within about 45° in the frontal plane). Since depolarization and repolarization are electrically opposite processes, this normal QRS–T-wave vector concordance indicates that repolarization must normally proceed in the reverse direction from depolarization (i.e., from ventricular epicardium to endocardium). The normal U wave is a small, rounded deflection (≤1 mm) that follows the T wave and usually has the same polarity as the T wave. An abnormal increase in U-wave amplitude is most commonly due to drugs (e.g., dofetilide, amiodarone, sotalol, quinidine, procainamide, disopyramide) or to hypokalemia. Very prominent U waves are a marker of increased susceptibility to the *torsades de pointe* type of ventricular tachycardia (Chap. 226). Inversion of the U wave in the precordial leads is abnormal and may be a subtle sign of ischemia.

MAJOR ECG ABNORMALITIES

CARDIAC ENLARGEMENT AND HYPERTROPHY

Right atrial overload (acute or chronic) may lead to an increase in P-wave amplitude (≥2.5 mm) **(Fig. 221-8)**. Left atrial overload typically produces a biphasic P wave in V$_1$ with a broad negative component or a broad (≥120 ms), often notched P wave in one or more limb leads (Fig. 221-8). This pattern may also occur with left atrial conduction delays in the absence of actual atrial enlargement, leading to the more general designation of *left atrial abnormality*.

Right ventricular hypertrophy due to a pressure load (as from pulmonic valve stenosis or pulmonary artery hypertension) is characterized by a relatively tall R wave in lead V$_1$ (R ≥ S wave), usually with right axis deviation **(Fig. 221-9)**; alternatively, there may be a qR pattern in V$_1$ or V$_3$R. ST depression and T-wave inversion in the right to midprecordial leads are also often present. This pattern, formerly called right ventricu-

lar "strain," is attributed to repolarization abnormalities in acutely or chronically overloaded muscle. Prominent S waves may occur in the left lateral precordial leads. Right ventricular hypertrophy due to ostium secundum–type atrial septal defects, with the accompanying right ventricular volume overload, is commonly associated with an incomplete or complete right bundle branch block pattern with a rightward QRS axis.

Acute cor pulmonale due to pulmonary embolism (Chap. 256), for example, may be associated with a normal ECG or a variety of abnormalities. Sinus tachycardia is the most common arrhythmia, although other tachyarrhythmias, such as atrial fibrillation or flutter, may occur. The QRS axis may shift to the right, sometimes in concert with the so-called S$_1$Q$_3$T$_3$ pattern (prominence of the S wave in lead I, Q wave in lead III, with T-wave inversion in lead III). Acute right ventricular dilation may also be associated with slow R-wave progression and T-wave inversions in V$_1$ to V$_4$ simulating acute anterior infarction. A right ventricular conduction disturbance may appear.

Chronic cor pulmonale due to obstructive lung disease (Chap. 227) usually does not produce the classic ECG patterns of right ventricular hypertrophy noted above. Instead of tall right precordial R waves, chronic lung disease more typically is associated with small R waves in right-to-midprecordial leads (slow R-wave progression) due in part to downward displacement of the diaphragm and the heart. Low-voltage complexes are commonly present, owing to hyperaeration of the lungs.

A number of different voltage criteria for *left ventricular hypertrophy* (Fig. 221-9) have been proposed on the basis of the presence of tall left precordial R waves and deep right precordial S waves [e.g., SV$_1$ + (RV$_5$ or RV$_6$) > 35 mm]. Repolarization abnormalities (ST depression with T-wave inversions, formerly called the left ventricular "strain"

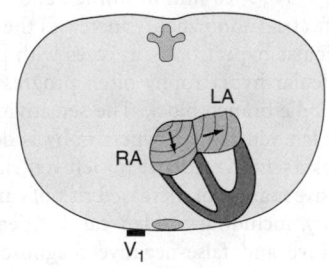

	Normal	Right	Left
II	RA ← → LA	RA (tall peaked) ← LA	RA ← → LA (notched)
V$_1$	RA / LA	RA / LA	RA / LA (biphasic)

FIGURE 221-8 Right atrial (RA) overload may cause tall, peaked P waves in the limb or precordial leads. Left atrial (LA) abnormality may cause broad, often notched P waves in the limb leads and a biphasic P wave in lead V1 with a prominent negative component representing delayed depolarization of the LA. (*After MK Park, WG Guntheroth: How to Read Pediatric ECGs, 4th ed. St. Louis, Mosby/Elsevier, 2006.*)

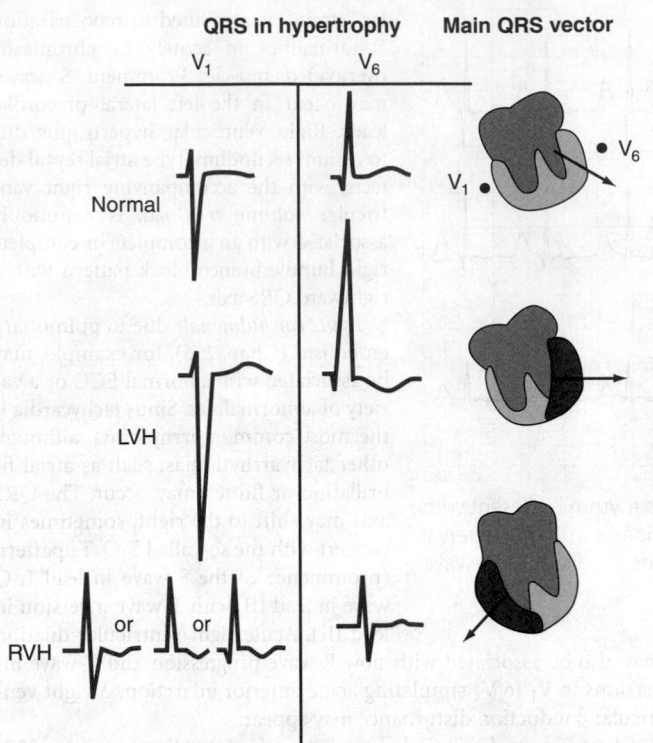

FIGURE 221-9 Left ventricular hypertrophy (LVH) increases the amplitude of electrical forces directed to the left and posteriorly. In addition, repolarization abnormalities may cause ST-segment depression and T-wave inversion in leads with a prominent R wave. Right ventricular hypertrophy (RVH) may shift the QRS vector to the right; this effect usually is associated with an R, RS, or qR complex in lead V_1. T-wave inversions may be present in right precordial leads.

pattern) may also appear in leads with prominent R waves. However, prominent precordial voltages may occur as a normal variant, especially in athletic or young individuals. Left ventricular hypertrophy may increase limb lead voltage with or without increased precordial voltage (e.g., $RaVL + SV_3 > 20$ mm in women and > 28 mm in men). The presence of left atrial abnormality increases the likelihood of underlying left ventricular hypertrophy in cases with borderline voltage criteria. Left ventricular hypertrophy often progresses to incomplete or complete left bundle branch block. The sensitivity of conventional voltage criteria for left ventricular hypertrophy is decreased in obese persons and in smokers. ECG evidence for left ventricular hypertrophy is a major noninvasive marker of increased risk of cardiovascular morbidity and mortality, including sudden cardiac death. However, because of false-positive and false-negative diagnoses, the ECG is of limited utility in diagnosing atrial or ventricular enlargement. More definitive information is provided by echocardiography (Chap. 222).

BUNDLE BRANCH BLOCKS

Intrinsic impairment of conduction in either the right or left bundle system (intraventricular conduction disturbances) leads to prolongation of the QRS interval. With complete bundle branch blocks, the QRS interval is ≥120 ms in duration; with incomplete blocks the QRS interval is between 100 and 120 ms. The QRS vector is usually oriented in the direction of the myocardial region where depolarization is delayed (Fig. 221-10). Thus, with right bundle branch block, the terminal QRS vector is oriented to the right and anteriorly (rSR′ in V_1 and qRS in V_6, typically). Left bundle branch block alters both early and later phases of ventricular depolarization. The major QRS vector is directed to the left and posteriorly. In addition, the normal early left-to-right pattern of septal activation is disrupted such that septal depolarization proceeds from right to left as well. As a result, left bundle branch block generates wide, predominantly negative (QS) complexes in lead V_1 and entirely positive (R) complexes in lead V_6. A pattern

FIGURE 221-10 Comparison of typical QRS-T patterns in right bundle branch block (RBBB) and left bundle branch block (LBBB) with the normal pattern in leads V_1 and V_6. Note the secondary T-wave inversions (*arrows*) in leads with an rSR′ complex with RBBB and in leads with a wide R wave with LBBB.

identical to that of left bundle branch block, preceded by a sharp spike, is seen in most cases of electronic right ventricular pacing because of the relative delay in left ventricular activation.

Bundle branch block may occur in a variety of conditions. In subjects without structural heart disease, right bundle branch block is seen more commonly than left bundle branch block. Right bundle branch block also occurs with heart disease, both congenital (e.g., atrial septal defect) and acquired (e.g., valvular, ischemic). Left bundle branch block is often a marker of one of four underlying conditions associated with increased risk of cardiovascular morbidity and mortality: coronary heart disease (frequently with impaired left ventricular function), hypertensive heart disease, aortic valve disease, and cardiomyopathy. Bundle branch blocks may be chronic or intermittent. A bundle branch block may be rate-related; for example, it often occurs when the heart rate exceeds some critical value.

Bundle branch blocks and depolarization abnormalities secondary to artificial pacemakers not only affect ventricular depolarization (QRS) but are also characteristically associated with *secondary repolarization* (ST-T) abnormalities. With bundle branch blocks, the T wave is typically opposite in polarity to the last deflection of the QRS (Fig. 221-10). This discordance of the QRS–T-wave vectors is caused by the altered sequence of repolarization that occurs secondary to altered depolarization. In contrast, *primary repolarization* abnormalities are independent of QRS changes and are related instead to actual alterations in the electrical properties of the myocardial fibers themselves (e.g., in the resting membrane potential or action potential duration), not just to changes in the sequence of repolarization. Ischemia, electrolyte imbalance, and drugs such as digitalis all cause such primary ST–T-wave changes. Primary and secondary T-wave changes may coexist. For example, T-wave inversions in the right precordial leads with left bundle branch block or in the left precordial leads with right bundle branch block may be important markers of underlying ischemia or other abnormalities. A distinctive abnormality simulating right bundle branch block with ST-segment elevations in the right chest leads is seen with the Brugada pattern (Chap. 226).

Partial blocks (fascicular or "hemiblocks") in the left bundle system (left anterior or posterior fascicular blocks) generally do not prolong the QRS duration substantially but instead are associated with shifts in

FIGURE 221-11 Acute ischemia causes a current of injury. With predominant subendocardial ischemia (**A**), the resultant ST vector will be directed toward the inner layer of the affected ventricle and the ventricular cavity. Overlying leads therefore will record ST depression. With ischemia involving the outer ventricular layer (**B**) (transmural or epicardial injury), the ST vector will be directed outward. Overlying leads will record ST elevation.

FIGURE 221-12 Severe anterior wall ischemia (with or without infarction) may cause prominent T-wave inversions in the precordial leads. This pattern is usually associated with a high-grade stenosis of the left anterior descending coronary artery.

the frontal plane QRS axis (leftward or rightward, respectively). More complex combinations of fascicular and bundle branch blocks may occur involving the left and right bundle system. Examples of *bifascicular block* include right bundle branch block and left posterior fascicular block, right bundle branch block with left anterior fascicular block, and complete left bundle branch block. Chronic bifascicular block in an asymptomatic individual is associated with a relatively low risk of progression to high-degree AV heart block. In contrast, new bifascicular block with acute anterior myocardial infarction carries a much greater risk of complete heart block. Alternation of right and left bundle branch block is a sign of *trifascicular disease*. However, the presence of a prolonged PR interval and bifascicular block does not necessarily indicate trifascicular involvement, since this combination may arise with AV node disease and bifascicular block. Intraventricular conduction delays can also be caused by extrinsic (toxic) factors that slow ventricular conduction, particularly hyperkalemia or drugs (e.g., class 1 antiarrhythmic agents, tricyclic antidepressants, phenothiazines).

Prolongation of QRS duration does not necessarily indicate a conduction delay but may be due to *preexcitation* of the ventricles via a bypass tract, as in Wolff-Parkinson-White (WPW) patterns (Chap. 226) and related variants. The diagnostic triad of WPW consists of a wide QRS complex associated with a relatively short PR interval and slurring of the initial part of the QRS (delta wave), the latter effect due to aberrant activation of ventricular myocardium. The presence of a bypass tract predisposes to reentrant supraventricular tachyarrhythmias.

MYOCARDIAL ISCHEMIA AND INFARCTION

(See also Chap. 239) The ECG is a cornerstone in the diagnosis of acute and chronic ischemic heart disease. The findings depend on several key factors: the nature of the process [reversible (i.e., ischemia) versus irreversible (i.e., infarction)], the duration (acute versus chronic), extent (transmural versus subendocardial), and localization (anterior versus inferoposterior), as well as the presence of other underlying abnormalities (ventricular hypertrophy, conduction defects).

Ischemia exerts complex time-dependent effects on the electrical properties of myocardial cells. Severe, acute ischemia lowers the resting membrane potential and shortens the duration of the action potential. Such changes cause a voltage gradient between normal and ischemic zones. As a consequence, current flows between these regions. These currents of injury are represented on the surface ECG by deviation of the ST segment (Fig. 221-11). When the acute ischemia is

transmural, the ST vector is usually shifted in the direction of the outer (epicardial) layers, producing ST elevations and sometimes, in the earliest stages of ischemia, tall, positive so-called hyperacute T waves over the ischemic zone. With ischemia confined primarily to the *subendocardium*, the ST vector typically shifts toward the subendocardium and ventricular cavity, so that overlying (e.g., anterior precordial) leads show ST-segment depression (with ST elevation in lead aVR). Multiple factors affect the amplitude of acute ischemic ST deviations. Profound ST elevation or depression in multiple leads usually indicates very severe ischemia. From a clinical viewpoint, the division of acute myocardial infarction into ST segment elevation and non-ST elevation types is useful since the efficacy of acute reperfusion therapy is limited to the former group.

The ECG leads are more helpful in localizing regions of ST elevation than non-ST elevation ischemia. For example, acute transmural anterior (including apical and lateral) wall ischemia is reflected by ST elevations or increased T-wave positivity in one or more of the precordial leads (V_1–V_6) and leads I and aVL. Inferior wall ischemia produces changes in leads II, III, and aVF. Posterior wall ischemia may be indirectly recognized by *reciprocal* ST depressions in leads V_1 to V_3. Prominent reciprocal ST depressions in these leads also occur with certain inferior wall infarcts, particularly those with posterior or lateral wall extension. Right ventricular ischemia usually produces ST elevations in right-sided chest leads (Fig. 221-5). When ischemic ST elevations occur as the earliest sign of acute infarction, they are typically followed within a period ranging from hours to days by evolving T-wave inversions and often by Q waves occurring in the same lead distribution. (T-wave inversions due to evolving or chronic ischemia correlate with prolongation of repolarization and are often associated with QT lengthening.) Reversible transmural ischemia, for example, due to coronary vasospasm (Prinzmetal's variant angina, and possibly the tako-tsubo cardiomyopathy syndrome), may cause transient ST-segment elevations without development of Q waves. Depending on the severity and duration of such ischemia, the ST elevations may either resolve completely in minutes or be followed by T-wave inversions that persist for hours or even days. Patients with ischemic chest pain who present with deep T-wave inversions in multiple precordial leads (e.g., V_1–V_4) with or without cardiac enzyme elevations typically have severe obstruction in the left anterior descending coronary artery system (Fig. 221-12). In contrast, patients whose baseline ECG already shows abnormal T-wave inversions may develop T-wave normalization (pseudonormalization) during episodes of acute transmural ischemia.

With infarction, depolarization (QRS) changes often accompany repolarization (ST-T) abnormalities. Necrosis of sufficient myocardial tissue may lead to decreased R-wave amplitude or abnormal Q waves in the anterior or inferior leads (Fig. 221-13). Previously, abnormal Q waves were considered to be markers of transmural myocardial infarction, while subendocardial infarcts were thought not to produce Q waves. However, careful ECG-pathology correlative studies have indicated that transmural infarcts may occur without Q waves and that subendocardial (nontransmural) infarcts may sometimes be associated with Q waves. Therefore, infarcts are more appropriately classified as "Q-wave" or "non-Q-wave." The major acute ECG changes in syndromes of ischemic heart disease are summarized schematically in Fig. 221-14. Loss of depolarization forces due to posterior or lateral infarction may cause reciprocal increases in R-wave amplitude in leads V_1 and V_2 without diagnostic Q waves in any of

FIGURE 221-13 Sequence of depolarization and repolarization changes with (**A**) acute anterior and (**B**) acute inferior wall Q-wave infarctions. With anterior infarcts, ST elevation in leads I, aVL, and the precordial leads may be accompanied by reciprocal ST depressions in leads II, III, and aVF. Conversely, acute inferior (or posterior) infarcts may be associated with reciprocal ST depressions in leads V_1 to V_3. (*After Goldberger, 2006.*)

the conventional leads. Atrial infarction may be associated with PR-segment deviations due to an atrial current of injury, changes in P-wave morphology, or atrial arrhythmias.

In the weeks and months following infarction, these ECG changes may persist or begin to resolve. Complete normalization of the ECG following Q-wave infarction is uncommon but may occur, particularly with smaller infarcts. In contrast, ST-segment elevations that persist for several weeks or more after a Q-wave infarct usually correlate with a severe underlying wall motion disorder (akinetic or dyskinetic zone), although not necessarily a frank ventricular aneurysm.

ECG changes due to ischemia may occur spontaneously or may be provoked by various exercise protocols (stress electrocardiography) (Chap. 237). In patients with severe ischemic heart disease, exercise testing is most likely to elicit signs of subendocardial ischemia (horizontal or downsloping ST depression in multiple leads). ST-segment elevation during exercise is most often observed after a Q-wave infarct. This repolarization change does not necessarily indicate active ischemia but correlates strongly with the presence of an underlying ventricular wall motion abnormality. However, in patients *without* prior infarction, transient ST-segment elevation with exercise is a reliable sign of transmural ischemia.

The ECG has important limitations in both sensitivity and specificity in the diagnosis of ischemic heart disease. Although a single normal ECG does not exclude ischemia or even acute infarction, a normal ECG *throughout* the course of an acute infarct is distinctly uncommon. Prolonged chest pain without diagnostic ECG changes, therefore, should always prompt a careful search for other noncoronary causes of chest pain (Chap. 13). Furthermore, the diagnostic changes of acute or evolving ischemia are often masked by the presence of left bundle branch block, electronic ventricular pacemaker patterns, and WPW preexcitation. On the other hand, clinicians may overdiagnose ischemia or infarction based on the presence of ST-segment elevations or depressions, T-wave inversions, tall positive T waves, or Q waves *not* related to ischemic heart disease (pseudoinfarct patterns). For example, ST-segment elevations simulating ischemia may occur with acute pericarditis or myocarditis, as a normal variant ("early repolarization" pattern), or in a variety of other conditions (Table 221-1). Similarly, tall, positive T waves do not invariably represent hyperacute ischemic changes but may also be caused by normal variants, hyperkalemia, cerebrovascular injury, and left ventricular volume overload due to mitral or aortic regurgitation, among other causes.

ST-segment elevations and tall, positive T waves are common findings in leads V_1 and V_2 in left bundle branch block or left ventricular hypertrophy in the absence of ischemia. The differential diagnosis of Q waves (Table 221-2) includes physiologic or positional variants, ventricular hypertrophy, acute or chronic noncoronary myocardial injury, hypertrophic cardiomyopathy, and ventricular conduction disorders. Digoxin, ventricular hypertrophy, hypokalemia, and a variety of other

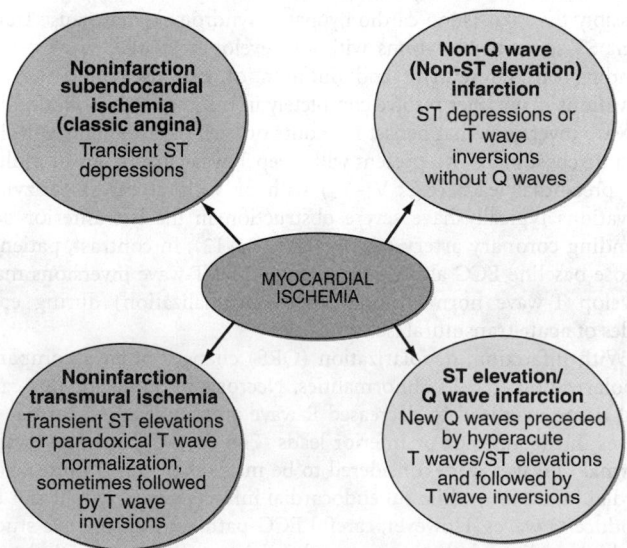

FIGURE 221-14 Variability of ECG patterns with acute myocardial ischemia. The ECG also may be normal or nonspecifically abnormal. Furthermore, these categorizations are not mutually exclusive. For example, a non-ST elevation infarct may evolve into a Q-wave infarct; ST elevations may be followed by a non-Q-wave infarct; or ST depressions and T-wave inversions may be followed by a Q-wave infarct. (*After Goldberger, 2006.*)

TABLE 221-1	DIFFERENTIAL DIAGNOSIS OF ST SEGMENT ELEVATIONS

Ischemia/myocardial infarction
    Noninfarction, transmural ischemia (Prinzmetal's angina, and possibly
        tako-tsubo syndrome)
    Acute myocardial infarction
    Postmyocardial infarction (ventricular aneurysm pattern)
Acute pericarditis
Normal variant ("early repolarization" pattern)
Left ventricular hypertrophy/left bundle branch block[a]
Other (rarer)
    Brugada pattern (right bundle branch block-like pattern with ST
        elevations in right precordial leads)[a]
    Class 1C antiarrhythmic drugs[a]
    DC cardioversion
    Hypercalcemia[a]
    Hyperkalemia[a]
    Hypothermia (J wave/Osborn waves)
    Myocardial injury
        Myocarditis
        Tumor invading left ventricle
        Trauma to ventricles

[a]Usually localized to V_1-V_2 or V_3.
Source: Modified from Goldberger, 2006.

TABLE 221-2	DIFFERENTIAL DIAGNOSIS OF Q WAVES (WITH SELECTED EXAMPLES)

Physiologic or positional factors
    Normal variant "septal" q waves
    Normal variant Q waves in V_1 to V_2, aVL, III, and aVF
    Left pneumothorax or dextrocardia: loss of lateral R-wave progression
Myocardial injury or infiltration
    Acute processes: myocardial ischemia or infarction, myocarditis,
        hyperkalemia
    Chronic processes: myocardial infarction, idiopathic cardiomyopathy,
        myocarditis, amyloid, tumor, sarcoid, scleroderma, Chagas' disease,
        echinococcus cyst
Ventricular hypertrophy/enlargement
    Left ventricular (slow R-wave progression[a])
    Right ventricular (reversed R-wave progression[b] or slow R-wave
        progression[a], particularly with chronic obstructive lung disease)
    Hypertrophic cardiomyopathy (may simulate anterior, inferior, posterior,
        or lateral infarcts)
Conduction abnormalities
    Left bundle branch block (slow R-wave progression[a])
    Wolff-Parkinson-White patterns

[a]Small or absent R waves in the right to midprecordial leads.
[b]Progressive decrease in R-wave amplitude from V_1 to the mid- or lateral precordial leads.
Source: After Goldberger, 2006.

factors may cause ST-segment depression mimicking subendocardial ischemia. Prominent T-wave inversion may occur with ventricular hypertrophy, cardiomyopathies, myocarditis, and cerebrovascular injury (particularly intracranial bleeds), among many other conditions.

METABOLIC FACTORS AND DRUG EFFECTS

A variety of metabolic and pharmacologic agents alter the ECG and, in particular, cause changes in repolarization (ST-T-U) and sometimes QRS prolongation. Certain life-threatening electrolyte disturbances may be diagnosed initially and monitored from the ECG. *Hyperkalemia* produces a sequence of changes (Fig. 221-15), usually beginning with narrowing and peaking (tenting) of the T waves. Further elevation of extracellular K^+ leads to AV conduction disturbances, diminution in P-wave amplitude, and widening of the QRS interval. Severe hyperkalemia eventually causes cardiac arrest with a slow sinusoidal type of mechanism ("sine-wave" pattern) followed by asystole. *Hypokalemia* (Fig. 221-16) prolongs ventricular repolarization, often with prominent U waves. Prolongation of the QT interval is also seen with drugs that increase the duration of the ventricular action potential—class 1A antiarrhythmic agents and related drugs

(e.g., quinidine, disopyramide, procainamide, tricyclic antidepressants, phenothiazines) and class III agents [amiodarone (Fig. 221-16), sotalol, ibutilide]. Marked QT prolongation, sometimes with deep, wide T-wave inversions, may occur with intracranial bleeds, particularly subarachnoid hemorrhage ("CVA T-wave" pattern) (Fig. 221-16). Systemic *hypothermia* also prolongs repolarization, usually with a distinctive convex elevation of the J point (Osborn wave). *Hypocalcemia* typically prolongs the QT interval (ST portion), while *hypercalcemia* shortens it (Fig. 221-17). Digitalis glycosides also shorten the QT interval, often with a characteristic "scooping" of the ST–T-wave complex (*digitalis effect*).

Many other factors are associated with ECG changes, particularly alterations in ventricular repolarization. T-wave flattening, minimal T-wave inversions, or slight ST-segment depression ("nonspecific ST–T-wave changes") may occur with a variety of electrolyte and acid-base disturbances, a variety of infectious processes, central nervous system disorders, endocrine abnormalities, many drugs, ischemia, hypoxia, and virtually any type of cardiopulmonary abnormality. While subtle ST–T-wave changes may be markers of ischemia, transient nonspecific repolariza-

Hyperkalemia

FIGURE 221-15 The earliest ECG change with hyperkalemia is usually peaking ("tenting") of the T waves. With further increases in the serum potassium concentration, the QRS complexes widen, the P waves decrease in amplitude and may disappear, and finally a sine-wave pattern leads to asystole unless emergency therapy is given. (*After Goldberger, 2006.*)

FIGURE 221-16 A variety of metabolic derangements, drug effects, and other factors may prolong ventricular repolarization with QT prolongation or prominent U waves. Prominent repolarization prolongation, particularly if due to hypokalemia, inherited "channelopathies," or certain pharmacologic agents, indicates increased susceptibility to *torsades des pointes*–type ventricular tachycardia (Chap. 226). Marked systemic hypothermia is associated with a distinctive convex "hump" at the J point (Osborn wave, *arrow*) due to altered ventricular action potential characteristics. Note QRS and QT prolongation along with sinus tachycardia in the case of tricyclic antidepressant overdose.

tion changes may also occur following a meal or with postural (orthostatic) change, hyperventilation, or exercise in healthy individuals.

ELECTRICAL ALTERNANS

Electrical alternans—a beat-to-beat alternation in one or more components of the ECG signal—is a common type of nonlinear cardiovascular response to a variety of hemodynamic and electrophysiologic perturbations. Total electrical alternans (P-QRS-T) with sinus tachycardia is a relatively specific sign of pericardial effusion, usually with cardiac tamponade. The mechanism relates to a periodic swinging motion of the heart in the effusion at a frequency exactly one-half the heart rate. Repolarization (ST-T or U wave) alternans is a sign of electrical instability and may precede ventricular tachyarrhythmias.

CLINICAL INTERPRETATION OF THE ECG

Accurate analysis of ECGs requires thoroughness and care. The patient's age, gender, and clinical status should always be taken into ac-

count. For example, T-wave inversions in leads V_1–V_3 are more likely to represent a normal variant in a healthy young adult woman ("persistent juvenile T-wave pattern") than in an elderly man with chest discomfort. Similarly, the likelihood that ST-segment depression during exercise testing represents ischemia depends partly on the prior probability of coronary artery disease.

Many mistakes in ECG interpretation are errors of omission. Therefore, a systematic approach is essential. The following 14 points should be analyzed carefully in every ECG: (1) standardization (calibration) and technical features (including lead placement and artifacts); (2) rhythm; (3) heart rate; (4) PR interval/AV conduction; (5) QRS interval; (6) QT/QT_c interval; (7) mean QRS electrical axis; (8) P waves; (9) QRS voltages; (10) precordial R-wave progression; (11) abnormal Q waves; (12) ST segments; (13) T waves; (14) U waves.

Only after analyzing all these points should the interpretation be formulated. Where appropriate, important clinical correlates or inferences should be mentioned. For example, the combination of left atrial abnormality (enlargement) and signs of right ventricular hypertrophy suggests mitral stenosis. Low voltage with sinus tachycardia raises the possibility of pericardial tamponade or chronic obstructive lung disease. Sinus tachycardia with QRS and QT-(U) prolongation, especially in the context of mental status changes, suggests tricyclic antidepressant overdose (Fig. 221-16). The triad of peaked T waves (hyperkalemia), a long QT due to ST segment lengthening (hypocalcemia) and left ventricular hypertrophy (systemic hypertension) suggests chronic renal failure. Comparison with previous ECGs is essential. The diagnosis and management of specific cardiac arrhythmias and conduction disturbances are discussed in Chaps. 225 and 226.

COMPUTERIZED ELECTROCARDIOGRAPHY

Computerized ECG systems are widely used. Digital systems provide for convenient storage and immediate retrieval of thousands of ECG records. Despite advances, computer interpretation of ECGs has important limitations. Incomplete or inaccurate readings are most likely with arrhythmias and complex abnormalities. Therefore, computerized interpretation (including measurements of basic ECG intervals) should not be accepted without careful clinician review.

FURTHER READINGS

ASHLEY EA et al: An evidence-based review of the resting electrocardiogram as a screening technique for heart disease. Prog Cardiovasc Dis 44:55, 2001

GOLDBERGER AL: *Clinical Electrocardiography: A Simplified Approach*, 7th ed. St. Louis, Mosby/Elsevier, 2006

GUGLIN MF, THATAI D: Common errors in computer electrocardiogram interpretation. Int J Cardiol 106:232, 2006

MIRVIS DM, GOLDBERGER AL: Electrocardiography, in *Braunwald's Heart Disease: A Textbook of Cardiovascular Medicine*, 8th ed, P Libby et al (eds). Philadelphia, Saunders, 2008

SURAWICZ B, KNILANS TK: *Chou's Electrocardiography in Clinical Practice*, 5th ed. Philadelphia, Saunders, 2001

FIGURE 221-17 Prolongation of the Q-T interval (ST-segment portion) is typical of hypocalcemia. Hypercalcemia may cause abbreviation of the ST segment and shortening of the QT interval.

222 Noninvasive Cardiac Imaging: Echocardiography, Nuclear Cardiology, and MRI/CT Imaging

Rick A. Nishimura, Raymond J. Gibbons,
James F. Glockner, A. Jamil Tajik

Cardiovascular imaging has significantly enhanced the practice of cardiology over the past few decades. Two-dimensional (2D) echocardiography is able to visualize the heart directly in real time using ultrasound, providing instantaneous assessment of the myocardium, cardiac chambers, valves, pericardium, and great vessels. Doppler echocardiography measures the velocity of moving red blood cells and has become a noninvasive alternative to cardiac catheterization for assessment of hemodynamics. Transesophageal echocardiography (TEE) provides a unique window for high-resolution imaging of posterior structures of the heart, particularly the left atrium, mitral valve, and aorta. Nuclear cardiology uses isotopes to assess myocardial perfusion and ventricular function and has contributed greatly to the evaluation of patients with ischemic heart disease. Cardiac MRI and CT can delineate cardiac structure and function with high resolution. They are particularly useful in the examination of cardiac masses, the pericardium, and the great vessels. MRI stress testing is now possible examining both ventricular function and perfusion. Detection of coronary calcification by CT as well as direct visualization of coronary arteries by CT angiography (CTA) are of growing utility in patients with suspected coronary artery disease (CAD). This chapter provides an overview of the basic concepts of these cardiac imaging modalities, as well as the clinical indications for each procedure. The illustrations in this chapter are supplemented by "real time" and other static images in **Chap. e20**, "The Atlas of Noninvasive Cardiac Imaging."

ECHOCARDIOGRAPHY

TWO-DIMENSIONAL ECHOCARDIOGRAPHY

Basic Principles 2D echocardiography uses the principle of ultrasound reflection off cardiac structures to produce images of the heart (Table 222-1). For a transthoracic echocardiogram (TTE), the imaging is performed with a handheld transducer placed directly on the chest wall. In selected patients, a TEE may be performed, in which an ultrasound transducer is mounted on the tip of an endoscope placed in the esophagus and directed toward the cardiac structures.

FIGURE 222-1 Two-dimensional echocardiographic still-frame images from a normal patient with a normal heart. *Top:* Parasternal long axis view during systole and diastole (*left*) and systole (*right*). During systole, there is thickening of the myocardium and reduction in the size of the left ventricle (LV). The valve leaflets are thin and open widely. *Bottom:* Parasternal short axis view during diastole (*left*) and systole (*right*) demonstrating a decrease in the left ventricular cavity size during systole as well as an increase in wall thickening. LA, left atrium; RV, right ventricle; Ao, aorta.

Current echocardiographic machines are portable and can be wheeled directly to the patient's bedside. Thus, a major advantage of echocardiography over other imaging modalities is the ability to obtain instantaneous images of the cardiac structures for immediate interpretation. Handheld echocardiographic units weighing 6 lb (<2.7 kg) have now become available, further enhancing the ease and portability of echocardiography. They are becoming an essential initial diagnostic modality for the critically ill patient in the emergency room and critical care setting.

A limitation of TTE is the inability to obtain high-quality images in all patients, especially those with a thick chest wall or severe lung disease, as ultrasound waves are poorly transmitted through lung parenchyma. New technology such as harmonic imaging and IV contrast agents (which traverse the pulmonary circulation) can now be used to enhance endocardial borders in patients with poor acoustic windows.

Chamber Size and Function 2D echocardiography is an ideal imaging modality for assessing left ventricular (LV) size and function (Fig. 222-1). A qualitative assessment of the cavity sizes of the ventricles and systolic function can be made directly from the 2D image by experienced observers. 2D echocardiography is useful in the diagnosis of LV hypertrophy and is the imaging modality of choice for the diagnosis of hypertrophic cardiomyopathy. Other chamber sizes are assessed by visual analysis, including the left atrium and right-sided chambers.

Valve Abnormalities (See Chap. 230) 2D echocardiography is the "gold standard" for imaging valve morphology and motion. Leaflet thickness and mobility, valve calcification, and the appearance of subvalvular and supravalvular structures can be assessed. Valve stenosis is reliably diagnosed by the thickening and decreased mobility of the valve. 2D echocardiography is also the gold standard for the diagnosis of mitral stenosis, which produces typical tethering and diastolic doming, and the severity of the stenosis can be ascertained from a direct

TABLE 222-1 CLINICAL USES OF ECHOCARDIOGRAPHY

Two-Dimensional Echocardiography	Doppler Echocardiography
Cardiac chambers	Valve stenosis
Chamber size	Gradient
Left ventricular	Valve area
Hypertrophy	Valve regurgitation
Regional wall motion	Semiquantitation
abnormalities	Intracardiac pressures
Valve	Volumetric flow
Morphology and motion	Diastolic filling
Pericardium	Intracardiac shunts
Effusion	**Transesophageal Echocardiography**
Tamponade	Inadequate transthoracic images
Masses	Aortic disease
Great vessels	Infective endocarditis
Stress Echocardiography	Source of embolism
Two-dimensional	Valve prosthesis
Myocardial ischemia	Intraoperative
Viable myocardium	
Doppler	
Valve disease	

FIGURE 222-2 Still frame two-dimensional echocardiographic image from the parasternal long axis view of a patient with aortic stenosis. The aortic valve is calcified with restricted opening during systole. Ao, aorta; RV, right ventricle; LA, left atrium; LV, left ventricle.

planimeter measurement of the mitral valve orifice. The presence and often the etiology of stenosis of the semilunar valves can be made by 2D echocardiography (Fig. 222-2), but evaluation of the severity of the stenosis requires Doppler echocardiography (see below). The diagnosis of valvular regurgitation must be made by Doppler echocardiography, but 2D echocardiography is valuable for determining the etiology of the regurgitation, as well as its effects on ventricular dimensions, shape, and function.

Pericardial Disease   (See Chap. 232) 2D echocardiography is the imaging modality of choice for the detection of pericardial effusion, which is easily visualized as a black echolucent ovoid structure surrounding the heart (Fig. 232-4). In the hemodynamically unstable patient with pericardial tamponade, typical echo findings include a dilated inferior vena cava, right atrial collapse, and then right ventricular collapse, usually at the base of the ventricle. Echocardiographically guided pericardiocentesis has now become a standard of care. A 2D echocardiogram can directly visualize the location of the pericardial fluid to guide the entry point of the needle.

Intracardiac Masses   (See Chap. 233) Intracardiac masses can be visualized on 2D echocardiography, provided that image quality is adequate. Solid masses appear as echo-dense structures, which can be located inside the cardiac chambers or infiltrating into the myocardium or pericardium. LV thrombus appears as an echo-dense structure, usually in the apical region associated with regional wall motion abnormalities. The appearance and mobility of the thrombus are predictive of embolic events. Vegetations appear as mobile linear echo densities attached to valve leaflets. Atrial myxoma can be diagnosed by the appearance of a well-circumscribed mobile mass with attachments to the atrial septum (Fig. 233-1). The high-resolution images provided by TEE may be required for further delineation of myocardial masses, especially those <1 cm in diameter.

Aortic Disease   (See Chap. 242) 2D echocardiography can provide extremely useful information on diseases of the aorta. The proximal ascending aorta, the arch, and the distal descending aorta can usually be visualized via the transthoracic ap-

proach. The definitive diagnosis of a suspected aortic dissection usually requires a TEE, which can rapidly provide high-resolution images of the proximal ascending and descending thoracic aorta (Fig. 222-3).

DOPPLER ECHOCARDIOGRAPHY

Basic Principles   Doppler echocardiography uses ultrasound reflecting off moving red blood cells to measure the velocity of blood flow across valves, within cardiac chambers, and through the great vessels. Normal and abnormal blood flow patterns can be assessed noninvasively. *Color-flow Doppler* imaging displays the blood velocities in real time superimposed upon a 2D echocardiographic image. The different colors indicate the direction of blood flow (red toward and blue away from the transducer), with green superimposed when there is turbulent flow. *Pulsed-wave Doppler* measures the blood flow velocity in a specific location on the 2D echocardiographic image. *Continuous-wave Doppler* echocardiography can measure high velocities of blood flow directed along the line of the Doppler beam, such as occur in the presence of valve stenosis, valve regurgitation, or intracardiac shunts. These high velocities can be used to determine intracardiac pressure gradients by a modified Bernoulli equation:

$$\text{Pressure change} = 4 \times (\text{velocity})^2$$

The derived pressure gradient can be used to determine intracardiac pressures and stenosis severity.

Tissue Doppler echocardiography measures the velocity of myocardial motion. The velocity of myocardium is several magnitudes lower than the velocity of moving red blood cells. Myocardial velocities can be used to determine myocardial strain rate, which is a quantitative measure of regional myocardial contraction and relaxation.

Valve Gradients   In the presence of valvular stenosis, there is an increase in the velocity of blood flow across the stenotic valve. A continuous-wave Doppler beam is used to determine an instantaneous gradient across the valve.

Valvular Regurgitation   Valvular regurgitation is diagnosed by Doppler echocardiography when there is abnormal retrograde flow across the valve. Color-flow imaging is the Doppler method used most frequently to detect valve regurgitation by visualization of a high-velocity turbulent jet in the chamber proximal to the regurgitant valve (Fig. 222-3). The size and extent of the color-flow jet into the receiving cardiac chamber provide a semiquantitative estimate of the severity of regurgitation.

Intracardiac Pressures   These can be calculated from the peak continuous-wave Doppler signal of a regurgitant lesion. The Bernoulli equa-

FIGURE 222-3 Transesophageal echocardiographic view of a patient with a dilated aorta, aortic dissection, and severe aortic regurgitation. **Left:** The long axis apex-down view of the black and white two-dimensional image in diastole. The arrow points to the intimal flap that is seen in the dilated ascending aorta. **Right:** Color-flow imaging that demonstrates a large mosaic jet of aortic regurgitation. Ao, aorta; RV, right ventricle; AR, aortic regurgitation.

FIGURE 222-4 Continuous-wave Doppler of tricuspid regurgitation in a patient with pulmonary hypertension. There is an increase in the velocity of flow from the right ventricle into the right atrium to 5.4 m/s. Using the modified Bernoulli equation, the peak pressure gradient between the right ventricle and right atrium during systole is 120 mmHg. Assuming a right atrial pressure of 10 mmHg, the right ventricular systolic pressure is 130 mmHg. In the absence of right ventricular outflow tract obstruction, this indicates there is severe pulmonary hypertension with a pulmonary artery systolic pressure of 130 mmHg.

tion is applied to the peak velocity to obtain the pressure gradient between two cardiac chambers. This is commonly applied to a tricuspid regurgitant jet, from which the systolic pressure gradient between the right atrium and right ventricle can be calculated. Adding an assumed right atrial pressure to this gradient will give a derived right ventricular systolic pressure. In the absence of right ventricular outflow tract obstruction, the latter provides the pulmonary artery systolic pressure (Fig. 222-4).

Cardiac Output   Volume flow rates (or stroke volume and cardiac output) can be reliably measured noninvasively by Doppler echocardiography. Flow is calculated as the product of the cross-sectional area of the vessel or chamber through which blood moves and the velocity of blood flow as assessed by continuous-wave Doppler determination. The time-velocity integral can be used to calculate pulsatile flow, and that integral multiplied by the cross-sectional area of, for example, the aortic root yields the stroke volume which, when multiplied by the heart rate, provides an estimate of the cardiac output.

Diastolic Filling   Doppler echocardiography allows noninvasive evaluation of ventricular diastolic filling. The transmitral velocity curves reflect the relative pressure gradients between the left atrium and ventricle throughout diastole. They are influenced by the rate of ventricular relaxation, the driving force across the valve, and the compliance of the ventricle. There is a progression of diastolic dysfunction, which can be assessed by Doppler flow velocity curves. In the early phase of diastolic dysfunction there is primarily an impairment of LV relaxation, with

reduced early transmitral flow and a compensatory increase in flow during atrial contraction (Fig. 222-5). As disease progresses, and ventricular compliance declines, left atrial pressure rises, resulting in a higher early transmitral velocity and shortening of the deceleration of flow in early diastole so that the filling pattern becomes normal, termed *pseudonormalization*. In patients with the most severe diastolic dysfunction and further elevation of left atrial pressure, early diastolic flow velocity rises further, termed the *restrictive filling pattern*. The addition of analysis of Doppler tissue velocities of annular motion provides further information concerning the diastolic properties.

Congenital Heart Disease   (See Chap. 229) 2D and Doppler echocardiography have been useful in the evaluation of patients with congenital heart disease. Congenital stenotic or regurgitant valve lesions can be assessed. The detection of intracardiac shunts is possible by 2D and Doppler echocardiography (Fig. 229-1). Patency of surgical shunts and conduits can be determined.

STRESS ECHOCARDIOGRAPHY

2D and Doppler echocardiography are usually performed with the patient in the resting state. Further information can be obtained by reimaging during either exercise or pharmacologic stress. The primary indications for stress echocardiography are to confirm the suspicion of ischemic heart disease and estimate its severity (see below).

A decrease in systolic contraction of an ischemic area of myocardium, termed a *regional wall motion abnormality*, occurs before symptoms or electrocardiographic changes. New regional wall motion abnormalities, a decline in ejection fraction, and an increase in end-systolic volume with stress are all indicators of myocardial ischemia. Exercise stress testing is usually done with exercise protocols using either upright treadmill or bicycle exercise. The echocardiographic imaging is done at baseline and then immediately after exercise. In patients who are not able to exercise, pharmacologic testing can be performed by infusion of dobutamine

FIGURE 222-5 Diagrammatic illustration indicating the progression of diastolic dysfunction. Top, left atrial and ventricular pressures; **Middle,** transmitral flow velocity as measured by Doppler echocardiography; **Bottom,** grade of diastolic dysfunction. LAD, left atrial pressure.

to increase myocardial oxygen demand. Dobutamine echocardiography has also been used to assess myocardial viability in patients with poor systolic function and concomitant CAD.

Doppler echocardiography can be used at rest and during exercise in patients with valvular heart disease to determine the hemodynamic response to stress. In patients with low-output, low-gradient aortic stenosis, the response of the gradient to dobutamine stimulation is of diagnostic and therapeutic value.

TRANSESOPHAGEAL ECHOCARDIOGRAPHY

When limited information is obtained from a TTE due to poor imaging windows, TEE can be useful. Diseases of the aorta, such as aortic dissection, can be readily diagnosed by TEE (Fig. 222-3). Defining the source of embolism is a common indication for TEE, as abnormalities such as atrial thrombi, patent foramen ovale, and aortic plaques can be detected. Other masses, particularly those in the atria, can be visualized. The presence of vegetations for the diagnosis of infective endocarditis and its complications can be assessed by TEE. This technique has been used before cardioversion in patients with atrial fibrillation to detect a thrombus in the left atrium or left atrial appendage. If no thrombus is present, cardioversion can be safely performed, as long as there is full-dose anticoagulation before, during, and after the procedure.

EMERGENCY ECHOCARDIOGRAPHY

A major advantage of echocardiography is the ability to obtain instantaneous images of the cardiac structures for immediate interpretation at the patient's bedside. Thus, echocardiography has become an ideal imaging modality for cardiac emergencies.

Unstable Hemodynamics   For the patient with unstable hemodynamics, echocardiography can determine LV size and function, right ventricular size and function, and the presence of acute valvular regurgitation and pericardial tamponade. Echocardiography is especially useful in the hemodynamically unstable patient following myocardial infarction (Chaps. 239 and 266), in whom acute mechanical complications (e.g., papillary muscle rupture, ventricular septal defect, myocardial perforation with tamponade, and right ventricular infarction) that need to be differentiated from severe LV systolic dysfunction can be diagnosed.

Chest Pain Syndromes   (See Chap. 13) Echocardiography can be useful in selected patients with chest pain syndromes. For those patients who have an equivocal electrocardiogram, the presence of regional wall motion abnormalities on an echocardiogram can lead to the diagnosis of myocardial ischemia as an etiology for the pain. Other etiologies of chest pain, such as acute dissection or pericarditis with effusion, can also be diagnosed by echocardiography.

NUCLEAR CARDIOLOGY

BASIC PRINCIPLES OF NUCLEAR CARDIOLOGY

All nuclear cardiology studies depend on the injection into the patient of an isotope that emits photons, generally gamma rays generated during radioactive decay when the nucleus of an isotope changes from one energy level to a lower one. Radionuclide imaging uses a special camera that images these photons.

ASSESSMENT OF VENTRICULAR FUNCTION

Equilibrium radionuclide angiography, also known as *multiple-gated blood pool imaging*, involves the imaging of ^{99m}Tc-labeled albumin or red cells that are uniformly distributed throughout the blood volume. Resting images of the blood pool of isotopes within the cardiac chambers are obtained by electrocardiographic gating through multiple cycles, so that sufficient counts can be detected to obtain an image. This requires that the heart rate be reasonably constant. It provides an accurate, reproducible method for assessment of LV function. It is most commonly used when echocardiography is technically difficult or when poor LV function requires accurate quantitation.

Gated single-photon emission computed tomography (SPECT) is the nuclear cardiology technique that is most commonly utilized to assess ejection fraction and regional wall motion. This is usually performed post-stress by gating the acquisition of SPECT myocardial perfusion images using ^{99m}Tc- labeled compounds (see below). An automated technique determines the endocardial borders of the LV cavity, and a geometric model is used to calculate the ejection fraction.

ASSESSMENT OF MYOCARDIAL PERFUSION BY SPECT

(See Chap. 237) Myocardial perfusion imaging by nuclear techniques is now widely applied for the evaluation of ischemic heart disease. Injection of radioisotopes at rest and during stress is performed to produce images of myocardial regional uptake proportional to regional blood flow. With maximal exercise, myocardial blood flow is increased up to fivefold above the resting condition. In the presence of a fixed coronary stenosis, there is an inability to increase myocardial perfusion in the territory supplied by the stenosis, creating a flow differential and inhomogeneous distribution of the isotope. In patients who are unable to exercise, pharmacologic agents are used to increase blood flow and create similar inhomogeneities. The preferred pharmacologic agents are adenosine or dipyridamole, which increase blood flow to a similar degree as exercise. In patients with bronchospastic lung disease, which is a contraindication to the use of adenosine or dipyridamole, dobutamine may be used as an alternative, although it does not increase myocardial blood flow to the same extent.

^{201}Tl (thallium) was the first isotope used for this purpose. It has been largely replaced by ^{99m}Tc, which has a higher photon energy and shorter half-life, permitting the injection of larger doses resulting in scans of higher quality (Fig. 222-6). Two technetium-labeled myocardium perfusion agents are in common use: tetrofosmin and sestamibi. Like thallium, both tetrofosmin and sestamibi distribute to the myocardium in relation to blood flow, and their uptake requires an intact cell membrane and a viable myocardial cell. Both agents are bound within the cell in a nearly irreversible fashion. As a result, these agents must generally be injected twice—once at rest and once during stress.

POSITRON EMISSION TOMOGRAPHY

The underlying physics of positron emission tomography (PET) scanning differs from that involved in the standard radionuclide techniques described above. Positron emission is a type of beta-decay of an unstable isotope. In this unstable isotope, a proton undergoes spontaneous decay into a neutron, a neutrino, and a β^+ particle (positron). The spontaneous release of positrons from these unstable nuclei leads to their interaction with electrons, which cause the release of gamma-radiation (photons) upon collision with tissue. It is this gamma emission that is detected by the gamma camera in the PET scanner. The very high energy of the photons results in far less scatter than with conventional nuclear cardiology techniques. PET cameras are considerably more expensive than conventional nuclear cardiology cameras. Rubidium-82 is the most commonly used positron emitter, as it is available from a generator and does not require a nearby cyclotron. Pharmacologic stress with dipyridamole, adenosine, or dobutamine is preferred for PET scanning.

Positron emitters can be employed to study both myocardial blood flow and myocardial metabolism. Nitrogen-13 ammonia, oxygen-15 water, and rubidium-82 have all been employed to assess myocardial blood flow. They permit measurement of absolute regional blood flows, in contrast to the relative blood flows that are assessed with ^{201}Tl- or ^{99m}Tc-labeled compounds. This advantage has been utilized for research purposes but has generally not been exploited clinically. Myocardial metabolism is most often assessed using fluorine-18 deoxyglucose. This agent permits the detection and quantification of exogenous glucose utilization in areas of hypoperfused myocardium.

The clinical application of PET scanning that has been best studied is the assessment of myocardial viability. The pattern of enhanced fluorodeoxyglucose uptake in regions of decreased perfusion (termed *glucose/blood flow "mismatch"*) indicates the presence of ischemic myocardium that has preferentially shifted its metabolic substrate toward

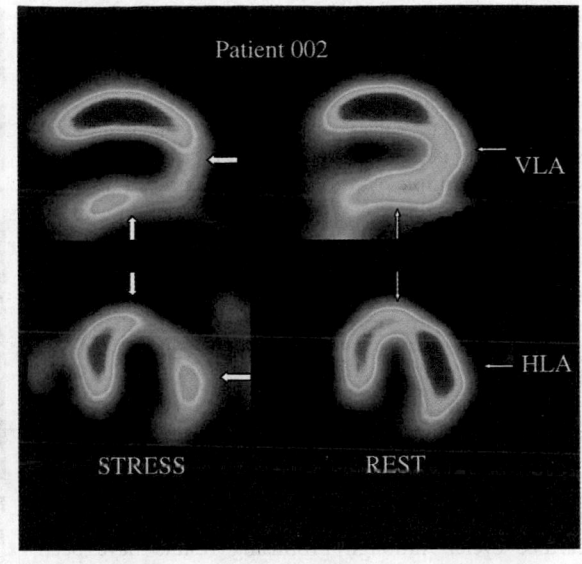

FIGURE 222-6 Exercise studies of atypical and typical angina.
A. Exercise ^{99m}Tc sestamibi study of a 71-year-old white female with atypical angina. **Left:** Stress images; **right:** rest images. The images are normal. There is uniform sestamibi uptake throughout the myocardium at rest and during stress. **B.** Exercise sestamibi study of a 75-year- old male with a history of typical angina. **Left:** Stress images; **right:** rest images. The stress images show a large defect involving the apex, lateral, and inferior walls (thick arrows), which improves at rest (thin arrows). Subsequent coronary angiography demonstrates severe three-vessel coronary artery disease.

glucose rather than fatty acid or lactate. This pattern identifies regions of ischemic or hibernating myocardium that are likely to improve in function after revascularization (Fig. 222-7).

Comparative studies have consistently shown the ability of PET to identify ischemic or hibernating myocardium in 10–20% of regions that would be classified as fibrotic (infarcted) by ^{201}Tl- or ^{99m}Tc-labeled compounds. For that reason, this technique is generally regarded as the gold standard for the assessment of myocardial viability. When large fixed defects (infarcts) are detected by ^{201}Tl- or ^{99m}Tc labeled compounds in patients who are candidates for coronary revascularization, PET imaging can help in the decision whether the risk of revascularization is justified by the potential benefit.

The technical limitations of both ^{201}Tl- and ^{99m}Tc-labeled compounds in obese patients, and the increasing prevalence of patient obesity, are contributing to the increasing use of PET scanning for the assessment of myocardial perfusion.

MRI AND CT IMAGING

MAGNETIC RESONANCE IMAGING

Basic Principles MRI is a technique based on the magnetic properties of hydrogen nuclei. In the presence of a large magnetic field, nuclear spin transitions from the ground state to excited states can be induced, and as the nuclei relax and return to their ground state, they release energy in the form of electromagnetic radiation that is detected and processed into an image. Contrast agents, such as gadolinium, are frequently employed to produce magnetic resonance angiograms (MRAs). These provide enhanced soft tissue contrast as well as the opportunity to obtain rapid angiographic images during the first pass of contrast through the vascular system. Cardiac MRI is particularly challenging because of the rapid motion of the heart and coronary arteries. Both static and cine images can be obtained using electrocardiographic triggering, often within a short breath-hold of 10–15 s. Cine images can be acquired in any plane with excellent blood-myocardial contrast, and these images can be used to quantify ejection fraction, end-systolic and end-diastolic volumes, and cardiac mass with high accuracy, reliability, and reproducibility, without the need for ionizing radiation.

Clinical Utility The multiplanar capabilities of MRI, coupled with excellent contrast and spatial

FIGURE 222-7 Positron emission tomography (PET). Short-axis PET resting ammonia image (**left**) and FDG image (**right**) of a 63-year-old diabetic female with dyspnea on exertion, a fixed SPECT defect, severe LV dysfunction, and severe coronary artery disease. The ammonia images show a very large apical, septal, anterior and lateral perfusion defect, which improves on the FDG images. This is consistent with hibernating myocardium. The patient underwent CABG with subsequent dramatic improvement in LV function. FDG, fluorodeoxyglucose; SPECT, single-photon emission CT; CABG, coronary artery bypass grafting; LV, left ventricular.

resolution, are often valuable in defining anatomic relationships in patients with complex congenital heart disease and cardiomyopathies (Fig. 231-2). Cardiac masses can be characterized and their relationship to normal anatomic structures defined. Likewise, MRI is often the examination of choice to determine whether a mediastinal or pulmonary mass has invaded the pericardium or heart. The entire pericardium can be visualized in multiple planes, and MRI has proved useful in characterizing pericardial effusions or pericardial thickening in patients with indeterminate results on echocardiography. Specialized pulse sequences have been designed to measure the velocity of blood in each pixel of the image, so that flow across valves and within blood vessels may be determined with accuracy. These techniques may allow characterization of the severity of valvular disease as well as quantification of shunt volumes.

MRA is a standard technique for imaging the aorta and large vessels of the chest and abdomen, with results essentially identical to conventional catheter-based angiography (Fig. 222-8). MRA of the coronary arteries is a much more difficult challenge, both because of the small size of these vessels and because of their rapid and complex motion during the cardiac cycle. Although promising results have been achieved, coronary MRA is not yet an accurate and reliable clinical technique.

MRI is a promising technology for the evaluation of patients with suspected or known coronary disease. Ventricular function and wall motion can be assessed at rest and during infusion of inotropic agents. Assessment of myocardial perfusion can be performed by injecting a bolus of gadolinium contrast and then continuously scanning the heart as the gadolinium passes through the cardiac chambers and into the myocardium. Relative perfusion deficits are reflected as regions of low signal intensity within the myocardium. Pharmacologic stress (typically achieved with vasodilators) can be applied during perfusion imaging to detect physiologically significant coronary artery lesions. Myocardial perfusion imaging with cardiac MRI is more sensitive then SPECT imaging for detecting subendocardial ischemia due to its enhanced spatial resolution. Myocardial viability may be determined by imaging the heart 10–20 min after gadolinium injection, as infarcted tissue retains contrast by virtue of its larger extracellular volume.

Limitations of MRI   Relative contraindications include the presence of pacemakers, internal defibrillators, or cerebral aneurysm clips. A small

FIGURE 222-8 Still frame of an MR angiogram showing a severe coarctation of the descending aorta, with abundant collateral arteries.

FIGURE 222-9 CT scan demonstrating calcium in a thickened pericardium in a patient with constrictive pericarditis. The calcium is shown as white densities.

percentage of patients are claustrophobic and unable to tolerate the examination within the relatively confined quarters of the magnet bore. However, open-bore magnets are now available to deal with this problem. Examination of clinically unstable patients is problematic, since close monitoring is difficult. Image quality in patients with significant arrhythmias is often limited.

COMPUTED TOMOGRAPHIC IMAGING
Basic Principles   CT is fast, simple, noninvasive, and provides images with excellent spatial resolution and good soft tissue contrast. Cardiac CT has long been technically challenging because image acquisition times for conventional CT were too long to freeze cardiac motion. The development of electron-beam CT and multislice spiral (helical) CT have led to improved temporal resolution and routine imaging of the beating heart.

Clinical Applications   Cardiac CT has several clinical applications. Pericardial calcification is an important sign of constrictive pericarditis and is easily detected by CT (Fig. 222-9). CT is useful in characterizing cardiac masses, particularly those containing fat or calcium. The ability to detect small amounts of fat with high spatial resolution makes CT an attractive technique for imaging patients with suspected arrhythmogenic right ventricular dysplasia (Chap. 231). Cine images can be used to evaluate wall motion and to determine ejection fraction, end-diastolic and end-systolic volumes, and cardiac mass.

CT angiography (CTA) has demonstrated accuracy similar to MRA in imaging the aorta and great vessels, and CTA is rapidly becoming the examination of choice in the evaluation of patients with suspected pulmonary embolus. CTA is an excellent imaging modality for the diagnosis of aortic dissection or penetrating ulcers. Visualization of the entire aorta is possible by CTA, so that the initial diagnosis as well as follow-up of patients with aortic aneurysmal disease can be done.

Coronary Calcification   Calcium in the coronary arteries occurs in atherosclerosis and is absent in the normal coronary artery. CT is very sensitive for the detection of coronary artery calcification and is being promoted as a noninvasive modality for the screening and diagnosis of CAD. The quantity of coronary calcification (coronary calcium score) is related to the severity of CAD. However, although CT has a very high sensitivity for the detection of CAD, it has a low specificity. The overall predictive accuracy for angiographic obstructive coronary disease in a typical population of patients with CAD is similar to other imaging modalities, such as SPECT. Due to its low specificity, CT should not be used for the diagnosis of obstructive coronary disease.

Contrast-Enhanced CT Angiography   With the high temporal and spatial resolution of multislice spiral CT, accurate assessment of luminal

FIGURE 222-10 Three-dimensional reconstruction of a CT angiogram demonstrating a normal main left coronary artery arising from the aorta, and its two branches, the left anterior descending artery (**left**) and the left circumflex artery (**right**).

narrowing in the major branches of the coronary arteries is possible in selected patients. Studies at experienced centers have shown a high sensitivity (>85%), and specificity (>90%) of CTA as compared to cardiac catheterization. The highest accuracy has been noted in the left main and the proximal portions of the left anterior descending and left circumflex arteries (Fig. 222-10), probably due to the rapid motion of the right and circumflex arteries. Fast, irregular heart rates and body motion limit the accuracy of CTA.

The concept of "noninvasive coronary angiography" has generated great interest in the widespread utility of CTA. However, at present, the major well-accepted indication for coronary CTA is in the evaluation of suspected coronary anomalies. CTA may also be of use in patients with chest pain syndromes who have an intermediate pretest probability of CAD who are unable to exercise or have an uninterpretable or equivocal stress test.

Limitations of CT Limitations of CT include its dependence on ionizing radiation (in contrast to MRI) and the need for iodinated contrast, which is problematic in patients with renal insufficiency or contrast allergy. While radiation doses for some applications (such as coronary calcification scoring) are relatively low, doses tend to increase as the spatial resolution improves, and the doses for coronary CTA generally exceed those delivered during standard diagnostic cardiac catheterization.

SELECTION OF IMAGING TESTS

BASIC PREMISE
The choice of the optimal imaging modality for a particular patient should be based upon the major problem being addressed, other concomitant clinical questions, as well as the local expertise and equipment available in an institution. The clinical urgency and costs need to be considered, due to the high costs of some of these modalities (Table 222-2).

Left Ventricular Size and Function 2D echocardiography is the primary imaging modality obtained for assessment of LV cavity size, systolic function, and wall thickness. It is widely available, portable, and provides an instantaneous view of the heart. Echocardiography can also provide concomitant information on valve function, pulmonary artery pressures, and diastolic filling, which are valuable in the patient presenting with possible heart failure. The disadvantage is poor endocardial resolution in some patients and the lack of reproducible quantitative measurements.

Equilibrium radionuclide angiography can provide an accurate quantitative measurement of LV function but is not widely available and cannot be used in patients with irregular rhythms. Gated SPECT can measure ejection fraction as a part of stress imaging. Both MRI and CT scanning provide the highest quality resolution of endocardial border and thus are the most accurate of all modalities. However, they are of higher cost, lack portability, and do not provide concomitant hemodynamic information as echocardiography does.

Valvular Heart Disease 2D and Doppler echocardiography provide both anatomic and hemodynamic information regarding valve disease, thus echocardiography is the first test of choice. MRI can also visualize valve motion and determine abnormal flow velocities across valves, but there is less validation of quantitative hemodynamic measurements in comparison to echocardiography.

Pericardial Disease Echocardiography is the first imaging modality of choice in patients with suspected pericardial effusion and tamponade, due to its rapid image display and portability. For patients with suspected constrictive pericarditis, either MRI or CT scanning is the imaging modality that best delineates pericardial thickness. Hemodynamic analysis of the enhancement of ventricular interaction that occurs in pericardial constriction can be assessed by Doppler echocardiography.

Aortic Disease Both CT scanning and MRI are the imaging modalities of choice for the evaluation of the stable patient with suspected aortic aneurysm or aortic dissection. In the acutely ill patient with suspected aortic dissection, either TEE or CT scanning is a reliable imaging modality.

TABLE 222-2 SELECTION OF IMAGING TESTS

	Echo	Nuclear	CT[a]	MRI[b]
LV Size/ function	Initial modality of choice Low cost, portable Provides ancillary structural and hemodynamic information	Available from gated SPECT stress imaging	Best resolution Highest cost	Best resolution Highest cost
Valve disease	Initial modality of choice Valve motion Doppler hemodynamics			Visualize valve motion Delineate abnormal flow
Pericardial disease	Pericardial effusion Doppler hemodynamics		Pericardial thickening	Pericardial thickening
Aortic disease	TEE rapid diagnosis[c] Acute dissection		Image entire aorta Acute aneurysm Aortic dissection	Image entire aorta Aortic aneurysm Chronic dissection
Cardiac masses	TTE—large intracardiac masses TEE—smaller intracardiac masses[c]		Extracardiac masses Myocardial masses	Extracardiac masses Myocardial masses

[a]Contrast required.
[b]Relative contraindication: pacemakers, metallic objects, claustrophobic.
[c]When not seen on TTE.
Note: Echo, echocardiography; SPECT, single-photon emission CT; TEE, transesophageal echocardiography; TTE, transthoracic echocardiogram.

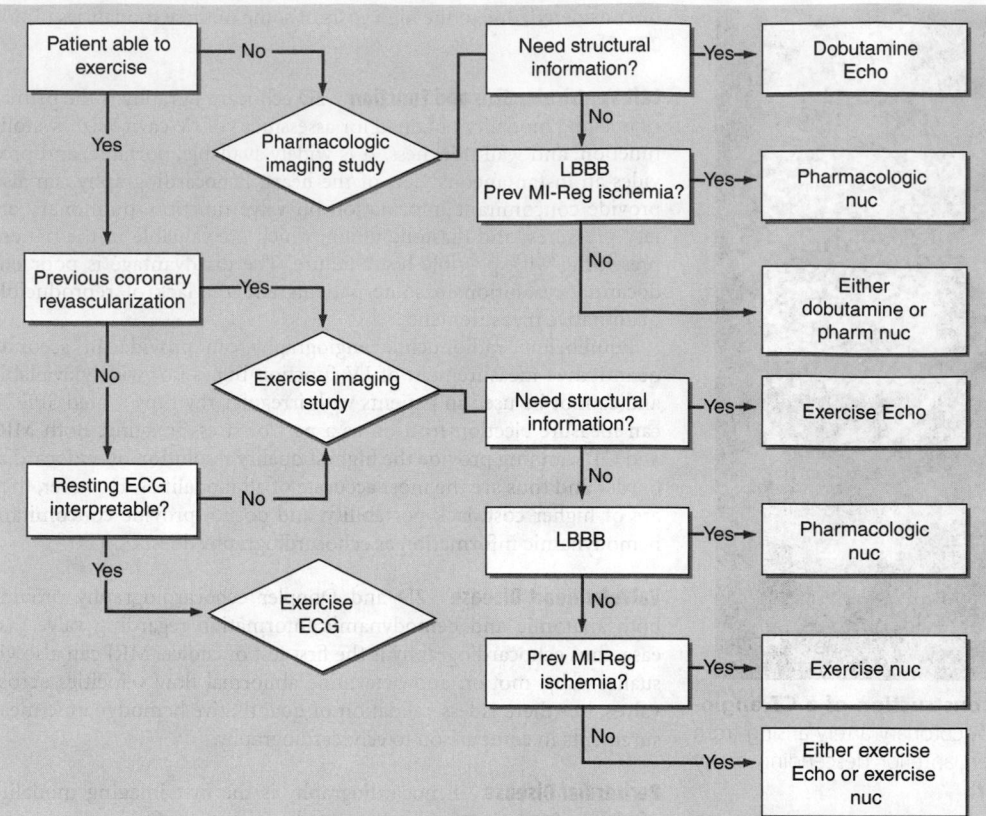

FIGURE 222-11 Flow diagram showing selection of initial stress test in a patient with chest pain. Patients who are able to exercise, without previous revascularization, and with an interpretable resting ECG can be tested with an exercise ECG. The appropriate imaging study for other patients depends on multiple factors (see text). LBBB, left bundle branch block; Prev MI-Reg ischemia, previous MI with a need to detect regional ischemia; Nuc, SPECT nuclear imaging study; Pharm, pharmacologic.

Cardiac Masses 2D TTE is the first test to rule out an intracardiac mass; masses >1.0 cm in diameter are usually well visualized. Intracardiac masses of smaller size may be visualized by TEE. CT scanning and MRI are optimal for evaluating masses extrinsic to the heart or involving the myocardium.

CHOOSING THE APPROPRIATE STRESS TEST

The choice of an initial stress testing modality should be based on the evaluation of the patient's resting electrocardiogram, the ability to perform exercise, and the available local expertise and technology (Fig. 222-11). For the standard assessment of CAD, the exercise electrocardiographic test should be the initial stress test in patients with an interpretable electrocardiogram who are able to exercise. If there are resting electrocardiographic abnormalities (ST depression >1 mm, LV hypertrophy, bundle branch block, paced rhythm, preexcitation), if the patient is taking digoxin, or if the patient has had a prior coronary revascularization, an imaging modality (either nuclear imaging or echocardiography) should be used for initial evaluation. Pharmacologic stress testing with imaging should be used in patients who are unable to exercise.

When an imaging modality is indicated, the decision to use an echocardiographic or a nuclear test depends not only on the clinical features but also on the available local expertise and technology. Both echocardiography and nuclear imaging require expertise in the performance and interpretation of the tests, and the patient is often best evaluated with the imaging modality for which the most expertise and experience are available. There are, however, certain situations in which one imaging modality has an advantage over the other.

Echocardiography provides additional structural information. Therefore, if there is a question of concomitant valve disease, pericardial disease, or aortic disease, echocardiography is able to provide information regarding these issues. The major limitation of echocardiography is the inability to obtain diagnostic images in all patients, especially those with chronic obstructive pulmonary disease or severe obesity. If there is inadequate definition of endocardial motion on the resting echocardiogram, stress echocardiography should not be performed unless contrast enhancement can be used. If the patient has had a previous infarction and one needs to determine whether a specific region of the myocardium is ischemic, nuclear imaging is the preferred modality. Nuclear imaging using ^{99m}Tc-labeled compounds is preferred in obese patients and those with severe lung disease. Nuclear imaging is more sensitive and less specific than echocardiography for the detection of myocardial ischemia.

The imaging tests can add prognostic information, especially when the results of an exercise electrocardiogram fall into an intermediate risk category. For nuclear imaging, a normal stress (exercise or pharmacologic) myocardial perfusion scan is highly predictive of the absence of significant artery disease and a low risk of subsequent cardiac death. Similarly, for stress (exercise or dobutamine) echocardiography, an increase in ejection fraction and a decrease in end-systolic volume at a high workload predict the absence of significant CAD and a low risk of subsequent cardiac death. On the other hand, for nuclear imaging, large or multiple stress-induced defects, or a large fixed defect with LV dilatation or increased ^{201}Tl lung uptake are high-risk findings. For stress echocardiography, patients with a decrease in ejection fraction, multiple new regional wall motion abnormalities, and an increase in end-systolic volume at a low workload are at high risk. Investigations are underway to determine the clinical value of stress MRI.

FURTHER READINGS

ACHENBACH S, DANIEL WG: Computed tomography of the heart, in P Libby et al (eds): *Braunwald's Heart Disease*, 8th ed, Philadelphia: Elsevier, 2008

CHEITLIN MD et al: ACC/AHA/ASE 2003 Guideline Update for the Clinical Application of Echocardiography: A Report of the American College of Cardiology/American Heart Association Task Force on Practice Guidelines (ACC/AHA/ASE Committee to Update the 1997 Guidelines for the Clinical Application of Echocardiography). Circulation 108:1146, 2003

CONSTANTINE G et al: Role of MRI in clinical cardiology. Lancet 363:2162, 2004

GIBBONS RJ et al: ACC/AHA 2002 Guideline Update for Exercise Testing: A Report of the American College of Cardiology/American Heart Association Task Force on Practice Guidelines (Committee on Exercise Testing). J Am Coll Cardiol 40:1531, 2002

HENDEL RC et al: ACCF Appropriateness criteria for cardiac computed tomography and cardiac magnetic resonance imaging: A report of the American College of Cardiology Foundation. J Am Coll Cardiol 48:1475, 2006

KLOCKE FJ et al: ACC/AHA/ASNC Guidelines for the Clinical Use of Cardiac Radionuclide Imaging-Executive Summary: A Report of the American College of Cardiology/American Heart Association Task Force on Practice Guidelines (ACC/AHA/ASNC Committee to Revise the 1995 Guidelines for the Clinical Use of Cardiac Radionuclide Imaging). J Am Coll Cardiol 42:1318, 2003

MARWICK TH: Measurement of strain and strain rate by echocardiography: Ready for prime time? J Am Coll Cardiol 47:1313, 2006

PENNELL D: Cardiovascular magnetic resonance, in P Libby et al (eds): *Braunwald's Heart Disease*, 8th ed, Philadelphia: Elsevier, 2008

223 Diagnostic Cardiac Catheterization and Angiography

Donald S. Baim*

Despite progressive improvements in noninvasive techniques, cardiac catheterization remains a key clinical tool for assessing the anatomy and physiology of the heart and its associated vasculature. It involves the insertion of catheters (2-mm diameter hollow plastic tubes) into a peripheral artery or vein under local anesthesia, and their passage into the heart for the purposes of intracardiac pressure measurement or the injection of a liquid radiographic contrast agent. The findings of diagnostic cardiac catheterization characterize the extent and severity of cardiac disease and thereby can help to determine the most appropriate plan for medical, surgical, or catheter-based treatment. While the majority of patients with coronary artery disease (CAD) or valvular disease can be managed medically using only clinical and noninvasive data (e.g., exercise testing, echocardiography, and MRI), >2 million patients each year undergo cardiac catheterization and angiographic procedures for diagnostic or interventional purposes, or both. This chapter focuses on the uses of cardiac catheterization as a diagnostic tool. For further discussion of catheter-based interventions, see Chap. 240.

BASIC PRINCIPLES

Given the expense and small but real risks of cardiac catheterization, this procedure is not indicated routinely whenever cardiac disease is diagnosed or suspected. Instead, cardiac catheterization is reserved for situations where there is a need to confirm the presence of a clinically suspected condition, define its anatomic and physiologic severity, and determine the presence or absence of important associated conditions. This situation arises most commonly when a patient experiences limiting or escalating symptoms of cardiac dysfunction (Chap. 227) that may include acute coronary syndromes, such as unstable angina or acute myocardial infarction (Chap. 238), or when objective measures (such as exercise testing or echocardiography) suggest that the patient has findings (such as an early positive exercise test or worsening ventricular function) that signal a high risk of progressing to rapid functional deterioration, myocardial infarction, or other adverse events. Under these circumstances, diagnostic catheterization may not only identify the culprit coronary lesions, but in ~40% of procedures may progress seamlessly into a catheter-based therapeutic procedure [percutaneous coronary intervention (PCI); Chap. 240] that can provide definitive correction. Alternatively, diagnostic catheterization may demonstrate only less critical lesions that can be managed medically or severe lesions poorly suited to PCI that may be referred for treatment by cardiac surgery (e.g., coronary bypass surgery, valve replacement, or valve repair).

While cardiac catheterization was once considered mandatory in *all* patients being considered for cardiac surgery, currently many patients with congenital or valvular heart disease undergo surgical correction based solely on clinical and noninvasive test data [e.g., echocardiography and MRI (Chap. 222)], with diagnostic coronary angiography

performed in older patients or those with risk factors for or non-invasive testing suggesting coronary disease, prior to surgery.

When there is a clinical "need to know," there are very few absolute contraindications to diagnostic cardiac catheterization in a patient who understands and accepts the associated risks. The risk of death from elective cardiac catheterization approaches 1 in 10,000 (0.01%), but the procedure does carry a small (~1 in 1000) risk of stroke or myocardial infarction, transient tachy- or bradyarrhythmias, or bruising or bleeding at the catheter insertion site. These complications respond to drug therapy, countershock, or vascular surgical repair, without long-term sequelae. About 1% of patients used to experience *allergic reactions* to iodinated contrast agents, ranging from urticaria to frank anaphylaxis in sensitive patients, but these have become rare events with current nonionic low-osmolar contrast agents.

Other patients (particularly those with baseline renal dysfunction or proteinuria) may develop transient deterioration in renal function, the chance of which may be further reduced by adequate prehydration (50% normal saline, or D$_5$W with 154 meq/L of sodium bicarbonate added, given at 3 mL/kg for 1 h prior to and 1 mL/kg for 6 h following the procedure, absent congestive heart failure), preprocedure administration of N-acetylcysteine (Mucomist, 600 mg orally before and twice a day after the procedure), or the use of an isoosmolar contrast agent (iodixanol). Newer low- or iso-osmolar contrast agents also reduce the chance of myocardial depression and other side effects (hypotension, nausea, bradycardia, or a sensation of marked warmth following injection) that were once common when earlier high-osmolar contrast agents were used.

Cardiac catheterization is generally performed with the patient fasting for the previous 6 h and awake but lightly sedated. The desired level of sedation may be achieved with preprocedure sedatives such as oral diazepam (Valium, 5–10 mg), or with IV conscious sedation using midazolam (Versed, 1 mg) or fentanyl (25–50 μg) following guidelines for conscious sedation. Most elective procedures are performed on an *outpatient* basis, with the patient discharged with instructions regarding maintenance of a liberal oral fluid intake, avoidance of strenuous activity, and self-monitoring for access site complications, following 2–4 h of postprocedure bed rest. If required by associated medical conditions or complications, or if a PCI has been performed, overnight hospitalization may be recommended.

To minimize the risks of bleeding at the local catheter insertion site, patients who have been anticoagulated chronically with warfarin should have this agent discontinued at least 48 h prior to the procedure, so that the INR falls below 2. Oral aspirin (325 mg/d) is routinely administered to patients undergoing diagnostic catheterization for suspected coronary disease, since aspirin pretreatment is desired if a coronary intervention is to be performed. Since cardiac catheterization is a sterile procedure, prophylactic antibiotics are not necessary.

Most (>95%) cardiac catheterizations are performed by the percutaneous femoral technique that begins with needle puncture of the common femoral artery or (for right heart catheterization) the femoral vein. A flexible guidewire is inserted through this needle and supports insertion of a vascular access sheath, through which the desired catheters can be advanced. This percutaneous technique can be adapted to other arterial sites such as (1) the brachial and radial artery in patients with peripheral vascular disease involving the abdominal aorta and iliac or femoral arteries or in whom immediate postprocedure ambulation is desired, or (2) the internal jugular vein for right heart catheterization in patients who may require prolonged hemodynamic monitoring.

Cardiac catheterization may include a variety of different measurements of pressure and flow (hemodynamics) as well as a variety of different contrast injections recorded as x-ray movies (angiography),

---

*At the time that Dr. Baim prepared this chapter he was a Professor of Medicine at Harvard Medical School and Senior Physician at Brigham and Women's Hospital. Since then, he has assumed the position of Senior Vice-President at Boston Scientific Co.

TABLE 223-1 NORMAL VALUES FOR HEMODYNAMIC PARAMETERS

Pressures (mmHg)	
Systemic arterial	
Peak systolic/end-diastolic	100–140/60–90
Mean	70–105
Left ventricle	
Peak systolic/end-diastolic	100–140/3–12
Left atrium (or pulmonary capillary wedge)	
Mean	2–10
a wave	3–15
v wave	3–15
Pulmonary artery	
Peak systolic/end-diastolic	15–30/4–12
Mean	9–18
Right ventricle	
Peak systolic/end-diastolic	15–30/2–8
Right atrium	
Mean	2–8
a wave	2–10
v wave	2–10
Resistances [(dyn·s)/cm^5]	
Systemic vascular resistance	700–1600
Pulmonary vascular resistance	20–130
Cardiac index [(L/min)/m^2]	2.6–4.2
Oxygen consumption index [(L/min)/m^2]	110–150
Arteriovenous oxygen difference (mL/L)	30–50

determined by the nature of the clinical problem being evaluated, and the extent of information available from prior noninvasive evaluation of left ventricular and valvular function. Full left and right heart hemodynamic studies are generally reserved for patients in whom the noninvasive data are unclear, or in whom intra- and postprocedural hemodynamic monitoring of unstable circulatory status may be desired.

Right Heart Catheterization This procedure involves measurement of the pressures in the right side of the heart. It was once a routine component of cardiac catheterization but is now used in <25% of procedures, especially when significant left and/or right ventricular dysfunction, valve disease, myopericardial disease, or intracardiac shunting is suspected. The right heart catheterization procedure is similar to the placement of a Swan-Ganz catheter at the bedside (except that it is performed under fluoroscopic guidance). A balloon flotation catheter is inserted percutaneously into a suitable vein (femoral, brachial, subclavian, or internal jugular) and advanced sequentially into the right atrium, right ventricle, pulmonary artery, and pulmonary artery wedge position. Pressure is recorded at each of these locations, and after recording the pulmonary wedge pressure (which approximates left atrial pressure), the balloon is deflated so that blood samples can be obtained for oxygen saturation measurement to screen for intracardiac shunts and to estimate the cardiac output by the Fick principle (Table 223-1). Alternatively, the cardiac output may be estimated by the thermodilution method, using a thermistor on the catheter to analyze the temperature deviations in the pulmonary artery that occur following a 10-mL bolus injection of room-temperature IV solution into the right atrium.

Left Heart Catheterization This procedure may be performed by percutaneous access of the femoral, brachial, or radial arteries. The left heart catheter is advanced under fluoroscopic guidance into the central aorta and then retrograde across the aortic valve into the left ventricle. If a right heart catheter is in place, simultaneous measurement and recording of left heart, right heart, and peripheral arterial pressures, together with a determination of cardiac output by either thermodilution or the Fick method, can capture a comprehensive hemodynamic profile. When valvular stenosis is present, the measurements of the pressures in the upstream and downstream chambers (e.g., in the left ventricle and ascending aorta for aortic stenosis, or the pulmonary capillary wedge pressure and left ventricle in mitral stenosis) can be combined with the measurement of flow from the cardiac output measurement to allow calculation of the stenotic valve orifice area.

FIGURE 223-1 Left ventricular (LV), radial artery, and pulmonary capillary wedge (PCW) pressures in a patient with normal cardiovascular function. Note the absence of a pressure gradient between the LV and radial artery in systole and between the LV and PCW in diastole.

An example of normal pressure tracings is shown in Fig. 223-1. In contrast, the characteristic hemodynamic tracings of mitral stenosis, with a diastolic pressure gradient between the left atrium (or pulmonary capillary wedge pressure) and the left ventricle, is seen in Fig. 223-2, and the findings of significant mitral regurgitation with a prominent *v* wave in the pulmonary capillary wedge pressure that in-

FIGURE 223-2 Pulmonary capillary wedge (PCW) and left ventricular (LV) pressure tracings in a 40-year-old woman with mitral stenosis. This patient also had systemic hypertension and significant elevation of her LV diastolic pressure. *[From BA Carabello, W Grossman, in Grossman's Cardiac Catheterization, Angiography, and Intervention, 7th ed, DS Baim (ed). Baltimore, Lippincott Williams & Wilkins, 2006.]*

FIGURE 223-3 Hemodynamic findings at rest and during exercise in a patient with mitral regurgitation. Left ventricular (LV), pulmonary capillary wedge (PCW), and radial artery pressure tracings are shown before (*left*) and during (*right*) the sixth minute of supine bicycle exercise. PCW mean pressure and *v* wave increase substantially with exercise. [*From W Grossman, in Grossman's Cardiac Catheterization, Angiography, and Intervention, 7th ed, DS Baim (ed). Baltimore, Lippincott Williams & Wilkins, 2006.*]

FIGURE 223-4 Severe aortic stenosis. Hemodynamic findings show the left ventricular (LV), and aortic (Ao) pressure with a slow systolic rise and large (96 mmHg) systolic gradient (shaded area) corresponding to critical aortic stenosis (aortic valve area 0.5 cm²). [*From BA Carabello, W Grossman, in Grossman's Cardiac Catheterization, Angiography, and Intervention, 7th ed, DS Baim (ed). Baltimore, Lippincott Williams & Wilkins, 2006.*]

FIGURE 223-5 Severe aortic regurgitation. There is equilibration between the left ventricular (LV) and aortic or femoral artery (FA) pressures in diastole. Also, LV diastolic pressure exceeds pulmonary capillary wedge (PCW) pressure early in diastole, indicating premature closure of the mitral valve (a characteristic feature of severe aortic regurgitation). [*From W Grossman, in Grossman's Cardiac Catheterization, Angiography, and Intervention, 7th ed, DS Baim, W Grossman (eds). Baltimore, Lippincott Williams & Wilkins, 2006.*]

creases substantially during modest exercise in Fig. 223-3. Severe *aortic stenosis* results in a systolic gradient between the left ventricular cavity and the ascending aorta, as shown in Fig. 223-4, while severe *aortic regurgitation* produces a widening of the aortic pulse pressure, with equilibration of aortic and left ventricular pressures in diastole as seen in Fig. 223-5. Valvular heart disease affecting the tricuspid or pulmonic valves results in similar deformities of the right-sided pressures, i.e., in patients with severe *tricuspid regurgitation*, the right atrial pressure resembles the right ventricular pressure closely in appearance, while in *tricuspid stenosis*, there is a pressure gradient between the right atrium and ventricle during diastole.

LEFT VENTRICULAR AND AORTIC ANGIOGRAPHY

If left ventricular size and function have not been previously assessed by noninvasive means, left ventriculography may be performed by power injection through a suitable catheter (usually a pigtail shape) of 30 to 45 mL of radiographic contrast material into the left ventricular chamber at a rate of 10–12 mL/s. The resulting radiographic images define the left ventricular cavity silhouette throughout the cardiac cycle, and tracing of that silhouette at end-diastole and end-systole permits calculation of the absolute left ventricular chamber volumes and the ejection fraction (the fraction of end diastolic volume ejected during systole; normally 50–80%), as well as qualitative assessment of regional wall motion abnormalities. Regional abnormalities of wall motion include diminished inward motion of a myocardial segment (*hypokinesis*), absence of inward movement of a myocardial segment (*akinesis*), and paradoxical systolic expansion of a regional myocardial segment (*dyskinesis*) (Fig. 223-6).

Mitral regurgitation is also easily visualized during left ventriculography as the leakage of radiographic contrast material back into the left atrium during left ventricular systole (Fig. 223-7). Its severity can be estimated qualitatively using a grading system of 1+ (mild; radio-

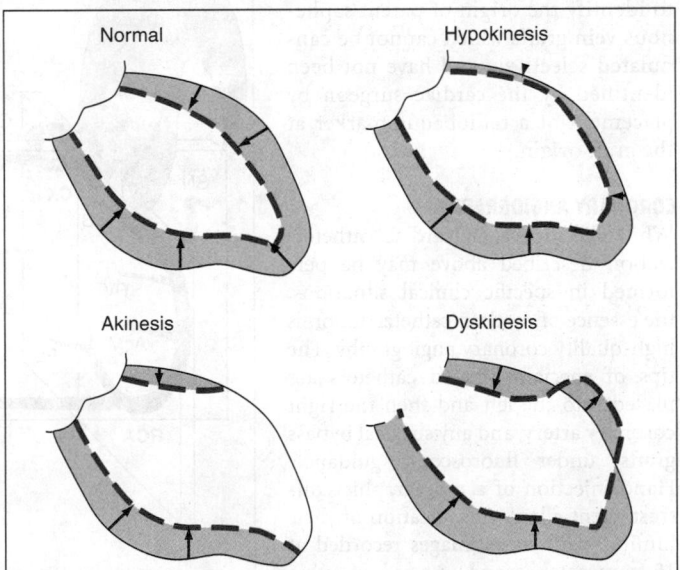

FIGURE 223-6 Diagrammatic representation of end-diastolic (*solid line*) and end-systolic (*dashed line*) silhouettes of left ventricular cineangiograms. These represent various forms of localized wall motion disorder in patients with coronary heart disease. Normal wall motion is symmetric; a patient with *hypokinesis* exhibits reduced contraction, seen here over the anterior and apical surfaces; a patient with *akinesis* exhibits absent wall motion, seen here over the anteroapical surface; a patient with *dyskinesis* exhibits paradoxic bulging of a small portion of the anterior wall with systole.

FIGURE 223-7 Left ventricular angiogram showing end-diastole (*left*) and end-systole (*right*). Left ventricular ejection fraction remains normal, but the calculated ventricular volumes are increased, due to severe chronic mitral regurgitation [note dense opacification of the left atrium (LA) and left atrial appendage (*arrow*) on the systolic frame]. *[From D Baim, in Grossman's Cardiac Catheterization, Angiography, and Intervention, 7th ed, DS Baim (ed). Baltimore, Lippincott Williams & Wilkins, 2006.]*

graphic contrast material clears with each beat and never opacifies the entire left atrium) to 4+ (severe; opacification of the entire left atrium occurs within one beat, and contrast material can be seen refluxing into the pulmonary veins).

Aortography involves rapid injection of radiographic contrast material into the ascending aorta, to detect abnormalities of the ascending aorta and aortic valve. It allows qualitative assessment abnormalities such as aortic regurgitation, which is graded using a 1+ to 4+ scale, similar to that used for mitral regurgitation (see above). Aortography can permit identification of aortic aneurysm and/or aortic dissection in which external compression of the aortic true lumen is caused by displacement of an intimal flap separating the true and false aortic lumina (Chap. 242). Aortography may also be used to identify the origin of patent saphenous vein grafts which cannot be cannulated selectively and have not been identified by the cardiac surgeon by placement of a radiopaque marker at the graft origin.

CORONARY ANGIOGRAPHY

While the aspects of cardiac catheterization described above may be performed in specific clinical situations, the essence of modern catheterization is high-quality coronary angiography. The tips of specially shaped catheters are placed into the left and then the right coronary artery, and any surgical bypass grafts, under fluoroscopic guidance. Hand injection of a radiographic contrast agent allows opacification of their lumina, with those images recorded at 15 frames per second on a radiographic image (*cine angiography*). Each coronary artery is usually viewed in several projections to permit assessment of the location and severity of any stenosis relative to the adjacent "normal" vessel segments (Fig. 223-8). In addition to the detection of coronary artery stenoses, coronary angiography evaluates the rapidity of coronary flow, the blush of

capillary filling in the myocardium, collateral pathways that perfuse myocardial territories supplied by an occluded vessel, the presence of congenital abnormalities of the coronary circulation (e.g., coronary fistulae), and patency of any previously constructed coronary artery bypass grafts.

The degree of stenosis is typically evaluated by visual estimation of percent diameter stenosis of each lesion relative to the "uninvolved" adjacent reference segment, with 50% diameter stenosis representing the minimal lesion severity that is capable of interfering with maximal increases in perfusion of the related myocardial territory during stress (Fig. 223-9). Borderline lesions (i.e., those between 40 and 70% diameter stenosis) that are not clearly related to the clinical ischemic syndrome may be further assessed by the following: (1) measurement of the pressure gradient between the segments proximal and distal to the stenosis; (2) measurement of the increase in distal coronary blood flow during maximal coronary vasodilatation using adenosine; and (3) use of intravascular ultrasound (IVUS), which has the advantage of imaging the underlying plaque as well as precisely measuring the luminal cross-sectional area at the point of a borderline lesion. Despite recent progress in multidetector computed tomography (MDCT) that suggests this evolving technique (Chap. 222) may ultimately replace screening pre-surgical coronary angiography (Fig. 223-10), coronary arteriography remains the most definitive diagnostic tool for evaluation of the *coronary anatomy* with sufficient precision to inform deci-

FIGURE 223-8 Representation of coronary anatomy relative to the interventricular and atrioventricular valve planes. Coronary branches are indicated as L main (left main), LAD (left anterior descending), D (diagonal), S (septal), CX (circumflex), OM (obtuse marginal), RCA (right coronary artery), CB (conus branch), SN (sinus node), AcM (acute marginal), PD (posterior descending), PL (posterolateral left ventricular). RAO, right anterior oblique, LAO, left anterior oblique. *[From DS Baim in Grossman's Cardiac Catheterization, Angiography, and Intervention, 7th ed, DS Baim (ed). Baltimore, Lippincott Williams & Wilkins, 2006.]*

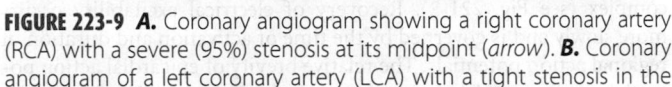

A

B

FIGURE 223-9 A. Coronary angiogram showing a right coronary artery (RCA) with a severe (95%) stenosis at its midpoint (*arrow*). **B.** Coronary angiogram of a left coronary artery (LCA) with a tight stenosis in the proximal left anterior descending (LAD) artery (*black arrow*) immediately prior to the origin of a large septal branch. The circumflex artery (CX) has two moderately severe stenoses (*white arrows*).

sions regarding coronary surgery vs. catheter-based interventions in patients with CAD.

POSTPROCEDURE CARE

The average diagnostic cardiac catheterization procedure takes ~30 min and ~60 mL of contrast (increased to ~90 mL by contrast left ventriculography). No anticoagulant agents are usually administered for a purely diagnostic procedure, and the vascular sheaths are removed at the end of the procedure. Hemostasis may be achieved by applying local pressure over the puncture site for 10–15 min, followed by a 2- to 4-h period of bed rest before ambulation and discharge. Alternatively, a variety of vascular closure devices (sutures or external clips or collagen plugs) are now available to seal the arterial puncture site, allowing a shorter period of bed rest and earlier ambulation. Most patients with suitable anatomy, however, will go on seamlessly to undergo PCI following the diagnostic catheterization procedure before the sheaths are removed, followed by an overnight hospital stay (Chap. 240).

FURTHER READINGS

BAIM DS (ed): *Grossman's Cardiac Catheterization, Angiography, and Intervention,* 7th ed. Baltimore, Lippincott Williams & Wilkins, 2006

BUDOFF MJ. Clinical utility of computed tomography and magnetic resonance techniques for noninvasive coronary angiography. *J Am Coll Cardiol* 42:1867, 2003

DAVIDSON CJ et al: Cardiac catheterization, in *Braunwald's Heart Disease,* 7th ed, D Zipes et al (eds). Philadelphia, Saunders, 2005

NICHOLLS SJ et al: Exploring the natural history of atherosclerosis with intravascular ultrasound. *Expert Rev Cardiovasc Ther* 5:295, 2007

RYAN TJ: The coronary angiogram and its seminal contributions to cardiovascular medicine over five decades. Circulation 106:752, 2002

FIGURE 223-10 Comparison of 64-slice multidetector CT imaging to contrast coronary angiography in a patient with severe stenosis of the proximal left anterior descending (*arrow*). This technique may supplant screening coronary angiography in patients who do not have clinical indications for percutaneous coronary intervention. *(Images provided by Thomas J. Brady, M.D.)*

224 Principles of Electrophysiology
Gordon F. Tomaselli

HISTORY AND INTRODUCTION

The field of cardiac electrophysiology was ushered in with the development of the electrocardiogram (ECG) by Einthoven at the turn of the twentieth century. The recording of cellular membrane currents revealed that the body surface ECG is the timed sum of the cellular action potentials in the atria and ventricles. In the late 1960s, the development of intracavitary recording, and in particular the ability to record His bundle electrograms with programmed stimulation of the heart, marked the beginning of contemporary clinical electrophysiology. Adoption of radiofrequency technology to ablate cardiac tissue in the early 1990s heralded the birth of interventional cardiac electrophysiology.

The clinical problem of sudden death caused by ventricular arrhythmias, most commonly in the setting of coronary obstruction, was recognized as early as the late nineteenth century. The problem was vexing and led to the development of pharmacologic and non-pharmacologic therapies, including transthoracic defibrillators, cardiac massage, and, most recently, implantable defibrillators. Over time the limitations of antiarrhythmic drug therapy have been repeatedly highlighted in clinical trials, such that ablation and devices are first-line therapy for a number of cardiac arrhythmias.

In the past decade the genetic basis of a number of heritable arrhythmias has been elucidated, revealing important insights into the mechanisms not only of these rare arrhythmias, but also of similar rhythm disturbances observed in more common forms of heart disease.

DESCRIPTIVE PHYSIOLOGY

The normal cardiac impulse is generated by pacemaker cells in the sinoatrial node located at the junction of the right atrium and superior vena cava (see Fig. 221-1). This impulse is slowly transmitted through nodal tissue to the anatomically complex atria, where it is more rapidly conducted to the atrioventricular node (AVN) inscribing the P wave of the ECG (see Fig. 221-2). There is a perceptible delay in conduction through the anatomically and functionally heterogeneous AVN. The time needed for activation of the atria and the AVN delay is represented as the PR interval of the ECG. The AVN is the only electrical connection between the atria and ventricles in the normal heart. The electrical impulse emerges from the AVN and is transmitted to the His-Purkinje system, specifically the common bundle of His, then the left and right bundle branches, and thence to the Purkinje network, facilitating activation of ventricular muscle. Under normal circumstances, the ventricles are rapidly activated in a well-defined fashion that is determined by the course of the Purkinje network and inscribes the QRS complex (see Fig. 221-2). Recovery of electrical excitability occurs more slowly and is governed by the time of activation and duration of regional action potentials. The relative brevity of epicardial action potentials in the ventricle results in repolarization occurring first on the epicardial surface then proceeding to the endocardium, which inscribes a T wave normally of the same polarity as the QRS complex. The duration of activation and recovery is determined by the action potential duration represented on the body surface ECG by the QT interval (see Fig. 221-2).

The gross anatomic features of the heart—the extracellular matrix and intramural vasculature—create both macro- and microanatomic barriers that are central to both the normal electrophysiology of the heart and clinically important arrhythmias. Cardiac myocytes exhibit a characteristically long action potential (200–400 ms) compared to neurons or skeletal muscle cells (1–5 ms). The action potential profile is sculpted by the orchestrated activity of multiple distinctive time- and voltage-dependent ionic currents (Fig. 224-1A). The currents, in turn, are carried by complex transmembrane proteins that passively conduct ions down their electrochemical gradients through selective pores (ion channels), actively transport ions against their electro-

FIGURE 224-1 A. Cellular atrial and ventricular action potentials. Schematic atrial and ventricular action potentials with the phases are shown in the top portion of the figure. Phases 0–4 are the rapid upstroke, early repolarization, plateau, late repolarization, and diastole respectively. The ionic currents and the genes that generate the currents with schematics of the current trajectories are shown above and below the action potentials. The active currents and their densities vary in atrial and ventricular myocytes. **B.** A ventricular action potential with a schematic of the ionic currents flowing during the phases of the action potential. Potassium current (I_{K1}) is the principal current during phase 4 and determines the resting membrane potential of the myocyte. Sodium current generates the upstroke of the action potential (phase 0), activation of I_{to} with inactivation of the Na current inscribes early repolarization (phase 1). The plateau phase (2) is generated by a balance of repolarizing potassium currents and depolarizing calcium current. Inactivation of the calcium current with persistent activation of potassium currents (predominantly I_{Kr} and I_{Ks}) cause phase 3 repolarization.

chemical gradient (pumps, transporters), or electrogenically exchange ionic species (exchangers).

Action potentials in the heart are regionally distinct. The regional variability in cardiac action potentials is the result of differences in the number and types of ion channel proteins expressed by different cell types in the heart. Further, unique sets of ionic currents are active in pacemaking and muscle cells, and the relative contributions of these currents may vary in the same cell type in different regions of the heart (Fig. 224-1A).

Ion channels are complex, multisubunit transmembrane glycoproteins that open and close in response to a number of biologic stimuli, including a change in membrane voltage, ligand binding (directly to the channel or to a G protein–coupled receptor), and mechanical deformation (Fig. 224-2). Other ion motive transmembrane proteins, such as exchangers and transporters, contribute importantly to cellular excitability in the heart. Ion pumps establish and maintain the ionic gradients across the cell membrane that serve as the driving force for current flow through ion channels. Transporters or exchangers that do not move ions in an electrically neutral manner (e.g., the sodium-calcium exchanger transports three Na^+ for one Ca^{2+}) are termed *electrogenic*, and contribute directly to the action potential profile.

The most abundant superfamily of ion channels expressed in the heart is voltage-gated. Several structural themes are common to all voltage-dependent ion channels. First, the architecture is modular, consisting either of four homologous subunits (e.g., K^+ channels) or of four internally homologous domains (e.g., Na^+ and Ca^{2+} channels). Second, the proteins fold around a central pore lined by amino acids that exhibit exquisite conservation within a given channel family of like selectivity (e.g., jellyfish, eel, fruit fly, and human Na channels have very similar P segments). Third, the general strategy for activation gating (opening and closing in response to changes in membrane voltage) is highly conserved: the fourth transmembrane segment (S4), studded with positively charged residues, lies within the membrane field and moves in response to depolarization, opening the channel. Fourth, most ion channel complexes include not only the pore-forming proteins (α subunits) but also auxiliary subunits (e.g., β subunits) that modify channel function (Fig. 224-2).

Na^+ and Ca^{2+} channels are the primary carriers of depolarizing current in both the atrium and ventricles; inactivation of these currents and activation of repolarizing K^+ currents hyperpolarize the heart cell, reestablishing the negative resting membrane potential (Fig. 224-1B). The *plateau phase* is a time when little current is flowing, and relatively minor changes in depolarizing or repolarizing currents can have profound effects on the action potential shape and duration. Mutations in subunits of these channel proteins produce arrhythmogenic alterations in the action potentials that cause long and short QT syndrome, idiopathic ventricular fibrillation, familial atrial fibrillation, and some forms of conduction system disease.

MECHANISMS OF CARDIAC ARRHYTHMIAS

Cardiac arrhythmias result from abnormalities of impulse generation, conduction, or both. It is, however, difficult to establish with certainty an underlying mechanism for many clinical arrhythmias. The response of a tachycardia to pacing (initiation, termination, entrainment) is used in the clinical electrophysiology laboratory to make the diagnosis of reentry. There are even fewer specific tools available to diagnose non-reentrant arrhythmias. It is clear that molecular changes in the heart predispose to the development of abnormalities of cardiac rhythm. However, an exclusively molecular approach to understanding arrhythmia mechanisms is limited by failure to include cellular and network properties of the heart. A summary of the cellular and molecular changes that underlie prototypic arrhythmias and their putative mechanisms is shown in Table 224-1.

Alterations in Impulse Initiation: Automaticity
Spontaneous (phase 4) diastolic depolarization underlies the property of automaticity (pacemaking) characteristic of cells in the sinoatrial (SA) and atrioventricu-

FIGURE 224-2 Topology and subunit composition of the voltage dependent ion channels. (***Top panel***) Potassium channels are formed by the tetramerization of α or pore-forming subunits and one or more β subunits, only single β subunits are shown for clarity. (***Bottom panel***) Sodium and calcium channels are composed of α subunits with four homologous domains and one or more ancillary subunits. In all channel types the loop of protein between the fifth and sixth membrane spanning repeat in each subunit or domain forms the ion-selective pore. In the case of the sodium channel, the channel is a target for phosphorylation, the linker between the third and fourth homologous domain is critical to inactivation, and the sixth membrane-spanning repeat in the fourth domain is important in local anesthetic antiarrhythmic drug binding.

lar (AV) nodes, His-Purkinje system, coronary sinus, and pulmonary veins. Phase 4 depolarization results from the concerted action of a number of ionic currents including the inward rectifier (I_{K1}) and delayed rectifier (rapid I_{Kr} and slow I_{Ks} components) K^+ currents, Ca^{2+} currents, electrogenic Na^+,K^+-ATPase, the Na^+-Ca^{2+} exchanger, and the so-called funny, or pacemaker, current (I_f); however, the relative importance of these currents remains controversial.

The rate of phase 4 depolarization and, therefore, the firing rate of pacemaker cells are dynamically regulated. Prominent among the factors that modulate phase 4 is autonomic nervous system tone. The

TABLE 224-1 ARRHYTHMIA MECHANISMS

Electrophysiologic Property	Molecular Components	Mechanism	Prototypic Arrhythmias
Cellular			
Impulse Initiation			
Automaticity	I_f, I_{Ca-L}, I_{Ca-T}, I_K, I_{K1}	Suppression/acceleration of phase 4	Sinus bradycardia, sinus tachycardia
Triggered automaticity	Calcium overload, I_{TI}	DADs	Digitalis toxicity, reperfusion VT
	I_{Ca-L}, I_K, I_{Na}	EADs	Torsades des pointes, congenital and acquired
Excitation	I_{Na}	Suppression of phase 0	Ischemic VF
	I_{K-ATP}	AP shortening, inexcitability	
	I_{Ca-L}	Suppression	AV block
Repolarization	I_{Na}, I_{Ca-L}, I_K, I_{K1}, Ca^{2+} homeostasis	AP prolongation, EADS, DADs	Polymorphic VT (HF, LVH)
	I_{Ca-L}, K channels, Ca^{2+} homeostasis	AP shortening	Atrial fibrillation
Multicellular			
Cellular coupling	Connexins (Cx43), I_{Na}, I_{K-ATP}	Decreased coupling	Ischemic VT/VF
Tissue Structure	Extracellular matrix, collagen	Excitable gap and functional reentry	Monomorphic VT, atrial fibrillation

Note: DAD, delayed afterdepolarization; VT, ventricular tachyarrhythmia; IVR, idioventricular rhythm; EAD, early afterdepolarization; VF, ventricular fibrillation; AV, atrioventricular; HF, heart failure; AP, action potential.

negative chronotropic effect of activation of the parasympathetic nervous system is the result of release of acetylcholine that binds to muscarinic receptors, releasing G protein βγ subunits that activate a potassium current (I_{KACh}) in nodal and atrial cells. The resulting increase in K^+ conductance opposes membrane depolarization, slowing the rate of rise of phase 4 of the action potential. Conversely, augmentation of sympathetic nervous system tone increases myocardial catecholamine concentrations, which activate both α and β receptors. The effect of β1-adrenergic stimulation predominates in pacemaking cells, augmenting both L-type Ca current (I_{Ca-L}) and I_f, thus increasing the slope of phase 4. Enhanced sympathetic nervous system activity can dramatically increase the rate of firing of SA nodal cells, producing sinus tachycardia with rates >200 beats/min. By contrast, the increased rate of firing of Purkinje cells is more limited, rarely producing ventricular tachyarrhythmias >120 beats/min.

Normal automaticity may be affected by a number other factors associated with heart disease. Hypokalemia and ischemia may reduce the activity of the Na^+,K^+-ATPase, thereby reducing the background repolarizing current and enhancing phase 4 diastolic depolarization. The end result would be an increase in the spontaneous firing rate of pacemaking cells. Modest increases in extracellular potassium may render the maximum diastolic potential more positive, thereby also increasing the firing rate of pacemaking cells. A more significant increase in $[K^+]_o$, however, renders the heart inexcitable by depolarizing the membrane potential.

Normal or enhanced automaticity of subsidiary latent pacemakers produces escape rhythms in the setting of failure of more dominant pacemakers. Suppression of a pacemaker cell by a faster rhythm leads to an increased intracellular Na^+ load ($[Na^+]_i$), and extrusion of Na^+ from the cell by the Na^+,K^+-ATPase produces an increased background repolarizing current that slows phase 4 diastolic depolarization. At slower rates, the $[Na^+]_i$ is decreased, as is the activity of the Na^+,K^+-ATPase, resulting in progressively more rapid diastolic depolarization and warm-up of the tachycardia rate. Overdrive suppression and warm-up are characteristic of, but may not be observed in, all automatic tachycardias. Abnormal conduction into tissue with enhanced automaticity (*entrance block*) may blunt or eliminate the phenomena of overdrive suppression and warm-up of automatic tissue.

Abnormal automaticity may underlie atrial tachycardia, accelerated idioventricular rhythms, and ventricular tachycardia, particularly that associated with ischemia and reperfusion. It has also been suggested that injury currents at the borders of ischemic myocardium may depolarize adjacent non-ischemic tissue, predisposing to automatic ventricular tachycardia.

Afterdepolarizations and Triggered Automaticity
Triggered automaticity or activity refers to impulse initiation that is dependent on afterdepolarizations (Fig. 224-3). Afterdepolarizations are membrane voltage oscillations that occur during (early afterdepolarizations, EAD) or following (delayed afterdepolarization, DADs) an action potential.

The cellular feature common to the induction of DADs is the presence of increased Ca^{2+} load in the cytosol and sarcoplasmic reticulum. Inhibition of the Na^+,K^+-ATPase by digitalis glycosides facilitates, but is not necessary for creating, the Ca^{2+} overload that predisposes to DADs. Catecholamines and ischemia sufficiently enhance Ca^{2+} loading to produce DADs. Accumulation of lysophospholipids in ischemic myocardium with consequent Na^+ and Ca^{2+} overload has been suggested as a mechanism for DADs and triggered automaticity. Cells from damaged areas or surviving a myocardial infarction may display spontaneous release of calcium from the sarcoplasmic reticulum, and this may generate "waves" of intracellular calcium elevation and arrhythmias.

EADs occur during the action potential and interrupt the orderly repolarization of the myocyte. It has been traditionally held that, unlike DADs, EADs do not depend on a rise in intracellular Ca^{2+}, and that, instead, action potential prolongation and reactivation of depolarizing currents are fundamental to their production. More recent experimental evidence suggests a previously unappreciated interrelationship between intracellular calcium loading and EADs. Cytosolic calcium may increase when action potentials are prolonged. This, in turn, appears to enhance L-type Ca current, further prolonging action potential dura-

FIGURE 224-3 Schematic action potentials with early (EAD) and delayed afterdepolarizations (DAD). Afterdepolarizations are spontaneous depolarizations in cardiac myocytes. EADs occur before the end of the action potential (phases 2 and 3), interrupting repolarization. DADs occur during phase 4 of the action potential after completion of repolarization. The cellular mechanisms of EADs and DADs differ (see text).

tion as well as providing the inward current driving EADs. Intracellular calcium loading by action potential prolongation may also enhance the likelihood of DADs. The interrelationship among intracellular [Ca²⁺], EADs, and DADs may be one explanation for the susceptibility of hearts that are calcium loaded (e.g., in ischemia or congestive heart failure) to develop arrhythmias, particularly on exposure to action potential–prolonging drugs.

EAD-triggered arrhythmias exhibit rate dependence. In general, the amplitude of an EAD is augmented at slow rates when action potentials are longer. Rapid pacing will shorten the action potential duration and reduce EAD amplitude, likely due to augmentation of delayed rectifier K⁺ currents and, perhaps, hastening of Ca²⁺-induced inactivation of L-type Ca currents. Similarly, catecholamines increase heart rate and decrease action potential duration and EAD amplitude, despite the well-described effect of β-adrenergic stimulation on increasing L-type Ca current. A fundamental condition that underlies the development of EADs is action potential and QT prolongation. Hypokalemia, hypomagnesemia, bradycardia, and, most commonly, drugs can predispose to the generation of EADs, invariably in the context of prolonging the action potential. Antiarrhythmics with class IA and III action (see below) produce action potential and QT prolongation intended to be therapeutic, but frequently causing arrhythmias. Noncardiac drugs, such as phenothiazines, nonsedating antihistamines, and some antibiotics can also prolong the action potential duration and predispose to EAD-mediated triggered arrhythmias. Decreased [K⁺]ₒ may paradoxically decrease membrane potassium currents (particularly I_{Kr}) in the ventricular myocyte, explaining why hypokalemia causes action potential prolongation and EADs. In fact, potassium infusions in patients with the congenital long QT syndrome (LQTS) and in those with drug-induced acquired QT prolongation shorten the QT interval.

EAD-mediated triggered activity likely underlies initiation of the characteristic polymorphic ventricular tachycardia, *torsades des pointes*, seen in patients with congenital and acquired forms of the LQTS. Structural heart disease, such as cardiac hypertrophy and failure, may also delay ventricular repolarization (so-called electrical remodeling) and predispose to arrhythmias related to abnormalities of repolarization. The abnormalities of repolarization in hypertrophy and failure are often magnified by concomitant drug therapy or electrolyte disturbances.

Abnormal Impulse Conduction: Reentry   The most common arrhythmia mechanism is reentry. Reentry is a property of networks of myocytes. Fundamentally, reentry is defined as circulation of an activation wave around an inexcitable obstacle. Thus, the requirements for reentry are two electrophysiologically dissimilar pathways for impulse propagation around an inexcitable region such that unidirectional block occurs in one of the pathways and a region of excitable tissue exists at the head of the propagating wavefront (Fig. 224-4). Structural and electrophysiologic properties of the heart may contribute to the development of the inexcitable obstacle and of unidirectional block. The complex geometry of muscle bundles in the heart and spatial heterogeneity of cellular coupling or other active membrane properties (i.e., ionic currents) appear to be critical.

A key feature in classifying reentrant arrhythmias, particularly for therapy, is the presence and size of an excitable gap. An excitable gap exists when the tachycardia circuit is longer than the tachycardia wavelength (λ = conduction velocity × refractory period, representing the size of the circuit that can sustain reentry), allowing appropriately timed stimuli to reset propagation in the circuit. Reentrant arrhythmias may exist in the heart in the absence of an excitable gap and with a tachycardia wavelength nearly the same size as the path length. In this case, the wavefront propagates through partially refractory tissue with no anatomic obstacle and no fully excitable gap; this is referred to as *leading circle reentry*, a form of functional reentry (reentry that depends on functional properties of the tissue). Unlike excitable gap reentry, there is no fixed anatomic circuit in leading circle reentry, and it may therefore not be possible to disrupt the tachycardia with pacing or destruction of a part of the circuit. Furthermore, the circuit in leading

FIGURE 224-4 Schematic diagram of reentry. A. The circuit comprises two limbs, one with slow conduction. **B.** A premature impulse blocks in the fast pathway and conducts over the slow pathway, allowing the fast pathway to recover so that the activation wave can reenter the fast pathway from the retrograde direction. **C.** During sustained reentry utilizing such a circuit, a gap (excitable gap) exists between the activating head of the wave and the recovering tail. **D.** One mechanism of termination of reentry is when the conduction and recovery characteristics of the circuit change, and the activating head of the wave collides with the tail, extinguishing the tachycardia.

circle reentry tends to be less stable than that in excitable gap reentrant arrhythmias, with large variations in cycle length and predilection to termination.

Anatomically determined, excitable gap reentry can explain several clinically important tachycardias, such as AV reentry, atrial flutter, bundle branch reentry ventricular tachycardia, and ventricular tachycardia in scarred myocardium. Atrial flutter represents an example of a reentrant tachycardia with a large excitable gap not always due to an anatomic constraint but to functional block (reflecting the special properties of the crista terminalis discussed above). There is strong evidence to suggest that arrhythmias, such as atrial and ventricular fibrillation, are associated with more complex activation of the heart and are due to functional reentry.

Structural heart disease is associated with changes in conduction and refractoriness that increase the risk of reentrant arrhythmias. Chronically ischemic myocardium exhibits a down-regulation of the gap junction channel protein (connexin 43) that carries intercellular ionic current. The border zones of infarcted and failing ventricular myocardium exhibit not only functional alterations of ionic currents but also remodeling of tissue and altered distribution of gap junctions. The changes in gap junction channel expression and distribution, in combination with macroscopic tissue alterations, support a role for slowed conduction in reentrant arrhythmias that complicate chronic coronary artery disease. Aged human atrial myocardium exhibits altered conduction, manifest as highly fractionated atrial electrograms, producing an ideal substrate for the reentry that may underlie the very common development of atrial fibrillation in the elderly.

APPROACH TO THE PATIENT:
Cardiac Arrhythmia

The evaluation of patients with suspected cardiac arrhythmias is highly individualized; however, two key features, the history and ECG, are pivotal in directing the diagnostic workup and therapy. Patients with cardiac arrhythmias exhibit a wide spectrum of clinical presentations from asymptomatic ECG abnormalities to survival from cardiac arrest. In general, the more severe the presenting symptoms, the more aggressive are the evaluation and treatment. Loss of consciousness that is believed to be of cardiac origin typically mandates an exhaustive search for the etiology and often requires invasive, device-based therapy. The presence of structural heart disease and prior myocardial infarction dictates a change in the approach to the management of syncope or ventricular arrhythmias. The presence of a family history of serious ventricular arrhythmias or premature sudden death will influence the evaluation of presumed heritable arrhythmias.

The physical examination is focused on determining if there is cardiopulmonary disease that is associated with specific cardiac arrhythmias. The absence of significant cardiopulmonary disease often, but not always, suggests benignity of the rhythm disturbance. In contrast, palpitations, syncope, or near syncope in the setting of significant heart or lung disease has more ominous implications. In addition, the physical examination may reveal the presence of a persistent arrhythmia such as atrial fibrillation.

The judicious use of noninvasive diagnostic tests is an important element in the evaluation of patients with arrhythmias, and there is none more important that the ECG, particularly if recorded at the time of symptoms. Uncommon but diagnostically important signatures of electrophysiologic disturbances may be unearthed on the resting ECG, such as delta waves in Wolff-Parkinson-White (WPW) syndrome, prolongation or shortening of the QT interval, right precordial ST-segment abnormalities in Brugada syndrome, and epsilon waves in arrhythmogenic right ventricular dysplasia. Variants of body surface ECG recording can provide important information about arrhythmia substrates and triggers. Holter monitoring and event recording, either continuous or intermittent, record the body surface ECG over longer periods of time, enhancing the possibility of observing the cardiac rhythm during symptoms. Implantable long-term monitors and commercial ambulatory ECG monitoring services exist that permit prolonged telemetric monitoring for both diagnosis and to assess the efficacy of therapy.

Long-term recordings permit the assessment of the time-varying behavior of the heart rhythm. Heart rate variability (HRV) and QT interval variability (QTV) provide noninvasive methods to assess autonomic nervous system influence on the heart. HRV arises because of subtle changes in sinus rate due to changes in sympathovagal input to the sinus node. Normal time domain, frequency domain, and geometric methods metrics have been established for HRV; a decrease in HRV and an increase in low-frequency power have been associated with increased sympathetic nervous system tone and increased mortality in patients after myocardial infarction. Signal-averaged electrocardiography (SAECG) uses signal-averaging techniques to amplify small potentials in the body surface ECG that are associated with slow conduction in the myocardium. The presence of these small potentials, referred to as *late potentials* because of their timing with respect to the QRS complex, and prolongation of the filtered (or averaged) QRS duration are indicative of slowed conduction in the ventricle and have been associated with an increased risk of ventricular arrhythmias after myocardial infarction. Exercise electrocardiography is important in determining the presence of myocardial demand ischemia; more recently, analysis of the morphology of the QT interval with exercise has been used to assess the risk of serious ventricular arrhythmias. Microscopic alterations in the T wave (T wave alternans, TWA) at low heart rates identify patients at risk for ventricular arrhythmias. A number of other tests of the variability in the T-wave morphology or duration of the QT interval have been used to assess instability in repolarization of the ventricle and an increased risk of arrhythmias.

Head-up tilt (HUT) testing is a useful in the evaluation of some patients with syncope. The physiologic response to HUT is incompletely understood; however, redistribution of blood volume and increased ventricular contractility occur consistently. Exaggerated activation of a central reflex in response to HUT produces a stereotypic response of an initial increase in heart rate, then a drop in blood pressure followed by a reduction in heart rate characteristic of neurally mediated hypotension. Other responses to HUT may be observed in patients with orthostatic hypotension and autonomic insufficiency. HUT is most often used in patients with recurrent syncope, although it may be useful in patients with single syncopal episodes with associated injury, particularly in the absence of structural heart disease. In patients with structural heart disease, HUT

may be indicated in those with syncope, in whom other causes (e.g., asystole, ventricular tachyarrhythmias) have been excluded. HUT has been suggested as a useful tool in the diagnosis and therapy of recurrent idiopathic vertigo, chronic fatigue syndrome, recurrent transient ischemic attacks, and repeated falls of unknown etiology in the elderly. Importantly, HUT is relatively contraindicated in the presence of severe coronary artery disease with proximal coronary stenoses, known severe cerebrovascular disease, severe mitral stenosis, and obstruction to left ventricular outflow (e.g., aortic stenosis). The method of HUT is variable, but the angle of tilt and the duration of upright posture are central to the diagnostic utility of the test. The use of pharmacologic provocation of orthostatic stress with isoproterenol, nitrates, adenosine, and edrophonium have been used to shorten the test and enhance specificity.

Electrophysiologic testing is central to the understanding and treatment of many cardiac arrhythmias. Indeed, most frequently electrophysiologic testing is interventional, providing both diagnosis and therapy. The components of the electrophysiologic test are baseline measurements of conduction under resting and stressed (rate or pharmacologic) conditions and maneuvers, both pacing and pharmacologic, to induce arrhythmias. A number of sophisticated electrical mapping and catheter-guidance techniques have been developed to facilitate catheter-based therapeutics in the electrophysiology laboratory.

℞ CARDIAC ARRHYTHMIAS

ANTIARRHYTHMIC DRUG THERAPY The interaction of antiarrhythmic drugs with cardiac tissues and the resulting electrophysiologic changes are complex. An incomplete understanding of the effects of these drugs has produced serious missteps that have had adverse effects on patient outcomes and the development of newer pharmacologic agents. Currently, antiarrhythmic drugs have been relegated to an ancillary role in the treatment of most cardiac arrhythmias.

There are several explanations for the complexity of antiarrhythmic drug action: the structural similarity of target ion channels; regional differences in the levels of expression of channels and transporters, which change with disease; time and voltage dependence of drug action; and the effect of these drugs on targets other than ion channels. Recognizing the limitations of any scheme to classify antiarrhythmic agents, a shorthand that is useful in describing the major mechanisms of action is of some utility. Such a classification scheme was proposed in 1970 by Vaughan-Williams and later modified by Singh and Harrison. The classes of antiarrhythmic action are: class I; local anesthetic effect due to blockade of Na+ current; class II, interference with the action of catecholamines at the β-adrenergic receptor; class III, delay of repolarization due to inhibition of K+ current or activation of depolarizing current; class IV, interference with calcium conductance **(Table 224-2)**. The limitations of the Vaughan-Williams classification scheme include multiple actions of most drugs, overwhelming consideration of antagonism as a mechanism of action, and the fact that several agents have none of the four classes of action in the scheme.

TABLE 224-2 ANTIARRHYTHMIC DRUG ACTIONS

Drug	Class Actions				Miscellaneous Action
	I	II	III	IV	
Quinidine	++		++		α-Adrenergic blockade
Procainamide	++		++		Ganglionic blockade
Flecainide	+++		+		
Propafenone	++	+			
Sotalol		++	+++		
Dofetilide			+++		
Amiodarone	++	++	+++	+	α-Adrenergic blockade
Ibutilide			+++		Na+ channel activator

FIGURE 224-5 Catheter ablation of cardiac arrhythmias. A. A schematic of the lead system and generator in a patient undergoing radiofrequency catheter ablation (RFA); the circuit involves the lead in the heart and a dispersive patch placed on the body surface (usually the back). The inset shows a diagram of the heart with a catheter located at the AV valve ring for ablation of an accessory pathway. **B.** A right anterior oblique fluoroscopic image of the catheter position for ablation of a left-sided accessory pathway. A catheter is placed in the atrial side of the mitral valve ring (abl) via a transseptal puncture, other catheters are placed in the coronary sinus to record intracardiac electrograms around the mitral annulus: a circumferential catheter in the right atrium (RA) and a catheter in the right ventricular apex (RV). **C.** Body surface ECG recordings (I, II, V1) and endocardial electrograms (HRA: high right atrium; HISp: proximal His bundle electrogram; CS 7,8 recordings from poles 7 and 8 of a decapolar catheter placed in the coronary sinus) during RFA of a left-sided accessory pathway in a patient with Wolff-Parkinson-White syndrome. The QRS narrows at the 4th complex, the arrow shows the His bundle electrogram, which becomes apparent with elimination of ventricular preexcitation over the accessory pathway.

CATHETER ABLATION   The use of catheter ablation is based on the principle that there is a critical anatomic region of impulse generation or propagation required for the initiation and maintenance of cardiac arrhythmias. Destruction of such a critical region results in the elimination of the arrhythmia. The use of radiofrequency (RF) energy in clinical medicine is nearly a century old. The first catheter ablation using a DC energy source was performed in the early 1980s by Scheinman and colleagues. By the early 1990s, RF had been adapted for use in catheter-based ablation in the heart (**Fig. 224-5**).

The RF frequency band (300–30,000 kHz) is used to generate energy for several biomedical applications, including coagulation and cauterizing tissues. Energy of this frequency will not stimulate skeletal muscle or the heart and heats tissue by a resistive mechanism, with the intensity of heating being proportional to the delivered power. The density of power in the tissue falls off rapidly (with the 4th power of the radius or distance), as does the temperature, allowing for the production of small-volume lesions. The applied power, energy, or current are not good predictors of lesion size; temperature at the electrode-tissue interface is the best predictor, with temperatures >55°C consistently producing tissue necrosis. The temperature rise at the tissue-electrode interface is rapid, but heating is slower in the tissue, and steady-state lesion size may be not achieved for ≥40 s of radiofrequency energy application. Notably, tissue temperature may remain high for many seconds despite cessation of energy delivery, producing undesired ablation of cardiac

structures. Alternative, less frequently used energy sources for catheter ablation of cardiac arrhythmias include microwaves (915 MHz or 2450 MHz), lasers, ultrasound, or freezing (cryoablation). In addition to RF energy, cryoablation is being used clinically and is a safe and effective alternative to RF, especially with ablation in the region of the AV node. At temperatures just below 32°C, membrane ion transport is disrupted, producing depolarization of cells, decreased action potential amplitude and duration, and slowed conduction velocity (resulting in local conduction block)—all of which are reversible, if the tissue is rewarmed in a timely fashion. Tissue cooling can be used for mapping and ablation. Cryomapping can be used to confirm the location of a desired ablation target, such as an accessory pathway in WPW syndrome, or can be used to determine the safety of ablation around the AV node by monitoring AV conduction during cooling. Another advantage of cryoablation is that once the catheter tip cools below freezing, it adheres to the tissue, increasing catheter stability independent of the rhythm or pacing.

FURTHER READINGS

AKAR FG, TOMASELLI GF: Genetic basis of cardiac arrhythmias, in *Hurst's The Heart*, 11th ed, V Fuster et al (eds). New York, McGraw-Hill, 2004

HILLE B: *Ion Channels of Excitable Membranes*, 3d ed. Sunderland, MA, Sinauer Associates, Inc, 2001, Chaps 1, 3, 4, 21, 22

JOSEPHSON ME: *Clinical Cardiac Electrophysiology: Techniques and Interpretations*, 3d ed. Philadelphia, Lippincott Williams & Wilkins, 2002

SAKSENA S, CAMM AJ (eds): *Electrophysiological Disorders of the Heart.* Philadelphia, Elsevier Churchill Livingstone, 2005

ZIPES DP, JALIFE J (eds): *Cardiac Electrophysiology: From Cell to Bedside*, 4th ed. Philadelphia, Elsevier, 2004

225 The Bradyarrhythmias
Gordon F. Tomaselli

Electrical activation of the heart normally originates in the sinoatrial (SA) node, the predominant pacemaker. Other subsidiary pacemakers in the atrioventricular (AV) node, specialized conducting system, and muscle may initiate electrical activation if the SA node is dysfunctional or suppressed. Typically subsidiary pacemakers discharge at a slower rate and, in the absence of an appropriate increase in stroke volume, may result in tissue hypoperfusion.

Spontaneous activation and contraction of the heart are the consequence of the specialized pacemaking tissue found within these anatomic locales. As described in Chap. 224, action potentials in the heart are regionally heterogeneous. The action potentials in cells isolated from nodal tissue are distinct from those recorded from atrial and ventricular myocytes (Fig. 225-1). The complement of ionic currents present in nodal cells results in a less negative resting membrane potential compared with atrial or ventricular myocytes. Electrical diastole in nodal cells is characterized by slow diastolic depolarization (phase 4), which generates an action potential as the membrane voltage reaches threshold. The action potential upstrokes (phase 0) are slow compared with atrial or ventricular myocytes, being mediated by calcium rather than sodium current. Cells with properties of SA and AV nodal tissue are electrically connected to the remainder of the myocardium by cells with an electrophysiologic phenotype between that of nodal cells and atrial or ventricular myocytes. Cells in the SA node exhibit the most rapid phase 4 depolarization and thus are the dominant pacemakers in the normal heart.

Bradycardia results from either a failure of impulse initiation or impulse conduction. Failure of impulse initiation may be caused by depressed automaticity resulting from a slowing or failure of phase 4 diastolic depolarization (Fig. 225-2), which may result from disease or exposure to drugs. Prominently, the autonomic nervous system modulates the rate of phase 4 diastolic depolarization and, thus, the firing rate of both primary (SA node) and subsidiary pacemakers. Failure of conduction of an impulse from nodal tissue to atrial or ventricular myocardium may produce bradycardia as a result of exit block. Conditions that alter activation and connectivity of cells (e.g., fibrosis) in the heart may result in failure of impulse conduction.

SA node dysfunction and AV conduction block are the most common causes of pathologic bradycardia. SA node dysfunction may be difficult to distinguish from physiologic sinus bradycardia, particularly in the young. SA node dysfunction increases in frequency between the

Depolarizing currents ↑ I_{Ca-T}, I_F, I_{Ca-L}

Repolarizing currents ↓ I_K, I_{K1}, $I_{K ACh}$

FIGURE 225-2 Schematics of nodal action potentials and the currents that contribute to phase 4 depolarization. Relative increases in depolarizing L- (I_{Ca-L}) and T- (I_{Ca-T}) type calcium and pacemaker currents (I_f) along with a reduction in repolarizing inward rectifier (I_{K1}) and delayed rectifier (I_K) potassium currents result in depolarization. Activation of ACh-gated (I_{KACh}) potassium current and beta blockade slows the rate of phase 4 and decreases the pacing rate. *(Modified from J Jalife et al: Basic Cardiac Electrophysiology for the Clinician, Blackwell Publishing, 1999.)*

fifth and sixth decades of life and should be considered in patients with fatigue, exercise intolerance, or syncope and sinus bradycardia. Transient AV block is common in the young and likely the result of the high vagal tone found in up to 10% of young adults. Acquired and persistent failure of AV conduction is decidedly rare in healthy adult populations, with an estimated incidence of ~200/million population per year.

Permanent pacemaking is the only reliable therapy for symptomatic bradycardia in the absence of extrinsic and reversible etiologies such as increased vagal tone, hypoxia, hypothermia, and drugs (Table 225-1). Approximately 50% of the 150,000 permanent pacemakers implanted in the United States and 20–30% of the 150,000 of those implanted in Europe were implanted for SA node disease.

SA NODE DISEASE
Structure and Physiology of the SA Node The SA node is composed of a cluster of small fusiform cells located in the sulcus terminalis on the epicardial surface of the heart at the right atrial–superior vena caval junction, where they envelop the SA nodal artery. The SA node is structurally heterogeneous, but the central prototypic nodal cells have fewer distinct myofibrils than the surrounding atrial myocardium, no intercalated disks visible on light microscopy, a poorly developed sarcoplasmic reticulum, and no T-tubules. Cells in the peripheral regions of the SA node are transitional in both structure and function. The SA nodal artery arises from the right coronary artery in 55–60% and left circumflex artery in 40–45% of persons. The SA node is richly innervated by sympathetic and parasympathetic nerves and ganglia.

Irregular and slow propagation of impulses from the SA node can be explained by the electrophysiology of nodal cells and the structure of the SA node itself. The action potentials of SA nodal cells are characterized by a relatively depolarized membrane potential (Fig. 225-1) of −40 to −60 mV, slow phase 0 upstroke, and relatively rapid phase 4 diastolic depolarization compared to the action potentials recorded in cardiac muscle cells. The relative absence of inward rectifier potassium current (I_{K1}) accounts for the depolarized membrane potential;

FIGURE 225-1 Action potential profiles recorded in cells isolated from SA or AV nodal tissue compared to that of cells from atrial or ventricular myocardium. Nodal cell action potentials exhibit more depolarized resting membrane potentials, slower phase 0 upstrokes, and phase 4 diastolic depolarization.

TABLE 225-1	ETIOLOGIES OF SA NODE DYSFUNCTION
Extrinsic	**Intrinsic**
Autonomic	Sick sinus syndrome (SSS)
Carotid sinus hypersensitivity	Coronary artery disease (chronic
Vasovagal (cardioinhibitory)	and acute MI)
stimulation	Inflammatory
Drugs	Pericarditis
Beta blockers	Myocarditis (including viral)
Calcium channel blockers	Rheumatic heart disease
Digoxin	Collagen vascular diseases
Antiarrhythmics (class I and III)	Lyme disease
Adenosine	Senile amyloidosis
Clonidine (other sympatholytics)	Congenital heart disease
Lithium carbonate	TGA/Mustard and Fontan repairs
Cimetidine	Iatrogenic
Amitriptyline	Radiation therapy
Phenothiazines	Post surgical
Narcotics (methadone)	Chest trauma
Pentamidine	Familial
Hypothyroidism	AD SSS, OMIM #163800
Sleep apnea	(15q24-25)
Hypoxia	AR SSS, OMIM #608567 (3p21)
Endotracheal suctioning (vagal	SA node disease with myopia,
maneuvers)	OMIM 182190
Hypothermia	Kearns-Sayre syndrome, OMIM
Increased intracranial pressure	#530000
	Myotonic dystrophy
	Type 1, OMIM #160900
	(19q13.2-13.3)
	Type 2, OMIM #602668
	(3q13.3-q24)
	Friedreich's ataxia, OMIM #229300
	(9q13, 9p23-p11)

Note: MI, myocardial infarction; TGA, transposition of the great arteries; AD, autosomal dominant; AR, autosomal recessive; OMIM, Online Mendelian Inheritance in Man (database).

the slow upstroke of phase 0 is the result of the absence of available fast sodium current (I_{Na}) and is mediated by L-type calcium current (I_{Ca-L}); and phase 4 depolarization is the result of the aggregate activity of a number of ionic currents. Prominently, both L- and T-type (I_{Ca-T}) calcium currents, the pacemaker current (so-called funny current, or I_f) formed by the tetramerization of hyperpolarization-activated cyclic nucleotide-gated channels, and the electrogenic sodium-calcium exchanger provide depolarizing current that is antagonized by delayed rectifier (I_{Kr}) and acetylcholine-gated (I_{KACh}) potassium currents. I_{Ca-L}, I_{Ca-T}, and I_f are modulated by β-adrenergic stimulation and I_{KACh} by vagal stimulation, explaining the exquisite sensitivity of diastolic depolarization to autonomic nervous system activity. The slow conduction within the SA node is explained by the absence of I_{Na} and poor electrical coupling of cells in the node, resulting from sizeable amounts of interstitial tissue and a low abundance of gap junctions. The poor coupling allows for graded electrophysiological properties within the node, with the peripheral transitional cells being silenced by electrotonic coupling to atrial myocardium.

Etiology of SA Nodal Disease SA nodal dysfunction has been classified as intrinsic or extrinsic. The distinction is important because extrinsic dysfunction is often reversible and should generally be corrected before considering pacemaker therapy (Table 225-1). The most common causes of extrinsic SA node dysfunction are drugs and autonomic nervous system influences that suppress automaticity and/or compromise conduction. Other extrinsic causes include hypothyroidism, sleep apnea, and conditions likely to occur in critically ill patients such as hypothermia, hypoxia, increased intracranial pressure (Cushing's response), and endotracheal suctioning via activation of the vagus nerve.

Intrinsic sinus node dysfunction is degenerative and often characterized pathologically by fibrous replacement of the SA node or its connections to the atrium. Acute and chronic coronary artery disease (CAD) may be associated with SA node dysfunction, although in the setting of acute myocardial infarction (MI; typically inferior), the ab-

normalities are transient. Inflammatory processes may alter SA node function, ultimately producing replacement fibrosis. Pericarditis, myocarditis, and rheumatic heart disease have been associated with SA nodal disease with sinus bradycardia, sinus arrest, and exit block. Carditis associated with systemic lupus erythematosus (SLE), rheumatoid arthritis (RA), and mixed connective tissue disorders (MCTDs) may also affect SA node structure and function. Senile amyloidosis is an infiltrative disorder in patients typically in their ninth decade of life; deposition of amyloid protein in the atrial myocardium can impair SA node function. Some SA node disease is iatrogenic and the result of surgical correction of congenital heart disease, particularly palliative repair of corrected transposition of the great arteries by the Mustard procedure.

Rare heritable forms of sinus node disease have been described, and several have been genetically characterized. Autosomal dominant sinus node dysfunction in conjunction with supraventricular tachycardia (i.e., tachycardia-bradycardia variant of sick-sinus syndrome, SSS) has been linked to mutations in the pacemaker current (I_f) subunit gene *HCN4* on chromosome 15. An autosomal recessive form of SSS with the prominent feature of atrial inexcitability and absence of P waves on the electrocardiogram (ECG) is caused by mutations in the cardiac sodium channel gene, *SCN5A*, on chromosome 3. SSS associated with myopia has been described but not genetically characterized. There are several neuromuscular diseases including Kearns-Sayre syndrome (ophthalmoplegia, pigmentary degeneration of the retina, and cardiomyopathy) and myotonic dystrophy that have a predilection for the conducting system and SA node.

SSS in both the young and the elderly is associated with an increase in fibrous tissue in the SA node. The onset of SSS may be hastened by coexisting disease, such as CAD, diabetes mellitus, hypertension, and valvular diseases and cardiomyopathies.

Clinical Features of SA Node Disease SA node dysfunction may be completely asymptomatic and manifest as an ECG anomaly such as sinus bradycardia; sinus arrest and exit block; or alternating supraventricular tachycardia, usually atrial fibrillation, and bradycardia. Symptoms associated with SA node dysfunction, and in particular tachycardia-bradycardia syndrome, may be related to both bradycardia and tachycardia. For example, tachycardia may be associated with palpitations, angina pectoris, and heart failure; and bradycardia may be associated with hypotension syncope, presyncope, fatigue, and weakness. In the setting of SSS, overdrive suppression of the SA node may result in prolonged pauses and syncope upon termination of the tachycardia. In many cases, symptoms associated with SA node dysfunction are the result of concomitant cardiovascular disease. A significant minority of patients with SSS will develop signs and symptoms of heart failure that may be related to slow or fast heart rates.

One-third to one-half of patients with SA node dysfunction will develop supraventricular tachycardia, usually atrial fibrillation or atrial flutter. The incidence of chronic atrial fibrillation in patients with SA node dysfunction increases with advanced age, hypertension, diabetes mellitus, left ventricular dilation, valvular heart disease, and ventricular pacing. Remarkably, some symptomatic patients may experience an improvement in symptoms with the development of atrial fibrillation, presumably from an increase in their average heart rate. Patients with the tachycardia-bradycardia variant of SSS, similar to patients with atrial fibrillation, are at risk for thromboembolism, and *those at greatest risk*, including patients ≥65 years, or patients with a prior history of stroke, valvular heart disease, left ventricular dysfunction, or atrial enlargement, should be treated with anticoagulants. Up to one-quarter of patients with SA node disease will have concurrent AV conduction disease; although only a minority will require specific therapy for high-grade AV block.

The natural history of SA node dysfunction is one of varying intensity of symptoms even in patients who present with syncope. Symptoms related to SA node dysfunction may be significant, but overall mortality is usually not compromised in the absence of other significant comorbid conditions. These features of the natural history need to be taken into account when considering therapy in these patients.

FIGURE 225-3 Sinus slowing and pauses on the ECG. The ECG is recorded during sleep in a young patient without heart disease. The heart rate before the pause is slow, and the PR interval is prolonged consistent with a physiologic response to an increase in vagal tone. The P waves have a morphology consistent with sinus rhythm.

Electrocardiography of SA Node Disease The electrocardiographic manifestations of SA node dysfunction include sinus bradycardia, sinus pauses, sinus arrest, sinus exit block, tachycardia (in SSS), and chronotropic incompetence. It is often difficult to distinguish pathologic from physiologic sinus bradycardia. By definition sinus bradycardia is a rhythm driven by the SA node with a rate of <60 beats/min; sinus bradycardia is very common and typically benign. Resting heart rates of <60 beats/min are very common in young healthy individuals and physically conditioned subjects. A sinus rate of <40 beats/min in the awake state in the absence of physical conditioning is generally considered abnormal. Sinus pauses and sinus arrest result from the failure of the SA node to discharge, producing a pause without P waves visible on the ECG (Fig. 225-3). Sinus pauses of up to 3 s are common in the awake athlete, and pauses of this duration or longer may be observed in asymptomatic elderly subjects. Intermittent failure of conduction from the SA node produces sinus exit block. The severity of sinus exit block may vary in a manner similar to that of AV block (see below). Prolongation of conduction from the sinus node will not be apparent on the ECG; second-degree SA block will produce intermittent conduction from the SA node and a regularly irregular atrial rhythm.

Type I second-degree SA block results from progressive prolongation of SA node conduction and appears on the ECG as a progressive lengthening of the P-R interval and progressive shortening of the R-R interval, followed by a pause (Fig. 225-4). In type II second-degree SA block there is no change in the P-R interval before the pause. Complete or third-degree SA block results in no P waves on the ECG. Tachycardia-bradycardia syndrome is manifest as alternating sinus bradycardia and atrial tachyarrhythmias. Although atrial tachycardia, atrial flutter, and atrial fibrillation may be observed, the latter is the most common tachycardia. Chronotropic incompetence is the inability to increase the heart rate in response to exercise or other stress appropriately and is defined in greater detail below.

Diagnostic Testing SA node dysfunction is most commonly a clinical or electrocardiographic diagnosis. Sinus bradycardia or pauses on the resting ECG are rarely sufficient to diagnose SA node disease, and longer-term recording and symptom correlation are generally required. Symptoms in the absence of sinus bradyarrhythmias may be sufficient to exclude a diagnosis of SA node dysfunction.

Electrocardiographic recording plays a central role in the diagnosis and management of SA node dysfunction. Despite the limitations of the resting ECG, longer-term recording employing Holter or event monitors may permit correlation of symptoms with the cardiac rhythm. Many contemporary event monitors may be automatically triggered to record the ECG when certain programmed heart rate criteria are met. Implantable ECG monitors permit long-term recording (12–18 months) in particularly challenging patients.

Failure to increase the heart rate with exercise is referred to as *chronotropic incompetence*. This is alternatively defined as a failure to reach 85% of predicted maximal heart rate at peak exercise, or failure to achieve a heart rate > 100 beats/min with exercise or a maximal heart rate with exercise less than two standard deviations below that of an age-matched control population. Exercise testing may be useful in discriminating chronotropic incompetence from resting bradycardia and may aid in the identification of the mechanism of exercise intolerance.

Autonomic nervous system testing is useful in diagnosing carotid sinus hypersensitivity; pauses >3 s are consistent with the diagnosis but may be present in asymptomatic elderly subjects. Determining the intrinsic heart rate (IHR) may distinguish SA node dysfunction from slow heart rates resulting from high vagal tone. The normal IHR after administration of 0.2 mg/kg propranolol and 0.04 mg/kg atropine is 117.2 – (0.53 × age) in beats/min; a low IHR is indicative of SA disease.

Electrophysiologic testing may play a role in the assessment of patients with presumed SA node dysfunction and in the evaluation of syncope, particularly in the setting of structural heart disease. In this circumstance, electrophysiologic testing is used to rule out more malignant etiologies of syncope such as ventricular tachyarrhythmias and AV conduction block. There are several ways to assess SA node function invasively. These include the sinus node recovery time (SNRT), defined as the longest pause after cessation of overdrive pacing of the right atrium near the SA node (normal: <1500 ms or, corrected for sinus cycle length, <550 ms); and the sinoatrial conduction time (SACT), defined as one-half the difference between the intrinsic sinus cycle length and a noncompensatory pause after a premature atrial stimulus (normal < 125 ms). The combination of an abnormal SNRT, an abnormal SACT, and a low IHR is a sensitive and specific indicator of intrinsic SA node disease.

℞ SINOATRIAL NODE DYSFUNCTION

Since SA node dysfunction is not associated with increased mortality, the aim of therapy is alleviation of symptoms. Exclusion of extrinsic causes of SA node dysfunction and correlation of the cardiac rhythm with symptoms is an essential part of patient management. Pacemaker implantation is the primary therapeutic intervention in patients with symptomatic SA node dysfunction. Pharmacologic considerations are important in the evaluation and management of patients with SA nodal disease. A number of drugs modulate SA node function and are extrinsic causes of dysfunction (Table 225-1).

Beta blockers and calcium channel blockers increase SNRT in patients with SA node dysfunction, and antiarrhythmic drugs with class I and III action may promote SA node exit block. In general such agents should be discontinued prior to making decisions regarding the need for permanent pacing in patients with SA node disease. Chronic pharmacologic therapy for sinus bradyarrhythmias is limited. Some pharmacologic agents may improve SA node function; digitalis, for example, has been shown to shorten SNRT in patients with SA node

FIGURE 225-4 Mobitz type I SA nodal exit block. A theoretical SA node electrogram (SAN EG) is shown. Note that there is grouped beating producing a regularly irregular heart rhythm. The SA node EG rate is constant with progressive delay in exit from the node, and activation of the atria, inscribing the P wave. This produces subtly decreasing P-P intervals prior to the pause, and the pause is less that twice the cycle length of the last sinus interval.

dysfunction. Isoproterenol or atropine administered IV may increase the sinus rate acutely. Theophylline has been used both acutely and chronically to increase heart rate but has liabilities when used in patients with tachycardia-bradycardia syndrome, increasing the frequency of supraventricular tachyarrhythmias; and in patients with structural heart disease, increasing the risk of potentially serious ventricular arrhythmias. At the current time, there is only a single randomized study of therapy for SA node dysfunction. In patients with resting heart rates <50 and >30 beats/min on a Holter monitor, patients who received dual-chamber pacemakers experienced significantly fewer syncopal episodes and had symptomatic improvement compared to patients randomized to theophylline or no treatment.

In certain circumstances, sinus bradycardia requires no specific treatment or only temporary rate support. Sinus bradycardia is common in patients with acute inferior or posterior MI and can be exacerbated by vagal activation induced by pain or the use of drugs such as morphine. Ischemia of the SA nodal artery probably occurs in acute coronary syndromes more typically with involvement with the right coronary artery, and even with infarction, the effect on SA node function is most often transient.

Sinus bradycardia is a prominent feature of carotid sinus hypersensitivity and neurally mediated hypotension associated with vasovagal syncope that responds to pacemaker therapy. Carotid hypersensitivity with recurrent syncope or presyncope associated with a predominant cardioinhibitory component responds to pacemaker implantation. Several randomized trials have demonstrated that patients with drug-refractory vasovagal syncope have fewer recurrences and longer time to recurrence of symptoms with permanent pacing.

The details of pacing modes and indications for pacing in SA node dysfunction are discussed below.

ATRIOVENTRICULAR CONDUCTION DISEASE

Structure and Physiology of the AV Node The AV conduction axis is structurally complex, involving the atria and ventricles as well as the AV node. Unlike the SA node, the AV node is a subendocardial structure originating in the transitional zone, which is composed of aggregates of cells in the posterior-inferior right atrium. Superior, medial, and posterior transitional atrionodal bundles converge on the compact AV node. The compact AV node (~1 × 3 × 5 mm) is located at the apex of the triangle of Koch, which is defined by the coronary sinus ostium posteriorly, the septal tricuspid valve annulus anteriorly, and the tendon of Todaro superiorly. The compact AV node continues as the penetrating AV bundle where it immediately traverses the central fibrous body and is in close proximity to the aortic, mitral, and tricuspid valve annuli; thus, it is subject to injury in the setting of valvular heart disease or its surgical treatment. The penetrating AV bundle continues through the annulus fibrosis and emerges along the ventricular septum adjacent to the membranous septum as the bundle of His. The right bundle branch (RBB) emerges from the distal AV bundle in a band that traverses the right ventricle (moderator band). In contrast, the left bundle branch (LBB) is a broad subendocardial sheet of tissue on the septal left ventricle. The Purkinje fiber network emerges from the RBB and LBB and extensively ramifies on the endocardial surfaces of the right and left ventricles, respectively.

The blood supply to the penetrating AV bundle is from the AV nodal artery and first septal perforator of the left anterior descending coronary artery. The bundle branches also have a dual blood supply from the septal perforators of the left anterior descending coronary artery and branches of the posterior descending coronary artery. The AV node is highly innervated with postganglionic sympathetic and parasympathetic nerves. The bundle of His and distal conducting system are minimally influenced by autonomic tone.

The cells that comprise the AV node complex are heterogeneous with a range of action potential profiles. In the transitional zones, the cells have an electrical phenotype between atrial myocytes and cells of the compact node (Fig. 225-1). Atrionodal transitional connections may exhibit *decremental conduction*, defined as slowing of conduction with increasingly rapid rates of stimulation. Fast and slow AV nodal pathways have been described, but controversy remains as to whether these two types of pathway are anatomically distinct or represent functional heterogeneities in different regions of the AV nodal complex.

Myocytes that comprise the compact node are depolarized (resting membrane potential ~ –60 mV); exhibit action potentials with low amplitudes, slow upstrokes of phase 0 (<10 V/s), and phase 4 diastolic depolarization; high-input resistance; and relative insensitivity to external [K$^+$]. The action potential phenotype is explained by the complement of ionic currents expressed. AV nodal cells lack I_{K1} and I_{Na}; I_{Ca-L} is responsible for phase 0; and phase 4 depolarization reflects the composite activity of the depolarizing currents I_f, I_{Ca-L}, I_{Ca-T}, and I_{NCX} and the repolarizing currents I_{Kr} and I_{KACh}. Electrical coupling between cells in the AV node is tenuous due to the relatively sparse expression of gap junction channels (predominantly connexin-40) and increased extracellular volume.

The His bundle and bundle branches are insulated from ventricular myocardium. The most rapid conduction in the heart is observed in these tissues. The action potentials exhibit very rapid upstrokes (phase 0), prolonged plateaus (phase 2), and modest automaticity (phase 4 depolarization). Gap junctions, composed largely of connexin-40, are abundant but bundles are poorly connected transversely to ventricular myocardium.

Etiology of AV Conduction Disease Conduction block from the atrium to the ventricle can occur for a variety of reasons in a number of clinical situations, and AV conduction block may be classified in a number of ways. The etiologies may be functional or structural, in part analogous to extrinsic and intrinsic causes of SA nodal dysfunction. The block may be classified by its severity from first to third degree or complete AV block, or by the location of block within the AV conduction system. Table 225-2 summarizes the etiologies of AV conduction

TABLE 225-2 ETIOLOGIES OF ATRIOVENTRICULAR BLOCK

Autonomic	
Carotid sinus hypersensitivity	Vasovagal
Metabolic/endocrine	
Hyperkalemia	Hypothyroidism
Hypermagnesemia	Adrenal insufficiency
Drug-related	
Beta blockers	Adenosine
Calcium channel blockers	Antiarrhythmics (class I & III)
Digitalis	Lithium
Infectious	
Endocarditis	Tuberculosis
Lyme disease	Diphtheria
Chagas disease	Toxoplasmosis
Syphilis	
Heritable/congenital	
Congenital heart disease	Facioscapulohumeral MD, OMIM
Maternal SLE	#158900 (4q35)
Kearns-Sayre syndrome, OMIM	Emery-Dreifuss MD, OMIM
#530000	#310300 (Xq28)
Myotonic dystrophy	Progressive familial heart block,
Type 1, OMIM #160900	OMIM #113900 (19q13.2-q13.3,
(19q13.2-13.3)	3p21)
Type 2, OMIM #602668	
(3q13.3-q24)	
Inflammatory	
SLE	MCTD
Rheumatoid arthritis	Scleroderma
Infiltrative	
Amyloidosis	Hemochromatosis
Sarcoidosis	
Neoplastic/traumatic	
Lymphoma	Radiation
Mesothelioma	Catheter ablation
Melanoma	
Degenerative	
Lev disease	Lenègre disease
Coronary artery disease	
Acute MI	

Note: SLE, systemic lupus erythematosus; OMIM, Online Mendelian Inheritance in Man (database); MCTD, mixed connective tissue disease; MI, myocardial infarction.

block, those that are functional (autonomic, metabolic/endocrine, and drug-related) tend to be reversible. Most other etiologies produce structural changes, typically fibrosis, in segments of the AV conduction axis that are generally permanent. Heightened vagal tone during sleep or in well-conditioned individuals can be associated with all grades of AV block. Carotid sinus hypersensitivity, vasovagal syncope, and cough and micturition syncope may be associated with SA node slowing and AV conduction block. Transient metabolic and endocrinologic disturbances as well as a number of pharmacologic agents may also produce reversible AV conduction block.

Several infectious diseases have a predilection for the conducting system. Lyme disease may involve the heart in up to 50% of cases; 10% of patients with Lyme carditis develop AV conduction block, which is generally reversible but may require temporary pacing support. Chagas disease, common in Latin America, and syphilis may produce more persistent AV conduction disturbances. Some autoimmune and infiltrative diseases may produce AV conduction block including SLE, RA, MCTD, scleroderma, amyloidosis (primary and secondary), sarcoidosis, and hemochromatosis; rare malignancies may also impair AV conduction.

FIGURE 225-5 First-degree AV block with slowing of conduction in the AV node as indicated by the prolonged atrial-to-His bundle electrogram (AH) interval, in this case 157 ms. The His bundle-to-earliest ventricular activation on the surface ECG (HV) interval is normal. The normal HV interval suggests normal conduction below the AV node to the ventricle. I and V1 are surface ECG leads, HIS is the recording of the endocavitary electrogram at the His bundle position. A, H, and V are labels for the atrial, His bundle, and right ventricular electrograms respectively.

Idiopathic progressive fibrosis of the conduction system is one of the more common and degenerative causes of AV conduction block. Aging is associated with degenerative changes in the summit of the ventricular septum, central fibrous body, and aortic and mitral annuli and has been described as "sclerosis of the left cardiac skeleton." The process typically begins in the fourth decade of life and may be accelerated by atherosclerosis, hypertension with arteriosclerosis, and diabetes mellitus. Accelerated forms of progressive familial heart block have been identified in families with mutations in the cardiac sodium channel gene (*SCN5A*) and a second locus that has been mapped to chromosome 19.

AV conduction block has been associated with heritable neuromuscular diseases, including the nucleotide repeat disease myotonic dystrophy, the mitochondrial myopathy Kearns-Sayre syndrome (Chap. 382), and several of the monogenic muscular dystrophies. Congenital AV block may be observed in complex congenital cardiac anomalies (Chap. 229), such as transposition of the great arteries, ostium primum atrial septal defects (ASD), ventricular septal defects (VSD), endocardial cushion defects, and some single ventricle defects. Congenital AV block in the setting of a structurally normal heart has been seen in children born to mothers with SLE. Iatrogenic AV block may occur during mitral or aortic valve surgery, rarely in the setting of thoracic radiation, and as a consequence catheter ablation. AV block is a decidedly rare complication of the surgical repair of VSDs or ASDs but may complicate Fontan or Mustard repairs of transposition of the great arteries.

CAD may produce transient or persistent AV block. In the setting of coronary spasm, ischemia, particularly in the right coronary artery distribution, may produce transient AV block. In acute MI, AV block transiently develops in 10–25% of patients; most commonly this is first- or second-degree AV block but complete heart block (CHB) may also occur. Second-degree and higher grade AV block tends to occur more often in inferior rather than anterior acute MI; however, the level of block in inferior MI tends to be in the AV node with more stable, narrow escape rhythms. In contrast, acute anterior MI is associated with block in the distal AV nodal complex, His bundle, or bundle

branches and results in wide complex, unstable escape rhythms and a worse prognosis with high mortality.

Electrocardiography and Electrophysiology of AV Conduction Block

Atrioventricular conduction block is typically diagnosed electrocardiographically which characterizes the severity of the conduction disturbance and allows one to draw inferences about the location of block. AV conduction block manifests as slow conduction in its mildest forms and failure to conduct, either intermittent or persistently, in more severe varieties. First-degree AV block (PR interval > 200 ms) is a slowing of conduction through the AV junction (Fig. 225-5). The site of delay is typically in the AV node but may be in the atria, AV node bundle of His, or His-Purkinje system; a wide QRS complex favors distal conduction and narrow QRS complex delay in the node proper or, less commonly, in the bundle of His. In second-degree AV block there is an intermittent failure of electrical impulse conduction from atrium to ventricle. Second-degree AV block is subclassified as Mobitz type 1 or Wenckebach and Mobitz type 2. The periodic failure of conduction in Mobitz type 1 block is characterized by a progressively lengthening PR interval, shortening of the RR interval, and a pause that is less than two times the immediately preceding RR interval on the ECG. The ECG complex after the pause exhibits a shorter PR interval that that immediately preceding the pause (Fig. 225-6). This ECG pattern most often arises because of decremental conduction of electrical impulses in the AV node.

It is important to distinguish type 1 from type 2 second-degree AV nodal block because the latter has more serious prognostic implications. Type 2 second-degree AV block is characterized by intermittent failure of conduction of the P wave without changes in the preceding PR or RR intervals. When AV block is 2:1 it may be difficult to distinguish type 1 from type 2 block. Type 2 second-degree AV block typically occurs in the distal or infra-His conduction system, is often associated with intraventricular conduction delays (e.g., bundle branch block), and is more likely to proceed to higher grades of AV block than is type 1 second-degree AV block. Second-degree AV block (particularly type 2) may be associated with a series of nonconducted P waves, referred to as *paroxysmal AV block* (Fig. 225-7), and implies significant

FIGURE 225-6 Mobitz type I second-degree AV block. The PR interval prolongs prior to the pause as shown in the ladder diagram. The ECG pattern results from slowing of conduction in the AV node.

FIGURE 225-7 Paroxysmal AV block. Multiple nonconducted P waves following a period of sinus bradycardia with a normal PR interval. This implies significant conduction system disease, requiring permanent pacemaker implantation.

conduction system disease and an indication for permanent pacing. Complete failure of conduction from atrium to ventricle is referred to as complete or third-degree AV block. AV block that is intermediate between second and third degree is referred to as high-grade AV block, and, as with CHB, implies advanced AV conduction system disease. In both cases, block is most often distal to the AV node, and the duration of the QRS complex can be helpful in determining the level of block. In the absence of a preexisting bundle branch block, a wide QRS escape rhythm (Fig. 225-8*B*) implies block in the distal His or bundle branches; in contrast, a narrow QRS rhythm implies block in the AV node or proximal His and an escape rhythm originating in the AV junction (Fig. 225-8*A*). Narrow QRS escape rhythms are typically faster and more stable than wide QRS escape rhythms and originate more proximally in the AV conduction system.

Diagnostic Testing Diagnostic testing in the evaluation of AV block is aimed at determining the level of conduction block, particularly in asymptomatic patients, since the prognosis and therapy depend upon whether block is in or below the AV node. Vagal maneuvers, carotid sinus massage, exercise, and administration of drugs such as atropine or isoproterenol may be diagnostically informative. Owing to the differences in innervation of the AV node and infranodal conduction system, vagal stimulation and carotid sinus massage slow conduction in the AV node but have less of an effect on

infranodal tissue and may even improve conduction due to a reduced rate of activation of distal tissues. Conversely, atropine, isoproterenol, and exercise improve conduction through the AV node and impair infranodal conduction. In patients with congenital CHB and a narrow QRS complex, exercise typically increases heart rate; by contrast, those with acquired CHB, particularly with wide QRS, do not respond to exercise with an increase in heart rate.

Additional diagnostic evaluation, including electrophysiologic testing, may be indicated in patients with syncope and suspected high-grade AV block. This is particularly relevant if noninvasive testing does not reveal the cause of syncope or if the patient has structural heart disease with ventricular tachyarrhythmias as a cause of symptoms. Electrophysiologic testing provides more precise information regarding the location of AV conduction block and permits studies of AV conduction under conditions of pharmacologic stress and exercise. Recording of the His bundle electrogram by a catheter positioned at the superior margin of the tricuspid valve annulus provides information about conduction at all levels of the AV conduction axis. A properly recorded His bundle electrogram reveals local atrial activity, the His electrogram, and local ventricular activation; when monitored simultaneously with recorded body surface electrocardiographic traces, intraatrial, AV nodal, and infranodal conduction times can be assessed (Fig. 225-5).

The *PA interval*, the time from the earliest onset of the P wave on the surface ECG to the onset of the atrial deflection on the His bundle catheter, is an index of intraatrial conduction time and should be ≤50 ms. The time from the most rapid deflection of the atrial electrogram in the His bundle recording to the His electrogram (*AH interval*) represents conduction through the AV node and is normally <130 ms. Finally, the time from the His electrogram to the earliest onset of the QRS on the surface ECG (*HV interval*) represents the conduction time through the His-Purkinje system and is normally ≤55 ms. Rate stress produced by pacing can unveil abnormal AV conduction. Mobitz I second-degree AV block at short atrial paced cycle lengths is a normal response; however, when it occurs at atrial cycle lengths > 500 ms

FIGURE 225-8 High-grade AV block. A. Multiple nonconducted P waves with a regular narrow complex QRS escape rhythm likely emanating from the AV junction. **B.** A wide complex QRS escape and a single PVC. In both cases there is no consistent temporal relationship between the P waves and QRS complexes.

(<120 beats/min) in the absence of high vagal tone, it is abnormal. Typically type I second-degree AV block is associated with prolongation of the AH interval representing conduction slowing and block in the AV node. Block below the node with prolongation of the HV interval or a His bundle electrogram with no ventricular activation (Fig. 225-9) is abnormal unless it is elicited at fast pacing rates or short coupling intervals with extra stimulation.

First-degree AV block is classically intranodal and is associated with a prolonged AH interval. Often, AH prolongation is due to the effect of drugs (beta blockers, calcium channel blockers, digitalis), or increased vagal tone. Atropine can be used to reverse high vagal tone; however, if AH prolongation and AV block at long pacing cycle lengths persist, intrinsic AV node disease is likely. Mobitz type 1 second-degree AV block is usually intranodal and type 2 second-degree block is infranodal, frequently in the His-Purkinje system. It is often difficult to determine the type of second-degree AV block when 2:1 conduction is present; however, the finding of a His bundle electrogram after every atrial electrogram indicates that block is occurring in the distal conduction system.

Intracardiac recording at electrophysiologic study that reveals the presence of His-Purkinje conduction block is associated with an increased risk of progression to higher grades of block and is generally an indication for pacing. In the setting of bundle branch block, the HV interval may reveal the condition of the unblocked bundle and the prognosis for developing more advanced AV conduction block. Prolongation of the HV interval in patients with asymptomatic bundle branch block is associated with an increased risk of developing higher-grade AV block. The risk increases with greater prolongation of the HV interval such that in patients with an HV interval > 100 ms, the annual incidence of complete AV block approaches 10%, indicating a need for pacing. In patients with acquired CHB, even if intermittent, there is little role for electrophysiologic testing, and pacemaker implantation is almost always indicated.

FIGURE 225-9 High-grade AV block below the His. The AH interval is normal and is not changing prior to block. Atrial and His bundle electrograms are recorded consistent with block below the distal AV junction. I, II, III, and V1 are surface ECG leads. HISp, HISd, RVA are the proximal HIS, distal HIS, and right ventricular apical electrical recordings. A, H, and V represent the atrial, His, and ventricular electrograms on the His bundle recording. (*Tracing courtesy of Dr. Joseph Marine; with permission.*)

℞ ATRIOVENTRICULAR CONDUCTION BLOCK

Temporary or permanent artificial pacing is the most reliable treatment for patients with symptomatic AV conduction system disease. However, exclusion of reversible causes of AV block and the need for temporary heart rate support based on the hemodynamic condition of the patient are essential considerations in each patient. Correction of electrolyte derangements and ischemia, inhibition of excessive vagal tone, and withholding drugs with AV nodal blocking properties may increase the heart rate. Adjunctive pharmacologic treatment with atropine or isoproterenol may be useful if block is in the AV node. Since most pharmacologic treatment may take some time to initiate and become effective, temporary pacing may be necessary. The most expeditious technique is the use of transcutaneous pacing, where pacing patches are placed anteriorly over the cardiac apex (cathode) and posteriorly between the spine and scapula or above the right nipple (anode). Acutely, transcutaneous pacing is highly effective, but its duration is limited by patient discomfort and longer-term failure to capture the ventricle owing to changes in lead impedance. If a patient requires more than a few minutes of pacemaker support, transvenous temporary pacing should be instituted. Temporary pacing leads can be placed from the jugular or subclavian venous system and advanced to the right ventricle, permitting stable temporary pacing for many days, if necessary. In most circumstances, in the absence of prompt resolution, conduction block distal to the AV node requires permanent pacemaking.

PERMANENT PACEMAKERS

Nomenclature and Complications The main therapeutic intervention in SA node dysfunction and AV conduction block is permanent pacing. Since the first implementation of permanent pacing in the 1950s, many advances in technology have resulted in miniaturization, increased longevity of pulse generators, improvement in leads, and increased functionality. In order to better understand pacemaker therapy of bradycardias, it is important to be familiar with fundamentals of pacemaking. Pacemaker modes and function are named using a five-letter code. The first letter indicates the chamber(s) that is paced (O, none; A, atrium; V, ventricle; D, dual; S, single), the second is the chamber(s) in which sensing occurs (O, none; A, atrium; V, ventricle; D, dual; S, single), the third is the response to a sensed event (O, none; I, inhibition; T, triggered; D, inhibition + triggered), the fourth letter refers to the programmability or rate response (R, rate responsive), and the fifth refers to the existence of antitachycardia functions if present (O, none; P, antitachycardia pacing; S, shock; D, pace + shock). Almost all modern pacemakers are multiprogrammable and have the capability for rate responsiveness using one of several rate sensors: activity or motion, minute ventilation, or QT interval. The most commonly programmed modes of implanted single- and dual-chamber pacemakers are VVIR and DDDR, respectively, although multiple modes can be programmed in modern pacemakers.

Although pacemakers are highly reliable, they are subject to a number of complications related to implantation and electronic function. In adults, permanent pacemakers are most commonly implanted with access to the heart by way of the subclavian–superior vena cava venous system. Rare, but possible, acute complications of transvenous pacemaker implantation include infection, hematoma, pneumothorax, cardiac perforation, diaphragmatic/phrenic nerve stimulation, and lead dislodgment. Limitations of chronic pacemaker therapy include infection, erosion, lead failure, and abnormalities resulting from inappropriate programming or interaction with the patient's native electrical cardiac function. Rotation of the pacemaker pulse generator in its subcutaneous pocket, either intentionally or inadvertently, often referred to as "twiddler's syndrome," can wrap the leads around the generator and produce dislodgment with failure to sense or pace the heart. The small size and light weight of contemporary pacemakers makes this a rare complication.

A common problem is pacemaker syndrome; a constellation of signs and symptoms associated with any mode of pacing that does not maintain or restore AV synchrony. The symptoms include neck pulsation, fatigue, palpitations, cough, confusion, exertional dyspnea, dizziness, and syncope, and they may be associated with an elevation in jugular venous pressure, canon A waves, and stigmata of congestive heart failure, including edema, rales, and a third heart sound. Often, there is a substantial drop in blood pressure with ventricular pacing. The management of pacemaker syndrome involves changing the pacing mode to restore AV synchrony.

Pacemaker Therapy in SA Node Dysfunction

Pacing in SA nodal disease is indicated to alleviate symptoms of bradycardia. Consensus guidelines published by the AHA/ACC/HRS outline the indications for the use of pacemakers, and categorize them by class based on levels of evidence. Class I conditions are those for which there is evidence or consensus of opinion that therapy is useful and effective. In class II conditions there is conflicting evidence or a divergence of opinion about the efficacy of a procedure or treatment; in class IIa conditions the weight of evidence or opinion favors treatment, and in class IIb conditions, efficacy is less well established by the evidence or opinion of experts. In class III conditions, the evidence or weight of opinion indicates that the therapy is not efficacious or useful, and may be harmful.

Class I indications for pacing in SA node dysfunction include documented symptomatic bradycardia, sinus node dysfunction–associated long-term drug therapy for which there is no alternative, or symptomatic chronotropic incompetence. Class IIa indications include those outlined previously in which sinus node dysfunction is suspected but not documented and for syncope of unexplained origin in the presence of major abnormalities of SA node dysfunction. Mildly symptomatic individuals with heart rates consistently <40 beats/min comprise a class IIb indication for pacing. Pacing is not indicated in patients with SA node dysfunction who do not have symptoms and in those in whom bradycardia is associated with the use of nonessential drugs (Table 225-3).

There is some controversy regarding the mode of pacing that should be employed in SA node disease. A number of randomized, single-blind trials of pacing mode have been performed. There are no trials that demonstrate an improvement in mortality with AV synchronous compared with single-chamber pacing in SA node disease. In some of these studies, the incidence of atrial fibrillation and thromboembolic events was reduced with AV synchronous pacing. In trials of patients with dual-chamber pacemakers designed to compare single-chamber with dual-chamber pacing by crossover design, the need for AV synchronous pacing due to pacemaker syndrome was common. Pacing modes that preserve AV synchrony appear to be associated with a reduction in the incidence of atrial fibrillation and improved quality of life. Because of the low but finite incidence of AV conduction disease, patients with SA node dysfunction will usually undergo dual-chamber pacemaker implantation.

Pacemaker Therapy in Carotid Sinus Hypersensitivity and Vasovagal Syncope

Carotid sinus hypersensitivity, if accompanied by a significant cardioinhibitory component, responds well to pacing. In this circumstance, pacing is only required intermittently and single-chamber

TABLE 225-3 SUMMARY OF GUIDELINES FOR PACEMAKER IMPLANTATION IN SA NODE DYSFUNCTION

Class I
1. SA node dysfunction with symptomatic bradycardia or sinus pauses
2. Symptomatic SA node dysfunction as a result of essential long-term drug therapy with no acceptable alternatives
3. Symptomatic chronotropic incompetence

Class IIa
1. SA node dysfunction with heart rates < 40 beats/min without a clear and consistent relationship between bradycardia and symptoms
2. SA node dysfunction with heart rates < 40 beats/min on an essential long-term drug therapy with no acceptable alternatives, without a clear and consistent relationship between bradycardia and symptoms
3. Syncope of unknown origin when major abnormalities of SA node dysfunction are discovered or provoked by electrophysiologic testing

Class IIb
1. Mildly symptomatic patients with waking chronic heart rates < 40 beats/min

Class III
1. SA node dysfunction in asymptomatic patients even those with heart rates < 40 beats/min
2. SA node dysfunction in which symptoms suggestive of bradycardia are not associated with a slow heart rate
3. SA node dysfunction with symptomatic bradycardia due to nonessential drug therapy

Source: Modified from Gregoratos et al, 1997, and Gregoratos et al, 2002.

ventricular pacing is often sufficient. The mechanism of vasovagal syncope is incompletely understood but appears to involve activation of cardiac mechanoreceptors with consequent activation of neural centers that mediate vagal activation and withdrawal of sympathetic nervous system tone. Several randomized clinical trials have been performed in patients with drug-refractory vasovagal syncope, with a reduction in the frequency and the time to recurrent syncope in patients who were paced compared to those who were not.

Pacemakers in AV Conduction Disease

There are no randomized trials that evaluate the efficacy of pacing in patients with AV block as there are no reliable therapeutic alternatives for AV block and untreated high-grade AV block is potentially lethal. The consensus guidelines for pacing in acquired AV conduction block in adults provide a general outline for situations in which pacing is indicated (Table 225-4). Pacemaker implantation should be performed in any patient with symptomatic bradycardia and irreversible second- or third-degree AV block, regardless of the cause or level of block in the conducting system. Symptoms may include those directly related to bradycardia and low cardiac output or to worsening heart failure, angina, or intolerance to an essential medication. Pacing in patients with asymptomatic AV block should be individualized; situations in which pacing should be considered are in those patients with acquired CHB, particularly in the setting of cardiac enlargement; left ventricular dysfunction; and waking heart rates of ≤40 beats/min. Patients who have asymptomatic second-degree AV block of either type should be considered for pacing if the block is demonstrated to be intra- or infraHis, or is associated with a wide QRS complex. Pacing may be indicated in asymptomatic patients under special circumstances; in patients with profound first-degree AV block and left ventricular dysfunction in whom a shorter AV interval produces hemodynamic improvement, and in the setting of milder forms of AV conduction delay (first-degree AV block, intraventricular conduction delay) in patients with neuromuscular diseases that have a predilection for the conduction system, such as myotonic dystrophy and other muscular dystrophies, and Kearns-Sayre syndrome.

Pacemaker Therapy in Myocardial Infarction

Atrioventricular block in acute MI is often transient, particularly in inferior infarction. The circumstances under which pacing is indicated in acute MI are persistent second- or third-degree AV block, particularly if symptomatic, and transient second- or third-degree AV block associated with bundle branch block (Table 225-5). Pacing is generally not indicated in the setting of transient AV block in the absence of intraventricular con-

TABLE 225-4 GUIDELINE SUMMARY FOR PACEMAKER IMPLANTATION IN ACQUIRED AV BLOCK

Class I
1. Third-degree or high-grade AV block at any anatomic level associated with:
   a. Symptomatic bradycardia
   b. Essential drug therapy that produces symptomatic bradycardia
   c. Periods of asystole > 3 s or any escape rate < 40 beats/min while awake
   d. Postoperative AV block not expected to resolve
   e. Catheter ablation of the AV junction
   f. Neuromuscular diseases such as myotonic dystrophy, Kearns-Sayre syndrome, Erb dystrophy, and peroneal muscular atrophy, regardless of the presence of symptoms
2. Second-degree AV block with symptomatic bradycardia
3. Type II second-degree AV block with a wide QRS complex with or without symptoms

Class IIa
1. Asymptomatic third-degree AV block regardless of level
2. Asymptomatic type II second-degree AV block with a narrow QRS complex
3. Asymptomatic type II second-degree AV block with block within or below the His at electrophysiologic study
4. First- or second-degree AV block with symptoms similar to pacemaker syndrome

Class IIb
1. Marked first-degree AV block (PR interval > 300 ms) in patients with LV dysfunction in whom shortening the AV delay would improve hemodynamics
2. Neuromuscular diseases, such as myotonic dystrophy, Kearns-Sayre syndrome, Erb dystrophy, and peroneal muscular atrophy, with any degree of AV block regardless of the presence of symptoms

Class III
1. Asymptomatic first-degree AV block
2. Asymptomatic type I second-degree AV block at the AV node level
3. AV block that is expected to resolve or is unlikely to recur (Lyme disease, drug toxicity)

Source: Modified from Gregoratos et al, 1997, and Gregoratos et al, 2002.

duction delays, or in the presence of fascicular block or first-degree AV block that develops in the setting of preexisting bundle branch block. Fascicular blocks that develop in acute MI in the absence of other forms of AV block also do not require pacing (Table 225-5 and Table 225-6).

Distal forms of AV conduction block may require pacemaker implantation in certain clinical settings. In patients with bifascicular or trifascicular block and symptoms, particularly syncope that is not attributable to other causes, should undergo pacemaker implantation.

TABLE 225-5 GUIDELINE SUMMARY FOR PACEMAKER IMPLANTATION IN AV CONDUCTION BLOCK IN ACUTE MYOCARDIAL INFARCTION (AMI)

Class I
1. Persistent second-degree AV block in the His-Purkinje system with bilateral bundle branch block or third-degree block within or below the His after AMI
2. Transient advanced (second- or third-degree) infranodal AV block and associated bundle branch block. If the site of block is uncertain, an electrophysiologic study may be necessary
3. Persistent and symptomatic second- or third-degree AV block

Class IIb
1. Persistent second- or third-degree AV block at the AV node level

Class III
1. Transient AV block in the absence of intraventricular conduction defects
2. Transient AV block in the presence of isolated left anterior fascicular block
3. Acquired left anterior fascicular block in the absence of AV block
4. Persistent first-degree AV block in the presence of bundle branch block that is old or age-indeterminate

Source: Modified from Gregoratos et al, 1997.

TABLE 225-6 INDICATIONS FOR PACEMAKER IMPLANTATION IN CHRONIC BIFASCICULAR AND TRIFASCICULAR BLOCK

Class I
1. Intermittent third-degree AV block
2. Type II second-degree AV block
3. Alternating bundle branch block

Class IIa
1. Syncope not demonstrated to be due to AV block when other likely causes (e.g., ventricular tachycardia) have been excluded
2. Incidental finding at electrophysiologic study of a markedly prolonged HV interval (>100 ms) in asymptomatic patients
3. Incidental finding at electrophysiologic study of pacing-induced infra-His block that is not physiologic

Class IIb
1. Neuromuscular diseases, such as myotonic dystrophy, Kearns-Sayre syndrome, Erb dystrophy, and peroneal muscular atrophy, with any degree of fascicular block regardless of the presence of symptoms, because there may be unpredictable progression of AV conduction disease

Class III
1. Fascicular block without AV block or symptoms
2. Fascicular block with first-degree AV block without symptoms

Source: Modified from Gregoratos et al, 1997, and Gregoratos et al, 2002.

Pacemaking is indicated in asymptomatic patients with bifascicular or trifascicular block who experience intermittent third-degree, type II second-degree AV block, or alternating bundle branch block. In patients with fascicular block who are undergoing electrophysiologic study, a markedly prolonged HV interval or block below the His at long cycle lengths may also constitute an indication for permanent pacing. In patients with fascicular block and the neuromuscular diseases previously described should also undergo pacemaker implantation (Table 225-6).

Selection of Pacing Mode In general, a pacing mode that maintains AV synchrony reduces complications of pacing such as pacemaker syndrome and pacemaker-mediated tachycardia. This is particularly true in younger patients, but the importance of dual-chamber pacing, especially in the elderly, is not well established. Several studies have failed to demonstrate a difference in mortality in older patients with AV block treated with a single- (VVI) compared to a dual- (DDD) chamber pacing mode. In some of these studies that randomized pacing mode, the risk of chronic atrial fibrillation and stroke risk decreased with physiologic pacing. In patients with sinus rhythm and AV block, the very modest increase in risk with dual-chamber pacemaker implantation appears to be justified to avoid the possible complications of single-chamber pacing.

FURTHER READINGS

BHARATI S et al: Sinus node dysfunction, in *Electrophysiological Disorders of the Heart*, S Saksena, AJ Camm (eds). Philadelphia, Elsevier Churchill Livingstone, 2005, Chap. 12

GOLDSCHLAGER N et al: Atrioventricular block, in *Electrophysiological Disorders of the Heart*, S Saksena, AJ Camm (eds). Philadelphia, Elsevier Churchill Livingstone, 2005, Chap. 13

GREGORATOS G et al: ACC/AHA Guidelines for implantation of cardiac pacemakers and antiarrhythmia devices: Executive summary. Circulation 97:1325, 1997

——— et al: ACC/AHA/NASPE 2002 Guideline Update for implantation of cardiac pacemakers and antiarrhythmia devices: Summary article. Circulation 106:2145, 2002

JOSEPHSON ME: *Clinical Cardiac Electrophysiology: Techniques and Interpretations*, 3d ed. Philadelphia, Lippincott Williams & Wilkins, 2002

VIJAYARAMAN P, ELLENBOGEN KA: Bradyarrhythmias and pacemakers, in *Hurst's The Heart*, 12th ed, V Fuster et al (eds). New York, McGraw-Hill, 2008, Chap. 40

226 The Tachyarrhythmias
Francis Marchlinski

Tachyarrhythmias typically refer to isolated premature complexes (depolarizations) or to nonsustained and sustained forms of tachycardia originating from myocardial foci or reentrant circuits. The standard definition of tachycardia is rhythm that produces a ventricular rate >100 beats/min. This definition has some limitations in that atrial rates can exceed 100 beats/min despite a slow ventricular rate. Furthermore, ventricular rates may exceed the baseline sinus rate and be <100 beats/min but still represent an important "tachycardia" response, such as is observed with accelerated ventricular rhythms.

SYMPTOMS DUE TO TACHYARRHYTHMIAS
Tachyarrhythmias classically produce symptoms of palpitations or racing of the pulse. For premature beats, skipping of the pulse or a pause may be experienced, and patients may even sense slowing of the heart rate. A more dramatic irregularity of the pulse will be experienced with chaotic rapid rhythms or tachyarrhythmias that originate in the atrium and conduct variably to the ventricles. For very rapid tachyarrhythmias, hemodynamic compromise can occur, as can dizziness or syncope due to a decrease in cardiac output or breathlessness due to a marked increase in cardiac filling pressures. Occasionally, chest discomfort may be experienced that mimics symptoms of myocardial ischemia. The underlying cardiac condition typically dictates the severity of symptoms at any specific heart rate. Even patients with normal systolic left ventricular (LV) function may experience severe symptoms if diastolic compliance due to hypertrophy or valvular obstruction is present. Hemodynamic collapse with the development of ventricular fibrillation (VF) can lead to sudden cardiac death (SCD) (Chap. 267). SCD remains one of the principal causes of death in the adult population, thus emphasizing the importance of appropriate tachyarrhythmia prevention as well as management.

DIAGNOSTIC TESTS IN EVALUATING TACHYARRHYTHMIAS
In patients who present with non-life-threatening symptoms, such as palpitations or dizziness, electrocardiogram (ECG) confirmation of an arrhythmia with the development of recurrent symptoms is essential. A 24-h Holter monitor should be considered only for patients with daily symptoms. For intermittent symptoms that are of a prolonged duration, a patient-activated event monitor can be used to obtain the ECG information without the need for continuous ECG lead attachment and recordings. A patient-activated monitor with a continuously recorded memory loop ("loop recorder") can be used to document short-lived episodes and the onset of the arrhythmia. This is the preferred monitoring technique for symptomatic patients with less frequent arrhythmia events but it requires continuous ECG recording. Patients with infrequent, severe symptoms that cannot be identified by intermittent ECG monitoring may receive an implanted loop ECG monitor that provides more extended periods of monitoring and automatic arrhythmia detection (Fig. 226-1).

In patients who present with more severe symptoms, such as syncope, outpatient monitoring may be insufficient. In patients with structural heart disease and syncope in whom there is suspicion of ventricular tachycardia (VT), hospitalization and diagnostic electrophysiologic testing are warranted, with strong consideration for an implantable cardioverter/defibrillator (ICD) device. The 12-lead ECG recorded in sinus rhythm should be carefully assessed in patients without structural heart disease for evidence of ST-segment elevation in leads V_1 and V_2 consistent with the Brugada syndrome, QT interval changes consistent with long

or short QT syndromes, or a short PR interval and delta wave consistent with Wolff-Parkinson-White (WPW) syndrome. These ECG patterns identify an arrhythmogenic substrate that may cause intermittent life-threatening symptoms and warrant further evaluation and therapy. The individual syndromes are discussed in detail later in this chapter.

Monitoring for asymptomatic tachyarrhythmias is indicated in several specific situations. In patients with a suspected tachycardia-induced cardiomyopathy marked by chamber dilatation and depression in systolic function, the demonstration of arrhythmia control is essential. Monitoring for asymptomatic ventricular premature complexes (VPCs) and nonsustained VT can be helpful in stratifying the risk of SCD in patients with depressed LV function after myocardial infarction. Finally, in patients with asymptomatic atrial fibrillation (AF), anticoagulation treatment strategies depend on an accurate assessment of the presence of this arrhythmia. The duration of monitoring for asymptomatic arrhythmias may vary. The transition from 24-h Holter monitoring to more extended periods of monitoring with technology capable of automatic arrhythmia detection improves the reliability of the monitoring information used in decision-making.

A 12-lead ECG recording during the tachycardia can be an important diagnostic tool in identifying the mechanism and the origin of a tachycardia not afforded by one- or two-lead ECG recordings. A 12-lead ECG of the tachyarrhythmia should be recorded and incorporated as a permanent part of the medical record whenever possible. For patients whose arrhythmias are provoked by exercise, an exercise test may provide the opportunity to obtain 12-lead ECG recordings of the arrhythmia and may obviate the need for more extended periods of monitoring.

Many paroxysmal supraventricular tachyarrhythmias are not associated with a significant risk of structural heart disease, and an evaluation for the presence of ischemic heart disease and cardiac function is uncommonly required unless dictated by the severity or characteristics of the symptoms. However in patients with focal or macroreentrant atrial tachycardias (ATs), atrial flutter (AFL), or AF, an evaluation of cardiac chamber size and function and of valve function is warranted. In patients with VT, an echocardiographic assessment of LV and right ventricular (RV) size and function should be the norm. VT occurring in the setting of depressed LV function should raise the suspicion of advanced coronary artery disease. Polymorphic VT in the absence of QT prolongation should always raise the concern for a potentially unstable ischemic process that may need to be corrected to effect VT control.

MECHANISMS OF TACHYARRHYTHMIAS
Tachycardias are due to abnormalities of impulse formation and/or abnormalities of impulse propagation (Fig. 226-2).

Abnormalities in Impulse Formation An increase in automaticity normally causes an increase in sinus rate and sinus tachycardia (Fig. 226-2A). Abnormal automaticity is due to an increase in the slope of phase 4 depolarization or a reduced threshold for action potential depolarization in myocardium other than the sinus node. Abnormal automaticity is thought to be responsible for most atrial premature complexes (APCs) and VPCs and some ATs. Pacing does not provoke automatic rhythms. Less commonly, abnormal impulse formation is

FIGURE 226-1 Spontaneous termination of atrial fibrillation at the time of a syncopal episode identified from implantable loop ECG recording.

09:22:49

09:22:59

▲A

09:23:09

FIGURE 226-2 Schematic representation of the different mechanisms for arrhythmias. A. Abnormal automaticity due to an increased slope of phase 4 of the action potential or a decrease in the threshold for phase 0. **B.** Triggered activity due to early afterdepolarizations (EADs) during phase 3 of the action potential due to alteration of plateau currents, or delayed afterdepolarizations (DADs) during phase 4 of the action potential due to intracellular calcium accumulation. **C.** Reentry with basic requirements of two pathways that have heterogeneous electrophysiologic properties which allows conduction to block in one pathway and to propagate slowly in the other, allowing for sufficient delay so that the blocked site has time for recovery to allow for reentry or circus movement tachycardia. Shown is typical schema for reentry in the AV node. (AV, atrioventricular; APC, atrial premature complex.)

due to the development of triggered activity. Triggered activity is related to cellular afterdepolarizations that occur at the end of the action potential, during phase 3, and are referred to as *early afterdepolarizations*, or they occur after the action potential, during phase 4, and are referred to as *late afterdepolarizations*. Afterdepolarizations are attributable to an increase in intracellular calcium accumulation. If sufficient afterdepolarization amplitude is achieved, repeated myocardial depolarization and a tachycardic response can occur. Early afterdepolarizations may be responsible for the VPCs that trigger the polymorphic ventricular arrhythmia known as *torsades des pointes* (TDP) (p. 1436). Late afterdepolarizations are thought to be responsible for atrial, junctional, and fascicular tachyarrhythmias caused by digoxin toxicity and also appear to be the basis for catecholamine-sensitive VT originating in the outflow tract. In contrast to automatic tachycardias, tachycardias due to triggered activity (Fig. 226-2B) can frequently be provoked with pacing maneuvers.

Abnormalities in Impulse Propagation Reentry is due to inhomogeneities in myocardial conduction and/or recovery properties. The presence of unidirectional block with slow conduction to allow for retrograde recovery of the blocked myocardium allows for a circuit to form that, if perpetuated, can sustain a tachycardia (Fig. 226-2C).

These inhomogeneities are somewhat inherent but minimized in normal myocardial activation/recovery. The inhomogeneities can be exaggerated by the presence of extra pathways, such as occurs with the WPW syndrome; generalized genetically determined myocardial ion channel abnormalities, such as occurs with long QT syndrome (LQTS); or by the interruption of normal myocardial patterns of activation due to the development of fibrosis.

Reentry appears to be the basis for most abnormal sustained supraventricular tachycardias (SVTs) and VTs. In general, reentry can be anatomically driven (fixed) based on the presence of "extra" pathways, natural anatomic barriers of conduction such as the crista terminalis, the vertical crest on the interior wall of the right atrium that separates the sinus of the vena cava and nontrabeculated posterior right atrium from the rest of the trabeculated right atrium located lateral to the structure, and/or extensive fibrosis created by underlying myocardial disease. This form of reentry seems to be more stable and results in a tachycardia that has a uniform (often monomorphic), repetitive appearance. Other forms of reentry appear to be more functional and are more dependent on dynamic changes in electrophysiologic properties of the myocardium. These tachycardias tend to be more unstable and may result in tachycardias that have a polymorphic appearance. Two classic examples of reentry that is primarily functional include VF due to acute myocardial ischemia and polymorphic VT in patients with genetically determined ion channel abnormalities, such as the Brugada syndrome, LQTS, or catecholaminergic polymorphic VT (p. 1441).

SUPRAVENTRICULAR TACHYARRHYTHMIAS

ATRIAL PREMATURE COMPLEXES

APCs are the most common arrhythmia identified during extended ECG monitoring. The incidence of APCs frequently increases with age and with the presence of structural heart diseases. APCs typically are asymptomatic, although some patients experience palpitations or an irregularity of the pulse.

ECG Diagnosis of APCs The ECG diagnosis of premature atrial complexes is based on the identification of a P wave that occurs prior to the anticipated sinus beat (**Figs. 226-3A** and **226-3B**). The source of the APC appears to parallel the typical sites of origin for ATs. The orifices of the superior vena cava and pulmonary veins, the coronary sinus, the crista terminalis, mitral and tricuspid valve annuli, and left and right atrial appendages are common sites of origin of APCs. The P wave contour differs from that noted during sinus rhythm, although APCs from the right atrial appendage, superior vena cava (SVC), and superior aspect of the crista terminalis in the region of the sinus node may mimic the sinus P wave morphology. In response to an APC, the PR interval lengthens, although APCs that originate near the atrioventricular (AV) nodal region may actually have a shorter PR interval because the atrial conduction time to the junction is shortened. A very early APC may not conduct to the ventricle and can create a pulse irregularity that may be perceived as a pause or "dropped beat." If the APC conducts rapidly through the AV node, a partially recovered His-Purkinje system will be encountered and a QRS pattern consistent with a right or left bundle branch block may occur. This wide QRS pattern and the failure to recognize the preceding P wave may result in the misdiagnosis of VPCs. APCs characteristically reset the sinus node. The resulting sum of the pre- and post-APC RR interval is less than two sinus PP intervals.

FIGURE 226-3 Atrial and ventricular premature complexes (APCs, VPCs). The APC resets the sinus node and no compensatory pause is present (**A**) even when conducted aberrantly in the ventricles with a bundle branch block type QRS pattern (**B**). VPCs tend not to reset the sinus activity (*arrows*) and will demonstrate a full compensatory pause (**C**).

℞ ATRIAL PREMATURE COMPLEXES

APCs uncommonly require intervention. For extremely symptomatic patients who do not respond to explanation and reassurance, an attempt can be made to suppress the APCs with pharmacologic agents. The repetitive focus can even be targeted for catheter ablation. Beta blockers are typical first-line therapy, but they may exacerbate symptoms if AV block occurs with the APC and irregularity of the pulse consequently becomes more profound. The use of class IC antiarrhythmic agents may eliminate the APCs but should be avoided if structural heart disease is present.

JUNCTIONAL PREMATURE COMPLEXES

Junctional premature complexes are extremely uncommon. The complexes originate from the AV node and His bundle region and may produce retrograde atrial activation with the P wave distorting the initial or terminal portions of the QRS complex producing pseudo Q or S waves in leads II, III, and aVF. Extrasystoles originating in the bundle of His that do not conduct to the ventricle and also block the atria can produce unexplained surface ECG PR prolongation that does not follow a typical Wenckebach periodicity, i.e., gradual PR prolongation culminating in atrial activity that fails to conduct to the ventricles. Intracardiac recordings can frequently identify a His depolarization, thus identifying the origin of the complex to the AV junction. Symptomatic patients may be typically treated with beta blockers or, if there is no structural heart disease, class IC antiarrhythmic agents.

SINUS TACHYCARDIA

Physiologic sinus tachycardia represents a normal or appropriate response to physiologic stress, such as occurs with exercise, anxiety, or fever. Pathologic conditions, such as thyrotoxicosis, anemia, or hypotension, may also produce sinus tachycardia. It is important to distinguish sinus tachycardia from other SVTs. Sinus tachycardia will produce a P wave contour consistent with its origin from the sinus node located in the superior-lateral and posterior aspect of the right atrium. The P wave is upright in leads II, III and aVF, and negative in lead aVR. The P wave morphology in lead V_1 characteristically has a biphasic, positive/negative contour. Onset of sinus tachycardia is gradual, and in response to carotid sinus pressure there may be some modest and transient slowing but no abrupt termination. Importantly, the diagnosis should not be based on the PR interval or the presence of a P wave before every QRS complex. The PR interval and the presence of 1:1 AV conduction properties are entirely determined by AV nodal and His-Purkinje conduction and, therefore, the PR interval can be dramatically prolonged while sinus tachycardia remains the mechanism of the atrial activity.

℞ PHYSIOLOGIC SINUS TACHYCARDIA

Treatment of physiologic sinus tachycardia is directed at the underlying condition causing the tachycardia response. Uncommonly, beta blockers are used to minimize the tachycardia response if it is determined to be potentially harmful, as may occur in a patient with ischemic heart disease and rate-related anginal symptoms.

Inappropriate sinus tachycardia represents an uncommon but important medical condition in which the heart rate increases either spontaneously or out of proportion to the degree of physiologic stress/exercise. Dizziness and even frank syncope can often accompany the sinus tachycardia and symptoms of palpitations. The syndrome can be quite disabling. Associated symptoms of chest pain, headaches, and gastrointestinal upset are common. In many patients, the syndrome occurs after a viral illness and may resolve spontaneously over the course of 3–12 months, suggesting a postviral dysautonomia.

Excluding the diagnosis of an automatic AT that originates in the region of the sinus node can be difficult and may require invasive electrophysiologic evaluation. Frequently, patients are misdiagnosed as having an anxiety disorder with physiologic sinus tachycardia.

℞ INAPPROPRIATE SINUS TACHYCARDIA

For symptomatic patients, maintaining an increased state of hydration, salt loading, and careful titration of beta blockers to the maximum tolerated dose, administered in divided doses, frequently minimizes symptoms. For severely symptomatic patients who are intolerant of or unresponsive to beta blockers, catheter ablation directed at modifying the sinus node may be effective. Because of the high recurrence rate after ablation and the frequent need for atrial pacing therapy, this intervention remains second-line treatment.

ATRIAL FIBRILLATION

(Fig. 226-4) AF is the most common sustained arrhythmia. It is marked by disorganized, rapid, and irregular atrial activation. The ventricular response to the rapid atrial activation is also irregular. In the untreated patient, the ventricular rate also tends to be rapid and is entirely dependent on the conduction properties of the AV junction. Although typically the rate will vary between 120 and 160 beats/min, in some patients it can be >200 beats/min. In other patients, because of heightened vagal tone or intrinsic AV nodal conduction properties, the ventricular response is <100 beats/min and occasionally even profoundly slow. The mechanism for AF initiation and maintenance, although still debated, appears to represent a complex interaction between drivers responsible for the initiation and the complex anatomic atrial substrate that promotes the maintenance of multiple wavelets of (micro)reentry. The drivers appears to originate predominantly from the atrialized musculature that enters the pulmonary veins and either represent focal abnormal automaticity or triggered firing that is somewhat modulated by autonomic influences. Sustained

FIGURE 226-4 Supraventricular tachycardias with irregular ventricular rates. Atrial fibrillation (**A**), atrial flutter (**B**), atrial tachycardia (**C**), and multifocal atrial tachycardia (MAT; **D**) are shown. The characteristics of the atrial activity with respect to the morphology and rate provide the clues to the diagnosis.

forms of microreentry as drivers have also been documented around the orifice of pulmonary veins; nonpulmonary vein drivers have also been demonstrated. The role these drivers play in maintaining the tachycardias may also be significant and may explain the success of pulmonary vein isolation procedures in eliminating more chronic or persistent forms of AF.

Although AF is common in the adult population, it is extremely unusual in children unless structural heart disease is present or there is another arrhythmia that precipitates the AF, such as paroxysmal SVT in patients with WPW syndrome. The incidence of AF increases with age such that >5% of the adult population over 70 will experience the arrhythmia. As many patients are asymptomatic with AF, it is anticipated that the overall incidence, particularly that noted in the elderly, may be more than double previously reported rates. Occasionally AF appears to have a well-defined etiology, such as acute hyperthyroidism, an acute vagotonic episode, or acute alcohol intoxication. Acute AF is particularly common during the acute or early recovery phase of major vascular, abdominal, and thoracic surgery where autonomic fluxes and/or direct mechanical irritation potentiate the arrhythmia. AF may also be triggered by other supraventricular tachycardias (p. 1433), such as AV nodal reentrant tachycardia (AVNRT), and elimination of these arrhythmias may prevent AF recurrence.

AF has clinical importance related to (1) the loss of atrial contractility, (2) the inappropriate fast ventricular response, and (3) the loss of atrial appendage contractility and emptying leading to the risk of clot formation and subsequent thromboembolic events.

Symptoms from AF vary dramatically. Many patients are asymptomatic and have no apparent hemodynamic consequences to the development of AF. Other patients experience only minor palpitations or sense irregularity of their pulse. Many patients, however, experience severe palpitations. The hemodynamic effect in patients can be quite dramatic, depending on the need for normal atrial contractility and the ventricular response. Hypotension, pulmonary congestion, and anginal symptoms may be severe in some patients. In patients with the LV diastolic dysfunction that occurs with hypertension, hypertrophic cardiomyopathy, or obstructive aortic valvular disease, symptoms may be even more dramatic, especially if the ventricular rate does not per-

mit adequate ventricular filling. Exercise intolerance and easy fatigability are the hallmarks of poor rate control with exertion. Occasionally, the only manifestation of AF is severe dizziness or syncope associated with the pause that occurs upon termination of AF before sinus rhythm resumes (Fig. 226-1).

The ECG in AF is characterized by the lack of organized atrial activity and the irregularly irregular ventricular response. Occasionally, one needs to record from multiple ECG leads simultaneously to identify the chaotic continuous atrial activation. Lead V_1 may frequently show the appearance of organized atrial activity that mimics AFL. This occurs because the crista terminalis serves as an effective anatomic barrier to electrical conduction, and the activation of the lateral right atrium may be represented by a more uniform activation wavefront that originates over the roof of the right atrium. ECG assessment of the PP interval (<200 ms) and the chaotic P wave morphology in the remaining ECG leads will confirm the presence of AF.

Evaluation of the patient with AF should include a search for reversible causes of the arrhythmia, such as hyperthyroidism or anemia. An echocardiogram should be performed to determine if there is structural heart disease. Persistent or labile hypertension should be identified and treated, and heart failure treatment should be optimized.

℞ ATRIAL FIBRILLATION

Treatment for AF must take into account the clinical situation in which the arrhythmia is encountered, the chronicity of the AF, the status of the patient's level of anticoagulation, risk factors for stroke, the patient's symptoms, the hemodynamic impact of the AF, and the ventricular rate.

ACUTE RATE CONTROL In the absence of hemodynamic compromise that might warrant emergent cardioversion to terminate the AF, the initial goals of therapy are (1) to establish control of the ventricular rate, and (2) to address anticoagulation status and begin IV heparin treatment if the duration of AF is >12 h and risk factors for stroke with AF are present **(Table 226-1)**. Ventricular rate control for acute AF is best established with beta blockers and/or calcium channel blocking agents, verapamil or diltiazem. The route of administration and dose will be dictated by the ventricular rate and clinical status. Digoxin may add to the rate-controlling benefit of the other agents but is uncommonly used as a stand-alone agent, especially in acute AF.

Anticoagulation is of particular importance in patients who have known risk factors for stroke associated with AF. Factors associated with the highest risk of stroke include a history of stroke, transient ischemic attack or systemic embolism, or the presence of rheumatic mitral stenosis. Other identified risk factors include age >65 years, history of congestive heart failure, diabetes mellitus, hypertension, LV dysfunction, and evidence of marked left atrial enlargement (>5.0 cm). Chronic anticoagulation with warfarin targeting an INR between 2.0 and 3.0 is recommended in patients with persistent or frequent and long-lived paroxysmal AF and risk factors. If patients have not been adequately anticoagulated and the AF is more

TABLE 226-1	RISK FACTORS FOR STROKE IN ATRIAL FIBRILLATION
History of stroke or transient ischemic attack	Age > 75 years
Mitral stenosis	Congestive heart failure
Hypertension	Left ventricular dysfunction
Diabetes mellitus	Marked left atrial enlargement (>5.0 cm)
	Spontaneous echo contrast

TABLE 226-2 COMMONLY USED ANTIARRHYTHMIC AGENTS—INTRAVENOUS DOSE RANGE/PRIMARY INDICATION

Drug	Loading	Maintenance	Primary Indication	Class[a]
Adenosine	6–18 mg (rapid bolus)	N/A	Terminate reentrant SVT involving AV node	—
Amiodarone	15 mg/min for 10 min, 1 mg/min for 6 h	0.5–1 mg/min	AF, AFL, SVT, VT/VF	III
Digoxin	0.25 mg q2h until 1.0 mg total	0.125–0.25 mg/d	AF/AFL rate control	—
Diltiazem	0.25 mg/kg over 3–5 min (max 20 mg)	5–15 mg/h	SVT, AF/AFL rate control	IV
Esmolol	500 µg/kg over 1 min	50 µg/kg per min	AF/AFL rate control	II
Ibutilide	1 mg over 10 min if over 60 kg	N/A	Terminate AF/AFL	III
Lidocaine	1–3 mg/kg at 20–50 mg/min	1–4 mg/min	VT	IB
Metoprolol	5 mg over 3–5 min times 3 doses	1.25–5 mg q6h	SVT, AF rate control; exercise-induced VT; long QT	II
Procainamide	15 mg/kg over 60 min	1–4 mg/min	Convert/prevent AF/VT	IA
Quinidine	6–10 mg/kg at 0.3–0.5 mg/kg per min	N/A	Convert/prevent AF/VT	IA
Verapamil	5–10 mg over 3–5 min	2.5–10 mg/h	SVT, AF rate control	IV

[a]Classification of antiarrhythmic drugs: Class I—agents that primarily block inward sodium current; class IA agents also prolong action potential duration; class II—antisympathetic agents; class III—agents that primarily prolong action potential duration; class IV—calcium channel-blocking agents.

Note: SVT, supraventricular tachycardia; AV, atrioventricular; AF, atrial fibrillation; AFL, atrial flutter; VT, ventricular tachycardia; VF, ventricular fibrillation.

than 24–48 h in duration, a transesophageal echocardiogram (TEE) can be performed to exclude the presence of a left atrial thrombus that might dislodge with the attempted restoration of sinus rhythm using either nonpharmacologic or pharmacologic therapy. Anticoagulation must be instituted coincident with the TEE and maintained for at least 1 month following restoration of sinus rhythm if the duration of AF has been prolonged or is unknown. Heparin is maintained routinely until the INR is 1.8 with the administration of warfarin after the TEE. For patients who do not warrant early cardioversion of AF, anticoagulation should be maintained for at least 3 weeks with the INR confirmed to be >1.8 on at least two separate occasions prior to attempts at cardioversion.

Termination of AF acutely may be warranted based on clinical parameters and/or hemodynamic status. Confirmation of appropriate anticoagulation status as described above must be documented unless symptoms and clinical status warrant emergent intervention. Direct current transthoracic cardioversion during short-acting anesthesia is a reliable way to terminate AF. Conversion rates using a 200-J biphasic shock delivered synchronously with the QRS complex typically are >90%. Pharmacologic therapy to terminate AF is less reliable. Oral and/or IV administration of amiodarone or procainamide have only modest success. The acute IV administration of ibutilide appears to be somewhat more effective and may be used in selected patients to facilitate termination with direct current (DC) cardioversion **(Tables 226-2** and **226-3)**.

Pharmacologic therapy to maintain sinus rhythm can be instituted once sinus rhythm has been established or in anticipation of cardioversion to attempt to maintain sinus rhythm (Table 226-3). A single episode of AF may not warrant any intervention or only a short course of beta blocker therapy. To prevent recurrent AF unresponsive to beta blockade, a trial of antiarrhythmic therapy may be warranted, particularly if the AF is associated with rapid rates and/or significant symptoms. The selection of antiarrhythmic agents should be dictated primarily by the presence or absence of coronary artery disease, depressed LV function not attributable to a reversible tachycardia-induced cardiomyopathy, and/or severe hypertension with evidence of marked LV hypertrophy. The presence of any significant structural heart disease typically narrows treatment to the use of sotalol, amiodarone, or dofetilide. Severely depressed LV function may preclude sotalol therapy or require only low-dose therapy be considered. Owing to the risk of QT prolongation and polymorphic VT, sotalol and dofetilide need to be initiated in hospital in most cases.

In patients without evidence of structural heart disease or hypertensive heart disease without evidence of severe hypertrophy, the use of the class IC antiarrhythmic agents flecainide or propafenone appears to be well tolerated and does not have significant proarrhythmia risk. It is important to recognize that no drug is uniformly effective, and arrhythmia recurrence should be anticipated in over half the patients during long-term follow-up regardless of type and number of agents tried. It is also important to recognize that although the maintenance of sinus rhythm has been associated with improved long-term survival, the survival outcome of patients randomized to the pharmacologic maintenance of sinus rhythm was not superior to those treated with rate control and anticoagulation in the

TABLE 226-3 COMMONLY USED ANTIARRHYTHMIC AGENTS—CHRONIC ORAL DOSING/PRIMARY INDICATIONS

Drug	Dosing Oral, mg, Maintenance	Half-Life, h	Primary Route(s) of Metabolism/Elimination	Most Common Indication	Class[a]
Acebutolol	200–400 mg q12h	6–7	Renal/hepatic	AF rate control/SVT Long QT/RVOT VT	II
Amiodarone	100–400 qd	40–55 d	Hepatic	AF/VT prevention	III
Atenolol	25–100 mg/d	6–9	Renal	AF rate control/SVT Long QT/RVOT VT	II
Digoxin	0.125–0.5 qd	38–48	Renal	AF rate control	—
Diltiazem	30–60 q6h	3–4.5	Hepatic	AF rate control/SVT	IV
Disopyramide	100–300 q6–8h	4–10	Renal 50%/hepatic	AF/SVT prevention	Ia
Dofetilide	125–500 q12h	10	Renal	AF prevention	III
Flecainide	50–200 q12h	7–22	Hepatic 75%/renal	AF/SVT/VT prevention	Ic
Metoprolol	25–100 q6h	3–8	Hepatic	AF rate control/SVT Long QT/RVOT VT	II
Mexiletine	150–300 q8–12h	10–14	Hepatic	VT prevention	Ib
Moricizine	100–400 q8h	3–13	Hepatic 60%/renal	AF prevention	Ic
Nadolol	40–240 mg/d	10–24	Renal	Same as metoprolol	II
Procainamide	250–500 q3–6h	3–5	Hepatic/renal	AF/SVT/VT prevention	Ia
Propafenone	150–300 q8h	2–8	Hepatic	AF/SVT/VT prevention	Ic
Quinidine	300–600 q6h	6–8	Hepatic 75%/renal	AF/SVT/VT prevention	Ia
Sotalol	80–160 q12h	12	Renal	AF/VT prevention	III
Verapamil	80–120 q6–8h	4.5–12	Hepatic/renal	AF rate control/RVOT VT Idiopathic LV VT	IV

[a]Classification of antiarrhythmic drugs: Class I—agents that primarily block inward sodium current; class II—antisympathetic agents; class III—agents that primarily prolong action potential duration; class IV—calcium channel-blocking agents.

Note: AF, atrial fibrillation; SVT, supraventricular tachycardia; RVOT, right ventricular outflow tract; VT, ventricular tachycardia; LV, left ventriclar.

TABLE 226-4	COMMON NONARRHYTHMIC TOXICITY OF MOST FREQUENTLY USED ANTIARRHYTHMIC AGENTS
Drug	**Common Nonarrhythmic Toxicity**
Amiodarone	Tremor, peripheral neuropathy, pulmonary inflammation, hypothyroidism and hyperthyroidism, photosensitivity
Adenosine	Cough, flushing
Digoxin	Anorexia, nausea, vomiting, visual changes
Disopyramide	Anticholinergic effects, decreased myocardial contractility
Dofetilide	Nausea
Flecainide	Dizziness, nausea, headache, decreased myocardial contractility
Ibutilide	Nausea
Lidocaine	Dizziness, confusion, delirium, seizures, coma
Mexiletine	Ataxia, tremor, gait disturbances, rash, nausea
Moricizine	Mood changes, tremor, loss of mental clarity, nausea,
Procainamide	Lupus erythematosus–like syndrome (more common in slow acetylators), anorexia, nausea, neutropenia
Propafenone	Taste disturbance, dyspepsia, nausea, vomiting
Quinidine	Diarrhea, nausea, vomiting, cinchonism, thrombocytopenia
Sotalol	Hypotension, bronchospasm

TABLE 226-5	PROARRHYTHMIC MANIFESTATIONS OF MOST FREQUENTLY USED ANTIARRHYTHMIC AGENTS
Drug	**Common Proarrhythmic Toxicity**
Amiodarone	Sinus bradycardia, AV block, increase in defibrillation threshold Rare: long QT and torsades des pointes, 1:1 ventricular conduction with atrial flutter
Adenosine	All arrhythmias potentiated by profound pauses, atrial fibrillation
Digoxin	High-grade AV block, fascicular tachycardia, accelerated junctional rhythm, atrial tachycardia
Disopyramide	Long QT and torsades des pointes, 1:1 ventricular response to atrial flutter; increased risk of some ventricular tachycardias in patients with structural heart disease
Dofetilide	Long QT and torsades des pointes
Flecainide	1:1 Ventricular response to atrial flutter; increased risk of some ventricular tachycardias in patients with structural heart disease; sinus bradycardia
Ibutilide	Long QT and torsades des pointes
Procainamide	Long QT and torsades des pointes, 1:1 ventricular response to atrial flutter; increased risk of some ventricular tachycardias in patients with structural heart disease
Propafenone	1:1 Ventricular response to atrial flutter; increased risk of some ventricular tachycardias in patients with structural heart disease; sinus bradycardia
Quinidine	Long QT and torsades des pointes, 1:1 ventricular response to atrial flutter; increased risk of some ventricular tachycardias in patients with structural heart disease
Sotalol	Long QT and torsades des pointes, sinus bradycardia

Note: AV, atrioventricular.

AFFIRM and RACE trials. The AFFIRM and RACE trials compared outcome with respect to survival and thromboembolic events in patients with AF and risk factors for stroke using the two treatment strategies. It is believed that the poor outcome related to pharmacologic therapy used to maintain sinus rhythm was primarily due to frequent inefficacy of such drug therapy and an increased incidence of asymptomatic AF. Many of the drugs used for rhythm control, including sotalol, amiodarone, propafenone, and flecainide, enhance slowing of AV nodal conduction. The absence of symptoms frequently leads to stopping anticoagulant therapy, and asymptomatic AF without anticoagulation increases stroke risk. Any consideration for stopping anticoagulation must, therefore, be accompanied by a prolonged period of ECG monitoring to document asymptomatic AF. It is also recommended that patients participate in monitoring by learning to take their pulse on a twice-daily basis and to reliably identify its regularity if discontinuing anticoagulant therapy is seriously contemplated.

It is clear that to reduce the risk of drug-induced complications when treating AF, a thorough understanding of the drug planned to be used is critical—its dosing, metabolism, and common side effects and important drug-drug interactions. This information has been summarized in Tables 226-2, 226-3, **226-4**, and **226-5** and serves as a starting point for a more complete review. When using antiarrhythmic agents that slow atrial conduction, strong consideration should be given to adding a beta blocker or a calcium channel blocker (verapamil or diltiazem) to the treatment regimen. This should help to avoid a rapid ventricular response if AF is converted to "slow" AF with the drug therapy **(Fig. 226-5)**.

CHRONIC RATE CONTROL This is an option in patients who are asymptomatic or symptomatic due to the resulting tachycardia. Rate control is frequently difficult to achieve in patients who have paroxysmal AF. In patients with more persistent forms of AF, rate control with beta blockers, calcium channel blockers, diltiazem or verapamil, and/or digoxin can frequently be achieved. Using the drugs in combination may avoid some of the common side effects seen with high-dose monotherapy. An effort should be made to document the adequacy of rate control to reduce the risk of a tachycardia-induced cardiomyopathy. Heart rates >80 beats/min at rest or 100 beats/min with very modest physical activity are indications that rate control is inadequate in persistent AF. Extended periods of ECG monitoring and assessment of heart rate with exercise should be considered.

In patients with symptoms resulting from inadequate rate control with pharmacologic therapy or worsening LV function due to the persistent tachycardia, a His bundle/AV junction ablation can be performed. The ablation must be coupled with the implantation of an activity sensor pacemaker to maintain a physiologic range of heart rates. Recent evidence that RV pacing can occasionally modestly depress LV function should be taken into consideration in identifying which patients are appropriate candidates for the "ablate and pace" treatment strategy. Occasionally, biventricular pacing may be used to minimize the degree of dyssynchronization that can occur with RV apical pacing alone. Rate control treatment options must be coupled with chronic anticoagulation therapy in all cases. Trials evaluating the elimination of embolic risk by surgical elimination or isolation of the left atrial appendage or by endovascular insertion of a left atrial appendage–occluding device are ongoing and may provide other treatment options that can eliminate the need for chronic anticoagulation.

CATHETER AND SURGICAL ABLATIVE THERAPY TO PREVENT RECURRENT AF Although the optimum ablation strategy has not been defined, most ablation strategies incorporate techniques that isolate the atrial muscle sleeves entering the pulmonary veins; these muscle sleeves have been identified as the source of the majority of triggers responsible for the initiation of AF. Ablation therapy is currently considered an alternative to pharmacologic therapy in patients with recurrent symptomatic AF. Elimination of AF in 50–80% of patients with a catheter-based ablation procedure should be anticipated, depending on the chronicity of the AF, with additional patients becoming responsive to previously ineffective medications.

FIGURE 226-5 Atrial fibrillation (**A**) transitions to "slow" atrial flutter during antiarrhythmic drug therapy. **B.** A rapid ventricular response with 1:1 atrioventricular conduction occurred with exercise, leading to (**C**) symptoms of dizziness.

Catheter ablative therapy also holds promise in patients with more persistent forms of AF and even those with severe atrial dilatation. If its efficacy is confirmed with additional study, it may also afford an important alternative to His bundle ablation and pacemaker insertion. Risks related to the left atrial ablation procedure, albeit low (overall 2–4%), include pulmonary vein stenosis, atrioesophageal fistula, systemic embolic events, and perforation/tamponade.

Surgical ablation of AF is typically performed at the time of other cardiac valve or coronary artery surgery and, less commonly, as a stand-alone procedure. The Cox surgical Maze procedure is designed to interrupt all macroreentrant circuits that might potentially develop in the atria, thereby precluding the ability of the atria to fibrillate. In an attempt to simplify the operation, the multiple incisions of the traditional Cox-Maze procedure have been replaced with linear lines of ablation and pulmonary vein isolation using a variety of energy sources.

Severity of AF symptoms and difficulties in rate and/or rhythm control with pharmacologic therapy will frequently dictate the optimum AF treatment strategy. Similar to the approach with pharmacologic rhythm control, a cautious approach to eliminating anticoagulant therapy is recommended after catheter or surgical ablation. Careful ECG monitoring for asymptomatic AF, particularly in patients with multiple risk factors for stroke, should be considered until guidelines are firmly established. If the left atrial appendage has been removed surgically, then the threshold for stopping anticoagulation should be lowered. Antiarrhythmic therapy typically can be discontinued after catheter or surgical ablation of AF. However, in selected patients, satisfactory AF control may require maintenance of previously ineffective drug therapy after the ablation intervention.

ATRIAL FLUTTER AND MACROREENTRANT ATRIAL TACHYCARDIAS

Macroreentrant arrhythmias involving the atrial myocardium are collectively referred to as AFL. The terms *AFL* and *macroreentrant AT* are frequently used interchangeably, with both denoting a nonfocal source of an atrial arrhythmia. The typical or most common AFL circuit rotates in a clockwise or counterclockwise direction in the right atrium around the tricuspid valve annulus. The posterior boundary of the right AFL circuit is defined by the crista terminalis, the Eustachian ridge, and the inferior and superior vena cavae. Counterclockwise right AFL represents ~80% of all AFL with superiorly directed activation of the interatrial septum, which produces the saw-toothed appearance of the P waves in ECG leads II, III, and aVF. Clockwise rotation of the same right atrial circuit produces predominantly positive P waves in leads II, III, and aVF (Fig. 226-4). Macroreentrant left AFL may also develop, albeit much less commonly. This type of arrhythmia may be the sequelae of surgical or catheter-based ablation procedures that create large anatomic barriers or promote slowing of conduction in the left atrium, especially around the mitral valve annulus. Atypical AFL or macroreentrant AT can also develop around incisions created during surgery for valvular or congenital heart disease or in and/or around large areas of atrial fibrosis.

Classic or typical right AFL has an atrial rate of 260–300 beats/min with a ventricular response that tends to be 2:1, or typically 130–150 beats/min. In the setting of severe atrial conduction disease and or antiarrhythmic drug therapy, the atrial rate can slow to <200 beats/min. In this setting, a 1:1 rapid ventricular response may occur, particularly with exertion, and produce adverse hemodynamic effects (Fig. 226-5). Atypical AFL or macroreentrant AT related to prior surgical incisions and atrial fibrosis demonstrates less predictability in terms of the atrial rate and is more likely to demonstrate slower rates that overlap with those identified with focal atrial tachycardias (p. 1432).

Because lead V_1 is frequently monitored in a hospitalized patient, coarse AF may be misdiagnosed as AFL. This occurs because in both typical right AFL and coarse AF the crista terminalis in the right atrium may serve as an effective anatomic barrier. The free wall of the right atrium, whose electrical depolarization is best reflected on the body surface by lead V_1, may demonstrate a uniform wavefront of atrial activation under both conditions. The timing of atrial activation is much more rapid in AF and always demonstrates variable atrial intervals with some intervals between defined P waves <200 ms (Fig. 226-6). A review of the other ECG leads demonstrates the disorganized atrial depolarization that is characteristic of AF. Frequently, an individual patient may alternate between AF and AFL or, less commonly, may manifest AF in one atria and AFL in the other, making the distinction more difficult.

℞ ATRIAL FLUTTER

Because of the anticipated rapid regular ventricular rate associated with AFL and the failure to respond to pharmacologic therapy directed at slowing the ventricular rate, patients are frequently treated with DC cardioversion. The organized atrial flutter activity can frequently be terminated with low-energy external cardioversion of 50–100 J. The risk of thromboembolic events associated with typical AFL is high, and anticoagulation must be managed similarly to that described for patients with AF (p. 1428).

Asymptomatic patients with AFL may develop heart failure symptoms with tachycardia-induced severe LV dysfunction. In all patients, an effort should be made to control the ventricular rate pharmacologically or restore sinus rhythm. Rate control with calcium antagonists (diltiazem or verapamil), beta blockers, and/or digoxin may be difficult. Even higher grade AV slowing, such as a 4:1 AV response, may only be transient and is easily overcome with activity or emotional stress. Owing to the typically faster ventricular rate, AFL tends to be poorly tolerated in comparison to AF.

In selected patients with high anesthestic risk, an attempt at pharmacologic cardioversion with procainamide, amiodarone, or ibutilide is appropriate. Antiarrhythmic drug therapy may also enhance the efficacy of direct current cardioversion and the maintenance of sinus rhythm after cardioversion. Recurrence rates of AFL with pharmacologic attempts at rhythm control exceed 80% by 1 year.

Patients who manifest recurrent AFL appear to be effectively treated with catheter ablative therapy. For typical right AFL, an isthmus ablation line from the tricuspid annulus to the opening of the inferior vena cava can permanently eliminate flutter, with an anticipated success rate of >90% in most experienced centers. In patients with macroreentrant atrial tachycardia or AFL involving prior surgical incisions or in areas of atrial fibrosis, detailed mapping of the arrhythmia circuit is required to design the best ablation strategy to interrupt the circuit. In selected patient with AF and typical right AFL, pharmacologic therapy may help to prevent the AF but not the AFL. In this type of patient, hybrid therapy with antiarrhythmic agents coupled with a right atrial isthmus ablation may produce AF and AFL control.

FIGURE 226-6 Atrial flutter/atrial fibrillation. Coarse atrial fibrillation (**A**) contrasted with organized atrial flutter (**B**).

MULTIFOCAL ATRIAL TACHYCARDIA

Multifocal AT (MAT) is the signature tachycardia of patients with significant pulmonary disease. The atrial rhythm is characterized by at least three distinct P wave morphologies and often at least three different PR intervals, and the associated atrial and ventricular rates are typically between 100 and 150 beats/min. The presence of an isoelectric baseline distinguishes this arrhythmia from AF (Fig. 226-4). The absence of any intervening sinus rhythm distinguishes MAT from normal sinus rhythm with frequent multifocal APCs, although this distinction may be moot as these processes define an electrophysiologic continuum.

℞ **MULTIFOCAL ATRIAL TACHYCARDIA**

Therapy for MAT should be directed at improving the underlying medical condition, which is typically, although not invariably, chronic obstructive or restrictive lung disease. Treatment with the calcium channel blocker, verapamil, may also provide some benefit. The judicious use of flecainide or propafenone may also decrease atrial arrhythmias. Patients should be screened for the presence of significant ventricular dysfunction or coronary artery disease before starting these agents. Low-dose amiodarone therapy may also control the arrhythmia and minimize the risk of pulmonary toxicity noted with the drug.

FOCAL ATRIAL TACHYCARDIAS

The two general mechanisms for focal ATs can be distinguished by observations made at AT initiation and in response to adenosine. *Automatic ATs* start with a "warm-up" period over the first 3–10 complexes and, similarly, slow in rate prior to termination. They may respond to adenosine not only with evidence of AV block but also with gradual slowing of the atrial rhythm and termination. The initiation of automatic ATs can frequently be provoked by isoproterenol infusion. The first P wave of the tachycardia has the same morphology as the remaining waves. Some of the ATs may be triggered or provoked by burst atrial pacing but are not reliably initiated by programmed atrial stimulation.

In contrast, evidence supporting a focal reentrant AT includes the initiation of the tachycardia with programmed atrial stimulation or spontaneous premature beats. The P wave initiating the tachycardia will characteristically have a different morphology than the P wave during the sustained AT. In response to adenosine, reentrant ATs will demonstrate AV block but typically do not slow and/or terminate. Most focal ATs in the absence of structural heart disease originate from specific anatomic locations. These anatomic locations appear to be associated with anatomic ridges, such as the crista terminalis, the valve annuli, or the limbus of the fossa ovalis. ATs also appear to originate from the muscular sleeves associated with the cardiac thoracic veins, i.e., the SVC, the coronary sinus, and the pulmonary veins. As indicated, repetitive firing of these foci appears to serve as the triggering mechanism for AF in most patients.

It is important to distinguish focal ATs from reentrant tachycardias that incorporate the AV node in the circuit (**Fig. 226-7**). The primary distinction is related to the persistence of the AT in the presence of AV block that occurs spontaneously or is created by carotid sinus massage or the administration of adenosine (Fig. 226-4). Atrial activity drives the ventricles in AT and all changes in the PP interval accompanied by correlative changes in the RR intervals; in addition, the V–A relationship changes when the atrial rate changes. The P wave in AT is characteristically distinct from the sinus P wave morphology, and, unless there is significant AV nodal conduction delay, the PR interval is shorter than the measured RP interval when there is a 1:1 relationship between atria and ventricles (Fig. 226-7).

The P wave for ATs depends on the anatomic site of origin. In addition to attempting to create AV block to establish the diagnosis of AT, analysis of the P wave morphology on the 12-lead ECG may help to exclude AV nodal reentry, AV bypass tract–mediated reentrant tachycardias, and physiologic or inappropriate sinus tachycardia (Fig. 226-7).

FIGURE 226-7 Pattern of atrial and ventricular activation and characteristic relationship of P wave and QRS complex as recorded in leads II and V₁ during regular supraventricular tachycardias. *A.* Sinus tachycardia. *B.* Atrial tachycardia from top of the atria. *C.* Atrioventricular nodal reentry. *D.* Accessory pathway–mediated orthodromic supraventricular tachycardia.

The ECG distinction between focal automatic or microreentrant AT and macroreentrant AT or atypical AFL is not always possible. Although sustained focal ATs tend to be slower, the atrial rates will frequently overlap. Focal ATs, which are more common in the absence of structural heart disease, will tend to demonstrate an isolectric baseline between P waves, whereas macroreentrant ATs represent atrial activation that is continuous and an isoelectric baseline between P waves may be frequently absent. In patients with a history of prior atrial surgery, one must suspect a macroreentrant mechanism. These distinctions are less important with respect to acute management but have importance related to ablation strategies and anticipated outcome (p. 1431).

℞ ATRIAL TACHYCARDIA

Pharmacologic treatment of AT is generally approached in a similar fashion to that of AF and AFL. AV nodal blocking agents are administered in the setting of rapid ventricular rates. Acute IV administration of procainamide or amiodarone may terminate the tachycardia. Tachycardias not responding to pharmacologic therapy may be terminated with electrical cardioversion. Typically, anticoagulation prior to treatment is not needed unless there is evidence of severe atrial dilatation, >5 cm left atrial diameter with a high risk of AF, and/or a history of coincident paroxysmal AF. Most focal ATs are readily amenable to catheter ablative therapy. In patients who fail to respond to medical therapy or who are reluctant to take chronic drug therapy, this option should be considered, with an anticipated 90% cure rate. A para-Hisian location for the AT and/or focus that is located in the left atrium may modestly increase the risk related to the procedure, and, for this reason, every effort should be made to determine the likely origin of the AT based on an analysis of the P wave morphology on 12-lead ECG prior to the procedure.

AV NODAL TACHYCARDIAS

AV Nodal Reentrant Tachycardia AVNRT is the most common paroxysmal regular SVT. It is more commonly observed in women than men and is typically manifest in the second to fourth decades of life. In general, because AVNRT tends to occur in the absence of structural heart disease, it is usually well tolerated. In the presence of hypertension or other forms of structural heart disease that limit ventricular filing, hypotension or syncope may occur.

AVNRT develops because of the presence of two electrophysiologically distinct pathways for conduction in the complex syncytium of muscle fibers that make up the AV node. The fast pathway located in the more superior part of the node has a longer refractory period, while the pathway lower in the AV node region conducts more slowly but has a shorter refractory period. As a result of the inhomogeneities of conduction and refractoriness, a reentrant circuit can develop in response to premature stimulation. Although conduction occurs over both pathways during sinus rhythm, only the conduction over the fast pathway is manifest and, as a result, the PR interval is normal. APCs occurring at a critical coupling interval are blocked in the fast pathway because of the longer refractory period and are conducted slowly over the slow pathway. When sufficient conduction slowing occurs, the blocked fast pathway can recover excitability and atrial activation can occur over the fast pathway to complete the circuit. Repetitive activation down the slow and up the fast pathway results in typical AV nodal reentrant tachycardia (Fig. 226-7).

ECG FINDINGS IN AVNRT The APC initiating AVNRT is characteristically followed by a long PR interval consistent with conduction via the slow pathway. AVNRT is manifest typically as a narrow QRS complex tachycardia at rates that range from 120 to 250 beats/min. The QRS-P wave pattern associated with typical AVNRT is quite characteristic, with simultaneous activation of the atria and ventricles from the reentrant AV nodal circuit. The P wave will frequently be buried inside the QRS complex and either not be visible or will distort the initial or terminal portion of the QRS complex (Fig. 226-7). Because atrial activation originates in the region of the AV node, a negative deflection will be generated by retrograde atrial depolarization.

Occasionally, AVNRT occurs with activation in the reverse direction, conducting down the fast pathway and returning up the slow pathway. This form of AVNRT occurs much less commonly and produces a prolonged RP interval during the tachycardia with a negative P wave in leads 2, 3, and aVF. This atypical form of AVNRT is more easily precipitated by ventricular stimulation.

℞ ATRIOVENTRICULAR NODAL REENTRANT TACHYCARDIA

ACUTE TREATMENT Treatment is directed at altering conduction within the AV node. Vagal stimulation, such as occurs with the Valsalva maneuver or carotid sinus massage, can slow conduction in the AV node sufficiently to terminate AVNRT. In patients in whom physical maneuvers do not terminate the tachyarrhythmia, the administration of adenosine, 6–12 mg IV, frequently does so. Intravenous beta blockade or calcium channel therapy should be considered second-line agents. If hemodynamic compromise is present, R wave synchronous DC cardioversion using 100–200 J can terminate the tachyarrhythmia.

PREVENTION Prevention may be achieved with drugs that slow conduction in the antegrade slow pathway, such as digitalis, beta blockers, or calcium channel blockers. In patients who have a history of exercise-precipitated AVNRT, the use of beta blockers frequently eliminates symptoms. In patients who do not respond to drug therapy directed at the antegrade slow pathway, treatment with class IA or IC agents directed at altering conduction of the fast pathway may be considered.

Catheter ablation, directed at elimination or modification of slow pathway conduction, is very effective in permanently eliminating AVNRT. Patients with recurrent AVNRT that produces significant symptoms or heart rates >200 beats/min and patients reluctant to take chronic drug therapy should be considered for ablative therapy. Catheter ablation can cure AV nodal reentry in >95% of patients. The risk of AV block requiring a permanent pacemaker is ~1% with the ablation procedure. This risk may be further minimized with the use of cryoablation techniques when the slow pathway is in close proximity to the compact AV node.

AV Junctional Tachycardias These can also occur in the setting of enhanced normal automaticity, abnormal automaticity, or triggered activity. These tachycardias may or may not be associated with retrograde conduction to the atria, and the P waves may appear dissociated or produce intermittent conduction and early activation of the junction. These arrhythmias may occur as a manifestation of increased adrenergic tone or drug effect in patients with sinus node dysfunction or following surgical or catheter ablation. The arrhythmia may also be a manifestation of digoxin toxicity. The most common manifestation of digoxin intoxication is the sudden regularization of the response to AF. A junctional tachycardia due to digoxin toxicity typically does not manifest retrograde conduction. Sinus activity may appear dissociated or result in intermittent capture beats with a long PR interval. If the rate is >50 beats/min and <100 beats/min, the term *accelerated junctional rhythm* applies. Occasionally, automatic rhythms are mimicked by AVNRT that fails to conduct to the atrium. The triggering events associated with the onset of the tachycardia may provide a clue to the appropriate diagnosis. Initiation of the tachycardia without an atrial premature beat with a gradual acceleration in rate suggests an automatic focus.

℞ ATRIOVENTRICULAR JUNCTIONAL TACHYCARDIAS

Treatment of automatic/triggered junctional tachycardias is directed at decreasing adrenergic stimulation and reversing digoxin toxicity, if present. Digoxin therapy can be withheld if toxicity is suspected, and the administration of digoxin-specific antibody fragments can rapidly reverse digoxin toxicity if the tachycardia is producing significant symptoms and rapid termination is indicated. Junctional tachycardia due to abnormal automaticity can be treated pharmacologically with beta blockers. A trial of class IA or IC drugs may also be attempted. For incessant automatic junctional tachycardia, focal catheter ablation can be performed but is associated with an increased risk of AV block.

Tachycardias that involve accessory pathways (APs) between atria and ventricles commonly manifest a normal QRS complex with a short or long RP interval. They must be considered in the differential diagnosis of other narrow-complex tachycardias. Importantly, most tachycardias associated with APs involve a large macroreentrant circuit that includes the ventricles (Fig. 226-7). Thus, identifying these arrhythmias as "supraventricular" is actually a misnomer, and they deserve separate consideration.

APs are typically capable of conducting rapidly both in an antegrade and retrograde direction. In the absence of an AP, the sinus impulse normally activates the ventricles via the AV node and His-Purkinje system, resulting in a PR interval of 120–200 ms. When an antegradely conducting AP is present, the sinus impulse bypasses the AV node and can rapidly activate the ventricles, resulting in ventricular preexcitation. The resulting PR interval is shorter than anticipated. In addition, because the initial ventricular activation is due to muscle-to-muscle conduction, as opposed to rapid spread of activation via the His-Purkinje system, the initial portion of the QRS complex is slurred, creating the characteristic "delta wave." The remaining portion of the QRS complex in sinus rhythm is created by a fusion of the ventricular activation wavefront originating from the Purkinje network and the continued spread of activation from the site of insertion of the AP (Fig. 226-8). Evidence of ventricular preexcitation includes evidence in sinus rhythm of a short PR interval and a delta wave.

The most common AP connects the left atrium to the left ventricle, followed by posterior septal, right free wall, and anterior septal APs. APs typically insert from the atrium into the adjacent ventricular myocardium. However, occasionally pathways, particularly those originating from the right atrium, can have a ventricular insertion at a site distant from the AV groove in the fascicles. These pathways tend to be long, conduct more slowly, and are referred to as *atriofascicular accessory pathways*. Atriofascicular APs are unique in their tendency to demonstrate decremental antegrade conduction.

Other accessory pathway connections from the AV node to the fascicles may also exist. These pathways are referred to as *Mahaim fibers* and typically manifest a normal PR interval with a delta wave.

Patients with manifest preexcitation and WPW syndrome are typically subject to both macroreentrant tachycardias and a rapid response to AF (Fig. 226-8). The most common macroreentrant tachycardia associated with the WPW syndrome is referred to as *orthodromic AV reentry*. Ventricular activation occurs via the AV node and the His-Purkinje system. Conduction then returns or reenters the atria via retrograde conduction over the AP. The reentrant circuit develops because of the inhomogeneity in conduction and refractoriness in the AP and normal AV node.

Characteristically, the AP has more rapid conduction but a longer refractory period when compared to that of the AV node. Typical APs do not show evidence of antegrade decremental conduction. An APC can block in the AP and conduct sufficiently slowly or with decrement via the AV node to allow for retrograde recovery of activation of the AP and, in turn, of the atria (Fig. 226-7). This retrograde activation of the atria via the AP is referred to as an *echo beat*. If the pattern repeats itself, a tachycardia develops. Uncommonly, the reentrant circuit can be reversed so that the impulse reaches the ventricle via the AP and conducts retrogradely through to the atria via the His-Purkinje system and the AV node; this is referred to as *antidromic AV reentry* and/or *preexcitated macroreentry*, with the entire activation of the ventricle originating from the site of insertion of the AP. Although uncommon, it is important to recognize antidromic SVT. The ECG pattern during the tachycardia mimics VT originating from the site of ventricular insertion of the AP. The presence of a similar or lesser degree of manifest preexcitation in sinus rhythm provides a valuable clue to the diagnosis.

The second most common and potentially more serious arrhythmia associated with the WPW syndrome is rapidly conducting AF. Nearly 50% of patients with evidence of APs are predisposed to episodes of AF. In patients who have rapid antegrade conduction from the atria to the ventricles over the AP, the AP can conduct rapidly in response to AF, resulting in a faster ventricular rate than would occur normally via the AV node. The rapid ventricular rates can result in hemodynamic compromise and even precipitate VF. The QRS pattern during AF in patients with manifest preexcitation can appear quite bizarre and change on a beat-to-beat basis due to the variability in the degree of fusion from activation over the AV node (Fig. 226-8).

Concealed APs In ~50% of patients with APs, there is no antegrade conduction over the AP; however, retrograde conduction is preserved. As a result, the AP is not manifest in sinus rhythm and is only manifest during the sustained tachycardia. The presence of a concealed AP is suggested by the timing and pattern of atrial activation during the tachycardia: the P wave typically follows ventricular activation with a short RP wave interval (Fig. 226-7). Because many APs connect the left ventricle to the left atrium, the pattern of atrial activation during the tachycardia frequently produces negative P waves in leads I and aVL. The tachycardia circuit circuit, and, therefore, its ECG manifestation during orthodromic tachycardia, are identical both in patients with overt preexcitation in sinus rhythm and in those with concealed APs. Patients with concealed APs, although prone to episodes of AF, are not at risk for developing a rapid ventricular response to the AF.

Occasionally, APs conduct extremely slowly in a retrograde fashion, resulting in longer retrograde conduction and the development of a long RP interval during the tachycardia (*long RP tachycardia*). Because of the presence of this dramatically slowed conduction, additional conduction slowing created by premature atrial complexes is not required for tachycardia to ensue. These patients are more prone to frequent episodes of tachycardia and can present with "incessant" tachycardias and tachycardia-induced LV cardiomyopathy. The correct diagnosis of a long RP tachycardia may be suggested by the pattern of initiation and the P wave morphology. Frequently, however, an electrophysiologic evaluation is required to establish the diagnosis.

FIGURE 226-8 ***A.*** Sinus rhythm tracing of leads V₁–V₃ showing evidence of Wolff-Parkinson-White syndrome with short PR interval and delta wave. ***B.*** During atrial fibrillation, rapid conduction to the ventricles is observed producing a wide QRS complex tachycardia with marked irregularity of the ventricular response and morphology of the QRS complex.

℞ ACCESSORY PATHWAY–MEDIATED TACHYCARDIAS

Acute treatment of AP-mediated macroreentrant orthodromic tachycardias is similar to that for AV nodal reentry and is directed at altering conduction in the AV node. Vagal stimulation with the Valsalva maneuver and carotid sinus pressure may create sufficient AV nodal slowing to terminate the AVRT. Intravenous administration of adenosine, 6–12 mg, is first-line pharmacologic therapy; IV calcium channel blockers, verapamil or diltiazem, or beta blockers may also be effective. In patients who demonstrate manifest preexcitation and AF, therapy should be aimed at preventing a rapid ventricular response. In life-threatening situations, DC cardioversion should be used to terminate the AF. In non-life-threatening situations, procainamide at a dose of 15 mg/kg administered IV over 20–30 min will slow the ventricular response and may organize and terminate AF. Ibutilide can also be used to facilitate termination of AF. During AF there may be rapid conduction over the AV node as well as the AP. Caution should be used in attempting to slow AV nodal conduction with the use of digoxin or verapamil; when administered IV, these drugs may actually result in an acute increase in rate over the AP, placing the patient at risk for development of VF. Digoxin appears to shorten the refractory period of the AP directly and thus increases the ventricular rate. Verapamil appears to shorten the refractory period indirectly by causing vasodilatation and a reflex increase in sympathetic tone.

Chronic oral administration of beta blockers and/or verapamil or diltiazem may be used to prevent recurrent supraventricular reentrant tachycardias associated with APs. In patients with evidence of AF and a rapid ventricular response and in those with recurrences of SVT on AV nodal blocking drugs, strong consideration should be given to the administration of either a class IA or IC antiarrhythmic drug, such as quinidine, flecainide, or propafenone, that slow conduction and increase refractoriness in the AP.

Patients with a history of recurrent symptomatic SVT episodes, incessant SVT, and heart rates >200 beats/min with SVT should be given strong consideration for undergoing catheter ablation. Patients who have demonstrated rapid antegrade conduction over their AP or the potential for rapid conduction should also be considered for catheter ablation. Catheter ablation therapy has been demonstrated to be successful in >95% of patients with documented WPW syndrome and appears effective regardless of age. The risk of catheter ablative therapy is low and is dictated primarily by the location of the AP. Ablation of para-Hisian APs is associated with a risk of heart block, and ablation in the left atrium is associated with a small but definite risk of thromboembolic phenomenon. These risks must be weighed against the potential serious complications associated with hemodynamic compromise, the risk of VF, and the severity of the patient's symptoms with AP-mediated tachycardias.

Patients who demonstrate evidence of ventricular preexcitation in the absence of any prior arrhythmia history deserve special consideration. The first arrhythmia manifestation can be a rapid SVT or, albeit of low risk (<1%), of a life-threatening rapid response to AF. Patients who demonstrate intermittent preexcitation during ECG monitoring or an abrupt loss of AP conduction during exercise testing are at low risk of a life-threatening rapid response to AF. All other patients should be advised of their risks and therapeutic options in advance of a documented arrhythmia event.

VENTRICULAR TACHYARRHYTHMIAS

VENTRICULAR PREMATURE COMPLEXES (VPCs)

The origin of premature beats in the ventricle at sites remote from the Purkinje network produces slow ventricular activation and a wide QRS complex that is typically >140 ms in duration. VPCs are common and increase with age and the presence of structural heart disease. VPCs can occur with a certain degree of periodicity that has become incorporated into the lexicon of electrocardiography. VPCs may occur in patterns of *bigeminy*, in which every sinus beat is followed by a VPC, or *trigeminy*, in which two sinus beats are followed by a VPC. VPCs may have different morphologies and are thus referred to as *multiformed*. Two successive VPCs are termed *pairs* or *couplets*. Three or more consecutive VPCs are termed *VT* when the rate is >100 beats/min. If the repetitive VPCs terminate spontaneously and are more than three beats in duration, the arrhythmia is referred to as *nonsustained VT*.

APCs with aberrant ventricular conduction may also create a wide and early QRS complex. The premature P wave can occasionally be difficult to discern when it falls on the preceding T wave, and other

clues must be used to make the diagnosis. The QRS pattern for a VPC does not appear to follow a typical right or left bundle branch block pattern as the QRS morphology is associated with aberrant atrial conduction and can be quite bizarre. On occasion, VPCs can arise from the Purkinje network of the ventricles, in which case the QRS pattern mimics aberration. The 12-lead ECG recording of the VPC may be required to identify subtle morphologic clues regarding the QRS complex to confirm its ventricular origin. Most commonly, VPCs are associated with a "fully compensatory pause"; i.e., the duration between the last QRS before the PVC and the next QRS complex is equal to twice the sinus rate (Fig. 226-3). The VPC typically does not conduct to the atrium. If the VPC does conduct to the atrium, it may not be sufficiently early to reset the sinus node. As a result, sinus activity will occur and the antegrade wavefront from the sinus node may encounter some delay in the AV node or His-Purkinje system from the blocked VPC wavefront, or it may collide with the retrograde atrial wavefront. Sinus activity will continue undisturbed, resulting in a delay to the next QRS complex (Fig. 226-3). Occasionally the VPC can occur early enough and conduct retrograde to the atrium to reset the sinus node; the pause that results will be less than compensatory. VPCs that fail to influence the oncoming sinus impulse are termed *interpolated VPCs*. A ventricular focus that fires repetitively at a fixed interval may produce variably coupled VPCs, depending on the sinus rate. This type of focus is referred to as a *parasystolic focus* because its firing does not appear to be modulated by sinus activity and the conducted QRS complex. The ventricular ectopy will occur at a characteristic fixed integer or multiple of these intervals. The variability in coupling relative to the underlying QRS complex and a fixed interval between complexes of ventricular origin provide the diagnostic information necessary to identify a parasystolic focus.

℞ VENTRICULAR PREMATURE COMPLEXES

The threshold for treatment of VPCs is high, and the treatment is primarily directed at eliminating severe symptoms associated with palpitations. VPCs of sufficient frequency can cause a reversible cardiomyopathy. Depressed LV function in the setting of ventricular bigeminy and/or frequent nonsustained VT should raise the possibility of a cardiomyopathy that is reversible with control of the ventricular arrhythmia. In the absence of structural heart disease, VPCs do not appear to have prognostic significance. In patients with structural heart disease, frequent VPCs and runs of nonsustained VT have prognostic significance and may portend an increased risk of SCD. However, no study has documented that elimination of VPCs with antiarrhythmic drug therapy reduces the risk of arrhythmic death in patients with severe structural heart disease. In fact, drug therapies that slow myocardial conduction and/or enhance dispersion of refractoriness can actually increase the risk of life-threatening arrhythmias (drug-induced QT prolongation and TDP) despite being effective at eliminating VPCs.

ACCELERATED IDIOVENTRICULAR RHYTHM (AIVR)

AIVR refers to a ventricular rhythm that is characterized by three or more complexes at a rate >40 beats/min and <120 beats/min. The arrhythmia mechanism causing AIVR is thought to be due to abnormal automaticity. By definition there is an overlap between AIVR and "slow" VT; both rhythms can manifest rates between 90 and 120 beats/min. Because AIVR tends to be a benign rhythm with different therapeutic implications, it is worthwhile to attempt to distinguish it from "slow" VT. AIVR has a characteristic gradual onset and offset and more variability in cycle length. It is typically a brief, self-limiting arrhythmia. AIVR can be seen in the absence of any structural heart disease, but it is frequently present in the setting of acute myocardial infarction, cocaine intoxication, acute myocarditis, digoxin intoxication, and postoperative cardiac surgery. Sustained forms of AIVR can exist, particularly in the setting of acute myocardial infarction and postoperatively. In the setting of sustained AIVR, hemodynamic compromise can occur because of the loss of AV synchrony. Patients with RV infarction associated with proximal right coronary artery occlusion are most susceptible to associated bradyarrhythmias and the hemodynamic consequences of AIVR. In these patients, acceleration of the atrial rate, either by the cautious administration of atropine or by atrial pacing, may be an important treatment consideration.

VENTRICULAR TACHYCARDIA

VT originates below the bundle of His at a rate >100 beats/min; most have rates >120 beats/min. Sustained VT at rates <120 beats/min and even <100 beats/min can be observed, particularly in association with the administration of antiarrhythmic agents that can slow the rate. Because of the overlap in rates with AIVR, the arrhythmia ECG characteristics and the clinical circumstance can sometimes be used to distinguish the two forms of tachycardia. Slow sustained VT is less likely to show a marked warm-up in rate and the marked cycle-length oscillations seen with AIVR, and it is more likely to occur in the setting of chronic infarction or cardiomyopathy and less likely with acute infarction or myocarditis. Obviously, significant overlap may exist. Typically, slow VT will be initiated with programmed stimulation and is found to represent a large macroreentrant circuit in chronically diseased myocardium capable of supporting markedly slow conduction.

The QRS complex during VT may be uniform (monomorphic) or may vary from beat to beat (polymorphic). Polymorphic VT in patients who demonstrate a long QT interval during their baseline rhythm is typically referred to as *TDP*. The polymorphic VT associated with QT prolongation dramatically oscillates around the baseline on most of the monitored ECG leads, mimicking the "turning of the points" stitching pattern (Fig. 226-9).

Monomorphic VT suggests a stable tachycardia focus in the absence of structural heart disease or a fixed anatomic substrate that can create the substrate for a stable reentrant VT circuit when structural disease is present. Monomorphic VT tends to be a reproducible and recurrent phenomenon and may be initiated with pacing and programmed ventricular stimulation. In contrast, polymorphic VT suggests a more dynamic and/or unstable process and, by its very nature, is less reproducible. Polymorphic VT may be produced by acute ischemia, myocarditis, or dynamic changes in the QT interval and enhanced dispersion of ventricular refractoriness. Polymorphic VTs are not reliably initiated with pacing or programmed stimulation.

A time duration of 30 s is frequently used to distinguish sustained from nonsustained VT. Hemodynamically unstable VT that requires termination before 30 s or VT that is terminated by therapy from an implantable defibrillator is also typically classified as sustained. Ventricular flutter appears as a sine wave on the ECG and has a rate of >250 beats/min. A rapid rate coupled with the sine wave nature of the arrhythmia makes it impossible to identify a discrete QRS morphology. When antiarrhythmic drugs are being administered, a sine wave appearance of the QRS complex can be observed, even at rates of 200 beats/min. VF is characterized by completely disorganized ventricular activation on the surface ECG. Polymorphic ventricular arrhythmias, ventricular flutter, and VF always produce hemodynamic collapse if allowed to continue. The hemodynamic stability of a unimorphic VT depends on the presence and severity of the underlying structural

heart disease, the location of the site of origin of the arrhythmia, and the heart rate.

It is important to distinguish monomorphic VT from SVT with aberrant ventricular conduction due to right or left bundle branch block.

Importantly, the sinus or baseline 12-lead ECG tracing can provide important clues that help establish the correct diagnosis of a wide complex tachycardia. The presence of an aberrant QRS pattern that matches exactly that of the wide complex rhythm strongly supports the diagnosis of SVT. A right or left bundle branch block QRS pattern that does not match the QRS and/or that is wider in duration than the QRS during the wide complex tachycardia supports the diagnosis of VT. Most patients with VT have structural heart disease and show evidence of a prior Q wave myocardial infarction during sinus rhythm. Important exceptions to this rule are discussed (p. 1438). Finally, the presence of a preexcited QRS pattern on the 12-lead ECG in sinus rhythm suggests that the wide complex rhythm represents an atrial arrhythmia, such as AFL or a focal AT, with rapid conduction over an AP or antidromic macroreentrant tachycardia (Fig. 226-8). If the arrhythmia is irregular with changing QRS complexes, then the diagnosis of AF with ventricular preexcitation should be considered.

With the exception of some idiopathic outflow tract tachycardias, most VTs do not respond to vagal stimulation provoked by carotid sinus massage, the Valsalva maneuver, or adenosine administration. The IV administration of verapamil and/or adenosine is not recommended as a diagnostic test. Verapamil has been associated with hemodynamic collapse when administered to patients with structural heart disease and VT.

Patients with VT frequently demonstrate AV disassociation. Findings on physical examination of intermittent cannon *a* waves and variability of the first heart sound are consistent with AV dissociation. The presence of AV dissociation is characteristically marked by the presence of sinus capture or fusion beats. The presence of 1:1 ventriculoatrial conduction does not preclude a diagnosis of VT.

Additional characteristics of the 12-lead ECG during the tachycardia that suggest VT include (1) the presence of a QRS duration >140 ms in the absence of drug therapy, (2) a superior and rightward QRS frontal plane axis, (3) a bizarre QRS complex that does not mimic the characteristic QRS pattern associated with left or right bundle branch block, and (4) slurring of the initial portion of the QRS (Fig. 226-10). Table 226-6 provides a useful summary of ECG criteria that have evolved based on the described characteristics of VT.

℞ VENTRICULAR TACHYCARDIA/FIBRILLATION

Sustained polymorphic VT, ventricular flutter, and VF all lead to immediate hemodynamic collapse. Emergency asynchronous defibrillation is therefore required, with at least 200-J monophasic or 100-J biphasic shock. The shock should be delivered asynchronously to avoid delays related to sensing of the QRS complex. If the arrhythmia persists, repeated shocks with the maximum energy output of the defibrillator are essential to optimize the chance of successful resuscitation. Intravenous lidocaine and/or amiodarone should be administered but should not delay repeated attempts at defibrillation.

For any monomorphic wide complex rhythm that results in hemodynamic compromise, a prompt R wave synchronous shock is required. Conscious sedation should be provided if the hemodynamic status permits. For patients with a well-tolerated wide complex tachycardia, the appropriate diagnosis should be established based on strict ECG criteria (Table 226-6). Pharmacologic treatment to terminate monomorphic VT is not typically successful (<30%). Intravenous procainamide, lidocaine, or amiodarone can be utilized. If the arrhythmia persists, synchronous R wave cardioversion after the administration of conscious sedation is appropriate. Selected patients with focal outflow tract tachycardias (p. 1438) who demonstrate triggered or automatic VT may respond to IV beta blocker administration. Idiopathic LV septal VT (see p. 1438) appears to respond uniquely to IV verapamil administration.

VT in patients with structural heart disease is now almost always treated with the implantation of an ICD to manage anticipated VT recurrence. The ICD can provide rapid pacing and shock therapy to treat most VTs effectively (Fig. 226-11).

FIGURE 226-9 Sinus rhythm with long QT interval and the polymorphic ventricular arrhythmia torsades des pointes. Dramatic T wave alternans is present in sinus rhythm.

FIGURE 226-10 Ventricular tachycardia. ECG showing AV dissociation (arrows mark P waves), wide QRS > 200 ms, superior frontal plane axis, slurring of the initial portion of the QRS, and large S wave in V_6—all clues to the diagnosis of ventricular tachycardia.

Prevention of VT remains important, and >50% of patients with a history of VT and an ICD may need to be treated with adjunctive antiarrhythmic drug therapy to prevent VT recurrences or to manage atrial arrhythmias. Because of the presence of an ICD, there is more flexibility with respect to antiarrhythmic drug therapy selection. The use of sotalol or amiodarone represents first-line therapy for patients with a history of structural heart disease and life-threatening monomorphic or polymorphic VT not due to long QT syndrome. Importantly, sotalol has been associated with a decrease in the defibrillation threshold, which reflects the amount of energy necessary to terminate VF. Amiodarone may be better tolerated in patients with a more marginal hemodynamic status and systolic blood pressure. The risk of end organ toxicity from amiodarone must be weighed against the ease of use and general efficacy. Antiarrhythmic drug therapy with agents such as quinidine, procainamide, or propafenone, which might not normally be used in patients with structural heart disease because of the risk of proarrhythmia, may be considered in patients with an ICD and recurrent VT.

Catheter ablative therapy for VT in patients without structural heart disease results in cure rates >90%. In patients with structural heart disease, catheter ablation that includes a strategy for eliminating unmappable/rapid VT and one that incorporates endocardial as well as epicardial mapping and ablation should be employed. In most patients, catheter ablation can reduce or eliminate the requirement for toxic drug therapy and should be considered in any patient with recurrent VT. The utilization of ablative therapy to reduce the incidence of ICD shocks for VT in patients who receive the ICD as part of primary prevention for VT is being actively investigated.

MANAGEMENT OF VT STORM Repeated VT episodes requiring external cardioversion/defibrillation or repeated appropriate ICD shock therapy is referred to as *VT storm*. While a definition of more than two episodes in 24 h is used, most patients with VT storm will experience many more episodes. In the extreme form of VT storm, the tachycardia becomes incessant and the baseline rhythm is unable to be restored for any extended period. In patients with recurrent polymorphic VT in the absence of the long QT interval, one should have a high suspicion of active ischemic disease or fulminant myocarditis. Intravenous lidocaine or amiodarone administration should be coupled with prompt assessment of the status of the coronary anatomy. Endomyocardial biopsy, if indicated by clinical circumstance, may be used to confirm the diagnosis of myocarditis, although the diagnostic yield is low. In patients who demonstrate QT prolongation and recurrent pause-dependent polymorphic VT (TDP), removal of an offending QT-prolonging drug, correction of potassium or magnesium deficiencies, and emergency pacing to prevent pauses should be considered. Intravenous beta blockade therapy should be considered for polymorphic VT storm. A targeted treatment strategy should be employed if the diagnosis of the polymorphic VT syndrome can be established. For example, quinidine or isoproterenol can be used in the treatment of Brugada's syndrome (p. 1442). Intraaortic balloon counterpulsation or acute coronary angioplasty may be needed to stop recurrent polymorphic VT precipitated by acute ischemia. In selected patients with a repeating VPC trigger for their polymorphic VT, the VPC can be targeted for ablation to prevent recurrent VT.

In patients with recurrent monomorphic VT, acute IV administration of lidocaine, procainamide, or amiodarone can prevent recurrences. The use of such therapy is empirical, and a clinical response is not certain. Procainamide and amiodarone are more likely to slow the tachycardia and make it hemodynamically tolerated. Unfortunately, antiarrhythmic drugs, especially those that slow conduction (e.g., amiodarone, procainamide), can also facilitate recurrent VT or even result in incessant VT. VT catheter ablation can eliminate frequent recurrent or incessant VT and frequent ICD shocks.

TABLE 226-6 ECG CLUES SUPPORTING THE DIAGNOSIS OF VENTRICULAR TACHYCARDIA

AV dissociation (atrial capture, fusion beats)
QRS duration > 140 ms for RBBB type V_1 morphology; V_1 > 160 ms for LBBB type V1 morphology
Frontal plane axis −90° to 180°
Delayed activation during initial phase of the QRS complex
  LBBB pattern—R wave in V_1, V2 >40 ms
  RBBB pattern—onset of R wave to nadir of S > 100 ms
Bizarre QRS pattern that does not mimic typical RBBB or LBBB QRS complex
  Concordance of QRS complex in all precordial leads
  RS or dominant S in V_6 for RBBB VT
  Q wave in V_6 with LBBB QRS pattern
  Monophasic R or biphasic qR or R/S in V_1 with RBBB pattern

Note: AV, atrioventricular; RBBB/LBBB, right/left bundle branch block.

Chart speed 25.0 mm/sec

FIGURE 226-11 Ventricular tachycardia (VT) (*) during atrial fibrillation stopped by pacing (#) from an implantable cardioverter defibrillator (ICD) from recording stored by ICD. The atrial electrogram shows characteristic fibrillatory waves through the tracing. The ventricular electrogram shows an irregularly irregular response consistent with atrial fibrillation at the beginning of the tracing. The ventricular electrogram suddenly changes in morphology (*) and becomes regular, consistent with the diagnosis of VT. Pacing transiently accelerates the rate and interrupts the rapid VT. The patient was unaware of the life-threatening event.

Such therapy should be deployed earlier in the course of arrhythmia events to prevent adverse consequences of recurrent VT episodes and adverse effects from antiarrhythmic drugs.

UNIQUE VT SYNDROMES

Although most ventricular arrhythmias occur in the setting of coronary artery disease with prior myocardial infarction, a significant number of patients develop VT in other settings. A brief discussion of each unique VT syndrome is warranted. Information that illustrates a unique pathogenesis and enhances the ability to make the correct diagnosis and institute appropriate therapy will be highlighted.

Idiopathic Outflow Tract VT VT in the absence of structural heart disease is referred to as *idiopathic VT*. There are two major varieties of these VTs. Outflow tachycardias originate in the RV and LV outflow tract regions. Approximately 80% of outflow tract VTs originate in the RV and ~20% in the LV outflow tract regions. Outflow tract VTs appear to originate from anatomic sites that form an arc beginning just above the tricuspid valve and extending along the roof of the outflow tract region to include the free wall and septal aspect of the right ventricle just beneath the pulmonic valve, the aortic valve region, and then the anterior/superior margin of the mitral valve annulus. These arrhythmias appear more commonly in women. Importantly, these ventricular arrhythmias are *not* associated with SCD. Patients manifest symptoms of palpitations with exercise, stress, and caffeine ingestion. In women, the arrhythmia is more commonly associated with hormonal triggers and can frequently be timed to the premenstrual period, gestation, and menopause. Uncommonly, the VPCs and VTs can be of sufficient frequency and duration to cause a tachycardia-induced cardiomyopathy.

The pathogenesis of outflow tract VT remains unknown, and there is no definite anatomic abnormality identified with these VTs. Vagal maneuvers, adenosine, and beta blockers tend to terminate the VTs, whereas catecholamine infusion, exercise, and stress tend to potentiate the outflow tract VTs. Based on these observations, the mechanism of the arrhythmia is most likely calcium-dependent triggered activity. Preliminary data suggest that at least in some patients, a somatic mutation of the inhibitory G protein (Gα I2) may serve as the genetic basis for the VT. In contrast to VT in patients with coronary artery disease, outflow tract VTs are uncommonly initiated with programmed stimulation but are able to be initiated by rapid-burst atrial or ventricular pacing, particularly when coupled with the infusion of isoproterenol.

Outflow tract VT typically produces large monophasic R waves in the inferior frontal plane leads II, III, and aVF, and typically occurs as nonsustained bursts of VT and/or frequent premature beats. Cycle length oscillations during the tachycardia are common. Since most VT originates in the RV outflow tract, the VT typically has a left bundle branch block pattern in lead V_1 (negative QRS vector) (Fig. 226-12). Outflow tract VT, originating in the left ventricle, particularly those associated with an origin from the mitral valve annulus, have a right bundle branch block pattern in lead V_1 (positive QRS vector).

℞ IDIOPATHIC OUTFLOW TRACT VENTRICULAR TACHYCARDIA

Acute medical therapy for idiopathic outflow tract VT is rarely required because the VT is hemodynamically tolerated and is typically nonsustained. Intravenous beta blockers frequently terminate the tachycardia. Chronic therapy with beta or calcium channel blockers frequently prevents recurrent episodes of the tachycardia. The arrhythmia also appears to respond to treatment with class IA or IC agents or with sotalol. In patients who are reluctant to take long-term drug therapy or who have persistent symptoms despite drug therapy, catheter ablative therapy has been utilized successfully to eliminate the tachycardia with success rates >90%. Because of the absence of structural heart disease and the focal nature of these arrhythmias, the 12-lead ECG pattern during VT can help localize the site of origin of the arrhythmia and help facilitate catheter ablation. Efficacy of therapy is assessed with treadmill testing and/or ECG monitoring, and electrophysiologic study is performed only when the diagnosis is in question or to perform catheter ablation.

Idiopathic LV Septal/Fascicular VT The second most common idiopathic VT is linked anatomically to the Purkinje system in the left ventricle. The arrhythmia mechanism appears to be macroreentry involving calcium-dependent slow response fibers that are part of the Purkinje network, although automatic tachycardias have also been observed. A 12-lead ECG morphology of the VT shows a narrow right bundle branch block pattern and a superior leftward axis or an inferior rightward axis, depending upon whether the VT originates from the posterior or anterior fascicles (Fig. 226-12). Idiopathic LV septal VT is unique in its suppression with verapamil. Beta blockers have also been used with some success as primary or effective adjunctive therapy. Catheter ablation is very effective therapy for VT resistant to drug therapy or in patients reluctant to take daily therapy, with anticipated successful elimination of VT in >90% of patients.

FIGURE 226-12 Common idiopathic ventricular tachycardia (VT) ECG patterns. Right ventricular outflow tract (RVOT) VT with typical left bundle QRS pattern in V_1 and inferiorly directed frontal plane axis, and left ventricular septal VT from the inferior septum with a narrow QRS right bundle branch block pattern in V_1 and superior and leftward front plane QRS axis.

FIGURE 226-13 Bundle branch reentrant ventricular tachycardia (VT) showing typical QRS morphologies when ventricular tachycardia (VT) is initiated with stimulation from the right ventricle [left bundle branch block (LBBB) VT pattern] or left ventricle [right bundle branch block (RBBB) VT pattern] and schema for circuit involving the His-Purkinje network.

< 30%, data now support the implantation of a prophylactic ICD device to reduce the risk of SCD from the first VT/VF episode effectively.

Bundle Branch Reentrant VT Monomorphic VT in patients with idiopathic nonischemic cardiomyopathy or valvular cardiomyopathy is frequently due to a large macroreentrant circuit involving the various elements of the His-Purkinje network. The arrhythmia usually occurs in the presence of underlying His-Purkinje system disease. In sinus rhythm, an incomplete left bundle block is typically present and the time that it takes to traverse the His-Purkinje network is delayed; this slow conduction serves as the substrate for reentry. Characteristically, the VT circuit rotates in an antegrade direction down the right bundle and retrograde up the left posterior or anterior fascicles and left bundle branch. As a result, bundle branch reentrant VT typically has a QRS morphology that mimics RV apical pacing with a left bundle branch block type pattern and a leftward superior axis (Fig. 226-13). The circuit for bundle branch reentrant VT can occasionally rotate in the opposite direction, antegrade through the left bundle and retrograde through the right bundle, in which case a right bundle branch block pattern during VT will be manifest.

It is important to recognize bundle branch reentrant VT because it is readily amenable to ablative therapy that targets a component of the His-Purkinje system, typically the right bundle, to block the VT circuit. In most patients, because of the presence of severely depressed LV function and a high risk of SCD, ablative therapy is coupled with an ICD. Less commonly, bundle branch reentry may occur in the absence of structural heart disease or in the setting of coronary artery disease. The use of adjunctive ICD therapy is dictated by the ability to eliminate the VT successfully and the severity of the LV dysfunction.

VT Associated with Hypertrophic Cardiomyopathy (See also Chap. 231) VT/VF have also been associated with hypertrophic cardiomyopathy. In patients with hypertrophic cardiomyopathy and a history of sustained VT/VF, unexplained syncope, a strong family history of SCD, LV septal thickness > 30 mm, or nonsustained spontaneous VT, the risk of SCD is high and ICD implantation is usually indicated. Amiodarone, sotalol, and beta blockers have been used to control recurrent VT. Experience with ablative therapy is limited because of the infre-

VT Associated with LV Dilated Cardiomyopathy Monomorphic and polymorphic VTs may occur in patients with nonischemic dilated cardiomyopathy (Chap. 231). Although the myopathic process may be diffuse, there appears to be a predilection for the development of fibrosis around the mitral and aortic valvular regions. Most uniform sustained VT can be mapped to these regions of fibrosis. Drug therapy is usually ineffective in preventing VT, and empirical trials of sotalol or amiodarone are usually initiated only for recurrent VT episodes after ICD implantation. VT associated with nonischemic dilated cardiomyopathy appears to be less amenable to catheter ablative therapy from the endocardium; frequently, the VT originates from epicardial areas of fibrosis and catheter access to the epicardium can be gained via a percutaneous pericardial puncture to improve the outcome of ablation techniques. In patients with a history of depressed myocardial dysfunction due to a nonischemic cardiomyopathy with an LV ejection fraction

TABLE 226-7 **INFILTRATIVE/INFLAMMATORY AND NEUROMUSCULAR DISORDERS ASSOCIATED WITH AN INCREASED VENTRICULAR ARRHYTHMIA RISK**

Sarcoidosis[a]	Emery-Dreyfuss muscular dystrophy[a]
Chagas disease[a]	Limb-girdle muscular dystrophy[a]
Amyloidosis[a]	Duchenne's muscular dystrophy
Fabry disease	Becker's muscular dystrophy
Hemochromatosis	Kearn-Sayre syndrome[a]
Myotonic muscular dystrophy[a]	Friedreich's ataxia

[a]High frequency of ventricular arrhythmias noted.

quency with which the VT is tolerated hemodynamically. Ablation procedures that target the substrate for VT/VF and ablate areas of low voltage consistent with fibrosis appear to have promise in this setting. The WPW syndrome has been observed in patients with hypertrophic cardiomyopathy associated with *PRKAG2* mutations.

VT Associated with Other Infiltrative Cardiomyopathies and Neuromuscular Disorders

An increased arrhythmia risk has been identified when cardiac involvement occurs in a variety of infiltrative diseases and neuromuscular disorders (Table 226-7). Many patients manifest AV conduction disturbances and may require permanent pacemaker insertion. The decision to implant an ICD device should follow current established guidelines for patients with nonischemic cardiomyopathy, which include a history of syncope with depressed LV function, a history of severely depressed LV function, and LV ejection fraction < 35% with class 2 or 3 heart failure symptoms. Additional study will be required to determine if patients with lesser degrees of LV dysfunction may also warrant primary ICD implantation. A potential proarrhythmic risk of antiarrhythmic drug therapy should be acknowledged, and drug therapy should be reserved for symptomatic arrhythmias and limited to amiodarone or sotalol if an ICD is not present.

Arrhythmogenic RV Cardiomyopathy/Dysplasia (ARVCM/D)

(See also Chap. 231) ARVCM/D, due to a genetically determined dysplastic process or after a suspected viral myocarditis, is also associated with VT/VF. The sporadic nonfamilial/nondysplastic form of RV cardiomyopathy appears to be more common; however, this may vary based on ethnicity. In patients predisposed to VT, there appears to be a predominance of perivalvular fibrosis involving mostly the free wall of the right ventri-

cle in proximity to the tricuspid and pulmonic valves. The surface ECG leads that reflect RV activation, including V_1–V_3, may show terminal notching of the QRS complex and inverted T waves in sinus rhythm. When the terminal notching is distinct and appears separated from the QRS complex, it is referred to as an *epsilon wave* (Fig. 226-14). Epsilon waves are consistent with markedly delayed ventricular activation in the region of the RV free wall near the base of the tricuspid and pulmonic valves in areas of extensive fibrosis.

In patients with ARVCM/D, echocardiography demonstrates RV enlargement with RV wall motion abnormalities and RV apical aneurysm formation. MRI may show fatty replacement of the ventricle, thinning of the RV free wall with increased fibrosis, and associated wall motion abnormalities. Because of the presence of extensive amounts of fat normally covering the epicardium in the region of the RV, caution must be used to not overinterpret the MRI in trying to determine the appropriate diagnosis. Patients tend to have multiple VT morphologies. The VT will typically have a left bundle branch block type QRS pattern in V_1 and tend to have poor R wave progression in V_1 through V_6, consistent with an RV free-wall origin. Areas of low electrogram voltage, identified during RV catheter endocardial sinus rhythm voltage mapping, may be helpful in confirming the diagnosis. Importantly, endocardial biopsy may not identify the presence of fatty replacement or fibrosis unless directed to the basal RV free wall. The familial forms of this syndrome have been linked to a number of desmosomal protein mutations. A distinct genetic form of this syndrome, Naxos disease, consists of arrhythmogenic RV dysplasia coupled with palmar-plantar keratosis and woolly hair and is associated with a high risk of SCD in adolescents and young adults.

Rx ARRHYTHMOGENIC RIGHT VENTRICULAR CARDIOMYOPATHY/DYSPLASIA

The threshold for ICD implantation in patients with an established diagnosis of ARVCM/D is low. An ICD will typically be implanted in patients deemed to have a persistent VT risk, those who have had spontaneous or inducible rapid VTs, and those patients who show concomitant LV cardiomyopathy. Treatment options for recurrent VT in patients with ARVCM/D include the use of the antiarrhythmic agent sotalol. Beta blockers serve as useful adjunctive therapy when coupled with other antiarrhythmic agents. Catheter ablative therapy directed at mappable sustained ventricular arrhythmias is also highly successful in controlling recurrent VT. In selected patients with multiple VT morphologies and unstable VT, linear ablation le-

FIGURE 226-14 Leads V_1 to V_3 in sinus rhythm from a normal subject (**A**); from a patient with arrhythmogenic right ventricular cardiomyopathy showing epsilon waves (*arrow*) and T wave inversion (**B**); and from a patient with Brugada syndrome with ST-segment elevation in V_1 and V_2 (**C**).

sions directed at endocardial and, if required, epicardial scarring, defined by catheter-based bipolar voltage mapping, provide significant amelioration of the recurrent VT episodes.

VT After Operative Tetralogy of Fallot Repair   VT may also occur after surgical repair of tetralogy of Fallot. Patients typically develop VT many years after the surgery. VT tends to occur in patients with evidence of RV systolic dysfunction. The VT mechanism and location are typically a macroreentrant circuit around the right ventriculotomy scar to the valve annuli. Catheter ablation creating linear lesions that extend from either the pulmonic or tricuspid annuli to the ventriculotomy scar is typically effective in preventing arrhythmia recurrences. An ICD is usually implanted in patients who manifest rapid VT, have persistent inducible VT after ablation, or have concomitant LV dysfunction.

Fascicular Tachycardia Caused by Digoxin Toxicity   Digoxin toxicity can produce increased ventricular ectopy and, when coupled with bradyarrhythmias caused by digoxin toxicity, may predispose to sustained polymorphic ventricular arrhythmias and VF. The signature VT associated with digoxin toxicity is bidirectional VT (Fig. 226-15). This unique VT is due to triggered activity associated with calcium overload resulting from the inhibition of sodium/potassium ATPase by digoxin. Bidirectional VT originates from the left anterior and posterior fascicles, creating a relatively narrow QRS right bundle branch configuration with beat-to-beat alternating right and left frontal plane QRS axis. This VT is uncommonly observed in the absence of digoxin toxicity. Treatment for bidirectional

Disorder	Gene	Protein/Channel Affected
TABLE 226-8	**INHERITED ARRHYTHMIA DISORDERS—"CHANNELOPATHIES" WITH HIGH RISK OF VENTRICULAR ARRHYTHMIAS**	
LQT1	KCNQ1	I_{Ks} channel α subunit
LQT2	KCNH2 (HERG)	I_{Kr} channel α subunit
LQT3	SCN5A	I_{Na} channel α subunit
LQT4	ANK2	Ankyrin-B
LQT5	KCNE1	I_{Ks} channel β subunit
LQT6	KCNE2	I_{Kr} channel β subunit
LQT7	KCNJ2	I_{K1} channel α subunit
LQT8	CACNA1C	I_{Ca} channel α subunit
Jervell LN1	KCNQ1	I_{Ks} channel β subunit
Jervell LN2	KCNE1	I_{Kr} channel β subunit
Brugada syndrome	SCN5A	I_{Na} channel
Catecholaminergic VT	Ry R2	Ryanodine receptor, calsequestron receptor
SOTS1	KCNH2 (HERG)	I_{Kr} channel α subunit
SQTS2	KCNQ1(KvLQT1)	I_{Ks} channel α subunit
SQTS3	KCNJ2	I_{K1} channel

Note: LQT, long QT (interval); SQT, short QT (interval).

VT or other hemodynamically significant arrhythmias due to digoxin excess includes correction of electrolyte disorders and the IV infusion of digoxin-specific Fab fragments. The antibody fragments will, over the course of 1 h, bind digoxin and eliminate toxic effects. In the setting of normal renal function, the bound complex is secreted.

GENETICALLY DETERMINED ABNORMALITIES THAT PREDISPOSE TO POLYMORPHIC VENTRICULAR ARRHYTHMIAS

Ion channel defects that affect cardiac depolarization and repolarization may predispose to life-threatening polymorphic VT and SCD. These defects frequently produce unique ECG characteristics during sinus rhythm that facilitate the diagnosis.

Long QT Syndrome (LQTS)   The congenital form of the LQTS consists of defects in cardiac ion channels that are responsible for cardiac repolarization. Defects that enhance sodium or calcium inward currents or inhibit outward potassium currents during the plateau phase of the action potential lengthen action potential duration and, hence, the QT interval. Of the eight genetic mutations identified to date, five affect the α or β subunits of the three different potassium channels involved with repolarization (Table 226-8). Since many patients with QT prolongation do not have one of the defined mutations, it is anticipated that other genetic abnormalities affecting repolarization channel function will be identified.

The triggers for the ventricular arrhythmias are thought to be due to early afterdepolarizations potentiated by intracellular calcium accumulation from a prolonged action potential plateau. Heterogeneity of myocardial repolarization indexed by a longer QT interval predisposes to polymorphic ventricular arrhythmias in response to the triggers (Fig. 226-9).

In most patients with LQTS, the QT interval corrected for heart rate using Bazette's formula is 4 to 460 ms in men and 4 to 480 ms in women. Marked lengthening of the QT interval to > 500 ms is clearly associated with a greater arrhythmia risk in patients with the LQTS. Many affected individuals may have QT intervals that intermittently measure within a normal range or that fail to shorten appropriately with exercise. Some individuals will only manifest the syndrome when exposed to a drug, such as sotalol, that alters channel function.

The genotype associated with the LQTS appears to influence prognosis, and identification of the genotype appears to help to optimize clinical management. The first three genotypic designations of the mutations identified, LQT1, LQT2, and LQT3, appear to account for >99% of patients with clinically relevant LQTSs. Surface ECG characteristics may be helpful in distinguishing the three most common genotypes, with genetic testing being definitive.

LQT1 represents the most common genotypic abnormality. Patients with LQT1 fail to shorten or actually prolong their QT interval with exercise. The T wave in patients with LQT1 tends to be broad and

FIGURE 226-15 Digoxin toxic bidirectional fascicular tachycardia.

comprises the majority of the prolonged QT interval. The most common triggers for potentiating cardiac arrhythmias in patients with LQT1 are exercise followed by emotional stress.

More than 80% of male patients have their first cardiac event by age 20, so competitive exercise should be restricted and swimming avoided for these patients. Patients tend to respond to beta blocker therapy. Patients with two LQT1 alleles have the Jervell and Lange-Neilsen syndrome, with more dramatic QT prolongation and deafness and a worse arrhythmia prognosis.

LQT2 is the second most common genotypic abnormality. The T wave tends to be notched and bifid. In LQT2 patients, the most frequent precipitant is emotional stress, followed by sleep or auditory stimulation. Despite the occurrence during sleep, patients typically respond to beta blocker therapy.

LQT3 is due to a mutation in the gene that encodes the cardiac sodium channel located on chromosome 3. Prolongation of the action potential duration occurs because of failure to inactivate this channel. LQT3 patients either have late-onset peaked biphasic T waves or asymmetric peaked T waves. The arrhythmia events tend to be more life-threatening, and thus the prognosis for LQT3 is the poorest of all the LQTs. Male patients appear to have the worst prognosis in patients with LQT3. Most events in LQT3 patients occur during sleep, suggesting that they are at higher risk during slow heart rates. Beta blockers are not recommended, and exercise is not restricted in LQT3.

℞ LONG QT SYNDROME

The institution of ICD therapy should be strongly considered in any patient with LQTS who has demonstrated any life-threatening arrhythmia. Patients with syncope with a confirmed diagnosis based on unequivocal ECG criteria or positive genetic testing should also be given the same strong consideration. Primary prevention with prophylactic ICD implantation should be considered in male patients with LQT3 and in all patients with marked QT prolongation (>500 ms), particularly when coupled with an immediate family history of SCD. Future epidemiologic investigation may provide firmer guidelines to sort patients further based on risks such as age, gender, arrhythmia history, and genetic characteristics. In all patients with documented or suspected LQTS, drugs that prolong the QT interval must be avoided. For an updated list of drugs, see www.qtdrug.org.

Acquired LQTS Patients with a genetic predisposition related to what appear to be sporadic mutations and/or single nucleotide polymorphisms can develop marked QT prolongation in response to drugs that alter repolarization currents. The QT prolongation and associated polymorphic ventricular tachycardia (TDP) are more frequently seen in women and may be a manifestation of subclinical LQTS. Drug-induced long QT and TDP are frequently potentiated by the development of hypokalemia and bradycardia. The offending drugs typically block the potassium I_{Kr} channel (Table 226-5). Since most drug effects are dose-dependent, important drug-drug interactions that alter metabolism and/or alterations in elimination kinetics because of hepatic or renal dysfunction frequently contribute to the arrhythmias.

℞ ACQUIRED LONG QT SYNDROME

Acute therapy for acquired LQTS is directed at eliminating the offending drug therapy, reversing metabolic abnormalities by the infusion of magnesium and/or potassium, and preventing pause-dependent arrhythmias by temporary pacing or the cautious infusion of isoproterenol. Class IB antiarrhythmic agents (e.g., lidocaine), which do not cause QT prolongation, may also be used, though they are frequently ineffective. Supportive therapy to allay anxiety and prevent pain with required DC shock therapy for sustained arrhythmias as well as efforts to facilitate drug elimination are important.

Short QT Syndrome A gain in function of repolarization currents can result in a shortening of atrial and ventricular refractoriness and marked QT shortening on the surface ECG (Table 226-8). The T wave tends to be tall and peaked. A QT interval < 320 ms is required to establish the diagnosis of this uncommon syndrome. Mutations in the HERG, KvLQT1, and KCNJ2 genes have been identified. Patients with the syndrome are predisposed to both AF and VF. ICD implantation is recommended. Double counting of QRS and T waves may lead to inappropriate ICD shocks. Drug therapy with quinidine has been used to lengthen the QT interval and reduce the amplitude of the T wave. This therapy is currently being evaluated to determine long-term efficacy in preventing arrhythmias in this syndrome.

Brugada Syndrome Mutations of SCN5A genes resulting in diminished inward sodium current in the region of the RV outflow tract epicardium appear responsible for the Brugada syndrome (Table 226-8). A loss of the action potential dome in the RV epicardium due to unopposed I_{To} potassium outward current results in dramatic action potential shortening. The large potential difference between the normal endocardium and rapidly depolarized RV outflow epicardium gives rise to ST-segment elevation in V_1-V_3 in sinus rhythm and predisposes to local reentry and life-threatening ventricular arrhythmias in the absence of structural heart disease (Fig. 226-14). Although identified in both genders and all races, the arrhythmia syndrome is most common in young Asian male patients and is thought to be responsible for the sudden and unexpected nocturnal death syndrome (SUDS) previously described in Southeast Asian men.

℞ BRUGADA SYNDROME

Patients do not benefit from beta blocker therapy. Sodium channel-blocking drugs, such as procainamide and flecainide, can exacerbate the syndrome and are used as a provocative test to identify the presence of the abnormality in family members with a more limited expression of the genetic abnormality. This drug challenge may also be important to establish more firmly the diagnosis and the probable cause of unexplained syncope when the surface ECG is equivocal. Acute management of recurrent VT has been reported to respond to isoproterenol administration or quinidine, although the efficacy of this treatment requires more extensive study. ICD treatment to manage recurrences is recommended for all patients who have had documented arrhythmia episodes. Family members should be screened for the presence of the abnormality. A history of syncope, spontaneous ST-segment elevation, and inducibility of VT with programmed stimulation may identify family members also at risk for SCD who warrant prophylactic ICD therapy.

Catecholaminergic Polymorphic VT A mutation of the myocardial ryanodine release channel, which effectively creates a "leak" in calcium from the sarcoplasmic reticulum, has been identified in patients with catecholaminergic VT (Table 226-8). The accumulation of intracellular calcium potentiates delayed afterdepolarizations and triggered activity. Patients can manifest bidirectional VT, nonsustained polymorphic VT, or recurrent VF. Both an autosomal dominant familial and sporadic forms of the disease have been described. More recently, an autosomal recessive variant associated with a mutation in the sarcoplasmic reticulum calcium-buffering protein, calsequestrin, has also been identified. The arrhythmias are precipitated by exercise and emotional stress (Fig. 226-16).

FIGURE 226-16 Catecholaminergic polymorphic ventricular tachycardia noted during an exercise stress test.

Exercise restriction is warranted. Treatment with beta blockers and ICD implantation has been recommended. Prevention of inappropriate or easily triggered ICD shocks by proper ICD programming are essential to prevent VT storm from endogenous catecholamine release.

FURTHER READINGS

CAPPATO R et al: Worldwide survey on the methods, efficacy, and safety of catheter ablation for human atrial fibrillation. Circulation 111(9):1100, 2005

DELACRETAZ E: Clinical practice. Supraventricular tachycardia. N Engl J Med 354(10):1039, 2006

FUSTER V et al: ACC/AHA/ESC 2006 guidelines for the management of patients with atrial fibrillation. Circulation 114:e257, 2006

HAISSAGUERRE M et al: Spontaneous initiation of atrial fibrillation by ectopic beats originating in the pulmonary veins. N Engl J Med 339(10):659, 1998

JOSEPHSON ME: *Clinical Cardiac Electrophysiology: Techniques and Interpretations*, 3d ed. Philadelphia, Lippincott Williams & Wilkins, 2002

KEATING MJ, SANGUINETTI MC: Molecular and cellular mechanisms of cardiac arrhythmia. Cell 104:569, 2001

MARCHLINSKI FE et al: Electroanatomic substrate and outcome of catheter ablative therapy for ventricular tachycardia in setting of right ventricular cardiomyopathy. Circulation 110(16):2293, 2004

———— et al: Ventricular tachycardia/ventricular fibrillation ablation in the setting of ischemic heart disease. J Cardiovasc Electrophysiol 16(1):59, 2005

MILLER JM, ZIPES DP: Therapy for cardiac arrhythmias, in *Braunwald's Heart Disease: A Textbook of Cardiovascular Medicine*, 7th ed. DP Zipes et al (eds). Philadelphia, Saunders, 2005, pp 712–756

PAGE RL: Medical management of atrial fibrillation: Future directions. Heart Rhythm 4:580, 2007

PRIORI SG et al: Clinical and molecular characterization of patients with the catecholaminergic polymorphic ventricular tachycardia. Circulation 106:69, 2002

———— et al: Risk stratification in the long QT syndrome. N Engl J Med 348;1866, 2003

RODEN DM: Drug-induced prolongation of the QT interval. N Engl J Med 350:1013, 2004

TAYLOR FC et al: Systematic review of long term anticoagulation or antiplatelet treatment in patients with non-rheumatic atrial fibrillation. BMJ 322:321, 2001

VAN GELDER IC et al: Rate Control versus Electrical Cardioversion for Persistent Atrial Fibrillation Study Group. A comparison of rate control and rhythm control in patients with recurrent persistent atrial fibrillation. N Engl J Med 347(23):1834, 2002

WELLENS HJ: Contemporary management of atrial flutter. Circulation 106:649, 2002

WYSE DG et al: AFFIRM: A comparison of rate control and rhythm control in patients with atrial fibrillation. N Engl J Med 347:1825, 2002

ZIPES DP et al: ACC/AHA/ESC 2006 guidelines for management of patients with ventricular arrhythmias and the prevention of sudden cardiac death. Circulation 114:e385, 2006

SECTION 4 DISORDERS OF THE HEART

227 Heart Failure and Cor Pulmonale
Douglas L. Mann

HEART FAILURE

DEFINITION

Heart failure (HF) is a clinical syndrome that occurs in patients who, because of an inherited or acquired abnormality of cardiac structure and/or function, develop a constellation of clinical symptoms (dyspnea and fatigue) and signs (edema and rales) that lead to frequent hospitalizations, a poor quality of life, and a shortened life expectancy.

EPIDEMIOLOGY

HF is a burgeoning problem worldwide, with more than 20 million people affected. The overall prevalence of HF in the adult population in developed countries is 2%. HF prevalence follows an exponential pattern, rising with age, and affects 6–10% of people over the age of 65. Although the relative incidence of HF is lower in women than in men, women constitute at least half of the cases of HF because of their longer life expectancy. In North America and Europe, the lifetime risk of developing HF is approximately one in five for a 40-year-old. The overall prevalence of HF is thought to be increasing, in part because current therapies of cardiac disorders, such as myocardial infarction (MI), valvular heart disease, and arrhythmias, are allowing patients to survive longer. Very little is known with respect to the prevalence or risk of developing HF in emerging nations because of the lack of population-based studies in these countries. Although HF was once thought to arise primarily in the setting of a depressed left ventricular (LV) ejection fraction (EF), epidemiological studies have shown that approximately one-half of patients who develop HF have a normal or preserved EF (EF ≥40–50%). Accordingly, HF patients are now broadly categorized into one of two groups: (1) HF with a depressed EF (commonly referred to as *systolic failure*) or (2) HF with a preserved EF (commonly referred to as *diastolic failure*).

ETIOLOGY

As shown in Table 227-1, any condition that leads to an alteration in LV structure or function can predispose a patient to developing HF. Although the etiology of HF in patients with a preserved EF differs from that of those with depressed EF, there is considerable overlap between the etiologies of these two conditions. In industrialized countries, coronary artery disease (CAD) has become the predominant cause in men and women and is responsible for 60–75% of cases of HF. Hypertension contributes to the development of HF in 75% of patients, including most patients with CAD. Both CAD and hypertension interact to augment the risk of HF, as does diabetes mellitus.

In 20–30% of the cases of HF with a depressed EF, the exact etiologic basis is not known. These patients are referred to as having nonischemic, dilated, or idiopathic cardiomyopathy if the cause is unknown (Chap. 231). Prior viral infection or toxin exposure (e.g., alcoholic or chemotherapeutic) may also lead to a dilated cardiomyopathy. Moreover, it is becoming increasingly clear that a large number of the cases of dilated cardiomyopathy are secondary to specific genetic defects, most notably those in the cytoskeleton. Most of the forms of familial dilated cardiomyopathy are inherited in an autosomal dominant fashion. Mutations of genes encoding cytoskeletal proteins (desmin, cardiac myosin, vinculin) and nuclear membrane proteins (lamin) have been identified thus far. Dilated cardiomyopathy is also associated with Duchenne's, Becker's, and limb girdle muscular dystrophies. Conditions that lead to a high cardiac output (e.g., arteriovenous fistula, anemia) are seldom responsible for the development of HF in a normal heart. However, in the presence of underlying structural heart disease, these conditions can lead to overt HF.

TABLE 227-1 ETIOLOGIES OF HEART FAILURE

Depressed Ejection Fraction (<40%)

Coronary artery disease	Nonischemic dilated cardiomyopathy
Myocardial infarction[a]	Familial/genetic disorders
Myocardial ischemia[a]	Infiltrative disorders[a]
Chronic pressure overload	Toxic/drug-induced damage
Hypertension[a]	Metabolic disorder[a]
Obstructive valvular disease[a]	Viral
Chronic volume overload	Chagas' disease
Regurgitant valvular disease	Disorders of rate and rhythm
Intracardiac (left-to-right) shunting	Chronic bradyarrhythmias
Extracardiac shunting	Chronic tachyarrhythmias

Preserved Ejection Fraction (>40–50%)

Pathological hypertrophy	Restrictive cardiomyopathy
Primary (hypertrophic cardio-	Infiltrative disorders (amyloidosis,
myopathies)	sarcoidosis)
Secondary (hypertension)	Storage diseases (hemochroma-
Aging	tosis)
	Fibrosis
	Endomyocardial disorders

Pulmonary Heart Disease

Cor pulmonale
Pulmonary vascular disorders

High-Output States

Metabolic disorders	Excessive blood-flow requirements
Thyrotoxicosis	Systemic arteriovenous shunting
Nutritional disorders (beriberi)	Chronic anemia

[a]**Note:** Indicates conditions that can also lead to heart failure with a preserved injection fraction.

FIGURE 227-1 Pathogenesis of heart failure with a depressed ejection fraction. Heart failure begins after an index event produces an initial decline in the heart's pumping capacity. Following this initial decline in pumping capacity, a variety of compensatory mechanisms are activated, including the adrenergic nervous system, the renin-angiotensin-aldosterone system and the cytokine system. In the short term, these systems are able to restore cardiovascular function to a normal homeostatic range with the result that the patient remains asymptomatic. However, with time the sustained activation of these systems can lead to secondary end-organ damage within the ventricle, with worsening left-ventricular remodeling and subsequent cardiac decompensation. *(From D Mann: Circulation 100:999, 1999.)*

GLOBAL CONSIDERATIONS

Rheumatic heart disease remains a major cause of HF in Africa and Asia, especially in the young. Hypertension is an important cause of HF in the African and African-American populations. Chagas' disease is still a major cause of HF in South America. Not surprisingly, anemia is a frequent concomitant factor in HF in many developing nations. As developing nations undergo socioeconomic development, the epidemiology of HF is becoming similar to that of Western Europe and North America, with CAD emerging as the single most common cause of HF. Although the contribution of diabetes mellitus to HF is not well understood, diabetes accelerates atherosclerosis and is often associated with hypertension.

PROGNOSIS

Despite many recent advances in the evaluation and management of HF, the development of symptomatic HF still carries a poor prognosis. Community-based studies indicate that 30–40% of patients die within 1 year of diagnosis and 60–70% die within 5 years, mainly from worsening HF or as a sudden event (probably because of a ventricular arrhythmia). Although it is difficult to predict prognosis in an individual, patients with symptoms at rest [New York Heart Association (NYHA) class IV] have a 30–70% annual mortality rate, whereas patients with symptoms with moderate activity (NYHA class II) have an annual mortality rate of 5–10%. Thus, functional status is an important predictor of patient outcome (see Table 272-2).

PATHOGENESIS

Figure 227-1 provides a general conceptual framework for considering the development and progression of HF with a depressed EF. As shown, HF may be viewed as a progressive disorder that is initiated after an *index event* either damages the heart muscle, with a resultant loss of functioning cardiac myocytes, or alternatively disrupts the ability of the myocardium to generate force, thereby preventing the heart from contracting normally. This index event may have an abrupt onset, as in the case of a MI; it may have a gradual or insidious onset, as in the case of hemodynamic pressure or volume overloading; or it may be hereditary, as in the case of many of the genetic cardiomyopathies. Regardless of the

nature of the inciting event, the feature that is common to each of these index events is that they all, in some manner, produce a decline in the pumping capacity of the heart. In most instances patients remain asymptomatic or minimally symptomatic following the initial decline in pumping capacity of the heart, or develop symptoms only after the dysfunction has been present for some time. Thus, when viewed within this conceptual framework, LV dysfunction is necessary, but not sufficient, for the development of the syndrome of HF.

Although the precise reasons why patients with LV dysfunction may remain asymptomatic is not certain, one potential explanation is that a number of compensatory mechanisms become activated in the presence of cardiac injury and/or LV dysfunction, and they appear to be able to sustain and modulate LV function for a period of months to years. The list of compensatory mechanisms that have been described thus far include (1) activation of the renin-angiotensin-aldosterone (RAA) and adrenergic nervous systems, which are responsible for maintaining cardiac output through increased retention of salt and water (**Fig. 227-2**), and (2) increased myocardial contractility. In addition, there is activation of a family of countervailing vasodilatory molecules, including the atrial and brain natriuretic peptides (ANP and BNP), prostaglandins (PGE_2 and PGI_2), and nitric oxide (NO), that offset the excessive peripheral vascular vasoconstriction. Genetic background, gender, age, or environment may influence these compensatory mechanisms, which are able to modulate LV function within a physiologic/homeostatic range, such that the functional capacity of the patient is preserved or is depressed only minimally. Thus, patients may remain asymptomatic or minimally symptomatic for a period of years. However, at some point patients become overtly symptomatic, with a resultant striking increase in morbidity and mortality. Although the exact mechanisms that are responsible for this transition are not known, as will be discussed below, the transition to symptomatic HF is accompanied by increasing activation of neurohormonal, adrenergic, and cytokine systems that lead to a series of adaptive changes within the myocardium, collectively referred to as *LV remodeling*.

In contrast to our understanding of the pathogenesis of HF with a depressed EF, our understanding of the mechanisms that contribute to the development of HF with a preserved EF is still evolving. That is, al-autophagic cell death; (4) β-adrenergic desensitization; (5) abnormal myocardial energetics and metabolism; and (6) reorganization of the extracellular matrix with dissolution of the organized structural collagen weave surrounding myocytes and subsequent replacement by an interstitial collagen matrix that does not provide structural support to the myocytes. The biological stimuli for these profound changes include mechanical stretch of the myocyte, circulating neurohormones (e.g., norepinephrine, angiotensin II), inflammatory cytokines [e.g., tumor necrosis factor (TNF)], other peptides and growth factors (e.g., endothelin), and reactive oxygen species (e.g., superoxide, NO). Although these molecules are collectively referred to as *neurohormones*, this historical terminology is somewhat misleading insofar as the classical neurohormones, such as norepinephrine and angiotensin II, may also be synthesized directly within the myocardium and thus may also act in an autocrine and paracrine manner. Nonetheless, the overarching concept is that the sustained overexpression of these biologically active molecules contributes to the progression of HF by virtue of the deleterious effects that they exert on the heart and the circulation. Indeed, this insight forms the clinical rationale for using pharmacologic agents that antagonize these systems [e.g., angiotensin-converting enzyme (ACE) inhibitors and beta blockers] in treating patients with HF.

Systolic Dysfunction In order to understand how the changes that occur in the failing cardiac myocyte contribute to depressed LV systolic function in HF, it is instructive first to review the biology of the cardiac muscle cell (Chap. 217). Sustained neurohormonal activation results in transcriptional and posttranscriptional changes in the genes and proteins that regulate excitation-contraction coupling and cross-bridge interaction (see Fig. 217-7). Collectively, these changes impair the ability of the myocyte to contract and, therefore, contribute to the depressed LV systolic function observed in patients with HF.

Diastolic Dysfunction Myocardial relaxation is an ATP-dependent process that is regulated by uptake of cytoplasmic calcium into the sarcoplasmic reticulum (SR) by sarcoplasmic reticulum Ca^{2+} adenosine triphosphatase (SERCA2A) and extrusion of calcium by sarcolemmal pumps (see Fig. 217-7). Accordingly, reductions in ATP concentration, as occurs

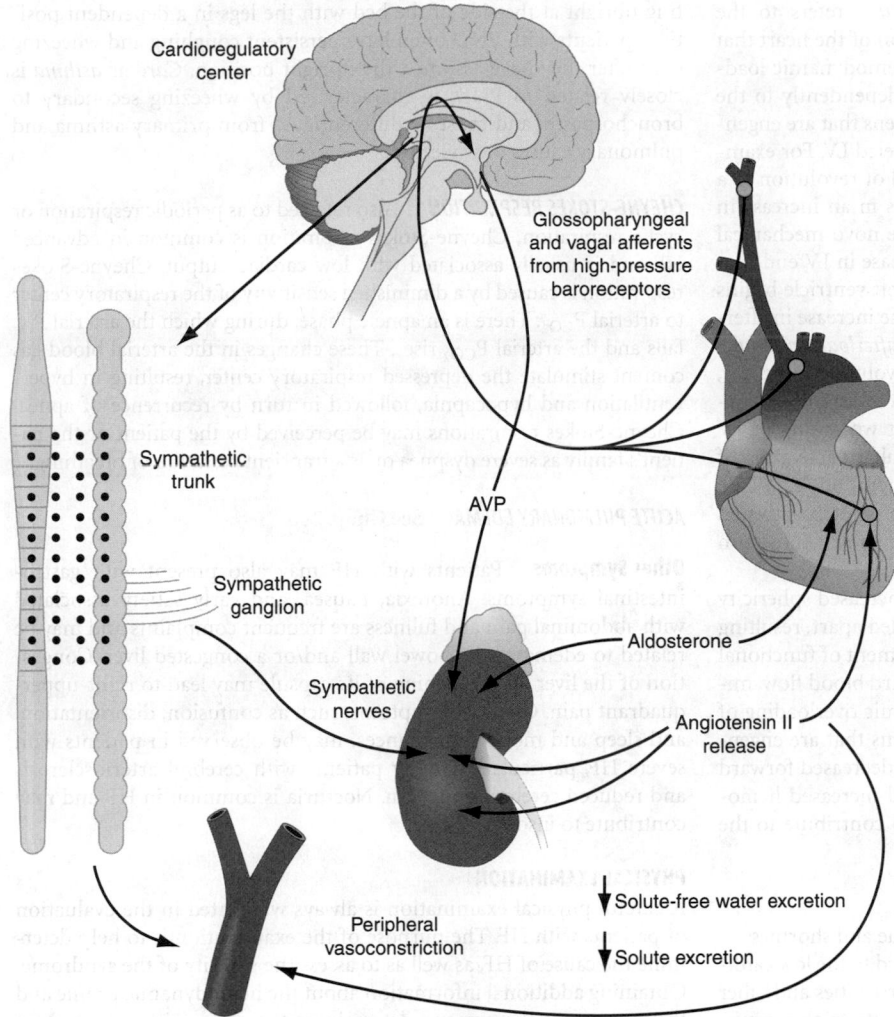

FIGURE 227-2 Activation of neurohormonal systems in heart failure. The decreased cardiac output in HF patients results in an "unloading" of high-pressure baroceptors (circles) in the left ventricle, carotid sinus, and aortic arch. This unloading leads to the generation of afferent signals to the central nervous system (CNS) that stimulate cardioregulatory centers in the brain which stimulate the release of arginine vasopression (AVP) from the posterior pituitary. AVP [or antidiuretic hormone (ADH)] is a powerful vasoconstrictor that increases the permeability of the renal collecting ducts, leading to the reabsorption of free water. These afferent signals to the CNS also activate efferent sympathetic nervous system pathways that innervate the heart, kidney, peripheral vasculature, and skeletal muscles.

Sympathetic stimulation of the kidney leads to the release of renin, with a resultant increase in the circulating levels of angiotensin II and aldosterone. The activation of the renin-angiotensin-aldosterone system promotes salt and water retention and leads to vasoconstriction of the peripheral vasculature, myocyte hypertrophy, myocyte cell death, and myocardial fibrosis. While these neurohormonal mechanisms facilitate short-term adaptation by maintaining blood pressure, and hence perfusion to vital organs, these same neurohormonal mechanisms are believed to contribute to end-organ changes in the heart and the circulation, and to the excessive salt and water retention in advanced HF. [*From E Braunwald: Pathophysiology of heart failure, in Braunwald's Heart Disease, 7th ed, D Zipes et al (eds). Philadelphia, Elsevier Saunders, pp 509–538, 2005; and adapted from Schrier RW, Abraham WT: N Engl J Med 341:577, 1999.*]

though diastolic dysfunction (see below) was thought to be the only mechanism responsible for the development of HF with a preserved EF, community-based studies suggest that additional mechanisms, such as increased vascular and ventricular (*ventricular-vascular*) stiffness, may also be important.

BASIC MECHANISMS OF HEART FAILURE
LV remodeling develops in response to a series of complex events that occur at the cellular and molecular levels. These changes include: (1) myocyte hypertrophy; (2) alterations in the contractile properties of the myocyte; (3) progressive loss of myocytes through necrosis, apoptosis, and

in ischemia, may interfere with these processes and lead to slowed myocardial relaxation. Alternatively, if LV filling is delayed because LV compliance is reduced (e.g., from hypertrophy or fibrosis), LV filling pressures will similarly remain elevated at end diastole (see Fig. 217-11). An increase in heart rate disproportionately shortens the time for diastolic filling, which may lead to elevated LV filling pressures, particularly in noncompliant ventricles. Elevated LV end-diastolic filling pressures result in increases in pulmonary capillary pressures, which can contribute to the dyspnea experienced by patients with diastolic dysfunction. Importantly, diastolic dysfunction can occur alone or in combination with systolic dysfunction in patients with HF.

Left Ventricular Remodeling *Ventricular remodeling* refers to the changes in LV mass, volume, shape, and composition of the heart that occur following cardiac injury and/or abnormal hemodynamic loading conditions. LV remodeling may contribute independently to the progression of HF by virtue of the mechanical burdens that are engendered by the changes in the geometry of the remodeled LV. For example, the change in LV shape from a prolate ellipsoid of revolution to a more spherical shape during LV remodeling results in an increase in meridional wall stress of the LV, which creates a de novo mechanical burden for the failing heart. In addition to the increase in LV end-diastolic volume, LV wall thinning also occurs as the left ventricle begins to dilate. The increase in wall thinning along with the increase in afterload created by LV dilation leads to a functional *afterload mismatch* that may contribute further to a decrease in stroke volume. Moreover, the high end-diastolic wall stress might be expected to lead to: (1) hypoperfusion of the subendocardium, with resultant worsening of LV function; (2) increased oxidative stress, with the resultant activation of families of genes that are sensitive to free radical generation (e.g., TNF and interleukin 1β); and (3) sustained expression of stretch-activated genes (angiotensin II, endothelin, and TNF) and/or stretch activation of hypertrophic signaling pathways.

A second important problem that results from increased sphericity of the ventricle is that the papillary muscles are pulled apart, resulting in incompetence of the mitral valve and the development of functional mitral regurgitation. In addition to the loss of forward blood flow, mitral regurgitation also results in further hemodynamic overloading of the ventricle. Taken together, the mechanical burdens that are engendered by LV remodeling can be expected to lead to decreased forward cardiac output, increased LV dilation (stretch), and increased hemodynamic overloading, all of which are sufficient to contribute to the progression of HF.

CLINICAL MANIFESTATIONS

Symptoms　The cardinal symptoms of HF are fatigue and shortness of breath. Although fatigue has been traditionally ascribed to the low cardiac output in HF, it is likely that skeletal-muscle abnormalities and other noncardiac comorbidities (e.g., anemia) also contribute to this symptom. In the early stages of HF, dyspnea is observed only during exertion; however, as the disease progresses, dyspnea occurs with less strenuous activity, and ultimately may occur even at rest. The origin of dyspnea in HF is likely multifactorial (Chap. 33). The most important mechanism is pulmonary congestion with accumulation of interstitial or intra-alveolar fluid, which activates juxtacapillary J receptors, which in turn stimulate rapid, shallow breathing characteristic of cardiac dyspnea. Other factors that contribute to dyspnea on exertion include reductions in pulmonary compliance, increased airway resistance, respiratory muscle and/or diaphragm fatigue, and anemia. Dyspnea may become less frequent with the onset of right ventricular (RV) failure and tricuspid regurgitation.

ORTHOPNEA　Orthopnea, which is defined as dyspnea occurring in the recumbent position, is usually a later manifestation of HF than is exertional dyspnea. It results from the redistribution of fluid from the splanchnic circulation and lower extremities into the central circulation during recumbency, with a resultant increase in pulmonary capillary pressure. Nocturnal cough is a frequent manifestation of this process and a frequently overlooked symptom of HF. Orthopnea is generally relieved by sitting upright or by sleeping with additional pillows. Although orthopnea is a relatively specific symptom of HF, it may occur in patients with abdominal obesity or ascites and in patients with pulmonary disease whose lung mechanics favor an upright posture.

PAROXYSMAL NOCTURNAL DYSPNEA (PND)　This term refers to acute episodes of severe shortness of breath and coughing that generally occur at night and awaken the patient from sleep, usually 1–3 h after the patient retires. PND may be manifest by coughing or wheezing, possibly because of increased pressure in the bronchial arteries leading to airway compression, along with interstitial pulmonary edema leading to increased airway resistance. Whereas orthopnea may be relieved by sit-

ting upright at the side of the bed with the legs in a dependent position, patients with PND often have persistent coughing and wheezing even after they have assumed the upright position. *Cardiac asthma* is closely related to PND, is characterized by wheezing secondary to bronchospasm, and must be differentiated from primary asthma and pulmonary causes of wheezing.

CHEYNE-STOKES RESPIRATION　Also referred to as periodic respiration or cyclic respiration, Cheyne-Stokes respiration is common in advanced HF and is usually associated with low cardiac output. Cheyne-Stokes respiration is caused by a diminished sensitivity of the respiratory center to arterial P_{CO_2}. There is an apneic phase, during which the arterial P_{O_2} falls and the arterial P_{CO_2} rises. These changes in the arterial blood gas content stimulate the depressed respiratory center, resulting in hyperventilation and hypocapnia, followed in turn by recurrence of apnea. Cheyne-Stokes respirations may be perceived by the patient or the patient's family as severe dyspnea or as a transient cessation of breathing.

ACUTE PULMONARY EDEMA　See Chap. 266.

Other Symptoms　Patients with HF may also present with gastrointestinal symptoms. Anorexia, nausea, and early satiety associated with abdominal pain and fullness are frequent complaints and may be related to edema of the bowel wall and/or a congested liver. Congestion of the liver and stretching of its capsule may lead to right-upper-quadrant pain. Cerebral symptoms, such as confusion, disorientation, and sleep and mood disturbances, may be observed in patients with severe HF, particularly elderly patients with cerebral arteriosclerosis and reduced cerebral perfusion. Nocturia is common in HF and may contribute to insomnia.

PHYSICAL EXAMINATION

A careful physical examination is always warranted in the evaluation of patients with HF. The purpose of the examination is to help determine the cause of HF, as well as to assess the severity of the syndrome. Obtaining additional information about the hemodynamic profile and the response to therapy and determining the prognosis are important additional goals of the physical examination.

General Appearance and Vital Signs　In mild or moderately severe HF, the patient appears in no distress at rest, except for feeling uncomfortable when lying flat for more than a few minutes. In more severe HF, the patient must sit upright, may have labored breathing, and may not be able to finish a sentence because of shortness of breath. Systolic blood pressure may be normal or high in early HF, but it is generally reduced in advanced HF because of severe LV dysfunction. The pulse pressure may be diminished, reflecting a reduction in stroke volume. Sinus tachycardia is a nonspecific sign caused by increased adrenergic activity. Peripheral vasoconstriction leading to cool peripheral extremities and cyanosis of the lips and nail beds is also caused by excessive adrenergic activity.

Jugular Veins　(See also Chap. 220) Examination of the jugular veins provides an estimation of right atrial pressure. The jugular venous pressure is best appreciated with the patient lying recumbent, with the head tilted at 45°. The jugular venous pressure should be quantified in centimeters of water (normal ≤8 cm) by estimating the height of the venous column of blood above the sternal angle in cm and then adding 5 cm. In the early stages of HF, the venous pressure may be normal at rest but may become abnormally elevated with sustained (~1 min) pressure on the abdomen (positive abdominojugular reflux). Giant *v* waves indicate the presence of tricuspid regurgitation.

Pulmonary Examination　Pulmonary crackles (rales or crepitations) result from the transudation of fluid from the intravascular space into the alveoli. In patients with pulmonary edema, rales may be heard widely over both lung fields and may be accompanied by expiratory wheezing (cardiac asthma). When present in patients without concomitant lung disease, rales are specific for HF. Importantly, rales are frequently absent in patients with chronic HF, even when LV filling pressures are elevated, because of increased lymphatic drainage of alveolar fluid. Pleural effusions result from the elevation of pleural capillary pressure and the resulting transudation of fluid into the pleural cavities. Since the pleural veins drain into both the systemic and pulmonary veins, pleural effusions occur most commonly with biventricular failure. Although pleural effusions are often bilateral in HF, when unilateral they occur more frequently in the right pleural space.

Cardiac Examination   Examination of the heart, although essential, frequently does not provide useful information about the severity of HF. If cardiomegaly is present, the point of maximal impulse (PMI) is usually displaced below the fifth intercostal space and/or lateral to the midclavicular line, and the impulse is palpable over two interspaces. Severe LV hypertrophy leads to a sustained PMI. In some patients, a third heart sound (S_3) is audible and palpable at the apex. Patients with enlarged or hypertrophied right ventricles may have a sustained and prolonged left parasternal impulse extending throughout systole. An S_3 (or *protodiastolic gallop*) is most commonly present in patients with volume overload who have tachycardia and tachypnea, and it often signifies severe hemodynamic compromise. A fourth heart sound (S_4) is not a specific indicator of HF but is usually present in patients with diastolic dysfunction. The murmurs of mitral and tricuspid regurgitation are frequently present in patients with advanced HF.

Abdomen and Extremities   Hepatomegaly is an important sign in patients with HF. When present, the enlarged liver is frequently tender and may pulsate during systole if tricuspid regurgitation is present. Ascites, a late sign, occurs as a consequence of increased pressure in the hepatic veins and the veins draining the peritoneum. Jaundice, also a late finding in HF, results from impairment of hepatic function secondary to hepatic congestion and hepatocellular hypoxia, and is associated with elevations of both direct and indirect bilirubin.

Peripheral edema is a cardinal manifestation of HF, but it is nonspecific and usually absent in patients who have been treated adequately with diuretics. Peripheral edema is usually symmetric and dependent in HF and occurs predominantly in the ankles and pretibial region in ambulatory patients. In bedridden patients, edema may be found in the sacral area (*presacral edema*) and the scrotum. Long-standing edema may be associated with indurated and pigmented skin.

Cardiac Cachexia   With severe chronic HF, there may be marked weight loss and cachexia. Although the mechanism of cachexia is not entirely understood, it is likely multifactorial and includes elevation of the resting metabolic rate; anorexia, nausea, and vomiting due to congestive hepatomegaly and abdominal fullness; elevation of circulating concentrations of cytokines such as TNF; and impairment of intestinal absorption due to congestion of the intestinal veins. When present, cachexia augers a poor overall prognosis.

DIAGNOSIS

The diagnosis of HF is relatively straightforward when the patient presents with classic signs and symptoms of HF; however, the signs and symptoms of HF are neither specific nor sensitive. Accordingly, the key to making the diagnosis is to have a high index of suspicion, particularly for high-risk patients. When these patients present with signs or symptoms of HF, additional laboratory testing should be performed.

Routine Laboratory Testing   Patients with new-onset HF and those with chronic HF and acute decompensation should have a complete blood count, a panel of electrolytes, blood urea nitrogen, serum creatinine, hepatic enzymes, and a urinalysis. Selected patients should have assessment for diabetes mellitus (fasting serum glucose or oral glucose tolerance test), dyslipidemia (fasting lipid panel), and thyroid abnormalities (thyroid-stimulating hormone level).

Electrocardiogram (ECG)   A routine 12-lead ECG is recommended. The major importance of the ECG is to assess cardiac rhythm, determine the presence of LV hypertrophy or a prior MI (presence or absence of Q waves), as well as to determine QRS width to ascertain whether the patient may benefit from resynchronization therapy (see below). A normal ECG virtually excludes LV systolic dysfunction.

Chest X-ray   This provides useful information about cardiac size and shape, as well as the state of the pulmonary vasculature, and may identify noncardiac causes of the patient's symptoms. Although patients with acute HF have evidence of pulmonary hypertension, interstitial edema, and/or pulmonary edema, the majority of patients with chronic HF do not. The absence of these findings in patients with chronic HF reflects the increased capacity of the lymphatics to remove interstitial and/or pulmonary fluid.

Assessment of LV Function   Noninvasive cardiac imaging (Chap. 222) is essential for the diagnosis, evaluation, and management of HF. The most useful test is the 2-D echocardiogram/Doppler, which can provide a semiquantitative assessment of LV size and function as well as the presence or absence of valvular and/or regional wall motion abnormalities (indicative of a prior MI). The presence of left atrial dilation and LV hypertrophy, together with abnormalities of LV diastolic filling provided by pulse-wave and tissue Doppler, are useful for the assessment of HF with a preserved EF. The 2-D echocardiogram/Doppler is also invaluable in assessing RV size and pulmonary pressures, which are critical in the evaluation and management of cor pulmonale (see below). MRI also provides a comprehensive analysis of cardiac anatomy and function and is now the gold standard for assessing LV mass and volumes.

The most useful index of LV function is the EF (stroke volume divided by end-diastolic volume). Because the EF is easy to measure by noninvasive testing and easy to conceptualize, it has gained wide acceptance among clinicians. Unfortunately, the EF has a number of limitations as a true measure of contractility, since it is influenced by alterations in afterload and/or preload. For example, the LV EF is increased in mitral regurgitation as a result of ejection of the blood into the low-pressure left atrium. Nonetheless, with the exceptions indicated above, when the EF is normal ($\geq 50\%$), systolic function is usually adequate, and when the EF is significantly depressed (<30–40%), contractility is usually also depressed.

Biomarkers   Circulating levels of natriuretic peptides are useful adjunctive tools in the diagnosis of patients with HF. Both B-type natriuretic peptide (BNP) and N-terminal pro-BNP, which are released from the failing heart, are relatively sensitive markers for the presence of HF with depressed EF; they are also elevated in HF patients with a preserved HF, albeit to a lesser degree. However, it is important to recognize that natriuretic peptide levels increase with age and renal impairment, are more elevated in women, and can be elevated in right HF from any cause. Levels can be falsely low in obese patients and may normalize in some patients following appropriate treatment. A normal concentration of natriuretic peptides in an untreated patient is extremely useful for excluding the diagnosis of HF. Other biomarkers, such as troponin T and I, C-reactive protein, TNF receptors, and uric acid, may be elevated in HF and provide important prognostic information. Serial measurements of one or more biomarkers may ultimately help to guide therapy in HF, but they are not currently recommended for this purpose.

Exercise Testing   Treadmill or bicycle exercise testing is not routinely advocated for patients with HF, but either is useful for assessing the need for cardiac transplantation in patients with advanced HF (Chap. 228). A peak oxygen uptake (V_{O_2}) <14 mL/kg per min is associated with a relatively poor prognosis. Patients with a V_{O_2} <14 mL/kg per min have been shown, in general, to have better survival when transplanted than when treated medically.

DIFFERENTIAL DIAGNOSIS

HF resembles but should be distinguished from (1) conditions in which there is circulatory congestion secondary to abnormal salt and water retention but in which there is no disturbance of cardiac structure or function (e.g., renal failure) and (2) noncardiac causes of pulmonary edema (e.g., acute respiratory distress syndrome). In most patients who present with classic signs and symptoms of HF, the diagnosis is relatively straightforward. However, even experienced clinicians have difficulty in differentiating the dyspnea that arises from cardiac and pulmonary causes (Chap. 33). In this regard, noninvasive cardiac imaging, biomarkers, pulmonary function testing, and chest x-ray may be useful. A very low BNP or N-terminal pro-BNP may be helpful in excluding a cardiac cause of dyspnea in this setting. Ankle edema may arise secondary to varicose veins, obesity, renal disease, or gravitational effects. When HF develops in patients with a preserved EF, it may be difficult to determine the relative contribution of HF to the dyspnea that occurs in chronic lung disease and/or obesity.

℞ HEART FAILURE

HF should be viewed as a continuum that is comprised of four interrelated stages. *Stage A* includes patients who are at high risk for developing HF but without structural heart disease or symptoms of HF (e.g., patients with diabetes mellitus or hypertension). *Stage B* includes patients who have structural heart disease but without symptoms of HF (e.g., patients with a previous MI and asymptomatic LV dysfunction). *Stage C* includes patients who have structural heart disease and have developed symptoms of HF (e.g., patients with a previous MI with dyspnea and fatigue). *Stage D* includes patients with refractory HF requiring special interventions (e.g., patients with refractory HF who are awaiting cardiac transplantation). In this continuum, every effort should be made to prevent HF, not only by treating the preventable causes of HF (e.g., hypertension) but by treating the patient in Stages B and C with drugs that prevent disease progression (e.g., ACE inhibitors and beta blockers) and by symptomatic management of patients in stage D.

DEFINING AN APPROPRIATE THERAPEUTIC STRATEGY FOR CHRONIC HF   Once patients have developed structural heart disease, their therapy depends on their NYHA functional classification (Table 227-2). Although this classification system is notoriously subjective and has large interobserver variability, it has withstood the test of time and continues to be widely applied to patients with HF. For patients who have developed LV systolic dysfunction but remain asymptomatic (class I), the goal should be to slow disease progression by blocking neurohormonal systems that lead to cardiac remodeling (see below). For patients who have developed symptoms (class II–IV), the primary goal should be to alleviate fluid retention, lessen disability, and reduce the risk of further disease progression and death. These goals generally require a strategy that combines diuretics (to control salt and water retention) with neurohormonal interventions (to minimize cardiac remodeling).

TABLE 227-2   NEW YORK HEART ASSOCIATION CLASSIFICATION

Functional Capacity	Objective Assessment
Class I	Patients with cardiac disease but without resulting limitation of physical activity. Ordinary physical activity does not cause undue fatigue, palpitations, dyspnea, or anginal pain.
Class II	Patients with cardiac disease resulting in slight limitation of physical activity. They are comfortable at rest. Ordinary physical activity results in fatigue, palpitation, dyspnea, or anginal pain.
Class III	Patients with cardiac disease resulting in marked limitation of physical activity. They are comfortable at rest. Less than ordinary activity causes fatigue, palpitation, dyspnea, or anginal pain.
Class IV	Patients with cardiac disease resulting in inability to carry on any physical activity without discomfort. Symptoms of heart failure or the anginal syndrome may be present even at rest. If any physical activity is undertaken, discomfort is increased.

Source: Adapted from New York Heart Association, Inc., *Diseases of the Heart and Blood Vessels: Nomenclature and Criteria for Diagnosis,* 6th ed. Boston, Little Brown, 1964, p. 114.

MANAGEMENT OF HF WITH DEPRESSED EJECTION FRACTION (<40%)   General Measures   Clinicians should aim to screen for and treat comorbidities such as hypertension, CAD, diabetes mellitus, anemia, and sleep-disordered breathing, as these conditions tend to exacerbate HF. HF patients should be advised to stop smoking and to limit alcohol consumption to two standard drinks per day in men or one per day in women. Patients suspected of having an alcohol-induced cardiomyopathy should be urged to abstain from alcohol consumption indefinitely. Extremes of temperature and heavy physical exertion should be avoided (Table 227-3). For example, nonsteroidal anti-inflammatory drugs, including cyclooxygenase 2 inhibitors, are not recommended in patients with chronic HF because the risk of renal failure and fluid retention is markedly increased in the presence of reduced renal function or ACE inhibitor therapy. Patients should receive immunization with influenza and pneumococcal vaccines to prevent respiratory infections. It is equally important to educate the patient and family about HF, the importance of proper diet, as well the importance of compliance with the medical regimen. Supervision of outpatient care by a specially trained nurse or physician assistant and/or in specialized HF clinics have all been found to be helpful, particularly in patients with advanced disease.

Activity   Although heavy physical labor is not recommended in HF, routine modest exercise has been shown to be beneficial in patients with NYHA class I–III HF. For euvolemic patients, regular isotonic exercise such as walking or riding a stationary-bicycle ergometer, as tolerated, should be encouraged. Some trials of exercise training have led to encouraging results with reduced symptoms, increased exercise capacity, and improved quality and duration of life. The benefits of weight loss by restriction of caloric intake have not been clearly established.

Diet   Dietary restriction of sodium (2–3 g daily) is recommended in all patients with HF and preserved or depressed EF. Further restriction (<2 g daily) may be considered in moderate to severe HF. Fluid restriction is generally unnecessary unless the patient develops hyponatremia (<130 meq/L), which may develop because of activation of the renin-angiotensin system, excessive secretion of antidiuretic hormone, or loss of salt in excess of water from diuretic use. Fluid restriction (<2 L/day) should be considered in hyponatremic patients or for those whose fluid retention is difficult to control despite high doses of diuretics and sodium restriction. Caloric supplementation is recommended for patients with advanced HF and unintentional weight loss or muscle wasting (cardiac cachexia); however, anabolic steroids are not recommended for these patients because of the potential problems with volume retention. The use of dietary supplements ("nutriceuticals") should be avoided in the management of symptomatic HF because of the lack of proven benefit and the potential for significant (adverse) interactions with proven HF therapies.

Diuretics   Many of the clinical manifestations of moderate to severe HF result from excessive salt and water retention that leads to volume expansion and congestive symptoms. Diuretics (Table 227-4) are the only pharmacologic agents that can adequately control fluid retention in advanced

TABLE 227-3   FACTORS THAT MAY PRECIPITATE ACUTE DECOMPENSATION IN PATIENTS WITH CHRONIC HEART FAILURE

Dietary indiscretion
Myocardial ischemia/infarction
Arrhythmias (tachycardia or bradycardia)
Discontinuation of HF therapy
Infection
Anemia
Initiation of medications that worsen HF
    Calcium antagonists (verapamil, diltiazem)
    Beta blockers
    Nonsteroidal anti-inflammatory drugs
    Antiarrhythmic agents [all class I agents, sotalol (class III)]
    Anti-TNF antibodies
Alcohol consumption
Pregnancy
Worsening hypertension
Acute valvular insufficiency

Note: HF, heart failure; TNF, tumor necrosis factor.

TABLE 227-4 DRUGS FOR THE TREATMENT OF CHRONIC HEART FAILURE (EF <40%)

	Initiating Dose	Maximal Dose
Diuretics		
Furosemide	20–40 mg qd or bid	400 mg/d[a]
Torsemide	10–20 mg qd bid	200 mg/d[a]
Bumetanide	0.5–1.0 mg qd or bid	10 mg/d[a]
Hydrochlorthiazide	25 mg qd	100 mg/d[a]
Metolazone	2.5–5.0 mg qd or bid	20 mg/d[a]
Angiotensin-Converting Enzyme Inhibitors		
Captopril	6.25 mg tid	50 mg tid
Enalapril	2.5 mg bid	10 mg bid
Lisinopril	2.5–5.0 mg qd	20–35 mg qd
Ramipril	1.25–2.5 mg bid	2.5–5 mg bid
Trandolapril	0.5 mg qd	4 mg qd
Angiotensin Receptor Blockers		
Valsartan	40 mg bid	160 mg bid
Candesartan	4 mg qd	32 mg qd
Irbesartan	75 mg qd	300 mg qd[b]
Losartan	12.5 mg qd	50 mg qd
β Receptor Blockers		
Carvedilol	3.125 mg bid	25–50 mg bid
Bisoprolol	1.25 mg qd	10 mg qd
Metoprolol succinate CR	12.5–25 mg qd	Target dose 200 mg qd
Additional Therapies		
Spironolactone	12.5–25 mg qd	25–50 mg qd
Eplerenone	25 mg qd	50 mg qd
Combination of hydrala- zine/isosorbide dinitrate	10–25 mg/10 mg tid	75 mg/40 mg tid
Fixed dose of hydralazine/ isosorbide dinitrate	37.5/20 mg (one tablet) tid	75 mg/40 mg (two tablets) tid
Digoxin	0.125 mg qd	≤0.375 mg/d[b]

[a]Dose must be titrated to reduce the patient's congestive symptoms.
[b]Target dose not established.

HF, and they should be used to restore and maintain normal volume status in patients with congestive symptoms (dyspnea, orthopnea, edema) or signs of elevated filling pressures (rales, jugular venous distention, or peripheral edema). Furosemide, torsemide, and bumetanide act at the loop of Henle (*loop diuretics*) by reversibly inhibiting the reabsorption of Na$^+$, K$^+$, and Cl$^-$ in the thick ascending limb of Henle's loop; thiazides and metolazone reduce the reabsorption of Na$^+$ and Cl$^-$ in the first half of the distal convoluted tubule; and potassium-sparing diuretics such as spironolactone act at the level of the collecting duct.

Although all diuretics increase sodium excretion and urinary volume, they differ in their potency and pharmacologic properties. Whereas loop diuretics increase the fractional excretion of sodium by 20–25%, thiazide diuretics increase it by only 5–10% and tend to lose their effectiveness in patients with moderate or severe renal insufficiency (creatinine >2.5 mg/dL). Hence, loop diuretics are generally required to restore normal volume status in patients with HF. Diuretics should be initiated in low doses (Table 227-4) and then carefully titrated upward to relieve signs and symptoms of fluid overload in an attempt to obtain the patient's "dry weight." This typically requires multiple dose adjustments over many days and occasionally weeks in patients with severe fluid overload. Intravenous administration of diuretics may be necessary to relieve congestion acutely and can be done safely in the outpatient setting. Once the congestion has been relieved, treatment with diuretics should be continued to prevent the recurrence of salt and water retention.

Refractoriness to diuretic therapy may represent patient noncompliance, a direct effect of chronic diuretic use on the kidney or progression of underlying HF. The addition of thiazides or metolazone, once or twice daily, to loop diuretics may be considered in patients with persistent fluid retention despite high-dose loop diuretic therapy. Metolazone is generally more potent and much longer-acting than the thiazides in this setting as well as in patients with chronic renal insufficiency. However, chronic daily use, especially of metolazone, should be avoided if possible because of the po-

tential for electrolyte shifts and volume depletion. Ultrafiltration and dialysis may be used in cases of refractory fluid retention that are unresponsive to high doses of diuretics and have been shown to be helpful in the short term.

Adverse Effects Diuretics have the potential to produce electrolyte and volume depletion, as well as worsening azotemia. In addition, they may lead to worsening neurohormonal activation and disease progression. One of the most important adverse consequences of diuresis is alterations in potassium homeostasis (hypokalemia or hyperkalemia), which increases the risk of life-threatening arrhythmias. In general, both loop- and thiazide-type diuretics lead to hypokalemia, whereas spironolactone, eplerenone, and triamterene lead to hyperkalemia.

PREVENTING DISEASE PROGRESSION (TABLE 227-4) Drugs that interfere with the excessive activation of the RAA system and the adrenergic nervous system can relieve the symptoms of HF with a depressed EF by stabilizing and/or reversing cardiac remodeling. In this regard, ACE inhibitors and beta blockers have emerged as the cornerstones of modern therapy for HF with a depressed EF.

ACE Inhibitors There is overwhelming evidence that ACE inhibitors should be used in symptomatic and asymptomatic patients (**Figs. 227-3 and 227-4**) with a depressed EF (<40%). ACE inhibitors interfere with the renin-angiotensin system by inhibiting the enzyme that is responsible for the conversion of angiotensin I to angiotensin II. However, because ACE inhibitors also inhibit kininase II, they may lead to the upregulation of bradykinin, which may further enhance the beneficial effects of angiotensin suppression. ACE inhibitors stabilize LV remodeling, improve symptoms, reduce hospitalization, and prolong life. Because fluid retention can attenuate the effects of ACE inhibitors, it is preferable to optimize the dose of

FIGURE 227-3 Meta-analysis of angiotensin-converting enzyme (ACE) inhibitors in heart failure patients with a depressed ejection fraction. *A.* The Kaplan-Meier curves for mortality for 5966 HF patients with a depressed EF treated with an ACE inhibitor following acute myocardial infarction (three trials). ***B.*** The Kaplan-Meier curves for mortality for 12,763 HF patients with a depressed EF treated with an ACE inhibitor in five clinical trials, including postinfarction trials. The benefits of ACE inhibitors were observed early and persisted long-term. (*Modified from Flather et al: Lancet 355:1575, 2000.*)

FIGURE 227-4 Treatment algorithm for chronic heart failure patients with a depressed ejection fraction. After the clinical diagnosis of HF is made, it is important to treat the patient's fluid retention before starting an ACE inhibitor (or an ARB if the patient is ACE-intolerant). Beta blockers should be started after the fluid retention has been treated and/or the ACE inhibitor has been uptitrated. If the patient remains symptomatic, an ARB, aldosterone antagonist, or digoxin can be added as "triple therapy." The fixed-dose combination of hydralazine/isosorbide dinitrate should be added to an ACE inhibitor and beta blocker in African-American patients with NYHA class II–IV HF. Device therapy should be considered in addition to pharmacological therapy in appropriate patients. HF, heart failure; ACE, angiotensin-converting enzyme; ARB, angiotensin receptor blocker; NYHA, New York Heart Association; CRT, cardiac resynchronization therapy; ICD, implantable cardiac defibrillator.

diuretic before starting the ACE inhibitor. However, it may be necessary to reduce the dose of diuretic during the initiation of ACE inhibition in order to prevent symptomatic hypotension. ACE inhibitors should be initiated in low doses, followed by gradual increments if the lower doses have been well tolerated. The doses of ACE inhibitors should be increased until they are similar to those that have been shown to be effective in clinical trials (Table 227-4). Higher doses are more effective than lower doses in preventing hospitalization.

Adverse Effects The majority of adverse effects are related to suppression of the renin-angiotensin system. The decreases in blood pressure and mild azotemia that may occur during the initiation of therapy are generally well tolerated and do not require a decrease in the dose of the ACE inhibitor. However, if hypotension is accompanied by dizziness or if the renal dysfunction becomes severe, it may be necessary to reduce the dose of the inhibitor. Potassium retention may also become problematic if the patient is receiving potassium supplements or a potassium-sparing diuretic. Potassium retention that is not responsive to these measures may require a reduction in the dose of ACE inhibitor.

The side effects of ACE inhibitors related to kinin potentiation include a nonproductive cough (10–15% of patients) and angioedema (1% of patients). In patients who cannot tolerate ACE inhibitors because of cough or angioedema, angiotensin receptor block-

ers (ARBs) are the recommended first line of therapy (see below). Patients intolerant of ACE inhibitors because of hyperkalemia or renal insufficiency are likely to experience the same side effects with ARBs. In these cases, the combination of hydralazine and an oral nitrate should be considered (Table 227-4).

Angiotensin Receptor Blockers These drugs are well tolerated in patients who are intolerant of ACE inhibitors because of cough, skin rash, and angioedema. ARBs should be used in symptomatic and asymptomatic patients with an EF <40% who are ACE-intolerant for reasons other than hyperkalemia or renal insufficiency (Table 227-4). Although ACE inhibitors and ARBs inhibit the renin-angiotensin system, they do so by different mechanisms. Whereas ACE inhibitors block the enzyme responsible for converting angiotensin I to angiotensin II, ARBs block the effects of angiotensin II on the angiotensin type 1 receptor. Some clinical trials have demonstrated a therapeutic benefit for the addition of ARB to an ACE inhibitor in patients with chronic HF. When given in concert with beta blockers, ARBs reverse the process of LV remodeling, improve patient symptoms, prevent hospitalization, and prolong life.

Adverse Effects Both ACE inhibitors and ARBs have similar effects on blood pressure, renal function, and potassium. Therefore the problems of symptomatic hypotension, azotemia, and hyperkalemia are similar for both of these agents.

β-Adrenergic Receptor Blockers Beta-blocker therapy represents a major advance in the treatment of patients with a depressed EF **(Fig. 227-5)**. These drugs interfere with the harmful effects of sustained activation of the adrenergic nervous system by competitively antagonizing one or more adrenergic receptors (α_1, β_1, and β_2). Although there are a number of potential benefits to blocking all three receptors, most of the deleterious effects of adrenergic activation are mediated by the β_1 receptor. When given in concert with ACE inhibitors, beta blockers reverse the process of LV remodeling, improve patient symptoms, prevent hospitalization, and prolong life. Therefore beta blockers are indicated for patients with symptomatic or asymptomatic HF and a depressed EF <40%.

Analogous to the use of ACE inhibitors, beta blockers should be initiated in low doses (Table 227-4), followed by gradual increments in the dose if lower doses have been well tolerated. The dose of beta blocker should be increased until the doses used are similar to those that have been reported to be effective in clinical trials (Table 227-4). However, unlike ACE inhibitors, which may be titrated upward relatively rapidly, the titration of beta blockers should proceed no more rapidly than at 2-week intervals, be-

FIGURE 227-5 Meta-analysis of beta blockers on mortality in HF patients with a depressed EF. Effect of beta blockers vs. placebo in patients who were not (**A**) or who were (**B**) receiving an angiotensin-converting enzyme (ACE) inhibitor or an angiotensin receptor blocker (ARB) at baseline in six clinical trials. There was a similar impact of beta-blocker therapy on the endpoints of all-cause mortality as well as death and heart failure hospitalization in both the presence and absence of ACE inhibitor or ARB at baseline. BEST, Beta-blocker Evaluation of Survival Trial (bucindolol); CIBIS, Cardiac Insufficiency BIsoprolol Study (bisoprol); COPERNICUS, Carvedilol prOsPEctive RaNdomIzed Cumulative Survival (carvedilol); MERIT-HF, Metoprolol CR/XL Randomized Intervention Trial in Heart Failure (metoprolol CR/XL). *(Modified from Krum et al: Eur Heart J 26:2154, 2005.)*

cause the initiation and/or increased dosing of these agents may lead to worsening fluid retention consequent to the withdrawal of adrenergic support to the heart and the circulation. Thus, it is important to optimize the dose of diuretic before starting therapy with beta blockers. If worsening fluid retention does occur, it is likely to do so within 3–5 days of initiating therapy, and it will be manifest as an increase in body weight and/or symptoms of worsening HF. The increased fluid retention can usually be managed by increasing the dose of diuretics. In some patients the dose of the beta blocker may have to be reduced.

Contrary to early reports, the aggregate results of clinical trials suggest that beta-blocker therapy is well tolerated by the great majority (≥85%) of HF patients, including patients with comorbid conditions such as diabetes mellitus, chronic obstructive lung disease, and peripheral vascular disease. Nonetheless, there is a subset of patients (10–15%) who remain intolerant to beta blockers because of worsening fluid retention or symptomatic hypotension or bradycardia.

Adverse Effects The adverse effects of beta-blocker use are generally related to the predictable complications that arise from interfering with the adrenergic nervous system. These reactions generally occur within several days of initiating therapy and are generally responsive to adjusting concomitant medications, as described above. Therapy with beta blockers can lead to bradycardia and/or exacerbate heart block. Accordingly, the dose of beta blocker should be reduced if the heart rate decreases to <50 beats/min and/or second or third degree heart block or symptomatic hypotension develops. Beta blockers are not recommended for patients who have asthma with active bronchospasm. Beta blockers that also block the α_1 receptor can lead to vasodilatory side effects.

Aldosterone Antagonists Although classified as potassium-sparing diuretics, drugs that block the effects of aldosterone (spironolactone or eplerenone) have beneficial effects that are independent of the effects of these agents on sodium balance. Although ACE inhibition may transiently decrease aldosterone secretion, with chronic therapy there is a rapid return of aldosterone to levels similar to those before ACE inhibition. Accordingly, the administration of an aldosterone antagonist is recommended for patients with NYHA class IV or class III (previously class IV) HF who have a depressed EF (<35%) and who are receiving standard therapy, including diuretics, ACE inhibitors, and beta blockers. The dose of aldosterone antagonist should be increased until the doses used are similar to those that have been shown to be effective in clinical trials (Table 227-4).

Adverse Effects The major problem with the use of aldosterone antagonists is the development of life-threatening hyperkalemia, which is more prone to occur in patients who are receiving potassium supplements or who have underlying renal insufficiency. Aldosterone antagonists are not recommended when the serum creatinine is >2.5 mg/dL (or creatinine clearance is <30 mL/min) or when the serum potassium is >5.0 mmol/L. Painful gynecomastia may develop in 10–15% of patients who use spironolactone, in which case eplerenone may be substituted.

SPECIAL POPULATIONS The combination of hydralazine and isosorbide dinitrate (Table 227-4) is recommended as part of standard therapy in addition to beta blockers and ACE inhibitors for African Americans with NYHA class II–IV HF. Although the exact mechanism for the effects of this combination is not known, it is believed to be secondary to the beneficial effects of NO on the peripheral circulation. Recent studies suggest that the combination of hydralazine and isosorbide dinitrate may be more effective for patients who have variant genotypic markers (polymorphisms) for the genes that encode for endothelial nitric oxide synthase (NOS3) and aldosterone synthase.

MANAGEMENT OF PATIENTS WHO REMAIN SYMPTOMATIC As noted above, an ACE inhibitor (or an ARB) plus a beta blocker should be standard background therapy for HF patients with a depressed LV EF. Additional pharmacologic therapy should be considered in patients who have persistent symptoms or progressive worsening despite optimized therapy with an ACE inhibitor and beta blocker. Agents that may be considered as part of additional therapy include an ARB, spironolactone, the combination of hydralazine and isosorbide dinitrate, or digitalis. The optimal choice of additional drug therapy to further improve outcome has not been firmly established. Thus, the choice of specific agent will be influenced by clinical considerations, including renal function, serum potassium concentration,

blood pressure, and race. The triple combination of an ACE inhibitor, an ARB, and an aldosterone antagonist should not be used because of the high risk of hyperkalemia.

Digoxin is recommended for patients with symptomatic LV systolic dysfunction who have concomitant atrial fibrillation, and it should be considered for patients who have signs or symptoms of HF while receiving standard therapy, including ACE inhibitors and beta blockers. Therapy with digoxin is commonly initiated and maintained at a dose of 0.125–0.25 mg daily. For the great majority of patients, the dose should be 0.125 mg daily, and the serum digoxin level should be <1.0 ng/mL, especially in elderly patients, patients with impaired renal function, and a low lean body mass. Higher doses (and serum concentrations) appear to be less beneficial. There is no indication for using loading doses of digoxin to initiate therapy in patients with HF.

ANTICOAGULATION AND ANTIPLATELET THERAPY Patients with HF have an increased risk for arterial or venous thromboembolic events. In clinical HF trials, the rate of stroke ranges from 1.3 to 2.4% per year. Depressed LV function is believed to promote relative stasis of blood in dilated cardiac chambers with increased risk of thrombus formation. Treatment with warfarin [goal international normalized ratio (INR) 2.0–3.0] is recommended for patients with HF and chronic or paroxysmal atrial fibrillation, or with a history of systemic or pulmonary emboli, including stroke or transient ischemic attack. Patients with symptomatic or asymptomatic ischemic cardiomyopathy and documented recent large anterior MI or recent MI with documented LV thrombus should be treated with warfarin (goal INR 2.0–3.0) for the initial 3 months after MI, unless there are contraindications to its use.

Aspirin is recommended in HF patients with ischemic heart disease for the prevention of MI and death. However, lower doses of aspirin (75 or 81 mg) may be preferable because of the concern of worsening of HF at higher doses.

MANAGEMENT OF CARDIAC ARRHYTHMIAS (See also Chap. 226) Atrial fibrillation occurs in 15–30% of patients with HF and is a frequent cause of cardiac decompensation. Most antiarrhythmic agents, with the exception of amiodarone and dofetilide, have negative inotropic effects and are proarrhythmic. Amiodarone is a class III antiarrhythmic that has little or no negative inotropic and/or proarrhythmic effects and is effective against most supraventricular arrhythmias. Amiodarone is the preferred drug for restoring and maintaining sinus rhythm, and it may improve the success of electrical cardioversion in patients with HF. Amiodarone increases the level of phenytoin and digoxin and prolongs the INR in patients taking warfarin. Therefore it is often necessary to reduce the dose of these drugs by as much as 50% when initiating therapy with amiodarone. The risk of adverse events, such as hyperthyroidism, hypothyroidism, pulmonary fibrosis, and hepatitis, are relatively low, particularly when lower doses of amiodarone are used (100–200 mg/d).

Implantable cardiac defibrillators (ICDs; see below) are highly effective in treating recurrences of sustained ventricular tachycardia and/or ventricular fibrillation in HF patients with recurrent arrhythmias and/or cardiac syncope, and they may be used as stand-alone therapy or in combination with amiodarone and/or a beta blocker (Chap. 226). There is no role for treating ventricular arrhythmias with an antiarrhythmic agent without an ICD.

DEVICE THERAPY **Cardiac Resynchronization** Approximately one-third of patients with a depressed EF and symptomatic HF (NYHA class III–IV) manifest a QRS duration >120 ms. This ECG finding of abnormal inter- or intraventricular conduction has been used to identify patients with dyssynchronous ventricular contraction. The mechanical consequences of ventricular dyssynchrony include suboptimal ventricular filling, a reduction in LV contractility, prolonged duration (and therefore greater severity) of mitral regurgitation, and paradoxical septal wall motion. *Biventricular pacing*, also termed *cardiac resynchronization therapy* (CRT), stimulates both ventricles near-simultaneously, thereby improving the coordination of ventricular contraction and reducing the severity of mitral regurgitation. When CRT is added to optimal medical therapy in patients in sinus rhythm, there is a significant decrease in patient mortality and hospitalization, a reversal of LV remodeling, as well as improved quality of life and exercise capacity. Accordingly, CRT is recommended for patients in sinus rhythm with an EF <35% and a QRS >120 ms and those who remain symptomatic (NYHA III–IV) despite optimal medical therapy. The benefits of CRT in patients with atrial fibrillation have not been established.

Implantable Cardiac Defibrillators (See also Chap. 226) The prophylactic implantation of ICDs in patients with mild to moderate HF (NYHA class II–III) has been shown to reduce the incidence of sudden cardiac death in patients with ischemic or nonischemic cardiomyopathy. Accordingly, implantation of an ICD should be considered for patients in NYHA class II–III HF with a depressed EF of <30–35% who are already on optimal background therapy, including an ACE inhibitor (or ARB), a beta blocker, and an aldosterone antagonist. An ICD may be combined with a biventricular pacemaker in appropriate patients.

MANAGEMENT OF HF WITH A PRESERVED EJECTION

FRACTION (>40–50%) Despite the wealth of information with respect to the evaluation and management of HF with a depressed EF, there are no proven and/or approved pharmacologic or device therapies for the management of patients with HF and a preserved EF. Therefore, it is recommended that initial treatment efforts should be focused, wherever possible, on the underlying disease process (e.g., myocardial ischemia, hypertension) associated with HF with preserved EF. Precipitating factors, such as tachycardia or atrial fibrillation, should be treated as quickly as possible through rate control and restoration of sinus rhythm when appropriate. Dyspnea may be treated by reducing total blood volume (dietary sodium restriction and diuretics), decreasing central blood volume (nitrates), or blunting neurohormal activation with ACE inhibitors, ARBs, and/or beta blockers. Treatment with diuretics and nitrates should be initiated at low doses to avoid hypotension and fatigue.

ACUTE HF **Defining an Appropriate Therapeutic Strategy** The therapeutic goals for the management of acute HF therapy are to (1) stabilize the hemodynamic derangements that provoked the symptoms responsible for the hospitalization, (2) identify and treat the reversible factors that precipitated decompensation, and (3) reestablish an effective outpatient medical regimen that will prevent disease progression and relapse. In most instances this will require hospitalization, often in an intensive care unit (ICU) setting. Every effort should be made to identify the precipitating causes, such as infection, arrhythmias, dietary indiscretion, pulmonary embolism, infective endocarditis, occult myocardial ischemia/infarction, environmental and/or emotional or environmental stress (Table 227-3), since removal of these precipitating events is critical to the success of treatment.

The two primary hemodynamic determinants of acute HF are elevated LV filling pressures and a depressed cardiac output. Frequently the depressed cardiac output is accompanied by an increase in systemic vascular resistance (SVR) as a result of excessive neurohormonal activation. Because these hemodynamic derangements may occur singly or together, patients with acute HF generally present with one of four basic hemodynamic profiles **(Fig. 227-6)**: normal LV filling pressure with normal perfusion (Profile A), elevated LV filling pressure with normal perfusion (Profile B), elevated LV filling pressures with decreased perfusion (Profile C), and normal or low LV filling pressure with decreased tissue perfusion (Profile L).

Accordingly, the therapeutic approach to treating patients with acute HF should be tailored to reflect the patient's hemodynamic presentation. The goal should be, whenever possible, to restore the patient to a normal hemodynamic profile (Profile A). In many instances the patient's hemodynamic presentation can be approximated from the clinical examination. For example, patients with elevated LV filling pressures may have signs of fluid retention (rales, elevated neck veins, peripheral edema) and are referred to as being "wet," whereas patients with a depressed cardiac output and an elevated SVR generally have poor tissue perfusion manifested by cool distal extremities and are referred to as being "cold." Nonetheless, it should be emphasized that patients with chronic heart failure may not have rales or evidence of peripheral edema at the time of the initial presentation with acute decompensation, which may lead to the underrecognition of elevated filling pressures. In these patients, it may be appropriate to perform invasive hemodynamic monitoring.

Patients who are not congested and have normal tissue perfusion are referred to as being "dry" and "warm," respectively. When acute HF patients present to the hospital with profile A, their symptoms are often due to conditions other than HF (e.g., pulmonary or hepatic disease, or transient myocardial ischemia). More commonly, however, acute HF patients present with congestive symptoms ["warm and wet" (profile B)], in which case treatment of the elevated filling pressures with diuretics and vasodilators is warranted to reduce LV filling pressures. Profile B includes most patients with acute pulmonary edema. **The treatment of this life-threatening condition is described in Chap. 266.**

Patients may also present with congestion and a significant elevated SVR and reduction of cardiac output ["cold and wet" (Profile C)]. In these patients, cardiac output can be increased and LV filling pressures reduced using intravenous vasodilators. Intravenous inotropic agents with vasodilating action [dobutamine, low-dose dopamine, milrinone **(Table 227-5)**] augment cardiac output by stimulating myocardial contractility as well as by functionally unloading the heart.

Patients who present with profile L ("cold and dry") should be carefully evaluated by right-heart catheterization for the presence of an occult elevation of LV filling pressures. If LV filling pressures are low [pulmonary capillary wedge pressure (PCWP) <12 mmHg] a cautious trial of fluid repletion may be considered. The goals of further therapy depend on the clinical situation. Therapy to reach the aforementioned goals may not be possible in some patients, particularly if they have disproportionate RV dysfunction or if they develop cardiorenal syndrome, in which renal function deteriorates during aggressive diuresis. Worsening renal dysfunction occurs in approximately 25% of patients hospitalized with HF and is associated with prolonged hospital stays and higher mortality after discharge.

Pharmacologic Management of Acute HF (Table 227-5)

Vasodilators After diuretics, intravenous vasodilators are the most useful medications for the management of acute HF. By stimulating guanylyl

Elevated LV filling pressures?

FIGURE 227-6 Hemodynamic profiles in patients with acute heart failure. Most patients can be categorized into one of the four hemodynamic profiles by performing a brief bedside examination that includes examination of the neck veins, lungs, and peripheral extremities. More definitive hemodynamic information may be obtained by performing invasive hemodynamic monitoring, particularly if the patient is gravely ill or if the clinical presentation is unclear. This hemodynamic classification provides a useful guide for selecting the initial optimal therapies for the management of acute HF. LV, left ventricular; CO, cardiac output; SVR, systemic vascular resistance. *(Modified from Grady et al: Circulation 102:2443, 2000.)*

TABLE 227-5 DRUGS FOR THE TREATMENT FOR ACUTE HEART FAILURE

	Initiating Dose	Maximal Dose
Vasodilators		
Nitroglycerin	20 μg/min	40–400 μg/min
Nitroprusside	10 μg/min	30–350 μg/min
Nesiritide	Bolus 2 μg/kg	0.01–0.03 μg/kg per min[a]
Inotropes		
Dobutamine	1–2 μg/kg per min	2–10 μg/kg per min[b]
Milrinone	Bolus 50 μg/kg	0.1–0.75 μg/kg per min[b]
Dopamine	1–2 μg/kg per min	2–4 μg/kg per min[b]
Levosimendan	Bolus 12 μg/kg	0.1–0.2 μg/kg per min[c]
Vasoconstrictors		
Dopamine for hypotension	5 μg/kg per min	5–15 μg/kg per min
Epinephrine	0.5 μg/kg per min	50 μg/kg per min
Phenylephrine	0.3 μg/kg per min	3 μg/kg per min
Vasopression	0.05 units/min	0.1–0.4 units/min

[a]Usually <4 μg/kg/min.
[b]Inotropes will also have vasodilatory properties.
[c]Approved outside of the United States for the management of acute heart failure.

cyclase within smooth-muscle cells, nitroglycerin, nitroprusside, and nesiritide exert dilating effects on arterial resistance and venous capacitance vessels, which results in a lowering of LV filling pressure, a reduction in mitral regurgitation, and improved forward cardiac output, without increasing heart rate or causing arrhythmias.

Intravenous *nitroglycerin* is generally begun at 20 μg/min and is increased in 20 μg increments until patient symptoms are improved or PCWP is decreased to 16 mmHg without reducing systolic blood pressure below 80 mmHg. The most common side effect of intravenous or oral nitrates is headache, which, if mild, can be treated with analgesics and often resolves during continued therapy.

Nitroprusside is generally initiated at 10 μg/min and increased by 10–20 μg every 10–20 min as tolerated, with the same hemodynamic goals as described above. The rapidity of onset and offset, with a half-life of approximately 2 min, facilitates early establishment of an individual patient's optimal level of vasodilation in the ICU. The major limitation of nitroprusside is side effects from cyanide, which manifests predominantly as gastrointestinal and central nervous system manifestations. Cyanide is most likely to accumulate in patients with severely reduced hepatic perfusion and decreased hepatic function from low cardiac output, and it is more likely to develop in patients receiving >250 μg/min for over 48 h. Suspected cyanide toxicity is treated by decreasing or discontinuing the nitroprusside infusion. Long-term (>48 h) use of both nitroprusside and nitroglycerin is associated with hemodynamic tolerance.

Nesiritide, the newest vasodilator, is a recombinant form of brain-type natriuretic peptide (BNP), which is an endogenous peptide secreted primarily from the LV in response to an increase in wall stress. Nesiritide is given as a bolus (2 μg/kg) followed by a fixed-dose infusion (0.01–0.03 μg/kg per min). Nesiritide effectively lowers LV filling pressures and improves symptoms during the treatment of acute HF. Headache is less common with nesiritide than with nitroglycerin. Although termed a *natriuretic peptide*, nesiritide has not been associated with major diuresis when used alone in clinical trials. It does, however, appear to potentiate the effect of concomitant diuretics such that the total required diuretic dose may be slightly lower.

Hypotension is the most common side effect of all three vasodilating agents, although less so with nesiritide. Hypotension is frequently associated with bradycardia, particularly when nitroglycerin is used. All three drugs can cause pulmonary artery vasodilation, which can lead to worsening hypoxia in patients with underlying ventilation-perfusion abnormalities.

Inotropic Agents   Positive inotropic agents produce direct hemodynamic benefits by stimulating cardiac contractility, as well as by producing peripheral vasodilation. Collectively, these hemodynamic effects result in an improvement in cardiac output and a fall in LV filling pressures.

Dobutamine, which is the most commonly used inotropic agent for the treatment of acute HF, exerts its effects by stimulating β_1 and β_2 receptors, with little effect on α_1 receptors. Dobutamine is given as a continuous infusion, at an initial infusion rate of 1–2 μg/kg per min. Higher doses (>5 μg/kg per min) are frequently necessary for severe hypoperfusion; however, there is little added benefit to increasing the dose above 10 μg/kg per min. Patients maintained on chronic infusions for >72 h generally develop tachyphylaxis and require increasing doses.

Milrinone is a phosphodiesterase III inhibitor that leads to increased cAMP by inhibiting its breakdown. Milrinone may act synergistically with β-adrenergic agonists to achieve further increase in cardiac output than either agent alone, and it may also be more effective than dobutamine in increasing cardiac output in the presence of beta blockers. Milrinone may be administered as a bolus dose of 0.5 μg/kg per min, followed by a continuous infusion rate of 0.1–0.75 μg/kg per min. Because milrinone is a more effective vasodilator than dobutamine, it produces a greater reduction in LV filling pressures, albeit with a greater risk of hypotension.

Although short-term use of inotropes provides hemodynamic benefits, these agents are more prone to cause tachyarrhythmias and ischemic events than vasodilators. Therefore inotropes are most appropriately used in clinical settings in which vasodilators and diuretics are not helpful, such as in patients with poor systemic perfusion and/or cardiogenic shock, in patients requiring short-term hemodynamic support after a MI or surgery, and in patients awaiting cardiac transplantation, or as palliative care in patients with advanced HF. If patients require sustained use of intravenous inotropes, strong consideration should be given to the use of an ICD to safeguard against the proarrhythmic effects of these agents.

Vasoconstrictors   Vasoconstrictors are used to support systemic blood pressure in patients with HF. Of the three agents that are commonly used (Table 227-5), dopamine is generally the first choice for therapy in situations where modest inotropy and pressor support are required. Dopamine is an endogenous catecholamine that stimulates β_1, α_1 receptors, and dopaminergic receptors (DA_1 and DA_2) in the heart and circulation. The effects of dopamine are dose-dependent. Low doses of dopamine (<2 μg/kg per min) stimulate the DA_1 and DA_2 receptors and cause vasodilation of the splanchnic and renal vasculature. Moderate doses (2–4 μg/kg per min) stimulate the β_1 receptors and cause an increase in cardiac output with little or no change in heart rate or SVR. At higher doses (≥5 μg/kg per min) the effects of dopamine on the α_1 receptors overwhelm the dopaminergic receptors, and vasoconstriction ensues, leading to an increase in SVR, LV filling pressures, and heart rate.

Dopamine also causes release of norepinephrine from nerve terminals, which itself stimulates α_1 and β_1 receptors, thus raising blood pressure. Dopamine is most useful in the treatment of HF patients who have depressed cardiac output with poor tissue perfusion (Profile C). Significant additional inotropic and blood pressure support can be provided by epinephrine, phenylephrine, and vasopressin (Table 227-5); however, prolonged use of these agents can lead to renal and hepatic failure and can cause gangrene of the limbs. Therefore, these agents should not be administered except in true emergency situations.

Mechanical and Surgical Interventions   If pharmacologic interventions fail to stabilize the patient with refractory HF, mechanical and surgical interventions may provide effective circulatory support. These include intraaortic balloon counter pulsation, LV assist device, and cardiac transplantation (Chap. 228).

Planning for Hospital Discharge   Patient education should take place during the entire hospitalization, with a specific focus on salt and fluid status and obtaining daily weights, in addition to medication schedules. Whereas the majority of patients hospitalized with HF can be stabilized and returned to a good level of function on an oral regimen designed to maintain stability, 30–50% of patients discharged with a diagnosis of HF are rehospitalized within 3–6 months. Although there are multiple reasons for rehospitalization, failure to meet criteria for discharge is perhaps the most frequent. Criteria for discharge should include at least 24 h of stable fluid status, blood pressure, and renal function on the oral regimen planned for home. Patients should be free of dyspnea or symptomatic hypotension while at rest, washing, and walking on the ward.

COR PULMONALE

DEFINITION

Cor pulmonale, often referred to as *pulmonary heart disease*, is defined as dilation and hypertrophy of the right ventricle (RV) in response to diseases of the pulmonary vasculature and/or lung parenchyma. Historically, this definition has excluded congenital heart disease and those diseases in which the right heart fails secondary to dysfunction of the left side of the heart.

ETIOLOGY AND EPIDEMIOLOGY

Cor pulmonale develops in response to acute or chronic changes in the pulmonary vasculature and/or the lung parenchyma that are sufficient to cause pulmonary hypertension. The true prevalence of cor pulmonale is difficult to ascertain for two reasons. First, not all cases of chronic lung disease will develop cor pulmonale, and second, our ability to diagnose pulmonary hypertension and cor pulmonale by routine physical examination and laboratory testing is relatively insensitive. However, recent advances in 2-D echo/Doppler imaging and biomakers (BNP) make it easier to screen for and detect cor pulmonale.

Once patients with chronic pulmonary or pulmonary vascular disease develop cor pulmonale, their prognosis worsens. Although chronic obstructive pulmonary disease (COPD) and chronic bronchitis are responsible for approximately 50% percent of the cases of cor pulmonale in North America (Chap. 254), any disease that affects the pulmonary vasculature (Chap. 244) or parenchyma can lead to cor pulmonale. Table 227-6 provides a list of common diseases that may lead to cor pulmonale. In contrast to COPD, the elevation in pulmonary artery

TABLE 227-6 ETIOLOGY OF CHRONIC COR PULMONALE

Diseases Leading to Hypoxic Vasoconstriction

Chronic bronchitis
Chronic obstructive pulmonary disease
Cystic fibrosis
Chronic hypoventilation
  Obesity
  Neuromuscular disease
  Chest wall dysfunction
Living at high altitudes

Diseases That Cause Occlusion of the Pulmonary Vascular Bed

Recurrent pulmonary thromboembolism
Primary pulmonary hypertension
Venocclusive disease
Collagen vascular disease
Drug-induced lung disease

Diseases That Lead to Parenchymal Disease

Chronic bronchitis
Chronic obstructive pulmonary disease
Bronchiectasis
Cystic fibrosis
Pneumoconiosis
Sarcoid
Idiopathic pulmonary fibrosis

pressure appears to be substantially higher in the interstitial lung diseases (Chap. 255), in which there is an inverse correlation between pulmonary artery pressure and the diffusion capacity for carbon monoxide, as well as patient survival. Sleep-disordered breathing, once thought to be a major mechanism for cor pulmonale, is rarely the sole cause of pulmonary hypertension and RV failure. The combination of COPD and associated daytime hypoxemia is required to cause sustained pulmonary hypertension in obstructive sleep apnea (Chap. 259).

PATHOPHYSIOLOGY AND BASIC MECHANISMS

Although many conditions can lead to cor pulmonale, the common pathophysiologic mechanism in each case is pulmonary hypertension that is sufficient to lead to RV dilation, with or without the development of concomitant RV hypertrophy. The systemic consequences of cor pulmonale relate to alterations in cardiac output as well as salt and water homeostasis. Anatomically, the RV is a thin-walled, compliant chamber that is better suited to handle volume overload than pressure overload. Thus, the sustained pressure overload imposed by pulmonary hypertension and increased pulmonary vascular resistance eventually causes the RV to fail.

The response of the RV to pulmonary hypertension depends on the acuteness and severity of the pressure overload. Acute cor pulmonale occurs after a sudden and severe stimulus (e.g., massive pulmonary embolus), with RV dilatation and failure but no RV hypertrophy (Chap. 256). Chronic cor pulmonale, however, is associated with a more slowly evolving and slowly progressive pulmonary hypertension that leads to RV dilation and hypertrophy. The severity of the pulmonary artery hypertension and the onset of RV failure are influenced by multiple factors that occur intermittently, including hypoxia secondary to alterations in gas exchange, hypercapnia, and acidosis, as well as alterations in RV volume overload that are affected by exercise, heart rate, polycythemia, or increased salt and retention because of a fall in cardiac output (Fig. 227-2). The most common mechanisms that lead to pulmonary hypertension, including vasoconstriction, activation of the clotting cascade, and obliteration of pulmonary arterial vessels, are discussed in Chap. 244.

CLINICAL MANIFESTATIONS

Symptoms The symptoms of chronic cor pulmonale are generally related to the underlying pulmonary disorder. Dyspnea, the most common symptom, is usually the result of the increased work of breathing secondary to changes in elastic recoil of the lung (fibrosing

lung diseases) or altered respiratory mechanics (e.g., overinflation with COPD), both of which may be aggravated by increased hypoxic respiratory drive. The hypoxia that occurs in lung disease is the result of reduced capillary membrane permeability, ventilation-perfusion mismatch, and occasionally intracardiac or intrapulmonary shunting.

Orthopnea and paroxysmal nocturnal dyspnea are rarely symptoms of isolated right HF. However, when present, these symptoms usually reflect the increased work of breathing in the supine position that results from compromised excursion of the diaphragm. Tussive or effort-related syncope may occur in patients with cor pulmonale with severe pulmonary hypertension because of the inability of the RV to deliver blood adequately to the left side of the heart. The abdominal pain and ascites that occur with cor pulmonale are similar to the right heart failure that ensues in chronic HF. Lower-extremity edema may occur secondary to neurohormonal activation, elevated RV filling pressures, or increased levels of carbon dioxide and hypoxia, which can lead to peripheral vasodilation and edema formation. The symptoms of acute cor pulmonale with pulmonary embolus are reviewed in Chap. 256.

Signs Many of the signs that are encountered in cor pulmonale are also present in HF patients with a depressed EF, including tachypnea, elevated jugular venous pressures, hepatomegaly, and lower-extremity edema. Patients may have prominent v waves in the jugular venous pulse as a result of tricuspid regurgitation. Other cardiovascular signs include an RV heave palpable along the left sternal border or in the epigastrium. A systolic pulmonary ejection click may be audible to the left of the upper sternum. The increase in intensity of the holosystolic murmur of tricuspid regurgitation with inspiration ("Carvallo's sign") may be eventually lost as RV failure worsens. Cyanosis is a late finding in cor pulmonale and is secondary to a low cardiac output with systemic vasoconstriction and ventilation-perfusion mismatches in the lung.

DIAGNOSIS

The most common cause of right heart failure is not pulmonary parenchymal or vascular disease, but left heart failure. Therefore it is important to evaluate the patient for LV systolic and diastolic dysfunction. The ECG in severe pulmonary hypertension shows P pulmonale, right axis deviation, and RV hypertrophy. Radiographic examination of the chest may show enlargement of the main pulmonary artery, hilar vessels, and the descending right pulmonary artery. Spiral CT scans of the chest are useful in diagnosing acute thromboembolic disease; however, the ventilation-perfusion lung scan remains reliable in most centers for establishing the diagnosis of *chronic thromboembolic disease* (Chap. 256). A high-resolution CT scan of the chest is the most accurate means of diagnosing emphysema and interstitial lung disease.

Two-dimensional echocardiography is useful for measuring RV thickness and chamber dimensions as well as the anatomy of the pulmonary and tricuspid valves. The interventricular septum may move paradoxically during systole in the presence of pulmonary hypertension. As noted, Doppler echocardiography can be used to assess pulmonary artery pressures. MRI is also useful for assessing RV structure and function, particularly in patients who are difficult to image with 2-D echocardiography because of severe lung disease. Right-heart catheterization is useful for confirming the diagnosis of pulmonary hypertension and for excluding elevated left-heart pressures (measured as the PCWP) as a cause for right heart failure. BNP and N-terminal BNP levels are elevated in patients with cor pulmonale secondary to RV stretch and may be dramatically elevated in acute pulmonary embolism.

R̲x̲ COR PULMONALE

The primary treatment goal of cor pulmonale is to target the underlying pulmonary disease, since this will lead to a decrease in pulmonary vascular resistance and relieve the pressure overload on the RV. Most pulmonary diseases that lead to chronic cor pulmonale are far advanced and are, therefore, less amenable to treatment. General principles of treatment include decreasing the work of breathing using noninvasive mechanical ventilation, bronchodilation, and steroids, as well as treating any underlying infection (Chaps. 254, 255). Adequate oxygenation (oxygen saturation ≥90–92%) will also decrease pulmonary vascular resistance and reduce the demands on the RV. Patients should be transfused if they are anemic, and a phlebotomy should be performed to reduce pulmonary artery pressure if the hematocrit exceeds 65%.

Diuretics are effective in the treatment of RV failure, and the indications for their use are similar to those for chronic HF. One caveat of chronic diuretic use is that they may lead to contraction alkalosis and worsening hypercapnea. Digoxin is of uncertain benefit in the treatment of cor pulmonale and may lead to arrhythmias in the setting of tissue hypoxia and acidosis. Therefore, if digoxin is administered, it should be given at low doses and monitored carefully. **The treatment of the acute cor pulmonale that occurs with pulmonary embolus is described in Chap. 256. The treatment of pulmonary hypertension is discussed in Chap. 244.**

FURTHER READINGS

ASHRAFIAN H et al: Metabolic mechanisms in heart failure. Circulation 116:434, 2007

BARDY GH et al: Amiodarone or an implantable cardioverter-defibrillator for congestive heart failure. N Engl J Med 352:225, 2005

CHAPMAN HA: Disorders of lung matrix remodeling. J Clin Invest 113:148, 2004

CLELAND JG et al: The effect of cardiac resynchronization on morbidity and mortality in heart failure. N Engl J Med 352:1539, 2005

FRIEDRICH EB, BOHM M: Management of end stage heart failure. Heart 93:626, 2007

KESSLER R et al: "Natural history" of pulmonary hypertension in a series of 131 patients with chronic obstructive lung disease. Am J Respir Crit Care Med 164:219, 2001

MANN DL, BRISTOW MR: Mechanisms and models in heart failure: The biomechanical model and beyond. Circulation 111:2837, 2005

MAZHARI R, HARE JM: Advances in cell-based therapy for structural heart disease. Prog Cardiovasc Dis 49:387, 2007

MOSTERD A, HOES AW: Clinical epidemiology of heart failure. Heart 93:1137, 2007

PENGO V et al: Incidence of chronic thromboembolic pulmonary hypertension after pulmonary embolism. N Engl J Med 350:2257, 2004

228 Cardiac Transplantation and Prolonged Assisted Circulation
Sharon A. Hunt

Advanced or end-stage heart failure is an increasingly frequent sequela as progressively more effective palliation for the earlier stages of heart disease and prevention of sudden death associated with heart disease become more widely recognized and employed (Chap. 227). When patients with end-stage or refractory heart failure are identified, the physician is faced with the decision of advising compassionate end-of-life care or choosing to recommend extraordinary life-extending measures. For the occasional patient who is relatively young and without serious comorbidities, the latter may represent a reasonable option. Current therapeutic options are limited to cardiac transplantation (with the option of mechanical cardiac assistance as a "bridge" to transplantation) or (at least in theory) the option of permanent mechanical assistance of the circulation.

CARDIAC TRANSPLANTATION

Surgical techniques for orthotopic transplantation of the heart were devised in the 1960s and taken into the clinical arena in 1967. The procedure did not gain widespread clinical acceptance until the introduction of "modern" and more effective immunosuppression in the early 1980s. By the 1990s the demand for transplantable hearts met, and then exceeded, the available donor supply and leveled off at about 4000 heart transplants annually worldwide, according to data from the Registry of the International Society for Heart and Lung Transplantation (ISHLT). Subsequently heart transplant activity in the United States has remained stable at ~2200/year, but worldwide activity reported to this Registry has decreased some. This apparent decline in numbers may be a result of the fact that reporting is legally mandated in the United States, but not elsewhere, and several countries have started their own databases.

SURGICAL TECHNIQUE

Donor and recipient hearts are excised in virtually identical operations with incisions made across the atria and atrial septum at the midatrial level (leaving the posterior walls of the atria in place) and across the great vessels just above the semilunar valves. The donor heart is generally "harvested" in an anatomically identical manner by a separate surgical team and transported from the donor hospital in a bag of iced saline solution and then is reanastomosed into the waiting recipient in the orthotopic or normal anatomic position. The only change in surgical technique since this method was first described has been a movement in recent years to move the right atrial anastamosis back to the level of the superior and inferior vena cavae in order to better preserve right atrial geometry and prevent atrial arrhythmias. Both methods of implantation leave the recipient with a surgically denervated heart that does not respond to any direct sympathetic or parasympathetic stimuli but does respond to circulating catecholamines. The physiologic responses of the denervated heart to the demands of exercise are atypical but quite adequate to carry on normal physical activity.

DONOR ALLOCATION SYSTEM

In the United States the allocation of donor organs is accomplished under the supervision of the United Network for Organ Sharing (UNOS), a private organization under contract to the federal government. The United States is divided geographically into eleven regions for donor heart allocation. Allocation of donor hearts within a region is decided according to a system of priority that takes into account (1) the severity of illness, (2) geographic distance from the donor, and (3) patient time on the waiting list. A physiologic limit of ~3 h of "ischemic" (out of body) time for hearts precludes a national sharing of hearts. This allocation system design is reissued annually and is responsive to input from a variety of constituencies, including donor families and transplant professionals.

At the current time, highest priority according to severity of illness is assigned to patients requiring hospitalization at the transplant center for IV inotropic support with a pulmonary artery catheter in place for hemodynamic monitoring or to patients requiring mechanical circulatory support [i.e., intra-aortic balloon pump (IABP), right or left ventricular assist device (RVAD, LVAD), extracorporeal membrane oxygenation (ECMO), or mechanical ventilation]. Second highest priority is given to patients requiring ongoing inotropic support, but without a pulmonary artery catheter in place. All other patients have priority according to their time on the waiting list, and matching is achieved only according to ABO blood group compatibility and gross body size compatibility, although some patients who are "pre-sensitized" and have preexisting anti-HLA antibodies (commonly multiparous women or patients previously multiply transfused) undergo prospective crossmatching with the donor.

INDICATIONS/CONTRAINDICATIONS

Heart failure is an increasingly common cause of death, particularly in the elderly. Most patients who reach what has recently been categorized

FIGURE 228-1 Adult heart transplantation. Kaplan-Meier. Actuarial survival for heart transplants performed between 1982 and 2003 by era of transplantation. (*J Heart Lung Transplant 24:945, 2005. Data by permission from International Society for Heart and Lung Transplantation.*)

as stage D, or refractory end-stage heart failure, are appropriately treated with compassionate end-of-life care. A subset of such patients who are younger and without significant comorbidities can be considered as candidates for heart transplantation. Exact criteria vary in different centers but generally take into consideration the patient's physiologic age and the existence of comorbidities such as peripheral or cerebrovascular disease, obesity, diabetes, cancer, or chronic infection.

RESULTS

A registry organized by the ISHLT has tracked worldwide and U.S. survival rates after heart transplantation since 1982. The most recent update reveals 83% and 76% survival 1 and 3 years posttransplant, or a posttransplant "half-life" of 9.3 years (Fig. 228-1). The quality of life in these patients is generally excellent, with well over 90% of patients in the registry returning to normal and unrestricted function following transplantation.

IMMUNOSUPPRESSION

Medical regimens employed to provide suppression of the normal immune response to a solid organ allograft vary from center to center and are in a constant state of evolution as more effective agents with improved side-effect profiles and less toxicity are introduced. All currently used regimens are nonspecific, providing general hyporeactivity to foreign antigens rather than donor-specific hyporeactivity as well as the attendant, and unwanted, susceptibility to infections and malignancy. Most cardiac transplant programs currently use a three-drug regimen including a calcineurin inhibitor (cyclosporine or tacrolimus), an inhibitor of T cell proliferation or differentiation (azathioprine, mycophenolate mofetil, or sirolimus), and at least a short initial course of glucocorticoids. Many programs also include an initial "induction" course of polyclonal or monoclonal anti-T cell antibodies in the perioperative period to decrease the frequency or severity of early posttransplant rejection. Most recently introduced have been monoclonal antibodies (daclizumab and basiliximab), which block the interleukin 2 receptor and may provide prevention of allograft rejection without additional global immunosuppression.

Diagnosis of cardiac allograft rejection is usually made with the use of endomyocardial biopsy, either done on a surveillance basis or in response to clinical deterioration. Biopsy surveillance is performed on a regular basis in most programs for the first year postoperatively and for the first 5 years in many programs. Therapy consists of augmentation of immunosuppression, the intensity and duration of which is dictated by the severity of the rejection.

LATE POSTTRANSPLANT MANAGEMENT ISSUES

Increasing numbers of heart transplant patients are surviving for years following transplantation and constitute a population of patients with a number of long-term management issues.

Allograft Coronary Artery Disease Despite usually having young donor hearts, cardiac allograft recipients are prone to develop coronary artery disease (CAD). This CAD is generally a diffuse, concentric, and longitudinal process that is quite different from "ordinary" atherosclerotic CAD, which is more focal and often eccentric. The underlying etiology is most likely primarily immunologic injury of the vascular endothelium, but a variety of risk factors influence its existence and progression and include nonimmunologic factors such as dyslipidemia, diabetes, and cytomegalovirus (CMV) infection. It is hoped that newer and improved immunosuppressive modalities will reduce the incidence and impact of these devastating complications, which currently account for the majority of late posttransplant deaths. Thus far the newer immunosuppressive agents mycophenolate mofetil and the mammalian target of rapamycin (mTOR) inhibitors sirolimus and everolimus have been shown to be associated with short-term lesser incidence and extent of coronary intimal thickening; in anecdotal reports institution of sirolimus was associated with some reversal of the disease. The use of statins has also been shown to be associated with a reduced incidence of this vasculopathy, and these drugs are now almost universally used in transplant recipients unless contraindicated. Palliation of the disease with percutaneous interventions is probably safe and effective in the short term, although the disease often advances relentlessly. Because of the denervated status of the organ, patients rarely experience angina pectoris, even with advanced stages of the disease.

Retransplantation is the only definitive form of therapy for advanced allograft CAD, but the scarcity of donor hearts make the decision to pursue retransplantation a difficult one in an individual patient, as well as a difficult ethical issue.

Malignancy The occurrence of an increased incidence of malignancy is a well-recognized sequela of any program of chronic immunosuppression, and organ transplantation is no exception. Lymphoproliferative disorders are among the most frequent posttransplant complications and, in most cases, seem to be driven by the Epstein-Barr virus. Effective therapy includes reduction of immunosuppression (a clear "double-edged sword" in the setting of a life-sustaining organ), antiviral agents, and traditional chemo- and radiotherapy. Most recently, specific antilymphocyte (CD20) therapy has shown great promise. Cutaneous malignancies (both basal cell and squamous cell carcinomas) also occur with increased frequency in transplant recipients and can pursue very aggressive courses. The role of decreasing immunosuppression for treatment of these cancers is much less clear.

Infections The use of currently available nonspecific immunosuppressive modalities to prevent allograft rejection naturally results in an increased susceptibility to infectious complications in transplant recipients. Although their incidence has decreased since the introduction of cyclosporine, infections with unusual and opportunistic organisms remain the major cause of death during the first postoperative year and remain a threat to the chronically immunosuppressed patient throughout life. Effective therapy depends on careful surveillance for early signs and symptoms of opportunistic infection and an extremely aggressive approach to obtaining a specific diagnosis as well as expertise in recognizing the more common clinical presentations of CMV, *Aspergillus*, and other opportunistic infectious agents.

PROLONGED ASSISTED CIRCULATON

The modern era of mechanical circulatory support can be traced back to 1953 when cardiopulmonary bypass was first used in a clinical setting and ushered in the possibility of brief periods of circulatory support to permit open-heart surgery. There have subsequently been developed a variety of extracorporeal pumps to provide circulatory support for brief periods of time. The use of a mechanical device to support the circulation for more than a few hours got off to a slow start in the 1980s when the first artificial hearts were introduced with much publicity but failed to produce the hoped-for treatment of end-stage heart disease. Subsequently, technology evolved to provide mechanical assistance to (rather than replacement of) the failing ventricle, although newer versions of the total artificial heart are now once again in preliminary clinical trials.

Although conceived of initially as alternatives to biologic replacement of the heart, LVADs were introduced as, and are still employed primarily as, temporary "bridges" to heart transplantation in candidates who begin to fail medical therapy before a donor heart becomes available. Several devices are approved by the U.S. Food and Drug Administration (FDA) and are currently in widespread use. Those that are implantable within the body are compatible with hospital discharge and offer the patient chance for life at home while waiting for a donor heart. However successful such "bridging" is for the individual patient, it does nothing to alleviate the scarcity of donor hearts, and the ultimate goal in the field remains that of providing a reasonable alternative to biologic replacement of the heart—one that is widely and easily available and cost effective.

AVAILABLE DEVICES

In the United States there are currently three FDA-approved devices that are used as bridges to transplantation. There are a number of other devices that are approved only for short-term support for postcardiac surgery shock and these will not be considered here. None of the long-term devices as yet are totally implantable, and, because of this need for transcutaneous connections, all share a common problem with infectious complications. Likewise, all share some tendency to thromboembolic complications as well as the expected possibility of mechanical device failure common to any man-made machine.

The Thoratec LVAD (Thoratec Corp., Pleasanton, CA) is an extracorporeal pump that takes blood from a large cannula placed in the left ventricular apex and propels it forward through an outflow cannula inserted into the ascending aorta. The pump itself sits in the paracorporeal position on the abdomen and is attached to a device console cart with wheels, allowing for limited ambulation. The extracorporeal nature of this pump allows it to be used for small adults for whom the intracorporeal pumps would be too large.

The Novacor LVAD (WorldHeart Inc., Oakland, CA) also takes blood from the left ventricular apex through a cannula and propels it into the ascending aorta through a second cannula. With this device the pump itself is placed in a surgically created pocket in the preperitoneal fascia in the abdomen. A drive line that connects to the power source is tunneled subcutaneously and usually exits in the right upper quadrant of the abdomen.

The HeartMate LVAD (Thoratec Corp., Pleasanton, CA) uses a configuration identical to that of the Novacor device (Fig. 228-2). Differences between the two have to do with the materials used and the tendency for thromboembolic complications. Both commonly lead to hospital discharge and an outpatient wait for a donor heart.

Newer devices, currently in clinical trials, include several axial-flow pumps that have basically the same connections to the circulatory system but are considerably smaller, have fewer moving parts than previous devices, and provide non-pulsatile blood flow. All current axial-flow pumps continue to require transcutaneous connections.

RESULTS

The use of these devices in the United States is limited mainly to patients with postcardiac surgery shock and to those who are "bridged" to transplantation. The results of bridging to transplantation with the available devices are quite good, with nearly 75% of younger patients receiving a transplant by 1 year and those having excellent posttransplant survival rates.

Publication of the REMATCH (Randomized Evaluation of Mechanical Assistance in the Treatment of Heart Failure) trial in 2001 documented a somewhat improved survival in nontransplant candidates with end-stage heart disease randomized to a Heartmate LVAD (albeit with a high rate of complications, especially neurologic ones) as opposed to continued medical therapy; this led to renewed interest in also using the devices as non-biologic permanent replacement of heart function as well as to FDA approval of one device for this indication. This, in turn, led the ISHLT to initiate a Mechanical Circulatory Support database in 2002. This database

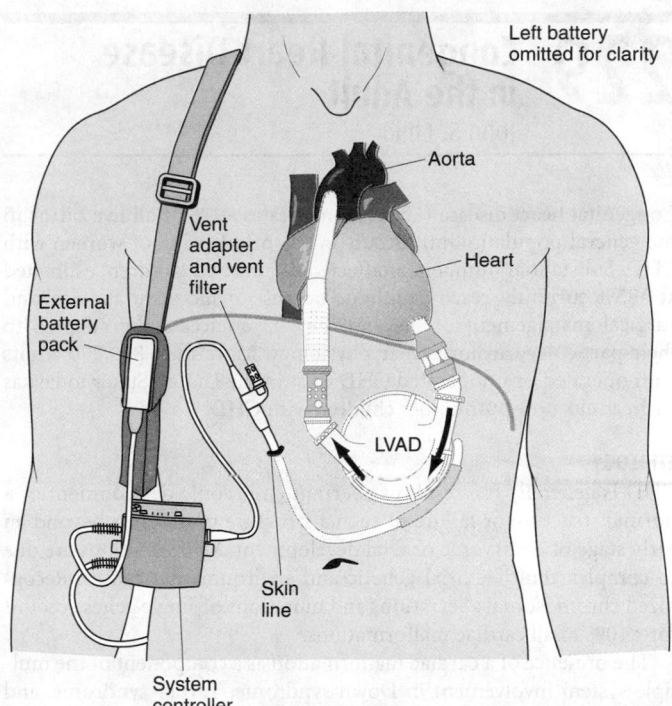

FIGURE 228-2 Diagram of HeartMate left ventricular assist device. (*Reprinted with permission from Thoratec Corp., Pleasanton, CA.*)

collects voluntary data from 60 international centers and contained data from 655 patients in its most recent publication. Only 12% of these had the device placed with the intention of permanent, or "destination," use, with survival rates of only 65% at 6 months and 34% at one year.

GOALS

Future developments in this field can be expected in two directions. First, newer generations of the pumps will likely be smaller and simpler mechanically and, most important, totally implantable. Second, increased use of the newer generations of pumps as "permanent" (destination) therapy in patients with end-stage heart failure who are not considered eligible for transplantation will likely happen in the near future. Eventually it is hoped that improved assist devices will be accepted as valid alternatives to biologic replacement of the heart even in transplant-eligible patients and help to modify the supply/demand mismatch for cardiac replacement therapy.

FURTHER READINGS

DENG MC et al: Mechanical circulatory support device database of the International Society for Heart and Lung Transplantation: Third annual report—2005. J Heart Lung Transplant 24:1182, 2005

GARNIER JL et al: Treatment of post-transplant lymphomas with anti-B-cell monoclonal antibodies. Recent Results Cancer Res 159:113, 2002

GRAY NA JR, SELZMAN CH: Current status of the total artificial heart. Am Heart J 152:4, 2006

HUNT SA et al: ACC/AHA 2005 guideline update for the diagnosis and management of chronic heart failure in the adult: A report of the American College of Cardiology/American Heart Association Task Force on Practice Guidelines (Writing committee to update the 2001 guidelines for the evaluation and management of heart failure). Available at *http://www.acc.org/clinical/guidelines/failure//index.pdf*

MANCINI D et al: Use of rapamycin slows progression of cardiac transplantation vasculopathy. Circulation 108:48, 2003

TAYLOR DO et al: Registry of the International Society for Heart and Lung Transplantation: Twenty-second official adult heart transplant report—2005. J Heart Lung Transplant 224:945, 2005

229 Congenital Heart Disease in the Adult

John S. Child

Congenital heart disease (CHD) complicates ~1% of all live births in the general population but occurs in 4% of offspring of women with CHD. Substantial numbers of affected infants and children, estimated at >85% currently, reach adulthood because of successful medical and surgical management or because they have successfully adapted to their particular cardiovascular physiology. More than 800,000 adults with operated or unoperated CHD exist in the United States today; as such, adults now outnumber children with CHD.

ETIOLOGY

CHD is generally the result of aberrant embryonic development of a normal structure or failure of such a structure to progress beyond an early stage of embryonic or fetal development. Malformations are due to complex multifactorial genetic and environmental causes. Recognized chromosomal aberrations and mutations of single genes account for <10% of all cardiac malformations.

The presence of a cardiac malformation as a component of the multiple system involvement in Down syndrome, Turner syndrome, and the trisomy 13-15(D1) and 17-18(E) syndromes may be anticipated in occasional pregnancies by detection of abnormal chromosomes in fetal cells obtained from amniotic fluid or chorionic villus biopsy. Identification in such cells of the enzyme disorders characteristic of Hurler's syndrome, homocystinuria, or type II glycogen storage disease may also allow one to predict cardiac disease.

PATHOPHYSIOLOGY

The anatomic and physiologic changes in the heart and circulation due to any specific CHD lesion are not static but, rather, progress from prenatal life to adulthood. Malformations that are benign or escape detection in childhood may become clinically significant in the adult. For example, a functionally normal congenitally bicuspid aortic valve may thicken and calcify with time, resulting in significant aortic stenosis; or a well-tolerated left-to-right shunt of an atrial septal defect may result in cardiac decompensation or pulmonary hypertension only after the fourth to fifth decade.

Pulmonary Hypertension The status of the pulmonary vascular bed is often a principal determinant of the clinical manifestations and course of a given lesion and of the feasibility of surgical repair. Increased pulmonary arterial pressure results from increased pulmonary blood flow and/or resistance, the latter usually the result of obstructive, obliterative structural changes within the pulmonary vascular bed. It is important to quantitate and compare pulmonary to systemic flows and resistances in patients with severe pulmonary hypertension. The causes of pulmonary vascular obstructive disease are unknown, although increased pulmonary blood flow, increased pulmonary arterial blood pressure, elevated pulmonary venous pressure, erythrocytosis, systemic hypoxemia, acidosis, and the bronchial circulation have been implicated. The term *Eisenmenger syndrome* is applied to patients with a large communication between the two circulations at the aortopulmonary, ventricular, or atrial levels and bidirectional or predominantly right-to-left shunts because of high-resistance and obstructive pulmonary hypertension. Pulmonary arterial vasodilators and both single lung transplantation with intracardiac defect repair and total heart-lung transplantation show promise for improvement in symptoms (Chaps. 228 and 260).

Erythrocytosis Chronic hypoxemia in cyanotic CHD results in secondary *erythrocytosis* due to increased erythropoietin production (Chap. 35). The commonly used term *polycythemia* is a misnomer because white cell counts are normal and platelet counts are normal to decreased. Cyanotic patients with erythrocytosis may have compensated or decompensated hematocrits. Compensated erythrocytosis with iron-replete equilibrium hematocrits rarely result in symptoms of hyperviscosity at hematocrits < 65% and occasionally not even with hematocrits ≥ 70%. Therapeutic phlebotomy is rarely required in compensated erythrocytosis. In contrast, patients with decompensated erythrocytosis fail to establish equilibrium with unstable, rising hematocrits and recurrent hyperviscosity symptoms. Therapeutic phlebotomy, a two-edged sword, allows temporary relief of symptoms but limits oxygen delivery, begets instability of the hematocrit, and compounds the problem by iron depletion. Iron-deficiency symptoms are usually indistinguishable from those of hyperviscosity; progressive symptoms after recurrent phlebotomy are usually due to iron depletion with hypochromic microcytosis. Iron depletion results in a larger number of smaller (microcytic) hypochromic red cells that are less capable of carrying oxygen. Because these microcytes are less deformable in the microcirculation and there are more of them relative to the plasma volume, the viscosity is greater than for an equivalent hematocrit with fewer, larger, iron-replete, deformable cells. As such, iron-depleted erythrocytosis results in increasing symptoms due to decreased oxygen delivery to the tissues.

Hemostasis is abnormal in cyanotic CHD, due in part to the increased blood volume and engorged capillaries, abnormalities in platelet function and sensitivity to aspirin or nonsteroidal anti-inflammatory agents, and abnormalities of the extrinsic and intrinsic coagulation system. Oral contraceptives are often contraindicated for cyanotic women because of the enhanced risk of vascular thrombosis.

The risk of stroke is greatest in children <4 years with cyanotic heart disease and iron deficiency, often with dehydration as an aggravating cause. Adults with cyanotic CHD do not appear to be at increased risk for stroke, unless there are excessive injudicious phlebotomies, inappropriate use of aspirin or anticoagulants, or the presence of atrial arrhythmias or infective endocarditis.

Symptoms of hyperviscosity can be produced in any cyanotic patient with erythrocytosis if dehydration reduces plasma volume. Phlebotomy for symptoms of hyperviscosity not due to dehydration or iron deficiency is a simple outpatient removal of 500 mL of blood over 45 min with isovolumetric replacement with isotonic saline. Acute phlebotomy without volume replacement is contraindicated. Iron repletion in decompensated iron-depleted erythrocytosis reduces iron-deficiency symptoms but must be done gradually to avoid an excessive rise in hematocrit and resultant hyperviscosity.

Pregnancy The physiologic alterations during normal gestation (Chap. 7) can create symptoms and physical findings that may be attributed erroneously to heart disease. The mother's health is most at risk if she has a cardiovascular lesion associated with pulmonary vascular disease and pulmonary hypertension (e.g., Eisenmenger physiology or mitral stenosis) or left ventricular (LV) outflow tract obstruction (e.g., aortic stenosis), but she is also at risk of death with any malformation that may cause heart failure or a hemodynamically important arrhythmia. The fetus is most at risk with maternal cyanosis, heart failure, or pulmonary hypertension. Women with aortic coarctation or Marfan syndrome risk aortic dissection. Patients with cyanotic heart disease, pulmonary hypertension, or Marfan syndrome with a dilated aortic root should not become pregnant; those with correctable lesions should be counseled about the risks of pregnancy with an uncorrected malformation versus repair and later pregnancy. The effect of pregnancy in postoperative patients depends on the outcome of the repair, including the presence and severity of residua, sequelae, or complications. Contraception is an important topic with such patients. Tubal ligation should be considered in those in whom pregnancy is strictly contraindicated.

INFECTIVE ENDOCARDITIS

(See also Chap. 118) Routine antimicrobial prophylaxis is recommended for most patients with CHD, whether operated on or not, for all dental procedures, gastrointestinal and genitourinary surgery, and

TABLE 229-1	COMPLEX ADULT CONGENITAL HEART DISEASE

Cyanotic congenital heart diseases (all forms)
Eisenmenger syndrome
Ebstein anomaly
Tetralogy of Fallot or pulmonary atresia (all forms)
Transposition of the great arteries
Single ventricle; tricuspid or mitral atresia
Double-outlet ventricle
Truncus arteriosus
Fontan or Rastelli procedures

TABLE 229-3	SIMPLE ADULT CONGENITAL HEART DISEASE

Native disease
  Uncomplicated congenital aortic valve disease
  Mild congenital mitral valve disease (e.g., except parachute valve, cleft leaflet)
  Uncomplicated small atrial septal defect
  Uncomplicated small ventricular septal defect
  Mild pulmonic stenosis
Repaired conditions
  Previously ligated or occluded ductus arteriosus
  Repaired secundum or sinus venosus atrial septal defect without residua
  Repaired ventricular septal defect without residua

some diagnostic procedures, e.g., sigmoidoscopy and cystoscopy. The clinical and bacteriologic profile of infective endocarditis in patients with CHD has changed with the advent of intracardiac surgery and of prosthetic devices. Two major predisposing causes of infective endocarditis are a susceptible cardiovascular substrate and a source of bacteremia. Prophylaxis includes both antimicrobial and hygienic measures. Meticulous dental and skin care is required.

EXERCISE

Advice on athletics and exercise is governed by the nature of the exercise and by the type and severity of the congenital cardiovascular lesion. Patients with LV outflow tract obstruction, if more than moderate, or pulmonary vascular disease risk syncope or sudden death. In unrepaired tetralogy of Fallot, isotonic exercise–induced decrease in systemic vascular resistance relative to the right ventricular (RV) outflow obstruction augments the right-to-left shunt, increases hypoxemia, and causes an increase in subjective breathlessness owing to the response of the respiratory center to the changes in blood gases and pH.

SPECIFIC CARDIAC DEFECTS

Tables 229-1, 229-2, and 229-3 list CHD malformations as complex, intermediate, or simple. The goal of these tables is to suggest when cardiology consultation or advanced CHD specialty care is needed. Patients with complex CHD (which includes most "named" surgeries that usually involve complex CHD) should virtually always be managed in conjunction with an experienced specialty adult CHD center. Intermediate lesions should have initial consultation and subsequent occasional intermittent follow-up with a cardiologist. Simple lesions may be managed by a well-informed internist, though consultation with a cardiologist is occasionally advisable.

ACYANOTIC CONGENITAL HEART DISEASE WITH A LEFT-TO-RIGHT SHUNT

Atrial Septal Defect This is a common cardiac anomaly that may be first encountered in the adult and occurs more frequently in females. The *sinus venosus* type occurs high in the atrial septum near the entry of the superior vena cava into the right atrium and is associated frequently with anomalous pulmonary venous connection from the right lung to the superior vena cava or right atrium. *Ostium primum* anomalies lie adjacent to the atrioventricular valves, either of which may be deformed and regurgitant. Ostium primum defects are common in Down's syndrome; the more complex atrioventricular septal defects with a common atrioventricular valve and a posterior defect of the

TABLE 229-2	INTERMEDIATE COMPLEXITY CONGENITAL HEART DISEASE

Ostium primum or sinus venosus atrial septal defect
Anomalous pulmonary venous drainage, partial or total
Atrioventricular canal defects (partial or complete)
Ventricular septal defect, complicated (e.g., absent or abnormal valves or with associated obstructive lesions, aortic regurgitation)
Coarctation of the aorta
Pulmonic valve stenosis (moderate to severe)
Infundibular right ventricular outflow obstruction of significance
Pulmonary valve regurgitation (moderate to severe)
Patent ductus arteriosus (non closed)—moderate to large
Sinus of Valsalva fistula/aneurysm
Subvalvular or supravalvular aortic stenosis

basal portion of the interventricular septum are more typical of this chromosomal defect. The most common *ostium secundum* type atrial septal defect involves the fossa ovalis and is midseptal in location. This type of defect should not be confused with a *patent foramen ovale*. Anatomic obliteration of the foramen ovale ordinarily follows its functional closure soon after birth, but residual "probe patency" is a normal variant; atrial septal defect denotes a true deficiency of the atrial septum and implies functional and anatomic patency.

The magnitude of the left-to-right shunt depends on the atrial septal defect size, ventricular diastolic properties, and the relative impedance in the pulmonary and systemic circulations. The left-to-right shunt causes diastolic overloading of the right ventricle and increased pulmonary blood flow.

Patients with atrial septal defect are usually asymptomatic in early life, although there may be some physical underdevelopment and an increased tendency for respiratory infections; cardiorespiratory symptoms occur in many older patients. Beyond the fourth decade, a significant number of patients develop atrial arrhythmias, pulmonary arterial hypertension, bidirectional and then right-to-left shunting of blood, and cardiac failure. Patients exposed to the chronic environmental hypoxia of high altitude tend to develop pulmonary hypertension at younger ages. In some older patients, left-to-right shunting across the defect increases as progressive systemic hypertension and/or coronary artery disease result in reduced compliance of the left ventricle.

PHYSICAL EXAMINATION Examination usually reveals a prominent RV impulse and palpable pulmonary artery pulsation. The first heart sound is normal or split, with accentuation of the tricuspid valve closure sound. Increased flow across the pulmonic valve is responsible for a midsystolic pulmonary outflow murmur. The second heart sound is widely split and is relatively fixed in relation to respiration. A mid-diastolic rumbling murmur, loudest at the fourth intercostal space and along the left sternal border, reflects increased flow across the tricuspid valve. In patients with ostium primum defects, an apical thrill and holosystolic murmur indicate associated mitral or tricuspid regurgitation or a ventricular septal defect.

The physical findings are altered when an increase in the pulmonary vascular resistance results in diminution of the left-to-right shunt. Both the pulmonary outflow and tricuspid inflow murmurs decrease in intensity, the pulmonic component of the second heart sound and a systolic ejection sound are accentuated, the two components of the second heart sound may fuse, and a diastolic murmur of pulmonic regurgitation appears. Cyanosis and clubbing accompany the development of a right-to-left shunt.

In adults with an atrial septal defect and atrial fibrillation, the physical findings may be confused with the findings of mitral stenosis with pulmonary hypertension because the tricuspid diastolic flow murmur and widely split second heart sound may be mistakenly thought to represent the diastolic murmur of mitral stenosis and the mitral "opening snap," respectively.

ELECTROCARDIOGRAM (ECG) In patients with an ostium secundum defect, the ECG usually shows right-axis deviation and an rSr′ pattern in the right precordial leads representing enlargement of the RV outflow tract. An ectopic atrial pacemaker or first-degree heart block may oc-

FIGURE 229-1 Secundum atrial septal defect. Transesophageal echocardiogram of secundum ASD and device closure. **A.** The atrial septal defect (ASD) between the left atrium (LA) and right atrium (RA) is shown. **B.** A percutaneous catheter–delivered device has occluded the defect. IVC, inferior vena cava; SVC, superior vena cava.

cur with defects of the sinus venous type. In ostium primum defect, the RV conduction defect is accompanied by left superior axis deviation and counterclockwise rotation of the frontal plane QRS loop. Varying degrees of RV and right atrial (RA) hypertrophy may occur with each type of defect, depending on the height of the pulmonary artery pressure. *Chest x-ray* reveals enlargement of the right atrium and right ventricle, dilatation of the pulmonary artery and its branches, and increased pulmonary vascular markings.

ECHOCARDIOGRAM Echocardiography reveals pulmonary arterial and RV and RA dilatation with abnormal (paradoxical) ventricular septal motion in the presence of a significant right heart volume overload. The atrial septal defect may be visualized directly by two-dimensional imaging, color flow imaging, or echocontrast. In most institutions, two-dimensional echocardiography plus color Doppler flow examination has supplanted cardiac catheterization. Transesophageal echocardiography is indicated if the transthoracic echocardiogram is ambiguous, which is often the case with sinus venosus defects, or during catheter device closure (**Fig. 229-1**). Cardiac catheterization is performed if inconsistencies exist in the clinical data, if significant pulmonary hypertension or associated malformations are suspected, or if coronary artery disease is a possibility.

℞ ATRIAL SEPTAL DEFECT

Operative repair, usually with a patch of pericardium or of prosthetic material, or percutaneous transcatheter device closure, if the defect is of an appropriate size and shape, should be advised for all patients with uncomplicated secundum atrial septal defects with significant left-to-right shunting, i.e., pulmonary-to-systemic flow ratios ≥2.0:1.0. Excellent results may be anticipated, at low risk, even in patients >40 years, in the absence of severe pulmonary hypertension. In ostium primum defects, cleft mitral valves may require repair in addition to patch closure of the atrial defect. Closure should not be carried out in patients with small defects and trivial left-to-right shunts or in those with severe pulmonary vascular disease without a significant left-to-right shunt.

Patients with atrial septal defect of the sinus venosus or ostium secundum types rarely die before the fifth decade. During the fifth and sixth decades, the incidence of progressive symptoms, often leading to severe disability, increases substantially. Medical management should include prompt treatment of respiratory tract infections, antiarrhythmic medications for atrial fibrillation or supraventricular tachycardia, and the usual measures for hypertension, coronary disease, or heart failure (Chap. 227), if these complications occur. The risk of infective endocarditis is quite low unless the defect is complicated by valvular regurgitation or has recently been repaired with a patch or device (Chap. 118).

Ventricular Septal Defect Defects of the ventricular septum are common as isolated defects or as a component of a combination of anomalies. The opening is usually single and situated in the membranous portion of the septum. The functional disturbance depends on its size and on the status of the pulmonary vascular bed. Only small or moderate-size defects are usually seen initially in adulthood as most patients with isolated large defects come to medical and, often, surgical attention early in life.

A wide spectrum exists in the natural history of ventricular septal defect, ranging from spontaneous closure to congestive cardiac failure and death in early infancy. Within this spectrum is the possible development of pulmonary vascular obstruction, RV outflow tract obstruction, aortic regurgitation, and infective endocarditis. Spontaneous closure is more common in patients born with a small ventricular septal defect and occurs in early childhood in most patients.

Patients with large ventricular septal defects and pulmonary hypertension are those at greatest risk for developing pulmonary vascular obstruction. Thus, large defects should be corrected surgically early in life when pulmonary vascular disease is still reversible or not yet developed. In patients with severe pulmonary vascular obstruction (Eisenmenger syndrome), symptoms in adult life consist of exertional dyspnea, chest pain, syncope, and hemoptysis. The right-to-left shunt leads to cyanosis, clubbing, and erythrocytosis. In all patients, the degree to which pulmonary vascular resistance is elevated before operation is a critical factor determining prognosis. If the pulmonary vascular resistance is one-third or less of the systemic value, progression of pulmonary vascular disease after operation is unusual. However, if a moderate to severe increase in pulmonary vascular resistance exists preoperatively, either no change or a progression of pulmonary vascular disease is common postoperatively.

RV outflow tract obstruction develops in ~5–10% of patients who present in infancy with a moderate to large left-to-right shunt. With time, as subvalvular RV outflow tract obstruction progresses, the findings in these patients whose VSD remains sizeable begin to resemble more closely those of the cyanotic tetralogy of Fallot.

In ~5% of patients, aortic valve regurgitation results from insufficient cusp tissue or prolapse of the cusp through the interventricular defect; the aortic regurgitation then complicates and dominates the clinical course.

Two-dimensional *echocardiography* with spectral and color Doppler examination defines the number and location of defects in the ventricular septum and associated anomalies and the hemodynamic physiology of the defect(s). Hemodynamic and angiographic study may be occasionally required to assess the status of the pulmonary vascular bed and clarify details of the altered anatomy.

℞ VENTRICULAR SEPTAL DEFECT

Surgery is not recommended for patients with normal pulmonary arterial pressures with small shunts (pulmonary-to-systemic flow ratios of <1.5 to 2.0:1.0). Operative correction or transcatheter closure is indicated when there is a moderate to large left-to-right shunt with a pulmonary-to-systemic flow ratio >1.5:1.0 or 2.0:1.0, in the absence of prohibitively high levels of pulmonary vascular resistance.

Patent Ductus Arteriosus The ductus arteriosus is a vessel leading from the bifurcation of the pulmonary artery to the aorta just distal to the left subclavian artery. Normally, the vascular channel is open in the fetus but closes immediately after birth. The flow across the ductus is determined by the pressure and resistance relationships between the systemic and pulmonary circulations and by the cross-sectional area and length of the ductus. In most adults with this anomaly, pulmonary pressures are normal and a gradient and shunt from aorta to pulmonary artery persist throughout the cardiac cycle, resulting in a characteristic thrill and a continuous "machinery" murmur with late systolic accentuation at the upper left sternal edge. In adults who were born with a large left-to-right shunt through the ductus arteriosus, pulmonary vascular obstruction (Eisenmenger syndrome) with pulmonary hypertension, right-to-left shunting, and cyanosis have usually developed. Severe pulmonary vascular disease results in reversal of flow through the ductus; unoxygenated blood is shunted to the descending aorta; and the toes, but not the fingers, become cyanotic and clubbed, a finding termed *differential cyanosis*. The leading causes of death in adults with patent ductus are cardiac failure and infective endocarditis; occasionally severe pulmonary vascular obstruction may cause aneurysmal dilatation, calcification, and rupture of the ductus.

℞ PATENT DUCTUS ARTERIOSUS

In the absence of severe pulmonary vascular disease and predominant left-to-right shunting of blood, the patent ductus should be surgically ligated or divided. Transcatheter closure using coils, buttons, plugs, and umbrellas has become commonplace for appropriately shaped defects. Thoracoscopic surgical approaches are considered experimental. Operation should be deferred for several months in patients treated successfully for infective endocarditis because the ductus may remain somewhat edematous and friable.

Aortic Root to Right Heart Shunts The three most common causes of aortic root to right heart shunts are congenital aneurysm of an aortic sinus of Valsalva with fistula, coronary arteriovenous fistula, and anomalous origin of the left coronary artery from the pulmonary trunk. *Aneurysm of an aortic sinus of Valsalva* consists of a separation or lack of fusion between the media of the aorta and the annulus of the aortic valve. Rupture usually occurs in the third or fourth decade of life; most often the aorticocardiac fistula is between the right coronary cusp and the right ventricle, but occasionally, when the noncoronary cusp is involved, the fistula drains into the right atrium. Abrupt rupture causes chest pain, bounding pulses, a continuous murmur accen-

tuated in diastole, and volume overload of the heart. Diagnosis is confirmed by two-dimensional and Doppler echocardiographic studies; cardiac catheterization quantitates the left-to-right shunt, and thoracic aortography visualizes the fistula. Medical management is directed at cardiac failure, arrhythmias, or endocarditis. At operation, the aneurysm is closed and amputated, and the aortic wall is reunited with the heart, either by direct suture or with a patch or prosthesis.

Coronary arteriovenous fistula, an unusual anomaly, consists of a communication between a coronary artery and another cardiac chamber, usually the coronary sinus, right atrium, or right ventricle. The shunt is usually of small magnitude and myocardial blood flow is not usually compromised; if the shunt is large, there may be a coronary "steal" syndrome with myocardial ischemia and possible angina or ventricular arrhythmias. Potential complications include infective endocarditis, thrombus formation with occlusion or distal embolization with myocardial infarction, rupture of an aneurysmal fistula, and, rarely, pulmonary hypertension and congestive failure. A loud, superficial, continuous murmur at the lower or midsternal border usually prompts a further evaluation of asymptomatic patients. Doppler echocardiography demonstrates the site of drainage; if the site of origin is proximal, it may be detectable by two-dimensional echocardiography. Angiography (classic catheterization, CT, or magnetic resonance angiography) permits identification of the size and anatomic features of the fistulous tract, which may be closed by suture or transcatheter obliteration.

The third anomaly causing a shunt from the aortic root to the right heart is *anomalous origin of the left coronary artery from the pulmonary artery*. Myocardial infarction and fibrosis commonly lead to death within the first year, although up to 20% of patients survive to adolescence and beyond without surgical correction. The diagnosis is supported by the ECG findings of an anterolateral myocardial infarction and LVH. Operative management of adults consists of coronary artery bypass with an internal mammary artery graft or saphenous vein–coronary artery graft.

ACYANOTIC CONGENITAL HEART DISEASE WITHOUT A SHUNT

Congenital Aortic Stenosis Malformations that cause obstruction to LV outflow include congenital valvular aortic stenosis, discrete subaortic stenosis, supravalvular aortic stenosis, and hypertrophic obstructive cardiomyopathy (Chap. 231).

VALVULAR AORTIC STENOSIS Bicuspid aortic valves are more common in males than in females. The congenital bicuspid aortic valve, which may initially be functionally normal, is one of the most common congenital malformations of the heart and may go undetected in early life. Because bicuspid valves may develop stenosis or regurgitation with time or be the site of infective endocarditis, the lesion may be difficult to distinguish in older adults from acquired rheumatic or degenerative calcific aortic valve disease. The dynamics of blood flow associated with a congenitally deformed, rigid aortic valve commonly lead to thickening of the cusps and, in later life, to calcification. Hemodynamically significant obstruction causes concentric hypertrophy of the LV wall. The ascending aorta is often dilated, misnamed "poststenotic" dilatation; this is due to histologic abnormalities of the aortic media similar to those in Marfan syndrome, and may result in aortic dissection. Diagnosis is best made by echocardiography, which can reveal the morphology of the aortic valve and aortic root and quantitate the degree of stenosis or regurgitation. The clinical manifestations and hemodynamic abnormalities are discussed in Chap. 230.

℞ VALVULAR AORTIC STENOSIS

The medical management of congenital valvular aortic stenosis includes prophylaxis against infective endocarditis and, in patients with diminished cardiac reserve, the administration of digoxin and diuretics and sodium restriction while awaiting operation. A dilated aortic root may require beta blockers. If severe aortic stenosis is present, strenuous physical activity should be avoided even when the patient is asymptomatic, and participation in competitive sports should probably be restricted in patients with milder degrees of obstruction. Aortic valve replacement is indicated in adults with critical obstruction, i.e., with an aortic valve area <0.45 cm^2/m^2, with symptoms secondary to LV dysfunction or myocardial ischemia, or with hemodynamic evidence of LV dysfunction. In asymptomatic children or adolescents or young adults with critical aortic stenosis without valvular calcification or these features, aortic balloon valvuloplasty is often useful (Chap. 240). If surgery is contraindicated in older patients because of a complicating medical problem such as malignancy or renal or hepatic failure, balloon valvuloplasty may provide short-term improvement. This procedure may serve as a bridge to aortic valve replacement in patients with severe heart failure.

SUBAORTIC STENOSIS The most common form of subaortic stenosis is the *idiopathic hypertrophic* variety, also termed *hypertrophic cardiomyopathy*, which is present at birth in about one-third of the patients and is discussed in Chap. 231. The *discrete* form of subaortic stenosis consists of a membranous diaphragm or fibromuscular ring encircling the LV outflow tract just beneath the base of the aortic valve. The jet impact from the subaortic stenotic jet on the underside of the aortic valve often begets progressive aortic valve fibrosis and valvular regurgitation. Echocardiography demonstrates the anatomy of the subaortic obstruction; Doppler studies show turbulence proximal to the aortic valve and can quantitate the pressure gradient and severity of aortic regurgitation. Treatment consists of complete excision of the membrane or fibromuscular ring.

SUPRAVALVULAR AORTIC STENOSIS This anomaly consists of a localized or diffuse narrowing of the ascending aorta originating just above the level of the coronary arteries at the superior margin of the sinuses of Valsalva. In contrast to other forms of aortic stenosis, the coronary arteries are subjected to elevated systolic pressures from the left ventricle, are often dilated and tortuous, and are susceptible to premature atherosclerosis. In most patients, a genetic defect for the anomaly is located in the same chromosomal region as elastin on chromosome 7.

Coarctation of the Aorta Narrowing or constriction of the lumen of the aorta may occur anywhere along its length but is most common distal to the origin of the left subclavian artery near the insertion of the ligamentum arteriosum. Coarctation occurs in ~7% of patients with congenital heart disease, is more common in males than females, and is particularly frequent in patients with gonadal dysgenesis (e.g., Turner syndrome). Clinical manifestations depend on the site and extent of obstruction and the presence of associated cardiac anomalies, most commonly a bicuspid aortic valve. Circle of Willis aneurysms may occur in up to 10% and pose a high risk of sudden rupture and death.

Most children and young adults with isolated, discrete coarctation are asymptomatic. Headache, epistaxis, cold extremities, and claudication with exercise may occur, and attention is usually directed to the cardiovascular system when a heart murmur or hypertension in the upper extremities and absence, marked diminution, or delayed pulsations in the femoral arteries are detected on physical examination. Enlarged and pulsatile collateral vessels may be palpated in the intercostal spaces anteriorly, in the axillae, or posteriorly in the interscapular area. The upper extremities and thorax may be more developed than the lower extremities. A midsystolic murmur over the left interscapular space may become continuous if the lumen is narrowed sufficiently to result in a high-velocity jet across the lesion throughout the cardiac cycle. Additional systolic and continuous murmurs over the lateral thoracic wall may reflect increased flow through dilated and tortuous collateral vessels. The ECG usually reveals LV hypertrophy. Chest x-ray may show a dilated left subclavian artery high on the left mediastinal border and a dilated ascending aorta. Indentation of the aorta at the site of coarctation and pre- and poststenotic dilatation (the "3" sign) along the left paramediastinal shadow are almost pathognomonic. Notching of the 3rd to 9th ribs, an important radiographic sign, is due to inferior rib erosion by dilated collateral vessels (**Figs. 229-2** and **229-3**). Two-dimensional echocardiography from para- or suprasternal windows identifies the site and length of coarctation, while Doppler quantitates the pressure gradient. Transesophageal echocardiography and MRI or

FIGURE 229-2 Aortic coarctation. The extensive collaterals (*left*) underneath the ribs and in the periscapular region are shown on a posterior view of a three-dimensional CT angiogram, which are responsible for rib notching on chest x-ray. dao, descending aorta.

three-dimensional CT allow visualization of the length and severity of the obstruction and the associated collateral arteries (Figs. 229-2 and 229-3). In adults, cardiac catheterization is indicated primarily to evaluate the coronary arteries or to perform catheter based intervention (angioplasty and stent of the coarctation).

The chief hazards of proximal aortic severe hypertension include cerebral aneurysms and hemorrhage, aortic dissection and rupture, premature coronary arteriosclerosis, and LV failure; infective endarteritis may occur on the coarctation site or endocarditis may settle on an associated bicuspid aortic valve.

℞ COARCTATION OF THE AORTA

Treatment is usually surgical, although percutaneous catheter balloon with stent dilatation is now a viable option for many patients. Late postopera-

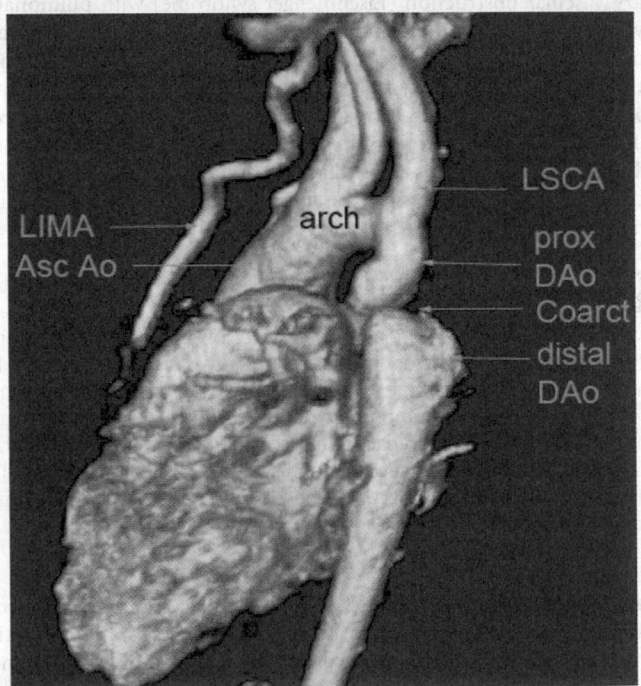

FIGURE 229-3 Aortic coarctation. The coarctation (Coarct) of the aorta is shown in the typical "adult" location in the descending aorta (DAo) just distal to the dilated left subclavian artery (LSCA) in this three-dimensional reconstruction of an MR angiogram. There is a post-coarct aneurysm that is in part due to intrinsic aortic medial tissue weakness. The left internal mammary artery (LIMA) is dilated. Asc Ao, ascending aorta; prox, proximal.

tive systemic hypertension in the absence of residual coarctation appears to be related to the duration of preoperative hypertension. Follow-up of rest and exercise blood pressures is important; in many only excessive systolic hypertension is seen during exercise, in part due to a diffuse vasculopathy. All operated or stented coarctation patients deserve a high-quality MRI or CT imaging procedure in follow-up.

Pulmonary Stenosis with Intact Ventricular Septum Obstruction to RV outflow may be localized to the supravalvular, valvular, or subvalvular levels or occur at a combination of these sites. Multiple sites of narrowing of the peripheral pulmonary arteries are a feature of *rubella embryopathy* and may occur with both the familial and sporadic forms of supravalvular aortic stenosis. Valvular pulmonic stenosis is the most common form of isolated RV obstruction.

The severity of the obstructing lesion, rather than the site of narrowing, is the most important determinant of the clinical course. In the presence of a normal cardiac output, a peak systolic transvalvular pressure gradient between 50 and 80 mmHg is considered to be moderate stenosis; levels below and above that range are classified as mild and severe, respectively. Patients with mild pulmonic stenosis are generally asymptomatic and demonstrate little or no progression in the severity of obstruction with age. In patients with more significant stenosis, the severity may increase with time. Symptoms vary with the degree of obstruction. Fatigue, dyspnea, RV failure, and syncope may limit the activity of older patients, in whom moderate or severe obstruction may prevent an augmentation of cardiac output with exercise. In patients with severe obstruction, the systolic pressure in the right ventricle may exceed that in the left ventricle, since the ventricular septum is intact. RV ejection is prolonged with moderate or severe stenosis, and the sound of pulmonary valve closure is delayed and soft. RV hypertrophy reduces the compliance of that chamber, and a forceful RA contraction is necessary to augment RV filling.

A fourth heart sound, prominent *a* waves in the jugular venous pulse, and, occasionally, presystolic pulsations of the liver reflect vigorous atrial contraction. The clinical diagnosis is supported by a left parasternal lift and harsh systolic crescendo-decrescendo murmur and thrill at the upper left sternal border, typically preceded by a systolic ejection sound if the obstruction is due to a mobile nondysplastic pulmonary valve. The holosystolic murmur of tricuspid regurgitation may accompany severe pulmonic stenosis, especially in the presence of congestive heart failure. Cyanosis usually reflects right-to-left shunting through a patent foramen ovale or atrial septal defect. In patients with supravalvular or peripheral pulmonary arterial stenosis, the murmur is systolic or continuous and is best heard over the area of narrowing, with radiation to the peripheral lung fields.

In mild cases, the ECG is normal, whereas moderate and severe stenoses are associated with RV hypertrophy. The chest x-ray with mild or moderate pulmonic stenosis shows a heart of normal size with normal lung vascularity. In pulmonary valvular stenosis, dilatation of the main and left pulmonary arteries occurs in part due to the direction of the PS jet and in part due to intrinsic tissue weakness. With severe obstruction, RV hypertrophy is generally evident. The pulmonary vascularity may be reduced with severe stenosis, RV failure, and/or a right-to-left shunt at the atrial level. Two-dimensional echocardiography visualizes pulmonary valve morphology; the outflow tract pressure gradient can be quantitated by Doppler echocardiography.

℞ PULMONARY STENOSIS

The cardiac catheter technique of balloon valvuloplasty (Chap. 223) is usually effective. Direct surgical relief of moderate and severe obstruction may be accomplished at a low risk. Multiple stenoses of the peripheral pulmonary arteries are usually inoperable, but narrowing of a proximal branch or at the bifurcation of the main pulmonary trunk may be surgically corrected or undergo balloon dilatation and stenting.

FIGURE 229-4 Tetralogy of Fallot. Magnetic resonance imaging angiogram. A mid-systolic frame showing the malaligned ventricular septal defect (VSD) with the aorta overriding the ventricular septal defect. LV, left ventricle; RVH, RV hypertrophy; VS, ventricular septum.

COMPLEX CONGENITAL HEART LESIONS
Tetralogy of Fallot The four components of the tetralogy of Fallot are malaligned ventricular septal defect, obstruction to RV outflow, aortic override of the ventricular septal defect, and RV hypertrophy due to the RV "seeing" aortic pressure via the large VSD (Fig. 229-4).

The severity of RV outflow obstruction determines the clinical presentation. The severity of hypoplasia of the RV outflow tract varies from mild to complete (pulmonary atresia). Pulmonary valve stenosis and supravalvular and peripheral pulmonary arterial obstruction may coexist; rarely there is unilateral absence of a pulmonary artery (usually the left). A right-sided aortic arch and descending thoracic aorta occur in ~25% of patients with tetralogy.

The relationship between the resistance of blood flow from the ventricles into the aorta and into the pulmonary vessels plays a major role in determining the hemodynamic and clinical picture. When the obstruction is severe, the pulmonary blood flow is reduced markedly, and a large volume of desaturated systemic venous blood is shunted from right to left across the ventricular septal defect. Severe cyanosis and erythrocytosis occur, and symptoms of systemic hypoxemia are prominent. In many infants and children the obstruction is mild but progressive.

The ECG shows RV hypertrophy. Chest x-ray shows a normal-sized, boot-shaped heart (*coeur en sabot*) with a prominent right ventricle and a concavity in the region of the pulmonary conus. Pulmonary vascular markings are typically diminished, and the aortic arch and knob may be on the right side. Two-dimensional echocardiography demonstrates the malaligned ventricular septal defect with the overriding aorta and the site and severity of pulmonary stenosis, which may be subpulmonic (fixed or dynamic), at the pulmonary valve or in the main or branch pulmonary arteries. Classic contrast angiography may provide details regarding the RV outflow tract, pulmonary valve and annulus, and caliber of the main branches of the pulmonary artery as well of possible associated aortopulmonary collaterals. Coronary arteriography identifies the anatomy and course of the coronary arteries. In experienced centers, these issues are often well demonstrated in adults by MR (Fig. 229-4) or CT angiography with 3-dimensional reconstruction.

℞ TETRALOGY OF FALLOT

For a variety of reasons, only a few adults with tetralogy of Fallot have not had some form of previous surgical intervention. Reoperation in adults is most commonly for severe pulmonary regurgitation. Long-term concerns about ventricular function persist. Ventricular and atrial arrhythmias may require medical treatment or electrophysiologic study and ablation. Interventional catheterization may be needed in selected patients (i.e., angioplasty and stenting of branch pulmonary stenosis). The aortic root has a medial tissue defect; it is commonly enlarged and associated with aortic regurgitation. Endocarditis remains a risk despite surgical repair.

Complete Transposition of the Great Arteries This condition is commonly called *dextro-* or *D-transposition of the great arteries*. The aorta arises rightward anteriorly from the right ventricle, and the pulmonary artery emerges leftward and posteriorly from the left ventricle, which results in two separate parallel circulations; some communication between them must exist after birth to sustain life. Most patients have an interatrial communication, two-thirds have a patent ductus arteriosus, and about one-third have an associated ventricular septal defect. Transposition is more common in males and accounts for ~10% of cyanotic heart disease.

The course is determined by the degree of tissue hypoxia, the ability of each ventricle to sustain an increased work load in the presence of reduced coronary arterial oxygenation, the nature of the associated cardiovascular anomalies, and the status of the pulmonary vascular bed. By the third decade of life, ~30% of patients will have developed decreased RV function and progressive tricuspid regurgitation, which may lead to congestive heart failure. Pulmonary vascular obstruction develops by 1 to 2 years of age in patients with an associated large ventricular septal defect or large patent ductus arteriosus in the absence of obstruction to LV outflow.

℞ TRANSPOSITION OF THE GREAT ARTERIES

The balloon or blade catheter or surgical creation or enlargement of an interatrial communication in the neonate is the simplest procedure for providing increased intracardiac mixing of systemic and pulmonary venous blood. Systemic–pulmonary artery anastomosis may be indicated in the patient with severe obstruction to LV outflow and diminished pulmonary blood flow. Intracardiac repair may be accomplished by rearranging the venous returns (intraatrial switch, i.e., Mustard or Senning operation) so that the systemic venous blood is directed to the mitral valve and thence to the left ventricle and pulmonary artery, while the pulmonary venous blood is diverted through the tricuspid valve and right ventricle to the aorta. The late survival after these repairs is good, but arrhythmias (e.g., atrial flutter) or conduction defects (e.g., sick sinus syndrome) occur in ~50% of such patients by 30 years after the intraatrial switch surgery. Progressive dysfunction of the systemic subaortic right ventricle, tricuspid regurgitation, ventricular arrhythmias or cardiac arrest and late sudden death are worrisome features. Preferably this malformation is corrected in infancy by transposing both coronary arteries to the posterior artery and transecting, contraposing, and anastomosing the aorta and pulmonary arteries (arterial switch operation). For those patients with a ventricular septal defect in whom it is necessary to bypass a severely obstructed LV outflow tract, corrective operation employs an intracardiac ventricular baffle and extracardiac prosthetic conduit to replace the pulmonary artery (Rastelli procedure).

Single Ventricle This is a family of complex lesions with both atrioventricular valves or a common atrioventricular valve opening to a single ventricular chamber. Associated anomalies include abnormal great artery positional relationships, pulmonic valvular or subvalvular stenosis, and subaortic stenosis.

Survival to adulthood depends on a relatively normal pulmonary blood flow, yet normal pulmonary resistance, and good ventricular function. Modifications of the Fontan approach are generally applied to carefully selected patients with creation of a pathway(s) from the systemic veins to the pulmonary arteries.

Tricuspid Atresia This malformation is characterized by atresia of the tricuspid valve, an interatrial communication, and, frequently, hypoplasia of the right ventricle and pulmonary artery. The clinical picture is usually dominated by severe cyanosis due to obligatory admixture of systemic and pulmonary venous blood in the left ventricle. The ECG characteristically shows RA enlargement, left-axis deviation, and LV hypertrophy.

Atrial septostomy and palliative operations to increase pulmonary blood flow, often by anastomosis of a systemic artery or vein to a pulmonary artery, may allow survival to the second or third decade. A Fontan atriopulmonary or total cavopulmonary connection may then allow functional correction in those patients with normal or low pulmonary arterial resistance pressure and good LV function.

Ebstein Anomaly Characterized by a downward displacement of the tricuspid valve into the right ventricle, due to anomalous attachment of the tricuspid leaflets, the Ebstein tricuspid valve tissue is dysplastic and results in tricuspid regurgitation. The abnormally situated tricuspid orifice produces an "atrialized" portion of the right ventricle lying between the atrioventricular ring and the origin of the valve, which is continuous with the RA chamber. Often the right ventricle is hypoplastic. Although the clinical manifestations are variable, some patients come to initial attention because of either (1) progressive cyanosis from right-to-left atrial shunting, (2) symptoms due to tricuspid regurgitation and RV dysfunction, or (3) paroxysmal atrial tachyarrhythmias with or without atrioventricular bypass tracts ("WPW" syndrome). Diagnostic findings by two-dimensional echocardiography include the abnormal positional relation between the tricuspid and mitral valves with abnormally increased apical displacement of the septal tricuspid leaflet. Tricuspid regurgitation is quantitated by Doppler examination. Surgical approaches include prosthetic replacement of the tricuspid valve when the leaflets are tethered or repair of the native valve.

Congenitally Corrected Transposition The two fundamental anatomic abnormalities in this malformation are transposition of the ascending aorta and pulmonary trunk and inversion of the ventricles. This arrangement results in desaturated systemic venous blood passing from the right atrium through the mitral valve to the left ventricle and into the pulmonary trunk, whereas oxygenated pulmonary venous blood flows from the left atrium through the tricuspid valve to the right ventricle and into the aorta. Thus, the circulation is corrected functionally. The clinical presentation, course, and prognosis of patients with congenitally corrected transposition vary depending on the nature and severity of any complicating intracardiac anomalies and of development of dysfunction of the systemic subaortic RV. Progressive RV dysfunction and tricuspid regurgitation may also develop in a third of patients by age 30; Ebstein-type anomalies of the left-side tricuspid atrioventricular valve are common. Ventricular septal defect or "pulmonary stenosis" due to obstruction to outflow from the right-sided subpulmonary (anatomic left) ventricle may coexist. Complete heart block occurs at a rate of 2–10% per decade. The diagnosis of the malformation and associated lesions can be established by comprehensive two-dimensional echocardiography and Doppler examination.

Malpositions of the Heart Positional anomalies refer to conditions in which the cardiac apex is in the right side of the chest (*dextrocardia*), or at the midline (*mesocardia*), or in which there is a normal location of the heart in the left side of the chest but abnormal position of the viscera (*isolated levocardia*). Knowledge of the position of the abdominal organs and of the branching pattern of the main stem bronchi is important in categorizing these malpositions. When dextrocardia occurs without situs inversus, when the visceral situs is indeterminate, or if isolated levocardia is present, associated, often complex, multiple cardiac anomalies are usually present. In contrast, mirror-image dextrocardia is usually observed with complete situs inversus, which occurs most frequently in individuals whose hearts are otherwise normal.

SURGICALLY MODIFIED CONGENITAL HEART DISEASE

Because of the enormous strides in cardiovascular surgical techniques that have occurred in the past 50 years, a large number of long-term survivors of corrective operations in infancy and childhood have reached adulthood. These patients are often challenging because of the diversity of anatomic, hemodynamic, and electrophysiologic residua and sequelae of cardiac operations.

The proper care of the survivor of operation for CHD requires that the clinician understand the details of the malformation before operation; pay meticulous attention to the details of the operative procedure; and recognize the postoperative residua (conditions left totally or partially uncorrected), the sequelae (conditions caused by surgery), and the complications that may have resulted from the operation. With the exception of ligation and division of an uncomplicated patent ductus arteriosus, almost every other surgical repair of an anomaly leaves behind or causes some abnormality of the heart and circulation that may range from trivial to serious. Intraoperative transesophageal echocardiography assists in detecting unsuspected lesions, in monitoring the repair, and in verifying a satisfactory result or directing further repair. Thus, even with results that are considered clinically to be good to excellent, continued long-term postoperative follow-up is advisable.

Cardiac operations importantly involving the atria, such as closure of atrial septal defect, repair of total or partial anomalous pulmonary venous return, or venous switch corrections of complete transposition of the great arteries (the Mustard or Senning operations), may be followed years later by sinus node or atrioventricular node dysfunction or by atrial arrhythmias (especially atrial flutter). Intraventricular surgery may also result in electrophysiologic consequences, including complete heart block necessitating pacemaker insertion to avoid sudden death. In addition, valvular problems may arise late after initial cardiac operation. An example is the progressive stenosis of an initially nonobstructive bicuspid aortic valve in the patient who underwent aortic coarctation repair. Such aortic valves may also be the site of infective endocarditis. After repair of the ostium primum atrial septal defect, the cleft mitral valve may become progressively regurgitant. Tricuspid regurgitation may also be progressive in the postoperative patient with tetralogy of Fallot if RV outflow tract obstruction was not relieved adequately at initial surgery. In many patients with surgically modified CHD, inadequate relief of an obstructive lesion, or a residual regurgitant lesion, or a residual shunt will cause or hasten the onset of clinical signs and symptoms of myocardial dysfunction. Despite a good hemodynamic repair, many patients with a subaortic right ventricle develop RV decompensation and signs of "left heart failure." In many patients, particularly those who were cyanotic for many years before operation, a preexisting compromise in ventricular performance is due to the original underlying malformation.

A final category of postoperative problems involves the use of prosthetic valves, patches, or conduits in the operative repair. The special risks include infective endocarditis, thrombus formation, and premature degeneration and calcification of the prosthetic materials. There are many patients in whom extracardiac conduits are required to correct the circulation functionally and often to carry blood to the lungs from the right atrium or right ventricle. These conduits may develop intraluminal obstruction, and, if they include a prosthetic valve, it may show progressive calcification and thickening.

FURTHER READINGS

ATTIE F et al: Surgical treatment for secundum atrial septal defects in patients >40 years old. A randomized clinical trial. J Am Coll Cardiol 38:2035, 2001

BASHORE T: Adult congenital heart disease: Right ventricular outflow tract lesions. Circulation 115:1933, 2007

CHILD JS: Transthoracic and transesophageal echocardiographic imaging: Anatomic and hemodynamic assessment, in *Congenital Heart Disease in Adults*, 2d ed, JK Perloff, JS Child (eds), Philadelphia, Saunders, 1998

FEDAK PWM et al: Clinical and pathophysiological implications of a bicuspid aortic valve. Circulation 106:900, 2002

LEWIN MB, OTTO CM: The bicuspid aortic valve: Adverse outcomes from infancy to old age. Circulation 111:832, 2005

MARSHALL AC, LOCK JE: Leaving neverland: A randomized trial for coarctation shows pediatric interventional cardiology is growing up. Circulation 111:3347, 2005

SALEHIAN O et al: Improvements in cardiac form and function after transcatheter closure of secundum atrial septal defects. J Am Coll Cardiol 45:499, 2005

WARNES CA: The adult with congenital heart disease: born to be bad? J Am Coll Cardiol 46:1, 2005

————: Bicuspid aortic valve and coarctation: Two villains part of a diffuse problem. Heart 89:965, 2003

WEBB G et al: Congenital heart disease, in: *Braunwald's Heart Disease: A Textbook of Cardiovascular Medicine*, 7th ed, Zipes D et al (eds), Philadelphia, Elsevier Saunders, 2005

WU JC, CHILD JS: Common congenital heart disorders in adults. Curr Probl Cardiol 29:641, 2004

230 Valvular Heart Disease
Patrick O'Gara, Eugene Braunwald

The role of the physical examination in the evaluation of patients with valvular heart disease is also considered in **Chaps. e8** and 220; of electrocardiography (ECG) in Chap. 221; of echocardiography and other noninvasive imaging techniques in Chap. 222; and of cardiac catheterization and angiography in Chap. 223.

MITRAL STENOSIS

ETIOLOGY AND PATHOLOGY

Rheumatic fever is the leading cause of mitral stenosis (MS) (Table 230-1). Other less common etiologies of obstruction to left atrial outflow include congenital mitral valve stenosis, cor triatriatum, mitral annular calcification with extension onto the leaflets, systemic lupus erythematosus, rheumatoid arthritis, left atrial myxoma, and infective endocarditis with large vegetations. Pure or predominant MS occurs in approximately 40% of all patients with rheumatic heart disease and a history of rheumatic fever (Chap. 315). In other patients with rheumatic heart disease, lesser degrees of MS may accompany mitral regurgitation (MR) and aortic valve disease. With reductions in the incidence of acute

rheumatic fever, particularly in temperate climates and developed countries, the incidence of MS has declined considerably over the past few decades. However, it remains a major problem in developing nations, especially in tropical and semitropical climates (see p. 1480).

In rheumatic MS, the valve leaflets are diffusely thickened by fibrous tissue and/or calcific deposits. The mitral commissures fuse, the chordae tendineae fuse and shorten, the valvular cusps become rigid, and these changes, in turn, lead to narrowing at the apex of the funnel-shaped ("fish-mouth") valve. Although the initial insult to the mitral valve is rheumatic, the later changes may be a nonspecific process resulting from trauma to the valve caused by altered flow patterns due to the initial deformity. Calcification of the stenotic mitral valve immobilizes the leaflets and narrows the orifice further. Thrombus formation and arterial embolization may arise from the calcific valve itself, but in patients with atrial fibrillation (AF), thrombi arise more frequently from the dilated left atrium (LA), particularly the left atrial appendage.

PATHOPHYSIOLOGY

In normal adults, the area of the mitral valve orifice is 4–6 cm^2. In the presence of significant obstruction, i.e., when the orifice area is reduced to < ~2 cm^2, blood can flow from the LA to the left ventricle (LV) only if propelled by an abnormally elevated left atrioventricular pressure gradient (see Fig. 223-2), the hemodynamic hallmark of MS. When the mitral valve opening is reduced to <1 cm^2, often referred to

TABLE 230-1 **MAJOR CAUSES OF VALVULAR HEART DISEASES**

Valve Lesion	Etiologies
Mitral stenosis	Rheumatic fever
	Congenital
	Severe mitral annular calcification
	SLE, RA
Mitral regurgitation	Acute
	Endocarditis
	Papillary muscle rupture (post-MI)
	Trauma
	Chordal rupture/Leaflet flail (MVP, IE)
	Chronic
	Myxomatous (MVP)
	Rheumatic fever
	Endocarditis (healed)
	Mitral annular calcification
	Congenital (cleft, AV canal)
	HOCM with SAM
	Ischemic (LV remodeling)
	Dilated cardiomyopathy
Aortic atenosis	Congenital (bicuspid, unicuspid)
	Degenerative calcific
	Rheumatic fever
Aortic regurgitation	Valvular
	Congenital (bicuspid)
	Endocarditis
	Rheumatic fever
	Myxomatous (prolapse)
	Traumatic
	Syphilis
	Ankylosing spondylitis
	Root disease
	Aortic dissection
	Cystic medial degeneration
	Marfan syndrome
	Bicuspid aortic valve
	Nonsyndromic familial aneurysm
	Aortitis
	Hypertension
Tricuspid stenosis	Rheumatic
	Congenital
Tricuspid regurgitation	Primary
	Rheumatic
	Endocarditis
	Myxomatous (TVP)
	Carcinoid
	Congenital (Ebstein's)
	Trauma
	Papillary muscle injury (post-MI)
	Secondary
	RV and tricuspid annular dilatation
	Multiple causes of RV enlargement (e.g.,
	long-standing pulmonary HTN)
	Chronic RV apical pacing
Pulmonic stenosis	Congenital
	Carcinoid
Pulmonic regurgitation	Valve disease
	Congenital
	Postvalvotomy
	Endocarditis
	Annular enlargement
	Pulmonary hypertension
	Idiopathic dilatation
	Marfan syndrome

Note: AV, atrioventricular; HOCM, hypertrophic obstructive cardiomyopathy; HTN, hypertension; IE, infective endocarditis; LV, left ventricular; MI, myocardial infarction; MVP, mitral valve prolapse; RA, rheumatoid arthritis; RV, right ventricular; SAM, systolic anterior motion of the anterior mitral valve leaflet; SLE, systemic lupus erythematosus; TVP, tricuspid valve prolapse.

as "severe" MS, a LA pressure of ~25 mmHg is required to maintain a normal cardiac output (CO). The elevated pulmonary venous and pulmonary arterial (PA) wedge pressures reduce pulmonary compliance, contributing to exertional dyspnea. The first bouts of dyspnea are usually precipitated by clinical events that increase the rate of blood flow across the mitral orifice, resulting in further elevation of the LA pressure (see below).

To assess the severity of obstruction hemodynamically, both the transvalvular pressure gradient and the flow rate must be measured (Chap. 223). The latter depends not only on the CO but on the heart rate as well. An increase in heart rate shortens diastole proportionately more than systole and diminishes the time available for flow across the mitral valve. Therefore, at any given level of CO, tachycardia including that associated with AF augments the transvalvular pressure gradient and elevates further the LA pressure. Similar considerations apply to the pathophysiology of tricuspid stenosis.

The LV diastolic pressure and ejection fraction (EF) are normal in isolated MS. In MS and sinus rhythm, the elevated LA and PA wedge pressures exhibit a prominent atrial contraction (a wave) and a gradual pressure decline after mitral valve opening (y descent) (see Fig. 223-2). In severe MS and whenever pulmonary vascular resistance is significantly increased, the pulmonary arterial pressure (PAP) is elevated at rest and rises further during exercise, often causing secondary elevations of right ventricular (RV) end-diastolic pressure and volume.

Cardiac Output In patients with moderate MS (mitral valve orifice 1.0 cm^2–1.5 cm^2), the CO is normal or almost so at rest but rises subnormally during exertion. In patients with severe MS (valve area <1.0 cm^2), particularly those in whom pulmonary vascular resistance is markedly elevated, the CO is subnormal at rest and may fail to rise or may even decline during activity.

Pulmonary Hypertension The clinical and hemodynamic features of MS are influenced importantly by the level of the PAP. Pulmonary hypertension results from: (1) passive backward transmission of the elevated LA pressure; (2) pulmonary arteriolar constriction, which presumably is triggered by LA and pulmonary venous hypertension (reactive pulmonary hypertension); (3) interstitial edema in the walls of the small pulmonary vessels; and (4) organic obliterative changes in the pulmonary vascular bed. Severe pulmonary hypertension results in RV enlargement, secondary tricuspid regurgitation (TR) and pulmonic regurgitation (PR), as well as right-sided heart failure.

SYMPTOMS

In temperate climates, the latent period between the initial attack of rheumatic carditis (in the increasingly rare circumstances in which a history of one can be elicited) and the development of symptoms due to MS is generally about two decades; most patients begin to experience disability in the fourth decade of life. Studies carried out before the development of mitral valvotomy revealed that once a patient with MS became seriously symptomatic, the disease progressed continuously to death within 2–5 years.

In patients whose mitral orifices are large enough to accommodate a normal blood flow with only mild elevations of LA pressure, marked elevations of this pressure leading to dyspnea and cough may be precipitated by sudden changes in the heart rate, volume status, or CO, as for example with severe exertion, excitement, fever, severe anemia, paroxysmal AF and other tachycardias, sexual intercourse, pregnancy, and thyrotoxicosis. As MS progresses, lesser stresses precipitate dyspnea, and the patient becomes limited in daily activities, and orthopnea and paroxysmal nocturnal dyspnea develop. The development of permanent AF often marks a turning point in the patient's course and is generally associated with acceleration of the rate at which symptoms progress.

Hemoptysis (Chap. 34) results from rupture of pulmonary-bronchial venous connections secondary to pulmonary venous hypertension. It occurs most frequently in patients who have elevated LA pressures without markedly elevated pulmonary vascular resistances and is almost never fatal. *Recurrent pulmonary emboli* (Chap. 256), sometimes with infarction, are an important cause of morbidity and mortality late in the course of MS. *Pulmonary infections*, i.e., bronchitis, bronchopneumonia, and lobar pneumonia, commonly complicate untreated MS, especially during the winter months. *Infective endocarditis* (Chap. 118) is rare in isolated MS.

Pulmonary Changes In addition to the aforementioned changes in the pulmonary vascular bed, fibrous thickening of the walls of the alveoli and pulmonary capillaries occurs commonly in MS. The vital capacity, total lung capacity, maximal breathing capacity, and oxygen uptake per unit of ventilation are reduced (Chap. 246). Pulmonary compliance falls further as pulmonary capillary pressure rises during exercise.

Thrombi and Emboli *Thrombi* may form in the left atria, particularly in the enlarged atrial appendages of patients with MS. Systemic embolization, the incidence of which is 10–20%, occurs more frequently in patients with AF, in older patients, and in those with a reduced CO. However, systemic embolization may be the presenting feature in otherwise asymptomatic patients with only mild MS.

PHYSICAL FINDINGS
(See also **Chaps. e8** and 220)

Inspection and Palpation In patients with severe MS, there may be a malar flush with pinched and blue facies. In patients with sinus rhythm and severe pulmonary hypertension or associated tricuspid stenosis (TS), the jugular venous pulse reveals prominent *a* waves due to vigorous right atrial systole. The systemic arterial pressure is usually normal or slightly low. An RV tap along the left sternal border signifies an enlarged RV. A diastolic thrill may be present at the cardiac apex, with the patient in the left lateral recumbent position.

Auscultation The first heart sound (S_1) is usually accentuated and slightly delayed. The pulmonic component of the second heart sound (P_2) also is often accentuated, and the two components of the second heart sound (S_2) are closely split. The opening snap (OS) of the mitral valve is most readily audible in expiration at, or just medial to, the cardiac apex. This sound generally follows the sound of aortic valve closure (A_2) by 0.05–0.12 s. The time interval between A_2 and OS varies inversely with the severity of the MS. The OS is followed by a low-pitched, rumbling, diastolic murmur, heard best at the apex with the patient in the left lateral recumbent position (see Fig. 220-4*B*). It is accentuated by mild exercise (e.g., a few rapid sit-ups) carried out just before auscultation. In general, the duration of this murmur correlates with the severity of the stenosis in patients with preserved CO. In patients with sinus rhythm, the murmur often reappears or becomes louder during atrial systole (presystolic accentuation). Soft grade I or II/VI systolic murmurs are commonly heard at the apex or along the left sternal border in patients with pure MS and do not necessarily signify the presence of MR. Hepatomegaly, ankle edema, ascites, and pleural effusion, particularly in the right pleural cavity, may occur in patients with MS and RV failure.

Associated Lesions With severe pulmonary hypertension, a pansystolic murmur produced by functional TR may be audible along the left sternal border. This murmur is usually louder during inspiration and diminishes during forced expiration (Carvallo's sign). When the CO is markedly reduced in MS, the typical auscultatory findings, including the diastolic rumbling murmur, may not be detectable (silent MS), but they may reappear as compensation is restored. The *Graham Steell murmur* of PR, a high-pitched, diastolic, decrescendo blowing murmur along the left sternal border, results from dilatation of the pulmonary valve ring and occurs in patients with mitral valve disease and severe pulmonary hypertension. This murmur may be indistinguishable from the more common murmur produced by aortic regurgitation (AR), though it may increase in intensity with inspiration and is accompanied by a loud P2.

LABORATORY EXAMINATION
ECG In MS and sinus rhythm, the P wave usually suggests LA enlargement (see Fig. 221-8). It may become tall and peaked in lead II and upright in lead V_1 when severe pulmonary hypertension or TS complicates MS and right atrial (RA) enlargement occurs. The QRS complex is usually normal. However, with severe pulmonary hypertension, right axis deviation and RV hypertrophy are often present.

Echocardiogram (See also Chap. 222) Transthoracic two-dimensional echocardiography (TTE) with color flow Doppler imaging provides critical information, including an estimate of the transvalvular peak and mean gradients and of mitral orifice size, the presence and severity of accompanying MR, the extent of restriction of valve leaflets and their thickness, the degree of distortion of the subvalvular apparatus, and the anatomic suitability for percutaneous mitral balloon valvotomy (PMBV; see below). In addition, TTE provides an assessment of the size of the cardiac chambers, an estimation of LV function, an estimation of the pulmonary artery pressure (PAP), and an indication of the presence and severity of associated valvular lesions. Transesophageal echocardiography (TEE) provides superior images and should be employed when TTE is inadequate for guiding therapy. TEE is especially indicated to exclude the presence of left atrial thrombi prior to PMBV.

Chest X-ray The earliest changes are straightening of the upper left border of the cardiac silhouette, prominence of the main pulmonary arteries, dilatation of the upper lobe pulmonary veins, and posterior displacement of the esophagus by an enlarged LA. Kerley B lines are fine, dense, opaque, horizontal lines that are most prominent in the lower and mid-lung fields and that result from distention of interlobular septae and lymphatics with edema when the resting mean LA pressure exceeds approximately 20 mmHg.

DIFFERENTIAL DIAGNOSIS
Like MS, significant MR may also be associated with a prominent diastolic murmur at the apex due to increased flow, but in MR this diastolic murmur commences slightly later than in patients with MS, and there is often clear-cut evidence of LV enlargement. An apical pansystolic murmur of at least grade III/VI intensity as well as an S_3 suggests significant associated MR. Similarly, the apical mid-diastolic murmur associated with severe AR (*Austin Flint murmur*) may be mistaken for MS but can be differentiated from it because it is not intensified in presystole. TS, which occurs rarely in the absence of MS, may mask many of the clinical features of MS or be clinically silent.

Atrial septal defect (Chap. 229) may be mistaken for MS; in both conditions there is often clinical, ECG, and chest x-ray evidence of RV enlargement and accentuation of pulmonary vascularity. However, the absence of LA enlargement and of Kerley B lines and the demonstration of fixed splitting of S_2 all favor atrial septal defect over MS.

Left atrial myxoma (Chap. 233) may obstruct LA emptying, causing dyspnea, a diastolic murmur, and hemodynamic changes resembling those of MS. However, patients with an LA myxoma often have features suggestive of a systemic disease, such as weight loss, fever, anemia, systemic emboli, and elevated serum IgG and interleukin 6 (IL-6) concentrations. The auscultatory findings may change markedly with body position. The diagnosis can be established by the demonstration of a characteristic echo-producing mass in the LA with TTE.

CARDIAC CATHETERIZATION
Left and right heart catheterization is useful when there is a discrepancy between the clinical and TTE findings that cannot be resolved with either TEE or cardiac magnetic resonance (CMR) imaging. The growing experience with CMR for the assessment of patients with valvular heart disease may decrease the need for invasive catheterization. Catheterization is helpful in assessing associated lesions such as aortic stenosis (AS) and AR. Catheterization and coronary arteriography are not usually necessary to aid in the decision about surgery in younger patients, with typical findings of severe obstruction on clinical examination and TTE. In males over 45 years of age, females over 55 years of age, and younger patients with coronary risk factors, especially those with positive noninvasive stress tests for myocardial ischemia, coronary angiography is advisable preoperatively to detect patients with critical coronary obstructions that should be bypassed at the time of

FIGURE 230-1 Management strategy for patients with mitral stenosis (MS) and mild symptoms. †There is controversy as to whether patients with severe MS (MVA <1.0 cm²) and severe pulmonary hypertension(PH) (PASP >60 mmHg) should undergo percutaneous mitral balloon valvotomy (PMBV) or mitral valve replacement (MVR) to prevent right ventricular failure. CXR, chest x-ray; ECG, electrocardiogram; echo, echocardiography; LA, left atrial; MR, mitral regurgitation; MVA, mitral valve area; MVG, mean mitral valve pressure gradient; NYHA, New York Heart Association; PASP, pulmonary artery systolic pressure; PAWP, pulmonary artery wedge pressure; 2D, 2-dimensional. *(From Bonow et al.)*

operation. Computed tomographic angiography (CTA) (Chap. 222) is now used in some centers to screen preoperatively for the presence of coronary artery disease (CAD) in patients with valvular heart disease. Catheterization and left ventriculography are also indicated in most patients who have undergone PMBV or previous mitral valve surgery and who have redeveloped serious symptoms, if questions remain after both TTE and TEE.

℞ MITRAL STENOSIS

(Fig. 230-1)
Penicillin prophylaxis of Group A β-hemolytic streptococcal infections (Chap. 315) to prevent rheumatic fever is important for at-risk patients with MS **(Table 230-2)**. Recommendations for infective endocarditis prophylaxis have recently changed. In symptomatic patients, some improvement usually occurs with restriction of sodium intake and maintenance doses of oral diuretics. Digitalis glycosides usually do not benefit patients with MS and sinus rhythm, but they are helpful in slowing the ventricular rate of patients with AF. Beta blockers and nondihydropyridine calcium channel blockers (e.g., verapamil or diltiazem) are also useful in this regard. Warfarin to an international normalized ration (INR) of 2–3 should be administered indefinitely to patients with MS who have AF or a history of thromboembolism. The routine use of warfarin in patients in sinus rhythm with LA enlargement (maximal dimension >5.5 cm) with or without spontaneous echo contrast is more controversial.

If AF is of relatively recent onset in a patient whose MS is not severe enough to warrant PMBV or surgical commissurotomy, reversion to sinus rhythm pharmacologically or by means of electrical countershock is indicated. Usually, cardioversion should be undertaken after the patient has had at least 3 consecutive weeks of anticoagulant treatment to a therapeutic INR. If cardioversion is indicated more urgently, then intravenous heparin should be provided and a TEE performed to exclude the presence of left atrial thrombus before the procedure. Conversion to sinus rhythm is rarely successful or sustained in patients with severe MS, particularly those in whom the LA is especially enlarged or in whom AF has been present for more than 1 year.

MITRAL VALVOTOMY Unless there is a contraindication, mitral valvotomy is indicated in symptomatic [New York Heart Association (NYHA) Functional Class II–IV] patients with isolated MS whose effective orifice (valve area) is < ~1.0 cm²/m² body surface area, or <1.5 cm² in normal-sized adults. Mitral valvotomy can be carried out by two techniques: PMBV and surgical valvotomy. In PMBV **(Figs. 230-2** and **230-3)**, a catheter is directed into the LA after transseptal puncture, and a single balloon is directed across the valve and inflated in the valvular orifice. Ideal patients have relatively pliable leaflets with little or no commissural calcium. In addition, the subvalvular structures should not be significantly scarred or thickened and there should be no left atrial thombus. The short- and long-term results of this procedure in appropriate patients are similar to those of surgical valvotomy, but with less morbidity and a lower periprocedural mortality rate. Event-free survival in younger (<45 years) patients with pliable valves is excellent, with rates as high as 80–90% over 3–7 years. Therefore, PMBV has become the procedure of choice for such patients when it can be performed by a skilled operator in a high-volume center.

Transthoracic echocardiography is helpful in identifying patients for the percutaneous procedure, and TEE is performed routinely to exclude left atrial thrombus. An "echo score" has been developed to help guide decision-making. The score accounts for the degree of leaflet thickening, calcification, and mobility, and for the extent of subvalvular thickening. A lower score predicts a higher likelihood of successful PMBV.

In patients in whom PMBV is not possible or unsuccessful, or in many patients with restenosis, an "open" valvotomy using cardiopulmonary bypass is necessary. In addition to

TABLE 230-2	MEDICAL THERAPY OF VALVULAR HEART DISEASE	
Lesion	**Symptom Control**	**Natural History**
Mitral stenosis	Beta blockers, nondihydropyridine calcium channel blockers, or digoxin for rate control of AF; cardioversion for new-onset AF and HF; diuretics for HF	Warfarin for AF or thromboembolism; PCN for RF prophylaxis
Mitral regurgitation	Diuretics for HF	Warfarin for AF or thromboembolism
	Vasodilators for acute MR	Vasodilators for HTN
Aortic stenosis	Diuretics for HF	No proven therapy
Aortic regurgitation	Diuretics and vasodilators for HF	Vasodilators for HTN

Note: Antibiotic prophylaxis is recommended according to current American Heart Association guidelines. For patients with these forms of valvular heart disease, prophylaxis is indicated for a prior history of endocarditis. HF is an indication for surgical or percutaneous treatment, and the recommendations here pertain to short-term therapy prior to definitive correction of the valve lesion. For patients whose comorbidities prohibit surgery, the medical therapies listed can be continued according to available guidelines for the management of HF. See text.

Abbreviations: AF, atrial fibrillation; HF, heart failure; HTN, systemic hypertension; PCN, penicillin; RF, rheumatic fever.

Source: Adapted from NA Boon, P Bloomfield: The medical management of valvular heart disease. Heart 87:395, 2002, with permission.

FIGURE 230-2 Inoue balloon technique for mitral balloon valvotomy. A. After transseptal puncture, the deflated balloon catheter is advanced across the inter-atrial septum, then across the mitral valve and into the left ventricle. **B.** The balloon is then inflated stepwise within the mitral orifice.

opening the valve commissures, it is important to loosen any subvalvular fusion of papillary muscles and chordae tendineae and to remove large deposits of calcium, thereby improving valvular function, as well as to remove atrial thrombi. The perioperative mortality rate is ~2%.

Successful valvotomy is defined by a 50% reduction in the mean mitral valve gradient and a doubling of the mitral valve area. Successful valvotomy, whether balloon or surgical, usually results in striking symptomatic and hemodynamic improvement and prolongs survival. However, there is no evidence that the procedure improves the prognosis of patients with

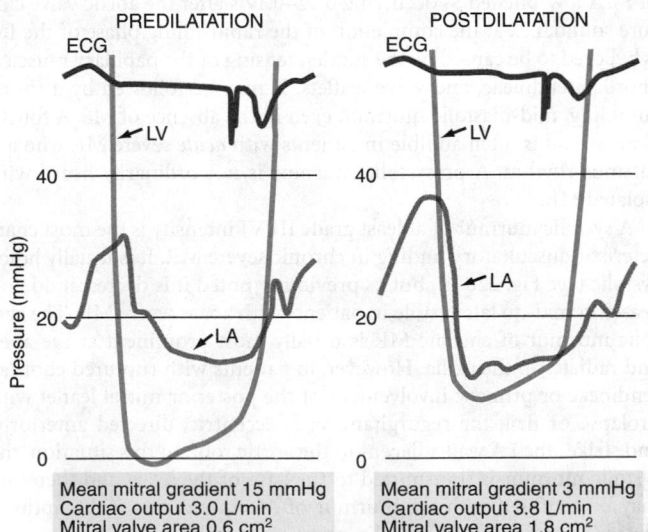

FIGURE 230-3 Simultaneous left atrial (LA) and left ventricular (LV) pressure before and after percutaneous mitral balloon valvuloplasty (PMBV) in a patient with severe mitral stenosis. *(Courtesy of Raymond G. McKay, MD; with permission.)*

TABLE 230-3	MORTALITY RATES AFTER VALVE SURGERY[a]	
Operation	**Number**	**Operative Mortality (%)**
AVR (isolated)	12,501	2.8
MVR (isolated)	3788	5.3
AVR + CAB	12,748	5.2
MVR + CAB	2683	10.3
AVR + MVR	1018	8.8
MVP	3982	1.0
MVP + CAB	4293	7.0
TV surgery	4358	9.6
PV surgery	432	5.2

[a]Data are for calendar year 2004, in which 594 sites reported a total of 232,050 procedures. Data are available from the Society of Thoracic Surgeons at http://www.sts.org/sections/stsnationaldatabase/publications/executive/article.html.

Abbreviations: AVR, aortic valve replacement; CAB, coronary artery bypass; MVR, mitral valve replacement; MVP, mitral valve repair; TV surgery, tricuspid valve repair and replacement; PV surgery, pulmonic valve repair and replacement.

slight or no functional impairment. Therefore, unless recurrent systemic embolization or severe pulmonary hypertension has occurred (PA systolic pressures >50 mmHg at rest or >60 mmHg with exercise), valvotomy is *not* recommended for patients who are entirely asymptomatic and/or who have mild stenosis (mitral valve area >1/5 cm^2). When there is little symptomatic improvement after valvotomy, it is likely that the procedure was ineffective, that it induced MR, or that associated valvular or myocardial disease was present. About half of all patients undergoing surgical mitral valvotomy require reoperation by 10 years. In the pregnant patient with MS, valvotomy should be carried out if pulmonary congestion occurs despite intensive medical treatment. PMBV is the preferred strategy in this setting and is performed with TEE and no or minimal x-ray exposure.

Mitral valve replacement (MVR) is necessary in patients with MS and significant associated MR, those in whom the valve has been severely distorted by previous transcatheter or operative manipulation, or those in whom the surgeon does not find it possible to improve valve function significantly. MVR is now routinely performed with preservation of the chordal attachments to optimize LV functional recovery. Perioperative mortality rates with MVR vary with age, LV function, the presence of CAD, and associated comorbidities. They average 5% overall but are lower in young patients and may be twice as high in older patients with comorbidities **(Table 230-3)**. Since there are also long-term complications of valve replacement (p. 1480), patients in whom preoperative evaluation suggests the possibility that MVR may be required should be operated on only if they have severe MS—i.e., an orifice area ≤1 cm^2—and are in NYHA Class III, i.e., symptomatic with ordinary activity despite optimal medical therapy. The overall 10-year survival of surgical survivors is ~70%. Long-term prognosis is worse in older patients and those with marked disability and marked depression of the CO preoperatively. Pulmonary hypertension and RV dysfunction are additional risk factors for poor outcome.

MITRAL REGURGITATION

ETIOLOGY

MR may result from an abnormality or disease process that affects any one or more of the five functional components of the mitral valve apparatus (leaflets, annulus, chordae tendineae, papillary muscles, and subjacent myocardium) (Table 230-1). Acute MR can occur in the setting of acute myocardial infarction (MI) with papillary muscle rupture (Chap. 239), following blunt chest wall trauma, or during the course of infective endocarditis. With acute MI, the posteromedial papillary muscle is involved much more frequently than the anterolateral papillary muscle because of its singular blood supply. Transient, acute MR can occur during periods of active ischemia and bouts of angina pectoris. Rupture of chordae tendineae can result in "acute on chronic MR" in patients with myxomatous degeneration of the valve apparatus.

Chronic MR can result from rheumatic disease, mitral valve prolapse (MVP) (p. 1472), extensive mitral annular calcification, congenital valve defects, hypertrophic obstructive cardiomyopathy (HOCM), and dilated cardiomyopathy (Chap. 231). Rheumatic heart disease is the cause of chronic MR in only about one-third of cases and occurs more frequently in males. The rheumatic process produces rigidity, deformity, and retraction of the valve cusps and commissural fusion, as well as shortening, contraction, and fusion of the chordae tendineae. The MR associated with both MVP and HOCM is usually dynamic in nature. MR in HOCM occurs as a consequence of anterior papillary muscle displacement and systolic anterior motion of the anterior mitral valve leaflet into the narrowed LV outflow tract. Annular calcification is especially prevalent among patients with advanced renal disease and is commonly observed in elderly women with hypertension and diabetes. MR may occur as a congenital anomaly (Chap. 229), most commonly as a defect of the endocardial cushions (atrioventricular cushion defects). A cleft anterior mitral valve leaflet accompanies primum atrial septal defect. Chronic MR is frequently secondary to ischemia and may occur as a consequence of ventricular remodeling, papillary muscle displacement, and leaflet tethering, or with fibrosis of a papillary muscle, in patients with healed myocardial infarction(s) and ischemic cardiomyopathy. Similar mechanisms of annular dilatation and ventricular remodeling contribute to the MR that occurs universally among patients with nonischemic forms of dilated cardiomyopathy once the left ventricular end-diastolic dimension reaches 6.0 cm.

Irrespective of cause, chronic severe MR is often progressive, since enlargement of the LA places tension on the posterior mitral leaflet, pulling it away from the mitral orifice and thereby aggravating the valvular dysfunction. Similarly, LV dilatation increases the regurgitation, which in turn enlarges the LA and LV further, causing chordal rupture and resulting in a vicious circle; hence the aphorism "mitral regurgitation begets mitral regurgitation."

PATHOPHYSIOLOGY

The resistance to LV emptying (LV afterload) is reduced in patients with MR. As a consequence, the LV is decompressed into the LA during ejection, and with the reduction in LV size during systole, there is a rapid decline in LV tension. The initial compensation to MR is more complete LV emptying. However, LV volume increases progressively with time as the severity of the regurgitation increases and as LV contractile function deteriorates. This increase in LV volume is often accompanied by a reduced forward CO, though LV compliance is often increased and thus LV diastolic pressure does not elevate until late in the course. The regurgitant volume varies directly with the LV systolic pressure and the size of the regurgitant orifice; as mentioned above, the latter, in turn, is influenced profoundly by the extent of LV and mitral annular dilatation. Since ejection fraction (EF) rises in severe MR in the presence of normal LV function, even a modest reduction in this parameter (<60%) reflects significant dysfunction.

During early diastole, as the distended LA empties, there is a particularly rapid y descent in the absence of accompanying MS. A brief, early diastolic LA-LV pressure gradient [often generating a rapid filling sound (S_3) and mid-diastolic murmur masquerading as MS] may occur in patients with pure MR as a result of the very rapid flow of blood across a normal-sized mitral orifice.

Quantitative estimates of left ventricular ejection fraction (LVEF), CO, PA pressure, regurgitant volume, regurgitant fraction (RF), and the effective regurgitant orifice area can be obtained during a careful Doppler echocardiographic examination. These measurements can also be obtained with CMR. Left and right heart catheterization with contrast ventriculography is utilized less frequently. Severe MR is defined by a regurgitant volume ≥60 mL/beat, regurgitant fraction (RF) ≥50%, and effective regurgitant orifice area ≥0.40 cm^2.

LA Compliance In acute severe MR, the regurgitant volume is delivered into a normal-sized LA having normal or reduced compliance. As a result, LA pressures rise markedly for any increase in LA volume. The v wave in the LA pressure pulse is usually prominent (see Fig. 223-3), LA and pulmonary venous pressures are markedly elevated, and pulmonary edema is common. Because of the rapid rise in LA pressures during ventricular systole, the murmur of acute MR is early in timing and decrescendo in configuration, as a reflection of the progressive

diminution in the LV-LA pressure gradient. LV systolic function in acute MR may be normal, hyperdynamic, or reduced, depending on the clinical context.

Patients with chronic severe MR, on the other hand, develop marked LA enlargement and *increased* LA compliance with little if any increase in LA and pulmonary venous pressures for any increase in LA volume. The LA v wave is relatively less prominent. The murmur of chronic MR is classically holosystolic in timing and plateau in configuration, as a reflection of the near-constant LV-LA pressure gradient. These patients usually complain of severe fatigue and exhaustion secondary to a low CO, while symptoms resulting from pulmonary congestion are less prominent initially; AF is almost invariably present once the LA dilates significantly.

Most common are patients whose clinical and hemodynamic features are intermediate between those in the two aforementioned groups.

SYMPTOMS

Patients with chronic mild-to-moderate isolated MR are usually asymptomatic. This form of LV volume overload is well tolerated. Fatigue, exertional dyspnea, and orthopnea are the most prominent complaints in patients with chronic severe MR. Palpitations are common and may signify the onset of AF. Right-sided heart failure, with painful hepatic congestion, ankle edema, distended neck veins, ascites, and secondary TR, occurs in patients with MR who have associated pulmonary vascular disease and marked pulmonary hypertension. On the other hand, acute pulmonary edema is common in patients with acute severe MR.

PHYSICAL FINDINGS

In patients with chronic severe MR, the arterial pressure is usually normal, though the arterial pulse may show a sharp upstroke. A systolic thrill is often palpable at the cardiac apex, the LV is hyperdynamic with a brisk systolic impulse and a palpable rapid-filling wave (S_3), and the apex beat is often displaced laterally.

In patients with acute severe MR, the arterial pressure may be reduced with a narrow pulse pressure, the jugular venous pressure and wave forms may be normal or increased and exaggerated, the apical impulse is not displaced, and signs of pulmonary congestion are prominent.

Auscultation The S_1 is generally absent, soft, or buried in the holosystolic murmur of chronic MR. In patients with severe MR, the aortic valve may close prematurely, resulting in wide but physiologic splitting of S_2. A low-pitched S_3 occurring 0.12–0.17 s after the aortic valve closure sound, i.e., at the completion of the rapid-filling phase of the LV, is believed to be caused by the sudden tensing of the papillary muscles, chordae tendineae, and valve leaflets. It may be followed by a short, rumbling, mid-diastolic murmur, even in the absence of MS. A fourth heart sound is often audible in patients with *acute* severe MR who are in sinus rhythm. A presystolic murmur is not ordinarily heard with isolated MR.

A systolic murmur of at least grade III/VI intensity is the most characteristic auscultatory finding in chronic severe MR. It is usually holosystolic (see Fig. 220-4), but as previously noted it is decrescendo and ceases in mid- to late systole in patients with acute severe MR. The systolic murmur of chronic MR is usually most prominent at the apex and radiates to the axilla. However, in patients with ruptured chordae tendineae or primary involvement of the posterior mitral leaflet with prolapse or flail, the regurgitant jet is eccentric, directed anteriorly, and strikes the LA wall adjacent to the aortic root. In this situation, the systolic murmur is transmitted to the base of the heart and therefore may be confused with the murmur of AS. In patients with ruptured chordae tendineae, the systolic murmur may have a cooing or "sea gull" quality, while a flail leaflet may cause a murmur with a musical quality. The systolic murmur of chronic MR not due to MVP is intensified by isometric exercise (handgrip) but is reduced during the strain phase of the Valsalva maneuver.

LABORATORY EXAMINATION

ECG In patients with sinus rhythm, there is evidence of LA enlargement, but RA enlargement also may be present when pulmonary hypertension is severe. Chronic severe MR is generally associated with AF. In many patients there is no clear-cut ECG evidence of enlargement of either ventricle. In others, the signs of LV hypertrophy are present.

Echocardiogram TTE with Doppler imaging is indicated to assess the mechanism of the MR and its hemodynamic severity. LV function can be assessed from LV end-diastolic and end-systolic volumes and EF. Observations can be made regarding leaflet structure and function, chordal integrity, LA and LV size, annular calcification, and regional and global LV systolic function. Doppler imaging should demonstrate the width or area of the color flow MR jet within the LA, the intensity of the continuous wave Doppler signal, the pulmonary venous flow contour, the early peak mitral inflow velocity, and the quantitative measures of regurgitant volume, RF, and effective regurgitant orifice area. In addition, the PA pressures can be estimated from the TR jet velocity. TTE is also indicated to follow the course of patients with chronic MR and to provide rapid assessment for any clinical change. The echocardiogram in patients with MVP is described in the next section. TEE provides greater detail than TTE (see Fig. 222-3).

Chest X-ray The LA and LV are the dominant chambers in chronic MR; late in the course of the disease, the former may be massively enlarged and forms the right border of the cardiac silhouette. Pulmonary venous congestion, interstitial edema, and Kerley B lines are sometimes noted. Marked calcification of the mitral leaflets occurs commonly in patients with longstanding combined MR and MS. Calcification of the mitral annulus may be visualized, particularly on the lateral view of the chest. Patients with acute severe MR may have asymmetric pulmonary edema if the regurgitant jet is directed predominantly to the orifice of an upper lobe pulmonary vein.

℞ MITRAL REGURGITATION

(Fig. 230-4)

MEDICAL (Table 230-2) The management of chronic severe MR depends to some degree on its cause. Warfarin should be provided once AF intervenes with a target INR of 2–3. Cardioversion should be considered depending on the clinical context and left atrial size. In contrast to the acute setting, there are no large, long-term prospective studies to substantiate the use of vasodilators for the treatment of chronic, isolated severe MR *in the absence of systemic hypertension*. The severity of MR in the setting of an ischemic or nonischemic dilated cardiomyopathy may diminish with aggressive, evidence-based treatment of heart failure, including the use of diuretics, beta blockers, ACE inhibitors, and digitalis. Asymptomatic patients with severe MR in sinus rhythm with normal LV size and systolic function should avoid isometric forms of exercise.

Patients with acute severe MR require urgent stabilization and preparation for surgery. Diuretics, intravenous vasodilators (particularly sodium nitroprusside), and even intraaortic balloon counterpulsation may be needed for patients with post-MI papillary muscle rupture or other forms of acute severe MR.

SURGICAL In the selection of patients with chronic severe MR for surgical treatment, the often slowly progressive nature of the condition must

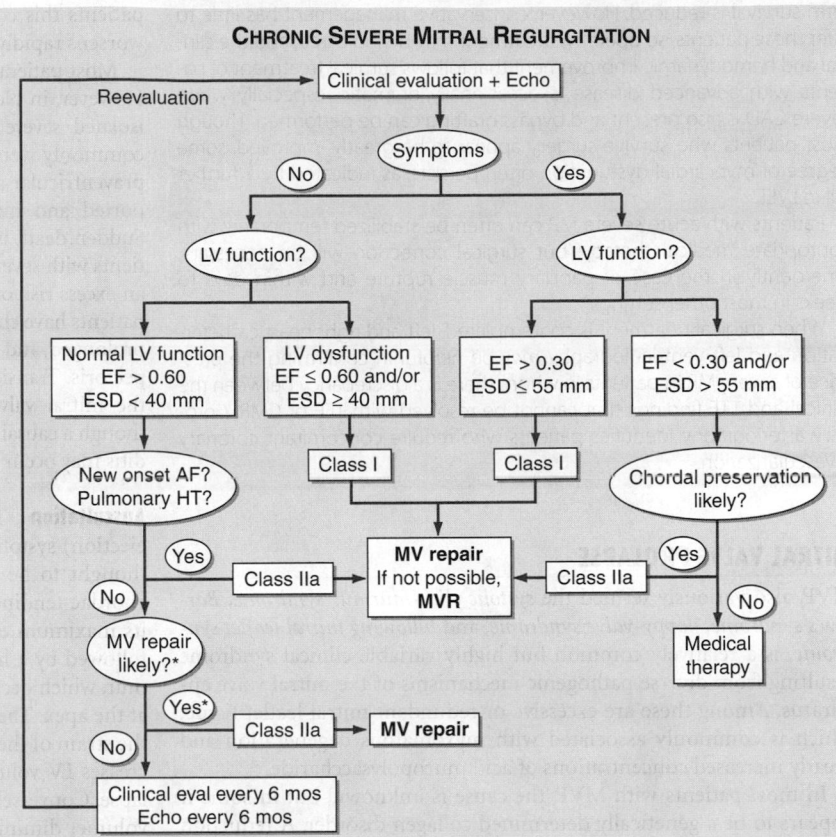

FIGURE 230-4 Management strategy for patients with chronic severe mitral regurgitation. *Mitral valve (MV) repair may be performed in asymptomatic patients with normal left ventricular (LV) function if performed by an experienced surgical team and if the likelihood of successful MV repair is >90%. AF, atrial fibrillation; Echo, echocardiography; EF, ejection fraction; ESD, end-systolic dimension; eval, evaluation; HT, hypertension; MVR, mitral valve replacement. *(From Bonow et al.)*

be balanced against the immediate and long-term risks associated with operation. These risks are significantly lower for primary valve repair than for valve replacement (Table 230-3). Repair usually consists of valve reconstruction utilizing a variety of valvuloplasty techniques and insertion of an annuloplasty ring. Repair spares the patient the long-term adverse consequences of valve replacement, i.e., thromboembolic and hemorrhagic complications in the case of mechanical prostheses and late valve failure necessitating repeat valve replacement in the case of bioprostheses (p. 1480). In addition, by preserving the integrity of the papillary muscles, subvalvular apparatus, and chordae tendineae, mitral repair and valvuloplasty maintain LV function to a relatively greater degree.

Surgery for chronic severe MR is indicated once symptoms occur, especially if valve repair is feasible (Fig. 230-4). Other indications for early consideration of mitral valve repair include recent-onset AF and pulmonary hypertension, defined as a PA pressure ≥50 mmHg at rest or ≥60 mmHg with exercise. Surgical treatment of chronic severe MR is indicated for asymptomatic patients when LV dysfunction is progressive, with LVEF declining below 60% and/or end-systolic cavity dimension on echocardiography rising above 40 mm. These aggressive recommendations for surgery are predicated on the outstanding results achieved with mitral valve repair, particularly when applied to patients with myxomatous disease. Indeed, primary valvuloplasty repair of patients younger than 75 years with normal LV systolic function and no CAD can now be performed by experienced surgeons with <1% perioperative mortality risk. Repair is feasible in up to 95% of patients with myxomatous disease. Long-term durability is excellent; the incidence of reoperative surgery for failed primary repair is ~1% per year for 10 years after surgery. For patients with AF, a left atrial Maze procedure or radiofrequency ablation of the pulmonary vein ostia is often performed to reduce the risk of recurrent AF.

In patients with significantly impaired LV function (EF <30%), the risk of surgery rises, the recovery of LV performance is incomplete, and the long-term survival is reduced. However, conservative management has little to offer these patients, so operative treatment may be indicated, and the clinical and hemodynamic improvement that follows surgical treatment of patients with advanced disease is occasionally dramatic, especially when severe CAD is also present and bypass grafting can be performed. Though most patients who survive surgery appear to be greatly improved, some degree of myocardial dysfunction often persists, as indicated by a further fall in LVEF.

Patients with acute severe MR can often be stabilized temporarily with appropriate medical therapy, but surgical correction will be necessary, emergently in the case of papillary muscle rupture and within days to weeks in most other settings.

When surgical treatment is contemplated, left and right heart catheterization and left ventriculography *may* be helpful in confirming the presence of severe MR in patients in whom there is a discrepancy between the clinical and TTE findings that cannot be resolved with TEE or CMR. Coronary arteriography identifies patients who require concomitant coronary revascularization.

MITRAL VALVE PROLAPSE

MVP, also variously termed the *systolic click-murmur syndrome, Barlow's syndrome, floppy-valve syndrome,* and *billowing mitral leaflet syndrome,* is a relatively common but highly variable clinical syndrome resulting from diverse pathogenic mechanisms of the mitral valve apparatus. Among these are excessive or redundant mitral leaflet tissue, which is commonly associated with myxomatous degeneration and greatly increased concentrations of acid mucopolysaccharide.

In most patients with MVP, the cause is unknown, but in some it appears to be a genetically determined collagen disorder. A reduction in the production of type III collagen has been incriminated, and electron microscopy has revealed fragmentation of collagen fibrils.

MVP is a frequent finding in patients with heritable disorders of connective tissue, including Marfan syndrome (Chap. 357), osteogenesis imperfecta, and Ehler-Danlos syndrome.

MVP may be associated with thoracic skeletal deformities similar to but not as severe as those in Marfan syndrome, encompassing a high-arched palate and alterations of the chest and thoracic spine, including the so-called straight back syndrome.

In most patients with MVP, myxomatous degeneration is confined to the mitral (or, less commonly, the tricuspid or aortic) valves without other clinical or pathologic manifestations of disease. The posterior leaflet is usually more affected than the anterior, and the mitral valve annulus is often greatly dilated. In many patients, elongated, redundant, or ruptured chordae tendineae cause or contribute to the regurgitation.

MVP also may occur rarely as a sequel to acute rheumatic fever, in ischemic heart disease, and in various cardiomyopathies, as well as in 20% of patients with ostium secundum atrial septal defect.

MVP may lead to excessive stress on the papillary muscles, which in turn leads to dysfunction and ischemia of the papillary muscles and the subjacent ventricular myocardium. Rupture of chordae tendineae and progressive annular dilatation and calcification also contribute to valvular regurgitation, which then places more stress on the diseased mitral valve apparatus, thereby creating a vicious circle. The ECG changes (see below) and ventricular arrhythmias appear to result from regional ventricular dysfunction related to increased stress placed on the papillary muscles.

CLINICAL FEATURES

MVP is more common in females and occurs most commonly between the ages of 15 and 30 years; the clinical course is often benign. MVP may also be observed in older (>50 years) patients, often males, in whom MR is often more severe and requires surgical treatment. There is an increased familial incidence for some patients, suggesting an autosomal dominant form of inheritance. MVP encompasses a broad spectrum of severities, ranging from only a systolic click and murmur and mild prolapse of the posterior leaflet of the mitral valve to severe MR due to chordal rupture and massive prolapse of both leaflets. In many

patients this condition progresses over years or decades. In others it worsens rapidly as a result of chordal rupture or endocarditis.

Most patients are asymptomatic and remain so for their entire lives. However, in North America MVP is now the most common cause of isolated severe MR requiring surgical treatment. Arrhythmias, most commonly ventricular premature contractions and paroxysmal supraventricular and ventricular tachycardia, as well as AF, have been reported and may cause palpitations, light-headedness, and syncope. Sudden death is a very rare complication and occurs most often in patients with severe MR and depressed LV systolic function. There may be an excess risk of sudden death among patients with a flail leaflet. Many patients have chest pain that is difficult to evaluate. It is often substernal, prolonged, and poorly related to exertion, and it rarely resembles angina pectoris. Transient cerebral ischemic attacks secondary to emboli from the mitral valve due to endothelial disruption have been reported, though a causal relationship has not been established. Infective endocarditis may occur in patients with MR and/or leaflet thickening.

Auscultation The most important finding is the mid- or late (non-ejection) systolic click, which occurs 0.14 s or more after the S_1 and is thought to be generated by the sudden tensing of slack, elongated chordae tendineae or by the prolapsing mitral leaflet when it reaches its maximum excursion. Systolic clicks may be multiple and may be followed by a high-pitched, late systolic crescendo-decrescendo murmur, which occasionally is "whooping" or "honking" and is heard best at the apex. The click and murmur occur earlier with standing, during the strain of the Valsalva maneuver, and with any intervention that decreases LV volume, exaggerating the propensity of mitral leaflet prolapse. Conversely, squatting and isometric exercises, which increase LV volume, diminish MVP, and the click-murmur complex is delayed, moves away from S1, and may even disappear. Some patients have a mid-systolic click without the murmur; others have the murmur without a click. Still others have both sounds at different times.

LABORATORY EXAMINATION

The ECG most commonly is normal but may show biphasic or inverted T waves in leads II, III, and aVF, and occasionally supraventricular or ventricular premature beats. *TTE* is particularly effective in identifying the abnormal position and prolapse of the mitral valve leaflets. A useful echocardiographic definition of MVP is systolic displacement (in the parasternal long axis view) of the mitral valve leaflets by at least 2 mm into the LA superior to the plane of the mitral annulus. Color flow and continuous wave Doppler imaging is helpful in revealing and evaluating associated MR. TEE is indicated when more accurate information is required and is performed routinely for intraoperative guidance for valve repair. Invasive left ventriculography is rarely necessary but can also show prolapse of the posterior and sometimes of both mitral valve leaflets.

℞ MITRAL VALVE PROLAPSE

Infective endocarditis prophylaxis is indicated only for patients with a prior history of endocarditis. Beta blockers sometimes relieve chest pain and control palpitations. If the patient is symptomatic from severe MR, mitral valve repair (or rarely, replacement) is indicated (Fig. 230-4). Antiplatelet agents such as aspirin should be given to patients with transient ischemic attacks, and if these are not effective, anticoagulants such as warfarin should be considered.

AORTIC STENOSIS

AS occurs in about one-fourth of all patients with chronic valvular heart disease; approximately 80% of adult patients with symptomatic valvular AS are male.

ETIOLOGY

(Table 230-1) AS in adults may be due to degenerative calcification of the aortic cusps. It may be congenital in origin or it may be secondary to rheumatic inflammation. *Age-related degenerative calcific AS* (also known as senile or sclerocalcific AS) is now the most common cause of AS in adults in North America and Western Europe. About 30% of persons >65 years exhibit aortic valve sclerosis; many of these have a systolic murmur of AS but without obstruction, while 2% exhibit frank stenosis. Aortic sclerosis is defined echocardiographically as focal thickening or calcification of the valve cusps with a peak Doppler transaortic velocity of ≤2.5 m/s. Aortic sclerosis appears to be a marker for an increased risk of coronary heart disease events. On histologic examination these valves frequently exhibit changes similar to those seen with atherosclerosis and vascular inflammation. Interestingly, risk factors for atherosclerosis, such as age, male sex, smoking, diabetes mellitus, hypertension, chronic kidney disease, increased LDL, reduced HDL cholesterol, and elevated C-reactive protein are all risk factors for aortic valve calcification.

The *congenitally affected valve* may be stenotic at birth (Chap. 229) and may become progressively more fibrotic, calcified, and stenotic. In other cases the valve may be congenitally deformed, usually bicuspid [bicuspid aortic valve (BAV)], without serious narrowing of the aortic orifice during childhood; its abnormal architecture makes its leaflets susceptible to otherwise ordinary hemodynamic stresses, which ultimately lead to valvular thickening, calcification, increased rigidity, and narrowing of the aortic orifice.

Rheumatic disease of the aortic leaflets produces commissural fusion, sometimes resulting in a bicuspid-appearing valve. This condition in turn makes the leaflets more susceptible to trauma and ultimately leads to fibrosis, calcification, and further narrowing. By the time the obstruction to LV outflow causes serious clinical disability, the valve is usually a rigid calcified mass, and careful examination may make it difficult or even impossible to determine the etiology of the underlying process. Rheumatic AS is almost always associated with involvement of the mitral valve and with AR.

OTHER FORMS OF OBSTRUCTION TO LEFT VENTRICULAR OUTFLOW

Besides valvular AS, three other lesions may be responsible for obstruction to LV outflow: *hypertrophic obstructive cardiomyopathy* (Chap. 231), *discrete congenital subvalvular AS*, and *supravalvular AS* (Chap. 229). The causes of left ventricular outflow obstruction can be differentiated on the basis of the cardiac examination and Doppler echocardiographic findings.

PATHOPHYSIOLOGY

The obstruction to LV outflow produces a systolic pressure gradient between the LV and aorta. When severe obstruction is suddenly produced experimentally, the LV responds by dilatation and reduction of stroke volume. However, in some patients the obstruction may be present at birth and/or increase gradually over the course of many years, and LV output is maintained by the presence of concentric LV hypertrophy. Initially, this serves as an adaptive mechanism because it reduces toward normal the systolic stress developed by the myocardium, as predicted by the Laplace relation ($S = Pr/h$, where S = systolic wall stress, P = pressure, r = radius, and h = wall thickness). A large transaortic valvular pressure gradient may exist for many years without a reduction in CO or LV dilatation; ultimately, however, excessive hypertrophy becomes maladaptive, and LV function declines.

A mean systolic pressure gradient >40 mmHg with a normal CO or an effective aortic orifice area < ~1.0 cm² (or ~<0.6 cm²/m² body surface area in a normal-sized adult)—i.e., less than approximately one-third of the normal orifice—is generally considered to represent severe obstruction to LV outflow (see Fig. 223-4). The elevated LV end-diastolic pressure observed in many patients with severe AS signifies the presence of LV dilatation and/or diminished compliance of the hypertrophied LV wall. Although the CO at rest is within normal limits in most patients with severe AS, it usually fails to rise normally during exercise. Loss of an appropriately timed, vigorous atrial contraction, as occurs in AF or atrioventricular dissociation, may cause rapid progression of symptoms. Late in the course, the CO and LV–aortic pressure gradient decline, and the mean LA, PA, and RV pressures rise.

The hypertrophied LV elevates myocardial oxygen requirements. In addition, even in the absence of obstructive CAD, there may be interference with coronary blood flow. This is because the pressure compressing the coronary arteries exceeds the coronary perfusion pressure, often causing ischemia (especially in the subendocardium), both in the presence and in the absence of coronary arterial narrowing.

SYMPTOMS

AS is rarely of clinical importance until the valve orifice has narrowed to approximately 1.0 cm². Even severe AS may exist for many years without producing any symptoms because of the ability of the hypertrophied LV to generate the elevated intraventricular pressures required for a normal stroke volume.

Most patients with pure or predominant AS have gradually increasing obstruction for years but do not become symptomatic until the sixth to eighth decades. Exertional dyspnea, angina pectoris, and syncope are the three cardinal symptoms. Often there is a history of insidious progression of fatigue and dyspnea associated with gradual curtailment of activities. *Dyspnea* results primarily from elevation of the pulmonary capillary pressure caused by elevations of LV diastolic pressures secondary to reduced left ventricular compliance. *Angina pectoris* usually develops somewhat later and reflects an imbalance between the augmented myocardial oxygen requirements and reduced oxygen availability; the former results from the increased myocardial mass and intraventricular pressure, while the latter may result from accompanying CAD, which is not uncommon in patients with AS, as well as from compression of the coronary vessels by the hypertrophied myocardium. Therefore, angina may occur in severe AS even without obstructive epicardial CAD. *Exertional syncope* may result from a decline in arterial pressure caused by vasodilatation in the exercising muscles and inadequate vasoconstriction in nonexercising muscles in the face of a fixed CO, or from a sudden fall in CO produced by an arrhythmia.

Since the CO at rest is usually well maintained until late in the course, marked fatigability, weakness, peripheral cyanosis, cachexia, and other clinical manifestations of a low CO are usually not prominent until this stage is reached. Orthopnea, paroxysmal nocturnal dyspnea, and pulmonary edema, i.e., symptoms of LV failure, also occur only in the advanced stages of the disease. Severe pulmonary hypertension leading to RV failure and systemic venous hypertension, hepatomegaly, AF, and TR are usually late findings in patients with isolated severe AS.

When AS and MS coexist, the reduction in CO induced by MS lowers the pressure gradient across the aortic valve and thereby masks many of the clinical findings produced by AS.

PHYSICAL FINDINGS

The rhythm is generally regular until late in the course; at other times, AF should suggest the possibility of associated mitral valve disease. The systemic arterial pressure is usually within normal limits. In the late stages, however, when stroke volume declines, the systolic pressure may fall and the pulse pressure narrow. The peripheral arterial pulse rises slowly to a delayed sustained peak (pulsus parvus et tardus; see Fig. 220-2). In the elderly, the stiffening of the arterial wall may mask this important physical sign. In many patients the *a* wave in the jugular venous pulse is accentuated. This results from the diminished distensibility of the RV cavity caused by the bulging, hypertrophied interventricular septum.

The LV impulse is usually displaced laterally. A double apical impulse may be recognized, particularly with the patient in the left lateral recumbent position. A systolic thrill is generally present at the base of the heart, in the suprasternal notch, and along the carotid arteries.

Auscultation An early systolic ejection sound is frequently audible in children and adolescents with congenital noncalcific valvular AS. This sound usually disappears when the valve becomes calcified and rigid. As AS increases in severity, LV systole may become prolonged so that the aortic valve closure sound no longer precedes the pulmonic valve closure sound, and the two components may become synchronous, or aortic valve closure may even follow pulmonic valve closure, causing paradoxic splitting of S_2 (Chap. 220). The sound of aortic valve closure can be heard most frequently in patients with AS who have pliable valves, and calcification diminishes the intensity of this sound. Frequently, an S_4 is audible at the apex and reflects the presence of LV hypertrophy and an elevated LV end-diastolic pressure; an S_3 generally occurs late in the course, when the LV dilates.

The murmur of AS is characteristically an ejection (mid) systolic murmur that commences shortly after the S_1, increases in intensity to reach a peak toward the middle of ejection, and ends just before aortic valve closure (see Fig. 220-4). It is characteristically low-pitched, rough and rasping in character, and loudest at the base of the heart, most commonly in the second right intercostal space. It is transmitted upward along the carotid arteries. Occasionally it is transmitted downward and to the apex, where it may be confused with the systolic murmur of MR (Gallavardin effect). In almost all patients with severe obstruction and preserved CO, the murmur is at least grade III/VI. In patients with mild degrees of obstruction or in those with severe stenosis with heart failure in whom the stroke volume and therefore the transvalvular flow rate are reduced, the murmur may be relatively soft and brief.

LABORATORY EXAMINATION

ECG In most patients with severe AS there is LV hypertrophy (see Fig. 221-9). In advanced cases, ST-segment depression and T-wave inversion (LV "strain") in standard leads I and aVL and in the left precordial leads are evident. However, there is no close correlation between the ECG and the hemodynamic severity of obstruction, and the absence of ECG signs of LV hypertrophy does not exclude severe obstruction.

Echocardiogram The key findings are LV hypertrophy and, in patients with valvular calcification (i.e., most adult patients with symptomatic AS), multiple, bright, thick, echoes from the valve (see Fig. 222-2). Eccentricity of the aortic valve cusps is characteristic of congenitally bicuspid valves. TEE imaging usually displays the obstructed orifice extremely well, but it is not routinely required for adequate characterization. The valve gradient and aortic valve area can be estimated by Doppler measurement of the transaortic velocity. Severe AS is defined by a valve area <1.0 cm^2, whereas moderate AS is defined by a valve area of 1.0–1.5 cm^2 and mild AS by a valve area of 1.5–2.0 cm^2. LV dilatation and reduced systolic shortening reflect impairment of LV function.

Echocardiography is useful for identifying coexisting valvular abnormalities such as MS and AR, which sometimes accompany AS; for differentiating valvular AS from other forms of outflow obstruction; and for measurement of the aortic root. Aneurysmal enlargement (maximal dimension >4.5 cm) of the root or ascending aorta can occur in up to 20% of patients with bicuspid aortic valve disease, independent of the severity of the valve lesion. Dobutamine stress echocardiography is useful for the evaluation of patients with severe AS and severe LV systolic dysfunction (EF <0.35).

Chest X-Ray The chest x-ray may show no or little overall cardiac enlargement for many years. Hypertrophy without dilatation may produce some rounding of the cardiac apex in the frontal projection and slight backward displacement in the lateral view; severe AS is often associated with poststenotic dilatation of the ascending aorta. As noted above, however, aortic enlargement may be an independent process and mediated by the same type of structural changes that occur in patients with Marfan syndrome. Aortic calcification is usually readily apparent on fluoroscopic examination or by echocardiography; the absence of valvular calcification in an adult suggests that severe valvular AS is *not* present. In later stages of the disease, as the LV dilates there is increasing roentgenographic evidence of LV enlargement, pulmonary congestion, and enlargement of the LA, PA, and right side of the heart.

Catheterization Right and left heart catheterization for invasive assessment of AS is performed infrequently but can be useful when there is a discrepancy between the clinical and echocardiographic findings. Con-

cerns have been raised that attempts to cross the aortic valve for measurement of left ventricular pressures are associated with a risk of cerebral embolization. Catheterization is also useful in three distinct categories of patients: (1) *patients with multivalvular disease*, in whom the role played by each valvular deformity should be defined to aid in the planning of definitive operative treatment; (2) *young, asymptomatic patients with noncalcific congenital AS*, to define with precision the severity of obstruction to LV outflow, since operation [which does not usually require aortic valve replacement (AVR)] or PABV may be indicated if severe AS is present, even in the absence of symptoms; balloon valvotomy may follow left heart catheterization immediately; and (3) *patients in whom it is suspected that the obstruction to LV outflow may not be at the aortic valve* but rather in the sub- or supravalvular regions.

Coronary angiography is indicated to detect or exclude CAD in patients >45 years old with severe AS who are being considered for operative treatment. The incidence of significant CAD for which bypass grafting is indicated at the time of AVR exceeds 50% among adult patients.

NATURAL HISTORY

Death in patients with severe AS occurs most commonly in the seventh and eighth decades. Based on data obtained at postmortem examination in patients before surgical treatment became widely available, the average time to death after the onset of various symptoms was as follows: angina pectoris, 3 years; syncope, 3 years; dyspnea, 2 years; congestive heart failure, 1.5–2 years. Moreover, in $>80\%$ of patients who died with AS, symptoms had existed for <4 years. Among adults dying with valvular AS, sudden death, which presumably resulted from an arrhythmia, occurred in 10–20%. However, most sudden deaths occurred in patients who had previously been symptomatic; thus, sudden death is very uncommon ($<1\%$ per year) in asymptomatic adult patients with severe AS. Obstructive calcific AS is a progressive disease, with an annual reduction in valve area averaging 0.1 cm^2/year and an annual increase in mean gradient averaging 7 mmHg/year.

℞ AORTIC STENOSIS

(Table 230-2, **Fig. 230-5**)

MEDICAL TREATMENT In patients with severe AS (<1.0 cm^2), strenuous physical activity should be avoided, even in the asymptomatic stage. Care must be taken to avoid dehydration and hypovolemia to protect against a significant reduction in CO. Medications used for the treatment of hypertension or CAD, including beta blockers and ACE inhibitors, are generally safe for asymptomatic patients with preserved left ventricular systolic function. Nitroglycerin is helpful in relieving angina pectoris. Retrospective studies have shown that patients with degenerative calcific AS who receive HMG-CoA reductase inhibitors ("statins") exhibit slower progression of leaflet calcification and aortic valve area reduction than those who do not. One prospective randomized clinical trial using high-dose atorvastatin failed to show a measurable benefit, although a more recent trial using rosuvastatin did show a beneficial effect. The role of statin medications may be more clearly defined with further study.

SURGICAL TREATMENT Asymptomatic patients with calcific AS and severe obstruction should be followed carefully for the development of symptoms and by serial echocardiograms for evidence of deteriorating LV function. Operation is indicated in patients with severe AS (valve area <1.0 cm^2 or 0.6 cm^2/m^2 body surface area) who are symptomatic, those who exhibit LV dysfunction (EF $<50\%$), as well as those with an aneurysmal or expanding aortic root (maximal dimension >4.5 cm or annual increase in size >0.5 cm/year), even if they are asymptomatic. In patients without heart failure, the operative risk of AVR is approximately 3% (Table 230-3). It is prudent to postpone operation in patients with severe calcific AS who are truly asymptomatic and who exhibit normal LV function, i.e., EF $>50\%$, since they may continue to do well for years. However, some advocate AVR in patients with severe valve calcification and rapid progression of obstruction. The risk of surgical mortality exceeds that of sudden death in asymptomatic patients. Exercise testing is em-

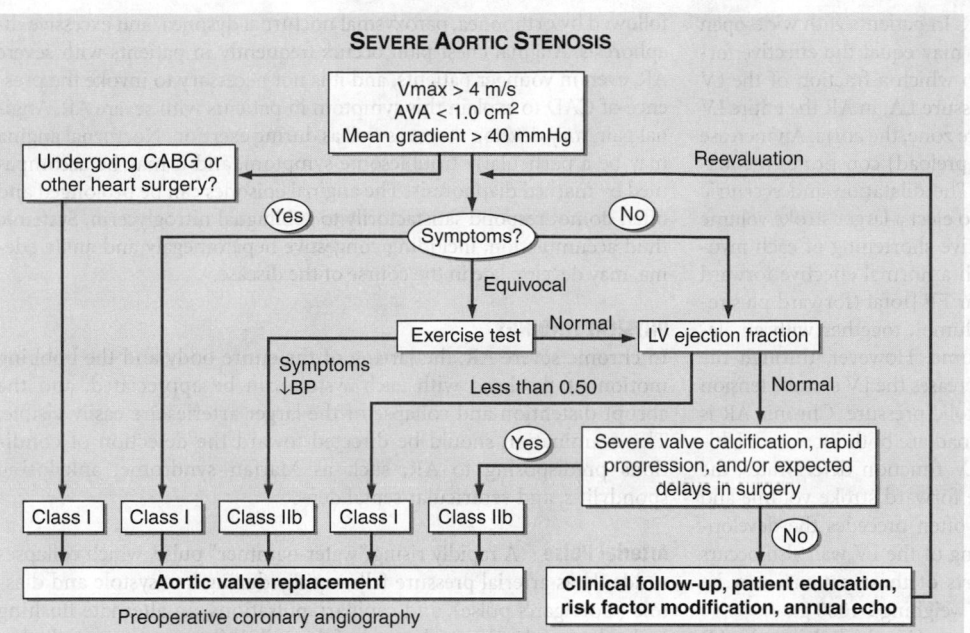

SEVERE AORTIC STENOSIS

Vmax > 4 m/s
AVA < 1.0 cm²
Mean gradient > 40 mmHg

Undergoing CABG or other heart surgery?

Reevaluation

Symptoms?

Yes / No

Equivocal

Exercise test — Normal — LV ejection fraction

Symptoms ↓BP

Less than 0.50

Normal

Yes

Severe valve calcification, rapid progression, and/or expected delays in surgery

No

Class I | Class I | Class IIb | Class I | Class IIb

Aortic valve replacement

Preoperative coronary angiography

Clinical follow-up, patient education, risk factor modification, annual echo

FIGURE 230-5 Management strategy for patients with severe aortic stenosis. Preoperative coronary angiography should be performed routinely as determined by age, symptoms, and coronary risk factors. Cardiac catheterization and angiography may also be helpful when there is discordance between clinical findings and echocardiography. AVA, aortic valve area; BP, blood pressure; CABG, coronary artery bypass graft surgery; echo, echocardiography; LV, left ventricle; Vmax, maximal velocity across aortic valve by Doppler echocardiography. *(From Bonow et al. Modified from CM Otto: J Am Coll Cardiol 47:2141, 2006.)*

ployed in many centers to assess objectively the functional capacity of asymptomatic patients for whom the history is ambiguous. As many as one-third of patients will show signs of functional impairment during exercise for which AVR should be considered. AVR is carried out in asymptomatic patients with severe or moderately severe stenosis who undergo coronary artery bypass grafting. AVR is also routinely performed in patients with moderate AS who are undergoing coronary bypass grafting or aortic root reconstruction.

Operation should, if possible, be carried out before frank LV failure develops; at this late stage, the aortic valve pressure gradient declines as the CO, stroke volume, and EF decline (low gradient, low output AS). In such patients the perioperative risk is high (15–20%), and evidence of myocardial disease may persist even when the operation is technically successful. Furthermore, long-term postoperative survival also correlates inversely with preoperative LV dysfunction. Nonetheless, in view of the even worse prognosis of such patients when they are treated medically, there is usually little choice but to advise surgical treatment, especially in patients in whom contractile reserve can be demonstrated by dobutamine echocardiography (defined by a ≥20% in stroke volume after dobutamine challenge). In patients in whom severe AS and CAD coexist, relief of the AS and revascularization of the myocardium by means of aortocoronary bypass grafting may result in striking clinical and hemodynamic improvement (Table 230-3).

Because many patients with calcific AS are elderly, particular attention must be directed to the adequacy of hepatic, renal, and pulmonary function before AVR is recommended. Age alone is not a contraindication to AVR for AS. The mortality rate depends to a substantial extent on the patient's preoperative clinical and hemodynamic state. The 10-year survival rate of patients with AVR is approximately 60%. Approximately 30% of bioprosthetic valves evidence primary valve failure in 10 years, requiring re-replacement, and an approximately equal percentage of patients with mechanical prostheses develop significant hemorrhagic complications as a consequence of treatment with anticoagulants (p. 1480).

PERCUTANEOUS BALLOON AORTIC VALVULOPLASTY This procedure is preferable to operation in children and young adults with congenital, noncalcific AS (Chap. 229). It is not commonly used in adults with severe calcific AS because of a very high restenosis rate and the risk of procedural complications, but on occasion it has been used successfully as

a "bridge to operation" in patients with severe LV dysfunction and shock who are too ill to tolerate surgery.

AORTIC REGURGITATION

ETIOLOGY

(Table 230-1) AR may be caused by primary valve disease or by primary aortic root disease.

Primary Valve Disease In approximately two-thirds of patients with valvular AR, the disease is rheumatic in origin, resulting in thickening, deformity, and shortening of the individual aortic valve cusps, changes that prevent their proper opening during systole and closure during diastole. A rheumatic origin is much less common in patients with isolated AR who do not have associated mitral valve disease. Patients with congenital BAV disease may develop predominant AR. Congenital fenestrations of the aortic valve occasionally produce mild AR. Membranous subaortic stenosis often leads to thickening and scarring of the aortic valve leaflets with secondary AR. Prolapse of an aortic cusp, resulting in progressive chronic AR, occurs in approximately 15% of patients with ventricular septal defect (Chap. 229) but may also occur as an isolated phenomenon or as a consequence of myxomatous degeneration sometimes associated with mitral (p. 1472) and/or tricuspid valve involvement.

AR may result from infective endocarditis, which can develop on a valve previously affected by rheumatic disease, a congenitally deformed valve, or, rarely, on a normal aortic valve, and may lead to perforation or erosion of one or more leaflets. The aortic valve leaflets may become scarred and retracted during the course of syphilis or ankylosing spondylitis and contribute further to the AR that derives primarily from the associated root disease. Although traumatic rupture or avulsion of the aortic valve is an uncommon cause of acute AR, it does represent the most frequent serious lesion in patients surviving nonpenetrating cardiac injuries. The coexistence of hemodynamically significant AS with AR usually excludes all the rarer forms of AR because it occurs almost exclusively in patients with rheumatic or congenital AR. In patients with AR due to primary valvular disease, dilatation of the aortic annulus may occur secondarily and intensify the regurgitation.

Primary Aortic Root Disease AR may also be due entirely to marked aortic dilatation, i.e., aortic root disease, without primary involvement of the valve leaflets; widening of the aortic annulus and separation of the aortic leaflets are responsible for the AR (Chap. 242). Cystic medial degeneration of the ascending aorta, which may or may not be associated with other manifestations of Marfan syndrome; idiopathic dilatation of the aorta; annulo-aortic ectasia; osteogenesis imperfecta; and severe hypertension may all widen the aortic annulus and lead to progressive AR. Occasionally AR is caused by retrograde dissection of the aorta involving the aortic annulus. Syphilis and ankylosing spondylitis, both of which may affect aortic valves, may also be associated with cellular infiltration and scarring of the media of the thoracic aorta, leading to aortic dilatation, aneurysm formation, and severe regurgitation. In syphilis of the aorta (Chap. 162), now a very rare condition, the involvement of the intima may narrow the coronary ostia, which in turn may be responsible for myocardial ischemia.

PATHOPHYSIOLOGY

The total stroke volume ejected by the LV (i.e., the sum of the effective forward stroke volume and the volume of blood that regurgitates back into the LV) is increased in patients with AR. In patients with wide-open (free) AR, the volume of regurgitant flow may equal the effective forward stroke volume. In contrast to MR, in which a fraction of the LV stroke volume is delivered into the low-pressure LA, in AR the entire LV stroke volume is ejected into a high-pressure zone, the aorta. An increase in the LV end-diastolic volume (increased preload) constitutes the major hemodynamic compensation for AR. The dilatation and eccentric hypertrophy of the LV allow this chamber to eject a larger stroke volume without requiring any increase in the relative shortening of each myofibril. Therefore, severe AR may occur with a normal effective forward stroke volume and a normal left ventricular EF [total (forward plus regurgitant) stroke volume/end-diastolic volume], together with an elevated LV end-diastolic pressure and volume. However, through the operation of Laplace's law, LV dilatation increases the LV systolic tension required to develop any given level of systolic pressure. Chronic AR is thus a state in which LV preload and afterload are both increased. Ultimately, these adaptive measures fail. As LV function deteriorates, the end-diastolic volume rises further and the forward stroke volume and EF decline. Deterioration of LV function often precedes the development of symptoms. Considerable thickening of the LV wall also occurs with chronic AR, and at autopsy the hearts of these patients may be among the largest encountered, sometimes weighing >1000 g.

The reverse pressure gradient from aorta to LV, which drives the AR flow, falls progressively during diastole (see Fig. 223-5), accounting for the decrescendo nature of the diastolic murmur. Equilibration between aortic and LV pressures may occur toward the end of diastole in patients with chronic severe AR, particularly when the heart rate is slow. In patients with acute severe AR, the LV is unprepared for the regurgitant volume load. LV compliance is normal or reduced, and LV diastolic pressures rise rapidly, occasionally to levels >40 mmHg. The LV pressure may exceed the LA pressure toward the end of diastole, and this reversed pressure gradient closes the mitral valve prematurely.

In patients with chronic severe AR, the effective forward CO usually is normal or only slightly reduced at rest, but often it fails to rise normally during exertion. Early signs of LV dysfunction include reduction in the EF. In advanced stages there may be considerable elevation of the LA, PA wedge, PA, and RV pressures and lowering of the forward CO at rest.

Myocardial ischemia may occur in patients with AR because myocardial oxygen requirements are elevated by LV dilatation, hypertrophy, and elevated LV systolic tension. However, a large fraction of coronary blood flow occurs during diastole, when arterial pressure is subnormal, thereby reducing coronary perfusion pressure. This combination of increased oxygen demand and reduced supply may cause myocardial ischemia, particularly of the subendocardium, even in the absence of concomitant CAD.

HISTORY

Approximately three-fourths of patients with pure or predominant valvular AR are males; females predominate among patients with primary valvular AR who have associated mitral valve disease. A history compatible with infective endocarditis may sometimes be elicited from patients with rheumatic or congenital involvement of the aortic valve, and the infection often precipitates or seriously aggravates preexisting symptoms.

In patients with *acute severe AR*, as may occur in infective endocarditis, aortic dissection, or trauma, the LV cannot dilate sufficiently to maintain stroke volume, and LV diastolic pressure rises rapidly with associated marked elevations of LA and PA wedge pressures. Pulmonary edema and/or cardiogenic shock may develop rapidly.

Chronic severe AR may have a long latent period, and patients may remain relatively asymptomatic for as long as 10–15 years. However, uncomfortable awareness of the heartbeat, especially on lying down, may be an early complaint. Sinus tachycardia, during exertion or with emotion, or premature ventricular contractions may produce particularly uncomfortable palpitations as well as head pounding. These complaints may persist for many years before the development of exertional dyspnea, usually the first symptom of diminished cardiac reserve. The dyspnea is

followed by orthopnea, paroxysmal nocturnal dyspnea, and excessive diaphoresis. Anginal chest pain occurs frequently in patients with severe AR, even in younger patients, and it is not necessary to invoke the presence of CAD to explain this symptom in patients with severe AR. Anginal pain may develop at rest as well as during exertion. Nocturnal angina may be a particularly troublesome symptom, and it may be accompanied by marked diaphoresis. The anginal episodes can be prolonged and often do not respond satisfactorily to sublingual nitroglycerin. Systemic fluid accumulation, including congestive hepatomegaly and ankle edema, may develop late in the course of the disease.

PHYSICAL FINDINGS

In chronic severe AR, the jarring of the entire body and the bobbing motion of the head with each systole can be appreciated, and the abrupt distention and collapse of the larger arteries are easily visible. The examination should be directed toward the detection of conditions predisposing to AR, such as Marfan syndrome, ankylosing spondylitis, and ventricular septal defect.

Arterial Pulse A rapidly rising "water-hammer" pulse, which collapses suddenly as arterial pressure falls rapidly during late systole and diastole (Corrigan's pulse), and capillary pulsations, an alternate flushing and paling of the skin at the root of the nail while pressure is applied to the tip of the nail (Quincke's pulse), are characteristic of free AR. A booming "pistol-shot" sound can be heard over the femoral arteries (Traube's sign), and a to-and-fro murmur (Duroziez's sign) is audible if the femoral artery is lightly compressed with a stethoscope.

The arterial pulse pressure is widened, and there is an elevation of the systolic pressure, sometimes to as high as 300 mmHg, and a depression of the diastolic pressure. The measurement of arterial diastolic pressure with a sphygmomanometer may be complicated by the fact that systolic sounds are frequently heard with the cuff completely deflated. However, the level of cuff pressure at the time of muffling of the Korotkoff sounds (Phase IV) generally corresponds fairly closely to the true intraarterial diastolic pressure. As the disease progresses and the LV end-diastolic pressure rises, the arterial diastolic pressure may actually rise as well, since the aortic diastolic pressure cannot fall below the LV end-diastolic pressure. For the same reason, acute severe AR may also be accompanied by only a slight widening of the pulse pressure. Such patients are invariably tachycardic as the heart rate increases in an attempt to preserve the CO.

Palpation In patients with chronic severe AR, the LV impulse is heaving and displaced laterally and inferiorly. The systolic expansion and diastolic retraction of the apex are prominent. A diastolic thrill is often palpable along the left sternal border, and a prominent systolic thrill may be palpable in the suprasternal notch and transmitted upward along the carotid arteries. This systolic thrill and the accompanying murmur do not necessarily signify the coexistence of AS. In many patients with pure AR or with combined AS and AR, the carotid arterial pulse is bisferiens, i.e., with two systolic waves separated by a trough (see Fig. 220-2D).

Auscultation In patients with severe AR, the aortic valve closure sound (A₂) is usually absent. An S₃ and systolic ejection sound are frequently audible, and occasionally an S₄ also may be heard. The murmur of chronic AR is typically a high-pitched, blowing, decrescendo diastolic murmur, heard best in the third intercostal space along the left sternal border (see Fig. 220-4B). In patients with mild AR, this murmur is brief but, as the severity increases, generally becomes louder and longer, indeed holodiastolic. When the murmur is soft, it can be heard best with the diaphragm of the stethoscope and with the patient sitting up, leaning forward, and with the breath held in forced expiration. In patients in whom the AR is caused by primary valvular disease, the diastolic murmur is usually louder along the left than the right sternal border. However, when the murmur is heard best along the right sternal border, it suggests that the AR is caused by aneurysmal dilatation of the aortic root. "Cooing" or musical diastolic murmurs suggest eversion of an aortic cusp vibrating in the regurgitant stream.

A mid-systolic ejection murmur is frequently audible in isolated AR. It is generally heard best at the base of the heart and is transmitted along the carotid vessels. This murmur may be quite loud without signifying aortic obstruction. A third murmur frequently heard in patients with severe AR is the *Austin Flint murmur*, a soft, low-pitched, rumbling mid-diastolic murmur. It is probably produced by the diastolic displacement of the anterior leaflet of the mitral valve by the AR stream but does not appear to be associated with hemodynamically significant mitral obstruction. The auscultatory features of AR are intensified by strenuous handgrip, which augments systemic resistance.

In acute severe AR, the elevation of LV end-diastolic pressure may lead to early closure of the mitral valve, an associated mid-diastolic sound, a soft or absent S_1, a pulse pressure that is not particularly wide, and a soft, short diastolic murmur of AR.

LABORATORY EXAMINATION

ECG In patients with chronic severe AR, the ECG signs of LV hypertrophy become manifest (Chap. 221). In addition, these patients frequently exhibit ST-segment depression and T-wave inversion in leads I, aVL, V_5, and V_6 ("LV strain"). Left axis deviation and/or QRS prolongation denote diffuse myocardial disease, generally associated with patchy fibrosis, and usually signify a poor prognosis.

Echocardiogram The extent and velocity of wall motion are normal or even supernormal, until myocardial contractility declines. A rapid, high-frequency fluttering of the anterior mitral leaflet produced by the impact of the regurgitant jet is a characteristic finding. The echocardiogram is also useful in determining the cause of AR, by detecting dilatation of the aortic annulus and root or aortic dissection (see Fig. 222-3). Thickening and failure of coaptation of the leaflets also may be noted. Color flow Doppler echocardiographic imaging is very sensitive in the detection of AR, and Doppler echocardiography is helpful in assessing its severity. With severe AR, the central jet width exceeds 65% of the left ventricular outflow tract, the regurgitant volume is ≥60 ml/beat, the regurgitant fraction is ≥50%, and there is diastolic flow reversal in the proximal descending thoracic aorta. The continuous wave Doppler profile shows a rapid deceleration time in patients with acute severe AR, due to the rapid increase in LV diastolic pressure. Serial two-dimensional echocardiography is valuable in assessing LV performance and in detecting progressive myocardial dysfunction.

Chest X-ray In chronic severe AR, the apex is displaced downward and to the left in the frontal projec-tion. In the left anterior oblique and lateral projections, the LV is displaced posteriorly and encroaches on the spine. When AR is caused by primary disease of the aortic root, aneurysmal dilatation of the aorta may be noted, and the aorta may fill the retrosternal space in the lateral view. Echocardiography and CT angiography are more sensitive than the chest x-ray for the detection of aortic root enlargement.

Cardiac Catheterization and Angiography When needed, right and left heart catheterization with contrast aortography can provide accurate confirmation of the magnitude of regurgitation and the status of LV function. Coronary angiography is performed routinely in appropriate patients prior to surgery.

℞ AORTIC REGURGITATION

(Fig. 230-6)

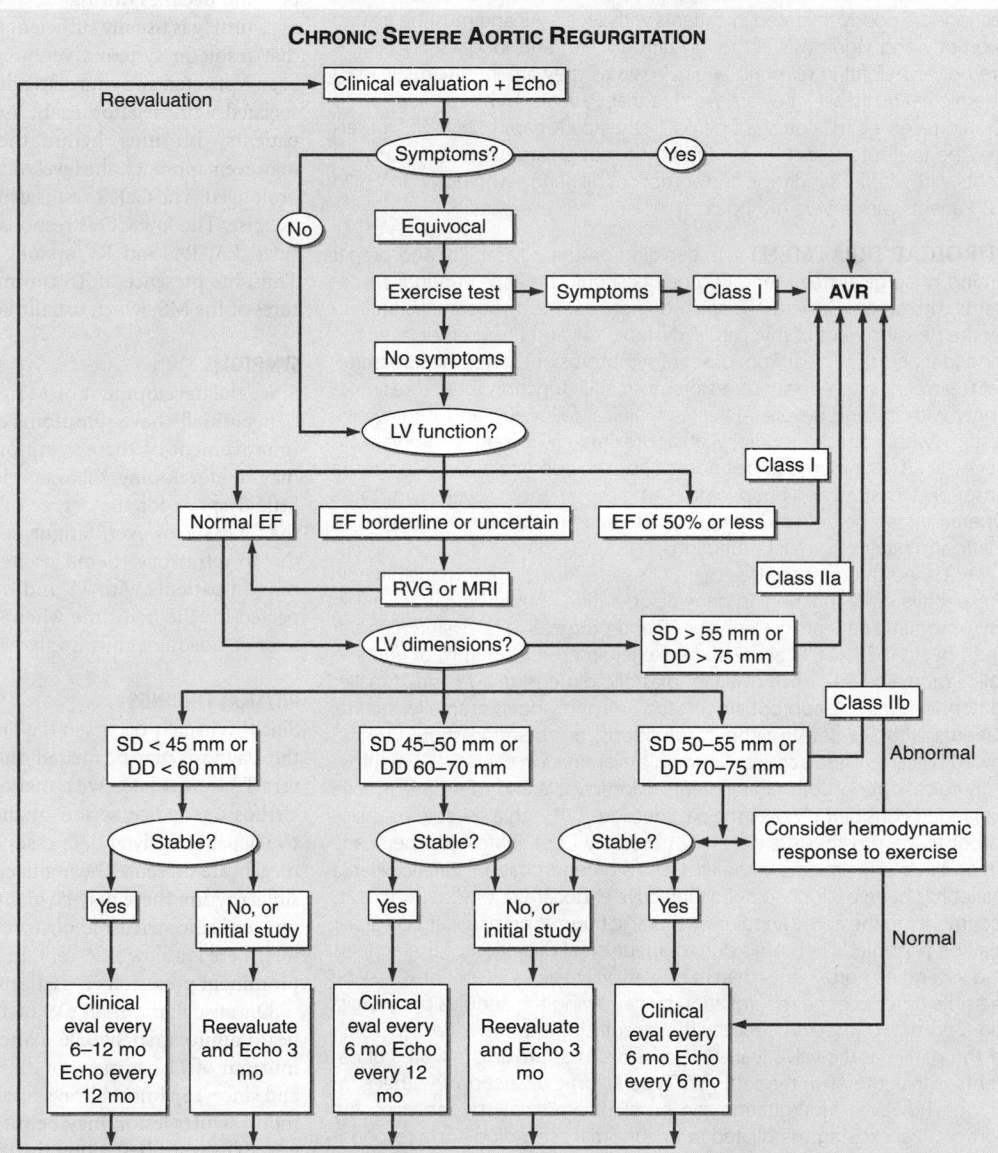

FIGURE 230-6 Management strategy for patients with chronic severe aortic regurgitation. Preoperative coronary angiography should be performed routinely, as determined by age, symptoms, and coronary risk factors. Cardiac catheterization and angiography may also be helpful when there is discordance between clinical findings and echocardiography. "Stable" refers to stable echocardiographic measurements. In some centers, serial follow-up may be performed with radionuclide ventriculography (RVG) or magnetic resonance imaging (MRI) rather than echocardiography (echo) to assess left ventricular (LV) volume and systolic function. AVR, aortic valve replacement; DD, end-diastolic dimension; EF, ejection fraction; eval, evaluation; SD, end-systolic dimension. (*Modified from Bonow et al.*)

ACUTE AORTIC REGURGITATION Patients with acute severe AR may respond to intravenous diuretics and vasodilators (such as sodium nitroprusside), but stabilization is usually short-lived and operation is indicated urgently. Intraaortic balloon counterpulsation is contraindicated. Beta-blockers are also best avoided so as not to reduce the CO further or slow the heart rate, which might allow proportionately more time in diastole for regurgitation to occur. Surgery is the treatment of choice.

CHRONIC AORTIC REGURGITATION Early symptoms of dyspnea and effort intolerance respond to treatment with diuretics and vasodilators (ACE inhibitors, dihydropyridine calcium channel blockers, or hydralazine) may be useful as well. Surgery can then be performed in more controlled circumstances. The use of vasodilators to extend the compensated phase of chronic severe AR before the onset of symptoms or the development of LV dysfunction is more controversial. Expert consensus is strong regarding the need to control systolic blood pressure (goal <140 mmHg) in patients with chronic AR, and vasodilators are an excellent first choice as antihypertensive agents. It is often difficult to achieve adequate control in such patients because of the increased stroke volume. Cardiac arrhythmias and systemic infections are poorly tolerated in patients with severe AR and must be treated promptly and vigorously. Although nitroglycerin and long-acting nitrates are not as helpful in relieving anginal pain as they are in patients with ischemic heart disease, they are worth a trial. Patients with syphilitic aortitis should receive a full course of penicillin therapy (Chap. 162). Beta blockers may be useful to retard the rate of aortic root enlargement in young patients with Marfan syndrome and aortic root dilatation with no or only mild AR. Patients with severe AR should avoid isometric exercises.

SURGICAL TREATMENT In deciding on the advisability and proper timing of surgical treatment, two points should be kept in mind: (1) patients with chronic severe AR usually do not become symptomatic until *after* the development of myocardial dysfunction; and (2) when delayed too long (defined as >1 year from onset of symptoms or LV dysfunction), surgical treatment often does not restore normal LV function. Therefore, in patients with chronic severe AR, careful clinical follow-up and noninvasive testing with echocardiography at approximately 6-month intervals are necessary if operation is to be undertaken at the optimal time, i.e., *after* the onset of LV dysfunction but *prior* to the development of severe symptoms. Operation can be deferred as long as the patient both remains asymptomatic and retains normal LV function.

AVR is indicated for the treatment of severe AR in symptomatic patients irrespective of LV function. In general, operation should be carried out in asymptomatic patients with severe AR and progressive LV dysfunction defined by an LVEF <50%, an LV end-systolic dimension >55mm or end-systolic volume >55 mL/m², or an LV diastolic dimension >75 mm. Smaller dimensions may be appropriate thresholds in individuals of smaller stature. Patients with severe AR without indications for operation should be followed by clinical and echocardiographic examination every 3–12 months.

Surgical options for management of aortic valve and root disease have expanded considerably over the past decade. AVR with a suitable mechanical or tissue prosthesis is generally necessary in patients with rheumatic AR and in many patients with other forms of regurgitation. Rarely, when a leaflet has been perforated during infective endocarditis or torn from its attachments to the aortic annulus by thoracic trauma, primary surgical repair may be possible. When AR is due to aneurysmal dilatation of the annulus and ascending aorta rather than to primary valvular involvement, it may be possible to reduce the regurgitation by narrowing the annulus or by excising a portion of the aortic root without replacing the valve. Resuspension of the native aortic valve leaflets is possible in approximately 50% of patients with acute AR in the setting of Type A aortic dissection. In other conditions, however, regurgitation can be eliminated only by replacing the aortic valve, excising the dilated or aneurysmal ascending aorta responsible for the regurgitation, and replacing it with a graft. This formidable procedure entails a higher risk than isolated AVR.

As in patients with other valvular abnormalities, both the operative risk and the late mortality are largely dependent on the stage of the disease and on myocardial function at the time of operation. The overall operative mortality for isolated AVR is about 3% (Table 230-3). However, patients with marked cardiac enlargement and prolonged LV dysfunction experience an operative mortality rate of approximately 10% and a late mortality rate of approximately 5% per year due to LV failure despite a technically satisfactory operation. Nonetheless, because of the very poor prognosis with medical management, even patients with LV failure should be considered for operation.

Patients with acute severe AR require prompt surgical treatment, which may be lifesaving.

TRICUSPID STENOSIS

TS, much less prevalent than MS in North America and Western Europe, is generally rheumatic in origin and is more common in females than in males. It does not occur as an isolated lesion and is usually associated with MS. Hemodynamically significant TS occurs in 5–10% of patients with severe MS; rheumatic TS is commonly associated with some degree of TR. Nonrheumatic causes of TS are rare.

PATHOPHYSIOLOGY

A diastolic pressure gradient between the RA and RV defines TS. It is augmented when the transvalvular blood flow increases during inspiration and declines during expiration. A mean diastolic pressure gradient of 4 mmHg is usually sufficient to elevate the mean RA pressure to levels that result in systemic venous congestion. Unless sodium intake has been restricted and diuretics administered, this venous congestion is associated with hepatomegaly, ascites, and edema, sometimes severe. In patients with sinus rhythm, the RA *a* wave may be extremely tall and may even approach the level of the RV systolic pressure. The *y* descent is prolonged. The CO at rest is usually depressed, and it fails to rise during exercise. The low CO is responsible for the normal or only slightly elevated LA, PA, and RV systolic pressures despite the presence of MS. Thus, the presence of TS can mask the hemodynamic and clinical features of the MS, which usually accompanies it.

SYMPTOMS

Since the development of MS generally precedes that of TS, many patients initially have symptoms of pulmonary congestion. Spontaneous improvement of these symptoms should raise the possibility that TS may be developing. Characteristically, patients complain of relatively little dyspnea for the degree of hepatomegaly, ascites, and edema that they have. However, fatigue secondary to a low CO and discomfort due to refractory edema, ascites, and marked hepatomegaly are common in patients with TS and/or TR. In some patients, TS may be suspected for the first time when symptoms of right-sided failure persist after an adequate mitral valvotomy.

PHYSICAL FINDINGS

Since TS usually occurs in the presence of other obvious valvular disease, the diagnosis may be missed unless it is considered and searched for. Severe TS is associated with marked hepatic congestion, often resulting in cirrhosis, jaundice, serious malnutrition, anasarca, and ascites. Congestive hepatomegaly and, in cases of severe tricuspid valve disease, splenomegaly are present. The jugular veins are distended, and in patients with sinus rhythm there may be giant *a* waves. The *v* waves are less conspicuous, and since tricuspid obstruction impedes RA emptying during diastole, there is a slow *y* descent. In patients with sinus rhythm there may be prominent presystolic pulsations of the enlarged liver as well.

On auscultation, an OS of the tricuspid valve may occasionally be heard approximately 0.06 s after pulmonic valve closure. The diastolic murmur of TS has many of the qualities of the diastolic murmur of MS, and since TS almost always occurs in the presence of MS, the less-common valvular lesion may be missed. However, the tricuspid murmur is generally heard best along the left lower sternal margin and over the xiphoid process, and it is most prominent during presystole in patients with sinus rhythm. The murmur of TS is augmented during inspiration, and it is reduced during expiration and particularly during the strain phase of the Valsalva maneuver, when tricuspid blood flow is reduced.

LABORATORY EXAMINATION

The ECG features of RA enlargement (see Fig. 221-8) include tall, peaked P waves in lead II, as well as prominent, upright P waves in lead V_1. The *absence* of ECG evidence of right ventricular hypertrophy

(RVH) in a patient with right-sided heart failure who is believed to have MS should suggest associated tricuspid valve disease. The chest x-ray in patients with combined TS and MS shows particular prominence of the RA and superior vena cava without much enlargement of the PA and with less evidence of pulmonary vascular congestion than occurs in patients with isolated MS. On echocardiographic examination, the tricuspid valve is usually thickened and domes in diastole; the transvalvular gradient can be estimated by Doppler echocardiography. TTE provides additional information regarding mitral valve structure and function, LV and RV size and function, and PA pressure.

℞ TRICUSPID STENOSIS

Patients with TS generally exhibit marked systemic venous congestion; intensive salt restriction, bed rest, and diuretic therapy are required during the preoperative period. Such a preparatory period may diminish hepatic congestion and thereby improve hepatic function sufficiently so that the risks of operation, particularly bleeding, are diminished. Surgical relief of the TS should be carried out, preferably at the time of surgical mitral valvotomy or MVR, in patients with moderate or severe TS who have mean diastolic pressure gradients exceeding ~4 mmHg and tricuspid orifice areas <1.5–2.0 cm². TS is almost always accompanied by significant TR. Operative repair may permit substantial improvement of tricuspid valve function. If repair cannot be accomplished, the tricuspid valve may have to be replaced with a prosthesis, preferably a large bioprosthetic valve. Mechanical valves in the tricuspid position are more prone to thromboembolic complications than in other positions.

TRICUSPID REGURGITATION

Most commonly, TR is functional and secondary to marked dilatation of the tricuspid annulus. Functional TR may complicate RV enlargement of any cause, including inferior wall infarcts that involve the RV. It is commonly seen in the late stages of heart failure due to rheumatic or congenital heart disease with severe pulmonary hypertension (pulmonary artery systolic pressure >55 mmHg), as well as in ischemic heart disease and dilated cardiomyopathy. It is reversible in part if pulmonary hypertension is relieved. Rheumatic fever may produce organic (primary) TR, often associated with TS. Infarction of RV papillary muscles, tricuspid valve prolapse, carcinoid heart disease, endomyocardial fibrosis, infective endocarditis, and trauma all may produce TR. Less commonly, TR results from congenitally deformed tricuspid valves, and it occurs with defects of the atrioventricular canal, as well as with Ebstein's malformation of the tricuspid valve (Chap. 229). TR also develops eventually in patients with chronic RV apical pacing.

As is the case for TS, the clinical features of TR result primarily from systemic venous congestion and reduction of CO. With the onset of TR in patients with pulmonary hypertension, symptoms of pulmonary congestion diminish, but the clinical manifestations of right-sided heart failure become intensified. The neck veins are distended with prominent *v* waves and rapid *y* descents, marked hepatomegaly, ascites, pleural effusions, edema, systolic pulsations of the liver, and a positive hepatojugular reflux. A prominent RV pulsation along the left parasternal region and a blowing holosystolic murmur along the lower left sternal margin, which may be intensified during inspiration and reduced during expiration or the strain of the Valsalva maneuver (Carvallo's sign), are characteristic findings; AF is usually present.

The ECG usually shows changes characteristic of the lesion responsible for the enlargement of the RV that leads to TR, e.g., inferior wall myocardial infarction or severe RVH. Echocardiography may be helpful by demonstrating RV dilatation and prolapsing, flail, scarred, or displaced tricuspid leaflets; the diagnosis of TR can be made by color flow Doppler echocardiography, and its severity can be estimated by Doppler examination (see Fig. 222-4). Severe TR is accompanied by hepatic vein systolic flow reversal. Continuous wave Doppler is also useful in estimating PA pressure. Roentgenographic examination usually reveals enlargement of both the RA and RV.

In patients with severe TR, the CO is usually markedly reduced, and the RA pressure pulse may exhibit no x descent during early systole but a prominent *c-v* wave with a rapid *y* descent. The mean RA and the RV end-diastolic pressures are often elevated.

℞ TRICUSPID REGURGITATION

Isolated TR, in the absence of pulmonary hypertension, such as that occurring as a consequence of infective endocarditis or trauma, is usually well tolerated and does not require operation. Indeed, even total excision of an infected tricuspid valve may be well tolerated for several years if the PA pressure is normal. Treatment of the underlying cause of heart failure usually reduces the severity of functional TR, by reducing the size of the tricuspid annulus. In patients with mitral valve disease and TR secondary to pulmonary hypertension and massive RV enlargement, effective surgical correction of the mitral valvular abnormality results in lowering of the PA pressures and gradual reduction or disappearance of the TR without direct treatment of the tricuspid valve. However, recovery may be much more rapid in patients with severe secondary TR if, at the time of mitral valve surgery, and especially when there is measurable enlargement of the tricuspid valve annulus, tricuspid annuloplasty (generally with the insertion of a plastic ring), open tricuspid valve repair, or, in the rare instance of severe organic tricuspid valve disease, tricuspid valve replacement is performed (Table 230-3). Tricuspid annuloplasty or replacement may be required for severe TR with primary involvement of the valve.

PULMONIC VALVE DISEASE

The pulmonic valve is affected by rheumatic fever far less frequently than are the other valves, and it is uncommonly the seat of infective endocarditis. The most common *acquired* abnormality affecting the pulmonic valve is regurgitation secondary to dilatation of the pulmonic valve ring as a consequence of severe pulmonary hypertension. This produces the *Graham Steell murmur*, a high-pitched, decrescendo, diastolic blowing murmur along the left sternal border, which is difficult to differentiate from the far more common murmur produced by AR. Pulmonic regurgitation is usually of little hemodynamic significance; indeed, surgical removal or destruction of the pulmonic valve by infective endocarditis does not produce heart failure unless serious pulmonary hypertension is also present.

The *carcinoid syndrome* may cause pulmonic stenosis and/or regurgitation. Pulmonic regurgitation occurs universally among patients who have undergone childhood repair of Tetralogy of Fallot with reconstruction of the RV outflow tract. **Congenital pulmonic stenosis is discussed in Chap. 229.**

VALVE REPLACEMENT

The results of replacement of any valve are dependent primarily on (1) the patient's myocardial function and general medical condition at the time of operation; (2) the technical abilities of the operative team and the quality of the postoperative care; and (3) the durability, hemodynamic characteristics, and thrombogenicity of the prosthesis. Increased perioperative mortality is associated with advanced age and comorbidity (e.g., pulmonary or renal disease, the need for nonvalvular cardiovascular surgery, diabetes mellitus) as well as with greater levels of preoperative functional disability and pulmonary hypertension. Late complications of valve replacement include paravalvular leakage, thromboemboli, bleeding due to anticoagulants, structural deterioration of the prosthesis, and infective endocarditis.

The considerations involved in the choice between a bioprosthetic (tissue) and artificial mechanical valve are similar in the mitral and aortic positions and in the treatment of stenotic, regurgitant, or mixed lesions. All patients who have undergone replacement of any valve with a mechanical prosthesis are at risk of thromboembolic complications and must be maintained permanently on anticoagulants, a treatment that imposes a hazard of hemorrhage. The primary advantage of bioprostheses over mechanical prostheses is the virtual absence of thromboembolic complications 3 months after implantation, and except for patients with chronic AF, few such instances have been associated with their use. The major disadvantage of bioprosthetic valves is their structural deterioration, the incidence of which is inversely proportional to the patient's age. This deterioration results in the need to replace the prosthesis in up to 30% of patients by 10 years and in 50% by 15 years. Rates of structural valve deterioration are higher for mitral than for aortic bioprostheses. This phenomenon may be due in part to the greater closing pressure to which a mitral prosthesis is exposed.

Traditionally, a mechanical prosthesis was considered preferable for a patient under age 65 who could take anticoagulation reliably. Bioprostheses were recommended for older patients (>65 years) who did not otherwise have an indication for anticoagulation (for example, AF). However, more recent surveys of cardiac surgery in the United States, as reflected in the Society of Thoracic Surgeons database, show a clear and progressive trend favoring the implantation of bioprosthetic valves in younger (<65 years) patients. Reasons for this development include improved durability of newer generation bioprostheses, decreased risk at time of reoperation, the aggregate risks of long-term anticoagulation, and patient preference to avoid anticoagulation. Patient preference should be factored into any decision regarding the type of valve replacement. A mechanical prosthesis is reasonable for aortic or mitral valve replacement in patients <65 years without a contraindication to anticoagulation. A bioprosthesis is equally reasonable for aortic or mitral valve replacement in patients <65 years who elect this strategy for lifestyle reasons with full knowledge of the likely need for reoperation over time.

Bioprostheses remain the preferred valve choice for patients >65 years, in both the aortic and mitral position. Bioprosthetic valves are also indicated for women who expect to become pregnant, as well as for others who refuse to take anticoagulation or for whom anticoagulation may be contraindicated. Types of bioprostheses include xenografts (i.e., porcine aortic valves; cryopreserved, mounted bovine pericardium), homograft (allograft) aortic valves obtained from cadavers, as well as pulmonary autografts transplanted into the aortic position. Homograft replacement may be preferred for the management of complicated aortic valve infective endocarditis.

In patients without contraindications to anticoagulants, particularly those under 65 years, a mechanical prosthesis is reasonable. Many surgeons now select the St. Jude prosthesis, a double-disk tilting prosthesis, for replacement of both aortic and mitral valves because of favorable hemodynamic characteristics and possible association with lower thrombogenicity.

GLOBAL BURDEN OF VALVULAR HEART DISEASE

Primary valvular heart disease ranks well below coronary heart disease, stroke, hypertension, obesity, and diabetes as major threats to the public health. Nevertheless, it is the source of significant morbidity and mortality. Rheumatic fever (Chap. 315) is the dominant cause of valvular heart disease in developing countries. Its prevalence has been estimated to range from as low as 1.0 per 100,000 school-age children in Costa Rica to as high as 150 per 100,000 in China. Rheumatic heart disease accounts for 12–65% of hospital admissions related to cardiovascular disease and 2–10% of hospital discharges in some developing countries. Prevalence and mortality rates vary among communities even within the same country as a function of crowding and the availability of medical resources and population-wide programs for detection and treatment of Group A streptococcal pharyngitis. In economically deprived areas, tropical and subtropical climates (particularly on the Indian subcontinent), Central America, and the Middle East, rheumatic valvular disease progresses more rapidly than in more-developed nations and frequently causes serious symptoms in patients <20 years of age. This accelerated natural history may be due to repeated infections with more virulent strains of rheumatogenic streptococci.

TS, a relatively uncommon valvular lesion in North America and Western Europe, is more common in tropical and subtropical climates, especially in southern Asia and in Latin America.

As of the year 2000, worldwide death rates for rheumatic heart disease approximated 5.5 per 100,000 population ($n = 332,000$), with the highest rates reported from Southeast Asia. Although there have been reports of recent isolated outbreaks of streptococcal infection in North America, valve disease in developed countries is now dominated by degenerative or inflammatory processes that lead to valve thickening, calcification, and dysfunction. The prevalence of valvular heart disease increases with age. Important left-sided valve disease may affect as many as 12–13% of adults over the age of 75.

The incidence of infective endocarditis (Chap. 118) has increased with the aging of the population, the more widespread prevalence of vascular grafts and intracardiac devices, the emergence of more virulent multidrug-resistant microorganisms, and the growing epidemic of diabetes. Infective endocarditis has become a more frequent cause of acute valvular regurgitation.

Bicuspid aortic valve disease affects as many as 1–2% of the population, and an increasing number of childhood survivors of congenital heart disease present later in life with valvular dysfunction. The past several years have witnessed significant improvements in surgical outcomes with progressive refinement of relatively less-invasive techniques. Percutaneous heart valve replacement or repair is under active clinical investigation.

FURTHER READINGS

Bonow RO et al: ACC/AHA 2006 Guidelines for the management of patients with valvular heart disease: Executive summary. Circulation 114:450, 2006

Coats L, Bonhoeffer P: New percutaneous treatments for valve disease. Heart 93:639, 2007

Enriquez-Sarano M, Tajik AJ: Aortic regurgitation. N Engl J Med 351:1539, 2004

Hara H et al: Percutaneous balloon aortic valvuloplasty revisited: Time for a renaissance? Circulation 115:e334, 2007

Nkomo VT et al: Burden of valvular heart diseases: A population-based study. Lancet 368:1005, 2006

Otto CM (ed): *Valvular Heart Disease,* 2d ed. Philadelphia, Saunders, 2003

———, Bonow RO: Valvular heart disease, in P Libby et al (eds): *Braunwald's Heart Disease,* 8th ed. Philadelphia, Saunders, 2008

Pellikka PA et al: Outcome of 622 adults with asymptomatic, hemodynamically significant aortic stenosis during prolonged follow-up. Circulation 111:3290, 2005

Quere JP et al: Influence of left ventricular preoperative contractile reserve on postoperative ejection fraction in low-gradient aortic stenosis. Circulation 113:1738, 2006

Rosenhek R et al: Outcome of watchful waiting in asymptomatic severe mitral regurgitation. Circulation 113:2238, 2006

Society of Thoracic Surgeons: STS Adult Cardiovascular National Surgery Database—Fall 2005 executive summary. Available online at *http://www.sts.org/documents/pdf/STS-ExecutiveSummaryFall2005.pdf*

———: STS national database risk calculator. Available online at *http://www.sts.org/sections/stsnationaldatabase/riskcalculator/*

Wilson W et al: Prevention of infective endocarditis. Guidelines from the American Heart Association Rheumatic Fever, Endocarditis, and Kawasaki Disease Committee, Council on Cardiovascular Disease in the Young, and the Council on Clinical Cardiology, Council on Cardiovascular Surgery and Anesthesia and the Quality of Care and Outcomes Research Interdisciplinary Working Group. Published April 2007, online at *http://circ.ahajournals.org*

World Health Organization: WHO expert consultation on rheumatic fever and rheumatic heart disease. Geneva, Switzerland, WHO technical report series: 923, 2001

231 Cardiomyopathy and Myocarditis

Joshua Wynne, Eugene Braunwald

The cardiomyopathies are a group of diseases that primarily affect the heart muscle and are *not* the result of congenital, acquired valvular, hypertensive, coronary arterial, or pericardial abnormalities. The diffuse myocardial fibrosis that accompanies multiple myocardial scars produced by myocardial infarctions can impair left ventricular (LV) function and is frequently referred to as *ischemic cardiomyopathy*. This colloquial use of the term *cardiomyopathy* should be avoided; instead, the term should be restricted to a condition *primarily* involving the myocardium.

Two fundamental forms of cardiomyopathy are recognized: (1) a primary type, consisting of heart muscle disease predominantly involving the myocardium and/or of unknown cause; and (2) a secondary type, consisting of myocardial disease of known cause or associated with a systemic disease such as amyloidosis or chronic alcohol use (Table 231-1). In many cases it is not possible to arrive at a specific etiologic diagnosis, and thus it is often more desirable to classify the cardiomyopathies into one of three morphologic types (dilated, restrictive, and hypertrophic) on the basis of differences in their pathophysiology and clinical presentation (Fig. 231-1; Tables 231-2 and 231-3). In some patients, two of these types may be present simultaneously or sequentially. An important additional consideration is whether or not the particular cardiomyopathy in question (whether primary or secondary) has a genetic basis.

DILATED CARDIOMYOPATHY

About one in three cases of congestive heart failure (CHF; Chap. 227) is due to dilated cardiomyopathy (DCM). LV and/or right ventricular (RV) systolic pump function is impaired, leading to progressive cardiac dilatation (remodeling). Symptoms of heart failure (HF) typically appear only after remodeling has been ongoing for some time (months or even years).

Normal   **Dilated cardiomyopathy**

Hypertrophic cardiomyopathy   **Restrictive cardiomyopathy**

FIGURE 231-1 Drawing comparing the morphologic classes of cardiomyopathies. Ao, aorta; LA, left atrium; LV, left ventricle. *(From BF Waller: J Am Soc Echocardiogr 1:4, 1988.)*

Although no cause is apparent in many cases, DCM is either familial or the end result of myocardial damage produced by a variety of known or unknown infectious, metabolic, or toxic agents. DCM may be the late consequence of acute viral myocarditis (see below), possibly mediated in part through an immunologic mechanism. Although DCM may occur at any age, it most commonly becomes apparent clinically in the third or fourth decades. A reversible form of DCM may be found with alcohol abuse (see below), pregnancy (see below), thyroid disease, cocaine use (see below), and chronic uncontrolled tachycardia.

GENETIC CONSIDERATIONS One-fifth to one-third of patients have familial forms of DCM. Mutations in >20 genes that are transmitted in an autosomal dominant fashion have been described. Most common are mutations in genes encoding sarcomeric proteins, such as α-cardiac actin; β- and α-myosin; heavy chain α-tropomyosin; and troponins T, I, and C. It is believed that the abnormal proteins cause contractile dysfunction by impairing the production and/or transmission of force.

Patients with genetic DCM may also exhibit skeletal myopathies, particularly Duchenne's and Emery-Dreyfuss muscular dystrophy (see below). Mutations in the gene encoding the nuclear envelope protein lamin A/C are also inherited in an autosomal dominant manner; they are responsible for the development of DCM associated with atrioventricular (AV) conduction disorder and other electrophysiologic disturbances that may cause sudden cardiac death (SCD). An X-linked autosomal recessive disorder caused by the dystrophin gene occurs in young males and is associated with a rapid downhill course; mutations in mitochondrial genes have also been reported in DCM.

CLINICAL FEATURES

Symptoms of left- and right-sided CHF usually develop gradually (Chap. 227). Some patients have LV dilatation for months or even years

TABLE 231-1 CLASSIFICATION OF CARDIOMYOPATHIES

Primary Myocardial Involvement

Idiopathic (D,R,H)
Familial (D,R,H)
Eosinophilic endomyocardial disease (R)
Endomyocardial fibrosis (R)

Secondary Myocardial Involvement

Infective (D)	Connective tissue disorders (D)
Viral myocarditis	Systemic lupus erythematosus
Bacterial myocarditis	Polyarteritis nodosa
Fungal myocarditis	Rheumatoid arthritis
Protozoal myocarditis	Progressive systemic sclerosis
Metazoal myocarditis	Dermatomyositis
Spirochetal	Infiltrations and granulomas (R,D)
Rickettsial	Amyloidosis
Metabolic (D)	Sarcoidosis
Familial storage disease (D,R)	Malignancy
Glycogen storage disease	Neuromuscular (D)
Mucopolysaccharidoses	Muscular dystrophy
Hemochromatosis	Myotonic dystrophy
Fabry's disease	Friedreich's ataxia (H,D)
Deficiency (D)	Sensitivity and toxic reactions (D)
Electrolytes	Alcohol
Nutritional	Radiation
	Drugs
	Peripartum heart disease (D)

Note: The principal clinical manifestation(s) of each etiologic grouping is denoted by D (dilated), R (restrictive), or H (hypertrophic) cardiomyopathy.
Source: Adapted from the WHO/ISFC task force report on the definition and classification of cardiomyopathies, 1980 and 1995.

TABLE 231-2 CLINICAL CLASSIFICATION OF CARDIOMYOPATHIES

1. Dilated: Left and/or right ventricular enlargement, impaired systolic function, congestive heart failure, arrhythmias, emboli
2. Restrictive: Endomyocardial scarring or myocardial infiltration resulting in restriction to left and/or right ventricular filling
3. Hypertrophic: Disproportionate left ventricular hypertrophy, typically involving septum more than free wall, with or without an intraventricular systolic pressure gradient; usually of a nondilated left ventricular cavity

TABLE 231-3 LABORATORY EVALUATION OF THE CARDIOMYOPATHIES

	Dilated	Restrictive	Hypertrophic
Chest roentgenogram	Moderate to marked cardiac silhouette enlargement Pulmonary venous hypertension	Mild cardiac silhouette enlargement	Mild to moderate cardiac silhouette enlargement
Electrocardiogram	ST-segment and T-wave abnormalities	Low voltage, conduction defects	ST-segment and T-wave abnormalities Left ventricular hypertrophy Abnormal Q waves
Echocardiogram	Left ventricular dilatation and dysfunction	Increased left ventricular wall thickness Normal or mildly reduced systolic function	Asymmetric septal hypertrophy (ASH) Systolic anterior motion (SAM) of the mitral valve
Radionuclide studies	Left ventricular dilatation and dysfunction (RVG)	Normal or mildly reduced systolic function (RVG)	Vigorous systolic function (RVG) Perfusion defect (^{201}Tl or technetium sestamibi)
Cardiac catheterization	Left ventricular dilatation and dysfunction Elevated left- and often right-sided filling pressures Diminished cardiac output	Normal or mildly reduced systolic function Elevated left- and right-sided filling pressures	Vigorous systolic function Dynamic left ventricular outflow obstruction Elevated left- and right-sided filling pressures

Note: RVG, radionuclide ventriculogram; ^{201}Tl, thallium 201.

before becoming symptomatic. Although vague chest pain may be present, typical angina pectoris is unusual and suggests the presence of ischemic heart disease. Syncope due to arrhythmias and systemic embolism (often emanating from a ventricular thrombus) may occur.

PHYSICAL EXAMINATION

Variable degrees of cardiac enlargement and findings of CHF (Chap. 227) are noted. In patients with advanced disease, the pulse pressure is narrow and the jugular venous pressure is elevated. Third and fourth heart sounds are common, and mitral or tricuspid regurgitation may occur.

LABORATORY EXAMINATIONS

The chest roentgenogram demonstrates enlargement of the cardiac silhouette due to LV dilatation, although generalized cardiomegaly is often seen. The lung fields may demonstrate pulmonary vascular redistribution and interstitial or, in advanced cases, alveolar edema. The electrocardiogram (ECG) often shows sinus tachycardia or atrial fibrillation, ventricular arrhythmias, left atrial abnormality, low voltage, diffuse nonspecific ST-T-wave abnormalities, and sometimes intraventricular and/or AV conduction defects. Echocardiography, computed tomographic imaging (CTI), and cardiac magnetic resonance imaging (CMRI) show LV dilatation, with normal, minimally thickened, or thinned walls, and systolic dysfunction. Circulating levels of brain natriuretic peptide are usually elevated.

Cardiac catheterization and coronary angiography are often performed to exclude ischemic heart disease, and bedside hemodynamic monitoring may be helpful in the management of selected acutely decompensated patients. Angiography reveals a dilated, diffusely hypokinetic left ventricle, often with some degree of mitral regurgitation. Cardiac CTI may distinguish between DCM and proximal coronary artery disease and, thereby, reduce the need for invasive procedures. Transvenous endomyocardial biopsy is usually not necessary in idiopathic or familial DCM; however, it may be helpful in the recognition of secondary cardiomyopathies, such as amyloidosis and acute myocarditis (see below).

℞ DILATED CARDIOMYOPATHY

Most patients pursue an inexorably downhill course, and the majority, particularly those >55 years, die within 4 years of the onset of symptoms. Patients of African ancestry are more likely to suffer more rapidly progressive CHF and death than Caucasians. Spontaneous improvement or stabilization occurs in about one-quarter of patients. Death is due to either progressive

HF or ventricular tachy- or bradyarrhythmia; SCD is a constant threat. Systemic embolization is a concern, and patients should be considered for chronic anticoagulation. Standard therapy of HF, as described in Chap. 227, is indicated. Alcohol should be avoided because of its cardiotoxic effects (see below), as should calcium channel blockers and nonsteroidal anti-inflammatory drugs. Antiarrhythmic agents are best avoided owing to the risk of proarrhythmia. Cardiac resynchronization therapy and insertion of an implantable cardioverter defibrillator (ICD) should be employed in DCM as in HF of other etiologies. In patients with advanced disease who are refractory to other therapies, cardiac transplantation should be considered (Chap. 228).

ALCOHOLIC CARDIOMYOPATHY

Individuals who consume large quantities (>90 g/d) of alcohol over many years may develop a clinical picture resembling idiopathic or familial DCM. The risk of developing cardiomyopathy is partially determined genetically. A polymorphism of the gene encoding the alcohol metabolizing enzyme, alcohol dehydrogenase (*ALDH2*2*), as well as the DD form of the angiotensin-converting enzyme (*ACE*) gene increase the predilection for the development of alcoholic cardiomyopathy. Patients with advanced alcoholic cardiomyopathy and severe CHF have a poor prognosis, particularly if they continue to drink; fewer than one-quarter of such patients survive 3 years. Management consists of abstention, which may halt the progression or even reverse the course of this disease.

A second presentation of alcoholic cardiotoxicity may be found in individuals without overt HF and consists of recurrent supraventricular or ventricular tachyarrhythmias. Termed the *holiday heart syndrome*, it typically appears after a drinking binge; atrial fibrillation is seen most frequently, followed by atrial flutter and frequent ventricular premature depolarizations.

In contrast to the adverse cardiac effects of excessive alcohol consumption, moderate consumption (20–30 g/d) appears to be cardioprotective; it raises high-density lipoprotein (HDL) cholesterol and is associated with a reduced incidence of ischemic heart disease, ischemic stroke, and metabolic syndrome.

PERIPARTUM CARDIOMYOPATHY

(See also Chap. 7) Cardiac dilatation and CHF may develop during the last trimester of pregnancy or within 6 months of delivery. The cause is unknown, although inflammatory myocarditis, immune activation, and gestational hypertension have all been incriminated. The patient who develops peripartum cardiomyopathy typically is multiparous, of African ancestry, and >30 years, although the disease may be found in a wide spectrum of patients. The symptoms, signs, and treatment are similar to those in patients with idiopathic DCM, the latter including implantation of an ICD or cardiac transplantation if the criteria for these therapies are satisfied. The mortality rate of this disorder is around 10%.

The prognosis is related to whether the heart size returns to normal after the first episode of CHF. If it does, subsequent pregnancies may sometimes be tolerated, albeit with an increased risk of recurrent CHF; if the heart remains enlarged, and/or the LV ejection fraction (EF) remains depressed after 6 months, the prognosis is poor, and further pregnancies frequently produce additional myocardial damage, ultimately leading to refractory CHF. Patients who recover from peripartum cardiomyopathy should be encouraged to avoid further pregnancies, particularly if LV dysfunction persists.

NEUROMUSCULAR DISEASE

(See also Chap. 382) Cardiac involvement is common in many of the muscular dystrophies. In *Duchenne's progressive muscular dystrophy*, mutations in a gene that encodes a cardiac structural protein (*dystrophin*) lead to myocyte death. Myocardial involvement is most frequently indicated by a distinctive and unique ECG pattern consisting of tall R waves in the right precordial leads with an R/S ratio > 1.0, often associated with deep Q waves in the limb and lateral precordial leads. A variety of supraventricular and ventricular arrhythmias is frequently found. Rapidly progressive HF may develop despite extended periods of apparent circulatory stability.

Myotonic dystrophy is characterized by a variety of ECG abnormalities, especially disorders of impulse formation and AV conduction, but other overt clinical evidence of heart disease is uncommon. Because of these abnormalities, syncope and sudden death are major hazards. In appropriate patients, insertion of an ICD and/or permanent pacemaker may be effective.

DRUGS

A variety of pharmacologic agents may damage the myocardium acutely, producing a pattern of inflammation (myocarditis, see below), or they may lead to chronic damage of the type seen with DCM. Certain drugs produce only ECG abnormalities, while others may precipitate fulminant CHF and death.

The anthracycline derivatives, particularly doxorubicin (Adriamycin), are powerful antineoplastic agents. Systolic dysfunction and ventricular arrhythmias occur in a dose-dependent manner with a dose >450 mg/m^2 and are frequent with doses >550 mg/m^2. The development of these complications appears to be related to damage to the inner mitochondrial membrane and interference with the synthesis of adenosine triphosphate. This development is related not only to the dose of the drug but also to the presence or absence of several risk factors, which include cardiac irradiation, underlying heart disease, hypertension, and concurrent treatment with cyclophosphamide. At any dose of doxorubicin, patients with these risk factors have a greater frequency of developing HF than do patients lacking them. Doxorubicin cardiotoxicity may occur acutely but more commonly develops a median of 3 months after the last dose. In others, late contractile dysfunction may develop years after doxorubicin administration.

By measuring cardiac-specific troponin and monitoring LV function with radionuclide ventriculography or echocardiography, usually combined with exercise stress, it is possible to document preclinical deterioration of LV function and allow appropriate dose adjustments. Also, monitoring may make it possible to continue doxorubicin even in patients at high risk for developing HF. Efforts to modify the dose schedule by giving the drug more slowly, along with the selective use of potentially cardioprotective agents such as the iron-chelator dexrazoxone, have reduced the risk of cardiotoxicity. Some patients have demonstrated recovery of cardiac function with aggressive management using ACE inhibitors.

Trastuzumab (*Herceptin*), used in the treatment of breast cancer, causes cardiomyopathy in 7% of patients when used as monotherapy and four times as frequently when combined with doxorubicin. High-dose *cyclophosphamide* may produce CHF acutely or within 2 weeks of administration; a characteristic histopathologic feature is myocardial edema and hemorrhagic necrosis. LV dysfunction has also been reported with the administration of the nonreceptor tyrosine kinase inhibitor *imatinib mesylate* (Gleevec), used in the treatment of chronic myeloid leukemia.

ECG changes and arrhythmias may result from treatment with tricyclic antidepressants, the phenothiazines, emetine, lithium, and various aerosol propellants. *Cocaine abuse* (Chap. 389) is associated with a variety of life-threatening cardiac complications, including SCD, myocarditis, DCM, and acute myocardial infarction (resulting from coronary spasm and/or thrombosis with or without underlying coronary artery disease). Nitrates, calcium channel blockers, antiplatelet agents, and benzodiazepines have been used to treat cocaine-induced cardiotoxicities.

ARRHYTHMOGENIC RIGHT VENTRICULAR CARDIOMYOPATHY/DYSPLASIA (ARVC/D)

ARVC/D is a familial cardiomyopathy characterized by progressive fibrofatty replacement of the right ventricle and, to a much lesser degree, of the LV myocardium. It is most commonly inherited in an autosomal dominant manner and is caused by multiple mutations of several genes encoding proteins that constitute desmosomes, structures that maintain normal contacts between cells. It has been suggested that abnormalities in the desmosomes cause detachment of myocytes with consequent myocyte apoptosis and fibrofatty replacement. Among the desmosomal protein genes, the most common gene mutation occurs in plakophilin-2 (*PKP-2*). Mutations in the cardiac ryanodine receptor gene (*RyR2*) and other genes have also been described.

On clinical examination, patients may manifest RV failure with jugular venous distention, hepatomegaly, and edema. Clinical manifestations usually develop during the second decade and include ventricular tachyarrhythmias as well as varying degrees of RV failure; both of these complications may be fatal.

The ECG typically shows QRS prolongation localized to the right precordial leads and left bundle branch block–type ventricular tachycardia. CTI and CMRI typically show RV dilatation, RV aneurysm, and fatty replacement (Fig. 231-2).

Restriction from competitive sports and antiarrhythmic therapy with beta blockers or amiodarone may be useful. Implantation of an ICD may be required (Chap. 226). If RV failure becomes intractable, cardiac transplantation (Chap. 228) may be necessary.

TAKO-TSUBO (STRESS) CARDIOMYOPATHY

Also known as *apical ballooning syndrome*, this uncommon cardiac syndrome is characterized by the abrupt onset of severe chest discomfort preceded by a very stressful emotional or physical event. It occurs most commonly in women >50 years and is accompanied by ST-segment elevations and/or deep T-wave inversions in the precordial leads. No obstruction in the epicardial coronary arteries is noted on angiography.

FIGURE 231-2 CMRI showing right ventricular (RV) enlargement (*left*) and fatty replacement of the RV myocardium (*black arrows*) of a patient with arrhythmogenic RV dysplasia. (*From S Sen-Chowdhry et al: Am J Med 117:685, 2004; with permission.*)

There is severe akinesia of the distal portion of the left ventricle with reduction of the EF. Troponins are usually mildly elevated. Cardiac imaging typically shows "ballooning" of the left ventricle in end-systole, especially of the LV apex. All of these changes, which are often quite dramatic, are reversible within 3–7 days and do not cause long-term cardiac dysfunction or disability.

The mechanism responsible for Tako-tsubo cardiomyopathy is not clear, although it is likely that an adrenergic surge that includes circulating catecholamines, acting on the epicardial coronary vessels and/or coronary microcirculation, is involved. Although beta blockers are used in therapy, there is no definitive evidence that they are beneficial.

LEFT VENTRICULAR NONCOMPACTION

Left ventricular noncompaction (LVNC) is a recently characterized uncommon congenital cardiomyopathy that may present at any age with symptoms of CHF, thromboembolism, or ventricular arrhythmias. It results from the arrest of normal embryogenesis, with the persistence of the deep recesses and sinusoids in the myocardium that characterize the embryonic heart. These sinusoids and associated spongy network of myocardial fibers ordinarily undergo organization and "compaction" early in embryonic life; when this fails to occur, LVNC results. This condition is diagnosed on echocardiography by the demonstration of multiple deep trabeculations into the myocardium, all of which communicate with the ventricular cavity, associated with LV contractile dysfunction. Standard therapy for CHF is routinely employed, typically along with chronic anticoagulation.

HYPERTROPHIC CARDIOMYOPATHY

Hypertrophic cardiomyopathy (HCM) is characterized by LV hypertrophy, typically of a nondilated chamber, without obvious cause, such as hypertension or aortic stenosis. It is found in about 1 in 500 of the general population. Two features of HCM have attracted the greatest attention: (1) asymmetric LV hypertrophy, often with preferential hypertrophy of the interventricular septum; and (2) a dynamic LV outflow tract pressure gradient, related to narrowing of the subaortic area. About one-third of patients with HCM demonstrate an outflow tract pressure gradient at rest and a similar fraction develop one with provocation. The ubiquitous pathophysiologic abnormality is *diastolic* dysfunction, which can be detected by Doppler tissue imaging and results in elevated LV end-diastolic pressures; the latter may be present despite a hyperdynamic, nondilated LV.

The pattern of hypertrophy is distinctive in HCM and usually differs from that seen in secondary hypertrophy (as in hypertension or aortic stenosis). Most patients have striking regional variations in the extent of hypertrophy in different portions of the left ventricle, and the majority demonstrate a ventricular septum whose thickness is disproportionately increased when compared with the free wall. Other patients may demonstrate symmetric hypertrophy, while others have mid-ventricular cavity obstruction or disproportionate involvement of the apex or LV free wall. In the disproportionately hypertrophied portions of the left ventricle, there is a bizarre and disorganized arrangement of myocytes, with disorganization of the myofibrillar architecture, along with a variable degree of myocardial fibrosis and thickening of the small intramural coronary arteries.

GENETIC CONSIDERATIONS About half of all patients with HCM have a positive family history compatible with autosomal dominant transmission. More than 400 mutations of 11 different genes that encode sarcomeric proteins have been identified; these account for ~60% of cases. The most common are mutations of the cardiac β-myosin heavy chain gene on chromosome 14. Others involve α-myosin heavy chains; cardiac troponins C, I, and T; cardiac myosin-binding protein C; actin; myosin light chains; and titin. Certain mutations are associated with more malignant prognoses. Many sporadic cases of HCM probably represent spontaneous mutations. Echocardiographic studies have confirmed that by the age of 20, when full expression has usually occurred, about one-half of the first-degree relatives of patients with familial HCM have evidence of the disease. However, in many of these relatives the extent of hypertrophy is mild, no outflow tract pressure gradient is present, and symptoms are not prominent. Since the hypertrophic characteristics may not be apparent in childhood, a single normal echocardiogram in a child does not exclude the presence of the disease. Screening by echocardiography of first-degree relatives between the ages of 12 and 20 should be carried out every 12–24 months, unless the diagnosis is established or excluded by genetic testing.

Genetic Testing Although not yet routinely available, genetic testing may allow a definitive diagnosis of HCM with a genetic cause to be established by identifying a mutation in a gene encoding a sarcomeric protein. Genetic testing can identify family members who are at risk for developing HCM and who, therefore, require echocardiographic screening and follow-up. It can also exclude the disease in family members.

CLINICAL FEATURES

The clinical course of HCM is highly variable. Many patients are asymptomatic or mildly symptomatic and may be relatives of patients with known disease. Unfortunately, the first clinical manifestation may be SCD, frequently occurring in children and young adults during or after physical exertion. Indeed, HCM is the most common cause of SCD in young competitive athletes. In symptomatic patients, the most common complaint is dyspnea, largely due to diastolic ventricular dysfunction, which impairs ventricular filling and leads to elevated LV diastolic, left atrial, and pulmonary capillary pressures. Other symptoms include syncope, angina pectoris, and fatigue. Symptoms are not closely related to the presence or severity of an outflow pressure gradient.

PHYSICAL EXAMINATION

Most patients demonstrate a double or triple apical precordial impulse and a fourth heart sound. Those with intraventricular pressure gradients may have a rapidly rising arterial pulse. The hallmark of obstructive HCM is a systolic murmur, which is typically harsh, diamond-shaped, and usually begins well after the first heart sound. The murmur is best heard at the lower left sternal border as well as at the apex, where it is often more holosystolic and blowing in quality, no doubt due to the mitral regurgitation that usually accompanies obstructive HCM.

HEMODYNAMICS

In contrast to the obstruction produced by a fixed narrowed orifice, such as valvular aortic stenosis, the pressure gradient in HCM, when present, is dynamic and may change between examinations and even from beat to beat. Obstruction appears to result from narrowing of the LV outflow tract by systolic anterior movement (SAM) of the mitral valve against the hypertrophied septum.

Three basic mechanisms are involved in the production and intensification of the dynamic intraventricular obstruction: (1) increased LV contractility, (2) decreased ventricular preload, and (3) decreased aortic impedance and pressure (afterload). Interventions that increase myocardial contractility, such as exercise and sympathomimetic amines, and those that reduce ventricular preload, such as the strain phase of the Valsalva maneuver, sudden standing, or nitroglycerin, reduce LV end-diastolic volume and, thereby, may cause an increase in the gradient and the murmur. Conversely, elevation of arterial pressure by squatting, sustained handgrip, augmentation of venous return by passive leg raising, and expansion of the blood volume (as during pregnancy) all increase ventricular volume and ameliorate the gradient and murmur.

LABORATORY EVALUATION

The ECG commonly shows LV hypertrophy and widespread deep, broad Q waves. The latter suggest an old myocardial infarction but actually reflect severe septal hypertrophy. Many patients demonstrate arrhythmias, both atrial (supraventricular tachycardia or atrial fibrillation) and ventricular (ventricular tachycardia), during ambulatory (Holter) monitoring. *Chest roentgenography* may be normal, although a mild to moderate increase in the cardiac silhouette is common.

The mainstay of the diagnosis of HCM is the *echocardiogram*, which demonstrates LV hypertrophy, often with the septum ≥1.3 times the thickness of the posterior LV free wall. The septum may demonstrate an unusual "ground-glass" appearance, probably related to its myocardial fibrosis. SAM of the mitral valve, often accompanied by mitral regurgitation, is found in patients with pressure gradients. The LV cavity typically is small in HCM, with vigorous motion of the posterior wall but with reduced septal excursion. An uncommon form of cardiomyopathy, characterized by apical hypertrophy, is associated with giant negative T waves on the ECG and a "spade-shaped" LV cavity; it usually has a benign clinical course. CMRI is superior to echocardiography in providing accurate measurements of regional hypertrophy and in identifying sites of regional fibrosis.

Although cardiac catheterization is not required to diagnose HCM, the two typical *hemodynamic* features are an elevated LV diastolic pressure due to diminished compliance and, in some patients, a systolic pressure gradient, usually between the body of the left ventricle and the subaortic region. When a gradient is not present, it can be induced in some patients by provocative maneuvers, such as infusion of isoproterenol, inhalation of amyl nitrite, the Valsalva maneuver, or a premature ventricular contraction.

℞ HYPERTROPHIC CARDIOMYOPATHY

Since SCD often occurs during or just after physical exertion, competitive sports and very strenuous activities should be proscribed. Dehydration should be avoided, and diuretics used with caution. β-Adrenergic blockers ameliorate angina pectoris and syncope in one-third to one-half of patients. Although resting intraventricular pressure gradients are usually unchanged, these drugs may limit the increase in the gradient that occurs during exercise. It does not appear that β-adrenergic blockers offer any protection against SCD. Amiodarone appears to be effective in reducing the frequency of supraventricular as well as of life-threatening ventricular arrhythmias, and anecdotal data suggest that it may reduce the risk of SCD. Nondihydropyridine calcium channel blockers (verapamil and diltiazem) may reduce the stiffness of the left ventricle, reduce the elevated diastolic pressures, increase exercise tolerance, and, in some instances, reduce the severity of outflow tract pressure gradients. Disopyramide has been used in some patients to reduce LV contractility and the outflow pressure gradient; it may reduce symptoms as well.

Digitalis, diuretics, nitrates, dihydropyridine calcium blockers, vasodilators, and β-adrenergic agonists are best avoided, particularly in patients with known LV outflow tract pressure gradients. Alcohol ingestion may produce sufficient vasodilatation to exacerbate an outflow pressure gradient.

Atrial fibrillation is poorly tolerated, and a strong effort should be made to restore and then maintain sinus rhythm. Slowing of the heart rate with a β-adrenergic blocker or ablation of the AV node and insertion of a pacemaker may be indicated when sinus rhythm cannot be sustained.

Surgical myotomy/myectomy of the hypertrophied septum usually abolishes intraventricular obstruction and provides lasting symptomatic improvement in about three-quarters of severely symptomatic patients with large pressure gradients who are unresponsive to medical management. Infarction of the interventricular septum induced by ethanol injections into the septal artery (alcohol septal ablation) can also reduce obstruction and improve symptoms. However, it should be carried out only by experts.

The insertion of an ICD should be considered in patients with a high-risk profile for SCD (see below).

PROGNOSIS

The natural history of HCM is variable, although many patients never exhibit any clinical manifestations. Atrial fibrillation is common late in the course of the disease; its onset often leads to the development of or an increase in symptoms. Infective endocarditis occurs in <10% of patients. However, endocarditis prophylaxis is currently recommended only in HCM patients with a prior episode of infective endocarditis. Progression of HCM to left ventricular dilatation and dysfunction (DCM) with wall thinning and disappearance of a preexisting outflow pressure gradient (so-called burnt out HCM) occurs in 5–10% of pa-

tients and may be associated with nonresponsive CHF requiring cardiac transplantation.

The major cause of mortality in HCM is SCD, which may occur in asymptomatic patients or interrupt an otherwise stable course in symptomatic ones. Patients at increased risk of SCD include those with a history of resuscitation, recurrent syncope, ventricular tachycardia on ambulatory monitoring or at electrophysiologic testing, marked ventricular hypertrophy (ventricular septal thickness >30 mm), failure of blood pressure to rise during exercise, a family history of SCD, and certain genetic mutations.

INHERITED METABOLIC CARDIOMYOPATHIES WITH LEFT VENTRICULAR HYPERTROPHY

Cardiac Danon Disease   This condition is caused by mutations in an X-linked lysosome-associated membrane protein (LAMP2). It is characterized by enlarged ventricular myocytes with periodic acid Schiff (PAS)–positive inclusions. Patients present in childhood with CHF and serious arrhythmias. The ECG shows severe LV hypertrophy and ventricular preexcitation.

Glycogen Storage Cardiomyopathy   (See also Chap. 356) This recently characterized condition is caused by a mutation in the γ_2 regulatory subunit (*PRKAG2*) of adenosine monophosphate–activated protein kinase (AMPK). It is characterized by ventricular hypertrophy resembling that observed in hypertrophic cardiomyopathies and enlarged myocytes with vacuoles in the myocytes that stain for glycogen.

Fabry Disease   (See also Chap. 355) This X-linked autosomal recessive lysosomal storage disorder is caused by deficiency of lysosomal α-galactoside A and can lead to the accumulation of glycosphingolipids in the heart, with ventricular hypertrophy resembling HCM. Because of severe impairment in ventricular filling, it is sometimes classified as a restrictive cardiomyopathy (see below). It may be associated with AV conduction abnormalities and ventricular tachyarrhythmias. CMRI is helpful in establishing the diagnosis. Treatment consists of enzyme replacement therapy with agalsidase β.

Friedreich's Ataxia   (See also Chap. 382) This is an autosomal recessive spinocerebellar degenerative disease caused by inadequate levels of frataxin, a protein involved in mitochondrial iron metabolism. Approximately one-half of the patients develop cardiac symptoms. The ECG most commonly demonstrates ST-segment and T-wave abnormalities. Echocardiography and other imaging studies (CTI, CMRI) usually show symmetric LV hypertrophy or asymmetric hypertrophy of the interventricular septum compared with the free wall. Although the gross morphologic appearance of the heart in Friedreich's ataxia may be similar to that in HCM (see above), cellular disarray is lacking.

RESTRICTIVE CARDIOMYOPATHY

The hallmark of the restrictive cardiomyopathies (RCMs) is abnormal diastolic function (Chap. 217); the ventricular walls are excessively rigid and impede ventricular filling. In late stages systolic function is also impaired. Myocardial fibrosis, hypertrophy, or infiltration due to a variety of causes is responsible. Myocardial involvement with *amyloid* is a common cause of secondary restrictive cardiomyopathy, although restriction is also seen in the transplanted heart, in hemochromatosis, glycogen deposition, endomyocardial fibrosis, sarcoidosis, hypereosinophilic disease, and scleroderma; following mediastinal irradiation; and in neoplastic infiltration and myocardial fibrosis of diverse causes. In many of these conditions, particularly those with substantial concomitant endocardial involvement, partial obliteration of the ventricular cavity by fibrous tissue and thrombus contributes to the abnormally increased resistance to ventricular filling. Thromboembolic complications are frequent in such patients.

CLINICAL FEATURES

The inability of the ventricles to fill limits cardiac output and raises filling pressures; thus, exercise intolerance and dyspnea are usually prominent. As a result of persistently elevated systemic venous pressure, these patients commonly have dependent edema, ascites, and an enlarged, tender, and often pulsatile liver. The jugular venous pressure is elevated and does not fall normally (or may rise) with inspiration (Kussmaul's sign). The heart sounds may be distant, and third and fourth heart sounds are common. In contrast to constrictive pericarditis (Chap. 232), which RCM resembles in many respects, the apex impulse is usually easily palpable, and mitral regurgitation is more common.

LABORATORY EXAMINATIONS

In patients with infiltrative cardiomyopathies, the ECG often shows low-voltage, nonspecific ST-T-wave abnormalities and various arrhythmias. Pericardial calcification on x-ray, which occurs in constrictive pericarditis, is absent. Echocardiography, CTI, and CMRI typically reveal symmetrically thickened LV walls and normal or slightly reduced ventricular volumes and systolic function; the atria are usually dilated. Doppler echocardiography typically shows diastolic dysfunction. Cardiac catheterization shows a reduced cardiac output, elevation of the RV and LV end-diastolic pressures, and a dip-and-plateau configuration of the diastolic portion of the ventricular pressure pulses resembling constrictive pericarditis.

Differentiation of RCM from constrictive pericarditis (Chap. 232) is of importance because the latter is often curable by surgery. Helpful in the differentiation of these two conditions are RV transvenous endomyocardial biopsy (by revealing myocardial infiltration or fibrosis in RCM) and CTI or CMRI (by demonstrating a thickened pericardium in constrictive pericarditis but not in RCM).

℞ RESTRICTIVE CARDIOMYOPATHY

Management is usually disappointing, except for hemochromatosis (see below) and Fabry's disease (see above). Chronic anticoagulation is often recommended to reduce the risk of embolization from the heart.

EOSINOPHILIC ENDOMYOCARDIAL DISEASE

Also called *Loeffler's endocarditis* and *fibroplastic endocarditis*, this condition occurs in temperate climates. It appears to be a subcategory of the hypereosinophilic syndrome (Chap. 249) in which the heart is predominantly involved, with cardiac damage the apparent result of the toxic effects of eosinophilic proteins. Typically, the endocardium of either or both ventricles is thickened markedly, with involvement of the underlying myocardium. Cardiac imaging typically reveals ventricular thickening, especially of the posterobasal LV wall. Mitral regurgitation is frequently present on Doppler echocardiography. Large mural thrombi may develop in either ventricle, thereby compromising the size of the ventricular cavity and serving as a source of pulmonary and systemic emboli. Hepatosplenomegaly and localized eosinophilic infiltration of other organs are usually present. Management usually includes diuretics, afterload-reducing agents, and anticoagulation. The use of glucocorticoids and hydroxyurea appears to improve survival. Surgical treatment with resection of fibrotic tissue and mitral valve repair or replacement may be helpful in selected patients.

CARDIAC AMYLOIDOSIS

(See also Chap. 324) Involvement of the heart is the most frequent cause of death in *primary amyloidosis* (AL) and *hereditary amyloidosis* (ATTR), with deposition of amyloid in the cardiac interstitium. On gross pathologic examination, the heart is firm, rubbery, and noncompliant and has a waxy appearance. Clinically significant cardiac involvement is uncommon in the secondary form. Focal deposits of amyloid in the hearts of elderly persons (*senile cardiac amyloidosis*), although common, are usually clinically insignificant.

Four clinical presentations (alone or in combination) are seen: (1) diastolic dysfunction, (2) systolic dysfunction, (3) arrhythmias and conduction disturbances, and (4) orthostatic hypotension. The two-dimensional echocardiogram may be helpful in establishing the diagnosis of amyloidosis and may show a thickened myocardial wall with a diffuse, hyperrefractile "speckled" appearance. CMRI typically shows late gadolinium enhancement of the subendocardium. Aspiration of abdominal fat or biopsy of the myocardium or other organs permits the ante mortem diagnosis to be established in over three-quarters of cases.

Chemotherapy, often with alkylating agents such as melphalan, together with glucocorticoids, appears to have improved survival in individual cases. Heart transplantation (often combined with bone marrow transplantation or liver or kidney transplantation for hereditary amyloidosis) may help selected patients. However, the overall prognosis is poor, especially in the primary form with advanced cardiac involvement.

OTHER RESTRICTIVE CARDIOMYOPATHIES

Iron-overload cardiomyopathy (hemochromatosis) (Chap. 351) is often the result of multiple transfusions or a hemoglobinopathy, most frequently β-thalassemia; the familial (autosomal recessive) form should be suspected if cardiomyopathy occurs in the presence of diabetes mellitus, hepatic cirrhosis, and increased skin pigmentation. The diagnosis may be confirmed by endomyocardial biopsy. CMRI shows a reduced $T2^*$ signal as iron levels rise. Phlebotomy may be of some benefit if employed early in the course of the disease. Continuous subcutaneous administration of deferoxamine or other iron chelators may reduce body iron stores and result in clinical improvement.

Myocardial *sarcoidosis* (Chap. 322) is generally associated with other manifestations of systemic disease. It may cause restrictive as well as congestive features, since cardiac infiltration by sarcoid granulomas results not only in increased stiffness of the myocardium but also in diminished systolic contractile function. A variety of arrhythmias, including high-grade AV block, have been noted. A common cardiac manifestation of systemic sarcoidosis is RV overload due to pulmonary hypertension as a result of parenchymal pulmonary involvement. Many patients are treated empirically with glucocorticoids.

The *carcinoid syndrome* (Chap. 230) results in endocardial fibrosis and stenosis and/or regurgitation of the tricuspid and/or pulmonary valve; morphologically similar lesions have been seen with the use of the anorexic agents fenfluramine and phentermine.

MYOCARDITIS

Myocarditis, i.e., cardiac inflammation, is most commonly the result of an infectious process, frequently complicated by autoimmunity. Myocarditis may also result from hypersensitivity to drugs (most commonly tricyclic antidepressants, antibiotics, and antipsychotics) or it may be caused by irradiation, chemicals, or physical agents. While almost every infective agent is capable of producing myocarditis (Table 231-1), clinically significant acute myocarditis in the United States is caused most commonly by viruses, especially Coxsackievirus B, adenovirus, hepatitis C virus, and HIV. Symptomatic viral myocarditis may be secondary to continued viral replication and/or autoimmune activation following viral infection.

CLINICAL FEATURES

Patients with viral myocarditis may give a history of a preceding upper respiratory febrile illness or a flulike syndrome, and viral nasopharyngitis or tonsillitis may be evident. The clinical spectrum ranges from an asymptomatic state, with the presence of myocarditis inferred only by the finding of transient electrocardiographic ST-T-wave abnormalities, to a fulminant condition with arrhythmias, acute CHF, and early death. In some patients, myocarditis simulates an acute coronary syndrome (Chap. 238), with chest pain, ECG changes, and elevated serum levels of troponin, but it typically occurs in patients younger than those with coronary atherosclerosis.

The *physical examination* is often normal, although more severe cases may show a muffled first heart sound, along with a third heart sound and a murmur of mitral regurgitation. A pericardial friction rub may be audible in patients with associated pericarditis. The isolation of virus from the stool, pharyngeal washings, or other body fluids and changes in specific antibody titers may be helpful clinically. Endomyocardial biopsy, carried out early in the illness, may show round-cell infiltration and necrosis of adjacent myocytes. CMRI frequently exhibits contrast enhancement (Chap. 222) and is valuable in identifying sites likely to exhibit typical histologic changes on biopsy, as well as in monitoring the activity of the disease.

Although viral myocarditis is most often self-limited and without sequelae, severe involvement may recur. Acute viral myocarditis, especially when accompanied by severe LV dysfunction (LVEF < 35%), may progress to a chronic form and to DCM.

Rx MYOCARDITIS

Exercise may be deleterious in patients with acute myocarditis, and strenuous activity should be proscribed until the ECG and LV function have returned to normal. Patients who develop CHF should be treated with the usual measures (Chap. 227). Arrhythmias are common and are occasionally difficult to manage. Deaths attributed to CHF, tachyarrhythmias, and AV block have been reported; the ECG should be monitored during the acute illness and in patients with arrhythmias.

Patients with fulminant myocarditis may require mechanical cardiopulmonary support or cardiac transplantation; however, the majority of these patients survive, and many demonstrate substantial recovery of LV function.

MYOCARDITIS IN PATIENTS WITH HIV

(See also Chap. 182) Many HIV-infected patients have subclinical cardiac involvement, including pericardial effusion, right-sided chamber enlargement, arrhythmias, and neoplastic involvement. Overt clinical manifestations are seen in 10% of HIV patients. The most common finding is LV dysfunction that in some cases appears to be due to infection of the myocardium by the virus itself. In other patients, the heart is affected by one of the various opportunistic infections common in HIV-AIDS, such as toxoplasmosis; by cardiac involvement by neoplastic disorders; or by toxicity from anti-HIV drugs. CHF in HIV myocarditis may respond, at least transiently, to standard anti-HIV therapy.

BACTERIAL MYOCARDITIS

Bacterial involvement of the heart is uncommon, but when it does occur, it is usually as a complication of infective endocarditis (Chap. 118) in which abscess formation involves the valve rings and interventricular septum.

Diphtheritic myocarditis develops in over one-quarter of patients with diphtheria (Chap. 131); it is one of the more serious complications and the most common cause of death in this infection. Cardiac damage is due to the liberation of a toxin that inhibits protein synthesis and leads to a dilated, flabby, hypocontractile heart. The conduction system is frequently involved, as well. Cardiomegaly and severe CHF typically appear after the first week of illness. Prompt therapy with antitoxin is critical; antibiotic therapy is also indicated but is of less urgency.

GIANT CELL MYOCARDITIS

This rare myocarditis of unknown cause is characterized by rapidly progressive CHF and ventricular tachyarrhythmia and occurs most commonly in the third or fourth decades; approximately two-thirds of patients die within 1 year. At necropsy, the distinctive features include cardiac enlargement, ventricular thrombi, grossly visible serpiginous areas of necrosis in both ventricles, and microscopic evidence of giant cells within an extensive inflammatory infiltrate. The etiology of giant cell myocarditis has not been identified, although an autoimmune cause appears to be likely. While treatment with immunosuppressive therapy may help some patients, cardiac transplantation is often necessary.

LYME CARDITIS

(See also Chap. 166) Lyme disease is caused by a tick-borne spirochete and is most common in the Northeast, upper Midwest, and Pacific Coastal regions of the United States during the summer months. About 10% of patients develop symptomatic cardiac involvement during the acute phase of the disease. AV conduction abnormalities are the most common manifestations of involvement and may lead to syncope. Concomitant myopericarditis is not uncommon, and mild, asymptomatic LV dysfunction may occur.

Intravenous ceftriaxone or penicillin is indicated in all but the mildest forms of Lyme carditis, in which case oral amoxicillin or doxycycline is employed. Hospitalization with ECG monitoring is indicated in patients with second- or third-degree AV block. A temporary pacemaker may be needed for symptomatic AV block, but permanent pacing is rarely required. Although glucocorticoids are often given, their effectiveness in reversing AV block is uncertain. Long-term cardiac manifestations of Lyme disease are uncommon.

GLOBAL CONSIDERATIONS

CHAGAS HEART DISEASE

(See also Chaps. 206 and e37) Chagas disease, caused by the protozoan *Trypanosoma cruzi* and transmitted by an insect vector, the reduvid bug, produces an extensive myocarditis that typically becomes evident years after the initial infection. It is one of the more common causes of heart disease encountered in Central and South America; in rural endemic areas, 20–75% of the population may be affected. It has been estimated that ~18 million persons are affected, with 200,000 new cases each year. An increasing number of cases are found in the United States as patients migrate from endemic areas; in rare cases, it has been transmitted by transfusion and organ donation.

About 1% of infected individuals have an acute illness, which may include acute myocarditis that usually resolves in 2–3 months. After a quiescent, asymptomatic period, the so-called *indeterminate phase*, approximately one-third of infected persons develop chronic myocardial damage. A combination of infection by the parasite as well as autoimmune reactions are responsible for the cardiac manifestations. Cardiac involvement in chronic Chagasic heart disease varies widely, from asymptomatic to severe cardiac failure involving the left ventricle, and sometimes the right ventricle, and/or AV block. This condition, which is more frequent in males, is characterized by dilatation of several cardiac chambers, fibrosis and thinning of the ventricular wall, aneurysm formation in the left ventricle (Fig. 231-3), and mural thrombi. Survival is poor in patients who develop overt CHF. The cause of death is either intractable CHF or SCD secondary to an arrhythmia, with a minority of patients dying from embolic phenomena.

FIGURE 231-3 Left ventriculogram of a 55-year-old woman with chronic Chagas disease. Multiple left ventricular aneurysms are noted in inferobasal, anterior, and inferior aspects of left ventricle (circled). *(From P Venegoni, HS Bhatia: Circulation 96:1363, 1997.)*

The ECG is abnormal in most patients and typically shows low voltage, along with right bundle branch block and left anterior hemiblock, and may progress to complete AV block. The chest roentgenogram may show LV enlargement. Echocardiography may reveal hypokinesis of the posterior LV wall and relatively preserved septal motion. Ventricular arrhythmias are common and are seen on Holter monitoring, especially during and after exertion.

℞ CHAGAS HEART DISEASE

Therapy is directed toward amelioration of the CHF and ventricular tachyarrhythmias; oral amiodarone appears to be particularly effective in treating the latter. Progressive conduction system disease and AV block may require implantation of a pacemaker. Anticoagulation reduces the risk of thromboembolism. Medical therapy is often unsatisfactory or unavailable (especially in poor rural areas); however, a more promising tactic in endemic areas is the use of insecticides to eliminate the vector.

CARDIOMYOPATHY IN AFRICA

Endomyocardial Fibrosis   This is a progressive disease that presents as a RCM. It occurs most commonly in children and young adults residing in tropical and subtropical Africa, particularly Uganda and Nigeria, as well as in tropical Asia and South America. It is related and similar to hypereosinophilic endomyocardial disease (see above), although the eosinophilia is less severe and the course more chronic in endomyocardial fibrosis. Endomyocardial fibrosis is a frequent cause of CHF in Africa, accounting for up to one-quarter of deaths due to heart disease. The condition is characterized by severe fibrosis of the endocardium, with involvement of the inflow portion of the right or left ventricle (or both). Endomyocardial fibrosis often involves the AV valves, producing valvular regurgitation. The apex of the ventricles may be obliterated by a mass of thrombus and fibrous tissue.

The clinical picture depends on which ventricle and AV valve shows predominant involvement; left-sided involvement results in symptoms of pulmonary congestion, while predominant right-sided disease presents features of systemic venous congestion. Medical treatment is often disappointing, and surgical excision of the fibrotic endocardium and replacement of the involved AV valve have led to substantial symptomatic improvement in some patients.

Dilated Cardiomyopathy   DCM is a common cause of heart failure in Africa and has been reported in up to one-half of patients hospitalized with CHF. The etiology of DCM in Africa is multifactorial. Infection with *Toxoplasma gondii* and *Coxsackievirus B* has been reported to be common in DCM patients in Nigeria, while *African trypanosomiasis* appears to be a common cause in Cameroon. Excess alcohol ingestion is considered to be causal or an important contributory factor in almost one-half of cases of DCM; severe thiamine deficiency may be present in some of these patients as well.

Peripartum cardiomyopathy is far more common in Africa than in North America or Europe; the incidence has been reported to be especially high in Nigeria. Pathogenetic factors that may be operative include low socioeconomic status, high parity, prolonged lactation, excessive dietary salt intake, and selenium deficiency.

CARDIOMYOPATHY IN ASIA

Thiamine (vitamin B_1) deficiency (Chap. 71) occurs in Asian countries, especially China, where polished rice, deficient in thiamine, is a major component of the diet and flour is not enriched with thiamine, as it is in the West. However, thiamine deficiency in the West may occur in patients with severe alcoholism.

So-called *wet beri-beri heart disease* is an important clinical manifestation of serious thiamine deficiency. It is characterized by cardiac failure secondary to a high cardiac output state caused by arteriolar vasodilation; it is associated with tachycardia, wide pulse pressure, a third heart sound, and warm extremities. ECG findings include reduced voltage, diffuse T-wave abnormalities and prolongation of the QT interval. On chest x-ray, the heart appears diffusely enlarged with pulmonary congestion. The response to thiamine is usually dramatic, but it should be accompanied by diuretics.

Selenium deficiency (Chap. 71) is also most common in China. It may cause *Keshan's disease*, a dilated cardiomyopathy with cardiomegaly, ventricular arrhythmias, and heart failure.

FURTHER READINGS

CORRADO D, THIENE G: Arrhythmogenic right ventricular cardiomyopathy/dysplasia: Clinical impact of molecular genetic studies. Circulation 113:1634, 2006

DUTRA WO et al: The clinical immunology of human Chagas disease. Trends Parasitol 21:581, 2005

FALK RH: Diagnosis and management of the cardiac amyloidoses. Circulation 112:2047, 2005

HO CY, SEIDMAN CE: A contemporary approach to hypertrophic cardiomyopathy. Circulation 113:e858, 2006

LUCAS DL et al: Alcohol and the cardiovascular system. J Am Coll Cardiol 45:1916, 2005

MAGNANI JW, DEC GW: Myocarditis: Current trends in diagnosis and treatment. Circulation 113:876, 2006

MARON BJ et al: Contemporary definitions and classification of the cardiomyopathies: An American Heart Association Scientific Statement. Circulation 113:1807, 2006

MCCROHON JA et al: Differentiation of heart failure related to dilated cardiomyopathy and coronary artery disease using gadolinium-enhanced cardiovascular magnetic resonance. Circulation 108:54, 2003

RASSI A JR et al: Development and validation of a risk score for predicting death in Chagas' heart disease. N Engl J Med 355:799, 2006

SEIDMAN CE et al: Genetic factors in myocardial disease, in *Braunwald's Heart Disease*, 8th ed, P Libby et al (eds). Philadelphia, Saunders, 2008

SLIWA K et al: Epidemiology and etiology of cardiomyopathy in Africa. Circulation 112:3577, 2005

——— et al: Peripartum cardiomyopathy. Lancet 368:687, 2006

SUDANO I et al: Cardiovascular disease in HIV infection. Am Heart J 151:1147, 2006

WEIFORD BC et al: Noncompaction of the ventricular myocardium. Circulation 109:2965, 2004

232 Pericardial Disease
Eugene Braunwald

NORMAL FUNCTIONS OF THE PERICARDIUM

The normal pericardium is a double-layered sac; the visceral pericardium is a serous membrane that is separated by a small quantity (15–50 mL) of fluid, an ultrafiltrate of plasma, from the fibrous parietal pericardium. The normal pericardium, by exerting a restraining force, prevents sudden dilation of the cardiac chambers, especially of the right atrium and ventricle, during exercise and with hypervolemia. It also restricts the anatomic position of the heart, minimizes friction between the heart and surrounding structures, prevents displacement of the heart and kinking of the great vessels, and probably retards the spread of infections from the lungs and pleural cavities to the heart. Notwithstanding the foregoing, total absence of the pericardium, either congenital or following surgery, does not produce obvious clinical disease. In partial left pericardial defects, the main pulmonary artery and left atrium may bulge through the defect; very rarely, herniation and subsequent strangulation of the left atrium may cause sudden death.

ACUTE PERICARDITIS

Acute pericarditis, by far the most common pathologic process involving the pericardium, may be classified both clinically and etiologically (Table 232-1). Pain, a pericardial friction rub, electrocardiographic changes, and pericardial effusion with cardiac tamponade and paradoxical pulse are cardinal manifestations of many forms of acute pericarditis.

Chest pain is an important but not invariable symptom in various forms of acute pericarditis (Chap. 13); it is usually present in the acute infectious types and in many of the forms presumed to be related to hypersensitivity or autoimmunity. Pain is often absent in slowly developing tuberculous, postirradiation, neoplastic, or uremic pericarditis. The pain of acute pericarditis is often severe, retrosternal and left precordial, and referred to the neck, arms, or the left shoulder. Often the pain is pleuritic, consequent to accompanying pleural inflammation, i.e., sharp and aggravated by inspiration, coughing, and changes in body position, but sometimes it is a steady, constricting pain that radiates into either arm or both arms and resembles that of myocardial ischemia; therefore, confusion with acute myocardial infarction (AMI) is common. Characteristically, however, pericardial pain may be relieved by sitting up and leaning forward and is intensified by lying supine. The differentiation of AMI from acute pericarditis becomes perplexing when, with acute pericarditis, serum biomarkers of myocardial damage such as creatine kinase and troponin rise, presumably because of concomitant involvement of the epicardium in the inflammatory process (an epi-myocarditis) with resulting myocyte necrosis. However, these elevations, if they occur, are quite modest, given the extensive electrocardiographic ST-segment elevation in pericarditis. This dissociation is useful in the differentiation between these conditions.

The *pericardial friction rub*, audible in about 85% of patients, may have up to three components per cardiac cycle, is high-pitched, and is described as rasping, scratching, or grating (Chap. 220); it can be elicited sometimes only when the diaphragm of the stethoscope is applied firmly to the chest wall at the left lower sternal border. It is heard most frequently at end-expiration with the patient upright and leaning forward. The rub is often inconstant, and the loud to-and-fro leathery sound may disappear within a few hours, possibly to reappear on the following day. A pericardial rub is heard throughout the respiratory cycle, while a pleural rub disappears when respiration is suspended.

The *electrocardiogram* (ECG) in acute pericarditis without massive effusion usually displays changes secondary to acute subepicardial inflammation (see Fig. 232-1). It typically evolves through four stages. In stage 1, there is widespread elevation of the ST segments, often with upward concavity, involving two or three standard limb leads and V_2 to V_6, with reciprocal depressions only in aVR and sometimes V_1, as well as PR-segment depression. Usually there are no significant changes in QRS complexes. In stage 2, after several days, the ST segments return to normal, and only then, or even later, do the T waves become inverted (stage 3). Ultimately, weeks or months after the onset of acute pericarditis, the ECG returns to normal in stage 4. In contrast, in AMI, ST elevations are convex, and reciprocal depression is usually more prominent; QRS changes occur, particularly the development of Q waves, as well as notching and loss of R-wave amplitude; and T-wave inversions are usually seen within hours *before* the ST segments have become isoelectric. Sequential ECGs are useful in distinguishing acute pericarditis from AMI. In the latter, elevated ST segments return to normal within hours.

Early repolarization is a normal variant and may also be associated with widespread ST-segment elevation, most prominent in left precordial leads. However, in this condition the T waves are usually tall and the ST/T ratio is <0.25; importantly, this ratio is higher in acute pericarditis. Depression of the PR segment (below the TP segment) is also common and reflects atrial involvement.

PERICARDIAL EFFUSION

In acute pericarditis, effusion is usually associated with pain and/or the above-mentioned ECG changes, as well as with an enlargement of the cardiac silhouette. Pericardial effusion is especially important clinically when it develops within a relatively short time as it may lead to cardiac

TABLE 232-1 CLASSIFICATION OF PERICARDITIS

Clinical Classification

I. Acute pericarditis (<6 weeks)
   A. Fibrinous
   B. Effusive (serous or sanguineous)
II. Subacute pericarditis (6 weeks to 6 months)
   A. Effusive-constrictive
   B. Constrictive
III. Chronic pericarditis (>6 months)
   A. Constrictive
   B. Effusive
   C. Adhesive (nonconstrictive)

Etiologic Classification

I. Infectious pericarditis
   A. Viral (coxsackievirus A and B, echovirus, mumps, adenovirus, hepatitis, HIV)
   B. Pyogenic (pneumococcus, streptococcus, staphylococcus, *Neisseria, Legionella*)
   C. Tuberculous
   D. Fungal (histoplasmosis, coccidioidomycosis, *Candida,* blastomycosis)
   E. Other infections (syphilitic, protozoal, parasitic)
II. Noninfectious pericarditis
   A. Acute myocardial infarction
   B. Uremia
   C. Neoplasia
     1. Primary tumors (benign or malignant, mesothelioma)
     2. Tumors metastatic to pericardium (lung and breast cancer, lymphoma, leukemia)
   D. Myxedema
   E. Cholesterol
   F. Chylopericardium
   G. Trauma
     1. Penetrating chest wall
     2. Nonpenetrating
   H. Aortic dissection (with leakage into pericardial sac)
   I. Postirradiation
   J. Familial Mediterranean fever
   K. Familial pericarditis
     1. Mulibrey nanism[a]
   L. Acute idiopathic
   M. Whipple's disease
   N. Sarcoidosis
III. Pericarditis presumably related to hypersensitivity or autoimmunity
   A. Rheumatic fever
   B. Collagen vascular disease (SLE, rheumatoid arthritis, ankylosing spondylitis, scleroderma, acute rheumatic fever, Wegener's granulomatosis)
   C. Drug-induced (e.g., procainamide, hydralazine, phenytoin, isoniazide, minoxidil, anticoagulants, methysergide)
   D. Postcardiac injury
     1. Postmyocardial infarction (Dressler's syndrome)
     2. Postpericardiotomy
     3. Posttraumatic

[a]An autosomal recessive syndrome, characterized by growth failure, muscle hypotonia, hepatomegaly, ocular changes, enlarged cerebral ventricles, mental retardation, ventricular hypertrophy, and chronic constrictive pericarditis.

tamponade (see below). Differentiation from cardiac enlargement may be difficult on physical examination, but heart sounds may be fainter with pericardial effusion. The friction rub may disappear, and the apex impulse may vanish, but sometimes it remains palpable, albeit medial to the left border of cardiac dullness. The base of the left lung may be compressed by pericardial fluid, producing *Ewart's sign*, a patch of dullness and increased fremitus (and egophony) beneath the angle of the left scapula. The chest roentgenogram may show a "water bottle" configuration of the cardiac silhouette (Fig. 232-2) but may also be normal.

Diagnosis *Echocardiography* (Chap. 222) is the most effective imaging technique available since it is sensitive, specific, simple, noninvasive, may be performed at the bedside, and can identify accompanying cardiac tamponade (see below) (Fig. 232-3). The presence of pericardial fluid is recorded by two-dimensional transthoracic echocardiography

FIGURE 232-1 Acute pericarditis often produces diffuse ST-segment elevations (in this case in leads I, II, aVF, and V_2 to V_6) due to a ventricular current of injury. Note also the characteristic PR-segment deviation (opposite in polarity to the ST segment) due to a concomitant atrial injury current.

as a relatively echo-free space between the posterior pericardium and left ventricular epicardium in patients with small effusions, and as a space between the anterior right ventricle and the parietal pericardium just beneath the anterior chest wall in those with larger effusions. In the latter the heart may swing freely within the pericardial sac. When severe, the extent of this motion alternates and may be associated with electrical alternans. Echocardiography allows localization and estimation of the quantity of pericardial fluid.

The diagnosis of pericardial fluid or thickening may be confirmed by computed tomography (CT) or magnetic resonance imaging (MRI) (**Fig. 232-4**). These techniques may be superior to echocardiography in detecting loculated pericardial effusions, pericardial thickening, and the presence of pericardial masses.

CARDIAC TAMPONADE

The accumulation of fluid in the pericardial space in a quantity sufficient to cause serious obstruction to the inflow of blood to the ventricles results in cardiac tamponade. This complication may be fatal if it is not rec-

ognized and treated promptly. The three most common causes of tamponade are neoplastic disease, idiopathic pericarditis, and pericardial effusion secondary to renal failure. Tamponade may also result from bleeding into the pericardial space either following cardiac operations and trauma (including cardiac perforation during cardiac catheterization, percutaneous coronary intervention, or insertion of pacemaker wires) or from tuberculosis and hemopericardium. The latter may occur when a patient with any form of acute pericarditis is treated with anticoagulants.

The three principal features of tamponade (*Beck's triad*) are hypotension, soft or absent heart sounds, and jugular venous distention with a prominent *x* descent but an absent *y* descent. There are both limitation of ventricular filling and reduction of cardiac output. The quantity of fluid necessary to produce this critical state may be as small as 200 mL when the fluid develops rapidly or >2000 mL in slowly developing effusions when the pericardium has had the opportunity to stretch and adapt to an increasing volume. The volume of fluid required to produce tamponade also varies directly with the thickness of the ventricular myocardium and inversely with the thickness of the parietal pericardium.

Tamponade may also develop more slowly, and under these circumstances the clinical manifestations may resemble those of heart failure, including dyspnea, orthopnea, and hepatic engorgement. A high index of suspicion for cardiac tamponade is required since, in many instances, no obvious cause for pericardial disease is apparent, and it should be considered in any patient with hypotension and elevation of jugular venous pressure. Otherwise unexplained enlargement of the cardiac silhouette (especially in subacute or chronic tamponade), reduction in

FIGURE 232-2 Chest radiogram from a patient with a pericardial effusion showing typical "water bottle" heart. There is also a right pleural effusion. [*From SS Kabbani, M LeWinter, in MH Crawford et al (eds): Cardiology. London, Mosby, 2001.*]

FIGURE 232-3 Apical four-chamber echocardiogram recorded in a patient with a moderate pericardial effusion and evidence of hemodynamic compromise. The frame is recorded in early ventricular systole, immediately after atrial contraction. Note that the right atrial wall is indented inward and its curvature is frankly reversed (*arrow*), implying elevated intrapericardial pressure above right atrial pressure. LA, left atrium; LV, left ventricle; RV, right ventricle. [*From WF Armstrong: Echocardiography, in DP Zipes et al (eds): Braunwald's Heart Disease, 7th ed. Philadelphia, Elsevier, 2005.*]

FIGURE 232-4 Chronic pericardial effusion in a 54-year-old female patient with Hodgkin's disease seen in contrast-enhanced 64-slice CT. The arrows point at the pericardial effusion (LV, left ventricle; RV, right ventricle; RA, right atrium). Due to the timing of the scan relative to contrast injection, only the blood in the left ventricle is contrast-enhanced, hence the low attenuation in the right-sided chambers. *(Courtesy of Stephan Achenbach, MD; with permission.)*

amplitude of the QRS complexes, and *electrical alternans* of the P, QRS, or T waves each should raise the suspicion of cardiac tamponade.

Table 232-2 lists the features that distinguish acute cardiac tamponade from constrictive pericarditis.

Paradoxical Pulse This important clue to the presence of cardiac tamponade consists of a greater than normal (10 mmHg) inspiratory decline in systolic arterial pressure. When severe, it may be detected by palpating weakness or disappearance of the arterial pulse during inspi-

ration, but usually sphygmomanometric measurement of systolic pressure during slow respiration is required.

Since both ventricles share a tight incompressible covering, i.e., the pericardial sac, the inspiratory enlargement of the right ventricle in cardiac tamponade compresses and reduces left ventricular volume; leftward bulging of the interventricular septum further reduces the left ventricular cavity as the right ventricle enlarges during inspiration. Thus, in cardiac tamponade the normal inspiratory augmentation of right ventricular volume causes an exaggerated reciprocal reduction in left ventricular volume. Also, respiratory distress increases the fluctuations in intrathoracic pressure, which exaggerates the mechanism just described. Right ventricular infarction (Chap. 239) may resemble cardiac tamponade with hypotension, elevated jugular venous pressure, an absent *y* descent in the jugular venous pulse, and, occasionally, pulsus paradoxus. The differences between these two conditions are shown in Table 232-2.

Paradoxical pulse occurs not only in cardiac tamponade but also in approximately one-third of patients with constrictive pericarditis (see below). This physical finding is not pathognomonic of pericardial disease because it may be observed in some cases of hypovolemic shock, acute and chronic obstructive airways disease, and pulmonary embolus.

Low-pressure tamponade refers to mild tamponade in which the intrapericardial pressure is increased from its slightly subatmospheric levels to +5 to +10 mmHg; in some instances, hypovolemia coexists. As a consequence, the central venous pressure is normal or only slightly elevated, while arterial pressure is unaffected and there is no paradoxical pulse. The patients are asymptomatic or complain of mild weakness and dyspnea. The diagnosis is aided by echocardiography, and both hemodynamic and clinical manifestations improve following pericardiocentesis.

Diagnosis Since immediate treatment of cardiac tamponade may be lifesaving, prompt measures to establish the diagnosis by echocardiography should be undertaken (Fig. 232-2). When pericardial effusion causes tamponade, Doppler ultrasound shows that tricuspid and pulmonic valve flow velocities increase markedly during inspiration, while pulmonic vein, mitral, and aortic flow velocities diminish. Often the right ventricular cavity is reduced in diameter, and there is late diastolic inward motion (collapse) of the right ventricular free wall and of the right atrium. Transesophageal echocardiography may be necessary to diagnose a loculated or hemorrhagic effusion responsible for cardiac tamponade.

TABLE 232-2 FEATURES THAT DISTINGUISH CARDIAC TAMPONADE FROM CONSTRICTIVE PERICARDITIS AND SIMILAR CLINICAL DISORDERS

Characteristic	Tamponade	Constrictive Pericarditis	Restrictive Cardiomyopathy	RVMI
Clinical				
Pulsus paradoxus	Common	Usually absent	Rare	Rare
Jugular veins				
Prominent y descent	Absent	Usually present	Rare	Rare
Prominent x descent	Present	Usually present	Present	Rare
Kussmaul's sign	Absent	Present	Absent	Present
Third heart sound	Absent	Absent	Rare	May be present
Pericardial knock	Absent	Often present	Absent	Absent
Electrocardiogram				
Low ECG voltage	May be present	May be present	May be present	Absent
Electrical alternans	May be present	Absent	Absent	Absent
Echocardiography				
Thickened pericardium	Absent	Present	Absent	Absent
Pericardial calcification	Absent	Often present	Absent	Absent
Pericardial effusion	Present	Absent	Absent	Absent
RV size	Usually small	Usually normal	Usually normal	Enlarged
Myocardial thickness	Normal	Normal	Usually increased	Normal
Right atrial collapse and RVDC	Present	Absent	Absent	Absent
Increased early filling, ↑ mitral flow velocity	Absent	Present	Present	May be present
Exaggerated respiratory variation in flow velocity	Present	Present	Absent	Absent
CT/MRI				
Thickened/calcific pericardium	Absent	Present	Absent	Absent
Cardiac catheterization				
Equalization of diastolic pressures	Usually present	Usually present	Usually absent	Absent or present
Cardiac biopsy helpful?	No	No	Sometimes	No

Abbreviations: RV, right ventricle; RVMI, right ventricular myocardial infarction; RVDC, right ventricular diastolic collapse; ECG, electrocardiograph.　　**Source:** From GM Brockington et al, Cardiol Clin 8:645, 1990, with permission.

℞ CARDIAC TAMPONADE

Patients with acute pericarditis should be observed frequently for the development of an effusion; if a large effusion is present, the patient should be hospitalized and watched closely for signs of tamponade. Arterial and venous pressures and heart rate should be monitored or followed carefully and serial echocardiograms obtained.

PERICARDIOCENTESIS If manifestations of tamponade appear, echocardiographically guided pericardiocentesis using an apical, parasternal, or, most commonly, a subxiphoid approach must be carried out at once as reduction of the elevated intrapericardial pressure may be lifesaving. Intravenous saline may be administered as the patient is being readied for the procedure. Intrapericardial pressure should be measured before fluid is withdrawn, and the pericardial cavity should be drained as completely as possible. A small, multiholed catheter advanced over the needle inserted into the pericardial cavity may be left in place to allow draining of the pericardial space if fluid reaccumulates. Surgical drainage through a limited (subxiphoid) thoracotomy may be required in recurrent tamponade, when it is necessary to remove loculated effusions, and/or when it is necessary to obtain tissue for diagnosis.

Pericardial fluid obtained from an effusion often has the physical characteristics of an exudate. Bloody fluid is most commonly due to neoplasm in the United States and tuberculosis in developing nations but may also be found in the effusion of rheumatic fever, post-cardiac injury, and postmyocardial infarction, as well as in the pericarditis associated with renal failure or dialysis. Transudative pericardial effusions may occur in heart failure.

The pericardial fluid should be analyzed for red and white blood cells, and cytologic studies for cancer, microscopic studies, and cultures should be obtained. The presence of DNA of *Mycobacterium tuberculosis* determined by polymerase chain reaction or an elevated adenosine deaminase activity (>30 U/L) strongly supports the diagnosis of tuberculous pericarditis (Chap. 158).

VIRAL OR IDIOPATHIC FORM OF ACUTE PERICARDITIS

In some cases of this common disorder, coxsackievirus A or B or the virus of influenza, echovirus, mumps, herpes simplex, chickenpox, adenovirus, cytomegalovirus, Epstein-Barr, or HIV has been isolated from pericardial fluid and/or appropriate elevations in viral antibody titers have been noted. In many instances, acute pericarditis occurs in association with illnesses of known viral origin and, presumably, are caused by the same agent. Commonly, there is an antecedent infection of the respiratory tract, but in many patients such an association is not evident, and viral isolation and serologic studies are negative. Pericardial effusion is a common cardiac manifestation of HIV; it is usually secondary to infection (often mycobacterial) or neoplasm, most frequently lymphoma. In full-blown AIDS, pericardial effusion is associated with a shortened survival (Chap. 182).

Most frequently, a viral causation cannot be established; the term *idiopathic acute pericarditis* is then appropriate. Viral or idiopathic acute pericarditis occurs at all ages but is more frequent in young adults, and is often associated with pleural effusions and pneumonitis. The almost simultaneous development of fever and precordial pain, often 10 to 12 days after a presumed viral illness, constitutes an important feature in the differentiation of acute pericarditis from AMI, in which pain precedes fever. The constitutional symptoms are usually mild to moderate, and a pericardial friction rub is often audible. The disease ordinarily runs its course in a few days to 4 weeks. The ST-segment alterations in the ECG usually disappear after 1 or more weeks, but the abnormal T waves may persist for several years and be a source of confusion in persons without a clear history of pericarditis.

Pleuritis and pneumonitis frequently accompany pericarditis. Accumulation of some pericardial fluid is common, and both tamponade and constrictive pericarditis are possible complications. Recurrent (relapsing) pericarditis occurs in about one-fourth of patients with acute idiopathic pericarditis. In a smaller number, there are multiple recurrences.

℞ IDIOPATHIC ACUTE PERICARDITIS

Hyperimmune globulin has been reported to be beneficial in cytomegalovirus, adenovirus, and parvovirus pericarditis, while interferon α has been re-

ported to be so in coxsackie B pericarditis. In acute idiopathic pericarditis there is no specific therapy, but bed rest and anti-inflammatory treatment with aspirin (2–4 mg/d) may be given. If this is ineffective, one of the nonsteroidal anti-inflammatory drugs (NSAIDs), such as ibuprofen (400–800 mg qid) or colchicine (0.6 mg bid), is often effective. Glucocorticoids (e.g., prednisone, 40–80 mg daily) usually suppress the clinical manifestations of the acute illness and may be useful in patients in whom purulent bacterial pericarditis has been excluded and in patients with pericarditis secondary to connective tissue disorders and renal failure (see below). Anticoagulants should be avoided since their use could cause bleeding into the pericardial cavity and tamponade.

After the patient has been asymptomatic and afebrile for about a week, the dose of the NSAID may be tapered gradually. Colchicine may prevent recurrences, but when recurrences are multiple, frequent, disabling, continue beyond 2 years, and are not controlled by pulses of high doses of glucocorticoids, pericardiectomy may be carried out in an attempt to terminate the illness.

Postcardiac Injury Syndrome Acute pericarditis may appear under a variety of circumstances that have one common feature: previous injury to the myocardium with blood in the pericardial cavity. The syndrome may develop after a cardiac surgery (postpericardiotomy syndrome); after cardiac trauma, blunt or penetrating (Chap. 233); or after perforation of the heart with a catheter. Rarely, it follows AMI.

The clinical picture mimics acute viral or idiopathic pericarditis. The principal symptom is the pain of acute pericarditis, which usually develops 1 to 4 weeks following the cardiac injury (1 to 3 days following AMI) but sometimes appears only after an interval of months. Recurrences are common and may occur up to 2 years or more after the injury. Fever with temperature up to 40°C, pericarditis, pleuritis, and pneumonitis are the outstanding features, and the bout of illness usually subsides in 1 or 2 weeks. The pericarditis may be of the fibrinous variety or it may be a pericardial effusion, which is often serosanguineous, but rarely causes tamponade. Leukocytosis, an increased sedimentation rate, and electrocardiographic changes typical of acute pericarditis may also occur.

The mechanisms responsible for this syndrome have not been identified, but they are probably the result of a hypersensitivity reaction to antigen which originates from injured myocardial tissue and/or pericardium. Circulating myocardial antisarcolemmal and antifibrillar autoantibodies occur frequently, but their precise role has not been defined. Viral infection may also play an etiologic role, since antiviral antibodies are often elevated in patients who develop this syndrome following cardiac surgery.

Often no treatment is necessary aside from aspirin and analgesics. The management of pericardial effusion and tamponade is discussed above. When the illness is followed by a series of disabling recurrences, therapy with an NSAID, colchicine, or a glucocorticoid is usually effective.

DIFFERENTIAL DIAGNOSIS

Since there is no specific test for *acute idiopathic pericarditis*, the diagnosis is one of exclusion. Consequently, all other disorders that may be associated with acute fibrinous pericarditis must be considered. A common diagnostic error is mistaking acute viral or idiopathic pericarditis for AMI and vice versa. When acute fibrinous pericarditis is associated with AMI (Chap. 239), it is characterized by fever, pain, and a friction rub in the first 4 days following the development of the infarct. ECG abnormalities (such as the appearance of Q waves, brief ST-segment elevations with reciprocal changes, and earlier T-wave changes in AMI) and the extent of the elevations of myocardial enzymes are helpful in differentiating pericarditis from AMI.

Pericarditis secondary to post-cardiac injury is differentiated from acute idiopathic pericarditis chiefly by timing. If it occurs within a few days or weeks of an AMI, a chest blow, a cardiac perforation, or cardiac operation, it may be justified to conclude that the two are probably related. If the infarct has been silent or the chest blow forgotten, the relationship to the pericarditis may not be recognized.

It is important to distinguish *pericarditis due to collagen vascular disease* from acute idiopathic pericarditis. Most important in the differential diagnosis is the pericarditis due to systemic lupus erythematosus (SLE; Chap. 313) or drug-induced (procainamide or hydralazine) lupus. Pain is often present in pericarditis due to collagen vascular disease. Sometimes in SLE the pericarditis appears as an asymptomatic effusion and, rarely, tamponade develops. When pericarditis occurs in the absence of any obvious underlying disorder, the diagnosis of SLE may be suggested by a rise in the titer of antinuclear antibodies. Acute pericarditis is an occasional complication of *rheumatoid arthritis*, *scleroderma*, and *polyarteritis nodosa*, and other evidence of these diseases is usually obvious. Asymptomatic pericardial effusion is also frequent in these disorders. It is important to question every patient with acute pericarditis about the ingestion of procainamide, hydralazine, isoniazid, cromolyn, and minoxidil, since these drugs can cause this syndrome. The pericarditis of *acute rheumatic fever* is generally associated with evidence of severe pancarditis and with cardiac murmurs (Chap. 315).

Pyogenic (purulent) pericarditis is usually secondary to cardiothoracic operations, by extension of infection from the lungs or pleural cavities, from rupture of the esophagus into the pericardial sac, or rupture of a ring abscess in a patient with infective endocarditis, or can occur if septicemia complicates aseptic pericarditis. It is accompanied by fever, chills, septicemia, and evidence of infection elsewhere and generally has a poor prognosis. The diagnosis is made by examination of the pericardial fluid. Acute pericarditis may also complicate the viral, pyogenic, mycobacterial, and fungal infections that occur with HIV infection.

Pericarditis of renal failure (Chap. 274) occurs in up to one-third of patients with chronic uremia *(uremic pericarditis)*, is also seen in patients undergoing chronic dialysis with normal levels of blood urea and creatinine, and is termed *dialysis-associated pericarditis*. These two forms of pericarditis may be fibrinous and are generally associated with an effusion that may be sanguineous. A friction rub is common, but pain is usually absent or mild. Treatment with a nonsteroidal anti-inflammatory drug and intensification of dialysis are usually adequate. Occasionally, tamponade occurs and pericardiocentesis is required. When the pericarditis of renal failure is recurrent or persistent, a pericardial window should be created or pericardiectomy may be necessary.

Pericarditis due to *neoplastic diseases* results from extension or invasion of metastatic tumors (most commonly carcinoma of the lung and breast, malignant melanoma, lymphoma, and leukemia) to the pericardium; pain, atrial arrhythmias, and tamponade are complications that occur occasionally. Diagnosis is made by pericardial fluid cytology or pericardial biopsy. *Mediastinal irradiation* for neoplasm may cause acute pericarditis and/or chronic constrictive pericarditis after eradication of the tumor. Unusual causes of acute pericarditis include syphilis, fungal infection (histoplasmosis, blastomycosis, aspergillosis, and candidiasis), and parasitic infestation (amebiasis, toxoplasmosis, echinococcosis, trichinosis).

CHRONIC PERICARDIAL EFFUSIONS

Chronic pericardial effusions are sometimes encountered in patients without an antecedent history of acute pericarditis. They may cause few symptoms per se, and their presence may be detected by finding an enlarged cardiac silhouette on chest roentgenogram. Tuberculosis is a common cause (Chap. 158).

Other Causes *Myxedema* may be responsible for chronic pericardial effusion that is sometimes massive but rarely, if ever, causes cardiac tamponade. The cardiac silhouette is markedly enlarged, and an echocardiogram distinguishes cardiomegaly from pericardial effusion. The diagnosis of myxedema can be confirmed by tests for thyroid function (Chap. 335). Myxedematous pericardial effusion responds to thyroid hormone replacement.

Neoplasms, SLE, rheumatoid arthritis, mycotic infections, radiation therapy to the chest, pyogenic infections, and chylopericardium may also cause chronic pericardial effusion and should be considered and specifically sought in such patients.

Aspiration and analysis of the pericardial fluid are often helpful in diagnosis. Pericardial fluid should be analyzed as described on p. 1492.

Grossly sanguineous pericardial fluid results most commonly from a neoplasm, tuberculosis, renal failure, or slow leakage from an aortic aneurysm. Pericardiocentesis may resolve large effusions, but pericardiectomy may be required with recurrence. Intrapericardial instillation of sclerosing agents or antineoplastic agents (e.g., bleomycin) may be used to prevent reaccumulation of fluid.

CHRONIC CONSTRICTIVE PERICARDITIS

This disorder results when the healing of an acute fibrinous or serofibrinous pericarditis or the resorption of a chronic pericardial effusion is followed by obliteration of the pericardial cavity with the formation of granulation tissue. The latter gradually contracts and forms a firm scar, encasing the heart and interfering with filling of the ventricles. In developing nations where the condition is prevalent, a high percentage of cases is of tuberculous origin, but in North America this is now an infrequent cause. Chronic constrictive pericarditis may follow acute or relapsing viral or idiopathic pericarditis, trauma with organized blood clot, cardiac surgery of any type, mediastinal irradiation, purulent infection, histoplasmosis, neoplastic disease (especially breast cancer, lung cancer, and lymphoma), rheumatoid arthritis, SLE, and chronic renal failure with uremia treated by chronic dialysis. In many patients the cause of the pericardial disease is undetermined, and in them an asymptomatic or forgotten bout of viral pericarditis, acute or idiopathic, may have been the inciting event.

The basic physiologic abnormality in patients with chronic constrictive pericarditis is the inability of the ventricles to fill because of the limitations imposed by the rigid, thickened pericardium or the tense pericardial fluid. In constrictive pericarditis, ventricular filling is unimpeded during early diastole but it is reduced abruptly when the elastic limit of the pericardium is reached, while in cardiac tamponade, ventricular filling is impeded throughout diastole. In both conditions, ventricular end-diastolic and stroke volumes are reduced and the end-diastolic pressures in both ventricles and the mean pressures in the atria, pulmonary veins, and systemic veins are all elevated to similar levels, i.e., within 5 mmHg of one another. Despite these hemodynamic changes, myocardial function may be normal or only slightly impaired in chronic constrictive pericarditis. However, the fibrotic process may extend into the myocardium and cause myocardial scarring, and atrophy, and venous congestion may then be due to the combined effects of the pericardial and myocardial lesions.

In constrictive pericarditis, the right and left atrial pressure pulses display an M-shaped contour, with prominent *x* and *y* descents; the *y* descent, which is absent or diminished in cardiac tamponade, is the most prominent deflection in constrictive pericarditis; it reflects rapid early filling of the ventricles. The *y* descent is interrupted by a rapid rise in atrial pressure during early diastole, when ventricular filling is impeded by the constricting pericardium. These characteristic changes are transmitted to the jugular veins, where they may be recognized by inspection. In constrictive pericarditis, the ventricular pressure pulses in both ventricles exhibit characteristic "square root" signs during diastole. These hemodynamic changes, although characteristic, are not pathognomonic of constrictive pericarditis and may also be observed in cardiomyopathies characterized by restriction of ventricular filling (Chap. 231) (Table 232-2).

CLINICAL AND LABORATORY FINDINGS

Weakness, fatigue, weight gain, increased abdominal girth, abdominal discomfort, a protuberant abdomen, and edema are common. The patient often appears chronically ill, and in advanced cases there are anasarca, skeletal muscle wasting, and cachexia. Exertional dyspnea is common, and orthopnea may occur, although it is usually not severe. Acute left ventricular failure (acute pulmonary edema) is very uncommon. The cervical veins are distended and may remain so even after intensive diuretic treatment, and venous pressure may fail to decline during inspiration (*Kussmaul's sign*). The latter is frequent in chronic pericarditis but may also occur in tricuspid stenosis, right ventricular infarction, and restrictive cardiomyopathy.

FIGURE 232-5 Constrictive pericarditis Doppler schema of respirophasic changes in mitral and tricuspid inflow. Reciprocal patterns of ventricular filling are assessed on pulsed Doppler examination of mitral (MV) and tricuspid (TV) inflow. *(Courtesy of Bernard E. Bulwer, MD; with permission.)*

The pulse pressure is normal or reduced. In about one-third of the cases, a paradoxical pulse (p. 1491) can be detected. Congestive hepatomegaly is pronounced and may impair hepatic function and cause jaundice; ascites is common and is usually more prominent than dependent edema. The apical pulse is reduced and may retract in systole (*Broadbent's sign*). The heart sounds may be distant; an early third heart sound, i.e., a pericardial knock, occurring 0.09 to 0.12 s after aortic valve closure at the cardiac apex, is often conspicuous; it occurs with the abrupt cessation of ventricular filling. A systolic murmur of tricuspid regurgitation may be present.

The *ECG* frequently displays low voltage of the QRS complexes and diffuse flattening or inversion of the T waves. Atrial fibrillation is present in about one-third of patients. The *chest roentgenogram* shows a normal or slightly enlarged heart; pericardial calcification is most common in tuberculous pericarditis.

Inasmuch as the usual physical signs of cardiac disease (murmurs, cardiac enlargement) may be inconspicuous or absent in chronic constrictive pericarditis, hepatic enlargement and dysfunction associated with jaundice and intractable ascites may lead to a mistaken diagnosis of hepatic cirrhosis. This error can be avoided if the neck veins are inspected carefully in patients with ascites and hepatomegaly. Given a clinical picture resembling hepatic cirrhosis, but with the added feature of distended neck veins, careful search for thickening of the pericardium by CT (Fig. 222-8) or MRI should be carried out and may disclose this curable or remediable form of heart disease.

The two-dimensional transthoracic *echocardiogram* typically shows pericardial thickening, dilatation of the inferior vena cava and hepatic veins, and a sharp halt in ventricular filling in early diastole, with normal ventricular systolic function and flattening of the left ventricular posterior wall. Atrial enlargement may be seen, especially in patients with long-standing constrictive physiology. There is a distinctive pattern of transvalvular flow velocity on Doppler flow-velocity echocardiography. During inspiration there is an exaggerated reduction in blood flow velocity in the pulmonary veins and across the mitral valve and a leftward shift of the ventricular septum; the opposite occurs during expiration. Diastolic flow velocity in the vena cavae into the right atrium and across the tricuspid valve increases in an exaggerated manner during inspiration and declines during expiration (Fig. 232-5). However, echocardiography cannot definitively exclude the diagnosis of constrictive pericarditis. MRI and CT scanning (Fig. 232-6) are more accurate than echocardiography in establishing or excluding the presence of a thickened pericardium. Pericardial thickening and even pericardial calcification, however, are not synonymous with constrictive pericarditis since they may occur without seriously impairing ventricular filling.

DIFFERENTIAL DIAGNOSIS

Like chronic constrictive pericarditis, cor pulmonale (Chap. 227) may be associated with severe systemic venous hypertension but little pulmonary congestion; the heart is usually not enlarged, and a paradoxical pulse may be present. However, in cor pulmonale, advanced parenchymal pulmonary disease is usually obvious and venous pressure *falls* during inspiration, i.e., Kussmaul's sign is negative. *Tricuspid stenosis* (Chap. 230) may also simulate chronic constrictive pericarditis; congestive hepatomegaly, splenomegaly, ascites, and venous distention may be equally prominent. However, in tricuspid stenosis, a characteristic murmur as well as the murmur of accompanying mitral stenosis are usually present. In tricuspid stenosis, a paradoxical pulse and a steep, deep *y* descent in the jugular venous pulse do *not* occur, serving to differentiate it from chronic constrictive pericarditis.

Because constrictive pericarditis can be corrected surgically, it is important to distinguish chronic constrictive pericarditis from restrictive cardiomyopathy (Chap. 231), which has a similar physiologic abnormality, i.e., restriction of ventricular filling. In many of these patients the ventricular wall is thickened on echocardiographic examination (Table 232-2). The features favoring the diagnosis of restrictive cardiomyopathy over chronic constrictive pericarditis include a well-defined apex beat, cardiac enlargement, and pronounced orthopnea with attacks of acute left ventricular failure, left ventricular hypertrophy, gallop sounds (in place of a pericardial knock), bundle branch block, and in some cases abnormal Q waves on the ECG. The typical echocardiographic features of constrictive pericarditis (see above) are useful in the differential diagnosis in chronic constrictive pericarditis (Fig. 232-5). CT scanning (usually with contrast) and MRI are key in distinguishing between restrictive cardiomyopathy and chronic constrictive pericarditis. In the former, the ventricular walls are hypertrophied, while in the latter the pericardium is thickened and sometimes calcified. When a patient has progressive, disabling, and unresponsive congestive heart failure and displays any of the features of constrictive heart disease, Doppler echocardiography to record respiratory effects on transvalvular flow, and an MRI or CT scan should be obtained to detect or exclude constrictive pericarditis, since the latter is usually curable.

℞ CONSTRICTIVE PERICARDITIS

Pericardial resection is the only definitive treatment of constrictive pericarditis, but dietary sodium restriction and diuretics are useful during pre-

FIGURE 232-6 Cardiovascular magnetic resonance in a patient with constrictive pericarditis. On the right is a basal short-axis view of the ventricles showing a thickened pericardium encasing the heart (*arrows*). On the left is a transaxial view, again showing the thickened pericardium, particularly over the right heart, but also a pleural effusion (Pl Eff). LV, left ventricle; RV, right ventricle. *[From D Pennell: Cardiovascular magnetic resonance, in DP Zipes et al (eds): Braunwald's Heart Disease, 7th ed. Philadelphia, Elsevier, 2005.]*

operative preparation. Coronary arteriography should be carried out preoperatively in patients older than 50 years to exclude unsuspected coronary disease. The benefits derived from cardiac decortication are usually progressive over a period of months. The risk of this operation depends on the extent of penetration of the myocardium by the calcific process, by the severity of myocardial atrophy, by the extent of secondary impairment of hepatic and/or renal function, and by the patient's general condition. Operative mortality is in the range of 5 to 10%; the patients with the most severe disease are at highest risk. Therefore, surgical treatment should be carried out relatively early in the course.

Subacute Effusive-Constrictive Pericarditis This form of pericardial disease is characterized by the combination of a tense effusion in the pericardial space and constriction of the heart by thickened pericardium. It shares a number of features both with chronic pericardial effusion producing cardiac compression and with pericardial constriction. It may be caused by tuberculosis (see below), multiple attacks of acute idiopathic pericarditis, radiation, traumatic pericarditis, renal failure, scleroderma, and neoplasms. The heart is generally enlarged, and a paradoxical pulse and a prominent x descent (without a prominent y descent) are present in the atrial and jugular venous pressure pulses. Following pericardiocentesis, the physiologic findings may change from those of cardiac tamponade to those of pericardial constriction, with a "square root" sign in the ventricular pressure pulse and a prominent y descent in the atrial and jugular venous pressure pulses. Furthermore, the intrapericardial pressure and the central venous pressure may decline, but not to normal. The diagnosis can be established by pericardiocentesis followed by pericardial biopsy. In many patients the condition progresses to the chronic constrictive form of the disease. Wide excision of both the visceral and parietal pericardium is usually effective therapy.

Tuberculous Pericardial Disease This chronic infection is a common cause of chronic pericardial effusion, although less so in the United States than in Africa, Asia, the Middle East, and other parts of the developing world where active tuberculosis is endemic (Chap. 158). The clinical picture is that of a chronic, systemic illness in a patient with pericardial effusion. It is important to consider this diagnosis in a patient with known tuberculosis, with HIV, and with fever, chest pain, weight loss, and enlargement of the cardiac silhouette of undetermined origin. Inasmuch as treatment is quite effective, overlooking a tuberculous pericardial effusion may have serious consequences. If the etiology of chronic pericardial effusion remains obscure, despite detailed analysis of the pericardial fluid (see above), a pericardial biopsy,

preferably by a limited thoracotomy, should be performed. If definitive evidence is then still lacking but the specimen shows granulomata with caseation, antituberculous chemotherapy (Chap. 158) is indicated.

If the biopsy specimen shows a thickened pericardium, pericardiectomy should be carried out in order to prevent the development of constriction, a serious complication of tuberculosis that occurs in about one-half of patients with tuberculous pericardial effusion despite treatment with chemotherapy and glucocorticoids. Tubercular cardiac constriction should be treated surgically while the patient is receiving antituberculous chemotherapy. In many patients, subacute effusive-constrictive pericarditis develops.

OTHER DISORDERS OF THE PERICARDIUM

Pericardial cysts appear as rounded or lobulated deformities of the cardiac silhouette, most commonly at the right cardiophrenic angle. They do not cause symptoms, and their major clinical significance lies in the possibility of confusion with a tumor, ventricular aneurysm, or massive cardiomegaly. *Tumors* involving the pericardium are most commonly secondary to malignant neoplasms originating in or invading the mediastinum, including carcinoma of the bronchus and breast, lymphoma, and melanoma. The most common *primary* malignant tumor is the mesothelioma. The usual clinical picture of malignant pericardial tumor is an insidiously developing, often bloody, pericardial effusion. Surgical exploration is required to establish a definitive diagnosis and to carry out definitive or, more commonly, palliative treatment.

FURTHER READINGS

AXEL L: Assessment of pericardial disease by magnetic resonance and computed tomography. J Magn Reson Imaging 19:816, 2004

HOIT BD: Management of effusive and constrictive pericardial heart disease. Circulation 105:2939, 2002

LANGE RA, HILLIS LD: Acute pericarditis. N Engl J Med 351:2195, 2004

LEWINTER M, KABBANI S: Pericardial diseases, in *Braunwald's Heart Disease*, 8th ed, D Zipes et al (eds). Philadelphia, Saunders, 2008

MAISCH B et al: Guidelines on the diagnosis and management of pericardial diseases executive summary: the Task Force on the Diagnosis and Management of Pericardial Diseases of the European Society of Cardiology. Eur Heart J 25:587, 2004

MAYOSI BM et al: Tuberculous pericarditis. Circulation 112:3608, 2005

RAJAGOPALAN N et al: Comparison of new Doppler echocardiographic methods to differentiate constrictive pericardial heart disease and restrictive cardiomyopathy. Am J Cardiol 87:86, 2001

233 Tumors and Trauma of the Heart
Eric H. Awtry, Wilson S. Colucci

TUMORS OF THE HEART

PRIMARY TUMORS

Primary tumors of the heart are rare. Approximately three-quarters are histologically benign, over half of which are myxomas. Malignant tumors, almost all of which are sarcomas, account for 25% of primary cardiac tumors (Table 233-1). All cardiac tumors, regardless of pathologic type, have the potential to cause life-threatening complications. Many tumors are now curable by surgery; thus, early diagnosis is imperative.

Clinical Presentation Cardiac tumors may present with a wide array of cardiac and noncardiac manifestations, which depend in large part on the location and size of the tumor. Many of the manifestations are non-

specific features of more common forms of heart disease, such as chest pain, syncope, heart failure, murmurs, arrhythmias, conduction disturbances, and pericardial effusion with or without tamponade. Additionally, embolic phenomena and constitutional symptoms may occur.

Myxoma Myxomas are the most common type of primary cardiac tumor in all age groups, accounting for one-third to one-half of all cases at postmortem and for about three-quarters of the tumors treated surgically. They occur at all ages, most commonly in the third through sixth decades, with a female predilection. Approximately 90% of myxomas are sporadic; the remainder are familial with autosomal dominant transmission. The familial variety often occurs as part of a syndrome complex (Carney complex) that comprises (1) myxomas (cardiac, skin, and/or breast), (2) lentigines and/or pigmented nevi, and (3) endocrine overactivity (primary nodular adrenal cortical disease with or without Cushing's syndrome, testicular tumors, and/or pituitary adenomas with gigantism or acromegaly). Certain constellations of findings have been referred to as the *NAME* syndrome (nevi, atrial myxoma, myxoid neurofibroma, and ephelides) or the *LAMB* syndrome (lentigines, atrial myxoma, and blue nevi), although these likely represent subsets of the Carney complex. The genetic basis of

TABLE 233-1	RELATIVE INCIDENCE OF PRIMARY TUMORS OF THE HEART	
Type	**Number**	**Percent**
Benign	199	58.0
Myxoma	114	33.2
Rhabdomyoma	20	5.8
Fibroma	20	5.8
Hemangioma	17	5.0
Atrioventricular nodal	10	2.9
Granular cell	4	1.2
Lipoma	2	0.6
Paraganglioma	2	0.6
Myocytic hamartoma	2	0.6
Histiocytoid cardiomyopathy	2	0.6
Inflammatory psuedotumor	2	0.6
Other benign tumors	4	1.2
Malignant	144	42.0
Sarcoma	137	39.9
Lymphoma	7	2.1

Source: Modified from A Burke, R Virmani: *Atlas of Tumor Pathology. Tumors of the Heart and Great Vessels.* Washington, DC, Armed Forces Institute of Pathology 1996, p 231; with permission.

FIGURE 233-2 Cardiac MRI demonstrating a rounded mass (M) within the left atrium (LA). Pathologic evaluation at the time of surgery revealed it to be an atrial myxoma. LV, left ventricle; RA, right atrium; RV, right ventricle.

this complex has not been completely elucidated; however, patients frequently have mutations in the tumor-suppressor gene *PRKAR1A*, which encodes the protein kinase A type I-α regulatory subunit.

Pathologically, myxomas are gelatinous structures consisting of myxoma cells embedded in a stroma rich in glycosaminoglycans. Most are pedunculated on a fibrovascular stalk and average 4–8 cm in diameter. Most are solitary and located in the atria, particularly the left atrium, where they usually arise from the interatrial septum in the vicinity of the fossa ovalis. In contrast to sporadic tumors, familial or myxoma syndrome tumors tend to occur in younger individuals, are often multiple, may be ventricular in location, and are more likely to recur after initial resection.

Myxomas commonly present with obstructive signs and symptoms. The most common clinical presentation mimics that of mitral valve disease—either stenosis owing to tumor prolapse into the mitral orifice or regurgitation resulting from tumor-induced valvular trauma. Ventricular myxomas may cause outflow obstruction similar to that caused by subaortic or subpulmonic stenosis. The symptoms and signs of myxoma may be sudden in onset or positional in nature, owing to the effects of gravity on tumor position. A characteristic low-pitched sound, referred to as a "tumor plop," may be appreciated on auscultation during early or mid-diastole and is thought to result from the im-

pact of the tumor against the mitral valve or ventricular wall. Myxomas may also present with peripheral or pulmonary emboli or with constitutional signs and symptoms, including fever, weight loss, cachexia, malaise, arthralgias, rash, digital clubbing, Raynaud's phenomenon, hypergammaglobulinemia, anemia, polycythemia, leukocytosis, elevated erythrocyte sedimentation rate, thrombocytopenia, or thrombocytosis. Not surprisingly, patients with myxomas are frequently misdiagnosed as having endocarditis, collagen vascular disease, or a paraneoplastic syndrome.

Two-dimensional transthoracic or omniplane transesophageal echocardiography is useful in the diagnosis of cardiac myxoma and allows assessment of tumor size and determination of the site of tumor attachment, both important considerations in the planning of surgical excision (Fig. 233-1). CT and MRI may provide important information regarding size, shape, composition, and surface characteristics of the tumor (Fig. 233-2).

Although cardiac catheterization and angiography were previously performed routinely prior to tumor resection, they are no longer considered mandatory when adequate noninvasive information is available and other cardiac disorders (e.g., coronary artery disease) are not considered likely. Additionally, catheterization of the chamber from which the tumor arises carries the risk of tumor embolization. Because myxomas may be familial, echocardiographic screening of first-degree relatives is appropriate, particularly if the patient is young and has multiple tumors or evidence of myxoma syndrome.

℞ PRIMARY TUMOR

Surgical excision utilizing cardiopulmonary bypass is indicated, regardless of tumor size, and is generally curative. Myxomas recur in ~12–22% of familial cases but in only 1–2% of sporadic cases. Tumor recurrence is most likely due to multifocal lesions in the former and inadequate resection in the latter.

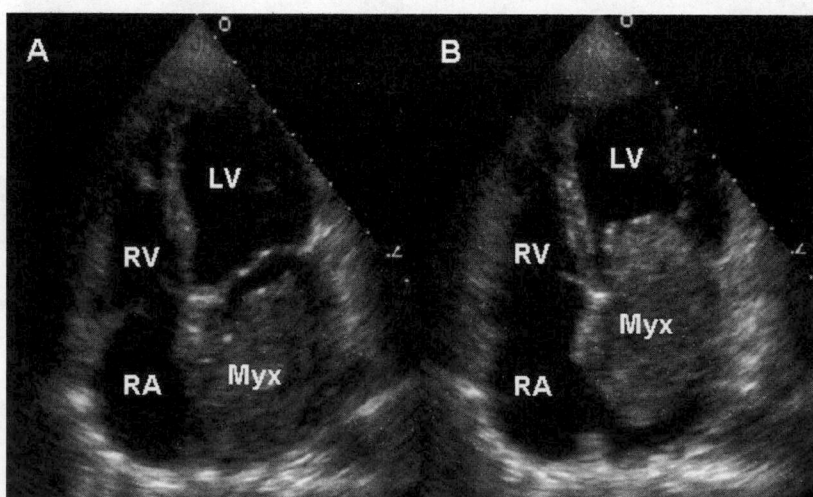

FIGURE 233-1 Transthoracic echocardiogram demonstrating a large atrial myxoma. The myxoma (Myx) fills the entire left atrium in systole (*panel A*) and prolapses across the mitral valve and into the left ventricle (LV) during diastole (*panel B*). RA, right atrium; RV, right ventricle. (*Courtesy of Dr. Michael Tsang; with permission.*)

Other Benign Tumors Cardiac *lipomas*, although relatively common, are usually incidental findings at postmortem examination; however, they may grow as large as 15 cm and may present with symptoms owing to mechanical interference with cardiac function, arrhythmias, or conduction disturbances, or as an abnormality of the cardiac silhouette on chest x-ray. *Papillary fibroelastomas* are the most common tumors of the cardiac valves. Although usually clinically silent, they can cause valve dysfunction and may embolize distally, resulting in transient ischemic attacks, stroke, or myocardial infarction. Therefore, these tumors should be resected even when asymptomatic. *Rhabdomyomas* and *fibromas* are the most common cardiac tumors in infants and children and usually occur in the ventricles where they may produce mechanical obstruction to blood flow, thereby mimicking valvular stenosis, congestive heart failure (CHF), restrictive or hypertrophic cardiomyopathy, or pericardial constriction. Rhabdomyomas are probably hamartomatous growths, are multiple in 90% of cases, and are strongly associated with tuberous sclerosis. These tumors have a tendency to regress completely or partially; only those tumors that cause obstruction require surgical resection. Fibromas are usually single, are often calcified, tend to grow and cause obstructive symptoms, and should be resected. *Hemangiomas* and *mesotheliomas* are generally small tumors, most often intramyocardial in location, and may cause atrioventricular (AV) conduction disturbances and even sudden death as a result of their propensity to develop in the region of the AV node. Other benign tumors arising from the heart include *teratoma, chemodectoma, neurilemoma, granular cell myoblastoma,* and *bronchogenic cysts.*

Sarcoma Almost all primary cardiac malignancies are sarcomas, which may be of several histologic types. In general, these tumors are characterized by rapid progression culminating in the patient's death within weeks to months from the time of presentation, as a result of hemodynamic compromise, local invasion, or distant metastases. Sarcomas commonly involve the right side of the heart, are characterized by rapid growth, frequently invade the pericardial space, and may obstruct the cardiac chambers or vena cavae. Sarcomas may also occur on the left side of the heart and may be mistaken for myxomas.

℞ SARCOMA

At the time of presentation these tumors have often spread too extensively to allow for surgical excision. Although scattered reports exist of palliation with surgery, radiotherapy, and/or chemotherapy, the response of cardiac sarcomas to these therapies is generally poor. The one exception appears to be cardiac lymphosarcomas, which may respond to a combination of chemo- and radiotherapy.

TUMORS METASTATIC TO THE HEART

Tumors metastatic to the heart are much more common than primary tumors, and their incidence is likely to increase as the life expectancy of patients with various forms of malignant neoplasms is extended by more effective therapy. Although cardiac metastases occur in 1–20% of all tumor types, the relative incidence is especially high in malignant melanoma and, to a somewhat lesser extent, in leukemia and lymphoma. In absolute terms, the most common primary originating sites of cardiac metastases are carcinoma of the breast and lung, reflecting the high incidence of these cancers. Cardiac metastases almost always occur in the setting of widespread primary disease, and most often either primary or metastatic disease exists elsewhere in the thoracic cavity. Nevertheless, cardiac metastasis may occasionally be the initial presentation of an extrathoracic tumor.

Cardiac metastases may occur via hematogenous or lymphangitic spread or by direct tumor invasion. They generally manifest as small, firm nodules; diffuse infiltration may also occur, especially with sarcomas or hematologic neoplasms. The pericardium is most often involved, followed by myocardial involvement of any chamber, and, rarely, by involvement of the endocardium or cardiac valves.

Cardiac metastases are clinically apparent only ~10% of the time, are usually not the cause of the patient's presentation, and rarely are the cause of death. The vast majority occur in the setting of a previously recognized malignant neoplasm. When symptomatic, cardiac metastases may result in a variety of clinical features, including dyspnea, acute pericarditis, cardiac tamponade, ectopic tachyarrhythmias, heart block, CHF, and rapid enlargement of the cardiac silhouette on chest x-ray. As with primary cardiac tumors, the clinical presentation reflects more the location and size of the tumor rather than its histologic type. Many of these signs and symptoms may also result from myocarditis, pericarditis, or cardiomyopathy induced by radiotherapy or chemotherapy.

Electrocardiographic (ECG) findings are nonspecific. On chest x-ray, the cardiac silhouette is most often normal but may be enlarged or exhibit a bizarre contour. Echocardiography is useful for identifying pericardial effusions and for visualizing larger metastases, although CT and radionuclide imaging with gallium or thallium may more clearly define the tumor burden. Cardiac MRI offers superb image quality and plays a central role in the diagnostic evaluation of cardiac metastases and cardiac tumors in general. Pericardiocentesis may allow for a specific cytologic diagnosis in patients with malignant pericardial effusions. Angiography is rarely necessary but may delineate discrete lesions.

℞ TUMORS METASTATIC TO THE HEART

Most patients with cardiac metastases have advanced malignant disease; thus, therapy is generally palliative and consists of treatment of the primary tumor. Symptomatic malignant pericardial effusions should be drained by pericardiocentesis. Concomitant instillation of a sclerosing agent (e.g., tetracycline) may delay or prevent reaccumulation of the effusion, while creation of a pericardial window allows drainage of the effusion to the pleural space.

TRAUMATIC CARDIAC INJURY

Traumatic cardiac injury may be caused by either penetrating or nonpenetrating trauma. *Penetrating injuries* most often result from gunshot or knife wounds, and the site of entry is usually obvious. *Nonpenetrating injuries* most often occur during motor vehicle accidents, either from a rapid deceleration injury or from impact of the chest against the steering wheel, and may be associated with significant cardiac injury even in the absence of external signs of thoracic trauma.

Myocardial contusions are the most common form of nonpenetrating cardiac injury and may initially be overlooked in trauma patients as the clinical focus is directed toward other more obvious injuries. Myocardial necrosis may occur as a direct result of the blunt injury or as a result of traumatic coronary laceration or thrombosis. The contused myocardium is pathologically similar to infarcted myocardium and may be associated with atrial or ventricular arrhythmias, conduction disturbances including bundle branch block, or ECG abnormalities resembling those of infarction or pericarditis. Thus, it is important to consider contusion as a cause of otherwise unexplained ECG changes in a trauma patient. Serum creatine kinase (CK-MB) isoenzyme levels are increased in ~20% of patients suffering blunt chest trauma but may be falsely elevated in the presence of massive skeletal muscle injury. Cardiac troponin levels are more specific for identifying cardiac injury in this setting. Echocardiography is useful in detecting structural and functional sequelae of contusion, including wall motion abnormalities, pericardial effusion, valvular dysfunction, and ventricular rupture. Although radionuclide scanning can detect myocardial contusion, its role is limited, given the ease and availability of echocardiography.

Rupture of the cardiac valves or their supporting structures, most commonly of the tricuspid or mitral valve, leads to acute valvular incompetence. This complication is usually heralded by the development of a loud murmur, may be associated with rapidly progressive heart failure, and can be diagnosed by either transthoracic or transesophageal echocardiography.

The most serious consequence of nonpenetrating injury is myocardial rupture, which may result in hemopericardium and tamponade (free wall rupture) or intracardiac shunting (ventricular septal rupture). Although generally fatal, up to 40% of patients with cardiac rupture have been reported to survive long enough to reach a specialized trauma center. Hemopericardium may also result from traumatic rupture of a pericardial vessel or a coronary artery. Additionally, a pericardial effusion may develop weeks or even months after blunt chest trauma as a manifestation of the post-cardiac injury syndrome, which resembles the post-pericardiotomy syndrome (Chap. 232).

Blunt, nonpenetrating, often innocent-appearing injuries to the chest may trigger ventricular fibrillation even in absence of overt signs of injury. This syndrome, referred to as *commotio cordis*, occurs most often in adolescents during sporting events (e.g., baseball, hockey, football, and lacrosse) and likely results from an impact to the chest wall overlying the heart during the susceptible phase of repolarization just prior to the peak of the T wave. Survival depends on prompt defibrillation.

Sudden emotional or physiologic trauma may precipitate a transient cardiomyopathy that is characterized by dysfunction of the mid-portion and apex of the left ventricle with hyperdynamic function at the ventricular base. This syndrome, referred to as *Tako-Tsubo syndrome* or the *apical ballooning syndrome*, is more common in women and usually presents with chest pain, anterior ST-segment elevation, and mildly elevated cardiac enzymes despite the absence of significant epicardial coronary artery disease. The pathophysiology of this syndrome likely relates to catecholamine excess, and possibly to coronary vasospasm. The prognosis is favorable, and complete and spontaneous resolution of the ventricular dysfunction usually occurs within several weeks.

Rupture of the aorta, usually just above the aortic valve or at the site of the ligamentum arteriosum, is a common consequence of nonpenetrating chest trauma and is the most common vascular deceleration injury. The clinical presentation is similar to that of aortic dissection (Chap. 242). The arterial pressure and pulse amplitude may be increased in the upper extremities and decreased in the lower extremities, and chest x-ray may reveal mediastinal widening. Occasionally, aortic rupture is contained by the aortic adventitia, resulting in a false, or *pseudo-*, aneurysm that may be discovered months or years after the initial injury.

Penetrating injuries of the heart produced by knife or bullet wounds usually result in rapid clinical deterioration and frequently in death as a result of hemopericardium/pericardial tamponade or massive hemorrhage. Nonetheless, up to half of such patients may survive long enough to reach a specialized trauma center if immediate resuscitation is performed. Prognosis in these patients relates to the mechanism of injury, their clinical condition at presentation, and the specific cardiac chamber(s) involved. Iatrogenic cardiac or coronary arterial perforation may occur as a complication during placement of central venous or intracardiac catheters, pacemaker leads, or intracoronary stents and is associated with a better prognosis than other forms of penetrating cardiac trauma.

Traumatic rupture of a great vessel from penetrating injury is usually associated with hemothorax and, less often, hemopericardium. Lo-

cal hematoma formation may compress major vessels and produce ischemic symptoms, and AV fistulae may develop, occasionally resulting in high-output CHF.

Occasionally, patients who survive penetrating cardiac injuries may subsequently present with a new cardiac murmur or CHF as a result of mitral regurgitation or an intracardiac shunt (i.e., ventricular or atrial septal defect, aortopulmonary fistula, or coronary AV fistula) that was undetected at the time of their initial injury or developed subsequently. Therefore, trauma patients should be carefully examined several weeks after their injury. If a mechanical complication is suspected, it can be confirmed by echocardiography or cardiac catheterization.

Rx TRAUMATIC CARDIAC INJURY

The treatment of an uncomplicated myocardial contusion is similar to that for a myocardial infarction, except that anticoagulation is contraindicated, and should include monitoring for the development of arrhythmias and mechanical complications such as cardiac rupture (Chap. 239). Acute myocardial failure resulting from traumatic valve rupture usually requires urgent operative correction. Immediate thoracotomy should be carried out for most cases of penetrating injury or if there is evidence of cardiac tamponade and/or shock regardless of the type of trauma. Pericardiocentesis may be lifesaving in patients with tamponade but is usually only a temporizing maneuver while they await definitive surgical therapy. Pericardial hemorrhage often leads to constriction (Chap. 232), which must be treated by decortication.

FURTHER READINGS

MATTOX KL: Traumatic heart disease, in *Braunwald's Heart Disease*, 7th ed, DP Zipes et al (eds). Philadelphia, Saunders, 2005

PRETRE R, CHILCOTT M: Blunt trauma to the heart and great vessels. N Engl J Med 336:626, 1997

REYMAN K: Cardiac myxomas. N Engl J Med 333:1610, 1995

RHEE PM et al: Penetrating cardiac injuries: A population-based study. J Trauma 45:366, 1998

SABATINE M, SCHOEN F: Primary tumors of the heart, in *Braunwald's Heart Disease*, 7th ed, DP Zipes et al (eds). Philadelphia, Saunders, 2005

SIMMERS TA et al: Traumatic papillary muscle rupture. Ann Thorac Surg 72:257, 2001

SYBRANDY KC et al: Diagnosing cardiac contusion: Old wisdom and new insights. Heart 89:485, 2003

TYBURSKI JG et al: Factors affecting prognosis with penetrating wounds of the heart. J Trauma 48:587, 2000

VAUGHAN CJ et al: Tumors and the heart: Molecular genetic advances. Curr Opin Cardiol 16:195, 2001

234 Cardiac Manifestations of Systemic Disease
Eric H. Awtry, Wilson S. Colucci

The common systemic disorders that have associated cardiac manifestations are summarized in Table 234-1.

DIABETES MELLITUS
(See also Chap. 338) Diabetes mellitus, both insulin- and non-insulin-dependent, is an independent risk factor for coronary artery disease (CAD; Chap. 235), accounting for 14–50% of new cases of cardiovascular disease. Furthermore, CAD is the most common cause of death in adults with diabetes mellitus. In the diabetic population the incidence of CAD relates to the duration of diabetes and the level of glycemic control, and its pathogenesis involves endothelial dysfunction,

increased lipoprotein peroxidation, increased inflammation, a prothrombotic state, and associated metabolic abnormalities.

Diabetic patients are more likely to suffer a myocardial infarction, have a greater burden of CAD, have larger infarct size, and suffer more postinfarct complications, including heart failure, shock, and death, than nondiabetics. Importantly, diabetic patients are more likely to have atypical ischemic symptoms; nausea, dyspnea, pulmonary edema, arrhythmias, heart block, or syncope may be their anginal equivalent. Additionally, "silent ischemia," resulting from autonomic nervous system dysfunction, is more common in diabetics, accounting for up to 90% of their ischemic episodes. Thus, one must have a low threshold for suspecting CAD in diabetic patients. The treatment of diabetics with CAD must include aggressive risk factor management (Chap. 338). Pharmacologic therapy and revascularization are similar in diabetics and nondiabetics, excepting that diabetics have greater morbidity and mortality associated with revascularization, have an increased risk of restenosis after percutaneous coronary intervention (PCI), and likely have improved survival when treated with surgical bypass compared with PCI for multivessel CAD.

TABLE 234-1 COMMON SYSTEMIC DISORDERS AND THEIR ASSOCIATED CARDIAC MANIFESTATIONS

Systemic Disorder	Common Cardiac Manifestations	Chapter
Diabetes mellitus	CAD, atypical angina, CMP, systolic or diastolic CHF	338
Protein-calorie malnutrition	Dilated CMP, CHF	72
Thiamine deficiency	High-output failure, dilated CMP	71
Hyperhomocysteinemia	Premature atherosclerosis	71
Obesity	CMP, systolic or diastolic CHF	74
Hyperthyroidism	Palpitations, SVT, atrial fibrillation, hypertension	335
Hypothyroidism	Hypotension, bradycardia, dilated CMP, CHF, pericardial effusion	335
Malignant carcinoid	Tricuspid and pulmonary valve disease, right heart failure	344
Pheochromocytoma	Hypertension, palpitations, CHF	337
Acromegaly	Systolic or diastolic heart failure	333
Rheumatoid arthritis	Pericarditis, pericardial effusions, coronary arteritis, myocarditis, valvulitis	314
Seronegative arthropathies	Aortitis, aortic and mitral insufficiency, conduction abnormalities	318
Systemic lupus erythematosus	Pericarditis, Libman-Sacks endocarditis, myocarditis, arterial and venous thrombosis	313
HIV	Myocarditis, dilated CMP, pericardial effusion	182
Amyloidosis	CHF, restrictive CMP, valvular regurgitation, pericardial effusion	324
Sarcoidosis	CHF, dilated or restrictive CMP, ventricular arrhythmias, heart block	322
Hemochromatosis	CHF, arrhythmias, heart block	351
Marfan syndrome	Aortic aneurysm and dissection, aortic insufficiency, mitral valve prolapse	357
Ehlers-Danlos syndrome	Aortic and coronary aneurysms, mitral and tricuspid valve prolapse	357

Note: CAD, coronary artery disease; CHF, congestive heart failure; CMP, cardiomyopathy; SVT, supraventricular tachycardia.

Patients with diabetes mellitus may also have abnormal left ventricular systolic and diastolic function, reflecting concomitant epicardial CAD and hypertension, coronary microvascular disease, endothelial dysfunction, ventricular hypertrophy, and autonomic dysfunction. A restrictive cardiomyopathy may be present with abnormal myocardial relaxation and elevated ventricular filling pressures. Histologically, interstitial fibrosis is seen, and intramural arteries may demonstrate intimal thickening, hyaline deposition, and inflammatory changes. Diabetic patients have an increased risk of developing clinical heart failure, which likely contributes to their excessive cardiovascular morbidity and mortality. There is some evidence that insulin therapy may ameliorate diabetes-related myocardial dysfunction.

MALNUTRITION AND VITAMIN DEFICIENCY

Malnutrition (See also Chap. 72) In patients whose intake of protein, calories, or both is severely deficient, the heart may become thin, pale, and hypokinetic with myofibrillar atrophy and interstitial edema. The systolic pressure and cardiac output fall, and the pulse pressure narrows. Generalized edema is common and relates to a variety of factors, including reduced serum oncotic pressure and myocardial dysfunction. Such profound states of protein and calorie malnutrition, termed *kwashiorkor* and *marasmus*, respectively, are most common in underdeveloped countries. However, significant nutritional heart disease may also occur in developed nations, particularly in patients with chronic diseases such as AIDS, in patients with anorexia nervosa, and in patients with severe cardiac failure in whom gastrointestinal hypoperfusion and venous congestion may lead to anorexia and malabsorption. Open-heart surgery poses increased risk in malnourished patients, and they may benefit from preoperative hyperalimentation.

Thiamine Deficiency (Beriberi) (See also Chap. 71) Generalized malnutrition is often accompanied by thiamine deficiency, although this hypovitaminosis may also occur in the presence of an adequate protein and caloric intake, particularly in the Far East where polished rice deficient in thiamine may be a major dietary component. In Western nations where the use of thiamine-enriched flour is widespread, clinical thiamine deficiency is limited primarily to alcoholics, food faddists, and patients receiving chemotherapy. Nonetheless, when thiamine stores are measured using the thiamine-pyrophosphate effect (TPPE), thiamine deficiency has been found in 20–90% of patients with chronic heart failure. This deficiency appears to result from both reduced dietary intake and a diuretic-induced increase in the urinary excretion of thiamine. The acute administration of thiamine to these patients increases the left ventricular ejection fraction and the excretion of salt and water.

Clinically, patients with thiamine deficiency usually have evidence of generalized malnutrition, peripheral neuropathy, glossitis, and anemia. The classic cardiovascular syndrome is characterized by high-output heart failure, tachycardia, and often elevated left and right ventricular filling pressures. The major cause of the high-output state is vasomotor depression leading to reduced systemic vascular resistance, the precise mechanism of which is not understood. The cardiac examination reveals a wide pulse pressure, tachycardia, a third heart sound, and, frequently, an apical systolic murmur. The ECG may reveal decreased voltage, a prolonged QT interval, and T-wave abnormalities. The chest x-ray generally reveals cardiomegaly and signs of congestive heart failure (CHF). The response to thiamine is often dramatic, with an increase in systemic vascular resistance, a decrease in cardiac output, clearing of pulmonary congestion, and a reduction in heart size often occurring in 12–48 h. Although the response to inotropes and diuretics may be poor before thiamine therapy, these agents may be important *after* thiamine is given, since the left ventricle may not be able to handle the increased work load presented by the return of vascular tone.

Vitamin B₆, B₁₂, and Folate Deficiency (See also Chap. 71) Vitamin B_6, B_{12}, and folate are cofactors in the metabolism of homocysteine. Their deficiency probably contributes to the majority of cases of hyperhomocysteinemia, a disorder associated with increased atherosclerotic risk. Supplementation of these vitamins has reduced the incidence of hyperhomocysteinemia in the United States; however, the clinical cardiovascular benefit of normalizing elevated homocysteine levels remains unproven.

OBESITY

(See also Chap. 74) Severe obesity, especially abdominal obesity, is associated with an increase in cardiovascular morbidity and mortality. Although obesity itself is not considered a disease, it is associated with an increased prevalence of hypertension, glucose intolerance, and atherosclerotic CAD. In addition, obese patients have a distinct cardiovascular abnormality characterized by increased total and central blood volumes, cardiac output, and left ventricular filling pressure. The elevated cardiac output appears to be required to support the metabolic needs of the excess adipose tissue. Left ventricular filling pressure is often at the upper limits of normal at rest and rises excessively with exercise. As a result of chronic volume overload, eccentric cardiac hypertrophy with cardiac dilatation and ventricular dysfunction may develop. Pathologically, there are left and, in some cases, right ventricular hypertrophy and generalized cardiac dilatation. Pulmonary congestion, peripheral edema, and exercise intolerance may all ensue; however, the recognition of these findings may be difficult in massively obese patients.

Weight reduction is the most effective therapy and results in reduction in blood volume and in the return of cardiac output toward normal. However, rapid weight reduction may be dangerous, as cardiac arrhythmias and sudden death owing to electrolyte imbalance have been described. Treatment with angiotensin-converting enzyme inhibitors, sodium restriction, and diuretics may be useful to control heart failure symptoms. This form of heart disease should be distinguished from the Pickwickian syndrome (Chap. 258), which may share several of the cardiovascular features of heart disease secondary to severe obesity but, in addition, frequently has components of central apnea, hypoxemia, pulmonary hypertension, and cor pulmonale.

THYROID DISEASE

(See also Chap. 335) Thyroid hormone exerts a major influence on the cardiovascular system by a number of direct and indirect mechanisms and, not surprisingly, cardiovascular effects are prominent in both hypo- and hyperthyroidism. Thyroid hormone causes increases in total-body metabolism and oxygen consumption that indirectly increase the cardiac workload. In addition, thyroid hormone exerts direct inotropic, chronotropic, and dromotropic effects that are similar to those seen with adrenergic stimulation (e.g., tachycardia, increased cardiac output); they are mediated at least partly by both transcriptional and non-transcriptional effects of thyroid hormone on myosin, calcium-activated ATPase, Na$^+$,K$^+$-ATPase, and myocardial β-adrenergic receptors.

Hyperthyroidism Common cardiovascular manifestations of hyperthyroidism include palpitations, systolic hypertension, and fatigue. Sinus tachycardia is present in ~40% of patients and atrial fibrillation in ~15%. Physical examination may reveal a hyperdynamic precordium, a widened pulse pressure, increases in the intensity of the first heart sound and the pulmonic component of the second heart sound, and a third heart sound. An increased incidence of mitral valve prolapse has been described in hyperthyroid patients, in which case a midsystolic murmur may be heard at the left sternal border with or without a systolic ejection click. A systolic pleuropericardial friction rub (*Means-Lerman scratch*) may be heard at the left second intercostal space during expiration and is thought to result from the hyperdynamic cardiac motion.

Elderly patients with hyperthyroidism may present with only cardiovascular manifestations of thyrotoxicosis, such as sinus tachycardia, atrial fibrillation, and hypertension, all of which may be resistant to therapy until the hyperthyroidism is controlled. Angina pectoris and CHF are unusual with hyperthyroidism unless there is coexistent heart disease; in such cases, symptoms often resolve with treatment of the hyperthyroidism.

Hypothyroidism Cardiac manifestations of hypothyroidism include a reduction in cardiac output, stroke volume, heart rate, blood pressure, and pulse pressure. Pericardial effusions are present in about one-third of patients, rarely progress to tamponade, and likely result from increased capillary permeability. Other clinical signs include cardiomegaly, bradycardia, weak arterial pulses, distant heart sounds, and pleural effusions. Although the signs and symptoms of myxedema may mimic those of CHF, in the absence of other cardiac disease, myocardial failure is uncommon. The electrocardiogram (ECG) generally reveals sinus bradycardia and low voltage, and may show prolongation of the QT interval, decreased P-wave voltage, prolonged AV conduction time, intraventricular conduction disturbances, and nonspecific ST-T wave abnormalities. Chest x-ray may show cardiomegaly, often with a "water bottle" configuration, pleural effusions, and, in some cases, evidence of CHF. Pathologically, the heart is pale and dilated, and often demonstrates myofibrillar swelling, loss of striations, and interstitial fibrosis.

Patients with hypothyroidism frequently have elevations of cholesterol and triglycerides, resulting in premature atherosclerotic CAD. Before treatment with thyroid hormone, patients with hypothyroidism frequently do not have angina pectoris, presumably because of the low metabolic demands caused by their condition. However, angina and myocardial infarction may be precipitated during initiation of thyroid hormone replacement, especially in elderly patients with underlying heart disease. Therefore, replacement should be done with care, starting with low doses that are increased gradually.

MALIGNANT CARCINOID

(See also Chap. 344) Carcinoid tumors most often originate in the small bowel and elaborate a variety of vasoactive amines (e.g., serotonin), kinins, indoles, and prostaglandins that are believed to be responsible for the diarrhea, flushing, and labile blood pressure that characterize the carcinoid syndrome. Some 50% of patients with carcinoid syndrome have cardiac involvement, usually manifesting as abnormalities of the right-sided cardiac structures. These patients invariably have hepatic metastases allowing vasoactive substances to circumvent hepatic metabolism. Left-sided cardiac involvement is rare and indicates either pulmonary carcinoid or an intracardiac shunt. Pathologically, carcinoid lesions are fibrous plaques that consist of smooth-muscle cells embedded in a stroma of glycosaminoglycans and collagen. They occur on the cardiac valves where they cause valvular dysfunction, as well as on the endothelium of the cardiac chambers and great vessels.

Carcinoid heart disease most often presents as tricuspid regurgitation, pulmonic stenosis, or both. In some cases a high cardiac output state may occur, presumably as a result of a decrease in systemic vascular resistance resulting from vasoactive substances released by the tumor. Treatment with somatostatin analogues (e.g., octreotide) or interferon-α improves symptoms and survival in patients with carcinoid heart disease but does not appear to improve valvular abnormalities. In some severely symptomatic patients, valve replacement is indicated. Coronary artery spasm, presumably due to a circulating vasoactive substance, may occur in patients with carcinoid syndrome.

PHEOCHROMOCYTOMA

(See also Chap. 337) In addition to causing labile or sustained hypertension, the high circulating levels of catecholamines resulting from a pheochromocytoma may also cause direct myocardial injury. Focal myocardial necrosis and inflammatory cell infiltration are present in ~50% of patients who die with pheochromocytoma and may contribute to clinically significant left ventricular failure and pulmonary edema. In addition, associated hypertension results in left ventricular hypertrophy. Left ventricular dysfunction and CHF may resolve after removal of the tumor.

ACROMEGALY

(See also Chap. 333) Exposure of the heart to excessive growth hormone may cause CHF as a result of high cardiac output, diastolic dysfunction owing to ventricular hypertrophy (with increased left ventricular chamber size or wall thickness), or global systolic dysfunction. Hypertension occurs in up to one-third of patients with acromegaly and is characterized by suppression of the renin-angiotensin-aldosterone axis and increases in total-body sodium and plasma volume. Some form of cardiac disease occurs in about one-third of patients with acromegaly and is associated with a doubling of the risk of cardiac death.

RHEUMATOID ARTHRITIS AND THE COLLAGEN VASCULAR DISEASES

Rheumatoid Arthritis (See also Chap. 314) Rheumatoid arthritis may be associated with inflammatory changes in any or all cardiac structures, although pericarditis is the most common clinical entity. Pericardial effusions may be found echocardiographically in 10–50% of patients with rheumatoid arthritis, particularly those with subcutaneous nodules. Nonetheless, only a small fraction of these patients have symptomatic pericarditis and, when present, it usually follows a benign course, only occasionally progressing to cardiac tamponade or constrictive pericarditis. The pericardial fluid is generally exudative, with decreased concentrations of complement and glucose and elevated cholesterol. Coronary arteritis with intimal inflammation and edema is present in ~20% of cases but only rarely results in angina pectoris or myocardial infarction. Inflammation and granuloma formation may affect the cardiac valves, most often the mitral and aortic, and may cause clinically significant regurgitation owing to valve deformity. Myocarditis is uncommon and rarely results in cardiac dysfunction.

Treatment is directed at the underlying rheumatoid arthritis and may include glucocorticoids. Urgent pericardiocentesis should be performed in patients with tamponade, while pericardiectomy is usually required in cases of pericardial constriction.

Seronegative Arthropathies (See also Chap. 318) The seronegative arthropathies, including ankylosing spondylitis, reactive arthritis, psoriatic arthritis, and the arthritides associated with ulcerative colitis and regional enteritis, are all strongly associated with the HLA-B27 histocompatibility antigen and may be accompanied by a pancarditis and proximal aortitis. The aortic inflammation is usually limited to the aortic root but may extend to involve the aortic valve, mitral valve, and ventricular myocardium, resulting in aortic and mitral regurgitation, conduction abnormalities, and ventricular dysfunction. One-tenth of patients have significant aortic insufficiency and one-third have conduction disturbances; both are more common in patients with peripheral joint involvement and long-standing disease. Treatment with aortic valve replacement and permanent pacemaker placement may be required. Occasionally, aortic regurgitation precedes the onset of arthritis, and, therefore, the diagnosis of a seronegative arthritis should be considered in young males with isolated aortic regurgitation.

Systemic Lupus Erythematosus (SLE)   (See also Chap. 313) A significant percentage of patients with SLE have cardiac involvement. Pericarditis is common, occurring in about two-thirds of patients, and generally follows a benign course, although rarely tamponade or constriction may result. The characteristic endocardial lesions of SLE are verrucous valvular abnormalities, known as *Libman Sacks endocarditis*. They are most often located on the left-sided cardiac valves, particularly on the ventricular surface of the posterior mitral leaflet, and are made up almost entirely of fibrin. These lesions may embolize or become infected but rarely cause hemodynamically important valvular regurgitation. Myocarditis generally parallels the activity of the disease

and, although common histologically, seldom results in clinical heart failure unless associated with hypertension. While arteritis of epicardial coronary arteries may occur, it rarely results in myocardial ischemia. There is, however, an increased incidence of coronary atherosclerosis that likely is related more to associated risk factors and glucocorticoid use than to SLE itself. Patients with the antiphospholipid antibody syndrome may have a higher incidence of cardiovascular abnormalities, including valvular regurgitation, venous and arterial thrombosis, premature stroke, myocardial infarction, pulmonary hypertension, and cardiomyopathy.

FURTHER READINGS

BRUCE IN: "Not only…but also": Factors that contribute to accelerated atherosclerosis and premature coronary artery disease in systemic lupus erythematosus. Rheumatology 44:1492, 2005

FOX DJ, KHATTAR RS: Carcinoid heart disease: Presentation, diagnosis, and management. Heart 90:1224, 2004

GRUNDY SM et al: Prevention Conference VI: Diabetes and cardiovascular disease, executive summary. Circulation 105:2231, 2002

HOFFMAN GS: Rheumatic diseases and the heart, in *Braunwald's Heart Disease*, 7th ed, DP Zipes et al (eds). Philadelphia, Saunders, 2005

KENCHAIAH S et al: Obesity and the risk of heart failure. N Engl J Med 347:305, 2002

KLEIN I, OJAMAA K: Thyroid hormone and the cardiovascular system. N Engl J Med 344:501, 2001

SECTION 5   VASCULAR DISEASE

235   The Pathogenesis, Prevention, and Treatment of Atherosclerosis
Peter Libby

PATHOGENESIS

Atherosclerosis remains the major cause of death and premature disability in developed societies. Moreover, current predictions estimate that by the year 2020 cardiovascular diseases, notably atherosclerosis, will become the leading global cause of total disease burden. Although many generalized or systemic risk factors predispose to its development, atherosclerosis affects various regions of the circulation preferentially and yields distinct clinical manifestations depending on the particular circulatory bed affected. Atherosclerosis of the coronary arteries commonly causes myocardial infarction (Chap. 239) and angina pectoris (Chap. 237). Atherosclerosis of the arteries supplying the central nervous system frequently provokes strokes and transient cerebral ischemia (Chap. 364). In the peripheral circulation, atherosclerosis causes intermittent claudication and gangrene and can jeopardize limb viability. Involvement of the splanchnic circulation can cause mesenteric ischemia. Atherosclerosis can affect the kidneys either directly (e.g., renal artery stenosis) or as a frequent site of atheroembolic disease (Chap. 242).

Even within a given arterial bed, stenoses due to atherosclerosis tend to occur focally, typically in certain predisposed regions. In the coronary circulation, for example, the proximal left anterior descending coronary artery exhibits a particular predilection for developing atherosclerotic disease. Likewise, atherosclerosis preferentially affects the proximal portions of the renal arteries and, in the extracranial circulation to the brain, the carotid bifurcation. Indeed, atherosclerotic lesions often form at branching points of arteries, regions of disturbed

blood flow. Not all manifestations of atherosclerosis result from stenotic, occlusive disease. Ectasia and development of aneurysmal disease, for example, frequently occur in the aorta (Chap. 242). In addition to focal, flow-limiting stenoses, nonocclusive intimal atherosclerosis also occurs diffusely in affected arteries, as shown by intravascular ultrasound and postmortem studies.

Atherogenesis in humans typically occurs over a period of many years, usually many decades. Growth of atherosclerotic plaques probably does not occur in a smooth, linear fashion, but rather discontinuously, with periods of relative quiescence punctuated by periods of rapid evolution. After a generally prolonged "silent" period, atherosclerosis may become clinically manifest. The clinical expressions of atherosclerosis may be *chronic*, as in the development of stable, effort-induced angina pectoris or of predictable and reproducible intermittent claudication. Alternatively, a dramatic *acute* clinical event, such as myocardial infarction, a stroke, or sudden cardiac death, may first herald the presence of atherosclerosis. Other individuals may never experience clinical manifestations of arterial disease despite the presence of widespread atherosclerosis demonstrated post-mortem.

INITIATION OF ATHEROSCLEROSIS

An integrated view of experimental results in animals and studies of human atherosclerosis suggests that the "fatty streak" represents the initial lesion of atherosclerosis. These early lesions most often seem to arise from focal increases in the content of lipoproteins within regions of the intima. This accumulation of lipoprotein particles may not result simply from an increased permeability, or "leakiness," of the overlying endothelium (Fig. 235-1). Rather, these lipoproteins may collect in the intima of arteries because they bind to constituents of the extracellular matrix, increasing the residence time of the lipid-rich particles within the arterial wall. Lipoproteins that accumulate in the extracellular space of the intima of arteries often associate with glycosaminoglycans of the arterial extracellular matrix, an interaction that may slow the egress of these lipid-rich particles from the intima. Lipoprotein particles in the

FIGURE 235-1 Cross-sectional view of an artery depicting steps in development of an atheroma, from left to right. The *upper panel* shows a detail of the boxed area below. The endothelial monolayer overlying the intima contacts blood. Hypercholesterolemia promotes accumulation of LDL particles (light spheres) in the intima. The lipoprotein particles often associate with constituents of the extracellular matrix, notably proteoglycans. Sequestration within the intima separates lipoproteins from some plasma antioxidants and favors oxidative modification. Such modified lipoprotein particles (darker spheres) may trigger a local inflammatory response responsible for signaling subsequent steps in lesion formation. The augmented expression of various adhesion molecules for leukocytes recruits monocytes to the site of a nascent arterial lesion.

Once adherent, some white blood cells will migrate into the intima. The directed migration of leukocytes probably depends on chemoattractant factors including modified lipoprotein particles themselves and chemoattractant cytokines depicted by the smaller spheres, such as the chemokine macrophage chemoattractant protein-1 produced by vascular wall cells in response to modified lipoproteins. Leukocytes in the evolving fatty streak can divide and exhibit augmented expression of receptors for modified lipoproteins (scavenger receptors). These mononuclear phagocytes ingest lipids and become foam cells, represented by a cytoplasm filled with lipid droplets. As the fatty streak evolves into a more complicated atherosclerotic lesion, smooth-muscle cells migrate from the media (*bottom of lower panel*), through the internal elastic membrane (*solid wavy line*), and accumulate within the expanding intima where they lay down extracellular matrix that forms the bulk of the advanced lesion (*bottom panel, right-hand side*).

extracellular space of the intima, particularly those retained by binding to matrix macromolecules, may undergo oxidative modifications. Considerable evidence supports a pathogenic role for products of oxidized lipoproteins in atherogenesis. Lipoproteins sequestered from plasma antioxidants in the extracellular space of the intima become particularly susceptible to oxidative modification, giving rise to hydroperoxides, lysophospholipids, oxysterols, and aldehydic breakdown products of fatty acids and phospholipids. Modifications of the apoprotein moieties may include breaks in the peptide backbone as well as derivatization of certain amino acid residues. Local production of hypochlorous acid by myeloperoxidase associated with inflammatory cells within the plaque yields chlorinated species such as chlorotyrosyl moieties. Considerable evidence supports the presence of such oxidation products in atherosclerotic lesions.

Leukocyte Recruitment Accumulation of leukocytes characterizes the formation of early atherosclerotic lesions (Fig. 235-1). Thus, from its very inception, atherogenesis involves elements of inflammation, a process that now provides a unifying theme in the pathogenesis of this disease. The inflammatory cell types typically found in the evolving atheroma include monocyte-derived macrophages and lymphocytes. A number of adhesion molecules or receptors for leukocytes expressed on the surface of the arterial endothelial cell likely participate in the recruitment of leukocytes to the nascent atheroma. Constituents of oxidatively modified low-density lipoprotein (LDL) can augment expression of leukocyte adhesion molecules. This example illustrates how the accumulation of lipoproteins in the arterial intima may link mechanistically with leukocyte recruitment, a key event in lesion formation.

Laminar shear forces such as those encountered in most regions of normal arteries can also suppress the expression of leukocyte adhesion molecules. Sites of predilection for atherosclerotic lesions (e.g., branch points) often have disturbed laminar flow. Ordered, pulsatile laminar shear of normal blood flow augments the production of nitric oxide by endothelial cells. This molecule, in addition to its vasodilator properties, can act at the low levels constitutively produced by arterial endothelium as a local anti-inflammatory autacoid, e.g., limiting local adhesion molecule expression. Exposure of endothelial cells to laminar shear stress increases the transcription of Kruppel-like factor 2 (KLF2) and reduces the expression of a thioredoxin-interacting protein (Txnip) that inhibits the activity of thioredoxin. KLF2 augments the activity of endothelial nitric oxide synthase, and reduced Txnip levels boost the function of the endogenous antioxidant thioredoxin. Laminar shear stress also stimulates endothelial cells to produce superoxide dismutase, an antioxidant enzyme. These examples indicate how hemodynamic forces may influence the cellular events that underlie atherosclerotic lesion initiation and provide a potential explanation for the favored localization of atherosclerotic lesions at sites that experience disturbance to laminar shear stress.

Once captured on the surface of the arterial endothelial cell by adhesion receptors, the monocytes and lymphocytes penetrate the endothelial layer and take up residence in the intima. In addition to products of modified lipoproteins, cytokines (protein mediators of inflammation) can regulate the expression of adhesion molecules involved in leukocyte recruitment. For example, interleukin 1 (IL-1) or tumor necrosis factor α (TNF-α) induces or augments the expression of leukocyte adhesion molecules on endothelial cells. Because products of lipoprotein oxidation can induce cytokine release from vascular wall cells, this pathway may provide an additional link between arterial accumulation of lipoproteins and leukocyte recruitment. Chemoattractant cytokines such as monocyte chemoattractant protein 1 appear to direct the migration of leukocytes into the arterial wall.

Foam Cell Formation Once resident within the intima, the mononuclear phagocytes mature into macrophages and become lipid-laden foam cells, a conversion that requires the uptake of lipoprotein particles by receptor-mediated endocytosis. One might suppose that the well-recognized "classical" receptor for LDL mediates this lipid uptake; however, patients or animals lacking effective LDL receptors due to genetic alterations (e.g., familial hypercholesterolemia) have abundant arterial lesions and extraarterial xanthomata rich in macrophage-derived foam cells. In addition, the exogenous cholesterol suppresses expression of the LDL receptor; thus, the level of this cell-surface receptor for LDL decreases under conditions of cholesterol excess. Candidates for alternative receptors that can mediate lipid-loading of foam cells include a growing number of macrophage "scavenger" receptors, which preferentially endocytose modified lipoproteins, and other receptors for oxidized LDL or beta very low density lipoprotein (β-VLDL). Monocyte attachment to the endothelium, migration into the intima, and maturation to form lipid-laden macrophages thus represent key steps in the formation of the fatty streak, the precursor of fully formed atherosclerotic plaques.

ATHEROMA EVOLUTION AND COMPLICATIONS

Although the fatty streak commonly precedes the development of a more advanced atherosclerotic plaque, not all fatty streaks progress to form complex atheromata. By ingesting lipids from the extracellular space, the mononuclear phagocytes bearing such scavenger receptors may remove lipoproteins from the developing lesion. Some lipid-laden macrophages may leave the artery wall, exporting lipid in the process. Lipid accumulation, and hence propensity to form atheroma, ensues if the amount of lipid entering the artery wall exceeds that removed by mononuclear phagocytes or other pathways.

Export by phagocytes may constitute one response to local lipid overload in the evolving lesion. Another mechanism, reverse cholesterol transport mediated by high-density lipoproteins (HDL), probably provides an independent pathway for lipid removal from atheroma. This transfer of cholesterol from the cell to the HDL particle involves specialized cell surface molecules such as the ATP binding cassette (ABC) transporters. *ABCA1*, the gene mutated in Tangier disease, a condition characterized by very low HDL levels, transfers cholesterol from cells to nascent HDL particles and ABCG1 to mature HDL particles. "Reverse cholesterol transport" mediated by these ABC transporters allows HDL loaded with cholesterol to deliver it to hepatocytes by binding to scavenger receptor B 1 or other receptors. The liver cell can metabolize the sterol to bile acids that can be excreted. This export pathway from macrophage foam cells to peripheral cells such as hepatocytes explains part of HDL's antiatherogenic action. (Anti-inflammatory and antioxidant properties may also contribute to HDL's atheroprotective effects.) Thus, macrophages may play a vital role in the dynamic economy of lipid accumulation in the arterial wall during atherogenesis.

Some lipid-laden foam cells within the expanding intimal lesion perish. Some foam cells may die as a result of programmed cell death, or *apoptosis*. This death of mononuclear phagocytes results in formation of the lipid-rich center, often called the *necrotic core*, in established atherosclerotic plaques. Macrophages loaded with modified lipoproteins may elaborate cytokines and growth factors that can further signal some of the cellular events in lesion complication. While accumulation of lipid-laden macrophages characterizes the fatty streak, build-up of fibrous tissue formed by extracellular matrix typifies the more advanced atherosclerotic lesion. The smooth-muscle cell synthesizes the bulk of the extracellular matrix of the complex atherosclerotic lesion. A number of growth factors or cytokines elaborated by mononuclear phagocytes can stimulate smooth-muscle cell proliferation and production of extracellular matrix. Cytokines found in the plaque, including IL-1 or TNF-α, can induce local production of growth factors, including forms of platelet-derived growth factor (PDGF), fibroblast growth factors, and others, that may contribute to plaque evolution and complication. Other cytokines, notably interferon γ (IFN-γ) derived from activated T cells within lesions, can limit the synthesis of interstitial forms of collagen by smooth-muscle cells. These examples illustrate how atherogenesis involves a complex mix of mediators that in the balance determines the characteristics of particular lesions.

The arrival of smooth-muscle cells and their elaboration of extracellular matrix probably provides a critical transition, yielding a fibrofatty lesion in place of a simple accumulation of macrophage-derived foam cells. For example, PDGF elaborated by activated platelets, macrophages, and endothelial cells can stimulate the migration of smooth-muscle cells normally resident in the tunica media into the intima. Such growth factors and cytokines produced locally can stimulate the proliferation of resident smooth-muscle cells in the intima as well as those that have migrated from the media. Transforming growth factor β (TGF-β), among other mediators, potently stimulates interstitial collagen production by smooth-muscle cells.

These mediators may arise not only from neighboring vascular cells or leukocytes (a "paracrine" pathway) but also, in some instances, from the same cell that responds to the factor (an "autocrine" pathway). Together, these alterations in smooth-muscle cells, signaled by these mediators acting at short distances, can hasten transformation of the fatty streak into a more fibrous smooth-muscle cell and extracellular matrix-rich lesion.

In addition to locally produced mediators, products of blood coagulation and thrombosis likely contribute to atheroma evolution and complication. This involvement justifies the use of the term *atherothrombosis* to convey the inextricable links between atherosclerosis and thrombosis. Fatty streak formation begins beneath a morphologically intact endothelium. In advanced fatty streaks, however, microscopic breaches in endothelial integrity may occur. Microthrombi rich in platelets can form at such sites of limited endothelial denudation owing to exposure of the thrombogenic extracellular matrix of the underlying basement membrane. Activated platelets release numerous factors that can promote the fibrotic response, including PDGF and TGF-β. Thrombin itself generates fibrin, not only during coagulation but also through protease-activated receptors that can signal smooth-muscle migration, proliferation, and extracellular matrix production. Many arterial mural microthrombi resolve without clinical manifestation by a process of local fibrinolysis, resorption, and endothelial repair, yet can lead to lesion progression by stimulating these pro-fibrotic functions of smooth-muscle cells (Fig. 235-2D).

Microvessels As atherosclerotic lesions advance, abundant plexuses of microvessels develop in connection with the artery's vasa vasorum. Newly developing microvascular networks may contribute to lesion complications in several ways. These blood vessels provide an abundant surface area for leukocyte trafficking and may serve as the portal of entry and exit of white blood cells from the established atheroma. Microvessels in the plaques may also furnish foci for intraplaque hemorrhage. Like the neovessels in the diabetic retina, microvessels in the atheroma may be friable and prone to rupture and can produce focal hemorrhage. Such a vascular leak leads to thrombosis in situ and thrombin generation from prothrombin. In addition to its role in blood coagulation, thrombin can modulate many aspects of vascular cell function, as described above. Atherosclerotic plaques often contain fibrin and hemosiderin, an indication that episodes of intraplaque hemorrhage contribute to plaque complications.

CALCIFICATION As they advance, atherosclerotic plaques also accumulate *calcium*. Proteins usually found in bone also localize in atherosclerotic lesions, e.g., osteocalcin, osteopontin, and bone morphogenetic proteins. Mineralization of the atherosclerotic plaque recapitulates many aspects of bone formation.

Plaque Evolution Although atherosclerosis research has focused much attention on proliferation of smooth-muscle cells, as in the case of macrophages, smooth-muscle cells can also undergo apoptosis in the atherosclerotic plaque. Indeed, complex atheromata often have a mostly fibrous character and lack the hypercellularity of less advanced lesions. This relative paucity of smooth-muscle cells in advanced atheromata may result from the predominance of cytostatic mediators such as TGF-β or IFN-γ (which can inhibit smooth-muscle cell proliferation) and also from smooth-muscle cell apoptosis. Some of the same pro-inflammatory cytokines that activate atherogenic functions of vascular wall cells can also sensitize these cells to undergo apoptosis.

Thus, during the evolution of the atherosclerotic plaque, a complex balance between entry and egress of lipoproteins and leukocytes, cell proliferation and cell death, extracellular matrix production and remodeling as well as calcification and neovascularization contribute to lesion formation. Multiple and often competing signals regulate these various cellular events. Increasingly, we appreciate links between atherogenic risk factors, inflammation, and the altered behavior of intrinsic vascular wall cells and infiltrating leukocytes that underlie the complex pathogenesis of these lesions.

FIGURE 235-2 Plaque rupture, thrombosis, and healing. A. Arterial remodeling during atherogenesis. During the initial part of the life history of an atheroma, growth is often outward, preserving the caliber of lumen. This phenomenon of "compensatory enlargement" accounts in part for the tendency of coronary arteriography to underestimate the degree of atherosclerosis. **B.** Rupture of the plaque's fibrous cap causes thrombosis. Physical disruption of the atherosclerotic plaque commonly causes arterial thrombosis by allowing blood coagulant factors to contact thrombogenic collagen found in the arterial extracellular matrix and tissue factor produced by macrophage-derived foam cells in the lipid core of lesions. In this manner, sites of plaque rupture form the nidus for thrombi. The normal artery wall possesses several fibrinolytic or antithrombotic mechanisms that tend to resist thrombosis and lyse clots that begin to form in situ. Such antithrombotic or thrombolytic molecules include thrombomodulin, tissue and urokinase-type plasminogen activators, heparan sulfate proteoglycans, prostacyclin, and nitric oxide. **C.** When the clot overwhelms the endogenous fibrinolytic mechanisms, it may propagate and lead to arterial occlusion. The consequences of this occlusion depend on the degree of existing collateral vessels. In a patient with chronic multivessel, occlusive coronary artery disease, collateral channels have often formed. In such circumstances, even a total arterial occlusion may not lead to myocardial infarction, or it may produce an unexpectedly modest or a non-ST-segment elevation infarct because of collateral flow. In the patient with less advanced disease and without substantial stenotic lesions to provide a stimulus to collateral vessel formation, sudden plaque rupture and arterial occlusion commonly produces ST-segment elevation infarction. These are the types of patients who may present with myocardial infarction or sudden death as a first manifestation of coronary atherosclerosis. In some cases, the thrombus may lyse or organize into a mural thrombus without occluding the vessel. Such instances may be clinically silent. **D.** The subsequent thrombin-induced fibrosis and healing causes a fibroproliferative response that can lead to a more fibrous lesion, one that can produce an eccentric plaque that causes a hemodynamically significant stenosis. In this way, a nonocclusive mural thrombus, even if clinically silent or causing unstable angina rather than infarction, can provoke a healing response that can promote lesion fibrosis and luminal encroachment. Such a sequence of events may convert a "vulnerable" atheroma with a thin fibrous cap prone to rupture into a more "stable" fibrous plaque with a reinforced cap. Angioplasty of unstable coronary lesions may "stabilize" the lesions by a similar mechanism, producing a wound followed by healing.

CLINICAL SYNDROMES OF ATHEROSCLEROSIS

Atherosclerotic lesions occur ubiquitously in Western societies. Most atheromata produce no symptoms, and many never cause clinical manifestations. Numerous patients with diffuse atherosclerosis may succumb to unrelated illnesses without ever having experienced a clinically significant manifestation of atherosclerosis. What accounts for this variability in the clinical expression of atherosclerotic disease?

Arterial remodeling during atheroma formation (Fig. 235-2A) represents a frequently overlooked but clinically important feature of lesion evolution. During the initial phases of atheroma development, the plaque usually grows outward, in an abluminal direction. Vessels affected by atherogenesis tend to increase in diameter, a phenomenon known as *compensatory enlargement*, in a type of vascular remodeling. The growing atheroma does not encroach upon the arterial lumen until the burden of atherosclerotic plaque exceeds ~40% of the area encompassed by the internal elastic lamina. Thus, during much of its life history, an atheroma will not cause stenosis that can limit tissue perfusion.

Flow-limiting stenoses commonly form later in the history of the plaque. Many such plaques cause stable syndromes such as demand-induced angina pectoris or intermittent claudication in the extremities. In the coronary and other circulations, even total vascular occlusion by atheroma does not invariably lead to infarction. The hypoxic stimulus of repeated bouts of ischemia characteristically induces formation of collateral vessels in the myocardium, mitigating the consequences of an acute occlusion of an epicardial coronary artery. By contrast, we now appreciate that many lesions that cause acute or unstable atherosclerotic syndromes, particularly in the coronary circulation, may arise from atherosclerotic plaques that do not produce a flow-limiting stenosis. Such lesions may produce only minimal luminal irregularities on traditional angiograms and often do not meet the traditional criteria for "significance" by arteriography. Instability of such nonocclusive stenoses may explain the frequency of myocardial infarction as an initial manifestation of coronary artery disease (in at least one-third of cases) in patients who report no prior history of angina pectoris, a syndrome usually caused by flow-limiting stenoses.

Plaque Instability and Rupture Postmortem studies afford considerable insight into the microanatomic substrate underlying the "instability" of plaques that do not cause critical stenoses. A superficial erosion of the endothelium or a frank plaque rupture or fissure usually produces the thrombus that causes episodes of unstable angina pectoris or the occlusive and relatively persistent thrombus that causes acute myocardial infarction (Fig. 235-2B). In the case of carotid atheromata, a deeper ulceration that provides a nidus for formation of platelet thrombi may cause transient cerebral ischemic attacks.

Rupture of the plaque's fibrous cap (Fig. 235-2C) permits contact between coagulation factors in the blood with highly thrombogenic tissue factor expressed by macrophage foam cells in the plaque's lipid-rich core. If the ensuing thrombus is nonocclusive or transient, the episode of plaque disruption may not cause symptoms or may result in episodic ischemic symptoms such as rest angina. Occlusive thrombi that endure will often cause acute myocardial infarction, particularly in the absence of a well-developed collateral circulation supplying the affected territory. Repetitive episodes of plaque disruption and healing provide one likely mechanism of transition of the fatty streak to a more complex fibrous lesion (Fig. 235-2D). The healing process in arteries, as in skin wounds, involves the laying down of new extracellular matrix and fibrosis.

Not all atheromata exhibit the same propensity to rupture. Pathologic studies of culprit lesions that have caused acute myocardial infarction reveal several characteristic features. Plaques that have caused fatal thromboses tend to have thin fibrous caps, relatively large lipid cores, and a high content of macrophages. Morphometric studies of such culprit lesions show that at sites of plaque rupture macrophages and T lymphocytes predominate and contain relatively few smooth-muscle cells. The cells that concentrate at sites of plaque rupture bear markers of inflammatory activation. The presence of the transplantation, or histocompatibility, antigen HLA-DR provides one convenient gauge of the degree of inflammation in cells in atheroma. Resting cells in normal arteries seldom express this transplantation antigen. However, macrophages and smooth-muscle cells at sites of human coronary artery plaque disruption do bear this inducible cell-surface marker. Therefore, the presence of HLA-DR-positive macrophages and T cells indicates an ongoing inflammatory response at sites of plaque rupture. In addition, patients with active atherosclerosis and acute coronary syndromes display signs of disseminated inflammation. For example, atherosclerotic plaques and even microvascular endothelial cells at sites remote from the "culprit" lesion of an acute coronary syndrome can exhibit markers of activation such as HLA-DR.

Inflammatory mediators regulate processes that govern the integrity of the plaque's fibrous cap and hence its propensity to rupture. For example, the T cell–derived cytokine IFN-γ, found in atherosclerotic plaques and required to induce the HLA-DR present at sites of rupture, can inhibit growth and collagen synthesis of smooth-muscle cells, as noted above. Cytokines derived from activated macrophages and lesional T cells can elicit the expression of genes encoding proteolytic enzymes that can degrade the extracellular matrix of the plaque's fibrous cap. Thus, inflammatory mediators can impair collagen synthesis required for maintenance and repair of the fibrous cap and trigger degradation of extracellular matrix macromolecules, processes that weaken the plaque's fibrous cap and enhance its vulnerability to rupture. In contrast to plaques with these features of vulnerability, those with a dense extracellular matrix and relatively thick fibrous cap without substantial tissue factor-rich lipid cores seem generally resistant to rupture and unlikely to provoke thrombosis.

Features of the biology of the atheromatous plaque in addition to its degree of luminal encroachment influence the clinical manifestations of this disease. This enhanced understanding of plaque biology provides insight into the diverse ways in which atherosclerosis can present clinically and why the disease may remain silent or stable for prolonged periods, punctuated by acute complications at certain times. Increased understanding of atherogenesis provides new insight into the mechanisms linking it to the risk factors discussed below, indicates the ways in which current therapies may improve outcomes, and also suggests new targets for future intervention.

PREVENTION AND TREATMENT

THE CONCEPT OF ATHEROSCLEROTIC RISK FACTORS

The systematic study of risk factors for atherosclerosis emerged from a coalescence of experimental results as well as cross-sectional and ultimately longitudinal studies in humans. The prospective, community-based Framingham Heart Study provided rigorous support for the concept that hypercholesterolemia, hypertension, and other factors correlated with cardiovascular risk. Similar observational studies performed worldwide bolstered the concept of "risk factors" for cardiovascular disease.

From a practical viewpoint, the cardiovascular risk factors that have emerged from such studies fall into two categories: those modifiable by lifestyle and/or pharmacotherapy and those such as age and gender that are immutable. The weight of evidence supporting various risk factors differs. For example, hypercholesterolemia and hypertension certainly predict coronary risk, but other so-called nontraditional risk factors, such as levels of homocysteine, lipoprotein (a) [Lp(a)], or infection, remain controversial. Moreover, the causality of some biomarkers that predict cardiovascular risk, such as C-reactive protein (CRP), remains uncertain. Table 235-1 lists the risk factors recognized by the current National Cholesterol Education Project Adult Treatment Panel III (ATP III). The

TABLE 235-1 MAJOR RISK FACTORS (EXCLUSIVE OF LDL CHOLESTEROL) THAT MODIFY LDL GOALS

Cigarette smoking
Hypertension (BP ≥140/90 mmHg or on antihypertensive medication)
Low HDL cholesterol[a] [<1.0 mmol/L (<40 mg/dL)]
Diabetes mellitus
Family history of premature CHD
   CHD in male first-degree relative <55 years
   CHD in female first-degree relative <65 years
Age (men ≥45 years; women ≥55 years)
Lifestyle risk factors
   Obesity (BMI ≥30 kg/m^2)
   Physical inactivity
   Atherogenic diet
Emerging risk factors
   Lipoprotein(a)
   Homocysteine
   Prothrombotic factors
   Proinflammatory factors
   Impaired fasting glucose
   Subclinical atherogenesis

[a]HDL cholesterol ≥1.6 mmol/L (≥60 mg/dL) counts as a "negative" risk factor; its presence removes one risk factor from the total count.
Note: LDL, low-density lipoprotein; BP, blood pressure; HDL, high-density lipoprotein; CHD, coronary heart disease; BMI, body-mass index.
Source: Modified from Expert Panel on Detection, Evaluation, and Treatment of High Blood Cholesterol in Adults (Adult Treatment Panel III). JAMA 285:2486, 2001.

sections below will consider some of these risk factors and approaches to their modification.

Lipid Disorders Abnormalities in plasma lipoproteins and derangements in lipid metabolism rank among the most firmly established and best understood risk factors for atherosclerosis. Chap. 350 describes the lipoprotein classes and provides a detailed discussion of lipoprotein metabolism. Current ATP III guidelines recommend lipid screening in all adults >20 years. The screen should include a fasting lipid profile (total cholesterol, triglycerides, LDL cholesterol, and HDL cholesterol) repeated every 5 years.

ATP III guidelines strive to match the intensity of treatment to an individual's risk. A quantitative estimate of risk places individuals in one of three treatment strata (Table 235-2). The first step in applying these guidelines involves counting an individual's risk factors (Table 235-1). Individuals with fewer than two risk factors fall into the lowest treatment intensity stratum [LDL goal <4.1 mmol/L (<160 mg/dL)]. In those with two or more risk factors, the next step involves a simple

TABLE 235-2 LDL CHOLESTEROL GOALS AND CUTPOINTS FOR THERAPEUTIC LIFESTYLE CHANGES (TLC) AND DRUG THERAPY IN DIFFERENT RISK CATEGORIES

	LDL Level, mmol/L (mg/dL)		
Risk Category	**Goal**	**Initiate TLC**	**Consider Drug Therapy**
Very high ACS, or CHD w/DM, or mult CRF	<1.8 (<70)	≥1.8 (≥70)	≥1.8 (≥70)
High CHD or CHD risk equivalents (10-year risk > 20%) If LDL < 2.6 (<100)	<2.6 (<100) [optional goal: <1.8 (<70)] <1.8 (<70)	≥2.6 (≥100)	≥2.6 (≥100) [<2.6 (<100): consider drug Rx]
Moderately high 2+ risk factors (10-year risk, 10–20%)	<2.6 (<100)	≥3.4 (≥130)	≥3.4 (≥130) [2.6–3.3 (100–129): consider drug Rx]
Moderate 2+ risk factors (risk < 10%)	<3.4 (<130)	≥3.4 (≥130)	≥4.1 (≥160)
Lower 0–1 risk factor	<4.1 (<160)	≥4.1 (≥160)	≥4.9 (≥190)

Note: LDL, low-density lipoprotein; ACS, acute coronary syndrome; CHD, coronary heart disease; DM, diabetes mellitus; CRF, coronary risk factors.
Source: Adapted from S Grundy et al: Circulation 110:227, 2004.

calculation that estimates the 10-year risk of developing coronary heart disease (CHD) (Table 235-2); see also *http://www.nhlbi.nih.gov/guidelines/cholesterol/* for the algorithm and a downloadable risk calculator. Those with a 10-year risk ≤20% fall into the intermediate stratum [LDL goal <3.4 mmol/L (<130 mg/dL)]. Those with a calculated 10-year CHD risk of >20%, any evidence of established atherosclerosis, or diabetes (now considered a CHD risk-equivalent) fall into the most intensive treatment group [LDL goal <2.6 mmol/L (<100 mg/dL)]. Members of the ATP III panel have recently suggested 1.8 mmol/L (70 mg/dL) as a goal for very high risk and as an optional goal for high-risk patients based on recent clinical trial data (Table 235-2).

The first maneuver to achieve the LDL goal involves therapeutic lifestyle changes (TLC), including specific diet and exercise recommendations established by the guidelines. According to ATP III criteria, those with LDL levels exceeding goal for their risk group by >0.8 mmol/L (>30 mg/dL) merit consideration for drug therapy. In patients with triglycerides > 2.6 mmol/L (>200 mg/dL), ATP III guidelines specify a secondary goal for therapy, "non-HDL cholesterol" (simply, the HDL cholesterol level subtracted from the total cholesterol). Cutpoints for therapeutic decision for non-HDL cholesterol are 0.8 mmol/L (30 mg/dL) more than those for LDL.

An extensive and growing body of rigorous evidence now supports the effectiveness of aggressive management of dyslipidemia. Addition of drug therapy to dietary and other nonpharmacologic measures reduces cardiovascular risk in patients with established coronary atherosclerosis and also in individuals who have not previously suffered CHD events (Fig. 235-3). As guidelines often lag the emerging clinical trial evidence base, the practitioner may elect to exercise clinical judgment in making therapeutic decisions in individual patients.

LDL-lowering therapies do not appear to exert their beneficial effect on cardiovascular events by causing a marked "regression" of obstructive coronary lesions. Angiographically monitored studies of lipid lowering have shown at best a modest reduction in coronary artery stenoses over the duration of study. Yet these same studies consistently show substantial decreases in coronary events. These results suggest that the beneficial mechanism of lipid lowering does not require a substantial reduction in the fixed stenoses. Rather, the benefit may derive from "stabilization" of atherosclerotic lesions without decreased stenosis. Such stabilization of atherosclerotic lesions and the attendant decrease in coronary events may result from the egress of lipids or by favorably influencing aspects of the biology of atherogenesis discussed above. In addition, as sizeable lesions may protrude abluminally rather than into the lumen due to complementary enlargement, shrinkage of such plaques might not be apparent on angiograms. The consistent benefit of LDL lowering by 3-hydroxy-3-methylgluatryl coenzyme A (HMG-CoA) reductase inhibitors (statins) observed in many risk groups may depend not only on their salutary effects on the lipid profile but also on direct modulation of plaque biology independent of lipid lowering.

A new class of LDL-lowering medications reduces cholesterol absorption from the proximal small bowel by targeting an enterocyte cholesterol transporter with the unwieldy name Niemann-Pick C1-like 1 protein (NPC1L1). The NPC1L1 inhibitor ezetimibe provides a useful adjunct to current therapies to achieve LDL goals; however, no clinical trial evidence yet demonstrates that ezetimibe benefits CHD outcomes.

As the mechanism by which elevated LDL levels promote atherogenesis likely involves oxidative modification, several trials have tested the possibility that antioxidant vitamin therapy might reduce CHD events. Rigorous and well-controlled clinical trials have failed to demonstrate that antioxidant vitamin therapy improves CHD outcomes. Therefore, the current evidence base does *not* support the use of antioxidant vitamins for this indication.

The clinical use of effective pharmacologic strategies for lowering LDL has markedly reduced cardiovascular events, but even their optimal utilization in clinical trials prevents only a minority of these endpoints. Hence other aspects of the lipid profile have become tempting targets for addressing the residual burden of cardiovascular disease that persists despite aggressive LDL lowering. Indeed, in the "post-

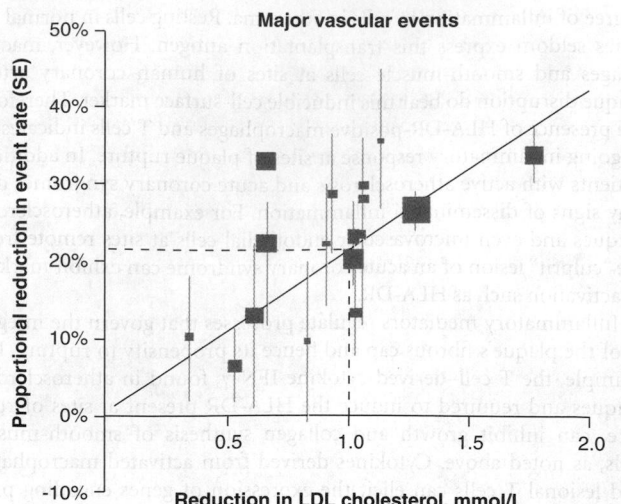

FIGURE 235-3 Lipid lowering reduces coronary events, as reflected on this graph showing the reduction in major cardiovascular events as a function of LDL level in a compendium of clinical trials with statins. *(Adapted from CTT Collaborators, Lancet 366:1267, 2005.)* The Management of Elevated Cholesterol in the Primary Prevention Group of Adult Japanese (MEGA), Treating to New Targets (TNT), and Incremental Decrease in Endpoints through Aggressive Lipid Lowering (IDEAL) studies have been added.

statin" era, patients with LDL levels at or below target not infrequently present with acute coronary syndromes. Low levels of HDL remain a prevalent problem in patients with coronary artery disease. Blood HDL levels vary inversely with those of triglycerides, and the independent role of triglycerides as a cardiovascular risk factor remains unsettled. For these reasons, approaches to raising HDL have emerged as a prominent next hurdle in the management of dyslipidemia. Weight loss and physical activity can raise HDL. Nicotinic acid, particularly in combination with statins, can robustly raise HDL. Some clinical trial data support the effectiveness of nicotinic acid in cardiovascular risk reduction. However, flushing and pruritus remain a challenge to patient acceptance, even with improved dosage forms of nicotinic acid. The identification of a cell-surface receptor for nicotinic acid may speed understanding of its mechanism of action and spur the development of new approaches to raising HDL.

Agonists of nuclear receptors that raise HDL levels provide another potential avenue to cardiovascular risk reduction. Peroxisome proliferator–activated receptor alpha (PPAR-α) agonists effectively raise HDL (by increasing transcription of its major apolipoprotein, AI) and lower triglyceride levels (by decreasing transcription of apolipoprotein CIII, an inhibitor of lipoprotein lipase, hence augmenting catabolism of triglyceride-rich lipoproteins). Cardiovascular outcome trials with PPAR-α and -γ agonists have yielded mixed results to date. Other agents in clinical development raise HDL levels by inhibiting cholesteryl ester transfer protein. Clinical studies currently underway will assess the effectiveness of this strategy to increase HDL in improvement of patient outcomes.

Hypertension
(See also Chap. 241) A wealth of epidemiologic data support a relationship between hypertension and atherosclerotic risk, and extensive clinical trial evidence has established that pharmacologic treatment of hypertension can reduce the risk of stroke, heart failure, and CHD events.

Diabetes Mellitus, Insulin Resistance, and the Metabolic Syndrome
(See also Chap. 338) Most patients with diabetes mellitus die of atherosclerosis and its complications. Aging and rampant obesity in the U.S. population underlie a current epidemic of type 2 diabetes mellitus. The abnormal lipoprotein profile associated with insulin resistance, known as *diabetic dyslipidemia*, accounts for part of the elevated car-

diovascular risk in patients with type 2 diabetes. While diabetic patients often have LDL cholesterol levels near average, the LDL particles tend to be smaller and denser, and, therefore, more atherogenic. Other features of diabetic dyslipidemia include low HDL and elevated triglyceride levels. Hypertension also frequently accompanies obesity, insulin resistance, and dyslipidemia. Indeed, the ATP III guidelines now recognize this cluster of risk factors and provide criteria for diagnosis of the "metabolic syndrome" (Table 235-3). Despite legitimate concerns regarding whether clustered components confer more risk than an individual component, the metabolic syndrome concept has considerable clinical utility.

Therapeutic objectives for intervention in these patients include addressing the underlying causes, including obesity and low physical activity, by initiating TLC. The ATP III guidelines provide an explicit step-by-step plan for implementing TLC, and treatment of the component risk factors should accompany TLC. Establishing that strict glycemic control reduces the risk of macrovascular complications of diabetes has proven much more elusive than the established beneficial effects on microvascular complications such as retinopathy or renal disease. In the absence of clear-cut evidence that tight glycemic control reduces coronary risk in patients with type 2, attention to other aspects of risk in this patient population assumes even greater importance. In this regard, multiple clinical trials, including the recent Collaborative Atorvastatin Diabetes Study (CARDS) that addressed specifically the diabetic population, have demonstrated unequivocal benefit of HMG-CoA reductase inhibitor therapy in diabetic patients over all ranges of LDL cholesterol levels. The Veterans Affairs HDL Intervention Trial (VA-HIT) showed that gemfibrozil, a PPAR-α agonist, reduced CHD and stroke in a population of men, many of whom had features of the metabolic syndrome. The recent Fenofibrate Intervention and Event Lowering in Diabetes (FIELD) trial did not meet its primary endpoint of reduced CHD death or nonfatal myocardial infarction but did show a significant reduction in a composite endpoint of total cardiovascular events. A cardiovascular endpoint study in diabetic patients with the PPAR-γ agonist pioglitazone likewise did not meet its multipartite primary endpoint but did show a significant reduction in a secondary composite endpoint of all-cause mortality, nonfatal myocardial infarction, and stroke. In view of the consistent benefit for diabetic populations of statin treatment, and the thus far equivocal results with PPAR agonists, the current stance of the American Diabetic Association that statins be considered for persons with diabetes older than 40 who have a total cholesterol level ≥ 135 appears amply justified. Among the oral hypoglycemic agents, metformin possesses the best evidence base for cardiovascular event reduction.

Diabetic populations appear to derive particular benefit from antihypertensive strategies that block the action of angiotensin II. Thus, the antihypertensive regimen for patients with the metabolic syndrome should include angiotensin-converting enzyme inhibitors or angiotensin receptor blockers when possible. Most of these individuals will require more than one antihypertensive agent to achieve the recently updated American Diabetes Association blood pressure goal of 130/80 mmHg.

Male Gender/Postmenopausal State Decades of observational studies have verified excess coronary risk in men compared with premenopausal women. After menopause, however, coronary risk accelerates in women. At least part of the apparent protection against CHD in premenopausal women derives from their relatively higher HDL levels compared with those of men. After menopause, HDL values fall in concert with increased coronary risk. Estrogen therapy lowers LDL cholesterol and raises HDL cholesterol, changes that should decrease coronary risk.

Multiple observational and experimental studies suggested that estrogen therapy reduces coronary risk. However, a spate of recent clinical trials has failed to demonstrate a net benefit of estrogen with or without progestins on CHD outcomes. In the Heart and Estrogen/Progestin Replacement Study (HERS), postmenopausal female survivors of acute myocardial infarction were randomized to an estrogen/progestin combination or to placebo. This study showed no overall reduction in recurrent coronary events in the active treatment arm. Indeed, early in the 5-year course of this trial, there was a trend toward an actual increase in vascular events in the treated women. Extended follow-up of this cohort did not disclose an accrual of benefit in the treatment group. The Women's Health Initiative (WHI) study arm using a similar estrogen plus progesterone regimen was halted due to a small but significant hazard of cardiovascular events, stroke, and breast cancer. The estrogen without progestin arm of WHI (conducted in women without a uterus) ceased early due to an increase in strokes, and failed to afford protection from myocardial infarction or CHD death during observation over 7 years. The excess cardiovascular events in these trials may result from an increase in thromboembolism (Chap. 342). Physicians should work with women to provide information and help weigh the small but evident CHD risk of estrogen ± progestin vs. the benefits on postmenopausal symptoms and osteoporosis, taking personal preferences into account. Post hoc analyses of observational studies suggest that estrogen therapy in women younger than or closer to menopause than the women enrolled in WHI might confer cardiovascular benefit. Thus, the timing in relation to menopause or age at which estrogen therapy begins may influence its risk/benefit balance.

The lack of efficacy of estrogen therapy in cardiovascular risk reduction highlights the need for redoubled attention to known modifiable risk factors in women. In the recent clinical trials with HMG-CoA reductase inhibitors, women, when included, have derived benefits at least commensurate with those seen in men.

Dysregulated Coagulation or Fibrinolysis Thrombosis ultimately causes the gravest complications of atherosclerosis. The propensity to form thrombi and/or to lyse clots once they form clearly influences the manifestations of atherosclerosis. Thrombosis provoked by atheroma rupture and subsequent healing may promote plaque growth. Certain individual characteristics can influence thrombosis or fibrinolysis and have received attention as potential coronary risk factors. For example, fibrinogen levels correlate with coronary risk and provide information regarding coronary risk independent of the lipoprotein profile. Elevated fibrinogen levels might promote thrombosis. As an acute-phase reactant, fibrinogen may also serve as a marker of inflammation.

The stability of an arterial thrombus depends on the balance between fibrinolytic factors, such as plasmin, and inhibitors of the fibrinolytic system, such as plasminogen activator inhibitor 1 (PAI-1). However, the levels of tissue plasminogen activator and PAI-1 in plasma have not proved to add considerable information beyond the lipid profile to the assessment of cardiovascular risk. Lp(a) (Chap. 350) may modulate fibrinolysis, and although individuals with elevated Lp(a) levels have increased CHD risk, Lp(a) levels do not potently predict risk in the population at large.

TABLE 235-3	CLINICAL IDENTIFICATION OF THE METABOLIC SYNDROME—ANY THREE RISK FACTORS	
Risk Factor		**Defining Level**
Abdominal obesity[a]		
Men (waist circumference)[b]		>102 cm (>40 in.)
Women		>88 cm (>35 in.)
Triglycerides		>1.7 mmol/L (>150 mg/dL)
HDL cholesterol		
Men		<1.0 mmol/L (<40 mg/dL)
Women		<1.3 mmol/L (<50 mg/dL)
Blood pressure		≥130/≥85 mmHg
Fasting glucose		>6.1 mmol/L (>110 mg/dL)

[a]Overweight and obesity are associated with insulin resistance and the metabolic syndrome. However, the presence of abdominal obesity is more highly correlated with the metabolic risk factors than is an elevated body-mass index (BMI). Therefore, the simple measure of waist circumference is recommended to identify the BMI component of the metabolic syndrome.

[b]Some male patients can develop multiple metabolic risk factors when the waist circumference is only marginally increased, e.g., 94–102 cm (37–39 in.). Such patients may have a strong genetic contribution to insulin resistance. They should benefit from life-style changes, similarly to men with categorical increases in waist circumference.

Aspirin reduces CHD events in several contexts. Chap. 237 discusses aspirin therapy in stable ischemic heart disease, Chap. 238 reviews recommendations for aspirin treatment in acute coronary syndromes, and Chap. 364 describes aspirin's role in preventing recurrent ischemic stroke. In primary prevention, pooled trial data show that low-dose aspirin treatment (81 mg qd to 325 mg alternate days) can reduce risk of first myocardial infarction in men. Although the recent Women's Health Study (WHS) showed that aspirin (100 mg alternate days) reduced strokes by 17%, it did not prevent myocardial infarction in women. Current American Heart Association (AHA) guidelines recommend the use of low-dose aspirin (75–160 mg/d) in women with high cardiovascular risk (≥20% 10-year risk), for men with a ≥10% 10-year risk of CHD, and for all aspirin-tolerant patients with established cardiovascular disease who lack contraindications.

Homocysteine   A large body of literature suggests a relationship between hyperhomocysteinemia and coronary events. Several mutations in the enzymes involved in homocysteine accumulation correlate with thrombosis and, in some studies, coronary risk. Prospective studies have not shown a robust utility of hyperhomocysteinemia in CHD risk stratification. Clinical trials have not shown that intervention to lower homocysteine levels reduces CHD events. Fortification of the U.S. diet with folic acid to reduce neural tube defects has lowered homocysteine levels in the population at large. Measurement of homocysteine levels should be reserved for individuals with atherosclerosis at a young age or out of proportion to established risk factors. Physicians who advise consumption of supplements containing folic acid should consider that this treatment might mask pernicious anemia.

Inflammation   An accumulation of clinical evidence shows that markers of inflammation correlate with coronary risk. For example, plasma levels of CRP, as measured by a high-sensitivity assay, prospectively predict risk of myocardial infarction. CRP levels also correlate with outcome of patients with acute coronary syndromes. In contrast to several other novel risk factors, CRP adds predictive information to that derived from established risk factors, such as those included in the Framingham score (Fig. 235-4). Elevated levels of the acute-phase reactant CRP may reflect merely ongoing inflammation rather than a direct etiologic role for CRP in coronary artery disease.

Elevations in acute-phase reactants such as fibrinogen or CRP could reflect overall atherosclerotic burden and/or extravascular inflammation that potentiate atherosclerosis or its complications. In all likelihood, both lesional and extravascular factors contribute to elevation of inflammatory markers in patients at risk for coronary events. Visceral adipose tissue releases pro-inflammatory cytokines that drive CRP production and may represent a major extravascular stimulus to elevation of inflammatory markers in obese and overweight individuals. Indeed, CRP levels rise with body mass index (BMI), and weight reduction lowers CRP levels. Infectious agents might also furnish in-

FIGURE 235-5 Evidence that both LDL-lowering and anti-inflammatory actions contribute to the benefit of statin therapy in survivors of acute coronary syndrome. See text for explanation. hs-CRP, high-sensitivity measurement of C-reactive protein (CRP); MI, myocardial infarction. (*Adapted from PM Ridker et al: N Engl J Med 352:20, 2005.*)

flammatory stimuli related to cardiovascular risk. However, the results of recent sufficiently powered randomized clinical trials do not support the use of antibiotics to reduce CHD risk.

Intriguing evidence suggests that lipid-lowering therapy reduces coronary events in part by muting the inflammatory aspects of the pathogenesis of atherosclerosis. A prespecified analysis of the Pravastatin or Atorvastatin Evaluation and Infection Therapy (PROVE-IT) trial, conducted in patients stabilized after acute coronary syndromes, showed that participants who achieved both below median LDL and CRP had fewer recurrent cardiovascular events than those who fell below only one of these cut points (Fig. 235-5). Those with both LDL and CRP above the median fared worst of all. The anti-inflammatory effect of statins appears independent of LDL lowering, as these two variables correlated very poorly in individual subjects in multiple clinical trials.

Lifestyle Modification   The prevention of atherosclerosis presents a long-term challenge to all health care professionals and for public health policy as well. Both individual practitioners and organizations providing health care should strive to help patients optimize their risk factor profile long before atherosclerotic disease becomes manifest. The current accumulation of cardiovascular risk in youth and in certain minority populations presents a particularly vexing concern from a public health perspective.

The care plan for all patients seen by internists should include measures to assess and minimize cardiovascular risk. Physicians must counsel patients regarding the health risks of tobacco use and provide guidance and resources regarding smoking cessation. Likewise, physicians should advise all patients about prudent dietary and physical activity habits for maintaining ideal body weight. Both National Institutes of Health and AHA statements recommend at least 30 min of moderate-intensity physical activity per day. Obesity, particularly the male pattern of centripetal or visceral fat accumulation, can contribute to the elements of the metabolic syndrome (Table 235-3). Physicians should encourage their patients to take personal responsibility for behavior related to modifiable risk factors for development of premature atherosclerotic disease. Conscientious counseling and patient education may forestall the need for pharmacologic measures intended to reduce coronary risk.

Issues in Risk Assessment   A growing panel of markers of coronary risk presents a perplexing array to the practitioner. Markers measured in peripheral blood include size fractions of LDL particles and concentrations of homocysteine, Lp(a), fibrinogen, CRP, PAI-1, myeloperoxidase, and lipoprotein-associated phospholipase A_2, among many others. In general, such specialized tests add little to the information

FIGURE 235-4 C-reactive protein (CRP) level adds to the predictive value of the Framingham score. hs-CRP, high-sensitivity measurement of CRP. (*Adapted from PM Ridker et al: Circulation 109:2818, 2004.*)

available from a careful history and physical examination combined with measurement of a plasma lipoprotein profile and fasting blood glucose. The high-sensitivity CRP measurement may well prove an exception in view of its robustness in risk prediction, its ease of reproducible and standardized measurement, its relative stability in individuals over time, and, most importantly, its ability to add to the risk information disclosed by standard measurements such as the components of the Framingham risk score (Fig. 235-4). Given the utility of high-sensitivity CRP measurement in predicting a gamut of important cardiovascular outcomes, this simple blood test may prove useful in the future in guiding therapy, particularly in primary prevention. Current advisories, however, recommend the use of this test only in individuals with intermediate risk of a CHD event (10–20%, 10-year risk). Clinical trials now under way will test the hypothesis that CRP levels can guide therapy. Results such as those from PROVE-IT (Fig. 235-5) suggest that CRP may prove a valid target of therapy, a proposition that requires more investigation before general adoption in practice.

Similar concerns pertain to the use of specialized radiographic estimations of coronary artery calcification and of the rapidly emerging computed tomographic coronary angiograms (CTA). Accumulating information indicates that the amount of calcium determined by such techniques as electron beam CT correlates with coronary risk; however, the utility of using such estimates of coronary artery calcium content as a guide to therapy remains unproven, particularly in asymptomatic individuals. Multidetector CTA provides visually appealing images of the epicardial coronary arteries yet still requires rigorous validation as a cardiovascular risk marker or guide to therapy. Inappropriate use of such imaging modalities might promote excessive invasive diagnostic and therapeutic procedures. Widespread application of such modalities for screening should await proof that clinical benefit derives from their application.

Progress in human genetics holds considerable promise for risk prediction and for individualization of cardiovascular therapy. Many reports have identified single nucleotide polymorphisms in candidate genes as predictors of cardiovascular risk. To date, the validation of such genetic markers of risk and drug-responsiveness in multiple populations has often proved disappointing. The advent of technology that permits relatively rapid and inexpensive genome-wide screens, and of powerful bioinformatics tools, should spur haplotype analyses and unbiased identification of risk and therapy-response genotypes in the future.

THE CHALLENGE OF IMPLEMENTATION: CHANGING PHYSICIAN AND PATIENT BEHAVIOR

Despite declining age-adjusted rates of coronary death, cardiovascular mortality is on the rise due to the overall aging of the population. There is a powerful global trend toward increased atherosclerotic disease. Enormous challenges remain regarding translation of the current evidence base into practice. We must learn how to help individuals adopt a healthy lifestyle and how to deploy our increasingly powerful pharmacologic tools most economically and effectively. The obstacles to implementation of current evidence-based prevention and treatment of atherosclerosis include economics, education, physician awareness, and patient adherence to recommended regimens. Future goals in the field of treatment of atherosclerosis should include more widespread implementation of the current evidence-based guidelines regarding risk-factor management and, when appropriate, drug therapy.

FURTHER READINGS

BAIGENT C et al: Efficacy and safety of cholesterol-lowering treatment: Prospective meta-analysis of data from 90,056 participants in 14 randomised trials of statins. Lancet 366:1267, 2005

BERLINER JA, WATSON AD: A role for oxidized phospholipids in atherosclerosis. N Engl J Med 353:9, 2005

GRODSTEIN F et al: Hormone therapy and coronary artery disease: The role of time since menopause and age at hormone initiation. J Women's Health 15:35, 2006

GRUNDY SM et al: Implications of recent clinical trials for the National Cholesterol Education Program Adult Treatment Panel III guidelines. Circulation 110:227, 2004

———— et al: Diagnosis and management of the metabolic syndrome: An American Heart Association/National Heart, Lung, and Blood Institute scientific statement. Circulation 112:2735, 2005

LIBBY P: The vascular endothelium and atherosclerosis, in *The Handbook of Experimental Pharmacology,* S Moncada, EA Higgs (eds), Berlin-Heidelberg, Springer-Verlag, 2006

————, RIDKER PM: Inflammation and atherothrombosis: From population biology and bench research to clinical practice. J Am Coll Cardiol 48(9 Suppl):A33–46, 2006

————, THEROUX P: Pathophysiology of coronary artery disease. Circulation 111:3481, 2005

MILLER DT et al: Atherosclerosis: The path from genomics to therapeutics. J Am Coll Cardiol 49:1589, 2007

236 The Metabolic Syndrome
Robert H. Eckel

The metabolic syndrome (syndrome X, insulin resistance syndrome) consists of a constellation of metabolic abnormalities that confer increased risk of cardiovascular disease (CVD) and diabetes mellitus (DM). The criteria for the metabolic syndrome have evolved since the original definition by the World Health Organization in 1998, reflecting growing clinical evidence and analysis by a variety of consensus conferences and professional organizations. The major features of the metabolic syndrome include central obesity, hypertriglyceridemia, low HDL cholesterol, hyperglycemia, and hypertension (Table 236-1).

EPIDEMIOLOGY

Prevalence of the metabolic syndrome varies across the globe, in part reflecting the age and ethnicity of the populations studied and the diagnostic criteria applied. In general, the prevalence of metabolic syndrome increases with age. The highest recorded prevalence worldwide is in Native Americans, with nearly 60% of women ages 45–49 and 45% of men ages 45–49 meeting National Cholesterol Education Program, Adult Treatment Panel III (NCEP:ATPIII) criteria. In the United States, metabolic syndrome is less common in African-American men but more common in Mexican-American women. Based on data from the National Health and Nutrition Examination Survey (NHANES) III, the age-adjusted prevalence of the metabolic syndrome in the United States is 34% for men and 35% for women. In France, a 30–64-year-old cohort shows a <10% prevalence for each gender, although 17.5% are affected in the 60–64 age range. Greater industrialization worldwide is associated with rising rates of obesity, which is anticipated to dramatically increase prevalence of the metabolic syndrome, especially as the population ages. Moreover, the rising prevalence and severity of obesity in children is initiating features of the metabolic syndrome in a younger population.

The frequency distribution of the five components of the syndrome for the U.S. population (NHANES III) is summarized in Fig. 236-1. Increases in waist circumference predominate in women whereas fasting triglycerides >150 mg/dL and hypertension are more likely in men.

RISK FACTORS

Overweight/Obesity Although the first description of the metabolic syndrome occurred in the early twentieth century, the worldwide overweight/obesity epidemic has been the driving force for more recent rec-

TABLE 236-1   NCEP:ATPIII 2001 AND IDF CRITERIA FOR THE METABOLIC SYNDROME

NCEP:ATPIII 2001	IDF Criteria for Central Adiposity[a]		
Three or more of the following:	**Waist Circumference**		
Central obesity: Waist circumference >102 cm (M), >88 cm (F)	**Men**	**Women**	**Ethnicity**
Hypertriglyceridemia: Triglycerides ≥150 mg/dL or specific medication	≥94 cm	≥80 cm	Europid, Sub-Saharan African, Eastern & Middle Eastern
Low HDL cholesterol: <40 mg/dL and <50 mg/dL, respectively, or specific medication	≥90 cm	≥80 cm	South Asian, Chinese, and ethnic South & Central American
Hypertension: Blood pressure ≥130 mm systolic or ≥85 mm diastolic or specific medication	≥85 cm	≥90 cm	Japanese
Fasting plasma glucose ≥100 mg/dL or specific medication or previously diagnosed type 2 diabetes	**Two or more of the following:**		
	Fasting triglycerides >150 mg/dL or specific medication		
	HDL cholesterol <40 mg/dL and <50 mg/dL for men and women, respectively, or specific medication		
	Blood pressure >130 systolic or >85 mm diastolic or previous diagnosis or specific medication		
	Fasting plasma glucose ≥100 mg/dL or previously diagnosed type 2 diabetes		

[a]In this analysis, the following thresholds for waist circumference were used: White men, ≥94 cm; African-American men, ≥94 cm; Mexican-American men, ≥90 cm; white women, ≥80 cm; African-American women, ≥80 cm; Mexican-American women, ≥80 cm. For participants whose designation was "other race—including multiracial," thresholds that were once based on Europid cut points (≥94 cm for men and ≥80 cm for women) and once based on South Asian cut points (≥90 cm for men and ≥80 cm for women) were used. For participants who were considered "other Hispanic," the IDF thresholds for ethnic South and Central Americans were used.

Abbreviations: NCEP:ATPIII, National Cholesterol Education Program, Adult Treatment Panel III; IDF, International Diabetes Foundation HDL, high-density lipoprotein.

ognition of the syndrome. Central adiposity is a key feature of the syndrome, reflecting the fact that the syndrome's prevalence is driven by the strong relationship between waist circumference and increasing adiposity. However, despite the importance of obesity, patients who are normal weight may also be insulin-resistant and have the syndrome.

Sedentary Lifestyle   Physical inactivity is a predictor of CVD events and related mortality. Many components of the metabolic syndrome are associated with a sedentary lifestyle, including increased adipose tissue (predominantly central); reduced HDL cholesterol; and a trend toward increased triglycerides, blood pressure, and glucose in the genetically susceptible. Compared with individuals who watched television or videos or used their computer <1 h daily, those who carried out these behaviors for >4 h daily have a twofold increased risk of the metabolic syndrome.

FIGURE 236-1 Prevalence of the metabolic syndrome components, from NHANES III. NHANES, National Health and Nutrition Examination Survey; TG, triglyceride; HDL, high-density lipoprotein; BP, blood pressure. *(From ES Ford et al: JAMA 287:356, 2002; with permission.)*

Aging   The metabolic syndrome affects 44% of the U.S. population older than age 50. A greater percentage of women older than age 50 have the syndrome than men. The age dependency of the syndrome's prevalence is seen in most populations around the world.

Diabetes Mellitus   DM is included in both the NCEP and International Diabetes Foundation (IDF) definitions of the metabolic syndrome. It is estimated that the large majority (~75%) of patients with type 2 diabetes or impaired glucose tolerance (IGT) have the metabolic syndrome. The presence of the metabolic syndrome in these populations relates to a higher prevalence of CVD compared to patients with type 2 diabetes or IGT without the syndrome.

Coronary Heart Disease   The approximate prevalence of the metabolic syndrome in patients with coronary heart disease (CHD) is 50%, with a prevalence of 37% in patients with premature coronary artery disease (≤ age 45), particularly in women. With appropriate cardiac rehabilitation and changes in lifestyle (e.g., nutrition, physical activity, weight reduction, and, in some cases, pharmacologic agents), the prevalence of the syndrome can be reduced.

Lipodystrophy   Lipodystrophic disorders in general are associated with the metabolic syndrome. Both genetic (e.g., Berardinelli-Seip congenital lipodystrophy, Dunnigan familial partial lipodystrophy) and acquired (e.g., HIV-related lipodystrophy in patients treated with highly active antiretroviral therapy) forms of lipodystrophy may give rise to severe insulin resistance and many of the metabolic syndrome's components.

ETIOLOGY

Insulin Resistance   The most accepted and unifying hypothesis to describe the pathophysiology of the metabolic syndrome is insulin resistance, caused by an incompletely understood defect in insulin action (Chap. 338). The onset of insulin resistance is heralded by postprandial hyperinsulinemia, followed by fasting hyperinsulinemia and, ultimately, hyperglycemia.

An early major contributor to the development of insulin resistance is an overabundance of circulating fatty acids (Fig. 236-2). Plasma albumin-bound free fatty acids (FFAs) are derived predominantly from adipose tissue triglyceride stores released by hormone-sensitive lipase. Fatty acids are also derived through the lipolysis of triglyceride-rich lipoproteins in tissues by lipoprotein lipase (LPL). Insulin mediates both antilipolysis and the stimulation of LPL in adipose tissue. Of note, the inhibition of lipolysis in adipose tissue is the most sensitive pathway of insulin action. Thus, when insulin resistance develops, increased lipolysis produces more fatty acids, which further decrease the antilipolytic effect of insulin. Excessive fatty acids enhance substrate availability and create insulin resistance by modifying downstream signaling. Fatty acids impair insulin-mediated glucose uptake and accumulate as triglycerides in both skeletal and cardiac muscle, whereas increased glucose production and triglyceride accumulation are seen in liver.

The oxidative stress hypothesis provides unifying theory for aging and the predisposition to the metabolic syndrome. In studies carried out in insulin-resistant subjects with obesity or type 2 diabetes, in the offspring of patients with type 2 diabetes, and in the elderly, a defect has been identified in mitochondrial oxidative phosphorylation, leading to the accumulation of triglycerides and related lipid molecules in muscle. The accumulation of lipids in muscle is associated with insulin resistance.

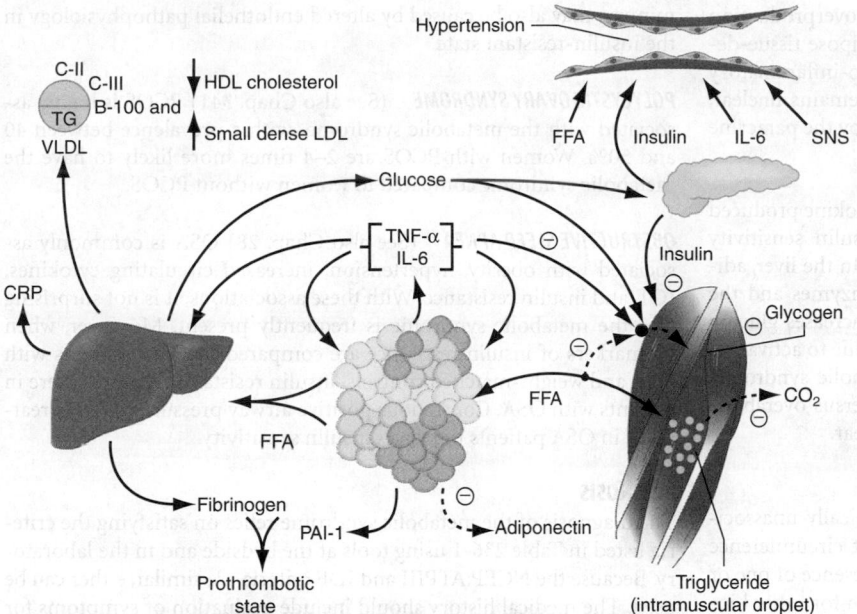

FIGURE 236-2 Pathophysiology of the metabolic syndrome. Free fatty acids (FFAs) are released in abundance from an expanded adipose tissue mass. In the liver, FFAs result in an increased production of glucose, triglycerides and secretion of very low density lipoproteins (VLDLs). Associated lipid/lipoprotein abnormalities include reductions in high-density lipoprotein (HDL) cholesterol and an increased density of low-density lipoproteins (LDLs). FFAs also reduce insulin sensitivity in muscle by inhibiting insulin-mediated glucose uptake. Associated defects include a reduction in glucose partitioning to glycogen and increased lipid accumulation in triglyceride (TG). Increases in circulating glucose, and to some extent FFA, increase pancreatic insulin secretion, resulting in hyperinsulinemia. Hyperinsulinemia may result in enhanced sodium reabsorption and increased sympathetic nervous system (SNS) activity and contribute to the hypertension, as might increased levels of circulating FFAs. The proinflammatory state is superimposed and contributory to the insulin resistance produced by excessive FFAs. The enhanced secretion of interleukin 6 (IL-6) and tumor necrosis factor α (TNF-α) produced by adipocytes and monocyte-derived macrophages results in more insulin resistance and lipolysis of adipose tissue triglyceride stores to circulating FFAs. IL-6 and other cytokines also enhance hepatic glucose production, VLDL production by the liver, and insulin resistance in muscle. Cytokines and FFAs also increase the hepatic production of fibrinogen and adipocyte production of plasminogen activator inhibitor 1 (PAI-1), resulting in a prothrombotic state. Higher levels of circulating cytokines also stimulate the hepatic production of C-reactive protein (CRP). Reduced production of the anti-inflammatory and insulin sensitizing cytokine adiponectin are also associated with the metabolic syndrome. *(Reprinted from Eckel et al., with permission from Elsevier.)*

Increased Waist Circumference Waist circumference is an important component of the most recent and frequently applied diagnostic criteria for the metabolic syndrome. However, measuring waist circumference does not reliably distinguish between a large waist due to increases in subcutaneous adipose tissue vs. visceral fat; this distinction requires CT or MRI. With increases in visceral adipose tissue, adipose tissue-derived FFAs are directed to the liver. On the other hand, increases in abdominal subcutaneous fat release lipolysis products into the systemic circulation and avoid more direct effects on hepatic metabolism. Relative increases in visceral versus subcutaneous adipose tissue with increasing waist circumference in Asians and Asian Indians may explain the greater prevalence of the syndrome in these populations compared to African-American men in whom subcutaneous fat predominates. It is also possible that visceral fat is a marker for, but not the source of, excess postprandial FFAs in obesity.

Dyslipidemia (See also Chap. 350) In general, FFA flux to the liver is associated with increased production of apoB–containing, triglyceride-rich very low density lipoproteins (VLDLs). The effect of insulin on this process is complex, but *hypertriglyceridemia* is an excellent marker of the insulin-resistant condition.

The other major lipoprotein disturbance in the metabolic syndrome is a *reduction in HDL cholesterol*. This reduction is a consequence of changes in HDL composition and metabolism. In the presence of hypertriglyceridemia, a decrease in the cholesterol content of HDL is a consequence of reduced cholesteryl ester content of the lipoprotein core in combination with cholesteryl ester transfer protein–mediated alterations in triglyceride making the particle small and dense. This change in lipoprotein composition also results in an increased clearance of HDL from the circulation. The relationships of these changes in HDL to insulin resistance are likely indirect, occurring in concert with the changes in triglyceride-rich lipoprotein metabolism.

In addition to HDL, LDLs are also modified in composition. With fasting serum triglycerides >2.0 mM (~180 mg/dL), there is almost always a predominance of small dense LDLs. Small dense LDLs are thought to be more atherogenic. They may be toxic to the endothelium, and they are able to transit through the endothelial basement membrane and adhere to glycosaminoglycans. They also have increased susceptibility to oxidation and are selectively bound to scavenger receptors on monocyte-derived macrophages. Subjects with increased small dense LDL particles and hypertriglyceridemia also have increased cholesterol content of both VLDL1 and VLDL2 subfractions. This relatively cholesterol-rich VLDL particle may also contribute to the atherogenic risk in patients with metabolic syndrome.

Glucose Intolerance (See also Chap. 338) The defects in insulin action lead to impaired suppression of glucose production by the liver and kidney and reduced glucose uptake and metabolism in insulin-sensitive tissues, i.e., muscle and adipose tissue. The relationship between impaired fasting glucose (IFG) or impaired glucose tolerance (IGT) and insulin resistance is well supported by human, nonhuman primate, and rodent studies. To compensate for defects in insulin action, insulin secretion and/or clearance must be modified to sustain euglycemia. Ultimately, this compensatory mechanism fails, usually because of defects in insulin secretion, resulting in progress from IFG and/or IGT to DM.

Hypertension The relationship between insulin resistance and hypertension is well established. Paradoxically, under normal physiologic conditions, insulin is a vasodilator with secondary effects on sodium reabsorption in the kidney. However, in the setting of insulin resistance, the vasodilatory effect of insulin is lost, but the renal effect on sodium reabsorption is preserved. Sodium reabsorption is increased in Caucasians with the metabolic syndrome but not in Africans or Asians. Insulin also increases the activity of the sympathetic nervous system, an effect that may also be preserved in the setting of the insulin resistance. Finally, insulin resistance is characterized by pathway-specific impairment in phosphatidylinositol 3-kinase signaling. In the endothelium, this may cause an imbalance between the production of nitric oxide and secretion of endothelin-1, leading to decreased blood flow. Although these mechanisms are provocative, when insulin action is assessed by levels of fasting insulin or by the Homeostasis Model Assessment (HOMA), insulin resistance contributes only modestly to the increased prevalence of hypertension in the metabolic syndrome.

Proinflammatory Cytokines The increases in proinflammatory cytokines, including interleukin (IL) 1, IL-6, IL-18, resistin, tumor necrosis factor (TNF) α, and C-reactive protein (CRP), reflect overproduction by the expanded adipose tissue mass (Fig. 236-2). Adipose tissue-derived macrophages may be the primary source of pro-inflammatory cytokines locally and in the systemic circulation. It remains unclear, however, how much of the insulin resistance is caused by the paracrine vs. endocrine effects of these cytokines.

Adiponectin Adiponectin is an anti-inflammatory cytokine produced exclusively by adipocytes. Adiponectin enhances insulin sensitivity and inhibits many steps in the inflammatory process. In the liver, adiponectin inhibits the expression of gluconeogenic enzymes and the rate of glucose production. In muscle, adiponectin increases glucose transport and enhances fatty acid oxidation, partially due to activation of AMP kinase. Adiponectin is reduced in the metabolic syndrome. The relative contribution of adiponectin deficiency versus overabundance of the proinflammatory cytokines remains unclear.

CLINICAL FEATURES
Symptoms and Signs The metabolic syndrome is typically unassociated with symptoms. On physical examination, waist circumference may be expanded and blood pressure elevated. The presence of one or either of these signs should alert the clinician to search for other biochemical abnormalities that may be associated with the metabolic syndrome. Less frequently, lipoatrophy or acanthosis nigricans is found on exam. Because these physical findings are typically associated with severe insulin resistance, other components of the metabolic syndrome should be expected.

Associated Diseases · *CARDIOVASCULAR DISEASE* The relative risk for new-onset CVD in patients with the metabolic syndrome, in the absence of diabetes, averages between 1.5- and threefold. In an 8-year follow-up of middle-aged men and women in the Framingham Offspring Study (FOS), the population attributable risk for patients with the metabolic syndrome to develop CVD was 34% in men and 16% in women. In the same study, both the metabolic syndrome and diabetes predicted ischemic stroke with greater risk for patients with the metabolic syndrome than for diabetes alone (19% vs 7%), particularly in women (27% vs 5%). Patients with metabolic syndrome are also at increased risk for peripheral vascular disease.

TYPE 2 DIABETES Overall, the risk for type 2 diabetes in patients with the metabolic syndrome is increased three- to fivefold. In the FOS's 8-year follow-up of middle-aged men and women, the population-attributable risk for developing type 2 diabetes was 62% in men and 47% in women.

Other Associated Conditions In addition to the features specifically associated with metabolic syndrome, insulin resistance is accompanied by other metabolic alterations. These included increases in apoB and C III, uric acid, prothrombotic factors (fibrinogen, plasminogen activator inhibitor 1), serum viscosity, asymmetric dimethylarginine, homocysteine, white blood cell count, pro-inflammatory cytokines, CRP, microalbuminuria, nonalcoholic fatty liver disease (NAFLD) and/or nonalcoholic steatohepatitis (NASH), polycystic ovarian disease (PCOS), and obstructive sleep apnea (OSA).

NONALCOHOLIC FATTY LIVER DISEASE (See also Chap. 303) Fatty liver is relatively common. However, in NASH, both triglyceride accumulation and inflammation coexist. NASH is now present in 2–3% of the population in the United States and other Western countries. As the prevalence of overweight/obesity and the metabolic syndrome increases, NASH may become one of the more frequent causes of end-stage liver disease and hepatocellular carcinoma.

HYPERURICEMIA (See also Chap. 353) Hyperuricemia reflects defects in insulin action on the renal tubular reabsorption of uric acid, whereas the increase in asymmetric dimethylarginine, an endogenous inhibitor of nitric oxide synthase, relates to endothelial dysfunction. Microalbu-

minuria may also be caused by altered endothelial pathophysiology in the insulin-resistant state.

POLYCYSTIC OVARY SYNDROME (See also Chap. 341) PCOS is highly associated with the metabolic syndrome, with a prevalence between 40 and 50%. Women with PCOS are 2–4 times more likely to have the metabolic syndrome compared to women without PCOS.

OBSTRUCTIVE SLEEP APNEA (See also Chap. 28) OSA is commonly associated with obesity, hypertension, increased circulating cytokines, IGT, and insulin resistance. With these associations, it is not surprising that the metabolic syndrome is frequently present. Moreover, when biomarkers of insulin resistance are compared between patients with OSA and weight-matched controls, insulin resistance is more severe in patients with OSA. Continuous positive airway pressure (CPAP) treatment in OSA patients improves insulin sensitivity.

DIAGNOSIS
The diagnosis of the metabolic syndrome relies on satisfying the criteria listed in Table 236-1 using tools at the bedside and in the laboratory. Because the NCEP:ATPIII and IDF criteria are similar, either can be used. The medical history should include evaluation of symptoms for OSA in all patients and PCOS in premenopausal women. Family history will help determine risk for CVD and DM. Blood pressure and waist circumference measurements provide information necessary for the diagnosis.

Laboratory Tests Fasting lipids and glucose are needed to determine if the metabolic syndrome is present. The measurement of additional biomarkers associated with insulin resistance must be individualized. Such tests might include apo B, high-sensitivity CRP, fibrinogen, uric acid, urinary microalbumin, and liver function tests. A sleep study should be performed if symptoms of OSA are present. If PCOS is suspected based on clinical features and anovulation, testosterone, luteinizing hormone, and follicle-stimulating hormone should be measured.

℞ THE METABOLIC SYNDROME

LIFESTYLE (See also Chap. 75) Obesity is the driving force behind the metabolic syndrome. Thus, weight reduction is the primary approach to the disorder. With weight reduction, the improvement in insulin sensitivity is often accompanied by favorable modifications in many components of the metabolic syndrome. In general, recommendations for weight loss include a combination of caloric restriction, increased physical activity, and behavior modification. For weight reduction, caloric restriction is the most important component, whereas increases in physical activity are important for maintenance of weight loss. Some, but not all, evidence suggests that the addition of exercise to caloric restriction may promote relatively greater weight loss from the visceral depot. The tendency for weight regain after successful weight reduction underscores the need for long-lasting behavioral changes.

Diet Before prescribing a weight-loss diet, it is important to emphasize that it takes a long time for a patient to achieve an expanded fat mass; thus, the correction need not occur quickly. On the basis of ~3500 kcal = one lb of fat, ~500 kcal restriction daily equates to a weight reduction of 1 lb per week. Diets restricted in carbohydrate typically provide a rapid initial weight loss. However, after one year, the amount of weight reduction is usually unchanged. Thus, adherence to the diet is more important than which diet is chosen. Moreover, there is concern about diets enriched in saturated fat, particularly for patients at risk for CVD. Therefore, a high quality of the diet—i.e., enriched in fruits, vegetables, whole grains, lean poultry, and fish—should be encouraged to provide the maximum overall health benefit.

Physical Activity Before a physical activity recommendation is provided to patients with the metabolic syndrome, it is important to ensure that this increased activity does not incur risk. Some high-risk patients should undergo formal cardiovascular evaluation before initiating an exercise program. For the inactive participant, gradual increases in physical activity should be encouraged to enhance adherence and to avoid injury. Although increases in physical activity can lead to modest weight reduction, 60–90 min of daily activity is required to achieve this goal. Even if an overweight or obese adult is unable to achieve this level of activity, they still derive a significant health benefit from at least 30 min of moderate intensity daily activity. The caloric value of 30 min of a variety of activities can be found at *http://www.americanheart.org/presenter.jhtml?identifier=3040364*. Of note, a variety of routine activities—such as gardening, walking, and housecleaning—require moderate caloric expenditure. Thus, physical activity need not be defined solely in terms of formal exercise such as jogging, swimming, or tennis.

Obesity (See also Chap. 75) In some patients with the metabolic syndrome, treatment options need to extend beyond lifestyle intervention. Weight-loss drugs come in two major classes: appetite suppressants and absorption inhibitors. Appetite suppressants approved by the Food and Drug Administration include phentermine (for short-term use only, 3 months) and sibutramine. Orlistat inhibits fat absorption by ~30% and is moderately effective compared to placebo (~5% weight loss). Orlistat has been shown to reduce the incidence of type 2 diabetes, an effect that was especially evident in patients with baseline IGT.

Bariatric surgery is an option for patients with the metabolic syndrome who have a body mass index (BMI) of >40 kg/m^2 or >35 kg/m^2 with comorbidities. Gastric bypass results in a dramatic weight reduction and improvement in the features of metabolic syndrome. At present, however, a survival benefit has yet to be realized.

LDL CHOLESTEROL (See also Chap. 350) The rationale for the NCEP:ATP III panel to develop criteria for the metabolic syndrome was to go beyond LDL cholesterol in identifying and reducing risk for CVD. The working assumption by the panel was that LDL cholesterol goals had already been achieved, and increasing evidence supports a linear reduction in CVD events with progressive lowering of LDL cholesterol. For patients with the metabolic syndrome and diabetes, LDL cholesterol should be reduced to <100 mg/dL and perhaps further in patients with a history of CVD events. For patients with the metabolic syndrome without diabetes, the Framingham risk score may predict a 10-year CVD risk that exceeds 20%. In these subjects, LDL cholesterol should also be reduced to <100 mg/dL. With a 10-year risk of < 20%, however, the targeted LDL cholesterol goal is < 130 mg/dL.

Diets restricted in saturated fats (<7% of calories), trans fat (as few as possible), and cholesterol (<200 mg daily) should be applied aggressively. If LDL cholesterol remains above goal, then pharmacologic intervention is needed. Statins (HMG-CoA reductase inhibitors), which produce a 20–60% lowering of LDL cholesterol, are generally the first choice for medication intervention. Of note, for each doubling of the statin dose, there is only ~6% additional lowering of LDL cholesterol. Side effects are rare and include an increase in hepatic transaminases and/or myopathy. The cholesterol absorption inhibitor ezetimibe is well tolerated and should be the second choice. Ezetimibe typically reduces LDL cholesterol by 15–20%. The bile acid sequestrants cholestyramine and colestipol are more effective than ezetimibe but must be used with caution in patients with the metabolic syndrome because they often increase triglycerides. In general, bile sequestrants should not be administered when fasting triglycerides are >200 mg/dL. Side effects include gastrointestinal symptoms (palatability, bloating, belching, constipation, anal irritation). Nicotinic acid has modest LDL cholesterol–lowering capabilities (<20%). Fibrates are best employed to lower LDL cholesterol when both LDL cholesterol and nontriglycerides are elevated. Fenofibrate may be more effective than gemfibrozil in this group.

TRIGLYCERIDES The NCEP:ATPIII has focused on non-HDL cholesterol rather than triglycerides. However, a fasting triglyceride value of <150 mg/dL is recommended. In general, the response of fasting triglycerides relates to the amount of weight reduction achieved. A weight reduction of >10% is necessary to lower fasting triglycerides.

A fibrate (gemfibrozil or fenofibrate) is the drug of choice to lower fasting triglycerides and typically achieve a 35–50% reduction. Concomitant administration with drugs metabolized by the 3A4 cytochrome P450 system (including some statins) greatly increases the risk of myopathy. In these cases, fenofibrate may be preferable to gemfibrozil. In the Veterans Affairs HDL Intervention Trial (VA-HIT), gemfibrozil was administered to men with known CHD and levels of HDL cholesterol <40 mg/dL. A coro-

nary disease event and mortality benefit was experienced predominantly in men with hyperinsulinemia and/or diabetes, many of whom retrospectively had the metabolic syndrome. Of note, the amount of triglyceride lowering in the VA-HIT did not predict benefit. Although levels of LDL cholesterol did not change, a decrease in LDL particle number related to benefit. Although several additional clinical trials have been performed, these have not shown clear evidence that fibrates reduce CVD risk as a consequence of triglyceride lowering.

Other drugs that lower triglycerides include statins, nicotinic acid, and high doses of omega-3 fatty acids. When choosing a statin for this purpose, the dose must be high for the "less potent" statins (lovastatin, pravastatin, fluvastatin) or intermediate for the "more potent" statins (simvastatin, atorvastatin, rosuvastatin). The effect of nicotinic acid on fasting triglycerides is dose-related and less than fibrates (~20–40%). In patients with the metabolic syndrome and diabetes, nicotinic acid may increase fasting glucose. Omega-3 fatty acid preparations that include high doses of docosahexaenoic acid and eicosapentaenoic acid (~3.0–4.5 g daily) lower fasting triglycerides by ~40%. No interactions with fibrates or statins occur, and the main side effect is eructation with a fishy taste. This can be partially blocked by ingesting the nutraceutical after freezing. Clinical trials of nicotinic acid or high-dose omega-3 fatty acids in patients with the metabolic syndrome have not been reported.

HDL CHOLESTEROL Beyond weight reduction, there are very few lipid-modifying compounds that increase HDL cholesterol. Statins, fibrates, and bile acid sequestrants have modest effects (5–10%), and there is no effect on HDL cholesterol with ezetimibe or omega-3 fatty acids. Nicotinic acid is the only currently available drug with predictable HDL cholesterol-raising properties. The response is dose-related and can increase HDL cholesterol ~30% above baseline. There is little evidence at present that raising HDL has a benefit on CVD events independent of lowering LDL cholesterol, particularly in patients with the metabolic syndrome.

BLOOD PRESSURE (See also Chap. 241) The direct relationship between blood pressure and all-cause mortality has been well established, including patients with hypertension (>140/90) versus prehypertension (>120/80 but <140/90) versus individuals with normal blood pressure (<120/80). In patients with the metabolic syndrome without diabetes, the best choice for the first antihypertensive should usually be an ACE inhibitor or an angiotensin II receptor blocker, as these two classes of drugs appear to reduce the incidence of new-onset type 2 diabetes. In all patients with hypertension, a sodium-restricted diet enriched in fruits and vegetables and low-fat dairy products should be advocated. Home monitoring of blood pressure may assist in maintaining good blood pressure control.

IMPAIRED FASTING GLUCOSE (See also Chap. 338) In patients with the metabolic syndrome and type 2 diabetes, aggressive glycemic control may favorably modify fasting triglycerides and/or HDL cholesterol. In those patients with IFG without a diagnosis of diabetes, a lifestyle intervention that includes weight reduction, dietary fat restriction, and increased physical activity has been shown to reduce the incidence of type 2 diabetes. Metformin has also been shown to reduce the incidence of diabetes, although the effect was less than that seen with lifestyle intervention.

INSULIN RESISTANCE (See also Chap. 338) Several drug classes [biguanides, thiazolidinediones (TZDs)] increase insulin sensitivity. If insulin resistance is the primary pathophysiologic mechanism for the metabolic syndrome, then representative drugs in these classes should reduce its prevalence. Both metformin and TZDs enhance insulin action in the liver and suppress endogenous glucose production. TZDs, but not metformin, also improve insulin-mediated glucose uptake in muscle and adipose tissue. Benefits of both drugs have also been seen in patients with NAFLD and PCOS, and they have been shown to reduce markers of inflammation and small dense LDL. In general, the beneficial effects of TZDs appear superior to those of metformin.

FURTHER READINGS

ALBERTI KG et al: The IDF Epidemiology Task Force Consensus Group. The metabolic syndrome—a new worldwide definition. Lancet 366:1059, 2005

ECKEL RH et al: The metabolic syndrome. Lancet 365:1415, 2005

EXPERT PANEL ON DETECTION EVALUATION, AND TREATMENT OF HIGH BLOOD CHOLESTEROL IN ADULTS: Executive summary of the third report of the National Cholesterol Education Program (NCEP) expert panel on detection, evaluation, and treatment of high blood cholesterol in adults (Adult Treatment Panel III). JAMA 285:2486, 2001

FORD ES: Prevalence of the metabolic syndrome defined by the International Diabetes Federation among adults in the U.S. Diabetes Care 28:2745, 2005

GRUNDY SM et al: Diagnosis and management of the metabolic syndrome. An American Heart Association/National Heart, Lung, and Blood Institute Scientific statement. Circulation 112:2735, 2005

———: Metabolic syndrome: Connecting and reconciling cardiovascular and diabetes worlds. J Am Coll Cardiol 47(6):1093, 2006

KAHN R et al: The metabolic syndrome: Time for a critical appraisal. Joint statement from the American Diabetes Association and the European Association for the Study of Diabetes. Diabetes Care 28:2289, 2005

237 Ischemic Heart Disease

Elliott M. Antman, Andrew P. Selwyn, Eugene Braunwald, Joseph Loscalzo

Ischemic heart disease (IHD) is a condition in which there is an inadequate supply of blood and oxygen to a portion of the myocardium; it typically occurs when there is an imbalance between myocardial oxygen supply and demand. The most common cause of myocardial ischemia is atherosclerotic disease of an epicardial coronary artery (or arteries) sufficient to cause a regional reduction in myocardial blood flow and inadequate perfusion of the myocardium supplied by the involved coronary artery.

EPIDEMIOLOGY

IHD causes more deaths and disability and incurs greater economic costs than any other illness in the developed world. IHD is the most common, serious, chronic, life-threatening illness in the United States, where 13 million persons have IHD, >6 million have angina pectoris, and >7 million have sustained a myocardial infarction (MI). A high-fat and energy-rich diet, smoking, and a sedentary lifestyle are associated with the emergence of IHD (Chap. 235). In the United States and western Europe, it is growing among low-income groups rather than high-income groups (who are adopting more healthful lifestyles), while primary prevention has delayed the disease to later in life in all socioeconomic groups.

Obesity, insulin resistance, and type 2 diabetes mellitus are increasing and are powerful risk factors for IHD. With urbanization in the developing world, the prevalence of risk factors for IHD is increasing rapidly in these regions such that a majority of the global burden of IHD is now occurring in low-income and middle-income countries. Population subgroups that appear to be particularly affected are men in South Asian countries, especially India. Given the projection of large increases in IHD throughout the world, IHD is likely to become the most common cause of death worldwide by 2020.

PATHOPHYSIOLOGY

Central to an understanding of the pathophysiology of myocardial ischemia is the concept of myocardial supply and demand. Under normal conditions, for any given level of a demand for oxygen, the myocardium will be supplied with oxygen-rich blood to prevent underperfusion of myocytes and the subsequent development of ischemia and infarction. The major determinants of myocardial oxygen demand (MVO$_2$) are heart rate, myocardial contractility, and myocardial wall tension (stress). An adequate supply of oxygen to the myocardium requires a satisfactory level of oxygen-carrying capacity of the blood (determined by the inspired level of oxygen, pulmonary function, and hemoglobin concentration and function) and an adequate level of coronary blood flow. Blood flows through the coronary arteries in a phasic fashion, with the majority occurring during diastole. About 75% of the total coronary resistance to flow occurs across three sets of arteries: (1) large epicardial arteries (Resistance 1 = R$_1$), (2) prearteriolar vessels (R$_2$), and (3) arteriolar and intramyocardial capillary vessels (R$_3$). In the absence of significant flow-limiting atherosclerotic obstructions, R$_1$ is trivial; the major determinant of coronary resistance is found in R$_2$ and R$_3$.

The normal coronary circulation is dominated and controlled by the heart's requirements for oxygen. This need is met by the ability of the coronary vascular bed to vary its resistance (and, therefore, blood flow) considerably while the myocardium extracts a high and relatively fixed percentage of oxygen. Normally, intramyocardial resistance vessels demonstrate an immense capacity for dilation (R$_2$ and R$_3$ decrease). For example, the changing oxygen needs of the heart with exercise and emotional stress affect coronary vascular resistance and in this manner regulate the supply of oxygen and substrate to the myocardium (*metabolic regulation*). The coronary resistance vessels also adapt to physiologic alterations in blood pressure in order to maintain coronary blood flow at levels appropriate to myocardial needs (*autoregulation*).

By reducing the lumen of the coronary arteries, atherosclerosis limits appropriate increases in perfusion when the demand for flow is augmented, as occurs during exertion or excitement. When the luminal reduction is severe, myocardial perfusion in the basal state is reduced. Coronary blood flow can also be limited by spasm (see "Prinzmetal's Variant Angina" in Chap. 238), arterial thrombi, and, rarely, coronary emboli as well as by ostial narrowing due to aortitis. Congenital abnormalities, such as origin of the left anterior descending coronary artery from the pulmonary artery, may cause myocardial ischemia and infarction in infancy, but this cause is very rare in adults.

Myocardial ischemia can also occur if myocardial oxygen demands are markedly increased and when coronary blood flow may be limited, as occurs in severe left ventricular (LV) hypertrophy due to aortic stenosis. The latter can present with angina that is indistinguishable from that caused by coronary atherosclerosis largely owing to subendocardial ischemia (Chap. 230). A reduction in the oxygen-carrying capacity of the blood, as in extremely severe anemia or in the presence of carboxyhemoglobin, rarely causes myocardial ischemia by itself but may lower the threshold for ischemia in patients with moderate coronary obstruction.

Not infrequently, two or more causes of ischemia coexist, such as an increase in oxygen demand due to LV hypertrophy secondary to hypertension and a reduction in oxygen supply secondary to coronary atherosclerosis and anemia. Abnormal constriction or failure of normal dilation of the coronary resistance vessels can also cause ischemia. When it causes angina, this condition is referred to as *microvascular angina*.

CORONARY ATHEROSCLEROSIS

Epicardial coronary arteries are the major site of atherosclerotic disease. The major risk factors for atherosclerosis [high plasma low-density lipoprotein (LDL), low plasma high-density lipoprotein (HDL), cigarette smoking, hypertension, and diabetes mellitus] (Chap. 235) disturb the normal functions of the vascular endothelium. These functions include local control of vascular tone, maintenance of an antithrombotic surface, and impairment of inflammatory cell adhesion and diapedesis. The loss of these defenses leads to inappropriate constriction, luminal thrombus formation, and abnormal interactions with blood leukocytes, especially monocytes, and platelets. Monocyte interaction ultimately results in the subintimal collections of fat, smooth-muscle cells, fibroblasts, and intercellular matrix (i.e., atherosclerotic plaques), which develop at irregular rates in different segments of the epicardial coronary tree and lead eventually to segmental reductions in cross-sectional area.

There is also a predilection for atherosclerotic plaques to develop at sites of increased turbulence in coronary flow, such as at branch points in the epicardial arteries. When a stenosis reduces the diameter of an epicardial artery by 50%, there is a limitation on the ability to increase flow to meet increased myocardial demand. When the diameter is reduced by ~80%, blood flow at rest may be reduced, and further minor decreases in the stenotic orifice area can reduce coronary flow dramatically and cause myocardial ischemia.

Segmental atherosclerotic narrowing of epicardial coronary arteries is caused most commonly by the formation of a plaque, which is subject to rupture or erosion of the cap separating the plaque from the bloodstream. Upon exposure of the plaque contents to blood, two important and interrelated processes are set in motion: (1) platelets are activated and aggregate; and (2) the coagulation cascade is activated, leading to deposition of fibrin strands. A thrombus composed of platelet aggregates and fibrin strands traps red blood cells and can reduce coronary blood flow, leading to the clinical manifestations of myocardial ischemia.

The location of the obstruction influences the quantity of myocardium rendered ischemic and determines the severity of the clinical manifestations. Thus, critical obstructions in vessels, such as the left main coronary artery or the proximal left anterior descending coronary artery, are particularly hazardous. Severe coronary narrowing and myocardial ischemia are frequently accompanied by the development of collateral vessels, especially when the narrowing develops gradually. When well developed, such vessels can, by themselves, provide sufficient blood flow to sustain the viability of the myocardium at rest but not during conditions of increased demand.

With progressive worsening of a proximal epicardial artery stenosis, the distal resistance vessels (when they function normally) dilate to reduce vascular resistance and maintain coronary blood flow. A pressure gradient develops across the proximal stenosis, and poststenotic pressure falls. When the resistance vessels are maximally dilated, myocardial blood flow becomes dependent on the pressure in the coronary artery distal to the obstruction. In these circumstances, ischemia, manifest clinically by angina or electrocardiographically by ST-segment deviation, can be precipitated by increases in myocardial oxygen demand caused by physical activity, emotional stress, and/or tachycardia. Changes in the caliber of the stenosed coronary artery due to physiologic vasomotion, loss of endothelial control of dilation (as occurs in diabetes mellitus), pathologic spasm (Prinzmetal's angina), or small platelet-rich plugs can also upset the critical balance between oxygen supply and demand and thereby precipitate myocardial ischemia.

EFFECTS OF ISCHEMIA
During episodes of inadequate perfusion caused by coronary atherosclerosis, myocardial tissue oxygen tension falls and may cause transient disturbances of the mechanical, biochemical, and electrical functions of the myocardium. Coronary atherosclerosis is a focal process that usually causes nonuniform ischemia. Regional disturbances of ventricular contractility cause segmental akinesia or, in severe cases, bulging (dyskinesia), which can greatly reduce myocardial pump function.

The abrupt development of severe ischemia, as occurs with total or subtotal coronary occlusion, is associated with almost instantaneous failure of normal muscle contraction and relaxation. The relatively poor perfusion of the subendocardium causes more intense ischemia of this portion of the wall (compared with the subepicardial region). Ischemia of large portions of the ventricle causes transient LV failure, and if the papillary muscle apparatus is involved, mitral regurgitation can occur. When ischemia is transient, it may be associated with angina pectoris; when it is prolonged, it can lead to myocardial necrosis and scarring with or without the clinical picture of acute MI (Chap. 239).

A wide range of abnormalities in cell metabolism, function, and structure underlie these mechanical disturbances during ischemia. The normal myocardium metabolizes fatty acids and glucose to carbon dioxide and water. With severe oxygen deprivation, fatty acids cannot be oxidized, and glucose is degraded to lactate; intracellular pH is reduced, as are the myocardial stores of high-energy phosphates, i.e., ATP and creatine phos-

phate. Impaired cell membrane function leads to the leakage of potassium and the uptake of sodium by myocytes, as well as an increase in cytosolic calcium. The severity and duration of the imbalance between myocardial oxygen supply and demand determine whether the damage is reversible (≤20 min for total occlusion in the absence of collaterals) or whether it is permanent, with subsequent myocardial necrosis (>20 min).

Ischemia also causes characteristic changes in the electrocardiogram (ECG) such as repolarization abnormalities, as evidenced by inversion of T waves and, when more severe, by displacement of ST segments (Chap. 221). Transient T-wave inversion likely reflects nontransmural, intramyocardial ischemia; transient ST-segment depression often reflects subendocardial ischemia; and ST-segment elevation is thought to be caused by more severe transmural ischemia. Another important consequence of myocardial ischemia is electrical instability, which may lead to isolated ventricular premature beats or even ventricular tachycardia or ventricular fibrillation (Chap. 226). Most patients who die suddenly from IHD do so as a result of ischemia-induced ventricular tachyarrhythmias (Chap. 267).

ASYMPTOMATIC VERSUS SYMPTOMATIC IHD
Postmortem studies on accident victims and military casualties in western countries have shown that coronary atherosclerosis often begins to develop prior to age 20 and is widespread even among adults who were asymptomatic during life. Exercise stress tests in asymptomatic persons may show evidence of silent myocardial ischemia, i.e., exercise-induced ECG changes not accompanied by angina pectoris; coronary angiographic studies of such persons may reveal coronary artery plaques and previously unrecognized obstructions (Chap. 223). Postmortem examination of patients with such obstructions without a history of clinical manifestations of myocardial ischemia often shows macroscopic scars secondary to MI in regions supplied by diseased coronary arteries, with or without collateral circulation. According to population studies, ~25% of patients who survive acute MI may not come to medical attention, and these patients carry the same adverse prognosis as those who present with the classic clinical picture of acute MI (Chap. 239). Sudden death may be unheralded and is a common presenting manifestation of IHD (Chap. 267).

Patients with IHD can also present with cardiomegaly and heart failure secondary to ischemic damage of the LV myocardium that may have caused no symptoms prior to the development of heart failure; this condition is referred to as *ischemic cardiomyopathy*. In contrast to the asymptomatic phase of IHD, the symptomatic phase is characterized by chest discomfort due to either angina pectoris or acute MI (Chap. 239). Having entered the symptomatic phase, the patient may exhibit a stable or progressive course, revert to the asymptomatic stage, or die suddenly.

STABLE ANGINA PECTORIS

This episodic clinical syndrome is due to transient myocardial ischemia. Males constitute ~70% of all patients with angina pectoris and an even greater fraction of those less than 50 years of age. Various diseases that cause myocardial ischemia as well as the numerous forms of discomfort with which it may be confused are discussed in Chap. 13.

HISTORY
The typical patient with angina is a man older than 50 years or a woman older than 60 years of age who complains of chest discomfort, usually described as heaviness, pressure, squeezing, smothering, or choking, and only rarely as frank pain. When the patient is asked to localize the sensation, he or she will typically place their hand over the sternum, sometimes with a clenched fist, to indicate a squeezing, central, substernal discomfort (Levine's sign). Angina is usually crescendo-decrescendo in nature, typically lasts 2–5 min, and can radiate to either shoulder and to both arms (especially the ulnar surfaces of the forearm and hand). It can also arise in or radiate to the back, interscapular region, root of the neck, jaw, teeth, and epigastrium. Angina is rarely

localized below the umbilicus or above the mandible. A useful finding in assessing the patient with chest discomfort is the fact that myocardial ischemic discomfort does not radiate to the trapezius muscles; such a radiation pattern is more typical of pericarditis.

Although episodes of angina are typically caused by exertion (e.g., exercise, hurrying, or sexual activity) or emotion (e.g., stress, anger, fright, or frustration) and are relieved by rest, they may also occur at rest (Chap. 238) and while the patient is recumbent (angina decubitus). The patient may be awakened at night by typical chest discomfort and dyspnea. Nocturnal angina may be due to episodic tachycardia, diminished oxygenation as the respiratory pattern changes during sleep, or expansion of the intrathoracic blood volume that occurs with recumbency; the latter causes an increase in cardiac size (end-diastolic volume), in wall tension, and in myocardial oxygen demand that lead to ischemia and transient LV failure.

The threshold for the development of angina pectoris may vary by time of day and emotional state. Many patients report a fixed threshold for angina, which occurs predictably at a certain level of activity, such as climbing two flights of stairs at a normal pace. In these patients, coronary stenosis and myocardial oxygen supply are fixed, and ischemia is precipitated by an increase in myocardial oxygen demand; they are said to have *stable exertional angina*. In other patients, the threshold for angina may vary considerably within any given day and from day to day. In such patients, variations in myocardial oxygen supply, most likely due to changes in coronary vascular tone, may play an important role in defining the pattern of angina. A patient may report symptoms upon minor exertion in the morning (a short walk or shaving), yet, by midday, may be capable of much greater effort without symptoms. Angina may also be precipitated by unfamiliar tasks, a heavy meal, exposure to cold, or a combination.

Exertional angina is typically relieved by slowing or ceasing activities in 1–5 min and even more rapidly by rest and sublingual nitroglycerin (see below). Indeed, the diagnosis of angina should be suspect if it does not respond to the combination of these measures. The severity of angina can be conveniently summarized by the Canadian Cardiac Society functional classification (Table 237-1). Its impact on the patient's functional capacity can be described using the New York Heart Association functional classification (Table 237-1).

Sharp, fleeting chest pain or a prolonged, dull ache localized to the left submammary area is rarely due to myocardial ischemia. However, especially in women and diabetics, angina pectoris may be atypical in location and not strictly related to provoking factors. In addition, this symptom may exacerbate and remit over days, weeks, or months. Its occurrence can be seasonal, being more frequent in the winter in temperate climates. Anginal "equivalents" are symptoms of myocardial ischemia other than angina. These include dyspnea, nausea, fatigue, and faintness, and are more common in the elderly and in diabetic patients.

Systematic questioning of the patient with suspected IHD is important to uncover the features of an unstable syndrome associated with increased risk, such as angina occurring with less exertion than in the past or occurring at rest or awakening the patient from sleep. Since coronary atherosclerosis is often accompanied by similar lesions in other arteries, the patient with angina should be questioned and examined for peripheral arterial disease (intermittent claudication, Chap. 243), stroke, or transient ischemic attacks (Chap. 364). It is also important to uncover a family history of premature IHD (<45 years in first-degree male relatives and <55 in female relatives) and the presence of diabetes mellitus, hyperlipidemia, hypertension, cigarette smoking, and other risk factors for coronary atherosclerosis (Chap. 235). The history of typical angina pectoris establishes the diagnosis of IHD until proven otherwise. In patients with atypical angina (Chap. 13), the coexistence of advanced age, male gender, the postmenopausal state, and risk factors for atherosclerosis increase the likelihood of hemodynamically significant coronary disease.

PHYSICAL EXAMINATION

This is often normal in patients with stable angina when they are asymptomatic, but it may reveal evidence of atherosclerotic disease at

TABLE 237-1 CARDIOVASCULAR DISEASE CLASSIFICATION CHART

Class	New York Heart Association Functional Classification	Canadian Cardiovascular Society Functional Classification
I	Patients have cardiac disease but *without* the resulting *limitations* of physical activity. Ordinary physical activity does not cause undue fatigue, palpitation, dyspnea, or anginal pain.	Ordinary physical activity, such as walking and climbing stairs, *does not cause angina*. Angina present with strenuous or rapid or prolonged exertion at work or recreation.
II	Patients have cardiac disease resulting in *slight limitation* of physical activity. They are comfortable at rest. Ordinary physical activity results in fatigue, palpitation, dyspnea, or anginal pain.	*Slight limitation* of ordinary activity. Walking or climbing stairs rapidly, walking uphill, walking or stair climbing after meals, in cold, or when under emotional stress or only during the few hours after awakening. Walking more than two blocks on the level and climbing more than one flight of stairs at a normal pace and in normal conditions.
III	Patients have cardiac disease resulting in *marked limitation* of physical activity. They are comfortable at rest. Less than ordinary physical activity causes fatigue, palpitation, dyspnea, or anginal pain.	*Marked limitation* of ordinary physical activity. Walking one to two blocks on the level and climbing more than one flight of stairs in normal conditions.
IV	Patients have cardiac disease resulting in *inability* to carry on any physical activity without discomfort. Symptoms of cardiac insufficiency or of the anginal syndrome may be present even at rest. If any physical activity is undertaken, discomfort is increased.	*Inability* to carry on any physical activity without discomfort—anginal syndrome may be present at rest.

Source: Modified from L Goldman et al: Circulation 64:1227, 1981.

other sites, such as an abdominal aortic aneurysm, carotid arterial bruits, and diminished arterial pulse in the lower extremities, or of risk factors for atherosclerosis, such as xanthelasmas and xanthomas (Chap. 235). Examination of the fundi may reveal an increased light reflex and arteriovenous nicking as evidence of hypertension. There may also be signs of anemia, thyroid disease, and nicotine stains on the fingertips from cigarette smoking. Palpation may reveal cardiac enlargement and abnormal contraction of the cardiac impulse (left ventricular akinesia or dyskinesia).

Auscultation can uncover arterial bruits, a third and/or fourth heart sound, and, if acute ischemia or previous infarction has impaired papillary muscle function, an apical systolic murmur due to mitral regurgitation. These auscultatory signs are best appreciated with the patient in the left lateral decubitus position. Aortic stenosis, aortic regurgitation (Chap. 230), pulmonary hypertension (Chap. 244), and hypertrophic cardiomyopathy (Chap. 231) must be excluded, since these disorders may cause angina in the absence of coronary atherosclerosis. Examination during an anginal attack is useful, since ischemia can cause transient LV failure with the appearance of a third and/or fourth heart sound, a dyskinetic cardiac apex, mitral regurgitation, and even pulmonary edema. Tenderness of the chest wall, localization of the discomfort with a single fingertip on the chest, or reproduction of the pain with palpation of the chest makes it unlikely that it is caused by myocardial ischemia.

LABORATORY EXAMINATION

Although the diagnosis of IHD can be made with a high degree of confidence from the clinical examination, a number of simple laboratory tests can be helpful. The urine should be examined for evidence of diabetes mellitus and renal disease (including microalbuminuria) since these conditions accelerate atherosclerosis. Similarly, examination of the blood should include measurements of lipids (cholesterol—total, LDL, HDL—and triglycerides), glucose, creatinine, hematocrit, and, if indicated based on the physical examination, thyroid function. A chest x-ray is important as it may show the consequences of IHD, i.e., cardiac enlargement, ventricular aneurysm, or signs of heart failure. These signs can support the diagnosis of IHD and are important in assessing the degree of cardiac damage.

ELECTROCARDIOGRAM

A 12-lead ECG recorded at rest may be normal in patients with typical angina pectoris, but there may also be signs of an old myocardial infarction (Chap. 221). Although repolarization abnormalities—i.e., ST-segment and T-wave changes—as well as LV hypertrophy and intraventricular conduction disturbances are suggestive of IHD, they are nonspecific since they can also occur in pericardial, myocardial, and valvular heart disease or, in the case of the former, transiently with anxiety, changes in posture, drugs, or esophageal disease. Dynamic ST-segment and T-wave changes that accompany episodes of angina pectoris and disappear thereafter are more specific.

STRESS TESTING

Electrocardiographic The most widely used test for both the diagnosis of IHD and estimating the prognosis involves recording the 12-lead ECG before, during, and after exercise, usually on a treadmill (Fig. 237-1). The test consists of a standardized incremental increase in external workload (Table 237-2) while the symptoms, ECG, and arm blood pressure are monitored. Performance is usually symptom-limited, and the test is discontinued upon evidence of chest discomfort, severe shortness of breath, dizziness, severe fatigue, ST-segment depression >0.2 mV (2 mm), a fall in systolic blood pressure >10 mmHg, or the development of a ventricular tachyarrhythmia. This test seeks to discover any limitation in exercise performance, to detect typical ECG signs of myocardial ischemia, and to establish their relationship to chest discomfort. The ischemic ST-segment response is generally defined as flat or downsloping depression of the ST segment >0.1 mV below baseline (i.e., the PR segment) and lasting longer than 0.08 s (Fig. 237-1). Upsloping or junctional ST-segment changes are not

A

Rest

Stress

B

FIGURE 237-1 Evaluation of the patient with known or suspected ischemic heart disease. At the top of the figure is an algorithm for identifying patients who should be referred for stress testing and the decision pathway for determining if a standard treadmill exercise with ECG monitoring alone is adequate. A specialized imaging study is necessary if the patient cannot exercise adequately (pharmacologic challenge is given) or if there are confounding features on the resting ECG (symptom limited treadmill exercise may be used to stress the coronary circulation). At the bottom of the figure are examples of the data obtained with ECG monitoring and specialized imaging procedures. IHD, ischemic heart disease; EBCT, electron beam computed tomography; ECG, electrocardiogram; MR, magnetic resonance; PET, positron emission tomography; ECHO, echocardiography; MIBI, methoxyisobutyl isonitrite; CMR, cardiac magnetic resonance.
A. Lead V$_4$ at rest (*top*) and after 4^1/$_2$ min of exercise (*bottom*). There is 3 mm (0.3 mV) of horizontal ST-segment depression, indicating a positive test for ischemia. [*Modified from BR Chaitman, in E Braunwald et al (eds): Heart Disease, 6th ed. Philadelphia, Saunders, 2001.*]
B. 45-year-old avid jogger who began experiencing classic substernal chest pressure underwent an exercise echo study. With exercise the patient's heart rate increased from 52 to 153 bpm. The left ventricular chamber dilated with exercise, and the septal and apical portions became akinetic to dyskinetic (*red arrow*). These findings are strongly suggestive of a significant flow limiting stenosis in the proximal left anterior descending coronary artery, which was confirmed at coronary angiography. [*Modified from SD Solomon, in E. Braunwald et al (eds): Primary Cardiology, 2d ed. Philadelphia, Saunders, 2003.*] *(continued)*

C

D

FIGURE 237-1 *(Continued)* **C.** Stress and rest myocardial perfusion SPECT images obtained with Tc99m sestamibi in a patient with chest pain and dyspnea on exertion. The images demonstrate a medium size and severe stress perfusion defect involving the inferolateral and basal inferior walls, showing near complete reversibility, consistent with moderate ischemia in the right coronary artery territory (*red arrows*). *(Images provided by Dr. Marcello Di Carli, Nuclear Medicine Division, Brigham and Women's Hospital, Boston, MA.)*

D. A patient with a prior myocardial infarction presented with recurrent chest discomfort. On CMR cine imaging a large area of anterior akinesia was noted (marked by the arrows in the top left and right images, systolic frame only). This area of akinesia was matched by a larger extent of late gadolinium-DTPA enhancements consistent with a large transmural myocardial infarction (marked by arrows in the middle left and right images). Resting (*bottom left*) and adenosine vasodilating stress (*bottom right*) first-pass perfusion images revealed reversible perfusion abnormality that extends to the inferior septum. This patient was found to have an occluded proximal left anterior descending coronary artery with extensive collateral formation. This case illustrates the utility of different modalities in a CMR examination in characterizing ischemic and infarcted myocardium. CMR, cardiac magnetic resonance; DTPA, diethylenetriamine pentaacetic acid *(Images provided by Dr. Raymond Kwong, Cardiovascular Division, Brigham and Women's Hospital, Boston, MA.)*

E. Stress and rest myocardial perfusion PET images obtained with rubidium-82 in a patient with chest pain on exertion. The images demonstrate a large and severe stress perfusion defect involving the mid and apical anterior, anterolateral, and anteroseptal walls, and the LV apex, showing complete reversibility, consistent with extensive and severe ischemia in the mid left anterior descending coronary artery territory (*red arrows*). *(Images provided by Dr. Marcello Di Carli, Nuclear Medicine Division, Brigham and Women's Hospital, Boston, MA.)*

E

TABLE 237-2 RELATION OF METS TO STAGES IN VARIOUS TESTING PROTOCOLS

NYHA Functional Class	Clinical Status	O₂ Cost mL/kg per min	METS	BRUCE Modified 3 min Stages MPH	%GR	BRUCE 3 min Stages MPH	%GR
				6.0	22	6.0	22
				5.5	20	5.5	20
				5.0	18	5.0	18
Normal and I	Healthy, dependent on age, activity	56.0	16				
		52.5	15				
		49.0	14				
		45.5	13	4.2	16	4.2	16
		42.0	12				
		38.5	11	3.4	14	3.4	14
	Sedentary healthy	35.0	10				
		31.5	9				
		28.0	8				
		24.5	7	2.5	12	2.5	12
		21.0	6				
II	Limited	17.5	5	1.7	10	1.7	10
		14.0	4				
III	Symptomatic	10.5	3	1.7	5		
		7.0	2	1.7	0		
IV		3.5	1				

Source: Modified from GF Fletcher et al: Circulation 104:1694, 2001.

considered characteristic of ischemia and do not constitute a positive test. Although T-wave abnormalities, conduction disturbances, and ventricular arrhythmias that develop during exercise should be noted, they are also not diagnostic. Negative exercise tests in which the target heart rate (85% of maximal predicted heart rate for age and sex) is not achieved are considered to be nondiagnostic.

When interpreting ECG stress tests, the probability that coronary artery disease (CAD) exists in the patient or population under study (i.e., pretest probability) should be considered. Overall, false-positive or false-negative results occur in one-third of cases. However, a positive result on exercise indicates that the likelihood of CAD is 98% in males >50 years with a history of typical angina pectoris and who develop chest discomfort during the test. The likelihood decreases if the patient has atypical or no chest pain by history and/or during the test.

The incidence of false-positive tests is significantly increased in patients with low probabilities of IHD, such as asymptomatic men under the age of 40 or in premenopausal women with no risk factors for premature atherosclerosis. It is also increased in patients taking cardioactive drugs, such as digitalis and antiarrhythmic agents, or in those with intraventricular conduction disturbances, resting ST-segment and T-wave abnormalities, ventricular hypertrophy, or abnormal serum potassium levels. Obstructive disease limited to the circumflex coronary artery may result in a false-negative stress test since the lateral portion of the heart which this vessel supplies is not well represented on the surface 12-lead ECG. Since the overall sensitivity of exercise stress electrocardiography is only ~75%, a negative result does not exclude CAD, although it makes the likelihood of three-vessel or left main CAD extremely unlikely.

The physician should be present throughout the exercise test, and it is important to measure total duration of exercise, the times to the onset of ischemic ST-segment change and chest discomfort, the external work performed (generally expressed as the stage of exercise), and the internal cardiac work performed, i.e., by the heart rate–blood pressure product. The depth of the ST-segment depression and the time needed for recovery of these ECG changes are also important. Because the risks of exercise testing are small but real—estimated at one fatality and two nonfatal complications per 10,000 tests—equipment for resuscitation should be available. Modified (heart rate–limited rather than symptom-limited) exercise tests can be performed safely in patients as early as 6 days after uncomplicated MI (Table 237-2). Contraindications to exercise stress testing include rest angina within 48 h, unstable rhythm, severe aortic stenosis, acute myocarditis, uncontrolled heart failure, severe pulmonary hypertension, and active infective endocarditis.

The normal response to graded exercise includes progressive increases in heart rate and blood pressure. Failure of the blood pressure to increase or an actual decrease with signs of ischemia during the test is an important adverse prognostic sign, since it may reflect ischemia-induced global LV dysfunction. The development of angina and/or severe (>0.2 mV) ST-segment depression at a low workload, i.e., before completion of stage II of the Bruce protocol, and/or ST-segment depression that persists for >5 min after the termination of exercise increases the specificity of the test and suggests severe IHD and a high risk of future adverse events.

Cardiac Imaging (See also Chap. 222) When the resting ECG is abnormal (e.g., preexcitation syndrome, >1 mm of resting ST-segment depression, left bundle branch block, paced ventricular rhythm), information gained from an exercise test can be enhanced by stress myocardial radionuclide perfusion imaging after the intravenous administration of thallium 201 or technetium 99m (⁹⁹ᵐTc) sestamibi during exercise (or a pharmacologic) stress. Recent data also suggest positron emission tomography (PET) imaging (with exercise or pharmacologic stress) using N-13 ammonia or rubidium-82 nuclide as another technique for assessing perfusion. Images obtained immediately after cessation of exercise to detect regional ischemia are compared with those obtained at rest to confirm reversible ischemia and regions of persistent absent uptake that signify infarction.

A sizable fraction of patients who need noninvasive stress testing to identify myocardial ischemia and increased risk of coronary events cannot exercise because of peripheral vascular or musculoskeletal disease, exertional dyspnea, or deconditioning. In these circumstances an intravenous pharmacologic challenge is used in place of exercise. For example, dipyridamole or adenosine can be given to create a coronary "steal" by temporarily increasing flow in nondiseased segments of the coronary vasculature at the expense of diseased segments. Alternatively, a graded incremental infusion of dobutamine may be administered to increase MVO₂. A variety of imaging options are available to accompany these pharmacologic stressors (Fig. 237-1). The development of a transient perfusion defect with a tracer such as radioactive thallium or ⁹⁹ᵐTc sestamibi is used to detect myocardial ischemia.

Two-dimensional echocardiography can assess both global and regional wall motion abnormalities of the left ventricle due to MI or persistent ischemia. Stress (exercise or dobutamine) echocardiography may cause the emergence of regions of akinesis or dyskinesis not present at rest. Stress echocardiography, like stress myocardial perfusion imaging, is more sensitive than exercise electrocardiography in the diagnosis of IHD. Cardiac magnetic resonance (CMR) stress testing is also evolving as an alternative to radionuclide, PET, or echocardiographic stress imaging. CMR stress testing performed with dobutamine infusion can be used to assess wall motion abnormalities accompanying ischemia, and myocardial perfusion CMR can be used to provide rather complete ventricular evaluation using multislice MR imaging studies. Ambulatory monitoring of the ECG can assess myocardial ischemia as episodes of ST-segment depression. Echocardiography or radionuclide angiography should be carried out to assess LV function in patients with chronic stable angina and in patients with a history of a prior MI, pathologic Q waves, or clinical evidence of heart failure.

Atherosclerotic plaques become progressively calcified over time, and coronary calcification in general increases with age. For this reason, methods for detecting coronary calcium have been developed as a measure of the presence of coronary atherosclerosis. These methods involve computed tomography (CT) applications that achieve rapid acquisition of images [ultrafast or electron beam (EBCT) and multidetector (MDCT)]. Coronary calcium detected by these imaging techniques is quantified using the Agatston score most commonly, which is based on the area and density of calcification. Although the diagnostic accuracy of this imaging method is high (sensitivity, 90–94%; specificity, 95–97%; negative predictive value, 93–99%), its prognostic utility and its role in the evaluative algorithm of patients with stable angina pectoris have not yet been defined.

CORONARY ARTERIOGRAPHY

(See also Chap. 223) This diagnostic method outlines the lumina of the coronary arteries and can be used to detect or exclude serious coronary obstruction. However, coronary arteriography provides no information regarding the arterial wall, and severe atherosclerosis that does not encroach on the lumen may go undetected. Of note, atherosclerotic plaques characteristically grow progressively in the intima and media of an epicardial coronary artery, at first without encroaching on the lumen, causing an outward bulging of the artery—a process referred to as negative remodeling (Chap. 235). Later in the course of the disease, further growth causes luminal narrowing.

Indications Coronary arteriography is indicated in (1) patients with chronic stable angina pectoris who are severely symptomatic despite medical therapy and who are being considered for revascularization, i.e., a percutaneous coronary intervention (PCI) or coronary artery bypass grafting (CABG); (2) patients with troublesome symptoms that present diagnostic difficulties in whom there is a need to confirm or rule out the diagnosis of IHD; (3) patients with known or possible angina pectoris who have survived cardiac arrest; (4) patients with angina or evidence of ischemia on noninvasive testing with clinical or laboratory evidence of ventricular dysfunction; and (5) patients judged to be at high risk of sustaining coronary events based on signs of severe ischemia on noninvasive testing, regardless of the presence or severity of symptoms (see below). Examples of other indications include:

1. Patients with chest discomfort suggestive of angina pectoris but a negative or nondiagnostic stress test who require a definitive diagnosis for guiding medical management, alleviating psychological stress, career or family planning, or insurance purposes.

2. Patients who have been admitted repeatedly to the hospital for a suspected acute coronary syndrome (Chaps. 238 and 239) but in whom this diagnosis has not been established and in whom the presence or absence of CAD should be determined.

3. Patients with careers that involve the safety of others (e.g., pilots, firefighters, police) who have questionable symptoms or suspicious or positive noninvasive tests, and in whom there are reasonable doubts about the state of the coronary arteries.

4. Patients with aortic stenosis or hypertrophic cardiomyopathy and angina in whom the chest pain could be due to IHD.

5. Male patients >45 years and females >55 years who are to undergo a cardiac operation, such as valve replacement or repair, and who may or may not have clinical evidence of myocardial ischemia.

6. Patients following myocardial infarction, especially those who are at high risk after MI because of the recurrence of angina or the presence of heart failure, frequent ventricular premature contractions, or signs of ischemia on the stress test.

7. Patients with angina pectoris, regardless of severity, in whom noninvasive testing indicates a high risk of coronary events.

8. Patients in whom coronary spasm or another nonatherosclerotic cause of myocardial ischemia (e.g., coronary artery anomaly, Kawasaki's disease) is suspected.

Noninvasive alternatives to diagnostic coronary arteriography include CT angiography and cardiac MR angiography (Chap. 222). While these new imaging techniques can provide information about obstructive lesions in the epicardial coronary arteries, their exact role in clinical practice has not yet been rigorously defined. Important aspects of their use that should be noted include the substantially higher radiation exposure with CT angiography compared to conventional diagnostic arteriography and the limitations on cardiac MR imposed by cardiac movement during the cardiac cycle, especially at high heart rates.

PROGNOSIS

The principal prognostic indicators in patients known to have IHD are age, the functional state of the left ventricle, the location(s) and severity of coronary artery narrowing, and the severity or activity of myocardial ischemia. Angina pectoris of recent onset, unstable angina (Chap. 238), early postmyocardial infarction angina, and angina that is unresponsive or poorly responsive to medical therapy or is accompanied by symptoms of congestive heart failure all indicate an increased risk for adverse coronary events. The same is true for the physical signs of heart failure, episodes of pulmonary edema, transient third heart sounds, or mitral regurgitation, and for echocardiographic or radioisotopic (or roentgenographic) evidence of cardiac enlargement and reduced (<0.40) ejection fraction.

Most importantly, any of the following signs during noninvasive testing indicate a high risk for coronary events: inability to exercise for 6 min, i.e., stage II (Bruce protocol) of the exercise test; a strongly positive exercise test showing onset of myocardial ischemia at low workloads (≥0.1 mV ST-segment depression before completion of stage II; ≥0.2 mV ST depression at any stage; ST depression for >5 min following the cessation of exercise; a decline in systolic pressure >10 mmHg during exercise; the development of ventricular tachyarrhythmias during exercise); the development of large or multiple perfusion defects or increased lung uptake during stress radioisotope perfusion imaging; and a decrease in LV ejection fraction (LVEF) during exercise on radionuclide ventriculography or during stress echocardiography. Conversely, patients who can complete stage III of the Bruce exercise protocol and have a normal stress perfusion scan or negative stress echocardiographic evaluation are at very low risk of future coronary events.

On cardiac catheterization, elevations of LV end-diastolic pressure and ventricular volume and reduced ejection fraction are the most important signs of LV dysfunction and are associated with a poor prognosis. Patients with chest discomfort but normal LV function and normal coronary arteries have an excellent prognosis. Obstructive lesions of the left main (>50% luminal diameter) or left anterior descending coronary artery proximal to the origin of the first septal artery are associated with a greater risk than are lesions of the right or left circumflex coronary artery because of the greater quantity of myocardium at risk. Atherosclerotic plaques in epicardial arteries with fissuring or filling defects indicate increased risk. These lesions go through phases of inflammatory cellular activity, degeneration, endothelial dysfunction, abnormal vasomotion, platelet aggregation, and fissuring or hemorrhage. These factors can temporarily worsen the stenosis and cause abnormal reactivity of the vessel wall, thus exacerbating the manifestations of ischemia. The recent onset of symptoms, the development of severe ischemia during stress testing (see above), and unstable angina pectoris (Chap. 238) all reflect episodes of rapid progression in coronary lesions.

With any degree of obstructive CAD, mortality is greatly increased when LV function is impaired; conversely, at any level of LV function, the prognosis is influenced importantly by the quantity of myocardium perfused by critically obstructed vessels. Therefore, it is useful to collect all the evidence substantiating past myocardial damage (evidence of MI on ECG, echocardiography, radioisotope imaging, or left ventriculography), residual LV function (ejection fraction and wall motion), and risk of future damage from coronary events (extent of coronary disease and severity of ischemia defined by noninvasive stress testing). The larger the quantity of established myocardial necrosis, the less the heart is able to withstand additional damage and the poorer the prognosis. All the above signs of past damage plus the risk of future damage should be considered indicators of risk.

The greater the number and severity of risk factors for coronary atherosclerosis [advanced age (>75 years), diabetes, morbid obesity, accompanying peripheral and/or cerebrovascular disease, previous MI], the worse the prognosis of the angina patient. Evidence exists that elevated levels of C-reactive protein in the plasma, extensive coronary calcification on EBCT (see above), and increased carotid intimal thickening on ultrasound examination also indicate an increased risk of coronary events.

℞ STABLE ANGINA PECTORIS

Each patient must be evaluated individually with respect to his or her expectations and goals, control of symptoms, and prevention of adverse clinical outcomes, such as MI and premature death. The degree of disability as well as the physical and emotional stress that precipitates angina must be carefully recorded in order to set treatment goals. The management plan should include the following components: (1) explanation of the problem and reassurance about the ability to formulate a treatment plan, (2) identification and treatment of aggravating conditions, (3) recommendations for adaptation of activity as needed, (4) treatment of risk factors that will decrease the occurrence of adverse coronary outcomes, (5) drug therapy for angina, and (6) consideration of revascularization.

EXPLANATION AND REASSURANCE Patients with IHD need to understand their condition and to realize that a long and productive life is possible even though they suffer from angina pectoris or have experienced and recovered from an acute MI. Offering results of clinical trials showing improved outcomes can be of great value when encouraging patients to resume or maintain activity and return to their occupation. A planned program of rehabilitation can encourage patients to lose weight, improve exercise tolerance, and control risk factors with more confidence.

IDENTIFICATION AND TREATMENT OF AGGRAVATING CONDITIONS A number of conditions may either increase oxygen demand or decrease oxygen supply to the myocardium and may precipitate or exacerbate angina in patients with IHD. Aortic valve disease and hypertrophic cardiomyopathy may cause or contribute to angina and should be excluded or treated. Obesity, hypertension, and hyperthyroidism should be treated aggressively in order to reduce the frequency and severity of anginal episodes. Decreased myocardial oxygen supply may be due to reduced oxygenation of the arterial blood (e.g., in pulmonary disease or, when carboxyhemoglobin is present, due to cigarette or cigar smoking) or decreased oxygen-carrying capacity (e.g., in anemia). Correction of these abnormalities, if present, may reduce or even eliminate angina pectoris.

ADAPTATION OF ACTIVITY Myocardial ischemia is caused by a discrepancy between the demand of the heart muscle for oxygen and the ability of the coronary circulation to meet this demand. Most patients can be helped to understand this concept and utilize it in the rational programming of activity. Many tasks that ordinarily evoke angina may be accomplished without symptoms simply by reducing the speed at which they are performed. Patients must appreciate the diurnal variation in their tolerance of certain activities and should reduce their energy requirements in the morning, immediately after meals, and in cold or inclement weather.

On occasion, it may be necessary to recommend a change in employment or residence to avoid physical stress. However, with the exception of manual laborers, most patients with IHD can continue to function merely by allowing more time to complete each task. In some patients, anger and frustration may be the most important factors precipitating myocardial ischemia. If these cannot be avoided, training in stress management may be useful. A treadmill exercise test to determine the approximate heart rate at which ischemic ECG changes or symptoms develop may be helpful in the development of a specific exercise program.

Physical conditioning usually improves the exercise tolerance of patients with angina and exerts substantial psychological benefits. A regular program of isotonic exercise that is within the limits of each patient's threshold for the development of angina pectoris and does not exceed 80% of the heart rate associated with ischemia on exercise testing should be strongly encouraged. Based on the results of an exercise test, the number of METS performed at the onset of ischemia can be estimated (Table 237-2) and a practical exercise prescription can be formulated to permit daily activities that will fall below the ischemic threshold **(Table 237-3)**.

TREATMENT OF RISK FACTORS A *family history* of premature IHD is an important indicator of increased risk and should trigger a search for treatable risk factors such as hyperlipidemia, hypertension, and diabetes mellitus. *Obesity* impairs the treatment of other risk factors and increases the risk of adverse coronary events. In addition, obesity is often accompanied by three other risk factors—diabetes mellitus, hypertension, and hyperlipidemia. The treatment of obesity and these accompanying risk factors is an important component of any management plan. A diet low in saturated and *trans*-unsaturated fatty acids and a caloric intake to achieve optimal body weight is a cornerstone in the management of chronic IHD.

Cigarette smoking accelerates coronary atherosclerosis in both sexes and at all ages and increases the risk of thrombosis, plaque instability, MI,

TABLE 237-3	ENERGY REQUIREMENTS FOR SOME COMMON ACTIVITIES			
Less than 3 METs	**3–5 METs**	**5–7 METs**	**7–9 METs**	**More than 9 METs**
Self-care				
Washing/shaving	Cleaning windows	Easy digging in	Heavy shoveling	Carrying loads
Dressing	Raking	garden	Carrying objects	upstairs (objects
Light housekeeping	Power lawn mowing	Level hand lawn	(60–90 lb)	more than 90 lb)
Desk work	Bed making/stripping	mowing		Climbing stairs
Driving auto	Carrying objects	Carrying objects		(quickly)
	(15–30 lb)	(30–60 lb)		Shoveling heavy
				snow
Occupational				
Sitting (clerical/	Stocking shelves	Carpentry	Digging ditches	Heavy labor
assembly)	(light objects)	(exterior)	(pick and shovel)	
Desk work	Light welding/	Shoveling dirt		
Standing	carpentry	Sawing wood		
(store clerk)				
Recreational				
Golf (cart)	Dancing (social)	Tennis (singles)	Canoeing	Squash
Knitting	Golf (walking)	Snow skiing	Mountain	Ski touring
	Sailing	(downhill)	climbing	Vigorous
	Tennis (doubles)	Light backpacking		basketball
		Basketball		
		Stream fishing		
Physical Conditioning				
Walking (2 mph)	Level walking	Level walking	Level jogging	Running (>6 mph)
Stationary bike	(3–4 mph)	(4.5–5.0 mph)	(5 mph)	Bicycling
Very light	Level biking	Bicycling (9–10	Swimming (crawl	(>13 mph)
calisthenics	(6–8 mph)	mph)	stroke)	Rope jumping
	Light calisthenics	Swimming,	Rowing machine	Walking uphill
		breast stroke	Heavy	(5 mph)
			calisthenics	
			Bicycling	
			(12 mph)	

Source: Modified from WL Haskell: Rehabilitation of the coronary patient, in NK Wenger, HK Hellerstein (eds): *Design and Implementation of Cardiac Conditioning Program.* New York, Churchill Livingstone. 1978.

and death (Chap. 235). In addition, by increasing myocardial oxygen needs and reducing oxygen supply, it aggravates angina. Smoking cessation studies have demonstrated important benefits with a significant decline in the occurrence of these adverse outcomes. The physician's message must be clear and strong and supported by programs that achieve and monitor abstinence (Chap. 390). *Hypertension* (Chap. 241) is associated with increased risk of adverse clinical events from coronary atherosclerosis as well as stroke. In addition, the LV hypertrophy that results from sustained hypertension aggravates ischemia. There is evidence that long-term, effective treatment of hypertension can decrease the occurrence of adverse coronary events. *Diabetes mellitus* (Chap. 338) accelerates coronary and peripheral atherosclerosis and is frequently associated with dyslipidemias and increases in the risk of angina, MI, and sudden coronary death. Aggressive control of the dyslipidemia (target LDL cholesterol <70 mg/dL) and hypertension (target BP 120/80 or less) that are frequently found in diabetic patients is essential, as described below.

DYSLIPIDEMIA   The treatment of dyslipidemia is central when aiming for long-term relief from angina, reduced need for revascularization, and reduction in myocardial infarction and death. The control of lipids can be achieved by the combination of a diet low in saturated and *trans*-unsaturated fatty acids, exercise, and weight loss. Frequently, HMG-CoA reductase inhibitors (statins) are required and can lower LDL cholesterol (25–50%), raise HDL cholesterol (5–9%), and lower triglycerides (5–30%). Niacin or fibrates can be used to raise HDL cholesterol and lower triglycerides (Chaps. 235 and 350). Controlled trials with lipid-regulating regimens have shown equal proportional benefit for men, women, the elderly, diabetics, and even smokers.

Compliance with regard to the health-promoting behaviors listed above is generally very poor, and the conscientious physician must not underestimate the major effort required to meet this challenge. Fewer than one-half of patients in the United States discharged from the hospital with proven coronary disease receive treatment for dyslipidemia. Given the proof that treating dyslipidemia brings major benefits, physicians need to secure treatment pathways, monitor compliance, and follow up.

RISK REDUCTION IN WOMEN WITH IHD   The incidence of clinical IHD in premenopausal women is very low; however, following the menopause, the atherogenic risk factors increase (e.g., increased LDL, reduced HDL) and the rate of clinical coronary events accelerates to the levels observed in men. Women have not given up cigarette smoking as effectively as have men. Diabetes mellitus, which is more common in women, greatly increases the occurrence of clinical IHD and amplifies the deleterious effects of hypertension, hyperlipidemia, and smoking. Cardiac catheterization and coronary revascularization are often applied more sparingly in women and at a later, and more severe, stage of the disease than in men. When cholesterol lowering, beta blockers after MI, and CABG are applied in the appropriate patient groups, women enjoy the same benefits of improved outcome as do men.

DRUG THERAPY   The commonly used drugs for the treatment of angina pectoris are summarized in Tables 237-4–237-6. Pharmacotherapy for IHD is designed to reduce the frequency of anginal episodes and blunt the surge in the patient's heart rate and blood pressure with exertion so that they can perform daily activities without approaching the heart rate–blood pressure threshold that provokes ischemia. Antiplatelet therapy with aspirin is also used to reduce thrombotic events that may occur with destabilization of atherosclerotic plaques.

Nitrates   The organic nitrates are a valuable class of drugs in the management of angina pectoris that have been in clinical use for over 125 years **(Table 237-4)**. Their major mechanisms of action include systemic venodilation with concomitant reduction in LV end-diastolic volume and pressure, thereby reducing myocardial wall tension and oxygen requirements; dilation of epicardial coronary vessels; and increased blood flow in collateral vessels. The organic nitrates, when

metabolized release nitric oxide (NO) which binds to guanylyl cyclase in vascular smooth-muscle cells, leading to an increase in cyclic guanosine monophosphate, which causes relaxation of vascular smooth muscle. Nitrates also exert antithrombotic activity by NO-dependent activation of platelet guanylyl cyclase and impairment of intraplatelet calcium flux, and platelet activation.

The absorption of these agents is most rapid and complete through the mucous membranes. For this reason, nitroglycerin is most commonly administered sublingually in tablets of 0.4 or 0.6 mg. Patients with angina should be instructed to take the medication both to relieve angina and also approximately 5 min before stress that is likely to induce an episode. The value of this prophylactic use of the drug cannot be overemphasized.

A pulsating feeling in the head or headache is the most common side effect of nitroglycerin and fortunately is only rarely disturbing at the doses usually required to relieve or prevent angina. Postural dizziness has also been reported. Nitroglycerin deteriorates with exposure to air, moisture, and sunlight, so that if the drug neither relieves discomfort nor produces a slight sensation of tingling at the sublingual site of absorption, the preparation may be inactive and a fresh supply should be obtained. If relief is not achieved by rest and within 2 or 3 min after up to three nitroglycerin tablets, the patient should consult a physician or report promptly to a hospital emergency room for evaluation of possible unstable angina or acute MI (Chap. 239).

Nitrates improve exercise tolerance in patients with chronic angina and relieve ischemia in patients with unstable angina as well as in patients with Prinzmetal's variant angina (Chap. 238). A diary of angina and nitroglycerin use may be valuable for detecting changes in the frequency, severity, or threshold for discomfort that may signify the development of unstable angina pectoris and/or herald an impending MI.

Long-Acting Nitrates   None of the long-acting nitrates is as effective as sublingual nitroglycerin for the acute relief of angina. These organic nitrate preparations can be swallowed, chewed, or administered as a patch or paste by the transdermal route (Table 237-4). They can provide effective plasma levels for up to 24 h, but the therapeutic response is highly variable. Different preparations and/or administration during the daytime should be tried only to prevent discomfort while avoiding side effects such as headache and dizziness. Individual dose titration is important in order to prevent side effects.

Useful preparations include isosorbide dinitrate (10–60 mg orally bid or tid) or mononitrate (30–120 mg orally qd), nitroglycerin ointment (0.5–2.0 in. qid), or sustained-release transdermal patches (5–25 mg/d). Tolerance with loss of efficacy develops within 12–24 h of continuous exposure to all of the long-acting nitrates. The mechanism of development of nitrate tolerance is incompletely understood, but leading hypotheses include inadequate generation of reduced sulfhydryl groups required for biotransformation to NO, inhibition of mitochondrial aldehyde dehydrogenase (responsible for formation of NO), counterregulatory neurohormonal activation with vasoconstric-

TABLE 237-4	NITROGLYCERIN AND NITRATES FOR PATIENTS WITH ISCHEMIC HEART DISEASE		
Compound	**Route**	**Dose**	**Duration of Effect**
Nitroglycerin	Sublingual tablets	0.3–0.6 mg up to 1.5 mg	Approximately 10 min
	Spray	0.4 mg as needed	Similar to sublingual tablets
	Ointment	2% 6 × 6 in; 15 × 15 cm 7.5-40 mg	Effect up to 7 h
	Transdermal	0.2–0.8 mg/h every 12 h	8–12 h during intermittent therapy
	Oral sustained release	2.5–13 mg	4–8 h
	Intravenous	5–200 µg/min	Tolerance may be seen in 7–8 h
Isosorbide dinitrate	Sublingual	2.5–10 mg	Up to 60 min
	Oral	5–80 mg, 2–3 times daily	Up to 8 h
	Spray	1.25 mg daily	2–3 min
	Chewable	5 mg	2–2 1/2 h
	Oral slow release	40 mg 1–2 daily	Up to 8 h
	Intravenous	1.25–5.0 mg/h	Tolerance in 7–8 h
	Ointment	100 mg/24 h	Not effective
Isosorbide mononitrate	Oral	20 mg twice daily 60–240 mg once daily	12–24 h
Pentaerythritol tetranitrate	Sublingual	10 mg as needed	Not known

Source: Modified from RJ Gibbons et al.

| **TABLE 237-5** | **PROPERTIES OF BETA BLOCKERS IN CLINICAL USE FOR ISCHEMIC HEART DISEASE** | | | |

Drugs	Selectivity	Partial Agonist Activity	Usual Dose for Angina
Acebutolol	β1	Yes	200–600 mg twice daily
Atenolol	β1	No	50–200 mg/d
Betaxolol	β1	No	10–20 mg/d
Bisoprolol	β1	No	10 mg/d
Esmolol (intravenous)*a*	β1	No	50–300 µg/kg per min
Labetalol*b*	None	Yes	200–600 mg twice daily
Metoprolol	β1	No	50–200 mg twice daily
Nadolol	None	No	40–80 mg/d
Pindolol	None	Yes	2.5–7.5 mg 3 times daily
Propranolol	None	No	80–120 mg twice daily
Timolol	None	No	10 mg twice daily

Note: This list of β blockers that may be used to treat patients with angina pectoris is arranged alphabetically. The agents for which there is the greatest clinical experience include atenolol, metoprolol, and propranolol. It is preferable to use a sustained release formulation that may be taken once daily to improve the patient's compliance with the regimen.

*a*Esmolol is an ultrashort acting β blocker that is administered as a continuous intravenous infusion. Its rapid offset of action makes esmolol an attractive agent to use in patients with relative contraindications to β blockade.

*b*Labetolol is a combined alpha- and β blocker.

Source: Modified from RJ Gibbons et al.

tion and fluid retention, and production of oxygen free radical species that inactivate NO and increase the sensitivity of vascular smooth muscle to circulating vasoconstrictors.

In order to minimize the effects of tolerance, the minimum effective dose should be used and a minimum of 8 h each day kept free of the drug so as to restore any useful response(s).

β-Adrenergic Blockers These drugs represent an important component of the pharmacologic treatment of angina pectoris **(Table 237-5)**. They reduce myocardial oxygen demand by inhibiting the increases in heart rate, arterial pressure, and myocardial contractility caused by adrenergic activation. Beta blockade reduces these variables most strikingly during exercise while causing only small reductions at rest. Long-acting beta-blocking drugs or sustained release formulations offer the advantage of once daily dosage (Table 237-5). The therapeutic aims include relief of angina and ischemia. These drugs can also reduce mortality and reinfarction in patients after MI and are moderately effective antihypertensive agents.

Relative contraindications include asthma and reversible airway obstruction in patients with chronic lung disease, atrioventricular conduction disturbances, severe bradycardia, Raynaud's phenomenon, and a history of mental depression. Side effects include fatigue, reduced exercise tolerance, nightmares, impotence, cold extremities, intermittent claudication, bradycardia (sometimes severe), impaired atrioventricular conduction, LV failure, bronchial asthma, worsening claudication, and intensification of the hypoglycemia produced by oral hypoglycemic agents and insulin. Reducing the dose or even discontinuation may be necessary if these side effects develop and persist. Since sudden discontinuation can intensify ischemia, the doses should be tapered over 2 weeks.

Beta blockers with relative β$_1$-receptor specificity, such as metoprolol and atenolol, may be preferable in patients with mild bronchial obstruction and insulin-requiring diabetes mellitus.

Calcium Channel Blockers Calcium channel blockers **(Table 237-6)** are coronary vasodilators

that produce variable and dose-dependent reductions in myocardial oxygen demand, contractility, and arterial pressure. These combined pharmacologic effects are advantageous and make these agents as effective as beta blockers in the treatment of angina pectoris. They are indicated when beta blockers are contraindicated, poorly tolerated, or ineffective. Verapamil and diltiazem may produce symptomatic disturbances in cardiac conduction and bradyarrhythmias. They also exert negative inotropic actions and are more likely to aggravate LV failure, particularly when used in patients with LV dysfunction, especially if they are also receiving beta blockers. Although useful effects are usually achieved when calcium channel blockers are combined with beta blockers and nitrates, careful individual titrations of the doses are essential with these combinations. Variant (Prinzmetal's) angina responds particularly well to calcium channel blockers (especially members of the dihydropyridine class), supplemented when necessary by nitrates (Chap. 238).

Verapamil should not ordinarily be combined with beta blockers because of the combined effects on heart rate and contractility. Diltiazem can be combined with beta blockers in patients with normal ventricular function and no conduction disturbances. Amlodipine and beta blockers have complementary actions on coronary blood supply and myocardial oxygen demands. While the former decreases blood pressure and dilates coronary arteries, the latter slows heart rate and decreases contractility. Amlodipine and the other second-generation dihydropyridine calcium antagonists (nicardipine, isradipine, long-acting nifedipine, and felodipine) are potent vasodilators and useful in the simultaneous treatment of angina and hypertension. Short-acting dihydropyridines should be avoided because of the risk of precipitating infarction, particularly in the absence of beta blockers.

Choice between Beta Blockers and Calcium Channel Blockers for Initial Therapy Since beta blockers have been shown to improve life expectancy following acute MI (Chaps. 238 and 239) while calcium channel blockers have not, the former may also be preferable in patients with chronic IHD. However, calcium channel blockers are indicated in patients with the following: (1) inadequate responsiveness to the combination of beta blockers and nitrates; many such patients do well with a combination of a beta blocker and a dihydropyridine calcium channel blocker; (2) ad-

| **TABLE 237-6** | **CALCIUM CHANNEL BLOCKERS IN CLINICAL USE FOR ISCHEMIC HEART DISEASE** | | |

Drugs	Usual Dose	Duration of Action	Side Effects
Dihydropyridines			
Amlodipine	5–10 mg qd	Long	Headache, edema
Felodipine	5–10 mg qd	Long	Headache, edema
Isradipine	2.5–10 mg bid	Medium	Headache, fatigue
Nicardipine	20–40 mg tid	Short	Headache, dizziness, flushing, edema
Nifedipine	Immediate release:*a* 30–90 mg/d orally Slow release: 30–180 mg orally	Short	Hypotension, dizziness, flushing, nausea, constipation, edema
Nisoldipine	20–40 mg qd	Short	Similar to nifedipine
Nondihydropyridines			
Diltiazem	Immediate release: 30–80 mg 4 times daily	Short	Hypotension, dizziness, flushing, bradycardia, edema
	Slow release: 120–320 mg qd	Long	
Verapamil	Immediate release: 80–160 mg tid	Short	Hypotension, myocardial depression, heart failure, edema, bradycardia
	Slow release: 120–480 mg qd	Long	

Note: This list of calcium channel blockers that may be used to treat patients with angina pectoris is divided into two broad classes, dihydropyridines and nondihydropyridines, and arranged alphabetically within each class. Among the dihydropyridines, the greatest clinical experience has been obtained with amlodipine and nifedipine. After the initial period of dose titration with a short-acting formulation, it is preferable to switch to a sustained release formulation that may be taken once daily to improve patient compliance with the regimen.

*a*May be associated with increased risk of mortality if administered during acute myocardial infarction.

Source: Modified from RJ Gibbons et al.

verse reactions to beta blockers such as depression, sexual disturbances, and fatigue; (3) angina and a history of asthma or chronic obstructive pulmonary disease; (4) sick-sinus syndrome or significant atrioventricular conduction disturbances; (5) Prinzmetal's angina; or (6) symptomatic peripheral arterial disease.

Antiplatelet Drugs Aspirin is an irreversible inhibitor of platelet cyclooxygenase activity and thereby interferes with platelet activation. Chronic administration of 75–325 mg orally per day has been shown to reduce coronary events in asymptomatic adult men, patients with chronic stable angina, and patients with or who have survived unstable angina and MI. There is a dose-dependent increase in bleeding when aspirin is used chronically. It is preferable to use an enteric-coated formulation in the range of 75–162 mg/d. Administration of this drug should be considered in all patients with IHD in the absence of gastrointestinal bleeding, allergy, or dyspepsia. Clopidogrel (300–600 mg loading and 75 mg/d maintenance) is an oral agent that blocks ADP receptor–mediated platelet aggregation. It provides similar benefits as aspirin in patients with stable chronic IHD and may be substituted for aspirin if aspirin causes the side effects listed above. Clopidogrel combined with aspirin reduces death and coronary ischemic events in patients with an acute coronary syndrome (Chap. 238) and also reduces the risk of thrombus formation in patients undergoing implantation of a stent in a coronary artery (Chap. 240). (In order to reduce the risk of gastrointestinal bleeding, it is recommended that a proton pump inhibitor be prescribed to patients taking a combination of clopidogrel and aspirin.) While combined treatment with clopidogrel and aspirin for at least a year is recommended in patients with an acute coronary syndrome and following implantation of a drug-eluting stent, studies have not shown any benefit of the routine addition of clopidogrel to aspirin in patients with chronic stable IHD.

OTHER THERAPIES Angiotensin-converting enzyme (ACE) inhibitors are widely used in the treatment of survivors of MI; patients with hypertension or chronic IHD, including angina pectoris; and those at high risk of vascular disease, such as diabetes. The benefits of ACE inhibitors are most evident in IHD patients at increased risk, especially if diabetes mellitus or LV dysfunction is present, and in those who have not achieved adequate control of blood pressure and LDL cholesterol on beta blockers and statins. However, the routine administration of ACE inhibitors to IHD patients with normal LV function and who have achieved blood pressure and LDL goals on other therapies does not reduce events and therefore is not cost-effective.

Despite treatment with nitrates, beta blockers, or calcium channel blockers, some patients with IHD continue to experience angina, and additional medical therapy is now available to alleviate their symptoms. Ranolazine, a piperazine derivative, was approved for use in January 2006 for patients with chronic angina who continue to be symptomatic despite a standard medical regimen. The mechanism of the antianginal effect of ranolazine is not firmly established, but the leading theory is that the drug inhibits the late inward sodium current (I_{Na}). The benefits of I_{Na} inhibition include limitation of the Na overload of ischemic myocytes and prevention of Ca^{2+} overload via the Na^+-Ca^{2+} exchanger. Prevention of Ca^{2+} overload minimizes diastolic tension and blunts the reduction in coronary nutrient flow that results from compression of the intramyocardial arterioles. A dose of 500–1000 mg orally twice daily is usually well tolerated. Ranolazine is contraindicated in patients with hepatic impairment, with conditions or drugs associated with QT_C prolongation, and when drugs that inhibit the CYP3A metabolic system (e.g., ketoconazole, diltiazem, verapamil, macrolide antibiotics, HIV protease inhibitors, and large quantities of grapefruit juice) are being taken by the patient.

Use of nonsteroidal anti-inflammatory drugs (NSAIDs) in patients with IHD may be associated with a small but finite increased risk of MI and mortality. For this reason, they should generally be avoided in IHD patients. If they are required for symptom relief, it is advisable to coadminister aspirin and strive to use the lowest NSAID dose required for the shortest period of time.

Another class of agents that may be considered are potassium channel openers. These agents open ATP-sensitive potassium channels in myocytes, leading to hyperpolarization of the cell membrane and a reduction of free intracellular calcium ions. The major drug in this class is nicorandil, which is typically administered in a dose of 20 mg twice daily orally for prevention of angina. (Nicorandil is not available for use in the United States but is used in several other countries.) Tolerance to nicorandil's anti-anginal effect may develop with chronic dosing, but there is no cross-tolerance to the organic nitrates.

Angina and Heart Failure Transient LV failure with angina can be controlled by the use of nitrates. For patients with established congestive heart failure, the increased LV wall tension raises myocardial oxygen demand. Treatment of congestive heart failure with an angiotensin-converting enzyme inhibitor, diuretic, and digoxin (Chap. 227) reduces heart size, wall tension, and myocardial oxygen demand, which in turn helps to control angina and ischemia. If the symptoms and signs of heart failure are controlled, an effort should be made to use beta blockers not only for angina but because trials in heart failure have shown significant improvement in survival. A trial of the intravenous ultrashort acting beta blocker esmolol may be useful to establish the safety of beta blockade in individual patients. Nocturnal angina can often be relieved by the treatment of heart failure. Nitrates are useful and can simultaneously improve the disturbed hemodynamics of congestive heart failure by vasodilatation, thereby reducing preload, and relieve angina by preventing or reversing myocardial ischemia. The combination of congestive heart failure and angina in patients with IHD usually indicates a poor prognosis and warrants serious consideration of cardiac catheterization and coronary revascularization.

CORONARY REVASCULARIZATION

While the basic management of patients with IHD is medical, as described above, many patients are improved by coronary revascularization procedures. *These interventions should be employed in conjunction with but do not replace the continuing need to modify risk factors and medical therapy.* An algorithm for integrating medical therapy and revascularization options in patients with IHD is shown in **Fig. 237-2**.

PERCUTANEOUS CORONARY INTERVENTION
(See also Chap. 240) PCI, involving balloon dilatation usually accompanied by coronary stenting, is widely used to achieve revascularization of the myocardium in patients with symptomatic IHD and suitable stenoses of epicardial coronary arteries. Whereas patients with stenosis of the left main coronary artery and those with three-vessel IHD (especially with diabetes and/or impaired LV function) who require revascularization are best treated with CABG, PCI is widely employed in patients with symptoms and evidence of ischemia due to stenoses of one or two vessels, and even in selected patients with three-vessel disease, and may offer many advantages over surgery.

Indications and Patient Selection The most common clinical indication for PCI is angina pectoris, despite medical therapy, accompanied by evidence of ischemia during a stress test. PCI is more effective than medical therapy for the relief of angina. Whereas PCI improves outcomes in patients with unstable angina and MI, the value of this procedure in reducing the occurrence of coronary death and MI in patients with chronic stable angina has not been established. PCI can be used to treat stenoses in native coronary arteries as well as in bypass grafts in patients who have recurrent angina following CABG.

Risks When coronary stenoses are discrete and symmetric, two and even three vessels can be dilated in sequence. However, case selection is essential in order to avoid a prohibitive risk of complications, which are usually due to dissection or thrombosis with vessel occlusion, uncontrolled ischemia, and ventricular failure (Chap. 240). Oral aspirin, clopidogrel, and an antithrombin are given to reduce coronary thrombus formation. Left main coronary artery stenosis is generally regarded as a contraindication to PCI; such patients should be treated with CABG. In rare cases, such as patients with prohibitive surgical risks, PCI of an unprotected left main can be considered, but such a procedure should only be performed by a highly skilled operator; importantly, there are regional differences in the use of this approach internationally.

Efficacy Primary success—i.e., adequate dilation (an increase in luminal diameter >20% to a residual diameter obstruction <50%) with relief of angina—is achieved in >95% of cases. Recurrent stenosis of the dilated vessels occurs in ~20% of cases within 6 months of PCI with bare metal stents, and angina will recur within 6 months in 10% of cas-

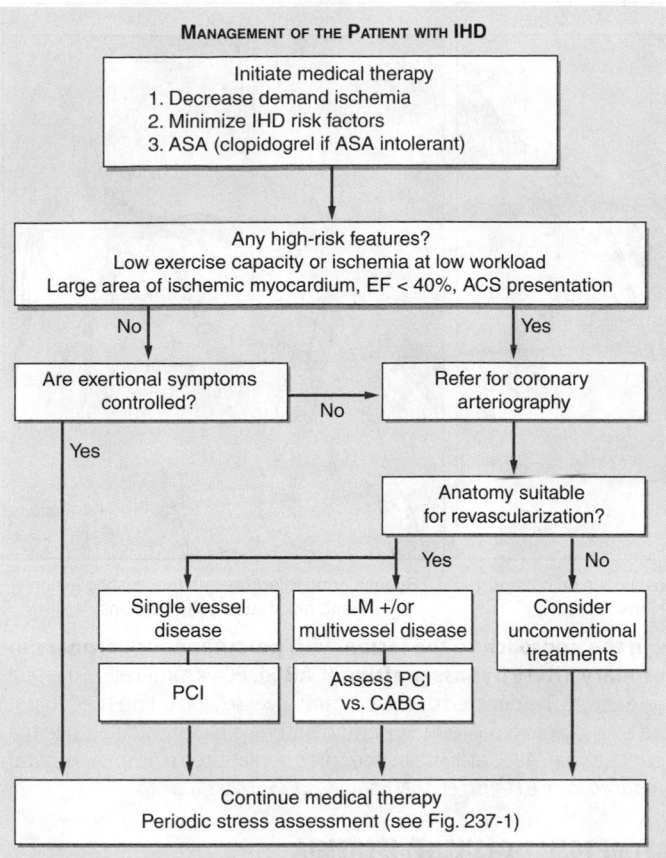

MANAGEMENT OF THE PATIENT WITH IHD

Initiate medical therapy
1. Decrease demand ischemia
2. Minimize IHD risk factors
3. ASA (clopidogrel if ASA intolerant)

Any high-risk features?
Low exercise capacity or ischemia at low workload
Large area of ischemic myocardium, EF < 40%, ACS presentation

No — Yes

Are exertional symptoms controlled? — No — Refer for coronary arteriography

Yes

Anatomy suitable for revascularization?

Yes — No

Single vessel disease | LM +/or multivessel disease | Consider unconventional treatments

PCI | Assess PCI vs. CABG

Continue medical therapy
Periodic stress assessment (see Fig. 237-1)

FIGURE 237-2 Algorithm for management of the patient with ischemic heart disease. All patients should receive the core elements of medical therapy as shown at the top of the algorithm. If high-risk features are present, as established by the clinical history, exercise test data, and imaging studies, the patient should be referred for coronary arteriography. Based on the number and location of the diseased vessels and their suitability for revascularization, the patient is treated with either a percutaneous coronary intervention (PCI), coronary artery bypass graft (CABG) surgery, or should be considered for unconventional treatments. See text for further discussion. IHD, ischemic heart disease; ASA, aspirin; EF, ejection fraction; ACS, acute coronary syndrome; LM, left main.

es. Restenosis is more common in patients with diabetes mellitus, arteries with small caliber, incomplete dilation of the stenosis, occluded vessels, obstructed vein grafts, dilation of the left anterior descending coronary artery, and stenoses containing thrombi. In diseased vein grafts, procedural success has been improved by the use of capture devices or filters that prevent embolization, ischemia, and infarction.

It is usual clinical practice to administer aspirin indefinitely and clopidogrel for 1–3 months after the implantation of a bare metal stent. Although aspirin and the antiplatelet drug clopidogrel may help prevent coronary thrombosis during and shortly following PCI with stenting, there is no evidence that these medications reduce the incidence of restenosis. The use of drug-eluting stents that locally deliver antiproliferative drugs such as rapamycin or paclitaxel can reduce restenosis to near zero within the stent and 3–7% at its edges. Advances in PCI, especially the availability of drug-eluting stents, have vastly extended the use of this revascularization option in patients with IHD. Of note, however, the delayed endothelial healing in the region of a drug-eluting stent also extends the period during which the patient is at risk for subacute stent thrombosis. Current recommendations are to administer aspirin indefinitely and clopidogrel daily for at least 1 year after implantation of a drug-eluting stent. When a situation arises where temporary discontinuation of antiplatelet therapy is desirable, the clinical circumstances should be reviewed with the operator who performed the PCI and a co-

ordinated plan should be established for minimizing the risk of late stent thrombus. Central to this plan is the discontinuation of antiplatelet therapy for the shortest acceptable period of time.

Successful PCI produces effective relief of angina in >95% of cases and has been shown to be more effective than medical therapy for up to 2 years. More than one-half of patients with symptomatic IHD who require revascularization can be treated initially by PCI. Successful PCI is less invasive and expensive than CABG, usually requires only 1–2 days in the hospital, and permits savings in the initial cost of care. Successful PCI also allows earlier return to work and the resumption of an active life. However, this economic benefit is reduced over time because of the greater need for follow-up and for repeat procedures.

CORONARY ARTERY BYPASS GRAFTING

Anastomosis of one or both of the internal mammary arteries or a radial artery to the coronary artery distal to the obstructive lesion is carried out. For additional obstructions that cannot be bypassed by an artery, a section of a vein (usually the saphenous) is used to form a connection between the aorta and the coronary artery distal to the obstructive lesion.

Although some indications for CABG are controversial, certain areas of agreement exist:

1. The operation is relatively safe, with mortality rates <1% in patients without serious comorbid disease and normal LV function, and when the procedure is performed by an experienced surgical team.

2. Intraoperative and postoperative mortality increase with the severity of ventricular dysfunction, comorbidities, age >80 years, and lack of surgical experience. The effectiveness and risk of CABG vary widely depending on case selection and the skill and experience of the surgical team.

3. Occlusion of *venous* grafts is observed in 10–20% of patients during the first postoperative year, in approximately 2% per year during 5- to 7-year follow-up, and in 4% per year thereafter. Long-term patency rates are considerably higher for internal mammary and radial artery implantations than saphenous vein grafts. In patients with left anterior descending coronary artery obstruction, survival is better when coronary bypass involves the internal mammary artery rather than a saphenous vein. Graft patency and outcomes are improved by meticulous treatment of risk factors, particularly dyslipidemia.

4. Angina is abolished or greatly reduced in ~90% of patients following complete revascularization. Although this is usually associated with graft patency and restoration of blood flow, the pain may also have been alleviated as a result of infarction of the ischemic segment or a placebo effect. Within 3 years, angina recurs in about one-fourth of patients but is rarely severe.

5. Survival may be improved by operation in patients with stenosis of the left main coronary artery as well as in patients with three- or two-vessel disease with significant obstruction of the proximal left anterior descending coronary artery. The survival benefit is greater in patients with abnormal LV function (ejection fraction <50%). Survival *may* also be improved in the following patients: (1) those with obstructive CAD who have survived sudden cardiac death or sustained ventricular tachycardia; (2) those who have undergone previous CABG and who have multiple saphenous vein graft stenoses, especially of a graft supplying the left anterior descending coronary artery; and (3) those with recurrent stenosis following PCI and high-risk criteria on noninvasive testing.

6. Minimally invasive CABG through a small thoracotomy and/or off-pump surgery can reduce morbidity and shorten convalescence in suitable patients but does not appear to significantly reduce the risk of neurocognitive dysfunction postoperatively.

Indications for CABG are usually based on the severity of symptoms, coronary anatomy, and ventricular function. The ideal candidate is male, is <80 years of age, has no other complicating disease, has troublesome or disabling angina that is not adequately controlled by medical therapy or does not tolerate medical therapy and wishes to lead a more active life, and has severe stenoses of two or three epicardial coronary arteries with objective evidence of myocardial ischemia as a cause of the chest discomfort. Great symptomatic benefit can be anticipated in such patients. Congestive heart failure and/or LV dysfunction, advanced age (>80 years), reoperation, urgent need for surgery, and the presence of diabetes mellitus are all associated with a higher perioperative mortality.

LV dysfunction can be due to noncontractile or hypocontractile segments that are viable but are chronically ischemic (hibernating myocardium). As a consequence of chronic reduction in myocardial blood flow these segments downregulate their contractile function. These can be detected by using radionuclide scans of myocardial perfusion and metabolism, PET, CMR imaging, or delayed scanning with thallium-201; or by improvement of regional functional impairment, provoked by low-dose dobutamine. In such patients, revascularization improves myocardial blood flow, can return function, and can improve survival.

The Choice between PCI and CABG A number of randomized clinical trials have compared PCI and CABG in patients with multivessel CAD who were suitable technically for both procedures. The redevelopment of angina requiring repeat coronary angiography and repeat revascularization is higher with PCI. This is a result of restenosis in the stented segment (a problem largely solved with drug-eluting stents) and the development of new stenoses in unstented portions of the coronary vasculature. It has been argued that PCI with stenting focuses on culprit lesions while a bypass graft to the target vessel also provides a conduit around future culprit lesions proximal to the anastomosis of the graft to the native vessel (Fig. 237-3).

Comparison of mortality rates in patients treated with CABG versus PCI is a complex issue. There is an early increased risk of mortality with CABG, but when considering a longer time horizon, such as 5 years, mortality is lower with CABG compared with PCI.

Based on available evidence, it is now recommended that patients with an unacceptable level of angina despite optimal medical management be considered for coronary revascularization. Patients with single- or two-vessel disease with normal LV function and anatomically suitable lesions are ordinarily advised to undergo PCI (Chap. 240). Patients with three-vessel disease (or two-vessel disease that includes the proximal left descending coronary artery) and impaired global LV function (LVEF <50%) or diabetes mellitus or those with left main coronary artery disease or other lesions unsuitable for catheter-based procedures should be considered for CABG as the initial method of revascularization.

UNCONVENTIONAL TREATMENTS FOR IHD

On occasion clinicians will encounter a patient with persistent disabling angina despite maximally tolerated medical therapy for whom revascularization is not an option (e.g., small diffusely diseased vessels not amenable to stent implantation or acceptable targets for bypass grafting). In such situations unconventional treatments should be considered.

Enhanced external counterpulsation utilizes pneumatic cuffs on the lower extremities to provide diastolic augmentation and systolic unloading of blood pressure in order to decrease cardiac work and oxygen consumption while enhancing coronary blood flow. Clinical trials have shown that regular application improves angina, exercise capacity, and regional myocardial perfusion.

Additional options include *transmyocardial laser revascularization* (to increase intramyocardial channels of blood flow), and the currently experimental approaches of gene and stem cell therapies are under study.

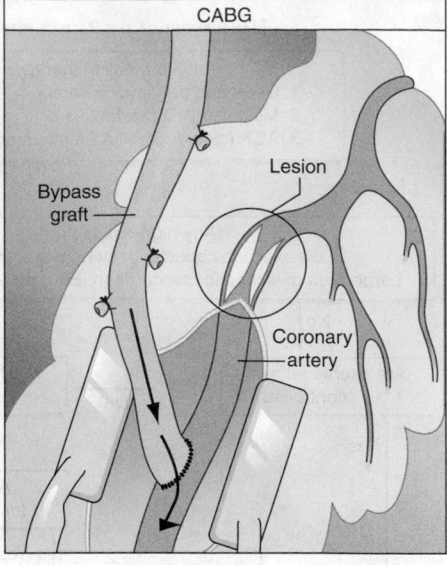

Stent addresses the existing lesion but not future lesions.

Bypass grafting addresses the existing lesion and also future culprit lesions.

FIGURE 237-3 Difference in the approach to the lesion with percutaneous coronary intervention (PCI) and coronary artery bypass grafting (CABG). PCI is targeted at the "culprit" lesion or lesions, whereas CABG is directed at the epicardial vessel, including the "culprit" lesion or lesions and future culprits, proximal to the insertion of the vein graft, a difference that may account for the superiority of CABG, at least in the intermediate term, in patients with multivessel disease. *(Reproduced from BJ Gersh et al: N Engl J Med 352:2235, 2005.)*

ASYMPTOMATIC (SILENT) ISCHEMIA

Obstructive CAD, acute MI, and transient myocardial ischemia are frequently asymptomatic. During continuous ambulatory ECG monitoring, the majority of ambulatory patients with typical chronic stable angina are found to have objective evidence of myocardial ischemia (ST-segment depression) during episodes of chest discomfort while they are active outside the hospital, but many of these patients have more frequent episodes of asymptomatic ischemia. In addition, there is a large (but as yet unknown) number of totally asymptomatic persons with severe coronary atherosclerosis who exhibit ST-segment changes during activity. Some of these patients exhibit higher thresholds to electrically induced pain, others show higher endorphin levels, and still others may be diabetics with autonomic dysfunction.

Frequent episodes of ischemia (symptomatic and asymptomatic) during daily life appear to be associated with an increased likelihood of adverse coronary events (death and MI). In addition, patients with asymptomatic ischemia after suffering a myocardial infarction are at greater risk for a second coronary event. The widespread use of exercise ECG during routine examinations has also identified some of these heretofore unrecognized patients with asymptomatic CAD. Longitudinal studies have demonstrated an increased incidence of coronary events in asymptomatic patients with positive exercise tests.

℞ ASYMPTOMATIC ISCHEMIA

The management of patients with asymptomatic ischemia must be individualized. Thus, the physician should consider the following: (1) the degree of positivity of the stress test, particularly the stage of exercise at which ECG signs of ischemia appear, the magnitude and number of the ischemic zones of myocardium on imaging, and the change in LVEF which occurs on radionuclide ventriculography or echocardiography during ischemia and/or during exercise; (2) the ECG leads showing a positive response, with changes in the anterior precordial leads indicating a less favorable prognosis than changes in the inferior leads; and (3) the patient's age, occupation, and general medical condition.

Most would agree that an asymptomatic 45-year-old commercial airline pilot with 0.4-mV ST-segment depression in leads V_1 to V_4 during mild exercise should undergo coronary arteriography, whereas the asymptomatic, sedentary 75-year-old retiree with 0.1-mV ST-segment depression in leads II and III during maximal activity need not. However, there is no consensus about the appropriate procedure in the large majority of patients for whom the situation is less extreme. Asymptomatic patients with silent ischemia, three-vessel CAD, and impaired LV function may be considered appropriate candidates for CABG.

The treatment of risk factors, particularly lipid lowering as described above, and the use of aspirin, beta blockers, and statins have been shown to reduce events and improve outcomes in asymptomatic as well as symptomatic patients with ischemia and proven CAD. While the incidence of asymptomatic ischemia can be reduced by treatment with beta blockers, calcium channel blockers, and long-acting nitrates, it is not clear whether this is necessary or desirable in patients who have not suffered a myocardial infarction.

FURTHER READINGS

ANTMAN EM et al: Use of nonsteroidal antiinflammatory drugs: An update for clinicians: A scientific statement from the American Heart Association. Circulation 115:1634, 2007; *http://circ.ahajournals.org/cgi/content/full/115/12/1634*

BHATT DL et al: Clopidogrel and aspirin versus aspirin alone for the prevention of atherothrombotic events. N Engl J Med 354:1706, 2006

CHAITMAN BR: Ranolazine for the treatment of chronic angina and potential use in other cardiovascular conditions. Circulation 113:2462, 2006

CLEEMAN JI et al: Executive summary of the Third Report of the National Cholesterol Education Program (NCEP) Expert Panel on Detection, Evaluation, and Treatment of High Blood Cholesterol in Adults (Adult Treatment Panel III). JAMA 285:2486, 2001

DEFEYTER PJ et al: Bypass surgery versus stenting for the treatment of multivessel disease in patients with unstable angina compared with stable angina. Circulation 105:2367, 2002

GIBBONS RJ et al: ACC/AHA 2002 guideline update for the management of patients with chronic stable angina: A report of the American College of Cardiology/American Heart Association Task Force on Practice Guidelines (Committee to Update the 1999 Guidelines for the Management of Patients with Chronic Stable Angina), 2002. *http://acc.org/qualityandscience/clinical/guidelines/stable/update_index.htm*

GOLDSCHMIDT-CLERMONT PJ et al: Atherosclerosis 2005: Recent discoveries and novel hypotheses. Circulation 112:3348, 2005

KIM MC et al: Refractory angina pectoris. Mechanism and therapeutic options. J Am Coll Cardiol 39:923, 2002

LEE TH et al: Noninvasive tests in patients with stable coronary artery disease. N Engl J Med 344:1840, 2001

MORROW D et al: Chronic ischemic heart disease, in *Braunwald's Heart Disease,* 7th ed, D Zipes et al (eds). Philadelphia, Saunders, 2005

OPIE LH et al: Controversies in stable coronary artery disease. Lancet 367:69, 2006

PRETRE R et al: Choice of revascularization strategy for patients with coronary artery disease. JAMA 285:992, 2001

SMITH SC JR et al: ACC/AHA/SCAI 2005 guideline update for percutaneous coronary intervention: A report of the American College of Cardiology/American Heart Association Task Force on Practice Guidelines (ACC/AHA/SCAI Writing Committee to Update the 2001 Guidelines for Percutaneous Coronary Intervention). American College of Cardiology web site. *http://acc.org/qualityandscience/clinical/guidelines/percutaneous/update/index.pdf*

VAN DEN BRAND MJBM et al: The effect of completeness of revascularization on event-free survival at one year in the ARTS trial. J Am Coll Cardiol 39:559, 2002

238 Unstable Angina and Non-ST-Elevation Myocardial Infarction
Christopher P. Cannon, Eugene Braunwald

Patients with ischemic heart disease fall into two large groups: patients with chronic coronary artery disease (CAD) who most commonly present with stable angina (Chap. 237) and patients with acute coronary syndromes (ACSs). The latter group, in turn, is composed of patients with acute myocardial infarction (MI) with ST-segment elevation on their presenting electrocardiogram (STEMI; Chap. 239) and those with unstable angina and non-ST-segment elevation MI (UA/NSTEMI; see Fig. 239-1). Every year in the United States, ~1.3 million patients are admitted to hospitals with UA/NSTEMI as compared with ~300,000 patients with acute STEMI. The relative incidence of UA/NSTEMI compared to STEMI appears to be increasing. Almost one-half of patients with UA/NSTEMI are women, while more than three-fourths of patients with STEMI are men.

DEFINITION

The diagnosis of UA is based largely on the clinical presentation. *Stable* angina pectoris is characterized by chest or arm discomfort that may not be described as pain but is reproducibly associated with physical exertion or stress and is relieved within 5–10 min by rest and/or sublingual nitroglycerin (Chaps. 13 and 237). UA is defined as angina pectoris or equivalent ischemic discomfort with at least one of three features: (1) it occurs at rest (or with minimal exertion), usually lasting >10 min; (2) it is severe and of new onset (i.e., within the prior 4–6 weeks); and/or (3) it occurs with a crescendo pattern (i.e., distinctly more severe, prolonged, or frequent than previously). The diagnosis of NSTEMI is established if a patient with the clinical features of UA develops evidence of myocardial necrosis, as reflected in elevated cardiac biomarkers.

PATHOPHYSIOLOGY

UA/NSTEMI is most commonly caused by a reduction in oxygen supply and/or by an increase in myocardial oxygen demand superimposed on an atherosclerotic coronary plaque, with varying degrees of obstruction. Four pathophysiologic processes that may contribute to the development of UA/NSTEMI have been identified: (1) plaque rupture or erosion with superimposed nonocclusive thrombus, believed to be the most common cause—NSTEMI may occur with downstream embolization of platelet aggregates and/or atherosclerotic debris; (2) dynamic obstruction [e.g., coronary spasm, as in Prinzmetal's variant angina (p. 1531)]; (3) progressive mechanical obstruction [e.g., rapidly advancing coronary atherosclerosis or restenosis following percutaneous coronary intervention (PCI)]; and (4) secondary UA related to increased myocardial oxygen demand and/or decreased supply (e.g., tachycardia, anemia). More than one of these processes may be involved.

Among patients with UA/NSTEMI studied at angiography, approximately 5% have left main stenosis, 15% have three-vessel CAD, 30% have two-vessel disease, 40% have single-vessel disease, and 10% have no critical coronary stenosis; some of the latter have Prinzmetal's variant angina (see below). The "culprit lesion" on angiography may show an eccentric stenosis with scalloped or overhanging edges and a narrow neck. Angioscopy may reveal "white" (platelet-rich) thrombi, as opposed to "red" thrombi, more often seen in patients with acute STEMI. Patients with UA/NSTEMI often have multiple plaques vulnerable to disruption.

CLINICAL PRESENTATION
History and Physical Examination The clinical hallmark of UA/NSTEMI is chest pain, typically located in the substernal region or sometimes in the epigastrium, that radiates to the neck, left shoulder, and left arm (Chap. 13). This discomfort is usually severe enough to be considered painful. Anginal "equivalents" such as dyspnea and epigastric discomfort may also occur, and these appear to occur more often in women. The examination resembles that in patients with stable an-

gina (Chap. 237) and may be unremarkable. If the patient has a large area of myocardial ischemia or a large NSTEMI, the physical findings can include diaphoresis, pale cool skin, sinus tachycardia, a third and/or fourth heart sound, basilar rales, and sometimes hypotension, resembling the findings of large STEMI.

Electrocardiogram In UA, ST-segment depression, transient ST-segment elevation, and/or T-wave inversion occur in 30–50% of patients, depending on the severity of the clinical presentation. In patients with the clinical features of UA, the presence of new ST-segment deviation, even of only 0.05 mV, is an important predictor of adverse outcome. T-wave changes are sensitive for ischemia but less specific, unless they are new, deep T-wave inversions (≥0.3 mV).

Cardiac Biomarkers Patients with UA who have elevated biomarkers of necrosis, such as CK-MB and troponin (a much more specific and sensitive marker of myocardial necrosis), are at increased risk for death or recurrent MI. Elevated levels of these markers distinguish patients with NSTEMI from those with UA. There is a direct relationship between the degree of troponin elevation and mortality. However, in patients *without* a clear clinical history of myocardial ischemia, minor troponin elevations have been reported and can be caused by congestive heart failure, myocarditis, or pulmonary embolism, or they may be false-positive readings. Thus, in patients with an *unclear* history, small troponin elevations may not be diagnostic of an ACS.

DIAGNOSTIC EVALUATION

(See also Chap. 13) Approximately 6–7 million persons per year in the United States present to hospital emergency departments (EDs) with a complaint of chest pain or other symptoms suggestive of ACS. A diagnosis of an ACS is established in 20–25% of such patients. The first step in evaluating patients with possible UA/NSTEMI is to determine the *likelihood* that CAD is the cause of the presenting symptoms. The American College of Cardiology/American Heart Association (ACC/AHA) Guidelines include, among the factors associated with a high likelihood of ACS, a clinical history typical of ischemic discomfort, a history of established CAD by angiography, prior MI, congestive heart failure, new electrocardiographic (ECG) changes, or elevated cardiac biomarkers. Factors associated with an intermediate likelihood of ACS in patients with the clinical features of this condition but without the above high-risk factors are: age >70 years, male gender, diabetes mellitus, known peripheral arterial or cerebrovascular disease, and old ECG abnormalities.

Diagnostic Pathways Four major diagnostic tools are used in the diagnosis of UA/NSTEMI in the ED: the clinical history, the ECG, cardiac markers, and stress testing. The goals are to (1) recognize or exclude MI (using cardiac markers), (2) evaluate for rest ischemia (chest pain at rest, serial or continuous ECGs), and (3) evaluate for significant CAD (using provocative stress testing). Typical pathways begin with assessment of the likelihood that the presenting symptoms are due to ischemia. Patients with a low likelihood of ischemia are usually managed with an ED-based critical pathway (which in some institutions is carried out in a "chest pain unit" (Fig. 238-1). Evaluation of such patients includes clinical monitoring for recurrent ischemic discomfort, serial ECGs, and cardiac markers, typically performed at baseline and at 4–6 h and 12 h after presentation. If new elevations in cardiac markers (CK-MB and/or troponin) or ECG changes are noted, the patient is admitted to the hospital. If the patient remains pain-free and the markers are negative, the patient may go on to stress testing. This may be performed as early as 6 h after presentation in the ED or chest pain center, or on an outpatient basis within 72 h. For most patients, standard treadmill ECG stress testing is used, but for patients with fixed abnormalities on the ECG (e.g., left bundle branch block), perfusion or echocardiographic imaging is used. For patients who cannot walk, pharmacologic stress is used. By demonstrating normal myocardial perfusion, sestamibi or thallium imaging can reduce unnecessary hospitalizations by excluding acute ischemia. CT angiography is used with increasing frequency to exclude obstructive CAD (Chap. 222).

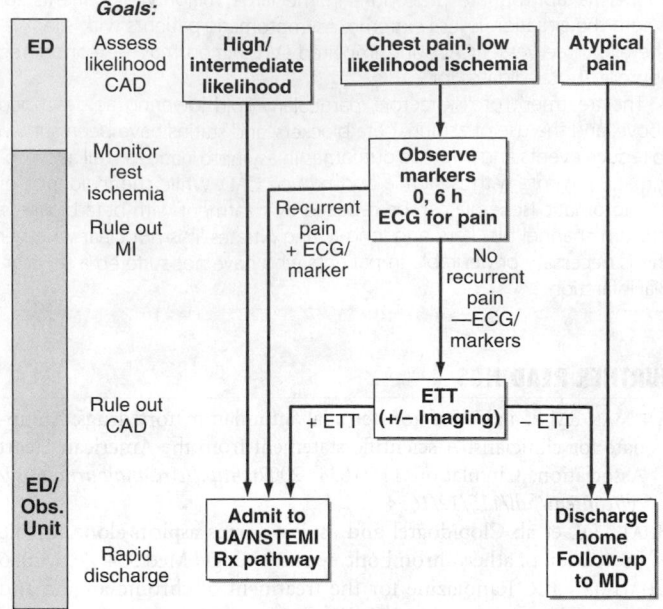

FIGURE 238-1 Diagnostic evaluation of patients presenting with suspected UA/NSTEMI. The first step is to assess the likelihood of coronary artery disease (CAD). Patients at *high* or *intermediate* likelihood are admitted to the hospital. Those with clearly atypical chest pain are sent home. Patients with a *low* likelihood of ischemia enter the pathway and are observed in a monitored bed in the emergency department (ED) or observation unit over a period of 6 h, and 12-lead electrocardiograms are performed if the patient has recurrent chest discomfort. A panel of cardiac markers (e.g., troponin and CK-MB) is drawn at baseline and 6 h later. If the patient develops recurrent pain, has ST-segment or T-wave changes, or has positive cardiac markers, he/she is admitted to the hospital and treated for UA/NSTEMI. If the patient has negative markers and no recurrence of pain, he/she is sent for exercise treadmill testing, with imaging reserved for patients with abnormal baseline electrocardiograms (e.g., left bundle branch block or left ventricular hypertrophy). If positive, the patient is admitted; if negative, the patient is discharged, with follow-up to his/her primary physician. ETT, exercise tolerance test; MI, myocardial infarction. [*Adapted from CP Cannon, E Braunwald, in Heart Disease: A Textbook of Cardiovascular Medicine, 6th ed, E Braunwald et al (eds). Philadelphia, Saunders, 2001.*]

RISK STRATIFICATION AND PROGNOSIS

Patients with documented UA/NSTEMI exhibit a wide spectrum of early (30 days) risk of death, ranging from 1 to 10%, and of new or recurrent infarction of 3–10%. Assessment of "global risk" can be accomplished by clinical risk scoring systems such as that developed from in the Thrombolysis in Myocardial Infarction (TIMI) Trials, which includes seven independent risk factors: age ≥ 65 years, three or more risk factors for CAD, documented CAD at catheterization, development of UA/NSTEMI while on aspirin, more than two episodes of angina within the preceding 24 h, ST deviation ≥0.5 mm, and an elevated cardiac marker (Fig. 238-2). Other risk factors include diabetes mellitus, left ventricular dysfunction, and elevated levels of creatinine, atrial natriuretic peptides, and C-reactive protein.

Early risk assessment (especially using troponin, ST-segment changes, and/or a global risk scoring system) is useful both in predicting the risk of recurrent cardiac events and in identifying those patients who would derive the greatest benefit from antithrombotic therapies more potent than unfractionated heparin, such as low-molecular-weight heparin (LMWH) and glycoprotein (GP)IIb/IIIa inhibitors, and from an early invasive strategy. For example, in the TACTICS-TIMI 18 Trial, an early invasive strategy conferred a 40% reduction in recurrent cardiac events in patients with a positive troponin

FIGURE 238-2 The TIMI Risk Score for UA/NSTEMI, a simple but comprehensive clinical risk stratification score to identify increasing risk of death, myocardial infarction, or urgent revascularization to day 14. CAD, coronary artery disease; ASA, aspirin. *(Adapted from Antman et al.)*

level, whereas no benefit was observed in those with a negative troponin level.

C-reactive protein, a marker of vascular inflammation, and B-type natriuretic peptide, a marker of increased myocardial wall tension, correlate independently with increased mortality (and, in some studies, recurrent cardiac events) in patients presenting with UA/NSTEMI. Multimarker strategies are now gaining favor both to define the pathophysiologic mechanisms underlying a given patient's presentation more fully and to stratify the patient's risk further.

℞ UNSTABLE ANGINA AND NON-ST ELEVATION MYOCARDIAL INFARCTION

MEDICAL TREATMENT   Patients with UA/NSTEMI should be placed at bed rest with continuous ECG monitoring for ST-segment deviation and cardiac rhythm. Ambulation is permitted if the patient shows no recurrence of ischemia (discomfort or ECG changes) and does not develop a biomarker of necrosis for 12–24 h. Medical therapy involves simultaneous anti-ischemic treatment and antithrombotic treatment.

ANTI-ISCHEMIC TREATMENT   (**Table 238-1**) In order to provide relief and prevention of recurrence of chest pain, initial treatment should include bed rest, nitrates, and beta blockers.

Nitrates   Nitrates should first be given sublingually or by buccal spray (0.3–0.6 mg) if the patient is experiencing ischemic pain. If pain persists after three doses given 5 min apart, intravenous nitroglycerin (5–10 µg/min using nonabsorbing tubing) is recommended. The rate of the infusion may be increased by 10 µg/min every 3–5 min until symptoms are relieved or systolic

| TABLE 238-1 | DRUGS COMMONLY USED IN INTENSIVE MEDICAL MANAGEMENT OF PATIENTS WITH UNSTABLE ANGINA AND NON-ST ELEVATION MI |

Drug Category	Clinical Condition	When to Avoid[a]	Dosage
Nitrates	Administer intravenously when symptoms are not fully relieved with three sublingual nitroglycerin tablets and initiation of beta-blocker therapy	Hypotension Patient receiving sildenafil or other PDE-5 inhibitor	5–10 µg/min by continuous infusion Titrated up to 75–100 µg/min until relief of symptoms or limiting side effects (headache or hypotension with a systolic blood pressure <90 mmHg or more than 30% below starting mean arterial pressure levels if significant hypertension is present) Topical, oral, or buccal nitrates are acceptable alternatives for patients without ongoing or refractory symptoms

Beta blockers[b]	Unstable angina	PR interval (ECG) >0.24 s
		2° or 3° atrioventricular block
		Heart rate <60 beats/min
		Blood pressure <90 mmHg
		Shock
		Left ventricular failure with congestive heart failure
		Severe reactive airway disease
			Metoprolol[c]
			  5-mg increments by slow (over 1–2 min IV administration)
			  Repeated every 5 min for a total initial dose of 15 mg
			  Followed in 1–2 h by 25–50 mg by mouth every 6 h
			  If a very conservative regimen is desired, initial doses can be reduced to 1–2 mg
			Esmolol[c]
			  Starting maintenance dose of 0.1 mg/kg per min IV
			  Titration in increments of 0.05 mg/kg per min every 10–15 min as tolerated by blood pressure until the desired therapeutic response has been obtained, limiting symptoms develop, or a dose of 0.20 mg/kg per min is reached
			  Optional loading dose of 0.5 mg/kg may be given by slow IV administration (2–5 min) for more rapid onset of action

Calcium channel blockers	Patients whose symptoms are not relieved by adequate doses of nitrates and beta blockers or in patients unable to tolerate adequate doses of one or both of these agents or in patients with variant angina	Pulmonary edema Evidence of left ventricular dysfunction (for diltiazem or verapamil)	Dependent on specific agent
Morphine sulfate	Patients whose symptoms are not relieved after three serial sublingual nitroglycerin tablets or whose symptoms recur with adequate anti-ischemic therapy	Hypotension Respiratory depression Confusion Obtundation	2–5 mg IV dose May be repeated every 5–30 min as needed to relieve symptoms and maintain patient comfort

[a]Allergy or prior intolerance is a contraindication for all categories of drugs listed in this chart.
[b]Choice of the specific agent is not as important as ensuring that appropriate candidates receive this therapy. If there are concerns about patient intolerance owing to existing pulmonary disease, especially asthma, left ventricular dysfunction, risk of hypotension or severe bradycardia, initial selection should favor a short-acting agent, such as propranolol or metoprolol or the ultra-short-acting agent esmolol. Mild wheezing or a history of chronic obstructive pulmonary disease should prompt a trial of a short-acting agent at a reduced dose (e.g., 2.5 mg IV metoprolol, 12.5 mg oral metoprolol, or 25 µg/kg per min esmolol as initial doses) rather than complete avoidance of beta-blocker therapy.

[c]Metoprolol and esmolol are two of several beta blockers that may be employed.
Note: Some of the recommendations in this guide suggest the use of agents for purposes or in doses other than those specified by the U.S. Food and Drug Adminstration. Such recommendations are made after consideration of concerns regarding nonapproved indications. Where made such recommendations are based on more recent clinical trials or expert consensus.
IV, intravenous; aPTT, activated partial thromboplastin time; ECG, electrocardiogram; 2°, second-degree; 3°, third-degree.
Source: Modified from E Braunwald et al: Circulation 1994;90:613–622.

TABLE 238-2 CLINICAL USE OF ANTITHROMBOTIC THERAPY

Oral Antiplatelet Therapy

Aspirin	Initial dose of 162–325 mg nonenteric formulation followed by 75–162 mg/d of an enteric or a nonenteric formulation
Clopidogrel (Plavix)	Loading dose of 300 mg followed by 75 mg/d

Intravenous Antiplatelet Therapy

Abciximab (ReoPro)	0.25 mg/kg bolus followed by infusion of 0.125 μg/kg per min (maximum 10 μg/min) for 12 to 24 h
Eptifibatide (Integrilin)	180 μg/kg bolus followed by infusion of 2.0 μg/kg per min for 72 to 96 h
Tirofiban (Aggrastat)	0.4 μg/kg per min for 30 min followed by infusion of 0.1 μg/kg per min for 48 to 96 h

Heparins[a]

Heparin (UFH)	Bolus 60–70 U/kg (maximum 5000 U) IV followed by infusion of 12–15 U/kg per h (initial maximum 1000 U/h) titrated to a PTT 50–70 s
Enoxaparin (Lovenox)	1 mg/kg SC every 12 h; the first dose may be preceded by a 30-mg IV bolus; renal adjustment to 1 mg/kg once daily if creatine Cl < 30 cc/min
Fondaparinux	2.5 mg SQ qd
Bivalirudin	Initial bolus intravenous bolus of 0.1 mg/kg and an infusion of 0.25 mg/kg per hour. Before PCI, an additional intravenous bolus of 0.5 mg/kg was administered, and the infusion was increased to 1.75 mg/kg per hour.

[a]Other LMWH exist beyond those listed.
Note: IV, intravenous; SC, subcutaneously; UFH, unfractionated heparin.
Source: Modified from E Braunwald et al: J Am Coll Cardiol 2000;36:970–1056.

arterial pressure falls to <100 mmHg. Topical or oral nitrates (Chap. 237) can be used once the pain has resolved, or they may replace intravenous nitroglycerin when the patient has been pain-free for 12–24 h. The only absolute contraindications to the use of nitrates are hypotension or the use of sildenafil (Viagra) or other drugs in that class within the previous 24 h.

β-Adrenergic Blockade These agents are the other mainstay of antiischemic treatment. Intravenous beta blockade followed by oral beta blockade targeted to a heart rate of 50–60 beats/min is recommended. Heart rate–slowing calcium channel blockers, e.g., verapamil or diltiazem, are recommended in patients who have persistent or recurrent symptoms after treatment with full-dose nitrates and beta blockers and in patients with contraindications to beta blockade. Additional medical therapy includes angiotensin-converting enzyme (ACE) inhibition and HMG-CoA reductase inhibitors (statins) for long-term secondary prevention.

If pain persists despite intravenous nitroglycerin and beta blockade, morphine sulfate, 1–5 mg intravenously, can be administered every 5–30 min as needed.

ANTITHROMBOTIC THERAPY (Table 238-2) This is the other main component of treatment for UA/NSTEMI. Initial treatment should begin with the platelet cyclooxygenase inhibitor aspirin (Fig. 238-3). The typical initial dose is 325 mg daily, with lower doses (75–162 mg daily) recommended for long-term therapy. "Aspirin resistance" has been noted in research studies in 5–10% of patients and more frequently in patients treated with lower doses of aspirin. No clear guidelines are available regarding evaluation or treatment, but the use of higher doses of aspirin and/or a thienopyridine (clopidogrel) appears to be logical in this situation.

The thienopyridine clopidogrel, which blocks the platelet $P2Y_{12}$ (adenosine) receptor (in combination with aspirin), was shown in the CURE trial to confer a 20% relative reduction in cardiovascular death, MI, or stroke, compared with aspirin alone in both low- and high-risk patients with UA/NSTEMI, but to be associated with a moderate (absolute 1%) increase in major bleeding, which is more common in patients who undergo coronary artery bypass grafting. Pretreatment with clopidogrel (a 300 or 600 mg loading dose, followed by 75 mg qd) has also been shown in three studies to reduce adverse outcomes associated with and following PCI and has a Class I, Grade A evidence recommendation in the PCI Guidelines (Chap. 240). Continued benefit of long-term (~1 year) treatment with the combination of clopidogrel and

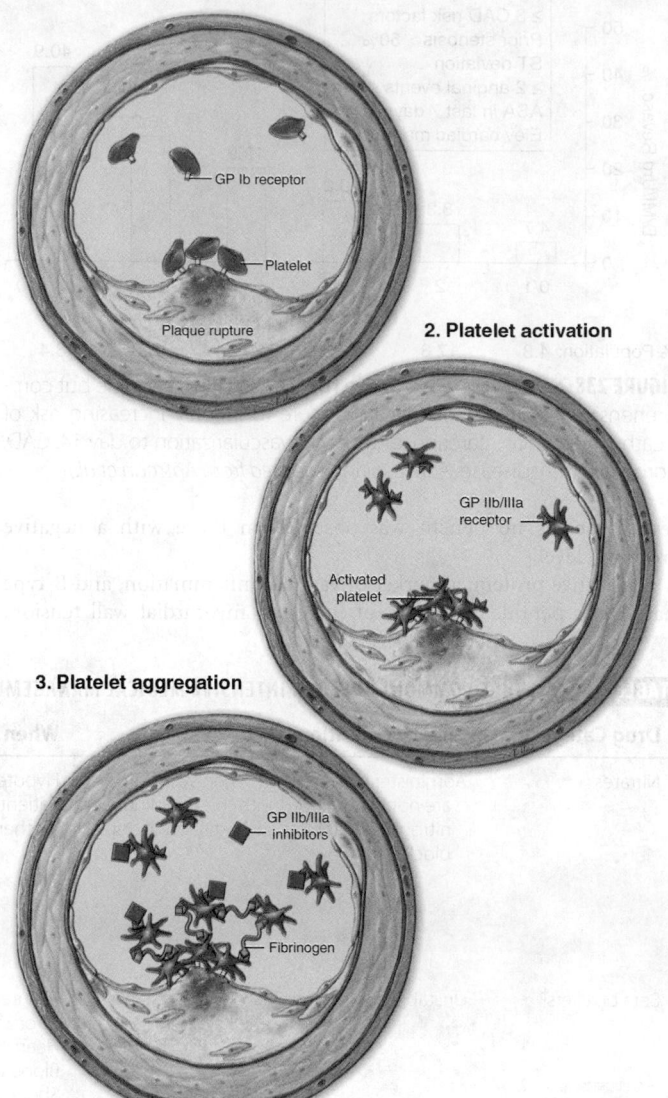

FIGURE 238-3 Platelets initiate thrombosis at the site of a ruptured plaque with denuded endothelium: *platelet adhesion* occurs via (1) the GP 1b receptor in conjunction with von Willebrand factor. This is followed by *platelet activation* (2), which leads to a shape change in the platelet, degranulation of the alpha and dense granules, and expression of glycoprotein IIb/IIIa receptors on the platelet surface with activation of the receptor, such that it can bind fibrinogen. The final step is *platelet aggregation* (3), in which fibrinogen (or von Willebrand factor) binds to the activated GP IIb/IIIa receptors. Aspirin (ASA) and clopidogrel act to decrease platelet activation, whereas the GP IIb/IIIa inhibitors inhibit the final step of platelet aggregation. GP, glycoprotein. [*Modified from CP Cannon, E Braunwald, in Heart Disease: A Textbook of Cardiovascular Medicine, 8th ed, P Libby et al (eds). Philadelphia, Saunders, 2008.*]

aspirin has been observed both in patients treated conservatively and in those who underwent a PCI. This combination is recommended for all patients with UA/NSTEMI who are not at excessive risk for bleeding.

Four options are available for anticoagulation therapy to be added to aspirin and clopidogrel. Unfractionated heparin (UFH) is the mainstay of therapy. The LMWH enoxaparin has been shown in several studies to be superior to UFH in reducing recurrent cardiac events, especially in conservatively managed patients. The Factor Xa inhibitor fondaparinux is equivalent for early efficacy compared with enoxaparin but appears to have a lower risk of major bleeding and thus may have the best benefit risk ratio. However, UFH, LMWH, or a direct thrombin inhibitor such as bivalirudin should be used during cardiac catheterization or PCI. Preliminary data indicate that bivalirudin is equivalent (for both efficacy and safety) to either UFH or enoxaparin among patients treated with a GP IIb/IIIa inhibitor, but use of bivalirudin alone had less bleeding than the combination of a heparin and GP IIb/IIIa inhibitor in patients with UA/NSTEMI undergoing PCI.

Intravenous GP IIb/IIIa inhibitors have also been shown to be beneficial in treating UA/NSTEMI. For "upstream" management of high-risk patients in whom an invasive management is intended (i.e., initiating therapy when the patient first presents to the hospital), the small molecule inhibitors eptifibatide and tirofiban show benefit, while the monoclonal antibody abciximab appears not to be effective in patients treated conservatively, (i.e., in those not undergoing coronary angiography or PCI). However, abciximab has been shown to be beneficial in patients with UA/NSTEMI undergoing PCI, even among troponin positive patients pretreated with clopidogrel. The ACC/AHA Guidelines note that these agents can be started either in the ED or during PCI. As with all antithrombotic agents, bleeding is the most important adverse effect of antiplatelet drugs, especially their combination. Thus, patients with a history of bleeding must be screened carefully and given fewer antithrombotic agents.

INVASIVE VERSUS CONSERVATIVE STRATEGY   Multiple clinical trials have shown the benefit of an early invasive strategy in high-risk patients, i.e., patients with multiple clinical risk factors, ST-segment deviation, and/or positive biomarkers (**Table 238-3**). In this strategy, following treatment with anti-ischemic and antithrombotic agents, coronary arteriography is carried out within ~48 h of admission, followed by coronary revascularization (PCI or coronary artery bypass grafting), depending on the coronary anatomy.

In low-risk patients, the outcomes from an invasive strategy are similar to those obtained from a conservative strategy, which consists of anti-ischemic and antithrombotic therapy followed by "watchful waiting," in which coronary arteriography is carried out only if rest pain or ST-segment changes recur or there is evidence of ischemia on a stress test.

LONG-TERM MANAGEMENT

The time of hospital discharge is a "teachable moment" for the patient with UA/NSTEMI, when the physician can review and optimize the medical regimen. Risk factor modification is key, and the physician should discuss with the patient the importance of smoking cessation, achieving optimal weight, daily exercise following an appropriate diet, blood pressure control, tight control of hyperglycemia (for diabetic patients), and lipid management, as recommended for patients with chronic stable angina (Chap. 237).

There is evidence of benefit with long-term therapy with five classes of drugs that are directed at different components of the atherothrombotic process. Beta blockers are appropriate anti-ischemic therapy and may help decrease triggers for MI. Statins (at a high dose, e.g., atorvastatin 80 mg/d) and ACE inhibitors are recommended for long-term plaque stabilization. Antiplatelet therapy, now recommended to be the combination of aspirin and clopidogrel for at least 9–12 months, with aspirin continued thereafter, prevents or reduces the severity of any thrombosis that would occur if a plaque does rupture. Thus, a multifactorial approach to long-term medical therapy is directed at preventing the various components of atherothrombosis. This therapy should be begun early, i.e. within a week of the event, whenever possible.

Observational registries have shown that patients with UA/NSTEMI at high risk, including women and the elderly as well as racial minorities, are less likely to receive evidence-based pharmacologic and interventional therapies with resultant poorer clinical outcomes and quality of life.

PRINZMETAL'S VARIANT ANGINA

In 1959 Prinzmetal et al. described a syndrome of ischemic pain that occurs at rest but not usually with exertion and is associated with transient ST-segment elevation. This syndrome is due to focal spasm of an epicardial coronary artery, leading to severe myocardial ischemia. The exact cause of the spasm is not well defined, but it may be related to hypercontractility of vascular smooth muscle due to vasoconstrictor mitogens, leukotrienes, or serotonin. In some patients it is a manifestation of a vasospastic disorder and is associated with migraine, Raynaud's phenomenon, or aspirin-induced asthma.

TABLE 238-3	CLASS I RECOMMENDATIONS FOR USE OF AN EARLY INVASIVE STRATEGY[a]

Class I (level of evidence: A) indications
Recurrent angina at rest/low-level activity despite Rx
Elevated TnT or TnI
New ST-segment depression
Rec. angina/ischemia with CHF symptoms, rales, MR
Positive stress test
EF < 0.40
Decreased BP
Sustained VT
PCI < 6 months, prior CABG

[a]Any one of the high-risk indicators.
Abbreviations: TnT, troponin T; TnI, troponin I; Rec, recurrent; CHF, congestive heart failure; MR, mitral regurgitation; EF, ejection fraction; BP, blood pressure; VT, ventricular tachycardia; PCI, percutaneous coronary intervention; CABG, coronary artery bypass grafting.
Source: E Braunwald et al: Circulation 106:1893, 2002.

Clinical and Angiographic Manifestations   Patients with variant angina are generally younger and have fewer coronary risk factors (with the exception of cigarette smoking) than patients with UA secondary to coronary atherosclerosis. The anginal discomfort is often extremely severe and has usually not progressed from a period of chronic stable angina. Cardiac examination is usually normal in the absence of ischemia.

The clinical diagnosis of variant angina is made with the detection of transient ST-segment *elevation* with rest pain. Many patients also exhibit multiple episodes of asymptomatic ST-segment elevation (*silent ischemia*). Small elevations of CK-MB and troponin may occur in patients with prolonged attacks of variant angina. Exercise testing in patients with variant angina is of limited value because the patients can demonstrate ST elevation, depression, or no ST changes.

Coronary angiography demonstrates transient coronary spasm as the diagnostic hallmark of Prinzmetal's angina. Atherosclerotic plaques, which do not usually cause critical obstruction, in at least one proximal coronary artery occur in the majority of patients, and in them spasm usually occurs within 1 cm of the plaque. Focal spasm is most common in the right coronary artery, and it may occur at one or more sites in one artery or in multiple arteries simultaneously. Ergonovine, acetylcholine, other vasoconstrictor medications, and hyperventilation have been used to provoke and demonstrate focal coronary stenosis to establish the diagnosis. Hyperventilation has also been used to provoke rest angina, ST-segment elevation, and spasm on coronary arteriography.

℞ PRINZMETAL'S VARIANT ANGINA

Nitrates and calcium channel blockers are the main treatments for patients with variant angina. Sublingual or intravenous nitroglycerin often abolishes episodes of variant angina promptly, and long-acting nitrates are useful in preventing recurrences. Calcium antagonists are extremely effective in preventing the coronary artery spasm of variant angina, and they should be prescribed in maximally tolerated doses. Similar efficacy rates have been noted among the various types of calcium antagonists. Prazosin, a selective α-adrenoreceptor blocker, has also been found to be of value in some patients, while aspirin may actually increase the severity of ischemic episodes. The response to beta blockers is variable. Coronary revascularization may be helpful in patients with variant angina who also have discrete, proximal fixed obstructive lesions.

Prognosis   Many patients with Prinzmetal's angina pass through an acute, active phase, with frequent episodes of angina and cardiac events during the first 6 months after presentation. Long-term survival at 5 years is excellent (~90–95%). Patients with no or mild fixed coronary obstruction tend to experience a more benign course than do patients with associated severe obstructive lesions. Nonfatal MI occurs in up to 20% of patients by 5 years. Patients with variant angina who develop serious arrhythmias during spontaneous episodes of pain are at a higher risk for sudden death. In most patients who survive an infarction or the initial 3–6-month period of frequent episodes, the condition stabilizes, and there is a tendency for symptoms and cardiac events to diminish with time.

FURTHER READINGS

ANTMAN EM et al: The TIMI risk score for unstable angina/non-ST elevation MI: A method for prognostication and therapeutic decision making. JAMA 284:835, 2000

BRAUNWALD E et al: ACC/AHA 2002 guideline update for the management of patients with unstable angina and non-ST segment elevation myocardial infarction: A report of the American College of Cardiology/American Heart Association Task Force on Practice Guidelines (Committee on the Management of Unstable Angina). URL: *http://www.acc.org/qualityandscience/clinical/guidelines/unstable/ update_index.htm*

CANNON CP, BRAUNWALD E: Unstable angina, in *Braunwald's Heart Disease*, 8th ed, P Libby et al (eds). Philadelphia, Saunders, 2008

———— et al: Intensive versus moderate lipid lowering with statins after acute coronary syndromes. N Engl J Med 350:1495, 2004

CLOPIDOGREL IN UNSTABLE ANGINA TO PREVENT RECURRENT EVENTS TRIAL INVESTIGATORS: Effects of clopidogrel in addition to aspirin in patients with acute coronary syndromes without ST-segment elevation. N Engl J Med 345:494, 2001

GIUGLIANO RP, BRAUNWALD E: The year in non-ST segment elevation acute coronary syndromes. J Am Coll Cardiol (in press)

KASTRATI A et al: Abciximab in patients with acute coronary syndromes undergoing percutaneous coronary intervention after clopidogrel pretreatment: The ISAR-REACT 2 randomized trial. JAMA 295:1531, 2006

MEHTA SR et al: Routine vs selective invasive strategies in patients with acute coronary syndromes: A collaborative meta-analysis of randomized trials. JAMA 293:2908, 2005

YUSUF S et al. Comparison of fondaparinux and enoxaparin in acute coronary syndromes. N Engl J Med 354:1464, 2006

239 ST-Segment Elevation Myocardial Infarction
Elliott M. Antman, Eugene Braunwald

Acute myocardial infarction (AMI) is one of the most common diagnoses in hospitalized patients in industrialized countries. In the United States, approximately 650,000 patients experience a new AMI and 450,000 experience a recurrent AMI each year. The early (30-day) mortality rate from AMI is ~30%, with more than half of these deaths occurring before the stricken individual reaches the hospital. Although the mortality rate after admission for AMI has declined by ~30% over the past two decades, approximately 1 of every 25 patients who survives the initial hospitalization dies in the first year after AMI. Mortality is approximately fourfold higher in elderly patients (over age 75) compared with younger patients.

When patients with prolonged ischemic discomfort at rest are first seen, the working clinical diagnosis is that they are suffering from an acute coronary syndrome (Fig. 239-1). The 12-lead electrocardiogram (ECG) is a pivotal diagnostic and triage tool since it is at the center of the decision pathway for management. It permits distinction of those patients presenting with ST-segment elevation from those presenting without ST-segment elevation. Serum cardiac biomarkers are obtained to distinguish unstable angina (UA) from non-ST-segment MI (NSTEMI) and to assess the magnitude of an ST-segment elevation MI (STEMI). This chapter focuses on the evaluation and management of patients with STEMI, while Chapter 238 discusses UA/NSTEMI.

PATHOPHYSIOLOGY: ROLE OF ACUTE PLAQUE RUPTURE

STEMI usually occurs when coronary blood flow decreases abruptly after a thrombotic occlusion of a coronary artery previously affected by atherosclerosis. Slowly developing, high-grade coronary artery stenoses do not typically precipitate STEMI because of the development of a rich collateral network over time. Instead, STEMI occurs when a coronary artery thrombus develops rapidly at a site of vascular injury. This injury is produced or facilitated by factors such as cigarette smoking, hypertension, and lipid accumulation. In most cases, STEMI occurs when the surface of an atherosclerotic plaque becomes disrupted (exposing its contents to the blood) and conditions (local or systemic) favor thrombogenesis. A mural thrombus forms at the site of plaque disruption, and the involved coronary artery becomes occluded. Histologic studies indicate that the coronary plaques prone to disruption are those with a rich lipid core and a thin fibrous cap (Chap. 235). After an initial platelet monolayer forms at the site of the disrupted plaque, various agonists (collagen, ADP, epinephrine, serotonin) promote platelet activation. After agonist stimulation of platelets, thromboxane A$_2$ (a

FIGURE 239-1 Acute coronary syndromes. Following disruption of a vulnerable plaque, patients experience ischemic discomfort resulting from a reduction of flow through the affected epicardial coronary artery. The flow reduction may be caused by a completely occlusive thrombus (**right**) or subtotally occlusive thrombus (**left**). Patients with ischemic discomfort may present with or without ST-segment elevation. Of patients with ST-segment elevation, the majority (*wide red arrow*) ultimately develop a Q-wave on the ECG (QwMI), while a minority (*thin red arrow*) do not develop Q-wave and in older literature where said to have sustained a non-Q-wave MI (NQMI). Patients who present without ST-segment elevation are suffering from either unstable angina or a non-ST-segment elevation MI (NSTEMI) (*wide green arrows*), a distinction that is ultimately made on the presence or absence of a serum cardiac marker such as CKMB or a cardiac troponin detected in the blood. The majority of patients presenting with NSTEMI do not develop a Q-wave on the ECG; a minority develop a QwMI (*thin green arrow*). (*Adapted from CW Hamm et al: Lancet 358:1533, 2001, and MJ Davies: Heart 83:361, 2000; with permission from the BMJ Publishing Group.*)

potent local vasoconstrictor) is released, further platelet activation occurs, and potential resistance to fibrinolysis develops.

In addition to the generation of thromboxane A$_2$, activation of platelets by agonists promotes a conformational change in the glycoprotein IIb/IIIa receptor (Chap. 109). Once converted to its functional state, this receptor develops a high affinity for amino acid sequences on soluble adhesive proteins (i.e., integrins) such as fibrinogen. Since fibrinogen is a multivalent molecule, it can bind to two different platelets simultaneously, resulting in platelet cross-linking and aggregation.

The coagulation cascade is activated on exposure of tissue factor in damaged endothelial cells at the site of the disrupted plaque. Factors

VII and X are activated, ultimately leading to the conversion of pro-thrombin to thrombin, which then converts fibrinogen to fibrin (Chap. 110). Fluid-phase and clot-bound thrombin participate in an autoamplification reaction leading to further activation of the coagulation cascade. The culprit coronary artery eventually becomes occluded by a thrombus containing platelet aggregates and fibrin strands.

In rare cases STEMI may be due to coronary artery occlusion caused by coronary emboli, congenital abnormalities, coronary spasm, and a wide variety of systemic—particularly inflammatory—diseases. The amount of myocardial damage caused by coronary occlusion depends on (1) the territory supplied by the affected vessel, (2) whether or not the vessel becomes totally occluded, (3) the duration of coronary occlusion, (4) the quantity of blood supplied by collateral vessels to the affected tissue, (5) the demand for oxygen of the myocardium whose blood supply has been suddenly limited, (6) native factors that can produce early spontaneous lysis of the occlusive thrombus, and (7) the adequacy of myocardial perfusion in the infarct zone when flow is restored in the occluded epicardial coronary artery.

Patients at increased risk of developing STEMI include those with multiple coronary risk factors (Chap. 235) and those with unstable angina (Chap. 238). Less common underlying medical conditions predisposing patients to STEMI include hypercoagulability, collagen vascular disease, cocaine abuse, and intracardiac thrombi or masses that can produce coronary emboli.

CLINICAL PRESENTATION

In up to one-half of cases, a precipitating factor appears to be present before STEMI, such as vigorous physical exercise, emotional stress, or a medical or surgical illness. Although STEMI may commence at any time of the day or night, circadian variations have been reported such that clusters are seen in the morning within a few hours of awakening.

Pain is the most common presenting complaint in patients with STEMI. The pain is deep and visceral; adjectives commonly used to describe it are *heavy*, *squeezing*, and *crushing*, although occasionally it is described as stabbing or burning (Chap. 13). It is similar in character to the discomfort of angina pectoris (Chap. 237) but commonly occurs at rest, is usually more severe, and lasts longer. Typically the pain involves the central portion of the chest and/or the epigastrium, and on occasion it radiates to the arms. Less common sites of radiation include the abdomen, back, lower jaw, and neck. The frequent location of the pain beneath the xiphoid and epigastrium and the patients' denial that they may be suffering a heart attack are chiefly responsible for the common mistaken impression of indigestion. The pain of STEMI may radiate as high as the occipital area but not below the umbilicus. It is often accompanied by weakness, sweating, nausea, vomiting, anxiety, and a sense of impending doom. The pain may commence when the patient is at rest, but when it begins during a period of exertion, it does not usually subside with cessation of activity, in contrast to angina pectoris.

The pain of STEMI can simulate pain from acute pericarditis (Chap. 232), pulmonary embolism (Chap. 256), acute aortic dissection (Chap. 242), costochondritis, and gastrointestinal disorders. These conditions should therefore be considered in the differential diagnosis. Radiation of discomfort to the trapezius is not seen in patients with STEMI and may be a useful distinguishing feature that suggests pericarditis is the correct diagnosis. However, *pain is not uniformly present in patients with STEMI.* The proportion of painless STEMIs is greater in patients with diabetes mellitus, and it increases with age. In the elderly, STEMI may present as sudden-onset breathlessness, which may progress to pulmonary edema. Other less common presentations, with or without pain, include sudden loss of consciousness, a confusional state, a sensation of profound weakness, the appearance of an arrhythmia, evidence of peripheral embolism, or merely an unexplained drop in arterial pressure.

PHYSICAL FINDINGS

Most patients are anxious and restless, attempting unsuccessfully to relieve the pain by moving about in bed, altering their position, and stretching. Pallor associated with perspiration and coolness of the ex-

tremities occurs commonly. The combination of substernal chest pain persisting for >30 min and diaphoresis strongly suggests STEMI. Although many patients have a normal pulse rate and blood pressure within the first hour of STEMI, about one-fourth of patients with anterior infarction have manifestations of sympathetic nervous system hyperactivity (tachycardia and/or hypertension), and up to one-half with inferior infarction show evidence of parasympathetic hyperactivity (bradycardia and/or hypotension).

The precordium is usually quiet, and the apical impulse may be difficult to palpate. In patients with anterior wall infarction, an abnormal systolic pulsation caused by dyskinetic bulging of infarcted myocardium may develop in the periapical area within the first days of the illness and then may resolve. Other physical signs of ventricular dysfunction include fourth and third heart sounds, decreased intensity of the first heart sound, and paradoxical splitting of the second heart sound (Chap. 220). A transient midsystolic or late systolic apical systolic murmur due to dysfunction of the mitral valve apparatus may be present. A pericardial friction rub is heard in many patients with transmural STEMI at some time in the course of the disease, if they are examined frequently. The carotid pulse is often decreased in volume, reflecting reduced stroke volume. Temperature elevations up to 38°C may be observed during the first week after STEMI. The arterial pressure is variable; in most patients with transmural infarction, systolic pressure declines by approximately 10–15 mmHg from the preinfarction state.

LABORATORY FINDINGS

Myocardial infarction (MI) progresses through the following temporal stages: (1) acute (first few hours–7 days), (2) healing (7–28 days), and (3) healed (≥29 days). When evaluating the results of diagnostic tests for STEMI, the temporal phase of the infarction must be considered. The laboratory tests of value in confirming the diagnosis may be divided into four groups: (1) ECG, (2) serum cardiac biomarkers, (3) cardiac imaging, and (4) nonspecific indices of tissue necrosis and inflammation.

ELECTROCARDIOGRAM

The electrocardiographic manifestations of STEMI are described in Chap. 221. During the initial stage, total occlusion of an epicardial coronary artery produces ST-segment elevation. Most patients initially presenting with ST-segment elevation ultimately evolve Q waves on the ECG (Fig. 239-1; see Fig. 221-13). However, Q waves in the leads overlying the infarct zone may vary in magnitude and even appear only transiently, depending on the reperfusion status of the ischemic myocardium and restoration of transmembrane potentials over time. A small proportion of patients initially presenting with ST-segment elevation will not develop Q waves when the obstructing thrombus is not totally occlusive, obstruction is transient, or if a rich collateral network is present. Among patients presenting with ischemic discomfort but *without* ST-segment elevation, if a serum cardiac biomarker of necrosis (see below) is detected, the diagnosis of NSTEMI is ultimately made (Fig. 239-1). A minority of patients who present initially without ST-segment elevation may develop a Q-wave MI. Previously it was believed that transmural MI is present if the ECG demonstrates Q waves or loss of R waves, and nontransmural MI may be present if the ECG shows only transient ST-segment and T-wave changes. However, electrocardiographic-pathologic correlations are far from perfect and terms such as *Q-wave MI, non-Q-wave MI, transmural MI,* and *nontransmural MI,* have been replaced by STEMI and NSTEMI (Fig. 239-1).

SERUM CARDIAC BIOMARKERS

Certain proteins, called serum cardiac biomarkers, are released from necrotic heart muscle after STEMI. The rate of liberation of specific proteins differs depending on their intracellular location, their molecular weight, and the local blood and lymphatic flow. Cardiac biomarkers become detectable in the peripheral blood once the capacity of the cardiac lymphatics to clear the interstitium of the infarct zone is exceeded and spillover into the venous circulation occurs. The temporal pattern of protein release is of diagnostic importance, but contemporary urgent reperfusion strategies necessitate making a decision (based largely on a combination of clinical and ECG findings) before the results of blood tests have returned from the laboratory. Rapid whole-blood bedside assays for serum cardiac markers are now available and may facilitate management decisions, particularly in patients with nondiagnostic ECGs.

Cardiac-specific troponin T (cTnT) and *cardiac-specific troponin I* (cTnI) have amino acid sequences different from those of the skeletal muscle forms of these proteins. These differences permitted the development of quantitative assays for cTnT and cTnI with highly specific monoclonal antibodies. Since cTnT and cTnI are not normally detectable in the blood of healthy individuals but may increase after STEMI to levels >20 times higher than the upper reference limit (the highest value seen in 99% of a reference population not suffering from MI), the measurement of cTnT or cTnI is of considerable diagnostic usefulness, and they are now the preferred biochemical markers for MI (Fig. 239-2). The cardiac troponins are particularly valuable when there is clinical suspicion of either skeletal muscle injury or a small MI that may be below the detection limit for CK and CKMB measurements, and they are therefore of particular value in distinguishing UA from NSTEMI. Levels of cTnI and cTnT may remain elevated for 7–10 days after STEMI.

Creatine phosphokinase (CK) rises within 4–8 h and generally returns to normal by 48–72 h (Fig. 239-2). An important drawback of total CK measurement is its lack of specificity for STEMI, as CK may be elevated with skeletal muscle disease or trauma, including intramuscular injection. The MB isoenzyme of CK has the advantage over total CK that it is not present in significant concentrations in extracardiac tissue and therefore is considerably more specific. However, cardiac surgery, myocarditis, and electrical cardioversion often result in elevated serum levels of the MB isoenzyme. A ratio (relative index) of CKMB mass:CK activity ≥2.5 suggests but is not diagnostic of a myocardial rather than a skeletal muscle source for the CKMB elevation.

Many hospitals are using cTnT or cTnI rather than CKMB as the routine serum cardiac marker for diagnosis of STEMI, although any of these analytes remains clinically acceptable. It is *not* cost-effective to measure both a cardiac-specific troponin and CKMB at all time points in every patient.

While it has long been recognized that the total quantity of protein released correlates with the size of the infarct, the peak protein concentration correlates only weakly with infarct size. Recanalization of a coronary artery occlusion (either spontaneously or by mechanical or pharmacologic means) in the early hours of STEMI causes earlier and higher peaking (at about 8–12 h after reperfusion) of serum cardiac biomarkers (Fig. 239-2) because of a rapid washout from the interstitium of the infarct zone, quickly overwhelming lymphatic clearance of the proteins.

The *nonspecific reaction* to myocardial injury is associated with polymorphonuclear leukocytosis, which appears within a few hours after the onset of pain and persists for 3–7 days; the white blood cell count often reaches levels of 12,000–15,000/μL. The erythrocyte sedimentation rate rises more slowly than the white blood cell count, peaking during the first week and sometimes remaining elevated for 1 or 2 weeks.

CARDIAC IMAGING

Abnormalities of wall motion on *two-dimensional echocardiography* (Chap. 222) are almost universally present. Although acute STEMI cannot be distinguished from an old myocardial scar or from acute severe ischemia by echocardiography, the ease and safety of the procedure make its use appealing as a screening tool in the Emergency Department setting. When the ECG is not diagnostic of STEMI, early detection of the presence or absence of wall motion abnormalities by echocardiography can aid in management decisions, such as whether the patient should receive reperfusion therapy [e.g., fibrinolysis or a percutaneous coronary intervention (PCI)]. Echocardiographic estimation of left ventricular (LV) function is useful prognostically; detection of reduced function serves as an indication for therapy with an inhibitor of the renin-angiotensin-aldosterone system. Echocardiography may also identify the presence of right ventricular (RV) infarction, ventricular aneurysm, pericardial effusion, and LV thrombus. In addi-

FIGURE 239-2 Typical cardiac biomarkers that are used to evaluate patients with STEMI include the MB isoenzyme of CK (CKMB) and cardiac-specific troponins. The black horizontal line depicts the upper reference limit (URL) for the cardiac biomarker in the clinical chemistry laboratory. The kinetics of release of CKMB and cardiac troponin in patients who do not undergo reperfusion are shown in the solid green and red curves as multiples of the URL. When patients with STEMI undergo reperfusion, as depicted in the dashed green and red curves, the cardiac biomarkers are detected sooner, rise to a higher peak value, but decline more rapidly, resulting in a smaller area under the curve and limitation of infarct size. (*Adapted from JS Alpert et al: J Am Coll Cardiol 36:959, 2000, and AH Wu et al: Clin Chem 45:1104, 1999.*)

tion, Doppler echocardiography is useful in the detection and quantitation of a ventricular septal defect and mitral regurgitation, two serious complications of STEMI.

Several *radionuclide imaging techniques* (Chap. 222) are available for evaluating patients with suspected STEMI. However, these imaging modalities are used less often than echocardiography because they are more cumbersome and lack sensitivity and specificity in many clinical circumstances. Myocardial perfusion imaging with ^{201}Tl or ^{99m}Tc-sestamibi, which are distributed in proportion to myocardial blood flow and concentrated by viable myocardium (Chap. 237), reveal a defect ("cold spot") in most patients during the first few hours after development of a transmural infarct. Although perfusion scanning is extremely sensitive, it cannot distinguish acute infarcts from chronic scars and thus is not specific for the diagnosis of *acute* MI. Radionuclide ventriculography, carried out with ^{99m}Tc-labeled red blood cells, frequently demonstrates wall motion disorders and reduction in the ventricular ejection fraction in patients with STEMI. While of value in assessing the hemodynamic consequences of infarction and in aiding in the diagnosis of RV infarction when the RV ejection fraction is depressed, this technique is nonspecific, as many cardiac abnormalities other than MI alter the radionuclide ventriculogram.

Myocardial infarction can be detected accurately with high-resolution cardiac magnetic resonance imaging (Chap. 222) using a technique referred to as late enhancement. A standard imaging agent (gadolinium) is administered and images are obtained after a 10-min delay. Since little gadolinium enters normal myocardium where there are tightly packed myocytes, but does percolate into the expanded intercellular region of the infarct zone, there is a bright signal in areas of infarction that appears in stark contrast to the dark areas of normal myocardium.

INITIAL MANAGEMENT

PREHOSPITAL CARE

The prognosis in STEMI is largely related to the occurrence of two general classes of complications: (1) electrical complications (arrhythmias) and (2) mechanical complications ("pump failure"). Most out-of-hospital deaths from STEMI are due to the sudden development of ventricular fibrillation. The vast majority of deaths due to ventricular fibrillation occur within the first 24 h of the onset of symptoms, and of these, over half occur in the first hour. Therefore, the major elements of prehospital care of patients with suspected STEMI include (1) recognition of symptoms by the patient and prompt seeking of medical attention; (2) rapid deployment of an emergency medical team capable of performing resuscitative maneuvers, including defibrillation; (3) expeditious transportation of the patient to a hospital facility that is continuously staffed by physicians and nurses skilled in managing arrhythmias and providing advanced cardiac life support; and (4) expeditious implementation of reperfusion therapy (Fig. 239-3). The biggest delay usually occurs not during transportation to the hospital but rather between the onset of pain and the patient's decision to call for help. This delay can best be reduced by health care professionals educating the public concerning the significance of chest discomfort and the importance of seeking early medical attention. Regular office visits with patients having a history of or who are at risk for ischemic heart disease are important "teachable moments" for clinicians to review the symptoms of STEMI and the appropriate action plan.

Increasingly, monitoring and treatment are carried out by trained personnel in the ambulance, further shortening the time between the onset of the infarction and appropriate treatment. General guidelines for initiation of fibrinolysis in the prehospital setting include the ability to transmit 12-lead ECGs to confirm the diagnosis, the presence of paramedics in the ambulance, training of paramedics in the interpretation of ECGs and management of STEMI, and online medical command and control that can authorize the initiation of treatment in the field.

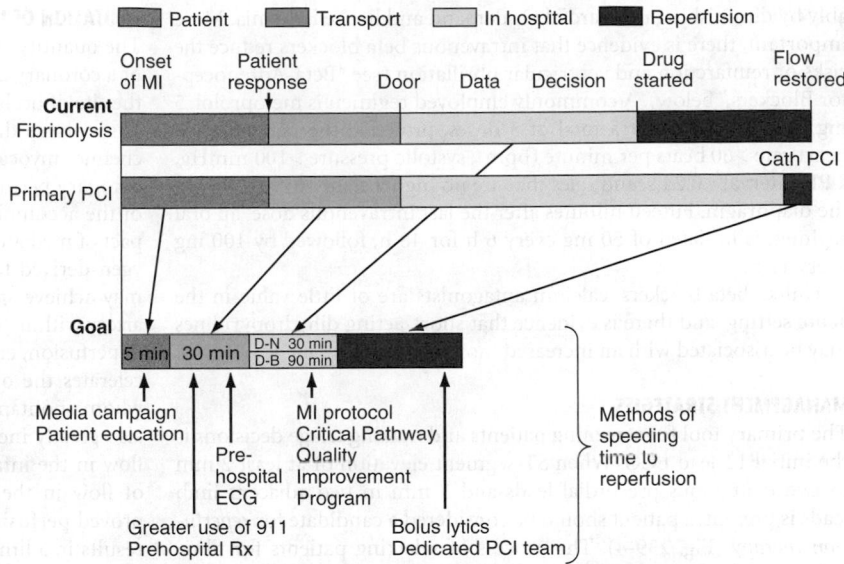

FIGURE 239-3 Major components of time delay between onset of symptoms from STEMI and restoration of flow in the infarct-related artery. Plotted sequentially from left to right are shown the times for patients to recognize symptoms and seek medical attention, transportation to the hospital, in-hospital decision-making, implementation of reperfusion strategy, and restoration of flow once the reperfusion strategy has been initiated. The time to initiate fibrinolytic therapy is the "door-to-needle" (D-N) time; this is followed by the period of time required for pharmacologic restoration of flow. More time is required to move the patient to the catheterization laboratory for a percutaneous coronary interventional (PCI) procedure, referred to as the "door-to-balloon" (D-B) time, but restoration of flow in the epicardial infarct-related artery occurs promptly after PCI. At the bottom are shown a variety of methods for speeding the time to reperfusion along with the goals for the time intervals for the various components of the time delay. (*Adapted from CP Cannon et al: J Thromb Thrombol 1:27, 1994.*)

MANAGEMENT IN THE EMERGENCY DEPARTMENT

In the Emergency Department, the goals for the management of patients with suspected STEMI include control of cardiac discomfort, rapid identification of patients who are candidates for urgent reperfusion therapy, triage of lower-risk patients to the appropriate location in the hospital, and avoidance of inappropriate discharge of patients with STEMI. Many aspects of the treatment of STEMI are initiated in the Emergency Department and then continued during the in-hospital phase of management.

Aspirin is essential in the management of patients with suspected STEMI and is effective across the entire spectrum of acute coronary syndromes (Fig. 239-1). Rapid inhibition of cyclooxygenase-1 in platelets followed by a reduction of thromboxane A_2 levels is achieved by buccal absorption of a chewed 160–325 mg tablet in the Emergency Department. This measure should be followed by daily oral administration of aspirin in a dose of 75–162 mg.

In patients whose arterial O_2 saturation is normal, supplemental O_2 is of limited if any clinical benefit and therefore is not cost-effective. However, when hypoxemia is present, O_2 should be administered by nasal prongs or face mask (2–4 L/min) for the first 6–12 h after infarction; the patient should then be reassessed to determine if there is a continued need for such treatment.

CONTROL OF DISCOMFORT

Sublingual *nitroglycerin* can be given safely to most patients with STEMI. Up to three doses of 0.4 mg should be administered at about 5-min intervals. In addition to diminishing or abolishing chest discomfort, nitroglycerin may be capable of both decreasing myocardial oxygen demand (by lowering preload) and increasing myocardial oxy-

gen supply (by dilating infarct-related coronary vessels or collateral vessels). In patients whose initially favorable response to sublingual nitroglycerin is followed by the return of chest discomfort, particularly if accompanied by other evidence of ongoing ischemia such as further ST-segment or T-wave shifts, the use of intravenous nitroglycerin should be considered. Therapy with nitrates should be avoided in patients who present with low systolic arterial pressure (<90 mmHg) or in whom there is clinical suspicion of right ventricular infarction (inferior infarction on ECG, elevated jugular venous pressure, clear lungs, and hypotension). Nitrates should not be administered to patients who have taken the phosphodiesterase-5 inhibitor sildenafil for erectile dysfunction within the preceding 24 h since it may potentiate the hypotensive effects of nitrates. An idiosyncratic reaction to nitrates, consisting of sudden marked hypotension, sometimes occurs but can usually be reversed promptly by the rapid administration of intravenous atropine.

Morphine is a very effective analgesic for the pain associated with STEMI. However, it may reduce sympathetically mediated arteriolar and venous constriction, and the resulting venous pooling may reduce cardiac output and arterial pressure. These hemodynamic disturbances usually respond promptly to elevation of the legs, but in some patients volume expansion with intravenous saline is required. The patient may experience diaphoresis and nausea, but these events usually pass and are replaced by a feeling of well-being associated with the relief of pain. Morphine also has a vagotonic effect and may cause bradycardia or advanced degrees of heart block, particularly in patients with posteroinferior infarction. These side effects usually respond to atropine (0.5 mg intravenously). Morphine is routinely administered by repetitive (every 5 min) intravenous injection of small doses (2–4 mg) rather than by the subcutaneous administration of a larger quantity, because absorption may be unpredictable by the latter route.

Intravenous *beta blockers* are also useful in the control of the pain of STEMI. These drugs control pain effectively in some patients, presumably by diminishing myocardial O_2 demand and hence ischemia. More important, there is evidence that intravenous beta blockers reduce the risks of reinfarction and ventricular fibrillation (see "Beta-Adrenoceptor Blockers," below). A commonly employed regimen is metoprolol, 5 mg every 2–5 min for a total of 3 doses, provided the patient has a heart rate >60 beats per minute (bpm), systolic pressure >100 mmHg, a PR interval <0.24 s, and rales that are no higher than 10 cm up from the diaphragm. Fifteen minutes after the last intravenous dose, an oral regimen is initiated of 50 mg every 6 h for 48 h, followed by 100 mg every 12 h.

Unlike beta blockers, calcium antagonists are of little value in the acute setting, and there is evidence that short-acting dihydropyridines may be associated with an increased mortality risk.

MANAGEMENT STRATEGIES

The primary tool for screening patients and making triage decisions is the initial 12-lead ECG. When ST-segment elevation of at least 2 mm in two contiguous precordial leads and 1 mm in two adjacent limb leads is present, a patient should be considered a candidate for *reperfusion therapy* (Fig. 239-4). The process of selecting patients for fibrinolysis versus primary PCI (angioplasty, or stenting; Chap. 240) is discussed below. In the absence of ST-segment elevation, fibrinolysis is not helpful, and evidence exists suggesting that it may be harmful.

LIMITATION OF INFARCT SIZE

The quantity of myocardium that becomes necrotic as a consequence of a coronary artery occlusion is determined by factors other than just the site of occlusion. While the central zone of the infarct contains necrotic tissue that is irretrievably lost, the fate of the surrounding ischemic myocardium may be improved by timely restoration of coronary perfusion, reduction of myocardial O_2 demands, prevention of the accumulation of noxious metabolites, and blunting of the impact of mediators of reperfusion injury (e.g., calcium overload and oxygen-derived free radicals). Up to one-third of patients with STEMI may achieve *spontaneous* reperfusion of the infarct-related coronary artery within 24 h and experience improved healing of infarcted tissue. Reperfusion, either pharmacologically (by fibrinolysis) or by PCI, accelerates the opening of infarct-related arteries in those patients in whom spontaneous fibrinolysis ultimately would have occurred and also greatly increases the number of patients in whom restoration of flow in the infarct-related artery is accomplished. Timely restoration of flow in the epicardial infarct–related artery combined with improved perfusion of the downstream zone of infarcted myocardium results in a limitation of infarct size. Protection of the ischemic myocardium by the maintenance of an optimal balance between myocardial O_2 supply and demand through pain control, treatment of congestive heart failure (CHF), and minimization of tachycardia and

FIGURE 239-4 Options for transportation of patients with STEMI and initial reperfusion treatment. Patient transported by EMS after calling 911: Reperfusion in patients with STEMI can be accomplished by the pharmacologic (fibrinolysis) or catheter-based (primary PCI) approaches. Implementation of these strategies varies based on the mode of transportation of the patient and capabilities at the receiving hospital. Transport time to the hospital is variable from case to case, but the goal is to keep total ischemic time within 120 min. There are three possibilities. (1) If EMS has fibrinolytic capability and the patient qualifies for therapy, prehospital fibrinolysis should be started within 30 min of EMS arrival on scene. (2) If EMS is not capable of administering prehospital fibrinolysis and the patient is transported to a non–PCI-capable hospital, the hospital door-to-needle time should be within 30 min for patients in whom fibrinolysis is indicated. (3) If EMS is not capable of administering prehospital fibrinolysis and the patient is transported to a PCI-capable hospital, the hospital door-to-balloon time should be within 90 min. *Interhospital transfer*: It is also appropriate to consider emergency interhospital transfer of the patient to a PCI-capable hospital for mechanical revascularization if: (1) there is a contraindication to fibrinolysis; (2) PCI can be initiated promptly (within 90 minutes after the patient presented to the initial receiving hospital or within 60 min compared to when fibrinolysis with a fibrin-specific agent could be initiated at the initial receiving hospital); (3) fibrinolysis is administered and is unsuccessful (i.e., "rescue PCI"). Secondary nonemergency interhospital transfer can be considered for recurrent ischemia. *Patient self-transport*: Patient self-transportation is discouraged. If the patient arrives at a non-PCI–capable hospital, the door-to-needle time should be within 30 min. If the patient arrives at a PCI-capable hospital, the door-to-balloon time should be within 90 min. The treatment options and time recommended after first hospital arrival are the same. *(Reproduced with permission from Antman et al: ACC/AHA guidelines for the management of patients with ST-elevation myocardial infarction: A report of the American College of Cardiology/American Heart Association Task Force on Practice Guidelines (Committee to Revise the 1999 Guidelines for the Management of Patients with Acute Myocardial Infarction). Available at www.acc.org/clinical/guidelines/stemi/index.pdf.)*

hypertension extends the "window" of time for the salvage of myocardium by reperfusion strategies.

Glucocorticoids and nonsteroidal anti-inflammatory agents, with the exception of aspirin, should be avoided in patients with STEMI. They can impair infarct healing and increase the risk of myocardial rupture, and their use may result in a larger infarct scar. In addition, they can increase coronary vascular resistance, thereby potentially reducing flow to ischemic myocardium.

Primary Percutaneous Coronary Intervention   (See also Chap. 240) PCI, usually angioplasty and/or stenting without preceding fibrinolysis, referred to as *primary PCI*, is effective in restoring perfusion in STEMI when carried out on an emergency basis in the first few hours of MI. It has the advantage of being applicable to patients who have contraindications to fibrinolytic therapy (see below) but otherwise are considered appropriate candidates for reperfusion. It appears to be more effective than fibrinolysis in opening occluded coronary arteries and, *when performed by experienced operators [≥75 PCI cases (not necessarily primary) per year] in dedicated medical centers (≥36 primary PCI cases per year)*, is associated with better short-term and long-term clinical outcomes. Compared with fibrinolysis, primary PCI is generally preferred when the diagnosis is in doubt, cardiogenic shock is present, bleeding risk is increased, or symptoms have been present for at least 2–3 h when the clot is more mature and less easily lysed by fibrinolytic drugs. However, PCI is expensive in terms of personnel and facilities, and its applicability is limited by its availability, around the clock, in only a minority of hospitals.

Fibrinolysis   If no contraindications are present (see below), fibrinolytic therapy should ideally be initiated within 30 min of presentation (i.e., door-to-needle time ≤30 min). The principal goal of fibrinolysis is prompt restoration of full coronary arterial patency. The fibrinolytic agents tissue plasminogen activator (tPA), streptokinase, tenecteplase (TNK), and reteplase (rPA) have been approved by the U.S. Food and Drug Administration for intravenous use in patients with STEMI. These drugs all act by promoting the conversion of plasminogen to plasmin, which subsequently lyses fibrin thrombi. Although considerable emphasis was first placed on a distinction between more fibrin-specific agents, such as tPA, and non-fibrin-specific agents, such as streptokinase, it is now recognized that these differences are only relative, as some degree of systemic fibrinolysis occurs with the former agents. TNK and rPA are referred to as *bolus fibrinolytics* since their administration does not require a prolonged intravenous infusion.

When assessed angiographically, flow in the culprit coronary artery is described by a simple qualitative scale called the *thrombolysis in myocardial infarction (TIMI) grading system*: grade 0 indicates complete occlusion of the infarct-related artery; grade 1 indicates some penetration of the contrast material beyond the point of obstruction but without perfusion of the distal coronary bed; grade 2 indicates perfusion of the entire infarct vessel into the distal bed but with flow that is delayed compared with that of a normal artery; and grade 3 indicates full perfusion of the infarct vessel with normal flow. The latter is the goal of reperfusion therapy, because full perfusion of the infarct-related coronary artery yields far better results in terms of limiting infarct size, maintenance of LV function, and reduction of both short- and long-term mortality rates. Additional methods of angiographic assessment of the efficacy of fibrinolysis include counting the number of frames on the cine film required for dye to flow from the origin of the infarct-related artery to a landmark in the distal vascular bed (*TIMI frame count*) and determining the rate of entry and exit of contrast dye from the microvasculature in the myocardial infarct zone (*TIMI myocardial perfusion grade*). These methods have an even tighter correlation with outcomes after STEMI than the more commonly employed TIMI flow grade.

Fibrinolytic therapy can reduce the relative risk of in-hospital death by up to 50% when administered within the first hour of the onset of symptoms of STEMI, and much of this benefit is maintained for at least 10 years. When appropriately used, fibrinolytic therapy appears to reduce infarct size, limit LV dysfunction, and reduce the incidence of serious complications such as septal rupture, cardiogenic shock, and malignant ventricular arrhythmias. Since myocardium can be salvaged only before it has been irreversibly injured, the timing of reperfusion therapy, by fibrinolysis or a catheter-based approach, is of extreme importance in achieving maximum benefit. While the upper time limit depends on specific factors in individual patients, it is clear that "every minute counts" and that patients treated within 1–3 h of the onset of symptoms generally benefit most. Although reduction of the mortality rate is more modest, the therapy remains of benefit for many patients seen 3–6 h after the onset of infarction, and some benefit appears to be possible up to 12 h, especially if chest discomfort is still present and ST segments remain elevated. Compared with PCI for STEMI (primary PCI), fibrinolysis is generally the preferred reperfusion strategy for patients presenting in the first hour of symptoms, if there are logistical concerns about transportation of the patient to a suitable PCI center (experienced operator and team with a track record for a "door-to-balloon" time of <2 h), or there is an anticipated delay of at least 1 h between the time that fibrinolysis could be started versus implementation of PCI. Although patients <75 years achieve a greater relative reduction in the mortality rate with fibrinolytic therapy than do older patients, the higher *absolute* mortality rate (15–25%) in the latter results in similar absolute reductions in the mortality rates for both age groups.

tPA and the other relatively fibrin-specific plasminogen activators, rPA and TNK, are more effective than streptokinase at restoring full perfusion—i.e., TIMI grade 3 coronary flow—and have a small edge in improving survival as well. The current recommended regimen of tPA consists of a 15 mg bolus followed by 50 mg intravenously over the first 30 min, followed by 35 mg over the next 60 min. Streptokinase is administered as 1.5 million units (MU) intravenously over 1 h. rPA is administered in a double-bolus regimen consisting of a 10-MU bolus given over 2–3 min, followed by a second 10-MU bolus 30 min later. TNK is given as a single weight-based intravenous bolus of 0.53 mg/kg over 10 s. In addition to the fibrinolytic agents discussed above, pharmacologic reperfusion typically involves adjunctive antiplatelet and antithrombotic drugs, as discussed subsequently.

Alternative pharmacologic regimens for reperfusion combine an intravenous glycoprotein IIb/IIIa inhibitor with a reduced dose of a fibrinolytic agent. Compared with fibrinolytic agents that involve a prolonged infusion (e.g., tPA), such combination reperfusion regimens facilitate the rate and extent of fibrinolysis by inhibiting platelet aggregation, weakening the clot structure, and allowing penetration of the fibrinolytic agent deeper into the clot. However, combination reperfusion regimens have similar efficacy as compared with bolus fibrinolytics and are associated with an increased risk of bleeding, especially in patients >75 years. Therefore, combination reperfusion regimens are not recommended for routine use. Glycoprotein IIb/IIIa inhibitors given alone (i.e., without any fibrinolytic agent) are being investigated as a preparatory pharmacologic regimen in STEMI patients who are referred promptly for PCI—an experimental strategy called *facilitated PCI*. Another experimental strategy that has been proposed but not yet rigorously evaluated is a *pharmacoinvasive* approach where STEMI patients are first treated with a pharmacologic reperfusion regimen followed by routine angiography and PCI after a delay of 12–24 h to minimize the risks of performing PCI while the effects of the lytic agent are still present.

Contraindications and Complications   Clear contraindications to the use of fibrinolytic agents include a history of cerebrovascular hemorrhage at any time, a nonhemorrhagic stroke or other cerebrovascular event within the past year, marked hypertension (a reliably determined systolic arterial pressure >180 mmHg and/or a diastolic pressure >110 mmHg) at any time during the acute presentation, suspicion of aortic dissection, and active internal bleeding (excluding menses). While advanced age is associated with an increase in hemorrhagic complications, the benefit of fibrinolytic therapy in the elderly appears to justify its use if no other contraindications are present and the amount of myocardium in jeopardy appears to be substantial.

Relative contraindications to fibrinolytic therapy, which require assessment of the risk:benefit ratio, include current use of anticoagulants (international normalized ratio ≥2), a recent (<2 weeks) invasive or surgical procedure or prolonged (>10 min) cardiopulmonary resuscitation, known bleeding diathesis, pregnancy, a hemorrhagic ophthalmic condition (e.g., hemorrhagic diabetic retinopathy), active peptic ulcer disease, and a history of severe hypertension that is currently adequately controlled. Because of the risk of an allergic reaction, patients should not receive streptokinase if that agent had been received within the preceding 5 days to 2 years.

Allergic reactions to streptokinase occur in ~2% of patients who receive it. While a minor degree of hypotension occurs in 4–10% of patients given this agent, marked hypotension occurs, although rarely, in association with severe allergic reactions.

Hemorrhage is the most frequent and potentially the most serious complication. Because bleeding episodes that require transfusion are more common when patients require invasive procedures, unnecessary venous or arterial interventions should be avoided in patients receiving fibrinolytic agents. Hemorrhagic stroke is the most serious complication and occurs in ~0.5–0.9% of patients being treated with these agents. This rate increases with advancing age, with patients >70 years experiencing roughly twice the rate of intracranial hemorrhage as those <65 years. Large-scale trials have suggested that the rate of intracranial hemorrhage with tPA or rPA is slightly higher than with streptokinase.

Cardiac catheterization and coronary angiography should be carried out after fibrinolytic therapy if there is evidence of either (1) failure of reperfusion (persistent chest pain and ST-segment elevation >90 min), in which case a *rescue PCI* should be considered; or (2) coronary artery reocclusion (re-elevation of ST segments and/or recurrent chest pain) or the development of recurrent ischemia (such as recurrent angina in the early hospital course or a positive exercise stress test before discharge), in which case an *urgent PCI* should be considered. The potential benefits of routine angiography and *elective* PCI even in asymptomatic patients following administration of fibrinolytic therapy are controversial, but such an approach may have merit given the numerous technological advances that have occurred in the catheterization laboratory and the increasing number of skilled interventionalists. Coronary artery bypass surgery should be reserved for patients whose coronary anatomy is unsuited to PCI but in whom revascularization appears to be advisable because of extensive jeopardized myocardium or recurrent ischemia.

HOSPITAL PHASE MANAGEMENT

CORONARY CARE UNITS

These units are routinely equipped with a system that permits continuous monitoring of the cardiac rhythm of each patient and hemodynamic monitoring in selected patients. Defibrillators, respirators, noninvasive transthoracic pacemakers, and facilities for introducing pacing catheters and flow-directed balloon-tipped catheters are also usually available. Equally important is the organization of a highly trained team of nurses who can recognize arrhythmias; adjust the dosage of antiarrhythmic, vasoactive, and anticoagulant drugs; and perform cardiac resuscitation, including electroshock, when necessary.

Patients should be admitted to a coronary care unit early in their illness when it is expected that they will derive benefit from the sophisticated and expensive care provided. The availability of electrocardiographic monitoring and trained personnel outside the coronary care unit has made it possible to admit lower-risk patients (e.g., those not hemodynamically compromised and without active arrhythmias) to "intermediate care units."

The duration of stay in the coronary care unit is dictated by the ongoing need for intensive care. If symptoms are controlled with oral therapy, patients may be transferred out of the coronary care unit. Also, patients who have a confirmed STEMI but who are considered to be at low risk (no prior infarction and no persistent chest discomfort, CHF, hypotension, or cardiac arrhythmias) may be safely transferred out of the coronary care unit within 24 h.

Activity   Factors that increase the work of the heart during the initial hours of infarction may increase the size of the infarct. Therefore, pa-

tients with STEMI should be kept at bed rest for the first 12 h. However, in the absence of complications, patients should be encouraged, under supervision, to resume an upright posture by dangling their feet over the side of the bed and sitting in a chair within the first 24 h. This practice is psychologically beneficial and usually results in a reduction in the pulmonary capillary wedge pressure. In the absence of hypotension and other complications, by the second or third day patients typically are ambulating in their room with increasing duration and frequency, and they may shower or stand at the sink to bathe. By day 3 after infarction, patients should be increasing their ambulation progressively to a goal of 185 m (600 ft) at least three times a day.

Diet   Because of the risk of emesis and aspiration soon after STEMI, patients should receive either nothing or only clear liquids by mouth for the first 4–12 h. The typical coronary care unit diet should provide ≤30% of total calories as fat and have a cholesterol content of ≤300 mg/d. Complex carbohydrates should make up 50–55% of total calories. Portions should not be unusually large, and the menu should be enriched with foods that are high in potassium, magnesium, and fiber but low in sodium. Diabetes mellitus and hypertriglyceridemia are managed by restriction of concentrated sweets in the diet.

Bowels   Bed rest and the effect of the narcotics used for the relief of pain often lead to constipation. A bedside commode rather than a bedpan, a diet rich in bulk, and the routine use of a stool softener such as dioctyl sodium sulfosuccinate (200 mg/d) are recommended. If the patient remains constipated despite these measures, a laxative can be prescribed. Contrary to prior belief, it is safe to perform a gentle rectal examination on patients with STEMI.

Sedation   Many patients require sedation during hospitalization to withstand the period of enforced inactivity with tranquillity. Diazepam (5 mg), oxazepam (15–30 mg), or lorazepam (0.5–2 mg), given three or four times daily, is usually effective. An additional dose of any of the above medications may be given at night to ensure adequate sleep. Attention to this problem is especially important during the first few days in the coronary care unit, where the atmosphere of 24-h vigilance may interfere with the patient's sleep. However, sedation is no substitute for reassuring, quiet surroundings. Many drugs used in the coronary care unit, such as atropine, H$_2$ blockers, and narcotics, can produce delirium, particularly in the elderly. This effect should not be confused with agitation, and it is wise to conduct a thorough review of the patient's medications before arbitrarily prescribing additional doses of anxiolytics.

PHARMACOTHERAPY

ANTITHROMBOTIC AGENTS

The use of antiplatelet and antithrombin therapy during the initial phase of STEMI is based on extensive laboratory and clinical evidence that thrombosis plays an important role in the pathogenesis of this condition. The primary goal of treatment with antiplatelet and antithrombin agents is to establish and maintain patency of the infarct-related artery, in conjunction with reperfusion strategies. A secondary goal is to reduce the patient's tendency to thrombosis and thus the likelihood of mural thrombus formation or deep venous thrombosis, either of which could result in pulmonary embolization. The degree to which antiplatelet and antithrombin therapy achieves these goals partly determines how effectively it reduces the risk of mortality from STEMI.

As noted previously (see "Management in the Emergency Department," above), aspirin is the standard antiplatelet agent for patients with STEMI. The most compelling evidence for the benefits of antiplatelet therapy (mainly with aspirin) in STEMI is found in the comprehensive overview by the Antiplatelet Trialists' Collaboration. Data from nearly 20,000 patients with MI enrolled in 15 randomized trials were pooled and revealed a relative reduction of 27% in the mortality rate, from 14.2% in control patients to 10.4% in patients receiving antiplatelet agents.

Inhibitors of the P2Y$_{12}$ ADP receptor prevent activation and aggregation of platelets. The addition of the P2Y$_{12}$ inhibitor clopidogrel to

Number of events

Days	0–6	7–13	14–20	21–28
Clopidogrel	1403	223	69	31
Placebo	1487	246	89	23

FIGURE 239-5 Panel A: Effect of the addition of clopidogrel on in-hospital mortality after STEMI. These time-to-event curves show a 0.6% reduction in mortality in the group receiving clopidogrel plus aspirin (N = 22,961) compared to placebo plus aspirin (N = 22,891) in the COMMIT trial. (*Reproduced with permission from ZM Chen et al: Lancet 366:1607, 2005.*) **Panel B:** Effects of the addition of clopidogrel in patients receiving fibrinolysis for STEMI. Patients in the clopidogrel group (N = 1752) had a 36% reduction in the odds of dying, sustaining a recurrent infarction, or having an occluded infarct artery compared to the placebo group (N = 1739) in the CLARITY-TIMI 28 trial (p <.001). (*Adapted from Sabatine MS et al: New Engl J Med 352:1179, 2005.*)

background treatment with aspirin to STEMI patients reduces the risk of clinical events (death, reinfarction, stroke) and in patients receiving fibrinolytic therapy has been shown to prevent reocclusion of a successfully reperfused infarct artery (Fig. 239-5). Glycoprotein IIb/IIIa receptor inhibitors appear useful for preventing thrombotic complications in patients with STEMI undergoing PCI.

The standard antithrombin agent used in clinical practice is unfractionated heparin (UFH). The available data suggest that when UFH is added to a regimen of aspirin and a non-fibrin-specific thrombolytic agent such as streptokinase, additional mortality benefit occurs (about five lives saved per 1000 patients treated). It appears that the immediate administration of intravenous UFH, in addition to a regimen of aspirin and relatively fibrin-specific fibrinolytic agents (tPA, rPA, or TNK), helps to maintain patency of the infarct-related artery. This effect is achieved at the cost of a small increased risk of bleeding. The recommended dose of UFH is an initial bolus of 60 U/kg (maximum 4000 U) followed by an initial infusion of 12 U/kg per hour (maximum 1000 U/h). The activated partial thromboplastin time during maintenance therapy should be 1.5–2 times the control value.

An alternative to UFH for anticoagulation of patients with STEMI are the low-molecular-weight heparin (LMWH) preparations, which are formed by enzymatic or chemical depolymerization to produce saccharide chains of varying length but with a mean molecular weight of about 5000 Da. Advantages of LMWHs include high bioavailability permitting administration subcutaneously, reliable anticoagulation without monitoring, and greater antiXa:IIa activity. Enoxaparin has been shown to significantly reduce the composite endpoints of death/nonfatal reinfarction (Fig. 239-6) and death/nonfatal reinfarction/urgent revascularization compared with UFH in STEMI patients who receive fibrinolysis. Although treatment with enoxaparin is associated with higher rates of serious bleeding, net clinical benefit—a composite endpoint that combines efficacy and safety—strongly favors enoxaparin over UFH.

Patients with an anterior location of the infarction, severe LV dysfunction, heart failure, a history of embolism, two-dimensional echocardiographic evidence of mural thrombus, or atrial fibrillation are at increased risk of systemic or pulmonary thromboembolism. Such individuals should receive full therapeutic levels of antithrombin therapy (LMWH or UFH) while hospitalized, followed by at least 3 months of warfarin therapy.

BETA-ADRENOCEPTOR BLOCKERS

The benefits of beta blockers in patients with STEMI can be divided into those that occur immediately when the drug is given acutely and those that accrue over the long term when the drug is given for secondary pre-

FIGURE 239-6 Enoxaparin is superior to unfractionated heparin in STEMI patients receiving fibrinolysis. In the ExTRACT-TIMI 25 trial, patients receiving the low-molecular-weight heparin enoxaparin in addition to a fibrinolytic agent plus aspirin (N = 10,256) had a significantly lower rate of the composite endpoint of death or nonfatal reinfarction compared to patients receiving unfractionated heparin in combination with a fibrinolytic plus aspirin (N = 10,223). RRR, relative risk reduction. (*Reproduced with permission from EM Antman et al: New Engl J Med 354:1477, 2006.*)

vention after an infarction. Acute intravenous beta blockade improves the myocardial O_2 supply-demand relationship, decreases pain, reduces infarct size, and decreases the incidence of serious ventricular arrhythmias. In patients who undergo fibrinolysis soon after the onset of chest pain, no incremental reduction in mortality rate is seen with beta blockers, but recurrent ischemia and reinfarction are reduced.

Thus, beta blocker therapy after STEMI is useful for most patients (including those treated with an ACE inhibitor) except those in whom it is specifically contraindicated (patients with heart failure or severely compromised LV function, heart block, orthostatic hypotension, or a history of asthma) and perhaps those whose excellent long-term prognosis (defined as an expected mortality rate of <1% per year, patients <55 years, no previous MI, with normal ventricular function, no complex ventricular ectopy, and no angina) markedly diminishes any potential benefit.

INHIBITION OF THE RENIN-ANGIOTENSIN-ALDOSTERONE SYSTEM

Angiotensin-converting enzyme (ACE) inhibitors reduce the mortality rate after STEMI, and the mortality benefits are additive to those achieved with aspirin and beta blockers. The maximum benefit is seen in high-risk patients (those who are elderly or who have an anterior infarction, a prior infarction, and/or globally depressed LV function), but evidence suggests that a short-term benefit occurs when ACE inhibitors are prescribed unselectively to all hemodynamically stable patients with STEMI (i.e., those with a systolic pressure >100 mmHg). The mechanism involves a reduction in ventricular remodeling after infarction (see "Ventricular Dysfunction," below) with a subsequent reduction in the risk of congestive heart failure (CHF). The rate of recurrent infarction may also be lower in patients treated chronically with ACE inhibitors after infarction.

Before hospital discharge, LV function should be assessed with an imaging study. ACE inhibitors should be continued indefinitely in patients who have clinically evident CHF, in patients in whom an imaging study shows a reduction in global LV function or a large regional wall motion abnormality, or in those who are hypertensive.

Angiotensin receptor blockers (ARBs) should be administered to STEMI patients who are intolerant of ACE inhibitors and who have either clinical or radiological signs of heart failure. Long-term aldosterone blockade should be prescribed for STEMI patients without significant renal dysfunction (creatinine ≥2.5 mg/dL in men and ≥2.0 mg/dL in women) or hyperkalemia (potassium ≥5.0 mEq/L) who are already receiving therapeutic doses of an ACE inhibitor, an LV ejection fraction ≤40 percent, and either symptomatic heart failure or diabetes mellitus. A multidrug regimen for inhibiting the renin-angiotensin-aldosterone system has been shown to reduce both heart failure-related and sudden cardiac death-related cardiovascular mortality after STEMI, but has not been as thoroughly explored as ACE inhibitors in STEMI patients.

OTHER AGENTS

Favorable effects on the ischemic process and ventricular remodeling (see below) previously led many physicians to routinely use *intravenous nitroglycerin* (5–10 µg/min initial dose and up to 200 µg/min as long as hemodynamic stability is maintained) for the first 24–48 h after the onset of infarction. However, the benefits of routine use of intravenous nitroglycerin are less in the contemporary era where beta-adrenoceptor blockers and ACE inhibitors are routinely prescribed for patients with STEMI.

Results of multiple trials of different calcium antagonists have failed to establish a role for these agents in the treatment of most patients with STEMI. Therefore, the routine use of calcium antagonists cannot be recommended. Strict control of blood glucose in diabetic patients with STEMI has been shown to reduce the mortality rate. Serum magnesium should be measured in all patients on admission, and any demonstrated deficits should be corrected to minimize the risk of arrhythmias.

COMPLICATIONS AND THEIR MANAGEMENT

VENTRICULAR DYSFUNCTION

After STEMI, the left ventricle undergoes a series of changes in shape, size, and thickness in both the infarcted and noninfarcted segments.

This process is referred to as *ventricular remodeling* and generally precedes the development of clinically evident CHF in the months to years after infarction. Soon after STEMI, the left ventricle begins to dilate. Acutely, this results from expansion of the infarct, i.e., slippage of muscle bundles, disruption of normal myocardial cells, and tissue loss within the necrotic zone, resulting in disproportionate thinning and elongation of the infarct zone. Later, lengthening of the noninfarcted segments occurs as well. The overall chamber enlargement that occurs is related to the size and location of the infarct, with greater dilation following infarction of the anterior wall and apex of the left ventricle and causing more marked hemodynamic impairment, more frequent heart failure, and a poorer prognosis. Progressive dilation and its clinical consequences may be ameliorated by therapy with ACE inhibitors and other vasodilators (e.g., nitrates). In patients with an ejection fraction <40%, regardless of whether or not heart failure is present, ACE inhibitors or ARBs should be prescribed (see "Inhibition of the Renin-Angiotensin-Aldosterone System," above).

HEMODYNAMIC ASSESSMENT

Pump failure is now the primary cause of in-hospital death from STEMI. The extent of infarction correlates well with the degree of pump failure and with mortality, both early (within 10 days of infarction) and later. The most common clinical signs are pulmonary rales and S_3 and S_4 gallop sounds. Pulmonary congestion is also frequently seen on the chest roentgenogram. Elevated LV filling pressure and elevated pulmonary artery pressure are the characteristic hemodynamic findings, but these findings may result from a reduction of ventricular compliance (diastolic failure) and/or a reduction of stroke volume with secondary cardiac dilation (systolic failure) (Chap. 227).

A classification originally proposed by Killip divides patients into four groups: class I, no signs of pulmonary or venous congestion; class II, moderate heart failure as evidenced by rales at the lung bases, S_3 gallop, tachypnea, or signs of failure of the right side of the heart, including venous and hepatic congestion; class III, severe heart failure, pulmonary edema; and class IV, shock with systolic pressure <90 mmHg and evidence of peripheral vasoconstriction, peripheral cyanosis, mental confusion, and oliguria. When this classification was established in 1967, the expected hospital mortality rate of patients in these classes was as follows: class I, 0–5%; class II, 10–20%; class III, 35–45%; and class IV, 85–95%. With advances in management, the mortality rate in each class has fallen, perhaps by as much as one-third to one-half.

Hemodynamic evidence of abnormal global LV function appears when contraction is seriously impaired in 20–25% of the left ventricle. Infarction of ≥40% of the left ventricle usually results in cardiogenic shock (Chap. 266). Positioning of a balloon flotation (Swan-Ganz) catheter in the pulmonary artery permits monitoring of LV filling pressure; this technique is useful in patients who exhibit hypotension and/or clinical evidence of CHF. Cardiac output can also be determined with a pulmonary artery catheter. With the addition of intraarterial pressure monitoring, systemic vascular resistance can be calculated as a guide to adjusting vasopressor and vasodilator therapy. Some patients with STEMI have markedly elevated LV filling pressures (>22 mmHg) and normal cardiac indices [2.6–3.6 L/(min/m^2)], while others have relatively low LV filling pressures (<15 mmHg) and reduced cardiac indices. The former patients usually benefit from diuresis, while the latter may respond to volume expansion.

HYPOVOLEMIA This is an easily corrected condition that may contribute to the hypotension and vascular collapse associated with STEMI in some patients. It may be secondary to previous diuretic use, to reduced fluid intake during the early stages of the illness, and/or to vomiting associated with pain or medications. Consequently, hypovolemia should be identified and corrected in patients with STEMI and hypotension before more vigorous forms of therapy are begun. Central venous pressure reflects RV rather than LV filling pressure and is an inadequate guide for adjustment of blood volume, since LV function is almost always affected much more adversely than RV function in patients with STEMI. The optimal LV filling or pulmonary artery wedge pressure may vary considerably among patients. Each patient's ideal level (generally ~20 mmHg) is reached by cautious fluid administration during careful monitoring of oxygenation and cardiac output. Eventually the cardiac output level plateaus, and further increases in LV filling pressure only increase congestive symptoms and decrease systemic oxygenation without raising arterial pressure.

℞ CONGESTIVE HEART FAILURE

The management of CHF in association with STEMI is similar to that of acute heart failure secondary to other forms of heart disease (avoidance of hypoxemia, diuresis, afterload reduction, inotropic support) (Chap. 227), except that the benefits of digitalis administration to patients with STEMI are unimpressive. By contrast, diuretic agents are extremely effective, as they diminish pulmonary congestion in the presence of systolic and/or diastolic heart failure. LV filling pressure falls and orthopnea and dyspnea improve after the intravenous administration of furosemide or other loop diuretics. These drugs should be used with caution, however, as they can result in a massive diuresis with associated decreases in plasma volume, cardiac output, systemic blood pressure, and hence coronary perfusion. Nitrates in various forms may be used to decrease preload and congestive symptoms. Oral isosorbide dinitrate, topical nitroglycerin ointment, or intravenous nitroglycerin all have the advantage over a diuretic of lowering preload through venodilation without decreasing the total plasma volume. In addition, nitrates may improve ventricular compliance if ischemia is present, as ischemia causes an elevation of LV filling pressure. Vasodilators must be used with caution to prevent serious hypotension. As noted earlier, ACE inhibitors are an ideal class of drugs for management of ventricular dysfunction after STEMI, especially for the long term. (See "Inhibition of the Renin-Angiotensin-Aldosterone System," above.)

CARDIOGENIC SHOCK

Prompt reperfusion, efforts to reduce infarct size, and treatment of ongoing ischemia and other complications of MI appear to have reduced the incidence of cardiogenic shock from 20% to about 7%. Only 10% of patients with this condition present with it on admission, while 90% develop it during hospitalization. Typically, patients who develop cardiogenic shock have severe multivessel coronary artery disease with evidence of "piecemeal" necrosis extending outward from the original infarct zone. The evaluation and management of cardiogenic shock and severe power failure after STEMI are discussed in detail in Chap. 266.

RIGHT VENTRICULAR INFARCTION

Approximately one-third of patients with inferior infarction demonstrate at least a minor degree of RV necrosis. An occasional patient with inferoposterior LV infarction also has extensive RV infarction, and rare patients present with infarction limited primarily to the RV. Clinically significant RV infarction causes signs of severe RV failure [jugular venous distention, Kussmaul's sign, hepatomegaly (Chap. 220)] with or without hypotension. ST-segment elevations of right-sided precordial ECG leads, particularly lead V_4R, are frequently present in the first 24 h in patients with RV infarction. Two-dimensional echocardiography is helpful in determining the degree of RV dysfunction. Catheterization of the right side of the heart often reveals a distinctive hemodynamic pattern resembling constrictive pericarditis (steep right atrial "y" descent and an early diastolic dip and plateau in RV waveforms) (Chap. 232). Therapy consists of volume expansion to maintain adequate RV preload and efforts to improve LV performance with attendant reduction in pulmonary capillary wedge and pulmonary arterial pressures.

ARRHYTHMIAS

(See also Chaps. 225 and 226) The incidence of arrhythmias after STEMI is higher in patients seen early after the onset of symptoms. The mechanisms responsible for infarction-related arrhythmias include autonomic nervous system imbalance, electrolyte disturbances, ischemia, and slowed conduction in zones of ischemic myocardium. An arrhythmia can usually be managed successfully if trained personnel and appropriate equipment are available when it develops. Since most deaths from arrhythmia occur during the first few hours after infarction, the effectiveness of treatment relates directly to the speed with which patients come under medical observation. The prompt management of arrhythmias constitutes a significant advance in the treatment of STEMI.

Ventricular Premature Beats Infrequent, sporadic ventricular premature depolarizations occur in almost all patients with STEMI and do not require therapy. Whereas in the past, frequent, multifocal, or early diastolic ventricular extrasystoles (so-called warning arrhythmias) were routinely treated with antiarrhythmic drugs to reduce the risk of development of ventricular tachycardia and ventricular fibrillation, pharmacologic therapy is now reserved for patients with sustained ventricular arrhythmias. Prophylactic antiarrhythmic therapy (either intravenous lidocaine early or oral agents later) is contraindicated for ventricular premature beats in the absence of clinically important ventricular tachyarrhythmias, as such therapy may actually increase the mortality rate. Beta-adrenoceptor blocking agents are effective in abolishing ventricular ectopic activity in patients with STEMI and in the prevention of ventricular fibrillation. As described above (see "Beta-Adrenoceptor Blockers," above), they should be used routinely in patients without contraindications. In addition, hypokalemia and hypomagnesemia are risk factors for ventricular fibrillation in patients with STEMI; the serum potassium concentration should be adjusted to approximately 4.5 mmol/L and magnesium to about 2.0 mmol/L.

Ventricular Tachycardia and Fibrillation Within the first 24 h of STEMI, ventricular tachycardia and fibrillation can occur without prior warning arrhythmias. The occurrence of ventricular fibrillation can be reduced by prophylactic administration of intravenous lidocaine. However, prophylactic use of lidocaine has not been shown to reduce overall mortality from STEMI. In fact, in addition to causing possible noncardiac complications, lidocaine may predispose to an excess risk of bradycardia and asystole. For these reasons, and with earlier treatment of active ischemia, more frequent use of beta-blocking agents, and the nearly universal success of electrical cardioversion or defibrillation, routine prophylactic antiarrhythmic drug therapy *is no longer recommended*.

Sustained ventricular tachycardia that is well tolerated hemodynamically should be treated with an intravenous regimen of amiodarone (bolus of 150 mg over 10 min, followed by infusion of 1.0 mg/min for 6 h and then 0.5 mg/min); or procainamide (bolus of 15 mg/kg over 20–30 min; infusion of 1–4 mg/min); if it does not stop promptly, electroversion should be used (Chap. 226). An unsynchronized discharge of 200–300 J (monophasic wave form; approximately 50% of these energies with biphasic wave forms) is used immediately in patients with ventricular fibrillation or when ventricular tachycardia causes hemodynamic deterioration. Ventricular tachycardia or fibrillation that is refractory to electroshock may be more responsive after the patient is treated with epinephrine (1 mg intravenously or 10 mL of a 1:10,000 solution via the intracardiac route), or amiodarone (a 75–150 mg bolus).

Ventricular arrhythmias, including the unusual form of ventricular tachycardia known as torsades des pointes (Chap. 226), may occur in patients with STEMI as a consequence of other concurrent problems (such as hypoxia, hypokalemia, or other electrolyte disturbances) or of the toxic effects of an agent being administered to the patient (such as digoxin or quinidine). A search for such secondary causes should always be undertaken.

Although the in-hospital mortality rate is increased, the long-term survival is excellent in patients who survive to hospital discharge after *primary* ventricular fibrillation, i.e., ventricular fibrillation that is a primary response to acute ischemia that occurs during the first 48 h and is not associated with predisposing factors such as CHF, shock, bundle branch block, or ventricular aneurysm. This result is in sharp contrast to the poor prognosis for patients who develop ventricular fibrillation *secondary* to severe pump failure. For patients who develop

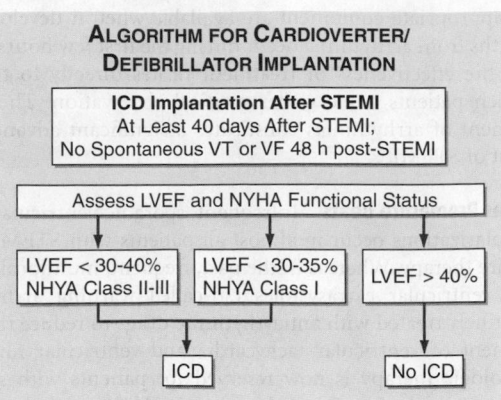

FIGURE 239-7 Algorithm for assessment of need for implantation of a cardioverter/defibrillator. The appropriate management is selected based upon measurement of left ventricular ejection fraction and assessment of the NYHA functional class. Patients with depressed left ventricular function at least 40 days post-STEMI are referred for insertion of an implantable cardioverter/defibrillator (ICD) if the LVEF is <30–40% and they are in NYHA class II–III or if the LVEF is <30–35% and they are in NYHA class I functional status. Patients with preserved left ventricular function (LVEF >40%) do not receive an ICD regardless of NYHA functional class. All patients are treated with medical therapy post-STEMI. [Adapted from data contained in Zipes DP, Camm AJ, et al: ACC/AHA/ESC 2006 guidelines for management of patients with ventricular arrhythmias and the prevention of sudden cardiac death; a report of the American College of Cardiology/American Heart Association Task Force and the European Society of Cardiology Committee for Practice Guidelines (Writing Committee to Develop Guidelines for Management of Patients with Ventricular Arrhythmias and the Prevention of Sudden Cardiac Death). J Am Coll Cardiol 48:1064, 2006.]

ventricular tachycardia or ventricular fibrillation late in their hospital course (i.e., after the first 48 h), the mortality rate is increased both in-hospital and during long-term follow-up. Such patients should be considered for electrophysiologic study and implantation of a cardioverter/defibrillator (ICD) (Chap. 226). A more challenging issue is the prevention of sudden cardiac death from ventricular fibrillation late after STEMI in patients who have not exhibited sustained ventricular tachyarrhythmias during their index hospitalization. An algorithm for selection of patients who warrant prophylactic implantation of an ICD is shown in Fig. 239-7.

Accelerated Idioventricular Rhythm Accelerated idioventricular rhythm (AIVR, "slow ventricular tachycardia"), a ventricular rhythm with a rate of 60–100 bpm, occurs in 25% of patients with STEMI. It often occurs transiently during fibrinolytic therapy at the time of reperfusion. For the most part, AIVR is benign and does not presage the development of classic ventricular tachycardia. Most episodes of AIVR do not require treatment if the patient is monitored carefully, as degeneration into a more serious arrhythmia is rare.

Supraventricular Arrhythmias Sinus tachycardia is the most common supraventricular arrhythmia. If it occurs secondary to another cause (such as anemia, fever, heart failure, or a metabolic derangement), the primary problem should be treated first. However, if it appears to be due to sympathetic overstimulation (e.g., as part of a hyperdynamic state), then treatment with a beta blocker is indicated. Other common arrhythmias in this group are atrial flutter and atrial fibrillation, which are often secondary to LV failure. Digoxin is usually the treatment of choice for supraventricular arrhythmias if heart failure is present. If heart failure is absent, beta blockers, verapamil, or diltiazem are suitable alternatives for controlling the ventricular rate, as they may also help to control ischemia. If the abnormal rhythm persists for >2 h with a ventricular rate >120 bpm, or if tachycardia induces heart failure, shock, or ischemia (as manifested by recurrent pain or ECG

changes), a synchronized electroshock (100–200 J monophasic wave form) should be used.

Accelerated junctional rhythms have diverse causes but may occur in patients with inferoposterior infarction. Digitalis excess must be ruled out. In some patients with severely compromised LV function, the loss of appropriately timed atrial systole results in a marked reduction of cardiac output. Right atrial or coronary sinus pacing is indicated in such instances.

Sinus Bradycardia Treatment of sinus bradycardia is indicated if hemodynamic compromise results from the slow heart rate. Atropine is the most useful drug for increasing heart rate and should be given intravenously in doses of 0.5 mg initially. If the rate remains <50–60 bpm, additional doses of 0.2 mg, up to a total of 2.0 mg, may be given. Persistent bradycardia (<40 bpm) despite atropine may be treated with electrical pacing. Isoproterenol should be avoided.

Atrioventricular and Intraventricular Conduction Disturbances (See also Chap. 225) Both the in-hospital mortality rate and the post-discharge mortality rate of patients who have complete atrioventricular (AV) block in association with anterior infarction are markedly higher than those of patients who develop AV block with inferior infarction. This difference is related to the fact that heart block in inferior infarction is commonly a result of increased vagal tone and/or the release of adenosine and therefore is transient. In anterior wall infarction, however, heart block is usually related to ischemic malfunction of the conduction system, which is commonly associated with extensive myocardial necrosis.

Temporary electrical pacing provides an effective means of increasing the heart rate of patients with bradycardia due to AV block. However, acceleration of the heart rate may have only a limited impact on prognosis in patients with anterior wall infarction and complete heart block in whom the large size of the infarct is the major factor determining outcome. It should be carried out if it improves hemodynamics. Pacing does appear to be beneficial in patients with inferoposterior infarction who have complete heart block associated with heart failure, hypotension, marked bradycardia, or significant ventricular ectopic activity. A subgroup of these patients, those with RV infarction, often respond poorly to ventricular pacing because of the loss of the atrial contribution to ventricular filling. In such patients, dual-chamber AV sequential pacing may be required.

External noninvasive pacing electrodes should be positioned in a "demand" mode for patients with sinus bradycardia (rate <50 bpm) that is unresponsive to drug therapy, Mobitz II second-degree AV block, third-degree heart block, or bilateral bundle branch block (e.g., right bundle branch block plus left anterior fascicular block). Retrospective studies suggest that permanent pacing may reduce the long-term risk of sudden death due to bradyarrhythmias in the rare patient who develops combined persistent bifascicular and transient third-degree heart block during the acute phase of MI.

OTHER COMPLICATIONS
Recurrent Chest Discomfort Recurrent angina develops in ~25% of patients hospitalized for STEMI. This percentage is even higher in patients who undergo successful fibrinolysis. Since recurrent or persistent ischemia often heralds extension of the original infarct or reinfarction in a new myocardial zone and is associated with a near tripling of mortality after STEMI, patients with these symptoms should be referred for prompt coronary arteriography and mechanical revascularization. Repeat administration of a fibrinolytic agent is an alternative to early mechanical revascularization.

Pericarditis (See also Chap. 232) Pericardial friction rubs and/or pericardial pain are frequently encountered in patients with STEMI involving the epicardium. This complication can usually be managed with aspirin (650 mg four times daily). It is important to diagnose the chest pain of pericarditis accurately, since failure to recognize it may lead to the erroneous diagnosis of recurrent ischemic pain and/or infarct extension, with resulting inappropriate use of anticoagulants, nitrates, beta blockers, or coronary arteriography. When it occurs, complaints of pain radiating to either trapezius muscle is helpful since such a pattern of discomfort is typical of pericarditis but rarely occurs with ischemic discomfort. Anticoagulants potentially could cause tamponade in the presence of acute pericarditis (as manifested by either pain or persistent rub) and therefore should not be used unless there is a compelling indication.

Thromboembolism Clinically apparent thromboembolism complicates STEMI in ~10% of cases, but embolic lesions are found in 20% of patients in necropsy series, suggesting that thromboembolism is often clinically silent. Thromboembolism is considered to be an important contributing cause of death in 25% of patients with STEMI who die after admission to the hospital. Arterial emboli originate from LV mural thrombi, while most pulmonary emboli arise in the leg veins.

Thromboembolism typically occurs in association with large infarcts (especially anterior), CHF, and a LV thrombus detected by echocardiography. The incidence of arterial embolism from a clot originating in the ventricle at the site of an infarction is small but real. Two-dimensional echocardiography reveals LV thrombi in about one-third of patients with anterior wall infarction but in few patients with inferior or posterior infarction. Arterial embolism often presents as a major complication, such as hemiparesis when the cerebral circulation is involved or hypertension if the renal circulation is compromised. When a thrombus has been clearly demonstrated by echocardiographic or other techniques or when a large area of regional wall motion abnormality is seen even in the absence of a detectable mural thrombus, systemic anticoagulation should be undertaken (in the absence of contraindications), as the incidence of embolic complications appears to be markedly lowered by such therapy. The appropriate duration of therapy is unknown, but 3–6 months is probably prudent.

Left Ventricular Aneurysm The term *ventricular aneurysm* is usually used to describe *dyskinesis* or local expansile paradoxical wall motion. Normally functioning myocardial fibers must shorten more if stroke volume and cardiac output are to be maintained in patients with ventricular aneurysm; if they cannot, overall ventricular function is impaired. True aneurysms are composed of scar tissue and neither predispose to nor are associated with cardiac rupture.

The complications of LV aneurysm do not usually occur for weeks to months after STEMI; they include CHF, arterial embolism, and ventricular arrhythmias. Apical aneurysms are the most common and the most easily detected by clinical examination. The physical finding of greatest value is a double, diffuse, or displaced apical impulse. Ventricular aneurysms are readily detected by two-dimensional echocardiography, which may also reveal a mural thrombus in an aneurysm.

Rarely, myocardial rupture may be contained by a local area of pericardium, along with organizing thrombus and hematoma. Over time, this *pseudoaneurysm* enlarges, maintaining communication with the LV cavity through a narrow neck. Because a pseudoaneurysm often ruptures spontaneously, it should be surgically repaired if recognized.

POSTINFARCTION RISK STRATIFICATION AND MANAGEMENT

Many clinical and laboratory factors have been identified that are associated with an increase in cardiovascular risk after initial recovery from STEMI. Some of the most important factors include persistent ischemia (spontaneous or provoked), depressed LV ejection fraction (<40%), rales above the lung bases on physical examination or congestion on chest radiograph, and symptomatic ventricular arrhythmias. Other features associated with increased risk include a history of previous MI, age >75, diabetes mellitus, prolonged sinus tachycardia, hypotension, ST-segment changes at rest without angina ("silent ischemia"), an abnormal signal-averaged ECG, nonpatency of the infarct-related coronary artery (if angiography is undertaken), and persistent advanced heart block or a new intraventricular conduction abnormality on the ECG. Therapy must be individualized on the basis of the relative importance of the risk(s) present.

The goal of preventing reinfarction and death after recovery from STEMI has led to strategies to evaluate risk after infarction. In stable patients, submaximal exercise stress testing may be carried out before hospital discharge to detect residual ischemia and ventricular ectopy and to provide the patient with a guideline for exercise in the early recovery period. Alternatively, or in addition, a maximal (symptom-limited) exercise stress test may be carried out 4–6 weeks after infarction. Evaluation of LV function is usually warranted as well. Recognition of a depressed LV ejection fraction by echocardiography or radionuclide ventriculography identifies patients who should receive medications to inhibit the renin-angiotensin-aldosterone system. Patients in whom angina is induced at relatively low workloads, those who have a large reversible defect on perfusion imaging or a depressed ejection fraction, those with demonstrable ischemia, and those in whom exercise provokes symptomatic ventricular arrhythmias should be considered at high risk for recurrent MI or death from arrhythmia (Fig. 239-7). Cardiac catheterization with coronary angiography and/or invasive electrophysiologic evaluation is advised.

Exercise tests also aid in formulating an individualized exercise prescription, which can be much more vigorous in patients who tolerate exercise without any of the above-mentioned adverse signs. Additionally, predischarge stress testing may provide an important psychological benefit, building the patient's confidence by demonstrating a reasonable exercise tolerance.

In many hospitals a cardiac rehabilitation program with progressive exercise is initiated in the hospital and continued after discharge. Ideally, such programs should include an educational component that informs patients about their disease and its risk factors.

The usual duration of hospitalization for an uncomplicated STEMI is about 5 days. The remainder of the convalescent phase may be accomplished at home. During the first 1–2 weeks, the patient should be encouraged to increase activity by walking about the house and outdoors in good weather. Normal sexual activity may be resumed during this period. After 2 weeks, the physician must regulate the patient's activity on the basis of exercise tolerance. Most patients will be able to return to work within 2–4 weeks.

SECONDARY PREVENTION

Various secondary preventive measures are at least partly responsible for the improvement in the long-term mortality and morbidity rates after STEMI. Long-term treatment with an antiplatelet agent (usually aspirin) after STEMI is associated with a 25% reduction in the risk of recurrent infarction, stroke, or cardiovascular mortality (36 fewer events for every 1000 patients treated). An alternative antiplatelet agent that may be used for secondary prevention in patients intolerant of aspirin is clopidogrel (75 mg orally daily). ACE inhibitors or ARBs and, in appropriate patients, aldosterone antagonists should be used indefinitely by patients with clinically evident heart failure, a moderate decrease in global ejection fraction, or a large regional wall motion abnormality to prevent late ventricular remodeling and recurrent ischemic events.

The chronic routine use of oral beta-adrenoceptor blockers for at least 2 years after STEMI is supported by well-conducted, placebo-controlled trials.

Evidence suggests that warfarin lowers the risk of late mortality and the incidence of reinfarction after STEMI. Most physicians prescribe aspirin routinely for all patients without contraindications and add warfarin for patients at increased risk of embolism (see "Thromboembolism," above). Several studies suggest that in patients <75 years a low dose of aspirin (75–81 mg/d) in combination with warfarin administered to achieve an INR >2.0 is more effective than aspirin alone for preventing recurrent MI and embolic cerebrovascular accident. However, there is an increased risk of bleeding and a high rate of discontinuation of warfarin that has limited clinical acceptance of combination antithrombotic therapy. There is increased risk of bleeding when warfarin is added to dual antiplatelet therapy (aspirin and clopidogrel). However, patients who have had a stent implanted and have an indication for anticoagulation should receive dual antiplatelet therapies in combination with warfarin. Such patients should also receive a proton pump inhibitor to minimize the risk of gastrointestinal bleeding and should have regular monitoring of their hemoglobin levels and stool hematest while on combination antithrombotic therapy.

Finally, risk factors for *atherosclerosis* (Chap. 217) should be discussed with the patient, and, when possible, favorably modified.

FURTHER READINGS

AMERICAN HEART ASSOCIATION: *Heart and Stroke Facts: 2005 Statistical Supplement*. Dallas, American Heart Association, 2006

ANTMAN EM, BRAUNWALD E: Acute myocardial infarction, in *Braunwald's Heart Disease*, 8th ed, P Libby et al (eds). Philadelphia, Saunders, 2008

BOERSMA E et al: Acute myocardial infarction. Lancet 361:847, 2003

FALK E et al: Coronary plaque disruption. Circulation 92:657, 1995

MICHAELS AD, GOLDSCHLAGER N: Risk stratification after acute myocardial infarction in the reperfusion era. Prog Cardiovasc Dis 42:273, 2000

MONTALESCOT G et al: Platelet glycoprotein IIb/IIIa inhibition with coronary stenting for acute myocardial infarction. N Engl J Med 344:1895, 2001

240 Percutaneous Coronary Intervention

Donald S. Baim*

The introduction of *percutaneous transluminal coronary angioplasty* (PTCA) by Andreas Gruntzig in 1977 established this form of catheter-based therapy as an alternative to bypass surgery for providing coronary revascularization in selected patients. The limitations of early equipment, however, meant that PTCA was applicable to <10% of all coronary revascularization candidates. By 1990, progressive improvements in PTCA equipment led to improved results, expanded indications for use, and an explosive growth in the annual number of PTCA procedures (to ~300,000 in the United States), roughly matching the coronary revascularization provided by surgical bypass operations. Newer interventional devices including atherectomy (plaque removal), stents (plaque scaffolding), and drug-eluting stents were introduced subsequently, further improving the acute success, safety, and long-term durability of percutaneous coronary intervention (PCI). Today, >1 million procedures are performed annually, representing twice the annual number of coronary bypass operations. This dominant role of catheter-based intervention in the treatment of coronary artery disease (CAD) has led to creation of a separate area within the field of cardiovascular diseases known as *interventional cardiology*, with incremental fellowship requirements and Board certification of additional qualification based on training, ongoing experience, and a written examination.

All catheter-based interventions are derivatives of diagnostic cardiac catheterization (Chap. 223), in which catheters are introduced into the arterial circulation by needle puncture, advanced into the heart under fluoroscopic guidance, and used for pressure measurements and injections of radiopaque liquid contrast agents. Interventional procedures differ in that the catheter placed into the ostium of the narrowed coronary artery is then used to advance a flexible, steerable guidewire (diameter < 0.4 mm) down the coronary artery lumen, through the narrowing, and into the vessel beyond. This guidewire then serves as a "rail" over which angioplasty balloons or other therapeutic devices can be advanced and used to enlarge the narrowed segment of coronary artery. Because PCI is performed under local anesthesia and requires only a short (1-day) hospitalization, its use in suitable patients can greatly decrease recovery time and expense compared to coronary bypass surgery.

While not all types of coronary narrowing are well suited to catheter-based intervention, PCI is the treatment of choice for the majority of patients with symptomatic coronary disease. To decide which patients should undergo revascularization (as opposed to continued medical management) and to select which patients should undergo

catheter-based rather than surgical revascularization requires a detailed understanding of both clinical and coronary angiographic features, as well as the capabilities of various interventional techniques. The remaining anatomic restrictions relate to dealing with diffuse disease, chronic total occlusions, and bifurcation lesions, but even these challenges are yielding to improved interventional devices and techniques. Deciding between PCI and bypass surgery thus requires balancing the individual patient's coronary anatomy and technical challenges against any factors that limit potential completeness of surgical revascularization or increase its risk (advanced age, poor left ventricular function, and concomitant medical problems). Both patient and physician need to be aware that while catheter-based intervention is done under local anesthesia and has a lower elective mortality rate than bypass surgery (0.4–1.0%, compared to a rate of 1–3%), it is still an invasive procedure whose risks and benefits need to be weighed carefully for each individual patient.

INDICATIONS

The fundamental indication for PCI is the presence of one or more coronary stenoses thought to be responsible for a clinical syndrome, that warrant revascularization, are approachable by catheter-based techniques, with risks and benefits that compare favorably with those of bypass surgery. For most patients with stable angina, the main goal of either surgical or catheter-based revascularization is the relief of angina rather than improved survival. In patients with multivessel CAD, particularly those with reduced left ventricular function or diabetes, there may also be a survival advantage to surgical revascularization. Trials randomizing patients with multivessel disease in whom either balloon angioplasty or bypass surgery is possible have suggested that the two procedures have essentially equivalent in-hospital and 3- to 5-year mortality rates (except for patients with diabetes mellitus, in whom surgical treatment appears to offer improved 5- to 7-year survival compared to PCI). These trials, however, showed that up to 20% of patients who underwent balloon angioplasty needed a second revascularization procedure to treat renarrowing at the initial treatment site (restenosis). Recent advances in PCI technology (particularly drug-eluting stents) have dramatically reduced the incidence of repeat procedures to treat restenosis to <5%, and have made the durability of symptomatic relief by PCI nearly identical to that of surgery in anatomically suitable patients. Even patients with ostial or mid-shaft left main coronary artery lesions and near normal left ventricular function have 1 year event rates <3% with drug-eluting stenting, although bypass surgery is still the preferred revascularization modality in patients without factors that increase surgical risk.

The current clinical indications for PCI cover the spectrum of ischemic heart disease, from patients with silent ischemia to patients with unstable angina or acute myocardial infarction (MI). The detailed indications are summarized in the recent ACC/AHA guidelines, and the following discussion is thus more conceptual in nature. One clear indication for PCI is moderately *chronic stable angina*, which persists despite medical antianginal therapy and is caused by anatomically suitable lesions (Chap. 237). If multiple severe lesions are present, these can generally be treated during a single procedure. In patients with *acute coronary syndromes*, the benefits of PCI include reduced

---

*At the time that Dr. Baim prepared the chapter he was a Professor of Medicine at Harvard Medical School and Senior Physician at Brigham and Women's Hospital. Since then he has assumed the position of Chief Medical and Scientific Officer at Boston Scientific Co.

death and MI. In *unstable angina* and *non-ST-elevation MI* (STEMI) (Chap. 238), recent studies employing platelet IIb/IIIa receptor blockers and coronary stenting have shown >20% reduction in death or MI at 6 months, with a parallel reduction in hospital readmission, compared to a conservative strategy in which PCI was reserved for strongly positive exercise test results. In patients with *acute STEMI* (Chap. 239), trials comparing thrombolysis to primary angioplasty have consistently shown lower mortality (5.0 vs. 7.0%, $p = .0002$), less non-fatal reinfarction (3.0% vs. 7.0%, $p = .0003$, and less hemorrhagic stroke (0.05% vs. 1%, $p = .0001$), with primary angioplasty (both PTCA and stenting). The current PCI guidelines thus recommend that primary PCI should be performed in patients with STEMI who present within 12 h of symptom onset, if performed in a timely fashion (medical contact-to-balloon or door-to-balloon time within 90 min) by persons skilled in the procedure, working in an appropriate laboratory environment.

As the clinical indications for PCI have broadened, so have its anatomic capabilities. Largely through the introduction of newer interventional devices, PCI has advanced well beyond the treatment of proximal, discrete, subtotal, concentric, non-calcified lesions. Calcified, complex, or diffuse lesions respond well to coronary stent placement, sometimes after pretreatment with rotational atherectomy. Even chronically totally occluded coronary arteries can be crossed and dilated effectively and, when treated with drug-eluting stents, have a 90% long-term patency rate. In addition to lesions in the native coronary tree, obstructions in the saphenous vein bypass grafts can also be dilated successfully to treat recurrent post-bypass angina, making use of distal embolic protection devices to reduce the incidence of peri-procedural MI caused by the tendency of atheroembolic debris to be liberated during stenting of such lesions.

CURRENT TECHNIQUES

While conventional balloon angioplasty (PTCA) offered anatomic versatility and acceptable short- and long-term results, it had limited efficacy in certain anatomic lesion types (e.g., calcified eccentric, ostial, thrombus-containing, or bifurcation lesions). It was also plagued by the problems of elastic recoil (Fig. 240-1), *intimal dissection* (which led to abrupt closure of the dilated segment in 3% of cases requiring emergency bypass surgery), and *restenosis* of 30–40% of the dilated segments within 6 months of initially successful treatment due to a combination of exaggerated neointimal hyperplasia and overall vessel contraction in response to the interventional injury (Fig. 240-2). These problems motivated the development of a number of newer, non-balloon techniques that entered routine clinical practice

FIGURE 240-2 Mechanisms of restenosis. Cross section of a restenotic lesion in the left anterior descending artery 5 months after initial coronary angioplasty shows the original atherosclerotic plaque (AS), the crack in the medial layer induced by the original procedure (star), and the proliferation of fibrocellular tissues (FC) that constitutes the restenotic lesion. In stent restenosis, the mechanism is purely such proliferation, whereas in non-stent interventions such as balloon angioplasty there is frequently also a component due to shrinkage of the overall vessel diameter (unfavorable remodeling) at the treatment site. *(From PW Serruys, et al: Am J Cardiol 54:482, 1984.)*

during the early 1990s. Stents (see below) increased acute procedural success to 98%, reduced the incidence of emergency surgery to 0.1%, and reduced the incidence of restenosis to 15–20%. The incidence of restenosis has been further reduced to 5% by the introduction of drug-eluting stents in 2003. In parallel, improvements in adjunctive pharmacotherapy (especially the acute use of platelet glycoprotein IIb/IIIa receptor blockers, and longer-term thienopyridine, i.e., clopidogrel) use has helped produce significant improvements in procedural safety. In large part, the progressive improvements in PCI results over the past 30 years, and thereby the growth of PCI to become the dominant coronary revascularization modality, lies in the progressive improvements in PCI devices and adjunctive pharmacology.

Stents   Stents are metallic scaffolds that are inserted into a diseased vessel segment in their collapsed form and are then deployed by balloon inflation. They overcome two of the principal limitations of balloon dilatation—local dissection of the plaque and elastic recoil of the vessel wall—allowing stents to consistently provide an essentially normal-appearing vessel lumen in the treated segment. In 1994, the first two balloon-expandable stent designs were approved by the U.S. Food and Drug Administration (FDA), with a number of second- and third-generation stent designs introduced subsequently that offered easier delivery into tortuous or distal lesions (Fig. 240-3). In the early experience, metallic stents proved prone to thrombotic occlusion, either acute (<24 h) or subacute (1–14 days with a peak at 6 days), which was ameliorated by greater attention to full initial deployment and the use of dual antiplatelet therapy [aspirin indefinitely, plus the platelet P_2Y_{12}-receptor blockers (ticlopidine or clopidogrel) for 2–4 weeks]. In addition to controlling complications related to abrupt vessel closure, the fact that stenting provided a larger acute luminal area than balloon angioplasty alone reduced the incidence of subsequent restenosis. When in-stent restenosis did occur as the result of excessive neointimal hyperplasia with-

FIGURE 240-1 Proposed mechanism of angioplasty. A. Deflated balloon positioned across stenosis. **B.** Inflation of the balloon catheter within the stenotic segment causes cracking of the intimal plaque, stretching of the media and adventitia, and expansion of the outer diameter of the vessel. **C.** Following balloon deflation, there is partial elastic recoil of the vessel wall, leaving a residual stenosis of 30% and local plaque disruption that would be evident as haziness of the lumen contours on angiography. *[From JT Willerson (ed): Treatment of Heart Diseases, New York, Gower Medical, 1992.]*

FIGURE 240-3 Examples of various coronary stent designs. Each design is shown in the expanded state. *[Modified from GW Stone. In D Baim (ed). Cardiac Catheterization, Angiography and Intervention, 7th ed, Philadelphia, Lippincott Williams & Wilkins, 2006.]*

in the stent, this could be treated by balloon dilatation followed by catheter-delivered local β or γ radiation (i.e., brachytherapy) to suppress subsequent neointimal regrowth. Despite the limitations of subacute stent thrombosis and in-stent restenosis, the major improvements in outcome led to the dominance of stent placement in catheter-based coronary revascularization, with placement of one or more stents in 85% of all procedures.

Since 2004, the concept of using stents as a local drug delivery platform to favorably modulate the neointimal healing process has entered clinical practice (Fig. 240-4). A wide variety of cytostatic, cytotoxic, and anti-inflammatory and antiproliferative agents have been studied, but current drug-eluting stents utilize either sirolimus (or a derivative thereof) or paclitaxel released from a polymer coating applied to the stent surface. *Sirolimus* is a naturally occurring and immunosuppressive agent that arrests cell proliferation in the G_1 phase, and has been shown to reduce target-vessel failure (target vessel revascularization, death, or MI) to 8.6% vs. 21.0% for bare metal stents. *Paclitaxel* is an inhibitor of microtubules that can arrest cell division at the M phase in high concentrations, but can have cytostatic G_1, anti-migratory, and anti-inflammatory effects on smooth-muscle cells at lower concentrations. It has also been shown to reduce the incidence of ischemia-driven target-vessel revascularization at 12 months, to 7.1% vs. 17.1% for bare metal stents.

Subsequent trials and registries with both drug-eluting stents have supported their use in various vessel sizes and lesion lengths, total occlusions, vein grafts, as well as in patients with diabetes, with target lesion revascularization rates generally in the 4–6% range, and has brought the durability of PCI up to arguably match that of bypass surgery (Fig. 240-5). One consequence of the reduced neointimal hyperplasia with drug-eluting stents, however, is vulnerability to late stent thrombosis, extending to 3 years after implantation, and perhaps even longer. It is thus standard practice to prolong dual antiplatelet therapy (aspirin and clopidogrel) for at least 12 months after placement of a drug-eluting stent, to minimize the small (0.2–0.6% per year) risk of this potentially serious late complication. The risk of late stent thrombosis should always be kept in mind, however, should antiplatelet therapy need to be interrupted for bleeding or a noncardiac surgical procedure within the first year after drug-eluting stent implantation.

Other PCI Technologies Whereas both balloon angioplasty and stent placement enlarge the coronary lumen by displacing plaque, *atherectomy catheters* enlarge the lumen by removing plaque mass from the treated lesion. Several mechanical atherectomy devices were developed in the 1990s, including directional, rotational, extraction, and laser atherectomy. Although each has certain applications, the greater technical difficulty and procedural complications associated with atherectomy compared to stenting has relegated these devices to niche roles (< 5% adjunctive use during current PCI). Various *thrombectomy* devices may be useful when large intracoronary thrombi are present (Fig. 240-6), although their routine use in acute MI PCI has failed to show any benefit in ST-segment resolution or final myocardial infarct size, and in one study their use has been associated with increased adverse events. *Embolic protection devices* (distal filters or occlusion/aspiration devices) may be useful adjuncts during the treatment of saphenous vein graft or other lesions prone to the liberation of debris that may compromise the distal myocardial microcircu-

FIGURE 240-4 Long-term results from one of the first patients to receive a sirolimus-eluting stent in the early Sao Paulo experience. A high-grade stenosis in the proximal left anterior descending artery is stented with a single 3.0 mm sirolimus-eluting stent. Serial angiography shows sustained vessel patency with minimal late loss over a 4-year period. *[From GW Stone, in D Baim (ed): Cardiac Catheterization, Angiography and Intervention, 7th ed. Philadelphia, Lippincott Williams & Wilkins, 2006.]*

FIGURE 240-5 Improving results of percutaneous coronary intervention (PCI) compared to coronary artery bypass grafting (CABG). In a series of trials spanning a decade from 1994–2004, the 180-day event-free survival of bypass surgery has remained 91%. This was markedly superior to percutaneous transluminal coronary angioplasty (PTCA) in the CABRI trial (32% absolute difference) due to the effect of restenosis. In the ARTS trial, this deficit improved to 11% with the use of bare metal stenting. In the ARTS 2 trial, the event-free survival of drug-eluting stents was actually superior to that of bypass by 2.6%. Although the patient groups are not exactly comparable, the significant improvement in repeat revascularization with the drug-eluting stents may shift the balance further towards PCI. (Courtesy of Prof. Patrick Serruys; with permission.)

lation. Again, study of the routine use of distal embolic protection in STEMI has failed to show any improvement in myocardial salvage.

THE PCI PROCEDURE

The procedure begins with percutaneous insertion of an arterial sheath and coronary angiography (Chap. 223). The target lesions for PCI are identified, and the sequencing and strategy for each is planned. Anticoagulation is achieved using either unfractionated heparin [50–70 IU/kg, to an activated clotting time of 250–300 s (slightly less if a glycoprotein IIb/IIIa inhibitor is used concomitantly)] or a direct thrombin inhibitor such as bivalirudin. Aspirin pretreatment (325 mg/d) is begun before the procedure, and clopidogrel loading (300–600 mg) is administered either just before a planned PCI or otherwise at its conclusion. A guiding catheter, which may have the same 6 F (2 mm) outer diameter as a diagnostic coronary angiography catheter but a larger inner lumen to permit balloon and stent advancement, is placed in the involved coronary artery ostium. Under fluoroscopic guidance, a steerable 0.4-mm (0.014-in.) guidewire is advanced across the target stenosis and into the distal vessel beyond, to permit the advancement of a predilating balloon that is ~0.5 mm smaller than the estimated normal caliber of the target vessel, across the lesion. This

balloon is inflated with dilute radiographic contrast to a pressure (usually 6–16 atm) to relieve any deformity in the balloon outline and thus partially relieve the stenosis.

If the lesion is heavily calcified, simple balloon predilation may be insufficient, and rotational atherectomy may be required to remove superficial luminal calcification and thereby improve lesion compliance. The guidewire is left in place as the predilating balloon is removed and a drug-eluting stent of appropriate size and length to cover the diseased segment plus a 5-mm margin on either side of the lesion is advanced into position. The angioplasty balloon on which the stent is mounted is then inflated to 14–16 atm to deploy the stent, which can then be further expanded at high pressure with a postdilating balloon as needed. The quality of the result is assessed with repeat angiography (and sometimes intravascular ultrasound) before moving on to treat other significant lesions. Lesions involving bifurcations may be treated either by placing a drug-eluting stent in the main vessel and "rescuing" a compromised branch by balloon dilation, or by any of several strategies to place drug-eluting stents in the main vessel and side branch.

A typical PCI may take 60–90 min, and utilize 150–250 mL of radiographic contrast, depending on the number and complexity of the lesions to be treated. At the end of the procedure, no further antithrombin therapy (heparin or bivalirudin) is given, although a IIb/IIIa receptor blocker may be continued for up to 18 h. The intraarterial sheath may be removed with manual pressure once the anticoagulated state has subsided (usually 2–4 after the procedure) or may be removed immediately through the aid of a vascular entry sealing device (one of several collagen plugs, suture, or external clip devices). The patient is returned to an inpatient unit for overnight observation, before discharge the following day on dual antiplatelet therapy. A predischarge electrocardiogram (ECG) and biomarkers (CK-MB fraction) assessment are obtained to monitor for the occurrence of periprocedural non-Q wave myocardial necrosis. Elevation of CK-MB <5 times the laboratory upper limit of normal occur in 3–5% of procedures and should be noted, but it generally does not require changes in subsequent therapy. Larger elevations or the development of ECG changes, particularly if in the setting of ongoing or recurrent postprocedural chest pain, suggest a procedural complication such as vessel closure or loss of a side branch within the stented segment and may mandate repeat diagnostic coronary angiography to evaluate, exclude, or treat such problems.

Upon discharge, the need for ongoing dual antiplatelet therapy is reemphasized to the patient, who can generally return to work within 2–3 days. No specific follow-up of the interventional result is usually performed in the absence of a recurrence in chest pain suggestive of myocardial ischemia, but it is crucial to modify any existing coronary risk factors (generally including optimization of lipid status). The

FIGURE 240-6 Diagnosis and treatment of an acute anterior wall myocardial infarction. In this patient, there is a subocclusive filling defect in the left anterior descending artery (**left**), which is removed by thrombectomy to show the underlying lesion (**center**), which is then treated by bifurcation stenting in the left anterior descending artery and the involved diagonal branch (**right**).

Risk factor	Integer coefficient
Age, 90–99 years	6
Preprocedural shock	5
Left main coronary artery disease	5
Age, 80–89 years	5
Age, 70–79 years	4
Renal disease	3
Age, 60–69 years	3
Nonelective procedure	2
NYHA class III or greater	2
Thrombus	2
Age, 50–59 years	2
Age, 40–49 years	1
Risk score, typical	0–25

At risk, %: 39.3 → 39.9 → 14.8 → 3.8 → 2.1

FIGURE 240-7 The Mayo Clinic risk score for mortality. This score assigns integer coefficients for each named clinical variable so that one can read the estimated mortality risk that corresponds to the total of the integer coefficients from the curve and the value on the y axis. The 2% of patients with a total score >14 thus have an expected procedural mortality of 25%. (*From M Singh et al, J Am Coll Cardiol 40:387, 2002, with permission.*)

main cause of recurrent events in the 5 years after a successful stent-based PCI is, in fact, progression of disease at other (non-stented) coronary sites.

Serious complications of modern PCI are uncommon, with a mortality < 0.3% for elective procedures (Fig. 240-7). As intervention has moved into more complex situations (multivessel disease, bifurcation lesions, vein graft, or unprotected left main lesions) in patients with acute coronary syndromes or poor baseline ventricular function, the average mortality of PCI has remained 1–1.5%. Abrupt vessel closure with emergency surgery has fallen to 0.1%, but current PCI guidelines still call for elective PCI to be performed in institutions that have on-site cardiac surgery support. Perforation of a coronary artery was an extremely rare complication of conventional balloon angioplasty but may occur in up to 1% of patients undergoing aggressive atherectomy procedures and may be seen with stenting. Even small perforations of the distal vessel by the angioplasty guidewire may lead to significant hemopericardium, requiring urgent pericardiocentesis in the setting of intense anticoagulant and antiplatelet therapy. PCI operators should thus be skilled in the management of such perforations using immediate balloon tamponade, placement of embolic vascular coils for small branch perforations, and placement of membrane-covered stents for perforations of major vessels. Finally, catheter-based interventions are subject to all of the complications of diagnostic catheterization, including local entry site complications, stroke, and contrast nephropathy in sensitive patients. For most patients, however, catheter-based coronary revascularization offers a safe and effective alternative to surgical revascularization.

NONCORONARY INTERVENTIONS

Because atherosclerosis is a systemic disease (i.e., not limited to the coronary arteries), it is increasingly common for analogous percutaneous interventions to be performed in the carotid, renal, or lower extremity arteries. These procedures may be combined with PCI when clinically indicated. Catheter-based interventions may also be used to treat structural cardiac defects (e.g., atrial septal defect, patent foramen ovale) or valvular heart disease. Balloon valvuloplasty is now the dominant treatment for rheumatic mitral stenosis (Chap. 230), and various catheter-based modalities are being developed for percutaneous mitral valve repair for mitral regurgitation and for percutaneous aortic valve replacement for severe aortic stenosis in patients at prohibitive risk for surgical aortic valve replacement.

SUMMARY

The past 30 years have seen the development of new techniques (such as stent placement), new drug regimens, and refinements in practice driven by "evidence-based" medicine, allowing catheter-based revascularization (PCI) to develop from a procedural curiosity to what is now the dominant form of coronary revascularization. As short- and long-term results have improved and the number of procedures has continued to grow, the pace of development continues to accelerate. Similar catheter techniques are now being used elsewhere in the arterial circulation and for the correction of structural heart disease in selected patients.

FURTHER READINGS

ANTMAN EM et al: ACC/AHA guidelines for the management of patients with ST-elevation myocardial infarction—executive summary. A report of the American College of Cardiology/American Heart Association Task Force on Practice Guidelines (Writing Committee to revise the 1999 guidelines for the management of patients with acute myocardial infarction). J Am Coll Cardiol 44:671, 2004

BAIM DS: Percutaneous balloon angioplasty and general coronary intervention, in *Cardiac Catheterization, Angiography, and Intervention*, 7th ed, D Baim (ed). Philadelphia, Lippincott Williams & Wilkins, 2006

HIRSH AT et al: ACC/AHA 2005 practice guidelines for the management of patients with peripheral arterial disease (lower extremity, renal, mesenteric and abdominal aortic): Executive summary. Circulation 113, 1474, 2006

KEELEY EC et al: Should patients with acute myocardial infraction be transferred to a tertiary center for primary angioplasty or receive it at qualified hospitals in the community? The case for emergency transfer for primary percutaneous coronary intervention. Circulation 112:3520, 2005

MORENO R et al: Drug-eluting stent thrombosis: Results from a pooled analysis including 10 randomized studies. J Am Coll Cardiol 45:954, 2005

RESNIC F et al: Percutaneous coronary and valvular intervention, in *Braunwald's Heart Disease*, 8th ed, P Libby et al (eds). Philadelphia, Elsevier Saunders, 2008 (in press)

SERRUYS PW et al: Coronary-artery stents. N Engl J Med 354: 483, 2006

SMITH SC et al: ACC/AHA/SCAI 2005 guideline update for percutaneous coronary intervention—summary article. A report of the American College of Cardiology/American Heart Association Task Force on Practice Guidelines (ACC/AHA/SCAI Writing Committee to Update the 2001 Guidelines for Percutaneous Coronary Intervention). Circulation 113: 156, 2006

WHITE CJ: Catheter-based therapy for atherosclerotic renal artery stenosis. Circulation 113:1464, 2006

YADAV JS et al: Protected carotid-artery stenting versus endarterectomy in high-risk patients. N Eng J Med 351:1493, 2004

241 Hypertensive Vascular Disease
Theodore A. Kotchen

Hypertension doubles the risk of cardiovascular diseases, including coronary heart disease (CHD), congestive heart failure (CHF), ischemic and hemorrhagic stroke, renal failure, and peripheral arterial disease. Hypertension is often associated with additional cardiovascular disease risk factors, and the risk of cardiovascular disease increases with the total burden of risk factors. Although antihypertensive therapy clearly reduces the risks of cardiovascular and renal disease, large segments of the hypertensive population are either untreated or inadequately treated.

EPIDEMIOLOGY

Blood pressure levels, the rate of age-related blood pressure increase, and the prevalence of hypertension vary among countries and among subpopulations within a country. Hypertension is present in all populations except for a small number of individuals living in primitive, culturally isolated societies. It has been estimated that hypertension accounts for 6% of deaths worldwide. In industrialized societies, blood pressure increases steadily during the first two decades. In children and adolescents, blood pressure is associated with growth and maturation. Blood pressure "tracks" over time in children and between adolescence and young adulthood. In the United States, average systolic blood pressure is higher for men than for women during early adulthood, although among older individuals the age-related rate of rise is steeper for women. Consequently, among individuals age 60 and older, systolic blood pressures of women are higher than those of men. Among adults, diastolic blood pressure also increases progressively with age until ~55 years, after which it tends to decrease. The consequence is a widening of pulse pressure (the difference between systolic and diastolic blood pressure) beyond age 60.

In the United States, based on results of the National Health and Nutrition Examination Survey (NHANES), 28.7% (age-adjusted prevalence) of U.S. adults, or ~58.4 million individuals, have hypertension (defined as any one of the following: systolic blood pressure ≥140 mmHg; diastolic blood pressure ≥90 mmHg; taking antihypertensive medications). Hypertension prevalence is 33.5% in non-Hispanic blacks, 28.9% in non-Hispanic whites, and 20.7% in Mexican Americans. The burden of hypertension increases with age, and among individuals aged ≥60, hypertension prevalence is 65.4%. Recent evidence suggests that the prevalence of hypertension in the United States may be increasing, possibly as a consequence of increasing obesity. The prevalence of hypertension and stroke mortality rates are higher in the southeastern United States than in other regions. In African Americans, hypertension appears earlier, is generally more severe, and results in higher rates of morbidity and mortality from stroke, left ventricular hypertrophy, CHF, and end-stage renal disease (ESRD) than in Caucasian Americans.

Both environmental and genetic factors may contribute to regional and racial variations of blood pressure and hypertension prevalence. Studies of societies undergoing "acculturation" and studies of migrants from a less to a more urbanized setting indicate a profound environmental contribution to blood pressure. Obesity and weight gain are strong, independent risk factors for hypertension. It has been estimated that 60% of hypertensives are >20% overweight. Among populations, hypertension prevalence is related to dietary NaCl intake, and the age-related increase of blood pressure may be augmented by a high NaCl intake. Low dietary intakes of calcium and potassium may also contribute to the risk of hypertension. Additional environmental factors that may contribute to hypertension include alcohol consumption, psychosocial stress, and low levels of physical activity.

Adoption, twin, and family studies document a significant heritable component to blood pressure levels and hypertension. Family studies

FIGURE 241-1 Determinants of arterial pressure.

controlling for a common environment indicate that blood pressure heritabilities are in the range of 15–35%. In twin studies, heritability estimates of blood pressure are ~60% for males and 30–40% for females. High blood pressure before age 55 occurs 3.8 times more frequently among persons with a positive family history of hypertension. Although specific genetic etiologies have been identified for relatively rare causes of hypertension, this has not been the case for the large majority of hypertensive patients. For most individuals, it is likely that hypertension represents a polygenic disorder in which a single gene or combination of genes act in concert with environmental exposures to contribute only a modest effect on blood pressure.

GENETIC CONSIDERATIONS Although specific genetic variants have been identified in rare Mendelian forms of hypertension (Table 241-5), these variants are not applicable to the vast majority (>98%) of patients with essential hypertension. Blood pressure levels reflect the contributions of many susceptibility genes interacting with each other and with the environment. Essential hypertension is a polygenic disorder, and different patients may carry different subsets of genes that lead to elevated blood pressure and to different phenotypes associated with hypertension, e.g., obesity, dyslipidemia, insulin resistance.

Several strategies are being utilized in the search for specific hypertension-related genes. Animal models (including selectively bred rats and congenic rat strains) provide a powerful approach for evaluating genetic loci and genes associated with hypertension. Comparative mapping strategies allow for the identification of syntenic genomic regions between the rat and human genome that may be involved in blood pressure regulation. In linkage studies, polymorphic genetic markers are examined at regular distances along each chromosome. Linkage information is gathered family by family, and the minimum family unit comprises at least two relatives, often a pair of siblings. To date, genome scans for hypertension have yielded inconsistent results. In complementary association studies, different alleles (or combinations of alleles at different loci) of specific genes or chromosomal regions are compared in hypertensive patients and normotensive control subjects. Current evidence suggests that genes encoding components of the renin-angiotensin-aldosterone system, and angiotensinogen and angiotensin-converting enzyme (ACE) polymorphisms, may be related to hypertension and to blood pressure sensitivity to dietary NaCl. The alpha-adducin gene is also thought to be associated with increased renal tubular absorption of sodium, and variants of this gene may also be associated with hypertension and salt sensitivity of blood pressure. Other genes possibly related to hypertension include genes encoding the AT_1 receptor, aldosterone synthase, and the β_2-adrenoreceptor.

Preliminary evidence suggests that there may also be genetic determinants of target organ damage attributed to hypertension. Family studies indicate significant heritability of left ventricular mass, and there is considerable individual variation in the responses of the heart to hypertension. Family studies and variations in candidate genes associated with renal damage suggest that genetic factors may also contribute to hypertensive nephropathy. Specific genetic variants have been linked to CHD and stroke.

In the future, it is possible that DNA analysis will predict individual risk for hypertension and target organ damage and will identify responders to specific classes of antihypertensive agents. However, with the exception of the rare, monogenic hypertensive diseases, the genetic variants associated with hypertension remain to be confirmed, and the intermediate steps by which these variants affect blood pressure remain to be determined.

MECHANISMS OF HYPERTENSION

To provide a framework for understanding the pathogenesis and treatment options of hypertensive disorders, it is useful to understand factors involved in the regulation of both normal and elevated arterial pressure. Cardiac output and peripheral resistance are the two determinants of arterial pressure (Fig. 241-1). Cardiac output is determined by stroke volume and heart rate; stroke volume is related to myocardial contractility and to the size of the vascular compartment. Peripheral resistance is determined by functional and anatomic changes in small arteries (lumen diameter 100–400 μm) and arterioles.

INTRAVASCULAR VOLUME

Vascular volume is a primary determinant of arterial pressure over the long term. Although the extracellular fluid space is composed of vascular and interstitial spaces, in general, alterations in total extracellular fluid volume are associated with proportional changes of blood volume. Sodium is predominantly an extracellular ion and is a primary determinant of the extracellular fluid volume. When NaCl intake exceeds the capacity of the kidney to excrete sodium, vascular volume initially expands and cardiac output increases. However, many vascular beds (including kidney and brain) have the capacity to autoregulate blood flow, and if constant blood flow is to be maintained in the face of increased arterial pressure, resistance within that bed must increase, since:

$$\text{Blood flow} = \frac{\text{pressure across the vascular bed}}{\text{vascular resistance}}$$

The initial elevation of blood pressure in response to vascular volume expansion is related to an increase of cardiac output; however, over time, peripheral resistance increases and cardiac output reverts toward normal. The effect of sodium on blood pressure is related to the provision of sodium with chloride; non-chloride salts of sodium have little or no effect on blood pressure. As arterial pressure increases in response to a high NaCl intake, urinary sodium excretion increases and sodium balance is maintained at the expense of an increase in arterial pressure. The mechanism for this "pressure-natriuresis" phenomenon may involve a subtle increase of glomerular filtration rate, decreased absorbing capacity of the renal tubules, and possibly hormonal factors such as atrial natriuretic factor. In individuals with an impaired capacity to excrete sodium, greater increases of arterial pressure are required to achieve natriuresis and sodium balance.

NaCl-dependent hypertension may be a consequence of a decreased capacity of the kidney to excrete sodium, due to either intrinsic renal disease or to increased production of a salt-retaining hormone (mineralocorticoid) resulting in increased renal tubular reabsorption of sodium. Renal tubular sodium reabsorption may also be augmented by increased neural activity to the kidney. In each of these situations, a higher arterial pressure may be required to achieve sodium balance, i.e., the pressure-natriuresis phenomenon. Conversely, salt-wasting disorders are associated with low blood pressure levels. ESRD is an extreme example of volume-dependent hypertension. In ~80% of these patients, vascular volume and hypertension can be controlled with adequate dialysis; in the other 20%, the mechanism of hypertension is related to increased activity of the renin-angiotensin system and is likely to be responsive to pharmacologic blockade of renin-angiotensin.

AUTONOMIC NERVOUS SYSTEM

The autonomic nervous system maintains cardiovascular homeostasis via pressure, volume, and chemoreceptor signals. Adrenergic reflexes modulate blood pressure over the short term, and adrenergic function, in concert with hormonal and volume-related factors, contributes to the long-term regulation of arterial pressure. The three endogenous catecholamines are norepinephrine, epinephrine, and dopamine. All three

play important roles in tonic and phasic cardiovascular regulation. Adrenergic neurons synthesize norepinephrine and dopamine (a precursor of norepinephrine), which are stored in vesicles within the neuron. When the neuron is stimulated, these neurotransmitters are released into the synaptic cleft and to receptor sites on target tissues. Subsequently, the transmitter is either metabolized or taken up into the neuron by an active reuptake process. Epinephrine is synthesized in the adrenal medulla and released into the circulation upon adrenal stimulation.

The activities of the adrenergic receptors are mediated by guanosine nucleotide-binding regulatory proteins (G proteins) and by intracellular concentrations of downstream second messengers. In addition to receptor affinity and density, physiologic responsiveness to catecholamines may also be altered by the efficiency of receptor-effector coupling at a site "distal" to receptor binding. The receptor sites are relatively specific both for the transmitter substance and for the response that occupancy of the receptor site elicits. Norepinephrine and epinephrine are agonists for all adrenergic receptor subtypes, although with varying affinities. Based on their physiology and pharmacology, adrenergic receptors have been divided into two principal types: α and β. These types have been further differentiated into α_1, α_2, β_1, and β_2 receptors. Recent molecular cloning studies have identified several additional subtypes. α Receptors are more avidly occupied and activated by norepinephrine than by epinephrine, and the reverse is true for β receptors. α_1 Receptors are located on postsynaptic cells in smooth muscle and elicit vasoconstriction. α_2 Receptors are localized on presynaptic membranes of postganglionic nerve terminals that synthesize norepinephrine. When activated by catecholamines, α_2 receptors act as negative feedback controllers, inhibiting further norepinephrine release. Different classes of antihypertensive agents either inhibit α_1 receptors or act as agonists of α_2 receptors and reduce systemic sympathetic outflow. Activation of myocardial β_1 receptors stimulates the rate and strength of cardiac contraction, and consequently increases cardiac output. β_1 Receptor activation also stimulates renin release from the kidney. Another class of antihypertensive agents acts by inhibiting β_1 receptors. Activation of β_2 receptors by epinephrine relaxes vascular smooth muscle and results in vasodilation.

Circulating catecholamine concentrations may affect the number of adrenoreceptors in various tissues. Downregulation of receptors may be a consequence of sustained high levels of catecholamines and provides an explanation for decreasing responsiveness, or tachyphylaxis, to catecholamines. For example, orthostatic hypotension is frequently observed in patients with pheochromocytoma, possibly due to the lack of norepinephrine-induced vasoconstriction with assumption of the upright posture. Conversely, with chronic reduction of neurotransmitter substances, adrenoreceptors may increase in number, or be upregulated, resulting in increased responsiveness to the neurotransmitter. Chronic administration of agents that block adrenergic receptors may result in upregulation, and withdrawal of these agents may produce a condition of temporary hypersensitivity to sympathetic stimuli. For example, clonidine is an antihypertensive agent that is a centrally acting α_2 agonist that inhibits sympathetic outflow. Rebound hypertension may occur with the abrupt cessation of clonidine therapy, probably as a consequence of upregulation of α_1 receptors.

Several reflexes modulate blood pressure on a minute-to-minute basis. One arterial baroreflex is mediated by stretch-sensitive sensory nerve endings located in the carotid sinuses and the aortic arch. The rate of firing of these baroreceptors increases with arterial pressure, and the net effect is a decrease of sympathetic outflow, resulting in decreases of arterial pressure and heart rate. This is a primary mechanism for rapid buffering of acute fluctuations of arterial pressure that may occur during postural changes, behavioral or physiologic stress, and changes in blood volume. However, the activity of the baroreflex declines or adapts to sustained increases of arterial pressure such that the baroreceptors are reset to higher pressures. Patients with autonomic neuropathy and impaired baroreflex function may have extremely labile blood pressures with difficult-to-control episodic blood pressure spikes.

Pheochromocytoma is the most obvious example of hypertension related to increased catecholamine production, in this instance by a tumor. Blood pressure can be reduced by surgical excision of the tumor or by pharmacologic treatment with an α_1 receptor antagonist or with an inhibitor of tyrosine hydroxylase, the rate-limiting step in catecholamine biosynthesis. Increased sympathetic activity may contribute to other forms of hypertension. Drugs that block the sympathetic nervous system are potent antihypertensive agents, indicating that the sympathetic nervous system plays a permissive, although perhaps not a causative, role in the maintenance of increased arterial pressure.

RENIN-ANGIOTENSIN-ALDOSTERONE

The renin-angiotensin-aldosterone system contributes to the regulation of arterial pressure primarily via the vasoconstrictor properties of angiotensin II and the sodium-retaining properties of aldosterone. Renin is an aspartyl protease that is synthesized as an enzymatically inactive precursor, prorenin. Most renin in the circulation is synthesized in the segment of the renal afferent renal arteriole (juxtaglomerular cells) that abuts the glomerulus and a group of sensory cells located at the distal end of the loop of Henle, the macula densa. Prorenin may be secreted directly into the circulation or may be activated within secretory cells and released as active renin. Although human plasma contains two- to fivefold times more prorenin than renin, there is no evidence that prorenin contributes to the physiologic activity of this system. There are three primary stimuli for renin secretion: (1) decreased NaCl transport in the thick ascending limb of the loop of Henle (macula densa mechanism), (2) decreased pressure or stretch within the renal afferent arteriole (baroreceptor mechanism), and (3) sympathetic nervous system stimulation of renin-secreting cells via β_1 adrenoreceptors. Conversely, renin secretion is inhibited by increased NaCl transport in the thick ascending limb of the loop of Henle, by increased stretch within the renal afferent arteriole, and by β_1 receptor blockade. In addition, renin secretion may be modulated by a number of humoral factors, including angiotensin II. Angiotensin II directly inhibits renin secretion due to angiotensin II type 1 receptors on juxtaglomerular cells, and renin secretion increases in response to pharmacologic blockade of either ACE or angiotensin II receptors.

Once released into the circulation, active renin cleaves a substrate, angiotensinogen, to form an inactive decapeptide, angiotensin I (Fig. 241-2). A converting enzyme, located primarily but not exclusively in the pulmonary circulation, converts angiotensin I to the active octapeptide, angiotensin II, by releasing the C-terminal histidyl-leucine dipeptide. The same converting enzyme cleaves a number of other peptides, including and thereby inactivating the vasodilator bradykinin. Acting primarily through angiotensin II type 1 (AT_1) receptors located on cell membranes, angiotensin II is a potent pressor substance, the primary trophic factor for the secretion of aldosterone by the adrenal zona glomerulosa, and a potent mitogen stimulating vascular smooth-muscle cell and myocyte growth. Independent of its hemodynamic effects, angiotensin II may play a role in the pathogenesis of atherosclerosis through a direct cellular action on the vessel wall. An angiotensin II type 2 (AT_2) receptor has been characterized. It is widely distributed in the kidney and has the opposite functional effects of the AT_1 receptor. The AT_2 receptor induces vasodilation, sodium excretion, and inhibition of cell growth and matrix formation. Experimental evidence suggests that the AT_2 receptor improves vascular remodeling by stimulating smooth-muscle cell apoptosis and contributes to the regulation of glomerular filtration rate. AT_1 receptor blockade induces an increase in AT_2 receptor activity. Currently, the AT_2 receptor has a less well defined functional role than the AT_1 receptor.

Renin-secreting tumors are clear examples of renin-dependent hypertension. In the kidney, these include benign hemangiopericytomas of the juxtaglomerular apparatus, and infrequently renal carcinomas, including Wilms' tumors. Renin-producing carcinomas have also been described in lung, liver, pancreas, colon, and adrenals. In these instances, in addition to excision and/or ablation of the tumor, treatment of hypertension includes pharmacologic therapies targeted to inhibit angiotensin II production or action. Renovascular hypertension is another renin-mediated form of hypertension. Obstruction of the renal artery leads to decreased renal perfusion pressure, thereby stimulating

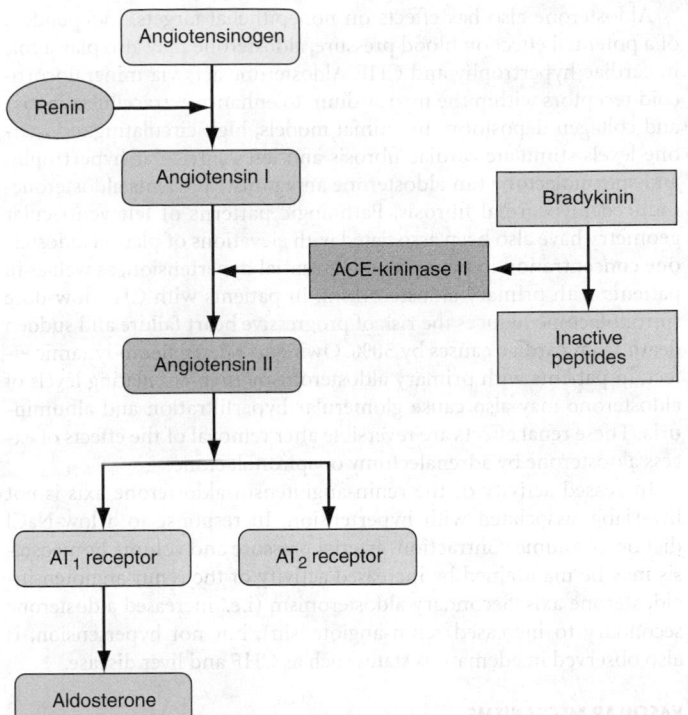

FIGURE 241-2 Renin-angiotensin-aldosterone axis.

renin secretion. Over time, as a consequence of secondary renal damage, this form of hypertension may become less renin dependent.

Angiotensinogen, renin, and angiotensin II are also synthesized locally in many tissues, including the brain, pituitary, aorta, arteries, heart, adrenal glands, kidneys, adipocytes, leukocytes, ovaries, testes, uterus, spleen, and skin. Angiotensin II in tissues may be formed by the enzymatic activity of renin or by other proteases, e.g., tonin, chymase, and cathepsins. In addition to regulating local blood flow, tissue angiotensin II is a mitogen that stimulates growth and contributes to modeling and repair. Excess tissue angiotensin II may contribute to atherosclerosis, cardiac hypertrophy, and renal failure and consequently may be a target for pharmacologic therapy to prevent target organ damage.

Angiotensin II is the primary trophic factor regulating the synthesis and secretion of aldosterone by the zona glomerulosa of the adrenal cortex. Aldosterone synthesis is also dependent on potassium, and aldosterone secretion may be decreased in potassium-depleted individuals. Although acute elevations of adrenocorticotropic hormone (ACTH) levels also increase aldosterone secretion, ACTH is not an important trophic factor for the chronic regulation of aldosterone.

Aldosterone is a potent mineralocorticoid that increases sodium reabsorption by amiloride-sensitive epithelial sodium channels (ENaC) on the apical surface of the principal cells of the renal cortical collecting duct (Chap. 271). Electric neutrality is maintained by exchanging sodium for potassium and hydrogen ions. Consequently, increased aldosterone secretion may result in hypokalemia and alkalosis. Because potassium depletion may inhibit aldosterone synthesis, clinically, hypokalemia should be corrected before evaluating a patient for hyperaldosteronism.

Mineralocorticoid receptors are also expressed in the colon, salivary glands, and sweat glands. Cortisol also binds to these receptors but normally functions as a less potent mineralocorticoid than aldosterone because cortisol is converted to cortisone by the enzyme 11 β-hydroxysteroid dehydrogenase type 2. Cortisone has no affinity for the mineralocorticoid receptor. Primary aldosteronism is a compelling example of mineralocorticoid-mediated hypertension. In this disorder, adrenal aldosterone synthesis and release are independent of renin-angiotensin, and renin release is suppressed by the resulting volume expansion.

Aldosterone also has effects on nonepithelial targets. Independent of a potential effect on blood pressure, aldosterone may also play a role in cardiac hypertrophy and CHF. Aldosterone acts via mineralocorticoid receptors within the myocardium to enhance extracellular matrix and collagen deposition. In animal models, high circulating aldosterone levels stimulate cardiac fibrosis and left ventricular hypertrophy, and spironolactone (an aldosterone antagonist) prevents aldosterone-induced myocardial fibrosis. Pathologic patterns of left ventricular geometry have also been associated with elevations of plasma aldosterone concentration in patients with essential hypertension, as well as in patients with primary aldosteronism. In patients with CHF, low-dose spironolactone reduces the risk of progressive heart failure and sudden death from cardiac causes by 30%. Owing to a renal hemodynamic effect, in patients with primary aldosteronism, high circulating levels of aldosterone may also cause glomerular hyperfiltration and albuminuria. These renal effects are reversible after removal of the effects of excess aldosterone by adrenalectomy or spironolactone.

Increased activity of the renin-angiotensin-aldosterone axis is not invariably associated with hypertension. In response to a low-NaCl diet or to volume contraction, arterial pressure and volume homeostasis may be maintained by increased activity of the renin-angiotensin-aldosterone axis. Secondary aldosteronism (i.e., increased aldosterone secondary to increased renin-angiotensin), but not hypertension, is also observed in edematous states such as CHF and liver disease.

VASCULAR MECHANISMS

Vascular radius and compliance of resistance arteries are also important determinants of arterial pressure. Resistance to flow varies inversely with the fourth power of the radius, and consequently small decreases in lumen size significantly increase resistance. In hypertensive patients, structural, mechanical, or functional changes may reduce lumen diameter of small arteries and arterioles. Remodeling refers to geometric alterations in the vessel wall without changing vessel volume. Hypertrophic (increased cell number, increased cell size, and increased deposition of intercellular matrix) or eutrophic (no change in the amount of material in the vessel wall) vascular remodeling results in decreased lumen size and hence contributes to increased peripheral resistance. Apoptosis, low-grade inflammation, and vascular fibrosis also contribute to remodeling. Lumen diameter is also related to elasticity of the vessel. Vessels with a high degree of elasticity can accommodate an increase of volume with relatively little change of pressure, whereas in a semi-rigid vascular system, a small increment in volume induces a relatively large increment of pressure.

Hypertensive patients have stiffer arteries, and arteriosclerotic patients may have particularly high systolic blood pressures and wide pulse pressures as a consequence of decreased vascular compliance due to structural changes in the vascular wall. Recent evidence suggests that arterial stiffness has independent predictive value for cardiovascular events. Clinically, a number of devices are available to evaluate arterial stiffness or compliance, including ultrasound and MRI.

Ion transport by vascular smooth-muscle cells may contribute to hypertension-associated abnormalities of vascular tone and vascular growth, both of which are modulated by intracellular pH (pH_i). Three ion transport mechanisms participate in the regulation of pH_i: (1) Na^+-H^+ exchange, (2) Na^+-dependent HCO_3^--Cl^- exchange, and (3) cation-independent HCO_3^--Cl^- exchange. Based on measurements in cell types that are more accessible than vascular smooth muscle (e.g., leukocytes, erythrocytes, platelets, skeletal muscle), activity of the Na^+-H^+ exchanger is increased in hypertension, and this may result in increased vascular tone by two mechanisms. First, increased sodium entry may lead to increased vascular tone by activating Na^+-Ca^{2+} exchange and thereby increasing intracellular calcium. Second, increased pH_i enhances calcium sensitivity of the contractile apparatus, leading to an increase in contractility for a given intracellular calcium concentration. Additionally, increased Na^+-H^+ exchange might stimulate vascular smooth-muscle cell growth by enhancing sensitivity to mitogens.

Vascular endothelial function also modulates vascular tone. The vascular endothelium synthesizes and releases a spectrum of vasoactive substances, including nitric oxide, a potent vasodilator. Endothelium-dependent vasodilation is impaired in hypertensive patients. This impairment is often assessed with high-resolution ultrasonography as flow-mediated vasodilation of the brachial artery. Alternatively, endothelium-dependent vasodilation may be assessed with venous occlusion plethysmography in response to an intraarterially infused endothelium-dependent vasodilator, e.g., acetylcholine.

Presently, it is not known if these hypertension-related vascular abnormalities of ion transport and endothelial function are primary alterations or secondary consequences of elevated arterial pressure. Limited evidence suggests that vascular compliance and endothelium-dependent vasodilation may be improved by aerobic exercise, weight loss, and antihypertensive agents. It remains to be determined whether these interventions affect arterial structure and stiffness via a blood pressure–independent mechanism and whether different classes of antihypertensive agents preferentially affect vascular structure and function.

PATHOLOGIC CONSEQUENCES OF HYPERTENSION

Hypertension is a risk factor for all clinical manifestations of atherosclerosis. It is an independent predisposing factor for heart failure, coronary artery disease, stroke, renal disease, and peripheral arterial disease (PAD).

HEART

Heart disease is the most common cause of death in hypertensive patients. Hypertensive heart disease is the result of structural and functional adaptations leading to left ventricular hypertrophy, diastolic dysfunction, CHF, abnormalities of blood flow due to atherosclerotic coronary artery disease and microvascular disease, and cardiac arrhythmias.

Both genetic and hemodynamic factors contribute to left ventricular hypertrophy. Clinically, left ventricular hypertrophy can be diagnosed by electrocardiogram, although echocardiography provides a more sensitive measure of left ventricular wall thickness. Individuals with left ventricular hypertrophy are at increased risk for CHD, stroke, CHF, and sudden death. Aggressive control of hypertension can regress or reverse left ventricular hypertrophy and reduce the risk of cardiovascular disease. It is not clear if different classes of antihypertensive agents have an added impact on reducing left ventricular mass, independent of their blood pressure–lowering effect.

Abnormalities of diastolic function, ranging from asymptomatic heart disease to overt heart failure, are common in hypertensive patients. Patients with diastolic heart failure have a preserved ejection fraction, which is a measure of systolic function. Approximately one-third of patients with CHF have normal systolic function but abnormal diastolic function. Diastolic dysfunction is an early consequence of hypertension-related heart disease and is exacerbated by left ventricular hypertrophy and ischemia. Clinically, cardiac catheterization provides the most accurate assessment of diastolic function; however, this is an invasive procedure and generally not indicated for the assessment of diastolic function. Alternatively, diastolic function can be evaluated by several noninvasive methods, including echocardiography and radionuclide angiography.

BRAIN

Hypertension is an important risk factor for brain infarction and hemorrhage. Approximately 85% of strokes are due to infarction and the remainder are due to hemorrhage, either intracerebral hemorrhage or subarachnoid hemorrhage. The incidence of stroke rises progressively with increasing blood pressure levels, particularly systolic blood pressure in individuals >65 years. Treatment of hypertension convincingly decreases the incidence of both ischemic and hemorrhagic strokes.

Hypertension is also associated with impaired cognition in an aging population, and longitudinal studies support an association between mid-life hypertension and late-life cognitive decline. Hypertension-related cognitive impairment and dementia may be a consequence of a single infarct due to occlusion of a "strategic" larger vessel or multiple lacunar infarcts due to occlusive small vessel disease resulting in sub-cortical white matter ischemia. Several clinical trials suggest that anti-hypertensive therapy has a beneficial effect on cognitive function, although this remains an active area of investigation.

Cerebral blood flow remains unchanged over a wide range of arterial pressures (mean arterial pressure of 50–150 mmHg) through a process termed *autoregulation* of blood flow. In patients with the clinical syndrome of malignant hypertension, encephalopathy is related to failure of autoregulation of cerebral blood flow at the upper pressure limit, resulting in vasodilation and hyperperfusion. Signs and symptoms of hypertensive encephalopathy may include severe headache, nausea and vomiting (often of a projectile nature), focal neurologic signs, and alterations in mental status. Untreated, hypertensive encephalopathy may progress to stupor, coma, seizures, and death within hours. It is important to distinguish hypertensive encephalopathy from other neurologic syndromes that may be associated with hypertension, e.g., cerebral ischemia, hemorrhagic or thrombotic stroke, seizure disorder, mass lesions, pseudotumor cerebri, delirium tremens, meningitis, acute intermittent porphyria, traumatic or chemical injury to the brain, and uremic encephalopathy.

KIDNEY

Primary renal disease is the most common etiology of secondary hypertension. Conversely, hypertension is a risk factor for renal injury and ESRD. The increased risk associated with high blood pressure is graded, continuous, and present throughout the entire distribution of blood pressure above optimal. Renal risk appears to be more closely related to systolic than to diastolic blood pressure, and black men are at greater risk than white men for developing ESRD at every level of blood pressure.

The atherosclerotic, hypertension-related vascular lesions in the kidney primarily affect the preglomerular arterioles, resulting in ischemic changes in the glomeruli and postglomerular structures. Glomerular injury may also be a consequence of direct damage to the glomerular capillaries due to glomerular hyperperfusion. Glomerular pathology progresses to glomerulosclerosis, and eventually the renal tubules may also become ischemic and gradually atrophic. The renal lesion associated with malignant hypertension consists of fibrinoid necrosis of the afferent arterioles, sometimes extending into the glomerulus, and may result in focal necrosis of the glomerular tuft.

Clinically, macroalbuminuria (a random urine albumin/creatinine ratio > 300 mg/g) or microalbuminuria (a random urine albumin/creatinine ratio 30–300 mg/g) are early markers of renal injury. These are also risk factors for renal disease progression and for cardiovascular disease.

PERIPHERAL ARTERIES

In addition to contributing to the pathogenesis of hypertension, blood vessels may be a target organ for atherosclerotic disease secondary to long-standing elevated blood pressure. Hypertensive patients with arterial disease of the lower extremities are at increased risk for future cardiovascular disease. Although patients with stenotic lesions of the lower extremities may be asymptomatic, intermittent claudication is the classic symptom of PAD. This is characterized by aching pain in the calves or buttocks while walking that is relieved by rest. The ankle-brachial index is a useful approach for evaluating PAD and is defined as the ratio of noninvasively assessed ankle to brachial (arm) systolic blood pressure. An ankle-brachial index < 0.90 is considered diagnostic of PAD and is associated with >50% stenosis in at least one major lower limb vessel. Several studies suggest that an ankle-brachial index < 0.80 is associated with elevated blood pressure, particularly systolic blood pressure.

DEFINING HYPERTENSION

From an epidemiologic perspective, there is no obvious level of blood pressure that defines hypertension. In adults, there is a continuous, incremental risk of cardiovascular disease, stroke, and renal disease across levels of both systolic and diastolic blood pressure. The Multiple

TABLE 241-1   BLOOD PRESSURE CLASSIFICATION

Blood Pressure Classification	Systolic, mmHg	Diastolic, mmHg
Normal	<120	*and* <80
Prehypertension	120–139	*or* 80–89
Stage 1 hypertension	140–159	*or* 90–99
Stage 2 hypertension	≥160	*or* ≥100
Isolated systolic hypertension	≥140	*and* <90

Source: Adapted from Chobanian et al.

Risk Factor Intervention Trial (MRFIT), which included >350,000 male participants, demonstrated a continuous and graded influence of both systolic and diastolic blood pressure on CHD mortality, extending down to systolic blood pressures of 120 mmHg. Similarly, results of a meta-analysis involving almost 1 million participants indicate that ischemic heart disease mortality, stroke mortality, and mortality from other vascular causes are directly related to the height of the blood pressure, beginning at 115/75 mmHg, without evidence of a threshold. Cardiovascular disease risk doubles for every 20-mmHg increase in systolic and 10-mmHg increase in diastolic pressure. Among older individuals, systolic blood pressure and pulse pressure are more powerful predictors of cardiovascular disease than diastolic blood pressure.

Clinically, hypertension might be defined as that level of blood pressure at which the institution of therapy reduces blood pressure–related morbidity and mortality. Current clinical criteria for defining hypertension are generally based on the average of two or more seated blood pressure readings during each of two or more outpatient visits. A recent classification recommends blood pressure criteria for defining normal blood pressure, prehypertension, hypertension (stages I and II), and isolated systolic hypertension, which is a common occurrence among the elderly (Table 241-1). In children and adolescents, hypertension is generally defined as systolic and/or diastolic blood pressure consistently >95th percentile for age, gender, and height. Blood pressures between the 90th and 95th percentiles are considered prehypertensive and are an indication for lifestyle interventions.

Home blood pressure and average 24-h ambulatory blood pressure measurements are generally lower than clinic blood pressures. Because ambulatory blood pressure recordings yield multiple readings throughout the day and night, they provide a more comprehensive assessment of the vascular burden of hypertension than a limited number of office readings. Increasing evidence suggests that home blood pressures, including 24-h blood pressure recordings, more reliably predict target organ damage than office blood pressures. Blood pressure tends to be higher in the early morning hours, soon after waking, than at other times of day. Myocardial infarction and stroke are more frequent in the early morning hours. Nighttime blood pressures are generally 10–20% lower than daytime blood pressures, and an attenuated nighttime blood pressure "dip" is associated with increased cardiovascular disease risk. Blunting of the day-night blood pressure pattern occurs in several clinical conditions, including sleep apnea and autonomic neuropathy, and in certain populations, including African Americans. Recommended criteria for a diagnosis of hypertension are average awake blood pressure ≥135/85 mmHg and asleep blood pressure ≥120/75 mmHg. These levels approximate a clinic blood pressure of 140/90 mmHg.

Approximately 15–20% of patients with stage 1 hypertension (as defined in Table 241-1) based on office blood pressures have average ambulatory readings <135/85 mmHg. This phenomenon, so-called white coat hypertension, may also be associated with an increased risk of target organ damage (e.g., left ventricular hypertrophy, carotid atherosclerosis, overall cardiovascular morbidity), although to a lesser extent than individuals with elevated office and ambulatory readings. Individuals with white coat hypertension are also at increased risk for developing sustained hypertension.

CLINICAL DISORDERS OF HYPERTENSION

Depending on methods of patient ascertainment, ~80–95% of hypertensive patients are diagnosed as having "essential" hypertension (also

TABLE 241-2 SYSTOLIC HYPERTENSION WITH WIDE PULSE PRESSURE

1. Decreased vascular compliance (arteriosclerosis)
2. Increased cardiac output
   a. Aortic regurgitation
   b. Thyrotoxicosis
   c. Hyperkinetic heart syndrome
   d. Fever
   e. Arteriovenous fistula
   f. Patent ductus arteriosus

TABLE 241-3 SECONDARY CAUSES OF SYSTOLIC AND DIASTOLIC HYPERTENSION

Renal	Parenchymal diseases, renal cysts (including polycystic kidney disease), renal tumors (including renin-secreting tumors), obstructive uropathy
Renovascular	Arteriosclerotic, fibromuscular dysplasia
Adrenal	Primary aldosteronism, Cushing's syndrome, 17α-hydroxylase deficiency, 11β-hydroxylase deficiency, 11-hydroxysteroid dehydrogenase deficiency (licorice), pheochromocytoma
Aortic coarctation	
Obstructive sleep apnea	
Preeclampsia/eclampsia	
Neurogenic	Psychogenic, diencephalic syndrome, familial dysautonomia, polyneuritis (acute porphyria, lead poisoning), acute increased intracranial pressure, acute spinal cord section
Miscellaneous endocrine	Hypothyroidism, hyperthyroidism, hypercalcemia, acromegaly
Medications	High-dose estrogens, adrenal steroids, decongestants, appetite suppressants, cyclosporine, tricyclic antidepressants, monamine oxidase inhibitors, erythropoietin, nonsteroidal anti-inflammatory agents, cocaine
Mendelian forms of hypertension	See Table 241-4

referred to as primary or idiopathic hypertension). In the remaining 5–20% of hypertensive patients, a specific underlying disorder causing the elevation of blood pressure can be identified (Tables 241-2 and 241-3). In individuals with "secondary" hypertension, a specific mechanism for the blood pressure elevation is often more apparent.

ESSENTIAL HYPERTENSION

Essential hypertension tends to be familial and is likely to be the consequence of an interaction between environmental and genetic factors. The prevalence of essential hypertension increases with age, and individuals with relatively high blood pressures at younger ages are at increased risk for the subsequent development of hypertension. It is likely that essential hypertension represents a spectrum of disorders with different underlying pathophysiologies. In the majority of patients with established hypertension, peripheral resistance is increased and cardiac output is normal or decreased; however, in younger patients with mild or labile hypertension, cardiac output may be increased and peripheral resistance may be normal.

When plasma renin activity (PRA) is plotted against 24-h sodium excretion, ~10–15% of hypertensive patients have high PRA and 25% have low PRA. High-renin patients may have a vasoconstrictor form of hypertension, whereas low-renin patients may have a volume-dependent hypertension. Inconsistent associations between plasma aldosterone and blood pressure have been described in patients with essential hypertension. The association between aldosterone and blood pressure is more striking in African Americans, and PRA tends to be low in hypertensive African Americans. This raises the possibility that subtle increases of aldosterone may contribute to hypertension in at least some groups of patients who do not have overt primary aldosteronism. Furthermore, spironolactone, an aldosterone antagonist, may be a particularly effective antihypertensive agent for some patients with essential hypertension, including some patients with "drug-resistant" hypertension.

METABOLIC SYNDROME

(See also Chap. 236) Hypertension and dyslipidemia frequently occur together and in association with resistance to insulin-stimulated glucose uptake. This clustering of risk factors is often, but not invariably, associated with obesity, particularly abdominal obesity. Insulin resistance is also associated with an unfavorable imbalance in the endothelial production of mediators that regulate platelet aggregation, coagulation, fibrinolysis, and vessel tone. When these risk factors cluster, the risks for CHD, stroke, diabetes, and cardiovascular disease mortality are further increased.

Depending on the populations studied and the methodologies for defining insulin resistance, ~25–50% of non-obese, non-diabetic hypertensive persons are insulin resistant. The constellation of insulin resistance, hypertension, and dyslipidemia has been designated as the *metabolic syndrome*. As a group, first-degree relatives of patients with essential hypertension are also insulin resistant, and hyperinsulinemia (a surrogate marker of insulin resistance) may predict the eventual development of hypertension and cardiovascular disease. Although the metabolic syndrome may in part be heritable as a polygenic condition, the expression of the syndrome is modified by environmental factors, such as degree of physical activity and diet. Insulin sensitivity increases and blood pressure decreases in response to weight loss. The recognition that cardiovascular disease risk factors tend to cluster within individuals has important implications for the evaluation and treatment of

hypertension. Evaluation of both hypertensive patients and individuals at risk for developing hypertension should include assessment of overall cardiovascular disease risk. Similarly, introduction of lifestyle modification strategies and drug therapies should address overall risk, and not simply focus on hypertension.

RENAL PARENCHYMAL DISEASES

Virtually all disorders of the kidney may cause hypertension (Table 241-3), and renal disease is the most common cause of secondary hypertension. Hypertension is present in >80% of patients with chronic renal failure. In general, hypertension is more severe in glomerular diseases than in interstitial diseases, such as chronic pyelonephritis. Conversely, hypertension may cause nephrosclerosis, and in some instances it may be difficult to determine whether hypertension or renal disease was the initial disorder. Proteinuria > 1000 mg/day and an active urine sediment are indicative of primary renal disease. In either instance, the goals are to control blood pressure and retard the rate of progression of renal dysfunction.

Renovascular Hypertension Hypertension due to obstruction of a renal artery, renovascular hypertension, is a potentially curable form of hypertension. The mechanism of hypertension is generally related to activation of the renin-angiotensin system. Two groups of patients are at risk for this disorder: older arteriosclerotic patients who have a plaque obstructing the renal artery, frequently at its origin, and patients with fibromuscular dysplasia. Although fibromuscular dysplasia may occur at any age, it has a strong predilection for young Caucasian women. The prevalence in females is eightfold that in males. There are several histologic variants of fibromuscular dysplasia, including medial fibroplasia, perimedial fibroplasia, medial hyperplasia, and intimal fibroplasia. Medial fibroplasia is the most common variant and accounts for approximately two-thirds of patients. The lesions of fibromuscular dysplasia are frequently bilateral, and in contrast to atherosclerotic renovascular disease, tend to affect more distal portions of the renal artery.

In addition to the age and gender of the patient, several clues from the history and physical examination suggest a diagnosis of renovascular hypertension. Patients should first be evaluated for evidence of atherosclerotic vascular disease. Although response to antihypertensive therapy does not exclude the diagnosis, severe or refractory hypertension, recent loss of hypertension control or recent onset of moderately severe hypertension, and unexplained deterioration of renal function or deterioration of renal function associated with an ACE inhibitor should raise the possibility of renovascular hypertension. Approximately 50% of patients with renovascular hypertension have an abdominal or flank bruit, and the bruit is more likely to be hemodynamically significant if it lateralizes or extends throughout systole into diastole.

If blood pressure is adequately controlled with a simple antihypertensive regimen and renal function remains stable, there may be little impetus to pursue an evaluation for renal artery stenosis, particularly in an older patient with atherosclerotic disease and comorbid conditions. Patients with long-standing hypertension, advanced renal insufficiency, or diabetes mellitus are less likely to benefit from renal vascular repair. The most effective medical therapies include an ACE inhibitor or an angiotensin II receptor blocker; however, these agents decrease glomerular filtration rate in the stenotic kidney owing to efferent renal arteriolar dilation. In the presence of bilateral renal artery stenosis or renal artery stenosis to a solitary kidney, progressive renal insufficiency may result from the use of these agents. Importantly, the renal insufficiency is generally reversible following discontinuation of the offending drug.

If renal artery stenosis is suspected, and if the clinical condition warrants an intervention such as percutaneous transluminal renal angioplasty (PTRA), placement of a vascular endoprosthesis (stent), or surgical renal revascularization, imaging studies should be the next step in the evaluation. As a screening test, renal blood flow may be evaluated with a radionuclide [^{131}I]-orthoiodohippurate (OIH) scan or glomerular filtration rate may be evaluated with [^{99m}Tc]-diethylen-etriamine pentaacetic acid (DTPA) scan, before and after a single dose of captopril (or other ACE inhibitor). The following are consistent with a positive study: (1) decreased relative uptake by the involved kidney, which contributes <40% of total renal function; (2) delayed uptake on the affected side; or (3) delayed washout on the affected side. In patients with normal, or near-normal, renal function, a normal captopril renogram essentially excludes functionally significant renal artery stenosis; however its usefulness is limited in patients with renal insufficiency (creatinine clearance < 20 mL/min) or bilateral renal artery stenosis. Additional imaging studies are indicated if the scan is positive. Doppler ultrasound of the renal arteries produces reliable estimates of renal blood flow velocity and offers the opportunity to track a lesion over time. Positive studies are usually confirmed at angiography, whereas false-negative results occur frequently, particularly in obese patients. Gadolinium-contrast magnetic resonance angiography offers clear images of the proximal renal artery but may miss distal lesions. An advantage is the opportunity to image the renal arteries with an agent that is not nephrotoxic. Contrast arteriography remains the "gold standard" for evaluation and identification of renal artery lesions. Potential risks include nephrotoxicity, particularly in patients with diabetes mellitus or preexisting renal insufficiency.

Some degree of renal artery obstruction may be observed in almost 50% of patients with atherosclerotic disease, and there are several approaches for evaluating the functional significance of such a lesion to predict the effect of vascular repair on blood pressure control and renal function. Each approach has varying degrees of sensitivity and specificity, and no single test is sufficiently reliable to determine a causal relationship between a renal artery lesion and hypertension. On angiography, the presence of collateral vessels to the ischemic kidney suggests a functionally significant lesion. A lateralizing renal vein renin ratio (ratio > 1.5 of affected side/contralateral side) has a 90% predictive value for a lesion that would respond to vascular repair; however, the false-negative rate for blood pressure control is 50–60%. Measurement of the pressure gradient across a renal artery lesion does not reliably predict the response to vascular repair.

In the final analysis, a decision concerning vascular repair vs. medical therapy and the type of repair procedure should be individualized for each patient. Patients with fibromuscular disease have more favorable outcomes than patients with atherosclerotic lesions, presumably owing to their younger age, shorter duration of hypertension, and less systemic disease. Because of its low risk-versus-benefit ratio and high success rate (improvement or cure of hypertension in 90% of patients

and restenosis rate of 10%), PTRA is the initial treatment of choice for these patients. Surgical revascularization may be undertaken if PTRA is unsuccessful or if a branch lesion is present. In atherosclerotic patients, vascular repair should be considered if blood pressure cannot be adequately controlled with medical therapy or if renal function deteriorates. Surgery may be the preferred initial approach for younger atherosclerotic patients without comorbid conditions; however, for most atherosclerotic patients, depending on the location of the lesion, the initial approach may be PTRA and/or stenting. Surgical revascularization may be indicated if these approaches are unsuccessful, if the vascular lesion is not amenable to PTRA or stenting, or if concomitant aortic surgery is required, e.g., to repair an aneurysm.

PRIMARY ALDOSTERONISM

Excess aldosterone production due to primary aldosteronism is a potentially curable form of hypertension. In patients with primary aldosteronism, increased aldosterone production is independent of the renin-angiotensin system, and the consequences are sodium retention, hypertension, hypokalemia, and low PRA. The reported prevalence of this disorder varies from <2% to ~15% of hypertensive individuals. In part, this variation is related to the intensity of screening and to the criteria for establishing the diagnosis.

History and physical examination provide little information about the diagnosis. The age at the time of diagnosis is generally in the third through fifth decades. Hypertension is usually mild to moderate but occasionally may be severe; primary aldosteronism should be considered in all patients with refractory hypertension. Hypertension in these patients may be associated with glucose intolerance. Most patients are asymptomatic, although, infrequently, polyuria, polydypsia, paresthesias, or muscle weakness may be present as a consequence of hypokalemic alkalosis. The simplest screening test is measurement of serum potassium concentration. In a hypertensive patient with unprovoked hypokalemia (i.e., unrelated to diuretics, vomiting, or diarrhea), the prevalence of primary aldosteronism approaches 40–50%. In patients on diuretics, serum potassium <3.1 mmol/L (<3.1 meq/L) also raises the possibility of primary aldosteronism; however, serum potassium is an insensitive and nonspecific screening test. On initial presentation, serum potassium is normal in ~25% of patients subsequently found to have an aldosterone-producing adenoma, and higher percentages of patients with other etiologies of primary aldosteronism are not hypokalemic. Additionally, hypokalemic hypertension may be a consequence of secondary aldosteronism, other mineralocorticoid- and glucocorticoid-induced hypertensive disorders, and pheochromocytoma.

The ratio of plasma aldosterone to plasma renin activity (PA/PRA) is a useful screening test. These measurements are preferably obtained in ambulatory patients in the morning. A ratio >30:1 in conjunction with a plasma aldosterone concentration > 555 pmol/L (>20 ng/dL) reportedly has a sensitivity of 90% and a specificity of 91% for an aldosterone-producing adenoma. In a Mayo Clinic series, an aldosterone-producing adenoma was subsequently surgically confirmed in >90% of hypertensive patients with a PA/PRA ratio ≥20 and a plasma aldosterone concentration ≥415 pmol/L (≥15 ng/dL). There are, however, several caveats to interpreting the ratio. The cutoff for a "high" ratio is laboratory- and assay-dependent. Although some antihypertensive agents may affect the ratio (e.g., aldosterone antagonists, angiotensin receptor antagonists, and ACE inhibitors may increase renin; aldosterone antagonists may increase aldosterone), the ratio has been reported to be useful as a screening test in measurements obtained with patients taking their usual antihypertensive medications. A high ratio in the absence of an elevated plasma aldosterone level is considerably less specific for primary aldosteronism since many patients with essential hypertension have low renin levels in this setting, particularly African Americans and elderly patients. In patients with renal insufficiency, the ratio may also be elevated because of decreased aldosterone clearance. In patients with an elevated PA/PRA ratio, the diagnosis of primary aldosteronism can be confirmed by demonstrating failure to suppress plasma aldosterone to <277 pmol/L (<10 ng/dL) after IV infusion of 2 L of isotonic saline over 4 h.

Several adrenal abnormalities may culminate in the syndrome of primary aldosteronism, and appropriate therapy depends on the specific etiology. Some 60–70% of patients have an aldosterone-producing adrenal adenoma. The tumor is almost always unilateral, and most measure <3 cm in diameter. Most of the remainder have bilateral adrenocortical hyperplasia (idiopathic hyperaldosteronism). Rarely, primary aldosteronism may be caused by an adrenal carcinoma or an ectopic malignancy, e.g., ovarian arrhenoblastoma. Most aldosterone-producing carcinomas, in contrast to adrenal adenomas and hyperplasia, produce excessive amounts of other adrenal steroids in addition to aldosterone. Functional differences in hormone secretion may assist in the differential diagnosis. Aldosterone biosynthesis is more responsive to ACTH in patients with adenoma and more responsive to angiotensin in patients with hyperplasia. Consequently, patients with adenoma tend to have higher plasma aldosterone in the early morning that decreases during the day, reflecting the diurnal rhythm of ACTH, whereas plasma aldosterone tends to increase with upright posture in patients with hyperplasia, reflecting the normal postural response of the renin-angiotensin-aldosterone axis.

Adrenal CT or MRI should be carried out in all patients diagnosed with primary aldosteronism. High-resolution CT may identify tumors as small as 0.3 cm and is positive for an adrenal tumor 90% of the time. If the CT or MRI is not diagnostic, an adenoma may be detected by adrenal scintigraphy with 6 β-[I^{131}]iodomethyl-19-norcholesterol after dexamethasone suppression (0.5 mg every 6 h for 7 days); however, this technique has decreased sensitivity for adenomas < 1 cm. When results of functional and anatomic studies are inconclusive, bilateral adrenal venous sampling for aldosterone and cortisol levels in response to ACTH stimulation should be carried out. An ipsilateral/contralateral aldosterone ratio >10, with symmetric ACTH-stimulated cortisol levels, is diagnostic of an aldosterone-producing adenoma.

Hypertension is generally responsive to surgery in patients with adenoma but not in patients with bilateral adrenal hyperplasia. Unilateral adrenalectomy, often done via a laparoscopic approach, is curative in 40–70% of patients with an adenoma. Surgery should be undertaken after blood pressure has been controlled and hypokalemia corrected. Transient hypoaldosteronism may occur for up to 3 months postoperatively, resulting in hyperkalemia. Potassium should be monitored during this time, and hyperkalemia should be treated with potassium-wasting diuretics and with fludrocortisone, if needed. Patients with bilateral hyperplasia should be treated medically. The drug regimen for these patients, as well as for patients with an adenoma who are poor surgical candidates, should include an aldosterone antagonist and, if necessary, other potassium-sparing diuretics.

Glucocorticoid-remediable hyperaldosteronism is a rare, monogenic autosomal dominant disorder characterized by moderate to severe hypertension, often at an early age. Hypokalemia is usually mild or absent. Normally, angiotensin II stimulates aldosterone production by the adrenal zona glomerulosa, whereas ACTH stimulates cortisol production in the zona fasciculata. Owing to a chimeric gene on chromosome 8, ACTH also regulates aldosterone secretion by the zona fasciculata in patients with glucocorticoid-remediable hyperaldosteronism. The consequence is overproduction in the zona fasciculata of both aldosterone and hybrid steroids (18-hydroxycortisol and 18-oxocortisol) due to oxidation of cortisol. The diagnosis may be established by urine excretion rates of these hybrid steroids that are twenty to thirty times normal or by direct genetic testing. Therapeutically, suppression of ACTH with low-dose glucocorticoids corrects the hyperaldosteronism, hypertension, and hypokalemia. Spironolactone is also a therapeutic option.

CUSHING'S SYNDROME

(See also Chap. 336) Hypertension occurs in 75–80% of patients with Cushing's syndrome. The mechanism of hypertension may be related to stimulation of mineralocorticoid receptors by cortisol and increased secretion of other adrenal steroids. If clinically suspected, in patients not taking exogenous glucocorticoids, laboratory screening may be carried out with measurement of 24-h excretion rates of urine free cortisol or an overnight dexamethasone-suppression test. Recent evidence suggests that late night salivary cortisol is a sensitive and convenient screening test. Further evaluation is required to confirm the diagnosis and to identify the specific etiology of Cushing's syndrome. Appropriate therapy depends on the etiology.

PHEOCHROMOCYTOMA

(See also Chap. 337) Catecholamine-secreting tumors are located in the adrenal medulla (pheochromocytoma) or in extra-adrenal paraganglion tissue (paraganglioma) and account for hypertension in ~0.05% of patients. Approximately 20% of pheochromocytomas are familial with an autosomal dominant inheritance. Inherited pheochromocytomas may be associated with multiple endocrine neoplasia (MEN) type 2A and type 2B (Table 241-4). If unrecognized, pheochromocytoma may result in lethal cardiovascular consequences. Clinical manifestations, including hypertension, are primarily related to increased circulating catecholamines, although some of these tumors may secrete a number of other vasoactive substances. In a small percent of patients, epinephrine is the predominant catecholamine secreted by the tumor, and these patients may present with hypotension rather than hypertension. The initial suspicion of the diagnosis is based on symptoms and/or the association of pheochromocytoma with other disorders (Table 241-4). Laboratory testing consists of measuring catecholamines in either urine or plasma. Genetic screening is also available for evaluating patients and relatives suspected of harboring a pheochromocytoma associated with a familial syndrome. Surgical excision is the definitive treatment of pheochromocytoma and results in cure in ~90% of patients.

MISCELLANEOUS CAUSES OF HYPERTENSION

Hypertension due to *obstructive sleep apnea* is being recognized with increasing frequency (Chap. 259). Independent of obesity, hypertension occurs in >50% of individuals with obstructive sleep apnea, the severe end of the sleep-disordered breathing syndrome. The severity of hypertension correlates with the severity of sleep apnea. Approximately 70% of patients with obstructive sleep apnea are obese. Hypertension related to obstructive sleep apnea should also be considered in patients with drug-resistant hypertension and in patients with a history of snoring. The diagnosis can be confirmed by polysomnography. In obese patients, weight loss may alleviate or cure sleep apnea and related hypertension. Continuous positive airway pressure (CPAP) administered during sleep is an effective therapy for obstructive sleep apnea. With CPAP, patients with apparently drug-resistant hypertension may be more responsive to antihypertensive agents.

Coarctation of the aorta is the most common congenital cardiovascular cause of hypertension (Chap. 229). The incidence is 1–8 per 1000 live births. It is usually sporadic but occurs in 35% of children with Turner's syndrome. Even when the anatomic lesion is surgically corrected in infancy, up to 30% of patients develop subsequent hypertension and are at risk of accelerated coronary artery disease and cerebrovascular events. Patients with less severe lesions may not be diagnosed until young adulthood. The physical findings are diagnostic, and include diminished and delayed femoral pulses and a systolic pressure gradient between the right arm and the legs, and, depending on the location of the coarctation, between the right and left arms. A blowing systolic murmur may be heard in the posterior left interscapular areas. The diagnosis may be confirmed by chest x-ray and transesophageal echocardiogram. Therapeutic options include surgical repair or balloon angioplasty, with or without placement of an intravascular stent. Subsequently, many patients do not have a normal life expectancy but may have persistent hypertension with death due to ischemic heart disease, cerebral hemorrhage, or aortic aneurysm.

Several additional endocrine disorders, including *thyroid diseases* and *acromegaly*, cause hypertension. Mild diastolic hypertension may be a consequence of hypothyroidism, whereas hyperthyroidism may result in systolic hypertension. *Hypercalcemia* of any etiology, the most common being primary hyperparathyroidism, may result in hypertension. Hypertension may also be related to a number of prescribed or over-the-counter *medications*.

TABLE 241-4 RARE MENDELIAN FORMS OF HYPERTENSION

Disease	Phenotype	Genetic Cause
Glucocorticoid-remediable hyperaldosteronism	Autosomal dominant Absent or mild hypokalemia	Chimeric 11β-hydroxylase/aldsoterone gene on chromosome 8
17α-hydroxylase deficiency	Autosomal recessive Males: pseudohermaphroditism Females: primary amenorrhea, absent secondary sexual characteristics	Random mutations of the CYP17 gene on chromosome 10
11β-hydroxylase deficiency	Autosomal recessive Masculinization	Mutations of the CYP11B1 gene on chromosome 8q21-q22
11β-hydroxysteroid dehydrogenase deficiency (apparent mineralocorticoid excess syndrome)	Autosomal recessive Hypokalemia, low renin, low aldosterone	Mutations in the 11β-hydroxysteroid dehydrogenase gene
Liddle's syndrome	Autosomal dominant Hypokalemia, low renin, low aldosterone	Mutation subunits of the epithelial sodium channel SCNN1B and SCNN1C genes
Pseudohypoaldosteronism type II (Gordon's syndrome)	Autosomal dominant Hyperkalemia, normal glomerular filtration rate	Linkage to chromosomes 1q31-q42 and 17p11-q21
Hypertension exacerbated in pregnancy	Autosomal dominant Severe hypertension in early pregnancy	Missense mutation with substitution of leucine for serine at codon 810 (MR$_{L810}$)
Polycystic kidney disease	Autosomal dominant Large cystic kidneys, renal failure, liver cysts, cerebral aneurysms, valvular heart disease	Mutations in the PKD1 gene on chromosome 16 and PKD2 gene on chromosome 4
Pheochromocytoma	Autosomal dominant	
	(a) Multiple endocrine neoplasia, type 2A Medullary thyroid carcinoma, hyperparathyroidism	(a) Mutations in the RET protooncogene
	(b) Multiple endocrine neoplasia, type 2B Medullary thyroid carcinoma, mucosal neuromas, thickened corneal nerves, alimentary ganglioneuromatoses, marfanoid habitus	(b) Mutations in the RET protooncogene
	(c) von Hippel–Lindau disease Retinal angiomas, hemangioblastomas of the cerebellum and spinal cord, renal cell carcinoma	(c) Mutations in the VHL tumor-suppressor gene
	(d) Neurofibromatosis type 1 Multiple neurofibromas, café au lait spots	(d) Mutations in the NF1 tumor-suppressor gene

MONOGENIC HYPERTENSION

A number of rare forms of monogenic hypertension have been identified (Table 241-4). These disorders may be recognized by their characteristic phenotypes, and in many instances the diagnosis may be confirmed by genetic analysis. Several inherited defects in adrenal steroid biosynthesis and metabolism result in mineralocorticoid-induced hypertension and hypokalemia. In patients with a 17α-hydroxylase deficiency, synthesis of sex hormones and cortisol is decreased (Fig. 241-3). Consequently, these individuals do not mature sexually; males may present with pseudohermaphroditism and females with primary amenorrhea and absent secondary sexual characteristics. Because cortisol-induced negative feedback on pituitary ACTH production is diminished, ACTH-stimulated adrenal steroid synthesis proximal to the enzymatic block is increased. Hypertension and hypokalemia are consequences of increased synthesis of mineralocorticoids proximal to the enzymatic block, particularly desoxycorticosterone. Increased steroid production and, hence, hypertension may be treated with low-dose glucocorticoids. An 11β-hydroxylase deficiency results in a salt-retaining adrenogenital syndrome, occurring in 1 in 100,000 live births. This enzymatic defect results in decreased cortisol synthesis, increased synthesis of mineralocorticoids (e.g., desoxycorticosterone), and shunting of steroid biosynthesis into the androgen pathway. In the severe form, the syndrome may present early in life, including the newborn period, with virilization and ambiguous genitalia in females and penile enlargement in males, or in older children as precocious puberty and short stature. Acne, hirsutism, and menstrual irregularities may be the presenting features when the disorder is first recognized in adolescence or early adulthood. Hypertension is less common in the late-onset forms. Patients with an 11β-hydroxysteroid dehydrogenase deficiency have an impaired capacity to metabolize cortisol to its inactive metabolite, cortisone, and hypertension is related to activation of mineralocorticoid receptors by cortisol. This defect may be inherited or acquired, due to licorice-containing glyccherizic acid. This same substance is present in the paste of several brands of chewing tobacco. The defect in Liddle's syndrome (Chaps. 46 and 336) results from constitutive activation of amiloride-sensitive epithelial sodium channels (ENaC) on the distal renal tubule, resulting in excess sodium reabsorption; the syndrome is ameliorated by amiloride. Hypertension exacerbated in pregnancy (Chap. 7) is due to activation of the mineralocorticoid receptor by progesterone. Approximately 20% of pheochromocytomas are familial and may be associated with distinctive phenotypes.

APPROACH TO THE PATIENT:
Hypertension

HISTORY The initial assessment of the hypertensive patient should include a complete history and physical examination to confirm a diagnosis of hypertension, screen for other cardiovascular disease risk factors, screen for secondary causes of hypertension, identify cardiovascular consequences of hypertension and other comorbidities, assess blood pressure–related lifestyles, and determine the potential for intervention.

Most patients with hypertension have no specific symptoms referable to their blood pressure elevation. Although popularly considered a symptom of elevated arterial pressure, headache generally occurs only in patients with severe hypertension. Characteristically, a "hypertensive headache" occurs in the morning and is localized to the occipital region. Other nonspecific symptoms that may be related to elevated blood pressure include dizziness, palpitations, easy fatigability, and impotence. When symptoms are present, they are generally related to hypertensive cardiovascular disease or to manifestations of secondary hypertension. Table 241-5 lists salient features that should be addressed in obtaining a history from a hypertensive patient.

MEASUREMENT OF BLOOD PRESSURE Reliable measurements of blood pressure depend on attention to the details of the technique and conditions of the measurement. Owing to recent regulations preventing the use of mercury because of concerns about its potential toxicity, most office measurements are made with aneroid instruments. The accuracy of automated blood pressure instruments should be confirmed. Before taking the blood pressure measurement, the individual should be seated quietly for 5 min in a private, quiet setting with a comfortable room temperature. The center of

FIGURE 241-3 Adrenal enzymatic defects.

Mineralocorticoid   Glucocorticoid   Androgen

the cuff should be at heart level, and the width of the bladder cuff should equal at least 40% of the arm circumference; the length of the cuff bladder should encircle at least 80% of the arm circumference. It is important to pay attention to cuff placement, stethoscope placement, and the rate of deflation of the cuff (2 mmHg/s). Systolic blood pressure is the first of at least two regular "tapping" Korotkoff sounds, and diastolic blood pressure is the point at which the last regular Korotkoff sound is heard. In current practice, a diagnosis of hypertension is generally based on seated, office measurements.

Currently available ambulatory monitors are fully automated, use the oscillometric technique, and typically are programmed to take readings every 15–30 min. Ambulatory blood pressure monitoring is not, however, routinely used in clinical practice and is generally reserved for patients in whom white coat hypertension is suspected. The Seventh Report of the Joint National Committee on Prevention, Detection, Evaluation, and Treatment of High Blood Pressure (JNC 7) has also recommended ambulatory monitoring for treatment resistance, symptomatic hypotension, autonomic failure, and episodic hypertension.

TABLE 241-5 PATIENT'S RELEVANT HISTORY

Duration of hypertension
Previous therapies: responses and side effects
Family history of hypertension and cardiovascular disease
Dietary and psychosocial history
Other risk factors: weight change, dyslipidemia, smoking, diabetes, physical inactivity
Evidence of secondary hypertension: history of renal disease; change in appearance; muscle weakness; spells of sweating, palpitations, tremor; erratic sleep, snoring, daytime somnolence; symptoms of hypo- or hyperthyroidism; use of agents that may increase blood pressure
Evidence of target organ damage: history of TIA, stroke, transient blindness; angina, myocardial infarction, congestive heart failure; sexual function
Other comorbidities

Note: TIA, transient ischemic attack.

PHYSICAL EXAMINATION Body habitus, including weight and height, should be noted. At the initial examination, blood pressure should be measured in both arms, and preferably in the supine, sitting, and standing positions to evaluate for postural hypotension. Even if the femoral pulse is normal to palpation, arterial pressure should be measured at least once in the lower extremity in patients in whom hypertension is discovered before age 30. Heart rate should also be recorded. Hypertensive individuals have an increased prevalence of atrial fibrillation. The neck should be palpated for an enlarged thyroid gland, and patients should be assessed for signs of hypo- and hyperthyroidism. Examination of blood vessels may provide clues about underlying vascular disease and should include funduscopic examination, auscultation for bruits over the carotid and femoral arteries, and palpation of femoral and pedal pulses. The retina is the only tissue in which arteries and arterioles can be examined directly. With increasing severity of hypertension and atherosclerotic disease, progressive funduscopic changes include increased arteriolar light reflex, arteriovenous crossing defects, hemorrhages and exudates, and, in patients with malignant hypertension, papilledema. Examination of the heart may reveal a loud second heart sound due to closure of the aortic valve and an S_4 gallop, attributed to atrial contraction against a noncompliant left ventricle. Left ventricular hypertrophy may be detected by an enlarged, sustained, and laterally displaced apical impulse. An abdominal bruit, particularly a bruit that lateralizes and extends throughout systole into diastole, raises the possibility of renovascular hypertension. Kidneys of patients with polycystic kidney disease may be palpable in the abdomen. The physical examination should also include evaluation for signs of CHF and a neurologic examination.

LABORATORY TESTING   Table 241-6 lists recommended laboratory tests in the initial evaluation of hypertensive patients. Repeat measurements of renal function, serum electrolytes, fasting glucose, and lipids may be obtained after introducing a new antihypertensive agent and then annually, or more frequently if clinically indicated. More extensive laboratory testing is appropriate for patients with apparent drug-resistant hypertension or when the clinical evaluation suggests a secondary form of hypertension.

TABLE 241-6 BASIC LABORATORY TESTS FOR INITIAL EVALUATION

System	Test
Renal	Microscopic urinalysis, albumin excretion, serum BUN and/or creatinine
Endocrine	Serum sodium, potassium, calcium, ?TSH
Metabolic	Fasting blood glucose, total cholesterol, HDL and LDL (often computed) cholesterol, triglycerides
Other	Hematocrit, electrocardiogram

Note: BUN, blood urea nitrogen; TSH, thyroid-stimulating hormone; HDL, LDL, high-/low-density lipoprotein.

TABLE 241-7 LIFESTYLE MODIFICATIONS TO MANAGE HYPERTENSION

Weight reduction	Attain and maintain BMI < 25 kg/m²
Dietary salt reduction	< 6 g NaCl/d
Adapt DASH-type dietary plan	Diet rich in fruits, vegetables, and low-fat dairy products with reduced content of saturated and total fat
Moderation of alcohol consumption	For those who drink alcohol, consume ≤2 drinks/day in men and ≤1 drink/day in women
Physical activity	Regular aerobic activity, e.g., brisk walking for 30 min/d

Note: BMI, body mass index; DASH, Dietary Approaches to Stop Hypertension (trial).

℞ HYPERTENSION

LIFESTYLE INTERVENTIONS Implementation of lifestyles that favorably affect blood pressure has implications for both the prevention and treatment of hypertension. Health-promoting lifestyle modifications are recommended for individuals with pre-hypertension and as an adjunct to drug therapy in hypertensive individuals. These interventions should address overall cardiovascular disease risk. Although the impact of lifestyle interventions on blood pressure is more pronounced in persons with hypertension, in short-term trials, weight loss and reduction of dietary NaCl have also been shown to prevent the development of hypertension. In hypertensive individuals, even if these interventions do not produce a sufficient reduction of blood pressure to avoid drug therapy, the number of medications or dosages required for blood pressure control may be reduced. Dietary modifications that effectively lower blood pressure are weight loss, reduced NaCl intake, increased potassium intake, moderation of alcohol consumption, and an overall healthy dietary pattern **(Table 241-7)**.

Prevention and treatment of obesity are important for reducing blood pressure and cardiovascular disease risk. In short-term trials, even modest weight loss can lead to a reduction of blood pressure and an increase of insulin sensitivity. Average blood pressure reductions of 6.3/3.1 mmHg have been observed with a reduction in mean body weight of 9.2 kg. Regular physical activity facilitates weight loss, decreases blood pressure, and reduces the overall risk of cardiovascular disease. Blood pressure may be lowered by 30 min of moderately intense physical activity, such as brisk walking, 6–7 days a week, or by more intense, less frequent workouts.

There is individual variability in the sensitivity of blood pressure to NaCl, and this variability may have a genetic basis. Based on results of meta-analyses, lowering of blood pressure by limiting daily NaCl intake to 4.4–7.4 g (75–125 meq) results in blood pressure reductions of 3.7–4.9/0.9–2.9 mmHg in hypertensive and lesser reductions in normotensive individuals. Diets deficient in potassium, calcium, and magnesium are associated with higher blood pressures and a higher prevalence of hypertension. The urine sodium-to-potassium ratio is a stronger correlate of blood pressure than either sodium or potassium alone. Potassium and calcium supplementation have inconsistent, modest antihypertensive effects, and, independent of blood pressure, potassium supplementation may be associated with reduced stroke mortality. Alcohol use in persons consuming three or more drinks per day (a standard drink contains ~14 g ethanol) is associated with higher blood pressures, and a reduction of alcohol consumption is associated with a reduction of blood pressure. Mechanisms by which dietary potassium, calcium, or alcohol may affect blood pressure have not been established.

The DASH (Dietary Approaches to Stop Hypertension) trial convincingly demonstrated that over an 8-week period a diet high in fruits, vegetables, and low-fat dairy products lowers blood pressure in individuals with high-normal blood pressures or mild hypertension. Reduction of daily NaCl intake to <6 g (100 meq) augmented the effect of this diet on blood pressure. Fruits and vegetables are enriched sources of potassium, magnesium, and fiber, and dairy products are an important source of calcium.

PHARMACOLOGIC THERAPY Drug therapy is recommended for individuals with blood pressures ≥140/90 mmHg. The degree of benefit derived from antihypertensive agents is related to the magnitude of the blood pressure reduction. Lowering systolic blood pressure by 10–12 mmHg and diastolic blood pressure by 5–6 mmHg confers relative risk reductions of 35–40% for stroke and 12–16% for CHD within 5 years of initiating treatment. Risk of heart failure is reduced by >50%. There is considerable variation in individual responses to different classes of antihypertensive agents, and the magnitude of response to any single agent may be limited by activation of counterregulatory mechanisms that oppose the hypotensive effect of the agent. Selection of antihypertensive agents, and combinations of agents, should be individualized, taking into account age, severity of hypertension, other cardiovascular disease risk factors, comorbid conditions, and practical considerations related to cost, side effects, and frequency of dosing **(Table 241-8)**.

Diuretics Low-dose thiazide diuretics are often used as first-line agents, alone or in combination with other antihypertensive drugs. Thiazides inhibit the Na^+/Cl^- pump in the distal convoluted tubule and, hence, increase sodium excretion. Long term, they may also act as vasodilators. Thiazides are safe, efficacious, and inexpensive and reduce clinical events. They provide additive blood pressure–lowering effects when combined with beta blockers, ACE inhibitors, or angiotensin receptor blockers. In contrast, addition of a diuretic to a calcium channel blocker is less effective. Usual doses of hydrochlorothiazide range from 6.25–50 mg/d. Owing to an increased incidence of metabolic side effects (hypokalemia, insulin resistance, increased cholesterol), higher doses are generally not recommended. Two potassium-sparing diuretics, amiloride and triamterene, act by inhibiting epithelial sodium channels in the distal nephron. These agents are weak antihypertensive agents but may be used in combination with a thiazide to protect against hypokalemia. The main pharmacologic target for loop diuretics is the $Na^+-K^+-2Cl^-$ cotransporter in the thick ascending limb of the loop of Henle. Loop diuretics are generally reserved for hypertensive patients with reduced glomerular filtration rates [reflected in serum creatinine > 220 μmol/L (>2.5 mg/dL)], CHF, or sodium retention and edema for some other reason such as treatment with a potent vasodilator, e.g., minoxidil.

Blockers of the Renin-Angiotensin System ACE inhibitors decrease the production of angiotensin II, increase bradykinin levels, and reduce sympathetic nervous system activity. Angiotensin II receptor blockers provide selective blockade of AT_1 receptors, and the effect of angiotensin II on unblocked AT_2 receptors may augment the hypotensive effect. Both classes of agents are effective antihypertensive agents that may be used as monotherapy or in combination with diuretics, calcium antagonists, and alpha-blocking agents. Side effects of ACE inhibitors and angiotensin receptor blockers include functional renal insufficiency due to efferent renal arteriolar dilatation in a kidney with a stenotic lesion of the renal artery. Additional predisposing conditions to renal insufficiency induced by these agents include dehydration, CHF, and use of nonsteroidal anti-inflammatory drugs. Dry cough occurs in ~15% of patients, and angioedema occurs in <1% of patients taking ACE inhibitors. Angioedema occurs most commonly in individuals of Asian origin and more commonly in African Americans than in Caucasians. Hyperkalemia due to hypoaldosteronism is an occasional side effect of both ACE inhibitors and angiotensin receptor blockers.

Aldosterone Antagonists Spironolactone is a nonselective aldosterone antagonist that may be used alone or in combination with a thiazide diuretic. It may be a particularly effective agent in patients with low-renin essential hypertension, resistant hypertension, and primary aldosteronism. In patients with CHF, low-dose spironolactone reduces mortality and hospitalizations for heart failure when given in addition to conventional therapy with ACE inhibitors, digoxin, and loop diuretics. Because spironolactone binds to progesterone and androgen receptors, side effects may include gynecomastia, impotence, and menstrual abnormalities. These side effects are circumvented by a newer agent, eplerenone, which is a selective aldosterone antagonist. Eplerenone has recently been approved in the United States for the treatment of hypertension.

Beta Blockers β-Adrenergic receptor blockers lower blood pressure by decreasing cardiac output, due to a reduction of heart rate and contractility. Other proposed mechanisms by which beta blockers lower blood pressure include a central nervous system effect, and inhibition of renin release. Beta blockers are particularly effective in hypertensive patients with tachycardia, and their hypotensive potency is enhanced by coadministration with a diuretic. In lower doses, some beta blockers selectively inhibit cardiac $β_1$ receptors and have less influence on $β_2$ receptors on bronchial and vascular smooth muscle cells; however, there seems to be no difference in

PART 9

Disorders of the Cardiovascular System

TABLE 241-8 EXAMPLES OF ORAL DRUGS USED IN TREATMENT OF HYPERTENSION

Drug Class	Examples	Usual Total Daily Dose[a] (Dosing Frequency/Day)	Other Indications	Contraindications/Cautions
Diuretics				
Thiazides	Hydrochlorothiazide	6.25–50 mg (1–2)		Diabetes, dyslipidemia, hyperuricemia, gout, hypokalemia
	Chlorthalidone	25–50 mg (1)		
Loop diuretics	Furosemide	40–80 mg (2–3)	CHF, renal failure	Diabetes, dyslipidemia, hyperuricemia, gout, hypokalemia
	Ethacrynic acid	50–100 mg (2–3)		
Aldosterone antagonists	Spironolactone	25–100 mg (1–2)	CHF, primary aldosteronism	Renal failure, hyperkalemia
	Eplerenone	50–100 mg (1–2)		
K+ retaining	Amiloride	5–10 mg (1–2)		Renal failure, hyperkalemia
	Triamterene	50–100 mg (1–2)		
Beta blockers				Asthma, COPD, 2nd or 3rd degree heart block, sick-sinus syndrome
Cardioselective	Atenolol	25–100 mg (1)	Angina, CHF, post-MI, sinus tachycardia, ventricular tachyarrhythmias	
	Metoprolol	25–100 mg (1–2)		
Nonselective	Propranolol	40–160 mg (2)		
	Propranolol LA	60–180 (1)		
Combined alpha/beta	Labetalol	200–800 mg (2)	? Post-MI, CHF	
	Carvedilol	12.5–50 mg (2)		
Alpha antagonists				
Selective	Prazosin	2–20 mg (2–3)	Prostatism	
	Doxazosin	1–16 mg (1)		
	Terazosin	1–10 mg (1–2)		
Nonselective	Phenoxybenzamine	20–120 mg (2–3)	Pheochromocytoma	
Sympatholytics				
Central	Clonidine	0.1–0.6 mg (2)		
	Clonidine patch	0.1–0.3 mg (1/week)		
	Methyldopa	250–1000 mg (2)		
	Reserpine	0.05–0.25 mg (1)		
	Guanfacine	0.5–2 mg (1)		
ACE inhibitors	Captopril	25–200 mg (2)	Post-MI, CHF, nephropathy	Renal failure, bilateral renal artery stenosis, pregnancy, hyperkalemia
	Lisinopril	10–40 mg (1)		
	Ramipril	2.5–20 mg (1–2)		
Angiotensin II antagonists	Losartan	25–100 mg (1–2)	CHF, diabetic nephropathy, ACE inhibitor cough	Renal failure, bilateral renal artery stenosis, pregnancy, hyperkalemia
	Valsartan	80–320 mg (1)		
	Candesartan	2–32 mg (1–2)		
Calcium antagonists				Heart failure, 2d or 3d degree heart block
Dihydropyridines	Nifedipine (long acting)	30–60 mg (1)	Angina	
Nondihydropyridines	Verapamil (long acting)	120–360 mg (1–2)	Post-MI, supraventricular tachycardias, angina	
	Diltiazem (long-acting)	180-420 mg (1)		
Direct vasodilators	Hydralazine	25–100 mg (2)		Severe coronary artery disease
	Minoxidil	2.5–80 mg (1–2)		

[a]At the initiation of therapy, lower doses may be preferable for elderly patients and for select combinations of antihypertensive agents.

Note: CHF, congestive heart failure; COPD, chronic obstructive pulmonary disease; MI, myocardial infarction; ACE, angiotensin-converting enzyme.

the antihypertensive potencies of cardio-selective and non-selective beta blockers. Certain beta blockers have intrinsic sympathomimetic activity, and it is uncertain whether this constitutes an overall advantage or disadvantage in cardiac therapy. Beta blockers without intrinsic sympathomimetic activity decrease the rate of sudden death, overall mortality, and recurrent myocardial infarction. In patients with CHF, beta blockers have been shown to reduce the risks of hospitalization and mortality. Carvedilol and labetalol block both β receptors and peripheral α-adrenergic receptors. The potential advantages of combined β- and α-adrenergic blockade in treating hypertension remain to be determined.

α-Adrenergic Blockers Postsynaptic, selective α-adrenoreceptor antagonists lower blood pressure by decreasing peripheral vascular resistance. They are effective antihypertensive agents, used either as monotherapy or in combination with other agents. However, in clinical trials of hypertensive patients, alpha blockade has not been shown to reduce cardiovascular morbidity and mortality or to provide as much protection against CHF as other classes of antihypertensive agents. These agents are also effective in treating lower urinary tract symptoms in men with prostatic hypertrophy. Nonselective α-adrenoreceptor antagonists bind to postsynaptic and presynaptic receptors and are primarily used for the management of patients with pheochromocytoma.

Sympatholytic Agents Centrally acting α_2 sympathetic agonists decrease peripheral resistance by inhibiting sympathetic outflow. They may be particularly useful in patients with autonomic neuropathy who have wide variations in blood pressure due to baroreceptor denervation. Drawbacks include somnolence, dry mouth, and rebound hypertension on withdrawal. Peripheral sympatholytics decrease peripheral resistance and venous constriction by depleting nerve terminal norepinephrine. Although potentially effective antihypertensive agents, their usefulness is limited by orthostatic hypotension, sexual dysfunction, and numerous drug-drug interactions.

Calcium Channel Blockers Calcium antagonists reduce vascular resistance through L-channel blockade, which reduces intracellular calcium and blunts vasoconstriction. This is a heterogeneous group of agents that includes drugs in the following three classes: phenylalkylamines (verapamil), benzothiazepines (diltiazem), and 1,4-dihydropyridines (nifedipine-like). Used alone and in combination with other agents (ACE inhibitors, beta blockers, α_1-adrenergic blockers), calcium antagonists effectively lower blood pressure; however, it is unclear if adding a diuretic to a calcium blocker results in a further lowering of blood pressure. Side effects of flushing, headache, and edema with dihydropyridine use are related to their potencies as arteriolar dilators; edema is due to an increase in transcapillary pressure gradients, not to net salt and water retention.

Direct Vasodilators These agents decrease peripheral resistance and concomitantly activate mechanisms that defend arterial pressure, notably the sympathetic nervous system, the renin-angiotensin-aldosterone system, and sodium retention. Usually, they are not considered first-line agents but are most effective when added to a combination that includes a diuretic and a beta blocker. Hydralazine is a potent direct vasodilator that has antioxidant and nitric-oxide enhancing actions, and minoxidil is a particularly potent agent and is most frequently used in patients with renal insufficiency who are refractory to all other drugs. Hydralazine may induce a lupus-like syndrome, and side effects of minoxidil include hypertrichosis and pericardial effusion.

COMPARISONS OF ANTIHYPERTENSIVES Based on pooling results from clinical trials, meta-analyses of the efficacy of different classes of antihypertensive agents suggest essentially equivalent blood pressure–lowering effects of the following six major classes of antihypertensive agents when used as monotherapy: thiazide diuretics, beta blockers, ACE inhibitors, angiotensin II receptor blockers, calcium antagonists, and α_2 blockers. On average, standard doses of most antihypertensive agents reduce blood pressure by 8–10/4–7 mmHg; however, there may be subgroup differences in responsiveness. Younger patients may be more responsive to beta blockers and ACE inhibitors, whereas patients over age 50 may be more responsive to diuretics and calcium antagonists. There is a limited relationship between plasma renin and blood pressure response. Patients with high-renin hypertension may be more responsive to ACE inhibitors and angiotensin II receptor blockers than to other classes of agents, whereas patients with low-renin hypertension are more responsive to diuretics and calcium antagonists. Hypertensive African Americans tend to have low renin and may require higher doses of ACE inhibitors and angiotensin II receptor blockers than whites for optimal blood pressure control, although this difference is abolished when these agents are combined with a diuretic. Beta blockers also appear to be less effective than thiazide diuretics in African Americans than in non-African Americans.

A number of clinical trials have evaluated the possibility that different classes of antihypertensive agents have cardiovascular and renal protective effects not totally accounted for by their capacity to lower blood pressure. ACE inhibitors may have particular advantages, beyond that of blood pressure control, in reducing cardiovascular and renal outcomes. ACE inhibitors and angiotensin II receptor blockers decrease proteinuria and retard the rate of progression of renal insufficiency in both diabetic and nondiabetic renal diseases. The renoprotective effect of these agents, compared with other antihypertensive drugs, is less obvious at lower blood pressures. In both hypertensive and normotensive individuals, ACE inhibitors improve symptomatology and risk of death from CHF and reduce morbidity and mortality in the post-myocardial infarction patient. Similar benefits in cardiovascular morbidity and mortality in patients with CHF have also been observed with the use of angiotensin II receptor blockers. ACE inhibitors provide better coronary protection than calcium channel blockers, whereas calcium channel blockers provide more stroke protection than either ACE inhibitors or beta blockers.

In most patients with hypertension and heart failure due to systolic and/or diastolic dysfunction, the use of diuretics, ACE inhibitors or angiotensin II receptor antagonists, and beta blockers is recommended to improve survival. Although the optimal target blood pressure in patients with heart failure has not been established, a reasonable goal is the lowest blood pressure that is not associated with evidence of hypoperfusion.

A recent summary compared the results of 15 large clinical trials on the effects of antihypertensive treatment with different classes of agents on cardiovascular morbidity and mortality. In 13 of these trials, the incidence of cardiovascular events was similar between treatment groups, and in the remaining 2 trials, the difference was only marginally significant. It is possible that drug-related differences in cardiovascular outcomes are minimized in these large trials because of patient dropout, unplanned crossover of patients between groups, and insufficient statistical power to detect subgroup differences. Nevertheless, it is clear that the greatest cardiovascular and renal protective effects of antihypertensive therapy are related to adequate control of hypertension.

BLOOD PRESSURE GOALS OF ANTIHYPERTENSIVE THERAPY

Based on clinical trial data, the maximum protection against combined cardiovascular endpoints is achieved with pressures <135–140 mmHg for systolic blood pressure and <80–85 mmHg for diastolic blood pressure; however, treatment has not reduced cardiovascular disease risk to the level in nonhypertensive individuals. More aggressive blood pressure targets for blood pressure control (e.g., office or clinic blood pressure < 130/80 mmHg) may be appropriate for patients with diabetes, CHD, chronic kidney disease, or with additional cardiovascular disease risk factors. In diabetic patients, effective blood pressure control reduces the risk of cardiovascular events and death as well as the risk for microvascular disease (nephropathy, retinopathy). Risk reduction is greater in diabetic than in nondiabetic individuals.

To achieve recommended blood pressure goals, the majority of individuals with hypertension will require treatment with more than one drug. Three or more drugs are frequently needed in patients with diabetes and renal insufficiency. For most agents, reduction of blood pressure at half-standard doses is only ~20% less than at standard doses. Appropriate combinations of agents at these lower doses may have additive or almost additive effects on blood pressure with a lower incidence of side effects.

Despite theoretical concerns about decreasing cerebral, coronary, and renal blood flow by overly aggressive antihypertensive therapy, clinical tri-

als have found no evidence for a "J-curve" phenomenon, i.e., at blood pressure reductions achieved in clinical practice, there does *not* appear to be a lower threshold for increasing cardiovascular risk. Even among patients with isolated systolic hypertension, further lowering of the diastolic blood pressure does not result in harm. However, relatively little information is available concerning the risk/benefit ratio of antihypertensive therapy in individuals >80 years, and, in this population, gradual blood pressure reduction to less aggressive target levels of control may be appropriate.

The term *resistant hypertension* refers to patients with blood pressures persistently >140/90 mmHg despite taking three or more antihypertensive agents, including a diuretic, in reasonable combination and at full doses. Resistant or difficult-to-control hypertension is more common in patients >60 years than in younger patients. Resistant hypertension may be related to "pseudoresistance" (high office blood pressures and lower home blood pressures), nonadherence to therapy, identifiable causes of hypertension (including obesity and excessive alcohol intake), and use of any of a number of nonprescription and prescription drugs (Table 241-3). Rarely, in older patients, pseudohypertension may be related to the inability to measure blood pressure accurately in severely sclerotic arteries. This condition is suggested if the radial pulse remains palpable despite occlusion of the brachial artery by the cuff (Osler maneuver). The actual blood pressure can be determined by direct intraarterial measurement. Evaluation of patients with resistant hypertension might include home blood pressure monitoring to determine if office blood pressures are representative of the usual blood pressure. A more extensive evaluation for a secondary form of hypertension should be undertaken if no other explanation for hypertension resistance becomes apparent.

HYPERTENSIVE EMERGENCIES Probably due to the widespread availability of antihypertensive therapy, in the United States there has been a decline in the numbers of patients presenting with "crisis levels" of blood pressure. Most patients who present with severe hypertension are chronically hypertensive, and in the absence of acute, end-organ damage, precipitous lowering of blood pressure may be associated with significant morbidity and should be avoided. The key to successful management of severe hypertension is to differentiate hypertensive crises from hypertensive urgencies. The degree of target organ damage, rather than the level of blood pressure alone, determines the rapidity with which blood pressure should be lowered. **Tables 241-9** and **241-10** list a number of hypertension-related emergencies and recommended therapies.

Malignant hypertension is a syndrome associated with an abrupt increase of blood pressure in a patient with underlying hypertension or related to the sudden onset of hypertension in a previously normotensive individual. The absolute level of blood pressure is not as important as its rate of rise. Pathologically, the syndrome is associated with diffuse necrotizing vasculitis, arteriolar thrombi, and fibrin deposition in arteriolar walls. Fibrinoid necrosis has been observed in arterioles of kidney, brain, retina, and other organs. Clinically, the syndrome is recognized by progressive retinopathy (arteriolar spasm, hemorrhages, exudates, and papilledema), deteriorating renal function with proteinuria, microangiopathic hemolytic anemia, and encephalopathy. In these patients, historic inquiry should include questions about the use of monamine oxidase inhibitors and recreational drugs (e.g., cocaine, amphetamines).

TABLE 241-9	PREFERRED PARENTERAL DRUGS FOR SELECTED HYPERTENSIVE EMERGENCIES
Hypertensive encephalopathy	Nitroprusside, nicardipine, labetalol
Malignant hypertension (when IV therapy is indicated)	Labetalol, nicardipine, nitroprusside, enalaprilat
Stroke	Nicardipine, labetalol, nitroprusside
Myocardial infarction/unstable angina	Nitroglycerin, nicardipine, labetalol, esmolol
Acute left ventricular failure	Nitroglycerin, enalaprilat, loop diuretics
Aortic dissection	Nitroprusside, esmolol, labetalol
Adrenergic crisis	Phentolamine, nitroprusside
Postoperative hypertension	Nitroglycerin, nitroprusside, labetalol, nicardipine
Preeclampsia/eclampsia of pregnancy	Hydralazine, labetalol, nicardipine

Source: Adapted from DG Vidt, in S Oparil, MA Weber (eds): *Hypertension*, 2d ed. Philadelphia, Elsevier Saunders, 2005.

TABLE 241-10 USUAL INTRAVENOUS DOSES OF ANTIHYPERTENSIVE AGENTS USED IN HYPERTENSIVE EMERGENCIES[a]

Antihypertensive Agent	Intravenous Dose
Nitroprusside	Initial 0.3 (μg/kg)/min; usual 2–4 (μg/kg)/min; maximum 10 (μg/kg)/min for 10 min
Nicardipine	Initial 5 mg/h; titrate by 2.5 mg/h at 5–15 min intervals; max 15 mg/h
Labetalol	2 mg/min up to 300 mg or 20 mg over 2 min, then 40–80 mg at 10-min intervals up to 300 mg total
Enalaprilat	Usual 0.625–1.25 mg over 5 min every 6–8 h; maximum 5 mg/dose
Esmolol	Initial 80–500 μg/kg over 1 min, then 50–300 (μg/kg)/min
Phentolamine	5–15 mg bolus
Nitroglycerin	Initial 5 μg/min, then titrate by 5 μg/min at 3–5 min intervals; if no response is seen at 20 μg/min, incremental increases of 10–20 μg/min may be used
Hydralazine	10–50 mg at 30-min intervals

[a]Constant blood pressure monitoring is required. Start with the lowest dose. Subsequent doses and intervals of administration should be adjusted according to the blood pressure response and duration of action of the specific agent.

Although blood pressure should be lowered rapidly in patients with hypertensive encephalopathy, there are inherent risks of overly aggressive therapy. In hypertensive individuals, the upper and lower limits of autoregulation of cerebral blood flow are shifted to higher levels of arterial pressure, and rapid lowering of blood pressure to below the lower limit of autoregulation may precipitate cerebral ischemia or infarction as a consequence of decreased cerebral blood flow. Renal and coronary blood flows may also decrease with overly aggressive acute therapy. The initial goal of therapy is to reduce mean arterial blood pressure by no more than 25% within minutes to 2 h or to a blood pressure in the range of 160/100–110 mmHg. This may be accomplished with IV nitroprusside, a short-acting vasodilator with a rapid onset of action that allows for minute-to-minute control of blood pressure. Parenteral labetalol and nicardipine are also effective agents for the treatment of hypertensive encephalopathy.

In patients with malignant hypertension without encephalopathy or some other catastrophic event, it is preferable to reduce blood pressure over hours or longer rather than minutes. This goal may effectively be achieved initially with frequent dosing of short-acting oral agents, such as captopril, clonidine, or labetalol.

Acute, transient blood pressure elevations, lasting days to weeks, frequently occur following thrombotic and hemorrhagic strokes. Autoregulation of cerebral blood flow is impaired in ischemic cerebral tissue, and higher arterial pressures may be required to maintain cerebral blood flow. Although specific blood pressure targets have not been defined for patients with acute cerebrovascular events, aggressive reductions of blood pressure are to be avoided. With the increasing availability of improved methods for measuring cerebral blood flow (using CT technology), studies are in progress to evaluate the effects of different classes of antihypertensive agents on both blood pressure and cerebral blood flow following an acute stroke. Currently, in the absence of other indications for acute therapy, for patients with cerebral infarction who are not candidates for thrombolytic therapy, one recommended guideline is to institute antihypertensive therapy only for those patients with a systolic blood pressure > 220 mmHg or a diastolic blood pressure > 130 mmHg. If thrombolytic therapy is to be used, the recommended goal blood pressure is <185 mmHg systolic pressure

and <110 mmHg diastolic pressure. In patients with hemorrhagic stroke, suggested guidelines for initiating antihypertensive therapy are systolic > 180 mmHg or diastolic pressure > 130 mmHg. The management of hypertension after subarachnoid hemorrhage is controversial. Cautious reduction of blood pressure is indicated if mean arterial pressure is >130 mmHg.

In addition to pheochromocytoma, an adrenergic crisis due to catecholamine excess may be related to cocaine or amphetamine overdose, clonidine withdrawal, acute spinal cord injuries, and an interaction of tyramine-containing compounds with monamine oxidase inhibitors. These patients may be treated with phentolamine or nitroprusside.

Treatment of hypertension in patients with acute aortic dissection is discussed in Chap. 242, and treatment of hypertension in pregnancy is discussed in Chap. 7.

FURTHER READINGS

ADROGUE JH, MADIAS NE: Sodium and potassium in the pathogenesis of hypertension. N Engl J Med 356:1966, 2007

ALLHAT COLLABORATIVE RESEARCH GROUP: Major outcomes in high-risk hypertensive patients randomized to angiotensin converting enzyme inhibitor or calcium channel blocker vs. diuretic: The Antihypertensive and Lipid-Lowering Treatment to Prevent Heart Attack Trial (ALLHAT). JAMA 288:2981, 2002

APPEL LJ et al: Dietary approaches to prevent and treat hypertension: A scientific statement from the American Heart Association. Hypertension 47:296, 2006

BATH PMW, SPRIGGS N: Control of blood pressure after stroke. Hypertension 48:203, 2006

BLOOD PRESSURE LOWERING TREATMENT TRIALISTS' COLLABORATION: Effects of ACE inhibitors, calcium antagonists, and other blood pressure-lowering drugs: Results of prospectively designed overviews of randomised trials. Lancet 355:1955, 2000

CASAS JP et al: Effect of inhibitors of the renin-angiotensin system and other antihypertensive drugs on renal outcomes: Systematic review and meta-analysis. Lancet 366:2026, 2005

CHOBANIAN AV et al: The Seventh Report of the Joint National Committee on Prevention, Detection, Evaluation, and Treatment of High Blood Pressure: The JNC 7 Report. JAMA 289:2560, 2003

HAAJAR IM, KOTCHEN TA: Trends in prevalence, awareness, treatment, and control of hypertension in the United States, 1988–2000. JAMA 290:199, 2003

LAW MR et al: Value of low dose combination treatment with blood pressure lowering drugs: Analysis of 354 randomised trials. BMJ 326:1427, 2003

LIU W et al: Genome scan meta-analysis for hypertension. Am J Hypertens 17:1100, 2004

MANCIA G: Role of outcome trials in providing information on antihypertensive treatment: Importance and limitations. Am J Hypertens 19:1, 2006

MOSER M, SETANO JF: Resistant or difficult-to-control hypertension. N Engl J Med 355:385, 2006

PICKERING TG et al: Ambulatory blood-pressure monitoring. N Engl J Med 3554:2368, 2006

STAESSEN JA et al: Cardiovascular prevention and blood pressure reduction: A quantitative overview updated until 1 March 2003. J Hypertens 21:1055, 2003

WU J et al: A summary of the effects of antihypertensive medications on measured blood pressure. Am J Hypertens 18:935, 2005

242 Diseases of the Aorta

Mark A. Creager, Joseph Loscalzo

The aorta is the conduit through which the blood ejected from the left ventricle is delivered to the systemic arterial bed. In adults, its diameter is approximately 3 cm at the origin and in the ascending portion, 2.5 cm in the descending portion in the thorax, and 1.8–2 cm in the abdomen. The aortic wall consists of a thin intima composed of endothelium, subendothelial connective tissue, and an internal elastic lamina; a thick tunica media composed of smooth-muscle cells and extracellular matrix; and an adventitia composed primarily of connective tissue enclosing the vasa vasorum and nervi vascularis. In addition to its conduit function, the viscoelastic and compliant properties of the aorta also subserve a buffering function. The aorta is distended during systole to enable a portion of the stroke volume and elastic energy to be stored, and it recoils during diastole so that blood continues to flow to the periphery. Because of its continuous exposure to high pulsatile pressure and shear stress, the aorta is particularly prone to injury and disease resulting from mechanical trauma (Table 242-1). The aorta is also more prone to rupture than any other vessel, especially with the development of aneurysmal dilatation, since its wall tension, as governed by Laplace's law (i.e., proportional to the product of pressure and radius), will be increased.

AORTIC ANEURYSM

An *aneurysm* is defined as a pathologic dilatation of a segment of a blood vessel. A *true aneurysm* involves all three layers of the vessel wall

TABLE 242-1 DISEASES OF THE AORTA: ETIOLOGY AND ASSOCIATED FACTORS

Aortic aneurysm
  Degenerative/atherosclerosis
    Aging
    Cigarette smoking
    Male gender
    Family history
  Cystic medial necrosis
    Marfan syndrome
    Ehlers-Danlos syndrome type IV
    Familial etiology
    Bicuspid aortic valve
  Chronic aortic dissection
  Infective (see below)
  Trauma

Acute aortic syndromes (aortic dissection, acute intramural hematoma, penetrating atherosclerotic ulcer)
  Atherosclerosis
  Cystic medial necrosis (see above)
  Hypertension
  Vasculitis (see below)
  Pregnancy
  Trauma

Aortic occlusion
  Atherosclerosis
  Thromboembolism

Aortitis
  Vasculitis
    Takayasu's arteritis
    Giant cell arteritis
  Rheumatic
    HLA-B27–associated spondyloarthropathies
    Behçet's syndrome
    Cogan's syndrome
  Idiopathic retroperitoneal fibrosis
  Infective
    Syphilis
    Tuberculosis
  Mycotic (*Salmonella*, staphylococcal, streptococcal, fungal)

and is distinguished from a *pseudoaneurysm*, in which the intimal and medial layers are disrupted and the dilatation is lined by adventitia only and, at times, by perivascular clot. Aneurysms may also be classified according to their gross appearance. A *fusiform aneurysm* affects the entire circumference of a segment of the vessel, resulting in a diffusely dilated artery. In contrast, a *saccular aneurysm* involves only a portion of the circumference, resulting in an outpouching of the vessel wall. Aortic aneurysms are also classified according to location, i.e., abdominal versus thoracic. Aneurysms of the descending thoracic aorta are usually contiguous with infradiaphragmatic aneurysms and are referred to as *thoracoabdominal aortic aneurysms*.

ETIOLOGY

Aortic aneurysms result from conditions that cause degradation or abnormal production of the aortic wall's structural components, elastin and collagen. The causes of aortic aneurysms may be broadly categorized as degenerative diseases, inherited or developmental diseases, infections, vasculitis, and trauma (Table 242-1). Inflammation, proteolysis, and biomechanical wall stress contribute to the degenerative processes that characterize most aneurysms of the abdominal and descending thoracic aorta. These are mediated by B and T cell lymphocytes, macrophages, inflammatory cytokines, and matrix metalloproteinases that degrade elastin and collagen and alter the tensile strength and ability of the aorta to accommodate pulsatile stretch. The associated histopathology demonstrates destruction of elastin and collagen, decreased vascular smooth muscle, ingrowth of new blood vessels, and inflammation. Factors associated with degenerative aortic aneurysms include aging, cigarette smoking, hypercholesterolemia, male gender, and a family history of aortic aneurysms.

The most common pathologic condition associated with degenerative aortic aneurysms is *atherosclerosis*. Many patients with aortic aneurysms have coexisting risk factors for atherosclerosis (Chap. 235), as well as atherosclerosis in other blood vessels.

Cystic medial necrosis is the histopathologic term used to describe the degeneration of collagen and elastic fibers in the tunica media of the aorta, as well as the loss of medial cells that are replaced by multiple clefts of mucoid material. Cystic medial necrosis characteristically affects the proximal aorta, results in circumferential weakness and dilatation, and leads to the development of fusiform aneurysms involving the ascending aorta and the sinuses of Valsalva. This condition is particularly prevalent in patients with Marfan syndrome, Ehlers-Danlos syndrome type IV (Chap. 357), hypertension, congenital bicuspid aortic valves, and familial thoracic aortic aneurysm syndromes. Sometimes it appears as an isolated condition in patients without any other apparent disease.

Familial clusterings of aortic aneurysms occur in 20% of patients, suggesting a hereditary basis for the disease. Mutations of the genes encoding fibrillin-1 and type III procollagen have been implicated in some cases of Marfan and Ehlers-Danlos type IV syndromes, respectively. Linkage analysis has identified loci on chromosomes 5q13–14, 11q23.3–q24, and 3p24–25 in several families, although the specific alleles have not been described.

The infectious causes of aortic aneurysms include syphilis, tuberculosis, and other bacterial infections. *Syphilis* (Chap. 162) is a relatively uncommon cause of aortic aneurysm. Syphilitic periaortitis and mesoaortitis damage elastic fibers, resulting in thickening and weakening of the aortic wall. Approximately 90% of syphilitic aneurysms are located in the ascending aorta or aortic arch. *Tuberculous aneurysms* (Chap. 158) typically affect the thoracic aorta and result from direct extension of infection from hilar lymph nodes or contiguous abscesses, or from bacterial seeding. Loss of aortic wall elasticity results from granulomatous destruction of the medial layer. A *mycotic aneurysm* is a rare condition that develops as a result of staphylococcal, streptococcal, *Salmonella* or other bacterial or fungal infections of the aorta, usually at an atherosclerotic plaque. These aneurysms are usually saccular. Blood cultures are often positive and reveal the nature of the infecting agent.

Vasculitides associated with aortic aneurysm include Takayasu's arteritis and giant cell arteritis, which may cause aneurysms of the aortic arch and descending thoracic aorta. Spondyloarthropathies, such as ankylosing spondylitis, rheumatoid arthritis, psoriatic arthritis, relapsing polychondritis, and Reiter's syndrome, are associated with dilatation of the ascending aorta. Behçet's syndrome (Chap. 320) causes thoracic and abdominal aortic aneurysms. *Traumatic aneurysms* may occur after penetrating or nonpenetrating chest trauma and most commonly affect the descending thoracic aorta just beyond the site of insertion of the ligamentum arteriosum. Chronic aortic dissections are associated with weakening of the aortic wall that may lead to the development of aneurysmal dilatation.

THORACIC AORTIC ANEURYSMS

The clinical manifestations and natural history of thoracic aortic aneurysms depend on their location. Cystic medial necrosis is the most common cause of ascending aortic aneurysms, whereas atherosclerosis is the condition most frequently associated with aneurysms of the aortic arch and descending thoracic aorta. The average growth rate of thoracic aneurysms is 0.1–0.2 cm per year. Thoracic aortic aneurysms associated with Marfan syndrome or aortic dissection may expand at a greater rate. The risk of rupture is related to the size of the aneurysm and the presence of symptoms, ranging approximately from 2–3% per year for thoracic aortic aneurysms <4.0 cm in diameter to 7% per year for those >6 cm in diameter. Most thoracic aortic aneurysms are asymptomatic; however, compression or erosion of adjacent tissue by aneurysms may cause symptoms such as chest pain, shortness of breath, cough, hoarseness, or dysphagia. Aneurysmal dilatation of the ascending aorta may cause congestive heart failure as a consequence of aortic regurgitation, and marked compression of the superior vena cava may produce congestion of the head, neck, and upper extremities.

A chest x-ray may be the first test to suggest the diagnosis of a thoracic aortic aneurysm (Fig. 242-1). Findings include widening of the mediastinal shadow and displacement or compression of the trachea or left mainstem bronchus. Two-dimensional echocardiography, particularly transesophageal echocardiography, can be used to assess the proximal ascending aorta and descending thoracic aorta. Contrast-enhanced computed tomography (CT), magnetic resonance imaging (MRI), and conventional invasive aortography are sensitive and specific tests for assessment of aneurysms of the thoracic aorta and involvement of branch vessels (Fig. 242-2). In asymptomatic patients whose aneurysms are too small to justify surgery, noninvasive testing with either contrast-enhanced CT or MRI should be performed at least every 6–12 months to monitor expansion.

FIGURE 242-1 **A chest x-ray** of a patient with a thoracic aortic aneurysm.

FIGURE 242-2 **An aortogram** demonstrating a large fusiform aneurysm of the descending thoracic aorta.

℞ THORACIC AORTIC ANEURYSMS

Patients with thoracic aortic aneurysms, and particularly patients with Marfan syndrome who have evidence of aortic root dilatation, should receive long-term beta-blocker therapy. Additional medical therapy should be given, as necessary, to control hypertension. Operative repair with placement of a prosthetic graft is indicated in patients with symptomatic thoracic aortic aneurysms, and in those in whom the aortic diameter is >5.5–6 cm or has increased by >1 cm per year. In patients with Marfan syndrome or bicuspid aortic valve, thoracic aortic aneurysms >5 cm should be considered for surgery.

ABDOMINAL AORTIC ANEURYSMS

Abdominal aortic aneurysms occur more frequently in males than in females, and the incidence increases with age. Abdominal aortic aneurysms ≥4.0 cm may affect 1–2% of men older than 50 years. At least 90% of all abdominal aortic aneurysms >4.0 cm are related to atherosclerotic disease, and most of these aneurysms are below the level of the renal arteries. Prognosis is related to both the size of the aneurysm and the severity of coexisting coronary artery and cerebrovascular disease. The risk of rupture increases with the size of the aneurysm: the 5-year risk for aneurysms <5 cm is 1–2%, whereas it is 20–40% for aneurysms >5 cm in diameter. The formation of mural thrombi within aneurysms may predispose to peripheral embolization.

An abdominal aortic aneurysm commonly produces no symptoms. It is usually detected on routine examination as a palpable, pulsatile, expansile, and nontender mass, or it is an incidental finding during an abdominal x-ray or ultrasound study performed for other reasons. As abdominal aortic aneurysms expand, however, they may become painful. Some patients complain of strong pulsations in the abdomen; others experience pain in the chest, lower back, or scrotum. Aneurysmal pain is usually a harbinger of rupture and represents a medical emergency. More often, acute rupture occurs without any prior warning, and this complication is always life-threatening. Rarely, there is leakage of the aneurysm with severe pain and tenderness. Acute pain and hypotension occur with rupture of the aneurysm, which requires emergency operation.

Abdominal radiography may demonstrate the calcified outline of the aneurysm; however, about 25% of aneurysms are not calcified and cannot be visualized by plain x-ray. An abdominal ultrasound can delineate the transverse and longitudinal dimensions of an abdominal aortic aneurysm and may detect mural thrombus. Abdominal ultrasound is useful for serial documentation of aneurysm size and can be

FIGURE 242-3 A computed tomographic angiogram (CTA) depicting a fusiform abdominal aortic aneurysm that has been treated with a bifurcated stent graft.

used to screen patients at risk for developing aortic aneurysm, such as those with affected siblings, peripheral atherosclerosis, or peripheral artery aneurysms. In one large study, ultrasound screening of men age 65–74 years was associated with a risk reduction in aneurysm-related death by 42%. CT with contrast and MRI are accurate, noninvasive tests to determine the location and size of abdominal aortic aneurysms and to plan endovascular or open surgical repair (Fig. 242-3). Contrast aortography may be used for the evaluation of patients with aneurysms, but the procedure carries a small risk of complications, such as bleeding, allergic reactions, and atheroembolism. Since the presence of mural thrombi may reduce the luminal size, aortography may underestimate the diameter of an aneurysm.

℞ ABDOMINAL AORTIC ANEURYSMS

Operative repair of the aneurysm and insertion of a prosthetic graft are indicated for abdominal aortic aneurysms of any size that are expanding rapidly or are associated with symptoms. For asymptomatic aneurysms, operation is indicated if the diameter is >5.5 cm. In randomized trials of patients with abdominal aortic aneurysms <5.5 cm, there was no difference in the long-term (5- to 8-year) mortality rate between those followed with ultrasound surveillance and those undergoing elective aneurysm repair. Thus, serial noninvasive follow-up of smaller aneurysms (<5 cm) is an alternative to immediate surgery. Percutaneous placement of endovascular stent grafts (Fig. 242-3) for treatment of infrarenal abdominal aortic aneurysms is available for selected patients and is associated with lower short-term morbidity but comparable long-term mortality, compared with open surgical reconstruction.

In surgical candidates, careful preoperative cardiac and general medical evaluations (followed by appropriate therapy of complicating conditions) are essential. Preexisting coronary artery disease, congestive heart failure, pulmonary disease, diabetes, and advanced age add to the risk of surgery. β-adrenergic blockers decrease perioperative cardiovascular morbidity and mortality. With careful preoperative cardiac evaluation and postoperative care, the operative mortality rate approximates 1–2%. After acute rupture, the mortality rate of emergent operation is 45–50%. Endovascular repair with stent placement is an emerging approach but, at the current time, is associated with a mortality rate of approximately 40%.

ACUTE AORTIC SYNDROMES

The four major acute aortic syndromes include aortic rupture (discussed above), aortic dissection, intramural hematoma, and penetrating atherosclerotic ulcer. Aortic dissection is caused by a circumferential or, less frequently, transverse tear of the intima. It often occurs along the right lateral wall of the ascending aorta where the hydraulic shear stress is high. Another common site is the descending thoracic aorta just below the ligamentum arteriosum. The initiating event is either a primary intimal tear with secondary dissection into the media or a medial hemorrhage that dissects into and disrupts the intima. The pulsatile aortic flow then dissects along the elastic lamellar plates of the aorta and creates a false lumen. The dissection usually propagates distally down the descending aorta and into its major branches, but it may also propagate proximally. Distal propagation may be limited by atherosclerotic plaque. In some cases, a secondary distal intimal disruption occurs, resulting in the reentry of blood from the false to the true lumen.

There are at least two important pathologic and radiologic variants of aortic dissection: intramural hematoma without an intimal flap and penetrating atherosclerotic ulcer. Acute intramural hematoma is thought to result from rupture of the vasa vasorum with hemorrhage into the wall of the aorta. Most occur in the descending thoracic aorta. Acute intramural hematomas may progress to dissection and rupture. Penetrating atherosclerotic ulcers are caused by erosion of a plaque into the aortic media, are usually localized, and are not associated with extensive propagation. They are found primarily in the mid and distal portions of the descending thoracic aorta and are associated with extensive atherosclerotic disease. The ulcer can erode beyond the internal elastic lamina, leading to medial hematoma, and may progress to false aneurysm formation or rupture.

Several classification schemes have been developed for thoracic aortic dissections. DeBakey and colleagues initially classified aortic dissections as type I, in which an intimal tear occurs in the ascending aorta but involves the descending aorta as well; type II, in which the dissection is limited to the ascending aorta; and type III, in which the intimal tear is located in the descending aorta with distal propagation of the dissection (Fig. 242-4). Another classification (Stanford) is that of type A, in which the dissection involves the ascending aorta (proximal dissection), and type B, in which it is limited to the descending aorta (distal dissection). From a management standpoint, classification of aortic dissections and intramural hematomas into type A or B is more practical and useful, since DeBakey types I and II are managed in a similar manner.

The factors that predispose to aortic dissection include systemic hypertension, a coexisting condition in 70% of patients, and cystic medial necrosis. Aortic dissection is the major cause of morbidity and mortality in patients with Marfan syndrome (Chap. 357) and similarly may affect patients with Ehlers-Danlos syndrome. The incidence is also increased in patients with inflammatory aortitis (i.e., Takayasu's arteritis, giant cell arteritis), congenital aortic valve anomalies (e.g., bicuspid valve), coarctation of the aorta, and a history of aortic trauma. In addition, the risk of dissection is increased in otherwise normal women during the third trimester of pregnancy.

CLINICAL MANIFESTATIONS

The peak incidence of aortic dissection is in the sixth and seventh decades. Men are more affected than women by a ratio of 2:1. The presentations of aortic dissection and its variants are the consequences of intimal tear, dissecting hematoma, occlusion of involved arteries, and compression of adjacent tissues. Acute aortic dissection presents with the sudden onset of pain (Chap. 13), which is often described as very severe and tearing and is associated with diaphoresis. The pain may be localized to the front or back of the chest, often the interscapular region, and typically migrates with propagation of the dissection. Other symptoms include syncope, dyspnea, and weakness. Physical findings may include hypertension or hypotension, loss of pulses, aortic regurgitation, pulmonary edema, and neurologic findings due to carotid artery obstruction (hemiplegia, hemianesthesia) or spinal cord ischemia

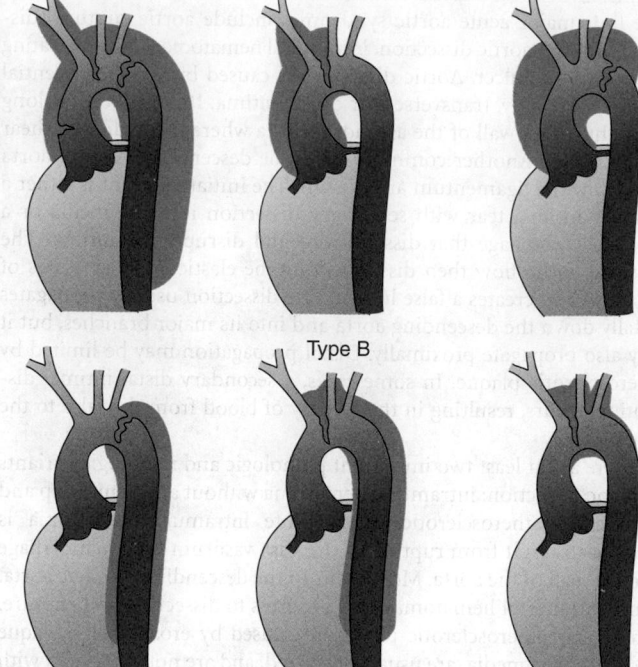

FIGURE 242-4 Classification of aortic dissections. Stanford classification: Type A dissections (*top panels*) involve the ascending aorta independent of site of tear and distal extension; type B dissections (*bottom panels*) involve transverse and/or descending aorta without involvement of the ascending aorta. DeBakey classification: Type I dissection involves ascending to descending aorta (*top left*); type II dissection is limited to ascending or transverse aorta, without descending aorta (*top center + top right*); type III dissection involves descending aorta only (*bottom left*). [From DC Miller, in RM Doroghazi, EE Slater (eds): Aortic Dissection. New York, McGraw-Hill, 1983, with permission.]

(paraplegia). Bowel ischemia, hematuria, and myocardial ischemia have all been observed. These clinical manifestations reflect complications resulting from the dissection occluding the major arteries. Furthermore, clinical manifestations may result from the compression of adjacent structures (e.g., superior cervical ganglia, superior vena cava, bronchus, esophagus) by the expanding dissection causing aneurysmal dilatation, and include Horner's syndrome, superior vena cava syndrome, hoarseness, dysphagia, and airway compromise. Hemopericardium and cardiac tamponade may complicate a type A lesion with retrograde dissection. Acute aortic regurgitation is an important and common (>50%) complication of proximal dissection. It is the outcome of either a circumferential tear that widens the aortic root or a disruption of the annulus by dissecting hematoma that tears a leaflet(s) or displaces it, inferior to the line of closure. Signs of aortic regurgitation include bounding pulses, a wide pulse pressure, a diastolic murmur often radiating along the right sternal border, and evidence of congestive heart failure. The clinical manifestations depend on the severity of the regurgitation.

In dissections involving the ascending aorta, the chest x-ray often reveals a widened superior mediastinum. A pleural effusion (usually left-sided) also may be present. This effusion is typically serosanguineous and not indicative of rupture unless accompanied by hypotension and falling hematocrit. In dissections of the descending thoracic aorta, a widened mediastinum may also be observed on chest x-ray. In addition, the descending aorta may appear to be wider than the ascending portion. An electrocardiogram that shows no evidence of myocardial ischemia is helpful in distinguishing aortic dissection from myocardial infarction. Rarely, the dissection involves the right or, less commonly, left coronary ostium and causes acute myocardial infarction.

The diagnosis of aortic dissection can be established by noninvasive techniques such as echocardiography, CT, or MRI. Aortography is

used less commonly because of the accuracy of these noninvasive techniques. Transthoracic echocardiography can be performed simply and rapidly and has an overall sensitivity of 60–85% for aortic dissection. For diagnosing proximal ascending aortic dissections, its sensitivity exceeds 80%; it is less useful for detecting dissection of the arch and descending thoracic aorta. Transesophageal echocardiography requires greater skill and patient cooperation but is very accurate in identifying dissections of the ascending and descending thoracic aorta, but not the arch, achieving 98% sensitivity and approximately 90% specificity. Echocardiography also provides important information regarding the presence and severity of aortic regurgitation and pericardial effusion. CT and MRI are both highly accurate in identifying the intimal flap and the extent of the dissection and involvement of major arteries; each has a sensitivity and specificity >90%. They are useful in recognizing intramural hemorrhage and penetrating ulcers. MRI can also detect blood flow, which may be useful in characterizing antegrade versus retrograde dissection. The relative utility of transesophageal echocardiography, CT, and MRI depends on the availability and expertise in individual institutions as well as on the hemodynamic stability of the patient, with CT and MRI obviously less suitable for unstable patients.

℞ AORTIC DISSECTION

Medical therapy should be initiated as soon as the diagnosis is considered. The patient should be admitted to an intensive care unit for hemodynamic monitoring. Unless hypotension is present, therapy should be aimed at reducing cardiac contractility and systemic arterial pressure, and thereby shear stress. For acute dissection, unless contraindicated, β-adrenergic blockers should be administered parenterally, using intravenous propranolol, metoprolol, or the short-acting esmolol to achieve a heart rate of approximately 60 beats/min. This should be accompanied by sodium nitroprusside infusion to lower systolic blood pressure to ≤120 mmHg. Labetalol (Chap. 242), a drug with both β- and α-adrenergic blocking properties, may also be used as a parenteral agent in the acute therapy of dissection.

The calcium channel antagonists verapamil and diltiazem may be used intravenously if nitroprusside or β-adrenergic blockers cannot be employed. The addition of a parenteral angiotensin-converting enzyme (ACE) inhibitor, such as enalaprilat, to a β-adrenergic blocker also may be considered. Isolated use of direct vasodilators, such as diazoxide and hydralazine, is contraindicated because these agents can increase hydraulic shear and may propagate dissection.

Emergent or urgent surgical correction is the preferred treatment for acute ascending aortic dissections and intramural hematomas (type A) and for complicated type B dissections, including those characterized by propagation, compromise of major aortic branches, impending rupture, or continued pain. Surgery involves excision of the intimal flap, obliteration of the false lumen, and placement of an interposition graft. A composite valve-graft conduit is used if the aortic valve is disrupted. The overall in-hospital mortality rate after surgical treatment of patients with aortic dissection is reported to be 15–25%. The major causes of perioperative mortality and morbidity include myocardial infarction, paraplegia, renal failure, tamponade, hemorrhage, and sepsis. Reports of the use of endoluminal stent grafts in selected patients with type B dissection are encouraging. Other transcatheter techniques, such as fenestration of the intimal flaps and stenting of narrowed branch vessels to increase flow to compromised organs, are investigational approaches used in selected patients. For uncomplicated and stable distal dissections and intramural hematomas (type B), medical therapy is the preferred treatment. The in-hospital mortality rate of medically treated patients with type B dissection is 10–20%. Long-term therapy for patients with aortic dissection and intramural hematomas (with or without surgery) consists of the control of hypertension and reduction of cardiac contractility with the use of beta blockers plus other antihypertensive agents, such as ACE inhibitors or calcium antagonists. Patients with chronic type B dissection and intramural hematomas should be followed on an outpatient basis every 6–12 months by contrast-enhanced CT or MRI to detect propagation or expansion. Patients with Marfan syndrome are at high risk for postdissection complications. The long-term prognosis for patients with treated dissections is generally good with careful follow-up; the 10-year survival rate is approximately 60%.

AORTIC OCCLUSION

CHRONIC ATHEROSCLEROTIC OCCLUSIVE DISEASE

Atherosclerosis may affect the thoracic and abdominal aorta. Occlusive aortic disease caused by atherosclerosis is usually confined to the distal abdominal aorta below the renal arteries. Frequently the disease extends to the iliac arteries (Chap. 243). Claudication characteristically involves the buttocks, thighs, and calves and may be associated with impotence in males (Leriche syndrome). The severity of the symptoms depends on the adequacy of collaterals. With sufficient collateral blood flow, a complete occlusion of the abdominal aorta may occur without the development of ischemic symptoms. The physical findings include absence of femoral and other distal pulses bilaterally, and the detection of an audible bruit over the abdomen (usually at or below the umbilicus) and the common femoral arteries. Atrophic skin, loss of hair, and coolness of the lower extremities are usually observed. In advanced ischemia, rubor on dependency and pallor on elevation can be seen.

The diagnosis is usually established by physical examination and noninvasive testing, including leg pressure measurements, Doppler velocity analysis, pulse volume recordings, and duplex ultrasonography. The anatomy may be defined by MRI, CT, or conventional aortography, typically performed when considering revascularization. Catheter-based endovascular or operative treatment is indicated in patients with lifestyle-limiting or debilitating symptoms of claudication and in patients with critical limb ischemia.

ACUTE OCCLUSION

Acute occlusion in the distal abdominal aorta constitutes a medical emergency because it threatens the viability of the lower extremities; it usually results from an occlusive embolus that almost always originates from the heart. Rarely, acute occlusion may occur as the result of in situ thrombosis in a preexisting severely narrowed segment of the aorta.

The clinical picture is one of acute ischemia of the lower extremities. Severe rest pain, coolness, and pallor of the lower extremities and the absence of distal pulses bilaterally are the usual manifestations. Diagnosis should be established rapidly by MRI, CT, or aortography. Emergency thrombectomy or revascularization is indicated.

AORTITIS

Aortitis, a term referring to inflammatory disease of the aorta, may be caused by large vessel vasculitides such as Takayasu's arteritis and giant cell arteritis, rheumatic and HLA-B27–associated spondyloarthropathies, Behçet's syndrome, ANCA-associated vasculitides, Cogan's syndrome, and infections, such as syphilis, tuberculosis, and *Salmonella*, or may be associated with retroperitoneal fibrosis. Aortitis may result in aneurysmal dilatation and aortic regurgitation, occlusion of the aorta and its branch vessels, or acute aortic syndromes.

TAKAYASU'S ARTERITIS

This inflammatory disease often affects the ascending aorta and aortic arch, causing obstruction of the aorta and its major arteries. Takayasu's arteritis is also termed *pulseless disease* because of the frequent occlusion of the large arteries originating from the aorta. It may also involve the descending thoracic and abdominal aorta and occlude large branches such as the renal arteries. Aortic aneurysms may also occur. The pathology is a panarteritis, characterized by mononuclear cells and occasionally giant cells, with marked intimal hyperplasia, medial and adventitial thickening, and, in the chronic form, fibrotic occlusion. The disease is most prevalent in young females of Asian descent but does occur in women of other geographic and ethnic origins and also in young men. During the acute stage, fever, malaise, weight loss, and other systemic symptoms may be evident. Elevations of the erythrocyte sedimentation rate and C-reactive protein are common. The chronic stages of the disease, which is intermittently active, present with symptoms related to large artery occlusion, such as upper extremity claudication, cerebral ischemia, and syncope. Since the process is progressive and there is no definitive therapy, the prognosis is usually poor. Glucocorticoids and immunosuppressive agents have been reported to be effective in some patients during the acute phase. Surgical bypass or endovascular intervention of a critically stenotic artery may be necessary.

GIANT CELL ARTERITIS

(See also Chap. 319) This vasculitis occurs in older individuals and affects women more often than men. Primarily large and medium-sized arteries are affected. The pathology is that of focal granulomatous lesions involving the entire arterial wall; it may be associated with polymyalgia rheumatica. Obstruction of medium-sized arteries (e.g., temporal and ophthalmic arteries) and of major branches of the aorta and the development of aortitis and aortic regurgitation are important complications of the disease. High-dose glucocorticoid therapy may be effective when given early.

RHEUMATIC AORTITIS

Rheumatoid arthritis (Chap. 314), ankylosing spondylitis (Chap. 318), psoriatic arthritis (Chap. 318), Reiter's syndrome (Chap. 318), relapsing polychondritis, and inflammatory bowel disorders may all be associated with aortitis involving the ascending aorta. The inflammatory lesions usually involve the ascending aorta and may extend to the sinuses of Valsalva, the mitral valve leaflets, and adjacent myocardium. The clinical manifestations are aneurysm, aortic regurgitation, and involvement of the cardiac conduction system.

SYPHILITIC INFECTIVE AORTITIS

Infective aortitis may result from direct invasion of the aortic wall by bacterial pathogens, such as *Staphylococcus*, *Streptococcus*, and *Salmonella*, or by fungi. These bacteria cause aortitis by infecting the aorta at sites of atherosclerotic plaque. Bacterial proteases lead to degradation of collagen, and the ensuing destruction of the aortic wall leads to formation of a saccular aneurysm, referred to as a mycotic aneurysm. Mycotic aneurysms have a predilection for the suprarenal abdominal aorta. The pathologic characteristics of the aortic wall include acute and chronic inflammation, abscesses, hemorrhage, and necrosis. Mycotic aneurysms typically affect the elderly and occur in men three times more frequently than in women. Patients may present with fever, sepsis, and chest, back, or abdominal pain; there may have been a preceding diarrheal illness. Blood cultures are positive in the majority of patients. Both CT and MRI are useful to diagnose mycotic aneurysms. Treatment includes antibiotic therapy and surgical removal of the affected part of the aorta, and revascularization of the lower extremities with grafts placed in uninfected tissue.

Syphilitic aortitis is a late manifestation of luetic infection (Chap. 162) that usually affects the proximal ascending aorta, particularly the aortic root, resulting in aortic dilatation and aneurysm formation. Syphilitic aortitis may occasionally involve the aortic arch or the descending aorta. The aneurysms may be saccular or fusiform and are usually asymptomatic, but compression of and erosion into adjacent structures may result in symptoms; rupture may also occur.

The initial lesion is an obliterative endarteritis of the vasa vasorum, especially in the adventitia. This is an inflammatory response to the invasion of the adventitia by the spirochetes. Destruction of the aortic media occurs as the spirochetes spread into this layer, usually via the lymphatics accompanying the vasa vasorum. Destruction of collagen and elastic tissues leads to dilation of the aorta, scar formation, and calcification. These changes account for the characteristic radiographic appearance of linear calcification of the ascending aorta.

The disease typically presents as an incidental chest radiographic finding 15–30 years after initial infection. Symptoms may result from aortic regurgitation, narrowing of coronary ostia due to syphilitic aortitis, compression of adjacent structures (e.g., esophagus), or rupture. Diagnosis is established by a positive serologic test, i.e., rapid plasmin reagin (RPR) or fluorescent treponemal antibody. Treatment includes penicillin and surgical excision and repair.

FURTHER READINGS

ASHTON HA et al: The Multicentre Aneurysm Screening Study (MASS) into the effect of abdominal aortic aneurysm screening on mortality in men: A randomized controlled trial. The Multicentre Aneurysm Screening Study Group. Lancet 360:1531, 2002

BARIL DT et al: Surgery insight: Advances in endovascular repair of abdominal aortic aneurysm. Nat Clin Pract Cardiovasc Med 4:206, 2007

BLANKENSTEIJN JD et al: Two-year outcomes after conventional or endovascular repair of abdominal aortic aneurysms. N Engl J Med 352:2398, 2005

CREAGER MA et al (eds): *Vascular Medicine: A Companion to Braunwald's Heart Disease*, 1st ed. Philadelphia, Saunders, 2006

FLEMING C et al: Screening for abdominal aortic aneurysm: A best-evidence systematic review for the U.S. Preventive Services Task Force. Ann Intern Med 142:203, 2005

GRECO C et al: Outcomes of endovascular treatment of ruptured abdominal aortic aneurysms. J Vasc Surg 43:453, 2006

HAGAN PG et al: The International Registry of Acute Aortic Dissection (IRAD): New insights into an old disease. JAMA 283:897, 2000

HIRSCH AT et al: ACC/AHA 2005 Practice Guidelines for the management of patients with peripheral arterial disease (lower extremity, renal, mesenteric, and abdominal aortic). Circulation 113:e463, 2006

ISSELBACHER EM: Thoracic and abdominal aortic aneurysms. Circulation 111:816, 2005

LEDERLE FA et al: Immediate repair compared with surveillance of small abdominal aortic aneurysms. The Aneurysm Detection and Management Veterans Affairs Cooperative Study Group. N Engl J Med 346:1437, 2002

UNITED KINGDOM SMALL ANEURYSM TRIAL PARTICIPANTS: Long-term outcomes of immediate repair compared with surveillance of small abdominal aortic aneurysms. N Engl J Med 346:1445, 2002

TSAI TT et al: Acute aortic syndromes. Circulation 112:3802, 2005

243 Vascular Diseases of the Extremities

Mark A. Creager, Joseph Loscalzo

ARTERIAL DISORDERS

PERIPHERAL ARTERIAL DISEASE

Peripheral arterial disease (PAD) is defined as a clinical disorder in which there is a stenosis or occlusion in the aorta or arteries of the limbs. Atherosclerosis is the leading cause of PAD in patients > 40 years old. Other causes include thrombosis, embolism, vasculitis, fibromuscular dysplasia, entrapment, cystic adventitial disease, and trauma. The highest prevalence of atherosclerotic PAD occurs in the sixth and seventh decades of life. As in patients with atherosclerosis of the coronary and cerebral vasculature, there is an increased risk of developing PAD in cigarette smokers and in persons with diabetes mellitus, hypercholesterolemia, hypertension, or hyperhomocysteinemia.

Pathology (See also Chap. 235) Segmental lesions causing stenosis or occlusion are usually localized to large and medium-sized vessels. The pathology of the lesions includes atherosclerotic plaques with calcium deposition, thinning of the media, patchy destruction of muscle and elastic fibers, fragmentation of the internal elastic lamina, and thrombi composed of platelets and fibrin. The primary sites of involvement are the abdominal aorta and iliac arteries (30% of symptomatic patients), the femoral and popliteal arteries (80–90% of patients), and the more distal vessels, including the tibial and peroneal arteries (40–50% of patients). Atherosclerotic lesions occur preferentially at arterial branch points, sites of increased turbulence, altered shear stress, and intimal injury. Involvement of the distal vasculature is most common in elderly individuals and patients with diabetes mellitus.

Clinical Evaluation Fewer than 50% of patients with PAD are symptomatic, although many have a slow or impaired gait. The most common *symptom* is intermittent claudication, which is defined as a pain, ache, cramp, numbness, or a sense of fatigue in the muscles; it occurs during exercise and is relieved by rest. The site of claudication is distal to the location of the occlusive lesion. For example, buttock, hip, and thigh discomfort occur in patients with aortoiliac disease, whereas calf claudication develops in patients with femoral-popliteal disease. Symptoms are far more common in the lower than in the upper extremities because of the higher incidence of obstructive lesions in the former region. In patients with severe arterial occlusive disease in whom resting blood flow cannot accommodate basal nutritional needs of the tissues, critical limb ischemia may develop. Patients will complain of rest pain or a feeling of cold or numbness in the foot and toes. Frequently, these symptoms occur at night when the legs are horizon-

tal and improve when the legs are in a dependent position. With severe ischemia, rest pain may be persistent.

Important *physical findings* of PAD include decreased or absent pulses distal to the obstruction, the presence of bruits over the narrowed artery, and muscle atrophy. With more severe disease, hair loss, thickened nails, smooth and shiny skin, reduced skin temperature, and pallor or cyanosis are frequent physical signs. In patients with critical limb ischemia, ulcers or gangrene may occur. Elevation of the legs and repeated flexing of the calf muscles produce pallor of the soles of the feet, whereas rubor, secondary to reactive hyperemia, may develop when the legs are dependent. The time required for rubor to develop or for the veins in the foot to fill when the patient's legs are transferred from an elevated to a dependent position is related to the severity of the ischemia and the presence of collateral vessels. Patients with severe ischemia may develop peripheral edema because they keep their legs in a dependent position much of the time. Ischemic neuropathy can result in numbness and hyporeflexia.

Noninvasive Testing The history and physical examination are often sufficient to establish the diagnosis of PAD. An objective assessment of the presence and severity of disease is obtained by noninvasive techniques. Arterial pressure can be recorded noninvasively in the legs by placement of sphygmomanometric cuffs at the ankles and use of a Doppler device to auscultate or record blood flow from the dorsalis pedis and posterior tibial arteries. Normally, systolic blood pressure in the legs and arms is similar. Indeed, ankle pressure may be slightly higher than arm pressure due to pulse-wave amplification. In the presence of hemodynamically significant stenoses, the systolic blood pressure in the leg is decreased. Thus, the ratio of the ankle and brachial artery pressures (termed the *ankle:brachial index*, or ABI) is ≥1.0 in normal individuals and <1.0 in patients with peripheral arterial disease; a ratio of <0.5 is consistent with severe ischemia.

Other noninvasive tests include segmental pressure measurements, pulse volume recordings, Doppler flow velocity waveform analysis, duplex ultrasonography (which combines B-mode imaging and pulse-wave Doppler examination), transcutaneous oximetry, and stress testing (usually using a treadmill). Placement of pneumatic cuffs enables assessment of systolic pressure along the legs. The presence of pressure gradients between sequential cuffs provides evidence of the presence and location of hemodynamically significant stenoses. Also, the volume displacement in the leg is decreased with each pulse, and the Doppler velocity contour becomes progressively blunted in the presence of significant PAD. Duplex ultrasonography is used to image and detect stenotic lesions in native arteries and bypass grafts.

Treadmill testing allows the physician to assess functional limitations objectively. Decline of the ABI immediately after exercise provides further support for the diagnosis of PAD in patients with equivocal symptoms and findings on examination.

Magnetic resonance angiography (MRA), computed tomographic angiography, and conventional contrast angiography should not be used for routine diagnostic testing but are performed prior to potential revascularization. Each test is useful in defining the anatomy to assist planning for catheter-based and surgical revascularization procedures.

Prognosis The natural history of patients with PAD is influenced primarily by the extent of coexisting coronary artery and cerebrovascular disease. Approximately one-third to one-half of patients with symptomatic PAD have evidence of coronary artery disease based on clinical presentation and electrocardiogram, and over one-half have significant coronary artery disease by coronary angiography. Patients with PAD have a 15–30% 5-year mortality rate and a two- to sixfold increased risk of death from coronary heart disease. Mortality is highest in those with the most severe PAD. The likelihood of symptomatic progression of PAD appears less than the chance of succumbing to coronary artery disease. Approximately 75–80% of nondiabetic patients who present with mild to moderate claudication remain symptomatically stable. Deterioration is likely to occur in the remainder, with approximately 1–2% of the group ultimately developing critical limb ischemia. Approximately 25–30% of patients with critical limb ischemia survive and undergo amputation within 1 year. The prognosis is worse in patients who continue to smoke cigarettes or who have diabetes mellitus.

℞ PERIPHERAL ARTERIAL DISEASE

Patients with PAD should receive therapies to reduce the risk of associated cardiovascular events, such as myocardial infarction and death, and to improve limb symptoms, prevent progression to critical limb ischemia, and preserve limb viability. Risk factor modification and antiplatelet therapy should be initiated to improve cardiovascular outcomes. The importance of discontinuing cigarette smoking cannot be overemphasized. The physician must assume a major role in this lifestyle modification. Counseling and adjunctive drug therapy with the nicotine patch, bupropion, or varenicline increase smoking cessation rates and reduce recidivism. It is important to control blood pressure in hypertensive patients. Angiotensin-converting enzyme inhibitors may reduce the risk of cardiovascular events in patients with symptomatic PAD. β-Adrenergic blockers do not worsen claudication and may be used to treat hypertension, especially in patients with coexistent coronary artery disease. Treatment of hypercholesterolemia with statins is advocated to reduce the risk of myocardial infarction, stroke and death. The National Cholesterol Education Program Adult Treatment Panel considers PAD to be a coronary heart disease equivalent and recommends treatment to reduce LDL cholesterol to <100 mg/dL. Platelet inhibitors, particularly aspirin, reduce the risk of adverse cardiovascular events in patients with peripheral atherosclerosis. Clopidogrel, a drug that inhibits platelet aggregation via its effect on adenosine diphosphate–dependent platelet-fibrinogen binding, appears to be more effective than aspirin in reducing cardiovascular morbidity and mortality in patients with PAD. There is insufficient evidence of efficacy to support the routine use of dual antiplatelet therapy with both aspirin and clopidogrel in patients with PAD. The anticoagulant warfarin is not indicated to improve outcome in patients with chronic PAD.

Therapies for intermittent claudication and critical limb ischemia include supportive measures, medications, nonoperative interventions, and surgery. Supportive measures include meticulous care of the feet, which should be kept clean and protected against excessive drying with moisturizing creams. Well-fitting and protective shoes are advised to reduce trauma. Elastic support hose should be avoided, as they reduce blood flow to the skin. In patients with critical limb ischemia, shock blocks under the head of the bed together with a canopy over the feet may improve perfusion pressure and ameliorate some of the rest pain.

Patients with claudication should be encouraged to exercise regularly and at progressively more strenuous levels. Supervised exercise training programs for 30–45 min sessions, three to five times per week for at least 12 weeks, prolong walking distance. Patients also should be advised to walk until near-maximum claudication discomfort occurs, then resting until the symptoms resolve before resuming ambulation. Pharmacologic treatment of PAD has not been as successful as the medical treatment of coronary artery disease (Chap. 237). In particular, vasodilators as a class have not proved to be beneficial. During exercise, peripheral vasodilation occurs distal to sites of significant arterial stenoses. As a result, perfusion pressure falls, often to levels less than that generated in the interstitial tissue by the exercising muscle. Drugs such as α-adrenergic blocking agents, calcium channel antagonists, papaverine, and other vasodilators have not been shown to be effective in patients with PAD.

Cilostazol, a phosphodiesterase inhibitor with vasodilator and antiplatelet properties, increases claudication distance by 40–60% and improves measures of quality of life. The mechanism of action accounting for its beneficial effects is not known. Pentoxifylline, a substituted xanthine derivative, has been reported to decrease blood viscosity and to increase red cell flexibility, thereby increasing blood flow to the microcirculation and enhancing tissue oxygenation. Although several placebo-controlled studies have found that pentoxifylline increases the duration of exercise in patients with claudication, its efficacy has not been confirmed in all clinical trials. Statins and propionyl-L-carnitine, a drug that affects skeletal muscle metabolic function, appear promising for treatment of intermittent claudication in initial clinical trials.

Several studies have suggested that long-term parenteral administration of vasodilator prostaglandins decreases pain and facilitates healing of ulcers in patients with critical limb ischemia. Clinical trials of angiogenic growth factors are proceeding. Intramuscular gene transfer of DNA encoding vascular endothelial growth factor, basic fibroblast growth factor, hepatocyte growth factor, or hypoxia-inducible factor-1α, and also administration of endothelial progenitor cells, may promote collateral blood vessel growth in patients with critical limb ischemia. Some trial results have been negative and others encouraging. The outcome of ongoing studies will further elucidate the potential role of therapeutic angiogenesis for PAD.

Revascularization Revascularization procedures, including catheter-based and surgical interventions, are usually indicated for patients with disabling, progressive, or severe symptoms of intermittent claudication despite medical therapy, and for those with critical limb ischemia. MRA, CT, or conventional contrast angiography should be performed to assess vascular anatomy in patients who are being considered for revascularization. Nonoperative interventions include percutaneous transluminal angiography (PTA), stent placement, and atherectomy (Chap. 240). PTA and stenting of the iliac artery are associated with higher success rates than PTA and stenting of the femoral and popliteal arteries. Approximately 90–95% of iliac PTAs are initially successful, and the 3-year patency rate is >75%. Patency rates may be higher if a stent is placed in the iliac artery. The initial success rates for femoral-popliteal PTA and stenting are approximately 80%, with 60% 3-year patency rates. Patency rates are influenced by the severity of pretreatment stenoses; the prognosis of occlusive lesions is worse than that of nonocclusive stenotic lesions. The role of drug-eluting stents in PAD is currently unclear.

Several operative procedures are available for treating patients with aortoiliac and femoral-popliteal artery disease. The preferred operative procedure depends on the location and extent of the obstruction(s) and general medical condition of the patient. Operative procedures for aortoiliac disease include aortobifemoral bypass, axillofemoral bypass, femoral-femoral bypass, and aortoiliac endarterectomy. The most frequently used procedure is the aortobifemoral bypass using knitted Dacron grafts. Immediate graft patency approaches 99%, and 5- and 10-year graft patency in survivors is >90% and 80%, respectively. Operative complications include myocardial infarction and stroke, infection of the graft, peripheral embolization, and sexual dysfunction from interruption of autonomic nerves in the pelvis. Operative mortality ranges from 1–3%, mostly due to ischemic heart disease.

Operative therapy for femoral-popliteal artery disease includes in situ and reverse autogenous saphenous vein bypass grafts, placement of polytetrafluoroethylene (PTFE) or other synthetic grafts, and thromboendarterectomy. Operative mortality ranges from 1–3%. The long-term patency rate depends on the type of graft used, the location of the distal anastomosis, and the patency of runoff vessels beyond the anastomosis. Patency rates of femoral-popliteal saphenous vein bypass grafts approach 90% at 1 year and 70–80% at 5 years. Five-year patency rates of infrapopliteal saphenous vein bypass grafts are 60–70%. In contrast, 5-year patency rates of infrapopliteal PTFE grafts are <30%. Lumbar sympathectomy alone or as an adjunct to aortofemoral reconstruction has fallen into disfavor.

Preoperative cardiac risk assessment may identify individuals especially likely to experience an adverse cardiac event during the perioperative period. Patients with angina, prior myocardial infarction, ventricular ectopy, heart failure, or diabetes are among those at increased risk. Noninvasive tests, such as treadmill testing (if feasible), dipyridamole or adenosine radionuclide myocardial perfusion imaging, dobutamine echocardiography, and ambulatory ischemia monitoring permit further stratification of patient risk (Chap. 240). Patients with abnormal test results require close supervision and adjunctive management with anti-ischemic medications. β-Adrenergic blockers reduce the risk of postoperative cardiovascular complications. Coronary angiography and coronary artery revascularization are not indicated in most patients undergoing peripheral vascular surgery, but cardiac catheterization should be considered in patients with unstable angina and angina refractory to medical therapy, as well as those suspected of having left main or three-vessel coronary artery disease.

FIBROMUSCULAR DYSPLASIA

This is a hyperplastic disorder affecting medium-sized and small arteries. It occurs predominantly in females and usually involves renal and carotid arteries but can affect extremity vessels, such as the iliac and subclavian arteries. The histologic classification includes intimal fibroplasia, medial dysplasia, and adventitial hyperplasia. Medial dysplasia is subdivided into medial fibroplasia, perimedial fibroplasia, and medial hyperplasia. Medial fibroplasia is the most common type and is characterized by alternating areas of thinned media and fibromuscular ridges. The internal elastic lamina is usually preserved. The iliac arteries are the limb arteries most likely to be affected by fibromuscular dysplasia. It is identified angiographically by a "string of beads" appearance caused by thickened fibromuscular ridges contiguous with thin, less-involved portions of the arterial wall. When limb vessels are involved, clinical manifestations are similar to those for atherosclerosis, including claudication and rest pain. PTA and surgical reconstruction have been beneficial in patients with debilitating symptoms or threatened limbs.

THROMBOANGIITIS OBLITERANS

Thromboangiitis obliterans (Buerger's disease) is an inflammatory occlusive vascular disorder involving small and medium-sized arteries and veins in the distal upper and lower extremities. Cerebral, visceral, and coronary vessels may be affected rarely. This disorder develops most frequently in men <40 years. The prevalence is higher in Asians and individuals of eastern European descent. While the cause of thromboangiitis obliterans is not known, there is a definite relationship to cigarette smoking in patients with this disorder.

In the initial stages of thromboangiitis obliterans, polymorphonuclear leukocytes infiltrate the walls of the small and medium-sized arteries and veins. The internal elastic lamina is preserved, and a cellular, inflammatory, thrombus develops in the vascular lumen. As the disease progresses, mononuclear cells, fibroblasts, and giant cells replace the neutrophils. Later stages are characterized by perivascular fibrosis, organized thrombus, and recanalization.

The clinical features of thromboangiitis obliterans often include a triad of claudication of the affected extremity, Raynaud's phenomenon, and migratory superficial vein thrombophlebitis. Claudication is usually confined to the calves and feet or the forearms and hands because this disorder primarily affects distal vessels. In the presence of severe digital ischemia, trophic nail changes, painful ulcerations, and gangrene may develop at the tips of the fingers or toes. The physical examination shows normal brachial and popliteal pulses but reduced or absent radial, ulnar, and/or tibial pulses. Arteriography is helpful in making the diagnosis. Smooth, tapering segmental lesions in the distal vessels are characteristic, as are collateral vessels at sites of vascular occlusion. Proximal atherosclerotic disease is usually absent. The diagnosis can be confirmed by excisional biopsy and pathologic examination of an involved vessel.

There is no specific treatment except abstention from tobacco. The prognosis is worse in individuals who continue to smoke, but results are discouraging even in those who do stop smoking. Arterial bypass of the larger vessels may be used in selected instances, as well as local debridement, depending on the symptoms and severity of ischemia. Antibiotics may be useful; anticoagulants and glucocorticoids are not helpful. If these measures fail, amputation may be required.

VASCULITIS

Other vasculitides may affect the arteries supplying the upper and lower extremities. Takayasu's arteritis and giant cell (temporal) arteritis are discussed in Chap. 319.

ACUTE ARTERIAL OCCLUSION

This results in the sudden cessation of blood flow to an extremity. The severity of ischemia and the viability of the extremity depend on the location and extent of the occlusion and the presence and subsequent development of collateral blood vessels. There are two principal causes of acute arterial occlusion: embolism and thrombus in situ.

The most common sources of arterial emboli are the heart, aorta, and large arteries. Cardiac disorders that cause thromboembolism include atrial fibrillation, both chronic and paroxysmal; acute myocardial infarction; ventricular aneurysm; cardiomyopathy; infectious and marantic endocarditis; thrombi associated with prosthetic heart valves; and atrial myxoma. Emboli to the distal vessels may also originate from proximal sites of atherosclerosis and aneurysms of the aorta and large vessels. Less frequently, an arterial occlusion results paradoxically from a venous thrombus that has entered the systemic circulation via a patent foramen ovale or other septal defect. Arterial emboli tend to lodge at vessel bifurcations because the vessel caliber decreases at these sites; in the lower extremities, emboli lodge most frequently in the femoral artery, followed by the iliac artery, aorta, and popliteal and tibioperoneal arteries.

Acute arterial thrombosis in situ occurs most frequently in atherosclerotic vessels at the site of an atherosclerotic plaque or aneurysm and in arterial bypass grafts. Trauma to an artery may also result in the formation of an acute arterial thrombus. Arterial occlusion may complicate arterial punctures and placement of catheters. Less-frequent causes include thoracic outlet compression syndrome, which causes subclavian artery occlusion, and entrapment of the popliteal artery by abnormal placement of the medial head of the gastrocnemius muscle. Polycythemia and hypercoagulable disorders (Chaps. 103 and 112) are also associated with acute arterial thrombosis.

Clinical Features The symptoms of an acute arterial occlusion depend on the location, duration, and severity of the obstruction. Often, severe pain, paresthesia, numbness, and coldness develop in the involved extremity within 1 h. Paralysis may occur with severe and persistent ischemia. Physical findings include loss of pulses distal to the occlusion, cyanosis or pallor, mottling, decreased skin temperature, muscle stiffening, loss of sensation, weakness, and/or absent deep tendon reflexes. If acute arterial occlusion occurs in the presence of an adequate collateral circulation, as is often the case in acute graft occlusion, the symptoms and findings may be less impressive. In this situation, the patient complains about an abrupt decrease in the distance walked before claudication occurs or of modest pain and paresthesia. Pallor and coolness are evident, but sensory and motor functions are generally preserved. The diagnosis of acute arterial occlusion is usually apparent from the clinical presentation. Arteriography is useful for confirming the diagnosis and demonstrating the location and extent of occlusion.

℞ ACUTE ARTERIAL OCCLUSION

Once the diagnosis is made, the patient should be anticoagulated with intravenous heparin to prevent propagation of the clot. In cases of severe ischemia of recent onset, and particularly when limb viability is jeopardized, immediate intervention to ensure reperfusion is indicated. Endovascular or surgical thromboembolectomy or arterial bypass procedures are used to restore blood flow to the ischemic extremity promptly, particularly when a large proximal vessel is occluded.

Intraarterial thrombolytic therapy with recombinant tissue plasminogen activator or urokinase is often effective when acute arterial occlusion is caused by a thrombus in an atherosclerotic vessel or arterial bypass graft. Thrombolytic therapy may also be indicated when the patient's overall condition contraindicates surgical intervention or when smaller distal vessels are occluded, thus preventing surgical access. Meticulous observation for hemorrhagic complications is required during intraarterial thrombolytic therapy. Another endovascular approach for thrombus removal is percutaneous mechanical thrombectomy using devices that employ hydrodynamic forces or rotating baskets to fragment and remove the clot. These may be used alone but are usually used in conjunction with pharmacologic thrombolysis.

FIGURE 243-1 Atheroembolism causing cyanotic discoloration and impending necrosis of the toes (blue toe syndrome).

If the limb is not in jeopardy, a more conservative approach that includes observation and administration of anticoagulants may be taken. Anticoagulation prevents recurrent embolism and reduces the likelihood of thrombus propagation; it can be initiated with intravenous heparin and followed by oral warfarin. Recommended dosages are the same as those used for deep vein thrombosis (see below). Emboli resulting from infective endocarditis, the presence of prosthetic heart valves, or atrial myxoma often require surgical intervention to remove the cause.

ATHEROEMBOLISM

Atheroembolism constitutes a subset of acute arterial occlusion. In this condition, multiple small deposits of fibrin, platelets, and cholesterol debris embolize from proximal atherosclerotic lesions or aneurysmal sites. Large protruding aortic atheromas are a source of emboli that may lead to stroke and renal insufficiency as well as limb ischemia. Atheroembolism may occur after intraarterial procedures. Since the emboli tend to lodge in the small vessels of the muscle and skin and may not occlude the large vessels, distal pulses usually remain palpable. Patients complain of acute pain and tenderness at the site of embolization. Digital vascular occlusion may result in ischemia and the "blue toe" syndrome; digital necrosis and gangrene may develop (Fig. 243-1). Localized areas of tenderness, pallor, and livedo reticularis (see below) occur at sites of emboli. Skin or muscle biopsy may demonstrate cholesterol crystals.

Ischemia resulting from atheroemboli is notoriously difficult to treat. Usually neither surgical revascularization procedures nor thrombolytic therapy is helpful because of the multiplicity, composition, and distal location of the emboli. Some evidence suggests that platelet inhibitors prevent atheroembolism. Surgical intervention to remove or bypass the atherosclerotic vessel or aneurysm that causes the recurrent atheroemboli may be necessary.

THORACIC OUTLET COMPRESSION SYNDROME

This is a symptom complex resulting from compression of the neurovascular bundle (artery, vein, or nerves) at the thoracic outlet as it courses through the neck and shoulder. Cervical ribs, abnormalities of the scalenus anticus muscle, proximity of the clavicle to the first rib, or abnormal insertion of the pectoralis minor muscle may compress the subclavian artery, subclavian vein (see below), and brachial plexus as these structures pass from the thorax to the arm. Depending on the structures affected, thoracic outlet compression syndrome may be divided into arterial, venous, and neurogenic forms. Patients with neurogenic thoracic outlet compression may develop shoulder and arm pain, weakness, and paresthesias. Patients with arterial compression may experience claudication, Raynaud's phenomenon, and even ischemic tissue loss and gangrene. Venous compression may cause thrombosis of the subclavian and axillary veins; this is often associated with effort and referred to as *Paget-Schroetter syndrome*.

APPROACH TO THE PATIENT:
Thoracic Outlet Compression Syndrome

Examination of the patient with thoracic outlet compression syndrome is often normal unless provocative maneuvers are performed. Occasionally, distal pulses are decreased or absent and digital cyanosis and ischemia may be evident. Tenderness may be present in the supraclavicular fossa. In patients with axillo-subclavian venous thrombosis, the affected extremity typically is swollen. Dilated collateral veins may be apparent around the shoulder and upper arm.

Several maneuvers that support the diagnosis of thoracic outlet compression syndrome may be used to precipitate symptoms, cause a subclavian artery bruit, and diminish arm pulses. These include the abduction and external rotation test, in which the affected arm is abducted by 90° and the shoulder is externally rotated; the scalene maneuver (extension of the neck and rotation of the head to the side of the symptoms); the costoclavicular maneuver (posterior rotation of shoulders); and the hyperabduction maneuver (raising the arm 180°). A chest x-ray will indicate the presence of cervical ribs. Duplex ultrasonography, MRA, and contrast angiography can be performed during provocative maneuvers to demonstrate thoracic outlet compression of the subclavian artery. Duplex ultrasography, magnetic resonance venography, or contrast venography can be used to diagnose axillo-subclavian vein thrombosis. Neurophysiologic tests such as the electromyogram, nerve conduction studies, and somatosensory evoked potentials may be abnormal if the brachial plexus is involved, but the diagnosis of neurogenic thoracic outlet syndrome is not necessarily excluded if these tests are normal owing to their low sensitivity.

℞ THORACIC OUTLET COMPRESSION SYNDROME

Most patients can be managed conservatively. They should be advised to avoid the positions that cause symptoms. Many patients benefit from shoulder girdle exercises. Surgical procedures such as removal of the first rib or resection of the scalenus anticus muscle are necessary occasionally for relief of symptoms or treatment of ischemia.

ARTERIOVENOUS FISTULA

Abnormal communications between an artery and a vein, bypassing the capillary bed, may be congenital or acquired. Congenital arteriovenous fistulas are the result of persistent embryonic vessels that fail to differentiate into arteries and veins; they may be associated with birthmarks, can be located in almost any organ of the body, and frequently occur in the extremities. Acquired arteriovenous fistulas are either created to provide vascular access for hemodialysis or occur as a result of a penetrating injury such as a gunshot or knife wound or as complications of arterial catheterization or surgical dissection. An infrequent cause of arteriovenous fistula is rupture of an arterial aneurysm into a vein.

The clinical features depend on the location and size of the fistula. Frequently, a pulsatile mass is palpable, and a thrill and bruit lasting throughout systole and diastole are present over the fistula. With longstanding fistulas, clinical manifestations of chronic venous insufficiency, including peripheral edema; large, tortuous varicose veins; and stasis pigmentation become apparent because of the high venous pressure. Evidence of ischemia may occur in the distal portion of the extremity. Skin temperature is higher over the arteriovenous fistula. Large arteriovenous fistulas may result in an increased cardiac output with consequent cardiomegaly and high-output heart failure (Chap. 227).

Diagnosis The diagnosis is often evident from the physical examination. Compression of a large arteriovenous fistula may cause reflex slowing of the heart rate (Nicoladoni-Branham sign). Duplex ultrasonography may detect an arteriovenous fistula, especially that which affects the femoral artery and vein at the site of catheter access. Computed tomographic and conventional angiography can confirm the diagnosis and are useful in demonstrating the site and size of the arteriovenous fistula.

℞ ARTERIOVENOUS FISTULA

Management of arteriovenous fistulas may involve surgery, radiotherapy, or embolization. Congenital arteriovenous fistulas are often difficult to treat because the communications may be numerous and extensive, and new ones frequently develop after ligation of the most obvious ones. Many of these lesions are best treated conservatively using elastic support hose to reduce the consequences of venous hypertension. Occasionally, embolization with autologous material, such as fat or muscle, or with hemostatic agents, such as gelatin sponges or silicon spheres, is used to obliterate the fistula. Acquired arteriovenous fistulas are usually amenable to surgical treatment that involves division or excision of the fistula. Occasionally, autogenous or synthetic grafting is necessary to reestablish continuity of the artery and vein.

RAYNAUD'S PHENOMENON

Raynaud's phenomenon is characterized by episodic digital ischemia, manifested clinically by the sequential development of digital blanching, cyanosis, and rubor of the fingers or toes following cold exposure and subsequent rewarming. Emotional stress may also precipitate Raynaud's phenomenon. The color changes are usually well demarcated and are confined to the fingers or toes. Typically, one or more digits will appear white when the patient is exposed to a cold environment or touches a cold object. The blanching, or pallor, represents the ischemic phase of the phenomenon and results from vasospasm of digital arteries. During the ischemic phase, capillaries and venules dilate, and cyanosis results from the deoxygenated blood that is present in these vessels. A sensation of cold or numbness or paresthesia of the digits often accompanies the phases of pallor and cyanosis.

With rewarming, the digital vasospasm resolves, and blood flow into the dilated arterioles and capillaries increases dramatically. This "reactive hyperemia" imparts a bright red color to the digits. In addition to rubor and warmth, patients often experience a throbbing, painful sensation during the hyperemic phase. Although the triphasic color response is typical of Raynaud's phenomenon, some patients may develop only pallor and cyanosis; others may experience only cyanosis.

Pathophysiology   Raynaud originally proposed that cold-induced episodic digital ischemia was secondary to exaggerated reflex sympathetic vasoconstriction. This theory is supported by the fact that α-adrenergic blocking drugs as well as sympathectomy decrease the frequency and severity of Raynaud's phenomenon in some patients. An alternative hypothesis is that the digital vascular responsiveness to cold or to normal sympathetic stimuli is enhanced. It is also possible that normal reflex sympathetic vasoconstriction is superimposed on local digital vascular disease or that there is enhanced adrenergic neuroeffector activity.

Raynaud's phenomenon is broadly separated into two categories: the idiopathic variety, termed *Raynaud's disease*, and the secondary variety, which is associated with other disease states or known causes of vasospasm (Table 243-1).

Raynaud's Disease   This appellation is applied when the secondary causes of Raynaud's phenomenon have been excluded. Over 50% of patients with Raynaud's phenomenon have Raynaud's disease. Women are affected about five times more often than men, and the age of presentation is usually between 20 and 40 years. The fingers are involved more frequently than the toes. Initial episodes may involve only one or two fingertips, but subsequent attacks may involve the entire finger and may include all the fingers. The toes are affected in 40% of patients. Although vasospasm of the toes usually occurs in patients with symptoms in the fingers, it may happen alone. Rarely, the earlobes, the tip of the nose, and the penis are involved. Raynaud's phenomenon occurs frequently in patients who also have migraine headaches or variant angina. These associations suggest that there may be a common predisposing cause for the vasospasm.

TABLE 243-1   CLASSIFICATION OF RAYNAUD'S PHENOMENON

Primary or idiopathic Raynaud's phenomenon: Raynaud's disease
Secondary Raynaud's phenomenon
   Collagen vascular diseases: scleroderma, systemic lupus erythematosus, rheumatoid arthritis, dermatomyositis, polymyositis
   Arterial occlusive diseases: atherosclerosis of the extremities, thromboangiitis obliterans, acute arterial occlusion, thoracic outlet syndrome
   Pulmonary hypertension
   Neurologic disorders: intervertebral disk disease, syringomyelia, spinal cord tumors, stroke, poliomyelitis, carpal tunnel syndrome
   Blood dyscrasias: cold agglutinins, cryoglobulinemia, cryofibrinogenemia, myeloproliferative disorders, Waldenström's macroglobulinemia
   Trauma: vibration injury, hammer hand syndrome, electric shock, cold injury, typing, piano playing
   Drugs: ergot derivatives, methysergide, β-adrenergic receptor blockers, bleomycin, vinblastine, cisplatin

Results of physical examination are often entirely normal; the radial, ulnar, and pedal pulses are normal. The fingers and toes may be cool between attacks and may perspire excessively. Thickening and tightening of the digital subcutaneous tissue (*sclerodactyly*) develop in 10% of patients. Angiography of the digits for diagnostic purposes is not indicated.

In general, patients with Raynaud's disease appear to have the milder forms of Raynaud's phenomenon. Fewer than 1% of these patients lose a part of a digit. After the diagnosis is made, the disease improves spontaneously in approximately 15% of patients and progresses in about 30%.

Secondary Causes of Raynaud's Phenomenon   Raynaud's phenomenon occurs in 80–90% of patients with systemic sclerosis (scleroderma) and is the presenting symptom in 30% (Chap. 316). It may be the only symptom of scleroderma for many years. Abnormalities of the digital vessels may contribute to the development of Raynaud's phenomenon in this disorder. Ischemic fingertip ulcers may develop and progress to gangrene and autoamputation. About 20% of patients with systemic lupus erythematosus (SLE) have Raynaud's phenomenon (Chap. 313). Occasionally, persistent digital ischemia develops and may result in ulcers or gangrene. In most severe cases, the small vessels are occluded by a proliferative endarteritis. Raynaud's phenomenon occurs in about 30% of patients with dermatomyositis or polymyositis (Chap. 383). It frequently develops in patients with rheumatoid arthritis and may be related to the intimal proliferation that occurs in the digital arteries.

Atherosclerosis of the extremities is a frequent cause of Raynaud's phenomenon in men >50 years. Thromboangiitis obliterans is an uncommon cause of Raynaud's phenomenon but should be considered in young men, particularly those who are cigarette smokers. The development of cold-induced pallor in these disorders may be confined to one or two digits of the involved extremity. Occasionally, Raynaud's phenomenon may follow acute occlusion of large and medium-sized arteries by a thrombus or embolus. Embolization of atheroembolic debris may cause digital ischemia. The latter situation often involves one or two digits and should not be confused with Raynaud's phenomenon. In patients with thoracic outlet compression syndrome, Raynaud's phenomenon may result from diminished intravascular pressure, stimulation of sympathetic fibers in the brachial plexus, or a combination of both. Raynaud's phenomenon occurs in patients with primary pulmonary hypertension (Chap. 244); this is more than coincidental and may reflect a neurohumoral abnormality that affects both the pulmonary and digital circulations.

A variety of blood dyscrasias may be associated with Raynaud's phenomenon. Cold-induced precipitation of plasma proteins, hyperviscosity, and aggregation of red cells and platelets may occur in patients with cold agglutinins, cryoglobulinemia, or cryofibrinogenemia. Hyperviscosity syndromes that accompany myeloproliferative disorders and Waldenström's macroglobulinemia should also be considered in the initial evaluation of patients with Raynaud's phenomenon.

Raynaud's phenomenon occurs often in patients whose vocations require the use of vibrating hand tools, such as chain saws or jackhammers.

The frequency of Raynaud's phenomenon also seems to be increased in pianists and keyboard operators. Electric shock injury to the hands or frostbite may lead to the later development of Raynaud's phenomenon.

Several drugs have been causally implicated in Raynaud's phenomenon. These include ergot preparations; methysergide; β-adrenergic receptor antagonists; and the chemotherapeutic agents bleomycin, vinblastine, and cisplatin.

℞ RAYNAUD'S PHENOMENON

Most patients with Raynaud's phenomenon experience only mild and infrequent episodes. These patients need reassurance and should be instructed to dress warmly and avoid unnecessary cold exposure. In addition to gloves and mittens, patients should protect the trunk, head, and feet with warm clothing to prevent cold-induced reflex vasoconstriction. Tobacco use is contraindicated.

Drug treatment should be reserved for the severe cases. Dihydropyridine calcium channel antagonists, such as nifedipine, isradipine, felodipine, and amlodipine, decrease the frequency and severity of Raynaud's phenomenon. Diltiazem may be considered but is less effective. The postsynaptic α_1-adrenergic antagonist prazosin has been used with favorable responses; doxazosin and terazosin may also be effective. Other sympatholytic agents, such as methyldopa, guanethidine, and phenoxybenzamine, may be useful in some patients, as may topical glyceryl trinitrate. Digital sympathectomy is helpful in some patients who are unresponsive to medical therapy.

ACROCYANOSIS

In this condition, there is arterial vasoconstriction and secondary dilation of the capillaries and venules with resulting persistent cyanosis of the hands and, less frequently, the feet. Cyanosis may be intensified by exposure to a cold environment. Acrocyanosis may be categorized as primary or secondary to an underlying condition. In primary acrocyanosis, women are affected much more frequently than men, and the age of onset is usually <30 years. Generally, patients are asymptomatic but seek medical attention because of the discoloration. The prognosis is favorable, and pain, ulcers, and gangrene do not occur. Examination reveals normal pulses, peripheral cyanosis, and moist palms. Trophic skin changes and ulcerations do *not* occur. The disorder can be distinguished from Raynaud's phenomenon because it is persistent and not episodic, the discoloration extends proximally from the digits, and blanching does not occur. Ischemia secondary to arterial occlusive disease can usually be excluded by the presence of normal pulses. Central cyanosis and decreased arterial oxygen saturation are not present. Patients should be reassured and advised to dress warmly and avoid cold exposure. Pharmacologic intervention is not indicated.

Secondary acrocyanosis may result from hypoxemia, connective tissue diseases, atheroembolism, antiphospholipid antibodies, cold agglutinins, or cryoglobulins, and is associated with anorexia nervosa and orthostatic tachycardia syndrome. Treatment should be directed at the underlying disorder.

LIVEDO RETICULARIS

In this condition, localized areas of the extremities develop a mottled or rete (net-like) appearance of reddish to blue discoloration. The mottled appearance may be more prominent following cold exposure. There are primary and secondary forms of livedo reticularis. The primary, or idiopathic, form of this disorder may be benign or associated with ulcerations. The benign form occurs more frequently in women than in men, and the most common age of onset is in the third decade. Patients with the benign form are usually asymptomatic and seek attention for cosmetic reasons. These patients should be reassured and advised to avoid cold environments. No drug treatment is indicated. Primary livedo reticularis with ulceration is also called *atrophie blanche en plaque*. The ulcers are painful and may take months to heal. Secondary livedo reticularis can occur with atheroembolism (see above), SLE and other vasculitides, anticardiolipin antibodies, hyperviscosity, cryoglobulinemia, and Sneddon's syndrome (ischemic stroke and livedo reticularis). Rarely, skin ulcerations develop.

PERNIO (CHILBLAINS)

This is a vasculitic disorder associated with exposure to cold; acute forms have been described. Raised erythematous lesions develop on the lower part of the legs and feet in cold weather. These are associated with pruritus and a burning sensation, and they may blister and ulcerate. Pathologic examination demonstrates angiitis characterized by intimal proliferation and perivascular infiltration of mononuclear and polymorphonuclear leukocytes. Giant cells may be present in the subcutaneous tissue. Patients should avoid exposure to cold, and ulcers should be kept clean and protected with sterile dressings. Sympatholytic drugs may be effective in some patients.

ERYTHROMELALGIA

This disorder is characterized by burning pain and erythema of the extremities. The feet are involved more frequently than the hands, and males are affected more frequently than females. Erythromelalgia may occur at any age but is most common in middle age. It may be primary (also termed erythermalgia) or secondary. The most common causes of secondary erythromelalgia are myeloproliferative disorders such as polycythemia vera and essential thrombocytosis. Less-common causes include drugs, such as calcium channel blockers, bromocriptine, and pergolide; neuropathies; connective tissue diseases, such as systemic lupus erythematosus; and paraneoplastic syndromes. Patients complain of burning in the extremities that is precipitated by exposure to a warm environment and aggravated by a dependent position. The symptoms are relieved by exposing the affected area to cool air or water or by elevation. Erythromelalgia can be distinguished from ischemia secondary to peripheral arterial disorders and peripheral neuropathy because the peripheral pulses are present and the neurologic examination is normal. There is no specific treatment; aspirin may produce relief in patients with erythromelalgia secondary to myeloproliferative disease. Treatment of associated disorders in secondary erythromelalgia may be helpful.

FROSTBITE

In this condition, tissue damage results from severe environmental cold exposure or from direct contact with a very cold object. Tissue injury results from both freezing and vasoconstriction. Frostbite usually affects the distal aspects of the extremities or exposed parts of the face, such as the ears, nose, chin, and cheeks. Superficial frostbite involves the skin and subcutaneous tissue. Patients experience pain or paresthesia, and the skin appears white and waxy. After rewarming, there is cyanosis and erythema, wheal-and-flare formation, edema, and superficial blisters. Deep frostbite involves muscle, nerves, and deeper blood vessels. It may result in edema of the hand or foot, vesicles and bullae, tissue necrosis, and gangrene.

Initial treatment is rewarming, performed in an environment where reexposure to freezing conditions will not occur. Rewarming is accomplished by immersion of the affected part in a water bath at temperatures of 40°–44°C (104°–111°F). Massage, application of ice water, and extreme heat are contraindicated. The injured area should be cleansed with soap or antiseptic and sterile dressings applied. Analgesics are often required during rewarming. Antibiotics are used if there is evidence of infection. The efficacy of sympathetic blocking drugs is not established. Following recovery, the affected extremity may exhibit increased sensitivity to cold.

DISORDERS OF THE VEINS AND LYMPHATICS

VENOUS DISORDERS

Veins in the extremities can be broadly classified as either superficial or deep. In the lower extremity, the superficial venous system includes the greater and lesser saphenous veins and their tributaries. The deep veins of the leg accompany the major arteries. Perforating veins connect the superficial and deep systems at multiple locations. Bicuspid valves are present throughout the venous system to direct the flow of venous blood centrally.

Venous Thrombosis The presence of thrombus within a superficial or deep vein and the accompanying inflammatory response in the vessel wall is termed *venous thrombosis* or *thrombophlebitis*. Initially the thrombus is composed principally of platelets and fibrin. Red cells become interspersed with fibrin, and the thrombus tends to propagate in the direction of blood flow. The inflammatory response in the vessel wall may be minimal or characterized by granulocyte infiltration, loss of endothelium, and edema.

The factors that predispose to venous thrombosis were initially described by Virchow in 1856 and include stasis, vascular damage, and hypercoagulability. Accordingly, a variety of clinical situations are associated with increased risk of venous thrombosis (Table 243-2). Venous thrombosis may occur in >50% of patients having orthopedic surgical procedures, particularly those involving the hip or knee, and in 10–40% of patients who undergo abdominal or thoracic operations. The prevalence of venous thrombosis is particularly high in patients with cancer of the pancreas, lungs, genitourinary tract, stomach, and breast. Approximately 10–20% of patients with idiopathic deep vein thrombosis have or develop clinically overt cancer; there is no consensus on whether these individuals should be subjected to intensive diagnostic workup to search for occult malignancy.

The risk of thrombosis is increased following trauma, such as fractures of the spine, pelvis, femur, and tibia. Immobilization, regardless of the underlying disease, is a major predisposing cause of venous thrombosis. This fact may account for the relatively high incidence in patients with acute myocardial infarction or congestive heart failure. The incidence of venous thrombosis is increased during pregnancy, particularly in the third trimester and in the first month postpartum, and in individuals who use oral contraceptives, postmenopausal hormone replacement therapy, or selective estrogen receptor modulators. A variety of clinical disorders that produce systemic hypercoagulability, including resistance to activated protein C (factor V Leiden); prothrombin G20210A gene mutation; antithrombin III, protein C, and protein S deficiencies; antiphospholipid syndrome; hyperhomocysteinemia; SLE; myeloproliferative diseases; dysfibrinogenemia; and disseminated intravascular coagulation, are associated with venous thrombosis. Venulitis occurring in thromboangiitis obliterans, Behçet's syndrome, and homocystinuria may also cause venous thrombosis.

Deep Venous Thrombosis   See Chapter 256.

Superficial Vein Thrombosis   Thrombosis of the greater or lesser saphenous veins or their tributaries—i.e., superficial vein thrombosis—does not result in pulmonary embolism. It is associated with intravenous catheters and infusions, occurs in varicose veins, and may develop in association with deep venous thrombosis (DVT). Migrating superficial vein thrombosis is often a marker for a carcinoma and

TABLE 243-2   CONDITIONS ASSOCIATED WITH AN INCREASED RISK FOR DEVELOPMENT OF VENOUS THROMBOSIS

Surgery
   Orthopedic, thoracic, abdominal, and genitourinary procedures
Neoplasms
   Pancreas, lung, ovary, testes, urinary tract, breast, stomach
Trauma
   Fractures of spine, pelvis, femur, or tibia; spinal cord injuries
Immobilization
   Acute myocardial infarction, congestive heart failure, stroke, postoperative convalescence
Pregnancy
Estrogen
   For replacement or contraception;
      Selective estrogen replacement modulators
Hypercoagulable states
   Resistance to activated protein C; prothrombin or 20210 A gene mutation deficiencies of antithrombin III, protein C, or protein S; antiphospholipid antibodies; myeloproliferative diseases; dysfibrinogenemia; disseminated intravascular coagulation
Venulitis
   Thromboangiitis obliterans, Behçet's disease, homocysteinuria
Previous deep vein thrombosis

may also occur in patients with vasculitides, such as thromboangiitis obliterans. The clinical features of superficial vein thrombosis are easily distinguished from those of DVT. Patients complain of pain localized to the site of the thrombus. Examination reveals a reddened, warm, and tender cord extending along a superficial vein. The surrounding area may be red and edematous.

℞ SUPERFICIAL VEIN THROMBOSIS

Treatment is primarily supportive. Initially, patients can be placed at bed rest with leg elevation and application of warm compresses. Nonsteroidal anti-inflammatory drugs may provide analgesia but may also obscure clinical evidence of thrombus propagation. If a thrombosis of the greater saphenous vein develops in the thigh and extends toward the saphenofemoral vein junction, it is reasonable to consider anticoagulant therapy to prevent extension of the thrombus into the deep system and a possible pulmonary embolism.

Varicose Veins   Varicose veins are dilated, tortuous superficial veins that result from defective structure and function of the valves of the saphenous veins, from intrinsic weakness of the vein wall, from high intraluminal pressure, or, rarely, from arteriovenous fistulas. Varicose veins can be categorized as primary or secondary. Primary varicose veins originate in the superficial system and occur two to three times as frequently in women as in men. Approximately half of patients have a family history of varicose veins. Secondary varicose veins result from deep venous insufficiency and incompetent perforating veins or from deep venous occlusion causing enlargement of superficial veins that are serving as collaterals.

Patients with venous varicosities are often concerned about the cosmetic appearance of their legs. Symptoms consist of a dull ache or pressure sensation in the legs after prolonged standing; it is relieved with leg elevation. The legs feel heavy, and mild ankle edema develops occasionally. Extensive venous varicosities may cause skin ulcerations near the ankle. Superficial venous thrombosis may be a recurring problem, and, rarely, a varicosity ruptures and bleeds. Visual inspection of the legs in the dependent position usually confirms the presence of varicose veins.

Varicose veins can usually be treated with conservative measures. Symptoms often decrease when the legs are elevated periodically, when prolonged standing is avoided, and when elastic support hose are worn. External compression stockings provide a counterbalance to the hydrostatic pressure in the veins. Ablative procedures, including sclerotherapy, endovenous radiofrequency or laser ablation, and surgery may be considered to treat varicose veins in selected patients who have persistent symptoms, suffer recurrent superficial vein thrombosis, and/or develop skin ulceration. Ablative therapy may also be indicated for cosmetic reasons. Small, symptomatic varicose veins can be treated with sclerotherapy, in which a sclerosing solution is injected into the involved varicose vein and a compression bandage is applied. Percutaneous, endovenous delivery of radiofrequency or laser energy can be used to treat incompetent greater saphenous veins. Surgical therapy usually involves ligation and stripping of the greater and lesser saphenous veins.

Chronic Venous Insufficiency   Chronic venous insufficiency may result from DVT and/or valvular incompetence. Following DVT, the delicate valve leaflets become thickened and contracted so that they cannot prevent retrograde flow of blood; the vein becomes rigid and thick-walled. Although most veins recanalize after an episode of thrombosis, the large proximal veins may remain occluded. Secondary incompetence develops in distal valves because high pressures distend the vein and separate the leaflets. Primary deep venous valvular dysfunction may also occur without previous thrombosis. Patients with venous insufficiency often complain of a dull ache in the leg that worsens with prolonged standing and resolves with leg elevation. Examination demonstrates increased leg circumference, edema, and superficial varicose veins. Erythema, dermatitis, and hyperpigmentation develop along the distal aspect of the leg, and skin ulceration may occur near the me-

TABLE 243-3	CAUSES OF LYMPHEDEMA
Primary	Secondary
Congenital (includes Milroy's disease)	Recurrent lymphangitis
	Filariasis
Lymphedema praecox (includes Meige's disease)	Tuberculosis
	Neoplasm
Lymphedema tarda	Surgery
	Radiation therapy

dial and lateral malleoli. Cellulitis may be a recurring problem. Patients should be advised to avoid prolonged standing or sitting; frequent leg elevation is helpful. Graduated compression stockings should be worn during the day. These efforts should be intensified if skin ulcers develop. Ulcers should be treated with applications of wet to dry dressings or occlusive hydrocolloid dressings. Commercially available compressive dressings comprising paste with zinc oxide, calamine, glycerin, and gelatin may be applied and should be changed weekly until healing occurs. Recurrent ulceration and severe edema may be treated by surgical interruption of incompetent communicating veins. Subfascial endoscopic perforator surgery (SEPS) is a minimally invasive technique to interrupt incompetent communicating veins. Rarely, surgical valvuloplasty and bypass of venous occlusions are employed.

LYMPHATIC DISORDERS

Lymphatic capillaries are blind-ended tubes formed by a single layer of endothelial cells. The absent or widely fenestrated basement membrane of lymphatic capillaries allows access to interstitial proteins and particles. Lymphatic capillaries merge to form larger vessels that contain smooth muscle and are capable of vasomotion. Small and medium-sized lymphatic vessels empty into progressively larger channels, most of which drain into the thoracic duct. The lymphatic circulation is involved in the absorption of interstitial fluid and in the response to infection.

Lymphedema Lymphedema may be categorized as primary or secondary (Table 243-3). The prevalence of primary lymphedema is approximately 1 per 10,000 individuals. Primary lymphedema may be secondary to agenesis, hypoplasia, or obstruction of the lymphatic vessels. It may be associated with Turner's syndrome, Klinefelter's syndrome, Noonan's syndrome, yellow nail syndrome, intestinal lymphangiectasia syndrome, and lymphangiomyomatosis. Women are affected more frequently than men. There are three clinical subtypes: congenital lymphedema, which appears shortly after birth; lymphedema praecox, which has its onset at the time of puberty; and lymphedema tarda, which usually begins after age 35. Familial forms of congenital lymphedema (Milroy's disease) and lymphedema praecox (Meige's disease) may be inherited in an autosomal dominant manner with variable penetrance; autosomal or sex-linked recessive forms are less common.

Secondary lymphedema is an acquired condition resulting from damage to or obstruction of previously normal lymphatic channels (Table 243-3). Recurrent episodes of bacterial lymphangitis, usually caused by streptococci, are a very common cause of lymphedema. The most common cause of secondary lymphedema worldwide is filariasis (Chap. 211). Tumors, such as prostate cancer and lymphoma, can also obstruct lymphatic vessels. Both surgery and radiation therapy for breast carcinoma may cause lymphedema of the upper extremity. Less-common causes include tuberculosis, contact dermatitis, lymphogranuloma venereum, rheumatoid arthritis, pregnancy, and self-induced or factitious lymphedema following application of tourniquets.

Lymphedema is generally a painless condition, but patients may experience a chronic dull, heavy sensation in the leg, and most often they are concerned about the appearance of the leg. Lymphedema of the lower extremity, initially involving the foot, gradually progresses up the leg so that the entire limb becomes edematous. In the early stages, the edema is soft and pits easily with pressure. In the chronic stages, the limb has a woody texture, and the tissues become indurated and fibrotic. At this point the edema may no longer be pitting. The limb loses its normal contour, and the toes appear square. Lymphedema should be distinguished from other disorders that cause unilateral leg swelling, such as DVT and chronic venous insufficiency. In the latter condition, the edema is softer, and there is often evidence of a stasis dermatitis, hyperpigmentation, and superficial venous varicosities.

The evaluation of patients with lymphedema should include diagnostic studies to clarify the cause. Abdominal and pelvic ultrasound and CT can be used to detect obstructing lesions such as neoplasms. MRI may reveal edema in the epifascial compartment and identify lymph nodes and enlarged lymphatic channels. Lymphoscintigraphy and lymphangiography are rarely indicated, but either can be used to confirm the diagnosis or to differentiate primary from secondary lymphedema. Lymphoscintigraphy involves the injection of radioactively labeled technetium-containing colloid into the distal subcutaneous tissue of the affected extremity. In lymphangiography, contrast material is injected into a distal lymphatic vessel that has been isolated and cannulated. In primary lymphedema, lymphatic channels are absent, hypoplastic, or ectatic. In secondary lymphedema, lymphatic channels are usually dilated, and it may be possible to determine the level of obstruction.

℞ LYMPHEDEMA

Patients with lymphedema of the lower extremities must be instructed to take meticulous care of their feet to prevent recurrent lymphangitis. Skin hygiene is important, and emollients can be used to prevent drying. Prophylactic antibiotics are often helpful, and fungal infection should be treated aggressively. Patients should be encouraged to participate in physical activity; frequent leg elevation can reduce the amount of edema. Physical therapy, including massage to facilitate lymphatic drainage, may be helpful. Patients can be fitted with graduated compression hose to reduce the amount of lymphedema that develops with upright posture. Occasionally, intermittent pneumatic compression devices can be applied at home to facilitate reduction of the edema. Diuretics are contraindicated and may cause depletion of intravascular volume and metabolic abnormalities. Microsurgical lymphatico-venous anastomotic procedures have been performed to rechannel lymph flow from obstructed lymphatic vessels into the venous system.

FURTHER READINGS

CREAGER MA et al (eds): *Vascular Medicine*. Philadelphia, Saunders Elsevier, 2006

FAXON DP et al: Atherosclerotic Vascular Disease Conference: Executive summary: Atherosclerotic Vascular Disease Conference proceeding for healthcare professionals from a special writing group of the American Heart Association. Circulation 109:2595, 2004

GOLOMB BA et al: Peripheral arterial disease: Morbidity and mortality implications. Circulation 114:688, 2006

HANKEY GJ et al: Medical treatment of peripheral arterial disease. JAMA 295:547, 2006

HIRSCH AT et al: ACC/AHA 2005 guidelines for the management of patients with peripheral arterial disease (lower extremity, renal, mesenteric, and abdominal aortic). J Am Coll Cardiol 47:1239, 2006

MCDERMOTT MM et al: The ankle brachial index is associated with leg function and physical activity: The Walking and Leg Circulation Study. Ann Intern Med 136:873, 2002

OLIN JW: Thromboangiitis obliterans (Buerger's disease). N Engl J Med 343:864, 2000

ROCKSON SG: Lymphedema. Current Treat Options Cardiovasc Med 8:129, 2006

WHITE C: Clinical practice. Intermittent claudication. N Engl J Med 356:1241, 2007

WIGLEY FM: Clinical practice. Raynaud's phenomenon. N Engl J Med 347:1001, 2002

244 Pulmonary Hypertension
Stuart Rich

Pulmonary hypertension, an abnormal elevation in pulmonary artery pressure, may be the result of left heart failure, pulmonary parenchymal or vascular disease, thromboembolism, or a combination of these factors. Whether the pulmonary hypertension arises from cardiac, pulmonary, or intrinsic vascular disease, it generally is a feature of advanced disease. Because the causes of pulmonary hypertension are so diverse, it is essential that the etiology underlying the pulmonary hypertension be clearly determined before embarking on treatment.

Cor pulmonale (Chap. 227) is a term used to indicate right ventricular (RV) enlargement secondary to any underlying cardiac or pulmonary disease. Pulmonary hypertension is the most common cause of cor pulmonale. Advanced cor pulmonale is associated with the development of RV failure.

PATHOPHYSIOLOGY

The right ventricle responds to an increase in resistance within the pulmonary circulation by increasing RV systolic pressure as necessary to preserve cardiac output. Over time, chronic changes occur in the pulmonary circulation that result in progressive remodeling of the vasculature, which can sustain or promote pulmonary hypertension even if the initiating factor is removed.

The ability of the RV to adapt to increased vascular resistance is influenced by several factors, including age and the rapidity of the development of pulmonary hypertension. For example, a large acute pulmonary thromboembolism can result in RV failure and shock, whereas chronic thromboembolic disease of equal severity may result in only mild exercise intolerance. Coexisting hypoxemia can impair the ability of the ventricle to compensate. Several studies support the concept that RV failure occurs in pulmonary hypertension when the RV myocardium becomes ischemic due to excessive demands and inadequate right ventricular coronary blood flow to the RV. The onset of clinical RV failure, usually manifest by peripheral edema, is associated with a poor outcome.

DIAGNOSIS

The most common symptom attributable to pulmonary hypertension is exertional dyspnea. Other common symptoms are fatigue, angina pectoris that may represent RV ischemia, syncope, near syncope, and peripheral edema.

The physical examination typically reveals increased jugular venous pressure, a reduced carotid pulse, and a palpable RV impulse. Most patients have an increased pulmonic component of the second heart sound, a right-sided fourth heart sound, and tricuspid regurgitation (Chap. 220). Peripheral cyanosis and/or edema tend to occur in later stages of the disease.

Laboratory Findings (Fig. 244-1) The chest x-ray generally shows enlarged central pulmonary arteries. The lung fields may or may not reveal other pathology. The electrocardiogram usually shows right axis deviation and RV hypertrophy. The echocardiogram commonly demonstrates RV and right atrial enlargement, a reduction in left ventricular (LV) cavity size, and a tricuspid regurgitant jet that can be used to estimate RV systolic pressure. Pulmonary function tests are helpful in documenting underlying obstructive airways disease, whereas high-resolution chest CT is preferred to diagnose restrictive lung disease. Hypoxemia and an abnormal diffusing capacity for carbon monoxide are common features of pulmonary hypertension of many causes. A perfusion lung scan is almost always abnormal in patients with thromboembolic pulmonary hypertension (Chap. 256). However, diffuse defects of a nonsegmental nature can often be seen in long-standing pulmonary hypertension in the absence of thromboemboli. Laboratory tests should include antinuclear antibody and HIV testing. Because of the high frequency of thyroid abnormalities in patients with idio-

pathic pulmonary hypertension, it is recommended that the thyroid-stimulating hormone level be determined periodically.

Cardiac Catheterization This procedure is mandatory for accurate measurement of pulmonary artery pressure, cardiac output, and LV filling pressure, as well as for exclusion of an underlying cardiac shunt. Care should be taken to measure pressures only at end expiration. It is also recommended that patients with pulmonary arterial hypertension undergo drug testing with a short-acting pulmonary vasodilator at the time of cardiac catheterization to determine the extent of pulmonary vasodilator reactivity (Fig. 244-2). Inhaled nitric oxide, intravenous adenosine, and intravenous epoprostenol appear to have comparable effects in reducing pulmonary artery pressure acutely. Nitric oxide is administered via inhalation in 10–20 parts per million. Adenosine is given in doses of 50 μg/kg per min and increased every 2 min until side effects develop. Epoprostenol is given in doses of 2 ng/kg per min and increased every 30 min until side effects develop. Patients who respond can often be treated with calcium channel blockers and have a more favorable prognosis.

PULMONARY ARTERIAL HYPERTENSION

There are many causes of pulmonary arterial hypertension (PAH) (Table 244-1). Patients with PAH share a common histopathology characterized by medial hypertrophy, eccentric and concentric intimal fibrosis, recanalized thrombi appearing as fibrous webs, and plexiform lesions.

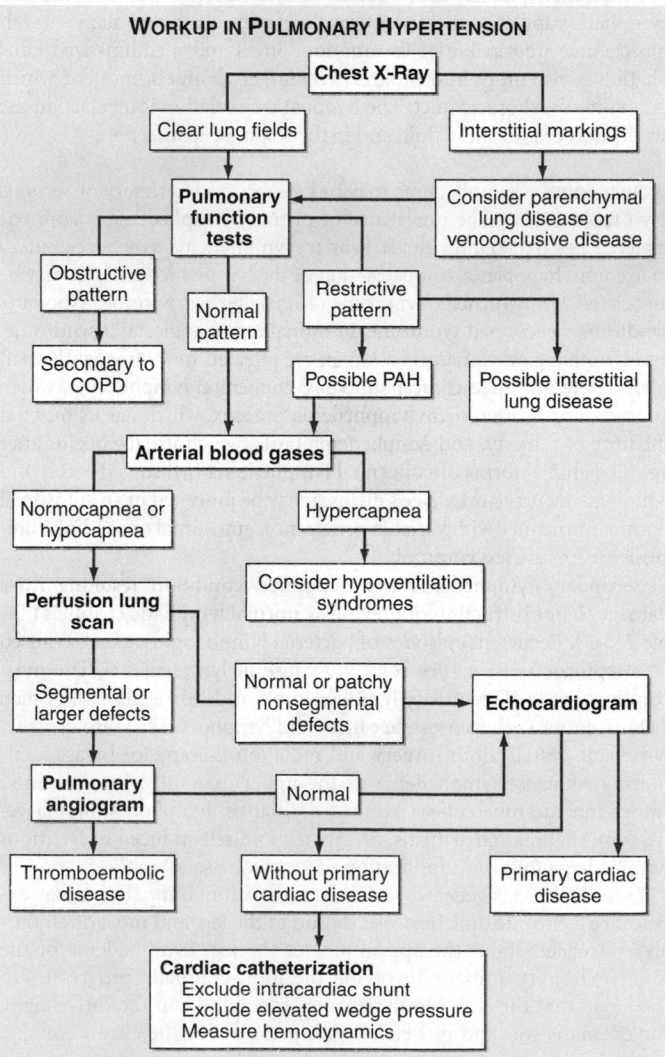

FIGURE 244-1 An algorithm for the workup of a patient with unexplained pulmonary hypertension. *(Adapted with permission from Rich.)*

ALGORITHM FOR DRUG TREATMENT SELECTION

FIGURE 244-2 An algorithm for the selection of optimal drug treatment of a patient with pulmonary arterial hypertension. A marked reduction in pulmonary artery pressure from acute vasodilator testing is defined as a fall in mean pulmonary artery pressure (MPAP) ≥ 10 mmHg and a final MPAP that is <40 mmHg. (*Adapted with permission from Rich.*)

PATHOBIOLOGY

Abnormalities in molecular pathways regulating the pulmonary vascular endothelial and smooth-muscle cells have been described as underlying PAH. These include inhibition of the voltage-regulated potassium channel, mutations in the bone morphogenetic protein-2 receptor, increased serotonin uptake in the smooth-muscle cells, increased angiopoietin expression in the smooth-muscle cells, and excessive thrombin deposition related to a procoagulant state. As a result there appears to be loss of apoptosis of the smooth-muscle cells allowing their proliferation, and the emergence of apoptosis-resistant endothelial cells which can obliterate the vascular lumen.

IDIOPATHIC PULMONARY ARTERIAL HYPERTENSION

Idiopathic pulmonary arterial hypertension (IPAH), formerly referred to as primary pulmonary hypertension is uncommon, with an estimated incidence of two cases per million. There is a strong female predominance, with most patients presenting in the fourth and fifth decades, although the age range is from infancy to >60 years.

Familial IPAH accounts for up to 20% of cases of IPAH and is characterized by autosomal dominant inheritance, variable age of onset, and incomplete penetrance. The clinical and pathologic features of familial and sporadic IPAH are identical. Heterozygous germline mutations that involve the gene coding the type II bone morphogenetic protein receptor (BMPR II), a member of the transforming growth factor (TGF)β superfamily, appear to account for most cases of familial IPAH. The TGF-β superfamily comprise multifunctional proteins that initiate diverse cellular responses by binding to and activating serine/threonine kinase receptors. The low gene penetrance suggests that other risk factors or abnormalities are necessary to manifest clinical disease. Germline mutations in the activin-like kinase gene and endoglin gene, which have been linked to hereditary hemorrhagic telangiectasia (HHT) have been described to coexist in some patients with familial IPAH (Fig. 244-3).

NATURAL HISTORY

The natural history of IPAH is uncertain, and because the predominant symptom is dyspnea, which can have an insidious onset, the dis-

ease is typically diagnosed late in its course. Prior to current therapies, a mean survival of 2–3 years from the time of diagnosis was reported. Functional class remains a strong predictor of survival, with patients who are in New York Heart Association (NYHA) functional class IV having a mean survival of <6 months. The cause of death is usually RV failure, which is manifest by progressive hypoxemia, tachycardia, hypotension, and edema.

℞ PULMONARY ARTERIAL HYPERTENSION

Pulmonary arterial hypertension (PAH) refers to a variety of diseases, which includes idiopathic (I)PAH, as noted in Table 244-1. The regulatory authorities have approved several treatments for PAH (reviewed below) without making a distinction between the different types. However, physicians need to be mindful that the efficacy and side effects of these drugs might not be the same in all types of PAH (**Fig. 244-4**). Because the pulmonary artery pressure in PAH increases dramatically with exercise, patients should be cautioned against participating in activities that demand increased physical stress. Diuretic therapy relieves peripheral edema and may be useful in reducing RV volume overload in the presence of tricuspid regurgitation. Resting and exercise pulse oximetry should be obtained, as O_2 supplementation helps to alleviate dyspnea and RV ischemia in patients whose arterial O_2 saturation is reduced. Anticoagulant therapy is advocated for all patients with PAH based on retrospective and prospective studies demonstrating that warfarin increases survival of patients with PAH. The dose of warfarin is generally titrated to achieve an INR of 2–3 times control.

CALCIUM CHANNEL BLOCKERS Patients who have substantial reductions in pulmonary arterial pressure in response to short-acting vasodilators at the time of cardiac catheterization (a fall in mean pulmonary arterial pressure ≥10 mmHg and a final mean pressure <40 mmHg) should be treated initially with calcium channel blockers. Typically, patients require high doses (e.g., nifedipine, 240 mg/d, or amlodipine, 20 mg/d). Patients who respond favorably usually have dramatic reductions in pulmonary artery pressure and

---

TABLE 244-1 CLINICAL CLASSIFICATION OF PULMONARY HYPERTENSION

1. **Pulmonary arterial hypertension (PAH)**
   1.1. Idiopathic (IPAH) (formerly PPH)
   1.2. Familial (FPAH)
   1.3. Associated with (APAH):
      1.3.1. Collagen vascular disease
      1.3.2. Congenital systemic-to-pulmonary shunts
      1.3.3. Portal hypertension
      1.3.4. HIV infection
      1.3.5. Drugs and toxins
      1.3.6. Other (thyroid disorders, glycogen storage disease, Gaucher disease, hereditary hemorrhagic telangiectasia, hemoglobinopathies, myeloproliferative disorders, splenectomy)
   1.4. Associated with significant venous or capillary involvement
      1.4.1. Pulmonary veno-occlusive disease (PVOD)
      1.4.2. Pulmonary capillary hemangiomatosis (PCH)
   1.5. Persistent pulmonary hypertension of the newborn
2. **Pulmonary hypertension with left heart disease**
   2.1. Left-sided atrial or ventricular heart disease
   2.2. Left-sided valvular heart disease
3. **Pulmonary hypertension associated with lung diseases and/or hypoxemia**
   3.1. Chronic obstructive pulmonary disease
   3.2. Interstitial lung disease
   3.3. Sleep-disordered breathing
   3.4. Alveolar hypoventilation disorders
   3.5. Chronic exposure to high altitude
   3.6. Developmental abnormalities
4. **Pulmonary hypertension due to chronic thrombotic and/or embolic disease**
   4.1. Thromboembolic obstruction of proximal pulmonary arteries
   4.2. Thromboembolic obstruction of distal pulmonary arteries
   4.3. Nonthrombotic pulmonary embolism (tumor, parasites, foreign material)
5. **Miscellaneous**
   Sarcoidosis, histiocytosis X, lymphangiomatosis, compression of pulmonary vessels (adenopathy, tumor, fibrosing mediastinitis)

Source: From G Simonneau et al: Clinical classification of pulmonary hypertension. J Am Coll Cardiol 43:S5, 2004.

FIGURE 244-3 Mechanistic pathways promoting pulmonary arterial hypertension (PAH). External stimuli, such as hypoxia or anorexigens, can stimulate a serotoninergic pathway which, in concert with internal stimuli involving the TGF-β receptor pathway can produce PAH. 5-HT2B, serotonin receptor; 5-HTT, serotonin transporter; TGF-β, transforming growth factor β; TIE2, angiopoietein-1 receptor; BMPR1A, bone morphogenetic protein receptor 1A; mBMPR2, mutant form of bone morphogenetic protein receptor 2; mALK1, activin-receptor-like kinase. (*From Farber and Loscalzo, with permission.*)

pulmonary vascular resistance associated with improved symptoms, regression of RV hypertrophy, and improved survival now documented to exceed 20 years. However, <20% of patients respond to calcium channel blockers in the long term. These drugs should not be given to patients who are unresponsive, as they can result in hypotension, hypoxemia, tachycardia, and worsening right heart failure. These agents have not been approved for the treatment of PAH by the U.S. Food and Drug Administration.

ENDOTHELIN RECEPTOR ANTAGONISTS The nonselective endothelin receptor antagonist *bosentan* is an approved treatment of PAH for patients who are NYHA functional classes III and IV. In randomized clinical trials, bosentan improved symptoms and exercise tolerance as measured by an increase in 6-min walking distance. Therapy is initiated at 62.5 mg bid for the first month and then increased to 125 mg bid thereafter. Because of the high frequency of abnormal hepatic function tests associated with drug use, primarily an increase in transaminases, it is recommended that liver function be monitored monthly throughout the duration of use. Bosentan is also contraindicated in patients who are on cyclosporine or glyburide concurrently.

PHOSPHODIESTERASE-5 INHIBITORS *Sildenafil,* a phosphodiesterase-5 inhibitor, is approved for the treatment of PAH patients who are NYHA functional classes II and III. Phosphodiesterase-5 is responsible for the hydrolysis of cyclic GMP in pulmonary vascular smooth muscle, the mediator through which nitric oxide lowers pulmonary artery pressure and inhibits pulmonary vascular growth. Randomized clinical trials have shown that sildenafil improves symptoms and exercise tolerance in PAH. The recommended dose is 20 mg tid. The most common side effect is headache. Sildenafil should not be given to patients who are taking nitrate compounds.

PROSTACYCLINS *Iloprost,* a prostacyclin analogue, is approved via inhalation for PAH patients who are NYHA functional classes III and IV. It has been shown to improve symptoms and exercise tolerance. Therapy can be given at either 2.5 or 5 mcg per inhalation treatment. The inhaler must be given by a dedicated nebulizer. The most common side effects are flushing and cough. Because of the very short half-life (<30 min) it is recommended to administer treatments as often as every 2 h.

Epoprostenol is approved for the treatment of PAH patients who are NYHA functional class III or IV. Clinical trials have demonstrated an improve-

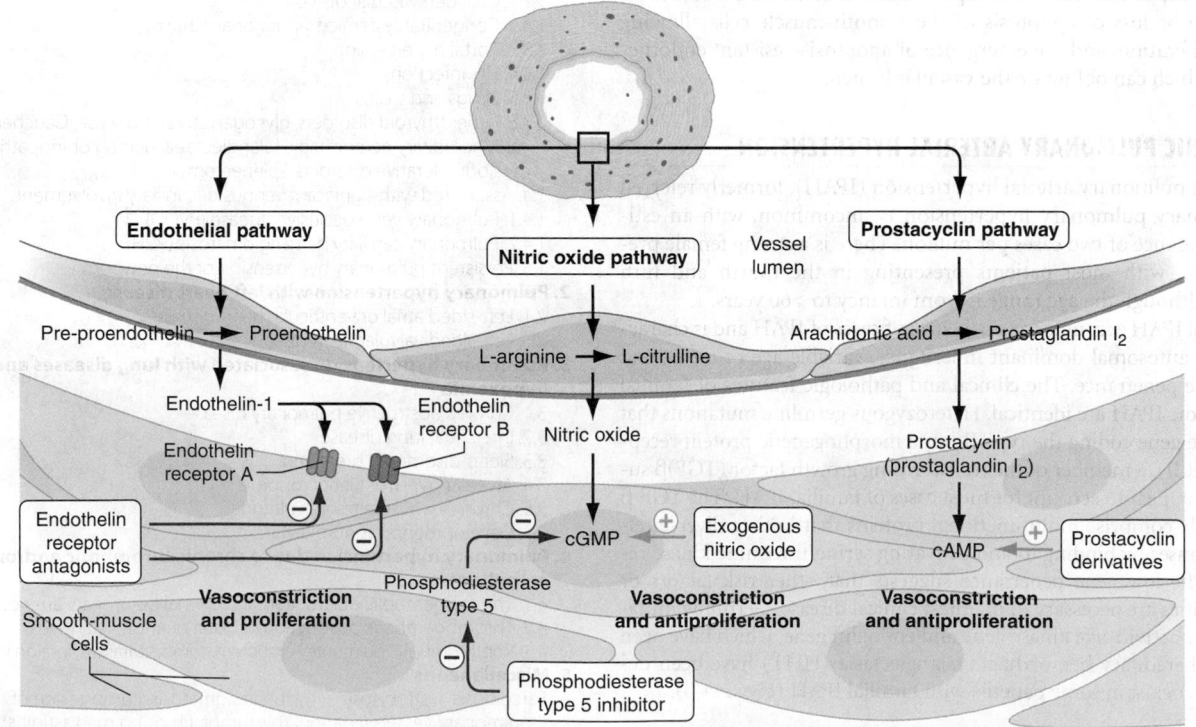

FIGURE 244-4 Current therapies target multiple growth factor pathways that appear to be involved in the pathogenesis of PAH. Whether treating multiple pathways simultaneously will yield better results is unknown. (*From Humbert et al., with permission.*)

ment in symptoms, exercise tolerance, and survival even if no acute hemodynamic response to drug challenge occurs. The drug is administered intravenously and requires placement of a permanent central venous catheter and infusion through an ambulatory infusion pump system. Side effects include flushing, jaw pain, and diarrhea, which are generally tolerated by most patients.

Treprostinil, an analogue of epoprostenol, is approved for patients with PAH who are NYHA functional classes II–IV. Treprostinil has a longer half-life than epoprostenol (4 h), is stable at room temperature, and may be given intravenously or subcutaneously through a small infusion pump that was originally developed for insulin. Clinical trials have demonstrated an improvement in symptoms and exercise capacity. The major problem with the subcutaneous administration has been local pain at the infusion site, which has caused many patients to discontinue therapy. Side effects are similar to those seen with epoprostenol.

The intravenous prostacyclins have the greatest efficacy as treatments for PAH, and are often effective in patients who have failed all other treatments. Favorable properties include vasodilation, platelet inhibition, inhibition of vascular smooth-muscle growth, and inotropic effects. It generally takes several months to titrate the dose of epoprostenol or treprostinil upwards to optimal clinical efficacy, which can be determined by symptoms, exercise testing, and catheterization. The optimal doses of these drugs have not been determined, but the typical doses of epoprostenol range from 25 to 40 ng/kg/min, and from 50 to 100 ng/kg/min for treprostinil. The major problem with intravenous therapy is infection related to the venous catheter, which requires close monitoring and diligence on behalf of the patient.

Although most clinical trials have focused on patients with advanced symptoms, it is recommended that every patient diagnosed with PAH be treated (Fig. 244-2). While no treatment has been demonstrated to be superior as first-line therapy, patients often prefer to initiate their treatment with an oral or inhaled form of therapy. In the trials using bosentan, sildenafil, and iloprost, full clinical benefit was generally manifest within the first 2 months of therapy. Patients who fail to adequately improve should have the treatment discontinued and started on a different therapy. Equally important is that delaying a more effective treatment may allow the disease to progress and become less responsive. The use of these drugs in combination has become popular, but there are no randomized clinical trials demonstrating beneficial effects in combination.

LUNG TRANSPLANTATION   (See also Chap. 260) Lung transplantation is considered for patients who, while on an intravenous prostacyclin, continue to manifest right heart failure. Acceptable results have been achieved with heart-lung, bilateral lung, and single-lung transplant. The availability of donor organs often influences the choice of procedure.

CONDITIONS ASSOCIATED WITH PULMONARY HYPERTENSION

COLLAGEN VASCULAR DISEASE

All of the collagen vascular diseases may be associated with PAH. This complication occurs commonly with the CREST syndrome (calcinosis, Raynaud's phenomenon, esophageal involvement, sclerodactyly, and telangiectasia) and in scleroderma (Chap. 316), and less frequently in systemic lupus erythematosus (Chap. 313), Sjögren's syndrome (Chap. 317), dermatomyositis, polymyositis (Chap. 319), and rheumatoid arthritis (Chap. 314). It is usual for these patients to have some element of coexistent interstitial pulmonary fibrosis even though it may not be apparent on chest x-ray, CT, or pulmonary function tests. Consequently, these patients tend to have hypoxemia as an important clinical feature, along with the other classic findings of pulmonary hypertension.

Treatment of these patients is identical to that of patients with IPAH (see above) but is less effective. The treatment of the pulmonary hypertension, however, does not affect the natural history of the underlying collagen vascular disease.

CONGENITAL SYSTEMIC TO PULMONARY SHUNTS

It is common for large post-tricuspid cardiac shunts (e.g., ventricular septal defect, patent ductus arteriosus) to produce severe PAH (Chap. 229). Although less common, it may also occur in pre-tricuspid shunts (e.g., atrial septal defect, anomalous pulmonary venous drainage). In

patients with uncorrected shunts, the clinical features include those associated with right-to-left shunting such as hypoxemia and peripheral cyanosis, which worsen dramatically with exertion (Chap. 35). PAH may occur years or even decades after surgical correction of these lesions, in which case there will be no associated right-to-left shunting. These patients present similarly to patients with IPAH but tend to have better long-term survival. The treatments are similar to those for IPAH.

PORTAL HYPERTENSION

Portal hypertension is associated with PAH, but the mechanism remains unknown. Patients with advanced cirrhosis can have the combined features of a high-output cardiac state in association with the features of pulmonary hypertension and RV failure. Thus, a normal cardiac output may actually reflect a marked impairment of RV function. The etiology of ascites and edema can be confusing in these patients since it can have both cardiac and hepatic causes. Patients with mild pulmonary hypertension who have a favorable response to epoprostenol have undergone successful liver transplantation with improvement of the pulmonary vascular disease.

ANOREXIGENS

A causal relationship has been established between exposure to several anorexigens, including aminorex and the fenfluramines, and the development of PAH. Often the pulmonary hypertension will not develop until years after the last exposure. While the clinical features are identical to those of IPAH, the patients appear to be less responsive to medical treatments and have a poorer prognosis.

PULMONARY VENOOCCLUSIVE DISEASE

Pulmonary venoocclusive disease is a rare and distinct pathologic entity found in <10% of patients who present with unexplained pulmonary hypertension. Histologically it is manifest by intimal proliferation and fibrosis of the intrapulmonary veins and venules, occasionally extending to the arteriolar bed. The pulmonary venous obstruction explains the increase in pulmonary capillary wedge pressure observed in patients with advanced disease. These patients may develop orthopnea that can mimic LV failure. The therapy of this condition is not established.

PULMONARY CAPILLARY HEMANGIOMATOSIS

Pulmonary capillary hemangiomatosis is a very rare form of pulmonary hypertension. Histologically it is characterized by the presence of infiltrating thin-walled blood vessels throughout the pulmonary interstitium and walls of the pulmonary arteries and veins. The presenting symptoms are usually those of IPAH but often with hemoptysis as a clinical feature. The diagnosis can be made with pulmonary angiography. The clinical course is usually one of progressive deterioration leading to death. There is no established therapy.

PULMONARY VENOUS HYPERTENSION

Pulmonary hypertension occurs as a result of increased resistance to pulmonary venous drainage. It is often associated with diastolic dysfunction of the left ventricle; diseases affecting the pericardium or mitral or aortic valves; or rare entities such as cor triatriatum, left atrial myxoma, extrinsic compression of the central pulmonary veins from fibrosing mediastinitis, and pulmonary venoocclusive disease. Pulmonary venous hypertension affects the pulmonary veins and venules, producing arterialization of the external elastic lamina, medial hypertrophy, and focal eccentric intimal fibrosis. Microcirculatory lesions include capillary congestion, focal alveolar edema, and dilatation of the interstitial lymphatics. Although these lesions are potentially reversible, regression may take years after the underlying cause is removed. In some patients pulmonary venous hypertension triggers reactive vasoconstriction in the pulmonary arterial bed and results in proliferative changes of the intima and media that can produce severe elevations in pulmonary artery pressure. Clinically it may be confusing and appear as if two separate disease processes are occurring simultaneously. The distinction is important, however, as treatments that are effective in PAH may make patients with pulmonary venous hypertension worse.

LEFT VENTRICULAR DIASTOLIC DYSFUNCTION

Pulmonary hypertension as a result of LV diastolic failure is common but often unrecognized (Chap. 227). It can occur with or without LV systolic failure. The most common causes are hypertensive heart disease; coronary artery disease; or impaired LV compliance related to age, diabetes, obesity, and hypoxemia. Symptoms of orthopnea and paroxysmal nocturnal dyspnea are prominent. Many patients improve considerably if LV end-diastolic pressure is lowered.

MITRAL VALVE DISEASE

Mitral stenosis and mitral regurgitation represent important causes of pulmonary hypertension (Chap. 230). These patients often have reactive pulmonary vasoconstriction resulting in marked elevations in pulmonary artery pressures. An echocardiogram usually shows abnormalities such as thickened mitral valve leaflets with reduced mobility or severe mitral regurgitation documented by Doppler echocardiography (Chap. 222). At cardiac catheterization, a pressure gradient between the pulmonary capillary wedge pressure and LV end-diastolic pressure is diagnostic of mitral stenosis.

In patients with mitral stenosis, corrective surgery of the mitral valve or mitral balloon valvuloplasty predictably results in a reduction in pulmonary artery pressure and pulmonary vascular resistance. Patients with mitral regurgitation, however, may not have as dramatic a response from surgery due to persistent elevations in LV end-diastolic pressure.

PULMONARY HYPERTENSION ASSOCIATED WITH LUNG DISEASE AND HYPOXEMIA

The mechanism of hypoxic pulmonary vasoconstriction involves the inhibition of potassium currents and membrane depolarization of pulmonary vascular smooth muscle as a result of the change in membrane sulfhydryl redox status. Increased calcium entry into the vascular smooth-muscle cells mediates hypoxic pulmonary vasoconstriction. Pulmonary vascular remodeling in response to chronic hypoxia is also mediated by a reduction in nitric oxide production; an increase in endothelin 1; and increased expression of platelet-derived growth factors, vascular endothelial growth factor, and angiotensin II. Chronic hypoxia results in muscularization of the arterioles with minimal effects on the intima. When it occurs as an isolated entity, the changes produced are potentially reversible.

Although chronic hypoxia is an established cause of pulmonary hypertension, it rarely leads to an increase in the systolic pulmonary artery pressure >50 mmHg. Polycythemia in response to the hypoxemia is a characteristic finding. Hypoxia may also occur in conjunction with other causes of pulmonary hypertension associated with more extensive vascular changes. Clinically, the hypoxia tends to have an added adverse effect. Patients with chronic hypoxia who have a marked elevation in pulmonary pressure should be evaluated for other causes of the pulmonary hypertension.

CHRONIC OBSTRUCTIVE LUNG DISEASE

Chronic obstructive lung disease (COLD) is associated with mild pulmonary hypertension in the advanced stages (Chap. 254). Pulmonary hypertension has been attributed to multiple factors, including hypoxic pulmonary vasoconstriction, acidemia, hypercapnia, the mechanical effects of high lung volume on pulmonary vessels, the loss of small vessels in the vascular bed, and regions of emphysematous lung destruction.

The presence of pulmonary hypertension in patients with COLD confers a worse outcome. The only effective therapy is supplemental oxygen. Several large clinical trials have documented that continuous oxygen therapy relieves some of the pulmonary vasoconstriction, relieves chronic ischemia throughout the systemic and pulmonary vascular beds, and improves survival. Long-term oxygen therapy is indicated if the resting arterial P_{O_2} remains <55 mmHg.

INTERSTITIAL LUNG DISEASE

Pulmonary hypertension from interstitial lung disease is often associated with obliteration of the pulmonary vascular bed by lung destruction and fibrosis (Chap. 255). In addition, hypoxemia and pulmonary vasculopathy can be contributory factors. Interstitial lung disease is often associated with the collagen vascular diseases. A large number of patients have pulmonary fibrosis of unknown etiology. Patients are commonly older than 50 years and report an insidious onset of progressive dyspnea and cough for months to years. It is uncommon for the mean pulmonary artery pressure to exceed 40 mmHg. While none of the medical treatments developed for PAH have been shown to be effective in these patients, their use may worsen the hypoxemia.

SLEEP-DISORDERED BREATHING

The incidence of pulmonary hypertension in the setting of *obstructive sleep apnea*, a common condition (Chap. 259), appears to be <20% and is generally mild. Some patients, however, present with severe pulmonary hypertension in conjunction with sleep apnea, which may or may not be related. It is recommended that the sleep apnea and the PAH be treated as coexisting problems.

ALVEOLAR HYPOVENTILATION

Pulmonary hypertension can occur in patients with chronic hypoventilation and hypoxia secondary to thoracovertebral deformities. Symptoms are slowly progressive and related to hypoxemia (Chap. 258). In patients with advanced disease, intermittent positive-pressure breathing and supplemental oxygen have been used successfully.

Pulmonary hypertension secondary to hypoxemia has been reported in patients with neuromuscular disease as a result of generalized weakness of the respiratory muscles and in patients with diaphragmatic paralysis, generally a result of trauma to the phrenic nerve. Patients with nontraumatic bilateral diaphragmatic paralysis may go unrecognized until they present with either respiratory failure or pulmonary hypertension.

PULMONARY HYPERTENSION DUE TO THROMBOEMBOLIC DISEASE

ACUTE PULMONARY THROMBOEMBOLISM
See Chap. 256.

CHRONIC THROMBOEMBOLIC PULMONARY HYPERTENSION

Patients appropriately treated for acute pulmonary thromboembolism with intravenous heparin and chronic oral warfarin therapy usually do not develop chronic pulmonary hypertension. However, some patients have impaired fibrinolytic resolution of the thromboembolism, which leads to organization and incomplete recanalization and chronic obstruction of the pulmonary vascular bed. The entity of chronic thromboembolic pulmonary hypertension has been well characterized and often mimics PAH. In many patients, the initial pulmonary thromboembolism was undetected or untreated. Many of these patients have underlying thrombophilic disorders, such as the lupus anticoagulant/anticardiolipin antibody syndrome, prothrombin gene mutation, or Factor V Leiden (Chap. 111).

Diagnosis   The physical examination is typical of pulmonary hypertension but may include bruits heard over areas of the lung, representing blood flow through vessels with partial occlusion. A perfusion lung scan or contrast-enhanced spiral CT scan usually reveals multiple thromboemboli. However, pulmonary angiography is necessary to determine the precise location and proximal extent of the thromboemboli, and hence the potential for operability.

℞ CHRONIC THROMBOEMBOLIC PULMONARY HYPERTENSION

Pulmonary thromboendarterectomy is an established surgical treatment in patients whose thrombi are accessible to surgical removal. The operative mortality is fairly high, at ~12% in experienced centers. Postoperative survivors who have a good result can expect to realize an improvement in functional class and exercise tolerance. Lifelong anticoagulation using warfarin is mandatory. Thrombolytic therapy is rarely of help in patients with chronic thromboembolic pulmonary hypertension and may expose these patients to the increased risk of bleeding without potential benefit.

SICKLE CELL DISEASE

Cardiovascular system abnormalities are prominent in the clinical spectrum of sickle cell disease, including pulmonary hypertension. The etiology is multifactorial, including hemolysis, impaired nitric oxide bioavailability, hypoxemia, thromboembolism, chronic high cardiac output, and chronic liver disease. Regardless of the mechanism(s), the presence of pulmonary hypertension in patients with sickle cell disease is associated with a higher morbidity and mortality. Intensification of sickle cell disease–specific therapy appears to reduce the morbidity. The use of drugs to treat pulmonary hypertension is under clinical trials, but their efficacy remains unknown.

OTHER DISORDERS DIRECTLY AFFECTING PULMONARY VASCULATURE

SARCOIDOSIS

Sarcoidosis can produce severe pulmonary hypertension as a result of chronic severe fibrocystic lung involvement (Chap. 322), or direct cardiovascular involvement. Consequently, patients with sarcoidosis who present with progressive dyspnea and clinical features of pulmonary hypertension need a thorough evaluation. There is a subset of patients with sarcoidosis who present with severe pulmonary hypertension believed to be due to direct pulmonary vascular involvement. Many of these patients exhibit a favorable response to intravenous epoprostenol therapy.

SCHISTOSOMIASIS

Although extremely rare in North America, schistosomiasis is the most common cause of pulmonary hypertension worldwide (Chap. 212). The development of pulmonary hypertension often occurs in the setting of hepatosplenic disease and portal hypertension. Schistosome ova can embolize from the liver to the lungs, where they result in an inflammatory pulmonary vascular reaction and chronic changes. The diagnosis is confirmed by finding the parasite ova in the urine or stools of patients with symptoms, which can be difficult. The efficacy of therapies directed toward pulmonary hypertension in these patients is unknown.

HIV INFECTION

The mechanism by which HIV infection produces pulmonary hypertension remains unknown (Chap. 182). Although it is uncommon for HIV infection to result in pulmonary hypertension, the marked rise in the prevalence of HIV infection worldwide could have a significant impact on the frequency that these entities are seen in combination. The evaluation and treatments are identical to those for IPAH. Treatment of the HIV infection does not appear to affect the severity or natural history of the underlying pulmonary hypertension.

FURTHER READINGS

DILLER GP, GATZOULIS MA: Pulmonary vascular disease in adults with congenital heart disease. Circulation 115:1039, 2007

FARBER HW, LOSCALZO J: Pulmonary arterial hypertension. N Engl J Med 351:1655, 2004

GALIE N, RUBIN LJ (eds): Pulmonary arterial hypertension. Epidemiology, pathobiology, assessment and therapy. J Amer Coll Cardiol 43:supplement S, 2004

HUMBERT M et al: Treatment of pulmonary arterial hypertension. N Engl J Med 351:1425, 2004

PENALOZA D, ARIAS-STELLA J: The heart and pulmonary circulation at high altitudes: Healthy highlanders and chronic mountain sickness. Circulation 115:1132, 2007

RAVIPATI G et al: Type 5 phosphodiesterase inhibitors in the treatment of erectile dysfunction and cardiovascular disease. Cardiol Rev 15:76, 2007

RICH S, MCLAUGHLIN VV: Pulmonary hypertension, in *Braunwald's Heart Disease: A Textbook of Cardiovascular Medicine,* 8th ed, P Libby et al (eds). Philadelphia, Elsevier Saunders, 2008

RICHTER A et al: Impaired transforming growth factor-beta signaling in idiopathic pulmonary arterial hypertension. Am J Respir Crit Care Med 170:1340, 2004

SITBON O et al: Long term response to calcium channel blockers in idiopathic pulmonary arterial hypertension. Circulation 111:3105, 2005

245 Approach to the Patient with Disease of the Respiratory System

David A. Lipson, Steven E. Weinberger

Patients with disease of the respiratory system generally present because of symptoms, an abnormality on a chest radiograph, or both. These findings often lead to a set of diagnostic possibilities; the differential diagnosis is then refined on the basis of additional information gleaned from the history and physical examination, pulmonary function testing, additional imaging studies, and bronchoscopic examination. This chapter will consider the approach to the patient based on the major patterns of presentation, focusing on the history, the physical examination, and the chest radiograph. For further discussion of pulmonary function testing, see Chap. 246, and of other diagnostic studies, see Chap. 247.

CLINICAL PRESENTATION

History Dyspnea (shortness of breath) and cough are nonspecific but common presenting symptoms for patients with respiratory system disease. Less common symptoms include hemoptysis (the coughing up of blood) and chest pain that often is pleuritic in nature.

DYSPNEA (See also Chap. 33) When evaluating a patient with shortness of breath, one should first determine the time course over which the symptom has become manifest. Patients who were well previously and developed *acute* shortness of breath (over a period of minutes to days) may have acute disease affecting either the upper or the intrathoracic airways (e.g., laryngeal edema or acute asthma, respectively), the pulmonary parenchyma (acute cardiogenic or noncardiogenic pulmonary edema or an acute infectious process such as a bacterial pneumonia), the pleural space (a pneumothorax), or the pulmonary vasculature (a pulmonary embolus). A *subacute* presentation (over days to weeks) can suggest an exacerbation of preexisting airways disease (asthma or chronic bronchitis), an indolent parenchymal infection (*Pneumocystis jiroveci* pneumonia in a patient with AIDS, mycobacterial or fungal pneumonia), a noninfectious inflammatory process that proceeds at a relatively slow pace (Wegener's granulomatosis, eosinophilic pneumonia, cryptogenic organizing pneumonia, and many others), neuromuscular disease (Guillain-Barré syndrome, myasthenia gravis), pleural disease (pleural effusion from a variety of possible causes), or chronic cardiac disease (congestive heart failure). A *chronic* presentation (over months to years) often indicates chronic obstructive lung disease, chronic interstitial lung disease, or chronic cardiac disease. Chronic diseases of airways (not only chronic obstructive lung disease but also asthma) are characterized by exacerbations and remissions. Patients often have periods when they are severely limited by shortness of breath, but these may be interspersed with periods in which symptoms are minimal or absent. In contrast, many of the diseases of the pulmonary parenchyma are characterized by slow but inexorable progression. Chronic respiratory symptoms may also be multifactorial in nature, as patients with chronic obstructive pulmonary disease may also have concomitant heart disease.

OTHER RESPIRATORY SYMPTOMS Cough (Chap. 34) may indicate the presence of lung disease, but cough per se is not useful for the differential diagnosis. The presence of sputum accompanying the cough often suggests airway disease and may be seen in asthma, chronic bronchitis, or bronchiectasis.

Hemoptysis (Chap. 34) can originate from disease of the airways, the pulmonary parenchyma, or the vasculature. Diseases of the airways can be inflammatory (acute or chronic bronchitis, bronchiectasis, or cystic fibrosis) or neoplastic (bronchogenic carcinoma or bronchial carcinoid tumors). Parenchymal diseases causing hemoptysis may be either localized (pneumonia, lung abscess, tuberculosis, or infection with *Aspergillus*) or diffuse (Goodpasture's syndrome, idiopathic pulmonary hemosiderosis). Vascular diseases potentially associated with hemoptysis include pulmonary thromboembolic disease and pulmonary arteriovenous malformations.

Chest pain (Chap. 13) caused by diseases of the respiratory system usually originates from involvement of the parietal pleura. As a result, the pain is accentuated by respiratory motion and is often referred to as pleuritic. Common examples include primary pleural disorders, such as neoplasm or inflammatory disorders involving the pleura, or pulmonary parenchymal disorders that extend to the pleural surface, such as pneumonia or pulmonary infarction.

ADDITIONAL HISTORIC INFORMATION Information about risk factors for lung disease should be explicitly explored to ensure a complete basis of historic data. A history of current and past smoking, especially of cigarettes, should be sought from all patients. The smoking history should include the number of years of smoking, the intensity (i.e., number of packs per day), and, if the patient no longer smokes, the interval since smoking cessation. The risk of lung cancer falls progressively in the decade following discontinuation of smoking, and loss of lung function above the expected age-related decline ceases with the discontinuation of smoking. Even though chronic obstructive lung disease and neoplasia are the two most important respiratory complications of smoking, other respiratory disorders (e.g., spontaneous pneumothorax, respiratory bronchiolitis–interstitial lung disease, pulmonary Langerhans cell histiocytosis, and pulmonary hemorrhage with Goodpasture's syndrome) are also associated with smoking. A history of significant secondhand (passive) exposure to smoke, whether in the home or at the workplace, should also be sought as it may be a risk factor for neoplasia or an exacerbating factor for airways disease.

The patient may have been exposed to other inhaled agents associated with lung disease, which act either via direct toxicity or through immune mechanisms (Chaps. 249 and 250). Such exposures can be either occupational or avocational, indicating the importance of detailed occupational and personal histories, the latter stressing exposures related to hobbies or the home environment. Important agents include the inorganic dusts associated with pneumoconiosis (especially asbestos and silica dusts) and organic antigens associated with hypersensitivity pneumonitis (especially antigens from molds and animal proteins). Asthma, which is more common in women than men, is often exacerbated by exposure to environmental allergens (dust mites, pet dander, or cockroach allergens in the home or allergens in the outdoor environment such as pollen and ragweed) or may be caused by occupational exposures (diisocyanates). Exposure to particular infectious agents can be suggested by contacts with individuals with known respiratory infections (especially tuberculosis) or by residence in an area with endemic pathogens (histoplasmosis, coccidioidomycosis, blastomycosis).

A history of coexisting nonrespiratory disease or of risk factors for or previous treatment of such diseases should be sought, as they may predispose a patient to both infectious and noninfectious respiratory system complications. Common examples include systemic rheumatic diseases that are associated with pleural or parenchymal lung disease (Chap. 314), metastatic neoplastic disease in the lung, or impaired host defense mechanisms and secondary infection, which occur in the case of immunoglobulin deficiency or with hematologic and lymph node malignancies. Risk factors for AIDS should be sought, as the lungs are not only the most common site of AIDS-defining infection but can also be involved by noninfectious complications of AIDS (Chap. 182). Treatment of nonrespiratory disease can be associated with respiratory complications, either because of effects on host defense mechanisms (immunosuppressive agents, cancer chemotherapy) with resulting infection or because of direct effects on the pulmonary parenchyma (cancer chemotherapy, radiation therapy, or treatment with other agents, such as amiodarone) or on the airways (beta-blocking agents causing airflow obstruction, angiotensin-converting enzyme inhibitors causing cough) (Chap. 249).

Family history is important for evaluating diseases that have a genetic component. These include disorders such as cystic fibrosis, α_1-antitrypsin deficiency, pulmonary hypertension, pulmonary fibrosis, and asthma.

Physical Examination The general principles of inspection, palpation, percussion, and auscultation apply to the examination of the respiratory system. However, the physical examination should be directed not only toward ascertaining abnormalities of the lungs and thorax but also toward recognizing other findings that may reflect underlying lung disease.

On *inspection*, the rate and pattern of breathing as well as the depth and symmetry of lung expansion are observed. Breathing that is unusually rapid, labored, or associated with the use of accessory muscles of respiration generally indicates either augmented respiratory demands or an increased work of breathing. Asymmetric expansion of the chest is usually due to an asymmetric process affecting the lungs, such as endobronchial obstruction of a large airway, unilateral parenchymal or pleural disease, or unilateral phrenic nerve paralysis. Visible abnormalities of the thoracic cage include kyphoscoliosis and ankylosing spondylitis, either of which can alter compliance of the thorax, increase the work of breathing, and cause dyspnea.

On *palpation*, the symmetry of lung expansion can be assessed, generally confirming the findings observed by inspection. Vibration produced by spoken sounds is transmitted to the chest wall and is assessed by the presence or absence and symmetry of tactile fremitus. Transmission of vibration is decreased or absent if pleural liquid is interposed between the lung and the chest wall or if an endobronchial obstruction alters sound transmission. In contrast, transmitted vibration may increase over an area of underlying pulmonary consolidation. Palpation may also reveal focal tenderness, as seen with costochondritis or rib fracture.

The relative resonance or dullness of the tissue underlying the chest wall is assessed by *percussion*. The normal sound of underlying air-containing lung is resonant. In contrast, consolidated lung or a pleural effusion sounds dull, while emphysema or air in the pleural space results in a hyperresonant percussion note.

On *auscultation* of the lungs, the examiner listens for both the quality and intensity of the breath sounds and for the presence of extra, or adventitious, sounds. Normal breath sounds heard through the stethoscope at the periphery of the lung are described as *vesicular breath sounds*, in which inspiration is louder and longer than expiration. If sound transmission is impaired by endobronchial obstruction or by air or liquid in the pleural space, breath sounds are diminished in intensity or absent. When sound transmission is improved through consolidated lung, the resulting *bronchial breath sounds* have a more tubular quality and a more pronounced expiratory phase. Sound transmission can also be assessed by listening to spoken or whispered sounds; when these are transmitted through consolidated lung, *bronchophony* and *whispered pectoriloquy*, respectively, are present. The sound of a spoken E becomes more like an A, although with a nasal or bleating quality, a finding that is termed *egophony*.

The primary adventitious (abnormal) sounds that can be heard include crackles (rales), wheezes, and rhonchi. *Crackles* are the discontinuous, typically inspiratory sound created when alveoli and small airways open and close with respiration. They are often associated with interstitial lung disease, microatelectasis, or filling of alveoli by liquid. *Wheezes*, which are generally more prominent during expiration than inspiration, reflect the oscillation of airway walls that occurs when there is airflow limitation, as may be produced by bronchospasm, airway edema or collapse, or intraluminal obstruction by neoplasm or secretions. *Rhonchi* is the term applied to the sounds created when there is free liquid or mucus in the airway lumen; the viscous interaction between the free liquid and the moving air creates a low-pitched vibratory sound. Other adventitious sounds include pleural friction rubs and stridor. The gritty sound of a *pleural friction rub* indicates inflamed pleural surfaces rubbing against each other, often during both inspiratory and expiratory phases of the respiratory cycle. *Stridor*, which occurs primarily during inspiration, represents flow through a narrowed upper airway, as occurs in an infant with croup.

A summary of the patterns of physical findings on pulmonary examination in common types of respiratory system disease is shown in Table 245-1.

A meticulous *general physical examination* is mandatory in patients with disorders of the respiratory system. Enlarged lymph nodes in the cervical and supraclavicular regions should be sought. Disturbances of mentation or even coma can occur in patients with acute carbon dioxide retention and hypoxemia. Telltale stains on the fingers point to heavy cigarette smoking; infected teeth and gums may occur in patients with aspiration pneumonitis and lung abscess.

Clubbing of the digits can be found in lung cancer, interstitial lung disease, and chronic infections in the thorax, such as bronchiectasis, lung abscess, and empyema. Clubbing can also be seen with congenital heart disease associated with right-to-left shunting and with a variety of chronic inflammatory or infectious diseases, such as inflammatory bowel disease and endocarditis. A number of systemic diseases, such as systemic lupus erythematosus, scleroderma, and rheumatoid arthritis,

TABLE 245-1 TYPICAL CHEST EXAMINATION FINDINGS IN SELECTED CLINICAL CONDITIONS

Condition	Percussion	Fremitus	Breath Sounds	Voice Transmission	Adventitious Sounds
Normal	Resonant	Normal	Vesicular (at lung bases)	Normal	Absent
Consolidation or atelectasis (with patent airway)	Dull	Increased	Bronchial	Bronchophony, whispered pectoriloquy, egophony	Crackles
Consolidation or atelectasis (with blocked airway)	Dull	Decreased	Decreased	Decreased	Absent
Asthma	Resonant	Normal	Vesicular	Normal	Wheezing
Interstitial lung disease	Resonant	Normal	Vesicular	Normal	Crackles
Emphysema	Hyperresonant	Decreased	Decreased	Decreased	Absent or wheezing
Pneumothorax	Hyperresonant	Decreased	Decreased	Decreased	Absent
Pleural effusion	Dull	Decreased	Decreased[a]	Decreased[a]	Absent or pleural friction rub

[a]May be altered by collapse of underlying lung, which will increase transmission of sound.

Source: Adapted from Weinberger, with permission.

may be associated with pulmonary complications, even though their primary clinical manifestations and physical findings are not primarily related to the lungs. Conversely, other diseases that most commonly affect the respiratory system, such as sarcoidosis, can have findings on physical examination not related to the respiratory system, including ocular findings (uveitis, conjunctival granulomas) and skin findings (erythema nodosum, cutaneous granulomas).

CHEST RADIOGRAPHY

Chest radiography is often the initial diagnostic study performed to evaluate patients with respiratory symptoms, but it can also provide the initial evidence of disease in patients who are free of symptoms. Perhaps the most common example of the latter situation is the finding of one or more nodules or masses when the radiograph is performed for a reason other than evaluation of respiratory symptoms.

A number of diagnostic possibilities are often suggested by the radiographic pattern (**Chap. e24**). A localized region of opacification involving the pulmonary parenchyma can be described as a nodule (usually <3 cm in diameter), a mass (usually ≥3 cm in diameter), or an infiltrate. Diffuse disease with increased opacification is usually characterized as having an alveolar, an interstitial, or a nodular pattern. In contrast, increased radiolucency can be localized, as seen with a cyst or bulla, or generalized, as occurs with emphysema. The chest radiograph is also particularly useful for the detection of pleural disease, especially if manifested by the presence of air or liquid in the pleural space. An abnormal appearance of the hila and/or the mediastinum can suggest a mass or enlargement of lymph nodes.

A summary of representative diagnoses suggested by these common radiographic patterns is presented in Table 245-2, and an atlas of chest radiographs and other chest images can be found in **Chap. e24**.

Additional Diagnostic Evaluation Further information for clarification of radiographic abnormalities is frequently obtained with CT scanning of the chest (see Figs. 247-1, 247-2; 255-1, 255-2; 262-3).

TABLE 245-2 MAJOR RESPIRATORY DIAGNOSES WITH COMMON CHEST RADIOGRAPHIC PATTERNS

Solitary circumscribed density—nodule (<3 cm) or mass (≥3 cm)
  Primary or metastatic neoplasm
  Localized infection (bacterial abscess, mycobacterial or fungal infection)
  Wegener's granulomatosis (one or several nodules)
  Rheumatoid nodule (one or several nodules)
  Vascular malformation
  Bronchogenic cyst
Localized opacification (infiltrate)
  Pneumonia (bacterial, atypical, mycobacterial, or fungal infection)
  Neoplasm
  Radiation pneumonitis
  Bronchiolitis obliterans with organizing pneumonia
  Bronchocentric granulomatosis
  Pulmonary infarction
Diffuse interstitial disease
  Idiopathic pulmonary fibrosis
  Pulmonary fibrosis with systemic rheumatic disease
  Sarcoidosis
  Drug-induced lung disease
  Pneumoconiosis
  Hypersensitivity pneumonitis
  Infection (*Pneumocystis*, viral pneumonia)
  Langerhans cell histiocytosis
Diffuse alveolar disease
  Cardiogenic pulmonary edema
  Acute respiratory distress syndrome
  Diffuse alveolar hemorrhage
  Infection (*Pneumocystis*, viral or bacterial pneumonia)
  Sarcoidosis
Diffuse nodular disease
  Metastatic neoplasm
  Hematogenous spread of infection (bacterial, mycobacterial, fungal)
  Pneumoconiosis
  Langerhans cell histiocytosis

This technique is more sensitive than plain radiography in detecting subtle abnormalities and can suggest specific diagnoses based on the pattern of abnormality. For further discussion of the use of other imaging studies, including MRI, scintigraphic studies, ultrasound, and angiography, see Chap. 247.

Alteration in the function of the lungs as a result of respiratory system disease is assessed objectively by pulmonary function tests, and effects on gas exchange are evaluated by measurement of arterial blood gases or by oximetry (Chap. 246). As part of pulmonary function testing, quantitation of forced expiratory flow assesses the presence of obstructive physiology, which is consistent with diseases affecting the structure or function of the airways, such as asthma and chronic obstructive lung disease. Measurement of lung volumes assesses the presence of restrictive disorders seen with diseases of the pulmonary parenchyma or respiratory pump and with space-occupying processes within the pleura. Bronchoscopy is useful in some settings for visualizing abnormalities of the airways and for obtaining a variety of samples from either the airway or the pulmonary parenchyma (Chap. 247).

INTEGRATION OF THE PRESENTING CLINICAL PATTERN AND DIAGNOSTIC STUDIES

Patients with respiratory symptoms but a normal chest radiograph often have diseases affecting the airways, such as asthma or chronic obstructive pulmonary disease. However, the latter diagnosis is also commonly associated with radiographic abnormalities, such as diaphragmatic flattening, an increase in the retrosternal air space, and attenuation of vascular markings. Other disorders of the respiratory system for which the chest radiograph is normal include disorders of the respiratory pump (either the chest wall or the neuromuscular apparatus controlling the chest wall) or pulmonary circulation and occasionally interstitial lung disease. Chest examination and pulmonary function tests are generally helpful in sorting out these diagnostic possibilities. Obstructive diseases associated with a normal or relatively normal chest radiograph are often characterized by findings on physical examination and pulmonary function testing that are typical for these conditions. Similarly, diseases of the respiratory pump or interstitial diseases may also be suggested by findings on physical examination or by particular patterns of restrictive disease seen on pulmonary function testing.

When respiratory symptoms are accompanied by radiographic abnormalities, diseases of the pulmonary parenchyma or the pleura are usually present. Either diffuse or localized parenchymal lung disease is generally visualized well on the radiograph, and both air and liquid in the pleural space (pneumothorax and pleural effusion, respectively) are usually readily detected by radiography.

Radiographic findings in the absence of respiratory symptoms often indicate localized disease affecting the airways or the pulmonary parenchyma. One or more nodules or masses can suggest intrathoracic malignancy, but they can also be the manifestation of a current or previous infectious process. Multiple nodules affecting only one lobe suggest an infectious etiology rather than malignancy, as metastatic disease would not have a predilection for only one discrete area of the lung. Patients with diffuse parenchymal lung disease on radiographic examination may be free of symptoms, as is sometimes the case with pulmonary sarcoidosis.

FURTHER READINGS

AMERICAN COLLEGE OF CHEST PHYSICIANS: Diagnosis and management of cough: ACCP evidence-based clinical practice guidelines. Chest 129: 1S, 2006

GOODMAN L: *Felson's Principles of Chest Roentgenology. A Programmed Text*, 2d ed. Philadelphia, Saunders, 1999

LEBLOND RF et al: *DeGowin & DeGowin's Diagnostic Examination*, 8th ed. New York, McGraw-Hill, 2004

WEINBERGER SE: *Principles of Pulmonary Medicine*, 4th ed. Philadelphia, Saunders, 2004

246 Disturbances of Respiratory Function

Steven E. Weinberger, Ilene M. Rosen

The respiratory system includes the lungs, the central nervous system (CNS), the chest wall (with the diaphragm and intercostal muscles), and the pulmonary circulation. The CNS controls the activity of the muscles of the chest wall, which constitute the pump of the respiratory system. Because these components of the respiratory system act in concert to achieve gas exchange, malfunction of an individual component or alteration of the relationships among components can lead to disturbances in function. In this chapter we consider three major aspects of disturbed respiratory function: (1) disturbances in ventilatory function, (2) disturbances in the pulmonary circulation, and (3) disturbances in gas exchange. **For further discussion of disorders relating to CNS control of ventilation, see Chap. 258.**

DISTURBANCES IN VENTILATORY FUNCTION

Ventilation is the process whereby the lungs replenish the gas in the alveoli. Measurements of ventilatory function in common diagnostic use consist of quantification of the gas volume contained in the lungs under certain circumstances and the rate at which gas can be expelled from the lungs. The two measurements of lung volume commonly used for respiratory diagnosis are (1) total lung capacity (TLC), the volume of gas contained in the lungs after a maximal inspiration; and (2) residual volume (RV), the volume of gas remaining in the lungs at the end of a maximal expiration. The volume of gas that is exhaled from the lungs in going from TLC to RV is the *vital capacity* (VC) (**Fig. 246-1**).

Common clinical measurements of airflow are obtained from maneuvers in which the subject inspires to TLC and then forcibly exhales to RV. Three measurements are commonly made from a recording of forced exhaled volume versus time—i.e., a *spirogram*: (1) the volume of gas exhaled during the first second of expiration [forced expiratory volume (FEV) in 1 s, or FEV_1], (2) the total volume exhaled [forced vital capacity (FVC)], and (3) the average expiratory flow rate during the middle 50% of the VC [forced expiratory flow (FEF) between 25 and 75% of the VC, or $FEF_{25-75\%}$, also called the maximal midexpiratory flow rate (MMFR)] (**Fig. 246-2**).

PHYSIOLOGIC FEATURES

The lungs are elastic structures, containing collagen and elastic fibers that resist expansion. For normal lungs to contain air, they must be distended either by a positive internal pressure—i.e., by a pressure in the airways and alveolar spaces—or by a negative external pressure—i.e., by a pressure outside the lung. The relationship between the vol-

ume of gas contained in the lungs and the distending pressure (the *transpulmonary pressure*, or P_{TP}, defined as alveolar pressure minus pleural pressure) is described by the pressure-volume curve of the lungs (**Fig. 246-3A**).

FIGURE 246-2 Spirographic tracings of forced expiration, comparing a normal tracing **(A)** and tracings in obstructive **(B)** and parenchymal restrictive **(C)** disease. Calculations of FVC, FEV_1, and $FEF_{25-75\%}$ are shown only for the normal tracing. Since there is no measure of absolute starting volume with spirometry, the curves are artificially positioned to show the relative starting lung volumes in the different conditions.

FIGURE 246-3 Pressure-volume curves. A. Pressure-volume curve of the lungs. **B.** Pressure-volume curve of the chest wall. **C.** Pressure-volume curve of the respiratory system, showing the superimposed component curves of the lungs and the chest wall. RV, residual volume; FRC, functional residual capacity; TLC, total lung capacity. (*From Weinberger, with permission.*)

FIGURE 246-1 Lung volumes, shown by block diagrams (*left*) and by a spirographic tracing (*right*). TLC, total lung capacity; VC, vital capacity; RV, residual volume; IC, inspiratory capacity; ERV, expiratory reserve volume; FRC, functional residual capacity; V_T, tidal volume. (*From Weinberger, with permission.*)

The chest wall is also an elastic structure, with properties similar to those of an expandable and compressible spring. The relationship between the volume enclosed by the chest wall and the distending pressure for the chest wall is described by the pressure-volume curve of the chest wall (Fig. 246-3B). For the chest wall to assume a volume different from its resting volume, the internal or external pressures acting on it must be altered.

At functional residual capacity (FRC), defined as the volume of gas in the lungs at the end of a normal exhalation, the tendency of the lungs to contract is opposed by the equal and opposite tendency of the chest wall to expand (Fig. 246-3C). For the lungs and the chest wall to achieve a volume other than this resting volume (FRC), either the pressures acting on them must be changed passively—e.g., by a mechanical ventilator that delivers positive pressure to the airways and alveoli—or the respiratory muscles must actively oppose the tendency of the lungs and the chest wall to return to FRC. During inhalation to volumes above FRC, the inspiratory muscles actively overcome the tendency of the respiratory system to decrease volume back to FRC. During active exhalation to volumes below FRC, expiratory muscle activity must overcome the tendency of the respiratory system to increase volume back to FRC.

At TLC, the maximal force applied by the inspiratory muscles to expand the lungs is opposed mainly by the inward recoil of the lungs. As a consequence, the major determinants of TLC are the stiffness of the lungs and inspiratory muscle strength. If the lungs become stiffer—i.e., less compliant and with increased inward recoil—TLC is decreased. If the lungs become less stiff (more compliant and with decreased inward recoil), TLC is increased. If the inspiratory muscles are significantly weakened, they are less able to overcome the inward elastic recoil of the lungs, and TLC is lowered.

At RV, the force exerted by the expiratory muscles to decrease lung volume further is balanced by the outward recoil of the chest wall, which becomes extremely stiff at low lung volumes. Two factors influence the volume of gas contained in the lungs at RV. The first is the ability of the subject to exert a prolonged expiratory effort, which is related to muscle strength and the ability to overcome sensory stimuli from the chest wall. The second is the ability of the lungs to empty to a small volume. In normal lungs, as P_{TP} is lowered, lung volume decreases. In lungs with diseased airways, as P_{TP} is lowered, flow limitation or airway closure may limit the amount of gas that can be expired. Consequently, either weak expiratory muscles or intrinsic airways disease can result in an elevation in measured RV.

Dynamic measurements of ventilatory function are made by having the subject inhale to TLC and then perform a forced expiration to RV. If a subject performs a series of such expiratory maneuvers using increasing muscular intensity, expiratory flow rates will increase until a certain level of effort is reached. Beyond this level, additional effort at any given lung volume will not increase the forced expiratory flow rate; this phenomenon is known as the *effort independence* of FEF. The physiologic mechanisms determining the flow rates during this effort-independent phase of FEF are the elastic recoil of the lung, the airflow resistance of the airways between the alveolar zone and the physical site of flow limitation, and the airway wall compliance up to the site of flow limitation. Physical processes that decrease elastic recoil, increase airflow resistance, or increase airway wall compliance decrease the flow rate that can be achieved at any given lung volume. Conversely, processes that increase elastic recoil, decrease resistance, or stiffen airway walls increase the flow rate that can be achieved at any given lung volume.

MEASUREMENT OF VENTILATORY FUNCTION

Ventilatory function is measured under static conditions for determination of lung volumes and under dynamic conditions for determination of FEF. VC, expiratory reserve volume (ERV), and inspiratory capacity (IC) (Fig. 246-1) are measured by having the patient breathe into and out of a spirometer, a device capable of measuring expired or inspired gas volume while plotting volume as a function of time. Other volumes—specifically, RV, FRC, and TLC—cannot be measured in this way because they include the volume of gas present in the lungs

even after a maximal expiration. Two techniques are commonly used to measure these volumes: helium dilution and body plethysmography. In the helium dilution method, the subject repeatedly breathes in and out from a reservoir with a known volume of gas containing a trace amount of helium. The helium is diluted by the gas previously present in the lungs and very little is absorbed into the pulmonary circulation. From knowledge of the reservoir volume and the initial and final helium concentrations, the volume of gas present in the lungs can be calculated. The helium dilution method may underestimate the volume of gas in the lungs if there are slowly communicating airspaces, such as bullae. In this situation, lung volumes can be measured more accurately with a body plethysmograph, a sealed box in which the patient sits while panting against a closed mouthpiece. Because there is no airflow into or out of the plethysmograph, the pressure changes in the thorax during panting cause compression and rarefaction of gas in the lungs and simultaneous rarefaction and compression of gas in the plethysmograph. By measuring the pressure changes in the plethysmograph and at the mouthpiece, the volume of gas in the thorax can be calculated using Boyle's law.

Lung volumes and measurements made during forced expiration are interpreted by comparing the values measured with the values expected given the age, height, sex, and race of the patient (Appendix, Table 14). Because there is some variability among normal individuals, values between 80 and 120% of the predicted value have traditionally been considered normal. Increasingly, calculated percentiles are used in determining normality. Specifically, values of individual measurements falling below the fifth percentile are considered to be below normal.

Obstructive lung disease is determined by a decreased FEV_1/VC ratio, where VC is defined as the largest of the FVC, SVC (slow vital capacity) or IVC (inspiratory vital capacity). Although a ratio <0.7 is typically considered abnormal, the normal value does vary with age. Historically, the FVC was the standard denominator for this ratio, and for most individuals the FVC, SVC, and IVC are very similar. However, in individuals with airways obstruction the SVC or IVC may be larger than the FVC. The $FEF_{25-75\%}$ is often considered a more sensitive measurement of early airflow obstruction, particularly in small airways. However, this measurement is less specific and must be interpreted cautiously in patients with abnormally small lungs (low TLC and VC). These patients exhale less air during forced expiration, and the $FEF_{25-75\%}$ may appear abnormal relative to the usual predicted value, even though it is normal relative to the size of the patient's lungs.

It is also a common practice to plot expiratory flow rates against lung volume (rather than against time); the close linkage of flow rates to lung volumes produces a typical *flow-volume curve* (Fig. 246-4). In addition, the spirometric values mentioned above can be calculated from the flow-volume curve. Commonly, flow rates during a maximal inspiratory effort performed as rapidly as possible are plotted as well, making the flow-volume curve into a *flow-volume loop*. At TLC, before expiratory flow starts, the flow rate is zero; once forced expiration has begun, a high peak flow rate is rapidly achieved. As expiration continues and lung volume approaches RV, the flow rate falls progressively, in a nearly linear fashion as a function of lung volume for a person with normal lung function. During maximal inspiration from RV to TLC, inspiratory flow is most rapid at the midpoint of inspiration, so the inspiratory portion of the loop is U-shaped or saddle-shaped. The flow rates achieved during maximal expiration can be analyzed quantitatively by comparing the flow rates at specified lung volumes with the predicted values, or qualitatively by analyzing the shape of the descending limb of the expiratory curve.

Assessing the strength of respiratory muscles is an additional part of the overall evaluation of some patients with respiratory dysfunction. When a patient exhales completely to RV and then tries to inspire maximally against an occluded airway, the pressure that can be generated is called the *maximal inspiratory pressure* (MIP). On the other hand, when a patient inhales to TLC and then tries to expire maximally against an occluded airway, the pressure generated is called the *maximal expiratory pressure* (MEP). In the proper clinical setting, these

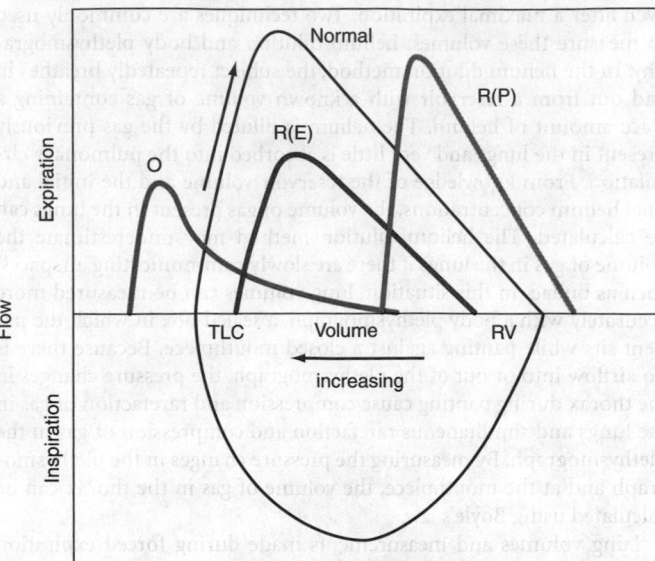

FIGURE 246-4 Flow-volume curves in different conditions: O, obstructive disease; R(P), parenchymal restrictive disease; R(E), extraparenchymal restrictive disease with limitation in inspiration and expiration. Forced expiration is plotted in all conditions; forced inspiration is shown only for the normal curve. TLC, total lung capacity; RV, residual volume. By convention, lung volume increases to the left on the abscissa. The arrow alongside the normal curve indicates the direction of expiration from TLC to RV.

studies may provide useful information regarding the cause of abnormal lung volumes and the possibility that respiratory muscle weakness may be causally related to the lung volume abnormalities.

PATTERNS OF ABNORMAL FUNCTION

The two major patterns of abnormal ventilatory function, as measured by static lung volumes and spirometry, are restrictive and obstructive patterns. In the *obstructive pattern*, the hallmark is a decrease in expiratory flow rates. With fully established disease, the ratio FEV_1/VC is decreased, as is the $FEF_{25-75\%}$ (Fig. 246-2, line *B*). The expiratory portion of the flow-volume loop demonstrates decreased flow rates for any given lung volume. Nonuniform emptying of airways is reflected by a coved (scooped) configuration of the descending part of the expiratory curve (Fig. 246-4). With early obstructive disease, which originates in the small airways, FEV_1/VC may be normal; the only abnormalities noted on routine testing of pulmonary function may be a depression in $FEF_{25-75\%}$ and an abnormal, i.e., coved, configuration in the terminal portion of the forced expiratory flow-volume curve.

In *obstructive* disease, the TLC is normal or increased. When helium equilibration tests are used to measure lung volumes, the measured volume may be less than the actual volume if helium was not well distributed to all regions of the lung. Residual volume is elevated as a result of airway closure during expiration, and the ratio RV/TLC is increased. VC is frequently decreased in obstructive disease because of the striking elevations in RV with only minor changes in TLC.

The hallmark of a *restrictive pattern* is a decrease in lung volumes, primarily TLC and VC. Disorders resulting in a restrictive pattern can be broadly divided into two subgroups, depending on the location of the pathology: pulmonary parenchymal and extraparenchymal. In pulmonary parenchymal disease, RV is also generally decreased, and FEF rates are preserved. In fact, when FEV_1 is considered as a percentage of the FVC, the flow rates are often supranormal, i.e., disproportionately high relative to the size of the lungs (Fig. 246-2, line *C*). The flow-volume curve may graphically demonstrate this disproportionate relationship between flow rates and lung volumes, since the expiratory portion of the curve appears relatively tall (preserved flow rates) but narrow (decreased lung volumes), as shown in Fig. 246-4.

With extraparenchymal disease, dysfunction can be due to neuromuscular disease with associated respiratory muscle weakness or to disorders of the chest wall or pleura (Table 246-1). In the extraparenchymal diseases, TLC is decreased due to inspiratory muscle weakness, a stiff chest wall, or a space-occupying process within the pleura. If inspiratory muscle weakness is the cause of this pattern, then RV is often not significantly affected, expiratory flow rates are preserved, and MIP is decreased. Alternatively, if the restrictive pattern is due to a deformed chest wall that is abnormally rigid at volumes below FRC, the ability to expire to a normal RV is also limited. Consequently, RV is often elevated, unlike the pattern observed in the other restrictive subcategories.

CLINICAL CORRELATIONS

Table 246-1 summarizes the typical patterns of altered ventilatory function as indicated by pulmonary function testing. This information can then be useful in diagnosis, as outlined in Table 246-2.

DISTURBANCES IN THE PULMONARY CIRCULATION

PHYSIOLOGIC FEATURES

The pulmonary vasculature must handle the entire output of the right ventricle, ~5 L/min in a normal adult at rest. The comparatively thin-walled vessels of the pulmonary arterial system provide relatively little resistance to flow and are capable of handling this large volume of blood at perfusion pressures that are low compared with those of the systemic circulation. The normal mean pulmonary artery pressure is 15 mmHg, as compared to ~95 mmHg for the normal mean aortic pressure. Regional blood flow in the lung is dependent on vascular geometry and on hydrostatic forces. In an upright person, perfusion is least at the apex of the lung and greatest at the base. When cardiac output increases, as occurs during exercise, the pulmonary vasculature is capable of recruiting previously unperfused vessels and distending underperfused vessels, thus responding to the increase in flow with a decrease in pulmonary vascular resistance. In consequence, the increase in mean pulmonary arterial pressure (PAP), even with a three- to fourfold increase in cardiac output, is small.

METHODS OF MEASUREMENT

Assessment of circulatory function in the pulmonary vasculature depends on measuring pulmonary vascular pressures and cardiac output. Clinically, these measurements are commonly made in intensive care units capable of invasive monitoring and in cardiac catheterization laboratories. With a flow-directed pulmonary arterial (Swan-Ganz) catheter, PAP and pulmonary capillary wedge pressure can be measured directly, and cardiac output can be obtained by the thermodilution method. Pulmonary vascular resistance (PVR) can then be calculated according to the equation

$$PVR = 80(PAP - PCW)/CO$$

where PVR = pulmonary vascular resistance (dyn · s/cm^5); PAP = mean pulmonary arterial pressure (mmHg); PCW = pulmonary capillary wedge pressure (mmHg); and CO = cardiac output (L/min).

The normal value for pulmonary vascular resistance is ~50–150 dyn · s/cm^5.

TABLE 246-1	ALTERATIONS IN VENTILATORY FUNCTION				
	TLC	**RV**	**VC**	**FEV$_1$/VC**	**MIP**
Obstructive	N to ↑	↑	↓ or N	↓	N
Restrictive					
Pulmonary parenchymal	↓	↓	↓	N to ↑	N
Extraparenchymal					
Neuromuscular weakness	↓	Variable[a]	↓	Variable[a]	↓
Chest wall deformity	↓	Variable[b]	↓	N	N

[a]Depends upon expiratory muscle strength.
[b]Depends upon specific chest wall disorder.

TABLE 246-2	**COMMON RESPIRATORY DISEASES BY DIAGNOSTIC CATEGORIES**

Obstructive
Asthma
Chronic obstructive lung disease (chronic bronchitis, emphysema)
Bronchiectasis
Cystic fibrosis
Bronchiolitis
Restrictive—Parenchymal
Sarcoidosis
Idiopathic pulmonary fibrosis
Pneumoconiosis
Drug- or radiation-induced interstitial lung disease
Restrictive—Extraparenchymal
Neuromuscular
  Diaphragmatic weakness/paralysis
  Myasthenia gravis
  Guillain-Barré syndrome
  Muscular dystrophies
  Cervical spine injury
Chest wall
  Kyphoscoliosis
  Obesity
  Ankylosing spondylitis

MECHANISMS OF ABNORMAL FUNCTION (See also Chap. 244)

PVR may increase by a variety of mechanisms. Pulmonary arterial and arteriolar vasoconstriction is a prominent response to alveolar hypoxia. PVR also increases if intraluminal thrombi or proliferation of smooth muscle in vessel walls diminishes the luminal cross-sectional area. If small pulmonary vessels are destroyed, either by scarring or by loss of alveolar walls (as in chronic obstructive lung disease), the total cross-sectional area of the pulmonary vascular bed diminishes, and PVR increases. When PVR is elevated, either PAP rises to maintain normal cardiac output or cardiac output falls if PAP does not increase.

CLINICAL CORRELATIONS

Disturbances in the function of the pulmonary vasculature as a result of primary cardiac disease, either congenital heart disease or conditions that elevate left atrial pressure, such as mitral stenosis, are beyond the scope of this chapter and are discussed in Chaps. 229 and 230, respectively. Instead, the focus will be on the pulmonary vasculature as its function is affected by diseases primarily involving the respiratory system, including the pulmonary vessels themselves.

All diseases of the respiratory system causing hypoxemia are potentially capable of increasing PVR, since alveolar hypoxia is a very potent stimulus for pulmonary vasoconstriction. The more prolonged and intense the hypoxic stimulus, the more likely it is that a significant increase in PVR producing pulmonary hypertension will result. In practice, patients with hypoxemia caused by chronic obstructive lung disease, interstitial lung disease, chest wall disease, and the obesity hypoventilation–sleep apnea syndrome are particularly prone to developing pulmonary hypertension. If there are additional structural changes in the pulmonary vasculature secondary to the underlying process, these will increase the likelihood of developing pulmonary hypertension.

With diseases directly affecting the pulmonary vessels, a decrease in the cross-sectional area of the pulmonary vascular bed is primarily responsible for increased PVR, while hypoxemia generally plays a lesser role. In the case of recurrent pulmonary emboli, parts of the pulmonary arterial system are occluded by intraluminal thrombi originating in the systemic venous system. With primary pulmonary hypertension (Chap. 244) or with pulmonary vascular disease secondary to scleroderma, the small pulmonary arteries and arterioles are affected by a generalized obliterative process that narrows and occludes these vessels. PVR increases, and significant pulmonary hypertension often results.

DISTURBANCES IN GAS EXCHANGE

PHYSIOLOGIC FEATURES

The primary functions of the respiratory system are to remove the appropriate amount of CO_2 from blood entering the pulmonary circulation and to provide adequate O_2 to blood leaving the pulmonary circulation. For these functions to be carried out properly, there must be adequate provision of fresh air to the alveoli for delivery of O_2 and removal of CO_2 (ventilation), adequate circulation of blood through the pulmonary vasculature (perfusion), adequate movement of gas between alveoli and pulmonary capillaries (diffusion), and appropriate contact between alveolar gas and pulmonary capillary blood (ventilation-perfusion matching).

A normal individual at rest inspires ~12–16 times per minute, each breath having a tidal volume of ~500 mL. A portion (~30%) of the fresh air inspired with each breath does not reach the alveoli but remains in the conducting airways of the lung. This component of each breath, which is not generally available for gas exchange, is called the *anatomic dead space* component. The remaining 70% reaches the alveolar zone, mixes rapidly with the gas already there, and can participate in gas exchange. In this example, the total ventilation each minute is ~7 L, composed of 2 L/min of dead space ventilation and 5 L/min of alveolar ventilation. In certain diseases, some alveoli are ventilated but not perfused, so that some ventilation in addition to the anatomic dead space component is wasted. If total dead space ventilation is increased but total minute ventilation is unchanged, then alveolar ventilation must fall correspondingly.

Gas exchange is dependent on alveolar ventilation rather than total minute ventilation, as outlined below. The partial pressure of CO_2 in arterial blood (Pa_{CO_2}) is directly proportional to the amount of CO_2 produced per minute ($\dot{V}_{CO_2}$) and inversely proportional to alveolar ventilation ($\dot{V}A$), according to the relationship

$$Pa_{CO_2} = 0.863 \times \dot{V}_{CO_2}/\dot{V}A$$

where $\dot{V}_{CO_2}$ is expressed in mL/min, $\dot{V}A$ in L/min, and Pa_{CO_2} in mmHg. At fixed $\dot{V}_{CO_2}$, when alveolar ventilation increases, Pa_{CO_2} falls, and when alveolar ventilation decreases, Pa_{CO_2} rises. Maintaining a normal level of O_2 in the alveoli (and consequently in arterial blood) also depends on provision of adequate alveolar ventilation to replenish alveolar O_2. This principle will become more apparent from consideration of the alveolar gas equation below.

Diffusion of O_2 and CO_2 Both O_2 and CO_2 diffuse readily down their respective concentration gradients through the alveolar wall and pulmonary capillary endothelium. Under normal circumstances, this process is rapid, and equilibration of both gases is complete within one-third of the transit time of erythrocytes through the pulmonary capillary bed. Even in disease states in which diffusion of gases is impaired, the impairment is unlikely to be severe enough to prevent equilibration of CO_2 and O_2. Consequently, a diffusion abnormality rarely results in arterial hypoxemia at rest. If erythrocyte transit time in the pulmonary circulation is shortened, as occurs with exercise, and diffusion is impaired, then diffusion limitation may contribute to hypoxemia. Exercise testing can often demonstrate such physiologically significant abnormalities due to impaired diffusion. Even though diffusion limitation rarely makes a clinically significant contribution to resting hypoxemia, clinical measurements of what is known as *diffusing capacity* (see below) can be a useful measure of the integrity of the alveolar-capillary membrane.

Ventilation-Perfusion Matching In addition to the absolute levels of alveolar ventilation and perfusion, gas exchange depends critically on the proper matching of ventilation and perfusion. The spectrum of possible ventilation-perfusion ($\dot{V}/\dot{Q}$) ratios in an alveolar-capillary unit ranges from zero, in which ventilation is totally absent and the unit behaves as a shunt, to infinity, in which perfusion is totally absent and the unit behaves as dead space. The P_{O_2} and P_{CO_2} of blood leaving each alveolar-capillary unit depend on the gas tension (of blood and air) entering that unit and on the particular $\dot{V}/\dot{Q}$ ratio of the unit. At one extreme, when an alveolar-capillary unit has a $\dot{V}/\dot{Q}$ ratio of 0 and behaves as a shunt, blood leaving the unit has the composition of mixed venous blood entering the pulmonary capillaries, i.e., $P\bar{v}_{O_2} \approx 40$ mmHg and $P\bar{v}_{CO_2} \approx 46$ mmHg. At the other extreme, when an alveolar-capillary unit has a high $\dot{V}/\dot{Q}$ ratio, it behaves almost like dead space, and the small amount of blood leaving the unit has partial pressures of O_2 and CO_2 ($P_{O_2} \approx 150$ mmHg, $P_{CO_2} \approx 0$ mmHg while breathing room air) approaching the composition of inspired gas.

In the ideal situation, all alveolar-capillary units have equal matching of ventilation and perfusion, i.e., a ratio of ~1 when each is expressed in L/min. However, even in the normal individual, some $\dot{V}/\dot{Q}$ mismatching is present, since there is normally an increasing gradient of blood flow from the apices to the bases of the lungs. There is a similar gradient of ventilation from the apices to the bases, but it is less marked than the perfusion gradient. As a result, ventilation-perfusion ratios are higher at the lung apices than at the lung bases. Therefore, blood coming from the apices has a higher P_{O_2} and lower P_{CO_2} than blood coming from the bases. The net P_{O_2} and P_{CO_2} of the blood mixture coming from all areas of the lung is a flow-weighted average of the individual components, which reflects both the relative amount of blood from each unit and the O_2 and CO_2 *content* of the blood coming from each unit. Because of the sigmoid shape of the oxyhemoglobin dissociation curve (see Fig. 99-2), it is important to distinguish between the partial pressure and the content of O_2 in blood. Hemoglobin is almost fully (~90%) saturated at a P_{O_2} of 60 mmHg, and little additional O_2 is carried by hemoglobin even with a substantial elevation of P_{O_2} >60 mmHg. On the other hand, significant O_2 desaturation of hemoglobin occurs once P_{O_2} falls to <60 mmHg and onto the steep descending limb of the curve. As a result, blood coming from regions of the lung with a high $\dot{V}/\dot{Q}$ ratio and a high P_{O_2} has only a small elevation in O_2 content and cannot compensate for blood coming from regions with a low $\dot{V}/\dot{Q}$ ratio and a low P_{O_2}, which has a significantly decreased O_2 content. Although $\dot{V}/\dot{Q}$ mismatching can influence P_{CO_2}, this effect is less marked and is often overcome by an increase in overall minute ventilation.

MEASUREMENT OF GAS EXCHANGE

Arterial Blood Gases   The most commonly used measures of gas exchange are the partial pressures of O_2 and CO_2 in arterial blood, i.e., Pa_{O_2} and Pa_{CO_2}, respectively. These partial pressures do not measure directly the quantity of O_2 and CO_2 in blood but rather the driving pressure for the gas in blood. The actual quantity or content of a gas in blood also depends on the solubility of the gas in plasma and the ability of any component of blood to react with or bind the gas of interest. Since hemoglobin is capable of binding large amounts of O_2, oxygenated hemoglobin is the primary form in which O_2 is transported in blood. The actual content of O_2 in blood therefore depends both on the hemoglobin concentration and on the Pa_{O_2}. The Pa_{O_2} determines what percentage of hemoglobin is saturated with O_2, based on the position on the oxyhemoglobin dissociation curve. Oxygen content in normal blood (at 37°C, pH 7.4) can be determined by adding the amount of O_2 dissolved in plasma to the amount bound to hemoglobin, according to the equation

$$O_2 \text{ content} = 1.34 \times [\text{hemoglobin}] \times \text{saturation} + 0.0031 \times P_{O_2}$$

since each gram of hemoglobin is capable of carrying 1.34 mL O_2 when fully saturated, and the amount of O_2 that can be dissolved in plasma is proportional to the P_{O_2}, with 0.0031 mL O_2 dissolved per deciliter of blood per mmHg P_{O_2}. In arterial blood, the amount of O_2 transported dissolved in plasma (~0.3 mL O_2 per deciliter of blood) is trivial compared with the amount bound to hemoglobin (~20 mL O_2 per deciliter of blood).

Most commonly, P_{O_2} is the measurement used to assess the effect of respiratory disease on the oxygenation of arterial blood. Direct measurement of O_2 saturation in arterial blood by oximetry is also important in selected clinical conditions. For example, in patients with carbon mon-

oxide intoxication, carbon monoxide preferentially displaces O_2 from hemoglobin, essentially making a portion of hemoglobin unavailable for binding to O_2. In this circumstance, carbon monoxide saturation is high and O_2 saturation is low, even though the driving pressure for O_2 to bind to hemoglobin, reflected by P_{O_2}, is normal. Measurement of O_2 saturation is also important for the determination of O_2 content when mixed venous blood is sampled from a pulmonary arterial catheter to calculate cardiac output by the Fick technique. In mixed venous blood, the P_{O_2} is normally ~40 mmHg, but small changes in P_{O_2} may reflect relatively large changes in O_2 saturation.

A useful calculation in the assessment of oxygenation is the alveolar-arterial O_2 difference ($PA_{O_2} - Pa_{O_2}$), commonly called the *alveolar-arterial O_2 gradient* (or A – a gradient). This calculation takes into account the fact that alveolar and, hence, arterial P_{O_2} can be expected to change depending on the level of alveolar ventilation, reflected by the arterial P_{CO_2}. When a patient hyperventilates and has a low P_{CO_2} in arterial blood and alveolar gas, alveolar and arterial P_{O_2} will rise; conversely, hypoventilation and a high P_{CO_2} are accompanied by a decrease in alveolar and arterial P_{O_2}. These changes in arterial P_{O_2} are independent of abnormalities in O_2 transfer at the alveolar-capillary level and reflect only the dependence of alveolar P_{O_2} on the level of alveolar ventilation.

In order to determine the alveolar-arterial O_2 difference, the alveolar P_{O_2} (PA_{O_2}) must first be calculated. The equation most commonly used for this purpose, a simplified form of the alveolar gas equation, is

$$PA_{O_2} = FI_{O_2} \times (P_B - P_{H_2O}) - Pa_{CO_2}/R$$

where FI_{O_2} = fractional concentration of inspired O_2 (0.21 when breathing room air); P_B = barometric pressure (~760 mmHg at sea level); P_{H_2O} = water vapor pressure (47 mmHg when air is fully saturated at 37°C); and R = respiratory quotient (the ratio of CO_2 production to O_2 consumption, usually assumed to be 0.8). If the preceding values are substituted into the equation for the patient breathing air at sea level, the equation becomes

$$PA_{O_2} = 150 - 1.25 \times Pa_{CO_2}$$

The alveolar-arterial O_2 difference can then be calculated by subtracting measured Pa_{O_2} from calculated PA_{O_2}. In a healthy young person breathing room air, the $PA_{O_2} - Pa_{O_2}$ is normally <15 mmHg; this value increases with age and may be as high as 30 mmHg in elderly patients.

The adequacy of CO_2 elimination is measured by the partial pressure of CO_2 in arterial blood, i.e., Pa_{CO_2}. A more complete understanding of the mechanisms and chronicity of abnormal levels of P_{CO_2} also requires measurement of pH and/or bicarbonate (HCO_3^-), since P_{CO_2} and the patient's acid-base status are so closely intertwined (Chap. 48).

Pulse Oximetry   Because measurement of Pa_{O_2} requires arterial puncture, it is not ideal either for office use or for routine or frequent measurement in the inpatient setting. Additionally, because it provides intermittent rather than continuous data about the patient's oxygenation, it is not ideal for close monitoring of unstable patients. Pulse oximetry, an alternative method for assessing oxygenation, is readily available in many clinical settings. Using a probe usually clipped over a patient's finger, the pulse oximeter calculates oxygen saturation (rather than Pa_{O_2}) based on measurements of absorption of two wavelengths of light by hemoglobin in pulsatile, cutaneous arterial blood. Because of differential absorption of the two wavelengths of light by oxygenated and nonoxygenated hemoglobin, the percentage of hemoglobin that is saturated with oxygen, i.e., the Sa_{O_2}, can be calculated and displayed instantaneously.

Although the pulse oximeter is widely used in the noninvasive assessment and monitoring of oxygenation, there are several issues and potential problems concerning its use. First, the clinician must be aware of the relationship between oxygen saturation and tension as shown by the oxyhemoglobin dissociation curve (see Fig. 99-2). Because the curve becomes relatively flat above an arterial P_{O_2} of 60

APPROACH TO PATIENT WITH HYPOXEMIA

FIGURE 246-5 Flow diagram outlining the diagnostic approach to the patient with hypoxemia ($Pa_{O_2} < 80$ mmHg). $PA_{O_2} - Pa_{O_2}$ is usually <15 mmHg for subjects ≤30 years old and increases by ~3 mmHg per decade after age 30. COPD, chronic obstructive pulmonary disease.

mmHg (corresponding to $Sa_{O_2} = 90\%$), the oximeter is relatively insensitive to changes in Pa_{O_2} above this level. In addition, the position of the curve and therefore the specific relationship between Pa_{O_2} and Sa_{O_2} may change depending on factors such as temperature, pH, and the erythrocyte concentration of 2,3-diphosphoglycerate. Second, when cutaneous perfusion is decreased, e.g., owing to low cardiac output or the use of vasoconstrictors, the signal from the oximeter may be less reliable or even unobtainable. Third, other forms of hemoglobin, such as carboxyhemoglobin and methemoglobin, are not distinguishable from oxyhemoglobin when only two wavelengths of light are used. The Sa_{O_2} values reported by the pulse oximeter are not reliable in the presence of significant amounts of either of these forms of hemoglobin. In contrast, the device used to measure oxygen saturation in samples of arterial blood, called the CO-oximeter, uses at least four wavelengths of light and is capable of distinguishing oxyhemoglobin, deoxygenated hemoglobin, carboxyhemoglobin, and methemoglobin. Finally, the clinician must remember that the often-used goal of $Sa_{O_2} \geq 90\%$ does not indicate anything about CO_2 elimination and therefore does not ensure a clinically acceptable P_{CO_2}.

Diffusing Capacity The ability of gas to diffuse across the alveolar-capillary membrane is ordinarily assessed by the diffusing capacity of the lung for carbon monoxide (DL_{CO}). In this test, a small concentration of carbon monoxide (0.3%) is inhaled, usually in a single breath that is held for ~10 s. During the breath hold, the carbon monoxide is diluted by the gas already present in the alveoli and is also taken up by hemoglobin as the erythrocytes course through the pulmonary capillary system. The concentration of carbon monoxide is then measured in the gas exhaled after the breath hold, and DL_{CO} is calculated as the quantity of carbon monoxide absorbed per minute per mmHg pressure gradient from the alveoli to the pulmonary capillaries. The value obtained for DL_{CO} depends on the alveolar-capillary surface area available for gas exchange and on the pulmonary capillary blood volume. In addition, the thickness of the alveolar-capillary membrane, the degree of $\dot{V}/\dot{Q}$ mismatching, and the patient's hemoglobin level will affect the measurement. Because of this effect of hemoglobin levels on DL_{CO}, the measured DL_{CO} is frequently corrected to take the patient's hemoglobin level into account. The value for DL_{CO}, ideally corrected for hemoglobin, can then be compared with a predicted value, based either on age, height, and gender or on the alveolar volume (VA) at which the value was obtained. Alternatively, the DL_{CO} can be divided by VA and the resulting value for DL_{CO}/VA compared with a predicted value.

APPROACH TO THE PATIENT:
Disturbance of Respiratory Function

ARTERIAL BLOOD GASES Hypoxemia is a common manifestation of a variety of diseases affecting the lungs or other parts of the respiratory system. The broad clinical problem of hypoxemia is often best characterized according to the underlying mechanism. The four basic, and not mutually exclusive, mechanisms of hypoxemia are (1) a decrease in inspired P_{O_2}, (2) hypoventilation, (3) shunting, and (4) $\dot{V}/\dot{Q}$ mismatching. A fifth potential mechanism of hypoxemia, due to decreased diffusion, occurs only under selected clinical circumstances and is not usually included among the general categories of hypoxemia. Determining the underlying mechanism for hypoxemia depends on measurement of the Pa_{CO_2}, calculation of $PA_{O_2} - Pa_{O_2}$, and knowledge of the response to supplemental O_2. A flowchart summarizing the approach to the hypoxemic patient is given in Fig. 246-5. See also Chap. 35.

A decrease in the inspired P_{O_2} and hypoventilation both cause hypoxemia by lowering PA_{O_2} and therefore Pa_{O_2}. In each case, gas exchange at the alveolar-capillary level occurs normally, and $PA_{O_2} - Pa_{O_2}$ is not elevated. Hypoxemia due to decreased inspired P_{O_2} can be diagnosed from knowledge of the clinical situation. Inspired P_{O_2} is lowered either because the patient is at a high altitude, where barometric pressure is low, or, much less commonly, because the patient is breathing a gas mixture containing <21% O_2. The hallmark of hypoventilation as a cause of hypoxemia is an elevation in Pa_{CO_2}. This is associated with an increase in PA_{CO_2} and a fall in PA_{O_2}. When hypoxemia is due purely to a low inspired P_{O_2} or to alveolar hypoventilation, $PA_{O_2} - Pa_{O_2}$ is normal. If $PA_{O_2} - Pa_{O_2}$ and Pa_{CO_2} are both elevated, then an additional mechanism, such as $\dot{V}/\dot{Q}$ mismatching or shunting, is contributing to hypoxemia.

Shunting is a cause of hypoxemia when desaturated blood effectively bypasses oxygenation at the alveolar-capillary level. This situation occurs either because a structural problem allows desaturated blood to bypass the normal site of gas exchange or because perfused alveoli are not ventilated. Shunting is associated with an elevation in the $PA_{O_2} - Pa_{O_2}$ value. When shunting is an important contributing factor to hypoxemia, the lowered Pa_{O_2} is relatively refractory to improvement by supplemental O_2.

Finally, the largest clinical category of hypoxemia is $\dot{V}/\dot{Q}$ mismatching. With $\dot{V}/\dot{Q}$ mismatching, regions with low $\dot{V}/\dot{Q}$ ratios contribute blood with a low P_{O_2} and a low O_2 content. Corresponding regions with high $\dot{V}/\dot{Q}$ ratios contribute blood with a high P_{O_2}. However, because blood is already almost fully saturated at a normal P_{O_2}, elevation of the P_{O_2} to a high value does not significantly increase O_2 saturation or content and therefore cannot compensate for the reduction of O_2 saturation and content in blood coming from regions with a low $\dot{V}/\dot{Q}$ ratio. When $\dot{V}/\dot{Q}$ mismatch is the primary cause of hypoxemia, $PA_{O_2} - Pa_{O_2}$ is elevated, and P_{CO_2} generally is normal. Supplemental O_2 corrects the hypoxemia by raising the P_{O_2} in blood coming from regions with a low $\dot{V}/\dot{Q}$ ratio; this response distinguishes hypoxemia due to $\dot{V}/\dot{Q}$ mismatching from that due to true shunt.

The essential mechanism underlying all cases of hypercapnia is alveolar ventilation that is inadequate for the amount of CO_2 produced. It is conceptually useful to characterize CO_2 retention further, based on a more detailed examination of the potential contributing factors. These include (1) increased CO_2 production; (2) decreased ventilatory drive ("won't breathe"); (3) malfunction of the respiratory pump or increased airways resistance, which makes it more difficult to sustain adequate ventilation ("can't breathe"); and (4) inefficiency of gas exchange (increased dead space or $\dot{V}/\dot{Q}$ mismatch) necessitating a compensatory increase in overall minute ventilation. In practice, more than one of these mechanisms is commonly responsible for hypercapnia, since increased minute ventilation is capable of compensating for increased CO_2 production and for inefficiencies of gas exchange.

DIFFUSING CAPACITY Although abnormalities in diffusion are rarely responsible for hypoxemia, clinical measurement of diffusing capacity is frequently used to assess the functional integrity of the alveolar-capillary membrane, which includes the pulmonary capillary bed. Diseases that affect solely the airways generally do not lower DL_{CO}, whereas diseases that affect the alveolar walls or the pulmonary capillary bed will have an effect on DL_{CO}. Even though DL_{CO} is a useful marker for assessing whether disease affecting the alveolar-capillary bed is present, an abnormal DL_{CO} does not necessarily imply that diffusion limitation is responsible for hypoxemia in a particular patient.

CLINICAL CORRELATIONS

Useful clinical correlations can be made with the mechanisms underlying hypoxemia (Fig. 246-5). A lowered inspired P_{O_2} contributes to hypoxemia if either the patient is at high altitude or the concentration of inspired O_2 is <21%. The latter problem occurs if a patient receiving anesthesia or ventilatory support is inadvertently given a gas mixture to breathe containing <21% O_2 or if O_2 is consumed from the ambient gas, as can occur during smoke inhalation from a fire. The primary feature of hypoventilation as a cause of hypoxemia is an elevation in arterial P_{CO_2}. For further discussion of the clinical correlations with hypoventilation, see Chap. 258.

Shunting as a cause of hypoxemia can reflect transfer of blood from the right to the left side of the heart without passage through the pulmonary circulation, as occurs with an intracardiac shunt. This problem is most common in the setting of cyanotic congenital heart disease, when an interatrial or interventricular septal defect is associated with pulmonary hypertension so that shunting is in the right-to-left rather than the left-to-right direction. Shunting of blood through the pulmonary parenchyma is most frequently due to disease causing absence of ventilation to perfused alveoli. This can occur if the alveoli

are atelectatic or if they are filled with fluid, as in pulmonary edema (both cardiogenic and noncardiogenic), or with extensive intraalveolar exudation of fluid due to pneumonia. Less commonly, vascular anomalies with arteriovenous shunting in the lung can cause hypoxemia. These anomalies can be hereditary, as found with hereditary hemorrhagic telangiectasia (Osler-Rendu-Weber syndrome), or acquired, as in pulmonary vascular malformations secondary to hepatic cirrhosis, which are similar to the commonly recognized cutaneous vascular malformations ("spider hemangiomas").

Ventilation-perfusion mismatch is the most common cause of hypoxemia clinically. Most of the processes affecting either the airways or the pulmonary parenchyma are distributed unevenly throughout the lungs and do not necessarily affect ventilation and perfusion equally. Some areas of lung may have good perfusion and poor ventilation, whereas others may have poor perfusion and relatively good ventilation. Important examples of airways diseases in which $\dot{V}/\dot{Q}$ mismatch causes hypoxemia are asthma and chronic obstructive lung disease. Parenchymal lung diseases causing $\dot{V}/\dot{Q}$ mismatch and hypoxemia include interstitial lung disease and pneumonia.

Clinically important alterations in CO_2 elimination range from excessive ventilation and hypocapnia to inadequate CO_2 elimination and hypercapnia. For further discussion of these clinical problems, see Chap. 258.

Diffusing Capacity Measurement of DL_{CO} may be useful for assessing disease affecting the alveolar-capillary bed or the pulmonary vasculature. In practice, three main categories of disease are associated with lowered DL_{CO}: interstitial lung disease, emphysema, and pulmonary vascular disease. With interstitial lung disease, scarring of alveolar-capillary units diminishes the area of the alveolar-capillary bed as well as pulmonary blood volume. With emphysema, alveolar walls are destroyed, so the surface area of the alveolar-capillary bed is again diminished. In patients with disease causing a decrease in the cross-sectional area and volume of the pulmonary vascular bed, such as recurrent pulmonary emboli or primary pulmonary hypertension, DL_{CO} is commonly diminished.

Diffusing capacity may be elevated if pulmonary blood volume is increased, as may be seen in congestive heart failure. However, once interstitial and alveolar edema ensues, the net DL_{CO} depends on the opposing influences of increased pulmonary capillary blood volume elevating DL_{CO} and pulmonary edema decreasing it. Finding an elevated DL_{CO} may be useful in the diagnosis of alveolar hemorrhage, as in Goodpasture's syndrome. Hemoglobin contained in erythrocytes in the alveolar lumen is capable of binding carbon monoxide, so the exhaled carbon monoxide concentration is diminished and the measured DL_{CO} is increased.

ACKNOWLEDGMENT

We acknowledge the contribution of Dr. Jeffrey M. Drazen to this chapter in previous editions.

FURTHER READINGS

CELLI BR: The importance of spirometry in COPD and asthma: Effect on approach to management. Chest 117:15S, 2000

CHUPP GL (ed): Pulmonary function testing. Clin Chest Med 22:599, 2001

PELLEGRINO R et al: Interpretative strategies for lung function tests. Eur Respir J 26:948, 2005

ROSE BD, POST T: *Clinical Physiology of Acid-Base and Electrolyte Disorders*, 5th ed. New York, McGraw-Hill, 2000

SCHWARTZSTEIN RM, PARKER MJ: *Respiratory Physiology: A Clinical Approach.* Philadelphia, Lippincott Williams & Wilkins, 2006

WEINBERGER SE: *Principles of Pulmonary Medicine*, 4th ed. Philadelphia, Saunders, 2004

247 Diagnostic Procedures in Respiratory Disease

Scott Manaker, Steven E. Weinberger

The diagnostic modalities available for assessing the patient with suspected or known respiratory system disease include imaging studies and techniques for acquiring biologic specimens, some of which involve direct visualization of part of the respiratory system. Methods to characterize the functional changes developing as a result of disease, including pulmonary function tests and measurements of gas exchange, are discussed in Chap. 246.

IMAGING STUDIES

Routine Radiography Routine chest radiography, generally including both posteroanterior and lateral views, is an integral part of the diagnostic evaluation of diseases involving the pulmonary parenchyma, the pleura, and, to a lesser extent, the airways and the mediastinum (see **Chap. e24**). Lateral decubitus views are often useful for determining whether pleural abnormalities represent freely flowing fluid, whereas apical lordotic views can often visualize disease at the lung apices better than the standard posteroanterior view. Portable equipment, which is often used for acutely ill patients who either cannot be transported to a radiology suite or cannot stand for posteroanterior and lateral views, generally yields a single radiograph taken in the anteroposterior direction. Common radiographic patterns and their clinical correlates are reviewed in **Chap. e24**.

Computed Tomography CT offers several advantages over routine chest radiography (**Figs. 247-1** and **247-2**; see also Figs. 255-3, 255-4, and 262-4). First, the use of cross-sectional images allows distinction between densities that would be superimposed on plain radiographs. Second, CT is far better than routine radiographic studies at characterizing tissue density, distinguishing subtle density differences between adjacent structures, and providing accurate size assessment of lesions. As a result, CT is particularly valuable in assessing hilar and mediastinal disease (which is often poorly characterized by plain radiography), in identifying and characterizing disease adjacent to the chest wall or spine (including pleural disease), and in identifying areas of fat density or calcification in pulmonary nodules (Fig. 247-1). Its utility in the assessment of mediastinal disease has made CT an important tool in the staging of lung cancer (Chap. 85), as an assessment of tumor involvement of mediastinal lymph nodes is critical to proper

FIGURE 247-1 CT scan demonstrating a mediastinal mass of heterogeneous density (*arrow*). CT is superior to plain radiography for the detection of abnormal mediastinal densities and the distinction of masses from adjacent vascular structures.

FIGURE 247-2 High-resolution CT scan from a patient with idiopathic pulmonary fibrosis. There are scattered reticular densities (arrows point to examples) that are especially prominent at the periphery of the lungs. This particular cross-section is from the base of the lungs, where the findings in idiopathic pulmonary fibrosis tend to be most marked.

staging. With the additional use of contrast material, CT also makes it possible to distinguish vascular from nonvascular structures, which is particularly important in distinguishing lymph nodes and masses from vascular structures primarily in the mediastinum.

Helical CT scanning allows the collection of continuous data over a larger volume of lung during a single breath-holding maneuver than is possible with conventional CT. With CT angiography, in which IV contrast is administered and images are acquired rapidly by helical scanning, pulmonary emboli can be detected in segmental and larger pulmonary arteries. With high-resolution CT (HRCT), the thickness of individual cross-sectional images is ~1–2 mm, rather than the usual 7–10 mm, and the images are reconstructed using high-spatial-resolution algorithms. The visible detail on HRCT scans allows better recognition of subtle parenchymal and airway disease, such as bronchiectasis, emphysema, and diffuse parenchymal disease (Fig. 247-2). Certain characteristic patterns have now been recognized for many of the interstitial lung diseases, such as lymphangitic carcinoma, idiopathic pulmonary fibrosis, sarcoidosis, and eosinophilic granuloma; however, it is not yet clear in what settings these patterns obviate the need for obtaining lung tissue.

Recent advances in computer processing of helical scanning data have provided the opportunity to display images in views and planes other than the traditional cross-sectional view, including sophisticated three-dimensional reconstructions, to produce images (called *virtual bronchoscopy*) mimicking direct visualization through a bronchoscope.

Magnetic Resonance Imaging The role of MR imaging in the evaluation of respiratory system disease is less well defined than that of CT. Because MR generally provides a less detailed view of the pulmonary parenchyma as well as poorer spatial resolution, its usefulness in the evaluation of parenchymal lung disease is limited at present. However, MR images can be reconstructed in sagittal and coronal as well as transverse planes, so that the technique is well suited for imaging abnormalities near the lung apex, the spine, and the thoracoabdominal junction. MR images depend on tissue characteristics other than density, unlike CT scanning. Therefore, in selected circumstances, MR images can better suggest the nature of abnormal tissue than can density-determined CT images. Finally, MR is particularly well-suited to evaluate intrathoracic cardiovascular pathology and to distinguish vascular from nonvascular structures without the need for contrast. Flowing blood does not produce a signal on MR imaging, so vessels appear as hollow tubular structures. This feature can be useful in determining whether abnormal hilar or mediastinal densities are vascular in origin and in defining aortic lesions, such as aneurysms or dissection. In addition, gadolinium can be used as an intravascular contrast agent for MR angiography.

Scintigraphic Imaging   Radioactive isotopes, administered by either IV or inhaled routes, allow the lungs to be imaged with a gamma camera. In the past, scintigraphic imaging in the form of ventilation-perfusion lung scanning was commonly performed for evaluation of pulmonary embolism. However, with advances in CT scanning, scintigraphic imaging has largely been replaced by CT angiography in patients with suspected pulmonary embolism. When injected intravenously, albumin macroaggregates labeled with technetium 99m become lodged in pulmonary capillaries; therefore, the distribution of the trapped radioisotope follows the distribution of blood flow. When inhaled, radiolabeled xenon gas can be used to demonstrate the distribution of ventilation. For example, pulmonary thromboembolism usually produces one or more regions of ventilation-perfusion mismatch, i.e., regions in which there is a defect in perfusion that follows the distribution of a vessel and that is not accompanied by a corresponding defect in ventilation (Chap. 256). Another common use of such radioisotope scans is in a patient with impaired lung function who is being considered for lung resection. The distribution of the isotope(s) can be used to assess the regional distribution of blood flow and ventilation, allowing the physician to estimate the level of postoperative lung function.

Positron Emission Tomographic Scanning   Positron emission tomographic (PET) scanning is increasingly being used to identify malignant lesions in the lung based on their increased uptake and metabolism of glucose. The technique involves injection of a radiolabeled glucose analogue, [^{18}F]-fluoro-2-deoxyglucose (FDG), which is taken up by metabolically active malignant cells. However, FDG is trapped within the cell following phosphorylation, and the unstable fluorine 18 decays by emission of positrons, which can be detected by a specialized PET camera or by a gamma camera that has been adapted for imaging of positron-emitting nuclides. This technique has been used in the evaluation of solitary pulmonary nodules and as an aid to staging lung cancer through identification of mediastinal lymph node involvement by malignancy.

Pulmonary Angiography   The pulmonary arterial system can be visualized by pulmonary angiography, in which radiopaque contrast medium is injected through a catheter previously placed in the pulmonary artery. When performed in cases of pulmonary embolism, pulmonary angiography demonstrates the consequences of an intravascular thrombus—either a defect in the lumen of a vessel (a "filling defect") or an abrupt termination ("cutoff") of the vessel. Other, less common indications for pulmonary angiography include visualization of a suspected pulmonary arteriovenous malformation and assessment of pulmonary arterial invasion by a neoplasm. However, with advances in CT scanning, traditional pulmonary angiography has largely been replaced by CT angiography. The latter allows rapid acquisition of images with a less invasive procedure, since the radiocontrast material is injected intravenously rather than into a pulmonary artery.

Ultrasound   Because ultrasound energy is rapidly dissipated in air, ultrasound imaging is not useful for evaluation of the pulmonary parenchyma. However, ultrasound is helpful in the detection and localization of pleural abnormalities and is often used as a guide to placement of a needle for sampling of pleural liquid (i.e., for thoracentesis). Endobronchial ultrasound, in which the ultrasound probe is passed through a bronchoscope, is emerging as a valuable adjunct to bronchoscopy, allowing identification and localization of pathology adjacent to airway walls or within the mediastinum.

TECHNIQUES FOR OBTAINING BIOLOGIC SPECIMENS
Collection of Sputum   Sputum can be collected either by spontaneous expectoration or after inhalation of an irritating aerosol, such as hypertonic saline. The latter method, called *sputum induction*, is commonly used to obtain sputum for diagnostic studies, either because sputum is not spontaneously being produced or because of an expected higher yield of certain types of findings. Knowledge of the appearance and quality of the sputum specimen obtained is especially important when one is interested in Gram's staining and culture. Because sputum consists mainly of secretions from the tracheobronchial tree rather than the upper airway, the finding of alveolar macrophages and other inflammatory cells is consistent with a lower respiratory tract origin of the sample, whereas the presence of squamous epithelial cells in a "sputum" sample indicates contamination by secretions from the upper airways.

In addition to processing for routine bacterial pathogens by Gram's staining and culture, sputum can be processed for a variety of other pathogens, including staining and culture for mycobacteria or fungi, culture for viruses, and staining for *Pneumocystis jiroveci*. In the specific case of sputum obtained for evaluation of *P. jiroveci* pneumonia in a patient infected with HIV, for example, sputum should be collected by induction rather than spontaneous expectoration, and an immunofluorescent stain should be used to detect the organisms. Cytologic staining of sputum for malignant cells, using the traditional Papanicolaou method, allows noninvasive evaluation for suspected lung cancer. Traditional stains and cultures are now also being supplemented in some cases by immunologic techniques and by molecular biologic methods, including the use of polymerase chain reaction amplification and DNA probes.

Percutaneous Needle Aspiration   A needle can be inserted through the chest wall into a pulmonary lesion to aspirate material for analysis by cytologic or microbiologic techniques. The procedure is usually carried out under CT guidance to assist positioning of the needle and assure localization in the lesion. The low potential risk of this procedure (intrapulmonary bleeding or creation of a pneumothorax with collapse of the underlying lung) in experienced hands is usually acceptable owing to the information obtained. However, a limitation of the technique is sampling error due to the small size of the tissue sample. Thus, findings other than a specific cytologic or microbiologic diagnosis are of limited clinical value.

Thoracentesis   Sampling of pleural liquid by thoracentesis is commonly performed for diagnostic purposes or, in the case of a large effusion, for palliation of dyspnea. Diagnostic sampling, either by blind needle aspiration or after localization by ultrasound, allows the collection of liquid for microbiologic and cytologic studies. Analysis of the fluid obtained for its cellular composition and chemical constituents, including glucose, protein, and lactate dehydrogenase, allows the effusion to be classified as either exudative or transudative (Chap. 257).

Bronchoscopy   Bronchoscopy is the process of direct visualization of the tracheobronchial tree. Although bronchoscopy is now performed almost exclusively with flexible fiberoptic instruments, rigid bronchoscopy, generally performed in an operating room on a patient under general anesthesia, still has a role in selected circumstances, primarily because of a larger suction channel and the fact that the patient can be ventilated through the bronchoscope channel. These situations include the retrieval of a foreign body and the suctioning of a massive hemorrhage, for which the small suction channel of the bronchoscope may be insufficient.

FLEXIBLE FIBEROPTIC BRONCHOSCOPY   This outpatient procedure is usually performed in an awake but sedated patient. The bronchoscope is passed through either the mouth or the nose, between the vocal cords, and into the trachea. The ability to flex the scope makes it possible to visualize virtually all airways to the level of subsegmental bronchi. The bronchoscopist is able to identify endobronchial pathology, including tumors, granulomas, bronchitis, foreign bodies, and sites of bleeding. Samples from airway lesions can be taken by several methods, including washing, brushing, and biopsy. Washing involves instillation of sterile saline through a channel of the bronchoscope and onto the surface of a lesion. A portion of the liquid is collected by suctioning through the bronchoscope, and the recovered material can be analyzed for cells (cytology) or organisms (by standard stains and cultures). Brushing or biopsy of the surface of the lesion, using a small brush or biopsy forceps at the end of a long cable inserted through a channel of the bronchoscope, allows recovery of cellular material or tissue for analysis by standard cytologic and histopathologic methods.

The bronchoscope can be used to sample material not only from the regions that can be directly visualized (i.e., the airways) but also from the more distal pulmonary parenchyma. With the bronchoscope wedged into a subsegmental airway, aliquots of sterile saline can be instilled through the scope, allowing sampling of cells and organisms even from alveolar spaces. This procedure, called *bronchoalveolar lavage*, has been particularly useful for the recovery of organisms such as *P. jiroveci* in patients with HIV infection.

Brushing and biopsy of the distal lung parenchyma can also be performed with the same instruments that are used for endobronchial sampling. These instruments can be passed through the scope into small airways, where they penetrate the airway wall, allowing biopsy of peribronchial alveolar tissue. This procedure, called *transbronchial biopsy*, is used when there is either relatively diffuse disease or a localized lesion of adequate size. With the aid of fluoroscopic imaging, the bronchoscopist is able to determine not only whether and when the instrument is in the area of abnormality, but also the proximity of the instrument to the pleural surface. If the forceps are too close to the pleural surface, there is a risk of violating the visceral pleura and creating a pneumothorax; the other potential complication of transbronchial biopsy is pulmonary hemorrhage. The incidence of these complications is less than several percent.

Another procedure involves use of a hollow-bore needle passed through the bronchoscope for sampling of tissue adjacent to the trachea or a large bronchus. The needle is passed through the airway wall, and cellular material can be aspirated from mass lesions or enlarged lymph nodes, generally in a search for malignant cells. This procedure can facilitate the staging of lung cancer by identifying mediastinal lymph node involvement and in some cases obviates the need for a more invasive procedure. Other promising new techniques that are not yet widely available include fluorescence bronchoscopy (to detect early endobronchial malignancy) and endobronchial ultrasound (to better identify and localize peribronchial and mediastinal pathology).

The bronchoscope may provide the opportunity for treatment as well as diagnosis. For example, an aspirated foreign body may be retrieved with an instrument passed through the scope, and bleeding may be controlled with a balloon catheter similarly introduced. Newer interventional techniques performed through a bronchoscope include methods for achieving and maintaining patency of airways that are partially or completely occluded, especially by tumors. These techniques include laser therapy, cryotherapy, argon plasma coagulation, electrocautery, and stent placement.

Video-Assisted Thoracic Surgery Advances in video technology have allowed the development of thoracoscopy, or video-assisted thoracic surgery (VATS), for the diagnosis and management of pleural as well as parenchymal lung disease. This procedure involves the passage of a rigid scope with a distal lens through a trocar inserted into the pleura. A high-quality image is shown on a monitor screen, allowing the operator to manipulate instruments passed into the pleural space through separate small intercostal incisions. With these instruments, the operator can biopsy lesions of the pleura under direct vision. In addition, this procedure is now used commonly to biopsy peripheral lung tissue or to remove peripheral nodules, for both diagnostic and therapeutic purposes. This much less invasive procedure has largely supplanted the traditional "open lung biopsy" performed by thoracotomy.

Thoracotomy Although frequently replaced by VATS, thoracotomy remains an option for the diagnostic sampling of lung tissue. It provides the largest amount of material, and it can be used to biopsy and/or excise lesions that are too deep or too close to vital structures for removal by VATS. The choice between VATS and thoracotomy needs to be made on a case-by-case basis.

Mediastinoscopy and Mediastinotomy Tissue biopsy is often critical for the diagnosis of mediastinal masses or enlarged mediastinal lymph nodes. Although CT and PET scanning are useful for determining the size and nature of mediastinal lymph nodes as part of the staging of lung cancer, confirmation that enlarged lymph nodes are actually involved with tumor generally requires biopsy and histopathologic examination. The two major procedures used to obtain specimens from masses or nodes in the mediastinum are mediastinoscopy (via a suprasternal approach) and mediastinotomy (via a parasternal approach). Both procedures are performed under general anesthesia by a qualified surgeon. In the case of suprasternal mediastinoscopy, a rigid mediastinoscope is inserted at the suprasternal notch and passed into the mediastinum along a pathway just anterior to the trachea. Tissue can be obtained with biopsy forceps passed through the scope, sampling masses or nodes that are in a paratracheal or pretracheal position. Left paratracheal and aortopulmonary lymph nodes are not accessible by this route and thus are commonly sampled by parasternal mediastinotomy (the Chamberlain procedure). This approach involves either a right or left parasternal incision and dissection directly down to a mass or node that requires biopsy.

FURTHER READINGS

DETTERBECK FC et al: Seeking a home for a PET. Defining the appropriate place for positron emission tomography imaging in the diagnosis of pulmonary nodules or masses. Chest 125:2294, 2300, 2004

DE WEVER W et al: Multidetector CT-generated virtual bronchoscopy: An illustrated review of the potential clinical indications. Eur Respir J 23:776, 2004

ERNST A et al: Interventional pulmonary procedures: Guidelines from the American College of Chest Physicians. Chest 123:1693, 2003

FELLER-KOPMAN D et al: Autofluorescence bronchoscopy and endobronchial ultrasound: A practical review. Ann Thorac Surg 80:2395, 2005

LIN J, IANNETTONI MD: The role of thoracoscopy in the management of lung cancer. Surgical Oncol 12:195, 2003

PATEL S, KAZEROONI EA: Helical CT for the evaluation of acute pulmonary embolism. AJR Am J Roentgenol 185:135, 2005

WEINBERGER SE: *Principles of Pulmonary Medicine*, 4th ed. Philadelphia, Saunders, 2004

248 Asthma
Peter J. Barnes

Asthma is a syndrome characterized by airflow obstruction that varies markedly, both spontaneously and with treatment. Asthmatics harbor a special type of inflammation in the airways that makes them more responsive than nonasthmatics to a wide range of triggers, leading to excessive narrowing with consequent reduced airflow and symptomatic wheezing and dyspnea. Narrowing of the airways is usually reversible, but in some patients with chronic asthma there may be an element of irreversible airflow obstruction. The increasing global prevalence of asthma, the large burden it now imposes on patients, and the high health care costs have led to extensive research into its mechanisms and treatment.

PREVALENCE

Asthma is one of the most common chronic diseases globally and currently affects ~300 million people. The prevalence of asthma has risen in affluent countries over the last 30 years but now appears to have stabilized, with ~10–12% of adults and 15% of children affected by the disease. In developing countries where the prevalence of asthma had been much lower, there is a rising incidence that appears to be associated with increased urbanization. The prevalence of atopy and other allergic diseases has also increased over the same time, suggesting that the reasons for the increase are likely to be systemic rather than confined to the lungs. This epidemiologic observation suggests that there is a maximum number of individuals in the community who are liable to be affected by asthma, likely by genetic predisposition. Most patients with asthma in affluent countries are atopic, with allergic sensitization to the house dust mite *Dermatophagoides pteronyssinus* and other environmental allergens.

Asthma is both common and frequently complicated by the effects of smoking on the lungs; hence, it is difficult to be certain about the natural history of the disease in adults. Asthma can present at any age with a peak age of 3 years. In childhood, twice as many males as females are asthmatic, but by adulthood the sex ratio has equalized. The commonly held belief that children "grow out of their asthma" is justified to some extent. Long-term studies that have followed children until they reach the age of 40 years suggest that many with asthma become asymptomatic during adolescence but that asthma returns in some during adult life, particularly in children with persistent symptoms and severe asthma. Adults with asthma, including those with onset during adulthood rarely become permanently asymptomatic. The severity of asthma does not vary significantly within a given patient; those with mild asthma rarely progress to more severe disease, whereas those with severe asthma usually have severe disease at the onset.

Deaths from asthma are uncommon and have been steadily declining in many affluent countries over the last decade. A rise in asthma mortality seen in several countries during the 1960s was associated with increased use of short-acting β_2-adrenergic agonists (as rescue therapy), but there is now compelling evidence that the more widespread use of inhaled corticosteroids (ICSs) in patients with persistent asthma is responsible for the decrease in mortality in recent years. Major risk factors for asthma deaths are poorly controlled disease with frequent use of bronchodilator inhalers, lack of corticosteroid therapy, and previous admissions to the hospital with near-fatal asthma.

It has proved difficult to agree on a definition of asthma, but there is good agreement on the description of the clinical syndrome and disease pathology. Until the etiologic mechanisms of the disease are better understood, it will be difficult to provide an accurate definition.

ETIOLOGY

Asthma is a heterogeneous disease with interplay between genetic and environmental factors. Several risk factors have been implicated (Table 248-1).

ATOPY

Atopy is the major risk factor for asthma, and nonatopic individuals have a very low risk of developing asthma. Patients with asthma commonly suffer from other atopic diseases, particularly allergic rhinitis, which may be found in over 80% of asthmatic patients, and atopic dermatitis (eczema). Atopy may be found in 40–50% of the population in affluent countries, with only a proportion of atopic individuals becoming asthmatic. This observation suggests that some other environmental or genetic factor(s) predispose to the development of asthma in atopic individuals. The allergens that lead to sensitization are usually proteins that have protease activity, and the commonest allergens are derived from house dust mites, cat and dog fur, cockroaches, grass and tree pollens, and rodents (in laboratory workers). Atopy is due to the genetically determined production of specific IgE antibody, with many patients showing a family history of allergic diseases.

INTRINSIC ASTHMA

A minority of asthmatic patients (approximately 10%) have negative skin test to common inhalant allergens and normal serum concentrations of IgE. These patients, with nonatopic or intrinsic asthma, usually show later onset of disease (adult-onset asthma), commonly have concomitant nasal polyps, and may be aspirin-sensitive. They usually have more severe, persistent asthma. Little is understood about mechanism, but the immunopathology in bronchial biopsies and sputum appears to be identical to that found in atopic asthma. There is recent evidence for increased local production of IgE in the airways, suggesting that there may be common IgE mediated mechanisms.

INFECTIONS

Although viral infections are common as triggers of asthma exacerbations, it is uncertain whether they play a role in etiology. There is some association between respiratory syncytial virus infection in infancy and the development of asthma, but the specific pathogenesis is difficult to elucidate, as this infection is very common in children. More recently, atypical bacteria such as *Mycoplasma* and *Chlamydia* have been implicated in the mechanism of severe asthma, but thus far evidence of a true association is not very convincing.

TABLE 248-1	**RISK FACTORS AND TRIGGERS INVOLVED IN ASTHMA**
Endogenous Factors	**Environmental Factors**
Genetic predisposition	Indoor allergens
Atopy	Outdoor allergens
Airway hyperresponsiveness	Occupational sensitizers
Gender	Passive smoking
Ethnicity?	Respiratory infections
	Obesity?
	Early viral infections?
Triggers	
Allergens	
Upper respiratory tract viral infections	
Exercise and hyperventilation	
Cold air	
Sulfur dioxide	
Drugs (β blockers, aspirin)	
Stress	
Irritants (household sprays, paint fumes)	

GENETIC CONSIDERATIONS The familial association of asthma and a high degree of concordance for asthma in identical twins indicate a genetic predisposition to the disease; however, whether or not the genes predisposing to asthma are similar or in addition to those predisposing of atopy is not yet clear. It now seems likely that different genes may also contribute to asthma specifically, and there is increasing evidence that the severity of asthma is also genetically determined. Genetic screens with classical linkage analysis and single nucleotide polymorphisms of various candidate genes indicate that asthma is polygenic, with each gene identified having a small effect that is often not replicated in different populations. This observation suggests that the interaction of many genes is important, and these may differ in different populations. The most consistent findings have been associations with polymorphisms of genes on chromosome 5q, including the T helper 2 (T_H2) cells interleukin (IL) 4, IL-5, IL-9, and IL-13, which are associated with atopy. There is increasing evidence for a complex interaction between genetic polymorphisms and environmental factors that will require very large population studies to unravel. Novel genes that have been associated with asthma, including ADAM-33, DPP-10, and GPRA, have also been identified by positional cloning, but their function in disease pathogenesis is thus far obscure. Genetic polymorphisms may also be important in determining the response to asthma therapy. For example, the Arg-Gly-16 variant in the β_2-receptor is associated with reduced response to β_2-agonists, and repeats of an Sp1 recognition sequence in the promoter region of 5-lipoxygenase may affect the response to antileukotrienes.

ENVIRONMENTAL FACTORS

It is likely that environmental factors in early life determine which atopic individuals become asthmatic. The increasing prevalence of asthma, particularly in developing countries, over the last few decades also indicates the importance of environmental mechanisms interacting with a genetic predisposition.

Hygiene Hypothesis The observation that allergic sensitization and asthma were less common in children with older siblings first suggested that lower levels of infection may be a factor in affluent societies that increase the risks of asthma. This "hygiene hypothesis" proposes that lack of infections in early childhood preserves the T_H2 cell bias at birth, whereas exposure to infections and endotoxin results in a shift toward a predominant protective T_H1 response. Children brought up on farms who are exposed to a high level of endotoxin are less likely to develop allergic sensitization than children raised on dairy farms. Intestinal parasite infection may also be associated with a reduced risk of asthma. While there is considerable epidemiologic support for the hygiene hypothesis, it cannot account for the parallel increase in T_H1-driven diseases, such as diabetes mellitus, over the same period.

Diet The role of dietary factors is controversial. Observational studies have shown that diets low in antioxidants, such as vitamin C and vitamin A, magnesium, selenium, and omega-3 polyunsaturated fats (fish oil), or high in sodium and omega-6 polyunsaturates are associated with an increased risk of asthma. However, interventional studies have not supported an important role for these dietary factors. Obesity is also an independent risk factor for asthma, particularly in women, but the mechanisms are thus far unknown.

Air Pollution There is no doubt that air pollutants, such as sulfur dioxide, ozone, and diesel particulates, may trigger asthma symptoms, but the role of different air pollutants in the etiology of the disease is much less certain. Most evidence argues against an important role for air pollution as asthma is no more prevalent in cities with a high ambient level of traffic pollution than in rural areas with low levels of pollution. Asthma had a much lower prevalence in East Germany compared to West Germany despite a much higher level of air pollution, but since reunification these differences have decreased as eastern Germa-

ny has become more affluent. Indoor air pollution may be more important with exposure to nitrogen oxides from cooking stoves and exposure to passive cigarette smoke. There is some evidence that maternal smoking is a risk factor for asthma, but it is difficult to dissociate this from an increased risk of respiratory infections.

Allergens Inhaled allergens are common triggers of asthma symptoms and have also been implicated in allergic sensitization. Exposure to house dust mites in early childhood is a risk factor for allergic sensitization and asthma, but rigorous allergen avoidance has not shown any evidence for a reduced risk of developing asthma. The increase in house dust mites in centrally heated, poorly ventilated homes with fitted carpets has been implicated in the increasing prevalence of asthma in affluent countries. Domestic pets, particularly cats, have also been associated with allergic sensitization, but early exposure to cats in the home may be protective through the induction of tolerance.

Occupational Exposure Occupational asthma is relatively common and may affect up to 10% of young adults. Over 200 sensitizing agents have been identified. Chemicals, such as toluene diisocyanate and trimellitic anhydride, may lead to sensitization independent of atopy. Individuals may also be exposed to allergens in the workplace, such as small animal allergens in laboratory workers and fungal amylase in wheat flour in bakers.

OTHER FACTORS

Several other factors have been implicated in the etiology of asthma, including lower maternal age, duration of breast-feeding, prematurity and low birth weight, and inactivity, but are unlikely to contribute to the recent global increase in asthma prevalence. There is also an association with acetaminophen (paracetamol) consumption, which remains unexplained.

PATHOGENESIS

Asthma is associated with a specific chronic inflammation of the mucosa of the lower airways. One of the main aims of treatment is to reduce this inflammation.

PATHOLOGY

The pathology of asthma has been revealed through examining the lungs at autopsy in patients who have died of asthma and from bronchial biopsies in patients with usually mild asthma. The airway mucosa is infiltrated with activated eosinophils and T lymphocytes, and there is activation of mucosal mast cells. The degree of inflammation is poorly related to disease severity and may be found in atopic patients without asthma symptoms. The inflammation is reduced by treatment with ICSs. A characteristic finding is thickening of the basement membrane due to subepithelial collagen deposition. This feature is also found in patients with eosinophilic bronchitis presenting as cough who do not have asthma; it is therefore likely to be a marker of eosinophilic inflammation in the airway, as eosinophils release fibrogenic factors. The epithelium is often shed or friable, with reduced attachments to the airway wall and increased numbers of epithelial cells in the lumen. The airway wall itself may be thickened and edematous, particularly in fatal asthma. Another common finding in fatal asthma is occlusion of the airway lumen by a mucous plug, which is composed of mucus glycoproteins secreted from goblet cells and plasma proteins from leaky bronchial vessels (Fig. 248-1). There is also vasodilatation and increased numbers of blood vessels (angiogenesis). Direct observation by bronchoscopy indicates that the airways may be narrowed, reddened, and edematous. The pathology of asthma is remarkably uniform in different types of asthma, including atopic, nonatopic, occupational, aspirin-sensitive, and pediatric asthma. These pathologic changes are found in all airways but do not extend to the lung parenchyma; small airway inflammation is found particularly in patients with severe asthma. The involvement of airways may be patchy, and this is consistent with bronchographic findings of uneven narrowing of the airways.

- Mucous plug with trapped inflammatory cells
- Goblet cell metaplasia
- Inflammatory cell infiltrate in submucosal layer
- Thickened basement membrane
- Thickened airway smooth muscle
- Normal parenchymal attachments

FIGURE 248-1 Histopathology of a small airway in fatal asthma. The lumen is occluded with a mucous plug, there is goblet cell metaplasia, and the airway wall is thickened, with an increase in basement membrane thickness and airway smooth muscle. *(Courtesy of Dr. J. Hogg, University of British Colombia; with permission.)*

INFLAMMATION

There is inflammation in the respiratory mucosa from trachea to terminal bronchioles, but with a predominance in the bronchi (cartilaginous airways). Considerable research has identified the major cellular components of inflammation, but it is still uncertain how inflammatory cells interact and how inflammation translates into the symptoms of asthma (Fig. 248-2). There is good evidence that the specific pattern of airway inflammation in asthma is associated with airway hyperresponsiveness (AHR), the physiologic abnormality of asthma that is correlated with variable airflow obstruction. The pattern of inflammation in asthma is characteristic of allergic diseases, with similar inflammatory cells seen in the nasal mucosa in rhinitis. However, an indistinguishable pattern of inflammation is found in intrinsic asthma, although this may reflect local rather than systemic IgE production. Although most attention has focused on the acute inflammatory changes seen in asthma, this is a chronic condition, with inflammation persisting over many years in most patients. The mechanisms involved in persistence of inflammation in asthma are still poorly understood. Superimposed on this chronic inflammatory state are acute inflammatory episodes, which correspond to exacerbations of asthma. Many inflammatory cells are known to be involved in asthma, with no predominant key cell (Fig. 248-3).

Mast Cells Mast cells are important in initiating the acute bronchoconstrictor responses to allergens and several other indirectly acting stimuli, such as exercise and hyperventilation (via osmolality or thermal changes), as well as fog. In biopsies from asthmatic patients, mast cells are localized to the airway smooth muscle layer; they are not found in normal subjects or in patients with eosinophilic cough. Mast cells are activated by allergens through an IgE-dependent mechanism, and binding of specific IgE to mast cells renders them more sensitive to activation. The importance of IgE in the pathophysiology of asthma has been highlighted by clinical studies with humanized anti-IgE antibodies, which inhibit IgE-mediated effects, reduce asthma symptoms, and prevent exacerbations. There are, however, uncertainties about the role of mast cells in more chronic allergic inflammatory events. Mast cells release several bronchoconstrictor mediators, including histamine and cysteinyl-leukotrienes, but also several cytokines, chemokines, growth factors, and neurotrophins.

Macrophages and Dendritic Cells Macrophages, which are derived from blood monocytes, may traffic into the airways in asthma and may be activated by allergens via low-affinity IgE receptors (Fc$_\varepsilon$RII). Macrophages have the capacity to initiate a type of inflammatory response via the release of a certain pattern of cytokines, but these cells also release anti-inflammatory mediators, such as IL-10, and thus their role in asthma is

uncertain. Dendritic cells are specialized macrophage-like cells in the airway epithelium, which are the major antigen-presenting cells. Dendritic cells take up allergens, process them to peptides, and migrate to local lymph nodes where they present the allergenic peptides to uncommitted T-lymphocytes to program the production of allergen-specific T cells. Immature dendritic cells in the respiratory tract promote T_H2 cell differentiation and require cytokines, such as IL-12 and TNF-α, to promote the normally preponderant T_H1 response.

Eosinophils Eosinophil infiltration is a characteristic feature of asthmatic airways. Allergen inhalation results in a marked increase in activated eosinophils in the airways at the time of the late reaction. Eosinophils are linked to the development of airway hyperresponsiveness through the release of basic proteins and oxygen-derived free radicals. Eosinophil recruitment involves adhesion of eosinophils to vascular endothelial cells in the airway circulation due to interaction between adhesion molecules, migration into the submucosa under the direction of chemokines, and their subsequent activation and prolonged survival. Blocking antibodies to IL-5 cause a profound and prolonged reduction in circulating and sputum eosinophils, but they are not associated with reduced AHR or asthma symptoms, thus questioning the pivotal role of eosinophils in asthma. Furthermore, eosinophilic inflammation is also found in patients with chronic cough who do not have any clinical features of asthma or AHR. Increasing evidence suggests that eosinophils may be more important in release of growth factors involved in airway remodeling than in AHR.

Neutrophils Increased numbers of activated neutrophils are found in sputum and airways of some patients with severe asthma and during exacerbations, although there is a proportion of patients even with mild or moderate asthma that have a predominance of neutrophils. The role of neutrophils in asthma, which are resistant to the anti-inflammatory effects of corticosteroids, is currently unknown.

T Lymphocytes T lymphocytes play a very important role in coordinating the inflammatory response in asthma through the release of specific patterns of cytokines, resulting in the recruitment and survival of eosinophils and in the maintenance of a mast cell population in the airways. The naïve immune system and the immune system of asthmatics are skewed to express the T_H2 phenotype, whereas in normal airways T_H1 cells predominate. T_H2 cells, through the release of IL-5, are associated with eosinophilic inflammation and, through the release of IL-4 and IL-

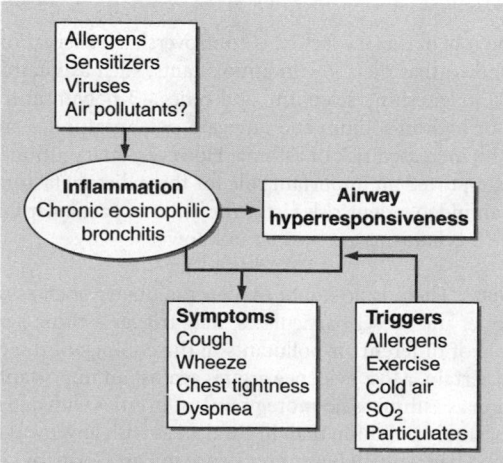

Allergens
Sensitizers
Viruses
Air pollutants?

↓

Inflammation
Chronic eosinophilic bronchitis → **Airway hyperresponsiveness**

↓ ↓

Symptoms
Cough
Wheeze
Chest tightness
Dyspnea

Triggers
Allergens
Exercise
Cold air
SO_2
Particulates

FIGURE 248-2 Inflammation in the airways of asthmatic patients leads to airway hyperresponsiveness and symptoms.

FIGURE 248-3 The pathophysiology of asthma is complex, with participation of several interacting inflammatory cells, resulting in acute and chronic inflammatory effects on the airway.

13, are associated with increased IgE formation. Recently, bronchial biopsies have demonstrated a preponderance of natural killer CD4+ T lymphocytes, which express high levels of IL-4. Regulatory T cells play an important role in determining the expression of other T cells, and there is evidence for a reduction in a certain subset of regulatory T cells (CD4+CD25+) in asthma, which is associated with increased T_H2 cells.

Structural Cells   Structural cells of the airways, including epithelial cells, fibroblasts and airway smooth-muscle cells, are also an important source of inflammatory mediators, such as cytokines and lipid mediators, in asthma. Indeed, because structural cells far outnumber inflammatory cells, they may become the major source of mediators driving chronic inflammation in asthmatic airways. In addition, epithelial cells may have a key role in translating inhaled environmental signals into an airway inflammatory response, and are probably a major target cell for ICSs.

INFLAMMATORY MEDIATORS

Many different mediators have been implicated in asthma, and they may have a variety of effects on the airways that could account for the pathologic features of asthma (Fig. 248-4). Mediators such as his-

tamine, prostaglandins, and cysteinyl-leukotrienes contract airway smooth muscle, increase microvascular leakage, increase airway mucus secretion, and attract other inflammatory cells. Because each mediator has many effects, the role of individual mediators in the pathophysiology of asthma is not yet clear. Although the multiplicity of mediators makes it unlikely that preventing the synthesis or action of a single mediator will have a major impact in clinical asthma, recent clinical studies with antileukotrienes suggest that cysteinyl-leukotrienes have a clinically important effect.

Cytokines   Multiple cytokines regulate the chronic inflammation of asthma. The T_H2 cytokines IL-4, IL-5, and IL-13 mediate allergic inflammation, whereas proinflammatory cytokines, such as tumor necrosis factor α (TNF-α) and IL-1β, amplify the inflammatory response and play a role in more severe disease. Thymic stromal lymphopoietin is an upstream cytokine released from epithelial cells of asthmatics that orchestrates the release of chemokines, which selectively attract T_H2 cells. Some cytokines, such as IL-10 and IL-12, are anti-inflammatory and may be deficient in asthma.

Chemokines   Chemokines are involved in attracting inflammatory cells from the bronchial circulation into the airways. Eotaxin (CCL11) is selectively attractant to eosinophils via CCR3 and is expressed by epithelial cells of asthmatics, whereas CCL17 (TARC) and CCL22 (MDC) from epithelial cells attract T_H2 cells via CCR4 (Fig. 248-5).

Oxidative Stress   There is increased oxidative stress in asthma as activated inflammatory cells, such as macrophages and eosinophils, produce reactive oxygen species. Evidence for increased oxidative stress in asthma is provided by the increased concentrations of 8-isoprostane (a product of oxidized arachidonic acid) in exhaled breath condensates

FIGURE 248-4 Many cells and mediators are involved in asthma and lead to several effects on the airways.

Inflammatory cells	Mediators	Effects
Mast cells	Histamine	Bronchospasm
Eosinophils	Leukotrienes	Plasma exudation
T_H2 cells	Prostanoids	Mucus secretion
Basophils	PAF	AHR
Neutrophils	Kinins	Structural changes
Platelets	Adenosine	
Structural cells	Endothelins	
Epithelial cells	Nitric oxide	
Sm muscle cells	Cytokines	
Endothelial cells	Chemokines	
Fibroblast	Growth factors	
Nerves		

FIGURE 248-5 Chemokines in asthma. Tumor necrosis factor α (TNF-α) and other triggers of airway epithelial cells release thymus and activation-regulated chemokine (TARC, CCL17) and macrophage-derived chemokine (MDC, CCL22) from epithelial cells, which attract T_H2 cells via activation of their CCR4 receptors. These promote eosinophilic inflammation directly through the release of interleukin 5 (IL-5) and indirectly via the release of IL-4 and IL-13, which induce eotaxin (CCL11) formation in airway epithelial cells.

and increased ethane (a product of lipid peroxidation) in the expired air of asthmatic patients. Increased oxidative stress is related to disease severity, may amplify the inflammatory response, and may reduce responsiveness to corticosteroids.

Nitric Oxide   Nitric oxide (NO) is produced by several cells in the airway by NO synthases, particularly airway epithelial cells and macrophages. The level of NO in the expired air of patients with asthma is higher than normal and is related to the eosinophilic inflammation. Increased NO may contribute to the bronchial vasodilation observed in asthma. Exhaled NO is increasingly used in the diagnosis and monitoring of asthmatic inflammation, although it is not used routinely in clinical practice.

Transcription Factors   Proinflammatory transcription factors, such as nuclear factor κB (NFκB) and activator protein 1 (AP-1), are activated in asthmatic airways and orchestrate the expression of multiple inflammatory genes. More-specific transcription factors that are involved include nuclear factor of activated T cells and GATA-3, which regulate the expression of T_H2 cytokines in T cells.

EFFECTS OF INFLAMMATION

The chronic inflammatory response has several effects on the target cells of the airways, resulting in the characteristic pathophysiologic changes associated with asthma. Asthma may be regarded as a disease with continuous inflammation and repair proceeding simultaneously. Important advances continue to be made in our understanding of these changes, but despite these new insights, the relationship between chronic inflammatory processes and asthma symptoms is often not clear.

Airway Epithelium   Airway epithelial shedding may be important in contributing to AHR and may explain how several mechanisms, such as ozone exposure, virus infections, chemical sensitizers, and allergen exposure, can lead to its development, as all of these stimuli may lead to epithelial disruption. Epithelial damage may contribute to AHR in a number of ways, including loss of its barrier function to allow penetration of allergens; loss of enzymes (such as neutral endopeptidase) that normally degrade inflammatory mediators; loss of a relaxant factor (so called epithelial-derived relaxant factor); and exposure of sensory nerves, which may lead to reflex neural effects on the airway.

Fibrosis   In all asthmatic patients, the basement membrane is apparently thickened due to subepithelial fibrosis with deposition of types III and V collagen below the true basement membrane, and it is associated with eosinophil infiltration, presumably through the release of profibrotic mediators, such as transforming growth factor β. Mechanical manipulations can alter the phenotype of airway epithelial cells in a profibrotic fashion. In more severe patients, there is also fibrosis within the airway wall, which may contribute to irreversible narrowing of the airways.

Airway Smooth Muscle   There is still debate about the role of abnormalities in airway smooth muscle is asthmatic airways. In vitro airway smooth muscle from asthmatic patients usually shows no increased responsiveness to constrictors. Reduced responsiveness to β-agonists has also been reported in post-mortem or surgically removed bronchi from asthmatics, although the number of β-receptors is not reduced, suggesting that β-receptors have been uncoupled. These abnormalities of airway smooth muscle may be secondary to the chronic inflammatory process. Inflammatory mediators may modulate the ion channels that serve to regulate the resting membrane potential of airway smooth-muscle cells, thus altering the level of excitability of these cells. In asthmatic airways there is also a characteristic hypertrophy and hyperplasia of airway smooth muscle, which is presumably the result of stimulation of airway smooth-muscle cells by various growth factors, such as platelet-derived growth factor or endothelin 1, released from inflammatory or epithelial cells.

Vascular Responses   There is increased airway mucosal blood flow in asthma. The bronchial circulation may play an important role in regulating airway caliber, since an increase in the vascular volume may contribute to airway narrowing. Increased airway blood flow may be important in removing inflammatory mediators from the airway and may play a role in the development of exercise-induced asthma. There is an increase in the number of blood vessels in asthmatic airways as a result of angiogenesis in response to growth factors, particularly vascular-endothelial growth factor. Microvascular leakage from postcapillary venules in response to inflammatory mediators is observed in asthma, resulting in airway edema and plasma exudation into the airway lumen.

Mucus Hypersecretion   Increased mucus secretion contributes to the viscid mucus plugs that occlude asthmatic airways, particularly in fatal asthma. There is evidence for hyperplasia of submucosal glands that are confined to large airways and of increased numbers of epithelial goblet cells. IL-4 and IL-13 induce mucus hypersecretion in experimental models of asthma.

Neural Effects   Various defects in autonomic neural control may contribute to AHR in asthma, but these are likely to be secondary to the disease, rather than primary defects. Cholinergic pathways, through the release of acetylcholine acting on muscarinic receptors, cause bronchoconstriction and may be activated reflexly in asthma. Inflammatory mediators may activate sensory nerves, resulting in reflex cholinergic bronchoconstriction or release of inflammatory neuropeptides. Inflammatory products may also sensitize sensory nerve endings in the airway epithelium, such that the nerves become hyperalgesic. Neurotrophins, which may be released from various cell types in peripheral tissues, may cause proliferation and sensitization of airway sensory nerves. Airway nerves may also release neurotransmitters, such as substance P, which have inflammatory effects.

AIRWAY REMODELING

Several changes in the structure of the airway are characteristically found in asthma, and these may lead to irreversible narrowing of the airways. Population studies have shown a greater decline in lung function over time than in normal subjects; however, most patients with asthma preserve normal or near-normal lung function throughout life if appropriately treated. This observation suggests that the accelerated decline in lung function occurs in a smaller proportion of asthmatics, and these are usually patients with more severe disease. There is debate about whether the early use of ICSs may reduce the decline in lung function. The characteristic structural changes are increased airway smooth muscle, fibrosis, angiogenesis, and mucus hyperplasia.

ASTHMA TRIGGERS

Several stimuli trigger airway narrowing, wheezing, and dyspnea in asthmatic patients. While the previous view held that these should be avoided, it is now seen as evidence for poor control and an indicator of the need to increase controller therapy.

ALLERGENS

Inhaled allergens are able to activate mast cells with bound IgE directly leading to the immediate release of bronchoconstrictor mediators, resulting in the early response reversed by bronchodilators. Often, experimental allergen challenge is followed by a late response when there is airway edema and an acute inflammatory response with increased eosinophils and neutrophils that is not very reversible with bronchodilators. The most common allergen to trigger asthma is *Dermatophagoides* sp., and environmental exposure leads to low-grade chronic symptoms that are perennial. Perennial allergens are derived from cats and other domestic pets, as well as cockroaches. Other allergens, including grass pollen, ragweed, tree pollen, and fungal spores, are seasonal. Pollens usually cause allergic rhinitis rather than asthma, but in thunderstorms the pollen grains are disrupted, and the particles that may be released can trigger severe asthma exacerbations (thunderstorm asthma).

VIRUS INFECTIONS

Upper respiratory tract virus infections, such as rhinovirus, respiratory syncytial virus, and coronavirus, are the commonest triggers of acute severe exacerbations. The mechanism whereby these viruses cause exacerbations is poorly understood, but there is an increase in airway inflammation with increased numbers of eosinophils and neutrophils. There is evidence for reduced production of type I interferons by epithelial cells from asthmatic patients, resulting in increased susceptibility to these viral infections and a greater inflammatory response.

PHARMACOLOGIC AGENTS

Several drugs may trigger asthma. β-adrenergic blockers commonly worsen asthma, and their use may be fatal. The mechanisms are not clear but are mediated through increased cholinergic bronchoconstriction. All beta blockers need to be avoided, and even selective β$_2$ blocker or topical application (e.g., timolol eye drops) may be dangerous. Angiotensin-converting enzyme inhibitors are theoretically detrimental as they inhibit breakdown of kinins, which are bronchoconstrictors; however, they rarely worsen asthma and the characteristic cough is no more frequent in asthmatics than nonasthmatics. Aspirin may worsen asthma in some patients (aspirin-sensitive asthma is discussed below under "Special Considerations").

EXERCISE

Exercise is a common trigger of asthma, particularly in children. The mechanism is linked to hyperventilation, which results in increased osmolality in airway lining fluids and triggers mast cell mediator release, resulting in bronchoconstriction. Exercise-induced asthma (EIA) typically begins after exercise has ended and recovers spontaneously within about 30 min. EIA is worse in cold, dry climates than in hot, humid conditions. It is therefore more common in sports such as cross-country running in cold weather, overland skiing, and ice hockey than in swimming. It may be prevented by prior administration of β$_2$-agonists and antileukotrienes, but is best prevented by regular treatment with inhaled glucocorticoids, which reduce the population of surface mast cells required for this response.

PHYSICAL FACTORS

Cold air and hyperventilation may trigger asthma through the same mechanisms as exercise. Laughter may also be a trigger. Many patients report worsening of asthma in hot weather and when the weather changes. Some asthmatics become worse when exposed to strong smells or perfumes, but the mechanism of this response is uncertain.

FOOD

There is little evidence that allergic reactions to food lead to increased asthma symptoms, despite the belief of many patients that their symptoms are triggered by particular food constituents. Exclusion diets are usually unsuccessful at reducing the frequency of episodes. Some foods, such as shellfish and nuts, may induce anaphylactic reactions that may include wheezing. Patients with aspirin-induced asthma may benefit from a salicylate-free diet, but these are difficult to maintain. Certain food additives may trigger asthma. Metabisulfite, which is used as a food preservative, may trigger asthma through the release of sulfur dioxide gas in the stomach. Tartrazine, a food yellow-coloring agent, was believed to be a trigger for asthma, but there is little convincing evidence for this.

AIR POLLUTION

Increased ambient levels of sulfur dioxide, ozone, and nitrogen oxides are associated with increased asthma symptoms.

OCCUPATIONAL FACTORS

Several substances found in the workplace may act as sensitizing agents, as discussed above, but may also act as triggers of asthma symptoms.

Occupational asthma is characteristically associated with symptoms at work with relief on weekends and holidays. If removed from exposure within the first 6 months of symptoms there is usually complete recovery. More persistent symptoms lead to irreversible airway changes, and therefore early detection and avoidance are important.

HORMONAL FACTORS

Some women show premenstrual worsening of asthma, which can occasionally be very severe. The mechanisms are not completely understood but are related to a fall in progesterone and in severe cases may be improved by treatment with high doses of progesterone or gonadotropin-releasing factors. Thyrotoxicosis and hypothyroidism can both worsen asthma, although the mechanisms are uncertain.

GASTROESOPHAGEAL REFLUX

Gastroesophageal reflux is common in asthmatic patients as it is increased by bronchodilators. While acid reflux might trigger reflex bronchoconstriction, it rarely causes asthma symptoms, and anti-reflux therapy fails to reduce asthma symptoms in most patients.

STRESS

Many asthmatics report worsening of symptoms with stress. There is no doubt that psychological factors can induce bronchoconstriction through cholinergic reflex pathways. Paradoxically, very severe stress, such as bereavement, usually does not worsen, and may even improve, asthma symptoms.

PATHOPHYSIOLOGY

Limitation of airflow is due mainly to bronchoconstriction, but airway edema, vascular congestion, and luminal occlusion with exudate may also contribute. This results in a reduction in forced expiratory volume in 1 s (FEV$_1$), FEV$_1$/forced vital capacity (FVC) ratio, and peak expiratory flow (PEF), as well as an increase in airway resistance. Early closure of peripheral airway results in lung hyperinflation (air trapping), and increased residual volume, particularly during acute exacerbations. In more severe asthma, reduced ventilation and increased pulmonary blood flow result in mismatching of ventilation and perfusion and in bronchial hyperemia. Ventilatory failure is very uncommon, even in patients with severe asthma, and arterial Pa$_{CO_2}$ tends to be low due to increased ventilation.

AIRWAY HYPERRESPONSIVENESS

AHR is the characteristic physiologic abnormality of asthma, and describes the excessive bronchoconstrictor response to multiple inhaled triggers that would have no effect on normal airways. The increase in AHR is linked to the frequency of asthma symptoms; thus, an important aim of therapy is to reduce AHR. Increased bronchoconstrictor responsiveness is seen with *direct* bronchoconstrictors, such as histamine and methacholine, which contract airway smooth muscle, but it is characteristically also seen with many *indirect* stimuli, which release bronchoconstrictors from mast cells or activate sensory neural reflexes. Most of the triggers for asthma symptoms appear to act indirectly, including allergens, exercise, hyperventilation, fog (via mast cell activation), irritant dusts, and sulfur dioxide (via cholinergic reflex).

CLINICAL FEATURES AND DIAGNOSIS

The characteristic symptoms of asthma are wheezing, dyspnea, and coughing which are variable, both spontaneously and with therapy. Symptoms may be worse at night, and patients typically awake in the early morning hours. Patients may report difficulty in filling their lungs with air. There is increased mucus production in some patients, with typically tenacious mucus that is difficult to expectorate. There may be increased ventilation and use of accessory muscles of ventilation. Prodromal symptoms may precede an attack, with itching under the chin, discomfort between the scapulae, or inexplicable fear (impending doom).

Typical physical signs are inspiratory, and to a great extent expiratory, rhonchi throughout the chest, and there may be hyperinflation. Some patients, particularly children, may present with a predominant nonproductive cough (cough-variant asthma). There may be no abnormal physical findings when asthma is under control.

DIAGNOSIS

The diagnosis of asthma is usually apparent from the symptoms of variable and intermittent airways obstruction, but is usually confirmed by objective measurements of lung function.

Lung Function Tests   Simple spirometry confirms airflow limitation with a reduced FEV_1, FEV_1/FVC ratio, and PEF. Reversibility is demonstrated by a >12% or 200 mL increase in FEV_1 15 min after an inhaled short-acting β_2-agonist or, in some patients, by a 2- to 4-week trial of oral glucocorticoids (prednisone or prednisolone 30–40 mg daily). Measurements of PEF twice daily may confirm the diurnal variations in airflow obstruction. Flow-volume loops show reduced peak flow and reduced maximum expiratory flow. Further lung function tests are rarely necessary, but whole body plethysmography shows increased airway resistance and may show increased total lung capacity and residual volume. Gas diffusion is usually normal but there may be a small increase in gas transfer in some patients.

Airway Responsiveness   The increased AHR is normally measured by methacholine or histamine challenge with calculation of the provocative concentration that reduces FEV_1 by 20% (PC_{20}). This is rarely useful in clinical practice, but can be used in the differential diagnosis of chronic cough and when the diagnosis is in doubt in the setting of normal pulmonary function tests. Occasionally exercise testing is done to demonstrate the post-exercise bronchoconstriction if there is a predominant history of EIA. Allergen challenge is rarely necessary, and should only be undertaken by a specialist if specific occupational agents are to be identified.

Hematologic Tests   Blood tests are not usually helpful. Total serum IgE and specific IgE to inhaled allergens (RAST) may be measured in some patients.

Imaging   Chest roentgenography is usually normal but may show hyperinflated lungs in more severe patients. In exacerbations, there may be evidence of a pneumothorax. Lung shadowing usually indicates pneumonia or eosinophilic infiltrates in patients with bronchopulmonary aspergillosis. High-resolution CT may show areas of bronchiectasis in patients with severe asthma, and there may be thickening of the bronchial walls, but these changes are not diagnostic of asthma.

Skin Tests   Skin prick tests to common inhalant allergens are positive in allergic asthma and negative in intrinsic asthma, but are not helpful in diagnosis. Positive skin responses may be useful in persuading patients to undertake allergen avoidance measures.

DIFFERENTIAL DIAGNOSIS

It is usually not difficult to differentiate asthma from other conditions that cause wheezing and dyspnea. Upper airway obstruction by a tumor or laryngeal edema can mimic severe asthma, but patients typically present with stridor localized to large airways. The diagnosis is confirmed by a flow-volume loop, which shows a reduction in inspiratory as well as expiratory flow, and bronchoscopy to demonstrate the site of upper airway narrowing. Persistent wheezing in a specific area of the chest may indicate endobronchial obstruction with a foreign body. Left ventricular failure may mimic the wheezing of asthma but basilar crackles are present in contrast to asthma.

Eosinophilic pneumonias and systemic vasculitis, including Churg-Strauss syndrome and polyarteritis nodosa, may be associated with wheezing. Chronic obstructive pulmonary disease (COPD) is usually easy to differentiate from asthma as symptoms show less variability, never completely remit, and show much less (or no) reversibility to bron-

TABLE 248-2   AIMS OF ASTHMA THERAPY

Minimal (ideally no) chronic symptoms, including nocturnal
Minimal (infrequent) exacerbations
No emergency visits
Minimal (ideally no) use of as-required β_2-agonist
No limitations on activities, including exercise
PEF circadian variation <20%
(Near) normal PEF
Minimal (or no) adverse effects from medicine

Note: PEF, peak expiratory flow.

chodilators. Approximately 10% of COPD patients have features of asthma, with increased sputum eosinophils and a response to oral corticosteroids; these patients probably have both diseases concomitantly.

℞ ASTHMA

The treatment of asthma is straightforward and the majority of patients are now managed by internists with effective and safe therapies. There are several aims of therapy (Table 248-2). Most emphasis has been placed on drug therapy, but several nonpharmacologic approaches have also been used. The main drugs for asthma can be divided into *bronchodilators*, which give rapid relief of symptoms mainly through relaxation of airway smooth muscle, and *controllers*, which inhibit the underlying inflammatory process.

BRONCHODILATOR THERAPIES   Bronchodilators act primarily on airway smooth muscle to reverse the bronchoconstriction of asthma. This gives rapid relief of symptoms but has little or no effect on the underlying inflammatory process. Thus, bronchodilators are not sufficient to control asthma in patients with persistent symptoms. There are three classes of bronchodilator in current use: β_2-adrenergic agonists, anticholinergics, and theophylline; of these, β_2-agonists are by far the most effective.

β_2-Agonists β_2-Agonists activate β_2-adrenergic receptors, which are widely expressed in the airways. β_2-Receptors are coupled through a stimulatory G protein to adenylyl cyclase, resulting in increased intracellular cyclic AMP, which relaxes smooth-muscle cells and inhibits certain inflammatory cells.

Mode of Action   The primary action of β_2-agonists is to relax airway smooth-muscle cells of all airways, where they act as functional antagonists, reversing and preventing contraction of airway smooth-muscle cells by all known bronchoconstrictors. This generalized action is likely to account for their great efficacy as bronchodilators in asthma. There are also additional non-bronchodilator effects that may be clinically useful, including inhibition of mast cell mediator release, reduction in plasma exudation, and inhibition of sensory nerve activation (Table 248-3). Inflammatory cells express small numbers of β_2-receptors, but these are rapidly down-regulated with β_2-agonist activation so that, in contrast to corticosteroids, there are no effects on inflammatory cells in the airways and there is no reduction in AHR.

Clinical Use β_2-Agonists are usually given by inhalation to reduce side effects. Short-acting β_2-agonists (SABAs), such as albuterol and terbutaline, have a duration of action of 3–6 hours. They have a rapid onset of bronchodilation and are therefore used as needed for symptom relief. Increased use of SABAs indicates that asthma is not controlled. They are also useful in preventing EIA if taken prior to exercise. SABAs are used in high doses by nebulizer or via a metered dose inhaler with a spacer. Long-acting β_2-agonists (LABAs) include salmeterol and formoterol, both of which have a duration of action over 12 hours and are given twice daily. LABAs have replaced the regular use of SABAs, but LABAs should not be given in the

TABLE 248-3   EFFECTS OF β-ADRENERGIC AGONISTS ON AIRWAYS

Relaxation of airway smooth muscle (proximal and distal airways)
Inhibition of mast cell mediator release
Inhibition of plasma exudation and airway edema
Increased mucociliary clearance
Increased mucus secretion
Decreased cough
No effect on chronic inflammation

absence of ICS therapy as they do not control the underlying inflammation. They do, however, improve asthma control and reduce exacerbations when added to ICS, which allows asthma to be controlled at lower doses of corticosteroids. This observation has led to the widespread use of fixed combination inhalers that contain a corticosteroid and a LABA, which have proved to be highly effective in the control of asthma.

Side Effects Adverse effects are not usually a problem with β_2-agonists when given by inhalation. The most common side effects are muscle tremor and palpitations, which are seen more commonly in elderly patients. There is a small fall in plasma potassium due to increased uptake by skeletal muscle cells, but this effect does not usually cause a clinical problem.

Tolerance Tolerance is a potential problem with any agonist given chronically, but while there is downregulation of β_2-receptors, this does not reduce the bronchodilator response as there is a large receptor reserve in airway smooth-muscle cells. By contrast, mast cells become rapidly tolerant, but their tolerance may be prevented by concomitant administration of ICS.

Safety The safety of β_2-agonists has been an important issue. There is an association between asthma mortality and the amount of SABA used, but careful analysis demonstrates that the increased use of rescue SABAs reflects poor asthma control, which is a risk factor for asthma death. The slight excess in mortality that has been associated with the use of LABAs is related to the lack of use of concomitant ICS, as the LABA therapy does not deal with the underlying inflammation. This highlights the importance of always using an ICS when LABAs are given, which is most conveniently achieved by using a combination inhaler.

Anti-Cholinergics Muscarinic receptor antagonists, such as ipratropium bromide, prevent cholinergic nerve–induced bronchoconstriction and mucus secretion. They are much less effective than β_2-agonists in asthma therapy as they inhibit only the cholinergic reflex component of bronchoconstriction, whereas β_2-agonists prevent all bronchoconstrictor mechanisms. Anticholinergics are therefore only used as an additional bronchodilator in patients with asthma that is not controlled on other inhaled medications. High doses may be given by nebulizer in treating acute severe asthma but should only be given following β_2-agonists since they have a slower onset of bronchodilation.

Side effects are not usually a problem as there is little or no systemic absorption. The most common side effect is dry mouth; in elderly patients, urinary retention and glaucoma may also be observed.

Theophylline Theophylline was widely prescribed as an oral bronchodilator several years ago, especially as it was inexpensive. It has now fallen out of favor as side effects are common and inhaled β_2-agonists are much more effective as bronchodilators. The bronchodilator effect is due to inhibition of phosphodiesterases in airway smooth-muscle cells, which increases cyclic AMP, but doses required for bronchodilation commonly cause side effects that are mediated mainly by phosphodiesterase inhibition. There is increasing evidence that theophylline at lower doses has antiinflammatory effects, and these are likely to be mediated through different molecular mechanisms. There is evidence that theophylline activates the key nuclear enzyme histone deacetylase-2, which is a critical mechanism for switching off activated inflammatory genes.

Clinical Use Oral theophylline is usually given as a slow-release preparation once or twice daily as this gives more stable plasma concentrations than normal theophylline tablets. It may be used as an additional bronchodilator in patients with severe asthma when plasma concentrations of 10–20 mg/L are required, although these concentrations are often associated with side effects. Low doses of theophylline, giving plasma concentrations of 5–10 mg/L, have additive effects to ICSs and are particularly useful in patients with severe asthma. Indeed, withdrawal of theophylline from these patients may result in marked deterioration in asthma control. The drug is well tolerated at low doses. Intravenous aminophylline (a soluble salt of theophylline) was used for the treatment of severe asthma but has now been largely supplemented by inhaled SABAs, which are more effective and have fewer side effects. Aminophylline is occasionally used (via slow intravenous infusion) in patients with severe exacerbations that are refractory to high-dose SABAs.

Side Effects Oral theophylline is well absorbed and is largely inactivated in the liver. Side effects are related to plasma concentrations; measurement

TABLE 248-4	**FACTORS AFFECTING CLEARANCE OF THEOPHYLLINE**

Increased Clearance

Enzyme induction (rifampicin, phenobarbitone, ethanol)
Smoking (tobacco, marijuana)
High protein, low carbohydrate diet
Barbecued meat
Childhood

Decreased Clearance

Enzyme inhibition (cimetidine, erythromycin, ciprofloxacin, allopurinol, zileuton, zafirlukast)
Congestive heart failure
Liver disease
Pneumonia
Viral infection and vaccination
High carbohydrate diet
Old age

of plasma theophylline may be useful in determining the correct dose. The most common side effects—nausea, vomiting, and headaches—are due to phosphodiesterase inhibition. Diuresis and palpitations may also occur, and at high concentrations cardiac arrhythmias, epileptic seizures, and death may occur due to adenosine receptor antagonism. Theophylline side effects are related to plasma concentration and are rarely observed at plasma concentrations below 10 mg/L. Theophylline is metabolized by CYP450 in the liver, and thus plasma concentrations may be elevated by drugs that block CYP450, such as erythromycin and allopurinol. Other drugs may also reduce clearance by other mechanisms leading to increased plasma concentrations **(Table 248-4)**.

CONTROLLER THERAPIES **Inhaled Corticosteroids** ICSs are by far the most effective controllers for asthma, and their early use has revolutionized asthma therapy.

Mode of Action ICSs are the most effective anti-inflammatory agents used in asthma therapy, reducing the number of inflammatory cells and their activation in the airways. ICSs reduce eosinophils in the airways and sputum, and numbers of activated T lymphocytes and surface mast cells in the airway mucosa. These effects may account for the reduction in AHR that is seen with chronic ICS therapy.

The molecular mechanism of action of corticosteroids involves several effects on the inflammatory process. The major effect of corticosteroids is to switch off the transcription of multiple activated genes that encode inflammatory proteins, such as cytokines, chemokines, adhesion molecules, and inflammatory enzymes. This effect involves several mechanisms, including inhibition of the transcription factors NFκB and AP-1, but an important mechanism is recruitment of histone deacetylase-2 to the inflammatory gene complex, which reverses the histone acetylation associated with increased gene transcription. Corticosteroids also activate antiinflammatory genes, such as mitogen-activated protein (MAP) kinase phosphatase-1, and increase the expression of β_2-receptors. Most of the metabolic and endocrine side effects of corticosteroids are also mediated through transcriptional activation.

Clinical Use ICSs are by far the most effective controllers in the management of asthma and are beneficial in treating asthma of any severity and age. ICSs are usually given twice daily, but some may be effective once daily in mildly symptomatic patients. ICSs rapidly improve the symptoms of asthma, and lung function improves over several days. They are effective in preventing asthma symptoms, such as EIA and nocturnal exacerbations, but also prevent severe exacerbations. ICSs reduce AHR, but maximal improvement may take several months of therapy. Early treatment with ICSs appears to prevent irreversible changes in airway function that occur with chronic asthma. Withdrawal of ICSs results in slow deterioration of asthma control, indicating that they suppress inflammation and symptoms but do not cure the underlying condition. ICSs are now given as first-line therapy for patients with persistent asthma, but if they do not control symptoms at low doses, it is usual to add an LABA as the next step.

Side Effects Local side effects include hoarseness (dysphonia) and oral candidiasis, which may be reduced with the use of a large-volume spacer device. There has been concern about systemic side effects from lung absorption, but many studies have demonstrated that ICSs have minimal systemic effects **(Fig. 248-6)**. At the highest recommended doses, there may

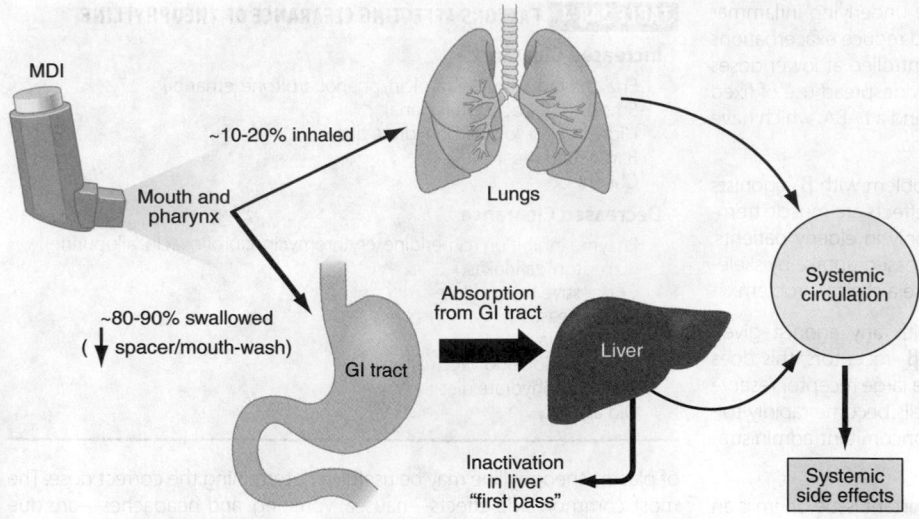

FIGURE 248-6 Pharmacokinetics of inhaled corticosteroids.

be some suppression of plasma and urinary cortisol concentrations, but there is no convincing evidence that long-term treatment leads to impaired growth in children or to osteoporosis in adults. Indeed, effective control of asthma with ICSs reduces the number of courses of oral corticosteroids that are needed and thus reduces systemic exposure to ICSs.

Systemic Corticosteroids Corticosteroids are used intravenously (hydrocortisone or methylprednisolone) for the treatment of acute severe asthma, although several studies now show that oral corticosteroids are as effective and easier to administer. A course of oral corticosteroids (usually prednisone or prednisolone 30–45 mg od for 5–10 days) is used to treat acute exacerbations of asthma; no tapering of the dose is needed. Approximately 1% of asthma patients may require maintenance treatment with oral corticosteroids; the lowest dose necessary to maintaining control needs to be determined. Systemic side effects, including truncal obesity, bruising, osteoporosis, diabetes, hypertension, gastric ulceration, proximal myopathy, depression, and cataracts may be a major problem, and steroid-sparing therapies may be considered if side effects are a significant problem. If patients require maintenance treatment with oral corticosteroids, it is important to monitor bone density so that preventive treatment with bisphosphonates, or estrogen in postmenopausal women, may be initiated if bone density is low. Intramuscular triamcinolone acetonide is a depot preparation that is occasionally used in noncompliant patients, but proximal myopathy is a major problem with this therapy.

Antileukotrienes Cysteinyl-leukotrienes are potent bronchoconstrictors, cause microvascular leakage, and increase eosinophilic inflammation through the activation of cys-LT_1-receptors. These inflammatory mediators are produced predominantly by mast cells and, to a lesser extent, eosinophils in asthma. Antileukotrienes, such as montelukast and zafirlukast, block cys-LT_1-receptors and provide modest clinical benefit in asthma. They are less effective than ICSs in controlling asthma and have less effect on airway inflammation, but are useful as an add-on therapy in some patients not controlled with low doses of inhaled corticosteroids (although they are less effective than LABAs). They are given orally once or twice daily and are well tolerated. Some patients show a better response than others to antileukotrienes, but this has not been convincingly linked to any genomic differences in the leukotriene pathway.

Cromones Cromolyn sodium and nedocromil sodium are asthma controller drugs that appear to inhibit mast cell and sensory nerve activation, and are therefore effective in blocking trigger-induced asthma, such as EIA, and allergen- and sulfur dioxide–induced symptoms. Cromones have relatively little benefit in the long-term control of asthma due to their short duration of action (at least 4 times daily by inhalation). They are very safe, and though they were popular in the treatment of childhood asthma, low doses of ICSs are now preferred as they are more effective and have a proven safety profile.

Steroid-Sparing Therapies Various immunomodulatory treatments have been used to reduce the requirement for oral corticosteroids in patients with severe asthma who have serious side effects with this therapy. Methotrexate, cyclosporine, azathioprine, gold, and intravenous gamma globulin have all been used as steroid-sparing therapies, but none of these treatments has any long-term benefit and each is associated with a relatively high risk of side effects.

Anti-IgE Omalizumab is a blocking antibody that neutralizes circulating IgE without binding to cell-bound IgE; it thus inhibits IgE-mediated reactions. This treatment has been shown to reduce the number of exacerbations in patients with severe asthma and may improve asthma control. However, the treatment is very expensive and only suitable for highly selected patients who are not controlled on maximal doses of inhaler therapy and have a circulating IgE within a specified range. Patients should be given a 3–4 month trial of therapy to show objective benefit. Omalizumab is usually given as a subcutaneous injection every 2–4 weeks and appears not to have significant side effects.

Immunotherapy Specific immunotherapy using injected extracts of pollens or house dust mite has not been very effective in controlling asthma and may cause anaphylaxis. Side effects may be reduced by sublingual dosing. It is not recommended in most asthma treatment guidelines because of lack of evidence of clinical efficacy.

Alternative Therapies Nonpharmacologic treatments, including hypnosis, acupuncture, chiropraxy, breathing control, yoga, and speleotherapy, may be popular with some patients. However, placebo-controlled studies have shown that each of these treatments lacks efficacy and cannot be recommended. However, they are not detrimental and may be used as long as conventional pharmacologic therapy is continued.

Future Therapies It has proved very difficult to discover novel pharmaceutical therapies, particularly as current therapy with corticosteroids and β_2-agonists is so effective in the majority of patients. There, however, is a need for the development of new therapies for patients with refractory asthma who have side effects with systemic corticosteroids. Antagonists of specific mediators have little or no benefit in asthma, apart from antileukotrienes, which have a rather weak effect, presumably reflecting the fact that multiple mediators are involved. Antagonists of chemokine receptors, particularly CCR3, are in development and may be more effective. Novel anti-inflammatory treatments that are in clinical development include inhibitors of phosphodiesterase-4, NFκB, p38 MAP kinase and phosphoinositide-3 kinase. However, these drugs, which act on signal transduction pathways common to many cells, are likely to have troublesome side effects, necessitating their delivery by inhalation. Safer and more effective immunotherapy using T cell peptide fragments of allergens or DNA vaccination are also being investigated. Bacterial products, such as CpG oligonucleotides that stimulate T_H1 immunity or regulatory T cells, are also currently under evaluation.

MANAGEMENT OF CHRONIC ASTHMA There are several aims of chronic therapy in asthma (Table 248-2). It is important to establish the diagnosis objectively using spirometry or PEF measurements at home. Triggers that worsen asthma control, such as allergens or occupational agents, should be avoided, whereas triggers such as exercise and fog, which result in transient symptoms, provide an indication that more controller therapy is needed.

Stepwise Therapy For patients with mild, intermittent asthma, a short-acting β_2-agonist is all that is required (Fig. 248-7). However, use of a reliever medication more than three times a week indicates the need for regular controller therapy. The treatment of choice for all patients is an ICS given twice daily. It is usual to start with an intermediate dose [e.g., 200 μg bid of beclomethasone dipropionate (BDP) or equivalent] and to decrease the dose if symptoms are controlled after 3 months. If symptoms are not controlled, an LABA should be added, most conveniently by switching to a combination inhaler. The dose of controller should be adjusted accordingly, as judged by the need for a rescue inhaler. Low doses of theophylline or

				OCS
			LABA	LABA
		LABA	ICS High dose	ICS High dose
ICS Low dose	ICS Low dose			

Short-acting β₂-agonist as required for symptom relief

| Mild
intermittent | Mild
persistent | Moderate
persistent | Severe
persistent | Very severe
persistent |

FIGURE 248-7 Step-wise approach to asthma therapy according to the severity of asthma and ability to control symptoms. ICS, inhaled corticosteroid; LABA, long-acting β₂-agonists; OCS, oral corticosteroid.

an antileukotriene may also be considered as an add-on therapy, but these are less effective than LABAs. In patients with severe asthma, low-dose oral theophylline is also helpful, and when there is irreversible airway narrowing, the long-acting anticholinergic tiotropium bromide may be tried. If asthma is not controlled despite the maximal recommended dose of inhaled therapy, it is important to check compliance and inhaler technique. In these patients, maintenance treatment with an oral corticosteroid may be needed, and the lowest dose that maintains control should be used. Occasionally omalizumab may be tried in steroid-dependent asthmatics who are not well controlled. Once asthma is controlled, it is important to slowly decrease therapy in order to find the optimal dose to control symptoms.

Education Patients with asthma need to understand how to use their medications and the difference between reliever and controller therapies. Education may improve compliance, particularly with ICSs. All patients should be taught how to use their inhalers correctly. In particular, they need to understand how to recognize worsening of asthma and how to step up therapy. Written action plans have been shown to reduce hospital admissions and morbidity in adults and children and are recommended particularly in patients with unstable disease who have frequent exacerbations.

ACUTE SEVERE ASTHMA

Exacerbations of asthma are feared by patients and may be life-threatening. One of the main aims of controller therapy is to prevent exacerbations; in this respect, ICS and combination inhalers are very effective.

CLINICAL FEATURES

Patients are aware of increasing chest tightness, wheezing, and dyspnea that are often not or poorly relieved by their usual reliever inhaler. In severe exacerbations patients may be so breathless that they are unable to complete sentences and may become cyanotic. Examination usually shows increased ventilation, hyperinflation, and tachycardia. Pulsus paradoxus may be present, but this is rarely a useful clinical sign. There is a marked fall in spirometric values and PEF. Arterial blood gases on air show hypoxia and Pa_{CO_2} is usually low due to hyperventilation. A normal or rising Pa_{CO_2} is an indication of impending respiratory failure and requires immediate monitoring and therapy. A chest roentgenogram is not usually informative, but may show pneumonia or pneumothorax.

℞ ACUTE SEVERE ASTHMA

A high concentration of oxygen should be given by face mask to achieve oxygen saturation of >90%. The mainstay of treatment is high doses of short-acting inhaled β₂-agonists that are given either by nebulizer or via a metered dose inhaler with a spacer. In severely ill patients with impending respiratory failure, intravenous β₂-agonists may be given. An inhaled anticholinergic may be added if there is not a satisfactory response to β₂-agonists alone, as there are additive effects. In patients who are refractory to inhaled therapies, a slow infusion of aminophylline may be effective, but it is important to monitor blood levels especially if patients have already been treated with oral theophylline. Magnesium sulfate given intravenously or by nebulizer has also been shown to be effective when added to inhaled β₂-agonists, and is relatively well tolerated but is not routinely recom-

mended. Prophylactic intubation may be indicated for impending respiratory failure, when the Pa_{CO_2} is normal or rises. For patients with respiratory failure, it is necessary to intubate and institute ventilation. These patients may benefit from an anesthetic, such as halothane, if they have not responded to conventional bronchodilators. Sedatives should never be given as they may depress ventilation. Antibiotics should not be used routinely unless there are signs of pneumonia.

REFRACTORY ASTHMA

Although most patients with asthma are easily controlled with appropriate medication, a small proportion of patients (approximately 5% of asthmatics) are difficult to control despite maximal inhaled therapy. Some of these patients will require maintenance treatment with oral corticosteroids. In managing these patients, it is important to investigate and correct any mechanisms that may be aggravating asthma. There are two major patterns of difficult asthma: some patients have persistent symptoms and poor lung function, despite appropriate therapy, whereas others may have normal or near-normal lung function but intermittent, severe (sometimes life-threatening) exacerbations.

MECHANISMS

The most common reason for poor control of asthma is noncompliance with medication, particularly ICS. Compliance with ICS may be low because patients do not feel any immediate clinical benefit or may be concerned about side effects. Compliance with ICS is difficult to monitor as there are no useful plasma measurements that can be made. Compliance may be improved by giving the ICS as a combination with an LABA that gives symptom relief. Compliance with oral corticosteroids may be measured by suppression of plasma cortisol and the expected concentration of prednisone/prednisolone in the plasma. There are several factors that may make asthma more difficult to control, including exposure to high, ambient levels of allergens or unidentified occupational agents. Severe rhinosinusitis may make asthma more difficult to control; upper airway disease should be vigorously treated. Gastroesophageal reflux is common among asthmatics due to bronchodilator therapy, but there is little evidence that it is a significant factor in worsening asthma, and treatment of the reflux is not usually effective at improving asthma symptoms. Some patients may have chronic infection with *Mycoplasma pneumoniae* or *Chlamydophila pneumoniae* and benefit from treatment with a macrolide antibiotic. Drugs such as β-adrenergic blockers, aspirin, and other cyclooxygenase (COX) inhibitors may worsen asthma. Some women develop severe premenstrual worsening of asthma, which is unresponsive to corticosteroids and requires treatment with progesterone or gonadotropin-releasing factors. Few systemic diseases make asthma more difficult to control, but hyper- and hypothyroidism may increase asthma symptoms and should be investigated if suspected.

Relatively little is known about the pathology of refractory asthma, as biopsy studies are more difficult in these patients. Some patients show the typical eosinophilic pattern of inflammation, whereas others have a predominantly neutrophilic pattern. There may be an increase in T_H1 cells and CD8 lymphocytes compared to mild asthma and increased expression of TNF-α. Structural changes in the airway, including fibrosis, angiogenesis, and airway smooth-muscle thickening, are more commonly seen in these patients.

DIFFERENTIAL DIAGNOSIS

Some patients who apparently have difficult-to-control asthma also have vocal cord dysfunction, resulting in wheezing or stridor. This symptom is thought to be an attention-seeking hysterical conversion syndrome and may lead to escalating doses of asthma therapy, with some patients taking high doses of oral corticosteroids. It may be recognized by the characteristic discrepancy between tests of forced expiration, such as FEV_1 and PEF, and relatively normal airway resistance. Direct inspection by laryngoscopy may confirm adduction of the vocal cords at the time of symptoms. This condition is usually difficult to manage, but it is important that patients be weaned off oral and inhaled corticosteroids. Speech therapy is sometimes beneficial. Some patients with COPD may be diagnosed as asthmatic and may show the characteristic poor response to corticosteroids and bronchodilators, but this situation is complicated by the fact that some patients with COPD also have concomitant asthma.

CORTICOSTEROID-RESISTANT ASTHMA

A few patients with asthma show a poor response to corticosteroid therapy and may have various molecular abnormalities that impair the anti-inflammatory action of corticosteroids. Complete resistance to corticosteroids is extremely uncommon and affects <1 in 1000 patients. It is defined by a failure to respond to a high dose of oral prednisone/prednisolone (40 mg od over 2 weeks), ideally with a 2-week run-in with matched placebo. More common is reduced responsiveness to corticosteroids where control of asthma requires oral corticosteroids (corticosteroid-dependent asthma). In all patients with poor responsiveness to corticosteroids, there is a reduction in the response of circulating monocytes and lymphocytes to the anti-inflammatory effects of corticosteroids in vitro and reduced skin blanching in response to topical corticosteroids. There are several mechanisms that have been described, including an excess of the transcription factor AP-1, an increase in the alternatively spliced form of the glucocorticoid receptor GR-β, an abnormal pattern of histone acetylation in response to corticosteroids, a defect in IL-10 production, and a reduction in histone deacetylase activity (as in COPD). These observations suggest that there are likely to be heterogeneous mechanisms for corticosteroid resistance; whether these mechanisms are genetically determined has yet to be determined.

BRITTLE ASTHMA

Some patients show chaotic variations in lung function despite taking appropriate therapy. Some show a persistent pattern of variability and may require oral corticosteroids or, at times, continuous infusion of β_2-agonists (type I brittle asthma), whereas others have generally normal or near-normal lung function but precipitous, unpredictable falls in lung function that may result in death (type 2 brittle asthma). These latter patients are difficult to manage as they do not respond well to corticosteroids, and the worsening of asthma does not reverse well with inhaled bronchodilators. The most effective therapy is subcutaneous epinephrine, which suggests that the worsening is likely to be a localized airway anaphylactic reaction with edema. In some of these patients, there may be allergy to specific foods. These patients should be taught to self-administer epinephrine and should carry a medical warning accordingly.

Rx REFRACTORY ASTHMA

Refractory asthma is difficult to control, by definition. It is important to check compliance and the correct use of inhalers and to identify and eliminate any underlying triggers. Low doses of theophylline may be helpful in some patients, and theophylline withdrawal has been found to worsen many patients. Most of these patients will require maintenance treatment with oral corticosteroids, and the minimal dose that achieves satisfactory control should be determined by careful dose titration. Steroid-sparing therapies are rarely effective. In some patients with allergic asthma, omalizumab is effective, particularly when there are frequent exacerbations. There is some evidence that anti-TNF therapy may be effective, but this is controversial and very expensive. A few patients may benefit from infusions of β_2-agonists. New therapies are needed for these patients, who currently consume a disproportionate amount of health care spending.

SPECIAL CONSIDERATIONS

Although asthma is usually straightforward to manage, there are some situations that may require additional investigation and different therapy.

ASPIRIN-SENSITIVE ASTHMA

A small proportion (approximately 1%) of asthmatics become worse with aspirin and other COX inhibitors, although this is much more commonly seen in severe patients and in those with frequent hospital admission. Aspirin-sensitive asthma is a well-defined subtype of asthma that is usually preceded by perennial rhinitis and nasal polyps in nonatopic patients with a late onset of the disease. Aspirin, even in small doses, characteristically provokes rhinorrhea, conjunctival irritation, facial flushing, and wheezing. There is a genetic predisposition to increased production of cysteinyl-leukotrienes with functional polymorphism of cys-leukotriene synthase. Asthma is triggered by COX inhibitors but is persistent even in their absence. All nonselective COX inhibitors should be avoided, but selective COX-2 inhibitors are apparently safe to use when an anti-inflammatory analgesic is needed. Aspirin-sensitive asthma responds to usual therapy with an ICS. Although antileukotrienes should be effective in these patients, they are no more effective than in allergic asthma. Occasionally aspirin desensitization is necessary, but this should only be undertaken in specialized centers.

ASTHMA IN THE ELDERLY

Asthma may start at any age, including in elderly patients. The principles of management are the same as in other asthmatics, but side effects of therapy may be a problem, including muscle tremor with β_2-agonists and more systemic side effects with ICSs. Comorbidities are more frequent in this age group, and interactions with drugs such as β_2 blockers, COX inhibitors, and agents that may affect theophylline metabolism need to be considered. COPD is more likely in elderly patients and may coexist with asthma. A trial of oral corticosteroids may be very useful in documenting the steroid responsiveness of asthma.

PREGNANCY

Approximately one-third of asthmatic patients who are pregnant improve during the course of a pregnancy, one-third deteriorate, and one-third are unchanged. It is important to maintain good control of asthma since poor control may have adverse effects on fetal development. Compliance may be a problem as there is often concern about the effects of anti-asthma medications on fetal development. The drugs that have been used for many years in asthma therapy have now been shown to be safe and without teratogenic potential. These drugs include short-acting β_2-agonists, ICSs, and theophylline; there is less safety information about newer classes of drugs such as LABAs, antileukotrienes, and anti-IgE. If an oral corticosteroid is needed, it is better to use prednisone rather than prednisolone as it cannot be converted to the active prednisolone by the fetal liver, thus protecting the fetus from systemic effects of the corticosteroid. There is no contraindication to breast-feeding when patients are using these drugs.

CIGARETTE SMOKING

Approximately 20% of asthmatics smoke, which may adversely affect asthma in several ways. Smoking asthmatics have more severe disease, more frequent hospital admissions, a faster decline in lung function, and a higher risk of death from asthma than nonsmoking asthmatics. There is evidence that smoking interferes with the anti-inflammatory actions of corticosteroids, necessitating higher doses for asthma control. Smoking cessation improves lung function and reverses the steroid resistance; thus, vigorous smoking cessation strategies should be used. Some patients report a temporary worsening of asthma when they first stop smoking, which could be due to the loss of the bronchodilating effect of nitric oxide in cigarette smoke.

SURGERY

If asthma is well-controlled, there is no contraindication to general anesthesia and intubation. Patients who are treated with oral corticosteroids will have adrenal suppression and should be treated with an increased dose of oral corticosteroid immediately prior to surgery. Patients with FEV$_1$ <80% of their normal levels should also be given a boost of oral corticosteroids prior to surgery. High maintenance doses of corticosteroids may be a contraindication to surgery because of increased risks of infection and delayed wound healing.

BRONCHOPULMONARY ASPERGILLOSIS

Bronchopulmonary aspergillosis (BPA) is uncommon and results from an allergic pulmonary reaction to inhaled spores of *Aspergillus fumigatus* and, occasionally, other *Aspergillus* species. A skin prick test to *A. fumigatus* is always positive, whereas serum *Aspergillus* precipitins are low or undetectable. Characteristically, there are fleeting eosinophilic infiltrates in the lungs, particularly in the upper lobes. As airways become blocked with mucoid plugs rich in eosinophils, patients may cough up brown plugs and have hemoptysis. BPA may result in bronchiectasis, particularly affecting central airways, if not suppressed by corticosteroids. Asthma is controlled in the usual way by ICSs, but it is necessary to give a course of oral corticosteroids if there is any sign of worsening or pulmonary shadowing is found. Treatment with the oral antifungal itraconazole is beneficial in preventing exacerbations.

FURTHER READINGS

ASHER MI et al: Worldwide time trends in the prevalence of symptoms of asthma, allergic rhinoconjunctivitis, and eczema in childhood: ISAAC Phases One and Three repeat multicountry cross-sectional surveys. Lancet 368:733, 2006

BARNES PJ: New drugs for asthma. Nat Rev Drug Discov 3:831, 2004

——, ADCOCK IM: How do corticosteroids work in asthma? Ann Intern Med 139:359, 2003

—— et al: *Asthma and COPD*. London, Academic Press, 2002

—— et al: Inflammatory mediators of asthma: An update. Pharmacol Rev 50:515, 1998

BUSSE WW, LEMANSKE RF: Asthma. N Engl J Med 344:350, 2001

COOKSON W, MOFFATT M: Making sense of asthma genes. N Engl J Med 351:1794, 2004

EDER W et al: The asthma epidemic. N Engl J Med 355:2226, 2006

HEANEY LG, ROBINSON DS: Severe asthma treatment: Need for characterising patients. Lancet 365:974, 2005

MAPP CE et al: Occupational asthma. Am J Respir Crit Care Med 172:280, 2005

O'BYRNE PM, PARAMESWARAN K: Pharmacological management of mild or moderate persistent asthma. Lancet 368:794, 2006

SZCZEKLIK A, STEVENSON DD: Aspirin-induced asthma: Advances in pathogenesis, diagnosis, and management. J Allergy Clin Immunol 111:913, 2003

WENZEL SE: Asthma: Defining of the persistent adult phenotypes. Lancet 368:804, 2006

249 Hypersensitivity Pneumonitis and Pulmonary Infiltrates with Eosinophilia

Joel N. Kline, Gary W. Hunninghake

HYPERSENSITIVITY PNEUMONITIS

First described in 1874, hypersensitivity pneumonitis (HP), or extrinsic allergic alveolitis, is an inflammatory disorder of the lung, involving alveolar walls and terminal airways, that is induced, in a susceptible host, by repeated inhalation of a variety of organic agents. Factors responsible for the expression of HP include both those related to the host (susceptibility) and the inciting agent. Causes of HP are typically designated with colorful names denoting the occupational or avocational risk associated with the disease; "farmer's lung" is the term most commonly used for HP due to inhalation of antigens present in moldy hay, such as thermophilic actinomyces, *Micropolyspora faeni*, and *Aspergillus* species. The frequency of HP varies with the environmental exposure and the specific antigen involved.

ETIOLOGY

Agents implicated as causes of HP are diverse and include those listed in Table 249-1. In the United States, the most common types of HP are farmer's lung, bird fancier's lung, and chemical worker's lung. In *farmer's lung*, inhalation of proteins such as thermophilic bacteria and fungal spores that are present in moldy bedding and feed are most commonly responsible for the development of HP. These antigens are probably also responsible for the etiology of *mushroom worker's disease* (moldy composted growth medium is the source of the proteins) and bagassosis (moldy sugar cane is the source). *Bird fancier's lung* (and the related disorders of duck fever, turkey handler's lung, and dove pillow's lung) is a response to inhalation of proteins from feathers and droppings. *Chemical worker's lung* is an example of how simple chemicals, such as isocyanates, may also cause immune-mediated diseases.

PATHOGENESIS

The finding that precipitating antibodies against extracts of moldy hay were demonstrable in most patients with farmer's lung led to the early conclusion that HP was an immune complex–mediated reaction. Subsequent investigations of HP in human beings and animal models provided evidence for the importance of cell-mediated hypersensitivity.

The very early (acute) reaction is characterized by an increase in polymorphonuclear leukocytes in the alveoli and small airways. This early lesion is followed by an influx of mononuclear cells into the lung and the formation of granulomas that appear to be the result of a classic delayed (T cell–mediated) hypersensitivity reaction to repeated inhalation of antigen and adjuvant-active materials. Studies in animal models suggest that the disease is a T_H1-mediated immune response to antigen, with interferon γ, interleukin (IL) 12, and possibly IL-18 contributing to disease expression. Most likely, multiple cytokines [including also IL-1β, transforming growth factor (TGF) β, tumor necrosis factor (TNF) α and others] interact to promote HP; their source includes both alveolar macrophages and T lymphocytes in the lung. Recent data support a genetic predisposition to the development of HP; certain polymorphisms of the TNF-α promoter region reportedly confer an enhanced susceptibility to pigeon breeder's disease.

The attraction and accumulation of inflammatory cells in the lung may be due to one or more of the following mechanisms: induction of the adhesion molecules L-selectin and E-selectin, elaboration by dendritic cells of CC chemokine 1 (DC-CK-1/CCL18), and increased expression of CXCR3/CXCL10 by CD4+ and CD8+ lymphocytes. Increased levels of Fas protein and FasL in the lung (which would be expected to suppress inflammation by induction of T cell apoptosis) is counterbalanced by increased expression of the inducible antiapoptotic gene Bcl-xL, resulting in a lower overall level of pulmonary lymphocyte apoptosis in HP patients.

Bronchoalveolar lavage (BAL) in patients with HP consistently demonstrates an increase in T lymphocytes in lavage fluid (a finding that is also observed in patients with other granulomatous lung disorders). Patients with recent or continual exposure to antigen may have an increase in polymorphonuclear leukocytes in lavage fluid; this has been associated with lung fibrosis. A role for oxidant injury has been proposed in HP. Several markers of oxidative stress are reported to be increased during exacerbation of HP and are reduced by treatment with glucocorticoids.

CLINICAL PRESENTATION

The clinical picture is that of an interstitial pneumonitis, which varies from patient to patient and seems related to the frequency and intensity of exposure to the causative antigen and perhaps other host factors. The presentation can be acute, subacute, or chronic. In the *acute* form, symptoms such as cough, fever, chills, malaise, and dyspnea may occur 6 to 8 h after exposure to the antigen and usually clear within a few days if there is no further exposure to antigen. The *subacute* form often appears insidiously over a period of weeks marked by cough and dyspnea and may progress to cyanosis and severe dyspnea requiring hospitalization. In

TABLE 249-1 SELECTED EXAMPLES OF HYPERSENSITIVITY PNEUMONITIS (HP)

Disease	Antigen	Source of Antigen
Bagassosis	Thermophilic actinomycetes[a]	"Moldy" bagasse (sugar cane)
Bird fancier's, breeder's, or handler's lung[b]	Parakeet, pigeon, chicken, turkey proteins	Avian droppings or feathers
Cephalosporium HP	Contaminated basement (sewage)	*Cephalosporium*
Cheese washer's lung	*Penicillium casei*	Moldy cheese
Chemical worker's lung[b]	Isocyanates	Polyurethane foam, varnishes, lacquer
Coffee worker's lung	Coffee bean dust	Coffee beans
Compost lung	*Aspergillus*	Compost
Detergent worker's disease	*Bacillus subtilis* enzymes (subtilisins)	Detergent
Familial HP	*Bacillus subtilis*	Contaminated wood dust in walls
Farmer's lung[b]	Thermophilic actinomycetes[a]	"Moldy" hay, grain, silage
Fish food lung	Unknown	Fish food
Fish meal worker's lung	Fish meal dust	Fish meal
Furrier's lung	Animal fur dust	Animal pelts
Hot tub lung	*Cladosporium* spp., *Mycobacterium avium* complex	Mold on ceiling; contaminated water
Humidifier or air-conditioner lung (ventilation pneumonitis)	*Aureobasidium pullulans, Candida albicans,* Thermophilic actinomycetes[a], mycobacterium spp., other microorganisms	Contaminated water in humidification or forced-air air-conditioning systems
Japanese summer-type HP	*Trichosporon cutaneum, T. asahii,* and *T. mucoides*	House dust? Bird droppings
Laboratory worker's HP	Male rat urine	Laboratory rat
Lycoperdonosis	*Lycoperdon* puffballs	Puffball spores
Malt worker's lung	*Aspergillus fumigatus* or *A. clavatus*	Moldy barley
Maple bark disease	*Cryptostroma corticale*	Maple bark
Metalworking fluid lung	*Mycobacterium* spp., *Pseudomonas* spp.	Contaminated metalworking fluid
Miller's lung	*Sitophilus granarius* (wheat weevil)	Infested wheat flour
Miscellaneous medication	Amiodarone, bleomycin, efavirenz, gemcitabine, hydralazine, hydroxyurea, isoniazid, methotrexate, paclitaxel, penicillin, procarbazine, propranolol, riluzole, sirolimus, sulfasalazine	Medication
Mushroom worker's lung	Thermophilic actinomycetes,[a] *Hypsizigus marmoreus, Bunashimeji,* and other exotic mushrooms	Mushroom compost; mushrooms
Pituitary snuff taker's lung	Animal proteins	Heterologous pituitary snuff
Potato riddler's lung	Thermophilic actinomycetes,[a] *Aspergillus*	"Moldy" hay around potatoes
Sauna taker's lung	*Aureobasidium* spp., other	Contaminated sauna water
Sausage worker's lung	*Penicillium nalgiovense*	Dry sausage mold
Sequoiosis	*Aureobasidium, Graphium* spp.	Redwood sawdust
Streptomyces albus HP	*Streptomyces albus*	Contaminated fertilizer
Suberosis	*Penicillium glabrum* and *Chrysonilia sitophila*	Cork dust
Tap water lung	*Mycobacteria* spp.	Contaminated tap water
Thatched roof disease	*Sacchoromonospora viridis*	Dried grasses and leaves
Tobacco worker's disease	*Aspergillus* spp.	Mold on tobacco
Winegrower's lung	*Botrytis cinerea*	Mold on grapes
Wood trimmer's disease	*Rhizopus* spp., *Mucor* spp.	Contaminated wood trimmings
Woodman's disease	*Penicillium* spp.	Oak and maple trees
Woodworker's lung	Wood dust, *Alternaria*	Oak, cedar, pine, and mahogany dusts

[a]Thermophilic actinomycetes species include *Micropolyspora faeni, Thermoactinomyces vulgaris, T. saccharrii, T. viridis,* and *T. candidus.*

[b]Most common causes of hypersensitivity pneumonitis in the United States.

some patients, a subacute form of the disease may persist after an acute presentation of the disorder, especially if there is continued exposure to antigen. In most patients with the acute or subacute form of HP, the symptoms, signs, and other manifestations of HP disappear within days, weeks, or months if the causative agent is no longer inhaled. Transformation to a chronic form of the disease may occur in patients with continued antigen exposure, but the frequency of such progression is uncertain.

The *chronic* form of HP may be clinically indistinguishable from pulmonary fibrosis due to a wide variety of causes. Physical examination may reveal clubbing. This stage may progressively worsen, resulting in dependence on supplemental oxygen, pulmonary hypertension, and respiratory failure. Pulmonary fibrosis is the clinical manifestation of HP with the greatest predictive value for mortality. An indolent, gradually progressive form of the disease can be associated with cough and exertional dyspnea without a prior history consistent with acute or subacute manifestations. Such a gradual onset frequently occurs with low-dose exposure to the antigen.

DIAGNOSIS

All forms of the disease may be associated with elevations in erythrocyte sedimentation rate, C-reactive protein, rheumatoid factor, and serum immunoglobulins. Following acute exposure to antigen, neutrophilia and lymphopenia are frequently present. Eosinophilia is not a feature. Examination for *serum precipitins* against suspected antigens, such as those listed in Table 249-1, is an important part of the diagnostic workup and should be performed on any patient with interstitial lung disease, especially if a suggestive exposure history is elicited. If found, precipitins indicate sufficient exposure to the causative agent for generation of an immunologic response. The diagnosis of HP is not established solely by the presence of precipitins, however, as precipitins are found in sera of many individuals exposed to appropriate antigens who demonstrate no other evidence of HP. False-negative results may occur because of poor-quality antigens or an inappropriate choice of antigens. Extraction of antigens from the suspected source may at times be helpful.

Chest x-ray shows no specific or distinctive changes in HP. It can be normal even in symptomatic patients. The acute or subacute phases may be associated with poorly defined, patchy, or diffuse infiltrates or with discrete, nodular infiltrates. In the chronic phase, the chest x-ray usually shows a diffuse reticulonodular infiltrate. Honeycombing may eventually develop as the condition progresses. Apical sparing is common, suggesting that disease severity correlates with inhaled antigen

FIGURE 249-1 Chest CT scan of a patient with acute hypersensitivity pneumonitis in which scattered regions of ground glass and nodular infiltrates are seen bilaterally. *(Courtesy of JS Wilson; with permission.)*

load, but no particular distribution or pattern is classic for HP. Abnormalities rarely seen in HP include pleural effusion or thickening, and hilar adenopathy. High-resolution chest computed tomography (CT) has become the procedure of choice for imaging of HP, and a consensus is developing as to the typical appearance of the disease. Although pathognomonic features have not been identified, acute HP may appear with confluent alveolar opacification. In subacute disease, centrilobular nodules and "ground glass" changes predominate in the lower lobes, and expiratory views may demonstrate air trapping; this pattern is more common in individuals whose exposure to antigen continues rather than those in whom removal from antigen exposure has occurred. In chronic HP, patchy emphysema is seen more often than interstitial fibrosis; subpleural linear opacities and honeycombing are common, and these changes may be found throughout the lung. Hilar or mediastinal adenopathy is not associated with HP (Fig. 249-1).

Pulmonary function studies in all forms of HP may show a restrictive or an obstructive pattern with loss of lung volumes, impaired diffusion capacity, decreased compliance, and exercise-induced hypoxemia. Resting hypoxemia may also be found. Bronchospasm and bronchial hyperreactivity are sometimes found in acute HP. With antigen avoidance, the pulmonary function abnormalities are usually reversible, but they may gradually increase in severity or may occur rapidly following acute or subacute exposure to antigen.

BAL is used in some centers to aid in diagnostic evaluation. A marked lymphocytic alveolitis on BAL is almost universal, although not pathognomonic. Lymphocytes typically have a decreased helper/suppressor ratio and are activated. Alveolar neutrophilia is also prominent acutely but tends to fade in the absence of recurrent exposure. Bronchoalveolar mastocytosis may correlate with disease activity.

Lung biopsy, obtained through flexible bronchoscopy, open-lung procedures, or thoracoscopy, may be diagnostic. Although the histopathology is distinctive, it may not be pathognomonic of HP (Fig. 249-2). When the biopsy is taken during the active phase of disease, typical findings include an interstitial alveolar infiltrate consisting of plasma cells, lymphocytes, and occasional eosinophils and neutrophils, usually accompanied by loose, noncaseating peribronchial granulomas. Interstitial fibrosis may be present but most often is mild in earlier stages of the disease. Some degree of bronchiolitis is found in about half the cases. Rarely, bronchiolitis obliterans with organizing pneumonia (BOOP) (Chap. 255) may be present. The triad of mononuclear bronchiolitis; interstitial infiltrates of lymphocytes and plasma cells; and single, nonnecrotizing, and randomly scattered parenchymal granulomas without mural vascular involvement is consistent with but not specific for HP.

A *prediction rule* for the clinical diagnosis of HP has been developed by the International HP Study Group. Six significant predictors of HP (exposure to a known antigen, positive predictive antibodies to the antigen, recurrent episodes of symptoms, inspiratory crackles, symptoms developing 4–8 h after exposure, and weight loss) were retrospectively developed then validated in a separate cohort. This diagnostic paradigm has a high predictive value in the diagnosis of HP, without the need for invasive testing. In cases where only a subset of the criteria are fulfilled, the diagnosis is less clearly established. It is clear, however, that the diagnosis of HP is established by (1) consistent symptoms, physical findings, pulmonary function tests, and radiographic tests; (2) a history of exposure to a recognized antigen; and (3) ideally, identification of an antibody to that antigen. In some circumstances, BAL and/or lung biopsy may be needed. The most important tool in diagnosing HP continues to be a high index of suspicion!

DIFFERENTIAL DIAGNOSIS

Chronic HP may often be difficult to distinguish from a number of other interstitial lung disorders (Chap. 255). A negative history for use of relevant drugs and no evidence of a systemic disorder usually exclude the presence of drug-induced lung disease or a collagen vascular disorder. BAL often shows predominance of neutrophils in idiopathic pulmonary fibrosis and a predominance of CD4+ lymphocytes in sarcoidosis. Hilar/paratracheal lymphadenopathy or evidence of multisystem involvement also favors the diagnosis of sarcoidosis. In some patients, a lung biopsy may be required to differentiate chronic HP from other interstitial diseases. The lung disease associated with acute or subacute HP may clinically resemble other disorders that present with systemic symptoms and recurrent pulmonary infiltrates, including the allergic bronchopulmonary mycoses and other eosinophilic pneumonias. Gene cluster analysis of DNA from lung biopsies of patients with fibrotic lung disease has shown a significantly different gene expression profile in HP and idiopathic pulmonary fibrosis (IPF). HP biopsies expressed T cell and other genes related to inflammation, whereas the IPF patients had greater expression of genes associated with pulmonary remodeling, especially epithelial and myofibroblast genes. While this finding may be related to the disease stage in which the disorders were diagnosed, they suggest that such analyses may be clinically useful in the future.

Eosinophilic pneumonia is often associated with asthma and is typified by peripheral eosinophilia; neither of these is a feature of HP. Allergic bronchopulmonary aspergillosis (ABPA) is the most common example of the allergic bronchopulmonary mycoses and is sometimes confused with HP because of the presence of precipitating antibodies

FIGURE 249-2 Open-lung biopsy from a patient with acute hypersensitivity pneumonitis demonstrating loose, nonnecrotizing granulomas and thickened interstitium with an associated interstitial inflammatory response. *(Courtesy of B DeYoung; with permission.)*

to *Aspergillus fumigatus*. ABPA is associated with allergic (atopic) asthma. Acute HP may be confused with *organic dust toxic syndrome* (ODTS), a condition that is more common than HP. ODTS follows heavy exposure to organic dusts and is characterized by transient fever and muscle aches, with or without dyspnea and cough. Serum precipitins are absent, and the chest x-ray is usually normal. This distinction is important, as ODTS is a self-limited disorder without significant long-term sequelae, whereas continued antigen exposure in HP can result in permanent disability. Massive exposure to moldy silage may result in a syndrome termed *pulmonary mycotoxicosis*, with fever, chills, and cough and the presence of pulmonary infiltrates within a few hours of exposure. No previous sensitization is required, and precipitins are absent to *Aspergillus*, the suspected causative agent.

℞ HYPERSENSITIVITY PNEUMONITIS

Because effective treatment depends largely on avoiding the antigen, identification of the causative agent and its source is essential. This is usually possible if the physician takes a careful environmental and occupational history or, if necessary, visits the patient's environment. The simplest way to avoid the incriminated agent is to remove the patient from the environment or the source of the agent from the patient's environment. This recommendation cannot be taken lightly when it completely changes the lifestyle or livelihood of the patient. In many cases, however, the source of exposure (birds, humidifiers) can easily be removed. Pollen masks, personal dust respirators, airstream helmets, and ventilated helmets with a supply of fresh air are increasingly efficient means of purifying inhaled air. If symptoms recur or physiologic abnormalities progress in spite of these measures, then more effective measures to avoid antigen exposure must be pursued. The chronic form of HP typically results from low-grade or recurrent exposure over many months to years, and the lung disease may already be partially or completely irreversible. These patients are usually advised to avoid all possible contact with the offending agent.

Patients with the *acute*, recurrent form of HP usually recover without need for glucocorticoids. *Subacute* HP may be associated with severe symptoms and marked physiologic impairment and may continue to progress for several days despite hospitalization. Urgent establishment of the diagnosis and prompt institution of glucocorticoid treatment are indicated in such patients. Prednisone at a dosage of 1 mg/kg per day or its equivalent is continued for 7 to 14 days and then tapered over the ensuing 2 to 6 weeks at a rate that depends on the patient's clinical status. Patients with *chronic* HP may gradually recover without therapy following environmental control. In many patients, however, a trial of prednisone may be useful to obtain maximal reversibility of the lung disease. Following initial prednisone therapy (1 mg/kg per day for 2 to 4 weeks), the drug is tapered to the lowest dosage that will maintain the functional status of the patient. Many patients will not require or benefit from long-term therapy if there is no further exposure to antigen. Regrettably, available studies demonstrate no effect of glucocorticoid therapy on long-term prognosis of farmer's lung.

PULMONARY INFILTRATES WITH EOSINOPHILIA

Pulmonary infiltrates with eosinophilia (PIE, eosinophilic pneumonias) include distinct individual syndromes characterized by eosinophilic pulmonary infiltrates and, commonly, peripheral blood eosinophilia. Since Loeffler's initial description of a transient, benign syndrome of migratory pulmonary infiltrates and peripheral blood eosinophilia of unknown cause, this group of disorders has been enlarged to include several diseases of both known and unknown etiology (Table 249-2). These diseases may be considered as immunologically mediated lung diseases but are not to be confused with HP, in which eosinophilia is *not* a feature.

When an eosinophilic pneumonia is associated with bronchial asthma, it is important to determine if the patient has atopic asthma and has wheal-and-flare skin reactivity to *Aspergillus* or other relevant fungal antigens. If so, other criteria should be sought for the diagnosis of allergic bronchopulmonary aspergillosis (ABPA) (Table 249-3) or other, rarer examples of allergic bronchopulmonary mycosis such as those caused by *Penicillium*, *Candida*, *Curvularia*, or *Helminthosporium* spp.

TABLE 249-2	PULMONARY INFILTRATES WITH EOSINOPHILIA

Etiology Known

Allergic bronchopulmonary mycoses
Parasitic infestations
Drug reactions
Eosinophilia-myalgia syndrome

Idiopathic

Loeffler's syndrome
Acute eosinophilic pneumonia
Chronic eosinophilic pneumonia
Allergic granulomatosis of Churg and Strauss
Hypereosinophilic syndrome

A. fumigatus is the most common cause of ABPA. The chest roentgenogram in ABPA may show transient, recurrent infiltrates or may suggest the presence of proximal bronchiectasis. High-resolution chest CT is a sensitive, noninvasive technique for the recognition of proximal bronchiectasis. The bronchial asthma of ABPA likely involves an IgE-mediated hypersensitivity, whereas the bronchiectasis associated with this disorder is thought to result from a deposition of immune complexes in proximal airways. Adequate treatment usually requires the long-term use of systemic glucocorticoids.

A travel history or evidence of recent immigration should prompt the consideration of parasite-associated disorders. *Tropical eosinophilia* is usually caused by filarial infection; however, eosinophilic pneumonias also occur with other parasites such as *Ascaris*, *Ancyclostoma* sp., *Toxocara* sp., and *Strongyloides stercoralis*. Tropical eosinophilia due to *Wuchereria bancrofti* or *W. malayi* occurs most commonly in southern Asia, Africa, and South America and is treated successfully with diethylcarbamazine. Even in cases of known foreign travel, identification of the causative agent is not always possible, as exemplified by 18 cases (2 fatal) of acute eosinophilic pneumonia reported among U.S. military personnel deployed in Iraq.

In the United States, *drug-induced eosinophilic pneumonias* are the most common cause of eosinophilic pulmonary infiltrates. These are exemplified by acute reactions to nitrofurantoin, which may begin 2 h to 10 days after nitrofurantoin is started, with symptoms of dry cough, fever, chills, and dyspnea; an eosinophilic pleural effusion accompanying patchy or diffuse pulmonary infiltrates may also occur. Other drugs associated with eosinophilic pneumonias include sulfonamides, penicillin, chlorpropamide, thiazides, tricyclic antidepressants, hydralazine, gold salts, isoniazid, indomethacin, and others. One report has identified anti-TNF-α monoclonal antibody therapy as a cause of eosinophilic pneumonitis. Treatment consists of withdrawal of the incriminated drugs and the use of glucocorticoids, if necessary.

The group of idiopathic eosinophilic pneumonias consists of diseases of varying severity. *Loeffler's syndrome* was originally reported as a benign, acute eosinophilic pneumonia of unknown cause characterized by migrating pulmonary infiltrates and minimal clinical manifestations. In some patients, these clinical characteristics may prove to be

TABLE 249-3	DIAGNOSTIC FEATURES OF ALLERGIC BRONCHOPULMONARY ASPERGILLOSIS (ABPA)

Main Diagnostic Criteria

Bronchial asthma
Pulmonary infiltrates
Peripheral eosinophilia (>1000/μL)
Immediate wheal-and-flare response to *Aspergillus fumigatus*
Serum precipitins to *A. fumigatus*
Elevated serum IgE
Central bronchiectasis

Other Diagnostic Features

History of brownish plugs in sputum
Culture of *A. fumigatus* from sputum
Elevated IgE (and IgG) class antibodies specific for *A. fumigatus*

secondary to parasites or drugs. *Acute eosinophilic pneumonia* is an idiopathic acute febrile illness of <7 days' duration with severe hypoxemia, pulmonary infiltrates, and no history of asthma. *Chronic eosinophilic pneumonia* presents with significant systemic symptoms including fever, chills, night sweats, cough, anorexia, and weight loss of several weeks' to months' duration. The chest x-ray classically shows peripheral infiltrates. Some patients also have bronchial asthma of the intrinsic or nonallergic type. Dramatic clearing of symptoms and chest x-rays is often noted within 48 h after initiation of glucocorticoid therapy.

The *hypereosinophilic syndrome* is characterized by presence of >1500 eosinophils per microliter of peripheral blood for 6 months or longer; lack of evidence for parasitic, allergic, or other known causes of eosinophilia; and signs or symptoms of multisystem organ dysfunction. Consistent features are blood and bone marrow eosinophilia with tissue infiltration by relatively mature eosinophils. The heart may be involved with tricuspid valve abnormalities or endomyocardial fibrosis and a restrictive, biventricular cardiomyopathy (Chap. 231). Other organs affected typically include the lungs, liver, spleen, skin, and nervous system. Therapy of the disorder consists of glucocorticoids and/or hydroxyurea, plus therapy as needed for cardiac dysfunction, which is frequently responsible for much of the morbidity and mortality in this syndrome. Pulmonary eosinophilia has also been associated with T cell lymphoma and has been reported following *lung* and *bone marrow transplantation*.

GLOBAL PICTURE OF HYPERSENSITIVITY PNEUMONITIS AND PULMONARY INFILTRATES WITH EOSINOPHILIA

HP is more prevalent outside of the United States than within, and the range of antigen responses is somewhat different. Internationally, bird-breeder's lung is the most common form of HP. Rather than being associated with avocational exposures, bird-raising practices, highlighted by the emerging threat of avian influenza, lead to substantial exposure to workers involved in poultry husbandry and processing. This increases antigen exposure enormously, in comparison to U.S. workers, and enhances the risk of HP. Importantly, it is the most common cause of pediatric HP and has been reported in individuals as young as 4 years, when it has presented as a chronic cough.

Farmer's lung, one of the earliest reported causes of HP, is now more prevalent outside the United States than within, but it appears to be waning world-wide. This is likely in response to changing agricultural practices; increased use of impermeable barriers in hay storage has reduced the proliferation of thermophilic bacteria, and thus HP.

In certain cases, the international manifestations of HP resemble those of the U.S. disease. Many industrialized nations have increasingly reported HP due to mycobacteria and pseudomonads in contaminated metalworking fluids; the prevalence of these environmental contaminants greatly depends on workplace hygiene practices. Some forms of HP are almost exclusively geographically limited; an example of this is summer-type hypersensitivity pneumonitis in Japan. Likewise, cork worker's pneumonitis (suberosis), caused by exposure to contaminated corks, is almost exclusively seen in Spain and southern Europe, because of the regional cork industry. However, one of the causative antigens (*Chrysonilia sitophila*) is also reported to be an antigen in lung diseases associated with logging in Canada. In Spain, esparto, a member of the grass family, is used as a fiber for the weaving of mats, baskets, and ropes; it is also incorporated into traditional plaster construction. In both of its uses, it has been associated with HP (most likely due to contamination with *A. fumigatus*), again geographically limited because of the utility of the product, though not of the underlying fungal antigen. Exposure to exotic mushrooms is greater in Asia than in the United States, and this has recently been linked to cases of HP.

Pulmonary infiltrates with eosinophilia are also a greater international than U.S. health burden. In this case, parasitic infestation is far more common than drug-induced lung disease, but the manifestations are similar.

FURTHER READINGS

ALLEN JN: Drug-induced eosinophilic lung disease. Clin Chest Med 25:77, 2004

BECKETT W et al: Hypersensitivity pneumonitis associated with environmental mycobacteria. Environ Health Perspect 113: 767, 2005

COORAY JH, ISMAIL MM: Re-examination of the diagnostic criteria of tropical pulmonary eosinophilia. Respir Med 93:655, 1999

FINK JN et al: Needs and opportunities for research in hypersensitivity pneumonitis. Am J Respir Crit Care Med 171: 792, 2005

LACASSE Y et al: Clinical diagnosis of hypersensitivity pneumonitis. Am J Respir Crit Care Med 168: 962, 2003

SELMAN M et al: Gene expression profiles distinguish idiopathic pulmonary fibrosis from hypersensitivity pneumonitis. Am J Respir Crit Care Med, 173:188, 2006

SHORR AF et al: Acute eosinophilic pneumonia among U.S. military personnel deployed in or near Iraq. JAMA 292: 2997, 2004

SILVA CI et al: Hypersensitivity pneumonitis: Spectrum of high-resolution CT and pathologic findings. Am J Roentgenol 188:334, 2007

ZACHARISEN MC et al: The long-term outcome in acute, subacute, and chronic forms of pigeon breeder's disease hypersensitivity pneumonitis. Ann Allergy Asthma Immunol 88:175, 2002

250 Environmental Lung Disease

Frank E. Speizer, John R. Balmes

This chapter provides perspectives on ways to assess pulmonary diseases for which environmental or occupational causes are suspected. This assessment is important because removal of the patient from harmful exposure is often the only intervention that might prevent further significant deterioration or lead to improvement in a patient's condition. Furthermore, the identification of an environment-associated disease in a single patient may lead to primary preventive strategies affecting other similarly exposed people who have not yet developed disease.

The exact magnitude of the problem is unknown, but there is no question that large numbers of individuals are at risk for developing serious respiratory disease as a result of occupational or environmental exposures. For example, for the populations over age 15, 15–20% of the burden of asthma and chronic obstructive pulmonary disease (COPD) has been estimated to be due to occupational factors.

HISTORY AND PHYSICAL EXAMINATION

The patient's history is of paramount importance in assessing any potential occupational or environmental exposure. Inquiry into specific work practices should include questions about specific contaminants involved, the availability and use of personal respiratory protection devices, the size and ventilation of workspaces, and whether co-workers have similar complaints. The temporal association of exposure at work and symptoms may provide clues to occupation-related disease. In addition, the patient must be questioned about alternative sources for exposure to potentially toxic agents, including hobbies, home characteristics, exposure to secondhand smoke, and proximity to traffic or industrial facilities. Short-term and long-term exposures to potential toxic agents in the distant past must also be considered.

Many employees are aware of the potential hazards in their workplaces, and many states require that employees be informed about potentially hazardous exposures. These requirements include the provision of specific information about potential hazardous agents in products being used (Material Safety Data Sheets) and training in personal protective equipment and environmental control procedures. Reminders posted in the workplace may warn workers about hazardous substances. Protective clothing, lockers, and shower facilities may be considered necessary parts of the job. However, the introduction of new processes and/or new chemical compounds may change exposure significantly, and often only the employee on the production line is aware of the change. For the physician who regularly sees patients from a particular industry, a visit to the work site can be very instructive. Alternatively, physicians can request inspections by appropriate federal and/or state authorities.

The physical examination of patients with environment-related lung diseases may help to determine the nature and severity of the pulmonary condition. Unfortunately, these findings do not typically point to the specific causative agent, and other types of information must be used to arrive at an etiologic diagnosis.

PULMONARY FUNCTION TESTS AND CHEST IMAGING

Many mineral dusts produce characteristic alterations in the mechanics of breathing and lung volumes that clearly indicate a restrictive pattern (Chap. 246). Similarly, exposures to a number of organic dusts or chemical agents may result in occupational asthma or COPD. Measurement of change in forced expiratory volume (FEV_1) before and after a working shift can be used to detect an acute bronchoconstrictive or inflammatory response. For example, an acute decrement of FEV_1 over the first work shift of the week is a characteristic feature of cotton textile workers with byssinosis (an obstructive airway disorder with features of both asthma and chronic bronchitis).

The chest radiograph is useful in detecting and monitoring the pulmonary response to mineral dusts, certain metals, and organic dusts capable of inducing hypersensitivity pneumonitis. The International Labour Organisation (ILO) International Classification of Radiographs of Pneumoconioses classifies chest radiographs according to the nature and size of opacities seen and the extent of involvement of the parenchyma. In general, small rounded opacities are seen in silicosis or coal worker's pneumoconiosis and small, linear opacities are seen in asbestosis. The profusion of such opacities is rated using a 12-point scheme. Although useful for epidemiologic studies and screening large numbers of workers, the ILO system can be problematic when applied to an individual worker's chest radiograph. With dusts causing rounded opacities, the degree of involvement on the chest radiograph may be extensive, while pulmonary function may be only minimally impaired. In contrast, in pneumoconiosis causing linear, irregular opacities like those seen in asbestosis, the radiograph may lead to underestimation of the severity of the impairment until relatively late in the disease. For the individual patient with a history of exposure, conventional CT and high-resolution CT (HRCT) have improved the sensitivity of identifying diffuse parenchymal abnormalities of the lung as well as pleural thickening characteristic of asbestos exposure.

Other procedures that may be of use in identifying the role of environment exposures in causing lung disease include evaluation of heavy metal concentrations in urine (cadmium in battery plant workers); skin prick testing or specific IgE antibody titers for evidence of immediate hypersensitivity to agents capable of inducing occupational asthma (flour antigens in bakery workers); specific IgG precipitating antibody titers for agents capable of causing hypersensitivity pneumonitis (pigeon antigens in bird handlers); or assays for specific cell-mediated immune responses (beryllium lymphocyte proliferation testing in nuclear workers or tuberculin skin testing in health care workers). Sometimes, a bronchoscopy to obtain bronchoalveolar lavage fluid and transbronchial biopsy of lung tissue may be required for histologic diagnosis (chronic beryllium disease). Rarely, video-assisted thoracoscopic surgery to obtain a larger sample of lung tissue may be required to determine the specific diagnosis of environment-induced lung disease (hypersensitivity pneumonitis or giant cell interstitial pneumonitis due to cobalt exposure).

MEASUREMENT OF EXPOSURE

If reliable environmental sampling data are available, this information should be used in assessing a patient's exposure. Since many of the chronic diseases result from exposure over many years, current environmental measurements should be combined with work histories to arrive at estimates of past exposure.

In situations where individual exposure to specific agents—either in a work setting or via ambient air pollutants—has been determined, the chemical and physical characteristics of these agents affect both inhaled dose and site of deposition in the respiratory tract. Water-soluble gases such as ammonia or sulfur dioxide are absorbed in the lining fluid of the upper and proximal airways and thus tend to produce irritative and bronchoconstrictive responses. In contrast, nitrogen dioxide and phosgene, which are less soluble, may penetrate to the bronchioles and alveoli in sufficient quantities to produce acute chemical pneumonitis that can be life-threatening (acute respiratory distress syndrome with noncardiogenic pulmonary edema).

Particle size of air contaminants must also be considered. Particles >10–15 μm in diameter, because of their settling velocities in air, do not penetrate beyond the upper airways. Particles <10 μm in size are deposited below the larynx and are primarily created by the burning of fossil fuels or high-temperature industrial processes resulting in condensation products from gases, fumes, or vapors. These particles are divided into three size fractions on the basis of their size characteristics and sources. Particles of ~2.5–10 μm (coarse-mode fraction) contain crustal elements, such as silica, aluminum, and iron. These particles mostly deposit relatively high in the tracheobronchial tree. Although the total mass of an ambient sample is dominated by these larger respirable particles, the number of particles, and therefore the surface area on which potential toxic agents can deposit and be carried to the lower airways, is dominated by particles <2.5 μm (fine-mode fraction). The smallest particles, those <0.1 μm in size, represent the ultrafine fraction and make up the largest number of particles, which tend to remain in the airstream and deposit in the lung only on a random basis as they come into contact with the alveolar walls. Besides the size characteristics of particles and the solubility of gases, the actual chemical composition, mechanical properties, and immunogenicity or infectivity of inhaled material determine in large part the nature of the diseases found among exposed persons.

OCCUPATIONAL EXPOSURES AND PULMONARY DISEASE

Table 250-1 provides broad categories of exposure in the workplace and diseases associated with chronic exposure in these industries.

ASBESTOS-RELATED DISEASES

Asbestos is a generic term for several different mineral silicates, including chrysolite, amosite, anthophyllite, and crocidolite. In addition to workers involved in the production of asbestos products (mining, milling, and manufacturing), many workers in the ship-building and construction trades, including pipe fitters and boilermakers, were occupationally exposed because asbestos was widely used for its thermal and electrical insulation properties. Asbestos also was used in the manufacture of fire-smothering blankets and safety garments, as filler for plastic materials, in cement and floor tiles, and in friction materials, such as brake and clutch linings.

Exposure to asbestos is not limited to persons who directly handle the material. Cases of asbestos-related diseases have been encountered in individuals with only bystander exposure, such as the painter or electrician who worked alongside the insulation worker in a shipyard. Community exposure resulted from the use of asbestos-containing mine or mill tailings as landfill, road surface, and playground material. Finally, exposure can also occur from the disturbance of naturally occurring asbestos (e.g., from increasing residential development in the foothills of the Sierra Mountains in California).

Asbestos was first used extensively in the 1930s. Starting in 1975 it was mostly replaced with synthetic mineral fibers, such as fiberglass or slag wool, but it continues to be used increasingly in the developing world.

TABLE 250-1 CATEGORIES OF OCCUPATIONAL EXPOSURE AND ASSOCIATED RESPIRATORY CONDITIONS

Occupational Exposures	Nature of Respiratory Responses	Comment
Inorganic Dusts		
Asbestos: mining, processing, construction, ship repair	Fibrosis (asbestosis), pleural disease, cancer, mesothelioma	Virtually all new mining and construction with asbestos done in developing countries
Silica: mining, stone cutting, sandblasting, quarrying	Fibrosis (silicosis), PMF, cancer, silicotuberculosis, COPD	Improved protection in United States, persistent risk in developing countries
Coal dust: mining	Fibrosis (coal workers' pneumoconiosis), PMF, COPD	Risk dropping in United States, increasing where new mines open
Beryllium: processing alloys for high-tech industries	Acute pneumonitis, chronic granulomatous disease, lung cancer (highly suspect)	Risk in high-tech industries persists
Other metals: aluminum, chromium, cobalt, nickel, titanium, tungsten carbide, or "hard metal" (contains cobalt)	Wide variety of conditions from acute pneumonitis to lung cancer and asthma	New diseases appear with new process development
Organic Dusts		
Cotton dust: milling, processing	Byssinosis (an asthma-like syndrome), chronic bronchitis, COPD	Increasing risk in developing countries with drop in United States as jobs shift overseas
Grain dust: elevator agents, dock workers, milling, bakers	Asthma, chronic bronchitis, COPD	Risk shifting more to migrant labor pool
Other agricultural dusts: fungal spores, vegetable products, insect fragments, animal dander, bird and rodent feces, endotoxins, microorganisms, pollens	Hypersensitivity pneumonitis (farmers' lung), asthma, chronic bronchitis	Important in migrant labor pool but also resulting from in-home exposures
Toxic chemicals: wide variety of industries, see Table 250-2	Chronic bronchitis, COPD, hypersensitivity pneumonitis, pneumoconiosis, and cancer	Reduced risk with recognized hazards; increasing risk for developing countries where controlled labor practices are less stringent
Other respiratory environmental agents (proven or highly suspect): uranium and radon daughters, environmental tobacco smoke, polycyclic hydrocarbons, biomass fuels, diesel exhaust, welding fumes, woods or wood finishing products	Estimates vary from ~3 to 10% of all lung cancers; in addition chronic bronchitis, COPD, and fibrosis	In-home exposures important, in developing countries disease rates as high or higher in females compared to males

Despite current regulations mandating adequate training for any worker potentially exposed to asbestos, exposure continues among inadequately trained and protected demolition workers. The major health effects from exposure to asbestos are pleural and pulmonary fibrosis and cancers of the respiratory tract, the pleura, and (in rare cases) the peritoneum.

Asbestosis is a diffuse interstitial fibrosing disease of the lung that is directly related to the intensity and duration of exposure. The disease resembles other forms of diffuse interstitial fibrosis (Chap. 255). Usually, moderate to severe exposure has taken place for at least 10 years before the disease becomes manifest and may occur following exposure to any of the asbestiform fiber types.

Physiologic studies reveal a restrictive pattern with a decrease in both lung volumes and diffusing capacity. There may also be evidence of mild airflow obstruction (due to peribronchiolar fibrosis).

The fibrotic lesions are the end result of oxidative injury due to the generation of reactive oxygen species by the transition metals on the surface of the fibers as well as from cells engaged in phagocytosis.

Diagnosis The chest radiograph can be used to detect a number of manifestations of asbestos exposure. Past exposure is specifically indicated by pleural plaques, which are characterized by either thickening or calcification along the parietal pleura, particularly along the lower lung fields, the diaphragm, and the cardiac border. Without additional manifestations, pleural plaques imply only exposure, not pulmonary impairment. Benign pleural effusions may also occur. The fluid is typ-

ically a serous or bloody exudate. The effusion may be slowly progressive or may resolve spontaneously. Irregular or linear opacities, usually first noted in the lower lung fields and spreading into the middle and upper lung fields, occur as the disease progresses. An indistinct heart border or a "ground glass" appearance in the lung fields is seen in some cases. In cases in which the x-ray changes are less obvious, HRCT may show distinct changes of subpleural curvilinear lines 5–10 mm in length that appear to be parallel to the pleural surface (Fig. 250-1).

No specific therapy is available for the management of patients with asbestosis. The supportive care is the same as that given to any patient with diffuse interstitial fibrosis from any cause. In general, newly diagnosed cases will have resulted from exposure levels that were present many years before and, in spite of the patients' having left the industry, are attributable to that former exposure. Since the patient may be eligible for compensation within a specific time frame after the diagnosis of an asbestos-related disease is made, the physician making the diagnosis should be certain to inform the patient promptly. On occasion, the physician may have reason to suspect ongoing exposure from a patient's current job description. Such a patient needs to wear appropriate respiratory protective gear according to federal regulation. Casual, nonoccupational exposure to undisturbed sources of asbestos-containing materials—e.g., in walls of schools or other buildings—represents virtually no hazard of asbestosis.

Lung cancer (Chap. 85) is the most frequent cancer associated with asbestos exposure. The excess frequency of lung cancer (all histologic types) in asbestos workers is associated with a minimum latency of 15–19 years between first exposure and development of the disease. Persons with more exposure are at greater risk of disease. In addition, there is a significant multiplicative effect of smoking and asbestos exposure than would be expected from the additive effect of each factor. The use of HRCT in such at-risk individuals to detect lung cancer at an earlier stage is currently under investigation.

Mesotheliomas (Chap. 257), both pleural and peritoneal, are also associated with asbestos exposure. In contrast to lung cancers, these tumors do not appear to be associated with smoking. Relatively short-term asbestos exposures of ≤ 1–2 years or less, occurring up to 40 years in the past, have been associated with the development of mesotheliomas (an observation that emphasizes the importance of obtaining a complete environmental exposure history). While the risk of mesothelioma is much less than for lung cancer among asbestos-exposed workers, over 2,000 cases were reported in the U.S. per year at the start of the 21st century.

Although ~50% of mesotheliomas metastasize, the tumor generally is locally invasive, and death usually results from local extension. Most patients present with effusions that may obscure the underlying pleural tumor. In contrast to the findings in effusion due to other causes, because of the restriction placed on the chest wall, no shift of mediastinal structures toward the opposite side of the chest will be seen. The major diagnostic problem is differentiation from peripherally spreading pulmonary adenocarcinoma or from adenocarcinoma metastasized to pleura from

A

B

FIGURE 250-1 Asbestosis: A. Frontal chest radiograph shows bilateral calcified pleural plaques consistent with asbestos-related pleural disease. Poorly defined linear and reticular abnormalities are seen in the lower lobes bilaterally. **B.** Axial high-resolution CT of the thorax obtained through the lung bases shows bilateral, subpleural reticulation (*black arrows*), representing fibrotic lung disease due to asbestosis. Subpleural lines are also present (*arrowheads*), characteristic of, though not specific for, asbestosis. Calcified pleural plaques representing asbestos-related pleural disease (*white arrows*) are also evident.

an extrathoracic primary site. Although cytologic examination of pleural fluid may suggest the diagnosis, biopsy of pleural tissue, generally with video-assisted thoracic surgery, and special immunohistochemical staining is usually required. There is no effective therapy.

Since epidemiologic studies have shown that >80% of mesotheliomas may be associated with asbestos exposure, documented mesothelioma in a patient with occupational or environmental exposure to asbestos may be compensable.

SILICOSIS

In spite of the technical adequacy of existing protective equipment, *free silica* (SiO$_2$), or crystalline quartz, is still a major occupational hazard. The major occupational exposures include: mining; stonecutting; employment

FIGURE 250-2 Acute silicosis. The high-resolution CT scan shows multiple small nodules consistent with silicosis but also diffuse ground-glass densities with thickened intralobular and interlobular septa, producing polygonal shapes. This has been referred to as "crazy paving."

in abrasive industries, such as stone, clay, glass, and cement manufacturing; foundry work; packing of silica flour; and quarrying, particularly of granite. Most often, pulmonary fibrosis due to silica exposure (silicosis) occurs in a dose-response fashion after many years of exposure.

Workers heavily exposed through sandblasting in confined spaces, tunneling through rock with high quartz content (15–25%), or the manufacture of abrasive soaps may develop acute silicosis with as little as 10 months' exposure. The clinical and pathological features of acute silicosis are similar to those of pulmonary alveolar proteinosis (Chap. 255). The chest radiograph may show profuse miliary infiltration or consolidation and there is a characteristic HRCT pattern known as "crazy paving" (**Fig. 250-2**). The disease may be quite severe and progressive, despite the discontinuation of exposure. Whole-lung lavage may provide symptomatic relief and slow progression.

With long-term, less intense exposure, small rounded opacities in the upper lobes may appear on the chest radiograph after 15–20 years of exposure (*simple silicosis*). Calcification of hilar nodes may occur in as many as 20% of cases and produces a characteristic "eggshell" pattern. Silicotic nodules may be identified more readily by HCRT (**Fig. 250-3**). The nodular fibrosis may be progressive in the absence of further exposure, with coalescence and formation of nonsegmental conglomerates of irregular masses >1 cm in diameter (*complicated silicosis*). These masses can become quite large and when this occurs the term *progressive massive fibrosis* (PMF) is applied. Significant functional impairment with both restrictive and obstructive components may be associated with this form of silicosis.

Because silica is cytotoxic to alveolar macrophages, patients with silicosis are at greater risk of acquiring lung infections that involve these cells as a primary defense (*Mycobacterium tuberculosis*, atypical mycobacteria and fungi). Because of the increased risk of active tuberculosis, the recommended treatment of latent tuberculosis in these patients is longer. Another potential clinical complication of silicosis is autoimmune connective tissue disorders such as rheumatoid arthritis or scleroderma. In addition, there are sufficient epidemiologic data that the International Agency for Research on Cancer lists silica as a probable lung carcinogen.

Other less hazardous silicates include Fuller's earth, kaolin, mica, diatomaceous earths, silica gel, soapstone, carbonate dusts, and ce-

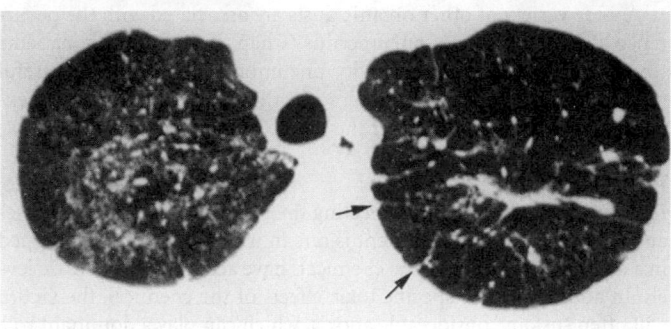

FIGURE 250-3 Chronic silicosis. A. Frontal chest radiograph in a patient with silicosis shows variably sized, poorly defined nodules (*arrows*) predominating in the upper lobes, **B.** Axial thoracic CT image through the lung apices shows numerous small nodules, more pronounced in the right upper lobe. A number of the nodules are subpleural in location (*arrows*).

ment dusts. The production of fibrosis in workers exposed to these agents is believed to be related either to the free silica content of these dusts or, for substances that contain no free silica, to the potentially large dust loads to which these workers may be exposed.

Other silicates, including *talc dusts*, may be contaminated with asbestos and/or free silica. Fibrosis and/or pleural or lung cancer have been associated with chronic exposure to commercial talc.

COAL WORKER'S PNEUMOCONIOSIS (CWP)

Occupational exposure to *coal dust* can lead to CWP, which has enormous social, economic, and medical significance in every nation in which coal mining is an important industry. Simple radiographically identified CWP is seen in ~10% of all coal miners and in as many as 50% of anthracite miners with more than 20 years' work on the coal face. The prevalence of disease is lower in workers in bituminous coal mines. Since much western U.S. coal is bituminous, CWP is less prevalent in that region.

With prolonged exposure to coal dust (i.e., 15–20 years), small, rounded opacities similar to those of silicosis may develop. As in silicosis, the presence of these nodules (*simple CWP*) is not usually associated with pulmonary impairment. Much of the symptomatology associated with simple CWP appears to be due to the effects of coal dust on the development of chronic bronchitis and COPD (Chap. 254). The effects of coal dust are additive to those of cigarette smoking.

Complicated CWP is manifested by the appearance on the chest radiograph of nodules ranging from 1 cm in diameter to the size of an entire lobe, generally confined to the upper half of the lungs. As in sili-

cosis, this condition can progress to PMF which is accompanied by severe lung function deficits and associated with premature mortality.

Caplan's syndrome (Chap. 314), first described in coal miners but subsequently found in patients with silicosis, includes seropositive rheumatoid arthritis with characteristic pneumoconiotic nodules. Silica has immunoadjuvant properties and is often present in anthracitic coal dust.

CHRONIC BERYLLIUM DISEASE

Beryllium is a light-weight metal with tensile strength, has good electrical conductivity, and is valuable in the control of nuclear reactions through its ability to quench neutrons. Although beryllium may produce an acute pneumonitis, it is far more commonly associated with a chronic granulomatous inflammatory disease that is similar to sarcoidosis (Chap. 322). Unless one inquires specifically about occupational exposures to beryllium in the manufacture of alloys, ceramics, or high-technology electronics in a patient with sarcoidosis, one may miss entirely the etiologic relationship to the occupational exposure. What distinguishes chronic beryllium disease (CBD) from sarcoidosis is evidence of a specific cell-mediated immune response (i.e., delayed hypersensitivity) to beryllium.

The test that usually provides this evidence is the beryllium lymphocyte proliferation test (BeLPT). The BeLPT uses the in vitro proliferation of lymphocytes from blood or bronchoalveolar lavage in the presence of beryllium salts as compared to that of unstimulated cells. Proliferation is usually measured by lymphocyte uptake of radiolabeled thymidine.

Chest imaging findings are similar to those of sarcoidosis (nodules along septal lines) except that hilar adenopathy is somewhat less common. Like sarcoidosis, pulmonary function test results may show restrictive and/or obstructive ventilatory deficits and decreased diffusing capacity. With early disease, both chest imaging studies and pulmonary function tests may be normal. Fiberoptic bronchoscopy with transbronchial lung biopsy is usually required to make the diagnosis of CBD. In a beryllium-sensitized individual, the presence of noncaseating granulomas or monocytic infiltration in lung tissue establishes the diagnosis. Accumulation of beryllium-specific CD4+ T cells occurs in the granulomatous inflammation seen on lung biopsy.

Chronic beryllium disease is one of the best studied examples of gene-environment interaction. Susceptibility to CBD is highly associated with HLA-DP alleles possessing a glutamic acid in position 69 of the β chain. In addition, there is also evidence that a polymorphism in position 308 of the promoter region of tumor necrosis factor α is involved in mediating the severity of the inflammatory response in patients with CBD.

Other metals, including aluminum and titanium dioxide, have been rarely associated with a sarcoid-like reaction in lung tissue. Exposure to dust containing tungsten carbide, also known as "hard metal," may produce giant cell interstitial pneumonitis. Cobalt is a constituent of tungsten carbide and is the likely etiologic agent of both the interstitial pneumonitis and the occupational asthma that may occur. The most common exposures to tungsten carbide occur in tool and dye, saw blade, and drill bit manufacture. Diamond polishing may also involve exposure to cobalt dust. The same Glu69 polymorphism of the HLA-DP β chain that confers increased risk of CBD also appears to increase risk of cobalt-induced giant cell interstitial pneumonitis.

In patients with interstitial lung disease, one should always inquire about exposure to metal fumes and/or dusts. Especially when sarcoidosis appears to be the diagnosis, one should always consider possible CBD.

OTHER INORGANIC DUSTS

Most of the inorganic dusts discussed thus far are associated with the production of either dust macules or interstitial fibrotic changes in the lung. Other inorganic and organic dusts (see categories in Table 250-1), along with some of the dusts previously discussed, are associated with chronic mucous hypersecretion (chronic bronchitis), with or without reduction of expiratory flow rates. Cigarette smoking is the major cause of these conditions and any effort to attribute some component of the disease to occupational and environmental exposures must take cigarette smoking into account. Most studies suggest an additive effect of dust exposure and smoking. The pattern of the irritant dust effect is similar to that of cigarette smoking, suggesting that small airway inflammation may be the initial site of pathologic response in those cases and continued exposure may lead to chronic bronchitis and COPD.

ORGANIC DUSTS

Some of the specific diseases associated with organic dusts are discussed in detail in the chapters on asthma (Chap. 248) and hypersensitivity pneumonitis (Chap. 249). Many of these diseases are named for the specific setting in which they are found, e.g., farmer's lung, malt worker's disease, or mushroom worker's disease. Often the temporal relation of symptoms to exposure furnishes the best evidence for the diagnosis. Three occupational groups are singled out for discussion because they represent the largest proportion of people affected by the diseases resulting from organic dusts.

Cotton Dust (Byssinosis)   Many persons are exposed occupationally to cotton, flax, or hemp in the production of yarns for cotton, linen, and rope making. Although this discussion focuses on cotton, the same syndrome—albeit somewhat less severe—has been reported in association with exposure to flax, hemp, and jute.

Exposure occurs throughout the manufacturing process but is most pronounced in those portions of the factory involved with the treatment of the cotton prior to spinning—i.e., blowing, mixing, and carding (straightening of fibers). Risk of byssinosis is associated with both cotton dust and endotoxin levels in the workplace environment. Attempts to control dust levels by use of exhaust hoods, general increases in ventilation, and wetting procedures in some settings have been highly successful. However, respiratory protective equipment appears to be required during certain operations to prevent workers from being exposed to levels of cotton dust that exceed the current U.S. permissible exposure level.

Byssinosis is characterized clinically as occasional (early stage) and then regular (late stage) chest tightness toward the end of the first day of the workweek ("Monday chest tightness"). In epidemiologic studies, depending on the level of exposure via the carding room air, up to 80% of employees may show a significant drop in their FEV_1 over the course of a Monday shift.

Initially the symptoms do not recur on subsequent days of the week. However, in 10–25% of workers, the disease may be progressive, with chest tightness recurring or persisting throughout the workweek. After >10 years of exposure, workers with recurrent symptoms are more likely to have an obstructive pattern on pulmonary function testing. The highest grades of impairment are generally seen in smokers.

Reduction of dust exposure is of primary importance to the management of byssinosis. All workers with persistent symptoms or significantly reduced levels of pulmonary function should be moved to areas of lower risk of exposure. Regular surveillance of pulmonary function in cotton dust–exposed workers using spirometry before and after the workshift is required by the Occupational Safety and Health Administration (OSHA) of the U.S. government.

Grain Dust   Although the exact number of workers at risk in the United States is not known, at least 500,000 people work in grain elevators, and >2 million farmers are potentially exposed to grain dust. The presentation of obstructive airway disease in grain dust-exposed workers is virtually identical to the characteristic findings in cigarette smokers, i.e., persistent cough, mucous hypersecretion, wheeze and dyspnea on exertion, and reduced FEV_1 and FEV_1/FVC ratio (Chap. 246).

Dust concentrations in grain elevators vary greatly but appear to be >10,000 μg/m^3; approximately one-third of the particles, by weight, are in the respirable range. The effect of grain dust exposure is additive to that of cigarette smoking, with ~50% of workers who smoke having symptoms. Among nonsmoking grain elevator operators, approximately one-quarter have mucous hypersecretion, about five times the num-

ber that would be expected in unexposed nonsmokers. Smoking grain dust–exposed workers are more likely to have obstructive ventilatory deficits on pulmonary function testing. As in byssinosis, endotoxin may play a role in grain dust–induced chronic bronchitis and COPD.

Farmer's Lung   This condition results from exposure to moldy hay containing spores of thermophilic actinomycetes that produce a hypersensitivity pneumonitis (Chap. 249). There are few good population-based estimates of the frequency of occurrence of this condition in the United States. However, among farmers in Great Britain, the rate of disease ranges from approximately 10–50 per 1000. The prevalence of disease varies in association with rainfall, which determines the amount of fungal growth, and with differences in agricultural practices related to turning and stacking hay.

The patient with acute farmer's lung presents 4–8 h after exposure with fever, chills, malaise, cough, and dyspnea without wheezing. The history of exposure is obviously essential to distinguish this disease from influenza or pneumonia with similar symptoms. In the chronic form of the disease, the history of repeated attacks after similar exposure is important in differentiating this syndrome from other causes of patchy fibrosis (e.g., sarcoidosis).

A wide variety of other organic dusts are associated with the occurrence of hypersensitivity pneumonitis (Chap. 249). For those patients who present with hypersensitivity pneumonitis, specific and careful inquiry about occupations, hobbies, or other home environmental exposures is necessary to uncover the source of the etiologic agent.

TOXIC CHEMICALS

Exposure to toxic chemicals affecting the lung generally involves gases and vapors. A common accident is one in which the victim is trapped in a confined space where the chemicals have accumulated to toxic levels. In addition to the specific toxic effects of the chemical, the victim will often sustain considerable anoxia, which can play a dominant role in determining whether the individual survives.

Table 250-2 lists a variety of toxic agents that can produce acute and sometimes life-threatening reactions in the lung. All these agents in sufficient concentrations have been demonstrated, at least in animal studies, to affect the lower airways and disrupt alveolar architecture, either acutely or as a result of chronic exposure. Some of these agents may be generated acutely in the environment (see below).

Firefighters and fire victims are at risk of *smoke inhalation*, a numerically important cause of acute cardiorespiratory failure. Smoke inhalation kills more fire victims than does thermal injury. Carbon monoxide poisoning with resulting significant hypoxemia can be life-threatening (**Chap. e35**). The use of synthetic materials (plastic, polyurethanes), which, when burned, may release a variety of other toxic agents (such as cyanide or hydrochloric acid), must be considered when evaluating smoke inhalation victims. Exposed victims may suffer some degree of lower respiratory tract inflammation and/or pulmonary edema.

Exposure to certain highly reactive, low-molecular-weight agents used in the manufacture of synthetic polymers, paints, and coatings (*diisocyanates* in polyurethanes; *aromatic amines* and *acid anhydrides* in epoxies) are associated with a high risk of occupational asthma. Although this occupational asthma manifests clinically as if sensitization has occurred, there is little evidence that an IgE antibody–mediated mechanism is involved. Hypersensitivity pneumonitis–like reactions also have been described in diisocyanate and acid anhydride–exposed workers.

Fluoropolymers, such as Teflon, which at normal temperatures produce no reaction, upon heating become volatilized. The inhaled agents cause a characteristic syndrome of fever, chills, malaise, and occasionally mild wheezing leading to the diagnosis of *polymer fume fever*. A similar self-limited, influenza-like syndrome—*metal fume fever*—results from acute exposure to fumes or smoke containing zinc oxide. The syndrome may begin several hours after work and resolves within 24 h, only to return on repeated exposure. Welding of galvanized steel is the most common exposure leading to metal fume fever.

Two other agents have been recently associated with potentially severe interstitial lung disease. Occupational exposure to nylon flock has

TABLE 250-2   SELECTED COMMON TOXIC CHEMICAL AGENTS AFFECTING THE LUNG

Agent(s)	Selected Exposures	Acute Effects from High or Accidental Exposure	Chronic Effects from Relatively Low Exposure
Acid fumes: H_2SO_4, HNO_3	Manufacture of fertilizers, chlorinated organic compounds, dyes, explosives, rubber products, metal etching, plastics	Mucous membrane irritation, followed by chemical pneumonitis 2–3 days later	Bronchitis and suggestion of mildly reduced pulmonary function in children with lifelong residential exposure to high levels; clinical significance unknown
Acrolein and other aldehydes	By-product of burning plastics, woods, tobacco smoke	Mucous membrane irritant, decrease in lung function	Mutagen in animals, no human data
Ammonia	Refrigeration; petroleum refining; manufacture of fertilizers, explosives, plastics, and other chemicals	Same as for acid fumes	Chronic bronchitis
Anhydrides	Manufacture of resin esters, polyester resins, thermoactivated adhesives	Nasal irritation, cough	Asthma, chronic bronchitis, hypersensitivity pneumonitis
Cadmium fumes	Smelting, soldering, battery production	Mucous membrane irritant, acute respiratory distress syndrome (ARDS)	COPD
Formaldehyde	Manufacture of resins, leathers, rubber, metals, and woods; laboratory workers, embalmers; emission from urethane foam insulation	Same as for acid fumes	Cancers in one species; no data on humans
Halides and acid salts (Cl, Br, F)	Bleaching in pulp, paper, textile industry; manufacture of chemical compounds; synthetic rubber, plastics, disinfectant, rocket fuel, gasoline	Mucous membrane irritation, pulmonary edema; possible reduced FVC 1–2 yrs after exposure	Dryness of mucous membrane, epistaxis, dental fluorosis, tracheobronchitis
Hydrogen sulfide	By-product of many industrial processes, oil, other petroleum processes and storage	Increase in respiratory rate followed by respiratory arrest, lactic acidosis, pulmonary edema, death	Conjunctival irritation, chronic bronchitis, recurrent pneumonitis
Isocyanates (TDI, HDI, MDI)	Production of polyurethane foams, plastics, adhesives, surface coatings	Mucous membrane irritation, dyspnea, cough, wheeze, pulmonary edema	Upper respiratory tract irritation, cough, asthma, allergic alveolitis
Nitrogen dioxide	Silage, metal etching, explosives, rocket fuels, welding, by-product of burning fossil fuels	Cough, dyspnea, pulmonary edema may be delayed 4–12 h; possible result from acute exposure: bronchiolitis obliterans in 2–6 wks	Emphysema in animals, ?chronic bronchitis, associated with reduced lung function in children with lifelong residential exposure, clinical significance unknown
Ozone	Arc welding, flour bleaching, deodorizing, emissions from copying equipment, photochemical air pollutant	Mucous membrane irritant, pulmonary hemorrhage and edema, reduced pulmonary function transiently in children and adults, and increased hospitalization with exposure to summer haze	Chronic eye irritation and slight excess in cardiopulmonary mortality in susceptible individuals
Phosgene	Organic compound, metallurgy, volatilization of chlorine-containing compounds	Delayed onset of bronchiolitis and pulmonary edema	Chronic bronchitis
Sulfur dioxide	Manufacture of sulfuric acid, bleaches, coating of nonferrous metals, food processing, refrigerant, burning of fossil fuels, wood pulp industry	Mucous membrane irritant, epistaxis	?Chronic bronchitis

been shown to induce a lymphocytic bronchiolitis, and workers exposed to diacetyl used to provide "butter" flavor in the manufacture of microwave popcorn have developed bronchiolitis obliterans (Chap. 255).

World Trade Center Disaster   A consequence of the attack on the World Trade Center (WTC) on September 11, 2001, was relatively heavy exposure of a large number of firefighters and other rescue workers to the dust generated by the collapse of the buildings. Environmental monitoring and chemical characterization of WTC dust has revealed a wide variety of potentially toxic constituents, although much of the dust was pulverized cement. Possibly because of the high alkalinity of WTC dust significant cough, wheeze, and phlegm production occurred among firefighters and clean-up crews. New cough and wheeze syndromes also occurred among local residents. Initial longitudinal follow-up of New York firefighters suggests that heavier exposure to WTC dust is associated with accelerated decline of lung function.

ENVIRONMENTAL RESPIRATORY CARCINOGENS
In addition to asbestos exposures, other occupational exposures associated with either proven or suspected respiratory carcinogens include those to acrylonitrile, arsenic compounds, beryllium, bis(chloromethyl) ether, chromium (hexavalent), formaldehyde (nasal), isopropyl oil

(nasal sinuses), mustard gas, the various ores used to produce pure nickel, polyaromatic hydrocarbons (coke oven emissions and diesel exhaust), secondhand tobacco smoke, silica (both mining and processing), talc (possible asbestos contamination in both mining and milling), vinyl chloride (sarcomas), wood (nasal cancer only), and uranium. The occurrence of excess cancers in uranium miners raises the possibility that a large number of workers are at risk by virtue of exposure to similar radiation hazards. This number includes not only workers involved in processing uranium but also workers exposed in underground mining operations where radon daughters may be emitted from rock formations.

ASSESSMENT OF DISABILITY
Patients who have lung disease may have difficulty continuing to work in their usual jobs because of respiratory symptoms. Such patients frequently seek assistance from their physicians in obtaining compensation for loss of income. *Disability* is the term used to describe the decreased ability to work due to the effects of a medical condition. Physicians are generally able to assess physiologic dysfunction, or *impairment*, but the rating of disability also involves non-medical factors such as the education and employability of the individual. The disability rating scheme differs with the compensation-

granting agency. For example, the U.S. Social Security Administration requires that an individual be unable to do any work (i.e., *total* disability) before he/she will receive income replacement payments. Many state workers' compensation systems allow for payments for *partial* disability. In the Social Security scheme no determination of cause is done, while work-relatedness must be established in workers' compensation systems.

Most commonly the need for disability assessment comes about because of the patient's complaint of shortness of breath. It is important to remember that dyspnea may result from cardiac, hematologic, or neuromuscular diseases in addition to respiratory diseases. For respiratory disability, resting pulmonary function tests (spirometry and diffusing capacity) are used as the initial assessment tool, with cardiopulmonary exercise testing (to assess maximal oxygen consumption) used if the results of the resting tests do not correlate with the patient's symptoms. Methacholine challenge (to assess airways reactivity) can also be useful in patients with asthma who have normal spirometry when evaluated. Some compensation agencies (e.g., Social Security) have proscribed disability classification schemes based on pulmonary function test results. When no specific scheme is proscribed, the *Guidelines of the American Medical Association* should be used.

Evaluating relation to work exposure requires a detailed work history, as previously discussed in this chapter. Occasionally, as with some cases of suspected occupational asthma, challenge to the putative agent in the work environment with repeated pulmonary function measures may be required.

GENERAL ENVIRONMENTAL EXPOSURES

OUTDOOR AIR POLLUTION

In 1971, the U.S. government established national air quality standards for several pollutants believed to be responsible for excess cardiorespiratory diseases. Primary standards regulated by the Environmental Protection Agency (EPA) designed to protect the public health with an adequate margin of safety exist for sulfur dioxide, particulates matter, nitrogen dioxide, ozone, lead, and carbon monoxide. Standards for each of these pollutants are updated regularly through an extensive review process conducted by the EPA. (For details on current standards—*http://www.epa.gov/air/criteria.html*.)

Pollutants are generated from both stationary sources (power plants and industrial complexes) and mobile sources (automobiles), and none of the pollutants occurs in isolation. Furthermore, pollutants may be changed by chemical reactions after being emitted. For example, reducing agents, such as sulfur dioxide and particulate matter from a power plant stack, may react in air to produce acid sulfates and aerosols, which can be transported long distances in the atmosphere. Oxidizing substances, such as oxides of nitrogen and oxidants from automobile exhaust, may react with sunlight to produce ozone. Although originally a problem confined to the southwestern part of the United States, in recent years, at least during the summertime, elevated ozone and acid aerosol levels have been documented throughout the United States. Both acute and chronic effects of these exposures have been documented in large population studies.

The symptoms and diseases associated with air pollution are the same as conditions commonly associated with cigarette smoking. In addition, respiratory illness in early childhood has been associated with chronic exposure to only modestly elevated levels of traffic-related gases and respirable particles. Multiple population-based time-series studies within cities have demonstrated excess cardiopulmonary hospitalizations and mortality. In addition, cohort studies comparing cities that have relatively high levels of particulate exposures with less polluted communities suggest excess morbidity and mortality from cardiorespiratory conditions in long-term residents of the former. These findings have led to stricter U.S. ambient air quality standards for particulate matter as well as greater emphasis on publicizing pollution alerts to encourage individuals with significant cardiopulmonary impairment to stay indoors during high pollution episodes.

INDOOR EXPOSURES

Environmental tobacco smoke (Chap. 390), radon gas, wood smoke, and other biologic agents generated indoors need to be considered. Several studies have shown that the respirable particulate load in any household is directly proportional to the number of cigarette smokers living in the home. Increases in prevalence of respiratory illnesses and reduced levels of pulmonary function measured with simple spirometry have been found in children of smoking parents in a number of studies. Recent meta-analyses for lung cancer, and cardiopulmonary diseases, combining data from the best of the environmental tobacco smoke exposure studies, suggest an ~25% increase in relative risk for each condition, even after adjustment for major potential confounders.

Radon gas is believed to be a risk factor for lung cancer. The main radon product (radon 222) is a gas that results from the decay series of uranium 238, with the immediate precursor being radium 226. The amount of radium in earth materials determines how much radon gas will be emitted. Outdoors, the concentrations are trivial. Indoors, levels are dependent on the sources, the ventilation rate of the space, and the size of the space into which the gas is emitted. Levels associated with excess lung cancer risk may be present in as many as 10% of the houses in the United States. When smokers reside in the household, the problem is potentially greater, since the molecular size of radon particles allows them to readily attach to smoke particles that are inhaled. Fortunately, technology is available for assessing and reducing the level of exposure.

Other indoor exposures associated with an increased risk of atopy and asthma include those to such specific recognized putative biologic agents as cockroach antigen, dust mites, and pet danders. Other indoor chemical agents include formaldehyde, perfumes, and latex particles. Nonspecific responses associated with "tight-building syndrome," in which no particular agent has been implicated, have included a wide variety of complaints, among them respiratory symptoms that are relieved only by avoiding exposure in the building in question. The degree to which "smells" or other sensory stimuli are involved in the triggering of potentially incapacitating psychological or physical responses has yet to be determined, and the long-term consequences of such environmental exposures are as yet unknown.

PORTAL OF ENTRY

The lung is a primary point of entry into the body for a number of toxic agents that affect other organ systems. For example, the lung is a route of entry for benzene (bone marrow), carbon disulfide (cardiovascular and nervous systems), cadmium (kidney), and metallic mercury (kidney, central nervous system). Thus, in any disease state of obscure origin, it is important to consider the possibility of inhaled environmental agents. Such consideration can sometimes furnish the clue needed to identify a specific external cause for a disorder that might otherwise be labeled "idiopathic."

Global Considerations Indoor exposure to *biomass smoke* (wood, dung, crop residues, charcoal) is estimated to be responsible for 2.7% of worldwide disability adjusted life-years (DALYs) lost, due to acute lower respiratory infections in children and COPD and lung cancer in women. This burden of disease places indoor exposure to biomass smoke as the second leading environmental hazard for poor health, just behind unsafe water, sanitation, and hygiene; and is 3.5 times larger than the burden attributed to outdoor air pollution.

More than one-half of the world's population uses biomass fuel for cooking, heating or baking. This occurs predominantly in the rural areas of developing countries. Because many families burn biomass fuels in open stoves, which are highly inefficient, and inside homes with poor ventilation, women and young children are exposed on a daily basis to high levels of smoke. In these homes, 24-h mean levels of fine particulate matter, a component of biomass smoke, have been reported to be 2–30 times higher than the National Ambient Air Quality Standards set by the U.S. EPA.

Epidemiologic studies have consistently shown associations between exposure to biomass smoke and both chronic bronchitis and COPD,

FIGURE 250-4 Histopathologic features of biomass smoke-induced interstitial lung disease. A. Anthracitic pigment is seen accumulating along alveolar septae (*arrow heads*) and within a pigmented dust macule (*single arrow*), **B.** A high-power photomicrograph contains a mixture of fibroblasts and carbon-laden macrophages.

with odds ratios ranging between 3 and 10 and increasing with longer exposures. In addition to the common occupational exposure to biomass smoke of women in developing countries, men from such countries may also be occupationally exposed. Because of increased migration to the United States from developing countries, clinicians need to be aware of the chronic respiratory effects of exposure to biomass smoke, which can also include interstitial lung disease (Fig. 250-4).

FURTHER READINGS

BALMES JR et al: ATS Statement: Occupational contribution to the burden of airway disease. Am J Respir Crit Care Med 167:787, 2003

CASTRANOVA V, VALLYATHAN V: Silicosis and coal workers' pneumoconiosis. Environ Health Perspect 108 (Suppl 4):675, 2000

CHEN TM et al: Outdoor air pollution: Overview and historical perspective. Am J Med Sci 333:230, 2007

DIAZ JV et al: A case of wood smoke–related pulmonary disease. Environ Health Perspect 114:759, 2006

D'MANNETJE A et al: Exposure-response analysis and risk assessment for silica and silicosis mortality in a pooled analysis of six cohorts. Occup Environ Med 59:723, 2002

EKICI A et al: Obstructive airway diseases in women exposed to biomass smoke. Environ Res 99: 93, 2005

FONTENOT AP, MAIER LA: Genetic susceptibility and immune-mediated destruction in beryllium-induced disease. Trends Immunol 26:543, 2005

KUSAKA Y et al (eds): *International Classification of HRCT for Occupational and Environmental Respiratory Diseases.* Tokyo, New York, Springer, 2005, 145

LANDRIGAN PJ et al. Health and environmental consequences of the World Trade Center disaster. Environ Health Perspect 112:731, 2004

NEWMAN LS et al: Beryllium sensitization progresses to chronic beryllium disease: A longitudinal study of disease risk. Am J Respir Crit Care Med 171:54, 2005

O'REILLY KM et al: Asbestos-related lung disease. Am Fam Physician 75:683, 2007

POPE CA III et al: Cardiovascular mortality and long-term exposure to particulate air pollution: Epidemiological evidence of general pathophysiological pathways of disease. Circulation 109:71, 2004

251 Pneumonia
Lionel A. Mandell, Richard Wunderink

DEFINITION

Pneumonia is an infection of the pulmonary parenchyma. Despite being the cause of significant morbidity and mortality, pneumonia is often misdiagnosed, mistreated, and underestimated.

In the past, pneumonia was typically classified as community-acquired, hospital-acquired, or ventilator-associated. Over the last decade or two, however, patients presenting to the hospital have often been found to be infected with multidrug-resistant (MDR) pathogens previously associated with hospital-acquired pneumonia. Factors responsible for this phenomenon include the development and widespread use of potent oral antibiotics, earlier transfer of patients out of acute-care hospitals to their homes or various lower-acuity facilities, increased use of outpatient IV antibiotic therapy, general aging of the population, and more extensive immunomodulatory therapies. The potential involvement of these MDR pathogens has led to a revised classification system in which infection is categorized as either community-acquired pneumonia (CAP) or health care–associated pneumonia (HCAP), with subcategories of HCAP including hospital-acquired pneumonia (HAP) and ventilator-associated pneumonia (VAP). The conditions associated with HCAP and the likely pathogens are listed in Table 251-1.

Although the new classification system has been helpful in designing empirical antibiotic strategies, it is not without disadvantages. For instance, not all MDR pathogens are associated with all risk factors (Table 251-1). Therefore, this system represents a distillation of multiple risk factors, and each patient must be considered individually. For

TABLE 251-1 CLINICAL CONDITIONS ASSOCIATED WITH AND LIKELY PATHOGENS IN HEALTH CARE–ASSOCIATED PNEUMONIA

Condition	Pathogen			
	MRSA	*Pseudomonas aeruginosa*	*Acinetobacter* spp.	MDR Enterobacteriaceae
Hospitalization for ≥48 h	X	X	X	X
Hospitalization for ≥2 days in prior 3 months	X	X	X	X
Nursing home or extended-care facility residence	X	X	X	X
Antibiotic therapy in preceding 3 months		X		X
Chronic dialysis	X			
Home infusion therapy	X			
Home wound care	X			
Family member with MDR infection	X			X

Note: MDR, multidrug-resistant; MRSA, methicillin-resistant *Staphylococcus aureus*.

example, the risk of infection with MDR pathogens for a nursing home resident with dementia who can independently dress, ambulate, and eat is quite different from the risk for a patient who is in a chronic vegetative state with a tracheostomy and a percutaneous feeding tube in place. In addition, risk factors for MDR infection do not preclude the development of pneumonia caused by the usual CAP pathogens.

This chapter deals with pneumonia in patients who are not considered to be immunocompromised. Pneumonia in immunocompromised patients is discussed in other chapters, including Chaps. 82, 126, and 182.

PATHOPHYSIOLOGY

Pneumonia results from the proliferation of microbial pathogens at the alveolar level and the host's response to those pathogens. Microorganisms gain access to the lower respiratory tract in several ways. The most common is by aspiration from the oropharynx. Small-volume aspiration occurs frequently during sleep (especially in the elderly) and in patients with decreased levels of consciousness. Many pathogens are inhaled as contaminated droplets. Rarely, pneumonia occurs via hematogenous spread (e.g., from tricuspid endocarditis) or by contiguous extension from an infected pleural or mediastinal space.

Mechanical factors are critically important in host defense. The hairs and turbinates of the nares catch larger inhaled particles before they reach the lower respiratory tract, and the branching architecture of the tracheobronchial tree traps particles on the airway lining, where mucociliary clearance and local antibacterial factors either clear or kill the potential pathogen. The gag reflex and the cough mechanism offer critical protection from aspiration. In addition, the normal flora adhering to mucosal cells of the oropharynx, whose components are remarkably constant, prevents pathogenic bacteria from binding and thereby decreases the risk of pneumonia caused by these more virulent bacteria.

When these barriers are overcome or when the microorganisms are small enough to be inhaled to the alveolar level, resident alveolar macrophages are extremely efficient at clearing and killing pathogens. Macrophages are assisted by local proteins (e.g., surfactant proteins A and D) that have intrinsic opsonizing properties or antibacterial or antiviral activity. Once engulfed, the pathogens—even if they are not killed by macrophages—are eliminated via either the mucociliary elevator or the lymphatics and no longer represent an infectious challenge. Only when the capacity of the alveolar macrophages to ingest or kill the microorganisms is exceeded does clinical pneumonia become manifest. In that situation, the alveolar macrophages initiate the inflammatory response to bolster lower respiratory tract defenses. The host inflammatory response, rather than the proliferation of microorganisms, triggers the clinical syndrome of pneumonia. The release of inflammatory mediators, such as interleukin (IL) 1 and tumor necrosis factor (TNF), results in fever. Chemokines, such as IL-8 and granulocyte colony-stimulating factor, stimulate the release of neutrophils and their attraction to the lung, producing both peripheral leukocytosis and increased purulent secretions. Inflammatory mediators released by macrophages and the newly recruited neutrophils create an alveolar capillary leak equivalent to that seen in the acute respiratory distress syndrome (ARDS), although in pneumonia this leak is localized (at least initially). Even erythrocytes can cross the alveolar-capillary membrane, with consequent hemoptysis. The capillary leak results in a radiographic infiltrate and rales detectable on auscultation, and hypoxemia results from alveolar filling. Moreover, some bacterial pathogens appear to interfere with the hypoxic vasoconstriction that would normally occur with fluid-filled alveoli, and this interference can result in severe hypoxemia. Increased respiratory drive in the systemic inflammatory response syndrome (SIRS) leads to respiratory alkalosis. Decreased compliance due to capillary leak, hypoxemia, increased respiratory drive, increased secretions, and occasionally infection-related bronchospasm all lead to dyspnea. If severe enough, the changes in lung mechanics secondary to reductions in lung volume and compliance and the intrapulmonary shunting of blood may cause the patient's death.

PATHOLOGY

Classic pneumonia evolves through a series of pathologic changes. The initial phase is one of *edema*, with the presence of a proteinaceous exudate—and often of bacteria—in the alveoli. This phase is rarely evident in clinical or autopsy specimens because it is so rapidly followed by a *red hepatization* phase. The presence of erythrocytes in the cellular intraalveolar exudate gives this second stage its name, but neutrophils are also present and are important from the standpoint of host defense. Bacteria are occasionally seen in cultures of alveolar specimens collected during this phase. In the third phase, *gray hepatization*, no new erythrocytes are extravasating, and those already present have been lysed and degraded. The neutrophil is the predominant cell, fibrin deposition is abundant, and bacteria have disappeared. This phase corresponds with successful containment of the infection and improvement in gas exchange. In the final phase, *resolution*, the macrophage is the dominant cell type in the alveolar space, and the debris of neutrophils, bacteria, and fibrin has been cleared, as has the inflammatory response.

This pattern has been described best for pneumococcal pneumonia and may not apply to pneumonias of all etiologies, especially viral or *Pneumocystis* pneumonia. In VAP, respiratory bronchiolitis may precede the development of a radiologically apparent infiltrate. Because of the microaspiration mechanism, a bronchopneumonia pattern is most common in nosocomial pneumonias, whereas a lobar pattern is more common in bacterial CAP. Despite the radiographic appearance, viral and *Pneumocystis* pneumonias represent alveolar rather than interstitial processes.

COMMUNITY-ACQUIRED PNEUMONIA

ETIOLOGY

The extensive list of potential etiologic agents in CAP includes bacteria, fungi, viruses, and protozoa. Newly identified pathogens include hantaviruses, metapneumoviruses, the coronavirus responsible for the severe acute respiratory syndrome (SARS), and community-acquired strains of methicillin-resistant *Staphylococcus aureus* (MRSA). Most cases of CAP, however, are caused by relatively few pathogens (Table 251-2). Although *Streptococcus pneumoniae* is most common, other organisms must also be considered in light of the patient's risk factors and severity of illness. In most cases, it is most useful to think of the potential causes as either "typical" bacterial pathogens or "atypical" organisms. The former category includes *S. pneumoniae*, *Haemophilus influenzae*, and (in selected patients) *S. aureus* and gram-negative bacilli such as *Klebsiella pneumoniae* and *Pseudomonas aeruginosa*. The "atypical" organisms include *Mycoplasma pneumoniae*, *Chlamydophila pneumoniae*, and *Legionella* spp. as well as respiratory viruses such as influenza viruses, adenoviruses, and respiratory syncytial viruses (RSVs). Data suggest that a virus may be responsible in up to 18% of cases of CAP that require admission to the hospital. The atypical organisms cannot be cultured on standard media, nor can they be seen on Gram's stain. The frequency and importance of atypical pathogens such as *M. pneumoniae* and *C. pneumoniae* in outpatients and *Legionella* in inpa-

TABLE 251-2	**MICROBIAL CAUSES OF COMMUNITY-ACQUIRED PNEUMONIA, BY SITE OF CARE**	

	Hospitalized Patients	
Outpatients	**Non-ICU**	**ICU**
Streptococcus pneumoniae	*S. pneumoniae*	*S. pneumoniae*
Mycoplasma pneumoniae	*M. pneumoniae*	*Staphylococcus aureus*
Haemophilus influenzae	*Chlamydophila pneumoniae*	*Legionella* spp.
C. pneumoniae		Gram-negative bacilli
Respiratory viruses[a]	*H. influenzae*	*H. influenzae*
	Legionella spp.	
	Respiratory viruses[a]	

Note: Pathogens are listed in descending order of frequency. ICU, intensive care unit.
[a]Influenza A and B viruses, adenoviruses, respiratory syncytial viruses, parainfluenza viruses.

TABLE 251-3 EPIDEMIOLOGIC FACTORS SUGGESTING POSSIBLE CAUSES OF COMMUNITY-ACQUIRED PNEUMONIA

Factor	Possible Pathogen(s)
Alcoholism	Streptococcus pneumoniae, oral anaerobes, Klebsiella pneumoniae, Acinetobacter spp., Mycobacterium tuberculosis
COPD and/or smoking	Haemophilus influenzae, Pseudomonas aeruginosa, Legionella spp., S. pneumoniae, Moraxella catarrhalis, Chlamydophila pneumoniae
Structural lung disease (e.g., bronchiectasis)	P. aeruginosa, Burkholderia cepacia, Staphylococcus aureus
Dementia, stroke, decreased level of consciousness	Oral anaerobes, gram-negative enteric bacteria
Lung abscess	CA-MRSA, oral anaerobes, endemic fungi, M. tuberculosis, atypical mycobacteria
Travel to Ohio or St. Lawrence river valleys	Histoplasma capsulatum
Travel to southwestern United States	Hantavirus, Coccidioides spp.
Travel to Southeast Asia	Burkholderia pseudomallei, avian influenza virus
Stay in hotel or on cruise ship in previous 2 weeks	Legionella spp.
Local influenza activity	Influenza virus, S. pneumoniae, S. aureus
Exposure to bats or birds	H. capsulatum
Exposure to birds	Chlamydophila psittaci
Exposure to rabbits	Francisella tularensis
Exposure to sheep, goats, parturient cats	Coxiella burnetii

Note: CA-MRSA, community-acquired methicillin-resistant Staphylococcus aureus; COPD, chronic obstructive pulmonary disease.

tients have significant implications for therapy. These organisms are intrinsically resistant to all β-lactam agents and must be treated with a macrolide, a fluoroquinolone, or a tetracycline. In the ~10–15% of CAP cases that are polymicrobial, the etiology often includes a combination of typical and atypical pathogens.

Anaerobes play a significant role only when an episode of aspiration has occurred days to weeks before presentation for pneumonia. The combination of an unprotected airway (e.g., in patients with alcohol or drug overdose or a seizure disorder) and significant gingivitis constitutes the major risk factor. Anaerobic pneumonias are often complicated by abscess formation and significant empyemas or parapneumonic effusions.

S. aureus pneumonia is well known to complicate influenza infection. Recently, however, MRSA strains have been reported as primary causes of CAP. While this entity is still relatively uncommon, clinicians must be aware of its potentially serious consequences, such as necrotizing pneumonia. Two important developments have led to this problem: the spread of MRSA from the hospital setting to the community and the emergence of genetically distinct strains of MRSA in the community. These novel community-acquired MRSA (CA-MRSA) strains have infected healthy individuals who have had no association with health care.

Unfortunately, despite a careful history and physical examination as well as routine radiographic studies, it is usually impossible to predict the pathogen in a case of CAP with any degree of certainty; in more than half of cases, a specific etiology is never determined. Nevertheless, it is important to consider epidemiologic and risk factors that might suggest certain pathogens (Table 251-3).

EPIDEMIOLOGY

In the United States, ~80% of the 4 million CAP cases that occur annually are treated on an outpatient basis, and ~20% are treated in the hospital. CAP results in more than 600,000 hospitalizations, 64 million days of restricted activity, and 45,000 deaths annually. The overall yearly cost associated with CAP is estimated at $9–10 billion (U.S.). The incidence rates are highest at the extremes of age. Although the overall annual figure in the United States is 12 cases per 1000 persons, the figure is 12–18 per 1000 among children <4 years of age and 20 per 1000 among persons >60 years of age.

The risk factors for CAP in general and for pneumococcal pneumonia in particular have implications for treatment regimens. Risk factors for CAP include alcoholism, asthma, immunosuppression, institutionalization, and an age of ≥70 years versus 60–69 years. Risk factors for pneumococcal pneumonia include dementia, seizure disorders, heart failure, cerebrovascular disease, alcoholism, tobacco smoking, chronic obstructive pulmonary disease, and HIV infection. CA-MRSA infection is more likely in Native Americans, homeless youths, men who have sex with men, prison inmates, military recruits, children in daycare centers, and athletes such as wrestlers. The Enterobacteriaceae tend to affect patients who have recently been hospitalized and/or received antibiotic therapy or who have comorbidities such as alcoholism, heart failure, or renal failure. P. aeruginosa may also infect these patients as well as those with severe structural lung disease. Risk factors for Legionella infection include diabetes, hematologic malignancy, cancer, severe renal disease, HIV infection, smoking, male gender, and a recent hotel stay or ship cruise. (Many of these risk factors would now reclassify as HCAP some cases that were previously designated CAP.)

CLINICAL MANIFESTATIONS

CAP can vary from indolent to fulminant in presentation and from mild to fatal in severity. The various signs and symptoms, which depend on the progression and severity of the infection, include both constitutional findings and manifestations limited to the lung and its associated structures. In light of the pathobiology of the disease, many of the findings are to be expected.

The patient is frequently febrile, with a tachycardic response, and may have chills and/or sweats and cough that is either nonproductive or productive of mucoid, purulent, or blood-tinged sputum. In accordance with the severity of infection, the patient may be able to speak in full sentences or may be very short of breath. If the pleura is involved, the patient may experience pleuritic chest pain. Up to 20% of patients may have gastrointestinal symptoms such as nausea, vomiting, and/or diarrhea. Other symptoms may include fatigue, headache, myalgias, and arthralgias.

Findings on physical examination vary with the degree of pulmonary consolidation and the presence or absence of a significant pleural effusion. An increased respiratory rate and use of accessory muscles of respiration are common. Palpation may reveal increased or decreased tactile fremitus, and the percussion note can vary from dull to flat, reflecting underlying consolidated lung and pleural fluid, respectively. Crackles, bronchial breath sounds, and possibly a pleural friction rub may be heard on auscultation. The clinical presentation may not be so obvious in the elderly, who may initially display new-onset or worsening confusion and few other manifestations. Severely ill patients who have septic shock secondary to CAP are hypotensive and may have evidence of organ failure.

DIAGNOSIS

When confronted with possible CAP, the physician must ask two questions: Is this pneumonia, and, if so, what is the etiology? The former question is typically answered by clinical and radiographic methods, whereas the latter requires the aid of laboratory techniques.

Clinical Diagnosis The differential diagnosis includes both infectious and noninfectious entities such as acute bronchitis, acute exacerbations of chronic bronchitis, heart failure, pulmonary embolism, and radiation pneumonitis. The importance of a careful history cannot be overemphasized. For example, known cardiac disease may suggest worsening pulmonary edema, while underlying carcinoma may suggest lung injury secondary to radiation. Epidemiologic clues, such as recent travel to areas with known endemic pathogens, may alert the physician to specific possibilities (Table 251-3).

Unfortunately, the sensitivity and specificity of the findings on physical examination are less than ideal, averaging 58% and 67%, respectively. Therefore, chest radiography is often necessary to help differentiate CAP from other conditions. Radiographic findings serve as a baseline and may include risk factors for increased severity (e.g., cavitation or multilobar involvement). Occasionally, radiographic results suggest an etiologic diagnosis. For example, pneumatoceles suggest infection with *S. aureus*, and an upper-lobe cavitating lesion suggests tuberculosis. CT is rarely necessary but may be of value in a patient with suspected post-obstructive pneumonia caused by a tumor or foreign body. For cases managed on an outpatient basis, the clinical and radiologic assessment is usually all that is done before treatment is started since most laboratory test results are not available soon enough to influence initial management. In certain cases, however (e.g., influenza virus infection), the availability of rapid point-of-care diagnostic tests and access to specific drugs for treatment and prevention can be very important.

Etiologic Diagnosis   The etiology of pneumonia usually cannot be determined on the basis of clinical presentation; instead, the physician must rely upon the laboratory for support. Except for the 2% of CAP patients who are admitted to the intensive care unit (ICU), no data exist to show that treatment directed at a specific pathogen is statistically superior to empirical therapy. The benefits of establishing a microbial etiology can therefore be questioned, particularly in light of the cost of diagnostic testing. However, a number of reasons can be advanced for attempting an etiologic diagnosis. Identification of an unexpected pathogen allows narrowing of the initial empirical regimen, which decreases antibiotic selection pressure and may lessen the risk of resistance. Pathogens with important public safety implications, such as *Mycobacterium tuberculosis* and influenza virus, may be found in some cases. Finally, without culture and susceptibility data, trends in resistance cannot be followed accurately, and appropriate empirical therapeutic regimens are harder to devise.

GRAM'S STAIN AND CULTURE OF SPUTUM   The main purpose of the sputum Gram's stain is to ensure that a sample is suitable for culture. However, Gram's staining may also help to identify certain pathogens (e.g., *S. pneumoniae*, *S. aureus*, and gram-negative bacteria) by their characteristic appearance. To be adequate for culture, a sputum sample must have >25 neutrophils and <10 squamous epithelial cells per low-power field. The sensitivity and specificity of the sputum Gram's stain and culture are highly variable; even in cases of proven bacteremic pneumococcal pneumonia, the yield of positive cultures from sputum samples is ≤50%.

Some patients, particularly elderly individuals, may not be able to produce an appropriate expectorated sputum sample. Others may already have started a course of antibiotics, which can interfere with results, at the time a sample is obtained. The inability to produce sputum can be a consequence of dehydration, and the correction of this condition may result in increased sputum production and a more obvious infiltrate on chest radiography. For patients admitted to the ICU and intubated, a deep-suction aspirate or bronchoalveolar lavage sample should be sent to the microbiology laboratory as soon as possible. Since the etiologies in severe CAP are somewhat different from those in milder disease (Table 251-2), the greatest benefit of staining and culturing respiratory secretions is to alert the physician of unsuspected and/or resistant pathogens and to permit appropriate modification of therapy. Other stains and cultures may be useful as well. For suspected tuberculosis or fungal infection, specific stains are available. Cultures of pleural fluid obtained from effusions >1 cm in height on a lateral decubitus chest radiograph may also be helpful.

BLOOD CULTURES   The yield from blood cultures, even those obtained before antibiotic therapy, is disappointingly low. Only ~5–14% of cultures of blood from patients hospitalized with CAP are positive, and the most frequently isolated pathogen is *S. pneumoniae*. Since recommended empirical regimens all provide pneumococcal coverage, a blood culture positive for this pathogen has little, if any, effect on clinical outcome. However, susceptibility data may allow a switch from a broader-spectrum regimen (e.g., a fluoroquinolone or β-lactam plus a macrolide) to penicillin in appropriate cases. Because of the low yield and the lack of significant impact on outcome, blood cultures are no longer considered *de rigueur* for all hospitalized CAP patients. Certain

high-risk patients—including those with neutropenia secondary to pneumonia, asplenia, or complement deficiencies; chronic liver disease; or severe CAP—should have blood cultured.

ANTIGEN TESTS   Two commercially available tests detect pneumococcal and certain *Legionella* antigens in urine. The test for *Legionella pneumophila* detects only serogroup 1, but this serogroup accounts for most community-acquired cases of Legionnaires' disease. The sensitivity and specificity of the *Legionella* urine antigen test are as high as 90% and 99%, respectively. The pneumococcal urine antigen test is also quite sensitive and specific (80% and >90%, respectively). Although false-positive results can be obtained with samples from colonized children, the test is generally reliable. Both tests can detect antigen even after the initiation of appropriate antibiotic therapy and after weeks of illness. Other antigen tests include a rapid test for influenza virus and direct fluorescent antibody tests for influenza virus and RSV, although the test for RSV is only poorly sensitive.

POLYMERASE CHAIN REACTION   Polymerase chain reaction (PCR) tests are available for a number of pathogens, including *L. pneumophila* and mycobacteria. In addition, a multiplex PCR can detect the nucleic acid of *Legionella* spp., *M. pneumoniae*, and *C. pneumoniae*. However, the use of these PCR assays is generally limited to research studies.

SEROLOGY   A fourfold rise in specific IgM antibody titer between acute- and convalescent-phase serum samples is generally considered diagnostic of infection with the pathogen in question. In the past, serologic tests were used to help identify atypical pathogens as well as some typical but relatively unusual organisms, such as *Coxiella burnetii*. Recently, however, they have fallen out of favor because of the time required to obtain a final result for the convalescent-phase sample.

℞ COMMUNITY-ACQUIRED PNEUMONIA

SITE OF CARE   The decision to hospitalize a patient with CAP must take into consideration diminishing health care resources and rising costs of treatment. The cost of inpatient management exceeds that of outpatient treatment by a factor of 20 and accounts for most CAP-related expenditures. Certain patients clearly can be managed at home, and others clearly require treatment in the hospital, but the choice is sometimes difficult. Tools that objectively assess the risk of adverse outcomes, including severe illness and death, may minimize unnecessary hospital admissions and help to identify patients who will benefit from hospital care. There are currently two sets of criteria: the Pneumonia Severity Index (PSI), a prognostic model used to identify patients at low risk of dying; and the CURB-65 criteria, a severity-of-illness score.

To determine the PSI, points are given for 20 variables, including age, coexisting illness, and abnormal physical and laboratory findings. On the basis of the resulting score, patients are assigned to one of five classes with the following mortality rates: class 1, 0.1%; class 2, 0.6%; class 3, 2.8%; class 4, 8.2%; and class 5, 29.2%. Clinical trials have demonstrated that routine use of the PSI results in lower admission rates for class 1 and class 2 patients. Patients in classes 4 and 5 should be admitted to the hospital, while those in class 3 should ideally be admitted to an observation unit until a further decision can be made.

The CURB-65 criteria include five variables: confusion (C); urea >7 mmol/L (U); respiratory rate ≥30/min (R); blood pressure, systolic ≤90 mmHg or diastolic ≤60 mmHg (B); and age ≥65 years (65). Patients with a score of 0, among whom the 30-day mortality rate is 1.5%, can be treated outside the hospital. With a score of 2, the 30-day mortality rate is 9.2%, and patients should be admitted to the hospital. Among patients with scores of ≥3, mortality rates are 22% overall; these patients may require admission to an ICU.

At present, it is difficult to say which assessment tool is superior. The PSI is less practical in a busy emergency-room setting because of the need to assess 20 variables. While the CURB-65 criteria are easily remembered, they have not been studied as extensively. Whichever system is used, these objective criteria must always be tempered by careful consideration of factors relevant to individual patients, including the ability to comply reliably with an oral antibiotic regimen and the resources available to the patient outside the hospital.

RESISTANCE Antimicrobial resistance is a significant problem that threatens to diminish our therapeutic armamentarium. Misuse of antibiotics results in increased antibiotic selection pressure that can affect resistance locally or even globally by clonal dissemination. For CAP, the main resistance issues currently involve *S. pneumoniae* and CA-MRSA.

S. pneumoniae In general, pneumococcal resistance is acquired (1) by direct DNA incorporation and remodeling resulting from contact with closely related oral commensal bacteria, (2) by the process of natural transformation, or (3) by mutation of certain genes.

Pneumococcal strains are classified as sensitive to penicillin if the minimal inhibitory concentration (MIC) is ≤ 0.06 μg/mL, as intermediate if the MIC is 0.1–1.0 μg/mL, and as resistant if the MIC is ≥ 2 μg/mL. Strains resistant to drugs from three or more antimicrobial classes with different mechanisms of action are considered MDR isolates. Pneumococcal resistance to β-lactam drugs is due solely to the presence of low-affinity penicillin-binding proteins. The propensity for pneumococcal resistance to penicillin to be associated with reduced susceptibility to other drugs, such as macrolides, tetracyclines, and trimethoprim-sulfamethoxazole (TMP-SMX), is of concern. In the United States, 58.9% of penicillin-resistant pneumococcal isolates from blood cultures are also resistant to macrolides. Penicillin is an appropriate agent for the treatment of pneumococcal infection caused by strains with MICs of ≤ 1 μg/mL. For infections caused by pneumococcal strains with penicillin MICs of 2–4 μg/mL, the data are conflicting; some studies suggest no increase in treatment failure with penicillin, while others suggest increased rates of death or complications. For strains of *S. pneumoniae* with intermediate levels of resistance, higher doses of the drug should be used. Risk factors for drug-resistant pneumococcal infection include recent antimicrobial therapy, an age of <2 years or >65 years, attendance at day-care centers, recent hospitalization, and HIV infection. Fortunately, resistance to penicillin appears to be reaching a plateau.

In contrast, resistance to macrolides is increasing through several mechanisms, including target-site modification and the presence of an efflux pump. Target-site modification is caused by ribosomal methylation in 23S rRNA encoded by the *ermB* gene and results in resistance to macrolides, lincosamides, and streptogramin B–type antibiotics. This *MLS$_B$ phenotype* is associated with high-level resistance, with typical MICs of ≥ 64 μg/mL. The efflux mechanism encoded by the *mef* gene (*M phenotype*) is usually associated with low-level resistance (MICs, 1–32 μg/mL). These two mechanisms account for ~45% and ~65%, respectively, of resistant pneumococcal isolates in the United States. Some pneumococcal isolates with both the *erm* and *mef* genes have been identified, but the exact significance of this finding is unknown. High-level resistance to macrolides is more common in Europe, whereas lower-level resistance seems to predominate in North America. Although clinical failures with macrolides have been reported, many experts think that these drugs still have a role to play in the management of pneumococcal pneumonia in North America.

Pneumococcal resistance to fluoroquinolones (e.g., ciprofloxacin and levofloxacin) has been reported. Changes can occur in one or both target sites (topoisomerases II and IV); changes in these two sites usually result from mutations in the *gyrA* and *parC* genes, respectively. The increasing number of pneumococcal isolates that, although susceptible to fluoroquinolones, already have a mutation in one target site is of concern. Such organisms may be more likely to undergo a second step mutation that will render them fully resistant to fluoroquinolones. In addition, an efflux pump may play a role in pneumococcal resistance to fluoroquinolones.

CA-MRSA CAP due to MRSA may be caused by infection with the classic hospital-acquired strains or with the more recently identified, genotypically and phenotypically distinct community-acquired strains. Most infections with the former strains have been acquired either directly or indirectly by contact with the health care environment and, although classified as HAP in the past, would now be classified as HCAP. In some hospitals, CA-MRSA strains are displacing the classic hospital-acquired strains—a trend suggesting that the newer strains may be more robust.

Methicillin resistance in *S. aureus* is determined by the *mecA* gene, which encodes for resistance to all β-lactam drugs. At least five *staphylococcal chromosomal cassette mec* (*SCCmec*) types have been described. The typical hospital-acquired strain usually has type II or III, whereas CA-MRSA has a type IV *SCCmec* element. CA-MRSA isolates tend to be less resistant than the older hospital-acquired strains and are often susceptible to TMP-SMX, clindamycin, and tetracycline in addition to vancomycin and linezo-

lid. However, CA-MRSA strains may also carry genes for superantigens, such as enterotoxins B and C and Panton-Valentine leukocidin, a membrane-tropic toxin that can create cytolytic pores in polymorphonuclear neutrophils, monocytes, and macrophages.

Gram-Negative Bacilli A detailed discussion of resistance among gram-negative bacilli is beyond the scope of this chapter (see Chap. 143). Fluoroquinolone resistance among isolates of *Escherichia coli* from the community appears to be increasing. *Enterobacter* spp. are typically resistant to cephalosporins; the drugs of choice for use against these bacteria are usually fluoroquinolones or carbapenems. Similarly, when infections due to bacteria producing extended-spectrum β-lactamases (ESBLs) are documented or suspected, a fluoroquinolone or a carbapenem should be used; these MDR strains are more likely to be involved in HCAP.

INITIAL ANTIBIOTIC MANAGEMENT Since the physician rarely knows the etiology of CAP at the outset of treatment, initial therapy is usually empirical and is designed to cover the most likely pathogens (**Table 251-4**). In all cases, antibiotic treatment should be initiated as expeditiously as possible.

The CAP treatment guidelines in the United States (summarized in Table 251-4) represent joint statements from the Infectious Diseases Society of America (IDSA) and the American Thoracic Society (ATS); the Canadian guidelines come from the Canadian Infectious Disease Society and the Canadian Thoracic Society. In these guidelines, coverage is always provided

---

TABLE 251-4 EMPIRICAL ANTIBIOTIC TREATMENT OF COMMUNITY-ACQUIRED PNEUMONIA

Outpatients
  Previously healthy and no antibiotics in past 3 months
  • A macrolide [clarithromycin (500 mg PO bid) or azithromycin (500 mg PO once, then 250 mg od)] **or**
  • Doxycycline (100 mg PO bid)
  Comorbidities or antibiotics in past 3 months: select an alternative from a different class
  • A respiratory fluoroquinolone [moxifloxacin (400 mg PO od), gemifloxacin (320 mg PO od), levofloxacin (750 mg PO od)] **or**
  • A β-lactam [preferred: high-dose amoxicillin (1 g tid) or amoxicillin/clavulanate (2 g bid); alternatives: ceftriaxone (1–2 g IV od), cefpodoxime (200 mg PO bid), cefuroxime (500 mg PO bid)] *plus* a macrolide^a
  In regions with a high rate of "high-level" pneumococcal macrolide resistance,^{b} consider alternatives listed above for patients with comorbidities.

Inpatients, non-ICU
  • A respiratory fluoroquinolone [moxifloxacin (400 mg PO or IV od), gemifloxacin (320 mg PO od), levofloxacin (750 mg PO or IV od)]
  • A β-lactam^c [cefotaxime (1–2 g IV q8h), ceftriaxone (1–2 g IV od), ampicillin (1–2 g IV q4–6h), ertapenem (1 g IV od in selected patients)] **plus** a macrolide^d [oral clarithromycin or azithromycin (as listed above for previously healthy patients) or IV azithromycin (1 g once, then 500 mg od)]

Inpatients, ICU
  • A β-lactam^e [cefotaxime (1–2 g IV q8h), ceftriaxone (2 g IV od), ampicillin-sulbactam (2 g IV q8h)] **plus**
  • Azithromycin or a fluoroquinolone (as listed above for inpatients, non-ICU)

Special concerns
  If *Pseudomonas* is a consideration
  • An antipneumococcal, antipseudomonal β-lactam [piperacillin/tazobactam (4.5 g IV q6h), cefepime (1–2 g IV q12h), imipenem (500 mg IV q6h), meropenem (1 g IV q8h)] *plus* either ciprofloxacin (400 mg IV q12h) or levofloxacin (750 mg IV od)
  • The above β-lactams *plus* an aminoglycoside [amikacin (15 mg/kg od) or tobramycin (1.7 mg/kg od) and azithromycin]
  • The above β-lactams^f *plus* an aminoglycoside *plus* an antipneumococcal fluoroquinolone
  If CA-MRSA is a consideration
  • Add linezolid (600 mg IV q12h) or vancomycin (1 g IV q12h)

Note: CA-MRSA, community-acquired methicillin-resistant *Staphylococcus aureus*; ICU, intensive care unit.
^{a}Doxycycline (100 mg PO bid) is an alternative to the macrolide.
^{b}MICs of >16 μg/mL in 25% of isolates.
^{c}A respiratory fluoroquinolone should be used for penicillin-allergic patients.
^{d}Doxycycline (100 mg IV q12h) is an alternative to the macrolide.
^{e}For penicillin-allergic patients, use a respiratory fluoroquinolone and aztreonam (2 g IV q8h).
^{f}For penicillin-allergic patients, substitute aztreonam.

for the pneumococcus and the atypical pathogens. In contrast, guidelines from some European countries do not always include atypical coverage based on local epidemiologic data. The U.S.-Canadian approach is supported by retrospective data from almost 13,000 patients >65 years of age. Atypical pathogen coverage provided by a macrolide or a fluoroquinolone has been associated with a significant reduction in mortality rates compared with those for β-lactam coverage alone.

Therapy with a macrolide or a fluoroquinolone within the previous 3 months is associated with an increased likelihood of infection with a macrolide- or fluoroquinolone-resistant strain of *S. pneumoniae*. For this reason, a fluoroquinolone-based regimen should be used for patients recently given a macrolide, and vice versa (Table 251-4). Telithromycin, a ketolide derived from the macrolide class, differs from the macrolides in that it binds to bacteria more avidly and at two sites rather than one. This drug is active against pneumococci resistant to penicillins, macrolides, and fluoroquinolones. Its future role in the outpatient management of CAP will depend on the evaluation of its safety by the U.S. Food and Drug Administration.

Once the etiologic agent(s) and susceptibilities are known, therapy may be altered to target the specific pathogen(s). However, this decision is not always straightforward. If blood cultures yield *S. pneumoniae* sensitive to penicillin after 2 days of treatment with a macrolide plus a β-lactam or a fluoroquinolone, should therapy be switched to penicillin? Penicillin alone would not be effective in the potential 15% of cases with atypical co-infection. No standard approach exists. Some experts would argue that pneumococcal coverage by a switch to penicillin is appropriate, while others would opt for continued coverage of both the pneumococcus and atypical pathogens. One compromise would be to continue atypical coverage with either a macrolide or a fluoroquinolone for a few more days and then to complete the treatment course with penicillin alone. In all cases, the individual patient and the various risk factors must be considered.

Management of bacteremic pneumococcal pneumonia is also controversial. Data from nonrandomized studies suggest that combination therapy (e.g., with a macrolide and a β-lactam) is associated with a lower mortality rate than monotherapy, particularly in severely ill patients. The exact reason is unknown, but explanations include possible atypical co-infection or the immunomodulatory effects of the macrolides.

For patients with CAP who are admitted to the ICU, the risk of infection with *P. aeruginosa* or CA-MRSA is increased, and coverage should be considered when a patient has risk factors or a Gram's stain suggestive of these pathogens (Table 251-4). The main risk factors for *P. aeruginosa* infection are structural lung disease (e.g., bronchiectasis) and recent treatment with antibiotics or glucocorticoids. If CA-MRSA infection is suspected, either linezolid or vancomycin should be added to the initial empirical regimen.

Although hospitalized patients have traditionally received initial therapy by the IV route, some drugs—particularly the fluoroquinolones—are very well absorbed and can be given orally from the outset to select patients. For patients initially treated IV, a switch to oral treatment is appropriate as long as the patient can ingest and absorb the drugs, is hemodynamically stable, and is showing clinical improvement.

The duration of treatment for CAP has recently generated considerable interest. Patients have usually been treated for 10–14 days, but recent studies with fluoroquinolones and telithromycin suggest that a 5-day course is sufficient for otherwise uncomplicated CAP. A longer course is required for patients with bacteremia, metastatic infection, or infection with a particularly virulent pathogen, such as *P. aeruginosa* or CA-MRSA. Longer-term therapy should also be considered if initial treatment was ineffective and in most cases of severe CAP. Data from studies with azithromycin, which suggest 3–5 days of treatment for outpatient-managed CAP, cannot be extrapolated to other drugs because of the extremely long half-life of azithromycin.

Patients may be discharged from the hospital once they are clinically stable and have no active medical problems requiring ongoing hospital care. The site of residence after discharge (in a nursing home, at home with family, at home alone) is an important consideration, particularly for elderly patients.

GENERAL CONSIDERATIONS In addition to appropriate antimicrobial therapy, certain general considerations apply in dealing with either CAP or HAP. Adequate hydration, oxygen therapy for hypoxemia, and assisted ventilation when necessary are critical to the success of therapy. Patients with severe CAP who remain hypotensive despite fluid resuscitation may have adrenal insufficiency and may respond to glucocorticoid treatment. Immunomodulatory therapy in the form of drotrecogin alfa (activated) should

be considered for CAP patients with persistent septic shock and APACHE II scores of ≥25, particularly if the infection is caused by *S. pneumoniae*.

Failure to Improve Patients who are slow to respond to therapy should be reevaluated at about day 3 (sooner if their condition is worsening rather than simply not improving), and a number of possible scenarios should be considered. (1) Is this a noninfectious condition? (2) If this is an infection, is the correct pathogen being targeted? (3) Is this a superinfection with a new nosocomial pathogen? A number of noninfectious conditions can mimic pneumonia, including pulmonary edema, pulmonary embolism, lung carcinoma, radiation and hypersensitivity pneumonitis, and connective tissue disease involving the lungs. If the patient has CAP and treatment is aimed at the correct pathogen, the lack of response may be explained in a number of ways. The pathogen may be resistant to the drug selected, or a sequestered focus (e.g., a lung abscess or empyema) may be blocking access of the antibiotic(s) to the pathogen. Alternatively, the patient may be getting either the wrong drug or the correct drug at the wrong dose or frequency of administration. It is also possible that CAP is the correct diagnosis but that a different pathogen (e.g., *M. tuberculosis* or a fungus) is the cause. In addition, nosocomial superinfections—both pulmonary and extrapulmonary—are possible explanations for persistence. In all cases of delayed response or deteriorating condition, the patient must be carefully reassessed and appropriate studies initiated. These studies may include such diverse procedures as CT and bronchoscopy.

Complications As in other severe infections, common complications of severe CAP include respiratory failure, shock and multiorgan failure, bleeding diatheses, and exacerbation of comorbid illnesses. Three particularly noteworthy conditions are metastatic infection, lung abscess, and complicated pleural effusion. Metastatic infection (e.g., brain abscess or endocarditis), although unusual, deserves immediate attention by the physician, with a detailed workup and proper treatment. Lung abscess may occur in association with aspiration or with infection caused by a single CAP pathogen, such CA-MRSA, *P. aeruginosa*, or (rarely) *S. pneumoniae*. Aspiration pneumonia is typically a mixed polymicrobial infection involving both aerobes and anaerobes. In either scenario, drainage should be established, and antibiotics that cover the known or suspected pathogens should be administered. A significant pleural effusion should be tapped for both diagnostic and therapeutic purposes. If the fluid has a pH of <7, a glucose level of <2.2 mmol/L, and a lactate dehydrogenase concentration of >1000 U/L or if bacteria are seen or cultured, then the fluid should be drained; a chest tube is usually required.

Follow-Up Fever and leukocytosis usually resolve within 2 and 4 days, respectively, in otherwise healthy patients with CAP, but physical findings may persist longer. Chest radiographic abnormalities are slowest to resolve and may require 4–12 weeks to clear, with the speed of clearance depending on the patient's age and underlying lung disease. For a patient whose condition is improving and who (if hospitalized) has been discharged, a follow-up radiograph can be done ~4–6 weeks later. If relapse or recurrence is documented, particularly in the same lung segment, the possibility of an underlying neoplasm must be considered.

PROGNOSIS

The prognosis of CAP depends on the patient's age, comorbidities, and site of treatment (inpatient or outpatient). Young patients without comorbidity do well and usually recover fully after ~2 weeks. Older patients and those with comorbid conditions can take several weeks longer to recover fully. The overall mortality rate for the outpatient group is <1%. For patients requiring hospitalization, the overall mortality rate is estimated at 10%, with ~50% of the deaths directly attributable to pneumonia.

PREVENTION

The main preventive measure is vaccination. The recommendations of the Advisory Committee on Immunization Practices should be followed for influenza and pneumococcal vaccines. In the event of an influenza outbreak, unprotected patients at risk from complications should be vaccinated immediately and given chemoprophylaxis with either oseltamivir or zanamivir for 2 weeks—i.e., until vaccine-induced antibody levels are sufficiently high. Because of an increased risk of pneumococcal infection, even among patients without obstructive lung disease, smokers should be strongly encouraged to stop smoking.

HEALTH CARE–ASSOCIATED PNEUMONIA

VENTILATOR-ASSOCIATED PNEUMONIA

Most research on VAP has focused on illness in the hospital setting. However, the information and principles based on this research can be applied to HCAP not associated with ventilator use as well. The main rationale for the new designation *HCAP* is that the pathogens and treatment strategies for VAP are more similar to those for HAP than to those for pure CAP. The greatest difference between VAP and HCAP/HAP—and the greatest similarity of VAP to CAP—is the return to dependence on expectorated sputum for a microbiologic diagnosis, which is further complicated by the frequent colonization with pathogens among patients in the hospital or other health care–associated settings.

Etiology Potential etiologic agents of VAP include both MDR and non-MDR bacterial pathogens (Table 251-5). The non-MDR group is nearly identical to the pathogens found in severe CAP (Table 251-2); it is not surprising that such pathogens predominate if VAP develops in the first 5–7 days of the hospital stay. However, if patients have other risk factors for HCAP, MDR pathogens are a consideration, even early in the hospital course. The relative frequency of individual MDR pathogens can vary significantly from hospital to hospital and even between different critical care units within the same institution. Many hospitals have problems with *P. aeruginosa* and MRSA, but other MDR pathogens are often institution-specific.

Less commonly, fungal and viral pathogens cause VAP, most frequently affecting severely immunocompromised patients. Rarely, community-associated viruses cause miniepidemics, usually when introduced by ill health care workers.

Epidemiology Pneumonia is a common complication among patients requiring mechanical ventilation. Prevalence estimates vary between 6 and 52 cases per 100 patients, depending on the population studied. On any given day in the ICU, an average of 10% of patients will have pneumonia—VAP in the overwhelming majority of cases. The frequency of diagnosis is not static but changes with the duration of mechanical ventilation, with the highest hazard ratio in the first 5 days and a plateau in additional cases (1% per day) after ~2 weeks. However, the cumulative rate among patients who remain ventilated for as long as 30 days is as high as 70%. These rates often do not reflect the recurrence of VAP in the same patient. Once a ventilated patient is transferred to a chronic care facility or to home, the incidence of pneumonia drops significantly, especially in the absence of other risk factors for pneumonia.

Three factors are critical in the pathogenesis of VAP: colonization of the oropharynx with pathogenic microorganisms, aspiration of these organisms from the oropharynx into the lower respiratory tract, and compromise of the normal host defense mechanisms. Most risk factors

TABLE 251-5 MICROBIOLOGIC CAUSES OF VENTILATOR-ASSOCIATED PNEUMONIA

Non-MDR Pathogens	MDR Pathogens
Streptococcus pneumoniae	*Pseudomonas aeruginosa*
Other *Streptococcus* spp.	MRSA
Haemophilus influenzae	*Acinetobacter* spp.
MSSA	Antibiotic-resistant Enterobacteriaceae
Antibiotic-sensitive Enterobacteriaceae	*Enterobacter* spp.
Escherichia coli	ESBL-positive strains
Klebsiella pneumoniae	*Klebsiella* spp.
Proteus spp.	*Legionella pneumophila*
Enterobacter spp.	*Burkholderia cepacia*
Serratia marcescens	*Aspergillus* spp.

Note: ESBL, extended-spectrum β-lactamase; MDR, multidrug-resistant; MRSA, methicillin-resistant *Staphylococcus aureus*; MSSA, methicillin-sensitive *S. aureus*.

TABLE 251-6 PATHOGENIC MECHANISMS AND CORRESPONDING PREVENTION STRATEGIES FOR VENTILATOR-ASSOCIATED PNEUMONIA

Pathogenic Mechanism	Prevention Strategy
Oropharyngeal colonization with pathogenic bacteria	
Elimination of normal flora	Avoidance of prolonged antibiotic courses
Large-volume oropharyngeal aspiration around time of intubation	Short course of prophylactic antibiotics for comatose patients[a]
Gastroesophageal reflux	Postpyloric enteral feeding[b]; avoidance of high gastric residuals, prokinetic agents
Bacterial overgrowth of stomach	Avoidance of gastrointestinal bleeding due to prophylactic agents that raise gastric pH[b]; selective decontamination of digestive tract with nonabsorbable antibiotics[b]
Cross-infection from other colonized patients	Hand washing, especially with alcohol-based hand rub; intensive infection control education[a]; isolation; proper cleaning of reusable equipment
Large-volume aspiration	Endotracheal intubation; avoidance of sedation; decompression of small-bowel obstruction
Microaspiration around endotracheal tube	
Endotracheal intubation	Noninvasive ventilation[a]
Prolonged duration of ventilation	Daily awakening from sedation,[a] weaning protocols[a]
Abnormal swallowing function	Early percutaneous tracheostomy[a]
Secretions pooled above endotracheal tube	Head of bed elevated[a]; continuous aspiration of subglottic secretions with specialized endotracheal tube[a]; avoidance of reintubation; minimization of sedation and patient transport
Altered lower respiratory host defenses	Tight glycemic control[a]; lowering of hemoglobin transfusion threshold; specialized enteral feeding formula

[a]Strategies demonstrated to be effective in at least one randomized controlled trial.
[b]Strategies with negative randomized trials or conflicting results.

and their corresponding prevention strategies pertain to one of these three factors (Table 251-6).

The most obvious risk factor is the endotracheal tube (ET), which bypasses the normal mechanical factors preventing aspiration. While the presence of an ET may prevent large-volume aspiration, microaspiration is actually enhanced by secretions pooling above the cuff. The ET and the concomitant need for suctioning can damage the tracheal mucosa, thereby facilitating tracheal colonization. In addition, pathogenic bacteria can form a glycocalyx biofilm on the ET surface that protects them from both antibiotics and host defenses. The bacteria can also be dislodged during suctioning and can reinoculate the trachea, or tiny fragments of glycocalyx can embolize to distal airways, carrying bacteria with them.

In a high percentage of critically ill patients, the normal oropharyngeal flora is replaced by pathogenic microorganisms. The most important risk factors are antibiotic selection pressure, cross-infection from other infected/colonized patients or contaminated equipment, and malnutrition.

How the lower respiratory tract defenses become overwhelmed remains poorly understood. Almost all intubated patients experience microaspiration and are at least transiently colonized with pathogenic bacteria. However, only around one-third of colonized patients develop VAP. Severely ill patients with sepsis and trauma appear to enter a state of immunoparalysis several days after admission to the ICU—a time that corresponds to the greatest risk of developing VAP. The mechanism of this immunosuppression is not clear, although several factors have been suggested. Hyperglycemia affects neutrophil function, and recent trials suggest that keeping the blood sugar close to normal with exogenous insulin may have beneficial effects, including a decreased risk of infection. More frequent transfusions, especially of leukocyte-depleted red blood cells, also affect the immune response positively.

Clinical Manifestations The clinical manifestations of VAP are generally the same as for all other forms of pneumonia: fever, leukocytosis, increase in respiratory secretions, and pulmonary consolidation on physical examination, along with a new or changing radiographic infiltrate. The frequency of abnormal chest radiographs before the onset of pneumonia in intubated patients and the limitations of portable radiographic technique make interpretation of radiographs more difficult than in patients who are not intubated. Other clinical features may include tachypnea, tachycardia, worsening oxygenation, and increased minute ventilation.

Diagnosis No single set of criteria is reliably diagnostic of pneumonia in a ventilated patient. The inability to identify such patients compromises efforts to prevent and treat VAP and even calls into question estimates of the impact of VAP on mortality rates.

Application of clinical criteria consistently results in overdiagnosis of VAP, largely because of three common findings in at-risk patients: (1) tracheal colonization with pathogenic bacteria in patients with ETs, (2) multiple alternative causes of radiographic infiltrates in mechanically ventilated patients, and (3) the high frequency of other sources of fever in critically ill patients. The differential diagnosis of VAP includes a number of entities, such as atypical pulmonary edema, pulmonary contusion and/or hemorrhage, hypersensitivity pneumonitis, ARDS, and pulmonary embolism. Clinical findings in ventilated patients with fever and/or leukocytosis may have alternative causes, including antibiotic-associated diarrhea, sinusitis, urinary tract infection, pancreatitis, and drug fever. Conditions mimicking pneumonia are often documented in patients in whom VAP has been ruled out by accurate diagnostic techniques. Most of these alternative diagnoses do not require antibiotic treatment; require antibiotics different from those used to treat VAP; or require some additional intervention, such as surgical drainage or catheter removal, for optimal management.

This diagnostic dilemma has led to debate and controversy. The major question is whether a quantitative-culture approach as a means of eliminating false-positive clinical diagnoses is superior to the clinical approach enhanced by principles learned from quantitative-culture studies. The recent IDSA/ATS guidelines for HCAP suggest that either approach is clinically valid.

QUANTITATIVE-CULTURE APPROACH The essence of the quantitative-culture approach is to discriminate between colonization and true infection by determining the bacterial burden. The more distal in the respiratory tree the diagnostic sampling, the more specific the results and therefore the lower the threshold of growth necessary to diagnose pneumonia and exclude colonization. For example, a quantitative endotracheal aspirate yields proximate samples, and the diagnostic threshold is 10^6 cfu/mL. The protected specimen brush method, in contrast, obtains distal samples and has a threshold of 10^3 cfu/mL. Conversely, sensitivity declines as more distal secretions are obtained, especially when they are collected blindly (i.e., by a technique other than bronchoscopy). Additional tests that may increase the diagnostic yield include Gram's stain, differential cell counts, staining for intracellular organisms, and detection of local protein levels elevated in response to infection.

Several studies have compared patient cohorts managed by the various quantitative-culture methods. While these studies documented issues of relative sensitivity and specificity, outcomes were not significantly different for the various groups of patients. The IDSA/ATS guidelines have suggested that all these methods are appropriate and that the choice depends on availability and local expertise.

The Achilles heel of the quantitative approach is the effect of antibiotic therapy. With sensitive microorganisms, a single antibiotic dose can reduce colony counts below the diagnostic threshold. Recent

TABLE 251-7 CLINICAL PULMONARY INFECTION SCORE (CPIS)	
Criterion	Score
Fever (°C)	
≥38.5 but ≤38.9	1
>39 or < 36	2
Leukocytosis	
<4000 or >11,000/μL	1
Bands > 50%	1 (additional)
Oxygenation (mmHg)	
Pa_{O_2}/Fl_{O_2} <250 and no ARDS	2
Chest radiograph	
Localized infiltrate	2
Patchy or diffuse infiltrate	1
Progression of infiltrate (no ARDS or CHF)	2
Tracheal aspirate	
Moderate or heavy growth	1
Same morphology on Gram's stain	1 (additional)
Maximal score[a]	12

[a]The progression of the infiltrate is not known and tracheal aspirate culture results are often unavailable at the time of the original diagnosis; thus, the maximal score is initially 8–10.

Note: ARDS, acute respiratory distress syndrome; CHF, congestive heart failure.

changes in antibiotic therapy are the most significant. After ≥3 days of consistent antibiotic therapy for another infection prior to suspicion of pneumonia, the accuracy of diagnostic tests for pneumonia is unaffected. Conversely, colony counts above the diagnostic threshold during antibiotic therapy suggest that the current antibiotics are ineffective. Even the normal host response may be sufficient to reduce quantitative-culture counts below the diagnostic threshold by the time of sampling. In short, expertise in quantitative-culture techniques is critical, with a specimen obtained as soon as pneumonia is suspected and before antibiotic therapy is initiated or changed.

In a study comparing the quantitative with the clinical approach, use of bronchoscopic quantitative cultures resulted in significantly less antibiotic use at 14 days after study entry and lower rates of mortality and severity-adjusted mortality at 28 days. In addition, more alternative sites of infection were found in patients randomized to the quantitative-culture strategy. A critical aspect of this study was that antibiotic treatment was initiated only in patients whose gram-stained respiratory sample was positive or who displayed signs of hemodynamic instability. Fewer than half as many patients were treated for pneumonia in the bronchoscopy group, and only one-third as many microorganisms were cultured.

CLINICAL APPROACH The lack of specificity of a clinical diagnosis of VAP has led to efforts to improve the diagnostic criteria. The Clinical Pulmonary Infection Score (CPIS) was developed by weighting of the various clinical criteria usually used for the diagnosis of VAP (Table 251-7). Use of the CPIS allows the selection of low-risk patients who may need only short-course antibiotic therapy or no treatment at all. Moreover, studies have demonstrated that the absence of bacteria in gram-stained endotracheal aspirates makes pneumonia an unlikely cause of fever or pulmonary infiltrates. These findings, coupled with a heightened awareness of the alternative diagnoses possible in patients with suspected VAP, can prevent inappropriate treatment for this disease. Furthermore, data show that the absence of an MDR pathogen in tracheal aspirate cultures eliminates the need for MDR coverage when empirical antibiotic therapy is narrowed. Since the most likely explanations for the mortality benefit of bronchoscopic quantitative cultures are decreased antibiotic selection pressure (which reduces the risk of subsequent infection with MDR pathogens) and identification of alternative sources of infection, a clinical diagnostic approach that incorporates such principles may result in similar outcomes.

℞ VENTILATOR-ASSOCIATED PNEUMONIA

Many studies have demonstrated higher mortality rates with inappropriate than with appropriate empirical antibiotic therapy. The key to appropriate

TABLE 251-8 EMPIRICAL ANTIBIOTIC TREATMENT OF HEALTH CARE–ASSOCIATED PNEUMONIA

Patients without Risk Factors for MDR Pathogens

Ceftriaxone (2 g IV q24h) *or*
Moxifloxacin (400 mg IV q24h), ciprofloxacin (400 mg IV q8h), or levofloxacin (750 mg IV q24h) *or*
Ampicillin/sulbactam (3 g IV q6h) *or*
Ertapenem (1 g IV q24h)

Patients with Risk Factors for MDR Pathogens

1. A β-lactam:
Ceftazidime (2 g IV q8h) or cefepime (2 g IV q8–12h) *or*
Piperacillin/tazobactam (4.5 g IV q6h), imipenem (500 mg IV q6h or 1 g IV q8h), or meropenem (1 g IV q8h) *plus*
2. A second agent active against gram-negative bacterial pathogens:
Gentamicin or tobramycin (7 mg/kg IV q24h) or amikacin (20 mg/kg IV q24h) *or*
Ciprofloxacin (400 mg IV q8h) or levofloxacin (750 mg IV q24h) *plus*
3. An agent active against gram-positive bacterial pathogens:
Linezolid (600 mg IV q12h) *or*
Vancomycin (15 mg/kg, up to 1 g IV, q12h)

Note: MDR, multidrug-resistant.

antibiotic management of VAP is an appreciation of the patterns of resistance of the most likely pathogens in any given patient.

RESISTANCE If it were not for the risk of infection with MDR pathogens (Table 251-1), VAP could be treated with the same antibiotics used for severe CAP. However, antibiotic selection pressure leads to the frequent involvement of MDR pathogens by selecting either for drug-resistant isolates of common pathogens (MRSA and ESBL-positive Enterobacteriaceae) or for intrinsically resistant pathogens (*P. aeruginosa* and *Acinetobacter* spp.). Frequent use of β-lactam drugs, especially cephalosporins, appears to be the major risk factor for infection with MRSA and ESBL-positive strains.

P. aeruginosa has demonstrated the ability to develop resistance to all routinely used antibiotics. Unfortunately, even if initially sensitive, *P. aeruginosa* isolates have also shown a propensity to develop resistance during treatment. Occasionally, derepression of resistance genes may be the cause of the selection of resistant clones within the large bacterial inoculum associated with most pneumonias. *Acinetobacter*, *Stenotrophomonas maltophilia*, and *Burkholderia cepacia* are intrinsically resistant to many of the empirical antibiotic regimens listed in **Table 251-8**. VAP caused by these pathogens emerges during treatment of other infections, and resistance is always evident at initial diagnosis.

EMPIRICAL THERAPY Recommended options for empirical therapy are listed in Table 251-8. Treatment should be started once diagnostic specimens have been obtained. The major factor in the selection of agents is the presence of risk factors for MDR pathogens. Choices among the various options listed depend on local patterns of resistance and the patient's prior antibiotic exposure.

The majority of patients *without* risk factors for MDR infection can be treated with a single agent. The major difference from CAP is the markedly lower incidence of atypical pathogens in VAP; the exception is *Legionella*, which can be a nosocomial pathogen, especially when there are deficiencies in the treatment of a hospital's potable water supply.

The standard recommendation for patients *with* risk factors for MDR infection is for three antibiotics: two directed at *P. aeruginosa* and one at MRSA. The choice of a β-lactam agent provides the greatest variability in coverage, yet the use of the broadest-spectrum agent—a carbapenem—still represents inappropriate initial therapy in 10–15% of cases.

SPECIFIC TREATMENT Once an etiologic diagnosis is made, broad-spectrum empirical therapy can be modified to address the known pathogen specifically. For patients with MDR risk factors, antibiotic regimens can be reduced to a single agent in more than half of cases and to a two-drug combination in more than one-quarter. Only a minority of cases require a complete course with three drugs. A negative tracheal-aspirate culture or growth below the threshold for quantitative cultures, especially if the sample was obtained before any antibiotic change, strongly suggests that antibiotics should be discontinued. Identification of other confirmed or suspected sites of infection may require ongoing antibiotic therapy, but

the spectrum of pathogens (and the corresponding antibiotic choices) may be different from those for VAP. If the CPIS decreases over the first 3 days, antibiotics should be stopped after 8 days. An 8-day course of therapy is just as effective as a 2-week course and is associated with less frequent emergence of antibiotic-resistant strains.

The major controversy regarding specific therapy for VAP concerns the need for ongoing combination treatment of *Pseudomonas* infection. No randomized controlled trials have demonstrated a benefit of combination therapy with a β-lactam and an aminoglycoside, nor have subgroup analyses in other trials found a survival benefit with such a regimen. The unacceptably high rates of clinical failure and death for VAP caused by *P. aeruginosa* despite combination therapy (see "Failure to Improve," below) indicate that better regimens are needed—including, perhaps, aerosolized antibiotics.

VAP caused by MRSA is associated with a 40% clinical failure rate when treated with standard-dose vancomycin. One proposed solution is the use of high-dose individualized treatment, but the risk-to-benefit ratio of this approach is not known. Linezolid appears to be more efficacious than the standard dose of vancomycin, especially in patients with renal insufficiency.

FAILURE TO IMPROVE Treatment failure is not uncommon in VAP, especially in that caused by MDR pathogens. In addition to the 40% failure rate for MRSA infection treated with vancomycin, VAP due to *Pseudomonas* has a 50% failure rate, no matter what the regimen. The causes of clinical failure vary with the pathogen(s) and the antibiotic(s). Inappropriate therapy can usually be minimized by use of the recommended triple-drug regimen (Table 251-8). However, the emergence of β-lactam resistance during therapy is an important problem, especially in infection with *Pseudomonas* and *Enterobacter* spp. Recurrent VAP caused by the same pathogen is possible because the biofilm on ETs allows reintroduction of the microorganism. However, studies of VAP caused by *Pseudomonas* show that approximately half of recurrent cases are caused by a new strain. Inadequate local levels of vancomycin are the likely cause of treatment failure in VAP due to MRSA.

Treatment failure is very difficult to diagnose. Pneumonia due to a new superinfection, the presence of extrapulmonary infection, and drug toxicity must be considered in the differential diagnosis of treatment failure. Serial CPIS appears to track the clinical response accurately, while repeat quantitative cultures may clarify the microbiologic response. A persistently elevated or rising CPIS value by day 3 of therapy is likely to indicate failure. The most sensitive component of the CPIS is improvement in oxygenation.

COMPLICATIONS Apart from death, the major complication of VAP is prolongation of mechanical ventilation, with corresponding increases in length of stay in the ICU and in the hospital. In most studies, an additional week of mechanical ventilation because of VAP is common. The additional expense of this complication warrants costly and aggressive efforts at prevention.

In rare cases, some types of necrotizing pneumonia (e.g., that due to *P. aeruginosa*) result in significant pulmonary hemorrhage. More commonly, necrotizing infections result in the long-term complications of bronchiectasis and parenchymal scarring leading to recurrent pneumonias. The long-term complications of pneumonia are underappreciated. Pneumonia results in a catabolic state in a patient already nutritionally at risk. The muscle loss and general debilitation from an episode of VAP often require prolonged rehabilitation and, in the elderly, commonly result in an inability to return to independent function and the need for nursing home placement.

FOLLOW-UP Clinical improvement, if it occurs, is usually evident within 48–72 h of the initiation of antimicrobial treatment. Because findings on chest radiography often worsen initially during treatment, they are less helpful than clinical criteria as an indicator of clinical response in severe pneumonia. Although no hard and fast rules govern the frequency of follow-up chest radiography in seriously ill patients with pneumonia, assessment every few days in a responding patient seems appropriate. Once the patient has improved substantially and has stabilized, follow-up radiographs may not be necessary for a few weeks.

Prognosis VAP is associated with significant mortality. Crude mortality rates of 50–70% have been reported, but the real issue is attributable mortality. Many patients with VAP have underlying diseases that would result in death even if VAP did not occur. Attributable mortality exceeded 25% in one matched-cohort study. Patients who develop VAP are at least twice as likely to die as those who do not. Some of the variability in reported figures is clearly related to the type of patient and ICU studied. VAP in trauma patients is not associated with attributable mortality, possibly because many of the patients were otherwise healthy before being injured. However, the causative pathogen also plays a major role. Generally, MDR pathogens are associated with significantly greater attributable mortality than non-MDR pathogens. Pneumonia caused by some pathogens (e.g., *S. maltophilia*) is simply a marker for a patient whose immune system is so compromised that death is almost inevitable.

Prevention   (Table 251-6) Because of the significance of the ET as a risk factor for VAP, the most important preventive intervention is to avoid endotracheal intubation or at least to minimize its duration. Successful use of noninvasive ventilation via a nasal or full-face mask avoids many of the problems associated with ETs. Strategies that minimize the duration of ventilation have also been highly effective in preventing VAP.

Unfortunately, a tradeoff in risks is sometimes required. Aggressive attempts to extubate early may result in reintubation(s), which pose a risk of VAP. Heavy continuous sedation increases the risk, but self-extubation because of too little sedation is also a risk. The tradeoff is probably best illustrated by antibiotic therapy. Short-course antibiotic prophylaxis can decrease the risk of VAP in comatose patients requiring intubation, and data suggest that antibiotics decrease VAP rates in general. However, the major benefit appears to be a decrease in the incidence of early-onset VAP, which is usually caused by the less pathogenic non-MDR microorganisms. Conversely, prolonged courses of antibiotics consistently increase the risk of VAP caused by the more lethal MDR pathogens. Despite its virulence and associated mortality, VAP caused by *Pseudomonas* is rare among patients who have not recently received antibiotics.

Minimizing the amount of microaspiration around the ET cuff is also a strategy for avoidance of VAP. Simply elevating the head of the bed (at least 30° above horizontal but preferably 45°) decreases VAP rates. Specially modified ETs that allow removal of the secretions pooled above the cuff may also prevent VAP. The risk-to-benefit ratio of transporting the patient outside the ICU for diagnostic tests or procedures should be carefully considered, since VAP rates are increased among transported patients.

Emphasis on the avoidance of agents that raise gastric pH and on oropharyngeal decontamination has been diminished by the equivocal and conflicting results of more recent clinical trials. The role in the pathogenesis of VAP that is played by the overgrowth of bacterial components of the bowel flora in the stomach has also been downplayed. MRSA and the nonfermenters *P. aeruginosa* and *Acinetobacter* spp. are not normally part of the bowel flora but reside primarily in the nose and on the skin, respectively. Therefore, an emphasis on controlling overgrowth of the bowel flora may be relevant only in certain populations, such as liver transplant recipients and patients who have undergone other major intraabdominal procedures or who have bowel obstruction.

In outbreaks of VAP due to specific pathogens, the possibility of a breakdown in infection control measures (particularly contamination of reusable equipment) should be investigated. Even high rates of pathogens that are already common in a particular ICU may be a result of cross-infection. Education and reminders of the need for consistent infection control practices can minimize this risk.

HOSPITAL-ACQUIRED PNEUMONIA

While significantly less well studied than VAP, HAP in nonintubated patients, both inside and outside the ICU, is similar to VAP. The main differences are in the higher frequency of non-MDR pathogens and the better underlying host immunity in nonintubated patients. The lower frequency of MDR pathogens allows monotherapy in a larger proportion of cases of HAP than of VAP.

The only pathogens that may be more common in the non-VAP population are anaerobes. The greater risk of macroaspiration by nonintubated patients and the lower oxygen tensions in the lower respiratory tract of these patients increase the likelihood of a role for anaerobes. As in the management of CAP, specific therapy targeting anaerobes probably is not indicated unless gross aspiration is a concern.

Diagnosis is even more difficult for HAP in the nonintubated patient than for VAP. Lower respiratory tract samples appropriate for culture are considerably more difficult to obtain from nonintubated patients. Many of the underlying diseases that predispose a patient to HAP are also associated with an inability to cough adequately. Since blood cultures are infrequently positive (<15% of cases), the majority of patients with HAP do not have culture data on which antibiotic modifications can be based. Therefore, de-escalation of therapy is less likely in patients with risk factors for MDR pathogens. Despite these difficulties, the better host defenses in non-ICU patients result in lower mortality rates than are documented for VAP. In addition, the risk of antibiotic failure is lower in HAP.

FURTHER READINGS

AMERICAN THORACIC SOCIETY/INFECTIOUS DISEASES SOCIETY OF AMERICA: Guidelines for the management of adults with hospital-acquired, ventilator-associated, and healthcare-associated pneumonia. Am J Respir Crit Care Med 171:388, 2005

CHASTRE J, FAGON JY: Ventilator-associated pneumonia. Am J Respir Crit Care Med 165:867, 2002

FAGON JY et al: Invasive and noninvasive strategies for management of suspected ventilator-associated pneumonia. A randomized trial. Ann Intern Med 132:621, 2000

FINE MJ et al: A prediction rule to identify low-risk patients with community-acquired pneumonia. N Engl J Med 336:243, 1997

LIM WS et al: Defining community acquired pneumonia severity on presentation to hospital: An international derivation and validation study. Thorax 58:377, 2003

MANDELL LA et al: Infectious Diseases Society of America/American Thoracic Society consensus guidelines on the management of community-acquired pneumonia. Clin Infect Dis 44(Suppl 2):S27, 2007

SINGH N et al: Short-course empiric antibiotic therapy for patients with pulmonary infiltrates in the intensive care unit. A proposed solution for indiscriminate antibiotic prescription. Am J Respir Crit Care Med 162:505, 2000

VANDERKOOI OG et al: Predicting antimicrobial resistance in invasive pneumococcal infections. Clin Infect Dis 40:1288, 2005

252 Bronchiectasis and Lung Abscess

Gregory Tino, Steven E. Weinberger

BRONCHIECTASIS

DEFINITION

Bronchiectasis is an abnormal and permanent dilatation of bronchi. It may be either focal, involving airways supplying a limited region of pulmonary parenchyma, or diffuse, involving airways in a more widespread distribution. Recent studies have estimated there to be about 110,000 patients with bronchiectasis in the United States. It is a disorder that typically affects older individuals; approximately two-thirds of patients are women.

PATHOLOGY

The bronchial dilatation of bronchiectasis is associated with destructive and inflammatory changes in the walls of medium-sized airways, often at the level of segmental or subsegmental bronchi. Airway inflammation is primarily mediated by neutrophils and results in upregulation of enzymes such as elastase and matrix metalloproteinases. The normal structural components of the wall, including cartilage, muscle, and elastic tissue, are destroyed and may be replaced by fibrous tissue. The dilated airways frequently contain pools of thick, purulent material, while more peripheral airways are often occluded by secretions or obliterated and replaced by fibrous tissue. Additional microscopic features include bronchial and peribronchial inflammation and fibrosis, ulceration of the bronchial wall, squamous metaplasia, and mucous gland hyperplasia. The parenchyma normally supplied by the affected airways is abnormal, containing varying combinations of fibrosis, emphysema, bronchopneumonia, and atelectasis. As a result of the inflammation, vascularity of the bronchial wall increases, with associated enlargement of the bronchial arteries and anastomoses between the bronchial and pulmonary arterial circulations.

Three different patterns of bronchiectasis have been described. In *cylindrical bronchiectasis*, the involved bronchi appear uniformly dilated and end abruptly at the point that smaller airways are obstructed by secretions. In *varicose bronchiectasis*, the affected bronchi have an irregular or beaded pattern of dilatation resembling varicose veins. In *saccular (cystic) bronchiectasis*, the bronchi have a ballooned appearance at the periphery, ending in blind sacs without recognizable bronchial structures distal to the sacs.

ETIOLOGY AND PATHOGENESIS

Bronchiectasis is a consequence of inflammation and destruction of the structural components of the bronchial wall. Infection is the usual cause of the inflammation; microorganisms such as *Pseudomonas aeruginosa* and *Haemophilus influenzae* produce pigments, proteases, and other toxins that injure the respiratory epithelium and impair mucociliary clearance. The host inflammatory response induces epithelial injury, largely as a result of mediators released from neutrophils. As protection against infection is compromised, the dilated airways become more susceptible to colonization and growth of bacteria. Thus, a reinforcing cycle can result, with inflammation producing airway damage, impaired clearance of microorganisms, and further infection, which then completes the cycle by inciting more inflammation.

Infectious Causes Adenovirus and influenza virus are the main viruses that cause bronchiectasis in association with lower respiratory tract involvement. Virulent bacterial infections, especially with potentially necrotizing organisms such as *Staphylococcus aureus*, *Klebsiella*, and anaerobes, remain important causes of bronchiectasis when antibiotic treatment of a pneumonia is not given or is significantly delayed. Infection with *Bordetella pertussis*, particularly in childhood, has also been classically associated with chronic suppurative airways disease.

Bronchiectasis has been reported in patients with HIV infection, perhaps at least partly due to recurrent bacterial infection. Tuberculosis, a major cause of bronchiectasis worldwide, can produce airway dilatation by a necrotizing effect on pulmonary parenchyma and airways and indirectly as a consequence of airway obstruction from bronchostenosis or extrinsic compression by lymph nodes. Nontuberculous mycobacteria are frequently cultured from patients with bronchiectasis, often as secondary infections or colonizing organisms. However, it has also been recognized that these organisms, especially those of the *Mycobacterium avium* complex, can serve as primary pathogens associated with the development and/or progression of bronchiectasis.

Impaired host defense mechanisms are often involved in the predisposition to recurrent infections. The major cause of localized impairment of host defenses is endobronchial obstruction. Bacteria and secretions cannot be cleared adequately from the obstructed airway, which develops recurrent or chronic infection. Slowly growing endobronchial neoplasms such as carcinoid tumors may be associated with bronchiectasis. Foreign-body aspiration is another important cause of endobronchial obstruction, particularly in children. Airway obstruction can also result from bronchostenosis, from impacted secretions, or from extrinsic compression by enlarged lymph nodes.

Generalized impairment of pulmonary defense mechanisms occurs with immunoglobulin deficiency, primary ciliary disorders, or cystic fibrosis (CF). Infections and bronchiectasis are therefore often more diffuse. With panhypogammaglobulinemia, the best described of the immunoglobulin disorders associated with recurrent infection and bronchiectasis, patients often also have a history of sinus or skin infections. Selective deficiency of an IgG subclass, especially IgG2, has also been described in a small number of patients with bronchiectasis.

The primary disorders associated with ciliary dysfunction, termed *primary ciliary dyskinesia*, are responsible for 5–10% of cases of bronchiectasis. Primary ciliary dyskinesia is inherited in an autosomal recessive fashion. Numerous defects are encompassed under this category, including structural abnormalities of the dynein arms, radial spokes, and microtubules; mutations in heavy and intermediate chain dynein have been described in a small number of patients. The cilia become dyskinetic; their coordinated, propulsive action is diminished, and bacterial clearance is impaired. The clinical effects include recurrent upper and lower respiratory tract infections, such as sinusitis, otitis media, and bronchiectasis. Because normal sperm motility also depends on proper ciliary function, males are generally infertile (Chap. 340). Additionally, since visceral rotation during development depends upon proper ciliary motion, the positioning of normally lateralized organs becomes random. As a result, approximately half of patients with primary ciliary dyskinesia fall into the subgroup of *Kartagener's syndrome*, in which situs inversus accompanies bronchiectasis and sinusitis.

In CF (Chap. 253), the tenacious secretions in the bronchi are associated with impaired bacterial clearance, resulting in colonization and recurrent infection with a variety of organisms, particularly mucoid strains of *P. aeruginosa* but also *S. aureus*, *H. influenzae*, *Escherichia coli*, and *Burkholderia cepacia*.

Noninfectious Causes Some cases of bronchiectasis are associated with exposure to a toxic substance that incites a severe inflammatory response. Examples include inhalation of a toxic gas such as ammonia or aspiration of acidic gastric contents, though the latter problem is often also complicated by aspiration of bacteria. An immune response in the airway may also trigger inflammation, destructive changes, and bronchial dilatation. This mechanism is presumably important for bronchiectasis with allergic bronchopulmonary aspergillosis (ABPA), which is due at least in part to an immune response to *Aspergillus* organisms that have colonized the airway (Chap. 249).

In α_1-antitrypsin deficiency, the usual respiratory complication is the early development of panacinar emphysema, but affected individuals may occasionally have bronchiectasis. In the *yellow nail syndrome*, which is due to hypoplastic lymphatics, the triad of lymphedema, pleural effusion, and yellow discoloration of the nails is accompanied by bronchiectasis in approximately 40% of patients.

Patients typically present with persistent or recurrent cough and purulent sputum production. Repeated, purulent respiratory tract infections should raise clinical suspicion for bronchiectasis. Hemoptysis occurs in 50–70% of cases and can be due to bleeding from friable, inflamed airway mucosa (Chap. 34). More significant, even massive bleeding is often a consequence of bleeding from hypertrophied bronchial arteries. Systemic symptoms such as fatigue, weight loss, and myalgias can also occur.

When a specific infectious episode initiates bronchiectasis, patients may describe a severe pneumonia followed by chronic cough and sputum production. Alternatively, patients without a dramatic initiating event often describe the insidious onset of symptoms. In some cases, patients are either asymptomatic or have a nonproductive cough, often associated with "dry" bronchiectasis in an upper lobe. Dyspnea or wheezing generally reflects either widespread bronchiectasis or underlying chronic obstructive pulmonary disease. With exacerbations of infection, the amount of sputum increases, and it becomes more purulent and often more bloody; systemic symptoms, including fever, may also be prominent.

Physical examination of the chest overlying an area of bronchiectasis is quite variable. Any combination of crackles, rhonchi, and wheezes may be heard, all of which reflect the damaged airways containing significant secretions. As with other types of chronic intrathoracic infection, clubbing may be present. Patients with severe diffuse disease, particularly those with chronic hypoxemia, may have associated cor pulmonale and right ventricular failure.

RADIOGRAPHIC AND LABORATORY FINDINGS

Though the chest radiograph is important in the evaluation of suspected bronchiectasis, the findings are often nonspecific. At one extreme, the radiograph may be normal with mild disease. Alternatively, patients with saccular bronchiectasis may have prominent cystic spaces, either with or without air-liquid levels, corresponding to the dilated airways. These may be difficult to distinguish from enlarged airspaces due to bullous emphysema or from regions of honeycombing in patients with severe interstitial lung disease. Other findings are due to dilated airways with thickened walls, which result from peribronchial inflammation. These dilated airways are often crowded together in parallel. When seen longitudinally, the airways appear as "tram tracks"; when seen in cross-section, they produce "ring shadows." Because the dilated airways may be filled with secretions, the lumen may appear dense rather than radiolucent, producing an opaque tubular or branched tubular structure.

CT, especially with high-resolution images 1.0–1.5 mm thick, provides an excellent view of dilated airways (Fig. 252-1). Consequently, it

FIGURE 252-1 High-resolution CT scan of bronchiectasis showing dilated airways in both lower lobes and in the lingula. When seen in cross-section, the dilated airways have a ringlike appearance. *(From SE Weinberger: Principles of Pulmonary Medicine, 4th ed. Philadelphia, Saunders, 2004, with permission.)*

FIGURE 252-2 Diagnostic approach to bronchiectasis. AFB, acid-fast bacilli; CXR, chest X-ray; GERD, gastroesophageal reflux disease; HRCT, high-resolution computed tomography; PFT, pulmonary function testing.

is now the standard technique for detecting or confirming the diagnosis of bronchiectasis.

Examination of sputum often reveals an abundance of neutrophils and colonization or infection with a variety of possible organisms. Appropriate staining and culturing of sputum often provide a guide to antibiotic therapy.

When bronchiectasis is focal, fiberoptic bronchoscopy may reveal an underlying endobronchial obstruction. In other cases, upper lobe involvement may be suggestive of either tuberculosis or ABPA. With more widespread disease, measurement of sweat chloride levels for CF, structural or functional assessment of nasal or bronchial cilia or sperm for primary ciliary dyskinesia, and quantitative assessment of immunoglobulins may explain recurrent airway infection.

Pulmonary function tests may demonstrate airflow obstruction as a consequence of diffuse bronchiectasis or associated chronic obstructive lung disease. Bronchial hyperreactivity, e.g., to methacholine challenge, and some reversibility of the airflow obstruction with inhaled bronchodilators are relatively common.

Figure 252-2 illustrates a diagnostic approach based on clinical suspicion and radiographic findings. As the differential diagnosis for focal versus diffuse bronchiectasis is different, the radiographic distribution of disease can serve as a starting point of the diagnostic workup. This algorithm should not imply that all studies be obtained in all patients with bronchiectasis. Rather, the workup should be dictated by a careful assessment of the clinical scenario. In a patient with focal bronchiectasis, for example, documentation of a prior pneumonia in the same location may suffice. Evaluation for immunoglobulin deficiency and CF should be considered for young patients with bronchiectasis and sino-pulmonary disease.

℞ BRONCHIECTASIS

Therapy has several major goals: (1) treatment of infection, particularly during acute exacerbations; (2) improved clearance of tracheobronchial secretions; (3) reduction of inflammation; and (4) treatment of an identifiable underlying problem.

Antibiotics are the cornerstone of bronchiectasis management. For patients with infrequent exacerbations characterized by an increase in quantity and purulence of the sputum, antibiotics are used only during acute episodes. Although choice of an antibiotic should be guided by Gram's stain and culture of sputum, empiric coverage (e.g., with amoxicillin, trimethoprim-sulfamethoxazole, or levofloxacin) is often given initially. Infection with *P. aeruginosa* is of particular concern, as it appears to be associated with greater rate of deterioration of lung function and worse quality of life. When *Pseudomonas* is present, oral therapy with a quinolone or parenteral therapy with an aminoglycoside, carbapenem, or third-generation cephalosporin is appropriate based on antibiotic sensitivity patterns. There are no firm guidelines for length of therapy, but a 10–14 day course or longer is typically administered.

A variety of mechanical methods and devices accompanied by appropriate positioning can facilitate drainage in patients with copious secretions. Though commonly employed and probably beneficial, these airway-clearance techniques have been poorly studied, and their efficacy is not proven. Pharmacologic agents are also employed to promote bronchopulmonary hygiene. Mucolytic agents to thin secretions and allow better clearance are controversial. Aerosolized recombinant DNase, which decreases viscosity of sputum by breaking down DNA released from neutrophils, has been shown to improve pulmonary function in CF but may be deleterious and should be avoided in bronchiectasis not associated with CF. Bronchodilators to improve obstruction and aid clearance of secretions are particularly useful in patients with airway hyperreactivity and reversible airflow obstruction.

Although surgical therapy was common in the past, more effective antibiotic and supportive therapy has largely replaced surgery. However, when bronchiectasis is localized and the morbidity is substantial despite adequate medical therapy, surgical resection of the involved region of lung should be considered.

When massive hemoptysis, often originating from the hypertrophied bronchial circulation, does not resolve with conservative therapy, including rest and antibiotics, therapeutic options are either surgical resection or bronchial arterial embolization (Chap. 34). Although resection may be successful if disease is localized, embolization is preferable with widespread disease.

LUNG ABSCESS

Lung abscess is defined as pulmonary parenchymal necrosis and cavitation resulting from infection. The development of a lung abscess implies a high microorganism burden as well as inadequate microbial clearance from the airways. Aspiration is the most common cause; factors that portend an increased risk of aspiration include esophageal dysmotility, seizure disorders, and neurologic conditions causing bulbar dysfunction. Other predisposing conditions for lung abscess include periodontal disease and alcoholism.

MICROBIOLOGY

Anaerobic bacteria are the most common causative organisms for lung abscess. Aerobic or facultative bacteria such as *S. aureus*, *Klebsiella pneumoniae*, *Nocardia sp.*, and gram-negative organisms, as well as nonbacterial pathogens like fungi and parasites, may also cause abscess formation. In the immunocompromised host, aerobic bacteria and opportunistic pathogens may predominate. Multiple isolates are more commonly seen in all patients when anaerobic and aerobic cultures are done.

CLINICAL MANIFESTATIONS

The symptoms of lung abscess are typical of pulmonary infection in general and may include cough, purulent sputum production, pleuritic chest pain, fever, and hemoptysis. In anaerobic infection, the clinical course may evolve over an extended period of time, and some patients may be asymptomatic. More acute presentations are typical of infection with aerobic bacteria.

Physical examination is often unrevealing. Rales or evidence of consolidation may be present. Fetid breath and poor dentition may be diagnostic clues. Clubbing or hypertrophic pulmonary osteoarthropathy may occur in chronic cases.

The chest radiograph classically reveals one or two thick-walled cavities in dependent areas of the lung, particularly the upper lobes and posterior segments of the lower lobes (Fig. 252-3). An air-fluid level is often present. CT of the chest is helpful in defining the size and location of the abscess, as well as to evaluate for additional cavities and the presence of pleural disease. Cavitary lesions in nondependent regions like

FIGURE 252-3 Cross-sectional CT image from a patient with an anaerobic lung abscess showing two contiguous thick-walled cavitary lesions in the right lower lobe with air-fluid levels. *(From WT Miller Jr: Diagnostic Thoracic Imaging. New York, McGraw-Hill, 2006, with permission.)*

the right middle lobe or anterior segments of the upper lobes should raise the possibility of other etiologies, including malignancy.

Laboratory studies may reveal leukocytosis, anemia, and an elevated erythrocyte sedimentation rate.

DIAGNOSIS

The diagnosis of lung abscess is based on clinical symptoms, identification of predisposing conditions, and chest radiographic findings. The differential diagnosis includes mycobacterial infection, pulmonary sequestration, malignancy, pulmonary infarction, and an infected bulla.

Identification of a causative organism is an ideal but challenging goal. Anaerobic bacteria are particularly difficult to isolate. Blood, sputum cultures, and, when appropriate, pleural fluid cultures should be obtained from patients with lung abscess. The role of fiberoptic bronchoscopy with bronchoalveolar lavage or protected-specimen brush for diagnosis or drainage of lung abscess is controversial. The relatively low yield, especially with anaerobic lung abscess, should be balanced against the risk of rupture of the abscess cavity with spillage into the airways. Bronchoscopy is perhaps most useful to rule out airway obstruction, mycobacterial infection, or malignancy. Other less commonly utilized methods for microbiologic sampling are transtracheal or transthoracic aspiration.

℞ LUNG ABSCESS

For many years, penicillin was the mainstay of empiric antibiotic therapy for lung abscess. Due to the emergence of β-lactamase–producing organisms, clindamycin (150 mg–300 mg every 6 h) is now standard therapy. Other agents, such as carbapenems and β-lactam/β-lactamase inhibitor combinations, may be useful in selected cases. Metronidazole alone is associated with a high treatment failure rate. When possible, the choice of antibiotics should be guided by microbiologic results.

The duration of treatment for lung abscess is controversial. Four to six weeks of antibiotic therapy is typically employed, though a more extended course is favored by some experts. Treatment failure suggests the possibility of a noninfectious etiology.

While surgery has had a limited role in treatment in the antibiotic era, indications include refractory hemoptysis, inadequate response to medical therapy, or the need for a tissue diagnosis when there is concern for a noninfectious etiology.

In general, outcomes for patients with classic anaerobic lung abscess are favorable, with a 90–95% cure rate. Higher mortality rates have been reported in immunocompromised patients, those with significant comorbidities, and infection with *P. aeruginosa*, *S. aureus*, and *K. pneumoniae*.

FURTHER READINGS

BARKER AF: Bronchiectasis. N Engl J Med 346:1383, 2002

MANSHARAMANI N et al: Lung abscess in adults: Clinical comparison of immunocompromised to non-immunocompromised patients. Respir Med 96:178, 2002

MANSHARAMANI N, KOZIEL H: Chronic lung sepsis: Lung abscess, bronchiectasis, and empyema. Curr Opin Pulm Med 9:181, 2003

NOONE PG et al: Primary ciliary dyskinesia: Diagnostic and phenotypic features. Am J Respir Crit Care Med 169:459, 2004

PASTEUR MC et al: An investigation into causative factors in patients with bronchiectasis. Am J Respir Crit Care Med 162:1277, 2000

ROSEN MJ: Chronic cough due to bronchiectasis. ACCP evidence-based clinical practice guidelines. Chest 129:122S, 2006

SCHEINBERG P, SHORE E: A pilot study of the safety and efficacy of tobramycin solution for inhalation in patients with severe bronchiectasis. Chest 127:1420, 2005

WEYCKER D et al: Prevalence and economic burden of bronchiectasis. Clin Pulm Med 12:205, 2005

WILLS P, GREENSTONE M: Inhaled hyperosmolar agents for bronchiectasis. Cochrane Database Syst Rev 2:CD002996, 2006

253 Cystic Fibrosis
Richard C. Boucher

Cystic fibrosis (CF) is a monogenic disorder that presents as a multisystem disease. The first signs and symptoms typically occur in childhood, but about 5% of patients in the United States are diagnosed as adults. Due to improvements in therapy, >41% of patients are now adults (≥18 years old) and 13% are past the age of 30. The median survival is >41 years for patients with CF. Thus, CF is no longer only a pediatric disease, and internists must be prepared to recognize and treat its many complications. This disease is characterized by chronic bacterial infection of the airways that ultimately leads to bronchiectasis and bronchiolectasis, exocrine pancreatic insufficiency and intestinal dysfunction, abnormal sweat gland function, and urogenital dysfunction.

PATHOGENESIS

GENETIC CONSIDERATIONS CF is an autosomal recessive disease resulting from mutations in the gene that encodes the CF transmembrane conductance regulator (CFTR) protein located on chromosome 7. The mutations in the CFTR gene fall into four major classes, as depicted in **Fig. 253-1**. Classes I–III mutations are considered "severe," as indexed by pancreatic insufficiency and high sweat NaCl values (see below). Class IV mutations can be "mild," i.e., associated with pancreatic sufficiency and intermediate/normal sweat NaCl values. Of note, Class I mutations that encode for premature stop codons are important to identify, as they may in the future be treated with agents that promote "read-through" of the stop codon with production of functional CFTR.

The prevalence of CF varies with the ethnic origin of a population. CF is detected in approximately 1 in 3000 live births in the Caucasian population of North America and northern Europe, 1 in 17,000 live births of African Americans, and 1 in 90,000 live births of the Asian population of Hawaii. The most common mutation in the CF gene (~70% of CF chromosomes) is a 3-bp deletion (a Class III mutation) that results in an absence of phenylalanine at amino acid position 508 (ΔF_{508}) of the CF gene protein product, known as CFTR. The large number (>1400) of relatively uncommon (<2% each) mutations identified in the CF gene makes it difficult to use DNA diagnostic technologies for identifying heterozygotes in populations at large.

CFTR PROTEIN

The CFTR protein is a single polypeptide chain, containing 1480 amino acids, that appears to function both as a cyclic AMP–regulated Cl⁻ channel and, as its name implies, a regulator of other ion channels. The fully processed form of CFTR is found in the plasma membrane in normal epithelia. Biochemical studies indicate that the ΔF_{508} mutation leads to improper processing and intracellular degradation of the CFTR protein. Thus, absence of CFTR in the plasma membrane is

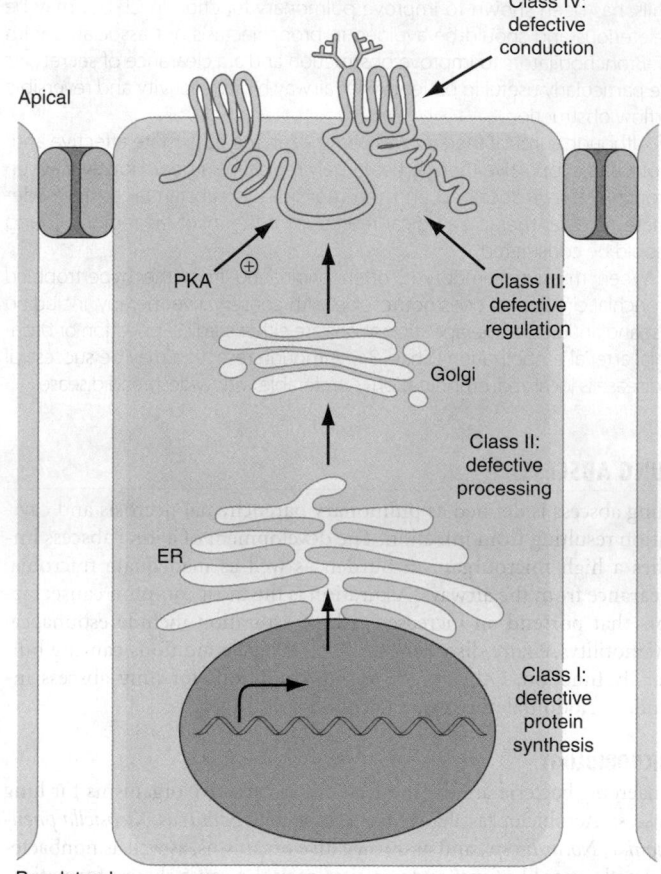

FIGURE 253-1 Schema describing classes of genetic mutations in *CFTR* gene and effects on CFTR protein/function. Note the ΔF_{508} mutation is a Class II mutation and, like Class I mutations, would be predicted to produce no mature CFTR protein in the apical membrane. CFTR, cystic fibrosis transmembrane conductance regulator.

central to the molecular pathophysiology of the ΔF_{508} mutation and other Classes I–II mutations. However, Classes III–IV mutations produce CFTR proteins that are fully processed but are nonfunctional or only partially functional in the plasma membrane.

EPITHELIAL DYSFUNCTION

The epithelia affected by CF exhibit different functions in their native state, i.e., some are volume-absorbing (airways and distal intestinal epithelia), and some are salt- but not volume-absorbing (sweat duct), whereas others are volume-secretory (proximal intestine and pancreas). Given this diversity of native activities, it is not surprising that CF produces organ-specific effects on electrolyte and water transport. However, the unifying concept is that all affected tissues express abnormal ion transport function.

ORGAN-SPECIFIC PATHOPHYSIOLOGY

Lung The diagnostic biophysical hallmark of CF airway epithelia is the raised transepithelial electric potential difference (PD). The transepithelial PD reflects both the rate of active ion transport and epithelial resistance to ion flow. CF airway epithelia exhibit abnormalities in both active Na^+ absorption and active Cl^- secretion (**Fig. 253-2**). The Cl^- secretory defect reflects the absence of cyclic AMP–dependent kinase and protein kinase C–regulated Cl^- transport mediated by CFTR itself. An important observation is that there is also a molecularly distinct Ca^{2+}-activated Cl^- channel (CaCC) expressed in the apical membrane. This channel can substitute for CFTR with regard to Cl^- secretion and may be a potential therapeutic target.

Abnormal regulation of Na^+ absorption is a key feature of CF airway epithelia. This abnormality reflects a second function of CFTR, its function as a tonic inhibitor of the epithelial Na^+ channel. The molecular mechanisms mediating this action of CFTR remain unknown.

Mucus clearance is the primary innate airways defense mechanism against infection by inhaled bacteria. Normal airways vary the rates of active Na^+ absorption and Cl^- secretion to adjust the volume of liquid (water), i.e., "hydration," on airway surfaces for efficient mucus clearance. The central hypothesis of CF airways pathophysiology is that the faulty regulation of Na^+ absorption and inability to secrete Cl^- via CFTR reduce the volume of liquid on airway surfaces; i.e., they are "dehydrated." Both

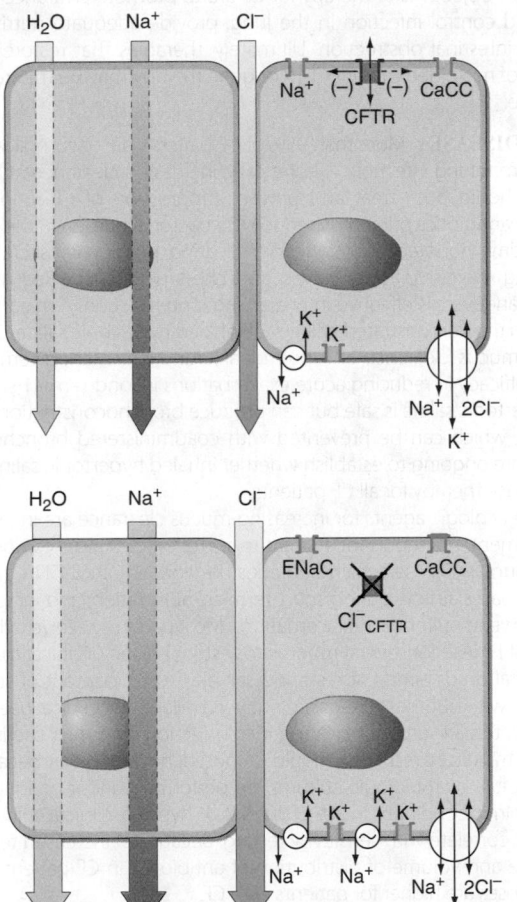

FIGURE 253-2 Comparison of ion transport properties of normal (*top*) and CF (*bottom*) airway epithelia. The vectors describe routes and magnitudes of Na^+ and Cl^- transport that is accompanied by osmotically driven water flow. The normal basal pattern for ion transport is absorption of Na^+ from the lumen via an amiloride-sensitive Na^+ channel. This process is accelerated in CF. The capacity to initiate cyclic AMP–mediated Cl^- secretion is diminished in CF airway epithelia due to absence/dysfunction of the CFTR Cl^- channel. The accelerated Na^+ absorption in CF reflects the absence of CFTR inhibitory effects on Na^+ channels.

the thickening of mucus and the depletion of the periciliary liquid lead to adhesion of mucus to the airway surface. Mucus adhesion leads to a failure to clear mucus from the airways both by ciliary and airflow-dependent (cough) mechanisms. The absence of a strict correspondence between gene mutation class and severity of lung disease suggests important roles for modifier genes and gene-environmental interactions.

The infection that characterizes CF airways involves the mucus layer rather than epithelial or airway wall invasion. The predisposition of CF airways to chronic infection by *Staphylococcus aureus* and *Pseudomonas aeruginosa* is consistent with failure to clear mucus. Recently it has been demonstrated that the O_2 tension is very low in CF mucus, and adaptations to hypoxia are important determinants of the physiology of bacteria in the CF lung. Indeed, both mucus stasis and mucus hypoxia may contribute to the propensity for *Pseudomonas* to grow in biofilm colonies within mucus plaques adherent to CF airway surfaces.

Gastrointestinal Tract The gastrointestinal effects of CF are diverse. In the exocrine pancreas, the absence of the CFTR Cl^- channel in the apical membrane of pancreatic ductal epithelia limits the function of an apical membrane Cl^--HCO_3^- exchanger to secrete bicarbonate and Na^+ (by a passive process) into the duct. The failure to secrete Na^+ HCO_3^- and water leads to retention of enzymes in the pancreas and ultimately destruction of virtually all pancreatic tissue. The CF intestinal epithelium, because of the lack of Cl^- and water secretion, fails to flush secreted mucins and other macromolecules from intestinal crypts. The diminished CFTR-mediated secretion of liquid may be exacerbated by excessive absorption of liquid, reflecting abnormalities of CFTR-mediated regulation of Na^+ absorption (both mediated by Na^+ channels and possibly other Na^+ transporters, e.g., Na^+-H^+ exchangers). Both dysfunctions lead to desiccated intraluminal contents and obstruction of both the small and large intestine. In the hepatobiliary system, defective hepatic ductal salt (Cl^-) and water secretion causes thickened biliary secretions, focal biliary cirrhosis, and bile duct proliferation in approximately 25–30% of patients with CF. The inability of the CF gallbladder epithelium to secrete salt and water can lead to both chronic cholecystitis and cholelithiasis.

Sweat Gland CF patients secrete nearly normal volumes of sweat in the sweat acinus. However, CF patients are not able to absorb NaCl from sweat as it moves through the sweat duct due to the inability to absorb Cl^- across the ductal epithelial cells. This dysfunction in the sweat gland is typically measured by collecting sweat after iontophoresing a cholinergic agonist into the forearm.

CLINICAL FEATURES

Most patients with CF present with signs and symptoms of the disease in childhood. Approximately 20% of patients present within the first 24 h of life with gastrointestinal obstruction, termed *meconium ileus*. Other common presentations within the first year or two of life include respiratory tract symptoms, most prominently cough and/or recurrent pulmonary infiltrates, and failure to thrive. A significant proportion of patients (~5%), however, are diagnosed after age 18.

RESPIRATORY TRACT

Upper respiratory tract disease is almost universal in patients with CF. Chronic sinusitis is common in childhood and leads to nasal obstruction and rhinorrhea. The occurrence of nasal polyps approaches 25% and often requires treatment with topical steroids and/or surgery.

In the lower respiratory tract, the first symptom of CF is cough. With time, the cough becomes persistent and produces viscous, purulent, often greenish-colored sputum. Inevitably, periods of clinical stability are interrupted by "exacerbations," defined by increased cough, weight loss, low-grade fever, increased sputum volume, and decrements in pulmonary function. Over the course of years, the exacerbations become more frequent and the recovery of lost lung function incomplete, leading to respiratory failure.

CF patients exhibit a characteristic sputum microbiology. *Haemophilus influenzae* and *S. aureus* are often the first organisms recovered from lung secretions in newly diagnosed patients with CF. *P. aeruginosa*, often mucoid and antibiotic-resistant, is typically cultured from lower respiratory tract secretions thereafter. *Burkholderia* (formerly *Pseudomonas cepacia*) is also recovered from CF sputum and is pathogenic. Patient-to-patient spread of certain strains of this organism mandates strict infection control in the hospital. Other gram-negative rods recovered from CF sputum include *Alcaligenes xylosoxidans*, *B. gladioli*, and occasionally mucoid forms of *Proteus*, *Escherichia coli*, and *Klebsiella*. Up to 50% of CF patients have *Aspergillus fumigatus* in their sputum, and up to 10% of these patients exhibit the syndrome of allergic bronchopulmonary aspergillosis. *Mycobacterium tuberculosis* is rare in patients with CF. However, 10–20% of adult patients with CF have sputum cultures positive for nontuberculous mycobacteria, and in some patients these microorganisms are associated with disease.

The first lung-function abnormalities observed in CF children, increased ratios of residual volume to total lung capacity, suggest that small-airways disease is the first functional lung abnormality in CF. As the disease progresses, both reversible and irreversible changes in forced vital capacity (FVC) and forced expiratory volume in 1 s (FEV_1) develop. The reversible component reflects the accumulation of intraluminal secretions and/or airway reactivity, which occurs in 40–60% of patients with CF. The irreversible component reflects chronic destruction of the airway wall and bronchiolitis.

The earliest chest x-ray change in CF lungs is hyperinflation, reflecting small-airways obstruction. Later, signs of luminal mucus impaction, bronchial cuffing, and finally bronchiectasis, e.g., ring shadows, are noted. For reasons that remain speculative, the right upper lobe displays the earliest and most severe changes.

CF pulmonary disease is associated with many intermittent complications. Pneumothorax is common (>10% of patients). The production of small amounts of blood in sputum is common in CF patients with advanced pulmonary disease. Massive hemoptysis is life-threatening. With advanced lung disease, digital clubbing appears in virtually all patients with CF. As late events, respiratory failure and cor pulmonale are prominent features of CF.

GASTROINTESTINAL TRACT

The syndrome of meconium ileus in infants presents with abdominal distention, failure to pass stool, and emesis. The abdominal flat plate can be diagnostic, with small-intestinal air-fluid levels, a granular appearance representing meconium, and a small colon. In children and young adults, a syndrome termed *meconium ileus equivalent* or *distal intestinal obstruction syndrome* (DIOS) occurs. The syndrome presents with right lower quadrant pain, loss of appetite, occasionally emesis, and often a palpable mass. The syndrome can be confused with appendicitis, whose frequency is not increased in CF patients.

Exocrine pancreatic insufficiency occurs in >90% of patients with CF. Insufficient pancreatic enzyme secretion yields the typical pattern of protein and fat malabsorption, with frequent, bulky, foul-smelling stools. Signs and symptoms of malabsorption of fat-soluble vitamins, including vitamins E and K, are also noted. Pancreatic beta cells are spared early, but function decreases with age. This effect, plus inflammation-induced insulin resistance, causes hyperglycemia and a requirement for insulin in >15% of older patients with CF (>35 years).

GENITOURINARY SYSTEM

Late onset of puberty is common in both males and females with CF. The delayed maturational pattern is likely secondary to the effects of chronic lung disease and inadequate nutrition on reproductive endocrine function. More than 95% of male patients with CF are azoospermic, reflecting obliteration of the vas deferens due to defective liquid secretion. Some 20% of CF women are infertile due to effects of chronic lung disease on the menstrual cycle; thick, tenacious cervical mucus that blocks sperm migration; and possibly fallopian tube/uterine wall abnormalities in liquid transport. Most pregnancies produce viable infants, and women with CF are able to breast-feed infants normally.

DIAGNOSIS

The diagnosis of CF rests on the combination of clinical criteria and abnormal CFTR function as demonstrated by sweat tests, nasal PD measurements, and CFTR mutation analysis. Elevated sweat Cl^- values are nearly pathognomonic for CF. The values for the Cl^- (and Na^+) concentrations in sweat vary with age, but typically in adults a Cl^- concentration of >70 meq/L discriminates between patients with CF and those with other lung diseases. DNA analysis of the most common mutations can identify CF mutations in >90% of affected patients. The nasal PD measurement can document CFTR dysfunction if the sweat Cl^- test is normal or borderline and two CF mutations are not identified. DNA analysis is performed routinely in patients with CF because pancreatic genotype-phenotype relationships have been identified, and mutation class-specific treatments are being developed.

Between 1 and 2% of patients with the clinical syndrome of CF have normal sweat Cl^- values. In most of these patients, the nasal transepithelial PD is raised into the diagnostic range for CF, and sweat acini do not secrete in response to injected β-adrenergic agonists. A single mutation of the CFTR gene, 3849 + 10 kb C→T, is associated with most CF patients with normal sweat Cl^- values.

℞ CYSTIC FIBROSIS

The major objectives of therapy for CF are to promote clearance of secretions and control infection in the lung, provide adequate nutrition, and prevent intestinal obstruction. Ultimately, therapies that restore the processing of misfolded mutant CFTR or gene therapy may be the treatments of choice.

LUNG DISEASE More than 95% of CF patients die of complications resulting from lung infection. Theoretically, increasing clearance of adherent mucus should both treat and prevent progression of CF lung disease, whereas antibiotics principally reduce the bacterial burden in the CF lung.

The time-honored techniques for clearing pulmonary secretions are breathing exercises, flutter valves, and chest percussion. Regular use of these maneuvers is effective in preserving lung function. A major advance has been the demonstrated efficacy of inhaled hypertonic saline (7%) in restoring mucus clearance and pulmonary function in short-term studies and its efficacy in reducing acute exacerbations in long-term (1 year) studies. Hypertonic saline is safe but can produce bronchoconstriction in some patients, which can be prevented with coadministered bronchodilators. Studies are ongoing to establish whether inhaled hypertonic saline should be the base therapy for all CF patients.

Pharmacologic agents for increasing mucus clearance are in use and in development. An important adjunct to secretion clearance can be recombinant human DNAse, which degrades the concentrated DNA in CF sputum, increases airflow during short-term administration, and increases the time between pulmonary exacerbations. Most patients receive a therapeutic trial of DNAse for several months to test for efficacy. Clinical trials of experimental drugs aimed at restoring salt and water content of secretions are underway, but these drugs are not yet available for clinical use.

Antibiotics are used for treating lung infection, and their use is guided by sputum culture results. It should be noted, however, that because routine hospital microbiologic cultures are performed under conditions that do not mimic conditions in the CF lung, e.g., hypoxia, clinical efficacy often does not correlate with sensitivity testing. Because of increased total-body clearance and volume of distribution of antibiotics in CF patients, the required doses are higher for patients with CF.

Early intervention with antibiotics in infants with infection may eradicate *P. aeruginosa* for extended periods. In older patients with established infection, suppression of bacterial growth is the therapeutic goal. Azithromycin (250 mg daily or 500 mg three times weekly) is often used chronically, although it is unclear whether its actions are antimicrobial or anti-inflammatory. Inhaled aminoglycosides, e.g., tobramycin 300 mg bid, for alternating monthly intervals are also used. "Mild exacerbations," as defined by increased cough and mucus production, are treated with additional oral antibiotics. Oral agents used to treat *Staphylococcus* include a semisynthetic penicillin or a cephalosporin. Oral ciprofloxacin may reduce pseudomonal bacterial counts and control symptoms, but its clinical utility may be limited by rapid emergence of resistant organisms. Accordingly, it is often used with an inhaled antibiotic, either tobramycin or colistin (75 mg bid). More severe exacerbations, or exacerbations associated with bacteria resistant to oral antibiotics, require intravenous antibiotics. Intravenous therapy is given both in the hospital and in the outpatient setting. Usually, two drugs with different mechanisms of action (e.g., a cephalosporin and an aminoglycoside) are used to treat *P. aeruginosa* to minimize emergence of resistant organisms. Drug dosage should be monitored so that levels for gentamicin or tobramycin peak at ranges of ~10 μg/mL and exhibit troughs of <2 μg/mL. Antibiotics directed at *Staphylococcus* and/or *H. influenzae* are added, depending on culture results.

Inhaled β-adrenergic agonists can be useful to control airways constriction, but long-term benefit has not been shown. Oral glucocorticoids may reduce airways inflammation, but their long-term use is limited by adverse side effects; however, they may be useful for treating allergic bronchopulmonary aspergillosis.

The chronic damage to airway walls reflects in part the destructive activities of inflammatory enzymes generated in part by inflammatory cells. Specific therapies with antiproteases have not been developed. However, a subset of adolescents with CF may benefit from long-term, high-dose nonsteroidal (ibuprofen) therapy.

A number of pulmonary complications require acute interventions. Atelectasis requires treatment with inhaled hypertonic saline, chest physiotherapy, and antibiotics. Pneumothoraces involving ≤10% of the lung can be observed, but chest tubes are required to expand collapsed, diseased lung. Small-volume hemoptysis typically requires treatment of lung infection and assessment of coagulation and vitamin K status. For massive hemoptysis, bronchial artery embolization should be performed. The most ominous complications of CF are respiratory failure and cor pulmonale. The most effective conventional therapy for these conditions is vigorous medical management of the lung disease and O_2 supplementation. Ultimately, the only effective treatment for respiratory failure in CF is lung transplantation (Chap. 260). The 2-year survival for lung transplantation exceeds 60%, and transplant patient deaths result principally from graft rejection, often involving obliterative bronchiolitis. The transplanted lungs do not develop a CF-specific phenotype.

GASTROINTESTINAL DISEASE Maintenance of adequate nutrition is critical for the health of the CF patient. Most (>90%) CF patients require pancreatic enzyme replacement. Capsules generally contain between 4000 and 20,000 units of lipase. The dose of enzymes (typically no more than 2500 units/kg per meal, to avoid risk of fibrosing colonopathy) should be adjusted on the basis of weight, abdominal symptomatology, and stool character. Replacement of fat-soluble vitamins, particularly vitamins E and

K, is usually required. Hyperglycemia most often becomes manifest in the adult and typically requires insulin treatment.

For treatment of the distal intestinal obstruction syndrome, megalodiatrizoate or other hypertonic radiocontrast materials delivered by enema to the terminal ileum are utilized. For control of symptoms, adjustment of pancreatic enzymes and use of salt solutions containing osmotically active agents, e.g. propyleneglycol, is recommended. Persistent symptoms may indicate a diagnosis of gastrointestinal malignancy, which is increased in incidence in patients with CF.

Cholestatic liver disease occurs in about 8% of CF patients. Treatment with urodeoxycholic acid is typically initiated if there is an increase in alkaline phosphatase and gammaglutamyl transpeptidase (GGT) (3× normal), but this treatment has not been shown to influence the course of hepatic disease. End-stage liver disease occurs in about 5% of CF patients and can be treated by transplantation.

OTHER ORGAN COMPLICATIONS Dehydration due to heat-induced salt loss from sweat ducts occurs more readily in CF patients. CF patients also have an increased incidence of osteoarthropy, renal stones, and osteoporosis, particularly following transplant.

PSYCHOSOCIAL FACTORS CF imposes a tremendous burden on patients, and depression is common. Health insurance, career options, family planning, and life expectancy become major issues. Thus, assisting patients with the psychosocial adjustments required by CF is critical.

FURTHER READINGS

DAVIS PB: Cystic fibrosis since 1938. Am J Respir Crit Care Med 173:475, 2006

GROMAN JD et al: Phenotypic and genetic characterization of patients with features of "nonclassic" forms of cystic fibrosis. J Pediatr 146:675, 2006

GUGGINO WB, STANTON BA: New insights into cystic fibrosis: molecular switches that regulate CFTR. Nat Rev Mol Cell Biol 7:426, 2006

PRINCE AS: Biofilms, antimicrobial resistance, and airway infection. N Engl J Med 347:1110, 2002

ROWE SM et al: Cystic fibrosis. N Engl J Med 352:1992, 2005

WORLITSCH D et al: Effects of reduced mucus oxygen concentration in airway pseudomonas infections of cystic fibrosis patients. J Clin Invest 109:317, 2002

254 Chronic Obstructive Pulmonary Disease

John J. Reilly, Jr., Edwin K. Silverman, Steven D. Shapiro

Chronic obstructive pulmonary disease (COPD) has been defined by the Global Initiative for Chronic Obstructive Lung Disease (GOLD), an international collaborative effort to improve awareness, diagnosis, and treatment of COPD, as a disease state characterized by airflow limitation that is not fully reversible (*http://www.goldcopd.com/*). COPD includes *emphysema*, an anatomically defined condition characterized by destruction and enlargement of the lung alveoli; *chronic bronchitis*, a clinically defined condition with chronic cough and phlegm; and *small airways disease*, a condition in which small bronchioles are narrowed. COPD is present only if chronic airflow obstruction occurs; chronic bronchitis *without* chronic airflow obstruction is *not* included within COPD.

COPD is the fourth leading cause of death and affects >16 million persons in the United States. COPD is also a disease of increasing public health importance around the world. GOLD estimates suggest that

COPD will rise from the sixth to the third most common cause of death worldwide by 2020.

RISK FACTORS

CIGARETTE SMOKING

By 1964, the Advisory Committee to the Surgeon General of the United States had concluded that cigarette smoking was a major risk factor for mortality from chronic bronchitis and emphysema. Subsequent longitudinal studies have shown accelerated decline in the volume of air exhaled within the first second of the forced expiratory maneuver (FEV_1) in a dose-response relationship to the intensity of cigarette smoking, which is typically expressed as pack-years (average number of packs of cigarettes smoked per day multiplied by the total number of years of smoking). This dose-response relationship between reduced pulmonary function and cigarette smoking intensity accounts for the higher prevalence rates for COPD with increasing age. The historically higher rate of smoking among males is the likely explanation for the higher prevalence of COPD among males; however, the prevalence of COPD among females is increasing as the gender gap in smoking rates has diminished in the past 50 years.

Although the causal relationship between cigarette smoking and the development of COPD has been absolutely proved, there is considerable

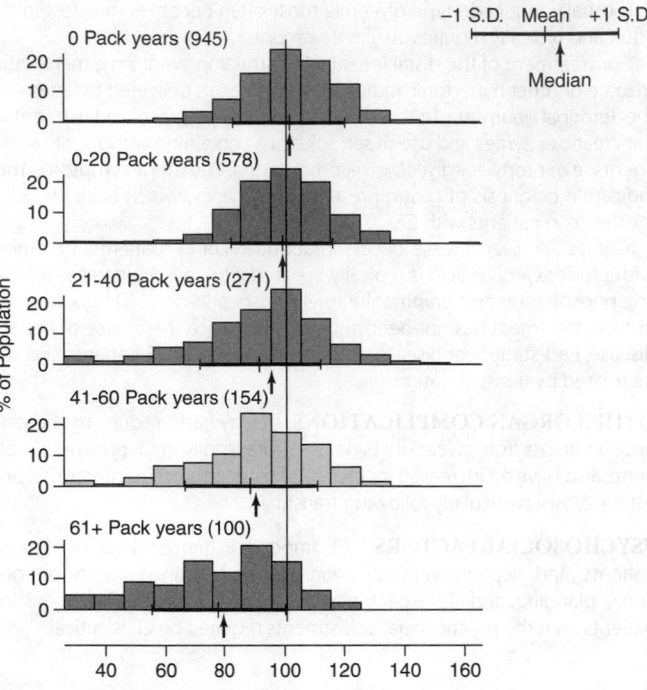

FIGURE 254-1 Distributions of forced expiratory volume in 1 s (FEV$_1$) values in a general population sample, stratified by pack-years of smoking. Means, medians, and ± 1 standard deviation of percent predicted FEV$_1$ are shown for each smoking group. Although a dose-response relationship between smoking intensity and FEV$_1$ was found, marked variability in pulmonary function was observed among subjects with similar smoking histories. (*From R Burrows et al: Am Rev Respir Dis 115:95, 1977; with permission.*)

variability in the response to smoking. Although pack-years of cigarette smoking is the most highly significant predictor of FEV$_1$ (**Fig. 254-1**), only 15% of the variability in FEV$_1$ is explained by pack-years. This finding suggests that additional environmental and/or genetic factors contribute to the impact of smoking on the development of airflow obstruction.

Although cigar and pipe smoking may also be associated with the development of COPD, the evidence supporting such associations is less compelling, likely related to the lower dose of inhaled tobacco byproducts during cigar and pipe smoking.

AIRWAY RESPONSIVENESS AND COPD

A tendency for increased bronchoconstriction in response to a variety of exogenous stimuli, including methacholine and histamine, is one of the defining features of asthma (Chap. 248). However, many patients with COPD also share this feature of airway hyperresponsiveness. The considerable overlap between persons with asthma and those with COPD in airway responsiveness, airflow obstruction, and pulmonary symptoms led to the formulation of the Dutch hypothesis. This suggests that asthma, chronic bronchitis, and emphysema are variations of the same basic disease, which is modulated by environmental and genetic factors to produce these pathologically distinct entities. The alternative British hypothesis contends that asthma and COPD are fundamentally different diseases: Asthma is viewed as largely an allergic phenomenon, while COPD results from smoking-related inflammation and damage. Determination of the validity of the Dutch hypothesis vs. the British hypothesis awaits identification of the genetic predisposing factors for asthma and/or COPD, as well as the interactions between these postulated genetic factors and environmental risk factors.

Longitudinal studies that compared airway responsiveness at the beginning of the study to subsequent decline in pulmonary function have demonstrated that increased airway responsiveness is clearly a significant predictor of subsequent decline in pulmonary function. Thus, airway hyperresponsiveness is a risk factor for COPD.

RESPIRATORY INFECTIONS

These have been studied as potential risk factors for the development and progression of COPD in adults; childhood respiratory infections have also been assessed as potential predisposing factors for the eventual development of COPD. The impact of adult respiratory infections on decline in pulmonary function is controversial, but significant long-term reductions in pulmonary function are not typically seen following an episode of bronchitis or pneumonia. The impact of the effects of childhood respiratory illnesses on the subsequent development of COPD has been difficult to assess due to a lack of adequate longitudinal data. Thus, although respiratory infections are important causes of exacerbations of COPD, the association of both adult and childhood respiratory infections to the development and progression of COPD remains to be proven.

OCCUPATIONAL EXPOSURES

Increased respiratory symptoms and airflow obstruction have been suggested as resulting from general exposure to dust at work. Several specific occupational exposures, including coal mining, gold mining, and cotton textile dust, have been suggested as risk factors for chronic airflow obstruction. However, although nonsmokers in these occupations developed some reductions in FEV$_1$, the importance of dust exposure as a risk factor for COPD, independent of cigarette smoking, is not certain. Among workers exposed to cadmium (a specific chemical fume), FEV$_1$, FEV$_1$/FVC, and DL$_{CO}$ were significantly reduced (FVC, forced vital capacity; DL$_{CO}$, carbon monoxide diffusing capacity of the lung; Chap. 246), consistent with airflow obstruction and emphysema. Although several specific occupational dusts and fumes are likely risk factors for COPD, the magnitude of these effects appears to be substantially less important than the effect of cigarette smoking.

AMBIENT AIR POLLUTION

Some investigators have reported increased respiratory symptoms in those living in urban compared to rural areas, which may relate to increased pollution in the urban settings. However, the relationship of air pollution to chronic airflow obstruction remains unproven. Prolonged exposure to smoke produced by biomass combustion—a common mode of cooking in some countries—also appears to be a significant risk factor for COPD among women in those countries. However, in most populations, ambient air pollution is a much less important risk factor for COPD than cigarette smoking.

PASSIVE, OR SECOND-HAND, SMOKING EXPOSURE

Exposure of children to maternal smoking results in significantly reduced lung growth. In utero tobacco smoke exposure also contributes to significant reductions in postnatal pulmonary function. Although passive smoke exposure has been associated with reductions in pulmonary function, the importance of this risk factor in the development of the severe pulmonary function reductions in COPD remains uncertain.

 GENETIC CONSIDERATIONS Although cigarette smoking is the major environmental risk factor for the development of COPD, the development of airflow obstruction in smokers is highly variable. Severe α$_1$ antitrypsin (α$_1$AT) deficiency is a proven genetic risk factor for COPD; there is increasing evidence that other genetic determinants also exist.

α$_1$ ANTITRYPSIN DEFICIENCY Many variants of the protease inhibitor (PI or SERPINA1) locus that encodes α$_1$AT have been described. The common M allele is associated with normal α$_1$AT levels. The S allele, associated with slightly reduced α$_1$AT levels, and the Z allele, associated with markedly reduced α$_1$AT levels, also occur with frequencies >1% in most Caucasian populations. Rare individuals inherit null alleles, which lead to the absence of any α$_1$AT production through a heterogeneous collection of mutations. Individuals with two Z alleles or one Z and one null allele are referred to as Pi^Z, which is the most common form of severe α$_1$AT deficiency.

Although only 1–2% of COPD patients are found to have severe α$_1$AT deficiency as a contributing cause of COPD, these patients demonstrate that genetic factors can have a profound influence on the susceptibility for developing COPD. Pi^Z individuals often develop early-onset COPD, but the ascertainment bias in the published series of Pi^Z individuals—which have usually included many Pi^Z subjects who were tested for α_1AT deficiency because they had COPD—means that the fraction of Pi^Z individuals who will develop COPD and the age-of-onset distribution for the development of COPD in Pi^Z subjects remain unknown. Approximately 1 in 3000 individuals in the United States inherits severe α_1AT deficiency, but only a small minority of these individuals has been recognized. The clinical laboratory test used most frequently to screen for α_1AT deficiency is measurement of the immunologic level of α_1AT in serum (see "Laboratory Findings," below).

A significant percentage of the variability in pulmonary function among Pi^Z individuals is explained by cigarette smoking; cigarette smokers with severe α_1AT deficiency are more likely to develop COPD at early ages. However, the development of COPD in Pi^Z subjects, even among current or ex-smokers, is not absolute. Among Pi^Z nonsmokers, impressive variability has been noted in the development of airflow obstruction. Other genetic and/or environmental factors likely contribute to this variability.

Specific treatment in the form of α_1AT augmentation therapy is available for severe α_1AT deficiency as a weekly intravenous infusion (see "Treatment," below).

The risk of lung disease in heterozygous Pi^MZ individuals, who have intermediate serum levels of α_1AT (~60% of Pi^MM levels), is controversial. Although previous general population surveys have not typically shown increased rates of airflow obstruction in Pi^MZ compared to Pi^MM individuals, case-control studies that compared COPD patients to control subjects have usually found an excess of Pi^MZ genotypes in the COPD patient group. Several recent large population studies have suggested that Pi^MZ subjects are at slightly increased risk for the development of airflow obstruction, but it remains unclear if all Pi^MZ subjects are at slightly increased risk for COPD or if a subset of Pi^MZ subjects are at substantially increased risk for COPD due to other genetic or environmental factors.

OTHER GENETIC RISK FACTORS Studies of pulmonary function measurements performed in general population samples have suggested that genetic factors other than PI type influence variation in pulmonary function. Familial aggregation of airflow obstruction within families of COPD patients has also been demonstrated.

Association studies have compared the distribution of variants in genes hypothesized to be involved in the development of COPD in COPD patients and control subjects. However, the results have been quite inconsistent, and no genetic determinants of COPD other than severe α_1AT deficiency have been definitively proven using this approach. Genome scan linkage analyses of early-onset COPD families have found evidence for linkage of spirometric phenotypes to several chromosomal regions, but the specific genetic determinants in those regions have yet to be definitively identified.

NATURAL HISTORY

The effects of cigarette smoking on pulmonary function appear to depend on the intensity of smoking exposure, the timing of smoking exposure during growth, and the baseline lung function of the individual; other environmental factors may have similar effects. Although rare individuals may demonstrate precipitous declines in pulmonary function, most individuals follow a steady trajectory of increasing pulmonary function with growth during childhood and adolescence, followed by a gradual decline with aging. Individuals appear to track in their quartile of pulmonary function based upon environmental and genetic factors that put them on different tracks. The risk of eventual mortality from COPD is closely associated with reduced levels of FEV$_1$. A graphic depiction of the natural history of COPD is shown as a function of the influences on tracking curves of FEV$_1$ in Fig. 254-2. Death or disability from COPD can result from a normal rate of decline after a reduced growth phase (curve C), an early initiation of pulmonary function decline after normal growth (curve B), or an accelerated decline after normal growth (curve D). The rate of decline in pulmonary function can be modified by changing environmental exposures (i.e., quitting smoking), with smoking cessation at an earlier age providing a more beneficial effect than smoking cessation after marked reductions in pulmonary function have already developed. Genetic factors likely contribute to the level of pulmonary function

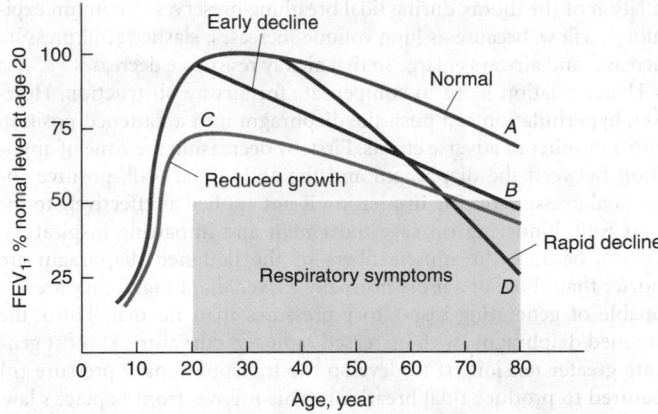

FIGURE 254-2 Hypothetical tracking curves of FEV$_1$ for individuals throughout their life spans. The normal pattern of growth and decline with age is shown by curve A. Significantly reduced FEV$_1$ (<65% of predicted value at age 20) can develop from a normal rate of decline after a reduced pulmonary function growth phase (curve C), early initiation of pulmonary function decline after normal growth (curve B), or accelerated decline after normal growth (curve D). (*From B Rijcken: Doctoral dissertation, p 133, University of Groningen, 1991; with permission.*)

achieved during growth and to the rate of decline in response to smoking and potentially to other environmental factors as well.

PATHOPHYSIOLOGY

Persistent reduction in forced expiratory flow rates is the most typical finding in COPD. Increases in the residual volume and the residual volume/total lung capacity ratio, nonuniform distribution of ventilation, and ventilation-perfusion mismatching also occur.

AIRFLOW OBSTRUCTION

Airflow limitation, also known as airflow obstruction, is typically determined by spirometry, which involves forced expiratory maneuvers after the subject has inhaled to total lung capacity (see Fig. 246-4). Key phenotypes obtained from spirometry include FEV$_1$ and the total volume of air exhaled during the entire spirometric maneuver (FVC). Patients with airflow obstruction related to COPD have a chronically reduced ratio of FEV$_1$/FVC. In contrast to asthma, the reduced FEV$_1$ in COPD seldom shows large responses to inhaled bronchodilators, although improvements up to 15% are common. Asthma patients can also develop chronic (not fully reversible) airflow obstruction. Maximal inspiratory flow can be relatively well preserved in the presence of a markedly reduced FEV$_1$.

Airflow during forced exhalation is the result of the balance between the elastic recoil of the lungs promoting flow and the resistance of the airways limiting flow. In normal lungs, as well as in lungs affected by COPD, maximal expiratory flow diminishes as the lungs empty because the lung parenchyma provides progressively less elastic recoil and because the cross-sectional area of the airways falls, raising the resistance to airflow. The decrease in flow coincident with decreased lung volume is readily apparent on the expiratory limb of a flow-volume curve. In the early stages of COPD, the abnormality in airflow is only evident at lung volumes at or below the functional residual capacity (closer to residual volume), appearing as a scooped-out lower part of the descending limb of the flow-volume curve. In more advanced disease the entire curve has decreased expiratory flow compared to normal.

HYPERINFLATION

Lung volumes are also routinely assessed in pulmonary function testing. In COPD there is often "air trapping" (increased residual volume and increased ratio of residual volume to total lung capacity) and progressive hyperinflation (increased total lung capacity) late in the disease. Hyperinflation of the thorax during tidal breathing preserves maximum expiratory airflow, because as lung volume increases, elastic recoil pressure increases and airways enlarge so that airway resistance decreases.

Hyperinflation helps to compensate for airway obstruction. However, hyperinflation can push the diaphragm into a flattened position with a number of adverse effects. First, by decreasing the zone of apposition between the diaphragm and the abdominal wall, positive abdominal pressure during inspiration is not applied as effectively to the chest wall, hindering rib cage movement and impairing inspiration. Second, because the muscle fibers of the flattened diaphragm are shorter than those of a more normally curved diaphragm, they are less capable of generating inspiratory pressures than normal. Third, the flattened diaphragm (with increased radius of curvature, r) must generate greater tension (t) to develop the transpulmonary pressure (p) required to produce tidal breathing. This follows from Laplace's law, $p = 2t/r$. Also, because the thoracic cage is distended beyond its normal resting volume, during tidal breathing the inspiratory muscles must do work to overcome the resistance of the thoracic cage to further inflation instead of gaining the normal assistance from the chest wall recoiling outward toward its resting volume.

GAS EXCHANGE

Although there is considerable variability in the relationships between the FEV_1 and other physiologic abnormalities in COPD, certain generalizations may be made. The Pa_{O_2} usually remains near normal until the FEV_1 is decreased to ~50% of predicted, and even much lower FEV_1s can be associated with a normal Pa_{O_2}, at least at rest. An elevation of Pa_{CO_2} is not expected until the FEV_1 is <25% of predicted and even then may not occur. Pulmonary hypertension severe enough to cause cor pulmonale and right ventricular failure due to COPD occurs only in those individuals who have marked decreases in FEV_1 (<25% of predicted) together with chronic hypoxemia (Pa_{O_2} <55 mmHg), although earlier in the course some elevation of pulmonary artery pressure, particularly with exercise, may occur (Chap. 244).

Nonuniform ventilation and ventilation-perfusion mismatching are characteristic of COPD, reflecting the heterogeneous nature of the disease process within the airways and lung parenchyma. Nitrogen wash-out while breathing 100% oxygen is delayed due to regions that are poorly ventilated, and the profile of the nitrogen wash-out curve is consistent with multiple parenchymal compartments having different wash-out rates due to regional differences in compliance and airway resistance. Ventilation/perfusion mismatching accounts for essentially all of the reduction in Pa_{O_2} that occurs in COPD; shunting is minimal. This finding explains the effectiveness of modest elevations of inspired oxygen in treating hypoxemia due to COPD and therefore the need to consider problems other than COPD when hypoxemia is difficult to correct with modest levels of supplemental oxygen in the patient with COPD.

PATHOLOGY

Cigarette smoke exposure may affect the large airways, small airways (≤2 mm diameter), and alveolar space. Changes in large airways cause cough and sputum, while changes in small airways and alveoli are responsible for physiologic alterations. Emphysema and small airway pathology are both present in most persons with COPD, and their relative contributions to obstruction vary from one person to another.

LARGE AIRWAY

Cigarette smoking often results in mucous gland enlargement and goblet cell hyperplasia. These changes are proportional to cough and mucus production that define chronic bronchitis, but these abnormalities are not related to airflow limitation. Goblet cells not only increase in number but in extent through the bronchial tree. Bronchi also undergo squamous metaplasia, which not only predisposes to carcinogenesis but also disrupts mucociliary clearance. Although not as prominent as in asthma, patients may have smooth-muscle hypertrophy and bronchial hyperreactivity leading to airflow limitation. Neutrophil influx has been associated with purulent sputum of upper

respiratory tract infections that hamper patients with COPD. Independent of its proteolytic activity, neutrophil elastase is among the most potent secretagogues identified.

SMALL AIRWAYS

The major site of increased resistance in most individuals with COPD is in airways ≤2 mm diameter. Characteristic cellular changes include goblet cell metaplasia and replacement of surfactant-secreting Clara cells with mucus-secreting and infiltrating mononuclear inflammatory cells. Smooth-muscle hypertrophy may also be present. These abnormalities may cause luminal narrowing by excess mucus, edema, and cellular infiltration. Reduced surfactant may increase surface tension at the air-tissue interface, predisposing to airway narrowing or collapse. Fibrosis in the wall may cause airway narrowing directly or, as in asthma, predispose to hyperreactivity. Respiratory bronchiolitis with mononuclear inflammatory cells collecting in distal airway tissues may cause proteolytic destruction of elastic fibers in the respiratory bronchioles and alveolar ducts where the fibers are concentrated as rings around alveolar entrances.

Because small airway patency is maintained by the surrounding lung parenchyma that provides radial traction on bronchioles at points of attachment to alveolar septa, loss of bronchiolar attachments as a result of extracellular matrix destruction may cause airway distortion and narrowing in COPD. Although the significance of alveolar attachments is not resolved, the concept of decreased alveolar attachments leading to small airway obstruction is appealing because it underscores the mechanistic relationship between loss of elastic recoil and increased resistance to airflow in small airways.

LUNG PARENCHYMA

Emphysema is characterized by destruction of gas-exchanging airspaces, i.e., the respiratory bronchioles, alveolar ducts, and alveoli. Their walls become perforated and later obliterated with coalescence of small distinct airspaces into abnormal and much larger airspaces. Macrophages accumulate in respiratory bronchioles of essentially all young smokers. Bronchoalveolar lavage fluid from such individuals contains roughly five times as many macrophages as lavage from nonsmokers. In smokers' lavage fluid, macrophages comprise >95% of the total cell count, and neutrophils, nearly absent in nonsmokers' lavage, account for 1–2% of the cells. T lymphocytes, particularly CD8+ cells, are also increased in the alveolar space of smokers.

Emphysema is classified into distinct pathologic types, the most important being centriacinar and panacinar. *Centriacinar emphysema*, the type most frequently associated with cigarette smoking, is characterized by enlarged airspaces found (initially) in association with respiratory bronchioles. Centriacinar emphysema is most prominent in the upper lobes and superior segments of lower lobes and is often quite focal. *Panacinar emphysema* refers to abnormally large airspaces evenly distributed within and across acinar units. Panacinar emphysema is usually observed in patients with α_1AT deficiency, which has a predilection for the lower lobes. Distinctions between centriacinar and panacinar emphysema are interesting and may ultimately be shown to have different mechanisms of pathogenesis. However, garden-variety smoking-related emphysema is usually mixed, particularly in advanced cases, and these pathologic classifications are not helpful in the care of patients with COPD.

PATHOGENESIS

Airflow limitation, the major physiologic change in COPD, can result from both small airway obstruction and emphysema, as discussed above. Pathologic findings that can contribute to small airway obstruction are described above, but their relative importance is unknown. Fibrosis surrounding the small airways appears to be a significant contributor. Mechanisms leading to collagen accumulation around the airways in the face of increased collagenase activity remain an enigma. Although seemingly counterintuitive, there are several potential mechanisms whereby a proteinase can predispose to fibrosis,

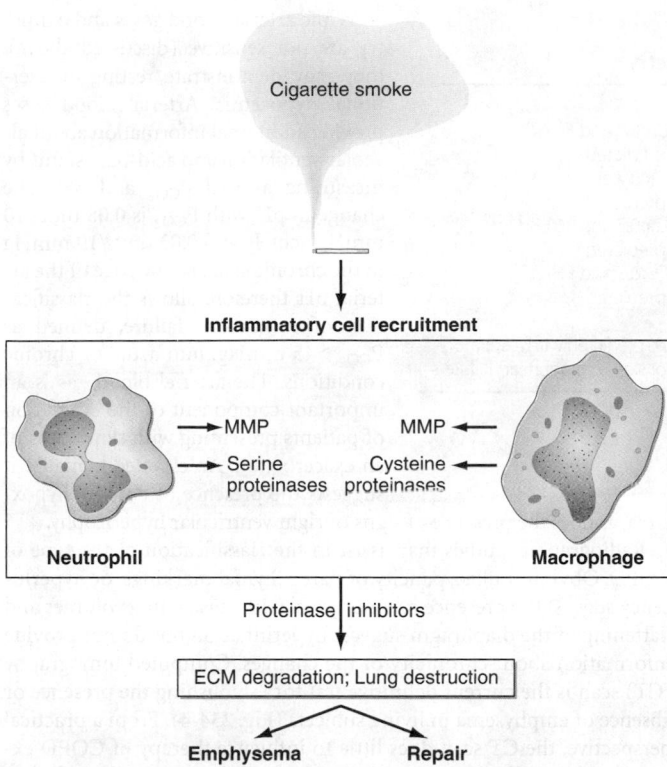

Cigarette smoke

↓

Inflammatory cell recruitment

Neutrophil →MMP MMP←
→Serine   Cysteine←
proteinases proteinases
Macrophage

Proteinase inhibitors

↓

ECM degradation; Lung destruction

Emphysema   **Repair**

FIGURE 254-3 Pathogenesis of emphysema. Upon long-term exposure to cigarette smoke, inflammatory cells are recruited to the lung; they release proteinases in excess of inhibitors, and if repair is abnormal, this leads to airspace destruction and enlargement or emphysema.

including proteolytic activation of transforming growth factor β (TGF-β) and insulin-like growth factor (IGF) binding protein degradation releasing profibrotic IGF. Largely due to availability of suitable animal models, we know much more about mechanisms involved in emphysema than small airway obstruction.

The pathogenesis of emphysema can be dissected into four interrelated events (Fig. 254-3): (1) Chronic exposure to cigarette smoke may lead to inflammatory cell recruitment within the terminal airspaces of the lung. (2) These inflammatory cells release elastolytic proteinases which damage the extracellular matrix of the lung. (3) Loss of matrix-cell attachment leads to apoptosis of structural cells of the lung. (4) Ineffective repair of elastin and perhaps other extracellular matrix components result in airspace enlargement that defines pulmonary emphysema.

The Elastase:Antielastase Hypothesis Elastin, the principal component of elastic fibers, is a highly stable component of the extracellular matrix that is critical to the integrity of both the small airways and the lung parenchyma. The elastase:antielastase hypothesis proposed in the mid-1960s states that the balance of elastin-degrading enzymes and their inhibitors determines the susceptibility of the lung to destruction resulting in airspace enlargement. This hypothesis was based on the clinical observation that patients with genetic deficiency in α_1AT, the inhibitor of the serine proteinase neutrophil elastase, were at increased risk of emphysema, and that instillation of elastases, including neutrophil elastase, to experimental animals results in emphysema. To this day, the elastase:antielastase hypothesis is the prevailing mechanism for the development of emphysema. However, a complex network of inflammatory cells and additional proteinases that contribute to emphysema have subsequently been identified.

Inflammation and Extracellular Matrix Proteolysis Macrophages patrol the lower airspace under normal conditions. Upon exposure to oxidants from cigarette smoke, histone deacetylase-2 is inactivated, shifting the balance toward acetylated or loose chromatin, exposing nuclear factor κB sites and resulting in transcription of matrix metal-

loproteinase-9, proinflammatory cytokines interleukin 8 (IL-8), and tumor necrosis factor α (TNF-α); this leads to neutrophil recruitment. CD8+ T-cells are also recruited in response to cigarette smoke and release interferon inducible protein-10 (IP-10, CXCL-7) that in turn leads to macrophage production of macrophage elastase [matrix metalloproteinase-12 (MMP-12)]. Matrix metalloproteinases and serine proteinases, most notably neutrophil elastase, work together by degrading the inhibitor of the other, leading to lung destruction. Proteolytic cleavage products of elastin also serve as a macrophage chemokine, fueling this destructive positive feedback loop.

Concomitant cigarette smoke-induced loss of cilia in the airway epithelium predisposes to bacterial infection with neutrophilia. Surprisingly, in end-stage lung disease, long after smoking cessation there remains an exuberant inflammatory response, suggesting that mechanisms of cigarette smoke-induced inflammation that initiate the disease differ from mechanisms that sustain inflammation after smoking cessation.

Collagen turnover in COPD is complex. The three collagenases (MMP-1, MMP-8, and MMP-13) that initiate the cleavage of interstitial collagens are also induced in both inflammatory cells and structural cells in COPD. While collagen is disrupted as alveolar units are obliterated, overall there is a net increase in collagen content in the COPD lung, with prominent accumulation in the airway submucosa.

Cell Death Airspace enlargement with loss of alveolar units obviously requires disappearance of both extracellular matrix and cells. Traditional theories suggest that inflammatory cell proteinases degrade lung extracellular matrix as the primary event, with subsequent loss of cell anchoring leading to apoptosis. Animal models have used endothelial and epithelial cell death as a means to generate transient airspace enlargement. Whether apoptosis is a primary or secondary event in COPD remains to be determined.

Ineffective Repair The ability of the adult lung to repair damaged alveoli appears limited. Whether the process of septation that is responsible for alveogenesis during lung development can be reinitiated is not clear. In animal models, treatment with all-trans retinoic acid has resulted in some repair. Also, lung resection results in compensatory lung growth in the remaining lung in animal models. In addition to restoring cellularity following injury, it appears difficult for an adult to completely restore an appropriate extracellular matrix, particularly functional elastic fibers.

CLINICAL PRESENTATION

HISTORY

The three most common symptoms in COPD are cough, sputum production, and exertional dyspnea. Many patients have such symptoms for months or years before seeking medical attention. Although the development of airflow obstruction is a gradual process, many patients date the onset of their disease to an acute illness or exacerbation. A careful history, however, usually reveals the presence of symptoms prior to the acute exacerbation. The development of exertional dyspnea, often described as increased effort to breathe, heaviness, air hunger, or gasping, can be insidious. It is best elicited by a careful history focused on typical physical activities and how the patient's ability to perform them has changed. Activities involving significant arm work, particularly at or above shoulder level, are particularly difficult for patients with COPD. Conversely, activities that allow the patient to brace the arms and use accessory muscles of respiration are better tolerated. Examples of such activities include pushing a shopping cart, walking on a treadmill, or pushing a wheelchair. As COPD advances, the principal feature is worsening dyspnea on exertion with increasing intrusion on the ability to perform vocational or avocational activities. In the most advanced stages, patients are breathless doing simple activities of daily living.

Accompanying worsening airflow obstruction is an increased frequency of exacerbations (described below). Patients may also develop resting hypoxemia and require institution of supplemental oxygen.

GOLD Stage	Severity	Symptoms	Spirometry
0	At Risk	Chronic cough, sputum production	Normal
I	Mild	With or without chronic cough or sputum production	FEV_1/FVC <0.7 and FEV_1 ≥80% predicted
IIA	Moderate	With or without chronic cough or sputum production	FEV_1/FVC <0.7 and 50%≤ FEV_1 <80% predicted
III	Severe	With or without chronic cough or sputum production	FEV_1/FVC <0.7 and 30%≤ FEV_1 <50% predicted
IV	Very Severe	With or without chronic cough or sputum production	FEV_1/FVC <0.7 and FEV_1 <30% predicted *or* FEV_1 <50% predicted with respiratory failure or signs of right heart failure

TABLE 254-1 GOLD CRITERIA FOR COPD SEVERITY

Note: GOLD, Global Initiative for Chronic Obstructive Pulmonary Disease (COPD).
Source: From Pauwels et al.

PHYSICAL FINDINGS

In the early stages of COPD, patients usually have an entirely normal physical examination. Current smokers may have signs of active smoking, including an odor of smoke or nicotine staining of fingernails. In patients with more severe disease, the physical examination is notable for a prolonged expiratory phase and expiratory wheezing. In addition, signs of hyperinflation include a barrel chest and enlarged lung volumes with poor diaphragmatic excursion as assessed by percussion. Patients with severe airflow obstruction may also exhibit use of accessory muscles of respiration, sitting in the characteristic "tripod" position to facilitate the actions of the sternocleidomastoid, scalene, and intercostal muscles. Patients may develop cyanosis, visible in the lips and nail beds.

Although traditional teaching is that patients with predominant emphysema, termed "pink puffers," are thin and noncyanotic at rest and have prominent use of accessory muscles, and patients with chronic bronchitis are more likely to be heavy and cyanotic ("blue bloaters"), current evidence demonstrates that most patients have elements of both bronchitis and emphysema and that the physical examination does not reliably differentiate the two entities.

Advanced disease may be accompanied by systemic wasting, with significant weight loss, bitemporal wasting, and diffuse loss of subcutaneous adipose tissue. This syndrome has been associated with both inadequate oral intake and elevated levels of inflammatory cytokines (TNF-α). Such wasting is an independent poor prognostic factor in COPD. Some patients with advanced disease have paradoxical inward movement of the rib cage with inspiration (Hoover's sign), the result of alteration of the vector of diaphragmatic contraction on the rib cage as a result of chronic hyperinflation.

Signs of overt right heart failure, termed *cor pulmonale*, are relatively infrequent since the advent of supplemental oxygen therapy.

Clubbing of the digits is not a sign of COPD, and its presence should alert the clinician to initiate an investigation for causes of clubbing. In this population, the development of lung cancer is the most likely explanation for newly developed clubbing.

LABORATORY FINDINGS

The hallmark of COPD is airflow obstruction (discussed above). Pulmonary function testing shows airflow obstruction with a reduction in FEV_1 and FEV_1/FVC (Chap. 246). With worsening disease severity, lung volumes may increase, resulting in an increase in total lung capacity, functional residual capacity, and residual volume. In patients with emphysema, the diffusing capacity may be reduced, reflecting the parenchymal destruction characteristic of the disease. The degree of airflow obstruction is an important prognostic factor in COPD and is the basis for the GOLD disease classification (Table 254-1). More recently it has been shown that a multifactorial index incorporating airflow obstruction, exercise performance, dyspnea, and body mass index is a better predictor of mortality than pulmonary function alone.

While arterial blood gases and oximetry are not sensitive (discussed above), they may demonstrate resting or exertional hypoxemia. Arterial blood gases provide additional information about alveolar ventilation and acid-base status by measuring arterial P_{CO_2} and pH. The change in pH with P_{CO_2} is 0.08 units/10 mmHg acutely and 0.03 units/10 mmHg in the chronic state. Knowledge of the arterial pH therefore allows the classification of ventilatory failure, defined as P_{CO_2} >45 mmHg, into acute or chronic conditions. The arterial blood gas is an important component of the evaluation of patients presenting with symptoms of an exacerbation. An elevated hematocrit suggests the presence of chronic hypoxemia, as does the presence of signs of right ventricular hypertrophy.

Radiographic studies may assist in the classification of the type of COPD. Obvious bullae, paucity of parenchymal markings, or hyperlucency suggest the presence of emphysema. Increased lung volumes and flattening of the diaphragm suggest hyperinflation but do not provide information about chronicity of the changes. Computed tomography (CT) scan is the current definitive test for establishing the presence or absence of emphysema in living subjects (Fig. 254-4). From a practical perspective, the CT scan does little to influence therapy of COPD except in those individuals considering surgical therapy for their disease (described below).

Recent guidelines have suggested testing for α_1AT deficiency in all subjects with COPD or asthma with chronic airflow obstruction. Measurement of the serum α_1AT level is a reasonable initial test. For subjects with low α_1AT levels, the definitive diagnosis of α_1AT deficiency requires PI type determination. This is typically performed by isoelectric focusing of serum, which reflects the genotype at the PI locus for the common alleles and many of the rare PI alleles as well. Molecular genotyping of DNA can be performed for the common PI alleles (M, S, and Z).

FIGURE 254-4 Chest CT scan of a patient with COPD who underwent a left single-lung transplant. Note the reduced parenchymal markings in the right lung (*left side of figure*) as compared to the left lung, representing emphysematous destruction of the lung, and mediastinal shift to the left, indicative of hyperinflation.

℞ CHRONIC OBSTRUCTIVE PULMONARY DISEASE

STABLE PHASE COPD Only three interventions—smoking cessation, oxygen therapy in chronically hypoxemic patients, and lung volume reduction surgery in selected patients with emphysema—have been demonstrated to influence the natural history of patients with COPD. There is currently suggestive, but not definitive, evidence that the use of inhaled glucocorticoids may alter mortality (but not lung function). All other current therapies are directed at improving symptoms and decreasing the frequency and severity of exacerbations. The institution of these therapies should involve an assessment of symptoms, potential risks, costs, and benefits of therapy. This should be followed by an assessment of response to therapy, and a decision should be made whether or not to continue treatment.

PHARMACOTHERAPY   Smoking Cessation (See also Chap. 390) It has been shown that middle-aged smokers who were able to successfully stop smoking experienced a significant improvement in the rate of decline in pulmonary function, returning to annual changes similar to that of nonsmoking patients. Thus, all patients with COPD should be strongly urged to quit and educated about the benefits of quitting. An emerging body of evidence demonstrates that combining pharmacotherapy with traditional supportive approaches considerably enhances the chances of successful smoking cessation. There are two principal pharmacologic approaches to the problem: bupropion, originally developed as an antidepressant medication, and nicotine replacement therapy. The latter is available as gum, transdermal patches, inhaler, and nasal spray. Current recommendations from the U.S. Surgeon General are that all adult, nonpregnant smokers considering quitting be offered pharmacotherapy, in the absence of any contraindication to treatment.

Bronchodilators In general, bronchodilators are used for symptomatic benefit in patients with COPD. The inhaled route is preferred for medication delivery as the incidence of side effects is lower than that seen with the use of parenteral medication delivery.

Anticholinergic Agents While regular use of ipratropium bromide does not appear to influence the rate of decline of lung function, it improves symptoms and produces acute improvement in FEV_1. Tiotropium, a long-acting anticholinergic, has been shown to improve symptoms and reduce exacerbations. Side effects are minor, and a trial of inhaled anticholinergics is recommended in symptomatic patients with COPD.

Beta Agonists These provide symptomatic benefit. The main side effects are tremor and tachycardia. Long-acting inhaled β agonists, such as salmeterol, have benefits comparable to ipratropium bromide. Their use is more convenient than short-acting agents. The addition of a β agonist to inhaled anticholinergic therapy has been demonstrated to provide incremental benefit. A recent report in asthma suggests that those patients, particularly African Americans, using a long-acting β agonist without concomitant inhaled corticosteroids have an increased risk of deaths from respiratory causes. The applicability of these data to patients with COPD is unclear.

Inhaled Glucocorticoids Several trials have failed to find a beneficial effect for the regular use of inhaled glucocorticoids on the rate of decline of lung function, as assessed by FEV_1. Patients studied included those with mild to severe airflow obstruction and current and ex-smokers. Patients with significant acute response to inhaled β agonists were excluded from these trials. Their use has been associated with increased rates of oropharyngeal candidiasis and an increased rate of loss of bone density. Some analyses suggest that inhaled glucocorticoids reduce exacerbation frequency by ~25%. A more recent meta-analysis suggests that they may also reduce mortality by ~25%. A definitive conclusion regarding the mortality benefits awaits the results of ongoing prospective trials. A trial of inhaled glucocorticoids should be considered in patients with frequent exacerbations, defined as two or more per year, and in patients who demonstrate a significant amount of acute reversibility in response to inhaled bronchodilators.

Oral Glucocorticoids The chronic use of oral glucocorticoids for treatment of COPD is not recommended because of an unfavorable benefit/risk ratio. The chronic use of oral glucocorticoids is associated with significant side effects, including osteoporosis, weight gain, cataracts, glucose intolerance, and increased risk of infection. A recent study demonstrated that patients tapered off chronic low-dose prednisone (~10 mg/d) did not experience any adverse effect on the frequency of exacerbations, health-related quality of life, or lung function. On average, patients lost ~4.5 kg (~10 lb) when steroids were withdrawn.

Theophylline Theophylline produces modest improvements in expiratory flow rates and vital capacity and a slight improvement in arterial oxygen and carbon dioxide levels in patients with moderate to severe COPD. Nausea is a common side effect; tachycardia and tremor have also been reported.

Oxygen Supplemental O_2 is the only pharmacologic therapy demonstrated to decrease mortality in patients with COPD. For patients with resting hypoxemia (resting O_2 saturation <88% or <90% with signs of pulmonary hypertension or right heart failure), the use of O_2 has been demonstrated to have a significant impact on mortality. Patients meeting these criteria should be on continual oxygen supplementation, as the mortality benefit is proportional to the number of hours/day oxygen is used. Various delivery systems are available, including portable systems that patients may carry to allow mobility outside the home.

Supplemental O_2 is commonly prescribed for patients with exertional hypoxemia or nocturnal hypoxemia. Although the rationale for supplemental O_2 in these settings is physiologically sound, the benefits of such therapy are not well substantiated.

Other Agents N-acetyl cysteine has been used in patients with COPD for both its mucolytic and antioxidant properties. A prospective trial failed to find any benefit with respect to decline in lung function or prevention of exacerbations. Specific treatment in the form of intravenous α_1AT augmentation therapy is available for individuals with severe α_1AT deficiency. Despite sterilization procedures for these blood-derived products and the absence of reported cases of viral infection from therapy, some physicians recommend hepatitis B vaccination prior to starting augmentation therapy. Although biochemical efficacy of α_1AT augmentation therapy has been shown, a randomized controlled trial of α_1AT augmentation therapy has never proven the efficacy of augmentation therapy in reducing decline of pulmonary function. Eligibility for α_1AT augmentation therapy requires a serum α_1AT level <11 μM (approximately 50 mg/dL). Typically, Pi^Z individuals will qualify, although other rare types associated with severe deficiency (e.g., null-null) are also eligible. Since only a fraction of individuals with severe α_1AT deficiency will develop COPD, α_1AT augmentation therapy is not recommended for severely α_1AT-deficient persons with normal pulmonary function and a normal chest CT scan.

NONPHARMACOLOGIC THERAPIES   General Medical Care Patients with COPD should receive the influenza vaccine annually. Polyvalent pneumococcal vaccine is also recommended, although proof of efficacy in this patient population is not definitive.

Pulmonary Rehabilitation This refers to a treatment program that incorporates education and cardiovascular conditioning. In COPD, pulmonary rehabilitation has been demonstrated to improve health-related quality of life, dyspnea, and exercise capacity. It has also been shown to reduce rates of hospitalization over a 6–12-month period.

Lung Volume Reduction Surgery (LVRS) Surgery to reduce the volume of lung in patients with emphysema was first introduced with minimal success in the 1950s and was reintroduced in the 1990s. The operation may be performed via either a median sternotomy or a thoracoscopic approach. Patients are excluded if they have significant pleural disease, a pulmonary artery systolic pressure >45 mmHg, extreme deconditioning, congestive heart failure, or other severe comorbid conditions. Recent data demonstrate that patients with an FEV_1 <20% of predicted and either diffusely distributed emphysema on CT scan or DL_{CO} <20% of predicted have an increased mortality after the procedure and thus are not candidates for LVRS.

The National Emphysema Treatment trial demonstrated that LVRS offers both a mortality benefit and a symptomatic benefit in certain patients with emphysema. The anatomic distribution of emphysema and postrehabilitation exercise capacity are important prognostic characteristics. Patients with upper lobe–predominant emphysema and a low postrehabilitation exercise capacity are most likely to benefit from LVRS.

Lung Transplantation (See also Chap. 260) COPD is the single leading indication for lung transplantation (Fig. 254-4). Current recommendations are that candidates for lung transplantation should be <65 years; have severe disability despite maximal medical therapy; and be free of comorbid conditions such as liver, renal, or cardiac disease. In contrast to

LVRS, the anatomic distribution of emphysema and the presence of pulmonary hypertension are not contraindications to lung transplantation. Unresolved issues concerning lung transplantation and COPD include whether single- or double-lung transplant is the preferred procedure.

EXACERBATIONS OF COPD   Exacerbations are a prominent feature of the natural history of COPD. Exacerbations are commonly considered to be episodes of increased dyspnea and cough and change in the amount and character of sputum. They may or may not be accompanied by other signs of illness, including fever, myalgias, and sore throat. Self-reported health-related quality of life correlates with frequency of exacerbations more closely than it does with the degree of airflow obstruction. Economic analyses have shown that >70% of COPD-related health care expenditures go to emergency department visits and hospital care; this translates to >$10 billion annually in the United States. The frequency of exacerbations increases as airflow obstruction increases; patients with moderate to severe airflow obstruction [GOLD stages III,IV (Table 254-1)] have 1–3 episodes per year.

The approach to the patient experiencing an exacerbation includes an assessment of the severity of the patient's illness, both acute and chronic components; an attempt to identify the precipitant of the exacerbation; and the institution of therapy.

Precipitating Causes and Strategies to Reduce Frequency of Exacerbations   A variety of stimuli may result in the final common pathway of airway inflammation and increased symptoms that are characteristic of COPD exacerbations. Bacterial infections play a role in many, but by no means all, episodes. Viral respiratory infections are present in approximately one-third of COPD exacerbations. In a significant minority of instances (20–35%), no specific precipitant can be identified.

Despite the frequent implication of bacterial infection, chronic suppressive or "rotating" antibiotics are not beneficial in patients with COPD. This is in contrast to their apparent efficacy in patients with significant bronchiectasis. In patients with bronchiectasis due to cystic fibrosis, suppressive antibiotics have been shown to reduce frequency of hospital admissions.

The role of anti-inflammatory therapy in reducing exacerbation frequency is less well studied. Chronic oral glucocorticoids are not recommended for this purpose. Inhaled glucocorticoids did reduce the frequency of exacerbations by 25–30% in some analyses. The use of inhaled glucocorticoids should be considered in patients with frequent exacerbations or those who have an asthmatic component, i.e., significant reversibility on pulmonary function testing or marked symptomatic improvement after inhaled bronchodilators.

Patient Assessment   An attempt should be made to establish the severity of the exacerbation as well as the severity of preexisting COPD. The more severe either of these two components, the more likely that the patient will require hospital admission. The history should include quantification of the degree of dyspnea by asking about breathlessness during activities of daily living and typical activities for the patient. The patient should be asked about fever; change in character of sputum; any ill contacts; and associated symptoms such as nausea, vomiting, diarrhea, myalgias, and chills. Inquiring about the frequency and severity of prior exacerbations can provide important information.

The physical examination should incorporate an assessment of the degree of distress of the patient. Specific attention should be focused on tachycardia, tachypnea, use of accessory muscles, signs of perioral or peripheral cyanosis, the ability to speak in complete sentences, and the patient's mental status. The chest examination should establish the presence or absence of focal findings, degree of air movement, presence or absence of wheezing, asymmetry in the chest examination (suggesting large airway obstruction or pneumothorax mimicking an exacerbation), and the presence or absence of paradoxical motion of the abdominal wall.

Patients with severe underlying COPD who are in moderate or severe distress or those with focal findings should have a chest x-ray. Approximately 25% of x-rays in this clinical situation will be abnormal, with the most frequent findings being pneumonia and congestive heart failure. Patients with advanced COPD, those with a history of hypercarbia, those with mental status changes (confusion, sleepiness), or those in significant distress should have an arterial blood gas measurement. The presence of hypercarbia, defined as a P_{CO_2} >45 mmHg, has important implications for treatment (discussed below). In contrast to its utility in the management of exacerbations of asthma, measurement of pulmonary function has not been demonstrated to be helpful in the diagnosis or management of exacerbations of COPD.

There are no definitive guidelines concerning the need for inpatient treatment of exacerbations. Patients with respiratory acidosis and hypercarbia, significant hypoxemia, or severe underlying disease or those whose living situation is not conducive to careful observation and the delivery of prescribed treatment should be admitted to the hospital.

ACUTE EXACERBATIONS   **Bronchodilators**   Typically, patients are treated with an inhaled β agonist, often with the addition of an anticholinergic agent. These may be administered separately or together, and the frequency of administration depends on the severity of the exacerbation. Patients are often treated initially with nebulized therapy, as such treatment is often easier to administer in older patients or to those in respiratory distress. It has been shown, however, that conversion to metered-dose inhalers is effective when accompanied by education and training of patients and staff. This approach has significant economic benefits and also allows an easier transition to outpatient care. The addition of methylxanthines (such as theophylline) to this regimen can be considered, although convincing proof of its efficacy is lacking. If added, serum levels should be monitored in an attempt to minimize toxicity.

Antibiotics   Patients with COPD are frequently colonized with potential respiratory pathogens and it is often difficult to identify conclusively a specific species of bacteria responsible for a particular clinical event. Bacteria frequently implicated in COPD exacerbations include *Streptococcus pneumoniae*, *Haemophilus influenzae*, and *Moraxella catarrhalis*. In addition, *Mycoplasma pneumoniae* or *Chlamydia pneumoniae* are found in 5–10% of exacerbations. The choice of antibiotic should be based on local patterns of antibiotic susceptibility of the above pathogens as well as the patient's clinical condition. Most practitioners treat patients with moderate or severe exacerbations with antibiotics, even in the absence of data implicating a specific pathogen.

Glucocorticoids   Among patients admitted to the hospital, the use of glucocorticoids has been demonstrated to reduce the length of stay, hasten recovery, and reduce the chance of subsequent exacerbation or relapse for a period of up to 6 months. One study demonstrated that 2 weeks of glucocorticoid therapy produced benefit indistinguishable from 8 weeks of therapy. The GOLD guidelines recommend 30–40 mg of oral prednisolone or its equivalent for a period of 10–14 days. Hyperglycemia, particularly in patients with preexisting diagnosis of diabetes, is the most frequently reported acute complication of glucocorticoid treatment.

Oxygen   Supplemental O_2 should be supplied to keep arterial saturations ≥90%. Hypoxic respiratory drive plays a small role in patients with COPD. Studies have demonstrated that in patients with both acute and chronic hypercarbia, the administration of supplemental O_2 does not reduce minute ventilation. It does, in some patients, result in modest increases in arterial P_{CO_2}, chiefly by altering ventilation-perfusion relationships within the lung. This should not deter practitioners from providing the oxygen needed to correct hypoxemia.

Mechanical Ventilatory Support   The initiation of noninvasive positive pressure ventilation (NIPPV) in patients with respiratory failure, defined as Pa_{CO_2} >45 mmHg, results in a significant reduction in mortality, need for intubation, complications of therapy, and hospital length of stay. Contraindications to NIPPV include cardiovascular instability, impaired mental status or inability to cooperate, copious secretions or the inability to clear secretions, craniofacial abnormalities or trauma precluding effective fitting of mask, extreme obesity, or significant burns.

Invasive (conventional) mechanical ventilation via an endotracheal tube is indicated for patients with severe respiratory distress despite initial therapy, life-threatening hypoxemia, severe hypercapnia and/or acidosis, markedly impaired mental status, respiratory arrest, hemodynamic instability, or other complications. The goal of mechanical ventilation is to correct the aforementioned conditions. Factors to consider during mechanical ventilatory support include the need to provide sufficient expiratory time in patients with severe airflow obstruction and the presence of auto-PEEP (positive end-expiratory pressure) which can result in patients having to generate significant respiratory effort to trigger a breath during a demand mode of ventilation. The mortality of patients requiring mechanical ventilatory support is 17–30% for that particular hospitalization. For patients age >65 admitted to the intensive care unit for treatment, the mortality doubles over the next year to 60%, regardless of whether mechanical ventilation was required.

FURTHER READINGS

AMERICAN THORACIC SOCIETY/EUROPEAN RESPIRATORY SOCIETY TASK FORCE: Standards for the diagnosis and management of patients with COPD [Internet]. Version 1.2. New York: American Thoracic Society; 2004 [updated 2005 September 8]. Available from: *http://www-test.thoracic.org/copd/*

FIORE MC et al: *Treating Tobacco Use and Dependence*, Clinical Practice Guideline. Rockville, MD: U.S. Department of Health and Human Services. Public Health Service, June 2000

ITO K et al: Decreased histone deacetylase activity in chronic obstructive pulmonary disease. N Engl J Med 352:1967, 2005

MANNINO DM, BUIST AS: Global burden of COPD: Risk factors, prevalence, and future trends. Lancet 370:765, 2007

RABE KF et al: Global strategy for the diagnosis, management and prevention of chronic obstructive pulmonary disease: GOLD executive summary. Am J Respir Crit Care Med 176:532, 2007

——— et al: Update in chronic obstructive pulmonary disease 2006. Am J Respir Crit Care Med 175:1222, 2007

SIN DD et al: Inhaled corticosteroids and mortality in chronic obstructive pulmonary disease. Thorax 60:992, 2005

WISE RA, TASHKIN DP: Optimizing treatment of chronic obstructive pulmonary disease: An assessment of current therapies. Am J Med 120:S4, 2007

255 Interstitial Lung Diseases
Talmadge E. King, Jr.

Patients with interstitial lung diseases (ILDs) come to medical attention mainly because of the onset of progressive exertional dyspnea or a persistent, nonproductive cough. Hemoptysis, wheezing, and chest pain may be present. Often, the identification of interstitial opacities on chest x-ray focuses the diagnostic approach toward one of the ILDs.

ILDs represent a large number of conditions that involve the parenchyma of the lung—the alveoli, the alveolar epithelium, the capillary endothelium, and the spaces between these structures, as well as the perivascular and lymphatic tissues. This heterogeneous group of disorders is classified together because of similar clinical, roentgenographic, physiologic, or pathologic manifestations. These disorders are often associated with considerable morbidity and mortality, and there is little consensus regarding the best management of most of them.

ILDs have been difficult to classify because > 200 known individual diseases are characterized by diffuse parenchymal lung involvement, either as the primary condition or as a significant part of a multiorgan process, as may occur in the connective tissue diseases (CTDs). One useful approach to classification is to separate the ILDs into two groups based on the major underlying histopathology: (1) those associated with predominant inflammation and fibrosis, and (2) those with a predominantly granulomatous reaction in interstitial or vascular areas (Table 255-1). Each of these groups can be further subdivided according to whether the cause is known or unknown. For each ILD there may be an acute phase, and there is usually a chronic one as well. Rarely, some are recurrent, with intervals of subclinical disease.

Sarcoidosis (Chap. 322), idiopathic pulmonary fibrosis (IPF), and pulmonary fibrosis associated with CTDs (Chaps. 313–319) are the most common ILDs of unknown etiology. Among the ILDs of known cause, the largest group comprises occupational and environmental exposures, especially the inhalation of inorganic dusts, organic dusts, and various fumes or gases (Chaps. 249 and 250) (Table 255-2). A clinical diagnosis is possible for many forms of ILD, especially if an occupational and environmental history is aggressively pursued. For other forms, tissue examination, usually obtained by thoracoscopic lung biopsy, is critical to confirmation of the diagnosis. High-resolution computed tomography (HRCT) scanning improves diagnostic accuracy as experience with histologic-image correlation is perfected.

PATHOGENESIS

The ILDs are nonmalignant disorders and are not caused by identified infectious agents. The precise pathway(s) leading from injury to fibrosis is not known. Although there are multiple initiating agent(s) of in-

---

TABLE 255-1   MAJOR CATEGORIES OF ALVEOLAR AND INTERSTITIAL INFLAMMATORY LUNG DISEASE

Lung Response: Alveolitis, Interstitial Inflammation, and Fibrosis

Known Cause

Asbestos	Radiation
Fumes, gases	Aspiration pneumonia
Drugs (antibiotics, amiodarone, gold) and chemotherapy drugs	Residual of adult respiratory distress syndrome

Unknown Cause

Idiopathic interstitial pneumonias	Pulmonary alveolar proteinosis
Idiopathic pulmonary fibrosis (usual interstitial pneumonia)	Lymphocytic infiltrative disorders (lymphocytic interstitial pneumonitis associated with connective tissue disease)
Desquamative interstitial pneumonia	Eosinophilic pneumonias
Respiratory bronchiolitis-associated interstitial lung disease	Lymphangioleiomyomatosis
Acute interstitial pneumonia (diffuse alveolar damage)	Amyloidosis
Cryptogenic organizing pneumonia (bronchiolitis obliterans with organizing pneumonia)	Inherited diseases
Nonspecific interstitial pneumonia	Tuberous sclerosis, neurofibromatosis, Niemann-Pick disease, Gaucher's disease, Hermansky-Pudlak syndrome
Connective tissue diseases	Gastrointestinal or liver diseases (Crohn's disease, primary biliary cirrhosis, chronic active hepatitis, ulcerative colitis)
Systemic lupus erythematosus, rheumatoid arthritis, ankylosing spondylitis, systemic sclerosis, Sjögren's syndrome, polymyositis-dermatomyositis	Graft-vs.-host disease (bone marrow transplantation; solid organ transplantation)
Pulmonary hemorrhage syndromes	
Goodpasture's syndrome, idiopathic pulmonary hemosiderosis, isolated pulmonary capillaritis	

Lung Response: Granulomatous

Known Cause

Hypersensitivity pneumonitis (organic dusts)	Inorganic dusts: beryllium, silica

Unknown Cause

Sarcoidosis	Bronchocentric granulomatosis
Langerhans' cell granulomatosis (eosinophilic granuloma of the lung)	Lymphomatoid granulomatosis
Granulomatous vasculitides	
Wegener's granulomatosis, allergic granulomatosis of Churg-Strauss	

TABLE 255-2 ESTIMATED RELATIVE FREQUENCY OF THE INTERSTITIAL LUNG DISEASES

Diagnosis	Relative Frequency, %
Idiopathic interstitial pneumonias	40
Idiopathic pulmonary fibrosis	55
Nonspecific interstitial pneumonia	25
Respiratory bronchiolitis—ILD and desquamative interstitial pneumonia	15
Cryptogenic organizing pneumonia	3
Acute interstitial pneumonia	<1
Occupational and environmental	26
Sarcoidosis	10
Connective tissue diseases	9
Drug and radiation	1
Pulmonary hemorrhage syndromes	<1
Other	13

Source: From DB Coultas, R Hubbard, in JP Lynch III (ed): *Lung Biology in Health and Disease.* New York, Marcel Dekker, 2004; and S Garantziotis et al: J Clin Invest 114:319, 2004.

jury, the immunopathogenic responses of lung tissue are limited, and the mechanisms of repair have common features (Fig. 255-1).

As mentioned above, the two major histopathologic patterns are a granulomatous pattern and a pattern in which inflammation and fibrosis predominate.

Granulomatous Lung Disease This process is characterized by an accumulation of T lymphocytes, macrophages, and epithelioid cells organized into discrete structures (granulomas) in the lung parenchyma. The granulomatous lesions can progress to fibrosis. Many patients with granulomatous lung disease remain free of severe impairment of lung function, or, when symptomatic, they improve after treatment. The main differential diagnosis is between sarcoidosis (Chap. 322) and hypersensitivity pneumonitis (Chap. 249).

Inflammation and Fibrosis The initial insult is an injury to the epithelial surface causing inflammation in the air spaces and alveolar walls (Fig. 255-2). If the disease becomes chronic, inflammation spreads to adjacent portions of the interstitium and vasculature and eventually causes interstitial fibrosis. Important histopathologic patterns found in the ILDs include: usual interstitial pneumonia (UIP), nonspecific interstitial pneumonia, respiratory bronchiolitis, organizing pneumonia [bronchiolitis obliterans with organizing pneumonia (BOOP) pattern], diffuse alveolar damage (acute or organizing), desquamative interstitial pneumonia, and lymphocytic interstitial pneumonia. The development of irreversible scarring (fibrosis) of alveolar walls, airways, or vasculature is the most feared outcome in all of these conditions because it is often progressive and leads to significant derangement of ventilatory function and gas exchange.

History • *DURATION OF ILLNESS* *Acute presentation* (days to weeks), while unusual, occurs with allergy (drugs, fungi, helminths), acute interstitial pneumonia (AIP), eosinophilic pneumonia, and hypersensitivity pneumonitis. These conditions may be confused with atypical pneumonias because of diffuse alveolar opacities on chest x-ray. *Subacute presentation* (weeks to months) may occur in all ILDs but is seen especially in sarcoidosis, drug-induced ILDs, the alveolar hemorrhage syndromes, cryptogenic organizing pneumonia (COP), and the acute immunologic pneumonia that complicates systemic lupus erythematosus (SLE) or polymyositis. In most ILDs the symptoms and signs form a *chronic presentation* (months to years). Examples include IPF, sarcoidosis, pulmonary Langerhans cell histiocytosis (PLCH) (also known as Langerhans cell granulomatosis, eosinophilic granuloma, or histiocytosis X), pneumoconioses, and CTDs. *Episodic presentations* are unusual and include eosinophilic pneumonia, hypersensitivity pneumonitis, COP, vasculitides, pulmonary hemorrhage, and Churg-Strauss syndrome.

AGE Most patients with sarcoidosis, ILD associated with CTD, lymphangioleiomyomatosis (LAM), PLCH, and inherited forms of ILD (familial IPF, Gaucher's disease, Hermansky-Pudlak syndrome) present between the ages of 20 and 40 years. Most patients with IPF are older than 50 years.

GENDER LAM and pulmonary involvement in tuberous sclerosis occur exclusively in premenopausal women. Also, ILD in Hermansky-Pudlak syndrome and in the CTDs is more common in women; an exception is ILD in rheumatoid arthritis (RA), which is more common in men. Because of occupational exposures, pneumoconioses also occur more frequently in men.

FAMILY HISTORY Family associations (with an autosomal dominant pattern) have been identified in tuberous sclerosis and neurofibromatosis. An autosomal recessive pattern of inheritance occurs in Niemann-Pick disease, Gaucher's disease, and the Hermansky-Pudlak syndrome. Familial clustering has been increasingly identified in sarcoidosis. Familial lung fibrosis has been associated with mutations in the surfactant protein C gene and is characterized by several patterns of interstitial pneumonia, including nonspecific interstitial pneumonia, desquamative interstitial pneumonia, and UIP.

SMOKING HISTORY Two-thirds to 75% of patients with IPF have a history of smoking. Patients with PLCH, desquamative interstitial pneumonia (DIP), Goodpasture's syndrome, respiratory bronchiolitis, and pulmonary alveolar proteinosis are almost always current or former smokers.

OCCUPATION AND ENVIRONMENTAL HISTORY A strict chronologic listing of the patient's lifelong employment must be sought, including specific duties and known exposures. In hypersensitivity pneumonitis (see Fig. 249-1), respiratory symptoms, fever, chills, and an abnormal chest roentgenogram are often temporally related to a hobby (pigeon breeder's disease) or to the workplace (farmer's lung) (Chap. 249). Symptoms may diminish or disappear after the patient leaves the site of exposure for several days; similarly, symptoms may reappear on returning to the exposure site.

FIGURE 255-1 Proposed mechanism for the pathogenesis of pulmonary fibrosis. The lung is naturally exposed to repetitive injury from a variety of exogenous and endogenous stimuli. Several local and systemic factors (e.g., fibroblasts, circulating fibrocytes, chemokines, growth factors, and clotting factors) contribute to tissue healing and functional recovery. Dysregulation of this intricate network through genetic predisposition, autoimmune conditions, or superimposed diseases can lead to aberrant wound healing with the result of pulmonary fibrosis. Alternatively, excessive injury to the lung may overwhelm even intact reparative mechanisms and lead to pulmonary fibrosis. (*From S Garantziotis, et al: J Clin Invest 114:319, 2004.*)

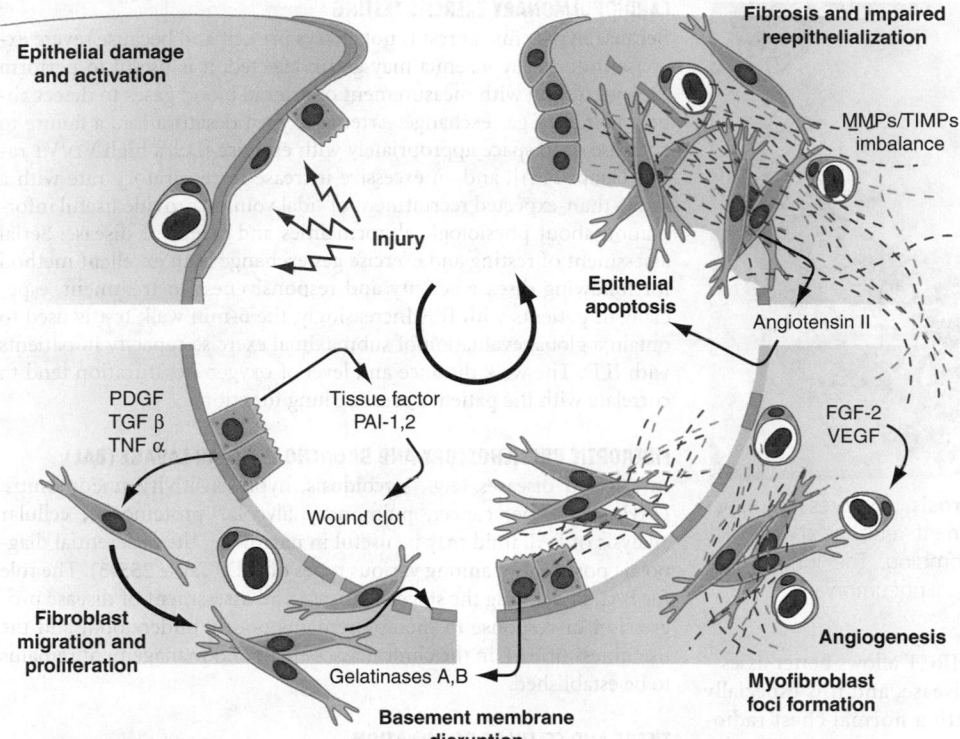

FIGURE 255-2 Cellular bases for the pathogenesis of interstitial lung disease. Multiple microinjuries damage and activate alveolar epithelial cells (*top left*), which in turn induce an antifibrinolytic environment in the alveolar spaces, enhancing wound clot formation. Alveolar epithelial cells secrete growth factors and induce migration and proliferation of fibroblasts and differentiation into myofibroblasts (*bottom left*). Subepithelial myofibroblasts and alveolar epithelial cells produce gelatinases that may increase basement membrane disruption and allow fibroblast–myofibroblast migration (*bottom right*). Angiogenic factors induce neovascularization. Both intraalveolar and interstitial myofibroblasts secrete extracellular matrix proteins, mainly collagens. An imbalance between interstitial collagenases and tissue inhibitors of metalloproteinases provokes the progressive deposit of extracellular matrix (*top right*). Signals responsible for myofibroblast apoptosis seem to be absent or delayed in usual interstitial pneumonia, increasing cell survival. Myofibroblasts produce angiotensinogen that as angiotensin II provokes alveolar epithelial cell death, further impairing reepithelialization. Abbreviations: FGF-2, fibroblast growth factor 2; MMPs, metalloproteinases; PAI-1, PAI-2, plasminogen activator inhibitor 1, 2; PDGF, platelet-derived growth factor; TGF-β, transforming growth factor β; TIMPs, tissue inhibitors of metalloproteinases; TNF-α, tumor necrosis factor α; VEGF, vascular endothelial growth factor. (*From M Selman et al: Ann Intern Med 134:136, 2001; with permission.*)

OTHER IMPORTANT PAST HISTORY   Parasitic infections may cause pulmonary eosinophilia, and therefore a travel history should be taken in patients with known or suspected ILD. History of risk factors for HIV infection should be elicited from all patients with ILD because several processes may occur at the time of initial presentation or during the clinical course, e.g., HIV infection, BOOP, AIP, lymphocytic interstitial pneumonitis, or diffuse alveolar hemorrhage.

RESPIRATORY SYMPTOMS AND SIGNS

Dyspnea is a common and prominent complaint in patients with ILD, especially the idiopathic interstitial pneumonias, hypersensitivity pneumonitis, COP, sarcoidosis, eosinophilic pneumonias, and PLCH. Some patients, especially patients with sarcoidosis, silicosis, PLCH, hypersensitivity pneumonitis, lipoid pneumonia, or lymphangitis carcinomatosis, may have extensive parenchymal lung disease on chest x-ray without significant dyspnea, especially early in the course of the illness. Wheezing is an uncommon manifestation of ILD but has been described in patients with chronic eosinophilic pneumonia, Churg-Strauss syndrome, respiratory bronchiolitis, and sarcoidosis. Clinically significant chest pain is uncommon in most ILDs. However, substernal discomfort is common in sarcoidosis. Sudden worsening of dyspnea, especially if associated with acute chest pain, may indicate a spontaneous pneumothorax, which occurs in PLCH, tuberous sclerosis, LAM,

and neurofibromatosis. Frank hemoptysis and blood-streaked sputum are rarely presenting manifestations of ILD but can be seen in the diffuse alveolar hemorrhage (DAH) syndromes, LAM, tuberous sclerosis, and the granulomatous vasculitides. Fatigue and weight loss are common in all ILDs.

PHYSICAL EXAMINATION

The findings are usually not specific. Most commonly, physical examination reveals tachypnea and bibasilar end-inspiratory dry crackles, which are common in most forms of ILD associated with inflammation but are less likely to be heard in the granulomatous lung diseases. Crackles may be present in the absence of radiographic abnormalities on the chest radiograph. Scattered late inspiratory high-pitched rhonchi—so-called inspiratory squeaks—are heard in patients with bronchiolitis. The cardiac examination is usually normal except in the mid or late stages of the disease, when findings of pulmonary hypertension and cor pulmonale may become evident (Chap. 244). Cyanosis and clubbing of the digits occur in some patients with advanced disease.

LABORATORY

Antinuclear antibodies and anti-immunoglobulin antibodies (rheumatoid factors) are identified in some patients, even in the absence of a defined CTD. A raised lactate dehydrogenase (LDH) level is a nonspecific finding common to ILDs. Elevation of the serum angiotensin-converting enzyme level is common in sarcoidosis. Serum precipitins confirm exposure when hypersensitivity pneumonitis is suspected, although they are not diagnostic of the process. Antineutrophil cytoplasmic or anti-basement membrane antibodies are useful if vasculitis is suspected. The electrocardiogram is usually normal unless pulmonary hypertension is present; then it demonstrates right-axis deviation, right ventricular hypertrophy, or right atrial enlargement or hypertrophy. Echocardiography also reveals right ventricular dilatation and/or hypertrophy in the presence of pulmonary hypertension.

CHEST IMAGING STUDIES

Chest X-ray   ILD may be first suspected based on an abnormal chest radiograph, which most commonly reveals a bibasilar reticular pattern. A nodular or mixed pattern of alveolar filling and increased reticular markings may also be present. A subgroup of ILDs exhibit nodular opacities with a predilection for the upper lung zones [sarcoidosis, PLCH, chronic hypersensitivity pneumonitis, silicosis, berylliosis, RA (necrobiotic nodular form), ankylosing spondylitis]. The chest x-ray correlates poorly with the clinical or histopathologic stage of the disease. The radiographic finding of honeycombing correlates with pathologic findings of small cystic spaces and progressive fibrosis; when present, it portends a poor prognosis. In most cases, the chest radiograph is nonspecific and usually does not allow a specific diagnosis.

Computed Tomography   High-resolution computed tomography (HRCT) is superior to the plain chest x-ray for early detection and confirma-

FIGURE 255-3 Idiopathic pulmonary fibrosis. High-resolution CT image shows bibasal, peripheral predominant reticular abnormality with traction bronchiectasis and honeycombing. The lung biopsy showed the typical features of usual interstitial pneumonia.

tion of suspected ILD (Fig. 255-3). Also, HRCT allows better assessment of the extent and distribution of disease, and it is especially useful in the investigation of patients with a normal chest radiograph. Coexisting disease is often best recognized on HRCT scanning, e.g., mediastinal adenopathy, carcinoma, or emphysema. In the appropriate clinical setting HRCT may be sufficiently characteristic to preclude the need for lung biopsy in IPF, sarcoidosis, hypersensitivity pneumonitis, asbestosis, lymphangitic carcinoma, and PLCH. When a lung biopsy is required, HRCT scanning is useful for determining the most appropriate area from which biopsy samples should be taken.

PULMONARY FUNCTION TESTING

Spirometry and Lung Volumes Measurement of lung function is important in assessing the extent of pulmonary involvement in patients with ILD. Most forms of ILD produce a restrictive defect with reduced total lung capacity (TLC), functional residual capacity, and residual volume (Chap. 246). Forced expiratory volume in one second (FEV_1) and forced vital capacity (FVC) are reduced, but these changes are related to the decreased TLC. The FEV_1/FVC ratio is usually normal or increased. Lung volumes decrease as lung stiffness worsens with disease progression. A few disorders produce interstitial opacities on chest x-ray and obstructive airflow limitation on lung function testing (uncommon in sarcoidosis and hypersensitivity pneumonitis, while common in tuberous sclerosis and LAM). Pulmonary function studies have proven to have prognostic value in patients with idiopathic interstitial pneumonias, particularly, IPF or nonspecific interstitial pneumonia (NSIP).

Diffusing Capacity A reduction in the diffusing capacity of the lung for carbon monoxide (DL_{CO}) is a common but nonspecific finding in most ILDs. This decrease is due, in part, to effacement of the alveolar capillary units but, more importantly, to mismatching of ventilation and perfusion ($\dot{V}/\dot{Q}$). Lung regions with reduced compliance due to either fibrosis or cellular infiltration may be poorly ventilated but may still maintain adequate blood flow, and the ventilation-perfusion mismatch in these regions acts like true venous admixture. The severity of the reduction in DL_{CO} does not correlate with disease stage.

Arterial Blood Gas The resting arterial blood gas may be normal or reveal hypoxemia (secondary to a mismatching of ventilation to perfusion) and respiratory alkalosis. A normal arterial O_2 tension (or saturation by oximetry) at rest does not rule out significant hypoxemia during exercise or sleep. CO_2 retention is rare and is usually a manifestation of end-stage disease.

CARDIOPULMONARY EXERCISE TESTING

Because hypoxemia at rest is not always present and because severe exercise-induced hypoxemia may go undetected, it is useful to perform exercise testing with measurement of arterial blood gases to detect abnormalities of gas exchange. Arterial oxygen desaturation, a failure to decrease dead space appropriately with exercise [i.e., a high VD/VT ratio (Chap. 246)], and an excessive increase in respiratory rate with a lower-than-expected recruitment of tidal volume provide useful information about physiologic abnormalities and extent of disease. Serial assessment of resting and exercise gas exchange is an excellent method for following disease activity and responsiveness to treatment, especially in patients with IPF. Increasingly, the 6-min walk test is used to obtain a global evaluation of submaximal exercise capacity in patients with ILD. The walk distance and level of oxygen desaturation tend to correlate with the patient's baseline lung function.

FIBEROPTIC BRONCHOSCOPY AND BRONCHOALVEOLAR LAVAGE (BAL)

In selected diseases (e.g., sarcoidosis, hypersensitivity pneumonitis, DAH syndrome, cancer, pulmonary alveolar proteinosis), cellular analysis of BAL fluid may be useful in narrowing the differential diagnostic possibilities among various types of ILD (Table 255-3). The role for BAL in defining the stage of disease and assessment of disease progression or response to therapy remains poorly understood, and the usefulness of BAL in the clinical assessment and management remains to be established.

TISSUE AND CELLULAR EXAMINATION

Lung biopsy is the most effective method for confirming the diagnosis and assessing disease activity. The findings may identify a more treatable process than originally suspected, particularly chronic hypersensitivity pneumonitis, COP, respiratory bronchiolitis–associated ILD, or sarcoidosis. Biopsy should be obtained before initiation of treatment. A definitive diagnosis avoids confusion and anxiety later in the clinical course if the patient does not respond to therapy or suffers serious side effects from it.

TABLE 255-3	DIAGNOSTIC VALUE OF BRONCHOALVEOLAR LAVAGE IN INTERSTITIAL LUNG DISEASE
Condition	**Bronchoalveolar Lavage Finding**
Sarcoidosis	Lymphocytosis; CD4:CD8 ratio >3.5 most specific of diagnosis
Hypersensitivity pneumonitis	Marked lymphocytosis (>50%)
Organizing pneumonia	Foamy macrophages; mixed pattern of increased cells characteristic; decreased CD4:CD8 ratio
Eosinophilic lung disease	Eosinophils >25%
Diffuse alveolar bleeding	Hemosiderin-laden macrophages, red blood cells
Diffuse alveolar damage, drug toxicity	Atypical hyperplastic type II pneumocytes
Opportunistic infections	*Pneumocystis carinii*, fungi, cytomegalovirus-transformed cells
Lymphangitic carcinomatosis, alveolar cell carcinoma, pulmonary lymphoma	Malignant cells
Alveolar proteinosis	Milky effluent, foamy macrophages and lipoproteinaceous intraalveolar material (periodic acid–Schiff stain positive)
Lipoid pneumonia	Fat globules in macrophages
Pulmonary Langerhans' cell histiocytosis	Increased CD1+ Langerhans' cells; Electron microscopy demonstrating Birbeck granule in lavaged macrophage (expensive and difficult to perform)
Asbestos-related pulmonary disease	Dust particles, ferruginous bodies
Berylliosis	Positive lymphocyte transformation test to beryllium
Silicosis	Dust particles by polarized light microscopy
Lipoidosis	Accumulation of specific lipopigment in alveolar macrophages

Fiberoptic bronchoscopy with multiple transbronchial lung biopsies (four to eight biopsy samples) is often the initial procedure of choice, especially when sarcoidosis, lymphangitic carcinomatosis, eosinophilic pneumonia, Goodpasture's syndrome, or infection is suspected. If a specific diagnosis is not made by transbronchial biopsy, then surgical lung biopsy by video-assisted thoracic surgery or open thoracotomy is indicated. Adequate-sized biopsies from multiple sites, usually from two lobes, should be obtained. Relative contraindications to lung biopsy include serious cardiovascular disease, honeycombing and other roentgenographic evidence of diffuse end-stage disease, severe pulmonary dysfunction, or other major operative risks, especially in the elderly.

Rx INTERSTITIAL LUNG DISEASE

Although the course of ILD is variable, progression is common and often insidious. All treatable possibilities should be carefully considered. Since therapy does not reverse fibrosis, the major goals of treatment are permanent removal of the offending agent, when known, and early identification and aggressive suppression of the acute and chronic inflammatory process, thereby reducing further lung damage.

Hypoxemia (Pa_{O_2} < 55 mmHg) at rest and/or with exercise should be managed by supplemental oxygen. If cor pulmonale develops, diuretic therapy and phlebotomy may occasionally be required (Chaps. 227 and 244).

DRUG THERAPY Glucocorticoids are the mainstay of therapy for suppression of the alveolitis present in ILD, but the success rate is low. There have been no placebo-controlled trials of glucocorticoids in ILD, so there is no direct evidence that steroids improve survival in many of the diseases for which they are commonly used. Glucocorticoid therapy is recommended for symptomatic ILD patients with eosinophilic pneumonias, COP, CTD, sarcoidosis, acute inorganic dust exposures, acute radiation pneumonitis, DAH, and drug-induced ILD. In organic dust disease, glucocorticoids are recommended for both the acute and chronic stages.

The optimal dose and proper length of therapy with glucocorticoids in the treatment of most ILDs are not known. A common starting dose is prednisone, 0.5–1 mg/kg in a once-daily oral dose (based on the patient's lean body weight). This dose is continued for 4–12 weeks, at which time the patient is reevaluated. If the patient is stable or improved, the dose is tapered to 0.25–0.5 mg/kg and is maintained at this level for an additional 4–12 weeks depending on the course. Rapid tapering or a shortened course of glucocorticoid treatment can result in recurrence. If the patient's condition continues to decline while on glucocorticoids, a second agent (see below) is often added and the prednisone dose is lowered to or maintained at 0.25 mg/kg per day.

Cyclophosphamide and azathioprine (1–2 mg/kg lean body weight per day), with or without glucocorticoids, have been tried with variable success in IPF, vasculitis, and other ILDs. An objective response usually requires at least 8–12 weeks to occur. In situations in which these drugs have failed or could not be tolerated, other agents, including methotrexate, colchicine, penicillamine, and cyclosporine, have been tried. However, their role in the treatment of ILDs remains to be determined.

Many cases of ILD are chronic and irreversible despite the therapy discussed above, and lung transplantation may then be considered (Chap. 260).

INDIVIDUAL FORMS OF ILD

IDIOPATHIC PULMONARY FIBROSIS

IPF is the most common form of idiopathic interstitial pneumonia. Separating IPF from other forms of lung fibrosis is an important step in the evaluation of all patients presenting with ILD. IPF has a distinctly poor response to therapy and a bad prognosis.

Clinical Manifestations Exertional dyspnea, a nonproductive cough, and inspiratory crackles with or without digital clubbing may be present on physical examination. The HRCT lung scans typically show patchy, predominantly basilar, subpleural reticular opacities, often associated with traction bronchiectasis and honeycombing (Fig. 255-3).

Atypical findings that should suggest an alternative diagnosis include: extensive ground-glass abnormality, nodular opacities, upper or midzone predominance, and prominent hilar or mediastinal lymphadenopathy. Pulmonary function tests often reveal a restrictive pattern, a reduced DL_{CO}, and arterial hypoxemia that is exaggerated or elicited by exercise.

Histologic Findings Confirmation of the presence of the UIP pattern on histologic examination is essential to confirm this diagnosis. Transbronchial biopsies are not helpful in making the diagnosis of UIP, and surgical biopsy is usually required. The histologic hallmark and chief diagnostic criterion of UIP is a heterogeneous appearance at low magnification with alternating areas of normal lung, interstitial inflammation, foci of proliferating fibroblasts, dense collagen fibrosis, and honeycomb changes. These histologic changes affect the peripheral, subpleural parenchyma most severely. The interstitial inflammation is usually patchy and consists of a lymphoplasmacytic infiltrate in the alveolar septa, associated with hyperplasia of type 2 pneumocytes. The fibrotic zones are composed mainly of dense collagen, although scattered foci of proliferating fibroblasts are a consistent finding. The extent of fibroblastic proliferation is predictive of disease progression. Areas of honeycomb change are composed of cystic fibrotic air spaces that are frequently lined by bronchiolar epithelium and filled with mucin. Smooth-muscle hyperplasia is commonly seen in areas of fibrosis and honeycomb change. A fibrotic pattern with some features similar to UIP may be found in the chronic stage of several specific disorders such as: pneumoconioses (e.g., asbestosis), radiation injury, certain drug-induced lung diseases (e.g., nitrofurantoin), chronic aspiration, sarcoidosis, chronic hypersensitivity pneumonitis, organized chronic eosinophilic pneumonia, and PLCH. Commonly, other histopathologic features are present in these situations thus allowing separation of these lesions from the UIP-like pattern. Consequently, the term *UIP* is used for those patients in whom the lesion is idiopathic and not associated with another condition.

Patients with IPF may suffer acute deterioration secondary to infections, pulmonary embolism, pneumothorax, or heart failure. These patients also commonly suffer an accelerated phase of rapid clinical decline that is associated with a poor prognosis (so-called acute exacerbations of IPF). These acute exacerbations are defined by: worsening of dyspnea within a few days to 4 weeks; newly developing diffuse radiographic opacities; worsening hypoxemia; and absence of infectious pneumonia, heart failure, and sepsis. The rate of these acute exacerbations ranges from 10–57%, apparently depending on the length of follow-up. During these episodes, the histopathologic pattern of diffuse alveolar damage is often found on the background of UIP.

Rx IDIOPATHIC PULMONARY FIBROSIS

No therapy has been found to be effective in the management of acute exacerbations of IPF. Often mechanical ventilation is required but is usually not successful, with a hospital mortality rate of up to three-fourths of the patients. In those that survive, a recurrence of acute exacerbation is common and usually results in death at those times.

Lung transplantation should be considered for those patients who experience progressive deterioration despite optimal medical management and who meet the established criteria (Chap. 260).

NONSPECIFIC INTERSTITIAL PNEUMONIA (NSIP)

This condition defines a subgroup of the idiopathic interstitial pneumonias that can be distinguished clinically and pathologically from UIP, desquamative interstitial pneumonia (DIP), AIP, and idiopathic BOOP. Importantly, many cases with this histopathologic pattern occur in the context of an underlying disorder, such as a connective tissue disease, drug-induced ILD, or chronic hypersensitivity pneumonitis. Idiopathic NSIP is a subacute restrictive process with a presentation similar to IPF but usually at a younger age, most commonly in women who have never smoked. It is often associated with a febrile illness. HRCT shows bilateral, subpleural ground-glass opacities, often

FIGURE 255-4 Nonspecific interstitial pneumonia. High-resolution CT through the lower lung shows volume loss with extensive ground-glass abnormality, reticular abnormality and traction bronchiectasis. There is sparing on the lung immediately adjacent to the pleura. Histology showed a combination of inflammation and mild fibrosis.

associated with lower lobe volume loss (Fig. 255-4). Patchy areas of airspace consolidation and reticular abnormalities may be present, but honeycombing is unusual. The key histopathologic features of NSIP are the uniformity of interstitial involvement across the biopsy section, and this may be predominantly cellular or fibrosing. There is less temporal and spatial heterogeneity than in UIP and little or no honeycombing is found. The cellular variant is rare. Unlike patients with IPF (UIP), the majority of patients with NSIP have a good prognosis (5-year mortality rate estimated at <15%) with most showing improvement after treatment with glucocorticoids, often used in combination with azathioprine.

ACUTE INTERSTITIAL PNEUMONIA (AIP, HAMMAN-RICH SYNDROME)

AIP is a rare, fulminant form of lung injury characterized histologically by diffuse alveolar damage on lung biopsy. Most patients are older than 40 years. AIP is similar in presentation to the acute respiratory distress syndrome (ARDS) (Chap. 262) and probably corresponds to the subset of cases of idiopathic ARDS. The onset is usually abrupt in a previously healthy individual. A prodromal illness, usually lasting 7–14 days before presentation, is common. Fever, cough, and dyspnea are frequent manifestations at presentation. Diffuse, bilateral, air-space opacification is present on chest radiograph. HRCT scans show bilateral, patchy, symmetric areas of ground-glass attenuation. Bilateral areas of air-space consolidation may also be present. A predominantly subpleural distribution may be seen. The diagnosis of AIP requires the presence of a clinical syndrome of idiopathic ARDS and pathologic confirmation of organizing diffuse alveolar damage. Therefore, lung biopsy is required to confirm the diagnosis. Most patients have moderate to severe hypoxemia and develop respiratory failure. Mechanical ventilation is often required. The mortality rate is high (>60%), with most patients dying within 6 months of presentation. Recurrences have been reported. However, those who recover often have substantial improvement in lung function. The main treatment is supportive. It is not clear that glucocorticoid therapy is effective.

CRYPTOGENIC ORGANIZING PNEUMONIA

Also known as *idiopathic BOOP*, COP is a clinicopathologic syndrome of unknown etiology. The onset is usually in the fifth and sixth decades. The presentation may be of a flulike illness with cough, fever, malaise, fatigue, and weight loss. Inspiratory crackles are frequently present on examination. Pulmonary function is usually impaired, with a restrictive defect and arterial hypoxemia being most common. The

roentgenographic manifestations are distinctive, revealing bilateral, patchy, or diffuse alveolar opacities in the presence of normal lung volume. Recurrent and migratory pulmonary opacities are common. HRCT shows areas of air-space consolidation, ground-glass opacities, small nodular opacities, and bronchial wall thickening and dilation. These changes occur more frequently in the periphery of the lung and in the lower lung zone. Lung biopsy shows granulation tissue within small airways, alveolar ducts, and airspaces, with chronic inflammation in the surrounding alveoli. Glucocorticoid therapy induces clinical recovery in two-thirds of patients. A few patients have rapidly progressive courses with fatal outcomes despite glucocorticoids.

Foci of organizing pneumonia (i.e., a "BOOP pattern") is a nonspecific reaction to lung injury found adjacent to other pathologic processes or as a component of other primary pulmonary disorders (e.g., cryptococcosis, Wegener's granulomatosis, lymphoma, hypersensitivity pneumonitis, and eosinophilic pneumonia). Consequently, the clinician must carefully reevaluate any patient found to have this histopathologic lesion to rule out these possibilities.

ILD ASSOCIATED WITH CIGARETTE SMOKING

Desquamative Interstitial Pneumonia DIP is a rare but distinct clinical and pathologic entity found exclusively in cigarette smokers. The histologic hallmark is the extensive accumulation of macrophages in intraalveolar spaces with minimal interstitial fibrosis. The peak incidence is in the fourth and fifth decades. Most patients present with dyspnea and cough. Lung function testing shows a restrictive pattern with reduced DL_{CO} and arterial hypoxemia. The chest x-ray and HRCT scans usually show diffuse hazy opacities. Clinical recognition of DIP is important because the process is associated with a better prognosis (10-year survival rate is ~70%) and a better response to smoking cessation and systemic glucocorticoids than IPF.

Respiratory Bronchiolitis–Associated ILD Respiratory bronchiolitis–associated ILD (RB-ILD) is considered to be a subset of DIP and is characterized by the accumulation of macrophages in peribronchial alveoli. The clinical presentation is similar to DIP. Rales are often heard on chest examination and occur throughout inspiration; sometimes they continue into expiration. The process is seen best on HRCT lung scanning which shows bronchial wall thickening, centrilobular nodules, ground-glass opacity, and emphysema with air trapping. RB-ILD appears to resolve in most patients following smoking cessation alone.

Pulmonary Langerhans Cell Histiocytosis (PLCH) This is a rare, smoking-related, diffuse lung disease that primarily affects men between the ages of 20 and 40 years. The clinical presentation varies from an asymptomatic state to a rapidly progressive condition. The most common clinical manifestations at presentation are cough, dyspnea, chest pain, weight loss, and fever. Pneumothorax occurs in ~25% of patients. Hemoptysis and diabetes insipidus are rare manifestations. The radiographic features vary with the stage of the disease. The combination of ill-defined or stellate nodules (2–10 mm in diameter), reticular or nodular opacities, bizarre-shaped upper zone cysts, preservation of lung volume, and sparing of the costophrenic angles are characteristics of PLCH. HRCT that reveals a combination of nodules and thin-walled cysts is virtually diagnostic of PLCH. The most frequent pulmonary function abnormality is a markedly reduced DL_{CO}, although varying degrees of restrictive disease, airflow limitation, and diminished exercise capacity may occur. The characteristic histopathologic finding in PLCH is the presence of nodular sclerosing lesions that contain Langerhans' cells accompanied by mixed cellular infiltrates. The nodular lesions are poorly defined and are distributed in a bronchiolocentric fashion with intervening normal lung parenchyma. As the disease progresses, fibrosis progresses to involve adjacent lung tissue leading to pericicatricial airspace enlargement, which accounts for the concomitant cystic changes. Discontinuance of smoking is the key treatment, resulting in clinical improvement in one-third of patients. Most patients with PLCH suffer persistent or progressive disease. Death due to respiratory failure occurs in ~10% of patients.

ILD ASSOCIATED WITH CONNECTIVE TISSUE DISORDERS

Clinical findings suggestive of a CTD (musculoskeletal pain, weakness, fatigue, fever, joint pains or swelling, photosensitivity, Raynaud's phenomenon, pleuritis, dry eyes, dry mouth) should be sought in any patient with ILD. The CTDs may be difficult to rule out since the pulmonary manifestations occasionally precede the more typical systemic manifestations by months or years. The most common form of pulmonary involvement is the nonspecific interstitial pneumonia histopathologic pattern. However, determining the precise nature of lung involvement in most of the CTDs is difficult due to the high incidence of lung involvement caused by disease-associated complications of esophageal dysfunction (predisposing to aspiration and secondary infections), respiratory muscle weakness (atelectasis and secondary infections), complications of therapy (opportunistic infections), and associated malignancies.

Progressive Systemic Sclerosis (PSS)

(See also Chap. 316) Clinical evidence of ILD is present in about one-half of patients with PSS, and pathologic evidence in three-quarters. Pulmonary function tests show a restrictive pattern and impaired diffusing capacity, often before any clinical or radiographic evidence of lung disease appears. Pulmonary vascular disease alone or in association with pulmonary fibrosis, pleuritis, or recurrent aspiration pneumonitis is strikingly resistant to current modes of therapy.

Rheumatoid Arthritis (RA)

(See also Chap. 314) ILD associated with RA is more common in men. Pulmonary manifestations of RA include pleurisy with or without effusion, ILD in up to 20% of cases, necrobiotic nodules (nonpneumoconiotic intrapulmonary rheumatoid nodules) with or without cavities, Caplan's syndrome (rheumatoid pneumoconiosis), pulmonary hypertension secondary to rheumatoid pulmonary vasculitis, BOOP, and upper airway obstruction due to crico-arytenoid arthritis.

Systemic Lupus Erythematosus (SLE)

(See also Chap. 313) Lung disease is a common complication in SLE. Pleuritis with or without effusion is the most common pulmonary manifestation. Other lung manifestations include the following: atelectasis, diaphragmatic dysfunction with loss of lung volumes, pulmonary vascular disease, pulmonary hemorrhage, uremic pulmonary edema, infectious pneumonia, and BOOP. Acute lupus pneumonitis characterized by pulmonary capillaritis leading to alveolar hemorrhage is uncommon. Chronic, progressive ILD is uncommon. It is important to exclude pulmonary infection. Although pleuropulmonary involvement may not be evident clinically, pulmonary function testing, particularly $D_{L_{CO}}$, reveals abnormalities in many patients with SLE.

Polymyositis and Dermatomyositis (PM/DM)

(See also Chap. 383) ILD occurs in ~10% of patients with PM/DM. Diffuse reticular or nodular opacities with or without an alveolar component occur radiographically, with a predilection for the lung bases. ILD occurs more commonly in the subgroup of patients with an anti-Jo-1 antibody that is directed to histidyl tRNA synthetase. Weakness of respiratory muscles contributing to aspiration pneumonia may be present. A rapidly progressive illness characterized by diffuse alveolar damage may cause respiratory failure.

Sjögren's Syndrome

(See also Chap. 317) General dryness and lack of airways secretion cause the major problems of hoarseness, cough, and bronchitis. Lymphocytic interstitial pneumonitis, lymphoma, pseudolymphoma, bronchiolitis, and bronchiolitis obliterans are associated with this condition. Lung biopsy is frequently required to establish a precise pulmonary diagnosis. Glucocorticoids have been used in the management of ILD associated with Sjögren's syndrome with some degree of clinical success.

DRUG-INDUCED ILD

Many classes of drugs have the potential to induce diffuse ILD, which is manifest most commonly as exertional dyspnea and nonproductive cough. A detailed history of the medications taken by the patient is needed to identify drug-induced disease, including over-the-counter medications, oily nose drops, or petroleum products (mineral oil). In most cases, the pathogenesis is unknown, although a combination of direct toxic effects of the drug (or its metabolite) and indirect inflammatory and immunologic events are likely. The onset of the illness may be abrupt and fulminant, or it may be insidious, extending over weeks to months. The drug may have been taken for several years before a reaction develops (e.g., amiodarone), or the lung disease may occur weeks to years after the drug has been discontinued (e.g., carmustine). The extent and severity of disease are usually dose-related. Treatment consists of discontinuation of any possible offending drug and supportive care.

EOSINOPHILIC PNEUMONIA
(See Chap. 249)

PULMONARY ALVEOLAR PROTEINOSIS (PAP)

Although not strictly an ILD, PAP resembles and is therefore considered with these conditions. It has been proposed that a defect in macrophage function, more specifically an impaired ability to process surfactant, may play a role in the pathogenesis of PAP. This diffuse disease is characterized by the accumulation of an amorphous, periodic acid–Schiff-positive lipoproteinaceous material in the distal air spaces. There is little or no lung inflammation, and the underlying lung architecture is preserved. Mutant mice lacking the gene for granulocyte-macrophage colony-stimulating factor (GM-CSF) have a similar accumulation of surfactant and surfactant apoprotein in the alveolar spaces. Moreover, reconstitution of the respiratory epithelium of GM-CSF knockout mice with the GM-CSF gene completely corrects the alveolar proteinosis. Data from BAL studies in patients suggest that PAP is an autoimmune disease with neutralizing antibody of immunoglobulin G isotype against GM-CSF. These findings suggest that neutralization of GM-CSF bioactivity by the antibody causes dysfunction of alveolar macrophages, which results in reduced surfactant clearance. There are three distinct classes of PAP: acquired (>90% of all cases), congenital, and secondary. *Congenital PAP* is transmitted in an autosomal recessive manner and is caused by homozygosity for a frame shift mutation (121ins2) in the *SP-B* gene, which leads to an unstable SP-B mRNA, reduced protein levels, and *secondary disturbances of SP-C processing. Secondary PAP* is rare among adults and is caused by lysinuric protein intolerance, acute silicosis and other inhalational syndromes, immunodeficiency disorders, and malignancies (almost exclusively of hematopoietic origin) and hematopoietic disorders.

The typical age of presentation is 30–50 years, and males predominate. The clinical presentation is usually insidious and manifested by progressive exertional dyspnea, fatigue, weight loss, and low-grade fever. A nonproductive cough is common, but occasionally expectoration of "chunky" gelatinous material may occur. Polycythemia, hypergammaglobulinemia, and increased LDH levels are frequent. Markedly elevated serum levels of lung surfactant proteins A and D have been found in PAP. Radiographically, bilateral symmetric alveolar opacities located centrally in mid and lower lung zones result in a "bat-wing" distribution. HRCT shows a ground-glass opacification and thickened intralobular structures and interlobular septa. Whole-lung lavage(s) through a double-lumen endotracheal tube provides relief to many patients with dyspnea or progressive hypoxemia and also may provide long-term benefit.

PULMONARY LYMPHANGIOLEIOMYOMATOSIS

Pulmonary LAM is a rare condition that afflicts premenopausal women and should be suspected in young women with "emphysema," recurrent pneumothorax, or chylous pleural effusion. It is often misdiagnosed as asthma or chronic obstructive pulmonary disease. Pathologically, LAM is characterized by the proliferation of atypical pulmonary interstitial smooth muscle and cyst formation. The immature-appearing smooth-muscle cells react with monoclonal antibody HMB45, which recognizes a 100-kDa glycoprotein (gp100) originally found in human melanoma cells. Caucasians are affected much more commonly than members of other racial groups. The disease accelerates during pregnancy and abates after oophorectomy. Common complaints at presentation are dyspnea, cough, and chest pain. Hemoptysis may be life threatening. Spontaneous pneumothorax occurs in 50% of patients; it may be bilateral and necessitate pleurodesis. Meningioma and renal angiomyolipomas (hamartomas), characteristic findings in the genetic disorder tuberous sclerosis, are also common in patients with LAM. Chylothorax, chyloperitoneum (chylous ascites), chyluria, and chylopericardium are other complications. Pulmonary function testing usually reveals an obstructive or mixed obstructive-restrictive pattern, and gas exchange is often abnormal. HRCT shows thin-walled cysts surrounded by normal lung without zonal predominance. Progression is common, with a median survival of 8–10 years from diagnosis. Progesterone (10 mg/d) and luteinizing hormone–releasing hormone analogues have been used. Oophorectomy is no longer recommended and estrogen-containing drugs should be discontinued. Lung transplantation offers the only hope for cure despite reports of recurrent disease in the transplanted lung.

SYNDROMES OF ILD WITH DIFFUSE ALVEOLAR HEMORRHAGE

Injury to arterioles, venules, and the alveolar septal (alveolar wall or interstitial) capillaries can result in hemoptysis secondary to disruption of the alveolar-capillary basement membrane. This results in bleeding into the alveolar spaces, which characterizes DAH. Pulmonary capillaritis, characterized by a neutrophilic infiltration of the alveolar septae, may lead to necrosis of these structures, loss of capillary structural integrity, and the pouring of red blood cells into the alveolar space. Fibrinoid necrosis of the interstitium and red blood cells within the interstitial space are sometimes seen. Bland pulmonary hemorrhage (i.e., DAH without inflammation of the alveolar structures) may also occur.

The clinical onset is often abrupt, with cough, fever, and dyspnea. Severe respiratory distress requiring ventilatory support may be evident at initial presentation. Although hemoptysis is expected, it can be absent at the time of presentation in one-third of the cases. For patients without hemoptysis, new alveolar opacities, a falling hemoglobin level, and hemorrhagic BAL fluid point to the diagnosis. The chest radiograph is non-specific and most commonly shows new patchy or diffuse alveolar opacities. Recurrent episodes of DAH may lead to pulmonary fibrosis, resulting in interstitial opacities on the chest radiograph. An elevated white blood cell count and falling hematocrit are frequent. Evidence for impaired renal function caused by focal segmental necrotizing glomerulonephritis, usually with crescent formation, may also be present.

Varying degrees of hypoxemia may occur and are often severe enough to require ventilatory support. The $D_{L_{CO}}$ may be increased, resulting from the increased hemoglobin within the alveoli compartment. Evaluation of either lung or renal tissue by immunofluorescent techniques indicates an absence of immune complexes (pauci-immune) in Wegener's granulomatosis, microscopic polyangiitis pauci-immune glomerulonephritis, and isolated pulmonary capillaritis. A granular pattern is found in the CTDs, particularly SLE, and a characteristic linear deposition is found in Goodpasture's syndrome. Granular deposition of IgA-containing immune complexes is present in Henoch-Schönlein purpura.

The mainstay of therapy for the DAH associated with systemic vasculitis, CTD, Goodpasture's syndrome, and isolated pulmonary capillaritis is IV methylprednisolone, 0.5–2.0 g daily in divided doses for up to 5 days, followed by a gradual tapering, and then maintenance on an oral preparation. Prompt initiation of therapy is important, particularly in the face of renal insufficiency, since early initiation of therapy has the best chance of preserving renal function. The decision to start other immunosuppressive therapy (cyclophosphamide or azathioprine) acutely depends on the severity of illness.

Goodpasture's Syndrome   Pulmonary hemorrhage and glomerulonephritis are features in most patients with this disease. Autoantibodies to renal glomerular and lung alveolar basement membranes are present. This syndrome can present and recur as DAH without an associated glomerulonephritis. In such case, circulating anti-basement membrane antibody is often absent, and the only way to establish the diagnosis is by demonstrating linear immunofluorescence in lung tissue. The underlying histology may be bland hemorrhage or DAH associated with capillaritis. Plasmapheresis has been recommended as adjunctive treatment.

INHERITED DISORDERS ASSOCIATED WITH ILD

Pulmonary opacities and respiratory symptoms typical of ILD can develop in related family members and in several inherited diseases. These include the phakomatoses, tuberous sclerosis and neurofibromatosis (Chap. 374), and the lysosomal storage diseases, Niemann-Pick disease and Gaucher's disease (Chap. 355). The Hermansky-Pudlak syndrome is an autosomal recessive disorder in which granulomatous colitis and ILD may occur. It is characterized by oculocutaneous albinism, bleeding diathesis secondary to platelet dysfunction, and the accumulation of a chromolipid, lipofuscin material in cells of the reticuloendothelial system. A fibrotic pattern is found on lung biopsy, but the alveolar macrophages may contain cytoplasmic ceroid-like inclusions.

ILD WITH A GRANULOMATOUS RESPONSE IN LUNG TISSUE OR VASCULAR STRUCTURES

Inhalation of organic dusts, which cause hypersensitivity pneumonitis, or of inorganic dust, such as silica, which elicits a granulomatous inflammatory reaction leading to ILD, produces diseases of known etiology (Table 255-1) that are discussed in Chaps. 249 and 250. Sarcoidosis (Chap. 322) is prominent among granulomatous diseases of unknown cause in which ILD is an important feature.

Granulomatous Vasculitides   (See also Chap. 319) The granulomatous vasculitides are characterized by pulmonary angiitis (i.e., inflammation and necrosis of blood vessels) with associated granuloma formation (i.e., infiltrates of lymphocytes, plasma cells, epithelioid cells, or histiocytes, with or without the presence of multinucleated giant cells, sometimes with tissue necrosis). The lungs are almost always involved, although any organ system may be affected. Wegener's granulomatosis and allergic angiitis and granulomatosis (Churg-Strauss syndrome) primarily affect the lung but are associated with a systemic vasculitis as well. The granulomatous vasculitides generally limited to the lung include necrotizing sarcoid granulomatosis and benign lymphocytic angiitis and granulomatosis. Granulomatous infection and pulmonary angiitis due to irritating embolic material (e.g., talc) are important known causes of pulmonary vasculitis.

LYMPHOCYTIC INFILTRATIVE DISORDERS

This group of disorders features lymphocyte and plasma cell infiltration of the lung parenchyma. The disorders either are benign or can behave as low-grade lymphomas. Included are angioimmunoblastic lymphadenopathy with dysproteinemia, a rare lymphoproliferative disorder characterized by diffuse lymphadenopathy, fever, hepatosplenomegaly, and hemolytic anemia, with ILD in some cases.

Lymphocytic Interstitial Pneumonitis   This rare form of ILD occurs in adults, some of whom have an autoimmune disease or dysproteinemia. It has been reported in patients with Sjögren's syndrome and HIV infection.

Lymphomatoid Granulomatosis   This multisystem disorder of unknown etiology is an angiocentric malignant (T cell) lymphoma characterized by a polymorphic lymphoid infiltrate, an angiitis, and granulomatosis. Although it may affect virtually any organ, it is most frequently characterized by pulmonary, skin, and central nervous system involvement.

BRONCHOCENTRIC GRANULOMATOSIS

Rather than a specific clinical entity, bronchocentric granulomatosis (BG) is a descriptive histologic term that describes an uncommon and nonspecific pathologic response to a variety of airway injuries. There is evidence that BG is caused by a hypersensitivity reaction to *Aspergillus* or other fungi in patients with asthma. About half of the patients described have chronic asthma with severe wheezing and peripheral blood eosinophilia. In patients with asthma, BG probably represents one pathologic manifestation of allergic bronchopulmonary aspergillosis or another allergic mycosis. In patients without asthma, BG has been associated with RA and a variety of infections, including tuberculosis, echinococcosis, histoplasmosis, coccidioidomycosis, and nocardiosis. The chest roentgenogram reveals irregularly shaped nodular or mass lesions with ill-defined margins, which are usually unilateral and solitary, with upper-lobe predominance. Glucocorticoids are the treatment of choice, often with excellent outcome, although recurrences may occur as therapy is tapered or stopped.

GLOBAL CONSIDERATIONS

Limited epidemiologic data exists describing the prevalence or incidence of ILD in the general population. With a few exceptions, e.g., sarcoidosis, certain occupational and environmental exposures, there appear to be no significant differences in the prevalence or incidence of ILD among various populations. For sarcoidosis, there are important environmental, racial, and genetic differences (Chap. 322).

FURTHER READINGS

AMERICAN THORACIC SOCIETY/EUROPEAN RESPIRATORY SOCIETY: Idiopathic pulmonary fibrosis: Diagnosis and treatment. International consensus statement. Am J Respir Crit Care Med 161:646, 2000

————: International multidisciplinary consensus classification of the idiopathic interstitial pneumonias. Am J Respir Crit Care Med 165:277, 2002

EL-ZAMMAR OA, KATZENSTEIN AL: Pathological diagnosis of granulomatous lung disease: A review. Histopathology 50:289, 2007

FREEMER M, KING TE JR: Connective tissue disease, in *Interstitial Lung Diseases*, 4th ed, MI Schwarz, TE King, Jr (eds). Hamilton, Ontario, BC Decker, 2003, pp 535–598

KING TE JR: Clinical advances in the diagnosis and therapy of the interstitial lung diseases. Am J Respir Crit Care Med 172:268, 2005

MARTINEZ FJ: Idiopathic interstitial pneumonias: Usual interstitial pneumonia versus nonspecific interstitial pneumonia. Proc Am Thorac Soc 3:81, 2006

SELMAN M et al: Idiopathic pulmonary fibrosis: Prevailing and evolving hypotheses about its pathogenesis and implications for therapy. Ann Intern Med 134:136, 2001

SEYMOUR JF, PRESNEILL JJ: Pulmonary alveolar proteinosis: Progress in the first 44 years. Am J Respir Crit Care Med 166:215, 2002

WALTER N et al: Current perspectives on the treatment of pulmonary fibrosis. Proc Am Thorac Soc 3:330, 2006

256 Deep Venous Thrombosis and Pulmonary Thromboembolism
Samuel Z. Goldhaber

EPIDEMIOLOGY

A quiet revolution has occurred in the field of venous thromboembolism (VTE), which encompasses deep venous thrombosis (DVT) and pulmonary embolism (PE). VTE is no longer an orphan disease. Its adverse public health impact has been acknowledged in the United States by the National Quality Forum, the Joint Commission for Accreditation of Hospitals, the National Comprehensive Cancer Network, and the Surgeon General's Office. Public service announcements have educated laypersons on the definition and medical consequences of DVT and PE, along with risk factors and warning signs. VTE-related deaths in the United States are estimated at 300,000 annually: 7% diagnosed with VTE and treated, 34% sudden fatal PE, and 59% as undetected PE. Approximately two-thirds of symptomatic VTE events are hospital acquired, and the remainder are community acquired. Residents of skilled nursing facilities are especially vulnerable. The most recent estimates of hospitalized patients at risk for VTE in the United States total 13.4 million (M) patients annually: 5.8 M surgical patients at moderate–high risk and 7.6 M medical patients with comorbidities such as heart failure, cancer, and stroke. These new data provide the rationale for changing the prophylaxis paradigm from voluntary to mandatory compliance with guidelines to prevent VTE among hospitalized patients.

VTE is also a major European health problem, with an estimated 370,000 per year PE-related deaths, when data in France, Germany, Spain, Italy, Sweden, and the United Kingdom are combined. The estimated direct cost for VTE-associated care in Europe exceeds 3 billion euros per year.

Though DVT and PE encompass one disease entity, VTE, there are important differences. DVT occurs about 3 times more often than PE. The major adverse outcome of DVT alone, without PE, is the development of *postphlebitic syndrome*, which occurs in more than half of patients with DVT. Postphlebitic syndrome is a late adverse effect of DVT that is caused by permanent damage to the venous valves of the leg, which become incompetent and permit abnormal exudation of interstitial fluid from the venous system. It may not become clinically manifest until several years after the initial DVT. There is no effective medical therapy for this condition, which impairs quality of life and disables. Most patients describe chronic ankle swelling and calf swelling and aching, especially after prolonged standing. In its most severe form, postphlebitic syndrome causes skin ulceration, especially in the medial malleolus of the leg. PE can be fatal or can cause chronic thromboembolic pulmonary hypertension, with breathlessness at rest or with mild exertion. Patients with PE are more likely to suffer recurrent VTE than patients with DVT alone.

Genetic and acquired factors contribute to the likelihood of VTE. The two most common autosomal dominant genetic mutations are the factor V Leiden and the prothrombin gene mutations (Chap. 59). However, only a minority of patients with VTE have identifiable predisposing genetic factors. The majority of patients with predisposing genetic factors will not develop clinical evidence of clotting. Acquired predispositions include long-haul air travel, obesity, cigarette smoking, oral contraceptives, pregnancy, postmenopausal hormone replacement, surgery, trauma, and medical conditions such as antiphospholipid antibody syndrome, cancer, systemic arterial hypertension, and chronic obstructive pulmonary disease. Thrombophilia contributes to the risk of venous thrombosis, often due to an inherited risk factor in combination with an acquired predisposition.

PATHOPHYSIOLOGY

Embolization When venous thrombi dislodge from their site of formation, they embolize to the pulmonary arterial circulation or, paradoxically, to the arterial circulation through a patent foramen ovale or atrial septal defect. About half of patients with pelvic vein thrombosis or proximal leg DVT develop PE, which is usually asymptomatic. Isolated calf vein thrombi pose a much lower risk of PE, but they are the most common source of paradoxical embolism. These tiny thrombi can cross a small patent foramen ovale or atrial septal defect, unlike larger, more proximal leg thrombi. With increased use of chronic indwelling central venous catheters for hyperalimentation and chemotherapy, as well as more frequent insertion of permanent pacemakers and internal cardiac defibrillators, upper extremity venous thrombosis is becoming a more common problem. These thrombi rarely embolize and cause PE.

Physiology The most common gas exchange abnormalities are hypoxemia (decreased arterial P_{O_2}) and an increased alveolar-arterial O_2 tension gradient, which represents the inefficiency of O_2 transfer across the lungs. Anatomic dead space increases because breathed gas does not enter gas exchange units of the lung. Physiologic dead space increases because ventilation to gas exchange units exceeds venous blood flow through the pulmonary capillaries.

Other pathophysiological abnormalities include:

1. *Increased pulmonary vascular resistance* due to vascular obstruction or platelet secretion of vasoconstricting neurohumoral agents such

as serotonin. Release of vasoactive mediators can produce ventilation-perfusion mismatching at sites remote from the embolus, thereby accounting for a potential discordance between a small PE and a large alveolar-arterial O_2 gradient.

2. *Impaired gas exchange* due to increased alveolar dead space from vascular obstruction, hypoxemia from alveolar hypoventilation relative to perfusion in the nonobstructed lung, right-to-left shunting, and impaired carbon monoxide transfer due to loss of gas exchange surface.

3. *Alveolar hyperventilation* due to reflex stimulation of irritant receptors

4. *Increased airway resistance* due to constriction of airways distal to the bronchi

5. *Decreased pulmonary compliance* due to lung edema, lung hemorrhage, or loss of surfactant

Right Ventricular (RV) Dysfunction Progressive right heart failure is the usual cause of death from PE. In the International Cooperative Pulmonary Embolism Registry (ICOPER), the presence of RV dysfunction on baseline echocardiography of PE patients who presented with a systolic blood pressure >90 mmHg was associated with a doubling of the 3-month mortality rate. As pulmonary vascular resistance increases, RV wall tension rises and causes further RV dilatation and dysfunction. RV contraction continues even after the left ventricle (LV) starts relaxing at end-systole. Consequently, the interventricular septum bulges into and compresses an intrinsically normal left ventricle. Diastolic LV impairment develops, attributable to septal displacement, and results in reduced LV distensibility and impaired LV filling during diastole. Increased RV wall tension also compresses the right coronary artery, diminishes subendocardial perfusion, limits myocardial oxygen supply, and may precipitate myocardial ischemia and RV infarction. Underfilling of the LV may lead to a fall in left ventricular cardiac output and systemic arterial pressure, thereby provoking myocardial ischemia due to compromised coronary artery perfusion. Eventually, circulatory collapse and death may ensue.

DIAGNOSIS
Clinical Evaluation The diagnosis is challenging because symptoms and signs are nonspecific. VTE mimics other illnesses, and PE is known as "The Great Masquerader."

For patients who have DVT, the most frequent history is a cramp in the lower calf that persists for several days and that becomes more uncomfortable as time progresses. For patients who have PE, the most frequent history is unexplained breathlessness.

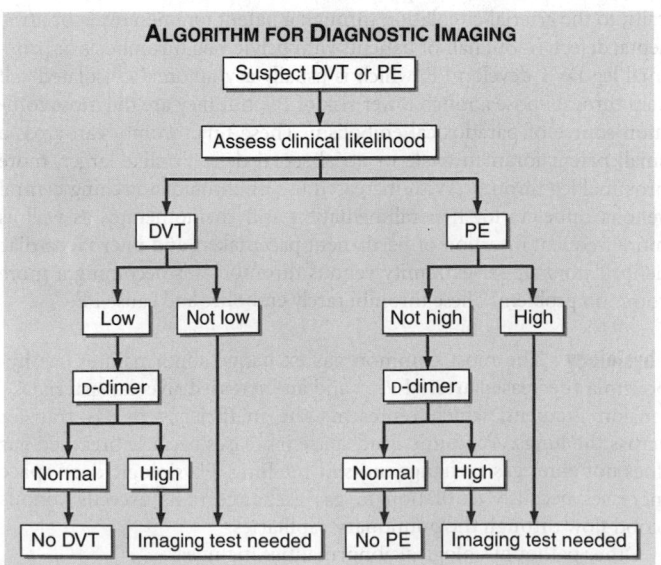

FIGURE 256-1 How to decide whether diagnostic imaging is needed. For assessment of clinical likelihood, see Table 256-1.

TABLE 256-1	CLINICAL DECISION RULES

Low Clinical Likelihood of DVT If the Point Score Is Zero or Less

Clinical Variable	Score
Active cancer	1
Paralysis, paresis, or recent cast	1
Bedridden for >3 days; major surgery <12 weeks	1
Tenderness along distribution of deep veins	1
Entire leg swelling	1
Unilateral calf swelling >3 cm	1
Pitting edema	1
Collateral superficial nonvaricose veins	1
Alternative diagnosis at least as likely as DVT	−2

High Clinical Likelihood of PE if the Point Score Exceeds 4

Clinical Variable	Score
Signs and symptoms of DVT	3.0
Alternative diagnosis less likely than PE	3.0
Heart rate >100/min	1.5
Immobilization >3 days; surgery within 4 weeks	1.5
Prior PE or DVT	1.5
Hemoptysis	1.0
Cancer	1.0

When evaluating patients with possible DVT, the initial task is to decide whether the clinical likelihood for DVT is low. When evaluating possible PE, the initial task is to decide whether the clinical likelihood is high. Patients with low likelihood of DVT or non-high (i.e., low/moderate) likelihood of PE can undergo initial diagnostic evaluation with D-dimer testing alone (see below) without obligatory imaging tests (Fig. 256-1).

Point score methods are useful for estimating the clinical likelihood of DVT and PE (Table 256-1).

Clinical Syndromes The differential diagnosis is critical because not all leg pain is due to DVT and not all dyspnea is due to PE (Table 256-2). Sudden, severe calf discomfort suggests a ruptured Baker's cyst. Fever and chills usually herald cellulitis rather than DVT, though DVT may be present concomitantly. Physical findings, if present at all, may simply consist of mild palpation discomfort in the lower calf. Massive DVT is much easier to recognize. The patient presents with severe thigh swelling and marked tenderness when palpating the inguinal area and common femoral vein. In extreme cases, patients will be unable to walk or may require a cane, crutches, or walker.

If the leg is diffusely edematous, DVT is unlikely. Much more common is an acute exacerbation of venous insufficiency due to postphlebitic syndrome. Upper extremity venous thrombosis may present with asymmetry in the supraclavicular fossa or in the circumference of the upper arms. A prominent superficial venous pattern may be evident on the anterior chest wall.

Patients with *massive PE* present with systemic arterial hypotension and usually have anatomically widespread thromboembolism. Those with *moderate to large PE* have RV hypokinesis on echocardiography but normal systemic arterial pressure. Patients with *small to moderate PE*

TABLE 256-2	DIFFERENTIAL DIAGNOSIS

DVT
  Ruptured Baker's cyst
  Cellulitis
  Postphlebitic syndrome/venous insufficiency
PE
  Pneumonia, asthma, chronic obstructive pulmonary disease
  Congestive heart failure
  Pericarditis
  Pleurisy: "viral syndrome," costochondritis, musculoskeletal discomfort
  Rib fracture, pneumothorax
  Acute coronary syndrome
  Anxiety

have both normal right heart function and normal systemic arterial pressure. They have an excellent prognosis with adequate anticoagulation.

The presence of *pulmonary infarction* usually indicates a small PE, but one that is exquisitely painful, because it lodges peripherally, near the innervation of pleural nerves. Pleuritic chest pain is more common with small, peripheral emboli. However, larger, more central PEs can occur concomitantly with peripheral pulmonary infarction.

Nonthrombotic PE may be easily overlooked. Possible etiologies include fat embolism after blunt trauma and long bone fractures, tumor embolism, bone marrow, or air embolism. Cement embolism and bony fragment embolism can occur after total hip or knee replacement. Intravenous drug users may inject themselves with a wide array of substances, such as hair, talc, or cotton. *Amniotic fluid embolism* occurs when fetal membranes leak or tear at the placental margin. Pulmonary edema in this syndrome is probably due to alveolar capillary leakage.

Dyspnea is the most frequent symptom of PE, and tachypnea is its most frequent sign. Whereas dyspnea, syncope, hypotension, or cyanosis indicates a massive PE, pleuritic pain, cough, or hemoptysis often suggests a small embolism located distally near the pleura. On physical examination, young and previously healthy individuals may appear anxious but otherwise seem deceptively well, even with an anatomically large PE. They may only have dyspnea with moderate exertion. They often lack "classic" signs such as tachycardia, low-grade fever, neck vein distension, or an accentuated pulmonic component of the second heart sound. Sometimes paradoxical bradycardia occurs.

Some patients have occult PE and an overt coexisting illness such as pneumonia or heart failure. In such circumstances, clinical improvement often fails to occur despite standard medical treatment of the concomitant illness. This situation can serve as a clinical clue to the possible coexistence of PE.

Nonimaging Diagnostic Modalities Nonimaging tests are best utilized in combination with clinical likelihood of DVT or PE (Fig. 256-1).

BLOOD TESTS The quantitative *plasma D-dimer enzyme-linked immunosorbent assay (ELISA)* rises in the presence of DVT or PE because of plasmin's breakdown of fibrin. Elevation of D-dimer indicates endogenous although often clinically ineffective thrombolysis. The sensitivity of the D-dimer is greater than 80% for DVT (including isolated calf DVT) and greater than 95% for PE. The D-dimer is less sensitive for DVT than PE because the DVT thrombus size is smaller. The D-dimer is a useful "rule out" test. It is normal (<500 ng/mL) in more than 95% of patients without PE. In patients with low clinical suspicion of DVT, it is normal in more than 90% without DVT.

The D-dimer assay is not specific. Levels increase in patients with myocardial infarction, pneumonia, sepsis, cancer, the postoperative state, and second or third trimester of pregnancy. Therefore, it rarely has a useful role among hospitalized patients because their D-dimers are frequently elevated due to some systemic illness.

Contrary to classic teaching, *arterial blood gases* lack diagnostic utility for PE, even though both the P_{O_2} and P_{CO_2} often decrease. Among patients suspected of PE, neither the room air arterial P_{O_2} nor calculation of the alveolar-arterial O_2 gradient can reliably differentiate or triage patients who actually have PE at angiography.

ELEVATED CARDIAC BIOMARKERS Serum troponin levels increase in RV microinfarction. Myocardial stretch often results in elevation of brain natriuretic peptide or NT-pro-brain natriuretic peptide. Elevated cardiac biomarkers predict an increase in major complications and mortality from PE.

ELECTROCARDIOGRAM The most cited abnormality, in addition to sinus tachycardia, is the S1Q3T3 sign: an S wave in lead I, Q wave in lead III, and inverted T wave in lead III (Chap. 221). This finding is relatively specific but insensitive. Perhaps the most frequent abnormality is T-wave inversion in leads V_1 to V_4.

TABLE 256-3	ULTRASONOGRAPHY OF THE DEEP LEG VEINS

Criteria for Establishing the Diagnosis of Acute DVT

Lack of vein compressibility (the principal criterion)
Vein does not "wink" when gently compressed in cross-section
Failure to appose the walls of the vein due to passive distension

Direct Visualization of Thrombus

Homogenous
Low echogenicity

Abnormal Doppler Flow Dynamics

Normal response: calf compression augments Doppler flow signal and confirms vein patency proximal and distal to Doppler
Abnormal response: flow blunted rather than augmented with calf compression

Noninvasive Imaging Modalities • *VENOUS ULTRASONOGRAPHY*
Ultrasonography of the deep venous system (Table 256-3) relies upon loss of vein compressibility as the primary criterion for DVT. When a normal vein is imaged in cross-section, it readily collapses with gentle manual pressure from the ultrasound transducer. This creates the illusion of a "wink." With acute DVT, the vein loses its compressibility because of passive distension by acute thrombus. The diagnosis of acute DVT is even more secure when thrombus is directly visualized. It appears homogeneous and has low echogenicity (Fig. 256-2). The vein itself often appears mildly dilated, and collateral channels may be absent.

Venous flow dynamics can be examined with Doppler imaging. Normally, manual calf compression causes augmentation of the Doppler flow pattern. Loss of normal respiratory variation is caused by obstructing DVT or by any obstructive process within the pelvis. Because DVT and PE are so closely related and are both treated with anticoagulation (see below), confirmed DVT is usually an adequate surrogate for PE. In contrast, a normal venous ultrasound does not exclude PE. The majority of patients with PE have no imaging evidence of DVT, probably because the clot has already embolized to the lung or is in the pelvic veins, where ultrasonography is usually inadequate. In patients without DVT, the ultrasound examination may identify other reasons for leg discomfort such as a Baker's cyst (also known as a popliteal or synovial cyst) or a hematoma. For patients with a technically poor or nondiagnostic venous ultrasound, consider alternative imaging modalities for DVT such as CT or magnetic resonance imaging.

FIGURE 256-2 Acute DVT on venous ultrasound examination. The vein is not compressible and thrombus (*far left arrow*) is visualized directly in the deep venous system. SFV, superficial femoral vein (which is a deep vein, despite the terminology "superficial"); DFV, deep femoral vein (synonymous with profunda femoral vein). (*From the personal collection of Samuel Z. Goldhaber, MD; with permission.*)

CHEST ROENTGENOGRAPHY A normal or near-normal chest x-ray in a dyspneic patient often occurs in PE. Well-established abnormalities include focal oligemia (Westermark's sign), a peripheral wedged-shaped density above the diaphragm (Hampton's hump), or an enlarged right descending pulmonary artery (Palla's sign).

CHEST CT Computed tomography (CT) of the chest with intravenous contrast is the principal imaging test for the diagnosis of PE (Fig. 256-3). Multidetector-row spiral CT acquires all chest images with ≤1 mm resolution during a short breath hold. This generation of CT scanners can image small peripheral emboli. Sixth-order branches can be visualized with resolution superior to conventional invasive contrast pulmonary angiography. The CT scan also obtains excellent images of the RV and LV and can be used for a risk stratification as well as a diagnostic tool. In patients with PE, RV enlargement on chest CT indicates a fivefold increased likelihood of death within the next 30 days compared with PE patients with normal RV size on chest CT. When imaging is continued below the chest to the knee, pelvic and proximal leg DVT can also be diagnosed by CT scanning. In patients without PE, the lung parenchymal images may establish alternative diagnoses not apparent on chest x-ray that explain the presenting symptoms and signs, such as pneumonia, emphysema, pulmonary fibrosis, pulmonary mass, or aortic pathology. Sometimes asymptomatic early stage lung cancer is diagnosed incidentally.

LUNG SCANNING Lung scanning is now a second-line diagnostic test for PE. It is mostly used for patients who cannot tolerate intravenous contrast. Small particulate aggregates of albumin labeled with a gamma-emitting radionuclide are injected intravenously and are trapped in the pulmonary capillary bed. The perfusion scan defect indicates absent or decreased blood flow, possibly due to PE. Ventilation scans, obtained with radiolabeled inhaled gases such as xenon or krypton, improve the specificity of the perfusion scan. Abnormal ventilation scans indicate abnormal nonventilated lung, thereby providing possible explanations for perfusion defects other than acute PE, such as asthma or chronic obstructive pulmonary disease. A high probability scan for PE is defined as having two or more segmental perfusion defects in the presence of normal ventilation.

The diagnosis of PE is very unlikely in patients with normal and near-normal scans but is about 90% certain in patients with high-probability scans. Unfortunately, most patients have nondiagnostic scans, and fewer than half of patients with angiographically confirmed PE have a high-probability scan. As many as 40% of patients with high clinical suspicion for PE and "low-probability" scans do, in fact, have PE at angiography.

MAGNETIC RESONANCE (MR) (CONTRAST-ENHANCED) When ultrasound is equivocal, MR venography is an excellent imaging modality to diagnose DVT. MR utilizes gadolinium contrast agent, which, unlike iodinated contrast agents used in venography or CT angiography, is not nephrotoxic. MR imaging should be considered for suspected DVT or PE patients with renal insufficiency or contrast dye allergy. MR pulmonary angiography detects large proximal PE but is not reliable for smaller segmental and subsegmental PE.

ECHOCARDIOGRAPHY Echocardiography is *not* a reliable diagnostic imaging tool for acute PE because most patients with PE have normal echocardiograms. However, echocardiography is a very useful diagnostic tool for detecting conditions that might mimic PE, such as acute myocardial infarction, pericardial tamponade, or aortic dissection.

Transthoracic echocardiography rarely images thrombus directly. The best-known indirect sign of PE on transthoracic echocardiography is McConnell's sign, hypokinesis of the RV free wall with normal motion of the RV apex.

Transesophageal echocardiography should be considered when CT scanning facilities are not available or when a patient has renal failure or severe contrast allergy that precludes administration of contrast despite premedication with high dose steroids. This imaging modality can directly visualize large proximal PE.

Invasive Diagnostic Modalities · PULMONARY ANGIOGRAPHY Chest CT with contrast (see above) has virtually replaced invasive pulmonary angiography as a diagnostic test. Invasive catheter-based diagnostic testing is reserved for patients with technically unsatisfactory chest CTs or for those in whom an interventional procedure such as catheter-directed thrombolysis or embolectomy is planned. A definitive diagnosis of PE depends upon visualization of an intraluminal filling defect in more than one projection. Secondary signs of PE include abrupt occlusion ("cut-off") of vessels, segmental oligemia or avascularity, a prolonged arterial phase with slow filling, or tortuous, tapering peripheral vessels.

CONTRAST PHLEBOGRAPHY Venous ultrasonography has virtually replaced contrast phlebography as the diagnostic test for suspected DVT.

Integrated Diagnostic Approach An integrated diagnostic approach (Fig. 256-1) streamlines the workup of suspected DVT and PE (Fig. 256-4).

℞ DEEP VENOUS THROMBOSIS

PRIMARY THERAPY VERSUS SECONDARY PREVENTION *Primary therapy* consists of clot dissolution with thrombolysis or removal of PE by embolectomy. Anticoagulation with heparin and warfarin or placement of an inferior vena caval filter constitutes *secondary prevention* of recurrent PE rather than primary therapy.

RISK STRATIFICATION Rapid and accurate risk stratification is critical in determining optimal treatment strategy. The presence of hemodynamic instability, RV dysfunction, or elevation of the troponin level due to RV microinfarction can identify high-risk patients. Detection of RV hypokinesis on echocardiography is the most widely used approach to risk stratification. However, RV enlargement on chest CT also predicts an increased mortality rate from PE. The combination of RV dysfunction plus elevated biomarkers such as troponin portends an especially ominous prognosis.

Primary therapy should be reserved for patients at high risk of an adverse clinical outcome. When RV function remains normal in a hemodynamically stable patient, a good clinical outcome is highly likely with anticoagulation alone (Fig. 256-5).

FIGURE 256-3 Large bilateral proximal PE on chest CT following radical prostatectomy.

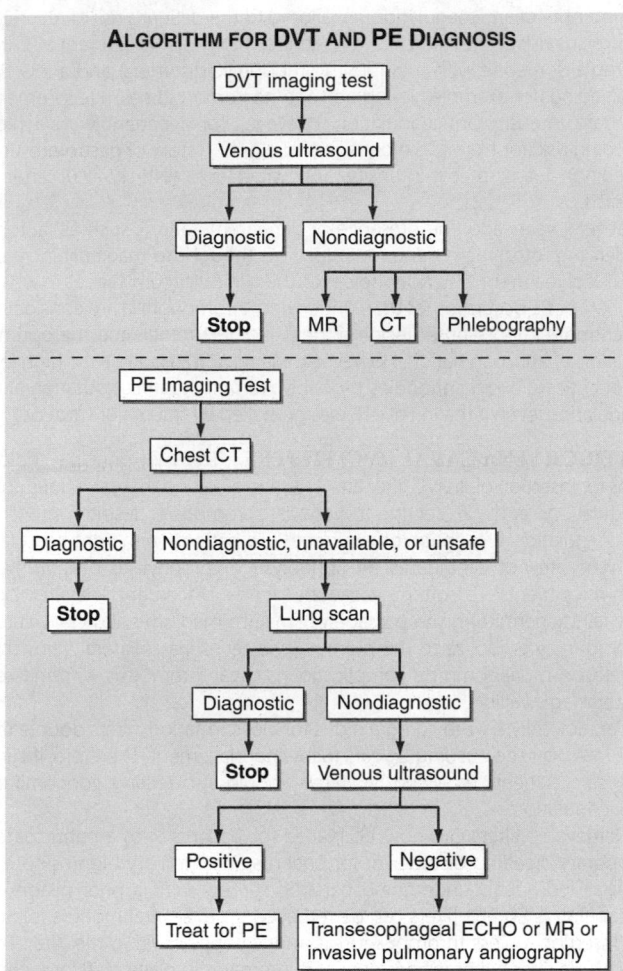

ALGORITHM FOR DVT AND PE DIAGNOSIS

DVT imaging test
↓
Venous ultrasound
↓
- Diagnostic → **Stop**
- Nondiagnostic → MR | CT | Phlebography

- - - - - - - - - - - - - - - -

PE Imaging Test
↓
Chest CT
- Diagnostic → **Stop**
- Nondiagnostic, unavailable, or unsafe
  ↓
  Lung scan
  - Diagnostic → **Stop**
  - Nondiagnostic
    ↓
    Venous ultrasound
    - Positive → Treat for PE
    - Negative → Transesophageal ECHO or MR or invasive pulmonary angiography

FIGURE 256-4 Imaging tests to diagnose DVT and PE.

Rx MASSIVE PULMONARY EMBOLISM

ANTICOAGULATION   Anticoagulation is the foundation for successful treatment of DVT and PE **(Table 256-4)**. Immediately effective anticoagulation is initiated with a parenteral drug: unfractionated heparin (UFH), low molecular weight heparin (LMWH), or fondaparinux. These parenteral drugs (see below) are continued as a transition or "bridge" to stable, long-term anticoagulation with a vitamin K antagonist (exclusively warfarin in the United States). The first dose of warfarin may be given as soon as several hours after the bridging anticoagulant if LMWH or fondaparinux are used. Otherwise, with UFH a therapeutic aPTT must first be documented. Warfarin requires 5–7 days to achieve a therapeutic effect. During that period, the parenteral and oral agents are overlapped. After 5–7 days of anticoagulation, residual thrombus begins to become endothelialized in the vein or pulmonary artery. However, anticoagulants do *not* directly dissolve thrombus that already exists.

ALGORITHM FOR PE MANAGEMENT

Risk stratify
- Normotension plus normal RV → Secondary prevention → Anticoagulation alone | IVC filter
- Normotension plus RV hypokinesis → Individualize therapy → Anticoagulation plus thrombolysis
- Hypotension → Primary therapy → Embolectomy: Catheter/surgical

FIGURE 256-5 Acute management of pulmonary thromboembolism. RV, right ventricular; IVC, inferior vena cava.

TABLE 256-4   ANTICOAGULATION OF VTE
Immediate Parenteral Anticoagulation
Unfractionated heparin, bolus and continuous infusion, to achieve aPTT 2–3 times the upper limit of the laboratory normal, or
Enoxaparin 1 mg/kg twice daily with normal renal function, or
Tinzaparin 175 units/kg once daily with normal renal function, or
Fondaparinux weight based once daily; adjust for impaired renal function
Warfarin Anticoagulation
Usual start dose is 5–10 mg.
Titrate to INR, target 2.0–3.0.
Continue parenteral anticoagulation for a minimum of 5 days and until 2 sequential INR values, at least 1 day apart, return in the target range.

Unfractionated Heparin   Unfractionated heparin (UFH) anticoagulates by binding to and accelerating the activity of antithrombin III, thus preventing additional thrombus formation and permitting endogenous fibrinolytic mechanisms to lyse clot that has already formed. UFH is dosed to achieve a target activated partial thromboplastin time (aPTT) that is 2–3 times the upper limit of the laboratory normal. This is usually equivalent to an aPTT of 60–80 s. For UFH, a typical intravenous bolus is 5000–10,000 units followed by a continuous infusion of 1000–1500 units/h. Nomograms based upon a patient's weight may assist in adjusting the dose of heparin. The most popular nomogram utilizes an initial bolus of 80 units/kg, followed by an initial infusion rate of 18 units/kg per hour.

The major advantage of UFH is that it has a short half-life. Its anticoagulant effect abates after several hours. This is especially useful if the patient will undergo an invasive procedure such as surgical embolectomy.

The major disadvantage of UFH is that achieving the target aPTT can be difficult and may require repeated blood sampling and heparin dose adjustment every 4–6 h. Furthermore, by using UFH, patients are at risk of developing heparin-induced thrombocytopenia.

Low Molecular Weight Heparins   These fragments of UFH exhibit less binding to plasma proteins and endothelial cells and consequently have greater bioavailability, a more predictable dose response, and a longer half-life than UFH. No monitoring or dose adjustment is needed unless the patient is markedly obese or has renal insufficiency.

Enoxaparin 1 mg/kg twice daily and *tinzaparin* 175 units/kg once daily have received U.S. Food and Drug Administration (FDA) approval for treatment of patients who present with DVT. The weight-adjusted doses must be adjusted downward in renal insufficiency because the kidneys excrete LMWH.

Fondaparinux   Fondaparinux, an anti-Xa pentasaccharide, is administered by once-daily subcutaneous injection and has been approved by the FDA to treat DVT and PE. No laboratory monitoring is required. Patients weighing <50 kg receive 5 mg, 50–100 kg patients receive 7.5 mg, and patients weighing >100 kg receive 10 mg. The dose must be adjusted downward for patients with renal dysfunction because the drug is excreted by the kidneys.

Warfarin   This vitamin K antagonist prevents carboxylation activation of coagulation factors II, VII, IX, and X. The full effect of warfarin requires at least 5 days, even if the prothrombin time, used for monitoring, becomes elevated more rapidly. If warfarin is initiated as monotherapy during an acute thrombotic illness, a paradoxical exacerbation of hypercoagulability can increase the likelihood of thrombosis rather than prevent it. Overlapping UFH, LMWH, or fondaparinux with warfarin for at least 5 days can counteract the early procoagulant effect of unopposed warfarin.

Dosing   In an average-sized adult, warfarin is usually initiated in a dose of 5 mg. Doses of 7.5 or 10 mg can be used in obese or large-framed young patients who are otherwise healthy. Patients who are malnourished or who have received prolonged courses of antibiotics are probably deficient in vitamin K and should receive smaller initial doses of warfarin, such as 2.5 mg. The prothrombin time is standardized with the INR, which assesses the anticoagulant effect of warfarin (Chap. 59). The target INR is usually 2.5, with a range of 2.0–3.0.

The warfarin dose is titrated to achieve the target INR. Proper dosing is difficult because hundreds of drug-drug and drug-food interactions affect warfarin metabolism. Furthermore, variables such as increasing age and comorbidities such as systemic illness, malabsorption, and diarrhea reduce the warfarin-dosing requirement.

No reliable nomogram has been established to predict how individual patients will respond to warfarin. Therefore, dosing is adjusted according to an "educated guess." Centralized anticoagulation clinics have improved the efficacy and safety of warfarin dosing. Based upon a meta-analysis of trials comparing anticoagulation clinic care versus self-monitoring, patients benefit if they can self-monitor their INR with a home point-of-care fingerstick machine. The subgroup with the best results also learns to self-adjust warfarin doses.

Pharmacogenomics may provide the gateway to rational dosing of warfarin. A recent discovery is that five polymorphisms of the vitamin K receptor gene explain 25% of the variance in warfarin dosing. These polymorphisms can stratify patients into low, intermediate, and high-dose warfarin groups. An additional 10% of dosing variance can be explained by allelic variants of the cytochrome P-450 enzyme 2C9. These mutations decrease warfarin dosing because they impair the metabolism of the S-enantiomer of warfarin. In the future, if rapid turnaround of genetic testing becomes possible, warfarin could be dosed according to specific pharmacogenomic profiles.

Complications of Anticoagulants The most important adverse effect of anticoagulation is hemorrhage. For life-threatening or intracranial hemorrhage due to heparin or LMWH, protamine sulfate can be administered. There is no specific antidote for bleeding from fondaparinux.

Major bleeding from warfarin is traditionally managed with cryoprecipitate or fresh-frozen plasma (usually 2–4 units) to achieve rapid hemostasis. Recombinant human coagulation factor VIIa (rFVIIa), FDA-approved for bleeding in hemophiliacs, is widely used off-label to manage catastrophic bleeding from warfarin. The optimal dose appears to be 40 mcg/kg. The greatest risk of this therapy is rebound thromboembolism. For minor bleeding, or to manage an excessively high INR in the absence of bleeding, a small 2.5 mg dose of oral vitamin K may be administered.

Heparin-induced thrombocytopenia (HIT) and osteopenia are far less common with LMWH than with UFH. Thrombosis due to HIT should be managed with a direct thrombin inhibitor: argatroban for patients with renal insufficiency or lepirudin for patients with hepatic failure. In the setting of percutaneous coronary intervention, administer bivalirudin.

The most common nonbleeding side effect of warfarin is alopecia. A rare complication is warfarin-induced skin necrosis, which may be related to warfarin-induced reduction of protein C.

During pregnancy, warfarin should be avoided if possible because of warfarin embryopathy, which is most common with exposure during the 6th through 12th week of gestation. However, women can take warfarin postpartum and breast-feed safely. Warfarin can also be administered safely during the second trimester.

Duration of Hospital Stay Acute DVT patients with good family and social support, permanent residence, telephone, and no hearing or language impairment can often be managed as outpatients. They or a family member or a visiting nurse can administer a parenteral anticoagulant. Warfarin dosing can be titrated to the INR and adjusted on an outpatient basis.

Acute PE patients, who traditionally have required 5-7 day hospital stays for intravenous heparin as a "bridge" to warfarin, can be considered for abbreviated hospitalization if they have an excellent prognosis. The latter are characterized by clinical stability, absence of chest pain or shortness of breath, normal right ventricular size and function, and normal levels of cardiac biomarkers.

Duration of Anticoagulation Patients with PE following surgery or trauma ordinarily have a low rate of recurrence after 3–6 months of anticoagulation. For DVT isolated to an upper extremity or calf that has been provoked by surgery or trauma, 3 months of anticoagulation suffices. For provoked proximal leg DVT or PE, 6 months of anticoagulation is sufficient.

However, among patients with "idiopathic," unprovoked DVT or PE, the recurrence rate is surprisingly high after cessation of anticoagulation. VTE that occurs during long-haul air travel is considered unprovoked.

Current American College of Chest Physicians (ACCP) guidelines recommend anticoagulation for an indefinite duration with a target INR between 2.0 and 3.0 for patients with idiopathic VTE. However, I recommend that the intensity of anticoagulation be tailored to the patient's risk of recurrent VTE versus risk of bleeding. For a patient at high risk of recurrent VTE (for example, someone with multiple thrombophilic disorders) and a low risk of bleeding (for example, young age and no comorbidities), I recommend standard intensity anticoagulation. However, for a patient with a high bleeding risk (for example, older age and a prior history of gastrointestinal bleeding), I advise low-intensity anticoagulation (INR 1.5–2.0) after 6 months.

Several years ago, the presence of genetic mutations such as factor V Leiden or prothrombin gene mutation was thought to markedly increase the risk of recurrent VTE. Now, however, the clinical circumstances in which the DVT or PE occurs rather than underlying thrombophilia are considered much more important in deciding the risk of recurrence and the optimal duration of anticoagulation. However, patients with moderate or high levels of anticardiolipin antibodies probably warrant indefinite duration anticoagulation, even if the initial VTE was provoked by trauma or surgery.

INFERIOR VENA CAVAL (IVC) FILTERS The two principal indications for insertion of an IVC filter are (1) active bleeding that precludes anticoagulation, and (2) recurrent venous thrombosis despite intensive anticoagulation. Prevention of recurrent PE in patients with right heart failure who are not candidates for fibrinolysis or prophylaxis of extremely high-risk patients are "softer" indications for filter placement. The filter itself may fail by permitting the passage of small to medium-sized clots. Large thrombi may embolize to the pulmonary arteries via collateral veins that develop. A more common complication is caval thrombosis with marked bilateral leg swelling.

Paradoxically, by providing a nidus for clot formation, filters double the DVT rate over the ensuing 2 years following placement. Therefore, if clinically safe, patients receiving IVC filters should also receive concomitant anticoagulation.

Retrievable filters can now be placed for patients with an anticipated temporary bleeding disorder or for patients at temporary high risk of PE, such as individuals undergoing bariatric surgery with a prior history of perioperative PE. The filters can be retrieved up to several months following insertion, unless thrombus forms and is trapped within the filter. The retrievable filter becomes permanent if it remains in place or if, for technical reasons such as rapid endothelialization, it cannot be removed.

MAINTAINING ADEQUATE CIRCULATION For patients with massive PE and hypotension, the most common initial approach is administration of 500–1,000 ml of normal saline. However, fluids should be used with extreme caution. Excessive fluid administration exacerbates RV wall stress, causes more profound RV ischemia, and worsens LV compliance and filling by causing further interventricular septal shift toward the LV. Dopamine and dobutamine are first-line inotropic agents for treatment of PE-related shock. There should be a low threshold to initiate these pressors. However, a "trial and error" approach may be necessary with other agents such as norepinephrine, vasopressin, or phenylephrine.

FIBRINOLYSIS Successful fibrinolytic therapy rapidly reverses right heart failure and leads to a lower rate of death and recurrent PE. Thrombolysis usually (1) dissolves much of the anatomically obstructing pulmonary arterial thrombus; (2) prevents the continued release of serotonin and other neurohumoral factors that exacerbate pulmonary hypertension; and (3) dissolves much of the source of the thrombus in the pelvic or deep leg veins, thereby decreasing the likelihood of recurrent PE.

The preferred fibrinolytic regimen is 100 mg of recombinant tissue plasminogen activator (tPA) administered as a continuous peripheral intravenous infusion over 2 h. Patients appear to respond to fibrinolysis for up to 14 days after the PE has occurred.

Contraindications to fibrinolysis include intracranial disease, recent surgery, or trauma. The overall major bleeding rate is about 10%, including a 1–3% risk of intracranial hemorrhage. Careful screening of patients for contraindications to fibrinolytic therapy (Chap. 239) is the best way to minimize bleeding risk.

The only FDA-approved indication for PE fibrinolysis is massive PE. For patients with preserved systolic blood pressure and submassive PE, guidelines recommend individual patient risk assessment of the thrombotic burden versus bleeding risk. I concur with these guidelines. Younger patients with submassive PE but without comorbidities are generally excellent candidates for fibrinolysis. For older patients (>70 yrs) with risk of intracranial hemorrhage, a "watch and wait" approach is suitable, with frequent serial evaluation of RV function by echocardiography; fibrinolysis should be considered in those with deterioration of RV function.

PULMONARY EMBOLECTOMY The risk of intracranial hemorrhage with fibrinolysis has prompted the renaissance of surgical embolectomy for acute PE. At Brigham and Women's Hospital, 47 patients with massive PE underwent emergency surgery in 53 months, with a 94% survival rate. This high survival rate may be attributed to improved surgical technique, rapid diagnosis and triage, and careful patient selection. A possible alternative to open surgical embolectomy is catheter embolectomy. New generation catheters are under development.

PULMONARY THROMBOENDARTERECTOMY Chronic thromboembolic pulmonary hypertension is caused by vascular obstruction at the capillary level, not direct thromboembolic occlusion. It used to be considered a rare complication (about 1 of 500) of acute PE. Now, however, it appears that chronic thromboembolic pulmonary hypertension is a more common development, occurring in approximately 4% of patients who develop acute PE. Therefore, PE patients should be followed to ensure that if they have initial pulmonary hypertension, it abates over time (usually 6 weeks).

Patients severely impaired with dyspnea due to chronic thromboembolic pulmonary hypertension should be considered for pulmonary thromboendarterectomy, which, if successful, can markedly reduce and at times even cure pulmonary hypertension (Chap. 244). The operation requires median sternotomy, cardiopulmonary bypass, deep hypothermia, and periods of hypothermic circulatory arrest. The fibrotic, thromboembolic material is grasped with a forceps and circumferentially dissected from the vessel wall. The mortality rate at experienced centers is approximately 5%. The two most common complications are (1) "pulmonary steal," where blood rushes from previously perfused areas to newly revascularized areas of the lung; and (2) reperfusion pulmonary edema.

EMOTIONAL SUPPORT Many patients with VTE will appear healthy and fit. They may be burdened with fear about the possible genetic implications of DVT or PE. They often feel overwhelmed when advised to continue lifelong anticoagulation. Many patients in whom anticoagulation is discontinued after 3–6 months of therapy feel vulnerable to a future recurrent VTE. They may be reluctant to discontinue warfarin. Support groups are useful. Responses to frequently asked questions by these patients have been posted on the following website: *http://web.mit.edu/karen/www/faq.html*.

PREVENTION OF POSTPHLEBITIC SYNDROME The only therapy to prevent postphlebitic syndrome is daily use of below-knee 30–40 mmHg vascular compression stockings. They halve the rate of developing postphlebitic syndrome. These vascular compression stockings should be prescribed as soon as DVT is diagnosed, and the stockings should be fitted carefully to maximize their benefit. When patients are in bed, the stockings need not be worn.

PREVENTION OF VTE

Prophylaxis is of paramount importance because VTE is difficult to detect and poses an excessive medical and economic burden. Mechanical and pharmacologic measures often succeed in preventing this complication (Table 256-5). Patients at high risk can receive a combination of mechanical and pharmacologic modalities. Graduated compression stockings and pneumatic compression devices may complement mini-dose unfractionated heparin (5000 units subcutaneously twice or preferably three times daily), low molecular weight heparin, a pentasaccharide (fondaparinux 2.5 mg daily), or warfarin administration. Computerized reminder systems can increase the use of preventive measures and at Brigham and Women's Hospital reduced the symptomatic VTE rate by more than 40%. Patients who have undergone total hip replacement, total knee replacement, or cancer surgery will benefit from extended pharmacologic prophylaxis for a total of 4–6 weeks.

TABLE 256-5	**PREVENTION OF VENOUS THROMBOEMBOLISM**
Condition	**Prophylaxis Strategy**
High-risk general surgery	Mini-UFH + GCS *or* LMWH + GCS
Thoracic surgery	Mini-UFH + IPC
Cancer surgery, including gynecologic cancer surgery	LMWH, consider 1 month of prophylaxis
Total hip replacement, total knee replacement, hip fracture surgery	LMWH, fondaparinux (a pentasaccharide) 2.5 mg sc, once daily *or* (except for total knee replacement) warfarin (target INR 2.5)
Neurosurgery	GCS + IPC
Neurosurgery for brain tumor	Mini-UFH *or* LMWH, + IPC, + predischarge venous ultrasonography
Benign gynecologic surgery	Mini-UFH + GCS
Medically ill patients	Mini-UFH *or* LMWH
Anticoagulation contraindicated	GCS + IPC
Long-haul air travel	Consider LMWH for very high risk patients

Note: Mini-UFH, minidose unfractionated heparin, 5000 units subcutaneously twice (less effective) or three times daily (more effective); GCS, graduated compression stockings, usually 10–18 mm Hg; LMWH, low-molecular-weight heparin, typically in the United States, enoxaparin, 40 mg once daily, or dalteparin, 2500 or 5000 units once daily; IPC, intermittent pneumatic compression devices.

FURTHER READINGS

BLAIVAS M: Ultrasound in the detection of venous thromboembolism. Crit Care Med 35:S224, 2007

FIUMARA K et al: Predictors of Major Hemorrhage Following Fibrinolysis for Acute Pulmonary Embolism. Am J Cardiol 97:127, 2006

GEERTS WH et al: Prevention of venous thromboembolism: The Seventh ACCP Conference on Antithrombotic and Thrombolytic Therapy. Chest 126:338S, 2004

HILL J, TREASURE T: Reducing the risk of venous thromboembolism (deep vein thrombosis and pulmonary embolism) in patients having surgery: Summary of NICE guidance. BMJ 334:1053, 2007

KUCHER N et al: Electronic alerts to prevent venous thromboembolism among hospitalized patients. N Engl J Med 352:969, 2005

——— et al: Prognostic role of echocardiography among patients with acute pulmonary embolism and a systolic arterial pressure of 90 mm Hg or higher. Arch Intern Med 165:1777, 2005

——— et al: Percutaneous catheter thrombectomy device for acute pulmonary embolism: in vitro and in vivo testing. Radiology 236:852, 2005

KUCHER N, GOLDHABER SZ: Management of massive pulmonary embolism. Circulation 112:e28, 2005

LEACCHE M et al: Modern surgical treatment of massive pulmonary embolism: Results in 47 consecutive patients after rapid diagnosis and aggressive surgical approach. J Thorac Cardiovasc Surg 129:1018, 2005

RIDKER P et al: Long-term, low-intensity warfarin therapy for the prevention of recurrent venous thromboembolism. N Engl J Med 348:1425, 2003

RIEDER MJ et al: Effect of VKORC1 haplotypes on transcriptional regulation and warfarin dose. N Engl J Med 352:2285, 2005

SEGAL JB et al: Management of venous thromboembolism: A systematic review for a practice guideline. Ann Intern Med 146:211, 2007

WELLS PS et al: Does this patient have deep vein thrombosis? JAMA 295:199, 2006

WRITING GROUP FOR THE CHRISTOPHER INVESTIGATORS: Effectiveness of managing suspected pulmonary embolism using an algorithm combining clinical probability, D-dimer testing, and computed tomography. JAMA 295:172, 2006

257 Disorders of the Pleura and Mediastinum

Richard W. Light

DISORDERS OF THE PLEURA

PLEURAL EFFUSION

The pleural space lies between the lung and chest wall and normally contains a very thin layer of fluid, which serves as a coupling system. A pleural effusion is present when there is an excess quantity of fluid in the pleural space.

Etiology Pleural fluid accumulates when pleural fluid formation exceeds pleural fluid absorption. Normally, fluid enters the pleural space from the capillaries in the parietal pleura and is removed via the lymphatics situated in the parietal pleura. Fluid can also enter the pleural space from the interstitial spaces of the lung via the visceral pleura or from the peritoneal cavity via small holes in the diaphragm. The lymphatics have the capacity to absorb 20 times more fluid than is normally formed. Accordingly, a pleural effusion may develop when there is excess pleural fluid formation (from the interstitial spaces of the lung, the parietal pleura, or the peritoneal cavity) or when there is decreased fluid removal by the lymphatics.

Diagnostic Approach When a patient is found to have a pleural effusion, an effort should be made to determine the cause (Fig. 257-1). The first step is to determine whether the effusion is a transudate or an exudate. A *transudative pleural effusion* occurs when *systemic factors* that influence the formation and absorption of pleural fluid are altered. The leading causes of transudative pleural effusions in the United States are left ventricular failure and cirrhosis. An *exudative pleural effusion* occurs when *local factors* that influence the formation and absorption of pleural fluid are altered. The leading causes of exudative pleural effusions are bacterial pneumonia, malignancy, viral infection, and pulmonary embolism. The primary reason to make this differentiation is that additional diagnostic procedures are indicated with exudative effusions to define the cause of the local disease.

Transudative and exudative pleural effusions are distinguished by measuring the lactate dehydrogenase (LDH) and protein levels in the pleural fluid. Exudative pleural effusions meet at least one of the following criteria, whereas transudative pleural effusions meet none:

1. pleural fluid protein/serum protein >0.5
2. pleural fluid LDH/serum LDH >0.6
3. pleural fluid LDH more than two-thirds normal upper limit for serum

The above criteria misidentify ~25% of transudates as exudates. If one or more of the exudative criteria are met and the patient is clinically thought to have a condition producing a transudative effusion, the difference between the protein levels in the serum and the pleural fluid should be measured. If this gradient is greater than 31 g/L (3.1 g/dL), the exudative categorization by the above criteria can be ignored because almost all such patients have a transudative pleural effusion.

If a patient has an exudative pleural effusion, the following tests on the pleural fluid should be obtained: description of the fluid, glucose level, differential cell count, microbiologic studies, and cytology.

Effusion Due to Heart Failure The most common cause of pleural effusion is left ventricular failure. The effusion occurs because the increased amounts of fluid in the lung interstitial spaces exit in part across the visceral pleura. This overwhelms the capacity of the lymphatics in the parietal pleura to remove fluid. Isolated right-sided pleural effusions are more common than left-sided effusions in heart failure. A diagnostic thoracentesis should be performed if the effusions are not bilateral and comparable in size, if the patient is febrile, or if the patient has pleuritic chest pain, to verify that the patient has a transudative effusion. Otherwise the patient is best treated with di-

FIGURE 257-1 Approach to the diagnosis of pleural effusions. CHF, congestive heart failure; CT, computed tomography; LDH, lactate dehydrogenase; PE, pulmonary embolism; TB, tuberculosis; PF, pleural fluid.

uretics. If the effusion persists despite diuretic therapy, a diagnostic thoracentesis should be performed. A pleural fluid N-terminal pro-brain natriuretic peptide (NT-proBNP) >1500 pg/mL is virtually diagnostic of an effusion secondary to congestive heart failure.

Hepatic Hydrothorax Pleural effusions occur in ~5% of patients with cirrhosis and ascites. The predominant mechanism is the direct movement of peritoneal fluid through small openings in the diaphragm into the pleural space. The effusion is usually right-sided and frequently is large enough to produce severe dyspnea.

Parapneumonic Effusion Parapneumonic effusions are associated with bacterial pneumonia, lung abscess, or bronchiectasis and are probably the most common cause of exudative pleural effusion in the United States. *Empyema* refers to a grossly purulent effusion.

Patients with aerobic bacterial pneumonia and pleural effusion present with an acute febrile illness consisting of chest pain, sputum production, and leukocytosis. Patients with anaerobic infections present with a subacute illness with weight loss, a brisk leukocytosis, mild anemia, and a history of some factor that predisposes them to aspiration.

The possibility of a parapneumonic effusion should be considered whenever a patient with a bacterial pneumonia is initially evaluated. The presence of free pleural fluid can be demonstrated with a lateral decubitus radiograph, computed tomography (CT) of the chest, or ultrasound. If the free fluid separates the lung from the chest wall by >10 mm, a therapeutic thoracentesis should be performed. Factors indicating the likely need for a procedure more invasive than a thoracentesis (in increasing order of importance) include:

1. loculated pleural fluid
2. pleural fluid pH < 7.20
3. pleural fluid glucose < 3.3 mmol/L (<60 mg/dL)
4. positive Gram stain or culture of the pleural fluid
5. the presence of gross pus in the pleural space

If the fluid recurs after the initial therapeutic thoracentesis, and if any of the above characteristics are present, a repeat thoracentesis should be performed. If the fluid cannot be completely removed with the therapeutic thoracentesis, consideration should be given to inserting a chest tube and instilling a fibrinolytic (e.g., streptokinase, 250,000 units) or performing thoracoscopy with the breakdown of adhesions. Decortication should be considered when the above are ineffective.

Effusion Secondary to Malignancy Malignant pleural effusions secondary to metastatic disease are the second most common type of exudative pleural effusion. The three tumors that cause ~75% of all malignant pleural effusions are lung carcinoma, breast carcinoma, and lymphoma. Most patients complain of dyspnea, which is frequently out of proportion to the size of the effusion. The pleural fluid is an exudate, and its glucose level may be reduced if the tumor burden in the pleural space is high.

The diagnosis is usually made via cytology of the pleural fluid. If the initial cytologic examination is negative, then thoracoscopy is the best next procedure if malignancy is strongly suspected. At the time of thoracoscopy, a procedure such as pleural abrasion should be performed to effect a pleurodesis. If thoracoscopy is unavailable, then needle biopsy of the pleura should be performed.

Patients with a malignant pleural effusion are treated symptomatically for the most part, since the presence of the effusion indicates disseminated disease and most malignancies associated with pleural effusion are not curable with chemotherapy. The only symptom that can be attributed to the effusion itself is dyspnea. If the patient's lifestyle is compromised by dyspnea, and if the dyspnea is relieved with a therapeutic thoracentesis, then one of the following procedures should be considered: (1) insertion of a small indwelling catheter; or (2) tube thoracostomy with the instillation of a sclerosing agent such as doxycycline, 500 mg.

Mesothelioma Malignant mesotheliomas are primary tumors that arise from the mesothelial cells that line the pleural cavities; most are related to asbestos exposure. Patients with mesothelioma present with chest pain and shortness of breath. The chest radiograph reveals a pleural effusion, generalized pleural thickening, and a shrunken hemithorax. Thoracoscopy or open pleural biopsy is usually necessary to establish the diagnosis. Chest pain should be treated with opiates and shortness of breath with oxygen and/or opiates.

Effusion Secondary to Pulmonary Embolization The diagnosis most commonly overlooked in the differential diagnosis of a patient with an undiagnosed pleural effusion is pulmonary embolism. Dyspnea is the most common symptom. The pleural fluid is almost always an exudate. The diagnosis is established by spiral CT scan or pulmonary arteriography (Chap. 256). Treatment of the patient with a pleural effusion secondary to pulmonary embolism is the same as for any patient with pulmonary emboli. If the pleural effusion increases in size after anticoagulation, the patient probably has recurrent emboli or another complication such as a hemothorax or a pleural infection.

Tuberculous Pleuritis (See also Chap. 158) In many parts of the world, the most common cause of an exudative pleural effusion is tu-

berculosis (TB), but tuberculous effusions are relatively uncommon in the United States. Tuberculous pleural effusions are usually associated with primary TB and are thought to be due primarily to a hypersensitivity reaction to tuberculous protein in the pleural space. Patients with tuberculous pleuritis present with fever, weight loss, dyspnea, and/or pleuritic chest pain. The pleural fluid is an exudate with predominantly small lymphocytes. The diagnosis is established by demonstrating high levels of TB markers in the pleural fluid (adenosine deaminase > 40 IU/L, interferon γ > 140 pg/mL, or positive polymerase chain reaction (PCR) for tuberculous DNA). Alternatively, the diagnosis can be established by culture of the pleural fluid, needle biopsy of the pleura, or thoracoscopy. The recommended treatment of pleural and pulmonary TB is identical (Chap. 158).

Effusion Secondary to Viral Infection Viral infections are probably responsible for a sizable percentage of undiagnosed exudative pleural effusions. In many series, no diagnosis is established for ~20% of exudative effusions, and these effusions resolve spontaneously with no long-term residua. The importance of these effusions is that one should not be too aggressive in trying to establish a diagnosis for the undiagnosed effusion, particularly if the patient is improving clinically.

AIDS (See also Chap. 182) Pleural effusions are uncommon in such patients. The most common cause is Kaposi's sarcoma, followed by parapneumonic effusion. Other common causes are TB, cryptococcosis, and primary effusion lymphoma. Pleural effusions are very uncommon with *Pneumocystis carinii* infection.

Chylothorax A chylothorax occurs when the thoracic duct is disrupted and chyle accumulates in the pleural space. The most common cause of chylothorax is trauma, but it also may result from tumors in the mediastinum. Patients with chylothorax present with dyspnea, and a large pleural effusion is present on the chest radiograph. Thoracentesis reveals milky fluid, and biochemical analysis reveals a triglyceride level that exceeds 1.2 mmol/L (110 mg/dL). Patients with chylothorax and no obvious trauma should have a lymphangiogram and a mediastinal CT scan to assess the mediastinum for lymph nodes. The treatment of choice for most chylothoraces is insertion of a chest tube plus the administration of octreotide. If these modalities fail, a pleuroperitoneal shunt should be placed unless the patient has chylous ascites. Patients with chylothoraces should not undergo prolonged tube thoracostomy with chest tube drainage because this will lead to malnutrition and immunologic incompetence.

Hemothorax When a diagnostic thoracentesis reveals bloody pleural fluid, a hematocrit should be obtained on the pleural fluid. If the hematocrit is more than half of that in the peripheral blood, the patient is considered to have a hemothorax. Most hemothoraces are the result of trauma; other causes include rupture of a blood vessel or tumor. Most patients with hemothorax should be treated with tube thoracostomy, which allows continuous quantification of bleeding. If the bleeding emanates from a laceration of the pleura, apposition of the two pleural surfaces is likely to stop the bleeding. If the pleural hemorrhage exceeds 200 mL/h, consideration should be given to thoracoscopy or thoracotomy.

Miscellaneous Causes of Pleural Effusion There are many other causes of pleural effusion (Table 257-1). Key features of some of these conditions are as follows: If the pleural fluid amylase level is elevated, the diagnosis of esophageal rupture or pancreatic disease is likely. If the patient is febrile, has predominantly polymorphonuclear cells in the pleural fluid, and has no pulmonary parenchymal abnormalities, an intraabdominal abscess should be considered. The diagnosis of an asbestos pleural effusion is one of exclusion. Benign ovarian tumors can produce ascites and a pleural effusion (Meigs' syndrome), as can the ovarian hyperstimulation syndrome. Several drugs can cause pleural effusion; the associated fluid is usually eosinophilic. Pleural effusions commonly occur following coronary artery bypass surgery. Effusions occurring within the first

TABLE 257-1 DIFFERENTIAL DIAGNOSES OF PLEURAL EFFUSIONS

Transudative Pleural Effusions

1. Congestive heart failure	5. Peritoneal dialysis
2. Cirrhosis	6. Superior vena cava obstruction
3. Pulmonary embolization	7. Myxedema
4. Nephrotic syndrome	8. Urinothorax

Exudative Pleural Effusions

1. Neoplastic diseases	6. Post-coronary artery bypass surgery
a. Metastatic disease	
b. Mesothelioma	7. Asbestos exposure
2. Infectious diseases	8. Sarcoidosis
a. Bacterial infections	9. Uremia
b. Tuberculosis	10. Meigs' syndrome
c. Fungal infections	11. Yellow nail syndrome
d. Viral infections	12. Drug-induced pleural disease
e. Parasitic infections	a. Nitrofurantoin
3. Pulmonary embolization	b. Dantrolene
4. Gastrointestinal disease	c. Methysergide
a. Esophageal perforation	d. Bromocriptine
b. Pancreatic disease	e. Procarbazine
c. Intraabdominal abscesses	f. Amiodarone
d. Diaphragmatic hernia	13. Trapped lung
e. After abdominal surgery	14. Radiation therapy
f. Endoscopic variceal sclerotherapy	15. Post-cardiac injury syndrome
g. After liver transplant	16. Hemothorax
5. Collagen-vascular diseases	17. Iatrogenic injury
a. Rheumatoid pleuritis	18. Ovarian hyperstimulation syndrome
b. Systemic lupus erythematosus	
c. Drug-induced lupus	19. Pericardial disease
d. Immunoblastic lymphadenopathy	20. Chylothorax
e. Sjögren's syndrome	
f. Wegener's granulomatosis	
g. Churg-Strauss syndrome	

weeks are typically left-sided and bloody, with large numbers of eosinophils, and respond to one or two therapeutic thoracenteses. Effusions occurring after the first few weeks are typically left-sided and clear yellow, with predominantly small lymphocytes, and tend to recur. Other medical manipulations that induce pleural effusions include abdominal surgery; radiation therapy; liver, lung, or heart transplantation; or the intravascular insertion of central lines.

PNEUMOTHORAX

Pneumothorax is the presence of gas in the pleural space. A *spontaneous pneumothorax* is one that occurs without antecedent trauma to the thorax. A *primary spontaneous pneumothorax* occurs in the absence of underlying lung disease, while a *secondary pneumothorax* occurs in its presence. A *traumatic pneumothorax* results from penetrating or nonpenetrating chest injuries. A *tension pneumothorax* is a pneumothorax in which the pressure in the pleural space is positive throughout the respiratory cycle.

Primary Spontaneous Pneumothorax
Primary spontaneous pneumothoraces are usually due to rupture of apical pleural blebs, small cystic spaces that lie within or immediately under the visceral pleura. Primary spontaneous pneumothoraces occur almost exclusively in smokers, which suggests that these patients have subclinical lung disease. Approximately one-half of patients with an initial primary spontaneous pneumothorax will have a recurrence. The initial recommended treatment for primary spontaneous pneumothorax is simple aspiration. If the lung does not expand with aspiration, or if the patient has a recurrent pneumothorax, thoracoscopy with stapling of blebs and pleural abrasion is indicated. Thoracoscopy or thoracotomy with pleural abrasion is almost 100% successful in preventing recurrences.

Secondary Pneumothorax
Most secondary pneumothoraces are due to chronic obstructive pulmonary disease, but pneumothoraces have been reported with virtually every lung disease. Pneumothorax in patients with lung disease is more life-threatening than it is in normal individuals because of the lack of pulmonary reserve in these patients. Nearly all patients with secondary pneumothorax should be treated with tube thoracostomy. Most should also be treated with thoracoscopy or thoracotomy with the stapling of blebs and pleural abrasion. If the patient is not a good operative candidate or refuses surgery, then pleurodesis should be attempted by the intrapleural injection of a sclerosing agent such as doxycycline.

Traumatic Pneumothorax
Traumatic pneumothoraces can result from both penetrating and nonpenetrating chest trauma. Traumatic pneumothoraces should be treated with tube thoracostomy unless they are very small. If a hemopneumothorax is present, one chest tube should be placed in the superior part of the hemithorax to evacuate the air, and another should be placed in the inferior part of the hemithorax to remove the blood. Iatrogenic pneumothorax is a type of traumatic pneumothorax that is becoming more common. The leading causes are transthoracic needle aspiration, thoracentesis, and the insertion of central intravenous catheters. Most can be managed with supplemental oxygen or aspiration, but if these are unsuccessful a tube thoracostomy should be performed.

Tension Pneumothorax
This condition usually occurs during mechanical ventilation or resuscitative efforts. The positive pleural pressure is life-threatening both because ventilation is severely compromised and because the positive pressure is transmitted to the mediastinum, which results in decreased venous return to the heart and reduced cardiac output.

Difficulty in ventilation during resuscitation or high peak inspiratory pressures during mechanical ventilation strongly suggests the diagnosis. The diagnosis is made by physical examination showing an enlarged hemithorax with no breath sounds, hyperresonance to percussion, and shift of the mediastinum to the contralateral side. Tension pneumothorax must be treated as a medical emergency. If the tension in the pleural space is not relieved, the patient is likely to die from inadequate cardiac output or marked hypoxemia. A large-bore needle should be inserted into the pleural space through the second anterior intercostal space. If large amounts of gas escape from the needle after insertion, the diagnosis is confirmed. The needle should be left in place until a thoracostomy tube can be inserted.

DISORDERS OF THE MEDIASTINUM

The mediastinum is the region between the pleural sacs. It is separated into three compartments. The *anterior mediastinum* extends from the sternum anteriorly to the pericardium and brachiocephalic vessels posteriorly. It contains the thymus gland, the anterior mediastinal lymph nodes, and the internal mammary arteries and veins. The *middle mediastinum* lies between the anterior and posterior mediastina and contains the heart; the ascending and transverse arches of the aorta; the venae cavae; the brachiocephalic arteries and veins; the phrenic nerves; the trachea, main bronchi, and their contiguous lymph nodes; and the pulmonary arteries and veins. The *posterior mediastinum* is bounded by the pericardium and trachea anteriorly and the vertebral column posteriorly. It contains the descending thoracic aorta, esophagus, thoracic duct, azygos and hemiazygos veins, and the posterior group of mediastinal lymph nodes.

MEDIASTINAL MASSES

The first step in evaluating a mediastinal mass is to place it in one of the three mediastinal compartments, since each has different characteristic lesions. The most common lesions in the anterior mediastinum are thymomas, lymphomas, teratomatous neoplasms, and thyroid masses. The most common masses in the middle mediastinum are vascular masses, lymph node enlargement from metastases or granulomatous disease, and pleuropericardial and bronchogenic cysts. In the posterior mediastinum, neurogenic tumors, meningoceles, meningomyeloceles, gastroenteric cysts, and esophageal diverticula are commonly found.

CT scanning is the most valuable imaging technique for evaluating mediastinal masses and is the only imaging technique that should be done in most instances. Barium studies of the gastrointestinal tract are indicated in many patients with posterior mediastinal lesions, since hernias, diverticula, and achalasia are readily diagnosed in this manner. An ^{131}I scan can efficiently establish the diagnosis of intrathoracic goiter.

A definite diagnosis can be obtained with mediastinoscopy or anterior mediastinotomy in many patients with masses in the anterior or middle mediastinal compartments. A diagnosis can be established without thoracotomy via percutaneous fine-needle aspiration biopsy or endoscopic transesophageal or endobronchial ultrasound-guided biopsy of mediastinal masses in most cases. Alternative ways to establish the diagnosis are video-assisted thoracoscopy, mediastinoscopy, or mediastinotomy. In many cases the diagnosis can be established and the mediastinal mass removed with video-assisted thoracoscopy.

ACUTE MEDIASTINITIS

Most cases of acute mediastinitis either are due to esophageal perforation or occur after median sternotomy for cardiac surgery. Patients with esophageal rupture are acutely ill with chest pain and dyspnea due to the mediastinal infection. The esophageal rupture can occur spontaneously or as a complication of esophagoscopy or the insertion of a Blakemore tube. Appropriate treatment is exploration of the mediastinum with primary repair of the esophageal tear and drainage of the pleural space and the mediastinum.

The incidence of mediastinitis following median sternotomy is 0.4–5.0%. Patients most commonly present with wound drainage. Other presentations include sepsis or a widened mediastinum. The diagnosis is usually established with mediastinal needle aspiration. Treatment includes immediate drainage, debridement, and parenteral antibiotic therapy, but the mortality still exceeds 20%.

CHRONIC MEDIASTINITIS

The spectrum of chronic mediastinitis ranges from granulomatous inflammation of the lymph nodes in the mediastinum to fibrosing mediastinitis. Most cases are due to TB or histoplasmosis, but sarcoidosis, silicosis, and other fungal diseases are at times causative. Patients with granulomatous mediastinitis are usually asymptomatic. Those with fibrosing mediastinitis usually have signs of compression of some mediastinal structure such as the superior vena cava or large airways, phrenic or recurrent laryngeal nerve paralysis, or obstruction of the pulmonary artery or proximal pulmonary veins. Other than antituberculous therapy for tuberculous mediastinitis, no medical or surgical therapy has been demonstrated to be effective for mediastinal fibrosis.

PNEUMOMEDIASTINUM

In this condition, there is gas in the interstices of the mediastinum. The three main causes are: (1) alveolar rupture with dissection of air into the mediastinum; (2) perforation or rupture of the esophagus, trachea, or main bronchi; and (3) dissection of air from the neck or the abdomen into the mediastinum. Typically, there is severe substernal chest pain with or without radiation into the neck and arms. The physical examination usually reveals subcutaneous emphysema in the suprasternal notch and *Hamman's sign*, which is a crunching or clicking noise synchronous with the heartbeat and best heard in the left lateral decubitus position. The diagnosis is confirmed with the chest radiograph. Usually no treatment is required, but the mediastinal air will be absorbed faster if the patient inspires high concentrations of oxygen. If mediastinal structures are compressed, the compression can be relieved with needle aspiration.

FURTHER READINGS

Light RW: *Pleural Diseases*, 5th ed. Philadelphia, Lippincott Williams & Wilkins, 2006

———: Pleural effusion. N Engl J Med 346:1971, 2002

Porcel JM: The use of probrain natriuretic peptide in pleural fluid for the diagnosis of pleural effusions resulting from heart failure. Curr Opin Pulm Med 11:329, 2005

Rahman NM et al: Investigating suspected malignant pleural effusion. BMJ 334:206, 2007

Tremblay A et al: Single-center experience with 250 tunnelled pleural catheter insertions for malignant pleural effusion. Chest 129:362, 2006

Vilmann P et al: Transesophageal endoscopic ultrasound-guided fine-needle aspiration and endobronchial ultrasound-guided transbronchial needle aspiration biopsy: A combined approach in the evaluation of mediastinal lesions. Endoscopy 37:833, 2005

258 Disorders of Ventilation
Eliot A. Phillipson

HYPOVENTILATION

DEFINITION AND ETIOLOGY

Alveolar hypoventilation exists by definition when arterial P_{CO_2} (Pa_{CO_2}) increases above the normal range of 37–43 mmHg, but in clinically important hypoventilation syndromes Pa_{CO_2} is generally in the range of 50–80 mmHg. Hypoventilation disorders can be acute or chronic. This chapter deals with chronic hypoventilation syndromes. The acute disorders, which represent life-threatening emergencies, are discussed in Chap. 262.

Chronic hypoventilation can result from numerous disease entities (Table 258-1), but in all cases the underlying mechanism involves a defect in either the metabolic respiratory control system, the respiratory neuromuscular system, or the ventilatory apparatus. Disorders associated with impaired respiratory drive, defects in the respiratory neuromuscular system, some chest wall disorders such as obesity, and upper airway obstruction produce an increase in Pa_{CO_2}, despite normal lungs, because of a reduction in overall minute volume of ventilation and hence in alveolar ventilation. In contrast, most disorders of the chest wall and disorders of the lower airways and lungs may produce an increase in Pa_{CO_2}, despite a normal or even increased minute volume of ventilation, because of severe ventilation-perfusion mismatching that results in net alveolar hypoventilation.

Several hypoventilation syndromes involve combined disturbances in two elements of the respiratory system. For example, patients with chronic obstructive pulmonary disease may hypoventilate not simply because of impaired ventilatory mechanics but also because of a reduced central respiratory drive, which can be inherent or secondary to a coexisting metabolic alkalosis (related to diuretic and steroid therapy).

PHYSIOLOGIC AND CLINICAL FEATURES

Regardless of cause, the hallmark of all alveolar hypoventilation syndromes is an increase in alveolar P_{CO_2} (PA_{CO_2}) and therefore in Pa_{CO_2} (Fig. 258-1). The resulting respiratory acidosis eventually leads to a compensatory increase in plasma HCO_3^- concentration and a decrease in Cl^- concentration. The increase in PA_{CO_2} produces an obligatory decrease in PA_{O_2}, resulting in hypoxemia. If severe, the hypoxemia manifests clinically as cyanosis and can stimulate erythropoiesis and induce secondary polycythemia. The combination of chronic hypoxemia and hypercapnia may also induce pulmonary vasoconstriction, leading eventually to pulmonary hypertension, right ventricular hypertrophy, and congestive heart failure. The disturbances in arterial blood gases are typically magnified during sleep because of a further reduction in central respiratory drive. The resulting increased nocturnal hypercapnia may cause cerebral vasodilation leading to morning headache; sleep quality may also be severely impaired, resulting in morning fatigue, daytime somnolence, mental confusion, and intellectual impairment. Other clinical features associated with hypoventilation syndromes are related to the specific underlying disease (Table 258-1).

TABLE 258-1 **CHRONIC HYPOVENTILATION SYNDROMES**

Mechanism	Site of Defect	Disorder
Impaired respiratory drive	Peripheral and central chemoreceptors	Carotid body dysfunction, trauma Prolonged hypoxia Metabolic alkalosis
	Brainstem respiratory neurons	Bulbar poliomyelitis, encephalitis Brainstem infarction, hemorrhage, trauma Brainstem demyelination, degeneration Chronic drug administration Hypothyroidism Primary alveolar hypoventilation syndrome
Defective respiratory neuromuscular system	Spinal cord and peripheral nerves	High cervical trauma Poliomyelitis Motor neuron disease Peripheral neuropathy
	Respiratory muscles	Myasthenia gravis Muscular dystrophy Chronic myopathy
Impaired ventilatory apparatus	Chest wall	Kyphoscoliosis Fibrothorax Thoracoplasty Ankylosing spondylitis Obesity hypoventilation
	Airways and lungs	Laryngeal and tracheal stenosis Obstructive sleep apnea Cystic fibrosis Chronic obstructive pulmonary disease

Source: From EA Phillipson, AS Slutsky in JF Murray, JA Nadel (eds), *Textbook of Respiratory Medicine*, 3d ed. Philadelphia, Saunders, 2000; with permission.

FIGURE 258-1 Physiologic and clinical features of alveolar hypoventilation. Hb, hemoglobin; Pa_{CO_2}, arterial P_{CO_2}; Pa_{O_2}, arterial P_{O_2}. *[After EA Phillipson, AS Slutsky, in JF Murray, JA Nadel (eds), Textbook of Respiratory Medicine, 3d ed. Philadelphia, Saunders, 2000.]*

DIAGNOSIS

Investigation of the patient with chronic hypoventilation involves several laboratory tests that will usually localize the disorder to either the metabolic respiratory control system, the neuromuscular system, or the ventilatory apparatus **(Fig. 258-2)**. Defects in the control system impair responses to chemical stimuli, including ventilatory, occlusion pressure, and diaphragmatic electromyographic (EMG) responses. During sleep, hypoventilation is usually more marked, and central apneas and hypopneas are common. However, because the behavioral

respiratory control system (which is anatomically distinct from the metabolic control system), the neuromuscular system, and the ventilatory apparatus are intact, such patients can usually hyperventilate voluntarily, generate normal inspiratory and expiratory muscle pressures (PI_{max}, PE_{max}, respectively) against an occluded airway, generate normal lung volumes and flow rates on routine spirometry, and have normal respiratory system resistance and compliance and a normal alveolar-arterial $P_{O_2}[(A–a)P_{O_2}]$ difference.

Patients with defects in the respiratory neuromuscular system also have impaired responses to chemical stimuli but in addition are unable to hyperventilate voluntarily or to generate normal static respiratory muscle pressures, lung volumes, and flow rates. However, at least in the early stages of the disease, the resistance and compliance of the respiratory system and the alveolar-arterial oxygen difference are normal.

Site of defect	Responses to CO_2, hypoxia			Sleep studies	Voluntary hyperventil.	PI_{max} PE_{max}	Volume flow rates	Resistance, compliance	$(A–a) P_{O_2}$
	Ventil.	P.1	EMGdi						
Metabolic control system (chemoreceptors, brainstem integrating neurons)	↓	↓	↓	↑ Hypoventil, central apneas	N	N	N	N	N
Respiratory neuromuscular system (brainstem motoneurons, spinal cord, respiratory nerves, and muscles)	↓	↓	↓	↑ Hypoventil, central apneas	↓	↓	↓	N	N
Ventilatory apparatus (chest wall, lungs, airways)	↓	N	N	Variable	↓	N	Abnormal	Abnormal	↑

FIGURE 258-2 Pattern of laboratory test results in alveolar hypoventilation syndromes, based on the site of defect. Ventil, ventilation; P.1, mouth pressure generated after 0.1 s of inspiration against an occluded airway; EMGdi, diaphragmatic EMG; PI_{max}, PE_{max}, maximum inspiratory or expiratory pressure that can be generated against an occluded airway; $(A–a)P_{O_2}$, alveolar-arterial P_{O_2} difference; N, normal. Defects in the metabolic control system impair central respiratory drive in response to chemical stimuli (CO_2 or hypoxia); therefore responses of EMGdi, P.1, and minute volume of ventilation are reduced and hypoventilation during sleep is aggravated. In contrast, tests of voluntary respira-

tory control, muscle strength, lung mechanics, and gas exchange [(A–a)P_{O_2}] are normal. Defects in the respiratory neuromuscular system impair muscle strength; therefore all tests dependent on muscular activity (voluntary or in response to metabolic stimuli) are abnormal, but lung resistance, lung compliance, and gas exchange are normal. Defects in the ventilatory apparatus usually impair gas exchange. Because resistance and compliance are also impaired, all tests dependent on ventilation (whether voluntary or in response to chemical stimuli) are abnormal; in contrast, tests of muscle activity or strength that do not involve airflow (i.e., P.1, EMGdi, PI_{max}, PE_{max}) are normal. *(After Phillipson and Duffin.)*

In contrast to patients with disorders of the respiratory control or neuromuscular systems, patients with disorders of the chest wall, lungs, and airways typically demonstrate abnormalities of respiratory system resistance and compliance and have a widened $(A-a)P_{O_2}$. Because of the impaired mechanics of breathing, routine spirometric tests are abnormal, as is the ventilatory response to chemical stimuli. However, because the neuromuscular system is intact, tests that are independent of resistance and compliance are usually normal, including tests of respiratory muscle strength and respiratory control that do not involve airflow.

℞ HYPOVENTILATION

The management of chronic hypoventilation must be individualized to the patient's particular disorder, circumstances, and needs and should include measures directed toward the underlying disease. Coexistent metabolic alkalosis should be corrected, including elevations of HCO_3^- that are inappropriately high for the degree of chronic hypercapnia. Administration of supplemental oxygen is effective in attenuating hypoxemia, polycythemia, and pulmonary hypertension but can aggravate CO_2 retention and the associated neurologic symptoms. For this reason, supplemental oxygen must be prescribed judiciously and the results monitored carefully. Pharmacologic agents that stimulate respiration, such as progesterone and methylxanthines, are of benefit in some patients, but results are generally disappointing.

Most patients with chronic hypoventilation related to impairment of respiratory drive or neuromuscular disease eventually require mechanical ventilatory assistance for effective management. When hypoventilation is severe, treatment may be required on a 24-h basis, but in most patients ventilatory assistance only during sleep produces dramatic improvement in clinical features and daytime arterial blood gases. In patients with reduced respiratory drive but intact respiratory lower motor neurons, phrenic nerves, and respiratory muscles, diaphragmatic pacing through an implanted phrenic electrode can be very effective. However, for patients with defects in the respiratory nerves and muscles, electrophrenic pacing is contraindicated. Such patients can usually be managed effectively with either intermittent negative-pressure ventilation in a cuirass or intermittent positive-pressure ventilation delivered through a tracheostomy or nose mask. For patients who require ventilatory assistance only during sleep, positive-pressure ventilation through a nose mask is the preferred method because it obviates a tracheostomy and avoids the problem of upper airway occlusion that can arise in a negative-pressure ventilator. Hypoventilation related to restrictive disorders of the chest wall (Table 258-1) can also be managed effectively with nocturnal intermittent positive-pressure ventilation through a nose mask or tracheostomy.

HYPOVENTILATION SYNDROMES

PRIMARY ALVEOLAR HYPOVENTILATION

Primary alveolar hypoventilation (PAH) is a disorder of unknown cause characterized by chronic hypercapnia and hypoxemia in the absence of identifiable neuromuscular disease or mechanical ventilatory impairment. The disorder is thought to arise from a defect in the metabolic respiratory control system, but few neuropathologic studies have been reported in such patients. Studies in animals suggest an important role for genetic factors in the pathogenesis of hypoventilation, and familial cases in humans have been described. Isolated PAH is relatively rare, and although it occurs in all age groups, the majority of reported cases in adults have been in males ages 20–50 years. The disorder typically develops insidiously and often first comes to attention when severe respiratory depression follows administration of standard doses of sedatives or anesthetics. As the degree of hypoventilation increases, patients typically develop lethargy, fatigue, daytime somnolence, disturbed sleep, and morning headaches; eventually cyanosis, polycythemia, pulmonary hypertension, and congestive heart failure occur (Fig. 258-1). Despite severe arterial blood gas derangements, dyspnea is uncommon, presumably because of impaired chemoreception and ventilatory drive. If left untreated, PAH is usually progressive over a period of months to years and ultimately fatal.

The key diagnostic finding in PAH is a chronic respiratory acidosis in the absence of respiratory muscle weakness or impaired ventilatory mechanics (Fig. 258-2). Because patients can hyperventilate voluntarily and reduce Pa_{CO_2} to normal or even hypocapnic levels, hypercapnia may not be demonstrable in a single arterial blood sample, but the presence of an elevated plasma HCO_3^- level should draw attention to the underlying chronic disturbance. Despite normal ventilatory mechanics and respiratory muscle strength, ventilatory responses to chemical stimuli are reduced or absent (Fig. 258-2), and breath-holding time may be markedly prolonged without any sensation of dyspnea.

Patients with PAH maintain rhythmic respiration when awake, although the level of ventilation is below normal. However, during sleep, when breathing is critically dependent on the metabolic control system, there is typically a further deterioration in ventilation, with frequent episodes of central hypopnea or apnea.

PAH must be distinguished from other central hypoventilation syndromes that are secondary to underlying neurologic disease of the brainstem or chemoreceptors (Table 258-1). This distinction requires a careful neurologic investigation for evidence of brainstem or autonomic disturbances. Unrecognized respiratory neuromuscular disorders, particularly those that produce diaphragmatic weakness, are often misdiagnosed as PAH. However, such disorders can usually be suspected on clinical grounds (see below) and can be confirmed by the finding of reduced voluntary hyperventilation, as well as PI_{max} and PE_{max}.

Patients with PAH must be cautioned against the use of sedative medications, which may readily induce acute respiratory failure. Some patients respond favorably to respiratory stimulant medications and to supplemental oxygen. However, the majority eventually require mechanical ventilatory assistance. Excellent long-term benefits can be achieved with diaphragmatic pacing by electrophrenic stimulation or with negative- or positive-pressure mechanical ventilation. The administration of such treatment only during sleep is sufficient in most patients.

RESPIRATORY NEUROMUSCULAR DISORDERS

Several primary disorders of the spinal cord, peripheral respiratory nerves, and respiratory muscles produce a chronic hypoventilation syndrome (Table 258-1). Hypoventilation usually develops gradually over a period of months to years and often first comes to attention when a relatively trivial increase in mechanical ventilatory load (such as mild airways obstruction) produces severe respiratory failure. In some of the disorders (such as motor neuron disease, myasthenia gravis, and muscular dystrophy), involvement of the respiratory nerves or muscles is usually a later feature of a more widespread disease. In other disorders, respiratory involvement can be an early or even isolated feature, and hence the underlying problem is often not suspected. Included in this category are the postpolio syndrome (a form of chronic respiratory insufficiency that develops 20–30 years following recovery from poliomyelitis), the myopathy associated with adult acid maltase deficiency, and idiopathic diaphragmatic paralysis.

Generally, respiratory neuromuscular disorders do not result in chronic hypoventilation unless there is significant weakness of the diaphragm. Distinguishing features of bilateral diaphragmatic weakness include orthopnea, paradoxical movement of the abdomen in the supine posture, and paradoxical diaphragmatic movement under fluoroscopy. However, the absence of these features does not exclude diaphragmatic weakness. Important laboratory features are a fall in forced vital capacity in the supine, compared to the upright, posture; a rapid deterioration of ventilation during a maximum voluntary ventilation maneuver; and reduced PI_{max} and PE_{max} (Fig. 258-2). More sophisticated investigations reveal reduced or absent transdiaphragmatic pressures, calculated from simultaneous measurement of esophageal and gastric pressures; reduced diaphragmatic EMG responses (recorded from an esophageal electrode) to transcutaneous phrenic nerve stimulation; and marked hypopnea and arterial oxygen desaturation during rapid eye movement sleep, when there is normally a physiologic inhibition of all nondiaphragmatic respiratory muscles and breathing becomes critically dependent on diaphragmatic activity.

The management of chronic alveolar hypoventilation due to respiratory neuromuscular disease involves treatment of the underlying disorder, where feasible, and mechanical ventilatory assistance as described for the PAH syndrome. However, electrophrenic diaphragmatic pacing is contraindicated in these disorders, except for high cervical spinal cord lesions in which the phrenic lower motor neurons and nerves are intact.

OBESITY-HYPOVENTILATION SYNDROME

Massive obesity represents a mechanical load to the respiratory system because the added weight on the rib cage and abdomen serves to reduce the compliance of the chest wall. As a result, the functional residual capacity (i.e., end-expiratory lung volume) is reduced, particularly in the recumbent posture. An important consequence of breathing at a low lung volume is that some airways, particularly those in the lung bases, may be closed throughout part or even all of each tidal breath, resulting in underventilation of the lung bases and widening of the $(A-a)P_{O_2}$. Nevertheless, in the majority of obese individuals, central respiratory drive is increased sufficiently to maintain a normal Pa_{CO_2}. However, a small proportion of obese patients develop chronic hypercapnia, hypoxemia, and eventually polycythemia, pulmonary hypertension, and right-sided heart failure. Studies in mice demonstrate that genetically obese mice lacking circulating leptin also develop chronic hypoventilation that can be reversed by leptin infusions. In humans with obesity-hypoventilation syndrome, serum leptin levels are elevated, suggesting that leptin resistance may play a role in the pathogenesis of the disorder.

In many patients, obstructive sleep apnea (Chap. 259) is a prominent feature, and even in those patients without sleep apnea, sleep-induced hypoventilation is an important element of the disorder and contributes to its progression. Most patients demonstrate a decrease in central respiratory drive, which may be inherent or acquired, and many have mild to moderate degrees of airflow obstruction, usually related to smoking. Based on these considerations, several therapeutic measures can be of considerable benefit, including weight loss, cessation of smoking, elimination of obstructive sleep apnea, and enhancement of respiratory drive by medications such as progesterone.

HYPERVENTILATION AND ITS SYNDROMES

DEFINITION AND ETIOLOGY

Alveolar hyperventilation exists when Pa_{CO_2} decreases below the normal range of 37–43 mmHg. *Hyperventilation* is not synonymous with *hyperpnea*, which refers to an increased minute volume of ventilation without reference to Pa_{CO_2}. Although hyperventilation is frequently associated with dyspnea, patients who are hyperventilating do not necessarily complain of shortness of breath; and conversely, patients with dyspnea need not be hyperventilating.

Numerous disease entities can be associated with alveolar hyperventilation (Table 258-2), but in all cases the underlying mechanism involves an increase in respiratory drive that is mediated through either the behavioral or the metabolic respiratory control systems (Fig. 258-3). Thus, hypoxemia drives ventilation by stimulating the peripheral chemoreceptors, and several pulmonary disorders and congestive heart failure drive ventilation by stimulating afferent vagal receptors in the lungs and airways. Low cardiac output and hypotension stimulate the peripheral chemoreceptors and inhibit the baroreceptors, both of which increase ventilation. Metabolic acidosis, a potent respiratory stimulant, excites both the peripheral and central chemoreceptors and increases the sensitivity of the peripheral chemoreceptors to coexistent hypoxemia. Hepatic failure can also produce hyperventilation, presumably as a result of metabolic stimuli acting on the peripheral and central chemoreceptors.

Several neurologic and psychological disorders are thought to drive ventilation through the behavioral respiratory control system. Included in this category are psychogenic or anxiety hyperventilation and severe cerebrovascular insufficiency, which may interfere with the inhibitory influence normally exerted by cortical structures on the

TABLE 258-2	HYPERVENTILATION SYNDROMES

1. Hypoxemia
  a. High altitude
  b. Pulmonary disease
  c. Cardiac shunts
2. Pulmonary disorders
  a. Pneumonia
  b. Interstitial pneumonitis, fibrosis, edema
  c. Pulmonary emboli, vascular disease
  d. Bronchial asthma
  e. Pneumothorax
  f. Chest wall disorders
3. Cardiovascular disorders
  a. Congestive heart failure
  b. Hypotension
4. Metabolic disorders
  a. Acidosis (diabetic, renal, lactic)
  b. Hepatic failure
	5. Neurologic and psychogenic disorders
	  a. Psychogenic or anxiety hyperventilation
	  b. Central nervous system infection, tumors
	6. Drug-induced
	  a. Salicylates
	  b. Methylxanthine derivatives
	  c. β-Adrenergic agonists
	  d. Progesterone
	7. Miscellaneous
	  a. Fever, sepsis
	  b. Pain
	  c. Pregnancy

brainstem respiratory neurons. Rarely, disorders of the midbrain and hypothalamus induce hyperventilation, and it is conceivable that fever and sepsis also cause hyperventilation through effects on these structures. Several drugs cause hyperventilation by stimulating the central or peripheral chemoreceptors or by direct action on the brainstem respiratory neurons. Chronic hyperventilation is a normal feature of pregnancy and results from the effects of progesterone and other hormones acting on the respiratory neurons.

PHYSIOLOGIC AND CLINICAL FEATURES

Because hyperventilation is associated with increased respiratory drive, muscle effort, and minute volume of ventilation, the most frequent symptom associated with hyperventilation is dyspnea. However, there is considerable discrepancy between the degree of hyperventilation, as measured by Pa_{CO_2}, and the degree of associated dyspnea. From a physiologic standpoint, hyperventilation is beneficial in patients who are hypoxemic, because the alveolar hypocapnia is associated with an increase in alveolar and arterial P_{O_2}. Conversely, hyperventilation can also be detrimental. In particular, the alkalemia associated with hypocapnia may produce neurologic symptoms, including dizziness, visual impairment, syncope, and seizure activity (secondary to cerebral vasoconstriction); paresthesia, carpopedal spasm, and tetany (secondary to decreased free serum calcium); and muscle weakness (secondary to hypophosphatemia). It may also be associated with panic attacks, and severe alkalemia can induce cardiac arrhythmias and evidence of myocardial ischemia. Patients with a primary respiratory alkalosis are also prone to periodic breathing and central sleep apnea (Chap. 259).

FIGURE 258-3 Schematic diagram of the mechanisms involved in alveolar hyperventilation. *[From EA Phillipson, AS Slutsky, in JF Murray, JA Nadel (eds), Textbook of Respiratory Medicine, 3d ed. Philadelphia, Saunders, 2000.]*

DIAGNOSIS

In most patients with a hyperventilation syndrome, the cause is readily apparent on the basis of history, physical examination, and knowledge of coexisting medical disorders (Table 258-2). In patients in whom the cause is not clinically apparent, investigation begins with arterial blood gas analysis, which establishes the presence of alveolar hyperventilation (decreased Pa_{CO_2}) and its severity. Equally important is the arterial pH, which generally allows the disorder to be classified as either a primary respiratory alkalosis (elevated pH) or a primary metabolic acidosis (decreased pH). Also of importance is the Pa_{O_2} and calculation of the $(A–a)P_{O_2}$, since a widened alveolar-arterial oxygen difference suggests a pulmonary disorder as the underlying cause. The finding of a reduced plasma HCO_3^- level establishes the chronic nature of the disorder and points toward an organic cause. Measurements of ventilation and arterial or transcutaneous P_{CO_2} during sleep are very useful in suspected psychogenic hyperventilation, since such patients do not maintain the hyperventilation during sleep.

The disorders that most frequently give rise to unexplained hyperventilation are pulmonary vascular disease (particularly chronic or recurrent thromboembolism) and psychogenic or anxiety hyperventilation. Hyperventilation due to pulmonary vascular disease is associated with exertional dyspnea, a widened $(A–a)P_{O_2}$ and maintenance of hyperventilation during exercise. In contrast, patients with psychogenic hyperventilation typically complain of dyspnea at rest, but not during mild exercise, and of the need to sigh frequently. They are also more likely to complain of dizziness, sweating, palpitations, and paresthesia. During mild to moderate exercise, their hyperventilation tends to disappear and $(A–a)P_{O_2}$ is normal, but heart rate and cardiac output may be increased relative to metabolic rate.

℞ HYPERVENTILATION

Mild alveolar hyperventilation is usually of relatively minor clinical consequence and therefore is generally managed by appropriate treatment of the underlying cause. In the few patients in whom alkalemia is thought to be inducing significant cerebral vasoconstriction, paresthesia, tetany, or cardiac disturbances, acute inhalation of a low concentration of CO_2 can be very beneficial. For patients with disabling psychogenic hyperventilation, careful explanation of the basis of their symptoms can be reassuring and is often sufficient. Others have benefited from β-adrenergic antagonists or an exercise program. Specific treatment for anxiety may also be indicated.

FURTHER READINGS

ANNANE D et al: Nocturnal mechanical ventilation for chronic hypoventilation in patients with neuromuscular and chest wall disorders. Cochrane Database Sys Rev 2:CD001941, 2000

FANBURG BL, SICILIAN L (eds): Respiratory dysfunction in neuromuscular disease. Clin Chest Med 15:607, 1994

LAFFEY JG, KAVANAGH BP: Hypocapnia. N Engl J Med 347:43, 2002

O'DONNELL CP et al: Leptin prevents respiratory depression in obesity. Am J Respir Crit Care Med 159:1477, 1999

OLSON AL, ZWILLICH C: The obesity hypoventilation syndrome. Am J Med 118:948, 2005

PHILLIPSON EA, DUFFIN J: Hypoventilation and hyperventilation syndromes, in Murray and Nadel's Textbook of Respiratory Medicine, 4th ed, RJ Mason et al (eds). Philadelphia, Saunders, 2005, pp 2069–2091

PHIPPS PR: Association of serum leptin with hypoventilation in human obesity. Thorax 57:75, 2002

TANKERSLEY CG et al: Genetic control of differential baseline breathing pattern. J Appl Physiol 82:874, 1997

259 Sleep Apnea
Neil J. Douglas

OBSTRUCTIVE SLEEP APNEA

Obstructive sleep apnea/hypopnea syndrome (OSAHS) is one of the most important medical conditions identified in the last 50 years. It is a major cause of morbidity, a significant cause of mortality throughout the world, and the most common medical cause of daytime sleepiness. Central sleep apnea is a less common clinical problem. Other sleep disorders are discussed in Chap. 28.

DEFINITION

OSAHS may be defined as the coexistence of unexplained excessive daytime sleepiness with at least five obstructed breathing events (apnea or hypopnea) per hour of sleep (Table 259-1). This event threshold may need to be refined upward in the elderly. Apneas are defined in adults as breathing pauses lasting ≥10 s and hypopneas as ≥10 s events where there is continued breathing but the ventilation is reduced by at least 50% from the previous baseline during sleep. As a syndrome, OSAHS is the association of a clinical picture with specific abnormalities on testing; asymptomatic individuals with abnormal breathing during sleep should not be labeled as having OSAHS.

MECHANISM OF OBSTRUCTION

Apneas and hypopneas are caused by the airway being sucked closed on inspiration during sleep. This occurs as the upper-airway dilating muscles—like all striated muscles—normally relax during sleep. In patients with OSAHS, the dilating muscles can no longer successfully oppose negative pressure within the airway during inspiration. The primary defect is not in the upper-airway muscles, which function normally in OSAHS patients when awake. These patients have narrow upper airways already during wakefulness, but when they are awake their airway dilating muscles have higher than normal activity, which ensures airway patency. However, when they are asleep, muscle tone falls and the airway narrows; snoring may commence before the airway occludes, and apnea results. Apneas and hypopneas terminate when the subject arouses, i.e., wakens briefly, from sleep. This arousal is sometimes too subtle to be seen on the electroencephalogram but may be detected by cardiac acceleration, blood pressure elevation, or sympathetic tone increase. The arousal results in return of upper-airway dilating muscle tone, and thus airway patency is resumed.

The factors predisposing to OSAHS by narrowing the pharynx include obesity—around 50% have a body mass index (BMI) >30 kg/m² in western populations—and shortening of the mandible and/or maxilla. This change in jaw shape may be subtle and can be familial. Hypothyroidism and acromegaly predispose to OSAHS by narrowing the

TABLE 259-1 CLINICAL INDICATORS IN THE SLEEPY PATIENT

	OSAHS	Narcolepsy	IHS
Age of onset (years)	35–60	10–30	10–30
Cataplexy	No	Yes	No
Night sleep			
Duration	Normal	Normal	Long
Awakenings	Occasional	Frequent	Rare
Snoring	Yes, loud	Occasional	Occasional
Morning drunkenness	Occasional	Occasional	Common
Daytime naps			
Frequency	Usually few	Many	Few
Time of day	Afternoon/ evening	Afternoon/ evening	Morning
Duration	<1 h	<1 h	>1 h

Note: Features suggesting obstructive sleep apnea/hypopnea syndrome (OSAHS), narcolepsy, or idiopathic hypersomnolence (IHS).

upper airway with tissue infiltration. Other predisposing factors for OSAHS include male gender and middle age (40–65 years), myotonic dystrophy, Ehlers Danlos syndrome, and perhaps also smoking.

EPIDEMIOLOGY

Broadly, the frequency of OSAHS is in the range of 1–4% of the middle-aged male population; it is around half as common in women. The syndrome also occurs in childhood–usually associated with tonsil or adenoid enlargement–and in the elderly, although the frequency is slightly lower in old age. Irregular breathing during sleep *without* daytime sleepiness is much more common, occurring in perhaps one-fourth of the middle-aged male population. However, as these individuals are asymptomatic, they do not have OSAHS and there is no evidence at present that these events are harmful.

CLINICAL FEATURES

Randomized controlled treatment trials have shown that OSAHS causes daytime sleepiness; impaired vigilance, cognitive performance, and driving; depression; disturbed sleep; and hypertension. Daytime sleepiness may range from mild to irresistible, and the sleep attacks can be indistinguishable from those in narcolepsy (Chap. 28). The sleepiness may result in inability to work effectively and may damage interpersonal relationships and prevent socializing. The somnolence is dangerous when driving, with a three- to sixfold risk in accidents on the road or when operating machinery. Experiments with normal subjects repeatedly aroused from sleep indicate that the sleepiness results, at least in part, from the repetitive sleep disruption associated with the breathing abnormality. The possible contribution from the recurrent hypoxemia requires further evaluation.

Other symptoms include difficulty concentrating, unrefreshing nocturnal sleep, nocturnal choking, nocturia, and decreased libido. Partners report nightly loud snoring in all postures, which may be punctuated by the silence of apneas. Partners often give a markedly different assessment of the extent of sleepiness.

Cardiovascular and Cerebrovascular Events
OSAHS raises 24-h mean blood pressure. The increase is greater in those with recurrent nocturnal hypoxemia, is at least 4–5 mmHg, and may be as great as 10 mmHg in those with >20% arterial oxygen desaturations per hour of sleep. This rise probably results from a combination of surges in blood pressure accompanying each arousal from sleep that end each apnea or hypopnea and from the associated 24-h increases in sympathetic tone.

Epidemiologic data in normal populations indicate that this rise in blood pressure would increase the risk of myocardial infarction by around 20% and stroke by about 40%. While there are no long-term randomized controlled trials to indicate whether this is true in OSAHS patients—and such studies would not be ethically defensible—observational studies suggest an increase in the risk of myocardial infarction and stroke in untreated OSAHS. Furthermore, epidemiologic studies suggest, but do not prove, increased vascular risk in normal subjects with raised apneas and hypopneas during sleep. Patients with recent stroke have a high frequency of apneas and hypopneas during sleep. These seem largely to be a consequence, not a cause, of the stroke and to decline over the weeks after the vascular event. There is no evidence that treating the apneas and hypopneas improves stroke outcome.

There has been debate for decades whether OSAHS is an adult form of sudden infant death syndrome. Although earlier studies showed no increase in sudden nocturnal deaths in OSAHS, a recent large study reported excess nocturnal deaths in subjects previously shown to have apneas and hypopneas during sleep.

Diabetes Mellitus
The association of OSAHS with diabetes mellitus is not just due to obesity being common in both conditions. Recent data suggest that increased apneas and hypopneas during sleep are associated with insulin resistance independent of obesity. In addition, uncontrolled trials suggest that OSAHS can aggravate diabetes and that treatment of OSAHS in patients who also have diabetes decreases their insulin requirements.

Liver
Hepatic dysfunction has also been associated with irregular breathing during sleep. Non-alcohol drinking subjects with apneas and hypopneas during sleep were found to have raised liver enzymes and more steatosis and fibrosis on liver biopsy, independent of body weight.

Anesthestic Risk
Patients with OSAHS are at increased risk perioperatively as their upper airway may obstruct during the recovery period or as a consequence of sedation. Patients whose anesthesiologists have difficulty intubating are much more likely to have irregular breathing during sleep. Anesthesiologists should thus take sleep histories on patients preoperatively and take the appropriate precautions with those who might have OSAHS. This should include referring patients suspected of having OSAHS for investigation, and some elective operations may need to be postponed until the OSAHS is treated.

Differential Diagnosis
(See also Chap. 28) Causes of sleepiness which may need to be distinguished include (Table 259-1):

- *Insufficient sleep:* this can usually be diagnosed by history.
- *Shift work:* this is a major cause of sleepiness, especially in those over 40 years old on either rotating shift or night shift work patterns.
- *Psychological/psychiatric causes:* depression is a major cause of sleepiness.
- *Drugs:* both stimulant and sedative drugs can produce sleepiness.
- *Narcolepsy:* around 50 times less common than OSAHS, narcolepsy is usually evident from childhood or teens and is associated with cataplexy.
- *Idiopathic hypersomnolence:* this is an ill-defined condition typified by long sleep duration and sleepiness.
- *Phase alteration syndromes:* both the phase delay and the less-common phase advancement syndromes are characterized by sleepiness at the characteristic time of day.

Who to Refer for Diagnosis
Anyone whose troublesome sleepiness is not readily explained and rectified by considering the above differential diagnosis should be referred to a sleep specialist. The guideline I use for patients with troublesome sleepiness includes those with an Epworth Sleepiness Score >11 (Table 259-2), and those for whom sleepiness during work or driving poses problems. However, the Epworth Score is not a perfect measure for detecting troublesome sleepiness, as many whose life is troubled by frequently fighting sleepiness but who never doze will correctly score themselves as having a low Epworth Score. The patient and his/her partner often give divergent scores for the patient's sleepiness, and in such cases the higher of the two scores should be used.

TABLE 259-2 EPWORTH SLEEPINESS SCORE

How often are you likely to doze off or fall asleep in the following situations, in contrast to feeling just tired? This refers to your usual way of life in recent times. Even if you have not done some of these things recently, try to work out how they would have affected you. Use the following scale to choose the *most appropriate number* for each situation:

0 = would *never* doze
1 = *slight* chance of dozing
2 = *moderate* chance of dozing
3 = *high* chance of dozing

Sitting and reading	....
Watching TV	....
Sitting, inactive in a public place (e.g., a theater or a meeting)	....
As a passenger in a car for an hour without a break	....
Lying down to rest in the afternoon when circumstances permit	....
Sitting and talking to someone	....
Sitting quietly after lunch without alcohol	....
In a car, while stopped for a few minutes in traffic	....
TOTAL	....

Source: From MW Johns: Sleep 14:540, 1991.

Diagnosis OSAHS is a condition requiring lifelong treatment, and the diagnosis needs to be made or excluded with certainty, when possible, by a specialist. This will hinge on obtaining a good sleep history from the patient and partner, including asking both to complete sleep questionnaires, including the Epworth Sleepiness Score (Table 259-2). Physical examination must include assessment of obesity, jaw structure, the upper airway, blood pressure, and possible predisposing causes, including hypothyroidism and acromegaly (see above).

In those with appropriate clinical features, the diagnostic test must demonstrate recurrent breathing pauses during sleep. This may be a full polysomnographic examination with recording of multiple respiratory and neurophysiologic signals during sleep (Chap. 28). Increasingly, and especially outside the United States, most diagnostic tests are "limited studies"—recording respiratory and oxygenation patterns overnight without neurophysiologic recording. Such approaches in expert hands produce good patient outcomes and are cost-effective. It is sensible to use such limited sleep studies as the first-line diagnostic test and then allow positively diagnosed patients to proceed to treatment. However, a reasonable approach at present is for patients with troublesome sleepiness but negative limited studies to then have polysomnography to exclude or confirm OSAHS.

℞ OBSTRUCTIVE SLEEP APNEA

WHOM TO TREAT There is evidence obtained from robust randomized controlled trials (RCT) that treatment improves symptoms, sleepiness, driving, cognition, mood, quality of life, and blood pressure in patients who have an Epworth score of >11, troublesome sleepiness while driving or working, and >15 apneas + hypopneas per hour of sleep. For those with similar degrees of sleepiness and 5–15 events per hour of sleep, RCTs indicate improvements in symptoms, including subjective sleepiness, with less strong evidence indicating gains in cognition and quality of life. There is no evidence of blood pressure improvements in this group, nor is there is evidence that treating nonsleepy subjects improves their symptoms, function, or blood pressure. Thus, treatment cannot be advocated for this large group.

HOW TO TREAT All patients diagnosed with OSAHS should have the condition and its significance explained to them and to their partner. This should be accompanied by provision of written and/or web-based information and a discussion of the implications of the local regulations for driving. Rectifiable predispositions should be discussed; this often includes weight loss and sometimes reduction of alcohol consumption to reduce caloric intake and because alcohol acutely decreases upper-airway dilating muscle tone, thus predisposing to obstructed breathing. Sedative drugs, which also affect airway tone, should be carefully withdrawn.

Continuous Positive Airway Pressure (CPAP) CPAP therapy works by blowing the airway open during sleep, usually with pressures of 5–20 cmHg. CPAP has been shown in randomized placebo-controlled trials to improve breathing during sleep, sleep quality, sleepiness, blood pressure, vigilance, cognition, and driving ability, as well as mood and quality of life in patients with OSAHS. However, this is obtrusive therapy, and care must be taken to explain the need for the treatment to the patient and his/her partner, and to support all patients on CPAP intensively, providing access to telephone support and regular follow-up. Initiation should include finding the most comfortable mask from the ranges of several manufacturers and trying the system for at least 30 min during the daytime to prepare for the overnight trial. An overnight monitored trial of CPAP is used to identify the pressure required to keep the patient's airway patent. The development of pressure-varying CPAP machines may make the in-lab CPAP night trial unnecessary, but treatment must be initiated in a supportive environment. Thereafter, patients can be treated with fixed-pressure CPAP machines set at the determined pressure or by a self-adjusting, intelligent CPAP device. The main side effect of CPAP is airway drying, which can be countered using an integral heated humidifier. CPAP use, like that of all therapies, is imperfect, but around 94% of patients with severe OSAHS are still using their therapy after 5 years on objective monitoring.

Mandibular Repositioning Splint (MRS) Also called oral devices, MRSs work by holding the lower jaw and the tongue forward, thereby widening the pharyngeal airway. MRSs have been shown in RCTs to improve

OSAHS patients' breathing during sleep, daytime somnolence, and blood pressure. As there are many devices of differing design with unknown relative efficacy, these results cannot be generalized to all MRSs. Self-reports of the use of devices long-term suggest high dropout rates.

Surgery Four forms of surgery have a role in OSAHS, although it must always be remembered that these patients have a raised perioperative risk. Bariatric surgery can be curative in the morbidly obese. Tonsillectomy can be highly effective in children but rarely in adults. Tracheostomy is curative but rarely used because of the associated morbidity; nevertheless, it should not be overlooked in extremely advanced cases. Jaw advancement surgery—particularly maxillo-mandibular osteotomy—is effective in those with retrognathia (posterior displacement of the mandible) and should be particularly considered in young and thin patients. There is no robust evidence that pharyngeal surgery, including uvulopalatopharyngoplasty (whether by scalpel, laser, or thermal techniques) helps OSAHS.

Drugs Unfortunately, no drugs are clinically useful in the prevention or reduction of apneas and hypopneas. A marginal improvement in sleepiness in patients who remain sleepy despite CPAP can be produced by modafinil, but the clinical value is debatable and the financial cost significant.

CHOICE OF TREATMENT CPAP and MRS are the two most widely used and best evidence-based therapies. Direct comparisons in RCTs indicate better outcomes with CPAP in terms of apneas and hypopneas, nocturnal oxygenation, symptoms, quality of life, mood, and vigilance. Adherence to CPAP is generally better than to an MRS, and there is evidence that CPAP improves driving, whereas there are no such data on MRSs, Thus, CPAP is the current treatment of choice. However, MRSs are evidence-based second-line therapy in those who fail CPAP. In younger, thinner patients, maxillo-mandibular advancement should be considered.

HEALTH RESOURCES Untreated OSAHS patients are heavy users of health care and dangerous drivers; they also work beneath their potential. Treatment of OSAHS with CPAP is cost-effective in terms of reducing health care costs of associated illness and associated accidents.

CENTRAL SLEEP APNEA

Central sleep apneas (CSAs) are respiratory pauses caused by lack of respiratory effort. These occur occasionally in normal subjects, particularly at sleep onset and in REM sleep, and are transiently increased following ascent to altitude. Recurrent CSA is most commonly found in the presence of cardiac failure or neurologic disease, especially stroke. Spontaneous central sleep syndrome is rare and can be classified on the basis of the arterial P_{CO_2}.

Hypercapnic CSA occurs in conjunction with diminished ventilatory drive in Ondine's curse (central alveolar hypoventilation). Patients with normocapnic spontaneous CSA have a normal or low arterial P_{CO_2} when awake, with brisk ventilatory responses to hypercapnia. This combination results in unstable ventilatory control, with subjects breathing close to or below their apneic threshold for P_{CO_2} during sleep; this apneic tendency is compounded by cycles of arousal-induced hyperventilation, inducing further hypocapnia.

CLINICAL FEATURES

Patients may present with sleep maintenance insomnia, which is relatively unusual in OSAHS. Daytime sleepiness may occur.

INVESTIGATION

Many apneas previously labeled central because of absent thoracoabdominal movement are actually obstructive, identification of movement being particularly difficult in the very obese. CSA can only be identified with certainty if either esophageal pressure or respiratory muscle electromyography is recorded and shown to be absent during the events.

℞ CENTRAL SLEEP APNEA

Patients with underlying cardiac failure should have their failure treated appropriately. CPAP may improve outcome but is difficult to initiate and has not been shown to improve survival. Patients with spontaneous normocapnic CSA may be successfully treated with acetazolamide. In a minority of patients, CPAP is effective, perhaps because in some patients with OSAHS, pharyngeal collapse initiates reflex inhibition of respiration, and these episodes are prevented by CPAP. Oxygen and nocturnal nasal positive/pressure ventilation may also be tried.

FURTHER READINGS

DOUGLAS NJ: *Clinicians' Guide to Sleep Medicine.* London, Arnold, 2002

————: Home diagnosis of the obstructive sleep apnoea/hypopnoea syndrome. Sleep Med Rev 7:53, 2003

ECKERT DJ et al: Central sleep apnea: Pathophysiology and treatment. Chest 131:595, 2007

ENGLEMAN HM et al: Randomized crossover trial of two treatments for sleep apnea/hypopnea syndrome: Continuous positive airway pressure and mandibular repositioning splint. Am J Respir Crit Care Med 165:855, 2002

MARIN JM et al: Long-term cardiovascular outcomes in men with obstructive sleep apnoea-hypopnoea with or without treatment with continuous positive airway pressure: An observational study. Lancet 365:1046, 2005

PACK AL et al: Risk factors for excessive sleepiness in older adults. Ann Neurol 59:893, 2006

SUNDARAM S et al: Surgery for obstructive sleep apnoea. Cochrane Database Syst Rev 2005, CD001004

WHITELAW WA et al: Clinical usefulness of home oximetry compared with polysomnography for assessment of sleep apnea. Am J Respir Crit Care Med 171:188, 2005

YAGGI HK et al: Obstructive sleep apnea as a risk factor for stroke and death. N Engl J Med 353:2034, 2005

260 Lung Transplantation
Elbert P. Trulock

Lung transplantation is a therapeutic consideration for patients with most nonmalignant end-stage lung diseases. After an initial period of rapid growth from 1990 through 1995, activity has increased slowly to ~1700 transplants per year worldwide. The demand for transplantation exceeds the supply of donor organs, and the waiting time is often lengthy. Recognizing the window of opportunity for transplantation in the clinical course of various lung diseases is crucial because deaths while awaiting transplantation are not unusual. However, in appropriately selected recipients, transplantation prolongs survival and improves quality of life, but it is also associated with significant morbidity and mortality.

INDICATIONS

The indications for lung transplantation span the gamut of lung diseases (Table 260-1). The distribution reflects the prevalence and natural history of the diseases, and the most common indications are chronic obstructive pulmonary disease (COPD), idiopathic pulmonary fibrosis (IPF), cystic fibrosis (CF), α_1-antitrypsin deficiency emphysema, and primary pulmonary hypertension (PPH). "Others" in Table 260-1 comprise many less prevalent lung diseases.

RECIPIENT SELECTION

Transplantation should be considered when other therapeutic options have been exhausted and when the patient's prognosis will be improved by the procedure. Survival rates after transplantation can be compared with predictive indices for the underlying disease, but each patient's clinical course must be integrated into the assessment, too. In any case, projected survival after transplantation should exceed life expectancy without the procedure. Quality of life is the primary motive for transplantation for many patients, and the prospect of an improved quality-adjusted survival is often attractive, even if the survival advantage itself might be marginal.

Disease-specific guidelines for referring patients for transplantation are summarized in Table 260-2, and these are intended to identify patients who may benefit from transplantation. Candidates for lung transplantation are thoroughly screened for any comorbidity that might adversely affect the outcome. Suitable candidates should have clinically and physiologically severe lung disease, but otherwise they must be in reasonably good health. The upper age limit is ~65 years at most centers.

Typical exclusions include HIV infection, chronic hepatitis B antigenemia or chronic active hepatitis C infection, uncured malignancy, active cigarette smoking, drug or alcohol dependency or abuse, uncontrolled or untreatable pulmonary or extrapulmonary infection, irreversible physical deconditioning, chronic noncompliance with medical care, and significant disease of any vital organ other than the lungs. Other problems that might increase the risk of complications or might be aggravated by the posttransplantation medical regimen constitute relative contraindications. Some typical issues are ventilator-dependent respiratory failure, previous thoracic surgical procedures, osteoporosis, systemic hypertension, diabetes mellitus, obesity or cachexia, and psychosocial problems. Chronic infection with antibiotic-resistant *Pseudomonas* species, some *Burkholderia* species, *Aspergillus* species, or nontuberculous mycobacteria is a unique concern in some patients with CF or other diseases that have a component of bronchiectasis or chronic bronchitis. The potential impact of these and many other factors has to be judged in clinical context to determine an individual candidate's suitability for transplantation.

WAITING LIST AND ORGAN ALLOCATION

Organ allocation policies are influenced by ethical, medical, geographical, and political factors, and systems vary from country to country. Re-

TABLE 260-1	INDICATIONS FOR ADULT LUNG TRANSPLANTATION (1995–2004)					
Diagnosis	**Single Lung Transplantation** (n = 6731)		**Bilateral Lung Transplantation** (n = 6276)		**Total (n = 13,007)**	
Chronic obstructive pulmonary disease	3541	52.6%	1462	23.3%	5003	38.5%
Idiopathic pulmonary fibrosis	1618	24.0%	639	10.0%	2257	17.4%
Cystic fibrosis	151	2.2%	2002	31.9%	2153	16.6%
α_1-Antitrypsin deficiency emphysema	554	8.2%	571	9.1%	1125	8.6%
Primary pulmonary hypertension	79	1.2%	436	6.9%	515	4.0%
Sarcoidosis	157	2.3%	166	2.6%	323	2.5%
Bronchiectasis	45	0.7%	309	4.9%	354	2.7%
Eisenmenger's syndrome	13	0.2%	118	1.9%	131	1.0%
Lymphoangioleiomyomatosis	55	0.8%	83	1.3%	138	1.0%
Retransplantation	129	1.9%	104	1.7%	233	1.8%
Others	389	5.8%	386	6.2%	775	6.0%

Source: Adapted from Trulock et al.

TABLE 260-2	DISEASE-SPECIFIC GUIDELINES FOR SELECTING CANDIDATES FOR LUNG TRANSPLANTATION

COPD and α_1-antitrypsin deficiency emphysema
  FEV_1 < 25% of predicted normal value (post-bronchodilator)
  Pa_{CO_2} ≥ 55 mmHg
  Pulmonary arterial hypertension (mean pulmonary artery pressure > 25 mmHg)

Cystic fibrosis/bronchiectasis
  FEV_1 < 30% of predicted normal value
  Pa_{CO_2} > 50 mmHg
  Pa_{O_2} < 50 mmHg (on room air)
  Pulmonary arterial hypertension
  Adverse clinical course in spite of optimal medical management
    Increasing hospitalizations
    Recurrent, massive hemoptysis
    Rapidly declining FEV_1

Idiopathic pulmonary fibrosis
  VC or TLC < 60–70% of predicted normal value
  DL_{CO} < 50–60% of predicted normal value
  Pulmonary arterial hypertension
  Hypoxemia (Pa_{O_2} < 60 mmHg or Sp_{O_2} < 90%) at rest or with activity (on room air)
  Progressive disease in spite of drug therapy

Primary pulmonary hypertension
  New York Heart Association functional class III or IV in spite of optimal drug therapy
  Unfavorable hemodynamic profile
    Right atrial pressure > 15 mmHg
    Mean pulmonary artery pressure > 55 mmHg
    Cardiac index < 2 (L/min)/m²

Abbreviations: VC, vital capacity; TLC, total lung capacity; FEV_1, forced expiratory volume in 1 s; DL_{CO}, diffusing capacity for carbon monoxide; Pa_{O_2} and Pa_{CO_2}, partial pressure of oxygen and carbon dioxide, respectively, in arterial blood; Sp_{O_2}, oxygen saturation by pulse oximetry.
Source: Modified from International Guidelines for the Selection of Lung Transplant Candidates: Am J Respir Crit Care Med 158:335, 1998.

gardless of the system, potential recipients are placed on a waiting list and must be matched for blood group compatibility and, with some latitude, for lung size with an acceptable donor. In the United States a priority algorithm for allocating donor lungs was implemented in May 2005. Priority is determined by a lung allocation score that weighs both the patient's risk of death on the waiting list and the likelihood of survival after transplantation. Both the type and the severity of lung disease affect the allocation score; relevant parameters must be updated periodically but can be submitted whenever the patient's condition changes. However, this priority system does not diminish the importance of timely referral.

The impact of the priority allocation scheme on key outcome measures has not been analyzed yet; however, this information will be forthcoming and may lead to further refinement of the allocation system. Under the previous seniority system, the median time to transplantation was 1104 days for patients who initially registered on the national waiting list in 1998. Approximately 10% of the patients on the waiting list died before transplantation, but the death rate while waiting was much higher for patients with IPF, PPH, or CF than for those with COPD or α_1-antitrypsin deficiency emphysema.

TRANSPLANT PROCEDURE

Bilateral transplantation is mandatory for bronchiectasis because the risk of spillover infection from a remaining native lung precludes single lung transplantation. Heart-lung transplantation is obligatory for Eisenmenger's syndrome with complex anomalies that cannot be readily repaired in conjunction with lung transplantation and for concomitant end-stage lung and heart disease. However, cardiac replacement is not necessary for cor pulmonale because right ventricular function will recover when pulmonary vascular afterload is normalized by lung transplantation.

Either bilateral or single lung transplantation is an acceptable alternative for other diseases unless there is a special consideration. Bilateral transplantation provides more reserve lung function as a buffer against complications, and it has been increasingly utilized for many indications. In recipients with COPD and α_1-antitrypsin deficiency emphysema, survival has been significantly better after bilateral transplantation, but there has not been a significant difference in survival between the two procedures for other diseases.

Living donor lobar transplantation has a limited role in adult lung transplantation. It has been performed predominantly in teenagers or young adults with CF. A right lower lobe is obtained from one living donor and a left lower lobe from another, and these lobes are implanted to replace the right and left lungs, respectively, in the recipient. Since a lobe must replace a whole lung, donor-recipient size considerations are crucial. The results have been comparable to those with transplantation from cadaveric donors. The usual morbidities associated with a lobectomy have been encountered in the donors, but no death has yet been reported. Because of ethical concerns, this approach is usually restricted to patients who are unlikely to survive the wait for a cadaveric donor.

POSTTRANSPLANTATION MANAGEMENT

Induction therapy with an antilymphocyte globulin or an interleukin 2 receptor antagonist is utilized by some centers, and a three-drug maintenance immunosuppressive regimen that includes a calcineurin inhibitor (cyclosporine or tacrolimus), a purine synthesis antagonist (azathioprine or mycophenolate mofetil), and prednisone is customary. Subsequently, other drugs such as sirolimus may be substituted in the maintenance regimen for various reasons. Prophylaxis for *Pneumocystis jiroveci* pneumonia is standard, and prophylaxis against cytomegalovirus (CMV) infection is prescribed in many protocols. The dose of cyclosporine or tacrolimus is adjusted by blood-level monitoring. Both are metabolized by the hepatic cytochrome P450 system, and interactions with medications that affect this pathway can significantly alter the clearance and blood levels of these key immunosuppressants.

Routine management is designed to monitor the allograft, to regulate immunosuppressive therapy, and to detect problems or complications expeditiously. The techniques include periodic contact with a transplant nurse coordinator, appointments with a physician, chest radiographs, blood tests, spirometry, and bronchoscopy. Lung function rapidly improves and then stabilizes by 3–6 months after transplantation. Subsequently, the coefficient of variation in spirometric measurements is small, and a sustained decline of 10–15% or more signals a potentially significant problem.

OUTCOMES

Survival   Major registries publish survival (Table 260-3) and other outcomes annually, and these reports are accessible via the Internet (*www.ishlt.org; www.ustransplant.org*).

The main sources of perioperative mortality include technical complications of the operation, primary graft dysfunction, and infections.

TABLE 260-3	RECIPIENT SURVIVAL, BY PRETRANSPLANTATION DIAGNOSIS (1994–2003)

		Survival Rate, %				
Diagnosis	n	3 Months	1 Year	3 Years	5 Years	10 Years
Chronic obstructive pulmonary disease	4888	90	81	63	48	19
α_1-Antitrypsin deficiency emphysema	1127	86	76	60	51	31
Cystic fibrosis	1934	88	81	65	54	32
Idiopathic pulmonary fibrosis	2058	81	69	54	42	15
Primary pulmonary hypertension	553	73	65	56	46	26

Source: Data from Trulock et al.

Acute rejection and CMV infection are common problems in the first year, but neither is usually fatal. Beyond the first year, chronic rejection and non-CMV infections cause the majority of deaths.

Function Regardless of the disease, successful transplantation impressively restores cardiopulmonary function. After bilateral transplantation standard pulmonary function tests are typically normal; after single lung transplantation the remaining diseased lung typically contributes a mild abnormality. Formal exercise testing usually demonstrates some impairment in maximum work rate and maximum oxygen uptake, but few recipients report any limitation to activity.

Quality of Life Both overall and health-related quality of life are enhanced. With multidimensional profiles, improvements extend across most domains and are sustained longitudinally unless chronic rejection or some other complication develops. Other problems that detract from quality of life include renal dysfunction and drug side effects.

Cost The cost of transplantation depends on the health care system, other health care policies, and economic factors that vary from country to country. In the 1990s transplant hospitalization costs in the range of $160,000 were reported from two centers in the United States. At one of these centers, the average charge for posttransplantation care was ~$132,000 in the first year and $54,000 in subsequent years. The distribution of costs after lung transplantation was estimated by a center in the United Kingdom: 57% for routine care including medications, clinic appointments, and tests; 17% for rejection episodes; and 26% for infectious complications.

Complications Lung transplantation can be complicated by a variety of problems. Aside from those that are unique to transplantation, side effects and toxicities of the immunosuppressive medications can cause new medical problems or aggravate preexisting conditions (Table 260-4).

Graft Dysfunction Primary graft dysfunction is an acute lung injury that is a manifestation of insults that are inherent in the transplantation process, and it has been referred to as *reperfusion edema, reimplantation response,* and *ischemia-reperfusion injury*. The principal clinical features are diffuse pulmonary infiltrates and hypoxemia within 72 h of transplantation, but the severity is variable. Pulmonary venous obstruction and hyperacute rejection can produce a similar pattern, and cardiogenic pulmonary edema and pneumonia must be excluded, too. The treatment is the conventional, supportive paradigm for acute lung injury, but inhaled nitric oxide and extracorporeal membrane oxygenation have been used successfully in severe cases. Most recipients recover, but severe primary graft dysfunction is a leading cause of early morbidity and mortality.

Airway Complications The bronchial blood supply to the donor lung is disrupted, and bronchial revascularization is not widely practiced. Consequently, when the lung is implanted in the recipient, the bronchus is dependent on retrograde bronchial blood flow through the pulmonary circulation and is vulnerable to ischemia.

The prevalence of major airway complications—dehiscence, stenosis, and bronchomalacia—has ranged from 4–20%, but the associated mortality has been very low. Bronchoscopic debridement or dilatation is sufficient in many cases, but stent placement is often necessary if a stricture or bronchomalacia evolves.

Acute Rejection This is an immunologic response to alloantigen recognition, and it is characterized by arteriolar and bronchiolar lymphocytic inflammation. With current immunosuppressive regimens, ~50% recipients have at least one episode of acute rejection in the first year. Acute rejection can be clinically silent, or it can be manifested by nonspecific symptoms or signs that may include cough, low-grade fever, dyspnea, hypoxemia, inspiratory crackles, interstitial infiltrates, and declining lung function; however, clinical impression is not reliable. The diagnosis should be confirmed by transbronchial biopsy, and a standardized pathologic

TABLE 260-4	MAJOR POTENTIAL COMPLICATIONS OF LUNG TRANSPLANTATION AND POSTTRANSPLANTATION IMMUNOSUPPRESSION
Category	**Complication**
Allograft	Acute graft dysfunction; anastomotic dehiscence or stenosis; ischemic airway injury with bronchostenosis or bronchomalacia; rejection; infections
Thoracic	Phrenic nerve injury—diaphragmatic dysfunction; recurrent laryngeal nerve injury—vocal cord dysfunction; cervical ganglia injury—Horner's syndrome; chylothorax; pneumothorax; pleural effusion
Cardiovascular	Air embolism; postoperative pericarditis; venous thromboembolism; supraventricular dysrhythmias; systemic hypertension
Gastrointestinal	Esophagitis (especially *Candida* species or CMV); gastroparesis; gastroesophageal reflux; *C. difficile* toxin diarrhea or pseudomembranous colitis
Hepatobiliary	Hepatitis (especially CMV or drug-induced)
Renal	Calcineurin inhibitor nephropathy; hemolytic-uremic syndrome (thrombotic microangiopathy)
Neurologic	Tremors; seizures; reversible posterior leukoencephalopathy; headaches
Musculoskeletal	Steroid myopathy; rhabdomyolysis (cyclosporine + HMG-CoA reductase inhibitor treatment); osteoporosis; avascular necrosis
Metabolic	Obesity; diabetes mellitus; hyperlipidemia; idiopathic hyperammonemia
Hematologic	Anemia; leukopenia; thrombocytopenia; thrombotic microangiopathy
Oncologic	Lymphoproliferative disease and lymphoma; skin cancers; other malignancies

classification scheme for rejection is used to grade the biopsies. Treatment usually includes a short course of high-dose steroid therapy and adjustment of the maintenance immunosuppressive regimen, but more intensive therapy may be necessary for persistent or recurrent episodes.

Chronic Rejection This complication is the main impediment to better medium-term survival rates, and it is the source of substantial morbidity because of its impact on lung function and quality of life. The pathogenesis is still a conundrum, but both alloimmune inflammatory and nonalloimmune fibroproliferative mechanisms are probably important.

Clinically, chronic rejection is a form of graft dysfunction that is synonymous with bronchiolitis obliterans syndrome (BOS). BOS is characterized physiologically by airflow limitation and pathologically by bronchiolitis obliterans. Transbronchial biopsies are relatively insensitive for detecting bronchiolitis obliterans, and the diagnosis of BOS is usually based on a sustained decrement ($\geq 20\%$) in the FEV_1. A smaller decline in FEV_1 ($\geq 10\%$) or a decrease in the $FEF_{25-75\%}$ may presage BOS.

The prevalence of BOS approaches 50% by 5 years after transplantation. Both antecedent acute rejection and lymphocytic bronchiolitis are risk factors for subsequent BOS, and CMV pneumonitis has been implicated inconsistently. BOS is usually treated with augmented immunosuppression. While immunosuppressive therapy may stabilize lung function, the overall results of treatment have been disappointing, probably because the fibroproliferative process is already well established. Retransplantation may be an option in ambulatory recipients without other complications, but in many cases the risk is prohibitive.

Infection The lung allograft is especially susceptible to infection, and infection has been one of the leading causes of death. In addition to a blunted immune response from the immunosuppressive drugs, other normal defenses are breached; the cough reflex is diminished, and mucociliary clearance is impaired in the transplanted lung. The spectrum of infections includes both opportunistic and nonopportunistic pathogens.

Bacterial bronchitis or pneumonia can occur at any time but are almost universal in the postoperative period. Later, episodes of bronchitis are quite common, especially in recipients with BOS, and

Pseudomonas aeruginosa or methicillin-resistant *Staphylococcus aureus* is often the culprit.

CMV is the most frequent viral infection. Although gastroenteritis, colitis, and hepatitis can occur, CMV viremia and CMV pneumonia are the main illnesses. Most episodes occur in the first 6 months, and treatment with ganciclovir is effective unless resistance develops with repeated exposure. Other community-acquired viruses such as influenza, parainfluenza, and respiratory syncytial virus also contribute to respiratory complications. *Aspergillus* species have been the most problematic fungal infection.

Other Complications   Other potential complications are summarized in Table 260-4, and many of these are related to side effects or toxicities of the immunosuppressive drugs. Management of most of these general medical problems is guided by standard practices for the condition, but the complex milieu of transplantation dictates close collaboration and good communication among health care providers.

ACKNOWLEDGMENT

Dr. G. Alexander Patterson and Dr. Joel D. Cooper were co-authors of this chapter in the 16th edition. Some of the materials have been carried over into this edition.

FURTHER READINGS

ESTENNE M et al: Bronchiolitis obliterans syndrome 2001: An update of the diagnostic criteria. J Heart Lung Transplant 21:297, 2002

KOTLOFF RM, AHYA VN: Medical complications of lung transplantation. Eur Respir J 23:334; 2004

LANDE JD et al: Novel insights into lung transplant rejection by microarray analysis. Proc Am Thorac Soc 4:44, 2007

TRULOCK EP et al: Registry of the International Society for Heart and Lung Transplantation: Twenty-second official adult lung and heart-lung transplant report—2005. J Heart Lung Transplant 24:956, 2005

CHAPTER 260

Lung Transplantation

261 Principles of Critical Care Medicine

John P. Kress, Jesse B. Hall

The care of critically ill patients requires a thorough understanding of pathophysiology and is centered initially around resuscitation of patients at extremes of physiologic deterioration. This resuscitation is often fast-paced and may occur in early stages without a detailed awareness of patients' chronic medical problems. While physiologic stabilization is taking place, intensivists attempt to gather important background medical information to supplement the real-time assessment of the patients' current physiologic conditions. Numerous tools are available to assist intensivists in the accurate assessment of pathophysiology and to support incipient organ failures, thus offering a window of opportunity for diagnosing and treating underlying disease(s) in a stabilized patient. Indeed, the use of invasive interventions such as mechanical ventilation and renal replacement therapy as well as diagnostic tools such as central venous catheters are commonplace in the intensive care unit. An appreciation of the risks and benefits of such aggressive and often invasive interventions is vital to assure an optimal patient outcome. Notwithstanding, intensivists must recognize when patients' chances for recovery are remote or impossible and work to counsel and comfort dying patients and their significant others. Critical care physicians must often redirect the goals of care from resuscitation and cure to comfort when the resolution of an underlying illness is not possible.

ASSESSMENT OF SEVERITY OF ILLNESS

Categorization of a patient's illness into grades of severity occurs frequently in the intensive care unit (ICU). There are numerous severity-of-illness scoring systems that have been developed and validated over the past two decades. While these scoring systems have been validated as tools to accurately assess populations of critically ill patients, their utility in predicting individual patient outcomes is not clear.

Severity-of-illness scoring systems are important for defining populations of critically ill patients. This allows effective comparison of groups of patients enrolled in clinical trials. To be assured that a purported benefit of a therapy is real, investigators must be assured that different groups involved in a clinical trial have similar illness severities. Severity-of-illness scores are also useful in guiding hospital administrative policies. Allocation of resources, such as nursing and ancillary care, can be directed by such scoring systems. Severity-of-illness scoring systems can also assist in the assessment of quality of ICU care over time. Scoring system validations are based on the premise that increasing age, presence of chronic medical illnesses, and increasingly severe derangements from normal physiology are each associated with increased mortality. All currently existing severity-of-illness scoring systems are derived from patients who have been already admitted to the ICU. There are no established scoring systems available that allege to direct clinicians' decision-making regarding what constitute criteria for admission to an ICU.

Currently, the most commonly utilized scoring systems are the APACHE (acute physiology and chronic health evaluation) system, the MPM (mortality probability model), and the SAPS (simplified acute physiology score) system. These were all designed to predict outcomes in critical illness and use severity-of-illness scoring systems with common variables. These include age; vital signs; assessments of respiratory, renal, and neurologic function; and an evaluation of chronic medical illnesses.

APACHE II SCORING SYSTEM

The APACHE II system is the most commonly used severity-of-illness scoring system in North America. Age, type of ICU admission (after elective surgery vs. nonsurgical or after emergency surgery), a chronic health problem score, and 12 physiologic variables (the most severely abnormal of each in the first 24 h of ICU admission) are used to derive a score. The predicted hospital mortality is derived from a formula that takes into account the APACHE II score, the need for emergency surgery, and a weighted, disease-specific diagnostic category (Table 261-1). The relationship between APACHE II score and mortality is illustrated in Fig. 261-1. More recently, the APACHE III scoring system has been released. This scoring system is similar to APACHE II, in that it is based upon age, physiologic abnormalities, and chronic medical comorbidities. The database from which this score was derived is larger.

THE SAPS AND MPM SCORING SYSTEM

The SAPS II score, used more frequently in Europe, was derived in a manner similar to the APACHE scores. This score is not disease specific but rather incorporates three underlying disease variables (AIDS, metastatic cancer, and hematologic malignancy). The MPM can be used to calculate a direct probability of death in patients admitted to the ICU.

Severity-of-illness scoring systems suffer from the problem of inability to predict survival in individual patients. Accordingly, the use of these scoring systems to direct therapy and clinical decision-making cannot be recommended at present. Rather, these tools should be used as important data to complement clinical bedside decision-making.

SHOCK (See also Chap. 264)

INITIAL EVALUATION

Shock is a common condition necessitating admission to the ICU or occurring in the course of critical care. Shock is defined by the presence of multisystem end-organ hypoperfusion. Clinical indicators include reduced mean arterial pressure (MAP), tachycardia, tachypnea, cool skin and extremities, acute altered mental status, and oliguria. Hypotension is usually, though not always, present. The end result of multiorgan hypoperfusion is tissue hypoxia, often clinically manifested by lactic acidosis. Since the MAP is the product of the cardiac output (CO) and the systemic vascular resistance (SVR), reductions in blood pressure can be caused by decreased CO and/or decreased SVR. Accordingly, the initial evaluation of a hypotensive patient should evaluate the adequacy of the CO. This should be part of the earliest assessment of the patient by the clinician at the bedside once shock is contemplated (Fig. 261-2). Clinical evidence of *diminished* CO includes a narrow pulse pressure—a marker that correlates with stroke volume—and cool extremities with delayed capillary refill. Signs of *increased* CO include a widened pulse pressure (particularly with a reduced diastolic pressure), warm extremities with bounding pulses, and rapid capillary refill. If a hypotensive patient has clinical signs of increased CO, one can infer that the reduced blood pressure is a result of decreased SVR.

In hypotensive patients with clinical signs of a reduced CO, an assessment of intravascular and cardiac volume status is appropriate. A hypotensive patient with decreased intravascular and cardiac volume status may have a history suggesting hemorrhage or other volume

TABLE 261-1 CALCULATION OF ACUTE PHYSIOLOGY AND CHRONIC HEALTH EVALUATION II (APACHE II)[a]

Acute Physiology Score

Score	4	3	2	1	0	1	2	3	4
Rectal temperature, °C	≥41	39.0–40.9		38.5–38.9	36.0–38.4	34.0–35.9	32.0–33.9	30.0–31.9	≤29.9
Mean blood pressure, mmHg	≥160	130–159	110–129		70–109		50–69		≤49
Heart rate	≥180	140–179	110–139		70–109		55–69	40–54	≤39
Respiratory rate	≥50	35–49		25–34	12–24	10–11	6–9		≤5
Arterial pH	≥7.70	7.60–7.69		7.50–7.59	7.33–7.49		7.25–7.32	7.15–7.24	<7.15
Oxygenation									
If F_{IO_2} > 0.5, use (A − a) D_{O_2}	≥500	350–499	200–349		<200				
If F_{IO_2} ≤ 0.5, use Pa_{O_2}					>70	61–70		55–60	<55
Serum sodium, meq/L	≥180	160–179	155–159	150–154	130–149		120–129	111–119	≤110
Serum potassium, meq/L	≥7.0	6.0–6.9		5.5–5.9	3.5–5.4	3.0–3.4	2.5–2.9		<2.5
Serum creatinine, mg/dL	≥3.5	2.0–3.4	1.5–1.9		0.6–1.4		<0.6		
Hematocrit	≥60		50–59.9	46–49.9	30–45.9		20–29.9		<20
WBC count, 10^3/mL	≥40		20–39.9	15–19.9	3–14.9		1–2.9		<1

Glasgow Coma Score[b,c]

Eye Opening	Verbal (Nonintubated)	Verbal (Intubated)	Motor Activity
4—Spontaneous	5—Oriented and talks	5—Seems able to talk	6—Verbal command
3—Verbal stimuli	4—Disoriented and talks	3—Questionable ability to talk	5—Localizes to pain
2—Painful stimuli	3—Inappropriate words	1—Generally unresponsive	4—Withdraws to pain
1—No response	2—Incomprehensible sounds		3—Decorticate
	1—No response		2—Decerebrate
			1—No response

Points Assigned to Age and Chronic Disease as Part of the APACHE II Score

Age, Years	Score
<45	0
45–54	2
55–64	3
65–74	5
≥75	6

Chronic Health (History of Chronic Conditions)[d]	Score
None	0
If patient is admitted after elective surgery	2
If patient is admitted after emergency surgery or for reason other than after elective surgery	5

[a]APACHE II score is the sum of the acute physiology score (vital signs, oxygenation, laboratory values), Glasgow coma score, age, and chronic health points. Worst values during first 24 h in the ICU should be used.
[b]Glasgow coma score (GCS) = eye-opening score + verbal (intubated or nonintubated) score + motor score.
[c]For GCS component of acute physiology score, subtract GCS from 15 to obtain points assigned.

[d]Chronic health conditions: liver, cirrhosis with portal hypertension or encephalopathy; cardiovascular, class IV angina (at rest or with minimal self-care activities); pulmonary, chronic hypoxemia or hypercapnia, polycythemia, ventilator dependent; kidney, chronic peritoneal or hemodialysis; immune, immunocompromised host.
Note: (A − a) D_{O_2}, alveolar-arterial oxygen difference; WBC, white blood (cell) count.

losses (e.g., vomiting, diarrhea, polyuria). The jugular venous pressure (JVP) is often reduced in such a patient, while the change in pulse pressure as a function of respiration is increased. A hypotensive patient with increased intravascular volume status and cardiac dysfunction may have S₃ and/or S₄ gallops on cardiac examination, increased JVP, extremity edema, and crackles on lung auscultation. The chest x-ray may show cardiomegaly, widening of the vascular pedicle, Kerley B lines, and pulmonary edema. Chest pain and electrocardiographic changes consistent with ischemia may also be noted (Chap. 266).

In hypotensive patients with clinical evidence of increased CO, a search for causes of decreased SVR is appropriate. The most common cause of high cardiac output hypotension is sepsis (Chap. 265). Other causes of high CO hypotension include liver failure, severe pancreatitis, burns and other trauma that elicit the systemic inflammatory response syndrome (SIRS), anaphylaxis, thyrotoxicosis, and peripheral arteriovenous shunts.

In summary, the three most common categories of shock are hypovolemic, cardiogenic, and high CO with decreased SVR (high-output hypotension). Certainly these categories may overlap and occur simultaneously (e.g., hypovolemic and septic shock, septic and cardiogenic shock).

The initial assessment of a patient in shock as outlined above should take only a few minutes. It is important that aggressive, early

resuscitation be instituted based on the initial assessment, particularly since early resuscitation of septic and cardiogenic shock may improve survival (see below). If the initial bedside assessment yields equivocal or confounding data, more objective assessments such as echocardiography and/or invasive vascular monitoring may be useful. The goal of early resuscitation is to reestablish adequate tissue perfusion to prevent or minimize end-organ injury.

MECHANICAL VENTILATORY SUPPORT

(See also Chap. 263) During the initial resuscitation of patients in shock, principles of advanced cardiac life support should be followed. Since patients in shock may be obtunded and unable to protect the airway, an early assessment of the patient's airway is mandatory during resuscitation from shock. Early intubation and mechanical ventilation are often required. Reasons for institution of endotracheal intubation and mechanical ventilation include acute hypoxemic respiratory failure as well as ventilatory failure, which frequently accompany shock. Acute hypoxemic respiratory failure may occur in patients with cardiogenic shock and pulmonary edema (Chap. 266) as well as in those in septic shock with pneumonia or acute respiratory distress syndrome (ARDS) (Chap. 265). Ventilatory failure often occurs as a result of an increased load on the respiratory system. This load may present

FIGURE 261-1 APACHE II survival curve. Blue, nonoperative; green, postoperative.

in the form of acute metabolic acidosis (often lactic acidosis) or decreased compliance of the lungs ("stiff" lungs) as a result of pulmonary edema. Inadequate perfusion to respiratory muscles in the setting of shock may be another reason for early intubation and mechanical ventilation. Normally, the respiratory muscles receive a very small percentage of the CO. However, in patients who are in shock with respiratory distress for the reasons listed above, the percentage of CO

dedicated to respiratory muscles may increase tenfold or more. Lactic acid production from inefficient respiratory muscle activity presents an additional ventilatory load.

Mechanical ventilation may relieve the patient of the work of breathing and allow redistribution of a limited CO to other vital organs, often with an improvement in lactic acidosis. Patients demonstrate signs of respiratory muscle fatigue with a number of clinical signs including inability to speak full sentences, accessory respiratory muscle use, paradoxical abdominal muscle activity, extreme tachypnea (> 40 breaths/min), and decreasing respiratory rate despite an increasing drive to breathe. When patients with shock are treated with mechanical ventilation, a major goal of ventilator settings is to assume all or the majority of work of breathing, facilitating a state of minimal respiratory muscle work. With the institution of mechanical ventilation for shock, further worsening of MAP is frequently seen. The reasons for this include impedance of venous return with positive-pressure ventilation, reduced endogenous catecholamine secretion once the stress associated with respiratory failure is abated, and drugs used to facilitate endotracheal intubation (e.g., barbiturates, benzodiazepines, opiates), all of which may result in hypotension. Accordingly, hypotension should be anticipated after endotracheal intubation and positive-pressure ventilation. Many of these patients have a component of hypovolemia, which may respond to IV volume administration. Fig. 261-2 summarizes the diagnosis and treatment of different types of shock. **For further discussion of individual forms of shock, see Chaps. 264, 265, and 266.**

RESPIRATORY FAILURE

Respiratory failure is one of the most common reasons patients are admitted to the ICU. In some ICU settings, ≥75% of patients require mechanical ventilation during their ICU stay. Respiratory failure can be categorized mechanistically, based on pathophysiologic derangements in respiratory function. Accordingly, four different types of respiratory failure can be described, based upon these pathophysiologic derangements.

Type I, or Acute Hypoxemic, Respiratory Failure This occurs when alveolar flooding and subsequent intrapulmonary shunt physiology occurs. Alveolar flooding may be a consequence of pulmonary edema, pneumonia, or alveolar hemorrhage. Pulmonary edema can be further categorized as occurring due to elevated intravascular pressures seen in heart failure and intravascular volume overload, or acute lung injury ("low-pressure pulmonary edema"; Chap. 266). ARDS (Chap. 262) represents an extreme degree of lung injury. This syndrome is defined by diffuse bilateral airspace edema seen by chest radiography, the absence of left atrial hypertension, and profound shunt physiology (Fig. 262-2), in a clinical setting in which this syndrome is known to occur. This includes sepsis, gastric aspiration, pneumonia, near drowning, multiple blood transfusions, and pancreatitis. The mortality rate of patients with ARDS was traditionally very high (50–70%), though recent changes in ventilator management strategy have led to reports of mortality in the low 30% range (see below).

For many years, physicians have suspected that mechanical ventilation of patients with acute lung injury and ARDS may propagate lung injury. Cyclical collapse and reopening of alveoli may be partly responsible for this. As seen in **Fig. 261-3**, the pressure-volume relationship of the lung in ARDS is not linear. Alveoli may collapse at very low lung volumes. Animal studies have suggested that stretching and overdistention of injured alveoli during mechanical ventilation can further injure the lung. Concern over this alveolar overdistention, termed *ventilator induced "volutrauma,"* led to a multicenter, randomized, prospective trial to compare traditional ventilator strategies for acute lung injury and ARDS (large tidal volume—12 mL/kg ideal body weight) to a low tidal volume (6 mL/kg ideal body weight). This study showed a dramatic reduction in mortality in the low tidal volume group (large tidal volume—39.8% mortality versus low tidal volume—31% mortality) and confirmed that ventilator management could impact outcomes in these patients. In addition, a "fluid conservative" man-

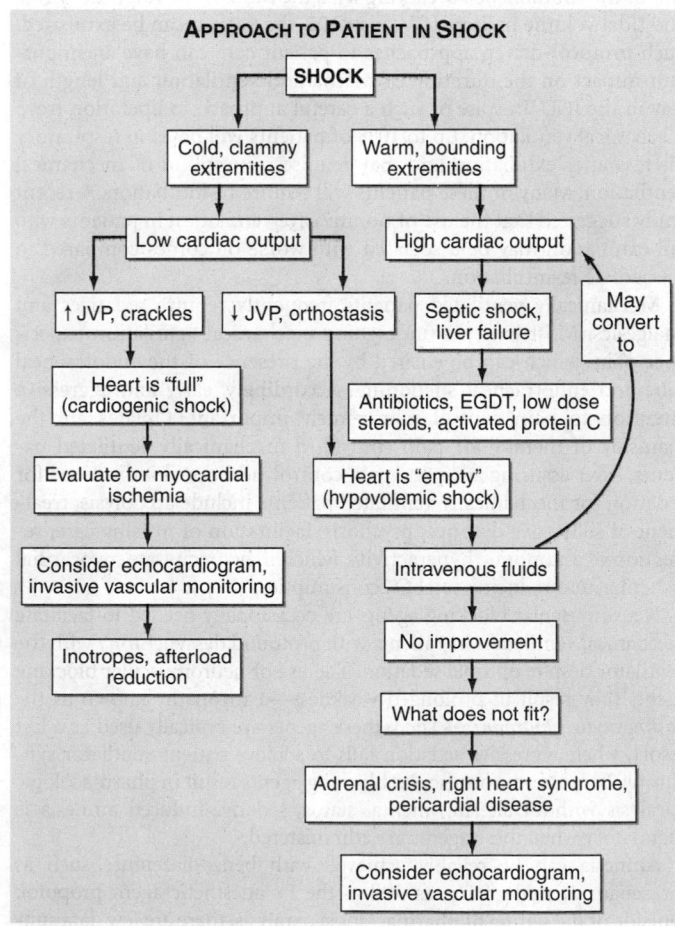

FIGURE 261-2 Approach to patient in shock. JVP, jugular venous pulse; EGDT, early goal-directed therapy.

FIGURE 261-3 Pressure-volume relationship of the lungs of a patient with ARDS. At the lower inflection point, collapsed alveoli begin to open, and the lung compliance changes. At the upper deflection point, alveoli become overdistended. The shape and size of alveoli are illustrated at the top.

agement strategy [maintaining a relatively low central venous pressure (CVP) or pulmonary capillary wedge pressure (PCWP)] is associated with the need for fewer days of mechanical ventilation when compared to a "fluid liberal" management strategy (maintaining a relatively high CVP or PCWP) in acute lung injury and ARDS.

Type II Respiratory Failure This type of respiratory failure occurs as a result of alveolar hypoventilation and results in the inability to eliminate carbon dioxide effectively. Mechanisms by which this occurs are categorized by impaired central nervous system (CNS) drive to breathe, impaired strength with failure of neuromuscular function in the respiratory system, and increased load(s) on the respiratory system. Reasons for diminished CNS drive to breathe include drug overdose, brainstem injury, sleep-disordered breathing, and hypothyroidism. Reduced strength can be due to impaired neuromuscular transmission (e.g., myasthenia gravis, Guillain-Barré syndrome, amyotrophic lateral sclerosis, phrenic nerve injury) or respiratory muscle weakness (e.g., myopathy, electrolyte derangements, fatigue).

The overall load on the respiratory system can be classified into increased resistive loads (e.g., bronchospasm), loads due to reduced lung compliance [e.g., alveolar edema, atelectasis, intrinsic positive end-expiratory pressure (autoPEEP)—see below], loads due to reduced chest wall compliance (e.g., pneumothorax, pleural effusion, abdominal distention), and loads due to increased minute ventilation requirements (e.g., pulmonary embolus with increased dead space fraction, sepsis).

The mainstays of therapy for type II respiratory failure are treatments directed at reversing the underlying cause(s) of ventilatory failure. Noninvasive positive-pressure ventilation using a mechanical ventilator with a tight-fitting face or nasal mask that avoids endotracheal intubation can often stabilize these patients. This approach has been shown to be beneficial in treating patients with exacerbations of chronic obstructive pulmonary disease. Noninvasive ventilation has been tested less extensively in other types of type II respiratory failure, but may be attempted nonetheless, in the absence of contraindications (hemodynamic instability, inability to protect airway, respiratory arrest).

Type III Respiratory Failure This form of respiratory failure occurs as a result of lung atelectasis. Because atelectasis occurs so commonly in the perioperative period, this is also called perioperative respiratory failure. After general anesthesia, decreases in functional residual capacity lead to collapse of dependent lung units. Such atelectasis can be treated by frequent changes in position, chest physiotherapy, upright positioning, and aggressive control of incisional and/or abdominal pain. Noninvasive positive-pressure ventilation may also be used to reverse regional atelectasis.

Type IV Respiratory Failure This form occurs due to hypoperfusion of respiratory muscles in patients in shock. Normally, respiratory muscles consume <5% of the total CO and O_2 delivery. Patients in shock often suffer respiratory distress due to pulmonary edema (e.g., patients in cardiogenic shock), lactic acidosis, and anemia. In this setting, up to 40% of the CO may be distributed to the respiratory muscles. Intubation and mechanical ventilation can allow redistribution of the CO away from the respiratory muscles and back to vital organs while the shock is treated.

CARE OF THE MECHANICALLY VENTILATED PATIENT (See also Chap. 263)

While a thorough understanding of the pathophysiology of respiratory failure is essential in order to optimize patient care, recognition of a patient's readiness to be liberated from mechanical ventilation is similarly important. Several studies have shown that subjecting patients to daily spontaneous breathing trials can identify those ready for extubation. Accordingly, all intubated, mechanically ventilated patients should undergo a daily screening of respiratory function. If oxygenation is stable (i.e., $Pa_{O_2}/FI_{O_2} > 200$ and PEEP ≤ 5 cmH_2O), cough and airway reflexes are intact, and no vasopressor agents or sedatives are being administered, the patient has passed the screening test and should undergo a spontaneous breathing trial. This trial consists of a period of breathing through the endotracheal tube without ventilator support [both continuous positive airway pressure (CPAP) of 5 cmH_2O and an open T-piece breathing system can be used] for 30–120 min. The spontaneous breathing trial is declared a failure and stopped if *any* of the following occur: (1) respiratory rate > 35/min for >5 min, (2) O_2 saturation < 90%, (3) heart rate > 140/min or a 20% increase or decrease from baseline, (4) systolic blood pressure < 90 mmHg or >180 mmHg, (5) increased anxiety or diaphoresis. If, at the end of the spontaneous breathing trial, the ratio of the respiratory rate and tidal volume in liters (f/V_T) is <105, the patient can be extubated. Such protocol-driven approaches to patient care can have an important impact on the duration of mechanical ventilation and length of stay in the ICU. In spite of such a careful approach to liberation from mechanical ventilation, up to 10% of patients will develop respiratory distress after extubation and may require resumption of mechanical ventilation. Many of these patients will require re-intubation. A recent study suggested that the use of noninvasive ventilation in patients who fail extubation may be associated with worse outcomes compared to immediate re-intubation.

Mechanically ventilated patients frequently require sedatives and analgesics. Most patients undergoing mechanical ventilation experience pain, which can be elicited by the presence of the endotracheal tube and endotracheal suctioning. Accordingly, early and aggressive attention to pain control is extremely important. Opiates are the mainstay of therapy for pain control in mechanically ventilated patients. After assuring adequate pain control, additional indications for sedation for mechanically ventilated patients include anxiolysis; treatment of subjective dyspnea; psychosis; facilitation of nursing care; reduction of autonomic hyperactivity, which may precipitate myocardial ischemia; and reducing total O_2 consumption (V_{O_2}).

Neuromuscular blocking agents are occasionally needed to facilitate mechanical ventilation in patients with profound dyssynchrony with the ventilator despite optimal sedation. The use of neuromuscular blocking agents may result in prolonged weakness—a myopathy known as the *postparalytic syndrome*. As such, these agents are typically used as a last resort, when aggressive sedation fails to achieve patient-ventilator synchrony. Because neuromuscular blocking agents result in pharmacologic paralysis without altering mental status, sedative-induced amnesia is mandatory when these agents are administered.

Amnesia can be reliably achieved with benzodiazepines such as lorazepam or midazolam, as well as the IV anesthetic agent propofol. Outside of the setting of pharmacologic paralysis, there are few data supporting the idea that amnesia is mandatory in all patients who require intubation and mechanical ventilation. Since many of these patients have impaired hepatic and renal function, sedatives and opiates may accumulate in critically ill patients when they are given for prolonged periods of time. A protocol-driven approach to sedation of mechanically ventilated patients with daily interruption of sedative infusions has been shown to prevent excessive drug accumulation and shorten the durations of mechanical ventilation and length of stay in the ICU.

MULTIORGAN SYSTEM FAILURE

The syndrome of multiorgan system failure is a common problem associated with critical illness. This syndrome is defined by the simultaneous presence of physiologic dysfunction and/or failure of two or more organs. Typically, this occurs in the setting of severe sepsis, shock of any kind, as well as severe inflammatory conditions such as pancreatitis, and trauma. That multiorgan system failure occurs commonly in the ICU is a testament to our current ability to stabilize and support single organ failure. The ability to support single organ failure aggressively (e.g., mechanical ventilation for respiratory failure, renal replacement therapy for acute renal failure) has impacted early mortality in critical illness greatly. As such, it is uncommon for critically ill patients to die in the initial stages of resuscitation. Instead, many patients succumb to critical illness later in the ICU stay, after the initial presenting problem has been stabilized.

While there is debate regarding specific definitions of organ failure, several general principles governing the syndrome of multiorgan system failure apply. First, organ failure, no matter how defined, must persist beyond 24 h. Second, mortality risk increases as patients accrue additional organ failures. Third, prognosis is worsened by increased duration of organ failure. These observations remain true across various critical care settings (e.g., medical versus surgical). SIRS is a common basis for multiorgan system failure. Though infection is a common cause of SIRS, "sterile" triggers such as pancreatitis, trauma, and burns are often invoked to explain multiorgan system failure.

MONITORING IN THE ICU

Because respiratory failure occurs commonly in critically ill patients, monitoring of the respiratory and cardiovascular systems is undertaken frequently in the ICU. Evaluation of respiratory gas exchange is routine in critical illness. The "gold standard" remains arterial blood-gas analysis, where pH, partial pressures of O_2 and CO_2, and O_2 saturation are measured directly. With arterial blood-gas analysis, the two main functions of the lung—oxygenation of arterial blood and elimination of CO_2—can be directly assessed. Importantly, the blood pH, which has a profound effect on the drive to breathe, can be assessed only by sampling of arterial blood. Though sampling of arterial blood is generally safe, it may be painful and cannot provide continuous information for clinicians routinely. Given these limitations, noninvasive monitoring of respiratory function is often employed in the critical care setting.

PULSE OXIMETRY

This is the most commonly utilized noninvasive monitor of respiratory function. This technique takes advantage of differences in the absorptive properties of oxygenated and deoxygenated hemoglobin. At wavelengths of 660 nm, oxyhemoglobin reflects light more effectively than deoxyhemoglobin, whereas the reverse is true in the infrared spectrum (940 nm). A pulse oximeter passes both wavelengths of light through a perfused digit such as a finger, and the relative intensity of light transmission at these two wavelengths is recorded. This allows the derivation of the relative percent of oxyhemoglobin. Since arterial pulsations produce phasic changes in the intensity of transmitted light, the pulse oximeter is designed to detect only light of alternating intensity. This allows distinction of arterial and venous blood O_2 saturations.

Respiratory System Mechanics These can be measured in patients during mechanical ventilation (Chap. 263). When volume-controlled modes of mechanical ventilation are used, accompanying airway pres-

sures can be easily measured. The peak airway pressure is determined by two variables—the airways resistance and respiratory system compliance. At the end of inspiration, inspiratory flow can be stopped transiently. This end-inspiratory pause (*plateau pressure*) is a static measurement, impacted only by respiratory system compliance, not airways resistance. Therefore, during volume-controlled ventilation, the difference between the peak (airways resistance + respiratory system compliance) and plateau (respiratory system compliance only) airway pressures provides a quantitative assessment of airways resistance. Accordingly, during volume-controlled ventilation, patients with increases in airways resistance typically have increased airway pressures as well as abnormally high gradients between peak and plateau airway pressures (typically >15 cmH$_2$O). The compliance of the respiratory system is defined by the change in pressure of the respiratory system per unit change in volume.

The respiratory system can be divided further into two components—the lungs and the chest wall. Normally, the respiratory system compliance is ~100 mL per cmH$_2$O. Pathophysiologic processes such as pleural effusions, pneumothorax, or increased abdominal girth from ascites or obesity all reduce chest wall compliance. Lung compliance may be reduced by pneumonia, pulmonary edema from any cause, or autoPEEP. Accordingly, patients with abnormalities in compliance of the respiratory system (lungs and/or chest wall) typically have elevated peak *and* plateau airway pressures but a normal gradient between peak and plateau airway pressures. AutoPEEP occurs when there is insufficient time for emptying of alveoli prior to the next inspiratory cycle. Since the alveoli have not decompressed completely, alveolar pressure remains positive at end-exhalation (functional residual capacity). This phenomenon occurs most commonly due to critical narrowing of distal airways in disease processes such as asthma and chronic obstructive pulmonary disease. AutoPEEP with resulting alveolar overdistention may result in diminished lung compliance, reflected by abnormally increased plateau airway pressures. Modern mechanical ventilators allow breath-to-breath display of pressure and flow, which may allow detection of problems such as patient-ventilator dyssynchrony, airflow obstruction, and autoPEEP (**Fig. 261-4**).

CIRCULATORY STATUS

Monitors to characterize the circulation status of critically ill patients are used commonly in the ICU. One of the most frequently used is the pulmonary artery catheter, also known as the right heart catheter or Swan-Ganz catheter. This catheter was originally designed as a tool to

FIGURE 261-4 Increased airway resistance with autoPEEP. The top waveform (airway pressure vs. time) shows a large difference between the peak airway pressure (80 cmH$_2$O) and the plateau airway pressure (20 cmH$_2$O). The bottom waveform (flow vs. time) demonstrates airflow throughout expiration (reflected by the flow tracing on the negative portion of the abscissa) that persists up to the next inspiratory effort.

guide therapy in acute myocardial infarction but is currently used in the ICU for evaluation and treatment of a variety of other conditions such as ARDS, septic shock, congestive heart failure, and acute renal failure. This device has never been validated as a tool associated with reduction in morbidity and mortality. Indeed, in spite of numerous prospective studies, there has been no report of mortality or morbidity benefit associated with the use of the pulmonary artery catheter in any setting.

Pulmonary artery catheters are invasive monitors and may be associated with a number of complications. Since the catheter is inserted via a central vein, all of the complications associated with central venous catheterization are present. These include central venous catheter–related infections, pneumothorax, arterial puncture with or without cannulation, bleeding, air embolism, venous thrombosis, and catheter embolism. The insertion of the pulmonary artery catheter also carries a number of risks, including dysrhythmias, heart block, cardiac perforation, and balloon fragmentation. After the catheter is placed, pulmonary infarction, pulmonary artery rupture, and pulmonic valve insufficiency may occur. Fortunately, most of these complications are quite rare. Indeed, misinterpretation of data derived from central venous and pulmonary artery catheters may be the most common "complication" seen with these monitors. Pressure measurements in various cardiac chambers require careful zeroing of the pressure transducer relative to atmospheric pressure. In addition, the transducer must also be at the same level as the cardiac chamber whose pressure is being measured. If the transducer is either higher or lower by several centimeters, the value recorded may be quite inaccurate.

Atrial pressure measurements should be made at end-expiration when there is no movement of air in or out of the thorax. It is during this period, with the lungs at functional residual capacity (cessation of gas flow), that gas flow in or out of the chest cannot complicate measurements of the atrial pressure. Many critically ill patients with respiratory distress may never come to a point where airflow in and out of the thorax ceases, instead breathing with continuous inspiratory and expiratory movements. In such patients, atrial pressure may be difficult to measure accurately. Failure to recognize this limitation may lead to reliance on inaccurate data obtained from the central venous or pulmonary artery catheter. Indeed, studies have shown that many clinicians are unable to obtain and interpret data from such catheters accurately. Accordingly, it appears that the routine use of pulmonary artery catheterization is not indicated as a monitor to characterize the circulatory status in most critically ill patients.

Oxygen delivery (Q_{O_2}) is a function of CO and the content of O_2 in the arterial blood (Ca_{O_2}). The Ca_{O_2} is determined by the hemoglobin concentration, the arterial hemoglobin saturation, and dissolved O_2 not bound to hemoglobin. For normal adults:

$$Q_{O_2} = 50 \text{ dL/min} \times [1.39 \times 15 \text{ g/dL (hemoglobin concentration)} \times 1.0$$
$$\text{(hemoglobin \% saturation)} + 0.0031 \times 100 \text{ (Pa}_{O_2})]$$
$$= 50 \text{ dL/min (CO)} \times 21.16 \text{ mL } O_2 \text{ per dL blood (Ca}_{O_2})$$
$$= 1058 \text{ mL } O_2 \text{ per min}$$

It is apparent that the vast majority of O_2 delivered to tissues is bound to hemoglobin and that the dissolved O_2 (Pa$_{O_2}$) contributes very little to O_2 content in arterial blood or O_2 delivery. Normally, the content of O_2 in mixed venous blood ($C\bar{v}_{O_2}$) is 15.95 mL O_2 per dL blood, since the mixed venous blood is 75% saturated. Therefore, the normal tissue extraction ratio for O_2 is $Ca_{O_2} - C\bar{v}_{O_2}/Ca_{O_2}$ (21.16 − 15.95/21.16) or ~25%. A pulmonary artery catheter allows measurements of O_2 delivery and O_2 extraction ratio.

The mixed venous O_2 saturation allows assessment of global tissue perfusion. A reduced mixed venous O_2 saturation may be caused by inadequate cardiac output, reduced hemoglobin concentration, and/or reduced arterial O_2 saturation. An abnormally high O_2 consumption (V_{O_2}) may also lead to a reduced mixed venous O_2 saturation if O_2 delivery is not concomitantly increased. Abnormally increased V_{O_2} by peripheral tissues may be caused by a multitude of problems such as fever, agitation, shivering, or thyrotoxicosis.

PREVENTION OF COMPLICATIONS OF CRITICAL ILLNESS

Sepsis in the Critical Care Unit (See also Chap. 265) Sepsis is a significant problem in the care of critically ill patients. It is the leading cause of death in noncoronary ICUs in the United States. Current estimates suggest that >750,000 patients are affected with this condition each year, and these numbers are expected to increase as the population continues to age and a greater percentage of persons vulnerable to infection seek medical care.

Many therapeutic interventions in the ICU are invasive and predispose patients to infectious complications. These interventions include endotracheal intubation, indwelling vascular catheters, nasally placed enteral feeding tubes, transurethral bladder catheters, and other catheters placed into sterile body cavities (e.g., tube thoracostomy, percutaneous intraabdominal drainage catheters). The longer such devices remain in place, the more prone to these infections patients become. For example, ventilator-associated pneumonia correlates strongly with the duration of intubation and mechanical ventilation. Therefore, an important aspect of preventive care is the timely removal of invasive devices as soon as they as no longer needed. Multidrug resistant organisms are commonplace in the ICU.

An important aspect of critical care is infection control in the ICU. Simple measures such as frequent handwashing are effective but underutilized strategies. Protective isolation of patients with colonization or infection by drug-resistant organisms is another frequently used strategy in the critical care setting. Antibiotic-coated vascular catheters or endotracheal tubes with specialized suction ports above the cuff to decrease pooling and aspiration of oral secretions are other strategies that may be used, with varying degrees of effectiveness reported. Surveillance programs monitoring adherence to infection control practices such as those described here may reduce the incidence of nosocomial infections.

Deep Venous Thromboses (DVTs) All ICU patients are at high risk for this complication given their predilection toward immobility. Therefore, all ICU patients should receive some form of prophylaxis against DVT. The most commonly employed forms of prophylaxis are subcutaneous low-dose heparin injections and sequential compression devices for the lower extremities. Observational studies report an alarming incidence of the occurrence of DVTs despite the use of these standard prophylactic regimens. Heparin prophylaxis may result in heparin-induced thrombocytopenia (HIT)—another relatively common nosocomial complication in critically ill patients.

Low-molecular-weight heparins such as enoxaparin are more effective than unfractionated heparin for DVT prophylaxis in high-risk patients, such as those undergoing orthopedic surgery, and they have a lower incidence of HIT. Fondaparinux, a selective factor Xa inhibitor, is even more effective than enoxaparin in high-risk orthopedic patients.

Stress Ulcers Prophylaxis against stress ulcers is frequently administered in most ICUs. Typically, histamine-2 antagonists are administered. Currently available data suggest that high-risk patients, such as those with coagulopathy, shock, or respiratory failure requiring mechanical ventilation, benefit from such prophylactic treatment.

Nutrition and Glycemic Control These are important issues in critically ill patients that may be associated with respiratory failure, impaired wound healing, and dysfunctional immune response. Early enteral feeding is reasonable, though no data are available to suggest that this improves patient outcome *per se*. Certainly, enteral feeding, if possible, is preferred over parenteral nutrition, which is associated with numerous complications including hyperglycemia, fatty liver, cholestasis, and sepsis. In addition to this, enteral feeding may prevent bacterial translocation across the gut mucosa. Intensive insulin therapy to normalize glucose levels is associated with improved survival in surgical ICU patients.

ICU-Acquired Weakness This occurs frequently in patients who survive critical illness. It is particularly common in those with SIRS and/or sepsis. Neuropathies and myopathies both have been described, most commonly after ~1 week in the ICU. The mechanisms behind ICU-acquired weakness syndromes are poorly understood. Intensive insulin therapy may reduce polyneuropathy of critical illness. Apart from this, no preventative measures against this complication of critical illness have been described.

Anemia This is a common problem in critically ill patients. Studies have shown that the vast majority of ICU patients are anemic. Furthermore, most suffer from anemia of chronic inflammation. Phlebotomy contributes significantly to anemia in ICU patients. Studies have demonstrated that erythropoietin levels are inappropriately reduced in most ICU patients and that exogenous erythropoietin administration may reduce transfusion requirements in the ICU. The hemoglobin level that merits transfusion in critically ill patients has been a long-standing area of controversy. A large, multicenter study involving patients in many different ICU settings challenged the conventional notion that a hemoglobin level of 100 g/L (10 g/dL) is needed in critically ill patients. Red blood cell transfusion is associated with impairment of immune function and increased risk of infections, as well as acute lung injury and volume overload—all of which may explain the findings in this study. A conservative transfusion strategy should be the rule in managing critically ill patients who are not actively hemorrhaging.

Acute Renal Failure (See also Chap. 273) This occurs in a significant percentage of critically ill patients. The most common underlying etiology is acute tubular necrosis, usually precipitated by hypoperfusion and/or nephrotoxic agents. Currently, there are no pharmacologic agents available for prevention of renal injury in critical illness. A recent study showed convincingly that low-dose dopamine is *not* effective in protecting the kidneys from acute injury.

NEUROLOGIC DYSFUNCTION IN CRITICALLY ILL PATIENTS

Neurologic dysfunction is common in critically ill patients.

Delirium (See also Chap. 26 and Chap. 268) This state is defined by: (1) an acute onset of changes or fluctuations in the course of mental status, (2) inattention, (3) disorganized thinking, and (4) an altered level of consciousness (i.e., other than alert). Delirium has been reported to occur in >80% of a cohort of patients admitted to the ICU. A rapid test—the Confusion Assessment Method (CAM)—to assess critically ill patients for delirium is available and has been validated. This assessment asks patients to answer simple questions and perform simple tasks and can be completed by the bedside nurse in ~2 min. The differential diagnosis of delirium in the ICU patient is broad and includes infectious etiologies (including sepsis), medications (particularly sedatives and analgesics), drug withdrawal, metabolic/electrolyte derangements, intracranial pathology (e.g., stroke, intracranial hemorrhage), seizures, hypoxia, hypertensive crisis, shock, and vitamin deficiencies (particularly thiamine).

Anoxic Cerebral Injury (See also Chap. 269) This condition is common after cardiac arrest and often results in severe and permanent brain injury in patients whose cardiac arrest is resuscitated. Active cooling of patients after cardiac arrest has been shown to improve neurologic outcomes. As such, patients who present to the ICU after circulatory arrest from ventricular fibrillation or pulseless ventricular tachycardia should be actively cooled with cooling blankets and ice packs if necessary to achieve a core body temperature of 32–34°C.

Stroke (See also Chap. 364) This is a common cause of neurologic critical illness. Hypertension must be managed carefully, since abrupt reductions in blood pressure may be associated with further brain ischemia and injury. Acute ischemic stroke treated with tissue plasminogen activator (tPA) shows improved neurologic outcome when treatment is given within 3 h of onset of symptoms. Mortality is not improved when tPA is compared to placebo, despite improved neurologic outcome. Cerebral hemorrhage is significantly higher in patients

given tPA. A treatment benefit is not seen when tPA therapy is given beyond 3 h. Heparin has not been shown to demonstrate improved outcomes convincingly in patients with acute ischemic stroke.

Subarachnoid Hemorrhage (See also Chap. 364) This may occur secondary to aneurysm rupture and is often complicated by cerebral vasospasm, rebleeding, and hydrocephalus. Vasospasm can be detected by either transcranial Doppler assessment or cerebral angiography; it is typically treated with the calcium channel blocker nimodipine, aggressive IV fluid administration, and therapy aimed at increasing the blood pressure, typically with vasoactive drugs such as phenylephrine. The IV fluids and vasoactive drugs (hypertensive hypervolemic therapy) are used to overcome the cerebral vasospasm. Early surgical clipping of aneurysms is advocated by most authorities to prevent complications related to rebleeding. Hydrocephalus, typically heralded by a decreased level of consciousness, may require ventriculostomy drainage.

Status Epilepticus (See also Chap. 363) Recurrent or relentless seizure activity is a medical emergency. Cessation of seizure activity is required to prevent irreversible neurologic injury. Lorazepam is the most effective benzodiazepine for treating status epilepticus and is the treatment of choice for controlling seizures acutely. Phenytoin or fosphenytoin should be given concomitantly since lorazepam has a short half-life. Other drugs such as gabapentin, carbamazepine, and phenobarbital should be reserved for patients with contraindications to phenytoin (e.g., allergy or pregnancy) or ongoing seizures despite phenytoin.

Brain Death (See also Chap. 269) Though critically ill patients usually die from irreversible cessation of circulatory and respiratory function, a diagnosis of death may also be established by irreversible cessation of all functions of the entire brain, including the brainstem, even if circulatory and respiratory function remains intact by artificial life support. Patients must demonstrate absence of cerebral function (unresponsive to all external stimuli) and brainstem functions [e.g., unreactive pupils, absent ocular movement to head turning or ice water irrigation of ear canals, positive apnea test (no drive to breathe)]. Absence of brain function must have an established cause and be permanent without possibility of recovery (e.g., must confirm the absence of sedative effect, hypothermia, hypoxemia, neuromuscular paralysis, or severe hypotension). If there is uncertainty about the cause of coma, studies of cerebral blood flow and electroencephalography should be performed.

WITHHOLDING AND WITHDRAWING CARE (See also Chap. 11)

The withholding and withdrawing of care occurs commonly in the ICU setting. The Task Force on Ethics of the Society of Critical Care Medicine reported that it is ethically sound to withhold or withdraw care if a patient or surrogate makes such a request or if the goals of therapy are not achievable according to the physician. Since all medical treatments are justified by their expected benefits, the loss of such an expectation justifies the act of withdrawing or withholding such a treatment. As such, the act of withdrawing care is fundamentally similar to the act of withholding care. An underlying stipulation derived from this Task Force report is that the informed patient should have his or her wishes respected with regard to life-sustaining therapy. Implicit in this stipulation is the need to ensure that patients are thoroughly and accurately informed regarding the plausibility and expected results of various therapies.

The act of informing patients and/or surrogate decision makers is the responsibility of the physician and other health care providers. In the event a patient or surrogate desires therapy deemed futile by the treating physician, the latter is not obligated ethically to provide such treatment. Rather, arrangements may be made to transfer the patient's care to another care provider. Critical care providers should meet regularly with patients and/or surrogates to discuss prognosis when the withholding or withdrawal of care is being considered. After a consensus amongst caregivers has been reached regarding withholding or withdrawal of care, this should be relayed to the patient and/or surrogate decision maker. If a decision to withhold or withdraw life-sustaining care for a patient has been reached, aggressive attention to analgesia and anxiolysis is needed. Opiates and benzodiazepines are typically used to achieve these goals.

FURTHER READINGS

ABRAHAM E et al: Drotrecogin alfa (activated) for adults with severe sepsis and a low risk of death. N Engl J Med 353:1332, 2005

COOK DJ et al: Deep venous thrombosis in medical-surgical critically ill patients: Prevalence, incidence, and risk factors. Crit Care Med 33:1565, 2005

ESTEBAN A et al: Noninvasive positive-pressure ventilation for respiratory failure after extubation. N Engl J Med 350:2452, 2004

SHAH MR et al: Impact of the pulmonary artery catheter in critically ill patients: Meta-analysis of randomized clinical trials. JAMA 294:1664, 2005

TASK FORCE ON ETHICS OF THE SOCIETY OF CRITICAL CARE MEDICINE: Consensus report on the ethics of forgoing life-sustaining treatments in the critically ill. Crit Care Med 18:1424, 1990

THE ACUTE RESPIRATORY DISTRESS SYNDROME NETWORK: Ventilation with lower tidal volumes as compared with traditional tidal volumes for acute lung injury and the acute respiratory distress syndrome. N Engl J Med 342:1301, 2000

THE HYPOTHERMIA AFTER CARDIAC ARREST STUDY GROUP: Mild therapeutic hypothermia to improve the neurologic outcome after cardiac arrest. N Engl J Med 346:549, 2002

THE NATIONAL HEART, LUNG, AND BLOOD INSTITUTE ACUTE RESPIRATORY DISTRESS SYNDROME (ARDS) CLINICAL TRIALS NETWORK: Comparison of two fluid-management strategies in acute lung injury. N Engl J Med 354:2564, 2006

VAN DEN BERGHE G et al: Intensive insulin therapy in the medical ICU. N Engl J Med 354:449, 2006

262 Acute Respiratory Distress Syndrome

Bruce D. Levy, Steven D. Shapiro

Acute respiratory distress syndrome (ARDS) is a clinical syndrome of severe dyspnea of rapid onset, hypoxemia, and diffuse pulmonary infiltrates leading to respiratory failure. ARDS is caused by diffuse lung injury from many underlying medical and surgical disorders. The lung injury may be direct, as occurs in toxic inhalation, or indirect, as occurs in sepsis (Table 262-1). The clinical features of ARDS are listed in Table 262-2. Acute lung injury (ALI) is a less severe disorder but has the potential to evolve into ARDS (Table 262-2). The arterial (a) P_{O_2} (in mmHg)/F_{IO_2} (inspiratory O_2 fraction) <200 mmHg is characteristic of ARDS, while a Pa_{O_2}/F_{IO_2} between 200 and 300 identifies patients with ALI who are likely to benefit from aggressive therapy.

The annual incidences of ALI and ARDS are estimated to be up to 80/100,000 and 60/100,000, respectively. Approximately 10% of all intensive care unit (ICU) admissions suffer from acute respiratory failure, with ~20% of these patients meeting criteria for ALI or ARDS.

ETIOLOGY

While many medical and surgical illnesses have been associated with the development of ALI and ARDS, most cases (>80%) are caused by a relatively small number of clinical disorders, namely, severe sepsis syndrome and/or bacterial pneumonia (~40–50%), trauma, multiple transfusions, aspiration of gastric contents, and drug overdose. Among patients with trauma, pulmonary contusion, multiple bone fractures, and chest wall trauma/flail chest are the most frequently reported surgical conditions in ARDS, whereas head trauma, near-drowning, toxic inhalation, and burns are rare causes. The risks of de-

TABLE 262-1 CLINICAL DISORDERS COMMONLY ASSOCIATED WITH ARDS

Direct Lung Injury	Indirect Lung Injury
Pneumonia	Sepsis
Aspiration of gastric contents	Severe trauma
Pulmonary contusion	Multiple bone fractures
Near-drowning	Flail chest
Toxic inhalation injury	Head trauma
	Burns
	Multiple transfusions
	Drug overdose
	Pancreatitis
	Post-cardiopulmonary bypass

TABLE 262-2 DIAGNOSTIC CRITERIA FOR ALI AND ARDS

Oxygenation	Onset	Chest Radiograph	Absence of Left Atrial Hypertension
ALI: Pa_{O_2}/F_{IO_2} ≤ 300 mmHg ARDS: Pa_{O_2}/F_{IO_2} ≤ 200 mmHg	Acute	Bilateral alveolar or interstitial infiltrates	PCWP ≤ 18 mmHg or no clinical evidence of increased left atrial pressure

Note: ALI, acute lung injury; ARDS, acute respiratory distress syndrome; Pa_{O_2}, arterial partial pressure of O_2; F_{IO_2}, inspired O_2 percentage; PCWP, pulmonary capillary wedge pressure.

veloping ARDS are increased in patients suffering from more than one predisposing medical or surgical condition; e.g., the risk for ARDS increases from 25% in patients with severe trauma to 56% in patients with trauma and sepsis.

Several other clinical variables have been associated with the development of ARDS. These include older age, chronic alcohol abuse, metabolic acidosis, and severity of critical illness. Trauma patients with an acute physiology and chronic health evaluation (APACHE) II score ≥16 (Chap. 261) have a 2.5-fold increase in the risk of developing ARDS, and those with a score >20 have an incidence of ARDS that is more than threefold greater than those with APACHE II scores ≤9.

CLINICAL COURSE AND PATHOPHYSIOLOGY

The natural history of ARDS is marked by three phases—exudative, proliferative, and fibrotic—each with characteristic clinical and pathologic features (Fig. 262-1).

Exudative Phase (Fig. 262-2) In this phase, alveolar capillary endothelial cells and type I pneumocytes (alveolar epithelial cells) are in-

Exudative	Proliferative	Fibrotic
Hyaline Membranes	Interstitial Inflammation	Fibrosis
Edema		

Day: 0 2   7   14   21 . . .

FIGURE 262-1 Diagram illustrating the time course for the development and resolution of ARDS. The exudative phase is notable for early alveolar edema and neutrophil-rich leukocytic infiltration of the lungs with subsequent formation of hyaline membranes from diffuse alveolar damage. Within 7 days, a proliferative phase ensues with prominent interstitial inflammation and early fibrotic changes. Approximately 3 weeks after the initial pulmonary injury, most patients recover. However, some patients enter the fibrotic phase, with substantial fibrosis and bullae formation.

FIGURE 262-2 A representative anteroposterior (AP) chest x-ray in the exudative phase of ARDS that shows diffuse interstitial and alveolar infiltrates, which can be difficult to distinguish from left ventricular failure.

jured, leading to the loss of the normally tight alveolar barrier to fluid and macromolecules. Edema fluid that is rich in protein accumulates in the interstitial and alveolar spaces. Significant concentrations of cytokines (e.g., interleukin 1, interleukin 8, and tumor necrosis factor α) and lipid mediators (e.g., leukotriene B_4) are present in the lung in this acute phase. In response to proinflammatory mediators, leukocytes (especially neutrophils) traffic into the pulmonary interstitium and alveoli. In addition, condensed plasma proteins aggregate in the air spaces with cellular debris and dysfunctional pulmonary surfactant to form hyaline membrane whorls. Pulmonary vascular injury also occurs early in ARDS, with vascular obliteration by microthrombi and fibrocellular proliferation (**Fig. 262-3**).

Alveolar edema predominantly involves *dependent* portions of the lung, leading to diminished aeration and atelectasis. Collapse of large sections of dependent lung markedly decreases lung compliance. Consequently, intrapulmonary shunting and hypoxemia develop and the work of breathing rises, leading to dyspnea. The pathophysiologic alterations in alveolar spaces are exacerbated by microvascular occlusion, which leads to reductions in pulmonary arterial blood flow to ventilated portions of the lung, increasing the dead space, and pulmonary hypertension. Thus, in addition to severe hypoxemia, hypercapnia secondary to an increase in pulmonary dead space is also prominent in early ARDS.

The exudative phase encompasses the first 7 days of illness after exposure to a precipitating ARDS risk factor, with the patient experiencing the onset of respiratory symptoms. Although usually present within 12–36 h after the initial insult, symptoms can be delayed by 5–7 days. Dyspnea develops with a sensation of rapid shallow breathing and an inability to get enough air. Tachypnea and increased work of breathing frequently result in respiratory fatigue and ultimately in respiratory failure. Laboratory values are generally nonspecific and primarily indicative of underlying clinical disorders. The chest radiograph usually reveals alveolar and interstitial opacities involving at least three-quarters of the lung fields (Fig. 262-2). While characteristic for ARDS or ALI, these radiographic findings are not specific and can be indistinguishable from cardiogenic pulmonary edema (Chap. 266). Unlike the latter, however, the chest x-ray in ARDS rarely shows cardiomegaly, pleural effusions, or pulmonary vascular redistribution. Chest computed tomography (CT) scanning in ARDS reveals extensive heterogeneity of lung involvement (**Fig. 262-4**).

Because the early features of ARDS and ALI are nonspecific, alternative diagnoses must be considered. In the differential diagnosis of ARDS, the most common disorders are cardiogenic pulmonary ede-

ma, diffuse pneumonia, and alveolar hemorrhage. Less frequent diagnoses to consider include acute interstitial lung diseases [e.g., acute interstitial pneumonitis (Chap. 255)], acute immunologic injury [e.g., hypersensitivity pneumonitis (Chap. 249)], toxin injury (e.g., radiation pneumonitis), and neurogenic pulmonary edema.

Proliferative Phase   This phase of ARDS usually lasts from day 7 to day 21. Most patients recover rapidly and are liberated from mechanical ventilation during this phase. Despite this improvement, many still experience dyspnea, tachypnea, and hypoxemia. Some patients develop progressive lung injury and early changes of pulmonary fibrosis during the proliferative phase. Histologically, the first signs of resolution are often evident in this phase with the initiation of lung repair, organization of alveolar exudates, and a shift from a neutrophil to a lymphocyte-predominant pulmonary infiltrate. As part of the reparative process, there is a proliferation of type II pneumocytes along alveolar basement membranes. These specialized epithelial cells synthesize new pulmonary surfactant and differentiate into type I pneumocytes. The presence of alveolar type III procollagen peptide, a marker of pulmonary fibrosis, is associated with a protracted clinical course and increased mortality from ARDS.

Fibrotic Phase   While many patients with ARDS recover lung function 3–4 weeks after the initial pulmonary injury, some will enter a fibrotic phase that may require long-term support on mechanical ventilators and/or supplemental oxygen. Histologically, the alveolar edema and inflammatory exudates of earlier phases are now converted to extensive alveolar duct and interstitial fibrosis. Acinar architecture is markedly disrupted, leading to emphysema-like changes with large bullae. Intimal fibroproliferation in the pulmonary microcirculation leads to progressive vascular occlusion and pulmonary hypertension. The physiologic consequences include an increased risk of pneumothorax, reductions in lung compliance, and increased pulmonary dead space. Patients in this late phase experience a substantial burden of excess morbidity. Lung biopsy evidence for pulmonary fibrosis in any phase of ARDS is associated with increased mortality.

℞ ACUTE RESPIRATORY DISTRESS

GENERAL PRINCIPLES   Recent reductions in ARDS/ALI mortality are largely the result of general advances in the care of critically ill patients (Chap. 261). Thus, caring for these patients requires close attention to: (1) the recognition and treatment of the underlying medical and surgical disorders (e.g., sepsis, aspiration, trauma); (2) minimizing procedures and their complications; (3) prophylaxis against venous thromboembolism, gastrointestinal bleeding, and central venous catheter infections; (4) the prompt recognition of nosocomial infections; and (5) provision of adequate nutrition.

MANAGEMENT OF MECHANICAL VENTILATION   (See also Chap. 263) Patients meeting clinical criteria for ARDS frequently fatigue from increased work of breathing and progressive hypoxemia, requiring mechanical ventilation for support.

Ventilator-Induced Lung Injury   Despite its life-saving potential, mechanical ventilation can aggravate lung injury. Experimental models have demonstrated that ventilator-induced lung injury appears to require two processes: repeated alveolar overdistention and recurrent alveolar collapse. Clearly evident by chest CT (Fig. 262-4), ARDS is a heterogeneous disorder, principally involving dependent portions of the lung with relative sparing of other regions. Because of their differing compliance, attempts to fully inflate the consolidated lung may lead to overdistention and injury to the more "normal" areas of lung. Ventilator-induced injury can be demonstrated in experimental models of ALI, with high tidal volume ventilation resulting in additional, synergistic alveolar damage. These findings led to the hypothesis that ventilating patients suffering from ALI or ARDS with lower tidal volumes would protect against ventilator-induced lung injury and improve clinical outcomes.

A large-scale, randomized controlled trial sponsored by the National Institutes of Health and conducted by the ARDS Network compared low tid-

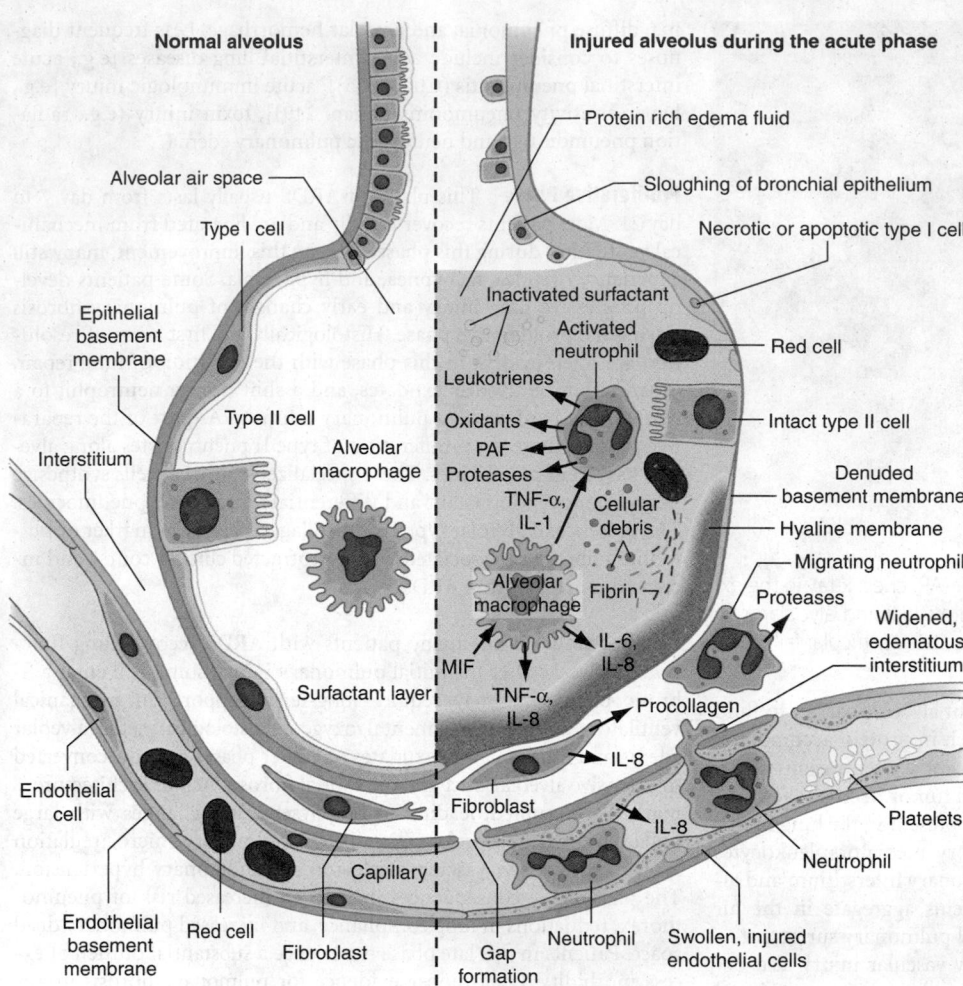

Normal alveolus

- Alveolar air space
- Type I cell
- Epithelial basement membrane
- Type II cell
- Interstitium
- Alveolar macrophage
- Surfactant layer
- Endothelial cell
- Endothelial basement membrane
- Red cell
- Fibroblast
- Capillary
- Gap formation

Injured alveolus during the acute phase

- Protein rich edema fluid
- Sloughing of bronchial epithelium
- Necrotic or apoptotic type I cell
- Inactivated surfactant
- Activated neutrophil
- Leukotrienes
- Red cell
- Oxidants
- PAF
- Intact type II cell
- Proteases
- TNF-α, IL-1
- Cellular debris
- Denuded basement membrane
- Hyaline membrane
- Alveolar macrophage
- Fibrin
- Migrating neutrophil
- Proteases
- MIF
- IL-6, IL-8
- Widened, edematous interstitium
- TNF-α, IL-8
- Procollagen
- Fibroblast
- IL-8
- Platelets
- IL-8
- Neutrophil
- Neutrophil
- Swollen, injured endothelial cells

FIGURE 262-3 The normal alveolus (left-hand side) and the injured alveolus in the acute phase of acute lung injury and the acute respiratory distress syndrome (right-hand side). In the acute phase of the syndrome (right-hand side), there is sloughing of both the bronchial and alveolar epithelial cells, with the formation of protein-rich hyaline membranes on the denuded basement membrane. Neutrophils are shown adhering to the injured capillary endothelium and marginating through the interstitium into the air space, which is filled with protein-rich edema fluid. In the air space, an alveolar macrophage is secreting cytokines, interleukin 1, 6, 8, and 10 (IL-1, 6, 8, and 10) and tumor necrosis factor α (TNF-α), which act locally to stimulate chemotaxis and activate neutrophils. Macrophages also secrete other cytokines, including interleukin 1, 6, and 10. Interleukin 1 can also stimulate the production of extracellular matrix by fibroblasts. Neutrophils can release oxidants, proteases, leukotrienes, and other proinflammatory molecules, such as platelet-activating factor (PAF). A number of anti-inflammatory mediators are also present in the alveolar milieu, including interleukin 1–receptor antagonist, soluble tumor necrosis factor receptor, autoantibodies against interleukin 8, and cytokines such as interleukin 10 and 11 (not shown). The influx of protein-rich edema fluid into the alveolus has led to the inactivation of surfactant. MIF denotes macrophage inhibitory factor. (*From Ware and Matthay, with permission.*)

al volume (6 mL/kg predicted body weight) ventilation to conventional tidal volume (12 mL/kg predicted body weight) ventilation. Mortality was significantly lower in the low tidal volume patients (31%) compared to the conventional tidal volume patients (40%). This improvement in survival represents the most substantial benefit in ARDS mortality demonstrated for *any* therapeutic intervention in ARDS to date.

Prevention of Alveolar Collapse   In ARDS, the presence of alveolar and interstitial fluid and the loss of surfactant can lead to a marked reduction of lung compliance. Without an increase in end-expiratory pressure, significant alveolar collapse can occur at end-expiration, impairing oxygenation. In most clinical settings, positive end-expiratory pressure (PEEP) is empirically set to minimize F_{IO_2} and maximize Pa_{O_2}. On most modern mechanical ventilators, it is possible to construct a static pressure–volume curve for the respiratory system. The lower inflection point on the curve represents alveolar opening (or "recruitment"). The pressure at this point, usually 12–15 mmHg in ARDS, is a theoretical "optimal PEEP" for alveolar recruitment. Titration of the PEEP to the lower inflection point on the static pressure–volume curve has been hypothesized to keep the lung open, improving oxygenation and protecting against lung injury. ARDS Network investigators compared low-to-high PEEP (8.3–13.2 cmH₂O) in over 500 patients with ARDS ventilated at low tidal volumes (6 mL/kg PBW). No significant differences in mortality, ventilator-free days, or ICU stay were observed. Until more data become available on the clinical utility of high PEEP, it is advisable to set PEEP to minimize F_{IO_2} and optimize Pa_{O_2} (Chap. 263).

Oxygenation can also be improved by increasing mean airway pressure with "inverse ratio ventilation." In this technique, the inspiratory (*I*) time is lengthened so that it is longer than the expiratory (*E*) time (*I:E* > 1:1). With diminished time to exhale, dynamic hyperinflation leads to increased end-expiratory pressure, similar to ventilator-prescribed PEEP. This mode of ventilation has the advantage of improving oxygenation with lower peak pressures than conventional ventilation. Although inverse ratio ventilation can improve oxygenation and help reduce F_{IO_2} to ≤0.60 to avoid possible oxygen toxicity, no mortality benefit in ARDS has been demonstrated.

In several randomized trials, mechanical ventilation in the prone position improved arterial oxygenation, but its effect on survival and other important clinical outcomes remains uncertain. Moreover, unless the critical-care team is experienced in "proning," repositioning critically ill patients can be hazardous, leading to accidental endotracheal extubation, loss of central venous catheters, and orthopedic injury. Until validation of its efficacy, prone-position ventilation should be reserved for only the most critically ill ARDS patients.

FIGURE 262-4 A representative computed tomographic scan of the chest during the exudative phase of ARDS in which *dependent* alveolar edema and atelectasis predominate.

Other Strategies in Mechanical Ventilation Several additional mechanical ventilation strategies that utilize specialized equipment have been tested in ARDS patients, most with mixed or disappointing results in adults. These include high-frequency ventilation (HFV), i.e., ventilating at extremely high respiratory rates (5–20 cycles per second) and low tidal volumes (1–2 mL/kg). Also, lung-replacement therapy with extracorporeal membrane oxygenation (ECMO), which provides a clear survival benefit in neonatal respiratory distress syndrome, has yet to have proven survival benefit in adults with ARDS. Ongoing research on partial liquid ventilation (PLV) with perfluorocarbon, an inert, high-density liquid that easily solubilizes oxygen and carbon dioxide, has revealed promising preliminary data on pulmonary function in patients with ARDS, but also without survival benefit.

Data in support of the efficacy of "adjunctive" ventilator therapies (e.g., high PEEP, inverse ratio ventilation, prone positioning, HFV, ECMO, and PLV) remain incomplete, so these modalities are not routinely used.

FLUID MANAGEMENT (See also Chap. 261) Increased pulmonary vascular permeability leading to interstitial and alveolar edema rich in protein is a central feature of ARDS. In addition, impaired vascular integrity augments the normal increase in extravascular lung water that occurs with increasing left atrial pressure. Maintaining a normal or low left atrial filling pressure minimizes pulmonary edema and prevents further decrements in arterial oxygenation and lung compliance, improves pulmonary mechanics, shortens ICU stay and the duration of mechanical ventilation, and is associated with a lower mortality. Thus, aggressive attempts to reduce left atrial filling pressures with fluid restriction and diuretics should be an important aspect of ARDS management, limited only by hypotension and hypoperfusion of critical organs, such as the kidneys.

GLUCOCORTICOIDS Inflammatory mediators and leukocytes are abundant in the lungs of patients with ARDS. Many attempts have been made to treat both early and late ARDS with glucocorticoids to reduce this potentially deleterious pulmonary inflammation. Few studies have shown any benefit. Current evidence does *not* support the use of glucocorticoids in the care of ARDS patients. However, the ARDS Network is currently conducting a large-scale study of glucocorticoids in the late phase of ARDS.

OTHER THERAPIES Clinical trials of surfactant replacement therapy have proved disappointing. Similarly, although several randomized clinical trials of inhaled nitric oxide (NO) in ARDS have demonstrated improved oxygenation, no significant improvement in survival or decrements in time on mechanical ventilation has been observed. Therefore, the use of NO is *not* currently recommended in ARDS.

RECOMMENDATIONS Many clinical trials have been undertaken to improve the outcome of patients with ARDS; most have been unsuccessful in modifying the natural history. The large number and uncertain clinical efficacy of ARDS therapies can make it difficult for clinicians to select a rational treatment plan, and these patients' critical illness can tempt physicians to try unproven and potentially harmful therapies. While results of large clinical trials must be judiciously administered to *individual* patients, evidence-based recommendations are summarized in **Table 262-3**, and an algorithm for the initial therapeutic goals and limits in ARDS management is provided in **Fig. 262-5**.

PROGNOSIS
Mortality Recent mortality estimates for ARDS range from 41 to 65%. There is substantial variability, but a trend toward improved ARDS outcomes appears evident. Of interest, mortality in ARDS is largely attributable to nonpulmonary causes, with sepsis and nonpulmonary organ failure accounting for >80% of deaths. Thus, improvement in survival is likely secondary to advances in the care of septic/infected patients and those with multiple organ failure (Chap. 261).

Several risk factors for mortality to help estimate prognosis have been identified. Similar to the risk factors for developing ARDS, the major risk factors for ARDS mortality are also nonpulmonary. Advanced age is an important risk factor. Patients >75 years have a substantially increased mortality (~60%) compared to those <45 (~20%). Also, patients >60 years with ARDS and sepsis have a threefold higher mortality compared to those <60. Preexisting organ dysfunction from chronic medical illness is an important additional risk factor for increased mor-

TABLE 262-3 EVIDENCE-BASED RECOMMENDATIONS FOR ARDS THERAPIES

Treatment	Recommendation[a]
Mechanical ventilation:	
Low tidal volume	A
High-PEEP or "open-lung"	C
Prone position	C
Recruitment maneuvers	C
High-frequency ventilation and ECMO	D
Minimize left atrial filling pressures	B
Glucocorticoids	C
Surfactant replacement, inhaled nitric oxide, and other antiinflammatory therapy (e.g., ketoconazole, PGE$_1$, NSAIDs)	D

[a]**A**, recommended therapy based on strong clinical evidence from randomized clinical trials; **B**, recommended therapy based on supportive but limited clinical data; **C**, indeterminate evidence: recommended only as alternative therapy; **D**, not recommended based on clinical evidence against efficacy of therapy.
Note: PEEP, positive end-expiratory pressure; ECMO, extracorporeal membrane oxygenation; PGE$_1$, prostaglandin E$_1$; NSAIDs, nonsteroidal antiinflammatory drugs.

tality. In particular, chronic liver disease, cirrhosis, chronic alcohol abuse, chronic immunosuppression, sepsis, chronic renal disease, any nonpulmonary organ failure, and increased APACHE II scores (Chap. 261) have also been linked to increased ARDS mortality. Several factors related to the presenting clinical disorders also increase risk for ARDS mortality. Patients with ARDS from direct lung injury (including pneumonia, pulmonary contusion, and aspiration; Table 262-1) have nearly twice the mortality of those with indirect causes of lung injury, while surgical and trauma patients with ARDS, especially those without direct lung injury, have a better survival rate than other ARDS patients.

Surprisingly, there is little value in predicting ARDS mortality from the extent of hypoxemia and any of the following measures of the severity of lung injury: the level of PEEP used in mechanical ventilation, the respiratory compliance, the extent of alveolar infiltrates on chest radiography, and the lung injury score (a composite of all these variables). However, recent data indicate that an early (within 24 h of presentation) elevation in dead space may predict increased mortality from ARDS.

Functional Recovery in ARDS Survivors While it is common for patients with ARDS to experience prolonged respiratory failure and re-

INITIAL MANAGEMENT OF ARDS

Initiate volume/pressure-limited ventilation →

Goals and Limits:
Tidal volume ≤ 6 ml/kg PBW
Plateau pressure ≤ 30 cmH$_2$O
RR ≤ 35 bpm

Oxygenate →
FiO$_2$ ≤ 0.6
PEEP ≤ 10 cmH$_2$O
SpO$_2$ 88 – 95%

Minimize acidosis →
pH ≥ 7.30
RR ≤ 135 bpm

Diuresis →
MAP ≥ 65 mmHg
Avoid hypoperfusion

FIGURE 262-5 Algorithm for the initial management of ARDS. Clinical trials have provided evidence-based therapeutic goals for a step-wise approach to the early mechanical ventilation, oxygenation, correction of acidosis and diuresis of critically ill patients with ARDS.

main dependent on mechanical ventilation for survival, it is a testament to the resolving powers of the lung that the majority of patients recover nearly normal lung function. Patients usually recover their maximum lung function within 6 months. One year after endotracheal extubation, over a third of ARDS survivors have normal spirometry values and diffusion capacity. Most of the remaining patients have only mild abnormalities in their pulmonary function. Unlike the risk for mortality, recovery of lung function is strongly associated with the extent of lung injury in early ARDS. Low static respiratory compliance, high levels of required PEEP, longer durations of mechanical ventilation, and high lung injury scores are all associated with worse recovery of pulmonary function. When caring for ARDS survivors it is important to be aware of the potential for a substantial burden of emotional and respiratory symptoms. There are significant rates of depression and posttraumatic stress disorder in ARDS survivors.

FURTHER READINGS

FAN EDM et al: Ventilatory management of acute lung injury and acute respiratory distress syndrome. JAMA 294:2889, 2005

TOMASHEFSKI JF JR.: Pulmonary pathology of acute respiratory distress syndrome. Clin Chest Med 21:435, 2000

WARE LB, MATTHAY MA: The acute respiratory distress syndrome. N Engl J Med 342:1334, 2000

263 Mechanical Ventilatory Support
Edward P. Ingenito

Ventilators are special pumps that can support the ventilatory function of the respiratory system and improve oxygenation through application of high oxygen content gas and positive pressure (Chap. 261).

INDICATIONS FOR MECHANICAL VENTILATION

The primary indication for initiation of mechanical ventilation is respiratory failure, of which there are two basic types.

1. *Hypoxemic respiratory failure* most commonly results from conditions such as pneumonia, pulmonary edema, pulmonary hemorrhage, and respiratory distress syndrome that cause ventilation-perfusion ($\dot{V}/\dot{Q}$) mismatch and shunt. Hypoxemic respiratory failure is present when arterial O_2 saturation (Sa_{O_2}) < 90% occurs despite an inspired O_2 fraction (Fi_{O_2}) > 0.6. The goal of ventilator treatment in this setting is to provide adequate Sa_{O_2} through a combination of supplemental O_2 and specific patterns of ventilation that improve $\dot{V}/\dot{Q}$ matching and reduce intrapulmonary shunt.

2. *Hypercarbic respiratory failure* results from conditions that decrease minute ventilation or increase physiologic dead space such that alveolar ventilation is inadequate to meet metabolic demands. Clinical conditions associated with hypercarbic respiratory failure include neuromuscular diseases, such as myasthenia gravis, ascending polyradiculopathy, and myopathies, and diseases that cause respiratory muscle fatigue due to increased workload, such as asthma, chronic obstructive pulmonary disease, and restrictive lung disease. *Acute* hypercarbic respiratory failure is characterized by arterial P_{CO_2} values > 50 mmHg and an arterial pH < 7.30.

Mechanical ventilation generally should be instituted in acute hypercarbic respiratory failure. In contrast, initiation of ventilator support when components of both acute and chronic hypercarbic respiratory failure are present depends on blood gas parameters and clinical evaluation. If a patient is not in respiratory distress and is not mentally impaired by CO_2 accumulation, it is not mandatory to initiate mechanical ventilation while other forms of treatment are being administered. The goal of ventilator treatment in hypercarbic respiratory failure is to normalize arterial pH through changes in CO_2 tensions. In patients with severe obstructive or restrictive lung disease, potentially injurious elevation in airway pressures may limit tidal volumes such that normalization of pH is not possible, a situation known as *permissive hypercapnia*. This strategy generally requires sufficient sedation to prevent tachypnea and dyssynchrony between patient and ventilator.

Accepted therapeutic applications of mechanical ventilation include controlled hyperventilation to reduce cerebral blood flow in patients with increased intracranial pressure (ICP) or to improve pulmonary hemodynamics in patients with postoperative pulmonary hypertension. Mechanical ventilation has also been used to reduce the work of breathing and decrease cardiac preload and afterload in patients with congestive heart failure or myocardial ischemia. Ventilator support is also frequently used in conjunction with endotracheal intubation to prevent aspiration of gastric contents in otherwise unstable patients during gastric lavage for suspected drug overdose or during upper gastrointestinal endoscopy. In the critically ill patient, intubation and mechanical ventilation are indicated before essential diagnostic or therapeutic studies if it appears that respiratory failure may occur during these maneuvers.

PHYSIOLOGY OF MECHANICAL VENTILATION

Mechanical ventilators provide warmed and humidified gas to the airway in conformance with various specific volume, pressure, and time patterns. The ventilator serves as the energy source for inspiration, replacing the muscles of the diaphragm and chest wall. Expiration is passive, driven by the recoil of the lungs and chest wall; at the completion of inspiration, internal ventilator circuitry vents the airway to atmospheric pressure or a specified level of positive end-expiratory pressure (PEEP).

PEEP helps maintain patency of alveoli and small airways in the presence of destabilizing factors, improving matching of ventilation and perfusion by reversing atelectasis. PEEP levels between 0 and 10 cmH_2O are generally safe and effective; higher levels can be used with caution in the management of significant refractory hypoxemia unresponsive to increments in Fi_{O_2} up to 0.6, but increase the risk of barotrauma and hypotension.

Positive-pressure ventilation affects the cardiovascular system through transmission of intrathoracic pressures to the heart and great vessels. Initiation of positive-pressure ventilation decreases both preload and afterload, while discontinuation increases both. The potential clinical impact of these effects should be considered when modifying ventilator support in hemodynamically tenuous patients.

ESTABLISHING AND MAINTAINING AN AIRWAY

A cuffed endotracheal tube is often inserted to allow positive-pressure ventilators to deliver conditioned gas, at pressures above atmospheric pressure, to the lungs. If neuromuscular paralysis is employed during intubation, the use of agents whose mechanism of action includes depolarization at the neuromuscular junction, such as succinylcholine chloride, should be avoided in patients with renal failure, tumor lysis syndrome, crush injuries, medical conditions associated with elevated serum potassium levels, and muscular dystrophy syndromes. Opiates and benzodiazepines can have a deleterious effect on hemodynamics in patients with depressed cardiac function or low systemic vascular resistance. Morphine can promote histamine release from tissue mast cells and may worsen bronchospasm in patients with asthma; fentanyl, sufentanil, and alfentanil are acceptable alternatives. Ketamine may increase systemic arterial pressure as well as ICP and has been associated with hallucinatory responses; it should be used with caution in patients with hypertensive crisis, increased ICP, or a history of psychiatric disorders. Newer agents such as etomidate and propofol have also been used for both induction and maintenance of anesthesia in ventilated patients. They are shorter acting, and etomidate has fewer adverse hemodynamic effects, but both agents are significantly more expensive than older agents.

Although definitive guidelines for performing a tracheostomy in the ventilated patient have not been established, in current clinical

TABLE 263-1 **CLINICAL CHARACTERISTICS OF COMMONLY USED MODES OF MECHANICAL VENTILATION**

Ventilator Mode	Independent Variables (Set by User)	Dependent Variables (Monitored by User)	Trigger/Cycle Limit	Advantages	Disadvantages	Initial Settings
ACMV[a]	FI_{O_2} Tidal volume Ventilator rate Level of PEEP Inspiratory flow pattern Peak inspiratory flow Pressure limit	Peak airway pressure, Pa_{O_2}, Pa_{CO_2} Mean airway pressure I/E ratio	Patient/timer Pressure limit	Timer backup Patient-vent synchrony Patient controls minute ventilation	Not useful for weaning Potential for dangerous respiratory alkalosis	$FI_{O_2} = 1.0$[b] $V_t = 10–15$ mL/kg[a] $f = 12–15$/min PEEP = 0–5 cmH$_2$O Inspiratory flow = 60 L/min
SIMV[a]	Same as for ACMV	Same as for ACMV	Same as for ACMV	Timer backup useful for weaning	Potential dyssynchrony	Same as for ACMV[a]
CPAP	FI_{O_2} Level of CPAP	Tidal volume Rate, flow pattern Airway pressure Pa_{O_2}, Pa_{CO_2}, I/E ratio	No trigger Pressure limit	Allows assessment of spontaneous function Helps prevent atelectasis	No backup	$FI_{O_2} = 0.5–1.0$[b] CPAP = 5–15 cmH$_2$O
PCV[a]	FI_{O_2} Inspiratory pressure level Ventilator rate Level of PEEP Pressure limit I/E ratio	Tidal volume Flow rate, pattern Minute ventilation Pa_{O_2}, Pa_{CO_2}	Timer/patient Timer/pressure limit	System pressures regulated Useful for barotrauma treatment Timer backup	Requires heavy sedation Not useful for weaning	$FI_{O_2} = 1.0$[b] PC = 20–40 cmH$_2$O[a] PEEP = 5–10 cmH$_2$O $f = 12–15$/min I/E = 0.7/1–4/1
PSV	FI_{O_2} Inspiratory pressure level PEEP Pressure limit	Same as for PCV + I/E ratio	Inspiratory flow Pressure limit	Assures synchrony Good for weaning	No timer backup	$FI_{O_2} = 0.5–1.0$[b] PS = 10–30 cmH$_2$O 5 cmH$_2$O usually the level used PEEP = 0–5 cmH$_2$O

[a]Open lung ventilation (OLV) involves the use of any of these specific modes with tidal volumes (or applied pressures) to achieve 5–6 mL/kg, and positive end-expiratory pressures achieve maximal alveolar recruitment.

[b]FI_{O_2} is usually set to 1.0 initially, unless there is a specific clinical indication to minimize FI_{O_2}, such as history of chemotherapy with bleomycin. Once adequate oxygenation is documented by blood gas analysis, FI_{O_2} should be decreased in decrements of 0.1–0.2 as tolerated, until the lowest FI_{O_2} required for an $Sa_{O_2} > 90\%$ is achieved.

Abbreviations: *f*, frequency; I/E, inspiration/expiration; FI_{O_2}, inspired O_2; PEEP, positive end-expiratory pressure; for ventilator modes, see text; V_t, tidal ventilation.

practice patients who are likely to require ventilator therapy for >3 weeks should be considered for this procedure. While it does not clearly reduce the incidence of laryngeal injury or tracheal stenosis, tracheostomy has been associated with improved patient comfort and enhanced ability to partake in rehabilitation-oriented activities.

VENTILATOR OPERATION

Terminology *Mode* refers to the manner in which ventilator breaths are triggered, cycled, and limited; commonly used modes of mechanical ventilation are given in Table 263-1. The *trigger*, either an inspiratory effort or a time-based signal, defines what the ventilator senses to initiate an assisted breath. *Cycle* refers to the factors that determine the end of inspiration. For example, in volume-cycled ventilation, inspiration ends when a specific tidal volume is delivered. Other types of cycling include pressure cycling, time cycling, and flow cycling. *Limiting factors* are operator-specified values, such as airway pressure, that are monitored by transducers internal to the ventilator circuit throughout the respiratory cycle; if the specified values are exceeded, inspiratory flow is terminated, and the ventilator circuit is vented to atmospheric pressure or the specified PEEP.

ASSIST CONTROL MODE VENTILATION (ACMV)

An inspiratory cycle is initiated either by the patient's inspiratory effort or, if none is detected within a specified time window, by a timer signal within the ventilator. Every breath delivered, whether patient or timer triggered, consists of the operator-specified tidal volume. Ventilatory rate is determined either by the patient or by the operator-specified backup rate, whichever is of higher frequency (Fig. 263-1A). ACMV is commonly used for initiation of mechanical ventilation because it ensures a backup minute ventilation in the absence of an intact respiratory drive and allows for synchronization of the ventilator cycle with the patient's inspiratory effort.

Problems can arise when ACMV is used in patients with tachypnea due to nonrespiratory or nonmetabolic factors such as anxiety, pain, or airway irritation. Respiratory alkalemia may develop and trigger myoclonus or seizures. Dynamic hyperinflation (so-called auto-PEEP) may occur if the patient's respiratory mechanics are such that inadequate time is available for complete exhalation between inspiratory cycles. Auto-PEEP can limit venous return, decrease cardiac output, and increase airway pressures, predisposing to barotrauma. ACMV is not effective for weaning patients from mechanical ventilation because it provides full ventilator assistance on each breath.

SYNCHRONIZED INTERMITTENT MANDATORY VENTILATION (SIMV)

The major difference between SIMV and ACMV is that in the former the patient is allowed to breathe spontaneously, i.e., without ventilator assist, between delivered ventilator breaths. However, mandatory breaths are delivered in synchrony with the patient's inspiratory efforts at a frequency determined by the operator. If the patient fails to initiate a breath, the ventilator delivers a fixed-tidal-volume breath and resets the internal timer for the next inspiratory cycle (Fig. 263-1B). SIMV differs from ACMV in that only the preset number of breaths is ventilator-assisted.

SIMV allows patients with an intact respiratory drive to exercise inspiratory muscles between assisted breaths, making it useful for both supporting and weaning intubated patients. SIMV may be difficult to use in patients with tachypnea because they may attempt to exhale during the ventilator-programmed inspiratory cycle. When this occurs, the airway pressure may exceed the inspiratory pressure limit, the ventilator-assisted breath will be aborted, and minute volume may drop below that programmed by the operator. In this setting, if the tachypnea is in response to respiratory or metabolic acidosis, a change to ACMV will increase minute ventilation and help normalize pH while the underlying process is further evaluated and treated.

FIGURE 263-1 Airway pressure and lung volume versus time profiles. A. During assist control mode ventilation (ACMV). Assisted breaths are triggered by the patient's effort. Controlled breaths are triggered by the ventilator timer. Every breath, whether triggered by the patient or by the timer, is a complete volume-cycled breath, with airway pressure as a dependent variable. The pressure limit is set above the peak inspiratory pressure. **B.** During synchronized intermittent mandatory ventilation (SIMV). Spontaneous breaths occur between patient-triggered assisted breaths and timer-triggered breaths. The tidal volume of the spontaneous breaths is determined by the patient's effort and lung impedance. Assisted and controlled breaths are volume cycled. **C.** During continuous positive airway pressure (CPAP). Breathing is spontaneous, and no ventilator assist is provided. The spontaneous profile is superimposed on an elevated mean airway pressure that the user specifies. FRC, functional residual capacity.

CONTINUOUS POSITIVE AIRWAY PRESSURE (CPAP)

This is not a true support-mode of ventilation, inasmuch as all ventilation occurs through the patient's spontaneous efforts. The ventilator provides fresh gas to the breathing circuit with each inspiration and charges the circuit to a constant, operator-specified pressure that can range from 0 to 20 cmH₂O (Fig. 263-1C). CPAP is used to assess extubation potential in patients who have been effectively weaned and are requiring little ventilator support and in patients with intact respiratory system function who require an endotracheal tube for airway protection.

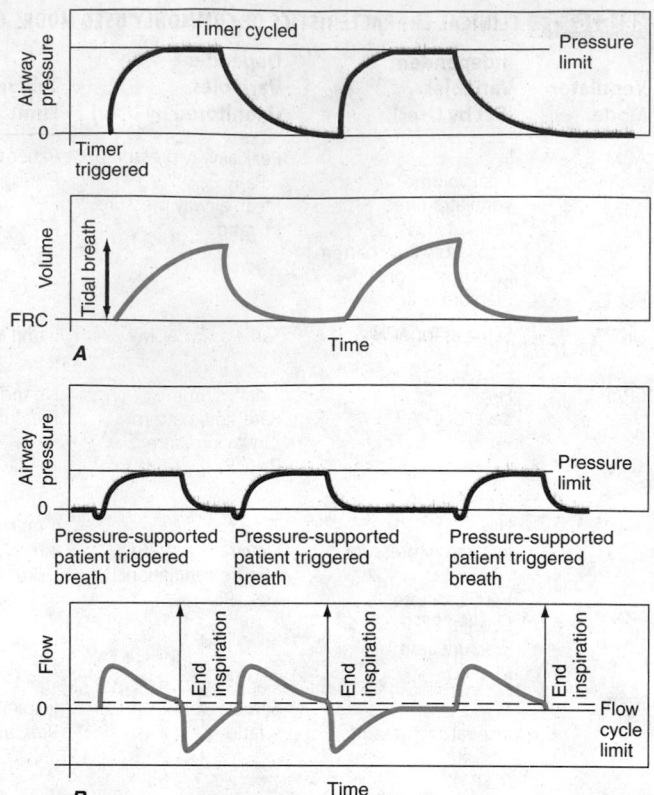

FIGURE 263-2 A. Airway pressure and lung volume versus time profiles during pressure-control ventilation (PCV). All breaths are timer triggered, timer cycled, and pressure limited. Peak airway pressure is set by the operator, and tidal volume is a dependent variable. The profiles shown here display the pressure limit as slightly higher than pressure-control level. This need not be the case, but it is appropriate to set the pressure limit only slightly above the pressure-control level when using this mode of ventilation for management of the patient with barotrauma. **B.** Airway pressure and airway flow versus time profiles during pressure-support ventilation (PSV). All breaths are patient triggered and flow cycled. Inspiration is cycled off when the inspiratory flow drops below a predetermined threshold internally set in the ventilator circuit. In the example shown, the pressure limit is slightly greater than the pressure-support level. Since each can be set independently, this need not be the case. FRC, functional residual capacity.

PRESSURE-CONTROL VENTILATION (PCV)

This form of ventilation is time triggered, time cycled, and pressure limited. During the inspiratory phase, a specified pressure is imposed at the airway opening throughout inspiration (Fig. 263-2A). Since inspiratory airway pressure is specified by the operator, tidal volume and inspiratory flow rate are *dependent* rather than *independent* variables and are not user specified. PCV is the preferred mode of ventilation for patients in whom it is desirable to regulate peak airway pressures, such as those with preexisting barotrauma or postoperative thoracic surgical patients, in whom the shear forces across a fresh suture line should be limited. When PCV is used, minute ventilation and tidal volume must be monitored; minute ventilation is altered through changes in rate or in the pressure-control value, which changes tidal volume.

PCV with the use of a prolonged inspiratory time has been applied to patients with severe hypoxemic respiratory failure. This approach, called inverse inspiratory-to-expiratory ratio ventilation (IRV), increases mean distending pressures without increasing peak airway pressures. It is thought to work in conjunction with PEEP to open collapsed alveoli and improve oxygenation, although there are no conclusive data to show that IRV improves outcomes in clinical trials.

PRESSURE-SUPPORT VENTILATION (PSV)

This form of ventilation is patient triggered, flow cycled, and pressure limited; it is specifically designed for use in the weaning process. During PSV, the inspiration is terminated when inspiratory airflow falls below a certain level; in most ventilators this flow rate cannot be adjusted by the operator. When PSV is used, patients receive ventilator assist only when the ventilator detects an inspiratory effort (Fig. 263-2*B*). PSV can also be used in combination with SIMV to ensure volume-cycled backup for patients whose respiratory drive is depressed.

PSV is well tolerated by most patients who are being weaned; PSV parameters can be set to provide full or nearly full ventilatory support and can be withdrawn slowly over a period of days in a systematic fashion to gradually load the respiratory muscles.

NONINVASIVE VENTILATION (NIV) Noninvasive ventilator support through a tight-fitting face mask or nasal mask, traditionally used for treatment of sleep apnea, has recently been used as primary ventilator support in patients with impending respiratory failure. NIV is most frequently employed using PSV or bi-level positive airway pressure ventilation, inasmuch as both of these modes are well tolerated by the conscious patient and optimize patient-ventilator synchrony. NIV has met with varying degrees of success when applied to patients with acute or chronic respiratory failure. The major limitation to its widespread application has been patient intolerance, because the tight-fitting mask required for NIV can cause both physical and emotional discomfort.

NONCONVENTIONAL VENTILATION STRATEGIES Several nonconventional ventilator strategies have been evaluated for their ability to improve oxygenation and reduce mortality in advanced hypoxemic respiratory failure. These include high-frequency oscillatory ventilation (HFOV), extracorporeal membrane oxygenation (ECMO), and partial liquid ventilation using perfluorocarbons. Although case reports and small uncontrolled cohort studies have shown benefit, randomized controlled trials have failed to demonstrate consistent improvements in outcome with any of these strategies. Currently, these approaches should be considered as "salvage" techniques and considered for patients with hypoxemia refractory to conventional therapy.

Interventions Used with Ventilator Support • *OPEN LUNG VENTILATION (OLV)* OLV is not a distinct mode of ventilation, but rather a strategy for applying either volume-cycled or pressure-control ventilation to patients with severe hypoxemic respiratory failure. In OLV, the primary objectives of ventilator support are maintenance of adequate oxygenation and avoidance of cyclic opening and closing of alveolar units by selecting a tidal volume and level of PEEP that allows the majority of units to remain inflated during tidal ventilation. Achievement of eucapnia and normal blood pH are of lower priority, and permissive hypercapnia is accepted. Current data suggest that a small tidal volume (i.e., 6 mL/kg) provides adequate ventilatory support with a lower incidence of adverse effects than more conventional tidal volumes of 10 to 15 mL/kg. Hypercapnia and consequent respiratory acidosis tend to be well tolerated physiologically, except in patients with significant hemodynamic compromise, ventricular dysfunction, cardiac dysrhythmias, or increased ICP. OLV has been used most extensively in the management of patients with hypoxemic respiratory failure due to acute lung injury. Several randomized clinical trials of OLV have been performed and suggest that this strategy reduces mortality and improves gas exchange in patients with acute lung injury.

PRONE POSITIONING DURING MECHANICAL VENTILATION Patients with acute respiratory distress syndrome (ARDS) experience hypoxemia as a result of intrapulmonary shunting due to regional atelectasis (Chap. 262). Collapse occurs most extensively in dependent regions of the lung. Prone positioning increases transdiaphragmatic pressures in these regions by altering their position relative to the hydrostatic pressures generated by abdominal contents. Thus, prone positioning increases distending pressures in these areas without the need to apply additional airway pressures that can overdistend less damaged areas of lung and

potentially cause additional lung damage. While conceptually appealing and simple to implement, a randomized trial in patients with acute lung injury failed to demonstrate a survival advantage with prone positioning despite demonstration of transient physiologic benefit.

NITRIC OXIDE ADMINISTRATION Nitric oxide (NO) gas has bronchodilator and pulmonary vasodilator effects when delivered through the airways and has been shown to improve arterial oxygenation in many patients with advanced hypoxemic respiratory failure. While physiologic benefits have been demonstrated in small cohort studies, randomized controlled trials have failed to confirm that therapeutic administration of NO reduces mortality in patients with advanced hypoxemic respiratory failure.

VENTILATOR MANAGEMENT PRINCIPLES

Most patients who are started on ventilator support receive ACMV or SIMV, because these modes ensure user-specified backup minute ventilation. Once the intubated patient has been stabilized with respect to oxygenation, definitive therapy for the underlying process responsible for respiratory failure is initiated. Subsequent modifications in ventilator therapy must be provided in parallel with changes in the patient's clinical status. As improvement in respiratory function is noted, the first priorities are to reduce PEEP and supplemental O_2. Once a patient can achieve adequate arterial saturation with an $F_{I_{O_2}} \leq 0.5$ and 5 cmH$_2$O PEEP, attempts should be made to reduce the level of mechanical ventilatory support. Patients previously on full ventilator support should be switched to a mode that allows for weaning, such as SIMV, PSV, or SIMV combined with PSV. Ventilator therapy can then be gradually removed, as outlined in the section on weaning. Patients whose condition continues to deteriorate after ventilator support is initiated may require increased O_2, PEEP, and alternative modes of ventilation such as IRV or OLV.

GENERAL SUPPORT DURING VENTILATION

Patients started on mechanical ventilation usually require sedation and analgesia to maintain an acceptable level of comfort. Often, this consists of a combination of a benzodiazepine and opiate administered intravenously. Medications commonly used for this purpose include lorazepam, midazolam, diazepam, morphine, and fentanyl.

Immobilized patients in the intensive care unit on mechanical ventilator support are at increased risk for deep venous thrombosis and decubitus ulcers. To prevent venous thrombosis, prophylaxis in the form of subcutaneous heparin and/or pneumatic compression boots is frequently prescribed. Fractionated low-molecular-weight heparin appears to be equally effective for this purpose. To help prevent decubitus ulcers, frequent changes in body position, and use of soft mattress overlays and air mattresses are employed.

Prophylaxis against diffuse gastrointestinal mucosal injury is indicated for patients who have suffered a neurologic insult or those with severe respiratory failure in association with ARDS. Histamine receptor antagonists (H$_2$-receptor antagonists), antacids, and cytoprotective agents such as carafate have all been used for this purpose and appear to be effective. Recent data suggest that carafate use may be associated with a reduction in the incidence of nosocomial pneumonias, since it does not affect stomach pH and is less likely to permit colonization of the gastrointestinal tract by pathogenic organisms.

Nutrition support by enteral feeding through either a nasogastric or an orogastric tube should be maintained in all intubated patients whenever possible. In patients with a normal baseline nutritional state, support should be initiated within 7 days. In malnourished patients, nutrition support should be initiated within 72 h. Delayed gastric emptying is common in critically ill patients on sedative medications but often responds to promotility agents such as metoclopramide. Parenteral nutrition is an alternative to enteral nutrition in patients with severe gastrointestinal pathology.

Endotracheal intubation and positive-pressure mechanical ventilation have direct and indirect effects on the lung and upper airways, the cardiovascular system, and the gastrointestinal system. Pulmonary complications include barotrauma, nosocomial pneumonia, oxygen toxicity, tracheal stenosis, and deconditioning of respiratory muscles. *Barotrauma*, which occurs when high pressures (i.e., >50 cmH_2O) overdistend and disrupt lung tissue, is clinically manifest by interstitial emphysema, pneumomediastinum, subcutaneous emphysema, or pneumothorax. Although the first three conditions may resolve spontaneously through the reduction of airway pressures, clinically significant pneumothorax requires tube thoracostomy.

Patients intubated for >72 h are at high risk for ventilator-associated pneumonia (VAP) as a result of aspiration from the upper airways through small leaks around the endotracheal tube cuff; the most common organisms responsible for this condition are *Pseudomonas aeruginosa*, enteric gram-negative rods, and *Staphylococcus aureus*. The diagnosis of VAP requires "protected brush" bronchoscopic sampling of airway secretions coupled with quantitative microbiologic techniques since this approach avoids sample contamination with bacteria that colonize the upper airways. Because this condition is associated with high mortality, early initiation of empirical antibiotics directed against likely pathogens is recommended.

Hypotension resulting from elevated intrathoracic pressures with decreased venous return is almost always responsive to intravascular volume repletion. In patients judged to have hypotension or respiratory failure on the basis of alveolar edema, hemodynamic monitoring with a pulmonary arterial catheter may be of value in optimizing O_2 delivery via manipulation of intravascular volume and FI_{O_2} and PEEP levels.

Gastrointestinal effects of positive-pressure ventilation include *stress ulceration* and *mild to moderate cholestasis*. It is common practice to provide prophylaxis with H_2-receptor antagonists or sucralfate for stress-related ulcers. Mild cholestasis [i.e., total bilirubin values ≤ 68 μmol/L (≤ 4.0 mg/dL)] attributable to the effects of increased intrathoracic pressures on portal vein pressures is common and generally self-limited. Cholestasis of a more severe degree should not be attributed to a positive-pressure ventilation response and is more likely due to a primary hepatic process.

WEANING FROM MECHANICAL VENTILATION

Removal of mechanical ventilator support requires that a number of criteria be met. Upper airway function must be intact for a patient to remain extubated but is difficult to assess in the intubated patient. Therefore, if a patient can breathe on his or her own through an endotracheal tube but develops stridor or recurrent aspiration once the tube is removed, upper airway dysfunction or an abnormal swallowing mechanism should be suspected and evaluated. Respiratory drive and chest wall function are assessed by observation of respiratory rate, tidal volume, inspiratory pressure, and vital capacity. The weaning index, defined as the ratio of breathing frequency to tidal volume (breaths per minute per liter), is both sensitive and specific for predicting the likelihood of successful extubation. When this ratio is <105 with the patient breathing without mechanical assistance through an endotra-

cheal tube, successful extubation is likely. Alveolar ventilation is deemed adequate when elimination of CO_2 is sufficient to maintain arterial pH in the range of 7.35 to 7.40, and an $Sa_{O_2} > 90\%$ can be achieved with an $FI_{O_2} < 0.5$ and a PEEP ≤ 5 cmH_2O. Although many patients may not meet all criteria for weaning, the likelihood of successful extubation increases as more criteria are met.

Many approaches to weaning patients from ventilator support have been advocated. T-piece and CPAP weaning are best tolerated by patients who have undergone mechanical ventilation for brief periods and require little respiratory muscle reconditioning, whereas SIMV and PSV are best for patients intubated for extended periods likely to require gradual respiratory-muscle reconditioning.

T-piece and CPAP weaning involve brief spontaneous breathing trials with supplemental O_2. These trials are usually initiated for 5 min/h followed by a 1-h interval of rest. Trials are increased in 5- to 10-min/h increments until the patient can remain ventilator independent for periods of several hours. Extubation can then be attempted.

Weaning by means of SIMV involves gradually tapering the mandatory backup rate in increments of 2 to 4 breaths per minute while monitoring blood gas parameters and respiratory rates. Rates of >25 breaths per minute on withdrawal of mandatory ventilator breaths generally indicate respiratory muscle fatigue and the need to combine periods of exercise with rest. Exercise periods are gradually increased until a patient remains stable on SIMV at ≤ 4 breaths per minute. A CPAP or T-piece trial can then be attempted before extubation.

PSV, as described in detail above, is used primarily for weaning from mechanical ventilation. PSV is usually initiated at a level adequate for full ventilator support (PSV_{max}); i.e., PSV is set slightly below the peak inspiratory pressures required by the patient during volume-cycled ventilation. The level of pressure support is then gradually withdrawn in increments of 3–5 cmH_2O until a level is reached at which the respiratory rate increases to 25 breaths per minute. At this point, intermittent periods of higher-pressure support are alternated with periods of lower-pressure support to provide muscle reconditioning while avoiding diaphragmatic fatigue. Gradual withdrawal of PSV continues until the level of support is just adequate to overcome the resistance of the endotracheal tube (~5 to 10 cmH_2O). Support can be discontinued and the patient extubated.

FURTHER READINGS

BROWER RG et al: Higher versus lower positive end-expiratory pressures in patients with the acute respiratory distress syndrome. N Engl J Med 351(4):327, 2004

FAN E et al: Ventilatory management of acute lung injury and acute respiratory distress syndrome. JAMA 294(22):2889, 2005

MACINTYRE NR: Current issues in mechanical ventilation for respiratory failure. Chest 128(Suppl 2):561S, 2005

MICHAEL JR et al: Inhaled nitric oxide versus conventional therapy. Am J Respir Crit Care Med 157(5):1372, 1998

PARK JE, GRIFFITHS MJ: Recent advances in mechanical ventilation. Clin Med 5:441, 2005

SCALISE PJ, VOTTO JJ: Weaning from long term mechanical ventilation. Chron Respir Dis 2:99, 2005

SECTION 2 | SHOCK AND CARDIAC ARREST

264 Approach to the Patient with Shock
Ronald V. Maier

Shock is the clinical syndrome that results from inadequate tissue perfusion. Irrespective of cause, the hypoperfusion-induced imbalance between the delivery of and requirements for oxygen and substrate leads to cellular dysfunction. The cellular injury created by the inadequate delivery of oxygen and substrates also induces the production and release of inflammatory mediators that further compromise perfusion through functional and structural changes within the microvasculature. This leads to a vicious circle in which impaired perfusion is responsible for cellular injury, which causes maldistribution of blood flow, further compromising cellular perfusion; the latter causes multiple organ failure and, if the process is not interrupted, leads to death. The clinical manifestations of shock are the result, in part, of autonomic neuroendocrine responses to hypoperfusion as well as the breakdown in organ function induced by severe cellular dysfunction (Fig. 264-1).

When very severe and/or persistent, inadequate oxygen delivery leads to irreversible cell injury; thus, only rapid restoration of oxygen delivery can reverse the progression of the shock state. The fundamental approach to management, therefore, is to recognize overt and impending shock in a timely fashion and to intervene emergently to restore perfusion. This often requires the expansion or reexpansion of intravascular blood volume. Control of any inciting pathologic process, e.g., continued hemorrhage, impairment of cardiac function, or infection, must occur simultaneously.

Clinical shock is usually accompanied by hypotension, i.e., a mean arterial pressure <60 mmHg in previously normotensive persons. Multiple classification schemes have been developed in an attempt to synthesize the seemingly dissimilar processes leading to shock. Strict adherence to a classification scheme may be difficult from a clinical standpoint because of the frequent combination of two or more causes of shock in any individual patient, but the classification shown in

TABLE 264-1	CLASSIFICATION OF SHOCK
Hypovolemic	Septic
Traumatic	Hyperdynamic
Cardiogenic	Hypodynamic
Intrinsic	Neurogenic
Compressive	Hypoadrenal

Table 264-1 provides a useful reference point from which to discuss and further delineate the underlying processes.

PATHOGENESIS AND ORGAN RESPONSE

MICROCIRCULATION

Normally when cardiac output falls, systemic vascular resistance rises to maintain a level of systemic pressure that is adequate for perfusion of the heart and brain at the expense of other tissues such as muscle, skin, and especially the gastrointestinal tract. Systemic vascular resistance is determined primarily by the luminal diameter of arterioles. The metabolic rates of the heart and brain are high, and their stores of energy substrate are low. These organs are critically dependent on a continuous supply of oxygen and nutrients, and neither tolerates severe ischemia for more than brief periods. Autoregulation, i.e., the maintenance of blood flow over a wide range of perfusion pressures, is critical in sustaining cerebral and coronary perfusion despite significant hypotension. However, when mean arterial pressure drops to ≤60 mmHg, flow to these organs falls, and their function deteriorates.

Arteriolar vascular smooth muscle has both α- and β-adrenergic receptors. The α_1 receptors mediate vasoconstriction, while the β_2 receptors mediate vasodilation. Efferent sympathetic fibers release norepinephrine, which acts primarily on α_1 receptors in one of the most fundamental compensatory responses to reduced perfusion pressure. Other constrictor substances that are increased in most forms of shock include angiotensin II, vasopressin, endothelin 1, and thromboxane A_2. Both norepinephrine and epinephrine are released by the adrenal medulla, and the concentrations of these catecholamines in the bloodstream rise. Circulating vasodilators in shock include prostacyclin [prostaglandin (PG) I_2], nitric oxide (NO), and, importantly, products of local metabolism such as adenosine that match flow to the tissue's metabolic needs. The balance between these various vasoconstrictor and vasodilator influences acting upon the microcirculation determines local perfusion.

Transport to cells depends on microcirculatory flow; capillary permeability; the diffusion of oxygen, carbon dioxide, nutrients, and products of metabolism through the interstitium; and the exchange of these products across cell membranes. Impairment of the microcirculation, which is central to the pathophysiologic responses in the late stages of all forms of shock, results in the derangement of cellular metabolism, which is ultimately responsible for organ failure.

The endogenous response to mild or moderate hypovolemia is an attempt at restitution of intravascular volume through alterations in hydrostatic pressure and osmolarity. Constriction of arterioles leads to reductions in both the capillary hydrostatic pressure and the number of capillary beds perfused, thereby limiting the capillary surface area across which filtration occurs. When filtration is reduced while intravascular oncotic pressure remains constant or rises, there is net reabsorption of fluid into the vascular bed, in accord with Starling's law

FIGURE 264-1 Shock-induced vicious circle.

of capillary-interstitial liquid exchange. Metabolic changes (including hyperglycemia and elevations in the products of glycolysis, lipolysis, and proteolysis) raise extracellular osmolarity, leading to an osmotic gradient between cells and interstitium that increases interstitial and intravascular volume at the expense of intracellular volume.

CELLULAR RESPONSES

Interstitial transport of nutrients is impaired in shock, leading to a decline of intracellular high-energy phosphate stores. Mitochondrial dysfunction and uncoupling of oxidative phosphorylation are the most likely causes for decreased amounts of ATP. As a consequence, there is an accumulation of hydrogen ions, lactate, and other products of anaerobic metabolism. As shock progresses, these vasodilator metabolites override vasomotor tone, causing further hypotension and hypoperfusion. Dysfunction of cell membranes is thought to represent a common end-stage pathophysiologic pathway in the various forms of shock. Normal cellular transmembrane potential falls, and there is an associated increase in intracellular sodium and water, leading to cell swelling, which interferes further with microvascular perfusion. In a preterminal event, homeostasis of calcium via membrane channels is lost with flooding of calcium intracellularly and a concomitant extracellular hypocalcemia. There is also increasing evidence for a widespread but selective apoptotic loss of cells, contributing to organ and immune failure.

NEUROENDOCRINE RESPONSE

Hypovolemia, hypotension, and hypoxia are sensed by baroreceptors and chemoreceptors, which contribute to an autonomic response that attempts to restore blood volume, maintain central perfusion, and mobilize metabolic substrates. Hypotension disinhibits the vasomotor center, resulting in increased adrenergic output and reduced vagal activity. Release of norepinephrine from adrenergic neurons induces peripheral and splanchnic vasoconstriction, a major contributor to the maintenance of central organ perfusion, while reduced vagal activity increases the heart rate and cardiac output. Vagal tone is also recognized to downregulate the innate immunity inflammatory response. The effects of circulating epinephrine released by the adrenal medulla in shock are largely metabolic, causing increased glycogenolysis and gluconeogenesis and reduced pancreatic insulin release. Epinephrine also inhibits production and release of inflammatory mediators through stimulation of β-adrenergic receptors on innate immune cells.

Severe pain and other severe stress cause the hypothalamic release of adrenocorticotropic hormone (ACTH). This stimulates cortisol secretion, which contributes to decreased peripheral uptake of glucose and amino acids, enhances lipolysis, and increases gluconeogenesis. Increased pancreatic secretion of glucagon during stress accelerates hepatic gluconeogenesis and further elevates blood glucose concentration. These hormonal actions act synergistically to increase blood glucose in the maintenance of blood volume. Many critically ill patients have recently been shown to exhibit low plasma cortisol levels and an impaired response to ACTH stimulation. Low levels of cortisol in response to stimulation are linked to a decrease in survival. The importance of the cortisol response to stress is illustrated by the profound circulatory collapse that occurs in patients with adrenal cortical insufficiency (Chap. 336).

Renin release is increased in response to adrenergic discharge and reduced perfusion of the juxtaglomerular apparatus in the kidney. Renin induces the formation of angiotensin I, which is then converted to angiotensin II, an extremely potent vasoconstrictor and stimulator of aldosterone release by the adrenal cortex and of vasopressin by the posterior pituitary. Aldosterone contributes to the maintenance of intravascular volume by enhancing renal tubular reabsorption of sodium, resulting in the excretion of a low-volume, concentrated, sodium-free urine. Vasopressin has a direct action on vascular smooth muscle, contributing to vasoconstriction, and acts on the distal renal tubules to enhance water reabsorption.

CARDIOVASCULAR RESPONSE

Three variables—ventricular filling (preload), the resistance to ventricular ejection (afterload), and myocardial contractility—are paramount in controlling stroke volume (Chap. 217). Cardiac output, the major determinant of tissue perfusion, is the product of stroke volume and heart rate. Hypovolemia leads to decreased ventricular preload, which in turn reduces the stroke volume. An increase in heart rate is a useful but limited compensatory mechanism to maintain cardiac output. A shock-induced reduction in myocardial compliance is frequent, reducing ventricular end-diastolic volume and hence stroke volume at any given ventricular filling pressure. Restoration of intravascular volume may return stroke volume to normal but only at elevated filling pressures. Increased filling pressures also stimulate release of brain natriuretic peptide (BNP) to secrete sodium and volume to relieve the pressure on the heart. Levels of BNP correlate with outcome following severe stress. In addition, sepsis, ischemia, myocardial infarction, severe tissue trauma, hypothermia, general anesthesia, prolonged hypotension, and acidemia may all impair myocardial contractility and also reduce the stroke volume at any given ventricular end-diastolic volume. The resistance to ventricular ejection is significantly influenced by the systemic vascular resistance, which is elevated in most forms of shock. However, resistance is depressed in the early hyperdynamic stage of septic shock (Chap. 265), thereby initially allowing the cardiac output to be maintained or elevated.

The venous system contains nearly two-thirds of the total circulating blood volume, most in the small veins, and serves as a dynamic reservoir for autoinfusion of blood. Active venoconstriction as a consequence of α-adrenergic activity is an important compensatory mechanism for the maintenance of venous return and therefore of ventricular filling during shock. On the other hand, venous dilatation, as occurs in neurogenic shock, reduces ventricular filling and hence stroke volume and cardiac output (see below).

PULMONARY RESPONSE

The response of the pulmonary vascular bed to shock parallels that of the systemic vascular bed, and the relative increase in pulmonary vascular resistance, particularly in septic shock, may exceed that of the systemic vascular resistance. Shock-induced tachypnea reduces tidal volume and increases both dead space and minute ventilation. Relative hypoxia and the subsequent tachypnea induce a respiratory alkalosis. Recumbency and involuntary restriction of ventilation secondary to pain reduce functional residual capacity and may lead to atelectasis. Shock is recognized as a major cause of acute lung injury and subsequent acute respiratory distress syndrome (ARDS; Chap. 262). These disorders are characterized by noncardiogenic pulmonary edema secondary to diffuse pulmonary capillary endothelial and alveolar epithelial injury, hypoxemia, and bilateral diffuse pulmonary infiltrates. Hypoxemia results from perfusion of underventilated and nonventilated alveoli. Loss of surfactant and lung volume in combination with increased interstitial and alveolar edema reduces lung compliance. The work of breathing and the oxygen requirements of respiratory muscles increase.

RENAL RESPONSE

Acute renal failure (Chap. 273), a serious complication of shock and hypoperfusion, occurs less frequently than heretofore because of early aggressive volume repletion. Acute tubular necrosis is now more frequently seen as a result of the interactions of shock, sepsis, the administration of nephrotoxic agents (such as aminoglycosides and angiographic contrast media), and rhabdomyolysis; the latter may be particularly severe in skeletal muscle trauma. The physiologic response of the kidney to hypoperfusion is to conserve salt and water. In addition to decreased renal blood flow, increased afferent arteriolar resistance accounts for diminished glomerular filtration rate, which together with increased aldosterone and vasopressin is responsible for reduced urine formation. Toxic injury causes necrosis of tubular epithelium and tubular obstruction by cellular debris with back-leak of filtrate. The depletion of renal ATP stores that occurs with prolonged renal hypoperfusion contributes to subsequent impairment of renal function.

METABOLIC DERANGEMENTS

During shock, there is disruption of the normal cycles of carbohydrate, lipid, and protein metabolism. Through the citric acid cycle, al-

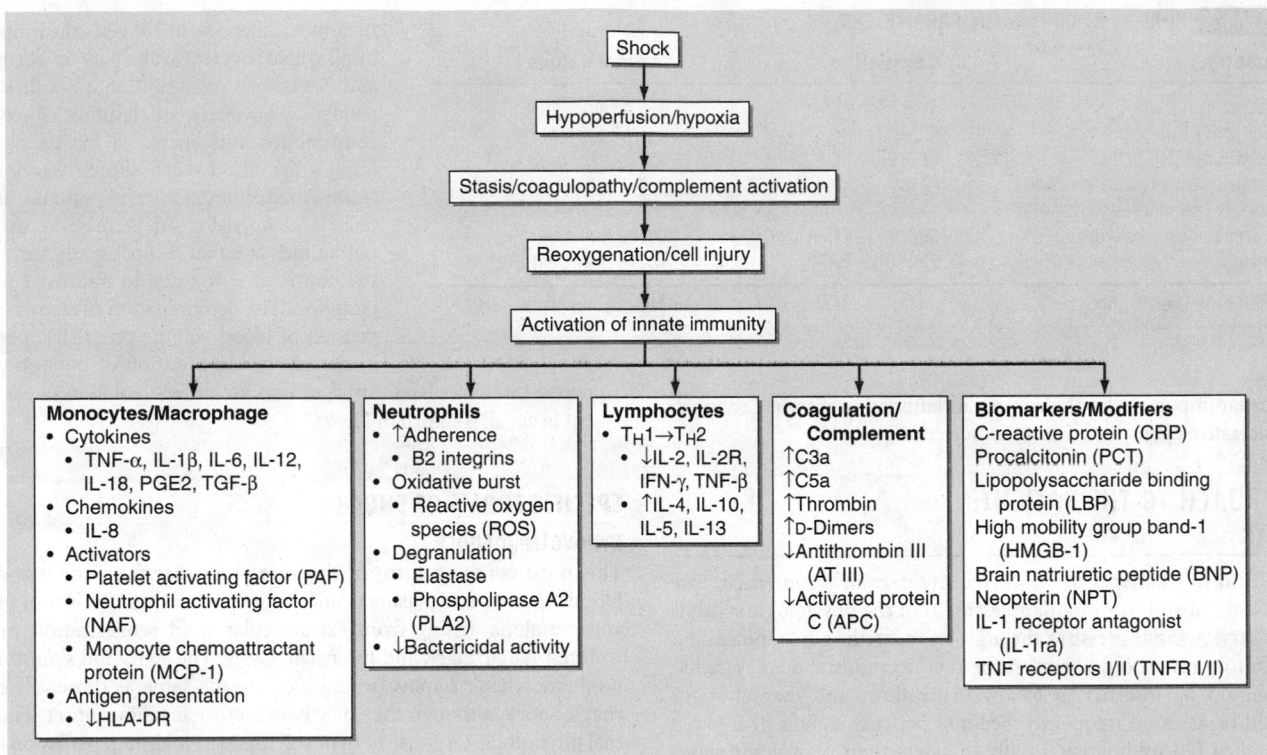

FIGURE 264-2 A schematic of the host immunoinflammatory response to shock.

anine in conjunction with lactate (which is converted from pyruvate in the periphery in the presence of oxygen deprivation) enhances the hepatic production of glucose. With reduced availability of oxygen, the breakdown of glucose to pyruvate and ultimately lactate represents an inefficient cycling of substrate with minimal net energy production. An elevated plasma lactate/pyruvate ratio is consistent with anaerobic metabolism and reflects inadequate tissue perfusion. Decreased clearance of exogenous triglycerides coupled with increased hepatic lipogenesis causes a significant rise in serum triglyceride concentrations. There is increased protein catabolism, a negative nitrogen balance, and, if the process is prolonged, severe muscle wasting.

INFLAMMATORY RESPONSES

Activation of an extensive network of proinflammatory mediator systems plays a significant role in the progression of shock and contributes importantly to the development of organ injury and failure (Fig. 264-2). In those surviving the acute insult, there is a delayed endogenous counterregulatory response to "turn off" the excessive proinflammatory response. If balance is restored, the patient does well. If the immunosuppressive response is excessive, the patient is highly susceptible to secondary nosocomial infections, which can then drive the inflammatory response and lead to delayed multiple organ failure.

Multiple humoral mediators are activated during shock and tissue injury. The complement cascade, activated through both the classic and alternate pathways, generates the anaphylatoxins C3a and C5a (Chap. 308). Direct complement fixation to injured tissues can progress to the C5-C9 attack complex, causing further cell damage. Activation of the coagulation cascade (Chap. 110) causes microvascular thrombosis, with subsequent fibrinolysis leading to repeated episodes of ischemia and reperfusion. Components of the coagulation system, such as thrombin, are potent proinflammatory mediators that cause expression of adhesion molecules on endothelial cells and activation of neutrophils, leading to microvascular injury. Coagulation also activates the kallikrein-kininogen cascade, contributing to hypotension.

Eicosanoids are vasoactive and immunomodulatory products of arachidonic acid metabolism that include cyclooxygenase-derived PGs and thromboxane A_2 as well as lipoxygenase-derived leukotrienes and lipoxins. Thromboxane A_2 is a potent vasoconstrictor that contributes to the pulmonary hypertension and acute tubular necrosis of shock. PGI_2 and PGE_2 are potent vasodilators that enhance capillary permeability and edema formation. The cysteinyl leukotrienes LTC_4 and LTD_4 are pivotal mediators of the vascular sequelae of anaphylaxis as well as of shock states resulting from sepsis or tissue injury. LTB_4 is a potent neutrophil chemoattractant and secretagogue that stimulates the formation of reactive oxygen species. Platelet-activating factor, an ether-linked, arachidonyl-containing phospholipid mediator, causes pulmonary vasoconstriction, bronchoconstriction, systemic vasodilation, increased capillary permeability, and the priming of macrophages and neutrophils to produce enhanced levels of inflammatory mediators.

Tumor necrosis factor α (TNF-α), produced by activated macrophages, reproduces many components of the shock state, including hypotension, lactic acidosis, and respiratory failure. Interleukin 1β (IL-1β), produced by tissue-fixed macrophages, is critical to the inflammatory response. Both are significantly elevated immediately following trauma and shock. IL-6, also produced predominantly by the macrophage, has a slightly delayed peak response but is the best predictor of prolonged recovery and development of multiple organ failure following shock. Chemokines such as IL-8 are potent neutrophil chemoattractants and activators that upregulate adhesion molecules on the neutrophil to enhance aggregation, adherence, and damage to the vascular endothelium. While the endothelium normally produces NO, the inflammatory response stimulates the inducible isoform of NO synthase (iNOS), which is overexpressed and produces toxic nitrosyl- and oxygen-derived free radicals that contribute to the hyperdynamic cardiovascular response in sepsis.

Multiple inflammatory cells, including neutrophils, macrophages, and platelets, are a major contributor to inflammation-induced injury. Margination of activated neutrophils in the microcirculation is a common pathologic finding in shock, causing secondary injury due to the release of toxic oxygen radicals, lipases, and proteases. Tissue-fixed macrophages produce virtually all major components of the inflammatory response and orchestrate the progression and duration of the inflammatory response. A major source of activation of the monocyte/macrophage is through the highly conserved membrane Toll-like receptors (TLRs), which recognize damage-associated molecular patterns (DAMPs) and pathogen-associated molecular patterns (PAMPs) released following tissue injury and by pathogenic microbial organisms, respectively. TLRs

TABLE 264-2 NORMAL HEMODYNAMIC PARAMETERS

Parameter	Calculation	Normal Values
Cardiac output (CO)	SV × HR	4–8 L/min
Cardiac index (CI)	CO/BSA	2.6–4.2 (L/min)/m²
Stroke volume (SV)	CO/HR	50–100 mL/beat
Systemic vascular resistance (SVR)	[(MAP – RAP)/CO] × 80	700–1600 dynes · s/cm⁵
Pulmonary vascular resistance (PVR)	[(PAP$_m$ – PCWP)/CO] × 80	20–130 dynes · s/cm⁵
Left ventricular stroke work (LVSW)	SV(MAP – PCWP) × 0.0136	60–80 g-m/beat
Right ventricular stroke work (RVSW)	SV(PAP$_m$ – RAP)	10–15 g-m/beat

Note: HR, heart rate; BSA, body surface area; MAP, mean arterial pressure; RAP, right atrial pressure; PAP$_m$, pulmonary artery pressure—mean; PCWP, pulmonary capillary wedge pressure.

also appear important for the chronic inflammation seen in Crohn's disease, ulcerative colitis, and transplant rejection.

APPROACH TO THE PATIENT:
Shock

MONITORING Patients in shock require care in an intensive care unit. Careful and continuous assessment of the physiologic status is necessary. Arterial pressure through an indwelling line, pulse, and respiratory rate should be monitored continuously; a Foley catheter should be inserted to follow urine flow; and mental status should be assessed frequently. Sedated patients should be allowed to awaken ("drug holiday") daily to assess their neurologic status and to shorten duration of ventilator support.

There is ongoing debate as to the indications for using the flow-directed pulmonary artery catheter (PAC, Swan-Ganz catheter). Most patients in the intensive care unit can be safely managed without the use of a PAC. However, in patients with significant ongoing blood loss, fluid shifts, and underlying cardiac dysfunction, a PAC may be useful. The PAC is placed percutaneously via the subclavian or jugular vein through the central venous circulation and right heart into the pulmonary artery. There are ports both proximal in the right atrium and distal in the pulmonary artery to provide access for infusions and for cardiac output measurements. Right atrial and pulmonary artery pressures are measured, and the pulmonary capillary wedge pressure (PCWP) serves as an approximation of the left atrial pressure. Normal hemodynamic parameters are shown in Table 223-1 and Table 264-2.

Cardiac output is determined by the thermodilution technique, and high-resolution thermistors can also be used to determine right ventricular end-diastolic volume to monitor further the response of the right heart to fluid resuscitation. A PAC with an oximeter port offers the additional advantage of on-line monitoring of the mixed venous oxygen saturation, an important index of tissue perfusion. Systemic and pulmonary vascular resistances are calculated as the ratio of the pressure drop across these vascular beds to the cardiac output (Chap. 223). Determinations of oxygen content in arterial and venous blood, together with cardiac output and hemoglobin concentration, allow calculation of oxygen delivery, oxygen consumption, and oxygen-extraction ratio (Table 264-3). The hemodynamic patterns associated with the various forms of shock are shown in Table 264-4.

In resuscitation from shock, it is critical to restore tissue perfusion and optimize oxygen delivery, hemodynamics, and cardiac function rapidly. A reasonable goal of therapy is to achieve normal mixed venous oxygen saturation and arteriovenous oxygen-extraction ratio. To enhance oxygen delivery, red cell mass, arterial oxygen saturation, and cardiac output may be augmented singly or simultaneously. An increase in oxygen delivery not accompanied by an increase in oxygen consumption implies that oxygen availability is adequate and that oxygen consumption is not flow-dependent. Conversely, an elevation of oxygen consumption with increased cardiac output implies that the oxygen supply was inadequate. A reduction in systemic vascular resistance accompanying an increase in cardiac output indicates that compensatory vasoconstriction is reversing due to improved tissue perfusion. The determination of stepwise expansion of blood volume on cardiac performance allows identification of the optimum preload (Starling's law). An algorithm for the resuscitation of the patient in shock is shown in Fig. 264-3.

SPECIFIC FORMS OF SHOCK

HYPOVOLEMIC SHOCK

This most common form of shock results either from the loss of red blood cell mass and plasma from hemorrhage or from the loss of plasma volume alone arising from extravascular fluid sequestration or gastrointestinal, urinary, and insensible losses. The signs and symptoms of nonhemorrhagic hypovolemic shock are the same as those of hemorrhagic shock, although they may have a more insidious onset. The normal physiologic response to hypovolemia is to maintain perfusion of the brain and heart while restoring an effective circulating blood volume. There is an increase in sympathetic activity, hyperventilation, collapse of venous capacitance vessels, release of stress hormones, and an attempt to limit the loss of intravascular volume through the recruitment of interstitial and intracellular fluid and reduction of urine output.

Mild hypovolemia (≤20% of the blood volume) generates mild tachycardia but relatively few external signs, especially in a supine resting young patient (Table 264-5). With moderate hypovolemia (~20–40% of the blood volume), the patient becomes increasingly anxious and tachycardic; although normal blood pressure may be maintained in the supine position, there may be significant postural hypotension and tachycardia. If hypovolemia is severe (≥40% of the blood volume), the classic signs of shock appear; the blood pressure declines and becomes unstable even in the supine position, and the patient develops marked tachycardia, oliguria, and agitation or confusion. Perfusion of the central nervous system is well maintained until shock becomes severe. Hence, mental obtundation is an ominous clinical sign. The transition from mild to severe hypovolemic shock can be insidious or extremely rapid. If severe shock is not reversed rapidly, especially in elderly patients and those with comorbid illnesses, death is imminent. A very narrow time frame separates the derangements found in severe shock that

TABLE 264-3 OXYGEN TRANSPORT CALCULATIONS

Parameter	Calculation	Normal Values
Oxygen-carrying capacity of hemoglobin		1.39 mL/g
Plasma O₂ concentration	P$_{O_2}$ × 0.0031	
Arterial O₂ concentration (Ca$_{O_2}$)	1.39 Sa$_{O_2}$ + 0.0031 Pa$_{O_2}$	20 vol%
Venous O₂ concentration (Cv$_{O_2}$)	1.39 Sv$_{O_2}$ + 0.0031 Pv$_{O_2}$	15.5 vol%
Arteriovenous O₂ difference (Ca$_{O_2}$ – Cv$_{O_2}$)	1.39 (Sa$_{O_2}$ – Sv$_{O_2}$) + 0.0031 (Pa$_{O_2}$ – Pv$_{O_2}$)	3.5 vol%
Oxygen delivery (D$_{O_2}$)	Ca$_{O_2}$ × CO (L/min) × 10 (dL/L) 1.39 Sa$_{O_2}$ × CO × 10	800–1600 mL/min
Oxygen uptake (V$_{O_2}$)	(Ca$_{O_2}$ – Cv$_{O_2}$) × CO × 10 1.39 (Sa$_{O_2}$ – Sv$_{O_2}$) × CO × 10	150–400 mL/min
Oxygen delivery index (D$_{O_2}$I)	D$_{O_2}$/BSA	520–720 (mL/min)/m²
Oxygen uptake index (V$_{O_2}$I)	V$_{O_2}$/BSA	115–165 (mL/min)/m²
Oxygen extraction ratio (O₂ER)	[1 – (V$_{O_2}$/D$_{O_2}$)] × 100	22–32%

Note: P$_{O_2}$, partial pressure of oxygen; Sa$_{O_2}$, saturation of hemoglobin with O₂ in arterial blood; Pa$_{O_2}$, partial pressure of O₂ in arterial blood; Sv$_{O_2}$, saturation of hemoglobin with O₂ in venous blood; Pv$_{O_2}$, partial pressure of O₂ in venous blood; CO, cardiac output; BSA, body surface area.

TABLE 264-4 PHYSIOLOGIC CHARACTERISTICS OF THE VARIOUS FORMS OF SHOCK

Type of Shock	CVP and PCWP	Cardiac Output	Systemic Vascular Resistance	Venous O₂ Saturation
Hypovolemic	↓	↓	↑	↓
Cardiogenic	↑	↓	↑	↓
Septic				
Hyperdynamic	↓↑	↑	↓	↑
Hypodynamic	↓↑	↓	↑	↑↓
Traumatic	↓	↓↑	↑↓	↓
Neurogenic	↓	↓	↓	↓
Hypoadrenal	↓↑	↓	=↓	↓

Note: CVP, central venous pressure; PCWP, pulmonary capillary wedge pressure.

TABLE 264-5 HYPOVOLEMIC SHOCK

Mild (<20% Blood Volume)	Moderate (20–40% Blood Volume)	Severe (>40% Blood Volume)
Cool extremities	Same, plus:	Same, plus:
Increased capillary refill time	Tachycardia	Hemodynamic instability
Diaphoresis	Tachypnea	Marked tachycardia
Collapsed veins	Oliguria	Hypotension
Anxiety	Postural changes	Mental status deterioration (coma)

can be reversed with aggressive resuscitation from those of progressive decompensation and irreversible cell injury.

Diagnosis Hypovolemic shock is readily diagnosed when there are signs of hemodynamic instability and the source of volume loss is obvious. The diagnosis is more difficult when the source of blood loss is occult, as into the gastrointestinal tract, or when plasma volume alone is depleted. After acute hemorrhage, hemoglobin and hematocrit values do not change until compensatory fluid shifts have occurred or ex-

ogenous fluid is administered. Thus, an initial normal hematocrit does not disprove the presence of significant blood loss. Plasma losses cause hemoconcentration, and free water loss leads to hypernatremia. These findings should suggest the presence of hypovolemia.

It is essential to distinguish between hypovolemic and cardiogenic shock (Chap. 266) because definitive therapy differs significantly. Both forms are associated with a reduced cardiac output and a compensatory sympathetic mediated response characterized by tachycardia and elevated systemic vascular resistance. However, the findings in cardiogenic shock of jugular venous distention, rales, and an S₃ gallop distinguish it from hypovolemic shock and signify that ongoing volume expansion is undesirable.

℞ HYPOVOLEMIC SHOCK

Initial resuscitation requires rapid reexpansion of the circulating intravascular blood volume along with interventions to control ongoing losses. In accordance with Starling's law (Chap. 217), stroke volume and cardiac output rise with the increase in preload. After resuscitation, the compliance of the ventricles may remain reduced due to increased interstitial fluid in the myocardium. Therefore elevated filling pressures are required to maintain adequate ventricular performance.

Volume resuscitation is initiated with the rapid infusion of isotonic saline (although care must be taken to avoid hyperchloremic acidosis from loss of bicarbonate buffering capacity and replacement with excess chloride) or a balanced salt solution such as Ringer's lactate through large-bore intravenous lines. No distinct benefit from the use of colloid has been demonstrated, and in trauma patients it is associated with a higher mortality, particularly in patients with traumatic brain injury. The infusion of 2–3 L of salt solution over 20–30 min should restore normal hemodynamic parameters. Continued hemodynamic instability implies that shock has not been reversed and/or that there are significant ongoing blood or volume losses. Continuing blood loss, with hemoglobin concentrations declining to ≤100 g/L (10 g/dL), should initiate blood transfusion, preferably as fully cross-matched blood. In extreme emergencies, type-specific or O-negative packed red cells may be transfused. In the presence of severe and/or prolonged hypovolemia, inotropic support with dopamine, vasopressin, or dobutamine may be required to maintain adequate ventricular performance *after* blood volume has been restored. Infusion of norepinephrine to increase arterial pressure by raising peripheral resistance is inappropriate, other than as a temporizing measure in severe shock while blood volume is reexpanded. Once hemorrhage is controlled and the patient has stabilized, blood transfusions should not be continued unless the hemoglobin is <~7g/dL. Studies have demonstrated an increased survival in patients treated with this restrictive blood transfusion protocol.

Successful resuscitation also requires support of respiratory function. Supplemental oxygen should be provided, and endotracheal intubation may be necessary to maintain arterial oxygenation. Following resuscitation from isolated hemorrhagic shock, end-organ

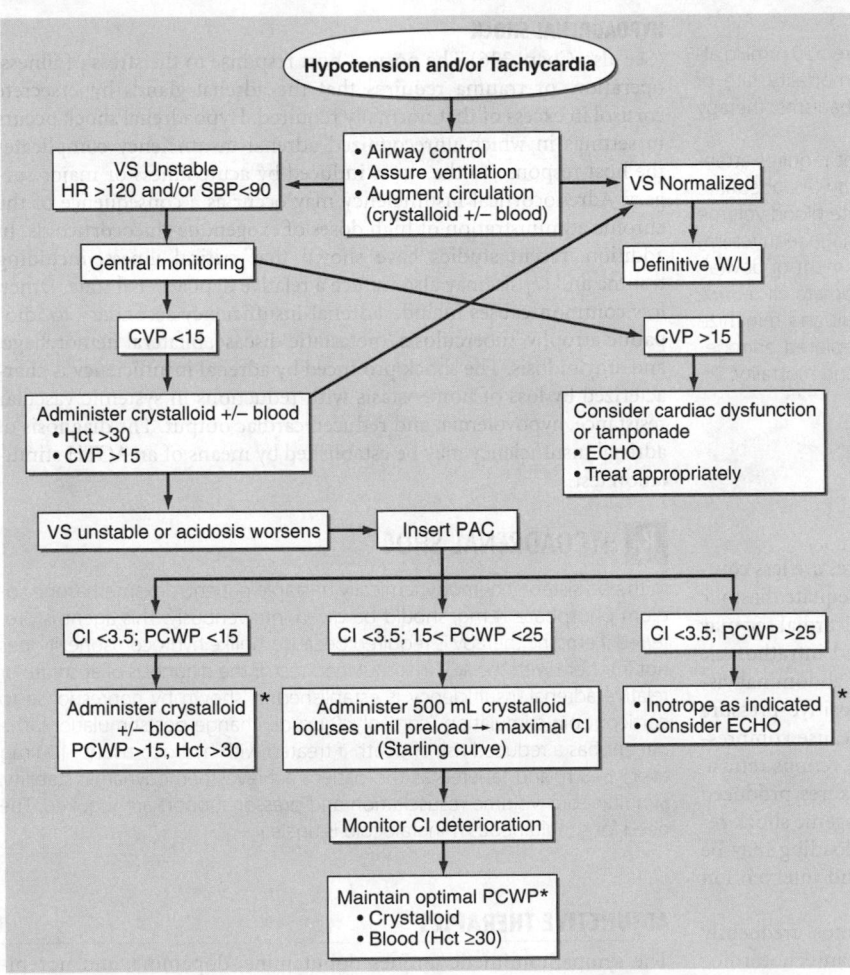

FIGURE 264-3 An algorithm for the resuscitation of the patient in shock. VS, vital signs; HR, heart rate; SBP, systolic blood pressure; W/U, work up; CVP, central venous pressure; Hct, hematocrit; ECHO, echocardiogram; PAC, pulmonary artery catheter; CI, cardiac index in (L/min) per m²; PCWP, pulmonary capillary wedge pressure in mmHg. *Monitor SV_{O₂}, SVRI, and RVEDVI as additional markers of correction for perfusion and hypovolemia. Consider age-adjusted CI. SV_{O₂}, saturation of hemoglobin with O₂ in venous blood; SVRI, systemic vascular resistance index; RVEDVI, right-ventricular end-diastolic volume index.

damage is frequently less than following septic or traumatic shock. This may be due to the absence of the massive activation of inflammatory mediator response systems and the consequent nonspecific organ injury seen in the latter conditions.

TRAUMATIC SHOCK

Shock following trauma is, in large measure, due to hypovolemia. However, even when hemorrhage has been controlled, patients can continue to suffer loss of plasma volume into the interstitium of injured tissues. These fluid losses are compounded by injury-induced inflammatory responses, which contribute to the secondary microcirculatory injury. Recent evidence demonstrates release of mediators induced by DAMPs from injured tissue that are recognized by the highly conserved membrane receptors of the TLR family (see "Inflammatory Responses," above). These receptors on the cells of the innate immune system, particularly the circulating monocyte, tissue-fixed macrophage, and dendritic cell, are potent activators of an excessive proinflammatory phenotype in response to cellular injury. This causes secondary tissue injury and maldistribution of blood flow, intensifying tissue ischemia and leading to multiple organ system failure. In addition, direct trauma to the heart, chest, or head can also contribute to the shock. For example, pericardial tamponade or tension pneumothorax impairs ventricular filling, while myocardial contusion depresses myocardial contractility.

Rx TRAUMATIC SHOCK

Inability of the patient to maintain a systolic blood pressure ≥90 mmHg after trauma-induced hypovolemia is associated with a mortality rate of ~50%. To prevent decompensation of homeostatic mechanisms, therapy must be promptly administered.

The initial management of the seriously injured patient requires attention to the "ABCs" of resuscitation: assurance of an *airway* (A), adequate ventilation (*breathing*, B), and establishment of an adequate blood volume to support the *circulation* (C). Control of ongoing hemorrhage requires immediate attention. Early stabilization of fractures, debridement of devitalized or contaminated tissues, and evacuation of hematomata all reduce the subsequent inflammatory response to the initial insult and minimize subsequent diffuse organ injury. Supplementation of depleted endogenous antioxidants also reduces subsequent organ failure and mortality.

CARDIOGENIC SHOCK

See Chap. 266.

COMPRESSIVE CARDIOGENIC SHOCK

With compression, the heart and surrounding structures are less compliant, and thus normal filling pressures generate inadequate diastolic filling. Blood or fluid within the poorly distensible pericardial sac may cause tamponade (Chap. 232). Any cause of increased intrathoracic pressure, such as tension pneumothorax, herniation of abdominal viscera through a diaphragmatic hernia, or excessive positive pressure ventilation to support pulmonary function, can also cause compressive cardiogenic shock while simultaneously impeding venous return. Although initially responsive to increased filling pressures produced by volume expansion, as compression increases, cardiogenic shock recurs. The window of opportunity gained by volume loading may be very brief until irreversible shock recurs. Diagnosis and intervention must occur urgently.

The diagnosis of compressive cardiogenic shock is most frequently based on clinical findings, the chest radiograph, and an echocardiogram. The diagnosis of compressive cardiac shock may be more difficult to establish in the setting of trauma when hypovolemia and cardiac compression are present simultaneously. The classic findings of pericardial tamponade include the triad of hypotension, neck vein distention, and muffled heart sounds (Chap. 232). Pulsus paradoxus, i.e., an inspiratory reduction in systolic pressure >10 mmHg, may also be noted. The diagnosis is confirmed by echocardiography, and treatment consists of immediate pericardiocentesis. A tension pneumothorax produces ipsilateral decreased breath sounds, tracheal deviation away from the affected thorax, and jugular venous distention. Radiographic findings include increased intrathoracic volume, depression of the diaphragm of the affected hemithorax, and shifting of the mediastinum to the contralateral side. Chest decompression must be carried out immediately. Release of air and restoration of normal cardiovascular dynamics are both diagnostic and therapeutic.

SEPTIC SHOCK
See Chap. 265.

NEUROGENIC SHOCK

Interruption of sympathetic vasomotor input after a high cervical spinal cord injury, inadvertent cephalad migration of spinal anesthesia, or devastating head injury may result in neurogenic shock. In addition to arteriolar dilatation, venodilation causes pooling in the venous system, which decreases venous return and cardiac output. The extremities are often warm, in contrast to the usual vasoconstriction-induced coolness in hypovolemic or cardiogenic shock. Treatment involves a simultaneous approach to the relative hypovolemia and to the loss of vasomotor tone. Excessive volumes of fluid may be required to restore normal hemodynamics if given alone. Once hemorrhage has been ruled out, norepinephrine or a pure α-adrenergic agent (phenylephrine) may be necessary to augment vascular resistance and maintain an adequate mean arterial pressure.

HYPOADRENAL SHOCK

(See also Chap. 336) The normal host response to the stress of illness, operation, or trauma requires that the adrenal glands hypersecrete cortisol in excess of that normally required. Hypoadrenal shock occurs in settings in which unrecognized adrenal insufficiency complicates the host response to the stress induced by acute illness or major surgery. Adrenocortical insufficiency may occur as a consequence of the chronic administration of high doses of exogenous glucocorticoids. In addition, recent studies have shown that critical illness, including trauma and sepsis, may also induce a relative hypoadrenal state. Other, less common causes include adrenal insufficiency secondary to idiopathic atrophy, tuberculosis, metastatic disease, bilateral hemorrhage, and amyloidosis. The shock produced by adrenal insufficiency is characterized by loss of homeostasis with reductions in systemic vascular resistance, hypovolemia, and reduced cardiac output. The diagnosis of adrenal insufficiency may be established by means of an ACTH stimulation test.

Rx HYPOADRENAL SHOCK

In the persistently hemodynamically unstable patient, dexamethasone sodium phosphate, 4 mg, should be given intravenously. This agent is preferred if empiric therapy is required because, unlike hydrocortisone, it does not interfere with the ACTH stimulation test. If the diagnosis of absolute or relative adrenal insufficiency is established as shown by nonresponse to corticotropin stimulation (cortisol ≤9 μg/dL change poststimulation), the patient has a reduced risk of death if treated with hydrocortisone, 100 mg every 6–8 h, and tapered as the patient achieves hemodynamic stability. Simultaneous volume resuscitation and pressor support are required. The need for simultaneous mineralocoid is unclear.

ADJUNCTIVE THERAPIES

The sympathomimetic amines dobutamine, dopamine, and norepinephrine are widely used in the treatment of all forms of shock. Dobutamine is inotropic with simultaneous afterload reduction, thus minimizing cardiac-oxygen consumption increases as cardiac output increases. Dopamine is an inotropic and chronotropic agent that also supports vascular resistance in those whose blood pressure will not tolerate peripheral vascular dilation. Norepinephrine primarily supports blood pressure through vasoconstriction and increases myocardial oxygen consumption while placing marginally perfused tissues, such as extremities and splanchnic organs, at risk for necrosis, but it is also inotropic without chronotropy. Arginine-vasopressin (antidiuretic hormone) is also being used increasingly and may better protect vital organ blood flow and prevent pathologic vasodilation.

POSITIONING

Positioning of the patient may be a valuable adjunct in the initial treatment of hypovolemic shock. Elevating the foot of the bed (i.e., placing it on "shock blocks") and assumption of the Trendelenburg position without flexion at the knees are effective but may increase work of breathing and risk for aspiration. Simply elevating both legs may be the optimal approach.

PNEUMATIC ANTISHOCK GARMENT (PASG)

The PASG and the military antishock trousers (MAST) are inflatable external compression devices that can be wrapped around the legs and abdomen and have been widely used in the prehospital setting as a means of providing temporary support of central hemodynamics in shock. However, they cause a significant increase in systemic vascular resistance and blood pressure by arterial compression, without causing a significant change in cardiac output or tissue perfusion. The most appropriate use appears to be as a means to tamponade and to prevent ongoing bleeding and augment hemostasis. Inflation of the suit provides splinting of fractures of the pelvis and lower extremities and helps to arrest hemorrhage.

REWARMING

Hypothermia is a potential adverse consequence of massive volume resuscitation. The infusion of large volumes of refrigerated blood products and room-temperature crystalloid solutions can rapidly drop core temperatures if fluid is not run through warming devices. Hypothermia may depress cardiac contractility and thereby further impair cardiac output and oxygen delivery. Hypothermia, particularly temperatures <35°C, directly impairs the coagulation pathway, sometimes causing a significant coagulopathy. Rapid rewarming to >35°C significantly decreases the requirement for blood products and produces an improvement in cardiac function. The most effective method for rewarming is endovascular countercurrent warmers through femoral vein cannulation. This process does not require a pump and can rewarm from 30° to 35°C in <30 min.

FURTHER READINGS

ANNANE D et al: Effect of treatment with low doses of hydrocortisone and fludrocortisone on mortality in patients with septic shock. JAMA 288:862, 2002

ANZICS CLINICAL TRIALS GROUP: Low-dose dopamine in patients with early renal dysfunction: A placebo-controlled randomized trial. Lancet 356:2139, 2000

ARDS CLINICAL TRIALS NETWORK: Pulmonary-artery versus central venous catheter to guide treatment of acute lung injury. N Engl J Med 354:2213, 2006

CHEN P: Vasopressin: New uses in critical care. Am J Med Sci 324:146, 2002

EGI M et al: Selecting a vasopressor drug for vasoplegic shock after adult cardiac surgery; a systematic literature review. Ann Thor Surg 83:715, 2007

FINFER S et al: A comparison of albumin and saline for fluid resuscitation in the intensive care unit. N Engl J Med 350:2247, 2004

HEBERT PC et al: Clinical consequence of anemia and red cell transfusion in the critically ill. Crit Care Clin 20:225, 2004

MOORE FA et al: The next generation in shock resuscitation. Lancet 363:1988, 2004

OSUCHOWSKI MF et al: Circulating cytokine/inhibitor profiles reshape the understanding of SIRS/CARS continuum in sepsis and predict mortality. J Immunol 177:1967, 2006

ROMICS L JR et al: The emerging role of toll-like receptor pathways in surgical diseases. Arch Surg 141:595, 2006

265 Severe Sepsis and Septic Shock
Robert S. Munford

DEFINITIONS

(See Table 265-1) Animals mount both local and systemic responses to microbes that traverse epithelial barriers and invade underlying tissues. Fever or hypothermia, leukocytosis or leukopenia, tachypnea, and tachycardia are the cardinal signs of the systemic response often called the *systemic inflammatory response syndrome* (SIRS). SIRS may have an infectious or a noninfectious etiology. If infection is suspected or proven, a patient with SIRS is said to have *sepsis*. When sepsis is associated with dysfunction of organs distant from the site of infection, the patient has *severe sepsis*. Severe sepsis may be accompanied by hypotension or evidence of hypoperfusion. When hypotension cannot be corrected by infusing fluids, the diagnosis is *septic shock*. These definitions were proposed by consensus conference committees in 1992 and 2001 and are now widely used; there is evidence that the different stages form a continuum. As sepsis progresses to septic shock, the risk of dying increases substantially. Sepsis is usually reversible, whereas patients with septic shock often succumb despite aggressive therapy.

ETIOLOGY

Severe sepsis can be a response to any class of microorganism. Microbial invasion of the bloodstream is not essential for the development of severe sepsis, since local inflammation can also elicit distant organ dysfunction and hypotension. In fact, blood cultures yield bacteria or fungi in only ~20–40% of cases of severe sepsis and 40–70% of cases of septic shock. Individual gram-negative or gram-positive bacteria account for ~70% of these isolates; the remainder are fungi or a mixture of microorganisms (Table 265-2). In patients whose blood cultures are negative, the etiologic agent is often established by culture or microscopic examination of infected material from a local site. In some case series, a majority of patients with a clinical picture of severe sepsis or septic shock have had negative microbiologic data.

EPIDEMIOLOGY

The septic response is a contributing factor in >200,000 deaths per year in the United States. The incidence of severe sepsis and septic shock has increased over the past 20 years, and the annual number of cases is now >700,000 (~3 per 1000 population). Approximately two-thirds of the cases occur in patients with significant underlying illness. Sepsis-related incidence and mortality rates increase with age and pre-existing comorbidity. The rising incidence of severe sepsis in the United States is attributable to the aging of the population, the increasing longevity of patients with chronic diseases, and the relatively high frequency with which sepsis develops in patients with AIDS. The widespread use of antimicrobial agents, immunosuppressive drugs, indwelling catheters and mechanical devices, and mechanical ventilation also plays a role.

Invasive bacterial infections are prominent causes of death around the world, particularly among young children. In sub-Saharan Africa, for example, careful screening for positive blood cultures found that community-acquired bacteremia accounted for at least one-fourth of deaths of children >1 year of age. Nontyphoidal *Salmonella* species, *Streptococcus pneumoniae*, *Haemophilus influenzae*, and *Escherichia coli* were the most commonly isolated bacteria. Bacteremic children often had HIV infection or were severely malnourished.

TABLE 265-1 DEFINITIONS USED TO DESCRIBE THE CONDITION OF SEPTIC PATIENTS

Bacteremia	Presence of bacteria in blood, as evidenced by positive blood cultures
Septicemia	Presence of microbes or their toxins in blood
Systemic inflammatory response syndrome (SIRS)	Two or more of the following conditions: (1) fever (oral temperature >38°C) or hypothermia (<36°C); (2) tachypnea (>24 breaths/min); (3) tachycardia (heart rate >90 beats/min); (4) leukocytosis (>12,000/μL), leukopenia (<4,000/μL), or >10% bands; may have a noninfectious etiology
Sepsis	SIRS that has a proven or suspected microbial etiology
Severe sepsis (similar to "sepsis syndrome")	Sepsis with one or more signs of organ dysfunction—for example:
	1. *Cardiovascular:* Arterial systolic blood pressure ≤90 mmHg or mean arterial pressure ≤70 mmHg that responds to administration of intravenous fluid
	2. *Renal:* Urine output <0.5 mL/kg per hour for 1 h despite adequate fluid resuscitation
	3. *Respiratory:* Pa_{O_2}/FI_{O_2} ≤250 or, if the lung is the only dysfunctional organ, ≤200
	4. *Hematologic:* Platelet count <80,000/μL or 50% decrease in platelet count from highest value recorded over previous 3 days
	5. *Unexplained metabolic acidosis:* A pH ≤7.30 or a base deficit ≥5.0 mEq/L and a plasma lactate level >1.5 times upper limit of normal for reporting lab
	6. *Adequate fluid resuscitation:* Pulmonary artery wedge pressure ≥12 mmHg or central venous pressure ≥8 mmHg
Septic shock	Sepsis with hypotension (arterial blood pressure <90 mmHg systolic, or 40 mmHg less than patient's normal blood pressure) for at least 1 h despite adequate fluid resuscitation; *or* Need for vasopressors to maintain systolic blood pressure ≥90 mmHg *or* mean arterial pressure ≥70 mmHg
Refractory septic shock	Septic shock that lasts for >1 h and does not respond to fluid or pressor administration
Multiple-organ dysfunction syndrome (MODS)	Dysfunction of more than one organ, requiring intervention to maintain homeostasis

Source: Adapted from the American College of Chest Physicians/Society of Critical Care Medicine Consensus Conference Committee and Bernard et al. Published in Crit Care Med, with permission.

PATHOPHYSIOLOGY

Most cases of severe sepsis are triggered by bacteria or fungi that do not ordinarily cause systemic disease in immunocompetent hosts (Table 265-2). These microbes probably exploit deficiencies in innate host defenses (e.g., phagocytes, complement, and natural antibodies) to survive within the body. Microbial pathogens, in contrast, are able to circumvent innate defenses by elaborating toxins or other virulence factors. In both cases, the body can fail to kill the invaders despite mounting a vigorous inflammatory reaction that can result in severe sepsis. The septic response may also be induced by microbial exotoxins that act as superantigens (e.g., toxic shock syndrome toxin 1; Chap. 129).

Host Mechanisms for Sensing Microbes Animals have exquisitely sensitive mechanisms for recognizing and responding to conserved microbial molecules. Recognition of the lipid A moiety of lipopolysaccharide (LPS, also called *endotoxin*; Chap. 114) is the best-studied example. A host protein (LPS-binding protein, or LBP) binds lipid A and transfers the LPS to CD14 on the surfaces of monocytes, macrophages, and neutrophils. LPS then is passed to MD-2, which interacts with Toll-like receptor (TLR) 4 to form a molecular complex that transduces the LPS recognition signal to the interior of the cell. This signal rapidly triggers the production and release of mediators, such as tumor necro-

TABLE 265-2 MICROORGANISMS INVOLVED IN EPISODES OF SEVERE SEPSIS AT EIGHT ACADEMIC MEDICAL CENTERS

Microorganisms	Episodes with Bloodstream Infection, % (n = 436)	Episodes with Documented Infection but No Bloodstream Infection, % (n = 430)	Total Episodes, % (n = 866)
Gram-negative bacteria[a]	35	44	40
Gram-positive bacteria[b]	40	24	31
Fungi	7	5	6
Polymicrobial	11	21	16
Classic pathogens[c]	<5	<5	<5

[a]Enterobacteriaceae, pseudomonads, *Haemophilus* spp., other gram-negative bacteria.
[b]*Staphylococcus aureus*, coagulase-negative staphylococci, enterococci, *Streptococcus pneumoniae*, other streptococci, other gram-positive bacteria.
[c]Such as *Neisseria meningitidis*, *S. pneumoniae*, *H. influenzae*, and *Streptococcus pyogenes*.
Source: Adapted from Sands et al.

sis factor (TNF; see below), that amplify the LPS signal and transmit it to other cells and tissues. Bacterial peptidoglycan and lipoteichoic acids elicit responses in animals that are generally similar to those induced by LPS; whereas these molecules also bind CD14, they interact with different TLRs. Having numerous TLR-based receptor complexes (10 different TLRs have been identified so far in humans) allows animals to recognize many conserved microbial molecules. The ability of some of the TLRs to serve as receptors for host ligands (e.g., hyaluronans, heparan sulfate, saturated fatty acids) raises the possibility that these molecules play a role in producing noninfectious sepsis-like states. Other host pattern-recognition proteins that are important for sensing microbial invasion and initiating host inflammation include the intracellular NOD1 and NOD2 proteins, which recognize discrete fragments of bacterial peptidoglycan; complement (principally the alternative pathway); mannose-binding lectin; and C-reactive protein.

The ability to recognize certain microbial molecules may influence both the potency of the host defense and the pathogenesis of severe sepsis. For example, MD-2–TLR4 best senses LPS that has a hexaacyl lipid A moiety (i.e., one with six fatty acyl chains). Most of the commensal aerobic and facultatively anaerobic gram-negative bacteria that trigger severe sepsis and shock (including *E. coli*, *Klebsiella*, and *Enterobacter*) make this lipid A structure. When they invade human hosts, often through breaks in an epithelial barrier, infection is typically localized to the subepithelial tissue. Bacteremia, if it occurs, is intermittent and low-grade, as these bacteria are efficiently cleared from the bloodstream by TLR4-expressing Kupffer cells and splenic macrophages. These mucosal commensals seem to induce severe sepsis most often by triggering severe local tissue inflammation rather than by circulating within the bloodstream. In contrast, gram-negative bacteria that do not make hexaacyl lipid A (*Yersinia pestis*, *Francisella tularensis*, *Vibrio vulnificus*, *Pseudomonas aeruginosa*, and *Burkholderia pseudomallei*, among others) are poorly recognized by MD-2–TLR4. These bacteria usually enter the body via nonmucosal routes—e.g., as a result of bites, cuts, or inhalation—and initially induce relatively little inflammation. When they do trigger severe sepsis, it is often in the setting of massive bacterial growth throughout the body. Engineering a virulent strain of *Y. pestis* to produce hexaacyl lipid A has rendered it avirulent in mice; this result attests to the importance of TLR4-based bacterial recognition in host defense. For most gram-negative bacteria, the pathogenesis of sepsis thus depends, at least in part, on whether the bacterium's LPS is sensed by the host receptor MD-2–TLR4.

Local and Systemic Host Responses to Invading Microbes Recognition of microbial molecules by tissue phagocytes triggers the production and/or release of numerous host molecules (cytokines, chemokines, prostanoids, leukotrienes, and others) that increase blood flow to the infected tissue, enhance the permeability of local blood vessels, recruit neutrophils to the site of infection, and elicit pain. These phenomena are familiar elements of local inflammation, the body's frontline innate immune mechanism for eliminating microbial invaders. Systemic responses are activated by neural and/or humoral communication with the hypothalamus and brainstem; these responses enhance local defenses by increasing blood flow to the infected area, augmenting the number of circulating neutrophils, and elevating blood levels of numerous molecules (such as the microbial recognition proteins discussed above) that have anti-infective functions.

CYTOKINES AND OTHER MEDIATORS   Cytokines can exert endocrine, paracrine, and autocrine effects (Chap. 308). TNF-α stimulates leukocytes and vascular endothelial cells to release other cytokines (as well as additional TNF-α), to express cell-surface molecules that enhance neutrophil-endothelial adhesion at sites of infection, and to increase prostaglandin and leukotriene production. Whereas blood levels of TNF-α are not elevated in individuals with localized infections, they increase in most patients with severe sepsis or septic shock. Moreover, IV infusion of TNF-α can elicit the characteristic abnormalities of SIRS. In animals, larger doses of TNF-α induce shock, disseminated intravascular coagulation (DIC), and death.

Although TNF-α is a central mediator, it is only one of many proinflammatory molecules that contribute to innate host defense. Chemokines, most prominently interleukin (IL) 8, attract circulating neutrophils to the infection site. IL-1β exhibits many of the same activities as TNF-α. TNF-α, IL-1β, interferon (IFN) γ, IL-12, and other cytokines probably interact synergistically with one another and with additional mediators. High-mobility group B-1, a transcription factor, can also be released from cells and interact with microbial products to induce host responses late in the course of the septic response.

COAGULATION FACTORS   Intravascular thrombosis, a hallmark of the local inflammatory response, may help wall off invading microbes and prevent infection and inflammation from spreading to other tissues. Intravascular fibrin deposition, thrombosis, and DIC can also be important features of the systemic response. IL-6 and other mediators promote intravascular coagulation initially by inducing blood monocytes and vascular endothelial cells to express tissue factor (Chap. 59). When tissue factor is expressed on cell surfaces, it binds to factor VIIa to form an active complex that can convert factors X and IX to their enzymatically active forms. The result is activation of both extrinsic and intrinsic clotting pathways, culminating in the generation of fibrin. Clotting is also favored by impaired function of the protein C–protein S inhibitory pathway and depletion of antithrombin and protein C, while fibrinolysis is prevented by increased plasma levels of plasminogen activator inhibitor 1. Thus, there may be a striking propensity toward intravascular fibrin deposition, thrombosis, and bleeding; this propensity has been most apparent in patients with intravascular endothelial infections such as meningococcemia (Chap. 136). Contact-system activation occurs during sepsis but contributes more to the development of hypotension than to DIC.

CONTROL MECHANISMS   Elaborate control mechanisms operate within both local sites of inflammation and the systemic circulation.

Local Control Mechanisms   Host recognition of invading microbes within subepithelial tissues typically ignites immune responses that rapidly kill the invader and then subside to allow tissue recovery. The anti-inflammatory forces that put out the fire and clean up the battleground include molecules that neutralize or inactivate microbial signals. Among these molecules are LPS; intracellular factors (e.g., suppressor of cytokine signaling 3) that diminish the production of proinflammatory mediators by neutrophils and macrophages; anti-inflammatory cytokines (IL-10, IL-4); and molecules derived from essential polyunsaturated fatty acids (lipoxins, resolvins, and protectins) that promote tissue restoration.

Systemic Control Mechanisms   The signaling apparatus that links microbial recognition to cellular responses in tissues is less active in the blood. For example, whereas LBP plays a role in recognizing the presence of LPS, in plasma it also prevents LPS signaling by transferring LPS molecules into plasma lipoprotein particles, which sequester the lipid A moiety so that it cannot interact with cells. At the high concentrations found in blood, LBP also inhibits monocyte responses to LPS, and the soluble (circulating) form of CD14 strips off LPS that has bound to monocyte surfaces.

Systemic responses to infection also diminish cellular responses to microbial molecules. Circulating levels of anti-inflammatory cytokines (e.g., IL-6 and IL-10) increase even in patients with mild infections. Glucocorticoids inhibit cytokine synthesis by monocytes in vitro; the increase in blood cortisol levels early in the systemic response presumably plays a similarly inhibitory role. Epinephrine inhibits the TNF-α response to endotoxin infusion in humans while augmenting and accelerating the release of IL-10; prostaglandin E_2 has a similar "reprogramming" effect on the responses of circulating monocytes to LPS and other bacterial agonists. Cortisol, epinephrine, IL-10, and C-reactive protein reduce the ability of neutrophils to attach to vascular endothelium, favoring their demargination and thus contributing to leukocytosis while preventing neutrophil-endothelial adhesion in uninflamed organs. The available evidence thus suggests that the body's systemic responses to injury and infection normally prevent inflammation within organs distant from a site of infection.

The acute-phase response increases the blood concentrations of numerous molecules that have anti-inflammatory actions. Blood levels of IL-1 receptor antagonist (IL-1Ra) often greatly exceed those of circulating IL-1β, for example, and this excess may result in inhibition of the binding of IL-1β to its receptors. High levels of soluble TNF receptors neutralize TNF-α that enters the circulation. Other acute-phase proteins are protease inhibitors; these may neutralize proteases released from neutrophils and other inflammatory cells.

Organ Dysfunction and Shock

As the body's responses to infection intensify, the mixture of circulating cytokines and other molecules becomes very complex: elevated blood levels of more than 50 molecules have been found in patients with septic shock. Although high concentrations of both pro- and anti-inflammatory molecules are found, the net mediator balance in the plasma of these extremely sick patients may actually be anti-inflammatory. For example, blood leukocytes from patients with severe sepsis are often hyporesponsive to agonists such as LPS. In patients with severe sepsis, persistence of leukocyte hyporesponsiveness has been associated with an increased risk of dying. Apoptotic death of B cells, follicular dendritic cells, and CD4+ T lymphocytes also may contribute significantly to the immunosuppressive state.

ENDOTHELIAL INJURY   Most investigators have favored widespread vascular endothelial injury as the major mechanism for multiorgan dysfunction. In keeping with this idea, one study found high numbers of vascular endothelial cells in the peripheral blood of septic patients. Leukocyte-derived mediators and platelet-leukocyte-fibrin thrombi may contribute to vascular injury, but the vascular endothelium also seems to play an active role. Stimuli such as TNF-α induce vascular endothelial cells to produce and release cytokines, procoagulant molecules, platelet-activating factor (PAF), nitric oxide, and other mediators. In addition, regulated cell-adhesion molecules promote the adherence of neutrophils to endothelial cells. While these responses can attract phagocytes to infected sites and activate their antimicrobial arsenals, endothelial cell activation can also promote increased vascular permeability, microvascular thrombosis, DIC, and hypotension.

Tissue oxygenation may decrease as the number of functional capillaries is reduced by luminal obstruction due to swollen endothelial cells, decreased deformability of circulating erythrocytes, leukocyte-platelet-fibrin thrombi, or compression by edema fluid. On the other hand, studies using orthogonal polarization spectral imaging of the microcirculation in the tongue found that sepsis-associated derangements in capillary flow could be reversed by applying acetylcholine to the surface of the tongue or giving nitroprusside intravenously; these observations suggest a neuroendocrine basis for the loss of capillary filling. Oxygen utilization by tissues may also be impaired by a state of "hibernation" in which ATP production is diminished as oxidative phosphorylation decreases because of mitochondrial dysfunction; nitric oxide or its metabolites may be responsible for inducing this response.

Remarkably, poorly functioning "septic" organs usually appear normal at autopsy. There is typically very little necrosis or thrombosis, and apoptosis is largely confined to lymphoid organs and the gastrointestinal tract. Moreover, organ function usually returns to normal if patients recover. These points suggest that organ dysfunction during severe sepsis has a basis that is principally biochemical, not anatomic.

SEPTIC SHOCK   The hallmark of septic shock is a decrease in peripheral vascular resistance that occurs despite increased levels of vasopressor catecholamines. Before this vasodilatory phase, many patients experience a period during which oxygen delivery to tissues is compromised by myocardial depression, hypovolemia, and other factors. During this "hypodynamic" period, the blood lactate concentration is elevated, and central venous oxygen saturation is low. Fluid administration is usually followed by the hyperdynamic, vasodilatory phase during which cardiac output is normal (or even high) and oxygen consumption is independent of oxygen delivery. The blood lactate level may be normal or increased, and normalization of the central venous oxygen saturation (SvO_2) may reflect either improved oxygen delivery or left-to-right shunting.

Prominent hypotensive molecules include nitric oxide, β-endorphin, bradykinin, PAF, and prostacyclin. Agents that inhibit the synthesis or action of each of these mediators can prevent or reverse endotoxic shock in animals. However, in clinical trials, neither a PAF receptor antagonist nor a bradykinin antagonist improved survival rates among patients with septic shock, and a nitric oxide synthetase inhibitor, L-N^G-methylarginine HCl, actually increased the mortality rate.

Severe Sepsis: A Single Pathogenesis?

In some cases, circulating bacteria and their products almost certainly elicit multiorgan dysfunction and hypotension by directly stimulating inflammatory responses within the vasculature. In patients with fulminant meningococcemia, for example, mortality rates have correlated well with blood endotoxin levels and with the occurrence of DIC (Chap. 136). In most patients with nosocomial infections, in contrast, circulating bacteria or bacterial molecules may reflect uncontrolled infection at a local tissue site and have little or no direct impact on distant organs; in these patients, inflammatory mediators or neural signals arising from the local site seem to be the key triggers for severe sepsis and septic shock. In a large series of patients with positive blood cultures, the risk of developing severe sepsis was strongly related to the site of primary infection: bacteremia arising from a pulmonary or abdominal source was eightfold more likely to be associated with severe sepsis than was bacteremic urinary tract infection, even after the investigators controlled for age, the kind of bacteria isolated from the blood, and other factors. A third pathogenesis may be represented by severe sepsis due to superantigen-producing *Staphylococcus aureus* or *Streptococcus pyogenes*, since the T cell activation induced by these toxins produces a cytokine profile that differs substantially from that elicited by gram-negative bacterial infection.

In summary, the pathogenesis of severe sepsis may differ according to the infecting microbe, the ability of the host's innate defense mechanisms to sense it, the site of the primary infection, the presence or absence of immune defects, and the prior physiologic status of the host. Genetic factors may also be important. For example, studies in different ethnic groups have identified associations between allelic polymorphisms in TLR4, caspase 12L, TNF-α, and IFN-γ genes and the risk of developing severe sepsis. Further studies in this area are needed.

CLINICAL MANIFESTATIONS

The manifestations of the septic response are usually superimposed on the symptoms and signs of the patient's underlying illness and primary infection. The rate at which signs and symptoms develop may differ from patient to patient, and there are striking individual variations in presentation. For example, some patients with sepsis are normo- or hypothermic; the absence of fever is most common in neonates, in elderly patients, and in persons with uremia or alcoholism.

Hyperventilation is often an early sign of the septic response. Disorientation, confusion, and other manifestations of encephalopathy may also develop early on, particularly in the elderly and in individuals with preexisting neurologic impairment. Focal neurologic signs are uncommon, although preexisting focal deficits may become more prominent.

Hypotension and DIC predispose to acrocyanosis and ischemic necrosis of peripheral tissues, most commonly the digits. Cellulitis, pustules, bullae, or hemorrhagic lesions may develop when hematogenous bacteria or fungi seed the skin or underlying soft tissue. Bacterial toxins may also be distributed hematogenously and elicit diffuse cutaneous reactions. On occasion, skin lesions may suggest specific pathogens. When sepsis is accompanied by cutaneous petechiae or purpura, infection with *Neisseria meningitidis* (or, less commonly, *H. influenzae*) should be suspected (Fig. 136-1); in a patient who has been bitten by a tick while in an endemic area, petechial lesions also suggest Rocky Mountain spotted fever (Fig. 167-1). A cutaneous lesion seen almost exclusively in neutropenic patients is ecthyma gangrenosum, usually caused by *P. aeruginosa*. It is a bullous lesion, surrounded by edema that undergoes central hemorrhage and necrosis (Fig. 145-1). Histopathologic examination shows bacteria in and around the wall of a small vessel, with little or no neutrophilic response. Hemorrhagic or bullous lesions in a septic patient who has recently eaten raw oysters suggest *V. vulnificus* bacteremia, while such lesions in a patient who has recently suffered a dog bite may indicate bloodstream infection due to *Capnocytophaga canimorsus* or *C. cynodegmi*. Generalized erythroderma in a septic patient suggests the toxic shock syndrome due to *S. aureus* or *S. pyogenes*.

Gastrointestinal manifestations such as nausea, vomiting, diarrhea, and ileus may suggest acute gastroenteritis. Stress ulceration can lead to upper gastrointestinal bleeding. Cholestatic jaundice, with elevated levels of serum bilirubin (mostly conjugated) and alkaline phosphatase, may precede other signs of sepsis. Hepatocellular or canalicular dysfunction appears to underlie most cases, and the results of hepatic function tests return to normal with resolution of the infection. Prolonged or severe hypotension may induce acute hepatic injury or ischemic bowel necrosis.

Many tissues may be unable to extract oxygen normally from the blood, so that anaerobic metabolism occurs despite near-normal mixed venous oxygen saturation. Blood lactate levels rise early because of increased glycolysis as well as impaired clearance of the resulting lactate and pyruvate by the liver and kidneys. The blood glucose concentration often increases, particularly in patients with diabetes, although impaired gluconeogenesis and excessive insulin release on occasion produce hypoglycemia. The cytokine-driven acute-phase response inhibits the synthesis of transthyretin while enhancing the production of C-reactive protein, fibrinogen, and complement components. Protein catabolism is often markedly accelerated. Serum albumin levels decline as a result of decreased hepatic synthesis and the movement of albumin into interstitial spaces, which is promoted by arterial vasodilation.

MAJOR COMPLICATIONS

Cardiopulmonary Complications   Ventilation-perfusion mismatching produces a fall in arterial P_{O_2} early in the course. Increasing alveolar capillary permeability results in an increased pulmonary water content, which decreases pulmonary compliance and interferes with oxygen exchange. Progressive diffuse pulmonary infiltrates and arterial hypoxemia (Pa_{O_2}/Fi_{O_2}, <200) indicate the development of the acute respiratory distress syndrome (ARDS). ARDS develops in ~50% of patients with severe sepsis or septic shock. Respiratory muscle fatigue can exacerbate hypoxemia and hypercapnia. An elevated pulmonary capillary wedge pressure (>18 mmHg) suggests fluid volume overload or cardiac failure rather than ARDS. Pneumonia caused by viruses or by *Pneumocystis* may be clinically indistinguishable from ARDS.

Sepsis-induced hypotension (see "Septic Shock," above) usually results initially from a generalized maldistribution of blood flow and blood volume and from hypovolemia that is due, at least in part, to diffuse capillary leakage of intravascular fluid. Other factors that may decrease effective intravascular volume include dehydration from antecedent disease or insensible fluid losses, vomiting or diarrhea, and polyuria. During early septic shock, systemic vascular resistance is usually elevated and cardiac output may be low. After fluid repletion, in contrast, cardiac output typically increases and systemic vascular resistance falls. Indeed, normal or increased cardiac output and decreased systemic vascular resistance distinguish septic shock from cardiogenic, extracardiac obstructive, and hypovolemic shock; other processes that can produce this combination include anaphylaxis, beriberi, cirrhosis, and overdoses of nitroprusside or narcotics.

Depression of myocardial function, manifested as increased end-diastolic and systolic ventricular volumes with a decreased ejection fraction, develops within 24 h in most patients with severe sepsis. Cardiac output is maintained despite the low ejection fraction because ventricular dilatation permits a normal stroke volume. In survivors, myocardial function returns to normal over several days. Although myocardial dysfunction may contribute to hypotension, refractory hypotension is usually due to a low systemic vascular resistance, and death results from refractory shock or the failure of multiple organs rather than from cardiac dysfunction per se.

Renal Complications   Oliguria, azotemia, proteinuria, and nonspecific urinary casts are frequently found. Many patients are inappropriately polyuric; hyperglycemia may exacerbate this tendency. Most renal failure is due to acute tubular necrosis induced by hypotension or capillary injury, although some patients also have glomerulonephritis, renal cortical necrosis, or interstitial nephritis. Drug-induced renal damage may complicate therapy, particularly when hypotensive patients are given aminoglycoside antibiotics.

Coagulopathy   Although thrombocytopenia occurs in 10–30% of patients, the underlying mechanisms are not understood. Platelet counts are usually very low (<50,000/μL) in patients with DIC; these low counts may reflect diffuse endothelial injury or microvascular thrombosis.

Neurologic Complications   When the septic illness lasts for weeks or months, "critical-illness" polyneuropathy may prevent weaning from ventilatory support and produce distal motor weakness. Electrophysiologic studies are diagnostic. Guillain-Barré syndrome, metabolic disturbances, and toxin activity must be ruled out.

LABORATORY FINDINGS

Abnormalities that occur early in the septic response may include leukocytosis with a left shift, thrombocytopenia, hyperbilirubinemia, and proteinuria. Leukopenia may develop. The neutrophils may contain toxic granulations, Döhle bodies, or cytoplasmic vacuoles. As the septic response becomes more severe, thrombocytopenia worsens (often with prolongation of the thrombin time, decreased fibrinogen, and the presence of D-dimers, suggesting DIC), azotemia and hyperbilirubinemia become more prominent, and levels of aminotransferases rise. Active hemolysis suggests clostridial bacteremia, malaria, a drug reaction, or DIC; in the case of DIC, microangiopathic changes may be seen on a blood smear.

During early sepsis, hyperventilation induces respiratory alkalosis. With respiratory muscle fatigue and the accumulation of lactate, metabolic acidosis (with increased anion gap) typically supervenes. Evaluation of arterial blood gases reveals hypoxemia, which is initially correctable with supplemental oxygen but whose later refractoriness to 100% oxygen inhalation indicates right-to-left shunting. The chest radiograph may be normal or may show evidence of underlying pneumonia, volume overload, or the diffuse infiltrates of ARDS. The electrocardiogram may show only sinus tachycardia or nonspecific ST–T-wave abnormalities.

Most diabetic patients with sepsis develop hyperglycemia. Severe infection may precipitate diabetic ketoacidosis, which may exacerbate hypotension (Chap. 338). Hypoglycemia occurs rarely. The serum albumin level, initially within the normal range, declines as sepsis continues. Hypocalcemia is rare.

DIAGNOSIS

There is no specific diagnostic test for the septic response. Diagnostically sensitive findings in a patient with suspected or proven infection include fever or hypothermia, tachypnea, tachycardia, and leukocytosis or leukopenia (Table 265-1); acutely altered mental status, thrombocytopenia, an elevated blood lactate level, or hypotension also should suggest the diagnosis. The septic response can be quite variable, however. In one study, 36% of patients with severe sepsis had a normal temperature, 40% had a normal respiratory rate, 10% had a normal pulse rate, and 33% had normal white blood cell counts. Moreover, the systemic responses of uninfected patients with other conditions may be similar to those characteristic of sepsis. Noninfectious etiologies of SIRS (Table 265-1) include pancreatitis, burns, trauma, adrenal insufficiency, pulmonary embolism, dissecting or ruptured aortic aneurysm, myocardial infarction, occult hemorrhage, cardiac tamponade, post–cardiopulmonary bypass syndrome, anaphylaxis, and drug overdose.

Definitive etiologic diagnosis requires isolation of the microorganism from blood or a local site of infection. At least two blood samples (10 mL each) should be obtained (from different venipuncture sites) for culture. Because gram-negative bacteremia is typically low-grade (<10 organisms/mL of blood), prolonged incubation of cultures may be necessary; *S. aureus* grows more readily and is detectable in blood cultures within 48 h in most instances. In many cases, blood cultures are negative; this result can reflect prior antibiotic administration, the presence of slow-growing or fastidious organisms, or the absence of microbial invasion of the bloodstream. In these cases, Gram's staining and culture of material from the primary site of infection or of infected cutaneous lesions may help establish the microbial etiology. The skin and mucosae should be examined carefully and repeatedly for lesions that might yield diagnostic information. With overwhelming bacteremia (e.g., pneumococcal sepsis in splenectomized individuals, fulminant meningococcemia, or infection with *V. vulnificus, B. pseudomallei,* or *Y. pestis*), microorganisms are sometimes visible on buffy coat smears of peripheral blood.

Rx SEVERE SEPSIS AND SEPTIC SHOCK

Patients in whom sepsis is suspected must be managed expeditiously. This task is best accomplished by personnel who are experienced in the care of the critically ill. Successful management requires urgent measures to treat the infection, to provide hemodynamic and respiratory support, and to eliminate the offending microorganism. Most emergency centers now aim to initiate these measures within 1 h of the patient's presentation with severe sepsis or shock. Rapid assessment and diagnosis are therefore essential.

ANTIMICROBIAL AGENTS   Antimicrobial chemotherapy should be initiated as soon as samples of blood and other relevant sites have been cultured. A large retrospective review of patients who developed septic shock found that the interval between the onset of hypotension and the administration of appropriate antimicrobial chemotherapy was the major determinant of outcome; a delay of as little as 1 h was associated with lower survival rates.

It is important, pending culture results, to initiate empirical antimicrobial therapy that is effective against both gram-positive and gram-negative bacteria **(Table 265-3)**. Maximal recommended doses of antimicrobial drugs should be given intravenously, with adjustment for impaired renal function when necessary. Available information about patterns of antimicrobial susceptibility among bacterial isolates from the community, the hospital, and the patient should be taken into account. When culture results become available, the regimen can often be simplified, as a single antimicrobial agent is usually adequate for the treatment of a known pathogen. Meta-analyses have concluded that, with one exception, combination antimicrobial therapy is not superior to monotherapy for treating gram-negative bacteremia; the exception is that aminoglycoside monotherapy for *P. aeruginosa* bacteremia is less effective than the combination of an aminoglycoside with an antipseudomonal β-lactam agent. Most pa-

TABLE 265-3 INITIAL ANTIMICROBIAL THERAPY FOR SEVERE SEPSIS WITH NO OBVIOUS SOURCE IN ADULTS WITH NORMAL RENAL FUNCTION

Clinical Condition	Antimicrobial Regimens (Intravenous Therapy)
Immunocompetent adult	The many acceptable regimens include (1) ceftriaxone (2 g q24h) *or* ticarcillin-clavulanate (3.1 g q4–6h) *or* piperacillin-tazobactam (3.375 g q4–6h); (2) imipenem-cilastatin (0.5 g q6h) *or* meropenem (1 g q8h) *or* cefepime (2 g q12h). Gentamicin *or* tobramycin (5–7 mg/kg q24h) may be *added* to either regimen. If the patient is allergic to β-lactam agents, use ciprofloxacin (400 mg q12h) *or* levofloxacin (500–750 mg q12h) *plus* clindamycin (600 mg q8h). If the institution or the community has a high prevalence of MRSA isolates, add vancomycin (15 mg/kg q12h) to each of the above regimens.
Neutropenia[a] (<500 neutrophils/μL)	Regimens include (1) imipenem-cilastatin (0.5 g q6h) *or* meropenem (1 g q8h) *or* cefepime (2 g q8h); (2) ticarcillin-clavulanate (3.1 g q4h) *or* piperacillin-tazobactam (3.375 g q4h) *plus* tobramycin (5–7 mg/kg q24h). Vancomycin (15 mg/kg q12h) should be added if the patient has an infected vascular catheter, if staphylococci are suspected, if the patient has received quinolone prophylaxis, if the patient has received intensive chemotherapy that produces mucosal damage, if the institution has a high incidence of MRSA infections, or if there is a high prevalence of MRSA isolates in the community.
Splenectomy	Cefotaxime (2 g q6–8h) *or* ceftriaxone (2 g q12h) should be used. If the local prevalence of cephalosporin-resistant pneumococci is high, *add* vancomycin. If the patient is allergic to β-lactam drugs, vancomycin (15 mg/kg q12h) *plus* ciprofloxacin (400 mg q12h) *or* levofloxacin (750 mg q12h) *or* aztreonam (2 g q8h) should be used.
IV drug user	Nafcillin or oxacillin (2 g q8h) *plus* gentamicin (5–7 mg/kg q24h). If the local prevalence of MRSA is high or if the patient is allergic to β-lactam drugs, vancomycin (15 mg/kg q12h) with gentamicin should be used.
AIDS	Cefepime (2 g q8h), ticarcillin-clavulanate (3.1 g q4h), *or* piperacillin-tazobactam (3.375 g q4h) *plus* tobramycin (5–7 mg/kg q24h) should be used. If the patient is allergic to β-lactam drugs, ciprofloxacin (400 mg q12h) *or* levofloxacin (750 mg q12h) *plus* vancomycin (15 mg/kg q12h) *plus* tobramycin should be used.

[a]Adapted in part from WT Hughes et al: Clin Infect Dis 25:551, 1997.
Note: MRSA, methicillin-resistant *Staphylococcus aureus*.

tients require antimicrobial therapy for at least 1 week; the duration of treatment is typically influenced by factors such as the site of tissue infection, the adequacy of surgical drainage, the patient's underlying disease, and the antimicrobial susceptibility of the bacterial isolate(s).

REMOVAL OF THE SOURCE OF INFECTION Removal or drainage of a focal source of infection is essential. Sites of occult infection should be sought carefully. Indwelling IV catheters should be removed and the tip rolled over a blood agar plate for quantitative culture; after antibiotic therapy has been initiated, a new catheter should be inserted at a different site. Foley and drainage catheters should be replaced. The possibility of paranasal sinusitis (often caused by gram-negative bacteria) should be considered if the patient has undergone nasal intubation. In patients with abnormalities on chest radiographs, CT of the chest may identify unsuspected parenchymal, mediastinal, or pleural disease. In the neutropenic patient, cutaneous sites of tenderness and erythema, particularly in the perianal region, must be carefully sought. In patients with sacral or ischial decubitus ulcers, it is important to exclude pelvic or other soft tissue pus collections with CT or MRI. In patients with severe sepsis arising from the urinary tract, sonography or CT should be used to rule out ureteral obstruction, perinephric abscess, and renal abscess.

HEMODYNAMIC, RESPIRATORY, AND METABOLIC SUPPORT The primary goals are to restore adequate oxygen and substrate delivery to the tissues as quickly as possible and to improve tissue oxygen utilization and cellular metabolism. Adequate organ perfusion is thus essential. Initial management of hypotension should include the administration of IV fluids, typically beginning with 1–2 L of normal saline over 1–2 h. To avoid pulmonary edema, the pulmonary capillary wedge pressure should be maintained at 12–16 mmHg or the central venous pressure at 8–12 cm H_2O. The urine output rate should be kept at >0.5 mL/kg per hour by continuing fluid administration; a diuretic such as furosemide may be used if needed. In about one-third of patients, hypotension and organ hypoperfusion respond to fluid resuscitation; a reasonable goal is to maintain a mean arterial blood pressure of >65 mmHg (systolic pressure, >90 mmHg) and a cardiac index of ≥4 L/min per m². If these guidelines cannot be met by volume infusion, vasopressor therapy is indicated. Circulatory adequacy is also assessed by clinical parameters (mentation, urine output, skin perfusion)

and, when possible, by measurements of oxygen delivery and consumption.

A study of "early goal-directed therapy" (EGDT) found that prompt resuscitation based on maintenance of the SvO_2 at >70% was associated with significantly improved survival of patients who were admitted to an emergency department with severe sepsis. The treatment algorithm included rapid administration of fluids, antibiotics, and vasopressor support; erythrocyte transfusion (to maintain the hematocrit above 30%); and administration of dobutamine if fluids, erythrocytes, and pressors did not result in an SvO_2 of >70%. The extent to which the different components of the EGDT algorithm contribute to the overall effect has not been examined in controlled trials. In particular, neither the use of SvO_2 to manage therapy nor the need for continuous SvO_2 monitoring with a pulmonary artery catheter has been formally confirmed. A multicenter study (sponsored by the National Institutes of Health) of the efficacy of the EGDT approach is in progress.

In patients with septic shock, plasma vasopressin levels increase transiently but then decrease dramatically. Studies have found that vasopressin infusion can reverse septic shock in some patients, reducing or eliminating the need for catecholamine pressors. An adequately powered and randomized trial of vasopressin infusion has not been performed. Vasopressin is a potent vasoconstrictor that may be most useful in patients who have vasodilatory shock and relative resistance to other pressor hormones.

Adrenal insufficiency is very likely when the plasma cortisol level is <15 μg/dL in a patient with severe sepsis. Generally accepted criteria for *partial* adrenal insufficiency have not been devised; major problems have been the inability to raise cortisol levels in extremely stressed individuals above high baseline values in response to cosyntropin (α^{1-24}–ACTH) (Chap. 336) and the high frequency of hypoalbuminemia, which decreases total but not free (active) plasma cortisol levels. Adrenal insufficiency should be strongly considered in septic patients with refractory hypotension, fulminant meningococcal bacteremia, disseminated tuberculosis, AIDS, or prior use of glucocorticoids, megestrol, etomidate, or ketoconazole. Hydrocortisone (50 mg IV every 6 h) may be given as a trial therapeutic intervention. If clinical improvement occurs over 24–48 h, most experts would continue hydrocortisone therapy, tapering and discontinuing it after 5–7 days. Improved recommendations regarding hydrocortisone therapy may come from the European CORTICUS trial.

Ventilator therapy is indicated for progressive hypoxemia, hypercapnia, neurologic deterioration, or respiratory muscle failure. Sustained tachypnea (respiratory rate, >30 breaths/min) is frequently a harbinger of impending respiratory collapse; mechanical ventilation is often initiated to ensure adequate oxygenation, to divert blood from the muscles of respiration, to prevent aspiration of oropharyngeal contents, and to reduce the cardiac afterload. The results of recent studies favor the use of low tidal volumes (6 mL/kg of ideal body weight, or as low as 4 mL/kg if the plateau pressure exceeds 30 cmH₂O). Patients undergoing mechanical ventilation require careful sedation, with daily interruptions; elevation of the head of the bed helps to prevent nosocomial pneumonia. Stress-ulcer prophylaxis with a histamine H₂-receptor antagonist may decrease the risk of gastrointestinal hemorrhage in ventilated patients.

The use of erythrocyte transfusion continues to be debated. In the study of EGDT, packed erythrocytes were given to raise the hematocrit to 30% if the patient's SvO_2 was <70%. The extent to which this intervention contributed to the improvement reported in patients who received the EGDT regimen is uncertain.

Bicarbonate is sometimes administered for severe metabolic acidosis (arterial pH <7.2), but there is little evidence that it improves either hemodynamics or the response to vasopressor hormones. DIC, if complicated by major bleeding, should be treated with transfusion of fresh-frozen plasma and platelets. Successful treatment of the underlying infection is essential to reverse both acidosis and DIC. Patients who are hypercatabolic and have acute renal failure may benefit greatly from hemodialysis or hemofiltration.

GENERAL SUPPORT In patients with prolonged severe sepsis (i.e., that lasting more than 2 or 3 days), nutritional supplementation may reduce the impact of protein hypercatabolism; the available evidence, which is not strong, favors the enteral delivery route. Prophylactic heparinization to prevent deep venous thrombosis is indicated for patients who do not have active bleeding or coagulopathy. Recovery is also assisted by preventing skin breakdown, nosocomial infections, and stress ulcers.

Investigators in Belgium reported in 2001 that maintaining blood glucose levels in the normal range (80–110 mg/dL) greatly improved survival rates among patients who had just undergone major surgery and had received IV glucose feeding for the previous 24 h. The same group then studied intensive glucose control in critically ill medical patients and found a survival benefit only for patients who remained in the intensive care unit for ≥3 days. Hypoglycemia was much more common in the intensive-insulin group. Until more experience with intensive glucose control is reported, it seems reasonable to maintain glucose levels of <150 mg/dL during the first 3 days of severe sepsis and then to target the normoglycemic range if the patient remains in the intensive care unit for a longer period. Frequent monitoring of blood glucose levels is indicated to avoid hypoglycemia during intensive insulin therapy.

OTHER MEASURES Despite aggressive management, many patients with severe sepsis or septic shock die. Numerous interventions have been tested for their ability to improve survival in patients with severe sepsis. The list includes endotoxin-neutralizing proteins, inhibitors of cyclooxygenase or nitric oxide synthase, anticoagulants, polyclonal immunoglobulins, glucocorticoids, and antagonists to TNF-α, IL-1, PAF, and bradykinin. Unfortunately, none of these agents has improved rates of survival among patients with severe sepsis/septic shock in more than one large, randomized, placebo-controlled clinical trial. This lack of reproducibility has had many contributing factors, including (1) heterogeneity in the patient populations studied and the inciting microbes and (2) the nature of the "standard" therapy also used. A dramatic example of this problem was seen in a trial of tissue factor pathway inhibitor (Fig. 265-1). Whereas the drug appeared to improve survival rates after 722 patients had been studied (*p* = .006), it did not do so in the next 1032 patients, and the overall result was negative. This inconsistency, even within a carefully selected patient population, argues strongly that a sepsis intervention should show significant survival benefit in more than one placebo-controlled clinical trial before it is accepted as part of routine clinical practice.

Recombinant activated protein C (aPC) was the first drug to be approved by the U.S. Food and Drug Administration (FDA) for the treatment of patients with severe sepsis or septic shock. In a single randomized controlled trial in which drug or placebo was given within 24 h of the patient's first sepsis-related organ dysfunction, 28-day mortality was significantly lower among recipients of aPC than among patients who received placebo (24.7% vs. 30.8%; *p* <.005). In addition, aPC recipients were more likely than placebo recipients to have severe bleeding (3.5% vs. 2%). Survival improved only for patients who had an APACHE II score of ≥25 during the 24 h before initiation of aPC infusion. Midtrial changes in the protocol and drug were followed by improvement in the apparent efficacy of aPC. The FDA approved aPC for use in adults (>18 years of age) who meet the APACHE II criterion and have a low risk of hemorrhage-related side effects.

aPC is administered as a constant IV infusion of 24 µg/kg per hour for 96 h. Each patient's clotting parameters must be monitored carefully. aPC should not be given to patients who have platelet counts of <30,000/µL or to patients who have dysfunction of one organ system and have had surgery during the previous 30 days. Treatment with aPC should not be started >24 h after the onset of severe sepsis, nor should it be used in the patient subsets—e.g., patients with pancreatitis or AIDS—that were excluded from the clinical trial.

Although the theoretical rationale for treating septic patients with anticoagulants is strong and studies have found that aPC may have anti-inflammatory and anti-apoptotic properties in vitro, two additional randomized, placebo-controlled trials of aPC were stopped when interim analyses showed lack of efficacy. One trial was in children, and the other was in

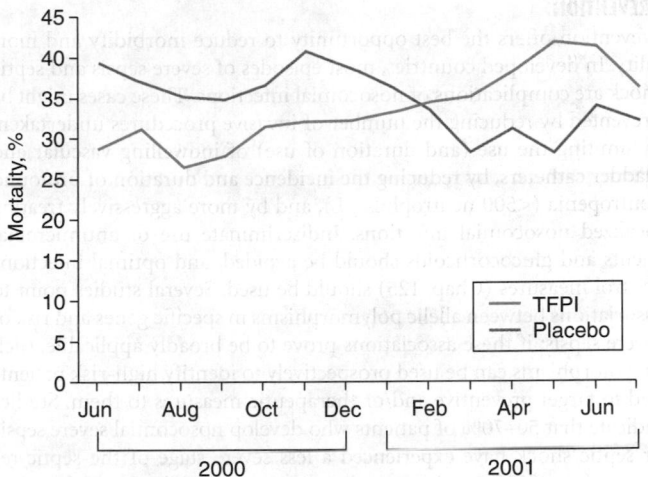

FIGURE 265-1 Mortality rates among patients who received tissue factor pathway inhibitor (TFPI) or placebo, shown as the running average over the course of the clinical trial. The drug seemed highly efficacious at the interim analysis in December 2000, but this trend reversed later in the trial. Demonstrating that therapeutic agents for sepsis have consistent, reproducible efficacy has been extremely difficult, even within well-defined patient populations. *(Reprinted with permission from Abraham et al.)*

adults with APACHE II scores of ≤25. aPC has not been tested again in the patient population for which it was approved by the FDA: adults with high APACHE II scores.

Some experts have advocated "bundling" of multiple therapeutic maneuvers into a unified, algorithmic approach to management that would become the standard of care for severe sepsis. The proposed *resuscitation* (6-h) bundle incorporates most of the elements discussed above for acute (EGDT) resuscitation. The *management* (24-h) bundle includes three measures of uncertain or marginal benefit: tight control of blood glucose, administration of low-dose hydrocortisone, and treatment with aPC. Bundling of therapies obscures the efficacy and toxicity of the individual interventions and allows little room for individualizing therapy. The use of bundling in an industry-sponsored marketing program for aPC (the Surviving Sepsis Campaign) has also been criticized.

A careful retrospective analysis found that the apparent efficacy of all sepsis therapeutics studied to date has been greatest among the patients at greatest risk of dying before treatment; conversely, use of many of these drugs has been associated with increased mortality rates among patients who are less ill. The authors proposed that neutralizing one of many different mediators may help patients who are very sick, whereas disrupting the mediator balance may be harmful to those whose adaptive defense mechanisms are still working. This analysis suggests that if more aggressive early resuscitation improves survival rates among sicker patients, it should become more difficult to show additional benefit from other therapies; that is, if early resuscitation improves patients' status, moving them into a "less severe illness" category, the addition of another agent is less likely to be beneficial.

PROGNOSIS

Approximately 20–35% of patients with severe sepsis and 40–60% of patients with septic shock die within 30 days. Others die within the ensuing 6 months. Late deaths often result from poorly controlled infection, immunosuppression, complications of intensive care, failure of multiple organs, or the patient's underlying disease.

Prognostic stratification systems such as APACHE II indicate that factoring in the patient's age, underlying condition, and various physiologic variables can yield estimates of the risk of dying of severe sepsis. Of the individual covariates, the severity of underlying disease most strongly influences the risk of dying. Septic shock is also a strong predictor of short- and long-term mortality. Case-fatality rates are similar for culture-positive and culture-negative severe sepsis.

Prevention offers the best opportunity to reduce morbidity and mortality. In developed countries, most episodes of severe sepsis and septic shock are complications of nosocomial infections. These cases might be prevented by reducing the number of invasive procedures undertaken, by limiting the use (and duration of use) of indwelling vascular and bladder catheters, by reducing the incidence and duration of profound neutropenia (<500 neutrophils/μL), and by more aggressively treating localized nosocomial infections. Indiscriminate use of antimicrobial agents and glucocorticoids should be avoided, and optimal infection-control measures (Chap. 125) should be used. Several studies point to associations between allelic polymorphisms in specific genes and risk of severe sepsis; if these associations prove to be broadly applicable, such polymorphisms can be used prospectively to identify high-risk patients and to target preventive and/or therapeutic measures to them. Studies indicate that 50–70% of patients who develop nosocomial severe sepsis or septic shock have experienced a less severe stage of the septic response (e.g., SIRS, sepsis) on at least one previous day in the hospital. Research is needed to develop adjunctive agents that can damp the septic response before organ dysfunction or hypotension occurs.

FURTHER READINGS

ABRAHAM E et al: Efficacy and safety of tifacogin (recombinant tissue factor pathway inhibitor) in severe sepsis: A randomized controlled trial. JAMA 290:238, 2003

ARAFAH BM: Hypothalamic pituitary adrenal function during critical illness: Limitations of current assessment methods. J Clin Endocrinol Metab 91:3725, 2006

BERKLEY JA et al: Bacteremia among children admitted to a rural hospital in Kenya. N Engl J Med 352:39, 2005

EICHACKER P et al: Risk and the efficacy of anti-inflammatory agents: Retrospective and confirmatory studies of sepsis. Am J Respir Crit Care Med 166:1197, 2002

HARBATH S et al: Does antibiotic selection impact patient outcome? Clin Infect Dis 44:87, 2007

HOTCHKISS RS, NICHOLSON DW: Apoptosis and caspases regulate death and inflammation in sepsis. Nat Rev Immunol 6:813, 2006

KUMAR A et al: Duration of hypotension before initiation of effective antimicrobial therapy is the critical determinant of survival in human septic shock. Crit Care Med 34:1589, 2006

MUNFORD RS: Severe sepsis and septic shock: The role of gram-negative bacteremia. Annu Rev Pathol Mech Dis 1:467, 2006

OTERO RM et al: Early goal-directed therapy in severe sepsis and septic shock revisited: Concepts, controversies, and contemporary findings. Chest 130:1579, 2006

RUSSELL JA: Management of sepsis. N Engl J Med 355:1699, 2006

SANDS KE et al: Epidemiology of sepsis syndrome in 8 academic medical centers. JAMA 278:234, 1997

TURGEON AF et al: Meta-analysis: Intravenous immunoglobulin in critically ill adult patients with sepsis. Ann Intern Med 146:193, 2007

266 Cardiogenic Shock and Pulmonary Edema
Judith S. Hochman, David H. Ingbar

Cardiogenic shock and pulmonary edema are life-threatening conditions that should be treated as medical emergencies. The most common etiology for both is severe left ventricular (LV) dysfunction, leading to pulmonary congestion and/or systemic hypoperfusion (**Fig. 266-1**). The pathophysiology of pulmonary edema and shock are discussed in Chaps. 33 and 264, respectively.

CARDIOGENIC SHOCK

Cardiogenic shock (CS) is characterized by systemic hypoperfusion due to severe depression of the cardiac index [<2.2 (L/min)/m²] and sustained systolic arterial hypotension (<90 mmHg), despite an elevated filling pressure [pulmonary capillary wedge pressure (PCWP) > 18 mmHg]. It is associated with in-hospital mortality rates >50%. The major causes of CS are listed in **Table 266-1**. Circulatory failure based on cardiac dysfunction may be caused by primary myocardial failure, most commonly secondary to acute myocardial infarction (MI) (Chap. 239), and less frequently by cardiomyopathy or myocarditis (Chap. 231) or cardiac tamponade (Chap. 232).

Incidence   CS is the leading cause of death of patients hospitalized with MI. Early reperfusion therapy for acute MI decreases the incidence of CS. The rate of CS complicating acute MI fell from 20% in the 1960s but has plateaued at ~8% for >20 years. Shock is typically associated with ST elevation MI (STEMI) and is less common with non-ST elevation MI (Chap. 239).

LV failure accounts for ~80% of the cases of CS complicating acute MI. Acute severe mitral regurgitation (MR), ventricular septal rupture (VSR), predominant right ventricular (RV) failure, and free wall rupture or tamponade account for the remainder.

Pathophysiology   CS is characterized by a vicious circle in which depression of myocardial contractility, usually due to ischemia, results in

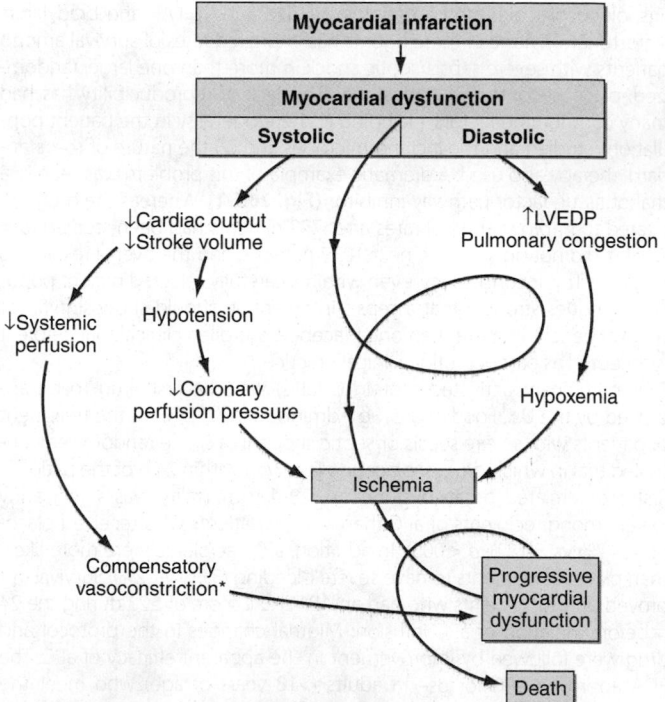

FIGURE 266-1 Pathophysiology of cardiogenic shock. Systolic and diastolic myocardial dysfunction result in a reduction in cardiac output and often pulmonary congestion. Systemic and coronary hypoperfusion occur, resulting in progressive ischemia. Although a number of compensatory mechanisms are activated in an attempt to support the circulation, these compensatory mechanisms may become maladaptive and produce a worsening of hemodynamics. *Release of inflammatory cytokines after myocardial infarction may lead to inducible nitrous oxide expression, excess NO, and inappropriate vasodilation. This causes further reduction in systemic and coronary perfusion. A vicious spiral of progressive myocardial dysfunction occurs that ultimately results in death if it is not interrupted. LVEDP, left ventricular end-diastolic pressure. (*From SM Hollenberg et al: Ann Intern Med 131:47, 1999.*)

TABLE 266-1 ETIOLOGIES OF CARDIOGENIC SHOCK (CS)ᵃ AND CARDIOGENIC PULMONARY EDEMA

Etiologies of Cardiogenic Shock or Pulmonary Edema

Acute myocardial infarction/ischemia
   LV failure
   VSR
   Papillary muscle/chordal rupture—severe MR
   Ventricular free wall rupture with subacute tamponade
   Other conditions complicating large MIs
      Hemorrhage
      Infection
      Excess negative inotropic or vasodilator medications
      Prior valvular heart disease
      Hyperglycemia/ketoacidosis
Post-cardiac arrest
Post-cardiotomy
Refractory sustained tachyarrhythmias
Acute fulminant myocarditis
End-stage cardiomyopathy
Left ventricular apical ballooning
Takotsubo cardiomyopathy
Hypertrophic cardiomyopathy with severe outflow obstruction
Aortic dissection with aortic insufficiency or tamponade
Pulmonary embolus
Severe valvular heart disease
   Critical aortic or mitral stenosis
   Acute severe aortic or MR
Toxic-metabolic
   Beta-blocker or calcium channel antagonist overdose

Other Etiologies of Cardiogenic Shockᵇ

RV failure due to:
   Acute myocardial infarction
   Acute coronary pulmonale
Refractory sustained bradyarrhythmias
Pericardial tamponade
Toxic/metabolic
   Severe acidosis, severe hypoxemia

ᵃThe etiologies of CS are listed. Most of these can cause pulmonary edema instead of shock or pulmonary edema with CS.
ᵇThese cause CS but not pulmonary edema.
Note: LV, left ventricular; VSR, ventricular septal rupture; MR, mitral regurgitation; RV, right ventricular.

reduced cardiac output and arterial pressure (BP), which result in hypoperfusion of the myocardium and further ischemia and depression of the cardiac output (Fig. 266-1). Systolic myocardial dysfunction reduces stroke volume and, together with diastolic dysfunction, leads to elevated LV end-diastolic pressure and PCWP as well as to pulmonary congestion. Reduced coronary perfusion leads to worsening ischemia and progressive myocardial dysfunction and a rapid downward spiral, which, if uninterrupted, is often fatal. A systemic inflammatory response syndrome may accompany large infarctions and shock. Inflammatory cytokines, inducible nitric oxide synthase, and excess nitric oxide and peroxynitrite may contribute to the genesis of CS as they do to other forms of shock (Chap. 264). Lactic acidosis from poor tissue perfusion and hypoxemia from pulmonary edema may result from pump failure and then contribute to the vicious circle by worsening myocardial ischemia and hypotension. Severe acidosis (pH < 7.25) reduces the efficacy of endogenous and exogenously administered catecholamines. Refractory sustained ventricular or atrial tachyarrhythmias can cause or exacerbate CS.

Autopsy specimens often reflect the stuttering course and piecemeal necrosis of the LV, showing varying stages of infarction. Reinfarction is apparent as new areas of necrosis contiguous with or remote from a slightly older infarct. Infarctions that extend through the full myocardial thickness and result in rupture of the interventricular septum, papillary muscle, or ventricular free wall may result in shock (Chap. 239).

Patient Profile In patients with acute MI, older age, female sex, prior MI, diabetes, and anterior MI location are all associated with increased risk of CS. Shock associated with a first inferior MI should prompt a search for a mechanical cause. Reinfarction soon after MI increases the risk of CS. Two-thirds of patients with CS have flow-limiting stenoses in all three major coronary arteries, and 20% have left main coronary artery stenosis. CS may rarely occur in the absence of significant stenosis, as seen in LV apical ballooning/Takotsubo cardiomyopathy, often in response to sudden severe emotional stress.

Timing Shock is present on admission in only one-quarter of patients who develop CS complicating MI; one-quarter develop it rapidly thereafter, within 6 h of MI onset. Another quarter develop shock later on the first day. Subsequent onset of CS may be due to reinfarction, marked infarct expansion, or a mechanical complication.

Diagnosis Due to the unstable condition of these patients, supportive therapy must be initiated simultaneously with diagnostic evaluation (Fig. 266-2). A focused history and physical examination should be performed, blood specimens sent to the laboratory, and an electrocardiogram (ECG) and chest x-ray obtained.

Echocardiography is an invaluable diagnostic tool in patients suspected of CS.

CLINICAL FINDINGS Most patients have continuing chest pain and dyspnea and appear pale, apprehensive, and diaphoretic. Mentation may be altered, with somnolence, confusion, and agitation. The pulse is typically weak and rapid, often in the range of 90–110 beats/min, or severe bradycardia due to high-grade heart block may be present. Systolic blood pressure (BP) is reduced (<90 mmHg) with a narrow pulse pressure (<30 mmHg), but occasionally BP may be maintained by very high systemic vascular resistance. Tachypnea, Cheyne-Stokes respirations, and jugular venous distention may be present. The precordium is typically quiet, with a weak apical pulse. S1 is usually soft, and an S3 gallop may be audible. Acute, severe MR and VSR are usually associated with characteristic systolic murmurs (Chap. 239). Rales are audible in most patients with LV failure causing CS. Oliguria (urine output < 30 mL/h) is common.

LABORATORY FINDINGS The white blood cell count is typically elevated with a left shift. In the absence of prior renal insufficiency, renal function is initially normal, but blood urea nitrogen and creatinine rise progressively. Hepatic transaminases may be markedly elevated due to liver hypoperfusion. Poor tissue perfusion may result in an anion gap acidosis and elevation of lactic acid level. Prior to support with supplemental O_2, arterial blood gases usually demonstrate hypoxemia and metabolic acidosis, which may be compensated by respiratory alkalosis. Cardiac markers, creatine phosphokinase and its MB fraction, are markedly elevated, as are troponins I and T.

ELECTROCARDIOGRAM In CS due to acute MI with LV failure, Q waves and/or >2-mm ST elevation in multiple leads or left bundle branch block are usually present. More than one-half of all infarcts associated with shock are anterior. Global ischemia due to severe left main stenosis is usually accompanied by severe (e.g., >3 mm) ST depressions in multiple leads.

CHEST ROENTGENOGRAM The chest x-ray typically shows pulmonary vascular congestion and often pulmonary edema, but these findings may be absent in up to a third of patients. The heart size is usually normal when CS results from a first MI but is enlarged when it occurs in a patient with a previous MI.

ECHOCARDIOGRAM A two-dimensional echocardiogram with color flow Doppler (Chap. 222) should be obtained promptly in patients with suspected CS to help define its etiology. Doppler mapping demonstrates a left-to-right shunt in patients with VSR and the severity of MR when the latter is present. Proximal aortic dissection with aortic regurgitation or tamponade may be visualized or evidence for pulmonary embolism obtained (Chap. 256).

ACUTE PULMONARY EDEMA, HYPOTENSION, SHOCK ALGORITHM

Clinical Signs: Shock, hypoperfusion, congestive heart failure, acute pulmonary edema
Most likely problem?

Acute pulmonary edema | Volume problem | Pump problem | Rate problem

First-line actions
• Oxygen and intubation as needed
• Nitroglycerin SL
• Furosemide IV 0.5 to 1.0 mg/kg[a]
• Morphine IV 2 to 4 mg

Administer
• Fluids
• Blood transfusions
• Cause-specific interventions
Consider vasopressors

Bradycardia[b] | Tachycardia[b]

Blood pressure?

Systolic BP defines 2nd line of action

Systolic BP: >100 mmHg

Systolic BP 70 to 100 mmHg No signs/symptoms of shock

Systolic BP 70 to 100 mmHg Signs/symptoms of shock

Systolic BP <70 mmHg Signs/symptoms of shock

Second-Line Actions — Acute pulmonary edema
• Nitroglycerin if SBP >100 mmHg
• Dopamine if SBP = 70 to100 mmHg, signs/symptoms of shock
• Dobutamine if SBP >100 mmHg, no signs/symptoms of shock

Nitroglycerin 10 to 20 μg/min IV

Dobutamine 2 to 20 μg/kg per min IV

Dopamine 2 to 20 μg/kg per min IV

Norepinephrine 0.5 to 30 μg/min IV

Further diagnostic/therapeutic considerations
• Identify and treat reversible causes
• Pulmonary artery catheterization
• Intra-aortic balloon pump
• Angiography and PCI
• Additional diagnostic studies
• Surgical interventions
• Additional drug therapy

FIGURE 266-2 The emergency management of patients with cardiogenic shock, acute pulmonary edema, or both is outlined. [a]Furosemide: <0.5 mg/kg for new-onset acute pulmonary edema without hypervolemia; 1 mg/kg for acute on chronic volume overload, renal insufficiency. [b]For management of bradycardia and tachycardia, see Chaps. 225 and 226. ACE, angiotensin-converting enzyme; BP, blood pressure; MI, myocardial infarction. [From J Fields et al (eds): Handbook of Emergency Cardiovascular Care for Healthcare Providers. Copyright 2006, American Heart Association, Inc. Reprinted with permission.]

PULMONARY ARTERY CATHETERIZATION There is controversy regarding the use of pulmonary artery (Swan-Ganz) catheters in patients with established or suspected CS (Chaps. 223 and 261). However, their use is generally recommended for measurement of filling pressures and cardiac output to confirm the diagnosis and optimize use of IV fluids, inotropic agents, and vasopressors (Table 266-2). Blood samples for O_2 saturation measurement should be obtained from the right atrium, right ventricle, and pulmonary artery to rule out a left-to-right shunt. Mixed venous O_2 saturations are low and arterial-venous O_2 differences are elevated, reflecting low cardiac index and high fractional O_2 extraction. The PCWP is elevated. However, use of sympathomimetic amines may return these measurements and the systemic BP toward normal. Systemic vascular resistance may be low, normal, or elevated in CS. Equalization of right- and left-sided filling pressures (right atrial and PCWP) suggests cardiac tamponade as the cause of CS (Chap. 232).

LEFT HEART CATHETERIZATION AND CORONARY ANGIOGRAPHY Measurement of LV pressure, definition of the coronary anatomy, and left ventriculography provide useful information and are indicated in most patients with CS complicating MI. Because of the procedural risk in this critically ill population, cardiac catheterization should be performed when there is a plan and capability for immediate coronary intervention (see below) or when a definitive diagnosis has not been made by other tests.

ACUTE MYOCARDIAL INFARCTION

GENERAL MEASURES (Fig. 266-2) In addition to the usual treatment of acute MI (Chap. 239), initial therapy is aimed at maintaining adequate systemic and coronary perfusion by raising systemic BP with vasopressors and adjusting volume status to a level that ensures optimum LV filling pressure. There is inter-patient variability, but the values that are generally associated with adequate perfusion are systolic BP of ~90 mmHg or mean BP > 60 mmHg and PCWP of ~20 mmHg. Hypoxemia and acidosis must be corrected; most patients require ventilatory support with either endotracheal intubation or bilevel positive airway pressure (Bi-PAP) to correct these abnormalities and reduce the work of breathing (see "Pulmonary Edema," below). Negative inotropic agents should be discontinued and the doses of renally cleared medications adjusted. Hyperglycemia should be corrected with continuous infusion of insulin. Bradyarrhythmias may require transvenous pacing. Recurrent ventricular tachycardia or rapid atrial fibrillation may require immediate treatment (Chap. 226).

TABLE 266-2 HEMODYNAMIC PATTERNS[a]

	RA, mmHg	RVS, mmHg	RVD, mmHg	PAS, mmHg	PAD, mmHg	PCW, mmHg	CI, (L/min)/m²	SVR, (dyn · s)/cm⁵
Normal values	< 6	< 25	0–12	< 25	0–12	< 6–12	≥ 2.5	(800–1600)
MI without pulmonary edema[b]	—	—	—	—	—	~13 (5–18)	~2.7 (2.2–4.3)	—
Pulmonary edema	↔↑	↔↑	↔↑	↑	↑	↑	↔↓	↑
Cardiogenic shock								
LV failure	↔↑	↔↑	↔↑	↔↑	↔↑↑	↑	↓	↔↑
RV failure[c]	↑	↓↔↑[d]	↑	↓↔↑[d]	↔↑↑[d]	↓↔↑[d]	↓	↑
Cardiac tamponade	↑	↔↑	↑	↔↑	↔↑	↔↑	↓	↑
Acute mitral regurgitation	↔↑	↑	↔↑	↑	↑	↑	↓	↔↑
Ventricular septal rupture	↑	↔↑	↑	↔↑	↔↑	↔↑	↑ PBF ↓ SBF	↑
Hypovolemic shock	↓	↔↓	↔↓	↓	↓	↓	↓	↑
Septic shock	↓	↔↓	↔↓	↓	↓	↓	↑	↓

[a]There is significant patient-to-patient variation. Pressure may be normalized if cardiac output is low.

[b]Forrester et al classified non-reperfused MI patients into four hemodynamic subsets. (From Forrester JS et al: N Engl J Med 295:1356, 1976.) PCWP and CI in clinically stable subset 1 patients are shown. Values in parentheses represent range.

[c]"Isolated" or predominant RV failure.

[d]PCW and PA pressures may rise in RV failure after volume loading due to RV dilation, right-to-left shift of the interventricular septum, resulting in impaired LV filling.

When biventricular failure is present, the patterns are similar to those shown for LV failure.

Note: RA, right atrium; RVS/D, right ventricular systolic/diastolic; PAS/D, pulmonary artery systolic/diastolic; PCW, pulmonary capillary wedge; CI, cardiac index; SVR, systemic vascular resistance; MI, myocardial infarction; P/SBF, pulmonary/systemic blood flow.

Source: Table prepared with the assistance of Krishnan Ramanathan, MD.

VASOPRESSORS Various IV drugs may be used to augment BP and cardiac output in patients with CS. All have important disadvantages, and none has been shown to change the outcome in patients with established shock. *Norepinephrine* is a potent vasoconstrictor and inotropic stimulant that increases myocardial O_2 consumption; it should be reserved for patients with CS and refractory hypotension, in particular those without elevated systemic vascular resistance. It should be started at a dosage of 2 to 4 µg/min and titrated upward as necessary. If systemic perfusion or systolic pressure cannot be maintained at >90 mmHg with a dosage of 15 µg/min, it is unlikely that a further increase will be beneficial.

Dopamine is useful in many patients; at low doses (≤ 2 µg/kg per min), it dilates the renal vascular bed; at moderate doses (2–10 µg/kg per min), it has positive chronotropic and inotropic effects as a consequence of β-adrenergic receptor stimulation. At higher doses, a vasoconstrictor effect results from α-receptor stimulation. It is started at an infusion rate of 2–5 µg/kg per min, and the dosage is increased every 2–5 min to a maximum of 20–50 µg/kg per min. *Dobutamine* is a synthetic sympathomimetic amine with positive inotropic action and minimal positive chronotropic activity at low doses (2.5 µg/kg per min), but moderate chronotropic activity at higher doses. Although the usual dosage is up to 10 µg/kg per min, its vasodilating activity precludes its use when a vasoconstrictor effect is required.

AORTIC COUNTERPULSATION In CS, mechanical assistance with an intraaortic balloon pumping (IABP) system capable of augmenting both arterial diastolic pressure and cardiac output is helpful in rapidly stabilizing patients. A sausage-shaped balloon is introduced percutaneously into the aorta via the femoral artery; the balloon is automatically inflated during early diastole, augmenting coronary blood flow. The balloon collapses in early systole, reducing the afterload against which the LV ejects. IABP improves hemodynamic status temporarily in most patients. In contrast to vasopressors and inotropic agents, myocardial O_2 consumption is reduced, ameliorating ischemia. IABP is useful as a stabilizing measure in patients with CS prior to and during cardiac catheterization and percutaneous coronary intervention (PCI) or prior to urgent surgery. IABP is contraindicated if aortic regurgitation is present or aortic dissection is suspected. Ventricular assist devices may be considered for eligible young patients with refractory shock as a bridge to cardiac transplantation (Chap. 228).

REPERFUSION-REVASCULARIZATION The rapid establishment of blood flow in the infarct-related artery is essential in the management of CS and forms the centerpiece of management. The randomized SHOCK Trial demonstrated 132 lives saved per 1000 patients treated with early revascularization with PCI or coronary artery bypass graft (CABG) compared to initial medical therapy including IABP with fibrinolytics followed by delayed revascularization **(Fig. 266-3)**. The benefit is seen across the risk strata and is sustained up to 11 years post MI. Early revascularization with PCI or CABG is a class I recommendation for patients age <75 years with ST elevation or left bundle branch block MI who develop CS within 36 h of MI and who can be revascularized within 18 h of development of CS. When mechanical revascularization is not possible, IABP and fibrinolytic therapy are recommended. Older patients who are suitable candidates for aggressive care should also be offered early revascularization.

Prognosis Within this high-risk condition, there is a wide range of expected death rates based on age, severity of hemodynamic abnormalities, severity of the clinical manifestations of hypoperfusion, and the performance of early revascularization. Independent risk factors are advanced age; depressed cardiac index, ejection fraction, and BP; more extensive coronary artery disease; and renal insufficiency.

SHOCK SECONDARY TO RIGHT VENTRICULAR INFARCTION
Although transient hypotension is common in patients with RV infarction and inferior MI (Chap. 239), persistent CS due to RV failure accounts for only 3% of CS complicating MI. The salient features of RV shock are absence of pulmonary congestion, high right atrial pressure (which may be seen only after volume loading), RV dilatation and dysfunction, only mildly or moderately depressed LV function, and predominance of single-vessel proximal right coronary artery occlusion. Management includes IV fluid administration to optimize right

FIGURE 266-3 Early revascularization (ERV) (percutaneous coronary intervention or coronary artery bypass graft) for cardiogenic shock complicating acute myocardial infarction resulted in substantially improved 1-year and long-term survival compared to initial mechanical stabilization (IMS), including intraaortic balloon pumping and fibrinolytic agents, followed by selective delayed revascularization in the SHOCK Trial (SHould we emergently revascularize Occluded coronaries for Cardiogenic shocK?). (*From JS Hochman et al: JAMA 295:2511–2515, 2006; reprinted with permission from JAMA.*)

atrial pressure (10–15 mmHg); avoidance of excess fluids, which cause a shift of the interventricular septum into the LV; sympathomimetic amines; IABP; and the early reestablishment of infarct-artery flow.

MITRAL REGURGITATION

(See also Chap. 239) Acute severe MR due to papillary muscle dysfunction and/or rupture may complicate MI and result in CS and/or pulmonary edema. This complication most often occurs on the first day, with a second peak several days later. The diagnosis is confirmed by echo-Doppler. Rapid stabilization with IABP is recommended, with administration of dobutamine as needed to raise cardiac output. Reducing the load against which the LV pumps (afterload) reduces the volume of regurgitant flow of blood into the left atrium. Mitral valve surgery is the definitive therapy and should be performed early in the course in suitable candidates.

VENTRICULAR SEPTAL RUPTURE

(See also Chap. 239) Echo-Doppler demonstrates shunting of blood from the left to the right ventricle and may visualize the opening in the interventricular septum. Timing and management are similar to that for MR with IABP support and surgical correction for suitable candidates.

FREE WALL RUPTURE

Myocardial rupture is a dramatic complication of STEMI that is most likely to occur during the first week after the onset of symptoms; its frequency increases with the age of the patient. First infarction, a history of hypertension, no history of angina pectoris, and a relatively large Q-wave infarct are associated with a higher incidence of cardiac rupture. The clinical presentation typically is a sudden loss of pulse, blood pressure, and consciousness but sinus rhythm on ECG (pulseless electrical activity). The myocardium continues to contract, but forward flow is not maintained as blood escapes into the pericardium. Cardiac tamponade (Chap. 232) ensues, and closed-chest massage is ineffective. This condition is almost universally fatal, although dramatic cases of urgent pericardiotensis followed by successful surgical repair have been reported. Free wall rupture may also result in subacute tamponade when the pericardium temporarily seals the rupture sites. Definitive surgical repair is required.

ACUTE FULMINANT MYOCARDITIS

(See also Chap. 231) Myocarditis can mimic acute MI with ST deviation or bundle branch block on the ECG and marked elevation of cardiac markers. Acute myocarditis causes CS in ~15% of cases. These patients are typically younger than those with CS due to acute MI and often do not have typical ischemic chest pain. Echocardiography usually shows global LV dysfunction. Initial management is the same as for CS complicating acute MI (Fig. 266-2) but of course does not involve coronary revascularization.

PULMONARY EDEMA

The etiologies and pathophysiology of pulmonary edema are discussed in Chap. 33.

Diagnosis Acute pulmonary edema usually presents with the rapid onset of dyspnea at rest, tachypnea, tachycardia, and severe hypoxemia. Rales and wheezing due to airway compression from peribronchial cuffing may be audible. Hypertension is usually present due to release of endogenous catecholamines.

It is often difficult to distinguish cardiogenic and noncardiogenic causes of acute pulmonary edema. *Echocardiography* may identify systolic and diastolic ventricular dysfunction and valvular lesions. Pulmonary edema associated with electrocardiographic ST elevation and evolving Q waves is usually diagnostic of acute MI and should prompt immediate institution of MI protocols and coronary artery reperfusion therapy (Chap. 239). Brain natriuretic peptide levels, when substantially elevated, support heart failure as the etiology of acute dyspnea with pulmonary edema (Chap. 227).

The use of a *Swan-Ganz catheter* permits measurement of PCWP and helps differentiate high pressure (cardiogenic) and normal pressure (noncardiogenic) causes of pulmonary edema. Pulmonary artery catheterization is indicated when the etiology of the pulmonary edema is uncertain, when it is refractory to therapy, or when it is accompanied by hypotension. Data derived from use of a catheter often alters the treatment plan, but impact on mortality has not been demonstrated.

℞ PULMONARY EDEMA

The treatment of pulmonary edema depends upon the specific etiology. Given the acute, life-threatening nature of the condition, a number of measures must be applied immediately to support the circulation, gas exchange, and lung mechanics. In addition, conditions that frequently complicate pulmonary edema, such as infection, acidemia, anemia, and renal failure, must be corrected.

SUPPORT OF OXYGENATION AND VENTILATION Patients with acute cardiogenic pulmonary edema generally have an identifiable cause of acute LV failure such as arrhythmia, ischemia/infarction, or myocardial decompensation (Chap. 227) that can be rapidly treated, with improvement in gas exchange. In contrast, noncardiogenic edema usually resolves much less quickly, and most patients require mechanical ventilation.

Oxygen Therapy Support of oxygenation is essential to ensure adequate O_2 delivery to peripheral tissues, including the heart.

Positive-Pressure Ventilation Pulmonary edema increases the work of breathing and the O_2 requirements of this work and may pose a significant physiologic stress on the heart. For patients with inadequate oxygenation or ventilation in spite of supplemental O_2, assisted ventilation by face or nasal mask or by endotracheal intubation should be initiated. Continuous or bilevel positive airway pressure (Chap. 263) can rest the respiratory muscles, improve oxygenation and cardiac function, and reduce the need for intubation. In refractory cases, mechanical ventilation can relieve the work of breathing more completely than noninvasive ventilation. Mechanical ventilation with positive end-expiratory pressure can have multiple beneficial effects on pulmonary edema: (1) it can decrease both preload and afterload, thereby improving cardiac function; (2) it can redistribute lung water from the intraalveolar to the extraalveolar space where the fluid does not interfere as much with gas exchange; and (3) it can increase lung volume to avoid atelectasis.

REDUCTION OF PRELOAD In most forms of pulmonary edema, the quantity of extravascular lung water is related to both the PCWP and the intravascular volume status.

Diuretics The "loop diuretics" furosemide, bumetanide, and torsemide are effective in most forms of pulmonary edema, even in the presence of hypoalbuminemia, hyponatremia, or hypochloremia. Furosemide is also a venodilator that can reduce preload rapidly, prior to any diuresis, and is the diuretic of choice. The initial dose of furosemide should be ≤ 0.5 mg/kg, but a higher dose (1 mg/kg) is required in patients with renal insufficiency, chronic diuretic use, or hypervolemia or after failure of a lower dose.

Nitrates Nitroglycerin and isosorbide dinitrate act predominantly as venodilators, with coronary vasodilating properties as well. They are rapid in onset and effective when administered by a variety of routes. Sublingual nitroglycerin (0.4 mg × 3 every 5 min) is first-line therapy for acute cardiogenic pulmonary edema. If pulmonary edema persists in the absence of hypotension, sublingual may be followed by IV nitroglycerin, commencing at 5–10 μg/min. IV nitroprusside (0.1–5 μg/kg per min) is a potent venous and arterial vasodilator. It is useful for patients with pulmonary edema and hypertension, but is not recommended in states of reduced coronary artery perfusion. It requires close monitoring and titration, including the use of an arterial catheter for continuous BP measurement in the intensive care unit.

Morphine Given in 2- to 4-mg IV boluses, morphine is a transient venodilator that reduces preload while relieving dyspnea and anxiety. These effects can diminish stress, catecholamine levels, tachycardia, and ventricular afterload in patients with pulmonary edema and systemic hypertension.

Angiotensin-Converting Enzyme (ACE) Inhibitors ACE inhibitors reduce both afterload and preload and are recommended in hypertensive patients. A low dose of a short-acting agent may be initiated and followed by increasing oral doses. In acute MI with heart failure, ACE inhibitors reduce short- and long-term mortality.

Other Preload-Reducing Agents   IV recombinant brain natriuretic peptide (nesiritide) is a potent vasodilator with diuretic properties and is effective in the treatment of cardiogenic pulmonary edema. It should be reserved for refractory patients and is not recommended in the setting of ischemia or MI.

Physical Methods   Reduction of venous return reduces preload. Patients without hypotension should be maintained in the sitting position with the legs dangling along the side of the bed.

Inotropic and Inodilator Drugs   The sympathomimetic amines dopamine and dobutamine (see above) are potent inotropic agents. The bipyridine phosphodiesterase-3 inhibitors (inodilators), such as milrinone (50 μg/kg followed by 0.25–0.75 μg/kg per min), stimulate myocardial contractility while promoting peripheral and pulmonary vasodilation. Such agents are indicated in patients with cardiogenic pulmonary edema and severe LV dysfunction.

Digitalis Glycosides   Once a mainstay of treatment because of their positive inotropic action (Chap. 227), digitalis glycosides are rarely used at present. However, they may be useful for control of ventricular rate in patients with rapid atrial fibrillation or flutter and LV dysfunction, since they do not have the negative inotropic effects of other drugs that inhibit atrioventricular nodal conduction.

Intraaortic Counterpulsation   IABP may help to relieve cardiogenic pulmonary edema. It is indicated as a stabilizing measure when acute severe mitral regurgitation or ventricular septal rupture causes refractory pulmonary edema, especially in preparation for surgical repair. IABP or LV-assist devices (Chap. 228) are useful as bridging therapy to cardiac transplantation in patients with refractory pulmonary edema secondary to myocarditis or cardiomyopathy.

Treatment of Tachyarrhythmias and Atrial-Ventricular Resynchronization   (See also Chap. 226) Sinus tachycardia or atrial fibrillation can result from elevated left atrial pressure and sympathetic stimulation. Tachycardia itself can also limit LV filling time and raise left atrial pressure further. While relief of pulmonary congestion will slow the sinus rate or ventricular response in atrial fibrillation, a primary tachyarrhythmia may require cardioversion. In patients with reduced LV function and without atrial contraction or with lack of synchronized atrioventricular contraction, placement of an atrioventricular sequential pacemaker should be considered (Chap. 225).

Stimulation of Alveolar Fluid Clearance   Recent mechanistic studies on alveolar epithelial ion transport have defined a variety of ways to upregulate the clearance of solute and water from the alveolar space. In patients with acute lung injury (noncardiogenic pulmonary edema) IV β-adrenergic agonist treatment decreases extravascular lung water.

SPECIAL CONSIDERATIONS   **The Risk of Iatrogenic Cardiogenic Shock**   In the treatment of pulmonary edema vasodilators lower BP, and, particularly when used in combination, their use may lead to hypotension, coronary artery hypoperfusion, and shock (Fig. 266-1). In general, patients with a *hypertensive* response to pulmonary edema tolerate and are benefit-

ed by these medications. In normotensive patients, low doses of single agents should be instituted sequentially, as needed.

Acute Coronary Syndromes   (See also Chap. 239) Acute STEMI complicated by pulmonary edema is associated with in-hospital mortality rates of 20–40%. After immediate stabilization, coronary artery blood flow must be reestablished rapidly. When available, primary PCI is preferable; alternatively, a fibrinolytic agent should be administered. Early coronary angiography and revascularization by PCI or CABG are also indicated for patients with non-ST elevation acute coronary syndrome. IABP use may be required to stabilize patients for coronary angiography if hypotension develops or for refractory pulmonary edema in patients with LV failure who are candidates for revascularization.

Unusual Types of Edema   Specific etiologies of pulmonary edema may require particular therapy. Reexpansion pulmonary edema can develop after removal of air or fluid that has been in the pleural space for some time. These patients may develop hypotension or oliguria resulting from rapid fluid shifts into the lung. In contrast to cardiogenic edema, diuretics and preload reduction are contraindicated, and intravascular volume repletion is often needed while supporting oxygenation and gas exchange.

High-altitude pulmonary edema can often be prevented by use of dexamethasone, calcium channel-blocking drugs, or long-acting inhaled β$_2$-adrenergic agonists. Treatment includes descent from altitude, bed rest, oxygen, and, if feasible, inhaled nitric oxide; nifedipine may also be effective.

For pulmonary edema resulting from upper airway obstruction, recognition of the obstructing cause is key, since treatment then is to relieve or bypass the obstruction.

FURTHER READINGS

ANTMAN EM: Treatment of ST elevation myocardial infarction, in *Braunwald's Heart Disease*, 8th ed, P Libby et al (eds). Philadelphia, Saunders, 2008

——— et al: ACC/AHA Guidelines for the management of patients with acute myocardial infarction. A report of the American College Of Cardiology/American Heart Association task force on practice guidelines (Committee on Management of Acute Myocardial Infarction). J Am Coll Cardiol 44:671, 2004

BABAEV A et al for the NRMI Investigators: National guidelines and trends in management of patients with acute myocardial infarction complicated by cardiogenic shock: Observations from the National Registry of Myocardial Infarction. J Am Med Assoc 294:448, 2005

HOCHMAN JS: Cardiogenic shock complicating acute myocardial infarction: Expanding the paradigm. Circulation 107:2998, 2003

——— et al: Early revascularization and long-term survival in cardiogenic shock complicating acute myocardial infarction. JAMA 295:2511, 2006

MATTHAY MA, INGBAR DH (eds): *Pulmonary Edema. Lung Biology in Health and Disease*, vol 116. New York, Marcel Dekker, 1998

OKUDA M: A multidisciplinary overview of cardiogenic shock. 25:557, 2006

WARE LB, MATTHAY MA: Clinical practice: Acute pulmonary edema. N Engl J Med 353(26):2788, 2005

267   Cardiovascular Collapse, Cardiac Arrest, and Sudden Cardiac Death

Robert J. Myerburg, Agustin Castellanos

OVERVIEW AND DEFINITIONS

The vast majority of naturally occurring sudden deaths are caused by cardiac disorders. The magnitude of sudden *cardiac* death (SCD) as a

public health problem is highlighted by the estimate that ~50% of all cardiac deaths are sudden and unexpected, at least two-thirds of which are first cardiac events or occur among population subsets with previously known heart disease considered to be relatively low risk. The total SCD burden is estimated to range from <200,000 to >450,000 deaths each year in the United States. SCD is a direct consequence of cardiac arrest, which may be reversible if responded to promptly. Since resuscitation techniques and emergency rescue systems are available to respond to victims of out-of-hospital cardiac arrest, which was uniformly fatal in the past, understanding the SCD problem has practical importance.

SCD must be defined carefully. In the context of time, "sudden" is defined, for most clinical and epidemiologic purposes, as 1 h or less

TABLE 267-1 DISTINCTION BETWEEN CARDIOVASCULAR COLLAPSE, CARDIAC ARREST, AND DEATH

Term	Definition	Qualifiers or Exceptions
Cardiovascular collapse	A sudden loss of effective blood flow due to cardiac and/or peripheral vascular factors which may reverse spontaneously (e.g., neurocardiogenic syncope; vasovagal syncope) or only with interventions (e.g., cardiac arrest)	Nonspecific term that includes cardiac arrest and its consequences and also events that characteristically revert spontaneously
Cardiac arrest	Abrupt cessation of cardiac pump function which may be reversible by a prompt intervention but will lead to death in its absence	Rare spontaneous reversions; likelihood of successful interventions relates to mechanism of arrest, clinical setting, and prompt return of circulation
Death	Irreversible cessation of all biologic functions	None

between a change in clinical status heralding the onset of the terminal clinical event and the cardiac arrest itself. An exception is unwitnessed deaths in which pathologists may expand the definition of time to 24 h after the victim was last seen to be alive and stable.

Because of community-based interventions, victims may remain biologically alive for days or even weeks after a cardiac arrest that has resulted in irreversible central nervous system damage. Confusion in terms can be avoided by adhering strictly to definitions of cardiovascular collapse, cardiac arrest, and death (Table 267-1). Death is biologically, legally, and literally an absolute and irreversible event. Death may be delayed in a survivor of cardiac arrest, but "survival after sudden death" is an irrational term. A generally accepted definition of SCD is *natural death due to cardiac causes*, heralded by abrupt loss of consciousness within *1 h* of the onset of acute symptoms, in an individual who may have known *preexisting* heart disease but in whom the *time* and *mode* of death are *unexpected*. When biologic death of the cardiac arrest victim is delayed because of interventions, the relevant pathophysiologic event remains the sudden and unexpected cardiac arrest that leads ultimately to death, even though delayed by artificial methods. The language used should reflect the fact that the index event was a cardiac arrest and that death was due to its delayed consequences. Accordingly, for statistical purposes, deaths that occur during hospitalization or within 30 days after resuscitated cardiac arrest are counted as sudden deaths.

CLINICAL DEFINITION OF FORMS OF CARDIOVASCULAR COLLAPSE

Cardiovascular collapse is a general term connoting loss of effective blood flow due to acute dysfunction of the heart and/or peripheral vasculature. Cardiovascular collapse may be caused by vasodepressor syncope (vasovagal syncope, postural hypotension with syncope, neurocardiogenic syncope; Chap. 21), a transient severe bradycardia, or cardiac arrest. The latter is distinguished from the transient forms of cardiovascular collapse in that it usually requires an intervention to achieve resuscitation. In contrast, vasodepressor syncope and other primary bradyarrhythmic syncopal events are transient and non-life-threatening, with spontaneous return of consciousness.

The most common electrical mechanism for cardiac arrest is ventricular fibrillation (VF), which is responsible for 50–80% of cardiac arrests. Severe persistent bradyarrhythmias, asystole, and pulseless electrical activity (PEA; an organized electrical activity without mechanical response, formerly called electromechanical dissociation) cause another 20–30%. Pulseless sustained ventricular tachycardia (VT) is a less-common mechanism. Acute low cardiac output states, having precipitous onset, may also present clinically as a cardiac arrest. These hemodynamic causes include massive acute pulmonary emboli, internal blood loss from ruptured aortic aneurysm, intense anaphylaxis, and cardiac rupture with tamponade after myocardial infarction (MI).

ETIOLOGY, INITIATING EVENTS, AND CLINICAL EPIDEMIOLOGY

Clinical and epidemiologic studies have identified population subgroups at high risk for SCD. In addition, a large body of pathologic data provides information on the underlying *structural abnormalities* in victims of SCD, and studies of clinical physiology have begun to identify a group of *transient functional factors* that may convert a long-standing underlying structural abnormality from a stable to an unstable state (Table 267-2).

Cardiac disorders constitute the most common causes of sudden *natural* death. After an initial peak incidence of sudden death between birth and 6 months of age (the sudden infant death syndrome), the incidence of sudden death declines sharply and remains low through childhood and adolescence. Among adolescents and young adults, the incidence of SCD is approximately 1 per 100,000 population per year. The incidence begins to increase in adults over the age of 30 years, reaching a second peak in the age range of 45–75 years, when the incidence approximates 1–2 per 1000 per year among the unselected adult population. Increasing age within this range is associated with increasing risk for sudden *cardiac* death (Fig. 267-1A). From 1 to 13 years of age, only one of five sudden *natural* deaths is due to cardiac causes. Between 14 and 21 years of age, the proportion increases to 30%, and then to 88% in the middle aged and elderly.

TABLE 267-2 CARDIAC ARREST AND SUDDEN CARDIAC DEATH

Structural Causes

I. Coronary heart disease
  A. Coronary artery abnormalities
    1. Chronic atherosclerotic lesions
    2. Acute (active) lesions (plaque fissuring, platelet aggregation, acute thrombosis)
    3. Anomalous coronary artery anatomy
  B. Myocardial infarction
    1. Healed
    2. Acute
II. Myocardial hypertrophy
  A. Secondary
  B. Hypertrophic cardiomyopathy
    1. Obstructive
    2. Nonobstructive
III. Dilated cardiomyopathy—primary muscle disease
IV. Inflammatory and infiltrative disorders
  A. Myocarditis
  B. Noninfectious inflammatory diseases
  C. Infiltrative diseases
  D. Right ventricular dysplasia
V. Valvular heart disease
VI. Electrophysiologic abnormalities, structural
  A. Anomalous pathways in Wolff-Parkinson-White syndrome
  B. Conducting system disease
VII. Inherited disorders of molecular structure associated with electrophysiologic abnormalities (e.g., congenital long QT syndromes, Brugada syndrome)

Functional Contributing Factors

I. Alterations of coronary blood flow
  A. Transient ischemia
  B. Reperfusion after ischemia
II. Low cardiac output states
  A. Heart failure
    1. Chronic
    2. Acute decompensation
  B. Shock
III. Systemic metabolic abnormalities
  A. Electrolyte imbalance (e.g., hypokalemia)
  B. Hypoxemia, acidosis
IV. Neurophysiologic disturbances
  A. Autonomic fluctuations: central, neural, humoral
  B. Receptor function
V. Toxic responses
  A. Proarrhythmic drug effects
  B. Cardiac toxins (e.g., cocaine, digitalis intoxication)
  C. Drug interactions

FIGURE 267-1 *Panel A demonstrates age-related risk for SCD.* For the general population age 35 years and older, SCD risk is 0.1–0.2 percent per year (1 per 500–1,000 population). Among the general population of adolescents and adults younger than the age of 30 years, the overall risk of SCD is 1 per 100,000 population, or 0.001 percent per year. The risk of SCD increases dramatically beyond the age of 35 years. The greatest rate of increase is between 40 and 65 years (vertical axis is discontinuous). Among patients older than 30 years of age, with advanced structural heart disease and markers of high risk for cardiac arrest, the event rate may exceed 25% per year, and age-related risk attenuates. *Panel B demonstrates the incidence of SCD in population subgroups* and the relation of total number of events per year to incidence figures. Approximations of subgroup incidence figures and the related population pool from which they are derived are presented. Approximately 50% of all cardiac deaths are sudden and unexpected. The incidence triangle on the left ("Percent/Year") indicates the approximate percentage of sudden and nonsudden deaths in each of the population subgroups indicated, ranging from the lowest percentage in unselected adult populations (0.1–2% per year) to the highest percentage in patients with VT or VF during convalescence after an MI (approximately 50% per year). The triangle on the right indicates the total number of events per year in each of these groups, to reflect incidence in context with the size of the population subgroups. The highest risk categories identify the smallest number of total annual events, and the lowest incidence category accounts for the largest number of events per year. EF, ejection fraction; VT, ventricular tachycardia; VF, ventricular fibrillation; MI, myocardial infarction. *[After RJ Myerburg et al, Circulation 85(Suppl 1):2, 1992. Reproduced with permission of the American Heart Association.]*

Young and middle aged men and women have different susceptibilities to SCD, but the gender differences decrease with advancing age. The difference in risk for SCD parallels the differences in age-related risks for other manifestations of coronary heart disease (CHD) between men and women. As the gender gap for manifestations of CHD closes in the sixth

to eighth decades of life, the excess risk of SCD in males progressively narrows. Despite the lower incidence among younger women, coronary risk factors such as cigarette smoking, diabetes, hyperlipidemia, and hypertension are highly influential, and SCD remains an important clinical and epidemiologic problem. The incidence of SCD among the African-American population appears to be higher than among the white population; the reasons remain uncertain.

Genetic factors contribute to the risk of SCD. In one sense, they contribute to familial predisposition to CHD and its expression as acute coronary syndromes. In addition, however, there are data suggesting a familial predisposition to SCD as a specific form of expression of CHD. A strong parental history of SCD as an initial coronary event increases the probability of a similar expression in the offspring. In a few syndromes, such as hypertrophic cardiomyopathy, congenital long QT interval syndromes, right ventricular dysplasia, and the syndrome of right bundle branch block and nonischemic ST-segment elevations (Brugada syndrome), there is a specific inherited risk of SCD (Chap. 226).

The structural causes of and functional factors contributing to the SCD syndrome are listed in Table 267-2. Worldwide, and especially in western cultures, coronary atherosclerotic heart disease is the most common structural abnormality associated with SCD in middle-aged and older adults. Up to 80% of all SCDs in the United States are due to the consequences of coronary atherosclerosis. The cardiomyopathies (dilated and hypertrophic, collectively; Chap. 231) account for another 10–15% of SCDs, and all the remaining diverse etiologies cause only 5–10% of all SCDs. The inherited arrhythmia syndromes (see above and Table 267-2) are more common causes in adolescents and young adults. For some of these syndromes, such as hypertrophic cardiomyopathy (Chap. 231), risk of SCD begins to increase after puberty.

Transient ischemia in the previously scarred or hypertrophied heart, hemodynamic and fluid and electrolyte disturbances, fluctuations in autonomic nervous system activity, and transient electrophysiologic changes caused by drugs or other chemicals (e.g., proarrhythmia) have all been implicated as mechanisms responsible for the transition from electrophysiologic stability to instability. In addition, reperfusion of ischemic myocardium may cause transient electrophysiologic instability and arrhythmias.

PATHOLOGY

Data from postmortem examinations of SCD victims parallel the clinical observations on the prevalence of CHD as the major structural etiologic factor. More than 80% of SCD victims have pathologic findings of CHD. The pathologic description often includes a combination of long-standing, extensive atherosclerosis of the epicardial coronary arteries and unstable coronary artery lesions, which include various permutations of fissured or ruptured plaques, platelet aggregates, hemorrhage, and/or thrombosis. As many as 70–75% of males who die suddenly have preexisting healed MIs, while only 20–30% have recent acute MIs, despite the prevalence of unstable plaques and thrombi. The latter suggests transient ischemia as the mechanism of onset. Regional or global left ventricular (LV) hypertrophy often coexists with prior MIs.

PREDICTION AND PREVENTION OF CARDIAC ARREST AND SUDDEN CARDIAC DEATH

SCD accounts for approximately one-half the total cardiovascular mortality rate. As shown in Fig. 267-1B, the very-high-risk subgroups provide more focused populations ("percent per year") for predicting cardiac arrest or SCD; but the impact of such subgroups on the overall problem of SCD, indicated by the absolute number of events ("events per year"), is relatively small. The requirements for achieving a major population impact are effective prevention of underlying diseases and/or new epidemiologic probes that will allow better resolution of subgroups at specific risk within the large general populations.

Strategies for predicting and preventing SCD are categorized as primary and secondary, in addition to responses intended to abort cardiac arrests. *Primary prevention*, as defined in various implantable defibrillator trials, refers to the attempt to identify individual patients at specific risk for SCD and institute preventive strategies. *Secondary prevention* refers to measures taken to prevent recurrent cardiac arrest or death in individuals who have survived a previous cardiac arrest. The primary prevention strategies currently used depend upon magnitude of risk among the various population subgroups. Because the annual incidence of SCD among the unselected adult population is limited to 1–2 per 1000 population per year (Fig. 267-1), and more than 30% of all SCDs due to coronary artery disease occur as the first clinical manifestation of the disease (Fig. 267-2*A*), the only practical strategies are profiling for risk of developing CHD and risk factor control (Fig. 267-2*B*). The most powerful long-term risk factors include age, cigarette smoking, elevated serum cholesterol, diabetes mellitus, elevated blood pressure, LV hypertrophy, and nonspecific electrocardiographic abnormalities. Markers of inflammation (e.g., C-reactive protein levels) that may predict plaque destabilization, have been added to risk classifications. The presence of multiple risk factors progressively increases incidence, but not sufficiently or specifically enough to warrant therapies targeted to potentially fatal arrhythmias (Fig. 267-1*A*). However, recent studies offer the hope that genetic markers for specific risk may become available. These studies suggest that a family history of SCD associated with acute coronary syndromes predicts a higher likelihood of cardiac arrest as the initial manifestation of coronary artery disease in first-degree family members.

After coronary artery disease has been identified in a patient, additional strategies for risk profiling become available (Fig. 267-2*B*), but the majority of SCDs occur among the large unselected groups rather than in the specific high-risk subgroups that become evident among populations with established disease (compare events per year with percent per year in Fig. 267-1*B*). Under most conditions of higher level of risk, particularly those indexed to a major recent cardiovascular event (e.g., MI, recent onset of heart failure, survival after out-of-hospital cardiac arrest), the highest risk of death occurs during the initial 6–18 months and then plateaus toward the baseline risk of the underlying disease. However, many of the early deaths are nonsudden, diluting the potential benefit of strategies targeted specifically to SCD. Thus, even though post-myocardial infarction beta-blocker therapy has an identifiable benefit for both early SCD and nonsudden mortality risk, a total mortality benefit for ICD therapy early after MI has not been observed.

Among patients in the acute, convalescent, and chronic phases of myocardial infarction (Chap. 239), subgroups at high absolute risk of SCD can be identified. During the acute phase, the potential risk of cardiac arrest from onset through the first 48 hours may be as high as 15%, emphasizing the importance for patients to respond promptly to the onset of symptoms. Those who survive acute-phase VF, however, are not at continuing risk for recurrent cardiac arrest indexed to that event. During the convalescent phase after MI (3 days to ~6 weeks), an episode of sustained VT or VF, associated with a large infarct, predicts a natural history mortality risk of up to 50% at 12 months. At least

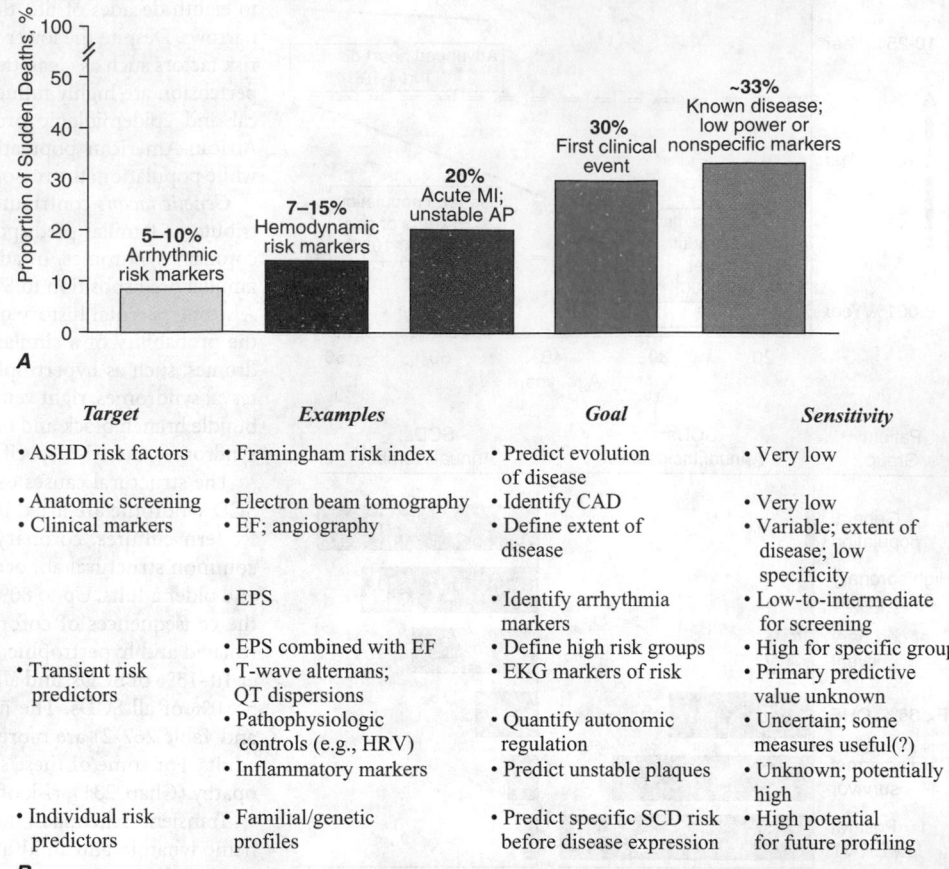

A

Target	Examples	Goal	Sensitivity
• ASHD risk factors	• Framingham risk index	• Predict evolution of disease	• Very low
• Anatomic screening	• Electron beam tomography	• Identify CAD	• Very low
• Clinical markers	• EF; angiography	• Define extent of disease	• Variable; extent of disease; low specificity
	• EPS	• Identify arrhythmia markers	• Low-to-intermediate for screening
	• EPS combined with EF	• Define high risk groups	• High for specific groups
• Transient risk predictors	• T-wave alternans; QT dispersions	• EKG markers of risk	• Primary predictive value unknown
	• Pathophysiologic controls (e.g., HRV)	• Quantify autonomic regulation	• Uncertain; some measures useful(?)
	• Inflammatory markers	• Predict unstable plaques	• Unknown; potentially high
• Individual risk predictors	• Familial/genetic profiles	• Predict specific SCD risk before disease expression	• High potential for future profiling

B

FIGURE 267-2 Population subsets, risk predictors, and distribution of sudden cardiac deaths (SCDs) according to clinical circumstances. *A.* The population subset with high-risk arrhythmia markers in conjunction with low ejection fraction is a group at high risk of SCD but accounts for <10% of the total SCD burden attributable to coronary artery disease. In contrast, nearly two-thirds of all SCD victims present with SCD as the first and only manifestation of underlying disease or have known disease but are considered relatively low-risk because of the absence of high-risk markers. ***B.*** Risk profile for prediction and prevention of SCD is difficult. The highest absolute numbers of events occur among the general population who may have risk factors for coronary heart disease or expressions of disease that do not predict high risk. This results in a low sensitivity for predicting and preventing SCD. New approaches that include epidemiologic modeling of transient risk factors and methods of predicting individual patient risk offer hope for greater sensitivity in the future. AP, angina pectoris; ASHD, arteriosclerotic heart disease; CAD, coronary artery disease; EPS, electrophysiologic study; HRV, heart rate variability. *(From Myerburg, reproduced with permission of the publisher.)*

50% of the deaths are sudden. Aggressive intervention techniques may reduce this incidence.

After passage into the chronic phase of MI, the longer-term risk for total and SCD mortality is predicted by a number of factors (Fig. 267-2*B*). The most important for both SCD and nonsudden death is the extent of myocardial damage sustained as a result of the acute MI. This is measured by the magnitude of reduction of the ejection fraction (EF), functional capacity, and/or the occurrence of heart failure. Various studies have demonstrated that ventricular arrhythmias identified by ambulatory monitoring contribute significantly to this risk, especially in patients with an EF <40%. In addition, inducibility of VT or VF during electrophysiologic testing of patients who have ambient ventricular arrhythmias [premature ventricular contractions (PVCs) and nonsustained VT] and an EF < 35 or 40% is a strong predictor of SCD risk. Patients in this subgroup are now considered candidates for implantable cardioverter defibrillators (ICDs) (see below). Risk falls off sharply with EFs >40% after MI and the absence of ambient arrhythmias, and conversely is high with EFs <30% even without the ambient arrhythmia markers.

The cardiomyopathies (dilated and hypertrophic, Chap. 231) are the second most common category of diseases associated with risk of SCD, following CHD (Table 267-2). Some risk factors have been identified, largely related to extent of disease, documented ventricular arrhythmias, and symptoms of arrhythmias (e.g., unexplained syncope). The less common causes of SCD include valvular heart disease (primarily aortic), and inflammatory and infiltrative disorders of the myocardium. The latter include viral myocarditis, sarcoidosis, and amyloidosis.

Among adolescents and young adults, rare inherited disorders, such as hypertrophic cardiomyopathy, the long QT interval syndromes, right ventricular dysplasia, and the Brugada syndrome, have received attention as important causes of SCD because of advances in genetics and the ability to identify some of those at risk before a fatal event. The subgroup of young competitive athletes has received special attention. The incidence of SCD among athletes appears to be higher than the general adolescent and young adult population, perhaps up to 1 in 75,000. Hypertrophic cardiomyopathy (Chap. 231) is the most common cause in the United States, compared to Italy, where more comprehensive screening programs remove potential victims from the population of athletes.

Secondary prevention strategies should be applied to surviving victims of a cardiac arrest that was not associated with an acute MI or a transient risk of SCD (e.g., drug exposures, correctable electrolyte imbalances). Multivessel coronary artery disease or dilated cardiomyopathy with left ventricular EF <40% or the presences of life-threatening arrhythmias with long QT syndromes or right ventricular dysplasia predict a 1–2-year risk of recurrence of a SCD or cardiac arrest of up to 30% in the absence of specific interventions (see below).

CLINICAL CHARACTERISTICS OF CARDIAC ARREST

PRODROME, ONSET, ARREST, DEATH

SCD may be presaged by days, weeks, or months of increasing angina, dyspnea, palpitations, easy fatigability, and other nonspecific complaints. However, these *prodromal complaints* are generally predictive of any major cardiac event; they are not specific for predicting SCD.

The *onset of the clinical transition*, leading to cardiac arrest, is defined as an acute change in cardiovascular status preceding cardiac arrest by up to 1 h. When the onset is instantaneous or abrupt, the probability that the arrest is cardiac in origin is >95%. Continuous ECG recordings, fortuitously obtained at the onset of a cardiac arrest, commonly demonstrate changes in cardiac electrical activity during the minutes or hours before the event. There is a tendency for the heart rate to increase and for advanced grades of PVCs to evolve. Most cardiac arrests that are caused by VF begin with a run of sustained or nonsustained VT, which then degenerates into VF.

The probability of achieving successful resuscitation from cardiac arrest is related to the interval from onset to institution of resuscitative efforts, the setting in which the event occurs, the mechanism (VF, VT, pulseless electrical activity, asystole), and the clinical status of the patient prior to the cardiac arrest. Return of circulation and survival rates as a result of defibrillation decrease linearly from the first minute to 10 min. By 5 min, survival rates are no better than 25–30% in out-of-hospital settings. Those settings in which it is possible to institute prompt cardiopulmonary resuscitation (CPR) with rapid defibrillation of VF provide a better chance of a successful outcome. However, the outcome in intensive care units and other in-hospital environments is heavily influenced by the patient's preceding clinical status. The immediate outcome is good for cardiac arrest occurring in the intensive care unit in the presence of an acute cardiac event or transient metabolic disturbance, but survival among patients with far-advanced chronic cardiac disease or advanced noncardiac diseases (e.g., renal failure, pneumonia, sepsis, diabetes, cancer) is low, and not much more successful in the in-hospital than in the out-of-hospital setting.

The success rate for initial resuscitation and survival to hospital discharge after an out-of-hospital cardiac arrest depends heavily on the mechanism of the event. When the mechanism is VT, the outcome is best; VF is the next most successful; and asystole and pulseless electrical activity (PEA) generate dismal outcome statistics. Advanced age also adversely influences the chances of successful resuscitation.

Progression to biologic death is a function of the mechanism of cardiac arrest and the length of the delay before interventions. VF or asystole without CPR within the first 4–6 min has a poor outcome even if defibrillation is successful, because of superimposed brain damage; there are few survivors among patients who had no life support activities for the first 8 min after onset. Outcome statistics are improved by lay bystander intervention (basic life support—see below) prior to definitive interventions (advanced life support), and even more by early defibrillation. In regard to the latter, evaluations of deployment of automatic external defibrillators (AEDs) in communities (e.g., police vehicles, large buildings, airports, and stadiums) are beginning to generate encouraging data. Increased deployment is to be encouraged.

Death during the hospitalization after a successfully resuscitated cardiac arrest relates closely to the severity of central nervous system injury. Anoxic encephalopathy and infections subsequent to prolonged respirator dependence account for 60% of the deaths. Another 30% occur as a consequence of low cardiac output states that fail to respond to interventions. Recurrent arrhythmias are the least common cause of death, accounting for only 10% of in-hospital deaths.

In the setting of acute MI (Chap. 239), it is important to distinguish between primary and secondary cardiac arrests. *Primary cardiac arrests* refer to those that occur in the absence of hemodynamic instability, and *secondary cardiac arrests* are those that occur in patients in whom abnormal hemodynamics dominate the clinical picture before cardiac arrest. The success rate for immediate resuscitation in primary cardiac arrest during acute MI in a monitored setting should approach 100%. In contrast, as many as 70% of patients with secondary cardiac arrest succumb immediately or during the same hospitalization.

℞ CARDIAC ARREST

The individual who collapses suddenly is managed in five stages: (1) the initial response and basic life support, (2) public access defibrillation (if available), (3) advanced life support, (4) postresuscitation care, and (5) long-term management. The initial response, including basic life support and public access defibrillation, can be carried out by physicians, nurses, paramedical personnel, and trained lay persons. There is a requirement for increasingly specialized skills as the patient moves through the stages of advanced life support, postresuscitation care, and long-term management.

INITIAL RESPONSE AND BASIC LIFE SUPPORT   The initial evaluation will confirm whether a sudden collapse is indeed due to a cardiac arrest. Observations of the state of consciousness, respiratory movements, skin color, and the presence or absence of pulses in the carotid or femoral arteries can promptly determine whether a life-threatening cardiac arrest has occurred. For lay responders, the pulse check is no longer recommended. As soon as a cardiac arrest is suspected, confirmed, or even considered to be impending, calling an emergency rescue system (e.g., 911) is the immediate priority. With the development of AEDs that are easily used by nonconventional emergency responders, an additional layer for response has evolved (see below).

Agonal respiratory movements may persist for a short time after the onset of cardiac arrest, but it is important to observe for severe stridor with a persistent pulse as a clue to aspiration of a foreign body or food. If this is suspected, a Heimlich maneuver (see below) may dislodge the obstructing body. A precordial blow, or "thump," delivered firmly by the clenched fist to the junction of the middle and lower third of the sternum may occasionally revert VT or VF, but there is concern about converting VT to VF. Therefore, it is recommended to use precordial thumps as an advanced life support technique when monitoring and defibrillation are available. This conservative application of the technique remains controversial.

The third action during the initial response is to clear the airway. The head is tilted back and chin lifted so that the oropharynx can be explored to clear the airway. Dentures or foreign bodies are removed, and the Heimlich maneuver is performed if there is reason to suspect that a foreign body is lodged in the oropharynx. If respiratory arrest precipitating cardiac arrest is suspected, a second precordial thump is delivered after the airway is cleared.

Basic life support, more popularly known as CPR, is intended to maintain organ perfusion until definitive interventions can be instituted. The elements of CPR are the maintenance of ventilation of the lungs and compression of the chest. Mouth-to-mouth respiration may be used if no specific rescue equipment is immediately available (e.g., plastic oropharyngeal airways, esophageal obturators, masked Ambu bag). Conventional ventilation techniques during single-responder CPR require the lungs to be inflated twice in succession every 30 chest compressions.

Chest compression is based on the assumption that cardiac compression allows the heart to maintain a pump function by sequential filling and emptying of its chambers, with competent valves maintaining forward direction of flow. The palm of one hand is placed over the lower sternum, with the heel of the other resting on the dorsum of the lower hand. The sternum is depressed, with the arms remaining straight, at a rate of approximately 100 per minute. Sufficient force is applied to depress the sternum 4–5 cm, and relaxation is abrupt.

AUTOMATED EXTERNAL DEFIBRILLATION (AED) AEDs that are easily used by nonconventional responders, such as nonparamedic firemen, police, ambulance drivers, trained security guards, and minimally trained or untrained lay persons, have been developed. This advance has inserted another level of response into the cardiac arrest paradigm. A number of studies have demonstrated that AED use by nonconventional and lay responders in strategic response systems can improve cardiac arrest survival rates. This strategy is based on shortening the time to first defibrillation attempt while awaiting arrival of advanced life support.

ADVANCED LIFE SUPPORT This is intended to achieve adequate ventilation, control cardiac arrhythmias, stabilize blood pressure and cardiac output, and restore organ perfusion. The activities carried out to achieve these goals include (1) defibrillation/cardioversion and/or pacing, (2) intubation with an endotracheal tube, and (3) insertion of an intravenous line. The speed with which defibrillation/cardioversion is carried out is an important element for successful resuscitation, both for restoration of spontaneous circulation and protection of the central nervous system. Immediate defibrillation should precede intubation and insertion of an intravenous line; CPR should be carried out while the defibrillator is being charged. As soon as a diagnosis of VF or VT is established, a shock of at least 300 J should be delivered. Additional shocks, up to a maximum of 360 J, are tried if the initial shock does not successfully abolish VT or VF, but it is now recommended that 60–90 s of CPR be carried out before repeated shocks, if the first shock fails to restore an organized rhythm, or before the first shock if 5 min has elapsed between the onset of cardiac arrest and ability to deliver a shock. Epinephrine, 1 mg intravenously, is given after failed defibrillation, and attempts to defibrillate are repeated. The dose of epinephrine may be repeated after intervals of 3–5 min **(Fig. 267-3A)**. Vasopressin (a single 40 Unit dose given IV) has been suggested as an alternative to epinephrine.

If the patient is less than fully conscious upon reversion, or if two or three attempts fail, prompt intubation, ventilation, and arterial blood gas analysis should be carried out. Ventilation with O₂ (room air if O₂ is not immediately available) may promptly reverse hypoxemia and acidosis. The patient who is persistently acidotic after successful defibrillation and intubation should be given 1 meq/kg NaHCO₃ initially and an additional 50% of the dose repeated every 10–15 min. However, it should not be used routinely.

After initial unsuccessful defibrillation attempts, or with persistent/recurrent electrical instability, antiarrhythmic therapy should be instituted. Intravenous amiodarone has emerged as the initial treatment of choice (150 mg over 10 min, followed by 1 mg/min for up to 6 h and 0.5 mg/min thereafter) (Fig. 267-3A). For cardiac arrest due to VF in the early phase of an acute coronary syndrome, a bolus of 1 mg/kg of lidocaine may be given intravenously as an alternative, and the dose may be repeated in 2 min. It also may be tried in those patients in whom amiodarone is unsuccessful. Intravenous procainamide (loading infusion of 100 mg/5 min to a total dose of 500–800 mg, followed by continuous infusion at 2–5 mg/min) is now rarely used in this setting but may be tried for persisting, hemodynamically stable arrhythmias. Intravenous calcium gluconate is no longer considered safe or necessary for routine administration. It is used only in patients in whom acute hyperkalemia is known to be the triggering event for resistant VF, in the presence of known hypocalcemia, or in patients who have received toxic doses of calcium channel antagonists.

Cardiac arrest secondary to bradyarrhythmias or asystole is managed differently (Fig. 267-3B). The patient is promptly intubated, CPR is continued, and an attempt is made to control hypoxemia and acidosis. Epinephrine and/or atropine are given intravenously or by an intracardiac route.

A

B

FIGURE 267-3 A. The algorithm of ventricular fibrillation or pulseless ventricular tachycardia begins with defibrillation attempts. If that fails, it is followed by epinephrine and then antiarrhythmic drugs. See text for details. **B. The algorithms for bradyarrhythmia/asystole** (left) or pulseless electrical activity (right) is dominated first by continued life support and a search for reversible causes. Subsequent therapy is nonspecific and accompanied by a low success rate. See text for details. CPR, cardiopulmonary resuscitation; MI, myocardial infarction.

External pacing devices are now available to attempt to establish a regular rhythm, but the prognosis is generally very poor in this form of cardiac arrest, even with successful electrical pacing. PEA is treated similarly to bradyarrhythmias, but its outcome is also dismal. The one exception is bradyarrhythmic/asystolic cardiac arrest secondary to airway obstruction.

This form of cardiac arrest may respond promptly to removal of foreign bodies by the Heimlich maneuver or, in hospitalized patients, by intubation and suctioning of obstructing secretions in the airway.

POSTRESUSCITATION CARE   This phase of management is determined by the clinical setting of the cardiac arrest. Primary VF in acute MI (Chap. 239) is generally very responsive to life-support techniques and easily controlled after the initial event. In the in-hospital setting, respirator support is usually not necessary or is needed for only a short time, and hemodynamics stabilize promptly after defibrillation or cardioversion. In secondary VF in acute MI (those events in which hemodynamic abnormalities predispose to the potentially fatal arrhythmia), resuscitative efforts are less often successful; and in those patients who are successfully resuscitated, the recurrence rate is high. The clinical picture and outcome are dominated by hemodynamic instability and the ability to control hemodynamic dysfunction. Bradyarrhythmias, asystole, and PEA are commonly secondary events in hemodynamically unstable patients. The in-hospital phase of care of the out-of-hospital cardiac arrest survivor is dictated by specific clinical circumstances. The most difficult is the presence of anoxic encephalopathy, which is a strong predictor of in-hospital death. A recent addition to the management of this condition is induced hypothermia to reduce metabolic demands and cerebral edema.

The outcome after in-hospital cardiac arrest associated with noncardiac diseases is poor, and in the few successfully resuscitated patients, the postresuscitation course is dominated by the nature of the underlying disease. Patients with end-stage cancer, renal failure, acute central nervous system disease, and uncontrolled infections, as a group, have a survival rate of <10% after in-hospital cardiac arrest. Some major exceptions are patients with transient airway obstruction, electrolyte disturbances, proarrhythmic effects of drugs, and severe metabolic abnormalities, most of whom may have an excellent chance of survival if they can be resuscitated promptly and maintained while the transient abnormalities are being corrected.

LONG-TERM MANAGEMENT AFTER SURVIVAL OF OUT-OF-HOSPITAL CARDIAC ARREST   Patients who survive cardiac arrest without irreversible damage to the central nervous system, and who achieve hemodynamic stability, should have extensive diagnostic testing and appropriate therapeutic interventions for their long-term management. This aggressive approach is driven by the fact that survival after out-of-hospital cardiac arrest was followed by a 25–30% mortality rate during the first 2 years after the event, and there are data suggesting that significant reductions in risk can be achieved by implantation of an internal cardiac defibrillator (ICD).

Among patients in whom an acute transmural MI is identified as the specific mechanism triggering an out-of-hospital cardiac arrest, the management is dictated in part by the transient nature of life-threatening arrhythmia risk in the acute phase of MI, and in part by the extent of permanent myocardial damage that results. Several clinical trials have now documented an improved survival among cardiac arrest survivors who have EFs <40% and receive ICDs.

For patients with cardiac arrest thought to be due to a transient ischemic mechanism, particularly with higher EFs, anti-ischemic therapy by pharmacologic or interventional methods is generally accepted as appropriate management. However, despite the absence of supportive clinical trial evidence, some adopt a more aggressive attitude about the use of ICDs in this group of cardiac arrest survivors as well, given the unpredictability of recurrent ischemia.

The principles guiding therapy for patients with coronary artery disease who survive a cardiac arrest generally apply to the other cardiac disorders as well, with the exception that there is less focus on the extent of disease in

certain disorders. Generally, cardiac arrest survivors from other categories of disease, such as the hypertrophic or dilated cardiomyopathies and various rare inherited disorders (e.g., RV dysplasia, long QT syndrome, Brugada syndrome, arrhythmic VF) are all considered ICD candidates.

PREVENTION OF SCD IN HIGH-RISK INDIVIDUALS WITHOUT PRIOR CARDIAC ARREST

Post-MI patients have been the subject of clinical trials for ICD benefit. It is now established that for post-MI patients with EFs <40%, ambient ventricular arrhythmias, and inducible ventricular tachyarrhythmias in the electrophysiology laboratory, ICDs provide a significant reduction in relative risk of SCD and total mortality. Total mortality benefits in the range of a 20–30% reduction over 2–3 years have been observed, and ICD has emerged as preferred therapy for such patients. One study suggests that when the EF <30%, electrophysiologic testing is not necessary to identify ICD benefit, and another demonstrates benefit for patients with Functional Class 2 or 3 heart failure and ejection fractions ≤35%, regardless of etiology (ischemic or nonischemic) or ambient or induced arrhythmias (see Chaps. 226 and 227).

Decision-making for primary prevention in disorders other than coronary artery disease and dilated cardiomyopathy is generally driven by observational data and judgment based on clinical observations. Controlled clinical trials providing evidence-based indicators for ICDs are lacking for these smaller population subgroups. In general, for the rare disorders listed above, indicators of arrhythmic risk such as syncope, documented ventricular tachyarrhythmias, aborted cardiac arrest or perhaps a family history of premature SCD, and a number of other clinical or ECG markers, may be used as indicators for ICDs.

FURTHER READINGS

GOLDBERGER Z, LAMPERT R: Implantable cardioverter-defibrillators: Expanding indications and technologies. JAMA 295:809, 2006

HUIKURI H et al: Sudden death due to cardiac arrhythmias. N Engl J Med 345:1473, 2001

INTERNATIONAL LIAISON COMMITTEE ON RESUSCITATION: 2005 International Consensus on Cardiopulmonary Resuscitation and Emergency Cardiovascular Care Science with Treatment Recommendations. Circulation 112(Suppl III):III-1–III-136, 2005

KOKOLIS S et al: Ventricular arrhythmias and sudden cardiac death. Prog Cardiovasc Dis 48:426, 2006

MARENCO JP et al: Improving survival from sudden cardiac arrest: The role of the automated external defibrillator. JAMA 285:1193, 2001

MARON BJ, PELLICCIA A: The heart of trained athletes: Cardiac remodeling and the risks of sports, including sudden death. Circulation 114:1633, 2006

MYERBURG RJ, CASTELLANOS A: Cardiac arrest and sudden cardiac death, in *Braunwald's Heart Disease*, 8th ed, P Libby et al (eds). Philadelphia, Saunders, 2008

ROBERTS R: Genomics and cardiac arrhythmias. J Am Coll Cardiol 47:9, 2006

WIK L et al: Delaying defibrillation to give basic cardiopulmonary resuscitation to patients with out-of-hospital ventricular fibrillation: a randomized trial. JAMA 289:1389, 2003

268 Coma
Allan H. Ropper

Coma is among the most common and striking problems in general medicine. It accounts for a substantial portion of admissions to emergency wards and occurs on all hospital services. Because coma demands immediate attention, the physician must employ an organized approach.

There is a continuum of states of reduced alertness, the severest form being *coma*, a deep sleeplike state from which the patient cannot be aroused. *Stupor* refers to a higher degree of arousability in which the patient can be awakened only by vigorous stimuli, accompanied by motor behavior that leads to avoidance of uncomfortable or aggravating stimuli. *Drowsiness*, which is familiar to all persons, simulates light sleep and is characterized by easy arousal and the persistence of alertness for brief periods. Drowsiness and stupor are usually attended by some degree of confusion (Chap. 26). A narrative description of the level of arousal and of the type of responses evoked by various stimuli, precisely as observed at the bedside, is preferable to ambiguous terms such as lethargy, semicoma, or obtundation.

Several other neurologic conditions render patients apparently unresponsive and thereby simulate coma, and certain subsyndromes of coma must be considered separately because of their special significance. Among the latter, the *vegetative state* signifies an awake but nonresponsive state. These patients have emerged from coma after a period of days or weeks to a state in which the eyelids are open, giving the appearance of wakefulness. Yawning, coughing, swallowing, as well as limb and head movements persist, but there are few, if any, meaningful responses to the external and internal environment—in essence, an "awake coma." Respiratory and autonomic functions are retained. The term "vegetative" is unfortunate as it is subject to misinterpretation by laypersons. The possibility of incorrectly attributing meaningful behavior to these patients has created inordinate problems. There are always accompanying signs that indicate extensive damage in both cerebral hemispheres, e.g., decerebrate or decorticate limb posturing and absent responses to visual stimuli (see below). In the closely related but less severe *minimally conscious state* the patient may make intermittent rudimentary vocal or motor responses. Cardiac arrest with cerebral hypoperfusion and head injuries are the most common causes of the vegetative and minimally conscious states (Chaps. 267 and 269). The prognosis for regaining mental faculties once the vegetative state has supervened for several months is very poor, and after a year, almost nil, hence the term *persistent vegetative state*. Most reports of dramatic recovery, when investigated carefully, are found to yield to the usual rules for prognosis, but there have been rare instances in which recovery has occurred to a demented condition and, in rare childhood cases, to an even better state.

Quite apart from the above conditions, certain syndromes that affect alertness are prone to be misinterpreted as stupor or coma. *Akinetic mutism* refers to a partially or fully awake state in which the patient is able to form impressions and think but remains virtually immobile and mute. The condition results from damage in the regions of the medial thalamic nuclei or the frontal lobes (particularly lesions situated deeply or on the orbitofrontal surfaces), or from hydrocephalus. The term *abulia* is in essence a milder form of akinetic mutism, used to describe mental and physical slowness and diminished ability to initiate activity. It is also generally the result of damage to the frontal lobe network (Chap. 27). *Catatonia* is a curious hypomobile and mute syndrome that arises as part of a major psychosis, usually schizophrenia or major depression. Catatonic patients make few voluntary or responsive movements, although they blink, swallow, and may not appear distressed. There are nonetheless signs that the patient is responsive, although it may take some ingenuity on the part of the examiner to demonstrate them. For example, eyelid elevation is actively resisted, blinking occurs in response to a visual threat, and the eyes move concomitantly with head rotation, all of which are inconsistent with the presence of a brain lesion. It is characteristic but not invariable in catatonia for the limbs to retain the postures in which they have been placed by the examiner ("waxy flexibility," or catalepsy). Upon recovery, such patients have some memory of events that occurred during their catatonic stupor. The appearance is superficially similar to akinetic mutism, but clinical evidence of cerebral damage such as Babinski signs and hypertonicity of the limbs is lacking. The singular problem of brain death is discussed below.

The *locked-in state* describes yet another type of pseudocoma in which an awake patient has no means of producing speech or volitional movement, but retains voluntary vertical eye movements and lid elevation, thus allowing the patient to signal with a clear mind. The pupils are normally reactive. Such individuals have written entire treatises using Morse code. The usual cause is an infarction or hemorrhage of the ventral pons, which transects all descending corticospinal and corticobulbar pathways. A similar awake but de-efferented state occurs as a result of total paralysis of the musculature in severe cases of Guillain-Barré syndrome (Chap. 380), critical illness neuropathy (Chap. 269), and pharmacologic neuromuscular blockade.

THE ANATOMY AND PHYSIOLOGY OF COMA

Almost all instances of diminished alertness can be traced to widespread abnormalities of the cerebral hemispheres or to reduced activity of a special thalamocortical alerting system termed the *reticular activating system*. The proper functioning of this system, its ascending projections to the cortex, and the cortex itself are required to maintain alertness and coherence of thought. It follows that the principal causes of coma are (1) lesions that damage the RAS or its projections; (2) destruction of large portions of both cerebral hemispheres; and (3) suppression of reticulocerebral function by drugs, toxins, or metabolic derangements such as hypoglycemia, anoxia, uremia, and hepatic failure.

The proximity of the RAS to structures that control pupillary function and eye movements permits clinical localization of the cause of coma in many cases. Pupillary enlargement with loss of light reaction and loss of vertical and adduction movements of the eyes suggests that the likely location of the lesion is in the upper brainstem. Conversely, preservation of pupillary reactivity and eye movements absolves the upper brainstem and indicates that widespread structural lesions or metabolic suppression of the cerebral hemispheres is responsible.

Coma Due to Cerebral Mass Lesions and Herniations   The cranial cavity is separated into compartments by infoldings of the dura. The two cerebral hemispheres are separated by the falx, and the anterior and posterior fossae by the tentorium. Herniation refers to displacement of brain tissue into a compartment that it normally does not occupy. Many of the signs associated with coma, and indeed coma itself, can be attributed to these tissue shifts, and certain clinical configurations are characteristic of specific herniations (Fig. 268-1). They are in essence "false localizing" signs since they derive from compression of brain structures at a distance from the mass.

The most common herniations are from the supratentorial to the infratentorial compartments through the tentorial opening, hence *transtentorial*. *Uncal transtentorial herniation* refers to impaction of the anterior medial temporal gyrus (the uncus) into the tentorial opening just anterior to and adjacent to the midbrain (Fig. 268-1, A). The displaced brain tissue compresses the third nerve as it traverses the subarachnoid space, and results in enlargement of the ipsilateral pupil ronal excitability (drug and alcohol intoxication, anesthesia, and epilepsy). The same metabolic abnormalities that produce coma may in milder form induce widespread cortical dysfunction and an acute confusional state. Thus, in metabolic encephalopathies, clouded consciousness and coma are in a continuum.

Cerebral neurons are fully dependent on cerebral blood flow (CBF) and the related delivery of oxygen and glucose. CBF is ~75 mL per 100g/min in gray matter and 30 mL per 100 g/min in white matter (mean = 55 mL per 100 g/min); oxygen consumption is 3.5 mL per 100 g/min, and glucose utilization is 5 mg per 100 g/min. Brain stores of glucose provide energy for ~2 min after blood flow is interrupted, and oxygen stores last 8–10 s after the cessation of blood flow. Simultaneous hypoxia and ischemia exhaust glucose more rapidly. The electroencephalogram (EEG) rhythm in these circumstances becomes diffusely slowed, typical of metabolic encephalopathies, and as conditions of substrate delivery worsen, eventually all recordable brain electrical activity ceases. In almost all instances of metabolic encephalopathy, the global metabolic activity of the brain is reduced in proportion to the degree of diminished consciousness.

Conditions such as hypoglycemia, hyponatremia, hyperosmolarity, hypercapnia, hypercalcemia, and hepatic and renal failure are associated with a variety of alterations in neurons and astrocytes. Unlike hypoxia-ischemia, which causes neuronal destruction, metabolic disorders generally cause only minor neuropathologic changes. The reversible effects of these conditions on the brain are not understood but may result from impaired energy supplies, changes in ion fluxes across neuronal membranes, and neurotransmitter abnormalities. For example, the high brain ammonia concentration of hepatic coma interferes with cerebral energy metabolism and with the Na^+, K^+-ATPase pump, increases the number and size of astrocytes, alters nerve cell function, and causes increased concentrations of potentially toxic products of ammonia metabolism; it may also result in abnormalities of neurotransmitters, including putative "false" neurotransmitters that are active at receptor sites. Apart from hyperammonemia, which of these mechanisms is of critical importance is not clear. The mechanism of the encephalopathy of renal failure is also not known. Unlike ammonia, urea itself does not produce central nervous system (CNS) toxicity. A multifactorial causation has been proposed, including increased permeability of the blood-brain barrier to toxic substances such as organic acids and an increase in brain calcium or cerebrospinal fluid (CSF) phosphate content.

FIGURE 268-1 Types of cerebral herniation. (A) uncal; (B) central; (C) transfalcial; (D) foraminal.

(putatively because the fibers subserving parasympathetic pupillary function are located peripherally in the nerve). The coma that follows is due to compression of the midbrain against the opposite tentorial edge by the displaced parahippocampal gyrus (Fig. 268-2). In some cases, the lateral displacement of the midbrain causes compression of the opposite cerebral peduncle, producing a Babinski sign and hemiparesis contralateral to the original hemiparesis (the Kernohan-Woltman sign). In addition to compressing the upper brainstem, tissue shifts, including herniations, may compress major blood vessels, particularly the anterior and posterior cerebral arteries as they pass over the tentorial reflections, thus producing brain infarctions. The distortions may also entrap portions of the ventricular system, resulting in regional hydrocephalus.

Central transtentorial herniation denotes a symmetric downward movement of the thalamic medial structures through the tentorial opening with compression of the upper midbrain (Fig. 268-1, B). Miotic pupils and drowsiness are the heralding signs. Both temporal and central herniations have classically been considered to cause a progressive compression of the brainstem from above in an orderly manner: first the midbrain, then the pons, and finally the medulla. The result is a sequence of neurologic signs that corresponds to each affected level. Other forms of herniation are *transfalcial herniation* (displacement of the cingulate gyrus under the falx and across the midline, Fig. 268-1, C), and *foraminal herniation* (downward forcing of the cerebellar tonsils into the foramen magnum, Fig. 268-1, D), which causes compression of the medulla and respiratory arrest.

A direct relationship between the various configurations of transtentorial herniations and coma is not always found. Drowsiness and stupor typically occur with moderate horizontal shifts at the level of the diencephalon (thalami) well before transtentorial or other herniations are evident. Lateral shift may be quantified on axial images of CT and MRI scans (Fig. 268-2). In cases of *acutely appearing masses*, horizontal displacement of the pineal calcification of 3–5 mm is generally associated with drowsiness, 6–8 mm with stupor, and >9 mm with coma. Intrusion of the medial temporal lobe into the tentorial opening may be apparent on MRI and CT scans by an obliteration of the cisterns that surround the upper brainstem.

Coma Due to Metabolic Disorders Many systemic metabolic abnormalities cause coma by interrupting the delivery of energy substrates (hypoxia, ischemia, hypoglycemia) or by altering neu-

FIGURE 268-2 Coronal (A) and axial (B) magnetic resonance images from a stuporous patient with a left third nerve palsy as a result of a large left-sided subdural hematoma (seen as a gray-white rim). The upper midbrain and lower thalamic regions are compressed and displaced horizontally away from the mass, and there is transtentorial herniation of the medial temporal lobe structures, including the uncus anteriorly. The lateral ventricle opposite to the hematoma has become enlarged as a result of compression of the third ventricle.

Coma and seizures are a common accompaniment of any large shifts in sodium and water balance in the brain. These changes in osmolarity arise from systemic medical disorders including diabetic ketoacidosis, the nonketotic hyperosmolar state, and hyponatremia from any cause (e.g., water intoxication, excessive secretion of antidiuretic hormone or atrial natriuretic peptides). Sodium levels <125 mmol/L induce confusion, and <115 mmol/L are associated with coma and convulsions. In hyperosmolar coma the serum osmolarity is generally >350 mosmol/L. Hypercapnia depresses the level of consciousness in proportion to the rise in CO_2 tension in the blood. *In all of these metabolic encephalopathies, the degree of neurologic change depends to a large extent on the rapidity with which the serum changes occur.* The pathophysiology of other metabolic encephalopathies such as hypercalcemia, hypothyroidism, vitamin B_{12} deficiency, and hypothermia are incompletely understood but must also reflect derangements of CNS biochemistry and membrane function.

Epileptic Coma Continuous, generalized electrical discharges of the cortex (*seizures*) are associated with coma even in the absence of epileptic motor activity (*convulsions*). The self-limited coma that follows seizures, termed the *postictal state*, may be due to exhaustion of energy reserves or effects of locally toxic molecules that are the byproduct of seizures. The postictal state produces a pattern of continuous, generalized slowing of the background EEG activity similar to that of other metabolic encephalopathies.

Toxic Drug-Induced Coma This common class of encephalopathy is in large measure reversible and leaves no residual damage providing hypoxia does not supervene. Many drugs and toxins are capable of depressing nervous system function. Some produce coma by affecting both the brainstem nuclei, including the RAS, and the cerebral cortex. The combination of cortical and brainstem signs, which occurs in certain drug overdoses, may lead to an incorrect diagnosis of structural brainstem disease. Overdose of medications that have atropinic actions produces physical signs such as dilated pupils, tachycardia, and dry skin.

Coma Due to Widespread Damage to the Cerebral Hemispheres This special category, comprising a number of unrelated disorders, results from widespread structural cerebral damage, thereby simulating a metabolic disorder of the cortex. The effect of prolonged hypoxia-ischemia is perhaps the best known and one in which it is not possible to distinguish the acute effects of hypoperfusion of the brain from the further effects of generalized neuronal damage. Similar bihemispheral damage is produced by disorders that occlude small blood vessels throughout the brain; examples include cerebral malaria, thrombotic thrombocytopenic purpura, and hyperviscosity. The presence of seizures and the bihemispheral damage are sometimes an indication of this class of disorder.

APPROACH TO THE PATIENT:
Coma

Acute respiratory and cardiovascular problems should be attended to prior to neurologic assessment. In most instances, a complete medical evaluation, except for vital signs, funduscopy, and examination for nuchal rigidity, may be deferred until the neurologic evaluation has established the severity and nature of coma. The approach to the patient with cranial trauma is discussed in Chap. 373.

HISTORY In many cases, the cause of coma is immediately evident (e.g., trauma, cardiac arrest, or known drug ingestion). In the remainder, certain points are especially useful: (1) the circumstances and rapidity with which neurologic symptoms developed; (2) the antecedent symptoms (confusion, weakness, headache, fever, seizures, dizziness, double vision, or vomiting); (3) the use of medications, illicit drugs, or alcohol; and (4) chronic liver, kidney, lung, heart, or other medical disease. Direct interrogation of family and observers on the scene, in person or by telephone, is an important part of the initial evaluation. Ambulance technicians often provide the most useful information.

GENERAL PHYSICAL EXAMINATION The temperature, pulse, respiratory rate and pattern, and blood pressure should be measured quickly. Fever suggests a systemic infection, bacterial meningitis, or encephalitis; only rarely is it attributable to a brain lesion that has disturbed hypothalamic temperature-regulating centers ("*central fever*"). A slight elevation in temperature may follow vigorous convulsions. High body temperature, 42–44°C, associated with dry skin should arouse the suspicion of heat stroke or anticholinergic drug intoxication. Hypothermia is observed with alcoholic, barbiturate, sedative, or phenothiazine intoxication; hypoglycemia; peripheral circulatory failure; or hypothyroidism. Hypothermia itself causes coma only when the temperature is <31°C. Tachypnea may indicate systemic acidosis or pneumonia. Aberrant respiratory patterns that reflect brainstem disorders are discussed below. Marked hypertension either indicates hypertensive encephalopathy or is the result of a rapid rise in intracranial pressure (ICP; the Cushing response) most often after cerebral hemorrhage or head injury. Hypotension is characteristic of coma from alcohol or barbiturate intoxication, internal hemorrhage, myocardial infarction, sepsis, profound hypothyroidism, or Addisonian crisis.

The funduscopic examination can detect subarachnoid hemorrhage (subhyaloid hemorrhages), hypertensive encephalopathy (exudates, hemorrhages, vessel-crossing changes, papilledema), and increased ICP (papilledema). Cutaneous petechiae suggest thrombotic thrombocytopenic purpura, meningococcemia, or a bleeding diathesis from which an intracerebral hemorrhage has arisen.

NEUROLOGIC EXAMINATION First, the patient should be observed without intervention by the examiner. Tossing about in the bed, reaching up toward the face, crossing legs, yawning, swallowing, coughing, or moaning denote a state close to normal awakeness. Lack of restless movements on one side or an outturned leg suggests a hemiplegia. Intermittent twitching movements of a foot, finger, or facial muscle may be the only sign of seizures. Multifocal myoclonus almost always indicates a metabolic disorder, particularly uremia, anoxia, or drug intoxication (lithium and haloperidol are particularly likely to cause this sign), or the rare conditions of a prion disease (Chap. 378) or "Hashimoto encephalopathy." In a drowsy and confused patient bilateral *asterixis* is a certain sign of metabolic encephalopathy or drug intoxication.

The terms *decorticate rigidity* and *decerebrate rigidity*, or "posturing," describe stereotyped arm and leg movements occurring spontaneously or elicited by sensory stimulation. Flexion of the elbows and wrists and supination of the arm (decortication) suggests bilateral damage rostral to the midbrain, whereas extension of the elbows and wrists with pronation (decerebration) indicates damage to motor tracts in the midbrain or caudal diencephalon. The less frequent combination of arm extension with leg flexion or flaccid legs is associated with lesions in the pons. These concepts have been adapted from animal work and cannot be applied with the same precision to coma in humans. In fact, acute and widespread disorders of any type, regardless of location, frequently cause limb extension, and almost all such extensor posturing becomes predominantly flexor as time passes. Posturing may also be unilateral and may coexist with purposeful limb movements, usually reflecting incomplete damage to the motor system.

LEVEL OF AROUSAL A sequence of increasingly intense stimuli is used to determine the threshold for arousal and the optimal motor response of each side of the body. The results of testing may vary from minute to minute and serial examinations are most useful. Tickling the nostrils with a cotton wisp is a moderate stimulus to arousal—all but deeply stuporous and comatose patients will move the head away and rouse to some degree. Using the hand to remove the offending stimulus represents an even greater degree of responsiveness. Stereotyped posturing in response to noxious stimuli indicates severe dysfunction of the corticospinal system. Abduction-avoidance movement of a limb is usually purposeful and denotes an intact

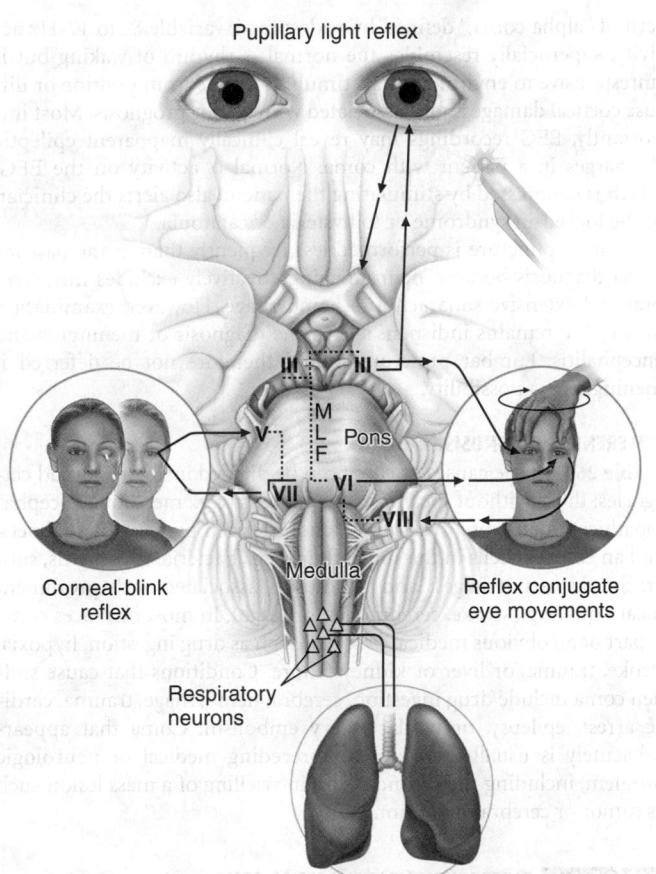

FIGURE 268-3 Examination of brainstem reflexes in coma. Midbrain and third nerve function are tested by pupillary reaction to light, pontine function by spontaneous and reflex eye movements and corneal responses, and medullary function by respiratory and pharyngeal responses. Reflex conjugate, horizontal eye movements are dependent on the medial longitudinal fasciculus (MLF) interconnecting the sixth and contralateral third nerve nuclei. Head rotation (oculocephalic reflex) or caloric stimulation of the labyrinths (oculovestibular reflex) elicits contraversive eye movements (for details see text).

corticospinal system. Pressure on the knuckles or bony prominences and pinprick stimulation are humane forms of noxious stimuli; pinching the skin causes unsightly ecchymoses and is generally not necessary but may be useful in eliciting abduction withdrawal movements of the limbs.

BRAINSTEM REFLEXES Assessment of brainstem function is essential to localization of the lesion in coma (**Fig. 268-3**). The brainstem reflexes that are conveniently examined are pupillary responses to light, spontaneous and elicited eye movements, corneal responses, and the respiratory pattern. As a rule, when these brainstem activities are preserved, particularly the pupil reactions and eye movements, coma must be ascribed to bilateral hemispheral disease. The converse, however, is not always true, as a mass in the hemispheres may be the underlying cause of coma but nonetheless produce brainstem signs by inducing transtentorial herniation.

Pupillary Signs Pupillary reactions are examined with a bright, diffuse light (not an ophthalmoscope); if the response is absent, this should be confirmed by observation through a magnifying lens. Normally reactive and round pupils of midsize (2.5–5 mm) essentially exclude midbrain damage, either primary or secondary to compression. Reaction to light is often difficult to appreciate in pupils < 2 mm in diameter, and bright room lighting mutes pupillary reactivity. One unreactive and enlarged pupil (>6 mm) or one that is poorly reactive signifies compression of the third nerve from the effects of a mass above. Enlargement of the pupil contralateral

to a mass may occur first but is infrequent. An oval and slightly eccentric pupil is a transitional sign that accompanies early midbrain–third nerve compression. The most extreme pupillary sign, bilaterally dilated and unreactive pupils, indicates severe midbrain damage, usually from compression by a supratentorial mass. Ingestion of drugs with anticholinergic activity, the use of mydriatic eye drops, and direct ocular trauma are among the causes of misleading pupillary enlargement.

Unilateral miosis in coma has been attributed to dysfunction of sympathetic efferents originating in the posterior hypothalamus and descending in the tegmentum of the brainstem to the cervical cord. It is an occasional finding with a large cerebral hemorrhage that affects the thalamus. Reactive and bilaterally small (1–2.5 mm) but not pinpoint pupils are seen in metabolic encephalopathies or in deep bilateral hemispheral lesions such as hydrocephalus or thalamic hemorrhage. Very small but reactive pupils (<1 mm) characterize narcotic or barbiturate overdoses but also occur with extensive pontine hemorrhage. The response to naloxone and the presence of reflex eye movements (see below) distinguish these.

Ocular Movements The eyes are first observed by elevating the lids and noting the resting position and spontaneous movements of the globes. Lid tone, tested by lifting the eyelids and noting their resistance to opening and the speed of closure, is reduced progressively as coma deepens. Horizontal divergence of the eyes at rest is normal in drowsiness. As coma deepens, the ocular axes may become parallel again.

Spontaneous eye movements in coma often take the form of conjugate horizontal roving. This finding alone exonerates the midbrain and pons and has the same significance as normal reflex eye movements (see below). Conjugate horizontal ocular deviation to one side indicates damage to the pons on the opposite side or alternatively, to the frontal lobe on the same side. This phenomenon is summarized by the following maxim: *The eyes look toward a hemispheral lesion and away from a brainstem lesion.* Seizures also drive the eyes to one side. On rare occasions, the eyes may turn paradoxically away from the side of a deep hemispheral lesion ("wrong-way eyes"). The eyes turn down and inward as a result of thalamic and upper midbrain lesions, typically with thalamic hemorrhage. "Ocular bobbing" describes brisk downward and slow upward movements of the eyes associated with loss of horizontal eye movements and is diagnostic of bilateral pontine damage, usually from thrombosis of the basilar artery. "Ocular dipping" is a slower, arrhythmic downward movement followed by a faster upward movement in patients with normal reflex horizontal gaze; it indicates diffuse cortical anoxic damage. Many other complex eye movements are known but do not have the same clinical importance as those mentioned earlier.

The oculocephalic reflexes depend on the integrity of the ocular motor nuclei and their interconnecting tracts that extend from the midbrain to the pons and medulla. These reflexes are elicited by moving the head from side to side or vertically and observing evoked eye movements in the direction opposite to the head movement (Fig. 268-3). The movements, called somewhat inappropriately "doll's eyes" (which refers more accurately to the reflex elevation of the eyelids with flexion of the neck), are normally suppressed in the awake patient. The ability to elicit them therefore indicates a reduced cortical influence on the brainstem. Furthermore, preservation of evoked reflex eye movements signifies the integrity of the brainstem and implies that the origin of unconsciousness lies in the cerebral hemispheres. The opposite, an absence of reflex eye movements, usually signifies damage within the brainstem but can be produced infrequently by profound overdoses of certain drugs. Normal pupillary size and light reaction distinguishes most drug-induced comas from structural brainstem damage.

Thermal, or "caloric," stimulation of the vestibular apparatus (oculovestibular response) provides a more intense stimulus for the oculocephalic reflex but gives fundamentally the same information. The test is performed by irrigating the external auditory canal with cool water in order to induce convection currents in the labyrinths. After a brief latency, the result is tonic deviation of both eyes to the side of cool-water irrigation and nystagmus in the opposite direction. (The acronym "COWS" has been used to remind generations of medical students of the direction of nystagmus—"cold water opposite, warm water same.") The loss of conjugate ocular movements indicates brainstem damage. The absence of nystagmus despite conjugate deviation of the globes indicates that the cerebral hemispheres are damaged or metabolically suppressed.

By touching the cornea with a wisp of cotton, a response consisting of brief bilateral lid closure is normally observed. The corneal reflexes depend on the integrity of pontine pathways between the fifth (afferent) and both seventh (efferent) cranial nerves; although rarely useful alone, in conjunction with reflex eye movements they are important clinical tests of pontine function. CNS depressant drugs diminish or eliminate the corneal responses soon after reflex eye movements are paralyzed but before the pupils become unreactive to light. The corneal (and pharyngeal) response may be lost for a time on the side of an acute hemiplegia.

Respiratory Patterns   These are of less localizing value in comparison to other brainstem signs. Shallow, slow, but regular breathing suggests metabolic or drug depression. Cheyne-Stokes respiration in its classic cyclic form, ending with a brief apneic period, signifies bihemispheral damage or metabolic suppression and commonly accompanies light coma. Rapid, deep (Kussmaul) breathing usually implies metabolic acidosis but may also occur with pontomesencephalic lesions. Agonal gasps are the result of lower brainstem (medullary) damage and are well known as the terminal respiratory pattern of severe brain damage. A number of other cyclic breathing variations have been described but are of lesser significance.

LABORATORY STUDIES AND IMAGING

The studies that are most useful in the diagnosis of coma are: chemical-toxicologic analysis of blood and urine, cranial CT or MRI, EEG, and CSF examination. Arterial blood-gas analysis is helpful in patients with lung disease and acid-base disorders. The metabolic aberrations commonly encountered in clinical practice require measurements of electrolytes, glucose, calcium, osmolarity, and renal (blood urea nitrogen) and hepatic (NH_3) function. Toxicologic analysis is necessary in any case of coma where the diagnosis is not immediately clear. However, the presence of exogenous drugs or toxins, especially alcohol, does not exclude the possibility that other factors, particularly head trauma, are also contributing to the clinical state. An ethanol level of 43 mmol/L (0.2 g/dL) in nonhabituated patients generally causes impaired mental activity and of >65 mmol/L (0.3 g/dL) is associated with stupor. The development of tolerance may allow the chronic alcoholic to remain awake at levels >87 mmol/L (0.4 g/dL).

The availability of CT and MRI has focused attention on causes of coma that are radiologically detectable (e.g., hemorrhages, tumors, or hydrocephalus). Resorting primarily to this approach, although at times expedient, is imprudent because most cases of coma (and confusion) are metabolic or toxic in origin. The notion that a normal CT scan excludes anatomic lesions as the cause of coma is also erroneous. Bilateral hemisphere infarction, acute brainstem infarction, encephalitis, meningitis, mechanical shearing of axons as a result of closed head trauma, sagittal sinus thrombosis, and subdural hematomas that are isodense to adjacent brain are some of the disorders that may not be detected. Nevertheless, if the source of coma remains unknown, a scan should be obtained.

The EEG is useful in metabolic or drug-induced states but is rarely diagnostic, except when coma is due to clinically unrecognized seizures, to herpesvirus encephalitis, or to prion (Creutzfeldt-Jakob) disease. The amount of background slowing of the EEG is a reflection of the severity of any diffuse encephalopathy. Predominant high-voltage slowing (δ or triphasic waves) in the frontal regions is typical of metabolic coma, as from hepatic failure, and widespread fast (β) activity implicates sedative drugs (e.g., diazepines, barbiturates). A special pattern of "alpha coma," defined by widespread, variable 8- to 12-Hz activity, superficially resembles the normal α rhythm of waking but is unresponsive to environmental stimuli. It results from pontine or diffuse cortical damage and is associated with a poor prognosis. Most importantly, EEG recordings may reveal clinically inapparent epileptic discharges in a patient with coma. Normal α activity on the EEG, which is suppressed by stimulating the patient, also alerts the clinician to the locked-in syndrome or to hysteria or catatonia.

Lumbar puncture is performed less frequently than in the past for coma diagnosis because neuroimaging effectively excludes intracerebral and extensive subarachnoid hemorrhage. However, examination of the CSF remains indispensable in the diagnosis of meningitis and encephalitis. Lumbar puncture should therefore not be deferred if meningitis is a possibility.

DIFFERENTIAL DIAGNOSIS OF COMA

(Table 268-1) The causes of coma can be divided into three broad categories: those without focal neurologic signs (e.g., metabolic encephalopathies); meningitis syndromes, characterized by fever or stiff neck and an excess of cells in the spinal fluid (e.g., bacterial meningitis, subarachnoid hemorrhage); and conditions associated with prominent focal signs (e.g., stroke, cerebral hemorrhage). In most instances coma is part of an obvious medical problem such as drug ingestion, hypoxia, stroke, trauma, or liver or kidney failure. Conditions that cause sudden coma include drug ingestion, cerebral hemorrhage, trauma, cardiac arrest, epilepsy, or basilar artery embolism. Coma that appears subacutely is usually related to a preceding medical or neurologic problem, including the secondary brain swelling of a mass lesion such as tumor or cerebral infarction.

TABLE 268-1   DIFFERENTIAL DIAGNOSIS OF COMA

1. Diseases that cause no focal or lateralizing neurologic signs, usually with normal brainstem functions; CT scan and cellular content of the CSF are normal
   a. Intoxications: alcohol, sedative drugs, opiates, etc.
   b. Metabolic disturbances: anoxia, hyponatremia, hypernatremia, hypercalcemia, diabetic acidosis, nonketotic hyperosmolar hyperglycemia, hypoglycemia, uremia, hepatic coma, hypercarbia, addisonian crisis, hypo- and hyperthyroid states, profound nutritional deficiency
   c. Severe systemic infections: pneumonia, septicemia, typhoid fever, malaria, Waterhouse-Friderichsen syndrome
   d. Shock from any cause
   e. Postseizure states, status epilepticus, subclinical epilepsy
   f. Hypertensive encephalopathy, eclampsia
   g. Severe hyperthermia, hypothermia
   h. Concussion
   i. Acute hydrocephalus
2. Diseases that cause meningeal irritation with or without fever, and with an excess of WBCs or RBCs in the CSF, usually without focal or lateralizing cerebral or brainstem signs; CT or MRI shows no mass lesion
   a. Subarachnoid hemorrhage from ruptured aneurysm, arteriovenous malformation, trauma
   b. Acute bacterial meningitis
   c. Viral encephalitis
   d. Miscellaneous: Fat embolism, cholesterol embolism, carcinomatous and lymphomatous meningitis, etc.
3. Diseases that cause focal brainstem or lateralizing cerebral signs, with or without changes in the CSF; CT and MRI are abnormal
   a. Hemispheral hemorrhage (basal ganglionic, thalamic) or infarction (large middle cerebral artery territory) with secondary brainstem compression
   b. Brainstem infarction due to basilar artery thrombosis or embolism
   c. Brain abscess, subdural empyema
   d. Epidural and subdural hemorrhage, brain contusion
   e. Brain tumor with surrounding edema
   f. Cerebellar and pontine hemorrhage and infarction
   g. Widespread traumatic brain injury
   h. Metabolic coma (see above) with preexisting focal damage
   i. Miscellaneous: cortical vein thrombosis, herpes simplex encephalitis, multiple cerebral emboli due to bacterial endocarditis, acute hemorrhagic leukoencephalitis, acute disseminated (postinfectious) encephalomyelitis, thrombotic thrombocytopenic purpura, cerebral vasculitis, gliomatosis cerebri, pituitary apoplexy, intravascular lymphoma, etc.

Note: CSF, cerebrospinal fluid; WBCs, white blood cells; RBCs, red blood cells.

Cerebrovascular diseases cause the greatest difficulty in coma diagnosis (Chap. 364). The most common categories are: (1) basal ganglia and thalamic hemorrhage (acute but not instantaneous onset, vomiting, headache, hemiplegia, and characteristic eye signs); (2) pontine hemorrhage (sudden onset, pinpoint pupils, loss of reflex eye movements and corneal responses, ocular bobbing, posturing, hyperventilation, and excessive sweating); (3) cerebellar hemorrhage (occipital headache, vomiting, gaze paresis, and inability to stand); (4) basilar artery thrombosis (neurologic prodrome or warning spells, diplopia, dysarthria, vomiting, eye movement and corneal response abnormalities, and asymmetric limb paresis); and (5) subarachnoid hemorrhage (precipitous coma after headache and vomiting). The most common stroke, infarction in the territory of the middle cerebral artery, does not generally cause coma, but edema surrounding large infarcts may expand during the first few days and act as a mass. The syndrome of acute hydrocephalus accompanies many intracranial diseases, particularly subarachnoid hemorrhage. It is characterized by headache and sometimes vomiting that may progress quickly to coma, with extensor posturing of the limbs, bilateral Babinski signs, small unreactive pupils, and impaired oculocephalic movements in the vertical direction.

If the history and examination do not indicate the cause of coma, then information obtained from CT or MRI may be needed. The majority of medical causes of coma can be established without a neuroimaging study.

BRAIN DEATH

This is a state of cessation of cerebral function while somatic function is maintained by artificial means and the heart continues to pump. It is the only type of brain damage that is recognized as equivalent to death. Several similar criteria have been advanced for the diagnosis of brain death, and it is essential to adhere to those standards endorsed by the local medical community. Ideal criteria are simple, can be assessed at the bedside, and allow no chance of diagnostic error. They contain three essential elements of clinical evidence: (1) widespread cortical destruction that is reflected by deep coma and unresponsiveness to all forms of stimulation; (2) global brainstem damage demonstrated by absent pupillary light reaction and by the loss of oculovestibular and corneal reflexes; and (3) destruction of the medulla manifested by complete apnea. The pulse rate is invariant and unresponsive to atropine. Diabetes insipidus is often present but may develop hours or days after the other clinical signs of brain death. The pupils are often enlarged but may be mid-sized; they should not, however, be constricted. The absence of deep tendon reflexes is not required because the spinal cord remains functional. There may or may not be Babinski signs.

Demonstration that apnea is due to irreversible medullary damage requires that the P_{CO_2} be high enough to stimulate respiration during a test of spontaneous breathing. *Apnea testing* can be done safely by the use of diffusion oxygenation prior to removing the ventilator. This is accomplished by preoxygenation with 100% oxygen, which is then sustained during the test by oxygen administered through a tracheal cannula. CO_2 tension increases ~0.3–0.4 kPa/min (2–3 mmHg/min) during apnea. At the end of the period of observation, typically several minutes, arterial P_{CO_2} should be at least >6.6–8.0 kPa (50–60 mmHg) for the test to be valid. Apnea is confirmed if no respiratory effort is observed in the presence of a sufficiently elevated P_{CO_2}.

The possibility of profound drug-induced or hypothermic depression of the nervous system should be excluded, and some period of observation, usually 6–24 h, is desirable during which the signs of brain death are sustained. It is advisable to delay clinical testing for at least 24 h if a cardiac arrest has caused brain death or if the inciting disease is not known. An isoelectric EEG may be used as a confirmatory test for total cerebral damage. Radionuclide brain scanning, cerebral angiography, or transcranial Doppler measurements may also be used to demonstrate the absence of cerebral blood flow but they have not been extensively correlated with pathologic changes.

Although it is largely accepted in western society that the respirator can be disconnected from a brain-dead patient, problems frequently arise because of poor communication and inadequate preparation of the family by the physician. Reasonable medical practice allows the removal of support or transfer out of an intensive care unit of patients who are not brain dead but whose condition is nonetheless hopeless and are likely to live for only a brief time.

Rx COMA

The immediate goal in a comatose patient is prevention of further nervous system damage. Hypotension, hypoglycemia, hypercalcemia, hypoxia, hypercapnia, and hyperthermia should be corrected rapidly. An oropharyngeal airway is adequate to keep the pharynx open in drowsy patients who are breathing normally. Tracheal intubation is indicated if there is apnea, upper airway obstruction, hypoventilation, or emesis, or if the patient is liable to aspirate because of coma. Mechanical ventilation is required if there is hypoventilation or a need to induce hypocapnia in order to lower ICP as described below. IV access is established, and naloxone and dextrose are administered if narcotic overdose or hypoglycemia are even remote possibilities; thiamine is given along with glucose to avoid provoking Wernicke disease in malnourished patients. In cases of suspected basilar thrombosis with brainstem ischemia, IV heparin or a thrombolytic agent is often utilized, after cerebral hemorrhage has been excluded by a neuroimaging study. Physostigmine may awaken patients with anticholinergic-type drug overdose but should be used only by experienced physicians and with careful monitoring; many physicians believe that it should only be used to treat anticholinergic overdose-associated cardiac arrhythmias. The use of benzodiazepine antagonists offers some prospect of improvement after overdoses of soporific drugs and has transient benefit in hepatic encephalopathy. IV administration of hypotonic solutions should be monitored carefully in any serious acute brain illness because of the potential for exacerbating brain swelling. Cervical spine injuries must not be overlooked, particularly prior to attempting intubation or evaluating of oculocephalic responses. Fever and meningismus indicate an urgent need for examination of the CSF to diagnose meningitis. If the lumbar puncture in a case of suspected meningitis is delayed for any reason, an antibiotic such as a third-generation cephalosporin should be administered as soon as possible, preferably after obtaining blood cultures. The management of raised ICP is discussed in Chap. 269.

PROGNOSIS

One hopes to avoid the emotionally painful, hopeless outcome of a patient who is left severely disabled or vegetative. The uniformly poor outcome of the persistent vegetative state has already been mentioned. Children and young adults may have ominous early clinical findings such as abnormal brainstem reflexes and yet recover, so that temporization in offering a prognosis in this group of patients is wise. Metabolic comas have a far better prognosis than traumatic ones. All systems for estimating prognosis in adults should be taken as approximations, and medical judgments must be tempered by factors such as age, underlying systemic disease, and general medical condition. In an attempt to collect prognostic information from large numbers of patients with head injury, the Glasgow Coma Scale was devised; empirically it has predictive value in cases of brain trauma (Table 373-2). For anoxic and metabolic coma, clinical signs such as the pupillary and motor responses after 1 day, 3 days, and 1 week have been shown to have predictive value (Fig. 269-4). The absence of the cortical waves of the somatosensory evoked potentials has also proved a strong indicator of poor outcome in coma from any cause.

FURTHER READINGS

LAUREYS S et al: Brain function in coma, vegetative state, and related disorders. Lancet Neurol 3:537, 2004

PARVIZI J AR: Neuroanatomical correlates of brainstem coma. Brain 126:1524, 2003

POSNER JB et al: *Plum and Posner's Diagnosis of Stupor and Coma*, 4th ed. New York and London, Oxford Univ Press, 2007

ROPPER AH: *Neurological and Neurosurgical Intensive Care*, 4th ed. New York, Lippincott Williams & Wilkins, 2004

WIJDICKS EFM: Current concepts: The diagnosis of brain death. N Engl J Med 344:1215, 2001

269 Neurologic Critical Care, Including Hypoxic-Ischemic Encephalopathy and Subarachnoid Hemorrhage

J. Claude Hemphill III, Wade S. Smith

Life-threatening neurologic illness may be caused by a primary disorder affecting any region of the neuraxis or may occur as a consequence of a systemic disorder such as hepatic failure, multisystem organ failure, or cardiac arrest (Table 269-1). Neurologic critical care focuses on preservation of neurologic tissue and prevention of secondary brain injury caused by ischemia, edema, and elevated intracranial pressure (ICP).

PATHOPHYSIOLOGY

Brain Edema Swelling, or edema, of brain tissue occurs with many types of brain injury. The two principal types of edema are vasogenic and cytotoxic. *Vasogenic edema* refers to the influx of fluid and solutes into the brain through an incompetent blood-brain barrier (BBB). In the normal cerebral vasculature, endothelial tight junctions associated with astrocytes create an impermeable barrier (the BBB), through which access into the brain interstitium is dependent upon specific transport mechanisms (Chap. 360). The BBB may be compromised in ischemia, trauma, infection, and metabolic derangements. Typically, vasogenic edema develops rapidly following injury. *Cytotoxic edema* refers to cellular swelling and occurs in a variety of settings including brain ischemia and trauma. Early astrocytic swelling is a hallmark of ischemia. Brain edema that is clinically significant usually represents a combination of vasogenic and cellular components. Edema can lead to increased ICP as well as tissue shifts and brain displacement from focal processes (Chap. 268). These tissue shifts can cause injury by mechanical distraction and compression in addition to the ischemia of impaired perfusion consequent to the elevated ICP.

Ischemic Cascade and Cellular Injury When delivery of substrates, principally oxygen and glucose, is inadequate to sustain cellular function, a series of interrelated biochemical reactions known as the *ischemic cascade* is initiated (see Fig. 364-2). The release of excitatory amino acids, especially glutamate, leads to influx of calcium and sodium ions, which disrupt cellular homeostasis. An increased intracellular calcium concentration may activate proteases and lipases, which then lead to lipid peroxidation and free radical–mediated cell membrane injury. Cytotoxic edema ensues, and ultimately necrotic cell death and tissue infarction occur. This pathway to irreversible cell death is common to ischemic stroke, global cerebral ischemia, and traumatic brain injury. *Penumbra* refers to ischemic brain tissue that has not yet undergone irreversible infarction, implying that the region is potentially salvageable if ischemia can be reversed. Factors that may exacerbate ischemic brain injury include systemic hypotension and hypoxia, which further reduce substrate delivery to vulnerable brain tissue, and fever, seizures, and hyperglycemia, which can increase cellular metabolism outstripping compensatory processes. Clinically, these events are known as *secondary brain insults* because they lead to exacerbation of the primary brain injury. Prevention, identification, and treatment of secondary brain insults are fundamental goals of management.

An alternative pathway of cellular injury is *apoptosis*. This process implies programmed cell death, which may occur in the setting of ischemic stroke, global cerebral ischemia, traumatic brain injury, and possibly intracerebral hemorrhage. Apoptotic cell death can be distinguished histologically from the necrotic cell death of ischemia and is mediated through a different set of biochemical pathways. At present, interventions for prevention and treatment of apoptotic cell death remain less well defined than those for ischemia. Excitotoxicity and mechanisms of cell death are discussed in more detail in Chap. 360.

TABLE 269-1 NEUROLOGIC DISORDERS IN CRITICAL ILLNESS

Localization Along Neuroaxis	Syndrome
Central Nervous System	
Brain: Cerebral hemispheres	Global encephalopathy
	Sepsis
	Organ failure—hepatic, renal
	Medication related
	Sedatives/hypnotics/analgesics
	H_2 blockers, antihypertensives
	Drug overdose
	Electrolyte disturbance—hyponatremia, hypoglycemia
	Hypotension/hypoperfusion
	Hypoxia
	Meningitis
	Subarachnoid hemorrhage
	Wernicke's disease
	Seizure—postictal or nonconvulsive status
	Hypertensive encephalopathy
	Hypothyroidism—myxedema
	Focal deficits
	Ischemic stroke
	Tumor
	Abscess, subdural empyema
	Subdural/epidural hematoma
Brainstem	Mass effect and compression
	Ischemic stroke, intraparenchymal hemorrhage
	Hypoxia
Spinal cord	Mass effect and compression
	Disc herniation
	Epidural hematoma
	Ischemia—hypotension/embolic
	Subdural empyema
	Trauma, central cord syndrome
Peripheral Nervous System	
Peripheral nerve	
Axonal	Critical illness polyneuropathy
	Possible neuromuscular blocking agent complication
	Metabolic disturbances, uremia, hyperglycemia
	Medication effects—chemotherapeutic, antiretroviral
Demyelinating	Guillian-Barré syndrome
	Chronic inflammatory demyelinating polyneuropathy
Neuromuscular junction	Prolonged effect of neuromuscular blockade
	Medication effects—aminoglycosides
	Myasthenia-gravis, Lambert-Eaton syndrome
Muscle	Critical illness myopathy
	Septic myopathy
	Cachectic myopathy—with or without disuse atrophy
	Electrolyte disturbances—hypokalemia/hyperkalemia, hypophosphatemia
	Acute quadriplegic myopathy

Cerebral Perfusion and Autoregulation Brain tissue requires constant perfusion in order to ensure adequate delivery of substrate. The hemodynamic response of the brain has the capacity to preserve perfusion across a wide range of systemic blood pressures. Cerebral perfusion pressure (CPP), defined as the mean systemic arterial pressure (MAP) minus the ICP, provides the driving force for circulation across the capillary beds of the brain. *Autoregulation* refers to the physiologic response whereby cerebral blood flow (CBF) remains relatively constant over a wide range of blood pressures as a consequence of alterations of cerebrovascular resistance (Fig. 269-1). If systemic blood pressure drops, cerebral perfusion is preserved through vasodilatation of arterioles in the brain; likewise, arteriolar vasoconstriction occurs at high systemic pressures to prevent hyperperfusion. At the extreme limits of MAP or CPP (high or low), flow becomes directly related to perfusion pressure. These autoregulatory changes occur in the microcirculation

FIGURE 269-1 Autoregulation of cerebral blood flow (solid line). Cerebral perfusion is constant over a wide range of systemic blood pressure. Perfusion is increased in the setting of hypoxia or hypercarbia. BP, blood pressure; CBF, cerebral blood flow. *(Reprinted with permission from Anesthesiology 43:447, 1975. Copyright 1975, Lippincott Company.)*

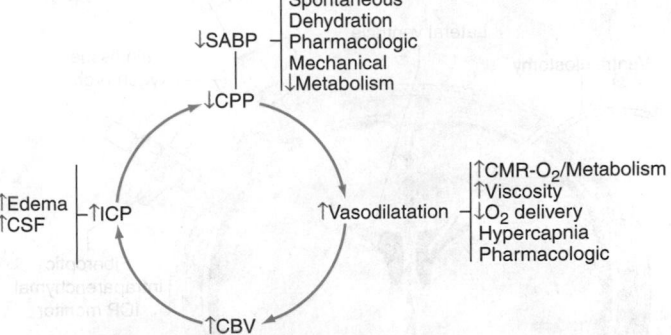

FIGURE 269-2 Ischemia and vasodilatation. Reduced cerebral perfusion pressure (CPP) leads to increased ischemia, vasodilatation, increased intracranial pressure (ICP), and further reductions in CPP, a cycle leading to further neurologic injury. CBV, cerebral blood volume; CMR, cerebral metabolic rate; CSF, cerebrospinal fluid; SABP, systolic arterial blood pressure. *(Adapted from MJ Rosner et al: J Neurosurg 83:949, 1995; with permission.)*

and are mediated by vessels below the resolution of those seen on angiography. CBF is also strongly influenced by pH and P_{CO_2}. CBF increases with hypercapnia and acidosis and decreases with hypocapnia and alkalosis. This forms the basis for the use of hyperventilation to lower ICP, and this effect on ICP is mediated through a decrease in intracranial blood volume. Cerebral autoregulation is critical to the normal homeostatic functioning of the brain, and this process may be disordered focally and unpredictably in disease states such as traumatic brain injury and severe focal cerebral ischemia.

Cerebrospinal Fluid and Intracranial Pressure The cranial contents consist essentially of brain, cerebrospinal fluid (CSF), and blood. CSF is produced principally in the choroid plexus of each lateral ventricle, exits the brain via the foramina of Luschka and Magendi, and flows over the cortex to be absorbed into the venous system along the superior sagittal sinus. Approximately 150 mL of CSF are contained within the ventricles and surrounding the brain and spinal cord; the cerebral blood volume is also ~150 mL. The bony skull offers excellent protection for the brain but allows little tolerance for additional volume. Significant increases in volume eventually result in increased ICP. Obstruction of CSF outflow, edema of cerebral tissue, or increases in volume from tumor or hematoma may increase ICP. Elevated ICP diminishes cerebral perfusion and can lead to tissue ischemia. Ischemia in turn may lead to vasodilatation via autoregulatory mechanisms designed to restore cerebral perfusion. However, vasodilatation also increases cerebral blood volume, which in turn then increases ICP, lowers CPP, and provokes further ischemia (Fig. 269-2). This vicious cycle is commonly seen in traumatic brain injury, massive intracerebral hemorrhage, and large hemispheric infarcts with significant tissue shifts.

APPROACH TO THE PATIENT:
Severe CNS Dysfunction

Critically ill patients with severe central nervous system dysfunction require rapid evaluation and intervention in order to limit primary and secondary brain injury. Initial neurologic evaluation should be performed concurrent with stabilization of basic respiratory, cardiac, and hemodynamic parameters. Significant barriers may exist to neurologic assessment in the critical care unit, including endotracheal intubation and the use of sedative or paralytic agents to facilitate procedures.

An impaired level of consciousness is common in critically ill patients. The essential first task in assessment is to determine whether the cause of dysfunction is related to a diffuse, usually metabolic, process or whether a focal, usually structural, process is implicated. Examples of diffuse processes include metabolic encephalopathies related to organ failure, drug overdose, or hypoxia-ischemia. Focal processes include ischemic and hemorrhagic stroke and traumatic brain injury, especially with intracranial hematomas. Since these two categories of disorders have fundamentally different causes, treatments, and prognoses, the initial focus is on making this distinction rapidly and accurately. The approach to the comatose patient is discussed in Chap. 268; etiologies are listed in Table 268-1.

Minor focal deficits may be present on the neurologic examination in patients with metabolic encephalopathies. However, the finding of prominent focal signs such as pupillary asymmetry, hemiparesis, gaze palsy, or paraplegia should suggest the possibility of a structural lesion. All patients with a decreased level of consciousness associated with focal findings should undergo an urgent neuroimaging procedure, as should all patients with coma of unknown etiology. CT scanning is usually the most appropriate initial study because it can be performed quickly in critically ill patients and demonstrates hemorrhage, hydrocephalus, and intracranial tissue shifts well. MRI may provide more specific information in some situations, such as acute ischemic stroke (diffusion-weighted imaging, DWI) and cerebral venous sinus thrombosis (magnetic resonance venography, MRV). Any suggestion of trauma from the history or examination should alert the examiner to the possibility of cervical spine injury and prompt an imaging evaluation using plain x-rays, MRI, or CT.

Other diagnostic studies are best utilized in specific circumstances, usually when neuroimaging studies fail to reveal a structural lesion and the etiology of the altered mental state remains uncertain. Electroencephalography (EEG) can be important in the evaluation of critically ill patients with severe brain dysfunction. The EEG of metabolic encephalopathy typically reveals generalized slowing. One of the most important uses of EEG is to help exclude inapparent seizures, especially nonconvulsive status epilepticus. Untreated continuous or frequently recurrent seizures may cause neuronal injury, making the diagnosis and treatment of seizures crucial in this patient group. Lumbar puncture (LP) may be necessary to exclude infectious processes, and an elevated opening pressure may be an important clue to cerebral venous sinus thrombosis. In patients with coma or profound encephalopathy, it is preferable to perform a neuroimaging study prior to LP. If bacterial meningitis is suspected, an LP may be performed first or antibiotics may be empirically administered before the diagnostic studies are completed. Standard laboratory evaluation of critically ill patients should include assessment of serum electrolytes (especially

Ventriculostomy

Lateral ventricle

Brain tissue oxygen probe

Fiberoptic intraparenchymal ICP monitor

FIGURE 269-3 Intracranial pressure and brain tissue oxygen monitoring. A ventriculostomy allows for drainage of cerebrospinal fluid to treat elevated intracranial pressure (ICP). Fiberoptic ICP and brain tissue oxygen monitors are usually secured using a screwlike skull bolt. Cerebral blood flow and microdialysis probes (not shown) may be placed in a manner similar to the brain tissue oxygen probe.

sodium and calcium), glucose, renal and hepatic function, complete blood count, and coagulation. Serum or urine toxicology screens should be performed in patients with encephalopathy of unknown cause. EEG, LP, and other specific laboratory tests are most useful when the mechanism of the altered level of consciousness is uncertain; they are not routinely performed in clear-cut cases of stroke or traumatic brain injury.

Monitoring of ICP can be an important tool in selected patients. In general, patients who should be considered for ICP monitoring are those with primary neurologic disorders, such as stroke or traumatic brain injury, who are at significant risk for secondary brain injury due to elevated ICP and decreased CPP. Included are patients with the following: severe traumatic brain injury [Glasgow Coma Scale (GCS) score ≤ 8 (Table 373-2)]; large tissue shifts from supratentorial ischemic or hemorrhagic stroke; or hydrocephalus from subarachnoid hemorrhage (SAH), intraventricular hemorrhage, or posterior fossa stroke. An additional disorder in which ICP monitoring can add important information is fulminant hepatic failure, in which elevated ICP may be treated with barbiturates or, eventually, liver transplantation. In general, ventriculostomy is preferable to ICP monitoring devices that are placed in the brain parenchyma, because ventriculostomy allows CSF drainage as a method of treating elevated ICP. However, parenchymal ICP monitoring is most appropriate for patients with diffuse edema and small ventricles (which may make ventriculostomy placement more difficult) or any degree of coagulopathy (in which ventriculostomy carries a higher risk of hemorrhagic complications) (Fig 269-3).

Treatment of Elevated ICP Elevated ICP may occur in a wide range of disorders including head trauma, intracerebral hemorrhage, SAH with hydrocephalus, and fulminant hepatic failure. Because CSF and blood volume can be redistributed initially, by the time elevated ICP occurs intracranial compliance is severely impaired. At this point, any small increase in the volume of CSF, intravascular blood, edema, or a mass lesion may result in a significant increase in ICP and a decrease in cerebral perfusion. This is a fundamental mechanism of secondary ischemic brain injury and constitutes an emergency that requires immediate attention. In general, ICP should be maintained at <20 mmHg and CPP should be maintained at ≤60 mmHg.

Interventions to lower ICP are ideally based on the underlying mechanism responsible for the elevated ICP (Table 269-2). For example, in hydrocephalus from SAH, the principal cause of elevated ICP is impairment of CSF drainage. In this setting, ventricular

TABLE 269-2   STEPWISE APPROACH TO TREATMENT OF ELEVATED INTRACRANIAL PRESSURE[a]

Insert ICP monitor—ventriculostomy versus parenchymal device
General goals: maintain ICP < 20 mmHg and CPP ≥ 60 mmHg
For ICP > 20–25 mmHg for >5 min:
1. Drain CSF via ventriculostomy (if in place)
2. Elevate head of the bed; midline head position
3. Osmotherapy—mannitol 25–100 g q4h as needed (maintain serum osmolality < 320 mosmol) or hypertonic saline (30 mL, 23.4% NaCl bolus)
4. Glucocorticoids—dexamethasone 4 mg q6h for vasogenic edema from tumor, abscess (avoid glucocorticoids in head trauma, ischemic and hemorrhagic stroke)
5. Sedation (e.g., morphine, propofol, or midazolam); add neuromuscular paralysis if necessary (patient will require endotracheal intubation and mechanical ventilation at this point, if not before)
6. Hyperventilation—to Pa$_{CO_2}$ 30–35 mmHg
7. Pressor therapy—phenylephrine, dopamine, or norepinephrine to maintain adequate MAP to ensure CPP ≥ 60 mmHg (maintain euvolemia to minimize deleterious systemic effects of pressors)
8. Consider second-tier therapies for refractory elevated ICP
   a. High-dose barbiturate therapy ("pentobarb coma")
   b. Aggressive hyperventilation to Pa$_{CO_2}$ < 30 mmHg
   c. Hypothermia
   d. Hemicraniectomy

[a]Throughout ICP treatment algorithm, consider repeat head CT to identify mass lesions amenable to surgical evacuation.
Note: CPP, cerebral perfusion pressure; CSF, cerebrospinal fluid; MAP, mean arterial pressure; Pa$_{CO_2}$, arterial partial pressure of carbon dioxide.

drainage of CSF is likely to be sufficient and most appropriate. In head trauma and stroke, cytotoxic edema may be most responsible, and the use of osmotic diuretics such as mannitol becomes an appropriate early step. As described above, elevated ICP may cause tissue ischemia, and, if cerebral autoregulation is intact, the resulting vasodilatation can lead to a cycle of worsening ischemia. Paradoxically, administration of vasopressor agents to increase mean arterial pressure may actually lower ICP by improving perfusion, thereby allowing autoregulatory vasoconstriction as ischemia is relieved and ultimately decreasing intracranial blood volume.

Early signs of elevated ICP include drowsiness and a diminished level of consciousness. Neuroimaging studies may reveal evidence of edema and mass effect. Hypotonic IV fluids should be avoided, and elevation of the head of the bed is recommended. Patients must be carefully observed for risk of aspiration and compromise of the airway as the level of alertness declines. Coma and unilateral pupillary changes are late signs and require immediate intervention. Emergent treatment of elevated ICP is most quickly achieved by intubation and hyperventilation, which causes vasoconstriction and reduces cerebral blood volume. In order to avoid provoking or worsening cerebral ischemia, hyperventilation is best used for short periods of time until a more definitive treatment can be instituted. Furthermore, the effects of hyperventilation on ICP are short-lived, often lasting only for several hours because of the buffering capacity of the cerebral interstitium, and rebound elevations of ICP may accompany abrupt discontinuation of hyperventilation. As the level of consciousness declines to coma, the ability to follow the neurologic status of the patient by examination deteriorates and measurement of ICP assumes greater importance. If a ventriculostomy device is in place, direct drainage of CSF to reduce ICP is possible. Finally, high-dose barbiturates, decompressive hemicraniectomy, or hypothermia are sometimes used for refractory elevations of ICP, although these have significant side effects and have not been proven to improve outcome.

Secondary Brain Insults Patients with primary brain injuries, whether due to trauma or stroke, are at risk for ongoing secondary ischemic brain injury. Because secondary brain injury can be a major determinant of a poor outcome, strategies for minimizing secondary brain insults are an integral part of the critical care of all patients. While elevated ICP may lead to secondary ischemia, most secondary brain injury is mediated through other clinical events that exacerbate the ischemic cascade already initiated by the primary brain injury. Episodes of secondary brain insults are usually not associated with apparent neurologic worsening. Rather, they lead to cumulative injury, which manifests as higher mortality or worsened long-term functional outcome. Thus, close monitoring of vital signs is important, as is early intervention to prevent secondary ischemia. Avoiding hypotension and hypoxia is critical, as significant hypotensive events (systolic blood pressure < 90 mmHg) as short as 10 min in duration have been shown to adversely influence outcome after traumatic brain injury. Even in patients with stroke or head trauma who do not require ICP monitoring, close attention to adequate cerebral perfusion is warranted. Hypoxia (pulse oximetry saturation < 90%), particularly in combination with hypotension, also leads to secondary brain injury. Likewise, fever and hyperglycemia both worsen experimental ischemia and have been associated with worsened clinical outcome after stroke and head trauma. Aggressive control of fever with a goal of normothermia is warranted but may be difficult to achieve with antipyretic medications and cooling blankets. The value of newer surface or intravascular temperature control devices for the management of refractory fever is under investigation. The use of IV insulin infusion is encouraged for control of hyperglycemia as this allows better regulation of serum glucose levels than subcutaneous insulin. A reasonable goal is to maintain the serum glucose level at <7.8 mmol/L (<140 mg/dL), although some have suggested that even tighter control is warranted. New cerebral monitoring tools that allow continuous evaluation of brain tissue oxygen tension, CBF, and metabolism (via microdialysis) may further improve the management of secondary brain injury.

CRITICAL CARE DISORDERS OF THE CENTRAL NERVOUS SYSTEM

HYPOXIC-ISCHEMIC ENCEPHALOPATHY

This occurs from lack of delivery of oxygen to the brain because of hypotension or respiratory failure. Causes include myocardial infarction, cardiac arrest, shock, asphyxiation, paralysis of respiration, and carbon monoxide or cyanide poisoning. In some circumstances, hypoxia may predominate. Carbon monoxide and cyanide poisoning are termed *histotoxic hypoxia* since they cause a direct impairment of the respiratory chain.

Clinical Manifestations Mild degrees of pure hypoxia, such as occur at high altitudes, cause impaired judgment, inattentiveness, motor incoordination, and, at times, euphoria. However, with hypoxia-ischemia, such as occurs with circulatory arrest, consciousness is lost within seconds. If circulation is restored within 3–5 min, full recovery may occur, but if hypoxia-ischemia lasts beyond 3–5 min, some degree of permanent cerebral damage is the rule. Except in extreme cases, it may be difficult to judge the precise degree of hypoxia-ischemia, and some patients make a relatively full recovery after even 8–10 min of global cerebral ischemia. The distinction between pure hypoxia and hypoxia-ischemia is important, since a Pa_{O_2} as low as 20 mmHg (2.7 kPa) can be well tolerated if it develops gradually and normal blood pressure is maintained, but short durations of very low or absent cerebral circulation may result in permanent impairment.

Clinical examination at different time points after a hypoxic-ischemic insult (especially cardiac arrest) is useful in assessing prognosis for long-term neurologic outcome. The prognosis is better for patients with intact brainstem function, as indicated by normal pupillary light responses and intact oculocephalic (doll's-eyes), oculovestibular (caloric), and corneal reflexes (Fig. 269-4). Absence of these reflexes and the presence of persistently dilated pupils that do not react to light are grave prognostic signs. A uniformly dismal prognosis from hypoxic-ischemic coma is conveyed by an absent pupillary light reflex or extensor or absent motor response to pain on day 3 following the injury. Electrophysiologically, the bilateral absence of the N20 component of

FIGURE 269-4 Prognostication of outcome in comatose survivors of cardiopulmonary resuscitation. Numbers in parentheses are 95% confidence intervals. Confounders could include use of sedatives or neuromuscular blocking agents, hypothermia therapy, organ failure, or shock. Tests denoted with an * may not be available in a timely and standardized manner. SSEP, somatosensory evoked potentials; NSE, neuron-specific enolase; FPR, false-positive rate (Chap. 3). *(From Wijdicks et al, with permission.)*

the somatosensory evoked response (SSEPs) in the first several days also conveys a poor prognosis. A very elevated serum level (>33 µg/L) of the biochemical marker neuron-specific enolase (NSE) is indicative of brain damage after resuscitation from cardiac arrest and predicts a poor outcome. However, at present, SSEPs and NSE levels may be difficult to obtain in a timely fashion, with SSEP testing requiring substantial expertise in interpretation and NSE measurements not yet standardized. Whether administration of mild hypothermia after cardiac arrest (see "Treatment") will alter the usefulness of these clinical and electrophysiologic predictors is unknown. Long-term consequences of hypoxic-ischemic encephalopathy include persistent coma or a vegetative state (Chap. 268), dementia, visual agnosia (Chap. 27), parkinsonism, choreoathetosis, cerebellar ataxia, myoclonus, seizures, and an amnestic state, which may be a consequence of selective damage to the hippocampus.

Pathology Principal histologic findings are extensive multifocal or diffuse laminar cortical necrosis (Fig. 269-5), with almost invariable involvement of the hippocampus. The hippocampal CA1 neurons are vulnerable to even brief episodes of hypoxia-ischemia, perhaps explaining why selective persistent memory deficits may occur after brief cardiac arrest. Scattered small areas of infarction or neuronal loss may be present in the basal ganglia, hypothalamus, or brainstem. In some cases, extensive bilateral thalamic scarring may affect pathways that mediate arousal, and this pathology may be responsible for the persistent vegetative state. A specific form of hypoxic-ischemic encephalopathy, so-called watershed infarcts, occurs at the distal territories between the major cerebral arteries and can cause cognitive deficits, including visual agnosia, and weakness that is greater in proximal than in distal muscle groups.

FIGURE 269-5 Cortical laminar necrosis in hypoxic-ischemic encephalopathy. T1-weighted postcontrast MRI shows cortical enhancement in a watershed distribution consistent with laminar necrosis.

Diagnosis Diagnosis is based upon the history of a hypoxic-ischemic event such as cardiac arrest. Blood pressure < 70 mmHg systolic or Pa_{O_2} < 40 mmHg is usually necessary, although both absolute levels as well as duration of exposure are important determinants of cellular injury. Carbon monoxide intoxication can be confirmed by measurement of carboxyhemoglobin and is suggested by a cherry red color of the skin, although the latter is an inconsistent clinical finding.

℞ HYPOXIC-ISCHEMIC ENCEPHALOPATHY

Treatment should be directed at restoration of normal cardiorespiratory function. This includes securing a clear airway, ensuring adequate oxygenation and ventilation, and restoring cerebral perfusion, whether by cardiopulmonary resuscitation, fluid, pressors, or cardiac pacing. Hypothermia may target the neuronal cell injury cascade and has substantial neuroprotective properties in experimental models of brain injury. In two trials, mild hypothermia (33°C) improved functional outcome in patients who remained comatose after resuscitation from a cardiac arrest. Treatment was initiated within minutes of cardiac resuscitation and continued for 12 h in one study and 24 h in the other. Potential complications of hypothermia include coagulopathy and an increased risk of infection. Based upon these studies, the International Liaison Committee on Resuscitation issued the following advisory statement in 2003: "Unconscious adult patients with spontaneous circulation after out-of-hospital cardiac arrest should be cooled to 32°–34°C for 12–24 h when the initial rhythm was ventricular fibrillation."

Severe carbon monoxide intoxication may be treated with hyperbaric oxygen. Anticonvulsants may be needed to control seizures, although these are not usually given prophylactically. Posthypoxic myoclonus may respond to oral administration of clonazepam at doses of 1.5–10 mg daily or valproate at doses of 300–1200 mg daily in divided doses. Myoclonic status epilepticus within 24 h after a primary circulatory arrest portends a universally poor prognosis, even if seizures are controlled.

DELAYED POSTANOXIC ENCEPHALOPATHY

Delayed postanoxic encephalopathy is an uncommon phenomenon in which patients appear to make an initial recovery from hypoxic-ischemic insult but then develop a relapse characterized by apathy, confusion, and agitation. Progressive neurologic deficits may include shuffling gait, diffuse rigidity and spasticity, persistent parkinsonism or myoclonus, and, on occasion, coma and death after 1–2 weeks. Widespread cerebral demyelination may be present.

Carbon monoxide and cyanide intoxication can also cause a delayed encephalopathy. Little clinical impairment is evident when the

patient first regains consciousness, but a parkinsonian syndrome characterized by akinesia and rigidity without tremor may develop. Symptoms can worsen over months, accompanied by increasing evidence of damage in the basal ganglia as seen on both CT and MRI.

METABOLIC ENCEPHALOPATHIES

Altered mental states, variously described as confusion, delirium, disorientation, and encephalopathy, are present in many patients with severe illness in an intensive care unit (ICU). Older patients are particularly vulnerable to delirium, a confusional state characterized by disordered perception, frequent hallucinations, delusions, and sleep disturbance. This is often attributed to medication effects, sleep deprivation, pain, and anxiety. The term *ICU psychosis* has been used to describe a mental state with profound agitation occurring in this setting. The presence of family members in the ICU may help to calm and orient agitated patients, and in severe cases, low doses of neuroleptics (e.g., haloperidol 0.5–1 mg) can be useful. Ultimately, the psychosis resolves with improvement in the underlying illness and a return to familiar surroundings.

In the ICU setting, several metabolic causes of an altered level of consciousness predominate. Hypercarbic encephalopathy can present with headache, confusion, stupor, or coma. Hypoventilation syndrome occurs most frequently in patients with a history of chronic CO_2 retention who are receiving oxygen therapy for emphysema or chronic pulmonary disease (Chap. 258). The elevated Pa_{CO_2} leading to CO_2 narcosis may have a direct anesthetic effect, and cerebral vasodilatation from increased Pa_{CO_2} can lead to increased ICP. Hepatic encephalopathy is suggested by asterixis and can occur in chronic liver failure or acute fulminant hepatic failure. Both hyperglycemia and hypoglycemia can cause encephalopathy, as can hypernatremia and hyponatremia. Confusion, impairment of eye movements, and gait ataxia are the hallmarks of acute Wernicke's disease (see below).

SEPTIC ENCEPHALOPATHY

Pathogenesis In patients with sepsis, the systemic response to infectious agents leads to the release of circulating inflammatory mediators that appear to contribute to encephalopathy. Critical illness, in association with the systemic inflammatory response syndrome (SIRS), can lead to multisystem organ failure. This syndrome can occur in the setting of apparent sepsis, severe burns, or trauma, even without clear identification of an infectious agent. Many patients with critical illness, sepsis, or SIRS develop encephalopathy without obvious explanation. This condition is broadly termed *septic encephalopathy*. While the specific mediators leading to neurologic dysfunction remain uncertain, it is clear that the encephalopathy is not simply the result of metabolic derangements of multiorgan failure. The cytokines tumor necrosis factor , interleukin (IL) 1, IL-2, and IL-6 are thought to play a role in this syndrome.

Diagnosis Septic encephalopathy presents clinically as a diffuse dysfunction of the brain without prominent focal findings. Confusion, disorientation, agitation, and fluctuations in level of alertness are typical. In more profound cases, especially with hemodynamic compromise, the decrease in level of alertness can be more prominent, at times resulting in coma. Hyperreflexia and frontal release signs such as a grasp or snout reflex (Chap. 27) can be seen. Abnormal movements such as myoclonus, tremor, or asterixis can occur. Septic encephalopathy is quite common, occurring in the majority of patients with sepsis and multisystem organ failure. Diagnosis is often difficult because of the multiple potential causes of neurologic dysfunction in critically ill patients and requires exclusion of structural, metabolic, toxic, and infectious (e.g., meningitis or encephalitis) causes. The mortality of patients with septic encephalopathy severe enough to produce coma approaches 50%, although this principally reflects the severity of the underlying critical illness and is not a singular result of the septic encephalopathy. Patients dying from severe sepsis or septic shock may have elevated levels of the serum brain injury biomarker S-100β and neuropathologic findings of neuronal apoptosis and cerebral ischemic

FIGURE 269-6 Central pontine myelinolysis. Axial T2-weighted MR scan through the pons reveals a symmetric area of abnormal high signal intensity within the basis pontis (*arrows*).

injury. However, successful treatment of the underlying critical illness almost always results in complete resolution of the encephalopathy, with profound long-term cognitive disability being uncommon.

CENTRAL PONTINE MYELINOLYSIS

This disorder typically presents in a devastating fashion as quadriplegia and pseudobulbar palsy. Predisposing factors include severe underlying medical illness or nutritional deficiency; most cases are associated with rapid correction of hyponatremia or with hyperosmolar states. The pathology consists of demyelination without inflammation in the base of the pons, with relative sparing of axons and nerve cells. MRI is useful in establishing the diagnosis (Fig. 269-6) and may also identify partial forms that present as confusion, dysarthria, and/or disturbances of conjugate gaze without quadriplegia. Occasional cases present with lesions outside of the brainstem. Therapeutic guidelines for the restoration of severe hyponatremia should aim for gradual correction, i.e., by ≥10 mmol/L (10 meq/L) within 24 h and 20 mmol/L (20 meq/L) within 48 h.

WERNICKE'S DISEASE

Wernicke's disease is a common and preventable disorder due to a deficiency of thiamine (Chap. 71). In the United States, alcoholics account for most cases, but patients with malnutrition due to hyperemesis, starvation, renal dialysis, cancer, AIDS, or rarely gastric surgery are also at risk. The characteristic clinical triad is that of ophthalmoplegia, ataxia, and global confusion. However, only one-third of patients with acute Wernicke's disease present with the classic clinical triad. Most patients are profoundly disoriented, indifferent, and inattentive, although rarely they have an agitated delirium related to ethanol withdrawal. If the disease is not treated, stupor, coma, and death may ensue. Ocular motor abnormalities include horizontal nystagmus on lateral gaze, lateral rectus palsy (usually bilateral), conjugate gaze palsies, and rarely ptosis. Gait ataxia probably results from a combination of polyneuropathy, cerebellar involvement, and vestibular paresis. The pupils are usually spared, but they may become miotic with advanced disease.

Wernicke's disease is usually associated with other manifestations of nutritional disease, such as polyneuropathy. Rarely, amblyopia or myelopathy occurs. Tachycardia and postural hypotension may be related to impaired function of the autonomic nervous system or to the coexistence of cardiovascular beriberi. Patients who recover show improvement in ocular palsies within hours after the administration of thiamine, but horizontal nystagmus may persist. Ataxia improves more slowly than the ocular motor abnormalities. Approximately half recover incompletely and are left with a slow, shuffling, wide-based gait and an inability to tandem walk. Apathy, drowsiness, and confusion improve more gradually. As these symptoms recede, an amnestic state with impairment in recent memory and learning may become more apparent (*Korsakoff's psychosis*). Korsakoff's psychosis is fre-

FIGURE 269-7 Wernicke's disease. Coronal T1-weighted postcontrast MRI reveals abnormal enhancement of the mammillary bodies (*arrows*), typical of acute Wernicke's encephalopathy.

quently persistent; the residual mental state is characterized by gaps in memory, confabulation, and disordered temporal sequencing.

Pathology   Periventricular lesions surround the third ventricle, aqueduct, and fourth ventricle, with petechial hemorrhages in occasional acute cases and atrophy of the mamillary bodies in most chronic cases. There is frequently endothelial proliferation, demyelination, and some neuronal loss. These changes may be detected by MRI scanning (Fig. 269-7). The amnestic defect is related to lesions in the dorsal medial nuclei of the thalamus.

Pathogenesis   Thiamine is a cofactor of several enzymes, including transketolase, pyruvate dehydrogenase, and α-ketoglutarate dehydrogenase. Thiamine deficiency produces a diffuse decrease in cerebral glucose utilization and results in mitochondrial damage. Glutamate accumulates owing to impairment of α-ketoglutarate dehydrogenase activity and, in combination with the energy deficiency, may result in excitotoxic cell damage.

℞ WERNICKE'S DISEASE

Wernicke's disease is a medical emergency and requires immediate administration of thiamine, in a dose of 100 mg either IV or IM. The dose should be given daily until the patient resumes a normal diet and should be begun prior to treatment with IV glucose solutions. Glucose infusions may precipitate Wernicke's disease in a previously unaffected patient or cause a rapid worsening of an early form of the disease. For this reason, thiamine should be administered to all alcoholic patients requiring parenteral glucose.

CRITICAL CARE DISORDERS OF THE PERIPHERAL NERVOUS SYSTEM

Critical illness with disorders of the peripheral nervous system (PNS) arises in two contexts: (1) primary neurologic diseases that require critical care interventions such as intubation and mechanical ventilation, and (2) secondary PNS manifestations of systemic critical illness, often involving multisystem organ failure. The former include acute polyneuropathies such as Guillain-Barré syndrome (Chap. 380), neuromuscular junction disorders including myasthenia gravis (Chap. 381) and botulism (Chap. 134), and primary muscle disorders such as polymyositis (Chap. 383). The latter result either from the systemic disease itself or as a consequence of interventions.

General principles of respiratory evaluation in patients with PNS involvement, regardless of cause, include assessment of pulmonary mechanics, such as maximal inspiratory force (MIF) and vital capacity (VC), and evaluation of strength of bulbar muscles. Regardless of the cause of weakness, endotracheal intubation should be considered when the MIF falls to <−25 cmH$_2$O or the VC is <1 L. Also, patients with severe palatal weakness may require endotracheal intubation in order to prevent acute upper airway obstruction or recurrent aspiration. Arterial blood gases and oxygen saturation from pulse oximetry are used to follow patients with potential respiratory compromise from PNS dysfunction. However, intubation and mechanical ventilation should be undertaken based on clinical assessment rather than waiting until oxygen saturation drops or CO$_2$ retention develops from hypoventilation. Noninvasive mechanical ventilation may be considered initially in lieu of endotracheal intubation but is generally insufficient in patients with severe bulbar weakness or ventilatory failure with hypercarbia. **Principles of mechanical ventilation are discussed in Chap. 263.**

NEUROPATHY

While encephalopathy may be the most obvious neurologic dysfunction in critically ill patients, dysfunction of the PNS is also quite common. It is typically present in patients with prolonged critical illnesses lasting several weeks and involving sepsis; clinical suspicion is aroused when there is failure to wean from mechanical ventilation despite improvement of the underlying sepsis and critical illness. *Critical illness polyneuropathy* refers to the most common PNS complication related to critical illness; it is seen in the setting of prolonged critical illness, sepsis, and multisystem organ failure. Neurologic findings include diffuse weakness, decreased reflexes, and distal sensory loss. Electrophysiologic studies demonstrate a diffuse, symmetric, distal axonal sensorimotor neuropathy, and pathologic studies have confirmed axonal degeneration. The precise mechanism of critical illness polyneuropathy remains unclear, but circulating factors such as cytokines, which are associated with sepsis and SIRS, are thought to play a role. It has been reported that up to 70% of patients with the sepsis syndrome have some degree of neuropathy, although far fewer have a clinical syndrome profound enough to cause severe respiratory muscle weakness requiring prolonged mechanical ventilation or resulting in failure to wean. Recent studies suggest that aggressive glycemic control with insulin infusions decreases the risk of critical illness polyneuropathy. Treatment is supportive, with specific intervention directed at treating the underlying illness. While spontaneous recovery is usually seen, the time course may extend over weeks to months and necessitate long-term ventilatory support and care even after the underlying critical illness has resolved.

DISORDERS OF NEUROMUSCULAR TRANSMISSION

A defect in neuromuscular transmission may be a source of weakness in critically ill patients. Myasthenia gravis may be a consideration; however, persistent weakness secondary to impaired neuromuscular junction transmission is almost always due to administration of drugs. A number of medications impair neuromuscular transmission; these include antibiotics, especially aminoglycosides, and beta-blocking agents. In the ICU, the nondepolarizing neuromuscular blocking agents (nd-NMBAs), also known as muscle relaxants, are most commonly responsible. Included in this group of drugs are such agents as pancuronium, vecuronium, rocuronium, and atracurium. They are often used to facilitate mechanical ventilation or other critical care procedures, but with prolonged use persistent neuromuscular blockade may result in weakness even after discontinuation of these agents hours or days earlier. Risk factors for this prolonged action of neuromuscular blocking agents include female sex, metabolic acidosis, and renal failure.

Prolonged neuromuscular blockade does not appear to produce permanent damage to the PNS. Once the offending medications are discontinued, full strength is restored, although this may take days. In general, the lowest dose of neuromuscular blocking agent should be used to achieve the desired result, and, when these agents are used in the ICU, a peripheral nerve stimulator should be used to monitor neuromuscular junction function.

MYOPATHY

Critically ill patients, especially those with sepsis, frequently develop muscle wasting, often in the face of seemingly adequate nutritional support. The assumption has been that this represents a catabolic myopathy brought about as a result of multiple factors, including elevated cortisol and catecholamine release and other circulating factors induced by the SIRS. In this syndrome, known as *cachectic myopathy*, serum creatine kinase levels and electromyography (EMG) are normal. Muscle biopsy shows type II fiber atrophy. Panfascicular muscle fiber necrosis may also occur in the setting of profound sepsis. This so-called *septic myopathy* is characterized clinically by weakness progressing to a profound level over just a few days. There may be associated elevations in serum creatine kinase and urine myoglobin. Both EMG and muscle biopsy may be normal initially but eventually show abnormal spontaneous activity and panfascicular necrosis with an accompanying inflammatory reaction. Both of these myopathic syndromes may be considered under the broader heading of *critical illness myopathy*.

Acute quadriplegic myopathy describes a clinical syndrome of severe weakness seen in the setting of glucocorticoid and nd-NMBA use. The most frequent scenario in which this is encountered is the asthmatic patient who requires high-dose glucocorticoids and nd-NMBA to facilitate mechanical ventilation. This muscle disorder is not due to prolonged action of nd-NMBAs at the neuromuscular junction but, rather, is an actual myopathy with muscle damage; it has occasionally been described with high-dose glucocorticoid use alone. Clinically this syndrome is most often recognized when a patient fails to wean from mechanical ventilation despite resolution of the primary pulmonary process. Pathologically, there may be vacuolar changes in both type I and type II muscle fibers with evidence of regeneration. Acute quadriplegic myopathy has a good prognosis. If patients survive their underlying critical illness, the myopathy invariably improves and most patients return to normal. However, because this syndrome is a result of true muscle damage, not just prolonged blockade at the neuromuscular junction, this process may take weeks or months, and tracheostomy with prolonged ventilatory support may be necessary. Some patients do have residual long-term weakness, with atrophy and fatigue limiting ambulation. At present, it is unclear how to prevent this myopathic complication, except by avoiding use of nd-NMBAs, a strategy not always possible. Monitoring with a peripheral nerve stimulator can help to avoid the overuse of these agents. However, this is more likely to prevent the complication of prolonged neuromuscular junction blockade than it is to prevent this myopathy.

SUBARACHNOID HEMORRHAGE

Subarachnoid hemorrhage (SAH) renders the brain critically ill from both primary and secondary brain insults. Excluding head trauma, the most common cause of SAH is rupture of a saccular aneurysm. Other causes include bleeding from a vascular malformation (arteriovenous malformation or dural arterial-venous fistula) and extension into the subarachnoid space from a primary intracerebral hemorrhage. Some idiopathic SAHs are localized to the perimesencephalic cisterns and are benign; they probably have a venous or capillary source, and angiography is unrevealing.

Saccular ("Berry") Aneurysm Autopsy and angiography studies have found that about 2% of adults harbor intracranial aneurysms, for a prevalence of 4 million persons in the United States; the aneurysm will rupture, producing SAH, in 25,000–30,000 cases per year. For patients who arrive alive at hospital, the mortality rate over the next month is about 45%. Of those who survive, more than half are left with major neurologic deficits as a result of the initial hemorrhage, cerebral vasospasm with infarction, or hydrocephalus. If the patient survives but the aneurysm is not obliterated, the rate of rebleeding is about 20% in the first 2 weeks, 30% in the first month, and about 3% per year afterwards. Given these alarming figures, the major therapeutic emphasis is on preventing the predictable early complications of the SAH.

Unruptured, asymptomatic aneurysms are much less dangerous than a recently ruptured aneurysm. The annual risk of rupture for aneurysms <10 mm in size is ~0.1%, and for aneurysms ≥10 mm in size is ~0.5–1%; the surgical morbidity far exceeds these percentages. Because of the longer length of exposure to risk of rupture, younger patients with aneurysms >10 mm in size may benefit from prophylactic treatment. As with the treatment of asymptomatic carotid stenosis, this risk-benefit strongly depends on the complication rate of treatment.

Giant aneurysms, those >2.5 cm in diameter, occur at the same sites (see below) as small aneurysms and account for 5% of cases. The three most common locations are the terminal internal carotid artery, middle cerebral artery (MCA) bifurcation, and top of the basilar artery. Their risk of rupture is ~6% in the first year after identification and may remain high indefinitely. They often cause symptoms by compressing the adjacent brain or cranial nerves.

Mycotic aneurysms are usually located distal to the first bifurcation of major arteries of the circle of Willis. Most result from infected emboli due to bacterial endocarditis causing septic degeneration of arteries and subsequent dilatation and rupture. Whether these lesions should be sought and repaired prior to rupture or left to heal spontaneously is controversial.

PATHOPHYSIOLOGY Saccular aneurysms occur at the bifurcations of the large to medium-sized intracranial arteries; rupture is into the subarachnoid space in the basal cisterns and often into the parenchyma of the adjacent brain. Approximately 85% of aneurysms occur in the anterior circulation, mostly on the circle of Willis. About 20% of patients have multiple aneurysms, many at mirror sites bilaterally. As an aneurysm develops, it typically forms a neck with a dome. The length of the neck and the size of the dome vary greatly and are factors that are important in planning neurosurgical obliteration or endovascular embolization. The arterial internal elastic lamina disappears at the base of the neck. The media thins, and connective tissue replaces smooth-muscle cells. At the site of rupture (most often the dome) the wall thins, and the tear that allows bleeding is often ≤0.5 mm long. Aneurysm size and site are important in predicting risk of rupture. Those >7 mm in diameter and those at the top of the basilar artery and at the origin of the posterior communicating artery are at greater risk of rupture.

CLINICAL MANIFESTATIONS Most unruptured intracranial aneurysms are completely asymptomatic. Symptoms are usually due to rupture and resultant SAH, although some present with mass effect on cranial nerves or brain parenchyma. At the moment of aneurysmal rupture with major SAH, the ICP suddenly rises. This may account for the sudden transient loss of consciousness that occurs in nearly half of patients. Sudden loss of consciousness may be preceded by a brief moment of excruciating headache, but most patients first complain of headache upon regaining consciousness. In 10% of cases, aneurysmal bleeding is severe enough to cause loss of consciousness for several days. In ~45% of cases, severe headache associated with exertion is the presenting complaint. The patient often calls the headache "the worst headache of my life"; however, the most important characteristic is sudden onset. Occasionally these ruptures may present as headache of only moderate intensity or as a change in the patient's usual headache pattern. The headache is usually generalized, often with neck stiffness, and vomiting is common.

Although sudden headache in the absence of focal neurologic symptoms is the hallmark of aneurysmal rupture, focal neurologic deficits may occur. Anterior communicating artery or MCA bifurcation aneurysms may rupture into the adjacent brain or subdural space and form a hematoma large enough to produce mass effect. The common deficits that result include hemiparesis, aphasia, and abulia.

Occasionally, prodromal symptoms suggest the location of a progressively enlarging unruptured aneurysm. A third cranial nerve palsy, particularly when associated with pupillary dilatation, loss of ipsilateral (but retained contralateral) light reflex, and focal pain above or behind the eye, may occur with an expanding aneurysm at the junction of the posterior communicating artery and the internal carotid artery. A sixth nerve palsy may indicate an aneurysm in the cavernous sinus, and visual field defects can occur with an expanding supraclinoid carotid or anterior cerebral artery aneurysm. Occipital and posterior cervical pain may signal a posterior inferior cerebellar artery or anteri-

Grade	Hunt-Hess Scale	World Federation of Neurosurgical Societies (WFNS) Scale
1	Mild headache, normal mental status, no cranial nerve or motor findings	Glasgow Coma Scale[a] (GCS) score 15, no motor deficits
2	Severe headache, normal mental status, may have cranial nerve deficit	GCS 13–14, no motor deficits
3	Somnolent, confused, may have cranial nerve or mild motor deficit	GCS 13–14, with motor deficits
4	Stupor, moderate to severe motor deficit, may have intermittent reflex posturing	GCS 7–12, with or without motor deficits
5	Coma, reflex posturing or flaccid	GCS 3–6, with or without motor deficits

[a]Glasgow Coma Scale: See Fig. 373-2.

or inferior cerebellar artery aneurysm. Pain in or behind the eye and in the low temple can occur with an expanding MCA aneurysm. Thunderclap headache is a variant of migraine that simulates a SAH. Before concluding that a patient with sudden, severe headache has thunderclap migraine, a definitive workup for aneurysm or other intracranial pathology is required.

Aneurysms can undergo small ruptures and leaks of blood into the subarachnoid space, so-called *sentinel bleeds*. Sudden unexplained headache at any location should raise suspicion of SAH and be investigated, because a major hemorrhage may be imminent.

The initial clinical manifestations of SAH can be graded using the Hunt-Hess or World Federation of Neurosurgical Societies classification schemes (Table 269-3). For ruptured aneurysms, prognosis for good outcomes falls as the grade increases. For example it is unusual for a Hunt-Hess grade 1 patient to die if the aneurysm is treated, but the mortality for grade 4 and 5 patients may be as high as 80%.

DELAYED NEUROLOGIC DEFICITS There are four major causes of delayed neurologic deficits: rerupture, hydrocephalus, vasospasm, and hyponatremia.

1. *Rerupture*. The incidence of rerupture of an untreated aneurysm in the first month following SAH is ~30%, with the peak in the first 7 days. Rerupture is associated with a 60% mortality and poor outcome. Early treatment eliminates this risk.
2. *Hydrocephalus*. Acute hydrocephalus can cause stupor and coma and can be mitigated by placement of an external ventricular drain. More often, subacute hydrocephalus may develop over a few days or weeks and causes progressive drowsiness or slowed mentation (abulia) with incontinence. Hydrocephalus is differentiated from cerebral vasospasm with a CT scan, CT angiogram, transcranial Doppler (TCD) ultrasound, or conventional x-ray angiography. Hydrocephalus may clear spontaneously or require temporary ventricular drainage. Chronic hydrocephalus may develop weeks to months after SAH and manifest as gait difficulty, incontinence, or impaired mentation. Subtle signs may be a lack of initiative in conversation or a failure to recover independence.
3. *Vasospasm*. Narrowing of the arteries at the base of the brain following SAH causes symptomatic ischemia and infarction in ~30% of patients and is the major cause of delayed morbidity and death. Signs of ischemia appear 4–14 days after the hemorrhage, most often at 7 days. The severity and distribution of vasospasm determine whether infarction will occur.

Delayed vasospasm is believed to result from direct effects of clotted blood and its breakdown products on the arteries within the subarachnoid space. In general, the more blood that surrounds the arteries, the greater the chance of symptomatic vasospasm. Spasm of major arteries produces symptoms referable to the appropriate vascular territory (Chap. 364). All of these focal symptoms may present abruptly, fluctuate, or develop over a few days. In most cases, focal spasm is preceded by a decline in mental status.

Vasospasm can be detected reliably with conventional x-ray angiography, but this invasive procedure is expensive and carries the risk of stroke and other complications. TCD ultrasound is based on the principle that the velocity of blood flow within an artery will rise as the lumen diameter is narrowed. By directing the probe along the MCA and proximal anterior cerebral artery (ACA), carotid terminus, and vertebral and basilar arteries on a daily or every-other-day basis, vasospasm can be reliably detected and treatments initiated to prevent cerebral ischemia (see below). CT angiography is another method that can detect vasospasm.

Severe cerebral edema in patients with infarction from vasospasm may increase the ICP enough to reduce cerebral perfusion pressure. Treatment may include mannitol, hyperventilation, and hemicraniectomy; moderate hypothermia may have a role as well.

4. *Hyponatremia.* Hyponatremia may be profound and can develop quickly in the first 2 weeks following SAH. There is both natriuresis and volume depletion with SAH, so that patients become both hyponatremic and hypovolemic. Both atrial natriuretic peptide and brain natriuretic peptide have a role in producing this "cerebral salt-wasting syndrome." Typically it clears over the course of 1–2 weeks and, in the setting of SAH, should not be treated with free-water restriction as this may increase the risk of stroke (see below).

LABORATORY EVALUATION AND IMAGING (Fig. 269-8) The hallmark of aneurysmal rupture is blood in the CSF. More than 95% of cases have enough blood to be visualized on a high-quality noncontrast CT scan obtained within 72 h. If the scan fails to establish the diagnosis of SAH and no mass lesion or obstructive hydrocephalus is found, a lumbar puncture should be performed to establish the presence of subarachnoid blood. Lysis of the red blood cells and subsequent conversion of hemoglobin to bilirubin stains the spinal fluid yellow within 6–12 h. This xanthochromic spinal fluid peaks in intensity at 48 h and lasts for 1–4 weeks, depending on the amount of subarachnoid blood.

The extent and location of subarachnoid blood on noncontrast CT scan help locate the underlying aneurysm, identify the cause of any neurologic deficit, and predict delayed vasospasm. A high incidence of symptomatic vasospasm in the MCA and ACA has been found when early CT scans show subarachnoid clots >5 × 3 mm in the basal cisterns or layers of blood >1 mm thick in the cerebral fissures. CT scans less reliably predict vasospasm in the vertebral, basilar, or posterior cerebral arteries.

Lumbar puncture prior to an imaging procedure is indicated only if a CT scan is not available at the time of the suspected SAH. Once the diagnosis of hemorrhage from a ruptured saccular aneurysm is suspected, four-vessel conventional x-ray angiography (both carotids and both vertebrals) is generally performed to localize and define the anatomic details of the aneurysm and to determine if other unruptured aneurysms exist (Fig. 269-8C). At some centers, the ruptured aneurysm can be treated using endovascular techniques at the time of the initial angiogram as a way to expedite treatment and minimize the number of invasive procedures. CT angiography is an alternative method for locating the aneurysm and may be sufficient to plan definitive therapy.

Close monitoring (daily or twice daily) of electrolytes is important because hyponatremia can occur precipitously during the first 2 weeks following SAH (see above).

The electrocardiogram (ECG) frequently shows ST-segment and T-wave changes similar to those associated with cardiac ischemia. Prolonged QRS complex, increased QT interval, and prominent "peaked" or deeply inverted symmetric T waves are usually secondary to the intracranial hemorrhage. There is evidence that structural myocardial lesions produced by circulating catecholamines and excessive discharge of sympathetic neurons may occur after SAH, causing these ECG changes and a reversible cardiomyopathy sufficient to cause shock or congestive heart failure. Echocardiography reveals a pattern of regional wall motion abnormalities that follow the distribution of

FIGURE 269-8 Subarachnoid hemorrhage. A. CT angiography revealing an aneurysm of the left superior cerebellar artery. **B.** Noncontrast CT scan at the level of the third ventricle revealing subarachnoid blood (bright) in the left sylvian fissure and within the left lateral ventricle. **C.** Conventional anteroposterior x-ray angiogram of the right vertebral and basilar artery showing the large aneurysm. **D.** Conventional angiogram following coil embolization of the aneurysm, whereby the aneurysm body is filled with platinum coils delivered through a microcatheter navigated from the femoral artery into the aneurysm neck.

sympathetic nerves rather than the major coronary arteries, with relative sparing of the ventricular wall apex. The sympathetic nerves themselves appear to be injured by direct toxicity from the excessive catecholamine release. An asymptomatic troponin elevation is common. Serious ventricular dysrhythmias are unusual.

℞ SUBARACHNOID HEMORRHAGE

Early aneurysm repair prevents rerupture and allows the safe application of techniques to improve blood flow (e.g., induced hypertension and hypervolemia) should symptomatic vasospasm develop. An aneurysm can be "clipped" by a neurosurgeon or "coiled" by an endovascular surgeon. Surgical repair involves placing a metal clip across the aneurysm neck, thereby immediately eliminating the risk of rebleeding. This approach requires craniotomy and brain retraction, which is associated with neurologic morbidity. Endovascular techniques involve placing platinum coils, or other embolic material, within the aneurysm via a catheter that is passed from the femoral artery. The aneurysm is packed tightly to enhance thrombosis and over time is walled-off from the circulation (Fig. 269-8D). The only prospective randomized trial of surgery versus endovascular treatment for ruptured aneurysm, the International Subarachnoid Aneurysm Trial (ISAT), was terminated early when 24% of patients treated with endovascular therapy were dead or dependent at 1 year compared to 31% treated with surgery, a significant 23% relative reduction. Follow-up for these patients, now complete, reveals that the benefit of endovascular therapy is durable. However, some aneurysms have a morphology that is not amenable to endovascular treatment. Thus, surgery remains an important treatment option. Centers that combine both endovascular and neurosurgical expertise likely offer the best outcomes for patients, and there are good data showing that centers that specialize in aneurysm treatment have improved mortality rates.

The medical management of SAH focuses on protecting the airway, managing blood pressure before and after aneurysm treatment, preventing rebleeding prior to treatment, managing vasospasm, treating hydrocephalus, treating hyponatremia, and preventing pulmonary embolus.

Intracranial hypertension following aneurysmal rupture occurs secondary to subarachnoid blood, parenchymal hematoma, acute hydrocephalus, or loss of vascular autoregulation. Patients who are stuporous should undergo emergent ventriculostomy to measure ICP and to treat high ICP in order to prevent cerebral ischemia. Medical therapies designed to combat raised ICP (e.g., mild hyperventilation, mannitol, and sedation) can also be used as needed. High ICP refractory to treatment is a poor prognostic sign.

Prior to definitive treatment of the ruptured aneurysm, care is required to maintain adequate cerebral perfusion pressure while avoiding excessive elevation of arterial pressure. If the patient is alert, it is reasonable to lower the blood pressure to normal using nicardipine, labetolol, or esmolol. If the patient has a depressed level of consciousness, ICP should be measured and the cerebral perfusion pressure targeted to 60–70 mmHg.

Because rebleeding is common, all patients who are not candidates for early aneurysm repair are put on bed rest in a quiet room and are given stool softeners to prevent straining. If headache or neck pain is severe, mild sedation and analgesia are prescribed. Extreme sedation is avoided because it can obscure changes in neurologic status. Adequate hydration is necessary to avoid a decrease in blood volume predisposing to brain ischemia.

Seizures are uncommon at the onset of aneurysmal rupture. The quivering, jerking, and extensor posturing that often accompany loss of consciousness with SAH are probably related to the sharp rise in ICP or, perhaps, acute generalized vasospasm rather than seizure. However, phenytoin is often given as prophylactic therapy since a seizure may promote rebleeding.

Glucocorticoids may help reduce the head and neck ache caused by the irritative effect of the subarachnoid blood. There is no good evidence that they reduce cerebral edema, are neuroprotective, or reduce vascular injury, and their routine use therefore is not recommended.

Antifibrinolytic agents are not routinely prescribed but may be considered in patients in whom aneurysm treatment cannot proceed immediately. They are associated with a reduced incidence of aneurysmal rerupture but may also increase the risk of delayed cerebral infarction and deep vein thrombosis (DVT).

Vasospasm remains the leading cause of morbidity and mortality following aneurysmal SAH. Treatment with the calcium channel antagonist nimodipine (60 mg PO every 4 h) improves outcome, perhaps by preventing ischemic injury rather than reducing the risk of vasospasm. Nimodipine can cause significant hypotension in some patients, which may worsen cerebral ischemia in patients with vasospasm. Symptomatic cerebral vasospasm can also be treated by increasing the cerebral perfusion pressure by raising mean arterial pressure through plasma volume expansion and the judicious use of IV vasopressor agents, usually phenylephrine or norepinephrine. Raised perfusion pressure has been associated with clinical improvement in many patients, but high arterial pressure may promote rebleeding in unprotected aneurysms. Treatment with induced hypertension and hypervolemia generally requires monitoring of arterial and central venous pressures; it is best to infuse pressors through a central venous line as well. Volume expansion helps prevent hypotension, augments cardiac output, and reduces blood viscosity by reducing the hematocrit. This method is called "triple-H" (hypertension, hemodilution, and hypervolemic) therapy.

If symptomatic vasospasm persists despite optimal medical therapy, intraarterial vasodilators and percutaneous transluminal angioplasty are considered. Vasodilatation by direct angioplasty appears to be permanent, allowing triple-H therapy to be tapered sooner. The pharmacologic vasodi-lators (verapamil and nicardipine) do not last more than 8–24 h, and therefore multiple treatments may be required until the subarachnoid blood is reabsorbed. Although intraarterial papaverine is an effective vasodilator, there is evidence that papaverine may be neurotoxic so its use should be reserved for refractory cases.

Acute hydrocephalus can cause stupor or coma. It may clear spontaneously or require temporary ventricular drainage. When chronic hydrocephalus develops, ventricular shunting is the treatment of choice.

Free-water restriction is contraindicated in patients with SAH at risk for vasospasm because hypovolemia and hypotension may occur and precipitate cerebral ischemia. Many patients continue to experience a decline in serum sodium despite receiving parenteral fluids containing normal saline. Frequently, supplemental oral salt coupled with normal saline will mitigate hyponatremia, but often patients also require hypertonic saline. Care must be taken not to correct serum sodium too quickly in patients with marked hyponatremia of several days' duration, as central pontine myelinolysis may occur.

All patients should have pneumatic compression stockings applied to prevent pulmonary embolism. Unfractionated heparin administered subcutaneously for DVT prophylaxis can be initiated immediately following endovascular treatment and within days following craniotomy and surgical clipping and is a useful adjunct to pneumatic compression stockings. Treatment of pulmonary embolus depends on whether the aneurysm has been treated and whether or not the patient has had a craniotomy. Systemic anticoagulation with heparin is contraindicated in patients with ruptured and untreated aneurysms. It is a relative contraindication following craniotomy for several days or perhaps weeks, and it may delay thrombosis of a coiled aneurysm. Following craniotomy, use of inferior vena cava filters is preferred to prevent further pulmonary emboli, while systemic anticoagulation with heparin is preferred following successful endovascular treatment.

FURTHER READINGS

Latronico N et al: Neuromuscular sequelae of critical illness. Curr Opin Crit Care 11:381, 2005

Liou AK et al: To die or not to die for neurons in ischemia, traumatic brain injury and epilepsy: A review on the stress-activated signaling pathways and apoptotic pathways. Prog Neurobiol 69:103, 2003

Molyneux A et al: International Subarachnoid Aneurysm Trial (ISAT) of neurosurgical clipping versus endovascular coiling in 2143 patients with ruptured intracranial aneurysms: A randomized trial. Lancet 360:1267, 2002

Nolan JP et al: Therapeutic Hypothermia After Cardiac Arrest: An Advisory Statement by the Advanced Life Support Task Force of the International Liaison Committee on Resuscitation. Circulation 108:118, 2003

Posner JB et al: *Plum and Posner's Diagnosis of Stupor and Coma*, 4th ed. New York, Oxford University Press, 2007

Safe Study Investigators et al: Saline or albumin for fluid resuscitation in patients with traumatic brain injury. N Engl J Med 357:874, 2007

Van den Berghe G et al: Insulin therapy protects the central and peripheral nervous system of intensive care patients. Neurology 64:1348, 2005

Wijdicks EFM et al: Practice parameter: Prediction of outcome in comatose survivors after cardiopulmonary resuscitation (an evidence-based review). Neurology 67:203, 2006

270 Oncologic Emergencies
Rasim Gucalp, Janice Dutcher

Emergencies in patients with cancer may be classified into three groups: pressure or obstruction caused by a space-occupying lesion, metabolic or hormonal problems (paraneoplastic syndromes, Chap. 96), and treatment-related complications.

STRUCTURAL-OBSTRUCTIVE ONCOLOGIC EMERGENCIES

SUPERIOR VENA CAVA SYNDROME

Superior vena cava syndrome (SVCS) is the clinical manifestation of superior vena cava (SVC) obstruction, with severe reduction in venous return from the head, neck, and upper extremities. Malignant tumors, such as lung cancer, lymphoma, and metastatic tumors, are responsible for the majority of SVCS cases. With the expanding use of intravascular devices (e.g., permanent central venous access catheters, pacemaker/defibrillator leads), the prevalence of benign causes of SVCS is increasing. Lung cancer, particularly of small cell and squamous cell histologies, accounts for approximately 85% of all cases of malignant origin. In young adults, malignant lymphoma is a leading cause of SVCS. Hodgkin's lymphoma involves the mediastinum more commonly than other lymphomas but rarely causes SVCS. When SVCS is noted in a young man with a mediastinal mass, the differential diagnosis is lymphoma vs primary mediastinal germ cell tumor. Metastatic cancers to the mediastinum, such as testicular and breast carcinomas, account for a small proportion of cases. Other causes include benign tumors, aortic aneurysm, thyromegaly, thrombosis, and fibrosing mediastinitis from prior irradiation or histoplasmosis.

Patients with SVCS usually present with neck and facial swelling (especially around the eyes), dyspnea, and cough. Other symptoms include hoarseness, tongue swelling, headaches, nasal congestion, epistaxis, hemoptysis, dysphagia, pain, dizziness, syncope, and lethargy. Bending forward or lying down may aggravate the symptoms. The characteristic physical findings are dilated neck veins, an increased number of collateral veins covering the anterior chest wall, cyanosis, and edema of the face, arms, and chest. More severe cases include proptosis, glossal and laryngeal edema, and obtundation. The clinical picture is milder if the obstruction is located above the azygos vein.

Signs and symptoms of cerebral and/or laryngeal edema, though rare, are associated with a poorer prognosis and require urgent evaluation. Seizures are more likely related to brain metastases than to cerebral edema from venous occlusion. Patients with small cell lung cancer and SVCS have a higher incidence of brain metastases than those without SVCS.

Cardiorespiratory symptoms at rest, particularly with positional changes, suggest significant airway and vascular obstruction and limited physiologic reserve. Cardiac arrest or respiratory failure can occur, particularly in patients receiving sedatives or undergoing general anesthesia.

The diagnosis of SVCS is a clinical one. The most significant chest radiographic finding is widening of the superior mediastinum, most commonly on the right side. Pleural effusion occurs in only 25% of patients, often on the right side. However, a normal chest radiograph is still compatible with the diagnosis if other characteristic findings are present. CT provides the most reliable view of the mediastinal anatomy. The diagnosis of SVCS requires diminished or absent opacification of central venous structures with prominent collateral venous circulation. MRI has no advantages over CT. Invasive procedures, including bronchoscopy, percutaneous needle biopsy, mediastinoscopy, and even thoracotomy, can be performed by a skilled clinician without any major risk of bleeding. For patients with a known cancer, a de-tailed workup usually is not necessary, and appropriate treatment may be started after obtaining a CT scan of the thorax. For those with no history of malignancy, a detailed evaluation is essential to rule out benign causes and determine a specific diagnosis to direct the appropriate therapy.

℞ SUPERIOR VENA CAVA SYNDROME

The one potentially life-threatening complication of a superior mediastinal mass is tracheal obstruction. Upper airway obstruction demands emergent therapy. Diuretics with a low-salt diet, head elevation, and oxygen may produce temporary symptomatic relief. Glucocorticoids may be useful at shrinking lymphoma masses; they are of no benefit in patients with lung cancer.

Radiation therapy is the primary treatment for SVCS caused by non-small cell lung cancer and other metastatic solid tumors. Chemotherapy is effective when the underlying cancer is small cell carcinoma of the lung, lymphoma, or germ cell tumor. SVCS recurs in 10–30% of patients; it may be palliated with the use of intravascular self-expanding stents (Fig. 270-1). Early stenting may be necessary in patients with severe symptoms; however, the prompt increase in venous return after stenting may precipitate heart failure and pulmonary edema. Surgery may provide immediate relief for patients in whom a benign process is the cause.

Clinical improvement occurs in most patients, although this improvement may be due to the development of adequate collateral circulation. The mortality associated with SVCS does not relate to caval obstruction, but rather to the underlying cause.

SVCS AND CENTRAL VENOUS CATHETERS IN ADULTS   The use of long-term central venous catheters has become common practice in patients with cancer. Major vessel thrombosis may occur. In these cases, catheter removal should be combined with anticoagulation to prevent embolization. SVCS in this setting, if detected early, can be treated by fibrinolytic therapy without sacrificing the catheter. The routine use of low-dose warfarin or low molecular weight heparin to prevent thrombosis related to permanent central venous access catheters in cancer patients is not recommended.

PERICARDIAL EFFUSION/TAMPONADE

Malignant pericardial disease is found at autopsy in 5–10% of patients with cancer, most frequently with lung cancer, breast cancer, leukemias, and lymphomas. Cardiac tamponade as the initial presentation of extrathoracic malignancy is rare. The origin is not malignancy in about 50% of cancer patients with symptomatic pericardial disease, but it can be related to irradiation, drug-induced pericarditis, hypothyroidism, idiopathic pericarditis, infection, or autoimmune diseases. Two types of radiation pericarditis occur: an acute inflammatory, effusive pericarditis occurring within months of irradiation, which usually resolves spontaneously, and a chronic effusive pericarditis that may appear up to 20 years after radiation therapy and is accompanied by a thickened pericardium.

Most patients with pericardial metastasis are asymptomatic. However, the common symptoms are dyspnea, cough, chest pain, orthopnea, and weakness. Pleural effusion, sinus tachycardia, jugular venous distension, hepatomegaly, peripheral edema, and cyanosis are the most frequent physical findings. Relatively specific diagnostic findings, such as paradoxical pulse, diminished heart sounds, pulsus alternans (pulse waves alternating between those of greater and lesser amplitude with successive beats), and friction rub are less common than with nonmalignant pericardial disease. Chest radiographs and ECG reveal abnormalities in 90% of patients, but half of these abnormalities are nonspecific. Echocardiography is the most helpful diagnostic test. Pericardial fluid may be serous, serosanguineous, or hemorrhagic, and cytologic examination of pericardial fluid is diagnostic in most pa-

FIGURE 270-1 Superior vena cava syndrome. A. Chest radiographs of a 59-year-old man with recurrent SVCS caused by non-small cell lung cancer showing right paratracheal mass with right pleural effusion. **B.** CT of same patient demonstrating obstruction of SVC with thrombosis (*arrow*) by the lung cancer (*square*) and collaterals (*arrowheads*). **C.** Balloon angioplasty (*arrowhead*) with walstent (*arrow*) in same patient.

tients. Cancer patients with pericardial effusion containing malignant cells on cytology have a very poor survival, about 7 weeks.

℞ PERICARDIAL EFFUSION/TAMPONADE

Pericardiocentesis with or without the introduction of sclerosing agents, the creation of a pericardial window, complete pericardial stripping, cardiac irradiation, or systemic chemotherapy are effective treatments. Acute pericardial tamponade with life-threatening hemodynamic instability requires immediate drainage of fluid. This can be quickly achieved by pericardiocentesis. The recurrence rate after percutaneous catheter drainage is around 20%. Sclerotherapy (pericardial instillation of bleomycin, mitomycin C, or tetracycline) may decrease recurrences. Alternatively, subxiphoid pericardiotomy can be performed in 45 min under local anesthesia. Thoracoscopic pericardial fenestration can be employed for benign causes; however, 60% of malignant pericardial effusions recur after this procedure.

INTESTINAL OBSTRUCTION

Intestinal obstruction and reobstruction are common problems in patients with advanced cancer, particularly colorectal or ovarian carcinoma. However, other cancers, such as lung or breast cancer and melanoma, can metastasize within the abdomen, leading to intestinal obstruction. Typically, obstruction occurs at multiple sites. Melanoma has a predilection to involve the small bowel; this involvement may be

isolated and resection may result in prolonged survival. Intestinal pseudoobstruction is caused by infiltration of the mesentery or bowel muscle by tumor, involvement of the celiac plexus, or paraneoplastic neuropathy in patients with small cell lung cancer. Paraneoplastic neuropathy is associated with IgG antibodies reactive to neurons of the myenteric and submucosal plexuses of the jejunum and stomach. Ovarian cancer can lead to authentic luminal obstruction or to pseudoobstruction that results when circumferential invasion of a bowel segment arrests the forward progression of peristaltic contractions.

The onset of obstruction is usually insidious. Pain is the most common symptom and is usually colicky in nature. Pain can also be due to abdominal distention, tumor masses, or hepatomegaly. Vomiting can be intermittent or continuous. Patients with complete obstruction usually have constipation. Physical examination may reveal abdominal distention with tympany, ascites, visible peristalsis, high-pitched bowel sounds, and tumor masses. Erect plain abdominal films may reveal multiple air-fluid levels and dilation of the small or large bowel. Acute cecal dilation to >12–14 cm is considered a surgical emergency because of the high likelihood of rupture. CT scan is useful in differentiating benign from malignant causes of obstruction in patients who have undergone surgery for malignancy. Malignant obstruction is suggested by a mass at the site of obstruction or prior surgery, adenopathy, or an abrupt transition zone and irregular bowel thickening at the obstruction site. Benign obstruction is more likely when CT shows mesenteric vascular changes, a large volume of ascites, or a smooth transition zone and smooth bowel thickening at the obstruction site. The prognosis for the patient with cancer who develops intestinal obstruction is poor; median survival is 3–4 months. About 25–30% of patients are found to have intestinal obstruction due to causes other than cancer. Adhesions from previous operations are a common benign cause. Ileus induced by vincristine or other drugs is another reversible cause.

Rx INTESTINAL OBSTRUCTION

The management of intestinal obstruction in patients with advanced malignancy depends on the extent of the underlying malignancy and the functional status of the major organs. The initial management should include surgical evaluation. Operation is not always successful and may lead to further complications with a substantial mortality rate (10–20%). Laparoscopy can diagnose and treat malignant bowel obstruction in some cases. Self-expanding metal stents placed in the gastric outlet, duodenum, proximal jejunum, colon, or rectum may palliate obstructive symptoms at those sites without major surgery. Patients known to have advanced intra-abdominal malignancy should receive a prolonged course of conservative management, including nasogastric decompression. Treatment with anti-emetics, antispasmodics, and analgesics may allow patients to remain outside the hospital. Octreotide may relieve obstructive symptoms through its inhibitory effect on gastrointestinal secretion.

URINARY OBSTRUCTION

Urinary obstruction may occur in patients with prostatic or gynecologic malignancies, particularly cervical carcinoma; metastatic disease from other primary sites such as carcinomas of the breast, stomach, lung, colon, and pancreas; or lymphomas. Radiation therapy to pelvic tumors may cause fibrosis and subsequent ureteral obstruction. Bladder outlet obstruction is usually due to prostate and cervical cancers and may lead to bilateral hydronephrosis and renal failure.

Flank pain is the most common symptom. Persistent urinary tract infection, persistent proteinuria, or hematuria in patients with cancer should raise suspicion of ureteral obstruction. Total anuria and/or anuria alternating with polyuria may occur. A slow, continuous rise in the serum creatinine level necessitates immediate evaluation. Renal ultrasound is the safest and cheapest way to identify hydronephrosis. The function of an obstructed kidney can be evaluated by a nuclear scan. CT scan can reveal the point of obstruction and identify a retroperitoneal mass or adenopathy.

Rx URINARY OBSTRUCTION

Obstruction associated with flank pain, sepsis, or fistula formation is an indication for immediate palliative urinary diversion. Internal ureteral stents can be placed under local anesthesia. Percutaneous nephrostomy offers an alternative approach for drainage. In the case of bladder outlet obstruction due to malignancy, a suprapubic cystostomy can be used for urinary drainage.

MALIGNANT BILIARY OBSTRUCTION

This common clinical problem can be caused by a primary carcinoma arising in the pancreas, ampulla of Vater, bile duct, or liver or by metastatic disease to the periductal lymph nodes or liver parenchyma. The most common metastatic tumors causing biliary obstruction are gastric, colon, breast, and lung cancers. Jaundice, light-colored stools, dark urine, pruritus, and weight loss due to malabsorption are usual symptoms. Pain and secondary infection are uncommon in malignant biliary obstruction. Ultrasound, CT scan, or percutaneous transhepatic or endoscopic retrograde cholangiography will identify the site and nature of the biliary obstruction.

Rx MALIGNANT BILIARY OBSTRUCTION

Palliative intervention is indicated only in patients with disabling pruritus resistant to medical treatment, severe malabsorption, or infection. Stenting under radiographic control, surgical bypass, or radiation therapy with or without chemotherapy may alleviate the obstruction. The choice of therapy should be based on the site of obstruction (proximal versus distal), the type of tumor (sensitive to radiotherapy, chemotherapy, or neither), and the general condition of the patient. In the absence of pruritus, biliary obstruction may be a largely asymptomatic cause of death.

SPINAL CORD COMPRESSION

Malignant spinal cord compression (MSCC) is defined as compression of the spinal cord and/or cauda equina by an extradural tumor mass. The minimum radiologic evidence for cord compression is indentation of the theca at the level of clinical features. Spinal cord compression occurs in 5–10% of patients with cancer. Epidural tumor is the first manifestation of malignancy in about 10% of patients. The underlying cancer is usually identified during the initial evaluation; lung cancer is the most common cause of MSCC.

Metastatic tumor involves the vertebral column more often than any other part of the bony skeleton. Lung, breast, and prostate cancer are the most frequent offenders. Multiple myeloma also has a high incidence of spine involvement. Lymphomas, melanoma, renal cell cancer, and genitourinary cancers also cause cord compression. The thoracic spine is the most common site (70%), followed by the lumbosacral spine (20%) and the cervical spine (10%). Involvement of multiple sites is most frequent in patients with breast and prostate carcinoma. Cord injury develops when metastases to the vertebral body or pedicle enlarge and compress the underlying dura. Another cause of cord compression is direct extension of a paravertebral lesion through the intervertebral foramen. These cases usually involve a lymphoma, myeloma, or pediatric neoplasm. Parenchymal spinal cord metastasis due to hematogenous spread is rare.

Expanding extradural tumors induce injury through several mechanisms. Obstruction of the epidural venous plexus leads to edema. Local production of inflammatory cytokines enhances blood flow and edema formation. Compression compromises blood flow leading to ischemia. Production of vascular endothelial growth factor is associated with spinal cord hypoxia and has been implicated as a potential cause of damage after spinal cord injury.

The most common initial symptom in patients with spinal cord compression is localized back pain and tenderness due to involvement of vertebrae by tumor. Pain is usually present for days or months before other neurologic findings appear. It is exacerbated by movement and by coughing or sneezing. It can be differentiated from the pain of disc disease by the fact that it worsens when the patient is supine. Radicular pain is less common than localized back pain and usually develops later. Radicular pain in the cervical or lumbosacral areas may be unilateral or bilateral. Radicular pain from the thoracic roots is often bilateral and is described by patients as a feeling of tight, band-like constriction around the thorax and abdomen. Typical cervical radicular pain radiates down the arm; in the lumbar region, the radiation is down the legs. *Lhermitte's sign*, a tingling or electric sensation down the back and upper and lower limbs upon flexing or extending the neck, may be an early sign of cord compression. Loss of bowel or bladder control may be the presenting symptom but usually occurs late in the course.

On physical examination, pain induced by straight leg raising, neck flexion, or vertebral percussion may help to determine the level of cord compression. Patients develop numbness and paresthesias in the extremities or trunk. Loss of sensibility to pinprick is as common as loss of sensibility to vibration or position. The upper limit of the zone of sensory loss is often one or two vertebrae below the site of compression. Motor findings include weakness, spasticity, and abnormal muscle stretching. An extensor plantar reflex reflects significant compression. Deep tendon reflexes may be brisk. Motor and sensory loss usually precedes sphincter disturbance. Patients with autonomic dysfunction may present with decreased anal tone, decreased perineal sensibility, and a distended bladder. The absence of the anal wink reflex or the bulbocavernosus reflex confirms cord involvement. In doubtful cases, evaluation of post-voiding urinary residual volume can be helpful. A residual volume of >150 mL suggests bladder dysfunction. Autonomic dysfunction is an unfavorable prognostic factor. Patients with progressive neurologic symptoms should

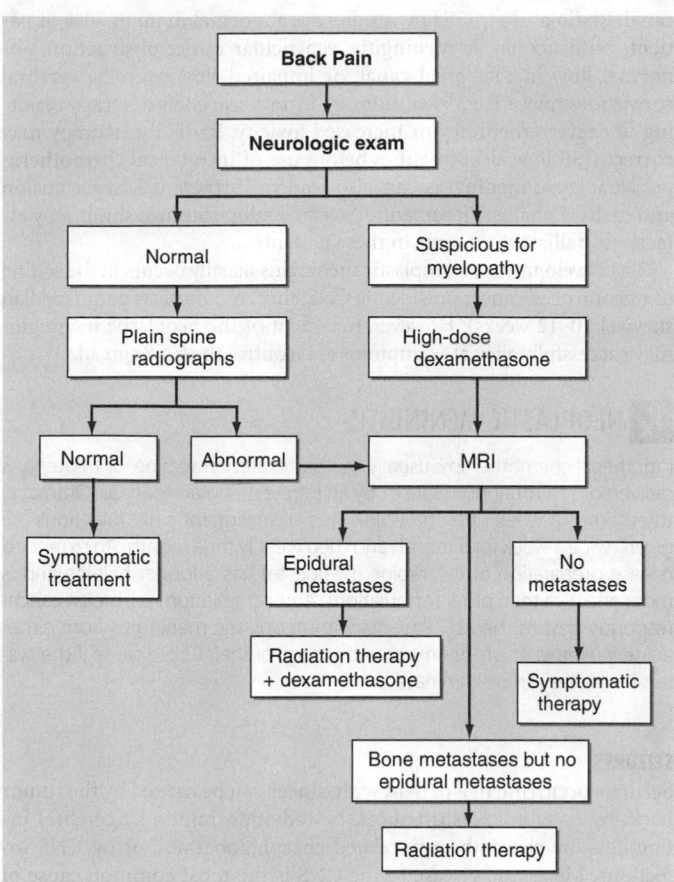

FIGURE 270-2 Management of cancer patients with back pain.

have frequent neurologic examinations and rapid therapeutic intervention. Other illnesses that may mimic cord compression include osteoporotic vertebral collapse, disc disease, pyogenic abscess or vertebral tuberculosis, radiation myelopathy, neoplastic leptomeningitis, benign tumors, epidural hematoma, and spinal lipomatosis.

Cauda equina syndrome is characterized by low back pain; diminished sensation over the buttocks; posterior-superior thighs; perineal area in a saddle distribution; rectal and bladder dysfunction; sexual impotence; absent bulbocavernous, patellar, and Achilles' reflexes; and variable amount of lower-extremity weakness. This reflects compression of nerve roots as they form the cauda equina after leaving the spinal cord.

Patients with cancer who develop back pain should be evaluated for spinal cord compression as quickly as possible (Fig. 270-2). Treatment is more often successful in patients who are ambulatory and still have sphincter control at the time treatment is initiated. Patients should have a neurologic examination and plain films of the spine. Those whose physical examination suggests cord compression should receive dexamethasone (24 mg intravenously every 6 h), starting immediately.

Erosion of the pedicles (the "winking owl" sign) is the earliest radiologic finding of vertebral tumor. Other radiographic changes include increased intrapedicular distance, vertebral destruction, lytic or sclerotic lesions, scalloped vertebral bodies, and vertebral body collapse. Vertebral collapse is not a reliable indicator of the presence of tumor; about 20% of cases of vertebral collapse, particularly those in older patients and postmenopausal women, are due not to cancer but to osteoporosis. Also, a normal appearance on plain films of the spine does not exclude the diagnosis of cancer. The role of bone scans in the detection of cord compression is not clear; this method is sensitive but less specific than spinal radiography.

The full-length image of the cord provided by MRI is useful. Multiple epidural metastases are noted in 25% of patients with cord compression, and their presence influences treatment plans. On T1-weighted images, good contrast is noted between the cord, cerebrospinal fluid, and extradural lesions. Owing to its sensitivity in demonstrating

the replacement of bone marrow by tumor, MRI can show which parts of a vertebra are involved by tumor. MRI also visualizes intraspinal extradural masses compressing the cord. T2-weighted images are most useful for the demonstration of intramedullary pathology. Gadolinium-enhanced MRI can help to delineate intramedullary disease. MRI is as good as or better than myelography plus postmyelogram CT scan in detecting metastatic epidural disease with cord compression. Myelography should be reserved for patients who have poor MR images or who cannot undergo MRI promptly. CT scan in conjunction with myelography enhances the detection of small areas of spinal destruction.

In patients with cord compression and an unknown primary tumor, a simple workup including chest radiography, mammography, measurement of prostate-specific antigen, and abdominal CT usually reveals the underlying malignancy.

℞ SPINAL CORD COMPRESSION

The treatment of patients with spinal cord compression is aimed at relief of pain and restoration/preservation of neurologic function (Fig. 270-2).

Radiation therapy plus glucocorticoids is generally the initial treatment of choice for most patients with spinal cord compression. Up to 75% of patients treated when still ambulatory remain ambulatory, but only 10% of patients with paraplegia recover walking capacity. Indications for surgical intervention include unknown etiology, failure of radiation therapy, a radioresistant tumor type (e.g., melanoma or renal cell cancer), pathologic fracture dislocation, and rapidly evolving neurologic symptoms. Laminectomy is done for tissue diagnosis and for the removal of posteriorly localized epidural deposits in the absence of vertebral body disease. Because most cases of epidural spinal cord compression are due to anterior or anterolateral extradural disease, resection of the anterior vertebral body along with the tumor, followed by spinal stabilization, has achieved good results. A randomized trial showed that patients who underwent an operation followed by radiotherapy (within 14 days) retained the ability to walk significantly longer than those treated with radiotherapy alone. Surgically treated patients also maintained continence and neurologic function significantly longer than patients in the radiation group. The length of survival was not significantly different in the two groups, although there was a trend toward longer survival in the surgery group. The study drew some criticism for the poorer than expected results in the patients who did not go to surgery. However, patients should be evaluated for surgery. Conventional radiotherapy has a role after surgery. Chemotherapy may have a role in patients with chemosensitive tumors who have had prior radiotherapy to the same region and who are not candidates for surgery. Most patients with prostate cancer who develop cord compression have already had hormonal therapy; however, for those who have not, androgen deprivation is combined with surgery and radiotherapy.

Patients with metastatic vertebral tumors may benefit from percutaneous vertebroplasty, the injection of acrylic cement into a collapsed vertebra to stabilize the fracture. Pain palliation is common, and local antitumor effects have been noted. Cement leakage may cause symptoms in about 10% of patients.

The histology of the tumor is an important determinant of both recovery and survival. Rapid onset and progression of signs and symptoms are poor prognostic features.

INCREASED INTRACRANIAL PRESSURE

About 25% of patients with cancer die with intracranial metastases. The cancers that most often metastasize to the brain are lung and breast cancers and melanoma. Brain metastases often occur in the presence of systemic disease, and they frequently cause major symptoms, disability, and early death. The initial presentation of brain metastases from a previously unknown primary cancer is common. Lung cancer is most commonly the primary malignancy. Chest CT scans and brain MRI as the initial diagnostic studies can identify a biopsy site in most patients.

The signs and symptoms of a metastatic brain tumor are similar to those of other intracranial expanding lesions: headache, nausea, vomiting, behavioral changes, seizures, and focal, progressive neurologic changes. Occasionally the onset is abrupt, resembling a stroke, with the sudden appearance of headache, nausea, vomiting, and neurologic deficits. This picture is usually due to hemorrhage into the metastasis. Melanoma, germ cell tumors, and renal cell cancers have a particularly high incidence of intracranial bleeding. The tumor mass and surrounding edema may cause obstruction of the circulation of cerebrospinal fluid, with resulting hydrocephalus. Patients with increased intracranial pressure may have papilledema with visual disturbances and neck stiffness. As the mass enlarges, brain tissue may be displaced through the fixed cranial openings, producing various herniation syndromes.

CT scan and MRI are equally effective in the diagnosis of brain metastases. CT scan with contrast should be used as a screening procedure. The CT scan shows brain metastases as multiple enhancing lesions of various sizes with surrounding areas of low-density edema. If a single lesion or no metastases are visualized by contrast-enhanced CT, MRI of the brain should be performed. Gadolinium-enhanced MRI is more sensitive than CT at revealing meningeal involvement and small lesions, particularly in the brainstem or cerebellum.

Intracranial hypertension secondary to tretinoin therapy has been reported.

Rx INCREASED INTRACRANIAL PRESSURE

If signs and symptoms of brain herniation (particularly headache, drowsiness, and papilledema) are present, the patient should be intubated and hyperventilated to maintain P_{CO_2} between 25 and 30 mmHg and should receive infusions of mannitol (1–1.5 g/kg) every 6 h. Dexamethasone is the best initial treatment for all symptomatic patients with brain metastases (see above). Patients with multiple lesions should receive whole-brain radiation therapy. Patients with a single brain metastasis and with controlled extracranial disease may be treated with surgical excision followed by whole-brain radiation therapy, especially if they are younger than 60 years. Radioresistant tumors should be resected if possible. Stereotactic radiosurgery is an effective treatment for inaccessible or recurrent lesions. With a gamma knife or linear accelerator, multiple small, well-collimated beams of ionizing radiation destroy lesions seen on MRI. Some patients with increased intracranial pressure associated with hydrocephalus may benefit from shunt placement. If neurological deterioration is not reversed with medical therapy, ventriculotomy to remove cerebrospinal fluid (CSF) or craniotomy to remove tumors or hematomas may be necessary.

NEOPLASTIC MENINGITIS

Tumor involving the leptomeninges is a complication of both primary central nervous system (CNS) tumors and tumors that metastasize to the CNS. The incidence is estimated at 3–8% of patients with cancer. Melanoma, breast and lung cancer, lymphoma (including AIDS-associated), and acute leukemia are the most common causes. Synchronous intraparenchymal brain metastases are evident in 11–31% of patients with neoplastic meningitis.

Patients typically present with multifocal neurologic signs and symptoms, including headache, gait abnormality, mental changes, nausea, vomiting, seizures, back or radicular pain, and limb weakness. Signs include cranial nerve palsies, extremity weakness, paresthesia, and decreased deep tendon reflexes.

Diagnosis is made by demonstrating malignant cells in the CSF; however, up to 40% of patients may have false negative CSF cytology. An elevated CSF protein level is nearly always present (except in HTLV-1–associated adult T cell leukemia). Patients with neurologic signs and symptoms consistent with neoplastic meningitis who have a negative CSF cytology but an elevated CSF protein level should have the spinal tap repeated at least three times for cytologic examination before the diagnosis is rejected. MRI findings suggestive of neoplastic meningitis include leptomeningeal, subependymal, dural, or cranial nerve enhancement; superficial cerebral lesions; and communicating hydrocephalus. Spinal cord imaging by MRI is a necessary component of the evaluation of nonleukemia neoplastic meningitis as ~20% of patients have cord abnormalities, including intradural enhancing nodules that are diagnostic for leptomeningeal involvement. Cauda equina lesions are common, but lesions may be seen anywhere in the spinal

canal. Radiolabeled CSF flow studies are abnormal in up to 70% of patients with neoplastic meningitis; ventricular outlet obstruction, abnormal flow in the spinal canal, or impaired flow over the cerebral convexities may affect distribution of intrathecal chemotherapy resulting in decreased efficacy or increased toxicity. Radiation therapy may correct CSF flow abnormalities before use of intrathecal chemotherapy. Neoplastic meningitis can also lead to intracranial hypertension and hydrocephalus. Placement of a ventriculoperitoneal shunt may effectively palliate symptoms in these patients.

The development of neoplastic meningitis usually occurs in the setting of uncontrolled cancer outside the CNS; thus, prognosis is poor (median survival 10–12 weeks). However, treatment of the neoplastic meningitis may successfully alleviate symptoms and control the CNS spread.

Rx NEOPLASTIC MENINGITIS

Intrathecal chemotherapy, usually methotrexate, cytarabine, or thiotepa, is delivered by lumbar puncture or by an intraventricular reservoir (Ommaya) three times a week until the CSF is free of malignant cells. Injections are given twice a week for a month and then weekly for a month. An extended release preparation of cytarabine (Depocyte) has a longer half-life and is more effective than other formulations. Among solid tumors, breast cancer responds best to therapy. Patients with neoplastic meningitis from either acute leukemia or lymphoma may be cured of their CNS disease if the systemic disease can be eliminated.

SEIZURES

Seizures occurring in a patient with cancer can be caused by the tumor itself, by metabolic disturbances, by radiation injury, by cerebral infarctions, by chemotherapy-related encephalopathies, or by CNS infections. Metastatic disease to the CNS is the most common cause of seizures in patients with cancer. However, seizures occur more frequently in primary brain tumors than in metastatic brain lesions. Seizures are a presenting symptom of CNS metastasis in 6–29% of cases. Approximately 10% of patients with CNS metastasis eventually develop seizures. The presence of frontal lesions correlates with early seizures, and the presence of hemispheric symptoms increases the risk for late seizures. Both early and late seizures are uncommon in patients with posterior fossa lesions. Seizures are also common in patients with CNS metastases from melanoma. Very rarely, cytotoxic drugs such as etoposide, busulfan, and chlorambucil cause seizures.

Rx SEIZURES

Patients in whom seizures due to CNS metastases have been demonstrated should receive anticonvulsive treatment with diphenylhydantoin. Prophylactic anticonvulsant therapy is not recommended unless the patient is at a high risk for late seizures (melanoma primary, hemorrhagic metastases, treatment with radiosurgery). In those patients, serum diphenylhydantoin levels should be monitored closely and the dosage adjusted according to serum levels. Phenytoin induces the hepatic metabolism of dexamethasone, reducing its half-life, while dexamethasone may decrease phenytoin levels. Most antiseizure medications induce CYP450, which alters the metabolism of antitumor agents, including irinotecan, taxanes, and etoposide as well as molecular targeted agents including imatinib, gefitinib, and tipifarnib.

PULMONARY AND INTRACEREBRAL LEUKOCYTOSTASIS

Hyperleukocytosis and the leukostasis syndrome associated with it is a potentially fatal complication of acute leukemia (particularly myeloid leukemia) that can occur when the peripheral blast cell count is >100,000/mL. The frequency of hyperleukocytosis is 5–13% in AML and 10–30% in acute lymphoid leukemia; however, leukostasis is rare in lymphoid leukemia. At such high blast cell counts, blood viscosity is increased, blood flow is slowed by aggregates of tumor cells, and the primitive myeloid leukemic cells are capable of invading through endothelium and causing hemorrhage. Brain and lung are most commonly affected. Patients with brain leukostasis may experience stupor, headache, dizziness, tinnitus, visual disturbances, ataxia, confusion, coma, or sudden death. Administration of 600 cGy of whole-brain irradiation can protect against this complication and can be followed by rapid institution of antileukemic therapy. Pulmonary leukostasis may present as respiratory distress, hypoxemia, and progress to respiratory failure. Chest radiographs may be normal but usually show interstitial or alveolar infiltrates. Arterial blood gas results should be interpreted cautiously. Rapid consumption of plasma oxygen by the markedly increased number of white blood cells can cause spuriously low arterial oxygen tension. Pulse oximetry is the most accurate way of assessing oxygenation in patients with hyperleukocytosis. Leukapheresis may be helpful in decreasing circulating blast counts. Treatment of the leukemia can result in pulmonary hemorrhage from lysis of blasts in the lung, called *leukemic cell lysis pneumopathy*. Intravascular volume depletion and unnecessary blood transfusions may increase blood viscosity and worsen the leukostasis syndrome. Leukostasis is not a feature of the high white cell counts associated with chronic lymphoid or chronic myeloid leukemia.

When acute promyelocytic leukemia is treated with differentiating agents like tretinoin and arsenic trioxide, cerebral or pulmonary leukostasis may occur as tumor cells differentiate into mature neutrophils. This complication can be largely avoided by using cytotoxic chemotherapy together with the differentiating agents.

HEMOPTYSIS

Hemoptysis may be caused by nonmalignant conditions, but lung cancer accounts for a large proportion of cases. Up to 20% of patients with lung cancer have hemoptysis some time in their course. Endobronchial metastases from carcinoid tumors, breast cancer, colon cancer, kidney cancer, and melanoma may also cause hemoptysis. The volume of bleeding is often difficult to gauge. Massive hemoptysis is defined as >600 mL of blood produced in 24 h. However, any hemoptysis should be considered massive if it threatens life. When respiratory difficulty occurs, hemoptysis should be treated emergently. The first priorities are to maintain the airway, optimize oxygenation, and stabilize the hemodynamic status. Often patients can tell where the bleeding is occurring. They should be placed bleeding side down and given supplemental oxygen. If large-volume bleeding continues or the airway is compromised, the patient should be intubated and undergo emergency bronchoscopy. If the site of bleeding is detected, either the patient undergoes a definitive surgical procedure or the lesion is treated with a neodymium:yttrium-aluminum-garnet (Nd:YAG) laser. The surgical option is preferred. Bronchial artery embolization may control brisk bleeding in 75–90% of patients, permitting the definitive surgical procedure to be done more safely. Embolization without definitive surgery is associated with rebleeding in 20–50% of patients.

Recurrent hemoptysis usually responds to a second embolization procedure. A post-embolization syndrome characterized by pleuritic pain, fever, dysphagia, and leukocytosis may occur; it lasts 5–7 days and resolves with symptomatic treatment. Bronchial or esophageal wall necrosis, myocardial infarction, and spinal cord infarction are rare complications.

Pulmonary hemorrhage with or without hemoptysis in hematologic malignancies is often associated with fungal infections, particularly *Aspergillus* sp. After granulocytopenia resolves, the lung infiltrates in aspergillosis may cavitate and cause massive hemoptysis. Thrombocytopenia and coagulation defects should be corrected, if possible. Surgical evaluation is recommended in patients with aspergillosis-related cavitary lesions.

AIRWAY OBSTRUCTION

Airway obstruction refers to a blockage at the level of the mainstem bronchi or above. It may result either from intraluminal tumor growth or from extrinsic compression of the airway. The most common cause of malignant upper airway obstruction is invasion from an adjacent primary tumor, most commonly lung cancer, followed by esophageal, thyroid, and mediastinal malignancies. Extrathoracic primary tumors such as renal, colon, or breast cancer can cause airway obstruction through endobronchial and/or mediastinal lymph node metastases. Patients may present with dyspnea, hemoptysis, stridor, wheezing, intractable cough, postobstructive pneumonia, or hoarseness. Chest radiographs usually demonstrate obstructing lesions. CT scans reveal the extent of tumor. Cool, humidified oxygen, glucocorticoids, and ventilation with a mixture of helium and oxygen (Heliox) may provide temporary relief. If the obstruction is proximal to the larynx, a tracheostomy may be lifesaving. For more distal obstructions, particularly intrinsic lesions incompletely obstructing the airway, bronchoscopy with laser treatment, photodynamic therapy, or stenting can produce immediate relief in most patients (**Fig. 270-3**). However, radiation therapy (either external-beam irradiation or brachytherapy) given together with glucocorticoids may open the airway. Symptomatic extrinsic compression may be palliated by stenting. Patients with primary airway tumors such as squamous cell carcinoma, carcinoid tumor, adenocystic carcinoma, or non-small cell lung cancer should have surgery.

METABOLIC EMERGENCIES

HYPERCALCEMIA

Hypercalcemia is the most common paraneoplastic syndrome. Its pathogenesis and management are fully discussed in Chaps. 96 and 347.

FIGURE 270-3 Airway obstruction. A. CT scan of a 62-year-old-man with tracheal obstruction caused by renal carcinoma showing paratracheal mass (*A*) with tracheal invasion/obstruction (*arrow*). **B.** Chest x-ray of same patient after stent (*arrows*) placement.

SYNDROME OF INAPPROPRIATE SECRETION OF ANTIDIURETIC HORMONE (SIADH)

Hyponatremia is a common electrolyte abnormality in cancer patients, and SIADH is the most common cause of hyponatremia among patients with cancer. SIADH is discussed fully in Chaps. 96 and 334.

LACTIC ACIDOSIS

Lactic acidosis is a rare and potentially fatal metabolic complication of cancer. Lactic acidosis associated with sepsis, and circulatory failure is a common preterminal event in many malignancies. Lactic acidosis in the absence of hypoxemia may occur in patients with leukemia, lymphoma, or solid tumors. Extensive involvement of the liver by tumor is present in most cases. Alteration of liver function may be responsible for the lactate accumulation. HIV-infected patients have an increased risk of aggressive lymphoma; lactic acidosis that occurs in such patients may be related either to the rapid growth of the tumor or from toxicity of nucleoside reverse transcriptase inhibitors. Symptoms of lactic acidosis include tachypnea, tachycardia, change of mental status, and hepatomegaly. The serum level of lactic acid may reach 10–20 meq/L (90–180 mg/dL). Treatment is aimed at the underlying disease. The danger from lactic acidosis is from the acidosis, not the lactate. Sodium bicarbonate should be added if acidosis is very severe or if hydrogen ion production is very rapid and uncontrolled. The prognosis is poor.

HYPOGLYCEMIA

Persistent hypoglycemia is occasionally associated with tumors other than pancreatic islet cell tumors. Usually these tumors are large; tumors of mesenchymal origin, hepatomas, or adrenocortical tumors may cause hypoglycemia. Mesenchymal tumors are usually located in the retroperitoneum or thorax. Obtundation, confusion, and behavioral aberrations occur in the postabsorptive period and may precede the diagnosis of the tumor. These tumors often secrete incompletely processed insulin-like growth factor II (IGF-II), a hormone capable of activating insulin receptors and causing hypoglycemia. Tumors secreting incompletely processed big IGF-II are characterized by an increased IGF-II to IGF-I ratio, suppressed insulin and C peptide level, and inappropriately low growth hormone and β-hydroxybutyrate concentrations. Rarely, hypoglycemia is due to insulin secretion by a non-islet cell carcinoma. The development of hepatic dysfunction from liver metastases and increased glucose consumption by the tumor can contribute to hypoglycemia. If the tumor cannot be resected, hypoglycemia symptoms may be relieved by the administration of glucose, glucocorticoids, or glucagon.

Hypoglycemia can be artifactual; hyperleukocytosis from leukemia, myeloproliferative diseases, leukemoid reactions, or colony stimulating factor treatment can increase glucose consumption in the test tube after blood is drawn, leading to pseudohypoglycemia.

ADRENAL INSUFFICIENCY

In patients with cancer, adrenal insufficiency may go unrecognized because the symptoms, such as nausea, vomiting, anorexia, and orthostatic hypotension, are nonspecific and may be mistakenly attributed to progressive cancer or to therapy. Primary adrenal insufficiency may develop owing to replacement of both glands by metastases (lung, breast, colon, or kidney cancer; lymphoma), to removal of both glands, or to hemorrhagic necrosis in association with sepsis or anticoagulation. Impaired adrenal steroid synthesis occurs in patients being treated for cancer with mitotane, ketoconazole, or aminoglutethimide or undergoing rapid reduction in glucocorticoid therapy. Rarely, metastatic replacement causes primary adrenal insufficiency as the first manifestation of an occult malignancy. Metastasis to the pituitary or hypothalamus is found at autopsy in up to 5% of patients with cancer, but associated secondary adrenal insufficiency is rare. Megesterol acetate, used to manage cancer and HIV-related cachexia, may suppress plasma levels of cortisol and adrenocorticotropic hormone (ACTH). Patients taking megesterol may develop adrenal insufficiency, and even those whose adrenal dysfunction is not symptomatic may have inadequate adrenal reserve if they become seriously ill. Cranial irradiation for childhood brain tumors may affect

the hypothalamus-pituitary-adrenal axis, resulting in secondary adrenal insufficiency.

Acute adrenal insufficiency is potentially lethal. Treatment of suspected adrenal crisis is initiated after the sampling of serum cortisol and ACTH levels (Chap. 336).

TREATMENT-RELATED EMERGENCIES

TUMOR LYSIS SYNDROME

Tumor lysis syndrome (TLS) is characterized by hyperuricemia, hyperkalemia, hyperphosphatemia, and hypocalcemia and is caused by the destruction of a large number of rapidly proliferating neoplastic cells. Acidosis may also develop. Acute renal failure occurs frequently.

TLS is most often associated with the treatment of Burkitt's lymphoma, acute lymphoblastic leukemia, and other high-grade lymphomas, but it also may be seen with chronic leukemias and, rarely, with solid tumors. This syndrome has been seen in patients with chronic lymphocytic leukemia after treatment with nucleosides. TLS has been observed with administration of glucocorticoids, hormonal agents such as letrozole and tamoxifen, and monoclonal antibodies such as rituximab and gemtuzumab. TLS usually occurs during or shortly (1–5 days) after chemotherapy. Rarely, spontaneous necrosis of malignancies causes TLS.

Hyperuricemia may be present at the time of chemotherapy. Effective treatment kills malignant cells and leads to increased serum uric acid levels from the turnover of nucleic acids. Owing to the acidic local environment, uric acid can precipitate in the tubules, medulla, and collecting ducts of the kidney, leading to renal failure. Lactic acidosis and dehydration may contribute to the precipitation of uric acid in the renal tubules. The finding of uric acid crystals in the urine is strong evidence for uric acid nephropathy. The ratio of urinary uric acid to urinary creatinine is >1 in patients with acute hyperuricemic nephropathy and <1 in patients with renal failure due to other causes.

Hyperphosphatemia, which can be caused by the release of intracellular phosphate pools by tumor lysis, produces a reciprocal depression in serum calcium, which causes severe neuromuscular irritability and tetany. Deposition of calcium phosphate in the kidney and hyperphosphatemia may cause renal failure. Potassium is the principal intracellular cation, and massive destruction of malignant cells may lead to hyperkalemia. Hyperkalemia in patients with renal failure may rapidly become life-threatening by causing ventricular arrhythmias and sudden death.

The likelihood that TLS will occur in patients with Burkitt's lymphoma is related to the tumor burden and renal function. Hyperuricemia and high serum levels of lactate dehydrogenase (LDH >1500 U/L), both of which correlate with total tumor burden, also correlate with the risk of TLS. In patients at risk for TLS, pretreatment evaluations should include a complete blood count, serum chemistry evaluation, and urine analysis. High leukocyte and platelet counts may artificially elevate potassium levels ("pseudohyperkalemia") due to lysis of these cells after the blood is drawn. In these cases, plasma potassium instead of serum potassium should be followed. In pseudohyperkalemia, no electrocardiographic abnormalities are present. In patients with abnormal baseline renal function, the kidneys and retroperitoneal area should be evaluated by sonography and/or CT to rule out obstructive uropathy. Urine output should be watched closely.

℞ TUMOR LYSIS SYNDROME

Recognition of risk and prevention are the most important steps in the management of this syndrome **(Fig. 270-4)**. The standard preventive approach consists of allopurinol, urinary alkalinization, and aggressive hydration. Intravenous allopurinol may be given in patients who cannot tolerate oral therapy. In some cases, uric acid levels cannot be lowered sufficiently with the standard preventive approach. Rasburicase can be effective in these instances. Urate oxidase is missing from primates and catalyzes the conversion of poorly soluble uric acid to readily soluble allantoin. Rasburicase acts rapidly, decreasing uric acid levels within hours; however, it may cause hypersensitivity reactions such as bronchospasm, hypoxemia, and hypotension. Rasburicase is contraindicated in patients with glucose-

FIGURE 270-4 Management of patients at high risk for the tumor lysis syndrome.

PT MANAGEMENT FOR TUMOR LYSIS

Maintain hydration by administration of normal or 1/2 normal saline at 3000 mL/m² per day
Keep urine pH at 7.0 or greater by administration of sodium bicarbonate
Administer allopurinol at 300 mg/m² per day
Monitor serum chemistry

If, after 24–48 h

Serum uric acid>8.0 mg/dL
Serum creatinine>1.6 mg/dL

Serum uric acid<8.0 mg/dL
Serum creatinine<1.6 mg/dL
Urine pH>7.0

Correct treatable renal failure (obstruction)
Start recombinant urate oxidase, 0.2 mg/kg IV daily

Start chemotherapy
Discontinue bicarbonate administration
Monitor serum chemistry every 6–12 h

Delay chemotherapy or start dialysis

If

Serum K⁺>6.0 meq/L
Serum uric acid>10 mg/dL
Serum creatinine>10 mg/dL
Serum phosphate>10 mg/dL or increasing
Symptomatic hypocalcemia present

Begin hemodialysis

6-phosphate dehydrogenase deficiency who are unable to break down hydrogen peroxide, an end product of the urate oxidase reaction. Despite aggressive prophylaxis, TLS and/or oliguric or anuric renal failure may occur. Care should be taken to prevent worsening of symptomatic hypocalcemia by induction of alkalosis during bicarbonate infusion. Administration of sodium bicarbonate may also lead to urinary precipitation of calcium phosphate, which is less soluble at alkaline pH. Dialysis is often necessary and should be considered early in the course. Hemodialysis is preferred. Hemofiltration offers a gradual, continuous method of removing cellular byproducts and fluid. The prognosis is excellent, and renal function recovers after the uric acid level is lowered to ≤10 mg/dL.

HUMAN ANTIBODY INFUSION REACTIONS

The initial infusion of human or humanized antibodies (e.g., rituximab, gemtuzumab, trastuzumab) is associated with fever, chills, nausea, asthenia, and headache in up to half of treated patients. Bronchospasm and hypotension occur in 1% of patients. The pathogenesis is thought to be activation of immune effector processes (cells and complement). In the presence of high levels of circulating lymphoid tumor cells, thrombocytopenia, a rapid fall in circulating tumor cells, and mild electrolyte evidence of TLS may also occur. In addition, increased liver enzymes, D-dimer, LDH, and prolongation of the prothrombin time may occur. This syndrome is related to release of inflammatory cytokines, such as tumor necrosis factor α and interleukin 6. Diphenhydramine and acetaminophen can often prevent or suppress the symptoms. If they occur, the infusion is stopped and restarted at half the initial infusion rate after the symptoms have abated.

HEMOLYTIC-UREMIC SYNDROME

Hemolytic-uremic syndrome (HUS) and, less commonly, thrombotic thrombocytopenic purpura (TTP) occurring after treatment with an-

tineoplastic drugs have been described. Mitomycin is by far the most common agent causing this peculiar syndrome. Other chemotherapeutic agents, including cisplatin, bleomycin, and gemcitabine, have also been reported to be associated with this syndrome. It occurs most often in patients with gastric, colorectal, pancreatic, and breast carcinoma. In one series, 35% of patients were without evident cancer at the time this syndrome appeared. Secondary HUS/TTP has also been reported as a rare but sometimes fatal complication of bone marrow transplantation.

HUS usually has its onset 4–8 weeks after the last dose of chemotherapy, but it is not rare to detect it several months later. HUS is characterized by microangiopathic hemolytic anemia, thrombocytopenia, and renal failure. Dyspnea, weakness, fatigue, oliguria, and purpura are also common initial symptoms and findings. Systemic hypertension and pulmonary edema frequently occur. Severe hypertension, pulmonary edema, and rapid worsening of hemolysis and renal function may occur after a blood or blood product transfusion. Cardiac findings include atrial arrhythmias, pericardial friction rub, and pericardial effusion. Raynaud's phenomenon is part of the syndrome in patients treated with bleomycin.

Laboratory findings include severe to moderate anemia associated with red blood cell fragmentation and numerous schistocytes on peripheral smear. Reticulocytosis, decreased plasma haptoglobin, and an LDH level document hemolysis. The serum bilirubin level is usually normal or slightly elevated. The Coombs' test is negative. The white cell count is usually normal, and thrombocytopenia (<100,000/μL) is almost always present. Most patients have a normal coagulation profile, although some have mild elevations in thrombin time and in level of fibrin degradation products. The serum creatinine level is elevated at presentation and shows a pattern of subacute worsening within weeks of the initial azotemia. The urinalysis reveals hematuria, proteinuria, and granular or hyaline casts; and circulating immune complexes may be present.

The basic pathologic lesion appears to be deposition of fibrin in the walls of capillaries and arterioles, and these deposits are similar to those seen in HUS due to other causes. These microvascular abnormalities involve mainly the kidneys and rarely occur in other organs. The pathogenesis of chemotherapy-related HUS is unknown. Other forms of HUS/TTP are related to a decrease in processing of von Willebrand factor by a protease called ADAMTS13.

The case fatality rate is high; most patients die within a few months. Plasmapheresis and plasma exchange may normalize the hematologic abnormalities, but renal failure is not reversed in most patients. Immunoperfusion over a staphylococcal protein A column is the most successful treatment. About half of the patients treated with immunoperfusion respond with resolution of thrombocytopenia, improvement in anemia, and stabilization of renal failure. Treatment is well tolerated. It is not clear how the treatment works.

NEUTROPENIA AND INFECTION

These remain the most common serious complications of cancer therapy. They are covered in detail in Chap. 82.

PULMONARY INFILTRATES

Patients with cancer may present with dyspnea associated with diffuse interstitial infiltrates on chest radiographs. Such infiltrates may be due to progression of the underlying malignancy, treatment-related toxicities, infection, and/or unrelated diseases. The cause may be multifactorial; however, most commonly they occur as a consequence of treatment. Infiltration of the lung by malignancy has been described in patients with leukemia, lymphoma, and breast and other solid cancers. Pulmonary lymphatics may be involved diffusely by neoplasm (pulmonary lymphangitic carcinomatosis), resulting in a diffuse increase in interstitial markings on chest radiographs. The patient is often mildly dyspneic at the onset, but pulmonary failure develops over a period of weeks. In some patients, dyspnea precedes changes on the chest radiographs and is accompanied by a nonproductive cough. This syndrome is characteristic of solid tumors. In patients with leukemia, diffuse microscopic neoplastic peribronchial and peribronchiolar infiltration is frequent but may be asymptomatic. However, some patients present with diffuse interstitial infiltrates, an alveolar capillary block syndrome, and respiratory distress. In these situations, glucocorticoids can provide symptomatic relief, but specific chemotherapy should always be started promptly.

Several cytotoxic agents, such as bleomycin, methotrexate, busulfan, and the nitrosoureas, may cause pulmonary damage. The most frequent presentations are interstitial pneumonitis, alveolitis, and pulmonary fibrosis. Some cytotoxic agents, including methotrexate and procarbazine, may cause an acute hypersensitivity reaction. Cytosine arabinoside has been associated with noncardiogenic pulmonary edema. Administration of multiple cytotoxic drugs, as well as radiotherapy and preexisting lung disease, may potentiate the pulmonary toxicity. Supplemental oxygen may potentiate the effects of drugs and radiation injury. Patients should always be managed with the lowest FI_{O_2} that is sufficient to maintain hemoglobin saturation.

The onset of symptoms may be insidious, with symptoms including dyspnea, nonproductive cough, and tachycardia. Patients may have bibasilar crepitant rales, end-inspiratory crackles, fever, and cyanosis. The chest radiograph generally shows an interstitial and sometimes an intraalveolar pattern that is strongest at the lung bases and may be symmetric. A small effusion may occur. Hypoxemia with decreased carbon monoxide diffusing capacity is always present. Glucocorticoids may be helpful in patients in whom pulmonary toxicity is related to radiation therapy or to chemotherapy. Treatment is otherwise supportive.

Molecular targeted agents, imatinib, erlotinib, and gefitinib are potent inhibitors of tyrosine kinases. These drugs may cause interstitial lung disease. In the case of gefitinib, preexisting fibrosis, poor performance status, and prior thoracic irradiation are independent risk factors; this complication has high fatality rate. In Japan, incidence of interstitial lung disease associated with gefitinib was about 4.5%.

Radiation pneumonitis and/or fibrosis is a relatively frequent side effect of thoracic radiation therapy. It may be acute or chronic. Radiation-induced lung toxicity is a function of the irradiated lung volume, dose per fraction, and radiation dose. The larger the irradiated lung field, the higher the risk for radiation pneumonitis. Radiation pneumonitis usually develops from 2 to 6 months after completion of radiotherapy. The clinical syndrome, which varies in severity, consists of dyspnea, cough with scanty sputum, low-grade fever, and an initial hazy infiltrate on chest radiographs. The infiltrate and tissue damage usually are confined to the radiation field. The patients subsequently may develop a patchy alveolar infiltrate and air bronchograms, which may progress to acute respiratory failure that is sometimes fatal. A lung biopsy may be necessary to make the diagnosis. Asymptomatic infiltrates found incidentally after radiation therapy need not be treated. However, prednisone should be administered to patients with fever or other symptoms. The dosage should be tapered slowly after the resolution of radiation pneumonitis, as abrupt withdrawal of glucocorticoids may cause an exacerbation of pneumonia. Delayed radiation fibrosis may occur years after radiation therapy and is signaled by dyspnea on exertion. Often it is mild, but it can progress to chronic respiratory failure. Therapy is supportive.

Classical radiation pneumonitis that leads to pulmonary fibrosis is due to radiation-induced production of local cytokines such as platelet-derived growth factor β, tumor necrosis factor, and transforming growth factor β in the radiation field. An immunologically mediated sporadic radiation pneumonitis occurs in about 10% of patients; bilateral alveolitis mediated by T cells results in infiltrates outside the radiation field. This form of radiation pneumonitis usually resolves without sequelae.

Pneumonia is a common problem in patients undergoing treatment for cancer. Bacterial pneumonia typically causes a localized infiltrate on chest radiographs. Therapy is tailored to the causative organism. When diffuse interstitial infiltrates appear in a febrile patient, the differential diagnosis is extensive and includes pneumonia due to infection with *Pneumocystis carinii*; viral infections including cytomegalovirus, adenovirus, herpes simplex virus, herpes zoster, respiratory syncytial virus, or intracellular pathogens such as *Mycoplasma* and *Legionella*; effects of drugs or radiation; tumor progression; nonspecific pneumonitis; and fungal disease. Detection of opportunistic pathogens in pulmonary infections is still a challenge. Diagnostic tools include chest radiographs, CT scans, bronchoscopy with bronchoalveolar lavage, brush cytology, transbronchial biopsy, fine-needle aspiration, and open lung biopsy. In addition to the culture, evaluation of bronchoalveolar lavage fluid for *P. carinii* by polymerase chain reaction (PCR) and aspergillus antigen improve the diagnostic yield. Patients with cancer who are neutropenic and have fever and local infiltrates on chest radiograph should be treated initially with broad spectrum antibiotics, such as ceftazidime or imipenem. A new or persistent focal infiltrate not responding to broad spectrum antibiotics argues for initiation of empiric antifungal therapy. When diffuse bilateral infiltrates develop in patients with febrile neutropenia, broad spectrum antibiotics plus trimethoprim-sulfamethoxazole, with or without erythromycin, should be initiated. Addition of an antiviral agent is necessary in some settings, such as patients undergoing allogeneic hematopoietic stem cell transplantation. The empiric administration of trimethoprim-sulfamethoxazole plus erythromycin to patients without neutropenia and these antibiotics plus ceftazidime to patients with neutropenia covers nearly every treatable diagnosis (except tumor progression) and gives as good overall survival as a strategy based on early invasive intervention with bronchoalveolar lavage or open lung biopsy. If the patient does not improve in 4 days, open lung biopsy is the procedure of choice. Bronchoscopy with bronchoalveolar lavage may be used in patients who are poor candidates for surgery.

In patients with pulmonary infiltrates who are afebrile, heart failure and multiple pulmonary emboli are in the differential diagnosis.

NEUTROPENIC ENTEROCOLITIS

Neutropenic enterocolitis (typhlitis) is the inflammation and necrosis of the cecum and surrounding tissues that may complicate the treatment of acute leukemia. This complication has also been seen in patients with other forms of cancer treated with taxanes and in patients receiving high-dose chemotherapy (Fig. 270-5). The patient develops right lower quadrant abdominal pain, often with rebound tenderness and a tense, distended abdomen, in a setting of fever and neutropenia. Watery diarrhea (often containing sloughed mucosa) and bacteremia are common, and bleeding may occur. Plain abdominal films are generally of little value in the diagnosis; CT scan may show marked bowel wall thickening, particularly in the cecum, with bowel wall edema. Patients with bowel wall thickness >10 mm on ultrasonogram have higher mortality rates. However, bowel wall thickening is significantly more prominent in patients with *Clostridium difficile* colitis. Pneumatosis intestinalis is a more specific finding, seen only in those with neutropenic enterocolitis and ischemia. The combined involvement of the small and large bowel suggests a diagnosis of neutropenic enterocolitis. Rapid institution of broad-spectrum antibiotics and nasogastric suction may reverse the process. Surgical intervention should be considered if no improvement is seen by 24 h after the start of antibiotic treatment. If the localized abdominal findings become diffuse, the prognosis is poor.

C. difficile colitis is increasing in incidence. Newer strains of *C. difficile* produce about 20 times more of toxins A and B compared to previously studied strains. *C. difficile* risk is also increased with chemotherapy. Antibiotic coverage for *C. difficile* should be added if pseudomembranous colitis cannot be excluded.

HEMORRHAGIC CYSTITIS

Hemorrhagic cystitis can develop in patients receiving cyclophosphamide or ifosfamide. Both drugs are metabolized to acrolein, which is a strong chemical irritant that is excreted in the urine. Prolonged contact or high concentrations may lead to bladder irritation and hemorrhage. Symptoms include gross hematuria, frequency, dysuria, burning, urgency, incontinence, and nocturia. The best management is prevention. Maintaining a high rate of urine flow minimizes exposure. In addition, 2-mercaptoethanesulfonate (mesna) detoxifies the process. In extreme cases, ligation of the hypogastric arteries, urinary diversion, or cystectomy may be necessary.

Hemorrhagic cystitis also occurs in patients who undergo bone marrow transplantation (BMT). In the BMT setting, early-onset hemorrhagic cystitis is related to drugs in the treatment regimen (e.g., cyclophosphamide) and late-onset hemorrhagic cystitis is usually due to the polyoma virus BKV or adenovirus type 11. BKV load in urine alone or in combination with acute graft-versus-host disease correlate with development of hemorrhagic cystitis. Viral causes are usually detected by PCR-based diagnostic tests. Treatment of viral hemorrhagic cystitis is largely supportive, with reduction in doses of immunosuppressive agents, if possible. No antiviral therapy is approved, though cidofovir is being tested.

HYPERSENSITIVITY REACTIONS TO ANTINEOPLASTIC DRUGS

Many antineoplastic drugs may cause hypersensitivity reaction (HSR). These reactions are unpredictable and potentially life-threatening. Most reactions occur during or within hours of parenteral drug administration. Taxanes; platinum compounds; asparginase; etoposide; and biologic agents including rituximab, bevacizumab, trastuzumab, gemtuzumab, cetuximab, and alemtuzumab are more commonly associated with acute HSR than are other agents. Acute hypersensitivity reactions to some drugs, such as taxanes, occur during the first or second dose administered. HSR from platinum compounds occurs after prolonged exposure. Skin testing may identify patients with high risk for HSR after carboplatin exposure. Premedication with histamine H1 and H2 receptor antagonists and glucocorticoids reduce the incidence of hypersensitivity reaction to taxanes, particularly paclitaxel. Despite premedication, HSR may still occur. In these cases, retreatment may be attempted with care, but use of alternative agents may be required.

FURTHER READINGS

ALBANELL J, BASELGA J: Systemic therapy emergencies. Semin Oncol 27:347, 2000

COIFFIER B, RIOUFFOL C: Management of tumor lysis syndrome in adults. Expert Rev Anticancer Ther 7:233, 2007

DAVIS MP et al: Modern management of cancer-related intestinal obstruction. Curr Oncol Rep 2:343, 2000

GLEISSNER B et al: Neoplastic meningitis. Lancet Neurol 5:443, 2006

GORNIK HL et al: Abnormal cytology predicts poor prognosis in cancer patients with pericardial effusion. J Clin Oncol 23:5211, 2005

GORSCHLUTER M et al: Neutropenic enterocolitis in adults: systematic analysis of evidence quality. Eur J Hematol 75:1, 2005

LOBLAW DA et al: Systematic review of the diagnosis and management of malignant extradural spinal cord compression: The Cancer Care Ontario Practice Guidelines Initiative's neuro-oncology disease site group. J Clin Oncol 23:2028, 2005

RICE TW et al: The superior vena cava syndrome: Clinical characteristics and evolving etiology. Medicine 85:37, 2006

RIPAMONTI C et al: Respiratory problems in advanced cancer. Support Care Cancer 10:204, 2002

ZANOTTI KM et al: Prevention and management of antineoplastic-induced hypersensitivity reactions; Drug Saf 24:767, 2001

FIGURE 270-5 Abdominal CT scans of a 72-year-old woman with neutropenic enterocolitis secondary to chemotherapy. A. Air in inferior mesenteric vein (*arrow*) and bowel wall with pneumatosis intestinalis. **B.** CT scans of upper abdomen demonstrating air in portal vein (*arrows*).

the metabolites and can be coadministered with the instigating drugs. Mesna usually is given three times on the day of ifosfamide administration in doses that are each 20% of the total ifosfamide dose. If hemorrhagic cystitis develops, the maintenance of a high urine flow may be sufficient supportive care. If conservative management is not effective, irrigation of the bladder with a 0.37–0.74% formalin solution for 10 min stops the bleeding in most cases. *N*-acetylcysteine may also be an effective irrigant. Prostaglandins (carboprost) can inhibit

271 Cellular and Molecular Biology of the Kidney

Alfred L. George, Jr., Eric G. Neilson

The kidney is one of the most highly differentiated organs in the body. Nearly 30 different cell types can be found in the renal interstitium or along segmented nephrons, blood vessels, and filtering capillaries at the conclusion of embryological development. This panoply of cells modulates a variety of complex physiologic processes. Endocrine functions, the regulation of blood pressure and intraglomerular hemodynamics, solute and water transport, acid-base balance, and removal of fuel or drug metabolites are all accomplished by intricate mechanisms of renal response. This breadth of physiology hinges on the clever ingenuity of nephron architecture that evolved as complex organisms came out of water to live on land.

EMBRYOLOGICAL DEVELOPMENT

The kidney develops from within the intermediate mesoderm under the timed or sequential control of a growing number of genes, described in Fig. 271-1. The transcription of these genes is guided by morphogenic cues that invite ureteric buds to penetrate the metanephric blastema, where they induce primary mesenchymal cells to form early nephrons. This induction involves a number of complex signaling pathways mediated by c-Met, fibroblast growth factor, transforming growth factor β, glial cell–derived neurotrophic factor, hepatocyte growth factor, epithelial growth factor, and the Wnt family of proteins. The ureteric buds derive from the posterior nephric ducts and mature into collecting ducts that eventually funnel to a renal pelvis and ureter. Induced mesenchyme undergoes mesenchymal-epithelia transitions to form comma-shape bodies at the proximal end of each ureteric bud leading to the formation of S-shape nephrons that cleft and enjoin with penetrating endothelial cells derived from sprouting angioblasts. Under the influence of vascular endothelial growth factor A, these penetrating cells form capillaries with surrounding mesangial cells that differentiate into a glomerular filter for plasma water and solute. The ureteric buds branch, and each branch produces a new set of nephrons. The number of branching events ultimately determines the total number of nephrons in each kidney. There are approximately 900,000 glomeruli in each kidney in normal-birth-weight adults and as few as 225,000 in low-birth-weight adults. In the latter case, a failure to complete the last one or two rounds of branching leads to smaller kidneys and increased risk for hypertension and cardiovascular disease later in life.

Glomeruli evolved as complex capillary filters with fenestrated endothelia. Outlining each capillary is a basement membrane covered by epithelial podocytes. Podocytes attach by special foot processes and share a slit-pore membrane with their neighbor. The slit-pore membrane is formed by the interaction of nephrin, annexin-4, CD2AP, FAT, ZO-1, P-cadherin, podocin, and neph 1–3 proteins. These glomerular capillaries seat in a mesangial matrix shrouded by parietal and proximal tubular epithelia forming Bowman's capsule. Mesangial cells have an embryonic lineage consistent with arteriolar or juxtaglomerular cells and contain contractile actin-myosin fibers. These cells make contact with glomerular capillary loops, and their matrix holds them in condensed arrangement. Between nephrons lies the renal interstitium. This region forms the functional space surrounding glomeruli and their downstream tubules, which are home to resident and trafficking cells, such as fibroblasts, dendritic cells, occasional lymphocytes, and lipid-laden macrophages. The cortical and medullary capillaries, which siphon off solute and water following tubular reclamation of glomerular filtrate, are also part of the interstitial fabric as well as a web of connective tissue that supports the kidney's emblematic architecture of folding tubules. The relational precision of these structures determines the unique physiology of the kidney.

Each nephron segments during embryological development into a proximal tubule, descending and ascending limbs of the loop of Henle, distal tubule, and the collecting duct. These classic tubular segments have subsegments recognized by highly unique epithelia serving regional physiology. All nephrons have the same structural components, but there are two types whose structure depends on their location within the kidney. The majority of nephrons are cortical, with glomeruli located in the mid-to-outer cortex. Fewer nephrons are juxtamedullary, with glomeruli at the boundary of the cortex and outer medulla. Cortical nephrons have short loops of Henle, whereas juxtamedullary nephrons have long loops of Henle. There are critical differences in blood supply as well. The peritubular capillaries surrounding cortical nephrons are shared among adjacent nephrons. By contrast, juxtamedullary nephrons use separate capillaries called *vasa recta*. Cortical nephrons

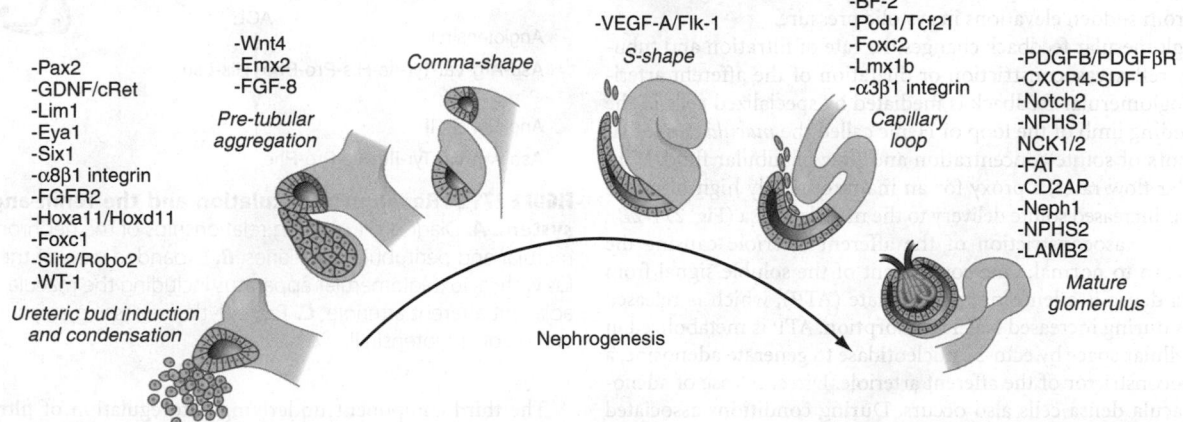

FIGURE 271-1 Genes controlling renal nephrogenesis. A growing number of genes have been identified at various stages of glomerulotubular development in mammalian kidney. The genes listed have been tested in various genetically modified mice, and their location corresponds to the classical stages of kidney development postulated by Saxen in 1987. GDNF, giant cell line–derived neutrophilic factor; FGFR2, fibroblast growth factor receptor 2; WT-1, Wilms tumor gene 1; FGF-8, fibroblast growth factor 8; VEGF–A/Flk-1, vascular endothelial growth factor–A/fetal liver kinase-1; PDGFB, platelet-derived growth factor B; PDGFβR, PDGFβ receptor; SDF-1, stromal-derived factor 1; NPHS1, nephrin; NCK1/2, NCK-adaptor protein; CD2AP, CD2-associated protein; NPHS2, podocin; LAMB2, laminin beta-2.

perform most of the glomerular filtration because there are more of them and because their afferent arterioles are larger than their respective efferent arterioles. The juxtamedullary nephrons, with longer loops of Henle, create a hyperosmolar gradient that allows for the production of concentrated urine. How developmental instructions specify the differentiation of all these unique epithelia among various tubular segments is still unknown.

DETERMINANTS AND REGULATION OF GLOMERULAR FILTRATION

Renal blood flow drains approximately 20% of the cardiac output, or 1000 mL/min. Blood reaches each nephron through the afferent arteriole leading into a glomerular capillary where large amounts of fluid and solutes are filtered as tubular fluid. The distal ends of the glomerular capillaries coalesce to form an efferent arteriole leading to the first segment of a second capillary network (peritubular capillaries) surrounding the cortical tubules (Fig. 271-2A). Thus, the cortical nephron has two capillary beds arranged in series separated by the efferent arteriole that regulates the hydrostatic pressure in both capillary beds. The peritubular capillaries empty into small venous branches, which coalesce into larger veins to eventually form the renal vein.

The hydrostatic pressure gradient across the glomerular capillary wall is the primary driving force for glomerular filtration. Oncotic pressure within the capillary lumen, determined by the concentration of unfiltered plasma proteins, partially offsets the hydrostatic pressure gradient and opposes filtration. As the oncotic pressure rises along the length of the glomerular capillary, the driving force for filtration falls to zero before reaching the efferent arteriole. Approximately 20% of the renal plasma flow is filtered into Bowman's space, and the ratio of glomerular filtration rate (GFR) to renal plasma flow determines the filtration fraction. Several factors, mostly hemodynamic, contribute to the regulation of filtration under physiologic conditions.

Although glomerular filtration is affected by renal artery pressure, this relationship is not linear across the range of physiologic blood pressures. Autoregulation of glomerular filtration is the result of three major factors that modulate either afferent or efferent arteriolar tone: these include an autonomous vasoreactive (myogenic) reflex in the afferent arteriole, *tubuloglomerular feedback,* and angiotensin II–mediated vasoconstriction of the efferent arteriole. The myogenic reflex is a first line of defense against fluctuations in renal blood flow. Acute changes in renal perfusion pressure evoke reflex constriction or dilatation of the afferent arteriole in response to increased or decreased pressure, respectively. This phenomenon helps protect the glomerular capillary from sudden elevations in systolic pressure.

Tubuloglomerular feedback changes the rate of filtration and tubular flow by reflex vasoconstriction or dilatation of the afferent arteriole. Tubuloglomerular feedback is mediated by specialized cells in the thick ascending limb of the loop of Henle called the *macula densa* that act as sensors of solute concentration and flow of tubular fluid. With high tubular flow rates, a proxy for an inappropriately high filtration rate, there is increased solute delivery to the macula densa (Fig. 271-2B), which evokes vasoconstriction of the afferent arteriole causing the GFR to return to normal. One component of the soluble signal from the macula densa is adenosine triphosphate (ATP), which is released by the cells during increased NaCl reabsorption. ATP is metabolized in the extracellular space by ecto-5′-nucleotidase to generate adenosine, a potent vasoconstrictor of the afferent arteriole. Direct release of adenosine by macula densa cells also occurs. During conditions associated with a fall in filtration rate, reduced solute delivery to the macula densa attenuates the tubuloglomerular response, allowing afferent arteriolar dilatation and restoring glomerular filtration to normal levels. Loop diuretics block tubuloglomerular feedback by interfering with NaCl reabsorption by macula densa cells. Angiotensin II and reactive oxygen species enhance, while nitric oxide blunts tubuloglomerular feedback.

A

B

C

FIGURE 271-2 Renal microcirculation and the renin-angiotensin system. A. Diagram illustrating relationships of the nephron with glomerular and peritubular capillaries. **B.** Expanded view of the glomerulus with its juxtaglomerular apparatus including the macula densa and adjacent afferent arteriole. **C.** Proteolytic processing steps in the generation of angiotensin II.

The third component underlying autoregulation of filtration rate involves angiotensin II. During states of reduced renal blood flow, renin is released from granular cells within the wall of the afferent arteriole near the macula densa in a region called the juxtaglomerular apparatus (Fig. 271-2B). Renin, a proteolytic enzyme, catalyzes the conversion of angiotensinogen to angiotensin I, which is subsequently converted to angiotensin II by angiotensin-converting enzyme (ACE) (Fig. 271-2C). Angiotensin II evokes vasoconstriction of the efferent

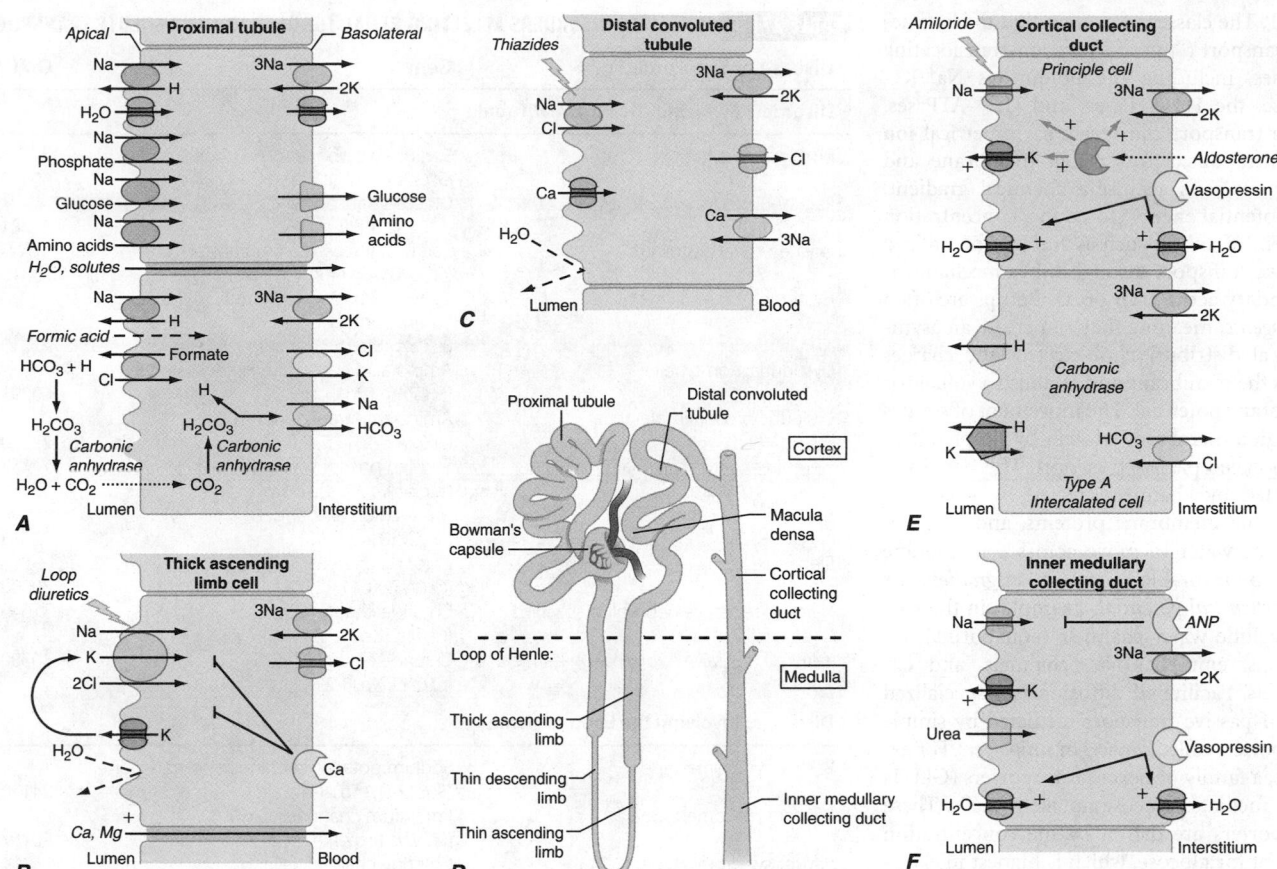

FIGURE 271-3 Transport activities of the major nephron segments. Representative cells from five major tubular segments are illustrated with the lumen side (apical membrane) facing left and interstitial side (basolateral membrane) facing right. **A.** Proximal tubular cells. **B.** Typical cell in the thick ascending limb of the loop of Henle. **C.** Distal convoluted tubular cell. **D.** Overview of entire nephron. **E.** Cortical collecting duct cells. **F.** Typical cell in the inner medullary collecting duct. The major membrane transporters, channels, and pumps are drawn with arrows indicating the direction of solute or water movement. For some events, the stoichiometry of transport is indicated by numerals preceding the solute. Targets for major diuretic agents are labeled. The actions of hormones are illustrated by arrows with plus signs for stimulatory effects and lines with perpendicular ends for inhibitory events. Dotted lines indicate free diffusion across cell membranes. The dashed line indicates water impermeability of cell membranes in the thick ascending limb and distal convoluted tubule.

arteriole, and the resulting increased glomerular hydrostatic pressure elevates filtration to normal levels.

MECHANISMS OF RENAL TUBULAR TRANSPORT

The renal tubules are composed of highly differentiated epithelia that vary dramatically in morphology and function along the nephron (Fig. 271-3). The cells lining the various tubular segments form monolayers connected to one another by a specialized region of the adjacent lateral membranes called the *tight junction*. Tight junctions form an occlusive barrier that separates the lumen of the tubule from the interstitial spaces surrounding the tubule. These specialized junctions also divide the cell membrane into discrete domains: the apical membrane faces the tubular lumen, and the basolateral membrane faces the interstitium. This physical separation of membranes allows cells to allocate membrane proteins and lipids asymmetrically to different regions of the membrane. Owing to this feature, renal epithelial cells are said to be *polarized*. The asymmetrical assignment of membrane proteins, especially proteins mediating transport processes, provides the structural machinery for directional movement of fluid and solutes by the nephron.

EPITHELIAL SOLUTE TRANSPORT

There are two types of epithelial transport. The movement of fluid and solutes sequentially across the apical and basolateral cell membranes (or vice versa) mediated by transporters, channels, or pumps is called *cellular transport*. By contrast, movement of fluid and solutes through the narrow passageway between adjacent cells is called *paracellular transport*. Paracellular transport occurs through tight junctions, indicating that they are not completely "tight." Indeed, some epithelial cell layers allow rather robust paracellular transport to occur (*leaky epithelia*), whereas other epithelia have more effective tight junctions (*tight epithelia*). In addition, because the ability of ions to flow through the paracellular pathway determines the electrical resistance across the epithelial monolayer, leaky and tight epithelia are also referred to as low- and high-resistance epithelia, respectively. The proximal tubule contains leaky epithelia, whereas distal nephron segments, such as the collecting duct, contain tight epithelia. Leaky epithelia are most well suited for bulk fluid reabsorption, whereas tight epithelia allow for more refined control and regulation of transport.

MEMBRANE TRANSPORT

Cell membranes are composed of hydrophobic lipids that repel water and aqueous solutes. The movement of solutes and water across cell membranes is made possible by discrete classes of integral membrane proteins, including channels, pumps, and transporters. These different components mediate specific types of transport activities, including *active transport* (pumps), *passive transport* (channels), *facilitated diffusion* (transporters), and *secondary active transport* (co-transporters). Different cell types in the mammalian nephron are endowed with distinct combinations of proteins that serve specific transport functions. Active transport requires metabolic energy generated by the hydrolysis of ATP. The classes of protein that mediate active transport ("pumps") are ion-translocating ATPases, including the ubiquitous Na^+/K^+-ATPase, the H^+-ATPases, and Ca^{2+}-ATPases. Active transport can create asymmetrical ion concentrations across a cell membrane and can move ions against a chemical gradient. The potential energy stored in a concentration gradient of an ion such as Na^+ can be utilized to drive transport through other mechanisms (secondary active transport). Pumps are often *electrogenic*, meaning they can create an asymmetrical distribution of electrostatic charges across the membrane and establish a voltage or membrane potential. The movement of solutes through a membrane protein by simple diffusion is called passive transport. This activity is mediated by channels created by selectively permeable membrane proteins, and it allows solute or water to move across a membrane driven by favorable *concentration gradients* or *electrochemical potential*. Examples in the kidney include water channels (aquaporins), K^+ channels, epithelial Na^+ channels, and Cl^- channels. Facilitated diffusion is a specialized type of passive transport mediated by simple transporters called *carriers* or *uniporters*. For example, a family of hexose transporters (GLUTs 1–13) mediates glucose uptake by cells. These transporters are driven by the concentration gradient for glucose, which is highest in extracellular fluids and lowest in the cytoplasm due to rapid metabolism. Many transporters operate by translocating two or more ions/solutes in concert either in the same direction (*symporters* or *co-transporters*) or in opposite directions (*antiporters* or *exchangers*) across the cell membrane. The movement of two or more ions/solutes may produce no net change in the balance of electrostatic charges across the membrane (*electroneutral*), or a transport event may alter the balance of charges (*electrogenic*). Several inherited disorders of renal tubular solute and water transport occur as a consequence of mutations in genes encoding a variety of channels, transporter proteins, and their regulators (Table 271-1).

SEGMENTAL NEPHRON FUNCTIONS

Each anatomic segment of the nephron has unique characteristics and specialized functions that enable selective transport of solutes and water (Fig. 271-3). Through sequential events of reabsorption and secretion along the nephron, tubular fluid is progressively conditioned into final urine for excretion. Knowledge of the major tubular mechanisms responsible for solute and water transport is critical for understanding hormonal regulation of kidney function and the pharmacologic manipulation of renal excretion.

PROXIMAL TUBULE

The proximal tubule is responsible for reabsorbing ~60% of filtered NaCl and water, as well as ~90% of filtered bicarbonate and most critical nutrients such as glucose and amino acids. The proximal tubule utilizes both cellu-

TABLE 271-1 INHERITED DISORDERS AFFECTING RENAL TUBULAR ION AND SOLUTE TRANSPORT		
Disease or Syndrome	**Gene**	**OMIM[a]**
Disorders Involving the Proximal Tubule		
Proximal renal tubular acidosis	Sodium bicarbonate co-transporter (*SLC4A4*, 4q21)	604278
Faconi-Bickel syndrome	Glucose transporter-2 (*SLC2A2* 3q26.1-q26.3)	227810
Isolated renal glycosuria	Sodium glucose co-transporter (*SLC5A2*,16p11.2)	233100
Cystinuria, type I	Cystine, dibasic and neutral amino acid transporter (*SLC3A1*, 2p16.3)	220100
Cystinuria, non-type I	Amino acid transporter, light subunit (*SLC7A9*, 19q13.1)	600918
Lysinuric protein intolerance	Amino acid transporter (*SLC7A7*, 4q11.2)	222700
Hereditary hypophosphatemic rickets with hypercalcemia	Sodium phosphate co-transporter (*SLC34A3*, 9q34)	241530
Renal hypouricemia	Urate-anion exchanger (*SLC22A12*, 11q13)	220150
Dent disease	Chloride channel, ClC-5 (*CLCN5*, Xp11.22)	300009
X-linked recessive nephrolithiasis with renal failure	Chloride channel, ClC-5 (*CLCN5*, Xp11.22)	310468
X-linked recessive hypophosphatemic rickets	Chloride channel, ClC-5 (*CLCN5*, Xp11.22)	307800
Disorders Involving the Loop of Henle		
Bartter syndrome, type 1	Sodium potassium-chloride co-transporter (*SLC12A1*,15q15-q21)	241200
Bartter syndrome, type 2	Potassium channel, ROMK (*KCNJ1*, 11q24)	601678
Bartter syndrome, type 3	Chloride channel, ClC-Kb (*CLCNKB*, 1p36)	602023
Bartter syndrome with sensorineural deafness	Chloride channel accessory subunit, barttin (*BSND*, 1p31)	602522
Autosomal dominant hypocalcemia with Bartter-like syndrome	Calcium-sensing receptor (*CASR*, 3q13.3-q21)	601199
Familial hypocalciuric hypercalcemia	Calcium-sensing receptor (*CASR*, 3q13.3-q21)	145980
Primary hypomagnesemia	Claudin-16 or paracellin-1 (*CLDN16* or *PCLN1*, 3q27)	248250
Isolated renal magnesium loss	Sodium potassium ATPase, γ_1-subunit (*ATP1G1*, 11q23)	154020
Primary hypomagnesemia with secondary hypocalcemia	Melastatin-related transient receptor potential cation channel 6 (*TRPM6*, 9q22)	602014
Disorders Involving the Distal Tubule and Collecting Duct		
Gitelman's syndrome	Sodium-chloride co-transporter (*SLC12A3*, 16q13)	263800
Pseudoaldosteronism (Liddle's syndrome)	Epithelial sodium channel β and γ subunits (*SCNN1B, SCNN1G*, 16p13-p12)	177200
Recessive pseudohypoaldosteronism type 1	Epithelial sodium channel, α, β, and γ subunits (*SCNN1A*, 12p13; *SCNN1B, SCNN1G*, 16p13-p12)	264350
Pseudohypoaldosteronism type 2 (Gordon hyperkalemia-hypertension syndrome)	Kinases WNK-1, WNK-4 (*WNK1*, 12p13; *WNK4*, 17q21-q22)	145260
X-Linked nephrogenic diabetes insipidus	Vasopressin V2 receptor (*AVPR2*, Xq28)	304800
Nephrogenic diabetes insipidus (autosomal)	Water channel, aquaporin-2 (*AQP2*, 12q13)	125800
Distal renal tubular acidosis, autosomal dominant	Anion exchanger-1 (*SLC4A1*, 17q21-q22)	179800
Distal renal tubular acidosis, autosomal recessive	Anion exchanger-1 (*SLC4A1*, 17q21-q22)	602722
Distal renal tubular acidosis with neural deafness	Proton ATPase, β1 subunit (*ATP6B1*,2cen-q13)	192132
Distal renal tubular acidosis with normal hearing	Proton ATPase, 116-kD subunit (*ATP6N1B*, 7q33-q34)	602722

[a]Online Mendelian Inheritance in Man database (*http://www.ncbi.nlm.nih.gov/Omim*).

lar and paracellular transport mechanisms. The apical membrane of proximal tubular cells has an expanded surface area available for reabsorptive work created by a dense array of microvilli called the *brush border*, and comparatively leaky tight junctions further enable high-capacity fluid reabsorption.

Solute and water pass through these tight junctions to enter the lateral intercellular space where absorption by the peritubular capillaries occurs. Bulk fluid reabsorption by the proximal tubule is driven by high oncotic pressure and low hydrostatic pressure within the peritubular capillaries. Physiologic adjustments in GFR made by changing efferent arteriolar tone cause proportional changes in reabsorption, a phenomenon known as *glomerulotubular balance*. For example, vasoconstriction of the efferent arteriole by angiotensin II will increase glomerular capillary hydrostatic pressure but lower pressure in the peritubular capillaries. At the same time, increased GFR and filtration fraction cause a rise in oncotic pressure near the end of the glomerular capillary. These changes, a lowered hydrostatic and increased oncotic pressure, increase the driving force for fluid absorption by the peritubular capillaries.

Cellular transport of most solutes by the proximal tubule is coupled to the Na$^+$ concentration gradient established by the activity of a basolateral Na$^+$/K$^+$-ATPase (Fig. 271-3*A*). This active transport mechanism maintains a steep Na$^+$ gradient by keeping intracellular Na$^+$ concentrations low. Solute reabsorption is coupled to the Na$^+$ gradient by Na$^+$-dependent co-transporters such as Na$^+$-glucose and the Na$^+$-phosphate. In addition to the paracellular route, water reabsorption also occurs through the cellular pathway enabled by constitutively active water channels (aquaporin-1) present on both apical and basolateral membranes. In addition, small, local *osmotic gradients* close to plasma membranes generated by cellular Na$^+$ reabsorption are likely responsible for driving directional water movement across proximal tubule cells.

Proximal tubular cells reclaim bicarbonate by a mechanism dependent on carbonic anhydrases. Filtered bicarbonate is first titrated by protons delivered to the lumen by Na$^+$/H$^+$ exchange. The resulting carbonic acid is metabolized by brush border carbonic anhydrase to water and carbon dioxide. Dissolved carbon dioxide then diffuses into the cell, where it is enzymatically hydrated by cytoplasmic carbonic anhydrase to reform carbonic acid. Finally, intracellular carbonic acid dissociates into free protons and bicarbonate anions, and bicarbonate exits the cell through a basolateral Na$^+$/HCO$_3^-$ co-transporter. This process is saturable, resulting in renal bicarbonate excretion when plasma levels exceed the physiologically normal range (24–26 meq/L). Carbonic anhydrase inhibitors such as acetazolamide, a class of weak diuretic agents, block proximal tubule reabsorption of bicarbonate and are useful for alkalinizing the urine.

Chloride is poorly reabsorbed throughout the first segment of the proximal tubule, and a rise in Cl$^-$ concentration counterbalances the removal of bicarbonate anion from tubular fluid. In later proximal tubular segments, cellular Cl$^-$ reabsorption is initiated by apical exchange of cellular formate for higher luminal concentrations of Cl$^-$. Once in the lumen, formate anions are titrated by H$^+$ (provided by Na$^+$/H$^+$ exchange) to generate neutral formic acid, which can diffuse passively across the apical membrane back into the cell where it dissociates a proton and is recycled. Basolateral Cl$^-$ exit is mediated by a K$^+$/Cl$^-$ co-transporter.

Reabsorption of glucose is nearly complete by the end of the proximal tubule. Cellular transport of glucose is mediated by apical Na$^+$-glucose co-transport coupled with basolateral, facilitated diffusion by a glucose transporter. This process is also saturable, leading to glycosuria when plasma levels exceed 180–200 mg/dL, as seen in untreated diabetes mellitus.

The proximal tubule possesses specific transporters capable of secreting a variety of organic acids (carboxylate anions) and bases (mostly primary amine cations). Organic anions transported by these systems include urate, ketoacid anions, and several protein-bound drugs not filtered at the glomerulus (penicillins, cephalosporins, and salicylates). Probenecid inhibits renal organic anion secretion and can be clinically useful for raising plasma concentrations of certain drugs

like penicillin and oseltamivir. Organic cations secreted by the proximal tubule include various biogenic amine neurotransmitters (dopamine, acetylcholine, epinephrine, norepinephrine, and histamine) and creatinine. Certain drugs like cimetidine and trimethoprim compete with endogenous compounds for transport by the organic cation pathways. These drugs elevate levels of serum creatinine, but this change does not reflect changes in the GFR.

The proximal tubule, through distinct classes of Na$^+$-dependent and Na$^+$-independent transport systems, reabsorbs amino acids efficiently. These transporters are specific for different groups of amino acids. For example, cystine, lysine, arginine, and ornithine are transported by a system comprising two proteins encoded by the *SLC3A1* and *SLC7A9* genes. Mutations in either *SLC3A1* or *SLC7A9* impair reabsorption of these amino acids and cause the disease cystinuria. Peptide hormones, such as insulin and growth hormone, β$_2$-microglobulin, and other small proteins, are taken up by the proximal tubule through a process of absorptive endocytosis and are degraded in acidified endocytic vesicles or lysosomes. Acidification of these vesicles depends on a "proton pump" (vacuolar H$^+$-ATPase) and a Cl$^-$ channel. Impaired acidification of endocytic vesicles because of mutations in a Cl$^-$ channel gene (*CLCN5*) causes low-molecular-weight proteinuria in Dent's disease. Renal ammoniagenesis from glutamine in the proximal tubule provides a major tubular fluid buffer to ensure excretion of secreted H$^+$ ion as NH$_4^+$ by the collecting duct. Cellular K$^+$ levels inversely modulate ammoniagenesis, and in the setting of high serum K$^+$ from hypoaldosteronism, reduced ammoniagenesis facilitates the appearance of Type IV renal tubular acidosis.

LOOP OF HENLE

The loop of Henle consists of three major segments: descending thin limb, ascending thin limb, and ascending thick limb. These divisions are based on cellular morphology and anatomic location, but also correlate well with specialization of function. Approximately 15–25% of filtered NaCl is reabsorbed in the loop of Henle, mainly by the thick ascending limb. The loop of Henle has a critically important role in urinary concentrating ability by contributing to the generation of a hypertonic medullary interstitium in a process called *countercurrent multiplication*. The loop of Henle is the site of action for the most potent class of diuretic agents (loop diuretics) and contributes to reabsorption of calcium and magnesium ions.

The descending thin limb is highly water-permeable owing to dense expression of constitutively active aquaporin-1 water channels. By contrast, water permeability is negligible in the ascending limb. In the thick ascending limb, there is a high level of secondary active salt transport enabled by the Na$^+$/K$^+$/2Cl$^-$ co-transporter on the apical membrane in series with basolateral Cl$^-$ channels and Na$^+$/K$^+$-ATPase (Fig. 271-3*B*). The Na$^+$/K$^+$/2Cl$^-$ co-transporter is the primary target for loop diuretics. Tubular fluid K$^+$ is the limiting substrate for this co-transporter (tubular concentration of K$^+$ is similar to plasma, about 4 meq/L), but it is maintained by K$^+$ recycling through an apical potassium channel. An inherited disorder of the thick ascending limb, Bartter's syndrome, results in a salt-wasting renal disease associated with hypokalemia and metabolic alkalosis. Loss-of-function mutations in one of four distinct genes encoding components of the Na$^+$/K$^+$/2Cl$^-$ co-transporter (*NKCC2*), apical K$^+$ channel (*KCNJ1*), or basolateral Cl$^-$ channel (*CLCNKB, BSND*) can cause the syndrome.

Potassium recycling also contributes to a positive electrostatic charge in the lumen relative to the interstitium, which promotes divalent cation (Mg^{2+} and Ca^{2+}) reabsorption through the paracellular pathway. A Ca^{2+}-sensing, G-protein coupled receptor (CaSR) on basolateral membranes regulates NaCl reabsorption in the thick ascending limb through dual signaling mechanisms utilizing either cyclic AMP or eicosanoids. This receptor enables a steep relationship between plasma Ca^{2+} levels and renal Ca^{2+} excretion. Loss-of-function mutations in CaSR cause familial hypercalcemic hypocalciuria because of a blunted response of the thick ascending limb to exocellular Ca^{2+}. Mutations in *CLDN16* encoding paracellin-1, a transmembrane protein located within the tight junction complex, leads to familial hypomagnesemia with hypercalcuria and nephrocalcinosis, suggesting that the ion conductance of the paracellular pathway in the thick limb is regulated. Mutations in *TRPM6* encoding a Mg^{2+} permeable ion channel also cause familial hypomagnesemia with hypocalcemia. A molecular complex of TRPM6 and TRPM7 proteins is critical for Mg^{2+} reabsorption in the thick ascending limb of Henle.

The loop of Henle contributes to urine concentrating ability by establishing a *hypertonic medullary interstitium*, which promotes water reabsorption by a more distal nephron segment, the inner medullary collecting duct. *Countercurrent multiplication* produces a hypertonic medullary interstitium using two countercurrent systems: the loop of Henle (opposing descending and ascending limbs) and the vasa recta (medullary peritubular capillaries enveloping the loop). The countercurrent flow in these two systems helps maintain the hypertonic environment of the inner medulla, but NaCl reabsorption by the thick ascending limb is the primary initiating event. Reabsorption of NaCl without water dilutes the tubular fluid and adds new osmoles to the interstitial fluid surrounding the thick ascending limb. Because the descending thin limb is highly water permeable, osmotic equilibrium occurs between the descending-limb tubular fluid and the interstitial space, leading to progressive solute trapping in the inner medulla. Maximum medullary interstitial osmolality also requires partial recycling of urea from the collecting duct.

DISTAL CONVOLUTED TUBULE

The distal convoluted tubule reabsorbs ~5% of the filtered NaCl. This segment is composed of a tight epithelium with little water permeability. The major NaCl transporting pathway utilizes an apical membrane, electroneutral thiazide-sensitive Na^+/Cl^- co-transporter in tandem with basolateral Na^+/K^+-ATPase and Cl^- channels (Fig. 271-3C). Apical Ca^{2+}-selective channels (TRPV5) and basolateral Na^+/Ca^{2+} exchange mediate calcium reabsorption in the distal convoluted tubule. Ca^{2+} reabsorption is inversely related to Na^+ reabsorption and is stimulated by parathyroid hormone. Blocking apical Na^+/Cl^- co-transport will reduce intracellular Na^+, favoring increased basolateral Na^+/Ca^{2+} exchange and passive apical Ca^{2+} entry. Loss-of-function mutations of *SLC12A3* encoding the apical Na^+/Cl^- co-transporter cause Gitelman's syndrome, a salt-wasting disorder associated with hypokalemic alkalosis and hypocalciuria. Mutations in genes encoding WNK kinases, WNK-1 and WNK-4, cause pseudohypoaldosteronism type II or Gordon's syndrome characterized by familial hypertension with hyperkalemia. WNK kinases influence the activity of several tubular ion transporters. Mutations in this disorder lead to overactivity of the apical Na^+/Cl^- co-transporter in the distal convoluted tubule as the primary stimulus for increased salt reabsorption, extracellular volume expansion, and hypertension. Hyperkalemia may be caused by diminished activity of apical K^+ channels in the collecting duct, a primary route for K^+ secretion.

COLLECTING DUCT

The collecting duct regulates the final composition of the urine. The two major divisions, the cortical collecting duct and inner medullary collecting duct, contribute to reabsorbing ~4–5% of filtered Na^+ and are important for hormonal regulation of salt and water balance. The cortical collecting duct contains a *high resistance epithelia* with two cell types. Principal cells are the main Na^+ reabsorbing cells and the site of action of aldosterone, K^+-sparing diuretics, and spironolactone. The other cells are type A and B intercalated cells. Type A intercalated cells mediate acid secretion and bicarbonate reabsorption. Type B intercalated cells mediate bicarbonate secretion and acid reabsorption.

Virtually all transport is mediated through the cellular pathway for both principal cells and intercalated cells. In principal cells, passive apical Na^+ entry occurs through the amiloride-sensitive, epithelial Na^+ channel with basolateral exit via the Na^+/K^+-ATPase (Fig. 271-3E). This Na^+ reabsorptive process is tightly regulated by aldosterone. Aldosterone enters the cell across the basolateral membrane, binds to a cytoplasmic mineralocorticoid receptor, and then translocates into the nucleus, where it modulates gene transcription, resulting in increased sodium reabsorption. Activating mutations in this epithelial Na^+ channel increase Na^+ reclamation and produce hypokalemia, hypertension, and metabolic alkalosis (Liddle's syndrome). The potassium-sparing diuretics amiloride and triamterene block the epithelial Na^+ channel causing reduced Na^+ reabsorption.

Principal cells secrete K^+ through an apical membrane potassium channel. Two forces govern the secretion of K^+. First, the high intracellular K^+ concentration generated by Na^+/K^+-ATPase creates a favorable concentration gradient for K^+ secretion into tubular fluid. Secondly, with reabsorption of Na^+ without an accompanying anion, the tubular lumen becomes negative relative to the cell interior, creating a favorable electrical gradient for secretion of cations. When Na^+ reabsorption is blocked, the electrical component of the driving force for K^+ secretion is blunted. K^+ secretion is also promoted by fast tubular fluid flow rates (which might occur during volume expansion or diuretics acting "upstream" of the cortical collecting duct), and the presence of relatively nonreabsorbable anions (including bicarbonate and penicillins) that contribute to the lumen-negative potential. Principal cells also participate in water reabsorption by increased water permeability in response to vasopressin; this effect is explained more fully below for the inner medullary collecting duct.

Intercalated cells do not participate in Na^+ reabsorption but instead mediate acid-base secretion. These cells perform two types of transport: active H^+ transport mediated by H^+-ATPase ("proton pump") and Cl^-/HCO_3^- exchanger. Intercalated cells arrange the two transport mechanisms on opposite membranes to enable either acid or base secretion. Type A intercalated cells have an apical proton pump that mediates acid secretion and a basolateral anion exchanger for mediating bicarbonate reabsorption (Fig. 271-3E). By contrast, type B intercalated cells have the anion exchanger on the apical membrane to mediate bicarbonate secretion while the proton pump resides on the basolateral membrane to enable acid reabsorption. Under conditions of acidemia, the kidney preferentially uses type A intercalated cells to secrete the excess H^+ and generate more HCO_3^-. The opposite is true in states of bicarbonate excess with alkalemia where the type B intercalated cells predominate. An extracellular protein called *hensin* mediates this adaptation.

Inner medullary collecting duct cells share many similarities with principal cells of the cortical collecting duct. They have apical Na^+ and K^+ channels that mediate Na^+ reabsorption and K^+ secretion, respectively (Fig. 271-3F). Inner medullary collecting duct cells also have vasopressin-regulated water channels (aquaporin-2 on the apical membrane, aquaporin-3 and 4 on the basolateral membrane). The antidiuretic hormone vasopressin binds to the V2 receptor on the basolateral membrane and triggers an intracellular signaling cascade through G-protein–mediated activation of adenylyl cyclase, resulting in an increase in levels of cyclic AMP. This signaling cascade ultimately stimulates the insertion of water channels into the apical membrane of the inner medullary collecting duct cells to promote increased water permeability. This increase in permeability enables water reabsorption and production of concentrated urine. In the absence of vasopressin, inner medullary collecting duct cells are water-impermeable, and urine remains dilute. Thus, the nephron separates NaCl from water so that considerations of volume or tonicity can determine whether to retain or excrete water.

Sodium reabsorption by inner medullary collecting duct cells is also inhibited by the natriuretic peptides called *atrial natriuretic peptide* or *renal natriuretic peptide* (urodilatin); the same gene encodes both peptides but uses different posttranslational processing of a common pre-prohormone to generate different proteins. Atrial natriuretic peptides are secreted by atrial myocytes in response to volume expansion, whereas urodilatin is secreted by renal tubular epithelia. Natriuretic peptides interact with either apical (urodilatin) or basolateral (atrial natriuretic peptides) receptors on inner medullary collecting duct cells to stimulate guanylyl cyclase and increase levels of cytoplasmic cGMP. This effect in turn reduces the activity of the apical Na^+ channel in these cells and attenuates net Na^+ reabsorption producing natriuresis. The inner medullary collecting duct is permeable to urea, allowing

FIGURE 271-4 Determinants of sodium and water balance. A. Plasma Na$^+$ concentration is a surrogate marker for plasma tonicity, the volume behavior of cells in a solution. Tonicity is determined by the number of effective osmols in the body divided by the total body H$_2$O (TB H$_2$0), which translates simply into the total body Na (TB Na$^+$) and anions outside the cell separated from the total body K (TB K$^+$) inside the cell by the cell membrane. Net water balance is determined by the integrated functions of thirst, osmoreception, Na reabsorption, vasopressin release, and the strength of the medullary gradient in the kidney, keeping tonicity within a narrow range of osmolality around 280 mosmol. When water metabolism is disturbed and total-body water increases, hyponatremia, hypotonicity, and water intoxication occurs; when total-body water decreases, hypernatremia, hypertonicity, and dehydration occurs. **B.** Extracellular blood volume and pressure are an integrated function of total body Na$^+$ (TB Na$^+$), total body H$_2$0 (TB H$_2$O), vascular tone, heart rate, and stroke volume that modulates volume and pressure in the vascular tree of the body. This extracellular blood volume is determined by net Na balance under the control of taste, baroreception, habit, Na$^+$ reabsorption, macula densa/tubuloglomerular feedback, and naturetic peptides. When Na$^+$ metabolism is disturbed and total body Na$^+$ increases, edema occurs; when total body Na$^+$ is decreased, volume depletion occurs. ADH, antidiuretic hormone; AP2, aquaporin-2.

urea to diffuse into the interstitium, where it contributes to the hypertonicity of the medullary interstitium. Urea is recycled by diffusing from the interstitium into the descending and ascending limbs of the loop of Henle.

HORMONAL REGULATION OF SODIUM AND WATER BALANCE

The balance of solute and water in the body is determined by the amounts ingested, distributed to various fluid compartments, and excreted by skin, bowel, and kidneys. *Tonicity,* the osmolar state determining the volume behavior of cells in a solution, is regulated by water balance (Fig. 271-4A), and *extracellular blood volume* is regulated by Na$^+$ balance (Fig. 271-4B). The kidney is a critical modulator for both of these physiologic processes.

WATER BALANCE

Tonicity depends on the variable concentration of *effective osmoles* inside and outside the cell that cause water to move in either direction across its membrane. Classic effective osmoles, like Na$^+$, K$^+$, and their anions, are solutes trapped on either side of a cell membrane, where they collectively partition and obligate water to move and find equilibrium in proportion to retained solute; Na$^+$/K$^+$-ATPase keeps most K$^+$ inside cells and most Na$^+$ outside. Normal tonicity (~280 mosmol/L) is rigorously defended by osmoregulatory mechanisms that control water balance to protect tissues from inadvertent *dehydration* (cell shrinkage) or *water intoxication* (cell swelling), both of which are deleterious to cell function (Fig. 271-4A).

The mechanisms that control osmoregulation are distinct from those governing extracellular volume, although there is some shared physiology in both processes. While cellular concentrations of K$^+$ have a determinant role in reaching any level of tonicity, the routine surrogate marker for assessing clinical tonicity is the concentration of serum Na$^+$. Any reduction in total body water, which raises the Na$^+$ concentration, triggers a brisk sense of thirst and conservation of water by decreasing renal water excretion mediated by release of vasopressin from the posterior pituitary. Conversely, a decrease in plasma Na$^+$ concentration triggers an increase in renal water excretion by suppressing the secretion of vasopressin. While all cells expressing mechanosensitive TRPV4 channels respond to changes in tonicity by altering their volume and Ca^{2+} concentration, only TRPV4$^+$ neuronal cells connected to the supraoptic and paraventricular nuclei in the hypothalamus are *osmoreceptive;* that is, they alone, because of their neural connectivity, modulate the release of vasopressin by the posterior lobe of the pituitary gland. Secretion is stimulated primarily by changing tonicity and secondarily by other nonosmotic signals, such as variable blood volume, stress, pain, and some drugs. The release of vasopressin by the posterior pituitary increases linearly as plasma tonicity rises above normal, although this varies depending on the perception of extracellular volume (one form of cross-talk between mechanisms that adjudicate blood volume and osmoregulation). Changing the intake or excretion of water provides a means for adjusting plasma tonicity; thus, osmoregulation governs water balance.

The kidneys play a vital role in maintaining water balance through their regulation of renal water excretion. The ability to concentrate urine to an osmolality exceeding that of plasma enables water conservation, while the ability to produce urine more dilute than plasma promotes excretion of excess water. Cell membranes are composed of lipids and other hydrophobic substances that are intrinsically impermeable to water. In order for water to enter or exit a cell, the cell membrane must express water channel aquaporins. In the kidney, aquaporin 1 is constitutively active in all water-permeable segments of the proximal and distal tubules, while aquaporins 2, 3, and 4 are regulated by vasopressin in the collecting duct. Vasopressin interacts with the V2 receptor on basolateral membranes of collecting duct cells and signals the insertion of new water channels into apical membranes to promote water permeability. Net water reabsorption is ultimately driven by the osmotic gradient between dilute tubular fluid and a hypertonic medullary interstitium.

SODIUM BALANCE

The perception of *extracellular blood volume* is determined, in part, by the integration of arterial tone, cardiac stroke volume, heart rate, and the water and solute content of the extracellular volume. Na^+ and its anions are the most abundant extracellular effective osmoles, and together they support a blood volume around which pressure is generated. Under normal conditions, this volume is regulated by sodium balance (Fig. 271-4B), and the balance between daily Na^+ intake and excretion is under the influence of *baroreceptors* in regional blood vessels and vascular hormone-sensors modulated by atrial naturetic peptides, the renin-angiotensin-aldosterone system, Ca^{2+} signaling, adenosine, vasopressin, and the neural adrenergic axis. If Na^+ intake exceeds Na^+ excretion (positive Na^+ balance), then an increase in blood volume will trigger a proportional increase in urinary Na^+ excretion. Conversely, when Na^+ intake is less than urinary excretion (negative Na^+ balance), blood volume will decrease and trigger enhanced renal Na^+ reabsorption, leading to decreased urinary Na^+ excretion.

The renin-angiotensin-aldosterone system is the best-understood hormonal system modulating renal Na^+ excretion. Renin is synthesized and secreted by granular cells in the wall of the afferent arteriole. Its secretion is controlled by several factors, including β_1-adrenergic stimulation to the afferent arteriole, input from the macula densa, and prostaglandins. Renin and ACE activity eventually produce angiotensin II, which directly or indirectly promotes renal Na^+ and water reabsorp-

tion. Stimulation of proximal tubular Na^+/H^+ exchange by angiotensin II directly increases Na^+ reabsorption. Angiotensin II also promotes Na^+ reabsorption along the collecting duct by stimulating aldosterone secretion by the adrenal cortex. Constriction of the efferent glomerular arteriole by angiotensin II indirectly increases the filtration fraction and raises peritubular capillary oncotic pressure to promote Na^+ reabsorption. Finally, angiotensin II inhibits renin secretion through a negative feedback loop.

Aldosterone is synthesized and secreted by granulosa cells in the adrenal cortex. It binds to cytoplasmic mineralocorticoid receptors in principal cells of the collecting duct that increase the activity of the apical membrane Na^+ channel, apical membrane K^+ channel, and basolateral Na^+/K^+-ATPase. These effects are mediated in part by aldosterone-stimulated transcription of the gene encoding serum/glucocorticoid-induced kinase 1 (SGK1). The activity of epithelial Na^+ channel is increased by SGK1-mediated phosphorylation of Nedd4-2, a protein that promotes recycling of the Na^+ channel from the plasma membrane. Phosphorylated Nedd4-2 has impaired interactions with epithelial Na^+ channel, leading to increased channel density at the plasma membrane and increased capacity for Na^+ reabsorption by the collecting duct.

Chronic overexpression of aldosterone causes a decrease in urinary Na^+ excretion lasting only a few days, after which Na^+ excretion returns to previous levels. This phenomenon, called *aldosterone escape*, is explained by decreased proximal tubular Na^+ reabsorption following blood volume expansion. Excess Na^+ that is not reabsorbed by the proximal tubule overwhelms the reabsorptive capacity of more distal nephron segments. This escape may be facilitated by atrial naturetic peptides, which lose their effectiveness in the clinical settings of heart failure, nephrotic syndrome, and cirrhosis, leading to severe Na^+ retention and volume overload.

FURTHER READINGS

BALLERMANN BJ: Glomerular endothelial cell differentiation. Kidney Int 67:1668, 2005

GIEBISCH G et al: New aspects of renal potassium transport. Pflugers Arch 446:289, 2003

KOPAN R et al: Molecular insights into segmentation along the proximal–distal axis of the nephron. J Am Soc Nephrol 18:2014, 2007

MANGE K et al: Language guiding therapy: The case of dehydration versus volume depletion. Ann Inten Med 127: 848, 1997

O'NEIL RG, HELLER S: The mechanosensitive nature of TRPV channels. Pflugers Arch-Eur J Physiol 451:193, 2005

RIBES D et al: Transcriptional control of epithelial differentiation during kidney development. J Am Soc Nephrol 14:S9, 2003

SCHRIER RW, ECDER T: Gibbs memorial lecture: Unifying hypothesis of body fluid volume regulation. Mt Sinai J Med 68: 350, 2001

WAGNER CA et al: Renal acid-base transport: Old and new players. Nephron Physiol 103:1, 2006

272 Adaptation of the Kidney to Renal Injury

Raymond C. Harris, Eric G. Neilson

The size of a kidney and the number of nephrons formed late in embryological development depend on the frequency with which the ureteric bud undergoes branching morphogenesis. Humans have between 225,000 and 900,000 nephrons in each kidney, a number that mathematically hinges on whether ureteric branching goes to completion or is prematurely terminated by one or two cycles. Although the signaling mechanism regulating cycle number is unknown, these final rounds of branching likely determine how well the kidney will adapt to the physio-

logic demands of blood pressure and body size, various environmental stresses, or unwanted inflammation leading to chronic renal failure.

One of the intriguing generalities made in the course of studying chronic renal failure is that residual nephrons hyperfunction to compensate for the loss of those nephrons falling to primary disease. This compensation depends on adaptive changes produced by renal hypertrophy and adjustments in *tubuloglomerular feedback* and *glomerulotubular balance,* as advanced in the *intact nephron hypothesis* by Neal Bricker in 1969. Some physiologic adaptations to nephron loss also produce unintended clinical consequences explained by Bricker's *trade-off hypothesis* in 1972, and eventually some adaptations accelerate the deterioration of residual nephrons, as described by Barry Brenner in his *hyperfiltration hypothesis* in 1982. These three important notions regarding chronic renal failure form a conceptual foundation for understanding common pathophysiology leading to uremia.

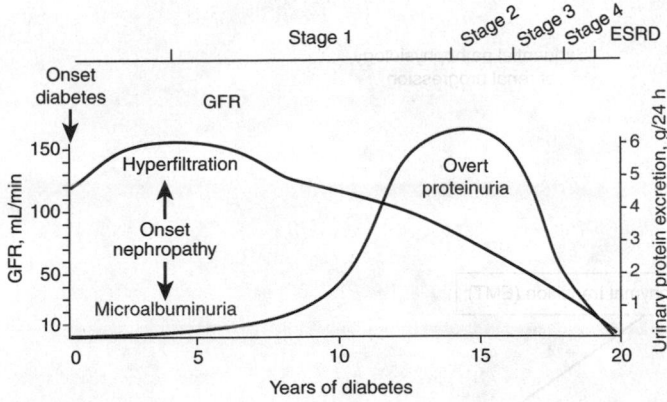

FIGURE 272-1 Progression of chronic renal injury. Although various types of renal injury have their own unique rates of progression, one of the best understood is that associated with type I diabetic nephropathy. Notice the early increase in glomerular filtration rate (GFR), followed by inexorable decline associated with increasing proteinuria. Also indicated is the National Kidney Foundation K/DOQI classification of the stages of chronic kidney disease. ESRD, end-stage renal disease.

COMMON MECHANISMS OF PROGRESSIVE RENAL DISEASE

When the initial complement of nephrons is reduced by a sentinel event, like unilateral nephrectomy, the remaining kidney adapts by enlarging and increasing its glomerular filtration rate (GFR). If the kidneys were initially normal, the GFR usually returns to 80% of normal for two kidneys. The remaining kidney grows by *compensatory renal hypertrophy* with very little cellular proliferation. This unique event is accomplished by increasing the size of each cell along the nephron, which is accommodated by the elasticity or growth of interstitial spaces and the renal capsule. The mechanism of this compensatory renal hypertrophy is only partially understood, but the signals for the remaining kidney to hypertrophy may rest with the local expression of angiotensin II; transforming growth factor β (TGF-β); p27kip1, a cell cycle protein that prevents tubular cells exposed to angiotensin II from proliferating; and epidermal growth factor (EGF), which induces the mammalian target of rapamycin (mTOR) to engage a transcriptome supporting new protein synthesis.

Hyperfiltration during pregnancy, or in humans born with one kidney or who lose one to trauma or transplantation, generally leads to no ill consequences. By contrast, experimental animals who undergo resection of 80% of their renal mass, or humans who have persistent injury that destroys a comparable amount of renal tissue, progress to end-stage disease (Fig. 272-1). Clearly there is a critical amount of primary nephron loss that produces a maladaptive deterioration in the remaining nephrons. This maladaptive response is referred to clinically as *renal progression*, and the pathologic correlate of renal progression is *relentless tubular atrophy* and *tissue fibrosis*. The mechanism for this maladaptive response has been the focus of intense investigation. A unified theory of renal progression is just starting to emerge, and, most importantly, this progression follows a final common pathway regardless of whether renal injury begins in glomeruli or within the tubulointerstitium.

There are six mechanisms that hypothetically unify this final common pathway. If injury begins in glomeruli, these sequential steps build on each other: (1) Persistent glomerular injury produces local hypertension in capillary tufts, increases their single-nephron GFR, and engenders protein leak into the tubular fluid. (2) Significant glomerular proteinuria, accompanied by increases in the local production of angiotensin II, facilitates (3) a downstream cytokine bath that induces an accumulation of interstitial mononuclear cells. (4) The initial appearance of interstitial neutrophils is quickly replaced by gathering macrophages and T lymphocytes that form a nephritogenic immune response producing interstitial nephritis. (5) Some tubular epithelia respond to this inflammation by disaggregating from their basement membrane and adjacent sister cells to undergo *epithelial-mesenchymal transitions* forming new interstitial fibroblasts. (6) Finally, surviving fi-

broblasts lay down a collagenous matrix that disrupts adjacent capillaries and tubular nephrons, eventually leaving an acellular scar. The details of these complex events are outlined below (Fig. 272-2).

Significant ablation of renal mass results in *hyperfiltration* characterized by an increase in the rate of *single-nephron glomerular filtration*. The remaining nephrons lose their ability to autoregulate, and systemic hypertension is transmitted to the glomerulus. Both the hyperfiltration and *intraglomerular hypertension* stimulate the eventual appearance of glomerulosclerosis. Angiotensin II acts as an essential mediator of increased *intraglomerular capillary pressure* by selectively increasing efferent arteriolar vasoconstriction relative to afferent arteriolar tone. Angiotensin II impairs glomerular size-selectivity, induces protein ultrafiltration, and increases intracellular Ca^{2+} in podocytes, which alters podocyte function. Diverse vasoconstrictor mechanisms, including blockade of nitric oxide synthase and activation of angiotensin II and thromboxane receptors, can also induce oxidative stress in surrounding renal tissue. Finally, the effects of aldosterone on increasing renal vascular resistance and glomerular capillary pressure, or stimulating plasminogen activator inhibitor-1, facilitate fibrogenesis and complement the detrimental activity of angiotensin II.

On occasion, inflammation that begins in the renal interstitium disables tubular reclamation of filtered protein, producing mild nonselective proteinuria. Renal inflammation that initially damages glomerular capillaries often spreads to the tubulointerstitium in association with heavier proteinuria. Many clinical observations support the association of worsening *glomerular proteinuria* with renal progression. The simplest explanation for this expansion is that increasingly severe proteinuria triggers a downstream inflammatory cascade around epithelia that line the nephron, producing interstitial nephritis, fibrosis, and tubular atrophy. As albumin is an abundant polyanion in plasma and can bind a variety of cytokines, chemokines, and lipid mediators, it might be that these small molecules carried by albumin initiate the tubular inflammation brought on by proteinuria. Furthermore, glomerular injury either adds activated mediators to the proteinuric filtrate or alters the balance of cytokine inhibitors and activators such that attainment of a critical level of activated cytokines eventually damages downstream tubular epithelia.

Tubular epithelia bathed in these complex mixtures of proteinuric cytokines respond by increasing their secretion of chemokines and relocating nuclear factor κB to the nucleus to induce proinflammatory release of TGF-β, platelet-derived growth factor B (PDGF-BB), and fibroblast growth factor 2 (FGF-2). Inflammatory cells are drawn into the renal interstitium by this cytokine milieu. This interstitial spreading reduces the likelihood that the kidney will survive. The immunologic mechanisms for spreading include loss of tolerance to parenchymal self, immune deposits that share cross-reactive epitopes in either compartment, or glomerular injury that reveals a new interstitial epitope. Drugs, infection, and metabolic defects may also induce autoimmunity through Toll-like receptors that bind to moieties with an immunologically distinct molecular pattern. Bacterial and viral ligands do so, but, interestingly, so do Tamm-Horsfall protein, bacterial CpG repeats, and RNA that is released nonspecifically from injured tubular cells. Dendritic cells and macrophages are subsequently activated, and circulating T cells engage in the formal cellular immunologic response.

Nephritogenic interstitial T cells are a mix of CD4+ helper and CD8+ cytotoxic lymphocytes. Presumptive evidence of antigen-driven T cells found by examining the DNA sequence of T cell receptors suggests a polyclonal expansion that responds to multiple epitopes. Some experimental interstitial lesions are histologically analogous to a cutaneous delayed-type hypersensitivity reaction, and more intense reactions sometimes induce granuloma formation. The cytotoxic activity of antigen-reactive T cells probably accounts for tubular cell destruction and atrophy. Cytotoxic T cells synthesize proteins with serine esterase activity as well as pore-forming proteins, which can affect membrane damage much like the activated membrane attack complex of the complement cascade. Such enzymatic activity provides a structural explanation for target cell lysis.

One long-term consequence of tubular epithelia exposed to cytokines is the profibrotic activation of *epithelial-mesenchymal transition*. Persis-

FIGURE 272-2 Mechanisms of renal progression. The general mechanisms of renal progression advance sequentially through six stages that include hyperfiltration, proteinuria, cytokine bath, mononuclear cell infiltration, epithelial-mesenchymal transition, and fibrosis. *(Modified from Harris and Neilson, 2006.)*

tent cytokine activity during renal inflammation and disruption of underlying basement membrane by local proteases initiates the process of transition. Rather than collapsing into the tubular lumens and dying, some epithelia become fibroblasts while translocating back into the interstitial space behind deteriorating tubules through holes in the ruptured basement membrane. Wnt proteins, integrin-linked kinases, insulin-like growth factors, EGF, FGF-2, and TGF-β are among the classic modulators of epithelial-mesenchymal transition. Fibroblasts that deposit collagen during fibrogenesis also replicate locally at sites of persistent inflammation. Estimates indicate that half of the total fibroblasts found in fibrotic renal tissues are products of the proliferation of newly transitioned or preexisting fibroblasts. Fibroblasts are stimulated to multiply by activation of cognate cell-surface receptors for PDGF and TGF-β.

Tubulointerstitial scars are composed principally of fibronectin, collagen types I and III, and tenascin, but other glycoproteins such as thrombospondin, SPARC, osteopontin, and proteoglycan may be also important. Although tubular epithelia can synthesize collagens I and III and are modulated by a variety of growth factors, these epithelia disappear through transition and tubular atrophy, leaving fibroblasts as the major contributor to matrix production. After fibroblasts acquire a synthetic phenotype, expand their population, and locally migrate around areas of inflammation, they begin to deposit fibronectin, which provides a scaffold for interstitial collagens. When fibroblasts outdistance their survival factors, they die from apoptosis, leaving an acellular scar.

RESPONSE TO REDUCTION IN NUMBERS OF FUNCTIONING NEPHRONS

The response to the loss of many functioning nephrons produces an increase in renal blood flow with glomerular hyperfiltration. Hyperfiltration is the result of increased vasoconstriction in postglomerular

efferent arterioles relative to preglomerular afferent arterioles, increasing the intraglomerular capillary pressure and filtration fraction. The discovery of this intraglomerular hypertension and the demonstration in experimental animals that maneuvers to decrease its effect will abrogate the further expression of glomerular and tubulointerstitial injury led to the formulation of the hyperfiltration hypothesis. The hypothesis explains why residual nephrons in the setting of persistent disease will first stabilize or increase the rate of glomerular filtration, only to succumb later to inexorable deterioration and progression to renal failure. Persistent intraglomerular hypertension is critical to this transition.

Although the hormonal and metabolic factors mediating hyperfiltration are not fully understood, a number of vasoconstrictive and vasodilatory substances have been implicated, chief among them being angiotensin II. Angiotensin II incrementally vasoconstricts the efferent arteriole, and studies in animals and humans demonstrate that interruption of the renin-angiotensin system with either angiotensin-converting inhibitors or angiotensin II receptor blockers will decrease intraglomerular capillary pressure, decrease proteinuria, and slow the rate of nephron destruction. The vasoconstrictive agent, endothelin, has also been implicated in hyperfiltration, and increases in afferent vasodilatation have been attributed, at least in part, to local prostaglandins and release of endothelium-derived nitric oxide. Finally, hyperfiltration may be mediated in part by a resetting of the kidney's intrinsic autoregulatory mechanism of glomerular filtration by a *tubuloglomerular feedback system*. This feedback originates from the macula densa and modulates renal blood flow and glomerular filtration (Chap. 271).

Even with the loss of functioning nephrons, there is some continued maintenance of *glomerulotubular balance*, by which the residual tubules adapt to increases in single-nephron glomerular filtration with appropriate alterations in reabsorption or excretion of filtered water and solutes in order to maintain homeostasis. Glomerulotubular balance results both from tubular hypertrophy and from regulatory adjustments in tubular oncotic pressure or solute transport along the proximal tubule. Some studies have indicated that these alterations in tubule size and function may themselves be maladaptive and, as a trade-off, predispose to further tubule injury.

TUBULAR FUNCTION IN CHRONIC RENAL FAILURE

SODIUM

Na^+ ions are reclaimed along most of the nephron by various transport mechanisms (Chap. 271). This transport function and its contribution to extracellular blood volume is usually maintained near normal until limitations from advanced renal disease can no longer keep up with dietary Na^+ intake. Prior to this point in the spectrum of renal progression, increasing the fractional excretion of Na^+ in final urine at reduced rates of glomerular filtration provides a mechanism of early adaptation. Na^+ excretion increases predominantly by decreasing Na^+ reabsorption in the loop of Henle and distal nephron. Increases in the osmotic obligation of residual nephrons lower the concentration of Na^+ in tubular fluid, and increased excretion of inorganic and organic anions obligates more Na^+ excretion. In addition, hormonal influences, notably increased expression of atrial natriuretic peptides that increase distal Na^+ excretion, as well as levels of GFR, play an important role in maintaining adequate Na^+ excretion. Although many details of these adjustments are only understood conceptually, it is an example of a trade-off by which initial adjustments following the loss of functioning nephrons lead to compensatory responses that maintain homeostasis. Eventually, with advancing nephron loss, the atrial natriuretic peptides lose their effectiveness, and Na^+ retention results in intravascular volume expansion, edema, and worsening hypertension.

URINARY DILUTION AND CONCENTRATION

Patients with progressive renal injury gradually lose the capacity either to dilute or concentrate their urine, and urine osmolality becomes relatively fixed around 350 mosmol/L (specific gravity approximating 1.010). Although the ability of a single nephron to excrete water free of solute may not be impaired, the reduced number of functioning nephrons obligates increased fractional solute excretion by residual nephrons, and this greater obligation impairs the ability to dilute tubular fluid maximally. Similarly, urinary concentrating ability falls due to the need for more water to hydrate the increased solute load. Tubulointerstitial damage also creates insensitivity to the antidiuretic effects of vasopressin along the collecting duct or loss of the medullary gradient, which eventually disturbs control of variation in urine osmolality. Patients with moderate degrees of chronic renal failure often complain of *nocturia* as a manifestation of this fixed urine osmolality and are prone to extracellular volume depletion if they do not keep up with the persistent loss of Na^+, or hypotonicity if they drink too much water.

POTASSIUM

Renal excretion is a major pathway for reducing excess total-body K^+. Normally, the kidney excretes 90% of dietary K^+, while 10% is excreted in the stool, with a trivial amount lost to sweat. Although the colon possesses some capacity to increase K^+ excretion—up to 30% of ingested K^+ may be excreted in the stool of patients with worsening renal failure—the majority of the K^+ load continues to be excreted by the kidneys due to elevation in levels of serum K^+ that increase this filtered load. Aldosterone also regulates collecting duct Na^+ reabsorption and K^+ secretion. Aldosterone is released from the adrenal cortex not only in response to the renin-angiotensin system but also in direct response to elevated levels of serum K^+, and for a while a compensatory increase in the capacity of the collecting duct to secrete K^+ keeps up with renal progression. As serum K^+ levels rise with renal failure, circulating levels of aldosterone also increase over what is required to maintain normal levels of blood volume.

ACID-BASE REGULATION

The kidneys excrete one meq/kg per day of noncarbonic H^+ ion on a normal diet. To do this, all of the filtered HCO_3^{2-} needs to be reabsorbed proximally so that H^+ pumps in the intercalated cells of the collecting duct can secrete H^+ ions that are subsequently trapped by urinary buffers, particularly phosphates and ammonia (Chap. 271). While remaining nephrons increase their solute load with loss of renal mass, the ability to maintain total-body H^+ excretion is often impaired by the gradual loss of H^+ pumps or with reductions in ammoniagenesis leading to development of a non-delta acidosis. Although hypertrophy of the proximal tubules initially increases their ability to reabsorb filtered HCO_3^{2-} and increase ammoniagenesis, with progressive loss of nephrons this compensation is eventually overwhelmed. In addition, with advancing renal failure, ammoniagenesis is further inhibited by elevation in levels of serum K^+, producing type IV renal tubular acidosis. Once the GFR falls below 25 mL/min, organic acids accumulate, producing a delta metabolic acidosis. Hyperkalemia can also inhibit tubular HCO_3^{2-} reabsorption, as can extracellular volume expansion and elevated levels of parathyroid hormone (PTH). Eventually, as the kidneys fail, the level of serum HCO_3^{2-} falls severely, reflecting the exhaustion of all body buffer systems, including bone.

CALCIUM AND PHOSPHATE

The kidney and gut play an important role in the regulation of serum levels of Ca^{2+} and PO_4^{2-}. With decreasing renal function and the appearance of tubulointerstitial nephritis, the expression of α_1-hydroxylase by the proximal tubule is reduced, lowering levels of calcitriol and Ca^{2+} absorption by the gut. Loss of nephron mass with progressive renal failure also gradually reduces the excretion of PO_4^{2-} and Ca^{2+}, and elevations in serum PO_4^{2-} further lower serum levels of Ca^{2+}, causing sustained secretion of PTH. Unregulated increases in levels of PTH cause Ca^{2+} mobilization from bone, Ca^{2+}/PO_4^{2-} precipitation in tissues, abnormal bone remodeling, decreases in tubular bicarbonate reabsorption, and increases in renal PO_4^{2-} excretion. While elevated serum levels of PTH initially maintain serum PO_4^{2-} near normal, with progressive nephron destruction the capacity for renal PO_4^{2-} excretion is overwhelmed, the serum PO_4^{2-} elevates, and bone is progressively demineralized from secondary hyperparathyroidism. These adaptations evoke another classic functional trade-off (Fig. 272-3).

MODIFIERS INFLUENCING THE PROGRESSION OF RENAL DISEASE

Well-described risk factors for the progressive loss of renal function include systemic hypertension, diabetes, and activation of the renin-angiotensin-aldosterone system (Table 272-1). Poor glucose control will aggravate renal progression in both diabetic and nondiabetic renal disease. Angiotensin II produces intraglomerular hypertension and stimulates fibrogenesis. Aldosterone also serves as an independent fibrogenic mediator of progressive nephron loss apart from its role in modulating Na^+ and K^+ homeostasis.

Lifestyle choices also have an impact on the progression of renal disease. Cigarette smoking has been shown to either predispose or accelerate the progression of nephron loss. Whether the effect of cigarettes is related to systemic hemodynamic alterations or specific damage to the renal microvasculature and/or tubules is unclear. Lipid oxidation associated with obesity or central adiposity can also accelerate cardiovascular disease and progressive renal damage. Recent epidemiologic studies confirm an association between high-protein diets and progression of renal disease. Progressive nephron loss in experimental animals, and possibly in humans, can be slowed by adherence to a low-protein diet. Although a large multicenter trial, the Modification of Diet in Renal Disease, did not provide conclusive evidence that dietary protein restriction could retard progression to renal failure, secondary analyses and a number of meta-analyses suggest a renoprotective effect from supervised low-protein diets in the range of 0.6–0.75 g/kg per day. Abnormal Ca^{2+} and PO_4^{2-} metabolism in chronic kidney disease also plays a role in renal progression, and administration of calcitriol or its analogues can attenuate progression in a variety of models of chronic kidney disease.

An intrinsic paucity in the number of functioning nephrons predisposes to the development of renal disease. A reduced number of nephrons can lead to permanent hypertension, either through direct renal

FIGURE 272-3 The "trade-off hypothesis" for Ca²⁺/PO₄²⁻ homeostasis with progressively declining renal function. A. How adaptation to maintain Ca²⁺/PO₄²⁻ homeostasis leads to increasing levels of parathyroid hormone ("classic" presentation from Slatopolsky E, Bricker

NS: The role of phosphorous restriction in the prevention of secondary hyperparathyroidism in chronic renal disease. Kidney Int 4:141, 1973). **B.** Current understanding of the underlying mechanisms for this Ca²⁺/PO₄²⁻ trade-off. GFR, glomerular filtration rate; PTH, parathyroid hormone.

damage or hyperfiltration producing glomerulosclerosis, or by primary induction of systemic hypertension that further exacerbates glomerular barotrauma. Younger individuals with hypertension who died suddenly as a result of trauma have 47% fewer glomeruli per kidney than age-matched controls.

A consequence of low birth weight is a relative deficit in the number of total nephrons; low birth weight is associated in adulthood with more hypertension and renal failure, among other abnormalities. In this regard, in addition to or instead of a genetic predisposition to development of a specific disease or condition such as low birth weight, different epigenetic phenomena may produce varying clinical phenotypes from a single genotype, depending on maternal exposure to different environmental stimuli during gestation, a phenomenon known as *developmental plasticity*. A specific clinical phenotype can also be selected in response to an adverse environmental exposure during critical periods of intrauterine development, also known as *fetal programming*. In the United States there is at least a twofold increased incidence of low birth weight among African Americans compared with Caucasians, much but not all of which can be attributed to maternal age, health, or socioeconomic status.

As in other conditions producing nephron loss, the glomeruli of low-birth-weight individuals are enlarged and associated with early hyperfiltration to maintain normal levels of renal function. With time, the resulting intraglomerular hypertension may initiate a progressive decline in residual hyperfunctioning nephrons, ultimately accelerating renal failure. In African Americans, as well as other populations at increased risk for kidney failure, such as Pima Indians and Australian aborigines, large glomeruli are seen at early stages of kidney disease. An association between low birth weight and the development of albuminuria and nephropathy has been reported for both diabetic and nondiabetic renal disease.

FURTHER READINGS

BRENNER BM: Remission of renal disease: Recounting the challenge, acquiring the goal. J Clin Invest 110:1753, 2002

HARRIS RC, NEILSON EG: Towards a unified theory of renal progression. Ann Rev Med 57:365, 2006

ISEKI K: Factors influencing the development of end-stage renal disease. Clin Exp Nephrol 9:5, 2005

LLACH F: Secondary hyperparathyroidism in renal failure: The trade-off hypothesis revisited. Am J. Kidney Dis 25:663, 1995

LUYCKX VA, BRENNER BM: Low birth weight, nephron number, and kidney disease. Kidney Int 68:S68, 2005

MEYER TW: Tubular injury in glomerular disease. Kidney Int 63:774, 2003

SLATOPOLSKY E et al: Calcium, phosphorus and vitamin D disorders in uremia. Contrib Nephrol 149:261, 2005

ZANDI-NEJAD K et al: Adult hypertension and kidney disease: The role of fetal programming. Hypertension 47:502, 2006

TABLE 272-1 POTENTIAL MODIFIERS OF RENAL DISEASE PROGRESSION

Hypertension	Hyperlipidemia
RAS activation	Abnormal calcium/phosphorus
Angiotensin II	homeostasis
Aldosterone	Cigarette smoking
Diabetes	Intrinsic paucity in nephron number
Obesity	Prematurity/low birth weight
Excessive dietary protein	Genetic predisposition
	Undefined genetic factors

273 Acute Renal Failure
Kathleen D. Liu, Glenn M. Chertow

Acute renal failure (ARF) is characterized by a rapid decline in glomerular filtration rate (GFR) over hours to days. Depending on the exact definition used, ARF complicates approximately 5–7% of hospital admissions and up to 30% of admissions to intensive care units. Retention of nitrogenous waste products, oliguria (urine output <400 mL/d contributing to extracellular fluid overload), and electrolyte and acid-base abnormalities are frequent clinical features. ARF is usually asymp-

tomatic and diagnosed when biochemical monitoring of hospitalized patients reveals a new increase in blood urea and serum creatinine concentrations. For purposes of diagnosis and management, causes of ARF are generally divided into three major categories: (1) diseases that cause renal hypoperfusion, resulting in decreased function without frank parenchymal damage (*prerenal ARF*, or azotemia) (~55%); (2) diseases that directly involve the renal parenchyma (*intrinsic ARF*) (~40%); and (3) diseases associated with urinary tract obstruction (*postrenal ARF*) (~5%). ARF is often considered to be reversible, although a return to baseline serum creatinine concentrations postinjury might not be sufficiently sensitive to detect clinically significant irreversible damage that may ultimately contribute to chronic kidney disease. ARF is associated with significant in-hospital morbidity and mortality, the latter in the range of 30–60%, depending on the clinical setting and presence or absence of nonrenal organ system failure.

ETIOLOGY AND PATHOPHYSIOLOGY

PRERENAL ARF (PRERENAL AZOTEMIA)

The most common form of ARF is prerenal ARF, which occurs in the setting of renal hypoperfusion. Prerenal ARF is generally reversible when renal perfusion pressure is restored. By definition, renal parenchymal tissue is not damaged. More severe or prolonged hypoperfusion may lead to ischemic injury, often termed *acute tubular necrosis*, or ATN. Thus, prerenal ARF and ischemic ATN fall along a spectrum of manifestations of renal hypoperfusion. As shown in Table 273-1, prerenal ARF can complicate any disease that induces hypovolemia, low cardiac output, systemic vasodilatation, or selective intrarenal vasoconstriction.

Hypovolemia leads to a fall in mean systemic arterial pressure, which is detected as reduced stretch by arterial (e.g., carotid sinus) and cardiac baroreceptors. In turn, this triggers a coordinated series of neurohormonal responses that aim to restore blood volume and arterial pressure. These include activation of the sympathetic nervous system and renin-angiotensin-aldosterone system, as well as release of arginine vasopressin. Relatively "nonessential" vascular beds (such as the musculocutaneous and splanchnic circulations) undergo vasoconstriction in an attempt to preserve cardiac and cerebral perfusion pressure. In addition, salt loss through sweat glands is inhibited, and thirst and salt appetite are stimulated. Renal salt and water retention also occur.

In states of mild hypoperfusion, glomerular perfusion and the filtration fraction are preserved through several compensatory mechanisms. In response to the reduction in perfusion pressure, stretch receptors in afferent arterioles trigger afferent arteriolar vasodilatation through a local myogenic reflex (autoregulation). Angiotensin II increases biosynthesis of vasodilator prostaglandins (e.g., prostaglandin E_2 and prostacyclin), also resulting in afferent arteriolar vasodilation. In addition, angiotensin II induces preferential constriction of efferent arterioles. As a result, the fraction of plasma flowing through glomerular capillaries that is filtered is increased (filtration fraction), intraglomerular pressure is maintained, and GFR is preserved. With more severe hypoperfusion, these compensatory responses are overwhelmed and GFR falls, leading to prerenal ARF.

Autoregulatory dilatation of afferent arterioles allows for maintenance of GFR despite systemic hypotension; however, when hypotension is severe or prolonged, these autoregulatory mechanisms fail, resulting in a precipitous decline in GFR. Lesser degrees of hypotension may provoke prerenal ARF in those at risk: the elderly and patients with diseases that affect the integrity of afferent arterioles (e.g., hypertensive nephrosclerosis, diabetic vasculopathy and other forms of occlusive (including atherosclerotic) renovascular disease). In addition, drugs that interfere with adaptive responses to hypoperfusion may convert compensated renal hypoperfusion into overt prerenal ARF or ATN. Pharmacologic inhibitors of renal prostaglandin biosynthesis [nonsteroidal anti-inflammatory drugs (NSAIDs)] or angiotensin-converting enzyme (ACE) activity (ACE inhibitors) and angiotensin II receptor blockers (ARBs) are major culprits. While NSAIDs do not compromise GFR in healthy individuals, these medications may precipitate prerenal ARF in patients with volume depletion or in those with chronic kidney disease (in whom GFR is maintained, in part, through prostaglandin-mediated hyperfiltration by the remaining functional nephrons). ACE inhibitors should be used with special care in patients with bilateral renal artery stenosis or unilateral stenosis in a solitary functioning kidney. In these settings, glomerular perfusion and filtration may be exquisitely dependent on the actions of angiotensin II. Angiotensin II preserves GFR in these circumstances by raising systemic arterial pressure and by triggering selective constriction of efferent arterioles. ACE inhibitors and ARBs blunt these responses and can precipitate ARF.

Hepatorenal Syndrome Hepatorenal syndrome (HRS) is a unique form of prerenal ARF that frequently complicates advanced cirrhosis as

TABLE 273-1 CLASSIFICATION AND MAJOR CAUSES OF ACUTE RENAL FAILURE

Prerenal ARF

I. Hypovolemia
  A. Increased extracellular fluid losses: hemorrhage
  B. Gastrointestinal fluid loss: vomiting, diarrhea, enterocutaneous fistula
  C. Renal fluid loss: diuretics, osmotic diuresis, hypoadrenalism, nephrogenic diabetes insipidus
  D. Extravascular sequestration: burns, pancreatitis, severe hypoalbuminemia (hypoproteinemia)
  E. Decreased intake: dehydration, altered mental status
II. Altered renal hemodynamics resulting in hypoperfusion
  A. Low cardiac output state: diseases of the myocardium, valves, and pericardium (including tamponade); pulmonary hypertension or massive pulmonary embolism leading to right and left heart failure; impaired venous return (e.g., abdominal compartment syndrome or positive pressure ventilation)
  B. Systemic vasodilation: sepsis, antihypertensives, afterload reducers, anaphylaxis
  C. Renal vasoconstriction: hypercalcemia, catecholamines, calcineurin inhibitors, amphotericin B
  D. Impairment of renal autoregulatory responses: cyclooxygenase inhibitors (e.g., nonsteroidal anti-inflammatory drugs), angiotensin-converting enzyme inhibitors, or angiotensin II receptor blockers
  E. Hepatorenal syndrome

Intrinsic ARF

I. Renovascular obstruction (bilateral, or unilateral in the setting of one kidney)
  A. Renal artery obstruction: atherosclerotic plaque, thrombosis, embolism, dissection aneurysm, large vessel vasculitis
  B. Renal vein obstruction: thrombosis or compression
II. Diseases of the glomeruli or vasculature
  A. Glomerulonephritis or vasculitis
  B. Other: thrombotic microangiopathy, malignant hypertension, collagen vascular diseases (systemic lupus erythematosus, scleroderma), disseminated intravascular coagulation, preeclampsia
III. Acute tubular necrosis
  A. Ischemia: causes are the same as for prerenal ARF, but generally the insult is more severe and/or more prolonged
  B. Infection, with or without sepsis syndrome
  C. Toxins:
    1. Exogenous: radiocontrast, calcineurin inhibitors, antibiotics (e.g., aminoglycosides), chemotherapy (e.g., cisplatin), antifungals (e.g., amphotericin B), ethylene glycol
    2. Endogenous: rhabdomyolysis, hemolysis
IV. Interstitial nephritis
  A. Allergic: antibiotics (β-lactams, sulfonamides, quinolones, rifampin), nonsteroidal anti-inflammatory drugs, diuretics, other drugs
  B. Infection: pyelonephritis (if bilateral)
  C. Infiltration: lymphoma, leukemia, sarcoidosis
  D. Inflammatory, nonvascular: Sjögren's syndrome, tubulointerstitial nephritis with uveitis
V. Intratubular obstruction
  A. Endogenous: myeloma proteins, uric acid (tumor lysis syndrome), systemic oxalalosis
  B. Exogenous: acyclovir, gancyclovir, methotrexate, indinavir

Postrenal ARF (Obstruction)

I. Ureteric (bilateral, or unilateral in the case of one kidney): calculi, blood clots, sloughed papillae, cancer, external compression (e.g., retroperitoneal fibrosis)
II. Bladder neck: neurogenic bladder, prostatic hypertrophy, calculi, blood clots, cancer
III. Urethra: stricture or congenital valves

well as acute liver failure. In HRS the kidneys are structurally normal but fail due to splanchnic vasodilation and arteriovenous shunting, resulting in profound renal vasoconstriction. Correction of the underlying liver disease (e.g., by liver transplantation) results in resolution of the acute renal failure. There are two forms of HRS, type I and type II, that differ in their clinical course. In type I HRS, the more aggressive form of the disease, ARF progresses even after optimization of systemic hemodynamics and carries a mortality rate of >90%. The diagnosis and management of this condition are discussed in Chap. 302.

Intrinsic causes of ARF can be conceptually divided based on the predominant compartment of the kidney that is affected: (1) ischemic or nephrotoxic tubular injury, (2) tubulointerstitial diseases, (3) diseases of the renal microcirculation and glomeruli, and (4) diseases of larger renal vessels (Table 273-1). Ischemia and nephrotoxins classically induce acute tubular injury. Although many patients with ischemic or nephrotoxic ARF do not have morphologic evidence of cellular necrosis, this disease is often referred to as *acute tubular necrosis*, or ATN. More recently, because of the important role of sublethal injury to tubular epithelial and other renal cells (e.g., endothelial cells) in the pathogenesis of this syndrome, the term *acute kidney injury* (AKI) has been proposed.

Etiology and Pathophysiology of Ischemic ATN Prerenal ARF and ischemic ATN are part of a spectrum of manifestations of renal hypoperfusion. In its most extreme form, ischemia leads to bilateral renal cortical necrosis and irreversible renal failure. ATN differs from prerenal ARF in that the renal tubular epithelial cells are injured in the latter. ATN occurs most frequently in patients undergoing major cardiovascular surgery or suffering severe trauma, hemorrhage, sepsis, and/or volume depletion (Table 273-1). Patients with other risk factors for ARF (e.g., exposure to nephrotoxins or preexisting chronic kidney disease) are at increased risk for ATN. Recovery typically takes 1–2 weeks after normalization of renal perfusion, as it requires repair and regeneration of renal cells.

The course of ischemic ATN is typically characterized by four phases: initiation, extension, maintenance, and recovery (Fig. 273-1). These phases are often preceded by a period of prerenal azotemia. During the *initiation phase* (lasting hours to days), GFR declines because (1) glomerular ultrafiltration pressure is reduced as renal blood flow falls, (2) the flow of filtrate within tubules is obstructed by casts comprised of shed epithelial cells and necrotic debris, and (3) there is backleak of glomerular filtrate through injured tubular epithelium. Ischemic injury is most prominent in the S$_3$ segment of the proximal tubule and the medullary portion of the thick ascending limb of the loop of Henle. These segments of the tubule are particularly sensitive to ischemia because of high rates of active (ATP-dependent) solute transport and location in the outer medulla, where the partial pressure of oxygen is low, even under basal conditions. Cellular ischemia results in ATP depletion, inhibition of active sodium transport, cytoskeletal disruption, loss of cell polarity, cell-cell and cell-matrix attachment, and oxygen free-radical formation. Renal injury may be limited by restoration of renal blood flow during this period. If severe, cell injury results in apoptosis or necrosis.

The *extension phase* follows the initiation phase and is characterized by continued ischemic injury and inflammation. It has been proposed that endothelial damage (resulting in vascular congestion) contributes to both of these processes. During the *maintenance phase* (typically 1–2 weeks), GFR stabilizes at its nadir (typically 5–10 mL/min), urine output is lowest, and uremic complications may arise (see below). It is not clear why the GFR remains low during this phase, despite correction of systemic hemodynamics. Proposed mechanisms include persistent intrarenal vasoconstriction and medullary ischemia triggered by dysregulated release of vasoactive mediators from injured endothelial cells, congestion of medullary blood vessels, and reperfusion injury induced by reactive oxygen species and inflammatory mediators released by leukocytes or renal parenchymal cells. In addition, epithelial cell injury may contribute to persistent intrarenal vasoconstriction through *tubuloglomerular feedback*. Specialized epithelial cells in the macula densa region of distal tubules detect increases in distal salt delivery that occur as a consequence of impaired reabsorption by more proximal nephron segments. Macula densa cells, in turn, stimulate constriction of adjacent afferent arterioles by a poorly defined mechanism and further compromise glomerular perfusion and filtration, thereby contributing to a vicious circle.

The *recovery phase* is characterized by tubular epithelial cell repair and regeneration as well as a gradual return of GFR toward premorbid levels. The recovery phase may be complicated by a marked diuretic phase due to delayed recovery of epithelial cell function (solute and water reabsorption) relative to glomerular filtration (see below).

	Systemic events	Renal events	
Initiation GFR falling	prolonged prerenal state hemorrhage sepsis vascular disruption (e.g.: trauma, coronary artery bypass grafting, aortic crossclamp) certain nephrotoxins, e.g. radiocontrast ↓ ischemia	polarized cell basolateral protein	
Extension GFR low/falling		depolarized cell	cellular apoptosis/necrosis ↓ disruption of normal epithelial integrity abnormal tubular function (filtration/clearance) cellular sloughing ↓ luminal obstruction inflammation ↓ capillary sludging and worsening ischemia
Maintenance GFR stable/low		dedifferentiated cell	cellular dedifferentiation proliferation ↓ reestablishment of tubular epithelium
Recovery GFR rising		polarized cell	cellular repolarization ↓ reestablishment of normal tubular function (filtration/clearance)

FIGURE 273-1 Four phases of acute tubular necrosis.

Etiology and Pathophysiology of Nephrotoxic ARF Nephrotoxic ATN may complicate exposure to many structurally diverse pharmacologic agents (Table 273-1). With most nephrotoxins, the incidence of ARF is increased in the elderly and in patients with preexisting chronic kidney disease, true or "effective" hypovolemia, or concomitant exposure to other toxins.

Radiocontrast agents, cyclosporine, and tacrolimus (FK506) cause kidney injury through intrarenal vasoconstriction. Consequently, ATN in association with these medications is characterized by an acute fall in renal blood flow and GFR, a relatively benign urine sediment, and a low fractional excretion of sodium (see below). Severe cases may show clinical or pathologic evidence of tubular cell necrosis. Contrast nephropathy is also thought to result from the generation of reactive oxygen species that are directly toxic to renal tubular epithelial cells. Contrast nephropathy classically presents as an acute (onset within 24–48 h) but reversible (peak 3–5 days, resolution within 1 week) rise in blood urea nitrogen and serum creatinine. Contrast nephropathy is most common in individuals with preexisting chronic kidney disease, diabetes mellitus, congestive heart failure, hypovolemia, or multiple myeloma. The type (low vs. isoosmolar contrast) and dose of contrast also influence the likelihood of injury associated with its administration.

Antibiotics and anticancer drugs typically cause ATN through direct toxicity to the tubular epithelial cells and/or intratubular obstruction. ARF complicates 10–30% of courses of *aminoglycoside antibiotics*. Aminoglycosides accumulate in renal tubular epithelial cells, where they cause oxidative stress and cell injury; thus, ARF usually occurs after several days of aminoglycoside therapy. Damage may occur in both the proximal and distal tubule; defects in the distal tubule may result in decreased concentrating ability. *Amphotericin B* causes dose-related ARF through intrarenal vasoconstriction and direct toxicity to proximal tubule epithelium. Newer (liposomal) formulations of amphotericin B may be associated with less nephrotoxicity. Acyclovir may precipitate in the renal tubules and cause acute renal failure. Foscarnet and pentamidine are less commonly prescribed antimicrobials also frequently associated with acute renal failure. Cisplatin and carboplatin, like the aminoglycosides, are accumulated by proximal tubule cells and typically provoke ARF after 7–10 days of exposure, typically in association with potassium and magnesium wasting. Ifosphamide administration may lead to hemorrhagic cystitis, manifested by hematuria, as well as acute and chronic renal failure. Type II renal tubular acidosis (Fanconi syndrome) often accompanies ifosphamide-associated ARF.

Endogenous nephrotoxins include calcium, myoglobin, hemoglobin, urate, oxalate, and myeloma light chains. Hypercalcemia can compromise GFR, predominantly by inducing intrarenal vasoconstriction as well as volume depletion from obligate water loss. Both *rhabdomyolysis* and *hemolysis* can induce ARF. Common causes of rhabdomyolysis include traumatic crush injury, acute muscle ischemia, prolonged seizure activity, excessive exercise, heat stroke or malignant hyperthermia, and infectious or metabolic disorders (e.g., hypophosphatemia, severe hypothyroidism). ARF due to hemolysis is relatively rare and is observed following blood transfusion reactions. It has been postulated that myoglobin and hemoglobin promote intrarenal oxidative stress, resulting in injury to tubular epithelial cells and inducing intratubular cast formation. In addition, cell-free hemoglobin and myoglobin are potent inhibitors of nitric oxide bioactivity and may trigger intrarenal vasoconstriction and ischemia. Hypovolemia or acidosis may further promote intratubular cast formation. Intratubular casts containing filtered immunoglobulin light chains and other proteins (including Tamm-Horsfall protein produced by thick ascending limb cells) cause ARF in patients with *multiple myeloma* (myeloma cast nephropathy). Light chains are also directly toxic to tubule epithelial cells. Intratubular obstruction is an important cause of ARF in patients with severe *hyperuricosuria* or *hyperoxaluria*. Acute uric acid nephropathy can complicate the treatment of selected lymphoproliferative or myeloproliferative disorders (e.g., Burkitt's lymphoma, acute myelogenous leukemia), especially after the administration of chemotherapy, resulting in increased cell lysis ("tumor lysis syndrome").

Pathology of Ischemic and Nephrotoxic ATN The classic pathologic features of ischemic ATN are patchy and focal necrosis of the tubular epithelium, with detachment of cells from the basement membrane, and occlusion of tubule lumens with casts composed of intact or degenerating epithelial cells, Tamm-Horsfall protein, and pigments. Leukocyte accumulation is frequently observed in vasa recta; however, the morphology of the glomeruli and renal vasculature is characteristically normal. Necrosis is most severe in the S3 segment of proximal tubules but may also affect the medullary thick ascending limb of the loop of Henle.

With exposure to nephrotoxins, morphologic changes tend to be most prominent in both the convoluted and straight portions of proximal tubules. Cellular necrosis is less pronounced than in ischemic ATN.

Other Causes of Intrinsic ARF Virtually any pharmacologic agent may trigger allergic interstitial nephritis, which is characterized by infiltration of the tubulointerstitium by granulocytes (typically but not invariably eosinophils), macrophages, and/or lymphocytes and by interstitial edema. The most common offenders are antibiotics (e.g., penicillins, cephalosporins, quinolones, sulfonamides, rifampin) and NSAIDs (Table 273-1).

Patients with advanced atherosclerosis can develop ARF after manipulation of the aorta or renal arteries during surgery or angiography, following trauma, or, rarely, spontaneously (atheroembolic ARF). Cholesterol crystals embolize to the renal vasculature, lodge in small- and medium-sized arteries, and incite a giant cell and fibrotic reaction in the vessel wall with narrowing or obstruction of the vessel lumen. Atheroembolic ARF is often associated with hypocomplementemia and eosinophiluria, and it is frequently irreversible. The acute glomerulonephritides are immune-mediated diseases characterized by proliferative or crescentic glomerular inflammation (glomerulonephritis). These diseases are discussed in detail in Chap. 277.

POSTRENAL ARF

(See also Chap. 283) Urinary tract obstruction accounts for fewer than 5% of cases of hospital-acquired ARF. Because one kidney has sufficient reserve to handle generated nitrogenous waste products, ARF from obstruction requires obstruction to urine flow between the external urethral meatus and bladder neck, bilateral ureteric obstruction, or unilateral ureteric obstruction in a patient with one functioning kidney or with significant preexisting chronic kidney disease. Bladder neck obstruction is the most common cause of postrenal ARF and is usually due to prostatic disease (e.g., hypertrophy, neoplasia, or infection), neurogenic bladder, or therapy with anticholinergic drugs. Less common causes of acute lower urinary tract obstruction include blood clots, calculi, and urethritis with spasm. Ureteric obstruction may result from intraluminal obstruction (e.g., calculi, blood clots, sloughed renal papillae), infiltration of the ureteric wall (e.g., neoplasia), or external compression (e.g., retroperitoneal fibrosis, neoplasia or abscess, inadvertent surgical ligature). During the early stages of obstruction (hours to days), continued glomerular filtration leads to increased intraluminal pressure upstream to the site of obstruction. As a result, there is gradual distention of the proximal ureter, renal pelvis, and calyces and a fall in GFR.

CLINICAL FEATURES AND DIFFERENTIAL DIAGNOSIS

The first step in evaluating a patient with renal failure is to determine if the disease is acute or chronic. If review of laboratory records demonstrates that the rise in blood urea nitrogen and creatinine is recent, this suggests that the process is acute. However, previous measurements are not always available. Findings that suggest chronic kidney disease (Chap. 274) include anemia, evidence of renal osteodystrophy (radiologic or laboratory), and small scarred kidneys. However, anemia may also complicate ARF (see below), and renal size may be normal or increased in several chronic renal diseases (e.g., diabetic nephropathy, amyloidosis, polycystic kidney disease, HIV associated nephropathy). Once a diagnosis of ARF has been established, the etiology of ARF needs to be determined. Depending on the cause, specific therapies may need to be instituted. If the etiology is felt to be an exogenous nephrotoxin (often a medication), the nephrotoxin should be eliminated or discontinued. Lastly, the prevention and management of complications should be instituted.

CLINICAL ASSESSMENT

Symptoms of *prerenal* ARF include thirst and orthostatic dizziness. Physical signs of orthostatic hypotension, tachycardia, reduced jugular venous pressure, decreased skin turgor and dry mucous membranes suggest prerenal ARF. Careful clinical examination may reveal stigmata of chronic liver disease and portal hypertension, advanced cardiac failure, sepsis, or other causes of reduced "effective" arterial blood volume (Table 273-1). Case records should be reviewed for documentation of a progressive fall in urine output and body weight and recent initiation of treatment with diuretics, NSAIDs, ACE inhibitors, or ARBs.

Hypovolemia, septic shock, and major surgery are important risk factors for ischemic ATN. The risk of ischemic ATN is increased further if ARF persists despite normalization of systemic hemodynamics. Diagnosis of nephrotoxic ATN requires careful review of the clinical data and records for evidence of recent exposure to nephrotoxic medications, radiocontrast agents, or endogenous toxins.

Although ischemic and nephrotoxic ATN account for >90% of cases of intrinsic ARF, other renal parenchymal diseases must be considered (Table 273-2). Fever, arthralgias, and a pruritic erythematous rash following exposure to a new drug suggest allergic interstitial nephritis, although systemic features of hypersensitivity are frequently absent. Flank pain may be a prominent symptom following occlusion of a renal artery or vein and with other parenchymal diseases distending the renal capsule (e.g., severe glomerulonephritis or pyelonephritis). Subcutaneous nodules, livedo reticularis, bright orange retinal arteriolar plaques, and digital ischemia ("purple toes"), despite palpable pedal pulses, suggest atheroembolization. ARF in association with oliguria, edema, and hypertension, with an "active" urine sediment (nephritic syndrome), suggests acute glomerulonephritis or vasculitis. Malignant hypertension may result in ARF, often in association with hypertensive injury to other organs (e.g., papilledema, neurologic dysfunction, left ventricular hypertrophy) and may mimic glomerulonephritis in its other clinical manifestations.

Postrenal ARF may present with suprapubic and flank pain due to distention of the bladder and of the renal collecting system and capsule, respectively. Colicky flank pain radiating to the groin suggests acute ureteric obstruction. Prostatic disease is likely if there is a history of nocturia, frequency, and hesitancy and enlargement of the prostate on rectal examination. Neurogenic bladder should be suspected in patients receiving anticholinergic medications or with physical evidence of autonomic dysfunction. Definitive diagnosis of postrenal ARF hinges on judicious use of radiologic investigations and rapid improvement in renal function following relief of obstruction.

URINALYSIS

(See also **Chap. e9**) Anuria suggests complete urinary tract obstruction but may complicate severe cases of prerenal or intrinsic renal ARF. Wide fluctuations in urine output raise the possibility of intermittent obstruction, whereas patients with partial urinary tract obstruction may present with polyuria due to impairment of urine concentrating mechanisms.

TABLE 273-2 EPIDEMIOLOGY, CLINICAL FEATURES, AND DIAGNOSTIC STUDIES FOR MAJOR CAUSES OF ACUTE RENAL FAILURE

Etiology	Epidemiology	Clinical Features	Serum Studies	Urine Studies	Other Testing
Prerenal ARF	Most common cause of community-acquired ARF; history of poor fluid intake, treatment with NSAIDs/ACE inhibitors/ARBs, worsening heart failure	Volume depletion (absolute/postural hypotension, low jugular venous pressure, dry mucus membranes) or decreased effective circulatory volume (e.g., heart failure or liver disease)	High BUN/CR ratio (≥20) is suggestive but not diagnostic	Hyaline casts FE_{Na} <1% U_{Na} <10 mmol/L SG >1.018	
Intrinsic ARF					
Diseases of large renal vessels					
Renal artery thrombosis	More common in those with atrial fibrillation or arterial thrombosis	Flank or abdominal pain	Elevated LDH	Mild proteinuria Occasional hematuria	Renal angiogram or MR angiogram are diagnostic
Atheroembolic disease	Vascular disease; classically occurs within days–weeks of manipulation of the aorta or other large vessels, often in the setting of anticoagulation	Retinal plaques, palpable purpura, livedo reticularis	Eosinophilia Hypocomplementemia	Eosinophiluria	Skin or renal biopsy
Renal vein thrombosis	History of nephrotic syndrome or pulmonary embolism	Flank pain		Mild proteinuria Occasional hematuria	Renal venogram or MR venogram are diagnostic
Diseases of small vessels and glomeruli					
Glomerulonephritis/vasculitis	Associated with recent infection (postinfectious or endocarditis), systemic lupus erythematosus, liver disease (hepatitis B or C) Anti-GBM disease: Typically men in their 20s–40s ANCA disease: Two peaks: 20s–30s and 50s–60s	New cardiac murmur (postinfectious) Skin rash/ulcers, arthralgias (lupus) Sinusitis (anti-GBM disease) Lung hemorrhage (anti-GBM, ANCA, lupus)	ANA, ANCA, anti-GBM antibody, hepatitis serologies, cryoglobulins, blood cultures, ASO, complements (positive tests depend on etiology)	Hematuria with red cell casts/dysmorphic red blood cells Granular casts Proteinuria (usually <1 g/d)	Renal biopsy

(continued)

TABLE 273-2 EPIDEMIOLOGY, CLINICAL FEATURES, AND DIAGNOSTIC STUDIES FOR MAJOR CAUSES OF ACUTE RENAL FAILURE (CONTINUED)

Etiology	Epidemiology	Clinical Features	Serum Studies	Urine Studies	Other Testing
Hemolytic-uremic syndrome/thrombotic thrombocytopenic	Recent GI infection (*E. coli*) or use of calcineurin inhibitors (FK506 and cyclosporine)	Fever, neurologic abnormalities	Schistocytes on peripheral blood smear, elevated LDH, anemia, thrombocytopenia	Hematuria Mild proteinuria Red cell casts (rare)	Renal biopsy
Malignant hypertension	Severe/uncontrolled hypertension	Evidence of damage to other organs: headache, papilledema, heart failure with LVH by echocardiography/ECG Typically resolves with blood pressure control		Hematuria with red cell casts/proteinuria	
Acute tubular necrosis Ischemia	Recent hemorrhage or severe hypotension			Muddy brown granular or tubular epithelial cell casts $FE_{Na} > 1\%$ $U_{Na} > 20$ mmol/L SG <1.015	
Exogenous toxins	Recent exposure to nephrotoxic antibiotics or chemotherapy, often in association with sepsis, or volume depletion			Muddy brown granular or tubular epithelial cell casts $FE_{Na} > 1\%$ $U_{Na} > 20$ mmol/L SG <1.015	
	Recent exposure to radiocontrast, often in association with volume depletion, diabetes or CKD			Muddy brown granular or tubular epithelial cell casts Urinalysis may be normal FE_{Na} often <1% U_{Na} often <20 mmol/L	
Endogenous toxins	Rhabdomyolysis	Post ictal state (seizures), evidence of trauma or prolonged immobilization	Increased myoglobin, creatine kinase	U/A positive for heme but no hematuria	
	Hemolysis: recent blood transfusion	Fever, other evidence of transfusion reaction	Pink plasma, increased LDH	Pink, heme-positive urine without hematuria	Transfusion reaction workup
	Tumor lysis: recent chemotherapy		Hyperuricemia, increased LDH	Urate crystals	
	Multiple myeloma	Individuals >60 years of age, ongoing constitutional symptoms (fatigue, malaise)	Circulating monoclonal spike, anemia	Dipstick-negative proteinuria, monoclonal spike on electrophoresis	Bone marrow or renal biopsy
	Ethylene glycol ingestion	History of alcohol abuse, altered mental status	Metabolic gap acidosis with osmolal gap, positive toxicology	Oxalate crystals	
Diseases of the tubulointerstitium Allergic interstitial nephritis	Recent medication exposure	Fever, rash, arthralgias	Eosinophilia	White cell casts, eosinophiluria	Renal biopsy
Acute bilateral pyelonephritis		Fever, flank pain and tenderness	Positive blood cultures	Leukocytes, proteinuria, positive urine culture	
Postrenal ARF	History of renal stones or prostatic disease	Palpable bladder, flank or abdominal pain		Usually normal; hematuria if due to stones	Imaging to assess obstruction: CT scan and/or ultrasound

Note: ACE, angiotensin-converting enzyme; ANA, antinuclear antibody; ANCA, antineutrophil cytoplasmic antibody; ARBs, angiotensin II receptor blockers; ARF, acute renal failure; ASO, antistreptolysin O; BUN, blood urea nitrogen; CKD, chronic kidney disease; CR, creatinine; CT, computed tomography; ECG, electrocardiogram; FE_{Na}, fractional excretion of sodium; GBM, glomerular basement membrane; GI, gastrointestinal; LDH, lactate dehydrogenase; LVH, left ventricular hypertrophy; MR, magnetic resonance; NSAIDs, nonsteroidal anti-inflammatory drugs; SG, specific gravity; U/A, urinalysis; U_{Na}, urine sodium concentration.

In prerenal ARF, the sediment is characteristically acellular and contains transparent hyaline casts ("bland," "benign," "inactive" urine sediment). Hyaline casts are formed in concentrated urine from normal constituents of urine—principally Tamm-Horsfall protein, which is secreted by epithelial cells of the loop of Henle. Postrenal ARF may also present with an inactive sediment, although hematuria and pyuria are common in patients with intraluminal obstruction or prostatic disease. Pigmented "muddy brown" granular casts and casts containing tubule epithelial cells are characteristic of ATN and suggest an ischemic or nephrotoxic etiology. These casts are usually found in association with mild "tubular" proteinuria (<1 g/d), reflecting impaired reabsorption and processing of filtered proteins by injured proximal tubules. Casts may be absent in 20–30% of patients with ATN and are not required for diagnosis. In general, red blood cell casts indicate glomerular injury or, less often, acute tubulointerstitial nephritis. White cell casts and nonpigmented granular casts suggest interstitial nephritis, whereas broad granular casts are characteristic of chronic kidney disease and probably reflect interstitial fibrosis and dilatation of tubules. Eosinophiluria (>5% of urine leukocytes) is a common finding (~90%) in antibiotic-induced allergic interstitial nephritis and can be detected with Hansel's stain; however, lymphocytes may predominate in allergic interstitial nephritis induced by NSAIDs and some other drugs (i.e., ampicillin, rifampicin, and interferon α). Occasional uric acid crystals (pleomorphic in shape) are common in the concentrated urine of prerenal ARF but suggest acute urate nephropathy if seen in abundance. Oxalate (envelope-shaped) and hippurate (needle-shaped) crystals raise the possibility of ethylene glycol ingestion and toxicity.

Proteinuria of >1 g/d suggests injury to the glomerular ultrafiltration barrier ("glomerular proteinuria") or excretion of myeloma light chains. The latter may not be detected by conventional dipstick analysis, and other tests may be needed (e.g., sulfosalicylic acid precipitation, immunoelectrophoresis). Hemoglobinuria or myoglobinuria should be suspected if urine is strongly positive for heme by dipstick but contains few red cells, and if the supernatant of centrifuged urine is positive for free heme. Bilirubinuria may provide a clue to the presence of HRS.

RENAL FAILURE INDICES

Analysis of urine and blood biochemistry may be useful for distinguishing prerenal ARF from ischemic or nephrotoxic intrinsic renal ARF. The fractional excretion of sodium (FE_{Na}) is most useful in this regard. The FE_{Na} relates sodium clearance to creatinine clearance. Sodium is reabsorbed avidly from glomerular filtrate in patients with prerenal ARF, in an attempt to restore intravascular volume. The FE_{Na} tends to be high in ischemic ATN but is often low in patients with sepsis-induced, pigment-induced, and some forms of nephrotoxic ATN (e.g., contrast-associated). In contrast, creatinine is not reabsorbed in either setting. Consequently, patients with prerenal ARF typically have a FE_{Na} of <1.0% (frequently <0.1%). In patients with metabolic alkalosis, where there may be obligate losses of sodium in the urine to maintain electroneutrality, the fractional excretion of chloride (FE_{Cl}) may be more sensitive than the FE_{Na} in detecting prerenal azotemia. The *urine sodium concentration* is a less-sensitive index for distinguishing prerenal ARF from ischemic and nephrotoxic ARF as values overlap between groups. Similarly, indices of urinary concentrating ability such as urine specific gravity, urine osmolality, urine-to-plasma urea ratio, and blood urea-to-creatinine ratio are of limited value in differential diagnosis.

Many caveats apply when interpreting biochemical renal failure indices. The FE_{Na} may be >1.0% in prerenal ARF if patients are receiving diuretics or with preexisting chronic kidney disease, certain salt-wasting syndromes, or adrenal insufficiency.

LABORATORY FINDINGS

Serial serum creatinine measurements can provide useful insights to the cause of ARF. Prerenal ARF is typified by fluctuating serum creatinine levels that parallel changes in hemodynamic status. Creatinine rises rapidly (within 24–48 h) in patients with ARF following renal is-

chemia, atheroembolization, and radiocontrast exposure. Peak serum creatinine concentrations are observed after 3–5 days with contrast nephropathy and return to baseline after 5–7 days. In contrast, serum creatinine concentrations typically peak later (7–10 days) in ATN and atheroembolic disease. The initial rise in serum creatinine is characteristically delayed until the second week of therapy with many tubular epithelial cell toxins (e.g., aminoglycosides, cisplatin) and is thought to reflect the need for accumulation of these agents within tubular epithelial cells to cause injury.

Hyperkalemia, hyperphosphatemia, hypocalcemia, and elevations in serum uric acid and creatine kinase (MM isoenzyme) levels at presentation suggest a diagnosis of rhabdomyolysis. Hyperuricemia [>890 μmol/L (>15 mg/dL)] in association with hyperkalemia, hyperphosphatemia, and increased circulating levels of intracellular enzymes such as lactate dehydrogenase may indicate acute urate nephropathy and tumor lysis syndrome following cancer chemotherapy. A wide anion and osmolal gap [the latter calculated as the difference between the observed (measured) serum osmolality minus the expected osmolality calculated from serum sodium, glucose, and urea concentrations] indicate the presence of an unusual anion or osmole in the circulation (e.g., ingestion of ethylene glycol or methanol). Severe anemia in the absence of hemorrhage raises the possibility of hemolysis, multiple myeloma, or thrombotic microangiopathy. Systemic eosinophilia suggests allergic interstitial nephritis but is also a feature of atheroembolic disease and polyarteritis nodosa.

RADIOLOGIC FINDINGS

Imaging of the urinary tract by ultrasonography is useful to exclude postrenal ARF. CT and MRI are alternative imaging modalities. Whereas pelvicalyceal dilatation is usual with urinary tract obstruction (98% sensitivity), dilatation may be absent immediately following obstruction or in patients with ureteric encasement (e.g., retroperitoneal fibrosis, neoplasia). Retrograde or anterograde pyelography are more definitive investigations in complex cases and provide precise localization of the site of obstruction. A plain film of the abdomen or unenhanced helical CT scan is a valuable initial screening technique in patients with suspected nephrolithiasis. Magnetic resonance angiography (MRA) is often used to assess patency of renal arteries and veins in patients with suspected vascular obstruction. Alternative methods include Doppler ultrasound (which is much more operator-dependent than MRA) and CT-based angiography. Catheter-based angiography may be required for definitive diagnosis and treatment.

RENAL BIOPSY

Biopsy is reserved for patients in whom prerenal and postrenal ARF have been excluded and the cause of intrinsic ARF is unclear. Renal biopsy is particularly useful when clinical assessment and laboratory investigations suggest diagnoses other than ischemic or nephrotoxic injury that may respond to disease-specific therapy. Examples include glomerulonephritis, vasculitis, and allergic interstitial nephritis.

COMPLICATIONS

ARF impairs renal excretion of sodium, potassium, and water and perturbs divalent cation homeostasis and urinary acidification mechanisms. As a result, ARF is frequently complicated by intravascular volume overload, hyponatremia, hyperkalemia, hyperphosphatemia, hypocalcemia, hypermagnesemia, and metabolic acidosis. In addition, patients are unable to excrete nitrogenous waste products and are prone to develop the uremic syndrome (Chap. 45). The speed of development and the severity of these complications reflect the degree of renal impairment and catabolic state of the patient.

Expansion of extracellular fluid volume is an inevitable consequence of diminished salt and water excretion in oliguric or anuric individuals. Whereas milder forms are characterized by weight gain, bibasilar lung rales, raised jugular venous pressure, and dependent edema, continued volume expansion may precipitate life-threatening pulmonary edema. Excessive administration of free water, either through ingestion and nasogastric administration or as hypotonic saline or isotonic dextrose solutions, can induce *hypoosmolality* and *hyponatremia*, which, if severe, lead to neurologic abnormalities, including seizures.

Hyperkalemia is a frequent complication of ARF. Coexistent metabolic acidosis may exacerbate hyperkalemia by promoting potassium efflux from cells. Hyperkalemia may be particularly severe, even at the time of diagnosis, in patients with rhabdomyolysis, hemolysis, and tumor lysis syndrome. Mild hyperkalemia (<6.0 mmol/L) is usually asymptomatic. Higher levels may trigger electrocardiographic abnormalities and/or arrhythmias.

ARF is typically complicated by *metabolic acidosis*, often with an increased anion gap (Chap. 48). Acidosis can be particularly severe when endogenous production of hydrogen ions is increased by other mechanisms (e.g., diabetic or fasting ketoacidosis; lactic acidosis complicating generalized tissue hypoperfusion, liver disease, or sepsis; metabolism of ethylene glycol or methanol).

Hyperphosphatemia is an almost invariable complication of ARF. Severe hyperphosphatemia may develop in highly catabolic patients or following rhabdomyolysis, hemolysis, or tissue ischemia. Metastatic deposition of calcium phosphate can lead to *hypocalcemia*, particularly with elevation of serum calcium (mg/dL) and phosphate (mg/dL) concentrations. Other factors that contribute to hypocalcemia include tissue resistance to the actions of parathyroid hormone and reduced levels of 1,25-dihydroxyvitamin D. Hypocalcemia is often asymptomatic but can cause perioral paresthesia, muscle cramps, seizures, altered mental status, prolongation of the QT interval and other nonspecific T-wave changes on electrocardiography.

Anemia develops rapidly in ARF and is usually multifactorial in origin. Contributing factors include impaired erythropoiesis, hemolysis, bleeding, hemodilution, and reduced red cell survival time. Prolongation of the *bleeding time* is also common. Common contributors to the bleeding diathesis include mild thrombocytopenia, platelet dysfunction, and/or clotting factor abnormalities (e.g., factor VIII dysfunction). *Infection* is a common and serious complication of ARF. It is unclear whether patients with ARF have a clinically significant defect in host immune responses or whether the high incidence of infection reflects repeated breaches of mucocutaneous barriers (e.g., intravenous cannulae, mechanical ventilation, bladder catheterization). *Cardiopulmonary complications* of ARF include arrhythmias, pericarditis and pericardial effusion, and pulmonary edema.

Protracted periods of severe ARF are invariably associated with the development of the *uremic syndrome* (Chap. 45).

A *vigorous diuresis* can occur during the recovery phase of ARF (see above), which may be inappropriate on occasion and lead to intravascular volume depletion. *Hypernatremia* can also complicate recovery if water losses via hypotonic urine are not replaced or if losses are inappropriately replaced by relatively hypertonic saline solutions. *Hypokalemia, hypomagnesemia, hypophosphatemia,* and *hypocalcemia* are less common metabolic complications during this period but may develop in response to injury associated with selected drugs (e.g., ifosphamide may lead to Fanconi syndrome or type II renal tubular acidosis associated with hypokalemia, acidosis, hypophosphatemia, and glycosuria).

Rx ACUTE RENAL FAILURE

PREVENTION   Because there are no specific therapies for ischemic or nephrotoxic ARF, prevention is of paramount importance. Many cases of ischemic ARF can be avoided by close attention to cardiovascular function and intravascular volume in high-risk patients, such as the elderly and those with preexisting chronic kidney disease. Indeed, aggressive restoration of intravascular volume has been shown to dramatically reduce the incidence of ischemic ARF after major surgery or trauma, burns, or cholera. The incidence of nephrotoxic ARF can be reduced by tailoring the administration (dose and frequency) of nephrotoxic drugs to body size and GFR. In this regard, it should be noted that serum creatinine is a relatively insensitive index of GFR and may overestimate GFR considerably in small or elderly patients. For purposes of drug dosing, it is advisable to estimate the GFR using the Cockcroft-Gault formula (which factors in age, sex, and weight) or the simplified Modification of Diet in Renal Disease (MDRD) equation

(which factors in age, sex, weight, and race) (Chap. 277). Of note, these equations cannot be used to estimate GFR when creatinine is not at steady state (e.g., during evolving ARF). Adjusting drug dosage according to circulating drug levels also appears to limit renal injury in patients receiving aminoglycoside antibiotics, cyclosporine, or tacrolimus. Diuretics, NSAIDs, ACE inhibitors, ARBs, and vasodilators should be used with caution in patients with suspected true or "effective" hypovolemia or renovascular disease as they may precipitate prerenal ARF or convert the latter to ischemic ARF. Allopurinol and forced alkaline diuresis are useful prophylactic measures in patients at high risk for acute urate nephropathy (e.g., cancer chemotherapy in hematologic malignancies) to limit uric acid generation and prevent precipitation of urate crystals in renal tubules. Rasburicase, a recombinant urate-oxidase enzyme, catalyzes enzymatic oxidation of uric acid into a soluble metabolite, allantoin. Forced alkaline diuresis may also prevent or attenuate ARF in patients receiving high-dose methotrexate or suffering from rhabdomyolysis. N-acetylcysteine limits acetaminophen-induced renal injury if given within 24 h of ingestion.

A number of preventive measures have been proposed for contrast nephropathy. It is clear that hydration is an effective preventive measure. Other measures that have been proposed include loop diuretics and mannitol, dopamine, fenoldopam, N-acetylcysteine, theophylline, and sodium bicarbonate. Despite favorable experimental data, there is insufficient evidence to support the use of loop diuretics or mannitol to prevent radiocontrast nephropathy or any other cause of ARF. Likewise, despite its widespread use, dopamine has proved ineffective as a prophylactic agent. Fenoldopam, a dopamine a-1 specific agonist approved for use as a parenteral antihypertensive agent, has been tested in several clinical trials and does not appear to reduce the incidence of contrast nephropathy. Moreover, fenoldopam is associated with significant side effects, including systemic hypotension, and its use as an agent to prevent radiocontrast nephropathy should be discouraged. In contrast, several (relatively small) randomized clinical trials (RCTs) have suggested a clinical benefit to the use of N-acetylcysteine, although meta-analyses have been inconclusive. However, aside from the potential hazards associated with a delay in radiographic imaging, N-acetylcysteine appears to be safe, and its use in patients at high risk for radiocontrast nephropathy is reasonable, based on its low side effect profile. Larger RCTs will be required to show definitive benefit. Theophylline and aminophylline (adenosine antagonists) offer the potential advantage of use immediately preceding radiocontrast administration, although the benefit, if present, appears marginal in most studies. Lastly, volume expansion with bicarbonate-containing intravenous fluids has been suggested to be superior to sodium chloride (saline) administration and showed a significant benefit in a single center RCT. Unlike N-acetylcysteine, the use of sodium bicarbonate does not obligate a delay in imaging (the published protocol began IV fluids 1 h before the imaging study was begun). Whether a combination of strategies (e.g., N-acetylcysteine + sodium bicarbonate) offers additive benefit and that patients require treatment remain unclear and warrant further study.

SPECIFIC THERAPIES   By definition, prerenal ARF is rapidly reversible upon correction of the primary hemodynamic abnormality, and postrenal ARF resolves upon relief of obstruction. To date there are no specific therapies for established AKI. Management of these disorders should focus on elimination of the causative hemodynamic abnormality or toxin, avoidance of additional insults, and prevention and treatment of complications. Specific treatment of other causes of intrinsic renal ARF depends on the underlying pathology.

Prerenal ARF   The composition of replacement fluids for treatment of prerenal ARF due to hypovolemia should be tailored according to the composition of the lost fluid. Severe hypovolemia due to hemorrhage should be corrected with packed red cells, whereas isotonic saline is usually appropriate replacement for mild to moderate hemorrhage or plasma loss (e.g., burns, pancreatitis). Urinary and gastrointestinal fluids can vary greatly in composition but are usually hypotonic. Hypotonic solutions (e.g., 0.45% saline) are usually recommended as initial replacement in patients with prerenal ARF due to increased urinary or gastrointestinal fluid losses, although isotonic saline may be more appropriate in severe cases. Subsequent therapy should be based on measurements of the volume and ionic content of excreted or drained fluids. Serum potassium and acid-base status should be monitored carefully, and potassium and bicarbonate supplemented as appropriate. Cardiac failure may require aggressive management with inotropic agents, preload and afterload reducing agents, antiarrhythmic drugs, and mechanical aids such as intraaortic balloon pumps. Invasive hemodynamic monitoring may be required in selected cases to guide therapy for complications in patients in whom clinical assessment of cardiovascular function and intravascular volume is difficult.

Fluid management may be particularly challenging in patients with cirrhosis complicated by ascites. In this setting, it is important to distinguish between full-blown HRS (Chap. 302), which carries a grave prognosis, and reversible ARF due to true or "effective" hypovolemia induced by overzealous use of diuretics or sepsis (e.g., spontaneous bacterial peritonitis). The contribution of hypovolemia to ARF can be definitively assessed only by administration of a fluid challenge. Fluids should be administered slowly and titrated to jugular venous pressure and, if necessary, central venous and pulmonary capillary wedge pressure. Patients with a reversible prerenal component typically have an increase in urine output and fall in serum creatinine with fluid challenge, whereas patients with HRS do not. Patients with HRS may suffer increased ascites formation and pulmonary compromise if not monitored closely during fluid challenge. Large volumes of ascitic fluid can usually be drained by paracentesis without deterioration in renal function if intravenous albumin is administered simultaneously. Indeed, "large-volume paracentesis" may afford an increase in GFR, likely by lowering intraabdominal pressure and improving flow in renal veins. Alternatively, for patients with refractory ascites, transjugular intrahepatic portosystemic shunting is an alternative. Older peritoneal-venous shunts (LaVeen or Denver shunt) have largely fallen out of favor. Transjugular intrahepatic portosystemic shunts may improve renal function through increased central blood volume and suppression of aldosterone and norepinephrine secretion.

Intrinsic ARF   Many different approaches to attenuate injury or hasten recovery have been tested in ischemic and nephrotoxic AKI. These include atrial natriuretic peptide, low-dose dopamine, endothelin antagonists, loop-blocking diuretics, calcium channel blockers, α-adrenoreceptor blockers, prostaglandin analogues, antioxidants, antibodies against leukocyte adhesion molecules, and insulin-like growth factor type I. Whereas many of these are beneficial in experimental models of ischemic or nephrotoxic ATN, they have either failed to confer consistent benefit or proved ineffective in humans.

ARF due to other intrinsic renal diseases such as acute glomerulonephritis or vasculitis may respond to immunosuppressive agents (glucocorticoids, alkylating agents, and/or plasmapheresis, depending on the primary pathology). Glucocorticoids also may hasten remission in allergic interstitial nephritis, although data are limited to small-case series. Aggressive control of systemic arterial pressure is of paramount importance in limiting renal injury in malignant hypertensive nephrosclerosis. Hypertension and ARF due to scleroderma may be exquisitely sensitive to treatment with ACE inhibitors.

Postrenal ARF   Management of postrenal ARF requires close collaboration between nephrologist, urologist, and radiologist. Obstruction of the urethra or bladder neck is usually managed initially by transurethral or suprapubic placement of a bladder catheter, which provides temporary relief while the obstructing lesion is identified and treated definitively. Similarly, ureteric obstruction may be treated initially by percutaneous catheterization of the dilated renal pelvis or ureter. Indeed, obstructing lesions can often be removed percutaneously (e.g., calculus, sloughed papilla) or bypassed by insertion of a ureteric stent (e.g., carcinoma). Most patients experience an appropriate diuresis for several days following relief of obstruction. Approximately 5% of patients develop a transient salt-wasting syndrome that may require administration of intravenous saline to maintain blood pressure.

SUPPORTIVE MEASURES   (**Table 273-3**) Following correction of hypovolemia, salt and water intake are tailored to match losses. Hypervolemia can usually be managed by restriction of salt and water intake and diuretics. Indeed, there is, as yet, no proven rationale for administration of diuretics in ARF except to treat this complication. Despite the fact that subpressor doses of dopamine may transiently promote salt and water excretion by increasing renal blood flow and GFR and by inhibiting tubule sodium reabsorption, subpressor ("low-dose," "renal-dose") dopamine has proved ineffective in clinical trials, may trigger arrhythmias, and should not be used as a renoprotective agent in this setting. Ultrafiltration or dialysis is used to treat severe hypervolemia when conservative measures fail. Hypo-

TABLE 273-3	MANAGEMENT OF ISCHEMIC AND NEPHROTOXIC ACUTE RENAL FAILURE[a]
Management Issue	**Therapy**
Reversal of Renal Insult	
Ischemic ATN	Restore systemic hemodynamics and renal perfusion through volume resuscitation and use of vasopressors
Nephrotoxic ATN	Eliminate nephrotoxic agents
	Consider toxin-specific measures: e.g., forced alkaline diuresis for rhabdomyolysis, allopurinol/rasburicase for tumor lysis syndrome
Prevention and Treatment of Complications	
Intravascular volume overload	Salt and water restriction
	Diuretics
	Ultrafiltration
Hyponatremia	Restriction of enteral free water intake
	Avoidance of hypotonic intravenous solutions, including dextrose-containing solutions
Hyperkalemia	Restriction of dietary K^+ intake
	Eliminate K^+ supplements and K^+-sparing diuretics
	Loop diuretics to promote K^+ excretion
	Potassium binding ion-exchange resins (e.g., sodium polystyrene sulfonate or Kayexalate)
	Insulin (10 units regular) and glucose (50 mL of 50% dextrose) to promote intracellular mobilization
	Inhaled β-agonist therapy to promote intracellular mobilization
	Calcium gluconate or calcium chloride (1 g) to stabilize the myocardium
	Dialysis
Metabolic acidosis	Sodium bicarbonate (maintain serum bicarbonate >15 mmol/L or arterial pH >7.2)
	Administration of other bases, e.g., THAM
	Dialysis
Hyperphosphatemia	Restriction of dietary phosphate intake
	Phosphate binding agents (calcium carbonate, calcium acetate, sevelamer hydrochloride, aluminum hydroxide)
Hypocalcemia	Calcium carbonate or gluconate (if symptomatic)
Hypermagnesemia	Discontinue Mg^{++} containing antacids
Hyperuricemia	Treatment usually not necessary if <890 μmol/L or <15mg/dL
	Allopurinol, forced alkaline diuresis, rasburicase
Nutrition	Protein and calorie intake to avoid net negative nitrogen balance
Dialysis	To prevent complications of acute renal failure
Choice of agents	Avoid other nephrotoxins: ACE inhibitors/ARBs, aminoglycosides, NSAIDs, radiocontrast unless absolutely necessary and no alternative
Drug dosing	Adjust doses and frequency of administration for degree of renal impairment

[a]Note that these are general recommendations and need to be tailored to the individual patient.
Abbreviations: ATN, acute tubular necrosis; THAM, tris(hydroxymethyl)aminomethane; ACE, angiotensin-converting enzyme; ARBs, angiotensin II receptor blockers; NSAIDs, nonsteroidal anti-inflammatory drugs.

free water intake. Conversely, hypernatremia is treated by administration of water or intravenous hypotonic saline or isotonic dextrose-containing solutions. **The management of hyperkalemia is described in Chap. 46.**

Metabolic acidosis is not usually treated unless serum bicarbonate concentration falls below 15 mmol/L or arterial pH falls below 7.2. More severe acidosis is corrected by oral or intravenous sodium bicarbonate. Initial rates of replacement are guided by estimates of bicarbonate deficit and adjusted thereafter according to serum levels (Chap. 48). Patients should be monitored for complications of sodium bicarbonate administration such as hypervolemia, metabolic alkalosis, hypocalcemia, and hypokalemia. From a practical point of view, most patients who require supplemental sodium bicarbonate administration will need emergency dialysis within days. Hyperphosphatemia is usually controlled by restriction of dietary phosphate and by oral phosphate binders (calcium carbonate, calcium acetate, sevelamer, and aluminum hydroxide) to reduce gastrointestinal absorption of phosphate. Hypocalcemia does not usually require treatment unless severe, as may occur with rhabdomyolysis or pancreatitis or following administration of bicarbonate. Hyperuricemia is typically mild [<890 µmol/L (<15 mg/dL)] and does not require intervention.

The objective of *nutritional management* during the maintenance phase of ARF is to provide sufficient calories and protein to minimize catabolism. Nutritional requirements will vary based on the underlying disease process; for example, those with sepsis-associated AKI are likely to be hypercatabolic. The presence of oliguria complicates nutritional management, and if the patient is not on dialysis, minimizing production of nitrogenous waste is a consideration. Often, the institution of dialysis facilitates the provision of adequate nutritional support. There is no clear benefit of parenteral nutrition compared with enteral nutrition; indeed, those supported with parenteral nutrition are at increased risk of complications, including infection.

Anemia may necessitate blood transfusion if severe. Recombinant human erythropoietin is rarely used in ARF because bone marrow resistance to erythropoietin is common, and more immediate treatment of anemia (if any) is required. Uremic bleeding may respond to administration of desmopressin or estrogens. Often dialysis is instituted to control bleeding that appears to be related to uremia. Gastrointestinal prophylaxis with histamine receptor (H2) antagonists or proton pump inhibitors should be prescribed, especially in the setting of critical illness. Meticulous care of intravenous and bladder catheters, and other invasive devices is mandatory to avoid infections.

Indications and Modalities of Dialysis (See also Chap. 275) During ARF, dialysis is often used to support renal function until renal repair/recovery occur. Absolute indications for dialysis include symptoms or signs of the uremic syndrome and management of refractory hypervolemia, hyperkalemia, or acidosis. Many nephrologists also initiate dialysis empirically for blood urea levels of >100 mg/dL; however, this approach has yet to be validated in controlled clinical trials. Although direct clinical comparisons are limited, hemodialysis appears to be somewhat more effective than peritoneal dialysis for management of ARF. Peritoneal dialysis may be useful when hemodialysis is unavailable or if it is impossible to obtain vascular access. However, peritoneal dialysis is associated with increased protein losses and is contraindicated in those patients who have undergone recent abdominal surgery or those with ongoing infection. Peritoneal dialysis access requires insertion of a cuffed catheter into the peritoneal cavity.

Vascular access for hemodialysis requires insertion of a temporary double-lumen hemodialysis catheter into the internal jugular or femoral vein. Insertion into the subclavian vein is generally avoided owing to the risk of subclavian stenosis. Hemodialysis may be provided in the form of intermittent hemodialysis (typically performed for 3–4 hours per day, 3–4 times per week), slow low-efficiency dialysis (performed for 6–12 hours per day, 3–6 times per week), or continuous renal replacement therapy (CRRT). CCRTs are particular valuable techniques in patients in whom intermittent therapy fails to control hypervolemia, uremia, or acidosis or in those who do not tolerate intermittent hemodialysis due to hemodynamic instability. In those patients where hemodynamic instability is a primary consideration, slow low-efficiency hemodialysis (SLED), a relatively new hybrid mode of dialysis, is an excellent alternative to CRRT.

Continuous arteriovenous modalities [continuous arteriovenous hemofiltration, hemodialysis, and hemodiafiltration (CAVH, CAVHD, and CAVHDF, respectively)] require both arterial and venous access. The patient's own blood pressure generates an ultrafiltrate of plasma across a porous biocompatible dialysis membrane. With the advent of peristaltic pumps, the arteriovenous modalities have fallen out of favor, in part because of the complications associated with cannulation of a large artery with a large bore catheter. In continuous venovenous hemodialysis (CVVHD), a blood pump generates ultrafiltration pressure across the dialysis membrane. In continuous venovenous hemofiltration (CVVH), the hemodialysis (diffusive clearance) component is eliminated, and an ultrafiltrate of plasma is removed across the dialysis membrane and replaced by a physiologic crystalloid solution (convective clearance). In continuous venovenous hemodiafiltration (CVVHDF), these two methods of clearance are combined. The bulk of evidence to date suggests that intermittent and continuous dialytic therapies are equally effective for the treatment of ARF. The choice of technique is currently tailored to the specific needs of the patient, the resources of the institution, and the expertise of the physician. Potential disadvantages of continuous techniques include the need for prolonged immobilization, systemic anticoagulation, and prolonged exposure of blood to synthetic (albeit biocompatible) dialysis membranes.

The optimal dose of dialysis for ARF remains unclear at present. Recent evidence (from a single center, nonrandomized trial) suggests that more intensive hemodialysis (e.g., daily rather than alternate-day intermittent dialysis) may be clinically superior and confers improved survival in ARF once dialysis is required. This conclusion may not be as intuitive as it first appears since dialysis itself has been postulated to prolong ARF by inducing hypotension and other adverse effects related to the blood-dialyzer contact (e.g., complement activation and inflammation). Similarly, data suggest that increased doses of continuous renal replacement therapy may be of benefit for ARF, although these results need to be confirmed in a larger, multicenter study.

OUTCOME AND LONG-TERM PROGNOSIS

The in-hospital mortality rate among patients with ARF ranges from 20 to 50% or more, depending on underlying conditions, and has declined only marginally over the past 15 years. Most patients who survive an episode of ARF recover sufficient renal function to remain dialysis-independent, although a fraction (roughly 10–20%) go on to require maintenance dialysis.

 Common etiologies for acute renal failure will vary, depending on the availability of health care in a given country. In general, the most common cause of community-acquired ARF is prerenal azotemia. However, in countries with less well-developed health care systems, infective etiologies for ARF predominate. In developed countries, postoperative and ischemic/nephrotoxic causes of ARF are more common.

ACKNOWLEDGMENT
We are grateful to Dr. Hugh Brady and Dr. Barry Brenner, authors of this chapter in the 16th edition, for contributions to this edition.

FURTHER READINGS

BRADY HR et al: Acute renal failure, in *Brenner and Rector's The Kidney*, 7th ed., BM Brenner (ed). Philadelphia, Saunders, 2004

LAMEIRE N: The pathophysiology of acute renal failure. Crit Care Clin 21:197, 2005

——— et al: Acute renal failure. Lancet 365:417, 2005

PANNU N et al: Prophylaxis strategies for contrast-induced nephropathy JAMA 295:2765, 2006

STAR RA: Treatment of acute renal failure. Kidney Int 54:1817, 1998

WEISBORD SD, PALEVSKY P: Radiocontrast-induced acute renal failure. J Intens Care Med 20:63, 2005

274 Chronic Kidney Disease
Joanne M. Bargman, Karl Skorecki

Chronic kidney disease (CKD) encompasses a spectrum of different pathophysiologic processes associated with abnormal kidney function, and a progressive decline in glomerular filtration rate (GFR). **Table** 274-1 provides a widely accepted classification, based on recent guidelines of the National Kidney Foundation [Kidney Dialysis Outcomes Quality Initiative (KDOQI)], in which stages of CKD are defined according to the estimated GFR.

The term *chronic renal failure* applies to the process of continuing significant irreversible reduction in nephron number, and typically corresponds to CKD stages 3–5. The pathophysiologic processes and adaptations associated with chronic renal failure will be the focus of

TABLE 274-1	CLASSIFICATION OF CHRONIC KIDNEY DISEASE (CKD)
Stage	**GFR, mL/min per 1.73 m²**
0	>90[a]
1	≥90[b]
2	60–89
3	30–59
4	15–29
5	<15

[a]With risk factors for CKD (see text).
[b]With demonstrated kidney damage (e.g., persistent proteinuria, abnormal urine sediment, abnormal blood and urine chemistry, abnormal imaging studies).
Note: GFR, glomerular filtration rate.
Source: Modified from National Kidney Foundation. K/DOQI Clinical Practice Guidelines for Chronic Kidney Disease: Evaluation, classification and stratification. Am J Kidney Dis 39:suppl 1, 2002.

TABLE 274-2	RECOMMENDED EQUATIONS FOR ESTIMATION OF GLOMERULAR FILTRATION RATE (GFR) USING SERUM CREATININE CONCENTRATION (P_Cr), AGE, SEX, RACE, AND BODY WEIGHT

1. Equation from the Modification of Diet in Renal Disease study[a]
   Estimated GFR (mL/min per 1.73 m²) = $1.86 \times (P_{Cr})^{-1.154} \times (age)^{-0.203}$
   Multiply by 0.742 for women
   Multiply by 1.21 for African Americans
2. Cockcroft-Gault equation
   Estimated creatinine clearance (mL/min)
   $$= \frac{(140 - age \times body\ weight,\ kg)}{72 \times PCr\ (mg/dL)}$$
   Multiply by 0.85 for women

[a]Equation is *available* in hand-held calculators and in tabular form.
Adapted from AS Levey et al: Am J Kidney Dis 39 (Suppl 1): S1, 2002, with permission.

this chapter. The dispiriting term *end-stage renal disease* represents a stage of CKD where the accumulation of toxins, fluid, and electrolytes normally excreted by the kidneys results in the *uremic syndrome*. This syndrome leads to death unless the toxins are removed by renal replacement therapy, using dialysis or kidney transplantation. These latter interventions are discussed in Chaps. 275 and 276. *End-stage renal disease* will be supplanted in this chapter by the term *stage 5 CKD*.

PATHOPHYSIOLOGY OF CHRONIC KIDNEY DISEASE

The pathophysiology of CKD involves two broad sets of mechanisms of damage: (1) initiating mechanisms specific to the underlying etiology (e.g., immune complexes and mediators of inflammation in certain types of glomerulonephritis, or toxin exposure in certain diseases of the renal tubules and interstitium); and (2) a set of progressive mechanisms, involving hyperfiltration and hypertrophy of the remaining viable nephrons, that are a common consequence following long-term reduction of renal mass, irrespective of underlying etiology (Chap. 272). The responses to reduction in nephron number are mediated by vasoactive hormones, cytokines, and growth factors. Eventually, these short-term adaptations of hypertrophy and hyperfiltration become maladaptive as the increased pressure and flow predisposes to sclerosis and dropout of the remaining nephrons. Increased intrarenal activity of the renin-angiotensin axis appears to contribute both to the initial adaptive hyperfiltration and to the subsequent maladaptive hypertrophy and sclerosis, the latter, in part, owing to the stimulation of transforming growth factor β (TGF-β). This process explains why a reduction in renal mass from an isolated insult may lead to a progressive decline in renal function over many years.

THE STAGES OF CKD AND IDENTIFICATION OF AT-RISK POPULATIONS

It is important to identify factors that increase the risk for CKD, even in individuals with normal GFR. Risk factors include hypertension, diabetes mellitus, autoimmune disease, older age, African ancestry, a family history of renal disease, a previous episode of acute renal failure, and the presence of proteinuria, abnormal urinary sediment, or structural abnormalities of the urinary tract.

In order to stage CKD, it is necessary to estimate the GFR. Two equations commonly used to estimate GFR are shown in Table 274-2, and incorporate the measured plasma creatinine concentration, age, sex, and ethnic origin. Many laboratories now report an estimated GFR, or "e-GFR," using one of these equations.

The normal annual mean decline in GFR with age from the peak GFR (~120 mL/min per 1.73 m²) attained during the third decade of life is ~1 mL/min per year per 1.73 m², reaching a mean value of 70 mL/min per 1.73 m² at age 70. The mean GFR is lower in women than in men. For example, a woman in her 80s with a normal serum creatinine may have a GFR of just 50 mL/min per 1.73 m². Thus, even a mild elevation in serum creatinine concentration [e.g., 130 μmol/L (1.5 mg/dL)], often signifies a substantial reduction in GFR in most individuals.

Measurement of albuminuria is also helpful for monitoring nephron injury and the response to therapy in many forms of CKD, espe-

cially chronic glomerular diseases. While an accurate 24-h urine collection is the "gold standard" for measurement of albuminuria, the measurement of albumin-to-creatinine ratio in a spot first-morning urine sample is often more practical to obtain and correlates well, but not perfectly, with 24-h urine collections. Persistence in the urine of >17 mg of albumin per gram of creatinine in adult males and 25 mg albumin per gram of creatinine in adult females usually signifies chronic renal damage. *Microalbuminuria* refers to the excretion of amounts of albumin too small to detect by urinary dipstick or conventional measures of urine protein. It is a good screening test for early detection of renal disease, in particular, and may be a marker for the presence of microvascular disease in general. If a patient has a large amount of excreted albumin, there is no reason to perform an assay for microalbuminuria.

Stages 1 and 2 CKD are usually not associated with any symptoms arising from the decrement in GFR. However, there may be symptoms from the underlying renal disease itself, such as edema in patients with nephrotic syndrome or signs of hypertension secondary to the renal parenchymal disease in patients with polycystic kidney disease, some forms of glomerulonephritis, and many other parenchymal and vascular renal diseases, even with well-preserved GFR. If the decline in GFR progresses to stages 3 and 4, clinical and laboratory complications of CKD become more prominent. Virtually all organ systems are affected, but the most evident complications include anemia and associated easy fatigability; decreasing appetite with progressive malnutrition, abnormalities in calcium, phosphorus, and mineral-regulating hormones, such as $1,25(OH)_2D_3$ (calcitriol) and parathyroid hormone (PTH); and abnormalities in sodium, potassium, water, and acid-base homeostasis. If the patient progresses to stage 5 CKD, toxins accumulate such that patients usually experience a marked disturbance in their activities of daily living, well-being, nutritional status, and water and electrolyte homeostasis, eventuating in the *uremic syndrome*. As discussed above, this state will culminate in death unless renal replacement therapy (dialysis or transplantation) is instituted.

ETIOLOGY AND EPIDEMIOLOGY

It has been estimated from population survey data that at least 6% of the adult population in the United States has chronic kidney disease at stages 1 and 2. An unknown subset of this group will progress to more advanced stages of CKD. An additional 4.5% of the U.S. population is estimated to have stages 3 and 4 CKD. The most frequent cause of CKD is diabetic nephropathy, most often secondary to type 2 diabetes mellitus. Hypertensive nephropathy is a common cause of CKD in the elderly, in whom chronic renal ischemia as a result of small and large vessel renovascular disease may be underrecognized. Progressive nephrosclerosis from vascular disease is the renal correlate of the same processes that lead to coronary heart disease and cerebrovascular disease. The increasing incidence of CKD in the elderly has been ascribed, in part, to decreased mortality from the cardiac and cerebral complications of atherosclerotic vascular disease in these individuals, enabling a greater segment of the population to manifest the renal component of generalized vascular disease. Nevertheless, it should be appreciated that overwhelmingly the vast majority of those with early stages of renal disease, especially of vascular origin, will succumb to the cardiovascular and cerebrovascular consequences of the vascular disease before they can progress to the most advanced stages of CKD. The early stage of CKD, manifesting as albuminuria and even a minor decrement in GFR, is now recognized as a major risk factor for cardiovascular disease.

The striking interindividual variability in the rate of progression to CKD has an important heritable component, and a number of genetic loci that contribute to the progression of CKD have been identified. Similarly, it has been noted that women of reproductive age are relatively protected against progression of many renal diseases, and sex-specific responses to angiotensin II and its blockade have been identified.

PATHOPHYSIOLOGY AND BIOCHEMISTRY OF UREMIA

Although serum urea and creatinine concentrations are used to measure the excretory capacity of the kidneys, accumulation of these two molecules themselves do not account for the many symptoms and signs that characterize the uremic syndrome in advanced renal failure. Hundreds of toxins that accumulate in renal failure have been implicated in the uremic syndrome. These include water-soluble, hydrophobic, protein-bound, charged, and uncharged compounds. Additional categories of nitrogenous excretory products include guanido compounds, urates and hippurates, products of nucleic acid metabolism, polyamines, myoinositol, phenols, benzoates, and indoles. Compounds with a molecular mass between 500 and 1500 Da, the so-called middle molecules, are also retained and contribute to morbidity and mortality. It is thus evident that the plasma concentrations of urea and creatinine should be viewed as being readily measured, but incomplete, surrogate markers for these compounds, and monitoring the levels of urea and creatinine in the patient with impaired kidney function represents a vast oversimplification of the uremic state.

The uremic syndrome and the disease state associated with advanced renal impairment involve more than renal excretory failure. A host of metabolic and endocrine functions normally undertaken by the kidneys are also impaired, and this results in anemia, malnutrition, and abnormal metabolism of carbohydrates, fats, and proteins. Furthermore, plasma levels of many hormones, including PTH, insulin, glucagon, sex hormones, and prolactin, change with renal failure as a result of urinary retention, decreased degradation, or abnormal regulation. Finally, progressive renal impairment is associated with worsening systemic inflammation. Elevated levels of C-reactive protein are detected along with other acute-phase reactants, while levels of so-called negative acute-phase reactants, such as albumin and fetuin, decline with progressive renal impairment. Thus, renal impairment is important in the malnutrition-inflammation-atherosclerosis/calcification syndrome, which contributes in turn to the acceleration of vascular disease and comorbidity associated with advanced renal disease.

In summary, the pathophysiology of the uremic syndrome can be divided into manifestations in three spheres of dysfunction: (1) those consequent to the accumulation of toxins normally undergoing renal excretion, including products of protein metabolism; (2) those consequent to the loss of other renal functions, such as fluid and electrolyte homeostasis and hormone regulation; and (3) progressive systemic inflammation and its vascular and nutritional consequences.

CLINICAL AND LABORATORY MANIFESTATIONS OF CHRONIC KIDNEY DISEASE AND UREMIA

Uremia leads to disturbances in the function of virtually every organ system. Chronic dialysis can reduce the incidence and severity of many of these disturbances, so that the overt and florid manifestations of uremia have largely disappeared in the modern health setting. However, as indicated in Table 274-3, even optimal dialysis therapy is not completely effective as renal replacement therapy, because some disturbances resulting from impaired renal function fail to respond to dialysis.

FLUID, ELECTROLYTE AND ACID-BASE DISORDERS
Sodium and Water Homeostasis In most patients with stable CKD, the total-body content of sodium and water is modestly increased, although this may not be apparent on clinical examination. Normal renal function guarantees that the tubular reabsorption of filtered sodium and water is adjusted so that urinary excretion matches net intake. Many forms of renal disease (e.g., glomerulonephritis) disrupt this glomerulotubular balance such that dietary intake of sodium exceeds its urinary excretion, leading to sodium retention and attendant extracellular fluid volume (ECFV) expansion. This expansion may contribute to hypertension, which itself can accelerate the nephron injury. As long as water intake does not exceed the capacity for water clearance, the ECFV expansion will be isotonic and the patient will have a normal plasma sodium concentration and effective osmolality (Chap. 272). Hyponatremia is not commonly seen in CKD patients but, when present, can respond to water restriction. If the patient has evidence of ECFV expansion (peripheral edema, sometimes hyperten-

TABLE 274-3   CLINICAL ABNORMALITIES IN UREMIA[a]

Fluid and electrolyte disturbances	Neuromuscular disturbances	Dermatologic disturbances
Volume expansion (I)	Fatigue (I)[b]	Pallor (I)[b]
Hyponatremia (I)	Sleep disorders (P)	Hyperpigmentation (I, P, or D)
Hyperkalemia (I)	Headache (P)	Pruritus (P)
Hyperphosphatemia (I)	Impaired mentation (I)[b]	Ecchymoses (I)
Endocrine-metabolic disturbances	Lethargy (I)[b]	Nephrogenic fibrosing dermopathy (D)
Secondary hyperparathyroidism (I or P)	Asterixis (I)	Uremic frost (I)
Adynamic bone (D)	Muscular irritability	**Gastrointestinal disturbances**
Vitamin D–deficient osteomalacia (I)	Peripheral neuropathy (I or P)	Anorexia (I)
Carbohydrate resistance (I)	Restless legs syndrome (I or P)	Nausea and vomiting (I)
Hyperuricemia (I or P)	Myoclonus (I)	Gastroenteritis (I)
Hypertriglyceridemia (I or P)	Seizures (I or P)	Peptic ulcer (I or P)
Increased Lp(a) level (P)	Coma (I)	Gastrointestinal bleeding (I, P, or D)
Decreased high-density lipoprotein level (P)	Muscle cramps (P or D)	Idiopathic ascites (D)
Protein-energy malnutrition (I or P)	Dialysis disequilibrium syndrome (D)	Peritonitis (D)
Impaired growth and development (P)	Myopathy (P or D)	**Hematologic and immunologic disturbances**
Infertility and sexual dysfunction (P)	**Cardiovascular and pulmonary disturbances**	Anemia (I)[b]
Amenorrhea (I/P)	Arterial hypertension (I or P)	Lymphocytopenia (P)
β_2-Microglobulin associated amyloidosis (P or D)	Congestive heart failure or pulmonary edema (I)	Bleeding diathesis (I or D)[b]
	Pericarditis (I)	Increased susceptibility to infection (I or P)
	Hypertrophic or dilated cardiomyopathy (I, P, or D)	Leukopenia (D)
	Uremic lung (I)	Thrombocytopenia (D)
	Accelerated atherosclerosis (P or D)	
	Hypotension and arrhythmias (D)	
	Vascular calcification (P or D)	

[a]Virtually all abnormalities in this table are completely reversed in time by successful renal transplantation. The response of these abnormalities to hemodialysis or peritoneal dialysis therapy is more variable. (I) denotes an abnormality that usually improves with an optimal program of dialysis and related therapy; (P) denotes an abnormality that tends to persist or even progress, despite an optimal program; (D) denotes an abnormality that develops only after initiation of dialysis therapy.
[b]Improves with dialysis and erythropoietin therapy.
Note: Lp(a), lipoprotein A.

sion poorly responsive to therapy) he or she should be counseled regarding salt restriction. Thiazide diuretics have limited utility in stages 3–5 CKD, such that administration of loop diuretics, including furosemide, bumetanide, or torsemide, may also be needed. Resistance to loop diuretics in renal failure often mandates use of higher doses than those used in patients with near-normal kidney function. The combination of loop diuretics with metolazone, which inhibits the sodium-chloride co-transporter of the distal convoluted tubule, can help effect renal salt excretion. Ongoing diuretic resistance with intractable edema and hypertension in advanced CKD may serve as an indication to initiate dialysis.

In addition to problems with salt and water excretion, some patients with CKD may also have impaired renal conservation of sodium and water. When an extrarenal cause for fluid loss, such as gastrointestinal (GI) loss, is present, these patients may be prone to ECFV depletion because of the inability of the failing kidney to reclaim filtered sodium adequately. Furthermore, depletion of ECFV, whether due to GI losses or over-zealous diuretic therapy, can further compromise kidney function on a "pre-renal" basis, lead to acute-on-chronic kidney failure and result in overt uremia. In this setting, cautious volume repletion with normal saline may return the ECFV to normal and restore renal function to baseline without having to intervene with dialysis.

Potassium Homeostasis In CKD, the decline in GFR is not necessarily accompanied by a parallel decline in urinary potassium excretion, which is predominantly mediated by aldosterone-dependent secretory events in the distal nephron segments. Another defense against potassium retention in these patients is augmented potassium excretion in the GI tract. Notwithstanding these two homeostatic responses, hyperkalemia may be precipitated in certain settings. These include increased dietary potassium intake, protein catabolism, hemolysis, hemorrhage, transfusion of stored red blood cells, and metabolic acidosis. In addition, a host of medications can inhibit potassium entry into cells and renal potassium excretion. The most important medications in this respect include the angiotensin-converting enzyme (ACE) inhibitors, angiotensin receptor blockers (ARBs), and spironolactone and other potassium-sparing diuretics such as amiloride, eplerenone, and triamterene.

Certain causes of CKD can be associated with earlier and more severe disruption of potassium-secretory mechanisms in the distal nephron, out of proportion to the decline in GFR. These include conditions associated with hyporeninemic hypoaldosteronism, such as diabetes, and renal diseases that preferentially affect the distal nephron, such as obstructive uropathy and sickle cell nephropathy.

Hypokalemia is not common in CKD and usually reflects markedly reduced dietary potassium intake, especially in association with excessive diuretic therapy or concurrent GI losses. Hypokalemia can also occur as a result of primary renal potassium wasting in association with other solute transport abnormalities, such as Fanconi's syndrome, renal tubular acidosis, or other forms of hereditary or acquired tubulointerstitial disease. However, even with these conditions, as the GFR declines, the tendency to hypokalemia diminishes and hyperkalemia may supervene. Therefore, the use of potassium supplements and potassium-sparing diuretics should be constantly reevaluated as GFR declines.

Metabolic Acidosis Metabolic acidosis is a common disturbance in advanced CKD. The majority of patients can still acidify the urine, but they produce less ammonia and, therefore, cannot excrete the normal quantity of protons in combination with this urinary buffer. Hyperkalemia, if present, further depresses ammonia production. The combination of hyperkalemia and hyperchloremic metabolic acidosis (known as type IV renal tubular acidosis, or hyporeninemic hypoaldosteronism) is often seen in patients with diabetic nephropathy or in those with predominant tubulointerstitial disease or obstructive uropathy; this is a non-anion-gap metabolic acidosis. Treatment of hyperkalemia may increase renal ammonia production, improve renal generation of bicarbonate, and improve the metabolic acidosis.

With worsening renal function, the total urinary net daily acid excretion is usually limited to 30–40 mmol, and the anions of retained organic acids can then lead to an anion-gap metabolic acidosis. Thus, the non-anion-gap metabolic acidosis that can be seen in earlier stages of CKD may be complicated by the addition of an anion-gap metabolic acidosis as CKD progresses. In most patients, the metabolic acidosis is mild; the pH is rarely <7.35 and can usually be corrected with oral sodium bicarbonate supplementation. Animal and human studies have suggested that even modest degrees of metabolic acidosis may be associated with the development of net protein catabolism, and it has been suggested that alkali supplementation be considered when the serum bicarbonate concentration falls below 20–23 mmol/L. The concomitant sodium load mandates careful attention to volume status and the potential need for diuretic agents.

℞ FLUID, ELECTROLYTE, AND ACID-BASE DISORDERS

Adjustments in the dietary intake of salt and use of loop diuretics, occasionally in combination with metolazone, may be needed to maintain euvolemia. In contrast, overzealous salt restriction or diuretic use can lead to ECFV depletion and precipitate a further decline in GFR. The rare patient with salt-losing nephropathy may require a sodium-rich diet or salt supplementation. Water restriction is indicated only if there is a problem with hyponatremia. Otherwise, patients with CKD and an intact thirst mechanism may be instructed to drink fluids in a quantity that keeps them just ahead of their thirst. Intractable ECFV expansion, despite dietary salt restriction and diuretic therapy, may be an indication to start renal replacement therapy. Hyperkalemia often responds to dietary restriction of potassium, avoidance of potassium supplements (including occult sources, such as dietary salt substitutes) or potassium-retaining medications (especially ACE inhibitors or ARBs), or the use of kaliuretic diuretics. Potassium-binding resins, such as calcium resonium or sodium polystyrene, can promote potassium loss through the GI tract and may reduce the incidence of hyperkalemia in CKD patients. Intractable hyperkalemia is an indication (although uncommon) to consider institution of dialysis in a CKD patient. The renal tubular acidosis and subsequent anion-gap metabolic acidosis in progressive CKD will respond to alkali supplementation, typically with sodium bicarbonate. Recent studies suggest that this replacement should be considered when the serum bicarbonate concentration falls to 20 mmol/L to avoid the protein catabolic state seen with even mild degrees of metabolic acidosis.

DISORDERS OF CALCIUM AND PHOSPHATE METABOLISM

The principal complications of abnormalities of calcium and phosphate metabolism in CKD occur in the skeleton and the vascular bed, with occasional severe involvement of extraosseous soft tissues. It is likely that disorders of bone turnover and disorders of vascular and soft tissue calcification are related to each other (Fig. 274-1).

Bone Manifestations of CKD The major disorders of bone disease can be classified into those associated with high bone turnover with increased PTH levels (including osteitis fibrosa cystica, the classic lesion of secondary hyperparathyroidism) and low bone turnover with low or normal PTH levels (adynamic bone disease and osteomalacia).

The pathophysiology of secondary hyperparathyroidism and the consequent high-turnover bone disease is related to abnormal mineral metabolism through the following events: (1) declining GFR leads to reduced excretion of phosphate, and, thus phosphate retention; (2) the retained phosphate stimulates increased synthesis of PTH and growth of parathyroid gland mass; and (3) decreased levels of ionized calcium, resulting from diminished calcitriol production by the failing kidney as well as phosphate retention, also stimulate PTH production. Low calcitriol levels contribute to hyperparathyroidism, both by leading to hypocalcemia and also by a direct effect on PTH gene transcription.

In addition to increased production of PTH from the parathyroid cells, the mass of the parathyroid glands increases progressively with CKD. The cell mass may assume one of the following growth patterns: (1) diffuse hyperplasia (polyclonal), (2) nodular growth (monoclonal) within diffuse hyperplasia, or (3) diffuse monoclonal hyperplasia ("ade-

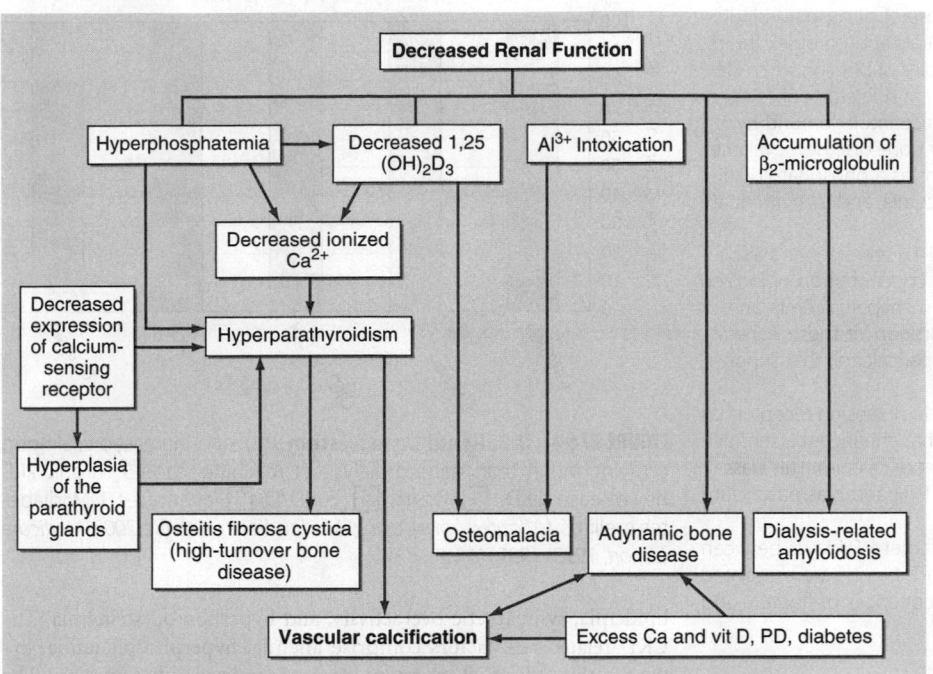

FIGURE 274-1 Flowchart for the development of bone, phosphate, and calcium abnormalities in chronic renal disease. PD, peritoneal dialysis.

noma" or tertiary autonomous hyperparathyroidism). Patients with the monoclonal ("autonomous") hyperplasia are especially prone to develop resistant hypercalcemia and may require surgical parathyroidectomy.

The hyperparathyroidism stimulates bone turnover and leads to osteitis fibrosa cystica. Bone histology shows abnormal osteoid, bone and bone marrow fibrosis, and formation of bone cysts, sometimes with hemorrhagic elements so that they appear brown in color, hence the term *brown tumor*. Clinical manifestations of severe hyperparathyroidism include bone pain and fragility, the brown tumors, rare compression syndromes caused by brown tumors, and erythropoietin resistance in part related to the bone marrow fibrosis. Furthermore, PTH is a uremic toxin, and high levels are associated with muscle weakness, fibrosis of cardiac muscle, and nonspecific constitutional symptoms.

Low-turnover bone disease can be grouped into two categories—adynamic bone disease and osteomalacia. In the latter condition, there is accumulation of unmineralized bone matrix that may be caused by vitamin D deficiency, excess aluminum deposition, or even metabolic acidosis. Adynamic bone disease is increasing in prevalence, especially among diabetics and the elderly. It is characterized by reduced bone volume and mineralization and may result from excessive suppression of PTH production. The latter can result from the use of vitamin D preparations or from excessive calcium exposure in the form of calcium-containing phosphate binders or high-calcium dialysis solutions. Complications of adynamic bone disease include an increased incidence of fracture and an association with increased vascular and cardiac calcification.

Calcium, Phosphorus, and the Cardiovascular System
Recent epidemiologic evidence has shown a strong association between hyperphosphatemia and increased cardiovascular mortality in patients with stage 5 CKD and even in patients with earlier stages of CKD. Hyperphosphatemia and hypercalcemia are associated with increased vascular calcification, but it is unclear whether the excessive mortality is mediated by this mechanism. Studies using CT and electron-beam CT scanning show that CKD patients have calcification of coronary arteries and even heart valves that appear to be orders of magnitude greater than that in patients without renal disease. The magnitude of the calcification is proportional to age and hyperphosphatemia and is also associated with low PTH levels and low bone turnover. It is possible that in patients with advanced kidney disease, ingested calcium intake cannot be deposited in

bones with low turnover and, therefore is deposited at extraosseous sites, such as the vascular bed and soft tissues. It is interesting in this regard that there is also an association between osteoporosis and vascular calcification in the general population. Finally, there is recent evidence indicating that hyperphosphatemia can induce a change in gene expression in vascular cells to an osteoblast-like profile.

Other Complications of Abnormal Mineral Metabolism
Calciphylaxis is a devastating condition seen almost exclusively in patients with advanced CKD. It is heralded by livedo reticularis and advances to patches of ischemic necrosis, especially on the legs, thighs, abdomen, and breasts (Fig. 274-2). Pathologically, there is evidence of vascular occlusion in association with extensive vascular calcification. It appears that this condition is increasing in incidence. Originally it was ascribed to severe abnormalities in calcium and phosphorus control in dialysis patients, usually associated with advanced hyperparathyroidism. However, more recently, calciphylaxis has been seen with increasing frequency in the absence of severe hyperparathyroidism. Other etiologies have been suggested, including the increased use of oral calcium as a phosphate binder. Warfarin is commonly used in hemodialysis patients, and one of the effects of warfarin therapy is to decrease the vitamin K–dependent regeneration of matrix GLA protein. This latter protein is important in preventing vascular calcification. Thus, warfarin treatment is considered a risk factor for calciphylaxis, and if a patient develops this syndrome, this medication should be discontinued and replaced with alternative forms of anticoagulation.

℞ DISORDERS OF CALCIUM AND PHOSPHATE METABOLISM

The optimal management of secondary hyperparathyroidism and osteitis fibrosa is prevention. Once the parathyroid gland mass is very large, it is difficult to control the disease. Careful attention should be paid to the plasma phosphate concentration in CKD patients, who should be counseled on a

FIGURE 274-2 Calciphylaxis. This peritoneal dialysis patient was on chronic warfarin therapy for prophylactic anticoagulation for a mechanical heart valve. She slept with the dialysis catheter pressed between her legs. A small abrasion was followed by progressive skin necrosis along the catheter tract on her inner thighs. Despite treatment with hyperbaric oxygen, intravenous thiosulfate, and discontinuation of warfarin, she succumbed to systemic complications of the necrotic process.

low-phosphate diet as well as the appropriate use of phosphate-binding agents. These are agents that are taken with meals and complex the dietary phosphate to limit its GI absorption. Examples of phosphate binders are calcium acetate and calcium carbonate. A major side effect of calcium-based phosphate binders is total-body calcium accumulation and hypercalcemia, especially in patients with low-turnover bone disease. Sevelamer, a non-calcium-containing polymer, also functions as a phosphate binder; it does not predispose CKD patients to hypercalcemia, and may attenuate calcium deposition in the vascular bed.

Calcitriol exerts a direct suppressive effect on PTH secretion and also indirectly suppresses PTH secretion by raising the concentration of ionized calcium. However, calcitriol therapy may result in hypercalcemia and/or hyperphosphatemia through increased GI absorption of these minerals. Certain analogues of calcitriol are available (e.g., paricalcitol) that suppress PTH secretion with less attendant hypercalcemia.

Recognition of the role of the extracellular calcium-sensing receptor has led to the development of calcimimetic agents that enhance the sensitivity of the parathyroid cell to the suppressive effect of calcium. This class of drug produces a dose-dependent reduction in PTH and plasma calcium concentration in some patients.

Current KDOQI recommendations call for a target PTH level between 150 and 300 pg/mL, recognizing that very low PTH levels are associated with adynamic bone disease and possible consequences of fracture and ectopic calcification.

CARDIOVASCULAR ABNORMALITIES

Cardiovascular disease is the leading cause of morbidity and mortality in patients at every stage of CKD. The incremental risk of cardiovascular disease in those with CKD compared to the age- and sex-matched general population ranges from 10- to 200-fold, depending on the stage of CKD (**Fig. 274-3**). Between 30 and 45% of patients reaching stage 5 CKD already have advanced cardiovascular complications. As a result, most patients with CKD succumb to cardiovascular disease (**Fig. 274-4**) before ever reaching stage 5 CKD. Thus, the focus of patient care in earlier CKD stages should be directed to prevention of cardiovascular complications.

Ischemic Vascular Disease   The presence of any stage of CKD is a major risk factor for ischemic cardiovascular disease, including occlusive coronary, cerebrovascular, and peripheral vascular disease. The increased prevalence of vascular disease in CKD patients derives from both traditional ("classic") and nontraditional (CKD-related) risk factors. Traditional risk factors include hypertension, hypervolemia, dys-

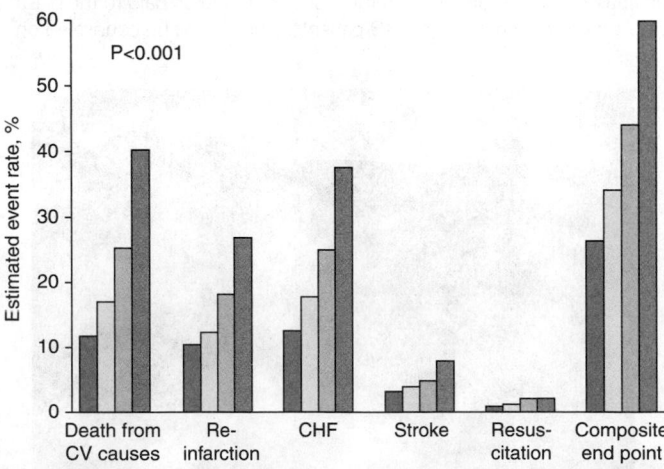

FIGURE 274-3 An analysis of the correlation between the decline in kidney function, as estimated by glomerular filtration rate (GFR), and the increasing incidence of cardiovascular (CV) complications and death from CV disease. Studies such as these suggest that a GFR that is less than normal should be considered a risk factor for CV events and mortality. CHF, congestive heart failure. Volume of GFR in mL/min per 1.73 m²: [1], ≥75.0; [2], 60.0–74.9; [3], 45.0–59.9; [4], < 45. *(From NS Anavekar et al: N Engl J Med 351:1285, 2004.)*

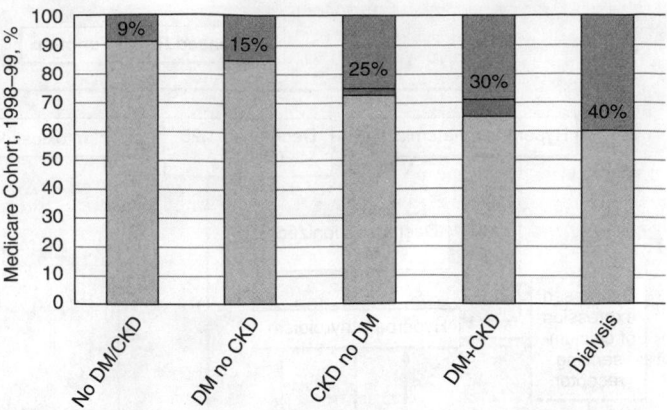

FIGURE 274-4 U.S. Renal Data System showing increased likelihood of dying rather than starting dialysis or reaching stage 5 chronic kidney disease (CKD). [1], Death; [2], ESRD/D; [3], event-free. DM; diabetes mellitus. *(Adapted from Collins, Adv Studies in Med (3c)2003, Medicare Cohort, 1998–1999.)*

lipidemia, sympathetic overactivity, and hyperhomocysteinemia. The CKD-related risk factors comprise anemia, hyperphosphatemia, hyperparathyroidism, sleep apnea, and generalized inflammation. The inflammatory state associated with a reduction in kidney function is reflected in increased circulating acute-phase reactants, such as inflammatory cytokines and C-reactive protein, with a corresponding fall in the "negative acute-phase reactants," such as serum albumin and fetuin. The inflammatory state appears to accelerate vascular occlusive disease, and low levels of fetuin may permit more rapid vascular calcification, especially in the face of hyperphosphatemia. Other abnormalities seen in CKD may augment myocardial ischemia, including left ventricular hypertrophy and microvascular disease. Coronary reserve, defined as the increase in coronary blood flow in response to greater demand, is also attenuated. There is diminished availability of nitric oxide because of increased concentration of asymmetric dimethyl-1-arginine and increased scavenging by reactive oxygen species. In addition, hemodialysis, with its attendant episodes of hypotension and hypovolemia, may further aggravate coronary ischemia.

Heart Failure   Abnormal cardiac function secondary to myocardial ischemia, left ventricular hypertrophy, and frank cardiomyopathy, in combination with the salt and water retention that can be seen with CKD, often results in heart failure or even episodes of pulmonary edema. Heart failure can be a consequence of diastolic or systolic dysfunction, or both. A form of "low-pressure" pulmonary edema can also occur in advanced CKD, manifesting as shortness of breath and a "bat wing" distribution of alveolar edema fluid on the chest x-ray. This finding can occur even in the absence of ECFV overload and is associated with normal or mildly elevated pulmonary capillary wedge pressure. This process has been ascribed to increased permeability of alveolar capillary membranes as a manifestation of the uremic state, and it responds to dialysis. Other CKD-related risk factors, including anemia and sleep apnea, may contribute to the risk of heart failure.

Hypertension and Left Ventricular Hypertrophy   Hypertension is one of the most common complications of CKD. It usually develops early during the course of CKD and is associated with adverse outcomes, including the development of ventricular hypertrophy and a more rapid loss of renal function. Many studies have shown a relationship between the level of blood pressure and the rate of progression of diabetic and non-diabetic kidney disease. Left ventricular hypertrophy and dilated cardiomyopathy are among the strongest risk factors for cardiovascular morbidity and mortality in patients with CKD and are thought to be related primarily, but not exclusively, to prolonged hypertension and ECFV overload. In addition, anemia and the placement of an arteriovenous fistula for hemodialysis can generate a high cardiac output state and consequent heart failure.

The absence of hypertension may signify the presence of a salt-wasting form of renal disease, the effect of antihypertensive therapy, or volume depletion or may signify poor left ventricular function. Indeed, in epidemiologic studies of dialysis patients, low blood pressure actually carries a worse prognosis than does high blood pressure. This mechanism, in part, accounts for the "reverse causation" seen in dialysis patients, wherein the presence of traditional risk factors, such as hypertension, hyperlipidemia, and obesity, appear to portend a better prognosis. Importantly, these observations derive from cross-sectional studies of late-stage CKD patients and should not be interpreted to discourage appropriate management of these risk factors in CKD patients, especially at early stages. In contrast to the general population, it is possible that in late-stage CKD, low blood pressure, reduced body mass index, and hypolipidemia indicate the presence of a malnutrition-inflammation state, with poor prognosis.

The use of exogenous erythropoietic products can increase blood pressure and the requirement for antihypertensive drugs. Chronic ECFV overload is also a contributor to hypertension, and improvement in blood pressure can often be seen with the use of oral sodium restriction, diuretics, and fluid removal with dialysis. Nevertheless, because of activation of the renin-angiotensin-aldosterone axis and other disturbances in the balance of vasoconstrictors and vasodilators, some patients remain hypertensive despite careful attention to ECFV status.

Rx CARDIOVASCULAR ABNORMALITIES

MANAGEMENT OF HYPERTENSION   There are two overall goals of therapy for hypertension in these patients: to slow the progression of the kidney disease itself, and to prevent the extrarenal complications of high blood pressure, such as cardiovascular disease and stroke. In all patients with CKD, blood pressure should be controlled to levels recommended by national guideline panels. In CKD patients with diabetes or proteinuria > 1 g per 24 h, blood pressure should be reduced to 125/75, if achievable without prohibitive adverse effects. Salt restriction and diuretics should be the first line of therapy. When volume management alone is not sufficient, the choice of antihypertensive agent is similar to that in the general population. The ACE inhibitors and ARBs slow the rate of decline of kidney function, even in dialysis patients, but their use may be complicated by the development of hyperkalemia. Often the concomitant use of a kaliuretic diuretic, such as metolazone, can improve potassium excretion in addition to improving blood pressure control. Potassium-sparing diuretics should be used with caution or avoided altogether in most patients.

MANAGEMENT OF CARDIOVASCULAR DISEASE   There are many strategies available to treat the traditional and nontraditional risk factors in CKD patients. While these have been proven effective in the general population, there is little evidence for their benefit in patients with advanced CKD, especially those on dialysis. Certainly hypertension, elevated serum levels of homocysteine, and dyslipidemia promote atherosclerotic disease and are treatable complications of CKD. Renal disease complicated by nephrotic syndrome is associated with a very atherogenic lipid profile and hypercoagulability, which increases the risk of occlusive vascular disease. Since diabetes mellitus and hypertension are the two most frequent causes of advanced CKD, it is not surprising that cardiovascular disease is the most frequent cause of death in dialysis patients. The role of "inflammation" may be quantitatively more important in patients with kidney disease, and the treatment of more traditional risk factors may result in only modest success. However, modulation of traditional risk factors may be the only weapon in the therapeutic armamentarium for these patients until the nature of inflammation in CKD and its treatment are better understood.

Lifestyle changes, including regular exercise, should be advocated but are not often implemented. Hyperhomocysteinemia may respond to vitamin therapy, including oral folate supplementation, but this therapy is of unproven benefit. Hyperlipidemia in patients with CKD should be managed according to national guidelines. If dietary measures are not sufficient, preferred lipid-lowering medications, such as statins, should be used. Again, the use of these agents has not been of proven benefit for patients with advanced CKD.

Pericardial Disease   Pericardial pain with respiratory accentuation, accompanied by a friction rub, is diagnostic of uremic pericarditis. Classic electrocardiographic abnormalities include PR-interval depression and diffuse ST-segment elevation. Pericarditis can be accompanied by pericardial effusion that is seen on echocardiography and can rarely lead to tamponade. However, the pericardial effusion can be asymptomatic, and pericarditis can be seen without significant effusion.

Pericarditis is observed in advanced uremia, and with the advent of timely initiation of dialysis, is not as common as it once was. It is now more often observed in underdialyzed, nonadherent patients than in those starting dialysis.

Rx PERICARDIAL DISEASE

Uremic pericarditis is an absolute indication for the urgent initiation of dialysis or for intensification of the dialysis prescription in those already receiving dialysis. Because of the propensity to hemorrhage in pericardial fluid, hemodialysis should be performed without heparin. A pericardial drainage procedure should be considered in patients with recurrent pericardial effusion. Nonuremic causes of pericarditis and effusion include viral, malignant, tuberculous, and autoimmune etiologies. It may also be seen after myocardial infarction and as a complication of treatment with minoxidil.

HEMATOLOGIC ABNORMALITIES

Anemia   A normocytic, normochromic anemia is observed as early as stage 3 CKD and is almost universal by stage 4. The primary cause in patients with CKD is insufficient production of erythropoietin (EPO) by the diseased kidneys. Additional factors include iron deficiency, acute and chronic inflammation with impaired iron utilization ("anemia of chronic disease"), severe hyperparathyroidism with consequent bone marrow fibrosis, and shortened red cell survival in the uremic environment. Less common causes include folate and vitamin B_{12} deficiency and aluminum toxicity. In addition, comorbid conditions such as hemoglobinopathy can worsen the anemia (Table 274-4).

The anemia of CKD is associated with a number of adverse pathophysiologic consequences, including decreased tissue xygen delivery and utilization, increased cardiac output, ventricular dilatation, and ventricular hypertrophy. Clinical manifestations include angina, heart failure, decreased cognition and mental acuity, and impaired host defense against infection. In addition, anemia may play a role in growth retardation in children with CKD. While many studies in CKD patients have found that anemia and resistance to exogenous EPO are associated with a poor prognosis, it is unclear as to how much the low hematocrit itself versus inflammation leads to a poor outcome.

Rx ANEMIA

The availability of recombinant human EPO and modified EPO products, such as darbopoetin-alpha, has been one of the most significant advances in the care of renal patients since the introduction of dialysis and renal transplantation. The routine use of these products has obviated the need for regular blood transfusions in severely anemic CKD patients, thus dramatically reducing the incidence of transfusion-associated infections and iron overload. Frequent blood transfusions in dialysis patients also led to the development of alloantibodies that could sensitize the patient to donor kidney antigens and make renal transplantation more problematic.

Adequate bone marrow iron stores should be available before treatment with EPO is initiated. Iron supplementation is ousually essential to

TABLE 274-4   CAUSES OF ANEMIA IN CKD

Relative deficiency of erythropoietin
Diminished red blood cell survival
Bleeding diathesis
Iron deficiency
Hyperparathyroidism/bone marrow fibrosis
"Chronic inflammation"
Folate or vitamin B_{12} deficiency
Hemoglobinopathy
Comorbid conditions: hypo/hyperthyroidism, pregnancy, HIV-associated
   disease, autoimmune disease, immunosuppressive drugs

ensure an adequate response to EPO in patients with CKD because the demand for iron by the marrow frequently exceeds the amount of iron that is immediately available for erythropoiesis (measured by percent transferrin saturation), as well as the amount in iron stores (measured by serum ferritin). For the CKD patient not yet on dialysis or the patient treated with peritoneal dialysis, oral iron supplementation should be attempted. If there is GI intolerance, the patient may have to undergo IV iron infusion, often during the dialysis session. In addition to iron, an adequate supply of other major substrates and cofactors for red cell production must be assured, including vitamin B_{12} and folate. Anemia resistant to recommended doses of EPO in the face of adequate iron stores may be due to some combination of the following: acute or chronic inflammation, inadequate dialysis, severe hyperparathyroidism, chronic blood loss or hemolysis, chronic infection, or malignancy. Patients with a hemoglobinopathy, such as sickle cell disease or thalassemia, will usually not respond normally to exogenous EPO; however, an increase in hemoglobin concentration is still seen in many of these patients. Blood transfusions may contribute to suppression of erythropoiesis in CKD; because they increase the risk of hepatitis, iron overload, and transplant sensitization, they should be avoided unless the anemia fails to respond to EPO and the patient is symptomatic.

Normalization of the hemoglobin concentration has not been demonstrated to be of incremental benefit to dialysis patients. Current practice is to target a hemoglobin concentration of 110 to 120 g/L.

Abnormal Hemostasis   Patients with later stages of CKD may have a prolonged bleeding time, decreased activity of platelet factor III, abnormal platelet aggregation and adhesiveness, and impaired prothrombin consumption. Clinical manifestations include an increased tendency to bleeding and bruising, prolonged bleeding from surgical incisions, menorrhagia, and spontaneous GI bleeding. Interestingly, CKD patients also have a greater susceptibility to thromboembolism, especially if they have renal disease that includes nephrotic-range proteinuria. The latter condition results in hypoalbuminemia and renal loss of anticoagulant factors, which can lead to a thrombophilic state.

℞ ABNORMAL HEMOSTASIS

Abnormal bleeding time and coagulopathy in patients with renal failure may be reversed temporarily with desmopressin (DDAVP), cryoprecipitate, IV conjugated estrogens, blood transfusions, and EPO therapy. Optimal dialysis will often correct a prolonged bleeding time.

Given the coexistence of bleeding disorders and a propensity to thrombosis that is unique in the CKD patient, decisions about anticoagulation that have a favorable risk-benefit profile in the general population may not be applicable to the patient with advanced CKD. One example is warfarin anticoagulation for atrial fibrillation: the decision to anticoagulate should be made on an individual basis in the CKD patient.

Certain anticoagulants, such as fractionated low-molecular-weight heparin, may need to be avoided or dose-adjusted in these patients, with monitoring of factor Xa activity where available. It is often more prudent to use conventional high-molecular-weight heparin, titrated to the measured partial thromboplastin time, in hospitalized patients requiring an alternative to warfarin anticoagulation.

NEUROMUSCULAR ABNORMALITIES

Central nervous system (CNS), peripheral, and autonomic neuropathy as well as abnormalities in muscle structure and function are all well-recognized complications of CKD. Retained nitrogenous metabolites and middle molecules, including PTH, contribute to the pathophysiology of neuromuscular abnormalities. Subtle clinical manifestations of uremic neuromuscular disease usually become evident at stage 3 CKD. Early manifestations of CNS complications include mild disturbances in memory and concentration and sleep disturbance. Neuromuscular irritability, including hiccups, cramps, and fasciculations or twitching of muscles, becomes evident at later stages. In advanced untreated kidney failure, asterixis, myoclonus, seizures, and coma can be seen.

Peripheral neuropathy usually becomes clinically evident after the patient reaches stage 4 CKD, although electrophysiologic and histolog-

ic evidence occurs earlier. Initially, sensory nerves are involved more than motor, lower extremities more than upper, and distal parts of the extremities more than proximal. The "restless leg syndrome" is characterized by ill-defined sensations of sometimes debilitating discomfort in the legs and feet relieved by frequent leg movement. If dialysis is not instituted soon after onset of sensory abnormalities, motor involvement follows, including muscle weakness. Evidence of peripheral neuropathy without another cause (e.g., diabetes mellitus) is a firm indication for starting renal replacement therapy. Many of the complications described above will resolve with dialysis, although subtle nonspecific abnormalities may persist. Successful renal transplantation may reverse residual neurologic changes.

GASTROINTESTINAL AND NUTRITIONAL ABNORMALITIES

Uremic fetor, a urine-like odor on the breath, derives from the breakdown of urea to ammonia in saliva and is often associated with an unpleasant metallic taste (dysgeusia). Gastritis, peptic disease, and mucosal ulcerations at any level of the GI tract occur in uremic patients and can lead to abdominal pain, nausea, vomiting, and GI bleeding. These patients are also prone to constipation, which can be worsened by the administration of calcium and iron supplements. The retention of uremic toxins also leads to anorexia, nausea, and vomiting.

Protein restriction may be useful to decrease nausea and vomiting; however, it may put the patient at risk for malnutrition and should be carried out, if possible, in consultation with a registered dietitian. Protein-energy malnutrition, a consequence of low protein and caloric intake, is common in advanced CKD and is often an indication for initiation of renal replacement therapy. In addition to diminished intake, these patients are resistant to the anabolic actions of insulin and other hormones and growth factors. Metabolic acidosis and the activation of inflammatory cytokines can promote protein catabolism. Assessment for protein-energy malnutrition should begin at stage 3 CKD. A number of indices are useful in this assessment and include dietary history, including diary and subjective global assessment; edema-free body weight; serum albumin concentration; and measurement of urinary protein nitrogen appearance. Dual-energy x-ray absorptiometry is now widely used to estimate lean body mass versus ECFV. Adjunctive tools include clinical signs, such as skinfold thickness, mid-arm muscle circumference, and additional laboratory tests such as serum pre-albumin and cholesterol levels. Nutritional guidelines for patients with CKD are summarized in the section below on "Principles of Treatment of CKD."

ENDOCRINE-METABOLIC DISTURBANCES

Glucose metabolism is impaired in CKD, as evidenced by a slowing of the rate at which blood glucose levels decline after a glucose load. However, fasting blood glucose is usually normal or only slightly elevated, and the mild glucose intolerance does not require specific therapy. Because the kidney contributes to insulin removal from the circulation, plasma levels of insulin are slightly to moderately elevated in most uremic patients, both in the fasting and postprandial states. Because of this diminished renal degradation of insulin, patients on insulin therapy may need progressive reduction in dose as their renal function worsens. Many hypoglycemic agents require dose reduction in renal failure, and some, such as metformin, are contraindicated when the GFR is less than half of normal.

In women with CKD, estrogen levels are low, and menstrual abnormalities and inability to carry pregnancies to term are common. When the GFR has declined to ~40 mL/min, pregnancy is associated with a high rate of spontaneous abortion, with only ~20% of pregnancies leading to live births, and pregnancy may hasten the progression of the kidney disease itself. Men with CKD have reduced plasma testosterone levels, and sexual dysfunction and oligospermia may supervene. Sexual maturation may be delayed or impaired in adolescent children with CKD, even among those treated with dialysis. Many of these abnormalities improve or reverse with intensive dialysis or successful renal transplantation.

DERMATOLOGIC ABNORMALITIES

Abnormalities of the skin are prevalent in progressive CKD. Anemic chromes. Pruritus and those with defective hemostasis may show dialysis, pruritus is quite common. In advanced CKD, to rule out unrelated skin is quite common. In advanced CKD, phosphate concentration. EPO is more pigmented, and this is felt prove uremic pruritus, although that is pigmented metabolites, or *uro*-moisturizers, mild topical glucocorticoids, oral antihistamines improve with traviolet radiation have been reported to be helpful.

A skin condition called *nephrogenic fibrosing dermopathy* has recently been reported in which *Progressive* cutaneous induration, especially on the arms and legs, is described. This condition is similar to scler-edema and is seen in patients with Condition is similar to scler- management are suggest that exposure to magnetic resonance precitate this syndrome.

MANAGEMENT OF PATIENTS WITH CKD

INITIAL APPROACH

History and Physical Examination Symptoms and overt signs of kidney disease are often absent until renal failure supervenes. Thus, the diagnosis of kidney disease often surprises patients and may be a cause of skepticism and denial. Particular aspects of the history that are germane to renal disease include a history of hypertension (which can cause CKD or be a reflection of CKD), diabetes mellitus, abnormal urinalyses, and problems with pregnancy such as preeclampsia or early pregnancy loss. A careful drug history should be elicited: patients may not volunteer use of analgesics, for example. Other drugs to consider include nonsteroidal anti-inflammatory agents, gold, penicillamine, antimicrobials, antiretroviral agents, proton pump inhibitors, and lithium. In evaluating the uremic syndrome, questions about appetite, weight loss, nausea, hiccups, peripheral edema, muscle cramps, pruritus, and restless legs are especially helpful.

The physical examination should focus on blood pressure and target organ damage from hypertension. Thus, funduscopy and precordial examination (left ventricular heave, a fourth heart sound) should be carried out. Funduscopy is important in the diabetic patient, seeking evidence of diabetic retinopathy, which is associated with nephropathy. Other physical examination manifestations of CKD include edema and sensory polyneuropathy. The finding of asterixis or a pericardial friction rub not attributable to other causes usually signifies the presence of the uremic syndrome.

Laboratory Investigation Laboratory studies should focus on a search for clues to an underlying causative or aggravating disease process and on the degree of renal damage and its consequences. If appropriate, tests for systemic lupus erythematosus and vasculitis should be performed. Serum and urine protein electrophoresis should be obtained in all patients >35 years with unexplained CKD, especially if there is associated anemia and elevated, or even inappropriately normal, serum calcium concentration in the face of renal insufficiency. In the presence of glomerulonephritis, underlying infectious etiologies such as hepatitis B and C and HIV should be assessed. Serial measurements of renal function should be obtained to determine the pace of renal deterioration and ensure that the disease is truly chronic rather than subacute and hence potentially reversible. Serum concentrations of calcium, phosphorus, and PTH should be measured to evaluate metabolic bone disease. Hemoglobin concentration, iron, B_{12}, and folate should also be evaluated. A 24-h urine collection may be helpful, as protein excretion > 300 mg may be an indication for therapy with ACE inhibitors or ARBs.

Imaging Studies The most useful imaging study is a renal ultrasound, which can verify the presence of two kidneys, determine if they are symmetric, provide an estimate of kidney size, and rule out renal masses and evidence of obstruction. Since it takes time for kidneys to shrink as a result of chronic disease, the finding of bilaterally small kidneys supports the diagnosis of CKD of long-standing duration, with an irreversible component of scarring. If the kidney size is normal, it is possible that the renal disease is acute or subacute. The exceptions are diabetic nephropathy where kidney size is increased at the outset of diabetic nephropathy before CKD with loss of GFR supervenes), amyloidosis, and HIV nephropathy, where kidney size may be normal in the face of renal failure will almost always present with enlarged the degree of renal failure (Chap. 278). A discrepancy >1 cm in kidneys with multiple cysts either a unilateral developmental abnormality or renovascular disease with arterial insufficiency affecting one kidney more than the other. The diagnosis of renovascular disease can be undertaken with different techniques, including Doppler sonography, nuclear medicine studies, or CT or MRI studies. If there is a suspicion of reflux nephropathy (recurrent childhood urinary tract infection, asymmetric renal size with scars on the renal poles, a voiding cystogram may be indicated. However, in most cases by the time the patient has CKD, the reflux has resolved, and even if still present, repair does not improve renal function. Radiographic contrast imaging studies are not particularly helpful in the investigation of CKD. Intravenous or intraarterial dye should be avoided where possible in the CKD patient, especially with diabetic nephropathy, because of the risk of radiographic contrast dye–induced renal failure. When unavoidable, appropriate precautionary measures include avoidance of hypovolemia at the time of contrast exposure, minimization of the dye load, and choice of radiographic contrast preparations with the least nephrotoxic potential.

Renal Biopsy In the patient with bilaterally small kidneys, renal biopsy is not advised because (1) it is technically difficult and has a greater likelihood of causing bleeding and other adverse consequences, (2) there is usually so much scarring that the underlying disease may not be apparent, and (3) the window of opportunity to render disease-specific therapy has passed. Other contraindications to renal biopsy include uncontrolled hypertension, active urinary tract infection, bleeding diathesis, and morbid obesity. Ultrasound-guided percutaneous biopsy is the favored approach, but a surgical or laparoscopic approach can be considered, especially in the patient with a single kidney where direct visualization and control of bleeding are crucial. In the CKD patient in whom a kidney biopsy is indicated (e.g., suspicion of a concomitant or superimposed active process, such as interstitial nephritis or accelerated loss of GFR), the bleeding time should be measured, and, if increased, desmopressin should be administered immediately prior to the procedure. A brief run of hemodialysis (without heparin) may also be considered prior to renal biopsy to normalize the bleeding time.

ESTABLISHING THE DIAGNOSIS AND ETIOLOGY OF CKD

The most important initial diagnostic step in the evaluation of a patient presenting with elevated serum creatinine is to distinguish newly diagnosed CKD from acute or subacute renal failure because the latter two conditions may respond to therapy specific to the disease. Previous measurements of plasma creatinine concentration are particularly helpful in this regard. Normal values from recent months or even years suggest that the current extent of renal dysfunction could be more acute, and hence reversible, than might otherwise be appreciated. In contrast, elevated plasma creatinine concentration in the past suggests that the renal disease represents the progression of a chronic process. Even if there is evidence of chronicity, there is the possibility of a superimposed acute process, such as ECFV depletion, supervening on the chronic condition. If the history suggests multiple systemic manifestations of recent onset (e.g., fever, polyarthritis, and rash) it should be assumed that renal insufficiency is part of the acute process.

Some of the laboratory tests and imaging studies outlined above can be helpful. Evidence of metabolic bone disease with hyperphosphatemia, hypocalcemia, and elevated PTH and bone alkaline phosphatase levels suggests chronicity. Normochromic, normocytic anemia suggests that the process has been ongoing for some time. The finding of bilaterally reduced kidney size (<8.5 cm in all but the smallest adults) favors CKD.

While renal biopsy can usually be performed in early CKD (stages 1–3), it is not always indicated. For example, in a patient with a history of type 1 diabetes mellitus for 15–20 years with retinopathy, nephrotic-range proteinuria, and absence of hematuria, the diagnosis of diabetic nephropathy is very likely and biopsy is not necessary. However, if there were some other finding not typical of diabetic nephrosis such as hematuria or white blood cell casts, some other diagnosis may be present and a biopsy may be indicated. Hypertension and progressive ischemic nephropathy are usually diagnosed clinically by the presence of long-standing hypertension (evidence of ischemic disease elsewhere (e.g., cardiac or peripheral vascular disease), and the finding of only mild (< 3g/d) proteinuria in the absence of urinary blood or red cell casts. It is important to consider progressive ischemic nephropathy because a small subset of these patients may respond to revascularization procedures although this remains controversial.

In the absence of a clinical diagnosis, renal biopsy may be the only recourse to establish an etiology in early stage CKD. However, as noted above, once the CKD is advanced and the kidneys are small and scarred, there is little utility and significant risk in attempting to arrive at a specific diagnosis.

℞ CHRONIC KIDNEY DISEASE

Treatments aimed at specific causes of CKD are discussed elsewhere. The optimal timing of therapy is usually well before there has been a measurable decline in GFR and certainly before CKD is established (Table 274-5). It is helpful to sequentially measure and plot the rate of decline of GFR in all patients. Any acceleration in the rate of decline should prompt a search for superimposed acute or subacute processes that may be reversible. These include ECFV depletion, uncontrolled hypertension, urinary tract infection, new obstructive uropathy, exposure to nephrotoxic agents [such as nonsteroidal anti-inflammatory drugs (NSAIDs) or radiographic dye], and reactivation or flare of the original disease, such as lupus or vasculitis.

SLOWING THE PROGRESSION OF CKD   There is variation in the rate of decline of GFR among patients with CKD. However, the following interventions should be considered in an effort to stabilize or slow the decline of renal function.

Protein Restriction   While protein restriction has been advocated to reduce symptoms associated with uremia, it may also slow the rate of renal decline at earlier stages of renal disease. This concept is based on clinical and experimental evidence that protein-mediated hyperfiltration contributes to ongoing decline in renal function in many different forms of renal

disease. A number of studies have shown that dietary protein restriction is effective in slowing the progression of chronic renal diseases. However, depending upon the study, the effect was unable to demonstrate proteinuria, and nutritional restriction of at least 50% of the protein intake below usual. As patients approach stage 5 CKD, spontaneous protein intake may be of concern, and patients may enter a state of protein-energy malnutrition; recommended, again, with a protein intake of up to 0.90 g/kg per day. Sufficient energy intake is important to prevent protein-calorie malnutrition, and 35 kcal/kg is recommended. Monitoring of parameters of nutritional status must accompany the dietary intervention as patients develop, as outlined above in the section on GI and nutritional.

Reducing Intraglomerular Hypertension   from different kidney diseases. The intraglomerulus of nephron promotes the ongoing decline of kidney, a response maladaptive, as it continues to respond even if the inciting process has been treated or spontaneously resolved. Control of systemic and glomerular hypertension is at least as important as dietary protein restriction in slowing the progression of CKD. Therefore in addition to reduction of cardiovascular disease risk, antihypertensive therapy in patients with CKD also aims to slow the progression of nephron injury by reducing intraglomerular hypertension. Elevated blood pressure increases proteinuria through its transmission to the glomerulus. Conversely, the renoprotective effect of antihypertensive medications is gauged through the consequent reduction of proteinuria. Thus, the more effective a given treatment is in lowering protein excretion, the greater the subsequent impact on protection from decline in GFR. This observation is the basis for the treatment guideline establishing 125/75 mmHg as the target blood pressure in proteinuric CKD patients.

ACE inhibitors and ARBs inhibit the angiotensin-induced vasoconstriction of the efferent arterioles of the glomerular microcirculation. This inhibition leads to a reduction in both intraglomerular filtration pressure and proteinuria. Several controlled studies have shown that these drugs are effective in slowing the progression of renal failure in patients with both diabetic and nondiabetic renal failure. This slowing in progression of CKD is strongly associated with their proteinuria-lowering effect. In the absence of an anti-proteinuric response with either agent alone, combined treatment with both ACE inhibitors and ARBs can be tried. Adverse effects from these agents include cough and angioedema with ACE inhibitors, anaphylaxis, and hyperkalemia with either class. A progressive increase in plasma creatinine concentration may suggest the presence of renovascular disease within the large or small arteries. Development of these side effects may mandate the use of second-line antihypertensive agents instead of the ACE inhibitors or ARBs. Among the calcium channel blockers, diltiazem and verapamil may exhibit superior antiproteinuric and renoprotective effects compared to the dihydropyridines. At least two different categories of response can be considered: one in which progression is strongly associated with systemic and intraglomerular hypertension and proteinuria (e.g., diabetic nephropathy, glomerular diseases) and in which ACE inhibitors and ARBs are likely to be the first choice; and another in which proteinuria is mild or absent initially (e.g., adult polycystic kidney disease and other tubulointerstitial diseases) and hence the contribution of intraglomerular hypertension less prominent, for which reason other antihypertensive agents can be useful for control of systemic hypertension.

SLOWING PROGRESSION OF DIABETIC RENAL DISEASE   (See also Chap. 338) Diabetic nephropathy is now the leading cause of CKD requiring renal replacement therapy in many parts of the world, and its prevalence is increasing disproportionately in the developing world. Furthermore, the prognosis of diabetic patients on dialysis is poor, with survival comparable to many forms of cancer. Accordingly, it is mandatory to develop strategies whose aim is to prevent or slow the progression of diabetic nephropathy in these patients.

Control of Blood Glucose   Excellent glycemic control reduces the risk of kidney disease and its progression in both type 1 and type 2 diabetes

TABLE 274-5   CLINICAL ACTION PLAN

Stage	Description	GFR, mL/min per 1.73 m²	Action[a]
1	Kidney damage with normal or ↑ GFR	≥90	Diagnosis and treatment, treatment of comorbid conditions, slowing progression, CVD risk reduction
2	Kidney damage with mild ↓ GFR	60–89	Estimating progression
3	Moderate ↓ GFR	30–59	Evaluating and treating complications
4	Severe ↓ GFR	15–29	Preparation for kidney replacement therapy
5	Kidney failure	<15 (or dialysis)	Kidney replacement (if uremia present)

[a]Includes actions from preceding stages.
Note: CVD, cardiovascular disease.
Source: National Kidney Foundation: Am J Kidney Dis 39(2 Suppl 1):S1, 2002.

PART 12

Disorders of the Kidney and Urinary Tract

DERMATOLOGIC ABNORMALITIES

Abnormalities of the skin are prevalent in progressive CKD. Anemic patients may be pale, and those with defective hemostasis may show multiple ecchymoses. Pruritus is quite common. In advanced CKD, even on dialysis, patients may become more pigmented, and this is felt to reflect the deposition of retained pigmented metabolites, or *urochromes*. Although many of the cutaneous abnormalities improve with dialysis, pruritus is often tenacious. The first lines of management are to rule out unrelated skin disorders, such as scabies, and to control phosphate concentration. EPO therapy was initially reported to improve uremic pruritus, although that is not always the case. Local moisturizers, mild topical glucocorticoids, oral antihistamines, and ultraviolet radiation have been reported to be helpful.

A skin condition called *nephrogenic fibrosing dermopathy* has recently been reported in which progressive subcutaneous induration, especially on the arms and legs, is described. The condition is similar to scleromyxedema and is seen in patients with CKD, most commonly on dialysis. Recent reports suggest that exposure to the magnetic resonance contrast agent, gadolinium, may precipitate this syndrome.

EVALUATION AND MANAGEMENT OF PATIENTS WITH CKD

INITIAL APPROACH

History and Physical Examination Symptoms and overt signs of kidney disease are often absent until renal failure supervenes. Thus, the diagnosis of kidney disease often surprises patients and may be a cause of skepticism and denial. Particular aspects of the history that are germane to renal disease include a history of hypertension (which can cause CKD or be a reflection of CKD), diabetes mellitus, abnormal urinalyses, and problems with pregnancy such as preeclampsia or early pregnancy loss. A careful drug history should be elicited: patients may not volunteer use of analgesics, for example. Other drugs to consider include nonsteroidal anti-inflammatory agents, gold, penicillamine, antimicrobials, antiretroviral agents, proton pump inhibitors, and lithium. In evaluating the uremic syndrome, questions about appetite, weight loss, nausea, hiccups, peripheral edema, muscle cramps, pruritus, and restless legs are especially helpful.

The physical examination should focus on blood pressure and target organ damage from hypertension. Thus, funduscopy and precordial examination (left ventricular heave, a fourth heart sound) should be carried out. Funduscopy is important in the diabetic patient, seeking evidence of diabetic retinopathy, which is associated with nephropathy. Other physical examination manifestations of CKD include edema and sensory polyneuropathy. The finding of asterixis or a pericardial friction rub not attributable to other causes usually signifies the presence of the uremic syndrome.

Laboratory Investigation Laboratory studies should focus on a search for clues to an underlying causative or aggravating disease process and on the degree of renal damage and its consequences. If appropriate, tests for systemic lupus erythematosus and vasculitis should be performed. Serum and urine protein electrophoresis should be obtained in all patients >35 years with unexplained CKD, especially if there is associated anemia and elevated, or even inappropriately normal, serum calcium concentration in the face of renal insufficiency. In the presence of glomerulonephritis, underlying infectious etiologies such as hepatitis B and C and HIV should be assessed. Serial measurements of renal function should be obtained to determine the pace of renal deterioration and ensure that the disease is truly chronic rather than subacute and hence potentially reversible. Serum concentrations of calcium, phosphorus, and PTH should be measured to evaluate metabolic bone disease. Hemoglobin concentration, iron, B$_{12}$, and folate should also be evaluated. A 24-h urine collection may be helpful, as protein excretion > 300 mg may be an indication for therapy with ACE inhibitors or ARBs.

Imaging Studies The most useful imaging study is a renal ultrasound, which can verify the presence of two kidneys, determine if they

are symmetric, provide an estimate of kidney size, and rule out renal masses and evidence of obstruction. Since it takes time for kidneys to shrink as a result of chronic disease, the finding of bilaterally small kidneys supports the diagnosis of CKD of long-standing duration, with an irreversible component of scarring. If the kidney size is normal, it is possible that the renal disease is acute or subacute. The exceptions are diabetic nephropathy (where kidney size is increased at the outset of diabetic nephropathy before CKD with loss of GFR supervenes), amyloidosis, and HIV nephropathy, where kidney size may be normal in the face of CKD. Polycystic kidney disease that has reached some degree of renal failure will almost always present with enlarged kidneys with multiple cysts (Chap. 278). A discrepancy >1 cm in kidney length suggests either a unilateral developmental abnormality or disease process or renovascular disease with arterial insufficiency affecting one kidney more than the other. The diagnosis of renovascular disease can be undertaken with different techniques, including Doppler sonography, nuclear medicine studies, or CT or MRI studies. If there is a suspicion of reflux nephropathy (recurrent childhood urinary tract infection, asymmetric renal size with scars on the renal poles), a voiding cystogram may be indicated. However, in most cases by the time the patient has CKD, the reflux has resolved, and even if still present, repair does not improve renal function. Radiographic contrast imaging studies are not particularly helpful in the investigation of CKD. Intravenous or intraarterial dye should be avoided where possible in the CKD patient, especially with diabetic nephropathy, because of the risk of radiographic contrast dye–induced renal failure. When unavoidable, appropriate precautionary measures include avoidance of hypovolemia at the time of contrast exposure, minimization of the dye load, and choice of radiographic contrast preparations with the least nephrotoxic potential.

Renal Biopsy In the patient with bilaterally small kidneys, renal biopsy is not advised because (1) it is technically difficult and has a greater likelihood of causing bleeding and other adverse consequences, (2) there is usually so much scarring that the underlying disease may not be apparent, and (3) the window of opportunity to render disease-specific therapy has passed. Other contraindications to renal biopsy include uncontrolled hypertension, active urinary tract infection, bleeding diathesis, and morbid obesity. Ultrasound-guided percutaneous biopsy is the favored approach, but a surgical or laparoscopic approach can be considered, especially in the patient with a single kidney where direct visualization and control of bleeding are crucial. In the CKD patient in whom a kidney biopsy is indicated (e.g., suspicion of a concomitant or superimposed active process, such as interstitial nephritis or accelerated loss of GFR), the bleeding time should be measured, and, if increased, desmopressin should be administered immediately prior to the procedure. A brief run of hemodialysis (without heparin) may also be considered prior to renal biopsy to normalize the bleeding time.

ESTABLISHING THE DIAGNOSIS AND ETIOLOGY OF CKD

The most important initial diagnostic step in the evaluation of a patient presenting with elevated serum creatinine is to distinguish newly diagnosed CKD from acute or subacute renal failure because the latter two conditions may respond to therapy specific to the disease. Previous measurements of plasma creatinine concentration are particularly helpful in this regard. Normal values from recent months or even years suggest that the current extent of renal dysfunction could be more acute, and hence reversible, than might otherwise be appreciated. In contrast, elevated plasma creatinine concentration in the past suggests that the renal disease represents the progression of a chronic process. Even if there is evidence of chronicity, there is the possibility of a superimposed acute process, such as ECFV depletion, supervening on the chronic condition. If the history suggests multiple systemic manifestations of recent onset (e.g., fever, polyarthritis, and rash) it should be assumed that renal insufficiency is part of the acute process.

Some of the laboratory tests and imaging studies outlined above can be helpful. Evidence of metabolic bone disease with hyperphosphatemia, hypocalcemia, and elevated PTH and bone alkaline phosphatase levels suggests chronicity. Normochromic, normocytic anemia suggests that the process has been ongoing for some time. The finding of bilaterally reduced kidney size (<8.5 cm in all but the smallest adults) favors CKD.

While renal biopsy can usually be performed in early CKD (stages 1–3), it is not always indicated. For example, in a patient with a history of type 1 diabetes mellitus for 15–20 years with retinopathy, nephrotic-range proteinuria, and absence of hematuria, the diagnosis of diabetic nephropathy is very likely and biopsy is not necessary. However, if there were some other finding not typical of diabetic nephropathy, such as hematuria or white blood cell casts, some other disease may be present and a biopsy may be indicated. Hypertensive nephrosclerosis and progressive ischemic nephropathy are usually diagnosed clinically by the presence of long-standing hypertension, evidence of ischemic disease elsewhere (e.g., cardiac or peripheral vascular disease), and the finding of only mild (< 3g/d) proteinuria in the absence of urinary blood or red cell casts. It is important to consider progressive ischemic nephropathy because a small subset of these patients may respond to revascularization procedures, although this remains controversial.

In the absence of a clinical diagnosis, renal biopsy may be the only recourse to establish an etiology in early-stage CKD. However, as noted above, once the CKD is advanced and the kidneys are small and scarred, there is little utility and significant risk in attempting to arrive at a specific diagnosis.

Rx CHRONIC KIDNEY DISEASE

Treatments aimed at specific causes of CKD are discussed elsewhere. The optimal timing of therapy is usually well before there has been a measurable decline in GFR and certainly before CKD is established **(Table 274-5)**. It is helpful to sequentially measure and plot the rate of decline of GFR in all patients. Any acceleration in the rate of decline should prompt a search for superimposed acute or subacute processes that may be reversible. These include ECFV depletion, uncontrolled hypertension, urinary tract infection, new obstructive uropathy, exposure to nephrotoxic agents [such as nonsteroidal anti-inflammatory drugs (NSAIDs) or radiographic dye], and reactivation or flare of the original disease, such as lupus or vasculitis.

SLOWING THE PROGRESSION OF CKD There is variation in the rate of decline of GFR among patients with CKD. However, the following interventions should be considered in an effort to stabilize or slow the decline of renal function.

Protein Restriction While protein restriction has been advocated to reduce symptoms associated with uremia, it may also slow the rate of renal decline at earlier stages of renal disease. This concept is based on clinical and experimental evidence that protein-mediated hyperfiltration contributes to ongoing decline in renal function in many different forms of renal disease. A number of studies have shown that protein restriction may be effective in slowing the progression of CKD, especially proteinuric and diabetic renal diseases. However, the Modification of Diet in Renal Disease study was unable to demonstrate a robust benefit in delaying progression to advanced stages of CKD with dietary restriction of protein intake. Nonetheless, restriction of dietary protein intake has been recommended for CKD patients. KDOQI clinical practice guidelines include a daily protein intake of between 0.60 and 0.75 g/kg per day, depending upon patient adherence, comorbid disease, presence of proteinuria, and nutritional status. It is further advised that at least 50% of the protein intake be of high biologic value. As patients approach stage 5 CKD, spontaneous protein intake tends to decrease, and patients may enter a state of protein-energy malnutrition. In these circumstances, a protein intake of up to 0.90 g/kg per day might be recommended, again, with an emphasis on proteins of high biologic value.

Sufficient energy intake is important to prevent protein-calorie malnutrition, and 35 kcal/kg is recommended. Monitoring of parameters of nutritional status must accompany the dietary intervention, using the parameters outlined above in the section on GI and nutritional abnormalities.

Reducing Intraglomerular Hypertension and Proteinuria Increased intraglomerular filtration pressures and glomerular hypertrophy develop as a response to loss of nephron number from different kidney diseases. This response is maladaptive, as it promotes the ongoing decline of kidney function even if the inciting process has been treated or spontaneously resolved. Control of systemic and glomerular hypertension is at least as important as dietary protein restriction in slowing the progression of CKD. Therefore, in addition to reduction of cardiovascular disease risk, antihypertensive therapy in patients with CKD also aims to slow the progression of nephron injury by reducing intraglomerular hypertension. Elevated blood pressure increases proteinuria through its transmission to the glomerulus. Conversely, the renoprotective effect of antihypertensive medications is gauged through the consequent reduction of proteinuria. Thus, the more effective a given treatment is in lowering protein excretion, the greater the subsequent impact on protection from decline in GFR. This observation is the basis for the treatment guideline establishing 125/75 mmHg as the target blood pressure in proteinuric CKD patients.

ACE inhibitors and ARBs inhibit the angiotensin-induced vasoconstriction of the efferent arterioles of the glomerular microcirculation. This inhibition leads to a reduction in both intraglomerular filtration pressure and proteinuria. Several controlled studies have shown that these drugs are effective in slowing the progression of renal failure in patients with both diabetic and nondiabetic renal failure. This slowing in progression of CKD is strongly associated with their proteinuria-lowering effect. In the absence of an anti-proteinuric response with either agent alone, combined treatment with both ACE inhibitors and ARBs can be tried. Adverse effects from these agents include cough and angioedema with ACE inhibitors, anaphylaxis, and hyperkalemia with either class. A progressive increase in plasma creatinine concentration may suggest the presence of renovascular disease within the large or small arteries. Development of these side effects may mandate the use of second-line antihypertensive agents instead of the ACE inhibitors or ARBs. Among the calcium channel blockers, diltiazem and verapamil may exhibit superior antiproteinuric and renoprotective effects compared to the dihydropyridines. At least two different categories of response can be considered: one in which progression is strongly associated with systemic and intraglomerular hypertension and proteinuria (e.g., diabetic nephropathy, glomerular diseases) and in which ACE inhibitors and ARBs are likely to be the first choice; and another in which proteinuria is mild or absent initially (e.g., adult polycystic kidney disease and other tubulointerstitial diseases) and hence the contribution of intraglomerular hypertension less prominent, for which reason other antihypertensive agents can be useful for control of systemic hypertension.

SLOWING PROGRESSION OF DIABETIC RENAL DISEASE (See also Chap. 338) Diabetic nephropathy is now the leading cause of CKD requiring renal replacement therapy in many parts of the world, and its prevalence is increasing disproportionately in the developing world. Furthermore, the prognosis of diabetic patients on dialysis is poor, with survival comparable to many forms of cancer. Accordingly, it is mandatory to develop strategies whose aim is to prevent or slow the progression of diabetic nephropathy in these patients.

Control of Blood Glucose Excellent glycemic control reduces the risk of kidney disease and its progression in both type 1 and type 2 diabetes

TABLE 274-5 CLINICAL ACTION PLAN

Stage	Description	GFR, mL/min per 1.73 m²	Action[a]
1	Kidney damage with normal or ↑ GFR	≥90	Diagnosis and treatment, treatment of comorbid conditions, slowing progression, CVD risk reduction
2	Kidney damage with mild ↓ GFR	60–89	Estimating progression
3	Moderate ↓ GFR	30–59	Evaluating and treating complications
4	Severe ↓ GFR	15–29	Preparation for kidney replacement therapy
5	Kidney failure	<15 (or dialysis)	Kidney replacement (if uremia present)

[a]Includes actions from preceding stages.
Note: CVD, cardiovascular disease.
Source: National Kidney Foundation: Am J Kidney Dis 39(2 Suppl 1):S1, 2002.

The absence of hypertension may signify the presence of a salt-wasting form of renal disease, the effect of antihypertensive therapy, or volume depletion or may signify poor left ventricular function. Indeed, in epidemiologic studies of dialysis patients, low blood pressure actually carries a worse prognosis than does high blood pressure. This mechanism, in part, accounts for the "reverse causation" seen in dialysis patients, wherein the presence of traditional risk factors, such as hypertension, hyperlipidemia, and obesity, appear to portend a better prognosis. Importantly, these observations derive from cross-sectional studies of late-stage CKD patients and should not be interpreted to discourage appropriate management of these risk factors in CKD patients, especially at early stages. In contrast to the general population, it is possible that in late-stage CKD, low blood pressure, reduced body mass index, and hypolipidemia indicate the presence of a malnutrition-inflammation state, with poor prognosis.

The use of exogenous erythropoietic products can increase blood pressure and the requirement for antihypertensive drugs. Chronic ECFV overload is also a contributor to hypertension, and improvement in blood pressure can often be seen with the use of oral sodium restriction, diuretics, and fluid removal with dialysis. Nevertheless, because of activation of the renin-angiotensin-aldosterone axis and other disturbances in the balance of vasoconstrictors and vasodilators, some patients remain hypertensive despite careful attention to ECFV status.

Rx CARDIOVASCULAR ABNORMALITIES

MANAGEMENT OF HYPERTENSION There are two overall goals of therapy for hypertension in these patients: to slow the progression of the kidney disease itself, and to prevent the extrarenal complications of high blood pressure, such as cardiovascular disease and stroke. In all patients with CKD, blood pressure should be controlled to levels recommended by national guideline panels. In CKD patients with diabetes or proteinuria > 1 g per 24 h, blood pressure should be reduced to 125/75, if achievable without prohibitive adverse effects. Salt restriction and diuretics should be the first line of therapy. When volume management alone is not sufficient, the choice of antihypertensive agent is similar to that in the general population. The ACE inhibitors and ARBs slow the rate of decline of kidney function, even in dialysis patients, but their use may be complicated by the development of hyperkalemia. Often the concomitant use of a kaliuretic diuretic, such as metolazone, can improve potassium excretion in addition to improving blood pressure control. Potassium-sparing diuretics should be used with caution or avoided altogether in most patients.

MANAGEMENT OF CARDIOVASCULAR DISEASE There are many strategies available to treat the traditional and nontraditional risk factors in CKD patients. While these have been proven effective in the general population, there is little evidence for their benefit in patients with advanced CKD, especially those on dialysis. Certainly hypertension, elevated serum levels of homocysteine, and dyslipidemia promote atherosclerotic disease and are treatable complications of CKD. Renal disease complicated by nephrotic syndrome is associated with a very atherogenic lipid profile and hypercoagulability, which increases the risk of occlusive vascular disease. Since diabetes mellitus and hypertension are the two most frequent causes of advanced CKD, it is not surprising that cardiovascular disease is the most frequent cause of death in dialysis patients. The role of "inflammation" may be quantitatively more important in patients with kidney disease, and the treatment of more traditional risk factors may result in only modest success. However, modulation of traditional risk factors may be the only weapon in the therapeutic armamentarium for these patients until the nature of inflammation in CKD and its treatment are better understood.

Lifestyle changes, including regular exercise, should be advocated but are not often implemented. Hyperhomocysteinemia may respond to vitamin therapy, including oral folate supplementation, but this therapy is of unproven benefit. Hyperlipidemia in patients with CKD should be managed according to national guidelines. If dietary measures are not sufficient, preferred lipid-lowering medications, such as statins, should be used. Again, the use of these agents has not been of proven benefit for patients with advanced CKD.

Pericardial Disease Pericardial pain with respiratory accentuation, accompanied by a friction rub, is diagnostic of uremic pericarditis. Classic electrocardiographic abnormalities include PR-interval depression and diffuse ST-segment elevation. Pericarditis can be accompanied by pericardial effusion that is seen on echocardiography and can rarely lead to tamponade. However, the pericardial effusion can be asymptomatic, and pericarditis can be seen without significant effusion.

Pericarditis is observed in advanced uremia, and with the advent of timely initiation of dialysis, is not as common as it once was. It is now more often observed in underdialyzed, nonadherent patients than in those starting dialysis.

Rx PERICARDIAL DISEASE

Uremic pericarditis is an absolute indication for the urgent initiation of dialysis or for intensification of the dialysis prescription in those already receiving dialysis. Because of the propensity to hemorrhage in pericardial fluid, hemodialysis should be performed without heparin. A pericardial drainage procedure should be considered in patients with recurrent pericardial effusion. Nonuremic causes of pericarditis and effusion include viral, malignant, tuberculous, and autoimmune etiologies. It may also be seen after myocardial infarction and as a complication of treatment with minoxidil.

HEMATOLOGIC ABNORMALITIES

Anemia A normocytic, normochromic anemia is observed as early as stage 3 CKD and is almost universal by stage 4. The primary cause in patients with CKD is insufficient production of erythropoietin (EPO) by the diseased kidneys. Additional factors include iron deficiency, acute and chronic inflammation with impaired iron utilization ("anemia of chronic disease"), severe hyperparathyroidism with consequent bone marrow fibrosis, and shortened red cell survival in the uremic environment. Less common causes include folate and vitamin B_{12} deficiency and aluminum toxicity. In addition, comorbid conditions such as hemoglobinopathy can worsen the anemia (Table 274-4).

The anemia of CKD is associated with a number of adverse pathophysiologic consequences, including decreased tissue xygen delivery and utilization, increased cardiac output, ventricular dilatation, and ventricular hypertrophy. Clinical manifestations include angina, heart failure, decreased cognition and mental acuity, and impaired host defense against infection. In addition, anemia may play a role in growth retardation in children with CKD. While many studies in CKD patients have found that anemia and resistance to exogenous EPO are associated with a poor prognosis, it is unclear as to how much the low hematocrit itself versus inflammation leads to a poor outcome.

Rx ANEMIA

The availability of recombinant human EPO and modified EPO products, such as darbopoetin-alpha, has been one of the most significant advances in the care of renal patients since the introduction of dialysis and renal transplantation. The routine use of these products has obviated the need for regular blood transfusions in severely anemic CKD patients, thus dramatically reducing the incidence of transfusion-associated infections and iron overload. Frequent blood transfusions in dialysis patients also led to the development of alloantibodies that could sensitize the patient to donor kidney antigens and make renal transplantation more problematic.

Adequate bone marrow iron stores should be available before treatment with EPO is initiated. Iron supplementation is ousually essential to

---

TABLE 274-4 CAUSES OF ANEMIA IN CKD

Relative deficiency of erythropoietin
Diminished red blood cell survival
Bleeding diathesis
Iron deficiency
Hyperparathyroidism/bone marrow fibrosis
"Chronic inflammation"
Folate or vitamin B_{12} deficiency
Hemoglobinopathy
Comorbid conditions: hypo/hyperthyroidism, pregnancy, HIV-associated disease, autoimmune disease, immunosuppressive drugs

ensure an adequate response to EPO in patients with CKD because the demand for iron by the marrow frequently exceeds the amount of iron that is immediately available for erythropoiesis (measured by percent transferrin saturation), as well as the amount in iron stores (measured by serum ferritin). For the CKD patient not yet on dialysis or the patient treated with peritoneal dialysis, oral iron supplementation should be attempted. If there is GI intolerance, the patient may have to undergo IV iron infusion, often during the dialysis session. In addition to iron, an adequate supply of other major substrates and cofactors for red cell production must be assured, including vitamin B_{12} and folate. Anemia resistant to recommended doses of EPO in the face of adequate iron stores may be due to some combination of the following: acute or chronic inflammation, inadequate dialysis, severe hyperparathyroidism, chronic blood loss or hemolysis, chronic infection, or malignancy. Patients with a hemoglobinopathy, such as sickle cell disease or thalassemia, will usually not respond normally to exogenous EPO; however, an increase in hemoglobin concentration is still seen in many of these patients. Blood transfusions may contribute to suppression of erythropoiesis in CKD; because they increase the risk of hepatitis, iron overload, and transplant sensitization, they should be avoided unless the anemia fails to respond to EPO and the patient is symptomatic.

Normalization of the hemoglobin concentration has not been demonstrated to be of incremental benefit to dialysis patients. Current practice is to target a hemoglobin concentration of 110 to 120 g/L.

Abnormal Hemostasis Patients with later stages of CKD may have a prolonged bleeding time, decreased activity of platelet factor III, abnormal platelet aggregation and adhesiveness, and impaired prothrombin consumption. Clinical manifestations include an increased tendency to bleeding and bruising, prolonged bleeding from surgical incisions, menorrhagia, and spontaneous GI bleeding. Interestingly, CKD patients also have a greater susceptibility to thromboembolism, especially if they have renal disease that includes nephrotic-range proteinuria. The latter condition results in hypoalbuminemia and renal loss of anticoagulant factors, which can lead to a thrombophilic state.

℞ ABNORMAL HEMOSTASIS

Abnormal bleeding time and coagulopathy in patients with renal failure may be reversed temporarily with desmopressin (DDAVP), cryoprecipitate, IV conjugated estrogens, blood transfusions, and EPO therapy. Optimal dialysis will often correct a prolonged bleeding time.

Given the coexistence of bleeding disorders and a propensity to thrombosis that is unique in the CKD patient, decisions about anticoagulation that have a favorable risk-benefit profile in the general population may not be applicable to the patient with advanced CKD. One example is warfarin anticoagulation for atrial fibrillation: the decision to anticoagulate should be made on an individual basis in the CKD patient.

Certain anticoagulants, such as fractionated low-molecular-weight heparin, may need to be avoided or dose-adjusted in these patients, with monitoring of factor Xa activity where available. It is often more prudent to use conventional high-molecular-weight heparin, titrated to the measured partial thromboplastin time, in hospitalized patients requiring an alternative to warfarin anticoagulation.

NEUROMUSCULAR ABNORMALITIES

Central nervous system (CNS), peripheral, and autonomic neuropathy as well as abnormalities in muscle structure and function are all well-recognized complications of CKD. Retained nitrogenous metabolites and middle molecules, including PTH, contribute to the pathophysiology of neuromuscular abnormalities. Subtle clinical manifestations of uremic neuromuscular disease usually become evident at stage 3 CKD. Early manifestations of CNS complications include mild disturbances in memory and concentration and sleep disturbance. Neuromuscular irritability, including hiccups, cramps, and fasciculations or twitching of muscles, becomes evident at later stages. In advanced untreated kidney failure, asterixis, myoclonus, seizures, and coma can be seen.

Peripheral neuropathy usually becomes clinically evident after the patient reaches stage 4 CKD, although electrophysiologic and histolog-

ic evidence occurs earlier. Initially, sensory nerves are involved more than motor, lower extremities more than upper, and distal parts of the extremities more than proximal. The "restless leg syndrome" is characterized by ill-defined sensations of sometimes debilitating discomfort in the legs and feet relieved by frequent leg movement. If dialysis is not instituted soon after onset of sensory abnormalities, motor involvement follows, including muscle weakness. Evidence of peripheral neuropathy without another cause (e.g., diabetes mellitus) is a firm indication for starting renal replacement therapy. Many of the complications described above will resolve with dialysis, although subtle nonspecific abnormalities may persist. Successful renal transplantation may reverse residual neurologic changes.

GASTROINTESTINAL AND NUTRITIONAL ABNORMALITIES

Uremic fetor, a urine-like odor on the breath, derives from the breakdown of urea to ammonia in saliva and is often associated with an unpleasant metallic taste (dysgeusia). Gastritis, peptic disease, and mucosal ulcerations at any level of the GI tract occur in uremic patients and can lead to abdominal pain, nausea, vomiting, and GI bleeding. These patients are also prone to constipation, which can be worsened by the administration of calcium and iron supplements. The retention of uremic toxins also leads to anorexia, nausea, and vomiting.

Protein restriction may be useful to decrease nausea and vomiting; however, it may put the patient at risk for malnutrition and should be carried out, if possible, in consultation with a registered dietitian. Protein-energy malnutrition, a consequence of low protein and caloric intake, is common in advanced CKD and is often an indication for initiation of renal replacement therapy. In addition to diminished intake, these patients are resistant to the anabolic actions of insulin and other hormones and growth factors. Metabolic acidosis and the activation of inflammatory cytokines can promote protein catabolism. Assessment for protein-energy malnutrition should begin at stage 3 CKD. A number of indices are useful in this assessment and include dietary history, including diary and subjective global assessment; edema-free body weight; serum albumin concentration; and measurement of urinary protein nitrogen appearance. Dual-energy x-ray absorptiometry is now widely used to estimate lean body mass versus ECFV. Adjunctive tools include clinical signs, such as skinfold thickness, mid-arm muscle circumference, and additional laboratory tests such as serum pre-albumin and cholesterol levels. Nutritional guidelines for patients with CKD are summarized in the section below on "Principles of Treatment of CKD."

ENDOCRINE-METABOLIC DISTURBANCES

Glucose metabolism is impaired in CKD, as evidenced by a slowing of the rate at which blood glucose levels decline after a glucose load. However, fasting blood glucose is usually normal or only slightly elevated, and the mild glucose intolerance does not require specific therapy. Because the kidney contributes to insulin removal from the circulation, plasma levels of insulin are slightly to moderately elevated in most uremic patients, both in the fasting and postprandial states. Because of this diminished renal degradation of insulin, patients on insulin therapy may need progressive reduction in dose as their renal function worsens. Many hypoglycemic agents require dose reduction in renal failure, and some, such as metformin, are contraindicated when the GFR is less than half of normal.

In women with CKD, estrogen levels are low, and menstrual abnormalities and inability to carry pregnancies to term are common. When the GFR has declined to ~40 mL/min, pregnancy is associated with a high rate of spontaneous abortion, with only ~20% of pregnancies leading to live births, and pregnancy may hasten the progression of the kidney disease itself. Men with CKD have reduced plasma testosterone levels, and sexual dysfunction and oligospermia may supervene. Sexual maturation may be delayed or impaired in adolescent children with CKD, even among those treated with dialysis. Many of these abnormalities improve or reverse with intensive dialysis or successful renal transplantation.

mellitus. It is recommended that plasma values for preprandial glucose be kept in the 5.0–7.2 mmol/L (90–130 mg/dL) range and hemoglobin A_{1C} should be < 7%. As the GFR decreases with progressive nephropathy, the use and dose of oral hypoglycemics needs to be reevaluated. For example, chlorpropamide may be associated with prolonged hypoglycemia in patients with decreased renal function; metformin has been reported to cause lactic acidosis in the patient with renal impairment and should be discontinued when the GFR is reduced; and the thiazolidinediones (e.g., rosiglitazone, pioglitazone, and others), may increase renal salt and water absorption and aggravate volume-overloaded states. Finally, as renal function declines, renal degradation of administered insulin will also decline, so that less insulin may be required for glycemic control.

Control of Blood Pressure and Proteinuria   Hypertension is found in the majority of type 2 diabetic patients at diagnosis. This finding correlates with the presence of albuminuria and is a strong predictor of cardiovascular events and nephropathy. Microalbuminuria, the finding of albumin in the urine not detectable by the urine dipstick, precedes the decline in GFR and heralds renal and cardiovascular complications. Testing for microalbumin is recommended in all diabetic patients, at least annually. If the patient already has established proteinuria, then testing for microalbumin is not necessary. Antihypertensive treatment reduces albuminuria and diminishes its progression even in normotensive diabetic patients. In addition to treatment of hypertension in general, the use of ACE inhibitors and ARBs in particular is associated with additional renoprotection. These salutary effects are mediated by reducing intraglomerular pressure and inhibition of angiotensin-driven sclerosing pathways, in part through inhibition of TGF-β-mediated pathways.

MANAGING OTHER COMPLICATIONS OF CHRONIC KIDNEY DISEASE   Medication Dose Adjustment   Although the loading dose of most drugs is not affected by CKD because no renal elimination is used in the calculation, the maintenance doses of many drugs will need to be adjusted. For those agents in which > 70% excretion is by a nonrenal route, such as hepatic elimination, dose adjustment may not be needed. Some drugs that should be avoided include metformin, meperidine, and oral hypoglycemics that are eliminated by the kidney. NSAIDs should be avoided because of the risk of further worsening of kidney function. Many antibiotics, antihypertensives, and antiarrhythmics may require a reduction in dosage or change in the dose interval. For a comprehensive, detailed listing of the dose adjustments for most of the commonly used medications, see "Drug Prescribing in Renal Failure" published by the American College of Physicians (see *www.acponline.org*).

Preparation for Renal Replacement Therapy   (See also Chap. 276) Temporary relief of symptoms and signs of impending uremia, such as anorexia, nausea, vomiting, lassitude, and pruritus, may sometimes be achieved with protein restriction. However, this carries a significant risk of protein-energy malnutrition, and thus plans for more long-term management should be in place.

The institution of maintenance dialysis and kidney transplantation has extended the lives of hundreds of thousands of patients with CKD worldwide. Clear indications for initiation of renal replacement therapy for patients with CKD include pericarditis, encephalopathy, intractable muscle cramping, anorexia, and nausea not attributable to reversible causes such as peptic ulcer disease, evidence of malnutrition, and fluid and electrolyte abnormalities, principally hyperkalemia, that are refractory to other measures.

Recommendations for the optimal time for initiation of renal replacement therapy have been established by the National Kidney Foundation in their KDOQI Guidelines and are based on recent evidence demonstrating that delaying initiation of renal replacement therapy until patients are malnourished or have severe uremic complications leads to a worse prognosis on dialysis or with transplantation. Because of the interindividual variability in the severity of uremic symptoms and renal function, it is ill-advised to assign an arbitrary urea nitrogen or creatinine level to the need to start dialysis. Moreover, patients may become accustomed to chronic uremia and deny symptoms, only to find that they feel better with dialysis and realize in retrospect how poorly they were feeling before its initiation.

Previous studies suggested that starting dialysis before the onset of severe symptoms and signs of uremia was associated with prolongation of survival. This lead to the concept of "healthy" start and is congruent with the philosophy that it is better to keep patients feeling well all along, rather than allowing them to become ill with uremia before trying to return them to better health with dialysis. Although recent studies have not confirmed a clear association of early-start dialysis with improved patient survival, there is still merit in this approach. On a practical level, advanced preparation may help to avoid problems with the dialysis process itself (e.g., a poorly functioning fistula for hemodialysis or malfunctioning peritoneal dialysis catheter) and thus preempt the morbidity associated with resorting to the insertion of temporary hemodialysis access with its attendant risks of sepsis, bleeding, and thrombosis.

Patient Education   Social, psychological, and physical preparation for the transition to renal replacement therapy and the choice of the optimal initial modality are best accomplished with a gradual approach involving a multidisciplinary team. Along with conservative measures discussed in the sections above, it is important to prepare patients with an intensive educational program, explaining the likelihood and timing of initiation of renal replacement therapy and the various forms of therapy available. The more knowledgeable that patients are about hemodialysis (both in-center and home-based), peritoneal dialysis, and kidney transplantation, the easier and more appropriate will be their decisions. Patients who are provided with educational programs are more likely to choose home-based dialysis therapy. This approach is of societal benefit because home-based therapy is less expensive and is associated with improved quality of life. The educational programs should be commenced no later than stage 4 CKD so that the patient has sufficient cognitive function to learn the important concepts.

Exploration of social service support is also important. In those who may perform home dialysis or undergo preemptive renal transplantation, early education of family members for selection and preparation of a home dialysis helper or a related (or unrelated) kidney donor should occur long before the onset of symptomatic renal failure.

Kidney transplantation (Chap. 276) offers the best potential for complete rehabilitation, because dialysis replaces only a small fraction of the kidneys' filtration function and none of the other renal functions, including endocrine and anti-inflammatory effects. Generally, kidney transplantation follows a period of dialysis treatment, although preemptive kidney transplantation (usually from a living donor) can be carried out if it is certain that the renal failure is irreversible.

IMPLICATIONS FOR GLOBAL HEALTH
In distinction to the natural decline and successful eradication of many devastating infectious diseases, there is rapid growth in the prevalence of hypertension and vascular disease in developing countries. Diabetes mellitus is becoming increasingly prevalent in these countries, perhaps due in part to change in dietary habits, diminished physical activity, and weight gain. Therefore, it follows that there will be a proportionate increase in vascular and renal disease. Healthcare agencies must plan for improved screening for early detection, prevention, and treatment plans in these nations and must start considering options for improved availability of renal replacement therapies.

FURTHER READINGS
GO A et al: Chronic kidney disease and the risks of death, cardiovascular events, and hospitalization. N Engl J Med 351:1296, 2004

KETTELER M et al: Calcification and cardiovascular health: New insights into an old phenomenon. Hypertension 47:1027, 2006

LEVEY AS et al: CKD: Common, harmful and treatable—World Kidney Day 2007. Am J Kidney Dis 49(2), 2007

NATIONAL KIDNEY FOUNDATION: Kidney Disease Outcomes Quality Initiative *Clinical Practice Guidelines for Nutrition in Chronic Renal Failure.* Am J Kidney Dis 35 (suppl 2): S1, 2000

NATIONAL KIDNEY FOUNDATION: K/DOQI Clinical Practice Guidelines for Chronic Kidney Disease: Evaluation, classification and stratification. Am J Kidney Dis 39 (suppl 1), 2000

SARNAK M et al: Kidney disease as a risk factor for development of cardiovascular disease: A statement from the American Heart Association Councils on Kidney in Cardiovascular Disease, High Blood Pressure Research, Clinical Cardiology, and Epidemiology and Prevention. Circulation 108:2154, 2003

STRONG K et al: Preventing chronic disease: How many lives can we save? Lancet 366:1578, 2005

275 Dialysis in the Treatment of Renal Failure

Kathleen D. Liu, Glenn M. Chertow

Dialysis may be required for the treatment of either acute or chronic kidney disease. The use of continuous renal replacement therapies (CRRT) and slow, low-efficiency dialysis (SLED) is specific to the management of acute renal failure and is discussed in Chap. 273. These modalities are performed continuously (CRRT) or over 6–12 hours per session (SLED), in contrast to the 3–4 hours of an intermittent hemodialysis session. Advantages and disadvantages of CRRT and SLED are discussed in Chap. 273.

Peritoneal dialysis is rarely used in developed countries for the treatment of acute renal failure because of the increased risk of infection and (as will be discussed in more detail below) less efficient clearance per unit of time. The focus of the majority of this chapter will be on the use of dialysis for end-stage renal disease (ESRD).

With the widespread availability of dialysis, the lives of hundreds of thousands of patients with ESRD have been prolonged. In the United States alone, there are now approximately 450,000 patients with ESRD, the vast majority of whom require dialysis. The incidence rate for ESRD is 330 cases per million population per year. The incidence of ESRD is disproportionately higher in African Americans (approximately 1000 per million population per year) as compared with white Americans (259 per million population per year). In the United States, the leading cause of ESRD is diabetes mellitus, currently accounting for nearly 45% of newly diagnosed cases of ESRD. Over one-quarter (27%) of patients have ESRD that has been attributed to hypertension, although it is unclear whether in these cases hypertension is the cause or a consequence of vascular disease or other unknown causes of kidney failure. Other important causes of ESRD include glomerulonephritis, polycystic kidney disease, and obstructive uropathy.

 Globally, mortality rates for patients with ESRD are lowest in Europe and Japan but very high in the developing world because of the limited availability of dialysis. In the United States, the mortality rate of patients on dialysis is approximately 18–20% per year, with a 5-year survival rate of approximately 30–35%. Deaths are due mainly to cardiovascular diseases and infections (approximately 50 and 15% of deaths, respectively). Older age, male sex, nonblack race, diabetes mellitus, malnutrition, and underlying heart disease are important predictors of death.

TREATMENT OPTIONS FOR ESRD PATIENTS

Commonly accepted criteria for initiating patients on maintenance dialysis include the presence of uremic symptoms, the presence of hyperkalemia unresponsive to conservative measures, persistent extracellular volume expansion despite diuretic therapy, acidosis refractory to medical therapy, a bleeding diathesis, and a creatinine clearance or estimated glomerular filtration rate (GFR) below 10 mL/min per 1.73 m^2 (see Chap. 274 for estimating equations). Timely referral to a nephrologist for advanced planning and creation of a dialysis access, education about ESRD treatment options, and management of the complications of advanced chronic kidney disease, including hypertension, anemia, acidosis, and secondary hyperparathyroidism, is advisable.

In ESRD, treatment options include hemodialysis (in center or at home); peritoneal dialysis, as either continuous ambulatory peritoneal dialysis (CAPD) or continuous cyclic peritoneal dialysis (CCPD); or transplantation (Chap. 276). Although there are geographic variations, hemodialysis remains the most common therapeutic modality for ESRD (>90% of patients) in the United States. In contrast to hemodialysis, peritoneal dialysis is continuous, but much less efficient, in terms of solute clearance. While no large-scale clinical trials have been completed comparing outcomes among patients randomized to either hemodialysis or peritoneal dialysis, outcomes associated with

both therapies are similar in most reports, and the decision of which modality to select is often based on personal preferences and quality-of-life considerations.

HEMODIALYSIS

Hemodialysis relies on the principles of solute diffusion across a semipermeable membrane. Movement of metabolic waste products takes place down a concentration gradient from the circulation into the dialysate. The rate of diffusive transport increases in response to several factors, including the magnitude of the concentration gradient, the membrane surface area, and the mass transfer coefficient of the membrane. The latter is a function of the porosity and thickness of the membrane, the size of the solute molecule, and the conditions of flow on the two sides of the membrane. According to the laws of diffusion, the larger the molecule, the slower its rate of transfer across the membrane. A small molecule, such as urea (60 Da), undergoes substantial clearance, whereas a larger molecule, such as creatinine (113 Da), is cleared less efficiently. In addition to diffusive clearance, movement of waste products from the circulation into the dialysate may occur as a result of ultrafiltration. Convective clearance occurs because of solvent drag, with solutes being swept along with water across the semipermeable dialysis membrane.

THE DIALYZER

There are three essential components to hemodialysis: the dialyzer, the composition and delivery of the dialysate, and the blood delivery system (Fig. 275-1). The dialyzer consists of a plastic device with the facility to perfuse blood and dialysate compartments at very high flow rates. The surface area of modern dialysis membranes in adult patients is usually in the range of 1.5–2.0 m^2. The hollow-fiber dialyzer is the most common in use in the United States. These dialyzers are composed of bundles of capillary tubes through which blood circulates while dialysate travels on the outside of the fiber bundle.

Recent advances have led to the development of many different types of membrane material. Broadly, there are four categories of dialysis membranes: cellulose, substituted cellulose, cellulosynthetic, and synthetic. Over the past three decades, there has been a gradual switch from cellulose-derived to synthetic membranes, because the latter are more "biocompatible." *Bioincompatibility* is generally defined as the ability of the membrane to activate the complement cascade. Cellulosic membranes are bioincompatible because of the presence of free hydroxyl groups on the membrane surface. In contrast, with the substituted cellulose membranes (e.g., cellulose acetate) or the cellulosynthetic membranes, the hydroxyl groups are chemically bound to either acetate or tertiary amino groups, resulting in limited complement activation. Synthetic membranes, such as polysulfone, polymethylmethacrylate, and polyacrylonitrile membranes, are even more biocompatible because of the absence of these hydroxyl groups. Polysulfone membranes are now used in >60% of the dialysis treatments in the United States.

Reprocessing and reuse of hemodialyzers are often employed for patients on maintenance hemodialysis in the United States. However, as the manufacturing costs for disposable dialyzers have declined, more and more outpatient dialysis facilities are no longer reprocessing dialyzers. In most centers employing reuse, only the dialyzer unit is reprocessed and reused, whereas in the developing world blood lines are also frequently reused. The reprocessing procedure can be either manual or automated. It consists of the sequential rinsing of the blood and dialysate compartments with water, a chemical cleansing step with reverse ultrafiltration from the dialysate to the blood compartment, the testing of the patency of the dialyzer, and, finally, disinfection of the dialyzer. Formaldehyde, peracetic acid–hydrogen peroxide, glutaraldehyde, and bleach have all been used as reprocessing agents.

DIALYSATE

The potassium concentration of dialysate may be varied from 0 to 4 mmol/L depending on the predialysis plasma potassium concentration. The usual dialysate calcium concentration in U.S. hemodialysis centers is

FIGURE 275-1 Schema for hemodialysis.

1.25 mmol/L (2.5 meq/L), although modification may be required in selected settings (e.g., higher dialysate calcium concentrations may be used in patients with hypocalcemia associated with secondary hyperparathyroidism or following parathyroidectomy). The usual dialysate sodium concentration is 140 mmol/L. Lower dialysate sodium concentrations are associated with a higher frequency of hypotension, cramping, nausea, vomiting, fatigue, and dizziness. In patients who frequently develop hypotension during their dialysis run, "sodium modeling" to counterbalance urea-related osmolar gradients is often used. When sodium modeling, the dialysate sodium concentration is gradually lowered from the range of 145–155 meq/L to isotonic concentrations (140 meq/L) near the end of the dialysis treatment, typically declining either in steps or in a linear or exponential fashion. Because patients are exposed to approximately 120 L of water during each dialysis treatment, water used for the dialysate is subjected to filtration, softening, deionization, and, ultimately, reverse osmosis. During the reverse osmosis process, water is forced through a semipermeable membrane at very high pressure to remove microbiologic contaminants and >90% of dissolved ions.

BLOOD DELIVERY SYSTEM

The blood delivery system is composed of the extracorporeal circuit in the dialysis machine and the dialysis access. The dialysis machine consists of a blood pump, dialysis solution delivery system, and various safety monitors. The blood pump moves blood from the access site, through the dialyzer, and back to the patient. The blood flow rate may range from 250–500 mL/min, depending largely on the type and integrity of the vascular access. Negative hydrostatic pressure on the dialysate side can be manipulated to achieve desirable fluid removal or *ultrafiltration*. Dialysis membranes have different ultrafiltration coefficients (i.e., mL removed/min per mmHg) so that along with hydrostatic changes, fluid removal can be varied. The dialysis solution delivery system dilutes the concentrated dialysate with water and monitors the temperature, conductivity, and flow of dialysate.

Dialysis Access The fistula, graft, or catheter through which blood is obtained for hemodialysis is often referred to as a *dialysis access*. A native fistula created by the anastomosis of an artery to a vein (e.g., the Brescia-Cimino fistula, in which the cephalic vein is anastomosed end-to-side to the radial artery) results in arterialization of the vein. This facilitates its subsequent use in the placement of large needles (typically 15 gauge) to access the circulation. Although fistulas have the highest long-term patency rate of all dialysis access options, fistulas are created in a minority of patients in the United States. Many patients undergo placement of an arteriovenous graft (i.e., the interposition of prosthetic material, usually polytetrafluoroethylene, between an artery and a vein) or a tunneled dialysis catheter. In recent years, nephrologists, vascular surgeons, and health care policy makers in the United States have encouraged creation of arteriovenous fistulas in a larger fraction of patients (the "fistula first" initiative). Unfortunately, even when created, arteriovenous fistulas may not mature sufficiently to provide reliable access to the circulation, or they may thrombose early in their development. Novel surgical approaches (e.g., brachiobasilic fistula creation with transposition of the basilic vein fistula to the arm surface) have increased options for "native" vascular access.

Grafts and catheters tend to be used among persons with smaller-caliber veins or persons whose veins have been damaged by repeated venipuncture, or after prolonged hospitalization. The most important complication of arteriovenous grafts is thrombosis of the graft and graft failure, due principally to intimal hyperplasia at the anastomosis between the graft and recipient vein. When grafts (or fistulas) fail, catheter-guided angioplasty can be used to dilate stenoses; monitoring of venous pressures on dialysis and of access flow, though not routinely performed, may assist in the early recognition of impending vascular access failure. In addition to an increased rate of access failure, grafts and (in particular) catheters are associated with much higher rates of infection than fistulas.

Intravenous large-bore catheters are often used in patients with acute and chronic kidney disease. For persons on maintenance hemodialysis, tunneled catheters (either two separate catheters or a single catheter with two lumens) are often used when arteriovenous fistulas and grafts have failed or are not feasible due to anatomical considerations. These catheters are tunneled under the skin; the tunnel reduces bacterial translocation from the skin, resulting in a lower infection rate than with nontunneled temporary catheters. Most tunneled catheters are placed in the internal jugular veins; the external jugular, femoral, and subclavian veins may also be used. Nephrologists, interventional radiologists, and vascular surgeons generally prefer to avoid placement of catheters into the subclavian veins; while flow rates are usually excellent, subclavian stenosis is a frequent complication and, if present, will likely prohibit permanent vascular access (i.e., a fistula or graft) in the ipsilateral extremity. Infection rates may be higher with femoral catheters. For patients with multiple vascular access complications and no other options for permanent vascular access, tunneled catheters may be the last "lifeline" for hemodialysis. Translumbar or transhepatic approaches into the inferior vena cava may be required if the superior vena cava or other central veins draining the upper extremities are stenosed or thrombosed.

GOALS OF DIALYSIS

The hemodialysis procedure is targeted at removing both low- and high-molecular-weight solutes. The procedure consists of pumping heparinized blood through the dialyzer at a flow rate of 300–500 mL/min, while dialysate flows in an opposite *counter-current* direction at 500–800 mL/min. The efficiency of dialysis is determined by blood and dialysate flow through the dialyzer as well as dialyzer characteristics (i.e., its efficiency in removing solute). The *dose* of dialysis, which is currently defined as a derivation of the fractional urea clearance during a single dialysis treatment, is further governed by patient size, residual kidney function, dietary protein intake, the degree of anabolism or catabolism, and the presence of comorbid conditions.

Since the landmark studies of Sargent and Gotch relating the measurement of the dose of dialysis using urea concentrations with morbidity in the National Cooperative Dialysis Study, the *delivered* dose of dialysis has been measured and considered as a quality assurance and improvement tool. While the fractional removal of urea nitrogen and derivations thereof are considered to be the standard methods by which "adequacy of dialysis" is measured, a large multicenter randomized clinical trial (the HEMO Study) failed to show a difference in mortality associated with a large difference in urea clearance. Still, multiple observational studies and widespread expert opinion have suggested that higher dialysis dose is warranted; current targets include a urea reduction ratio (the fractional reduction in blood urea nitrogen per hemodialysis session) of >65–70% and a body water–indexed clearance × time product (KT/V) above 1.3 or 1.05, depending on whether urea concentrations are "equilibrated."

For the majority of patients with ESRD, between 9 and 12 h of dialysis are required each week, usually divided into three equal sessions. Several studies have suggested that longer hemodialysis session lengths may be beneficial, although these studies are confounded by a variety of patient characteristics, including body size and nutritional status. Hemodialysis "dose" should be individualized, and factors other than the urea nitrogen should be considered, including the adequacy of ultrafiltration or fluid removal. Several authors have highlighted improved intermediate outcomes associated with more frequent hemodialysis (i.e., more than three times a week), although these studies are also confounded by multiple factors. A randomized clinical trial is currently underway to test whether more frequent dialysis results in differences in a variety of physiologic and functional markers.

COMPLICATIONS DURING HEMODIALYSIS

Hypotension is the most common acute complication of hemodialysis, particularly among diabetics. Numerous factors appear to increase the risk of hypotension, including excessive ultrafiltration with inadequate compensatory vascular filling, impaired vasoactive or autonomic responses, osmolar shifts, overzealous use of antihypertensive agents, and reduced cardiac reserve. Patients with arteriovenous fistulas and grafts may develop high output cardiac failure due to shunting of blood through the dialysis access; on rare occasions, this may necessitate ligation of the fistula or graft. Because of the vasodilatory and cardiodepressive effects of acetate, its use as the buffer in dialysate was once a common cause of hypotension. Since the introduction of bicarbonate-containing dialysate, dialysis-associated hypotension has become less common. The management of hypotension during dialysis consists of discontinuing ultrafiltration, the administration of 100–250 mL of isotonic saline or 10 mL of 23% saturated hypertonic saline, and administration of salt-poor albumin. Hypotension during dialysis can frequently be prevented by careful evaluation of the dry weight and by ultrafiltration modeling, such that more fluid is removed at the beginning rather than the end of the dialysis procedure. Additional maneuvers include the performance of sequential ultrafiltration followed by dialysis; the use of midodrine, a selective α_1-adrenergic pressor agent; cooling of the dialysate during dialysis treatment; and avoiding heavy meals during dialysis.

Muscle cramps during dialysis are also a common complication of the procedure. The etiology of dialysis-associated cramps remains obscure. Changes in muscle perfusion because of excessively aggressive volume removal, particularly below the estimated dry weight, and the use of low-sodium–containing dialysate, have been proposed as precipitants of dialysis-associated cramps. Strategies that may be used to prevent cramps include reducing volume removal during dialysis, ultrafiltration profiling, and the use of higher concentrations of sodium in the dialysate or sodium modeling (see above).

Anaphylactoid reactions to the dialyzer, particularly on its first use, have been reported most frequently with the bioincompatible cellulosic-containing membranes. With the gradual phasing out of cuprophane membranes in the United States, dialyzer reactions have become relatively uncommon. Dialyzer reactions can be divided into two types, A and B. Type A reactions are attributed to an IgE-mediated intermediate hypersensitivity reaction to ethylene oxide used in the sterilization of new dialyzers. This reaction typically occurs soon after the initiation of a treatment (within the first few minutes) and can progress to full-blown anaphylaxis if the therapy is not promptly discontinued. Treatment with steroids or epinephrine may be needed if symptoms are severe. The type B reaction consists of a symptom complex of nonspecific chest and back pain, which appears to result from complement activation and cytokine release. These symptoms typically occur several minutes into the dialysis run and typically resolve over time with continued dialysis.

Cardiovascular diseases constitute the major causes of death in patients with ESRD. Cardiovascular mortality and event rates are higher in dialysis patients than in patients posttransplantation, although rates are extraordinarily high in both populations. The underlying cause of cardiovascular disease is unclear but may be related to shared risk factors (e.g., diabetes mellitus), chronic inflammation, massive changes in extracellular volume (especially with high interdialytic weight gains), inadequate treatment of hypertension, dyslipidemia, anemia, dystrophic vascular calcification, hyperhomocysteinemia, and, perhaps, alterations in cardiovascular dynamics during the dialysis treatment. Few studies have targeted cardiovascular risk reduction in ESRD patients; none have demonstrated consistent benefit. Nevertheless, most experts recommend conventional cardioprotective strategies (e.g., lipid-lowering agents, aspirin, β-adrenergic antagonists) in dialysis patients based on the patients' cardiovascular risk profile, which appears to be increased by more than an order of magnitude relative to persons unaffected by kidney disease.

PERITONEAL DIALYSIS

In peritoneal dialysis, 1.5–3 L of a dextrose-containing solution is infused into the peritoneal cavity and allowed to dwell for a set period of time, usually 2–4 h. As with hemodialysis, toxic materials are removed through a combination of convective clearance generated through ultrafiltration and diffusive clearance down a concentration gradient. The clearance of solutes and water during a peritoneal dialysis exchange depends on the balance between the movement of solute and water into the peritoneal cavity versus absorption from the peritoneal cavity. The rate of diffusion diminishes with time and eventually stops when equilibration between plasma and dialysate is reached. Absorption of solutes and water from the peritoneal cavity occurs across the peritoneal membrane into the peritoneal capillary circulation and via peritoneal lymphatics into the lymphatic circulation. The rate of peritoneal solute transport varies from patient to patient and may be altered by the presence of infection (peritonitis), drugs, and physical factors such as position and exercise.

FORMS OF PERITONEAL DIALYSIS

Peritoneal dialysis may be carried out as continuous ambulatory peritoneal dialysis (CAPD), continuous cyclic peritoneal dialysis (CCPD), or a combination of both. In CAPD, dialysis solution is manually infused into the peritoneal cavity during the day and exchanged three to five times daily. A nighttime dwell is frequently instilled at bedtime and remains in the peritoneal cavity through the night. The drainage of spent dialysate is performed manually with the assistance of gravity to move fluid out of the abdomen. In CCPD, exchanges are performed in an automated fashion, usually at night; the patient is connected to an automated cycler that performs a series of exchange cycles while the patient sleeps. The number of exchange cycles required to optimize peritoneal solute clearance varies by the peritoneal membrane characteristics; as with hemodialysis, experts suggest careful tracking of solute clearances to ensure dialysis "adequacy."

Peritoneal dialysis solutions are available in volumes typically ranging from 1.5 to 3.0 L. Lactate is the preferred buffer in peritoneal dialysis solutions. The most common additives to peritoneal dialysis solutions are heparin to prevent obstruction of the dialysis catheter lumen with fibrin and antibiotics during an episode of acute peritonitis. Insulin may also be added in patients with diabetes mellitus.

ACCESS TO THE PERITONEAL CAVITY

Access to the peritoneal cavity is obtained through a peritoneal catheter. Catheters used for maintenance peritoneal dialysis are flexible, being made of silicon rubber with numerous side holes at the distal end. These catheters usually have two Dacron cuffs to promote fibroblast proliferation, granulation, and invasion of the cuff. The scarring that occurs around the cuffs anchors the catheter and seals it from bacteria tracking from the skin surface into the peritoneal cavity; it also prevents the external leakage of fluid from the peritoneal cavity. The cuffs are placed in the preperitoneal plane and ~2 cm from the skin surface.

The *peritoneal equilibrium test* is a formal evaluation of peritoneal membrane characteristics that measures the transfer rates of creatinine and glucose across the peritoneal membrane. Patients are classified as low, low–average, high–average, and high "transporters." Patients with rapid equilibration (i.e., high transporters) tend to absorb more glucose and lose efficiency of ultrafiltration with long daytime dwells. High transporters also tend to lose larger quantities of albumin and other proteins across the peritoneal membrane. In general, patients with rapid transporting characteristics require more frequent, shorter dwell time exchanges, nearly always obligating use of a cycler for feasibility. Slower (low and low–average) transporters tend to do well with fewer exchanges. The efficiency of solute clearance also depends on the volume of dialysate infused. Larger volumes allow for greater solute clearance, particularly with CAPD in patients with low and low–average transport characteristics. Interestingly, solute clearance also increases with physical activity, presumably related to more efficient flow dynamics within the peritoneal cavity.

As with hemodialysis, the optimal dose of peritoneal dialysis is unknown. Several observational studies have suggested that higher rates of urea and creatinine clearance (the latter generally measured in L/week) are associated with lower mortality rates and fewer uremic complications. However, a randomized clinical trial (ADEMEX) failed to show a significant reduction in mortality or complications with a relatively large increment in urea clearance. In general, patients on peritoneal dialysis do well when they retain residual kidney function. The rates of technique failure increase with years on dialysis and have been correlated with loss of residual function to a greater extent than loss of peritoneal membrane capacity. Recently, a nonabsorbable carbohydrate (icodextrin) has been introduced as an alternative osmotic agent. Studies have demonstrated more efficient ultrafiltration with icodextrin than with dextrose-containing solutions. Icodextrin is typically used as the "last fill" for patients on CCPD or for the longest dwell in patients on CAPD. For some patients in whom CCPD does not provide sufficient solute clearance, a hybrid approach can be adopted where one or more daytime exchanges are added to the CCPD regimen. While this approach can enhance solute clearance and prolong a patient's capacity to remain on peritoneal dialysis, the burden of the hybrid approach can be overwhelming to some.

COMPLICATIONS DURING PERITONEAL DIALYSIS

The major complications of peritoneal dialysis are peritonitis, catheter-associated nonperitonitis infections, weight gain and other meta-

bolic disturbances, and residual uremia (especially among patients with no residual kidney function).

Peritonitis typically develops when there has been a break in sterile technique during one or more of the exchange procedures. Peritonitis is usually defined by an elevated peritoneal fluid leukocyte count (100/mm³, of which at least 50% are polymorphonuclear neutrophils). The clinical presentation typically consists of pain and cloudy dialysate, often with fever and other constitutional symptoms. The most common culprit organisms are gram-positive cocci, including *Staphylococcus*, reflecting the origin from the skin. Gram-negative rod infections are less common; fungal and mycobacterial infections can be seen in selected patients, particularly after antibacterial therapy. Most cases of peritonitis can be managed either with intraperitoneal or oral antibiotics, depending on the organism; many patients with peritonitis do not require hospitalization. In cases where peritonitis is due to hydrophilic gram negative rods (e.g., *Pseudomonas* sp.) or yeast, antimicrobial therapy is usually not sufficient, and catheter removal is required to ensure complete eradication of infection. Nonperitonitis catheter-associated infections (often termed *tunnel infections*) vary widely in severity. Some cases can be managed with local antibiotic or silver nitrate administration, while others are severe enough to require parenteral antibiotic therapy and catheter removal.

Peritoneal dialysis is associated with a variety of metabolic complications. As noted above, albumin and other proteins can be lost across the peritoneal membrane in concert with the loss of metabolic wastes. The hypoproteinemia induced by peritoneal dialysis obligates a higher dietary protein intake in order to maintain nitrogen balance. Hyperglycemia and weight gain are also common complications of peritoneal dialysis. Several hundred calories in the form of dextrose are absorbed each day, depending on the concentration employed. Peritoneal dialysis patients, particularly those with type II diabetes mellitus, are then prone to other complications of insulin resistance, including hypertriglyceridemia. On the positive side, the continuous nature of peritoneal dialysis usually allows for a more liberal diet, due to continuous removal of potassium and phosphorus—two major dietary components whose accumulation can be hazardous in ESRD.

GLOBAL PERSPECTIVE

The incidence of ESRD is increasing worldwide with longer life expectancies and improved care of infectious and cardiovascular diseases. The management of ESRD varies widely by country and within country by region, and it is influenced by economic and other major factors. In general, peritoneal dialysis is more commonly performed in poorer countries owing to its lower expense and the high cost of establishing in-center hemodialysis units.

ACKNOWLEDGMENT
We are grateful to Dr. Ajay Singh and Dr. Barry Brenner, authors of "Dialysis in the Treatment of Renal Failure" in the 16th edition of Harrison's, for contributions to this chapter.

FURTHER READINGS

BURKART JM et al: Peritoneal dialysis, in *Brenner and Rector's The Kidney*, 7th ed, BM Brenner (ed). Philadelphia, Saunders, 2004

EKNOYAN G et al: Effect of dialysis dose and membrane flux in maintenance hemodialysis. N Engl J Med 346:2010, 2002

FORNI LG, HILTON PJ: Current concepts: Continuous hemofiltration in the treatment of acute renal failure. N Engl J Med 336:1303, 1997

HIMMELFARB J, KLIGER AS: End-stage renal disease measures of quality. Annu Rev Med 58:387, 2007

NATIONAL KIDNEY FOUNDATION: Kidney Disease Quality Initiative Clinical Practice Guidelines: Hemodialysis and peritoneal dialysis adequacy, 2001. Available online at *http://www.kidney.org/professionals/kdoqi/guidelines.cfm*

PANIAGUA R et al: Effects of increased peritoneal clearances on mortality rates in peritoneal dialysis: ADEMEX, a prospective, randomized, controlled trial. J Am Soc Nephrol 13:1307, 2002

RAYNER HC et al: Vascular access results from the Dialysis Outcomes and Practice Patterns Study (DOPPS): Performance against Kidney Disease Outcomes Quality Initiative (K/DOQI) Clinical Practice Guidelines. Am J Kidney Dis. 44:S22, 2004

U.S. RENAL DATA SYSTEM: USRDS 2005 Annual Data Report: Atlas of End-Stage Renal Disease in the United States. Bethesda, National Institutes of Health, National Institute of Diabetes and Digestive and Kidney Disease, 2005

276 Transplantation in the Treatment of Renal Failure

Charles B. Carpenter, Edgar L. Milford, Mohamed H. Sayegh

Transplantation of the human kidney is the treatment of choice for advanced chronic renal failure. Worldwide, tens of thousands of such procedures have been performed. When azathioprine and prednisone were initially used as immunosuppressive drugs in the 1960s, the results with properly matched familial donors were superior to those with organs from deceased donors—namely, 75–90% compared with 50–60% graft survival rates at 1 year. During the 1970s and 1980s, the success rate at the 1-year mark for deceased-donor transplants rose progressively. By the time cyclosporine was introduced in the early 1980s, deceased-donor grafts had a 70% 1-year survival and reached the 82% level in the mid-1990s. After the first year, graft survival curves show an exponential decline in numbers of functioning grafts from which a half-life ($t_{1/2}$) in years is calculated; this has increased by only 2 years since the 1980s.

Mortality rates after transplantation are highest in the first year and are age-related: 2% for ages 18–34 years, 3% for ages 35–49 years, and 6.8% for ages ≥50–60 years. These rates compare favorably with those in the chronic dialysis population, even after risk adjustments for age, diabetes, and cardiovascular status. Occasionally, acute irreversible rejection may occur after many months of good function, especially if the patient neglects to take the prescribed immunosuppressive drugs. Most grafts, however, succumb at varying rates to a chronic vascular obliterative process termed *chronic allograft nephropathy*, the pathogenesis of which is incompletely understood. Overall, transplantation returns most patients to an improved lifestyle and an improved life expectancy compared with patients on dialysis. There are at least 100,000 patients with functioning kidney transplants in the United States, and when one adds in the numbers of kidney transplants in centers around the world, the total activity is doubled.

RECENT ACTIVITY AND RESULTS

In 1994 there were more than 7000 deceased donor kidney transplants and 3000 living donor transplants in the United States. Table 276-1 shows an increase in numbers of transplants for deceased and living donors over the decade ending in 2003. Whereas deceased donor availability rose by 11%, the living donor rate more than doubled. The backlog of patients with end-stage renal disease (ESRD) has been increasing every year, and it always lags behind the number of available donors. In this decade, the size of the waiting list more than doubled, and the percentage of those on the waiting list receiving deceased donor transplants dropped from 28 to 14%. The increase in the living donor rate is in response to the demand; it continues to rise to exceed the number of deceased donor grafts. As there were 16,534 new registrants added to the waiting list in 1994 and 24,493 in 2003, demand will continue to exceed supply. Waiting lists continue to grow, and the average wait time for a cadaver kidney is now >4 years in many locations.

The overall results of transplantation are presented in Table 276-2 as the survival of grafts and of patients. At the 1-year mark, graft survival is higher for living donor recipients, most likely because those grafts are not subject to as much ischemic injury. The more powerful drugs now in use for immunosuppression have almost equalized the risk of graft rejection in all patients for the first year. At 5 and 10 years, however, there has been a steeper decline in survival of those with deceased-donor kidneys.

RECIPIENT SELECTION

There are few absolute contraindications to renal transplantation. The transplant procedure is relatively noninvasive, as the organ is placed in the inguinal fossa without entering the peritoneal cavity. Recipients without perioperative complications can often be discharged from the hospital in excellent condition within 5 days of the operation.

Virtually all patients with ESRD who receive a transplant have a higher life expectancy than risk-matched patients who remain on dialysis. Even though diabetics and older candidates have a higher mortality rate than other transplant recipients, their survival is improved with transplantation compared with remaining on dialysis. This global benefit of transplantation as a treatment modality poses substantial ethical issues for policy makers, as the number of deceased kidneys available is far from sufficient to meet the current needs of the candidates. The current standard of care is that the candidate should have a life expectancy of >5 years to be put on a deceased organ wait list. Even for living donation, the candidate should have >5 years of life expectancy. This standard has been established because the benefits of kidney transplantation over dialysis are realized only after a perioperative period in which the mortality is higher in transplanted patients than in dialysis patients with comparable risk profiles.

All candidates must have a thorough risk-versus-benefit evaluation prior to being approved for transplantation. In particular, an aggressive approach to diagnosis of correctable coronary artery disease, presence of latent or indolent infection (HIV, hepatitis B or C, tuberculosis), and

TABLE 276-1 GROWTH IN KIDNEY TRANSPLANTATION FROM 1994 TO 2003 IN THE UNITED STATES

	1994			2003		
	Number of Transplants	Size of Wait List	Patients Receiving Grafts, %	Number of Transplants	Size of Wait List	Patients Receiving Grafts, %
Deceased donor	7533	27,196	28	8389	57,211	14
Living donor	3007			6464		
Total	10,540			14,853		

Source: Data from Summary Tables, 2004 and 2005 Annual Reports, Scientific Registry of Transplant Recipients.

TABLE 276-2 MEAN RATES OF GRAFT AND PATIENT SURVIVALS FOR KIDNEYS TRANSPLANTED IN THE UNITED STATES FROM 1992 TO 2002[a]

	1-Year Follow-Up		5-Year Follow-Up		10-Year Follow-Up	
	Grafts, %	Patients, %	Grafts, %	Patients, %	Grafts, %	Patients, %
Deceased donor	89	95	67	81	41	61
Living donor	95	98	80	90	56	76

[a]All patients transplanted are included, and the follow-up unadjusted survival data from the 1-, 5-, and 10-year periods are presented to show the attrition rates over time within the two types of organ donors.
Source: Data from Summary Tables, 2004 and 2005 Annual Reports, Scientific Registry of Transplant Recipients.

neoplasm should be a routine part of the candidate workup. Most transplant centers consider overt AIDS and active hepatitis to be absolute contraindications to transplantation because of the high risk of opportunistic infection. Some centers are now transplanting individuals with hepatitis and even HIV infection under strict protocols to determine whether the risks and benefits favor transplantation over dialysis.

Among the few absolute "immunologic" contraindications to transplantation is the presence of a potentially harmful antibody against the donor kidney at the time of the anticipated transplant. Harmful antibodies that can cause very early graft loss include natural antibodies against the ABO blood group antigens and antibodies against human leukocyte antigen (HLA) class I (A, B, C) or class II (DR) antigens. These antibodies are routinely excluded by proper screening of the candidate's ABO compatibility, HLA typing of donor and recipient, and direct cross-matching of candidate serum with lymphocytes of the donor.

DONOR SELECTION

Donors can be deceased or volunteer living donors. The latter are usually family members selected to have at least partial compatibility for HLA antigens. Living volunteer donors should be normal on physical examination and of the same major ABO blood group, because crossing major blood group barriers prejudices survival of the allograft. It is possible, however, to transplant a kidney of a type O donor into an A, B, or AB recipient. Selective renal arteriography should be performed on donors to rule out the presence of multiple or abnormal renal arteries because the surgical procedure is difficult and the ischemic time of the transplanted kidney long when vascular abnormalities exist. Transplant surgeons are now using a laparoscopic method to isolate and remove the living donor kidney. This operation has the advantage of less evident surgical scars, and, because there is less tissue trauma, the laparoscopic donors have a substantially shorter hospital stay and less discomfort than those who have the traditional surgery. Deceased donors should be free of malignant neoplastic disease, hepatitis, and HIV because of possible transmission to the recipient. Increased risk of graft failure exists when the donor is elderly or has renal failure and when the kidney has a prolonged period of ischemia and storage.

In the United States, there is a coordinated national system of regulations, allocation support, and outcomes analysis for kidney transplantation called the Organ Procurement Transplant Network. It is now possible to remove deceased donor kidneys and to maintain them for up to 48 h on cold pulsatile perfusion or simple flushing and cooling. This approach permits adequate time for typing, cross-matching, transportation, and selection problems to be solved.

TISSUE TYPING AND CLINICAL IMMUNOGENETICS

Matching for antigens of the HLA major histocompatibility gene complex (Chap. 309) is an important criterion for selection of donors for renal allografts. Each mammalian species has a single chromosomal region that encodes the strong, or major, transplantation antigens, and this region on the human sixth chromosome is called *HLA*. HLA antigens have been classically defined by serologic techniques, but methods to define specific nucleotide sequences in genomic DNA are increasingly being used. Other "minor" antigens may play crucial roles, in addition to the ABH(O) blood groups and endothelial antigens that are not shared with lymphocytes. The Rh system is not expressed on graft tissue. Evidence for designation of HLA as the genetic region encoding major transplantation antigens comes from the success rate in living related donor renal and bone marrow transplantation, with superior results in HLA-identical sibling pairs. Nevertheless, 5% of HLA-identical renal allografts are rejected, often within the first weeks after transplantation. These failures represent states of prior sensitization to non-HLA antigens. Non-HLA minor antigens are relatively weak when initially encountered and are, therefore, suppressible by conventional immunosuppressive therapy. Once priming has occurred, however, secondary responses are much more refractory to treatment.

LIVING DONORS

When first-degree relatives are donors, graft survival rates at 1 year are 5–7% greater than those for deceased-donor grafts. The 5-year survival rates still favor the partially matched (3/6 HLA mismatched) family donor over a randomly selected cadaver donor (Table 276-3). In addition, living donors provide the advantage of immediate availability. For both living and deceased donors, the 5-year outcomes are poor if there is a complete (6/6) HLA mismatch.

The survival rate of living unrelated renal allografts is as high as that of perfectly HLA-matched cadaver renal transplants and comparable to that of kidneys from living relatives. This outcome is likely a consequence of both short cold ischemia time and the extra care taken to document that the condition and renal function of the donor are optimal before proceeding with a living unrelated donation. It is illegal in the United States to purchase organs for transplantation.

Concern has been expressed regarding the potential risk to a volunteer kidney donor of premature renal failure after several years of increased blood flow and hyperfiltration per nephron in the remaining kidney. There are a few reports of the development of hypertension, proteinuria, and even lesions of focal segmental sclerosis in donors over long-term follow-up. Difficulties in donors followed for ≥20 years are unusual, however, and it may be that having a single kidney becomes significant only when another condition, such as hypertension, is superimposed. It is also desirable to consider the risk of development of type 1 diabetes mellitus in a family member who is a potential donor to a diabetic renal failure patient. Anti-insulin and anti-islet cell antibodies should be measured, and glucose tolerance tests should be performed in such donors to exclude a prediabetic state.

PRESENSITIZATION

A positive cross-match of recipient serum with donor T lymphocytes representing anti-HLA class I is usually predictive of an acute vasculitic event termed *hyperacute rejection*. Patients with anti-HLA antibodies can be safely transplanted if careful cross-matching of donor blood lymphocytes with recipient serum is performed. The known sources of such sensitization are blood transfusion, prior transplant, and pregnancy. Patients sustained by dialysis often show fluctuating antibody titers and specificity patterns. At the time of assignment of a cadaveric kidney, cross-matches are performed with at least a current serum. Previously analyzed antibody specificities and additional cross-matches are performed accordingly. Techniques for cross-matching are not universally standardized; however, at least two techniques are employed in most laboratories. The minimal purpose for the cross-match is avoidance of hyperacute rejection mediated by recipient antibodies to donor HLA class I antigens. Sensitive tests, such as the use of flow cytometry, can be useful for avoidance of accelerated, and often untreatable, early graft rejection in patients receiving second or third transplants. Donor T lymphocytes, which express only class I antigens, are used as targets for detection of anti–class I (HLA-A and -B) antibodies. Preformed anti–class II (HLA-DR) antibod-

TABLE 276-3	EFFECT OF HLA-A, -B, -DR MISMATCHING ON KIDNEY GRAFT SURVIVAL	
Degree of Donor Mismatch	**1-Year Survival, %**	**5-Year Survival, %**
Cadaver donor (all)	89.2	61.3
0/6-HLA mismatch	91.3	68.2
3/6-HLA mismatch	90.1	60.8
6/6-HLA mismatch	85.2	55.3
Living related donor (all)	94.7	76.0
0/6-HLA mismatch	96.7	87.0
3/6-HLA mismatch	94.3	73.2
6/6-HLA mismatch	92.7	57.7
Living unrelated donor	95.3	77.4

Note: 0-mismatched related donor transplants are virtually all from HLA-identical siblings, while 3/6-mismatched transplants can be one haplotype mismatched (1-A, 1-B, and 1-DR antigen) from parent, child or sibling; 6/6-HLA-mismatched living related kidneys are derived from siblings or relatives outside of the nuclear family.

ies against the donor carry a higher risk of graft loss as well, particularly in recipients who have suffered early loss of a prior kidney transplant. B lymphocytes expressing both class I and class II antigens are used in these assays. Non-HLA antigens restricted in expression to endothelium and sometimes monocytes have been described, but clinical relevance is not well established. A series of minor histocompatibility antigens do not elicit antibodies, and sensitization to these is detectable only by cytotoxic T cells, an assay too cumbersome for routine use. Desensitization prior to transplantation by reducing the level of antidonor antibodies via plasmapheresis of blood, administration of large doses of immunoglobulin, or both has been useful in reducing the hazard of hyperacute rejection.

IMMUNOLOGY OF REJECTION

Both cellular and humoral (antibody-mediated) effector mechanisms can play roles in kidney transplant rejection. Antibodies can also initiate a form of antibody-dependent but cell-mediated cytotoxicity by recipient cells that bear receptors for the Fc portion of immunoglobulin.

Cellular rejection is mediated by lymphocytes that respond to HLA antigens expressed within the organ. The CD4+ lymphocyte responds to class II (HLA-DR) incompatibility by proliferating and releasing proinflammatory cytokines that augment the proliferative response of both CD4+ and CD8+ cells. CD8+ cytotoxic lymphocyte precursors respond primarily to class I (HLA-A, -B) antigens and mature into cytotoxic effector cells. The cytotoxic effector ("killer") T cells cause organ damage through direct contact and lysis of donor target cells. The natural role of HLA antigen molecules is to present processed peptide fragments of antigen to T lymphocytes, the fragments residing in a "groove" of the HLA molecule distal to the cell surface. T cells can be directly stimulated by intact non-self HLA molecules expressed on donor parenchymal cells and residual donor leukocytes residing in the kidney interstitium. In addition, donor HLA molecules can be processed by a variety of donor or recipient cells capable of antigen presentation of peptides and then presented to T cells in the same manner as most other antigens. The former mode of stimulation is sometimes called *direct presentation* and the latter mode called *indirect presentation* (Fig. 276-1). There is evidence that non-HLA antigens can also play a role in renal transplant rejection episodes. Recipients who receive a kidney from an HLA-identical sibling can have rejection episodes and require maintenance immunosuppression, while identical twin transplants require no immunosuppression. There are documented non-HLA antigens, such as an endothelial-specific antigen system with limited polymorphism and a tubular antigen, that can be targets of humoral or cellular rejection responses, respectively.

IMMUNOSUPPRESSIVE TREATMENT

Immunosuppressive therapy, as presently available, generally suppresses all immune responses, including those to bacteria, fungi, and even malignant tumors. In the 1950s when clinical renal transplantation began, sublethal total-body irradiation was employed. We have now reached the point where sophisticated pharmacologic immunosuppression is available, but it still has the hazard of promoting infection and malignancy. In general, all clinically useful drugs are more selective to primary than to memory immune responses. Agents to suppress the immune response are discussed in the following paragraphs, and those currently in clinical use are listed in Table 276-4.

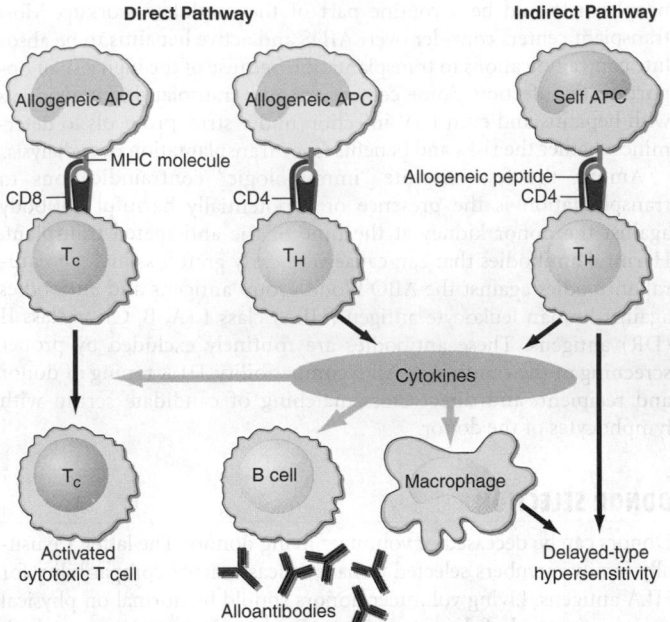

FIGURE 276-1 Recognition pathways for major histocompatibility complex (MHC) antigens. Graft rejection is initiated by CD4 helper T lymphocytes (T_H) having antigen receptors that bind to specific complexes of peptides and MHC class II molecules on antigen-presenting cells (APC). In transplantation, in contrast to other immunologic responses, there are two sets of T cell clones involved in rejection. In the direct pathway the class II MHC of donor allogeneic APCs is recognized by CD4 T_H cells that bind to the intact MHC molecule, and class I MHC allogeneic cells are recognized by CD8 T cells. The latter generally proliferate into cytotoxic cells (T_C). In the indirect pathway, the incompatible MHC molecules are processed into peptides that are presented by the self-APCs of the recipient. The indirect, but not the direct, pathway is the normal physiologic process in T cell recognition of foreign antigens. Once T_H cells are activated, they proliferate, and by secretion of cytokines and direct contact exert strong helper effects on macrophages, T_C, and B cells. *(From Sayegh and Turka, Copyright 1998, Massachusetts Medical Society. All rights reserved.)*

TABLE 276-4 MAINTENANCE IMMUNOSUPPRESSIVE DRUGS

Agent	Pharmacology	Mechanisms	Side Effects
Glucocorticoids	Increased bioavailability with hypoalbuminemia and liver disease; prednisone/prednisolone generally used	Binds cytosolic receptors and heat shock proteins. Blocks transcription of IL-1,-2,-3,-6, TNF-α, and IFN-γ	Hypertension, glucose intolerance, dyslipidemia, osteoporosis
Cyclosporine (CsA)	Lipid-soluble polypeptide, variable absorption, microemulsion more predictable	Trimolecular complex with cyclophilin and calcineurin → block in cytokine (e.g., IL-2) production; however, stimulates TGF-β production	Nephrotoxicity, hypertension, dyslipidemia, glucose intolerance, hirsutism/hyperplasia of gums
Tacrolimus (FK506)	Macrolide, well absorbed	Trimolecular complex with FKBP-12 and calcineurin → block in cytokine (e.g., IL-2) production; may stimulate TGF-β production	Similar to CsA, but hirsutism/hyperplasia of gums unusual, and diabetes more likely
Azathioprine	Mercaptopurine analogue	Hepatic metabolites inhibit purine synthesis	Marrow suppression (WBC > RBC > platelets)
Mycophenolate mofetil (MMF)	Metabolized to mycophenolic acid	Inhibits purine synthesis via inosine monophosphate dehydrogenase	Diarrhea/cramps; dose-related liver and marrow suppression is uncommon
Sirolimus	Macrolide, poor oral bioavailability	Complexes with FKBP-12 and then blocks p70 S6 kinase in the IL-2 receptor pathway for proliferation	Hyperlipidemia, thrombocytopenia

Note: IL, interleukin; TNF, tumor necrosis factor; IFN, interferon; TGF, transforming growth factor; FKBP-12, FK506 binding protein 12; WBC, white blood cells; RBC, red blood cells.

DRUGS

Azathioprine, an analogue of mercaptopurine, was for two decades the keystone to immunosuppressive therapy in humans but has now given way to more effective agents. This agent can inhibit synthesis of DNA, RNA, or both. Because cell division and proliferation are a necessary part of the immune response to antigenic stimulation, suppression by this agent may be mediated by the inhibition of mitosis of immunologically competent lymphoid cells, interfering with synthesis of DNA. Alternatively, immunosuppression may be brought about by blocking the synthesis of RNA (possibly messenger RNA), inhibiting processing of antigens prior to lymphocyte stimulation. Therapy with azathioprine in doses of 1.5–2.0 mg/kg per d is generally added to cyclosporine as a means of decreasing the requirements for the latter. Because azathioprine is rapidly metabolized by the liver, its dosage need not be varied directly in relation to renal function, even though renal failure results in retention of the metabolites of azathioprine. Reduction in dosage is required because of leukopenia and occasionally thrombocytopenia. Excessive amounts of azathioprine may also cause jaundice, anemia, and alopecia. If it is essential to administer allopurinol concurrently, the azathioprine dose must be reduced. As inhibition of xanthine oxidase delays degradation, this combination is best avoided.

Mycophenolate mofetil (MMF) is now used in place of azathioprine in most centers. It has a similar mode of action and a mild degree of gastrointestinal toxicity but produces minimal bone marrow suppression. Its advantage is its increased potency in preventing or reversing rejection. Patients with hyperuricemia can be given allopurinol without adjustment of the MMF dose. The usual dose is 2–3 g/d in divided doses.

Glucocorticoids are important adjuncts to immunosuppressive therapy. Of all the agents employed, prednisone has effects that are easiest to assess, and in large doses it is usually effective for the reversal of rejection. In general, 200–300 mg prednisone is given immediately prior to or at the time of transplantation, and the dosage is reduced to 30 mg within a week. The side effects of the glucocorticoids, particularly impairment of wound healing and predisposition to infection, make it desirable to taper the dose as rapidly as possible in the immediate postoperative period. Many centers have protocols for early discontinuance or avoidance of steroids because of long-term adverse effects on bone, skin, and glucose metabolism. For treatment of acute rejection, methylprednisolone, 0.5–1.0 g IV, is administered immediately upon diagnosis of beginning rejection and continued once daily for 3 days. When the drug is effective, the results are usually apparent within 96 h. Such "pulse" doses are not effective in chronic rejection. Most patients whose renal function is stable after 6 months or a year do not require large doses of prednisone; maintenance doses of 10–15 mg/d are the rule. Many patients tolerate an alternate-day course of steroids without an increased risk of rejection. A major effect of steroids is on the monocyte-macrophage system, preventing the release of interleukin (IL) 6 and IL-1.

Cyclosporine is a fungal peptide with potent immunosuppressive activity. It acts on the calcineurin pathway to block transcription of mRNA for IL-2 and other proinflammatory cytokines, thereby inhibiting T cell proliferation. Although it works alone, cyclosporine is more effective in conjunction with glucocorticoids and MMF. Clinical results with tens of thousands of renal transplants have been impressive. Of its toxic effects (nephrotoxicity, hepatotoxicity, hirsutism, tremor, gingival hyperplasia, diabetes), only nephrotoxicity presents a serious management problem and is further discussed below.

Tacrolimus (previously called FK506) is a fungal macrolide that has the same mode of action as cyclosporine, as well as a similar side-effect profile; it does not, however, produce hirsutism or gingival hyperplasia. De novo diabetes mellitus is more common with tacrolimus. The drug was first used in liver transplantation and may substitute for cyclosporine entirely or be tried as an alternative in renal patients whose rejections are poorly controlled by cyclosporine.

Sirolimus (previously called rapamycin) is another fungal macrolide but has a different mode of action, i.e., it inhibits T cell growth factor signaling pathways, preventing the response to IL-2 and other cytokines. Sirolimus can be used in conjunction with cyclosporine or tacrolimus, or with MMF, to avoid calcineurin inhibitors. Its use with tacrolimus alone shows promise as a steroid-sparing regimen, especially in patients who would benefit from pancreatic islet cell transplantation, where steroids have an adverse effect on islet survival.

ANTIBODIES TO LYMPHOCYTES

When serum from animals made immune to host lymphocytes is injected into the recipient, a marked suppression of cellular immunity to the tissue graft results. The action on cell-mediated immunity is greater than on humoral immunity. A globulin fraction of serum [antilymphocyte globulin (ALG)] is the agent generally employed. For use in humans, peripheral human lymphocytes, thymocytes, or lymphocytes from spleens or thoracic duct fistulas have been injected into horses, rabbits, or goats to produce antilymphocyte serum, from which the globulin fraction is then separated. A rabbit antithymocyte globulin (Thymoglobulin) is the most common agent currently in use. Monoclonal antibodies against defined lymphocyte subsets offer a more precise and standardized form of therapy. OKT3 is directed to the CD3 molecules that form a portion of the T cell antigen-receptor complex and is thus expressed on all mature T cells.

Another approach to more selective therapy is to target the 55-kDa alpha chain of the IL-2 receptor, expressed only on T cells that have been recently activated. Two such antibodies to the IL-2 receptor, in which either a chimeric protein has been made between mouse Fab with human Fc (basiliximab) or the antibody has been "humanized" by splicing the combining sites of the mouse into a molecule that is 90% human IgG (daclizumab), are in use for prophylaxis of acute rejection in the immediate posttransplant period. They are effective at decreasing the acute rejection rate and have few adverse side effects.

More recently, two new strategies have involved administration of engineered biologic agents: a depleting T cell antibody (alemtuzumab) as induction therapy to minimize maintenance immunosuppression, and a fusion protein (LEA29Y) to block B7 T cell co-stimulatory signals. The latter has shown promise in phase 2 trials and is currently being tested in phase 3 trials in kidney transplantation.

CLINICAL COURSE AND MANAGEMENT OF THE RECIPIENT

Adequate hemodialysis should be performed within 48 h of surgery, and care should be taken that the serum potassium level is not markedly elevated so that intraoperative cardiac arrhythmias can be averted. The diuresis that commonly occurs postoperatively must be carefully monitored; in some instances, it may be massive, reflecting the inability of ischemic tubules to regulate sodium and water excretion; with large diureses, massive potassium losses may occur. Most chronically uremic patients have some excess of extracellular fluid, and it is useful to maintain an expanded fluid volume in the immediate postoperative period. Acute tubular necrosis (ATN) may cause immediate oliguria or may follow an initial short period of graft function. ATN is most likely when cadaveric donors have been underperfused or if the interval between cessation of blood flow and organ harvest (warm ischemic time) is more than a few minutes. Recovery usually occurs within 3 weeks, although periods as long as 6 weeks have been reported. Superimposition of rejection on ATN is common, and the differential diagnosis may be difficult without a graft biopsy. Cyclosporine therapy prolongs ATN, and some patients do not diurese until the dose is drastically reduced. Many centers avoid starting cyclosporine for the first several days, using ALG or a monoclonal antibody along with MMF and prednisone until renal function is established. Figure 276-2 illustrates an algorithm followed by many transplant centers for early posttransplant management of recipients at high or low risk of early renal dysfunction.

THE REJECTION EPISODE

Early diagnosis of rejection allows prompt institution of therapy to preserve renal function and to prevent irreversible damage. Clinical evidence of rejection is rarely characterized by fever, swelling, and tenderness over the allograft. Rejection may present only with a rise in serum creatinine, with or without a reduction in urine volume. The focus should be on ruling out other causes of functional deterioration.

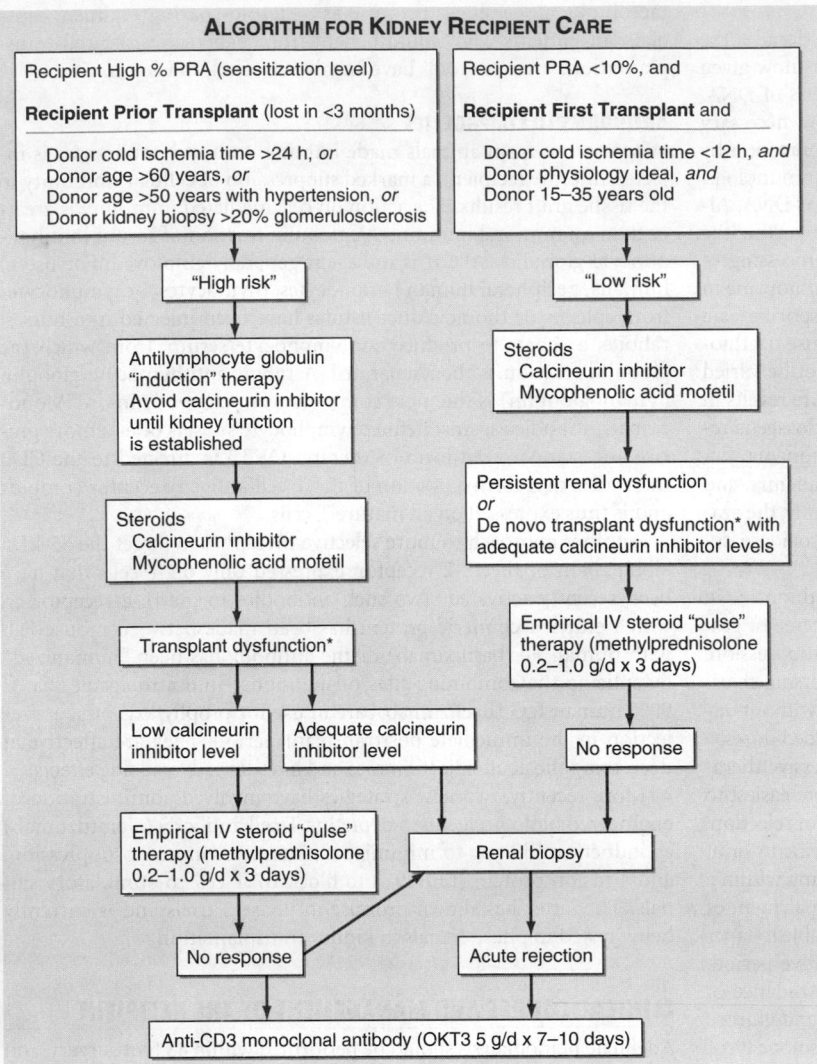

ALGORITHM FOR KIDNEY RECIPIENT CARE

Recipient High % PRA (sensitization level)

Recipient Prior Transplant (lost in <3 months)

Donor cold ischemia time >24 h, *or*
Donor age >60 years, *or*
Donor age >50 years with hypertension, *or*
Donor kidney biopsy >20% glomerulosclerosis

Recipient PRA <10%, and

Recipient First Transplant and

Donor cold ischemia time <12 h, *and*
Donor physiology ideal, *and*
Donor 15–35 years old

"High risk"

"Low risk"

Antilymphocyte globulin
"induction" therapy
Avoid calcineurin inhibitor
until kidney function
is established

Steroids
  Calcineurin inhibitor
  Mycophenolic acid mofetil

Steroids
  Calcineurin inhibitor
  Mycophenolic acid mofetil

Persistent renal dysfunction
or
De novo transplant dysfunction* with
adequate calcineurin inhibitor levels

Transplant dysfunction*

Empirical IV steroid "pulse"
therapy (methylprednisolone
0.2–1.0 g/d x 3 days)

Low calcineurin
inhibitor level

Adequate calcineurin
inhibitor level

No response

Empirical IV steroid "pulse"
therapy (methylprednisolone
0.2–1.0 g/d x 3 days)

Renal biopsy

No response

Acute rejection

Anti-CD3 monoclonal antibody (OKT3 5 g/d x 7–10 days)

FIGURE 276-2 A typical algorithm for early posttransplant care of the kidney recipient. If any of the recipient or donor "high-risk" factors exist, more aggressive management is called for. Low-risk patients can be treated with a standard immuno-suppressive regimen. Patients at higher risk of rejection or early ischemic and nephro-toxic transplant dysfunction are often induced with an antilymphocyte globulin to provide more potent early immunosuppression or to spare calcineurin nephrotoxicity. *When there is early transplant dysfunction, prerenal, obstructive, and vascular causes must be ruled out by ultrasonographic examination. The panel reactive antibody (PRA) is a quantitation of how much antibody is present in a candidate against a panel of cells representing the distribution of antigens in the donor pool.

Doppler ultrasonography or magnetic resonance angiography may be useful in ascertaining changes in the renal vasculature and in renal blood flow, even in the absence of changes in urinary flow. Thrombosis of the renal vein occurs rarely; it may be reversible if caused by technical factors and intervention is prompt. Diagnostic ultrasound is the procedure of choice to rule out urinary obstruction or to confirm the presence of peri-renal collections of urine, blood, or lymph. When renal function has been good initially, a rise in the serum creatinine level is the most sensitive and reliable indicator of possible rejection and may be the only sign.

Calcineurin inhibitors (cyclosporine or tacrolimus) may cause deterioration in renal function in a manner similar to a rejection episode. In fact, rejection processes tend to be more indolent with these inhibitors, and the only way to make a diagnosis may be by renal biopsy. Calcineurin inhibitors have an afferent arteriolar constrictor effect on the kidney and may produce permanent vascular and interstitial injury after sustained high-dose therapy. Addition of angiotensin-converting enzyme (ACE) inhibitors or nonsteroidal anti-inflammatory drugs are likely to raise serum creatinine levels. The former are generally safe to

use after the early months, while the latter are best avoided in all renal transplant patients. There is no universally accepted lesion that makes a diagnosis of calcineurin inhibitor toxicity, although interstitial fibrosis, isometric tubular vacuolization, and thickening of arteriolar walls have been noted by some. Basically, if the biopsy does not reveal moderate and active cellular rejection activity, the serum creatinine will most likely respond to a reduction in dose. Blood levels of drug can be useful if they are very high or very low but do not correlate precisely with renal function, although serial changes in a patient can be useful. If rejection activity is present in the biopsy, appropriate therapy is indicated. The first rejection episode is usually treated with IV administration of methylprednisolone, 500–1000 mg daily for 3 days. Failure to respond is an indication for antibody therapy, usually with OKT3 or antithymocyte globulin.

Biopsy may be necessary to confirm the presence of rejection; when evidence of antibody-mediated injury is present with endothelial injury and deposition of complement component C4d is detected by fluorescence labeling, one can usually detect the antibody in recipient blood. The prognosis is poor, and aggressive use of plasmapheresis, immunoglobulin infusions, or anti-CD20 monoclonal antibody (rituximab) that targets B lymphocytes is indicated.

MANAGEMENT PROBLEMS

The usual clinical manifestations of infection in the posttransplant period are blunted by immunosuppressive therapy. The major toxic effect of azathioprine is bone marrow suppression, which is less likely with MMF, while calcineurin inhibitors have no marrow effects. All drugs predispose to unusual opportunistic infections, however. The typical times after transplantation when the most common opportunistic infections occur are tabulated in Table 276-5. The signs and symptoms of infection may be masked or distorted. Fever without obvious cause is common, and only after days or weeks may it become apparent that it has a viral or fungal origin. Bacterial infections are most common during the first month after transplantation. The importance of blood cultures in such patients cannot be overemphasized because systemic infection without obvious foci is frequent, although wound infections with or without urinary fistulas are most common. Particularly ominous are rapidly occurring pulmonary lesions, which may result in death within 5 days of onset. When these become apparent, immunosuppressive agents should be discontinued, except for maintenance doses of prednisone.

Aggressive diagnostic procedures, including transbronchial and open lung biopsy, are frequently indicated. In the case of *Pneumocystis carinii*

TABLE 276-5	THE MOST COMMON OPPORTUNISTIC INFECTIONS IN THE RENAL TRANSPLANT RECIPIENT
Peritransplant (<1 month)	Late (>6 months)
Wound infections	*Aspergillus*
Herpesvirus	*Nocardia*
Oral candidiasis	BK virus (polyoma)
Urinary tract infection	Herpes zoster
Early (1–6 months)	Hepatitis B
Pneumocystis carinii	Hepatitis C
Cytomegalovirus	
Legionella	
Listeria	
Hepatitis B	
Hepatitis C	

PART 12

Disorders of the Kidney and Urinary Tract

(Chap. 200) infection, trimethoprim-sulfamethoxazole (TMP-SMX) is the treatment of choice; amphotericin B has been used effectively in systemic fungal infections. Prophylaxis against *P. carinii* with daily or alternate-day low-dose TMP-SMX is very effective. Involvement of the oropharynx with *Candida* (Chap. 196) may be treated with local nystatin. Tissue-invasive fungal infections require treatment with systemic agents such as fluconazole. Small doses (a total of 300 mg) of amphotericin given over a period of 2 weeks may be effective in fungal infections refractory to fluconazole. Macrolide antibiotics, especially ketoconazole and erythromycin, and some calcium channel blockers (diltiazem, verapamil) compete with calcineurin inhibitors for P450 catabolism and cause elevated levels of these immunosuppressive drugs. Analeptics, such as phenytoin and carbamazepine, will increase catabolism to result in low levels. *Aspergillus* (Chap. 197), *Nocardia* (Chap. 155), and especially cytomegalovirus (CMV) (Chap. 175) infections also occur.

CMV is a common and dangerous DNA virus in transplant recipients. It does not generally appear until the end of the first posttransplant month. Active CMV infection is sometimes associated, or occasionally confused, with rejection episodes. Patients at highest risk for severe CMV disease are those without anti-CMV antibodies who receive a graft from a CMV antibody–positive donor (15% mortality). Valganciclovir is a cost-effective and bioavailable oral form of ganciclovir that has been proven effective in both prophylaxis and treatment of CMV disease. Early diagnosis in a febrile patient with clinical suspicion of CMV disease can be made by determining CMV viral load in the blood. A rise in IgM antibodies to CMV is also diagnostic. Culture of CMV from blood may be less sensitive. Tissue invasion of CMV is common in the gastrointestinal tract and lungs. CMV retinopathy occurs late in the course, if untreated. Treatment of active CMV disease with valganciclovir is always indicated. In many patients immune to CMV, viral activation can occur with major immunosuppressive regimens.

The polyoma group (BK, JC, SV40) is another class of DNA viruses that can become dormant in kidneys and can be activated by immunosuppression. When reactivation occurs with BK there is a 50% chance of progressive fibrosis and loss of the graft within 1 year by the activated virus. The use of tacrolimus has been associated with the highest risk.

Renal biopsy is necessary for the diagnosis. There are promising results with leflunomide and cidofovir, but it is most important to reduce the immunosuppressive load.

The complications of glucocorticoid therapy are well known and include gastrointestinal bleeding, impairment of wound healing, osteoporosis, diabetes mellitus, cataract formation, and hemorrhagic pancreatitis. The treatment of unexplained jaundice in transplant patients should include cessation or reduction of immunosuppressive drugs if hepatitis or drug toxicity is suspected. Therapy in such circumstances often does not result in rejection of a graft, at least for several weeks. Acyclovir is effective in therapy of herpes simplex virus infections.

CHRONIC LESIONS OF THE TRANSPLANTED KIDNEY

While 1-year transplant survival is excellent, most recipients experience progressive decline in kidney function over time thereafter. Chronic renal transplant dysfunction can be caused by recurrent disease, hypertension, cyclosporine or tacrolimus nephrotoxicity, chronic immunologic rejection, secondary focal glomerulosclerosis, or a combination of these pathophysiologies. Chronic vascular changes with intimal proliferation and medial hypertrophy are commonly found. Control of systemic and intrarenal hypertension with ACE inhibitors is thought to have a beneficial influence on the rate of progression of chronic renal transplant dysfunction. Renal biopsy can distinguish subacute cellular rejection from recurrent disease or secondary focal sclerosis.

MALIGNANCY

The incidence of tumors in patients on immunosuppressive therapy is 5–6%, or approximately 100 times greater than that in the general population of the same age range. The most common lesions are cancer of the skin and lips and carcinoma in situ of the cervix, as well as lymphomas such as non-Hodgkin's lymphoma. The risks are increased in proportion

to the total immunosuppressive load administered and time elapsed since transplantation. Surveillance for skin and cervical cancers is necessary.

OTHER COMPLICATIONS

Hypercalcemia after transplantation may indicate failure of hyperplastic parathyroid glands to regress. Aseptic necrosis of the head of the femur is probably due to preexisting hyperparathyroidism, with aggravation by glucocorticoid treatment. With improved management of calcium and phosphorus metabolism during chronic dialysis, the incidence of parathyroid-related complications has fallen dramatically. Persistent hyperparathyroid activity may require subtotal parathyroidectomy.

Hypertension may be caused by (1) native kidney disease; (2) rejection activity in the transplant; (3) renal artery stenosis, if an end-to-end anastomosis was constructed with an iliac artery branch; and (4) renal calcineurin inhibitor toxicity. This toxicity may improve with reduction in dose. Whereas ACE inhibitors may be useful, calcium channel blockers are more frequently used initially. Amelioration of hypertension to the range of 120–130/70–80 mmHg should be the goal in all patients.

While most transplant patients have a robust production of erythropoietin and normalization of hemoglobin, *anemia* is commonly seen in the posttransplant period. Often the anemia is attributable to bone marrow–suppressant immunosuppressive medications such as azathioprine, MMF, or sirolimus. Gastrointestinal bleeding is a common side effect of high-dose and long-term steroid administration. Many transplant patients have creatinine clearances of 30–50 mL/min and can be considered in the same way as other patients with chronic renal insufficiency for anemia management, including supplemental erythropoietin.

Chronic hepatitis, particularly when due to hepatitis B virus, can be a progressive, fatal disease over a decade or so. Patients who are persistently hepatitis B surface antigen–positive are at higher risk, according to some studies, but the presence of hepatitis C virus is also a concern when one embarks on a course of immunosuppression in a transplant recipient.

Both chronic dialysis and renal transplant patients have a higher incidence of death from myocardial infarction and stroke than does the population at large, and this is particularly true in diabetic patients. Contributing factors are the use of glucocorticoids and sirolimus, as well as hypertension. Recipients of renal transplants have a high prevalence of coronary artery and peripheral vascular diseases. The percentage of deaths from these causes has been slowly rising as the numbers of transplanted diabetic patients and the average age of all recipients increase. More than 50% of renal recipient mortality is attributable to cardiovascular disease. In addition to strict control of blood pressure and blood lipid levels, close monitoring of patients for indications of further medical or surgical intervention is an important part of management.

FURTHER READINGS

CHANDRAKER A et al: Transplantation immunobiology, in *Brenner and Rector's The Kidney*, 7th ed, B Brenner (ed). Philadelphia, Saunders, 2004, pp 2759–2784

DENTON MD et al: Immunosuppressive strategies in renal transplantation. Lancet 353:1083, 1999

HIRSCH HH: Polyomavirus BK nephropathy: A (re-)emerging complication in renal transplantation. Am J Transplant 2:25, 2002

MAHONEY RJ et al: B-cell crossmatching and kidney allograft outcome in 9031 United States transplant recipients. Hum Immunol 63:324, 2002

PESCOVITZ MD, GOVANI M: Sirolimus and mycophenolate mofetil for calcineurin-free immunosuppression in renal transplant recipients. Am J Kidney Dis 38:S16, 2001

SAYEGH MH, CARPENTER CB: Transplantation 50 years later—progress, challenges and promises. N Engl J Med 351:2761, 2004

SAYEGH MH, TURKA LA: The role of T-cell costimulatory activation pathways in transplant rejection. N Engl J Med 338:1813, 1998

VELIDEDEOGLU E et al: Comparison of open, laparoscopic, and hand-assisted approaches to live-donor nephrectomy. Transplantation 74:169, 2002

VICENTI F: Immunosuppression minimization: Current and future trends in transplant immunosuppression. J Am Soc Nephrol 14:1940, 2003

277 Glomerular Diseases
Julia B. Lewis, Eric G. Neilson

Two human kidneys harbor nearly 1.8 million glomerular capillary tufts. Each glomerular tuft resides within Bowman's space. The capsule circumscribing this space is lined by parietal epithelial cells that transition into tubular epithelia forming the proximal nephron. The glomerular capillary tuft derives from an afferent arteriole that forms a branching capillary bed embedded in mesangial matrix (Fig. 277-1). This capillary network funnels into an efferent arteriole, which passes filtered blood into cortical peritubular capillaries or medullary vasa recta that supply and exchange with a folded tubular architecture. Hence the glomerular capillary tuft, fed and drained by arterioles, represents an arteriolar portal system. Fenestrated endothelial cells resting on a glomerular basement membrane (GBM) line glomerular capillaries. Delicate foot processes extending from epithelial podocytes shroud the outer surface of these capillaries, and podocytes interconnect to each other by slit-pore membranes forming a selective filtration barrier.

The glomerular capillaries filter 120–180 L/d of plasma water containing various solutes for reclamation or discharge by downstream tubules. Most large proteins and all cells are excluded from filtration by a physicochemical barrier governed by pore size and negative electrostatic charge. The mechanics of filtration and reclamation are quite complicated for many solutes (Chap. 271). For example, in the case of

serum albumin, the glomerulus is an imperfect barrier. Although albumin has a negative charge, which would tend to repel the negatively charged GBM, it only has a physical radius of 3.6 nm, while pores in the GBM and slit-pore membranes have a radius of 4 nm. Consequently, considerable amounts of albumin (estimates range from 4000 to 9000 mg/d) inevitably cross the filtration barrier to be reclaimed by megalin and cubilin receptors along the proximal tubule. Remarkably, humans with normal nephrons do not excrete more than 8–10 mg of albumin in daily voided urine. This amount of albumin, and other proteins, can rise to gram quantities following glomerular injury.

The breadth of diseases affecting the glomerulus is expansive because the glomerular capillaries can be injured in a variety of ways, producing many different lesions and several unique changes to the urinalysis. Some order to this vast subject is brought by grouping all of these diseases into a smaller number of clinical syndromes.

PATHOGENESIS OF GLOMERULAR DISEASE

There are many forms of glomerular disease with pathogenesis variably linked to the presence of genetic mutations, infection, toxin exposure, autoimmunity, atherosclerosis, hypertension, emboli, thrombosis, or diabetes mellitus. Even after careful study, however, the cause often remains unknown, and the lesion is called *idiopathic*. Specific or unique features of pathogenesis are mentioned with the description of each of the glomerular diseases later in this chapter.

Some glomerular diseases result from genetic mutations producing familial disease. (1) Congenital nephrotic syndrome from mutations in *NPHS1* (nephrin) and *NPHS2* (podocin) affect the slit-pore mem-

FIGURE 277-1 Glomerular architecture. A. The glomerular capillaries form from a branching network of renal arteries, arterioles, leading to an afferent arteriole, glomerular capillary bed (tuft), and a draining efferent arteriole (modified from Hypertension 5:8–16, 1983). **B.** Scanning electron micrograph of podocytes that line the outer surface of the glomerular capillaries (arrow shows foot process). **C.** Scanning electron micrograph of the fenestrated endothelia lining the glomerular capillary. **D.** The various normal regions of the glomerulus on light microscopy (*A–C, courtesy of Dr. Vincent Gattone, Indiana University; with permission*).

FIGURE 277-2 The glomerulus is injured by a variety of mechanisms. A. Preformed immune deposits can precipitate from the circulation and collect along the glomerular basement membrane (GBM) in the subendothelial space or can form in situ along the subepithelial space. **B.** Immunofluorescent staining of glomeruli with labeled anti-IgG demonstrating linear staining from a patient with anti-GBM disease or immune deposits from a patient with membranous glomerulonephritis. **C.** The mechanisms of glomerular injury have a complicated pathogenesis. Immune deposits and complement deposition classically draw macrophages and neutrophils into the glomerulus. T lymphocytes may follow to participate in the injury pattern as well. **D.** Amplification mediators as locally derived oxidants and proteases expand this inflammation, and, depending on the location of the target antigen and the genetic polymorphisms of the host, basement membranes are damaged with either endocapillary or extracapillary proliferation.

brane at birth, and *TRPC6* cation channel mutations in adulthood produce *focal segmental glomerulosclerosis* (FSGS). (2) Partial lipodystrophy from mutations in genes encoding lamin A/C or PPARγ cause a metabolic syndrome that can be associated with *membranoproliferative glomerulonephritis* (MPGN), which is sometimes accompanied by dense deposits and C3 nephritic factor. (3) Alport's syndrome, from mutations in the genes encoding for the α3, α4, or α5 chains of type IV collagen, produces *split-basement membranes* with *glomerulosclerosis*. (4) Lysosomal storage diseases, such as α-galactosidase A deficiency causing Fabry's disease and *N*-acetylneuraminic acid hydrolase deficiency causing nephrosialidosis, produce FSGS.

Systemic hypertension and atherosclerosis can produce pressure stress, ischemia, or lipid oxidants that lead to *chronic glomerulosclerosis*. *Malignant hypertension* can quickly complicate glomerulosclerosis with fibrinoid necrosis of arterioles and glomeruli, thrombotic microangiopathy, and acute renal failure. *Diabetic nephropathy* is an acquired sclerotic injury associated with thickening of the GBM secondary to the long-standing effects of hyperglycemia, advanced glycosylation endproducts, and reactive oxygen species.

Inflammation of the glomerular capillaries is called *glomerulonephritis*. Most glomerular or mesangial antigens involved in *immune-mediated glomerulonephritis* are unknown (Fig. 277-2). Glomerular epithelial or mesangial cells may shed them or express epitopes that mimic other

immunogenic proteins made elsewhere in the body. Bacteria, fungi, and viruses can directly infect the kidney producing their own antigens. Autoimmune diseases like idiopathic *membranous glomerulonephritis* (MGN) or MPGN are confined to the kidney, while systemic inflammatory diseases like *lupus nephritis* or *Wegener's granulomatosis* spread to the kidney, causing secondary glomerular injury. *Antiglomerular basement membrane disease* producing Goodpasture's syndrome primarily injures both the lung and kidney because of the narrow distribution of the α3 NC1 domain of type IV collagen that is the target antigen.

While the adaptive immune response is similar to that of other tissues, early T cell activation plays an important role in the mechanism of glomerulonephritis. Antigens presented by class II major histocompatibility complex (MHC) molecules on macrophages and dendritic cells in conjunction with associative recognition molecules engage the CD4/8 T cell repertoire. Local activation of Toll-like receptors on glomerular cells, deposition of immune complexes, or complement injury to glomerular structures induces mononuclear cell infiltration, which subsequently leads to an adaptive immune response attracted to the kidney by local release of chemokines. Neutrophils, macrophages, and T cells are drawn by chemokines into the glomerular tuft, where they react with antigens and epitopes on or near somatic cells or their structures, producing more cytokines and proteases that damage the mesangium, capillaries, and/or the GBM.

Mononuclear cells by themselves can injure the kidney, but autoimmune events that damage glomeruli classically produce a humoral immune response. *Poststreptococcal glomerulonephritis*, *lupus nephritis*, and idiopathic *membranous nephritis* typically are associated with immune deposits along the GBM, while anti-GBM antibodies are produced in anti-GBM disease. Preformed circulating immune complexes can precipitate along the subendothelial side of the GBM, while other immune deposits form in situ on the subepithelial side. These latter deposits accumulate when circulating autoantibodies find their antigen trapped along the subepithelial edge of the GBM. Immune deposits in the glomerular mesangium may result from the deposition of preformed circulating complexes or in situ antigen-antibody interactions. Immune deposits can stimulate the release of local proteases and activate the complement cascade, producing C_{5-9} attack complexes. In addition, local oxidants can damage glomerular structures, producing proteinuria and effacement of the podocytes. Overlapping etiologies or pathophysiologic mechanisms can produce similar glomerular lesions, suggesting that downstream molecular and cellular responses often converge towards common patterns of injury.

PROGRESSION OF GLOMERULAR DISEASE

Persistent glomerulonephritis that worsens renal function is always accompanied by interstitial nephritis, renal fibrosis, and tubular atrophy (**Fig. e9-25**). What is not so obvious, however, is that renal failure in glomerulonephritis best correlates histologically with the appearance of tubulointerstitial nephritis rather than with the type of inciting glomerular injury.

Loss of renal function due to interstitial damage can be explained hypothetically by several mechanisms. The simplest explanation is that urine flow is impeded by tubular obstruction as a result of interstitial inflammation and fibrosis. Thus, obstruction of the tubules with debris or by extrinsic compression results in aglomerular nephrons. A second mechanism suggests that interstitial changes, including interstitial edema or fibrosis, alter tubular and vascular architecture and thereby compromise the normal tubular transport of solutes and water from tubular lumen to vascular space. This failure increases the solute and water content of the tubule fluid, resulting in isothenuria and polyuria. Adaptive mechanisms related to tubuloglomerular feedback also fail, resulting in a reduction of renin output from the juxtaglomerular apparatus of glomeruli trapped by interstitial inflammation. Consequently, the local vasoconstrictive influence of angiotensin II on the glomerular arterioles decreases, and filtration drops owing to a generalized decrease in arteriolar tone. A third mechanism involves changes in vascular resistance due to damage of peritubular capillaries. The cross-sectional volume of these capillaries is decreased in areas of interstitial inflammation, edema, or fibrosis. These structural alterations in vascular resistance affect renal function through two mechanisms. First, tubular cells are very metabolically active, and, as a result, decreased perfusion could lead to ischemic injury. Second, impairment of glomerular arteriolar outflow leads to increased intraglomerular hypertension in less involved glomeruli; this selective intraglomerular hypertension aggravates and extends *mesangial sclerosis* and *glomerulosclerosis* to less-involved glomeruli. Regardless of the exact mechanism, early *acute tubulointerstitial nephritis* suggests potentially recoverable renal function, while the development of *chronic interstitial fibrosis* prognosticates a permanent loss.

Persistent damage to glomerular capillaries spreads to the tubulointerstitium in association with proteinuria. There is an untested hypothesis that efferent arterioles leading from inflamed glomeruli carry forward inflammatory mediators, which induces downstream interstitial nephritis, resulting in fibrosis. Glomerular filtrate from injured glomerular capillaries adherent to Bowman's capsule may also be misdirected to the periglomerular interstitium. Most nephrologists believe, however, that proteinuric glomerular filtrate forming tubular fluid is the primary route to downstream tubulointerstitial injury, although none of these hypotheses are mutually exclusive.

The simplest explanation for the effect of proteinuria on the development of interstitial nephritis is that increasingly severe proteinuria,

carrying activated cytokines and lipoproteins producing reactive oxygen species, triggers a downstream inflammatory cascade in and around epithelial cells lining the tubular nephron. These effects induce T lymphocyte and macrophage infiltrates in the interstitial spaces along with fibrosis and tubular atrophy. The details of this process are described in Chap. 272.

Tubules disappear following direct damage to their basement membranes, leading to decondensation and epithelial-mesenchymal transitions forming more interstitial fibroblasts at the site of injury. Transforming growth factor β (TGF-β), fibroblast growth factor 2, and platelet-derived growth factor (PDGF) are particularly active in this transition. With persistent nephritis, fibroblasts multiply and lay down tenascin and a fibronectin scaffold for the polymerization of new interstitial collagens I/III. These events form scar tissue through a process called fibrogenesis. In experimental studies, bone morphogenetic protein 7 and hematopoietic growth factor can reverse early fibrogenesis and preserve tubular architecture. When fibroblasts outdistance their survival factors, they apoptose, and the permanent renal scar becomes acellular, leading to irreversible renal failure.

APPROACH TO THE PATIENT:
Glomerular Disease

HEMATURIA, PROTEINURIA, AND PYURIA Patients with glomerular disease usually have some hematuria with varying degrees of proteinuria. Hematuria is typically asymptomatic. As little as 3–5 red blood cells in the spun sediment from first voided morning urine is suspicious. The diagnosis of glomerular injury can be delayed because patients will not realize they have *microscopic hematuria*, and only rarely with the exception of IgA nephropathy and sickle cell disease is *gross hematuria* present. When working up microscopic hematuria, perhaps accompanied by minimal proteinuria (<500 mg/24 h), it is important to exclude anatomic lesions, such as malignancy of the urinary tract, particularly in older men. Microscopic hematuria may also appear with the onset of benign prostatic hypertrophy, interstitial nephritis, papillary necrosis, renal stones, cystic kidney diseases, or renal vascular injury. However, when red blood cell casts (**Fig. e9-31**) or dysmorphic red blood cells are found in the sediment, glomerulonephritis is likely.

Sustained proteinuria >1–2 g/24 h is also commonly associated with glomerular disease. Patients often will not know they have proteinuria unless they become edematous or notice foamy urine on voiding. *Sustained proteinuria* has to be distinguished from lesser amounts of so-called *benign proteinuria* in the normal population (Table 277-1). This latter class of proteinuria is nonsustained, generally <1 g/24 h, and is sometimes called *functional* or *transient proteinuria*. Fever, exercise, obesity, sleep apnea, emotional stress, and congestive heart failure can explain transient proteinuria. Proteinuria only seen with upright posture is called *orthostatic proteinuria*. Occasionally, isolated proteinuria sustained over multiple clinic visits is found in diabetic nephropathy, *nil lesion, mesangioproliferative glomerulonephritis*, and FSGS. Proteinuria in most adults with glomerular disease is *nonselective*, containing albumin and a mixture of other serum proteins, while in children with nil

TABLE 277-1	URINE ASSAYS FOR ALBUMINURIA/PROTEINURIA			
	24-Hour Albumin[a] (mg/24 h)	Albumin[a]/ Creatinine Ratio (mg/G)	Dipstick Proteinuria	24-Hour Urine Protein[b] (mg/24 h)
Normal	8–10	<30	–	<150
Microalbuminuria	30-300	30–300	–/Trace/1+	–
Proteinuria	>300	>300	Trace–3+	>150

[a]Albumin detected by radioimmunoassay.
[b]Albumin represents 30–70% of the total protein excreted in the urine.

lesion from *minimal change disease*, the proteinuria is *selective* and largely composed of albumin.

Some patients with inflammatory glomerular disease, such as acute poststreptococcal glomerulonephritis or MPGN, may have *pyuria* caused by the presence of considerable numbers of leukocytes in the urine. This latter finding has to be distinguished from urine infected with bacteria.

CLINICAL SYNDROMES Various forms of glomerular injury can also be parsed into several distinct syndromes on clinical grounds (Table 277-2). These syndromes, however, are not always mutually exclusive. There is an *acute nephritic syndrome* producing 1–2 g/24 h of proteinuria, hematuria with red blood cell casts, pyuria, hypertension, fluid retention, and a rise in serum creatinine associated with a reduction in glomerular filtration. If glomerular inflammation develops slowly, the serum creatinine will rise gradually over many weeks, but if the serum creatinine rises quickly, particularly over a few days, acute nephritis is sometimes called *rapidly progressive glomerulonephritis* (RPGN); the histopathologic term *crescentic glomerulonephritis* refers to the clinical occurrence of RPGN in a patient with this characteristic glomerular lesion. When patients with RPGN present with lung hemorrhage from Goodpasture's syndrome, antineutrophil cytoplasmic antibodies (ANCA) small-vessel vasculitis, lupus erythematosus, or cryoglobulinemia, they are often diagnosed as having a *pulmonary-renal syndrome*. *Nephrotic syndrome* describes the onset of heavy proteinuria (>3.0 g/24 h), hypertension, hypercholesterolemia, hypoalbuminemia, edema/anasarca, and microscopic hematuria; if only large amounts of proteinuria are present without clinical manifestations, the condition is sometimes called *nephrotic-range proteinuria*. The glomerular filtration rate (GFR) in these patients may initially be normal or, rarely, higher than normal, but with persistent hyperfiltration and continued nephron loss, it typically declines over months to years. Patients with a *basement membrane syndrome* either have genetically abnormal basement membranes or an autoimmune response to basement membrane collagen IV associated with microscopic hematuria, mild to heavy proteinuria, and hypertension with variable elevations in serum creatinine. *Glomerular-vascular syndrome* describes patients with vascular injury producing hematuria and moderate proteinuria. Affected individuals can have vasculitis, thrombotic microangiopathy, antiphospholipid syndrome, or, more commonly, a systemic disease such as atherosclerosis, cholesterol emboli, hypertension, sickle cell anemia, and autoimmunity. *Infectious diseases-asso-*

TABLE 277-2 PATTERNS OF CLINICAL GLOMERULONEPHRITIS

Glomerular Syndromes	Proteinuria	Hematuria	Vascular Injury
Acute Nephritic Syndromes			
Poststreptococcal glomerulonephritis[a]	+/++	++/+++	–
Subacute bacterial endocarditis[a]	+/++	++	–
Lupus nephritis[a]	+/++	++/+++	–
Antiglomerular basement membrane disease[a]	++	++/+++	–
IgA nephropathy[a]	+/++	++/+++[c]	–
ANCA small-vessel vasculitis[a]			
Wegener's granulomatosis	+/++	++/+++	++++
Microscopic polyangiitis	+/++	++/+++	++++
Churg-Strauss syndrome	+/++	++/+++	++++
Henoch-Schönlein purpura[a]	+/++	++/+++	++++
Cryoglobulinemia[a]	+/++	++/+++	++++
Membranoproliferative glomerulonephritis[a]	++	++/+++	–
Mesangioproliferative glomerulonephritis	+	+/++	–
Pulmonary-Renal Syndromes			
Goodpasture's syndrome[a]	++	++/+++	–
ANCA small-vessel vasculitis[a]			
Wegener's granulomatosis	+/++	++/+++	++++
Microscopic polyangiitis	+/++	++/+++	++++
Churg-Strauss syndrome	+/++	++/+++	++++
Henoch-Schönlein purpura[a]	+/++	++/+++	++++
Cryoglobulinemia[a]	+/++	++/+++	++++
Nephrotic Syndromes			
Minimal change disease	++++	–	–
Focal segmental glomerulosclerosis	+++/++++	+	–
Membranous glomerulonephritis	++++	+	–
Diabetic nephropathy	++/++++	–/+	–
AL and AA amyloidosis	+++/++++	+	+/++
Light-chain deposition disease	+++	+	–
Fibrillary-immunotactoid disease	+++/++++	+	+
Fabry's disease	+	+	–
Basement Membrane Syndromes			
Anti-GBM disease[a]	++	++/+++	–
Alport's syndrome	++	++	–
Thin basement membrane disease	+	++	–
Nail-patella syndrome	++/+++	++	–
Glomerular Vascular Syndromes			
Atherosclerotic nephropathy	+	+	+++
Hypertensive nephropathy[b]	+/++	+/++	++
Cholesterol emboli	+/++	++	+++
Sickle cell disease	+/++	++[c]	+++
Thrombotic microangiopathies	++	++	+++
Antiphospholipid syndrome	++	++	+++
ANCA small-vessel vasculitis[a]			
Wegener's granulomatosis	+/++	++/+++	++++
Microscopic polyangiitis	+/++	++/+++	++++
Churg-Strauss syndrome	+++	++/+++	++++
Henoch-Schönlein purpura[a]	+/++	++/+++	++++
Cryoglobulinemia[a]	+/++	++/+++	++++
AL and AA amyloidosis	+++/++++	+	+/++
Infectious Disease–Associated Syndromes			
Poststreptococcal glomerulonephritis[a]	+/++	++/+++	–
Subacute bacterial endocarditis[a]	+/++	++	–
HIV	+++	+/++	–
Hepatitis B and C	+++	+/++	–
Syphilis	+++	+	–
Leprosy	+++	+	–
Malaria	+++	+/++	–
Schistosomiasis	+++	+/++	–

[a]Can present as rapidly progressive glomerulonephritis (RPGN); sometimes called crescentic glomerulonephritis.
[b]Can present as a malignant hypertensive crisis producing an aggressive fibrinoid necrosis in arterioles small arteries with microangiopathic hemolytic anemia.
[c]Can present with gross hematuria.
Abbreviations: ANCA, antineutrophil cytoplasmic antibodies; AL, amyloid L; AA, amyloid A; GBM, glomerular basement membrane.

ciated syndrome is most important if one has an international perspective. Save for subacute bacterial endocarditis in the Western Hemisphere, malaria and schistosomiasis may be the most common causes of glomerulonephritis throughout the world, closely followed by HIV and chronic hepatitis B and C. These infectious diseases produce a variety of inflammatory reactions in glomerular capillaries, ranging from nephrotic syndrome to acute nephritic injury, and yield urinalyses that demonstrate a combination of hematuria and proteinuria.

These six general categories of syndromes are usually determined at the bedside with the help of a history and physical examination, blood chemistries, renal ultrasound, and urinalysis. These initial studies help frame further diagnostic work up that typically involves some testing of the serum for the presence of various proteins (HIV and hepatitis B and C antigens), antibodies [anti-GBM, antiphospholipid, ASO, anti-DNAase, antihyaluronidase, ANCA, anti-DNA, cryoglobulins, anti-HIV, and anti-hepatitis B and C antibodies] or depletion of complement components (C_3 and C_4). The bedside history and physical examination can also help determine whether the glomerulonephritis is isolated to the kidney (primary glomerulonephritis) or is part of a systemic disease (secondary glomerulonephritis). When confronted with an abnormal urinalysis and elevated serum creatinine, with or without edema or congestive heart failure, one must consider whether the glomerulonephritis is acute or chronic. This assessment is best made by careful history (last known urinalysis or serum creatinine during pregnancy or insurance physical, evidence of infection, or use of medication or recreational drugs); the size of the kidneys on renal ultrasound examination; and how the patient feels at presentation. Chronic glomerular disease often presents with decreased kidney size. Patients who quickly develop renal failure are fatigued and weak; feel miserable; often have uremic symptoms associated with nausea, vomiting, fluid retention, and somnolence. Primary glomerulonephritis presenting with renal failure that has progressed slowly, however, can be remarkably asymptomatic, as are patients with acute glomerulonephritis without much loss in renal function. Once this initial information is collected, selected patients who are clinically stable, have adequate blood clotting parameters, and are willing to receive treatment are encouraged to have a renal biopsy. Biopsies can be done safely with an ultrasound-guided biopsy gun.

RENAL PATHOLOGY

A renal biopsy in the setting of glomerulonephritis can quickly identify the type of glomerular injury and often suggests a course of treatment. The biopsy is processed for light microscopy using stains for hematoxylin and eosin (H&E) to assess cellularity and architecture, periodic acid-Schiff (PAS) to stain carbohydrate moieties in the membranes of the glomerular tuft and tubules, Jones-methenamine silver to enhance basement membrane structure, Congo red for amyloid deposits, and Masson's trichrome to identify collagen deposition and assess the degree of glomerulosclerosis and interstitial fibrosis. Biopsies are also processed for direct immunofluorescence using conjugated antibodies against IgG, IgM, and IgA to detect the presence of "lumpy-bumpy" immune deposits or "linear" IgG or IgA antibodies bound to GBM, antibodies against trapped complement proteins (C_3 and C_4), or specific antibodies against a relevant antigen. High-resolution electron microscopy can clarify the principal location of immune deposits and the status of the basement membrane.

Each region of a renal biopsy is assessed separately. By light microscopy, glomeruli (at least 10 and ideally 20) are reviewed individually for discrete lesions; <50% involvement is considered focal, and >50% is diffuse. Injury in each glomerular tuft can be segmental, involving a portion of the tuft, or global, involving most of the glomerulus. Glomeruli can have proliferative characteristics, showing increased cellularity. When cells in the capillary tuft proliferate, it is called endocapillary, and when cellular proliferation extends into Bowman's

space, it is called extracapillary. Synechiae are formed when epithelial podocytes attach to Bowman's capsule in the setting of glomerular injury; crescents, which in some cases may be the extension of synechiae, develop when fibrocellular/fibrin collections fill all or part of Bowman's space; and sclerotic glomeruli show acellular, amorphous accumulations of proteinaceous material throughout the tuft with loss of functional capillaries and normal mesangium. Since age-related glomerulosclerosis is common in adults, one can estimate the background percentage of sclerosis by dividing the patient's age in half and subtracting 10. Immunofluorescent and electron microscopy can detect the presence and location of subepithelial, subendothelial, or mesangial immune deposits, or reduplication or splitting of the basement membrane. In the other regions of the biopsy, the vasculature surrounding glomeruli and tubules can show angiopathy, vasculitis, the presence of fibrils, or thrombi. The tubules can be assessed for adjacency to one another; separation can be the result of edema, tubular dropout, or collagen deposition resulting from interstitial fibrosis. Interstitial fibrosis is an ominous sign of irreversibility and progression to renal failure.

ACUTE NEPHRITIC SYNDROMES

Acute nephritic syndromes classically present with hypertension, hematuria, red blood cell casts, pyuria, and mild to moderate proteinuria. Extensive inflammatory damage to glomeruli can cause a fall in GFR and eventually produce uremic symptoms with salt and water retention, leading to edema and hypertension.

POSTSTREPTOCOCCAL GLOMERULONEPHRITIS

Poststreptococcal glomerulonephritis is prototypical for acute endocapillary proliferative glomerulonephritis. The incidence of poststreptococcal glomerulonephritis is decreasing in Western countries, and it is typically sporadic. Epidemic cases are still seen, though less commonly. Acute poststreptococcal glomerulonephritis typically affects children between the ages of 2 and 14 years, but 10% of cases are patients older than 40. It is more common in males, and the familial or cohabitant incidence is as high as 40%. Skin and throat infections with particular M types of streptococci (nephritogenic strains) antedate glomerular disease; M types 47, 49, 55, 2, 60, and 57 are seen following impetigo and M types 1, 2, 4, 3, 25, 49, and 12 with pharyngitis. Poststreptococcal glomerulonephritis due to impetigo develops 2–6 weeks after skin infection and 1–3 weeks after streptococcal pharyngitis.

The renal biopsy in poststreptococcal glomerulonephritis demonstrates hypercellularity of mesangial and endothelial cells, glomerular infiltrates of polymorphonuclear leukocytes, granular subendothelial immune deposits of IgG, IgM, C_3, C_4, and C_{5-9}, and subepithelial deposits (which appear as "humps") (**Fig. e9-4**). Poststreptococcal glomerulonephritis is an immune-mediated disease involving putative streptococcal antigens, circulating immune complexes, and activation of complement in association with cell-mediated injury. Many candidate antigens have been proposed over the years; three such candidates from nephritogenic streptococci are zymogen, a precursor of exotoxin B; glyceraldehyde phosphate dehydrogenase, also known as presorbing antigen (PA-Ag); and streptokinase. All have a biochemical affinity for GBMs, and in this location they may act as a target for antibodies.

The classic presentation is an acute nephritic picture with hematuria, pyuria, red blood cell casts, edema, hypertension, and oliguric renal failure, which may be severe enough to appear as RPGN. Systemic symptoms of headache, malaise, anorexia, and flank pain (due to swelling of the renal capsule) are reported in as many as 50% of cases. Five percent of children and 20% of adults have proteinuria in the nephrotic range. In the first week of symptoms, 90% of patients will have a depressed CH_{50} and decreased levels of C_3 with normal levels of C_4. Positive rheumatoid factor (30–40%), cryoglobulins and circulating immune complexes (60–70%), and ANCA against myeloperoxidase (10%) are also reported. Positive cultures for streptococcal infection are inconsistently present (10–70%), but increased titers of ASO (30%), anti-DNAase (70%) or antihyaluronidase antibodies (40%) can help confirm the diagnosis. Consequently, the diagnosis of poststreptococcal glomerulonephritis rarely requires a renal biopsy. A subclinical disease is reported in some series to be four to five times as common as clinical nephritis, and these latter cases are characterized by asymptomatic microscopic hematuria with low serum complement levels. Treatment is supportive, with control of hypertension, edema, and dialysis as needed. Antibiotic treatment for streptococcal infection should be given to all patients and their cohabitants. There is no role for immunosuppressive therapy, even in the setting of crescents. Recurrent poststreptococcal glomerulonephritis is rare despite repeated streptococcal infections. Early death is rare in children but does occur in the elderly. Overall, the prognosis is good, with permanent renal failure being very uncommon (1–3%), and even less so in children. Complete resolution of the hematuria and proteinuria in children occurs within 3–6 weeks of the onset of nephritis.

SUBACUTE BACTERIAL ENDOCARDITIS

Endocarditis-associated glomerulonephritis is typically a complication of subacute bacterial endocarditis, particularly in patients who remain untreated for a long time, have negative blood cultures, or have right-sided endocarditis. Glomerulonephritis is unusual in acute bacterial endocarditis because it takes 10–14 days to develop immune complex–mediated injury, by which time the patient has been treated, often with emergent surgery. Grossly, the kidneys in subacute bacterial endocarditis have subcapsular hemorrhages with a "flea-bitten" appearance, and microscopy on renal biopsy reveals a focal proliferation around foci of necrosis associated with abundant mesangial, subendothelial, and subepithelial immune deposits of IgG, IgM, and C_3. Patients who present with a clinical picture of RPGN have crescents. Embolic infarcts or septic abscesses may also be present. The pathogenesis hinges on the renal deposition of circulating immune complexes in the kidney with complement activation. Patients present with gross or microscopic hematuria, pyuria, and mild proteinuria or, less commonly, RPGN with rapid loss of renal function. A normocytic anemia, elevated erythrocyte sedimentation rate, hypocomplementemia, high titers of rheumatoid factor, type III cryoglobulins, and circulating immune complexes are often present. Levels of serum creatinine may be elevated at diagnosis, but with modern therapy there is little progression to chronic renal failure. Primary treatment is eradication of the infection with 4–6 weeks of antibiotics, and if accomplished expeditiously, the prognosis for renal recovery is good.

As variants of persistent bacterial infection in blood, glomerulonephritis can occur in patients with ventriculoatrial and ventriculoperitoneal shunts; pulmonary, intra-abdominal, pelvic, or cutaneous infections; and infected vascular prostheses. The clinical presentation of these conditions is variable and includes proteinuria, microscopic hematuria, and acute renal failure. Blood cultures are usually positive and serum complement levels low, and there may be elevated levels of C-reactive proteins, rheumatoid factor, antinuclear antibodies, and cryoglobulins. Renal lesions include membranoproliferative glomerulonephritis (MPGN), diffuse proliferative glomerulonephritis (DPGN), or mesangioproliferative glomerulonephritis, sometimes leading to RPGN. Treatment focuses on eradicating the infection, with most patients treated as if they have endocarditis.

LUPUS NEPHRITIS

Lupus nephritis is a common and serious complication of systemic lupus erythematosus (SLE) and most severe in African-American female adolescents. Thirty to fifty percent of patients will have clinical manifestations of renal disease at the time of diagnosis, and 60% of adults and 80% of children develop renal abnormalities at some point in the course of their disease. Lupus nephritis results from the deposition of circulating immune complexes, which activate the complement cascade leading to complement-mediated damage, leukocyte infiltration, activation of procoagulant factors, and release of various cytokines. In situ immune complex formation following glomerular binding of nuclear antigens may also play a role in renal injury. The presence of antiphospholipid antibodies may trigger a thrombotic microangiopathy in a minority of patients.

TABLE 277-3		CLASSIFICATION FOR LUPUS NEPHRITIS
Class I	Minimal mesangial	Normal histology with mesangial deposits
Class II	Mesangial proliferation	Mesangial hypercellularity with expansion of the mesangial matrix
Class III	Focal nephritis	Focal endocapillary ± extracapillary proliferation with focal subendothelial immune deposits and mild mesangial expansion
Class IV	Diffuse nephritis	Diffuse endocapillary ± extracapillary proliferation with diffuse subendothelial immune deposits and mesangial alterations
Class V	Membranous nephritis	Thickened basement membranes with diffuse subepithelial immune deposits; may occur with Class III or IV lesions and is sometimes called mixed membranous and proliferative nephritis
Class VI	Sclerotic nephritis	Global sclerosis of nearly all glomerular capillaries

Note: Revised in 2004 by the International Society of Nephrology-Renal Pathology Society Study Group.

The clinical manifestations, course of disease, and treatment of lupus nephritis are closely linked to the renal pathology. The most common clinical sign of renal disease is proteinuria, but hematuria, hypertension, varying degrees of renal failure, and an active urine sediment with red blood cell casts can all be present. Although significant renal pathology can be found on biopsy even in the absence of major abnormalities in the urinalysis, most nephrologists do not biopsy patients until the urinalysis is convincingly abnormal. The extrarenal manifestations of lupus are important in establishing a firm diagnosis of systemic lupus because, while serologic abnormalities are common in lupus nephritis, they are not diagnostic. Anti-dsDNA antibodies that fix complement correlate best with the presence of renal disease. Hypocomplementemia is common in patients with acute lupus nephritis (70–90%) and declining complement levels may herald a flare. Renal biopsy, however, is the only reliable method of identifying the morphologic variants of lupus nephritis.

The World Health Organization (WHO) workshop in 1974 first outlined several distinct patterns of lupus-related glomerular injury; these were modified in 1982. In 2004 the International Society of Nephrology in conjunction with the Renal Pathology Society again updated the classification. This latest version of lesions seen on biopsy (Table 277-3) best defines clinicopathologic correlations, provides valuable prognostic information, and forms the basis for modern treatment recommendations. Class I nephritis describes normal glomerular histology by any technique or normal light microscopy with minimal mesangial deposits on immunofluorescent or electron microscopy. Class II designates mesangial immune complexes with *mesangial proliferation*. Both Class I and II lesions are typically associated with minimal renal manifestation and normal renal function; nephrotic syndrome is rare. Patients with lesions limited to the renal mesangium have an excellent prognosis and generally do not need therapy for their lupus nephritis.

The subject of lupus nephritis is presented under acute nephritic syndromes because of the aggressive and important proliferative lesions seen in Class III–V renal disease. Class III describes *focal lesions with proliferation or scarring*, often involving only a segment of the glomerulus (**Fig. e9-10**). Class III lesions have the most varied course. Hypertension, an active urinary sediment, and proteinuria are common with nephrotic-range proteinuria in 25–33% of patients. Elevated serum creatinine is present in 25% of patients. Patients with mild proliferation involving a small percentage of glomeruli respond well to therapy with steroids alone, and fewer than 5% progress to renal failure over 5 years. Patients with more severe proliferation involving a greater percentage of glomeruli have a far worse prognosis and may have lower remission rates. Treatment of those patients is the same as that for Class IV lesions, as some nephrologists believe that Class III lesions are simply an early presentation of Class IV disease. Class IV describes *global, diffuse proliferative lesions* involving the vast majority of glomeruli. Patients with Class IV lesions commonly have high anti-DNA antibody titers, low serum complement, hematuria, red blood cell casts, proteinuria, hypertension, and decreased renal function; 50% of patients have nephrotic-range proteinuria. Patients with crescents on biopsy may have a rapidly progressive decline in renal function. Without treatment, this aggressive lesion has the worst renal prognosis. However, if a remission—defined as a return to near-normal renal function and proteinuria ≤330 mg/dL per day—is achieved with treatment, renal outcomes are excellent. Treatment must combine high-dose steroids with either cyclophosphamide or mycophenolate mofetil. Current evidence suggests that inducing a remission with administration of steroids and either cyclophosphamide or mycophenolate mofetil for 2–6 months, followed by maintenance therapy with lower doses of steroids and mycophenolate mofetil, may best balance the likelihood of successful remission with the side effects of therapy. There is no consensus on use of high-dose intravenous methylprednisolone versus oral prednisone, monthly intravenous cyclophosphamide versus daily oral cyclophosphamide, or other immunosuppressants such as cyclosporine or azathioprine. Nephrologists tend to avoid prolonged use of cyclophosphamide in patients of childbearing age without first banking eggs or sperm.

The Class V lesion describes subepithelial immune deposits producing a *membranous pattern;* a subcategory of Class V lesions is associated with proliferative lesions and is sometimes called *mixed membranous and proliferative disease;* this category of injury is treated like Class IV glomerulonephritis. Sixty percent of patients present with nephrotic syndrome or lesser amounts of proteinuria. Patients with lupus nephritis Class V, like patients with *idiopathic membranous nephropathy,* are predisposed to renal-vein thrombosis and other thrombolic complications. A minority of patients with Class V will present with hypertension and renal dysfunction. There are conflicting data on the clinical course, prognosis, and appropriate therapy for patients with Class V disease, which may reflect the heterogeneity of this group of patients. Patients with severe nephrotic syndrome, elevated serum creatinine, and a progressive course will probably benefit from therapy with steroids in combination with other immunosuppressive agents. Therapy with inhibitors of the renin-angiotensin system also may attenuate the proteinuria.

Patients with any of the above lesions also can transform to another lesion; hence patients often require reevaluation, including repeat renal biopsy. Lupus patients with Class VI lesions have greater than 90% *sclerotic glomeruli* and end-stage renal disease with interstitial fibrosis. As a group, approximately 20% of patients with lupus nephritis will reach end-stage disease, requiring dialysis or transplantation. Systemic lupus tends to become quiescent once there is renal failure, perhaps due to the immunosuppressant effects of uremia. Renal transplantation in renal failure from lupus, usually performed after approximately 6 months of inactive disease, results in allograft survival rates comparable to patients transplanted for other reasons.

ANTIGLOMERULAR BASEMENT MEMBRANE DISEASE

Patients who develop autoantibodies directed against glomerular basement antigens frequently develop a glomerulonephritis termed *antiglomerular basement membrane (anti-GBM) disease.* When they present with lung hemorrhage and glomerulonephritis, they have a pulmonary-renal syndrome called *Goodpasture's syndrome.* The target epitopes for this autoimmune disease lie in the quaternary structure of α3 NC1 domain of collagen IV. MHC-restricted T cells initiate the autoantibody response because humans are not tolerant to the epitopes created by this quaternary structure. The epitopes are normally sequestered in the collagen IV hexamer and can be exposed by infection, smoking, oxidants, or solvents. Goodpasture's syndrome appears in two age groups: in young men in their late 20s and in men and women in their 60–70s. Disease in the younger age group is usually explosive, with hemoptysis, a sudden fall in hemoglobin, fever, dyspnea, and hematuria. Hemoptysis is largely confined to smokers, and those who present with lung hemorrhage as a group do better than older populations who have prolonged, asymptomatic renal injury; presentation with oliguria is often associated with a particularly bad outcome. The performance of an urgent kidney biopsy is important in suspected cases of Goodpasture's syndrome to confirm the diagnosis and assess prognosis. Renal biopsies typically show *focal or segmental necrosis* that later, with aggressive destruction of the capillaries by cellular proliferation, leads to crescent formation in Bowman's space (**Fig. e9-12**). As these lesions progress, there is concomitant interstitial nephritis with fibrosis and tubular atrophy. The presence of anti-GBM antibodies and complement is recognized on biopsy by linear immunofluorescent staining for IgG (rarely IgA). In testing serum for anti-GBM antibodies, it is particularly important that the α3 NC1 domain of collagen IV alone be used as the target. This is because nonnephritic antibodies against the α1 NC1 domain are seen in paraneoplastic syndromes and cannot be discerned from assays that use whole basement membrane fragments as the binding target. Between 10–15% of sera from patients with Goodpasture's syndrome also contain ANCA antibodies against myeloperoxidase. This subset of patients has a vasculitis-associated variant, which has a surprisingly good prognosis with treatment. Prognosis at presentation is worse if there are >50% crescents on renal biopsy with advanced fibrosis, if serum creatinine is >5–6 mg/dL, if oliguria is present, or if there is a need for acute dialysis. Although frequently attempted, most of these latter patients will not respond to plasmapheresis and steroids. Patients with advanced renal failure who present with hemoptysis should still be treated for their lung hemorrhage, as it responds to plasmapheresis and can be lifesaving. Treated patients with less severe disease typically respond to 8–10 treatments of plasmapheresis accompanied by oral prednisone and cyclophosphamide in the first 2 weeks. Kidney transplantation is possible, but because there is risk of recurrence, experience suggests that patients should wait for 6 months and until serum antibodies are undetectable.

IgA NEPHROPATHY

Berger first described the glomerulonephritis termed *IgA nephropathy.* It is classically characterized by episodic hematuria associated with the deposition of IgA in the mesangium. IgA nephropathy is one of the most common forms of glomerulonephritis worldwide. There is a male preponderance, a peak incidence in the second and third decades of life, and rare familial clustering. There are geographic differences in the prevalence of IgA nephropathy, with 30% prevalence along the Asian and Pacific Rim and 20% in southern Europe, compared to lower prevalence in northern Europe and North America. It was initially hypothesized that variation in detection, in part, reflected regional differences in the recognition of asymptomatic microscopic hematuria or the frequency of renal biopsies. With clinical care in nephrology becoming more uniform and regional reports coming largely from larger cities, however, this variation in prevalence more likely reflects true differences among racial and ethnic groups. Clinical and laboratory evidence suggests close similarities between Henoch-Schönlein purpura and IgA nephropathy. Henoch-Schönlein purpura is distinguished clinically from IgA nephropathy by prominent systemic symptoms, a younger age (<20 years old), preceding infection, and abdominal complaints. Deposits of IgA are also found in the glomerular mesangium in a variety of systemic diseases, including chronic liver disease, Crohn's disease, gastrointestinal adenocarcinoma, chronic obstructive bronchiectasis, idiopathic interstitial pneumonia, dermatitis herpetiformis, mycosis fungoides, leprosy, ankylosing spondylitis, relapsing polychondritis, and Sjögren's syndrome. IgA deposition in these entities is not usually associated with clinically significant glomerular inflammation or renal dysfunction and thus is not called IgA nephropathy.

IgA nephropathy is an immune complex-mediated glomerulonephritis defined by the presence of diffuse mesangial IgA deposits often associated with mesangial hypercellularity. IgM, IgG, C_3, or immunoglobulin light chains may be codistributed with IgA. IgA deposited in the mesangium is typically polymeric and of the IgA1 subclass, the pathogenic significance of which is not clear. Abnormalities have been described in IgA production by plasma cells, particularly secretory

IgA; in IgA O-glycosylation; in IgA clearance, predominately by the liver; in mesangial IgA clearance and receptors for IgA; and in growth factor and cytokine-mediated events. Despite the presence of elevated serum IgA levels in 20–50% of patients, IgA deposition in skin biopsies in 15–55% of patients, or elevated levels of secretory IgA and IgA-fibronectin complexes, a renal biopsy is necessary to make the diagnosis. Although the immunofluorescent pattern of IgA on renal biopsy defines IgA nephropathy in the proper clinical context, a variety of histologic lesions may be seen on light microscopy (**Fig. e9-6**), including DPGN; *segmental sclerosis*; and, rarely, *segmental necrosis with cellular crescent formation*, which typically presents as RPGN.

The two most common presentations of IgA nephropathy are recurrent episodes of macroscopic hematuria during or immediately following an upper respiratory infection in children (Henoch-Schönlein purpura) or asymptomatic microscopic hematuria most often seen in adults. Between episodes, the urinalysis is normal. When the hematuria persists, one finds increasing amounts of proteinuria; nephrotic syndrome, however, is uncommon. The presence or absence of proteinuria at the time of diagnosis often determines whether patients with asymptomatic hematuria are biopsied, which reflects the bias in habits of clinical practice. Proteinuria can occur late in the course of the disease. Rarely, patients can present with acute renal failure and a rapidly progressive clinical picture. IgA nephropathy is a benign disease for the majority of patients, with progression to renal failure seen in only 25–30% over 20–25 years; in fact, 5–30% of patients go into complete remission. Risk factors for the loss of renal function include the presence of hypertension or proteinuria, the absence of episodes of macroscopic hematuria, male age, older age of onset, and more severe changes on renal biopsy.

There is no agreement on optimal treatment. Both large studies that include patients with multiple glomerular diseases or small studies of patients with IgA nephropathy support the use of angiotensin-converting enzyme (ACE) inhibitors in patients with proteinuria or declining renal function. Tonsillectomy, steroid therapy, and fish oil have all been suggested in small studies to benefit select patients with IgA nephropathy. When presenting as RPGN, patients typically receive steroids, cytotoxic agents, and plasmapheresis.

ANCA SMALL VESSEL VASCULITIS

A group of patients with small-vessel vasculitis (arterioles, capillaries, and venules; rarely small arteries) and glomerulonephritis have serum ANCA; the antibodies are of two types, anti-proteinase 3 (PR3) or anti-myeloperoxidase (MPO) (Chap. 319). ANCA are produced with the help of T cells and activate leukocytes and monocytes, which together damage the walls of small vessels. Endothelial injury also attracts more leukocytes and extends the inflammation. Wegener's granulomatosis, microscopic polyangiitis, and Churg-Strauss syndrome belong to this group because they are ANCA-positive and have a *pauci-immune glomerulonephritis* with few immune complexes in small vessels and glomerular capillaries. Patients with any of these three diseases can have any combination of the above serum antibodies, but anti-PR3 antibodies are more common in Wegener's and anti-MPO antibodies are more common in microscopic polyangiitis or Churg-Strauss. While each of these diseases have some unique clinical features, most features do not predict relapse or progression, and as a group they are generally treated in the same way. Only the presence of upper-airway involvement, persistent pulmonary injury, and anti-PR3 antibodies suggests that the course of disease will be more difficult. Induction therapy usually includes some combination of plasmapheresis, methylprednisolone, and cyclophosphamide. The benefit of plasmapheresis in this setting is uncertain. The steroids are tapered soon after acute inflammation subsides, and patients are maintained on cyclophosphamide or azathioprine for up to a year to minimize the risk of relapse.

Wegener's Granulomatosis
Patients with this disease classically present with fever, purulent rhinorrhea, nasal ulcers, sinus pain, polyarthralgias/arthritis, cough, hemoptysis, shortness of breath, microscopic hematuria, and 0.5–1 g/24 h of proteinuria; occasionally there

may be cutaneous purpura and mononeuritis multiplex. Presentation without renal involvement is termed *limited Wegener's granulomatosis*, although some of these patients will show signs of renal injury later. Chest x-ray often reveals nodules and persistent infiltrates, sometimes with cavities. Biopsy of involved tissue will show a small-vessel vasculitis and adjacent noncaseating granulomas. Renal biopsies during active disease demonstrate *segmental necrotizing glomerulonephritis* without immune deposits (**Fig. e9-11**). The cause of Wegner's granulomatosis is unknown. In case-controlled studies there is greater risk associated with exposure to silica dust. The disease is also more common in patients with α_1 antitrypsin deficiency, which is an inhibitor of PR3.

Microscopic Polyangiitis
Clinically, these patients look somewhat similar to those with Wegener's granulomatosis, except they rarely have significant lung disease or destructive sinusitis. The distinction is made on biopsy where the vasculitis in microscopic polyangiitis is without granulomas. Some patients will also have injury limited to the capillaries and venules.

Churg-Strauss Syndrome
When small-vessel vasculitis is associated with peripheral eosinophilia, cutaneous purpura, mononeuritis, asthma, and allergic rhinitis, a diagnosis of Churg-Strauss syndrome is considered. Hypergammaglobulinemia, elevated levels of serum IgE, or the presence of rheumatoid factor sometimes accompanies the allergic state. Lung inflammation, including fleeting cough and pulmonary infiltrates, often precedes the systemic manifestations of disease by years; lung manifestations are rarely absent. A third of patients may have exudative pleural effusions associated with eosinophils. Small-vessel vasculitis and *focal segmental necrotizing glomerulonephritis* can be seen on renal biopsy, usually absent eosinophils or granulomas. The cause of Churg-Strauss syndrome is autoimmune, but the inciting factors are unknown. Interestingly, some asthma patients treated with leukotriene receptor antagonists will develop this vasculitis.

MEMBRANOPROLIFERATIVE GLOMERULONEPHRITIS

MPGN is sometimes called *mesangiocapillary glomerulonephritis* or *lobar glomerulonephritis*. It is an immune-mediated glomerulonephritis characterized by thickening of the GBM with mesangioproliferative changes; 70% of patients have hypocomplementemia. MPGN is rare in African Americans, and idiopathic disease usually presents in childhood or young adulthood. MPGN is subdivided pathologically into Type I, Type II, and Type III disease. *Type I MPGN* is commonly associated with persistent hepatitis C infections, autoimmune diseases like lupus or cryoglobulinemia, or neoplastic diseases (Table 277-4). *Types II and III MPGN* are usually idiopathic, except in the presence of C_3 nephritic factor and/or in partial lipodystrophy producing Type II disease or complement receptor deficiency in Type III disease.

Type I MPGN, the most proliferative of the three types, shows mesangial proliferation with lobular segmentation on renal biopsy and

TABLE 277-4 MEMBRANOPROLIFERATIVE GLOMERULONEPHRITIS

Type I Disease (Most Common)

Idiopathic
Subacute bacterial endocarditis
Systemic lupus erythematosus
Hepatitis C ± cryoglobulinemia
Mixed cryoglobulinemia
Hepatitis B
Cancer: Lung, breast, and ovary (germinal)

Type II Disease (Dense Deposit Disease)

Idiopathic
C_3 nephritic factor-associated
Partial lipodystrophy

Type III Disease

Idiopathic
Complement receptor deficiency

mesangial interposition between the capillary basement membrane and endothelial cells, producing a double contour sometimes called *tram-tracking* (**Figs. e9-7** and **e9-9**). Subendothelial deposits with low serum levels of C_3 are typical, although 50% of patients have normal levels of C_3 and occasional intra-mesangial deposits. Low serum C_3 and a dense thickening of the GBM containing ribbons of dense deposits and C_3 characterize Type II MPGN, sometimes called *dense deposit disease* (**Fig. e9-8**). Classically, the glomerular tuft has a lobular appearance; intramesangial deposits are rarely present and subendothelial deposits are generally absent. Proliferation in Type III MPGN is less common than the other two types and is often focal; mesangial interposition is rare, and subepithelial deposits can occur along widened segments of the GBM that appear laminated and disrupted.

Type I MPGN is secondary to glomerular deposition of circulating immune complexes or their in situ formation. Types II and III MPGN may be related to "nephritic factors," which are autoantibodies that stabilize C_3 convertase and allow it to activate serum C_3. Patients with MPGN present with proteinuria, hematuria, and pyuria (30%), systemic symptoms of fatigue and malaise that are most common in children with Type I disease, or an acute nephritic picture with RPGN and a speedy deterioration in renal function in up to 25% of patients. Low serum C_3 levels are common. Fifty percent of patients with MPGN develop end-stage disease 10 years after diagnosis, and 90% have renal insufficiency after 20 years. Nephrotic syndrome, hypertension, and renal insufficiency all predict poor outcome. In the presence of proteinuria, treatment with inhibitors of the renin-angiotensin system is prudent. Evidence for treatment with dipyridamole, coumadin, or cyclophosphamide is not strongly established nor recommended. There is some evidence supporting the efficacy of treatment of *primary MPGN* with steroids, particularly in children. In *secondary MPGN*, treating the associated infection, autoimmune disease, or neoplasms is of demonstrated benefit. Although all primary renal diseases can recur over time in transplanted renal allografts, patients with MPGN are well known to be at risk for this adverse event.

MESANGIOPROLIFERATIVE GLOMERULONEPHRITIS

Mesangioproliferative glomerulonephritis is characterized by expansion of the mesangium, sometimes associated with mesangial hypercellularity; thin, single contoured capillary walls; and mesangial immune deposits. Clinically, it can present with varying degrees of proteinuria and, commonly, hematuria. Mesangioproliferative disease may be seen in IgA nephropathy, *P. falciparum* malaria, resolving postinfectious glomerulonephritis, and Class II nephritis from lupus, all of which can have a similar histologic appearance. With these secondary entities excluded, the diagnosis of *primary mesangioproliferative glomerulonephritis* is made in less than 15% of renal biopsies. As an immune-mediated renal lesion with deposits of IgM, C1q, and C_3, the clinical course is variable. Patients with isolated hematuria may have a very benign course, and those with heavy proteinuria occasionally progress to renal failure. There is little agreement on treatment, but some clinical reports suggest benefit from use of inhibitors of the renin-angiotensin system, steroid therapy, and even cytotoxic agents.

NEPHROTIC SYNDROME

Nephrotic syndrome classically presents with heavy proteinuria, minimal hematuria, hypoalbuminemia, hypercholesterolemia, edema, and hypertension. If left undiagnosed or untreated, some of these syndromes will progressively damage enough glomeruli to cause a fall in GFR, producing renal failure.

Therapies for various causes of nephrotic syndrome are noted under individual disease headings below. In general, all patients with hypercholesterolemia secondary to nephrotic syndrome should be treated with lipid-lowering agents since they are at increased risk for cardiovascular disease. Edema secondary to salt and water retention can be controlled with the judicious use of diuretics, avoiding intravascular volume depletion. Venous complications secondary to the hypercoagulable state associated with nephrotic syndrome can be treated with

anticoagulants. The losses of various serum binding proteins, such as thyroid-binding globulin, lead to alterations in functional tests. Lastly, proteinuria itself is hypothesized to be nephrotoxic, and treatment of proteinuria with inhibitors of the renin-angiotensin system can lower urinary protein excretion.

MINIMAL CHANGE DISEASE

MCD, sometimes known as *nil lesion*, causes 70–90% of nephrotic syndrome in childhood but only 10–15% of nephrotic syndrome in adults. MCD usually presents as a primary renal disease but can be associated with several other conditions, including Hodgkin's disease, allergies, or use of nonsteroidal anti-inflammatory agents; significant interstitial nephritis often accompanies cases associated with nonsteroidal use. MCD on renal biopsy shows no obvious glomerular lesion by light microscopy and is negative for deposits by immunofluorescent microscopy, or occasionally shows small amounts of IgM in the mesangium (**Fig. e9-1**). Electron microscopy, however, consistently demonstrates an effacement of the foot process supporting the epithelial podocytes with weakening of slit-pore membranes. The pathophysiology of this lesion is uncertain. Most agree there is a circulating cytokine, perhaps related to a T cell response that alters capillary charge and podocyte integrity. The evidence for cytokine-related immune injury is circumstantial and is suggested by the presence of preceding allergies, altered cell-mediated immunity during viral infections, and the high frequency of remissions with steroids.

MCD presents clinically with the abrupt onset of edema and nephrotic syndrome accompanied by acellular urinary sediment. Less common clinical features include hypertension (30% in children, 50% in adults), microscopic hematuria (20% in children, 33% in adults), atopy or allergic symptoms (40% in children, 30% in adults), and decreased renal function (<5% in children, 30% in adults). The appearance of acute renal failure in adults is usually caused by intrarenal edema (nephrosarca) that is responsive to intravenous albumin and diuretics. This presentation must be distinguished from acute renal failure secondary to hypovolemia. In children, the abnormal urine principally contains albumin with minimal amounts of higher molecular weight proteins, and is sometimes called *selective proteinuria*. Although up to 30% of children have a spontaneous remission, all children today are treated with steroids; only children who are nonresponders are biopsied in this setting. Primary responders are patients who have a complete remission (<0.2 mg/24 h of proteinuria) after a single course of prednisone; steroid-dependent patients relapse as their steroid dose is tapered. Frequent relapsers have two or more relapses in the 6 months following taper, and steroid-resistant patients fail to respond to steroid therapy. Ninety to 95% of children will develop a complete remission after 8 weeks of steroid therapy, and 80–85% of adults will achieve complete remission, but only after a longer course of 20–24 weeks. Patients with steroid resistance can develop FSGS on repeat biopsy. Some hypothesize that if the first renal biopsy does not have a sample of deeper glomeruli, then the correct early diagnosis of FSGS may be missed.

Relapses occur in 70–75% of children after the first remission, and early relapse predicts multiple subsequent relapses. The frequency of relapses decreases after puberty, although there is an increased risk of relapse following the rapid tapering of steroids in all groups. Relapses are less common in adults but are more resistant to subsequent therapy. Prednisone is first-line therapy, and other immunosuppressive drugs, such as cyclophosphamide, chlorambucil, and mycophenolate mofetil, are saved for frequent relapsers, steroid-dependent, or steroid-resistant patients. Cyclosporine can induce remission, but relapse is also common when cyclosporine is withdrawn. The long-term prognosis in adults is less favorable when acute renal failure or steroid resistance occurs.

FOCAL SEGMENTAL GLOMERULOSCLEROSIS

FSGS refers to a pattern of renal injury characterized by segmental glomerular scars that involve some but not all glomeruli; the clinical findings of FSGS largely manifest as proteinuria. When the secondary causes of FSGS are eliminated (Table 227-5), the remaining patients

TABLE 277-5 FOCAL SEGMENTAL GLOMERULOSCLEROSIS

Primary focal segmental glomerulosclerosis
Secondary focal segmental glomerulosclerosis
  Viruses: HIV/Hepatitis B/Parvovirus
  Hypertensive nephropathy
  Reflux nephropathy
  Cholesterol emboli
  Drugs: Heroin/analgesics
  Oligomeganephronia
  Renal dysgenesis
  Alport's syndrome
  Sickle cell disease
  Lymphoma
  Radiation nephritis
  Familial podocytopathies
    NPHS1 mutation/nephrin
    NPHS2 mutation/podocin
    TRPC6 mutation/cation channel
    ACTN4 mutation/Actinin
    α-Galactosidase A deficiency/Fabry's disease
    N-acetylneuraminic acid hydrolase deficiency/nephrosialidosis

TABLE 277-6 MEMBRANOUS GLOMERULONEPHRITIS

Primary/idiopathic membranous glomerulonephritis
Secondary membranous glomerulonephritis
  Infection: Hepatitis B and C, syphilis, malaria, schistosomiasis, leprosy, filariasis
  Cancer: Breast, colon, lung, stomach, kidney, esophagus, neuroblastoma
  Drugs: gold, mercury, penicillamine, nonsteroidal anti-inflammatory agents, probenecid
  Autoimmune diseases: systemic lupus erythematosus, rheumatoid arthritis, primary biliary cirrhosis, dermatitis herpetiformis, bullous pemphigoid, myasthenia gravis, Sjögren's syndrome, Hashimoto's thyroiditis
  Other systemic diseases: Fanconi's syndrome, sickle cell anemia, diabetes, Crohn's disease, sarcoidosis, Guillain-Barré syndrome, Weber-Christian disease, angiofollicular lymph node hyperplasia

are considered to have FSGS. The incidence of this disease is increasing, and it now represents up to one-third of cases of nephrotic syndrome in adults and one-half of cases of nephrotic syndrome in African Americans, in whom it is seen more commonly. The pathogenesis of FSGS is probably multifactorial. Possible mechanisms include a T cell–mediated circulating permeability factor, TGF-β–mediated cellular proliferation and matrix synthesis, and podocyte abnormalities associated with genetic mutations.

The pathologic changes of FSGS are most prominent in glomeruli located at the corticomedullary junction (**Fig. e9-2**), so if the renal biopsy specimen is from superficial tissue, the lesions can be missed, which sometimes leads to a misdiagnosis of MCD. In addition to focal and segmental scarring, other variants have been described, including cellular lesions with *endocapillary hypercellularity* and heavy proteinuria; *collapsing glomerulopathy* (**Fig. e9-3**) with segmental or global glomerular collapse and a rapid decline in renal function; or the *glomerular tip lesion*, which seems to have a better prognosis.

FSGS can present with any level of proteinuria, hematuria, hypertension, or renal insufficiency. Nephrotic range proteinuria, African-American race, and renal insufficiency are associated with a poor outcome, with 50% of patients reaching renal failure in 6–8 years. FSGS rarely remits spontaneously, but treatment-induced remission of proteinuria significantly improves prognosis. Treatment of patients with *primary FSGS* should include inhibitors of the renin-angiotensin system. Based on retrospective studies, patients with nephrotic range proteinuria can be treated with steroids but respond far less often than patients with MCD. Proteinuria remits in only 20–45% of patients receiving a course of steroids over 6–9 months. Limited evidence suggests that the use of cyclosporine in steroid-responsive patients helps ensure remissions, while other cytotoxic agents confer little added benefit over steroid therapy. Primary FSGS recurs in 25–40% of patients given allografts at end-stage disease, leading to graft loss in half of those cases. The treatment of *secondary FSGS* typically involves treating the underlying cause and controlling proteinuria. There is no role for steroids or other immunosuppressive agents in secondary FSGS.

MEMBRANOUS GLOMERULONEPHRITIS

MGN, or *membranous nephropathy* as it is sometimes called, accounts for approximately 30% of cases of nephrotic syndrome in adults, with a peak incidence between the ages of 30–50 years and a male to female ratio of 2:1. It is rare in childhood and by far the most common cause of nephrotic syndrome in the elderly. In 25–30% of cases, MGN is secondary to malignancy (solid tumors of the breast, lung, colon), infection (hepatitis B, malaria, schistosomiasis), or rheumatologic disorders like lupus or rarely rheumatoid arthritis (Table 277-6).

Uniform thickening of the basement membrane along the peripheral capillary loops is seen by light microscopy on renal biopsy (**Fig. e9-5**); this thickening needs to be distinguished from that seen in dia-

betes and amyloidosis. Immunofluorescence demonstrates diffuse granular deposits of IgG and C3, and electron microscopy typically reveals electron-dense subepithelial deposits. While different stages (I–V) of progressive membranous lesions have been described, some published analyses indicate the degree of tubular atrophy or interstitial fibrosis is more predictive of progression than is the stage of glomerular disease. The presence of subendothelial deposits or the presence of tubuloreticular inclusions strongly points to a diagnosis of membranous lupus nephritis, which may precede the extrarenal manifestations of lupus. Work in Heyman nephritis, an animal model of MGN, suggests that glomerular lesions result from in situ formation of immune complexes with megalin receptor–associated protein as the putative antigen. This antigen is not found in human podocytes, but human antibodies have been described against neutral endopeptidase expressed by podocytes, hepatitis antigens B/C, *Helicobacter pylori* antigens, tumor antigens, and thyroglobulin.

Eighty percent of patients with MGN present with nephrotic syndrome and nonselective proteinuria. Microscopic hematuria is seen in up to 50% of patients. Spontaneous remissions occur in 20–33% of patients and often occur late in the course after years of nephrotic syndrome. One-third of patients continue to have relapsing nephrotic syndrome but maintain normal renal function, and approximately another third of patients develop renal failure or die from the complications of nephrotic syndrome. Male gender, older age, hypertension, and the persistence of proteinuria are associated with worse prognosis. Although thrombotic complications are a feature of all nephrotic syndromes, MGN has the highest reported incidences of renal vein thrombosis, pulmonary embolism, and deep vein thrombosis. Prophylactic anticoagulation is controversial but has been recommended for patients with severe or prolonged proteinuria in the absence of risk factors for bleeding.

In addition to the treatment of edema, dyslipidemia, and hypertension, inhibition of the renin-angiotensin system is recommended. Therapy with immunosuppressive drugs is also recommended for patients with primary MGN and persistent proteinuria (>3.0 g/24 h). The choice of immunosuppressive drugs for therapy is controversial, but current recommendations based on small clinical studies are to treat with steroids and cyclophosphamide, chlorambucil, or cyclosporine. Experience with mycophenolate mofetil or anti-CD20 antibody is even more limited.

DIABETIC NEPHROPATHY

Diabetic nephropathy is the single most common cause of chronic renal failure in the United States, accounting for 45% of patients receiving renal replacement therapy, and is a rapidly growing problem worldwide. The dramatic increase in the number of patients with diabetic nephropathy reflects the epidemic increase in obesity, metabolic syndrome, and Type 2 diabetes mellitus. Approximately 40% of patients with Types 1 or 2 diabetes develop nephropathy, but due to the higher prevalence of Type 2 diabetes (90%) compared to Type 1 (10%), the majority of patients with diabetic nephropathy have Type 2 disease. Renal lesions are more common in African-American, Native American, Polynesian, and Maori populations. Risk factors for the development of diabetic nephropathy include hyperglycemia, hypertension, dyslipidemia, smoking, a family history of diabetic nephropathy, and gene polymorphisms affecting the activity of the renin-angiotensin-aldosterone axis.

Within 1–2 years after the onset of clinical diabetes, morphologic changes appear in the kidney. Thickening of the GBM is a sensitive indicator for the presence of diabetes but correlates poorly with the presence or absence of clinically significant nephropathy. The composition of the GBM is altered notably with a loss of heparan sulfate moieties that form the negatively charged filtration barrier. This change results in increased filtration of serum proteins into the urine, predominately negatively charged albumin. The expansion of the mesangium due to the accumulation of extracellular matrix correlates with the clinical manifestations of diabetic nephropathy. This expansion in mesangial matrix can be associated with the development of *mesangial sclerosis*. Some patients also develop eosinophilic, PAS$^+$ nodules called *nodular glomerulosclerosis* or *Kimmelstiel-Wilson nodules*. Immunofluorescence microscopy often reveals the nonspecific deposition of IgG (at times in a linear pattern) or complement staining without immune deposits on electron microscopy. Prominent vascular changes are frequently seen with hyaline and hypertensive arteriosclerosis. This is associated with varying degrees of chronic glomerulosclerosis and tubulointerstitial changes. Renal biopsies from patients with Types 1 and 2 diabetes are largely indistinguishable.

These pathologic changes are the result of a number of postulated factors. Multiple lines of evidence support an important role for increases in glomerular capillary pressure (intraglomerular hypertension) in alterations in renal structure and function. Direct effects of hyperglycemia on the actin cytoskeleton of renal mesangial and vascular smooth-muscle cells as well as diabetes-associated changes in circulating factors such as atrial naturetic factor, angiotensin II, and insulin-like growth factor (IGF) may account for this. Sustained glomerular hypertension increases matrix production, alterations in the GBM with disruption in the filtration barrier (and hence proteinuria) and glomerulosclerosis. A number of factors have also been identified which alter matrix production, including the accumulation of advanced glycosylation end products, circulating factors including growth hormone, IGF-I, angiotensin II, connective tissues growth factor, TGF-β, and dyslipidemia.

The natural history of diabetic nephropathy in patients with Types 1 and 2 diabetes is similar. However, since the onset of Type 1 diabetes is readily identifiable and the onset of Type 2 diabetes is not, a patient newly diagnosed with Type 2 diabetes may have renal disease for many years before nephropathy is discovered and presents as *advanced diabetic nephropathy*. At the onset of diabetes, renal hypertrophy and glomerular hyperfiltration are present. The degree of glomerular hyperfiltration correlates with the subsequent risk of clinically significant nephropathy. In the approximately 40% of patients with diabetes who develop diabetic nephropathy, the earliest manifestation is an increase in albuminuria detected by sensitive radioimmunoassay (Table 277-1). Albuminuria in the range of 30–300 mg/24 h is called *microalbuminuria*. In patients with Types 1 or 2 diabetes, microalbuminuria appears 5–10 years after the onset of diabetes. It is currently recommended to test patients with Type 1 disease for microalbuminuria 5 years after diagnosis of diabetes and yearly thereafter, and, because the time of onset of Type 2 diabetes is often unknown, to test Type 2 patients at the time of diagnosis of diabetes and yearly thereafter.

Patients with small rises in albuminuria increase their levels of urinary albumin excretion, typically reaching dipstick positive levels of proteinuria (>300 mg albuminuria) 5–10 years after the onset of early albuminuria. Microalbuminuria is a potent risk factor for cardiovascular events and death in patients with Type 2 diabetes. Many patients with Type 2 diabetes and microalbuminuria succumb to cardiovascular events before they progress to proteinuria or renal failure. Proteinuria in frank diabetic nephropathy can be variable, ranging from 500 mg to 25 g/24 h, and is often associated with nephrotic syndrome. More than 90% of patients with Type 1 diabetes and nephropathy have diabetic retinopathy, so the absence of retinopathy in Type 1 patients

with proteinuria should prompt consideration of a diagnosis other than diabetic nephropathy; only 60% of patients with Type 2 diabetes with nephropathy have diabetic retinopathy. There is a highly significant correlation between the presence of retinopathy and the presence of Kimmelstiel-Wilson nodules (**Fig. e9-18**). Also, characteristically, patients with advanced diabetic nephropathy have normal to enlarged kidneys, in contrast to other glomerular diseases where kidney size is usually decreased. Using the above epidemiologic and clinical data, and in the absence of other clinical or serologic data suggesting another disease, diabetic nephropathy is usually diagnosed without a renal biopsy. After the onset of proteinuria >500 mg/24 h, renal function inexorably declines, with 50% of patients reaching renal failure in 5–10 years; thus, from the earliest stages of microalbuminuria, it usually takes 10–20 years to reach end-stage renal disease. Hypertension may predict which patients develop diabetic nephropathy, as the presence of hypertension accelerates the rate of decline in renal function. Once renal failure appears, however, survival on dialysis is far shorter for patients with diabetes compared to other dialysis patients; some diabetics do better clinically if they are started on dialysis before they reach advanced renal failure. Survival is best for patients with Type 1 diabetes who receive a transplant from a living related donor.

Good evidence supports the benefits of blood sugar and blood pressure control as well as inhibition of the renin-angiotensin system in retarding the progression of diabetic nephropathy. In patients with Type 1 diabetes, intensive control of blood sugar clearly prevents the development or progression of diabetic nephropathy. The evidence in patients with Type 2 disease, although less compelling, also supports intensive control of blood sugar. Controlling systemic blood pressure to levels of 130/80 mmHg or less decreases renal and cardiovascular adverse events in this high-risk population. The vast majority of patients with diabetic nephropathy require three or more antihypertensive drugs to achieve this goal. Drugs that inhibit the renin-angiotensin system, independent of their effects on systemic blood pressure, have been repeatedly shown to slow the progression of diabetic nephropathy at early (microalbuminuria) and late (proteinuria with reduced glomerular filtration) stages, independent of any effect they may have on systemic blood pressure.

Since angiotensin II increases efferent arteriolar resistance and, hence, glomerular capillary pressure, one key mechanism for the efficacy of ACE inhibitors or angiotensin receptor blockers (ARBs) is reducing glomerular hypertension. Patients with Type 1 diabetes for 5 years who develop albuminuria or declining renal function should be treated with ACE inhibitors. Patients with Type 2 diabetes and microalbuminuria or proteinuria may be treated with ACE inhibitors or ARBs.

GLOMERULAR DEPOSITION DISEASES

Plasma cell dyscrasias producing excess light chain immunoglobulin sometimes lead to the formation of glomerular and tubular deposits that cause heavy proteinuria and renal failure; the same is true for the accumulation of serum amyloid A protein fragments seen in several inflammatory diseases. This broad group of proteinuric patients has *glomerular deposition disease*.

Light Chain Deposition Disease The biochemical characteristics of nephrotoxic light chains produced in light chain malignancies typically confers a specific pattern of renal injury in each individual patient; that of either cast nephropathy (**Fig. e9-15**), which causes renal failure but not heavy proteinuria, amyloidosis, or *light chain deposition disease* (**Fig. e9-14**), which produce nephrotic syndrome with renal failure. These latter patients produce kappa light chains that do not have the biochemical features necessary to form amyloid fibrils. Instead, they self-aggregate and form granular deposits along the glomerular capillary and mesangium, tubular basement membrane, and Bowman's capsule. When predominant in glomeruli, nephrotic syndrome develops, and about 70% of patients progress to dialysis. Light-chain deposits are not fibrillar and do not stain with Congo red, but they are easily detected with anti-light–chain antibody using immunofluorescence, or as granular deposits on electron microscopy. A combination of the light-chain rearrangement, self-aggregating properties at neutral pH, and abnormal metabolism probably contribute to the deposition. Treatment for light-chain deposition disease is treatment of the primary disease. As so many patients with light-chain deposition disease progress to renal failure, the overall prognosis is grim.

Renal Amyloidosis Most *renal amyloidosis* is either the result of primary fibrillar deposits of immunoglobulin light chains [amyloid L (AL)], or secondary to fibrillar deposits of serum amyloid A (AA) protein fragments (Chap. 324). Even though both occur for different reasons, their clinicopathophysiology is quite similar and will be discussed together. Amyloid infiltrates the liver, heart, peripheral nerves, carpal tunnel, upper pharynx, and kidney, producing restrictive cardiomyopathy, hepatomegaly, macroglossia, and heavy proteinuria sometimes associated with renal vein thrombosis. In systemic AL amyloidosis, also called *primary amyloidosis*, light chains produced in excess by clonal plasma cell dyscrasias are made into fragments by macrophages so they can self-aggregate at acid pH. A disproportionate number of these light chains (75%) are of the *lambda* class. About 10% of these patients have overt myeloma with lytic bone lesions and infiltration of the bone marrow with >30% plasma cells; nephrotic syndrome is common, and about 20% of patients progress to dialysis. AA amyloidosis is sometimes called *secondary amyloidosis* and also affects the kidney with nephrotic syndrome. It is due to deposition of β-pleated sheets of serum amyloid A protein, an acute phase reactant whose physiologic function is unknown. Forty percent of patients with AA amyloid have rheumatoid arthritis, and another 10% have ankylosing spondylitis or psoriatic arthritis; the rest derive from other lesser causes. Less common in Western countries but more common in Mediterranean regions, particularly in Sephardic and Iraqi Jews, is familial Mediterranean fever (FMF). FMF is caused by a mutation in the gene encoding pyrin, while Muckle-Wells syndrome, a related disorder, results from a mutation in cryopyrin; both proteins are important in the apoptosis of leukocytes early in inflammation. Receptor mutations in TNFR1–associated periodic syndrome also produce chronic inflammation and secondary amyloidosis. Fragments of serum amyloid A protein increase and self-aggregate by attaching to receptors for advanced glycation end products in the extracellular environment; nephrotic syndrome is common, and about 40–60% of patients progress to dialysis. AA and AL amyloid fibrils are detectable with Congo red or in more detail with electron microscopy (**Fig. e9-13**). Biopsy of involved liver or kidney is diagnostic 90% of the time when the pretest probability is high; abdominal fat pad aspirates are positive about 70% of the time, but apparently less so when looking for AA amyloid. Amyloid deposits are distributed along blood vessels and in the mesangial regions of the kidney. The treatment for primary amyloidosis is not particularly effective; melphalan and autologous hematopoietic stem cell transplantation can delay the course of disease in about 30% of patients. Secondary amyloidosis is also relentless unless the primary disease can be controlled. Some new drugs in development that disrupt the formation of fibrils may be available in the future.

Fibrillary-Immunotactoid Glomerulopathy There is no agreement on whether *fibrillary glomerulonephritis* and *immunotactoid glomerulonephritis* are different or one and the same. Both are hard to distinguish by clinical presentation but have some apparent differences with electron microscopy. Fibrillar/microtubular deposits of oligoclonal or oligotypic immunoglobulins and complement appear in the mesangium and along the glomerular capillary wall. In fibrillary glomerulonephritis the fibrils are smaller and more randomly distributed than in immunotactoid glomerulonephritis. Congo red stains are negative in both disorders. The cause of this "nonamyloid" glomerulopathy is mostly idiopathic; reports of immunotactoid glomerulonephritis describe an occasional association with chronic lymphocytic leukemia or B cell lymphoma. Both disorders appear in adults in the fourth decade with moderate to heavy proteinuria, hematuria, and a wide variety of histologic lesions, including DPGN, MPGN, MGN, or mesangioproliferative glomerulonephritis. Nearly half of patients will develop renal

failure over a few years. There is no consensus on treatment of this uncommon disorder.

FABRY'S DISEASE

Fabry's disease is an X-linked inborn error of globotriaosylceramide metabolism secondary to deficient lysosomal α-galactosidase A activity, resulting in excessive intracellular storage of globotriaosylceramide. Affected organs include the vascular endothelium, heart, brain, and kidneys. Classically, Fabry's disease presents in childhood in males with multi-organ involvement. Hemizygotes with hypomorphic mutations sometimes present in the fourth to sixth decade with single organ involvement. Rarely, dominant-negative α-galactosidase A mutations or female heterozygotes with unfavorable X inactivation present with mild single-organ involvement. Renal biopsy reveals enlarged glomerular visceral epithelial cells packed with small clear vacuoles containing globotriaosylceramide; vacuoles may also be found in parietal and tubular epithelia (**Fig. e9-16**). These vacuoles of electron-dense materials in parallel arrays (zebra bodies) are easily seen on electron microscopy. Ultimately, glomeruli develop FSGS. The nephropathy of Fabry's disease typically presents in the third decade as mild to moderate proteinuria, sometimes with microscopic hematuria or nephrotic syndrome. Urinalysis may reveal oval fat bodies and birefringent glycolipid globules under polarized light (Maltese cross). Renal biopsy is necessary for definitive diagnosis. Progression to renal failure occurs by the fourth or fifth decade. Treatment with recombinant α-galactosidase A has been demonstrated to clear microvascular endothelial deposits of globotriaosylceramide from the kidneys, heart, and skin.

PULMONARY-RENAL SYNDROMES

Several diseases can present with catastrophic hemoptysis and glomerulonephritis associated with varying degrees of renal failure. The usual causes include Goodpasture's syndrome, Wegener's granulomatosis, microscopic polyangiitis, Churg-Strauss vasculitis, and, rarely, Henoch-Schönlein purpura or cryoglobulinemia. Each of these diseases can also present without hemoptysis and are discussed in detail in "Acute Nephritic Syndromes," above. Pulmonary bleeding in this setting is life-threatening and often results in airway intubation, and acute renal failure requires dialysis in the intensive care unit. Diagnosis is difficult initially because biopsies and serologic testing take time. Treatment with plasmapheresis and methylprednisolone is often empiric and temporizing until results of testing are available.

BASEMENT MEMBRANE SYNDROMES

All kidney epithelia, including podocytes, rest on basement membranes assembled into a planar surface through the interweaving of collagen IV with laminins, nidogen, and sulfated proteoglycans. Structural abnormalities in GBMs associated with hematuria are characteristic of several familial disorders related to the expression of collagen IV genes. The extended family of collagen IV contains six chains, which are expressed in different tissues at different stages of embryonic development. All epithelial basement membranes early in human development are composed of interconnected triple-helical protomers rich in $\alpha1.\alpha1.\alpha2(IV)$ collagen. Some specialized tissues undergo a developmental switch replacing $\alpha1.\alpha1.\alpha2(IV)$ protomers with an $\alpha3.\alpha4.\alpha5(IV)$ collagen network; this switch occurs in the kidney (glomerular and tubular basement membrane), lung, testis, cochlea, and eye, while an $\alpha5.\alpha5.\alpha6(IV)$ network appears in skin, smooth muscle, and esophagus and along Bowman's capsule in the kidney. This switch probably occurs because the $\alpha3.\alpha4.\alpha5(IV)$ network is more resistant to proteases and ensures the structural longevity of critical tissues. When basement membranes are the target of glomerular disease, they produce moderate proteinuria, some hematuria, and progressive renal failure.

ANTI-GBM DISEASE

Autoimmune disease where antibodies are directed against the α3 NC1 domain of collagen IV produces an *anti-GBM disease* often associated with RPGN and/or a pulmonary-renal syndrome called *Goodpasture's syndrome*. Discussion of this disease is covered in "Acute Nephritic Syndromes," above.

ALPORT'S SYNDROME
Classically, patients with Alport's syndrome develop hematuria, thinning and splitting of the GBMs, mild proteinuria (<1–2 g/24 h), and chronic glomerulosclerosis, leading to renal failure in association with sensorineural deafness. Some patients develop lenticonus of the anterior lens capsule and, rarely, mental retardation or leiomyomatosis. Approximately 85% of patients with Alport's syndrome have an X-linked inheritance of mutations in the $\alpha5(IV)$ collagen chain on chromosome Xq22–24. Female carriers have variable penetrance depending on the type of mutation or the degree of mosaicism created by X inactivation. Fifteen percent of patients have autosomal recessive disease of the $\alpha3(IV)$ or $\alpha4(IV)$ chains on chromosome 2q35–37. Rarely, some kindred have an autosomal dominant inheritance of dominant-negative mutations in $\alpha3(IV)$ or $\alpha4(IV)$ chains.

Pedigrees with this syndrome are quite variable in their rate and frequency of tissue damage leading to organ failure. Patients with nonsense or missense mutations, reading frame shifts, or large deletions generally develop renal failure and sensorineural deafness by age 30 (juvenile form), while patients with splice variants, exon skipping, or missense mutations of α-helical glycines generally deteriorate after the age of 30 (adult form) with mild or late deafness. Early severe deafness or lenticonus suggest a poorer prognosis.

Alport's patients early in their disease typically have thin basement membranes on renal biopsy (**Fig. e9-17**), which thicken over time into multilamellations surrounding lucent areas that often contain granules of varying density—the so-called split basement membrane. In any Alport kidney there are areas of thinning mixed with splitting of the GBM. Tubules drop out, glomeruli scar, and the kidney eventually succumbs to interstitial fibrosis. Primary treatment is control of systemic hypertension and use of ACE inhibitors to slow renal progression. Although patients who receive renal allografts usually develop anti-GBM antibodies directed toward the collagen epitopes absent in their native kidney, overt Goodpasture's syndrome is uncommon and graft survival is good.

THIN BASEMENT MEMBRANE DISEASE
Some variants of Alport's syndrome are now recognized as a subpopulation of patients with *thin basement membrane disease*. Thin basement membranes are found in 5–10% of the so-called normal population. These subclinical patients have normal blood pressure and little proteinuria, and they rarely progress to renal failure. If they present with hematuria, they are often given the diagnosis of *benign familial hematuria*. Many of these patients have mutations in the same $\alpha3(IV)$ or $\alpha4(IV)$ collagen genes associated with autosomal recessive or dominant Alport's syndrome. Clearly, the boundary between nonprogressive Alport's syndrome and benign familial hematuria is quite variable, as there is a spectrum of clinical penetrance.

NAIL-PATELLA SYNDROME
Patients with nail-patella syndrome develop iliac horns on the pelvis and dysplasia of the dorsal limbs involving the patella, elbows, and nails, variably associated with neural-sensory hearing impairment, glaucoma, and abnormalities of the GBM and podocytes, leading to hematuria, proteinuria, and FSGS. The syndrome is autosomal-dominant, with haploinsufficiency for the LIM homeodomain transcription factor LMX1B; pedigrees are extremely variable in the penetrance for all features of the disease. LMX1B regulates the expression of genes encoding $\alpha3$ and $\alpha4$ chains of collagen IV, interstitial type III collagen, podocin, and CD2AP that help form the slit-pore membranes connecting podocytes. Mutations in the LIM domain region of LMX1B are associated with glomerulopathy, and renal failure appears in as many as 30% of patients. Proteinuria or isolated hematuria is discovered throughout life, but usually by the third decade, and is inexplicably more common in females. On renal biopsy there is lucent damage

to the lamina densa of the GBM, an increase in collagen III fibrils along glomerular capillaries and in the mesangium, and damage to the slit-pore membrane, producing heavy proteinuria not unlike that seen in congenital nephrotic syndrome. Patients with renal failure do well with transplantation.

GLOMERULAR-VASCULAR SYNDROMES
A variety of diseases result in classic vascular injury to the glomerular capillaries. Most of these processes also damage blood vessels elsewhere in the body. The group of diseases discussed here lead to vasculitis, renal endothelial injury, thrombosis, ischemia, and/or lipid-based occlusions.

ATHEROSCLEROTIC NEPHROPATHY
Aging in the developed world is commonly associated with the occlusion of coronary and systemic blood vessels. The reasons for this include obesity, insulin resistance, smoking, hypertension, and diets rich in lipids that deposit in the arterial and arteriolar circulation, producing local inflammation and fibrosis of small blood vessels. When the renal arterial circulation is involved, the glomerular microcirculation is damaged, leading to *chronic nephrosclerosis*. Patients with GFRs <60 mL/min have more cardiovascular events and hospitalizations than those with higher filtration rates. Several aggressive lipid disorders can accelerate this process, but most of the time atherosclerotic progression to chronic nephrosclerosis is associated with poorly controlled hypertension. Approximately 10% of glomeruli are normally sclerotic by age 40, rising to 20% by age 60 and 30% by age 80. Serum lipid profiles in humans are greatly affected by *apolipoprotein E* polymorphisms; the E4 allele is accompanied by increases in serum cholesterol and is more closely associated with atherogenic profiles in patients with renal failure. Mutations in E2 alleles, particularly in Japanese patients, produce a specific renal abnormality called *lipoprotein glomerulopathy* associated with glomerular lipoprotein thrombi and capillary dilation.

HYPERTENSIVE NEPHROSCLEROSIS
Uncontrolled systemic hypertension causes permanent damage to the kidneys in about 6% of patients with elevated blood pressure. As many as 27% of patients with end-stage kidney disease have hypertension as a primary cause. Although there is not a clear correlation between the extent or duration of hypertension and the risk of end-organ damage, *hypertensive nephrosclerosis* is fivefold more frequent in African Americans than Caucasians. Associated risk factors for progression to end-stage kidney disease include age, sex, race, smoking, hypercholesterolemia, duration of hypertension, low birth weight, and preexisting renal injury. Kidney biopsies in patients with hypertension, microhematuria, and moderate proteinuria demonstrate arteriolosclerosis, chronic nephrosclerosis, and interstitial fibrosis in the absence of immune deposits (**Fig. e9-19**). Today, based on a careful history, physical examination, urinalysis, and some serologic testing, the diagnosis of chronic nephrosclerosis is usually inferred without a biopsy. Treating hypertension is the best way to avoid progressive renal failure; most guidelines recommend lowering blood pressure to <130/80 mmHg if there is preexisting diabetes or kidney disease. In the presence of kidney disease, most patients begin therapy with two drugs, classically a thiazide diuretic and an ACE inhibitor; many will require three drugs. There is strong evidence in African Americans with hypertensive nephrosclerosis that therapy initiated with an ACE inhibitor can slow the rate of decline in renal function independent of systemic blood pressure. Patients with lower levels of hypertension are usually started on a thiazide diuretic or an ACE inhibitor alone. Malignant acceleration of hypertension can complicate the course of chronic nephrosclerosis, particularly in the setting of scleroderma (**Fig. e9-22**) or cocaine use. The hemodynamic stress of malignant hypertension causes fibrinoid necrosis of small blood vessels, thrombotic microangiography, a nephritic urinalysis, and acute renal failure. In the setting of renal failure, chest pain, or papilledema, the condition is treated as a hypertensive emergency. Slightly lowering the blood pressure often produces an immediate re-

duction in GFR that improves as the vascular injury attenuates and autoregulation of blood vessel tone is restored.

CHOLESTEROL EMBOLI

Aging patients with clinical complications from atherosclerosis sometimes shower cholesterol crystals into the circulation—either spontaneously or, more commonly, following an endovascular procedure with manipulation of the aorta—or with use of systemic anticoagulation. Spontaneous emboli may shower acutely or shower subacutely and somewhat more silently. Irregular emboli trapped in the microcirculation produce ischemic damage that induces an inflammatory reaction. Depending on the location of the atherosclerotic plaques releasing these cholesterol fragments, one may see cerebral transient ischemic attacks; livedo reticularis in the lower extremities; Hollenhorst plaques in the retina with visual field cuts; necrosis of the toes; and acute glomerular capillary injury leading to *focal glomerulosclerosis* sometimes associated with hematuria, mild proteinuria, and loss of renal function, which typically progresses over a few years. Occasional patients have fever, eosinophilia, or eosinophiluria. A skin biopsy of an involved area may be diagnostic. Since tissue fixation dissolves the cholesterol, one typically sees only residual, biconvex clefts in the vessel (**Fig. e9-20**). There is no therapy to reverse embolic occlusions, and steroids do not help. Controlling blood pressure and lipids and cessation of smoking are usually recommended for prevention.

SICKLE CELL DISEASE

Although individuals with SA-hemoglobin are usually asymptomatic, most will gradually develop hyposthenuria due to subclinical infarction of the renal medulla, thus predisposing them to volume depletion. Patients with homozygous SS-sickle cell disease develop chronic vasoocclusive disease in many organs. Polymers of deoxygenated SS-hemoglobin distort the shape of red blood cells. These cells attach to endothelia and obstruct small blood vessels, producing frequent, random, and painful sickle cell crises over time. Vessel occlusions in the kidney produce glomerular hypertension, FSGS, interstitial nephritis, and renal infarction associated with hyposthenuria, microscopic hematuria, and even gross hematuria; some patients also present with MPGN. By the second or third decade of life, persistent vasoocclusive disease in the kidney leads to varying degrees of renal failure, and some patients end up on dialysis. Treatment is directed to reducing the frequency of painful crises and administering ACE inhibitors in the hope of delaying a progressive decline in renal function. Sickle cell patients can have transplantations, and renal graft survival is comparable to African Americans given transplantations for other reasons.

THROMBOTIC MICROANGIOPATHIES

Thrombotic thrombocytopenic purpura (TTP) and *hemolytic-uremic syndrome* (HUS) represent a spectrum of thrombotic microangiopathies. TTP and HUS share the general features of idiopathic thrombocytopenic purpura, hemolytic anemia, fever, renal failure, and neurologic disturbances. When patients have more evidence of renal injury, their condition tends to be called HUS, and when there is more neurologic disease, it is considered to be TTP. In adults there is often a mixture of both, which is why they are often called TTP/HUS. On examination of kidney tissue there is evidence of *glomerular capillary endotheliosis* associated with platelet thrombi, damage to the capillary wall, and formation of fibrin material in and around glomeruli (**Fig. e9-21**). These tissue findings are similar to what is seen in preeclampsia/HELLP (hemolysis, elevated liver enzymes, and low platelet count syndrome), malignant hypertension, and the antiphospholipid syndrome. TTP/HUS is also seen in pregnancy; with the use of oral contraceptives or quinine; in renal transplant patients given OKT3 for rejection; in patients taking the calcineurin inhibitors cyclosporine and tacrolimus or in patients taking the antiplatelet agents ticlopidine and clopidogrel; or following HIV infection.

Although there is no agreement on how much they share a final common pathophysiology, two general groups of patients are recognized: childhood HUS associated with enterohemorrhagic diarrhea

and TTP-HUS in adults. Childhood HUS is caused by a toxin released by *Escherichia coli* O157:H7 and occasionally by *Shigella dysenteriae*. This shiga toxin (veratoxin) directly injures endothelia, enterocytes, and renal cells, causing apoptosis, platelet clumping, and intravascular hemolysis by binding to the glycolipid receptors (Gb3). These receptors are more abundant along endothelia in children compared to adults. In familial cases of adult TTP/HUS, there is a genetic deficiency of the ADAMTS13 metalloprotease that cleaves large multimers of von Willebrand's factor. Absent ADAMTS13, these large multimers cause platelet clumping and intravascular hemolysis. An antibody to ADAMTS13 is found in many sporadic cases of adult TTP/HUS, but not all; many patients also have antibodies to the thrombospondin receptor on selected endothelial cells in small vessels or increased levels of plasminogen-activator inhibitor 1 (PAI-1). The treatment of childhood HUS or adult TTP/HUS is daily plasmapheresis, which can be lifesaving. Plasmapheresis is given until the platelet count rises, but in relapsing patients it may need to be continued well after the platelet count improves, and in resistant patients twice-daily exchange may be helpful. Most patients respond within 2 weeks of daily plasmapheresis. Since TTP/HUS often has an autoimmune basis, there is an anecdotal role in relapsing patients for using splenectomy, steroids, immunosuppressive drugs, or anti-CD20 antibody. Patients with childhood HUS from infectious diarrhea are not given antibiotics, as antibiotics are thought to accelerate the release of the toxin and the diarrhea is usually self-limited.

ANTIPHOSPHOLIPID SYNDROME

Antiphospholipid syndrome develops in patients expressing antibodies to anionic phospholipids, particularly β_2 glycoprotein 1. Half of the patients have no obvious cause, a few are pregnant, some are already receiving hemodialysis or have a renal allograft, and the rest have a primary glomerulonephritis (nil lesion or membranous nephropathy) or a rheumatologic disease such as SLE. Lupus patients also often coexpress a lupus anticoagulant, with elevation in the activated partial tissue thromboplastin time. Clinical presentation of the catastrophic form of antiphospholipid syndrome appears as mixed thrombosis of the arterial and venous circulation with varying degrees of thrombocytopenia, hemolytic anemia, deep vein thrombosis, transient ischemic attacks, pulmonary embolism, and spontaneous abortions; lesser degrees of disease are more common. The kidneys are injured in this syndrome in approximately 25% of patients, particularly those with IgG antibodies. Some patients develop acute renal failure, while others suffer subclinical damage over time. Patients who present with acute flank pain and renal vein thrombosis in the setting of proteinuria should always be checked for antiphospholipid antibodies. Clinically, the antiphospholipid syndrome can wax and wane, and many patients have recurrences; <10% present with catastrophic multi-organ involvement and acute renal failure. Dialysis patients with antiphospholipid syndrome experience frequent occlusion of their arteriovenous graft. The urinalysis in most patients typically shows a mixed picture of moderate proteinuria (1–2 g/24 h) and hematuria. Glomerular capillaries and large and small renal arteries and veins occlude, accompanied by ischemic mesangiolysis and vessel hyperplasia, leading eventually to chronic glomerulosclerosis and interstitial fibrosis. Evidence of antiphospholipid syndrome on biopsy can usually be distinguished as an added complication of an underlying renal disease, particularly lupus nephritis. The mainstay of treatment for antiphospholipid syndrome is warfarin. There is also evidence of vasculitis in many patients due to complement-fixing antiphospholipid antibodies, which responds to the addition of steroids. Acute renal failure sometimes responds to removal of antiphospholipid antibodies with plasmapheresis and adjustment of immunosuppression where clinically indicated.

INFECTIOUS DISEASE–ASSOCIATED SYNDROMES

A number of infectious diseases will injure the glomerular capillaries as part of a systemic reaction producing an immune response or from direct infection of renal tissue. Evidence of this immune response is collected by glomeruli in the form of immune deposits that damage the kidney, producing moderate proteinuria and hematuria. Some of these infectious diseases represent the most common causes of glomerulonephritis worldwide.

POST-STREPTOCOCCAL GLOMERULONEPHRITIS

This form of glomerulonephritis is one of the classic complications of streptococcal infection. The discussion of this disease can be found in the section on *acute nephritic syndromes.*

SUBACUTE BACTERIAL ENDOCARDITIS

Renal injury from persistent bacteremia absent the continued presence of a foreign body, regardless of cause, is treated presumptively as if the patient has endocarditis. The discussion of this disease can be found in "Acute Nephritic Syndromes," above.

HUMAN IMMUNODEFICIENCY VIRUS

HIV-associated nephropathy is seen after an interval of approximately 2.5 years from discovery of HIV, and many patients have low CD4 counts. Most lesions on renal biopsy show FSGS followed by MPGN. Other less common renal lesions include DPGN, IgA nephropathy, MCD, and membranous or mesangioproliferative glomerulonephritis. The disease affects up to 10% of HIV-infected patients and is more commonly seen in African-American men than in Caucasians, and in intravenous drug users or homosexuals. The FSGS characteristically reveals collapse of the glomerular capillary tuft called *collapsing glomerulopathy,* visceral epithelial cell swelling, microcystic dilatation of renal tubules, and tubuloreticular inclusions. Renal epithelial cells express replicating HIV virus, but host immune responses also play a role in the pathogenesis. MPGN and DPGN have been reported more commonly in HIV-infected Caucasians and in patients co-infected with hepatitis B or C. HIV-associated TTP has also been reported.

HIV patients with FSGS typically present with nephrotic-range proteinuria and hypoalbuminemia, but unlike patients with other etiologies for nephrotic syndrome, they do not commonly have hypertension, edema, or hyperlipidemia. Renal ultrasound also reveals large, echogenic kidneys, and renal function in some patients declines rapidly. Treatment with inhibitors of the renin-angiotensin system decreases the proteinuria. Although evidence from large well-designed clinical trials is lacking, many feel that effective antiretroviral therapy benefits both the patient and the kidney. Dismal survival once renal failure is reached has improved, and many centers now offer renal allografts to select HIV patients.

HEPATITIS B AND C

Chronic hepatitis B infection can be associated with polyarteritis nodosa, more commonly in adults than children. Typically, however, infected patients only present with microscopic hematuria, nonnephrotic or nephrotic-range proteinuria, and hypertension. Alternatively, the hepatitis B carrier state can produce a MGN that is more common in children than adults or MPGN that is more common in adults than in children. Renal histology is indistinguishable from idiopathic MGN or Type I MPGN. There are no good treatment guidelines, but interferon α and lamivudine have been used to some effect in small studies. Children have a good prognosis, with 66% achieving spontaneous remission within 3 years. In contrast, 30% of adults have renal insufficiency and 10% have renal failure 5 years after diagnosis.

Up to 30% of patients with chronic hepatitis C infection have some renal manifestations. Patients often present with cryoglobulinemia and nephrotic syndrome, microscopic hematuria, abnormal liver function tests, depressed C3 levels, anti-HCV antibodies, and viral RNA in the blood. The renal lesions most commonly seen, in order of decreasing frequency, are *cryoglobulinemic glomerulonephritis, MGN, and Type I MPGN.* Treatment aims at reducing the level of the infection.

OTHER VIRUSES

Other viral infections are occasionally associated with glomerular lesions, but cause and effect are not well-established. These viral infec-

tions and their respective glomerular lesions include: cytomegalovirus producing MPGN; influenza and anti-GBM disease; measles-associated endocapillary proliferative glomerulonephritis, with measles antigen in the capillary loops and mesangium; parvovirus causing mild proliferative or mesangioproliferative glomerulonephritis; mumps and mesangioproliferative glomerulonephritis; Epstein-Barr virus producing MPGN, diffuse proliferative nephritis, or IgA nephropathy; dengue hemorrhagic fever causing endocapillary proliferative glomerulonephritis; and coxsackie virus producing *focal glomerulonephritis* or DPGN.

SYPHILIS

Secondary syphilis, with rash and constitutional symptoms, develops weeks to months after the chancre first appears and occasionally presents with the nephrotic syndrome from MGN caused by subepithelial immune deposits containing treponemal antigens. The diagnosis is confirmed with non-treponemal and treponemal tests for *Treponema pallidum.* The renal lesion responds to treatment with penicillin or an alternative drug, if allergic. Additional testing for other sexually transmitted diseases is an important part of disease management.

LEPROSY

Despite aggressive eradication programs, approximately 400,000 new cases of leprosy appear annually worldwide. The diagnosis is best made in patients with multiple skin lesions accompanied by sensory loss in affected areas, using skin smears showing paucibacillary or multibacillary infection (WHO criteria). Leprosy is caused by infection with *Mycobacterium leprae* and can be classified by Ridley-Jopling criteria into various types: tuberculoid, borderline tuberculoid, mid-borderline and borderline lepromatous, and lepromatous. In some series, all cases with borderline lepromatous and lepromatous types of leprosy have various forms of glomerulonephritis. Most common is focal glomerulonephritis followed by mesangioproliferative glomerulonephritis or renal amyloidosis; much less common are the renal lesions of DPGN and MPGN. Treatment with dapsone, rifampicin, and clofazimine can irradiate the infection in nearly all patients.

MALARIA

There are 300–500 million incident cases of malaria each year worldwide, and the kidney is commonly involved. Glomerulonephritis is due to immune complexes containing malarial antigens that are implanted in the glomerulus. In malaria from *P. falciparum,* mild proteinuria is associated with subendothelial deposits, mesangial deposits, and mesangioproliferative glomerulonephritis that usually resolve with treatment. In quartian malaria from infection with *P. malariae,* children are more commonly affected and renal involvement is more severe. Transient proteinuria and microscopic hematuria can resolve with treatment of the infection. However, resistant nephrotic syndrome with progression to renal failure over 3–5 years does happen, as <50% of patients respond to steroid therapy. Affected patients with nephrotic syndrome have thickening of the glomerular capillary walls, with subendothelial deposits of IgG, IgM, and C3 associated with a sparse membranoproliferative lesion. The rare mesangioproliferative glomerulonephritis reported with *P. vivax* or *P. ovale* typically has a benign course.

SCHISTOSOMIASIS

Schistosomiasis affects more than 300 million people worldwide and primarily involves the urinary and gastrointestinal tracts. Glomerular involvement varies with the specific strain of schistosomiasis; *Schistosoma mansoni* is most commonly associated with clinical renal disease, and the glomerular lesions can be classified: Class I is a *mesangioproliferative glomerulonephritis;* Class II is an *extracapillary proliferative glomerulonephritis;* Class III is a *membranoproliferative glomerulonephritis;* Class IV is a *focal segmental glomerulonephritis;* and Class V lesions have *amyloidosis.* Classes I–II often remit with treatment of the infection, but Classes III and IV lesions are associated with IgA immune deposits and progress despite antiparasitic and/or immunosuppressive therapy.

OTHER PARASITES

Renal involvement with toxoplasmosis infections is rare. When it occurs, patients present with nephrotic syndrome and have a histologic picture of MPGN. Fifty percent of patients with leishmaniasis will have mild to moderate proteinuria and microscopic hematuria, but renal insufficiency is rare. Acute DPGN, MGN, and mesangio-proliferative glomerulonephritis have all been observed on biopsy. The nematodes, filariasis and trichinosis, can be associated with glomerular injury presenting with proteinuria, hematuria, and a variety of histologic lesions that typically resolve with eradication of the infection.

FURTHER READINGS

CHADBAN SJ, ATKINS RC: Glomerulonephritis. Lancet 365:1797, 2005
CUNARD R, KELLY CJ: Immune-mediated renal disease. J Allergy Clin Immunol 111:S637, 2003
HUDSON BG et al: Alport and Goodpasture syndromes and the type IV collagen family. N Engl J Med 348:2543, 2003
HURTADO A, JOHNSON RJ: Hygiene hypothesis and the prevalence of glomerulonephritis. Kidney Int 68:S62, 2005
TRYGGVASON K et al: Hereditary proteinuria syndromes and mechanisms of proteinuria. N Engl J Med 354:1387, 2006

278 Polycystic Kidney Disease and Other Inherited Tubular Disorders

David J. Salant, Parul S. Patel

INTRODUCTION

The polycystic kidney diseases are among the most common life-threatening inherited diseases worldwide. They are equally prevalent in all ethnic and racial groups. Progressive expansion of numerous fluid-filled cysts results in massive enlargement of the kidneys (Fig. 278-1) and frequently causes kidney failure. Autosomal dominant polycystic kidney disease (ADPKD) is seen predominantly in adults, whereas autosomal recessive polycystic kidney disease (ARPKD) is mainly a disease of childhood. As shown in Table 278-1, renal cysts are also seen in several other hereditary kidney diseases, some of which may have defects in a common signaling pathway with ADPKD and ARPKD. Table 278-2 summarizes the gene defects and functional abnormalities in inherited tubular diseases that manifest primarily with alterations in fluid, electrolyte, acid-base, and mineral balance.

AUTOSOMAL DOMINANT POLYCYSTIC KIDNEY DISEASE

Etiology And Pathogenesis ADPKD is a systemic disorder resulting from mutations in either the *PKD-1* or *PKD-2* gene. The *PKD-1* encoded protein, polycystin-1, is a large receptor-like molecule, whereas the *PKD-2* gene product, polycystin-2, has features of an ion-channel protein. Both are transmembrane proteins present throughout all segments of the nephrin and are localized to the luminal surface of tubular cells in primary cilia, on the basal surface in focal adhesion complexes, and on the lateral surface in adherens junctions. The proteins are thought to function independently, or as a complex, to regulate fetal and adult epithelial cell gene transcription, apoptosis, differentiation, and cell-matrix interactions. Disruption of these processes leads to epithelial dedifferentiation, unregulated proliferation and apoptosis, altered cell polarity, disorganization of surrounding extracellular matrix, excessive fluid secretion, and abnormal expression of several genes, including some that encode growth factors. Vasopressin-mediated elevation of cyclic AMP (cAMP) levels in cyst epithelia plays a major role in cystogenesis by stimulating cell proliferation and fluid secretion into the cyst lumen through apical chloride and aquaporin channels. Cyst formation begins in utero from any point along the nephron, although <5% of total nephrons are thought to be involved. As the cysts accumulate fluid, they enlarge, separate entirely from the nephron, compress the neighboring renal parenchyma, and progressively compromise renal function.

GENETIC CONSIDERATIONS ADPKD occurs in 1:400–1:1,000 individuals worldwide and accounts for ~4% of end-stage renal disease (ESRD) in the United States. Over 90% of cases are inherited as an autosomal dominant trait, with the remainder likely representing spontaneous mutations. Mutations in the *PKD-1* gene on chromosome 16 (ADPKD-1) account for 85% of cases, whereas mutations in the *PKD-2* gene on chromosome 4 (ADPKD-2) represent the remainder. A few families appear to have a defect at a site that is different from either of these loci. Direct mutation analysis of isolated cysts suggests there is loss of heterozygosity, whereby a somatic mutation in the normal "wild-type" allele of a small number of tubular epithelial cells leads to unregulated clonal proliferation of the cells that ultimately form the cyst lining.

Clinical Features Phenotypic heterogeneity is a hallmark of ADPKD, as evidenced by family members who share the same mutation but have a different clinical course. Affected individuals are often asymptomatic

FIGURE 278-1 Renal ultrasonogram and contrast-enhanced abdominal CT scan in a 56-year-old woman with autosomal dominant polycystic kidney disease. **A.** Sonogram of the right kidney showing numerous cysts of varying sizes (*arrows*). **B.** Abdominal CT scan demonstrating bilaterally enlarged kidneys with large cysts (*arrows*). **C.** Multiple liver cysts (*arrowheads*) and renal cysts (*arrow*) are seen in an upper abdominal image.

TABLE 278-1 INHERITED CYSTIC KIDNEY DISEASES

Disease (OMIM)	Mode of Inheritance	Locus	Gene	Protein	Renal Abnormalities	Extra-Renal Abnormalities
Autosomal dominant polycystic kidney disease (601313, 173910)	AD	16p13	PKD1	polycystin-1	Cortical and medullary cysts	Cerebral aneurysms; liver cysts, other[a]
	AD	4q21	PKD2	polycystin-2	Cortical and medullary cysts	Cerebral aneurysms; liver cysts, other[a]
Autosomal recessive polycystic kidney disease (263200)	AR	6p21	PKDH1	fibrocystin	Distal tubule and collecting duct cysts	Hepatic fibrosis; Caroli syndrome
Nephronophthisis I (Juvenile/adolescent, 256100)	AR	2q13	NPHP1	nephrocystin	Small fibrotic kidneys; medullary cysts	Retinitis pigmentosa
Nephronophthisis II (Infantile, 602088)	AR	9q31	INVS	inversin	Large kidneys; widespread cysts	Situs inversus
Nephronophthisis III (Juvenile/Adolescent, 604387)	AR	3q22	NPHP3	nephrocystin-3	Small fibrotic kidneys; medullary cysts	Retinitis pigmentosa; hepatic fibrosis
Nephronophthisis IV (Juvenile/Adolescent, 606966)	AR	1p36	NPHP4	nephrocystin-4	Small fibrotic kidneys; medullary cysts	Retinitis pigmentosa
Nephronophthisis V (Juvenile/adolescent)	AR	3q13	NPHP5	nephrocystin-5	Small fibrotic kidneys; medullary cysts	Amaurosis
Medullary cystic kidney disease (174000, 603860)	AD	1q21	MCKD1	unknown	Small fibrotic kidneys; medullary cysts	None
	AD	16p12	UMOD	uromodulin (Tamm-Horsfall protein)	Small fibrotic kidneys; medullary cysts	Hyperuricemia and gout
Tuberous sclerosis (191100)	AD	9q34	TSC1	tuberin	Renal cysts; angiomyo-lipomas; renal cell carcinoma	Adenoma sebaceum; CNS hamartomas
	AD	16p13	TSC1	hamartin	Renal cysts; angiomyo-lipomas; renal cell carcinoma	Adenoma sebaceum; CNS hamartomas
Von Hippel-Lindau disease (608537)	AD	3p26-p25	VHL	pVHL	Renal cysts; renal cell carcinoma	Retinal angiomas; CNS hemangioblastomas; pheochromocytomas

Note: AD, autosomal dominant; AR, autosomal recessive; OMIM, online Mendelian inheritance in man.
[a]See text for details.

into the fourth or fifth decade. Presenting symptoms and signs include abdominal discomfort, hematuria, urinary tract infection, incidental discovery of hypertension, abdominal mass, elevated serum creatinine, or cystic kidneys on imaging studies (Fig. 278-1A and B). Frequently the diagnosis is made prior to the onset of symptoms, when asymptomatic members in affected families request screening. In most patients, renal function declines progressively over the course of 10–20 years from the time of diagnosis, but not everyone with ADPKD develops ESRD; it occurs in about 60% of patients by age 70. Those with ADPKD-2 tend to have later onset and slower progression. Hypertension is common and often precedes renal dysfunction, perhaps mediated by increased activity of the renin-angiotensin system. There is only mild proteinuria, and impaired urinary concentrating ability manifests early as polyuria and nocturia. Risk factors for progressive kidney disease include younger age at diagnosis, black race, male gender, presence of polycystin-1 mutation, and hypertension. There is a close correlation between the rate of kidney expansion and the rate of decline in kidney function. Dull, persistent flank and abdominal pain and early satiety and gastroesophageal reflux symptoms are common due to the mass effect of the enlarged kidneys. Cyst rupture or hemorrhage into a cyst may produce acute flank pain or symptoms and signs of localized peritonitis. Hematuria may result from cyst rupture into the collecting system or from uric acid or calcium oxalate kidney stones. Nephrolithiasis occurs in about 20% of patients. Urinary tract infection, including acute pyelonephritis, occurs with increased frequency in ADPKD. Infection in a kidney or liver cyst is a particularly serious complication. It is most often due to Gram-negative bacteria and presents with pain, fever, and chills. Blood cultures are frequently positive, but urine culture may be negative because infected kidney cysts do not communicate directly with the collecting system. Distinguishing between infection and cyst hemorrhage is often a challenge, and the diagnosis relies mainly on clinical and bacteriological findings. Radiological and nuclear imaging studies are generally not helpful.

Numerous extrarenal manifestations of ADPKD highlight the systemic nature of the disease and likely reflect a generalized abnormality in collagen and extracellular matrix. Patients with ADPKD have a fourfold increased risk of subarachnoid or cerebral hemorrhage from a ruptured intracranial aneurysm as compared to the general population. Saccular aneurysms of the anterior cerebral circulation may be detected in up to 10% of asymptomatic patients on MRA screening, but most are small, have a low risk of spontaneous rupture, and do not merit the risk of intervention. In general, hemorrhage tends to occur before the age of 50 years, in patients with a family history of intracranial hemorrhage, those who have survived a previous bleed, have aneurysms larger than 10 mm and have uncontrolled hypertension. Other vascular abnormalities include aortic root and annulus dilatation. Cardiac valvular abnormalities occur in 25% of patients, most commonly mitral valve prolapse and aortic regurgitation. Although most valvular lesions are asymptomatic, some may progress over time and warrant valve replacement. The incidence of hepatic cysts rises progressively up to 40% in patients over the age of 60 years. Most patients are asymptomatic with normal liver function tests, but hepatic cysts may bleed, become infected, rupture, and cause pain. Although the frequency of liver cysts is equal between genders, women are more likely to have massive cysts (Fig. 278-1C). Colonic diverticulae are common, with a higher incidence of perforation in patients with ADPKD. Abdominal wall and inguinal hernias also occur with a higher frequency than in the general population.

Diagnosis and Screening The sensitivity of renal ultrasonography for the detection of ADPKD is 100% for subjects 30 years or older with a positive family history. Diagnostic criteria require two or more cysts in one kidney and at least one cyst in the contralateral kidney in young subjects, but four or more in subjects older than 60 years because of the increased frequency of benign simple cysts. Most often, the diagnosis is made from a positive family history and imaging studies showing large kidneys with multiple bilateral cysts and possibly liver cysts (Fig. 278-1). Before the age of 30 years, CT scan or T2-weighted MRI is more sensitive for detecting presymptomatic disease because the sensitivity of ultrasound falls to 95% for ADPKD type 1 and <70% for ADPKD type 2. Genetic linkage analysis and mutational screening for *ADPKD-1* and *ADPKD-2* is available for equivocal cases, especially when a young adult from an affected family is being considered as a potential kidney donor. Genetic counseling is essential for those being screened. It is recommended that screening for asymptomatic intracranial aneurysms should be restricted to patients with a personal or family history of intracranial hemorrhage and those in high-risk occupations. Intervention should be limited to aneurysms larger than 10 mm.

℞ AUTOSOMAL DOMINANT POLYCYSTIC KIDNEY DISEASE

At present, treatment is largely supportive, as there is no single therapy that has been shown to prevent the decline in kidney function. Hypertension control with a target blood pressure of 130/85 or less is recommended according to Joint National Committee (JNC) VII guidelines; however, lower levels have been reported to slow the rate of loss of kidney function. A multidrug approach that includes agents to inhibit the renin-angiotensin system is frequently required. There is no compelling evidence to recommend a low-protein diet, especially in patients with advanced kidney dysfunction where optimizing nutritional status is important. Lipid-soluble antimicrobials, such as trimethoprim-sulfamethoxazole and quinolone antibiotics that have good tissue permeation, are the preferred therapy for infected kidney and liver cysts. Pain management occasionally requires cyst drainage by percutaneous aspiration, sclerotherapy with alcohol or, rarely, surgical drainage. Patients with ADPKD appear to have a survival advantage on either peritoneal or hemodialysis compared to patients with other causes of ESRD. Those undergoing kidney transplantation may require bilateral nephrectomy if the kidneys are massively enlarged or have been the site of infected cysts. Posttransplantation survival rates are similar to those of patients with other causes of kidney failure, but patients remain at risk for the extrarenal complications of ADPKD. Studies in animal models of inherited cystic diseases have identified promising therapeutic strategies, including vasopressin V2 receptor antagonists that suppress cyst growth by lowering intracellular cAMP and inhibitors of cell signaling that target the epidermal growth factor receptor tyrosine kinase to control cell proliferation.

AUTOSOMAL RECESSIVE POLYCYSTIC KIDNEY DISEASE

 GENETIC CONSIDERATIONS ARPKD is primarily a disease of infants and children. The incidence is 1:20,000 births. The kidneys are enlarged, with small cysts, <5 mm, limited to the collecting tubules.

The ARPKD gene on chromosome 6p21, *PKHD1* (polycystic kidney and hepatic disease 1), encodes several alternatively spliced transcripts (Table 278-1). The largest transcript produces a multidomain transmembrane protein termed *fibrocystin* (*polyductin*) that is found in the cortical and medullary collecting ducts and thick ascending limb of Henle's loop in the kidney as well as in biliary and pancreatic duct epithelia. Like the polycystins, fibrocystin has receptor-like features and may be involved in cell-cell and cell-matrix interactions. Fibrocystin, the polycystins, and several proteins involved in animal models of PKD are located in association with primary cilia on the tubular epithelial cell apical surface, which suggests that they may cooperate in a mechanosensory pathway. A large number of different mutations have been identified throughout *PKHD1* and are unique to individual families. Most patients are compound heterozygotes. Those with two truncating mutations frequently die shortly after birth, whereas those that survive beyond the neonatal period generally have at least one missense mutation. Mutations in *PKHD1* have also been identified in about 30% of children with congenital hepatic fibrosis (Caroli syndrome) without evident kidney involvement.

Clinical Features The clinical presentation of ARPKD is highly variable. Up to 50% of affected neonates die of pulmonary hypoplasia, the result

of oligohydramnios from severe intrauterine kidney disease. About 80% of those who survive the neonatal period are still alive after 10 years; however, one-third of them will have developed ESRD. Enlarged kidneys may be detected soon after birth as bilateral abdominal masses. Impaired urinary concentrating ability and metabolic acidosis ensue as tubular function deteriorates. Hypertension often occurs in the first few years of life. Kidney function deteriorates progressively from childhood into early adult life. Longer-term survivors frequently develop portal hypertension, esophageal varices, and hypersplenism from periportal fibrosis.

Diagnosis Ultrasonography reveals large, echogenic kidneys. The diagnosis can be made in utero after 24 weeks of gestation in severe cases, but cysts generally become visible only after birth. The absence of renal cysts in either parent on ultrasonography helps to distinguish ARPKD from ADPKD in older patients. The wide range of different mutations and the large size of the gene complicate molecular diagnosis, although prenatal diagnosis is possible by gene linkage to the *PKHD1* locus in families with a previous confirmed ARPKD birth.

℞ AUTOSOMAL RECESSIVE POLYCYSTIC KIDNEY DISEASE

No specific therapy exists for ARPKD. Improvements in mechanical ventilation, neonatal support, blood pressure management, dialysis, and kidney transplantation have led to survival well into adulthood. Complications of hepatic fibrosis may necessitate liver transplantation. Future therapies may target aberrant cell signaling mechanisms, as in ADPKD.

NEPHRONOPHTHISIS
Genetics and Pathogenesis Nephronophthisis (NPHP) is the most common genetic cause of ESRD in childhood and adolescence. Five distinct genetic mutations with autosomal recessive inheritance have been identified (Table 278-1). Although their precise functions are unclear, the defective protein products, named nephrocystins and inversin, localize to the primary cilium and associated basal body of renal epithelial cells, similar to the polycystins and fibrocystin. NPHP is classified into infantile, juvenile, and adolescent forms based on the age of ESRD onset. In juvenile NPHP, the most common form, the kidneys are shrunken and histology shows tubular atrophy, thickening of tubular basement membranes, diffuse interstitial fibrosis, and microscopic medullary cysts. In the infantile form, the kidneys are large and histology is similar to the juvenile form, except that medullary cysts are more prominent and develop earlier.

Clinical Features In juvenile NPHP, symptoms typically appear after one year of age. Impaired tubular function causes salt wasting and defective urinary concentration and acidification. Patients may present with polyuria, polydipsia, volume depletion, or systemic acidosis. Progressive kidney failure leads to growth retardation, anemia, and symptoms of uremia. On average, ESRD occurs by age 5 in the infantile form, age 13 in the juvenile form, and age 19 in the adolescent form. Up to 15% of patients with juvenile NPHP have extrarenal manifestations (Table 278-1), most commonly retinitis pigmentosa (Senior-Loken syndrome). Other abnormalities include blindness from amaurosis, oculomotor apraxia, cerebellar ataxia, mental retardation, hepatic fibrosis, and ventricular septal defect. Situs inversus is seen in some cases of infantile NPHP, consistent with mutation in *INVS*, a gene that is critical for left-right patterning in the embryo.

Diagnosis The diagnosis of NPHP should be considered in patients with a family history of kidney disease, early-onset progressive renal failure, and a bland urine sediment with minimal proteinuria. Ultrasonography reveals small hyperechoic kidneys in juvenile NPHP and large kidneys with cysts in the infantile form.

℞ NEPHRONOPHTHISIS

No specific therapy exists to prevent loss of kidney function in NPHP. Salt and water replacement are required for patients with salt wasting and polyuria. Therapy should include sodium bicarbonate or citrate for acidosis, control of secondary hyperparathyroidism, erythropoietin for anemia, and timely institution of dialysis and transplantation.

MEDULLARY CYSTIC KIDNEY DISEASE

 GENETIC CONSIDERATIONS The medullary cystic kidney diseases (MCKD) generally present in young adults. Two genetic loci have been defined, both with autosomal dominant transmission (Table 278-1). The locus for MCKD1 has been mapped to chromosome 1q21. Mutations in the uromodulin gene (*UMOD*) that encodes the Tamm-Horsfall mucoprotein on chromosome 16p12 have been identified in MCKD2.

Clinical Features Like NPHP, patients with MCKD have atrophic kidneys with diffuse interstitial fibrosis, cysts restricted to the renal medulla, salt wasting, and polyuria. Disease onset is later than NPHP. Consequently, there is no growth retardation, salt wasting is milder, and ESRD occurs later, usually between the ages of 20 and 60. There are no extrarenal manifestations in MCKD1. Most patients with MCKD2 and the genetically related familial juvenile hyperuricemic nephropathy also have severe hyperuricemia and precocious onset of gout.

Diagnosis The diagnosis of MCKD should be considered in young adults presenting with a family history suggesting dominant inheritance of kidney disease, progressive renal failure, bland urinalysis with little or no proteinuria, and small dense kidneys with medullary cysts on ultrasonography or CT. The presence of hyperuricemia and gout are further clues to the diagnosis of MCKD2. MCKD2 can be confirmed by mutation analysis of *UMOD*.

℞ MEDULLARY CYSTIC KIDNEY DISEASE

There is no specific therapy for MCKD. Allopurinol is indicated for patients with gout and makes sense for those with presymptomatic hyperuricemia, although there is no evidence that it prevents progressive renal failure in MCKD2. Dialysis and transplantation outcomes appear to be favorable.

TUBEROUS SCLEROSIS

Tuberous sclerosis (TS) is an autosomal dominant disorder affecting 1 out of 6000 people. It results from inactivating mutations in either the *TSC1* gene encoding tuberin or the *TSC2* gene encoding hamartin (Table 278-1). Hamartin and tubulin form a complex that is thought to negatively regulate the cell cycle. The presence of either mutation produces uncontrolled proliferation in numerous tissues, including the skin, central nervous system (CNS), heart, skeleton, and kidneys. CNS hamartomas can cause seizures, mental retardation, and autism. Expressivity is highly variable, but the kidneys are affected in 80% of patients. Renal TS occurs in three forms: renal cysts, renal angiomyolipomas, and renal cell carcinoma. Cysts are usually asymptomatic and are not evident on imaging studies until adulthood. Cysts may be large and numerous, sometimes leading to ESRD and producing a clinical scenario that can be confused with ADPKD, especially if there are few other systemic manifestations of TS. Angiomyolipomas are the most common renal abnormality, occur bilaterally, are often multiple, and are usually asymptomatic. Spontaneous bleeding can produce flank pain, nausea and vomiting, hematuria, and even life-threatening retroperitoneal hemorrhage. Large lesions, >4 cm, are most likely to cause pain and bleeding, and may require surgical excision. Multicentric renal cell carcinomas have been reported to occur with increased frequency in TS. Patients with TS should be screened for renal involvement at initial diagnosis with ultrasound or CT. Those with cysts or angiomyolipomas require regular imaging to monitor for the development of renal cell carcinoma.

VON HIPPEL-LINDAU DISEASE

Von Hippel-Lindau disease (VHL) is a rare autosomal dominant disease characterized by abnormal angiogenesis with benign and malignant tumors affecting multiple tissues. The disease is inherited as a mutation in one allele of the *VHL* tumor suppressor gene. Somatic mutation of the normal allele leads to retinal angiomas, CNS hemangioblastomas, pheochromocytomas and multicentric clear cell cysts, hemangiomas, and adenomas of the kidney. The kidneys are affected in three-quarters of patients, and half develop clear cell carcinomas in the renal cysts. Ten percent of patients present with symptoms of clear cell carcinoma. It is noteworthy that *VHL* mutations also account for 60% of spontaneous clear cell carcinomas of the kidney. The diagnosis of renal cell carcinoma in VHL disease is made at a mean age of 44 years, while 70% of patients who survive to age 60 develop renal carcinoma. The high risk of renal cell carcinoma mandates periodic surveillance (usually yearly in adults) by either CT or MRI. Routine screening and awareness of the natural history of lesions has enabled renal-sparing approaches to disease management. Tumors <3 cm in size require careful monitoring for growth, while partial nephrectomy is indicated in those >3 cm in the absence of metastasis. Nonsurgical renal-sparing strategies, including percutaneous radiofrequency ablation and selective arterial embolization, have shown promise in short-term trials.

MEDULLARY SPONGE KIDNEY

Pathology and Clinical Features Medullary sponge kidney (MSK) is a common, benign condition of unknown cause characterized by ectasia of the papillary collecting ducts of one or both kidneys. Urinary stasis in the dilated ducts, hypocitraturia, and, occasionally, incomplete distal renal tubular acidosis (dRTA) contribute to the formation of small calcium-containing calculi. Most cases are asymptomatic or are discovered during investigation of asymptomatic hematuria. Symptomatic patients typically present as young adults with renal colic and the passage of stones or recurrent urinary tract infections; however, MSK may cause hematuria and nephrolithiasis in children. Most cases are sporadic, although MSK has been found rarely in association with other congenital anomalies of the urinary tract and with congenital hepatic ductal ectasia and fibrosis (Caroli disease).

Diagnosis In patients with nephrolithiasis, MSK is characteristically seen as hyperdense papillae with clusters of small stones on renal ultrasonography or abdominal X-ray (Fig. 278-2). The classical "paintbrush-like" features of MSK, representing the ectatic collecting ducts, are best seen on intravenous urography. However, this procedure has been supplanted in many radiology departments by contrast-enhanced, high-resolution helical CT with digital reconstruction (Fig. 278-2).

℞ MEDULLARY SPONGE KIDNEY

No treatment is necessary in asymptomatic individuals aside from maintaining high fluid intake to reduce the risk of nephrolithiasis. Recurrent stone formation should prompt a metabolic evaluation and treatment as in any stone former (Chap. 281). In those patients with hypocitraturia and incomplete distal renal tubular acidosis, treatment with potassium citrate helps prevent new stone formation. Urinary tract infections should be treated promptly.

HEREDITARY DISORDERS OF SODIUM, POTASSIUM, AND MAGNESIUM HANDLING WITHOUT HYPERTENSION

Inherited forms of hypochloremic metabolic alkalosis and hypokalemia without hypertension are due to genetic mutations of various ion transporters and channels of the thick ascending limb (TAL) of Henle's loop and distal convoluted tubule (DCT) (Table 278-2 and Fig. 278-3). In 1962 Bartter and colleagues described two African-American patients with a syndrome of metabolic alkalosis, hypovolemia, hyposthenuria, and failure to thrive associated with juxtaglomerular apparatus hyperplasia, hyperaldosteronism, and normal blood pressure. Subsequently, Gitelman and colleagues identified a similar but milder syndrome accompanied by severe hypomagnesemia from urinary magnesium wasting and presenting in later childhood and adolescence. These disorders are now known to occur sporadically or

FIGURE 278-2 Radiographs of medullary sponge kidney disease. *A.* Plain x-ray film of a patient with a history of recurrent neph rolithiasis showing clusters of stones in the papillae (*arrows*). ***B–E.*** CT scan of an 18-year-old male patient investigated for persistent microscopic hematuria. ***B*** and ***C.*** CT without contrast showing a few small stones in the papillae (*arrows*). ***D*** and ***E.*** Contrast-enhanced CT of the same region shown in *B.* In addition to the stone (*arrow*), a blush of contrast is seen filling the ectatic collecting ducts (*arrowheads*).

from genetically heterogenous loss-of-function autosomal recessive mutations that cause salt-losing tubulopathy.

BARTTER'S SYNDROME AND GITELMAN'S SYNDROME
Genetics and Pathogenesis *Bartter's syndrome* may result from mutations affecting any of four ion transport proteins in the TAL. The proteins affected include the apical loop-diuretic sensitive sodium-potassium-chloride co-transporter NKCC2 (type 1), the apical potassium channel ROMK (type 2), and the basolateral chloride channel ClC-Kb (type 3). Bartter type 4 results from mutations in barttin, an essential subunit of ClC-Ka and ClC-Kb that enables transport of the chloride channels to the cell surface. Barttin is also expressed in the inner ear, which accounts for the deafness invariably associated with Bartter type 4. The TAL transporters function in an integrated manner to maintain both the electrical potential difference and sodium gradient between the lumen and the cell (Fig. 278-3). Loss of the lumen-positive electrical transport potential that normally drives the paracellular reabsorption of sodium, calcium, and magnesium causes NaCl wasting, hypercalciuria, and mild hypomagnesemia. As expected, the clinical syndrome mimics a state induced by chronic ingestion of a loop diuretic.

Gitelman's syndrome is due to mutations in the thiazide-sensitive Na-Cl co-transporter (NCCT) in the DCT. Defects in NCCT in Gitelman's syndrome impair sodium and chloride reabsorption in the DCT (Fig. 278-3) and, thus, resemble the effects of thiazide diuretics. It remains unclear how this defect leads to severe magnesium wasting. A Bartter-like phenotype (type 5) with associated hypocalcemia has also been described in a few patients with autosomal dominant gain-of-function mutations in the extracellular calcium-sensing receptor (CaSR). Unregulated activation of this G-protein–coupled receptor inhibits sodium reabsorption in the TAL.

In both Bartter's and Gitelman's syndromes, hypovolemia from impaired sodium and chloride reabsorption in either the TAL or DCT activates the renin-angiotensin-aldosterone system (RAS). The consequent hyperaldosteronism, together with increased distal flow and sodium delivery, stimulates increased sodium reabsorption in the collecting tubules via the epithelial sodium channel (ENaC). This promotes increased potassium and hydrogen ion secretion, causing hypokalemia and metabolic alkalosis. Additionally, in Bartter's syndrome, RAS activation causes increased levels of cyclooxygenase 2 (COX-2) and

marked overproduction of renal prostaglandins (PGE2), which exacerbates the polyuria and electrolyte abnormalities.

Clinical Features · *BARTTER'S SYNDROME* Bartter's syndrome is a rare disease that most often presents in the neonatal period or early childhood with polyuria, polydipsia, salt craving, and growth retardation. Blood pressure is normal or low. Metabolic abnormalities include hypokalemia, hypochloremic metabolic alkalosis, decreased urinary concentrating and diluting ability, hypercalciuria with nephrocalcinosis, mild hypomagnesemia, and increased urinary prostaglandin excretion. Hyperprostaglandin E syndrome is a particularly severe form of Bartter's syndrome in which neonates present with pronounced volume depletion and failure to thrive, as well as fever, vomiting, and diarrhea from PGE_2 overproduction. In the antenatal period, fetal polyuria may cause maternal polyhydramnios and premature labor. Sensorineural deafness occurs in those cases with barttin gene mutations. Patients with severe Bartter's syndrome that survive early childhood may develop chronic renal failure from nephrocalcinosis or from tubular atrophy and interstitial fibrosis from severe persistent hypokalemia. Patients with Bartter's syndrome type 3 have a phenotype intermediate between Bartter's and Gitelman's syndromes, consistent with mutation of the ClC-Kb chloride channel in both the TAL and DCT with preservation of the ClC-Ka chloride channel in the TAL. This disease occurs predominantly in African-American patients and resembles most closely the classical syndrome described by Bartter. Onset is generally later in childhood, patients have mild or no nephrocalcinosis, and prostaglandin excretion is normal.

GITELMAN'S SYNDROME Gitelman's syndrome is more common than Bartter's syndrome and has a generally milder clinical course with later age of presentation. It is characterized by hypocalciuria, severe hypomagnesemia, and prominent muscular symptoms and signs, including fatigue, weakness, carpopedal spasm, cramps, and tetany. Excess prostaglandin production does not typically occur in Gitelman's syndrome.

Diagnosis Hypokalemia and hypochloremic metabolic alkalosis without hypertension is more often due to surreptitious vomiting or diuretic abuse rather than Bartter's or Gitelman's syndromes. In contrast to the salt-losing tubulopathies, urinary chloride levels are very low or undetectable in patients with surreptitious vomiting. Diuretic abuse can be excluded by screening the urine for the offending drugs. Gitelman's

TABLE 278-2   INHERITED TUBULAR DISORDERS

Disease (OMIM)	Mode of Inheritance	Locus	Gene	Protein	Renal Abnormalities	Extra-Renal Abnormalities
Bartter's syndrome						
Type 1 (601678)	AR	15q15	SLC12A1	NKCC2	Salt wasting; hypokalemia	
Type 2 (241200)	AR	11q24	KCNJ1	ROMK	Salt wasting; hypokalemia	
Type 3 (607364)	AR	1p36	ClCNKb	CLCNKB	Salt wasting; hypokalemia	
Type 4 (602023)	AR	1p31	BSND	Barttin	Salt wasting; hypokalemia	Sensorineural deafness
Type 5 (601199)	AD	3q13	CASR	CASR	Salt wasting; hypokalemia	
Gitelman's syndrome (263800)	AR	16q13	SLC12A3	NCCT	Salt wasting; hypokalemia; hypomagnesemia	
Pseudohypoaldosteronism Type I (264350, 177735)	AR	16p13	SCNN1B	α, β, or γ subunits of ENaC	Hyperkalemia; salt wasting	Increased lung secretions and lung infections
		16p13	SCNN1G			
		12p13	SCNN1A			
	AD	4q31	NR3C2	Mineralocorticoid receptor (type I)	Hyperkalemia; salt wasting	
Primary hypomagnesemia (FHHNC, 248250)	AR	3q27	CLDN16	Claudin 16 (Paracellin-1)	Hypomagnesemia; nephrocalcinosis	
Hypomagnesemia with secondary hypocalcemia (602014)	AR	9q22	TRPM6	TRPM6	Hypomagnesemia; hypocalcemia	
Renal magnesium wasting (154020)	AD	11q23	FXYD2	FXYD2	Hypomagnesemia; hypocalciuria	
Autosomal dominant hypoparathyroidism (601199)	AD	3q13	CASR	CASR	Hypocalcemia; hypercalciuria; hypomagnesemia	
Liddle's syndrome (177200)	AD	16p13	SCNN1B	β and γ subunits of ENaC	Hypertension; hypokalemia; alkalosis	
Pseudohypoaldosteronism Type II (Gordon syndrome, 145260)	AD	12p13	WNK1	WNK 1	Hypertension; hyperkalemia	
		17q21	Wnk4	WNK 4		
Nephrogenic DI Type 1 (304800)	XL	Xq28	AVPR2	AVPR2	Renal concentrating defect	
Nephrogenic DI Type 2 (125800)	AR, AD	12q13	AQP2	AQP2	Renal concentrating defect	
Nephrogenic syndrome of inappropriate antidiuresis (300539)	XL	Xq28	AVPR2	AVPR2	Hyponatremia	
Distal renal tubular acidosis (267300, 602722, 259730, 179800)	AR	2cenq13	ATP6B1	H⁺-ATPase (B1)	Hyperchloremic metabolic acidosis; nephrocalcinosis	Sensorineural deafness (B1 defect only); growth retardation
		7q33	ATP6A4	H⁺-ATPase (α4)		
	AR	8q22	CA2	CA2	Proximal and distal RTA	
	AD	17q21	SLC4A1	AE1	Distal RTA	
Proximal renal tubular acidosis (604278)	AR	4q21	SLC4A4	NBC-1	Moderate hyperchloremic metabolic acidosis	Glaucoma; band keratopathy
Cystinuria (220100)	AR	2p16	SLC3A1	rBAT	Cystine stones; dibasic amino aciduria	
		19q13	SLC7A9	b⁰,⁺AT		
Hartnup disease (234500)	AR	5p15	SLC6A19	B⁰AT1	Neutral amino aciduria	Rash, dermatitis, ataxia; dementia
Dent's disease (300009)	XL	Xp11	CLCN5	CLC5	Proximal tubular dysfunction; nephrocalcinosis	Osteomalacia; rickets
Renal glucosuria (233100)	AR	16p11	SLC5A2	SGLT2	Glucosuria	
Hereditary hypophosphatemic rickets with hypercalciuria (HHRH, 241530)	AR	9q34	SLC34A3	Sodium-phosphate co-transporter	Hypophosphatemia; hypercalciuria	Rickets
Vitamin D–dependent rickets type I (VDDR I, 264700)	AR	12q14	CYP27B1	25-vitamin D3-1-α-hydroxylase	Hypocalcemia	Rickets

Note: OMIM, online Mendelian inheritance in man; AD, autosomal dominant; AR, autosomal recessive; XL, X-linked; DI, diabetes insipidus; NKCC2, Na-K-2Cl co-transporter; ROMK, renal outer medullary potassium channel; CLCNKb, chloride channel Kb; CASR, calcium-sensing receptor; NCCT, thiazide-sensitive Na-Cl co-transporter; ENaC, amiloride-sensitive epithelial sodium channel; FHHNC, familial hypomagnesemia with hypercalciuria and nephrocalcinosis; TRPM6, transient receptor potential cation channel, subfamily M, member 6; WNK, with no lysine (K); AVPR2, arginine vasopressin receptor 2; CA2, carbonic anhydrase II; AE1, anion exchanger 1; NBC, sodium-bicarbonate co-transporter; rBAT, renal basic amino acid transport glycoprotein; AT1, amino acid transporter; CLC5, chloride channel 5; SGLT2, sodium/glucose co-transporter.

syndrome is distinguished from most forms of Bartter's syndrome by the presence of severe hypomagnesemia and hypocalciuria.

℞ BARTTER'S SYNDROME AND GITELMAN'S SYNDROME

Both conditions require lifelong therapy with potassium and magnesium supplements and liberal salt intake. High doses of spironolactone or amiloride are necessary to treat the hypokalemia, alkalosis, and magnesium wasting. Nonsteroidal anti-inflammatory drugs (NSAIDs) reduce the polyuria and salt wasting in Bartter's syndrome but are ineffective in Gitelman's syndrome. They may be lifesaving in hyperprostaglandin E syndrome. COX-2 inhibitors are effective and justified because of the gastrointestinal complications that may arise from the long-term use of high doses of NSAIDs. In Gitelman's syndrome, magnesium repletion is essential to correct the hypokalemia and control

FIGURE 278-3 Schematic representation of channels, transporters, and enzymes associated with hereditary renal tubular disorders. AD, autosomal dominant; AR, autosomal recessive; DI, diabetes insipidus; NKCC2, Na-K-2Cl co-transporter; ROMK, renal outer medullary potassium channel; ClC-Kb, chloride channel Kb; CaR, calcium-sensing receptor 1; FHHNC, familial hypomagnesemia with hypercalciuria and nephrocalcinosis; NCCT, thiazide-sensitive Na-Cl co-transporter; ENaC, amiloride-sensitive epithelial sodium channel; TRPM6, transient receptor potential cation channel, subfamily M, member 6; WNK, with no lysine (K); V2R, arginine vasopressin receptor 2; MR, mineralocorticoid receptor; RTA, renal tubular acidosis; CA2, carbonic anhydrase II; AE1, anion exchanger 1; NBC1, sodium-bicarbonate co-transporter 1; rBAT, renal basic amino acid transport glycoprotein; AT1, amino acid transporter 1; CLC5, chloride channel 5; AA, amino acids; AA+, basic AA.

muscle weakness, tetany, and metabolic alkalosis; however, it may prove difficult in patients wasting large amounts of magnesium.

PSEUDOHYPOALDOSTERONISM TYPE I

Patients with type I pseudohypoaldosteronism present with severe renal salt wasting and hyperkalemia. Although these findings resemble mineralocorticoid deficiency, plasma renin activity and aldosterone levels are elevated. Defective salt handling is the result of autosomal recessive loss-of-function mutations of the α, β, or γ subunits of the ENaC or autosomal dominant mutations of one allele of the mineralocorticoid receptor (Table 278-2 and Fig. 278-3). The autosomal recessive form is a multisystem disorder with a severe phenotype, often manifesting in the neonatal period with renal salt wasting, vomiting, hyponatremia, hyperkalemia, acidosis, and failure to thrive. Impaired channel activity in the skin and lungs can produce excess sodium and chloride loss in sweat, excess fluid in the airways, and a propensity for lower respiratory tract infections mimicking cystic fibrosis. In contrast, the autosomal dominant form of type I pseudohypoaldosteronism has a more benign course that is limited mainly to renal salt wasting and hyperkalemia. Aggressive salt replacement and management of hyperkalemia can lead to survival into adulthood, and symptoms may become less severe with time, especially in the dominant form. In the latter, high-dose fludrocortisone or carbenoxolone provides additional benefit by raising intracellular mineralocorticoid activity and partly restoring the functional defect in the mutant receptor.

MAGNESIUM WASTING DISORDERS

In addition to Gitelman's syndrome, there are several hereditary disorders that cause urinary magnesium wasting (Table 278-2 and Fig. 278-3). These include autosomal recessive familial hypomagnesemia with hypercalciuria and nephrocalcinosis (FHHNC), autosomal recessive hypomagnesemia with secondary hypocalcemia (HSH), autosomal dominant hypomagnesemia, and autosomal dominant hypoparathyroidism (Chap. 347). Common clinical features are the early onset of spasms, tetany, and seizures, as well as associated or secondary disturbances in calcium homeostasis.

Familial Hypomagnesemia with Hypercalciuria and Nephrocalcinosis

FHHNC (also known as primary hypomagnesemia) is the first example of a disorder attributable to a defective protein involved in paracellular ion transport. *CLDCN16* encodes claudin 16 (previously known as paracellin-1), a member of the claudin family of proteins that are involved in tight junction formation. Claudin 16 is expressed in the TAL of Henle's loop and the DCT. Claudin 16 is thought to be an essential component of the paracellular pathway for Mg, and Ca to a lesser extent, reabsorption in the TAL. Clinical manifestations begin in infancy and include hypomagnesemia that is refractory to oral supplementation, hypercalciuria and nephrocalcinosis. Recurrent urinary tract infections and nephrolithiasis have also been observed, and some patients manifest ocular defects, including corneal calcifications and chorioretinitis.

Hypomagnesemia with Secondary Hypocalcemia
Hypomagnesemia in HSH results from a defect in the TRPM6 channel, a member of the transient receptor potential (TRP) family of proteins that are involved in cation transport. TRPM6 is expressed in intestinal epithelia and renal tubules and is thought to mediate transepithelial magnesium transport. Affected individuals have presented with symptoms attributable to hypomagnesemia with secondary impairment of parathyroid function and hypocalcemia. Seizures and muscle spasms occur in infancy, and restoration of magnesium and calcium levels requires high doses of oral magnesium supplementation.

Other Hereditary Hypomagnesemic Disorders
Mutations of the sodium-potassium-ATPase gamma-subunit can cause an autosomal dominant form of hypomagnesemia. Activating mutations of the CaSR in autosomal dominant hypoparathyroidism primarily manifests as hypocalcemia, but hypomagnesemia has been reported in 50% of patients.

HEREDITARY TUBULAR DISORDERS CAUSING HYPERTENSION DUE TO SALT RETENTION

LIDDLE'S SYNDROME
Liddle's syndrome mimics a state of aldosterone excess by the presence of early and severe hypertension, often accompanied by hypokalemia and metabolic alkalosis, but plasma aldosterone and renin levels are low. This disorder is due to unregulated sodium reabsorption by an overactive ENaC in the cortical collecting duct (Fig. 278-3). Deletional mutations of the intracellular domain of the β or γ subunit of ENaC (Table 278-2) prevent recycling from the apical membrane and an inability to downregulate the number of channels despite a high intracellular sodium concentration. Increased potassium and hydrogen ion secretion follow the lumen-negative electrical potential that results from chloride-independent sodium reabsorption. Amiloride or triamterene block ENaC and, combined with salt restriction, provide effective therapy for hypertension and hypokalemia.

FAMILIAL HYPERKALEMIC HYPERTENSION (PSEUDOHYPOALDOSTERONISM TYPE II; GORDON SYNDROME)
Familial hyperkalemic hypertension (FHHt) is a rare autosomal dominant disease that manifests in adolescence or early adulthood with thiazide-responsive low-renin hypertension, hyperkalemia, and metabolic acidosis with normal renal function. In some families, mutations have been identified in the WNK kinases 1 and 4 that lead to increased activity of the thiazide-sensitive sodium chloride co-transporter, NCCT. This causes hypertension from enhanced salt reabsorption in the DCT and impaired distal secretion of potassium and hydrogen ion, all of which can be corrected with thiazide diuretics.

INHERITED DISORDERS OF WATER HANDLING

HEREDITARY NEPHROGENIC DIABETES INSIPIDUS
Hereditary nephrogenic diabetes insipidus (NDI) is a rare monogenic disease that usually presents in infancy with severe vasopressin-resistant polyuria, dehydration, failure to thrive, and dilute urine despite the presence of hypernatremia.

Genetics and Pathogenesis
Vasopressin [antidiuretic hormone (ADH)]-stimulated water reabsorption in the collecting duct is mediated by the type 2 vasopressin receptor (V2R) on the basal surface of principal cells. Activation of the adenylyl cyclase-cAMP pathway phosphorylates vesicle-associated aquaporin-2 (AQP2) water channels and stimulates their insertion into the apical plasma membrane. Water enters the cells from the tubular lumen through AQP2 and exits along an osmotic gradient into the hypertonic medulla and vasa rectae via basal AQP3/4 channels (Fig. 278-3). X-linked mutations of V2R account for about 90% of cases of NDI, such that the expression of the receptor on the cell surface is impaired. The remaining cases are due to various autosomal recessive or dominant mutations of AQP2 that cause the water channels to be retained within the cytosol (Table 278-2). The effect of these mutations is an inability to concentrate the urine and conserve water despite high plasma levels of vasopressin. Penetrance is variable in heterozygous female carriers of X-linked NDI, and some have a moderate concentrating defect.

Clinical Features
Whereas NDI in adults is most often acquired from conditions such as hypercalcemia, lithium therapy, and partial chronic urinary obstruction, hereditary NDI typically presents in infancy. Unlike other polyuric syndromes such as Bartter's and Gitelman's syndromes, conservation of electrolytes is normal, and hypernatremia is entirely from the loss of water. Recurrent episodes of dehydration and hypernatremia can lead to seizures and mental retardation. Although renal function is otherwise normal, chronically high urine flow causes dilatation of the ureters and bladder and may cause bladder dysfunction and obstructive uropathy.

Diagnosis
The diagnosis in infants and children with hereditary NDI is usually apparent from the family history and clinical presentation. The diagnosis can be confirmed by the presence of high plasma levels of vasopressin in the face of polyuria and hypotonic urine. This may be especially useful in adults with partial NDI to distinguish the polyuric state from central diabetes insipidus or psychogenic polydipsia (Chap. 334). Genetic screening for mutations in *AVPR2* and *AQP2* is available in research centers and should be performed to identify affected infants from families at risk of NDI in order to begin treatment and avoid dehydration and its consequences.

℞ HEREDITARY NEPHROGENIC DIABETES INSIPIDUS

In families with high awareness of the condition, early diagnosis and treatment with abundant water intake has enabled many patients to live to adulthood with normal mental and physical development. Exogeneous vasopressin is ineffective, and because these patients can excrete up to 20 L of urine per day, maintaining adequate water intake is challenging. Thiazide diuretics and salt restriction can reduce urine output by inducing a state of mild volume contraction, thereby promoting increased proximal reabsorption of isotonic fluid and inhibiting the generation of free water. A combination thiazide-amiloride formulation will avoid thiazide-induced hypokalemia and alkalosis, and indomethacin may further reduce urine output by inhibiting prostaglandin synthesis.

NEPHROGENIC SYNDROME OF INAPPROPRIATE ANTIDIURESIS
Activating mutations of the V2R were recently described in two boys who presented with irritability and seizures within the first three months of life. Laboratory evaluation was significant for hyponatremia with inappropriately elevated urinary osmolality and undetectable vasopressin levels. Genomic analysis revealed missense mutations of *AVPR2* causing constitutive activation of V2R and inappropriate water reabsorption.

INHERITED RENAL TUBULAR ACIDOSIS
Nonanion gap (hyperchloremic) metabolic acidosis from proximal tubular bicarbonate wasting or impaired distal net acid excretion may be a primary (sporadic or inherited) tubular disorder or acquired secondary to a variety of conditions (Chap. 48). There are three forms of

renal tubular acidosis (RTA). Types 1 and 2 may be acquired or primarily whereas the most common form, type 4 RTA, is usually acquired in association with moderate renal dysfunction and is characterized by hyperkalemia.

TYPE 1 (DISTAL) RTA

Clinical Features and Diagnosis In primary distal RTA (dRTA), the kidneys are unable to acidify the urine to pH <5.5 in the presence of systemic metabolic acidosis or after acid loading as a result of impaired hydrogen ion secretion or bicarbonate reabsorption in the distal nephron. Other features are hypokalemia, hypocitraturia, hypercalciuria, nephrocalcinosis, and/or nephrolithiasis. Chronic untreated acidosis may cause rickets or osteomalacia. Inheritance of primary dRTA includes autosomal dominant and autosomal recessive forms with a broad spectrum of clinical expression. Autosomal recessive dRTA most often presents in infancy with severe acidosis, failure to thrive, impaired growth, and impaired kidney function from nephrocalcinosis. Many patients with autosomal dominant dRTA, and some with recessive disease, are asymptomatic, and RTA is discovered incidentally in adolescence or adulthood during evaluation for kidney stones. In the absence of systemic acidosis, the diagnosis of incomplete dRTA is suggested by hypocitraturia and hypercalciuria and can be confirmed by failure of the urine to acidify to pH <5.5 after acid loading with oral ammonium chloride or calcium chloride.

Genetics and Pathophysiology Primary dRTA may be hereditary or sporadic. Several kindreds with hereditary dRTA have been identified in Southeast Asia and in areas of the world where parental consanguinity is high. The cellular basis for dRTA lies in dysfunction at the level of the α type intercalated cell of the cortical collecting duct (Fig. 278-3). Mutations affecting subunits of the H$^+$-ATPase proton pump on the luminal surface impair hydrogen ion secretion, account for most forms of autosomal recessive dRTA, and are often associated with early-onset sensorineural hearing loss (Table 278-2). Autosomal dominant dRTA results from mutations involving the chloride-bicarbonate exchanger AE1, the gateway for bicarbonate exit into the blood. Anion exchange by the mutant AE1 is normal, but aberrant targeting of AE1 from the basal to apical plasma membrane is believed to cause bicarbonate loss into the urine instead of recovery. Bi-allelic mutations of AE1 may impair transport activity and account for some cases of recessive disease, sometimes associated with late-onset hearing loss (Table 278-2). A syndrome of osteopetrosis, short stature, and mental retardation, so-called "marble-brain disease" with dRTA, is due to mutations in carbonic anhydrase II. Urinary potassium wasting and defective urinary concentration are characteristic of dRTA, but the precise mechanisms are unclear. Calcium is released from bone in the process of buffering of acid and results in hypercalciuria. Enhanced proximal citrate absorption accounts for hypocitraturia and, together with hypercalciuria, predisposes to nephrocalcinosis and calcium phosphate stone formation.

Rx TYPE 1 (DISTAL) RTA

Early initiation of alkali replacement at doses equivalent to 1–3 mmol/kg/day of bicarbonate in divided doses will usually correct the acidosis, hypokalemia, and hypocitraturia, maintaining growth and preventing bone disease in early-onset dRTA. Citrate is generally tolerated better than sodium bicarbonate and can be given as potassium or sodium salt, depending on the severity of hypokalemia. In patients who present later with kidney stones, large fluid intake and sufficient alkali to restore normal acid-base balance corrects the hypocitraturia and reduces hypercalciuria, thereby inhibiting the formation of new stones.

TYPE 2 (PROXIMAL) RTA

Proximal RTA (pRTA) is the result of impaired bicarbonate reabsorption in the proximal tubular where the bulk of filtered bicarbonate is recovered (Fig. 278-3). It is most often secondary to various autoimmune, drug-induced, infiltrative, or other tubulopathies (Chap. 48) or a result of tubular injury from inherited diseases in which endogenous metabolites accumulate and produce tubular injury. Such inherited disorders include Wilson's disease, cystinosis, tyrosinemia, galactosemia, hereditary fructose intolerance, glycogen storage disease type I, and Lowe's syndrome. In this situation pRTA is but one of several abnormalities that constitute Fanconi syndrome. Other features are hyperphosphaturia, hyperuricosuria, hypercalciuria, nonselective amino aciduria and glycosuria. In addition to hyperchloremic acidosis, rickets or osteomalacia are the predominant effects of Fanconi syndrome.

A rare infantile form of primary pRTA with isolated proximal tubular bicarbonate wasting is due to homozygous mutations of the proximal tubule basolateral sodium-bicarbonate exchanger NBC1 (Table 278-2). This exchanger is the main mechanism by which bicarbonate moves from the proximal tubule cell back into the blood. Other manifestations include short stature and mental retardation. An ocular phenotype that includes bilateral glaucoma, cataracts, and band keratopathy reflects a role of NBC1 in maintaining normal fluid balance in the eye and clarity of the lens.

Patients with pRTA have severe metabolic acidosis, and it is difficult to restore normal acid-base balance despite large amounts of alkali. This is a consequence of their continuing to waste bicarbonate (fractional excretion >15%) until the serum level falls below a threshold level, usually about 15–17 mmol/L, at which time bicarbonate is completely reabsorbed and the urine is maximally acidified with pH <5.5. When the serum bicarbonate is raised above the threshold with alkali therapy, bicarbonate wasting recurs and causes hypokalemia by flooding the distal nephron with a nonreabsorbable anion.

Rx TYPE 2 (PROXIMAL) RTA

Treatment of pRTA requires 5–15 mmol/kg/day of bicarbonate together with supplemental potassium and vitamin D.

OTHER MONOGENIC DISORDERS OF PROXIMAL TUBULAR FUNCTION (Fig. 278-3)

CYSTINURIA

Cystinuria is an autosomal recessive disorder of cystine and dibasic amino acid (ornithine, arginine, and lysine) transport in the proximal tubule and intestinal epithelial cells. With a prevalence of about 1 in 7000, it represents one of the more common heritable diseases. Impaired tubular absorption leads to high concentrations of cystine, which is insoluble in the acid environment of the renal tubules. Clinical severity varies from asymptomatic cystine crystalluria in heterozygous carriers to the frequent passage of gravel and cystine stones, ureteral obstruction, recurrent urinary infections, and progressive kidney failure in homozygotes. The disease is due to mutations in one of two genes, SLC3A1 and SLC7A9 (Table 278-2). SLC3A1 encodes rBAT, a high-affinity, sodium-independent transporter for dibasic amino acids. The protein product of SLC7A9, b$^{0,+}$AT, is a catalytic subunit that associates with rBAT to form the active transporter. Diagnosis of cystinuria is established by a positive family history, the finding of hexagonal cystine crystals on urinalysis, and 24-hour urinary cystine excretion that exceeds 400 mg (normal less than 30 mg/d). Genetic analysis will probably become commonly available.

Rx CYSTINURIA

The mainstay of treatment is hydration to achieve a urine output of 2.5 L/day or more to reduce urine cystine concentration to <300mg/L, together with urine alkalinization to pH 7.0–7.5 with potassium citrate, and sodium restriction. Cystine is an oxidized dimer formed by linking two cysteine residues via a disulfide bond between the -SH groups. Thus, in intractable cases, thiol derivatives like penicillamine, captopril, and tiopronin may be added as second-line chelation therapy to dissociate the cystine molecule into more soluble disulfide compounds. Various stone removal and urinary drainage procedures are often required.

HARTNUP DISEASE

Hartnup disease is an autosomal recessive condition caused by a defect in intestinal and renal transport of neutral amino acids. The major clinical manifestations are cerebellar ataxia and pellagra-like skin lesions. Other than aminoaciduria, the kidneys are unaffected. The defective gene *SLC6A19* encodes a sodium-dependent and chloride-independent neutral amino acid transporter, which is expressed predominately in the intestine and renal tubules (Table 278-2). Amino acids such as tryptophan that are retained in the intestinal lumen are converted to indole compounds that are toxic to the CNS. Abnormal tryptophan metabolism also leads to niacin deficiency that accounts for the skin manifestations. Symptoms are aggravated by a protein-deficient diet and alleviated with a high-protein diet and nicotinamide supplements.

DENT'S DISEASE

Dent's disease and X-linked recessive nephrolithiasis are unusual forms of Fanconi syndrome due to X-linked recessive mutations of the gene encoding CLCN5, a channel belonging to a family of voltage-gated chloride channels (Table 278-2). The disorders are characterized by childhood onset of low-molecular-weight proteinuria, hypercalciuria, nephrocalcinosis and nephrolithiasis. Rickets or osteomalacia occurs in 30% of patients, and progressive renal failure from interstitial fibrosis, tubular atrophy, and glomerulosclerosis commonly develops in adulthood. CLCN5 serves to maintain the electrical gradient and acid environment established in proximal tubular cell endosomes by proton-ATPase, which is necessary for the degradation of low-molecular-weight proteins normally filtered by the glomerulus. Defects in CLCN5 appear to disrupt this process and lead to tubular cell dysfunction.

R_x DENT'S DISEASE

Treatment is directed at controlling hypercalciuria by dietary salt restriction and thiazide diuretics, which favor calcium reabsorption. Restriction of dietary calcium is not recommended.

RENAL GLUCOSURIA

Isolated glucosuria in the presence of a normal blood glucose concentration is due to mutations in *SLC5A2*, the gene encoding the high-capacity sodium-glucose co-transporter SGLT2 in the proximal renal tubule (Table 278-2). Subjects with this disorder are usually asymptomatic and do not have other features of proximal tubular dysfunction. Depending on the severity of the defect, the tubular maximum for glucose reabsorption may fall well within normal blood glucose levels and lead to >50 grams/day of glucosuria. Such patients may have polyuria from osmotic diuresis.

RENAL PHOSPHATE WASTING

Renal phosphate wasting resulting in hypophosphatemia and rickets or osteomalacia may be part of a generalized disorder of proximal tubular function, as in Fanconi syndrome, or an isolated phenomenon.

Isolated phosphaturia is most often due to the inhibition of renal tubular phosphate reabsorption by one or other phosphaturic hormone (Chap. 346). An exception is hereditary hypophosphatemic rickets with hypercalciuria (HHRH). HHRH is an autosomal recessive disorder due to mutations in *SLC34A3*, the gene encoding the proximal tubule sodium-phosphate co-transporter (Table 278-2). Defective phosphate reabsorption causes renal phosphate wasting and leads to stunted growth from rickets. The low serum phosphorus levels appropriately stimulate 1-hydroxylation of vitamin D, which increases intestinal calcium absorption, suppresses parathyroid hormone (PTH) secretion and results in hypercalciuria. High levels of 1,25-dihydroxy-vitamin D help distinguish HHRH from hormonal causes of hyperphosphaturia. Treatment is directed at phosphate repletion.

VITAMIN D–DEPENDENT RICKETS

Vitamin D–dependent rickets exists in two forms that manifest with hypocalcemia, hypophosphatemia, elevated PTH levels, and the skeletal abnormalities of rickets and osteomalacia. Tetany may be present in severe cases. Vitamin D–dependent rickets type I is an autosomal recessive disease resulting from mutations in *CYP27B1*, the gene that encodes $25(OH)D_3$-1α-hydroxylase, an enzyme in the proximal tubule that catalyzes the hydroxylation and activation of $25(OH)D_3$ into $1,25(OH)_2D_3$ (Table 278-2). It can be treated with physiologic replacement doses of $1,25(OH)_2D_3$. In contrast, vitamin D–dependent rickets type II is due to end-organ resistance to $1,25(OH)_2D_3$ as a result of mutations in the vitamin D receptor (Chap. 347).

FURTHER READINGS

COLE DE, QUAMME GA: Inherited disorders of renal magnesium handling. J Am Soc Nephrol 11:1937, 2000

DEVONALD MA, KARET FE: Renal epithelial traffic jams and one-way streets. J Am Soc Nephrol 15:1370, 2004

GUAY-WOODFORD L: Other cystic kidney diseases, in *Comprehensive Clinical Nephrology*, 2d ed, RJ Johnson and J Feehally (eds). New York, Saunders, 2003

HART TC et al: Mutations of the UMOD gene are responsible for medullary cystic kidney disease 2 and familial juvenile hyperuricaemic nephropathy. J Med Genet 39:882, 2002

JECK N et al: Salt handling in the distal nephron: Lessons learned from inherited human disorders. Am J Physiol Regul Integr Comp Physiol 288:R782, 2005

LAING CM et al: Renal tubular acidosis: Developments in our understanding of the molecular basis. Int J Biochem Cell Biol 37:1151, 2005

SANDS JM, BICHET DG: Nephrogenic diabetes insipidus. Ann Intern Med 144:186, 2006

SAUNIER S et al: Nephronophthisis. Curr Opin Genet Dev 15:324, 2005

TORRES VE, HARRIS PC: Mechanisms of disease: Autosomal dominant and recessive polycystic kidney diseases. Nat Clin Pract Nephrol 2:40, 2006

279 Tubulointerstitial Diseases of the Kidney
Alan S. L. Yu, Barry M. Brenner

Primary tubulointerstitial diseases of the kidney are characterized by histologic and functional abnormalities that involve the tubules and interstitium to a greater degree than the glomeruli and renal vasculature (Table 279-1). Secondary tubulointerstitial disease occurs as a consequence of progressive glomerular or vascular injury. Morphologically, acute forms of these disorders are characterized by interstitial edema, often associated with cortical and medullary infiltration by both mononuclear cells and polymorphonuclear leukocytes, and patchy areas of tubule cell necrosis. In more chronic forms, interstitial fibrosis predominates, inflammatory cells are typically mononuclear, and abnormalities of the tubules tend to be more widespread, as evidenced by atrophy, luminal dilatation, and thickening of tubule basement membranes. Because of the nonspecific nature of the histology, particularly in chronic tubulointerstitial diseases, biopsy specimens rarely provide a specific diagnosis. The urine sediment is also unlikely to be diagnostic, except in allergic forms of acute tubulointerstitial disease in which eosinophils may predominate in the urinary sediment.

Defects in renal function often accompany these alterations of tubule and interstitial structure (Table 279-2). Proximal tubule dysfunction may be manifested as selective reabsorptive defects leading to hypokalemia, aminoaciduria, glycosuria, phosphaturia, uricosuria, or

TABLE 279-1 PRINCIPAL CAUSES OF TUBULOINTERSTITIAL DISEASE OF THE KIDNEY

Acute Interstitial Nephritis

Drugs[a]
  Antibiotics (β-lactams, sulfonamides, quinolones, vancomycin, erythromycin, minocycline, rifampin, ethambutol, acyclovir)
  Nonsteroidal anti-inflammatory drugs, cyclooxygenase 2 inhibitors
  Diuretics (thiazides, furosemide, triamterene)
  Anticonvulsants (phenytoin, phenobarbital, carbamazepine, valproic acid)
  Miscellaneous (captopril, H$_2$ receptor blockers, proton pump inhibitors, mesalazine, indinavir, allopurinol)
Infection
  Bacteria (*Streptococcus, Staphylococcus, Legionella, Salmonella, Brucella, Yersinia, Corynebacterium diphtheriae*)
  Viruses (Epstein-Barr virus, cytomegalovirus, Hantavirus, polyomavirus, HIV)
  Miscellaneous (*Leptospira, Rickettsia, Mycoplasma*)
Idiopathic
  Tubulointerstitial nephritis–uveitis syndrome
  Anti-tubule basement membrane disease
  Sarcoidosis

Chronic Tubulointerstitial Diseases

Hereditary renal diseases
  Polycystic kidney disease[a] (Chap. 278)
  Medullary cystic disease (Chap. 278)
  Medullary sponge kidney (Chap. 278)
Exogenous toxins
  Analgesic nephropathy[a]
  Lead nephropathy
  Miscellaneous nephrotoxins (e.g. lithium[a], cyclosporine[a], heavy metals, slimming regimens with Chinese herbs)
Metabolic toxins
  Hyperuricemia[a]
  Hypercalcemia
  Miscellaneous metabolic toxins (e.g., hypokalemia, hyperoxaluria, cystinosis, Fabry's disease)
Autoimmune disorders
  Sjögren's syndrome
Neoplastic disorders
  Leukemia
  Lymphoma
  Multiple myeloma[a]
Miscellaneous disorders
  Sickle cell nephropathy
  Chronic pyelonephritis
  Chronic urinary tract obstruction
  Vesicoureteral reflux[a]
  Radiation nephritis
  Balkan nephropathy
  Tubulointerstitial disease secondary to glomerular and vascular disease

[a]Common.

bicarbonaturia [proximal or type II renal tubular acidosis (RTA); Chap. 278]. In combination, these defects constitute the *Fanconi syndrome*. Proteinuria, predominantly of low-molecular-weight proteins, is usually modest, rarely > 2 g/d.

Defects in urinary acidification and concentrating ability often represent the most troublesome of the tubule dysfunctions encountered in patients with tubulointerstitial disease. Hyperchloremic metabolic acidosis often develops at a relatively early stage in the course. Patients with this finding generally elaborate urine of maximal acidity (pH ≤ 5.3). In such patients the defect in acid excretion is usually caused by a reduced capacity to generate and excrete ammonia due to the reduction in renal mass. Preferential damage to the collecting ducts, as in amyloidosis or chronic obstructive uropathy, may also predispose to distal or type I RTA, characterized by high urine pH (≥ 5.5) during spontaneous or NH$_4$Cl-induced metabolic acidosis. Patients with tubulointerstitial diseases affecting predominantly medullary and papillary structures (such as analgesic nephropathy and sickle cell disease) may also exhibit concentrating defects, with resultant nocturia and polyuria.

TOXINS

Although the kidney is vulnerable to toxic injury, renal damage by a variety of nephrotoxins often goes unrecognized because the manifestations of such injury are usually nonspecific in nature and insidious in onset. Diagnosis largely depends on a history of exposure to a certain toxin. Particular attention should be paid to the occupational history, as well as to an assessment of exposure—current and remote—to drugs, especially antibiotics and analgesics, and to dietary supplements or herbal remedies. The recognition of a potential association between a patient's renal disease and exposure to a nephrotoxin is crucial, because, unlike many other forms of renal disease, progression of the functional and morphologic abnormalities associated with toxin-induced nephropathies may be prevented, and even reversed, by eliminating additional exposure.

Exogenous Toxins · *ANALGESIC NEPHROPATHY* A distinct syndrome has been described in heavy users of analgesic mixtures containing phenacetin (banned in the United States since 1983) in combination with aspirin, acetaminophen, or caffeine. Morphologically, analgesic nephropathy is characterized by papillary necrosis and tubulointerstitial inflammation. At an early stage, damage to the vascular supply of the inner medulla (vasa recta) leads to a local interstitial inflammatory reaction and, eventually, to papillary ischemia, necrosis, fibrosis, and calcification. The susceptibility of the renal papillae to damage by phenacetin is believed to be related to the establishment of a renal gradient for its acetaminophen metabolite, resulting in papillary tip concentrations tenfold higher than those in renal cortex.

In analgesic nephropathy, renal function usually declines gradually. Occasionally, papillary necrosis may be associated with hematuria and even renal colic owing to obstruction of a ureter by necrotic tissue. More than half of patients have sterile pyuria. Patients with analgesic nephropathy are usually unable to generate maximally concentrated urine, reflecting the underlying medullary and papillary damage. An acquired form of distal RTA (Chap. 278) may contribute to the development of *nephrocalcinosis*. The occurrence of anemia out of proportion to the degree of renal failure may also provide a clue to the diagnosis. When analgesic nephropathy has progressed to renal insufficiency, the kidneys usually appear bilaterally shrunken on intravenous pyelography, and the calyces are deformed. A "ring sign" on the pyelogram is pathognomonic of papillary necrosis and represents the radiolucent sloughed papilla surrounded by the radiodense contrast material in the calyx. CT may reveal papillary calcifications surrounding the central sinus complex in a "garland" pattern (Fig. 279-1). Transitional cell carcinoma may develop in the urinary pelvis or ureters as a late complication of analgesic abuse.

TABLE 279-2 FUNCTIONAL CONSEQUENCES OF TUBULOINTERSTITIAL DISEASE

Defect	Cause(s)
Reduced glomerular filtration rate[a]	Obliteration of microvasculature and obstruction of tubules
Fanconi syndrome	Damage to proximal tubular reabsorption of glucose, amino acids, phosphate, and bicarbonate
Hyperchloremic acidosis[a]	1. Reduced ammonia production 2. Inability to acidify the collecting duct fluid (distal renal tubular acidosis) 3. Proximal bicarbonate wasting
Tubular or small-molecular-weight proteinuria[a]	Failure of proximal tubule protein reabsorption
Polyuria, isosthenuria[a]	Damage to medullary tubules and vasculature
Hyperkalemia[a]	Potassium secretory defects including aldosterone resistance
Salt wasting	Distal tubular damage with impaired sodium reabsorption

[a]Common.

FIGURE 279-1 Radiologic appearance of analgesic nephropathy. A non-contrast CT scan shows an atrophic left kidney with papillary calcifications in a garland pattern. *(Reprinted by permission from Macmillan Publishers Ltd, MM Elseviers et al, Kidney International 48:1316, 1995.)*

Whether non-phenacetin analgesics, alone or in combination, cause renal disease is controversial. Recent cohort studies in individuals with normal baseline renal function suggest that the risk of moderate analgesic use, if any, is low. Until conclusive evidence is available, however, physicians should consider screening heavy users of acetaminophen and nonsteroidal anti-inflammatory drugs (NSAIDs) for evidence of renal disease and discouraging their use of these drugs.

LEAD NEPHROPATHY (See also **Chap. e33**) Lead intoxication may produce a chronic tubulointerstitial renal disease. Children who repeatedly ingest lead-based paints (pica) may develop kidney disease as adults. Significant occupational exposure may occur in workplaces where lead-containing metals or paints are heated to high temperatures, such as battery factories, smelters, salvage yards, and weapon firing ranges.

Tubule transport processes enhance the accumulation of lead within renal cells, particularly in the proximal convoluted tubule, leading to cell degeneration, mitochondrial swelling, and eosinophilic intranuclear inclusion bodies rich in lead. In addition, lead nephropathy is associated with ischemic changes in the glomeruli, fibrosis of the adventitia of small renal arterioles, and focal areas of cortical scarring. Eventually, the kidneys become atrophic. Urinary excretion of lead, porphyrin precursors such as δ-aminolevulinic acid and coproporphyrin, and urobilinogen may be increased. Patients with chronic lead nephropathy are characteristically *hyperuricemic*, a consequence of enhanced reabsorption of filtered urate. Acute gouty arthritis (so-called saturnine gout) develops in about 50% of patients with lead nephropathy, in striking contrast to other forms of chronic renal failure in which de novo gout is rare (Chap. 353). Hypertension is also a complication. Therefore, in any patient with slowly progressive renal failure, atrophic kidneys, gout, and hypertension, the diagnosis of lead intoxication should be considered. Features of acute lead intoxication (abdominal colic, anemia, peripheral neuropathy, and encephalopathy) are usually absent.

The diagnosis may be suspected by finding elevated serum levels of lead. However, because blood levels may not be elevated even in the presence of a toxic total-body burden of lead, the quantitation of lead excretion following infusion of the chelating agent calcium disodium edetate is a more reliable indicator of serious lead exposure. Urinary excretion of >0.6 mg/d of lead is indicative of overt toxicity, but even lead burdens of 0.08–0.6 mg/d may cause progressive loss of renal function.

℞ LEAD NEPHROPATHY

Treatment includes removing the patient from the source of exposure and augmenting lead excretion with a chelating agent such as calcium disodium edetate.

LITHIUM Use of lithium salts for bipolar disorder (Chap. 386) is associated with chronic tubulointerstitial nephropathy, generally manifest as the insidious development of chronic renal insufficiency. Nephrogenic diabetes insipidus, which may occur alone or in association with the renal insufficiency, is common. It manifests as polyuria and polydipsia and is due to lithium-induced downregulation of the vasopressin-regulated water channels in the collecting duct. Mild proteinuria and hypercalcemia due to lithium-induced hyperparathyroidism are common. The predominant finding on renal biopsy is tubular atrophy and interstitial fibrosis out of proportion to the extent of glomerular or vascular disease. Tubular cysts are common, and concomitant focal segmental glomerulosclerosis can be observed.

Renal function should be followed in patients taking this drug, and caution should be exercised if lithium is employed in patients with underlying renal disease. Once renal impairment occurs, lithium therapy should be stopped and an alternative agent substituted. Despite discontinuation of lithium, chronic renal disease in such patients is often irreversible and can progress to end-stage renal failure.

MISCELLANEOUS NEPHROTOXINS The immunosuppressant *cyclosporine* causes both acute and chronic renal injury. The acute injury and the use of cyclosporine in transplantation are discussed in Chap. 276. The chronic injury results in an irreversible reduction in glomerular filtration rate (GFR), with mild proteinuria and arterial hypertension. Hyperkalemia is a relatively common complication and results, in part, from tubule resistance to aldosterone. The histologic changes in renal tissue include patchy interstitial fibrosis and tubular atrophy. In addition, the intrarenal vasculature often demonstrates hyalinosis, and focal segmental glomerular sclerosis can be present as well. In patients receiving this drug for renal transplantation (Chap. 276), chronic graft dysfunction and recurrence of the primary disease may coincide with chronic cyclosporine injury, and, on clinical grounds, distinction among these may be difficult. Dose reduction appears to mitigate cyclosporine-associated renal fibrosis but may increase the risk of rejection and graft loss. Treatment of any associated arterial hypertension may lessen renal injury.

Chinese herbs nephropathy is characterized by rapidly progressive interstitial renal fibrosis in young women due to ingestion of weight-reduction pills containing Chinese herbs; at least one of the culprit ingredients is aristolochic acid. Clinically, patients present with progressive chronic renal insufficiency with sterile pyuria and anemia that is disproportionately severe relative to the level of renal function. The pathologic findings are interstitial fibrosis and tubular atrophy that affects the cortex in preference to the medulla, fibrous intimal thickening of the interlobular arteries, and a relative paucity of cellular infiltrates.

Metabolic Toxins • *ACUTE URIC ACID NEPHROPATHY* (See also Chap. 327) Acute overproduction of uric acid and extreme hyperuricemia often lead to a rapidly progressive renal insufficiency, so-called acute uric acid nephropathy. This tubulointerstitial disease is usually seen as part of the tumor lysis syndrome in patients given cytotoxic drugs for the treatment of lymphoproliferative or myeloproliferative disorders but may also occur in these patients before such treatment is begun. The pathologic changes are largely the result of deposition of uric acid crystals in the kidneys and their collecting systems, leading to partial or complete obstruction of collecting ducts, renal pelvis, or ureter. Since obstruction is often bilateral, patients typically follow the clinical course of acute renal failure, characterized by oliguria and rapidly rising serum creatinine concentration. In the early phase uric acid crystals can be found in urine, usually in association with microscopic or gross hematuria. Hyperuricemia can also be a consequence of renal failure of any etiology. The finding of a urine uric acid/creatinine ratio >1 mg/mg (0.7 mol/mol) distinguishes acute uric acid nephropathy from other causes of renal failure.

Prevention of hyperuricemia in patients at risk by treatment with allopurinol in doses of 200–800 mg/d prior to cytotoxic therapy reduces the danger of acute uric acid nephropathy. Once hyperuricemia develops, however, efforts should be directed to preventing deposition of uric acid within the urinary tract. Increasing urine volume with potent diuretics (furosemide or mannitol) effectively lowers intratubular uric acid concentrations, and alkalinization of the urine to pH ≥ 7 with sodium bicarbonate and/or a carbonic anhydrase inhibitor (acetazolamide) enhances uric acid solubility. If these efforts, together with allopurinol therapy, are ineffective in preventing acute renal failure, dialysis should be instituted to lower the serum uric acid concentration as well as to treat the acute manifestations of uremia.

GOUTY NEPHROPATHY (See also Chap. 327) Patients with less severe but prolonged forms of hyperuricemia are predisposed to a more chronic tubulointerstitial disorder, often referred to as *gouty nephropathy*. The severity of renal involvement correlates with the duration and magnitude of the elevation of the serum uric acid concentration. Histologically, the distinctive feature of gouty nephropathy is the presence of crystalline deposits of uric acid and monosodium urate salts in kidney parenchyma. These deposits not only cause intrarenal obstruction but also incite an inflammatory response, leading to lymphocytic infiltration, foreign-body giant cell reaction, and eventual fibrosis, especially of medullary and papillary regions of the kidney. Since patients with gout frequently suffer from hypertension and hyperlipidemia, degenerative changes of the renal arterioles may constitute a striking feature of the histologic abnormality, often out of proportion to other morphologic defects. Clinically, gouty nephropathy is an insidious cause of renal insufficiency. Early in its course, GFR may be near normal, often despite focal morphologic changes in medullary and cortical interstitium, proteinuria, and diminished urinary concentrating ability. Whether reducing serum uric acid levels with allopurinol exerts a beneficial effect on the kidney remains to be demonstrated. Although such undesirable consequences of hyperuricemia as gout and uric acid stones respond well to allopurinol, use of this drug in asymptomatic hyperuricemia has not been shown to improve renal function consistently. Uricosuric agents such as probenecid, which may increase uric acid stone production, are clearly contraindicated.

HYPERCALCEMIC NEPHROPATHY (See also Chap. 347) Chronic hypercalcemia, as occurs in primary hyperparathyroidism, sarcoidosis, multiple myeloma, vitamin D intoxication, or metastatic bone disease, can cause tubulointerstitial damage and progressive renal insufficiency. The earliest lesion is a focal degenerative change in renal epithelia, primarily in collecting ducts, distal convoluted tubules, and loops of Henle. Tubule cell necrosis leads to nephron obstruction and stasis of intrarenal urine, favoring local precipitation of calcium salts and infection. Dilatation and atrophy of tubules eventually occur, as do interstitial fibrosis, mononuclear leukocyte infiltration, and interstitial calcium deposition (nephrocalcinosis). Calcium deposition may also occur in glomeruli and the walls of renal arterioles.

Clinically, the most striking defect is an inability to concentrate the urine maximally, resulting in polyuria and nocturia. Reduced collecting duct responsiveness to vasopressin and defective transport of NaCl in the ascending limb of Henle's loop are responsible for this. Reductions in GFR and renal blood flow also occur, both in acute severe hypercalcemia and with prolonged hypercalcemia of lesser severity. Eventually, uncontrolled hypercalcemia leads to severe tubulointerstitial damage and overt renal failure. Abdominal x-rays may demonstrate nephrocalcinosis as well as nephrolithiasis, the latter due to the hypercalciuria that often accompanies hypercalcemia.

℞ HYPERCALCEMIC NEPHROPATHY

Treatment consists of reducing the serum calcium concentration toward normal and correcting the primary abnormality of calcium metabolism. The management of hypercalcemia is discussed in Chap. 347. Renal dysfunction of acute hypercalcemia may be completely reversible. Gradual, progressive renal insufficiency related to chronic hypercalcemia, however, may not improve even with correction of the calcium disorder.

RENAL PARENCHYMAL DISEASE ASSOCIATED WITH EXTRARENAL NEOPLASM

Except for the glomerulopathies associated with lymphomas and several solid tumors (Chap. 277), the renal manifestations of primary ex-

FIGURE 279-2 Histologic appearance of myeloma cast nephropathy. A hematoxylin-eosin-stained kidney biopsy shows many atrophic tubules filled with eosinophilic casts (consisting of Bence-Jones protein), which are surrounded by giant cell reactions. *(Courtesy of Dr. Michael N. Koss, University of Southern California Keck School of Medicine; with permission.)*

trarenal neoplastic processes are confined mainly to the interstitium and tubules. Although metastatic renal involvement by solid tumors is unusual, the kidneys are often invaded by neoplastic cells in hematologic malignancies. In postmortem studies of patients with *lymphoma* and *leukemia*, renal involvement is found in approximately half. Diffuse infiltration of the renal parenchyma with malignant cells is seen most commonly. There may be flank pain, and x-rays may show enlargement of one or both kidneys. Renal insufficiency occurs in a minority, and treatment of the primary disease may improve renal function in these cases.

Plasma Cell Dyscrasias Several glomerular and tubulointerstitial disorders may occur in association with plasma cell dyscrasias (Chap. 106). Infiltration of the kidneys with myeloma cells is infrequent. When it occurs, the process is usually focal, so renal insufficiency from this cause is also uncommon. The more usual lesion is *myeloma kidney*, characterized histologically by atrophic tubules, many with eosinophilic intraluminal casts, and numerous multinucleated giant cells within tubule walls and in the interstitium (Fig. 279-2). Bence-Jones proteins are thought to cause myeloma kidney through direct toxicity to renal tubule cells. In addition, Bence-Jones proteins may precipitate within the distal nephron where the high concentrations of these proteins and the acid composition of the tubule fluid favor intraluminal cast formation and intrarenal obstruction. Further precipitation of Bence-Jones proteins can be induced by dehydration, which should, therefore, be avoided. Multiple myeloma may also affect the kidneys indirectly. Hypercalcemia or hyperuricemia may lead to the nephropathies described above. Proximal tubule disorders are also seen occasionally, including type II proximal RTA and the Fanconi syndrome.

Amyloidosis (See also Chaps. 277 and 324) Glomerular pathology usually predominates and leads to heavy proteinuria and azotemia. However, tubule function may also be deranged, giving rise to a nephrogenic diabetes insipidus and to distal (type I) RTA. In several cases these functional abnormalities correlated with peritubular deposition of amyloid, particularly in areas surrounding vasa rectae, loops of Henle, and collecting ducts. Bilateral enlargement of the kidneys, especially in a patient with massive proteinuria and tubule dysfunction, should raise the possibility of amyloid renal disease.

IMMUNE DISORDERS
Allergic Interstitial Nephritis An acute diffuse tubulointerstitial reaction may result from hypersensitivity to a number of drugs, including

β-lactams, sulfonamides, fluoroquinolone antibiotics, and the antituberculous drugs isoniazid and rifampin. Acute tubulointerstitial damage has also occurred after use of thiazide and loop diuretics, allopurinol, NSAIDs, and cyclooxygenase 2 (COX-2) inhibitors. Of note, the tubulointerstitial nephropathy that develops in some patients taking NSAIDs and COX-2 inhibitors may be associated with nephrotic-range proteinuria and histologic evidence of either minimal change or membranous glomerulopathy. Proton-pump inhibitors are an increasingly recognized culprit and have recently been implicated in up to half of cases of biopsy-proven acute tubulointerstitial nephritis. The use of mesalazine for the treatment of inflammatory bowel disease is associated with a more subacute disorder in which a severe indolent interstitial nephritis occurs several months after the initiation of the drug. Grossly, the kidneys are usually enlarged. Histologically, the interstitium of the kidney reveals pronounced edema and infiltration with polymorphonuclear leukocytes, lymphocytes, plasma cells, and, in some cases, large numbers of eosinophils. If the process is severe, tubule cell necrosis and regeneration may also be apparent. Immunofluorescence studies have either been unrevealing or demonstrated a linear pattern of immunoglobulin and complement deposition along tubule basement membranes.

Most patients require several weeks of drug exposure before developing evidence of renal injury. Rare cases have occurred after only a few doses or after a year or more of use. Renal failure is usually present; a triad of fever, skin rash, and peripheral blood eosinophilia is highly suggestive of acute tubulointerstitial nephritis but is present in only 10% of patients. Examination of the urine sediment reveals hematuria and often pyuria; occasionally, eosinophils may be present. Proteinuria is usually mild to moderate, except in cases of NSAID- or COX-2 inhibitor–associated glomerulopathy. The clinical picture may be confused with acute glomerulonephritis, but when acute renal failure and hematuria are accompanied by eosinophilia, skin rash, and a history of drug exposure, acute tubulointerstitial nephritis should be regarded as the leading diagnostic possibility. Discontinuation of the drug usually results in complete reversal of the renal injury; rarely, renal damage may be irreversible. Glucocorticoids may accelerate renal recovery, but their value has not been definitively established.

Sjögren's Syndrome   (See also Chap. 317) When the kidneys are involved in this disorder, the predominant histologic findings are those of chronic tubulointerstitial disease. Interstitial infiltrates are composed primarily of lymphocytes, causing the histology of the renal parenchyma in these patients to resemble that of the salivary and lacrimal glands. Renal functional defects include diminished urinary concentrating ability and distal (type I) RTA. Urinalysis may show pyuria (predominantly lymphocyturia) and mild proteinuria.

Tubulointerstitial Abnormalities Associated with Glomerulonephritis   Primary glomerulopathies are often associated with damage to tubules and the interstitium. Occasionally, the primary disorder may affect glomeruli and tubules directly. For example, in more than half of patients with the nephropathy of systemic lupus erythematosus, deposits of immune complexes can be identified in tubule basement membranes, usually accompanied by an interstitial mononuclear inflammatory reaction. Similarly, in many patients with glomerulonephritis associated with anti-glomerular basement membrane antibody, the same antibody is reactive against tubule basement membranes as well. More frequently, tubulointerstitial damage is a secondary consequence of glomerular dysfunction. The extent of tubulointerstitial fibrosis correlates closely with the degree of renal impairment. Potential mechanisms by which glomerular disease might cause tubulointerstitial injury include glomerular leak of plasma proteins toxic to epithelial cells, activation of tubule epithelial cells by glomerulus-derived cytokines, reduced peritubular blood flow leading to downstream tubulointerstitial ischemia, and hyperfunction of remnant tubules.

MISCELLANEOUS DISORDERS

Vesicoureteral Reflux   (See also Chap. 283) When the function of the ureterovesical junction is impaired, urine may reflux into the ureters due to the high intravesical pressure that develops during voiding. Clinically, reflux is often detected on the voiding and postvoiding films obtained during intravenous pyelography, although voiding cystourethrography may be required for definitive diagnosis. Bladder infection may ascend the urinary tract to the kidneys through incompetent ureterovesical sphincters. Not surprisingly, therefore, reflux is often discovered in patients with acute and/or chronic urinary tract infections. With more severe degrees of reflux, characterized by dilatation of ureters and renal pelves, progressive renal damage often appears. Uncertainty exists as to the necessity of infection in producing the scarred kidney of reflux nephropathy. Substantial proteinuria is often present, and glomerular lesions similar to those of idiopathic focal glomerulosclerosis (Chap. 277) are often found in addition to the changes of chronic tubulointerstitial disease. Surgical correction of reflux is usually necessary only with the more severe degrees of reflux since renal damage correlates with the extent of reflux. Obviously, if extensive glomerulosclerosis already exists, urologic repair may no longer be warranted.

Radiation Nephritis   Renal dysfunction can be expected to occur if ≥23 Gy (2300 rad) of x-ray irradiation is administered to both kidneys. Histologic examination of the kidneys reveals hyalinized glomeruli and arterioles, atrophic tubules, and extensive interstitial fibrosis. Radiation nephritis can present acutely or chronically with renal failure, moderate to malignant hypertension, anemia, and proteinuria that may reach the nephrotic range. Malignant hypertension without renal failure may follow unilateral renal irradiation and resolve with ipsilateral nephrectomy. Radiation nephritis has all but vanished because of heightened awareness of its pathogenesis by radiotherapists.

GLOBAL CONSIDERATIONS

The spectrum of causes of chronic tubulointerstitial nephritis shows marked geographical variation. Chinese herb nephropathy has mostly been reported in Belgium and in parts of Asia. Analgesic nephropathy has been found worldwide but is a particularly frequent cause of chronic renal failure in Scotland, Belgium, and Australia. Balkan endemic nephropathy is a chronic, slowly progressive tubulointerstitial disease of unknown etiology that is exclusively confined to Bulgaria, Serbia, Croatia, Bosnia, and Romania. These differences in incidence probably reflect geographical variation in exposure to particular nephrotoxins but could also be explained by genetic factors or differing diagnostic criteria.

FURTHER READINGS

BAKER RJ, PUSEY CD: The changing profile of acute tubulointerstitial nephritis. Nephrol Dial Transplant 19:8, 2004

BATEMAN V: Proximal tubular injury in myeloma. Contrib Nephrol 153:87, 2007

CURHAN GC et al: Lifetime non-narcotic analgesic abuse and decline in renal function in women. Arch Intern Med 164:1519, 2004

HARRIS DC: Tubulointerstitial renal disease. Curr Opin Nephrol Hypertens 10:303, 2001

KELLY CJ, NEILSON EG: Tubulointerstitial diseases, in *Brenner and Rector's The Kidney*, 7th ed, BM Brenner (ed). Philadelphia, Saunders, 2004, pp 1483–1512

LIN JL et al: Environmental lead exposure and progression of chronic renal diseases in patients without diabetes. N Engl J Med 348:277, 2003

PRESNE C et al: Lithium-induced nephropathy: Rate of progression and prognostic factors. Kidney Int 64:585, 2003

SHAH SV et al: Oxidants in chronic kidney disease. J Am Soc Nephrol 18:16, 2007

280 Vascular Injury to the Kidney
Kamal F. Badr, Barry M. Brenner

Renal vasculature is commonly involved in atherosclerotic, hypertensive, embolic, inflammatory, and hematologic vascular disorders. Adequate delivery of blood to the glomerular capillary network is crucial for glomerular filtration and overall salt and water balance. Thus, in addition to threatening the viability of renal tissue, vascular injury to the kidney may compromise the maintenance of body fluid volume and composition. It is important to keep in mind the unique nature of the renal microvasculature, in particular the presence of a large network of (glomerular) capillaries which subserves the process of glomerular filtration.

ATHEROSCLEROSIS

Renal Vascular Injury in Systemic Atherosclerotic Vascular Disease (AVD)
• *MACROVASCULAR ATHEROSCLEROTIC DISEASE* As is the case in other vascular beds, the renal artery and its branches are potential sites for plaque formation, which may lead to ischemic renal disease and hypertension (see below).

MICROVASCULAR ATHEROSCLEROTIC DISEASE Numerous trials in cardiovascular medicine have focused attention on the clinical significance of the rate of urinary albumin excretion (UAE) as an early and powerful predictor of systemic AVD. As illustrated in Fig. 280-1, while both systemic and renal endothelial beds are subject to oxidant stress, inflammation, and hemodynamic injury, a measurable response (elevated UAE) is detectable in the renal microcirculation years before the emergence of systemic disease and/or adverse events in other vascular beds. The strong correlation between UAE and cardiovascular risk, and the parallel improvements noted in both with pharmacologic therapy, support the emerging concept of the renal circulation as an early detection site for atherosclerotic endothelial injury and an integrated marker of cardiovascular risk.

Atherosclerotic Renovascular Disease (ARVD) (Renal Artery Stenosis and Ischemic Nephropathy)
It is estimated that ~5% of cases of hypertension are caused by renal artery stenosis (RAS). In population-based studies, significant (>60%) stenosis is found in 9.1% of men and 5.5% of women over 65. The incidence, however, is considerably higher in those being studied for coronary (19%) or peripheral (35–50%) vascular disease. Autopsy studies in patients dying of stroke revealed that at least 1 renal artery is >75% stenosed in 10% of the patients studied. The common cause in the middle-aged and elderly is an atheromatous plaque at the origin of the renal artery. Bilateral involvement is present in half of the affected cases. Established plaques progress in >50% of cases over 5 years (15% to total occlusion). Renal hypotrophy is detectable in 20% of affected kidneys. In younger women (15–50 years), stenosis is due to intrinsic structural abnormalities of the arterial wall caused by *fibromuscular dysplasia*.

In addition to stimulation of renin release, renovascular disease is associated with increased sympathetic neural activity, resulting in frequently described flushing, loss of nocturnal blood pressure (BP) decrease, autonomic instability, and rapid BP swings. In most patients being evaluated for RAS, glomerular filtration rate (GFR) is <60 mL/min, with 85% having stage 3–5 chronic kidney disease. GFR in these ranges is a strong independent predictor of cardiovascular risk. Thus, patients with ARVD are more likely to suffer from stroke, heart failure, or myocardial infarction than to progress to end-stage renal disease.

DIAGNOSIS Diagnostic evaluation for significant RAS should begin with noninvasive approaches. An initial screening test is Doppler ultrasonography, which provides information on blood-flow velocity and pressure waveforms in the renal arteries and, when positive, is helpful (sensitivity is 70% at best). Its limitations, however, include significant operator dependence, technical difficulty in obese patients, and poor sensitivity in the presence of multiple renal arteries, distal stenoses, and total occlusion. Measurement of the intrarenal resistance index (RI) provides valuable information on the extent of parenchymal disease and, hence, on the prognosis for functional recovery following revascularization procedures. Absence of compensatory hypertrophy in the contralateral kidney should raise the suspicion of bilateral stenosis or superimposed parenchymal renal disease, most commonly hypertensive or diabetic nephropathy. Because angiotensin-converting enzyme (ACE) inhibitors magnify the impairment in renal blood flow and GFR caused by functionally significant renal artery stenosis, use of these drugs in association with ^{99m}Tc-labeled pentetic acid (DTPA) or ^{99m}Tc-labeled mertiatide (MAG$_3$) renography enhances diagnostic precision and is of additional predictive value. Gadolinium-enhanced three-dimensional magnetic resonance angiography (MRA) has replaced previous modalities as the most sensitive (>90%) and specific (95%) test for the diagnosis of RAS. The most definitive diagnostic procedure is contrast-enhanced arteriography. Intraarterial digital subtraction tech-

FIGURE 280-1 Comparative pathophysiology and clinical consequences of atherosclerosis-associated endothelial cell injury in systemic versus renal circulations. In contrast to the systemic endothelial bed in which early atherosclerotic injury is undetectable, the high volume of fluid filtered across the glomerular endothelium (140–180 L/day) markedly amplifies the functional consequence (increased albumin filtration) of early endothelial (and podocyte) injury in the glomerulus. The emergence of microalbuminuria thus unmasks systemic endothelial injury likely occurring simultaneously in other vascular beds, progressing silently to overt disease years later. CV, cardiovascular; ACS, acute coronary syndrome; MI, myocardial infarction; TIA, transient ischemic attack; HTN, hypertension; GFR, glomerular filtration rate; UAE, urinary albumin excretion.

niques minimize the requirements for contrast, reducing the risk of renal toxicity.

Rx RENAL ARTERY STENOSIS

When blood pressure is controlled and renal function is preserved, expectant therapy and careful follow-up form the best approach for managing RAS. This approach is justified by the devastating consequences of atheroembolic complications of percutaneous revascularization, including loss of renal function. Despite enthusiasm for revascularization procedures for tight RAS in the early to mid-nineties, the past decade has witnessed a significant change in management strategies, stressing more conservative approaches. Medical therapy is aimed at controlling BP and preserving GFR, and includes typically at least three drugs. Angiotensin antagonists (ACE inhibitors or angiotensin receptor blockers) and diuretics are required in most patients. When goal BPs are achieved, clinical outcomes and survival are comparable for medical and revascularization therapies. Revascularization therapy (angioplasty with stent placement) may improve the chances of attaining goal BP but should be considered only after optimal medical therapy has failed to achieve goal BP, or resulted in a >30% increase in serum creatinine. BP control and preservation of renal function following revascularization should not be expected when the RI of the targeted kidney is >80%. In experienced hands, the complications of angioplasty or stenting are acceptably low. Clinical studies suggest that percutaneous revascularization prevents additional deterioration or even improves renal function in selected patients. Despite technical advances in percutaneous renal revascularization, optimal technique is still evolving. Embolic protection devices may prove useful. **Table 280-1** lists current indications for revascularization in patients with RAS. Because of safety, cost, and long-term efficacy, surgical repair is now rarely indicated.

Success rates with conventional percutaneous transluminal angioplasty in young patients with fibromuscular dysplasia are 50% cure and improvement in BP control in another 30%.

Atheroembolic Renovascular Disease   Atheroembolic renal disease is part of a systemic syndrome characterized by cholesterol crystal embolization. Renal damage results from embolization of cholesterol crystals from atherosclerotic plaques present in large arteries, such as the aorta, to small arteries in the renal vasculature. Atheroembolic renal disease is an increasingly common and often underdiagnosed cause of renal insufficiency in the elderly. Autopsy studies identify cholesterol emboli in 2.4–4% of renal tissue samples, but the incidence increases significantly in elderly individuals, especially in those who had undergone abdominal arteriography or surgery. Male gender, older age, hypertension, and diabetes mellitus are important predisposing factors, present in 85% of cases. Patients with cholesterol embolization syndrome also often have a history of ischemic cardiovascular disease, aortic aneurysm, cerebrovascular disease, congestive heart failure, or renal insufficiency. A significant association is present between RAS and atheroembolic renal disease. Inciting events, which include vascular surgery, arteriography, angioplasty, anticoagulation with heparin, and thrombolytic therapy, can be identified in ~50% of

TABLE 280-1   INDICATIONS AND PREREQUISITES FOR REVASCULARIZATION IN RENAL ARTERY STENOSIS

Indications
   Uncontrolled BP despite maximal therapy
   Progressive rise in creatinine (other causes excluded)
   Intolerance to ACE-Is, ARBs (>30% increase in creatinine or severe hyperkalemia)
   Recurrent pulmonary edema, CHF, or volume overload

Prerequisites
   Experienced operator
   Presence of two kidneys
   RI < 0.80 in target kidney(s)

Note: BP, blood pressure; ACE-Is, angiotensin-converting enzyme inhibitors; ARBs, angiotensin receptor blockers; CHF, congestive heart failure; RI, renal index.

cases. Arteriographic procedures constitute the most common cause of cholesterol embolization.

Clinical manifestations usually appear 1–14 days after an inciting event, but their onset can be more insidious. Systemic manifestations occur in fewer than half of the patients and include fever, myalgias, headache, and weight loss. Cutaneous manifestations, such as livedo reticularis, "purple" toes, and toe gangrene, occur in 50–90% of patients and constitute the most common extrarenal findings. Other targets of cholesterol embolization include the retina, musculoskeletal system, nervous system, and gut. Accelerated or labile hypertension is present in one-half of patients; malignant hypertension has been described. Renal insufficiency is usually subacute and advances in a stepwise fashion over a period of several weeks. Renal failure, however, can be acute and oliguric. Uremic signs and symptoms requiring dialytic therapy develop in 40% of patients, only half of whom recover sufficient renal function to discontinue dialysis after 1 year. Renal infarction secondary to cholesterol embolization is rare. Cholesterol embolic disease in renal allografts has been reported and can be of donor or of recipient origin.

LABORATORY FINDINGS   In addition to rising blood urea nitrogen (BUN) and creatinine, laboratory findings may include eosinophilia (60–80%), eosinophiluria, leukocytosis, elevated sedimentation rate, anemia, and hypocomplementemia.

Antemortem diagnosis of atherosclerotic renal emboli is difficult. The demonstration of cholesterol emboli in the retina is helpful, but a firm diagnosis is established only by renal biopsy. Histologic examination of the occluded vessels reveals biconvex needle-shaped clefts representing the sites of cholesterol crystal deposition. The cholesterol crystals themselves are removed by the usual solvents of tissue fixation but can be visualized in frozen sections of fresh tissue as birefringent crystals under polarized light. They may also be seen in asymptomatic skeletal muscle or skin. Atheroembolic renal disease is associated with a 64–81% mortality rate.

Rx ATHEROEMBOLIC RENAL DISEASE

No effective therapy for atheroembolic renal disease is available. Withdrawal of anticoagulation may be beneficial. In some patients, kidney function improved even after a prolonged period of renal insufficiency. Cholesterol-lowering agents may also improve outcome. An aggressive therapeutic approach with patient-tailored supportive measures may be associated with more favorable clinical outcome. Numerous reports suggest a beneficial effect for steroid therapy, but controlled studies are lacking.

Thromboembolic Renovascular Disease   Thrombosis of the major renal arteries or their branches is an important cause of deterioration of renal function, especially in the elderly. It is often difficult to diagnose and, therefore, requires a high index of suspicion. Thrombosis may occur as a result of intrinsic pathology in the renal vessels (posttraumatic, atherosclerotic, or inflammatory) or as a result of emboli originating in distant vessels, most commonly fat emboli, emboli originating in the left heart (mural thrombi following myocardial infarction, bacterial endocarditis, or aseptic vegetations), or "paradoxical" emboli passing from the right side of the circulation via a patent foramen ovale or atrial septal defect. Renal emboli are bilateral in 15–30% of cases.

The clinical presentation is variable, depending on the time course and the extent of the occlusive event. Acute thrombosis and infarction, such as follows embolization, may result in sudden onset of flank pain and tenderness, fever, hematuria, leukocytosis, nausea, and vomiting. If infarction occurs, renal enzymes may be elevated, namely aspartate aminotransferase (AST), lactate dehydrogenase (LDH), and alkaline phosphatase, which rise and fall in the order listed. Urinary LDH and alkaline phosphatase may also increase after infarction. Renal function deteriorates acutely, leading in bilateral thrombosis to acute oliguric renal failure. More gradual (i.e., atherosclerotic) occlusion of a single renal artery may go undetected. A spectrum of clinical presentations lies between these two extremes. Hypertension usually follows renal infarction and results from renin release in the peri-infarction zone. Hypertension is usually transient but may be persistent. Diagnosis is established by renal arteriography.

℞ ACUTE RENAL ARTERIAL THROMBOSIS

Management options for *acute* renal arterial thrombosis include surgical intervention, anticoagulant therapy, intrarenal tissue plasminogen activator, percutaneous rheolytic thrombectomy, conservative and supportive therapy, and control of hypertension. The choice of treatment depends mainly on (1) the condition of the patient, in particular the patient's ability to withstand major surgery; and (2) the extent of renovascular occlusion and amount of renal mass at risk of infarction. In general, supportive care and anticoagulant therapy are indicated in unilateral disease. In *acute* bilateral thrombosis, medical and surgical therapies yield comparable results. About 25% of patients die during the acute episode, usually from extrarenal complications.

RENAL VASCULAR INJURY IN HYPERTENSION

Whether it is "essential" or of known etiology, hypertension results in development of intrinsic lesions of the renal arterioles (hyaline arteriolosclerosis) that eventually lead to loss of function (nephrosclerosis).

"Essential" Hypertension (Arteriolar Nephrosclerosis) Arteriolar nephrosclerosis is seen in patients who are hypertensive (BP > 150/90 mmHg) for an extended period of time but whose hypertension has not progressed to a malignant form (described below). Such patients, usually in the older age group, are often discovered to be hypertensive on routine physical examination or as a result of nonspecific symptomatology (e.g., headaches, weakness, palpitations).

The characteristic pathology is in the afferent arterioles, which have thickened walls due to deposition of homogeneous eosinophilic material (hyaline arteriolosclerosis). Narrowing of vascular lumina results, with consequent ischemic injury to glomeruli and tubules.

Physical examination may reveal changes in retinal vessels (arteriolar narrowing and/or flame-shaped hemorrhages), cardiac hypertrophy, and possibly signs of congestive heart failure. Renal disease may manifest as a mild to moderate elevation of serum creatinine concentration, microalbuminuria, or proteinuria.

"Malignant" Hypertension Patients with long-standing hypertension or patients not previously known to be hypertensive may develop malignant hypertension characterized by a sudden (accelerated) elevation of BP (diastolic BP often >130 mmHg) accompanied by papilledema, central nervous system manifestations, cardiac decompensation, and acute progressive deterioration of renal function. The absence of papilledema does not rule out the diagnosis in a patient with markedly elevated BP and rapidly declining renal function. The kidneys are characterized by a flea-bitten appearance resulting from hemorrhages in surface capillaries. Histologically, two distinct vascular lesions can be seen. The first, affecting arterioles, is fibrinoid necrosis, i.e., infiltration of arteriolar walls with eosinophilic material including fibrin, thickening of vessel walls, and, occasionally, an inflammatory infiltrate (necrotizing arteriolitis). The second lesion, involving the interlobular arteries, is a concentric hyperplastic proliferation of the cellular elements of the vascular wall with deposition of collagen to form a hyperplastic arteriolitis (onion-skin lesion). Fibrinoid necrosis occasionally extends into the glomeruli, which may also undergo proliferative changes or total necrosis. Most glomerular and tubular changes are secondary to ischemia and infarction. The sequence of events leading to the development of malignant hypertension is poorly defined. Two pathophysiologic alterations appear central in its initiation and/or perpetuation: (1) increased permeability of vessel walls to invasion by plasma components, particularly fibrin, which activates clotting mechanisms leading to a microangiopathic hemolytic anemia, thus perpetu-

ating the vascular pathology; and (2) activation of the renin-angiotensin-aldosterone system at some point in the disease process, which contributes to the acceleration and maintenance of BP elevation and, in turn, to vascular injury.

Malignant hypertension is most likely to develop in a previously hypertensive individual, usually in the third or fourth decade of life. There is a higher incidence among black men. Presenting symptoms are usually neurologic (dizziness, headache, blurring of vision, altered states of consciousness, and focal or generalized seizures). Cardiac decompensation and renal failure appear thereafter. Renal abnormalities include a rapid rise in serum creatinine, hematuria (at times macroscopic), proteinuria, and red and white blood cell casts in the sediment. Nephrotic syndrome may be present. Elevated plasma aldosterone levels cause hypokalemic metabolic alkalosis in the early phase. Uremic acidosis and hyperkalemia eventually obscure these early findings. Hematologic indices of microangiopathic hemolytic anemia (i.e., schistocytes) are often seen.

℞ HYPERTENSION

Control of hypertension is the principal goal of therapy. The time of initiation of therapy, its effectiveness, and patient compliance are crucial factors in arresting the progression of benign nephrosclerosis. Untreated, most of these patients succumb to the extrarenal complications of hypertension. In contrast, malignant hypertension is a medical emergency; its natural course includes a death rate of 80–90% within 1 year of onset, almost always due to uremia. Supportive measures should be instituted to control the neurologic, cardiac, and other complications of acute renal failure, but the mainstay of therapy is prompt and aggressive reduction of BP, which, if successful, can reverse all complications in the majority of patients. Presently, 5-year survival is 50%, and some patients have evidence of partial reversal of the vascular lesions and a return of renal function to near-normal levels.

RENAL VASCULAR INJURY IN SYSTEMIC DISEASES

Hemolytic Uremic Syndrome (HUS) and Thrombotic Thrombocytopenic Purpura (TTP) (See also Chap. 109) HUS and TTP, consumptive coagulopathies characterized by microangiopathic hemolytic anemia and thrombocytopenia, have a particular predilection for the kidney and the central nervous system. Previously, the overlap in clinical manifestations had prompted investigators to regard the two syndromes as a continuum of a single disease entity. Recent evidence, however, points to clearly distinct molecular basis for their pathophysiology.

RENAL INVOLVEMENT Evidence of renal involvement is present in the majority of patients with HUS/TTP. Microscopic hematuria (78%) and subnephrotic proteinuria (75%) are the most consistent findings. Male sex, hypertension, prolonged anuria, and hemoglobin levels <10 g/L at onset are associated with a higher risk of renal sequelae in children. Gross hematuria is rare. More than 90% of patients with HUS have significant renal failure, one-third of whom are anuric. The mean duration of renal failure is 2 weeks. Severe acute renal failure or anuria occurs in <10% of cases of classic TTP. The degree of elevation of BUN on presentation may be a prognostic indicator in patients with HUS/TTP.

PATHOLOGY The characteristic lesion in HUS/TTP is thrombotic microangiopathy. Microthrombi are demonstrated in renal arterioles and capillaries. In TTP, microthrombi are composed predominantly of platelet aggregates and a thin layer of fibrin and stain strongly for von Willebrand factor (vWF), which has been implicated in its pathogenesis. In contrast, microthrombi in HUS contain predominantly fibrin. Subendothelial hyaline deposits and endothelial cell swelling also contribute to vascular occlusion. Glomerular lesions are ischemic. The glomerular capillary walls are wrinkled, the glomerular tuft may be atrophied, and the Bowman capsule is thickened. Acute cortical or tubular necrosis may occur. Immunofluorescence studies invariably demonstrate fibrinogen along the glomerular capillary walls and in arterial thrombi. Granular deposits of C3 and IgM may be observed in vessel walls and glomeruli. Electron-microscopic studies demonstrate swelling of the glomerular endothelial cells and detachment from the glomerular basement membrane.

ETIOLOGY HUS Two forms of HUS have been described: (1) Diarrhea-associated HUS (D + HUS), the most common form in children, is associated with infection by Shiga toxin–producing *Escherichia coli* (most commonly O157;H7). This form has an excellent prognosis. Most cases occur in summer and autumn. (2) In contrast, non-Shiga toxin–associated HUS (D – HUS) typically affects adults but can occur at any age. It occurs in sporadic or familial forms, is noninfective, and is usually precipitated by drugs and pregnancy. Several studies have demonstrated genetic predisposition in atypical HUS, involving two regulatory proteins of the complement alternative pathway: factor H (FH) and membrane cofactor protein (MCP, or CD46).

TTP ADAMTS 13 is a member of the recently recognized ADAMTS (a disintegrin with thrombospondin type 1 motifs) zinc metalloproteinase family that cleaves vWF complexes and prevents vWF-platelet interaction. A *severe deficiency of ADAMTS 13* has been described in patients with TTP. Two forms have been identified: (1) In sporadic TTP, the deficiency appears to be *autoimmune suppression* of ADAMTS 13 by circulating IgG antibodies to the protein. (2) Schulman-Upshaw syndrome (a hereditary deficiency) is characterized by thrombocytopenia and microangiopathic hemolysis soon after birth, responding to plasma infusion. Most patients require plasma infusions every 2–4 weeks. Relapses are often triggered by fever, infection, pregnancy, or surgery.

Drug-induced HUS/TTP is well recognized in patients receiving chemotherapeutic agents, most commonly mitomycin C (cumulative dose of $\geq$20–30 mg/m^2). The onset of hemolytic anemia and renal failure is usually sudden, and mortality rate is high despite supportive therapy. Treatment with plasma exchange, glucocorticoids, immunosuppressive agents, and staphylococcal protein A immunoadsorption, however, are successful in some cases. Ticlopidine and clopidogrel use has also been associated with the disease. Cyclosporine-induced TTP was first reported following bone marrow transplantation but is more common in patients receiving renal transplants and other solid organs. In renal allograft recipients, cyclosporine-induced HUS occurs during the first week after transplantation as drug toxicity is dose-related. Renal failure reverses with the cessation of cyclosporine or reduction in its dose.

HUS/TTP may occur after bone marrow transplantation independent of prior radiation or cyclosporine therapy. TTP is commonly associated with pregnancy. Approximately 10–25% of patients with TTP are women who are either near-term pregnant or in the postpartum period; this is also the time for thrombotic events and the occurrence of preeclampsia, eclampsia, and HELLP syndrome (*h*emolysis, *e*levated *l*iver enzymes, and *l*ow *p*latelet count). These syndromes are difficult to distinguish from TTP-HUS. Decreased activity of ADAMTS 13 in late pregnancy may be an additional risk. Finally, thrombotic microangiopathy has been described in conjunction with vascular tumors, acute promyelocytic leukemia, and prostatic, gastric, and pancreatic carcinomas.

℞ HEMOLYTIC UREMIC SYNDROME

Supportive measures—including dialysis, antihypertensive medications, blood transfusions, and management of neurologic complications—have improved survival in patients with HUS/TTP. Adequate fluid balance and bowel rest are important in treating typical HUS associated with diarrhea. Antibiotics to treat infection caused by Shiga toxin–producing *E. coli* O157:H7 have been found to increase the risk of overt HUS by 17-fold, likely by favoring the acute release of large amounts of preformed toxin or by providing selective advantage to *E. coli* O157. Among the therapeutic modalities used to treat patients with HUS/TTP, plasma exchange (plasmapheresis combined with fresh-frozen plasma replacement) is currently the treatment of choice and is superior to plasma infusion alone. Plasmapheresis may remove the recently identified inhibitory autoantibodies against

vWF protease from the circulation and supply larger amounts of the protease enzyme. Plasma exchange should be performed daily until remission is achieved, remission being normalization of platelet count, or resolution of neurologic symptoms, or both. Hemoglobin level, percent schistocytosis, reticulocyte count, and renal indices do not appear to be determinants of initial response to therapy, as they may be abnormal for an undefined period after remission. Continuation of plasma exchange for several sessions after remission has been advocated to prevent relapses. Severe renal insufficiency resulting from HUS/TTP often requires dialysis. Renal transplantation has also been performed. HUS/TTP may recur in up to 17% of transplanted patients, independent of cyclosporine use. Higher recurrence rates have been reported for familial HUS.

SCLERODERMA (PROGRESSIVE SYSTEMIC SCLEROSIS)

(See also Chap. 316) Renal involvement in scleroderma can present in one of two ways, depending on whether malignant hypertension is superimposed on the renal pathology: (1) *Persistent urinary abnormalities* and an indolent clinical course characterized by proteinuria (15–36%), hypertension (24%), and mild azotemia (15%). Anti-RNA POL3 antibodies are strongly associated with scleroderma renal disease. (2) *Scleroderma renal crisis* (SRC) is a rapid deterioration in renal function, usually accompanied by malignant hypertension, oliguria, proteinuria, fluid retention, microangiopathic hemolytic anemia, and central nervous system involvement. It occurs in 10% of patients, most commonly in the first 4 years following diagnosis, particularly in patients with diffuse cutaneous involvement, 25% of whom develop SRC. SRC may occur in patients with previously undemonstrable or slowly progressive renal disease. Untreated, it leads to chronic renal failure within days to months. A significant association exists between antecedent glucocorticoid therapy and the development of SRC.

℞ SCLERODERMA

In SRC, ACE inhibitors have improved 5-year survival from 10% to 65%. Some 60% of SRC patients who receive ACE inhibitors require no dialysis (or temporary dialysis) with a survival rate at 8 years of 80–85%, similar to scleroderma patients who do not develop renal crisis. More than half of patients with SRC who require dialysis and are treated aggressively with ACE inhibitors are able to discontinue dialysis 3–18 months later, suggesting that patients should continue ACE inhibitor therapy even after beginning dialysis. Angiotensin receptor antagonists have not proven to be a satisfactory substitute for ACE inhibitors in patients with SRC. SRC patients who progress to end-stage renal disease can undergo hemodialysis or peritoneal dialysis, the latter being occasionally limited by compromised peritoneal clearance. A decrease in graft and overall survival has been noted in scleroderma patients following renal transplantation, as well recurrence of progressive sclerosis in the transplanted kidney, particularly in patients with aggressive disease.

SICKLE CELL NEPHROPATHY

(See also Chap. 99) Sickle cell disease causes renal complications as a result of sickling of red blood cells in the microvasculature. The hypertonic and relatively hypoxic environment of the renal medulla, coupled with the slow blood flow in the vasa recta, favors sickling of red blood cells, with resultant local infarction (papillary necrosis). Functional tubule defects in patients with sickle cell disease are likely the result of partial ischemic injury to the renal tubules.

In addition to the intrarenal microvascular pathology described above, the sickle cell disease in young patients is characterized by renal hyperperfusion, glomerular hypertrophy, and hyperfiltration. Many of these individuals eventually develop a glomerulopathy leading to glomerular proteinuria (present in as many as 30%) and, in some, the nephrotic syndrome. Co-inheritance of microdeletions in the α-globin gene (α thalassemia) appear to protect against the development of nephropathy and are associated with lower mean arterial pressure and less proteinuria.

Mild azotemia and hyperuricemia can also develop. Advanced renal failure and uremia occur in 10% of cases. Pathologic examination reveals the typical lesion of "hyperfiltration nephropathy," namely, focal segmental glomerular sclerosis. This finding has led to the suggestion that anemia-induced hyperfiltration in childhood is the principal cause of the adult glomerulopathy. Nephron loss secondary to ischemic injury also contributes to the development of azotemia in these patients.

In addition to the glomerulopathy described above, renal complications of sickle cell disease include *cortical infarcts* leading to loss of function, persistent hematuria, and perinephric hematomas. *Papillary infarcts*, demonstrable radiographically in 50% of patients with sickle trait, lead to an increased risk of bacterial infection in the scarred renal tissues and functional tubule abnormalities. Painless gross hematuria occurs with a higher frequency in sickle trait than in sickle cell disease and likely results from infarctive episodes in the renal medulla. *Functional tubule abnormalities* such as nephrogenic diabetes insipidus result from marked reduction in vasa recta blood flow, combined with ischemic tubule injury. This concentrating defect places these patients at increased risk of dehydration and, hence, sickling crises. The concentrating defect also occurs in individuals with sickle trait. Other tubule defects involve potassium and hydrogen ion excretion, occasionally leading to hyperkalemic metabolic acidosis and a defect in uric acid excretion which, combined with increased purine synthesis in the bone marrow, results in hyperuricemia.

Management of sickle nephropathy is not separate from that of overall patient management (Chap. 99). In addition, however, the use of ACE inhibitors has been associated with improvement of the hyperfiltration glomerulopathy. Three-year graft and patient survival in renal transplant recipients with sickle nephropathy is diminished as compared to those with other causes of end-stage renal disease.

RENAL VEIN THROMBOSIS (RVT)

Thrombosis of one or both main renal veins occurs in a variety of settings (Table 280-2). Nephrotic syndrome accompanying membranous glomerulopathy and certain carcinomas seems to predispose to the development of RVT, which occurs in 10–50% of patients with these disorders. RVT may exacerbate preexisting proteinuria but is infrequently the cause of the nephrotic syndrome.

The clinical manifestations depend on the severity and abruptness of its occurrence. Acute cases occur typically in children and are characterized by sudden loss of renal function, often accompanied by fever, chills, lumbar tenderness (with kidney enlargement), leukocytosis, and hematuria. Hemorrhagic infarction and renal rupture may lead to hypovolemic shock. In young adults RVT is usually suspected from an unexpected and relatively acute or subacute deterioration of renal function and/or exacerbation of proteinuria and hematuria in the appropriate clinical setting. In cases of gradual thrombosis, usually occurring in the elderly, the only manifestation may be recurrent pulmonary emboli or development of hypertension. A Fanconi-like syndrome and proximal renal tubular acidosis have been described. RVT is a potential cause of early graft dysfunction following renal transplantation, and its incidence may be decreased with prophylactic

TABLE 280-2   CONDITIONS ASSOCIATED WITH RENAL VEIN THROMBOSIS
Trauma
Extrinsic compression (lymph nodes, aortic aneurysm, tumor)
Invasion by renal cell carcinoma
Dehydration (infants)
Nephrotic syndrome
Pregnancy or oral contraceptives

low-dose aspirin. The definitive diagnosis can only be established through selective renal venography with visualization of the occluding thrombus. Short of angiography, Doppler ultrasound, contrast-enhanced CT, and MRI often provide evidence of thrombus.

℞ RENAL VEIN THROMBOSIS

Treatment consists of anticoagulation, the main purpose of which is prevention of pulmonary embolization, although some authors have also claimed improvement in renal function and proteinuria. Encouraging reports have appeared concerning the use of streptokinase. Spontaneous recanalization with clinical improvement has also been observed. Anticoagulant therapy is more rewarding in the acute thrombosis seen in younger individuals. Nephrectomy is advocated in infants with life-threatening renal infarction. Percutaneous mechanical thrombectomy is effective in some cases.

TOXEMIAS OF PREGNANCY

See also Chap. 7.

BILATERAL CORTICAL NECROSIS

Acute bilateral cortical necrosis is associated with septic abortions, abruptio placentae, and preeclampsia. Coagulation in cortical vessels and arterioles leads to renal tissue necrosis. Anuria and renal failure ensue and may be irreversible. In other cases, renal function returns partially, but on long-term follow-up most patients slowly progress to uremia.

FURTHER READINGS

CHONCHOL M, LINAS S: Diagnosis and management of ischemic nephropathy. Clin J Am Soc Nephrol 1:172, 2006

GAROVIC VD, TEXTOR SC: Renovascular hypertension and ischemic nephropathy. Circulation 112:1362, 2005

LAMMLE B et al: Thrombotic thrombocytopenic purpura. J Thromb Haemost 3:1663, 2005

SCHEINMAN JI: Sickle cell disease and the kidney. Semin Nephrol 23:66, 2003

STEEN VD: Scleroderma renal crisis. Rheum Dis Clin North Am 29:315, 2003

TEXTOR SC: Renovascular hypertension update. Curr Hypertens Rep 8:521, 2006

CHAPTER 281   Nephrolithiasis

281   Nephrolithiasis
John R. Asplin, Fredric L. Coe, Murray J. Favus

Kidney stones are one of the most common urological problems. In the United States, ~13% of men and 7% of women will develop a kidney stone during their lifetime, and the prevalence is increasing throughout the industrialized world.

TYPES OF STONES

Calcium salts, uric acid, cystine, and struvite ($MgNH_4PO_4$) are the basic constituents of most kidney stones in the western hemisphere (Chap. e24). Calcium oxalate and calcium phosphate stones make up

75–85% of the total (Table 281-1) and may be admixed in the same stone. Calcium phosphate in stones is usually hydroxyapatite [$Ca_5(PO_4)_3OH$] or, less commonly, brushite ($CaHPO_4H_2O$).

Calcium stones are more common in men; the average age of onset is the third to fourth decade. Approximately 50% of people who form a single calcium stone eventually form another within the next 10 years. The average rate of new stone formation in recurrent stone formers is about one stone every 2 or 3 years. *Uric acid stones* account for 5–10% of kidney stones and are also more common in men. Half of patients with uric acid stones have gout; uric acid lithiasis is usually familial whether or not gout is present. *Cystine stones* are uncommon, comprising ~1% of cases in most series of nephrolithiasis. *Struvite stones* are common and potentially dangerous. These stones occur mainly in women or patients who require chronic bladder catheterization and result from uri-

TABLE 281-1 MAJOR CAUSES OF RENAL STONES

Stone Type and Causes	Percent of all Stones[a]	Percent Occurrence of Specific Causes[a]	Ratio of Males to Females	Etiology	Diagnosis	Treatment
Calcium stones	75–85		2:1 to 3:1			
Idiopathic hypercalciuria		50–55	2:1	Hereditary (?)	Normocalcemia, unexplained hypercalciuria[b]	Low-sodium, low-protein diet; thiazide diuretics
Hyperuricosuria		20	4:1	Diet	Urine uric acid >750 mg per 24 h (women), >800 mg per 24 h (men)	Allopurinol or diet
Primary hyperparathyroidism		3–5	3:10	Neoplasia	Unexplained hypercalcemia	Surgery
Distal renal tubular acidosis		Rare	1:1	Hereditary	Hyperchloremic acidosis, minimum urine pH >5.5	Alkali replacement
Dietary hyperoxaluria		10–30	1:1	High oxalate diet or low calcium diet	Urine oxalate >50 mg per 24 h	Low oxalate diet
Enteric hyperoxaluria		~1–2	1:1	Bowel surgery	Urine oxalate >75 mg per 24 h	Cholestyramine or oral calcium loading
Primary hyperoxaluria		Rare	1:1	Hereditary	Urine oxalate and glycolic or l-glyceric acid increased	Fluids and pyridoxine
Hypocitraturia		20–40	1:1 to 2:1	Hereditary (?), diet	Urine citrate <320 mg per 24 h	Alkali supplements
Idiopathic stone disease		20	2:1	Unknown	None of the above present	Oral phosphate, fluids
Uric acid stones	5–10					
Gout		~50	3:1 to 4:1	Hereditary	Clinical diagnosis	Alkali and allopurinol
Idiopathic		~50	1:1	Hereditary (?)	Uric acid stones, no gout	Alkali and allopurinol if daily urine uric acid above 1000 mg
Dehydration		?	1:1	Intestinal, habit	History, intestinal fluid loss	Alkali, fluids, reversal of cause
Lesch-Nyhan syndrome		Rare	Males only	Hereditary	Reduced hypoxanthine-guanine phosphoribosyltransferase level	Allopurinol
Malignant tumors		Rare	1:1	Neoplasia	Clinical diagnosis	Allopurinol
Cystine stones	1		1:1	Hereditary	Stone type; elevated cystine excretion	Massive fluids, alkali, D-penicillamine if needed
Struvite stones	5–10		1:3	Infection	Stone type	Antimicrobial agents and judicious surgery

[a]Values are percent of patients who form a particular type of stone and who display each specific cause of stones.

[b]Urine calcium above 300 mg/24 h (men), 250 mg/24 h (women), or 4 mg/kg per 24 h either sex. Hyperthyroidism, Cushing syndrome, sarcoidosis, malignant tumors, im-mobilization, vitamin D intoxication, rapidly progressive bone disease, and Paget's disease all cause hypercalciuria and must be excluded in diagnosis of idiopathic hypercalciuria.

nary tract infection with urease-producing bacteria, usually *Proteus* species. The stones can grow to a large size and fill the renal pelvis and calyces to produce a "staghorn" appearance.

MANIFESTATIONS OF STONES

As stones grow on the surfaces of the renal papillae or within the collecting system, they need not produce symptoms. Asymptomatic stones may be discovered during the course of radiographic studies undertaken for unrelated reasons. Stones rank, along with benign and malignant neoplasms and renal cysts, among the common causes of isolated hematuria. Stones become symptomatic when they enter the ureter or occlude the ureteropelvic junction, causing pain and obstruction.

Stone Passage A stone can traverse the ureter without symptoms, but passage usually produces pain and bleeding. The pain begins gradually, usually in the flank, but increases over the next 20–60 min to become so severe that narcotic drugs may be needed for its control. The pain may remain in the flank or spread downward and anteriorly toward the ipsilateral loin, testis, or vulva. A stone in the portion of the ureter within the bladder wall causes frequency, urgency, and dysuria that may be confused with urinary tract infection. The vast majority of ureteral stones <0.5 cm in diameter will pass spontaneously.

It has been standard practice to diagnose acute renal colic by intravenous pyelography; however, helical CT scan without radiocontrast enhancement is now the preferred procedure. The advantages of CT include detection of uric acid stones in addition to the traditional radiopaque stones, no exposure to the risk of radiocontrast agents, and possible diagnosis of other causes of abdominal pain in a patient suspected of having renal colic from stones. Ultrasound is not as sensitive as CT in detecting renal or ureteral stones. Standard abdominal x-rays may be used to monitor patients for formation and growth of kidney stones, as they are less expensive and provide less radiation exposure than CT scans. Calcium, cystine, and struvite stones are all radiopaque on standard x-rays, whereas uric acid stones are radiolucent.

Other Syndromes • STAGHORN CALCULI Struvite, cystine, and uric acid stones often grow too large to enter the ureter. They gradually fill the renal pelvis and may extend outward through the infundibula to the calyces themselves. Very large staghorn stones can have surprisingly few symptoms and may lead to the eventual loss of kidney function.

NEPHROCALCINOSIS Calcium stones grow on the papillae. Most break loose and cause colic, but they may remain in place so that multiple papillary calcifications are found by x-ray, a condition termed *nephrocalcinosis*. Papillary nephrocalcinosis is common in hereditary distal renal tubular acidosis (RTA) and in other types of severe hypercalciuria. In medullary sponge kidney disease (Chap. 278), calcification may occur in dilated distal collecting ducts.

Infection Although urinary tract infection is not a direct consequence of stone disease, it can occur after instrumentation and surgery of the urinary tract, which are frequent in the treatment of stone disease. Stone disease and urinary tract infection can enhance their respective seriousness and interfere with treatment. Obstruction of an infected kidney by a stone may lead to sepsis and extensive damage of renal tissue, since it converts the urinary tract proximal to the obstruction into a closed, or partially closed, space that can become an abscess. Stones may harbor bacteria in the stone matrix, leading to recurrent urinary tract infection. On the other hand, infection due to bacteria that possess the enzyme urease can cause stones composed of struvite.

Activity of Stone Disease   Active disease means that new stones are forming or that preformed stones are growing. Sequential radiographs are needed to document the growth or appearance of new stones and to ensure that passed stones are actually newly formed, not preexistent.

PATHOGENESIS OF STONES

Urinary stones usually arise because of the breakdown of a delicate balance between solubility and precipitation of salts. The kidneys must conserve water, but they must excrete materials that have a low solubility. These two opposing requirements must be balanced during adaptation to diet, climate, and activity. The problem is mitigated to some extent by the fact that urine contains substances that inhibit crystallization. These protective mechanisms are less than perfect. When the urine becomes supersaturated with insoluble materials, because excretion rates are excessive and/or because water conservation is extreme, crystals form and may grow and aggregate to form a stone.

Supersaturation   A solution in equilibrium with crystals of calcium oxalate is said to be saturated with respect to calcium oxalate. If crystals are removed, and if either calcium or oxalate ions are added to the solution, the chemical activities increase, but no new crystals form. Such a solution is *metastably supersaturated*. If calcium oxalate crystals are now added, they will grow in size. Ultimately, as calcium or oxalate is added to the solution, supersaturation reaches a critical value at which a solid phase begins to develop spontaneously. This value is called the *upper limit of metastability*. Kidney stone growth requires a urine that, on average, is supersaturated. Excessive supersaturation is common in stone formation.

Calcium, oxalate, and phosphate form many soluble complexes among themselves and with other substances in urine, such as citrate. As a result, their free ion activities are below their chemical concentrations. Reduction in ligands such as citrate can increase ion activity and, therefore, supersaturation. Urine supersaturation can be increased by dehydration or by overexcretion of calcium, oxalate, phosphate, cystine, or uric acid. Urine pH is also important; phosphate and uric acid are acids that dissociate readily over the physiologic range of urine pH. Alkaline urine contains more dibasic phosphate, favoring deposits of brushite and apatite. Below a urine pH of 5.5, uric acid crystals (pK 5.47) predominate, whereas phosphate crystals are rare. The solubility of calcium oxalate is not influenced by changes in urine pH. Measurements of supersaturation in a 24-h urine sample probably underestimate the risk of precipitation. Transient dehydration, variation of urine pH, and postprandial bursts of overexcretion may cause values considerably above average.

Crystallization   When urine supersaturation exceeds the upper limit of metastability, crystals begin to nucleate. Cell debris and other crystals present in the urinary tract can serve as templates for crystal formation, a process known as *heterogeneous nucleation*. Heterogeneous nucleation lowers the level of supersaturation required for crystal formation. Once formed, crystal nuclei will grow in size if urine is supersaturated with respect to that crystal phase. Multiple crystals can then aggregate to form a kidney stone.

In order for a kidney stone to form, crystals must be retained in the renal pelvis long enough to grow and aggregate to a clinically significant size. The mechanism of crystal retention has been a matter of much debate. Recent studies have shown that common calcium oxalate kidney stones form as overgrowths on apatite plaques in the renal papillae. These plaques, called Randall's plaques, provide an excellent surface for heterogeneous nucleation of calcium oxalate salts. The

Randall's plaques begin in the deep medulla in the basement membrane of the thin limb of the loop of Henle and then spread through the interstitium to the basement membrane of the papillary urothelium. If the urothelium becomes damaged, the plaque is exposed to the urine, and calcium oxalate crystallization and stone formation begins.

Inhibitors of Crystal Formation   Urine contains potent inhibitors of nucleation, growth, and aggregation for calcium salts. Inorganic pyrophosphate is a potent inhibitor that appears to affect formation of calcium phosphate more than calcium oxalate crystals. Citrate inhibits crystal growth and nucleation, although most of the stone inhibitory activity of citrate is due to lowering urine supersaturation via complexation of calcium. Other urine components such as glycoproteins inhibit calcium oxalate crystallization.

EVALUATION AND TREATMENT OF PATIENTS WITH NEPHROLITHIASIS

Most patients with nephrolithiasis have remediable metabolic disorders that cause stones and can be detected by chemical analyses of serum and urine. Adults with recurrent kidney stones and children with even a single kidney stone should be evaluated. A practical outpatient evaluation consists of two 24-h urine collections, with a corresponding blood sample; measurements of serum and urine calcium, uric acid, electrolytes, and creatinine, and urine pH, volume, oxalate, and citrate should be made. Since stone risks vary with diet, activity, and environment, at least one urine collection should be made on a weekend when the patient is at home and another on a work day. When possible, the composition of kidney stones should be determined because treatment depends on stone type (Table 281-1). No matter what disorders are found, every patient should be counseled to avoid dehydration and to drink copious amounts of water. The efficacy of high fluid intake was confirmed in a prospective study of first-time stone formers. Increasing urine volume to 2.5 L per day resulted in a 50% reduction of stone recurrence compared to the control group.

℞ NEPHROLITHIASIS

The management of stones already present in the kidneys or urinary tract requires a combined medical and surgical approach. The specific treatment depends on the location of the stone, the extent of obstruction, the nature of the stone, the function of the affected and unaffected kidney, the presence or absence of urinary tract infection, the progress of stone passage, and the risks of operation or anesthesia given the clinical state of the patient. Medical therapy can enhance passage of ureteral stones. Oral α_1-adrenergic blockers relax ureteral muscle and have been shown to reduce time to stone passage and the need for surgical removal of small stones. In general, severe obstruction, infection, intractable pain, and serious bleeding are indications for removal of a stone.

Advances in urologic technology have rendered open surgery for stones a rare event. There are now three alternatives for stone removal. *Extracorporeal lithotripsy* causes the in situ fragmentation of stones in the kidney, renal pelvis, or ureter by exposing them to shock waves. The kidney stone is centered at a focal point of high-intensity shock waves. The waves are transmitted to the patient using water as a conduction medium, either by placing the patient in a water tank or by placing water-filled cushions between the patient and the shock wave generators. After multiple shock waves, most stones are reduced to powder that moves through the ureter into the bladder. *Percutaneous nephrolithotomy* requires the passage of a cystoscope-like instrument into the renal pelvis through a small incision in the flank. Stones are then disrupted by a small ultrasound transducer or holmium laser. The last method is *ureteroscopy* with stone disruption using a holmium laser. Ureteroscopy is generally used for stones in the ureter but some surgeons are now using ureteroscopy for stones in the renal pelvis as well.

Calcium Stones   ·   *IDIOPATHIC HYPERCALCIURIA*   (See also Chap. 347) This condition is the most common metabolic abnormality found in patients with nephrolithiasis (Table 281-1). It is familial and is likely a polygenic trait, although there are some rare monogenic causes of hypercalciuria and kidney stones such as Dent's disease, which is an X-linked disorder characterized by hypercalciuria, nephrocalcinosis, and progressive kidney failure. Idiopathic hypercalciuria is diagnosed by the presence of hypercalciuria without hypercalcemia and the absence of other systemic disorders known to affect mineral metabolism. In the past, the separation of "absorptive" and "renal" forms of hypercalciuria was used to guide treatment. However, these may not be distinct entities but the extremes of a continuum of behavior. Vitamin D overactivity, either through high calcitriol levels or excess vitamin D receptor, is a likely explanation for the hypercalciuria in many of these patients. Hypercalciuria contributes to stone formation by raising urine saturation with respect to calcium oxalate and calcium phosphate.

Rx HYPERCALCIURIA

For many years the standard therapy for hypercalciuria was dietary calcium restriction. However, recent studies have shown that low-calcium diets increase the risk of incident stone formation. Low-calcium diets may lead to stone formation by reducing the amount of calcium to bind oxalate in the intestine, thereby increasing urine oxalate levels. However, the mechanism by which a low-calcium diet increases stone risk has not been clearly defined. In addition, hypercalciuric stone formers have reduced bone mineral density and an increased risk of fracture compared to the non-stone-forming population. Low calcium intake likely contributes to the low bone mineral density. A 5-year prospective trial compared the efficacy of a low-calcium diet to a low-protein, low-sodium, normal-calcium diet in preventing stone recurrence in male calcium stone formers. The group on the low-calcium diet had a significantly greater rate of stone relapse. Low-calcium diets are of unknown efficacy in preventing stone formation and carry a long-term risk of bone disease in the stone-forming population. Low-sodium and low-protein diets are a superior option in stone formers. If diet therapy is not sufficient to prevent stones, then thiazide diuretics may be used. Thiazide diuretics lower urine calcium and are effective in preventing the formation of stones. Three 3-year randomized trials have shown a 50% decrease in stone formation in the thiazide-treated groups as compared to the placebo-treated controls. The drug effect requires slight contraction of the extracellular fluid volume, and high dietary NaCl intake reduces its therapeutic effect. Thiazide-induced hypokalemia should be aggressively treated since hypokalemia will reduce urine citrate, an important inhibitor of calcium crystallization.

HYPERURICOSURIA About 20% of calcium oxalate stone formers are hyperuricosuric, primarily because of an excessive intake of purine from meat, fish, and poultry. The mechanism of stone formation is probably due to salting out calcium oxalate by urate. A low-purine diet is desirable but difficult for many patients to achieve. The alternative is allopurinol, which has been shown to be effective in a randomized, controlled trial. A dose of 100 mg bid is usually sufficient.

PRIMARY HYPERPARATHYROIDISM (See also Chap. 347) The diagnosis of this condition is established by documenting that hypercalcemia that cannot be otherwise explained is accompanied by inappropriately elevated serum concentrations of parathyroid hormone. Hypercalciuria, usually present, raises the urine supersaturation of calcium phosphate and/or calcium oxalate (Table 281-1). Prompt diagnosis is important because parathyroidectomy should be carried out before renal damage or bone disease occurs.

DISTAL RENAL TUBULAR ACIDOSIS (See also Chap. 278) The defect in this condition seems to reside in the distal nephron, which cannot establish a normal pH gradient between urine and blood, leading to hyperchloremic acidosis. The diagnosis is suggested by a minimum urine pH >5.5 in the presence of systemic acidosis. If the diagnosis is in doubt because metabolic abnormalities are mild, an ammonium chloride loading test can be performed. Patients with distal RTA will not lower urine pH below 5.5. Hypercalciuria, an alkaline urine, and a low urine citrate level increase urine saturation with respect to calcium phosphate. Calcium phosphate stones form, nephrocalcinosis is common, and osteomalacia or rickets may occur. Renal damage is frequent, and glomerular filtration rate falls gradually.

Treatment with supplemental alkali reduces hypercalciuria and limits the production of new stones. The usual dose of sodium bicarbonate is 0.5–2.0 mmol/kg of body weight per day in four to six divided doses. An alternative is potassium citrate supplementation, given at the same dose per day but needing to be given only two to three times per day. In incomplete distal RTA, systemic acidosis is absent, but urine pH cannot be lowered below 5.5 after an exogenous acid load such as ammonium chloride. Incomplete RTA may develop in some patients who form calcium oxalate stones because of idiopathic hypercalciuria; the importance of RTA in producing stones in this situation is uncertain, and thiazide treatment is a reasonable alternative. Alkali can also be used in incomplete RTA. When treating patients with alkali, it is prudent to monitor changes in urine citrate and pH. If urine pH increases without an increase in citrate, then calcium phosphate supersaturation will increase and stone disease may worsen.

HYPEROXALURIA Oxalate is a metabolic end product in humans. Urine oxalate comes from diet and endogenous metabolic production, with ~40–50% originating from dietary sources. The upper limit of normal for oxalate excretion is generally considered to be 40–50 mg per day. Mild hyperoxaluria (50–80 mg/d) is usually caused by excessive intake of high-oxalate foods such as spinach, nuts, and chocolate. In addition, low-calcium diets may promote hyperoxaluria as there is less calcium available to bind oxalate in the intestine. Enteric hyperoxaluria is a consequence of small-bowel disease resulting in fat malabsorption. Oxalate excretion is often >100 mg per day. Enteric hyperoxaluria may be caused by jejunoileal bypass for obesity, pancreatic insufficiency, or extensive small-intestine involvement from Crohn's disease. With fat malabsorption, calcium in the bowel lumen is bound by fatty acids instead of oxalate, which is left free for absorption in the colon. Delivery of unabsorbed fatty acids and bile salts to the colon may injure the colonic mucosa and enhance oxalate absorption. Primary hyperoxaluria is a rare autosomal recessive disease that causes severe hyperoxaluria. Patients usually present with recurrent calcium oxalate stones during childhood. Primary hyperoxaluria type 1 is due to a deficiency in the peroxisomal enzyme alanine:glyoxylate aminotransferase. Type 2 is due to a deficiency of D-glyceric dehydrogenase. Severe hyperoxaluria from any cause can produce tubulointerstitial nephropathy (Chap. 279) and lead to stone formation.

Rx HYPEROXALURIA

Patients with mild to moderate hyperoxaluria should be treated with a diet low in oxalate and with a normal intake of calcium and magnesium to reduce oxalate absorption. Enteric hyperoxaluria can be treated with a low-fat, low-oxalate diet and calcium supplements, given with meals, to bind oxalate in the gut lumen. The oxalate-binding resin cholestyramine at a dose of 8–16 g/d, provides an additional form of therapy. Treatment for primary hyperoxaluria includes a high fluid intake, neutral phosphate, and pyridoxine (25–200 mg/d). Citrate supplementation may also have some benefit. Even with aggressive therapy, irreversible renal failure may occur. Liver transplantation, to correct the enzyme defect, combined with a kidney transplantation has been successfully utilized in patients with primary hyperoxaluria.

HYPOCITRATURIA Urine citrate prevents calcium stone formation by creating a soluble complex with calcium, effectively reducing free urine calcium. Hypocitraturia is found in 20–40% of stone formers, either as a single disorder or in combination with other metabolic abnormalities. It can be secondary to systemic disorders, such as RTA, chronic diarrheal illness, or hypokalemia, or it may be a primary disorder, in which case it is called *idiopathic hypocitraturia*.

Rx HYPOCITRATURIA

Treatment is with alkali, which increases urine citrate excretion; generally bicarbonate or citrate salts are used. Potassium salts are preferred as sodium loading increases urinary excretion of calcium, reducing the effectiveness of treatment. Two randomized, placebo-controlled trials have demonstrated the effectiveness of citrate supplements in calcium oxalate stone formers.

IDIOPATHIC CALCIUM LITHIASIS Some patients have no metabolic cause for stones despite a thorough metabolic evaluation (Table 281-1). The best treatment appears to be high fluid intake so that the urine specific gravity remains at ≤1.005 throughout the day and night. Thiazide diuretics, allopurinol, and citrate therapy may help reduce crystallization of calcium salts, but there are no prospective trials in this patient population. Oral phosphate at a dose of 2 g phosphorus daily may lower urine calcium and increase urine pyrophosphate and thereby reduce the rate of recurrence. Orthophosphate causes mild nausea and diarrhea, but tolerance may improve with continued intake.

Uric Acid Stones In gout, idiopathic uric acid lithiasis, and dehydration, the average urine pH is usually <5.4 and often below 5.0. Metabolic syndrome has also been found to be a cause of acidic urine as insulin resistance leads to a decrease in renal ammoniagenesis. When urine pH is low, the protonated form of uric acid predominates and is soluble in urine only in concentrations of 100 mg/L. Concentrations above this level represent supersaturation that causes crystals and stones to form. Hyperuricosuria, when present, increases supersaturation, but urine of low pH can be supersaturated with undissociated uric acid even though the daily excretion rate is normal. Myeloproliferative syndromes, chemotherapy of malignant tumors, and Lesch-Nyhan syndrome cause such massive production of uric acid and consequent hyperuricosuria that stones and uric acid sludge form even at a normal urine pH. Plugging of the renal collecting tubules by uric acid crystals can cause acute renal failure.

Rx URIC ACID LITHIASIS

The two goals of treatment are to raise urine pH and to lower excessive urine uric acid excretion to <1 g/d. Supplemental alkali, 1–3 mmol/kg of body weight per day, should be given in three or four divided doses, one of which should be given at bedtime. The goal of treatment should be a urine pH between 6.0 and 6.5 in a 24-h urine collection. Increasing urine pH above 6.5 will not provide additional benefit in preventing uric acid crystallization but does increase the risk of calcium phosphate stone formation. The form of the alkali may be important. Potassium citrate may reduce the risk of calcium salts crystallizing when urine pH is increased, whereas sodium citrate or sodium bicarbonate may increase the risk. A low-purine diet should be instituted in uric acid stone formers with hyperuricosuria. Patients who continue to form uric acid stones despite treatment with fluids, alkali, and a low-purine diet should have allopurinol added to their regimen.

Cystinuria and Cystine Stones (See also Chap. 358) In this inherited disorder, proximal tubular and jejunal transport of the dibasic amino acids cysteine (cysteine disulfide), lysine, arginine, and ornithine are defective, and excessive amounts are lost in the urine. Clinical disease is due solely to the insolubility of cystine, which forms stones.

PATHOGENESIS Cystinuria occurs because of defective transport of dibasic amino acids by the brush borders of renal tubule and intestinal epithelial cells. Disease-causing mutations have been identified in both the heavy and light chain of a heteromeric amino acid transporter found in the proximal tubule of the kidney. Cystinuria is classified into two main types, based on the urinary excretion of cystine in obligate heterozygotes. In type I cystinuria, heterozygotes have normal urine cystine excretion; thus type I has an autosomal recessive pattern of inheritance. A gene located on chromosome 2 and designated *SLC3A1* encodes the heavy chain of the transporter and has been found to be abnormal in type I. In non-type-I cystinuria, heterozygotes have moderately elevated urine cystine excretion, with homozygotes having a much higher urine cystine excretion. Non-type-I is inherited as a dominant trait with incomplete penetrance. Non-type-I is due to mutations in the *SLC7A9* gene on chromosome 19, which encodes the light chain of the heteromeric transporter. In rare cases, mutations of the *SLC7A9* gene can lead to a type I phenotype.

DIAGNOSIS Cystine stones are formed only by patients with cystinuria, but 10% of stones in cystinuric patients do not contain cystine; therefore, every stone former should be screened for the disease. The sediment from a first morning urine specimen in many patients with homozygous cystinuria reveals typical hexagonal, platelike cystine crystals. Cystinuria can also be detected using the urine sodium nitroprusside test. Because the test is sensitive, it is positive in many asymptomatic heterozygotes for cystinuria. A positive nitroprusside test or the finding of cystine crystals in the urine sediment should be evaluated by measurement of daily cystine excretion. Cystine stones seldom form in adults unless urine excretion is at least 300 mg/day.

Rx CYSTINURIA AND CYSTINE STONES

High fluid intake, even at night, is the cornerstone of therapy. Daily urine volume should exceed 3 L. Raising urine pH with alkali is helpful, provided the urine pH exceeds 7.5. A low-salt diet (100 mmol/d) can reduce cystine excretion up to 40%. Because side effects are frequent, drugs such as penicillamine and tiopronin, which form the mixed soluble disulfide cysteine-drug complexes, should be used only when fluid loading, salt reduction, and alkali therapy are ineffective. Low-methionine diets have not proved to be practical for clinical use, but patients should avoid protein gluttony.

Struvite Stones These stones are a result of urinary infection with bacteria, usually *Proteus* species, which possess urease, an enzyme that degrades urea to NH_3 and CO_2. The NH_3 hydrolyzes to NH_4^+ and raises urine pH to 8 or 9. The CO_2 hydrates to H_2CO_3 and then dissociates to CO_3^{2-} that precipitates with calcium as $CaCO_3$. The NH_4^+ precipitates PO_4^{3-} and Mg^{2+} to form $MgNH_4PO_4$ (struvite). The result is a stone of calcium carbonate admixed with struvite. Struvite does not form in urine in the absence of infection, because NH_4^+ concentration is low in urine that is alkaline in response to physiologic stimuli. Chronic *Proteus* infection can occur because of impaired urinary drainage, urologic instrumentation or surgery, and especially with chronic antibiotic treatment, which can favor the dominance of *Proteus* in the urinary tract. The presence of struvite crystals in urine, rectangular prisms said to resemble coffin lids, indicates infection with urease producing organisms.

Rx STRUVITE STONES

Complete removal of the stone with subsequent sterilization of the urinary tract is the treatment of choice for patients who can tolerate the procedures. Percutaneous nephrolithotomy is the preferred surgical approach for most patients. At times, extracorporeal lithotripsy may be used in combination with a percutaneous approach. Open surgery is rarely required. Irrigation of the renal pelvis and calyces with hemiacidrin, a solution that dissolves struvite, can reduce recurrence after surgery. Stone-free rates of 50–90% have been reported after surgical intervention. Antimicrobial treatment is best reserved for dealing with acute infection and for maintenance of a sterile urine after surgery. Urine cultures and culture of stone fragments removed at surgery should guide the choice of antibiotic. For patients who are not candidates for surgical removal of stone, acetohydroxamic acid, an inhibitor of urease, can be used. Unfortunately, acetohydroxamic acid has many side effects, such as headache, tremor, and thrombophlebitis, that limit its use.

FURTHER READINGS

ABATE N et al: The metabolic syndrome and uric acid nephrolithiasis: Novel features of renal manifestation of insulin resistance. Kidney Int 65:386, 2004

COE FL et al: Kidney stone disease. J Clin Invest 115:2598, 2005

1820 EVAN AP et al: Randall's plaque of patients with nephrolithiasis begins in basement membranes of thin loops of Henle. J Clin Invest 111:607, 2003

GAMBARO G et al: Genetics of hypercalciuria and calcium nephrolithiasis: From the rare monogenic to the common polygenic forms. Am J Kidney Dis 44:963, 2004

MILLER NL, Lingeman JE: Management of kidney stones. Br Med J 334:468, 2007

PREMINGER GM et al: AUA guideline on management of staghorn calculi: Diagnosis and treatment recommendations. J Urol 173:1991, 2005

STAMATELOU K et al: Time trends in reported prevalence of kidney stones in the United States: 1976–1994. Kidney Int 63:1817, 2003

282 Urinary Tract Infections, Pyelonephritis, and Prostatitis

Walter E. Stamm

DEFINITIONS

Acute infections of the urinary tract fall into two general anatomic categories: lower tract infection (urethritis and cystitis) and upper tract infection (acute pyelonephritis, prostatitis, and intrarenal and perinephric abscesses). Infections at various sites may occur together or independently and may either be asymptomatic or present as one of the clinical syndromes described in this chapter. Infections of the urethra and bladder are often considered superficial (or mucosal) infections, while prostatitis, pyelonephritis, and renal suppuration signify tissue invasion.

From a microbiologic perspective, urinary tract infection (UTI) exists when pathogenic microorganisms are detected in the urine, urethra, bladder, kidney, or prostate. In most instances, growth of $\geq 10^5$ organisms per milliliter from a properly collected midstream "clean-catch" urine sample indicates infection. However, significant bacteriuria is lacking in some cases of true UTI. Especially in symptomatic patients, fewer bacteria (10^2–10^4/mL) may signify infection. In urine specimens obtained by suprapubic aspiration or "in-and-out" catheterization and in samples from a patient with an indwelling catheter, colony counts of 10^2–10^4/mL generally indicate infection. Conversely, colony counts of $>10^5$/mL in midstream urine are occasionally due to specimen contamination, which is especially likely when multiple bacterial species are found.

Infections that recur after antibiotic therapy can be due to the persistence of the originally infecting strain (as judged by species, antibiogram, serotype, and molecular type) or to reinfection with a new strain. "Same-strain" recurrent infections that become evident within 2 weeks of cessation of therapy can be the result of unresolved renal or prostatic infection (termed *relapse*) or of persistent vaginal or intestinal colonization leading to rapid reinfection of the bladder.

Symptoms of dysuria, urgency, and frequency that are unaccompanied by significant bacteriuria have been termed the *acute urethral syndrome*. Although widely used, this term lacks anatomic precision because many cases so designated are actually bladder infections. Moreover, since the pathogen can usually be identified, the term *syndrome*—implying unknown causation—is inappropriate.

Chronic pyelonephritis refers to chronic interstitial nephritis believed to result from bacterial infection of the kidney (Chap. 279). Many noninfectious diseases also cause an interstitial nephritis that is indistinguishable pathologically from chronic pyelonephritis.

ACUTE UTIS: URETHRITIS, CYSTITIS, AND PYELONEPHRITIS

EPIDEMIOLOGY

Epidemiologically, UTIs are subdivided into catheter-associated (or nosocomial) infections and non-catheter-associated (or community-acquired) infections. Infections in either category may be symptomatic or asymptomatic. Acute community-acquired UTIs are very common and account for more than 7 million office visits annually in the United States. In the female population, these infections occur in 1–3% of schoolgirls and then increase markedly in incidence with the onset of sexual activity in adolescence. The vast majority of acute symptomatic infections involve young women; a prospective study demonstrated an annual incidence of 0.5–0.7 infections per patient-year in this group. In the male population, acute symptomatic UTIs occur in the first year of life (often in association with urologic abnormalities); thereafter, UTIs are unusual in male patients under the age of 50. The development of asymptomatic bacteriuria parallels that of symptomatic infection and is rare among men under 50 but common among women between 20 and 50. Asymptomatic bacteriuria is more common among elderly men and women, with rates as high as 40–50% in some studies. The incidence of acute uncomplicated pyelonephritis among community-dwelling women 18–49 years of age is 28 cases per 10,000 women.

ETIOLOGY

Many microorganisms can infect the urinary tract, but by far the most common agents are the gram-negative bacilli (Chap. 143). *Escherichia coli* causes ~80% of acute infections (both cystitis and pyelonephritis) in patients without catheters, urologic abnormalities, or calculi. Other gram-negative rods, especially *Proteus* and *Klebsiella* spp. and occasionally *Enterobacter* spp., account for a smaller proportion of uncomplicated infections. These organisms, along with *Serratia* spp. (Chap. 143) and *Pseudomonas* spp. (Chap. 145), assume increasing importance in recurrent infections and in infections associated with urologic manipulation, calculi, or obstruction. They play a major role in nosocomial, catheter-associated infections (see below). *Proteus* spp. (through the production of urease) and *Klebsiella* spp. (through the production of extracellular slime and polysaccharides) predispose to stone formation and are isolated more frequently from patients with calculi.

Gram-positive cocci play a lesser role in UTIs. However, *Staphylococcus saprophyticus* (Chap. 129)—a novobiocin-resistant, coagulase-negative species—accounts for 10–15% of acute symptomatic UTIs in young female patients. Enterococci occasionally cause acute uncomplicated cystitis in women. More commonly, enterococci (Chap. 130) and *Staphylococcus aureus* (Chap. 129) cause infections in patients with renal stones or with previous instrumentation or surgery. Isolation of *S. aureus* from the urine should arouse suspicion of bacteremic infection of the kidney. *Staphylococcus epidermidis* (Chap. 129) is a common cause of catheter-associated UTI.

About one-third of women with dysuria and frequency have either an insignificant number of bacteria in midstream urine cultures or completely sterile cultures and have been previously defined as having the urethral syndrome. About three-quarters of these women have pyuria, while one-quarter have no pyuria and little objective evidence of infection. In the women with pyuria, two groups of pathogens account for most infections. Low counts (10^2–10^4/mL) of typical bacterial uropathogens such as *E. coli*, *S. saprophyticus*, *Klebsiella*, or *Proteus* are found in midstream urine specimens from most of these women. These bacteria are probably the causative agents in these infections because they can usually be isolated from a suprapubic aspirate, are associated with pyuria, and respond to appropriate antimicrobial therapy. In other women with acute urinary symptoms, pyuria, and urine that is sterile (even when obtained by suprapubic aspiration), sexually transmitted urethritis-producing agents such as *Chlamydia trachomatis* (Chap. 169), *Neisseria gonorrhoeae* (Chap. 137), and herpes simplex virus (HSV; Chap. 172) are etiologically important. These agents are found most frequently in young, sexually active women with new sexual partners.

The causative role of several more unusual bacterial and nonbacterial pathogens in UTIs remains poorly defined. *Ureaplasma urealyticum* (Chap. 168) has frequently been isolated from the urethra and urine of patients with acute dysuria and frequency but is also found in specimens from many patients without urinary symptoms. Ureaplasmas and *Mycoplasma genitalium* (Chap. 168) probably account for some cases of urethritis and cystitis. *U. urealyticum* and *Mycoplasma hominis* have been isolated from prostatic and renal tissues of patients with acute prostatitis and pyelonephritis, respectively, and are probably responsible for some of these infections as well. Adenoviruses cause acute hemorrhagic cystitis in children and in some young adults, often in epidemics. Although other viruses can be isolated from urine (e.g., cytomegalovirus), they are thought not to cause acute UTI. Colonization of the urine of catheterized or diabetic patients by *Candida* and other fungal species is common and sometimes progresses to symptomatic invasive infection (Chap. 196). Mycobacterial infection of the genitourinary tract is discussed in Chap. 158.

PATHOGENESIS AND SOURCES OF INFECTION

The urinary tract should be viewed as a single anatomic unit that is united by a continuous column of urine extending from the urethra to the kidney. In the vast majority of UTIs, bacteria gain access to the bladder via the urethra. Ascent of bacteria from the bladder may follow and is probably the pathway for most renal parenchymal infections.

The vaginal introitus and distal urethra are normally colonized by diphtheroids, streptococcal species, lactobacilli, and staphylococcal species but not by the enteric gram-negative bacilli that commonly cause UTIs. In females prone to the development of cystitis, however, enteric gram-negative organisms residing in the bowel colonize the introitus, the periurethral skin, and the distal urethra before and during episodes of bacteriuria. The factors that predispose to periurethral colonization with gram-negative bacilli remain poorly understood, but alteration of the normal vaginal flora by antibiotics, other genital infections, or contraceptives (especially spermicide) appears to play an important role. Loss of the normally dominant H_2O_2-producing lactobacilli from the vaginal flora appears to facilitate colonization by *E. coli*. Small numbers of periurethral bacteria probably gain entry to the bladder frequently, and this process is facilitated in some cases by urethral massage during intercourse. Whether bladder infection ensues depends on interacting effects of strain pathogenicity, inoculum size, and local and systemic host defense mechanisms. Recent data from both animal models and human studies indicate that *E. coli* sometimes invades the bladder epithelium, forming intracellular colonies (biofilms) that may persist and become a source of recurrent infection.

Under normal circumstances, bacteria placed in the bladder are rapidly cleared, partly through the flushing and dilutional effects of voiding but also as a result of the antibacterial properties of urine and the bladder mucosa. Owing mostly to a high urea concentration and high osmolarity, the bladder urine of many healthy persons inhibits or kills bacteria. Prostatic secretions possess antibacterial properties as well. Bladder epithelial cells secrete cytokines and chemokines—primarily interleukin (IL) 6 and IL-8—upon interaction with bacteria, causing polymorphonuclear leukocytes to enter the bladder epithelium and the urine soon after infection arises and play a role in clearing bacteriuria. The role of locally produced antibody remains unclear.

Hematogenous pyelonephritis occurs most often in debilitated patients who are either chronically ill or receiving immunosuppressive therapy. Metastatic staphylococcal or candidal infections of the kidney may follow bacteremia or fungemia, spreading from distant foci of infection in the bone, skin, or vasculature or elsewhere.

CONDITIONS AFFECTING PATHOGENESIS

Gender and Sexual Activity The female urethra appears to be particularly prone to colonization with colonic gram-negative bacilli because of its proximity to the anus, its short length (~4 cm), and its termination beneath the labia. Sexual intercourse causes the introduction of bacteria into the bladder and is temporally associated with the onset of cystitis; it thus appears to be important in the pathogenesis of UTIs in both pre- and postmenopausal women. Voiding after intercourse reduces the risk of cystitis, probably because it promotes the clearance of bacteria introduced during intercourse. Use of spermicidal com-

pounds with a diaphragm or cervical cap or use of spermicide-coated condoms dramatically alters the normal introital bacterial flora and has been associated with marked increases in vaginal colonization with *E. coli* and in the risk of both cystitis and acute pyelonephritis. In healthy, community-dwelling postmenopausal women, the risk of UTI (both cystitis and pyelonephritis) is increased by a history of recent sexual activity, recent UTI, diabetes mellitus, and incontinence.

In male patients who are <50 years old and who have no history of heterosexual or homosexual insertive rectal intercourse, UTI is exceedingly uncommon, and this diagnosis should be questioned in the absence of clear documentation. An important factor predisposing to bacteriuria in men is urethral obstruction due to prostatic hypertrophy. Insertive rectal intercourse is also associated with an increased risk of cystitis in men. Men (and women) who are infected with HIV and who have CD4+ T cell counts of <200/μL are at increased risk of both bacteriuria and symptomatic UTI. Finally, lack of circumcision has been identified as a risk factor for UTI in both male neonates and young men.

Pregnancy UTIs are detected in 2–8% of pregnant women. Symptomatic upper tract infections, in particular, are unusually common during pregnancy; fully 20–30% of pregnant women with asymptomatic bacteriuria subsequently develop pyelonephritis. This predisposition to upper tract infection during pregnancy results from decreased ureteral tone, decreased ureteral peristalsis, and temporary incompetence of the vesicoureteral valves. Bladder catheterization during or after delivery causes additional infections. Increased incidences of low birth weight, premature delivery, and neonatal death result from UTIs (particularly upper tract infections) during pregnancy.

Obstruction Any impediment to the free flow of urine—tumor, stricture, stone, or prostatic hypertrophy—results in hydronephrosis and a greatly increased frequency of UTI. Infection superimposed on urinary tract obstruction may lead to rapid destruction of renal tissue. It is of utmost importance, therefore, when infection is present, to identify and repair obstructive lesions. On the other hand, when an obstruction is minor and is not progressive or associated with infection, great caution should be exercised in attempting surgical correction. The introduction of infection in such cases may be more damaging than an uncorrected minor obstruction that does not significantly impair renal function.

Neurogenic Bladder Dysfunction Interference with bladder enervation, as in spinal cord injury, tabes dorsalis, multiple sclerosis, diabetes, and other diseases, may be associated with UTI. The infection may be initiated by the use of catheters for bladder drainage and is favored by the prolonged stasis of urine in the bladder. An additional factor often operative in these cases is bone demineralization due to immobilization, which causes hypercalciuria, calculus formation, and obstructive uropathy.

Vesicoureteral Reflux Defined as reflux of urine from the bladder cavity up into the ureters and sometimes into the renal pelvis, vesicoureteral reflux occurs during voiding or with elevation of pressure in the bladder. In practice, this condition is detected as retrograde movement of radiopaque or radioactive material during a voiding cystourethrogram. An anatomically impaired vesicoureteral junction facilitates reflux of bacteria and thus upper tract infection. However, since—even in the healthy urinary system—a fluid connection between the bladder and the kidneys always exists, some retrograde movement of bacteria probably takes place during infection but is not detected by radiologic techniques.

Vesicoureteral reflux is common among children with anatomic abnormalities of the urinary tract or with anatomically normal but infected urinary tracts. In the latter group, reflux disappears with advancing age and is probably attributable to factors other than UTI. Long-term follow-up of children with UTI who have reflux has established that renal damage correlates with marked reflux, not with infection. Thus, it

FIGURE 282-1 Adherence of fluorescein-labeled uropathogenic *Escherichia coli* to a uroepithelial cell.

appears reasonable to search for reflux in children with unexplained failure of renal growth or with renal scarring, because UTI per se is an insufficient explanation for these abnormalities. On the other hand, it is doubtful that all children who have recurrent UTIs but whose urinary tract appears normal on pyelography should be subjected to voiding cystoureterography merely for the detection of the rare patient with marked reflux not revealed by intravenous pyelography.

Bacterial Virulence Factors   Not all strains of *E. coli* are equally capable of infecting the intact urinary tract. Bacterial virulence factors markedly influence the likelihood that a given strain, once introduced into the bladder, will cause UTI. Most *E. coli* strains that cause symptomatic UTIs in noncatheterized patients belong to a small number of specific O, K, and H serogroups. These uropathogenic clones have accumulated a number of virulence genes that are often closely linked on the bacterial chromosome in "pathogenicity islands." Bacterial adherence to uroepithelial cells is a critical first step in the initiation of infection (Fig. 282-1). For both *E. coli* and *Proteus* spp., fimbriae (hairlike proteinaceous surface appendages) mediate bacterial attachment to specific receptors on epithelial cells, which in turn initiates important events in the mucosal epithelial cell, including secretion of IL-6 and IL-8 (with subsequent chemotaxis of leukocytes to the bladder mucosa) and induction of apoptosis and epithelial cell desquamation. Besides fimbriae, uropathogenic *E. coli* strains usually produce cytotoxins, hemolysin, and aerobactin (a siderophore for scavenging iron) and are resistant to the bactericidal action of human serum. Nearly all *E. coli* strains causing acute pyelonephritis and most of those causing acute cystitis are uropathogenic strains possessing pathogenicity islands. In contrast, infections in patients with structural or functional abnormalities of the urinary tract are generally caused by bacterial strains that lack these uropathogenic properties; the implication is that these properties are not needed for infection of the compromised urinary tract.

Genetic Factors   Increasing evidence suggests that host genetic factors influence susceptibility to UTI. A maternal history of UTI is more often found among women who have experienced recurrent UTIs than among controls. The number and type of receptors on uroepithelial cells to which bacteria may attach are, at least in part, genetically determined. Many of these structures are components of blood group antigens and are present on both erythrocytes and uroepithelial cells. For example, P fimbriae mediate attachment of *E. coli* to P-positive erythrocytes and are found on nearly all strains causing acute uncomplicated pyelonephritis. Conversely, P blood group–negative individuals, who lack these receptors, are at decreased risk of pyelonephritis. Furthermore, nonsecretors of blood group antigens are at increased risk of recurrent UTI; this predisposition may relate to a different profile of genetically determined glycolipids on uroepithelial cells. Mutations in host genes integral to the immune response (e.g., Toll-like receptors, interferon γ receptors) may also affect susceptibility to UTI.

CLINICAL PRESENTATION
Localization of Infection   Unfortunately, available methods of distinguishing renal parenchymal infection from cystitis are neither reliable nor convenient enough for routine clinical use. Fever or an elevated C-reactive protein level often accompanies acute pyelonephritis and is found in rare cases of cystitis but also occurs in infections other than pyelonephritis.

Cystitis   Patients with cystitis usually report dysuria, frequency, urgency, and suprapubic pain. The urine often becomes grossly cloudy and malodorous and is bloody in ~30% of cases. White cells and bacteria can be detected by examination of unspun urine in most cases. However, some women with cystitis have only 10^2–10^4 bacteria per milliliter of urine, and in these instances bacteria cannot be seen in a Gram-stained preparation of unspun urine. Physical examination generally reveals only tenderness of the urethra or the suprapubic area. If a genital lesion or a vaginal discharge is evident, especially in conjunction with <10^5 bacteria per milliliter on urine culture, then pathogens that may cause urethritis, vaginitis, or cervicitis (e.g., *C. trachomatis*, *N. gonorrhoeae*, *Trichomonas*, *Candida*, and HSV) should be considered. Prominent systemic manifestations, such as a temperature of >38.3°C (>101°F), nausea, and vomiting, usually indicate concomitant renal infection, as does costovertebral angle tenderness. However, the absence of these findings does not ensure that infection is limited to the bladder and urethra.

Acute Pyelonephritis   Symptoms of acute pyelonephritis generally develop rapidly over a few hours or a day and include fever, shaking chills, nausea, vomiting, abdominal pain, and diarrhea. Symptoms of cystitis are sometimes present. Besides fever, tachycardia, and generalized muscle tenderness, physical examination generally reveals marked tenderness on deep pressure in one or both costovertebral angles or on deep abdominal palpation. The range of illness severity is broad. Some patients have mild disease; in others, signs and symptoms of gram-negative sepsis predominate. Most patients have significant leukocytosis and bacteria detectable in Gram-stained unspun urine. Leukocyte casts are present in the urine of some patients, and the detection of these casts is pathognomonic. Hematuria may be demonstrated during the acute phase of the disease; if it persists after acute manifestations of infection have subsided, a stone, a tumor, or tuberculosis should be considered.

Except in individuals with papillary necrosis, abscess formation, or urinary obstruction, the manifestations of acute pyelonephritis usually respond to appropriate therapy within 48–72 h. However, despite the absence of symptoms, bacteriuria or pyuria may persist. In severe pyelonephritis, fever subsides more slowly and may not disappear for several days, even after appropriate antibiotic treatment has been instituted. Persistence of fever or of symptoms and signs beyond 72 h suggests the need for urologic imaging.

Urethritis   Of women with acute dysuria, frequency, and pyuria, ~30% have midstream urine cultures with either no growth or insignificant bacterial growth. Clinically, these women cannot always be readily distinguished from those with cystitis. In this situation, a distinction should be made between women infected with sexually transmitted pathogens (e.g., *C. trachomatis*, *N. gonorrhoeae*, or HSV) and those with low-count *E. coli* or *S. saprophyticus* infection of the urethra and bladder. Chlamydial or gonococcal infection should be suspected in women with a gradual onset of illness, no hematuria, no suprapubic pain, and >7 days of symptoms. The additional history of a recent sex-partner change, especially if the partner has recently had chlamydial or gonococcal urethritis, should heighten the suspicion of a sexually transmitted infection, as should the finding of mucopurulent cervicitis (Chap. 124). Gross hematuria, suprapubic pain, an abrupt onset of illness, a duration of illness of <3 days, and a history of UTIs favor the diagnosis of *E. coli* UTI.

Catheter-Associated UTIs (See also Chap. 125) Bacteriuria develops in at least 10–15% of hospitalized patients with short-term indwelling urethral catheters. The risk of infection is ~3–5% per day of catheterization. *E. coli*, *Proteus*, *Pseudomonas*, *Klebsiella*, *Serratia*, staphylococci, enterococci, and *Candida* usually cause these infections. Many infecting strains display markedly broader antimicrobial resistance profiles than do organisms that cause community-acquired UTIs. Factors associated with an increased risk of catheter-associated UTI include female sex, prolonged catheterization, severe underlying illness, disconnection of the catheter and drainage tube, other types of faulty catheter care, and lack of systemic antimicrobial therapy.

Infection occurs when bacteria reach the bladder by one of two routes: migration through the column of urine in the catheter lumen (intraluminal route) or up the mucous sheath outside the catheter (periurethral route). Hospital-acquired pathogens can reach the patient's catheter or urine-collecting system on the hands of hospital personnel, in contaminated solutions or irrigants, and via contaminated instruments or disinfectants. Bacteria usually enter the catheter system at the catheter–collecting tube junction or at the drainage bag portal. The organisms then ascend intraluminally into the bladder within 24–72 h. Alternatively, the patient's own bowel flora may colonize the perineal skin and periurethral area and reach the bladder by ascending along the external surface of the catheter. Studies have shown the importance of bacterial attachment to and growth on the device's surfaces in the pathogenesis of catheter-associated UTI. Bacterial growth in biofilms on the catheter eventually produces encrustations consisting of bacteria, bacterial glycocalyces, host urinary proteins, and urinary salts. These encrustations provide a refuge for bacteria and may protect them from antimicrobial agents and phagocytes.

Clinically, catheter-associated infections usually cause minimal symptoms without fever and often resolve after withdrawal of the catheter. The frequency of upper tract infection associated with catheter-induced bacteriuria is unknown. Gram-negative bacteremia, which follows catheter-associated bacteriuria in 1–2% of cases, is the most significant recognized complication of catheter-induced UTIs. The catheterized urinary tract has repeatedly been shown to be the most common source of gram-negative bacteremia in hospitalized patients, generally accounting for ~30% of cases.

In patients catheterized for <2 weeks, catheter-associated UTIs can sometimes be prevented by use of a sterile closed collecting system, by attention to aseptic technique during catheter insertion and care, and by measures to minimize cross-infection. Other preventive approaches, including short courses of systemic antimicrobial therapy, topical application of periurethral antimicrobial ointments, use of preconnected catheter–drainage tube units, and addition of antimicrobial drugs to the drainage bag, have all been protective in at least one controlled trial but are not recommended for general use. The use of catheters impregnated with antimicrobial agents reduces the incidence of asymptomatic bacteriuria in patients catheterized for <2 weeks. Despite precautions, the majority of patients catheterized for >2 weeks eventually develop bacteriuria. For example, because of spinal cord injury, incontinence, or other factors, some patients in hospitals or nursing homes require long-term or semipermanent bladder catheterization. Measures intended to prevent infection have been largely unsuccessful in these chronically catheterized patients, essentially all of whom develop bacteriuria. If feasible, intermittent catheterization by a nurse or by the patient appears to reduce the incidence of bacteriuria and associated complications in such patients. Treatment should be provided when symptomatic infections arise, but treatment of asymptomatic bacteriuria in such patients has no apparent benefit.

DIAGNOSTIC TESTING

Determination of the number and type of bacteria in the urine is an extremely important diagnostic procedure. In symptomatic patients, bacteria are usually present in the urine in large numbers ($\geq 10^5$/mL). In asymptomatic patients, two consecutive urine specimens should be examined bacteriologically before therapy is instituted, and $\geq 10^5$ bacteria of a single species per milliliter should be demonstrable in both specimens. Since the large number of bacteria in the bladder urine is due in part to bacterial multiplication in the bladder cavity, samples of urine from the ureters or renal pelvis may contain $<10^5$ bacteria per milliliter and yet indicate infection. Similarly, the presence of bacteriuria of any degree in suprapubic aspirates or of $\geq 10^2$ bacteria per milliliter of urine obtained by catheterization usually indicates infection. In some circumstances (antibiotic treatment, high urea concentration, high osmolarity, low pH), urine inhibits bacterial multiplication, resulting in relatively low bacterial colony counts despite infection. For this reason, antiseptic solutions should not be used to wash the periurethral area before collection of the urine specimen. Water diuresis or recent voiding also reduces bacterial counts in urine.

Microscopy of urine from symptomatic patients can be of great diagnostic value. Microscopic bacteriuria, which is best assessed with Gram-stained uncentrifuged urine, is found in >90% of specimens from patients whose infections are associated with colony counts of at least 10^5/mL, and this finding is very specific. However, bacteria cannot usually be detected microscopically in infections with lower colony counts (10^2–10^4/mL). The detection of bacteria by urinary microscopy thus constitutes firm evidence of infection, but the absence of microscopically detectable bacteria does not exclude the diagnosis. When carefully sought by chamber-count microscopy, pyuria is a highly sensitive indicator of UTI in symptomatic patients. Pyuria is demonstrated in nearly all acute bacterial UTIs, and its absence calls the diagnosis into question. The leukocyte esterase "dipstick" method is less sensitive than microscopy in identifying pyuria but is a useful alternative when microscopy is not feasible. Pyuria in the absence of bacteriuria (sterile pyuria) may indicate infection with unusual agents such as *C. trachomatis*, *U. urealyticum*, or *Mycobacterium tuberculosis* or with fungi. Alternatively, sterile pyuria may be documented in noninfectious urologic conditions such as calculi, anatomic abnormality, nephrocalcinosis, vesicoureteral reflux, interstitial nephritis, or polycystic disease.

Although many authorities have recommended that urine culture and antimicrobial susceptibility testing be performed for any patient with a suspected UTI, it is more practical and cost-effective to manage women who have symptoms characteristic of acute uncomplicated cystitis without an initial urine culture. Two approaches to presumptive therapy have generally been used. In the first, treatment is initiated solely on the basis of a typical history and/or typical findings on physical examination. In the second, women with symptoms and signs of acute cystitis and without complicating factors are managed with urinary microscopy (or, alternatively, with a leukocyte esterase test). A positive result for pyuria and/or bacteriuria provides enough evidence of infection to omit urine culture and susceptibility testing and treat the patient empirically. Urine should be cultured, however, when a woman's symptoms and urine-examination findings leave the diagnosis of cystitis in question. Pretherapy cultures and susceptibility testing are also essential in the management of all patients with suspected upper tract infections and of those with complicating factors (including all men). In these situations, any of a variety of pathogens may be involved, and antibiotic therapy is best tailored to the individual organism.

UROLOGIC EVALUATION

Very few women with recurrent UTIs have correctable lesions discovered at cystoscopy or upon IV pyelography, and these procedures should not be undertaken routinely in such cases. Urologic evaluation should be performed for selected female patients—namely, women with relapsing infection, a history of childhood infections, stones or painless hematuria, or recurrent pyelonephritis. Most male patients with UTI should be considered to have complicated infection and thus should be evaluated urologically. Possible exceptions include young men who have cystitis associated with sexual activity, who are uncircumcised, or who have AIDS. Men or women presenting with acute infection and signs or symptoms suggestive of an obstruction or stones should undergo prompt urologic evaluation, generally by means of ultrasound.

℞ URINARY TRACT INFECTIONS

The following principles underlie the treatment of UTIs:

1. Except in acute uncomplicated cystitis in women, a quantitative urine culture or a comparable alternative diagnostic test should be performed to confirm infection before empirical treatment is begun, and antimicrobial sensitivity testing should be used to direct therapy.
2. Factors predisposing to infection, such as obstruction and calculi, should be identified and corrected if possible.
3. Relief of clinical symptoms does not always indicate bacteriologic cure.
4. Each course of treatment should be classified after its completion as a failure (symptoms and/or bacteriuria not eradicated during therapy or in the immediate posttreatment culture) or a cure (resolution of symptoms and elimination of bacteriuria). Recurrent infections should be classified as same-strain or different-strain and as early (occurring within 2 weeks of the end of therapy) or late.
5. In general, uncomplicated infections confined to the lower urinary tract respond to short courses of therapy, while upper tract infections require longer treatment. After therapy, early recurrences due to the same strain may result from an unresolved upper tract focus of infection but often (especially after short-course therapy for cystitis) result from persistent vaginal colonization. Recurrences >2 weeks after the cessation of therapy nearly always represent reinfection with a new strain or with the previously infecting strain that has persisted in the vaginal and rectal flora.
6. Despite increasing resistance, community-acquired infections (especially initial infections) are usually due to relatively antibiotic-sensitive strains.
7. In patients with repeated infections, instrumentation, or recent hospitalization, the presence of antibiotic-resistant strains should be suspected. Although many antimicrobial agents reach high concentrations in urine, in vitro resistance usually predicts a substantially higher failure rate.

The anatomic location of a UTI greatly influences the success or failure of a therapeutic regimen. Bladder bacteriuria (cystitis) can usually be eliminated with short courses or even single doses of antimicrobial agents. In the past, it was demonstrated that as little as a single 500-mg dose of intramuscular kanamycin eliminated bladder bacteriuria in most cases. With upper tract infections, however, single-dose therapy fails in the majority of cases, and 7- to 14-day courses are generally needed. Longer periods of treatment (2–6 weeks) aimed at eradicating a persistent focus of infection may be necessary in some cases.

ACUTE UNCOMPLICATED CYSTITIS Taken together, *E. coli* and *S. saprophyticus* cause >90–95% of cases of acute uncomplicated cystitis. Although resistance patterns vary geographically (both globally and within the United States), resistance has increased in many areas. Nevertheless, most strains are sensitive to several antibiotics. In most parts of the United States, more than one-quarter of *E. coli* strains causing acute cystitis are resistant to amoxicillin, sulfa drugs, and cephalexin; resistance to trimethoprim (TMP) and trimethoprim-sulfamethoxazole (TMP-SMX) is now approaching these levels in many areas. Substantially higher rates of resistance to TMP-SMX have been documented in some other countries, as has resistance to fluoroquinolones. Thus, knowledge of local resistance patterns is needed to guide empirical therapy.

Many have advocated single-dose treatment for acute cystitis. The advantages include less expense, ensured compliance, fewer side effects, and perhaps less intense pressure favoring the selection of resistant organisms in the intestinal, vaginal, or perineal flora. However, more frequent recurrences develop shortly after single-dose therapy than after 3-day treatment, and single-dose therapy does not eradicate vaginal colonization with *E. coli* as effectively as do longer regimens. A 3-day course of TMP-SMX, TMP, norfloxacin, ciprofloxacin, or levofloxacin appears to preserve the low rate of side effects of single-dose therapy while improving efficacy **(Table 282-1)**; thus 3-day regimens of these drugs are currently preferred for acute cystitis. In areas where TMP-SMX resistance exceeds 20%, either a fluoroquinolone or nitrofurantoin can be used (Table 282-1). Resistance to these agents among strains causing cystitis remains low. A 3-day regimen of amoxicillin/clavulanate was found to be significantly less effective than a 3-day regimen of ciprofloxacin in treating uncomplicated UTIs in women. Neither single-dose nor 3-day therapy should be used for women with symptoms or signs of pyelonephritis, urologic abnormalities or stones, or

TABLE 282-1 TREATMENT REGIMENS FOR BACTERIAL URINARY TRACT INFECTIONS

Condition	Characteristic Pathogens	Mitigating Circumstances	Recommended Empirical Treatment[a]
Acute uncomplicated cystitis in women	*Escherichia coli, Staphylococcus saprophyticus, Proteus mirabilis, Klebsiella pneumoniae*	None	3-Day regimens: oral TMP-SMX, TMP, quinolone; 7-day regimen: macrocrystalline nitrofurantoin[b]
		Diabetes, symptoms for >7 d, recent UTI, use of diaphragm, age >65 years	Consider 7-day regimen: oral TMP-SMX, TMP, quinolone[b]
		Pregnancy	Consider 7-day regimen: oral amoxicillin, macrocrystalline nitrofurantoin, cefpodoxime proxetil, or TMP-SMX[b]
Acute uncomplicated pyelonephritis in women	*E. coli, P. mirabilis, S. saprophyticus*	Mild to moderate illness, no nausea or vomiting; outpatient therapy	Oral[c] quinolone for 7–14 d (initial dose given IV if desired); or single-dose ceftriaxone (1 g) or gentamicin (3–5 mg/kg) IV followed by oral TMP-SMX[b] for 14 d
		Severe illness or possible urosepsis: hospitalization required	Parenteral[d] quinolone, gentamicin (± ampicillin), ceftriaxone, or aztreonam until defervescence; then oral[c] quinolone, cephalosporin, or TMP-SMX for 14 d
Complicated UTI in men and women	*E. coli, Proteus, Klebsiella, Pseudomonas, Serratia,* enterococci, staphylococci	Mild to moderate illness, no nausea or vomiting: outpatient therapy	Oral[c] quinolone for 10–14 d
		Severe illness or possible urosepsis: hospitalization required	Parenteral[d] ampicillin and gentamicin, quinolone, ceftriaxone, aztreonam, ticarcillin/clavulanate, or imipenem-cilastatin until defervescence; then oral[c] quinolone or TMP-SMX for 10–21 d

[a]Treatments listed are those to be prescribed before the etiologic agent is known; Gram's staining can be helpful in the selection of empirical therapy. Such therapy can be modified once the infecting agent has been identified. Fluoroquinolones should not be used in pregnancy. TMP-SMX, although not approved for use in pregnancy, has been widely used. Gentamicin should be used with caution in pregnancy because of its possible toxicity to eighth-nerve development in the fetus.

[b]Multiday oral regimens for cystitis are as follows: TMP-SMX, 160/800 mg q12h; TMP, 100 mg q12h; norfloxacin, 400 mg q12h; ciprofloxacin, 250 mg q12h; ofloxacin, 200 mg q12h; levofloxacin, 250 mg/d; gatifloxacin, 200 or 400 mg/d; moxifloxacin, 400 mg/d; lomefloxacin, 400 mg/d; enoxacin, 400 mg q12h; macrocrystalline nitrofurantoin, 100 mg qid; amoxicillin, 250 mg q8h; cefpodoxime proxetil, 100 mg q12h.

[c]Oral regimens for pyelonephritis and complicated UTI are as follows: TMP-SMX, 160/800 mg q12h; ciprofloxacin, 500 mg q12h; ofloxacin, 200–300 mg q12h; lomefloxacin, 400 mg/d; enoxacin, 400 mg q12h; gatifloxacin, 400 mg/d; levofloxacin, 200 mg q12h; moxifloxacin, 400 mg/d; amoxicillin, 500 mg q8h; cefpodoxime proxetil, 200 mg q12h.

[d]Parenteral regimens are as follows: ciprofloxacin, 400 mg q12h; ofloxacin, 400 mg q12h; gatifloxacin, 400 mg/d; levofloxacin, 500 mg/d; gentamicin, 1 mg/kg q8h; ceftriaxone, 1–2 g/d; ampicillin, 1 g q6h; imipenem-cilastatin, 250–500 mg q6–8h; ticarcillin/clavulanate, 3.2 g q8h; aztreonam, 1 g q8–12h.

Note: UTI, urinary tract infection; TMP, trimethoprim; TMP-SMX, trimethoprim-sulfamethoxazole.

previous infections due to antibiotic-resistant organisms. Male patients with UTI often have urologic abnormalities or prostatic involvement and hence are not candidates for single-dose or 3-day therapy. For empirical therapy, they should generally receive a 7- to 14-day course of a fluoroquinolone (Table 282-1).

ACUTE URETHRITIS   The choice of treatment for women with acute urethritis depends on the etiologic agent involved. In chlamydial infection, azithromycin (1 g in a single oral dose) or doxycycline (100 mg twice daily by mouth for 7 days) should be used. Women with acute dysuria and frequency, negative urine cultures, and no pyuria usually do not respond to antimicrobial agents.

ACUTE UNCOMPLICATED PYELONEPHRITIS   In women, most cases of acute uncomplicated pyelonephritis without accompanying clinical evidence of calculi or urologic disease are due to E. coli. Although the optimal route and duration of therapy have not been established, a 7- to 14-day course of a fluoroquinolone is usually adequate. Neither ampicillin nor TMP-SMX should be used as initial therapy because >25% of E. coli strains causing pyelonephritis are now resistant to these drugs in vitro. For at least the first few days of treatment, antibiotics should probably be given intravenously to most patients, but patients with mild symptoms can be treated for 7–14 days with an oral antibiotic (usually ciprofloxacin or levofloxacin), with or without an initial single parenteral dose (Table 282-1). Patients who fail to respond to treatment within 72 h or who relapse after therapy should be evaluated for unrecognized suppurative foci, calculi, or urologic disease.

COMPLICATED URINARY TRACT INFECTIONS   Complicated UTIs (those arising in a setting of catheterization, instrumentation, anatomic or functional urologic abnormalities, stones, obstruction, immunosuppression, renal disease, or diabetes) are typically due to hospital-acquired bacteria, including E. coli, Klebsiella, Proteus, Serratia, Pseudomonas, enterococci, and staphylococci. Many of the infecting strains are antibiotic-resistant. Empirical antibiotic therapy ideally provides broad-spectrum coverage against these pathogens. In patients with minimal or mild symptoms, oral therapy with a fluoroquinolone, such as ciprofloxacin or levofloxacin, can be administered until culture results and antibiotic sensitivities are known. In patients with more severe illness, including acute pyelonephritis or suspected urosepsis, hospitalization and parenteral therapy should be undertaken. In patients with diabetes, severe outcomes are more common and should be anticipated; they include renal suppurative foci, papillary necrosis, emphysematous infection, and unusual infecting agents. Commonly used empirical regimens include imipenem alone, an extended-spectrum penicillin or cephalosporin plus an aminoglycoside, and (when the involvement of enterococci is unlikely) ceftriaxone or ceftazidime. When information on the antimicrobial sensitivity pattern of the infecting strain becomes available, a more specific antimicrobial regimen can be selected. Therapy should generally be administered for 10–21 days, with the exact duration depending on the severity of the infection and the susceptibility of the infecting strain. Follow-up cultures should be performed 2–4 weeks after cessation of therapy to demonstrate cure.

ASYMPTOMATIC BACTERIURIA   The need for treatment as well as the optimal type and duration of treatment for catheterized patients with asymptomatic bacteriuria have not been established. Removal of the catheter in conjunction with a short course of antibiotics to which the organism is susceptible probably constitutes the best course of action and nearly always eradicates bacteriuria. Treatment of asymptomatic catheter-associated bacteriuria may be of greatest benefit to elderly women, who most often develop symptoms if left untreated. If the catheter cannot be removed, antibiotic therapy usually proves unsuccessful and may in fact result in infection with a more resistant strain. In this situation, the bacteriuria should be ignored unless the patient develops symptoms or is at high risk of developing bacteremia. In these cases, use of systemic antibiotics or urinary bladder antiseptics may reduce the degree of bacteriuria and the likelihood of bacteremia.

Asymptomatic bacteriuria in noncatheterized patients is common, especially among the elderly, but has not been linked to adverse outcomes in most circumstances other than pregnancy (see below). Thus antimicrobial therapy is unnecessary and may in fact promote the emergence of resistant strains in most patients with asymptomatic bacteriuria. High-risk patients with neutropenia, renal transplants, obstruction, or other compli-

cating conditions may require treatment when asymptomatic bacteriuria occurs. Seven days of therapy with an oral agent to which the organism is sensitive should be given initially. If bacteriuria persists, it can be monitored without further treatment in most patients. Longer-term therapy (4–6 weeks) may be necessary in high-risk patients with persistent asymptomatic bacteriuria.

TREATMENT DURING PREGNANCY   In pregnancy, acute cystitis can be managed with 7 days of treatment with amoxicillin, nitrofurantoin, or a cephalosporin. All pregnant women should be screened for asymptomatic bacteriuria during the first trimester and, if bacteriuric, should be treated with one of the regimens listed in Table 282-1. After treatment, a culture should be performed to ensure cure, and cultures should be repeated monthly thereafter until delivery. Acute pyelonephritis in pregnancy should be managed with hospitalization and parenteral antibiotic therapy, generally with a cephalosporin or an extended-spectrum penicillin. Continuous low-dose prophylaxis with nitrofurantoin should be given to women who have recurrent infections during pregnancy.

PROGNOSIS

In uncomplicated cystitis or pyelonephritis, treatment ordinarily results in complete resolution of symptoms. Lower tract infections in women are of concern mainly because they cause discomfort, morbidity, loss of time from work, and substantial health care costs. Cystitis may also result in upper tract infection or in bacteremia (especially during instrumentation), but little evidence suggests that renal impairment follows. When repeated episodes of cystitis occur, they are more commonly reinfections rather than relapses.

Acute uncomplicated pyelonephritis in adults rarely progresses to renal functional impairment and chronic renal disease. Repeated upper tract infections often represent relapse rather than reinfection, and renal calculi or an underlying urologic abnormality should be vigorously sought. If neither is found, 6 weeks of chemotherapy may be useful in eradicating an unresolved focus of infection.

Repeated symptomatic UTIs in children and in adults with obstructive uropathy, neurogenic bladder, structural renal disease, or diabetes progress to renal scarring and chronic renal disease with unusual frequency. Asymptomatic bacteriuria in these groups as well as in adults without urologic disease or obstruction predisposes to increased numbers of episodes of symptomatic infection but does not result in renal impairment in most instances.

PREVENTION

Women who experience frequent symptomatic UTIs (≥3 per year on average) are candidates for long-term administration of low-dose antibiotics directed at preventing recurrences. Such women should be advised to avoid spermicide use and to void soon after intercourse. Daily or thrice-weekly administration of a single dose of TMP-SMX (80/400 mg), TMP alone (100 mg), or nitrofurantoin (50 mg) has been particularly effective. Fluoroquinolones have also been used for prophylaxis. Prophylaxis should be initiated only after bacteriuria has been eradicated with a full-dose treatment regimen. The same prophylactic regimens can be used after sexual intercourse to prevent episodes of symptomatic infection in women in whom UTIs are temporally related to intercourse. Postmenopausal women who are not taking oral estrogen replacement therapy can effectively manage recurrent UTIs with topical intravaginal estrogen cream. Other patients for whom prophylaxis appears to have some merit include men with chronic prostatitis; patients undergoing prostatectomy, both during the operation and in the postoperative period; and pregnant women with asymptomatic bacteriuria. All pregnant women should be screened for bacteriuria in the first trimester and should be treated if bacteriuria is detected.

PAPILLARY NECROSIS

When infection of the renal pyramids develops in association with vascular diseases of the kidney or with urinary tract obstruction, renal papillary necrosis is likely to result. Patients with diabetes, sickle cell

TABLE 282-2 CLASSIFICATION OF PROSTATITIS

Classification	Clinical Presentation	Prostate	EPS	Etiologic Agent	Antibiotics
Acute bacterial prostatitis	Acute onset of fever, chills, dysuria, urgency	Tender, tense, boggy	PMNs, bacteria	*Escherichia coli*, other uropathogens	Fluoroquinolone, other (see text)
Chronic bacterial prostatitis	Recurrent UTIs, obstructive symptoms, perineal pain	Normal	PMNs, bacteria	*E. coli*, other uropathogens	Fluoroquinolone, other (see text)
Chronic pelvic pain syndrome					
Inflammatory	Perineal and low-back pain, obstructive symptoms, recent NGU	Normal	↑PMNs	*Ureaplasma*? *Mycoplasma*? *Chlamydia*?	4–6 weeks of oral macrolide, tetracycline, other (see text)
Noninflammatory	Same as above	Normal	No PMNs	Unknown	None

Note: EPS, expressed prostatic secretion; NGU, nongonococcal urethritis; PMNs, polymorphonuclear leukocytes.

disease, chronic alcoholism, and vascular disease seem peculiarly susceptible to this complication. Hematuria, pain in the flank or abdomen, and chills and fever are the most common presenting symptoms. Acute renal failure with oliguria or anuria sometimes develops. Rarely, sloughing of a pyramid may take place without symptoms in a patient with chronic UTI, and the diagnosis is made when the necrotic tissue is passed in the urine or identified as a "ring shadow" on pyelography. If renal function deteriorates suddenly in a diabetic individual or a patient with chronic obstruction, the diagnosis of renal papillary necrosis should be entertained, even in the absence of fever or pain. Renal papillary necrosis is often bilateral; when it is unilateral, however, nephrectomy may be a life-saving approach to the management of overwhelming infection.

EMPHYSEMATOUS PYELONEPHRITIS AND CYSTITIS

These unusual clinical entities almost always occur in diabetic patients, often in concert with urinary obstruction and chronic infection. Emphysematous pyelonephritis is usually characterized by a rapidly progressive clinical course, with high fever, leukocytosis, renal parenchymal necrosis, and accumulation of fermentative gases in the kidney and perinephric tissues. Most patients also have pyuria and glucosuria. *E. coli* causes most cases, but occasionally other Enterobacteriaceae are isolated. Gas in tissues is often seen on plain films and is best confirmed and localized by CT. Surgical resection of the involved tissue in addition to systemic antimicrobial therapy is usually needed to prevent a fatal outcome in emphysematous pyelonephritis.

Emphysematous cystitis also occurs primarily in diabetic patients, usually in association with *E. coli* or other facultative gram-negative rods and often in relation to bladder outlet obstruction. Patients with this condition generally are less severely ill and have less rapidly progressive disease than those with emphysematous pyelonephritis. The patient typically reports abdominal pain, dysuria, frequency, and (in some cases) pneumaturia. CT shows gas within both the bladder lumen and the bladder wall. Generally, conservative therapy with systemic antimicrobial agents and relief of outlet obstruction are effective, but some patients do not respond to these measures and require cystectomy.

RENAL AND PERINEPHRIC ABSCESS   See Chap. 121.

PROSTATITIS

The term *prostatitis* has been used for various inflammatory conditions affecting the prostate, including acute and chronic infections with specific bacteria and, more commonly, instances in which signs and symptoms of prostatic inflammation are present but no specific organisms can be detected. Patients with acute bacterial prostatitis can usually be identified readily on the basis of typical symptoms and signs, pyuria, and bacteriuria. To classify a patient with suspected chronic prostatitis correctly, a midstream urine specimen, a prostatic expressate, and a postmassage urine specimen should be quantitatively cultured and evaluated for numbers of leukocytes. On the basis of these studies and other considerations, patients with suspected chron-

ic prostatitis can be categorized as having chronic bacterial prostatitis or chronic pelvic pain syndrome, with or without inflammation (Table 282-2).

ACUTE BACTERIAL PROSTATITIS

When it occurs spontaneously, this disease generally affects young men; however, it may also be associated with an indwelling urethral catheter in older men. It is characterized by fever, chills, dysuria, and a tense or boggy, extremely tender prostate. Although prostatic massage usually produces purulent secretions with a large number of bacteria on culture, vigorous massage may cause bacteremia and should be avoided. The etiologic agent can usually be identified by Gram's staining and culture of urine. In cases not associated with catheters, the infection is generally due to common gram-negative urinary tract pathogens (*E. coli* or *Klebsiella*). Initially, an intravenous fluoroquinolone is the preferred antibiotic regimen; alternatively, a third-generation cephalosporin or an aminoglycoside can be administered. The response to antibiotics in acute bacterial prostatitis is usually prompt, perhaps because drugs penetrate readily into the acutely inflamed prostate. In catheter-associated cases, the spectrum of etiologic agents is broader, including hospital-acquired gram-negative rods and enterococci. The urinary Gram stain may be particularly helpful in such cases. Imipenem, an aminoglycoside, a fluoroquinolone, or a third-generation cephalosporin should be used for initial empirical therapy. The long-term prognosis is good, although in some instances acute infection may result in abscess formation, epididymoorchitis, seminal vesiculitis, septicemia, or residual chronic bacterial prostatitis. Since the advent of antibiotics, the frequency of acute bacterial prostatitis has diminished markedly.

CHRONIC BACTERIAL PROSTATITIS

This entity is now infrequent but should be considered in men with a history of recurrent bacteriuria. Symptoms are often lacking between episodes, and the prostate usually feels normal on palpation. Obstructive symptoms or perineal pain develops in some patients. Intermittently, infection spreads to the bladder, producing frequency, urgency, and dysuria. A pattern of relapsing infection in a middle-aged man strongly suggests chronic bacterial prostatitis. Classically, the diagnosis is established by culture of *E. coli*, *Klebsiella*, *Proteus*, or other uropathogenic bacteria from the expressed prostatic secretion or postmassage urine in higher quantities than are found in midstream urine. Antibiotics promptly relieve the symptoms associated with acute exacerbations but are less effective in eradicating the focus of chronic infection in the prostate. This relative ineffectiveness for long-term cure is due in part to the poor penetration of most antibiotics into the prostate. In this respect, fluoroquinolones are considerably more successful than other antimicrobial agents, but even they must generally be given for at least 12 weeks to be effective. Patients with frequent episodes of acute cystitis in whom attempts at curative therapy fail can be managed with prolonged suppressive courses of low-dose antimicrobial agents (usually a sulfonamide, TMP, or nitrofurantoin). Total prostatectomy obviously results in the cure of chronic prostatitis but is associated with considerable morbidity. Transurethral prostatectomy is safer but cures only one-third of patients.

CHRONIC PELVIC PAIN SYNDROME (FORMERLY NONBACTERIAL PROSTATITIS)

Patients who present with symptoms of prostatitis (intermittent perineal and low-back pain, obstructive voiding symptoms), few signs on examination, no bacterial growth in cultures, and no history of recurrent episodes of bacterial prostatitis are classified as having chronic pelvic pain syndrome (CPPS). Patients with CPPS are divided into inflammatory and noninflammatory subgroups based on the presence or absence of prostatic inflammation. Prostatic inflammation can be considered present when the expressed prostatic secretion and postmassage urine contain at least tenfold more leukocytes than midstream urine or when the expressed prostatic secretion contains ≥1000 leukocytes per microliter.

The likely etiology of CPPS associated with inflammation is an infectious agent, but the agent has not yet been identified. Evidence for a causative role of both *U. urealyticum* and *C. trachomatis* has been presented but is not conclusive. Since most cases of inflammatory CPPS occur in young, sexually active men and since many cases follow an episode of nonspecific urethritis, the causative agent may well be sexually transmitted. The effectiveness of antimicrobial agents in this condition is uncertain. Some patients benefit from a 4- to 6-week course of treatment with erythromycin, doxycycline, TMP-SMX, or a fluoroquinolone, but controlled trials are lacking. Patients who have symptoms and signs of prostatitis but who have no evidence of prostatic inflammation (normal leukocyte counts) and negative urine cultures are classified as having noninflammatory CPPS. Despite their symptoms, these patients most likely do not have prostatic infection and should not be given antimicrobial agents.

FURTHER READINGS

FIHN SD et al: Clinical practice: Acute uncomplicated urinary tract infection in women. N Engl J Med 349:259, 2003

GUPTA K et al: Increasing antimicrobial resistance and the management of uncomplicated community-acquired urinary tract infections. Ann Intern Med 135:41, 2001

HOOTON TM et al: Amoxicillin-clavulanate vs ciprofloxacin for the treatment of uncomplicated cystitis in women. A randomized trial. JAMA 293:949, 2005

—— et al: A prospective study of risk factors for symptomatic urinary tract infection in young women. N Engl J Med 335:468, 1996

JOHNSON JR et al: Systematic review. Antimicrobial urinary catheters to prevent catheter-associated UTI in hospitalized patients. Ann Intern Med 144:116, 2006

SCHOLES D et al: Risk factors associated with acute pyelonephritis in healthy women. Ann Intern Med 142:20, 2005

STAMM WE, SCHAEFFER AJ (eds): *The State of the Art in the Management of Urinary Tract Infections.* Am J Med 113(Suppl 1A):1S, 2002

TALAN DA et al: Comparison of ciprofloxacin (7 days) and trimethoprim-sulfamethoxazole (14 days) for acute uncomplicated pyelonephritis in women. JAMA 283:1583, 2000

WARREN JW et al: Guidelines for antimicrobial therapy of uncomplicated acute bacterial cystitis and acute pyelonephritis in women. Clin Infect Dis 29:745, 1999

283 Urinary Tract Obstruction

Julian L. Seifter, Barry M. Brenner

Obstruction to the flow of urine, with attendant stasis and elevation in urinary tract pressure, impairs renal and urinary conduit functions and is a common cause of acute and chronic renal failure. With early relief of obstruction, the defects in function usually disappear completely. However, chronic obstruction may produce permanent loss of renal mass (renal atrophy) and excretory capability, as well as enhanced susceptibility to local infection and stone formation. Early diagnosis and prompt therapy are, therefore, essential to minimize the otherwise devastating effects of obstruction on kidney structure and function.

ETIOLOGY

Obstruction to urine flow can result from *intrinsic* or *extrinsic mechanical blockade* as well as from *functional defects* not associated with fixed occlusion of the urinary drainage system. Mechanical obstruction can occur at any level of the urinary tract, from the renal calyces to the external urethral meatus. Normal points of narrowing, such as the ureteropelvic and ureterovesical junctions, bladder neck, and urethral meatus, are common sites of obstruction. When blockage is above the level of the bladder, unilateral dilatation of the ureter (*hydroureter*) and renal pyelocalyceal system (*hydronephrosis*) occur; lesions at or below the level of the bladder cause bilateral involvement.

Common forms of obstruction are listed in Table 283-1. Childhood causes include *congenital malformations,* such as narrowing of the ureteropelvic junction and anomalous (retrocaval) location of the ureter. Vesicoureteral reflux is a common cause of prenatal hydronephrosis and, if severe, can lead to recurrent urinary infections and renal scarring in childhood. Hydronephrosis in utero may be associated with oligohydramnios and associated fetal respiratory complications. Posterior urethral valves are the most common cause of bilateral hydronephrosis in boys. Bladder dysfunction may be secondary to congenital urethral stricture, urethral meatal stenosis, or bladder neck obstruction. Prenatal obstructive uropathy may lead to decreased tubular function and decreased nephron number, which may contribute to development of hypertension and chronic kidney disease later in life. In adults, urinary tract

TABLE 283-1 COMMON MECHANICAL CAUSES OF URINARY TRACT OBSTRUCTION

Ureter	Bladder Outlet	Urethra
Congenital		
Ureteropelvic junction narrowing or obstruction	Bladder neck obstruction	Posterior urethral valves
Ureterovesical junction narrowing or obstruction and reflux	Ureterocele	Anterior urethral valves
Ureterocele		Stricture
Retrocaval ureter		Meatal stenosis
		Phimosis
Acquired Intrinsic Defects		
Calculi	Benign prostatic hyperplasia	Stricture
Inflammation	Cancer of prostate	Tumor
Infection	Cancer of bladder	Calculi
Trauma	Calculi	Trauma
Sloughed papillae	Diabetic neuropathy	Phimosis
Tumor	Spinal cord disease	
Blood clots	Anticholinergic drugs and	
Uric acid crystals	α-adrenergic antagonists	
Acquired Extrinsic Defects		
Pregnant uterus	Carcinoma of cervix, colon	Trauma
Retroperitoneal fibrosis	Trauma	
Aortic aneurysm		
Uterine leiomyomata		
Carcinoma of uterus, prostate, bladder, colon, rectum		
Lymphoma		
Pelvic inflammatory disease, endometriosis		
Accidental surgical ligation		

TABLE 283-2 PATHOPHYSIOLOGY OF BILATERAL URETERAL OBSTRUCTION

Hemodynamic Effects	Tubule Effects	Clinical Features
Acute		
↑Renal blood flow ↓GFR ↓Medullary blood flow ↑Vasodilator prostaglandins	↑Ureteral and tubule pressures ↑Reabsorption of Na$^+$, urea, water	Pain (capsule distention) Azotemia Oliguria or anuria
Chronic		
↓Renal blood flow ↓↓GFR ↑Vasoconstrictor prostaglandins ↑Renin-angiotensin production	↓Medullary osmolarity ↓Concentrating ability Structural damage; parenchymal atrophy ↓Transport functions for Na$^+$, K$^+$, H$^+$	Azotemia Hypertension ADH-insensitive polyuria Natriuresis Hyperkalemic, hyperchloremic acidosis
Release of Obstruction		
Slow ↑ in GFR (variable)	↓Tubule pressure ↑Solute load per nephron (urea, NaCl) Natriuretic factors present	Postobstructive diuresis Potential for volume depletion and electrolyte imbalance due to losses of Na$^+$, K$^+$, PO$_4^{2-}$, Mg^{2+}, and water

Note: GFR, glomerular filtration rate.

obstruction (UTO) is due mainly to *acquired defects*. Pelvic tumors, calculi, and urethral stricture predominate. Ligation of, or injury to, the ureter during pelvic or colonic surgery can lead to hydronephrosis which, if unilateral, may remain relatively silent and undetected. *Schistosoma haematobium* and genitourinary tuberculosis are infectious causes of ureteral obstruction. Obstructive uropathy may also result from extrinsic neoplastic (carcinoma of cervix or colon) or inflammatory disorders. Retroperitoneal fibrosis, an inflammatory condition in middle-aged men, must be distinguished from other retroperitoneal causes of ureteral obstruction, particularly lymphomas and pelvic and colonic neoplasms.

Functional impairment of urine flow usually results from disorders that involve both the ureter and bladder. Causes include neurogenic bladder, often with adynamic ureter, and vesicoureteral reflux. Reflux of urine from bladder to ureter(s) is more common in children and may result in severe unilateral or bilateral hydroureter and hydronephrosis. Abnormal insertion of the ureter into the bladder is the most common cause. Vesicoureteral reflux in the absence of urinary tract infection or bladder neck obstruction usually does not lead to renal parenchymal damage and often resolves with age. Reinsertion of the ureter into the bladder is indicated if reflux is severe and unlikely to improve spontaneously, if renal function deteriorates, or if urinary tract infections recur despite chronic antimicrobial therapy. Urinary retention may be the consequence of levodopa, anticholinergic agents, and opiates. Diphenhydramine may decrease bladder emptying in the elderly patient and should be used with caution. Hydronephrosis is common in pregnancy, due both to ureteral compression by the enlarged uterus and to functional effects of progesterone.

CLINICAL FEATURES

The pathophysiology and clinical features of UTO are summarized in Table 283-2. *Pain*, the symptom that most commonly leads to medical attention, is due to distention of the collecting system or renal capsule. Pain severity is influenced more by the rate at which distention develops than by the degree of distention. Acute supravesical obstruction, as from a stone lodged in a ureter (Chap. 281), is associated with excruciating pain, known as *renal colic*. This pain is relatively steady and continuous, with little fluctuation in intensity, and often radiates to the lower abdomen, testes, or labia. By contrast, more insidious causes of obstruction, such as chronic narrowing of the ureteropelvic junction, may produce little or no pain and yet result in total destruction of the affected kidney. Flank pain that occurs only with micturition is pathognomonic of vesicoureteral reflux.

Azotemia develops when overall excretory function is impaired, often in the setting of bladder outlet obstruction, bilateral renal pelvic or ureteric obstruction, or unilateral disease in a patient with a solitary functioning kidney. Complete bilateral obstruction should be suspected when acute renal failure is accompanied by anuria. Any patient with renal failure otherwise unexplained, or with a history of nephrolithiasis, hematuria, diabetes mellitus, prostatic enlargement, pelvic surgery, trauma, or tumor should be evaluated for UTO.

In the acute setting, bilateral obstruction may mimic prerenal azotemia. However, with more prolonged obstruction, symptoms of *polyuria* and *nocturia* commonly accompany partial UTO and result from impaired renal concentrating ability. This defect usually does not improve with administration of vasopressin and is therefore a form of acquired nephrogenic diabetes insipidus. Disturbances in sodium chloride transport in the ascending limb of the loop of Henle and, in azotemic patients, the osmotic (urea) diuresis per nephron lead to decreased medullary hypertonicity and, hence, a concentrating defect. Partial obstruction, therefore, may be associated with increased rather than decreased urine output. Indeed, wide fluctuations in urine output in a patient with azotemia should always raise the possibility of intermittent or partial UTO. If fluid intake is inadequate, severe dehydration and hypernatremia may develop. Hesitancy and straining to initiate the urinary stream, postvoid dribbling, urinary frequency, and incontinence are common with obstruction at or below the level of the bladder.

Partial bilateral UTO often results in *acquired distal renal tubular acidosis*, *hyperkalemia*, and *renal salt wasting*. These defects in tubule function are often accompanied by renal tubulointerstitial damage. Initially the interstitium becomes edematous and infiltrated with mononuclear inflammatory cells. Later, interstitial fibrosis and atrophy of the papillae and medulla occur and precede these processes in the cortex.

UTO must always be considered in patients with urinary tract infections or urolithiasis. Urinary stasis encourages the growth of organisms. Urea-splitting bacteria are associated with magnesium ammonium phosphate (struvite) calculi. *Hypertension* is frequent in acute and subacute unilateral obstruction and is usually a consequence of increased release of renin by the involved kidney. Chronic hydronephrosis, in the presence of extracellular volume expansion, may result in significant hypertension. *Erythrocytosis*, an infrequent complication of obstructive uropathy, is probably secondary to increased erythropoietin production.

DIAGNOSIS

A history of difficulty in voiding, pain, infection, or change in urinary volume is common. Evidence for distention of the kidney or urinary bladder can often be obtained by palpation and percussion of the abdomen. A careful rectal examination may reveal enlargement or nodularity of the prostate, abnormal rectal sphincter tone, or a rectal or pelvic mass. The penis should be inspected for evidence of meatal stenosis or phimosis. In the female, vaginal, uterine, and rectal lesions responsible for UTO are usually revealed by inspection and palpation.

Urinalysis may reveal hematuria, pyuria, and bacteriuria. The urine sediment is often normal, even when obstruction leads to marked azotemia and extensive structural damage. An abdominal scout film may detect nephrocalcinosis or a radiopaque stone. As indicated in Fig. 283-1, if UTO is suspected, a bladder catheter should be inserted. If diuresis does not follow, then abdominal ultrasonography should be performed to evaluate renal and bladder size, as well as pyelocalyceal contour. Ultrasonography is approximately 90% specific and sensitive for detection of hydronephrosis. False-positive results are associated

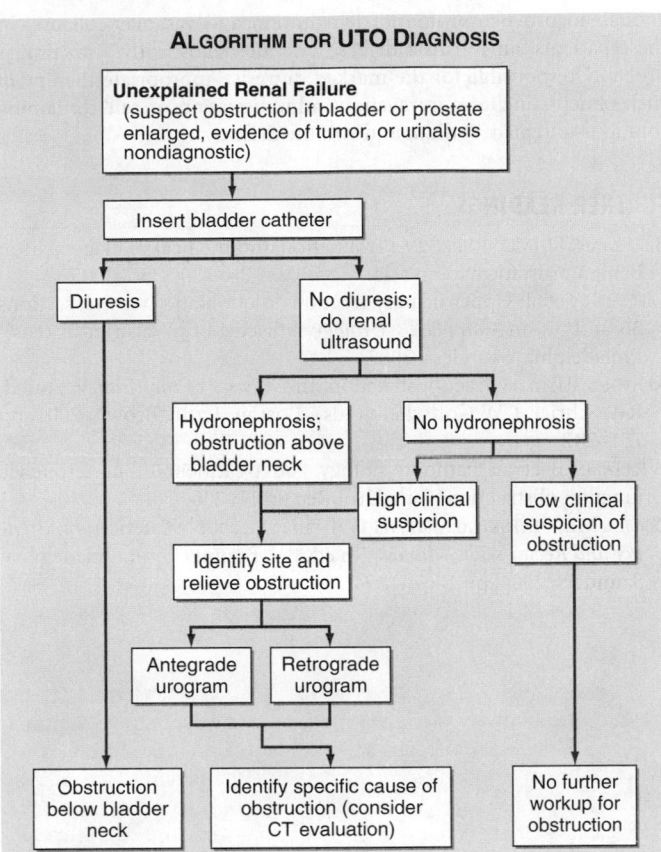

FIGURE 283-1 Diagnostic approach for urinary tract obstruction in unexplained renal failure. CT, computed tomography.

with diuresis, renal cysts, or the presence of an extrarenal pelvis, a normal congenital variant. Hydronephrosis may be absent on ultrasound when obstruction is associated with volume contraction, staghorn calculi, retroperitoneal fibrosis, or infiltrative renal disease. Duplex Doppler ultrasonography may detect an increased resistive index in urinary obstruction, but that finding is not specific. Ultrasound often does not allow visualization of the ureter.

In some cases, the intravenous urogram may define the site of obstruction. In the presence of obstruction, the appearance time of the nephrogram is delayed. Eventually the renal image becomes more dense than normal because of slow tubular fluid flow rate, which results in greater concentration of contrast medium. The kidney involved by an acute obstructive process is usually slightly enlarged, and there is dilatation of the calyces, renal pelvis, and ureter above the obstruction. The ureter is not tortuous as in chronic obstruction. In comparison with the nephrogram, the urogram may be faint, especially if the dilated renal pelvis is voluminous, causing dilution of the contrast medium. The radiographic study should be continued until the site of obstruction is determined or the contrast medium is excreted. Radionuclide scans, though sensitive for the detection of obstruction, define less anatomic detail than intravenous urography and, like the urogram, are of limited value when renal function is poor. They have a role in patients at high risk for reaction to intravenous contrast. Patients suspected of having intermittent ureteropelvic obstruction should have radiologic evaluation while in pain, since a normal urogram is commonly seen during asymptomatic periods. Hydration often helps to provoke a symptomatic attack.

To facilitate visualization of a suspected lesion in a ureter or renal pelvis, *retrograde* or *antegrade urography* should be attempted. These diagnostic studies may be preferable to the intravenous urogram in the azotemic patient, in whom poor excretory function precludes adequate visualization of the collecting system. Furthermore, intravenous urography carries the risk of contrast-induced acute renal failure in patients with proteinuria, renal insufficiency, diabetes mellitus, or multiple myeloma, particularly if they are dehydrated. The retrograde approach in-

volves catheterization of the involved ureter under cystoscopic control, while the antegrade technique necessitates placement of a catheter into the renal pelvis via a needle inserted percutaneously under ultrasonic or fluoroscopic guidance. While the antegrade approach may provide immediate decompression of a unilateral obstructing lesion, many urologists initially attempt the retrograde approach unless the catheterization is unsuccessful or general anesthesia is contraindicated.

Voiding cystourethrography is of value in the diagnosis of vesicoureteral reflux and bladder neck and urethral obstructions. Patients with obstruction at or below the level of the bladder exhibit thickening, trabeculation, and diverticula of the bladder wall. Postvoiding films reveal residual urine. If these radiographic studies fail to provide adequate information for diagnosis, endoscopic visualization by the urologist often permits precise identification of lesions involving the urethra, prostate, bladder, and ureteral orifices.

CT is useful in the diagnosis of specific intraabdominal and retroperitoneal causes of obstruction. The unenhanced helical CT is the preferred study to image obstructing urinary calculi in the patient with colic, and it is also useful in imaging nonobstructing calculi in the patient with hematuria. MRI may also be useful in the identification of specific obstructive causes.

℞ **URINARY TRACT OBSTRUCTION**

UTO complicated by infection requires relief of obstruction as soon as possible to prevent development of generalized sepsis and progressive renal damage. On a temporary basis, drainage is often satisfactorily achieved by nephrostomy, ureterostomy, or ureteral, urethral, or suprapubic catheterization. The patient with acute urinary tract infection and obstruction should be given appropriate antibiotics based on in vitro bacterial sensitivity and the ability of the drug to concentrate in the urine. Treatment may be required for 3–4 weeks. Chronic or recurrent infections in an obstructed kidney with poor intrinsic function may necessitate nephrectomy. When infection is not present, immediate surgery often is not required, even in the presence of complete obstruction and anuria because of the availability of dialysis, until acid-base, fluid and electrolyte, and cardiovascular status are restored. Nevertheless, the site of obstruction should be ascertained as soon as feasible, in part because of the possibility that sepsis may occur, a complication that necessitates prompt urologic intervention. Elective relief of obstruction is usually recommended in patients with urinary retention, recurrent urinary tract infections, persistent pain, or progressive loss of renal function. Benign prostatic hypertrophy may be treated medically with alpha adrenergic blockers and 5α-reductase inhibitors. Mechanical obstruction may be alleviated by radiation therapy in cases of retroperitoneal lymphoma. Functional obstruction secondary to neurogenic bladder may be decreased with the combination of frequent voiding and cholinergic drugs. **The approach to obstruction secondary to renal stones is discussed in Chap. 281.**

PROGNOSIS

With relief of obstruction, the prognosis regarding return of renal function depends largely on whether irreversible renal damage has occurred. When obstruction is not relieved, the course will depend mainly on whether the obstruction is complete or incomplete and bilateral or unilateral, as well as whether or not urinary tract infection is also present. Complete obstruction with infection can lead to total destruction of the kidney within days. Partial return of glomerular filtration rate may follow relief of complete obstruction of 1 and 2 weeks' duration, but after 8 weeks of obstruction, recovery is unlikely. In the absence of definitive evidence of irreversibility, every effort should be made to decompress the obstruction in the hope of restoring renal function at least partially. A renal radionuclide scan, performed after a prolonged period of decompression, may be used to predict the reversibility of renal dysfunction.

POSTOBSTRUCTIVE DIURESIS

Relief of bilateral, but not unilateral, complete obstruction commonly results in polyuria, which may be massive. The urine is usually hypotonic and may contain large amounts of sodium chloride, potassium, and magnesium. The natriuresis is due in part to the excretion of retained urea (osmotic diuresis). The increase in intratubular pressure very likely also contributes to the impairment in net sodium chloride reabsorption, especially in the terminal nephron segments. Natriuretic factors may also accumulate during uremia and depress salt and water reabsorption when urine flow is reestablished. In the majority of patients this diuresis results in the *appropriate* excretion of the excesses of retained salt and water. When extracellular volume and composition return to normal, the diuresis usually abates spontaneously. Therefore, replacement of urinary losses should only be done in the setting of hypovolemia, hypotension, or disturbances in serum electrolyte concentrations. Occasionally, iatrogenic expansion of extracellular volume is responsible for, or sustains, the diuresis observed in the postobstructive period. Replacement of no more than two-thirds of urinary volume losses per day is usually effective in avoiding this complication. The loss of electrolyte-free water with urea may result in hypernatremia. Serum and urine sodium and osmolal concentrations should guide the use of appropriate intravenous replacement. Often replacement with 0.45% saline is required. In a rare patient, relief of obstruction may be followed by urinary salt and water losses severe enough to provoke profound dehydration and vascular collapse. In these patients, an intrinsic defect in tubule reabsorptive function is probably responsible for the marked diuresis. Appropriate therapy in such patients includes intravenous administration of salt-containing solutions to replace sodium and volume deficits.

FURTHER READINGS

BECKMAN TJ, MYNDERSE LA: Evaluation and medical management of benign prostatic hyperplasia. Mayo Clin Proc 80:1356, 2005

GULMI FA et al: Upper urinary tract obstruction and trauma, sections 36 and 37, in *Campbell's Urology*, 9th ed., PC Walsh et al (eds). Philadelphia, Saunders, 2007

KLAHR S: Urinary tract obstruction, in *Diseases of the Kidney*, 7th ed, RW Schrier, CW Gottschalk (eds). Boston, Little, Brown, 2001, pp 751–787

WILLIAMS B et al: Pathophysiology and treatment of ureteropelvic junction obstruction. Curr Urol Rep 8:111, 2007

ZEIDEL ML, PIRTSKHALAISHVILI G: Urinary tract obstruction, in: *Brenner and Rector's The Kidney*, 7th ed, BM Brenner (ed). Philadelphia, Saunders, 2004, pp 1867–1894

284   Approach to the Patient with Gastrointestinal Disease

William L. Hasler, Chung Owyang

ANATOMIC CONSIDERATIONS

The gastrointestinal (GI) tract extends from the mouth to the anus and comprises several organs with distinct functions. Separating the organs are specialized independently controlled thickened sphincters that assist in gut compartmentalization. The gut wall is organized into well-defined layers that contribute to the functional activities in each region. The mucosa serves as a barrier to luminal contents or as a site for transfer of fluids or nutrients. Gut smooth muscle mediates propulsion from one region to the next. Many GI organs possess a serosal layer that provides a supportive foundation but that also permits external input.

Interactions with other organ systems serve the needs both of the gut and the body. Pancreaticobiliary conduits deliver bile and enzymes into the duodenum. A rich vascular supply is modulated by GI tract activity. Lymphatic channels assist in gut immune activities. Intrinsic gut wall nerves provide the basic controls for propulsion and fluid regulation. Extrinsic neural input provides volitional or involuntary control to degrees that are specific for each gut region.

FUNCTIONS OF THE GASTROINTESTINAL TRACT

The GI tract serves two main functions—assimilation of nutrients and elimination of waste. The gut anatomy is organized to serve these functions. In the mouth, food is processed, mixed with salivary amylase, and delivered to the luminal GI tract. The esophagus propels the bolus into the stomach, and the lower esophageal sphincter prevents oral reflux of gastric contents. The esophageal mucosa has a protective squamous histology that does not permit significant diffusion or absorption. The propulsive activities of the esophagus are exclusively aboral and are coordinated with relaxation of the upper and lower esophageal sphincters upon swallowing.

The stomach furthers food preparation by triturating and mixing the bolus with pepsin and acid. Gastric acid also sterilizes the upper gut. Gastric motor activities exhibit regional variability. The proximal stomach serves a storage function by relaxing to accommodate the meal. The distal stomach exhibits phasic contractions that propel solid food residue against the pylorus where it is repeatedly propelled proximally for further mixing before it is emptied into the duodenum. Finally, the stomach secretes intrinsic factor for vitamin B_{12} absorption.

The small intestine serves most of the nutrient absorptive function of the gut. The intestinal mucosa exhibits villous architecture to provide maximal surface area for absorption and is endowed with specialized enzymes and transporters. Triturated food from the stomach is mixed with pancreatic juice and bile in the proximal duodenum to facilitate digestion. Pancreatic juice contains the main enzymes for carbohydrate, protein, and fat digestion as well as bicarbonate to optimize the pH for activation of these enzymes. Bile secreted by the liver and stored in the gallbladder is essential for intestinal lipid digestion. The proximal intestine is optimized for rapid absorption of nutrient breakdown products and most minerals, while the ileum is better suited for absorption of vitamin B_{12} and bile acids. The small intestine also aids in waste elimination. Bile contains byproducts of erythrocyte degradation, toxins,

metabolized and unaltered medications, and cholesterol. Motor function of the small intestine delivers indigestible food residue and sloughed enterocytes into the colon for further processing. The small intestine terminates in the ileocecal junction, a sphincteric structure that prevents coloileal reflux and maintains small-intestinal sterility.

The colon prepares the waste material for controlled evacuation. The colonic mucosa dehydrates the stool, decreasing daily fecal volumes from 1000–1500 mL delivered from the ileum to 100–200 mL expelled from the rectum. The colonic lumen possesses a dense bacterial colonization that ferments undigested carbohydrates and short-chain fatty acids. Whereas transit times in the esophagus are on the order of seconds and times in the stomach and small intestine range from minutes to a few hours, propagation through the colon takes >1 day in most individuals. Colonic motor patterns exhibit a to-and-fro character that facilitates slow fecal desiccation. The proximal colon serves to mix and absorb fluid, while the distal colon exhibits peristaltic contractions and mass actions that function to expel the stool. The colon terminates in the anus, a structure with volitional and involuntary controls to permit retention of the fecal bolus until it can be released in a socially convenient setting.

EXTRINSIC MODULATION OF GUT FUNCTION

GI function is modified by influences outside of the gut. Unlike other organ systems, the gut is in physical continuity with the outside environment. Thus, protective mechanisms are vigilant against the deleterious effects of consumed foods, medications, toxins, and infectious organisms. Mucosal immune mechanisms include an indwelling lymphocyte and plasma cell population in the epithelial layer and lamina propria backed up by lymph node chains to prevent noxious agents from entering the circulation. All substances absorbed into the bloodstream are filtered through the liver via the portal venous circulation. In the liver, many drugs and toxins are detoxified by a variety of mechanisms. Although intrinsic nerves control most basic gut activities, extrinsic neural input affects a number of functions. The two activities under voluntary control are swallowing and defecation. Many normal GI reflexes involve extrinsic vagus or splanchnic nerve pathways. An active brain gut axis further alters function in regions not under volitional regulation. As an example, stress has potent effects on gut motor, secretory, and sensory function.

OVERVIEW OF GASTROINTESTINAL DISEASES

GI diseases develop as a consequence of abnormalities within or outside of the gut and range in severity from those that produce mild symptoms and no long-term morbidity to those with intractable symptoms or an adverse outcome. Diseases may be localized to a single organ or exhibit diffuse involvement at a number of sites.

CLASSIFICATION OF GI DISEASES

GI diseases are manifestations of alterations in nutrient assimilation or waste evacuation or in the activities supporting these main functions.

Impaired Digestion and Absorption   Diseases of the stomach, intestine, biliary tree, and pancreas can disrupt nutrient digestion and absorption. Gastric hypersecretory conditions such as Zollinger-Ellison syndrome damage the intestinal mucosa, impair pancreatic enzyme activation, and accelerate transit due to excess gastric acid. The most common intestinal maldigestion syndrome, lactase deficiency, produces gas and diarrhea after consumption of dairy products and has no adverse effect on survival. Other intestinal enzyme deficiencies produce similar symptoms with ingestion of other simple sugars. Conversely, celiac disease, bacterial overgrowth, infectious enteritis, Crohn's ileitis, and radiation damage, which affect digestion and/or absorption more diffusely, produce anemia, dehydration, electrolyte disorders, or malnutrition. Biliary obstruction from stricture or neoplasm may impair fat digestion. Impaired release of pancreatic enzymes in chronic pancreatitis or pancreatic cancer decreases intraluminal digestion and can lead to profound malnutrition.

Altered Secretion   Selected GI diseases result from dysregulation of gut secretion. Gastric acid hypersecretion occurs in Zollinger-Ellison syndrome, G cell hyperplasia, retained antrum syndrome, and some individuals with duodenal ulcer disease. Conversely, patients with atrophic gastritis or pernicious anemia release little or no gastric acid. Inflammatory and infectious small-intestinal and colonic diseases produce fluid loss through impaired absorption or enhanced secretion, but usually do not cause malnutrition. Common intestinal and colonic hypersecretory conditions cause diarrhea and these include acute bacterial or viral infection, chronic *Giardia* or *Cryptosporidia* infections, small-intestinal bacterial overgrowth, bile salt diarrhea, microscopic colitis, diabetic diarrhea, and abuse of certain laxatives. Less common causes include large colonic villous adenomas and endocrine neoplasias with tumor overproduction of secretagogue transmitters such as vasoactive intestinal polypeptide.

Altered Gut Transit   Alterations in gut transit may be due to mechanical obstruction. Esophageal occlusion often results from acid-induced stricture or neoplasm. Gastric outlet obstruction develops from peptic ulcer disease or gastric cancer. Small-intestinal obstruction most commonly results from adhesions but may also occur with Crohn's disease, radiation- or drug-induced strictures, and less likely malignancy. The most common cause of colonic obstruction is colon cancer, although inflammatory strictures develop in patients with inflammatory bowel disease, after certain infections, or with some drugs.

Retardation of propulsion also develops from disordered gut motor function. *Achalasia* is characterized by impaired esophageal body peristalsis and incomplete lower esophageal sphincter relaxation. *Gastroparesis* is the symptomatic delay in gastric emptying of solid or liquid meals secondary to impaired gastric motility. Intestinal pseudoobstruction causes marked delays in small-bowel transit due to injury to enteric nerves or intestinal smooth muscle. Slow-transit constipation is produced by diffusely impaired colonic propulsion. Constipation is also produced by outlet abnormalities such as rectal prolapse, intussusception, or failure of anal relaxation upon attempted defecation.

Disorders of rapid propulsion are less common than those with delayed transit. Rapid gastric emptying occurs in postvagotomy dumping syndrome, with gastric hypersecretion, and in some cases of functional dyspepsia and cyclic vomiting syndrome. Exaggerated intestinal or colonic motor patterns may be responsible for diarrhea in irritable bowel syndrome. Accelerated transit with hyperdefecation is noted in hyperthyroidism.

Immune Dysregulation   Many inflammatory GI conditions are consequences of altered gut immune function. The mucosal inflammation of celiac disease results from dietary ingestion of gluten-containing grains. Some patients with food allergy also exhibit altered immune populations. Eosinophilic esophagitis and eosinophilic gastroenteritis are inflammatory disorders with prominent mucosal eosinophils. Ulcerative colitis and Crohn's disease are disorders of uncertain etiology that produce mucosal injury primarily in the lower gut. The microscopic colitides, lymphocytic and collagenous colitis, exhibit colonic subepithelial infiltrates without visible mucosal damage. Bacterial, viral, and protozoal organisms may produce ileitis or colitis in selected patient populations.

Impaired Gut Blood Flow   Different GI regions are at variable risk for ischemic damage from impaired blood flow. Rare cases of gastroparesis result from blockage of the celiac and superior mesenteric arteries. More commonly encountered are intestinal and colonic ischemia, which are consequences of arterial embolus, arterial thrombosis, venous thrombosis, or hypoperfusion from dehydration, sepsis, hemorrhage, or reduced cardiac output. These may produce mucosal injury, hemorrhage, or even perforation. Some cases of radiation enterocolitis exhibit reduced mucosal blood flow.

Neoplastic Degeneration   All GI regions are susceptible to malignant degeneration to varying degrees. In the United States, colorectal cancer is most common and typically presents after age 50. Worldwide, gastric cancer is prevalent, especially in certain Asian regions. Esophageal cancer develops with chronic acid reflux or in those with an extensive alcohol or tobacco use history. Small-intestinal neoplasms are rare and occur with underlying inflammatory disease. Anal cancers may arise with prior anal infection or inflammation. Pancreatic and biliary cancers elicit severe pain, weight loss, and jaundice and have poor prognoses. Hepatocellular carcinoma usually arises in the setting of chronic viral hepatitis or cirrhosis secondary to other causes. Most GI cancers are carcinomas, but lymphomas and tumors of other cell types also are observed.

Disorders without Obvious Organic Abnormalities   The most common GI disorders show no abnormalities on biochemical or structural testing and include irritable bowel syndrome (IBS), functional dyspepsia, non-cardiac chest pain, and functional heartburn. These functional bowel disorders exhibit altered gut motor function; however, the pathogenic relevance of these abnormalities is uncertain. Exaggerated visceral sensory responses to noxious stimulation may cause discomfort in these disorders. Symptoms in other patients result from altered processing of visceral pain sensations in the central nervous system. Functional bowel patients with severe symptoms may exhibit significant emotional disturbances on psychometric testing.

Genetic Influences   Although many GI diseases result from environmental factors, others exhibit hereditary components. Family members of inflammatory bowel disease (IBD) patients show a genetic predisposition to disease development themselves. Colonic and esophageal malignancies arise in certain inherited disorders. Rare genetic dysmotility syndromes are described. Familial clustering is even observed in the functional bowel disorders, although this may be learned familial illness behavior rather than a true hereditary factor.

SYMPTOMS OF GASTROINTESTINAL DISEASE

The most common GI symptoms are abdominal pain, heartburn, nausea and vomiting, altered bowel habits, GI bleeding, and jaundice (Table 284-1). Others are dysphagia, anorexia, weight loss, fatigue, and extraintestinal symptoms.

Abdominal Pain   Abdominal pain results from GI disease and extraintestinal conditions involving the genitourinary tract, abdominal wall, thorax, or spine. Visceral pain generally is midline in location and vague in character, while parietal pain is localized and precisely described. Common inflammatory diseases with pain include peptic ulcer, appendicitis, diverticulitis, IBD, and infectious enterocolitis. Other intraabdominal causes of pain include gallstone disease and pancreatitis. Noninflammatory visceral sources include mesenteric ischemia and neoplasia. The most common causes of abdominal pain are IBS and functional dyspepsia.

Heartburn   Heartburn, a burning substernal sensation, is reported intermittently by at least 40% of the population. Classically, heartburn is felt to result from excess gastroesophageal reflux of acid. However, some cases exhibit normal esophageal acid exposure and may result from heightened sensitivity of esophageal mucosal nerves.

Nausea and Vomiting   Nausea and vomiting are caused by GI diseases, medications, toxins, acute and chronic infection, endocrine disor-

TABLE 284-1 COMMON CAUSES OF COMMON GI SYMPTOMS

Abdominal Pain	Nausea and Vomiting	Diarrhea	GI Bleeding	Obstructive Jaundice
Appendicitis	Medications	Infection	Ulcer disease	Bile duct stones
Gallstone disease	GI obstruction	Poorly absorbed	Esophagitis	Cholangio-
Pancreatitis	Motor disorders	sugars	Varices	carcinoma
Diverticulitis	Functional	Inflammatory	Vascular lesions	Cholangitis
Ulcer disease	bowel disorder	bowel disease	Neoplasm	Sclerosing
Esophagitis	Enteric infection	Microscopic	Diverticula	cholangitis
GI obstruction	Pregnancy	colitis	Hemorrhoids	Ampullary
Inflammatory	Endocrine	Functional	Fissures	stenosis
bowel disease	disease	bowel disorder	Inflammatory	Ampullary
Functional	Motion sickness	Celiac disease	bowel disease	carcinoma
bowel disorder	Central nervous	Pancreatic	Infectious colitis	Pancreatitis
Vascular disease	system disease	insufficiency		Pancreatic tumor
Gynecologic		Hyperthyroidism		
causes		Ischemia		
Renal stone		Endocrine tumor		

ders, labyrinthine conditions, and central nervous system disease. The best-characterized GI etiologies relate to mechanical obstruction of the upper gut; however, disorders of propulsion including gastroparesis and intestinal pseudoobstruction also elicit prominent symptoms. Nausea and vomiting also are commonly reported by patients with IBS and functional disorders of the upper gut (including chronic idiopathic nausea and functional vomiting).

Altered Bowel Habits Altered bowel habits are common complaints of patients with GI disease. Constipation is reported as infrequent defecation, straining with defecation, passage of hard stools, or a sense of incomplete fecal evacuation. Causes of constipation include obstruction, motor disorders of the colon, medications, and endocrine diseases such as hypothyroidism and hyperparathyroidism. Diarrhea is reported as frequent defecation, passage of loose or watery stools, fecal urgency, or a similar sense of incomplete evacuation. The differential diagnosis of diarrhea is broad and includes infections, inflammatory causes, malabsorption, and medications. IBS produces constipation, diarrhea, or an alternating bowel pattern. Fecal mucus is common in IBS, while pus characterizes inflammatory disease. Steatorrhea develops with malabsorption.

GI Bleeding Hemorrhage may develop from any gut organ. Most commonly, upper GI bleeding presents with melena or hematemesis, whereas lower GI bleeding produces passage of bright red or maroon stools. However, briskly bleeding upper sites can elicit voluminous red rectal bleeding, while slowly bleeding ascending colon sites may produce melena. Chronic slow GI bleeding may present with iron-deficiency anemia. The most common upper GI causes of bleeding are ulcer disease, gastroduodenitis, and esophagitis. Other etiologies include portal hypertension, malignancy, tears across the gastroesophageal junction, and vascular lesions. The most prevalent lower GI sources of hemorrhage include hemorrhoids, anal fissures, diverticula, ischemic colitis, and arteriovenous malformations. Other causes include neoplasm, IBD, infectious colitis, drug-induced colitis, and other vascular lesions.

Jaundice Jaundice results from prehepatic, intrahepatic, or posthepatic disease. Posthepatic causes of jaundice include biliary diseases such as choledocholithiasis, cholangitis, stricture, and neoplasm and pancreatic disorders such as acute and chronic pancreatitis, stricture, and malignancy.

Other Symptoms Other symptoms may be manifestations of GI disease. Dysphagia, odynophagia, and unexplained chest pain suggest esophageal disease. A globus sensation is reported with esophagopharyngeal conditions but also occurs with functional GI disorders. Weight loss, anorexia, and fatigue are nonspecific symptoms of neoplastic, inflammatory, gut motility, pancreatic, small-bowel mucosal,

and psychiatric conditions. Fever is reported with inflammatory illness, but malignancies also evoke febrile responses. GI disorders also produce extraintestinal symptoms. IBD is associated with hepatobiliary dysfunction, skin and eye lesions, and arthritis. Celiac disease may present with dermatitis herpetiformis. Jaundice can produce pruritus. Conversely, systemic diseases can have GI consequences. Systemic lupus may cause gut ischemia, presenting with pain or bleeding. Overwhelming stress or severe burns may lead to gastric ulcer formation.

EVALUATION OF THE PATIENT WITH GASTROINTESTINAL DISEASE

Evaluation of the patient with GI disease begins with a careful history and physical examination. Subsequent investigation with a variety of tools designed to test the structure or function of the gut is indicated in selected cases. Some patients exhibit normal findings on diagnostic testing. In these individuals, validated symptom profiles are employed for confident diagnosis of a functional bowel disorder.

HISTORY

The history of the patient with suspected GI disease has several components. Symptom timing can suggest specific etiologies. Symptoms of short duration commonly result from acute infection, toxin exposure, or abrupt inflammation or ischemia. Long-standing symptoms point to an underlying chronic inflammatory or neoplastic condition or a functional bowel disorder. Symptoms from mechanical obstruction, ischemia, IBD, and functional bowel disorders are worsened by meal ingestion. Conversely, ulcer symptoms may be relieved by eating or antacids. The symptom pattern and duration may suggest underlying etiologies. Ulcer pain occurs at intermittent intervals lasting weeks to months, whereas biliary colic has a sudden onset and lasts up to several hours. Pain from acute inflammation, as with acute pancreatitis, is severe and persists for days to weeks. Meals elicit diarrhea in some cases of IBD and IBS; defecation relieves discomfort in both. Functional bowel disorders are exacerbated by stress. Sudden awakening from sound sleep suggests organic disease rather than a functional bowel disorder. Diarrhea from malabsorption usually improves with fasting, while secretory diarrhea persists without oral intake.

Symptom relation to other factors narrows the list of diagnostic possibilities. Obstructive symptoms with prior abdominal surgery raise concern for adhesions, whereas loose stools after gastrectomy or gallbladder excision suggest dumping syndrome or post-cholecystectomy diarrhea. Symptom onset after travel prompts a search for enteric infection. Medications or food supplements may produce pain, altered bowel habits, or GI bleeding. Lower GI bleeding likely results from a neoplasm, diverticula, or vascular lesions in an older person and anorectal abnormalities or IBD in a younger individual. Celiac disease is prevalent in people of Irish descent, whereas IBD is more common in certain Jewish populations. A sexual history may raise concern for sexually transmitted diseases or immunodeficiency.

Over the past two decades, working groups have been convened to devise symptom criteria to improve the confident diagnosis of the functional bowel disorders and to minimize the numbers of unnecessary diagnostic tests performed. The most widely accepted symptom-based criteria are the *Rome criteria*. When tested against findings of structural investigations, the Rome criteria exhibit diagnostic specificities >90% for many of the functional bowel disorders.

PHYSICAL EXAMINATION

The physical examination complements information from the history. Abnormal vital signs provide diagnostic clues and determine the need for acute intervention. Fever suggests inflammation or neoplasm.

Orthostasis is found with significant blood loss, dehydration, sepsis, or autonomic neuropathy. Skin, eye, or joint findings may point to specific diagnoses. Neck examination with swallowing assessment evaluates dysphagia. Cardiopulmonary disease may present with abdominal pain or nausea; thus, lung and cardiac examinations are important. Pelvic examination tests for a gynecologic source of abdominal pain. Rectal examination may detect blood indicating gut mucosal injury or neoplasm or a palpable inflammatory mass in appendicitis. Metabolic conditions and gut motor disorders have associated peripheral neuropathy.

Inspection of the abdomen may reveal distention from obstruction, tumor, or ascites or vascular abnormalities with liver disease. Ecchymoses develop with severe pancreatitis. Auscultation can detect bruits or friction rubs from vascular disease or hepatic tumors. Loss of bowel sounds signifies ileus, while high-pitched, hyperactive sounds characterize intestinal obstruction. Percussion assesses liver size and can detect shifting dullness from ascites. Palpation assesses for hepatosplenomegaly as well as neoplastic or inflammatory masses. Abdominal examination is helpful in evaluating unexplained pain. Intestinal ischemia elicits severe pain but little tenderness. Patients with visceral pain may exhibit generalized discomfort, while those with parietal pain or peritonitis have directed pain, often with involuntary guarding, rigidity, or rebound. Patients with musculoskeletal abdominal wall pain may note tenderness exacerbated by Valsalva or straight leg lift maneuvers.

TOOLS FOR PATIENT EVALUATION

Laboratory, radiographic, and functional tests can assist in diagnosis of suspected GI disease. The GI tract is also amenable to internal evaluation with upper and lower endoscopy and to examination of luminal contents. Histopathologic examinations of gastrointestinal tissues complement these tests.

Laboratory   Selected laboratory tests facilitate the diagnosis of GI disease. Iron-deficiency anemia suggests mucosal blood loss, whereas vitamin B_{12} deficiency results from small-intestinal, gastric, or pancreatic disease. Either can also result from inadequate oral intake. Leukocytosis and increased sedimentation rates are found in inflammatory conditions, while leukopenia is seen in viremic illness. Severe vomiting or diarrhea elicits electrolyte disturbances, acid-base abnormalities, and elevated blood urea nitrogen. Pancreaticobiliary or liver disease is suggested by elevated pancreatic or liver chemistries. Thyroid chemistries, cortisol, and calcium levels are obtained to exclude endocrinologic causes of GI symptoms. Pregnancy testing is considered for young women with unexplained nausea. Serologies tests are available to screen for celiac disease, IBD, and rheumatologic diseases such as lupus or scleroderma. Hormone levels are obtained for suspected endocrine neoplasia. Intraabdominal malignancies produce tumor markers including the carcinoembryonic antigen CA 19-9 and α-fetoprotein. Paraneoplastic serology panels can be ordered for individuals with gut dysmotility that is believed to be a consequence of extraintestinal neoplasm. Other body fluids are sampled under certain circumstances. Ascitic fluid is analyzed for infection, malignancy, or findings of portal hypertension. Cerebrospinal fluid is obtained for suspected central nervous system causes of vomiting. Urine samples are screened for carcinoid, porphyria, and heavy metal intoxication.

Luminal Contents   Luminal contents can be examined for diagnostic clues. Stool samples are cultured for bacterial pathogens, examined for leukocytes and parasites, or tested for *Giardia* antigen. Duodenal aspirates can be examined for parasites or cultured for bacterial

overgrowth. Fecal fat is quantified in possible malabsorption. Stool electrolytes can be measured in diarrheal conditions. Laxative screens are done when laxative abuse is suspected. Gastric acid is quantified to rule out Zollinger-Ellison syndrome. Esophageal pH testing is done for refractory symptoms of acid reflux, whereas newer impedance techniques assess for nonacidic reflux. Pancreatic juice is analyzed for enzyme or bicarbonate content to exclude pancreatic exocrine insufficiency.

Endoscopy   The gut is accessible with endoscopy which can provide the diagnosis of the causes of bleeding, pain, nausea and vomiting, weight loss, altered bowel function, and fever. Table 284-2 lists the most common indications for the major endoscopic procedures. Upper endoscopy evaluates the esophagus, stomach, and duodenum, while colonoscopy assesses the colon and distal ileum. Upper endoscopy is advocated as the initial structural test performed in patients with suspected ulcer disease, esophagitis, neoplasm, malabsorption, and Barrett's metaplasia because of its ability to directly visualize as well as biopsy the abnormality. Colonoscopy is the procedure of choice for colon cancer screening and surveillance as well as diagnosis of colitis secondary to infection, ischemia, radiation, and IBD. Sigmoidoscopy examines the colon up to the splenic flexure and is currently used to exclude distal colonic inflammation or obstruction in young patients not at significant risk for colon cancer. For elusive GI bleeding due to arteriovenous malformations or superficial ulcers, small-intestinal examination is performed with push enteroscopy, capsule endoscopy, or the novel technique of double-balloon enteroscopy. Capsule endoscopy is also increasingly being employed to visualize small-intestinal Crohn's disease in individuals with negative barium radiography. Endoscopic retrograde cholangiopancreaticography (ERCP) provides diagnoses of pancreatic and biliary disease. Endoscopic ultrasound can evaluate the extent of disease in GI malignancy as well as exclude choledocholithiasis, evaluate pancreatitis, drain pancreatic pseudocysts, and assess anal continuity.

Radiography/Nuclear Medicine   Radiographic tests evaluate diseases of the gut and extraluminal structures. Oral or rectal contrast agents such as barium provide mucosal definition from the esophagus to the rectum. Contrast radiography also assesses gut transit and pelvic floor dysfunction. Barium swallow is the initial procedure for evaluation of dysphagia to exclude subtle rings or strictures and assess for achalasia, whereas small-bowel contrast radiology reliably diagnoses intestinal tumors and Crohn's ileitis. Contrast enemas are performed when colonoscopy is unsuccessful or contraindicated. Ultrasound and CT evaluate regions not accessible by endoscopy or contrast studies, including the liver, pancreas, gallbladder, kidneys, and retroperitoneum.

TABLE 284-2   COMMON INDICATIONS FOR ENDOSCOPY

Upper Endoscopy	Colonoscopy	Endoscopic Retrograde Cholangiopancreatography	Endoscopic Ultrasound
Dyspepsia despite treatment	Cancer screening	Jaundice	Staging of malignancy
Dyspepsia with signs of organic disease	Lower GI bleeding	Postbiliary surgery complaints	Characterize and biopsy submucosal mass
Refractory vomiting	Diarrhea	Cholangitis	
Dysphagia	Polypectomy	Gallstone pancreatitis	Bile duct stones
Upper GI bleeding	Obstruction	Pancreatic/biliary/ampullary tumor	Chronic pancreatitis
Anemia	Biopsy radiologic abnormality	Unexplained pancreatitis	Drain pseudocyst
Weight loss	Cancer surveillance: family history, prior polyp/cancer, colitis	Pancreatitis with unrelenting pain	Large gastric folds
Malabsorption		Fistulas	Anal continuity
Biopsy radiologic abnormality	Palliate neoplasm	Biopsy radiologic abnormality	
Polypectomy	Remove foreign body	Pancreaticobiliary drainage	
Place gastrostomy		Sample bile	
Barrett's surveillance		Sphincter of Oddi manometry	
Palliate neoplasm			
Sample duodenal tissue/fluid			
Remove foreign body			

These tests are useful for diagnosis of mass lesions, fluid collections, organ enlargement, and in the case of ultrasound gallstones. CT and MR colonography are being evaluated as alternatives to colonoscopy for colon cancer screening. MRI assesses the pancreaticobiliary ducts to exclude neoplasm, stones, and sclerosing cholangitis, and the liver to characterize benign and malignant tumors. Angiography excludes mesenteric ischemia and determines spread of malignancy. Angiographic techniques also access the biliary tree in obstructive jaundice. CT and MR techniques can be used to screen for mesenteric occlusion, thereby limiting exposure to angiographic dyes. Positron emission tomography is showing promise in distinguishing malignant from benign disease in several organ systems.

Scintigraphy both evaluates structural abnormalities and quantifies luminal transit. Radionuclide bleeding scans localize bleeding sites in patients with brisk hemorrhage so that therapy with endoscopy, angiography, or surgery may be directed. Radiolabeled leukocyte scans can search for intraabdominal abscesses not visualized on CT. Biliary scintigraphy is complementary to ultrasound in the assessment of cholecystitis. Scintigraphy to quantify esophageal and gastric emptying are well established, while techniques to measure small-intestinal or colonic transit are less widely used.

Histopathology Gut mucosal biopsies obtained at endoscopy evaluate for inflammatory, infectious, and neoplastic disease. Deep rectal biopsies assist with diagnosis of Hirschsprung's disease or amyloid. Liver biopsy is indicated in cases with abnormal liver chemistries, unexplained jaundice, following liver transplant to exclude rejection, and to characterize the degree of inflammation in patients with chronic viral hepatitis before initiating antiviral therapy. Biopsies obtained during CT or ultrasound can evaluate for other intraabdominal conditions not accessible by endoscopy.

Functional Testing Tests of gut function provide important data when structural testing is nondiagnostic. In addition to gastric acid and pancreatic function testing, functional testing of motor activity is provided by regional manometric techniques. Esophageal manometry is useful for suspected achalasia, whereas small-intestinal manometry tests for pseudoobstruction. In addition to scintigraphy, breath tests and capsule techniques are available for quantifying gastric emptying. Anorectal manometry with balloon expulsion testing is employed for unexplained incontinence or constipation from outlet dysfunction. Biliary manometry tests for sphincter of Oddi dysfunction with unexplained biliary pain. Electrogastrography measures gastric electrical activity in individuals with nausea and vomiting, whereas electromyography assesses anal function in fecal incontinence. Measurement of breath hydrogen while fasting and after oral mono- or oligosaccharide challenge can screen for carbohydrate intolerance and small-intestinal bacterial overgrowth.

℞ GASTROINTESTINAL DISEASE

Management options for the patient with GI disease depend on the cause of symptoms. Available treatments include modifications in dietary intake, medications, interventional endoscopy or radiology techniques, surgery, and therapies directed to external influences.

NUTRITIONAL MANIPULATION Dietary modifications for GI disease include treatments that only reduce symptoms, therapies that correct pathologic defects, and measures that replace normal food intake with enteral or parenteral formulations. Changes that improve symptoms but do not reverse an organic abnormality include lactose restriction for lactase deficiency, liquid meals in gastroparesis, carbohydrate restrictions in dumping syndrome, and high-fiber diets in IBS. The gluten-free diet for celiac disease exemplifies a modification that serves as primary therapy to reduce mucosal inflammation. Enteral medium-chain triglycerides replace normal fats with short-gut syndrome or severe ileal disease. Perfusion of liquid meals through a gastrostomy is performed in those who cannot swallow safely. Enteral feeding through a jejunostomy is considered for gastric dysmotility syndromes that preclude feeding into the stomach. Intravenous hyperalimentation is employed for individuals with generalized gut malfunction who cannot tolerate or who cannot be sustained with enteral nutrition.

PHARMACOTHERAPY Several medications are available to treat GI diseases. Considerable health care resources are expended on over-the-counter remedies. Many prescription drug classes are offered as short-term or continuous therapy of GI illness. A plethora of alternative treatments have gained popularity in GI conditions for which traditional therapies provide incomplete relief.

Over-the-Counter Agents Over-the-counter agents are reserved for mild GI symptoms. Antacids and histamine H_2 antagonists decrease symptoms in gastroesophageal reflux and dyspepsia, whereas antiflatulents and adsorbents reduce gaseous symptoms. More potent acid inhibitors such as proton pump inhibitors are now available over the counter for treatment of chronic gastrointestinal reflux disease. Fiber supplements, stool softeners, enemas, and laxatives are used for constipation. Laxatives are categorized as stimulants, saline cathartics, and poorly absorbed sugars. Nonprescription antidiarrheal agents include bismuth subsalicylate, kaolin pectin combinations, and loperamide. Supplemental enzymes include lactase pills for lactose intolerance and bacterial α-galactosidase to treat excess gas. In general, use of a nonprescription preparation for more than a short time for chronic persistent symptoms should be supervised by a health care provider.

Prescription Drugs Prescription drugs for GI diseases are a major focus of attention from pharmaceutical companies. Potent acid suppressants including drugs that inhibit the proton pump are advocated for acid reflux when over-the-counter preparations are inadequate. Cytoprotective agents sometimes are used for upper gut ulcers. Prokinetic drugs stimulate GI propulsion in gastroparesis, pseudoobstruction, and constipation as well as the functional bowel disorders. Prosecretory drugs and isotonic solutions containing polyethylene glycol are prescribed for constipation refractory to other agents. Prescription antidiarrheals include opiate drugs, anticholinergic antispasmodics, tricyclics, bile acid binders, and serotonin antagonists. Antispasmodics and tricyclic drugs are also useful for functional abdominal pain, whereas narcotics are used for pain control in organic conditions such as disseminated malignancy and chronic pancreatitis. Antiemetics in several classes reduce nausea and vomiting. Potent pancreatic enzymes decrease malabsorption and pain from pancreatic disease. Antisecretory drugs such as the somatostatin analogue octreotide treat hypersecretory states. Antibiotics treat ulcer disease secondary to *Helicobacter pylori*, infectious diarrhea, diverticulitis, intestinal bacterial overgrowth, and Crohn's disease. Anti-inflammatory and immunosuppressive drugs are used in ulcerative colitis, Crohn's disease, microscopic colitis, refractory celiac disease, and gut vasculitis. Chemotherapy with or without radiotherapy is offered for GI malignancies. Most GI carcinomas respond poorly to such therapy, whereas lymphomas may be cured with such intervention.

Alternative Therapies Alternative treatments are marketed to treat selected GI symptoms. Ginger, acupressure, and acustimulation have been advocated for nausea, while pyridoxine has been investigated for nausea of first-trimester pregnancy. Probiotics containing active bacterial cultures are used as adjuncts in some cases of refractory infectious diarrhea and are being advocated by some as primary therapy of IBS. Low-potency pancreatic enzyme preparations are sold as general digestive aids but have little evidence to support their efficacy.

ENTERIC THERAPIES/INTERVENTIONAL ENDOSCOPY AND RADIOLOGY Simple luminal interventions are commonly performed for GI diseases. Nasogastric tube suction decompresses the upper gut in ileus or mechanical obstruction. Nasogastric lavage of saline or water in the patient with upper GI hemorrhage determines the rate of bleeding and helps evacuate blood prior to endoscopy. Enteral feedings can be initiated through a nasogastric or nasoenteric tube. Enemas relieve fecal impaction or assist in gas evacuation in acute colonic pseudoobstruction. A rectal tube can be left in place to vent the distal colon in colonic pseudoobstruction and other colonic distention disorders.

In addition to its diagnostic role, endoscopy has therapeutic capabilities in certain settings (**Chap. e25**). Cautery techniques can stop hemorrhage from ulcers, vascular malformations, and tumors. Injection with vasoconstrictor substances or sclerosants is used for bleeding ulcers, vascular malformations, varices, and hemorrhoids. Endoscopic encirclement of varices and hemorrhoids with constricting bands stops hemorrhage from these sites, while endoscopically placed clips can occlude arterial bleeding sites. Endoscopy can remove polyps or debulk lumen-narrowing malignancies. Endoscopic sphincterotomy of the ampulla of Vater relieves symptoms of choledocholithiasis. Obstructions of the gut lumen and pancreaticobiliary tree are relieved by endoscopic dilation or placement of plastic or expandable metal stents. In cases of acute colonic pseudoobstruction, colonoscopy is employed to withdraw luminal gas. Finally, endoscopy is commonly used to insert feeding tubes.

Radiologic measures also are useful in GI disease. Angiographic embolization or vasoconstriction decrease bleeding from sites not amenable to endoscopic intervention. Dilation or stenting with fluoroscopic guidance relieves luminal strictures. Contrast enemas can reduce volvulus and evacuate air in acute colonic pseudoobstruction. CT and ultrasound help drain abdominal fluid collections, in many cases obviating the need for surgery. Percutaneous transhepatic cholangiography relieves biliary obstruction when ERCP is contraindicated. Lithotripsy can fragment gallstones in patients who are not candidates for surgery. In some instances, radiologic approaches offer advantages over endoscopy for gastroenterostomy placement. Finally, central venous catheters for parenteral nutrition may be placed using radiographic techniques.

SURGERY Surgery is performed to cure GI disease, control symptoms without cure, maintain nutrition, or palliate unresectable neoplasm. Medication-unresponsive ulcerative colitis, diverticulitis, cholecystitis, appendicitis, and intraabdominal abscess are curable with surgery, whereas only symptom control without cure is possible with Crohn's disease. Surgery is mandated for ulcer complications such as bleeding, obstruction, or perforation and intestinal obstructions that do not resolve with conservative care. Fundoplication of the gastroesophageal junction is performed for presentations ranging from ulcerative esophagitis to drug-refractory symptoms of acid reflux. Achalasia responds to operations to relieve lower esophageal sphincter pressure. Novel operative therapies for motility disorders have been introduced including implanted electrical stimulators for gastroparesis and electrical devices and artificial sphincters for fecal incontinence. Surgery may be needed to place a jejunostomy for long-term enteral feedings. The threshold for performing surgery depends on the clinical setting. In all cases, the benefits of operation must be weighed against the potential for postoperative complications.

THERAPY DIRECTED TO EXTERNAL INFLUENCES In some conditions, GI symptoms respond to treatments directed outside the gut. Psychological therapies including psychotherapy, behavior modification, hypnosis, and biofeedback have shown efficacy in functional bowel disorders. Patients with significant psychological dysfunction and those with little response to treatments targeting the gut are likely to benefit from this form of therapy.

FURTHER READINGS

AMERICAN SOCIETY FOR GASTROINTESTINAL ENDOSCOPY: Appropriate use of gastrointestinal endoscopy. Gastrointest Endo 52:831, 2000

LONGSTRETH GF et al: Functional bowel disorders. Gastroenterology 130:1480, 2006

WINAWER S et al: Colorectal cancer screening and surveillance: Clinical guidelines and rationale—Update based on new evidence. Gastroenterology 124:544, 2003

YAMADA T (ed): *Textbook of Gastroenterology and Hepatology*, 4th ed. Philadelphia, Lippincott Williams & Wilkins, 2003

285 Gastrointestinal Endoscopy
Louis Michel Wong-Kee-Song, Mark Topazian

Gastrointestinal endoscopy has been attempted for over 200 years, but the introduction of semirigid gastroscopes in the middle of the twentieth century marked the dawn of the modern endoscopic era. Since then, rapid advances in endoscopic technology have led to dramatic changes in the diagnosis and treatment of many digestive diseases. Innovative endoscopic devices and new endoscopic treatment modalities continue to expand the use of endoscopy in patient care.

Flexible endoscopes provide either an optical image (transmitted over fiberoptic bundles) or an electronic video image (generated by a charge-coupled device in the tip of the endoscope). Operator controls permit deflection of the endoscope tip; fiberoptic bundles bring light to the tip of the endoscope; and working channels allow washing, suctioning, and the passage of instruments. Progressive changes in the diameter and stiffness of endoscopes have improved the ease and patient tolerance of endoscopy.

ENDOSCOPIC PROCEDURES

UPPER ENDOSCOPY

Upper endoscopy, also referred to as esophagogastroduodenoscopy (EGD), is performed by passing a flexible endoscope through the mouth into the esophagus, stomach, bulb, and second duodenum. The procedure is the best method for examining the upper gastrointestinal mucosa. While the upper gastrointestinal radiographic series has similar accuracy for diagnosis of duodenal ulcer (Fig. 285-1), EGD is superior for detection of gastric ulcers (Fig. 285-2) and flat mucosal lesions such as Barrett's esophagus (Fig. 285-3), and it permits directed biopsy and endoscopic therapy. Intravenous conscious sedation is given to most patients in the United States to ease the anxiety and discomfort of the procedure, although in many countries EGD is routinely performed with topical pharyngeal anesthesia only.

A   *B*

FIGURE 285-1 Duodenal ulcers. A. Ulcer with a clean base. **B.** Ulcer with a visible vessel (*arrow*) in a patient with recent hemorrhage.

Patient tolerance of unsedated EGD is improved by the use of an ultrathin, 5-mm diameter endoscope that can be passed transorally or transnasally.

COLONOSCOPY

Colonoscopy is performed by passing a flexible colonoscope through the anal canal into the rectum and colon. The cecum is reached in >95% of

A   *B*

FIGURE 285-2 Gastric ulcers. A. Benign gastric ulcer. **B.** Malignant gastric ulcer involving greater curvature of stomach.

FIGURE 285-3 Barrett's esophagus. A. Pink tongues of Barrett's mucosa extending proximally from the gastro-esophageal junction. **B.** Barrett's esophagus with a suspicious nodule (*arrow*) identified during endoscopic surveillance. **C.** Histologic finding of intramucosal adenocarcinoma in the endoscopically resected nodule. Tumor extends into the esophageal submucosa (*arrow*). **D.** Barrett's esophagus with locally advanced adenocarcinoma.

cases, and the terminal ileum can often be examined. Colonoscopy is the "gold standard" for diagnosis of colonic mucosal disease. Colonoscopy has greater sensitivity than barium enema or CT for colitis (Fig. 285-4), polyps (Fig. 285-5), and cancer (Fig. 285-6). Conscious sedation is usually given before colonoscopy in the United States, although a willing patient and a skilled examiner can complete the procedure without sedation in many cases.

FLEXIBLE SIGMOIDOSCOPY

Flexible sigmoidoscopy is similar to colonoscopy but visualizes only the rectum and a variable portion of the left colon, typically to 60 cm from the anal verge. This procedure causes brief abdominal cramping and is usually performed without sedation. Flexible sigmoidoscopy is primarily used for evaluation of diarrhea and rectal outlet bleeding.

SMALL-BOWEL ENDOSCOPY

Three techniques are currently used to evaluate the small intestine, most often in patients presenting with presumed small-bowel bleeding. For *capsule endoscopy* the patient swallows a disposable capsule that contains a complementary metal oxide silicon (CMOS) chip camera. Color still images (Fig. 285-7) are transmitted wirelessly to an external receiver at several frames per second until the capsule's battery is exhausted or it is passed into the toilet. Although capsule endoscopy allows visualization of the jejunal and ileal mucosa beyond the reach of a conventional endoscope, it remains purely a diagnostic procedure at present.

Push enteroscopy is performed with a long endoscope similar in design to an upper endoscope. The enteroscope is pushed down the small bowel, sometimes with the help of a stiffening overtube that extends from the mouth to the small intestine. The mid-jejunum is usually reached, and the endoscope's instrument channel allows for biopsies or endoscopic therapy. In *double-balloon enteroscopy* (Fig. 285-8), a long overtube and endoscope are both equipped with balloons that, when inflated, appose the intestinal wall and allow for pleating of the small intestine over the endoscope and overtube. The double-balloon enteroscope may be passed orally or anally, and the entire small bowel can be visualized in some patients when both approaches are used.

FIGURE 285-5 Colonic polyps. A. Pedunculated colon polyp on a thick stalk covered with normal mucosa (*arrow*). **B.** Sessile rectal polyp.

FIGURE 285-4 Causes of colitis. A. Chronic ulcerative colitis with diffuse ulcerations and exudates. **B.** Severe Crohn's colitis with deep ulcers. **C.** Pseudomembranous colitis with yellow, adherent pseudomembranes. **D.** Ischemic colitis with patchy mucosal edema, subepithelial hemorrhage, and cyanosis.

FIGURE 285-6 Colon adenocarcinoma growing into the lumen.

FIGURE 285-7 Capsule endoscopy image of jejunal vascular ectasia.

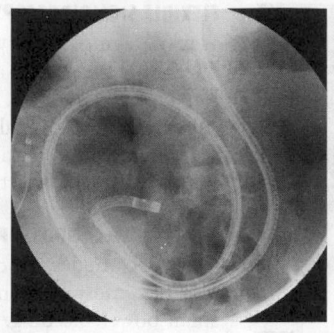

FIGURE 285-8 Radiograph of a double-balloon enteroscope in the small intestine. *(Image courtesy of Dr. Ananya Das; with permission.)*

Biopsies and endoscopic therapy can be performed throughout the visualized small bowel.

ENDOSCOPIC RETROGRADE CHOLANGIOPANCREATOGRAPHY (ERCP)

During ERCP, a side-viewing endoscope is passed through the mouth to the duodenum, the ampulla of Vater is identified and cannulated with a thin plastic catheter, and radiographic contrast material is injected into the bile duct and pancreatic duct under fluoroscopic guidance. When indicated, the sphincter of Oddi can be opened using the technique of endoscopic sphincterotomy (Fig. 285-9). Stones can be retrieved from the ducts (Fig. 285-10, Video e25-6), biopsies can be obtained, and strictures (Fig. 285-11) or ductal leaks (Fig. 285-12) can be dilated and stented. ERCP is often performed for therapy but remains important in diagnosis, especially for ductal strictures and bile duct stones.

ENDOSCOPIC ULTRASOUND (EUS)

EUS utilizes high-frequency ultrasound transducers incorporated into the tip of a flexible endoscope. Ultrasound images are obtained of the gut wall and adjacent organs, vessels, and lymph nodes. By sacrificing depth of ultrasound penetration and bringing the ultrasound transducer close to the area of interest via endoscopy, very-high-resolution images are obtained. EUS provides the most accurate preoperative local staging of esophageal, pancreatic, and rectal malignancies, although it does not detect most distant metastases. Examples of EUS tumor staging are shown in Fig. 285-13. EUS is also highly sensitive for diagnosis of bile duct stones, gallbladder disease, submucosal gastrointestinal lesions, and chronic pancreatitis. Fine-needle aspiration of masses and lymph nodes in the posterior mediastinum, abdomen, and pelvis can be performed under EUS guidance (Fig. 285-14).

FIGURE 285-10 Endoscopic sphincterotomy. A. A normal-appearing ampulla of Vater. **B.** Sphincterotomy is performed with electrocautery. **C.** Bile duct stones are extracted with a balloon catheter. **D.** Final appearance of the sphincterotomy.

RISKS OF ENDOSCOPY

All endoscopic procedures carry some risk of bleeding and gastrointestinal perforation. These risks are quite low with diagnostic upper endoscopy and colonoscopy (<1:1000 procedures), although the risk is as high as 2:100 when therapeutic procedures such as polypectomy, control of hemorrhage, or stricture dilation are performed. Bleeding and perforation are rare with flexible sigmoidoscopy. The risks for diagnostic EUS (without needle aspiration) are similar to the risks for diagnostic upper endoscopy.

Infectious complications are unusual with most endoscopic procedures. Some procedures carry a higher incidence of postprocedure bacteremia, and prophylactic antibiotics may be indicated for these procedures in some patients (Table 285-1).

ERCP carries additional risks. Pancreatitis occurs in about 5% of patients undergoing ERCP and in up to 25% of patients with sphincter of Oddi dysfunction. Young anicteric patients with normal ducts are at increased risk. Post-ERCP pancreatitis is usually mild and self-limited but may rarely result in prolonged hospitalization, surgery, diabetes, or death. Bleeding occurs in 1% of endoscopic sphincterotomies. Ascending cholangitis, pseudocyst infection, retroperitoneal perforation, and abscess formation may all occur as a result of ERCP.

The conscious sedation used during endoscopy may cause respiratory depression or allergic reactions. Percutaneous gastrostomy tube placement during EGD is associated with a 10–15% incidence of complications, most often wound infections. Fasciitis, pneumonia, bleeding, and colonic injury may result from gastrostomy tube placement.

FIGURE 285-9 Endoscopic retrograde cholangiopancreatography (ERCP) for bile duct stones with cholangitis. A. Faceted bile duct stones are demonstrated in the common bile duct. **B.** After endoscopic sphincterotomy, the stones are extracted with a Dormia basket. A small abscess communicates with the left hepatic duct.

URGENT ENDOSCOPY

ACUTE GASTROINTESTINAL HEMORRHAGE

Endoscopy is an important diagnostic and therapeutic technique for patients with acute gastrointestinal hemorrhage. Although most gastrointestinal bleeding stops spontaneous-

FIGURE 285-11 Endoscopic diagnosis, staging, and palliation of hilar cholangiocarcinoma. A. ERCP in a patient with obstructive jaundice demonstrates a malignant appearing stricture of the biliary confluence extending into the left and right intrahepatic ducts (*arrow*). **B.** Intraductal ultrasound of the biliary stricture demonstrates marked bile duct wall thickening due to tumor (T) with partial encasement of the hepatic artery (*arrow*). **C.** Intraductal biopsy obtained during ERCP demonstrates malignant cells infiltrating the submucosa of the bile duct wall (*arrow*). **D.** Endoscopic placement of bilateral self-expanding metal stents (*arrow*) relieves the biliary obstruction.

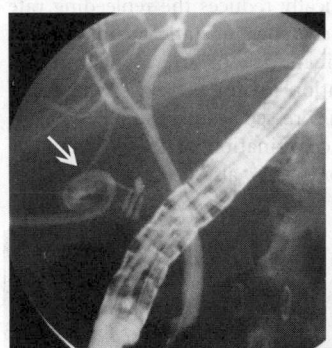

FIGURE 285-12 Bile leak (*arrow*) from a duct of Luschka after laparoscopic cholecystectomy. Contrast leaks from a small right intrahepatic duct into the gall-bladder fossa, then flows into the pigtail of a percutaneous drainage catheter.

FIGURE 285-14 Endoscopic ultrasound (EUS)–guided fine-needle aspiration (FNA). A. Ultrasound image of a 22-gauge needle passed through the duodenal wall and positioned in a hypoechoic pancreatic head mass. **B.** Micrograph of aspirated malignant cells. (*Image B courtesy of Dr. Mary S. Chacho; with permission.*)

ly, a minority of patients will have persistent or recurrent hemorrhage that may be life-threatening. Clinical predictors of rebleeding help identify patients most likely to benefit from urgent endoscopy and endoscopic, angiographic, or surgical hemostasis.

Initial Evaluation The initial evaluation of the bleeding patient focuses on the magnitude of hemorrhage as reflected by the postural vital signs, the frequency of hematemesis or melena, and (in some cases) findings on nasogastric lavage. Decreases in hematocrit and hemoglobin lag behind the clinical course and are not reliable gauges of the magnitude of acute bleeding. This initial evaluation, completed well before the bleeding source is confidently identified, guides immediate supportive care of the patient and helps determine the timing of endoscopy. The magnitude of the initial hemorrhage is the most important indication for urgent endoscopy, since a large initial bleed increases the likelihood of ongoing or recurrent bleeding. Patients with resting hypotension, repeated hematemesis, nasogastric aspirate that does not clear with large volume lavage, or orthostatic change in vital signs, or those requiring blood transfusions, should be considered for urgent endoscopy. In addition, patients with cirrhosis, coagulopathy, or respiratory or renal failure and those over 70 years are more likely to have significant rebleeding.

Bedside evaluation also suggests an upper or lower gastrointestinal source of bleeding in most patients. Over 90% of patients with melena are bleeding proximal to the ligament of Treitz, and about 90% of patients with hematochezia are bleeding from the colon. Melena can result from bleeding in the small bowel or right colon, especially in older patients with slow colonic transit. Conversely, some patients with massive hematochezia may be bleeding from an upper GI source, such as a gastric Dieulafoy's lesion or duodenal ulcer, with rapid intestinal transit. Early upper endoscopy should be considered in such patients.

FIGURE 285-13 Local staging of gastrointestinal cancers with endoscopic ultrasound. In each example the white arrowhead marks the primary tumor and the black arrow indicates the muscularis propria (mp) of the intestinal wall. "AO" indicates aorta. **A.** T1 gastric cancer. The tumor does not invade the mp. **B.** T2 esophageal cancer. The tumor invades the mp. **C.** T3 esophageal cancer. The tumor extends through the mp into the surrounding tissue, and focally abuts the aorta.

TABLE 285-1 ANTIBIOTIC PROPHYLAXIS FOR SELECTED ENDOSCOPIC PROCEDURES

Patient Condition	Procedure Contemplated	Antibiotic Prophylaxis[a]
High risk: Prosthetic valve, history of endocarditis, systemic-pulmonary shunt, synthetic vascular graft (<1 year old), complex cyanotic congenital heart disease	High risk[b] Low risk[c]	Recommended Optional (insufficient data)
Moderate risk: Most other congenital abnormalities, acquired valvular dis-function (rheumatic heart disease), hypertrophic cardiomyopathy, mitral valve prolapse with regurgitation or thickened leaflets	High risk Low risk	Optional (insufficient data) Not recommended[d]
Low risk: CABG, repaired septal defect or patent ductus, mitral valve pro-lapse without valvular regurgitation, pacemakers, implantable defibrillators	High or low risk	Not recommended
Obstructed bile duct	ERCP	Recommended
Pancreatic cystic lesion	ERCP, EUS-FNA	Recommended
Cirrhosis acute GI bleed	All endoscopic procedures	Recommended
Ascites, immunocompromised patients	High risk Low risk	No recommendation Not recommended
Prosthetic joints	All endoscopic procedures	Not recommended
All patients	Percutaneous endoscopic feed tube placement	Recommended (paren-teral cephalosporin or equivalent)

[a]Cardiac prophylaxis regimens include amoxicillin, 2 g PO, 1 h before; or ampicillin, 2 g IV, 30 min before procedure. In penicillin-allergic patients, may substitute clindamycin, 600 mg PO; or cephalexin or cefadroxil, 2 g PO; or azithro-mycin or clarithromycin 500 mg PO; or cefazolin 1 g IV or IM; or vancomycin 1 g IV. Regimens for noncardiac indica-tions vary.

[b]High-risk endoscopic procedures: stricture dilation, variceal sclerotherapy, ERCP/obstructed biliary tree.

[c]Low-risk endoscopic procedures: EGD and colonoscopy with or without biopsy and polyp removal, variceal ligation.

[d]Controversy exists and recommendations may vary. See, e.g., Dajani AS et al: Clin Infect Dis 25:1448, 1997.

Note: CABG, coronary artery bypass grafting; ERCP, endoscopic retrograde cholangiopancreatography; EUS, endo-scopic ultrasound; FNA, fine-needle aspiration; EGD, esophagogastroduodenoscopy.

Source: Adapted from WK Hirota et al: Guidelines for antibiotic prophylaxis for GI endoscopy. Gastrointest Endosc 58(4):475, 2003; with permission.

Endoscopy should be performed after the patient has been resusci-tated with intravenous fluids and transfusions as necessary. Marked coagulopathy or thrombocytopenia is usually treated before endosco-py, since correction of these abnormalities may lead to resolution of bleeding, and techniques for endoscopic hemostasis are limited in such patients. Metabolic de-rangements should also be ad-dressed. Tracheal intubation for airway protection should be considered before upper endos-copy in patients with repeated recent hematemesis and sus-pected variceal hemorrhage.

Most patients with impres-sive hematochezia can undergo colonoscopy after a rapid colon-ic purge with a polyethylene glycol solution; the preparation fluid may be administered via a nasogastric tube. Colonoscopy has a higher diagnostic yield than bleeding scans or angiog-raphy in lower gastrointestinal bleeding, and endoscopic ther-apy can be applied in some cas-es. In a minority of patients, endoscopic assessment is hin-dered by poor visualization due to persistent vigorous bleeding with recurrent hemodynamic

instability, and other techniques (such as bleeding scans, angiography, or emergency subtotal colectomy) must be employed. In such patients, massive bleeding originating from an upper GI source should be excluded by upper endoscopy. The anal and rectal mu-cosa should be visualized endoscopically early in the course of massive rectal bleeding, as bleeding lesions in or close to the anal canal may be identified that are often amenable to endoscopic or surgical transanal hemostatic techniques.

Peptic Ulcer The endoscopic appearance of peptic ulcers provides useful prognostic infor-mation and guides the need for endoscopic therapy in patients with acute hemorrhage (Fig. 285-15). A clean-based ulcer is associated with a low 3–5% risk of rebleeding; patients with melena and a clean-based ulcer are often dis-charged home from the emergency room or en-doscopy suite if they are young, reliable, and otherwise healthy. Flat red or purple spots in the ulcer base and large adherent clots covering the ulcer base have a 10 and 20% risk of re-bleeding, respectively. Endoscopic therapy is of-ten considered for an ulcer with an adherent clot. When a platelet plug is seen protruding from a vessel wall in the base of an ulcer (so-called sentinel clot or visible vessel), the risk of rebleeding from the ulcer is 40%. This finding generally leads to local endoscopic therapy to decrease the rebleeding rate. Occasionally, ac-tive spurting from an ulcer is seen with >90% risk of ongoing bleeding.

Endoscopic therapy of ulcers with high-risk stigmata typically reduces the rebleeding rate to 5–10%. Several hemostatic techniques are available, including injection of epinephrine or sclerosant into and around the vessel, "coaptive coagulation" of the vessel in the base of the ulcer using a thermal probe that is pressed against the site of bleed-ing, placement of hemoclips, or a combination of these modalities (**Video e25-1**). Proton pump inhibitor therapy also decreases the risk of

FIGURE 285-15 Stigmata of hemorrhage in peptic ulcers. A. Gastric antral ulcer with a clean base. **B.** Duodenal ulcer with flat pig-mented spots. **C.** Duodenal ulcer with a dense adherent clot. **D.** Gastric ulcer with a pig-mented protuberance/visible vessel. **E.** Duode-nal ulcer with active spurting (*arrow*).

FIGURE 285-16 Esophageal varices.

FIGURE 285-18   Mallory-Weiss tear at the gastroesophageal junction.

A   **B**

FIGURE 285-17 Dieulafoy's lesion. A. Actively spurting jejunal Dieulafoy's lesion. There is no underlying mucosal lesion. **B.** Histology of a gastric Dieulafoy's lesion. A persistent caliber artery (*arrows*) is present in the gastric submucosa, immediately beneath the mucosa.

recurrent hemorrhage and should be administered in patients with endoscopic stigmata of recent bleeding.

Varices   Two complementary strategies guide therapy of bleeding varices: local treatment of the bleeding vessel and treatment of the underlying portal hypertension. Local therapies, including endoscopic sclerotherapy, endoscopic band ligation, and balloon tamponade with a Sengstaken-Blakemore tube, effectively control acute hemorrhage in most patients and are the mainstay of acute treatment, although therapies that decrease portal pressures (pharmacologic treatment, surgical shunts, or radiologically placed intrahepatic shunts) also play an important role.

When feasible, endoscopic band ligation is the preferred local therapy for control of active esophageal variceal bleeding and for subsequent eradication of esophageal varices (Fig. 285-16). In this technique a varix is suctioned into a cap fitted on the end of the endoscope, and a rubber band is then released from the cap, ligating the varix (**Video e25-2**). Acute hemorrhage can be controlled in up to 90% of patients, and complications (such as sepsis, symptomatic esophageal ulceration, or esophageal stenosis) are uncommon. Endoscopic sclerotherapy is another technique in which a sclerosing, thrombogenic solution is injected into or next to the esophageal varices. Sclerotherapy also controls acute hemorrhage in most patients but has a higher complication rate. Bleeding from large gastric fundic varices is best treated by cyanoacrylate ("glue") injection (**Video e25-3**), since band ligation or sclerotherapy of these varices are associated with a high rebleeding rate. These techniques are used when varices are actively bleeding during endoscopy or (more commonly) when varices are the only identifiable cause of acute hemorrhage.

After treatment of the acute hemorrhage, an elective course of endoscopic therapy can be undertaken with the goal of eradicating esophageal varices and preventing rebleeding months to years later. This chronic therapy is less

successful, however, preventing long-term rebleeding in ~50% of patients. Pharmacologic therapies that decrease portal pressure have similar efficacy, and the two modalities may be combined.

Dieulafoy's Lesion   This lesion, also called *persistent caliber artery*, is a large-caliber arteriole that runs immediately beneath the gastrointestinal mucosa and bleeds through a pinpoint mucosal erosion (Fig. 285-17). Dieulafoy's lesion is seen most commonly on the lesser curvature of the proximal stomach, causes impressive arterial hemorrhage, and may be difficult to diagnose; it is often recognized only after repeated endoscopy for recurrent bleeding. Endoscopic therapy is typically effective for control of bleeding and ablation of the underlying vessel once the lesion has been identified (**Video e25-4**). Angiographic embolization or surgical oversewing is considered when endoscopic therapy has failed.

Mallory-Weiss Tear   A Mallory-Weiss tear is a linear mucosal rent near or across the gastroesophageal junction that is often associated with retching or vomiting (Fig. 285-18). When the tear disrupts a submucosal arteriole, brisk hemorrhage may result. Endoscopy is the best diagnostic method, and an actively bleeding tear can be treated endoscopically with epinephrine injection, coaptive coagulation, hemoclips, or band ligation. Unlike peptic ulcer, a Mallory-Weiss tear with a nonbleeding sentinel clot in its base rarely rebleeds and thus does not require endoscopic therapy.

Vascular Ectasias   Vascular ectasias are flat mucosal vascular anomalies that are best diagnosed by endoscopy. They usually cause slow intestinal blood loss and have several characteristic distributions in the gastrointestinal tract (Fig. 285-19). Cecal vascular ectasias (senile lesions), gastric antral vascular ectasias ("watermelon stomach"), and radiation-induced rectal ectasias are often responsive to local endoscopic ablative therapy, such as argon plasma coagulation (APC). Patients with diffuse small-bowel vascular ectasias (associated with chronic renal failure and hereditary hemorrhagic telangiectasia) may continue to bleed despite endoscopic treatment of easily accessible lesions by conventional endoscopy. These patients may benefit from double balloon enteroscopy with endoscopic therapy, pharmacologic treatment with octreotide or estrogen/progesterone therapy, or intraoperative enteroscopy.

A   **B**   **C**

FIGURE 285-19 Gastrointestinal vascular ectasias. A. Gastric antral vascular ectasias, or "watermelon stomach," characterized by prominent flat or raised red angioectatic stripes radiating in a spoke-like fashion from the pylorus to the antrum. **B.** Cecal vascular ectasias. **C.** Radiation-induced vascular ectasias of the rectum in a patient previously treated for prostate cancer.

Colonic Diverticula Diverticula form where nutrient arteries penetrate the muscular wall of the colon en route to the colonic mucosa. The artery found in the base or neck of a diverticulum may bleed, causing painless and impressive hematochezia. Colonoscopy is indicated in patients with hematochezia and suspected diverticular hemorrhage, since other causes of bleeding (such as vascular ectasias, colitis, and colon cancer) must be excluded. In addition, an actively bleeding diverticulum may be seen and treated during colonoscopy (**Video e25-5**).

GASTROINTESTINAL OBSTRUCTION AND PSEUDOOBSTRUCTION

Endoscopy is useful for evaluation and treatment of several causes of gastrointestinal obstruction. An important exception is small-bowel obstruction due to surgical adhesions, which is generally not diagnosed or treated endoscopically. Esophageal, gastroduodenal, and colonic obstruction or pseudoobstruction can all be diagnosed and often managed endoscopically.

Acute Esophageal Obstruction Esophageal obstruction by impacted food or an ingested foreign body is a potentially life-threatening event and represents an endoscopic emergency. Left untreated, the patient may develop esophageal ulceration, ischemia, and perforation. Patients with persistent esophageal obstruction often have hypersalivation and are usually unable to swallow water; endoscopy is generally the best initial test in such patients, since endoscopic removal of the obstructing material is usually possible, and the presence of underlying esophageal pathology can often be determined. Radiographs of the chest and neck should be considered before endoscopy in patients with fever, obstruction for ≥24 h, or ingestion of a sharp object such as a fishbone. Radiographic contrast studies interfere with subsequent endoscopy and are not advisable in most patients with a clinical picture of esophageal obstruction. Occasionally, sublingual nifedipine or nitrates, or intravenous glucagon, may resolve an esophageal food impaction, but in most patients an underlying web, ring, or stricture is present, and endoscopic removal of the obstructing food bolus is necessary.

Gastric Outlet Obstruction Obstruction of the gastric outlet is commonly caused by malignancy of the prepyloric gastric antrum or chronic peptic ulceration with stenosis of the pylorus. Patients vomit partially digested food many hours after eating. Gastric decompression with a nasogastric tube and subsequent lavage for removal of retained material is the first step in treatment. The diagnosis can then be confirmed with a saline load test, if desired. Endoscopy is useful for diagnosis and treatment. Patients with benign pyloric stenosis may be treated with endoscopic balloon dilation of the pylorus, and a course of endoscopic dilation results in long-term relief of symptoms in about 50% of patients. Malignant pyloric obstruction can be palliated with endoscopically placed expandable stents in a patient with an inoperable malignancy.

Colonic Obstruction and Pseudoobstruction These both present with abdominal distention and discomfort; tympany; and a dilated, air-filled colon on plain abdominal radiography. The radiographic appearance can be characteristic of a particular cause, such as sigmoid volvulus (Fig. 285-20). Both structural obstruction and pseudoobstruction may lead to colonic perforation if untreated. Acute colonic pseudoobstruction is a form of colonic ileus that is usually attributable to electrolyte disorders, narcotic and anticholinergic medications, immobility (as after surgery), and retroperitoneal hemorrhage or mass. Multiple causative factors are often present. Either colonoscopy or a water-soluble contrast enema may be used to look for an obstructing lesion and differentiate obstruction from pseudoobstruction. One of these diagnostic studies should be strongly considered if the patient does not have clear risk factors for pseudoobstruction, if radiographs do not show air in the rectum, or if the patient fails to improve when the underlying causes of pseudoobstruction have been addressed. The risk of cecal perforation in pseudoobstruction rises when the cecal diameter exceeds 12 cm, and in such patients decompression of the colon may be achieved using intravenous neostigmine, colonoscopic

FIGURE 285-20 Sigmoid volvulus with the characteristic radiological appearance of a "bent inner tube."

decompression, or placement of a cecostomy tube. Most patients should receive a trial of conservative therapy (with correction of electrolyte disorders, removal of offending medications, and increased mobilization) before undergoing an invasive decompressive procedure for colonic pseudoobstruction.

Colonic obstruction is an indication for urgent intervention. Emergency diverting colostomy may be performed with a subsequent second operation after bowel preparation to treat the underlying cause of obstruction. Colonoscopic placement of an expandable stent is an alternative that can relieve the malignant obstruction without emergency surgery and permit bowel preparation for an elective one-stage operation (Fig. 285-21).

ACUTE BILIARY OBSTRUCTION

The steady, severe pain that occurs when a gallstone acutely obstructs the common bile duct often brings patients to a hospital. The diagnosis of a ductal stone is suspected when the patient is jaundiced or when serum liver tests or pancreatic enzyme levels are elevated; it is confirmed by direct cholangiography (performed endoscopically, percutaneously, or during surgery). ERCP is currently the primary means of diagnosing and treating common bile duct stones in most hospitals in the United States (Figs. 285-9 and 285-10).

Bile Duct Imaging While transabdominal ultrasound diagnoses only a minority of bile duct stones, magnetic resonance cholangiopancreatography (MRCP) and EUS are >90% accurate and have an important role in diagnosis. Examples of these modalities are shown in Fig. 285-22.

If the suspicion for a bile duct stone is high and urgent treatment is required (as in a patient with jaundice and biliary sepsis), ERCP is the procedure of choice, since it remains the gold standard for diagnosis and provides immediate treatment (**Video e25-6**). If a persistent bile duct stone is unlikely (as in a patient with gallstone pancreatitis), ERCP may be supplanted by less-invasive, safer imaging techniques.

Ascending Cholangitis Charcot's triad of jaundice, abdominal pain, and fever is present in about 70% of patients with ascending cholangitis and biliary sepsis. Initially, such patients are managed with fluid resuscitation and intravenous antibiotics. Abdominal ultrasound is often done to look for gallbladder stones and bile duct dilation. However, the bile duct may not be dilated early in the course of acute biliary obstruction. Medical management usually improves the patient's clinical status, providing a window of approximately 24 h during which biliary drainage should be established, typically by ERCP. Undue delay can result in recrudescence of overt sepsis and increased

A

B

C

FIGURE 285-21 Obstructing colonic carcinoma. A. Colonic adenocarcinoma causing marked luminal narrowing of the descending colon. **B.** Endoscopic placement of a self-expanding metal stent. **C.** Radiograph of expanded stent across the obstructing tumor with a residual waist *(arrow). (Image A courtesy of Dr. Glenn Alexander; with permission.)*

morbidity. In addition to Charcot's triad, the presence of shock and confusion (Reynolds' pentad) should prompt urgent attempts at restoring biliary drainage.

Gallstone Pancreatitis Gallstones may cause acute pancreatitis as they pass through the ampulla of Vater. The occurrence of gallstone pancreatitis usually implies passage of a stone into the duodenum, and

only about 20% of patients harbor a persistent stone in the ampulla or the common bile duct. Retained stones are more common in patients with jaundice, rising serum liver tests following hospitalization, severe pancreatitis, or superimposed ascending cholangitis.

Urgent ERCP decreases the morbidity of gallstone pancreatitis in some subsets of patients. It remains unclear whether the benefit of ERCP is mainly attributable to treatment and prevention of ascending cholangitis or to relief of pancreatic duct obstruction. ERCP is warranted early in the course of gallstone pancreatitis if ascending cholangitis is also suspected, especially in a jaundiced patient. Urgent ERCP also appears to benefit patients predicted to have severe pancreatitis using a clinical index of severity such as the Glasgow or Ranson score.

ELECTIVE ENDOSCOPY

DYSPEPSIA AND REFLUX

Dyspepsia is a chronic or recurrent burning discomfort or pain in the upper abdomen that may be caused by diverse processes such as gastroesophageal reflux, peptic ulcer disease, and "nonulcer dyspepsia," a heterogeneous category that includes disorders of motility, sensation, and somatization. Gastric and esophageal malignancies are less-common causes of dyspepsia. Careful history-taking allows accurate differential diagnosis of dyspepsia in only about half of patients. In the remainder, endoscopy can be a useful diagnostic tool, especially in those patients whose symptoms are not resolved by an empirical trial of symptomatic treatment.

GASTROESOPHAGEAL REFLUX DISEASE (GERD)

When classic symptoms of gastroesophageal reflux are present, such as water brash and substernal heartburn, presumptive diagnosis and empirical treatment are often sufficient. Although endoscopy is sensitive for diagnosis of esophagitis (Fig. 285-23), it can miss cases of nonerosive reflux disease (NERD), since some patients have symptomatic reflux without esophagitis. The most sensitive test for diagnosis of GERD is 24-h ambulatory pH monitoring. To assess the esophagus and exclude other diseases, endoscopy is indicated in patients with reflux symptoms refractory to medical therapy; in those with alarm symptoms such as dysphagia, weight loss, or gastrointestinal bleeding; and in those with recurrent dyspepsia after treatment that is not clearly due to reflux on clinical grounds alone. Endoscopy may be indicated in patients with long-standing (≥10 years) frequent heartburn, who are at sixfold increased risk of Barrett's esophagus compared to a patient with <1 year of reflux symptoms. Patients with Barrett's esophagus (Fig. 285-3) usually enter a program of periodic endoscopy with biopsies to detect dysplasia or early carcinoma. Endoscopic treatments for GERD have been developed as alternatives to pharmacologic and

A

B

C

FIGURE 285-22 Methods of bile duct imaging. Arrows mark bile duct stones. Arrowheads indicate the common bile duct, and the asterisk marks the portal vein. **A.** Endoscopic ultrasound (EUS). **B.** Magnetic resonance cholangiopancreatography (MRCP). **C.** CT.

FIGURE 285-23 Causes of esophagitis. A. Severe reflux esophagitis with mucosal ulceration and friability. **B.** Cytomegalovirus esophagitis. **C.** Herpes simplex virus esophagitis with numerous shallow ulcerations. **D.** Candida esophagitis with white plaques adherent to the esophageal mucosa.

laparoscopic therapies, and their role in the treatment of patients is still being assessed.

PEPTIC ULCER

Peptic ulcer classically causes epigastric gnawing or burning, often occurring nocturnally and promptly relieved by food or antacids. Although endoscopy is the most sensitive diagnostic test for peptic ulcer, it is not a cost-effective strategy in young patients with ulcer-like dyspeptic symptoms unless endoscopy is available at low cost. Patients with suspected peptic ulcer should be evaluated for *Helicobacter pylori* infection. Serology (past or present infection), urea breath testing (current infection), and stool tests are less invasive and costly than endoscopy with biopsy. Patients with alarm symptoms and those with persistent symptoms despite treatment should undergo endoscopy to exclude gastric malignancy and other etiologies.

NONULCER DYSPEPSIA

Nonulcer dyspepsia may be associated with bloating and, unlike peptic ulcer, tends not to remit and recur. Most patients obtain little relief with acid-reducing, prokinetic, or anti-*Helicobacter* therapy, and they are typically referred for endoscopy to exclude a refractory ulcer and assess for other causes. Although endoscopy is useful for excluding other diagnoses, its impact on the treatment of patients with nonulcer dyspepsia is marginal.

DYSPHAGIA

About 50% of patients with difficulty swallowing have a mechanical obstruction; the remainder have a motility disorder, such as achalasia

FIGURE 285-25 Schatzki's ring at the gastroesophageal junction.

or diffuse esophageal spasm. Careful history-taking often suggests a diagnosis and leads to the appropriate use of diagnostic tests. Esophageal strictures (Fig. 285-24) typically cause progressive dysphagia, first for solids, then for liquids; motility disorders often cause intermittent dysphagia for both solids and liquids. Some underlying disorders have characteristic historic features: Schatzki's ring (Fig. 285-25) causes episodic dysphagia for solids, typically at the beginning of a meal; pharyngeal motor disorders are associated with difficulty initiating deglutition ("transfer dysphagia") and nasal reflux or coughing with swallowing; and achalasia may cause nocturnal regurgitation of undigested food.

When mechanical obstruction is suspected, endoscopy is a useful initial diagnostic test, since it permits immediate biopsy and/or dilation of strictures, masses, or rings. The presence of multiple corrugated rings throughout a narrowed esophagus should raise suspicion for eosinophilic esophagitis, an increasingly recognized cause of recurrent dysphagia and food impaction (Fig. 285-26). Blind or forceful passage of an endoscope may lead to perforation in a patient with stenosis of the cervical esophagus or a Zencker's diverticulum, but gentle passage of an endoscope under direct visual guidance is reasonably safe. Endoscopy can miss a subtle stricture or ring in some patients.

When a motility disorder is suspected, esophageal radiography and/or a video-swallow study are the best initial diagnostic tests. The pharyngeal swallowing mechanism, esophageal peristalsis, and the lower esophageal sphincter can all be assessed. In some disorders, subsequent esophageal manometry may also be important for diagnosis.

ANEMIA AND OCCULT BLOOD IN THE STOOL

Iron-deficiency anemia may be attributed to poor iron absorption (as in celiac sprue) or, more commonly, chronic blood loss. Intestinal bleeding should be strongly suspected in men and postmenopausal women with iron-deficiency anemia, and colonoscopy is indicated in such patients, even in the absence of detectable occult blood in the stool. Approximately 30% of patients will have colon polyps, 10% will have colorectal cancer, and a few additional patients will have colonic vascular lesions. When a convincing source of blood loss is not found in the colon, upper gastrointestinal endoscopy should be considered; if no lesion is found, duodenal biopsies should be obtained to exclude sprue (Fig. 285-27). Small bowel evaluation with capsule endoscopy may be appropriate if both EGD and colonoscopy are unrevealing (Fig. 285-28).

Tests for occult blood in the stool detect hemoglobin or the heme moiety and are most sensitive for colonic blood loss, although they will also detect larger amounts of upper gastrointestinal bleeding. Patients over age 50 with occult blood in normal-appearing stool should

FIGURE 285-24 Peptic esophageal stricture associated with ulceration and scarring of the distal esophagus.

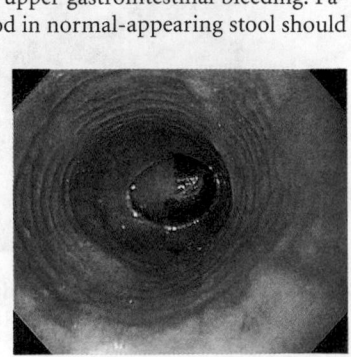

FIGURE 285-26 Eosinophilic esophagitis with multiple circular rings of the esophagus creating a corrugated appearance, and an impacted grape at the narrowed esophagogastric junction. The diagnosis requires biopsy with histologic finding of ≥20 eosinophils/high power field.

FIGURE 285-27 Scalloped duodenal folds in a patient with celiac sprue.

FIGURE 285-29 Innumerable colon polyps of various sizes in a patient with familial adenomatous polyposis syndrome.

undergo colonoscopy to diagnose or exclude colorectal neoplasia. The diagnostic yield is lower than in iron-deficiency anemia. Whether upper endoscopy is also indicated depends on the patient's symptoms.

The small intestine may be the source of chronic intestinal bleeding, especially if colonoscopy and upper endoscopy are not diagnostic. The utility of small-bowel evaluation varies with the clinical setting and is most important in patients in whom bleeding causes chronic or recurrent anemia. While small-bowel radiography is usually of low diagnostic yield, capsule endoscopy provides a specific diagnosis in about 50% of such patients (Fig. 285-28). The most common finding is mucosal vascular ectasias.

COLORECTAL CANCER SCREENING

The majority of colon cancers develop from preexisting colonic adenomas, and colorectal cancer can be largely prevented by the detection and removal of adenomatous polyps (**Video e25-7**). The choice of screening strategy for an asymptomatic person depends on his or her personal and family history. Individuals with inflammatory bowel disease, a history of colorectal polyps, family members with adenomatous polyps or cancer, or certain familial syndromes (Fig. 285-29) are at increased risk for colon cancer. An individual without these factors is generally considered at average risk.

Screening strategies are summarized in Table 285-2. While stool tests for occult blood have been shown to decrease mortality from colorectal cancer, they do not detect some cancers and many polyps, and direct visualization of the colon is a more effective screening strategy. Either sigmoidoscopy or colonoscopy may be used for cancer screening in asymptomatic average-risk patients. The use of sigmoidoscopy was based on the historic finding that the majority of colorectal cancers occurred in the rectum and left colon and that patients with right-sided colon cancers had left-sided polyps. Over the past several decades, however, the distribution of colon cancers has changed, with proportionally fewer rectal and left-sided cancers than in the past. Large studies of colonoscopy for screening of average-risk individuals show that cancers are roughly equally distributed between left and right colon, and half of patients with right-sided lesions have no polyps in the left colon. Visualization of the entire colon thus appears to be the optimal strategy for colorectal cancer screening and prevention.

Virtual colonoscopy (VC) is a radiologic technique that images the colon with CT following rectal insufflation of the colonic lumen. Computer rendering of CT images generates an electronic display of a virtual "flight" along the colonic lumen, simulating colonoscopy (Fig. 285-30). Most comparative studies of VC and conventional colonoscopy have shown that VC lacks adequate sensitivity for polyps, but technical refinements have improved its performance characteristics,

and in one study it detected more polyps than conventional colonoscopy. VC may become more widely used for colorectal cancer screening, particularly at institutions with demonstrated skill with this technique. Findings detected during VC often require subsequent conventional colonoscopy for confirmation and treatment.

DIARRHEA

Most cases of diarrhea are acute, self-limited, and due to infections or medication. Chronic diarrhea (lasting >6 weeks) is more often due to a primary inflammatory, malabsorptive, or motility disorder; is less likely to resolve spontaneously; and generally requires diagnostic evaluation. Patients with chronic diarrhea or severe, unexplained acute diarrhea often undergo endoscopy if stool tests for pathogens are unrevealing. The choice of endoscopic testing depends on the clinical setting.

Patients with colonic symptoms and findings such as bloody diarrhea, tenesmus, fever, or stool leukocytes generally undergo sigmoidoscopy or colonoscopy to search for colitis (Fig. 285-4). Sigmoidoscopy is often adequate and is the best initial test in most of these patients. On the other hand, patients with symptoms and findings suggestive of small-bowel disease, such as large-volume watery stools, substantial weight loss, and malabsorption of iron, calcium, or fat, may undergo upper endoscopy with duodenal biopsies and aspirates.

Many patients with chronic diarrhea do not fit either of these patterns. In the setting of a long-standing history of alternating constipation and diarrhea dating to early adulthood, without findings such as blood in the stool or anemia, a diagnosis of irritable bowel syndrome may be made without direct visualization of the bowel. Steatorrhea and upper abdominal pain may prompt evaluation of the pancreas rather than the gut. Patients whose chronic diarrhea is not easily categorized often undergo initial colonoscopy to examine the entire colon and terminal ileum for inflammatory or neoplastic disease.

MINOR HEMATOCHEZIA

Bright red blood passed with or on formed brown stool usually has a rectal, anal, or distal sigmoid source (Fig. 285-31). Patients with even trivial amounts of hematochezia should be investigated with flexible sigmoidoscopy and anoscopy to exclude large polyps or cancers in the distal bowel. Patients reporting red blood on the toilet tissue only, without blood in the toilet or on the stool, are generally bleeding from a lesion in the anal canal. Careful external inspection, digital examination, and anoscopy are sufficient for diagnosis in most cases.

PANCREATITIS

Approximately 20% of patients with pancreatitis have no identifiable cause after routine clinical investigation (including a review of medication and alcohol use, measurement of serum triglyceride and calcium levels, abdominal ultrasonography, and CT). Endoscopic techniques lead to a specific diagnosis in the majority of such patients, often altering clinical management. Endoscopic investigation is particularly appropriate if the patient has had more than one episode of pancreatitis.

Microlithiasis, or the presence of microscopic crystals in bile, is a leading cause of previously unexplained acute pancreatitis and is sometimes seen during abdominal ultrasonography as layering sludge or flecks of floating, echogenic material in the gallbladder. Gallbladder bile can be obtained for microscopic analysis by administering a cholecysto-

FIGURE 285-28 Capsule endoscopy images of a mildly scalloped jejunal fold (*left*) and an ileal tumor (*right*) in a patient with celiac sprue. (*Images courtesy of Dr. Elizabeth Rajan; with permission.*)

TABLE 285-2 COLORECTAL CANCER SCREENING STRATEGIES

	Recommendation	Comments
Average-Risk Patients		
Asymptomatic individuals ≥50 years of age	Annual fecal occult blood testing, two samples from each of three consecutive stools	Fails to detect many polyps and some cancers
	Flexible sigmoidoscopy every 5 years *or*	Fails to detect some polyps and cancers
	Colonoscopy every 10 years	CT colonography may become a reasonable alternative (see text)
	Double-contrast barium enema every 5 years	Less sensitivity than colonoscopy for polyps and cancer
High-Risk Patients		
Personal history: colon cancer	Evaluate entire colon around the time of resection, then colonoscopy in 3 years	
Personal history: advanced, large, or fewer than three adenomas, completely removed	Repeat colonoscopy in 3 years	
One or two small tubular adenomas	Repeat colonoscopy in 5 years	
Personal history: long-standing (>8 years) extensive ulcerative colitis or Chrohn's colitis, or left-sided ulcerative colitis >15 years' duration	Colonoscopy with biopsies every 1–3 years	
Family history: first-degree relative with colorectal cancer or adenomatous polyp at age ≥60 years, or two second-degree relatives with a history of colorectal cancer	Same as average risk, but start at age 40	
Family history: fewer than two first-degree relatives with colon cancer, or a single first-degree relative with colon cancer or adenomatous polyps diagnosed at an age <60 years	Colonoscopy every 5 years beginning at age 40 or 10 years younger than the earliest diagnosis in the family, whichever comes first	
Family history: one second-degree or third-degree relative with colorectal cancer	Same as average risk	
Family history: familial adenomatous polyposis	Sigmoidoscopy annually, beginning at age 10–12 years	Consider genetic counseling and testing
Family history: hereditary non-polyposis colorectal cancer (HNPCC)	Colonscopy every 1–2 years, beginning at age 20–25 years or 10 years younger than the earliest case in the family, whichever comes first	Consider genetic counseling and testing

Source: Adapted from S Winawer et al: Colorectal cancer screening and surveillance: clinical guidelines and rationale—update based on new evidence. Gastroenterology 124:544, 2003; with permission from the American Gastroenterological Association.

kinin analogue during endoscopy, causing contraction of the gallbladder. Bile is suctioned from the duodenum as it drains from the papilla, and the darkest fraction is examined for cholesterol crystals or bilirubinate granules. Combined EUS of the gallbladder and bile microscopy is probably the most sensitive means of diagnosing microlithiasis.

Previously undetected chronic pancreatitis, pancreatic malignancy, or pancreas divisum may be diagnosed by either ERCP or EUS. Sphincter of Oddi dysfunction probably causes some cases of pancreatitis and can be diagnosed by manometric studies performed during ERCP.

Severe pancreatitis often results in pancreatic fluid collections. Both pseudocysts and areas of organized pancreatic necrosis can be drained into the stomach or duodenum endoscopically, using transpapillary and transmural endoscopic techniques (**Video e25-8**).

CANCER STAGING

Local staging of esophageal, gastric, pancreatic, bile duct, and rectal cancers can be obtained with EUS (Fig. 285-13). EUS with fine-needle aspiration (Fig. 285-14) currently provides the most accurate preoperative assessment of local tumor and nodal staging, but it does not detect most distant metastases. Details of the local tumor stage can guide treatment decisions including resectability and need for neoadjuvant therapy. EUS with transesophageal needle biopsy may also be used to assess the presence of non-small cell lung cancer in mediastinal nodes.

OPEN-ACCESS ENDOSCOPY

Direct scheduling of endoscopic procedures by primary care physicians without preceding gastroenterology consultation, or *open-access endoscopy*, is an increasingly common practice. When the indications for endoscopy are clear-cut and appropriate, the procedural risks are low, and the patient understands what to expect, open-access endoscopy streamlines patient care and decreases costs.

Patients referred for open-access endoscopy should have a recent history, physical examination, and medication review. A copy of such an evaluation should be available when the patient comes to the endoscopy suite. Patients with unstable cardiovascular or respiratory conditions should not be referred directly for open-access endoscopy. Patients with selected cardiac conditions undergoing certain procedures should be prescribed prophylactic antibiotics prior to endoscopy (Table 285-1). In addition, patients on anticoagulants and antiplatelet drugs may require adjustment of these agents before endoscopy (Table 285-3). Most evidence suggests that, in the absence of a preexisting bleeding disorder, it is safe to perform endoscopic procedures in patients taking aspirin and nonsteroidal anti-inflammatory drugs. Little data are

FIGURE 285-30 Virtual colonoscopy image of a colon polyp (*arrow*). (Image courtesy of Dr. Jeff Fidler; with permission.)

FIGURE 285-31 Internal hemorrhoids with bleeding (*arrow*) as seen on a retroflexed view of the rectum.

Drug	Procedural Risk of Bleeding[a,b]	High Patient Risk of Thromboembolism[c]	Low Patient Risk of Thromboembolism[d]
Warfarin	High	Stop warfarin 3–5 days before the procedure; consider heparin while INR is below the therapeutic range	Stop warfarin 3–5 days before the procedure; restart warfarin after the procedure
	Low	No change in anticoagulation; elective procedures should be delayed while INR is in the supratherapeutic range	
Low molecular weight heparin	High	Consider discontinuation at least 8 h before procedure	
	Low	No change in therapy	
Clopidogrel or Ticlopidine	High	Consider discontinuation 5–10 days before procedure	
	Low	No change in therapy	
Aspirin	High or Low	No change in therapy	

TABLE 285-3 MANAGEMENT OF ANTICOAGULANTS AND ANTIPLATELET DRUGS BEFORE ENDOSCOPIC PROCEDURES

[a]High-risk procedures: Polypectomy, stricture dilation, treatment of varices, gastrostomy tube placement, biliary sphincterotomy, endoscopic ultrasound (EUS) with fine-needle aspiration (FNA), laser ablation and coagulation.
[b]Low-risk procedures: Diagnostic upper endoscopy, colonoscopy, or sigmoidoscopy, with or without biopsy; endoscopic retrograde cholangiopancreatography (ERCP) without endoscopic sphincterotomy; EUS without FNA.
[c]High-risk conditions: Atrial fibrillation associated with valvular heart disease, mechanical valve in the mitral position, mechanical valve and prior thromboembolic event.
[d]Low-risk conditions: Uncomplicated or paroxysmal nonvalvular atrial fibrillation, mechanical valve in the aortic position, bioprosthetic valve, deep vein thrombosis.
Note: INR, international normalized ratio.
Source: Adapted from G Eisen et al: Guideline on the management of anticoagulation and antiplatelet therapy for endoscopic procedures. Gastrointest Endosc 55:775, 2002; and from M Zuckerman et al: ASGE guideline: The management of low molecular weight heparin and nonaspirin antiplatelet agents for endoscopic procedures. Gastrointest Endosc 61:189, 2005; with permission.

available regarding the risks of hemorrhage in patients receiving clopidogrel who undergo endoscopic biopsy or therapy, but current guidelines advise discontinuation of this agent at least 5 days before elective endoscopic procedures.

Common indications for open-access EGD include dyspepsia resistant to a trial of appropriate therapy, gastrointestinal bleeding, and persistent anorexia or early satiety. Open-access colonoscopy is often requested in men or postmenopausal women with iron-deficiency anemia, in patients over age 50 with occult blood in the stool, in patients with a previous history of colorectal adenomatous polyps or cancer, and for colorectal cancer screening. Flexible sigmoidoscopy is commonly performed as an open-access procedure.

When patients are referred for open-access colonoscopy, the primary care provider may need to choose a colonic preparation. Commonly used oral preparations include polyethylene glycol lavage solution and oral sodium phosphate. Sodium phosphate may cause fluid and electrolyte abnormalities, especially in patients with renal failure or congestive heart failure and those over 70 years of age.

FURTHER READINGS

BARON TH: Expandable metal stents for the treatment of cancerous obstruction of the gastrointestinal tract. N Engl J Med 344:1681, 2001

HU WH et al: Comparison between empirical prokinetics, helicobacter test-and-treat and empirical endoscopy in primary-care patients presenting with dyspepsia: A one-year study. World J Gastroenterol 12:5010, 2006

IMPERIALE TF et al: Risk of advanced proximal neoplasms in asymptomatic adults according to the distal colorectal findings. N Engl J Med 343:169, 2000

JENSEN DM et al: Urgent colonoscopy for the diagnosis and treatment of severe diverticular hemorrhage. N Engl J Med 342:78, 2000

LIN S, ROCKEY DC: Obscure gastrointestinal bleeding. Gastroenterol Clin North Am 34:679-98, 2005

ROSMAN AS, HORSTEN MA: Meta-analysis comparing CT colonography, air contrast barium enema, and colonoscopy. Am J Med 120:203, 2007

286 Diseases of the Esophagus
Raj K. Goyal

Two major functions of the esophagus are transport of food bolus from the mouth to the stomach and prevention of retrograde flow of gastrointestinal contents. Esophageal transport function begins with the transfer of food from the mouth and pharynx through the opened upper esophageal sphincter (UES) into the esophagus, and it involves esophageal peristalsis and relaxation of the lower esophageal sphincter (LES). Retrograde flow from the stomach into the esophagus is prevented by the LES and from the esophagus into the pharynx by the UES. **Physiology of swallowing, esophageal motility, and oral and pharyngeal dysphagia are described in Chap. 38.**

Normally, the LES relaxes in association with esophageal peristalsis with swallowing. However, relaxation of the LES without esophageal peristalsis may occur during belching and gastric distention. Gastric distention–evoked transient lower esophageal sphincter relaxation (tLESR) is a vagovagal reflex. Reflex LES relaxation is augmented by phosphodiesterase-5 inhibitors such as sildenafil that increase cyclic guanosine monophosphate (cGMP) in the sphincter muscle, and it is inhibited by GABA-B agonists such as baclofen. Fatty meals, smoking, and beverages with high xanthine content (tea, coffee, cola) also cause a reduction in sphincter pressure. Many hormones and neurotransmitters can modify LES pressure. Muscarinic M_2 and M_3 receptor agonists, α-adrenergic agonists, gastrin, substance P, and prostaglandin $F_{2\alpha}$ all cause LES contraction. On the other hand, nicotine, β-adrenergic agonists, dopamine, cholecystokinin, secretin, vasoactive intestinal peptide (VIP), calcitonin gene–related peptide, adenosine, prostaglandin E, nitric oxide donors such as nitrates, and inhibitors of phosphodiesterase 5 reduce LES pressure.

SYMPTOMS

DYSPHAGIA
See Chap. 38.

HEARTBURN, ODYNOPHAGIA, AND ESOPHAGEAL PAIN
Heartburn, or pyrosis, is characterized by burning retrosternal discomfort that may move up and down the chest like a wave. When severe, it may radiate to the sides of the chest, the neck, and the angles of the jaw. Heartburn is a characteristic symptom of *reflux esophagitis* and may be associated with regurgitation or a feeling of warm fluid climbing up the throat. It is aggravated by bending forward, straining, or lying recumbent and is worse after meals. It is relieved by an upright posture, by the swallowing of saliva or water, and, more reliably, by antacids. Heartburn is produced by heightened mucosal sensitivity and can be reproduced by infusion of dilute (0.1 N) hydrochloric acid (Bernstein test) or neutral hyperosmolar solutions into the esophagus.

Odynophagia, or painful swallowing, is characteristic of nonreflux esophagitis (particularly monilial), herpes, and pill-induced esophagitis.

FIGURE 286-1 Radiographic appearance of some motor disorders of the esophagus. *(1)* Pharyngeal paralysis with tracheal aspiration *(arrow)*. *(2)* Cricopharyngeal achalasia. Note the prominent cricopharyngeus, which is recognized by its smoothness and location in the posterior wall. *(3)* Diffuse esophageal spasm. Note the typical corkscrew appearance of the lower part of the esophagus. *(4)* Achalasia, showing a dilated esophageal body with an air-fluid level and a closed lower esophageal sphincter. *(5)* Muscular (contractile) lower esophageal ring. The asymmetric contraction visible in *(5A)* has disappeared in *(5B)*, obtained during the same examination. *(6)* Scleroderma esophagus showing dilated esophagus with a stricture *(6A)* and reflux of barium from the stomach into the esophagus *(6B)*.

Odynophagia may occur with peptic ulcer of the esophagus (Barrett's ulcer), carcinoma with periesophageal involvement, caustic damage of the esophagus, and esophageal perforation. Odynophagia is unusual in uncomplicated reflux esophagitis. Crampy chest pain associated with a food bolus impaction should be distinguished from odynophagia.

Esophageal chest pain resembling cardiac pain is called *noncardiac chest pain* or *atypical chest pain*. Such pain is different from heartburn or odynophagia, and it may occur in gastroesophageal reflux disease (GERD) or esophageal motility disorders such as diffuse esophageal spasm (DES). Chest pain due to periesophageal involvement with carcinoma or peptic ulcer may be constant and agonizing. Sometimes different types of esophageal pains exist concomitantly in the same patient, and frequently patients are not able to describe the pain accurately enough to allow its classification. Coronary artery disease should always be excluded before the esophagus is considered as the origin of atypical chest pain. The most frequent esophageal cause of chest pain is reflux esophagitis. Therefore, studies to investigate GERD should be performed. A trial of proton pump inhibitors (PPIs) is usual; an esophageal motility study may be useful in these cases. A few patients with atypical chest pain are found to have DES or achalasia. However, achalasia usually has associated dysphagia. Some patients have nonspecific esophageal motor abnormalities of uncertain significance. Smooth-muscle relaxants may be tried in selected cases. However, a large number of these patients are thought to have esophageal hypersensitivity syndrome, which can be revealed by a low threshold of pain production by esophageal balloon distension. A low-dose antidepressant treatment may be helpful in these cases. Many of these patients also have behavioral and psychosomatic disorders such as depression, anxiety, or panic reactions.

REGURGITATION

Regurgitation is the effortless appearance of gastric or esophageal contents in the mouth. In distal esophageal obstruction and stasis, as in achalasia or the presence of a large diverticulum, the regurgitated material consists of tasteless mucoid fluid or undigested food. Regurgitation of sour or bitter-tasting material occurs in severe gastroesophageal reflux and is associated with incompetence of both the UES and the LES.

Regurgitation may result in chronic cough, laryngitis, and laryngeal aspiration, with spells of coughing and choking that may awaken the patient from sleep. It may also result in aspiration pneumonia. In some patients, regurgitation and rumination may be a behavioral problem. Water brash is reflex salivary hypersecretion that occurs in response to peptic esophagitis and should not be confused with regurgitation.

DIAGNOSTIC TESTS

RADIOLOGIC STUDIES

Barium swallow with fluoroscopy and an esophagogram is often used to evaluate both structural and motor disorders and is the initial test of choice in the motility disorders. Videofluoroscopic swallow study focuses on oral and pharyngeal phases of swallowing (Chap. 38). A finding of spontaneous reflux of barium from the stomach into the esophagus as an indicator of gastroesophageal reflux is unreliable. Esophageal peristalsis is best studied in the recumbent position, because in the upright position barium passage occurs largely by gravity alone. A double-contrast esophagogram, obtained by coating the esophageal mucosa with barium and distending the esophageal lumen with air using effervescent granules, is particularly useful in demonstrating mucosal ulcers and early cancers. A barium-soaked piece of bread or a 13-mm barium tablet is sometimes used to demonstrate an obstructive lesion. Figures 286-1 and 286-2 illustrate the radiographic appearance of some structural and motor disorders of the esophagus. CT examination of the chest may be helpful in assessing the esophageal wall and the structures surrounding the esophagus.

ESOPHAGOSCOPY

Esophagoscopy is the direct method of establishing the cause of mechanical dysphagia. It can identify mucosal lesions that may not be revealed by the usual barium swallow. Ultrathin endoscopes have been used when the lumen is markedly narrowed; on occasion, a stricture must be dilated before the examination can be completed. Endoscopy is usually performed under sedation. Unsedated esophagoscopy using an ultrathin endoscope is an alternative approach in patients without known stricture. Endoscopic biopsies are useful in diagnosing carcinoma, esophagitis, and

FIGURE 286-2 Selected structural lesions of the esophagus. *(1)* Carcinoma of the esophagus, with typical annular narrowing with overhanging margins and destruction of the mucosa. *(2)* Leiomyoma of the esophagus, with a smooth filling defect and right angles of origin from the esophageal wall. *(3)* Esophageal ulcer in columnar cell–lined esophagus (Barrett's esophagus). *(4)* Monilial esophagitis, with irregular plaque-like filling defects. *(5)* Long stricture secondary to lye ingestion. *(6)* Peptic stricture, short and tubular, with associated hiatal hernia. *(7)* Lower esophageal mucosal (Schatzki) ring. A thin, weblike annular constriction at the esophagogastric junction is associated with a small hiatal hernia.

other mucosal diseases such as eosinophilic esophagitis. Cells obtained by a cytology balloon or by brushing the mucosa can be evaluated for carcinoma. Endoscopic ultrasonography permits evaluation of intramural and periesophageal masses and staging of esophageal cancer.

ESOPHAGEAL MOTILITY

The study of esophageal motility entails simultaneous recording of pressures from different sites in the esophageal lumen with an assembly of pressure sensors positioned 5 cm apart. The UES and LES appear as zones of high pressure that relax on swallowing. The esophagus normally shows peristaltic waves with each swallow.

Esophageal motility studies are helpful in the diagnosis of esophageal motor disorders (achalasia, spasm, and scleroderma) (Fig. 286-3) but are of little value in the differential diagnosis of mechanical dysphagia. In patients with reflux esophagitis, esophageal manometry is useful in quantifying LES competence and providing information on the status of the esophageal body motor activity. Manometry provides quantitative data that cannot be obtained by barium swallow or endoscopy. Esophageal impedance testing identifies the nature (fluid or gas) and the direction of movement (oral or aboral) by measuring impedance across segments using a special catheter positioned in the esophagus. It may be helpful in the study of transit of the contents, particularly nonacid gastric contents. Other tests for reflux esophagitis are described later.

MOTOR DISORDERS

CERVICAL ESOPHAGUS

Motor disorders of the cervical esophagus (striated muscle) are accompanied by oral and pharyngeal dysphagia. Their clinical manifestations are described in Chap. 38.

THORACIC AND ABDOMINAL ESOPHAGUS

Achalasia Achalasia is a motor disorder of the esophageal smooth muscle and involves thoracic and abdominal parts of the esophagus. In achalasia, the esophageal body loses peristaltic contractions and the LES does not relax normally in response to swallowing.

PATHOPHYSIOLOGY The underlying abnormality is the loss of intramural neurons. Inhibitory neurons containing VIP and nitric oxide

FIGURE 286-3 Motility patterns in selected esophageal and pharyngeal disorders. In normal individuals, the upper and lower esophageal sphincters (UES and LES) appear as zones of high pressure. With a swallow (indicated by ↑), pressure in the sphincters falls and a contraction wave starts in the pharynx and progresses down the esophagus. In scleroderma, the thoracic esophagus (smooth muscle) shows reduced amplitude of contractions, which may be peristaltic or simultaneous in onset, and hypotension of the LES. In achalasia, the lower part of the esophagus shows contractions that are reduced in amplitude and simultaneous in onset. In contrast to scleroderma, the LES in achalasia is hypertensive and fails to relax in response to a swallow. In diffuse esophageal spasm, the lower part of the esophagus shows simultaneous-onset, large-amplitude, prolonged, repetitive contractions. In contrast, in motor disorders of the cervical esophagus, the cervical esophagus shows poor contractions while contractions in the thoracic esophagus are normal. Moreover, these cases also show poor pharyngeal contractions and a hypotensive UES that fails to fully relax on swallowing.

synthase are predominantly involved, but cholinergic neurons are also affected in advanced disease. Primary idiopathic achalasia accounts for most of the cases seen in the United States. Secondary achalasia may be caused by gastric carcinoma that infiltrates the esophagus, lymphoma, Chagas' disease, certain viral infections, eosinophilic gastroenteritis, and neurodegenerative disorders.

CLINICAL FEATURES Achalasia affects patients of all ages and both sexes. Dysphagia, chest pain, and regurgitation are the main symptoms. Dysphagia occurs early with both liquids and solids and is worsened by emotional stress and hurried eating. Various maneuvers designed to increase intraesophageal pressure, including the Valsalva maneuver, may aid the passage of the bolus into the stomach. Regurgitation and pulmonary aspiration occur because of retention of a large amount of saliva and ingested food in the esophagus. Patients may complain of difficulty belching. The presence of gastroesophageal reflux argues against achalasia; in patients with long-standing heartburn, cessation of heartburn and appearance of dysphagia may suggest development of achalasia, peptic stricture, or carcinoma on top of reflux esophagitis. The course is usually chronic, with progressive dysphagia and weight loss over months to years. Achalasia associated with carcinoma is characterized by severe weight loss and a rapid downhill course.

DIAGNOSIS A chest x-ray shows absence of the gastric air bubble and sometimes a tubular mediastinal mass beside the aorta. An air-fluid level in the mediastinum in the upright position represents retained food in the esophagus. Barium swallow shows esophageal dilation, and in advanced cases the esophagus may become sigmoid. On fluoroscopy with barium swallow, normal peristalsis is lost in the lower two-thirds of the esophagus. The terminal part of the esophagus shows a persistent beaklike narrowing representing the nonrelaxing LES (Fig. 286-1, panel 4).

Manometry shows the basal LES pressure to be normal or elevated, and swallow-induced relaxation either does not occur or is reduced in degree, duration, and consistency. The esophageal body shows an elevated resting pressure. In response to swallows, primary peristaltic waves are replaced by simultaneous contractions (Fig. 286-3). These contractions may be of poor amplitude (classic achalasia) or of large amplitude and long duration (vigorous achalasia). Cholecystokinin (CCK), which normally causes a fall in the sphincter pressure, paradoxically causes contraction of the LES (the CCK test). This paradoxical response occurs because, in achalasia, the neurally transmitted inhibitory effect of CCK is absent and the direct excitatory effect of CCK remains unopposed. Endoscopy is helpful in excluding the secondary causes of achalasia, particularly gastric carcinoma.

℞ ACHALASIA

Treatment with soft food, sedatives, and anticholinergics is usually unsatisfactory. Nitrates and calcium channel blockers provide short-term benefit, but their use may be limited by side effects. Nitroglycerin, 0.3–0.6 mg, is used sublingually before meals and as needed for chest pain. Isosorbide dinitrate, 2.5–5 mg sublingually or 10–20 mg orally before meals, can also be used. Nitrates are associated with headache and postural hypotension. The calcium channel blocker nifedipine, 10–20 mg orally or sublingually before meals, may be effective. Sildenafil provides symptomatic relief by increasing cGMP that may reduce LES pressure and augment swallow-induced relaxation. Botulinum toxin acts by blocking cholinergic excitatory nerves in the sphincter. Endoscopic intrasphincteric injection of botulinum toxin is effective with clinical improvement in 60% of patients at 6 months; it may be very useful in temporizing symptoms in elderly or high-risk patients. However, repeated injections may lead to fibrosis, complicating further operative therapy. Balloon dilatation reduces the basal LES pressure by tearing muscle fibers. In experienced hands, this technique is effective in ~85% of patients; perforation and bleeding are potential complications. Heller's extramucosal myotomy of the LES, in which the circular muscle layer is incised, is equally effective. Laparoscopic myotomy is currently the procedure of choice. Since reflux esophagitis and peptic stricture may follow after a successful treatment (more often with myotomy than with balloon dilatation), surgical myotomy is sometimes accompanied by partial fundoplication to lessen postoperative reflux.

Diffuse Esophageal Spasm and Hypertensive Motor Disorders DES is characterized by nonperistaltic contractions. The contraction may have low, normal, or large amplitude. The duration of contraction may be prolonged, and repetitive contractions may be present. The hypertensive disorders include nutcracker esophagus, hypercontracting LES, and hypertensive LES. In *nutcracker esophagus*, esophageal contractions are normally peristaltic but hypertensive. In *hypercontracting LES*, the normal sphincter relaxation is followed by hypertensive contraction. In *hypertensive LES*, basal LES pressure is elevated, but sphincter relaxation and contraction are normal.

PATHOPHYSIOLOGY Nonperistaltic contractions are due to dysfunction of inhibitory nerves. Histopathology shows patchy neural degeneration localized to nerve processes, rather than the prominent degeneration of nerve cell bodies seen in achalasia. DES may progress to achalasia. Hypertensive peristaltic contractions and hypertensive or hypercontracting LES may represent cholinergic or myogenic hyperactivity.

CLINICAL FEATURES DES and hypertensive motor disorders may present with chest pain. Chest pain is particularly marked in patients with esophageal contractions of large amplitude with long duration. It usually occurs at rest but may be brought on by swallowing or by emotional stress. The pain is retrosternal; it may radiate to the back, the sides of the chest, both arms, or the sides of the jaw and may last from a few seconds to several minutes. Pain may be acute and severe, mimicking the pain of myocardial ischemia. Dysphagia with solids and liquids may occur with or without chest pain and is correlated with simultaneous contractions.

DES and hypertensive esophageal motor disorders must be differentiated from other causes of chest pain, particularly ischemic heart disease with atypical angina. A complete cardiac workup should be done before a noncardiac etiology is considered. The presence of dysphagia in association with pain should point to the esophagus as the origin. Esophageal motility disorders are uncommon causes of noncardiac chest pain.

DIAGNOSIS In DES, barium swallow shows that normal sequential peristalsis below the aortic arch is replaced by uncoordinated simultaneous contractions that produce the appearance of curling or multiple ripples in the wall, sacculations, and pseudodiverticula—the "corkscrew" esophagus (Fig. 286-1, panel 3). Sometimes an esophageal contraction obliterates the lumen, and barium is pushed away in both directions. The barium swallow may be normal.

Diffuse esophageal spasm (Fig. 286-3) is best diagnosed by manometry. Because these abnormalities may be episodic, manometry may be normal at the time of the study. Several techniques are used to provoke esophageal spasm. Cold swallows produce chest pain but do not produce spasm on manometric studies. Solid boluses and pharmacologic agents, particularly edrophonium, may induce both chest pain and motor abnormalities. However, correlation between induction of pain and manometric changes is poor. The usefulness of pharmacologic provocative tests is limited.

℞ DIFFUSE ESOPHAGEAL SPASM AND HYPERTENSIVE MOTOR DISORDERS

Anticholinergics are usually of limited value. Agents that relax smooth muscle, such as sublingual nitroglycerin (0.3–0.6 mg) or longer-acting agents such as isosorbide dinitrate (10–30 mg orally before meals) or nifedipine (10–20 mg orally before meals) may be helpful. Reassurance and tranquilizers are helpful in allaying apprehension.

Scleroderma Esophagus The esophageal lesions in systemic sclerosis consist of atrophy of smooth muscle, manifested by weakness in the lower two-thirds of the esophagus and incompetence of the LES. The esophageal wall is atrophic and thin and may exhibit areas of patchy fibrosis. Patients usually present with dysphagia to solids. Liquids may cause dysphagia when the patient is recumbent. These patients usually also complain of heartburn, regurgitation, and other symptoms of

GERD. Barium swallow shows dilation and loss of peristaltic contractions in the middle and distal portions of the esophagus. The LES is patulous, and gastroesophageal reflux may occur freely (Fig. 286-1, panel 6). Mucosal changes due to esophageal ulceration and stricture may be present. Motility studies show a marked reduction in the amplitude of smooth-muscle contractions, which is usually peristaltic but may be nonperistaltic. The resting pressure of the LES is subnormal, but sphincter relaxation is normal (Fig. 286-3). Similar esophageal motor abnormalities are found in other collagen vascular diseases, including Raynaud's phenomenon. Dietary adjustments with the use of soft foods are helpful in management. GERD and its complications should be treated aggressively.

GASTROESOPHAGEAL REFLUX DISEASE

GERD is one of the most prevalent gastrointestinal disorders. Population-based studies show that up to 15% of individuals have heartburn and/or regurgitation at least once a week, and 7% have symptoms daily. Symptoms are caused by backflow of gastric acid and other gastric contents into the esophagus due to incompetent barriers at the gastroesophageal junction.

PATHOPHYSIOLOGY

The normal antireflux mechanisms consist of the LES, the crural diaphragm, and the anatomical location of the gastroesophageal junction below the diaphragmatic hiatus. Reflux occurs only when the gradient of pressure between the LES and the stomach is lost. It can be caused by a sustained or transient decrease in LES tone. A sustained hypotension of the LES may be due to muscle weakness that is often without apparent cause. Secondary causes of sustained LES incompetence include scleroderma-like diseases, myopathy associated with chronic intestinal pseudo-obstruction, pregnancy, smoking, anticholinergic drugs, smooth-muscle relaxants (β-adrenergic agents, aminophylline, nitrates, calcium channel blockers, and phosphodiesterase inhibitors), surgical damage to the LES, and esophagitis. tLESR without associated esophageal contraction is due to a vagovagal reflex in which LES relaxation is elicited by gastric distention. Increased episodes of tLESR are associated with GERD. A similar reflex operates during belching. Apart from incompetent barriers, gastric contents are most likely to reflux (1) when gastric volume is increased (after meals, in pyloric obstruction, in gastric stasis, during acid hypersecretion states), (2) when gastric contents are near the gastroesophageal junction (in recumbency, bending down, hiatal hernia), and (3) when gastric pressure is increased (obesity, pregnancy, ascites, tight clothes). Incompetence of the diaphragmatic crural muscle, which surrounds the esophageal hiatus in the diaphragm and functions as an external LES, also predisposes to GERD. Obesity is a risk factor for GERD.

Esophageal exposure to refluxed gastric contents depends on the amount of refluxed material per episode, the frequency of reflux episodes, and the rate of clearing of the esophagus by gravity and peristaltic contractions. When peristaltic contractions are impaired, esophageal clearance is impaired. Acid refluxed into the esophagus is neutralized by saliva. Thus, impaired salivary secretion also increases esophageal exposure time. If the refluxed material extends to the cervical esophagus and crosses the upper sphincter, it can enter the pharynx, larynx, and trachea.

Reflux esophagitis is a complication of reflux. It develops when mucosal defenses are unable to counteract the damage caused by acid, pepsin, and bile. *Mild esophagitis* involves microscopic changes of mucosal infiltration with granulocytes or small numbers of eosinophils, hyperplasia of basal cells, and elongation of dermal pegs. In nonerosive reflux disease (NERD), the mucosa may be normal or mildly erythematous. *Erosive esophagitis* reveals clear mucosal damage with redness, friability, superficial linear ulcers, and exudates. Histology shows polymorphonuclear or mild eosinophilic infiltrates and granulation tissue. *Peptic stricture* results from fibrosis that causes luminal constriction. These strictures occur in ~10% of patients with untreated GERD. Short strictures caused by spontaneous reflux are usually 1–3 cm long and are present in the distal esophagus near the squamocolumnar junction (Fig. 286-2, panel 6). Long, tubular peptic strictures can result from persistent vomiting or prolonged nasogastric intubation. Erosive esophagitis may heal by intestinal metaplasia (*Barrett's esophagus*), a risk factor for adenocarcinoma.

CLINICAL FEATURES

Heartburn and regurgitation of sour material into the mouth are the characteristic symptoms of GERD. Heartburn is induced by the contact of refluxed material with the sensitized or ulcerated esophageal mucosa. Angina-like or atypical chest pain occurs in some patients. Persistent dysphagia suggests development of a peptic stricture. Most patients with peptic stricture have a history of several years of heartburn preceding dysphagia. However, in one-third of patients, dysphagia is the presenting symptom. Rapidly progressive dysphagia and weight loss may indicate the development of adenocarcinoma in Barrett's esophagus. Bleeding occurs due to mucosal erosions or Barrett's ulcer. Many patients with GERD remain asymptomatic, while many symptomatic patients treat themselves and do not seek medical help until severe symptoms or complications occur.

Extraesophageal manifestations of GERD are due to reflux of gastric contents into the pharynx, larynx, tracheobronchial tree, nose, and mouth. It may cause chronic cough, laryngitis, and pharyngitis. Morning hoarseness may be noted. Recurrent pulmonary aspiration may cause or aggravate chronic bronchitis, asthma, pulmonary fibrosis, chronic obstructive pulmonary disease, or pneumonia. Chronic sinusitis and dental decay have also been ascribed to GERD.

DIAGNOSIS

The diagnosis can be made by history alone in many cases. A therapeutic trial with a PPI such as omeprazole, 40 mg bid for 1 week, provides support for the diagnosis of GERD.

Diagnostic studies are indicated in patients with persistent symptoms or symptoms while on therapy, or in those with complications. The diagnostic approach to GERD can be divided into three categories: (1) documentation of mucosal injury, (2) documentation and quantitation of reflux, and (3) definition of the pathophysiology.

Mucosal damage is documented by the use of barium swallow, esophagoscopy, and mucosal biopsy. Barium swallow is usually normal but may reveal an ulcer or a stricture. A high esophageal peptic stricture, a deep ulcer, or adenocarcinoma suggests Barrett's esophagus. Esophagoscopy may reveal the presence of erosions, ulcers, peptic strictures, or Barrett's metaplasia with or without ulcer, peptic stricture, or adenocarcinoma. A variety of in vivo imaging techniques that facilitate the identification of Barrett's mucosa, dysplasia, or carcinoma during the endoscopy are being developed. Esophagoscopy is not diagnostic of GERD; it is normal in NERD, which constitutes one-third to one-half of all cases of GERD. Mucosal biopsies and the Bernstein test may be helpful in the diagnosis of NERD. Mucosal biopsies may show early changes of esophagitis, including dilation of intracellular spaces. The mucosal biopsies should be performed at least 5 cm above the LES, as the esophageal mucosal changes of chronic esophagitis are quite frequent in the most distal esophagus in otherwise normal individuals. The Bernstein test involves the infusion of solutions of 0.1 N HCl or normal saline into the esophagus. In patients with symptomatic esophagitis, infusion of acid, but not of saline, reproduces the symptoms of heartburn. Infusion of acid in normal individuals usually produces no symptoms. Supraesophageal manifestations are documented by careful otolaryngologic and pulmonary examination.

Documentation and quantitation of reflux, when necessary, can be done by ambulatory long-term (24–48 h) esophageal pH recording. Long-term pH recording may be performed using a pH-sensitive capsule (BRAVO) that is anchored into the esophageal mucosa via an endoscope, rather than the traditional nasally placed pH probe. For evaluation of pharyngeal reflux, a system of recording simultaneously from pharyngeal and esophageal sites may be useful. The pH recordings are helpful only in the evaluation of acid reflux. Endoscopic esophagitis does not correlate with gastroesophageal reflux. Documentation of reflux is necessary only when the role of reflux in the symptom complex is unclear, particularly in evaluation of supraesophageal symptoms, in cases with NERD, and in cases with noncardiac chest pain. Reflux of nonacid contents may be responsible for symptoms of regurgitation and extraesophageal manifestations of GERD. Reflux of nonacid contents can be documented by the use of an impedance test.

Determination of pathophysiologic factors in GERD is sometimes indicated for management decisions such as antireflux surgery. Esophageal motility studies may provide useful quantitative information on the competence of the LES and on esophageal motor function. Determination of tLESR as a cause of GERD requires studies that are usually not available in the clinical laboratory.

℞ GASTROESOPHAGEAL REFLUX DISEASE

The goals of treatment are to provide symptom relief, heal erosive esophagitis, and prevent complications. The management of mild cases includes weight reduction, sleeping with the head of the bed elevated by about 4–6 in. with blocks, and elimination of factors that increase abdominal pressure. Patients should not smoke and should avoid consuming fatty foods, coffee, chocolate, alcohol, mint, orange juice, and certain medications (such as anticholinergic drugs, calcium channel blockers, and other smooth-muscle relaxants). They should also avoid ingesting large quantities of fluids with meals. The lifestyle change and over-the-counter antisecretory agents may be adequate. H_2 receptor blocking agents (cimetidine, 300 mg qid; ranitidine, 150 mg bid; famotidine, 20 mg bid; nizatidine, 150 mg bid) are effective in symptom relief. PPIs are more effective and more commonly used.

The PPIs are comparably effective: omeprazole (20 mg/d), lansoprazole (30 mg/d), pantoprazole (40 mg/d), esomeprazole (40 mg/d), or rabeprazole (20 mg/d) for 8 weeks can heal erosive esophagitis in up to 90% of patients. The PPI should be taken 30 min before breakfast. Refractory patients can double the dose. Since GERD is a chronic disease, long-term maintenance therapy is often required, and symptoms may relapse in up to 80% of patients within 1 year if therapy is discontinued. PPIs are most effective in preventing recurrences. The side effects of PPI therapy are generally minimal. However, aggressive acid suppression may cause hypergastrinemia but does not increase the risk for carcinoid tumors or gastrinomas. Vitamin B_{12} and calcium absorption may be compromised by the treatment. Patients on PPIs for prolonged periods have an increased incidence of hip fractures. Patients who have Barrett's esophagus with concomitant esophagitis should be treated similarly; however, acid suppression does not lead to resolution of the Barrett's metaplasia or cancer prevention. Patients who have an associated peptic stricture are treated with endoscopic dilation to relieve dysphagia, and such patients should be vigorously treated for reflux. Esophagoscopy should also be performed in patients suspected of other complications such as bleeding or development of cancer.

Antireflux surgery, in which the gastric fundus is wrapped around the esophagus (fundoplication), creates an antireflux barrier. The efficacy of the antireflux barrier depends on the type of surgery and experience of the operator. Open fundoplication has mostly been replaced by laparoscopic fundoplication, and endoscopic antireflux procedures are being vigorously tested. Laparoscopic or endoscopic antireflux procedures should be considered as alternatives in young patients who require long-term, high-dose PPIs. Ideal candidates for fundoplication are those who have classical GERD with good response to PPI therapy and in whom motility studies show poor LES pressures but normal peristaltic contractions in the esophageal body.

Symptomatic GERD patients with low or no acid or alkaline (bile) reflux are also considered candidates for antireflux operations. Nonoperative treatment of alkaline esophagitis includes general antireflux measures and neutralization of bile salts with cholestyramine, aluminum hydroxide, or sucralfate. Sucralfate is particularly useful in these cases, as it also serves as a mucosal protector.

BARRETT'S ESOPHAGUS

The metaplasia of esophageal squamous epithelium to columnar epithelium (Barrett's esophagus) is a complication of severe reflux esophagitis, and it is a risk factor for esophageal adenocarcinoma (Chap. 87). Metaplastic columnar epithelium develops during healing of erosive esophagitis with continued acid reflux because columnar epithelium is more resistant to acid-pepsin damage than is squamous epithelium. The metaplastic epithelium is a mosaic of different epithelial types, including goblet cells and columnar cells, which have features of both

secretory and absorptive cells. Finding intestinal metaplasia with goblet cells in the esophagus is diagnostic of Barrett's esophagus; this type of mucosa is thought to be at risk of cancer. Barrett's esophagus is arbitrarily divided into long-segment (>2–3 cm) and short-segment (<2–3 cm) groups; long-segment disease is diagnosed in about 1.5% and short-segment disease in 10–15% of the GERD population.

The rate of cancer development is 0.5% per year in long-segment disease, a 30- to 125-fold increased risk as compared to the general population. Short-segment Barrett's esophagus may also progress to cancer, but the actual risk in these cases is unclear.

Barrett's intestinal metaplasia progresses to adenocarcinoma through dysplastic stages, including low-grade dysplasia (LGD) and high-grade dysplasia (HGD). The sequence of disease progression is variable and inconsistent. Sampling error is a major problem in monitoring progression of the disease by mucosal biopsies. Therefore, optical methods of recognizing dysplasia during the endoscopy (laser-induced fluorescence spectroscopy, optical coherence tomography) are being developed. Moreover, an intense search for molecular markers of neoplastic progression is ongoing.

Barrett's esophagus can also lead to chronic peptic ulcer of the esophagus with high (midesophageal) and long strictures. Barrett's esophagus is more common in obese white men; its incidence increases with age. Usefulness of routine endoscopic population screening for Barrett's esophagus has not been established. However, a one-time esophagoscopy is recommended in patients with persistent GERD symptoms at age 50, particularly in white males. Over 90% of patients with esophageal adenocarcinoma are diagnosed during their first visit to a physician. When Barrett's esophagus is identified for the first time, no effort should be spared to exclude the presence of concurrent dysplasia or carcinoma. This effort may require a follow-up endoscopic study after aggressive treatment of esophagitis, with multiple esophageal mucosal biopsies.

The frequency of surveillance endoscopies in patients with established Barrett's esophagus depends on the initial endoscopic findings. HGD is often associated with concurrent carcinoma and progresses to cancer in about 20% of the cases. Currently, patients with HGD can be treated with esophagectomy, endoscopic mucosal resection, or photodynamic therapy with HGD. Close endoscopic follow-up (every 3 months) is recommended in all patients with HGD. In LGD, follow-up endoscopy is recommended at 6 and 12 months initially and yearly thereafter, as long as LGD persists. Patients with Barrett's esophagus without dysplasia should have two examinations within the first year and subsequently every 3 years. Acid suppression and fundoplication are indicated when active esophagitis is also present. Established metaplasia does not regress with antisecretory treatment.

INFLAMMATORY DISORDERS

INFECTIOUS ESOPHAGITIS

Infectious esophagitis can be due to viral, bacterial, fungal, or parasitic organisms. In severely immunocompromised patients, multiple organisms may coexist.

Viral Esophagitis *Herpes simplex virus* (HSV) type 1 occasionally causes esophagitis in immunocompetent individuals, but either HSV-1 or HSV-2 may afflict patients who are immunosuppressed (Chap. 172). Patients may complain of an acute onset of chest pain, odynophagia, and dysphagia. Bleeding may occur in severe cases; tracheoesophageal fistula and food impaction have been reported. Systemic manifestations such as nausea, vomiting, fever, chills, and mild leukocytosis may be present. Herpetic vesicles on the nose and lips may provide a clue to the diagnosis. Barium swallow is inadequate to detect early lesions and cannot reliably distinguish HSV infection from other types of infections. Endoscopy shows vesicles and small, discrete, punched-out ("volcano-like") superficial ulcerations with or without a fibrinous exudate. In later stages, a diffuse erosive esophagitis develops from enlargement and coalescence of the ulcers. Mucosal cells from a biopsy sample taken at the edge of an ulcer or from a cytologic smear show ballooning degeneration, ground-glass changes in the nuclei with eosinophilic intranuclear inclusions (Cowdry type A), and giant cell formation on routine stains. Culture for HSV becomes positive within days and is helpful in diagnosis and to identify acyclovir-resistant strains. PCR assays are more sensitive than viral cultures. Spontaneous resolution may occur in 1–2 weeks. Acyclovir (400 mg PO 5 times a day for 14–21 days) causes early resolution of symptoms. Valacyclovir (1 g PO tid for 7 days) may be more convenient and have better patient adherence. In patients with severe odynophagia, intravenous acyclovir, 5 mg/kg every 8 h for 7–14 days, is used. Symptoms usually resolve in 1 week, but large ulcerations may take longer to heal. Foscarnet (90 mg/kg intravenously bid for 2–4 weeks) is used if acyclovir resistance occurs. Oral famciclovir may be considered in patients who are able to swallow.

Varicella-zoster virus (VZV) (Chap. 173) sometimes produces esophagitis in children with chickenpox and adults with herpes zoster. Esophageal VZV can also be the source of disseminated VZV infection without skin involvement. In an immunocompromised host, VZV esophagitis causes vesicles and confluent ulcers and usually resolves spontaneously, but it may cause necrotizing esophagitis in severely compromised patients. On routine histologic examination of mucosal biopsy samples or cytology specimens, VZV is difficult to distinguish from HSV, but the distinction can be made immunohistologically or by culture. Acyclovir and valacyclovir reduce duration of symptoms and may be used in combination with glucocorticoids.

Cytomegalovirus (CMV) infections (Chap. 175) occur only in immunocompromised patients. CMV is usually activated from a latent stage or may be acquired from blood product transfusions. CMV lesions initially appear as serpiginous ulcers in an otherwise normal mucosa. These may coalesce to form giant ulcers, particularly in the distal esophagus. Patients present with odynophagia, persistent and focal chest pain, nausea, vomiting, and hematemesis. Diagnosis requires endoscopy and biopsies from the ulcer base. Mucosal brushings are not useful. Routine histologic examination shows intranuclear and small intracytoplasmic inclusions in large fibroblasts and endothelial cells. Immunohistology with monoclonal antibodies to CMV and in situ hybridization tests are useful for early diagnosis. Ganciclovir, 5 mg/kg every 12 h intravenously, is the treatment of choice. Valganciclovir (900 mg bid), an oral formulation of ganciclovir, can be used. Foscarnet (90 mg/kg every 12 h intravenously) may be used in resistant cases. Therapy is continued until healing occurs, which may take 3–6 weeks.

HIV (Chap. 182) may be associated with a self-limited syndrome of acute esophageal ulceration associated with oral ulcers and a maculopapular skin rash, which occurs at the time of HIV seroconversion. Some patients with advanced disease have deep, persistent esophageal ulcers requiring treatment with oral glucocorticoids or thalidomide. Some ulcers respond to local steroid injection.

Bacterial and Fungal Esophagitis

Bacterial esophagitis is unusual, but *Lactobacillus* and β-hemolytic streptococci can cause esophagitis in immunocompromised patients. In patients with profound granulocytopenia and patients with cancer, bacterial esophagitis is often overlooked because it is commonly present with other organisms, including viruses and fungi. In patients with AIDS, infection with *Cryptosporidium* or *Pneumocystis carinii* may cause nonspecific inflammation, and *Mycobacterium tuberculosis* infection may cause deep ulcerations of the distal esophagus. Very rarely, other types of fungi may cause esophagitis.

CANDIDA ESOPHAGITIS

Candida species are normal commensals in the throat but become pathogenic and produce esophagitis in a compromised host. Candida esophagitis can occur without any predisposing factors. Patients may be asymptomatic or complain of odynophagia and dysphagia. Oral thrush or other evidence of mucocutaneous candidiasis may be absent. Rarely, Candida esophagitis is complicated by esophageal bleeding, perforation, and stricture or by systemic invasion. Barium swallow may be normal or show multiple nodular filling defects of various sizes (Fig. 286-2, panel 4). Large nodular defects may resemble grape clusters. Endoscopy shows

small, yellow-white raised plaques with surrounding erythema in mild disease. Confluent linear and nodular plaques reflect extensive disease. Diagnosis is made by demonstration of yeast or hyphal forms in plaque smears and exudate stained with periodic acid–Schiff or Gomori silver stains. Histologic examination is often negative. Culture is not useful in diagnosis but may define the species and the drug sensitivities of the yeast; *Candida albicans* is most common (Chap. 196). Oral fluconazole (200 mg on the first day, followed by 100 mg daily) for 7–14 days is the preferred treatment. Patients refractory to fluconazole often respond to itraconazole. Patients who respond poorly or cannot swallow oral medications can be treated with an intravenous echinocandin such as caspofungin (50 mg daily for 7–21 days). Amphotericin B (10–15 mg IV infusion for 6 h daily to a total dose of 300–500 mg) is used in severe cases.

OTHER TYPES OF ESOPHAGITIS

Eosinophilic Esophagitis Eosinophilic esophagitis is characterized by eosinophilic inflammation and submucosal fibrosis. The eosinophil chemokine eotaxin-3 is involved in the pathogenesis of the disease. Clinically, eosinophilic esophagitis is more common in children and in males. Presenting symptoms vary with age. Younger children present with failure to thrive and refusal to swallow. Older children present with regurgitation, vomiting, and pain. Adolescents usually present with heartburn and dysphagia. Adults often present with intermittent dysphagia and food impaction. A history of allergic disease or mild peripheral eosinophilia is present in about half of patients. Barium esophagogram may show a small-caliber esophagus, isolated esophageal narrowing, or single or multiple esophageal rings. Esophagoscopy may reveal one or more longitudinal fissures, fixed or transient concentric rings, proximal strictures, and focal white specks (abscesses). Endoscopic ultrasound may show thickening of the esophageal wall. Differential diagnosis includes reflux esophagitis, eosinophilic gastroenteritis, and esophageal rings and strictures. Diagnosis is confirmed by esophageal mucosal biopsies that show increased eosinophils (>15) per high-power field or eosinophilic microabscesses. Treatment consists of a 12-week course of swallowed fluticasone propionate (440 μg bid) using a metered dose inhaler. Oral prednisone may also be used. Dietary management involves identification of the offending food and its elimination from the diet or a trial of elemental diet for 4 weeks. Food impaction requires endoscopic dislodging. Esophageal dilation should be performed with great care because of a high rate of esophageal perforation in these cases. Antibody to interleukin 5 is an effective therapy emerging from clinical trials.

Radiation esophagitis is a common occurrence during radiation treatment for thoracic cancers. The frequency and severity of esophagitis increase with the amount of radiation delivered and may be enhanced by radiosensitizing drugs like doxorubicin, bleomycin, cyclophosphamide, and cisplatin. Dysphagia and odynophagia may last several weeks to several months after therapy. The esophageal mucosa becomes erythematous, edematous, and friable. Superficial erosions coalesce to form larger ulcers. Submucosal fibrosis and degenerative changes in the blood vessels, muscles, and myenteric neurons may occur, and esophageal stricture may develop. The treatment aims to relieve the pain with viscous lidocaine during the acute phase; indomethacin treatment may reduce radiation damage. Esophageal stricture may need to be dilated.

Corrosive esophagitis is caused by the ingestion of caustic agents, such as strong alkali or acid. Severe corrosive injury may lead to esophageal perforation, bleeding, and death. Glucocorticoids are not useful in acute corrosive esophagitis. Healing is usually associated with stricture formation. Caustic strictures are usually long and rigid (Fig. 286-2, panel 5) and generally require dilatation with dilators passed over a guide wire through the stricture.

Pill-induced esophagitis is associated with the ingestion of certain types of pills. Antibiotics such as doxycycline, tetracycline, oxytetracycline, minocycline, penicillin, and clindamycin account for more than half the cases. Nonsteroidal anti-inflammatory agents such as aspirin, indomethacin, and ibuprofen may cause injury. Other commonly prescribed pills that cause esophageal injury include potassium chloride, ferrous sulfate or succinate, quinidine, alprenolol, theophylline, ascorbic acid, and pinaverium bromide. Bisphosphonates, particularly alendronate and pamidronate, are more common offenders. Pill-induced esophagitis can be prevented by avoiding the offending agents or taking pills in the upright position with copious amount of fluid.

Sclerotherapy for bleeding esophageal varices usually produces transient retrosternal chest pain and dysphagia; esophageal ulcer, stricture, hematoma, or perforation may occur. Variceal banding causes similar complications, but less frequently. Esophagitis associated with mucocutaneous and systemic diseases is usually associated with blister and bulla formation, epithelial desquamation, and thin, weblike, or dense esophageal strictures. Pemphigus vulgaris and bullous pemphigoid form intraepithelial and subepithelial bullae, respectively, and can be distinguished by specific immunohistology; both are characterized by sloughing of epithelium or the presence of esophageal casts. Glucocorticoid treatment is usually effective. Cicatricial pemphigoid, Stevens-Johnson syndrome, and toxic epidermolysis bullosa can produce esophageal bullous lesions and strictures requiring gentle dilatation. Graft-versus-host disease (GVHD) occurs in patients who have received allogeneic bone marrow or cord blood transplant. If it involves the esophagus, dysphagia and odynophagia are common symptoms. Radiologic findings include mid- and upper esophageal rings or webs and strictures. Esophageal ulcers may be seen. Behçet's syndrome and eosinophilic gastroenteritis may involve the esophagus and respond to glucocorticoid therapy. An erosive lichen planus can also involve the esophagus. Crohn's disease may cause inflammatory strictures, sinus tracts, filiform polyps, and fistulas in the esophagus.

OTHER ESOPHAGEAL DISORDERS

DIVERTICULA

Diverticula are outpouchings of the esophagus wall. A *Zenker's diverticulum* appears in the natural zone of weakness in the posterior hypopharyngeal wall (Killian's triangle) and causes halitosis and regurgitation of saliva and food that may have been consumed several days earlier. When it becomes large and filled with food, it can compress the esophagus and cause dysphagia or complete obstruction. Nasogastric intubation and endoscopy should be performed with utmost care in these patients, as the diverticulum may perforate. A *midesophageal diverticulum* may be caused by traction from old adhesions or by propulsion associated with esophageal motor abnormalities. An *epiphrenic diverticulum* may be associated with achalasia. Small or medium-sized diverticula and midesophageal and epiphrenic diverticula are usually asymptomatic. *Diffuse intramural esophageal diverticulosis* is due to dilation of the deep esophageal glands and may lead to chronic candidiasis or to the development of a stricture that is usually high up in the esophagus. These patients may present with dysphagia. Symptomatic Zenker's diverticula are treated by cricopharyngeal myotomy with or without diverticulectomy. Large symptomatic esophageal diverticula are removed surgically. Diverticula associated with DES or achalasia are treated with distal myotomy. Strictures associated with diffuse intramural diverticulosis are treated with rubber dilators.

WEBS AND RINGS

Weblike constrictions of the esophagus are usually congenital or inflammatory in origin. Asymptomatic hypopharyngeal webs are demonstrated in <10% of normal individuals. When concentric, they cause intermittent dysphagia to solids. The combination of symptomatic hypopharyngeal webs and iron-deficiency anemia in middle-aged women constitutes *Plummer-Vinson syndrome*. The clinical importance of this syndrome is uncertain. Midesophageal webs are rare. Often they are inflammatory in nature and may occur in mucocutaneous disorders, GVHD, and eosinophilic esophagitis. Multiple mucosal rings (feline esophagus) are characteristic of eosinophilic esophagitis.

A *lower esophageal mucosal ring* (Schatzki ring) is a thin, weblike constriction located at the squamocolumnar mucosal junction at or near the border of the LES (Fig. 286-2, panel 7). It may result from GERD or be congenital in origin. It invariably produces dysphagia when the lumen diameter is <1.3 cm. Dysphagia to solids is the only symptom, and it is usually episodic. A lower esophageal ring is one of the common causes of dysphagia. Asymptomatic rings may be present in ~10% of normal individuals. Symptomatic rings and webs are easily treated by dilatation.

A *lower esophageal muscular ring* (contractile ring) is located proximal to the site of mucosal rings and may represent an abnormal uppermost segment of the LES. These rings can be recognized by the fact that they are not constant in size and shape. They may also cause dysphagia and should be differentiated from peptic strictures, achalasia, and lower esophageal mucosal rings. Muscular rings do not respond well to dilatation.

HIATAL HERNIA

A *hiatal hernia* is a herniation of part of the stomach into the thoracic cavity through the esophageal hiatus in the diaphragm. A *sliding hiatal hernia* is one in which the gastroesophageal junction and fundus of the stomach slide upward. A sliding hernia may result from weakening of the anchors of the gastroesophageal junction to the diaphragm, from longitudinal contraction of the esophagus, or from increased intraabdominal pressure. Small sliding hernias can be demonstrated commonly during barium studies if intraabdominal pressure is increased. Incidence increases with age; in individuals in the sixth decade of life, the prevalence of such hernias is ~60%. Small sliding hiatal hernias alone probably produce no symptoms but can contribute to reflux esophagitis. A *paraesophageal hernia* is one in which the esophagogastric junction remains fixed in its normal location and a pouch of stomach is herniated beside the gastroesophageal junction through the esophageal hiatus. A paraesophageal or mixed paraesophageal and sliding hernia may become incarcerated and strangulated, leading to acute chest pain, dysphagia, and a mediastinal mass and requiring surgery. A herniated gastric pouch may cause dysphagia, gastritis, ulceration, or chronic blood loss. Large paraesophageal hernias should be surgically repaired.

MECHANICAL TRAUMA

Esophageal rupture may be caused by (1) iatrogenic damage from instrumentation of the esophagus or external trauma, (2) increased intraesophageal pressure associated with forceful vomiting or retching (*spontaneous rupture* or *Boerhaave's syndrome*), or (3) diseases of the esophagus such as corrosive esophagitis, esophageal ulcer, and neoplasm. The site of perforation depends on the cause. Instrumental perforation usually occurs in the pharynx or lower esophagus, just above the diaphragm in the posterolateral wall. Esophageal perforation causes severe retrosternal chest pain, which may be worsened by swallowing and breathing. Free air enters the mediastinum and spreads to neighboring structures, causing palpable subcutaneous emphysema in the neck, mediastinal crackling sounds on auscultation, and pneumothorax. With time, secondary infection supervenes, and mediastinal abscess may develop. Esophageal perforation associated with vomiting usually deposits gastric contents in the mediastinum and causes severe mediastinal complications. By contrast, instrumental perforation may be clinically mild and free of severe complications. Spontaneous rupture of the esophagus may mimic myocardial infarction, pancreatitis, or rupture of an abdominal viscus. Symptoms of chest pain may be mild, particularly in the elderly. Mediastinal emphysema may develop late. An x-ray of the chest shows abnormalities in most patients, but CT of the chest is more sensitive in detecting mediastinal air. Fluid from pleural effusions may have a high content of (salivary) amylase. The diagnosis is confirmed by swallow of radiopaque contrast material. Gastrografin is used initially, and if no leak is found, a small amount of thin barium is used to confirm the diagnosis. Treatment includes esophageal and gastric suction and parenteral broad-spectrum antibiotics. Surgical drainage and repair of the laceration should be performed as soon as possible. In patients with terminal carcinoma, surgical repair may not be feasible. Endoscopic clipping or stent placement may be indicated in some cases. Patients with minor instrumental perforation can be treated conservatively. Extensive corrosive damage may require esophageal diversion and excision of the damaged portion.

Mucosal Tear (Mallory-Weiss Syndrome) This tear is usually caused by vomiting, retching, or vigorous coughing. The tear usually involves the

gastric mucosa near the squamocolumnar mucosal junction. Patients present with upper gastrointestinal bleeding, which may be severe. In most patients, bleeding ceases spontaneously; continued bleeding may respond to vasopressin therapy or angiographic embolization. Surgery is rarely needed.

Intramural Hematoma Emetogenic injury, particularly in patients with bleeding abnormalities, can cause bleeding between the mucosal and muscle layers of the esophagus. The patients may develop sudden chest pain and dysphagia. The diagnosis is made by barium swallow and CT. Resolution is usually spontaneous.

FOREIGN BODIES AND FOOD IMPACTION

Foreign bodies may lodge in the cervical esophagus just beyond the UES, near the aortic arch, or above the LES. They usually require endoscopic removal. Impaction of food may occur when the esophageal lumen is narrowed due to stricture, carcinoma, lower esophageal ring, or eosinophilic esophagitis. Acute impaction may cause complete inability to swallow and severe chest pain. Impacted food is dislodged endoscopically. Use of a meat tenderizer to facilitate passage of a meat bolus is discouraged because of potential esophageal perforation and aspiration pneumonia. Glucagon (1.0 mg IV) is sometimes tried before endoscopic dislodgement. Esophageal dilation is needed to avoid recurrence. In eosinophilic esophagitis, esophageal dilation should be performed cautiously because of a high risk of perforation.

287 Peptic Ulcer Disease and Related Disorders
John Del Valle

PEPTIC ULCER DISEASE

Burning epigastric pain exacerbated by fasting and improved with meals is a symptom complex associated with peptic ulcer disease (PUD). An *ulcer* is defined as disruption of the mucosal integrity of the stomach and/or duodenum leading to a local defect or excavation due to active inflammation. Ulcers occur within the stomach and/or duodenum and are often chronic in nature. Acid peptic disorders are very common in the United States, with 4 million individuals (new cases and recurrences) affected per year. Lifetime prevalence of PUD in the United States is ~12% in men and 10% in women. Moreover, an estimated 15,000 deaths per year occur as a consequence of complicated PUD. The financial impact of these common disorders has been substantial, with an estimated burden on direct and indirect health care costs of ~$10 billion per year in the United States.

GASTRIC PHYSIOLOGY

Despite the constant attack on the gastroduodenal mucosa by a host of noxious agents (acid, pepsin, bile acids, pancreatic enzymes, drugs, and bacteria), integrity is maintained by an intricate system that provides mucosal defense and repair.

Gastric Anatomy The gastric epithelial lining consists of rugae that contain microscopic gastric pits, each branching into four or five gastric glands made up of highly specialized epithelial cells. The makeup of gastric glands varies with their anatomic location. Glands within the gastric cardia comprise <5% of the gastric gland area and contain mucous and endocrine cells. The 75% of gastric glands are found within the oxyntic mucosa and contain mucous neck, parietal, chief, endocrine, and enterochromaffin cells (Fig. 287-1). Pyloric glands contain mucous and endocrine cells (including gastrin cells) and are found in the antrum.

FURTHER READINGS

FORD CN: Evaluation and management of laryngopharyngeal reflux. JAMA 28:1534, 2005

HIRANO I: Pathophysiology of achalasia and diffuse esophageal spasm. GI Motility Online, *http://www.nature.com/gimo/contents/pt1/full/gimo22.html*, 2006

LOGEMANN JA: Medical and rehabilitative therapy of oral, pharyngeal motor disorders. GI Motility Online, *http://www.nature.com/gimo/contents/pt1/full/gimo50.html, 2006*

LOWE RC: Medical management of gastroesophageal reflux disease. GI Motility Online, *http://www.nature.com/gimo/contents/pt1/full/gimo54.html*, 2006

NURKO S, FURUTA GT: Eosinophilic esophagitis. GI Motility Online, *http://www.nature.com/gimo/contents/pt1/full/gimo49.html*, 2006

PEHLIVANOV N, PASRICHA PJ: Medical and endoscopic treatment of achalasia. GI Motility Online, *http://www.nature.com/gimo/contents/pt1/full/gimo52.html*, 2006

SPECHLER SJ: Clinical practice: Barrett's esophagus. N Engl J Med 346:836, 2002

SPECHLER SJ et al: Thoughts on the complex relationship between gastroesophageal reflux disease and eosinophilic esophagitis. Am J Gastroenterol 102:1301, 2007

WISE JL, MURRAY JA: Oral, pharyngeal and esophageal motility disorders in systemic diseases Systemic diseases. GI Motility Online, *http://www.nature.com/gimo/contents/pt1/full/gimo40.html*, 2006

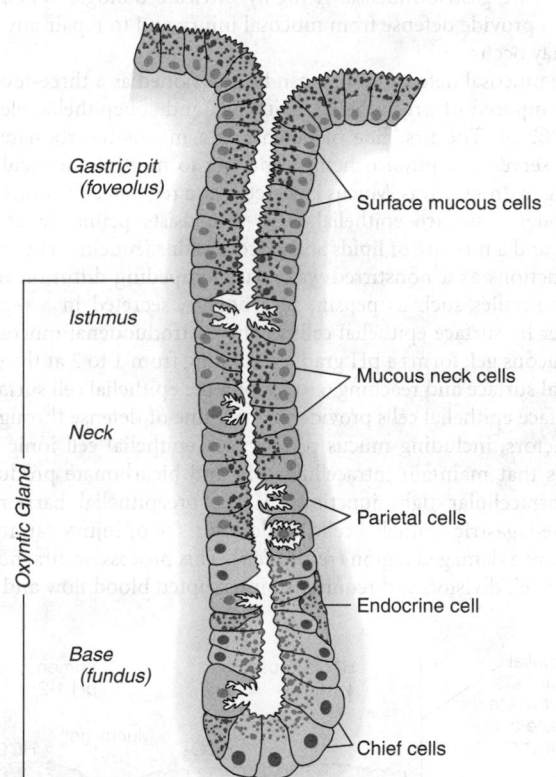

FIGURE 287-1 Diagrammatic representation of the oxyntic gastric gland. *(Adapted from S Ito, RJ Winchester: Cell Biol 16:541, 1963.)*

The parietal cell, also known as the oxyntic cell, is usually found in the neck, or isthmus, or in the oxyntic gland. The resting, or unstimulated, parietal cell has prominent cytoplasmic tubulovesicles and intracellular canaliculi containing short microvilli along its apical surface (Fig. 287-2). H+,K+-ATPase is expressed in the tubulovesicle membrane; upon cell stimulation, this membrane, along with apical membranes, transforms into a dense network of apical intracellular canaliculi containing long microvilli. Acid secretion, a process requir-

FIGURE 287-2 Gastric parietal cell undergoing transformation after secretagogue-mediated stimulation. *(Adapted from SJ Hersey, G Sachs: Physiol Rev 75:155, 1995.)*

ing high energy, occurs at the apical canalicular surface. Numerous mitochondria (30–40% of total cell volume) generate the energy required for secretion.

Gastroduodenal Mucosal Defense The gastric epithelium is under constant assault by a series of endogenous noxious factors, including HCl, pepsinogen/pepsin, and bile salts. In addition, a steady flow of exogenous substances such as medications, alcohol, and bacteria encounter the gastric mucosa. A highly intricate biologic system is in place to provide defense from mucosal injury and to repair any injury that may occur.

The mucosal defense system can be envisioned as a three-level barrier, composed of preepithelial, epithelial, and subepithelial elements (Fig. 287-3). The first line of defense is a mucus-bicarbonate layer, which serves as a physicochemical barrier to multiple molecules, including hydrogen ions. Mucus is secreted in a regulated fashion by gastroduodenal surface epithelial cells. It consists primarily of water (95%) and a mixture of lipids and glycoproteins (mucin). The mucous gel functions as a nonstirred water layer impeding diffusion of ions and molecules such as pepsin. Bicarbonate, secreted in a regulated manner by surface epithelial cells of the gastroduodenal mucosa into the mucous gel, forms a pH gradient ranging from 1 to 2 at the gastric luminal surface and reaching 6 to 7 along the epithelial cell surface.

Surface epithelial cells provide the next line of defense through several factors, including mucus production, epithelial cell ionic transporters that maintain intracellular pH and bicarbonate production, and intracellular tight junctions. If the preepithelial barrier were breached, gastric epithelial cells bordering a site of injury can migrate to restore a damaged region (*restitution*). This process occurs independent of cell division and requires uninterrupted blood flow and an al-

FIGURE 287-4 Schematic representation of the steps involved in synthesis of prostaglandin E$_2$ (PGE$_2$) and prostacyclin (PGI$_2$). Characteristics and distribution of the cyclooxygenase (COX) enzymes 1 and 2 are also shown. TXA$_2$, thromboxane A$_2$.

kaline pH in the surrounding environment. Several growth factors, including epidermal growth factor (EGF), transforming growth factor (TGF) α, and basic fibroblast growth factor (FGF), modulate the process of restitution. Larger defects that are not effectively repaired by restitution require cell proliferation. Epithelial cell regeneration is regulated by prostaglandins and growth factors such as EGF and TGF-α. In tandem with epithelial cell renewal, formation of new vessels (*angiogenesis*) within the injured microvascular bed occurs. Both FGF and vascular endothelial growth factor (VEGF) are important in regulating angiogenesis in the gastric mucosa.

An elaborate microvascular system within the gastric submucosal layer is the key component of the subepithelial defense/repair system, providing HCO$_3^-$, which neutralizes the acid generated by parietal cell. Moreover, this microcirculatory bed provides an adequate supply of micronutrients and oxygen while removing toxic metabolic by-products.

Prostaglandins play a central role in gastric epithelial defense/repair (Fig. 287-4). The gastric mucosa contains abundant levels of prostaglandins that regulate the release of mucosal bicarbonate and mucus, inhibit parietal cell secretion, and are important in maintaining mucosal blood flow and epithelial cell restitution. Prostaglandins are derived from esterified arachidonic acid, which is formed from phospholipids (cell membrane) by the action of phospholipase A$_2$. A key enzyme that controls the rate-limiting step in prostaglandin synthesis is cyclooxygenase (COX), which is present in two isoforms (COX-1, COX-2), each having distinct characteristics regarding structure, tissue distribution, and expression. COX-1 is expressed in a host of tissues, including the stomach, platelets, kidneys, and endothelial cells. This isoform is expressed in a constitutive manner and plays an important role in maintaining the integrity of renal function, platelet aggregation, and gastrointestinal mucosal integrity. In contrast, the expression of COX-2 is inducible by inflammatory stimuli, and it is expressed in macrophages, leukocytes, fibroblasts, and synovial cells. The beneficial effects of nonsteroidal anti-inflammatory drugs (NSAIDs) on tissue inflammation are due to inhibition of COX-2; the toxicity of these drugs (e.g., gastrointestinal mucosal ulceration and renal dysfunction) is related to inhibition of the COX-1 isoform. The highly COX-2–selective NSAIDs have the potential to provide the beneficial effect of decreasing tissue inflammation while minimizing toxicity in the gastrointestinal tract. Selective COX-2 inhibitors have had adverse effects on the cardiovascular system, leading to increased risk of myocardial infarction. Therefore, the FDA has removed two of these agents (valdecoxib and rofecoxib) from the market (see below).

FIGURE 287-3 Components involved in providing gastroduodenal mucosal defense and repair.

Nitric oxide (NO) is important in the maintenance of gastric mucosal integrity. The key enzyme NO synthase is constitutively expressed in the mucosa and contributes to cytoprotection by stimulating gastric mucus, increasing mucosal blood flow and maintaining epithelial cell barrier function.

Physiology of Gastric Secretion Hydrochloric acid and pepsinogen are the two principal gastric secretory products capable of inducing mucosal injury. Acid secretion should be viewed as occurring under basal and stimulated conditions. Basal acid production occurs in a circadian pattern, with highest levels occurring during the night and lowest levels during the morning hours. Cholinergic input via the vagus nerve and histaminergic input from local gastric sources are the principal contributors to basal acid secretion. Stimulated gastric acid secretion occurs primarily in three phases based on the site where the signal originates (cephalic, gastric, and intestinal). Sight, smell, and taste of food are the components of the cephalic phase, which stimulates gastric secretion via the vagus nerve. The gastric phase is activated once food enters the stomach. This component of secretion is driven by nutrients (amino acids and amines) that directly stimulate the G cell to release gastrin, which in turn activates the parietal cell via direct and indirect mechanisms. Distention of the stomach wall also leads to gastrin release and acid production. The last phase of gastric acid secretion is initiated as food enters the intestine and is mediated by luminal distention and nutrient assimilation. A series of pathways that inhibit gastric acid production are also set into motion during these phases. The gastrointestinal hormone somatostatin is released from endocrine cells found in the gastric mucosa (D cells) in response to HCl. Somatostatin can inhibit acid production by both direct (parietal cell) and indirect mechanisms [decreased histamine release from enterochromaffin-like (ECL) cells and gastrin release from G cells]. Additional neural (central and peripheral) and hormonal (secretin, cholecystokinin) factors play a role in counterbalancing acid secretion. Under physiologic circumstances, these phases occur simultaneously.

The acid-secreting parietal cell is located in the oxyntic gland, adjacent to other cellular elements (ECL cell, D cell) important in the gastric secretory process (Fig. 287-5). This unique cell also secretes intrinsic factor (IF). The parietal cell expresses receptors for several stimulants of acid secretion, including histamine (H_2), gastrin (cholecystokinin B/gastrin receptor), and acetylcholine (muscarinic, M_3). Binding of histamine to the H_2 receptor leads to activation of adenylate cyclase and an increase in cyclic AMP. Activation of the gastrin and muscarinic receptors results in activation of the protein kinase C/phosphoinositide signaling pathway. Each of these signaling pathways in turn regulates a series of downstream kinase cascades, which control the acid-secreting pump, H^+,K^+-ATPase. The discovery that different ligands and their corresponding receptors lead to activation of different signaling pathways explains the potentiation of acid secretion that occurs when histamine and gastrin or acetylcholine are combined. More importantly, this observation explains why blocking one receptor type (H_2) decreases acid secretion stimulated by agents that activate a different pathway (gastrin, acetylcholine). Parietal cells also express receptors for ligands that inhibit acid production (prostaglandins, somatostatin, and EGF).

The enzyme H^+,K^+-ATPase is responsible for generating the large concentration of H^+. It is a membrane-bound protein that consists of two subunits, α and β. The active catalytic site is found within the α subunit; the function of the β subunit is unclear. This enzyme uses the chemical energy of ATP to transfer H^+ ions from parietal cell cytoplasm to the secretory canaliculi in exchange for K^+. The H^+,K^+-ATPase is located within the secretory canaliculus and in nonsecretory cytoplasmic tubulovesicles. The tubulovesicles are impermeable to K^+, which leads to an inactive pump in this location. The distribution of pumps between the nonsecretory vesicles and the secretory canaliculus varies according to parietal cell activity (Fig. 287-2). Proton pumps are recycled back to the inactive state in cytoplasmic vesicles once parietal cell activation ceases.

The chief cell, found primarily in the gastric fundus, synthesizes and secretes pepsinogen, the inactive precursor of the proteolytic enzyme pepsin. The acid environment within the stomach leads to cleavage of the inactive precursor to pepsin and provides the low pH (<2.0) required for pepsin activity. Pepsin activity is significantly diminished at a pH of 4 and irreversibly inactivated and denatured at a pH of ≥7. Many of the secretagogues that stimulate acid secretion also stimulate pepsinogen release. The precise role of pepsin in the pathogenesis of PUD remains to be established.

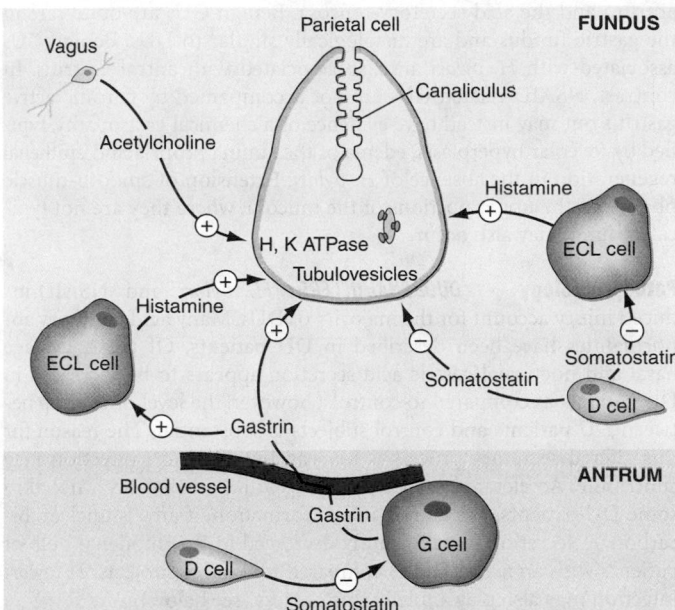

FIGURE 287-5 Regulation of gastric acid secretion at the cellular level. ECL cell, enterochromaffin-like cell.

PATHOPHYSIOLOGIC BASIS OF PEPTIC ULCER DISEASE

PUD encompasses both gastric and duodenal ulcers. *Ulcers* are defined as breaks in the mucosal surface >5 mm in size, with depth to the submucosa. Duodenal ulcers (DUs) and gastric ulcers (GUs); share many common features in terms of pathogenesis, diagnosis, and treatment, but several factors distinguish them from one another.

Epidemiology • DUODENAL ULCERS DUs are estimated to occur in 6–15% of the Western population. The incidence of DUs declined steadily from 1960 to 1980 and has remained stable since then. The death rates, need for surgery, and physician visits have decreased by >50% over the past 30 years. The reason for the reduction in the frequency of DUs is likely related to the decreasing frequency of *Helicobacter pylori*. Before the discovery of *H. pylori*, the natural history of DUs was typified by frequent recurrences after initial therapy. Eradication of *H. pylori* has greatly reduced these recurrence rates.

GASTRIC ULCERS GUs tend to occur later in life than duodenal lesions, with a peak incidence reported in the sixth decade. More than half of GUs occur in males and are less common than DUs, perhaps due to the higher likelihood of GUs being silent and presenting only after a complication develops. Autopsy studies suggest a similar incidence of DUs and GUs.

Pathology • DUODENAL ULCERS DUs occur most often in the first portion of duodenum (>95%), with ~90% located within 3 cm of the pylorus. They are usually ≤1 cm in diameter but can occasionally reach 3–6 cm (giant ulcer). Ulcers are sharply demarcated, with depth at times reaching the muscularis propria. The base of the ulcer often consists of a zone of eosinophilic necrosis with surrounding fibrosis. Malignant DUs are extremely rare.

GASTRIC ULCERS In contrast to DUs, GUs can represent a malignancy. Benign GUs are most often found distal to the junction between the antrum and the acid secretory mucosa. Benign GUs are quite rare in the gastric fundus and are histologically similar to DUs. Benign GUs associated with *H. pylori* are also associated with antral gastritis. In contrast, NSAID-related GUs are not accompanied by chronic active gastritis but may instead have evidence of a chemical gastropathy, typified by foveolar hyperplasia, edema of the lamina propria and epithelial regeneration in the absence of *H. pylori*. Extension of smooth-muscle fibers into the upper portions of the mucosa, where they are not typically found, may also occur.

Pathophysiology · *DUODENAL ULCERS* *H. pylori* and NSAID-induced injury account for the majority of DUs. Many acid secretory abnormalities have been described in DU patients. Of these, average basal and nocturnal gastric acid secretion appears to be increased in DU patients as compared to controls; however, the level of overlap between DU patients and control subjects is substantial. The reason for this altered secretory process is unclear, but *H. pylori* infection may contribute. Accelerated gastric emptying of liquids has been noted in some DU patients, but its role in DU formation, if any, is unclear. Bicarbonate secretion is significantly decreased in the duodenal bulb of patients with an active DU as compared to control subjects. *H. pylori* infection may also play a role in this process (see below).

GASTRIC ULCERS As in DUs, the majority of GUs can be attributed to either *H. pylori* or NSAID-induced mucosal damage. GUs that occur in the prepyloric area or those in the body associated with a DU or a duodenal scar are similar in pathogenesis to DUs. Gastric acid output (basal and stimulated) tends to be normal or decreased in GU patients. When GUs develop in the presence of minimal acid levels, impairment of mucosal defense factors may be present.

Abnormalities in resting and stimulated pyloric sphincter pressure with a concomitant increase in duodenal gastric reflux have been implicated in some GU patients. Although bile acids, lysolecithin, and pancreatic enzymes may injure gastric mucosa, a definite role for these in GU pathogenesis has not been established. Delayed gastric emptying of solids has been described in GU patients but has not been reported consistently.

H. PYLORI AND ACID PEPTIC DISORDERS Gastric infection with the bacterium *H. pylori* accounts for the majority of PUD. This organism also plays a role in the development of gastric mucosal-associated lymphoid tissue (MALT) lymphoma and gastric adenocarcinoma. Although the entire genome of *H. pylori* has been sequenced, it is still not clear how this organism, which resides in the stomach, causes ulceration in the duodenum, or whether its eradication will lead to a decrease in gastric cancer.

The Bacterium The bacterium, initially named *Campylobacter pyloridis*, is a gram-negative microaerophilic rod found most commonly in the deeper portions of the mucous gel coating the gastric mucosa or between the mucous layer and the gastric epithelium. It may attach to gastric epithelium but under normal circumstances does not appear to invade cells. It is strategically designed to live within the aggressive environment of the stomach. It is S-shaped (~0.5 × 3 μm in size) and contains multiple sheathed flagella. Initially, *H. pylori* resides in the antrum but, over time, migrates toward the more proximal segments of the stomach. The organism is capable of transforming into a coccoid form, which represents a dormant state that may facilitate survival in adverse conditions. The genome of *H. pylori* (1.65 million base pairs) encodes ~1500 proteins. Among this multitude of proteins there are factors that are essential determinants of *H. pylori*–mediated pathogenesis and colonization, such as the outer membrane protein (Hop proteins), urease, and the vacuolating cytotoxin (Vac A). Moreover, the majority of *H. pylori* strains contain a genomic fragment that encodes the cag pathogenicity island (cag-PAI). Several of the genes that make up cag-PAI encode components of a type IV secretion island that translocates Cag A into host cells. Once in the cell, Cag A activates a series of cellular events important in cell growth and cytokine pro-

duction. The first step in infection by *H. pylori* is dependent on the bacteria's motility and its ability to produce urease. Urease produces ammonia from urea, an essential step in alkalinizing the surrounding pH. Additional bacterial factors include catalase, lipase, adhesins, platelet-activating factor, and pic B (induces cytokines). Multiple strains of *H. pylori* exist and are characterized by their ability to express several of these factors (Cag A, Vac A, etc.). It is possible that the different diseases related to *H. pylori* infection can be attributed to different strains of the organism with distinct pathogenic features.

Epidemiology The prevalence of *H. pylori* varies throughout the world and depends largely on the overall standard of living in the region. In developing parts of the world, 80% of the population may be infected by the age of 20, whereas the prevalence is 20–50% in industrialized countries. In contrast, in the United States this organism is rare in childhood. The overall prevalence of *H. pylori* in the United States is ~30%, with individuals born before 1950 having a higher rate of infection than those born later. About 10% of Americans <30 are colonized with the bacteria. The rate of infection with *H. pylori* in industrialized countries has decreased substantially in recent decades. The steady increase in the prevalence of *H. pylori* noted with increasing age is due primarily to a cohort effect, reflecting higher transmission during a period in which the earlier cohorts were children. It has been calculated through mathematical models that improved sanitation during the latter half of the nineteenth century dramatically decreased transmission of *H. pylori*. Moreover, with the present rate of intervention, the organism will be ultimately eliminated from the United States. Two factors that predispose to higher colonization rates include poor socioeconomic status and less education. These factors, not race, are responsible for the rate of *H. pylori* infection in blacks and Hispanic Americans being double the rate seen in whites of comparable age. Other risk factors for *H. pylori* infection are (1) birth or residence in a developing country, (2) domestic crowding, (3) unsanitary living conditions, (4) unclean food or water, and (5) exposure to gastric contents of an infected individual.

Transmission of *H. pylori* occurs from person to person, following an oral-oral or fecal-oral route. The risk of *H. pylori* infection is declining in developing countries. The rate of infection in the United States has fallen by >50% when compared to 30 years ago.

Pathophysiology *H. pylori* infection is virtually always associated with a chronic active gastritis, but only 10–15% of infected individuals develop frank peptic ulceration. The basis for this difference is unknown. Initial studies suggested that >90% of all DUs were associated with *H. pylori*, but *H. pylori* is present in only 30–60% of individuals with GUs and 50–70% of patients with DUs. The pathophysiology of ulcers not associated with *H. pylori* or NSAID ingestion [or the rare Zollinger-Ellison syndrome (ZES)] is becoming more relevant as the incidence of *H. pylori* is dropping, particularly in the Western world (see below).

The particular end result of *H. pylori* infection (gastritis, PUD, gastric MALT lymphoma, gastric cancer) is determined by a complex interplay between bacterial and host factors (Fig. 287-6).

1. *Bacterial factors*: *H. pylori* is able to facilitate gastric residence, induce mucosal injury, and avoid host defense. Different strains of *H. pylori* produce different virulence factors. A specific region of the bacterial genome, the pathogenicity island, encodes the virulence factors Cag A and pic B. Vac A also contributes to pathogenicity, though it is not encoded within the pathogenicity island. These virulence factors, in conjunction with additional bacterial constituents, can cause mucosal damage. Urease, which allows the bacteria to reside in the acidic stomach, generates NH_3, which can damage epithelial cells. The bacteria produce surface factors that are chemotactic for neutrophils and monocytes, which in turn contribute to epithelial cell injury (see below). *H. pylori* makes proteases and phospholipases that break down the glycoprotein lipid complex of the mucous gel, thus reducing the efficacy of this first line of mucosal defense. *H. pylori* expresses adhesins, which facilitate attachment of the bacteria to gastric epithelial cells. Although lipopolysaccharide

FIGURE 287-6 Outline of the bacterial and host factors important in determining *H. pylori*–induced gastrointestinal disease. MALT, mucosal-associated lymphoid tissue.

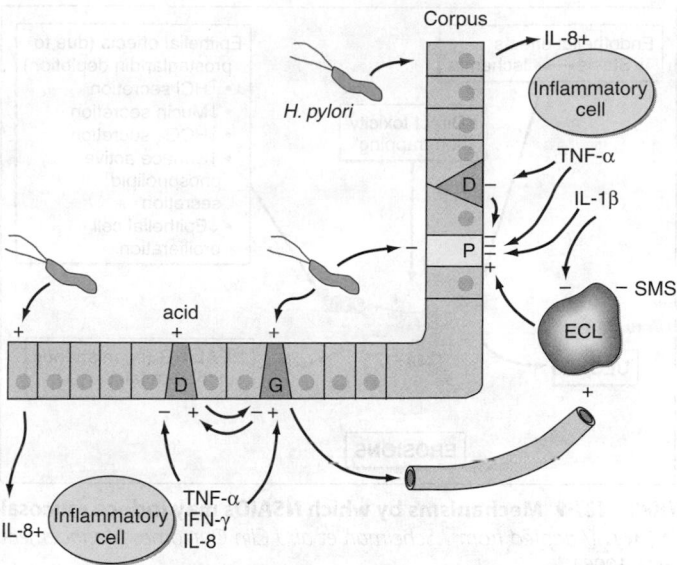

FIGURE 287-7 Summary of potential mechanisms by which *H. pylori* may lead to gastric secretory abnormalities. D, somatostatin cell; ECL, enterochromaffin-like cell; G, G cell; IFN, interferon; IL, interleukin; P, parietal cell; SMS, somatostatin; TNF, tumor necrosis factor. *(Adapted from J Calam et al: Gastroenterology 113:543, 1997.)*

(LPS) of gram-negative bacteria often plays an important role in the infection, *H. pylori* LPS has low immunologic activity compared to that of other organisms. It may promote a smoldering chronic inflammation.

2. *Host factors*: The inflammatory response to *H. pylori* includes recruitment of neutrophils, lymphocytes (T and B), macrophages, and plasma cells. The pathogen leads to local injury by binding to class II MHC molecules expressed on gastric epithelial cells, leading to cell death (*apoptosis*). Moreover, bacterial strains that encode cag-PAI can introduce Cag A into the host cells, leading to further cell injury and activation of cellular pathways involved in cytokine production. Elevated concentrations of multiple cytokines are found in the gastric epithelium of *H. pylori*–infected individuals, including interleukin (IL) 1α/β, IL-2, IL-6, IL-8, tumor necrosis factor (TNF) α and interferon (IFN-γ). *H. pylori* infection also leads to both a mucosal and a systemic humoral response, which does not lead to eradication of the bacteria but further compounds epithelial cell injury. Additional mechanisms by which *H. pylori* may cause epithelial cell injury include (1) activated neutrophil-mediated production of reactive oxygen or nitrogen species and enhanced epithelial cell turnover and (2) apoptosis related to interaction with T cells (T helper 1, or T$_H$1, cells) and IFN-γ.

The reason for *H. pylori*–mediated duodenal ulceration remains unclear. One potential explanation is that gastric metaplasia in the duodenum of DU patients permits *H. pylori* to bind to it and produce local injury secondary to the host response. Another hypothesis is that *H. pylori* antral infection could lead to increased acid production, increased duodenal acid, and mucosal injury. Basal and stimulated [meal, gastrin-releasing peptide (GRP)] gastrin release are increased in *H. pylori*–infected individuals, and somatostatin-secreting D cells may be decreased. *H. pylori* infection might induce increased acid secretion through both direct and indirect actions of *H. pylori* and proinflammatory cytokines (IL-8, TNF, and IL-1) on G, D, and parietal cells (Fig. 287-7). *H. pylori* infection has also been associated with decreased duodenal mucosal bicarbonate production. Data supporting and contradicting each of these interesting theories have been demonstrated. Thus, the mechanism by which *H. pylori* infection of the stomach leads to duodenal ulceration remains to be established.

In summary, the final effect of *H. pylori* on the gastrointestinal tract is variable and determined by microbial and host factors. The type and distribution of gastritis correlate with the ultimate gastric and duodenal pathology observed. Specifically, the presence of antral-predominant gastritis is associated with DU formation; gastritis involving primarily the corpus predisposes to the development of GUs, gastric atrophy, and ultimately gastric carcinoma (Fig. 287-8).

NSAID-INDUCED DISEASE   Epidemiology   NSAIDs represent a group of the most commonly used medications in the United States. More than 30 billion over-the-counter tablets and over 100 million prescriptions are sold yearly in the United States alone. In fact, after the introduction of COX-2 inhibitors in the year 2000, the number of prescriptions written for NSAIDs was >111 million at a cost of $4.8 billion. Side effects and complications due to NSAIDs are considered the most common drug-related toxicities in the United States. The spectrum of NSAID-induced morbidity ranges from nausea and dyspepsia (prevalence reported as high as 50–60%) to a serious gastrointestinal complication such as endoscopy-documented peptic ulceration (15–30% of individuals taking NSAIDs regularly) complicated by bleeding or perforation in as many as 1.5% of users per year. About 20,000 patients die each year from serious gastrointestinal complications from NSAIDs. Unfortunately, dyspeptic symptoms do not correlate with NSAID-induced pathology. Over 80% of patients with serious NSAID-related complications did not have preceding dyspepsia. In view of the lack of warning

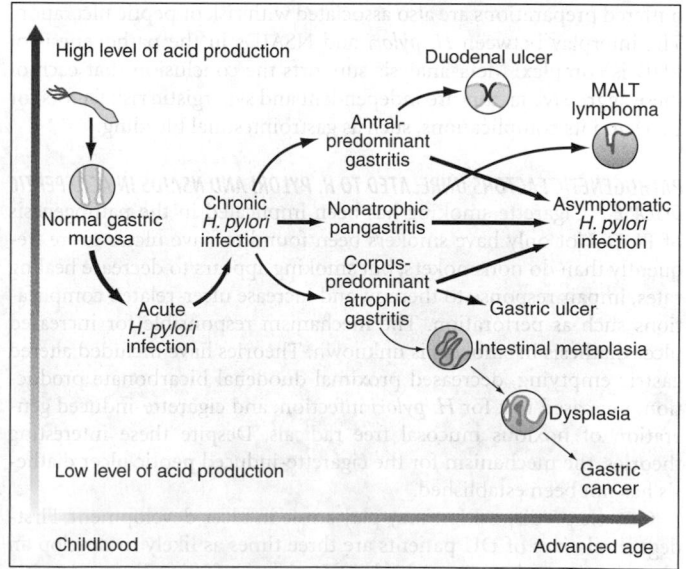

FIGURE 287-8 Natural history of *H. pylori* infection. *(Used with permission from Suerbaum and Michetti.)*

FIGURE 287-9 Mechanisms by which NSAIDs may induce mucosal injury. *(Adapted from J Scheiman et al: J Clin Outcomes Management 3:23, 1996.)*

signs, it is important to identify patients who are at increased risk for morbidity and mortality related to NSAID usage. Even 75 mg/d of aspirin may lead to serious gastrointestinal ulceration; thus, no dose of NSAID is completely safe. Established risk factors include advanced age, history of ulcer, concomitant use of glucocorticoids, high-dose NSAIDs, multiple NSAIDs, concomitant use of anticoagulants, and serious or multisystem disease. Possible risk factors include concomitant infection with *H. pylori*, cigarette smoking, and alcohol consumption.

Pathophysiology Prostaglandins play a critical role in maintaining gastroduodenal mucosal integrity and repair. It therefore follows that interruption of prostaglandin synthesis can impair mucosal defense and repair, thus facilitating mucosal injury via a systemic mechanism. A summary of the pathogenetic pathways by which systemically administered NSAIDs may lead to mucosal injury is shown in **Fig. 287-9**.

Injury to the mucosa also occurs as a result of the topical encounter with NSAIDs. Aspirin and many NSAIDs are weak acids that remain in a nonionized lipophilic form when found within the acid environment of the stomach. Under these conditions, NSAIDs migrate across lipid membranes of epithelial cells, leading to cell injury once trapped intracellularly in an ionized form. Topical NSAIDs can also alter the surface mucous layer, permitting back diffusion of H^+ and pepsin, leading to further epithelial cell damage. Moreover, enteric-coated or buffered preparations are also associated with risk of peptic ulceration. The interplay between *H. pylori* and NSAIDs in the pathogenesis of PUD is complex. Meta-analysis supports the conclusion that each of these aggressive factors are independent and synergistic risk factors for PUD and its complications, such as gastrointestinal bleeding.

PATHOGENETIC FACTORS UNRELATED TO H. PYLORI AND NSAIDS IN ACID PEPTIC DISEASE Cigarette smoking has been implicated in the pathogenesis of PUD. Not only have smokers been found to have ulcers more frequently than do nonsmokers, but smoking appears to decrease healing rates, impair response to therapy, and increase ulcer-related complications such as perforation. The mechanism responsible for increased ulcer diathesis in smokers is unknown. Theories have included altered gastric emptying, decreased proximal duodenal bicarbonate production, increased risk for *H. pylori* infection, and cigarette-induced generation of noxious mucosal free radicals. Despite these interesting theories, the mechanism for the cigarette-induced peptic ulcer diathesis has not been established.

Genetic predisposition may play a role in ulcer development. First-degree relatives of DU patients are three times as likely to develop an ulcer; however, the potential role of *H. pylori* infection in contacts is a major consideration. Increased frequency of blood group O and of the nonsecretor status have also been implicated as genetic risk factors for

peptic diathesis. However, *H. pylori* preferentially binds to group O antigens. The role of genetic predisposition in common PUD has not been established.

Psychological stress has been thought to contribute to PUD, but studies examining the role of psychological factors in its pathogenesis have generated conflicting results. Although PUD is associated with certain personality traits (neuroticism), these same traits are also present in individuals with nonulcer dyspepsia (NUD) and other functional and organic disorders. Although more work in this area is needed, no typical PUD personality has been found.

Diet has also been thought to play a role in peptic diseases. Certain foods can cause dyspepsia, but no convincing studies indicate an association between ulcer formation and a specific diet. This is also true for beverages containing alcohol and caffeine. Specific chronic disorders have been associated with PUD. Those with a strong association are (1) systemic mastocytosis, (2) chronic pulmonary disease, (3) chronic renal failure, (4) cirrhosis, (5) nephrolithiasis, and (6) α_1-antitrypsin deficiency. Those with a possible association are (1) hyperparathyroidism, (2) coronary artery disease, (3) polycythemia vera, and (4) chronic pancreatitis.

Multiple factors play a role in the pathogenesis of PUD. The two predominant causes are *H. pylori* infection and NSAID ingestion. PUD not related to *H. pylori* or NSAIDs is increasing. Other less common causes of PUD are shown in **Table 287-1**. These etiologic agents should be considered as the incidence of *H. pylori* is decreasing. Independent of the inciting or injurious agent, peptic ulcers develop as a result of an imbalance between mucosal protection/repair and aggressive factors. Gastric acid plays an essential role in mucosal injury.

CLINICAL FEATURES

History Abdominal pain is common to many gastrointestinal disorders, including DU and GU, but has a poor predictive value for the presence of either DU or GU. Up to 10% of patients with NSAID-induced mucosal disease can present with a complication (bleeding, perforation, and obstruction) without antecedent symptoms. Despite this poor correlation, a careful history and physical examination are essential components of the approach to a patient suspected of having peptic ulcers.

Epigastric pain described as a burning or gnawing discomfort can be present in both DU and GU. The discomfort is also described as an ill-defined, aching sensation or as hunger pain. The typical pain pattern in DU occurs 90 min to 3 h after a meal and is frequently relieved by antacids or food. Pain that awakes the patient from sleep (between

TABLE 287-1	CAUSES OF ULCERS NOT CAUSED BY *HELICOBACTER PYLORI* AND NSAIDS

Pathogenesis of Non-Hp and Non-NSAID Ulcer Disease

Infection
  Cytomegalovirus
  Herpes simplex virus
  Helicobacter heilmanni
Drug/Toxin
  Bisphosphonates
  Chemotherapy
  Clopidogrel
  Crack cocaine
  Glucocorticoids (when combined with NSAIDs)
  Mycophenolate mofetil
  Potassium chloride
Miscellaneous
  Basophilia in myeloproliferative disease
  Duodenal obstruction (e.g., annular pancreas)
  Infiltrating disease
  Ischemia
  Radiation therapy
  Sarcoidosis
  Crohn's disease
  Idiopathic hypersecretory state

Note: Hp, *Helicobacter pylori*; NSAID, nonsteroidal anti-inflammatory drug.

midnight and 3 A.M.) is the most discriminating symptom, with two-thirds of DU patients describing this complaint. Unfortunately, this symptom is also present in one-third of patients with NUD. The pain pattern in GU patients may be different from that in DU patients, where discomfort may actually be precipitated by food. Nausea and weight loss occur more commonly in GU patients. Endoscopy detects ulcers in <30% of patients who have dyspepsia.

The mechanism for development of abdominal pain in ulcer patients is unknown. Several possible explanations include acid-induced activation of chemical receptors in the duodenum, enhanced duodenal sensitivity to bile acids and pepsin, or altered gastroduodenal motility.

Variation in the intensity or distribution of the abdominal pain, as well as the onset of associated symptoms such as nausea and/or vomiting, may be indicative of an ulcer complication. Dyspepsia that becomes constant, is no longer relieved by food or antacids, or radiates to the back may indicate a penetrating ulcer (pancreas). Sudden onset of severe, generalized abdominal pain may indicate perforation. Pain worsening with meals, nausea, and vomiting of undigested food suggest gastric outlet obstruction. Tarry stools or coffee-ground emesis indicate bleeding.

Physical Examination Epigastric tenderness is the most frequent finding in patients with GU or DU. Pain may be found to the right of the midline in 20% of patients. Unfortunately, the predictive value of this finding is rather low. Physical examination is critically important for discovering evidence of ulcer complication. Tachycardia and orthostasis suggest dehydration secondary to vomiting or active gastrointestinal blood loss. A severely tender, boardlike abdomen suggests a perforation. Presence of a succussion splash indicates retained fluid in the stomach, suggesting gastric outlet obstruction.

PUD-Related Complications · *GASTROINTESTINAL BLEEDING* Gastrointestinal bleeding is the most common complication observed in PUD. It occurs in ~15% of patients and more often in individuals >60 years old. The higher incidence in the elderly is likely due to the increased use of NSAIDs in this group. Up to 20% of patients with ulcer-related hemorrhage bleed without any preceding warning signs or symptoms.

PERFORATION The second most common ulcer-related complication is perforation, being reported in as many as 6–7% of PUD patients. As in the case of bleeding, the incidence of perforation in the elderly appears to be increasing secondary to increased use of NSAIDs. *Penetration* is a form of perforation in which the ulcer bed tunnels into an adjacent organ. DUs tend to penetrate posteriorly into the pancreas, leading to pancreatitis, whereas GUs tend to penetrate into the left hepatic lobe. Gastrocolic fistulas associated with GUs have also been described.

GASTRIC OUTLET OBSTRUCTION Gastric outlet obstruction is the least common ulcer-related complication, occurring in 1–2% of patients. A patient may have relative obstruction secondary to ulcer-related inflammation and edema in the peripyloric region. This process often resolves with ulcer healing. A fixed, mechanical obstruction secondary to scar formation in the peripyloric areas is also possible. The latter requires endoscopic (balloon dilation) or surgical intervention. Signs and symptoms relative to mechanical obstruction may develop insidiously. New onset of early satiety, nausea, vomiting, increase of postprandial abdominal pain, and weight loss should make gastric outlet obstruction a possible diagnosis.

Differential Diagnosis The list of gastrointestinal and nongastrointestinal disorders that can mimic ulceration of the stomach or duodenum is quite extensive. The most commonly encountered diagnosis among patients seen for upper abdominal discomfort is NUD. NUD, also known as *functional dyspepsia* or *essential dyspepsia*, refers to a group of heterogeneous disorders typified by upper abdominal pain without the presence of an ulcer. Dyspepsia has been reported to occur in up to 30% of the U.S. population. Up to 60% of patients seeking medical care for dyspepsia have a negative diagnostic evaluation. The etiology of NUD is not established, and the potential role of *H. pylori* in NUD remains controversial.

Several additional disease processes that may present with "ulcer-like" symptoms include proximal gastrointestinal tumors, gastroesophageal reflux, vascular disease, pancreaticobiliary disease (biliary colic, chronic pancreatitis), and gastroduodenal Crohn's disease.

Diagnostic Evaluation In view of the poor predictive value of abdominal pain for the presence of a gastroduodenal ulcer and the multiple disease processes that can mimic this disease, the clinician is often confronted with having to establish the presence of an ulcer. Documentation of an ulcer requires either a radiographic (barium study) or an endoscopic procedure. However, a large percentage of patients with symptoms suggestive of an ulcer have NUD; empirical therapy is appropriate for individuals who are otherwise healthy and <45, before embarking on a diagnostic evaluation (Chap. 39).

Barium studies of the proximal gastrointestinal tract are still commonly used as a first test for documenting an ulcer. The sensitivity of older single-contrast barium meals for detecting a DU is as high as 80%, with a double-contrast study providing detection rates as high as 90%. Sensitivity for detection is decreased in small ulcers (<0.5 cm), presence of previous scarring, or in postoperative patients. A DU appears as a well-demarcated crater, most often seen in the bulb (Fig. 287-10A). A GU may represent benign or malignant disease. Typically, a benign GU also appears as a discrete crater with radiating mucosal folds originating from the ulcer margin (Fig. 287-10B). Ulcers >3 cm in size or those associated with a mass are more often malignant. Unfortunately, up to 8% of GUs that appear to be benign by radiographic appearance are malignant by endoscopy or surgery. Radiographic studies that show a GU must be followed by endoscopy and biopsy.

Endoscopy provides the most sensitive and specific approach for examining the upper gastrointestinal tract (Fig. 287-11). In addition to permitting direct visualization of the mucosa, endoscopy facilitates photographic documentation of a mucosal defect and tissue biopsy to rule out malignancy (GU) or *H. pylori*. Endoscopic examination is particularly helpful in identifying lesions too small to detect by radio-

A   *B*

FIGURE 287-10 Barium study demonstrating: *A.* a benign duodenal ulcer; *B.* a benign gastric ulcer.

FIGURE 287-11 Endoscopy demonstrating: *A.* a benign duodenal ulcer; ***B.*** a benign gastric ulcer.

graphic examination, for evaluation of atypical radiographic abnormalities, or to determine if an ulcer is a source of blood loss.

Although the methods for diagnosing *H. pylori* are outlined in Chap. 144, a brief summary will be included here (Table 287-2). Several biopsy urease tests have been developed (PyloriTek, Clotest, Hpfast, Pronto Dry) that have a sensitivity and specificity of >90–95%. Several noninvasive methods for detecting this organism have been developed. Three types of studies routinely used include serologic testing, the ^{13}C- or ^{14}C-urea breath test, and the fecal *H. pylori* (Hp) antigen test. A urinary Hp antigen test, as well as a refined monoclonal antibody stool antigen test, appears promising.

Occasionally, specialized testing such as serum gastrin and gastric acid analysis or sham feeding may be needed in individuals with complicated or refractory PUD (see "Zollinger-Ellison Syndrome," below). Screening for aspirin or NSAIDs (blood or urine) may also be necessary in refractory *H. pylori*–negative PUD patients.

℞ PEPTIC ULCER DISEASE

Before the discovery of *H. pylori*, the therapy of PUD was centered on the old dictum by Schwartz of "no acid, no ulcer." Although acid secretion is still important in the pathogenesis of PUD, eradication of *H. pylori* and therapy/

prevention of NSAID-induced disease is the mainstay of treatment. A summary of commonly used drugs for treatment of acid peptic disorders is shown in **Table 287-3**.

ACID NEUTRALIZING/INHIBITORY DRUGS Antacids Before we understood the important role of histamine in stimulating parietal cell activity, neutralization of secreted acid with antacids constituted the main form of therapy for peptic ulcers. They are now rarely, if ever, used as the primary therapeutic agent but instead are often used by patients for symptomatic relief of dyspepsia. The most commonly used agents are mixtures of aluminum hydroxide and magnesium hydroxide. Aluminum hydroxide can produce constipation and phosphate depletion; magnesium hydroxide may cause loose stools. Many of the commonly used antacids (e.g., Maalox, Mylanta) have a combination of both aluminum and magnesium hydroxide in order to avoid these side effects. The magnesium-containing preparation should not be used in chronic renal failure patients because of possible hypermagnesemia, and aluminum may cause chronic neurotoxicity in these patients.

Calcium carbonate and sodium bicarbonate are potent antacids with varying levels of potential problems. The long-term use of calcium carbonate (converts to calcium chloride in the stomach) can lead to milk-alkali syndrome (hypercalcemia, hyperphosphatemia with possible renal calcinosis and progression to renal insufficiency). Sodium bicarbonate may induce systemic alkalosis.

H$_2$ Receptor Antagonists Four of these agents are presently available (cimetidine, ranitidine, famotidine, and nizatidine), and their structures share homology with histamine. Although each has different potency, all will significantly inhibit basal and stimulated acid secretion to comparable levels when used at therapeutic doses. Moreover, similar ulcer-healing rates are achieved with each drug when used at the correct dosage. Presently, this class of drug is often used for treatment of active ulcers (4–6 weeks) in combination with antibiotics directed at eradicating *H. pylori* (see below).

Cimetidine was the first H$_2$ receptor antagonist used for the treatment of acid peptic disorders. The initial recommended dosing profile for cimetidine was 300 mg qid. Subsequent studies have documented the efficacy of using 800 mg at bedtime for treatment of active ulcer, with healing rates approaching 80% at 4 weeks. Cimetidine may have weak antiandrogenic side effects resulting in reversible gynecomastia and impotence, primarily in patients receiving high doses for prolonged periods of time (months to years, as in ZES). In view of cimetidine's ability to inhibit cytochrome P450, careful monitoring of drugs such as warfarin, phenytoin, and theophylline is indicated with long-term usage. Other rare reversible adverse effects re-

TABLE 287-2 TESTS FOR DETECTION OF *H. PYLORI*

Test	Sensitivity/Specificity, %	Comments
Invasive (Endoscopy/Biopsy Required)		
Rapid urease	80–95/95–100	Simple, false negative with recent use of PPIs, antibiotics, or bismuth compounds
Histology	80–90/>95	Requires pathology processing and staining; provides histologic information
Culture	—/—	Time-consuming, expensive, dependent on experience; allows determination of antibiotic susceptibility
Non-invasive		
Serology	>80/>90	Inexpensive, convenient; not useful for early follow-up
Urea breath test	>90/>90	Simple, rapid; useful for early follow-up; false negatives with recent therapy (see rapid urease test); exposure to low-dose radiation with ^{14}C test
Stool antigen	>90/>90	Inexpensive, convenient; not established for eradication but promising

Note: PPIs, proton pump inhibitors.

TABLE 287-3 DRUGS USED IN THE TREATMENT OF PEPTIC ULCER DISEASE

Drug Type/Mechanism	Examples	Dose
Acid-suppressing drugs		
Antacids	Mylanta, Maalox, Tums, Gaviscon	100–140 meq/L 1 and 3 h after meals and hs
H$_2$ receptor antagonists	Cimetidine	400 mg bid
	Ranitidine	300 mg hs
	Famotidine	40 mg hs
	Nizatidine	300 mg hs
Proton pump inhibitors	Omeprazole	20 mg/d
	Lansoprazole	30 mg/d
	Rabeprazole	20 mg/d
	Pantoprazole	40 mg/d
	Esomeprazole	20 mg/d
Mucosal protective agents		
Sucralfate	Sucralfate	1 g qid
Prostaglandin analogue	Misoprostol	200 μg qid
Bismuth-containing compounds	Bismuth subsalicylate (BSS)	See anti-*H. pylori* regimens (Table 287-4)

ported with cimetidine include confusion and elevated levels of serum aminotransferases, creatinine, and serum prolactin. Ranitidine, famotidine, and nizatidine are more potent H_2 receptor antagonists than cimetidine. Each can be used once a day at bedtime for ulcer prevention, which was commonly done before the discovery of *H. pylori* and the development of proton pump inhibitors (PPIs). Patients may develop tolerance to H_2 blockers, a rare event with PPIs (see below). Comparable nighttime dosing regimens are ranitidine 300 mg, famotidine 40 mg, and nizatidine 300 mg.

Additional rare, reversible systemic toxicities reported with H_2 receptor antagonists include pancytopenia, neutropenia, anemia, and thrombocytopenia, with a prevalence rate varying from 0.01 to 0.2%. Cimetidine and ranitidine (to a lesser extent) can bind to hepatic cytochrome P450; famotidine and nizatidine do not.

Proton Pump (H^+,K^+-ATPase) Inhibitors Omeprazole, esomeprazole, lansoprazole, rabeprazole, and pantoprazole are substituted benzimidazole derivatives that covalently bind and irreversibly inhibit H^+,K^+-ATPase. Esomeprazole, the newest member of this drug class, is the S-enantiomer of omeprazole, which is a racemic mixture of both S- and R-optical isomers. These are the most potent acid inhibitory agents available. Omeprazole and lansoprazole are the PPIs that have been used for the longest time. Both are acid-labile and are administered as enteric-coated granules in a sustained-release capsule that dissolves within the small intestine at a pH of 6. Lansoprazole is available in an orally disintegrating tablet that can be taken with or without water, an advantage for individuals who have significant dysphagia. Absorption kinetics are similar to the capsule. In addition, a lansoprazole-naproxen combination preparation that has been made available is targeted at decreasing NSAID-related gastrointestinal injury (see below). Omeprazole is available as non-enteric-coated granules mixed with sodium bicarbonate in a powder form which can be administered orally or via gastric tube. The sodium bicarbonate has two purposes: to protect the omeprazole from acid degradation and to promote rapid gastric alkalinization and subsequent proton pump activation, which facilitates rapid action of the PPI. Pantoprazole and rabeprazole are available as enteric-coated tablets. Pantoprazole is also available as a parenteral formulation for intravenous use. These agents are lipophilic compounds; upon entering the parietal cell, they are protonated and trapped within the acid environment of the tubulovesicular and canalicular system. These agents potently inhibit all phases of gastric acid secretion. Onset of action is rapid, with a maximum acid inhibitory effect between 2 and 6 h after administration and duration of inhibition lasting up to 72–96 h. With repeated daily dosing, progressive acid inhibitory effects are observed, with basal and secretagogue-stimulated acid production being inhibited by >95% after 1 week of therapy. The half-life of PPIs is ~18 h; thus, it can take between 2 and 5 days for gastric acid secretion to return to normal levels once these drugs have been discontinued. Because the pumps need to be activated for these agents to be effective, their efficacy is maximized if they are administered before a meal (except for the immediate-release formulation of omeprazole) (e.g., in the morning before breakfast). Mild to moderate hypergastrinemia has been observed in patients taking these drugs. Carcinoid tumors developed in some animals given the drugs preclinically; however, extensive experience has failed to demonstrate gastric carcinoid tumor development in humans. Serum gastrin levels return to normal levels within 1–2 weeks after drug cessation. Intrinsic factor (IF) production is also inhibited, but vitamin B_{12}-deficiency anemia is uncommon, probably because of the large stores of the vitamin. As with any agent that leads to significant hypochlorhydria, PPIs may interfere with absorption of drugs such as ketoconazole, ampicillin, iron, and digoxin. Hepatic cytochrome P450 can be inhibited by the earlier PPIs (omeprazole, lansoprazole). Rabeprazole, pantoprazole, and esomeprazole do not appear to interact significantly with drugs metabolized by the cytochrome P450 system. The overall clinical significance of this observation is not definitely established. Caution should be taken when using warfarin, diazepam, atazanavir, and phenytoin concomitantly with PPIs. Long-term acid suppression, especially with PPIs, has been associated with a higher incidence of community-acquired pneumonia. This observation requires confirmation but should alert the practitioner to take caution when recommending these agents for long-term use, especially in elderly patients at risk for developing pneumonia.

Two new formulations of acid inhibitory agents are being developed. Tenatoprazole is a PPI containing an imidazopyridine ring instead of a benzimidazole ring, which promotes irreversible proton pump inhibition. This agent has a longer half-life than the other PPIs and may be beneficial for in-

Drug	Dose
Triple Therapy	
1. Bismuth subsalicylate *plus*	2 tablets qid
Metronidazole *plus*	250 mg qid
Tetracycline[a]	500 mg qid
2. Ranitidine bismuth citrate *plus*	400 mg bid
Tetracycline *plus*	500 mg bid
Clarithromycin or metronidazole	500 mg bid
3. Omeprazole (lansoprazole) *plus*	20 mg bid (30 mg bid)
Clarithromycin *plus*	250 or 500 mg bid
Metronidazole[b] *or*	500 mg bid
Amoxicillin[c]	1 g bid
Quadruple Therapy	
Omeprazole (lansoprazole)	20 mg (30 mg) daily
Bismuth subsalicylate	2 tablets qid
Metronidazole	250 mg qid
Tetracycline	500 mg qid

[a]Alternative: use prepacked Helidac (see text).
[b]Alternative: use prepacked Prevpac (see text).
[c]Use either metronidazole or amoxicillin, not both.

hibiting nocturnal acid secretion, which has significant relevance in gastroesophageal reflux disease (GERD). A second new class of agents is the potassium-competitive acid pump antagonists (P-CABs). These compounds inhibit gastric acid secretion via potassium competitive binding of the H^+,K^+-ATPase.

CYTOPROTECTIVE AGENTS **Sucralfate** Sucralfate is a complex sucrose salt in which the hydroxyl groups have been substituted by aluminum hydroxide and sulfate. This compound is insoluble in water and becomes a viscous paste within the stomach and duodenum, binding primarily to sites of active ulceration. Sucralfate may act by several mechanisms: serving as a physicochemical barrier, promoting a trophic action by binding growth factors such as EGF, enhancing prostaglandin synthesis, stimulating mucous and bicarbonate secretion, and enhancing mucosal defense and repair. Toxicity from this drug is rare, with constipation being most common (2–3%). It should be avoided in patients with chronic renal insufficiency to prevent aluminum-induced neurotoxicity. Hypophosphatemia and gastric bezoar formation have also been reported rarely. Standard dosing of sucralfate is 1 g qid.

Bismuth-Containing Preparations Sir William Osler considered bismuth-containing compounds the drug of choice for treating PUD. The resurgence in the use of these agents is due to their effect against *H. pylori*. Colloidal bismuth subcitrate (CBS) and bismuth subsalicylate (BSS, Pepto-Bismol) are the most widely used preparations. The mechanism by which these agents induce ulcer healing is unclear. Potential mechanisms include ulcer coating; prevention of further pepsin/HCl-induced damage; binding of pepsin; and stimulation of prostaglandins, bicarbonate, and mucous secretion. Adverse effects with short-term usage include black stools, constipation, and darkening of the tongue. Long-term usage with high doses, especially with the avidly absorbed CBS, may lead to neurotoxicity. These compounds are commonly used as one of the agents in an anti-*H. pylori* regimen (see below).

Prostaglandin Analogues In view of their central role in maintaining mucosal integrity and repair, stable prostaglandin analogues were developed for the treatment of PUD. The mechanism by which this rapidly absorbed drug provides its therapeutic effect is through enhancement of mucosal defense and repair. Prostaglandin analogues enhance mucous bicarbonate secretion, stimulate mucosal blood flow, and decrease mucosal cell turnover. The most common toxicity noted with this drug is diarrhea (10–30% incidence). Other major toxicities include uterine bleeding and contractions; misoprostol is contraindicated in women who may be pregnant, and women of childbearing age must be made clearly aware of this potential drug toxicity. The standard therapeutic dose is 200 μg qid.

Miscellaneous Drugs A number of drugs aimed at treating acid peptic disorders have been developed over the years. In view of their limited utilization in the United States, if any, they will only be listed briefly. Anticholinergics, designed to inhibit activation of the muscarinic receptor in parietal cells, met with limited success due to their relatively weak acid-inhibiting effect and significant side effects (dry eyes, dry mouth, urinary retention). Tricyclic antidepressants have been suggested by some, but again the toxicity of these agents in comparison to the safe, effective drugs already described precludes their utility.

THERAPY OF *H. PYLORI* Extensive effort has been made into determining who of the many individuals with *H. pylori* infection should be treated. The common conclusion arrived at by multiple consensus conferences around the world is that *H. pylori* should be eradicated in patients with documented PUD. This holds true independent of time of presentation (first episode or not), severity of symptoms, presence of confounding factors such as ingestion of NSAIDs, or whether the ulcer is in remission. Some have advocated treating patients with a history of documented PUD who are found to be *H. pylori*–positive by serology or breath testing. Over half of patients with gastric MALT lymphoma experience complete remission of the tumor in response to *H. pylori* eradication. Treating patients with NUD, to prevent gastric cancer or patients with GERD requiring long-term acid suppression, remains controversial.

Multiple drugs have been evaluated in the therapy of *H. pylori*. No single agent is effective in eradicating the organism. Combination therapy for 14 days provides the greatest efficacy. A shorter course administration (7–10 days), although attractive, has not proved as successful as the 14-day regimens. The agents used with the greatest frequency include amoxicillin, metronidazole, tetracycline, clarithromycin, and bismuth compounds.

The physician's goal in treating PUD is to provide relief of symptoms (pain or dyspepsia), promote ulcer healing, and ultimately prevent ulcer recurrence and complications. The greatest impact of understanding the role of *H. pylori* in peptic disease has been the ability to prevent recurrence. Documented eradication of *H. pylori* in patients with PUD is associated with a dramatic decrease in ulcer recurrence to <10–20% as compared to 59% in GU patients and 67% in DU patients when the organism is not eliminated. Eradication of the organism may lead to diminished recurrent ulcer bleeding. The impact of its eradication on ulcer perforation is unclear.

Suggested treatment regimens for *H. pylori* are outlined in Table 287-4. Choice of a particular regimen will be influenced by several factors, including efficacy, patient tolerance, existing antibiotic resistance, and cost of the drugs. The aim for initial eradication rates should be 85–90%. Dual therapy [PPI plus amoxicillin, PPI plus clarithromycin, ranitidine bismuth citrate (Tritec) plus clarithromycin] are not recommended in view of studies demonstrating eradication rates of <80–85%. The combination of bismuth, metronidazole, and tetracycline was the first triple regimen found effective against *H. pylori*. The combination of two antibiotics plus either a PPI, H_2 blocker, or bismuth compound has comparable success rates. Addition of acid suppression assists in providing early symptom relief and may enhance bacterial eradication.

Triple therapy, although effective, has several drawbacks, including the potential for poor patient compliance and drug-induced side effects. Compliance is being addressed by simplifying the regimens so that patients can take the medications twice a day. Simpler (dual therapy) and shorter regimens (7 and 10 days) are not as effective as triple therapy for 14 days. Two anti-*H. pylori* regimens are available in prepackaged formulation: Prevpac (lansoprazole, clarithromycin, and amoxicillin) and Helidac (bismuth subsalicylate, tetracycline, and metronidazole). The contents of the Prevpac are to be taken twice per day for 14 days, whereas Helidac constituents are taken four times per day with an antisecretory agent (PPI or H_2 blocker), also for at least 14 days.

Side effects have been reported in up to 20–30% of patients on triple therapy. Bismuth may cause black stools, constipation, or darkening of the tongue. The most feared complication with amoxicillin is pseudomembranous colitis, but this occurs in <1–2% of patients. Amoxicillin can also lead to antibiotic-associated diarrhea, nausea, vomiting, skin rash, and allergic reaction. Tetracycline has been reported to cause rashes and, very rarely, hepatotoxicity and anaphylaxis.

One important concern with treating patients who may not need treatment is the potential for development of antibiotic-resistant strains. The incidence and type of antibiotic-resistant *H. pylori* strains vary worldwide. Strains resistant to metronidazole, clarithromycin, amoxicillin, and tetracycline have been described, with the latter two being uncommon. Antibiotic-resistant strains are the most common cause for treatment failure in compliant patients. Unfortunately, in vitro resistance does not predict outcome in patients. Culture and sensitivity testing of *H. pylori* is not performed routinely. Although resistance to metronidazole has been found in as many as 30% of isolates in North America and 80% in developing countries, triple therapy is effective in eradicating the organism in >50% of patients infected with a resistant strain. Clarithromycin resistance is seen in 13% of individuals in the United States, with resistance to amoxicillin being <1% and resistance to both metronidazole and clarithromycin in the 5% range.

Failure of *H. pylori* eradication with triple therapy in a compliant patient is usually due to infection with a resistant organism. Quadruple therapy (Table 287-4), where clarithromycin is substituted for metronidazole (or vice versa), should be the next step. The combination of pantoprazole, amoxicillin, and rifabutin for 10 days has also been used successfully (86% cure rate) in patients infected with resistant strains. Additional regimens considered for second-line therapy include levofloxin-based triple therapy (levofloxin, amoxicillin, PPI) for 10 days and furazolidone-based triple therapy (furazolidone, amoxicillin an PPI) for 14 days. Unfortunately, there is no universally accepted treatment regimen recommended for patients who have failed two courses of antibiotics. If eradication is still not achieved in a compliant patient, then culture and sensitivity of the organism should be considered. Additional factors that may lower eradication rates include the patient's country of origin (higher in Northeast Asia than other parts of Asia or Europe) and cigarette smoking.

In view of the observation that between 15 and 25% of patients treated with first-line therapy may still remain infected with the organism, new approaches to treatment have been explored. One promising approach is sequential therapy. This regimen consists of 5 days of amoxicillin and a PPI, followed by an additional 5 days of PPI plus tinidazole and clarithromycin. Initial studies have demonstrated eradication rates of >90% with good patient tolerance. Confirmation of these findings and applicability of this approach in the United States are needed.

Reinfection after successful eradication of *H. pylori* is rare in the United States (<1%/year). If recurrent infection occurs within the first 6 months after completing therapy, the most likely explanation is recrudescence as opposed to reinfection.

THERAPY OF NSAID-RELATED GASTRIC OR DUODENAL INJURY Medical intervention for NSAID-related mucosal injury includes treatment of an active ulcer and primary prevention of future injury. Recommendations for the treatment and primary prevention of NSAID-related mucosal injury are listed in **Table 287-5**. Ideally, the injurious agent should be stopped as the first step in the therapy of an active NSAID-induced ulcer. If that is possible, then treatment with one of the acid inhibitory agents (H_2 blockers, PPIs) is indicated. Cessation of NSAIDs is not always possible because of the patient's severe underlying disease. Only PPIs can heal GUs or DUs, independent of whether NSAIDs are discontinued.

The approach to primary prevention has included avoiding the agent, using NSAIDs that are theoretically less injurious, and/or the use of concomitant medical therapy to prevent NSAID-induced injury. Primary prevention of NSAID-induced ulceration can be accomplished by misoprostol (200 μg qid) or a PPI. High-dose H_2 blockers (famotidine, 40 mg bid) have also shown some promise in preventing endoscopically documented ulcers, although PPIs are superior. The highly selective COX-2 inhibitors, celecoxib and rofecoxib, are 100 times more selective inhibitors of COX-2 than standard NSAIDs, leading to gastric or duodenal mucosal injury that is comparable to placebo; their utilization led to an increase in cardiovascular events and withdrawal from the market. Additional caution was engen-

TABLE 287-5 **RECOMMENDATIONS FOR TREATMENT OF NSAID-RELATED MUCOSAL INJURY**

Clinical Setting	Recommendation
Active ulcer	
NSAID discontinued	H_2 receptor antagonist or PPI
NSAID continued	PPI
Prophylactic therapy	Misoprostol
	PPI
	Selective COX-2 inhibitor
H. pylori infection	Eradication if active ulcer present or there is a past history of peptic ulcer disease

Note: PPI, proton pump inhibitor; COX-2, isoenzyme of cyclooxygenase.

TABLE 287-6 **GUIDE TO NSAID THERAPY**

	No/Low NSAID GI Risk	NSAID GI Risk
No CV risk (no aspirin)	Traditional NSAID	Coxib or Traditional NSAID + PPI Consider non-NSAID therapy
CV risk (consider aspirin)	Traditional NSAID + PPI if GI risk warrants gastroprotection	A gastroprotective agent must be added if a traditional NSAID is prescribed
	Consider non-NSAID therapy	Consider non-NSAID therapy

Note: NSAID, nonsteroidal anti-inflammatory drug; GI, gastrointestinal; CV, cardiovascular; PPI, proton pump inhibitor.
Source: Adapted from AM Fendrick: Am J Manag Care 10:740, 2004.

dered when the CLASS study demonstrated that the advantage of celecoxib in preventing gastrointestinal complications was offset when low-dose aspirin was used simultaneously. Therefore, gastric protection therapy is required in individuals taking COX-2 inhibitors and aspirin prophylaxis. Finally, much of the work performed demonstrating the benefit of COX-2 inhibitors and PPIs on gastrointestinal injury has been performed in individuals of average risk; it is unclear if the same level of benefit will be achieved in high-risk patients. For example, concomitant use of warfarin and a COX-2 inhibitor was associated with rates of gastrointestinal bleeding similar to those observed in patients taking nonselective NSAIDs. A combination of factors, including withdrawal of the majority of COX-2 inhibitors from the market, the observation that low-dose aspirin appears to diminish the beneficial effect of COX-2 selective inhibitors, and the growing use of aspirin for prophylaxis of cardiovascular events, have significantly altered the approach to gastric protective therapy during the use of NSAIDs. A guide for the approach to the use of NSAIDs is shown in **Table 287-6**. Individuals who are not at risk for cardiovascular events, do not use aspirin, and are without risk for GI complications can receive nonselective NSAIDs without gastric protection. In those without cardiovascular risk factors but with a high potential risk for NSAID-induced GI toxicity, cautious use of a selective COX-2 inhibitor or a nonselective NSAID with gastric protection with a PPI is in order. Individuals with cardiovascular risk factors who require low-dose aspirin and have low potential for NSAID-induced toxicity should be considered for a non-NSAID agent or use of a traditional NSAID in combination with gastric protection, if warranted. Finally, individuals with cardiovascular and GI risks who require aspirin must be considered for non-NSAID therapy, but if that is not an option, then gastric protection with any type of NSAID must be considered.

APPROACH AND THERAPY: SUMMARY Controversy continues regarding the best approach to the patient who presents with dyspepsia (Chap. 39). The discovery of *H. pylori* and its role in pathogenesis of ulcers has added a new variable to the equation. Previously, if a patient <50 years old presented with dyspepsia and without alarming signs or symptoms suggestive of an ulcer complication or malignancy, an empirical therapeutic trial with acid suppression was commonly recommended. Although this approach is practiced by some today, an approach presently gaining approval for the treatment of patients with dyspepsia is outlined in **Fig. 287-12**. The referral to a gastroenterologist is for the potential need of endoscopy and subsequent evaluation and treatment if the endoscopy is negative.

Once an ulcer (GU or DU) is documented, the main issue at stake is whether *H. pylori* or an NSAID is involved. With *H. pylori* present, independent of the NSAID status, triple therapy is recommended for 14 days, followed by continued acid-suppressing drugs (H₂ receptor antagonist or PPIs) for a total of 4–6 weeks. Selection of patients for documentation of *H. pylori* eradication (organisms gone at least 4 weeks after completing antibiotics) is an area of some debate. The test of choice for documenting eradication is the urea breath test (UBT). The stool antigen assay may also hold promise for this purpose, but the data have not been as clear-cut as in the case of using the stool antigen test for primary diagnosis, especially if one considers patients who live in areas of low *H. pylori* prevalence. Further studies are warranted, but if the UBT is not available, a stool antigen should be considered to document eradication. The patient must be off antisecretory agents when being tested for eradication of *H. pylori* with UBT or stool antigen. Serologic testing is not useful for the purpose of documenting

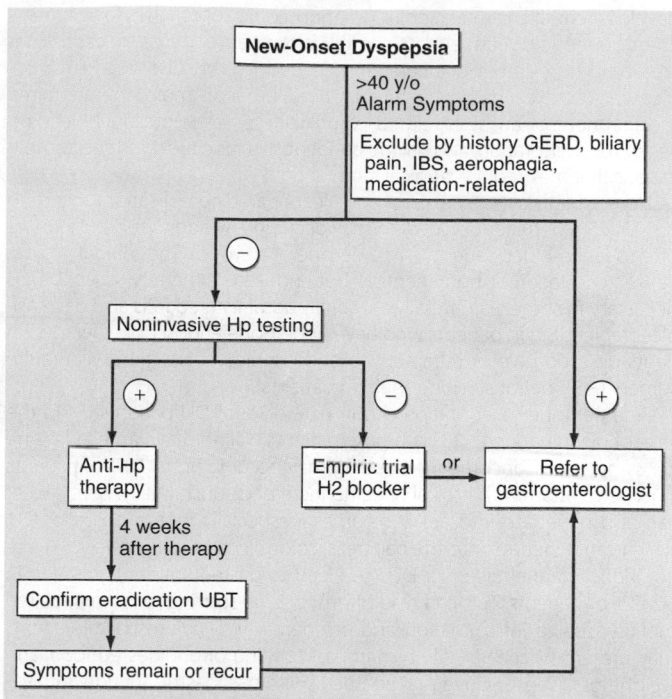

FIGURE 287-12 Overview of new-onset dyspepsia. Hp, *Helicobacter pylori*; UBT, urea breath test; IBS, irritable bowel syndrome. (*Adapted from BS Anand and DY Graham: Endoscopy 31:215, 1999.*)

eradication since antibody titers fall slowly and often do not become undetectable. Two approaches toward documentation of eradication exist: (1) test for eradication only in individuals with a complicated course or in individuals who are frail or with multisystem disease who would do poorly with an ulcer recurrence, and (2) test all patients for successful eradication. Some recommend that patients with complicated ulcer disease or who are frail should be treated with long-term acid suppression, thus making documentation of *H. pylori* eradication a moot point. In view of this discrepancy in practice, it would be best to discuss with the patient the different options available.

Several issues differentiate the approach to a GU versus a DU. GUs, especially of the body and fundus, have the potential of being malignant. Multiple biopsies of a GU should be taken initially; even if these are negative for neoplasm, repeat endoscopy to document healing at 8–12 weeks should be performed, with biopsy if the ulcer is still present. About 70% of GUs eventually found to be malignant undergo significant (usually incomplete) healing.

The majority (>90%) of GUs and DUs heal with the conventional therapy outlined above. A GU that fails to heal after 12 weeks and a DU that does not heal after 8 weeks of therapy should be considered refractory. Once poor compliance and persistent *H. pylori* infection have been excluded, NSAID use, either inadvertent or surreptitious, must be excluded. In addition, cigarette smoking must be eliminated. For a GU, malignancy must be meticulously excluded. Next, consideration should be given to a gastric acid hypersecretory state such as ZES (see "Zollinger-Ellison Syndrome," below) or the idiopathic form, which can be excluded with gastric acid analysis. Although a subset of patients have gastric acid hypersecretion of unclear etiology as a contributing factor to refractory ulcers, ZES should be excluded with a fasting gastrin or secretin stimulation test (see below). More than 90% of refractory ulcers (either DUs or GUs) heal after 8 weeks of treatment with higher doses of PPI (omeprazole, 40 mg/d; lansoprazole 30–60 mg/d). This higher dose is also effective in maintaining remission. Surgical intervention may be a consideration at this point; however, other rare causes of refractory ulcers must be excluded before recommending surgery. Rare etiologies of refractory ulcers that may be diagnosed by gastric or duodenal biopsies include ischemia, Crohn's disease, amyloidosis, sarcoidosis, lymphoma, eosinophilic gastroenteritis, or infection [cytomegalovirus (CMV), tuberculosis, or syphilis].

SURGICAL THERAPY Surgical intervention in PUD can be viewed as being either elective, for treatment of medically refractory disease, or as urgent/emergent, for the treatment of an ulcer-related complication. The development of pharmacologic and endoscopic approaches for the treatment of peptic disease and its complications has led to a substantial decrease in the number of operations needed for this disorder. Refractory ulcers are an exceedingly rare occurrence. Surgery is more often required for treatment of an ulcer-related complication. Gastrointestinal bleeding (Chap. 42), perforation, and gastric outlet obstruction are the three complications that may require surgical intervention.

Hemorrhage is the most common ulcer-related complication, occurring in ~15–25% of patients. Bleeding may occur in any age group but is most often seen in older patients (sixth decade or beyond). The majority of patients stop bleeding spontaneously, but endoscopic therapy (Chap. 285) is necessary in some. Parenterally and orally administered PPIs also decrease ulcer rebleeding in patients who have undergone endoscopic therapy. Patients unresponsive or refractory to endoscopic intervention will require surgery (~5% of transfusion-requiring patients).

Free peritoneal perforation occurs in ~2–3% of DU patients. As in the case of bleeding, up to 10% of these patients will not have antecedent ulcer symptoms. Concomitant bleeding may occur in up to 10% of patients with perforation, with mortality being increased substantially. Peptic ulcer can also penetrate into adjacent organs, especially with a posterior DU, which can penetrate into the pancreas, colon, liver, or biliary tree.

Pyloric channel ulcers or DUs can lead to gastric outlet obstruction in ~2–3% of patients. This can result from chronic scarring or from impaired motility due to inflammation and/or edema with pylorospasm. Patients may present with early satiety, nausea, vomiting of undigested food, and weight loss. Conservative management with nasogastric suction, intravenous hydration/nutrition, and antisecretory agents is indicated for 7–10 days with the hope that a functional obstruction will reverse. If a mechanical obstruction persists, endoscopic intervention with balloon dilation may be effective. Surgery should be considered if all else fails.

SPECIFIC OPERATIONS FOR DUODENAL ULCERS Surgical treatment is designed to decrease gastric acid secretion. Operations most commonly performed include (1) vagotomy and drainage (by pyloroplasty, gastroduodenostomy, or gastrojejunostomy), (2) highly selective vagotomy (which does not require a drainage procedure), and (3) vagotomy with antrectomy. The specific procedure performed is dictated by the underlying circumstances: elective vs. emergency, the degree and extent of duodenal ulceration, and the expertise of the surgeon. Moreover, the trend has been toward minimally invasive and anatomy-preserving operations.

Vagotomy is a component of each of these procedures and is aimed at decreasing acid secretion through ablating cholinergic input to the stomach. Unfortunately, both truncal and selective vagotomy (preserves the celiac and hepatic branches) result in gastric atony despite successful reduction of both basal acid output (BAO, decreased by 85%) and maximal acid output (MAO, decreased by 50%). Drainage through pyloroplasty or gastroduodenostomy is required in an effort to compensate for the vagotomy-induced gastric motility disorder. This procedure has an intermediate complication rate and a 10% ulcer recurrence rate. To minimize gastric dysmotility, highly selective vagotomy (also known as parietal cell, super-selective, or proximal vagotomy) was developed. Only the vagal fibers innervating the portion of the stomach that contains parietal cells is transected, thus leaving fibers important for regulating gastric motility intact. Although this procedure leads to an immediate decrease in both BAO and stimulated acid output, acid secretion recovers over time. By the end of the first postoperative year, basal and stimulated acid output are ~30 and 50%, respectively, of preoperative levels. Ulcer recurrence rates are higher with highly selective vagotomy (≥10%), although the overall complication rates are the lowest of the three procedures.

The procedure that provides the lowest rates of ulcer recurrence (1%) but has the highest complication rate is vagotomy (truncal or selective) in combination with antrectomy. Antrectomy is aimed at eliminating an additional stimulant of gastric acid secretion, gastrin. Two principal types of reanastomoses are used after antrectomy: gastroduodenostomy (Billroth I) or gastrojejunostomy (Billroth II) **(Fig. 287-13)**. Although Billroth I is often preferred over II, severe duodenal inflammation or scarring may preclude its performance.

Of these procedures, highly selective vagotomy may be the one of choice in the elective setting, except in situations where ulcer recurrence rates are high (prepyloric ulcers and those refractory to medical therapy). Selection of vagotomy and antrectomy may be more appropriate in these circumstances.

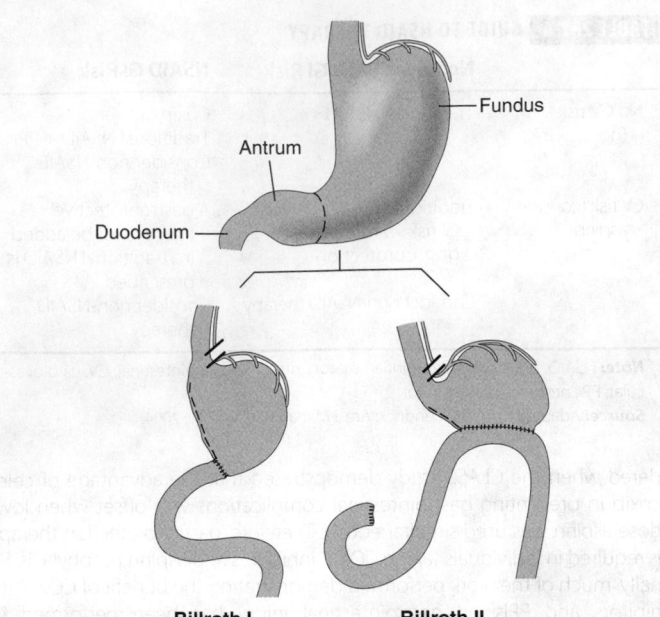

FIGURE 287-13 Schematic representation of Billroth I and II procedures.

These procedures have been traditionally performed by standard laparotomy. The advent of laparoscopic surgery has led several surgical teams to successfully perform highly selective vagotomy, truncal vagotomy/pyloroplasty, and truncal vagotomy/antrectomy through this approach. An increase in the number of laparoscopic procedures for treatment of PUD has occurred.

Specific Operations for Gastric Ulcers The location and the presence of a concomitant DU dictate the operative procedure performed for a GU. Antrectomy (including the ulcer) with a Billroth I anastomosis is the treatment of choice for an antral ulcer. Vagotomy is performed only if a DU is present. Although ulcer excision with vagotomy and drainage procedure has been proposed, the higher incidence of ulcer recurrence makes this a less desirable approach. Ulcers located near the esophagogastric junction may require a more radical approach, a subtotal gastrectomy with a Roux-en-Y esophagogastrojejunostomy (Csende's procedure). A less aggressive approach, including antrectomy, intraoperative ulcer biopsy, and vagotomy (Kelling-Madlener procedure), may be indicated in fragile patients with a high GU. Ulcer recurrence approaches 30% with this procedure.

Surgery-Related Complications Complications seen after surgery for PUD are related primarily to the extent of the anatomical modification performed. Minimal alteration (highly selective vagotomy) is associated with higher rates of ulcer recurrence and less gastrointestinal disturbance. More aggressive surgical procedures have a lower rate of ulcer recurrence but a greater incidence of gastrointestinal dysfunction. Overall, morbidity and mortality related to these procedures are quite low. Morbidity associated with vagotomy and antrectomy or pyloroplasty is ≤5%, with mortality ~1%. Highly selective vagotomy has lower morbidity and mortality rates of 1 and 0.3%, respectively.

In addition to the potential early consequences of any intraabdominal procedure (bleeding, infection, thromboembolism), gastroparesis, duodenal stump leak, and efferent loop obstruction can be observed.

Recurrent Ulceration The risk of ulcer recurrence is directly related to the procedure performed. Ulcers that recur after partial gastric resection tend to develop at the anastomosis (stomal or marginal ulcer). Epigastric abdominal pain is the most frequent presenting complaint (>90%). Severity and duration of pain tend to be more progressive than observed with DUs before surgery.

Ulcers may recur for several reasons, including incomplete vagotomy, inadequate drainage, retained antrum, and, less likely, persistent or recurrent *H. pylori* infection. ZES should have been excluded preoperatively. Surreptitious use of NSAIDs is an important reason for recurrent ulcers after surgery, especially if the initial procedure was done for an NSAID-induced ulcer. Once *H. pylori* and NSAIDs have been excluded as etiologic factors, the question of incomplete vagotomy or retained gastric antrum should be explored. For the latter, fasting plasma gastrin levels should be determined. If elevated, retained antrum or ZES (see below) should be considered. A combination of acid secretory analysis and secretin stimulation (see below) can assist in this differential diagnosis. Incomplete vagotomy can be ruled out by gastric acid analysis coupled with sham feeding. In this test, gastric acid output is measured while the patient sees, smells, and chews a meal (without swallowing). The cephalic phase of gastric secretion, which is mediated by the vagus, is being assessed with this study. An increase in gastric acid output in response to sham feeding is evidence that the vagus nerve is intact. A rise in serum pancreatic polypeptide >50% within 30 min of sham feeding is also suggestive of an intact vagus nerve.

Medical therapy with H_2 blockers will heal postoperative ulceration in 70–90% of patients. The efficacy of PPIs has not been fully assessed in this group, but one may anticipate greater rates of ulcer healing compared to those obtained with H_2 blockers. Repeat operation (complete vagotomy, partial gastrectomy) may be required in a small subgroup of patients who have not responded to aggressive medical management.

Afferent Loop Syndromes Two types of afferent loop syndrome can occur in patients who have undergone partial gastric resection with Billroth II anastomosis. The more common of the two is bacterial overgrowth in the afferent limb secondary to stasis. Patients may experience postprandial abdominal pain, bloating, and diarrhea with concomitant malabsorption of fats and vitamin B_{12}. Cases refractory to antibiotics may require surgical revision of the loop. The less-common afferent loop syndrome can present with severe abdominal pain and bloating that occur 20–60 min after meals. Pain is often followed by nausea and vomiting of bile-containing material. The pain and bloating may improve after emesis. The cause of this clinical picture is theorized to be incomplete drainage of bile and pancreatic secretions from an afferent loop that is partially obstructed. Cases refractory to dietary measures may need surgical revision.

Dumping Syndrome Dumping syndrome consists of a series of vasomotor and gastrointestinal signs and symptoms and occurs in patients who have undergone vagotomy and drainage (especially Billroth procedures). Two phases of dumping, early and late, can occur. Early dumping takes place 15–30 min after meals and consists of crampy abdominal discomfort, nausea, diarrhea, belching, tachycardia, palpitations, diaphoresis, light-headedness, and, rarely, syncope. These signs and symptoms arise from the rapid emptying of hyperosmolar gastric contents into the small intestine, resulting in a fluid shift into the gut lumen with plasma volume contraction and acute intestinal distention. Release of vasoactive gastrointestinal hormones (vasoactive intestinal polypeptide, neurotensin, motilin) is also theorized to play a role in early dumping.

The late phase of dumping typically occurs 90 min to 3 h after meals. Vasomotor symptoms (light-headedness, diaphoresis, palpitations, tachycardia, and syncope) predominate during this phase. This component of dumping is thought to be secondary to hypoglycemia from excessive insulin release.

Dumping syndrome is most noticeable after meals rich in simple carbohydrates (especially sucrose) and high osmolarity. Ingestion of large amounts of fluids may also contribute. Up to 50% of postvagotomy and drainage patients will experience dumping syndrome to some degree. Signs and symptoms often improve with time, but a severe protracted picture can occur in up to 1% of patients.

Dietary modification is the cornerstone of therapy for patients with dumping syndrome. Small, multiple (six) meals devoid of simple carbohydrates coupled with elimination of liquids during meals is important. Antidiarrheals and anticholinergic agents are complementary to diet. Guar and pectin, which increase the viscosity of intraluminal contents, may be beneficial in more symptomatic individuals. Acarbose, an α-glucosidase inhibitor that delays digestion of ingested carbohydrates, has also been shown to be beneficial in the treatment of the late phases of dumping. The somatostatin analogue octreotide has been successful in diet-refractory cases. This drug is administered subcutaneously (50 μg tid), titrated according to clinical response. A long-acting depot formulation of octreotide can be administered once every 28 days and provides symptom relief comparable to the short-acting agent. In addition, patient weight gain and quality of life appear to be superior with the long-acting form.

Postvagotomy Diarrhea Up to 10% of patients may seek medical attention for the treatment of postvagotomy diarrhea. This complication is most commonly observed after truncal vagotomy. Patients may complain of intermittent diarrhea that occurs typically 1–2 h after meals. Occasionally the symptoms may be severe and relentless. This is due to a motility disorder from interruption of the vagal fibers supplying the luminal gut. Other contributing factors may include decreased absorption of nutrients (see below), increased excretion of bile acids, and release of luminal factors that promote secretion. Diphenoxylate or loperamide is often useful in symptom control. The bile salt–binding agent cholestyramine may be helpful in severe cases. Surgical reversal of a 10-cm segment of jejunum may yield a substantial improvement in bowel frequency in a subset of patients.

Bile Reflux Gastropathy A subset of post-partial gastrectomy patients who present with abdominal pain, early satiety, nausea, and vomiting will have mucosal erythema of the gastric remnant as the only finding. Histologic examination of the gastric mucosa reveals minimal inflammation but the presence of epithelial cell injury. This clinical picture is categorized as bile or alkaline reflux gastropathy/gastritis. Although reflux of bile is implicated as the reason for this disorder, the mechanism is unknown. Prokinetic agents, cholestyramine, and sucralfate have been somewhat effective treatments. Severe refractory symptoms may require using either nuclear scanning with ^{99m}Tc-HIDA to document reflux or an alkaline challenge test, where 0.1 N NaOH is infused into the stomach in an effort to reproduce the patient's symptoms. Surgical diversion of pancreaticobiliary secretions away from the gastric remnant with a Roux-en-Y gastrojejunostomy consisting of a long (50–60 cm) Roux limb has been used in severe cases. Bilious vomiting improves, but early satiety and bloating may persist in up to 50% of patients.

Maldigestion and Malabsorption Weight loss can be observed in up to 60% of patients after partial gastric resection. A significant component of this weight reduction is due to decreased oral intake. However, mild steatorrhea can also develop. Reasons for maldigestion/malabsorption include decreased gastric acid production, rapid gastric emptying, decreased food dispersion in the stomach, reduced luminal bile concentration, reduced pancreatic secretory response to feeding, and rapid intestinal transit.

Decreased serum vitamin B_{12} levels can be observed after partial gastrectomy. This is usually not due to deficiency of IF, since a minimal amount of parietal cells (source of IF) are removed during antrectomy. Reduced vitamin B_{12} may be due to competition for the vitamin by bacterial overgrowth or inability to split the vitamin from its protein-bound source due to hypochlorhydria.

Iron-deficiency anemia may be a consequence of impaired absorption of dietary iron in patients with a Billroth II gastrojejunostomy. Absorption of iron salts is normal in these individuals; thus, a favorable response to oral iron supplementation can be anticipated. Folate deficiency with concomitant anemia can also develop in these patients. This deficiency may be secondary to decreased absorption or diminished oral intake.

Malabsorption of vitamin D and calcium resulting in osteoporosis and osteomalacia is common after partial gastrectomy and gastrojejunostomy (Billroth II). Osteomalacia can occur as a late complication in up to 25% of post-partial gastrectomy patients. Bone fractures occur twice as commonly in men after gastric surgery as in a control population. It may take years before x-ray findings demonstrate diminished bone density. Elevated alkaline phosphatase, reduced serum calcium, bone pain, and pathologic fractures may be seen in patients with osteomalacia. The high incidence of these abnormalities in this subgroup of patients justifies treating them with vitamin D and calcium supplementation indefinitely. Therapy is especially important in females.

Gastric Adenocarcinoma The incidence of adenocarcinoma in the gastric stump is increased 15 years after resection. Some have reported a four- to fivefold increase in gastric cancer 20–25 years after resection. The pathogenesis is unclear but may involve alkaline reflux, bacterial proliferation, or hypochlorhydria. The role of endoscopic screening is not clear, and most guidelines do not support its use.

RELATED CONDITIONS

ZOLLINGER-ELLISON SYNDROME

Severe peptic ulcer diathesis secondary to gastric acid hypersecretion due to unregulated gastrin release from a non-β cell endocrine tumor (gastrinoma) defines the components of ZES. Initially, ZES was typified by aggressive and refractory ulceration in which total gastrectomy provided the only chance for enhancing survival. Today it can be cured by surgical resection in up to 30% of patients.

Epidemiology The incidence of ZES varies from 0.1 to 1% of individuals presenting with PUD. Males are more commonly affected than females, and the majority of patients are diagnosed between ages 30 and 50. Gastrinomas are classified into sporadic tumors (more common) and those associated with multiple endocrine neoplasia (MEN) type I (see below).

Pathophysiology Hypergastrinemia originating from an autonomous neoplasm is the driving force responsible for the clinical manifestations in ZES. Gastrin stimulates acid secretion through gastrin receptors on parietal cells and by inducing histamine release from ECL cells. Gastrin also has a trophic action on gastric epithelial cells. Longstanding hypergastrinemia leads to markedly increased gastric acid secretion through both parietal cell stimulation and increased parietal cell mass. The increased gastric acid output leads to peptic ulcer diathesis, erosive esophagitis, and diarrhea.

Tumor Distribution Although early studies suggested that the vast majority of gastrinomas occurred within the pancreas, a significant number of these lesions are extrapancreatic. Over 80% of these tumors are found within the hypothetical gastrinoma triangle (confluence of the cystic and common bile ducts superiorly, junction of the second and third portions of the duodenum inferiorly, and junction of the neck and body of the pancreas medially). Duodenal tumors constitute the most common nonpancreatic lesion; between 50% and 75% of gastrinomas are found here. Duodenal tumors are smaller, slower-growing, and less likely to metastasize than pancreatic lesions. Less-common extrapancreatic sites include stomach, bones, ovaries, heart, liver, and lymph nodes. More than 60% of tumors are considered malignant, with up to 30–50% of patients having multiple lesions or metastatic disease at presentation. Histologically, gastrin-producing cells appear well-differentiated, expressing markers typically found in endocrine neoplasms (chromogranin, neuron-specific enolase).

Clinical Manifestations Gastric acid hypersecretion is responsible for the signs and symptoms observed in patients with ZES. Peptic ulcer is the most common clinical manifestation, occurring in >90% of gastrinoma patients. Initial presentation and ulcer location (duodenal bulb) may be indistinguishable from common PUD. Clinical situations that should create suspicion of gastrinoma are ulcers in unusual locations (second part of the duodenum and beyond), ulcers refractory to standard medical therapy, ulcer recurrence after acid-reducing surgery, ulcers presenting with frank complications (bleeding, obstruction, and perforation), or ulcers in the absence of *H. pylori* or NSAID ingestion. Symptoms of esophageal origin are present in up to two-thirds of patients with ZES, with a spectrum ranging from mild esophagitis to frank ulceration with stricture and Barrett's mucosa.

Diarrhea, the next most common clinical manifestation, is found in up to 50% of patients. Although diarrhea often occurs concomitantly with acid peptic disease, it may also occur independent of an ulcer. Etiology of the diarrhea is multifactorial, resulting from marked volume overload to the small bowel, pancreatic enzyme inactivation by acid, and damage of the intestinal epithelial surface by acid. The epithelial damage can lead to a mild degree of maldigestion and malabsorption of nutrients. The diarrhea may also have a secretory component due to the direct stimulatory effect of gastrin on enterocytes or the cosecretion of additional hormones from the tumor, such as vasoactive intestinal peptide.

Gastrinomas can develop in the presence of MEN I syndrome (Chaps. 344, 345) in ~25% of patients. This autosomal dominant disorder involves primarily three organ sites: the parathyroid glands (80–90%), pancreas (40–80%), and pituitary gland (30–60%). The genetic defect in MEN I is in the long arm of chromosome 11 (11q11-q13). In

---

TABLE 287-7	WHEN TO OBTAIN A FASTING SERUM GASTRIN LEVEL

Multiple ulcers
Ulcers in unusual locations; associated with severe esophagitis; resistant to therapy with frequent recurrences; in the absence of NSAID ingestion or *H. pylori* infection
Ulcer patients awaiting surgery
Extensive family history for peptic ulcer disease
Postoperative ulcer recurrence
Basal hyperchlorhydria
Unexplained diarrhea or steatorrhea
Hypercalcemia
Family history of pancreatic islet, pituitary, or parathyroid tumor
Prominent gastric or duodenal folds

---

view of the stimulatory effect of calcium on gastric secretion, the hyperparathyroidism and hypercalcemia seen in MEN I patients may have a direct effect on ulcer disease. Resolution of hypercalcemia by parathyroidectomy reduces gastrin and gastric acid output in gastrinoma patients. An additional distinguishing feature in ZES patients with MEN I is the higher incidence of gastric carcinoid tumor development (as compared to patients with sporadic gastrinomas). Gastrinomas tend to be smaller, multiple, and located in the duodenal wall more often than is seen in patients with sporadic ZES. Establishing the diagnosis of MEN I is critical not only from the standpoint of providing genetic counseling to the patient and his or her family but also to the surgical approach recommended.

Diagnosis The first step in the evaluation of a patient suspected of having ZES is to obtain a fasting gastrin level. A list of clinical scenarios that should arouse suspicion regarding this diagnosis is shown in Table 287-7. Fasting gastrin levels are usually <150 pg/mL. Virtually all gastrinoma patients will have a gastrin level >150–200 pg/mL. Measurement of fasting gastrin should be repeated to confirm the clinical suspicion.

Multiple processes can lead to an elevated fasting gastrin level: gastric hypochlorhydria or achlorhydria (the most frequent), with or without pernicious anemia; retained gastric antrum; G cell hyperplasia; gastric outlet obstruction; renal insufficiency; massive small-bowel obstruction; and conditions such as rheumatoid arthritis, vitiligo, diabetes mellitus, and pheochromocytoma. Gastric acid induces feedback inhibition of gastrin release. A decrease in acid production will subsequently lead to failure of the feedback inhibitory pathway, resulting in net hypergastrinemia. Gastrin levels will thus be high in patients using antisecretory agents for the treatment of acid peptic disorders and dyspepsia. *H. pylori* infection can also cause hypergastrinemia. Although a fasting gastrin >10 times normal is highly suggestive of ZE, two-thirds of patients will have fasting gastrin levels that overlap with levels found in the more common disorders outlined above.

The next step in establishing a biochemical diagnosis of gastrinoma is to assess acid secretion. Nothing further needs to be done if decreased acid output is observed. In contrast, normal or elevated gastric acid output suggests a need for additional tests. Up to 12% of patients with common PUD may have comparable levels of acid secretion. A BAO/MAO ratio >0.6 is highly suggestive of ZES, but a ratio <0.6 does not exclude the diagnosis. Pentagastrin is no longer available in the United States, making measurement of MAO virtually impossible. An endoscopic method for measuring gastric acid output has been developed but requires further validation. If the technology for measuring gastric acid secretion is not available, a basal gastric pH ≥3 virtually excludes a gastrinoma.

Gastrin provocative tests have been developed in an effort to differentiate between the causes of hypergastrinemia and are especially helpful in patients with indeterminate acid secretory studies. The tests are the secretin stimulation test and the calcium infusion study. The most sensitive and specific gastrin provocative test for the diagnosis of gastrinoma is the secretin study. An increase in gastrin of ≥200 pg within 15 min of secretin injection has a sensitivity and specificity of >90% for ZES. The calcium infusion study is less sensitive and specific

TABLE 287-8 SENSITIVITY OF IMAGING STUDIES IN ZOLLINGER-ELLISON SYNDROME

Study	Sensitivity, %	
	Primary Gastrinoma	Metastatic Gastrinoma
Ultrasound	21–28	14
CT scan	35–59	35–72
Selective angiography	35–68	33–86
Portal venous sampling	70–90	N/A
SASI	55–78	41
MRI	30–60	71
Octreoscan	67–86	80–100
EUS	80–100	N/A

Note: CT, computed tomography; SASI, selective arterial secretin injection; MRI, magnetic resonance imaging; octreoscan, imaging with ^{111}In-pentreotide; EUS, endoscopic ultrasonography.

than the secretin test, with a rise of >400 pg/mL observed in ~80% of gastrinoma patients. The lower accuracy, coupled with it being a more cumbersome study with greater potential for adverse effects, makes calcium infusion less useful. It is used in the rare cases where the patient's clinical characteristics are highly suggestive of ZES, but the secretin stimulation is inconclusive.

Tumor Localization Once the biochemical diagnosis of gastrinoma has been confirmed, the tumor must be located. Multiple imaging studies have been utilized in an effort to enhance tumor localization (Table 287-8). The broad range of sensitivity is due to the variable success rates achieved by the different investigative groups. Endoscopic ultrasound (EUS) permits imaging of the pancreas with a high degree of resolution (<5 mm). This modality is particularly helpful in excluding small neoplasms within the pancreas and in assessing the presence of surrounding lymph nodes and vascular involvement, but it is not very sensitive for finding duodenal lesions. Several types of endocrine tumors express cell-surface receptors for somatostatin. This permits the localization of gastrinomas by measuring the uptake of the stable somatostatin analogue ^{111}In-pentreotide (octreoscan) with sensitivity and specificity rates of >75%.

Up to 50% of patients have metastatic disease at diagnosis. Success in controlling gastric acid hypersecretion has shifted the emphasis of therapy toward providing a surgical cure. Detecting the primary tumor and excluding metastatic disease are critical in view of this paradigm shift. Once a biochemical diagnosis has been confirmed, the patient should first undergo an abdominal CT scan, MRI, or octreoscan (depending on availability) to exclude metastatic disease. Once metastatic disease has been excluded, an experienced endocrine surgeon may opt for exploratory laparotomy with intraoperative ultrasound or transillumination. In other centers, careful examination of the peripancreatic area with EUS, accompanied by endoscopic exploration of the duodenum for primary tumors, will be performed before surgery. Selective arterial secretin injection may be a useful adjuvant for localizing tumors in a subset of patients.

℞ ZOLLINGER-ELLISON SYNDROME

Treatment of functional endocrine tumors is directed at ameliorating the signs and symptoms related to hormone overproduction, curative resection of the neoplasm, and attempts to control tumor growth in metastatic disease.

PPIs are the treatment of choice and have decreased the need for total gastrectomy. Initial PPI doses tend to be higher than those used for treatment of GERD or PUD. The initial dose of omeprazole or lansoprazole should be in the range of 60 mg in divided doses in a 24-h period. Dosing can be adjusted to achieve a BAO <10 meq/h (at the drug trough) in surgery-naive patients and to <5 meq/h in individuals who have previously undergone an acid-reducing operation. Although the somatostatin analogue has inhibitory effects on gastrin release from receptor-bearing tumors and inhibits gastric acid secretion to some extent, PPIs have the advantage of reducing parietal cell activity to a greater degree. Despite this, octreotide may be considered as adjunctive therapy to the PPI in patients with tumors that express somatostatin receptors and have peptic symptoms that are difficult to control with high-dose PPI.

The ultimate goal of surgery would be to provide a definitive cure. Improved understanding of tumor distribution has led to 10-year disease-free intervals as high as 34% in sporadic gastrinoma patients undergoing surgery. A positive outcome is highly dependent on the experience of the surgical team treating these rare tumors. Surgical therapy of gastrinoma patients with MEN I remains controversial because of the difficulty in rendering these patients disease-free with surgery. In contrast to the encouraging postoperative results observed in patients with sporadic disease, only 6% of MEN I patients are disease-free 5 years after an operation. Some groups suggest surgery only if a clearly identifiable, nonmetastatic lesion is documented by structural studies. Others advocate a more aggressive approach, where all patients free of hepatic metastasis are explored and all detected tumors in the duodenum are resected; this is followed by enucleation of lesions in the pancreatic head, with a distal pancreatectomy to follow. The outcome of the two approaches has not been clearly defined. Laparoscopic surgical interventions may provide attractive approaches in the future.

Therapy of metastatic endocrine tumors in general remains suboptimal; gastrinomas are no exception. Medical approaches including chemotherapy (streptozotocin, 5-fluorouracil, and doxorubicin), IFN-α, and hepatic artery embolization lead to significant toxicity without a substantial improvement in overall survival. ^{111}In-pentetreotide has been used in the therapy of metastatic neuroendocrine tumors; further studies are needed. Several novel therapies are being explored, including radiofrequency or cryoablation of liver lesions and use of agents that block the vascular endothelial growth receptor pathway (bevacizumab, sunitinib) (Chap. 344).

Surgical approaches including debulking surgery and liver transplantation for hepatic metastasis have also produced limited benefit. Therefore, early recognition and surgery are the only chances for curing this disease.

The overall 5- and 10-year survival rates for gastrinoma patients are 62–75% and 47–53%, respectively. Individuals with the entire tumor resected or those with a negative laparotomy have 5- and 10-year survival rates >90%. Patients with incompletely resected tumors have 5- and 10-year survival of 43% and 25%, respectively. Patients with hepatic metastasis have <20% survival at 5 years. Favorable prognostic indicators include primary duodenal wall tumors, isolated lymph node tumor, and undetectable tumor upon surgical exploration. Poor outcome is seen in patients with shorter disease duration; higher gastrin levels (>10,000 pg/mL); large pancreatic primary tumors (>3 cm); metastatic disease to lymph nodes, liver, and bone; and Cushing's syndrome. Rapid growth of hepatic metastases is also predictive of poor outcome.

STRESS-RELATED MUCOSAL INJURY

Patients suffering from shock, sepsis, massive burns, severe trauma, or head injury can develop acute erosive gastric mucosal changes or frank ulceration with bleeding. Classified as stress-induced gastritis or ulcers, injury is most commonly observed in the acid-producing (fundus and body) portions of the stomach. The most common presentation is gastrointestinal bleeding, which is usually minimal but can occasionally be life-threatening. Respiratory failure requiring mechanical ventilation and underlying coagulopathy are risk factors for bleeding, which tends to occur 48–72 h after the acute injury or insult.

Histologically, stress injury does not contain inflammation or *H. pylori*; thus, "gastritis" is a misnomer. Although elevated gastric acid secretion may be noted in patients with stress ulceration after head trauma (Cushing's ulcer) and severe burns (Curling's ulcer), mucosal ischemia and breakdown of the normal protective barriers of the stomach also play an important role in the pathogenesis. Acid must contribute to injury in view of the significant drop in bleeding noted when acid inhibitors are used as prophylaxis for stress gastritis.

Improvement in the general management of intensive care unit patients has led to a significant decrease in the incidence of gastrointestinal bleeding due to stress ulceration. The estimated decrease in bleeding is from 20–30% to <5%. This improvement has led to some debate regarding the need for prophylactic therapy. The limited benefit of medical (endoscopic, angiographic) and surgical therapy in a patient with hemodynamically compromising bleeding associated with stress ulcer/gastritis supports the use of preventive measures in high-risk patients (mechanically ventilated, coagulopathy, multiorgan failure, or severe burns). Maintenance of gastric pH > 3.5 with continuous infusion of H_2 blockers or liquid antacids administered every 2–3 h are viable options. Tolerance to the H_2 blocker is likely to develop; thus, careful monitoring of the gastric pH and dose adjustment is important if H_2 blockers are used. Moreover, administration of antacids is cumbersome, requiring use of a gastric tube, and the agent may lead to diarrhea and electrolyte abnormalities. Sucralfate slurry (1 g every 4–6 h) has also been somewhat successful but requires a gastric tube and may lead to constipation and aluminum toxicity. Sucralfate use in endotracheal intubated patients has also been associated with aspiration pneumonia. PPIs are the treatment of choice for stress prophylaxis. Oral PPI is the best option if the patient can tolerate enteral administration. Pantoprazole is available as an intravenous formulation for individuals in whom enteral administration is not possible. If bleeding occurs despite these measures, endoscopy, intraarterial vasopressin, or embolization are options. If all else fails, then surgery should be considered. Although vagotomy and antrectomy may be used, the better approach would be a total gastrectomy, which has an exceedingly high mortality rate in this setting.

GASTRITIS

The term *gastritis* should be reserved for histologically documented inflammation of the gastric mucosa. Gastritis is not the mucosal erythema seen during endoscopy and is not interchangeable with "dyspepsia." The etiologic factors leading to gastritis are broad and heterogeneous. Gastritis has been classified based on time course (acute vs. chronic), histologic features, and anatomical distribution or proposed pathogenic mechanism (Table 287-9).

The correlation between the histologic findings of gastritis, the clinical picture of abdominal pain or dyspepsia, and endoscopic findings noted on gross inspection of the gastric mucosa is poor. Therefore, there is no typical clinical manifestation of gastritis.

Acute Gastritis The most common causes of acute gastritis are infectious. Acute infection with *H. pylori* induces gastritis. However, *H. pylori* acute gastritis has not been extensively studied. It is reported as presenting with sudden onset of epigastric pain, nausea, and vomiting, and limited mucosal histologic studies demonstrate a marked infiltrate of neutrophils with edema and hyperemia. If not treated, this picture will evolve into one of chronic gastritis. Hypochlorhydria lasting for up to 1 year may follow acute *H. pylori* infection.

The highly acidic gastric environment may be one reason why infectious processes of the stomach are rare. Bacterial infection of the stomach or phlegmonous gastritis is a rare, potentially life-threatening disorder characterized by marked and diffuse acute inflammatory infiltrates of the entire gastric wall, at times accompanied by necrosis. Elderly individuals, alcoholics, and AIDS patients may be affected. Potential iatrogenic causes include polypectomy and mucosal injection with India ink. Organisms associated with this entity include streptococci, staphylococci, *Escherichia coli*, *Proteus*, and *Haemophilus* sp. Failure of supportive measures and antibiotics may result in gastrectomy.

TABLE 287-9 CLASSIFICATION OF GASTRITIS

I. Acute gastritis	II. Chronic atrophic gastritis
A. Acute *H. pylori* infection	A. Type A: Autoimmune, body-predominant
B. Other acute infectious gastritides	B. Type B: *H. pylori*–related, antral-predominant
1. Bacterial (other than *H. pylori*)	C. Indeterminant
2. *Helicobacter helmanni*	III. Uncommon forms of gastritis
3. Phlegmonous	A. Lymphocytic
4. Mycobacterial	B. Eosinophilic
5. Syphilitic	C. Crohn's disease
6. Viral	D. Sarcoidosis
7. Parasitic	E. Isolated granulomatous gastritis
8. Fungal	

Other types of infectious gastritis may occur in immunocompromised individuals such as AIDS patients. Examples include herpetic (herpes simplex) or CMV gastritis. The histologic finding of intranuclear inclusions would be observed in the latter.

Chronic Gastritis Chronic gastritis is identified histologically by an inflammatory cell infiltrate consisting primarily of lymphocytes and plasma cells, with very scant neutrophil involvement. Distribution of the inflammation may be patchy, initially involving superficial and glandular portions of the gastric mucosa. This picture may progress to more severe glandular destruction, with atrophy and metaplasia. Chronic gastritis has been classified according to histologic characteristics. These include superficial atrophic changes and gastric atrophy.

The early phase of chronic gastritis is *superficial gastritis*. The inflammatory changes are limited to the lamina propria of the surface mucosa, with edema and cellular infiltrates separating intact gastric glands. Additional findings may include decreased mucus in the mucous cells and decreased mitotic figures in the glandular cells. The next stage is *atrophic gastritis*. The inflammatory infiltrate extends deeper into the mucosa, with progressive distortion and destruction of the glands. The final stage of chronic gastritis is *gastric atrophy*. Glandular structures are lost, and there is a paucity of inflammatory infiltrates. Endoscopically, the mucosa may be substantially thin, permitting clear visualization of the underlying blood vessels.

Gastric glands may undergo morphologic transformation in chronic gastritis. Intestinal metaplasia denotes the conversion of gastric glands to a small intestinal phenotype with small-bowel mucosal glands containing goblet cells. The metaplastic changes may vary in distribution from patchy to fairly extensive gastric involvement. Intestinal metaplasia is an important predisposing factor for gastric cancer (Chap. 87).

Chronic gastritis is also classified according to the predominant site of involvement. Type A refers to the body-predominant form (autoimmune) and type B is the antral-predominant form (*H. pylori*–related). This classification is artificial in view of the difficulty in distinguishing these two entities. The term *AB gastritis* has been used to refer to a mixed antral/body picture.

TYPE A GASTRITIS The less common of the two forms involves primarily the fundus and body, with antral sparing. Traditionally, this form of gastritis has been associated with pernicious anemia (Chap. 100) in the presence of circulating antibodies against parietal cells and IF; thus, it is also called *autoimmune gastritis*. *H. pylori* infection can lead to a similar distribution of gastritis. The characteristics of an autoimmune picture are not always present.

Antibodies to parietal cells have been detected in >90% of patients with pernicious anemia and in up to 50% of patients with type A gastritis. The parietal cell antibody is directed against H^+,K^+-ATPase. T cells are also implicated in the injury pattern of this form of gastritis.

Parietal cell antibodies and atrophic gastritis are observed in family members of patients with pernicious anemia. These antibodies are observed in up to 20% of individuals over age 60 and in ~20% of patients with vitiligo and Addison's disease. About half of patients with pernicious anemia have antibodies to thyroid antigens, and about 30% of patients with thyroid disease have circulating antiparietal cell antibodies. Anti-IF antibodies are more specific than parietal cell antibodies for type A gastritis, being present in ~40% of patients with pernicious anemia. Another parameter consistent with this form of gastritis being autoimmune in origin is the higher incidence of specific familial histocompatibility haplotypes such as HLA-B8 and -DR3.

The parietal cell–containing gastric gland is preferentially targeted in this form of gastritis, and achlorhydria results. Parietal cells are the source of IF, lack of which will lead to vitamin B_{12} deficiency and its sequelae (megaloblastic anemia, neurologic dysfunction).

Gastric acid plays an important role in feedback inhibition of gastrin release from G cells. Achlorhydria, coupled with relative sparing of the antral mucosa (site of G cells), leads to hypergastrinemia. Gastrin levels can be markedly elevated (>500 pg/mL) in patients with perni-

FIGURE 287-14 Chronic gastritis and *H. pylori* organisms. Steiner silver stain of superficial gastric mucosa, showing abundant darkly staining microorganisms layered over the apical portion of the surface epithelium. Note that there is no tissue invasion.

cious anemia. ECL cell hyperplasia with frank development of gastric carcinoid tumors may result from gastrin trophic effects. The role of gastrin in carcinoid development is confirmed by the observation that antrectomy leads to regression of these lesions. Hypergastrinemia and achlorhydria may also be seen in non-pernicious anemia–associated type A gastritis.

TYPE B GASTRITIS   Type B, or antral-predominant, gastritis is the more common form of chronic gastritis. *H. pylori* infection is the cause of this entity. Although described as "antral-predominant," this is likely a misnomer in view of studies documenting the progression of the inflammatory process toward the body and fundus of infected individuals. The conversion to a pan-gastritis is time-dependent–estimated to require 15–20 years. This form of gastritis increases with age, being present in up to 100% of persons over age 70. Histology improves after *H. pylori* eradication. The number of *H. pylori* organisms decreases dramatically with progression to gastric atrophy, and the degree of inflammation correlates with the level of these organisms. Early on, with antral-predominant findings, the quantity of *H. pylori* is highest and a dense chronic inflammatory infiltrate of the lamina propria is noted, accompanied by epithelial cell infiltration with polymorphonuclear leukocytes (Fig. 287-14).

Multifocal atrophic gastritis, gastric atrophy with subsequent metaplasia, has been observed in chronic *H. pylori*–induced gastritis. This may ultimately lead to development of gastric adenocarcinoma (Fig. 287-8; Chap. 87). *H. pylori* infection is now considered an independent risk factor for gastric cancer. Worldwide epidemiologic studies have documented a higher incidence of *H. pylori* infection in patients with adenocarcinoma of the stomach as compared to control subjects. Seropositivity for *H. pylori* is associated with a three- to sixfold increased risk of gastric cancer. This risk may be as high as ninefold after adjusting for the inaccuracy of serologic testing in the elderly. The mechanism by which *H. pylori* infection leads to cancer is unknown, but it appears to be related to the chronic inflammation induced by the organism. Eradication of *H. pylori* as a general preventative measure for gastric cancer is being evaluated but is not yet recommended.

Infection with *H. pylori* is also associated with development of a low-grade B cell lymphoma, gastric MALT lymphoma (Chap. 105). The chronic T cell stimulation caused by the infection leads to production of cytokines that promote the B cell tumor. The tumor should be initially staged with a CT scan of the abdomen and EUS. Tumor growth remains dependent on the presence of *H. pylori*, and its eradication is often associated with complete regression of the tumor. The tumor may take more than a year to regress after treating the infection. Such patients should be followed by EUS every 2–3 months. If the tumor is stable or decreasing in size, no other therapy is necessary. If the

tumor grows, it may have become a high-grade B cell lymphoma. When the tumor becomes a high-grade aggressive lymphoma histologically, it loses responsiveness to *H. pylori* eradication.

℞ CHRONIC GASTRITIS

Treatment in chronic gastritis is aimed at the sequelae and not the underlying inflammation. Patients with pernicious anemia will require parenteral vitamin B$_{12}$ supplementation on a long-term basis. Eradication of *H. pylori* is not routinely recommended unless PUD or a low-grade MALT lymphoma is present.

Miscellaneous Forms of Gastritis   *Lymphocytic gastritis* is characterized histologically by intense infiltration of the surface epithelium with lymphocytes. The infiltrative process is primarily in the body of the stomach and consists of mature T cells and plasmacytes. The etiology of this form of chronic gastritis is unknown. It has been described in patients with celiac sprue, but whether there is a common factor associating these two entities is unknown. No specific symptoms suggest lymphocytic gastritis. A subgroup of patients have thickened folds noted on endoscopy. These folds are often capped by small nodules that contain a central depression or erosion; this form of the disease is called *varioliform gastritis*. *H. pylori* probably plays no significant role in lymphocytic gastritis. Therapy with glucocorticoids or sodium cromoglycate has obtained unclear results.

Marked eosinophilic infiltration involving any layer of the stomach (mucosa, muscularis propria, and serosa) is characteristic of *eosinophilic gastritis*. Affected individuals will often have circulating eosinophilia with clinical manifestation of systemic allergy. Involvement may range from isolated gastric disease to diffuse eosinophilic gastroenteritis. Antral involvement predominates, with prominent edematous folds being observed on endoscopy. These prominent antral folds can lead to outlet obstruction. Patients can present with epigastric discomfort, nausea, and vomiting. Treatment with glucocorticoids has been successful.

Several systemic disorders may be associated with *granulomatous gastritis*. Gastric involvement has been observed in Crohn's disease. Involvement may range from granulomatous infiltrates noted only on gastric biopsies to frank ulceration and stricture formation. Gastric Crohn's disease usually occurs in the presence of small-intestinal disease. Several rare infectious processes can lead to granulomatous gastritis, including histoplasmosis, candidiasis, syphilis, and tuberculosis. Other unusual causes of this form of gastritis include sarcoidosis, idiopathic granulomatous gastritis, and eosinophilic granulomas involving the stomach. Establishing the specific etiologic agent in this form of gastritis can be difficult, at times requiring repeat endoscopy with biopsy and cytology. Occasionally a surgically obtained full-thickness biopsy of the stomach may be required to exclude malignancy.

MÉNÉTRIER'S DISEASE

Ménétrier's disease is a rare entity characterized by large, tortuous gastric mucosal folds. The differential diagnosis of large gastric folds includes ZES, malignancy, infectious etiologies (CMV, histoplasmosis, syphilis), and infiltrative disorders such as sarcoidosis. The mucosal folds in Ménétrier's disease are often most prominent in the body and fundus. Histologically, massive foveolar hyperplasia (hyperplasia of surface and glandular mucous cells) is noted, which replaces most of the chief and parietal cells. This hyperplasia produces the prominent folds observed. The pits of the gastric glands elongate and may become extremely tortuous. Although the lamina propria may contain a mild chronic inflammatory infiltrate, Ménétrier's disease is not considered a form of gastritis. The etiology of this unusual clinical picture is unknown. Overexpression of growth factors such as TGF-α may be involved in the process.

Epigastric pain, at times accompanied by nausea, vomiting, anorexia, and weight loss, are signs and symptoms in patients with Ménétrier's disease. Occult gastrointestinal bleeding may occur, but overt bleeding is unusual and, when present, is due to superficial mucosal erosions.

Twenty to 100% of patients (depending on time of presentation) develop a protein-losing gastropathy accompanied by hypoalbuminemia and edema. Gastric acid secretion is usually reduced or absent because of the replacement of parietal cells. Large gastric folds are readily detectable by either radiographic (barium meal) or endoscopic methods. Endoscopy with deep mucosal biopsy (and cytology) is required to establish the diagnosis and exclude other entities that may present similarly. A nondiagnostic biopsy may lead to a surgically obtained full-thickness biopsy to exclude malignancy.

Rx MÉNÉTRIER'S DISEASE

Medical therapy with anticholinergic agents, prostaglandins, PPIs, prednisone, and H$_2$ receptor antagonists yields varying results. Anticholinergics decrease protein loss. A high-protein diet should be recommended to replace protein loss in patients with hypoalbuminemia. Ulcers should be treated with a standard approach. Severe disease with persistent and substantial protein loss may require total gastrectomy. Subtotal gastrectomy is performed by some; it may be associated with higher morbidity and mortality secondary to the difficulty in obtaining a patent and long-lasting anastomosis between normal and hyperplastic tissues.

ACKNOWLEDGMENTS
The author acknowledges the contribution of material to this chapter by Dr. Lawrence Friedman and Dr. Walter Peterson from their chapter on this subject in the 14th edition of Harrison's.

FURTHER READINGS

BESWICK EJ et al: *H pylori* and host interactions that influence pathogenesis. World J Gastroenterol 12:5599, 2006

CHAN FK et al: Preventing recurrent upper gastrointestinal bleeding in patients with *Helicobacter pylori* infection who are taking low-dose aspirin or naproxen. N Engl J Med 344:967, 2001

CHAN FKL, LEUNG WK: Peptic-ulcer disease. Lancet 360:933, 2002

ERNST PB et al: The translation of *Helicobacter pylori* basic research to patient care. Gastroenterology 130:188, 2006

FOX JG, WANG TC: Inflammation, atrophy, and gastric cancer. J Clin Invest 117:60, 2007

LAI KC et al: Lansoprazole for the prevention of recurrences of ulcer complications from long-term low-dose aspirin use. N Engl J Med 346:2033, 2002

LAINE L: Approaches to nonsteroidal anti-inflammatory drug use in the high-risk patient. Gastroenterology 120:594, 2001

————: Gastrointestinal effects of NSAIDs and coxibs. J Pain Symptom Manage 25(Suppl 2):532, 2003

MOAYYEDI P et al: An update of the Cochrane systematic review of *Helicobacter pylori* eradication therapy in nonulcer dyspepsia: Resolving the discrepancy between systematic reviews. Am J Gastroenterol 98:2621, 2003

SUERBAUM S, MICHETTI P: *Helicobacter pylori* infection. N Engl J Med 347:1175, 2002

VILAICHONE RK et al: *Helicobacter pylori* diagnosis and management. Gastroenterol Clin North Am 35:229, 2006

288 Disorders of Absorption
Henry J. Binder

Disorders of absorption constitute a broad spectrum of conditions with multiple etiologies and varied clinical manifestations. Almost all of these clinical problems are associated with *diminished* intestinal absorption of one or more dietary nutrients and are often referred to as the *malabsorption syndrome*. This term is not ideal as it represents a pathophysiologic state, does *not* provide an etiologic explanation for the underlying problem, and should not be considered an adequate final diagnosis. The only clinical situations in which absorption is *increased* are hemochromatosis and Wilson's disease, in which absorption of iron and copper, respectively, are increased.

Most, but not all, malabsorption syndromes are associated with *steatorrhea*, an increase in stool fat excretion of >6% of dietary fat intake. Some malabsorption disorders are not associated with steatorrhea: primary lactase deficiency, a congenital absence of the small intestinal brush border disaccharidase enzyme lactase, is associated with lactose "malabsorption," and pernicious anemia is associated with a marked decrease in intestinal absorption of cobalamin (vitamin B$_{12}$) due to an absence of gastric parietal cell intrinsic factor required for cobalamin absorption.

Disorders of absorption must be included in the differential diagnosis of diarrhea (Chap. 40). First, diarrhea is frequently associated with and/or is a consequence of the diminished absorption of one or more dietary nutrients. The diarrhea may be secondary either to the intestinal process that is responsible for the steatorrhea or to steatorrhea per se. Thus, celiac sprue (see below) is associated with both extensive morphologic changes in the small intestinal mucosa and reduced absorption of several dietary nutrients; in contrast, the diarrhea of steatorrhea is the result of the effect of nonabsorbed dietary fatty acids on intestinal, usually colonic, ion transport. For example, oleic acid and ricinoleic acid (a bacterially hydroxylated fatty acid that is also the active ingredient in castor oil, a widely used laxative) induce active colonic Cl ion secretion, most likely secondary to increasing intracellular Ca. In addition, diarrhea per se may result in mild steator-

rhea (<11 g fat excretion while on a 100-g fat diet). Second, most patients will indicate that they have diarrhea, not that they have fat malabsorption. Third, many intestinal disorders that have diarrhea as a prominent symptom (e.g., ulcerative colitis, traveler's diarrhea secondary to an enterotoxin produced by *Escherichia coli*) do not necessarily have diminished absorption of any dietary nutrient.

Diarrhea as a *symptom* (i.e., when used by patients to describe their bowel movement pattern) may be either a decrease in stool consistency, an increase in stool volume, an increase in number of bowel movements, or any combination of these three changes. In contrast, diarrhea as a *sign* is a quantitative increase in stool water or weight of >200–225 mL, or gram per 24 h, when a western-type diet is consumed. Individuals consuming a diet with higher fiber content may normally have a stool weight of up to 400 g/24 h. Thus, the clinician must clarify what an individual patient means by diarrhea. Some 10% of patients referred to gastroenterologists for further evaluation of unexplained diarrhea do not have an increase in stool water when it is determined quantitatively. Such patients may have small, frequent, somewhat loose bowel movements with stool urgency that is indicative of proctitis but do not have an increase in stool weight or volume.

It is also critical to establish whether a patient's diarrhea is secondary to diminished absorption of one or more dietary nutrients, in contrast to diarrhea that is due to small- and/or large-intestinal fluid and electrolyte secretion. The former has often been termed *osmotic diarrhea*, while the latter has been referred to as *secretory diarrhea*. Unfortunately, both secretory and osmotic elements can be present simultaneously in the same disorder; thus, this separation is not always precise. Nonetheless, two studies—determination of stool electrolytes and observation of the effect of a fast on stool output—can help make this distinction.

The demonstration of the effect of prolonged (>24 h) fasting on stool output can be very effective in suggesting that a *dietary nutrient* is responsible for the individual's diarrhea. A secretory diarrhea associated with enterotoxin-induced traveler's diarrhea would not be affected by prolonged fasting, as enterotoxin-induced stimulation of intestinal fluid and electrolyte secretion is not altered by eating. In contrast, diarrhea secondary to lactose malabsorption in primary lactase deficiency would undoubtedly cease during a prolonged fast. Thus, a substantial decrease in stool output while fasting during a quantitative stool collection of at least 24 h is presumptive evidence that the diarrhea is related to malabsorption of a dietary nutrient. The persistence of stool output while fasting indicates that the diarrhea is likely secretory and that the cause of diarrhea is *not* a dietary nutrient. Either a luminal (e.g., *E. coli* enterotoxin) or circulating (e.g., vasoactive intestinal peptide) secretagogue could be responsible for the patient's diarrhea persisting unaltered during a prolonged fast. The observed effects of fasting can be compared and correlated with stool electrolyte and osmolality determinations.

Measurement of stool electrolytes and osmolality requires the comparison of stool Na$^+$ and K$^+$ concentrations determined in liquid stool to the stool osmolality to determine the presence or absence of a so-called stool osmotic gap. The following formula is used:

$$2 \times (\text{stool } [Na^+] + \text{stool } [K^+]) \leq \text{stool osmolality}$$

The cation concentrations are doubled to estimate stool anion concentrations. The presence of a significant osmotic gap suggests the presence in stool water of a substance (or substances) other than Na/K/anions that is presumably responsible for the patient's diarrhea. Originally, stool osmolality was measured, but it is almost invariably greater than the required 290–300 mosmol/kg H$_2$O, reflecting bacterial degradation of nonabsorbed carbohydrate either immediately before defecation or in the stool jar while awaiting chemical analysis, even when the stool is refrigerated. As a result, the stool osmolality should be assumed to be 300 mosmol/kg H$_2$O. A low stool osmolality (<290 mosmol/kg H$_2$O) reflects the addition of either dilute urine or water indicating either collection of urine and stool together or so-called factitious diarrhea, a form of Munchausen's syndrome. When the calculated difference is >50, an osmotic gap is present, suggesting that the diarrhea is due to a nonabsorbed dietary nutrient, e.g., a fatty acid and/or carbohydrate. When this difference is <25, it is presumed that a dietary nutrient is not responsible for the diarrhea. Since elements of both osmotic (i.e., malabsorption of a dietary nutrient) and secretory diarrhea may be present, this separation at times is less clearcut at the bedside than when used as a teaching example. Ideally, the presence of an osmotic gap will be associated with a marked decrease in stool output during a prolonged fast, while the absence of an osmotic gap will likely be present in an individual whose stool output had not been reduced substantially during a period of fasting.

NUTRIENT DIGESTION AND ABSORPTION

The lengths of the small intestine and colon are ~300 cm and ~80 cm, respectively. However, the effective functional surface area is approximately 600-fold greater than that of a hollow tube as a result of the presence of folds, villi (in the small intestine), and microvilli. The functional surface area of the small intestine is somewhat greater than that of a doubles tennis court. In addition to nutrient digestion and absorption, the intestinal epithelia have several other functions:

1. *Barrier and immune defense.* The intestine is exposed to a large number of potential antigens and enteric and invasive microorganisms, and it is extremely effective preventing the entry of almost all these agents. The intestinal mucosa also synthesizes and secretes secretory IgA.
2. *Fluid and electrolyte absorption and secretion.* The intestine absorbs ~7–8 L of fluid daily, comprising dietary fluid intake (1–2 L/d) and salivary, gastric, pancreatic, biliary, and intestinal fluid (6–7 L/d). Several stimuli, especially bacteria and bacterial enterotoxins, induce fluid and electrolyte secretion that may lead to diarrhea (Chap. 122).
3. *Synthesis and secretion of several proteins.* The intestinal mucosa is a major site for the production of proteins, including apolipoproteins.
4. *Production of several bioactive amines and peptides.* The intestine is one of the largest endocrine organs in the body and produces several amines and peptides that serve as paracrine and hormonal mediators of intestinal function.

The small and large intestines are distinct anatomically (villi are present in the small intestine but are absent in the colon) and func-

tionally (nutrient digestion and absorption take place in the small intestine but not in the colon). No precise anatomic characteristics separate duodenum, jejunum, and ileum, although certain nutrients are absorbed exclusively in specific areas of the small intestine. However, villous cells in the small intestine (and surface epithelial cells in the colon) and crypt cells have distinct anatomic and functional characteristics. Intestinal epithelial cells are continuously renewed, with new proliferating epithelial cells at the base of the crypt migrating over 48–72 h to the tip of the villus (or surface of the colon), where they are well-developed epithelial cells with digestive and absorptive function. This high rate of cell turnover explains the relatively rapid resolution of diarrhea and other digestive tract side effects during chemotherapy as new cells not exposed to these toxic agents are produced. Equally important is the paradigm of separation of villous/surface cell and crypt cell function: digestive hydrolytic enzymes are present primarily in the brush border of villous epithelial cells. Absorptive and secretory functions are also separated, with villous/surface cells primarily, but not exclusively, being the site for absorptive function, while secretory function is present in crypts of both the small and large intestine.

Nutrients, minerals, and vitamins are absorbed by one or more active transport mechanisms. Active transport mechanisms are energy-dependent and mediated by membrane transport proteins. These processes will result in the *net* movement of a substance against or in the absence of an electrochemical concentration gradient. Intestinal absorption of amino acids and monosaccharides, e.g., glucose, is also a specialized form of active transport—*secondary active transport*. The movement of these actively transported nutrients against a concentration gradient is Na$^+$-dependent and is due to a Na$^+$ gradient across the apical membrane. The Na$^+$ gradient is maintained by Na$^+$,K$^+$-ATPase, the so-called Na$^+$ pump located on the basolateral membrane, which extrudes Na$^+$ and maintains low intracellular [Na] as well as the Na$^+$ gradient across the apical membrane. As a result, active glucose absorption and glucose-stimulated Na$^+$ absorption require both the apical membrane transport protein, SGLT1, and the basolateral Na$^+$,K$^+$-ATPase. In addition to glucose absorption being Na$^+$-dependent, glucose also stimulates Na$^+$ and fluid absorption, which is the physiologic basis of oral rehydration therapy for the treatment of diarrhea (Chap. 40). The mechanisms of intestinal fluid and electrolyte absorption and secretion are discussed in Chap. 40.

Although the intestinal epithelial cells are crucial mediators of absorption and ion and water flow, the several cell types in the lamina propria (e.g., mast cells, macrophages, myofibroblasts) and the enteric nervous system interact with the epithelium to regulate mucosal cell function. The function of the intestine is the result of the integrated responses of and interactions between both intestinal epithelial cells and intestinal muscle.

ENTEROHEPATIC CIRCULATION OF BILE ACIDS

Bile acids are not present in the diet but are synthesized in the liver by a series of enzymatic steps that also include cholesterol catabolism. Indeed, interruption of the enterohepatic circulation of bile acids can reduce serum cholesterol levels by 10% before a new steady state is established. Bile acids are either primary or secondary: primary bile acids are synthesized in the liver from cholesterol, and secondary bile acids are synthesized from primary bile acids in the intestine by colonic bacterial enzymes. The two primary bile acids in humans are cholic acid and chenodeoxycholic acid; the two most abundant secondary bile acids are deoxycholic acid and lithocholic acid. Approximately 500-mg bile acids are synthesized in the liver daily, conjugated to either taurine or glycine to form tauro-conjugated or glyco-conjugated bile acids, respectively, and are secreted into the duodenum in bile. The primary functions of bile acids are (1) to promote bile flow, (2) to solubilize cholesterol and phospholipid in the gallbladder by mixed micelle formation, and (3) to enhance dietary lipid digestion and absorption by forming mixed micelles in the proximal small intestine.

Bile acids are primarily absorbed by an active, Na$^+$-dependent process that is located exclusively in the ileum, though bile acids can also be absorbed to a lesser extent by non-carrier-mediated transport processes in the jejunum, ileum, and colon. Conjugated bile acids that en-

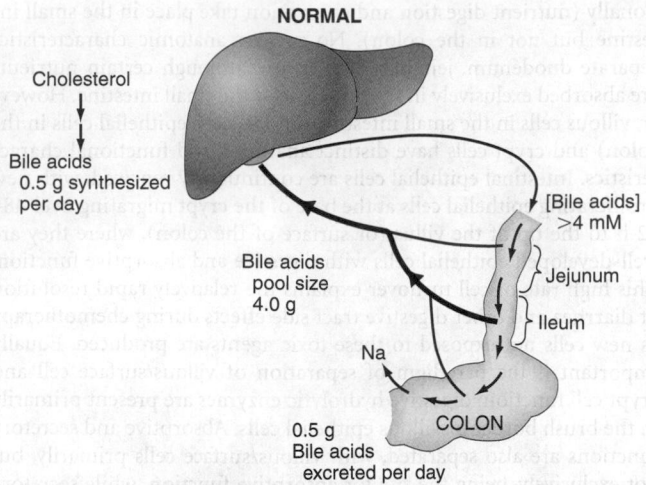

NORMAL

Cholesterol

Bile acids
0.5 g synthesized
per day

[Bile acids]
>4 mM

Bile acids
pool size
4.0 g

Jejunum

Ileum

Na

COLON

0.5 g
Bile acids
excreted per day

FIGURE 288-1 Schematic representation of the enterohepatic circulation of bile acids. Bile acid synthesis is cholesterol catabolism and occurs in the liver. Bile acids are secreted in bile and are stored in the gallbladder between meals and at night. Food in the duodenum induces the release of cholecystokinin, a potent stimulus for gallbladder contraction resulting in bile acid entry into the duodenum. Bile acids are primarily absorbed via a Na-dependent transport process that is located only in the ileum. A relatively small quantity of bile acids (~500 mg) is not absorbed in a 24-h period and is lost in stool. Fecal bile acid losses are matched by bile acid synthesis. The bile acid pool (the total amount of bile acids in the body) is ~4 g and is circulated twice during each meal or six to eight times in a 24-h period.

ter the colon are deconjugated by colonic bacterial enzymes to unconjugated bile acids and are rapidly absorbed. Colonic bacterial enzymes also dehydroxylate bile acids to secondary bile acids.

Bile acids absorbed from the intestine return to the liver via the portal vein where they are resecreted (Fig. 288-1). Bile acid synthesis is largely autoregulated by 7α-hydroxylase, the initial enzyme in cholesterol degradation. A decrease in the amount of bile acids returning to the liver from the intestine is associated with an increase in bile acid synthesis/cholesterol catabolism, which helps keep the bile acid pool size relatively constant. However, the capacity to increase bile acid synthesis is limited to about two to two and a half-fold (see below). The bile acid pool size is approximately 4 g and is circulated via the enterohepatic circulation about twice during each meal, or six to eight times during a 24-h period. A relatively small quantity of bile acids is not absorbed and is excreted in stool daily; this fecal loss is matched by hepatic bile acid synthesis.

Defects in any of the steps of the enterohepatic circulation of bile acids can result in a decrease in duodenal concentration of conjugated bile acids and, as a result, steatorrhea. Thus, steatorrhea can be caused by abnormalities in bile acid synthesis and excretion, their physical state in the intestinal lumen, and reabsorption (Table 288-1).

Synthesis Decreased bile acid synthesis and steatorrhea have been demonstrated in chronic liver disease, but steatorrhea is often not a major component of the illness of these patients.

Secretion Although bile acid secretion may be reduced or absent in biliary obstruction, steatorrhea is rarely a significant medical problem

in these patients. In contrast, primary biliary cirrhosis represents a defect in canalicular excretion of organic anions, including bile acids, and not infrequently is associated with steatorrhea and its consequences, e.g., chronic bone disease. Thus, the osteomalacia and other chronic bone abnormalities often present in patients with primary biliary cirrhosis and other cholestatic syndromes are secondary to steatorrhea that then leads to calcium and vitamin D malabsorption.

Maintenance of Conjugated Bile Acids In bacterial overgrowth syndromes associated with diarrhea, steatorrhea, and macrocytic anemia, a colonic type of bacterial flora is increased in the small intestine. The steatorrhea is primarily a result of the decrease in conjugated bile acids secondary to their deconjugation by colonic-type bacteria. Two complementary explanations account for the resulting impairment of micelle formation: (1) unconjugated bile acids are rapidly absorbed in the jejunum by nonionic diffusion, resulting in a reduced concentration of duodenal bile acids; and (2) the critical micellar concentration (CMC) of unconjugated bile acids is higher than that of conjugated bile acids, and therefore unconjugated bile acids are less effective than conjugated bile acids in micelle formation.

Reabsorption Ileal dysfunction caused by either Crohn's disease or surgical resection results in a decrease in bile acid reabsorption in the ileum and an *increase* in the delivery of bile acids to the large intestine. The resulting clinical consequences—diarrhea with or without steatorrhea—are determined by the *degree* of ileal dysfunction and the *response* of the enterohepatic circulation to bile acid losses (Table 288-2). Patients with limited ileal disease or resection will often have diarrhea but not steatorrhea. The diarrhea, a result of bile acids in the colon stimulating active Cl secretion, has been called *bile acid diarrhea*, or cholorrheic enteropathy, and responds promptly to cholestyramine, an anion-binding resin. Such patients do not develop steatorrhea because hepatic synthesis of bile acids increases to compensate for the rate of fecal bile acid losses, resulting in maintenance of both the bile acid pool size and the intraduodenal concentrations of bile acids. In contrast, patients with greater degrees of ileal disease and/or resection will often have diarrhea and steatorrhea that do not respond to cholestyramine. In this situation, ileal disease is also associated with increased amounts of bile acids entering the colon; however, hepatic synthesis can no longer increase sufficiently to maintain the bile acid pool size. As a consequence, the intraduodenal concentration of bile acids is also reduced to less than the CMC, resulting in impaired micelle formation and steatorrhea. This second situation is often called *fatty acid diarrhea*. Cholestyramine may not be effective (and may even increase the diarrhea by further depleting the intraduodenal bile acid concentration); however, a low-fat diet to reduce fatty acids entering the colon can be effective. Two clinical features, the length of ileum removed and the degree of steatorrhea, can predict whether an individual patient will respond to cholestyramine. Unfortunately, these predictors are imperfect, and a therapeutic trial of cholestyramine is often necessary to establish whether an individual patient will benefit from cholestyramine. Table 288-2 contrasts the characteristics of bile acid diarrhea (small ileal dysfunction) and fatty acid diarrhea (large ileal dysfunction).

TABLE 288-1 DEFECTS IN ENTEROHEPATIC CIRCULATION OF BILE ACIDS

Process	Pathophysiologic Defect	Disease Example
Synthesis	Decreased hepatic function	Cirrhosis
Biliary secretion	Altered canalicular function	Primary biliary cirrhosis
Maintenance of conjugated bile acids	Bacterial overgrowth	Jejunal diverticulosis
Reabsorption	Abnormal ileal function	Crohn's disease

TABLE 288-2 COMPARISON OF BILE ACID AND FATTY ACID DIARRHEA

	Bile Acid Diarrhea	Fatty Acid Diarrhea
Extent of ileal disease	Limited	Extensive
Ileal bile acid absorption	Reduced	Reduced
Fecal bile acid excretion	Increased	Increased
Fecal bile acid loss compensated by hepatic synthesis	Yes	No
Bile acid pool size	Normal	Reduced
Intraduodenal [bile acid]	Normal	Reduced
Steatorrhea	None or mild	>20 g
Response to cholestyramine	Yes	No
Response to low-fat diet	No	Yes

TABLE 288-3	COMPARISON OF DIFFERENT TYPES OF FATTY ACIDS		
	Long-Chain	Medium-Chain	Short-Chain
Carbon chain length	>12	8–12	<8
Present in diet	In large amounts	In small amounts	No
Origin	In diet as triglycerides	Only in small amounts in diet as triglycerides	Bacterial degradation in colon of nonabsorbed carbohydrate to fatty acids
Primary site of absorption	Small intestine	Small intestine	Colon
Requires pancreatic lipolysis	Yes	No	No
Requires micelle formation	Yes	No	No
Presence in stool	Minimal	No	Substantial

TABLE 288-4	DEFECTS IN LIPID DIGESTION AND ABSORPTION IN STEATORRHEA		
Phase: Process	Pathophysiologic Defect	Disease Example
---	---	---
Digestive		
Lipolysis formation	Decrease lipase secretion	Chronic pancreatitis
Micelle formation	Decreased intraduodenal bile acids	See Table 288-1
Absorptive		
Mucosal uptake and resterification	Mucosal dysfunction	Celiac sprue
Post-absorptive		
Chylomicron formation	Absent betalipoproteins	Abetalipoproteinemia
Delivery from intestine	Abnormal lymphatics	Intestinal lymphangiectasia

LIPIDS

Steatorrhea is caused by one or more defects in the digestion and absorption of dietary fat. Average intake of dietary fat in the United States is approximately 120–150 g/d, and fat absorption is linear to dietary fat intake. The total load of fat presented to the small intestine is considerably greater, as substantial amounts of lipid are secreted in bile each day. (See above for discussion of enterohepatic circulation of bile acids.) Three types of fatty acids compose fats: long-chain fatty acids (LCFAs), medium-chain fatty acids (MCFAs), and short-chain fatty acids (SCFAs) (Table 288-3). Dietary fat is exclusively composed of long-chain triglycerides (LCTs), i.e., glycerol that is bound via ester-linkages to three LCFAs. While the majority of dietary LCFAs have carbon chain lengths of 16 or 18, fatty acids of carbon chain length >12 are metabolized in the same manner; saturated and unsaturated fatty acids are handled identically.

Assimilation of dietary lipid requires three integrated processes: (1) an intraluminal, or digestive, phase; (2) a mucosal, or absorptive, phase; and (3) a delivery, or postabsorptive, phase. An abnormality at any site of this process can cause steatorrhea (Table 288-4). Therefore it is essential that any patient with steatorrhea be evaluated to identify the specific physiologic defect in overall lipid digestion-absorption, as therapy will be determined by the specific cause of the steatorrhea.

The digestive phase has two components, *lipolysis* and *micellar formation*. Although dietary lipid is in the form of LCTs, the intestinal mucosa does not absorb triglycerides; they must first be hydrolyzed (Fig. 288-2). The initial step in lipid digestion is the formation of emulsions of finely dispersed lipid, which is accomplished by mastication and gastric contractions. Lipolysis, the hydrolysis of triglycerides to free fatty acids, monoglycerides, and glycerol by lipase, is initiated in the stomach by a gastric lipase that has a pH optimum of 4.5–6.0. About 20–30% of total lipolysis occurs in the stomach. Lipolysis is completed in the duodenum and jejunum by pancreatic lipase, which is inactivated by a pH < 7.0. Pancreatic lipolysis is greatly enhanced by the presence of a second pancreatic enzyme, colipase, which facilitates the movement of lipase to the triglyceride.

Impaired lipolysis can lead to steatorrhea and can occur in the presence of pancreatic insufficiency due to chronic pancreatitis in adults or cystic fibrosis in children and adolescents. Normal lipolysis can be maintained by approximately 5% of maximal pancreatic lipase secretion; thus, steatorrhea is a late manifestation of these disorders. A reduction in intraduodenal pH can also result in altered lipolysis as pancreatic lipase is inactivated at pH <7. Thus, ~15% of patients with gastrinoma (Chap. 287)

with substantial increases in gastric acid secretion from ectopic production of gastrin (usually from an islet cell adenoma) have diarrhea, and some will have steatorrhea believed secondary to acid-inactivation of pancreatic lipase. Similarly, patients with chronic pancreatitis (who have reduced lipase secretion) often have a decrease in pancreatic bicarbonate secretion, which will also result in a decrease in intraduodenal pH and inactivation of endogenous pancreatic lipase or of therapeutically administered lipase.

Overlying the microvillus membrane of the small intestine is the so-called unstirred water layer, a relatively stagnant aqueous phase that must be traversed by the products of lipolysis that are primarily water-insoluble. Water-soluble mixed micelles provide a mechanism for the water-insoluble products of lipolysis to reach the luminal plasma membrane of villous epithelial cells, the site for lipid absorption. Mixed micelles are molecular aggregates composed of fatty acids, monoglycerides, phospholipids, cholesterol, and conjugated bile acids. Mixed micelles are formed when the concentration of conjugated bile acids is greater than its CMC, which differs among the several bile acids present in the small intestinal lumen. Conjugated bile acids, synthesized in the liver and excreted into the duodenum in bile, are regulated by the enterohepatic circulation (see above). Steatorrhea can result from impaired movement of fatty acids across the unstirred aqueous fluid layer in two situations: (1) an increase in the relative thickness of the unstirred water layer that occurs in bacterial overgrowth syndromes (see below) secondary to functional stasis (e.g., scleroderma); and (2) a decrease in the *duodenal* concentration of conjugated bile acids below its CMC, resulting in impaired micelle formation. Thus, steatorrhea can be caused by one or more defects in the enterohepatic circulation of bile acids.

Pancreas	Liver	Jejunal Mucosa	Lymphatics
Lipolysis	Micellar Solubilization with Bile Acid	Absorption	Delivery

FIGURE 288-2 Schematic representation of lipid digestion and absorption. Dietary lipid is in the form of long-chain triglycerides (LCTs). The overall process can be divided into (1) a digestive phase that includes both lipolysis and micelle formation requiring pancreatic lipase and conjugated bile acids, respectively, in the duodenum; (2) an absorptive phase for mucosal uptake and reesterification; and (3) a postabsorptive phase that includes chylomicron formation and exit from the intestinal epithelial cell via lymphatics. (*Courtesy of John M. Dietschy, MD; with permission.*)

Uptake and reesterification constitute the *absorptive phase* of lipid digestion-absorption. Although passive diffusion has been thought responsible, a carrier-mediated process may mediate fatty acid and monoglyceride uptake. Regardless of the uptake process, fatty acids and monoglycerides are reesterified by a series of enzymatic steps in the endoplasmic reticulum and Golgi to form triglycerides, the form in which lipid exits from the intestinal epithelial cell. Impaired lipid absorption as a result of either mucosal inflammation (e.g., celiac sprue) and/or intestinal resection can also lead to steatorrhea.

The reesterified triglycerides require the formation of *chylomicrons* to permit their exit from the small-intestinal epithelial cell and their delivery to the liver via the *lymphatics*. Chylomicrons are composed of β-lipoprotein and contain triglycerides, cholesterol, cholesterol esters, and phospholipids and enter the lymphatics, not the portal vein. Defects in the *postabsorptive phase* of lipid digestion-absorption can also result in steatorrhea, but these disorders are uncommon. Abetalipoproteinemia, or acanthocytosis, is a rare disorder of impaired synthesis of β-lipoprotein associated with abnormal erythrocytes (acanthocytes), neurologic problems, and steatorrhea. Lipolysis, micelle formation, and lipid uptake are all normal in patients with abetalipoproteinemia, but the reesterified triglyceride cannot exit from the epithelial cell because of the failure to produce chylomicrons. Small-intestinal biopsies of these rare patients in the postprandial state reveal lipid-laden small-intestinal epithelial cells that become perfectly normal in appearance following a 72–96 h fast. Similarly, abnormalities of intestinal lymphatics (e.g., intestinal lymphangiectasia) may also be associated with steatorrhea as well as protein loss (see below). Steatorrhea can result from defects at any of the several steps in lipid digestion-absorption.

The mechanism of lipid digestion-absorption outlined above is limited to *dietary* lipid that is almost exclusively in the form of LCTs (Table 288-3). Medium-chain triglycerides (MCTs), composed of fatty acids with carbon chain lengths of 8–10, are present in large amounts in coconut oil and are used as a nutritional supplement. MCTs can be digested and absorbed by a different pathway from LCTs and at one time held promise as an important treatment of steatorrhea of almost all etiologies. Unfortunately, their therapeutic effects have been less than expected because their use is often not associated with an increase in body weight for reasons that are not completely understood.

MCTs, in contrast to LCTs, do not require pancreatic lipolysis as the triglyceride can be absorbed intact by the intestinal epithelial cell. Further, micelle formation is not necessary for the absorption of MCTs or medium-chain fatty acids, if hydrolyzed by pancreatic lipase. MCTs are absorbed more efficiently than LCTs for the following reasons: (1) the rate of MCT absorption is greater than that of long-chain fatty acids; (2) medium-chain fatty acids following absorption are not reesterified; (3) following absorption, MCTs are hydrolyzed to medium-chain fatty acids; (4) MCTs do not require chylomicron formation for their exit from the intestinal epithelial cells; and (5) their route of exit is via the portal vein and not via lymphatics. Thus, the absorption of MCTs is greater than that of LCTs in pancreatic insufficiency, conditions with reduced intraduodenal bile acid concentrations, small-intestinal mucosal disease, abetalipoproteinemia, and intestinal lymphangiectasia.

SCFAs are not dietary lipids but are synthesized by colonic bacterial enzymes from nonabsorbed carbohydrate and are the anions in highest concentration in stool (between 80 and 130 m*M*). The SCFAs present in stool are primarily acetate, propionate, and butyrate, whose carbon chain lengths are 2, 3, and 4, respectively. Butyrate is the primary nutrient for colonic epithelial cells, and its deficiency may be associated with one or more colitides. SCFAs conserve calories and carbohydrate, because carbohydrates not completely absorbed in the small intestine will not be absorbed in the large intestine due to the absence of both disaccharidases and SGLT1, the transport protein that mediates monosaccharide absorption. In contrast, SCFAs are rapidly absorbed and stimulate colonic Na-Cl and fluid absorption. Most non–*Clostridium difficile* antibiotic-associated diarrhea is due to antibiotic suppression of colonic microflora, with a resulting decrease in SCFA production. As *C. difficile* accounts for about 10–15% of all antibiotic-associated diarrhea, a relative decrease in colonic production of SCFAs is likely the cause of most antibiotic-associated diarrhea.

The clinical manifestations of steatorrhea are a consequence of both the underlying disorder responsible for the development of steatorrhea and steatorrhea per se. Depending on the degree of steatorrhea and the level of dietary intake, significant fat malabsorption may lead to weight loss. Steatorrhea per se can be responsible for diarrhea; if the primary cause of the steatorrhea has not been identified, a low-fat diet can often ameliorate the diarrhea by decreasing fecal fat excretion. Steatorrhea is often associated with fat-soluble vitamin deficiency, which will require replacement with water-soluble preparations of these vitamins.

Disorders of absorption may also be associated with malabsorption of other dietary nutrients, most often carbohydrates, with or without a decrease in dietary lipid digestion and absorption. Therefore, knowledge of the mechanism of the digestion and absorption of carbohydrates, proteins, and other minerals and vitamins is useful in the evaluation of patients with altered intestinal nutrient absorption.

CARBOHYDRATES

Carbohydrates in the diet are present in the form of starch, disaccharides (sucrose and lactose), and glucose. Carbohydrates are absorbed only in the small intestine and only in the form of monosaccharides. Therefore, before their absorption, starch and disaccharides must first be digested by pancreatic amylase and intestinal brush border disaccharidases to monosaccharides. Monosaccharide absorption occurs by a Na-dependent process mediated by the brush border transport protein SGLT1.

Lactose malabsorption is the only clinically important disorder of carbohydrate absorption. Lactose, the disaccharide present in milk, requires digestion by brush border lactase to its two constituent monosaccharides, glucose and galactose. Lactase is present in almost all species in the postnatal period but then disappears throughout the animal kingdom, except in humans. Lactase activity persists in many individuals throughout life. Two different types of lactase deficiency exist—primary and secondary. In *primary lactase deficiency*, a genetically determined decrease or absence of lactase is noted, while all other aspects of both intestinal absorption and brush border enzymes are normal. In a number of non-Caucasian groups, primary lactase deficiency is common in adulthood. Table 288-5 presents the incidence of primary lactase deficiency in several ethnic groups. Northern European and North American Caucasians are the only groups to maintain small-intestinal lactase activity throughout adult life. The persistence of lactase is the abnormality due to a defect in the regulation of its maturation. In contrast, *secondary lactase deficiency* occurs in association with small-intestinal mucosal disease with abnormalities in both structure and function of other brush border enzymes and transport processes. Secondary lactase deficiency is often seen in celiac sprue.

As lactose digestion is rate-limiting compared to glucose/galactose absorption, lactase deficiency is associated with significant lactose malabsorption. Some individuals with lactose malabsorption develop symptoms such as diarrhea, abdominal pain, cramps, and/or flatus. Most individuals with primary lactase deficiency do not have symptoms. Since lactose intolerance may be associated with symptoms sug-

TABLE 288-5	PRIMARY LACTASE DEFICIENCY IN DIFFERENT ADULT ETHNIC GROUPS
Ethnic Group	**Prevalence of Lactase Deficiency, %**
Northern European	5–15
Mediterranean	60–85
African black	85–100
American black	45–80
American Caucasian	10–25
Native American	50–95
Mexican American	40–75
Asian	90–100

Source: From FJ Simons: Am J Dig Dis 23:963, 1978.

gestive of irritable bowel syndrome, persistence of such symptoms in an individual with lactose intolerance while on a strict lactose-free diet would suggest that the individual's symptoms were related to irritable bowel syndrome.

Development of symptoms of lactose intolerance is related to several factors:

1. *Amount of lactose in the diet.*
2. *Rate of gastric emptying.* Symptoms are more likely when gastric emptying is rapid than when gastric emptying is slower. Therefore it is more likely that skim milk will be associated with symptoms of lactose intolerance than will whole milk, as the rate of gastric emptying following skim milk intake is more rapid. Similarly, the diarrhea observed following subtotal gastrectomy is often a result of lactose intolerance, as gastric emptying is accelerated in patients with a gastrojejunostomy.
3. *Small-intestinal transit time.* Although the small and large intestine contribute to the development of symptoms, many of the symptoms of lactase deficiency are related to the interaction of colonic bacteria and nonabsorbed lactose. More rapid small-intestinal transit makes symptoms more likely.
4. *Colonic compensation by production of SCFAs from nonabsorbed lactose.* Reduced levels of colonic microflora, which can occur following antibiotic use, will also be associated with increased symptoms following lactose ingestion, especially in a lactase-deficient individual.

Glucose-galactose or monosaccharide malabsorption may also be associated with diarrhea and is due to a congenital absence of SGLT1. Diarrhea is present when individuals with this disorder ingest carbohydrates that contain actively transported monosaccharides (e.g., glucose, galactose) but not monosaccharides that are not actively transported (e.g., fructose). Fructose is absorbed by the brush border transport protein GLUT 5, a facilitated diffusion process that is not Na-dependent and is distinct from SGLT1. In contrast, some individuals develop diarrhea as a result of consuming large quantities of sorbitol, a sugar used in diabetic candy; sorbitol is only minimally absorbed due to the absence of an intestinal absorptive transport mechanism for sorbitol.

PROTEINS

Protein is present in food almost exclusively as polypeptides and requires extensive hydrolysis to di- and tripeptides and amino acids before absorption. Proteolysis occurs in both the stomach and small intestine; it is mediated by pepsin secreted as pepsinogen by gastric chief cells and trypsinogen and other peptidases from pancreatic acinar cells. These proenzymes, pepsinogen and trypsinogen, must be activated to pepsin (by pepsin in the presence of a pH <5) and trypsin (by the intestinal brush border enzyme enterokinase and subsequently by trypsin). Proteins are absorbed by separate transport systems for di- and tripeptides and for different types of amino acids, e.g., neutral and dibasic. Alterations in either protein or amino acid digestion and absorption are rarely observed clinically, even in the presence of extensive small-intestinal mucosal inflammation. However, three rare genetic disorders involve protein digestion-absorption: (1) *Enterokinase deficiency* is due to an absence of the brush border enzyme that converts the proenzyme trypsinogen to trypsin and is associated with diarrhea, growth retardation, and hypoproteinemia. (2) *Hartnup syndrome*, a defect in neutral amino acid transport, is characterized by a pellagra-like rash and neuropsychiatric symptoms. (3) *Cystinuria*, a defect in dibasic amino acid transport, is associated with renal calculi and chronic pancreatitis.

APPROACH TO THE PATIENT:
Malabsorption

The clues provided by the history, symptoms, and initial preliminary observations will serve to limit extensive, ill-focused, and expensive laboratory and imaging studies. For example, a clinician evaluating a patient with symptoms suggestive of malabsorption who recently had extensive small-intestinal resection for mesenter-

ic ischemia should direct the initial assessment almost exclusively to define whether a short bowel syndrome might explain the entire clinical picture. Similarly, the development of a pattern of bowel movements suggestive of steatorrhea in a patient with long-standing alcohol abuse and chronic pancreatitis should lead toward assessing pancreatic exocrine function.

The classic picture of malabsorption is rarely seen today in most parts of the United States. As a consequence, diseases with malabsorption must be suspected in individuals with less severe symptoms and signs and with subtle evidence of the altered absorption of only a *single* nutrient rather than obvious evidence of the malabsorption of multiple nutrients.

Although diarrhea can be caused by changes in fluid and electrolyte movement in either the small or the large intestine, dietary nutrients are absorbed almost exclusively in the small intestine. Therefore the demonstration of diminished absorption of a dietary nutrient provides unequivocal evidence of small-intestinal disease, although colonic dysfunction may also be present (e.g., Crohn's disease may involve both small and large intestine). Dietary nutrient absorption may be segmental or diffuse along the small intestine and is site-specific. Thus, for example, calcium, iron, and folic acid are exclusively absorbed by active transport processes in the proximal small intestine, especially the duodenum; in contrast, the active transport mechanisms for both cobalamin and bile acids are present only in the ileum. Therefore, in an individual who years previously had had an intestinal resection, the details of which are not presently available, a presentation with evidence of calcium, folic acid, and iron malabsorption but without cobalamin deficiency would make it likely that the duodenum and jejunum, but not ileum, had been resected.

Some nutrients, e.g., glucose, amino acids, and lipids, are absorbed throughout the small intestine, though their rate of absorption is greater in the proximal than in the distal segments. However, following segmental resection of the small intestine, the remaining segments undergo both morphologic and functional "adaptation" to enhance absorption. Such adaptation is secondary to the presence of luminal nutrients and hormonal stimuli and may not be complete in humans for several months following the resection. Adaptation is critical for survival in individuals who have undergone massive resection of the small intestine and/or colon.

Establishing the presence of steatorrhea and identifying its specific cause are often quite difficult. The "gold standard" still remains a timed, quantitative stool fat determination. On a practical basis, stool collections are invariably difficult and often incomplete, as nobody wants to handle stool. A qualitative test—Sudan III stain—has long been available to establish the presence of an increase in stool fat. This test is rapid and inexpensive but, as a qualitative test, does not establish the degree of fat malabsorption and is best used as a preliminary screening study. Many of the blood, breath, and isotopic tests that have been developed (1) do not directly measure fat absorption; (2) have excellent sensitivity when steatorrhea is obvious and severe but have poor sensitivity when steatorrhea is mild (e.g., stool chymotrypsin, elastase, that can potentially distinguish pancreatic from nonpancreatic etiologies of steatorrhea); or (3) have not survived the transition from the research laboratory to commercial application.

Despite this situation, the use of routine laboratory studies (i.e., complete blood count, prothrombin time, serum protein determination, alkaline phosphatase) may suggest the presence of dietary nutrient depletion, especially iron, folate, cobalamin, and vitamins D and K. Additional studies include measurement of serum carotene, cholesterol, albumin, iron, folate, and cobalamin levels. The serum carotene level can also be reduced if the patient has poor dietary intake of leafy vegetables.

If steatorrhea and/or altered absorption of other nutrients are suspected, the history, clinical observations, and laboratory testing can help detect deficiency of a nutrient, especially the fat-soluble vitamins A, D, E, or K. Thus, evidence of metabolic bone disease with elevated alkaline phosphatase and/or reduced serum calcium levels would suggest vitamin D malabsorption. A deficiency of vitamin K would be suggested by an elevated prothrombin time in an individual without liver disease who was not taking anticoagulants. Macrocytic anemia would lead to evaluation of whether cobalamin or folic acid malabsorption was present. The presence of iron-deficiency anemia in the absence of occult bleeding from the gastrointestinal tract in either a male or a nonmenstruating female would require evaluation of iron malabsorption and the exclusion of celiac sprue, as iron is absorbed exclusively in the proximal small intestine.

At times, however, a timed (72 h) quantitative stool collection, preferably on a defined diet, must be obtained to determine stool fat content and establish the presence of steatorrhea. The presence of steatorrhea then requires further assessment to establish the pathophysiologic process(es) responsible for the defect in dietary lipid digestion-absorption (Table 288-4). Some of the other studies include the Schilling test, D-xylose test, duodenal mucosal biopsy, small-intestinal radiologic examination, and tests of pancreatic exocrine function.

THE SCHILLING TEST This test is performed to determine the cause for cobalamin malabsorption. Since cobalamin absorption requires multiple steps, including gastric, pancreatic, and ileal processes, the Schilling test can also be used to assess the integrity of these other organs (Chap. 100). Cobalamin is present primarily in meat. Except in strict vegans, *dietary* cobalamin deficiency is exceedingly uncommon. Dietary cobalamin is bound in the stomach to a glycoprotein called *R-binder protein*, which is synthesized in both the stomach and salivary glands. This cobalamin–R binder complex is formed in the acid milieu of the stomach. Cobalamin absorption has an absolute requirement for intrinsic factor, another glycoprotein synthesized and released by gastric parietal cells, to promote its uptake by specific cobalamin receptors on the brush border of ileal enterocytes. Pancreatic protease enzymes split the cobalamin–R binder complex to release cobalamin in the proximal small intestine, where cobalamin is then bound by intrinsic factor.

As a consequence, cobalamin absorption may be abnormal in the following:

1. *Pernicious anemia*, a disease in which immunologically mediated atrophy of gastric parietal cells leads to an absence of both gastric acid and intrinsic factor secretion.
2. *Chronic pancreatitis* as a result of deficiency of pancreatic proteases to split the cobalamin–R binder complex. Although 50% of patients with chronic pancreatitis have been reported to have an abnormal Schilling test that was corrected by pancreatic enzyme replacement, the presence of a cobalamin-responsive macrocytic anemia in chronic pancreatitis is extremely rare. Although this probably reflects a difference in the digestion/absorption of cobalamin in food versus that in a crystalline form, the Schilling test can still be used to assess pancreatic exocrine function.
3. *Achlorhydria*, or absence of another factor secreted with acid that is responsible for splitting cobalamin away from the proteins in food to which it is bound. Up to one-third of individuals >60 years of age have marginal vitamin B_{12} absorption because of the inability to release cobalamin from food; these people have no defects in absorbing crystalline vitamin B_{12}.
4. *Bacterial overgrowth syndromes*, which are most often secondary to stasis in the small intestine, leading to bacterial utilization of cobalamin (often referred to as *stagnant bowel syndrome*; see below).
5. *Ileal dysfunction* (as a result of either inflammation or prior intestinal resection) due to impaired function of the mechanism of cobalamin–intrinsic factor uptake by ileal intestinal epithelial cells.

The Schilling test is performed by administering [58]Co-labeled cobalamin orally and collecting urine for 24 h, and it is dependent on normal renal and bladder function. Urinary excretion of cobalamin will reflect cobalamin absorption provided that intrahepatic

TABLE 288-6 DIFFERENTIAL RESULTS OF SCHILLING TEST IN SEVERAL DISEASES ASSOCIATED WITH COBALAMIN (CBL) MALABSORPTION

	[58]Co-Cbl	With Intrinsic Factor	With Pancreatic Enzymes	After 5 Days of Antibiotics
Pernicious anemia	Reduced	Normal	Reduced	Reduced
Chronic pancreatitis	Reduced	Reduced	Normal	Reduced
Bacterial overgrowth	Reduced	Reduced	Reduced	Normal
Ileal disease	Reduced	Reduced	Reduced	Reduced

binding sites for cobalamin are fully occupied. To ensure saturation of hepatic cobalamin binding sites so that all absorbed radiolabeled cobalamin will be excreted in urine, 1 mg cobalamin is administered intramuscularly 1 h following ingestion of the radiolabeled cobalamin. The Schilling test may be abnormal (usually defined as <10% excretion in 24 h) in pernicious anemia, chronic pancreatitis, blind loop syndrome, and ileal disease (Table 288-6). Therefore, whenever an abnormal Schilling test is found, [58]Co-labeled cobalamin should be administered on another occasion either bound to intrinsic factor, with pancreatic enzymes, or following a 5-day course of antibiotics (often tetracycline). A variation of the Schilling test can detect failure to split cobalamin from food proteins. The labeled cobalamin is cooked together with a scrambled egg and administered orally. People with achlorydria will excrete <10% of the labeled cobalamin in the urine. In addition to establishing the etiology for cobalamin deficiency, the Schilling test can be used to help delineate the pathologic process responsible for steatorrhea by assessing ileal, pancreatic, and small-intestinal luminal function. Unfortunately, the Schilling test is infrequently performed because of the unavailability of human intrinsic factor.

URINARY D-XYLOSE TEST The urinary D-xylose test for carbohydrate absorption provides an assessment of proximal small-intestinal mucosal function. D-Xylose, a pentose, is absorbed almost exclusively in the proximal small intestine. The D-xylose test is usually performed by giving 25 g D-xylose and collecting urine for 5 h. An abnormal test (<4.5 g excretion) primarily reflects the presence of duodenal/jejunal mucosal disease. The D-xylose test can also be abnormal in patients with blind loop syndrome (as a consequence primarily of abnormal intestinal mucosa) and, as a false-positive study, in patients with large collections of fluid in a third space (i.e., ascites, pleural fluid). The ease of obtaining a mucosal biopsy of the small intestine by endoscopy and the false-negative rate of the D-xylose test have led to its diminished use. When small-intestinal mucosal disease is suspected, a small-intestinal mucosal biopsy should be performed.

RADIOLOGIC EXAMINATION Radiologic examination of the small intestine using barium contrast (small-bowel series or study) can provide important information in the evaluation of the patient with presumed or suspected malabsorption. These studies are most often performed in conjunction with the examination of the esophagus, stomach, and duodenal bulb, and insufficient barium is given to the patient to permit an adequate examination of the small-intestinal mucosa, especially the ileum. As a result, many gastrointestinal radiologists alter the procedure of a barium contrast examination of the small intestine by performing either a small-bowel series in which a large amount of barium is given by mouth without concurrent examination of the esophagus and stomach or an enteroclysis study in which a large amount of barium is introduced into the duodenum via a fluoroscopically placed tube. In addition, many of the diagnostic features initially described by radiologists to denote the presence of small-intestinal disease (e.g., flocculation, segmentation) are rarely seen with current barium suspensions. Nonetheless, in skilled hands barium contrast examination of the small intestine can yield important information. For example, with extensive mucosal disease, dilation of intestine can be seen, as dilution of barium from increased intestinal fluid secretion (Fig. 288-3). A normal barium contrast study does *not* exclude the possibility of small-intestinal disease. However, a small-bowel series remains a useful examination to look for anatomical abnormalities, such as strictures and fistulas (as in Crohn's disease) or blind loop syndrome (e.g., multiple jejunal diverticula), and to define the extent of a previous surgical resection. Noninvasive capsule endoscopy and double-barrel enteroscopy are useful aids in the diagnostic assessment of small intestinal pathology.

BIOPSY OF SMALL-INTESTINAL MUCOSA A small-intestinal mucosal biopsy is essential in the evaluation of a patient with documented steatorrhea or chronic diarrhea (lasting >3 weeks) (Chap. 40). The ready availability of endoscopic equipment to examine the stomach and duodenum has led to its almost uniform use as the preferred method to obtain histologic material of proximal small-intestinal mucosa. The primary indications for a small-intestinal biopsy are (1) evaluation of a patient either with documented or suspected steatorrhea or with chronic diarrhea, and (2) diffuse or focal abnormalities of the small intestine defined on a small-intestinal series. Lesions seen on small-bowel biopsy can be classified into three different categories (Table 288-7):

1. *Diffuse, specific lesions.* Relatively few diseases associated with altered nutrient absorption have specific histopathologic abnormalities on small-intestinal mucosal biopsy, and they are uncommon. Whipple's disease is characterized by the presence of periodic acid-Schiff (PAS)–positive macrophages in the lamina propria, while the bacilli that are also present may require electron-microscopic examination for identification (Fig. 288-4). *Abetalipoproteinemia* is characterized by a normal mucosal appearance except for the presence of mucosal absorptive cells that contain lipid postprandially and disappear following a prolonged period of either fat-free intake or fasting. *Immune globulin deficiency* is associated with a variety of histopathologic findings on small-intestinal mucosal biopsy. The characteristic feature is the absence of or substantial reduction in the number of plasma cells in the lamina propria; the mucosal architecture may be either perfectly normal or flat (i.e., villous atrophy). As patients with immune globulin deficiency are often infected with *Giardia lamblia*, *Giardia* trophozoites may also be seen in the biopsy.
2. *Patchy, specific lesions.* Several diseases show abnormal small-intestinal mucosa with a patchy distribution. As a result, biopsies obtained randomly or in the absence of abnormalities visualized endoscopically may not reveal the diagnostic features. Intestinal *lymphoma* can at times be diagnosed on mucosal biopsy by the identification of malignant lymphoma cells in the lamina propria and submucosa (Chap. 105). The presence of dilated lymphat-

ics in the submucosa and sometimes in the lamina propria indicates the presence of *lymphangiectasia* associated with hypoproteinemia secondary to protein loss into the intestine. *Eosinophilic gastroenteritis* comprises a heterogeneous group of disorders with a spectrum of presentations and symptoms with an eosinophilic infiltrate of the lamina propria, with or without peripheral eosinophilia. The patchy nature of the infiltrate as well as its presence in the submucosa often leads to an absence of histopathologic findings on mucosal biopsy. As the involvement of the duodenum in *Crohn's disease* is also submucosal and not necessarily continuous, mucosal biopsies are not the most direct approach to the diagnosis of duodenal Crohn's disease (Chap. 289). Amyloid deposition can be identified by Congo Red stain in some patients with *amyloidosis* involving the duodenum (Chap. 324).

3. Several microorganisms can be identified on small-intestinal biopsies, establishing a correct diagnosis. Many of these microorganisms are associated with diarrhea that occurs in immunodeficient individuals, especially those with HIV infection, and include *Cryptosporidium*, *Isospora belli*, cytomegalovirus, *Mycobacterium avium-intracellulare*, and *G. lamblia*.
4. *Diffuse, nonspecific lesions.* Celiac sprue presents with a characteristic mucosal appearance on duodenal/proximal jejunal mucosal biopsy that is not diagnostic of the disease. The diagnosis of celiac sprue is established by clinical, histologic, and immu-

A. **B.** **C.** **D.**

FIGURE 288-3 Barium contrast small-intestinal radiologic examinations. A. Normal individual. **B.** Celiac sprue. **C.** Jejunal diverticulosis. **D.** Crohn's disease. *(Courtesy of Morton Burrell, MD, Yale University; with permission.)*

TABLE 288-7 **DISEASE THAT CAN BE DIAGNOSED BY SMALL-INTESTINAL MUCOSAL BIOPSIES**

Lesions	Pathologic Findings
Diffuse, specific	
Whipple's disease	Lamina propria contains macrophages containing PAS+ material
Agammaglobulinemia	No plasma cells; either normal or absent villi ("flat mucosa")
Abetalipoproteinemia	Normal villi; epithelial cells vacuolated with fat postprandially
Patchy, specific	
Intestinal lymphoma	Malignant cells in lamina propria and submucosa
Intestinal lymphangiectasia	Dilated lymphatics; clubbed villi
Eosinophilic gastroenteritis	Eosinophil infiltration of lamina propria and mucosa
Amyloidosis	Amyloid deposits
Crohn's disease	Noncaseating granulomas
Infection by one or more microorganisms (see text)	Specific organisms
Mastocytosis	Mast cell infiltration of lamina propria
Diffuse, nonspecific	
Celiac sprue	Short or absent villi; mononuclear infiltrate; epithelial cell damage; hypertrophy of crypts
Tropical sprue	Similar to celiac sprue
Bacterial overgrowth	Patchy damage to villi; lymphocyte infiltration
Folate deficiency	Short villi; decreased mitosis in crypts; megalocytosis
Vitamin B_{12} deficiency	Similar to folate deficiency
Radiation enteritis	Similar to folate deficiency
Zollinger-Ellison syndrome	Mucosal ulceration and erosion from acid
Protein-calorie malnutrition	Villous atrophy; secondary bacterial overgrowth
Drug-induced enteritis	Variable histology

Note: PAS+, periodic acid–Schiff positive.

nologic response to a gluten-free diet. *Tropical sprue* is associated with histologic findings similar to those of celiac sprue after a tropical or subtropical exposure but does not respond to gluten restriction; most often symptoms improve with antibiotics and folate administration.

Patients with steatorrhea require assessment of *pancreatic exocrine function*, which is often abnormal in chronic pancreatitis. The secretin test that collects pancreatic secretions by duodenal intubation following intravenous administration of secretin is the only test that directly measures pancreatic exocrine function and is available at few specialized centers. Endoscopic approaches provide excellent assessment of pancreatic duct anatomy but do *not* assess exocrine function (Chap. 306).

Table 288-8 summarizes the results of the D-xylose test, Schilling test, and small-intestinal mucosal biopsy in patients with five different causes of steatorrhea.

SPECIFIC DISEASE ENTITIES

CELIAC SPRUE

Celiac sprue is a common cause of malabsorption of one or more nutrients in Caucasians, especially those of European descent. Estimated incidence in the United States may be as high as 1:113 people. Celiac sprue has had several other names, including nontropical sprue, celiac disease (in children), adult celiac disease, and gluten-sensitive enteropathy. The etiology of celiac sprue is not known, but environmental, immunologic, and genetic factors are important. Celiac sprue has protean manifestations, almost all of which are secondary to nutrient malabsorption, and a varied natural history, with the onset of symptoms occurring at ages ranging from the first year of life through the eighth decade.

The hallmark of celiac sprue is the presence of an abnormal small-intestinal biopsy (Fig. 288-4) and the response of the condition—malabsorption and the histologic changes on the small-intestinal biopsy—to the elimination of gluten from the diet. The histologic changes have a proximal-to-distal intestinal distribution of severity, which probably reflects the exposure of the intestinal mucosa to varied amounts of dietary gluten; the symptoms correlate with histologic changes.

The symptoms of celiac sprue may appear with the introduction of cereals in an infant's diet, although spontaneous remissions often occur during the second decade of life that may be either permanent or followed by the reappearance of symptoms over several years. Alternatively, the symptoms of celiac sprue may first become evident at almost any age throughout adulthood. In many patients, frequent spontaneous remissions and exacerbations occur. The symptoms range from significant malabsorption of multiple nutrients, with diarrhea, steatorrhea, weight loss, and the consequences of nutrient depletion (i.e., anemia and metabolic bone disease), to the absence of any gastrointestinal symptoms but with evidence of the depletion of a single nutrient (e.g., iron or folate deficiency, osteomalacia, edema from protein loss). Asymptomatic relatives of patients with celiac sprue have been identified as having this disease either by small-intestinal biopsy or by serologic studies [e.g., antiendomysial antibodies, tissue transglutaminase (tTG)]. The availability of these "celiac serologies" has led to a substantial increase in the diagnosis of celiac sprue and the diagnosis is now being made primarily in patients without "classic" symptoms but with atypical and subclinical presentations.

Etiology The etiology of celiac sprue is not known, but environmental, immunologic, and genetic factors all appear to contribute to the disease. One *environmental* factor is the clear association of the disease with gliadin, a component of gluten that is present in wheat, barley, and rye. In addition to the role of gluten restriction in treatment, the instillation of gluten into both normal-appearing rectum and distal ileum of patients with celiac sprue results in morphologic changes within hours.

An *immunologic* component to etiology is suspected. Serum antibodies—IgA antigliadin, IgA antiendomysial, and IgA anti-tTG antibodies—are present, but it is not known whether such antibodies are primary or secondary to the tissue damage. The antiendomysial antibody has 90–95% sensitivity and 90–95% specificity; the antigen recognized by the antiendomysial antibody is tTG. Antibody studies are frequently used to identify patients with celiac sprue; patients with these antibodies should undergo duodenal biopsy. This autoantibody has not been linked to a pathogenetic mechanism (or mechanisms) responsible for celiac sprue. Nonetheless, this antibody is useful in establishing the true prevalence of celiac sprue in the general population. A 4-week treatment with prednisolone of a patient with celiac sprue who continues to eat gluten will induce a remission and convert the "flat" abnormal duodenal biopsy to a more normal-appearing one. In addition, gliadin peptides may interact with gliadin-specific T cells that may either mediate tissue injury or induce the release of one or more cytokines that cause tissue injury.

Genetic factor(s) also appear to be involved in celiac sprue. The incidence of celiac sprue varies widely in different population groups (high in Caucasians, low in blacks and Asians) and is 10% in first-degree relatives of celiac sprue patients. Furthermore, almost all patients with celiac sprue express the HLA-DQ2 allele, though only a minority of people expressing DQ2 have celiac sprue. Absence of DQ2 excludes the diagnosis of celiac sprue.

Diagnosis A small-intestinal biopsy is required to establish a diagnosis of celiac sprue (Fig. 288-4). A biopsy should be performed in patients with symptoms and laboratory findings suggestive of nutrient malabsorption and/or deficiency and with a positive tTG serology. Since the presentation of celiac sprue is often subtle, without overt evidence of malabsorption or nutrient deficiency, it is important to have a relatively low threshold to perform a biopsy. It is more prudent to

FIGURE 288-4 Small-intestinal mucosal biopsies. A. Normal individual. **B.** Untreated celiac sprue. **C.** Treated celiac sprue. **D.** Intestinal lymphangiectasia. **E.** Whipple's disease. **F.** Lymphoma. **G.** Giardiasis. *(Courtesy of Marie Robert, MD, Yale University; with permission.)*

clinical and histologic response following the institution of a gluten-free diet. If serologic studies have detected the presence of IgA anti-endomysial or tTG antibodies, they too should disappear after a gluten-free diet is started. The changes seen on duodenal/jejunal biopsy are restricted to the mucosa and include (1) absence or reduced height of villi, resulting in a flat appearance; (2) increased loss of villous cells in association with increased crypt cell proliferation, resulting in crypt hyperplasia and loss of villous structure, with consequent villous, but not mucosal, atrophy; (3) cuboidal appearance and nuclei that are no longer oriented basally in surface epithelial cells and increased intraepithelial lymphocytes; and (4) increased lymphocytes and plasma cells in the lamina propria (Fig. 288-4*B*). Although these features are characteristic of celiac sprue, they are *not* diagnostic because a similar appearance can be seen in tropical sprue, eosinophilic enteritis, and milk-protein intolerance in children and occasionally in lymphoma, bacterial overgrowth, Crohn's disease, and gastrinoma with acid hypersecretion. However, the presence of a characteristic histologic appearance that reverts toward normal following the initiation of a gluten-free diet establishes the diagnosis of celiac sprue (Fig. 288-4*C*). Readministration of gluten with or without an additional small-intestinal biopsy is not necessary.

Failure to Respond to Gluten Restriction

The most common cause of persistent symptoms in a patient who fulfills all the criteria for diagnosing celiac sprue is continued intake of gluten. Gluten is ubiquitous, and significant effort must be made to exclude all gluten from the diet. Use of rice in place of wheat flour is very helpful, and several support groups provide important aid to patients with celiac sprue and to their families. More than 90% of patients who have the characteristic findings of celiac sprue will respond to complete dietary gluten restriction. The remainder constitute a heterogeneous group (whose condition is often called *refractory sprue*) that includes some patients who (1) respond to restriction of other dietary protein, e.g., soy; (2) respond to glucocorticoids; (3) are "temporary" (i.e., the clinical and morphologic findings disappear after several months or years); or (4) fail to respond to all measures and have a fatal outcome, with or without documented complications of celiac sprue, such as development of intestinal T cell lymphoma.

Mechanism of Diarrhea The diarrhea in celiac sprue has several pathogenetic mechanisms. Diarrhea may be secondary to (1) steatorrhea, which is primarily a result of the changes in jejunal mucosal function; (2) secondary lactase deficiency, a consequence of changes in jejunal brush border enzymatic function; (3) bile acid malabsorption resulting in bile acid–induced fluid secretion in the colon, in cases with more extensive disease involving the ileum; and (4) endogenous fluid secretion resulting from crypt hyperplasia. Patients with more severe involvement with celiac sprue may obtain temporary improvement with *dietary lactose and fat restriction* while awaiting the full effects of total gluten restriction, which is primary therapy.

Associated Diseases Celiac sprue is associated with dermatitis herpetiformis (DH), though the association has not been explained. Pa-

perform a biopsy than to obtain another test of intestinal absorption, which can never completely exclude or establish this diagnosis.

The diagnosis of celiac sprue requires the presence of characteristic histologic changes on small-intestinal biopsy together with a prompt

TABLE 288-8 RESULTS OF DIAGNOSTIC STUDIES IN DIFFERENT CAUSES OF STEATORRHEA

	D-Xylose Test	Schilling Test	Duodenal Mucosal Biopsy
Chronic pancreatitis	Normal	50% abnormal; if abnormal, normal with pancreatic enzymes	Normal
Bacterial overgrowth syndrome	Normal or only modestly abnormal	Often abnormal; if abnormal, normal after antibiotics	Usually normal
Ileal disease	Normal	Abnormal	Normal
Celiac sprue	Decreased	Normal	Abnormal: probably "flat"
Intestinal lymphangiectasia	Normal	Normal	Abnormal: "dilated lymphatics"

tients with DH have characteristic papulovesicular lesions that respond to dapsone. Almost all patients with DH have histologic changes in the small intestine consistent with celiac sprue, although usually much milder and less diffuse in distribution. Most patients with DH have mild or no gastrointestinal symptoms. In contrast, relatively few patients with celiac sprue have DH.

Celiac sprue is also associated with diabetes mellitus type 1 and IgA deficiency. The clinical importance of the former association is that although severe watery diarrhea without evidence of malabsorption is most often seen in patients with "diabetic diarrhea" (Chap. 338), assay of antiendomysial antibodies and/or a small-intestinal biopsy must at times be considered to exclude this association.

Complications   The most important complication of celiac sprue is the development of cancer. An increased incidence of both gastrointestinal and nongastrointestinal neoplasms as well as intestinal lymphoma exists in patients with celiac sprue. For unexplained reasons the occurrence of lymphoma in patients with celiac sprue is higher in Ireland and the United Kingdom than in the United States. The possibility of lymphoma must be considered whenever a patient with celiac sprue previously doing well on a gluten-free diet is no longer responsive to gluten restriction or a patient who presents with clinical and histologic features consistent with celiac sprue does not respond to a gluten-free diet. Other complications of celiac sprue include the development of intestinal ulceration independent of lymphoma and so-called refractory sprue (see above) and collagenous sprue. In *collagenous sprue*, a layer of collagen-like material is present beneath the basement membrane; patients with collagenous sprue generally do not respond to a gluten-free diet and often have a poor prognosis.

TROPICAL SPRUE

Tropical sprue is a poorly understood syndrome that affects both expatriates and natives in certain but not all tropical areas and is manifested by chronic diarrhea, steatorrhea, weight loss, and nutritional deficiencies, including those of both folate and cobalamin. This disease affects 5–10% of the population in some tropical areas.

Chronic diarrhea in a tropical environment is most often caused by infectious agents including *G. lamblia*, *Yersinia enterocolitica*, *C. difficile*, *Cryptosporidium parvum*, and *Cyclospora cayetanensis*, among other organisms. Tropical sprue should not be entertained as a possible diagnosis until the presence of cysts and trophozoites has been excluded in three stool samples. Chronic infections of the gastrointestinal tract and diarrhea in patients with or without AIDS are discussed in Chaps. 122 and 182.

The small-intestinal mucosa in individuals living in tropical areas is not identical to that of individuals who reside in temperate climates. Biopsies reveal a mild alteration of villous architecture with a modest increase in mononuclear cells in the lamina propria, which on occasion can be as severe as that seen in celiac sprue. These changes are observed both in native residents and in expatriates living in tropical regions and are usually associated with mild decreases in absorptive function, but they revert to "normal" when an individual moves or returns to a temperate area. Some have suggested that the changes seen in tropical enteropathy and in tropical sprue represent different ends of the spectrum of a single entity, but convincing evidence to support this concept is lacking.

Etiology   Because tropical sprue responds to antibiotics, the consensus is that it may be caused by one or more infectious agents. Nonetheless, the etiology and pathogenesis of tropical sprue are uncertain. First, its occurrence is not evenly distributed in all tropical areas; rather, it is found in specific locations, including southern India, the Philippines, and several Caribbean islands (e.g., Puerto Rico, Haiti), but is rarely observed in Africa, Jamaica, or Southeast Asia. Second, an occasional individual will not develop symptoms of tropical sprue until long after having left an endemic area. This is the reason why the original term for celiac sprue was *nontropical sprue* to distinguish it from tropical sprue. Third, multiple microorganisms have been identified

on jejunal aspirate with relatively little consistency among studies. *Klebsiella pneumoniae*, *Enterobacter cloacae*, or *E. coli* have been implicated in some studies of tropical sprue, while other studies have favored a role for a toxin produced by one or more of these bacteria. Fourth, the incidence of tropical sprue appears to have decreased substantially during the past two decades. One speculation for the reduced occurrence is the wider use of antibiotics in acute diarrhea, especially in travelers to tropical areas from temperate countries. Fifth, the role of folic acid deficiency in the pathogenesis of tropical sprue requires clarification. Folic acid is absorbed exclusively in the duodenum and proximal jejunum, and most patients with tropical sprue have evidence of folate malabsorption and depletion. Although folate deficiency can cause changes in small-intestinal mucosa that are corrected by folate replacement, several earlier studies reporting that tropical sprue could be cured by folic acid did not provide an explanation for the "insult" that was initially responsible for folate malabsorption.

The clinical pattern of tropical sprue varies in different areas of the world (e.g., India vs Puerto Rico). Not infrequently, individuals in South India initially will report the occurrence of an acute enteritis before the development of steatorrhea and malabsorption. In contrast, in Puerto Rico a most insidious onset of symptoms and a more dramatic response to antibiotics is seen when compared to some other locations. Tropical sprue in different areas of the world may not be the same disease, and similar clinical entities may have different etiologies.

Diagnosis   The diagnosis of tropical sprue is best made by the presence of an abnormal small-intestinal mucosal biopsy in an individual with chronic diarrhea and evidence of malabsorption who is either residing or has recently lived in a tropical country. The small-intestinal biopsy in tropical sprue does not have pathognomonic features but resembles, and can often be indistinguishable from, that seen in celiac sprue (Fig. 288-4). The biopsy in tropical sprue will have less villous architectural alteration and more mononuclear cell infiltrate in the lamina propria. In contrast to celiac sprue, the histologic features of tropical sprue are present with a similar degree of severity throughout the small intestine, and a gluten-free diet does not result in either clinical or histologic improvement in tropical sprue.

℞ TROPICAL SPRUE

Broad-spectrum antibiotics and folic acid are most often curative, especially if the patient leaves the tropical area and does not return. Tetracycline should be used for up to 6 months and may be associated with improvement within 1–2 weeks. Folic acid alone will induce a hematologic remission as well as improvement in appetite, weight gain, and some morphologic changes in small intestinal biopsy. Because of the presence of marked folate deficiency, folic acid is most often given together with antibiotics.

SHORT BOWEL SYNDROME

This is a descriptive term for the myriad clinical problems that occur following resection of varying lengths of small intestine. The factors that determine both the type and degree of symptoms include (1) the specific segment (jejunum vs ileum) resected, (2) the length of the resected segment, (3) the integrity of the ileocecal valve, (4) whether any large intestine has also been removed, (5) residual disease in the remaining small and/or large intestine (e.g., Crohn's disease, mesenteric artery disease), and (6) the degree of adaptation in the remaining intestine. Short bowel syndrome can occur at any age from neonates through the elderly.

Three different situations in adults demand intestinal resections: (1) mesenteric vascular disease, including atherosclerosis, thrombotic phenomena, and vasculitides; (2) primary mucosal and submucosal disease, e.g., Crohn's disease; and (3) operations without preexisting small intestinal disease, such as trauma and jejunoileal bypass for obesity.

Following resection of the small intestine, the residual intestine undergoes adaptation of both structure and function that may last for up to 6–12 months. Continued intake of dietary nutrients and calories is required to stimulate adaptation via direct contact with intestinal mucosa, the release of one or more intestinal hormones, and pancreatic and biliary secretions. Thus, enteral nutrition and calorie administration must be maintained, especially in the early postoperative period, even if an extensive intestinal resection requiring total parenteral nutrition (TPN) had been performed. The subsequent ability of such patients to absorb nutrients will not be known for several months, until adaptation is completed.

Multiple factors besides the absence of intestinal mucosa (required for lipid, fluid, and electrolyte absorption) contribute to the diarrhea and steatorrhea in these patients. Removal of the ileum and especially the ileocecal valve is often associated with more severe diarrhea than jejunal resection. Without part or all of the ileum, diarrhea can be caused by an increase in bile acids entering the colon, leading to their stimulation of colonic fluid and electrolyte secretion. Absence of the ileocecal valve is also associated with a decrease in intestinal transit time and bacterial overgrowth from the colon. Lactose intolerance as a result of the removal of lactase-containing mucosa as well as gastric hypersecretion will also contribute to the diarrhea.

In addition to diarrhea and/or steatorrhea, a range of nonintestinal symptoms is also observed in some patients. A significant increase in renal calcium oxalate calculi is observed in patients with a small-intestinal resection with an intact colon and is due to an increase in oxalate absorption by the large intestine, with subsequent hyperoxaluria (called *enteric hyperoxaluria*). Two possible mechanisms for the increase in oxalate absorption in the colon have been suggested: (1) bile acids and fatty acids that increase colonic mucosal permeability, resulting in increased oxalate absorption; and (2) increased fatty acids that bind calcium, resulting in increased soluble oxalate that is then absorbed. Since oxalate is high in relatively few foods (e.g., spinach, rhubarb, tea), dietary restrictions alone are not adequate treatment. Cholestyramine, an anion-binding resin, and calcium have proved useful in reducing the hyperoxaluria. Similarly, an increase in cholesterol gallstones is related to a decrease in the bile acid pool size, which results in the generation of cholesterol supersaturation in gallbladder bile. Gastric hypersecretion of acid occurs in many patients following large resections of the small intestine. The etiology is unclear but may be related to either reduced hormonal inhibition of acid secretion or increased gastrin levels due to reduced small-intestinal catabolism of circulating gastrin. The resulting gastric acid secretion may be an important factor contributing to the diarrhea and steatorrhea. A reduced pH in the duodenum can inactivate pancreatic lipase and/or precipitate duodenal bile acids, thereby increasing steatorrhea, and an increase in gastric secretion can create a volume overload relative to the reduced small-intestinal absorptive capacity. Inhibition of gastric acid secretion with proton pump inhibitors can help in reducing the diarrhea and steatorrhea.

℞ SHORT BOWEL SYNDROME

Treatment of short bowel syndrome depends on the severity of symptoms and whether the individual is able to maintain caloric and electrolyte balance with oral intake alone. Initial treatment includes judicious use of opiates (including codeine) to reduce stool output and to establish an effective diet. An initial diet should be low-fat and high-carbohydrate to minimize the diarrhea from fatty acid stimulation of colonic fluid secretion. MCTs (see above), a low-lactose diet, and various fiber-containing diets should also be tried. In the absence of an ileocecal valve, the possibility of bacterial overgrowth must be considered and treated. If gastric acid hypersecretion is contributing to the diarrhea and steatorrhea, a proton pump inhibitor may be helpful. Usually none of these therapeutic approaches will provide an instant solution, but they can reduce disabling diarrhea.

The patient's vitamin and mineral status must also be monitored; replacement therapy should be initiated if indicated. Fat-soluble vitamins, folate, cobalamin, calcium, iron, magnesium, and zinc are the most critical factors to monitor on a regular basis. If these approaches are not successful, home TPN is an established therapy that can be maintained for many years. Intestinal transplantation is becoming established as a possible approach for individuals with extensive intestinal resection who cannot be maintained without TPN, which is often called "intestinal failure." Considerable attention has been

directed to the potential effectiveness of trophic hormones, e.g. glucagon-like peptide 2 (GLP-2) to improve absorptive function, and small-intestinal transplantation is also available in selected patients.

BACTERIAL OVERGROWTH SYNDROME

Bacterial overgrowth syndrome comprises a group of disorders with diarrhea, steatorrhea, and macrocytic anemia whose common feature is the proliferation of colonic-type bacteria within the small intestine. This bacterial proliferation is due to stasis caused by impaired peristalsis (*functional stasis*), changes in intestinal anatomy (*anatomic stasis*), or direct communication between the small and large intestine. These conditions have also been referred to as *stagnant bowel syndrome* or *blind loop syndrome*.

Pathogenesis The manifestations of bacterial overgrowth syndromes are a direct consequence of the presence of increased amounts of a colonic-type bacterial flora, such as *E. coli* or *Bacteroides*, in the small intestine. *Macrocytic anemia* is due to cobalamin, not folate, deficiency. Most bacteria require cobalamin for growth, and increasing concentrations of bacteria use up the relatively small amounts of dietary cobalamin. *Steatorrhea* is due to impaired micelle formation as a consequence of a reduced intraduodenal concentration of conjugated bile acids and the presence of unconjugated bile acids. Certain bacteria, e.g., *Bacteroides*, deconjugate conjugated bile acids to unconjugated bile acids. Unconjugated bile acids will be absorbed more rapidly than conjugated bile acids, and, as a result, the intraduodenal concentration of bile acids will be reduced. In addition, the CMC of unconjugated bile acids is higher than that of conjugated bile acids, resulting in a decrease in micelle formation. *Diarrhea* is due, at least in part, to the steatorrhea, when it is present. However, some patients manifest diarrhea *without* steatorrhea, and it is assumed that the colonic-type bacteria in these patients are producing one or more bacterial enterotoxins that are responsible for fluid secretion and diarrhea.

Etiology The etiology of these different disorders is bacterial proliferation in the small intestinal lumen secondary to either anatomical or functional stasis or to a communication between the relatively sterile small intestine and the colon with its high levels of aerobic and anaerobic bacteria. Several examples of *anatomical* stasis have been identified: (1) one or more diverticula (both duodenal and jejunal) (Fig. 288-3*C*); (2) fistulas and strictures related to Crohn's disease (Fig. 288-3*D*); (3) a proximal duodenal afferent loop following a subtotal gastrectomy and gastrojejunostomy; (4) a bypass of the intestine, e.g., jejunoileal bypass for obesity; and (5) dilation at the site of a previous intestinal anastomosis. These anatomical derangements are often associated with the presence of a segment (or segments) of intestine out of continuity of propagated peristalsis, resulting in stasis and bacterial proliferation. Bacterial overgrowth syndromes can also occur in the *absence* of an anatomical blind loop when *functional* stasis is present. Impaired peristalsis and bacterial overgrowth in the absence of a blind loop occur in scleroderma, where motility abnormalities exist in both the esophagus and small intestine (Chap. 316). Functional stasis and bacterial overgrowth can also occur in association with diabetes mellitus and in the small intestine when a direct connection exists between the small and large intestine, including an ileocolonic resection, or occasionally following an enterocolic anastomosis that permits entry of bacteria into the small intestine as a result of bypassing the ileocecal valve.

Diagnosis The diagnosis may be suspected from the combination of a low serum cobalamin level and an elevated serum folate level, as enteric bacteria frequently produce folate compounds that will be absorbed in the duodenum. Ideally, the diagnosis of the bacterial overgrowth syndrome is the demonstration of increased levels of aerobic and/or anaerobic colonic-type bacteria in a jejunal aspirate obtained by intubation. This specialized test is rarely available, and bacterial overgrowth is best established by a Schilling test (Table 288-6), which should be abnormal following the administration of ^{58}Co-labeled cobalamin, with or without the administration of intrinsic factor. Following the administration of tetracycline for 5 days, the Schilling test will become normal, confirming the diagnosis of bacterial overgrowth. Breath hydrogen testing or lactulose (nondigestible disaccharide) administration has also been used to detect bacterial overgrowth.

℞ BACTERIAL OVERGROWTH SYNDROME

Primary treatment should be directed, if at all possible, to the surgical correction of an anatomical blind loop. In the absence of functional stasis, it is important to define the anatomical relationships responsible for stasis and bacterial overgrowth. For example, bacterial overgrowth secondary to strictures, one or more diverticula, or a proximal afferent loop can potentially be cured by surgical correction of the anatomical state. In contrast, the functional stasis of scleroderma or certain anatomical stasis states (e.g., multiple jejunal diverticula), cannot be corrected surgically, and these conditions should be treated with broad-spectrum antibiotics. Tetracycline used to be the initial treatment of choice; due to increasing resistance, however, other antibiotics such as metronidazole, amoxicillin/clavulanic acid, and cephalosporins have been employed. The antibiotic should be given for approximately 3 weeks or until symptoms remit. Although the natural history of these conditions is chronic, antibiotics should not be given continuously. Symptoms usually remit within 2–3 weeks of initial antibiotic therapy. Therapy need not be repeated until symptoms recur. In the presence of frequent recurrences, several treatment strategies exist, but the use of antibiotics for 1 week per month, whether or not symptoms are present, is often most effective.

Unfortunately, therapy for bacterial overgrowth syndrome is largely empirical, with an absence of clinical trials on which to base decisions regarding the antibiotic choice, the duration of treatment, and/or the best approach for treating recurrences. Bacterial overgrowth may also occur as a component of another chronic disease, e.g., Crohn's disease, radiation enteritis, or short bowel syndrome. Treatment of the bacterial overgrowth in these settings will not cure the underlying problem but may be very important in ameliorating a subset of clinical problems that are related to bacterial overgrowth.

WHIPPLE'S DISEASE

Whipple's disease is a chronic multisystem disease associated with diarrhea, steatorrhea, weight loss, arthralgia, and central nervous system (CNS) and cardiac problems; it is caused by the bacteria *Tropheryma whipplei*. Until the identification of *T. whipplei* by polymerase chain reaction, the hallmark of Whipple's disease had been the presence of PAS-positive macrophages in the small intestine (Fig. 288-4E) and other organs with evidence of disease.

Etiology Whipple's disease is caused by a small gram-positive bacillus, *T. whipplei*. The bacillus, an actinobacterium, has low virulence but high infectivity, and relatively minimal symptoms are observed compared to the extent of the bacilli in multiple tissues.

Clinical Presentation The onset of Whipple's disease is insidious and is characterized by diarrhea, steatorrhea, abdominal pain, weight loss, migratory large-joint arthropathy, and fever as well as ophthalmologic and CNS symptoms. The development of dementia is a relatively late symptom and an extremely poor prognostic sign, especially in patients who relapse following the induction of a remission with antibiotics. For unexplained reasons, the disease occurs primarily in middle-aged Caucasian men. The steatorrhea in these patients is generally believed secondary to both small-intestinal mucosal injury and lymphatic obstruction secondary to the increased number of PAS-positive macrophages in the lamina propria of the small intestine.

Diagnosis The diagnosis of Whipple's disease is suggested by a multisystem disease in a patient with diarrhea and steatorrhea. Obtaining tissue biopsies from the small intestine and/or other organs that may be involved (e.g., liver, lymph nodes, heart, eyes, CNS, or synovial membranes), based on the patient's symptoms, is the primary approach to establish the diagnosis of Whipple's disease. The presence of

PAS-positive macrophages containing the characteristic small (0.25 × 1–2 mm) bacilli is suggestive of this diagnosis. However, Whipple's disease can be confused with the PAS-positive macrophages containing *M. avium* complex, which may be a cause of diarrhea in AIDS. The presence of the *T. whipplei* bacillus outside of macrophages is a more important indicator of active disease than is their presence within the macrophages. *T. whipplei* has now been successfully grown in culture.

℞ WHIPPLE'S DISEASE

The treatment for Whipple's disease is prolonged use of antibiotics. The current drug of choice is double-strength trimethoprim/sulfamethoxazole for approximately 1 year. PAS-positive macrophages can persist following successful treatment, and the presence of bacilli outside of macrophages is indicative of persistent infection or an early sign of recurrence. Recurrence of disease activity, especially with dementia, is an extremely poor prognostic sign and requires an antibiotic that crosses the blood-brain barrier. If trimethoprim/sulfamethoxazole is not tolerated, chloramphenicol is an appropriate second choice.

PROTEIN-LOSING ENTEROPATHY

Protein-losing enteropathy is not a specific disease but rather a group of gastrointestinal and nongastrointestinal disorders with hypoproteinemia and edema in the absence of either proteinuria or defects in protein synthesis, e.g., chronic liver disease. These diseases are characterized by excess protein loss into the gastrointestinal tract. Normally, about 10% of total protein catabolism occurs via the gastrointestinal tract. Evidence of increased protein loss into the gastrointestinal tract occurs in more than 65 different diseases, which can be classified into three groups: (1) mucosal ulceration, such that the protein loss primarily represents exudation across damaged mucosa, e.g., ulcerative colitis, gastrointestinal carcinomas, and peptic ulcer; (2) nonulcerated mucosa, but with evidence of mucosal damage so that the protein loss represents loss across epithelia with altered permeability, e.g., celiac sprue and Ménétrier's disease in the small intestine and stomach, respectively; and (3) lymphatic dysfunction, representing either primary lymphatic disease or secondary to partial lymphatic obstruction that may occur as a result of enlarged lymph nodes or cardiac disease.

Diagnosis The diagnosis of protein-losing enteropathy is suggested by the presence of peripheral edema and low serum albumin and globulin levels in the absence of renal and hepatic disease. It is extremely rare for an individual with protein-losing enteropathy to have selective loss of *only* albumin or *only* globulins. Therefore, marked reduction of serum albumin with normal serum globulins should not initiate an evaluation for protein-losing enteropathy but should suggest the presence of renal and/or hepatic disease. Likewise, reduced serum globulins with normal serum albumin levels are more likely a result of reduced globulin synthesis rather than enhanced globulin loss into the intestine. Documentation of an increase in protein loss into the gastrointestinal tract has been established by the administration of one of several radiolabeled proteins and its quantitation in stool during a 24- or 48-h period. Unfortunately, none of these radiolabeled proteins is available for routine clinical use. α_1-Antitrypsin, a protein that accounts for ~4% of total serum proteins and is resistant to proteolysis, can be used to document enhanced rates of serum protein loss into the intestinal tract but cannot be used to assess gastric protein loss due to its degradation in an acid milieu. α_1-Antitrypsin clearance is measured by determining stool volume and both stool and plasma α_1-antitrypsin concentrations. In addition to the loss of protein via abnormal and distended lymphatics, peripheral lymphocytes may also be lost via lymphatics, resulting in a relative lymphopenia. Thus, the presence of lymphopenia in a patient with hypoproteinemia supports the presence of increased loss of protein into the gastrointestinal tract.

Patients with increased protein loss into the gastrointestinal tract from lymphatic obstruction often have steatorrhea and diarrhea. The steatorrhea is a result of altered lymphatic flow as lipid-containing chylomicrons exit from intestinal epithelial cells via intestinal lymphatics

TABLE 288-9 CLASSIFICATION OF MALABSORPTION SYNDROMES

Inadequate digestion
  Postgastrectomy[a]
  Deficiency or inactivation of pancreatic lipase
    Exocrine pancreatic insufficiency
      Chronic pancreatitis
      Pancreatic carcinoma
      Cystic fibrosis
      Pancreatic insufficiency—congenital or acquired
    Gastrinoma—acid inactivation of lipase[a]
    Drugs—orlistat
Reduced intraduodenal bile acid concentration/impaired micelle formation
  Liver disease
    Parenchymal liver disease
    Cholestatic liver disease
  Bacterial overgrowth in small intestine:

Anatomic stasis	Functional stasis
Afferent loop stasis/	Diabetes[a]
blind loop/strictures/	Scleroderma[a]
fistulae	Intestinal pseudoobstruction

  Interrupted enterohepatic circulation of bile salts
    Ileal resection
    Crohn's disease[a]
  Drugs (bind or precipitate bile salts)—neomycin, cholestyramine, calcium carbonate
Impaired mucosal absorption/mucosal loss or defect
  Intestinal resection or bypass[a]
  Inflammation, infiltration, or infection:

Crohn's disease[a]	Celiac sprue
Amyloidosis	Collagenous sprue
Scleroderma[a]	Whipple's disease[a]
Lymphoma[a]	Radiation enteritis[a]
Eosinophilic enteritis	Folate and vitamin B$_{12}$ deficiency
Mastocytosis	Infections—giardiasis
Tropical sprue	Graft-vs.-host disease

  Genetic disorders
    Disaccharidase deficiency
    Agammaglobulinemia
    Abetalipoproteinemia
    Hartnup disease
    Cystinuria
Impaired nutrient delivery to and/or from intestine:

Lymphatic obstruction	Circulatory disorders
Lymphoma[a]	Congestive heart failure
Lymphangiectasia	Constrictive pericarditis
	Mesenteric artery atherosclerosis
	Vasculitis

Endocrine and metabolic disorders
  Diabetes[a]
  Hypoparathyroidism
  Adrenal insufficiency
  Hyperthyroidism
  Carcinoid syndrome

[a]Malabsorption caused by more than one mechanism.

TABLE 288-10 PATHOPHYSIOLOGY OF CLINICAL MANIFESTATIONS OF MALABSORPTION DISORDERS

Symptom or Sign	Mechanism
Weight loss/malnutrition	Anorexia, malabsorption of nutrients
Diarrhea	Impaired absorption or secretion of water and electrolytes; colonic fluid secretion secondary to unabsorbed dihydroxy bile acids and fatty acids
Flatus	Bacterial fermentation of unabsorbed carbohydrate
Glossitis, cheilosis, stomatitis	Deficiency of iron, vitamin B$_{12}$, folate, and vitamin A
Abdominal pain	Bowel distention or inflammation, pancreatitis
Bone pain	Calcium, vitamin D malabsorption, protein deficiency, osteoporosis
Tetany, paresthesia	Calcium and magnesium malabsorption
Weakness	Anemia, electrolyte depletion (particularly K$^+$)
Azotemia, hypotension	Fluid and electrolyte depletion
Amenorrhea, decreased libido	Protein depletion, decreased calories, secondary hypopituitarism
Anemia	Impaired absorption of iron, folate, vitamin B$_{12}$
Bleeding	Vitamin K malabsorption, hypoprothrombinemia
Night blindness/ xerophthalmia	Vitamin A malabsorption
Peripheral neuropathy	Vitamin B$_{12}$ and thiamine deficiency
Dermatitis	Deficiency of vitamin A, zinc, and essential fatty acid

and is characterized by large gastric folds, reduced gastric acid secretion, and, at times, enhanced protein loss into the stomach.

Rx PROTEIN-LOSING ENTEROPATHY

As excess protein loss into the gastrointestinal tract is most often secondary to a specific disease, treatment should be directed primarily to the underlying disease process and not to the hypoproteinemia. For example, if significant hypoproteinemia with resulting peripheral edema is secondary to either celiac sprue or ulcerative colitis, a gluten-free diet or mesalamine, respectively, would be the initial therapy. When enhanced protein loss is secondary to lymphatic obstruction, it is critical to establish the nature of this obstruction. Identification of mesenteric nodes or lymphoma may be possible by imaging studies. Similarly, it is important to exclude cardiac disease as a cause of protein-losing enteropathy either by echosonography or, on occasion, by a right-heart catheterization.

The increased protein loss that occurs in intestinal lymphangiectasia is a result of distended lymphatics associated with lipid malabsorption. Treatment of the hypoproteinemia is accomplished by a low-fat diet and the administration of MCTs (Table 288-3), which do not exit from the intestinal epithelial cells via lymphatics but are delivered to the body via the portal vein.

SUMMARY

A pathophysiologic classification of the many conditions that can produce malabsorption is given in Table 288-9. A summary of the pathophysiology of the various clinical manifestations of malabsorption is given in Table 288-10.

FURTHER READINGS

AMERICAN GASTROENTEROLOGICAL ASSOCIATION: AGA technical review on the evaluation and management of chronic diarrhea. Gastroenterology 116:1464, 1999

BUCHMAN AL: Etiology and initial management of short bowel syndrome. Gastroenterology 130:S5, 2006

COOK SI, SELLIN JH: Short chain fatty acids in health and disease. Aliment Pharmacol Ther 12:499, 1998

FENOLLER F et al: Whipple's disease. N Engl J Med 356:55, 2007

GREENBERGER NJ: Enzymatic therapy in patients with chronic pancreatitis. Gastroenterol Clin North Am 28:687, 1999

(Table 288-4; Fig. 288-4). In the absence of mechanical or anatomical lymphatic obstruction, intrinsic intestinal lymphatic dysfunction, with or without lymphatic dysfunction in the peripheral extremities, has been named *intestinal lymphangiectasia*. Similarly, about 50% of individuals with intrinsic peripheral lymphatic disease (Milroy disease) will also have intestinal lymphangiectasia and hypoproteinemia. Other than steatorrhea and enhanced protein loss into the gastrointestinal tract, all other aspects of intestinal absorptive function are normal in intestinal lymphangiectasia.

Other Causes Patients who appear to have idiopathic protein-losing enteropathy without any evidence of gastrointestinal disease should be examined for cardiac disease—especially right-sided valvular disease and chronic pericarditis (Chaps. 230 and 232). On occasion, hypoproteinemia can be the only presentation for these two types of heart disease. Ménétrier's disease (also called *hypertrophic gastropathy*) is an uncommon entity that involves the body and fundus of the stomach

JAMES S: Celiac disease: Proceedings of the NIH Consensus Conference on Celiac Disease. Gastroenterology 128:S1, 2005

HAREWOOD GC, MURRAY JA: Approaching the patient with chronic malabsorption syndrome. Semin Gastrointest Dis 10:138, 1999

KAGNOFF MF: Celiac disease: pathogenesis of a model immunogenetic disease. J Clin Invest 117:41, 2007

SHAW AD, DAVIES GJ: Lactose intolerance: Problems in diagnosis and treatment. J Clin Gastroenterol 28:208, 1999

289 Inflammatory Bowel Disease
Sonia Friedman, Richard S. Blumberg

Inflammatory bowel disease (IBD) is an immune-mediated chronic intestinal condition. Ulcerative colitis (UC) and Crohn's disease (CD) are the two major types of IBD.

EPIDEMIOLOGY

The incidence of IBD varies within different geographic areas. CD and UC both occur at the highest incidence in Europe, the United Kingdom, and North America. In North America, incidence rates range from 2.2 to 14.3 cases per 100,000 person-years for UC and from 3.1 to 14.6 cases per 100,000 person-years for CD (Table 289-1). Prevalence ranges from 37 to 246 cases per 100,000 person-years for UC and from 26 to 199 cases per 100,000 person-years for CD. In Europe, incidence ranges from 1.5 to 20.3 cases per 100,000 person-years for UC and from 0.7 to 9.8 cases per 100,000 person-years for CD; prevalence ranges from 21.4 to 243 cases for UC and from 8.3 to 214 cases per 100,000 person-years for CD. IBD has been rare in other areas except Israel, Australia, and South Africa. The incidence of IBD, especially UC, is rising in Japan, South Korea, Singapore, northern India, and Latin America, areas previously thought to have low incidence. The highest mortality is during the first years of disease and in long-duration disease due to the risk of colon cancer. In a Swedish population study, the standardized mortality ratios for CD and UC were 1.51 and 1.37, respectively.

The peak age of onset of UC and CD is between 15 and 30 years. A second peak occurs between the ages of 60 and 80. The male to female ratio for UC is 1:1 and for CD is 1.1–1.8:1. UC and CD have two- to fourfold increased frequency in Jewish populations in the United States, Europe, and South Africa. Furthermore, disease frequency differs within the Jewish populations. The prevalence of IBD in Ashkenazi Jews is about twice that of Israeli-born, Sephardic, or Oriental Jews. The prevalence decreases progressively in non-Jewish Caucasian, African-American, Hispanic, and Asian populations. Urban areas have a higher prevalence of IBD than rural areas, and high socioeconomic classes have a higher prevalence than lower socioeconomic classes.

The effects of cigarette smoking are different in UC and CD. The risk of UC in smokers is 40% that of nonsmokers. Additionally, former smokers have a 1.7-fold increased risk for UC than people who have never smoked. In contrast, smoking is associated with a twofold increased risk of CD. Oral contraceptives are also linked to CD; the odds ratio of CD for oral contraceptive users is about 1.4. Appendectomy is protective against UC but increases the risk of CD.

IBD runs in families. If a patient has IBD, the lifetime risk that a first-degree relative will be affected is ~10%. If two parents have IBD, each child has a 36% chance of being affected. In twin studies, 58% of monozygotic twins are concordant for CD and 6% are concordant for UC, whereas 4% of dizygotic twins are concordant for CD and none are concordant for UC. The risks of developing IBD are higher in first-degree relatives of Jewish versus non–Jewish patients: 7.8% versus 5.2% for CD and 4.5% versus 1.6% for UC. Anatomic site and clinical type of CD is also concordant within families.

Additional evidence for genetic predisposition to IBD comes from its association with certain genetic syndromes. UC and CD are both associated with Turner's syndrome, and Hermansky-Pudlak syndrome is associated with granulomatous colitis. Glycogen storage disease type 1b can present with Crohn's-like lesions of the large and small bowel. Other immunodeficiency disorders, such as hypogammaglobulinemia, selective IgA deficiency, and hereditary angioedema, also exhibit an increased association with IBD.

ETIOLOGY AND PATHOGENESIS

A consensus hypothesis is that in genetically predisposed individuals, both exogenous factors (e.g., normal luminal flora) and host factors (e.g., intestinal epithelial cell barrier function, innate and adaptive immune function) cause a chronic state of dysregulated mucosal immune function that is further modified by specific environmental factors (e.g., smoking). Although chronic activation of the mucosal immune system may represent an appropriate response to an unidentified infectious agent, a search for such an agent has thus far been unrewarding. As such, IBD is currently considered an inappropriate response to the endogenous microbial flora within the intestine, with or without some component of autoimmunity. Importantly, the normal intestine contains a large number of immune cells in a chronic state of so-called physiologic inflammation, in which the gut is poised for, but actively restrained from, full immunologic responses. During the course of infections in the normal host, full activation of the gut-associated lymphoid tissue occurs but is rapidly superseded by dampening the immune response and tissue repair. In IBD this process may not be regulated normally.

GENETIC CONSIDERATIONS IBD is a polygenic disorder that gives rise to multiple clinical subgroups within UC and CD. Genome-wide searches have shown disease-associated loci on many chromosomes (Table 289-2). Some loci are associated with both UC and CD, suggesting some overlap in pathogenesis. Specific gene associations are mostly undefined; however, several predisposing genes have been identified (Table 289-2). CARD15 (caspase-associated recruitment domain containing protein 15) on chromosome 16 is a cytosolic molecule that senses bacterial muramyl dipeptide and regulates intracellular signaling. CARD15 protein is expressed by intestinal epithelial cells, including Paneth cells, monocytes, macrophages, and dendritic cells. Loss-of-function mutations in CARD15 are highly associated with CD and may account for up to 10% of CD risk. CD-associated CARD15 alleles either allow excess NF-κB activation or decreased intestinal antimicrobial activity by diminishing defensin production by Paneth cells. Homozygosity for these mutant alleles confers up to a fortyfold increased risk for fibrostenosing CD, especially in the ileum.

IBD has also been associated with polymorphisms in DLG5 and the IL-23 receptor. These studies show the importance of both innate and adaptive immunity and the involvement of many different cell types, including the intestinal epithelium and lymphocytes, in IBD. Indeed, patients with IBD and their first-degree relatives may exhibit diminished intestinal epithelial cell barrier function.

TABLE 289-1	EPIDEMIOLOGY OF IBD	
	Ulcerative Colitis	**Crohn's Disease**
Incidence (North America) per person-years	2.2–14.3/100,000	3.1–14.6/100,000
Age of onset	15–30 & 60–80	15–30 & 60–80
Ethnicity	Jewish > Non-Jewish Caucasian > African American > Hispanic > Asian	
Male:female ratio	1:1	1.1–1.8:1
Smoking	May prevent disease	May cause disease
Oral contraceptives	No increased risk	Odds ratio 1.4
Appendectomy	Protective	Not protective
Monozygotic twins	6% concordance	58% concordance
Dizygotic twins	0% concordance	4% concordance

TABLE 289-2	REPLICATED GENETIC LOCI IN IBD		
IBD Locus[a]	**Chromosome**	**Gene**[b]	**Phenotype**
IBD1	16q	CARD15	CD
IBD2	12p	—	CD,UC
IBD3	6p	MHC?	CD
IBD4	14q	—	CD
IBD5	5q	OCTN?	CD
IBD6	19p	—	CD,UC
IBD7	1p	—	CD,UC
IBD8	16p	—	CD
IBD9	3p	—	CD
—	10q	DLG5	CD
—	1p	IL-23R	CD,UC
—	2q	ATG16L1	CD
—	5p	PTGER4	CD

[a]Taken from National Center for Biotechnology Information, Online Mendelian Inheritance in Man, *http://www.ncbi.nlm.nih.gov/entrez/query.fcgi?db=OMIM*.
[b]CARD15, caspase-associated recruitment domain containing protein 15; MHC, major histocompatibility complex; DLG5, Drosophila Discs Large Homolog 5; OCTN, novel organic cation transporter protein; IL-23R, Interleukin-23 receptor; ATG16L1, autophagy-related 16-like 1 gene; PTGER4, prostaglandin receptor EP4.
Source: Adapted from S Vermeire, P Rutgeerts: Genes Immun 6:637, 2005.

DEFECTIVE IMMUNE REGULATION IN IBD

The mucosal immune system is normally unreactive to luminal contents due to oral tolerance. When soluble antigens are administered orally rather than subcutaneously or intramuscularly, antigen-specific nonresponsiveness is induced. Multiple mechanisms are involved in the induction of oral tolerance and include deletion or anergy of antigen-reactive T cells or activation of CD4+ T cells that suppress gut inflammation through secretion of inhibitory cytokines, such as interleukin (IL) 10 and transforming growth factor β (TGF-β). Oral tolerance may be responsible for the lack of immune responsiveness to dietary antigens and the commensal flora in the intestinal lumen. In IBD this suppression of inflammation is altered, leading to uncontrolled inflammation. The mechanisms of this regulated immune suppression are incompletely known.

Gene knockout (–/–) or transgenic (Tg) mouse models of colitis have revealed that deleting specific cytokines (e.g., IL-2, IL-10, TGF-β) or their receptors, deleting molecules associated with T cell antigen recognition (e.g., T cell antigen receptors) or interfering with intestinal epithelial cell barrier function (e.g., deleting N-cadherin, mucus glycoprotein or NF-κB) leads to colitis or enteritis. Thus, a variety of specific alterations can lead to immune activation and inflammation directed at the colon in mice. How these relate to human IBD remains to be defined.

In both UC and CD, an inflammatory pathway emerges from the genetic predisposition in which activated CD4+ T cells in the lamina propria secrete inflammatory cytokines. Some activate other inflammatory cells (macrophages and B cells) and others act indirectly to recruit other lymphocytes, inflammatory leukocytes, and mononuclear cells from the blood stream into the gut through interactions between homing receptors on leukocytes (e.g., α4β7 integrin) and addressins on vascular endothelium (e.g., MadCAM1). CD4+ T cells are of three major types, all of which may be associated with colitis in animal models and humans: T_H1 cells [interferon (IFN) γ], T_H2 cells (IL-4, IL-5, IL-13), and T_H17 cells (IL-17). T_H1 cells induce transmural granulomatous inflammation that resembles CD, T_H2 cells and related natural killer T cells that secrete IL-13 induce superficial mucosal inflammation resembling UC, and T_H17 cells may be responsible for neutrophilic recruitment. The T_H1 cytokine pathway is initiated by IL-12, a key cytokine in the pathogenesis of experimental models of mucosal inflammation. IL-4 and IL-23, together with IL-6 and TGF-β, induce T_H2 and T_H17 cells, respectively. Activated macrophages secrete tumor necrosis factor (TNF). Thus, use of antibodies to block proinflammatory cytokines (e.g., anti-TNF, anti-IL-12, anti-IL-23, anti-IL-6, anti-IFN-γ) or molecules associated with leukocyte recruitment (e.g., anti-α4β7) or use of cytokines that inhibit inflammation and promote regulatory T cells (e.g., IL-10) or promote intestinal barrier function (e.g., granulocyte-macrophage colony-stimulating factor) may be beneficial to humans with colitis.

THE INFLAMMATORY CASCADE IN IBD

Once initiated in IBD, the immune inflammatory response is perpetuated by T-cell activation. A sequential cascade of inflammatory mediators extends the response; each step is a potential target for therapy. Inflammatory cytokines, such as IL-1, IL-6, and TNF, have diverse effects on tissues. They promote fibrogenesis, collagen production, activation of tissue metalloproteinases, and the production of other inflammatory mediators; they also activate the coagulation cascade in local blood vessels (e.g., increased production of von Willebrand's factor). These cytokines are normally produced in response to infection but are usually turned off or inhibited at the appropriate time to limit tissue damage. In IBD their activity is not regulated, resulting in an imbalance between the proinflammatory and anti-inflammatory mediators. Therapies such as the 5-ASA (5-aminosalicylic acid) compounds are potent inhibitors of these inflammatory mediators through inhibition of transcription factors such as NF-κB that regulate their expression.

EXOGENOUS FACTORS

IBD may have an as yet undefined infectious etiology. Observational studies suggest that multiple pathogens (e.g., *Salmonella* sp., *Shigella* sp., *Campylobacter* sp., *Clostridium difficile*) may initiate IBD by triggering an inflammatory response that the mucosal immune system may fail to control. However, in an IBD patient, the normal flora is likely perceived as if it were a pathogen. Anaerobic organisms, particularly *Bacteroides* and *Clostridia* species, and some aerobic species such as *Escherichia* may be responsible for the induction of inflammation. This notion is supported by the immune response in patients with CD to bacterial antigens such as I2, OmpC and flagellin. In addition, agents that alter the intestinal flora, such as metronidazole, ciprofloxacin, and elemental diets, may improve CD. CD also responds to fecal diversion, demonstrating the ability of luminal contents to exacerbate disease. On the other hand, other organisms, so-called probiotics (e.g., *Lactobacillus* sp., *Bifidobacterium* sp., *Taenia suis*, and *Saccharomyces boulardii*), may inhibit inflammation in animal models and humans.

Psychosocial factors can contribute to worsening of symptoms. Major life events such as illness or death in the family, divorce or separation, interpersonal conflict, or other major loss are associated with an increase in IBD symptoms such as pain, bowel dysfunction, and bleeding. Acute daily stress can worsen bowel symptoms even after controlling for major life events. When the sickness-impact profile, a measurement of overall psychological and physical functioning, is used, IBD patients have functional impairment greater than that of a normal population but less than that of patients with chronic back pain or amyotrophic lateral sclerosis.

PATHOLOGY

ULCERATIVE COLITIS: MACROSCOPIC FEATURES

UC is a mucosal disease that usually involves the rectum and extends proximally to involve all or part of the colon. About 40–50% of patients have disease limited to the rectum and rectosigmoid, 30–40% have disease extending beyond the sigmoid but not involving the whole colon, and 20% have a total colitis. Proximal spread occurs in continuity without areas of uninvolved mucosa. When the whole colon is involved, the inflammation extends 1–2 cm into the terminal ileum in 10–20% of patients. This is called *backwash ileitis* and is of little clinical significance. Although variations in macroscopic activity may suggest skip areas, biopsies from normal-appearing mucosa are usually abnormal. Thus, it is important to obtain multiple biopsies from apparently uninvolved mucosa, whether proximal or distal, during endoscopy.

With mild inflammation, the mucosa is erythematous and has a fine granular surface that looks like sandpaper. In more severe disease, the mucosa is hemorrhagic, edematous, and ulcerated (**Fig. 289-1**). In long-standing disease, inflammatory polyps (pseudopolyps) may be present as a result of epithelial regeneration. The mucosa may appear normal in remission, but in patients with many years of disease it appears atrophic and featureless and the entire colon becomes narrowed and shortened. Patients with fulminant disease can develop a toxic colitis or megacolon where the bowel wall thins and the mucosa is severely ulcerated; this may lead to perforation.

FIGURE 289-1 Pan-ulcerative colitis. Mucosa has a lumpy, bumpy appearance because of areas of inflamed but intact mucosa separated by ulcerated areas. *(Courtesy of Dr. KE Rosado and Dr. CA Parkos, Division of Gastrointestinal Pathology, Department of Pathology, Emory University, Atlanta, Georgia; with permission.)*

ULCERATIVE COLITIS: MICROSCOPIC FEATURES

Histologic findings correlate well with the endoscopic appearance and clinical course of UC. The process is limited to the mucosa and superficial submucosa, with deeper layers unaffected except in fulminant disease. In UC, two major histologic features suggest chronicity and help distinguish it from infectious or acute self-limited colitis. First, the crypt architecture of the colon is distorted; crypts may be bifid and reduced in number, often with a gap between the crypt bases and the muscularis mucosae. Second, some patients have basal plasma cells and multiple basal lymphoid aggregates. Mucosal vascular congestion, with edema and focal hemorrhage, and an inflammatory cell infiltrate of neutrophils, lymphocytes, plasma cells, and macrophages may be present. The neutrophils invade the epithelium, usually in the crypts, giving rise to cryptitis and, ultimately, to crypt abscesses (Fig. 289-2).

CROHN'S DISEASE: MACROSCOPIC FEATURES

CD can affect any part of the gastrointestinal tract from the mouth to the anus. Some 30–40% of patients have small-bowel disease alone, 40–55% have disease involving both the small and large intestines, and

FIGURE 289-3 Portion of colon with stricture in patient with CD. *(Courtesy of Dr. KE Rosado and Dr. CA Parkos, Division of Gastrointestinal Pathology, Department of Pathology, Emory University, Atlanta, Georgia; with permission.)*

15–25% have colitis alone. In the 75% of patients with small-intestinal disease, the terminal ileum is involved in 90%. Unlike UC, which almost always involves the rectum, the rectum is often spared in CD. CD is segmental with skip areas in the midst of diseased intestine (Fig. 289-3). Perirectal fistulas, fissures, abscesses, and anal stenosis are present in one-third of patients with CD, particularly those with colonic involvement. Rarely, CD may also involve the liver and the pancreas.

Unlike UC, CD is a transmural process. Endoscopically, aphthous or small superficial ulcerations characterize mild disease; in more active disease, stellate ulcerations fuse longitudinally and transversely to demarcate islands of mucosa that frequently are histologically normal. This "cobblestone" appearance is characteristic of CD, both endoscopically and by barium radiography. As in UC, pseudopolyps can form in CD.

Active CD is characterized by focal inflammation and formation of fistula tracts, which resolve by fibrosis and stricturing of the bowel. The bowel wall thickens and becomes narrowed and fibrotic, leading to chronic, recurrent bowel obstructions. Projections of thickened mesentery encase the bowel ("creeping fat"), and serosal and mesenteric inflammation promotes adhesions and fistula formation.

CROHN'S DISEASE: MICROSCOPIC FEATURES

The earliest lesions are aphthoid ulcerations and focal crypt abscesses with loose aggregations of macrophages, which form noncaseating granulomas in all layers of the bowel wall (Fig. 289-4). Granulomas can be seen in lymph nodes, mesentery, peritoneum, liver, and pancreas. Although granulomas are a pathognomonic feature of CD, they are rarely found on mucosal biopsies. Surgical resection reveals granulomas in about half of cases. Other histologic features of CD include submucosal or subserosal lymphoid aggregates, particularly away from areas of ulceration, gross and microscopic skip areas, and trans-

FIGURE 289-2 Medium power view of colonic mucosa in ulcerative colitis showing diffuse mixed inflammation, basal lymphoplasmacytosis, crypt atrophy and irregularity and superficial erosion. These features are typical of chronic active ulcerative colitis. *(Courtesy of Dr. R Odze, Division of Gastrointestinal Pathology, Department of Pathology, Brigham and Women's Hospital, Boston, Massachusetts; with permission.)*

FIGURE 289-4 Medium power view of Crohn's colitis showing mixed acute and chronic inflammation, crypt atrophy, and multiple small epithelioid granulomas in the mucosa. *(Courtesy of Dr. R Odze, Division of Gastrointestinal Pathology, Department of Pathology, Brigham and Women's Hospital, Boston, Massachusetts; with permission.)*

mural inflammation that is accompanied by fissures that penetrate deeply into the bowel wall and sometimes form fistulous tracts or local abscesses.

CLINICAL PRESENTATION

ULCERATIVE COLITIS

Signs and Symptoms The major symptoms of UC are diarrhea, rectal bleeding, tenesmus, passage of mucus, and crampy abdominal pain. The severity of symptoms correlates with the extent of disease. Although UC can present acutely, symptoms usually have been present for weeks to months. Occasionally, diarrhea and bleeding are so intermittent and mild that the patient does not seek medical attention.

Patients with proctitis usually pass fresh blood or blood-stained mucus, either mixed with stool or streaked onto the surface of a normal or hard stool. They also have tenesmus, or urgency with a feeling of incomplete evacuation, but rarely have abdominal pain. With proctitis or proctosigmoiditis, proximal transit slows, which may account for the constipation commonly seen in patients with distal disease.

When the disease extends beyond the rectum, blood is usually mixed with stool or grossly bloody diarrhea may be noted. Colonic motility is altered by inflammation with rapid transit through the inflamed intestine. When the disease is severe, patients pass a liquid stool containing blood, pus, and fecal matter. Diarrhea is often nocturnal and/or postprandial. Although severe pain is not a prominent symptom, some patients with active disease may experience vague lower abdominal discomfort or mild central abdominal cramping. Severe cramping and abdominal pain can occur with severe attacks of the disease. Other symptoms in moderate to severe disease include anorexia, nausea, vomiting, fever, and weight loss.

Physical signs of proctitis include a tender anal canal and blood on rectal examination. With more extensive disease, patients have tenderness to palpation directly over the colon. Patients with a toxic colitis have severe pain and bleeding, and those with megacolon have hepatic tympany. Both may have signs of peritonitis if a perforation has occurred. The classification of disease activity is shown in Table 289-3.

Laboratory, Endoscopic, and Radiographic Features Active disease can be associated with a rise in acute-phase reactants [C-reactive protein (CRP)], platelet count, erythrocyte sedimentation rate (ESR), and a decrease in hemoglobin. Fecal calprotectin levels correlate well with histological inflammation, predict relapses, and detect pouchitis. In severely ill patients, the serum albumin level will fall rather quickly. Leukocytosis may be present but is not a specific indicator of disease activity. Proctitis or proctosigmoiditis rarely causes a rise in CRP. Diagnosis relies upon the patient's history; clinical symptoms; negative stool examination for bacteria, *C. difficile* toxin, and ova and parasites; sigmoidoscopic appearance (see Fig. 285-4A); and histology of rectal or colonic biopsy specimens.

Sigmoidoscopy is used to assess disease activity and is often performed before treatment. If the patient is not having an acute flare, colonoscopy is used to assess disease extent and activity. Histologic features change more slowly than clinical features but can also be used to grade disease activity.

The earliest radiologic change of UC seen on single-contrast barium enema is a fine mucosal granularity (Fig. 289-5). With increasing severity, the mucosa becomes thickened, and superficial ulcers are seen. Deep ulcerations can appear as "collar-button" ulcers, which indicate that the ulceration has penetrated the mucosa. Haustral folds may be normal in mild disease, but as activity progresses they become edematous and thickened. Loss of haustration can occur, especially in patients with long-standing disease. In addition, the colon becomes shortened and narrowed. Polyps in the colon may be postinflammatory polyps or pseudopolyps, adenomatous polyps, or carcinoma.

TABLE 289-3	ULCERATIVE COLITIS: DISEASE PRESENTATION		
	Mild	**Moderate**	**Severe**
Bowel movements	<4 per day	4–6 per day	>6 per day
Blood in stool	Small	Moderate	Severe
Fever	None	<37.5°C mean	>37.5°C mean
Tachycardia	None	<90 mean pulse	>90 mean pulse
Anemia	Mild	>75%	≤75%
Sedimentation rate	<30 mm		>30 mm
Endoscopic appearance	Erythema, decreased vascular pattern, fine granularity	Marked erythema, coarse granularity, absent vascular markings, contact bleeding, no ulcerations	Spontaneous bleeding, ulcerations

CT scanning is not as helpful as endoscopy and barium enema in making the diagnosis of UC, but typical findings include mild mural thickening (<1.5 cm), inhomogeneous wall density, absence of small-bowel thickening, increased perirectal and presacral fat, target appearance of the rectum, and adenopathy.

Complications Only 15% of patients with UC present initially with catastrophic illness. Massive hemorrhage occurs with severe attacks of disease in 1% of patients, and treatment for the disease usually stops the bleeding. However, if a patient requires 6–8 units of blood within 24–48 h, colectomy is indicated. *Toxic megacolon* is defined as a transverse colon with a diameter of >5–6 cm, with loss of haustration in patients with severe attacks of UC. It occurs in about 5% of attacks and can be triggered by electrolyte abnormalities and narcotics. About 50% of acute dilations will resolve with medical therapy alone, but urgent colectomy is required for those that do not improve. Perforation is the most dangerous of the local complications, and the physical signs of peritonitis may not be obvious, especially if the patient is receiving glucocorticoids. Although perforation is rare, the mortality rate for perforation complicating a toxic megacolon is about 15%. In addition, patients can develop a toxic colitis and such severe ulcerations that the bowel may perforate without first dilating.

Strictures occur in 5–10% of patients and are always a concern in UC because of the possibility of underlying neoplasia. Although be-

FIGURE 289-5 Barium enema in a patient with acute ulcerative colitis: inflammation of the entire colon. (*Courtesy of Dr. JM Braver, Gastrointestinal Radiology, Department of Radiology, Brigham and Women's Hospital, Boston, Massachusetts; with permission.*)

nign strictures can form from the inflammation and fibrosis of UC, strictures that are impassable with the colonoscope should be presumed malignant until proven otherwise. A stricture that prevents passage of the colonoscope is an indication for surgery. UC patients occasionally develop anal fissures, perianal abscesses, or hemorrhoids, but the occurrence of extensive perianal lesions should suggest CD.

CROHN'S DISEASE

Signs and Symptoms Although CD usually presents as acute or chronic bowel inflammation, the inflammatory process evolves toward one of two patterns of disease: a fibrostenotic-obstructing pattern or a penetrating-fistulous pattern, each with different treatments and prognoses. The site of disease influences the clinical manifestations.

ILEOCOLITIS Because the most common site of inflammation is the terminal ileum, the usual presentation of ileocolitis is a chronic history of recurrent episodes of right lower quadrant pain and diarrhea. Sometimes the initial presentation mimics acute appendicitis with pronounced right lower quadrant pain, a palpable mass, fever, and leukocytosis. Pain is usually colicky; it precedes and is relieved by defecation. A low-grade fever is usually noted. High-spiking fever suggests intraabdominal abscess formation. Weight loss is common—typically 10–20% of body weight— and develops as a consequence of diarrhea, anorexia, and fear of eating.

An inflammatory mass may be palpated in the right lower quadrant of the abdomen. The mass is composed of inflamed bowel, adherent and indurated mesentery, and enlarged abdominal lymph nodes. Extension of the mass can cause obstruction of the right ureter or bladder inflammation, manifested by dysuria and fever. Edema, bowel wall thickening, and fibrosis of the bowel wall within the mass account for the radiographic "string sign" of a narrowed intestinal lumen.

Bowel obstruction may take several forms. In the early stages of disease, bowel wall edema and spasm produce intermittent obstructive manifestations and increasing symptoms of postprandial pain. Over several years, persistent inflammation gradually progresses to fibrostenotic narrowing and stricture. Diarrhea will decrease and be replaced by chronic bowel obstruction. Acute episodes of obstruction occur as well, precipitated by bowel inflammation and spasm or sometimes by impaction of undigested food or medication. These episodes usually resolve with intravenous fluids and gastric decompression.

Severe inflammation of the ileocecal region may lead to localized wall thinning, with microperforation and fistula formation to the adjacent bowel, the skin, or the urinary bladder, or to an abscess cavity in the mesentery. Enterovesical fistulas typically present as dysuria or recurrent bladder infections or, less commonly, as pneumaturia or fecaluria. Enterocutaneous fistulas follow tissue planes of least resistance, usually draining through abdominal surgical scars. Enterovaginal fistulas are rare and present as dyspareunia or as a feculent or foul-smelling, often painful vaginal discharge. They are unlikely to develop without a prior hysterectomy.

JEJUNOILEITIS Extensive inflammatory disease is associated with a loss of digestive and absorptive surface, resulting in malabsorption and steatorrhea. Nutritional deficiencies can also result from poor intake and enteric losses of protein and other nutrients. Intestinal malabsorption can cause hypoalbuminemia, hypocalcemia, hypomagnesemia, coagulopathy, and hyperoxaluria with nephrolithiasis in patients with an intact colon. Vertebral fractures are caused by a combination of vitamin D deficiency, hypocalcemia, and prolonged glucocorticoid use. Pellagra from niacin deficiency can occur in extensive small-bowel disease, and malabsorption of vitamin B_{12} can lead to megaloblastic anemia and neurologic symptoms.

Diarrhea is characteristic of active disease; its causes include (1) bacterial overgrowth in obstructive stasis or fistulization, (2) bile-acid malabsorption due to a diseased or resected terminal ileum, and (3) intestinal inflammation with decreased water absorption and increased secretion of electrolytes.

COLITIS AND PERIANAL DISEASE Patients with colitis present with low-grade fevers, malaise, diarrhea, crampy abdominal pain, and some-

times hematochezia. Gross bleeding is not as common as in UC and appears in about half of patients with exclusively colonic disease. Only 1–2% bleed massively. Pain is caused by passage of fecal material through narrowed and inflamed segments of large bowel. Decreased rectal compliance is another cause for diarrhea in Crohn's colitis patients. Toxic megacolon is rare but may be seen with severe inflammation and short-duration disease.

Stricturing can occur in the colon in 4–16% of patients and produce symptoms of bowel obstruction. If the endoscopist is unable to traverse a stricture in Crohn's colitis, surgical resection should be considered, especially if the patient has symptoms of chronic obstruction. Colonic disease may fistulize into the stomach or duodenum, causing feculent vomiting, or to the proximal or mid small bowel, causing malabsorption by "short circuiting" and bacterial overgrowth. Ten percent of women with Crohn's colitis will develop a rectovaginal fistula.

Perianal disease affects about one-third of patients with Crohn's colitis and is manifested by incontinence, large hemorrhoidal tags, anal strictures, anorectal fistulae, and perirectal abscesses. Not all patients with perianal fistula will have endoscopic evidence of colonic inflammation.

GASTRODUODENAL DISEASE Symptoms and signs of upper gastrointestinal tract disease include nausea, vomiting, and epigastric pain. Patients usually have a *H. pylori*–negative gastritis. The second portion of the duodenum is more commonly involved than the bulb. Fistulas involving the stomach or duodenum arise from the small or large bowel and do not necessarily signify the presence of upper gastrointestinal tract involvement. Patients with advanced gastroduodenal CD may develop a chronic gastric outlet obstruction.

Laboratory, Endoscopic, and Radiographic Features Laboratory abnormalities include elevated ESR and CRP. In more severe disease, findings include hypoalbuminemia, anemia, and leukocytosis.

Endoscopic features of CD include rectal sparing, aphthous ulcerations, fistulas, and skip lesions. Endoscopy is useful for biopsy of mass lesions or strictures, or for inspecting filling defects seen on barium enema. Colonoscopy allows examination and biopsy of the terminal ileum, and upper endoscopy is useful in diagnosing gastroduodenal involvement in patients with upper tract symptoms. Ileal or colonic strictures may be dilated with balloons introduced through the colonoscope. Wireless capsule endoscopy (WCE) allows direct visualization of the entire small-bowel mucosa (Fig. 289-6). The diagnostic yield of detecting lesions suggestive of active CD is higher with WCE than CT enterography or small-bowel series. WCE cannot be used in the setting of a small-bowel stricture. Capsule retention occurs in <1% of patients with suspected CD, but retention rates of 4–6% are seen in patients with established CD.

In CD, early radiographic findings in the small bowel include thickened folds and aphthous ulcerations. "Cobblestoning" from longitudi-

FIGURE 289-6 Wireless capsule endoscopy image in a patient with Crohn's disease of the ileum shows ulcerations and narrowing of the intestinal lumen. *(Courtesy of Dr. S Reddy, Gastroenterology Division, Department of Medicine, Brigham and Women's Hospital, Boston, Massachusetts; with permission.)*

nal and transverse ulcerations most frequently involves the small bowel. In more advanced disease, strictures, fistulas, inflammatory masses, and abscesses may be detected. The earliest macroscopic findings of colonic CD are aphthous ulcers. These small ulcers are often multiple and separated by normal intervening mucosa. As disease progresses, aphthous ulcers become enlarged, deeper, and occasionally connected to one another, forming longitudinal stellate, serpiginous, and linear ulcers (see Fig. 285-4*B*).

The transmural inflammation of CD leads to decreased luminal diameter and limited distensibility. As ulcers progress deeper, they can lead to fistula formation. The radiographic "string sign" represents long areas of circumferential inflammation and fibrosis, resulting in long segments of luminal narrowing. The segmental nature of CD results in wide gaps of normal or dilated bowel between involved segments.

CT enterography combines the improved spatial and temporal resolution of multidetector-row CT with large volumes of ingested neutral enteric contrast material to permit visualization of the entire small bowel and lumen. Unlike routine CT, which is used to detect the extraenteric complications of CD such as fistula and abscess, CT enterography clearly depicts the small-bowel inflammation associated with CD by displaying mural hyperenhancement, stratification, and thickening; engorged vasa recta; and perienteric inflammatory changes (Figs. 289-7 and 289-8). CT enterography is becoming the first-line test for the evaluation of suspected CD and its complications. MRI may prove superior for demonstrating pelvic lesions such as ischiorectal abscesses.

Complications Because CD is a transmural process, serosal adhesions develop that provide direct pathways for fistula formation and reduce the incidence of free perforation. Perforation occurs in 1–2% of pa-

FIGURE 289-8 Coronal contrast-enhanced MDCT image obtained after oral administration of 1350 cc of neutral oral contrast material shows mucosal hyperenhancement of the terminal ileum with narrowing and mild prestenotic dilatation. *(Courtesy of Dr. K Mortele, Gastrointestinal Radiology, Department of Radiology, Brigham and Women's Hospital, Boston, Massachusetts; with permission.)*

FIGURE 289-7 Coronal contrast-enhanced MDCT image obtained after oral administration of 1350 cc of neutral oral contrast material shows dilation of small-bowel loops, segmental mucosal hyperenhancement, and interloop sinus tracts *(white arrow)* and mesenteric fat stranding. *(Courtesy of Dr. K Mortele, Gastrointestinal Radiology, Department of Radiology, Brigham and Women's Hospital, Boston, Massachusetts; with permission.)*

tients, usually in the ileum but occasionally in the jejunum or as a complication of toxic megacolon. The peritonitis of free perforation, especially colonic, may be fatal. Intraabdominal and pelvic abscesses occur in 10–30% of patients with Crohn's disease at some time in the course of their illness. CT-guided percutaneous drainage of the abscess is standard therapy. Despite adequate drainage, most patients need resection of the offending bowel segment. Percutaneous drainage has an especially high failure rate in abdominal wall abscesses. Systemic glucocorticoid therapy increases the risk of intraabdominal and pelvic abscesses in CD patients who have never had an operation. Other complications include intestinal obstruction in 40%, massive hemorrhage, malabsorption, and severe perianal disease.

Serologic Markers Two antibodies that can be detected in the serum of IBD patients are perinuclear antineutrophil cytoplasmic antibodies (pANCAs) and anti-*Saccharomyces cerevisiae* antibodies (ASCAs). A distinct set of pANCAs is associated with UC. The antigens to which these antibodies are directed have not been identified, but they are distinct from those associated with vasculitis and likely represent cross-reactions with enteric bacterial antigens. pANCA positivity is found in about 60–70% of UC patients and 5–10% of CD patients; 5–15% of first-degree relatives of UC patients are pANCA positive, whereas only 2–3% of the general population is pANCA-positive. pANCA may also identify specific disease phenotypes. pANCA positivity is more often associated with pancolitis, early surgery, pouchitis, or inflammation of the pouch after ileal pouch–anal anastomosis (IPAA) and primary sclerosing cholangitis (PSC). pANCA in CD is associated with colonic disease that resembles UC.

ASCA antibodies recognize mannose sequences in the cell wall of *S. cerevisiae*; 60–70% of CD patients, 10–15% of UC patients, and up to 5% of non-IBD controls are ASCA-positive. The sensitivity and specificity of pANCA/ASCA vary depending upon the prevalence of IBD in a given population. In a patient population with a combined prevalence of UC and CD of 62%, pANCA/ASCA serology showed a sensitivity of 64% and a specificity of 94%. Positive and negative predictive values (PPV and NPV) for pANCA/ASCA also vary based on the prevalence of IBD in a given population. For the patient population with a prevalence of IBD of 62%, the PPV is 94% and the NPV is 63%.

In a referral center population, 55% of CD patients are seroreactive to outer membrane porin C (Omp C) of *E. coli*; 50–54% of CD patients are positive for antibody to I₂, a homologue of the bacterial transcription-factor families from a *Pseudomonas fluorescens*–associated sequence. Combining these diagnostic assays further improves the ability to diagnose CD. In a referral population of CD patients, 85% had an antibody to at least one antigen (pANCA, ASCA, Omp C, and I₂); only 4% responded to all four. Antibody positivity may help predict disease phenotype. ASCA positivity is associated with an increased rate of early CD complications; Omp C–positive patients are more likely to have internal perforating disease; and I₂ positive patients are more likely to have fibrostenosing disease. Patients positive for I₂, Omp C, and ASCA are the most likely to have undergone small-bowel surgery.

Cbir1 flagellin is an immunodominant antigen of the enteric microbial flora to which strong B cell and CD4+ T cell responses occur in colitic mice. Transfer of Cbir1-specific CD4+ T_H1 T cells to C3H/SCID mice generates a severe colitis dependent on exogenous expression of Cbir1 flagellin in the cecum and colon. Around 50% of patients with CD have serum reactivity to Cbir1, whereas UC patients have little or no reactivity to this flagellin. Anti-Cbir1 expression is associated with small-bowel disease, fibrostenosing, and internal penetrating disease. Children with CD positive for all four immune responses (ASCA+, Omp C+, I₂+ and anti-Cbir1+) may have more aggressive disease and a shorter time to progression to internal perforating and/or stricturing disease. In addition, these antibody tests may help decide whether a patient with indeterminate colitis should undergo an IPAA, because patients with predominant features of CD have a more difficult postoperative course.

Other serologic markers in IBD patients include antigoblet cell autoantibodies, pancreatic autoantibodies, and an autoantibody against tropomyosin isoform 5 found in colon epithelial cells. Antibodies to red cell membrane antigens that cross-react with enteropathogens such as *Campylobacter* sp. may be associated with hemolytic anemia in CD. None of these antibodies are useful in the diagnosis and management of patients with IBD.

DIFFERENTIAL DIAGNOSIS OF UC AND CD

UC and CD have similar features to many other diseases. In the absence of a key diagnostic test, a combination of features is used (Table 289-4). Once a diagnosis of IBD is made, distinguishing between UC and CD is impossible in up to 15% of cases. These are termed *indeterminate colitis*.

INFECTIOUS DISEASE

Infections of the small intestines and colon can mimic CD or UC. They may be bacterial, fungal, viral, or protozoal in origin (Table 289-5). *Campylobacter* colitis can mimic the endoscopic appearance of severe UC and can cause a relapse of established UC. *Salmonella* can cause watery or bloody diarrhea, nausea, and vomiting. Shigellosis causes watery diarrhea, abdominal pain, and fever followed by rectal tenesmus and by the passage of blood and mucus per rectum. All three are usually self-limited, but 1% of patients infected with *Salmonella* become asymptomatic carriers. *Yersinia enterocolitica* infection occurs mainly in the terminal ileum and causes mucosal ulceration, neutrophil invasion, and thickening of the ileal wall. Other bacterial infections that may mimic IBD include *C. difficile*, which presents with watery diarrhea, tenesmus, nausea, and vomiting; and *E. coli*, three categories of which can cause colitis. These are enterohemorrhagic, enteroinvasive, and enteroadherent *E. coli*, all of which can cause bloody diarrhea and abdominal tenderness. Diagnosis of bacterial colitis is made by sending stool specimens for bacterial culture and *C. difficile* toxin analysis. Gonorrhea, *Chlamydophila*, and syphilis can also cause proctitis.

Gastrointestinal involvement with mycobacterial infection occurs primarily in the immunosuppressed patient but may occur in patients with normal immunity. Distal ileal and cecal involvement predominates, and patients present with symptoms of small-bowel obstruction and a tender abdominal mass. The diagnosis is made most directly by colonoscopy with biopsy and culture. *Mycobacterium avium-intracellulare* complex infection occurs in advanced stages of HIV infection and in other immunocompromised states; it usually manifests as a systemic infection with diarrhea, abdominal pain, weight loss, fever, and malabsorption. Diagnosis is established by acid-fast smear and culture of mucosal biopsies.

TABLE 289-4	DIFFERENT CLINICAL, ENDOSCOPIC, AND RADIOGRAPHIC FEATURES	
	Ulcerative Colitis	Crohn's Disease
Clinical		
Gross blood in stool	Yes	Occasionally
Mucus	Yes	Occasionally
Systemic symptoms	Occasionally	Frequently
Pain	Occasionally	Frequently
Abdominal mass	Rarely	Yes
Significant perineal disease	No	Frequently
Fistulas	No	Yes
Small-intestinal obstruction	No	Frequently
Colonic obstruction	Rarely	Frequently
Response to antibiotics	No	Yes
Recurrence after surgery	No	Yes
ANCA-positive	Frequently	Rarely
ASCA-positive	Rarely	Frequently
Endoscopic		
Rectal sparing	Rarely	Frequently
Continuous disease	Yes	Occasionally
"Cobblestoning"	No	Yes
Granuloma on biopsy	No	Occasionally
Radiographic		
Small bowel significantly abnormal	No	Yes
Abnormal terminal ileum	Occasionally	Yes
Segmental colitis	No	Yes
Asymmetric colitis	No	Yes
Stricture	Occasionally	Frequently

Note: ANCA, antineutrophil cytoplasm antibody; ASCA, anti-*Saccharomyces cerevisiae* antibody.

TABLE 289-5	DISEASES THAT MIMIC IBD	
Infectious Etiologies		
Bacterial	**Mycobacterial**	**Viral**
Salmonella	Tuberculosis	Cytomegalovirus
Shigella	Mycobacterium	Herpes simplex
Toxigenic	avium	HIV
Escherichia coli	**Parasitic**	**Fungal**
Campylobacter	Amebiasis	Histoplasmosis
Yersinia	Isospora	Candida
Clostridium difficile	Trichuris trichura	Aspergillus
Gonorrhea	Hookworm	
Chlamydia trachomatis	Strongyloides	
Noninfectious Etiologies		
Inflammatory	**Neoplastic**	**Drugs and Chemicals**
Appendicitis	Lymphoma	NSAIDs
Diverticulitis	Metastatic carcinoma	Phosphasoda
Diversion colitis	Carcinoma of the ileum	Cathartic colon
Collagenous/lymphocytic colitis	Carcinoid	Gold
Ischemic colitis	Familial polyposis	Oral contraceptives
Radiation colitis/enteritis		Cocaine
Solitary rectal ulcer syndrome		Chemotherapy
Eosinophilc gastroenteritis		
Neutropenic colitis		
Beçhet's syndrome		
Graft-versus-host disease		

Note: NSAIDs, nonsteroidal anti-inflammatory drugs.

Although most of the patients with viral colitis are immunosuppressed, cytomegalovirus (CMV) and herpes simplex proctitis may occur in immunocompetent individuals. CMV occurs most commonly in the esophagus, colon, and rectum but may also involve the small intestine. Symptoms include abdominal pain, bloody diarrhea, fever, and weight loss. With severe disease, necrosis and perforation can occur. Diagnosis is made by identification of intranuclear inclusions in mucosal cells on biopsy. Herpes simplex infection of the gastrointestinal tract is limited to the oropharynx, anorectum, and perianal areas. Symptoms include anorectal pain, tenesmus, constipation, inguinal adenopathy, difficulty with urinary voiding, and sacral paresthesias. Diagnosis is made by rectal biopsy. HIV itself can cause diarrhea, nausea, vomiting, and anorexia. Small-intestinal biopsies show partial villus atrophy; small-bowel bacterial overgrowth and fat malabsorption may also be noted.

Protozoan parasites include *Isospora belli*, which can cause a self-limited infection in healthy hosts but causes a chronic profuse, watery diarrhea, and weight loss in AIDS patients. *Entamoeba histolytica* or related species infect about 10% of the world's population; symptoms include abdominal pain, tenesmus, frequent loose stools containing blood and mucus, and abdominal tenderness. Colonoscopy reveals focal punctate ulcers with normal intervening mucosa; diagnosis is made by biopsy or serum amebic antibodies. Fulminant amebic colitis is rare but has a mortality rate of >50%.

Other parasitic infections that may mimic IBD include hookworm (*Necator americanus*), whipworm (*Trichuris trichiura*), and *Strongyloides stercoralis*. In severely immunocompromised patients, *Candida* or *Aspergillus* can be identified in the submucosa. Disseminated histoplasmosis can involve the ileocecal area.

NONINFECTIOUS DISEASE

Diverticulitis can be confused with CD clinically and radiographically. Both diseases cause fever, abdominal pain, tender abdominal mass, leukocytosis, elevated ESR, partial obstruction, and fistulas. Perianal disease or ileitis on small-bowel series favors the diagnosis of CD. Significant endoscopic mucosal abnormalities are more likely in CD than in diverticulitis. Endoscopic or clinical recurrence following segmental resection favors CD. Diverticular-associated colitis is similar to CD, but mucosal abnormalities are limited to the sigmoid and descending colon.

Ischemic colitis is commonly confused with IBD. The ischemic process can be chronic and diffuse, as in UC, or segmental, as in CD. Colonic inflammation due to ischemia may resolve quickly or may persist and result in transmural scarring and stricture formation. Ischemic bowel disease should be considered in the elderly following abdominal aortic aneurysm repair or when a patient has a hypercoagulable state or a severe cardiac or peripheral vascular disorder. Patients usually present with sudden onset of left lower quadrant pain, urgency to defecate, and the passage of bright red blood per rectum. Endoscopic examination often demonstrates a normal-appearing rectum and a sharp transition to an area of inflammation in the descending colon and splenic flexure.

The effects of radiotherapy on the gastrointestinal tract can be difficult to distinguish from IBD. Acute symptoms can occur within 1–2 weeks of starting radiotherapy. When the rectum and sigmoid are irradiated, patients develop bloody, mucoid diarrhea and tenesmus, as in distal UC. With small-bowel involvement, diarrhea is common. Late symptoms include malabsorption and weight loss. Stricturing with obstruction and bacterial overgrowth may occur. Fistulas can penetrate the bladder, vagina, or abdominal wall. Flexible sigmoidoscopy reveals mucosal granularity, friability, numerous telangiectasias, and occasionally discrete ulcerations. Biopsy can be diagnostic.

Solitary rectal ulcer syndrome is uncommon and can be confused with IBD. It occurs in persons of all ages and may be caused by impaired evacuation and failure of relaxation of the puborectalis muscle. Single or multiple ulcerations may arise from anal sphincter overactivity, higher intrarectal pressures during defecation, and digital removal of stool. Patients complain of constipation with straining and pass blood and mucus per rectum. Other symptoms include abdominal pain, diarrhea, tenesmus, and perineal pain. Ulceration as large as 5 cm in diameter is usually seen anteriorly or anteriorlaterally 3–15 cm from the anal verge. Biopsies can be diagnostic.

Several types of colitis are associated with nonsteroidal anti-inflammatory drugs (NSAIDs), including de novo colitis, reactivation of IBD, and proctitis caused by use of suppositories. Most patients with NSAID-related colitis present with diarrhea and abdominal pain, and complications include stricture, bleeding, obstruction, perforation, and fistulization. Withdrawal of these agents is crucial, and in cases of reactivated IBD, standard therapies are indicated.

INDETERMINATE COLITIS

Cases of IBD that cannot be categorized as UC or CD are called *indeterminate colitis*. Long-term follow-up reduces the number of cases labeled indeterminate to about 10%. The disease course of indeterminate colitis is unclear, and surgical recommendations are difficult, especially since up to 20% of pouches fail, requiring permanent ileostomy. A multistage IPAA (the initial stage consisting of a subtotal colectomy with Hartmann pouch), with careful histologic evaluation of the resected specimen to exclude CD, is advised. Medical therapy is similar to that for UC and CD; most clinicians use 5-ASA drugs, glucocorticoids, and immunomodulators as necessary.

THE ATYPICAL COLITIDES

Two atypical colitides—collagenous colitis and lymphocytic colitis—have completely normal endoscopic appearances. Collagenous colitis has two main histologic components: increased subepithelial collagen deposition and colitis with increased intraepithelial lymphocytes. Female to male ratio is 9:1, and most patients present in the sixth or seventh decades of life. The main symptom is chronic watery diarrhea. Treatments range from sulfasalazine or mesalamine and Lomotil to bismuth to budesonide to prednisone for refractory disease.

Lymphocytic colitis has features similar to collagenous colitis, including age at onset and clinical presentation, but it has almost equal incidence in men and women and no subepithelial collagen deposition on pathologic section. However, intraepithelial lymphocytes are increased. The frequency of celiac disease is increased in lymphocytic colitis and ranges from 9 to 27%. Celiac disease should be excluded in all patients with lymphocytic colitis, particularly if diarrhea does not respond to conventional therapy. Treatment is similar to that of collagenous colitis with the exception of a gluten-free diet for those who have celiac disease.

Diversion colitis is an inflammatory process that arises in segments of the large intestine that are excluded from the fecal stream. It usually occurs in patients with ileostomy or colostomy when a mucus fistula or a Hartmann's pouch has been created. Clinically, patients have mucus or bloody discharge from the rectum. Erythema, granularity, friability, and, in more severe cases, ulceration can be seen on endoscopy. Histopathology shows areas of active inflammation with foci of cryptitis and crypt abscesses. Crypt architecture is normal, which differentiates it from UC. It may be impossible to distinguish from CD. Short-chain fatty acid enemas may help in diversion colitis, but the definitive therapy is surgical reanastomosis.

EXTRAINTESTINAL MANIFESTATIONS

Up to one-third of IBD patients have at least one extraintestinal disease manifestation.

DERMATOLOGIC

Erythema nodosum (EN) occurs in up to 15% of CD patients and 10% of UC patients. Attacks usually correlate with bowel activity; skin lesions develop after the onset of bowel symptoms, and patients frequently have concomitant active peripheral arthritis. The lesions of EN are hot, red, tender nodules measuring 1–5 cm in diameter and are found on the anterior surface of the lower legs, ankles, calves, thighs, and arms. Therapy is directed toward the underlying bowel disease.

Pyoderma gangrenosum (PG) is seen in 1–12% of UC patients and less commonly in Crohn's colitis. Although it usually presents after the diagnosis of IBD, PG may occur years before the onset of bowel symptoms, run a course independent of the bowel disease, respond poorly to colectomy, and even develop years after proctocolectomy. It is usually associated with severe disease. Lesions are commonly found on the dorsal surface of the feet and legs but may occur on the arms, chest, stoma, and even the face. PG usually begins as a pustule and then spreads concentrically to rapidly undermine healthy skin. Lesions then ulcerate, with violaceous edges surrounded by a margin of erythema. Centrally, they contain necrotic tissue with blood and exudates. Lesions may be single or multiple and grow as large as 30 cm. They are sometimes very difficult to treat and often require intravenous antibiotics, intravenous glucocorticoids, dapsone, azathioprine, thalidomide, intravenous cyclosporine, or infliximab.

Other dermatologic manifestations include pyoderma vegetans, which occurs in intertriginous areas; pyostomatitis vegetans, which involves the mucous membranes; Sweet's syndrome, a neutrophilic dermatosis; and metastatic CD, a rare disorder defined by cutaneous granuloma formation. Psoriasis affects 5–10% of patients with IBD and is unrelated to bowel activity. Perianal skin tags are found in 75–80% of patients with CD, especially those with colon involvement. Oral mucosal lesions, seen often in CD and rarely in UC, include aphthous stomatitis and "cobblestone" lesions of the buccal mucosa.

RHEUMATOLOGIC

Peripheral arthritis develops in 15–20% of IBD patients, is more common in CD, and worsens with exacerbations of bowel activity. It is asymmetric, polyarticular, and migratory and most often affects large joints of the upper and lower extremities. Treatment is directed at reducing bowel inflammation. In severe UC, colectomy frequently cures the arthritis.

Ankylosing spondylitis (AS) occurs in about 10% of IBD patients and is more common in CD than UC. About two-thirds of IBD patients with AS express the HLA-B27 antigen. The AS activity is not related to bowel activity and does not remit with glucocorticoids or colectomy. It most often affects the spine and pelvis, producing symptoms of diffuse low-back pain, buttock pain, and morning stiffness. The course is continuous and progressive, leading to permanent skeletal damage and deformity. Infliximab reduces spinal inflammation and improves functional status and quality of life.

Sacroiliitis is symmetric, occurs equally in UC and CD, is often asymptomatic, does not correlate with bowel activity, and does not always progress to AS. Other rheumatic manifestations include hypertrophic osteoarthropathy, pelvic/femoral osteomyelitis, and relapsing polychondritis.

OCULAR

The incidence of ocular complications in IBD patients is 1–10%. The most common are conjunctivitis, anterior uveitis/iritis, and episcleritis. Uveitis is associated with both UC and Crohn's colitis, may be found during periods of remission, and may develop in patients following bowel resection. Symptoms include ocular pain, photophobia, blurred vision, and headache. Prompt intervention, sometimes with systemic glucocorticoids, is required to prevent scarring and visual impairment. Episcleritis is a benign disorder that presents with symptoms of mild ocular burning. It occurs in 3–4% of IBD patients, more commonly in Crohn's colitis, and is treated with topical glucocorticoids.

HEPATOBILIARY

Hepatic steatosis is detectable in about half of the abnormal liver biopsies from patients with CD and UC; patients usually present with hepatomegaly. Fatty liver usually results from a combination of chronic debilitating illness, malnutrition, and glucocorticoid therapy. Cholelithiasis is more common in CD than UC and occurs in 10–35% of patients with ileitis or ileal resection. Gallstone formation is caused by malabsorption of bile acids, resulting in depletion of the bile salt pool and the secretion of lithogenic bile.

PSC shows both intrahepatic and extrahepatic bile duct inflammation and fibrosis, frequently leading to biliary cirrhosis and hepatic failure; 1–5% of patients with IBD have PSC, but 50–75% of patients with PSC have IBD. Although it can be recognized after the diagnosis of IBD, PSC can be detected earlier or even years after proctocolectomy. Most patients have no symptoms at the time of diagnosis; when symptoms are present, they consist of fatigue, jaundice, abdominal pain, fever, anorexia, and malaise. The traditional gold-standard diagnostic test is endoscopic retrograde cholangiopancreatography (ERCP) but magnetic resonance cholangiopancreatography (MRCP) is also sensitive and specific. MRCP is reasonable as an initial diagnostic test in children and can visualize irregularities, multifocal strictures, and dilatations of all levels of the biliary tree. In patients with PSC, both ERCP and MRCP demonstrate multiple bile duct strictures alternating with relatively normal segments.

The bile acid ursodeoxycholic acid (ursodiol) may reduce alkaline phosphatase and serum aminotransferase levels, but histologic improvement has been marginal. High doses (25–30 mg/kg per day) may decrease the risk of colorectal dysplasia and cancer in patients with UC and PSC. Endoscopic stenting may be palliative for cholestasis secondary to bile duct obstruction. Patients with symptomatic disease develop cirrhosis and liver failure over 5–10 years and eventually require liver transplantation. Ten percent of PSC patients develop cholangiocarcinoma and cannot be transplanted. Patients with IBD and PSC are at increased risk of colon cancer and should be surveyed yearly by colonoscopy and biopsy. Pericholangitis is a subset of PSC found in about 30% of IBD patients; it is confined to small bile ducts and is usually benign.

UROLOGIC

The most frequent genitourinary complications are calculi, ureteral obstruction, and fistulas. The highest frequency of nephrolithiasis (10–20%) occurs in patients with CD following small-bowel resection. Calcium oxalate stones develop secondary to hyperoxaluria, which results from increased absorption of dietary oxalate. Normally, dietary calcium combines with luminal oxalate to form insoluble calcium oxalate, which is eliminated in the stool. In patients with ileal dysfunction, however, nonabsorbed fatty acids bind calcium and leave oxalate unbound. The unbound oxalate is then delivered to the colon, where it is readily absorbed, especially in the presence of inflammation.

METABOLIC BONE DISORDERS

Low bone mass occurs in 3%–30% of IBD patients. The risk is increased by glucocorticoids, cyclosporine, methotrexate and total parenteral nutrition (TPN). Malabsorption and inflammation mediated by IL-1, IL-6, and TNF also contribute to low bone density. An increased incidence of hip, spine, wrist, and rib fractures has been noted: 36% in CD and 45% in UC. The absolute risk of an osteoporotic fracture is about 1% per person per year. Fracture rates, particularly in the spine and hip, were highest among the elderly (age >60). One study noted an odds ratio of vertebral fracture to be 1.72 and hip fracture 1.59. The disease severity predicted the risk of a fracture. Only 13% of IBD patients who had a fracture were on any kind of antifracture treatment. Up to 20% of bone mass can be lost per year with chronic glucocorticoid use. The effect is dosage-dependent. Budesonide may also suppress the pituitary-adrenal axis and thus carries a risk of causing osteoporosis.

Osteonecrosis is characterized by death of osteocytes and adipocytes and eventual bone collapse. The pain is aggravated by motion and swelling of the joints. It affects the hips more often than knees and shoulders, and in one series 4.3% of patients developed osteonecrosis within 6 months of starting glucocorticoids. Diagnosis is made by bone scan or MRI, and treatment consists of pain control, cord decompression, and arthroplasty.

THROMBOEMBOLIC DISORDERS

Patients with IBD have an increased risk of both venous and arterial thrombosis even if the disease is not active. Factors responsible for the hypercoagulable state have included abnormalities of the platelet-endothelial interaction, hyperhomocysteinemia, alterations in the coagulation cascade, impaired fibrinolysis, involvement of tissue factor-bearing microvesicles, disruption of the normal coagulation system by autoantibodies, as well as a genetic predisposition. A spectrum of vasculitides involving small, medium, and large vessels has also been observed.

OTHER DISORDERS

More common cardiopulmonary manifestations include endocarditis, myocarditis, pleuropericarditis, and interstitial lung disease. A secondary or reactive amyloidosis can occur in patients with long-standing IBD, especially in patients with CD. Amyloid material is deposited systemically and can cause diarrhea, constipation, and renal failure. The renal disease can be successfully treated with colchicine. Pancreatitis is a rare extraintestinal manifestation of IBD and results from duodenal fistulas; ampullary CD; gallstones; PSC; drugs such as 6-mercaptopurine, azathioprine, or, very rarely, 5-ASA agents; autoimmune pancreatitis; and primary CD of the pancreas.

TABLE 289-6 ORAL 5-ASA PREPARATIONS

Preparation	Formulation	Delivery	Dosing Per Day
Azo-bond			
Sulfasalazine (500 mg) (Azulfadine)	Sulfapyridine-5-ASA	Colon	3–6 g (acute) 2–4 g (maintenance)
Olsalazine (250 mg) (Dipentum)	5-ASA-5-ASA	Colon	1–3 g
Balsalazide (750 mg) (Colazal)	Aminobenzoyl-alanine-5-ASA	Colon	6.75–9 g
Delayed-Release			
Mesalamine (400, 800 mg) (Asacol)	Eudragit S (pH 7)	Distal ileum-colon	2.4–4.8 g (acute) 1.6–4.8 g (maintenance)
Claversal/Mesasal/Salofalk (250, 500 mg)	Eudragit L (pH 6)	Ileum-colon	1.5–3 g (acute) 1.5–3 g (maintenance)
Sustained-Release			
Mesalamine (250, 500, 1000 mg) (Pentasa)	Ethylcellulose microgranules	Stomach-colon	2–4 g (acute) 1.5–4 g (maintenance)
Extended-Release			
Mesalamine (1.2 gm) (under review by the FDA)	MMX mesalamine (SPD476)	Ileum-colon	2.4–4.8 (acute) 2.4–4.8 (maintenance)

℞ INFLAMMATORY BOWEL DISEASE

5-ASA AGENTS The mainstay of therapy for mild to moderate UC and Crohn's colitis is sulfasalazine and the other 5-ASA agents. These agents are effective at inducing remission in both UC and CD and in maintaining remission in UC; it remains unclear whether they have a role in remission maintenance in CD.

Sulfasalazine was originally developed to deliver both antibacterial (sulfapyridine) and anti-inflammatory (5-ASA) therapy into the connective tissues of joints and the colonic mucosa. The molecular structure provides a convenient delivery system to the colon by allowing the intact molecule to pass through the small intestine after only partial absorption, and to be broken down in the colon by bacterial azo reductases that cleave the azo bond linking the sulfa and 5-ASA moieties. Sulfasalazine is effective treatment for mild to moderate UC and Crohn's ileocolitis and colitis, but its high rate of side effects limits its use. Although sulfasalazine is more effective at higher doses, at 6 or 8 g/d up to 30% of patients experience allergic reactions or intolerable side effects such as headache, anorexia, nausea, and vomiting that are attributable to the sulfapyridine moiety. Hypersensitivity reactions, independent of sulfapyridine levels, include rash, fever, hepatitis, agranulocytosis, hypersensitivity pneumonitis, pancreatitis, worsening of colitis, and reversible sperm abnormalities. Sulfasalazine can also impair folate absorption, and patients should be given folic acid supplements.

Newer sulfa-free aminosalicylate preparations deliver increased amounts of the pharmacologically active ingredient of sulfasalazine (5-ASA, mesalamine) to the site of active bowel disease while limiting systemic toxicity. Peroxisome proliferator activated receptor γ (PPAR-γ) may mediate 5-ASA therapeutic action by regulating NF-κB. Sulfa-free aminosalicylate formulations include alternative azo-bonded carriers, 5-ASA dimers, pH-dependent tablets, and continuous-release preparations. Each has the same efficacy as sulfasalazine when equimolar concentrations are used. Olsalazine is composed of two 5-ASA radicals linked by an azo bond, which is split in the colon by bacterial reduction and two 5-ASA molecules are released. Olsalazine is similar in effectiveness to sulfasalazine in treating CD and UC, but up to 17% of patients experience nonbloody diarrhea caused by increased secretion of fluid in the small bowel. Balsalazide contains an azo bond binding mesalamine to the carrier molecule 4-aminobenzoyl-β-alanine; it is effective in the colon. Claversal is an enteric-coated form of 5-ASA that consists of mesalamine surrounded by an acrylic-based polymer resin and a cellulose coating that releases mesalamine at pH >6.0, a level that is present from the mid-jejunum continuously to the distal colon.

Asacol is also an enteric-coated form of mesalamine, but it has a slightly different release pattern, with 5-ASA liberated at pH >7.0. The disintegration of Asacol is variable, with complete breakup of the tablet occurring in many different parts of the gut ranging from the small intestine to the splenic flexure; it has increased gastric residence when taken with a meal.

Asacol is used to induce and maintain remission in UC and to induce remission in CD ileitis, ileocolitis, and colitis, but meta-analyses have not proven 5-ASA medications superior to placebo for the maintenance of remission in CD. Appropriate doses of Asacol and other 5-ASA compounds are shown in **Table 289-6**. Some 50–75% of patients with mild to moderate UC and CD improve when treated with 2 g/d of 5-ASA; the dose response continues up to at least 4.8 g/d. Doses of 1.5–4 g/d maintain remission in 50–75% of patients with UC.

Pentasa is another mesalamine formulation that uses an ethylcellulose coating to allow water absorption into small beads containing the mesalamine. Water dissolves the 5-ASA, which then diffuses out of the bead into the lumen. Disintegration of the capsule occurs in the stomach. The microspheres then disperse throughout the entire gastrointestinal tract from the small intestine through the distal colon in both fasted and fed conditions. Controlled trials of Pentasa and Asacol in active CD demonstrate a 40–60% clinical improvement or remission. 5-ASA agents may be effective in postoperative prophylaxis of CD.

Topical mesalamine enemas are effective in mild-to-moderate distal UC and CD. Clinical response occurs in up to 80% of UC patients with colitis distal to the splenic flexure. Combination therapy with mesalamine in both oral and enema form is more effective than either treatment alone for both distal and extensive UC. Mesalamine suppositories are effective in treating proctitis.

GLUCOCORTICOIDS The majority of patients with moderate to severe UC benefit from oral or parenteral glucocorticoids. Prednisone is usually started at doses of 40–60 mg/d for active UC that is unresponsive to 5-ASA therapy. Parenteral glucocorticoids may be administered as intravenous hydrocortisone, 300 mg/d, or methylprednisolone, 40–60 mg/d. Adrenocorticotropic hormone (ACTH) is occasionally preferred for glucocorticoid-naïve patients despite a risk of adrenal hemorrhage. ACTH has equivalent efficacy to intravenous hydrocortisone in both glucocorticoid-naïve and -experienced CD patients.

Topically applied glucocorticoids are also beneficial for distal colitis and may serve as an adjunct in those who have rectal involvement plus more proximal disease. Hydrocortisone enemas or foam may control active disease, although they have no proven role as maintenance therapy. These glucocorticoids are significantly absorbed from the rectum and can lead to adrenal suppression with prolonged administration. Topical 5-ASA therapy is more effective than topical steroid therapy in the treatment of distal UC.

Glucocorticoids are also effective for treatment of moderate-to-severe CD and induce a 60–70% remission rate compared to a 30% placebo response. The systemic effects of standard glucocorticoid formulations have led to the development of more potent formulations that are less well-absorbed and have increased first-pass metabolism. Controlled ileal-release budesonide has been nearly equal to prednisone for ileocolonic CD with fewer glucocorticoid side effects. Budesonide is used for 2–3 months at a dose of 9 mg/d, then tapered. Budesonide 6 mg/d is effective in reducing relapse rates at 3–6 months but not at 12 months in CD patients with a medically induced remission.

Glucocorticoids play no role in maintenance therapy in either UC or CD. Once clinical remission has been induced, they should be tapered according to the clinical activity, normally at a rate of no more than 5 mg/week. They can usually be tapered to 20 mg/d within 4–5 weeks but often take several months to be discontinued altogether. The side effects are numerous, including fluid retention, abdominal striae, fat redistribution, hyperglycemia, subcapsular cataracts, osteonecrosis, myopathy, emotional disturbances, and withdrawal symptoms. Most of these side effects, aside from osteonecrosis, are related to the dose and duration of therapy.

ANTIBIOTICS Antibiotics have no role in the treatment of active or quiescent UC. However, pouchitis, which occurs in about a third of UC patients after colectomy and IPAA, usually responds to treatment with metronidazole or ciprofloxacin.

Metronidazole is effective in active inflammatory, fistulous, and perianal CD and may prevent recurrence after ileal resection. The most effective dose is 15–20 mg/kg per day in three divided doses; it is usually continued for several months. Common side effects include nausea, metallic taste, and disulfiram-like reaction. Peripheral neuropathy can occur with prolonged administration (several months) and on rare occasions is permanent despite discontinuation. Ciprofloxacin (500 mg bid) is also beneficial for inflammatory, perianal, and fistulous CD. These two antibiotics should be used as second-line drugs in active CD after 5-ASA agents and as first-line drugs in perianal and fistulous CD. Rifaximin has modest activity in CD.

AZATHIOPRINE AND 6-MERCAPTOPURINE Azathioprine and 6-mercaptopurine (6-MP) are purine analogues commonly employed in the management of glucocorticoid-dependent IBD. Azathioprine is rapidly absorbed and converted to 6-MP, which is then metabolized to the active end product, thioinosinic acid, an inhibitor of purine ribonucleotide synthesis and cell proliferation. These agents also inhibit the immune response. Efficacy is seen at 3–4 weeks. Compliance can be monitored by measuring the levels of 6-thioguanine and 6-methyl-mercaptopurine, end products of 6-MP metabolism. Azathioprine (2.0–3.0 mg/kg per day) or 6-MP (1.0–1.5 mg/kg per day) have been employed successfully as glucocorticoid-sparing agents in up to two-thirds of UC and CD patients previously unable to be weaned from glucocorticoids. The role of these immunomodulators as maintenance therapy in UC and CD and for treating active perianal disease and fistulas in CD appears promising. In addition, 6-MP or azathioprine is effective for postoperative prophylaxis of CD.

Although azathioprine and 6-MP are usually well tolerated, pancreatitis occurs in 3–4% of patients, typically presents within the first few weeks of therapy, and is completely reversible when the drug is stopped. Other side effects include nausea, fever, rash, and hepatitis. Bone marrow suppression (particularly leukopenia) is dose-related and often delayed, necessitating regular monitoring of the complete blood cell count (CBC). Additionally, 1 in 300 individuals lacks thiopurine methyltransferase, the enzyme responsible for drug metabolism; an additional 11% of the population are heterozygotes with intermediate enzyme activity. Both are at increased risk of toxicity because of increased accumulation of thioguanine metabolites. Although 6-thioguanine and 6-methylmercaptopurine levels can be followed to determine correct drug dosing and reduce toxicity, weight-based dosing is an acceptable alternative. CBCs and liver function tests should be monitored frequently regardless of dosing strategy. IBD patients treated with azathioprine/6-MP are at a fourfold increased risk of developing a lymphoma. This increased risk could be a result of the medications, the underlying disease, or both.

METHOTREXATE Methotrexate (MTX) inhibits dihydrofolate reductase, resulting in impaired DNA synthesis. Additional anti-inflammatory properties may be related to decreased IL-1 production. Intramuscular or subcutaneous MTX (25 mg/week) is effective in inducing remission and reducing glucocorticoid dosage; 15 mg/week is effective in maintaining remission in active CD. Potential toxicities include leukopenia and hepatic fibrosis, necessitating periodic evaluation of CBCs and liver enzymes. The

role of liver biopsy in patients on long-term MTX is uncertain. Hypersensitivity pneumonitis is a rare but serious complication of therapy.

CYCLOSPORINE Cyclosporine (CSA) is a lipophilic peptide with inhibitory effects on both the cellular and humoral immune systems. CSA blocks the production of IL-2 by T-helper lymphocytes. CSA binds to cyclophilin, and this complex inhibits calcineurin, a cytoplasmic phosphatase enzyme involved in the activation of T cells. CSA also indirectly inhibits B cell function by blocking helper T cells. It has a more rapid onset of action than 6-MP and azathioprine.

CSA is most effective given at 2–4 mg/kg per day intravenously in severe UC that is refractory to intravenous glucocorticoids, with 82% of patients responding. CSA can be an alternative to colectomy. The long-term success of oral CSA is not as dramatic, but if patients are started on 6-MP or azathioprine at the time of hospital discharge, remission can be maintained. Intravenous CSA is effective in 80% of patients with refractory fistulas, but 6-MP or azathioprine must be used to maintain remission. Oral CSA alone is effective only at a higher dose (7.5 mg/kg per day) in active disease but is not effective in maintaining remission without 6-MP/azathioprine. For the 2 mg/kg dose, levels as measured by monoclonal radioimmunoassay or by the high performance liquid chromatography assay should be maintained between 150 and 350 ng/mL.

CSA may cause significant toxicity; renal function should be monitored frequently. Hypertension, gingival hyperplasia, hypertrichosis, paresthesias, tremors, headaches, and electrolyte abnormalities are common side effects. Creatinine elevation calls for dose reduction or discontinuation. Seizures may also complicate therapy, especially if the patient is hypomagnesemic or if serum cholesterol levels are <3.1 mmol/L (<120 mg/dL). Opportunistic infections, most notably *Pneumocystis carinii* pneumonia, may occur with combination immunosuppressive treatment; prophylaxis should be given.

TACROLIMUS Tacrolimus is a macrolide antibiotic with immunomodulatory properties similar to CSA. It is 100 times as potent as CSA and is not dependent on bile or mucosal integrity for absorption. These pharmacologic properties enable tacrolimus to have good oral absorption despite proximal small-bowel Crohn's involvement. It has shown efficacy in children with refractory IBD and in adults with extensive involvement of the small bowel. It is also effective in adults with steroid-dependent or refractory UC and CD as well as refractory fistulizing CD.

ANTI-TNF ANTIBODY TNF is a key inflammatory cytokine and mediator of intestinal inflammation. The expression of TNF is increased in IBD. Infliximab is a chimeric mouse-human monoclonal antibody against TNF that is effective in CD. It blocks TNF in the serum and at the cell surface and probably lyses TNF-producing macrophages and T cells through complement fixation and antibody-dependent cytotoxicity. Of active CD patients refractory to glucocorticoids, 6-MP, or 5-ASA, 65% will respond to intravenous infliximab (5 mg/kg); one-third will enter complete remission. Of the patients who experience an initial response, 40% will maintain remission for at least 1 year with repeated infusions of infliximab every 8 weeks.

Infliximab is also effective in CD patients with refractory perianal and enterocutaneous fistulas, with a 68% response rate (50% reduction in fistula drainage) and a 50% complete remission rate. Reinfusion, typically every 8 weeks, is necessary to continue therapeutic benefits in many patients.

The development of antibodies to infliximab (ATI) is associated with an increased risk of infusion reactions and a decreased response to treatment. Patients who receive on-demand or episodic infusions rather than periodic (every 8 weeks) infusions are more likely to develop ATI. If infliximab is used episodically for flares, patients must use concomitant immunosuppression with AZA, 6-MP, or methotrexate in therapeutic doses to decrease the clinical consequences of immunogenicity of the chimeric antibodies. Moreover, prophylaxis with hydrocortisone before each infusion of infliximab will also decrease the formation of antibodies to infliximab. ATI are generally responsible when the quality of response or the response duration to infliximab infusion decreases. Increasing the dosage to 10 mg/kg may restore the efficacy of the drug.

In the CD and rheumatoid arthritis (RA) trials, six lymphomas were diagnosed in 4148 patient-years of follow-up versus none for 691 placebo patient-years. All lymphomas occurred in patients treated with concomitant immunosuppression. Other morbidities of infliximab include acute infusion reactions, severe serum sickness, and increased risk of infections, particularly reactivation of latent tuberculosis. Rarely, infliximab has been associated with optic neuritis, seizures, new-onset or exacerbation of clinical symptoms, and radiographic evidence of central nervous system demyelinating disorders, including multiple sclerosis. It may exacerbate symptoms in patients with New York Heart Association functional class III/IV heart failure.

Infliximab has also shown efficacy in UC. In two large randomized, placebo-controlled trials, 37–49% of patients responded to infliximab and 22 and 20% of patients were able to maintain remission after 30 and 54 weeks, respectively. Patients received infliximab at 0, 2, and 6 weeks and then every 8 weeks until the end of the study.

Nutritional Therapies Dietary antigens may stimulate the mucosal immune response. Patients with active CD respond to bowel rest, along with total parenteral nutrition or TPN. Bowel rest and TPN are as effective as glucocorticoids at inducing remission of active CD but are not effective as maintenance therapy. Enteral nutrition in the form of elemental or peptide-based preparations are also as effective as glucocorticoids or TPN, but these diets are not palatable. Enteral diets may provide the small intestine with nutrients vital to cell growth and do not have the complications of TPN. In contrast to CD, dietary intervention does not reduce inflammation in UC. Standard medical management of UC and CD is shown in **Fig. 289-9**.

FIGURE 289-9 Medical management of IBD.

NEWER IMMUNOSUPPRESSIVE AGENTS Thalidomide has been shown to inhibit TNF production by monocytes and other cells. Thalidomide is effective in glucocorticoid-refractory and fistulous CD, but randomized controlled trials are needed.

Adalimumab is a recombinant human monoclonal IgG1 antibody containing only human peptide sequences and is injected subcutaneously. Adalimumab binds TNF-α and neutralizes its function by blocking the interaction between TNF and its cell-surface receptor. Therefore, it seems to have a similar mechanism of action to infliximab but with less immunogenicity. Adalimumab has recently been approved for treatment of CD. It has shown promise in treating CD in several trials and may be useful in infliximab-allergic patients.

Certolizumab Pegol is a PEGylated form of an anti-TNF antibody administered subcutaneously once monthly. Subcutaneous Certolizumab Pegol was effective for induction of clinical response in patients with active inflammatory CD.

SURGICAL THERAPY Ulcerative Colitis Nearly half of patients with extensive chronic UC undergo surgery within the first 10 years of their illness. The indications for surgery are listed in **Table 289-7**. Morbidity is about 20% in elective, 30% for urgent, and 40% for emergency proctocolectomy. The risks are primarily hemorrhage, contamination and sepsis, and neural injury. The operation of choice is an IPAA.

Because UC is a mucosal disease, the rectal mucosa can be dissected and removed down to the dentate line of the anus or about 2 cm proximal to it. The ileum is fashioned into a pouch that serves as a neorectum. This ileal pouch is then sutured circumferentially to the anus in an end-to-end

fashion. If performed carefully, this operation preserves the anal sphincter and maintains continence. The overall operative morbidity is 10%, with the major complication being bowel obstruction. Pouch failure necessitating conversion to permanent ileostomy occurs in 5–10% of patients. Some inflamed rectal mucosa is usually left behind, and thus endoscopic surveillance is necessary. Primary dysplasia of the ileal mucosa of the pouch has occurred rarely.

Patients with IPAAs usually have about six to eight bowel movements a day. On validated quality-of-life indices, they report better performance in sports and sexual activities than ileostomy patients. The most frequent late complication of IPAA is pouchitis in about one-third of patients with UC. This syndrome consists of increased stool frequency, watery stools, cramping, urgency, nocturnal leakage of stool, arthralgias, malaise, and fever. Pouch biopsies may distinguish true pouchitis from underlying CD. Al-

TABLE 289-7 INDICATIONS FOR SURGERY

Ulcerative Colitis	Crohn's Disease
Intractable disease	**Small Intestine**
Fulminant disease	Stricture and obstruction unresponsive
Toxic megacolon	to medical therapy
Colonic perforation	Massive hemorrhage
Massive colonic hemorrhage	Refractory fistula
Extracolonic disease	Abscess
Colonic obstruction	**Colon and Rectum**
Colon cancer prophylaxis	Intractable disease
Colon dysplasia or cancer	Fulminant disease
	Perianal disease unresponsive to
	medical therapy
	Refractory fistula
	Colonic obstruction
	Cancer prophylaxis
	Colon dysplasia or cancer

though pouchitis usually responds to antibiotics, 3–5% of patients are refractory and require pouch take-down. A highly concentrated probiotic preparation with four strains of *Lactobacillus*, three strains of *Bifidobacterium*, and one strain of *Streptococcus salivarius* can prevent onset of pouchitis when taken daily.

Crohn's Disease   Most patients with CD require at least one operation in their lifetime. The need for surgery is related to duration of disease and the site of involvement. Patients with small-bowel disease have an 80% chance of requiring surgery. Those with colitis alone have a 50% chance. Surgery is an option only when medical treatment has failed or complications dictate its necessity. The indications for surgery are shown in Table 289-7.

Small Intestinal Disease   Because CD is chronic and recurrent, with no clear surgical cure, as little intestine as possible is resected. Current surgical alternatives for treatment of obstructing CD include resection of the diseased segment and strictureplasty. Surgical resection of the diseased segment is the most frequently performed operation, and in most cases primary anastomosis can be done to restore continuity. If much of the small bowel has already been resected and the strictures are short, with intervening areas of normal mucosa, strictureplasties should be done to avoid a functionally insufficient length of bowel. The strictured area of intestine is incised longitudinally and the incision sutured transversely, thus widening the narrowed area. Complications of strictureplasty include prolonged ileus, hemorrhage, fistula, abscess, leak, and restricture.

Colorectal Disease   A greater percentage of patients with Crohn's colitis require surgery for intractability, fulminant disease, and anorectal disease. Several alternatives are available, ranging from the use of a temporary loop ileostomy to resection of segments of diseased colon or even the entire colon and rectum. For patients with segmental involvement, segmental colon resection with primary anastomosis can be performed. In 20–25% of patients with extensive colitis, the rectum is spared sufficiently to consider rectal preservation. Most surgeons believe that an IPAA is contraindicated in CD due to the high incidence of pouch failure. A diverting colostomy may help heal severe perianal disease or rectovaginal fistulas, but disease almost always recurs with reanastomosis. These patients often require a total proctocolectomy and ileostomy.

INFLAMMATORY BOWEL DISEASE AND PREGNANCY

Patients with quiescent UC and CD have normal fertility rates; the fallopian tubes can be scarred by the inflammatory process of CD, especially on the right side because of the proximity of the terminal ileum. In addition, perirectal, perineal, and rectovaginal abscesses and fistulae can result in dyspareunia. Infertility in men can be caused by sulfasalazine but reverses when treatment is stopped.

In mild or quiescent UC and CD, fetal outcome is nearly normal. Spontaneous abortions, stillbirths, and developmental defects are increased with increased disease activity, not medications. The courses of CD and UC during pregnancy mostly correlate with disease activity at the time of conception. Patients should be in remission for 6 months before conceiving. Most CD patients can deliver vaginally, but cesarean section may be the preferred route of delivery for patients with anorectal and perirectal abscesses and fistulas to reduce the likelihood of fistulas developing or extending into the episiotomy scar.

Sulfasalazine, mesalamine, and balsalazide are safe for use in pregnancy and nursing, but additional folate supplementation must be given with sulfasalazine. Topical 5-ASA agents are also safe during pregnancy and nursing. Glucocorticoids are generally safe for use during pregnancy and are indicated for patients with moderate to severe disease activity. The amount of glucocorticoids received by the nursing infant is minimal. The safest antibiotics to use for CD in pregnancy for short periods of time (weeks, not months) are ampicillin and cephalosporin. Metronidazole can be used in the second or third trimester. Ciprofloxacin causes cartilage lesions in immature animals and should be avoided because of the absence of data on its effects on growth and development in humans.

6-MP and azathioprine pose minimal or no risk during pregnancy, but experience is limited. If the patient cannot be weaned from the drug or has an exacerbation that requires 6-MP/azathioprine during pregnancy, she should continue the drug with informed consent. Their effects during nursing are unknown.

Little data exist on CSA in pregnancy. In a small number of patients with severe IBD treated with intravenous CSA during pregnancy, 80% of pregnancies were successfully completed without development of renal toxicity, congenital malformations, or developmental defects. However, because of the lack of data, CSA should probably be avoided unless the patient would otherwise require surgery. Methotrexate is contraindicated in pregnancy and nursing. No increased risk of stillbirths, miscarriages, or spontaneous abortions has been seen with infliximab.

Surgery in UC should be performed only for emergency indications, including severe hemorrhage, perforation, and megacolon refractory to medical therapy. Total colectomy and ileostomy carry a 50–60% risk of postoperative spontaneous abortion. Fetal mortality is also high in CD requiring surgery. Patients with IPAAs have increased nighttime stool frequency during pregnancy that resolves post-partum. Transient small-bowel obstruction or ileus has been noted in up to 8% of patients with ileostomies.

CANCER IN INFLAMMATORY BOWEL DISEASE

ULCERATIVE COLITIS

Patients with long-standing UC are at increased risk for developing colonic epithelial dysplasia and carcinoma (Fig. 289-9).

The risk of neoplasia in chronic UC increases with duration and extent of disease. The risk of cancer rises 0.5–1% per year after 8–10 years of disease in patients with pancolitis. The only prospective surveillance study reported a lower rate of cancer; 2.5% at 20 years of disease, 7.6% at 30 years of disease, and 10.8% at 40 years. The rates of colon cancer are higher than in the general population, and colonoscopic surveillance is the standard of care.

Annual or biennial colonoscopy with multiple biopsies is recommended for patients with >8–10 years of pancolitis or 12–15 years of left-sided colitis and has been widely employed to screen and survey for subsequent dysplasia and carcinoma. Risk factors for cancer in UC include long-duration disease, extensive disease, family history of colon cancer, PSC, a colon stricture, and the presence of postinflammatory pseudopolyps on colonoscopy.

CROHN'S DISEASE

Risk factors for developing cancer in Crohn's colitis are long-duration and extensive disease, bypassed colon segments, colon strictures, PSC, and family history of colon cancer. The cancer risks in CD and UC are probably equivalent for similar extent and duration of disease. In patients with extensive Crohn's colitis, 22% developed dysplasia or cancer by the fourth surveillance exam after a negative screening colonoscopy. Thus, the same endoscopic surveillance strategy used for UC is recommended for patients with chronic Crohn's colitis. A pediatric colonoscope can be used to pass narrow strictures in CD patients, but surgery should be considered in symptomatic patients with impassable strictures.

MANAGEMENT OF DYSPLASIA AND CANCER

Dysplasia can be flat or polypoid. If flat high-grade dysplasia (HGD) is encountered on colonoscopic surveillance, the usual treatment for UC is colectomy and for CD is either colectomy or segmental resection. If flat low-grade dysplasia (LGD) is found (Fig. 289-10), most investigators recommend immediate colectomy. Adenomas may occur coincidently in UC and CD patients with chronic colitis and can be removed endoscopically provided that biopsies of the surrounding mucosa are free of dysplasia.

IBD patients are also at greater risk for other malignancies. Patients with CD may have an increased risk of non-Hodgkin's lymphoma, leukemia, and myelodysplastic syndromes. Severe chronic, complicated perianal disease in CD patients may be associated with an increased risk of cancer in the lower rectum and anal canal (squamous cell cancers). Although the absolute risk of small-bowel adenocarcinoma in

FIGURE 289-10 Medium power view of low-grade dysplasia in a patient with chronic ulcerative colitis. Low-grade dysplastic crypts are interspersed among regenerating crypts. (*Courtesy of Dr. R Odze, Division of Gastrointestinal Pathology, Department of Pathology, Brigham and Women's Hospital, Boston, Massachusetts; with permission.*)

CD is low (2.2% at 25 years in one study), patients with long-standing, extensive, small-bowel disease should undergo screening.

QUALITY OF LIFE IN INFLAMMATORY BOWEL DISEASE

The assessment of health-related quality of life plays an important role in the evaluation and treatment of IBD patients. Although clinical trials have generally relied upon traditional disease activity indices such as the Crohn's Disease Activity Index to measure therapeutic efficacy, these measures do not reflect quality of life. The Inflammatory Bowel Disease Questionnaire is a validated, disease-specific instrument that has been used to measure quality of life. It is a 32-item questionnaire

290 Irritable Bowel Syndrome
Chung Owyang

Irritable bowel syndrome (IBS) is a functional bowel disorder characterized by abdominal pain or discomfort and altered bowel habits in the absence of detectable structural abnormalities. No clear diagnostic markers exist for IBS, thus the diagnosis of the disorder is based on clinical presentation. In 2006, the Rome II criteria for the diagnosis of IBS were revised (Table 290-1). IBS is one of the most common conditions encountered in clinical practice but one of the least well understood. Throughout the world, about 10–20% of adults and adolescents have symptoms consistent with IBS, and most studies show a female predominance. IBS symptoms tend to come and go over time and often overlap with other functional disorders such as fibromyalgia, headache, backache, and genitourinary symptoms. Severity of symptoms varies and can significantly impair quality of life, resulting in high health care costs. Advances in basic, mechanistic, and clinical investigations have improved our understanding of this disorder and its physiologic and psychosocial determinants. Altered gastrointestinal (GI) motility, visceral hyperalgesia, disturbance of brain-gut interaction, abnormal central processing, autonomic and hormonal events, genetic and environmental factors, and psychosocial disturbances are variably involved, depending on the individual. This progress may result in improved methods of treatment.

CLINICAL FEATURES

IBS is a disorder that affects all ages, although most patients have their first symptoms before age 45. Older individuals have a lower reporting frequency. Women are diagnosed with IBS two to three times as often

that measures global function, systemic and bowel symptoms, functional and social impairment, and emotional function. When compared to the general population, IBD patients have an impaired quality of life in all six categories. The most frequent concerns of UC patients are having an ostomy bag, developing cancer, effects of medication, the uncertain nature of the disease, and having surgery. The most frequent concerns of CD patients are the uncertain nature of the disease, impaired energy level, effects of medication, the need for surgery, and having an ostomy bag.

FURTHER READINGS

ABREU MT et al: Mutations in NOD2 are associated with fibrostenosing disease in patients with Crohn's disease. Gastroenterology 123(3):679, 2002

AUSTIN G et al: Positive and negative predictive values: Use of inflammatory bowel disease serologic markers. Am J Gastroenterology 101:413, 2006

BAUMGART DC, SANDBORN WJ: Inflammatory bowel disease: Clinical aspects and established and evolving therapies. Lancet 369:1641, 2007

ITZKOWITZ S et al: Consensus conference: Colorectal cancer screening and surveillance in inflammatory bowel disease. Inflamm Bowel Dis 11(3):314, 2005

KORNBLUTH A et al: Ulcerative colitis practice guidelines in adults. Am J Gastroenterol 99(7):1371, 2004

LOFTUS EV: Clinical epidemiology of inflammatory bowel disease: Incidence, prevalence, and environmental influences. Gastroenterology 126:1504, 2004

RUTGEERTS P et al: Optimizing anti-TNF treatment in inflammatory bowel disease. Gastroenterology 126:1593, 2004

RUTTER MD et al: Thirty-year analysis of a colonoscopic surveillance program for neoplasia in ulcerative colitis. Gastroenterology 130:1030, 2006

as men and make up 80% of the population with severe IBS. As indicated in Table 290-1, pain or abdominal discomfort is a key symptom for the diagnosis of IBS. These symptoms should be improved with defecation and/or have their onset associated with a change in frequency or form of stool. Painless diarrhea or constipation does not fulfill the diagnostic criteria to be classified as IBS. Supportive symptoms that are not part of the diagnostic criteria include defecation straining, urgency or a feeling of incomplete bowel movement, passing mucus, and bloating.

Abdominal Pain According to the current IBS diagnostic criteria, abdominal pain or discomfort is a prerequisite clinical feature of IBS. Abdominal pain in IBS is highly variable in intensity and location. Pain in IBS is localized to the hypogastrium in 25%, the right side in 20%, to the left side in 20%, and the epigastrium in 10% of patients. It is frequently episodic and crampy, but it may be superimposed on a background of constant ache. Pain may be mild enough to be ignored or it may interfere with daily activities. Despite this, malnutrition due to inadequate

TABLE 290-1 DIAGNOSTIC CRITERIA FOR IRRITABLE BOWEL SYNDROME[a]

Recurrent abdominal pain or discomfort[b] at least 3 days per month in the last 3 months associated with *two or more* of the following:
1. Improvement with defecation
2. Onset associated with a change in frequency of stool
3. Onset associated with a change in form (appearance) of stool

[a]Criteria fulfilled for the last 3 months with symptom onset at least 6 months prior to diagnosis.
[b]Discomfort means an uncomfortable sensation not described as pain. In pathophysiology research and clinical trials, a pain/discomfort frequency of at least 2 days a week during screening evaluation is required for subject eligibility.
Source: Adapted from Longstreth et al.

caloric intake is exceedingly rare with IBS. Sleep deprivation is also unusual because abdominal pain is almost uniformly present only during waking hours. However, patients with severe IBS frequently wake repeatedly during the night; thus, nocturnal pain is a poor discriminating factor between organic and functional bowel disease. Pain is often exacerbated by eating or emotional stress and improved by passage of flatus or stools. In addition, female patients with IBS commonly report worsening symptoms during the premenstrual and menstrual phases.

Altered Bowel Habits Alteration in bowel habits is the most consistent clinical feature in IBS. The most common pattern is constipation alternating with diarrhea, usually with one of these symptoms predominating. At first, constipation may be episodic, but eventually it becomes continuous and increasingly intractable to treatment with laxatives. Stools are usually hard with narrowed caliber, possibly reflecting excessive dehydration caused by prolonged colonic retention and spasm. Most patients also experience a sense of incomplete evacuation, thus leading to repeated attempts at defecation in a short time span. Patients whose predominant symptom is constipation may have weeks or months of constipation interrupted with brief periods of diarrhea. In other patients, diarrhea may be the predominant symptom. Diarrhea resulting from IBS usually consists of small volumes of loose stools. Most patients have stool volumes of < 200 mL. Nocturnal diarrhea does not occur in IBS. Diarrhea may be aggravated by emotional stress or eating. Stool may be accompanied by passage of large amounts of mucus; hence, the term *mucous colitis* has been used to describe IBS. This is a misnomer, since inflammation is not present. Bleeding is not a feature of IBS unless hemorrhoids are present, and malabsorption or weight loss does not occur.

Bowel pattern subtypes are highly unstable. In a patient population with ~33% prevalence rates of IBS-diarrhea predominant (IBS-D), IBS-constipation predominant (IBS-C), and IBS-mixed (IBS-M) forms, 75% of patients change subtypes and 29% switch between IBS-C and IBS-D over 1 year. The heterogeneity and variable natural history of bowel habits in IBS increase the difficulty of conducting pathophysiology studies and clinical trials.

Gas and Flatulence Patients with IBS frequently complain of abdominal distention and increased belching or flatulence, all of which they attribute to increased gas. Although some patients with these symptoms actually may have a larger amount of gas, quantitative measurements reveal that most patients who complain of increased gas generate no more than a normal amount of intestinal gas. Most IBS patients have impaired transit and tolerance of intestinal gas loads. In addition, patients with IBS tend to reflux gas from the distal to the more proximal intestine, which may explain the belching.

Upper Gastrointestinal Symptoms Between 25 and 50% of patients with IBS complain of dyspepsia, heartburn, nausea, and vomiting. This suggests that other areas of the gut apart from the colon may be involved. Prolonged ambulant recordings of small-bowel motility in patients with IBS show a high incidence of abnormalities in the small bowel during the diurnal (waking) period; nocturnal motor patterns are not different from those of healthy controls. The overlap between dyspepsia and IBS is great. The prevalence of IBS is higher among patients with dyspepsia (31.7%) than among those who reported no symptoms of dyspepsia (7.9%). Conversely, among patients with IBS, 55.6% reported symptoms of dyspepsia. In addition the functional abdominal symptoms can change over time. Those with predominant dyspepsia or IBS can flux between the two. Thus it is conceivable that functional dyspepsia and IBS are two manifestations of a single, more extensive digestive system disorder. Furthermore, IBS symptoms are prevalent in noncardiac chest pain patients, suggesting overlap with other functional gut disorders.

PATHOPHYSIOLOGY

The pathogenesis of IBS is poorly understood, although roles of abnormal gut motor and sensory activity, central neural dysfunction, psychological disturbances, stress, and luminal factors have been proposed.

Studies of colonic myoelectrical and motor activity under unstimulated conditions have not shown consistent abnormalities in IBS. In contrast, colonic motor abnormalities are more prominent under stimulated conditions in IBS. IBS patients may exhibit increased rectosigmoid motor activity for up to 3 h after eating. Similarly, inflation of rectal balloons both in IBS-D and IBS-C patients leads to marked distention-evoked contractile activity, which may be prolonged. Recordings from the transverse, descending, and sigmoid colon showed that the motility index and peak amplitude of high-amplitude propagating contractions (HAPCs) in diarrhea-prone IBS patients were greatly increased compared to those in healthy subjects and were associated with rapid colonic transit and accompanied by abdominal pain.

As with studies of motor activity, IBS patients frequently exhibit exaggerated sensory responses to visceral stimulation. Postprandial pain has been temporally related to entry of the food bolus into the cecum in 74% of patients. Rectal balloon inflation produces nonpainful and painful sensations at lower volumes in IBS patients than in healthy controls without altering rectal tension, suggestive of visceral afferent dysfunction in IBS. Similar studies show gastric and esophageal hypersensitivity in patients with nonulcer dyspepsia and noncardiac chest pain, raising the possibility that these conditions have a similar pathophysiologic basis. Lipids lower the thresholds for the first sensation of gas, discomfort, and pain in IBS patients. Furthermore, IBS patients have an increased area of referred pain after lipid ingestion that was not observed in healthy individuals. Hence, postprandial symptoms in IBS patients may be explained in part by a nutrient-dependent exaggerated sensory component of the gastrocolonic response. In contrast to enhanced gut sensitivity, IBS patients do not exhibit heightened sensitivity elsewhere in the body. Thus, the afferent pathway disturbances in IBS appear to be selective for visceral innervation with sparing of somatic pathways. The mechanisms responsible for visceral hypersensitivity are still under investigation. It has been proposed that these exaggerated responses may be due to: (1) increased end-organ sensitivity with recruitment of "silent" nociceptors; (2) spinal hyperexcitability with activation of nitric oxide and possibly other neurotransmitters; (3) endogenous (cortical and brainstem) modulation of caudad nociceptive transmission; and (4) over time, the possible development of long-term hyperalgesia due to development of neuroplasticity, resulting in permanent or semipermanent changes in neural responses to chronic or recurrent visceral stimulation (Table 290-2).

The role of central nervous system (CNS) factors in the pathogenesis of IBS is strongly suggested by the clinical association of emotional disorders and stress with symptom exacerbation and the therapeutic response to therapies that act on cerebral cortical sites. Functional brain imaging studies such as MRI have shown that in response to distal colonic stimulation, the mid-cingulate cortex, a brain region concerned with attention processes and response selection, shows greater activation in IBS patients. Modulation of this region is associated with changes in the subjective unpleasantness of pain. In addition, IBS patients also show preferential activation of the prefrontal lobe, which contains a vigilance network within the brain that increases alertness. These may represent a form of cerebral dysfunction leading to the increased perception of visceral pain.

Abnormal psychiatric features are recorded in up to 80% of IBS patients, especially in referral centers; however, no single psychiatric diagnosis predominates. Most of these patients demonstrated exaggerated symptoms in response to visceral distention, and this abnormality persists even after exclusion of psychological factors. Psychological factors

TABLE 290-2	PROPOSED MECHANISMS FOR VISCERAL HYPERSENSITIVITY
End-organ sensitivity	Long-term hyperalgesia
"Silent" nociceptors	Tonic cortical regulation
CNS modulation	Neuroplasticity
Cortex	
Brainstem	

Note: CNS, central nervous system.

FIGURE 290-1 Therapeutic targets for irritable bowel syndrome. Patients with mild to moderate symptoms usually have intermittent symptoms that correlate with altered gut physiology. Treatments include gut-acting pharmacologic agents such as antispasmodics, antidiarrheals, fiber supplements, and gut serotonin modulators. Patients who have severe symptoms usually have constant pain and psychosocial difficulties. This group of patients is best managed with antidepressants and other psychosocial treatments. CNS, central nervous system; ENS, enteric nervous system.

influence pain thresholds in IBS patients, as stress alters sensory thresholds. An association between prior sexual or physical abuse and development of IBS has been reported. The pathophysiologic relationship between IBS and sexual or physical abuse is unknown. Sexual abuse is not associated with lower pain threshold in IBS patients.

Thus, patients with IBS frequently demonstrate increased motor reactivity of the colon and small bowel to a variety of stimuli and altered visceral sensation associated with lowered sensation thresholds. These may result from CNS–enteric nervous system dysregulation (Fig. 290-1).

IBS may be induced by GI infection. In an investigation of 544 patients with confirmed bacterial gastroenteritis, one-quarter developed IBS subsequently. Conversely, about a third of IBS patients experienced an acute "gastroenteritis-like" illness at the onset of their chronic IBS symptomatology. This group of "postinfective" IBS occurs more commonly in females and affects younger rather than older patients and those who have a protracted acute diarrheal illness. The microbes involved in the initial infection are *Campylobacter*, *Salmonella*, and *Shigella*. Those patients with *Campylobacter* infection who are toxin-positive are more likely to develop postinfective IBS. Increased rectal mucosal enteroendocrine cells, T lymphocytes, and increased gut permeability are acute changes following *Campylobacter* enteritis that could persist for more than a year and may contribute to postinfective IBS.

The serotonin (5HT)-containing enterochromaffin cells in the colon are increased in a subset of IBS-D patients compared to healthy individuals or patients with ulcerative colitis. Furthermore, postprandial plasma 5HT plasma levels were significantly higher in this group of patients compared to healthy controls. Since serotonin plays an important role in the regulation of GI motility and visceral perception, the increased release of serotonin may contribute to the postprandial symptoms of these patients and provides a rationale for the use of serotonin antagonists in the treatment of this disorder.

APPROACH TO THE PATIENT:
Irritable Bowel Syndrome

Because IBS is a disorder for which no pathognomonic abnormalities have been identified, its diagnosis relies on recognition of positive clinical features and elimination of other organic diseases. A careful history and physical examination are frequently helpful in establishing the diagnosis. Clinical features suggestive of IBS include the following: recurrence of lower abdominal pain with altered bowel habits over a period of time without progressive deterioration, onset of symptoms during periods of stress or emotional upset, absence of other systemic symptoms such as fever and weight loss, and small-volume stool without any evidence of blood.

On the other hand, the appearance of the disorder for the first time in old age, progressive course from time of onset, persistent diarrhea after a 48-h fast, and presence of nocturnal diarrhea or steatorrheal stools argue against the diagnosis of IBS.

Because the major symptoms of IBS—abdominal pain, abdominal bloating, and alteration in bowel habits—are common complaints of many GI organic disorders, the list of differential diagnoses is a long one. The quality, location, and timing of pain may be helpful to suggest specific disorders. Pain due to IBS that occurs in the epigastric or periumbilical area must be differentiated from biliary tract disease, peptic ulcer disorders, intestinal ischemia, and carcinoma of the stomach and pancreas. If pain occurs mainly in the lower abdomen, the possibility of diverticular disease of the colon, inflammatory bowel disease (including ulcerative colitis and Crohn's disease), and carcinoma of the colon must be considered. Postprandial pain accompanied by bloating, nausea, and vomiting suggests gastroparesis or partial intestinal obstruction. Intestinal infestation with *Giardia lamblia* or other parasites may cause similar symptoms. When diarrhea is the major complaint, the possibility of lactase deficiency, laxative abuse, malabsorption, celiac sprue, hyperthyroidism, inflammatory bowel disease, and infectious diarrhea must be ruled out. On the other hand, constipation may be a side effect of many different drugs, such as anticholinergic, antihypertensive, and antidepressant medications. Endocrinopathies such as hypothyroidism and hypoparathyroidism must also be considered in the differential diagnosis of constipation, particularly if other systemic signs or symptoms of these endocrinopathies are present. In addition, acute intermittent porphyria and lead poisoning may present in a fashion similar to IBS, with painful constipation as the major complaint. These possibilities are suspected on the basis of their clinical presentations and are confirmed by appropriate serum and urine tests.

Few tests are required for patients who have typical IBS symptoms and no alarm features. Unnecessary investigations may be costly and even harmful. The American Gastroenterological Association has delineated factors to be considered when determining the aggressiveness of the diagnostic evaluation. These include the duration of symptoms, the change in symptoms over time, the age and sex of the patient, the referral status of the patient, prior diagnostic studies, a family history of colorectal malignancy, and the degree of psychosocial dysfunction. Thus, a younger individual with mild symptoms requires a minimal diagnostic evaluation, while an older person or an individual with rapidly progressive symptoms should undergo a more thorough exclusion of organic disease. Most patients should have a complete blood count and sigmoidoscopic examination; in addition, stool specimens should be examined for ova and parasites in those who have diarrhea. In those >40 years, an air-contrast barium enema or colonoscopy should also be performed. If the main symptoms are diarrhea and increased gas, the possibility of lactase deficiency should be ruled out with a hydrogen breath test or with evaluation after a 3-week lactose-free diet. Some patients with IBS-D may have undiagnosed celiac sprue. Because the symptoms of celiac sprue respond to a gluten-free diet, testing for celiac sprue in IBS may prevent years of morbidity and attendant expense. Decision-analysis studies show that serology testing for celiac sprue in patients with IBS-D has an acceptable cost when the prevalence of celiac sprue is >1% and is the dominant strategy when the prevalence is >8%. In patients with concurrent symptoms of dyspepsia, upper GI radiographs or esophagogastroduodenoscopy may be advisable. In patients with postprandial right upper quadrant pain, an ultrasonogram of the gallbladder should be obtained. Laboratory features that argue against IBS include evidence of anemia, elevated sedimentation rate, presence of leukocytes or blood in stool, and stool volume >200–300 mL/d. These findings would necessitate other diagnostic considerations.

℞ IRRITABLE BOWEL SYNDROME

PATIENT COUNSELING AND DIETARY ALTERATIONS Reassurance and careful explanation of the functional nature of the disorder and of how to avoid obvious food precipitants are important first steps in patient counseling and dietary change. Occasionally, a meticulous dietary history may reveal substances (such as coffee, disaccharides, legumes, and cabbage) that aggravate symptoms. Excessive fructose and artificial sweeteners, such as sorbitol or mannitol, may cause diarrhea, bloating, cramping or flatulence. As a therapeutic trial, patients should be encouraged to eliminate any foodstuffs that appear to produce symptoms. However patients should avoid nutritionally depleted diets.

Stool-Bulking Agents High-fiber diets and bulking agents, such as bran or hydrophilic colloid, are frequently used in treating IBS. Studies suggest that dietary fiber has multiple effects on colonic physiology. The water-holding action of fibers may contribute to increased stool bulk because of the ability of fiber to increase fecal output of bacteria. Fiber also speeds up colonic transit in most persons. In diarrhea-prone patients, whole-colonic transit is faster than average; however, dietary fiber can delay transit. Furthermore, because of their hydrophilic properties, stool-bulking agents bind water and thus prevent both excessive hydration or dehydration of stool. The latter observation may explain the clinical experience that a high-fiber diet relieves diarrhea in some IBS patients. More recently, fiber supplementation with psyllium has been shown to reduce perception of rectal distention, indicating that fiber may have positive affect on visceral afferent function.

The beneficial effects of dietary fiber on colonic physiology suggest that dietary fiber should be an effective treatment for IBS patients, but controlled trials of dietary fiber have produced variable results. This is not surprising since IBS is a heterogeneous disorder, with some patients being constipated and other having predominant diarrhea. Most investigations report increases in stool weight, decreases in colonic transit times, and improvement in constipation. Others have noted benefits in patients with alternating diarrhea and constipation, pain, and bloating. However, most studies observe no responses in patients with diarrhea- or pain-predominant IBS. It is possible that different fiber preparations may have dissimilar effects on selected symptoms in IBS. A cross-over comparison of different fiber preparations found that psyllium produced greater improvements in stool pattern and abdominal pain than bran. Furthermore psyllium preparations tend to produce less bloating and distention. Despite the equivocal data regarding efficacy, most gastroenterologists consider stool-bulking agents worth trying in patients with IBS-C.

Antispasmodics Clinicians have observed that anticholinergic drugs may provide temporary relief for symptoms such as painful cramps related to intestinal spasm. Although controlled clinical trials have produced mixed results, evidence generally supports beneficial effects of anticholinergic drugs for pain. A meta-analysis of 26 double-blind clinical trials of antispasmodic agents in IBS reported better global improvement (62%) and abdominal pain reductions (64%) compared to placebo (35% and 45%, respectively), suggesting efficacy in some patients. The drugs are most effective when prescribed in anticipation of predictable pain. Physiologic studies demonstrate that anticholinergic drugs inhibit the gastrocolic reflex; hence, postprandial pain is best managed by giving antispasmodics 30 min before meals so that effective blood levels are achieved shortly before the anticipated onset of pain. Most anticholinergics contain natural belladonna alkaloids, which may cause xerostomia, urinary hesitancy and retention, blurred vision, and drowsiness. They should be used in the elderly with caution. Some physicians prefer to use synthetic anticholinergics such as dicyclomine that have less effect on mucous membrane secretions and produce fewer undesirable side effects.

Antidiarrheal Agents Peripherally acting opiate-based agents are the initial therapy of choice for IBS-D. Physiologic studies demonstrate increases in segmenting colonic contractions, delays in fecal transit, increases in anal pressures, and reductions in rectal perception with these drugs. When diarrhea is severe, especially in the painless diarrhea variant of IBS, small doses of loperamide, 2–4 mg every 4–6 h up to a maximum of 12 g/d, can be prescribed. These agents are less addictive than paregoric, codeine, or tincture of opium. In general, the intestines do not become tolerant of the antidiarrheal effect of opiates, and increasing doses are not required to maintain antidiarrheal potency. These agents are most useful if taken before anticipated stressful events that are known to cause diarrhea. Another anti-diarrhea agent that may be used in IBS patients is the bile acid binder cholestyramine resin.

Antidepressant Drugs In addition to their mood-elevating effects, antidepressant medications have several physiologic effects that suggest they may be beneficial in IBS. In IBS-D patients, the tricyclic antidepressant imipramine slows jejunal migrating motor complex transit propagation and delays orocecal and whole-gut transit, indicative of a motor inhibitory effect. Some studies also suggest that tricyclic agents may alter visceral afferent neural function.

A number of studies indicate that tricyclic antidepressants may be effective in some IBS patients. In a 2-month study of desipramine, abdominal pain improved in 86% of patients compared to 59% given placebo. Another study of desipramine in 28 IBS patients showed improvement in stool frequency, diarrhea, pain, and depression. When stratified according to the predominant symptoms, improvements were observed in IBS-D patients with no improvement being noted in IBS-C patients. The beneficial effects of the tricyclic compounds in the treatment of IBS appear to be independent of their effects on depression. The therapeutic benefits for the bowel symptoms occur faster and at a lower dosage. The efficacy of antidepressant agents in other chemical classes in the management of IBS is less well-evaluated. In contrast to tricyclic agents, the selective serotonin reuptake inhibitor (SSRI) paroxetine accelerates orocecal transit, raising the possibility that this drug class may be useful in IBS-C patients. The SSRI citalopram blunts perception of rectal distention and reduces the magnitude of the gastrocolonic response in healthy volunteers. A small placebo-controlled study of citalopram in IBS patients reported reductions in pain. Mianserin, with serotonin 5-HT2 and 5-HT3 receptor antagonist and α_2-adrenoceptor antagonist effects, reduced pain, distress, and functional disability compared to placebo. Despite these preliminary results, the efficacy of SSRIs in the treatment of IBS needs further confirmation.

Antiflatulence Therapy The management of excessive gas is seldom satisfactory, except when there is obvious aerophagia or disaccharidase deficiency. Patients should be advised to eat slowly and not chew gum or drink carbonated beverages. Bloating may decrease if an associated gut syndrome such as IBS or constipation is improved. If bloating is accompanied by diarrhea and worsens after ingesting dairy products, fresh fruits, vegetables, or juices, further investigation or a dietary exclusion trial may be worthwhile. Avoiding flatogenic foods, exercising, losing excess weight, and taking activated charcoal are safe but unproven remedies. Data regarding the use of surfactants such as simethicone are conflicting. Antibiotics are unlikely to help, but trials of probiotics are encouraging. Beano, an over-the-counter oral β-glycosidase solution, may reduce rectal passage of gas without decreasing bloating and pain. Pancreatic enzymes reduce bloating, gas, and fullness during and after high-calorie, high-fat meal ingestion. Tegaserod improves bloating in some constipated female IBS patients.

Serotonin Receptor Agonist and Antagonists Serotonin receptor antagonists have been evaluated as therapies for IBS-D. Serotonin acting on 5-HT3 receptors enhances the sensitivity of afferent neurons projecting from the gut. In humans, a 5-HT3 receptor antagonist such as alosetron reduces perception of painful visceral stimulation in IBS. It also induces rectal relaxation, increases rectal compliance, and delays colonic transit. Large, 12-week placebo-controlled trials of alosetron reported reductions in discomfort and improvements in stool frequency, consistency, and urgency in nonconstipated IBS patients. A follow-up 48-week study confirmed the long-term efficacy of alosetron. For unclear reasons, women with IBS derived greater benefit than men. However, in postrelease surveillance, 84 cases of ischemic colitis were observed, including 44 cases that required surgery and 4 deaths. As a consequence, the medication was voluntarily withdrawn by the manufacturer in 2000. Alosetron has been reintroduced under a new risk-management program where patients have to sign a patient-physician agreement. This has significantly limited its usage.

Novel 5-HT4 receptor agonists such as tegaserod exhibit prokinetic activity by stimulating peristalsis. In IBS patients with constipation, tegaserod accelerated intestinal and ascending colon transit. Clinical trials involving >4000 IBS-C patients reported reductions in discomfort and improvements in constipation and bloating, compared to placebo. Diarrhea is the major side effect. However, tegaserod has been withdrawn from the market; a meta-analysis revealed an increase in serious cardiovascular events.

Chloride Channel Activators Lubiprostone is a bicyclic fatty acid that stimulates chloride channels in the apical membrane of intestinal epithelial cells. Chloride secretion induces passive movement of sodium and water into the bowel lumen and improves bowel function. The major side

TABLE 290-3	SPECTRUM OF SEVERITY IN IBS			
		Mild	Moderate	Severe
Clinical features				
Prevalence		70%	25%	5%
Correlations with gut physiology		+++	++	+
Symptoms constant		0	+	+++
Psychosocial difficulties		0	+	+++
Health care issues		+	++	+++
Practice type		Primary	Specialty	Referral

effects are nausea and diarrhea. Lubiprostone is a new class of compounds for treatment of chronic constipation with or without IBS.

SUMMARY The treatment strategy of IBS depends on the severity of the disorder **(Table 290-3)**. Most of the IBS patients have mild symptoms. They are usually cared for in primary care practices, have little or no psychosocial difficulties, and do not seek health care often. Treatment usually

TABLE 290-4	POSSIBLE DRUGS FOR A DOMINANT SYMPTOM IN IBS	
Symptom	Drug	Dose
Diarrhea	Loperamide	2–4 mg when necessary/maximum 12 g/d
	Cholestyramine resin	4 g with meals
	Alosetron[a]	0.5–1 mg bid (for severe IBS, women)
Constipation	Psyllium husk	3–4 g bid with meals, then adjust
	Methylcellulose	2 g bid with meals, then adjust
	Calcium polycarbophil	1 g qd to qid
	Lactulose syrup	10–20 g bid
	70% sorbitol	15 mL bid
	Polyethylene glycol 3350	17 g in 250 mL water qd
	Lubiprostone (Amitiza)	24 mg bid
	Magnesium hydroxide	30–60 mL qd
Abdominal pain	Smooth-muscle relaxant	qd to qid ac
	Tricyclic antidepressants	Start 25–50 mg hs, then adjust
	Selective serotonin reuptake inhibitors	Begin small dose, increase as needed

[a]Available only in the United States.
Source: Adapted from Longstreth GF et al.

involves education, reassurance, and dietary/lifestyle changes. A smaller portion have moderate symptoms that are usually intermittent and correlate with altered gut physiology, e.g., worsened with eating or stress and relieved by defecation. Treatments include gut-acting pharmacologic agents such as antispasmodics, antidiarrheals, fiber supplements, and the newer gut serotonin modulators **(Table 290-4)**. A small proportion of IBS patients have severe and refractory symptoms, are usually seen in referral centers, and frequently have constant pain and psychosocial difficulties (Fig. 290-1). This group of patients is best managed with antidepressants and other psychological treatments (Table 290-4).

FURTHER READINGS

DROSSMAN DA et al: AGA technical review on irritable bowel syndrome. Gastroenterology 123:2108, 2002

GERSHON MD, JACK J: The serotonin signaling system: From basic understanding to drug development for functional GI disorders. Gastroenterology 132:397, 2007

LONGSTRETH GF et al: Functional bowel disorders. Gastroenterology 130:1480, 2006

MAYER EA et al: Neuroimaging of the brain-gut axis: From basic understanding to treatment of functional GI disorders. Gastroenterology 131:1925, 2006

MERTZ H: Irritable bowel syndrome. N Engl J Med 349:2136, 2003

OWYANG C: Irritable bowel syndrome, in Textbook of Gastroenterology, 4th ed, T Yamada (ed). Philadelphia, Lippincott Williams and Wilkins, 2003, pp 1817–42

SPIEGEL BM et al: Testing for celiac sprue in irritable bowel syndrome with predominant diarrhea: A cost effectiveness analysis. Gastroenterology 126:1721, 2004

TALLEY NJ: Evaluation of drug treatment for irritable bowel syndrome. Br J Clin Pharmacol 56:362, 2003

291 Diverticular Disease and Common Anorectal Disorders
Susan L. Gearhart

DIVERTICULAR DISEASE

Incidence and Epidemiology Among western populations, diverticulosis of the colon affects nearly one-half of individuals over age 60. Fortunately, only 20% of patients with diverticulosis develop symptomatic disease. However, in the United States, diverticular disease results in >200,000 hospitalizations annually, making it the fifth most costly gastrointestinal disorder. The mean hospital stay is 9.7 days, with an average cost of $42,000 per patient. The mean age at presentation of the disease is 59 years. Although the prevalence among females and males is similar, males tend to present at a younger age. Diverticulosis is rare in underdeveloped countries, where diets include more fiber and roughage. However, shortly following migration to the United States, immigrants will develop diverticular disease at the same rate as U.S. natives.

Anatomy and Pathophysiology Two types of diverticula occur in the intestine: true and false, or pseudodiverticula. A true diverticulum is a saclike herniation of the entire bowel wall, whereas a pseudodiver-

ticulum involves only a protrusion of the mucosa through the muscularis propria of the colon (Fig. 291-1). The most common type of diverticulum affecting the colon is the pseudodiverticulum. The protrusion occurs at the point where the nutrient artery, or *vasa recti*, penetrates through the muscularis propria, resulting in a break in the integrity of the colonic wall. Diverticula commonly affect the sigmoid colon; only 5% of persons exhibit pancolonic diverticula. This anatomic restriction may be a result of the relative high-pressure zone within the muscular sigmoid colon. Thus, higher amplitude contractions combined with constipated, high-fat content stool within the sigmoid lumen results in the creation of these diverticula. *Diverticulitis*, or inflammation of a diverticulum, is related to the retention of particulate material within the diverticular sac and the formation of a fecalith. Consequently, the vasa recti is either compressed or eroded, leading to either perforation or bleeding.

Presentation, Evaluation, and Management of Diverticular Bleeding

Hemorrhage from a colonic diverticulum is the most common cause of hematochezia in patients >60 years, yet only 20% of patients with diverticulosis will have gastrointestinal bleeding. Patients at increased risk for bleeding tend to be hypertensive, have atherosclerosis, and regularly use nonsteroidal anti-inflammatory agents. Most bleeds are self-limited and stop spontaneously with bowel rest. The lifetime risk of rebleeding is 25%.

Localization of diverticular bleeding should include colonoscopy, which may be both diagnostic and therapeutic in the management of mild to moderate diverticular bleeding. If the patient is stable, massive

FIGURE 291-1 Gross and microscopic view of sigmoid diverticular disease. Arrows mark an inflamed diverticula with the diverticular wall made up only of mucosa.

bleeding is best managed by angiography. Mesenteric angiography can localize the bleeding site and occlude the bleeding vessel successfully with a coil in 80% of cases. The patient can then be followed closely with repetitive colonoscopy, if necessary, looking for evidence of colonic ischemia. Alternatively, a segmental resection of the colon can be undertaken to eliminate the risk of further bleeding. This may be advantageous in patients on chronic blood thinners. However, with newer techniques of highly selective coil embolization, the rate of colonic ischemia is <10% and the risk of acute rebleeding is <25%. As another alternative, a selective infusion of vasopressin can be given to stop the hemorrhage, although this has been associated with significant complications, including myocardial infarction and intestinal ischemia. Furthermore, bleeding recurs in 50% of patients once the infusion is stopped. Localization studies indicate that bleeding as a result of colonic diverticulosis is more often seen from the right colon. For this reason, patients with presumed bleeding from diverticular disease requiring emergent surgery without localization should undergo a total abdominal colectomy. If the patient is unstable or has had a 6-unit bleed within 24 h, current recommendations are that surgery should be performed. In patients without severe comorbidities, surgical resection can be performed with a primary anastomosis. A higher anastomotic leak rate has been reported in patients who received >10 units of blood.

Presentation, Evaluation, and Staging of Diverticulitis Acute uncomplicated diverticulitis characteristically presents with fever, anorexia, left lower quadrant abdominal pain, and obstipation (Table 291-1). In <25% of cases, patients may present with generalized peritonitis indicating the presence of a diverticular perforation. On examination, the patient may have abdominal distention and signs of localized or generalized peritonitis. Laboratory investigations will demonstrate a leukocytosis. Rarely, a patient may present with an air-fluid level in the left lower quadrant on plain abdominal film. This is a giant diverticulum

TABLE 291-1 PRESENTATION OF DIVERTICULAR DISEASE

Uncomplicated Diverticular Disease—75%
Abdominal pain
Fever
Leukocytosis
Anorexia/obstipation
Complicated Diverticular Disease—25%
Abscess 16%
Perforation 10%
Stricture 5%
Fistula 2%

of the sigmoid colon and is managed with resection to avoid impending perforation.

The diagnosis of diverticulitis is best made on CT with the following findings: sigmoid diverticula, thickened colonic wall >4 mm, and inflammation within the pericolic fat ± the collection of contrast material or fluid. In 16% of patients, an abdominal abscess may be present. Symptoms of irritable bowel syndrome (IBS) may mimic those of diverticulitis. Therefore, suspected diverticulitis that does not meet CT criteria or is not associated with a leukocytosis or fever is not diverticular disease. Other conditions that can mimic diverticular disease include an ovarian cyst, endometriosis, acute appendicitis, and pelvic inflammatory disease.

Barium enema or colonoscopy should not be performed in the acute setting because of the higher risk of colonic perforation associated with insufflation or insertion of barium-based contrast material under pressure. A sigmoid malignancy can masquerade as diverticular disease. Therefore, a barium enema or colonoscopy should be performed ~6 weeks after an attack of diverticular disease.

Complicated diverticular disease is defined as diverticular disease associated with an abscess or perforation and less commonly with a fistula (Table 291-1). Perforated diverticular disease is staged using the Hinchey classification system (Fig. 291-2). This staging system was developed to predict outcomes following the surgical management of complicated diverticular disease. In complicated diverticular disease with fistula formation, common locations include cutaneous, vaginal, or vesicle fistulae. These conditions present with either passage of stool through the skin or vagina or the presence of air in the urinary stream (pneumaturia). Colovaginal fistulae are more common in women who have undergone a hysterectomy.

Rx DIVERTICULAR DISEASE

MEDICAL MANAGEMENT Asymptomatic diverticular disease discovered on imaging studies or at the time of colonoscopy is best managed by diet alterations. Patients should be instructed to eat a fiber-enriched diet that includes 30 g of fiber each day. Supplementary fiber products such as Metamucil, Fibercon, or Citrucel are useful. The patient should also be instructed to avoid nuts and popcorn, which may obstruct the lumen of a diverticulum.

Symptomatic diverticular disease, defined as radiographic and hematologic confirmation of inflammation and infection within the colon, should be treated initially with antibiotics and bowel rest. Nearly 75% of patients hospitalized for acute diverticulitis will respond to nonoperative treatment with a suitable antimicrobial regimen. The current recommended antimi-

FIGURE 291-2 Hinchey classification of diverticulitis. Stage I: perforated diverticulitis with a confined paracolic abscess. Stage II: perforated diverticulitis that has closed spontaneously with distant abscess formation. Stage III: noncommunicating perforated diverticulitis with fecal peritonitis (the diverticular neck is closed off and therefore contrast will not freely expel on radiographic images). Stage IV: perforation and free communication with the peritoneum, resulting in fecal peritonitis.

crobial coverage is trimethoprim/sulfamethoxazole or ciprofloxacin and metronidazole targeting aerobic gram-negative rods and anaerobic bacteria. Unfortunately, these agents do not cover enterococci, and the addition of ampicillin to this regimen for nonresponders is recommended. Alternatively, single-agent therapy with a third-generation penicillin such as IV piperacillin or oral penicillin/clavulinic acid may be effective. The usual course of antibiotics is 7–10 d. Rifiximin (a poorly absorbed broad-spectrum antibiotic) in combination with fiber, is associated with less frequent recurrent symptoms from uncomplicated diverticular disease. Patients should remain on a limited diet until their pain resolves. A role for parenteral nutrition has not been established.

SURGICAL MANAGEMENT   Preoperative risk factors influencing postoperative mortality rates include higher American Society of Anesthesia (ASA) class and preexisting organ failure. In patients who are low risk (ASA I and II), surgical therapy can be offered to patients who have had at least two documented attacks of diverticulitis requiring hospitalization or those who do not rapidly improve on medical therapy. Studies indicate that medical therapy can be continued beyond two attacks without an increased risk of perforation requiring a colostomy, especially in those >50 years. In contrast, younger patients may experience a more aggressive form of the disease; therefore, waiting beyond two attacks is not recommended. Surgical therapy is indicated in all low surgical risk patients with complicated diverticular disease.

The goals of surgical management of diverticular disease include controlling sepsis, eliminating complications such as fistula or obstruction, removing the diseased colonic segment, and restoring intestinal continuity. These goals must be obtained while minimizing morbidity, length of hospitalization, and cost in addition to maximizing survival and quality of life. Table 291-2 lists the operation most commonly indicated based upon Hinchey classification and the predicted morbidity and mortality. Surgical objectives include removal of the diseased sigmoid down to the rectosigmoid junction. Failure to do this may result in recurrent disease. The current options for uncomplicated diverticular disease include an open sigmoid resection or a laparoscopic sigmoid resection. The benefits of laparoscopic resection over open surgical techniques include early discharge (by at least 1 day), less narcotic use, and an earlier return to work. However,

TABLE 291-2   OUTCOME FOLLOWING SURGICAL THERAPY FOR COMPLICATED DIVERTICULAR DISEASE

Hinchey Stage	Operative Procedure	Anastomotic Leak Rate, %	Overall Morbidity, %
I	Resection with primary anastomosis without diverting stoma	3.8	22
II	Resection with primary anastomosis +/– diversion	3.8	30
III	Hartmann's procedure vs. diverting colostomy and omental pedal graft	—	0 vs. 6 mortality
IV	Hartmann's procedure vs. diverting colostomy and omental pedicle graft	—	6 vs. 2 mortality

laparoscopic resection is associated with a longer operative procedure and is more costly. The complication rates between open and laparoscopic surgery are similar.

The options for the surgical management of complicated diverticular disease **(Fig. 291-3)** include the following: (1) proximal diversion of the fecal stream with an ileostomy or colostomy and sutured omental patch with drainage, (2) resection with colostomy and mucus fistula or closure of distal bowel with formation of a Hartmann's pouch, (3) resection with anastomosis (coloproctostomy), or (4) resection with anastomosis and diversion (coloproctostomy with loop ileostomy or colostomy). Laparoscopic techniques have been employed for complicated diverticular disease; however, higher conversion rates to open techniques have been reported.

Patients with Hinchey stages I and II disease are managed with percutaneous drainage followed by resection with anastomosis about 6 weeks later. Percutaneous drainage is recommended for abscesses ≥ 5 cm with a well-defined wall that is accessible. Paracolic abscesses < 5 cm in size may resolve with antibiotics alone. Contraindications to percutaneous drainage are no percutaneous access route, pneumoperitoneum, and fecal peritonitis. Urgent operative intervention is undertaken if patients develop gener-

FIGURE 291-3   Methods of surgical management of complicated diverticular disease. *(1)* Drainage, omental pedicle graft, and proximal diversion. *(2)* Hartman's procedure. *(3)* Sigmoid resection with coloproctostomy. *(4)* Sigmoid resection with coloproctostomy and proximal diversion.

alized peritonitis, and most will need to be managed with a Hartmann's procedure. In selected cases, nonoperative therapy may be considered. In one nonrandomized study, nonoperative management of isolated paracolic abscesses (Hinchey stage I) was associated with only a 20% recurrence rate at 2 years. Over 80% of patients with distant abscesses (Hinchey stage II) required surgical resection for recurrent symptoms.

Hinchey stage III disease is managed with a Hartman's procedure or with primary anastomosis and proximal diversion. If the patient has significant comorbidities, making operative intervention risky, a limited procedure including intraoperative peritoneal lavage (irrigation), omental patch to the oversewn perforation, and proximal diversion of the fecal stream with either an ileostomy or transverse colostomy can be performed. No anastomosis of any type should be attempted in Hinchey stage IV disease. A limited approach to these patients is associated with a decreased mortality.

Recurrent Symptoms   Recurrent abdominal symptoms following surgical resection for diverticular disease occurs in 10% of patients. Recurrent diverticular disease develops in patients following inadequate surgical resection. A retained segment of diseased rectosigmoid colon is associated with twice the incidence of recurrence. IBS may also cause recurrence of initial symptoms. Patients undergoing surgical resection for presumed diverticulitis and symptoms of abdominal cramping and irregular loose bowel movements consistent with IBS have functionally poorer outcomes.

COMMON DISEASES OF THE ANORECTUM

RECTAL PROLAPSE (PROCIDENTIA)
Incidence and Epidemiology   Rectal prolapse is six times more common in women than in men. The incidence of rectal prolapse peaks in women >60 years. Women with rectal prolapse have a higher incidence of associated pelvic floor disorders including urinary incontinence, rectocele, cystocele, and enterocele. About 20% of children with rectal prolapse will have cystic fibrosis. All children presenting with prolapse should undergo a sweat chloride test. Less common associations include Ehlers-Danlos syndrome, solitary rectal ulcer syndrome, congenital hypothyroidism, and Hirschsprung's disease.

Anatomy and Pathophysiology   Rectal prolapse (procidentia) is a circumferential, full-thickness protrusion of the rectal wall through the anal orifice. It is often associated with a redundant sigmoid colon, pelvic laxity, and a deep rectovaginal septum (pouch of Douglas). Initially, rectal prolapse was felt to be the result of early internal rectal intussusception, which occurs in the upper to mid rectum. This was considered to be the first step in an inevitable progression to full-thickness external prolapse. However, only 1 of 38 patients with internal prolapse followed for >5 years developed full-thickness prolapse. Others have suggested that full-thickness prolapse is the result of damage to the nerve supply to the pelvic floor muscles or pudendal nerves from repeated stretching with straining to defecate. Damage to the pudendal nerves would weaken the pelvic floor muscles, including the external anal sphincter muscles. Bilateral pudendal nerve injury is more significantly associated with prolapse and incontinence than unilateral injury.

Presentation and Evaluation   The majority of patient complaints include anal mass, bleeding per rectum, and poor perianal hygiene. Prolapse of the rectum usually occurs following defecation and will spontaneously reduce or require the patient to manually reduce the prolapse. Constipation occurs in ~30–67% of patients with rectal prolapse. Differing degrees of fecal incontinence occur in 50–70% of patients. Other associated findings include outlet obstruction (anismus) in 30%, colonic inertia in 10%, and solitary rectal ulcer syndrome in 12%.

Office evaluation is best performed after the patient has been given an enema, which enables the prolapse to protrude. An important distinction should be made between full-thickness rectal prolapse and isolated mucosal prolapse associated with hemorrhoidal disease (Fig. 291-4). Mucosal prolapse is known for radial grooves rather than circumferential folds around the anus and is due to increased laxity of the connective tis-

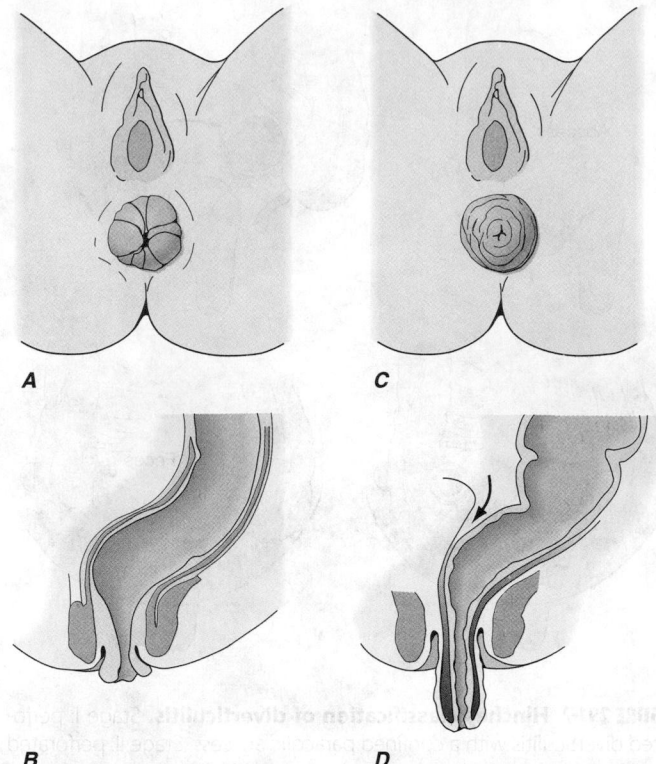

FIGURE 291-4 Degree of rectal prolapse. Mucosal prolapse only (**A, B,** sagittal view). Full-thickness prolapse associated with redundant rectosigmoid and deep pouch of Douglas (**C, D,** sagittal view).

sue between the submucosa and underlying muscle of the anal canal. The evaluation of prolapse should also include cystoproctography and colonoscopy. These examinations evaluate for associated pelvic floor disorders and rule out a malignancy or a polyp as the lead point for prolapse. If rectal prolapse is associated with chronic constipation, the patient should undergo a defecating proctogram and a sitzmark study. This will evaluate for the presence of anismus or colonic inertia. Anismus is the result of attempting to defecate against a closed pelvic floor and is also known as *nonrelaxing puborectalis*. This can be seen when straightening of the rectum fails to occur on fluoroscopy while the patient is attempting to defecate. In colonic inertia, a sitzmark study will demonstrate retention of >20% of markers on abdominal x-ray 5 days after swallowing. For patients with fecal incontinence, endoanal ultrasound and manometric evaluation, including pudendal nerve testing of their anal sphincter muscles, may be performed before surgery for prolapse (see "Fecal Incontinence," below).

℞ RECTAL PROLAPSE

The medical approach to the management of rectal prolapse is limited and includes stool-bulking agents or fiber supplementation to ease the process of evacuation. Surgical correction of rectal prolapse is the mainstay of therapy. Two approaches are commonly considered, transabdominal and transperineal. Transabdominal approaches have been associated with lower recurrence rates, but some patients with significant comorbidities are better served by a transperineal approach.

Common transperineal approaches include a transanal proctectomy (Altmeier procedure), mucosal proctectomy (Delorme procedure), or placement of a Tirsch wire encircling the anus. The goal of the transperineal approach is to remove the redundant rectosigmoid colon. Common transabdominal approaches include presacral suture or mesh rectopexy (Ripstein) with (Frykman-Goldberg) or without resection of the redundant sigmoid. Transabdominal procedures can be performed effectively with laparoscopic techniques without increased incidence of recurrence. The goal of the transabdominal approach is to restore normal anatomy by removing redundant bowel and reattaching the supportive tissue of the rectum to the presacral fascia. The final alternative is abdominal proctectomy with end-sigmoid colostomy. Colon resection, in general, is reserved for patients with constipation and outlet obstruction. If total colonic inertia is present, as defined by a history of constipation and a positive sitzmark study, a subtotal colectomy with an ileosigmoid or rectal anastomosis may be required at the time of rectopexy.

FECAL INCONTINENCE

Incidence and Epidemiology   The prevalence of fecal incontinence in the United States is 0.5–11%. The majority of patients are women. A higher incidence of incontinence is seen among parous women. One-half of patients with fecal incontinence also suffer from urinary incontinence. The majority of incontinence is a result of obstetric injury to the pelvic floor, either while carrying a fetus or during the delivery. Risk factors at the time of delivery include the use of forceps and the need for an episiotomy. Other causes include congenital abnormalities such as imperforate anus, trauma, or rectal prolapse.

Anatomy and Pathophysiology   The anal sphincter complex is made up of the internal and external anal sphincter. The internal sphincter is smooth muscle and a continuation of the circular fibers of the rectal wall. It is innervated by the intestinal myenteric plexus and is therefore not under voluntary control. The external anal sphincter is formed in continuation with the levator ani muscles and is under voluntary control. The pudendal nerve supplies motor innervation to the external anal sphincter. Obstetric injury may result in tearing of the muscle fibers anteriorly at the time of the delivery. This results in an obvious anterior defect on endoanal ultrasound. Injury may also be the result of stretching of the pudendal nerves. The majority of patients who suffer from fecal incontinence following obstetric injury do so several years following the birth of their last child.

Presentation and Evaluation   Patients may suffer with varying degrees of fecal incontinence. Minor incontinence includes incontinence to flatus and occasional seepage of liquid stool. Major incontinence is frequent inability to control solid waste. As a result of fecal incontinence, patients suffer from poor perianal hygiene. Beyond the immediate problems associated with fecal incontinence, these patients are often withdrawn and suffer from depression. For this reason, quality-of-life measures have become an important component in the evaluation of patients with fecal incontinence.

The evaluation of fecal incontinence should include a thorough history and physical examination, anal manometry, pudendal nerve terminal motor latency (PNTML), and endoanal ultrasound. Unfortunately, all of these investigations are user-dependent. Centers that care for patients with fecal incontinence will have an anorectal physiology laboratory that uses standardized methods of evaluating anorectal physiology. Anal manometry measures resting and squeeze pressures within the anal canal using an intraluminal water-perfused catheter. Pudendal nerve studies evaluate the function of the nerves innervating the anal canal using a finger electrode placed in the anal canal. Stretch injuries to these nerves will result in a delayed response of the sphincter muscle to a stimulus, indicating a prolonged latency. Finally, ultrasound will evaluate the extent of the injury to the sphincter muscles before surgical repair. Only PNTML has been shown to consistently predict outcome following surgical intervention.

Rarely does a pelvic floor disorder exist alone. The majority of patients with fecal incontinence will have a degree of urinary incontinence. Similarly, fecal incontinence is a part of the spectrum of pelvic organ prolapse. For this reason, patients may present with symptoms of obstructed defecation as well as fecal incontinence. Careful evaluation including cinedefography should be performed to search for other associated defects. Surgical repair of incontinence without attention to other associated defects may decrease the success of the repair.

℞ FECAL INCONTINENCE

The "gold standard" for the treatment of fecal incontinence with an isolated sphincter defect is overlapping sphincteroplasty. The external anal sphincter muscle and scar tissue as well as any identifiable internal sphincter muscle are dissected free from the surrounding adipose and connective tissue and then an overlapping repair is performed in an attempt to rebuild the muscular ring and restore its function. Other newer approaches include radiofrequency therapy to the anal canal to aid in the development of collagen fibers and provide tensile strength to the sphincter muscles. Sacral nerve stimulation and the artificial bowel sphincter are both adaptations of procedures developed for the management of urinary incontinence. Sacral nerve stimulation is ideally suited for patients with intact but weak anal sphincters. A temporary nerve stimulator is placed on the third sacral nerve. If there is at least a 50% improvement in symptoms, a permanent nerve stimulator is placed under the skin. The artificial bowel sphincter is a cuff and reservoir apparatus that allows for manual inflation of a cuff placed around the anus, increasing anal tone. This allows the patient to manually close off the anal canal until defecation is necessary.

Long-term results following overlapping sphincteroplasty show about a 50% failure rate over 5 years. Poorer outcome has been seen in patients with prolonged PNTML. Long-term results for sacral stimulation and the artificial bowel sphincter are limited. However, the artificial bowel sphincter has been associated with a 30% infection rate.

HEMORRHOIDAL DISEASE

Incidence and Epidemiology   Symptomatic hemorrhoids affect >1 million individuals in western civilization per year. The prevalence of hemorrhoidal disease is not selective for age or sex. However, age is known to have a deleterious effect on the anal canal. The prevalence of hemorrhoidal disease is less in underdeveloped countries. The typical low-fiber, high-fat western diet is associated with constipation and straining and the development of symptomatic hemorrhoids.

Anatomy and Pathophysiology   Hemorrhoidal cushions are a normal part of the anal canal. The vascular structures contained within this tissue aid in continence by preventing damage to the sphincter muscle. Three main hemorrhoidal complexes traverse the anal canal—the left lateral, the right anterior, and the right posterior. Engorgement and straining results in prolapse of this tissue into the anal canal. Over time, the anatomic support system of the hemorrhoidal complex weakens, exposing this tissue to the outside of the anal canal where it is susceptible to injury. Hemorrhoids are commonly classified as internal or external. Although small external cushions do exist, the standard classification of hemorrhoidal disease is based on the progression of the disease from their normal internal location to the prolapsing external position (Table 291-3).

Presentation and Evaluation   Patients commonly present to a physician for two reasons: bleeding and protrusion. Pain is less common than with fissures and, if present, is described as a dull ache from engorgement of the hemorrhoidal tissue. Severe pain may indicate a thrombosed hemorrhoid. Hemorrhoidal bleeding is described as bright red blood seen either in the toilet or upon wiping. Occasional patients can present with significant bleeding, which may be a cause of

TABLE 291-3   THE STAGING AND TREATMENT OF HEMORRHOIDS

Stage	Description of Classification	Treatment
I	Enlargement with bleeding	Fiber supplementation Cortisone suppository Sclerotherapy
II	Protrusion with spontaneous reduction	Fiber supplementation Cortisone suppository
III	Protrusion requiring manual reduction	Fiber supplementation Cortisone suppository Banding Operative hemorrhoidectomy (stapled or traditional)
IV	Irreducible protrusion	Fiber supplementation Cortisone suppository Operative hemorrhoidectomy

anemia; however, the presence of a colonic neoplasm must be ruled out. Patients who present with a protruding mass complain about inability to maintain perianal hygiene and are often concerned about the presence of a malignancy.

The diagnosis of hemorrhoidal disease is made on physical examination. Inspection of the perianal region for evidence of thrombosis or excoriation is performed, followed by a careful digital examination. Anoscopy is performed paying particular attention to the known position of hemorrhoidal disease. The patient is asked to strain. If this is difficult for the patient, the maneuver can be performed while sitting on a toilet. The physician is notified when the tissue prolapses. It is important to differentiate the circumferential appearance of a full-thickness rectal prolapse from the radial nature of prolapsing hemorrhoids (see "Rectal Prolapse," above). The stage and location of the hemorrhoidal complexes are defined.

℞ HEMORRHOIDAL DISEASE

The treatment for bleeding hemorrhoids is based upon the stage of the disease (Table 291-3). In all patients with bleeding, the possibility of other causes must be considered. In young patients without a family history of colorectal cancer, the hemorrhoidal disease may be treated first and a colonoscopic examination performed if the bleeding continues. Older patients who have not had colorectal cancer screening should undergo colonoscopy or flexible sigmoidoscopy.

With rare exceptions, the acutely thrombosed hemorrhoid can be excised within the first 72 h by performing an elliptical excision. Sitz baths, fiber, and stool softeners are prescribed. Additional therapy for bleeding hemorrhoids includes banding, sclerotherapy, excisional hemorrhoidectomy, and stapled hemorrhoidectomy. Sensation begins at the dentate line; therefore, banding or sclerotherapy can be performed without discomfort in the office. Bands are placed around the engorged tissue, causing ischemia and fibrosis. This aids in fixing the tissue proximally in the anal canal. Patients may complain of a dull ache for 24 h following band application. During sclerotherapy, 1–2 mL of a sclerosant (usually sodium tetradechol sulfate) is injected using a 25-gauge needle into the submucosa of the hemorrhoidal complex. Care must be taken not to inject the anal canal circumferentially or stenosis may occur. The sutured and stapled hemorrhoidectomy are equally effective in the treatment of symptomatic third- and fourth-degree hemorrhoids. However, because the sutured hemorrhoidectomy involves the removal of redundant tissue down to the anal verge, unpleasant anal skin tags are removed as well. The stapled hemorrhoidectomy is associated with less discomfort; however, this procedure does not remove anal skin tags. No procedures on hemorrhoids should be done in patients who are immunocompromised or who have active proctitis. Furthermore, emergent hemorrhoidectomy for bleeding hemorrhoids is associated with a higher complication rate.

Acute complications associated with the treatment of hemorrhoids include pain, infection, recurrent bleeding, and urinary retention. Care should be taken to place bands properly and to avoid overhydration in patients undergoing operative hemorrhoidectomy. Late complications include fecal incontinence as a result of injury to the sphincter during the dissection. Anal stenosis may develop from overzealous excision, with loss of mucosal skin bridges for reepithelialization. Finally, an *ectropion* (prolapse of rectal mucosa from the anal canal) may develop. Patients with an ectropion complain of a "wet" anus as a result of inability to prevent soiling once the rectal mucosa is exposed below the dentate line.

ANORECTAL ABSCESS
Incidence and Epidemiology The development of a perianal abscess is more common in men than women by a ratio of 3:1. The peak incidence is in the third to fifth decade of life. Perianal pain associated with the presence of an abscess accounts for 15% of office visits to a colorectal surgeon. The disease is more prevalent in immunocompromised patients such as diabetics, those with hematologic disorders or inflammatory bowel disease (IBD), and persons who are HIV positive. These disorders should be considered in patients with recurrent perianal infections.

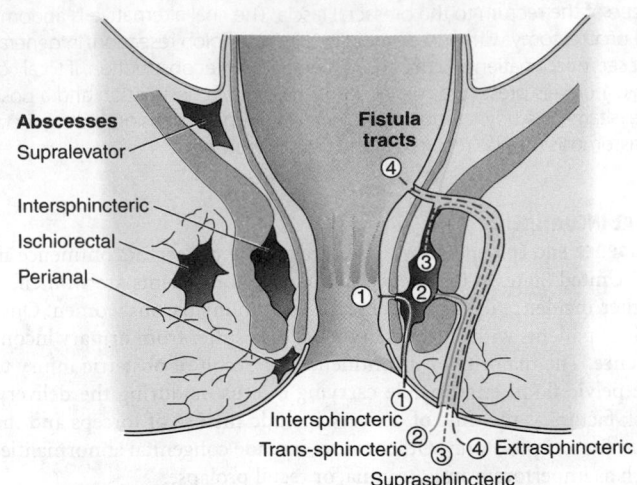

FIGURE 291-5 Common locations of anorectal abscess (left) and fistula in ano (right).

Anatomy and Pathophysiology An anorectal abscess is an abnormal fluid-containing cavity in the anorectal region. Anorectal abscess results from an infection involving the glands surrounding the anal canal. Normally, these glands release mucus into the anal canal, which aids in defecation. When stool accidentally enters the anal glands, the glands become infected and an abscess develops. Anorectal abscesses are perianal in 40–50% of patients, ischiorectal in 20–25%, intersphincteric in 2–5%, and supralevator in 2.5% (Fig. 291-5).

Presentation and Evaluation Perianal pain and fever are the hallmarks of an abscess. Patients may have difficulty voiding and have blood in the stool. A prostatic abscess may present with similar complaints including dysuria. Patients with a prostatic abscess will often have a history of recurrent sexually transmitted diseases. On physical examination, a large fluctuant area is usually readily visible. Routine laboratory evaluation shows an elevated white blood cell count. Diagnostic procedures are rarely necessary unless evaluating a recurrent abscess. A CT scan or MRI has an accuracy of 80% in determining incomplete drainage. If there is a concern about the presence of IBD, a rigid or flexible sigmoidoscopic examination may be done at the time of drainage to evaluate for inflammation within the rectosigmoid region. A more complete evaluation for Crohn's disease would include a full colonoscopy and small-bowel series.

℞ ANORECTAL ABSCESS

Office drainage of an uncomplicated anorectal abscess may suffice. A small incision close to the anal verge is made and a Mallenkot drain is advanced into the abscess cavity. For patients who have a complicated abscess or who are diabetic or immunocompromised, drainage should be performed in a operating room under anesthesia. These patients are at greater risk for developing necrotizing fasciitis. The course of antibiotics is controversial but should be at least 2 weeks in patients who are immunocompromised or have prosthetic heart valves, artificial joints, diabetes, or IBD.

FISTULA IN ANO
Incidence and Epidemiology The incidence and prevalence of fistulating perianal disease parallels the incidence of anorectal abscess. Some 30–40% of abscesses will give rise to fistula in ano. While the majority of the fistulas are cryptoglandular in origin, 10% are associated with IBD, tuberculosis, malignancy, and radiation.

Anatomy and Pathophysiology A fistula in ano is defined as a communication of an abscess cavity with an identifiable internal opening within the anal canal. This identifiable opening is most commonly located at the dentate line where the anal glands enter the anal canal. Patients experiencing continuous drainage following the treatment of a perianal abscess likely have a fistula in ano. These fistulas are classified by their relationship to the anal sphincter muscles, with 70% being intersphincteric, 23% transsphincteric, 5% suprasphincteric, and 2% extrasphincteric (Fig. 291-5).

Presentation and Evaluation A patient with a fistula in ano will complain of constant drainage from the perianal region. The drainage may increase with defecation. Perianal hygiene is difficult to maintain. Examination under anesthesia is the best way to evaluate a fistula. At the time of the examination, anoscopy is performed to look for an internal opening. Diluted hydrogen peroxide will aid in identifying such an opening. In lieu of anesthesia, MRI with an endoanal coil will also identify tracts in 80% of the cases. After drainage of an abscess with insertion of a Mallenkot catheter, a fistulagram through the catheter can be obtained in search of an occult fistula tract. Goodsall's rule states that a posterior external fistula will enter the anal canal in the posterior midline, whereas an anterior fistula will enter at the nearest crypt. A fistula exiting >3 cm from the anal verge may have a complicated upward extension and may not obey Goodsall's rule.

Rx FISTULA IN ANO

A newly diagnosed draining fistula is best managed with placement of a seton, a vessel loop or silk tie placed through the fistula tract, which maintains the tract open and quiets down the surrounding inflammation that occurs from repeated blockage of the tract. Once the inflammation is less, the exact relationship of the fistula tract to the anal sphincters can be ascertained. A simple fistulotomy can be performed for intersphincteric and low (less than one-third of the muscle) transphincteric fistulas without compromising continence. For a higher transphincteric fistula, an anorectal advancement flap in combination with a drainage catheter or fibrin glue may be used. Very long (>2 cm) and narrow tracts respond better to fibrin glue than shorter tracts. Patients should be maintained on stool-bulking agents, nonnarcotic pain medication, and sitz baths. Early complications from these procedures include urinary retention and bleeding. Later complications include temporary and permanent incontinence. Recurrence following fistulotomy is 0–18% and following anorectal advancement flap is 20–30% and is related to failure to excise and close the internal opening.

ANAL FISSURE

Incidence and Epidemiology Anal fissures occur at all ages but are more common in the third through the fifth decades. A fissure is the most common cause of rectal bleeding in infancy. The prevalence is equal in males and females. It is associated with constipation, diarrhea, infectious etiologies, perianal trauma, and Crohn's disease.

Anatomy and Pathophysiology Trauma to the anal canal occurs following defecation. This injury occurs in the anterior or, more commonly, the posterior anal canal. Irritation caused by the trauma to the anal canal results in an increased resting pressure of the internal sphincter. The blood supply to the sphincter and anal mucosa enters laterally. Therefore, increased anal sphincter tone results in a relative ischemia in the region of the fissure and leads to poor healing of the anal injury. A fissure that is not in the posterior or anterior position should raise suspicion for other causes, including tuberculosis, syphilis, Crohn's disease, and malignancy.

Presentation and Evaluation A fissure can be easily diagnosed on history alone. The classic complaint is pain, which is strongly associated with defecation and is relentless. The bright red bleeding that can be associated with a fissure is less extensive than that associated with hemorrhoids. On examination, most fissures are located in either the posterior or anterior position. A lateral fissure is worrisome as it may have a less benign nature, and systemic disorders should be ruled out. A chronic fissure is indicated by the presence of a hypertrophied anal papilla at the proximal end of the fissure and a sentinel pile or skin tag at the distal end. Often the circular fibers of the hypertrophied internal sphincter are visible within the base of the fissure. If anal manometry is performed, elevation in anal resting pressure and a sawtooth deformity with paradoxical contractions of the sphincter muscles are pathognomonic.

Rx ANAL FISSURE

The management of the acute fissure is conservative. Stool softeners for those with constipation, increased dietary fiber, topical anesthetics, glucocorticoids, and sitz baths are prescribed and will heal 60–90% of fissures. Chronic fissures are those present for >6 weeks. These can be treated with modalities aimed at decreasing the anal canal resting pressure including nifedipine or nitroglycerin ointment applied three times a day, and botulinum toxin type A, up to 20 units, injected into the internal sphincter on each side of the fissure. Surgical management includes anal dilation and lateral internal sphincterotomy. Usually, one-third of the internal sphincter muscle is divided; it is easily identified because it is hypertrophied. Recurrence rates from medical therapy are higher, but this is offset by a risk of incontinence following sphincterotomy. Lateral internal sphincterotomy more commonly leads to incontinence in women.

ACKNOWLEDGMENT

We would like to thank Cory Sandore for providing some illustrations for this chapter. Gregory Bulkley, MD, contributed to this chapter in the 16th edition.

FURTHER READINGS

COLECCHIA A et al: Diverticular disease of the colon: New perspectives in symptom development and treatment. World J Gastroenterol 9:1385, 2003

JANES S et al: Elective surgery after acute diverticulitis. Br J Surgery 92:133, 2005

KARULF R et al: Rectal prolapse. Curr Probl Surg 38:757, 2001

LINDSEY I et al: A randomized, controlled trial of fibrin glue vs. conventional treatment for anal fistula. Dis Colon Rectum 45:1608, 2002

STEIN E: Botulinum toxin and anal fissure. Curr Probl Dermatol 30:218, 2002

SUTHERLAND LM et al: A systematic review of stapled hemorrhoidectomy. Arch Surg 137:1395, 2002

WONG WD et al: Practice parameters for the treatment of sigmoid diverticulitis—supporting documentation. Dis Colon Rectum 43:290, 2000

292 Mesenteric Vascular Insufficiency

Susan L. Gearhart

INTESTINAL ISCHEMIA

Incidence and Epidemiology Intestinal ischemia is an uncommon vascular disease associated with a high mortality. It is categorized according to etiology: (1) arteriooclusive mesenteric ischemia (AOMI), (2) nonocclusive mesenteric ischemia (NOMI), and (3) mesenteric venous thrombosis (MVT). Acute intestinal ischemia is more common than its counterpart, chronic arterial ischemia. Risk factors for acute arterial ischemia include atrial fibrillation, recent myocardial infarction, valvular heart disease, and recent cardiac or vascular catheterization. The increased incidence of intestinal ischemia seen in western countries parallels the incidence of atherosclerosis and the aging population. With the exception of strangulated small-bowel obstruction, ischemic colitis is the most common form of acute ischemia and the most prevalent gastrointestinal disease complicating cardiovascular surgery. The incidence of ischemic colitis following elective aortic repair is 5–9%, and the incidence triples in patients following emergent repair. Other less common forms of intestinal ischemia include chronic mesenteric angina associated with atherosclerotic disease and MVT. The latter is associated with the presence of a hypercoagulable state including protein C or S deficiency, antithrombin III deficiency, polycythemia vera, and carcinoma.

Anatomy and Pathophysiology Intestinal ischemia occurs when insufficient perfusion to intestinal tissue produces ischemic tissue injury. The blood supply to the intestines is depicted in Fig. 292-1. To prevent ischemic injury, extensive collateralization occurs between major mesenteric trunks and branches of the mesenteric arcades (Table 292-1). Collateral vessels within the small bowel are numerous and meet within the duodenum and the bed of the pancreas. Collateral vessels within the colon meet at the splenic flexure and descending/sigmoid colon. These areas, which are inherently at risk for decreased blood flow, are known as *Griffiths' point* and *Sudeck's point*, respectively, and are the most common locations for colonic ischemia (Fig. 292-1, shaded area). The splanchnic circulation can receive up to 30% of the cardiac output. Protective responses to prevent intestinal ischemia include abundant collateralization, autoregulation of blood flow, and the ability to increase oxygen extraction from the blood.

Occlusive ischemia is a result of disruption of blood flow by an embolus or progressive thrombosis in a major artery supplying the intestine. Emboli originate from the heart in >75% of cases and lodge preferentially just distal to the origin of the middle colic artery from the superior mesenteric artery. Progressive thrombosis of at least two of the major vessels supplying the intestine is required for the development of chronic intestinal angina. Nonocclusive ischemia is disproportionate mesenteric vasoconstriction (arteriolar vasospasm) in response to a severe physiologic stress such as dehydration or shock. If left untreated, early mucosal stress ulceration will progress to full-thickness injury.

Presentation, Evaluation, and Management Intestinal ischemia remains one of the most challenging diagnoses. The mortality rate is >50%. The most significant indicator of survival is the timeliness of diagnosis and treatment. An overview of diagnosis and management of each form of intestinal ischemia is given in Table 292-2.

Acute mesenteric ischemia resulting from arterial embolus or thrombosis presents with severe acute, nonremitting abdominal pain strikingly out of proportion to the physical findings. Associated symptoms may include nausea and vomiting, transient diarrhea, and bloody stools. With the exception of minimal abdominal distention and hypoactive bowel sounds, early abdominal examination is unimpressive. Later findings will demonstrate peritonitis and cardiovascular collapse. In the evaluation of acute intestinal ischemia, routine laboratory tests should be obtained, including complete blood count, serum chemistry, coagulation profile, arterial blood gas, amylase, lipase, lactic acid, blood type and cross match, and cardiac enzymes. Regardless of the need for urgent surgery, emergent admission to a monitored bed or intensive care unit is recommended for resuscitation and further evaluation. If the diagnosis of intestinal ischemia is being considered, consultation with a surgical service is necessary.

Other diagnostic modalities that may be useful in diagnosis but should not delay surgical therapy include electrocardiogram (ECG), abdominal radiographs, CT, and mesenteric angiography. More recently, mesentery duplex scanning and visible light spectroscopy during colonoscopy have been demonstrated to be beneficial. The ECG may demonstrate an arrhythmia, indicating the possible source of the emboli. A plain abdominal film may show evidence of free intraperitoneal air, indicating a perforated viscus and the need for emergent exploration. Earlier features of intestinal ischemia seen on abdominal radiographs include bowel-wall edema, known as "thumbprinting." If the ischemia progresses, air can be seen within the bowel wall (*pneu-*

TABLE 292-1	COLLATERAL ARTERIAL INTESTINAL BLOOD FLOW		
Involved Circulation	**Mesenteric Artery**	**Adjoining Artery**	**Collateral Artery**
Systemic	Celiac	Descending aorta	Phrenic
Systemic	IMA	Hypogastric	Middle hemorrhoidal
Mesenteric	Celiac	SMA	Superior/inferior pancreaticoduodenal
Mesenteric	SMA	IMA	Arch of Riolan
Mesenteric	SMA	Celiac/IMA	Intramesenteric
Mesenteric	SMA	IMA	Marginal

Note: IMA, inferior mesenteric artery; SMA, superior mesenteric artery.

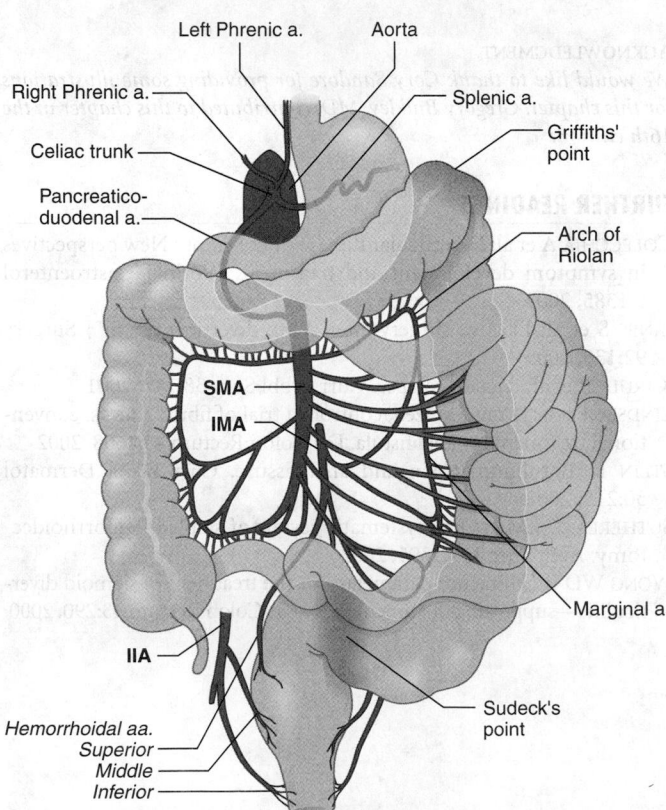

FIGURE 292-1 Blood supply to the intestines includes the celiac artery, superior mesenteric artery (SMA), inferior mesenteric artery (IMA), and branches of the internal iliac artery (IIA). Sudeck's and Griffiths' points, indicated by shaded area, are watershed areas within the colonic blood supply and common locations for ischemia.

Labels in figure: Left Phrenic a., Aorta, Right Phrenic a., Splenic a., Celiac trunk, Griffiths' point, Pancreatico-duodenal a., Arch of Riolan, SMA, IMA, Marginal a., IIA, Sudeck's point, Hemorrhoidal aa. Superior Middle Inferior

TABLE 292-2 OVERVIEW OF THE MANAGEMENT OF ACUTE INTESTINAL ISCHEMIA

Condition	Key to Early Diagnosis	Treatment of Underlying Cause	Treatment of Specific Lesion	Treatment of Systemic Consequences
Arterial embolus	Early laparotomy	Anticoagulation Cardioversion Proximal thrombectomy Aneurysmectomy	Laparotomy Embolectomy Vascular bypass Assess viability and resect dead bowel	Ensure hydration Give antibiotics Reverse acidosis Optimize oxygen delivery Support cardiac output Treat other embolic sites Avoid vasoconstrictors
Arterial thrombosis	Duplex ultrasound Angiography	Anticoagulation Hydration	Endovascular stent Endarterectomy/thrombectomy or vascular bypass Assess viability and resect dead bowel	Give antibiotics Reverse acidosis Optimize oxygen delivery Support cardiac output Avoid vasoconstrictors
Venous thrombosis	Spiral CT	Anticoagulation Massive hydration	Anticoagulation +/− laparotomy/thrombectomy/portasystemic shunt Assess viability and resect dead bowel	Give antibiotics Reverse acidosis Optimize oxygen delivery Support cardiac output Avoid vasoconstrictors
Nonocclusive mesenteric ischemia	Vasospasm: Angiography Hypoperfusion: Spiral CT or colonoscopy	Ensure hydration Support cardiac output Avoid vasoconstrictors Ablate renin-angiotensin axis	Vasospasm: Intraarterial vasodilators Hypoperfusion: Delayed laparotomy Assess viability and resect dead bowel	Ensure hydration Give antibiotics Reverse acidosis Optimize oxygen delivery Support cardiac output Avoid vasoconstrictors

Source: Modified from GB Bulkley, in JL Cameron (ed): *Current Surgical Therapy*, 2d ed. Toronto, BC Decker, 1986.

matosis intestinalis) and within the portal venous system. Other features include calcifications of the aorta and its tributaries, indicating atherosclerotic disease. With the administration of oral and IV contrast, dynamic CT with three-dimensional reconstruction is a highly sensitive test for intestinal ischemia. In acute embolic disease, mesenteric angiography is best performed intraoperatively. A mesenteric duplex scan demonstrating a high peak velocity of flow in the superior mesenteric artery (SMA) is associated with an ~80% positive predictive value of mesenteric ischemia. More significantly, a negative duplex scan virtually precludes the diagnosis of mesenteric ischemia. Duplex imaging serves as a screening test; further investigations with angiography are needed. Endoscopic techniques using visible light spectroscopy can be used in the diagnosis of chronic ischemia.

The "gold standard" for the diagnosis and management of acute arterial occlusive disease is laparotomy. Surgical exploration should not be delayed if suspicion of acute occlusive mesenteric ischemia is high or evidence of clinical deterioration or frank peritonitis is present. The goal of operative exploration is to resect compromised bowel and restore blood supply. Intraoperative or preoperative arteriography and systemic heparinization may assist the vascular surgeon in restoring blood supply to compromised bowel. The entire length of the small and large bowel beginning at the ligament of Treitz should be evaluated. The pattern of intestinal ischemia may indicate the level of arterial occlusion. In the case of SMA occlusion where the embolus usually lies just proximal to the origin of the middle colic artery, the proximal jejunum is often spared while the remainder of the small bowel to the transverse colon will be ischemic. The surgical management of acute mesenteric ischemia of the small bowel is attempted embolectomy via intraoperative angiography or arteriotomy. Although more commonly applied to chronic disease, acute thrombosis may be managed with angioplasty, with or without endovascular stent placement. If this is unsuccessful, a bypass from the aorta to the superior mesenteric artery is performed.

Nonocclusive or vasospastic mesenteric ischemia presents with generalized abdominal pain, anorexia, bloody stools, and abdominal distention. Often these patients are obtunded, and physical findings may not assist in the diagnosis. The presence of a leukocytosis, metabolic acidosis, elevated amylase or creatinine phosphokinase levels, and/or lactic acidosis are use-

ful in support of the diagnosis of advanced intestinal ischemia; however, these markers may not be indicative of either reversible ischemia or frank necrosis. Investigational markers for intestinal ischemia include D-dimer, glutathione S-transferase, platelet-activating factor (PAF), and mucosal pH monitoring. Regardless of the need for urgent surgery, emergent admission to a monitored bed or intensive care unit is recommended for resuscitation and further evaluation. Early manifestations of intestinal ischemia include fluid sequestration within the bowel wall leading to a loss of interstitial volume. Aggressive fluid resuscitation may be necessary. To optimize oxygen delivery, nasal O_2 and blood transfusions may be given. Broad-spectrum antibiotics should be given to provide sufficient coverage for enteric pathogens, including gram-negative and anaerobic organisms. Frequent monitoring of the patient's vital signs, urine output, blood gases, and lactate levels is paramount, as is frequent abdominal examination. All vaso-

constricting agents should be avoided; fluid resuscitation is the intervention of choice to maintain hemodynamics.

If ischemic colitis is a concern, colonoscopy should be performed to assess the integrity of the colon mucosa. Visualization of the rectosigmoid region may demonstrate decreased mucosal integrity, associated more commonly with nonocclusive mesenteric ischemia, or, on occasion, occlusive disease as a result of acute loss of inferior mesenteric arterial flow following aortic surgery. Ischemia of the colonic mucosa is graded as *mild* with minimal mucosal erythema or as *moderate* with pale mucosal ulcerations and evidence of extension to the muscular layer of the bowel wall. *Severe* ischemic colitis presents with severe ulcerations resulting in black or green discoloration of the mucosa, consistent with full-thickness bowel-wall necrosis. The degree of reversibility can be predicted from the mucosal findings: mild erythema is nearly 100% reversible, moderate ~50%, and frank necrosis is simply dead bowel. Follow-up colonoscopy can be performed to rule out progression of ischemic colitis.

Laparotomy for nonocclusive mesenteric ischemia is warranted for signs of peritonitis or worsening endoscopic findings and if the patient's condition does not improve with aggressive resuscitation. Ischemic colitis is optimally treated with resection of the ischemic bowel and formation of a proximal stoma. Primary anastomosis should not be performed in patients with acute intestinal ischemia.

Patients with MVT may present with a gradual or sudden onset. Symptoms include vague abdominal pain, nausea, and vomiting. Examination findings include abdominal distention with mild to moderate tenderness and signs of dehydration. The diagnosis of mesenteric thrombosis is frequently made on abdominal spiral CT with oral and IV contrast. Findings on CT include bowel-wall thickening and ascites. Intravenous contrast will demonstrate a delayed arterial phase and clot within the superior mesenteric vein. The goal of management is to optimize hemodynamics and correct electrolyte abnormalities with massive fluid resuscitation. Intravenous antibiotics as well as anticoagulation should be initiated. If laparotomy is performed and MVT is suspected, heparin anticoagulation is immediately initiated and compromised bowel is resected. Of all acute intestinal disorders, mesenteric venous insufficiency is associated with the best prognosis.

Chronic intestinal ischemia presents with intestinal angina or abdominal pain associated with need for increased blood flow to the intestine. Patients report abdominal cramping and pain following ingestion of a meal. Weight loss and chronic diarrhea may also be noted. Abdominal pain without weight loss is not chronic mesenteric angina. Physical examination will often reveal the presence of an abdominal bruit as well as other manifestations of atherosclerosis. Duplex ultrasound evaluation of the mesenteric vessels has gained in popularity. In the absence of obesity and an increased bowel gas pattern, the radiologist may be able to identify flow disturbances within the vessels or the lack of a vasodilation response to feeding. This tool is frequently used as a screening test for patients with symptoms suggestive of chronic mesenteric ischemia. The gold standard for confirmation of mesenteric arterial occlusion is mesenteric angiography. Evaluation with mesenteric angiography allows for identification and possible intervention for the treatment of thrombus within the vessel lumen and will also evaluate the patency of remaining mesenteric vessels. The use of mesenteric angiography may be limited in the presence of renal failure or contrast allergy. Magnetic resonance angiography is an alternative if the administration of contrast dye is contraindicated.

The management of chronic intestinal ischemia includes medical management of atherosclerotic disease by lipid-lowering medications, exercise, and cessation of smoking. A full cardiac evaluation should be performed before intervention. Newer endovascular procedures may avoid an operative intervention in selected patient populations. Angioplasty with endovascular stenting in the treatment of chronic mesenteric ischemia is associated with an 80% long-term success rate. In patients requiring surgical exploration, the approach used is determined by the mesenteric angiogram. The entire length of the small and large bowel should be evaluated, beginning at the ligament of Treitz. Restoration of blood flow at the time of laparotomy is accomplished with mesenteric bypass.

Determination of intestinal viability intraoperatively in patients with suspected intestinal ischemia can be challenging. After revascularization, the bowel wall should be observed for return of a pink color and peristalsis. Palpation of major arterial vessels can be performed as well as applying a doppler flowmeter to the antimesenteric border of the bowel wall, but neither is a definitive indicator of viability. In equivocal cases, 1 g of IV sodium fluorescein is administered and the pattern of bowel reperfusion is observed under ultraviolet illumination with a standard (3600 A) Wood's lamp. An area of nonfluorescence >5 mm in diameter suggests nonviability. If doubt persists, reexploration performed 24–48 h following surgery will allow demarcation of nonviable bowel. Primary intestinal anastomosis in patients with ischemic bowel is always worrisome, and reanastomosis should be deferred to the time of second-look laparotomy.

ACKNOWLEDGMENTS
We thank Cory Sandore for providing some illustrations for this chapter. Gregory Bulkley contributed to this chapter in the 16th edition.

FURTHER READINGS

HSU H et al: Impact of etiological factors and APACHE II and POSSUM scores in management and clinical outcomes of acute intestinal ischemic disease after surgical treatment. World J Surg 30(12):2152, 2006

MATSUMOTO AH et al: Percutaneous transluminal angioplasty and stenting in the treatment of chronic mesenteric ischemia: Results and long-term follow-up. J Am Coll Surg 194(Suppl):S22, 2002

MITCHELL EL, MONETA GL: Mesenteric duplex scanning. Perspect Vasc Surg Endovas Ther 18:175, 2006

SHIH MC et al: CTA and MRA in mesenteric ischemia: Part 2, normal findings and complications after surgical and endovascular treatment. AJR Am J Roentgenol 188:462, 2007

293 Acute Intestinal Obstruction
Susan L. Gearhart, William Silen

ETIOLOGY AND CLASSIFICATION

In 75% of patients, acute intestinal obstruction results from previous abdominal surgery secondary to adhesive bands or internal or external hernias. The incidence of acute intestinal obstruction requiring hospital admission within the first few post-operative weeks is 5–25%, and 10–50% of these patients will require surgical intervention. The incidence of postoperative intestinal obstruction may be lower following laparoscopic surgery than open procedures. However, the laparoscopic gastric bypass procedure may be associated with an unexpected high rate of intestinal obstruction, with a higher reoperative rate. The reason for this is unknown. Other causes of intestinal obstruction not related to previous abdominal surgery include lesions *intrinsic* to the wall of the intestine, e.g., diverticulitis, carcinoma, regional enteritis; and luminal obstruction, e.g., gallstone obstruction, intussusception.

Two other conditions that must be differentiated from acute intestinal obstruction include *adynamic ileus* and *primary intestinal pseudo-obstruction*. Adynamic ileus is mediated via the hormonal component of the sympathoadrenal system and may occur after any peritoneal insult; its severity and duration will be dependent to some degree on the type of peritoneal injury. Hydrochloric acid, colonic contents, and pancreatic enzymes are among the most irritating substances, whereas blood and urine are less so. Adynamic ileus occurs to some degree after any abdominal operation. Retroperitoneal hematoma, particularly associated with vertebral fracture, may cause severe adynamic ileus, and the latter may occur with other retroperitoneal conditions, such as ureteral calculus or severe pyelonephritis. Thoracic diseases, including lower-lobe pneumonia, fractured ribs, and myocardial infarction, frequently produce adynamic ileus, as do electrolyte disturbances, particularly potassium depletion. Finally, intestinal ischemia, whether from vascular occlusion or intestinal distention itself, may perpetuate an adynamic ileus. Intestinal pseudo-obstruction is a chronic motility disorder that frequently mimics mechanical obstruction. This condition is often exacerbated by narcotic use. Unnecessary operations in such patients should be avoided.

PATHOPHYSIOLOGY

Distention of the intestine is caused by the accumulation of gas and fluid proximal to and within the obstructed segment. Between 70 and 80% of intestinal gas consists of swallowed air, and because this is composed mainly of nitrogen, which is poorly absorbed from the intestinal lumen, removal of air by continuous gastric suction is a useful adjunct in the treatment of intestinal distention. The accumulation of fluid proximal to the obstructing mechanism results not only from ingested fluid, swallowed saliva, gastric juice, and biliary and pancreatic secretions but also from interference with normal sodium and water transport. During the first 12–24 h of obstruction, a marked depression of flux from lumen to blood occurs of sodium and consequently water in the distended proximal intestine. After 24 h, sodium and water move into the lumen, contributing further to the distention and fluid losses. Intraluminal pressure rises from a normal of 2–4 cmH_2O to 8–10 cmH_2O. The loss of fluids and electrolytes may be extreme, and unless replacement is prompt, hypovolemia, renal insufficiency, and shock may result. Vomiting, accumulation of fluids within the lumen, and the sequestration of fluid into the edematous intestinal wall and peritoneal cavity as a result of impairment of venous return from the intestine all contribute to massive loss of fluid and electrolytes.

The most feared complication of acute intestinal obstruction is the presence of a "closed loop." Closed-loop obstruction of the small intestine results when the lumen is occluded at two points by a single mechanism such as a fascial hernia or adhesive band, thus producing a closed loop whose blood supply is often occluded by the hernia or band as well. During peristalsis, when a "closed loop" is present, pressures reach 30–60 cmH$_2$O. Strangulation of the closed loop is common in association with marked distention proximal to the involved loop. A form of closed-loop obstruction is encountered when complete obstruction of the colon exists in the presence of a competent ileocecal valve (85% of individuals). Although the blood supply of the colon is not entrapped within the obstructing mechanism, distention of the cecum is extreme because of its greater diameter (Laplace's law), and impairment of the intramural blood supply is considerable, with consequent gangrene of the cecal wall. Once impairment of blood supply to the gastrointestinal tract occurs, bacterial invasion supervenes, and peritonitis develops. The systemic effects of extreme distention include elevation of the diaphragm with restricted ventilation and subsequent atelectasis. Venous return via the inferior vena cava may also be impaired.

SYMPTOMS

Mechanical intestinal obstruction is characterized by cramping midabdominal pain, which tends to be more severe the higher the obstruction. The pain occurs in paroxysms, and the patient is relatively comfortable in the intervals between the pains. Audible borborygmi are often noted by the patient simultaneously with the paroxysms of pain. The pain may become less severe as distention progresses, probably because motility is impaired in the edematous intestine. When strangulation is present, the pain is usually more localized and may be steady and severe without a colicky component, a fact that often causes delay in diagnosis of obstruction. Vomiting is almost invariable, and it is earlier and more profuse the higher the obstruction. The vomitus initially contains bile and mucus and remains as such if the obstruction is high in the intestine. With low ileal obstruction, the vomitus becomes feculent, i.e., orange-brown in color with a foul odor, which results from the overgrowth of bacteria proximal to the obstruction. Hiccups (singultus) are common. Obstipation and failure to pass gas by rectum are invariably present when the obstruction is complete, although some stool and gas may be passed spontaneously or after an enema shortly after onset of the complete obstruction. Diarrhea is occasionally observed in partial obstruction. Blood in the stool is rare but does occur in cases of intussusception.

In *adynamic ileus* as well as *colonic pseudo-obstruction*, colicky pain is absent and only discomfort from distention is evident. Vomiting may be frequent but is rarely profuse. Complete obstipation may or may not occur. Singultus (hiccups) is common.

PHYSICAL FINDINGS

Abdominal distention is the hallmark of all forms of intestinal obstruction. It is least marked in cases of obstruction high in the small intestine and most marked in colonic obstruction. In early obstruction of the small and large intestine, tenderness and rigidity are usually minimal; the temperature is rarely >37.8°C (100°F). The appearance of shock, tenderness, rigidity, and fever indicates that contamination of the peritoneum with infected intestinal content has occurred. Hernial orifices should always be carefully examined for the presence of a mass. Auscultation may reveal loud, high-pitched borborygmi coincident with colicky pain, but this finding is often absent late in strangulating or nonstrangulating obstruction. A quiet abdomen does not eliminate the possibility of obstruction, nor does it necessarily establish the diagnosis of adynamic ileus. The presence of a palpable abdominal mass usually signifies a closed-loop strangulating small-bowel obstruction; the tense fluid-filled loop is the palpable lesion.

LABORATORY AND X-RAY FINDINGS

Laboratory and radiographic studies are used to help differentiate the two important clinical aspects of this disorder: strangulation vs. non-

FIGURE 293-1 CT with oral and intravenous contrast demonstrating (**A**) evidence of small-bowel dilatation with air-fluid levels consistent with a small-bowel obstruction; (**B**) a partial small-bowel obstruction from an incarcerated ventral hernia (*arrow*); and (**C**) decompressed bowel seen distal to the hernia (*arrow*).

strangulation and partial vs. complete obstruction. Leukocytosis, with shift to the left, usually occurs when strangulation is present, but a normal white blood cell count does not exclude strangulation. Elevation of the serum amylase level is encountered occasionally in all forms of intestinal obstruction. Roentgenographic images demonstrating distention of fluid- and gas-filled loops of small intestine usually arranged in a "stepladder" pattern with air-fluid levels and an absence or paucity of colonic gas are pathognomonic for small-bowel obstruction. Complete obstruction is suggested when passage of gas or stool per rectum has ceased and when gas is absent in the distal intestine by x-ray. A general haze due to peritoneal fluid and sometimes a "coffee bean"–shaped mass are seen in strangulating closed loop obstruction. A thin barium upper gastrointestinal series may help to differentiate partial from complete obstruction. However, thick barium given by mouth should be avoided when the obstruction is considered to be high grade or complete since retained barium sulfate may become inspissated. CT is the most commonly used modality to evaluate postoperative patients for intestinal obstruction because of its ability in differentiating adynamic ileus, partial obstruction, and complete obstruction (Fig. 293-1). However, the sensitivity and specificity of CT for strangulating obstruction are low (50 and 80%, respectively).

Common causes of colonic obstruction can be seen on abdominal roentgenographic series. These films may demonstrate a "bird's beak" sign when a sigmoid volvulus has occurred or an enlarged cecum when a cecal torsion or bascule is present. Colonic obstruction with a competent ileocecal valve is easily recognized because distention with gas is mainly confined to the colon. Gastrografin enema may help in demonstrating a complete colonic obstruction. Furthermore, *barium should never be given by mouth to a patient with a possible colonic obstruction* until that possibility has been excluded.

℞ ACUTE INTESTINAL OBSTRUCTION

SMALL-INTESTINAL OBSTRUCTION The overall mortality rate for obstruction of the small intestine is about 10%. While the mortality rate for nonstrangulating obstruction is 5–8%, the mortality rate for a strangulating obstruction ranges from 20 to 75%. Since strangulating small-bowel obstruction is always complete, surgical interventions should always be undertaken in such patients after suitable preparation. Before operating, fluid and electrolyte balance should be restored and decompression instituted by means of a nasogastric tube. Replacement of potassium is especially important because intake is nil and losses in vomitus are large. There are few, if any, indications for the use of a long intestinal tube. Operative intervention may be undertaken successfully by laparoscopic techniques with a decreased incidence of wound complications. However, laparoscopic lysis of adhesions is associated with a longer operative time and higher conversion to open rate when compared to other laparoscopic procedures. Alternatively, lysis of adhesions can occur through an open abdominal incision. In general, >50% of adhesions that occur are found at the previous incision site. Purely nonoperative therapy is safe only in the presence of incomplete obstruction and is best utilized in patients without increasing abdominal pain or leukocytosis. The overall recurrence of small-bowel obstruction is 16%. Population-based studies show that although the surgical management of small-bowel obstruction is associated with longer hospital stays, the rate of readmission for obstruction is lower. However, regardless of treatment type, following the index admission, only 20% of patients required readmission within a 5-year follow-up period.

COLONIC OBSTRUCTION The mortality rate for colonic obstruction is about 20%. As in small-bowel obstruction, nonoperative treatment is contraindicated unless the obstruction is incomplete. Incomplete obstruction can be treated with colonoscopic decompression and placement of a metallic stent if a malignant lesion is present. The success rate approaches 90% depending on the location of the obstruction, with left-sided lesions being more successfully stented than right-sided lesions. In general, the colonic stent is considered to be a temporary solution or a "bridge to surgery," which allows for colonic preparation before surgical intervention. When obstruction is complete, early operation is mandatory, especially when the ileocecal valve is competent, because of the concern for cecal perforation. Cecal perforation is more likely if the cecal diameter is >10 cm on plain abdominal film.

Decisions regarding the operative management of colonic obstruction are based on the cause of the obstruction and the patient's overall well-being. For obstruction on the left side of the colon, operative management strategies include either decompression by cecostomy or transverse colostomy or resection with end-colostomy formation (Hartmann's procedure). Primary resection of obstructing left-sided lesions with on-table washout of the colon has also been accomplished safely. For a lesion of the right or transverse colon, primary resection and anastomosis can be performed safely because distention of the ileum with consequent discrepancy in size and hazard in suture are usually not present. Furthermore, the bacterial and stool content is less on the right side of the colon, decreasing the chance of infection.

ADYNAMIC ILEUS This type of ileus usually responds to nonoperative decompression and treatment of the primary disease. The prognosis is usually good. Correction of electrolyte abnormalities should be performed (i.e., potassium, magnesium). Successful decompression of a colonic ileus has been accomplished by repetitive colonoscopy. Neostigmine is also effective in cases of colonic ileus that have not responded to other conservative treatment. Rarely, adynamic colonic distention may become so great that cecostomy is required if cecal gangrene is feared.

FURTHER READINGS

DUBOIS A et al: Postoperative ileus: Physiopathology, etiology and treatment. Ann Surg 178:781, 1973

ESKELINEN M et al: Contributions of history-taking, physical examination, and computer assistance to diagnosis of acute small-bowel obstruction. A prospective study of 1333 patients with acute abdominal pain. Scand J Gastroenterol 29:715, 1994

FEVANG BT et al: Complications and death after surgical treatment of small bowel obstruction: A 35-year institutional experience. Ann Surg 231:529, 2000

JACKSON BR: The diagnosis of colonic obstruction. Dis Colon Rectum 25:603, 1982

SILEN W: *Cope's Early Diagnosis of the Acute Abdomen*, 21st ed. London, Oxford, 2005

294 Acute Appendicitis and Peritonitis

Susan L. Gearhart, William Silen

ACUTE APPENDICITIS

INCIDENCE AND EPIDEMIOLOGY

With more than 250,000 appendectomies performed annually, appendicitis is the most common abdominal surgical emergency in the United States. The peak incidence of acute appendicitis is in the second and third decades of life; it is relatively rare at the extremes of age. However, perforation is more common in infancy and in the elderly, during which periods mortality rates are highest. Males and females are equally affected, except between puberty and age 25, when males predominate in a 3:2 ratio. The incidence of appendicitis has remained stable in the United States over the last 30 years, while the incidence of appendicitis is much lower in underdeveloped countries, especially parts of Africa, and in lower socioeconomic groups. The mortality rate in the United States decreased eightfold between 1941 and 1970 but has remained at <1 per 100,000 since then.

PATHOGENESIS

Appendicitis is believed to occur as a result of appendiceal luminal obstruction. Obstruction is most commonly caused by a fecalith, which results from accumulation and inspissation of fecal matter around vegetable fibers. Enlarged lymphoid follicles associated with viral infections (e.g., measles), inspissated barium, worms (e.g., pinworms, *Ascaris*, and *Taenia*), and tumors (e.g., carcinoid or carcinoma) may also obstruct the lumen. Other common pathological findings include appendiceal ulceration. The cause of the ulceration is unknown, although a viral etiology has been postulated. Infection with *Yersinia* organisms may cause the disease, since high complement fixation antibody titers have been found in up to 30% of cases of proven appendicitis. Luminal bacteria multiply and invade the appendiceal wall as venous engorgement and subsequent arterial compromise result from the high intraluminal pressures. Finally, gangrene and perforation occur. If the process evolves slowly, adjacent organs such as the terminal ileum, cecum, and omentum may wall off the appendiceal area so that a localized abscess will develop, whereas rapid progression of vascular impairment may cause perforation with free access to the peritoneal cavity. Subsequent rupture of primary appendiceal abscesses may produce fistulas between the appendix and bladder, small intestine, sigmoid, or cecum. Occasionally, acute appendicitis may be the first manifestation of Crohn's disease.

While chronic infection of the appendix with tuberculosis, amebiasis, and actinomycosis may occur, a useful clinical aphorism states that *chronic appendiceal inflammation is not usually the cause of prolonged abdominal pain of weeks' or months' duration*. In contrast, recurrent acute appendicitis does occur, often with complete resolution of inflammation and symptoms between attacks. Recurrent acute appendicitis may also occur if a long appendiceal stump is left after initial appendectomy.

CLINICAL MANIFESTATIONS

The sequence of abdominal discomfort and anorexia associated with acute appendicitis is pathognomonic. The pain is described as being located in the periumbilical region initially and then migrating to the right lower quadrant. This classic sequence of symptoms occurs in only 66% of patients. However, in a male patient these symptoms are sufficient to advise surgical exploration. The differential diagnoses for periumbilical and right lower quadrant pain is listed in Table 294-1. The periumbilical abdominal pain is of the visceral type, resulting from distention of the appendiceal lumen. This pain is carried on slow-conducting C fibers and is usually poorly localized in the periumbilical or epigastric region. In general, this visceral pain is mild, often cramping and usually lasting 4–6 h, but it may not be noted by stoic individuals. As inflammation spreads to the parietal peritoneal surfaces, the pain becomes somatic, steady, and more severe and aggravated by motion or cough. Parietal afferent nerves are A delta fibers, which are fast-conducting and unilateral. These fibers localize the pain to the *right lower quadrant. Anorexia* is very common; a hungry patient does not have acute appendicitis. *Nausea* and *vomiting* occur in 50–60% of cases, but vomiting is usually self-limited. Change in bowel habit is of little diagnostic value, since any or no alteration may be observed, although the presence of diarrhea caused by an inflamed appendix in juxtaposition to the sigmoid may cause diagnostic difficulties. Urinary frequency and dysuria occur if the appendix lies adjacent to the bladder.

TABLE 294-1	THE ANATOMIC ORIGIN OF PERIUMBILICAL AND RIGHT LOWER QUADRANT PAIN IN THE DIFFERENTIAL DIAGNOSIS OF APPENDICITIS

Periumbilical

Appendicitis
Small-bowel obstruction
Gastroenteritis
Mesenteric ischemia

Right Lower Quadrant

Gastrointestinal causes	Gynecologic causes
Appendicitis	Ovarian tumor/torsion
Inflammatory bowel disease	Pelvic inflammatory disease
Right-sided diverticulitis	Renal causes
Gastroenteritis	Pyelonephritis
Inguinal hernia	Perinephritic abscess
	Nephrolithiasis

Physical findings vary with time after onset of the illness and according to the location of the appendix, which may be situated deep in the pelvic cul-de-sac; in the right lower quadrant in any relation to the peritoneum, cecum, and small intestine; in the right upper quadrant (especially during pregnancy); or even in the left lower quadrant. *The diagnosis cannot be established unless tenderness can be elicited*. While tenderness is sometimes absent in the early visceral stage of the disease, it ultimately always develops and is found in any location corresponding to the position of the appendix. Typically, tenderness to palpation will often occur at McBurney's point, anatomically located on a line one-third of the way between the anterior iliac spine and the umbilicus. Abdominal tenderness may be completely absent if a retrocecal or pelvic appendix is present, in which case the sole physical finding may be tenderness in the flank or on rectal or pelvic examination. Referred rebound tenderness is often present and is most likely to be absent early in the illness. Flexion of the right hip and guarded movement by the patient are due to parietal peritoneal involvement. Hyperesthesia of the skin of the right lower quadrant and a positive psoas or obturator sign are often late findings and are rarely of diagnostic value.

The temperature is usually normal or slightly elevated [37.2°–38°C (99°–100.5°F)], but a temperature >38.3°C (101°F) should suggest perforation. Tachycardia is commensurate with the elevation of the temperature. Rigidity and tenderness become more marked as the disease progresses to perforation and localized or diffuse peritonitis. Distention is rare unless severe diffuse peritonitis has developed. A mass may develop if localized perforation has occurred but will not usually be detectable before 3 days after onset. Earlier presence of a mass suggests carcinoma of the cecum or Crohn's disease. Perforation is rare before 24 h after onset of symptoms, but the rate may be as high as 80% after 48 h.

Although moderate leukocytosis of 10,000–18,000 cells/μL is frequent (with a concomitant left shift), the absence of leukocytosis does not rule out acute appendicitis. Leukocytosis of >20,000 cells/μL suggests probable perforation. Anemia and blood in the stool suggest a primary diagnosis of carcinoma of the cecum, especially in elderly individuals. The urine may contain a few white or red blood cells without bacteria if the appendix lies close to the right ureter or bladder. Urinalysis is most useful in excluding genitourinary conditions that may mimic acute appendicitis.

Radiographs are rarely of value except when an opaque fecalith (5% of patients) is observed in the right lower quadrant (especially in children). Consequently, abdominal films are not routinely obtained unless other conditions such as intestinal obstruction or ureteral calculus may be present. The diagnosis may also be established by the ultrasonic demonstration of an enlarged and thick-walled appendix. Ultrasound is most useful to exclude ovarian cysts, ectopic pregnancy, or tuboovarian abscess. Several studies have recently demonstrated the benefit of contrast-enhanced or nonenhanced CT over ultrasound and plain radiographs in the diagnosis of acute appendicitis. The findings on CT will include a thickened appendix with periappendiceal stranding and often the presence of a fecalith (Figs. 294-1 and 294-2). The reported positive predictive value of CT is 95–97% and the overall accuracy is 90–98%. Furthermore, nonvisualization of the appendix on CT is associated with the findings of a normal appendix 98% of the time. Free peritoneal air is uncommon, even in perforated appendicitis.

While the typical historic sequence and physical findings are present in 50–60% of cases, a wide variety of atypical patterns of disease are encountered, especially at the age extremes and during pregnancy. Infants under 2 years of age have a 70–80% incidence of perforation and generalized peritonitis. This is thought to be the result of a delay in diagnosis. Any infant or child with diarrhea, vomiting, and abdominal pain is highly suspect. Fever is much more common in this age group, and abdominal distention is often the only physical finding. In the elderly, pain and tenderness are often blunted, and thus the diagnosis is also frequently delayed and leads to a 30% incidence of perforation in patients over 70. Elderly patients often present initially with a slightly painful mass (a primary appendiceal abscess) or with

FIGURE 294-1 CT with oral and intravenous contrast of acute appendicitis. There is thickening of the wall of the appendix and periappendiceal stranding (*arrow*).

adhesive intestinal obstruction 5 or 6 days after a previously undetected perforated appendix.

Appendicitis occurs about once in every 500–2000 pregnancies and is the most common extrauterine condition requiring abdominal operation. The diagnosis may be missed or delayed because of the frequent occurrence of mild abdominal discomfort and nausea and vomiting during pregnancy and because of the gradual shift of the appendix from the right lower quadrant to the right upper quadrant during the second and third trimester of pregnancy. Appendicitis tends to be most common during the second trimester. The diagnosis is best made with ultrasound, which has an 80% accuracy; however, if perforation has already occurred, the accuracy of ultrasound decreases to 30%. Early intervention is warranted because the incidence of fetal loss with a normal appendix is 1.5%. With perforation, the incidence of fetal loss is 20–35%.

DIFFERENTIAL DIAGNOSIS

Acute appendicitis has been labeled the *masquerader*, and the diagnosis is often more difficult to make in young females. Obtaining a good history, including sexual activity and the presence of a vaginal discharge, will help differentiate acute appendicitis from pelvic inflammatory disease (PID). The presence of a malodorous vaginal discharge and gram-negative intracellular diplococci are pathognomonic for PID. Pain on movement of the cervix is also more specific for PID but may occur in appendicitis if perforation has occurred or if the appendix lies adjacent to the uterus or adnexa. *Rupture of a graafian follicle*

FIGURE 294-2 Appendiceal fecolith (*arrow*).

(mittelschmerz) occurs at midcycle and will produce pain and tenderness more diffuse and usually of a less severe degree than in appendicitis. *Rupture of a corpus luteum cyst* is identical clinically to rupture of a graafian follicle but develops about the time of menstruation. The presence of an adnexal mass, evidence of blood loss, and a positive pregnancy test help differentiate *ruptured tubal pregnancy*. *Twisted ovarian cyst* and *endometriosis* are occasionally difficult to distinguish from appendicitis. In all these female conditions, ultrasonography and laparoscopy may be of great value.

Acute mesenteric lymphadenitis and *acute gastroenteritis* are the diagnoses usually given when enlarged, slightly reddened lymph nodes at the root of the mesentery and a normal appendix are encountered at operation in a patient who usually has right lower quadrant tenderness. Retrospectively, these patients may have had a higher temperature, diarrhea, more diffuse pain and abdominal tenderness, and a lymphocytosis. Between cramps, the abdomen is completely relaxed. Children seem to be affected more frequently than adults. Some of these patients have infection with *Y. pseudotuberculosis* or *Y. enterocolitica*, in which case the diagnosis can be established by culture of the mesenteric nodes or by serologic titers (Chap. 152). In *Salmonella* gastroenteritis, the abdominal findings are similar, although the pain may be more severe and more localized, and fever and chills are common. The occurrence of similar symptoms among other members of the family may be helpful. *Regional enteritis* (Crohn's disease) is usually associated with a more prolonged history, often with previous exacerbations regarded as episodes of gastroenteritis unless the diagnosis has been established previously. Often an inflammatory mass is palpable. In addition, acute cholecystitis, perforated ulcer, acute pancreatitis, acute diverticulitis, strangulating intestinal obstruction, ureteral calculus, and pyelonephritis may present diagnostic difficulties.

℞ ACUTE APPENDICITIS

If the diagnosis is in question, 4–6 h of observation with serial abdominal exams is always more beneficial than harmful. Antibiotics should not be administered when the diagnosis is in question, since they will only mask the perforation. The treatment of presumed acute appendicitis is early operation and appendectomy as soon as the patient can be prepared. Appendectomy is frequently accomplished laparoscopically and is associated with less postoperative narcotic use and earlier discharge. It is acceptable to have a 15–20% incidence of a normal appendix at the time of appendectomy to avoid perforation. The use of early laparoscopy instead of close clinical observation has not shown a clinical benefit in the management of patients with nonspecific abdominal pain.

A different approach is indicated if a palpable mass is found 3–5 days after the onset of symptoms. This finding usually represents the presence of a phlegmon or abscess, and complications from attempted surgical excision are frequent. Such patients treated with broad-spectrum antibiotics, drainage of abscesses >3 cm, parenteral fluids, and bowel rest usually show resolution of symptoms within 1 week. *Interval appendectomy* can be performed safely 6–12 weeks later. A randomized clinical trial has demonstrated that antibiotics alone can effectively treat acute, nonperforated appendicitis in 86% of male patients. However, antibiotics alone were associated with a higher recurrence rate than surgical intervention. If the mass enlarges or the patient becomes more toxic, the abscess should be drained. Perforation is associated with generalized peritonitis and its complications, including subphrenic, pelvic, or other abscesses, and can be avoided by early diagnosis. The mortality rate for nonperforated appendicitis is 0.1%, little more than the risk of general anesthesia; for perforated appendicitis, mortality is 3% (and can reach 15% in the elderly).

ACUTE PERITONITIS

Peritonitis is an inflammation of the peritoneum; it may be localized or diffuse in location, acute or chronic in natural history, infectious or aseptic in pathogenesis. Acute peritonitis is most often infectious and is usually related to a perforated viscus (and called *secondary peritonitis*). When no intraabdominal source is identified, infectious peritonitis is called *primary* or *spontaneous*. Acute peritonitis is associated with

TABLE 294-2	CONDITIONS LEADING TO SECONDARY BACTERIAL PERITONITIS

Perforations of bowel	**Perforations or leaking of other organs**
Trauma, blunt or penetrating	Pancreas—pancreatitis
Inflammation	Gall bladder—cholecystitis
Appendicitis	Urinary bladder—trauma, rupture
Diverticulitis	Liver—bile leak after biopsy
Peptic ulcer disease	Fallopian tubes—salpingitis
Inflammatory bowel disease	Bleeding into the peritoneal cavity
Iatrogenic	**Disruption of integrity of peritoneal cavity**
Endoscopic perforation	
Anastomotic leaks	Trauma
Catheter perforation	Continuous ambulatory peritoneal
Vascular	dialysis (indwelling catheter)
Embolus	Intraperitoneal chemotherapy
Ischemia	Perinephric abscess
Obstructions	Iatrogenic—postoperative,
Adhesions	foreign body
Strangulated hernias	
Volvulus	
Intussusception	
Neoplasms	
Ingested foreign body, toothpick, fish bone	

decreased intestinal motor activity, resulting in distention of the intestinal lumen with gas and fluid. The accumulation of fluid in the bowel together with the lack of oral intake leads to rapid intravascular volume depletion with effects on cardiac, renal, and other systems.

ETIOLOGY

Infectious agents gain access to the peritoneal cavity through a perforated viscus, a penetrating wound of the abdominal wall, or external introduction of a foreign object that is or becomes infected (for example, a chronic peritoneal dialysis catheter). In the absence of immune compromise, host defenses are capable of eradicating small contaminations. The conditions that most commonly result in the introduction of bacteria into the peritoneum are ruptured appendix, ruptured diverticulum, perforated peptic ulcer, incarcerated hernia, gangrenous gall bladder, volvulus, bowel infarction, cancer, inflammatory bowel disease, or intestinal obstruction. However, a wide range of mechanisms may play a role (Table 294-2). Bacterial peritonitis can also occur in the apparent absence of an intraperitoneal source of bacteria (primary or spontaneous bacterial peritonitis). This condition occurs in the setting of ascites and liver cirrhosis in 90% of the cases, usually in patients with ascites with low protein concentration (<1 g/L) (Chap. 302). Bacterial peritonitis is discussed in detail in Chap. 121.

Aseptic peritonitis may be due to peritoneal irritation by abnormal presence of physiologic fluids (e.g., gastric juice, bile, pancreatic enzymes, blood, or urine) or sterile foreign bodies (e.g., surgical sponges or instruments, starch from surgical gloves) in the peritoneal cavity or as a complication of rare systemic diseases such as lupus erythematosus, porphyria, or familial Mediterranean fever (Chap. 323). Chemical irritation of the peritoneum is greatest for acidic gastric juice and pancreatic enzymes. In chemical peritonitis, a major risk of secondary bacterial infection exists.

CLINICAL FEATURES

The cardinal manifestations of peritonitis are acute abdominal pain and tenderness, usually with fever. The location of the pain depends on the underlying cause and whether the inflammation is localized or generalized. Localized peritonitis is most common in uncomplicated appendicitis and diverticulitis, and physical findings are limited to the area of inflammation. Generalized peritonitis is associated with widespread inflammation and diffuse abdominal tenderness and rebound. Rigidity of the abdominal wall is common in both localized and generalized peritonitis. Bowel sounds are usually absent. Tachycardia, hypotension, and signs of dehydration are common. Leukocytosis and marked acidosis are common laboratory findings. Plain abdominal films may show dilation of large and small bowel with edema of the bowel wall. Free air under the diaphragm is associated with a perforated viscus. CT and/or ultrasonography can identify the presence of free fluid or an abscess. When ascites is present, diagnostic paracentesis with cell count (>250 neutrophils/μL is usual in peritonitis), protein and lactate dehydrogenase levels, and culture is essential. In elderly and immunosuppressed patients, signs of peritoneal irritation may be more difficult to detect.

THERAPY AND PROGNOSIS

Treatment relies on rehydration, correction of electrolyte abnormalities, antibiotics, and surgical correction of the underlying defect. Mortality rates are <10% for uncomplicated peritonitis associated with a perforated ulcer or ruptured appendix or diverticulum in an otherwise healthy person. Mortality rates of ≥40% have been reported for elderly people, those with underlying illnesses, and when peritonitis has been present for >48 h.

FURTHER READINGS

ANDERSON RE: The natural history and traditional management of appendicitis revisited: Spontaneous resolution and predominance of prehospital perforations imply that a correct diagnosis is more important than an early diagnosis. World J Surg 31:86, 2007

CHEADLE WG, SPAIN DA: The continuing challenge of intraabdominal infection. Am J Surg 186(Suppl 1):15, 2003

FLUM DR et al: Has misdiagnosis of appendicitis decreased over time? A population-based analysis. JAMA 286:1748, 2001

GANGULI S et al: Right lower quadrant pain: Value of the nonvisualized appendix in patients at multidetector CT. Radiology 214:175, 2006

GRONROOS JM, GRONROOS P: Leucocyte count and C-reactive protein in the diagnosis of acute appendicitis. Br J Surg 86:501, 1999

MORINO M et al: Acute non-specific abdominal pain: A randomized controlled study comparing early laparoscopy vs. clinical observation. Ann Surg 241:881, 2006

STYRUD J et al: Appendectomy vs. antibiotic treatment in acute appendectomy: A prospective multicenter randomized controlled trial. World J Surg 30:1033, 2006

295   Approach to the Patient with Liver Disease

Marc Ghany, Jay H. Hoofnagle

In most instances, a diagnosis of liver disease can be made accurately by a careful history, physical examination, and application of a few laboratory tests. In some circumstances, radiologic examinations are helpful or, indeed, diagnostic. Liver biopsy is considered the "gold standard" in evaluation of liver disease but is now needed less for diagnosis than for grading and staging disease. This chapter provides an introduction to diagnosis and management of liver disease, briefly reviewing the structure and function of the liver; the major clinical manifestations of liver disease; and the use of clinical history, physical examination, laboratory tests, imaging studies, and liver biopsy.

LIVER STRUCTURE AND FUNCTION

The liver is the largest organ of the body, weighing 1–1.5 kg and representing 1.5–2.5% of the lean body mass. The size and shape of the liver vary and generally match the general body shape—long and lean or squat and square. The liver is located in the right upper quadrant of the abdomen under the right lower rib cage against the diaphragm and projects for a variable extent into the left upper quadrant. The liver is held in place by ligamentous attachments to the diaphragm, peritoneum, great vessels, and upper gastrointestinal organs. It receives a dual blood supply; ~20% of the blood flow is oxygen-rich blood from the hepatic artery, and 80% is nutrient-rich blood from the portal vein arising from the stomach, intestines, pancreas, and spleen.

The majority of cells in the liver are hepatocytes, which constitute two-thirds of the mass of the liver. The remaining cell types are Kupffer cells (members of the reticuloendothelial system), stellate (Ito or fat-storing) cells, endothelial cells and blood vessels, bile ductular cells, and supporting structures. Viewed by light microscopy, the liver appears to be organized in lobules, with portal areas at the periphery and central veins in the center of each lobule. However, from a functional point of view, the liver is organized into acini, with both hepatic arterial and portal venous blood entering the acinus from the portal areas (zone 1) and then flowing through the sinusoids to the terminal hepatic veins (zone 3); the intervening hepatocytes constitute zone 2. The advantage of viewing the acinus as the physiologic unit of the liver is that it helps to explain the morphologic patterns and zonality of many vascular and biliary diseases not explained by the lobular arrangement.

Portal areas of the liver consist of small veins, arteries, bile ducts, and lymphatics organized in a loose stroma of supporting matrix and small amounts of collagen. Blood flowing into the portal areas is distributed through the sinusoids, passing from zone 1 to zone 3 of the acinus and draining into the terminal hepatic veins ("central veins"). Secreted bile flows in the opposite direction, in a countercurrent pattern from zone 3 to zone 1. The sinusoids are lined by unique endothelial cells that have prominent fenestrae of variable size, allowing the free flow of plasma but not cellular elements. The plasma is thus in direct contact with hepatocytes in the subendothelial space of Disse.

Hepatocytes have distinct polarity. The basolateral side of the hepatocyte lines the space of Disse and is richly lined with microvilli; it demonstrates endocytotic and pinocytotic activity, with passive and active uptake of nutrients, proteins, and other molecules. The apical pole of the hepatocyte forms the cannicular membranes through which bile components are secreted. The canniculi of hepatocytes form a fine network, which fuses into the bile ductular elements near the portal areas. Kupffer cells usually lie within the sinusoidal vascular space and represent the largest group of fixed macrophages in the body. The stellate cells are located in the space of Disse but are not usually prominent unless activated, when they produce collagen and matrix. Red blood cells stay in the sinusoidal space as blood flows through the lobules, but white blood cells can migrate through or around endothelial cells into the space of Disse and from there to portal areas, where they can return to the circulation through lymphatics.

Hepatocytes perform numerous and vital roles in maintaining homeostasis and health. These functions include the synthesis of most essential serum proteins (albumin, carrier proteins, coagulation factors, many hormonal and growth factors), the production of bile and its carriers (bile acids, cholesterol, lecithin, phospholipids), the regulation of nutrients (glucose, glycogen, lipids, cholesterol, amino acids), and metabolism and conjugation of lipophilic compounds (bilirubin, anions, cations, drugs) for excretion in the bile or urine. Measurement of these activities to assess liver function is complicated by the multiplicity and variability of these functions. The most commonly used liver "function" tests are measurements of serum bilirubin, albumin, and prothrombin time. The serum bilirubin level is a measure of hepatic conjugation and excretion, and the serum albumin level and prothrombin time are measures of protein synthesis. Abnormalities of bilirubin, albumin, and prothrombin time are typical of hepatic dysfunction. Frank liver failure is incompatible with life, and the functions of the liver are too complex and diverse to be subserved by a mechanical pump; dialysis membrane; or concoction of infused hormones, proteins, and growth factors.

LIVER DISEASES

While there are many causes of liver disease (Table 295-1), they generally present clinically in a few distinct patterns, usually classified as hepatocellular, cholestatic (obstructive), or mixed. In *hepatocellular diseases* (such as viral hepatitis or alcoholic liver disease), features of liver injury, inflammation, and necrosis predominate. In *cholestatic diseases* (such as gall stone or malignant obstruction, primary biliary cirrhosis, some drug-induced liver diseases), features of inhibition of bile flow predominate. In a mixed pattern, features of both hepatocellular and cholestatic injury are present (such as in cholestatic forms of viral hepatitis and many drug-induced liver diseases). The pattern of onset and prominence of symptoms can rapidly suggest a diagnosis, particularly if major risk factors are considered, such as the age and sex of the patient and a history of exposure or risk behaviors.

Typical presenting symptoms of liver disease include jaundice, fatigue, itching, right upper quadrant pain, abdominal distention, and intestinal bleeding. At present, however, many patients are diagnosed with liver disease who have no symptoms and who have been found to have abnormalities in biochemical liver tests as a part of a routine physical examination or screening for blood donation or for insurance or employment. The wide availability of batteries of liver tests makes it relatively simple to demonstrate the presence of liver injury as well as to rule it out in someone suspected of liver disease.

Evaluation of patients with liver disease should be directed at (1) establishing the etiologic diagnosis, (2) estimating the disease severity (grading), and (3) establishing the disease stage (staging). *Diagnosis* should focus on the category of disease, such as hepatocellular, cholestatic, or mixed injury, as well as on the specific etiologic diagnosis. *Grading* refers to assessing the severity or activity of disease—active or inactive, and mild, moderate, or severe. *Staging* refers to estimating the place in the course of the natural history of the disease, whether acute or chronic; early or late; precirrhotic, cirrhotic, or end-stage.

The goal of this chapter is to introduce general, salient concepts in the evaluation of patients with liver disease that help lead to the diagnoses discussed in subsequent chapters.

TABLE 295-1 **LIVER DISEASES**

Inherited hyperbilirubinemia	Liver involvement in systemic diseases
Gilbert syndrome	Sarcoidosis
Crigler-Najjar syndrome, types I and II	Amyloidosis
Dubin-Johnson syndrome	Glycogen storage diseases
Rotor syndrome	Celiac disease
Viral hepatitis	Tuberculosis
Hepatitis A	*Mycobacterium avium intracellulare*
Hepatitis B	Cholestatic syndromes
Hepatitis C	Benign postoperative cholestasis
Hepatitis D	Jaundice of sepsis
Hepatitis E	Total parenteral nutrition (TPN)–induced jaundice
Others (mononucleosis, herpes, adenovirus	Cholestasis of pregnancy
hepatitis)	Cholangitis and cholecystitis
Cryptogenic hepatitis	Extrahepatic biliary obstruction (stone, stricture, cancer)
Immune and autoimmune liver diseases	Biliary atresia
Primary biliary cirrhosis	Caroli disease
Autoimmune hepatitis	Cryptosporidiosis
Sclerosing cholangitis	Drug-induced liver disease
Overlap syndromes	Hepatocellular patterns (isoniazid, acetaminophen)
Graft-vs-host disease	Cholestatic patterns (methyltestosterone)
Allograft rejection	Mixed patterns (sulfonamides, phenytoin)
Genetic liver diseases	Micro- and macrovesicular steatosis (methotrexate,
α_1 Antitrypsin deficiency	fialuridine)
Hemochromatosis	Vascular injury
Wilson disease	Venoocclusive disease
Benign recurrent intrahepatic cholestasis	Budd-Chiari syndrome
(BRIC)	Ischemic hepatitis
Progressive familial intrahepatic cholestasis	Passive congestion
(PFIC), types I–III	Portal vein thrombosis
Others (galactosemia, tyrosinemia, cystic	Nodular regenerative hyperplasia
fibrosis, Newman-Pick disease, Gaucher	Mass lesions
disease)	Hepatocellular carcinoma
Alcoholic liver disease	Cholangiocarcinoma
Acute fatty liver	Adenoma
Acute alcoholic hepatitis	Focal nodular hyperplasia
Laennec cirrhosis	Metastatic tumors
Nonalcoholic fatty liver	Abscess
Steatosis	Cysts
Steatohepatitis	Hemangioma
Acute fatty liver of pregnancy	

CLINICAL HISTORY

The clinical history should focus on the symptoms of liver disease—their nature, pattern of onset, and progression—and on potential risk factors for liver disease. The symptoms of liver disease include constitutional symptoms such as fatigue, weakness, nausea, poor appetite, and malaise and the more liver-specific symptoms of jaundice, dark urine, light stools, itching, abdominal pain, and bloating. Symptoms can also suggest the presence of cirrhosis, end-stage liver disease, or complications of cirrhosis such as portal hypertension. Generally, the constellation of symptoms and their pattern of onset rather than a specific symptom points to an etiology.

Fatigue is the most common and most characteristic symptom of liver disease. It is variously described as lethargy, weakness, listlessness, malaise, increased need for sleep, lack of stamina, and poor energy. The fatigue of liver disease typically arises after activity or exercise and is rarely present or severe in the morning after adequate rest (afternoon vs. morning fatigue). Fatigue in liver disease is often intermittent and variable in severity from hour to hour and day to day. In some patients, it may not be clear whether fatigue is due to the liver disease or to other problems such as stress, anxiety, sleep disturbance, or a concurrent illness.

Nausea occurs with more severe liver disease and may accompany fatigue or be provoked by odors of food or eating fatty foods. Vomiting can occur but is rarely persistent or prominent. Poor appetite with weight loss occurs commonly in acute liver diseases but is rare in chronic disease, except when cirrhosis is present and advanced. Diarrhea is uncommon in liver disease, except with severe jaundice, where lack of bile acids reaching the intestine can lead to steatorrhea.

Right upper quadrant discomfort or ache ("liver pain") occurs in many liver diseases and is usually marked by tenderness over the liver ar-

ea. The pain arises from stretching or irritation of Glisson's capsule, which surrounds the liver and is rich in nerve endings. Severe pain is most typical of gall bladder disease, liver abscess, and severe venoocclusive disease but is an occasional accompaniment of acute hepatitis.

Itching occurs with acute liver disease, appearing early in obstructive jaundice (from biliary obstruction or drug-induced cholestasis) and somewhat later in hepatocellular disease (acute hepatitis). Itching also occurs in chronic liver diseases, typically the cholestatic forms such as primary biliary cirrhosis and sclerosing cholangitis where it is often the presenting symptom, occurring before the onset of jaundice. However, itching can occur in any liver disease, particularly once cirrhosis is present.

Jaundice is the hallmark symptom of liver disease and perhaps the most reliable marker of severity. Patients usually report darkening of the urine before they notice scleral icterus. Jaundice is rarely detectable with a bilirubin level <43 μmol/L (2.5 mg/dL). With severe cholestasis there will also be lightening of the color of the stools and steatorrhea. Jaundice without dark urine usually indicates indirect (unconjugated) hyperbilirubinemia and is typical of hemolytic anemia and the genetic disorders of bilirubin conjugation, the common and benign form being Gilbert syndrome and the rare and severe form being Crigler-Najjar syndrome. Gilbert syndrome affects up to 5% of the population; the jaundice is more noticeable after fasting and with stress.

Major risk factors for liver disease that should be sought in the clinical history include details of alcohol use, medications (including herbal compounds, birth control pills, and over-the-counter medications), personal habits, sexual activity, travel, exposure to jaundiced or other high-risk persons, injection drug use, recent surgery, remote or recent transfusion with blood and blood products, occupation, accidental exposure to blood or needlestick, and familial history of liver disease.

For assessing the risk of viral hepatitis, a careful history of sexual activity is of particular importance and should include number of lifetime sexual partners and, for men, a history of having sex with men. Sexual exposure is a common mode of spread of hepatitis B but is rare for hepatitis C. A family history of hepatitis, liver disease, and liver cancer is also important. Maternal-infant transmission occurs with both hepatitis B and C. Vertical spread of hepatitis B can now be prevented by passive and active immunization of the infant at birth. Vertical spread of hepatitis C is uncommon, but there are no reliable means of prevention. Transmission is more common in HIV-co-infected mothers and is also linked to prolonged and difficult labor and delivery, early rupture of membranes, and internal fetal monitoring. A history of injection drug use, even in the remote past, is of great importance in assessing the risk for hepatitis B and C. Injection drug use is now the single most common risk factor for hepatitis C. Transfusion with blood or blood products is no longer an important risk factor for acute viral hepatitis. However, blood transfusions received before the introduction of sensitive enzyme immunoassays for antibody to hepatitis C virus (anti-HCV) in 1992 is an important risk factor for chronic hepatitis C. Blood transfusion before 1986, when screening for antibody to hepatitis B core antigen (anti-HBc) was introduced, is also a risk factor for hepatitis B. Travel to an underdeveloped area of the world, exposure to persons with jaundice, and exposure to young children in day-care centers are risk factors for hepatitis A. Hepatitis E is uncommon in the United States; however, it is one of the more common causes of jaundice in Asia and Africa. Tattooing and body piercing (for hepatitis B and C) and eating shellfish (for hepatitis A) are frequently mentioned but are actually quite rare types of exposure for acquiring hepatitis.

A history of alcohol intake is important in assessing the cause of liver disease and also in planning management and recommendations. In the United States, for example, at least 70% of adults drink alcohol to some degree, but significant alcohol intake is less common; in population-based surveys, only 5% have more than two drinks per day, the average drink representing 11–15 g alcohol. Alcohol consumption associated with an increased rate of alcoholic liver disease is probably more than two drinks (22–30 g) per day in women and three drinks (33–45 g) in men. Most patients with alcoholic cirrhosis have a much higher daily intake and have drunk excessively for ≥10 years before onset of liver disease. In assessing alcohol intake, the history should also focus upon whether alcohol abuse or dependence is present. Alcoholism is usually defined on the behavioral patterns and consequences of alcohol intake, not on the basis of the amount of alcohol intake. *Abuse* is defined by a repetitive pattern of drinking alcohol that has adverse effects on social, family, occupational, or health status. *Dependence* is defined by alcohol-seeking behavior, despite its adverse effects. Many alcoholics demonstrate both dependence and abuse, and dependence is considered the more serious and advanced form of alcoholism. A clinically helpful approach to diagnosis of alcohol dependence and abuse is the use of the CAGE questionnaire (Table 295-2), which is recommended in all medical history taking.

Family history can be helpful in assessing liver disease. Familial causes of liver disease include Wilson disease; hemochromatosis and α_1 antitrypsin (α_1AT) deficiency; and the more uncommon inherited pediatric liver diseases of familial intrahepatic cholestasis, benign recurrent intrahepatic cholestasis, and Alagille syndrome. Onset of severe liver disease in childhood or adolescence with a family history of liver disease or neuropsychiatric disturbance should lead to investigation for Wilson disease. A family history of cirrhosis, diabetes, or endocrine failure and the appearance of liver disease in adulthood should suggest hemochromatosis and lead to investigation of iron status. Patients with abnormal iron studies warrant genotyping of the *HFE* gene for the C282Y and H63D mutations typical of genetic hemochromatosis. A family history of emphysema should provoke investigation of α_1AT levels and, if low, for Pi genotype.

PHYSICAL EXAMINATION

The physical examination rarely demonstrates evidence of liver dysfunction in a patient without symptoms or laboratory findings, nor are most signs of liver disease specific to one diagnosis. Thus, the physical examination usually complements rather than replaces the need for other diagnostic approaches. In many patients, the physical examination is normal unless the disease is acute or severe and advanced. Nevertheless, the physical examination is important in that it can be the first evidence for the presence of hepatic failure, portal hypertension, and liver decompensation. In addition, the physical examination can reveal signs that point to a specific diagnosis, either in risk factors or in associated diseases or findings.

TABLE 295-2   CAGE QUESTIONS[a]

Acronym	Question
C	Have you ever felt you ought to *Cut* down on your drinking?
A	Have people *Annoyed* you by criticizing your drinking?
G	Have you ever felt *Guilty* or bad about your drinking?
E	Have you ever had a drink first thing in the morning to steady your nerves or get rid of a hangover (*Eyeopener*)?

[a]One "yes" response should raise suspicion of an alcohol use problem, and more than one is a strong indication that abuse or dependence exists.

Typical physical findings in liver disease are icterus, hepatomegaly, hepatic tenderness, splenomegaly, spider angiomata, palmar erythema, and excoriations. Signs of advanced disease include muscle-wasting, ascites, edema, dilated abdominal veins, hepatic fetor, asterixis, mental confusion, stupor, and coma. In males with cirrhosis, particularly when related to alcohol, signs of hyperestrogenemia such as gynecomastia, testicular atrophy, and loss of male-pattern hair distribution may be found.

Icterus is best appreciated by inspecting the sclera under natural light. In fair-skinned individuals, a yellow color of the skin may be obvious. In dark-skinned individuals, the mucous membranes below the tongue can demonstrate jaundice. Jaundice is rarely detectable if the serum bilirubin level is <43 μmol/L (2.5 mg/dL) but may remain detectable below this level during recovery from jaundice (because of protein and tissue binding of conjugated bilirubin).

Spider angiomata and palmar erythema occur in both acute and chronic liver disease and may be especially prominent in persons with cirrhosis, but they can occur in normal individuals and are frequently present during pregnancy. Spider angiomata are superficial, tortuous arterioles and, unlike simple telangiectases, typically fill from the center outwards. Spider angiomata occur only on the arms, face, and upper torso; they can be pulsatile and may be difficult to detect in dark-skinned individuals.

Hepatomegaly is not a very reliable sign of liver disease, because of the variability of the size and shape of the liver and the physical impediments to assessing liver size by percussion and palpation. Marked hepatomegaly is typical of cirrhosis, venoocclusive disease, infiltrative disorders such as amyloidosis, metastatic or primary cancers of the liver, and alcoholic hepatitis. Careful assessment of the liver edge may also demonstrate unusual firmness, irregularity of the surface, or frank nodules. Perhaps the most reliable physical finding in examining the liver is hepatic tenderness. Discomfort on touching or pressing on the liver should be carefully sought with percussive comparison of the right and left upper quadrants.

Splenomegaly occurs in many medical conditions but can be a subtle but significant physical finding in liver disease. The availability of ultrasound (US) assessment of the spleen allows for confirmation of the physical finding.

Signs of advanced liver disease include muscle-wasting and weight loss as well as hepatomegaly, bruising, ascites, and edema. Ascites is best appreciated by attempts to detect shifting dullness by careful percussion. US examination will confirm the finding of ascites in equivocal cases. Peripheral edema can occur with or without ascites. In patients with advanced liver disease, other factors frequently contribute to edema formation, including hypoalbuminemia, venous insufficiency, heart failure, and medications.

Hepatic failure is defined as the occurrence of signs or symptoms of hepatic encephalopathy in a person with severe acute or chronic liver disease. The first signs of hepatic encephalopathy can be subtle and nonspecific—change in sleep patterns, change in personality, irritability, and mental dullness. Thereafter, confusion, disorientation, stupor, and eventually coma supervene. In acute liver failure, excitability and mania may be present. Physical findings include asterixis and flapping tremors of the body and tongue. *Fetor hepaticus* refers to the slightly sweet, ammoniacal odor that can occur in patients with liver failure, particularly if there is portal-venous shunting of blood around the liver. Other causes of coma and confusion should be excluded, mainly electrolyte imbalances, sedative use, and renal or respiratory failure. The appearance of hepatic encephalopathy during acute hepatitis is the major criterion for diagnosis of fulminant hepatitis and indicates a poor prognosis. In chronic liver disease, encephalopathy is usually triggered by a medical complication, such as gastrointestinal bleeding, over-diuresis, uremia, dehydration, electrolyte imbalance, infection, constipation, or use of narcotic analgesics.

A helpful measure of hepatic encephalopathy is a careful mental status examination and use of the trail-making test, which consists of a series of 25 numbered circles that the patient is asked to connect as rapidly as possible using a pencil. The normal range for the connect-the-dot test is 15–30 s; it is considerably delayed in patients with early hepatic encephalopathy. Other tests include drawing abstract objects or comparison of a signature to previous examples. More sophisticated testing such as with electroencephalography and visual evoked potentials can detect mild forms of encephalopathy, but are rarely clinically useful.

Other signs of advanced liver disease include umbilical hernia from ascites, hydrothorax, prominent veins over the abdomen, and *caput medusa*, which consists of collateral veins seen radiating from the umbilicus and resulting from the recanalization of the umbilical vein. Widened pulse pressure and signs of a hyperdynamic circulation can occur in patients with cirrhosis as a result of fluid and sodium retention, increased cardiac output, and reduced peripheral resistance. Patients with long-standing cirrhosis and portal hypertension are prone to develop the hepatopulmonary syndrome, defined by the triad of liver disease, hypoxemia, and pulmonary arteriovenous shunting. The hepatopulmonary syndrome is characterized by platypnea and orthodeoxia, representing shortness of breath and oxygen desaturation that occur paradoxically upon assuming an upright position.

Several skin disorders and changes occur commonly in liver disease. Hyperpigmentation is typical of advanced chronic cholestatic diseases such as primary biliary cirrhosis and sclerosing cholangitis. In these same conditions, xanthelasma and tendon xanthomata occur as a result of retention and high serum levels of lipids and cholesterol. A slate-gray pigmentation to the skin also occurs with hemochromatosis if iron levels are high for a prolonged period. Mucocutaneous vasculitis with palpable purpura, especially on the lower extremities, is typical of cryoglobulinemia of chronic hepatitis C but can also occur in chronic hepatitis B.

Some physical signs point to specific liver diseases. Kayser-Fleischer rings occur in Wilson's disease and consist of a golden-brown copper pigment deposited in Descemet's membrane at the periphery of the cornea; they are best seen by slit-lamp examination. Dupuytren contracture and parotid enlargement are suggestive of chronic alcoholism and alcoholic liver disease. In metastatic liver disease or primary hepatocellular carcinoma, signs of cachexia and wasting may be prominent, as well as firm hepatomegaly and a hepatic bruit.

LABORATORY TESTING

Diagnosis in liver disease is greatly aided by the availability of reliable and sensitive tests of liver injury and function. A typical battery of blood tests used for initial assessment of liver disease includes measuring levels of serum alanine and aspartate aminotransferases (ALT and AST), alkaline phosphatase, direct and total serum bilirubin, and albumin and assessing prothrombin time. The pattern of abnormalities generally points to hepatocellular versus cholestatic liver disease and will help to decide whether the disease is acute or chronic and whether cirrhosis and hepatic failure are present. Based on these results, further testing over time may be necessary. Other laboratory tests may be helpful, such as γ-glutamyl transpeptidase (GGT) to define whether alkaline phosphatase elevations are due to liver disease; hepatitis serology to define the type of viral hepatitis; and autoimmune markers to diagnose primary biliary cirrhosis (antimitochondrial antibody; AMA), sclerosing cholangitis (peripheral antineutrophil cytoplasmic antibody; P-ANCA), and autoimmune hepatitis (antinuclear, smooth-muscle, and liver-kidney microsomal antibody). A simple delineation of laboratory abnormalities and common liver diseases is given in Table 295-3. The use and interpretation of liver function tests is summarized in Chap. 296.

DIAGNOSTIC IMAGING

There have been great advances made in hepatic imaging, although no method is suitably accurate in demonstrating underlying cirrhosis. There are many modalities available for imaging the liver. US, CT, and MRI are the most commonly employed and are complementary to each other. In general, US and CT have a high sensitivity for detecting biliary duct dilatation and are the first-line options for investigating the patient with suspected obstructive jaundice. Both US and CT can detect a fatty liver, which appears bright on both studies. Magnetic resonance cholangiopancreatography (MRCP) and endoscopic retrograde cholangiopancreatography (ERCP) are the procedures of choice

TABLE 295-3 IMPORTANT DIAGNOSTIC TESTS IN COMMON LIVER DISEASES

Disease	Diagnostic Test
Hepatitis A	Anti-HAV IgM
Hepatitis B	
Acute	HBsAg and anti-HBc IgM
Chronic	HBsAg and HBeAg and/or HBV DNA
Hepatitis C	Anti-HCV and HCV RNA
Hepatitis D (delta)	HBsAg and anti-HDV
Hepatitis E	Anti-HEV
Autoimmune hepatitis	ANA or SMA, elevated IgG levels, and compatible histology
Primary biliary cirrhosis	Mitochondrial antibody, elevated IgM levels, and compatible histology
Primary sclerosing cholangitis	P-ANCA, cholangiography
Drug-induced liver disease	History of drug ingestion
Alcoholic liver disease	History of excessive alcohol intake and compatible histology
Nonalcoholic steatohepatitis	Ultrasound or CT evidence of fatty liver and compatible histology
α_1 Antitrypsin disease	Reduced α_1 antitrypsin levels, phenotypes PiZZ or PiSZ
Wilson disease	Decreased serum ceruloplasmin and increased urinary copper; increased hepatic copper level
Hemochromatosis	Elevated iron saturation and serum ferritin; genetic testing for *HFE* gene mutations
Hepatocellular cancer	Elevated α-fetoprotein level >500; ultrasound or CT image of mass

Note: HAV, HBV, HCV, HDV, HEV: hepatitis A, B, C, D, or E virus; HBsAg, hepatitis B surface antigen; anti-HBc, antibody to hepatitis B core (antigen); HBeAg, hepatitis e antigen; ANA, antinuclear antibodies; SMA, smooth-muscle antibody; P-ANCA, peripheral antineutrophil cytoplasmic antibody.

for visualization of the biliary tree. MRCP offers several advantages over ERCP; there is no need for contrast media or ionizing radiation, images can be acquired faster, it is less operator dependent, and it carries no risk of pancreatitis. MRCP is superior to US and CT for detecting choledocholithiasis but less specific. It is useful in the diagnosis of bile duct obstruction and congenital biliary abnormalities, but ERCP is more valuable in evaluating ampullary lesions and primary sclerosing cholangitis. ERCP allows for biopsy, direct visualization of the ampulla and common bile duct, and intraductal ultrasonography. It also provides several therapeutic options in patients with obstructive jaundice, such as sphincterotomy, stone extraction, and placement of nasobiliary catheters and biliary stents. Doppler US and MRI are used to assess hepatic vasculature and hemodynamics and to monitor surgically or radiologically placed vascular shunts such as transjugular intrahepatic portosystemic shunts. CT and MRI are indicated for the identification and evaluation of hepatic masses, staging of liver tumors, and preoperative assessment. With regard to mass lesions, sensitivity of hepatic imaging continues to increase; unfortunately, specificity remains a problem, and often two and sometimes three studies are needed before a diagnosis can be reached. Recently, methods using elastography have been developed to measure hepatic stiffness as a means of assessing hepatic fibrosis. US elastography is now undergoing evaluation for its ability to detect different degrees of hepatic fibrosis and to obviate the need for liver biopsy in assessing disease stage. If found to be reliable, hepatic elastography may be an appropriate means of monitoring fibrosis and disease progression. Finally, interventional radiologic techniques allow the biopsy of solitary lesions, insertion of drains into hepatic abscesses, measurement of portal pressure, and creation of vascular shunts in patients with portal hypertension. Which modality to use depends on factors such as availability, cost, and experience of the radiologist with each technique.

LIVER BIOPSY

Liver biopsy remains the gold standard in the evaluation of patients with liver disease, particularly in patients with chronic liver diseases.

FIGURE 295-1 Algorithm for evaluation of abnormal liver tests. For patients with suspected liver disease, an appropriate approach to evaluation is initial testing for routine liver tests such as bilirubin, albumin, alanine aminotransferase (ALT), aspartate aminotransferase (AST), and alkaline phosphatase (AlkP). These results (sometimes complemented by testing of γ-glutamyl transpeptidase; GGT) will establish whether the pattern of abnormalities is hepatic, cholestatic, or mixed. In addition, the duration of symptoms or abnormalities will show whether the disease is acute or chronic. If the disease is acute and if history, laboratory tests, and imaging studies do not reveal a diagnosis, liver biopsy is appropriate to help to establish the diagnosis. If the disease is chronic, liver biopsy can be helpful not only for diagnosis but also to grade the activity and stage the progression of disease. This approach is largely applicable to patients without immune deficiency. In patients with HIV infection or after bone marrow or solid organ transplantation, diagnostic evaluation should also include evaluation of opportunistic infections (adenovirus, cytomegalovirus, coccidioidomycosis, etc.) as well as vascular and immunologic conditions (venoocclusive disease, graft-vs-host disease). HAV, HCV: hepatitis A or C virus; HBsAg, hepatitis B surface antigen; anti-HBc, antibody to hepatitis B core (antigen); ANA, antinuclear antibodies; SMA, smooth-muscle antibody; MRCP, magnetic resonance cholangiopancreatography; ERCP, endoscopic retrograde cholangiopancreatography; α_1AT, α_1 antitrypsin; AMA; antimitochondrial antibody; P-ANCA, peripheral antineutrophil cytoplasmic antibody.

In selected instances, liver biopsy is necessary for diagnosis but is more often useful in assessing the severity (grade) and stage of liver damage, in predicting prognosis, and in monitoring response to treatment. The size of the liver biopsy is an important determinant of its reliability; a length of 1.5–2 cm being necessary for accurate assessment of fibrosis. In the future, noninvasive means of assessing disease activity (batteries of blood tests) and fibrosis (elastography and fibrosis markers) may replace liver biopsy in assessing stage and grade of disease.

DIAGNOSIS OF LIVER DISEASE

The major causes of liver disease and key diagnostic features are outlined in Table 295-3, and an algorithm for evaluation of the patient with suspected liver disease is given in Fig. 295-1. Specifics of diagno-

sis are discussed in later chapters. The most common causes of acute liver disease are viral hepatitis (particularly hepatitis A, B, and C), drug-induced liver injury, cholangitis, and alcoholic liver disease. Liver biopsy is usually not needed in the diagnosis and management of acute liver disease, exceptions being situations where the diagnosis remains unclear despite thorough clinical and laboratory investigation. Liver biopsy can be helpful in the diagnosis of drug-induced liver disease and in establishing the diagnosis of acute alcoholic hepatitis.

The most common causes of chronic liver disease in general order of frequency are chronic hepatitis C, alcoholic liver disease, nonalcoholic steatohepatitis, chronic hepatitis B, autoimmune hepatitis, sclerosing cholangitis, primary biliary cirrhosis, hemochromatosis, and Wilson disease. Strict diagnostic criteria have not been developed for most liver diseases, but liver biopsy plays an important role in the diagnosis of autoimmune hepatitis, primary biliary cirrhosis, nonalcoholic and alcoholic steatohepatitis, and Wilson disease (with a quantitative hepatic copper level).

GRADING AND STAGING OF LIVER DISEASE

Grading refers to an assessment of the severity or activity of liver disease, whether acute or chronic; active or inactive; and mild, moderate, or severe. Liver biopsy is the most accurate means of assessing severity, particularly in chronic liver disease. Serum aminotransferase levels are used as a convenient and noninvasive means to follow disease activity, but aminotransferase levels are not always reliable in reflecting disease severity. Thus, normal serum aminotransferase levels in patients with hepatitis B surface antigen (HBsAg) in serum may indicate the inactive HBsAg carrier state or may reflect mild chronic hepatitis B or hepatitis B with fluctuating disease activity. Serum testing for hepatitis B e antigen and hepatitis B virus DNA can help resolve these different patterns, but these markers can also fluctuate and change over time. Similarly, in chronic hepatitis C, serum aminotransferase levels can be normal despite moderate activity of disease. Finally, in both alcoholic and nonalcoholic steatohepatitis, aminotransferase levels are quite unreliable in reflecting severity. In these conditions, liver biopsy is helpful in guiding management and recommending therapy, particularly if therapy is difficult, prolonged, and expensive as is often the case in chronic viral hepatitis. There are several well-verified numerical scales for grading activity in chronic liver disease, the most common being the histology activity index and the Ishak histology scale.

Liver biopsy is also the most accurate means of assessing stage of disease as early or advanced, precirrhotic, and cirrhotic. Staging of disease pertains largely to chronic liver diseases in which progression to cirrhosis and end-stage liver disease can occur, but which may require years or decades to develop. Clinical features, biochemical tests, and hepatic imaging studies are helpful in assessing stage but generally become abnormal only in the middle to late stages of cirrhosis. Noninvasive tests that suggest advanced fibrosis include mild elevations of bilirubin, prolongation of prothrombin time, slight decreases in serum albumin, and mild thrombocytopenia (which is often the first indication of worsening fibrosis). Combinations of blood test results have been used to create models for predicting advanced liver disease, but these are not reliable enough to use on a regular basis and they only separate advanced from early disease. Recently, elastography has been proposed as a means of detecting early stages of fibrosis, but its reliability and reproducibility remain to be proven. Thus, at present early stages of fibrosis are detectable only by liver biopsy. In assessing stage, the degree of fibrosis is usually used as its quantitative measure. The amount of fibrosis is generally staged on a 0 to 4+ (histology activity index) or 0 to 6+ scale (Ishak scale). The importance of staging relates primarily to prognosis and to guiding management of complications. Patients with cirrhosis are candidates for screening and surveillance for esophageal varices and hepatocellular carcinoma. Patients without advanced fibrosis need not undergo screening.

Cirrhosis can also be staged clinically. A reliable staging system is the modified Child-Pugh classification with a scoring system of 5–15: scores of 5 and 6 being Child-Pugh class A (consistent with "compensated cirrhosis"), scores of 7–9 indicating class B, and 10–15 class C (Table 295-4). This scoring system was initially devised to stratify patients into risk groups prior to undergoing portal decompressive surgery. The Child-Pugh score is a reasonably reliable predictor of survival in many liver diseases and predicts the likelihood of major complications of cirrhosis such as bleeding from varices and spontaneous bacterial peritonitis. It was used to assess prognosis in cirrhosis and to provide the standard criteria for listing for liver transplantation (Child-Pugh class B). Recently the Child-Pugh system has been replaced by the model for end-stage liver disease (MELD) score for assessing the need for liver transplantation. The MELD score is a prospectively derived scoring system designed to predict prognosis of patients with liver disease and portal hypertension. It is calculated using three noninvasive variables—the prothrombin time expressed as international normalized ratio (INR), serum bilirubin, and serum creatinine (http://www.unos.org/resources/meldPeldCalculator.asp).

MELD provides a more objective means of assessing disease severity and has less center-to-center variation than the Child-Pugh score and has a wider range of values. MELD is currently used to establish priority listing for liver transplantation in the United States. A similar system using bilirubin, INR, serum albumin, age, and nutritional status is used for children below the age of 12 (PELD).

Thus, liver biopsy is helpful not only in diagnosis but also in management of chronic liver disease and assessment of prognosis. Because liver biopsy is an invasive procedure and not without complications, it should be used only when it will contribute materially to management and therapeutic decisions.

NONSPECIFIC ISSUES IN MANAGEMENT OF PATIENTS WITH LIVER DISEASE

Specifics on management of different forms of acute or chronic liver disease are given in subsequent chapters, but certain issues are applicable to any patient with liver disease. These include advice regarding alcohol use, medications, vaccination, and surveillance for complications of liver disease. Alcohol should be used sparingly, if at all, by patients

TABLE 295-4 CHILD-PUGH CLASSIFICATION OF CIRRHOSIS				
Factor	Units	1	2	3
Serum bilirubin	μmol/L	<34	34–51	>51
	mg/dL	<2.0	2.0–3.0	>3.0
Serum albumin	g/L	>35	30–35	<30
	g/dL	>3.5	3.0–3.5	<3.0
Prothrombin time	seconds prolonged	0–4	4–6	>6
	INR	<1.7	1.7–2.3	>2.3
Ascites		None	Easily controlled	Poorly controlled
Hepatic encephalopathy		None	Minimal	Advanced

Note: The Child-Pugh score is calculated by adding the scores of the five factors and can range from 5–15. Child-Pugh class is either A (a score of 5–6), B (7–9), or C (10 or above). Decompensation indicates cirrhosis with a Child-Pugh score of 7 or more (class B). This level has been the accepted criterion for listing for liver transplantation.

with liver disease. Abstinence from alcohol should be encouraged for all patients with alcohol-related liver disease and in patients with cirrhosis and those receiving interferon-based therapy for hepatitis B or C. Regarding vaccinations, all patients with liver disease should receive hepatitis A vaccine and those with risk factors should receive hepatitis B vaccination as well. Influenza and pneumococcal vaccination should also be encouraged. Patients with liver disease should be careful in use of any medications, other than the most necessary. Drug-induced hepatotoxicity can mimic many forms of liver disease and can cause exacerbations of chronic hepatitis and cirrhosis; drugs should be suspected in any situation where the cause of exacerbation is unknown. Finally, consideration should be given to surveillance for complications of chronic liver disease such as variceal hemorrhage and hepatocellular carcinoma. Patients with cirrhosis warrant upper endoscopy to assess the presence of varices and should be given chronic therapy with beta blockers or offered endoscopic obliteration if large varices are found. Patients with cirrhosis also warrant screening and long-term surveillance for development of hepatocellular carcinoma. While the optimal regimen for such surveillance has not been established, an appropriate approach is US of the liver at 6- to 12-month intervals.

FURTHER READINGS

BOYER TD, WRIGHT TL, MANNS MP (eds): *Zakim and Boyer's Hepatology: A Textbook of Liver Disease*, 5th ed. Philadelphia, Saunders, 2006

CASTERA L et al: Prospective comparison of transient elastography, Fibrotest, APRI, and liver biopsy for the assessment of fibrosis in chronic hepatitis C. Gastroenterology 128:343, 2005

KAPLOWITZ N, DELEVE LD (eds): *Drug-Induced Liver Disease*. New York, Marcel Dekker, 2003

KLEINER DE: The liver biopsy in chronic hepatitis C: A view from the other side of the microscope. Semin Liver Dis 25:52, 2005

SAINI S: Imaging of the hepatobiliary tract. N Engl J Med 336:1880, 1997

WIESNER R et al: United Network for Organ Sharing Liver Disease Severity Score Committee. Model for end-stage liver disease (MELD) and allocation of donor livers. Gastroenterology 124:91:2003

296 Evaluation of Liver Function
Daniel S. Pratt, Marshall M. Kaplan

Several biochemical tests are useful in the evaluation and management of patients with hepatic dysfunction. These tests can be used to (1) detect the presence of liver disease, (2) distinguish among different types of liver disorders, (3) gauge the extent of known liver damage, and (4) follow the response to treatment.

Liver tests have shortcomings. They can be normal in patients with serious liver disease and abnormal in patients with diseases that do not affect the liver. Liver tests rarely suggest a specific diagnosis; rather, they suggest a general category of liver disease, such as hepatocellular or cholestatic, which then further directs the evaluation.

The liver carries out thousands of biochemical functions, most of which cannot be easily measured by blood tests. Laboratory tests measure only a limited number of these functions. In fact, many tests, such as the aminotransferases or alkaline phosphatase, do not measure liver function at all. Rather, they detect liver cell damage or interference with bile flow. Thus, no one test enables the clinician to accurately assess the liver's total functional capacity.

To increase both the sensitivity and the specificity of laboratory tests in the detection of liver disease, it is best to use them as a battery. Those tests usually employed in clinical practice include the bilirubin, aminotransferases, alkaline phosphatase, albumin, and prothrombin time tests. When more than one of these tests provide abnormal findings, or the findings are persistently abnormal on serial determinations, the probability of liver disease is high. When all test results are normal, the probability of missing occult liver disease is low.

When evaluating patients with liver disorders, it is helpful to group these tests into general categories. The classification we have found most useful is given below.

TESTS BASED ON DETOXIFICATION AND EXCRETORY FUNCTIONS

Serum Bilirubin (See also Chap. 43) Bilirubin, a breakdown product of the porphyrin ring of heme-containing proteins, is found in the blood in two fractions—conjugated and unconjugated. The unconjugated fraction, also termed the *indirect fraction*, is insoluble in water and is bound to albumin in the blood. The conjugated (direct) bilirubin fraction is water soluble and can therefore be excreted by the kidney. When measured by the original van den Bergh method, the normal total serum bilirubin concentration is <17 μmol/L (1 mg/dL). Up to 30%, or 5.1 μmol/L (0.3 mg/dL), of the total is direct-reacting (or conjugated) bilirubin.

Elevation of the unconjugated fraction of bilirubin is rarely due to liver disease. An isolated elevation of unconjugated bilirubin is seen primarily in hemolytic disorders and in a number of genetic conditions such as Crigler-Najjar and Gilbert's syndromes (Chap. 43). Isolated unconjugated hyperbilirubinemia (bilirubin elevated but <15% direct) should prompt a workup for hemolysis (Fig. 296-1). In the absence of hemolysis, an isolated unconjugated hyperbilirubinemia in an otherwise healthy patient can be attributed to Gilbert's syndrome and no further evaluation is required.

In contrast, conjugated hyperbilirubinemia almost always implies liver or biliary tract disease. The rate-limiting step in bilirubin metabolism is not conjugation of bilirubin, but rather the transport of conjugated bilirubin into the bile canaliculi. Thus, elevation of the conjugated fraction may be seen in any type of liver disease. In most liver diseases, both conjugated and unconjugated fractions of the bilirubin tend to be elevated. Except in the presence of a purely unconjugated hyperbilirubinemia, fractionation of the bilirubin is rarely helpful in determining the cause of jaundice.

Urine Bilirubin Unconjugated bilirubin always binds to albumin in the serum and is not filtered by the kidney. Therefore, any bilirubin found in the urine is conjugated bilirubin; the presence of bilirubinuria implies the presence of liver disease. A urine dipstick test can theoretically give the same information as fractionation of the serum bilirubin. This test is almost 100% accurate. Phenothiazines may give a false-positive reading with the Ictotest tablet. In patients recovering from jaundice, the urine bilirubin clears prior to the serum bilirubin.

Blood Ammonia Ammonia is produced in the body during normal protein metabolism and by intestinal bacteria, primarily those in the colon. The liver plays a role in the detoxification of ammonia by converting it to urea, which is excreted by the kidneys. Striated muscle also plays a role in detoxification of ammonia, which is combined with glutamic acid to form glutamine. Patients with advanced liver disease typically have significant muscle wasting, which likely contributes to hyperammonemia in these patients. Some physicians use the blood ammonia for detecting encephalopathy or for monitoring hepatic synthetic function, although its use for either of these indications has problems. There is very poor correlation between either the presence or the severity of acute encephalopathy and elevation of blood ammonia; it can be occasionally useful for identifying occult liver disease in patients with mental status changes. There is also a poor correlation of the blood serum ammonia and hepatic function. The ammonia can be elevated in patients with severe portal hypertension and portal blood shunting around the liver even in the presence of normal or near-normal hepatic function. Elevated arterial ammonia levels have been shown to correlate with outcome in fulminant hepatic failure.

Serum Enzymes The liver contains thousands of enzymes, some of which are also present in the serum in very low concentrations. These enzymes have no known function in the serum and behave like other serum proteins. They are distributed in the plasma and in interstitial fluid and have characteristic half-lives, usually measured in days. Very little is known about the catabolism of serum enzymes, although they are probably cleared by cells in the reticuloendothelial system. The elevation of a given enzyme activity in the serum is thought to primarily reflect its increased rate of entrance into serum from damaged liver cells.

Serum enzyme tests can be grouped into three categories: (1) enzymes whose elevation in serum reflects damage to hepatocytes, (2) enzymes whose elevation in serum reflects cholestasis, and (3) enzyme tests that do not fit precisely into either pattern.

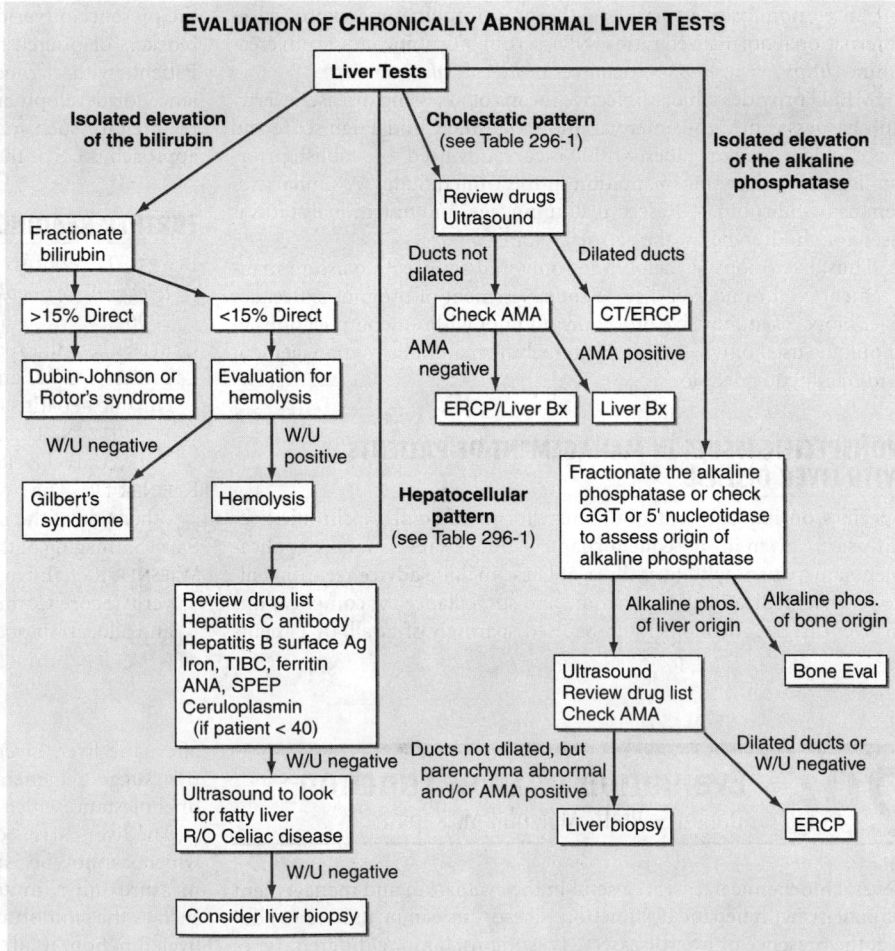

FIGURE 296-1 Algorithm for the evaluation of chronically abnormal liver tests. ERCP, endoscopic retrograde cholangiopancreatography; CT, computed tomography; AMA, antimitochondrial antibody; ANA, antinuclear antibody; SPEP, serum protein electrophoresis; TIBC, total iron-binding capacity; GGT, γ glutamyl transpeptidase; W/U, work up.

ENZYMES THAT REFLECT DAMAGE TO HEPATOCYTES The aminotransferases (transaminases) are sensitive indicators of liver cell injury and are most helpful in recognizing acute hepatocellular diseases such as hepatitis. They include the aspartate aminotransferase (AST) and the alanine aminotransferase (ALT). AST is found in the liver, cardiac muscle, skeletal muscle, kidneys, brain, pancreas, lungs, leukocytes, and erythrocytes in decreasing order of concentration. ALT is found primarily in the liver. The aminotransferases are normally present in the serum in low concentrations. These enzymes are released into the blood in greater amounts when there is damage to the liver cell membrane resulting in increased permeability. Liver cell necrosis is not required for the release of the aminotransferases, and there is a poor correlation between the degree of liver cell damage and the level of the aminotransferases. Thus, the absolute elevation of the aminotransferases is of no prognostic significance in acute hepatocellular disorders.

Any type of liver cell injury can cause modest elevations in the serum aminotransferases. Levels of up to 300 U/L are nonspecific and may be found in any type of liver disorder. Minimal ALT elevations in asymptomatic blood donors rarely indicate severe liver disease; studies have shown that fatty liver disease is the most likely explanation. Striking elevations—i.e., aminotransferases > 1000 U/L—occur almost exclusively in disorders associated with extensive hepatocellular injury such as (1) viral hepatitis, (2) ischemic liver injury (prolonged hypotension or acute heart failure), or (3) toxin- or drug-induced liver injury.

The pattern of the aminotransferase elevation can be helpful diagnostically. In most acute hepatocellular disorders, the ALT is higher than or equal to the AST. An AST:ALT ratio > 2:1 is suggestive while a ratio > 3:1 is highly suggestive of alcoholic liver disease. The AST in alcoholic liver disease is rarely >300 U/L and the ALT is often normal. A low level of ALT in the serum is due to an alcohol-induced deficiency of pyridoxal phosphate.

The aminotransferases are usually not greatly elevated in obstructive jaundice. One notable exception occurs during the acute phase of biliary obstruction caused by the passage of a gallstone into the common bile duct. In this setting, the aminotransferases can briefly be in the 1000–2000 U/L range. However, aminotransferase levels decrease quickly, and the liver function tests rapidly evolve into one typical of cholestasis.

ENZYMES THAT REFLECT CHOLESTASIS The activities of three enzymes—alkaline phosphatase, 5′-nucleotidase, and γ-glutamyl transpeptidase (GGT)—are usually elevated in cholestasis. Alkaline phosphatase and 5′-nucleotidase are found in or near the bile canalicular membrane of hepatocytes, while GGT is located in the endoplasmic reticulum and in bile duct epithelial cells. Reflecting its more diffuse localization in the liver, GGT elevation in serum is less specific for cholestasis than are elevations of alkaline phosphatase or 5′-nucleotidase. Some have advocated the use of GGT to identify patients with occult alcohol use. Its lack of specificity makes its use in this setting questionable.

The normal serum alkaline phosphatase consists of many distinct isoenzymes found in the liver, bone, placenta, and, less commonly, small intestine. Patients over age 60 can have a mildly elevated alkaline phosphatase (1–1½ times normal), while individuals with blood types O and B can have an elevation of the serum alkaline phosphatase after eating a fatty meal due to the influx of intestinal alkaline phosphatase into the blood. It is also nonpathologically elevated in children and adolescents undergoing rapid bone growth, because of bone alkaline phosphatase, and late in normal pregnancies due to the influx of placental alkaline phosphatase.

Elevation of liver-derived alkaline phosphatase is not totally specific for cholestasis, and a less than threefold elevation can be seen in almost any type of liver disease. Alkaline phosphatase elevations greater than four times normal occur primarily in patients with cholestatic liver disorders, infiltrative liver diseases such as cancer and amyloidosis, and bone conditions characterized by rapid bone turnover (e.g., Paget's disease). In bone diseases, the elevation is due to increased amounts of the bone isoenzymes. In liver diseases, the elevation is almost always due to increased amounts of the liver isoenzyme.

If an elevated serum alkaline phosphatase is the only abnormal finding in an apparently healthy person, or if the degree of elevation is higher than expected in the clinical setting, identification of the source of elevated isoenzymes is helpful (Fig. 296-1). This problem can be approached in several ways. First, and most precise, is the fractionation of the alkaline phosphatase by electrophoresis. The second approach is based on the observation that alkaline phosphatases from individual tissues differ in susceptibility to inactivation by heat. The finding of an elevated serum alkaline phosphatase level in a patient with a heat-stable fraction strongly suggests that the placenta or a tumor is the source of the elevated enzyme in serum. Susceptibility to inactivation by heat increases, respectively, for the intestinal, liver, and bone alkaline phosphatases, bone being by far the most sensitive. The third, best substantiated, and most available approach involves the measurement of serum 5′-nucleotidase or GGT. These enzymes are rarely elevated in conditions other than liver disease.

In the absence of jaundice or elevated aminotransferases, an elevated alkaline phosphatase of liver origin often, but not always, suggests early cholestasis and, less often, hepatic infiltration by tumor or granulomata. Other conditions that cause isolated elevations of the alkaline phosphatase include Hodgkin's disease, diabetes, hyperthyroidism, congestive heart failure, amyloidosis, and inflammatory bowel disease.

The level of serum alkaline phosphatase elevation is not helpful in distinguishing between intrahepatic and extrahepatic cholestasis. There is essentially no difference among the values found in obstructive jaundice due to cancer, common duct stone, sclerosing cholangitis, or bile duct stricture. Values are similarly increased in patients with intrahepatic cholestasis due to drug-induced hepatitis, primary biliary cirrhosis, rejection of transplanted livers, and, rarely, alcohol-induced steatonecrosis. Values are also greatly elevated in hepatobiliary disorders seen in patients with AIDS (e.g., AIDS cholangiopathy due to cytomegalovirus or cryptosporidial infection and tuberculosis with hepatic involvement).

TESTS THAT MEASURE BIOSYNTHETIC FUNCTION OF THE LIVER

Serum Albumin Serum albumin is synthesized exclusively by hepatocytes. Serum albumin has a long half-life: 18–20 days, with ~4% degraded per day. Because of this slow turnover, the serum albumin is not a good indicator of acute or mild hepatic dysfunction; only minimal changes in the serum albumin are seen in acute liver conditions such as viral hepatitis, drug-related hepatoxicity, and obstructive jaundice. In hepatitis, albumin levels < 3 g/dL should raise the possibility of chronic liver disease. Hypoalbuminemia is more common in chronic liver disorders such as cirrhosis and usually reflects severe liver damage and decreased albumin synthesis. One exception is the patient with ascites in whom synthesis may be normal or even increased, but levels are low because of the increased volume of distribution. However, hypoalbuminemia is not specific for liver disease and may occur in protein malnutrition of any cause, as well as protein-losing enteropathies, nephrotic syndrome, and chronic infections that are associated with prolonged increases in levels of serum interleukin 1 and/or tumor necrosis factor, cytokines that inhibit albumin synthesis. Serum albumin should not be measured for screening in patients in whom there is no suspicion of liver disease. A general medical clinic study of consecutive patients in whom no indications were present for albumin measurement showed that while 12% of patients had abnormal test results, the finding was of clinical importance in only 0.4%.

Serum Globulins Serum globulins are a group of proteins made up of γ globulins (immunoglobulins) produced by B lymphocytes and α and β globulins produced primarily in hepatocytes. γ Globulins are increased in chronic liver disease, such as chronic hepatitis and cirrhosis. In cirrhosis, the increased serum gamma globulin concentration is due to the increased synthesis of antibodies, some of which are directed against intestinal bacteria. This occurs because the cirrhotic liver fails to clear bacterial antigens that normally reach the liver through the hepatic circulation.

Increases in the concentration of specific isotypes of γ globulins are often helpful in the recognition of certain chronic liver diseases. Diffuse polyclonal increases in IgG levels are common in autoimmune hepatitis; increases >100% should alert the clinician to this possibility. Increases in the IgM levels are common in primary biliary cirrhosis, while increases in the IgA levels occur in alcoholic liver disease.

TABLE 296-1 LIVER TEST PATTERNS IN HEPATOBILIARY DISORDERS

Type of Disorder	Bilirubin	Aminotransferases	Alkaline Phosphatase	Albumin	Prothrombin Time
Hemolysis/Gilbert's syndrome	Normal to 86 μmol/L (5 mg/dL) 85% due to indirect fractions No bilirubinuria	Normal	Normal	Normal	Normal
Acute hepatocellular necrosis (viral and drug hepatitis, hepatotoxins, acute heart failure)	Both fractions may be elevated Peak usually follows aminotransferases Bilirubinuria	Elevated, often >500 IU ALT >AST	Normal to <3 times normal elevation	Normal	Usually normal. If >5X above control and not corrected by parenteral vitamin K, suggests poor prognosis
Chronic hepatocellular disorders	Both fractions may be elevated Bilirubinuria	Elevated, but usually <300 IU	Normal to <3 times normal elevation	Often decreased	Often prolonged Fails to correct with parenteral vitamin K
Alcoholic hepatitis Cirrhosis	Both fractions may be elevated Bilirubinuria	AST:ALT > 2 suggests alcoholic hepatitis or cirrhosis	Normal to <3 times normal elevation	Often decreased	Often prolonged Fails to correct with parenteral vitamin K
Intra- and extra-hepatic cholestasis (Obstructive jaundice)	Both fractions may be elevated Bilirubinuria	Normal to moderate elevation Rarely >500 IU	Elevated, often >4 times normal elevation	Normal, unless chronic	Normal If prolonged, will correct with parenteral vitamin K
Infiltrative diseases (tumor, granulomata); partial bile duct obstruction	Usually normal	Normal to slight elevation	Elevated, often >4 times normal elevation Fractionate, or confirm liver origin with 5' nucleotidase or γ glutamyl transpeptidase	Normal	Normal

COAGULATION FACTORS

With the exception of factor VIII, the blood clotting factors are made exclusively in hepatocytes. Their serum half-lives are much shorter than albumin, ranging from 6 h for factor VII to 5 days for fibrinogen. Because of their rapid turnover, measurement of the clotting factors is the single best acute measure of hepatic synthetic function and helpful in both the diagnosis and assessing the prognosis of acute parenchymal liver disease. Useful for this purpose is the *serum prothrombin time*, which collectively measures factors II, V, VII, and X. Biosynthesis of factors II, VII, IX, and X depends on vitamin K. The prothrombin time may be elevated in hepatitis and cirrhosis as well as in disorders that lead to vitamin K deficiency such as obstructive jaundice or fat malabsorption of any kind. Marked prolongation of the prothrombin time, >5 s above control and not corrected by parenteral vitamin K administration, is a poor prognostic sign in acute viral hepatitis and other acute and chronic liver diseases.

OTHER DIAGNOSTIC TESTS

While tests may direct the physician to a category of liver disease, additional radiologic testing and procedures are often necessary to make the proper diagnosis, as shown in Fig. 296-1. The two most commonly used ancillary tests are reviewed here.

Percutaneous Liver Biopsy Percutaneous biopsy of the liver is a safe procedure that can be easily performed at the bedside with local anesthesia. Liver biopsy is of proven value in the following situations: (1) hepatocellular disease of uncertain cause, (2) prolonged hepatitis with the possibility of chronic active hepatitis, (3) unexplained hepatomegaly, (4) unexplained splenomegaly, (5) hepatic filling defects by radiologic imaging, (6) fever of unknown origin, (7) staging of malignant lymphoma. Liver biopsy is most accurate in disorders causing diffuse changes throughout the liver and is subject to sampling error in focal infiltrative disorders such as hepatic metastases. Liver biopsy should not be the initial procedure in the diagnosis of cholestasis. The biliary tree should first be assessed for signs of obstruction. Contraindications to performing a percutaneous liver biopsy include significant ascites and prolonged INR. Under these circumstances the biopsy can be performed via the transjugular approach.

Ultrasonography Ultrasonography is the first diagnostic test to use in patients whose liver tests suggest cholestasis, to look for the presence of a dilated intrahepatic or extrahepatic biliary tree or to identify gallstones. In addition, it shows space-occupying lesions within the liver, enables the clinician to distinguish between cystic and solid masses, and helps direct percutaneous biopsies. Ultrasound with Doppler imaging can detect the patency of the portal vein, hepatic artery, and hepatic veins and determine the direction of blood flow. This is the first test ordered in patients suspected of having Budd-Chiari syndrome.

USE OF LIVER TESTS

As previously noted, the best way to increase the sensitivity and specificity of laboratory tests in the detection of liver disease is to employ a battery of tests that include the aminotransferases, alkaline phosphatase, bilirubin, albumin, and prothrombin time along with the judicious use of the other tests described in this chapter. Table 296-1 shows how patterns of liver tests can lead the clinician to a category of disease that will direct further evaluation. However, it is important to remember that no single set of liver tests will necessarily provide a diagnosis. It is often necessary to repeat these tests on several occasions over days to weeks for a diagnostic pattern to emerge. Figure 296-1 is an algorithm for the evaluation of chronically abnormal liver tests.

FURTHER READINGS

BHATIA V et al: Predictive value of arterial ammonia for complications and outcome in acute liver failure. Gut 55:98, 2006

BOSMA PJ et al: The genetic basis of the reduced expression of bilirubin UDP-glucuronosyltransferase 1 in Gilbert's syndrome. N Engl J Med 333:1171, 1995

PRATT DS, KAPLAN MM: Evaluation of abnormal liver-enzyme tests in the asymptomatic patient. N Engl J Med 342:1266, 2000

———, ———: Laboratory tests, in *Schiff's Diseases of the Liver*, 9th ed, ER Schiff et al (eds). Philadelphia, Lippincott Williams & Wilkins, 2003

TOREZAN-FILHO MA et al: Clinical significance of elevated alanine aminotransferase in blood donors: A follow-up study. Liver International 24:575, 2004

297 The Hyperbilirubinemias
Allan W. Wolkoff

BILIRUBIN METABOLISM

The details of bilirubin metabolism are presented in Chap. 43, "Jaundice." However, the hyperbilirubinemias are best understood in terms of perturbations of specific aspects of bilirubin metabolism and transport, and these will be briefly reviewed here as depicted in Fig. 297-1.

Bilirubin is the end product of heme degradation. From 70–90% of bilirubin is derived from degradation of the hemoglobin of senescent red blood cells. Bilirubin produced in the periphery is transported to the liver within the plasma, where, due to its insolubility in aqueous solutions, it is tightly bound to albumin. Under normal circumstances, bilirubin is removed from the circulation rapidly and efficiently by hepatocytes. Transfer of bilirubin from blood to bile involves four distinct but interrelated steps (Fig. 297-1):

1. *Hepatocellular uptake:* Uptake of bilirubin by the hepatocyte has carrier-mediated kinetics. Although a number of candidate bilirubin transporters have been proposed, the actual transporter remains elusive.
2. *Intracellular binding:* Within the hepatocyte, bilirubin is kept in solution by binding as a nonsubstrate ligand to several of the glutathione-S-transferases, formerly called ligandins.
3. *Conjugation:* Bilirubin is conjugated with one or two glucuronic acid moieties by a specific UDP-glucuronosyltransferase to form bilirubin mono- and diglucuronide, respectively. Conjugation disrupts the internal hydrogen bonding that limits aqueous solubility of bilirubin, and the resulting glucuronide conjugates are highly soluble in water. Conjugation is obligatory for excretion of bilirubin across the bile canalicular membrane into bile. The UDP-glucuronosyltransferases have been classified into gene families based on the degree of homology among the mRNAs for the various isoforms. Those that conjugate bilirubin and certain other substrates have been designated the *UGT1* family. These are expressed from a single gene complex by alternative promoter usage. This gene complex contains multiple substrate-specific first exons, designated A1, A2, etc. (Fig. 297-2), each with its own promoter and each encoding the amino-terminal half of a specific isoform. In addition, there are four common exons (exons 2–5) that encode the shared carboxyl-terminal half of all of the *UGT1* isoforms. The various first exons encode the specific aglycone substrate–binding sites for each isoform, while the shared exons encode the binding site for the sugar donor, UDP-glucuronic acid, and the transmembrane domain. Exon A1 and the four common exons, collectively designated the *UGT1A1* gene (Fig. 297-2), encode the physiologically critical enzyme bilirubin-UDP-glucuronosyltransferase (UGT1A1). A functional corollary of the organization of the *UGT1* gene is that a mutation in one of the first exons will affect only a single enzyme isoform. By contrast, a mutation in exons 2–5 will alter all isoforms encoded by the *UGT1* gene complex.
4. *Biliary excretion:* Bilirubin mono- and diglucuronides are excreted across the canalicular plasma membrane into the bile canaliculus by an ATP-dependent transport process mediated by a canalicular membrane protein called *multidrug resistance–associated protein 2* (MRP2). Mutations of MRP2 result in the Dubin-Johnson syndrome (see below).

FIGURE 297-1 Hepatocellular bilirubin transport. Albumin-bound bilirubin in sinusoidal blood passes through endothelial cell fenestrae to reach the hepatocyte surface, entering the cell by both facilitated and simple diffusional processes. Within the cell it is bound to glutathione-S-transferases and conjugated by bilirubin-UDP-glucuronosyltransferase (UGT1A1) to mono- and diglucuronides, which are actively transported across the canalicular membrane into the bile. ALB, albumin; UCB, unconjugated bilirubin, UGT1A1, bilirubin-UDP-glucuronosyltransferase; BMG, bilirubin monoglucuronide; GST, glutathione-S-transferase; MRP2, multidrug resistance–associated protein 2; BDG, bilirubin diglucuronide; BT, proposed bilirubin transporter.

EXTRAHEPATIC ASPECTS OF BILIRUBIN DISPOSITION

Bilirubin in the Gut Following secretion into bile, conjugated bilirubin reaches the duodenum and passes down the gastrointestinal tract without reabsorption by the intestinal mucosa. An appreciable fraction is converted by bacterial metabolism in the gut to the water-soluble colorless compound, urobilinogen. Urobilinogen undergoes enterohepatic cycling. Urobilinogen not taken up by the liver reaches the systemic circulation, from which some is cleared by the kidneys. Unconjugated bilirubin ordinarily does not reach the gut except in neonates or, by ill-defined alternative pathways, in the presence of severe unconjugated hyperbilirubinemia [e.g., Crigler-Najjar syndrome, type I (CN-I)]. Unconjugated bilirubin that reaches the gut is partly reabsorbed, amplifying any underlying hyperbilirubinemia. Recent reports suggest that oral administration of calcium phosphate with or without the lipase inhibitor orlistat may be an efficient means to interrupt bilirubin enterohepatic cycling to reduce serum bilirubin levels in this situation; however, this remains to be validated in larger clinical trials.

FIGURE 297-2 Structural organization of the human *UGT1* gene complex. This large complex on chromosome 2 contains at least 13 substrate-specific first exons (A1, A2, etc.). Since four of these are pseudogenes, nine UGT1 isoforms with differing substrate specificities are expressed. Each exon 1 has its own promoter and encodes the amino-terminal substrate-specific ~286 amino acids of the various *UGT1*-encoded isoforms, and common exons 2–5 that encode the 245 carboxyl-terminal amino acids common to all of the isoforms. mRNAs for specific isoforms are assembled by splicing a particular first exon such as the bilirubin-specific exon A1 to exons 2 to 5. The resulting message encodes a complete enzyme, in this particular case bilirubin-UDP-glucuronosyltransferase (UGT1A1). Mutations in a first exon affect only a single isoform. Those in exons 2–5 affect all enzymes encoded by the UGT1 complex.

Renal Excretion of Bilirubin Conjugates   Unconjugated bilirubin is not excreted in urine as it is too tightly bound to albumin for effective glomerular filtration and there is no tubular mechanism for its renal secretion. In contrast, the bilirubin conjugates are readily filtered at the glomerulus and can appear in urine in disorders characterized by increased bilirubin conjugates in the circulation.

DISORDERS OF BILIRUBIN METABOLISM LEADING TO UNCONJUGATED HYPERBILIRUBINEMIA

INCREASED BILIRUBIN PRODUCTION

Hemolysis   Increased destruction of erythrocytes leads to increased bilirubin turnover and unconjugated hyperbilirubinemia; the hyperbilirubinemia is usually modest in the presence of normal liver function. In particular, the bone marrow is only capable of a sustained eightfold increase in erythrocyte production in response to a hemolytic stress. Therefore, hemolysis alone cannot result in a sustained hyperbilirubinemia of more than ~68 μmol/L (4 mg/dL). Higher values imply concomitant hepatic dysfunction. When hemolysis is the only abnormality in an otherwise healthy individual, the result is a purely unconjugated hyperbilirubinemia, with the direct-reacting fraction as measured in a typical clinical laboratory being ≤15% of the total serum bilirubin. In the presence of systemic disease, which may include a degree of hepatic dysfunction, hemolysis may produce a component of conjugated hyperbilirubinemia in addition to an elevated unconjugated bilirubin concentration. Prolonged hemolysis may lead to the precipitation of bilirubin salts within the gall bladder or biliary tree, resulting in the formation of gallstones in which bilirubin, rather than cholesterol, is the major component. Such pigment stones may lead to acute or chronic cholecystitis, biliary obstruction, or any other biliary tract consequence of calculous disease.

Ineffective Erythropoiesis   During erythroid maturation, small amounts of hemoglobin may be lost at the time of nuclear extrusion, and a fraction of developing erythroid cells is destroyed within the marrow. These processes normally account for a small proportion of bilirubin that is produced. In various disorders, including thalassemia major, megaloblastic anemias due to folate or vitamin B_{12} deficiency, congenital erythropoietic porphyria, lead poisoning, and various congenital and acquired dyserythropoietic anemias, the fraction of total bilirubin production derived from ineffective erythropoiesis is increased, reaching as much as 70% of the total. This may be sufficient to produce modest degrees of unconjugated hyperbilirubinemia.

Miscellaneous   Degradation of the hemoglobin of extravascular collections of erythrocytes, such as those seen in massive tissue infarctions or large hematomas, may lead transiently to unconjugated hyperbilirubinemia.

DECREASED HEPATIC BILIRUBIN CLEARANCE

Decreased Hepatic Uptake   Decreased hepatic bilirubin uptake is believed to contribute to the unconjugated hyperbilirubinemia of Gilbert's syndrome (GS), although the molecular basis for this finding remains unclear (see below). Several drugs, including flavaspidic acid, novobiocin, rifampin, and various cholecystographic contrast agents, have been reported to inhibit bilirubin uptake. The resulting unconjugated hyperbilirubinemia resolves with cessation of the medication.

Impaired Conjugation · *PHYSIOLOGIC NEONATAL JAUNDICE*   Bilirubin produced by the fetus is cleared by the placenta and eliminated by the maternal liver. Immediately after birth, the neonatal liver must assume responsibility for bilirubin clearance and excretion. However, many hepatic physiologic processes are incompletely developed at birth. Levels of UGT1A1 are low, and alternative excretory pathways allow passage of unconjugated bilirubin into the gut. Since the intestinal flora that convert bilirubin to urobilinogen are also undeveloped, an enterohepatic circulation of unconjugated bilirubin ensues. As a consequence, most neonates develop mild unconjugated hyperbilirubinemia between days 2 and 5 after birth. Peak levels are typically <85–170 μmol/L (5–10 mg/

dL) and decline to normal adult concentrations within 2 weeks, as mechanisms required for bilirubin disposition mature. Prematurity, with more profound immaturity of hepatic function, or hemolysis, result in higher levels of unconjugated hyperbilirubinemia. A rapidly rising unconjugated bilirubin concentration, or absolute levels >340 μmol/L (20 mg/dL), puts the infant at risk for bilirubin encephalopathy, or kernicterus. Under these circumstances, bilirubin crosses an immature blood-brain barrier and precipitates in the basal ganglia and other areas of the brain. The consequences range from appreciable neurologic deficits to death. Treatment options include phototherapy, which converts bilirubin into water-soluble photoisomers that are excreted directly into bile, and exchange transfusion. The canalicular mechanisms responsible for bilirubin excretion are also immature at birth, and their maturation may lag behind that of UGT1A1; this can lead to transient conjugated neonatal hyperbilirubinemia, especially in infants with hemolysis.

ACQUIRED CONJUGATION DEFECTS   A modest reduction in bilirubin-conjugating capacity may be observed in advanced hepatitis or cirrhosis. However, in this setting, conjugation is better preserved than other aspects of bilirubin disposition, such as canalicular excretion. Various drugs, including pregnanediol, novobiocin, chloramphenicol, and gentamicin, may produce unconjugated hyperbilirubinemia by inhibiting UGT1A1 activity. Finally, bilirubin conjugation may be inhibited by certain fatty acids that are present in breast milk but not serum of mothers whose infants have excessive neonatal hyperbilirubinemia (*breast milk jaundice*). The pathogenesis of breast milk jaundice appears to differ from that of transient familial neonatal hyperbilirubinemia (Lucey-Driscoll syndrome), in which there is a UGT1A1 inhibitor in maternal serum.

HEREDITARY DEFECTS IN BILIRUBIN CONJUGATION

Three familial disorders characterized by differing degrees of unconjugated hyperbilirubinemia have long been recognized. The defining clinical features of each are described below (Table 297-1). While these disorders have been recognized for decades to reflect differing degrees of deficiency in the ability to conjugate bilirubin, recent advances in the molecular biology of the *UGT1* gene complex have elucidated their interrelationships and clarified previously puzzling features.

Crigler-Najjar Syndrome, Type I   CN-I is characterized by striking unconjugated hyperbilirubinemia of about 340–765 μmol/L (20–45 mg/dL) that appears in the neonatal period and persists for life. Other conventional hepatic biochemical tests such as serum aminotransferases and alkaline phosphatase are normal, and there is no evidence of hemolysis. Hepatic histology is also essentially normal except for the occasional presence of bile plugs within canaliculi. Bilirubin glucuronides are virtually absent from the bile, and there is no detectable constitutive expression of UGT1A1 activity in hepatic tissue. Neither UGT1A1 activity nor the serum bilirubin concentration responds to administration of phenobarbital or other enzyme inducers. In the absence of conjugation, unconjugated bilirubin accumulates in plasma, from which it is eliminated very slowly by alternative pathways that include direct passage into the bile and small intestine. These account for the small amounts of urobilinogen found in feces. No bilirubin is found in the urine. First described in 1952, the disorder is rare (estimated prevalence of 0.6–1.0 per million). Many patients are from geographically or socially isolated communities in which consanguinity is common, and pedigree analyses show an autosomal recessive pattern of inheritance. The majority of patients (type IA) exhibit defects in the glucuronide conjugation of a spectrum of substrates in addition to bilirubin, including various drugs and other xenobiotics. These individuals have mutations in one of the common exons (2–5) of the *UGT1* gene (Fig. 297-2). In a smaller subset (type IB), the defect is limited largely to bilirubin conjugation, and the causative mutation is in the bilirubin-specific exon A1. Estrogen glucuronidation is mediated by UGT1A1 and is defective in all CN-I patients. More than 30 different genetic lesions of *UGT1A1* responsible for CN-I have been identified, including deletions, insertions, alterations in intronic splice donor and acceptor sites, exon skipping, and point mutations that introduce pre-

TABLE 297-1 **PRINCIPAL DIFFERENTIAL CHARACTERISTICS OF GILBERT'S AND CRIGLER-NAJJAR SYNDROMES**

Feature	Crigler-Najjar Syndrome		Gilbert's Syndrome
	Type I	Type II	
Total serum bilirubin, μmol/L [mg/dL]	310–755 (usually >345) [18–45 (usually >20)]	100–430 (usually ≤345) [6–25 (usually ≤20)]	Typically ≤70 μmol/L (≤4 mg/dL) in absence of fasting or hemolysis
Routine liver tests	Normal	Normal	Normal
Response to phenobarbital	None	Decreases bilirubin by >25%	Decreases bilirubin to normal
Kernicterus	Usual	Rare	No
Hepatic histology	Normal	Normal	Usually normal; increased lipofuscin pigment in some
Bile characteristics			
Color	Pale or colorless	Pigmented	Normal dark color
Bilirubin fractions	>90% unconjugated	Largest fraction (mean: 57%) monoconjugates	Mainly diconjugates but monoconjugates increased (mean: 23%)
Bilirubin UDP-glucuronosyl-transferase activity	Typically absent; traces in some patients	Markedly reduced: 0–10% of normal	Reduced: typically 10–33% of normal
Inheritance (all autosomal)	Recessive	Predominantly recessive	Promoter mutation: recessive Missense mutations: 7 of 8 dominant; 1 reportedly recessive

mature stop codons or alter critical amino acids. Their common feature is that they all encode proteins with absent or, at most, traces of bilirubin-UDP-glucuronosyltransferase enzymatic activity.

Prior to the availability of phototherapy, most patients with CN-I died of bilirubin encephalopathy (*kernicterus*) in infancy or early childhood. A few lived as long as early adult life without overt neurologic damage, although more subtle testing usually indicated mild but progressive brain damage. In the absence of liver transplantation, death eventually supervened from late-onset bilirubin encephalopathy, which often followed a nonspecific febrile illness. Although isolated hepatocyte transplantation has been used in a small number of cases of CN-I, early liver transplantation (Chap. 304) remains the best hope to prevent brain injury and death.

Crigler-Najjar Syndrome, Type II (CN-II) This condition was recognized as a distinct entity in 1962 and is characterized by marked unconjugated hyperbilirubinemia in the absence of abnormalities of other conventional hepatic biochemical tests, hepatic histology, or hemolysis. It differs from CN-I in several specific ways (Table 297-1): (1) Although there is considerable overlap, average bilirubin concentrations are lower in CN-II; (2) accordingly, CN-II is only infrequently associated with kernicterus; (3) bile is deeply colored, and bilirubin glucuronides are present, with a striking, characteristic increase in the proportion of monoglucuronides; (4) UGT1A1 in liver is usually present at reduced levels (typically ≤10% of normal) but may be undetectable by older, less sensitive assays; (5) while typically detected in infancy, hyperbilirubinemia was not recognized in some cases until later in life and, in one instance, at age 34. As with CN-I, most CN-II cases exhibit abnormalities in the conjugation of other compounds, such as salicylamide and menthol, but in some instances the defect appears limited to bilirubin. Reduction of serum bilirubin concentrations by >25% in response to enzyme inducers such as phenobarbital distinguishes CN-II from CN-I, although this response may not be elicited in early infancy and often is not accompanied by measurable UGT1A1 induction. Bilirubin concentrations during phenobarbital administration do not return to normal but are typically in the range of 51–86 μmol/L (3–5 mg/dL). Although the incidence of kernicterus in CN-II is low, instances have occurred, not only in infants but also in adolescents and adults, often in the setting of an intercurrent illness, fasting, or another factor that temporarily raises the serum bilirubin concentration above baseline and reduces serum albumin levels. For this reason, phenobarbital therapy is widely recommended, a single bedtime dose often sufficing to maintain clinically safe plasma bilirubin concentrations.

Over 77 different mutations in the *UGT1* gene have been identified as causing CN-I or CN-II. It was found that missense mutations are more common in CN-II patients as would be expected in this less severe phenotype. Their common feature is that they encode for a bilirubin-UDP-glucuronosyltransferase with markedly reduced, but detectable, enzymatic activity. The spectrum of residual enzyme activity explains the spectrum of phenotypic severity of the resulting hyperbilirubinemia. Molecular analysis has established that a large majority of CN-II patients are either homozygotes or compound heterozygotes for CN-II mutations and that individuals carrying one mutated and one entirely normal allele have normal bilirubin concentrations.

Gilbert's Syndrome This syndrome is characterized by mild unconjugated hyperbilirubinemia, normal values for standard hepatic biochemical tests, and normal hepatic histology other than a modest increase of lipofuscin pigment in some patients. Serum bilirubin concentrations are most often <51 μmol/L (<3 mg/dL), although both higher and lower values are frequent. The clinical spectrum of hyperbilirubinemia fades into that of CN-II at serum bilirubin concentrations of 86–136 μmol/L (5–8 mg/dL). At the other end of the scale, the distinction between mild cases of GS and a normal state is often blurred. Bilirubin concentrations may fluctuate substantially in any given individual, and at least 25% of patients will exhibit temporarily normal values during prolonged follow-up. More elevated values are associated with stress, fatigue, alcohol use, reduced caloric intake, and intercurrent illness, while increased caloric intake or administration of enzyme-inducing agents produce lower bilirubin levels. GS is most often diagnosed at or shortly after puberty or in adult life during routine examinations that include multichannel biochemical analyses. UGT1A1 activity is typically reduced to 10–35% of normal, and bile pigments exhibit a characteristic increase in bilirubin monoglucuronides. Studies of radiobilirubin kinetics indicate that hepatic bilirubin clearance is reduced to an average of one-third of normal. Administration of phenobarbital normalizes both the serum bilirubin concentration and hepatic bilirubin clearance; however, failure of UGT1A1 activity to improve in many such instances suggests the possible coexistence of an additional defect. Compartmental analysis of bilirubin kinetic data suggests that GS patients have a defect in bilirubin uptake as well as in conjugation. Defect(s) in the hepatic uptake of other organic anions that at least partially share an uptake mechanism with bilirubin, such as sulfobromophthalein and indocyanine green (ICG), are observed in a minority of patients. The metabolism and transport of bile acids, which do not utilize the bilirubin uptake mechanism, are normal. The magnitude of changes in the plasma bilirubin concentration induced by provocation tests such as 48 h of fasting or the IV administration of nicotinic acid have been reported to be of help in separating GS patients from normal individuals. Other studies dispute this assertion. Moreover, on theoretical grounds, the results of such studies should provide no more information than simple measurements of the baseline plasma bilirubin concentration. Family studies indicate that GS and hereditary hemolytic anemias such as hereditary spherocytosis, glucose-6-phosphate dehydrogenase deficiency, and β-thalassemia trait sort independently. Reports of hemolysis in up to 50% of GS patients are believed to reflect better case finding, since patients with both GS and hemolysis have higher bilirubin concentrations, and are more likely to be jaundiced, than patients with either defect alone.

GS is common, with many series placing its prevalence at ≥8%. Males predominate over females by reported ratios ranging from 1.5:1 to >7:1. However, these ratios may have a large artifactual component since normal males have higher mean bilirubin levels than normal females, but the diagnosis of GS is often based on comparison to normal ranges established in men. The high prevalence of GS in the general population may explain the reported frequency of mild unconjugated hyperbilirubinemia in liver transplant recipients. The disposition of most xenobiotics metabolized by glucuronidation appears to be normal in GS, as is oxidative drug metabolism in the majority of reported studies. The principal exception is the metabolism of the antitumor agent irinotecan (CPT-11), whose active metabolite (SN-38) is glucuronidated specifically by bilirubin-UDP-glucuronosyltransferase. Administration of CPT-11 to patients with GS has resulted in several toxicities, including intractable diarrhea and myelosuppression. Some reports also suggest abnormal disposition of menthol, estradiol benzoate, acetaminophen, tolbutamide, and rifamycin SV. Although some of these studies have been disputed, and there have been no reports of clinical complications from use of these agents in GS, prudence should be exercised in prescribing them, or any agents metabolized primarily by glucuronidation, in this condition. It should also be noted that the HIV protease inhibitors indinavir and atazanavir (Chap. 182) can inhibit UGT1A1, resulting in hyperbilirubinemia that is most pronounced in patients with preexisting GS.

Most older pedigree studies of GS were consistent with autosomal dominant inheritance with variable expressivity. However, studies of the *UGT1* gene in GS have indicated a variety of molecular genetic bases for the phenotypic picture and several different patterns of inheritance. Studies in Europe and the United States found that nearly all patients had normal coding regions for UGT1A1 but were homozygous for the insertion of an extra TA (i.e., A[TA]$_7$TAA rather than A[TA]$_6$TAA) in the promoter region of the first exon. This appeared to be necessary, but not sufficient, for clinically expressed GS, since 15% of normal controls were also homozygous for this variant. While normal by standard criteria, these individuals had somewhat higher bilirubin concentrations than the rest of the controls studied. Heterozygotes for this abnormality had bilirubin concentrations identical to those homozygous for the normal A[TA]$_6$TAA allele. The prevalence of the A[TA]$_7$TAA allele in a general western population is 30%, in which case 9% would be homozygotes. This is slightly higher than the prevalence of GS based on purely phenotypic parameters. It was suggested that additional variables, such as mild hemolysis or a defect in bilirubin uptake, might be among the factors enhancing phenotypic expression of the defect.

Phenotypic expression of GS due solely to the A[TA]$_7$TAA promoter abnormality is inherited as an autosomal recessive trait. A number of CN-II kindreds have been identified in which there is also an allele containing a normal coding region but the A[TA]$_7$TAA promoter abnormality. CN-II heterozygotes who have the A[TA]$_6$TAA promoter are phenotypically normal, whereas those with the A[TA]$_7$TAA promoter express the phenotypic picture of GS. GS in such kindreds may also result from homozygosity for the A[TA]$_7$TAA promoter abnormality. Seven different missense mutations in the *UGT1* gene that reportedly cause GS with dominant inheritance have been found in Japanese individuals. Another Japanese patient with mild unconjugated hyperbilirubinemia was homozygous for a missense mutation in exon 5. GS in her family appeared to be recessive. Missense mutations causing GS have not been reported outside of certain Asian populations.

DISORDERS OF BILIRUBIN METABOLISM LEADING TO MIXED OR PREDOMINANTLY CONJUGATED HYPERBILIRUBINEMIA

In hyperbilirubinemia due to acquired liver disease (e.g., acute hepatitis, common bile duct stone), there are usually elevations in the serum concentrations of both conjugated and unconjugated bilirubin. Although biliary tract obstruction or hepatocellular cholestatic injury may present on occasion with a predominantly conjugated hyperbilirubinemia, it is generally not possible to differentiate intrahepatic from extrahepatic

causes of jaundice based upon the serum levels or relative proportions of unconjugated and conjugated bilirubin. The major reason for determining the amounts of conjugated and unconjugated bilirubin in the serum is for the initial differentiation of hepatic parenchymal and obstructive disorders (mixed conjugated and unconjugated hyperbilirubinemia) from the inheritable and hemolytic disorders discussed above that are associated with unconjugated hyperbilirubinemia.

FAMILIAL DEFECTS IN HEPATIC EXCRETORY FUNCTION

Dubin-Johnson Syndrome (DJS) This benign, relatively rare disorder is characterized by low-grade, predominantly conjugated hyperbilirubinemia (Table 297-2). Total bilirubin concentrations are typically between 34 and 85 μmol/L (2 and 5 mg/dL) but on occasion can be in the normal range or as high as 340–430 μmol/L (20–25 mg/dL) and can fluctuate widely in any given patient. The degree of hyperbilirubinemia may be increased by intercurrent illness, oral contraceptive use, and pregnancy. As the hyperbilirubinemia is due to a predominant rise in conjugated bilirubin, bilirubinuria is characteristically present. Aside from elevated serum bilirubin levels, other routine laboratory tests are normal. Physical examination is usually normal except for jaundice, although an occasional patient may have hepatosplenomegaly.

Patients with DJS are usually asymptomatic, although some may have vague constitutional symptoms. These latter patients have usually undergone extensive and often unnecessary diagnostic examinations for unexplained jaundice and have high levels of anxiety. In women, the condition may be subclinical until the patient becomes pregnant or receives oral contraceptives, at which time chemical hyperbilirubinemia becomes frank jaundice. Even in these situations, other routine liver function tests, including serum alkaline phosphatase and transaminase activities, are normal.

A cardinal feature of DJS is the accumulation in the lysosomes of centrilobular hepatocytes of dark, coarsely granular pigment. As a result, the liver may be grossly black in appearance. This pigment is thought to be derived from epinephrine metabolites that are not excreted normally. The pigment may disappear during bouts of viral hepatitis, only to reaccumulate slowly after recovery.

Biliary excretion of a number of anionic compounds is compromised in DJS. These include various cholecystographic agents, as well as sulfobromophthalein (Bromsulphalein, BSP), a synthetic dye formerly used in a test of liver function. In this test, the rate of disappearance of BSP from plasma was determined following bolus intravenous administration. BSP is conjugated with glutathione in the hepatocyte; the resulting conjugate is normally excreted rapidly into the bile canaliculus. Patients with DJS exhibit a characteristic rise in its plasma concentration at 90 min after injection, due to reflux of conjugated BSP into the circulation from the hepatocyte. Dyes such as ICG that are taken up by hepatocytes but are not further metabolized prior to biliary excretion do not show this reflux phenomenon. Continuous BSP infusion studies suggest a reduction in the t_{max} for biliary excretion. Bile acid disposition, including hepatocellular uptake and biliary excretion, is normal in DJS. These patients have normal serum and biliary bile acid concentrations and do not have pruritus.

By analogy with findings in several mutant rat strains, the selective defect in biliary excretion of bilirubin conjugates and certain other classes of organic compounds, but not of bile acids, that characterizes DJS in humans was found to reflect defective expression of MRP2, an ATP-dependent canalicular membrane transporter. Several different mutations in the *MRP2* gene produce the Dubin-Johnson phenotype, which has an autosomal recessive pattern of inheritance. Although MRP2 is undoubtedly important in the biliary excretion of conjugated bilirubin, the fact that this pigment is still excreted in the absence of MRP2 suggests that other, as yet uncharacterized, transport proteins may serve in a secondary role in this process.

Patients with DJS also have a diagnostic abnormality in urinary coproporphyrin excretion. There are two naturally occurring coproporphyrin isomers, I and III. Normally, ~75% of the coproporphyrin in urine is isomer III. In urine from DJS patients, total coproporphyrin content is normal, but >80% is isomer I. Heterozygotes for the syn-

TABLE 297-2 PRINCIPAL DIFFERENTIAL CHARACTERISTICS OF INHERITABLE DISORDERS OF BILE CANALICULAR FUNCTION

	DJS	Rotor	PFIC1	BRIC1	PFIC2	BRIC2	PFIC3
Gene	*ABCCA*	?	*ATP8B1*	*ATP8B1*	*ABCB11*	*ABCB11*	*ABCB4*
Protein	MRP2	?	FIC1	FIC1	BSEP	BSEP	MDR3
Cholestasis	No	No	Yes	Episodic	Yes	Episodic	Yes
Serum γ-GT	Normal	Normal	Normal	Normal	Normal	Normal	↑↑
Serum bile acids	Normal	Normal	↑↑	↑↑ during episodes	↑↑	↑↑ during episodes	↑↑
Clinical features	Mild conjugated hyperbilirubinemia; otherwise normal liver function; dark pigment in liver; characteristic pattern of urinary coproporphyrins	Mild conjugated hyperbilirubinemia; otherwise normal liver function; liver without abnormal pigmentation	Severe cholestasis beginning in childhood	Recurrent episodes of cholestasis beginning at any age	Severe cholestasis beginning in childhood	Recurrent episodes of cholestasis beginning at any age	Severe cholestasis beginning in childhood; decreased phospholipids in bile

Note: DJS, Dubin-Johnson syndrome; PFIC, progressive familial intrahepatic cholestasis; MRP2, multidrug resistance–associated protein 2; BSEP, bile salt excretory protein; γ-GT, γ-glutamyltransferase BRIC, benign recurrent intrahepatic cholestasis; ↑↑, increased.

drome show an intermediate pattern. The molecular basis for this phenomenon remains unclear.

Rotor Syndrome This benign, autosomal recessive disorder is clinically similar to DJS (Table 297-2), although it is seen even less frequently. A major phenotypic difference is that the liver in patients with Rotor syndrome has no increased pigmentation and appears totally normal. The only abnormality in routine laboratory tests is an elevation of total serum bilirubin, due to a predominant rise in conjugated bilirubin. This is accompanied by bilirubinuria. Several additional features differentiate Rotor syndrome and DJS. In Rotor syndrome, the gallbladder is usually visualized on oral cholecystography, in contrast to the nonvisualization that is typical of DJS. The pattern of urinary coproporphyrin excretion also differs. The pattern in Rotor syndrome resembles that of many acquired disorders of hepatobiliary function, in which coproporphyrin I, the major coproporphyrin isomer in bile, refluxes from the hepatocyte back into the circulation and is excreted in urine. Thus, total urinary coproporphyrin excretion is substantially increased in Rotor syndrome, in contrast to the normal levels seen in DJS. Although the fraction of coproporphyrin I in urine is elevated, it is usually <70% of the total, as compared to ≥80% in DJS. The disorders also can be distinguished by their patterns of BSP excretion. Although clearance of BSP from plasma is delayed in Rotor syndrome, there is no reflux of conjugated BSP back into the circulation as seen in DJS. Kinetic analysis of plasma BSP infusion studies suggests the presence of a defect in intrahepatocellular storage of this compound. This has never been demonstrated directly, and the molecular basis of Rotor syndrome remains unknown.

Benign Recurrent Intrahepatic Cholestasis (BRIC) This rare disorder is characterized by recurrent attacks of pruritus and jaundice. The typical episode begins with mild malaise and elevations in serum aminotransferase levels, followed rapidly by rises in alkaline phosphatase and conjugated bilirubin and onset of jaundice and itching. The first one or two episodes may be misdiagnosed as acute viral hepatitis. The cholestatic episodes, which may begin in childhood or adulthood, can vary in duration from several weeks to months, following which there is complete clinical and biochemical resolution. Intervals between attacks may vary from several months to years. Between episodes, physical examination is normal, as are serum levels of bile acids, bilirubin, transaminases, and alkaline phosphatase. The disorder is familial and has an autosomal recessive pattern of inheritance. BRIC is considered a benign disorder in that it does not lead to cirrhosis or end-stage liver disease. However, the episodes of jaundice and pruritus can be prolonged and debilitating, and some patients have undergone liver transplantation to relieve the intractable and disabling symptoms. Treatment during the cholestatic episodes is symptomatic; there is no specific treatment to prevent or shorten the occurrence of episodes.

A gene termed *FIC1* was recently identified and found to be mutated in patients with BRIC. Curiously, this gene is expressed strongly in the small intestine but only weakly in the liver. The protein encoded by *FIC1* shows little similarity to genes that have been shown to play a role in bile canalicular excretion of various compounds. Rather, it appears to be a member of a P-type ATPase family that transports aminophospholipids from the outer to the inner leaflet of a variety of cell membranes. Its relationship to the pathobiology of this disorder remains unclear. A second phenotypically identical form of BRIC, termed BRIC type 2, has been described resulting from mutations in the bile salt excretory protein (BSEP), the protein that is defective in progressive familial intrahepatic cholestasis type 2 (Table 297-2). How some mutations in this protein result in the episodic BRIC phenotype is unknown.

Progressive Familial Intrahepatic Cholestasis (FIC) This name is applied to three phenotypically related syndromes (Table 297-2). Progressive FIC type 1 (Byler disease) presents in early infancy as cholestasis that may be initially episodic. However, in contrast to BRIC, Byler disease progresses to malnutrition, growth retardation, and end-stage liver disease during childhood. This disorder is also a consequence of a *FIC1* mutation. The functional relationship of the FIC1 protein to the pathogenesis of cholestasis in these disorders is unknown. Two other types of progressive FIC (types 2 and 3) have been described. Progressive FIC type 2 is associated with a mutation in the protein named *sister of p-glycoprotein*, which is the major bile canalicular exporter of bile acids and is also known as *bile salt excretory protein* (BSEP). As noted above, some mutations of this protein are associated with BRIC type 2, rather than the progressive FIC type 2 phenotype. Progressive FIC type 3 has been associated with a mutation of MDR3, a protein that is essential for normal hepatocellular excretion of phospholipids across the bile canaliculus. Although all three types of progressive FIC have similar clinical phenotypes, only type 3 is associated with high serum levels of γ-glutamyltransferase activity. In contrast, activity of this enzyme is normal or only mildly elevated in symptomatic BRIC and progressive FIC types 1 and 2.

FURTHER READINGS

BOSMA P et al: The genetic basis of the reduced expression of bilirubin-UDP-glucuronosyltransferase 1 in Gilbert's syndrome. N Engl J Med 333:1171, 1995

BURCHELL B: Genetic variation of human UDP-glucuronosyltransferase: Implications in disease and drug glucuronidation. Am J Pharmacogenomics 3:37, 2003

HARRIS MJ et al: Progressive familial intrahepatic cholestasis: Genetic disorders of biliary transporters. J Gastroenterol Hepatol 20:807, 2005

JANSEN PL: Diagnosis and management of Crigler-Najjar syndrome. Eur J Pediatr 158:S89, 1999

VAN MIL SW et al: Benign recurrent intrahepatic cholestasis type 2 is caused by mutations in ABCB11. Gastroenterology 127:379, 2004

298 Acute Viral Hepatitis
Jules L. Dienstag

Acute viral hepatitis is a systemic infection affecting the liver predominantly. Almost all cases of acute viral hepatitis are caused by one of five viral agents: hepatitis A virus (HAV), hepatitis B virus (HBV), hepatitis C virus (HCV), the HBV-associated delta agent or hepatitis D virus (HDV), and hepatitis E virus (HEV). Other transfusion-transmitted agents, e.g., "hepatitis G" virus and "TT" virus, have been identified but do not cause hepatitis. All these human hepatitis viruses are RNA viruses, except for hepatitis B, which is a DNA virus. Although these agents can be distinguished by their molecular and antigenic properties, all types of viral hepatitis produce clinically similar illnesses. These range from asymptomatic and inapparent to fulminant and fatal acute infections common to all types, on the one hand, and from subclinical persistent infections to rapidly progressive chronic liver disease with cirrhosis and even hepatocellular carcinoma, common to the bloodborne types (HBV, HCV, and HDV), on the other.

VIROLOGY AND ETIOLOGY
Hepatitis A Hepatitis A virus is a nonenveloped 27-nm, heat-, acid-, and ether-resistant RNA virus in the hepatovirus genus of the picornavirus family (Fig. 298-1). Its virion contains four capsid polypeptides, designated VP1 to VP4, which are cleaved posttranslationally from the polyprotein product of a 7500-nucleotide genome. Inactivation of viral activity can be achieved by boiling for 1 min, by contact with formaldehyde and chlorine, or by ultraviolet irradiation. Despite nucleotide sequence variation of up to 20% among isolates of HAV, all strains of this virus are immunologically indistinguishable and belong to one serotype. Hepatitis A has an incubation period of ~4 weeks. Its replication is limited to the liver, but the virus is present in the liver, bile, stools, and blood during the late incubation period and acute preicteric phase of illness. Despite persistence of virus in the liver, viral shedding in feces, viremia, and infectivity diminish rapidly once jaundice becomes apparent. HAV can be cultivated reproducibly in vitro.

Antibodies to HAV (anti-HAV) can be detected during acute illness when serum aminotransferase activity is elevated and fecal HAV shedding is still occurring. This early antibody response is predominantly of the IgM class and persists for several months, rarely for 6–12 months. During convalescence, however, anti-HAV of the IgG class becomes the predominant antibody (Fig. 298-2). Therefore, the diagnosis of hepatitis A is made during acute illness by demonstrating anti-HAV of the IgM class. After acute illness, anti-HAV of the IgG class remains detectable indefinitely, and patients with serum anti-HAV are immune

FIGURE 298-2 Scheme of typical clinical and laboratory features of hepatitis A.

to reinfection. Neutralizing antibody activity parallels the appearance of anti-HAV, and the IgG anti-HAV present in immune globulin accounts for the protection it affords against HAV infection.

Hepatitis B Hepatitis B virus is a DNA virus with a remarkably compact genomic structure; despite its small, circular, 3200-bp size, HBV DNA codes for four sets of viral products with a complex, multiparticle structure. HBV achieves its genomic economy by relying on an efficient strategy of encoding proteins from four overlapping genes: S, C, P, and X (Fig. 298-3), as detailed below. Once thought to be unique among viruses, HBV is now recognized as one of a family of animal viruses, hepadnaviruses (hepatotropic DNA viruses), and is classified as hepadnavirus type 1. Similar viruses infect certain species of woodchucks, ground and tree squirrels, and Pekin ducks, to mention the most carefully characterized. Like HBV, all have the same distinctive three morphologic forms, have counterparts to the envelope and nucleocapsid virus antigens of HBV, replicate in the liver but exist in extrahepatic sites, contain their own endogenous DNA polymerase, have partially double-strand and partially single-strand genomes, are associated with acute and chronic hepatitis and hepatocellular carcinoma, and rely on a replicative strategy unique among DNA viruses but typical of retroviruses. Instead of DNA replication directly from a DNA template, hepadnaviruses rely on reverse transcription (effected by the DNA polymerase) of minus-strand DNA from a "pregenomic" RNA intermediate. Then plus-strand DNA is transcribed from the minus-strand DNA template by the DNA-dependent DNA polymerase and converted in the hepatocyte nucleus to a covalently closed circular DNA, which serves as a template for messenger RNA and pregenomic RNA. Viral proteins are translated by the messenger RNA, and the proteins and genome are packaged into virions and secreted from the hepatocyte. Although HBV is difficult to cultivate in vitro in the conventional sense from clinical material, several cell lines have been transfected with HBV DNA. Such transfected cells support in vitro replication of the intact virus and its component proteins.

VIRAL PROTEINS AND PARTICLES Of the three particulate forms of HBV (Table 298-1), the most numerous are the 22-nm particles, which appear as spherical or long filamentous forms; these are antigenically indistinguishable from the outer surface or envelope protein of HBV and are thought to represent excess viral envelope protein. Outnumbered in serum by a factor of 100 or 1000 to 1 compared with the spheres and tubules are large, 42-nm, double-shelled spherical particles, which repre-

FIGURE 298-1 Electron micrographs of hepatitis A virus particles and serum from a patient with hepatitis B. *Left:* 27-nm hepatitis A virus particles purified from stool of a patient with acute hepatitis A and aggregated by antibody to hepatitis A virus. *Right:* Concentrated serum from a patient with hepatitis B, demonstrating the 42-nm virions, tubular forms, and spherical 22-nm particles of hepatitis B surface antigen. 132,000×. (Hepatitis D resembles 42-nm virions of hepatitis B but is smaller, 35–37 nm; hepatitis E resembles hepatitis A virus but is slightly larger, 32–34 nm; hepatitis C has been visualized as a 55-nm particle.)

FIGURE 298-3 Compact genomic structure of HBV. This structure, with overlapping genes, permits HBV to code for multiple proteins. The S gene codes for the "major" envelope protein, HBsAg. Pre-S1 and pre-S2, upstream of S, combine with S to code for two larger proteins, "middle" protein, the product of pre-S2 + S, and "large" protein, the product of pre-S1 + pre-S2 + S. The largest gene, P, codes for DNA polymerase. The C gene codes for two nucleocapsid proteins, HBeAg, a soluble, secreted protein (initiation from the pre-C region of the gene) and HBcAg, the intracellular core protein (initiation after pre-C). The X gene codes for HBxAg, which can transactivate the transcription of cellular and viral genes; its clinical relevance is not known, but it may contribute to carcinogenesis by binding to p53.

sent the intact hepatitis B virion (Fig. 298-1). The envelope protein expressed on the outer surface of the virion and on the smaller spherical and tubular structures is referred to as *hepatitis B surface antigen* (HBsAg). The concentration of HBsAg and virus particles in the blood may reach 500 μg/mL and 10 trillion particles per milliliter, respectively. The envelope protein, HBsAg, is the product of the S gene of HBV.

A number of different HBsAg subdeterminants have been identified. There is a common group-reactive antigen, *a*, shared by all HBsAg isolates. In addition, HBsAg may contain one of several subtype-specific antigens, namely, *d* or *y*, *w* or *r*, as well as other more recently characterized specificities. Hepatitis B isolates fall into one of at least eight subtypes and eight genotypes (A–H). Geographic distribution of genotypes and subtypes varies; genotypes A (corresponding to subtype *adw*) and D (*ayw*) predominate in the United States and Europe, while genotypes B (*adw*) and C (*adr*) predominate in Asia. Clinical course and outcome are independent of subtype, but preliminary reports suggest that genotype B is associated with less rapidly progressive liver disease and a lower likelihood, or delayed appearance, of hepatocellular carcinoma than genotype C. Patients with genotype A appear to be more likely to clear circulating viremia and to achieve HBsAg seroconversion, both spontaneously and in response to antiviral therapy. In addition, "precore" mutations are favored by certain genotypes (see below).

Upstream of the S gene are the pre-S genes (Fig. 298-3), which code for pre-S gene products, including receptors on the HBV surface for polymerized human serum albumin and for hepatocyte membrane proteins. The pre-S region actually consists of both pre-S1 and pre-S2. Depending on where translation is initiated, three potential HBsAg gene products are synthesized. The protein product of the S gene is HBsAg (*major protein*), the product of the S region plus the adjacent pre-S2 region is the *middle protein*, and the product of the pre-S1 plus pre-S2 plus S regions is the *large protein*. Compared with the smaller spherical and tubular particles of HBV, complete 42-nm virions are enriched in the large protein. Both pre-S proteins and their respective antibodies can be detected during HBV infection, and the period of pre-S antigenemia appears to coincide with other markers of virus replication, as detailed below.

The intact 42-nm virion contains a 27-nm nucleocapsid core particle. Nucleocapsid proteins are coded for by the C gene. The antigen expressed on the surface of the nucleocapsid core is referred to as *hepatitis B core antigen* (HBcAg), and its corresponding antibody is anti-HBc. A third HBV antigen is *hepatitis B e antigen* (HBeAg), a soluble, nonparticulate, nucleocapsid protein that is immunologically distinct from intact HBcAg but is a product of the same C gene. The C gene has two initiation codons, a precore and a core region (Fig. 298-3). If translation is initiated at the precore region, the protein product is HBeAg, which has a signal peptide that binds it to the smooth endoplasmic reticulum and leads to its secretion into the circulation. If translation begins with the core region, HBcAg is the protein product; it has no signal peptide, it is not secreted, but it assembles into nucleocapsid particles, which bind to and incorporate RNA and which, ultimately, contain HBV DNA. Also packaged within the nucleocapsid core is a DNA polymerase, which directs replication and repair of HBV DNA. When packaging within viral proteins is complete, synthesis of the incomplete plus strand stops; this accounts for the single-strand gap and for differences in the size of the gap. HBcAg particles remain in the hepatocyte, where they are readily detectable by immunohistochemical staining, and are exported after encapsidation by an envelope of HBsAg. Therefore, naked core particles do not circulate in the serum. The secreted nucleocapsid protein, HBeAg, provides a convenient, readily detectable, qualitative marker of HBV replication and relative infectivity.

HBsAg-positive serum containing HBeAg is more likely to be highly infectious and to be associated with the presence of hepatitis B virions (and detectable HBV DNA, see below) than HBeAg-negative or anti-HBe-positive serum. For example, HBsAg carrier mothers who are HBeAg-positive almost invariably (>90%) transmit hepatitis B infection to their offspring, whereas HBsAg carrier mothers with anti-HBe rarely (10–15%) infect their offspring.

Early during the course of acute hepatitis B, HBeAg appears transiently; its disappearance may be a harbinger of clinical improvement and resolution of infection. Persistence of HBeAg in serum beyond the first 3 months of acute infection may be predictive of the development of chronic infection, and the presence of HBeAg during chronic hepatitis B is associated with ongoing viral replication, infectivity, and inflammatory liver injury.

The third of the HBV genes is the largest, the P gene (Fig. 298-3), which codes for the DNA polymerase; as noted above, this enzyme has both DNA-dependent DNA polymerase and RNA-dependent reverse transcriptase activities. The fourth gene, X, codes for a small, nonparticulate protein, *hepatitis B x antigen* (HBxAg), that is capable of transactivating the transcription of both viral and cellular genes (Fig. 298-3). In the cytoplasm, HBxAg effects calcium release (possibly from mitochondria), which activates signal-transduction pathways that lead to stimulation of HBV reverse transcription and HBV DNA replication. Such transactivation may enhance the replication of HBV, leading to the clinical association observed between the expression of HBxAg and antibodies to it in patients with severe chronic hepatitis and hepatocellular carcinoma. The transactivating activity can enhance the transcription and replication of other viruses besides HBV, such as HIV. Cellular processes transactivated by X include the human interferon γ gene and class I major histocompatibility genes; potentially, these effects could contribute to enhanced susceptibility of HBV-infected hepatocytes to cytolytic T cells. The expression of X can also induce programmed cell death (apoptosis).

SEROLOGIC AND VIROLOGIC MARKERS After a person is infected with HBV, the first virologic marker detectable in serum within 1–12 weeks, usually between 8–12 weeks, is HBsAg (Fig. 298-4). Circulating HBsAg precedes elevations of serum aminotransferase activity and clinical symptoms by 2–6 weeks and remains detectable during the entire icteric or symptomatic phase of acute hepatitis B and beyond. In typical cases, HBsAg becomes undetectable 1–2 months after the onset of jaundice and rarely persists beyond 6 months. After HBsAg disappears, antibody to HBsAg (anti-HBs) becomes detectable in serum and remains detectable indefinitely thereafter. Because HBcAg is intracellular and, when in the serum, sequestered within an HBsAg coat,

TABLE 298-1 NOMENCLATURE AND FEATURES OF HEPATITIS VIRUSES

Hepatitis Type	Virus Particle, nm	Morphology	Genome[a]	Classification	Antigen(s)	Antibodies	Remarks
HAV	27	Icosahedral non-enveloped	7.5-kb RNA, linear, ss, +	Hepatovirus	HAV	Anti-HAV	Early fecal shedding; Diagnosis: IgM anti-HAV; Previous infection: IgG anti-HAV
HBV	42	Double-shelled virion (surface and core) spherical	3.2-kb DNA, circular, ss/ds	Hepadnavirus	HBsAg HBcAg HBeAg	Anti-HBs Anti-HBc Anti-HBe	Bloodborne virus; carrier state; Acute diagnosis: HBsAg, IgM anti-HBc; Chronic diagnosis: IgG anti-HBc, HBsAg; Markers of replication: HBeAg, HBV DNA; Liver, lymphocytes, other organs
	27	Nucleocapsid core			HBcAg HBeAg	Anti-HBc Anti-HBe	Nucleocapsid contains DNA and DNA polymerase; present in hepatocyte nucleus; HBcAg does not circulate; HBeAg (soluble, nonparticulate) and HBV DNA circulate—correlate with infectivity and complete virions
	22	Spherical and filamentous; represents excess virus coat material			HBsAg	Anti-HBs	HBsAg detectable in >95% of patients with acute hepatitis B; found in serum, body fluids, hepatocyte cytoplasm; anti-HBs appears following infection—protective antibody
HCV	Approx. 40–60	Enveloped	9.4-kb RNA, linear, ss, +	Hepacivirus	HCV C100-3 C33c C22-3 NS5	Anti-HCV	Bloodborne agent, formerly labeled non-A, non-B hepatitis; Acute diagnosis: anti-HCV (C33c, C22-3, NS5), HCV RNA; Chronic diagnosis: anti-HCV (C100-3, C33c, C22-3, NS5) and HCV RNA; cytoplasmic location in hepatocytes
HDV	35–37	Enveloped hybrid particle with HBsAg coat and HDV core	1.7-kb RNA, circular, ss, −	Resembles viroids and plant satellite viruses	HBsAg HDV antigen	Anti-HBs Anti-HDV	Defective RNA virus, requires helper function of HBV (hepadnaviruses); HDV antigen present in hepatocyte nucleus; Diagnosis: anti-HDV, HDV RNA; HBV/HDV coinfection—IgM anti-HBc and anti-HDV; HDV superinfection—IgG anti-HBc and anti-HDV
HEV	32–34	Nonenveloped icosahedral	7.6-kb RNA, linear, ss, +	Hepevirus	HEV antigen	Anti-HEV	Agent of enterically transmitted hepatitis; rare in USA; occurs in Asia, Mediterranean countries, Central America; Diagnosis: IgM/IgG anti-HEV (assays being developed); virus in stool, bile, hepatocyte cytoplasm

[a]ss, single-strand; ss/ds, partially single-strand, partially double-strand; −, minus-strand; +, plus-strand.

naked core particles do not circulate in serum and, therefore, HBcAg is not detectable routinely in the serum of patients with HBV infection. By contrast, anti-HBc is readily demonstrable in serum, beginning within the first 1–2 weeks after the appearance of HBsAg and preceding detectable levels of anti-HBs by weeks to months. Because variability exists in the time of appearance of anti-HBs after HBV infection, occasionally a gap of several weeks or longer may separate the disappearance of HBsAg and the appearance of anti-HBs. During this "gap" or "window" period, anti-HBc may represent the only serologic evidence of current or recent HBV infection, and blood containing anti-HBc in the absence of HBsAg and anti-HBs has been implicated in the development of transfusion-associated hepatitis B. In part because the sensitivity of immunoassays for HBsAg and anti-HBs has increased, however, this window period is rarely encountered. In some persons, years after HBV infection, anti-HBc may persist in the circulation longer than anti-HBs. Therefore, isolated anti-HBc does not necessarily indicate active virus replication; most instances of isolated anti-HBc represent hepatitis B infection in the remote past. Rarely, however, isolated anti-HBc represents low-level hepatitis B viremia, with HBsAg below the detection threshold; occasionally, isolated anti-HBc represents a cross-reacting or false-positive immunologic specificity. Recent and remote HBV infections can be distinguished by determination of the immunoglobulin class of anti-HBc. Anti-HBc of the IgM class (IgM anti-HBc) predominates during the first 6 months after acute infection, whereas IgG anti-HBc is the predominant class of anti-HBc beyond 6 months. Therefore, patients with current or recent acute

hepatitis B, including those in the anti-HBc window, have IgM anti-HBc in their serum. In patients who have recovered from hepatitis B in the remote past as well as those with chronic HBV infection, anti-HBc is predominantly of the IgG class. Infrequently, in ≤1–5% of patients with acute HBV infection, levels of HBsAg are too low to be detected;

FIGURE 298-4 Scheme of typical clinical and laboratory features of acute hepatitis B.

in such cases, the presence of IgM anti-HBc establishes the diagnosis of acute hepatitis B. When isolated anti-HBc occurs in the rare patient with chronic hepatitis B whose HBsAg level is below the sensitivity threshold of contemporary immunoassays (a low-level carrier), the anti-HBc is of the IgG class. Generally, in persons who have recovered from hepatitis B, anti-HBs and anti-HBc persist indefinitely.

The temporal association between the appearance of anti-HBs and resolution of HBV infection as well as the observation that persons with anti-HBs in serum are protected against reinfection with HBV suggests that *anti-HBs are the protective antibody*. Therefore, strategies for prevention of HBV infection are based on providing susceptible persons with circulating anti-HBs (see below). Occasionally, in 10–20% of patients with chronic hepatitis B, low-level, low-affinity anti-HBs can be detected. This antibody is directed against a subtype determinant different from that represented by the patient's HBsAg; its presence is thought to reflect the stimulation of a related clone of antibody-forming cells, but it has no clinical relevance and does not signal imminent clearance of hepatitis B. These patients with HBsAg and such nonneutralizing anti-HBs should be categorized as having chronic HBV infection.

The other readily detectable serologic marker of HBV infection, HBeAg, appears concurrently with or shortly after HBsAg. Its appearance coincides temporally with high levels of virus replication and reflects the presence of circulating intact virions and detectable HBV DNA (with the notable exception of patients with precore mutations who cannot synthesize HBeAg—see "Molecular Variants," below). Pre-S1 and pre-S2 proteins are also expressed during periods of peak replication, but assays for these gene products are not routinely available. In self-limited HBV infections, HBeAg becomes undetectable shortly after peak elevations in aminotransferase activity, before the disappearance of HBsAg, and anti-HBe then becomes detectable, coinciding with a period of relatively lower infectivity (Fig. 298-4). Because markers of HBV replication appear transiently during acute infection, testing for such markers is of little clinical utility in typical cases of acute HBV infection. In contrast, markers of HBV replication provide valuable information in patients with protracted infections.

Departing from the pattern typical of acute HBV infections, in chronic HBV infection, HBsAg remains detectable beyond 6 months, anti-HBc is primarily of the IgG class, and anti-HBs is either undetectable or detectable at low levels (see "Laboratory Features," below) (Fig. 298-5). During early chronic HBV infection, HBV DNA can be detected both in serum and in hepatocyte nuclei, where it is present in free or episomal form. This *replicative stage* of HBV infection is the time of maximal infectivity and liver injury; HBeAg is a qualitative marker and HBV DNA a quantitative marker of this replicative phase, during which all three forms of HBV circulate, including intact virions. Over time, the replicative phase of chronic HBV infection gives way to a relatively *nonreplicative phase*. This occurs at a rate of ~10% per year and is accompanied by seroconversion from HBeAg-positive to anti-HBe-positive. In most cases, this seroconversion coincides with a transient, acute hepatitis-like elevation in aminotransferase activity, believed to reflect cell-mediated immune clearance of virus-infected hepatocytes. In the nonreplicative phase of chronic infection, when HBV DNA is demonstrable in hepatocyte nuclei, it tends to be integrated into the host genome. In this phase, only spherical and tubular forms of HBV, *not intact virions*, circulate, and liver injury tends to subside. Most such patients would be characterized as *inactive HBV carriers*. In reality, the designations *replicative* and *nonreplicative* are only relative; even in the so-called nonreplicative phase, HBV replication can be detected at levels of ~≤10^3 virions with highly sensitive amplification probes such as the polymerase chain reaction (PCR); below this replication threshold, liver injury and infectivity of HBV are limited to negligible. Still, the distinctions are pathophysiologically and clinically meaningful. Occasionally, nonreplicative HBV infection converts back to replicative infection. Such spontaneous reactivations are accompanied by reexpression of HBeAg and HBV DNA, and sometimes of IgM anti-HBc, as well as by exacerbations of liver injury. Because high-titer IgM anti-HBc can reappear during acute exacerbations of chronic hepatitis

FIGURE 298-5 Scheme of typical laboratory features of wild-type chronic hepatitis B. HBeAg and HBV DNA can be detected in serum during the *replicative phase* of chronic infection, which is associated with infectivity and liver injury. Seroconversion from the replicative phase to the *nonreplicative phase* occurs at a rate of ~10% per year and is heralded by an acute hepatitis–like elevation of ALT activity; during the nonreplicative phase, infectivity and liver injury are limited. In HBeAg-negative chronic hepatitis B associated with mutations in the precore region of the HBV genome, replicative chronic hepatitis B occurs in the absence of HBeAg.

B, relying on IgM anti-HBc versus IgG anti-HBc to distinguish between acute and chronic hepatitis B infection, respectively, may not always be reliable; in such cases, patient history is invaluable in helping to distinguish de novo acute hepatitis B infection from acute exacerbation of chronic hepatitis B infection.

MOLECULAR VARIANTS Variation occurs throughout the HBV genome, and clinical isolates of HBV that do not express typical viral proteins have been attributed to mutations in individual or even multiple gene locations. For example, variants have been described that lack nucleocapsid proteins, envelope proteins, or both. Two categories of naturally occurring HBV variants have attracted the most attention. One of these was identified initially in Mediterranean countries among patients with an unusual serologic-clinical profile. They have severe chronic HBV infection and detectable HBV DNA but with anti-HBe instead of HBeAg. These patients were found to be infected with an HBV mutant that contained an alteration in the precore region rendering the virus incapable of encoding HBeAg. Although several potential mutation sites exist in the pre-C region, the region of the C gene necessary for the expression of HBeAg (see "Virology and Etiology," above), the most commonly encountered in such patients is a single base substitution, from G to A, which occurs in the second to last codon of the pre-C gene at nucleotide 1896. This substitution results in the replacement of the TGG tryptophan codon by a stop codon (TAG), which prevents the translation of HBeAg. Another mutation, in the core-promoter region, prevents transcription of the coding region for HBeAg and yields an HBeAg-negative phenotype. Patients with such mutations in the precore region and who are unable to secrete HBeAg tend to have severe liver disease that progresses more rapidly to cirrhosis. Both "wild-type" HBV and precore-mutant HBV can coexist in the same patient, or mutant HBV may arise late during wild-type HBV infection. In addition, clusters of fulminant hepatitis B in Israel and Japan have been attributed to common-source infection with a precore mutant. Fulminant hepatitis B in North America and western Europe, however, occurs in patients infected with wild-type HBV, in the absence of precore mutants, and both precore mutants and other mutations throughout the HBV genome occur commonly even in patients with typical, self-limited, milder forms of HBV infection. HBeAg-negative chronic hepatitis with mutations in the precore region is now the most frequently encountered form of hepatitis B in Mediterranean countries and in Europe. In the United States, where HBV genotype A (less prone to G1896A mutation) is prevalent, precore-mutant HBV is much less common; however, as a result of immigration from Asia and Europe, the proportion of HBeAg-negative hepatitis B–infected individuals has increased in the United States, and they now represent approximately a third of patients with chronic hepatitis B. Characteristic of such HBeAg-negative chronic hepatitis B are lower levels of HBV DNA (usually ≤10^5 copies/mL) and one of several patterns of aminotransferase activity—persistent elevations, periodic fluctuations above the normal range, and periodic fluctuations between the normal and elevated range.

The second important category of HBV mutants consists of *escape mutants*, in which a single amino acid substitution, from glycine to arginine, occurs at position 145 of the immunodominant *a* determinant common to all subtypes of HBsAg. This change in HBsAg leads to a critical conformational change that results in a loss of neutralizing activity by anti-HBs. This specific HBV/*a* mutant has been observed in two situations, active and passive immunization, in which humoral immunologic pressure may favor evolutionary change ("escape") in the virus—in a small number of hepatitis B vaccine recipients who acquired HBV infection despite the prior appearance of neutralizing anti-HBs and in liver transplant recipients who underwent the procedure for hepatitis B and who were treated with a high-potency human monoclonal anti-HBs preparation. Although such mutants have not been recognized frequently, their existence raises a concern that may complicate vaccination strategies and serologic diagnosis. Different types of mutations emerge during antiviral therapy of chronic hepatitis B with nucleoside analogues; such "YMDD" and similar mutations in the polymerase motif of HBV are described in Chap. 300.

EXTRAHEPATIC SITES Hepatitis B antigens and HBV DNA have been identified in extrahepatic sites, including lymph nodes, bone marrow, circulating lymphocytes, spleen, and pancreas. Although the virus does not appear to be associated with tissue injury in any of these extrahepatic sites, its presence in these "remote" reservoirs has been invoked to explain the recurrence of HBV infection after orthotopic liver transplantation. A more complete understanding of the clinical relevance of extrahepatic HBV remains to be defined.

Hepatitis D The delta hepatitis agent, or HDV, is a defective RNA virus that coinfects with and requires the helper function of HBV (or other hepadnaviruses) for its replication and expression. Slightly smaller than HBV, delta is a formalin-sensitive, 35- to 37-nm virus with a hybrid structure. Its nucleocapsid expresses delta antigen, which bears no antigenic homology with any of the HBV antigens, and contains the virus genome. The delta core is "encapsidated" by an outer envelope of HBsAg, indistinguishable from that of HBV except in its relative compositions of major, middle, and large HBsAg component proteins. The genome is a small, 1700-nucleotide, circular, single-strand RNA (minus strand) that is nonhomologous with HBV DNA (except for a small area of the polymerase gene) but that has features and the rolling circle model of replication common to genomes of plant satellite viruses or viroids. HDV RNA contains many areas of internal complementarity; therefore, it can fold on itself by internal base pairing to form an unusual, very stable, rodlike structure. HDV RNA requires host RNA polymerase II for its replication via RNA-directed RNA synthesis by transcription of genomic RNA to a complementary antigenomic (plus strand) RNA; the antigenomic RNA, in turn, serves as a template for subsequent genomic RNA synthesis. Between the genomic and antigenomic RNAs of HDV, there are coding regions for nine proteins. Delta antigen, which is a product of the antigenomic strand, exists in two forms, a small, 195-amino-acid species, which plays a role in facilitating HDV RNA replication, and a large, 214-amino-acid species, which appears to suppress replication but is required for assembly of the antigen into virions. Delta antigens have been shown to bind directly to RNA polymerase II, resulting in stimulation of transcription. Although complete hepatitis D virions and liver injury require the cooperative helper function of HBV, intracellular replication of HDV RNA can occur without HBV. Genomic heterogeneity among HDV isolates has been described; however, pathophysiologic and clinical consequences of this genetic diversity have not been recognized.

HDV can either infect a person simultaneously with HBV (*co-infection*) or superinfect a person already infected with HBV (*superinfection*); when HDV infection is transmitted from a donor with one HBsAg subtype to an HBsAg-positive recipient with a different subtype, the HDV agent assumes the HBsAg subtype of the recipient, rather than the donor. Because HDV relies absolutely on HBV, the duration of HDV infection is determined by the duration of (and cannot outlast) HBV infection. HDV antigen is expressed primarily in hepatocyte nuclei and is occasionally detectable in serum. During acute HDV infection, anti-HDV of the IgM class predominates, and 30–40 days may elapse after symptoms appear before anti-HDV can be detected. In self-limited infection, anti-HDV is low titer and transient, rarely remaining detectable beyond the clearance of HBsAg and HDV antigen. In chronic HDV infection, anti-HDV circulates in high titer, and both IgM and IgG anti-HDV can be detected. HDV antigen in the liver and HDV RNA in serum and liver can be detected during HDV replication.

Hepatitis C Hepatitis C virus, which, before its identification was labeled "non-A, non-B hepatitis," is a linear, single-strand, positive-sense, 9600-nucleotide RNA virus, the genome of which is similar in organization to that of flaviviruses and pestiviruses; HCV is the only member of the genus *Hepacivirus* in the family Flaviviridae. The HCV genome contains a single large open reading frame (gene) that codes for a virus polyprotein of ~3000 amino acids, which is cleaved after translation to yield 10 viral proteins. The 5′ end of the genome consists of an untranslated region (containing an internal ribosomal entry site) adjacent to the genes for four structural proteins, the nucleocapsid core protein, C; two envelope glycoproteins, E1 and E2; and a membrane protein p7. The 5′ untranslated region and core gene are highly conserved among genotypes, but the envelope proteins are coded for by the hypervariable region, which varies from isolate to isolate and may allow the virus to evade host immunologic containment directed at accessible virus-envelope proteins. The 3′ end of the genome also includes an untranslated region and contains the genes for six nonstructural (NS) proteins NS2, NS3, NS4A, NS4B, NS5A, and NS5B. The NS2 cysteine protease cleaves NS3 from NS2, and the NS3-4A serine protease cleaves all the downstream proteins from the polyprotein. Important NS proteins involved in virus replication include the NS3 helicase, NS3-NS4A serine protease, and the NS5B RNA-dependent RNA polymerase (Fig. 298-6). Because HCV does not replicate via a DNA intermediate, it does not integrate into the host genome. Because HCV tends to circulate in relatively low titer, 10^3–10^7 virions/mL, visualization of virus particles, estimated to be 40–60 nm in diameter, remains difficult. Still, the replication rate of HCV is very high, 10^{12} virions per day; its half-life is 2.7 h. The chimpanzee is a helpful but cumbersome animal model. Although a robust, reproducible, small-animal model is lacking, HCV replication has been documented in an immunodeficient-mouse model containing explants of human liver and in transgenic mouse and rat models. Although in vitro replication has been difficult, hepatocellular carcinoma–derived cell lines have been described (replicon systems) that support replication of genetically manipulated, truncated or full-length HCV RNA (but not intact virions). Recently, complete replication of HCV and intact 55-nm virions has been described in cell culture systems. Preliminary data suggest that HCV gains entry into the hepatocyte via the CD81 receptor.

At least six distinct genotypes, as well as >50 subtypes within genotypes, of HCV have been identified by nucleotide sequencing. Genotypes differ one from another in sequence homology by ≥30%. Because divergence of HCV isolates within a genotype or subtype, and within the same host, may vary insufficiently to define a distinct genotype, these intragenotypic differences are referred to as *quasispecies* and differ in sequence homology by only a few percent. The genotypic and quasispecies diversity of HCV, resulting from its high mutation rate, interferes with effective humoral immunity. Neutralizing anti-

FIGURE 298-6 Organization of the hepatitis C virus genome and its associated, 3000-amino-acid (AA) proteins. The three structural genes at the 5′ end are the core region, C, which codes for the nucleocapsid, and the envelope regions, E1 and E2, which code for envelope glycoproteins. The 5′ untranslated region and the C region are highly conserved among isolates, while the envelope domain E2 contains the hypervariable region. Adjacent to the structural proteins is p7, a membrane protein that appears to function as an ion channel. At the 3′ end are six nonstructural (NS) regions, NS2, which codes for a cysteine protease; NS3, which codes for a serine protease and an RNA helicase; NS4 and NS4B; NS5A; and NS5B, which codes for an RNA-dependent RNA polymerase. After translation of the entire polyprotein, individual proteins are cleaved by both host and viral proteases.

bodies to HCV have been demonstrated, but they tend to be short-lived, and HCV infection does not induce lasting immunity against reinfection with different virus isolates or even the same virus isolate. Thus, neither *heterologous* nor *homologous* immunity appears to develop commonly after acute HCV infection. Some HCV genotypes are distributed worldwide, while others are more geographically confined (see "Epidemiology and Global Features," below). In addition, differences exist among genotypes in responsiveness to antiviral therapy; however, early reports of differences in pathogenicity among genotypes have not been corroborated.

Currently available, third-generation immunoassays, which incorporate proteins from the core, NS3, and NS5 regions, detect anti-HCV antibodies during acute infection. The most sensitive indicator of HCV infection is the presence of HCV RNA, which requires molecular amplification by PCR or transcription-mediated amplification (TMA) (Fig. 298-7). To allow standardization of the quantification of HCV RNA among laboratories and commercial assays, HCV RNA is reported as international units (IU) per milliliter; quantitative assays are available that allow detection of HCV RNA with a sensitivity as low as 5 IU/mL. HCV RNA can be detected within a few days of exposure to HCV, well before the appearance of anti-HCV, and tends to persist for the duration of HCV infection; however, occasionally in patients with chronic HCV infection, HCV RNA may be detectable only intermittently. Application of sensitive molecular probes for HCV RNA has revealed the presence of replicative HCV in peripheral blood lymphocytes of infected persons; however, as is the case for HBV in lymphocytes, the clinical relevance of HCV lymphocyte infection is not known.

Hepatitis E Previously labeled *epidemic* or *enterically transmitted non-A, non-B hepatitis*, HEV is an enterically transmitted virus that occurs primarily in India, Asia, Africa, and Central America; in those geographic areas, HEV is the most common cause of acute hepatitis. This agent, with epidemiologic features resembling those of hepatitis A, is a 32- to 34-nm, nonenveloped, HAV-like virus with a 7600-nucleotide, single-strand, positive-sense RNA genome. HEV has three open reading frames (ORF) (genes), the largest of which, *ORF1*, encodes nonstructural proteins involved in virus replication. A middle-sized gene, *ORF2*, encodes the nucleocapsid protein, and the smallest, *ORF3*, encodes a structural protein whose function remains undetermined. All HEV isolates appear to belong to a single serotype, despite genomic heterogeneity of up to 25% and the existence of five genotypes, only four of which have been detected in humans; genotypes 1 and 2 appear to be more virulent, while genotypes 3 and 4 are more attenuated and account for subclinical infections. Contributing to the perpetuation of this virus are animal reservoirs, most notably in swine.

There is no genomic or antigenic homology, however, between HEV and HAV or other picornaviruses; and HEV, although resembling caliciviruses, is sufficiently distinct from any known agent to merit a new classification of its own as a unique genus, *Hepevirus*, within the Hepeviridae family. The virus has been detected in stool, bile, and liver and is excreted in the stool during the late incubation period; immune responses to viral antigens occur very early during the course of acute infection. Both IgM anti-HEV and IgG anti-HEV can be detected, but both fall rapidly after acute infection, reaching low levels within 9–12 months. Currently, serologic testing for HEV infection is not available routinely.

PATHOGENESIS

Under ordinary circumstances, none of the hepatitis viruses is known to be directly cytopathic to hepatocytes. Evidence suggests that the clinical manifestations and outcomes after acute liver injury associated with viral hepatitis are determined by the immunologic responses of the host. Among the viral hepatitides, the immunopathogenesis of hepatitis B and C have been studied most extensively.

Hepatitis B For HBV, the existence of inactive hepatitis B carriers with normal liver histology and function suggests that the virus is not directly cytopathic. The fact that patients with defects in cellular immune competence are more likely to remain chronically infected rather than to clear HBV is cited to support the role of cellular immune responses in the pathogenesis of hepatitis B–related liver injury. The model that has the most experimental support involves cytolytic T cells sensitized specifically to recognize host and hepatitis B viral antigens on the liver cell surface. Laboratory observations suggest that nucleocapsid proteins (HBcAg and possibly HBeAg), present on the cell membrane in minute quantities, are the viral target antigens that, with host antigens, invite cytolytic T cells to destroy HBV-infected hepatocytes. Differences in the robustness of CD8+ cytolytic T cell responsiveness and in the elaboration of antiviral cytokines by T cells have been invoked to explain differences in outcomes between those who recover after acute hepatitis and those who progress to chronic hepatitis or between those with mild and those with severe (fulminant) acute HBV infection.

Although a robust cytolytic T cell response occurs and eliminates virus-infected liver cells during acute hepatitis B, >90% of HBV DNA has been found in experimentally infected chimpanzees to disappear from the liver and blood before maximal T cell infiltration of the liver and before most of the biochemical and histologic evidence of liver injury. This observation suggests that components of the innate immune

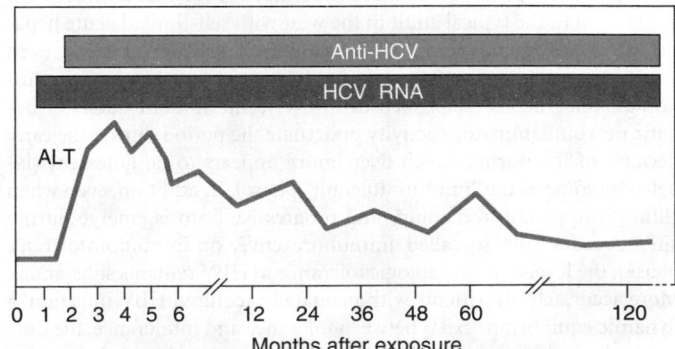

FIGURE 298-7 Scheme of typical laboratory features during acute hepatitis C progressing to chronicity. HCV RNA is the first detectable event, preceding ALT elevation and the appearance of anti-HCV.

system and inflammatory cytokines, independent of cytopathic antiviral mechanisms, participate in the early immune response to HBV infection; this effect has been shown to represent elimination of HBV replicative intermediates from the cytoplasm and covalently closed circular viral DNA from the nucleus of infected hepatocytes. Ultimately, HBV-HLA-specific cytolytic T cell responses of the adaptive immune system are felt to be responsible for recovery from HBV infection.

Debate continues over the relative importance of viral and host factors in the pathogenesis of HBV-associated liver injury and its outcome. As noted above, precore genetic mutants of HBV have been associated with the more severe outcomes of HBV infection (severe chronic and fulminant hepatitis), suggesting that, under certain circumstances, relative pathogenicity is a property of the virus, not the host. The fact that concomitant HDV and HBV infections are associated with more severe liver injury than HBV infection alone and the fact that cells transfected in vitro with the gene for HDV (delta) antigen express HDV antigen and then become necrotic in the absence of any immunologic influences are also consistent with a viral effect on pathogenicity. Similarly, in patients who undergo liver transplantation for end-stage chronic hepatitis B, occasionally, rapidly progressive liver injury appears in the new liver. This clinical pattern is associated with an unusual histologic pattern in the new liver, *fibrosing cholestatic hepatitis*, which, ultrastructurally, appears to represent a choking of the cell with overwhelming quantities of HBsAg. This observation suggests that under the influence of the potent immunosuppressive agents required to prevent allograft rejection, HBV may have a direct cytopathic effect on liver cells, independent of the immune system.

Although the precise mechanism of liver injury in HBV infection remains elusive, studies of nucleocapsid proteins have shed light on the profound immunologic tolerance to HBV of babies born to mothers with highly replicative (HBeAg-positive), chronic HBV infection. In HBeAg-expressing transgenic mice, in utero exposure to HBeAg, which is sufficiently small to traverse the placenta, induces T cell tolerance to both nucleocapsid proteins. This, in turn, may explain why, when infection occurs so early in life, immunologic clearance does not occur, and protracted, lifelong infection ensues.

An important distinction should be drawn between HBV infection acquired at birth, common in endemic areas, such as the Far East, and infection acquired in adulthood, common in the west. Infection in the neonatal period is associated with the acquisition of immunologic tolerance to HBV, absence of an acute-hepatitis illness, but the almost invariable establishment of chronic, often life-long infection. Neonatally acquired HBV infection can culminate decades later in cirrhosis and hepatocellular carcinoma (see "Complications and Sequelae," below.) In contrast, when HBV infection is acquired during adolescence or early adulthood, the host-immune response to HBV-infected hepatocytes tends to be robust, an acute hepatitis-like illness is the rule, and failure to recover is the exception. After adulthood-acquired infection, chronicity is uncommon, and the risk of hepatocellular carcinoma is very low. Based on these observations, some authorities categorize HBV infection into an "immunotolerant" phase, an "immunoreactive" phase, and an inactive phase. This somewhat simplistic formulation does not apply at all to the typical adult in the west with self-limited acute hepatitis B, in whom no period of immunologic tolerance occurs. Even among those with neonatally acquired HBV infection, in whom immunologic tolerance is established definitively, intermittent bursts of hepatic necroinflammatory activity punctuate the period during the early decades of life during which liver injury appears to be quiescent (labeled by some as the "immunotolerant" phase). In addition, even when clinically apparent liver injury and progressive fibrosis emerge during later decades (the so-called immunoreactive, or immunointolerant, phase), the level of immunologic tolerance to HBV remains substantial. More accurately, in patients with neonatally acquired HBV infection, a dynamic equilibrium exists between tolerance and intolerance, the outcome of which determines the clinical expression of chronic infection.

Hepatitis C Cell-mediated immune responses and elaboration by T cells of antiviral cytokines contribute to the containment of infection

and pathogenesis of liver injury associated with hepatitis C. Perhaps HCV infection of lymphoid cells plays a role in moderating immune responsiveness to the virus, as well. Intrahepatic HLA class I–restricted cytolytic T cells directed at nucleocapsid, envelope, and nonstructural viral protein antigens have been demonstrated in patients with chronic hepatitis C; however, such virus-specific cytolytic T cell responses do not correlate adequately with the degree of liver injury or with recovery. Yet, a consensus has emerged supporting a role in the pathogenesis of HCV-associated liver injury of virus-activated CD4 helper T cells that stimulate, via the cytokines they elaborate, HCV-specific CD8 cytotoxic T cells. These responses appear to be more robust (higher in number, more diverse in viral antigen specificity, more functionally effective, and more long-lasting) in those who recover from HCV than in those who have chronic infection. Several HLA alleles have been linked with self-limited hepatitis C, but such associations do not apply universally. Attention has been focused as well on adaptive immunity; the establishment of persistent infection correlates with failure of adaptive immune responses to HCV. Furthermore, HCV proteins have been shown to interfere with innate immunity by resulting in blocking of type 1 interferon responses and inhibition of interferon signaling and effector molecules in the interferon signaling cascade. Also shown to contribute to limiting HCV infection are natural killer cells of the innate immune system, which function when HLA class 1 molecules required for successful adaptive immunity are underexpressed. Of note, the emergence of substantial viral quasispecies diversity allows the virus to evade attempts by the host to contain HCV infection immunologically.

Finally, cross-reactivity between viral antigens (HCV NS3 and NS5A) and host autoantigens (cytochrome P450 2D6) has been invoked to explain the association between hepatitis C and a subset of patients with autoimmune hepatitis and antibodies to liver-kidney microsomal (LKM) antigen (anti-LKM) (Chap. 300).

EXTRAHEPATIC MANIFESTATIONS
Immune complex–mediated tissue damage appears to play a pathogenetic role in the extrahepatic manifestations of acute hepatitis B. The occasional prodromal serum sickness–like syndrome observed in acute hepatitis B appears to be related to the deposition in tissue blood vessel walls of HBsAg-anti-HBs circulating immune complexes, leading to activation of the complement system and depressed serum complement levels.

In patients with chronic hepatitis B, other types of immune-complex disease may be seen. Glomerulonephritis with the nephritic syndrome is occasionally observed; HBsAg, immunoglobulin, and C3 deposition has been found in the glomerular basement membrane. While polyarteritis nodosa develops in considerably fewer than 1% of patients with chronic HBV infection, 20–30% of patients with polyarteritis nodosa have HBsAg in serum (Chap. 319). In these patients, the affected small and medium-size arterioles have been shown to contain HBsAg, immunoglobulins, and complement components. Another extrahepatic manifestation of viral hepatitis, essential mixed cryoglobulinemia (EMC), was reported initially to be associated with hepatitis B. The disorder is characterized clinically by arthritis, cutaneous vasculitis (palpable purpura), and occasionally with glomerulonephritis and serologically by the presence of circulating cryoprecipitable immune complexes of more than one immunoglobulin class (Chaps. 277 and 319). Many patients with this syndrome have chronic liver disease, but the association with HBV infection is limited; instead, a substantial proportion has chronic HCV infection, with circulating immune complexes containing HCV RNA. Immune-complex glomerulonephritis is another recognized extrahepatic manifestation of chronic hepatitis C.

PATHOLOGY
The typical morphologic lesions of all types of viral hepatitis are similar and consist of panlobular infiltration with mononuclear cells, hepatic cell necrosis, hyperplasia of Kupffer cells, and variable degrees of cholestasis. Hepatic cell regeneration is present, as evidenced by numerous mitotic figures, multinucleated cells, and "rosette" or

"pseudoacinar" formation. The mononuclear infiltration consists primarily of small lymphocytes, although plasma cells and eosinophils occasionally are present. Liver cell damage consists of hepatic cell degeneration and necrosis, cell dropout, ballooning of cells, and acidophilic degeneration of hepatocytes (forming so-called Councilman or apoptotic bodies). Large hepatocytes with a ground-glass appearance of the cytoplasm may be seen in chronic but not in acute HBV infection; these cells contain HBsAg and can be identified histochemically with orcein or aldehyde fuchsin. In uncomplicated viral hepatitis, the reticulin framework is preserved.

In hepatitis C, the histologic lesion is often remarkable for a relative paucity of inflammation, a marked increase in activation of sinusoidal lining cells, lymphoid aggregates, the presence of fat (more frequent in genotype 3 and linked to increased fibrosis), and, occasionally, bile duct lesions in which biliary epithelial cells appear to be piled up without interruption of the basement membrane. Occasionally, microvesicular steatosis occurs in hepatitis D. In hepatitis E, a common histologic feature is marked cholestasis. A cholestatic variant of slowly resolving acute hepatitis A also has been described.

A more severe histologic lesion, *bridging hepatic necrosis*, also termed *subacute* or *confluent necrosis* or *interface hepatitis*, is occasionally observed in some patients with acute hepatitis. "Bridging" between lobules results from large areas of hepatic cell dropout, with collapse of the reticulin framework. Characteristically, the bridge consists of condensed reticulum, inflammatory debris, and degenerating liver cells that span adjacent portal areas, portal to central veins, or central vein to central vein. This lesion had been thought to have prognostic significance; in many of the originally described patients with this lesion, a subacute course terminated in death within several weeks to months, or severe chronic hepatitis and postnecrotic cirrhosis developed. Subsequent investigations have failed to uphold the association between bridging necrosis and such a poor prognosis in patients with acute hepatitis. Therefore, although demonstration of this lesion in patients with chronic hepatitis has prognostic significance (Chap. 300), its demonstration during acute hepatitis is less meaningful, and liver biopsies to identify this lesion are no longer undertaken routinely in patients with acute hepatitis. In *massive hepatic necrosis* (fulminant hepatitis, "acute yellow atrophy"), the striking feature at postmortem examination is the finding of a small, shrunken, soft liver. Histologic examination reveals massive necrosis and dropout of liver cells of most lobules with extensive collapse and condensation of the reticulin framework. When histologic documentation is required in the management of fulminant or very severe hepatitis, a biopsy can be done by the angiographically guided transjugular route, which permits the performance of this invasive procedure in the presence of severe coagulopathy.

Immunohistochemical and electron-microscopic studies have localized HBsAg to the cytoplasm and plasma membrane of infected liver cells. In contrast, HBcAg predominates in the nucleus, but occasionally, scant amounts are also seen in the cytoplasm and on the cell membrane. HDV antigen is localized to the hepatocyte nucleus, while HAV, HCV, and HEV antigens are localized to the cytoplasm.

EPIDEMIOLOGY AND GLOBAL FEATURES

Before the availability of serologic tests for hepatitis viruses, all viral hepatitis cases were labeled either as "infectious" or "serum" hepatitis. Modes of transmission overlap, however, and *a clear distinction among the different types of viral hepatitis cannot be made solely on the basis of clinical or epidemiologic features* (Table 298-2). The most accurate means to distinguish the various types of viral hepatitis involves specific serologic testing.

Hepatitis A *This agent is transmitted almost exclusively by the fecal-oral route.* Person-to-person spread of HAV is enhanced by poor personal hygiene and overcrowding; large outbreaks as well as sporadic cases have been traced to contaminated food, water, milk, frozen raspberries and strawberries, green onions imported from Mexico, and shellfish. Intrafamily and intrainstitutional spread are also common. Early epidemiologic observations supported a predilection for hepati-

---

TABLE 298-2 CLINICAL AND EPIDEMIOLOGIC FEATURES OF VIRAL HEPATITIS

Feature	HAV	HBV	HCV	HDV	HEV
Incubation (days)	15–45, mean 30	30–180, mean 60–90	15–160, mean 50	30–180, mean 60–90	14–60, mean 40
Onset	Acute	Insidious or acute	Insidious	Insidious or acute	Acute
Age preference	Children, young adults	Young adults (sexual and percutaneous), babies, toddlers	Any age, but more common in adults	Any age (similar to HBV)	Young adults (20–40 years)
Transmission					
Fecal-oral	+++	–	–	–	+++
Percutaneous	Unusual	+++	+++	+++	–
Perinatal	–	+++	±[a]	+	–
Sexual	±	++	±[a]	++	–
Clinical					
Severity	Mild	Occasionally severe	Moderate	Occasionally severe	Mild
Fulminant	0.1%	0.1–1%	0.1%	5–20%[b]	1–2%[e]
Progression to chronicity	None	Occasional (1–10%) (90% of neonates)	Common (85%)	Common[d]	None
Carrier	None	0.1–30%[c]	1.5–3.2%	Variable[f]	None
Cancer	None	+ (neonatal infection)	+	±	None
Prognosis	Excellent	Worse with age, debility	Moderate	Acute, good Chronic, poor	Good
Prophylaxis	IG Inactivated vaccine	HBIG Recombinant vaccine	None	HBV vaccine (none for HBV carriers)	Vaccine
Therapy	None	Interferon Lamivudine Adefovir Pegylated interferon Entecavir Telbivudine	Pegylated interferon plus ribavirin	Interferon ±	None

[a]Primarily with HIV co-infection and high-level viremia in index case; risk ~5%.
[b]Up to 5% in acute HBV/HDV co-infection; up to 20% in HDV superinfection of chronic HBV infection.
[c]Varies considerably throughout the world and in subpopulations within countries; see text.

[d]In acute HBV/HDV co-infection, the frequency of chronicity is the same as that for HBV; in HDV superinfection, chronicity is invariable.
[e]10–20% in pregnant women.
[f]Common in Mediterranean countries, rare in North America and western Europe.

tis A to occur in late fall and early winter. In temperate zones, epidemic waves have been recorded every 5–20 years as new segments of nonimmune population appeared; however, in developed countries, the incidence of hepatitis A has been declining, presumably as a function of improved sanitation, and these cyclic patterns are no longer observed. No HAV carrier state has been identified after acute hepatitis A; perpetuation of the virus in nature depends presumably on nonepidemic, inapparent subclinical infection and/or contamination linked to environmental reservoirs.

In the general population, anti-HAV, a marker for previous HAV infection, increases in prevalence as a function of increasing age and of decreasing socioeconomic status. In the 1970s, serologic evidence of prior hepatitis A infection occurred in ~40% of urban populations in the United States, most of whose members never recalled having had a symptomatic case of hepatitis. In subsequent decades, however, the prevalence of anti-HAV has been declining in the United States. In developing countries, exposure, infection, and subsequent immunity are almost universal in childhood. As the frequency of subclinical childhood infections declines in developed countries, a susceptible cohort of adults emerges. Hepatitis A tends to be more symptomatic in adults; therefore, paradoxically, as the frequency of HAV infection declines, the likelihood of clinically apparent, even severe, HAV illnesses increases in the susceptible adult population. Travel to endemic areas is a common source of infection for adults from nonendemic areas. More recently recognized epidemiologic foci of HAV infection include child-care centers, neonatal intensive care units, promiscuous men who have sex with men, and injection drug users. Although hepatitis A is rarely bloodborne, several outbreaks have been recognized in recipients of clotting factor concentrates. In the United States, the introduction of hepatitis A vaccination programs among children from high-incidence states has resulted in a >70% reduction in the annual incidence of new HAV infections and has shifted the burden of new infections from children to young adults.

Hepatitis B Percutaneous inoculation has long been recognized as a major route of hepatitis B transmission, but the outmoded designation "serum hepatitis" is an inaccurate label for the epidemiologic spectrum of HBV infection recognized today. As detailed below, most of the hepatitis transmitted by blood transfusion is not caused by HBV; moreover, in approximately two-thirds of patients with acute type B hepatitis, no history of an identifiable percutaneous exposure can be elicited. We now recognize that many cases of hepatitis B result from less obvious modes of nonpercutaneous or covert percutaneous transmission. HBsAg has been identified in almost every body fluid from infected persons, and at least some of these body fluids—most notably semen and saliva—are infectious, albeit less so than serum, when administered percutaneously or nonpercutaneously to experimental animals. Among the nonpercutaneous modes of HBV transmission, oral ingestion has been documented as a potential but inefficient route of exposure. By contrast, the two nonpercutaneous routes considered to have the greatest impact are intimate (especially sexual) contact and perinatal transmission.

In sub-Saharan Africa, intimate contact among toddlers is considered instrumental in contributing to the maintenance of the high frequency of hepatitis B in the population. Perinatal transmission occurs primarily in infants born to HBsAg carrier mothers or mothers with acute hepatitis B during the third trimester of pregnancy or during the early postpartum period. Perinatal transmission is uncommon in North America and western Europe but occurs with great frequency and is the most important mode of HBV perpetuation in the Far East and developing countries. Although the precise mode of perinatal transmission is unknown, and although ~10% of infections may be acquired in utero, epidemiologic evidence suggests that most infections occur approximately at the time of delivery and are not related to breast feeding. The likelihood of perinatal transmission of HBV correlates with the presence of HBeAg; 90% of HBeAg-positive mothers but only 10–15% of anti-HBe-positive mothers transmit HBV infection to their offspring. In most cases, acute infection in the neonate is clinically asymptomatic, but the child is very likely to become an HBsAg carrier.

The >350 million HBsAg carriers in the world constitute the main reservoir of hepatitis B in human beings. Serum HBsAg is infrequent (0.1–0.5%) in normal populations in the United States and western Europe. However, a prevalence of up to 5–20% has been found in the Far East and in some tropical countries; in persons with Down's syndrome, lepromatous leprosy, leukemia, Hodgkin's disease, polyarteritis nodosa; in patients with chronic renal disease on hemodialysis; and in injection drug users.

Other groups with high rates of HBV infection include spouses of acutely infected persons, sexually promiscuous persons (especially promiscuous men who have sex with men), health care workers exposed to blood, persons who require repeated transfusions especially with pooled blood product concentrates (e.g., hemophiliacs), residents and staff of custodial institutions for the developmentally handicapped, prisoners, and, to a lesser extent, family members of chronically infected patients. In volunteer blood donors, the prevalence of anti-HBs, a reflection of previous HBV infection, ranges from 5–10%, but the prevalence is higher in lower socioeconomic strata, older age groups, and persons—including those mentioned above—exposed to blood products. Because of highly sensitive virologic screening of donor blood, the risk of acquiring HBV infection from a blood transfusion is 1 in 230,000.

Prevalence of infection, modes of transmission, and human behavior conspire to mold geographically different epidemiologic patterns of HBV infection. In the Far East and Africa, hepatitis B, a disease of the newborn and young children, is perpetuated by a cycle of maternal-neonatal spread. In North America and western Europe, hepatitis B is primarily a disease of adolescence and early adulthood, the time of life when intimate sexual contact as well as recreational and occupational percutaneous exposures tend to occur. The introduction of hepatitis B vaccine in the early 1980s and adoption of universal childhood vaccination policies in many countries resulted in a dramatic, ~90%, decline in the incidence of new HBV infections in those countries as well as in the dire consequences of chronic infection.

Hepatitis D Infection with HDV has a worldwide distribution, but two epidemiologic patterns exist. In Mediterranean countries (northern Africa, southern Europe, the Middle East), HDV infection is endemic among those with hepatitis B, and the disease is transmitted predominantly by nonpercutaneous means, especially close personal contact. In nonendemic areas, such as the United States and northern Europe, HDV infection is confined to persons exposed frequently to blood and blood products, primarily injection drug users and hemophiliacs. HDV infection can be introduced into a population through drug users or by migration of persons from endemic to nonendemic areas. Thus, patterns of population migration and human behavior facilitating percutaneous contact play important roles in the introduction and amplification of HDV infection. Occasionally, the migrating epidemiology of hepatitis D is expressed in explosive outbreaks of severe hepatitis, such as those that have occurred in remote South American villages as well as in urban centers in the United States. Ultimately, such outbreaks of hepatitis D—either of co-infections with acute hepatitis B or of superinfections in those already infected with HBV—may blur the distinctions between endemic and nonendemic areas. On a global scale, HDV infection is declining. Even in Italy, an HDV-endemic area, public health measures introduced to control HBV infection resulted during the 1990s in a 1.5%/year reduction in the prevalence of HDV infection.

Hepatitis C Routine screening of blood donors for HBsAg and the elimination of commercial blood sources in the early 1970s reduced the frequency of, but did not eliminate, transfusion-associated hepatitis. During the 1970s, the likelihood of acquiring hepatitis after transfusion of voluntarily donated, HBsAg-screened blood was ~10% per patient (up to 0.9% per unit transfused); 90–95% of these cases were classified, based on serologic exclusion of hepatitis A and B, as "non-A, non-B" hepatitis. For patients requiring transfusion of pooled products, such as clotting factor concentrates, the risk was even higher, up to 20–30%.

During the 1980s, voluntary self-exclusion of blood donors with risk factors for AIDS and then the introduction of donor screening for anti-HIV reduced further the likelihood of transfusion-associated hepatitis to <5%. During the late 1980s and early 1990s, the introduction first of "surrogate" screening tests for non-A, non-B hepatitis [alanine aminotransferase (ALT) and anti-HBc, both shown to identify blood donors with a higher likelihood of transmitting non-A, non-B hepatitis to recipients] and, subsequently, after the discovery of HCV, first-generation immunoassays for anti-HCV reduced the frequency of transfusion-associated hepatitis even further. A prospective analysis of transfusion-associated hepatitis conducted between 1986 and 1990 showed that the incidence of transfusion-associated hepatitis at one urban university hospital fell from a baseline of 3.8% per patient (0.45% per unit transfused) to 1.5% per patient (0.19% per unit) after the introduction of surrogate testing and to 0.6% per patient (0.03% per unit) after the introduction of first-generation anti-HCV assays. The introduction of second-generation anti-HCV assays reduced the frequency of transfusion-associated hepatitis C to almost imperceptible levels, 1 in 100,000, and these gains were reinforced by the application of automated PCR testing of donated blood for HCV RNA, which has resulted in a reduction in the risk of transfusion-associated HCV infection to 1 in 2.3 million transfusions.

In addition to being transmitted by transfusion, hepatitis C can be transmitted by other percutaneous routes, such as injection drug use. In addition, this virus can be transmitted by occupational exposure to blood, and the likelihood of infection is increased in hemodialysis units. Although the frequency of transfusion-associated hepatitis C fell as a result of blood donor screening, the overall frequency of hepatitis C remained the same until the early 1990s, when the overall frequency fell by 80%, in parallel with a reduction in the number of new cases in injection drug users. After the exclusion of anti-HCV-positive plasma units from the donor pool, rare, sporadic instances have occurred of hepatitis C among recipients of immunoglobulin (IG) preparations for intravenous (but not intramuscular) use.

Serologic evidence for HCV infection occurs in 90% of patients with a history of transfusion-associated hepatitis (almost all occurring before 1992, when second-generation HCV-screening tests were introduced); hemophiliacs and others treated with clotting factors; injection drug users; 60–70% of patients with sporadic "non-A, non-B" hepatitis who lack identifiable risk factors; 0.5% of volunteer blood donors; and, in the most recent survey conducted in the United States between 1999 and 2000, 1.6% of the general population in the United States, which translates into 4.1 million persons (3.2 million with viremia). Comparable frequencies of HCV infection occur in most countries around the world, with 170 million persons infected worldwide, but extraordinarily high prevalences of HCV infection occur in certain countries, such as Egypt, where >20% of the population in some cities is infected. The high frequency in Egypt is attributable to contaminated equipment used for medical procedures and unsafe injection practices. In the United States, African Americans and Mexican Americans have higher frequencies of HCV infection than whites. Between 1988 and 1994, 30- to 40-year-old adult males had the highest prevalence of HCV infection; however, in a survey conducted between 1999 and 2000, the peak age decile had shifted to those age 40–49 years. Thus, despite an 80% reduction in new HCV infections during the 1990s, the prevalence of HCV infection in the population was sustained by an aging cohort that had acquired their infections two to three decades earlier, during the 1960s and 1970s, as a result predominantly of self inoculation with recreational drugs. Hepatitis C accounts for 40% of chronic liver disease, is the most frequent indication for liver transplantation, and is estimated to account for 8000–10,000 deaths per year in the United States.

The distribution of HCV genotypes varies in different parts of the world. World-wide, genotype 1 is the most common. In the United States, genotype 1 accounts for 70% of HCV infections, while genotypes 2 and 3 account for the remaining 30%; among African Americans, the frequency of genotype 1 is even higher, i.e., 90%. Genotype 4 predominates in Egypt; genotype 5 is localized to South Africa and genotype 6 to Hong Kong.

Most asymptomatic blood donors found to have anti-HCV and ~20–30% of persons with reported cases of acute hepatitis C do not fall into a recognized risk group; however, many such blood donors do recall risk-associated behaviors when questioned carefully.

As a bloodborne infection, HCV potentially can be transmitted sexually and perinatally; however, both of these modes of transmission are inefficient for hepatitis C. Although 10–15% of patients with acute hepatitis C report having potential sexual sources of infection, most studies have failed to identify sexual transmission of this agent. The chances of sexual and perinatal transmission have been estimated to be ~5%, well below comparable rates for HIV and HBV infections. Moreover, sexual transmission appears to be confined to such subgroups as persons with multiple sexual partners and sexually transmitted diseases; transmission of HCV infection is rare between stable, monogamous sexual partners. Breast feeding does not increase the risk of HCV infection between an infected mother and her infant. Infection of health workers is not dramatically higher than among the general population; however, health workers are more likely to acquire HCV infection through accidental needle punctures, the efficiency of which is ~3%. Infection of household contacts is rare as well.

Other groups with an increased frequency of HCV infection include patients who require hemodialysis and organ transplantation and those who require transfusions in the setting of cancer chemotherapy. In immunosuppressed individuals, levels of anti-HCV may be undetectable, and a diagnosis may require testing for HCV RNA. Although new acute cases of hepatitis C are rare, newly diagnosed cases are common among otherwise healthy persons who experimented briefly with injection drugs, as noted above, two or three decades earlier. Such instances usually remain unrecognized for years, until unearthed by laboratory screening for routine medical examinations, insurance applications, and attempted blood donation.

Hepatitis E   This type of hepatitis, identified in India, Asia, Africa, the Middle East, and Central America, resembles hepatitis A in its primarily enteric mode of spread. The commonly recognized cases occur after contamination of water supplies such as after monsoon flooding, but sporadic, isolated cases occur. An epidemiologic feature that distinguishes HEV from other enteric agents is the rarity of secondary person-to-person spread from infected persons to their close contacts. Infections arise in populations that are immune to HAV and favor young adults. In endemic areas, the prevalence of antibodies to HEV is ≤40%. In nonendemic areas of the world, such as the United States, clinically apparent acute hepatitis E is extremely rare; however, the prevalence of antibodies to HEV can be as high as 20% in such areas. In nonendemic areas, HEV does not account for any of the sporadic "non-A, non-B" cases of hepatitis; however, cases imported from endemic areas have been found in the United States. Several reports suggest a zoonotic reservoir for HEV in swine.

CLINICAL AND LABORATORY FEATURES
Symptoms and Signs   Acute viral hepatitis occurs after an incubation period that varies according to the responsible agent. Generally, incubation periods for hepatitis A range from 15–45 days (mean, 4 weeks), for hepatitis B and D from 30–180 days (mean, 8–12 weeks), for hepatitis C from 15–160 days (mean, 7 weeks), and for hepatitis E from 14–60 days (mean, 5–6 weeks). The *prodromal symptoms* of acute viral hepatitis are systemic and quite variable. Constitutional symptoms of anorexia, nausea and vomiting, fatigue, malaise, arthralgias, myalgias, headache, photophobia, pharyngitis, cough, and coryza may precede the onset of jaundice by 1–2 weeks. The nausea, vomiting, and anorexia are frequently associated with alterations in olfaction and taste. A low-grade fever between 38° and 39°C (100°–102°F) is more often present in hepatitis A and E than in hepatitis B or C, except when hepatitis B is heralded by a serum sickness–like syndrome; rarely, a fever of 39.5°–40°C (103°–104°F) may accompany the constitutional symptoms. Dark urine and clay-colored stools may be noticed by the patient from 1–5 days before the onset of clinical jaundice.

With the onset of *clinical jaundice*, the constitutional prodromal symptoms usually diminish, but in some patients mild weight loss (2.5–5 kg) is common and may continue during the entire icteric phase. The liver becomes enlarged and tender and may be associated with right upper quadrant pain and discomfort. Infrequently, patients present with a cholestatic picture, suggesting extrahepatic biliary obstruction. Splenomegaly and cervical adenopathy are present in 10–20% of patients with acute hepatitis. Rarely, a few spider angiomas appear during the icteric phase and disappear during convalescence. During the *recovery phase*, constitutional symptoms disappear, but usually some liver enlargement and abnormalities in liver biochemical tests are still evident. The duration of the posticteric phase is variable, ranging 2–12 weeks, and is usually more prolonged in acute hepatitis B and C. Complete clinical and biochemical recovery is to be expected 1–2 months after all cases of hepatitis A and E and 3–4 months after the onset of jaundice in three-quarters of uncomplicated, self-limited cases of hepatitis B and C (among healthy adults, acute hepatitis B is self-limited in 95–99% while hepatitis C is self-limited in only ~15%). In the remainder, biochemical recovery may be delayed. A substantial proportion of patients with viral hepatitis never become icteric.

Infection with HDV can occur in the presence of acute or chronic HBV infection; the duration of HBV infection determines the duration of HDV infection. When acute HDV and HBV infection occur simultaneously, clinical and biochemical features may be indistinguishable from those of HBV infection alone, although occasionally they are more severe. As opposed to patients with *acute* HBV infection, patients with *chronic* HBV infection can support HDV replication indefinitely. This can happen when acute HDV infection occurs in the presence of a nonresolving acute HBV infection. More commonly, acute HDV infection becomes chronic when it is superimposed on an underlying chronic HBV infection. In such cases, the HDV superinfection appears as a clinical exacerbation or an episode resembling acute viral hepatitis in someone already chronically infected with HBV. Superinfection with HDV in a patient with chronic hepatitis B often leads to clinical deterioration (see below).

In addition to superinfections with other hepatitis agents, acute hepatitis–like clinical events in persons with chronic hepatitis B may accompany spontaneous HBeAg–to–anti-HBe seroconversion or spontaneous reactivation, i.e., reversion from nonreplicative to replicative infection. Such reactivations can occur as well in therapeutically immunosuppressed patients with chronic HBV infection when cytotoxic/immunosuppressive drugs are withdrawn; in these cases, restoration of immune competence is thought to allow resumption of previously checked cell-mediated immune cytolysis of HBV-infected hepatocytes. Occasionally, acute clinical exacerbations of chronic hepatitis B may represent the emergence of a precore mutant (see "Virology and Etiology," above), and the subsequent course in such patients may be characterized by periodic exacerbations.

Laboratory Features The serum aminotransferases aspartate aminotransferase (AST) and ALT (previously designated SGOT and SGPT) show a variable increase during the prodromal phase of acute viral hepatitis and precede the rise in bilirubin level (Figs. 298-2 and 298-4). The acute level of these enzymes, however, does not correlate well with the degree of liver cell damage. Peak levels vary from 400–4000 IU or more; these levels are usually reached at the time the patient is clinically icteric and diminish progressively during the recovery phase of acute hepatitis. The diagnosis of anicteric hepatitis is based on clinical features and on aminotransferase elevations.

Jaundice is usually visible in the sclera or skin when the serum bilirubin value is >43 µmol/L (2.5 mg/dL). When jaundice appears, the serum bilirubin typically rises to levels ranging from 85–340 µmol/L (5–20 mg/dL). The serum bilirubin may continue to rise despite falling serum aminotransferase levels. In most instances, the total bilirubin is equally divided between the conjugated and unconjugated fractions. Bilirubin levels >340 µmol/L (20 mg/dL) extending and persisting late into the course of viral hepatitis are more likely to be associated with severe disease. In certain patients with underlying hemolytic anemia, however, such as glucose-6-phosphate dehydrogenase deficiency and sickle cell anemia, a high serum bilirubin level is common, resulting from superimposed hemolysis. In such patients, bilirubin levels >513 µmol/L (30 mg/dL) have been observed and are not necessarily associated with a poor prognosis.

Neutropenia and lymphopenia are transient and are followed by a relative lymphocytosis. Atypical lymphocytes (varying between 2 and 20%) are common during the acute phase. Measurement of the prothrombin time (PT) is important in patients with acute viral hepatitis, for a prolonged value may reflect a severe hepatic synthetic defect, signify extensive hepatocellular necrosis, and indicate a worse prognosis. Occasionally, a prolonged PT may occur with only mild increases in the serum bilirubin and aminotransferase levels. Prolonged nausea and vomiting, inadequate carbohydrate intake, and poor hepatic glycogen reserves may contribute to hypoglycemia noted occasionally in patients with severe viral hepatitis. Serum alkaline phosphatase may be normal or only mildly elevated, while a fall in serum albumin is uncommon in uncomplicated acute viral hepatitis. In some patients, mild and transient steatorrhea has been noted as well as slight microscopic hematuria and minimal proteinuria.

A diffuse but mild elevation of the γ globulin fraction is common during acute viral hepatitis. Serum IgG and IgM levels are elevated in about one-third of patients during the acute phase of viral hepatitis, but the serum IgM level is elevated more characteristically during acute hepatitis A. During the acute phase of viral hepatitis, antibodies to smooth muscle and other cell constituents may be present, and low titers of rheumatoid factor, nuclear antibody, and heterophil antibody can also be found occasionally. In hepatitis C and D, antibodies to LKM may occur; however, the species of LKM antibodies in the two types of hepatitis are different from each other as well as from the LKM antibody species characteristic of autoimmune hepatitis type 2 (Chap. 300). The autoantibodies in viral hepatitis are nonspecific and can also be associated with other viral and systemic diseases. In contrast, virus-specific antibodies, which appear during and after hepatitis virus infection, are serologic markers of diagnostic importance.

As described above, serologic tests are available with which to establish a diagnosis of hepatitis A, B, D, and C. Tests for fecal or serum HAV are not routinely available. Therefore, a diagnosis of hepatitis A is based on detection of IgM anti-HAV during acute illness (Fig. 298-2). Rheumatoid factor can give rise to false-positive results in this test.

A diagnosis of HBV infection can usually be made by detection of HBsAg in serum. Infrequently, levels of HBsAg are too low to be detected during acute HBV infection, even with contemporary, highly sensitive immunoassays. In such cases, the diagnosis can be established by the presence of IgM anti-HBc.

The titer of HBsAg bears little relation to the severity of clinical disease. Indeed, an inverse correlation exists between the serum concentration of HBsAg and the degree of liver cell damage. For example, titers are highest in immunosuppressed patients, lower in patients with chronic liver disease (but higher in mild chronic than in severe chronic hepatitis), and very low in patients with acute fulminant hepatitis. These observations suggest that, in hepatitis B, the degree of liver cell damage and the clinical course are related to variations in the patient's immune response to HBV rather than to the amount of circulating HBsAg. In immunocompetent persons, however, there is a correlation between markers of HBV *replication* and liver injury (see below).

Another serologic marker that may be of value in patients with hepatitis B is HBeAg. Its principal clinical usefulness is as an indicator of relative infectivity. Because HBeAg is invariably present during early acute hepatitis B, HBeAg testing is indicated primarily during followup of chronic infection.

In patients with hepatitis B surface antigenemia of unknown duration, e.g., blood donors found to be HBsAg-positive and referred to a physician for evaluation, testing for IgM anti-HBc may be useful to distinguish between acute or recent infection (IgM anti-HBc-positive) and chronic HBV infection (IgM anti-HBc-negative, IgG anti-HBc-positive). A false-positive test for IgM anti-HBc may be encountered in patients with high-titer rheumatoid factor.

TABLE 298-3 COMMONLY ENCOUNTERED SEROLOGIC PATTERNS OF HEPATITIS B INFECTION

HBsAg	Anti-HBs	Anti-HBc	HBeAg	Anti-HBe	Interpretation
+	–	IgM	+	–	Acute hepatitis B, high infectivity
+	–	IgG	+	–	Chronic hepatitis B, high infectivity
+	–	IgG	–	+	1. Late acute or chronic hepatitis B, low infectivity 2. HBeAg-negative ("precore-mutant") hepatitis B (chronic or, rarely, acute)
+	+	+	+/–	+/–	1. HBsAg of one subtype and heterotypic anti-HBs (common) 2. Process of seroconversion from HBsAg to anti-HBs (rare)
–	–	IgM	+/–	+/–	1. Acute hepatitis B 2. Anti-HBc "window"
–	–	IgG	–	+/–	1. Low-level hepatitis B carrier 2. Hepatitis B in remote past
–	+	IgG	–	+/–	Recovery from hepatitis B
–	+	–	–	–	1. Immunization with HBsAg (after vaccination) 2. Hepatitis B in the remote past (?) 3. False-positive

Anti-HBs is rarely detectable in the presence of HBsAg in patients with *acute* hepatitis B, but 10–20% of persons with *chronic* HBV infection may harbor low-level anti-HBs. This antibody is directed not against the common group determinant, *a*, but against the heterotypic subtype determinant (e.g., HBsAg of subtype *ad* with anti-HBs of subtype *y*). In most cases, this serologic pattern cannot be attributed to infection with two different HBV subtypes, and the presence of this antibody is not a harbinger of imminent HBsAg clearance. When such antibody is detected, its presence is of no recognized clinical significance (see "Virology and Etiology," above).

After immunization with hepatitis B vaccine, which consists of HBsAg alone, anti-HBs is the only serologic marker to appear. The commonly encountered serologic patterns of hepatitis B and their interpretations are summarized in Table 298-3. Tests for the detection of HBV DNA in liver and serum are now available. Like HBeAg, serum HBV DNA is an indicator of HBV replication, but tests for HBV DNA are more sensitive and quantitative. First-generation hybridization assays for HBV DNA had a sensitivity of $10^5–10^6$ virions/mL, a relative threshold below which infectivity and liver injury are limited and HBeAg is usually undetectable. Currently, testing for HBV DNA has shifted from insensitive hybridization assays to amplification assays, e.g., the PCR-based assay, which can detect as few as 10 or 100 virions/mL; among the commercially available PCR assays, the most useful are those with the highest sensitivity (5–10 IU/mL) and the largest dynamic range ($10^0–10^9$ IU/mL). With increased sensitivity, amplification assays remain reactive well below the threshold for infectivity and liver injury. These markers are useful in following the course of HBV replication in patients with chronic hepatitis B receiving antiviral chemotherapy, e.g., with interferon or nucleoside analogues (Chap. 300). In immunocompetent persons, a general correlation does appear to exist between the level of HBV replication, as reflected by the level of HBV DNA in serum, and the degree of liver injury. High serum HBV DNA levels, increased expression of viral antigens, and necroinflammatory activity in the liver go hand in hand unless immunosuppression interferes with cytolytic T cell responses to virus-infected cells; reduction of HBV replication with antiviral drugs tends to be accompanied by an improvement in liver histology. Among patients with chronic hepatitis B, high levels of HBV DNA increase the risk of cirrhosis, hepatic decompensation, and hepatocellular carcinoma (see "Complications and Sequelae," below).

In patients with hepatitis C, an episodic pattern of aminotransferase elevation is common. A specific serologic diagnosis of hepatitis C can be made by demonstrating the presence in serum of anti-HCV. When contemporary immunoassays are used, anti-HCV can be detected in acute hepatitis C during the initial phase of elevated aminotransferase activity. This antibody may never become detectable in 5–10% of patients with acute hepatitis C, and levels of anti-HCV may become undetectable after recovery (albeit rare) from acute hepatitis C. In patients with chronic hepatitis C, anti-HCV is detectable in >95% of cases. Nonspecificity can confound immunoassays for anti-HCV, especially in persons with a low prior probability of infection, such as volunteer blood donors, or in persons with circulating rheumatoid factor, which can bind nonspecifically to assay reagents; testing for HCV RNA can be used in such settings to distinguish between true-positive and false-positive anti-HCV determinations. Assays for HCV RNA are the most sensitive tests for HCV infection and represent the "gold standard" in establishing a diagnosis of hepatitis C. HCV RNA can be detected even before acute elevation of aminotransferase activity and before the appearance of anti-HCV in patients with acute hepatitis C. In addition, HCV RNA remains detectable indefinitely, continuously in most but intermittently in some, in patients with chronic hepatitis C (detectable as well in some persons with normal liver tests, i.e., inactive carriers). In the small minority of patients with hepatitis C who lack anti-HCV, a diagnosis can be supported by detection of HCV RNA. If all these tests are negative and the patient has a well-characterized case of hepatitis after percutaneous exposure to blood or blood products, a diagnosis of hepatitis caused by another agent, as yet unidentified, can be entertained.

Amplification techniques are required to detect HCV RNA, and two types are available. One is a branched-chain complementary DNA (bDNA) assay, in which the detection signal (a colorimetrically detectable enzyme bound to a complementary DNA probe) is amplified. The other involves target amplification, i.e., synthesis of multiple copies of the viral genome. This can be done by PCR or TMA, in which the viral RNA is reverse transcribed to complementary DNA and then amplified by repeated cycles of DNA synthesis. Both can be used as quantitative assays and a measurement of relative "viral load"; PCR and TMA, with a sensitivity of $10–10^2$ IU/mL, are more sensitive than bDNA, with a sensitivity of 10^3 IU/mL; assays are available with a wide dynamic range ($10–10^7$ IU/mL). Determination of HCV RNA level is not a reliable marker of disease severity or prognosis but is helpful in predicting relative responsiveness to antiviral therapy. The same is true for determinations of HCV genotype (Chap. 300).

A proportion of patients with hepatitis C have isolated anti-HBc in their blood, a reflection of a common risk in certain populations of exposure to multiple bloodborne hepatitis agents. The anti-HBc in such cases is almost invariably of the IgG class and usually represents HBV infection in the remote past (HBV DNA undetectable), rarely current HBV infection with low-level virus carriage.

The presence of HDV infection can be identified by demonstrating intrahepatic HDV antigen or, more practically, an anti-HDV seroconversion (a rise in titer of anti-HDV or de novo appearance of anti-HDV). Circulating HDV antigen, also diagnostic of acute infection, is detectable only briefly, if at all. Because anti-HDV is often undetectable once HBsAg disappears, retrospective serodiagnosis of acute self-limited, simultaneous HBV and HDV infection is difficult. Early diagnosis of acute infection may be hampered by a delay of up to 30–40 days in the appearance of anti-HDV.

When a patient presents with acute hepatitis and has HBsAg and anti-HDV in serum, determination of the class of anti-HBc is helpful in establishing the relationship between infection with HBV and HDV. Although IgM anti-HBc does not distinguish *absolutely* between acute and chronic HBV infection, its presence is a reliable indicator of recent infection and its absence a reliable indicator of infection in the remote past. In simultaneous acute HBV and HDV infections, IgM anti-HBc

TABLE 298-4 SIMPLIFIED DIAGNOSTIC APPROACH IN PATIENTS PRESENTING WITH ACUTE HEPATITIS

Serologic Tests of Patient's Serum				
HBsAg	IgM Anti-HAV	IgM Anti-HBc	Anti-HCV	Diagnostic Interpretation
+	−	+	−	Acute hepatitis B
+	−	−	−	Chronic hepatitis B
+	+	−	−	Acute hepatitis A superimposed on chronic hepatitis B
+	+	+	−	Acute hepatitis A and B
−	+	−	−	Acute hepatitis A
−	+	+	−	Acute hepatitis A and B (HBsAg below detection threshold)
−	−	+	−	Acute hepatitis B (HBsAg below detection threshold)
−	−	−	+	Acute hepatitis C

will be detectable, while in acute HDV infection superimposed on chronic HBV infection, anti-HBc will be of the IgG class.

Tests for the presence of HDV RNA are useful for determining the presence of ongoing HDV replication and relative infectivity. Diagnostic tests for hepatitis E are commercially available in several countries outside the United States; in the United States, diagnostic assays can be performed at the Centers for Disease Control and Prevention.

Liver biopsy is rarely necessary or indicated in acute viral hepatitis, except when the diagnosis is questionable or when clinical evidence suggests a diagnosis of chronic hepatitis.

A diagnostic algorithm can be applied in the evaluation of cases of acute viral hepatitis. A patient with acute hepatitis should undergo four serologic tests, HBsAg, IgM anti-HAV, IgM anti-HBc, and anti-HCV (Table 298-4). The presence of HBsAg, with or without IgM anti-HBc, represents HBV infection. If IgM anti-HBc is present, the HBV infection is considered acute; if IgM anti-HBc is absent, the HBV infection is considered chronic. A diagnosis of acute hepatitis B can be made in the absence of HBsAg when IgM anti-HBc is detectable. A diagnosis of acute hepatitis A is based on the presence of IgM anti-HAV. If IgM anti-HAV coexists with HBsAg, a diagnosis of simultaneous HAV and HBV infections can be made; if IgM anti-HBc (with or without HBsAg) is detectable, the patient has simultaneous acute hepatitis A and B, and if IgM anti-HBc is undetectable, the patient has acute hepatitis A superimposed on chronic HBV infection. The presence of anti-HCV supports a diagnosis of acute hepatitis C. Occasionally, testing for HCV RNA or repeat anti-HCV testing later during the illness is necessary to establish the diagnosis. Absence of all serologic markers is consistent with a diagnosis of "non-A, non-B, non-C" hepatitis, if the epidemiologic setting is appropriate.

In patients with chronic hepatitis, initial testing should consist of HBsAg and anti-HCV. Anti-HCV supports and HCV RNA testing establishes the diagnosis of chronic hepatitis C. If a serologic diagnosis of chronic hepatitis B is made, testing for HBeAg and anti-HBe is indicated to evaluate relative infectivity. Testing for HBV DNA in such patients provides a more quantitative and sensitive measure of the level of virus replication and, therefore, is very helpful during antiviral therapy (Chap. 300). In patients with chronic hepatitis B and normal aminotransferase activity in the absence of HBeAg, serial testing over time is often required to distinguish between inactive carriage and HBeAg-negative chronic hepatitis B with fluctuating virologic and necroinflammatory activity. In patients with hepatitis B, testing for anti-HDV is useful under the following circumstances: patients with severe and fulminant disease, patients with severe chronic disease, patients with chronic hepatitis B who have acute hepatitis-like exacerbations, persons with frequent percutaneous exposures, and persons from areas where HDV infection is endemic.

PROGNOSIS

Virtually all previously healthy patients with hepatitis A recover completely from their illness with no clinical sequelae. Similarly, in acute hepatitis B, 95–99% of previously healthy adults have a favorable course and recover completely. Certain clinical and laboratory features, however, suggest a more complicated and protracted course. Patients of advanced age and with serious underlying medical disorders may have a prolonged course and are more likely to experience severe hepatitis. Initial presenting features such as ascites, peripheral edema, and symptoms of hepatic encephalopathy suggest a poorer prognosis. In addition, a prolonged PT, low serum albumin level, hypoglycemia, and very high serum bilirubin values suggest severe hepatocellular disease. Patients with these clinical and laboratory features deserve prompt hospital admission. The case-fatality rate in hepatitis A and B is very low (~0.1%) but is increased by advanced age and underlying debilitating disorders. Among patients ill enough to be hospitalized for acute hepatitis B, the fatality rate is 1%. Hepatitis C is less severe during the acute phase than hepatitis B and is more likely to be anicteric; fatalities are rare, but the precise case-fatality rate is not known. In outbreaks of waterborne hepatitis E in India and Asia, the case-fatality rate is 1–2% and up to 10–20% in pregnant women. Patients with simultaneous acute hepatitis B and hepatitis D do not necessarily experience a higher mortality rate than do patients with acute hepatitis B alone; however, in several recent outbreaks of acute simultaneous HBV and HDV infection among injection drug users, the case-fatality rate has been ~5%. In the case of HDV superinfection of a person with chronic hepatitis B, the likelihood of fulminant hepatitis and death is increased substantially. Although the case-fatality rate for hepatitis D has not been defined adequately, in outbreaks of severe HDV superinfection in isolated populations with a high hepatitis B carrier rate, the mortality rate has been recorded in excess of 20%.

COMPLICATIONS AND SEQUELAE

A small proportion of patients with hepatitis A experience *relapsing hepatitis* weeks to months after apparent recovery from acute hepatitis. Relapses are characterized by recurrence of symptoms, aminotransferase elevations, occasionally jaundice, and fecal excretion of HAV. Another unusual variant of acute hepatitis A is *cholestatic hepatitis*, characterized by protracted cholestatic jaundice and pruritus. Rarely, liver test abnormalities persist for many months, even up to a year. Even when these complications occur, hepatitis A remains self-limited and does not progress to chronic liver disease. During the prodromal phase of acute hepatitis B, a serum sickness–like syndrome characterized by arthralgia or arthritis, rash, angioedema, and rarely hematuria and proteinuria may develop in 5–10% of patients. This syndrome occurs before the onset of clinical jaundice, and these patients are often diagnosed erroneously as having rheumatologic diseases. The diagnosis can be established by measuring serum aminotransferase levels, which are almost invariably elevated, and serum HBsAg. As noted above, EMC is an immune-complex disease that can complicate chronic hepatitis C and is part of a spectrum of B cell lymphoproliferative disorders, which, in rare instances, can evolve to B cell lymphoma (Chap. 105). Attention has been drawn as well to associations between hepatitis C and such cutaneous disorders as porphyria cutanea tarda and lichen planus. A mechanism for these associations is unknown.

The most feared complication of viral hepatitis is *fulminant hepatitis* (massive hepatic necrosis); fortunately, this is a rare event. Fulminant hepatitis is primarily seen in hepatitis B and D, as well as hepatitis E, but rare fulminant cases of hepatitis A occur primarily in older adults and in persons with underlying chronic liver disease, including, according to some reports, chronic hepatitis B and C. Hepatitis B accounts for >50% of fulminant cases of viral hepatitis, a sizable proportion of which are associated with HDV infection and another proportion with underlying chronic hepatitis C. Fulminant hepatitis is hardly ever seen in hepatitis C, but hepatitis E, as noted above, can be complicated by fatal fulminant hepatitis in 1–2% of all cases and in up to 20% of cases occurring in pregnant women. Patients usually present with signs and symptoms of encephalopathy that may evolve to deep coma. The liver is usually small and the PT excessively prolonged. The combination of rapidly shrinking liver size, rapidly rising bilirubin level, and marked prolongation of the PT, even as aminotransferase levels fall, together with clinical signs of confusion, disorientation, somnolence, ascites, and edema, indicates that the patient has hepatic failure with encephalopathy. Cerebral edema is common; brainstem compression, gastrointestinal bleeding, sepsis, respiratory failure, cardiovascular collapse, and renal failure are terminal events. The mortality rate is exceedingly high (>80% in patients with deep coma), but patients who survive may have a complete biochemical and histologic recovery. If a donor liver can be located in time, liver transplantation may be life-saving in patients with fulminant hepatitis (Chap. 304).

Documenting the disappearance of HBsAg after apparent clinical recovery from acute hepatitis B is particularly important. Before laboratory methods were available to distinguish between acute hepatitis and acute hepatitis–like exacerbations (*spontaneous reactivations*) of chronic hepatitis B, observations suggested that ~10% of previously healthy patients remained HBsAg-positive for >6 months after the onset of clinically apparent acute hepatitis B. Half of these persons cleared the antigen from their circulations during the next several years, but the other 5% remained chronically HBsAg-positive. More recent observations suggest that the true rate of chronic infection after clinically apparent acute hepatitis B is as low as 1% in normal, immunocompetent, young adults. Earlier, higher estimates may have been confounded by inadvertent inclusion of acute exacerbations in chronically infected patients; these patients, chronically HBsAg-positive before exacerbation, were unlikely to seroconvert to HBsAg-negative thereafter. Whether the rate of chronicity is 10 or 1%, such patients have anti-HBc in serum; anti-HBs is either undetected or detected at low titer against the opposite subtype specificity of the antigen (see "Laboratory Features," above). These patients may (1) be inactive carriers; (2) have low-grade, mild chronic hepatitis; or (3) have moderate to severe chronic hepatitis with or without cirrhosis. The likelihood of remaining chronically infected after acute HBV infection is especially high among neonates, persons with Down's syndrome, chronically hemodialyzed patients, and immunosuppressed patients, including persons with HIV infection.

Chronic hepatitis is an important late complication of acute hepatitis B occurring in a small proportion of patients with acute disease but more common in those who present with chronic infection without having experienced an acute illness, as occurs typically after neonatal infection or after infection in an immunosuppressed host (Chap. 300). Certain clinical and laboratory features suggest progression of acute hepatitis to chronic hepatitis: (1) lack of complete resolution of clinical symptoms of anorexia, weight loss, and fatigue and the persistence of hepatomegaly; (2) the presence of bridging/interface or multilobular hepatic necrosis on liver biopsy during protracted, severe acute viral hepatitis; (3) failure of the serum aminotransferase, bilirubin, and globulin levels to return to normal within 6–12 months after the acute illness; and (4) the persistence of HBeAg for >3 months or HBsAg for >6 months after acute hepatitis.

Although acute hepatitis D infection does not increase the likelihood of chronicity of simultaneous acute hepatitis B, hepatitis D has the potential for contributing to the severity of chronic hepatitis B. Hepatitis D superinfection can transform inactive or mild chronic hepatitis B into severe, progressive chronic hepatitis and cirrhosis; it also can accelerate the course of chronic hepatitis B. Some HDV superinfections in patients with chronic hepatitis B lead to fulminant hepatitis. Although HDV and HBV infections are associated with severe liver disease, mild hepatitis and even inactive carriage have been identified in some patients, and the disease may become indolent beyond the early years of infection. After acute HCV infection, the likelihood of remaining chronically *infected* approaches 85–90%. Although many patients with chronic hepatitis C have no symptoms, cirrhosis may develop in as many as 20% within 10–20 years of acute illness; in some series of cases reported by referral centers, cirrhosis has been reported in as many as 50% of patients with chronic hepatitis C. Although chronic hepatitis C accounts for at least 40% of cases of chronic liver disease and of patients undergoing liver transplantation for end-stage liver disease in the United States and Europe, in the majority of patients with chronic hepatitis C, morbidity and mortality are limited during the initial 20 years after the onset of infection. Progression of chronic hepatitis C may be influenced by age of acquisition, duration of infection, immunosuppression, coexisting excessive alcohol use, concomitant hepatic steatosis, other hepatitis virus infection, or HIV co-infection. In fact, instances of severe and rapidly progressive chronic hepatitis B and C are being recognized with increasing frequency in patients with HIV infection (Chap. 182). In contrast, neither HAV nor HEV causes chronic liver disease.

Rare complications of viral hepatitis include pancreatitis, myocarditis, atypical pneumonia, aplastic anemia, transverse myelitis, and peripheral neuropathy. Persons with chronic hepatitis B, particularly those infected in infancy or early childhood and especially those with HBeAg and/or high-level HBV DNA, have an enhanced risk of hepatocellular carcinoma. The risk of hepatocellular carcinoma is increased as well in patients with chronic hepatitis C, almost exclusively in patients with cirrhosis, and almost always after at least several decades, usually after three decades of disease (Chap. 88). In children, hepatitis B may present rarely with anicteric hepatitis, a nonpruritic papular rash of the face, buttocks, and limbs, and lymphadenopathy (papular acrodermatitis of childhood, or Gianotti-Crosti syndrome).

Rarely, autoimmune hepatitis (Chap. 300) can be triggered by a bout of otherwise self-limited acute hepatitis, as reported after acute hepatitis A, B, and C.

DIFFERENTIAL DIAGNOSIS

Viral diseases such as infectious mononucleosis; those due to cytomegalovirus, herpes simplex, and coxsackieviruses; and toxoplasmosis may share certain clinical features with viral hepatitis and cause elevations in serum aminotransferase and less commonly in serum bilirubin levels. Tests such as the differential heterophile and serologic tests for these agents may be helpful in the differential diagnosis if HBsAg, anti-HBc, IgM anti-HAV, and anti-HCV determinations are negative. Aminotransferase elevations can accompany almost any systemic viral infection; other rare causes of liver injury confused with viral hepatitis are infections with *Leptospira*, *Candida*, *Brucella*, *Mycobacteria*, and *Pneumocystis*. A complete drug history is particularly important, for many drugs and certain anesthetic agents can produce a picture of either acute hepatitis or cholestasis (Chap. 299). Equally important is a past history of unexplained "repeated episodes" of acute hepatitis. This history should alert the physician to the possibility that the underlying disorder is chronic hepatitis. Alcoholic hepatitis must also be considered, but usually the serum aminotransferase levels are not as markedly elevated and other stigmata of alcoholism may be present. The finding on liver biopsy of fatty infiltration, a neutrophilic inflammatory reaction, and "alcoholic hyaline" would be consistent with alcohol-induced rather than viral liver injury. Because acute hepatitis may present with right upper quadrant abdominal pain, nausea and vomiting, fever, and icterus, it is often confused with acute cholecystitis, common duct stone, or ascending cholangitis. Patients with acute viral hepatitis may tolerate surgery poorly; therefore, it is important to exclude this diagnosis, and in confusing cases, a percutaneous liver biopsy may be necessary before laparotomy. Viral hepatitis in the elderly is often misdiagnosed as obstructive jaundice resulting from a common duct stone or carcinoma of the pancreas. Because acute hepatitis in the elderly may be quite severe and the operative mortality high, a thorough evaluation including biochemical tests, radiographic studies of the biliary tree, and even liver biopsy may be necessary to exclude primary parenchymal liver disease. Another clinical constellation that may mimic acute hepatitis is right ventricular failure with passive hepatic congestion or hypoperfusion syndromes, such as those associated with shock, severe hypotension, and severe left ventricular failure. Also included in this general category is any disorder that interferes with venous return to the heart, such as right atrial myxoma, constrictive pericarditis, hepatic vein occlusion (Budd-Chiari syndrome), or venoocclusive disease. Clinical features are usually sufficient to distinguish between these vascular disorders and viral hepatitis. Acute fatty liver of pregnancy, cholestasis of pregnancy, eclampsia, and the HELLP syndrome (*h*emolysis, *e*levated *l*iver tests, and *l*ow *p*latelets) can be confused with viral hepatitis during pregnancy. Very rarely, malignancies metastatic to the liver can mimic acute or even fulminant viral hepatitis. Occasionally, genetic or metabolic liver disorders (e.g., Wilson's disease, α_1-antitrypsin deficiency) as well as nonalcoholic fatty liver disease are confused with viral hepatitis.

℞ ACUTE VIRAL HEPATITIS

In hepatitis B, among previously healthy adults who present with clinically apparent acute hepatitis, recovery occurs in ~99%; therefore, antiviral therapy is not likely to improve the rate of recovery and is not required. In rare instances of severe acute hepatitis B, treatment with a nucleoside analogue, such as lamivudine, at the 100-mg/d oral dose used to treat chronic hepatitis B (Chap. 300), has been attempted successfully. Although clinical trials have not been done to establish the efficacy of this approach, although severe acute hepatitis B is not an approved indication for therapy, and although the duration of therapy has not been determined, nonetheless, most authorities would recommend institution of antiviral therapy for severe, but not mild-moderate, acute hepatitis B. In typical cases of acute hepatitis C, recovery is rare, progression to chronic hepatitis is the rule, and meta-analyses of small clinical trials suggest that antiviral therapy with interferon α monotherapy (3 million units SC three times a week) is beneficial, reducing the rate of chronicity considerably by inducing sustained responses in 30–70% of patients. In a German multicenter study of 44 patients with acute symptomatic hepatitis C, initiation of intensive interferon α therapy (5 million units SC daily for 4 weeks, then three times a week for another 20 weeks) within an average of 3 months after infection resulted in a sustained virologic response rate of 98%. Although treatment of acute hepatitis C is recommended, the optimum regimen, duration of therapy, and time to initiate therapy remain to be determined. Many authorities now opt for a 24-week course (beginning within 2–3 months after onset) of the best regimen identified for the treatment of chronic hepatitis C, long-acting pegylated interferon plus the nucleoside analogue ribavirin, the efficacy of which is superior to that of standard interferon monotherapy regimens (see Chap. 300 for doses). Because of the marked reduction over the past two decades in the frequency of acute hepatitis C, opportunities to identify and treat patients with acute hepatitis C are rare indeed, except in injection drug users. Hospital epidemiologists, however, will encounter health workers who sustain hepatitis C–contaminated needle sticks; when monitoring for ALT elevations and HCV RNA after these accidents identifies acute hepatitis C (risk only ~3%), therapy should be initiated.

Notwithstanding these specific therapeutic considerations, in most cases of typical acute viral hepatitis, specific treatment generally is not necessary. Although hospitalization may be required for clinically severe illness, most patients do not require hospital care. Forced and prolonged bed rest is not essential for full recovery, but many patients will feel better with restricted physical activity. A high-calorie diet is desirable, and because many patients may experience nausea late in the day, the major caloric intake is best tolerated in the morning. Intravenous feeding is necessary in the acute stage if the patient has persistent vomiting and cannot maintain oral intake. Drugs capable of producing adverse reactions such as cholestasis and drugs metabolized by the liver should be avoided. If severe pruritus is present, the use of the bile salt–sequestering resin cholestyramine is helpful. Glucocorticoid therapy has no value in acute viral hepatitis, even in severe cases associated with *bridging necrosis*, and may be deleterious, even increasing the risk of chronicity (e.g., of acute hepatitis B).

Physical isolation of patients with hepatitis to a single room and bathroom is rarely necessary except in the case of fecal incontinence for hepatitis A and E or uncontrolled, voluminous bleeding for hepatitis B (with or without concomitant hepatitis D) and hepatitis C. Because most patients hospitalized with hepatitis A excrete little if any HAV, the likelihood of HAV transmission from these patients during their hospitalization is low. Therefore, burdensome *enteric precautions are no longer recommended*. Although gloves should be worn when the bedpans or fecal material of patients with hepatitis A are handled, these precautions do not represent a departure from sensible procedure and contemporary universal precautions for all hospitalized patients. For patients with hepatitis B and hepatitis C, emphasis should be placed on blood precautions, i.e., avoiding direct, ungloved hand contact with blood and other body fluids. Enteric precautions are unnecessary. The importance of simple hygienic precautions, such as hand washing, cannot be overemphasized. Universal precautions that have been adopted for all patients apply to patients with viral hepatitis.

Hospitalized patients may be discharged following substantial symptomatic improvement, a significant downward trend in the serum aminotransferase and bilirubin values, and a return to normal of the PT. Mild aminotransferase elevations should not be considered contraindications to the gradual resumption of normal activity.

In *fulminant hepatitis*, the goal of therapy is to support the patient by maintenance of fluid balance, support of circulation and respiration, control of bleeding, correction of hypoglycemia, and treatment of other complications of the comatose state in anticipation of liver regeneration and repair. Protein intake should be restricted, and oral lactulose or neomycin administered. Glucocorticoid therapy has been shown in controlled trials to be ineffective. Likewise, exchange transfusion, plasmapheresis, human cross-circulation, porcine liver cross-perfusion, hemoperfusion, and extracorporeal liver-assist devices have not been proved to enhance survival. Meticulous intensive care that includes prophylactic antibiotic coverage is the one factor that does appear to improve survival. Orthotopic liver transplantation is resorted to with increasing frequency, with excellent results, in patients with fulminant hepatitis (Chap. 304).

PROPHYLAXIS

Because application of therapy for acute viral hepatitis is limited, and because antiviral therapy for chronic viral hepatitis is cumbersome and costly but effective in only a proportion of patients (Chap. 300), emphasis is placed on prevention through immunization. The prophylactic approach differs for each of the types of viral hepatitis. In the past, immunoprophylaxis relied exclusively on passive immunization with antibody-containing globulin preparations purified by cold ethanol fractionation from the plasma of hundreds of normal donors. Currently, for hepatitis A and B, active immunization with vaccines is the preferable approach to prevention.

Hepatitis A Both passive immunization with IG and active immunization with killed vaccines are available. All preparations of IG contain anti-HAV concentrations sufficient to be protective. When administered before exposure or during the early incubation period, IG is effective in preventing clinically apparent hepatitis A. For postexposure prophylaxis of intimate contacts (household, sexual, institutional) of persons with hepatitis A, the administration of 0.02 mL/kg is recommended as early after exposure as possible; it may be effective even when administered as late as 2 weeks after exposure. Prophylaxis is not necessary for those who have already received hepatitis A vaccine, casual contacts (office, factory, school, or hospital), for most elderly persons, who are very likely to be immune, or for those known to have anti-HAV in their serum. In day-care centers, recognition of hepatitis A in children or staff should provide a stimulus for immunoprophylaxis in the center and in the children's family members. By the time most common-source outbreaks of hepatitis A are recognized, it is usually too late in the incubation period for IG to be effective; however, prophylaxis may limit the frequency of secondary cases. For travelers to tropical countries, developing countries, and other areas outside standard tourist routes, IG prophylaxis had been recommended, before a vaccine became available. When such travel lasted <3 months, 0.02 mL/kg was given; for longer travel or residence in these areas, a dose of 0.06 mL/kg every 4–6 months was recommended. Administration of plasma-derived globulin is safe; all contemporary lots of IG are subjected to viral inactivation steps and must be free of HCV RNA as determined by PCR testing. Administration of IM lots of IG has not been associated with transmission of HBV, HCV, or HIV.

Formalin-inactivated vaccines made from strains of HAV attenuated in tissue culture have been shown to be safe, immunogenic, and effective in preventing hepatitis A. Hepatitis A vaccines are approved for use in persons who are at least 1 year old and appear to provide adequate protection beginning 4 weeks after a primary inoculation. If it can be given within 4 weeks of an expected exposure, such as by travel to an endemic area, hepatitis A vaccine is the preferred approach to *preexposure* immunoprophylaxis. If travel is more imminent, IG (0.02 mL/kg) should be administered at a different injection site, along with the first dose of vaccine. Because vaccination provides long-lasting protection (protective levels of anti-HAV should last 20 years after vaccination), persons whose risk will be sustained (e.g., frequent travelers or those remaining in endemic areas for prolonged periods) should be vaccinated, and vaccine should supplant the need for repeated IG injections. Shortly after its introduction, hepatitis A vaccine was recommended for children living in communities with a high incidence of HAV infection; in 1999, this recommendation was extended to include all children living in states, counties, and communities with high rates of HAV infection. As of 2006, the Advisory Committee on Immunization Practices of the U.S. Public Health Service recommended *routine hepatitis A vaccination of all children*. Other groups considered to be at increased risk for HAV infection and who are candidates for hepatitis A vaccination include military personnel, populations with cyclic outbreaks of hepatitis A (e.g., Alaskan natives), employees of day-care centers, primate handlers, laboratory workers exposed to hepatitis A or fecal specimens, and patients with chronic liver disease. Because of an increased risk of fulminant hepatitis A—observed in some experiences but not confirmed in others—among patients with chronic hepatitis C, patients with chronic hepatitis C have been singled out as candidates for hepatitis A vaccination. Other populations whose recognized risk of hepatitis A is increased should be vaccinated, including men who have sex with men, injection drug users, and persons with clotting disorders who require frequent administration of clotting-factor concentrates. Recommendations for dose and frequency differ for the two approved vaccine preparations (Table 298-5); all injections are IM. Hepatitis A vaccine has been reported to be effective in preventing secondary household cases of acute hepatitis A, but its role in other instances of postexposure prophylaxis remains to be demonstrated.

Hepatitis B Until 1982, prevention of hepatitis B was based on *passive* immunoprophylaxis either with standard IG, containing modest levels of anti-HBs, or hepatitis B immune globulin (HBIG), containing high-titer anti-HBs. The efficacy of standard IG has never been established and remains questionable; even the efficacy of HBIG, demonstrated in several clinical trials, has been challenged, and its contribution appears to be in reducing the frequency of clinical *illness*, not in preventing *infection*. The first vaccine for *active* immunization, introduced in 1982, was prepared from purified, noninfectious 22-nm spherical forms of HBsAg derived from the plasma of healthy HBsAg carriers. In 1987, the plasma-derived vaccine was supplanted by a genetically engineered vaccine derived from recombinant yeast. The latter vaccine consists of HBsAg particles that are nonglycosylated but are otherwise indistinguishable from natural HBsAg; two recombinant vaccines are licensed for use in the United States. Current recommendations can be divided into those for preexposure and postexposure prophylaxis.

For *preexposure* prophylaxis against hepatitis B in settings of frequent exposure (health workers exposed to blood; hemodialysis patients and staff; residents and staff of custodial institutions for the developmentally handicapped; injection drug users; inmates of long-

TABLE 298-5 HEPATITIS A VACCINATION SCHEDULES

Age, years	No. of Doses	Dose	Schedule, months
HAVRIX (GlaxoSmithKline)[a]			
1–18	2	720 ELU[b] (0.5 mL)	0, 6–12
≥19	2	1440 ELU (1.0 mL)	0, 6–12
VAQTA (Merck)			
1–18	2	25 units (0.5 mL)	0, 6–18
≥19	2	50 units (1.0 mL)	0, 6–18

[a]A combination of this hepatitis A vaccine and hepatitis B vaccine, TWINRIX, is licensed for simultaneous protection against both of these viruses among adults (age ≥18 years). Each 1.0-mL dose contains 720 ELU[b] of hepatitis A vaccine and 20 μg of hepatitis B vaccine. These doses are recommended at months 0, 1, and 6.
[b]Enzyme-linked immunoassay units.

TABLE 298-6 PREEXPOSURE HEPATITIS B VACCINATION SCHEDULES

Target Group	No. of Doses	Dose	Schedule, months
RECOMBIVAX-HB (Merck)[a]			
Infants, children (<1–10 years)	3	5 μg (0.5 mL)	0, 1–2, 4–6
Adolescents (11–19 years)	3 or 4	5 μg (0.5 mL)	0–2, 1–4, 4–6 *or* 0, 12, 24 *or* 0, 1, 2, 12
	or		
	2	10 μg (1.0 mL)	0, 4–6 (age 11–15)
Adults (≥20 years)	3	10 μg (1.0 mL)	0–2, 1–4, 4–6
Hemodialysis patients[b]			
<20 years	3	5 μg (0.5 mL)	0, 1, 6
≥20 years	3	40 μg (4.0 mL)	0, 1, 6
ENGERIX-B (GlaxoSmithKline)[c]			
Infants, children (<1–10 years)	3 or 4	10 μg (0.5 mL)	0, 1–2, 4–6 *or* 0, 1, 2,12
Adolescents (10–19 years)	3 or 4	10 μg (0.5 mL)	0, 1–2, 4–6 *or* 0, 12, 24 *or* 0, 1, 2, 12
Adults (≥20 years)	3 or 4	20 μg (1.0 mL)	0–2, 1–4, 4–6 0, 1, 2, 12
Hemodialysis patients[b]			
<20 years	4	10 μg (0.5 mL)	0, 1, 2, 6
≥20 years	4	40 μg (2.0 mL)	0, 1, 2, 6

[a]This manufacturer produces a licensed combination of hepatitis B vaccine and vaccines against *Haemophilus influenzae* type b and *Neisseria meningitides*, Comvax, for use in infants and young children. Please consult product insert for dose and schedule.
[b]This group also includes other immunocompromised persons.
[c]This manufacturer produces two licensed combination hepatitis B vaccines: (1) Twinrix, recombinant hepatitis B vaccine plus inactivated hepatitis A vaccine, is licensed for simultaneous protection against both of these viruses among adults (age ≥ 18 years). Each 1.0-mL dose contains 720 ELU[b] of hepatitis A vaccine and 20 μg of hepatitis B vaccine. These doses are recommended at months 0, 1, and 6. (2) Pediatrix, recombinant hepatitis B vaccine plus diphtheria and tetanus toxoid, pertussis, and inactivated poliovirus, is licensed for use in infants and young children. Please consult product insert for doses and schedules.

term correctional facilities; persons with multiple sexual partners; persons such as hemophiliacs who require long-term, high-volume therapy with blood derivatives; household and sexual contacts of HBsAg carriers; persons living in or traveling extensively in endemic areas; unvaccinated children under the age of 18; and unvaccinated children who are Alaskan natives, Pacific Islanders, or residents in households of first-generation immigrants from endemic countries), three IM (deltoid, not gluteal) injections of hepatitis B vaccine are recommended at 0, 1, and 6 months (other, optional schedules are summarized in Table 298-6). Pregnancy is *not* a contraindication to vaccination. In areas of low HBV endemicity such as the United States, despite the availability of safe and effective hepatitis B vaccines, a strategy of vaccinating persons in high-risk groups has not been effective. The incidence of new hepatitis B cases continued to increase in the United States after introduction of vaccines; <10% of all targeted persons in high-risk groups have actually been vaccinated, and ~30% of persons with sporadic acute hepatitis B do not fall into any high-risk-group category. Therefore, to have an impact on the frequency of HBV infection in an area of low endemicity such as the United States, universal hepatitis B vaccination in childhood has been recommended. For unvaccinated children born after the implementation of universal infant vaccination, vaccination during early adolescence, at age 11–12 years, was recommended, and this recommendation has been extended to include all unvaccinated children age 0–19 years. In HBV-hyperendemic areas, e.g., Asia, universal vaccination of children has resulted in a marked 10- to 15-year decline in hepatitis B and its complications.

The two available recombinant hepatitis B vaccines are comparable, one containing 10 μg of HBsAg (Recombivax-HB) and the other containing 20 μg of HBsAg (Engerix-B), and recommended doses for each injection vary for the two preparations (Table 298-6). Combinations of hepatitis B vaccine with other childhood vaccines are available as well (Table 298-6).

For unvaccinated persons sustaining an exposure to HBV, *postexposure* prophylaxis with a combination of HBIG (for rapid achievement of high-titer circulating anti-HBs) and hepatitis B vaccine (for achievement of long-lasting immunity as well as its apparent efficacy in attenuating clinical illness after exposure) is recommended. For *perinatal* exposure of infants born to HBsAg-positive mothers, a single dose of HBIG, 0.5 mL, should be administered IM in the thigh *immediately after birth*, followed by a complete course of three injections of recombinant hepatitis B vaccine (see doses above) to be started within the first 12 h of life. For those experiencing a direct percutaneous inoculation or transmucosal exposure to HBsAg-positive blood or body fluids (e.g., accidental *needle stick*, other mucosal penetration, or ingestion), a single IM dose of HBIG, 0.06 mL/kg, administered as soon after exposure as possible, is followed by a complete course of hepatitis B vaccine to begin within the first week. For those exposed by *sexual* contact to a patient with acute hepatitis B, a single IM dose of HBIG, 0.06 mL/kg, should be given within 14 days of exposure, to be followed by a complete course of hepatitis B vaccine. When both HBIG and hepatitis B vaccine are recommended, they may be given at the same time but at separate sites.

The precise duration of protection afforded by hepatitis B vaccine is unknown; however, ~80–90% of immunocompetent vaccinees retain protective levels of anti-HBs for at least 5 years, and 60–80% for 10 years. Thereafter and even after anti-HBs becomes undetectable, protection persists against clinical hepatitis B, hepatitis B surface antigenemia, and chronic HBV infection. Currently, *booster* immunizations are not recommended routinely, except in immunosuppressed persons who have lost detectable anti-HBs or immunocompetent persons who sustain percutaneous HBsAg-positive inoculations after losing detectable antibody. Specifically, for hemodialysis patients, annual anti-HBs testing is recommended after vaccination; booster doses are recommended when anti-HBs levels fall to <10 mIU/mL. As noted above, for persons at risk of both hepatitis A and B, a combined vaccine is available containing 720 enzyme-linked immunoassay units of inactivated HAV and 20 μg of recombinant HBsAg (at 0, 1, and 6 months).

Hepatitis D Infection with hepatitis D can be prevented by vaccinating susceptible persons with hepatitis B vaccine. No product is available for immunoprophylaxis to prevent HDV superinfection in HBsAg carriers; for them, avoidance of percutaneous exposures and limitation of intimate contact with persons who have HDV infection are recommended.

Hepatitis C IG is ineffective in preventing hepatitis C and is no longer recommended for postexposure prophylaxis in cases of perinatal, needle stick, or sexual exposure. Although prototype vaccines that induce antibodies to HCV envelope proteins have been developed, currently, hepatitis C vaccination is not feasible practically. Genotype and quasispecies viral heterogeneity, as well as rapid evasion of neutralizing antibodies by this rapidly mutating virus, conspire to render HCV a difficult target for immunoprophylaxis with a vaccine. Prevention of transfusion-associated hepatitis C has been accomplished by the following successively introduced measures: Exclusion of commercial blood donors and reliance on a volunteer blood supply; screening donor blood with surrogate markers such as ALT (no longer recommended) and anti-HBc, markers that identify segments of the blood donor population with an increased risk of bloodborne infections; exclusion of blood donors in high-risk groups for AIDS and the introduction of anti-HIV screening tests; and progressively sensitive serologic and virologic screening tests for HCV infection.

In the absence of active or passive immunization, prevention of hepatitis C includes behavior changes and precautions to limit exposures to infected persons. Recommendations designed to identify patients with clinically inapparent hepatitis as candidates for medical management have as a secondary benefit the identification of persons whose contacts could be at risk of becoming infected. A so-called lookback program has been recommended to identify persons who were transfused before 1992 with blood from a donor found subsequently to have hepatitis C. In addition, anti-HCV testing is recommended for anyone who received a blood transfusion or a transplanted organ before the introduction of second-generation screening tests in 1992, those who ever used injection drugs, chronically hemodialyzed patients, persons with clotting disorders who received clotting factors made before 1987 from pooled blood products, persons with elevated aminotransferase levels, health workers exposed to HCV-positive blood or contaminated needles, and children born to HCV-positive mothers.

For stable, monogamous sexual partners, sexual transmission of hepatitis C is unlikely, and sexual barrier precautions are not recommended. For persons with multiple sexual partners or with sexually transmitted diseases, the risk of sexual transmission of hepatitis C is increased, and barrier precautions (latex condoms) are recommended. A person with hepatitis C should avoid sharing such items as razors, toothbrushes, and nail clippers with sexual partners and family members. No special precautions are recommended for babies born to mothers with hepatitis C, and breast feeding does not have to be restricted.

Hepatitis E Whether IG prevents hepatitis E remains undetermined. A recombinant vaccine has been developed and is undergoing clinical testing.

FURTHER READINGS

BLUM HE, MARCELLIN P: EASL Consensus Conference on Hepatitis B. J Hepatol 39(Suppl 1):1, 2003

CENTERS FOR DISEASE CONTROL AND PREVENTION: Updated U.S. Public Health Service guidelines for the management of occupational exposures to HBV, HCV, and HIV and recommendations for postexposure prophylaxis. MMWR 50(RR-11):1, 2001

———: General recommendations on immunization: Recommendations of the Advisory Committee on Immunization Practices and the American Academy of Family Physicians. MMWR 51(RR-2):1, 2002

CHEN CJ et al: Risk of hepatocellular carcinoma across a biological gradient of serum hepatitis B virus DNA level. JAMA 295:65, 2006

CHU C-J et al: Hepatitis B virus genotype B is associated with earlier HBeAg seroconversion compared with hepatitis B virus genotype C. Gastroenterology 122:1756, 2002

CONSENSUS STATEMENT: EASL International Consensus Conference on Hepatitis C. J Hepatol 30:956, 1999

DIENSTAG JL, McHUTCHISON JG: American Gastroenterological Association technical review on the management of hepatitis C. Gastroenterology 130:231, 2006

FERRARI C et al: Immunopathogenesis of hepatitis B. J Hepatol 39(Suppl 1):S36, 2003

GISH RG, LOCARNINI SA: Chronic hepatitis B: Current testing strategies. Clin Gastroenterol Hepatol 4:666, 2006

HADZIYANNIS SJ, VASSILOPOULOS D: Hepatitis B e antigen-negative chronic hepatitis B. Hepatology 34:617, 2001

JAECKEL E et al: Treatment of acute hepatitis C with interferon alfa-2b. N Engl J Med 345:1452, 2001

LAUER GM, WALKER BD: Medical progress: Hepatitis C virus infection. N Engl J Med 345:41, 2001

LOK ASF, McMAHON BJ: Chronic hepatitis B. Hepatology 34:1225, 2001

MARGOLIS HS et al (eds): *Viral Hepatitis and Liver Disease*. Atlanta/London, International Medical Press, 2002

PAWLOTSKY J-M: Molecular diagnosis of viral hepatitis. Gastroenterology 122:1554, 2002

REHERMANN B: Immune response in hepatitis B virus infection. Semin Liver Dis 23:21, 2003

SCHREIBER GB et al: The risk of transfusion-transmitted viral infection. N Engl J Med 334:1685, 1996

SEEFF LB: Natural history of chronic hepatitis C. Hepatology 36(Suppl 1):S35, 2002

STRADER DB et al: Diagnosis, management, and treatment of hepatitis C (AASLD practice guidelines). Hepatology 39:1147, 2004

THIMME R et al: Viral and immunological determinants of hepatitis C virus clearance, persistence, and disease. Proc Natl Acad Sci USA 99:15661, 2002

YANG H-I et al: Hepatitis B e antigen and the risk of hepatocellular carcinoma. N Engl J Med 347:168, 2002

299 Toxic and Drug-Induced Hepatitis

Jules L. Dienstag

Liver injury may follow the inhalation, ingestion, or parenteral administration of a number of pharmacologic and chemical agents. These include industrial toxins (e.g., carbon tetrachloride, trichloroethylene, and yellow phosphorus), the heat-stable toxic bicyclic octapeptides of certain species of *Amanita* and *Galerina* (hepatotoxic mushroom poisoning), and, more commonly, pharmacologic agents used in medical therapy. It is essential that any patient presenting with jaundice or altered biochemical liver tests be questioned carefully about exposure to chemicals used in work or at home, drugs taken by prescription or bought "over the counter," and herbal or alternative medicines. Hepatotoxic drugs can injure the hepatocyte directly, e.g., via a free-radical or metabolic intermediate that causes peroxidation of membrane lipids and that results in liver cell injury. Alternatively, the drug or its metabolite can distort cell membranes or other cellular molecules, bind covalently to intracellular proteins, activate apoptotic pathways, interfere with bile salt export proteins, or block biochemical pathways or cellular integrity. Interference with bile canalicular pumps can allow endogenous bile acids, which can injure the liver, to accumulate. Such injuries, in turn, may lead to necrosis of hepatocytes; injure bile ducts, producing cholestasis; or block pathways of lipid movement, inhibit protein synthesis, or impair mitochondrial oxidation of fatty acids, resulting in lactic acidosis and intracellular triglyceride accumulation (expressed histologically as microvesicular steatosis). In some cases, drug metabolites sensitize hepatocytes to toxic cytokines, and differences between susceptible and nonsusceptible drug recipients may be attributable to polymorphisms in elaboration of competing, protective cytokines, as has been suggested for acetaminophen hepatotoxicity (see below). Immunologically mediated liver injury has been postulated to represent another mechanism of drug hepatotoxicity (see below). In addition, a role has been shown for activation of nuclear transporters, such as the constitutive androstane receptor (CAR), in the induction of drug hepatotoxicity. In general, two major types of chemical hepatotoxicity have been recognized: (1) direct toxic type and (2) idiosyncratic type.

Most drugs, which are water-insoluble, undergo a series of hepatic metabolic transformation steps, culminating in a water-soluble form appropriate for renal or biliary excretion. This process begins with ox-idation or methylation initially mediated by the microsomal mixed-function oxygenases cytochrome P450 (phase I reaction), followed by glucuronidation or sulfation (phase II reaction) or inactivation by glutathione. Most drug hepatotoxicity is mediated by a phase I toxic metabolite, but glutathione depletion, precluding inactivation of harmful compounds by glutathione S-transferase, can contribute as well.

As shown in Table 299-1, direct toxic hepatitis occurs with predictable regularity in individuals exposed to the offending agent and is dose-dependent. The latent period between exposure and liver injury is usually short (often several hours), although clinical manifestations may be delayed for 24–48 h. Agents producing toxic hepatitis are generally systemic poisons or are converted in the liver to toxic metabolites. The direct hepatotoxins result in morphologic abnormalities that are reasonably characteristic and reproducible for each toxin. For example, carbon tetrachloride and trichloroethylene characteristically produce a centrilobular zonal necrosis, whereas yellow phosphorus poisoning typically results in periportal injury. The hepatotoxic octapeptides of *Amanita phalloides* usually produce massive hepatic necrosis; the lethal dose of the toxin is ~10 mg, the amount found in a single deathcap mushroom. Tetracycline, when administered in IV doses >1.5 g daily, leads to microvesicular fat deposits in the liver. Liver injury, which is often only one facet of the toxicity produced by the direct hepatotoxins, may go unrecognized until jaundice appears.

In idiosyncratic drug reactions, the occurrence of hepatitis is usually infrequent (1 in 10^3–10^5 patients) and unpredictable, the response is not dose-dependent, and liver injury may occur at any time during or shortly after exposure to the drug. Adding to the difficulty of predicting or identifying idiosyncratic drug hepatotoxicity is the occurrence of mild, transient, nonprogressive serum aminotransferase elevations that resolve with continued drug use. Such "adaptation," the mechanism of which is unknown, occurs in such drugs as isoniazid, valproate, phenytoin, and HMG-CoA reductase inhibitors (statins). Extrahepatic manifestations of hypersensitivity, such as rash, arthralgias, fever, leukocytosis, and eosinophilia, occur in about one-quarter of patients with idiosyncratic hepatotoxic drug reactions; this observation and the unpredictability of idiosyncratic drug hepatotoxicity contributed to the hypothesis that this category of drug reactions is immunologically mediated. More recent evidence, however, suggests that, in most cases, even idiosyncratic reactions represent direct hepatotoxicity but are caused by drug metabolites rather than by the intact compound. Even the prototypes of idiosyncratic hepatotoxicity reactions, halothane hepatitis and isoniazid hepatotoxicity, associated frequently with hypersensitivity manifestations, are now recognized to be mediated by toxic metabolites that damage liver cells directly. Current-

TABLE 299-1 SOME FEATURES OF TOXIC AND DRUG-INDUCED HEPATIC INJURY

Features	Direct Toxic Effect[a]		Idiosyncratic[a]			Other[a]
	(Carbon Tetrachloride)	(Acetaminophen)	(Halothane)	(Isoniazid)	(Chlorpromazine)	(Oral Contraceptive Agents)
Predictable and dose-related toxicity	+	+	0	0	0	+
Latent period	Short	Short	Variable	Variable	Variable	Variable
Arthralgia, fever, rash, eosinophilia	0	0	+	0	+	0
Liver morphology	Necrosis, fatty infiltration	Centrilobular necrosis	Similar to viral hepatitis	Similar to viral hepatitis	Cholestasis *with* portal inflammation	Cholestasis *without* portal inflammation, vascular lesions

[a]The drugs listed are typical samples.

ly, most idiosyncratic reactions are thought to result from differences in metabolic reactivity to specific agents; host susceptibility is mediated by the kinetics of toxic metabolite generation, which differs among individuals, probably mediated by genetic polymorphisms in drug-metabolizing pathways. Occasionally, however, the clinical features of an allergic reaction (prominent tissue eosinophilia, autoantibodies, etc.) are difficult to ignore. In vitro models have been described in which lymphocyte cytotoxicity can be demonstrated against rabbit hepatocytes altered by incubation with the potential offending drug. Furthermore, several instances of drug hepatotoxicity are associated with the appearance of autoantibodies, including a class of antibodies to liver-kidney microsomes, anti-LKM2, directed against a cytochrome P450 enzyme. Similarly, in selected cases, a drug or its metabolite has been shown to bind to a host cellular component forming a hapten; the immune response to this "neoantigen" is postulated to play a role in the pathogenesis of liver injury. Therefore, some authorities subdivide idiosyncratic drug hepatotoxicity into hypersensitivity (allergic) and "metabolic" categories. Several unusual exceptions notwithstanding, true drug allergy is difficult to support in most cases of idiosyncratic drug-induced liver injury.

Idiosyncratic reactions lead to a morphologic pattern that is more variable than those produced by direct toxins; a single agent is often capable of causing a variety of lesions, although certain patterns tend to predominate. Depending on the agent involved, idiosyncratic hepatitis may result in a clinical and morphologic picture indistinguishable from that of viral hepatitis (e.g., halothane) or may simulate extrahepatic bile duct obstruction clinically with morphologic evidence of cholestasis. Drug-induced cholestasis ranges from mild to increasingly severe: (1) bland cholestasis with limited hepatocellular injury (e.g., estrogens, 17,α-substituted androgens); (2) inflammatory cholestasis (e.g., phenothiazines, amoxicillin–clavulanic acid, oxacillin, erythromycin estolate); (3) sclerosing cholangitis (e.g., after intrahepatic infusion of the chemotherapeutic agent floxuridine for hepatic metastases from a primary colonic carcinoma); (4) disappearance of bile ducts, "ductopenic" cholestasis, similar to that observed in chronic rejection following liver transplantation (e.g., carbamazepine, chlorpromazine, tricyclic antidepressant agents). Cholestasis may result from binding of drugs to canalicular membrane transporters, accumulation of toxic bile acids resulting from canalicular pump failure, or genetic defects in canalicular transporter proteins. Morphologic alterations may also include bridging hepatic necrosis (e.g., methyldopa), or, infrequently, hepatic granulomas (e.g., sulfonamides). Some drugs result in macrovesicular or microvesicular steatosis or steatohepatitis, which in some cases has been linked to mitochondrial dysfunction and lipid peroxidation. Severe hepatotoxicity associated with steatohepatitis, most likely a result of mitochondrial toxicity, is being recognized with increasing frequency among patients receiving antiretroviral therapy with reverse transcriptase inhibitors (e.g., zidovudine, didanosine) or protease inhibitors (e.g., indinavir, ritonavir) for HIV infection (Chap. 182). Generally, such mitochondrial hepatotoxicity of these antiretroviral agents is reversible, but dramatic, nonreversible hepatotoxicity associated with mitochondrial injury (inhibition of DNA polymerase γ) was the cause of acute liver failure encountered during early clinical trials of now-abandoned fialuridine, a fluorinated pyrimidine analogue with potent antiviral activity against hepatitis B virus. Another potential target for idiosyncratic drug hepatotoxicity is sinusoidal lining cells; when these are injured, such as by high-dose chemotherapeutic agents (e.g., cyclophosphamide, melphalan, busulfan) administered prior to bone marrow transplantation, venoocclusive disease can result.

Not all adverse hepatic drug reactions can be classified as either toxic or idiosyncratic in type. For example, oral contraceptives, which combine estrogenic and progestational compounds, may result in impairment of hepatic tests and occasionally in jaundice; however, they do not produce necrosis or fatty change, manifestations of hypersensitivity are generally absent, and susceptibility to the development of oral contraceptive–induced cholestasis appears to be genetically determined. Such estrogen-induced cholestasis is more common in women with cholestasis of pregnancy, a disorder linked to genetic defects in multidrug resistance–

associated canalicular transporter proteins. Other instances of genetically determined drug hepatotoxicity have been identified. For example, ~10% of the population have an autosomally recessive trait associated with the absence of cytochrome P450 enzyme 2D6 and have impaired debrisoquine-4-hydroxylase enzyme activity. As a result, they cannot metabolize, and are at increased risk of hepatotoxicity resulting from, certain compounds such as desipramine, propranolol, and quinidine.

Some forms of drug hepatotoxicity are so rare, e.g., occurring in <1:10,000 recipients, that they do not become apparent during clinical trials, involving only several thousand recipients, conducted to obtain drug registration. An example of such rare, but serious, idiosyncratic drug hepatotoxicity followed the approval and generalized use of troglitazone, a peroxisomal, proliferator activator–receptor γ agonist, the first-introduced example of a thiazolidinedione insulin-sensitizing agent. This instance of drug hepatotoxicity was not recognized until well after the drug was introduced, underlining the importance of postmarketing surveillance in identifying toxic drugs and in leading to their withdrawal from use. Fortunately, such hepatotoxicity is not characteristic of the second-generation thiazolidinedione insulin-sensitizing agents rosiglitazone and pioglitazone; in clinical trials, the frequency of aminotransferase elevations in patients treated with these medications did not differ from that in placebo recipients, and isolated reports of liver injury among recipients are extremely rare.

Because drug-induced hepatitis is often a presumptive diagnosis and many other disorders produce a similar clinicopathologic picture, evidence of a causal relationship between the use of a drug and subsequent liver injury may be difficult to establish. The relationship is most convincing for the direct hepatotoxins, which lead to a high frequency of hepatic impairment after a short latent period. Idiosyncratic reactions may be reproduced, in some instances, when rechallenge, after an asymptomatic period, results in a recurrence of signs, symptoms, and morphologic and biochemical abnormalities. Rechallenge, however, is often ethically unfeasible, because severe reactions may occur.

Generally, drug hepatotoxicity is not more frequent in persons with underlying chronic liver disease. Reported exceptions include hepatotoxicity of aspirin, methotrexate, isoniazid (only in certain experiences), and antiretroviral therapy for HIV infection.

℞ TOXIC AND DRUG-INDUCED HEPATIC DISEASE

Treatment is largely supportive, except in acetaminophen hepatotoxicity (see below). In patients with fulminant hepatitis resulting from drug hepatotoxicity, liver transplantation may be life-saving (Chap. 304). Withdrawal of the suspected agent is indicated at the first sign of an adverse reaction. In the case of the direct toxins, liver involvement should not divert attention from renal or other organ involvement, which may also threaten survival. Glucocorticoids for drug hepatotoxicity with allergic features, silibinin for hepatotoxic mushroom poisoning, and ursodeoxycholic acid for cholestatic drug hepatotoxicity have never been shown to be effective and are not recommended.

In Table 299-2, several classes of chemical agents are listed, together with examples of the pattern of liver injury produced by them. Certain drugs appear to be responsible for the development of chronic as well as acute hepatic injury. For example, oxyphenisatin, methyldopa, and isoniazid have been associated with moderate to severe chronic hepatitis, and halothane and methotrexate have been implicated in the development of cirrhosis. A syndrome resembling primary biliary cirrhosis has been described following treatment with chlorpromazine, methyl testosterone, tolbutamide, and other drugs. Portal hypertension in the absence of cirrhosis may result from alterations in hepatic architecture produced by vitamin A or arsenic intoxication, industrial exposure to vinyl chloride, or administration of thorium dioxide. The latter three agents have also been associated with angiosarcoma of the liver. Oral contraceptives have been implicated in the development of hepatic adenoma and, rarely, hepatocellular carcinoma and hepatic vein occlusion (Budd-Chiari syndrome). Another unusual lesion, peliosis hepatis (blood cysts of the liver), has been

TABLE 299-2 PRINCIPAL ALTERATIONS OF HEPATIC MORPHOLOGY PRODUCED BY SOME COMMONLY USED DRUGS AND CHEMICALS[a]

Principal Morphologic Change	Class of Agent	Example
Cholestasis	Anabolic steroid	Methyl testosterone
	Antibiotic	Erythromycin estolate, nitrofurantoin, rifampin, amoxicillin-clavulanic acid, oxacillin
	Anticonvulsant	Carbamazine
	Antidepressant	Duloxetine, mirtazapine, tricyclic antidepressants
	Anti-inflammatory	Sulindac
	Antiplatelet	Clopidogrel
	Antihypertensive	Irbesartan
	Antithyroid	Methimazole
	Calcium channel blocker	Nifedipine, verapamil
	Immunosuppressive	Cyclosporine
	Lipid-lowering	Ezetimibe
	Oncotherapeutic	Anabolic steroids, busulfan, tamoxifen, irinotecan
	Oral contraceptive	Norethynodrel with mestranol
	Oral hypoglycemic	Chlorpropamide
	Tranquilizer	Chlorpromazine[b]
Fatty liver	Antiarrhythmic	Amiodarone
	Antibiotic	Tetracycline (high-dose, intravenous)
	Anticonvulsant	Valproic acid
	Antiviral	Dideoxynucleosides (e.g., zidovudine), protease inhibitors (e.g., indinavir, ritonavir)
	Oncotherapeutic	Asparaginase, methotrexate
Hepatitis	Anesthetic	Halothane[c]
	Antiandrogen	Flutamide
	Antibiotic	Isoniazid,[c] rifampicin, nitrofurantoin, telithromycin, minocycline, pyrazinamide, trovafloxacin[d]
	Anticonvulsant	Phenytoin, carbamazine
	Antidepressant	Iproniazid, amitriptyline, imipramine, trazodone, venlafaxine, fluoxetine, paroxetine, duloxetine, sertraline, nefazodone[d]
	Antifungal	Ketoconazole, fluconazole, itraconazole
	Antihypertensive	Methyldopa,[c] captopril, enalapril, lisinopril, losartan
	Anti-inflammatory	Ibuprofen, indomethacin, diclofenac, sulindac, bomfenac
	Antipsychotic	Risperidone
	Antiviral	Zidovudine, didanosine, stavudine, nevirapine, ritonavir, idinavir
	Calcium channel blocker	Nifedipine, verapamil, diltiazem
	Cholinesterase inhibitor	Tacrine
	Diuretic	Chlorothiazide
	Laxative	Oxyphenisatin[c,d]
	Norepinephrine-reuptake inhibitor	Atomoxetine
	Oral hypoglycemic	Troglitazone,[d] acarbose
Mixed hepatitis/ cholestatic	Antibiotic	Amoxicillin-clavulanic acid, trimethoprim-sulfamethoxazole
	Antifungal	Terbinafine
	Immunosuppressive	Azathioprine
	Lipid-lowering	Nicotinic acid, lovastatin, ezetimide
Toxic (necrosis)	Analgesic	Acetaminophen
	Hydrocarbon	Carbon tetrachloride
	Metal	Yellow phosphorus
	Mushroom	*Amanita phalloides*
	Solvent	Dimethylformamide
Granulomas	Antiarrhythmic	Quinidine, diltiazem
	Antibiotic	Sulfanomides
	Anticonvulsant	Carbamazine
	Anti-inflammatory	Phenylbutazone
	Xanthine oxidase inhibitor	Allopurinol

[a]Several agents cause more than one type of liver lesion and appear under more than one category.
[b]Rarely associated with primary biliary cirrhosis-like lesion.
[c]Occasionally associated with chronic hepatitis or bridging hepatic necrosis or cirrhosis.
[d]Withdrawn from use because of severe hepatotoxicity.

observed in some patients treated with anabolic steroids. The existence of these hepatic disorders expands the spectrum of liver injury induced by chemical agents and emphasizes the need for a thorough drug history in all patients with liver dysfunction.

The following are the patterns of adverse hepatic reactions for some prototypic agents.

ACETAMINOPHEN HEPATOTOXICITY (DIRECT TOXIN)

Acetaminophen can cause severe centrilobular hepatic necrosis when ingested in large amounts in suicide attempts or accidentally by children; in the United States and England, acetaminophen hepatotoxicity is the most common culprit among patients presenting with acute liver failure. A single dose of 10–15 g, occasionally less, may produce clinical evidence of liver injury. Fatal fulminant disease is usually (although not invariably) associated with ingestion of ≥25 g. Blood levels of acetaminophen correlate with the severity of hepatic injury (levels > 300 µg/mL 4 h after ingestion are predictive of the development of severe damage; levels < 150 µg/mL suggest that hepatic injury is highly unlikely). Nausea, vomiting, diarrhea, abdominal pain, and shock are early manifestations occurring 4–12 h after ingestion. Then 24–48 h later, when these features are abating, hepatic injury becomes apparent. Maximal abnormalities and hepatic failure may not be evident until 4–6 days after ingestion, and aminotransferase levels approaching 10,000 units are not uncommon, i.e., levels far exceeding those in patients with viral hepatitis. Renal failure and myocardial injury may be present.

Acetaminophen is metabolized predominantly by a phase II reaction to innocuous sulfate and glucuronide metabolites; however, a small proportion of acetaminophen is metabolized by a phase I reaction to a hepatotoxic metabolite formed from the parent compound by the cytochrome P450 CYP2E1. This metabolite, *N*-acetylbenzoquinone-imine (NAPQI), is detoxified by binding to "hepatoprotective" glutathione to become harmless, water-soluble mercapturic acid, which undergoes renal excretion. When excessive amounts of NAPQI are formed, or when glutathione levels are low, glutathione levels are depleted and overwhelmed, permitting covalent binding to nucleophilic hepatocyte macromolecules forming acetaminophen-protein "adducts." These adducts, which can be measured in serum by high-performance liquid chromatography, hold promise as diagnostic markers of acetaminophen hepatotoxicity. The binding of acetaminophen to hepatocyte macromolecules is believed to lead to hepatocyte necrosis; the precise sequence and mechanism are unknown. Hepatic injury may be potentiated by prior administration of alcohol, phenobarbital, isoniazid, or other drugs; by conditions that stimulate the mixed-function oxidase system; or by conditions such as starvation that reduce hepatic glutathione levels. The xenobiotic (environmental, exogenous substance) receptor CAR has been shown in a mouse model of acetaminophen hepatotoxicity to induce acetaminophen-metabolizing enzymes and, thereby, regulate and increase hepatotoxicity. Cimetidine, which inhibits P450 enzymes, has the potential to reduce generation of the toxic metabolite. Alcohol induces cytochrome P450 CYP2E1; consequently, increased levels of the toxic metabolite NAPQI are produced in chronic alcoholics after acetaminophen ingestion. In addition, alcohol suppresses hepatic glutathione production. Therefore, in chronic alcoholics, the toxic dose of acetaminophen may be as low as 2 g, and alcoholic patients should be warned specifically about the dangers of even standard doses of this commonly used

FIGURE 299-1 Nomogram to define risk of acetaminophen hepatotoxicity according to initial plasma acetaminophen concentration. *(After BH Rumack, H Matthew, Pediatrics 55:871, 1975.)*

drug. Such "therapeutic misadventures" also occur occasionally in patients with severe, febrile illnesses or pain syndromes; in such a setting, several days of anorexia and near-fasting coupled with regular administration of extra-strength acetaminophen formulations result in a combination of glutathione depletion and relatively high NAPQI levels in the absence of a history of recognized acetaminophen overdose. Recently, aminotransferase elevations were identified in 31–44% of normal subjects treated for 14 days with the maximal recommended dose of acetaminophen, 4 g daily (administered alone or as part of an acetaminophen/opioid combination). Ironically, in patients with nonalcoholic liver disease, acetaminophen taken in recommended doses, may be the safest analgesic/antipyretic.

℞ ACETAMINOPHEN OVERDOSAGE

Treatment includes gastric lavage, supportive measures, and oral administration of activated charcoal or cholestyramine to prevent absorption of residual drug. Neither of these agents appears to be effective if given >30 min after acetaminophen ingestion; if they are used, the stomach lavage should be done before other agents are administered orally. The chances of possible-, probable-, and high-risk hepatotoxicity can be derived from a nomogram plot **(Fig. 299-1)**, readily available in emergency departments, of acetaminophen plasma levels as a function of hours after ingestion. In patients with high acetaminophen blood levels (>200 mg/mL measured at 4 h or >100 mg/mL at 8 h after ingestion), the administration of sulfhydryl compounds (e.g., cysteamine, cysteine, or N-acetylcysteine) reduces the severity of hepatic necrosis. These agents appear to act by providing a reservoir of sulfhydryl groups to bind the toxic metabolites or by stimulating synthesis and repletion of hepatic glutathione. Therapy should be begun within 8 h of ingestion but may be effective even if given as late as 24–36 h after overdose. Later administration of sulfhydryl compounds is of uncertain value. Routine use of N-acetylcysteine has substantially reduced the occurrence of fatal acetaminophen hepatotoxicity. When given orally, N-acetylcysteine is diluted to yield a 5% solution. A loading dose of 140 mg/kg is given, followed by 70 mg/kg every 4 h for 15–20 doses. Whenever a patient with potential acetaminophen hepatotoxicity is encountered, a local poison control center should be contacted. Treatment can be stopped when plasma acetaminophen levels indicate that the risk of liver damage is low. If signs of hepatic failure (e.g., progressive jaundice, coagulopathy,

confusion) occur despite N-acetylcysteine therapy for acetaminophen hepatotoxicity, liver transplantation may be the only option. Preliminary data suggest that early arterial blood lactate levels among such patients with acute liver failure may distinguish patients highly likely to require liver transplantation (lactate levels > 3.5 mmol/L) from those likely to survive without liver replacement.

Survivors of acute acetaminophen overdose usually have no evidence of hepatic sequelae. In a few patients, prolonged or repeated administration of acetaminophen in therapeutic doses appears to have led to the development of chronic hepatitis and cirrhosis.

HALOTHANE HEPATOTOXICITY (IDIOSYNCRATIC REACTION)

Although, currently, halothane anesthesia is administered in only rare situations, halothane hepatotoxicity was one of the prototypical, and most intensively studied, examples of idiosyncratic drug hepatotoxicity. Administration of halothane, a nonexplosive fluorinated hydrocarbon anesthetic agent that is structurally similar to chloroform, results in severe hepatic necrosis in a small number of individuals, many of whom have previously been exposed to this agent. The failure to produce similar hepatic lesions reliably in animals, the rarity of hepatic impairment in human beings, and the delayed appearance of hepatic injury suggest that halothane is not a direct hepatotoxin but rather a sensitizing agent; however, manifestations of hypersensitivity are seen in <25% of cases. A genetic predisposition leading to an idiosyncratic metabolic reactivity has been postulated and appears to be the most likely mechanism of halothane hepatotoxicity. Adults (rather than children), obese people, and women appear to be particularly susceptible. Fever, moderate leukocytosis, and eosinophilia may occur in the first week following halothane administration. Jaundice is usually noted 7–10 days after exposure but may occur earlier in previously exposed patients. Nausea and vomiting may precede the onset of jaundice. Hepatomegaly is often mild, but liver tenderness is common, and serum aminotransferase levels are elevated. The pathologic changes at autopsy are indistinguishable from massive hepatic necrosis resulting from viral hepatitis. The case-fatality rate of halothane hepatitis is not known but may vary from 20–40% in cases with severe liver involvement. Patients in whom unexplained spiking fever, especially delayed fever, or jaundice develops after halothane anesthesia should not receive this agent again. Because cross-reactions between halothane and methoxyflurane have been reported, the latter agent should not be used after halothane reactions. Later-generation halogenated hydrocarbon anesthetics, which have supplanted halothane except in rare instances (e.g., certain types of thoracic surgery), are felt to be associated with a lower risk of hepatotoxicity.

METHYLDOPA HEPATOTOXICITY (TOXIC AND IDIOSYNCRATIC REACTION)

Minor alterations in liver tests are reported in ~5% of patients treated with this antihypertensive agent. These trivial abnormalities typically resolve despite continued drug administration. In <1% of patients, acute liver injury resembling viral or chronic hepatitis or, rarely, a cholestatic reaction is seen 1–20 weeks after methyldopa is started. In 50% of cases the interval is <4 weeks. A prodrome of fever, anorexia, and malaise may be noted for a few days before the onset of jaundice. Rash, lymphadenopathy, arthralgia, and eosinophilia are rare. Serologic markers of autoimmunity are detected infrequently, and <5% of patients have a Coombs-positive hemolytic anemia. In ~15% of patients with methyldopa hepatotoxicity, the clinical, biochemical, and histologic features are those of moderate to severe chronic hepatitis, with or without bridging necrosis and macronodular cirrhosis. With discontinuation of the drug, the disorder usually resolves. Although methyldopa is currently used infrequently, its hepatotoxicity is very well characterized. Among the currently popular antihypertensive agents, angiotensin-converting enzyme (ACE) inhibitors, such as captopril and enalapril, have been blamed, albeit rarely, for hepatotoxicity (primarily cholestasis and cholestatic hepatitis, but also hepatocellular injury). Angiotensin-II receptor antagonists, such as losartan, are unlikely hepatotoxins, although rare reports of liver injury in their recipients have appeared.

ISONIAZID HEPATOTOXICITY (TOXIC AND IDIOSYNCRATIC REACTION)

In ~10% of adults treated with the antituberculosis agent isoniazid, elevated serum aminotransferase levels develop during the first few weeks of therapy; this appears to represent an adaptive response to a toxic metabolite of the drug. Whether or not isoniazid is continued, these values (usually <200 units) return to normal in a few weeks. In ~1% of treated patients, an illness develops that is indistinguishable from viral hepatitis; approximately half of these cases occur within the first 2 months of treatment, while in the remainder, clinical disease may be delayed for many months. Liver biopsy reveals morphologic changes similar to those of viral hepatitis or bridging hepatic necrosis. The disease may be severe, with a case-fatality rate of 10%. Important liver injury appears to be age-related, increasing substantially after age 35; the highest frequency is in patients over age 50, the lowest under the age of 20. Even for patients >50 years monitored carefully during therapy, hepatotoxicity occurs in only ~2%, well below the risk estimate derived from earlier experiences. Isoniazid hepatotoxicity is enhanced by alcohol, rifampin, and pyrazinamide. Fever, rash, eosinophilia, and other manifestations of drug allergy are distinctly unusual. A reactive metabolite of acetylhydrazine, a metabolite of isoniazid, may be responsible for liver injury, and patients who are rapid acetylators would be more prone to such injury. Counterintuitively, in some reports, the opposite is true; slow acetylators are more likely to experience hepatotoxicity and more severe hepatotoxicity than rapid acetylators. Contrary to past reports, more recent studies suggest that hepatotoxicity due to isoniazid as well as to combination antituberculous therapy that includes isoniazid is more likely in patients with underlying chronic hepatitis B. A picture resembling chronic hepatitis has been observed in a few patients. Careful liver-test monitoring is advisable in patients being treated with isoniazid.

SODIUM VALPROATE HEPATOTOXICITY (TOXIC AND IDIOSYNCRATIC REACTION)

Sodium valproate, an anticonvulsant useful in the treatment of petit mal and other seizure disorders, has been associated with the development of severe hepatic toxicity and, rarely, fatalities, predominantly in children but also in adults. Asymptomatic elevations of serum aminotransferase levels have been recognized in as many as 45% of treated patients. These "adaptive" changes, however, appear to have no clinical importance, for major hepatotoxicity is not seen in the majority of patients despite continuation of drug therapy. In those rare patients in whom jaundice, encephalopathy, and evidence of hepatic failure are found, examination of liver tissue reveals microvesicular fat and bridging hepatic necrosis, predominantly in the centrilobular zone. Bile duct injury may also be apparent. Most likely, sodium valproate is not directly hepatotoxic, but its metabolite, 4-pentenoic acid, may be responsible for hepatic injury. Valproate hepatotoxicity is more common in persons with mitochondrial enzyme deficiencies and may be ameliorated by IV administration of carnitine, which valproate therapy can deplete.

PHENYTOIN HEPATOTOXICITY (IDIOSYNCRATIC REACTION)

Phenytoin, formerly diphenylhydantoin, a mainstay in the treatment of seizure disorders, has been associated in rare instances with the development of severe hepatitis-like liver injury leading to fulminant hepatic failure. In many patients the hepatitis is associated with striking fever, lymphadenopathy, rash (Stevens-Johnson syndrome or exfoliative dermatitis), leukocytosis, and eosinophilia, suggesting an immunologically mediated hypersensitivity mechanism. Despite these observations, evidence suggests that metabolic idiosyncrasy may be responsible for hepatic injury. In the liver, phenytoin is converted by the cytochrome P450 system to metabolites, which include the highly reactive electrophilic arene oxides. These metabolites are normally metabolized further by epoxide hydrolases. A defect (genetic or acquired) in epoxide hydrolase activity could permit covalent binding of arene oxides to hepatic macromolecules, thereby leading to hepatic injury. Regardless of the mechanism, hepatic injury is usually manifest within the first 2 months after beginning phenytoin therapy. With the exception of an abundance of eosinophils in the liver, the clinical, biochem-

ical, and histologic picture resembles that of viral hepatitis. In rare instances, bile duct injury may be the salient feature of phenytoin hepatotoxicity, with striking features of intrahepatic cholestasis. Asymptomatic elevations of aminotransferase and alkaline phosphatase levels have been observed in a sizable proportion of patients receiving long-term phenytoin therapy. These liver changes are believed by some authorities to represent the potent hepatic enzyme–inducing properties of phenytoin and are accompanied histologically by swelling of hepatocytes in the absence of necroinflammatory activity or evidence of chronic liver disease.

AMIODARONE HEPATOTOXICITY (TOXIC AND IDIOSYNCRATIC REACTION)

Therapy with this potent antiarrhythmic drug is accompanied in 15–50% of patients by modest elevations of serum aminotransferase levels that may remain stable or diminish despite continuation of the drug. Such abnormalities may appear days to many months after beginning therapy. A proportion of those with elevated aminotransferase levels have detectable hepatomegaly, and clinically important liver disease develops in <5% of patients. Features that represent a direct effect of the drug on the liver and that are common to the majority of long-term recipients are ultrastructural phospholipidosis, unaccompanied by clinical liver disease, and interference with hepatic mixed-function oxidase metabolism of other drugs. The cationic amphiphilic drug and its major metabolite desethylamiodarone accumulate in hepatocyte lysosomes and mitochondria and in bile duct epithelium. The relatively common elevations in aminotransferase levels are also considered a predictable, dose-dependent, direct hepatotoxic effect. On the other hand, in the rare patient with clinically apparent, symptomatic liver disease, liver injury resembling that seen in alcoholic liver disease is observed. The so-called pseudoalcoholic liver injury can range from steatosis, to alcoholic hepatitis-like neutrophilic infiltration and Mallory's hyaline, to cirrhosis. Electron-microscopic demonstration of phospholipid-laden lysosomal lamellar bodies can help to distinguish amiodarone hepatotoxicity from typical alcoholic hepatitis. This category of liver injury appears to be a metabolic idiosyncrasy that allows hepatotoxic metabolites to be generated. Rarely, an acute idiosyncratic hepatocellular injury resembling viral hepatitis or cholestatic hepatitis occurs. Hepatic granulomas have occasionally been observed. Because amiodarone has a long half-life, liver injury may persist for months after the drug is stopped.

ERYTHROMYCIN HEPATOTOXICITY (CHOLESTATIC IDIOSYNCRATIC REACTION)

The most important adverse effect associated with erythromycin, more common in children than adults, is the infrequent occurrence of a cholestatic reaction. Although most of these reactions have been associated with erythromycin estolate, other erythromycins may also be responsible. The reaction usually begins during the first 2 or 3 weeks of therapy and includes nausea, vomiting, fever, right upper quadrant abdominal pain, jaundice, leukocytosis, and moderately elevated aminotransferase levels. The clinical picture can resemble acute cholecystitis or bacterial cholangitis. Liver biopsy reveals variable cholestasis; portal inflammation comprising lymphocytes, polymorphonuclear leukocytes, and eosinophils; and scattered foci of hepatocyte necrosis. Symptoms and laboratory findings usually subside within a few days of drug withdrawal, and evidence of chronic liver disease has not been found on follow-up. The precise mechanism remains ill-defined.

ORAL CONTRACEPTIVE HEPATOTOXICITY (CHOLESTATIC REACTION)

The administration of oral contraceptive combinations of estrogenic and progestational steroids leads to intrahepatic cholestasis with pruritus and jaundice in a small number of patients weeks to months after taking these agents. Especially susceptible seem to be patients with recurrent idiopathic jaundice of pregnancy, severe pruritus of pregnancy, or a family history of these disorders. With the exception of liver biochemical tests, laboratory studies are normal, and extrahepatic manifestations of hypersensitivity are absent. Liver biopsy reveals cholestasis with bile plugs in dilated canaliculi and striking bilirubin staining of liver cells. In contrast to chlorpromazine-induced cholestasis, portal inflammation is absent. The lesion is reversible on withdrawal of the agent. The two steroid components appear to act synergistically on hepatic function, although the estrogen may be primarily responsible. Oral contraceptives are contraindicated in patients with a history of recurrent jaundice of pregnancy. Primarily benign, but rarely malignant, neoplasms of the liver, hepatic vein occlusion, and peripheral sinusoidal dilatation have also been associated with oral contraceptive therapy. Focal nodular hyperplasia of the liver is not more frequent among users of oral contraceptives.

17,α-ALKYL-SUBSTITUTED ANABOLIC STEROIDS (CHOLESTATIC REACTION)

In the majority of patients receiving these agents, used therapeutically mainly in the treatment of bone marrow failure but used surreptitiously and without medical indication by athletes to improve their performance, mild hepatic dysfunction develops. Impaired excretory function is the predominant defect, but the precise mechanism is uncertain. Jaundice, which appears to be dose-related, develops in only a minority of patients and may be the sole clinical manifestation of hepatotoxicity, although anorexia, nausea, and malaise may occur. Pruritus is not a prominent feature. Serum aminotransferase levels are usually <100 units, and serum alkaline phosphatase levels are normal, mildly elevated, or, in <5% of patients, three or more times the upper limit of normal. Examination of liver tissue reveals cholestasis without inflammation or necrosis. Hepatic sinusoidal dilatation and peliosis hepatis have been found in a few patients. The cholestatic disorder is usually reversible on cessation of treatment, although fatalities have been linked to peliosis. An association with hepatic adenoma and hepatocellular carcinoma has been reported.

TRIMETHOPRIM-SULFAMETHOXAZOLE HEPATOTOXICITY (IDIOSYNCRATIC REACTION)

This antibiotic combination is used routinely for urinary tract infections in immunocompetent persons and for prophylaxis against and therapy of *Pneumocystis carinii* pneumonia in immunosuppressed persons (transplant recipients, patients with AIDS). With its increasing use, its occasional hepatotoxicity is being recognized with growing frequency. Its likelihood is unpredictable, but when it occurs, trimethoprim-sulfamethoxazole hepatotoxicity follows a relatively uniform latency period of several weeks and is often accompanied by eosinophilia, rash, and other features of a hypersensitivity reaction. Biochemically and histologically, acute hepatocellular necrosis predominates, but cholestatic features are quite frequent. Occasionally, cholestasis without necrosis occurs, and very rarely, a severe cholangiolytic pattern of liver injury is observed. In most cases, liver injury is self-limited, but rare fatalities have been recorded. The hepatotoxicity is attributable to the sulfamethoxazole component of the drug and is similar in features to that seen with other sulfonamides; tissue eosinophilia and granulomas may be seen. The risk of trimethoprim-sulfamethoxazole hepatotoxicity is increased in persons with HIV infection.

HMG-COA REDUCTASE INHIBITORS (STATINS) (IDIOSYNCRATIC MIXED HEPATOCELLULAR AND CHOLESTATIC REACTION)

Between 1 and 2% of patients taking lovastatin, simvastatin, pravastatin, fluvastatin, or one of the newer statin drugs for the treatment of hypercholesterolemia experience asymptomatic, reversible elevations (>threefold) of aminotransferase activity. Acute hepatitis-like histologic changes, centrilobular necrosis, and centrilobular cholestasis have been described in several cases. In a larger proportion, minor aminotransferase elevations appear during the first several weeks of therapy. Careful laboratory monitoring can distinguish between patients with minor, transitory changes, who may continue therapy, and those with more profound and sustained abnormalities, who should discontinue therapy. Because clinically meaningful aminotransferase elevations are so rare after statin use, a panel of liver experts recommended to the National Lipid Association's Safety Task Force that liver-test monitoring was not necessary in patients treated with statins and that statin therapy need not be discontinued in patients found to

have asymptomatic isolated aminotransferase elevations during therapy. Statin hepatotoxicity is not increased in patients with chronic hepatitis C or hepatic steatosis, and statins can be used safely in these patients.

TOTAL PARENTERAL NUTRITION (STEATOSIS, CHOLESTASIS)

Total parenteral nutrition (TPN) is often complicated by cholestatic hepatitis attributable to either steatosis, cholestasis, or gallstones (or gallbladder sludge). Steatosis or steatohepatitis may result from the excess carbohydrate calories in these nutritional supplements and is the predominant form of TPN-associated liver disorder in adults. The frequency of this complication has been reduced substantially by the introduction of balanced TPN formulas that rely on lipid as an alternative caloric source. Cholestasis and cholelithiasis, caused by the absence of stimulation of bile flow and secretion resulting from the lack of oral intake, is the predominant form of TPN-associated liver disease in infants, especially in premature neonates. Often, cholestasis in such neonates is multifactorial, contributed to by other factors such as sepsis, hypoxemia, and hypotension; occasionally, TPN-induced cholestasis in neonates culminates in chronic liver disease and liver failure. When TPN-associated liver test abnormalities occur in adults, balancing the TPN formula with more lipid is the intervention of first recourse. In infants with TPN-associated cholestasis, the addition of oral feeding may ameliorate the problem. Therapeutic interventions suggested, but not shown to be of proven benefit, include cholecystokinin, ursodeoxycholic acid, S-adenosyl methionine, and taurine.

"ALTERNATIVE AND COMPLEMENTARY MEDICINES" (IDIOSYNCRATIC HEPATITIS, STEATOSIS)

The misguided popularity of herbal medications that are of scientifically unproven efficacy and that lack prospective safety oversight by regulatory agencies has resulted in occasional instances of hepatotoxicity. Included among the herbal remedies associated with toxic hepatitis are Jin Bu Huan (Chap. 10), xiao-chai-hu-tang, germander, chaparral, senna, mistletoe, skullcap, gentian, comfrey (containing pyrrolizidine alkaloids), Ma huang, bee pollen, valerian root, pennyroyal oil, kava, celandine, Impila (*Callilepsis laureaola*), LipoKinetix, Hyroxycut, and herbal teas. Well characterized are the acute hepatitis-like histologic lesions following Jin Bu Huan use: focal hepatocellular necrosis, mixed mononuclear portal tract infiltration, coagulative necrosis, apoptotic hepatocyte degeneration, tissue eosinophilia, and microvesicular steatosis. Megadoses of vitamin A can injure the liver, as can pyrrolizidine alkaloids, which often contaminate Chinese herbal preparations and can cause a venoocclusive injury leading to sinusoidal hepatic vein obstruction. Because some alternative medicines induce toxicity via active metabolites, alcohol and drugs that stimulate cytochrome P450 enzymes may enhance the toxicity of some of these products. Conversely, some alternative medicines also stimulate cytochrome P450 and may result in or amplify the toxicity of recognized drug hepatotoxins. Given the widespread use of such poorly defined herbal preparations, hepatotoxicity is likely to be encountered with increasing frequency; therefore, a drug history in patients with acute and chronic liver disease should include use of "alternative medicines" and other nonprescription preparations sold in so-called health food stores.

HIGHLY ACTIVE ANTIRETROVIRAL THERAPY (HAART) FOR HIV INFECTION (MITOCHONDRIAL TOXIC, IDIOSYNCRATIC, STEATOSIS; HEPATOCELLULAR, CHOLESTATIC, AND MIXED)

The recognition of drug hepatotoxicity in persons with HIV infection is complicated in this population by the many alternative causes of liver injury (chronic viral hepatitis, fatty infiltration, infiltrative disorders, mycobacterial infection, etc.), but drug hepatotoxicity associated with HAART is an emerging and common type of liver injury in HIV-infected persons (Chap. 182). Although no one antiviral agent is recognized as a potent hepatotoxin, combination regimens including reverse transcriptase and protease inhibitors cause hepatotoxicity in

~10% of treated patients. Implicated most frequently are combinations including nucleoside analogue reverse transcriptase inhibitors zidovudine, didanosine, and, to a lesser extent, stavudine; protease inhibitors ritonavir and indinavir (and amprenivir when used together with ritonavir); and nonnucleoside reverse transcriptase inhibitors nevirapine and, to a lesser extent, efavirenz. These drugs cause predominantly hepatocellular injury but cholestatic injury as well, and prolonged (>6 months) use of reverse transcriptase inhibitors has been associated with mitochondrial injury, steatosis, and lactic acidosis. Indirect hyperbilirubinemia, resulting from direct inhibition of bilirubin-conjugating activity by UDP-glucuronosyltransferase, usually without elevation of aminotransferase or alkaline phosphatase activities, occurs in ~10% of patients treated with the protease inhibitor indinavir. Distinguishing the impact of HAART hepatotoxicity in patients with HIV and hepatitis virus co-infection is made challenging by the following: (1) both chronic hepatitis B and hepatitis C can affect the natural history of HIV infection and the response to HAART, and (2) HAART can have an impact on chronic viral hepatitis. For example, immunologic reconstitution with HAART can result in immunologically mediated liver-cell injury in patients with chronic hepatitis B co-infection if treatment with an antiviral agent for hepatitis B, e.g., the nucleoside analogue lamivudine, is withdrawn or if nucleoside analogue resistance emerges. Infection with HIV, especially with low CD4+ T cell counts, has been reported to increase the rate of hepatic fibrosis associated with chronic hepatitis C, and HAART therapy can increase levels of serum aminotransferases and hepatitis C virus RNA in patients with hepatitis C co-infection.

ACKNOWLEDGMENT
Kurt J. Isselbacher, MD, contributed to this chapter in previous editions of Harrison's.

FURTHER READINGS

BISSELL DM et al: Drug-induced liver injury: Mechanisms and test systems. Hepatology 33:1009, 2001

FARRELL GC, LIDDLE C (guest eds.): Hepatotoxicity in the twenty-first century. Semin Liver Dis 22:109, 2002

KAPLOWITZ N, DELEVE LD (eds): *Drug-Induced Liver Disease.* New York, Marcel Dekker, 2002

LEE WM: Drug-induced hepatotoxicity. N Engl J Med 349:474, 2003

NAVARRO VJ, SENIOR JR: Drug-related hepatotoxicity. N Engl J Med 354:731, 2006

NOLAN CM et al: Hepatotoxicity associated with isoniazid preventive therapy. JAMA 281:1014, 1999

SCHMIDT LE et al: Acute versus chronic alcohol consumption in acetaminophen-induced hepatotoxicity. Hepatology 35:876, 2002

SULKOWSKI MS et al: Hepatotoxicity associated with antiretroviral therapy in adults infected with human immunodeficiency virus and the role of hepatitis C or B virus infection. JAMA 283:74, 2000

ZHANG J et al: Modulation of acetaminophen-induced hepatotoxicity by the xenobiotic receptor CAR. Science 298:422, 2002

ZIMMERMAN HJ et al: Drug-induced liver disease, in *Schiff's Diseases of the Liver*, 8th ed, E Schiff et al (eds). Philadelphia, Lippincott-Raven, 1999, p 973

300 Chronic Hepatitis
Jules L. Dienstag

Chronic hepatitis represents a series of liver disorders of varying causes and severity in which hepatic inflammation and necrosis continue for at least 6 months. Milder forms are nonprogressive or only slowly progressive, while more severe forms may be associated with scarring and architectural reorganization, which, when advanced, lead ultimately to cirrhosis. Several categories of chronic hepatitis have been recognized. These include chronic viral hepatitis, drug-induced chronic hepatitis (Chap. 299), and autoimmune chronic hepatitis. In many cases, clinical and laboratory features are insufficient to allow assignment into one of these three categories; these "idiopathic" cases are also believed to represent autoimmune chronic hepatitis. Finally, clinical and laboratory features of chronic hepatitis are observed occasionally in patients with such hereditary/metabolic disorders as Wilson's disease (copper overload) and even occasionally in patients with alcoholic liver injury (Chap. 301). Although all types of chronic hepatitis share certain clinical, laboratory, and histopathologic features, chronic viral and chronic autoimmune hepatitis are sufficiently distinct to merit separate discussions. For discussion of acute hepatitis, see Chap. 298.

CLASSIFICATION OF CHRONIC HEPATITIS

Common to all forms of chronic hepatitis are histopathologic distinctions based on localization and extent of liver injury. These vary from the milder forms, previously labeled *chronic persistent hepatitis* and *chronic lobular hepatitis*, to the more severe form, formerly called *chronic active hepatitis*. When first defined, these designations were felt to have prognostic implications, which have been challenged by more recent observations. Categorization of chronic hepatitis based primarily on histopathologic features has been replaced by a more informative classification based on a combination of clinical, serologic, and histologic variables. Classification of chronic hepatitis is based on (1) its *cause*; (2) its histologic activity, or *grade*; and (3) its degree of progression, or *stage*. Thus, neither clinical features alone nor histologic features—requiring liver biopsy—alone are sufficient to characterize and distinguish among the several categories of chronic hepatitis.

CLASSIFICATION BY CAUSE

Clinical and serologic features allow the establishment of a diagnosis of *chronic viral hepatitis*, caused by hepatitis B, hepatitis B plus D, or hepatitis C; *autoimmune hepatitis*, including several subcategories, I and II (perhaps III), based on serologic distinctions; *drug-associated chronic hepatitis*; and a category of unknown cause, or *cryptogenic chronic hepatitis* (Table 300-1). These are addressed in more detail below.

CLASSIFICATION BY GRADE

Grade, a histologic assessment of necroinflammatory activity, is based on examination of the liver biopsy. An assessment of important histologic features includes the degree of *periportal necrosis* and the disruption of the limiting plate of periportal hepatocytes by inflammatory cells (so-called *piecemeal necrosis* or *interface hepatitis*); the degree of confluent necrosis that links or forms bridges between vascular structures—between portal tract and portal tract or even more important bridges between portal tract and central vein—referred to as *bridging necrosis*; the degree of hepatocyte degeneration and focal necrosis within the lobule; and the degree of *portal inflammation*. Several scoring systems that take these histologic features into account have been devised, and the most popular are the histologic activity index (HAI) and the METAVIR score (Table 300-2). Based on the presence and degree of these features of histologic activity, chronic hepatitis can be graded as mild, moderate, or severe.

CLASSIFICATION BY STAGE

The stage of chronic hepatitis, which reflects the level of progression of the disease, is based on the degree of hepatic fibrosis. When fibrosis is so extensive that fibrous septa surround parenchymal nodules and alter the

TABLE 300-1 CLINICAL AND LABORATORY FEATURES OF CHRONIC HEPATITIS

Type of Hepatitis	Diagnostic Test(s)	Autoantibodies	Therapy
Chronic hepatitis B	HBsAg, IgG anti-HBc, HBeAg, HBV DNA	Uncommon	IFN-α, PEG IFN-α, lamivudine, adefovir, entecavir
Chronic hepatitis C	Anti-HCV, HCV RNA	Anti-LKM1[a]	PEG IFN-α plus ribavirin
Chronic hepatitis D	Anti-HDV, HDV RNA, HBsAg, IgG anti-HBc	Anti-LKM3	IFN-α, PEG IFN-α[b]
Autoimmune hepatitis	ANA[c] (homogeneous), anti-LKM1(±), Hyper-globulinemia	ANA, anti-LKM1, anti-SLA[d]	Prednisone, azathioprine
Drug-associated	—	Uncommon	Withdraw drug
Cryptogenic	All negative	None	Prednisone (?), azathioprine (?)

[a]Antibodies to liver-kidney microsomes type 1 (autoimmune hepatitis type II and some cases of hepatitis C).
[b]Clinical trials suggest benefit of IFN-α therapy or PEG IFN-α.
[c]Antinuclear antibody (autoimmune hepatitis type I).
[d]Antibodies to soluble liver antigen (autoimmune hepatitis type III).
Note: HBc, hepatitis B core; HBeAg, hepatitis B e antigen; HBsAg, hepatitis B surface antigen; HBV, hepatitis B virus; HCV, hepatitis C virus; HDV, hepatitis D virus; IFN-α, interferon α; IgG, immunoglobulin G; LKM, liver-kidney microsome; PEG-IFN-α, pegylated interferon α; SLA, soluble liver antigen.

normal architecture of the liver lobule, the histologic lesion is defined as *cirrhosis*. Staging is based on the degree of fibrosis as categorized on a numerical scale from 0–6 (HAI) or 0–4 (METAVIR) (Table 300-2).

CHRONIC VIRAL HEPATITIS

Both the enterically transmitted forms of viral hepatitis, hepatitis A and E, are self-limited and do not cause chronic hepatitis (rare reports notwithstanding in which acute hepatitis A serves as a trigger for the onset of autoimmune hepatitis in genetically susceptible patients). In contrast, the entire clinicopathologic spectrum of chronic hepatitis occurs in patients with chronic viral hepatitis B and C as well as in patients with chronic hepatitis D superimposed on chronic hepatitis B.

CHRONIC HEPATITIS B

The likelihood of chronicity after acute hepatitis B varies as a function of age. Infection at birth is associated with clinically silent acute infection but a 90% chance of chronic infection, while infection in young adulthood in immunocompetent persons is typically associated with clinically apparent acute hepatitis but a risk of chronicity of only approximately 1%. Most cases of chronic hepatitis B among adults, however, occur in patients who never had a recognized episode of clinically apparent viral hepatitis. The degree of liver injury (grade) in patients with chronic hepatitis B is variable, ranging from none in inactive carriers to mild to moderate to severe. Among adults with chronic hepatitis B, histologic features are of prognostic importance. In one long-term study of patients with chronic hepatitis B, investigators found a 5-year survival rate of 97% for patients with mild chronic hepatitis, 86% for patients with moderate to severe chronic hepatitis, and only 55% for patients with chronic hepatitis and postnecrotic cirrhosis. The 15-year survival in these cohorts was 77, 66, and 40%, respectively. On the other hand, more re-

cent observations do not allow us to be so sanguine about the prognosis in patients with mild chronic hepatitis; among such patients followed for 1–13 years, progression to more severe chronic hepatitis and cirrhosis has been observed in more than a quarter of cases.

More important to consider than histology alone in patients with chronic hepatitis B is the degree of hepatitis B virus (HBV) replication. As reviewed in Chap. 298, chronic HBV infection can occur in the presence or absence of serum hepatitis B e antigen (HBeAg), and generally, for both HBeAg-reactive and HBeAg-negative chronic hepatitis B, the level of HBV DNA correlates with the level of liver injury and risk of progression. In *HBeAg-reactive chronic hepatitis B*, two phases have been recognized based on the relative level of HBV replication. The relatively *replicative phase* is characterized by the presence in the serum of HBeAg and HBV DNA levels well in excess of 10^5–10^6 virions/mL, by the presence in the liver of detectable intrahepatocyte nucleocapsid antigens [primarily hepatitis B core antigen (HBcAg)], by high infectivity, and by accompanying liver injury. In contrast, the relatively *nonreplicative phase* is

TABLE 300-2 HISTOLOGIC GRADING AND STAGING IN CHRONIC HEPATITIS

Histologic Feature	Histologic Activity Index (HAI)[a]		METAVIR[b]	
	Severity	Score	Severity	Score
Necroinflammatory Activity (grade)				
Perioportal necrosis, including piecemeal necrosis (PN) and/or bridging necrosis (BN)	None	0	None	0
	Mild	1	Mild	1
	Mild/Moderate	2	Moderate	2
	Moderate	3	Severe	3
	Severe	4		
			Bridging necrosis	Yes
				No
Intralobular Confluent necrosis	—None	0	None or mild	0
	—Focal	1	Moderate	1
	—Zone 3 some	2	Severe	2
	—Zone 3 most	3		
	—Zone 3 + BN few	4		
	—Zone 3 + BN multiple	5		
	—Panacinar/multiacinar	6		
Focal	—None	0		
	—≤1 Focus/10× field	1		
	—2–4 Foci/10× field	2		
	—5–10 Foci/10× field	3		
	—>10 Foci/10× field	4		
Portal inflammation	None	0		
	Mild	1		
	Moderate	3		
	Moderate/marked	3		
	Marked	4		
	Total	0–18		A0–A3[c]
Fibrosis (stage)				
None		0		F0
Portal fibrosis—some		1		F1
Portal fibrosis—most		2		F1
Bridging fibrosis—few		3		F2
Bridging fibrosis—many		4		F3
Incomplete cirrhosis		5		F4
Cirrhosis		6		F4
	Total	6		4

[a]J Hepatol 22:696, 1995.
[b]Hepatology 24:289, 1996.
[c]Necroinflammatory grade: A0 = none; A1 = mild; A2 = moderate; A3 = severe.

characterized by the absence of the conventional serum marker of HBV replication (HBeAg), the appearance of anti-HBe, levels of HBV DNA below a threshold of ~10^3 virions/mL, the absence of intrahepatocytic HBcAg, limited infectivity, and minimal liver injury. Those patients in the replicative phase tend to have more severe chronic hepatitis, while those in the nonreplicative phase tend to have minimal or mild chronic hepatitis or to be inactive hepatitis B carriers; however, distinctions in HBV replication and in histologic category do not always coincide. The likelihood in a patient with HBeAg-reactive chronic hepatitis B of converting spontaneously from relatively replicative to nonreplicative infection is approximately 10–15% per year. In patients with HBeAg-reactive chronic HBV infection, especially when acquired at birth or in early childhood, as recognized commonly in Asian countries, a dichotomy is common between very high levels of HBV replication and negligible levels of liver injury. Yet despite the relatively immediate, apparently benign nature of liver disease for many decades in this population, patients with childhood-acquired HBV infection are the ones at ultimately increased risk later in life of cirrhosis and hepatocellular carcinoma (HCC) (Chap. 88). A discussion of the pathogenesis of liver injury in patients with chronic hepatitis B appears in Chap. 298.

HBeAg-negative chronic hepatitis B, i.e., chronic HBV infection with active virus replication, readily detectable HBV DNA but without HBeAg (anti-HBe-reactive), is more common than HBeAg-reactive chronic hepatitis B in Mediterranean and European countries and in Asia (and, correspondingly, in HBV genotypes other than A). Compared to patients with HBeAg-reactive chronic hepatitis B, patients with HBeAg-negative chronic hepatitis B have levels of HBV DNA that are several orders of magnitude lower (no more than 10^5–10^6 virions/mL) than those observed in the HBeAg-reactive subset. Most such cases represent precore or core-promoter mutations acquired late in the natural history of the disease (mostly early-life onset; age range 40–55 years, older than that for HBeAg-reactive chronic hepatitis B); these mutations prevent translation of HBeAg from the precore component of the HBV genome (precore mutants) or are characterized by down-regulated transcription of precore mRNA (core-promoter mutants; Chap. 298). Although their levels of HBV DNA tend to be lower than among patients with HBeAg-reactive chronic hepatitis B, patients with HBeAg-negative chronic hepatitis B can have progressive liver injury (complicated by cirrhosis and HCC) and experience episodic reactivation of liver disease reflected in fluctuating levels of aminotransferase activity ("flares"). The biochemical and histologic activity of HBeAg-negative disease tends to correlate closely with levels of HBV replication, unlike the case mentioned above of Asian patients with HBeAg-reactive chronic hepatitis B during the early decades of their HBV infection. An important point worth reiterating is the observation that the level of HBV replication is the most important risk factor for the ultimate development of cirrhosis and HCC in both HBeAg-reactive and HBeAg-negative patients. Although levels of HBV DNA are lower and more readily suppressed to undetectable levels in HBeAg-negative (compared to HBeAg-reactive) chronic hepatitis B, achieving sustained responses that permit discontinuation of antiviral therapy is less likely in HBeAg-negative patients (see below). Inactive carriers are patients with circulating hepatitis B surface antigen (HBsAg), normal serum aminotransferase levels, undetectable HBeAg, and levels of HBV DNA that are either undetectable or present at levels ≤10^3 virions/mL. This serologic profile can occur not only in inactive carriers but also in patients with HBeAg-negative chronic hepatitis B during periods of relative inactivity; distinguishing between the two requires sequential biochemical and virologic monitoring over many months.

The spectrum of *clinical features* of chronic hepatitis B is broad, ranging from asymptomatic infection to debilitating disease or even end-stage, fatal hepatic failure. As noted above, the onset of the disease tends to be insidious in most patients, with the exception of the very few in whom chronic disease follows failure of resolution of clinically apparent acute hepatitis B. The clinical and laboratory features associated with progression from acute to chronic hepatitis B are discussed in Chap. 298.

Fatigue is a common symptom, and persistent or intermittent *jaundice* is a common feature in severe or advanced cases. Intermittent deepening of jaundice and recurrence of malaise and anorexia, as well as worsening fatigue, are reminiscent of acute hepatitis; such exacerbations may occur spontaneously, often coinciding with evidence of virologic reactivation; may lead to progressive liver injury; and, when superimposed on well-established cirrhosis, may cause hepatic decompensation. Complications of cirrhosis occur in end-stage chronic hepatitis and include ascites, edema, bleeding gastroesophageal varices, hepatic encephalopathy, coagulopathy, or hypersplenism. Occasionally these complications bring the patient to initial clinical attention. Extrahepatic complications of chronic hepatitis B, similar to those seen during the prodromal phase of acute hepatitis B, are associated with deposition of circulating hepatitis B antigen–antibody immune complexes. These include arthralgias and arthritis, which are common, and the more rare purpuric cutaneous lesions (leukocytoclastic vasculitis), immune-complex glomerulonephritis, and generalized vasculitis (polyarteritis nodosa) (Chaps. 298 and 319).

Laboratory features of chronic hepatitis B do not distinguish adequately between histologically mild and severe hepatitis. Aminotransferase elevations tend to be modest for chronic hepatitis B but may fluctuate in the range of 100–1,000 units. As is true for acute viral hepatitis B, alanine aminotransferase (ALT) tends to be more elevated than aspartate aminotransferase (AST); however, once cirrhosis is established, AST tends to exceed ALT. Levels of alkaline phosphatase activity tend to be normal or only marginally elevated. In severe cases, moderate elevations in serum bilirubin [51.3–171 μmol/L (3–10 mg/dL)] occur. Hypoalbuminemia and prolongation of the prothrombin time occur in severe or end-stage cases. Hyperglobulinemia and detectable circulating autoantibodies are distinctly absent in chronic hepatitis B (in contrast to autoimmune hepatitis). Viral markers of chronic HBV infection are discussed in Chap. 298.

CHRONIC HEPATITIS B

Although progression to cirrhosis is more likely in severe than in mild or moderate chronic hepatitis B, all forms of chronic hepatitis B can be progressive, and progression occurs primarily in patients with active HBV replication. Moreover, in populations of patients with chronic hepatitis B who are at risk for HCC (Chap. 88), the risk is highest for those with continued, high-level HBV replication. Therefore, management of chronic hepatitis B is directed at suppressing the level of virus replication. To date, five drugs have been approved for treatment of chronic hepatitis B: injectable interferon (INF) α; pegylated interferon [long-acting IFN bound to polyethylene glycol (PEG), known as *PEG IFN*]; and the oral agents lamivudine, adefovir dipivoxil, and entecavir. Several other drugs, including emtricitabine, tenofovir, telbivudine, pradefovir, and clevudine, are in the process of efficacy testing in clinical trials.

Antiviral therapy for hepatitis B has evolved rapidly since the mid-1990s, as has the sensitivity of tests for HBV DNA. When IFN and lamivudine were evaluated in clinical trials, HBV DNA was measured by insensitive hybridization assays with detection thresholds of 10^5–10^6 virions/mL; when adefovir, entecavir, and PEG IFN were studied in clinical trials, HBV DNA was measured by sensitive amplification assays (polymerase chain reaction [PCR]) with detection thresholds of 10^2–10^3 virions/mL. Recognition of these distinctions is helpful when comparing results of clinical trials that established the efficacy of these therapies (reviewed below in chronological order of publication of these efficacy trials).

INTERFERON IFN-α was the first approved therapy for chronic hepatitis B. For immunocompetent adults with HBeAg-reactive chronic hepatitis B (who tend to have high-level HBV DNA [>10^5–10^6 virions/mL] and histologic evidence of chronic hepatitis on liver biopsy), a 16-week course of IFN given subcutaneously at a daily dose of 5 million units, or three times a week at a dose of 10 million units, results in a loss of HBeAg and hybridization-detectable HBV DNA (i.e., a reduction to levels below 10^5–10^6 virions/mL) in ~30% of patients, with a concomitant improvement in liver histology. Seroconversion from HBeAg to anti-HBe occurs in approximately 20%, and, in early trials, approximately 8% lost HBsAg. Successful INF therapy and seroconversion are often accompanied by an acute hepatitis-like elevation in aminotransferase activity, which has been postulated to result from enhanced cytolytic T cell clearance of HBV-infected hepatocytes. Relapse after successful therapy is rare (1 or 2%). The likelihood of responding to IFN is higher in patients with lower levels of HBV DNA and substantial elevations of ALT. Although children can respond as well as adults, IFN therapy has not been effective in very young children infected at birth. Similarly, IFN therapy has not been effective in immunosuppressed persons, Asian patients with minimal-to-mild ALT elevations, or patients with decompensated chronic hepatitis B (in whom such therapy can actually be detrimental, sometimes precipitating decompensation, often associated with severe adverse effects). Among patients with HBeAg loss during therapy, long-term follow-up has demonstrated that 80% experience eventual loss of HBsAg, i.e., all serologic markers of infection, and normalization of ALT over a 9-year posttreatment period. In addition, improved long-term and complication-free survival as well as a reduction in the frequency of HCC have been documented among interferon responders, supporting the conclusion that successful interferon therapy improves the natural history of chronic hepatitis B.

Retreatment of IFN nonresponders with another course of IFN may enhance response rates somewhat; currently, however, most would opt to address IFN nonresponders by offering them one of the newer, oral therapies.

Initial trials of brief-duration IFN therapy in patients with *HBeAg-negative chronic hepatitis B* were disappointing, suppressing HBV replication transiently during therapy but almost never resulting in sustained antiviral responses. In subsequent IFN trials among patients with HBeAg-negative chronic hepatitis B, however, more protracted courses, lasting up to a year and a half, have been reported to result in sustained remissions, with suppressed HBV DNA and aminotransferase activity, in ~20%.

Complications of IFN therapy include systemic "flu-like" symptoms; marrow suppression; emotional lability (irritability commonly, depression/anxiety less frequently); autoimmune reactions (especially autoimmune thyroiditis); and miscellaneous side effects such as alopecia, rashes, diarrhea, and numbness and tingling of the extremities. With the possible exception of autoimmune thyroiditis, all these side effects are reversible upon dose lowering or cessation of therapy.

Whether or not IFN remains competitive with the newer generation of antivirals, it did represent the first successful antiviral approach, and it set the standard against which subsequent drugs are measured—the achievement of durable virologic, serologic, biochemical, and histologic responses; consolidation of virologic and biochemical benefit in the ensuing years after therapy; and improvement in the natural history of chronic hepatitis B. For all practical purposes, standard IFN has been supplanted by long-acting PEG IFN (see below).

LAMIVUDINE The first of the nucleoside analogues to be approved, the dideoxynucleoside lamivudine, inhibits reverse transcriptase activity of both HIV and HBV and is a potent and effective agent for patients with chronic hepatitis B. In clinical trials among patients with HBeAg-reactive chronic hepatitis B, lamivudine therapy at daily doses of 100 mg for 48–52 weeks suppressed HBV DNA by a median of approximately 5.5 $\log_{10}$ copies/mL and to undetectable levels, as measured by PCR amplification assays, in approximately 40% of patients. Therapy was associated with HBeAg loss in 32–33%; HBeAg seroconversion (i.e., conversion from HBeAg-reactive to anti-HBe-reactive) in 16–21%; normalization of ALT in 40%–75%; improvement in histology in 50%–60%; retardation in fibrosis in 20–30%; and prevention of progression to cirrhosis. HBeAg responses can occur even in subgroups who are resistant to IFN (e.g., those with high-level HBV DNA) or who failed in the past to respond to it. As is true for IFN therapy of chronic hepatitis B, patients with near-normal ALT activity tend not to experience HBeAg responses (despite suppression of HBV DNA), and those with ALT levels exceeding five times the upper limit of normal can expect 1-year HBeAg seroconversion rates of 50–60%. Generally, HBeAg seroconversions are confined to patients who achieve suppression of HBV DNA to <10^4 genomes/mL. Among patients who undergo HBeAg responses during a yearlong course of therapy and in whom the response is sustained for 4–6 months after cessation of therapy, the response is durable thereafter in the vast majority, >80%; therefore, the achievement of an HBeAg response represents a viable stopping point in therapy. Reduced durability has been reported in some Asian experiences; however, in most western and Asian patient study populations, long-term durability of HBeAg responses is the rule, which, at least in Western patients, is accompanied by a posttreatment

HBsAg seroconversion rate comparable to that seen after IFN-induced HBeAg responses. If HBeAg is unaffected by lamivudine therapy, the current approach is to continue therapy until an HBeAg response occurs, but long-term therapy may be required to suppress HBV replication and, in turn, limit liver injury; HBeAg seroconversions can increase to a level of 50% after 5 years of therapy. Histologic improvement continues to accrue with therapy beyond the first year; after a cumulative course of 3 years of lamivudine therapy, necroinflammatory activity is reduced in the majority of patients, and even cirrhosis has been shown to regress to precirrhotic stages.

Losses of HBsAg have been few during the first year of lamivudine therapy, and this observation had been cited as an advantage of IFN over lamivudine; however, in head-to-head comparisons between standard IFN and lamivudine monotherapy, HBsAg losses were rare in both groups. Trials in which lamivudine and interferon were administered in combination failed to show a benefit of combination therapy over lamivudine monotherapy for either treatment-naïve patients or prior interferon nonresponders.

In patients with *HBeAg-negative chronic hepatitis B*, i.e., in those with precore and core-promoter HBV mutations, 1 year of lamivudine therapy results in HBV DNA suppression and normalization of ALT in three-quarters of patients and in histologic improvement in approximately two-thirds. Therapy has been shown to suppress HBV DNA by approximately 4.5 $\log_{10}$ copies/mL (baseline HBV DNA levels are lower than in patients with HBeAg-reactive hepatitis B) and to undetectable levels in 70%, as measured by sensitive PCR amplification assays. Lacking HBeAg at the outset, patients with HBeAg-negative chronic hepatitis B cannot achieve an HBeAg response—a stopping point in HBeAg-reactive patients; invariably, when therapy is discontinued, reactivation is the rule. Therefore, these patients require long-term therapy; with successive years, the proportion with suppressed HBV DNA and normal ALT increases.

Clinical and laboratory side effects of lamivudine are negligible, indistinguishable from those observed in placebo recipients. During lamivudine therapy, transient ALT elevations, resembling those seen during IFN therapy and during spontaneous HBeAg-to-anti-HBe seroconversions, occur in a quarter of patients. These ALT elevations may result from restored cytolytic T cell activation permitted by suppression of HBV replication. Similar ALT elevations, however, occur at an identical frequency in placebo recipients, but ALT elevations associated with HBeAg seroconversion are confined to lamivudine-treated patients. When therapy is stopped after a year of therapy, two- to threefold ALT elevations occur in 20–30% of lamivudine-treated patients, representing renewed liver-cell injury as HBV replication returns. Although these posttreatment flares are almost always transient and mild, rare severe exacerbations, especially in cirrhotic patients, have been observed, mandating close and careful clinical and virologic monitoring after discontinuation of treatment. Many authorities caution against discontinuing therapy in patients with cirrhosis, in whom posttreatment flares could precipitate decompensation.

Long-term monotherapy with lamivudine is associated with methionine-to-valine (M204V) or methionine-to-isoleucine (M204I) mutations, primarily at amino acid 204 in the tyrosine-methionine-aspartate-aspartate (YMDD) motif of HBV DNA polymerase, analogous to mutations that occur in HIV-infected patients treated with this drug. During a year of therapy, YMDD mutations occur in 15–30% of patients; the frequency increases with each year of therapy, reaching 70% at year 5. Although resistance to lamivudine may not lead to immediate loss of antiviral effect, patients with YMDD mutants ultimately experience degradation of clinical, biochemical, and histologic responses. Therefore, if treatment is begun with lamivudine monotherapy, the emergence of lamivudine resistance, reflected clinically by a breakthrough from suppressed levels of HBV DNA and ALT, is managed by adding another antiviral to which YMDD variants are sensitive (e.g., adefovir; see below).

Currently, although lamivudine is very safe and still used widely in other parts of the world, in the United States and Europe lamivudine has been eclipsed by more potent antivirals that have superior resistance profiles (see below). Still, as the first successful oral antiviral agent for use in hepatitis B, lamivudine has provided proof of the concept that polymerase inhibitors can achieve both virologic, serologic, biochemical, and histologic benefit. In addition, lamivudine has been shown to be effective in the treatment of patients with decompensated hepatitis B (for whom IFN is contraindicated), in some of whom decompensation can be reversed. Moreover, among patients with cirrhosis or advanced fibrosis, lamivudine has been shown to be effective in reducing the risk of progression to hepatic decompensation and, marginally, the risk of HCC.

Because lamivudine monotherapy can result universally in the rapid emergence of YMDD variants in persons with HIV infection, patients with chronic hepatitis B should be tested for anti-HIV prior to therapy; if HIV infection is identified, lamivudine monotherapy at the HBV daily dose of 100 mg is contraindicated. These patients should be treated with triple-drug antiretroviral therapy, including a lamivudine daily dose of 300 mg (Chap. 182). The safety of lamivudine during pregnancy has not been established; however, the drug is not teratogenic in rodents and has been used safely in pregnant women with HIV infection and with HBV infection. Limited data even suggest that administration of lamivudine during the last month of pregnancy to mothers with high-level hepatitis B viremia can reduce the likelihood of perinatal transmission of hepatitis B.

ADEFOVIR DIPIVOXIL The acyclic nucleotide analogue adefovir dipivoxil, the prodrug of adevovir, is a potent antiviral that, at an oral daily dose of 10 mg, reduces HBV DNA by approximately 3.5–4 $\log_{10}$ copies/mL and is equally effective in treatment-naïve patients and IFN nonresponders. In HBeAg-reactive chronic hepatitis B, a 48-week course of adefovir dipivoxil was shown to achieve histologic improvement (and reduce the progression of fibrosis) and normalization of ALT in half of patients, HBeAg seroconversion in 12%, HBeAg loss in 23%, and suppression to an undetectable level of HBV DNA in 20–30%, as measured by PCR. Similar to IFN and lamivudine, adefovir dipivoxil is more likely to achieve an HBeAg response in patients with high baseline ALT; for example, among adefovir-treated patients with ALT level >5 times the upper limit of normal, HBeAg seroconversions occurred in 25%. The durability of adefovir-induced HBeAg responses is high (91% in one study); therefore, HBeAg response can be relied upon as a stopping point for adefovir therapy. Although data on the impact of additional therapy beyond one year are limited, biochemical, serologic, and virologic outcomes improve progressively as therapy is continued.

In patients with *HBeAg-negative chronic hepatitis B*, a 48-week course of 10 mg/d of adefovir dipivoxil resulted in histologic improvement in two-thirds, normalization of ALT in three-quarters, and suppression of HBV DNA to PCR-undetectable levels in half. As was true for lamivudine, because HBeAg responses—a potential stopping point—cannot be achieved in this group, reactivation is the rule when adefovir therapy is discontinued, and indefinite, long-term therapy is required. Treatment beyond the first year consolidates the gain of the first year; after five years of therapy, improvement in hepatic inflammation and regression of fibrosis was observed in three-quarters of patients, ALT was normal in 70%, and HBV DNA was undetectable in almost 70%.

Adefovir contains a flexible acyclic linker instead of the L-nucleoside ring of lamivudine, avoiding steric hindrance by mutated amino acids. In addition, the molecular structure of phosphorylated adefovir is very similar to that of its natural substrate; therefore mutations to adefovir would also affect binding of the natural substrate, dATP. Hypothetically, these are among the reasons that resistance to adefovir dipivoxil is much less likely than resistance to lamivudine; no resistance was encountered in 1 year of clinical-trial therapy. In subsequent years, however, adefovir resistance begins to emerge [asparagine to threonine at amino acid 236 (N236T) and alanine to valine or threonine at amino acid 181 (A181V/T) primarily], occurring in 2.5% after 2 years, but in 29% after 5 years of therapy. Among patients co-infected with HBV and HIV and who have normal CD4+ T cell counts, adefovir dipivoxil is effective in suppressing HBV dramatically (by 5 $\log_{10}$ in one study). Moreover, adefovir dipivoxil is effective in lamivudine-resistant, YMDD-mutant HBV and can be used when such lamivudine-induced variants emerge. When lamivudine resistance occurs, authorities have debated whether to add adefovir or switch to adefovir; however, adding adefovir, i.e., maintaining lamivudine to preempt the emergence of adefovir resistance, appears to be the favored approach. In this vein, almost invariably, patients with adefovir-mutant HBV respond to lamivudine. When, in the past, adefovir had been evaluated as therapy for HIV infection, doses of 60–120 mg were required to suppress HIV, and at these doses the drug was nephrotoxic. Even at 30 mg/d, creatinine elevations of 44 μmol/L (0.5 mg/dL) occur in 10% of patients; however, at the HBV-effective dose of 10 mg, such elevations of creatinine are rarely encountered. If any nephrotoxicity does occur, it rarely appears before 6–8 months of therapy. Although renal tubular injury is a rare potential side effect, and although creatinine monitoring is recommended during treatment, the therapeutic index of adefovir dipivoxil is high, and the nephrotoxicity observed in clinical trials at higher doses was reversible. For patients with underlying renal disease, adefovir dipivoxil dose reductions are recommended: administration reduced to every 48 h for creatinine clearances of 20–49 mL/min, to every 72 h for creatinine clearances of 10–19 mL/min, and once a week, following dialysis, for patients undergoing hemodialysis. Adefovir dipivoxil is very well tolerated, and ALT elevations during and after withdrawal of therapy are similar to those observed and described above in clinical trials of lamivudine. An advantage of adefovir is its relatively favorable resistance profile; however, it is not as potent as the other approved oral agents, it does not suppress HBV DNA as rapidly or as uniformly as the others, and a small proportion of patients have no demonstrable response to the drug ("primary nonresponders").

PEGYLATED INTERFERON After long-acting PEG IFN was shown to be effective in the treatment of hepatitis C (see below), this more convenient drug was evaluated in the treatment of chronic hepatitis B. Preliminary trials documented that once-a-week PEG IFN was more effective than the more frequently administered, standard IFN, following which several large-scale trials were conducted among patients with HBeAg-reactive and HBeAg-negative chronic hepatitis B.

In HBeAg-reactive chronic hepatitis B, two large-scale studies were done, one with PEG IFN-α2b (100 μg weekly for 32 weeks, then 50 μg weekly for another 20 weeks for a total of 52 weeks, with a comparison arm of combination PEG IFN with oral lamivudine) in 307 subjects; the other involved PEG IFN-α2a (180 μg weekly for 48 weeks) in 814 primarily Asian patients confined to those with ALT $\geq$2 $\times$ the upper limit of normal, with comparison arms of lamivudine monotherapy and combination PEG IFN plus lamivudine. At the end of therapy (48–52 weeks) in the PEG IFN monotherapy arms, HBeAg loss occurred in approximately 30%, HBeAg seroconversion in 22%–27%, undetectable HBV DNA (<400 copies/mL by PCR) in 10–25%, normal ALT in 34–39%, and a mean reduction in HBV DNA of 2 $\log_{10}$ copies/mL (PEG IFN-α2b) to 4.5 $\log_{10}$ copies/mL (PEG IFN-α2a). Six months after completing PEG IFN monotherapy in these trials, HBeAg losses were present in approximately 35%, HBeAg seroconversion in approximately 30%, undetectable HBV DNA in 7–14%, normal ALT in 32–41%, and a mean reduction in HBV DNA of 2–2.4 $\log_{10}$ copies/mL. Although the combination of PEG IFN and lamivudine was superior at the end of therapy in one or more serologic, virologic, or biochemical outcomes, neither the combination arm (in both studies) nor the lamivudine monotherapy arm (in the PEG IFN-α2a trial) demonstrated any benefit compared to the PEG IFN monotherapy arms 6 months after therapy. Moreover, HBsAg seroconversion occurred in 3%–7% of PEG IFN recipients (with or without lamivudine); some of these seroconversions were identified by the end of therapy, but many were identified during the posttreatment follow-up period. The likelihood of HBeAg loss in PEG IFN–treated HBeAg-reactive patients is associated with HBV genotype A > B > C > D.

Based on these results, some authorities concluded that PEG IFN monotherapy should be the first-line therapy of choice in HBeAg-reactive chronic hepatitis B; however, this conclusion has been challenged. Although a finite, 1-year course of PEG IFN results in a higher rate of sustained response (6 months after treatment) than is achieved with oral nucleoside/nucleotide analogue therapy, the comparison is confounded by the fact that oral agents are not discontinued at the end of a year. Instead, taken orally and free of side effects, therapy with oral agents is extended indefinitely or until after the occurrence of an HBeAg response. The rate of HBeAg responses after two years of oral-agent therapy is at least as high as, if not higher than, that achieved with PEG IFN after 1 year; favoring oral agents is the absence of injections and difficult-to-tolerate side effects as well as lower direct and indirect medical costs and inconvenience. The association of HBsAg responses with PEG IFN therapy occurs in such a small proportion of patients that subjecting everyone to PEG IFN for the marginal gain of HBsAg responses during or immediately after therapy in such a very small minority is questionable. Moreover, HBsAg responses occur in a comparable proportion of nucleoside/nucleotide-treated patients in the years after therapy. Of course, resistance is not an issue during PEG IFN therapy, but the risk of resistance is much lower with new agents (none recorded after two years in previously treatment-naïve entecavir-treated patients; see below). Finally, the level of HBV DNA inhibition that can be achieved with the newer agents, and even with lamivudine, exceeds that which can be achieved with PEG IFN, in some cases by several orders of magnitude.

In HBeAg-negative chronic hepatitis B, a trial of PEG IFN-α2a (180 μg weekly for 48 weeks versus comparison arms of lamivudine monotherapy

TABLE 300-3 COMPARISON OF INTERFERON (PEG IFN), LAMIVUDINE, ADEFOVIR, AND ENTECAVIR THERAPY FOR CHRONIC HEPATITIS B[a]

Feature	PEG IFN[b]	Lamivudine	Adefovir	Entecavir
Route of administration	Subcutaneous injection	Oral	Oral	Oral
Duration of therapy[c]	48–52 weeks	≥52 weeks	≥48 weeks	≥48 weeks
Tolerability	Poorly tolerated	Well tolerated	Well tolerated; creatinine monitoring recommended	Well tolerated
HBeAg loss 1 year	29–30%	20–33%	23%	22%
HBeAg seroconversion				
1 year Rx	18–20%	16–21%	12%	21%
>1 year Rx	NA	Up to 50% @ 5 years	43% @ 3 years[d]	31% @ 2 years
HBeAg seroconversion if ALT >5 × normal	Not reported	>50%	21%	Not reported
Log$_{10}$ HBV DNA reduction (mean copies/mL)				
HBeAg-reactive	4.5	5.5	Median 3.5–5	6.9
HBeAg-negative	4.1	4.4–4.7	Median 3.5–3.9	5.0
HBV DNA PCR negative (<300–400 copies/mL; <1,000 copies/mL for adefovir) end of year 1				
HBeAg-reactive	10–25%	36–40%	12–21%	69% (80% @ 2 years)
HBeAg-negative	63%	39–73%	51% (79% @ 3 years)	90%
ALT normalization at end of year 1				
HBeAg-reactive	39%	41–75%	58% (81% @ year 3)	78%
HBeAg-negative	34–38%	62–79%	48% (69% @ year 3)	78%
HBsAg loss during year 1	0–7%	0–4%	0% (1–2% @ 2 years)	2% (5% @ 2 years)
HBsAg loss after therapy	3–7% after 6 months	23% after 2 years	Not reported	Not reported
Histologic improvement (≥2 point reduction in HAI) at year 1				
HBeAg-reactive	38% 6 months after	51–62%	53%	62%
HBeAg-negative	48% 6 months after	61–66%	64%	70%
Viral resistance	None	15–30% @ 1 year 70% @ 5 years	None @ 1 year 29% @ 5 years	None @ 2 years[e]
Durability of response 4–6 months after therapy[f]				
HBeAg-reactive	Limited data	70–80%	91%	82%
HBeAg-negative	36%	23–35%	Low	48%
Cost (U.S. $) for 1 year	~$18,000	~$2,500	~$6,500	~$8,700[g]

[a]Generally, these comparisons are based on data on each drug tested individually versus placebo in registration clinical trials. With rare exception, these comparisons are not based on head-to-head testing of these drugs, hence relative advantages and disadvantages should be interpreted cautiously.

[b]Although standard interferon α administered daily or three times a week is approved as therapy for chronic hepatitis B, it has been supplanted by pegylated interferon (PEG IFN), which is administered once a week and is more effective. Standard interferon has no advantages over PEG IFN.

[c]Duration of therapy in clinical efficacy trials; use in clinical practice may vary.

[d]Because of a computer-generated randomization error that resulted in misallocation of drug versus placebo during the second year of clinical-trial treatment, the frequency of

HBeAg serconversion beyond the first year is an estimate (Kaplan-Meier analysis) based on the small subset in whom adefovir was administered correctly.

[e]7% during a year of therapy (9% during two years) in lamivudine-resistant patients.

[f]In HBeAg-reactive patients, durability of HBeAg seroconversion; in HBeAg-negative patients, durability of virologic (HBV DNA undetectable by PCR) and biochemical (normal ALT) response.

[g]~17,400 for lamivudine-refractory patients.

Note: ALT, alanine aminotransferase; HAI, histologic activity index; HBeAg, hepatitis B e antigen; HBsAg, hepatitis B surface antigen; HBV, hepatitis B virus; NA, not applicable; Rx, therapy; PCR, polymerase chain reaction.

and of combination therapy) in 564 patients showed that PEG IFN monotherapy resulted at the end of therapy in suppression of HBV DNA by a mean of 4.1 log$_{10}$ copies/mL, undetectable HBV DNA (<400 copies/mL by PCR) in 63%, and normal ALT in 38%. Although lamivudine monotherapy and combination lamivudine–PEG IFN therapy were both superior to PEG IFN at the end of therapy, no advantage of lamivudine monotherapy or combination therapy was apparent over PEG IFN monotherapy 6 months after therapy—suppression of HBV DNA by a mean of 2.3 log$_{10}$ copies/mL, undetectable HBV DNA in 19%, and normal ALT in 59%. As was the case for standard IFN therapy in HBeAg-negative patients, after longer periods of post-PEG IFN treatment observation, sustained response rates fell substantially, raising questions about the value of a finite period of PEG IFN in these patients.

ENTECAVIR Entecavir, an oral guanosine analogue polymerase inhibitor, appears to be the most potent of the HBV antivirals and is just as well tolerated as lamivudine. In a 709-subject clinical trial among HBeAg-reactive patients, oral entecavir, 0.5 mg daily, was compared to lamivudine, 100 mg daily. At 48 weeks, entecavir was superior to lamivudine in suppression of HBV DNA, mean 6.9 versus 5.5 log$_{10}$ copies/mL and in percent with undetectable HBV DNA (<300 copies/mL by PCR), 67% versus 36%; histologic improvement (≥2-point improvement in necroinflammatory HAI score), 72% versus 62%; and normal ALT (68% versus 60%). The two treatments were indistinguishable in percent with HBeAg loss (22% versus 20%) and seroconversion (21% versus 18%). Among patients treated with entecavir for 96 weeks, HBV DNA was undetectable cumulatively in 80% (versus 39% for lamivudine), and HBeAg seroconversions had occurred in 31% (versus 26% for lamivudine). Similarly, in a 638-subject clinical trial among HBeAg-

negative patients, at week 48, oral entecavir, 0.5 mg daily, was superior to lamivudine, 100 mg daily, in suppression of HBV DNA, mean 5.0 versus 4.5 log$_{10}$ copies/mL and in percent with undetectable HBV DNA, 90% versus 72%; histologic improvement, 78% versus 71% and normal ALT, 68% versus 60%. No resistance mutations were encountered in previously treatment-naïve entecavir-treated patients during 96 weeks of therapy.

Entecavir is also effective against lamivudine-resistant HBV infection. In a trial of 286 lamivudine-resistant patients, entecavir, at a higher daily dose of 1.0 mg, was superior to lamivudine, as measured at week 48, in achieving suppression of HBV DNA (mean 5.1 versus 0.48 log$_{10}$ copies/mL); undetectable HBV DNA, in 72% versus 19%; normal ALT, in 61% versus 15%; HBeAg loss, in 10% versus 3%; and HBeAg seroconversion, in 8% versus 3%. In this population of lamivudine-experienced patients, however, entecavir resistance did emerge in 7% at 48 weeks and in 9% at 96 weeks. Therefore, entecavir is not as attractive a choice as adefovir (or off-label tenofovir) for patients with lamivudine-resistant hepatitis B.

At the end of two years of entecavir therapy in clinical trials among HBeAg-reactive patients, HBsAg seroconversion were observed in 5% (≤2% during the first year). In addition, on-treatment and posttreatment ALT flares are relatively uncommon and relatively mild in entecavir-treated patients.

A comparison of the four antiviral therapies in current use appears in Table 300-3.

COMBINATION THERAPY Although the combination of lamivudine and PEG IFN suppresses HBV DNA more profoundly during therapy than does monotherapy with either drug alone (and is much less likely to be associated with lamivudine resistance), this combination used for a year is no better than a year of PEG IFN in achieving sustained responses. To

TABLE 300-4 **RECOMMENDATIONS FOR TREATMENT OF CHRONIC HEPATITIS B** 1961

HBeAg Status	Clinical	HBV DNA (copies/mL)	ALT	Recommendation
HBeAg-reactive	[a]	<10^5	Normal (≤2 × ULN)[b]	No treatment; monitor
	Chronic hepatitis	≥10^5	Normal (≤2 × ULN)[b,c]	No treatment; current treatment of limited benefit (Some suggest liver biopsy and treating if abnormal)
	Chronic hepatitis	≥10^5	Elevated (>2 × ULN)[b]	Treat[d]
	Cirrhosis compensated	+ or –[e]	Normal or elevated	Treat[e] with oral agents,[f] not PEG IFN
	Cirrhosis decompensated	+ or –[e]	Normal or elevated	Treat[e] with oral agents,[g] not PEG IFN; refer for liver transplantation
HBeAg-negative	[a]	<10^4 or 10^{5h}	Normal (≤2 × ULN)[b]	Inactive carrier; treatment not necessary
	Chronic hepatitis	≥10^4 or 10^{5h}	Normal	Consider liver biopsy; treat if biopsy abnormal
	Chronic hepatitis	≥10^4 or 10^{5h} (>2 × ULN)[b]	Elevated	Treat[i]
	Cirrhosis compensated	+ or –	Elevated or normal	Treat with oral agents,[i] not PEG IFN (some authorites recommend either following or treating for HBV DNA <10^4 copies/mL)
	Cirrhosis decompensated	+ or –	Elevated or normal	Treat with oral agents,[i] not PEG IFN (some authorities would follow without therapy for undetectable HBV DNA; refer for liver transplantation)

[a]Liver disease tends to be mild or inactive clinically; most such patients do not undergo liver biopsy.

[b]In some guidelines, ALT categories are normal or elevated; in others, ALT categories are ≤ or > 2 times the upper limit of normal.

[c]Typical pattern in childhood-acquired infection, common in Asian populations.

[d]Any of the oral drugs (lamivudine, adefovir, entecavir) or PEG IFN can be used as first-line therapy (see text); although still used extensively in some parts of the world, lamivudine has been supplanted in some countries as first-line therapy because of its resistance profile. The oral agents, but not PEG IFN, should be used for interferon-refractory/intolerant and immunocompromised patients. PEG IFN is administered weekly by subcutaneous injection for a year; the oral agents are administered daily for at least a year and continued indefinitely or until at least 6 months after HBeAg seroconversion.

[e]Treating or monitoring without therapy are options for patients with HBV DNA <10^4 or <10^5 copies/mL.

[f]Some authorities would observe without treatment if HBV DNA is undetectable (<10^4 copies/mL), while others would treat regardless of the HBV DNA status. Lamivudine monotherapy is not an attractive choice because of its resistance profile.

[g]Some authorities recommend treating regardless of HBV DNA status, while others suggest referring for liver transplantation, without treatment, for those with undetectable HBV DNA (<10^5 copies/mL). Lamivudine is a less attractive choice because of its resistance profile. Because the emergence of resistance can lead to loss of antiviral benefit and further deterioration in decompensated cirrhosis, some authorities recommend combination therapy (e.g., lamivudine or entecavir plus adefovir) for patients with decompensated cirrhosis.

[h]Some authorities rely on a cutoff of 10^4 copies/mL, while others choose 10^5 copies/mL.

[i]Because HBeAg seroconversion is not an option, the goal of therapy is to suppress HBV DNA and maintain a normal ALT. Although any of the oral agents or PEG IFN can be used as first-line therapy, lamivudine is less favored because of its resistance profile and the need, in the vast majority of cases, for long-term therapy. PEG IFN is administered by subcutaneous injection weekly for a year (caution is warranted in relying on a 6-month posttreatment interval to define a sustained response; the majority of such responses are lost thereafter). Adefovir and entecavir are administered daily, usually indefinitely or, until, as occurs very rarely, virologic and biochemical responses are accompanied by an HBsAg seroconversion.

[j]Low-resistance regimen favored (i.e., adefovir or entecavir, not lamivudine) indefinitely.

Note: ALT, alanine aminotransferase; HBeAg, hepatitis B e antigen; HBsAg, hepatitis B surface antigen; HBV, hepatitis B virus; ULN, upper limits of normal; PEG IFN, pegylated interferon.

date, combinations of oral nucleoside/nucleotide agents have not achieved an enhancement in virologic, serologic, or biochemical efficacy over that achieved by the more potent of the combined drugs given individually. On the other hand, combining agents that are not cross-resistant (e.g., lamivudine and adefovir) has the potential to reduce the risk or perhaps even to preempt entirely the emergence of drug resistance. In the future, the treatment paradigm is likely to shift from the current approach of sequential monotherapy to preemptive combination therapy; clinical trials are warranted.

TREATMENT RECOMMENDATIONS Several learned societies and groups of expert physicians have issued treatment recommendations for patients with chronic hepatitis B. Although the recommendations differ slightly, a consensus has emerged on most of the important points (**Table 300-4**). No treatment is recommended or available for inactive "nonreplicative" hepatitis B carriers (undetectable HBeAg with normal ALT and HBV DNA <10^4 copies/mL documented serially over time). In patients with detectable HBeAg and HBV DNA levels ≥10^5 copies/mL, treatment is recommended for those with elevated ALT levels (some authorities require the elevation to be at least twice the upper limit of normal). For those patients with normal ALT (or ≤2 × the upper limit of normal), in whom sustained responses are not likely and who would require multiyear therapy, antiviral therapy is not recommended currently. For patients with HBeAg-negative chronic hepatitis B, elevated ALT (≥2 × the upper limit of normal according to some authorities), and HBV DNA ≥10^4 (or 10^5 according to some authorities) copies/mL, antiviral therapy is recommended. If HBV DNA is <10^4–10^5 and ALT is normal (or near normal), treatment is not recommended; however, if HBV DNA is ≥10^4 copies/mL but ALT is normal or near normal, some would recommend considering liver biopsy and basing a decision to treat on the presence of substantial liver injury.

For patients with compensated cirrhosis, because antiviral therapy has been shown to retard clinical progression, many authorities would choose to treat regardless of HBeAg status, HBV DNA level and ALT; however, some authorities favor monitoring without therapy for those with HBV DNA levels <10^4 copies/mL. For patients with decompensated cirrhosis, treatment is recommended by some authorities regardless of serologic, virologic, and biochemical status; however, other experts do not recommend therapy if HBV DNA is undetectable or low (<10^5 copies/mL). At the same time, patients with decompensated cirrhosis should be evaluated as candidates for liver transplantation.

Among the five available drugs for hepatitis B, PEG IFN has supplanted standard IFN. Because entecavir has been proved superior to lamivudine in clinical trials, entecavir has supplanted lamivudine in some countries. PEG IFN, lamivudine, adefovir, and entecavir can each be used as first-line therapy (Table 300-3). PEG IFN requires finite-duration therapy, achieves the highest rate of HBeAg responses after a year of therapy, and does not support viral mutations, but it requires subcutaneous injections and is associated with inconvenience and intolerability. Lamivudine, adefovir, and entecavir require long-term therapy in most patients, and when used alone, lamivudine fosters the emergence of viral mutations, adefovir much less so, and entecavir rarely at all, except in lamivudine-experienced patients. These oral agents do not require injections, are very well tolerated, lead to improved histology in 50–90% of patients, for the most part suppress HBV DNA more profoundly than does PEG IFN, and are effective even in patients who fail to respond to IFN-based therapy. Although these oral agents are less likely to result in HBeAg responses during the first year of therapy, as compared to PEG IFN, treatment with oral agents tends to be extended beyond the first year and, by the end of the second year, yields HBeAg responses (and even HBsAg responses) comparable in frequency to those achieved after 1 year of PEG IFN (and without the associated side effects). Although adefovir is safe, creatinine monitoring is recommended. Substantial experience with lamivudine during pregnancy (see above) has identified no teratogenicity. Standard IFN does not appear to cause congenital anomalies, and data on the safety of PEG IFN during pregnancy are not available. Adefovir during pregnancy has not been associated with birth defects; however, there may be an increased risk of spontaneous abortion. Data on the safety of entecavir during pregnancy have not been published. In general, except perhaps for lamivudine, and until additional data become available, the other antivirals for hepatitis B should be avoided or used with extreme caution during pregnancy.

As noted above, some physicians prefer to begin with PEG IFN, while other physicians and patients prefer oral agents as first-line therapy. For patients with decompensated cirrhosis, the emergence of resistance can result in further deterioration and loss of antiviral effectiveness. Therefore, in this patient subset, the threshold for relying on therapy with a very favorable resistance profile (e.g., entecavir) or on combination therapy (e.g., lamivudine or entecavir along with adefovir or the yet-to-be-approved tenofovir) is low. PEG IFN should not be used in patients with compensated or decompensated cirrhosis.

For patients with end-stage chronic hepatitis B who undergo liver transplantation, reinfection of the new liver is almost universal in the absence of antiviral therapy. The majority of patients become high-level viremic carriers with minimal liver injury. Before the availability of antiviral therapy, an unpredictable proportion experienced severe hepatitis B–related liver injury, sometimes a fulminant-like hepatitis, sometimes a rapid recapitulation of the original severe chronic hepatitis B (Chap. 304). Currently, however, prevention of recurrent hepatitis B after liver transplantation has been achieved definitively by *combining* hepatitis B immune globulin with one of the oral nucleoside or nucleotide analogues (lamivudine, adefovir, or entecavir) (Chap. 304).

Patients with HBV-HIV co-infection can have progressive HBV-associated liver disease and, occasionally, a severe exacerbation of hepatitis B resulting from immunologic reconstitution following highly active antiretroviral therapy. Lamivudine should never be used as monotherapy in patients with HBV-HIV infection, because HIV resistance emerges rapidly to both viruses. Adefovir and entecavir have been used successfully to treat chronic hepatitis B in HBV-HIV co-infected patients. Tenofovir and the combination of tenofovir and emtricitabine in one pill are approved therapies for HIV and represent excellent choices for treating HBV infection in HBV-HIV co-infected patients.

Patients with chronic hepatitis B who undergo cytotoxic chemotherapy for treatment of malignancies experience enhanced HBV replication and viral expression on hepatocyte membranes during chemotherapy coupled with suppression of cellular immunity. When chemotherapy is withdrawn, such patients are at risk for reactivation of hepatitis B, often severe and occasionally fatal. Such rebound reactivation represents restoration of cytolytic T-cell function against a target organ enriched in HBV expression. Preemptive treatment with lamivudine prior to the initiation of chemotherapy has been shown to reduce the risk of such reactivation. In all likelihood, the newer, more potent oral antiviral agents will work as well and with a lower risk of antiviral drug resistance. The optimal duration of antiviral therapy after completion of chemotherapy is not known, but some authorities have suggested 3 months.

NOVEL ANTIVIRALS AND STRATEGIES In addition to the five approved antiviral drugs for hepatitis B, several others are being evaluated in clinical trials, as listed in **Table 300-5**. Telbivudine, a cytosine analogue, appears to be similar in efficacy to entecavir but slightly less potent in suppressing HBV DNA, and it is associated with low-level resistance (M204I, not M204V mutations). This drug was approved in October 2006. Resistance mutations after 2 years of treatment occur in ~20%. Tenofovir, a nucleotide analogue, is similar to adefovir but more potent in suppressing HBV DNA and inducing HBeAg responses; it is highly active against both wild-type and lamivudine-resistant HBV and active in patients with primary nonresponse to adefovir. Its safety and resistance profile are very favorable as well; in all likelihood, it will supplant adefovir once comparisons in clinical trials are complete. Emtricitabine is a fluorinated cytosine analogue very similar to lamivudine in structure, efficacy, and resistance profile. A combination of emtricitabine and tenofovir is approved for the treatment

TABLE 300-5 NEW ANTIVIRAL DRUGS BEING DEVELOPED FOR THE TREATMENT OF CHRONIC HEPATITIS B

Telbivudine[a]	Emtricitabine (FTC)
Tenofovir[b]	Clevudine (L-MFAU)

[a]Approved in October 2006.
[b]Active against lamivudine-associated YMDD-mutant HBV. (YMDD, tyrosine-methionine-aspartate-aspartate.)

of HIV infection and is an appealing combination therapy for hepatitis B; however, neither emtricitabine nor the combination are approved yet for hepatitis B. Clevudine is a pyrimidine nucleoside analogue whose potency in the woodchuck model of hepatitis B is higher than that of any other antiviral agent; however, in human trials, maximal HBV DNA suppression has been 5 $\log_{10}$ copies/mL; after clevudine therapy, HBV DNA is much slower to rebound than after withdrawal of other agents. Because direct-acting antivirals have been so successful in the management of chronic hepatitis B, more unconventional approaches—e.g., immunologic or genetic manipulation—are not likely to be competitive. Finally, initial emphasis in the development of antiviral therapy for hepatitis B was placed on monotherapy; however, in the future, with or without additive or synergistic efficacy, combination therapy regimens that prevent resistance are likely to become the norm.

CHRONIC HEPATITIS D (DELTA HEPATITIS)

Chronic hepatitis D (HDV) may follow acute co-infection with HBV but at a rate no higher than the rate of chronicity of acute hepatitis B. That is, although HDV co-infection can increase the severity of acute hepatitis B, HDV does not increase the likelihood of progression to chronic hepatitis B. When, however, HDV superinfection occurs in a person who is already chronically infected with HBV, long-term HDV infection is the rule and a worsening of the liver disease the expected consequence. Except for severity, chronic hepatitis B plus D has similar clinical and laboratory features to those seen in chronic hepatitis B alone. Relatively severe chronic hepatitis, with or without cirrhosis, is the rule, and mild chronic hepatitis is the exception. Occasionally, mild hepatitis or even, rarely, inactive carriage occurs in patients with chronic hepatitis B plus D, and the disease may become indolent after several years of infection. A distinguishing serologic feature of chronic hepatitis D is the presence in the circulation of antibodies to liver-kidney microsomes (anti-LKM); however, the anti-LKM seen in hepatitis D, anti-LKM3, are directed against uridine diphosphate glucuronosyltransferase and are distinct from anti-LKM1 seen in patients with autoimmune hepatitis and in a subset of patients with chronic hepatitis C (see below). The clinical and laboratory features of chronic HDV infection are summarized in Chap. 298.

CHRONIC HEPATITIS D

Management is not well defined. Glucocorticoids are ineffective and are not used. Preliminary experimental trials of IFN-α suggested that conventional doses and durations of therapy lower levels of HDV RNA and aminotransferase activity only transiently during treatment but have no impact on the natural history of the disease. In contrast, high-dose IFN-α (9 million units three times a week) for 12 months may be associated with a sustained loss of HDV replication and clinical improvement in up to 50% of patients. Moreover, the beneficial impact of treatment has been observed to persist for 15 years and to be associated with a reduction in grade of hepatic necrosis and inflammation, reversion of advanced fibrosis (improved stage), and clearance of HDV RNA in some patients. A suggested approach to therapy has been high-dose, long-term IFN for at least a year and, in responders, extension of therapy until HDV RNA and HBsAg clearance. Although experience with PEG IFN in the treatment of chronic hepatitis D is limited, if future studies confirm its equivalence to, or superiority over, standard IFN, PEG IFN is likely to become a more convenient replacement for standard IFN. None of the new antiviral agents for hepatitis B—lamivudine, adefovir, entecavir—are effective in hepatitis D; however, preliminary indications in the woodchuck model of hepatitis B are that clevudine may be. In patients with end-stage liver disease secondary to chronic hepatitis D, liver transplantation has been effective. If hepatitis D recurs in the new liver without the expression of hepatitis B (an unusual serologic profile in immunocompetent persons but common in transplant patients), liver injury is limited. In fact, the outcome of transplantation for chronic hepatitis D is superior to that for chronic hepatitis B (Chap. 304).

CHRONIC HEPATITIS C

Regardless of the epidemiologic mode of acquisition of hepatitis C virus (HCV) infection, chronic hepatitis follows acute hepatitis C in 50–

70% of cases; chronic infection is common even in those with a return to normal in aminotransferase levels after acute hepatitis C, adding up to an 85% likelihood of chronic HCV infection after acute hepatitis C. Furthermore, in patients with chronic transfusion-associated hepatitis followed for 10–20 years, progression to cirrhosis occurs in about 20%. Such is the case even for patients with relatively clinically mild chronic hepatitis, including those without symptoms, with only modest elevations of aminotransferase activity and with mild chronic hepatitis on liver biopsy. Even in cohorts of well-compensated patients with chronic hepatitis C referred for clinical research trials (no complications of chronic liver disease and with normal hepatic synthetic function), the prevalence of cirrhosis may be as high as 50%. Most cases of hepatitis C are identified initially in asymptomatic patients who have no history of acute hepatitis C, e.g., those discovered while attempting to donate blood, while undergoing lab testing as part of an application for life insurance, or as a result of routine laboratory tests. The source of HCV infection in many of these cases is not defined, although a long-forgotten percutaneous exposure in the remote past can be elicited in a substantial proportion and probably accounts for most infections; most of these infections were acquired in the 1960s and 1970s, coming to clinical attention decades later.

Approximately a third of patients with chronic hepatitis C have normal or near-normal aminotransferase activity; although a third to a half of these patients have chronic hepatitis on liver biopsy, the grade of liver injury and stage of fibrosis tend to be mild in the vast majority. In some cases, more severe liver injury has been reported—even, rarely, cirrhosis, most likely the result of previous histologic activity. Among patients with persistent normal aminotransferase activity sustained over ≥5–10 years, histologic progression has been shown not to occur; however, approximately a quarter of patients with normal aminotransferase activity experience subsequent aminotransferase elevations, and histologic injury can be progressive once abnormal biochemical activity resumes. Therefore, continued clinical monitoring is indicated, even for patients with normal aminotransferase activity.

Despite this substantial rate of progression of chronic hepatitis C, and despite the fact that liver failure can result from end-stage chronic hepatitis C, the long-term prognosis for chronic hepatitis C in a majority of patients is relatively benign. Mortality over 10–20 years among patients with transfusion-associated chronic hepatitis C has been shown not to differ from mortality in a matched population of transfused patients in whom hepatitis C did not develop. Although death in the hepatitis group is more likely to result from liver failure, and although hepatic decompensation may occur in ~15% of such patients over the course of a decade, the majority (almost 60%) of patients remain asymptomatic and well compensated, with no clinical sequelae of chronic liver disease. Overall, then, chronic hepatitis C tends to be very slowly and insidiously progressive, if at all, in the vast majority of patients, while in approximately a quarter of cases, chronic hepatitis C will progress eventually to end-stage cirrhosis. In fact, because HCV infection is so prevalent, and because a proportion of patients progress inexorably to end-stage liver disease, hepatitis C is the most frequent indication for liver transplantation (Chap. 304). Referral bias may account for the more severe outcomes described in cohorts of patients reported from tertiary care centers (20-year progression of 20%) versus the more benign outcomes in cohorts of patients monitored from initial blood-product-associated acute hepatitis or identified in community settings (20-year progression of only 4–7%). Still unexplained, however, are the wide ranges in reported progression to cirrhosis, from 2% over 17 years in a population of women with hepatitis C infection acquired from contaminated anti-D immune globulin to 30% over ≤11 years in recipients of contaminated intravenous immune globulin.

Progression of liver disease in patients with chronic hepatitis C has been reported to be more likely in patients with older age, longer duration of infection, advanced histologic stage and grade, genotype 1, more complex quasispecies diversity, increased hepatic iron, concomitant other liver disorders (alcoholic liver disease, chronic hepatitis B, hemochromatosis, α_1-antitrypsin deficiency, and steatohepatitis), HIV infection,

and obesity. Among these variables, however, duration of infection appears to be the most important, and some of the others probably reflect disease duration to some extent (e.g., quasispecies diversity, hepatic iron accumulation). No other epidemiologic or clinical features of chronic hepatitis C (e.g., severity of acute hepatitis, level of aminotransferase activity, level of HCV RNA, presence or absence of jaundice during acute hepatitis) are predictive of eventual outcome. Despite the relatively benign nature of chronic hepatitis C over time in many patients, cirrhosis following chronic hepatitis C has been associated with the late development, after several decades, of HCC (Chap. 88); the annual rate of HCC in cirrhotic patients with hepatitis C is 1–4%, occurring primarily in patients who have had HCV infection for 30 or more years.

Perhaps the best prognostic indicator in chronic hepatitis C is liver histology; the rate of hepatic fibrosis may be slow, moderate, or rapid. Patients with mild necrosis and inflammation as well as those with limited fibrosis have an excellent prognosis and limited progression to cirrhosis. In contrast, among patients with moderate to severe necroinflammatory activity or fibrosis, including septal or bridging fibrosis, progression to cirrhosis is highly likely over the course of 10–20 years. Among patients with compensated cirrhosis associated with hepatitis C, the 10-year survival is close to 80%; mortality occurs at a rate of 2–6% per year, decompensation at a rate of 4–5% per year, and, as noted above, HCC at a rate of 1–4% per year.

Clinical features of chronic hepatitis C are similar to those described above for chronic hepatitis B. Generally, *fatigue* is the most common symptom; jaundice is rare. Immune complex–mediated extrahepatic complications of chronic hepatitis C are less common than in chronic hepatitis B (despite the fact that assays for immune complexes are often positive in patients with chronic hepatitis C), with the exception of essential mixed cryoglobulinemia (Chap. 298). In addition, chronic hepatitis C has been associated with extrahepatic complications unrelated to immune-complex injury. These include Sjögren's syndrome, lichen planus, and porphyria cutanea tarda.

Laboratory features of chronic hepatitis C are similar to those in patients with chronic hepatitis B, but aminotransferase levels tend to fluctuate more (the characteristic episodic pattern of aminotransferase activity) and to be lower, especially in patients with long-standing disease. An interesting and occasionally confusing finding in patients with chronic hepatitis C is the presence of autoantibodies. Rarely, patients with autoimmune hepatitis (see below) and hyperglobulinemia have false-positive immunoassays for anti-HCV. On the other hand, some patients with serologically confirmable chronic hepatitis C have circulating anti-LKM. These antibodies are anti-LKM1, as seen in patients with autoimmune hepatitis type 2 (see below), and are directed against a 33-amino-acid sequence of cytochrome P450 IID6. The occurrence of anti-LKM1 in some patients with chronic hepatitis C may result from the partial sequence homology between the epitope recognized by anti-LKM1 and two segments of the HCV polyprotein. In addition, the presence of this autoantibody in some patients with chronic hepatitis C suggests that autoimmunity may be playing a role in the pathogenesis of chronic hepatitis C. Histopathologic features of chronic hepatitis C, especially those that distinguish hepatitis C from hepatitis B, are described in Chap. 298.

℞ CHRONIC HEPATITIS C

Therapy for chronic hepatitis C has evolved substantially in the decade and a half since IFN-α was introduced for this indication. When first approved, IFN-α was administered via subcutaneous injection three times a week for 6 months but achieved a sustained virologic response (a reduction of HCV RNA to undetectable levels by PCR when measured ≥6 months after completion of therapy) below 10%. Doubling the duration of therapy—but not increasing the dose or changing IFN preparations—increased the sustained virologic response rate to ~20%, and addition to the regimen of daily ribavirin, an oral guanosine nucleoside, increased sustained virologic responses to 40%. When used alone, ribavirin is ineffective and does not reduce HCV RNA levels, but ribavirin enhances the efficacy of IFN by reducing the likelihood of virologic relapse after the achievement of an end-treatment response (response measured during, and maintained to the end of, treatment). Proposed mechanisms to explain the role of ribavirin include subtle direct reduction of HCV replication, inhibition of host inosine monophosphate dehydrogenase activity (and associated depletion of guanosine pools), immune modulation, and induction of virologic mutational catastrophe.

Many important lessons about antiviral therapy for chronic hepatitis C were learned from the experience with IFN monotherapy and combination IFN-ribavirin therapy. Even in the absence of biochemical and virologic responses, histologic improvement occurs in approximately three-quarters of all treated patients. In chronic hepatitis C, unlike the case in hepatitis B, responses to therapy are not accompanied by transient, acute hepatitis–like aminotransferase elevations. Instead, ALT levels fall precipitously during therapy. Up to 90% of virologic responses are achieved within the first 12 weeks of therapy; responses thereafter are rare. Most relapses occur within the first 12 weeks after treatment. Sustained virologic responses are very durable; normal ALT, improved histology, and absence of HCV RNA in serum and liver have been documented 5–6 years after successful therapy, and "relapses" 2 years after sustained responses are almost unheard of. Thus, sustained virologic responses to antiviral therapy of chronic hepatitis C are tantamount to cures.

Patient variables that tend to correlate with sustained virologic responsiveness to IFN include favorable genotype (genotypes 2 and 3 as opposed to genotypes 1 and 4), low baseline HCV RNA level (<2 million copies/mL, which is equivalent to ~800,000 international units/mL, the current convention of quantitation), histologically mild hepatitis and minimal fibrosis, age <40, absence of obesity, and female gender. Patients with cirrhosis can respond, but they are less likely to do so. Studies of combination IFN-ribavirin therapy showed conclusively that in patients with genotype 1, therapy should last a full year, while in those with genotypes 2 and 3, a 6-month course of therapy suffices. The response rate in African Americans is disappointingly low for reasons that remain obscure. Finally, the likelihood of a sustained response is best if adherence to the treatment regimen is high, i.e., if patients receive ≥80% of the IFN and ribavirin doses and if they continue treatment for ≥80% of the anticipated duration of therapy. Other variables reported to correlate with increased responsiveness include brief duration of infection, low HCV quasispecies diversity, immunocompetence, and low liver iron levels. High levels of HCV RNA, more histologically advanced liver disease, and high quasispecies diversity all go hand in hand with advanced duration of infection, which may be the single most important variable determining IFN responsiveness. The ironic fact, then, is that patients whose disease is least likely to progress are the ones *most* likely to respond to interferon and vice versa. Finally, among patients with genotype 1b, responsiveness to IFN is enhanced in those with amino-acid-substitution mutations in the nonstructural protein 5A gene.

Side effects of IFN therapy are described above in the section on treatment of chronic hepatitis B. The most pronounced side effect of ribavirin therapy is hemolysis; a reduction in hemoglobin of up to 2–3 g or in hematocrit of 5–10% can be anticipated. A small, unpredictable proportion of patients experience profound, brisk hemolysis, resulting in symptomatic anemia; therefore, close monitoring of blood counts is crucial, and ribavirin should be avoided in patients with anemia or hemoglobinopathies and in patients with coronary artery disease or cerebrovascular disease, in whom anemia can precipitate an ischemic event. When symptomatic anemia occurs, ribavirin dose reductions or addition of erythropoietin to boost red blood cell levels may be required. In addition, ribavirin, which is renally excreted, should not be used in patients with renal insufficiency; the drug is teratogenic, precluding its use during pregnancy and mandating the scrupulous use of efficient contraception during therapy.

Ribavirin can also cause nasal and chest congestion, pruritus, and precipitation of gout. Combination IFN-ribavirin therapy is more difficult to tolerate than IFN monotherapy. In one large clinical trial of combination therapy versus monotherapy, among those in the 1-year treatment group, 21% of the combination group (but only 14% of the monotherapy group) had to discontinue treatment, while 26% of the combination group (but only 9% of the monotherapy group) required dose reductions.

Studies of viral kinetics have shown that despite a virion half-life in serum of only 2–3 h, the level of HCV is maintained by a high replication rate of 10^{12} hepatitis C virions per day. IFN-α blocks virion production or release with an efficacy that increases with increasing drug doses; moreover, the calculated death rate for infected cells during IFN therapy is inversely related to viral load; patients with the most rapid death rate of infected hepatocytes are more likely to achieve undetectable HCV RNA at 3 months; achieving this landmark is predictive of a subsequent sustained response. Therefore, to achieve rapid viral clearance from serum and the liver, *high-dose induction therapy* has been advocated. In practice, however, high-dose induction therapy has not yielded higher sustained response rates.

TREATMENT OF CHOICE For the treatment of chronic hepatitis C, standard IFNs have now been supplanted by PEG IFNs. These have elimination times up to sevenfold longer than standard IFNs, i.e., a substantially longer half-life, and achieve prolonged concentrations, permitting administration once (rather than three times) a week. Instead of the frequent drug peaks (linked to side effects) and troughs (when drug is absent) associated with frequent administration of short-acting IFNs, administration of PEG IFNs results in drug concentrations that are more stable and sustained over time. Once-a-week PEG IFN monotherapy is twice as effective as monotherapy with its standard IFN counterpart, approaches the efficacy of combination standard IFN plus ribavirin, and is as well tolerated as standard IFNs, without more difficult-to-manage thrombocytopenia and leukopenia than standard IFNs. The current standard of care, however, is a combination of PEG IFN plus ribavirin.

Two PEG IFNs are available: PEG IFN-α2b and α2a. In the registration trial for PEG IFN-α2b plus ribavirin, the best regimen was 48 weeks of 1.5 μg/kg of PEG IFN once a week plus 800 mg of ribavirin daily. A post hoc analysis suggested that weight-based dosing of ribavirin would have been more effective than the fixed 800-mg dose used in the study. In the first registration trial for PEG IFN-α2a plus ribavirin, the best regimen was 48 weeks of 180 μg of PEG IFN plus 1000 mg (for patients <75 kg) to 1200 mg (for patients ≥75 kg) of ribavirin. Sustained virologic responses of 54 and 56% were reported in these two studies, respectively. A subsequent study of PEG IFN-α2a plus ribavirin showed that, for patients with genotypes 2 and 3, a duration of 6 months and a ribavirin dose of 800 mg was sufficient. Among the three studies, for patients in the optimal treatment arm, sustained response rates for patients with genotype 1 were 42–51% and for patients with genotypes 2 and 3 rates were 76–82%. Subsequent studies have shown that, in patients with genotypes 2 and 3, if HCV RNA is undetectable at 4 weeks ("rapid virologic response"), the total duration of therapy required to achieve a sustained virologic response can be as short as 12–16 weeks, especially for patients with genotype 2 (less so for those with genotype 3). These clinical trials of abbreviated treatment, however, were conducted with full, weight-based ribavirin doses rather than the current convention of uniform, 800-mg flat dosing; studies of abbreviated-duration therapy with flat ribavirin dosing in patients with genotypes 2 and 3 are awaited. Between genotypes 2 and 3, genotype 3 is somewhat more refractory, and some authorities would extend therapy for a full 48 weeks in patients with genotype 3, especially if they have advanced hepatic fibrosis or cirrhosis and/or high-level HCV RNA.

In the initial registration trials for combination PEG IFN plus ribavirin, both combination PEG IFN regimens were compared to standard IFN-α2b plus ribavirin. Side effects of the combination PEG IFN-α2b regimen were comparable to those for the combination standard IFN regimen; however, when the combination PEG IFN-α2a regimen was compared to the combination standard IFN-α2b regimen, flulike symptoms and depression were less common in the combination PEG IFN group. Although the two combination PEG IFN regimens were not tested head-to-head, and although ascertainment of side effects differed between studies of the two drugs, when each was tested against standard IFN-α2b plus ribavirin, combination PEG IFN-α2a plus ribavirin appeared to be better tolerated. Recommended doses for the two PEG IFNs plus ribavirin and other comparisons between the two therapies are shown in **Table 300-6**.

Unless ribavirin is contraindicated (see above), combination PEG IFN plus ribavirin is the recommended course of therapy—24 weeks for genotypes 2 and 3 and 48 weeks for genotype 1. Measurement of quantitative HCV RNA levels at 12 weeks is helpful in guiding therapy; if a 2-$\log_{10}$ drop in HCV RNA has not been achieved by this time, chances for a sustained virologic response are negligible. If the 12-week HCV RNA has fallen by two $\log_{10}$ ("early virologic response"), the chances for a sustained virologic response at the end of therapy are approximately two-thirds; if the 12-week HCV RNA is undetectable, the chances for a sustained virologic response exceed 80%. If the goal of therapy is sustained virologic response, failure to achieve a 12-week 2-$\log_{10}$ drop in HCV RNA may be used as a signal to discontinue therapy, es-

TABLE 300-6 PEGYLATED INTERFERON-α-2A AND α-2B FOR CHRONIC HEPATITIS C

	PEG IFN-α2b	PEG IFN-α2a
PEG size	12 kD linear	40 kD branched
Elimination half-life	54 h	65 h
Clearance	725 mL/h	60 mL/h
Best dose monotherapy[a]	1.0 μg/kg (weight-based)	180 μg
Best dose combination therapy	1.5 μg/kg (weight-based)	180 μg
Storage	Room temperature	Refrigerated
Ribavirin dose		
Genotype 1	800 mg[b]	1,000–1,200 mg[c]
Genotype 2/3	800 mg	800 mg
Duration of therapy		
Genotype 1	48 weeks	48 weeks
Genotype 2/3	48 weeks[d]	24 weeks
Efficacy of combination Rx[e]	54%	56%
Genotype 1	42%	46–51%
Genotype 2/3	82%	76–78%

[a]Reserved for patients in whom ribavirin is contraindicated or not tolerated.

[b]In the registration trial for PEG IFN-α2b plus ribavirin, the optimal regimen was 1.5 μg of PEG IFN plus 800 mg of ribavirin; however, a post hoc analysis of this study suggested that higher ribavirin doses are better. In addition, data from the study of PEG IFN-α2a supported weight-based dosing, 1000 mg (for patients weighing <75 kg) and 1200 mg (for patients weighing ≥75 kg) for genotype 1. Therefore, the higher ribavirin doses are recommended for both types of PEG IFN in patients with genotype 1.

[c]1000 mg for patients weighing <75 kg; 1200 mg for patients weighing ≥75 kg.

[d]In the registration trial for PEG IFN-α2b plus ribavirin, all patients were treated for 48 weeks; however, data from other trials of standard interferons and the other PEG IFN demonstrated that 24 weeks suffices for patients with genotypes 2 and 3. For patients with genotype 3 who have advanced fibrosis/cirrhosis and/or high-level HCV RNA, a full 48 weeks is preferable.

[e]To date, direct, head-to-head comparisons of the two PEG IFNs have not been reported. Attempts to compare the two PEG IFN preparations based on the results of registration clinical trials are confounded by differences between trials of the two agents in methodological details (different ribavirin doses, different methods for recording depression and other side effects) and study-population composition (different proportion with bridging fibrosis/cirrhosis, proportion from the United States versus international, mean weight, proportion with genotype 1, and proportion with high-level HCV RNA).

Note: HCV RNA, hepatitis C virus RNA; PEG, polyethylene glycol; PEG IFN, pegylated interferon.

pecially in those who do not tolerate the drugs well. Still, conceivably, some may achieve histologic benefit in the absence of a virologic response, and some clinicians choose to continue therapy even in the absence of a 2-log$_{10}$ HCV RNA reduction at 12 weeks. Studies are underway to determine whether, even in the absence of a virologic response, maintenance therapy with PEG IFN can slow histologic and clinical progression of hepatitis C.

Studies have suggested that the frequency of sustained virologic responses to PEG IFN/ribavirin therapy can be increased by raising the dose of ribavirin (if tolerated or supplemented by erythropoietin) or by tailoring treatment based on viral response to prolong the duration of viral clearance before discontinuing therapy, i.e., extending therapy from 48 to 72 weeks for patients with genotype 1 and a slow virologic response, i.e., those whose HCV RNA has not fallen rapidly to undetectable levels within 4 weeks (absence of "rapid virologic response"). Confirmatory studies are awaited. Tailoring therapy based on the kinetics of HCV RNA reduction has also been applied to abbreviating the duration of therapy in patients with genotype 1. The results of several clinical trials suggest that, in genotype 1 patients with a 4-week rapid virologic response, but only in the subset with a baseline low level of HCV RNA, 24 weeks of therapy with PEG IFN and weight-based ribavirin suffices, yielding sustained response rates comparable to those achieved with 48 weeks of therapy. Again, although regulatory agencies in Europe have adopted this treatment approach, broad adoption of this approach awaits confirmatory studies.

INDICATIONS FOR ANTIVIRAL THERAPY Patients with chronic hepatitis C who have detectable HCV RNA in serum and chronic hepatitis of at least moderate grade and stage (portal or bridging fibrosis) are candidates for antiviral therapy with PEG IFN plus ribavirin. Most authorities rec-

TABLE 300-7 INDICATIONS AND RECOMMENDATIONS FOR ANTIVIRAL THERAPY OF CHRONIC HEPATITIS C

Standard Indications for Therapy
Detectable HCV RNA (with or without elevated ALT)
Portal/bridging fibrosis or moderate to severe hepatitis on liver biopsy

Retreatment Recommended
Relapsers after a previous course of standard interferon monotherapy or combination standard interferon/ribavirin therapy
    A course of PEG IFN plus ribavirin
Nonresponders to a previous course of standard IFN monotherapy or combination standard IFN/ribavirin therapy
    A course of PEG IFN plus ribavirin—more likely to achieve a sustained virologic response in Caucasian patients without previous ribavirin therapy, with low baseline HCV RNA levels, with a 2-log$_{10}$ reduction in HCV RNA during previous therapy, with genotypes 2 and 3, and without reduction in ribavirin dose.

Antiviral Therapy Not Recommended Routinely but Management Decisions Made on an Individual Basis
Children (age <18 years)
Age >60
Mild hepatitis on liver biopsy

Long-Term Maintenance Therapy Recommended
Cutaneous vasculitis and glomerulonephritis associated with chronic hepatitis C

Long-Term Maintenance Therapy Being Assessed in Clinical Trials
Relapsers
Nonresponders

Antiviral Therapy Not Recommended
Decompensated cirrhosis
Pregnancy (teratogenicity of ribavirin)

Therapeutic Regimens
First-line treatment: PEG IFN subcutaneously once a week plus daily ribavirin orally
    HCV genotypes 1 and 4–48 weeks of therapy
    PEG IFN-α2a 180 μg weekly plus ribavirin 1,000 mg/d (weight <75 kg) to 1200 mg/d (weight ≥75 kg) or
    PEG IFN-α2b 1.5 μg/kg weekly plus ribavirin 800 mg/d (the dose used in registration clinical trials, but the higher, weight-based ribavirin doses above are recommended for both types of PEG IFN)
    HCV genotypes 2 and 3–24 weeks of therapy
    PEG IFN-α2a 180 μg weekly plus ribavirin 800 mg/d or
    PEG IFN-α2b 1.5 μg/kg weekly plus ribavirin 800 mg/d (for patients with genotype 3 who have advanced fibrosis and/or high-level HCV RNA, a full 48 weeks of therapy may be preferable)
Alternative regimen: PEG IFN (α2a 180 μg or α2b 1.0 μg/kg) subcutaneously once a week (primarily for patients in whom ribavirin is contraindicated or not tolerated) for 24 (genotypes 2 and 3) or 48 (genotypes 1 and 4) weeks
For HCV-HIV co-infected patients: 48 weeks, regardless of genotype, of weekly PEG IFN-α2a (180 μg) or PEG IFN-α2b (1.5 μg/kg) plus a daily ribavirin dose of at least 600–800 mg, up to full weight-based 1000–1200 mg dosing if tolerated

Features Associated with Reduced Responsiveness
Genotype 1
High-level HCV RNA (>2 million copies/mL or >800,000 IU/mL)
Advanced fibrosis (bridging fibrosis, cirrhosis)
Long-duration disease
Age >40
High HCV quasispecies diversity
Immunosuppession
African American
Obesity
Hepatic steatosis
Reduced adherence (lower drug doses and reduced duration of therapy)

Note: ALT, alanine aminotransferase; HCV, hepatitis C virus; IFN, interferon; PEG IFN, pegylated interferon; IU, international units (1 IU/mL is equivalent to ~2.5 copies/mL).

ommend 800 mg of ribavirin for patients with genotypes 2 and 3 and weight-based 1000–1200 mg for patients with genotype 1 (and 4) for both types of PEG IFN, unless ribavirin is contraindicated (Table 300-7). Although patients with persistently normal ALT activity tend not to progress histologically, they respond to antiviral therapy just as well as do patients with elevated ALT levels; therefore, while observation without therapy is an option, such patients are potential candidates for antiviral therapy. Therapy with IFN has been shown to improve survival and complication-free survival and to slow progression of fibrosis.

Prior to therapy, HCV genotype should be determined, and the genotype dictates the duration of therapy: 1 year (48 weeks) for patients with genotype 1; 6 months (24 weeks) for those with genotypes 2 and 3; and potentially only 12–16 weeks for patients with genotype 2 whose HCV RNA becomes undetectable within 4 weeks. As noted above, the absence of a 2-$\log_{10}$ drop in HCV RNA at week 12 (an *early virologic response*) weighs heavily against the likelihood of a sustained virologic response even if therapy is continued for the remainder of the planned full year. Therefore, measuring HCV RNA at baseline and at 12 weeks is recommended routinely, especially for patients with genotype 1. The consensus view is that therapy can be discontinued if an early virologic response is not achieved; however, histologic benefit may occur even in the absence of a virologic response. In addition, if current trials show that maintenance therapy can slow the progression of chronic hepatitis C, early virologic nonresponders may be identified as candidates for maintenance therapy; the results of these trials are awaited. Although response rates are lower in patients with certain pretreatment variables, selection for treatment should not be based on symptoms, genotype, HCV RNA level, mode of acquisition of hepatitis C, or advanced hepatic fibrosis. Patients with cirrhosis can respond and should not be excluded as candidates for therapy.

Patients who have relapsed after a course of IFN monotherapy are candidates for retreatment with PEG IFN plus ribavirin (i.e., a more effective treatment regimen is required). For nonresponders to a prior course of IFN monotherapy, retreatment with IFN monotherapy or combination IFN plus ribavirin therapy is unlikely to achieve a sustained virologic response; however, a trial of combination PEG IFN plus ribavirin may be worthwhile. End-treatment virologic responses as high as 40% can occur in this setting, but a sustained virologic response is the outcome in <15–20% of patients. Sustained virologic responses to retreatment of nonresponders are more frequent in those who had never received ribavirin in the past, those with genotypes 2 and 3, those with low pretreatment HCV RNA levels, and noncirrhotics, but less frequent in African Americans, those who failed to achieve a substantial reduction in HCV RNA during their previous course of therapy, and those who required ribavirin-dose reductions. Potential approaches to improving responsiveness to PEG IFN/ribavirin in prior nonresponders include longer duration of treatment; higher doses of either PEG IFN, ribavirin, or both; and switching to a different IFN preparation. However, none of these approaches is of proven efficacy.

Early treatment is indicated for persons with acute hepatitis C (Chap. 298). In patients with biochemically and histologically mild chronic hepatitis C, the rate of progression is slow, and monitoring without therapy is an option; however, such patients respond just as well to combination PEG IFN plus ribavirin therapy as those with elevated ALT and more histologically severe hepatitis. Therefore, therapy for these patients should be considered and the decision made based on such factors as patient motivation, genotype, stage of fibrosis, age, and comorbid conditions. A pretreatment liver biopsy to assess histologic grade and stage provides substantial information about progression of hepatitis C in the past and has prognostic value for future progression. As therapy has improved for patients with a broad range of histologic severity, and as noninvasive laboratory markers of fibrosis have gained popularity, some authorities have placed less value on pretreatment liver biopsies. On the other hand, serum markers of fibrosis are not considered sufficiently accurate, and histologic findings provide important prognostic information to physician and patient. Therefore, a pretreatment liver biopsy is still recommended in most cases.

Patients with compensated cirrhosis can respond to therapy, although their likelihood of a sustained response is lower than in noncirrhotics. Whether survival is improved after successful antiviral therapy in cirrhotics is controversial. Similarly, although several retrospective studies have suggested that antiviral therapy in cirrhotics with chronic hepatitis C reduces the frequency of HCC, less advanced disease in the treated cirrhotics, not treatment itself, may have accounted for the reduced frequency of HCC observed in the treated cohort; prospective studies to address this question are in progress. Patients with decompensated cirrhosis are not candidates for IFN-based antiviral therapy but should be referred for liver transplantation. Some liver transplantation centers have evaluated progressively escalated, low-dose antiviral therapy in an attempt to eradicate hepatitis C viremia prior to transplantation; however, data supporting this approach are limited. After liver transplantation, recurrent hepatitis C is the

rule, and the pace of disease progression is more accelerated than in immunocompetent patients (Chap. 304). Current therapy with PEG IFN and ribavirin is unsatisfactory in most patients, but attempts to minimize immunosuppression are beneficial. The cutaneous and renal vasculitis of HCV-associated essential mixed cryoglobulinemia (Chap. 298) may respond to antiviral therapy, but sustained responses are rare after discontinuation of therapy; therefore, prolonged, perhaps indefinite, therapy is recommended in this group. Anecdotal reports suggest that antiviral therapy may be effective in porphyria cutanea tarda or lichen planus associated with hepatitis C.

In patients with HCV/HIV co-infection, hepatitis C is more progressive and severe than in HCV-monoinfected patients. Although patients with HCV/HIV co-infection respond to antiviral therapy for hepatitis C, they do not respond as well as patients with HCV infection alone. Four large national and international trials of antiviral therapy among patients with HCV/HIV co-infection have shown that PEG IFN (both α2a and α2b) plus ribavirin (daily doses ranging from flat-dosed 600–800 mg to weight-based 1000/1200 mg) is superior to standard IFN regimens; however, sustained response rates were lower than in HCV-monoinfected patients, ranging from 14 to 38% for patients with genotypes 1 and 4 and from 44 to 73% for patients with genotypes 2 and 3. In the three largest trials, all patients, including those with genotypes 2 and 3, were treated for a full 48 weeks. In addition, tolerability of therapy was lower than in HCV-monoinfected patients; therapy was discontinued because of side effects in 12–39% of patients in these clinical trials. Based on these trials, weekly PEG IFN plus daily ribavirin at a daily dose of at least 600–800 mg, up to full weight-based doses if tolerated, is recommended for a full 48 weeks, regardless of genotype. An alternative recommendation for ribavirin doses was issued by a European Consensus Conference and consisted of standard, weight-based 1000–1200 mg for genotypes 1 and 4, but 800 mg for genotypes 2 and 3. In HCV/HIV-infected patients, ribavirin can potentiate the toxicity of—and should not be used together with—didanosine.

Persons with a history of injection-drug use and alcoholism can be treated successfully for chronic hepatitis C, preferably in conjunction with drug and alcohol treatment programs. Because ribavirin is excreted renally, patients with end-stage renal disease, including those undergoing dialysis (which does not clear ribavirin), are not candidates for ribavirin therapy. Rare reports suggest that reduced-dose ribavirin can be used, but the frequency of anemia is very high and data on efficacy are limited. In addition, the manufacturer of PEG IFN-α2a recommends a dose reduction from 180 to 135 μg daily in patients with renal failure. Neither the optimal regimen nor the efficacy of therapy is established in this population.

NOVEL ANTIVIRALS   Among the new approaches to antiviral therapy are direct antivirals (so-called specifically targeted antiviral therapy), including orally administered polymerase and protease inhibitors. For example, in preliminary studies among small numbers of subjects, one of the protease inhibitors being investigated has been shown to suppress HCV RNA by 4 $\log_{10}$ in 14 days when used as monotherapy, to suppress HCV RNA by 5.5 $\log_{10}$ in 14 days when combined with PEG IFN injections, and to suppress HCV RNA to undetectable levels in 12 of 12 subjects treated for 28 days when combined with PEG IFN and ribavirin. Because resistance to these oral agents used alone has been both anticipated and observed, polymerase and protease inhibitors are being evaluated in combinations with PEG IFN (± ribavirin) to preempt the emergence of resistance. Potentially, in the future, combinations of specifically targeted antiviral agents will be used in drug cocktails that may replace IFN-based regimens entirely.

AUTOIMMUNE HEPATITIS

DEFINITION

Autoimmune hepatitis is a chronic disorder characterized by continuing hepatocellular necrosis and inflammation, usually with fibrosis, which can progress to cirrhosis and liver failure. When fulfilling criteria of severity, this type of chronic hepatitis, when untreated, may have a 6-month mortality of as high as 40%. Based on contemporary estimates of the natural history of treated autoimmune hepatitis, the 10-year survival is 80–90%. The prominence of extrahepatic features of autoimmunity as well as seroimmunologic abnormalities in this disorder supports an autoimmune process in its pathogenesis; this concept is reflected in the labels *lupoid, plasma cell*, or *autoimmune hepatitis*. Autoantibodies and other typical features of autoimmunity, however, do not occur in all cases; among the broader categories of "idiopathic" or cryptogenic chronic hepatitis, many, perhaps the majority, are probably autoimmune in origin. Cases in which hepatotropic viruses, metabolic/genetic derangements, and hepatotoxic drugs have been excluded represent a spectrum of heterogeneous liver disorders of unknown cause, a proportion of which are most likely autoimmune hepatitis.

IMMUNOPATHOGENESIS

The weight of evidence suggests that the progressive liver injury in patients with autoimmune hepatitis is the result of a cell-mediated immunologic attack directed against liver cells. In all likelihood, predisposition to autoimmunity is inherited, while the liver specificity of this injury is triggered by environmental (e.g., chemical or viral) factors. For example, patients have been described in whom apparently self-limited cases of acute hepatitis A, B, or C led to autoimmune hepatitis, presumably because of genetic susceptibility or predisposition. Evidence to support an autoimmune pathogenesis in this type of hepatitis includes the following: (1) In the liver, the histopathologic lesions are composed predominantly of cytotoxic T cells and plasma cells; (2) circulating autoantibodies (nuclear, smooth muscle, thyroid, etc.; see below), rheumatoid factor, and hyperglobulinemia are common; (3) other autoimmune disorders—such as thyroiditis, rheumatoid arthritis, autoimmune hemolytic anemia, ulcerative colitis, membranoproliferative glomerulonephritis, juvenile diabetes mellitus, celiac disease, and Sjögren's syndrome—occur with increased frequency in patients who have autoimmune hepatitis and in their relatives; (4) histocompatibility haplotypes associated with autoimmune diseases, such as HLA-B1, -B8, -DR3, and -DR4 as well as extended haplotype DRB1 alleles, are common in patients with autoimmune hepatitis; and (5) this type of chronic hepatitis is responsive to glucocorticoid/immunosuppressive therapy, effective in a variety of autoimmune disorders.

Cellular immune mechanisms appear to be important in the pathogenesis of autoimmune hepatitis. In vitro studies have suggested that in patients with this disorder, lymphocytes are capable of becoming sensitized to hepatocyte membrane proteins and of destroying liver cells. Abnormalities of immunoregulatory control over cytotoxic lymphocytes (impaired regulatory CD4+CD25+ T cell influences) may play a role as well. Studies of genetic predisposition to autoimmune hepatitis demonstrate that certain haplotypes are associated with the disorder, as enumerated above. The precise triggering factors, genetic influences, and cytotoxic and immunoregulatory mechanisms involved in this type of liver injury remain poorly defined.

Intriguing clues into the pathogenesis of autoimmune hepatitis come from the observation that circulating autoantibodies are prevalent in patients with this disorder. Among the autoantibodies described in these patients are antibodies to nuclei [so-called antinuclear antibodies (ANAs), primarily in a homogeneous pattern] and smooth muscle (so-called anti-smooth-muscle antibodies, directed at actin), anti-LKM (see below), antibodies to "soluble liver antigen/liver pancreas antigen" (directed against a uracil-guanine-adenine transfer RNA suppressor protein), as well as antibodies to the liver-specific asialoglycoprotein receptor (or "hepatic lectin") and other hepatocyte membrane proteins. Although some of these provide helpful diagnostic markers, their involvement in the pathogenesis of autoimmune hepatitis has not been established.

Humoral immune mechanisms have been shown to play a role in the extrahepatic manifestations of autoimmune and idiopathic hepatitis. Arthralgias, arthritis, cutaneous vasculitis, and glomerulonephritis occurring in patients with autoimmune hepatitis appear to be mediated by the deposition of circulating immune complexes in affected tissue vessels, followed by complement activation, inflammation, and tissue injury. While specific viral antigen-antibody complexes can be identified in acute and chronic viral hepatitis, the nature of the immune complexes in autoimmune hepatitis has not been defined.

Many of the *clinical features* of autoimmune hepatitis are similar to those described for chronic viral hepatitis. The onset of disease may be insidious or abrupt; the disease may present initially like, and be confused with, acute viral hepatitis; a history of recurrent bouts of what had been labeled *acute hepatitis* is not uncommon. A subset of patients with autoimmune hepatitis has distinct features. Such patients are predominantly young to middle-aged women with marked hyperglobulinemia and high-titer circulating ANAs. This is the group with positive lupus erythematosus (LE) preparations (initially labeled "lupoid" hepatitis) in whom other autoimmune features are common. Fatigue, malaise, anorexia, amenorrhea, acne, arthralgias, and jaundice are common. Occasionally arthritis, maculopapular eruptions (including cutaneous vasculitis), erythema nodosum, colitis, pleurisy, pericarditis, anemia, azotemia, and sicca syndrome (keratoconjunctivitis, xerostomia) occur. In some patients, complications of cirrhosis, such as ascites and edema (associated with hypoalbuminemia), encephalopathy, hypersplenism, coagulopathy, or variceal bleeding may bring the patient to initial medical attention.

The course of autoimmune hepatitis may be variable. In those with mild disease or limited histologic lesions (e.g., piecemeal necrosis without bridging), progression to cirrhosis is limited. In those with severe symptomatic autoimmune hepatitis (aminotransferase levels >10 times normal, marked hyperglobulinemia, "aggressive" histologic lesions—bridging necrosis or multilobular collapse, cirrhosis), the 6-month mortality without therapy may be as high as 40%. Such severe disease accounts for only 20% of cases; the natural history of milder disease is variable, often accentuated by spontaneous remissions and exacerbations. Especially poor prognostic signs include the presence histologically of multilobular collapse at the time of initial presentation and failure of the bilirubin to improve after 2 weeks of therapy. Death may result from hepatic failure, hepatic coma, other complications of cirrhosis (e.g., variceal hemorrhage), and intercurrent infection. In patients with established cirrhosis, HCC may be a late complication but occurs less frequently than in cirrhosis associated with viral hepatitis (Chap. 88).

Laboratory features of autoimmune hepatitis are similar to those seen in chronic viral hepatitis. Liver biochemical tests are invariably abnormal but may not correlate with the clinical severity or histopathologic features in individual cases. Many patients with autoimmune hepatitis have normal serum bilirubin, alkaline phosphatase, and globulin levels with only minimal aminotransferase elevations. Serum AST and ALT levels are increased and fluctuate in the range of 100–1000 units. In severe cases, the serum bilirubin level is moderately elevated [51–171 μmol/L (3–10 mg/dL)]. Hypoalbuminemia occurs in patients with very active or advanced disease. Serum alkaline phosphatase levels may be moderately elevated or near normal. In a small proportion of patients, marked elevations of alkaline phosphatase activity occur; in such patients, clinical and laboratory features overlap with those of primary biliary cirrhosis (Chap. 302). The prothrombin time is often prolonged, particularly late in the disease or during active phases.

Hypergammaglobulinemia (>2.5 g/dL) is common in autoimmune hepatitis. Rheumatoid factor is common as well. As noted above, circulating autoantibodies are also prevalent. The most characteristic are ANAs in a homogeneous staining pattern. Smooth-muscle antibodies are less specific, seen just as frequently in chronic viral hepatitis. Because of the high levels of globulins achieved in the circulation of some patients with autoimmune hepatitis, occasionally the globulins may bind nonspecifically in solid-phase binding immunoassays for viral antibodies. This has been recognized most commonly in tests for antibodies to hepatitis C virus, as noted above. In fact, studies of autoantibodies in autoimmune hepatitis have led to the recognition of new categories of autoimmune hepatitis. *Type I autoimmune hepatitis* is the classic syndrome occurring in young women, associated with marked hyperglobulinemia, lupoid features, circulating ANAs, and HLA-DR3 or HLA-DR4. Also associated with type I autoimmune hepatitis are autoantibodies against actin as well as atypical perinuclear antineutrophilic cytoplasmic antibodies (pANCA).

Type II autoimmune hepatitis, often seen in children, more common in Mediterranean populations, and linked to HLA-DRB1 and HLA-

DQB1 haplotypes, is associated not with ANA but with anti-LKM. Actually, anti-LKM represent a heterogeneous group of antibodies. In type II autoimmune hepatitis, the antibody is anti-LKM1, directed against cytochrome P450 2D6. This is the same anti-LKM seen in some patients with chronic hepatitis C. Anti-LKM2 is seen in drug-induced hepatitis, and anti-LKM3 is seen in patients with chronic hepatitis D. Another autoantibody observed in type II autoimmune hepatitis is directed against liver cytosol formiminotransferase cyclodeaminase (anti-liver cytosol 1). Another type of autoimmune hepatitis has been recognized, *type III autoimmune hepatitis*. These patients lack ANA and anti-LKM1 but have circulating antibodies to soluble liver antigen/liver pancreas antigen. Most of these patients are women and have clinical features similar to, perhaps more severe than, those of patients with type I autoimmune hepatitis. Whether type III autoimmune hepatitis actually represents a distinct category or is part of the spectrum of type I autoimmune hepatitis remains controversial, and this subcategory has not been adopted by a consensus of international experts.

Liver biopsy abnormalities are similar to those described for chronic viral hepatitis. Expanding portal tracts and extending beyond the plate of periportal hepatocytes into the parenchyma (designated *interface hepatitis* or *piecemeal necrosis*) is a mononuclear cell infiltrate that, in autoimmune hepatitis, may include the presence of plasma cells. Necroinflammatory activity characterizes the lobular parenchyma, and evidence of hepatocellular regeneration is reflected by "rosette" formation, the occurrence of thickened liver cell plates, and regenerative "pseudolobules." Septal fibrosis, bridging fibrosis, and cirrhosis are frequent. Bile duct injury and granulomas are uncommon; however, a subgroup of patients with autoimmune hepatitis have histologic, biochemical, and serologic features overlapping those of primary biliary cirrhosis (Chap. 302).

DIAGNOSTIC CRITERIA

An international group has suggested a set of criteria for establishing a diagnosis of autoimmune hepatitis. Exclusion of liver disease caused by genetic disorders, viral hepatitis, drug hepatotoxicity, and alcohol are linked with such inclusive diagnostic criteria as hyperglobulinemia, autoantibodies, and characteristic histologic features. This international group has also suggested a comprehensive diagnostic scoring system that, rarely required for typical cases, may be helpful when typical features are not present. Factors that weigh in favor of the diagnosis include female gender; predominant aminotransferase elevation; presence and level of globulin elevation; presence of nuclear, smooth muscle, LKM1, and other autoantibodies; concurrent other autoimmune diseases; characteristic histologic features (interface hepatitis, plasma cells, rosettes); HLA DR3 or DR4 markers; and response to treatment (see below). Weighing against the diagnosis are predominant alkaline phosphatase elevation, mitochondrial antibodies, markers of viral hepatitis, history of hepatotoxic drugs or excessive alcohol, histologic evidence of bile duct injury, or such atypical histologic features as fatty infiltration, iron overload, and viral inclusions.

DIFFERENTIAL DIAGNOSIS

Early during the course of chronic hepatitis, autoimmune hepatitis may resemble typical *acute viral hepatitis*. Without histologic assessment, severe chronic hepatitis cannot be readily distinguished based on clinical or biochemical criteria from mild chronic hepatitis. In adolescence, *Wilson's disease* may present with features of chronic hepatitis long before neurologic manifestations become apparent and before the formation of Kayser-Fleischer rings. In this age group, serum ceruloplasmin and serum and urinary copper determinations plus measurement of liver copper levels will establish the correct diagnosis. *Postnecrotic* or *cryptogenic cirrhosis* and *primary biliary cirrhosis* share clinical features with autoimmune hepatitis, and both alcoholic hepatitis and nonalcoholic steatohepatitis may present with many features common to autoimmune hepatitis; historic, biochemical, serologic, and histologic assessments are usually sufficient to allow these entities to be distinguished from autoimmune hepatitis. Of course, the dis-

tinction between autoimmune and chronic viral hepatitis is not always straightforward, especially when viral antibodies occur in patients with autoimmune disease or when autoantibodies occur in patients with viral disease. Furthermore, the presence of extrahepatic features such as arthritis, cutaneous vasculitis, or pleuritis—not to mention the presence of circulating autoantibodies—may cause confusion with *rheumatologic disorders* such as rheumatoid arthritis and systemic lupus erythematosus. The existence of clinical and biochemical features of progressive necroinflammatory liver disease distinguishes chronic hepatitis from these other disorders, which are not associated with severe liver disease.

Finally, occasionally, features of autoimmune hepatitis overlap with features of autoimmune biliary disorders such as primary biliary cirrhosis, primary sclerosing cholangitis, or, even more rarely, mitochondrial antibody-negative autoimmune cholangitis. Such overlap syndromes are difficult to categorize, and often response to therapy may be the distinguishing factor that establishes the diagnosis.

℞ AUTOIMMUNE HEPATITIS

The mainstay of management in autoimmune hepatitis is glucocorticoid therapy. Several controlled clinical trials have documented that such therapy leads to symptomatic, clinical, biochemical, and histologic improvement as well as increased survival. A therapeutic response can be expected in up to 80% of patients. Unfortunately, therapy has not been shown to prevent ultimate progression to cirrhosis; however, instances of reversal of fibrosis and cirrhosis have been reported in patients responding to treatment. Although some advocate the use of prednisolone (the hepatic metabolite of prednisone), prednisone is just as effective and is favored by most authorities. Therapy may be initiated at 20 mg/d, but a popular regimen in the United States relies on an initiation dose of 60 mg/d. This high dose is tapered successively over the course of a month down to a maintenance level of 20 mg/d. An alternative but equally effective approach is to begin with half the prednisone dose (30 mg/d) along with azathioprine (50 mg/d). With azathioprine maintained at 50 mg/d, the prednisone dose is tapered over the course of a month down to a maintenance level of 10 mg/d. The advantage of the combination approach is a reduction, over the span of an 18-month course of therapy, in serious, life-threatening complications of steroid therapy from 66% down to under 20%. In combination regimens, 6-mercaptopurine may be substituted for its prodrug azathioprine, but this is rarely required. Azathioprine alone, however, is not effective in achieving remission, nor is alternate-day glucocorticoid therapy. Although therapy has been shown to be effective for severe autoimmune hepatitis (AST ≥10 times the upper limit of normal or ≥5 times the upper limit of normal in conjunction with serum globulin ≥ twice normal; bridging necrosis or multilobular necrosis on liver biopsy; presence of symptoms), therapy is not indicated for mild forms of chronic hepatitis, and the efficacy of therapy in mild or asymptomatic autoimmune hepatitis has not been established.

Improvement of fatigue, anorexia, malaise, and jaundice tends to occur within days to several weeks; biochemical improvement occurs over the course of several weeks to months, with a fall in serum bilirubin and globulin levels and an increase in serum albumin. Serum aminotransferase levels usually drop promptly, but improvements in AST and ALT alone do not appear to be a reliable marker of recovery in individual patients; histologic improvement, characterized by a decrease in mononuclear infiltration and in hepatocellular necrosis, may be delayed for 6–24 months. Still, if interpreted cautiously, aminotransferase levels are valuable indicators of relative disease activity, and many authorities do *not* advocate serial liver biopsies to assess therapeutic success or to guide decisions to alter or stop therapy. Therapy should continue for at least 12–18 months. After tapering and cessation of therapy, the likelihood of relapse is at least 50%, even if posttreatment histology has improved to show mild chronic hepatitis, and the majority of patients require therapy at maintenance doses indefinitely. Continuing azathioprine alone (2 mg/kg body weight daily) after cessation of prednisone therapy may reduce the frequency of relapse.

In medically refractory cases, an attempt should be made to intensify treatment with high-dose glucocorticoid monotherapy (60 mg daily) or combination glucocorticoid (30 mg daily) plus high-dose azathioprine (150 mg daily) therapy. After a month, doses of prednisone can be reduced by 10 mg a month, and doses of azathioprine can be reduced by 50 mg a month toward ultimate, conventional maintenance doses. Patients refractory to this regimen may be treated with cyclosporine, tacrolimus, or mycophenolate mofetil; however, to date only limited anecdotal reports support these approaches. If medical therapy fails, or when chronic hepatitis progresses to cirrhosis and is associated with life-threatening complications of liver decompensation, liver transplantation is the only recourse (Chap. 304); failure of the bilirubin to improve after 2 weeks of therapy should prompt early consideration of the patient for liver transplantation. Recurrence of autoimmune hepatitis in the new liver occurs rarely in most experiences but in as many as 35–40% of cases in others.

ACKNOWLEDGMENT

Kurt J. Isselbacher, MD, contributed to this chapter in previous editions of Harrison's.

FURTHER READINGS

BENHAMOU Y, SALMON D (guest ed): Proceedings of the 1st European consensus conference on the treatment of chronic hepatitis B and C in HIV co-infected patients. J Hepatol 44(Suppl 1):S1, 2006

CHANG T-T et al: A comparison of entecavir and lamivudine for HBeAg-positive chronic hepatitis B. N Engl J Med 354:1001, 2006

CZAJA AJ, FREESE DK: AASLD practice guidelines: Diagnosis and treatment of autoimmune hepatitis. Hepatology 36:479, 2002

DIENSTAG JL, MCHUTCHISON JG: American Gastroenterological Association technical review on the management of hepatitis C. Gastroenterology 130:231, 2006

———: American Gastroenterological Association medical position statement on the management of hepatitis C. Gastroenterology 130:225, 2006

EUROPEAN ASSOCIATION FOR THE STUDY OF THE LIVER: EASL Consensus Conference on Hepatitis B. J Hepatol 39(Suppl 1):S1, 2003

FUNG SK, LOK ASF: Treatment of chronic hepatitis B: Who to treat, what to use, and for how long? Clin Gastroenterol Hepatol 2:839, 2004

KRAWITT EL: Autoimmune hepatitis. N Engl J Med 354:54, 2006

LAI C-L et al: Entecavir versus lamivudine for patients with HBeAg-negative chronic hepatitis B. N Engl J Med 354:1011, 2006

LIAW Y-F et al: Asian-Pacific consensus statement on the management of chronic hepatitis B: A 2005 update. Liver International 25:472, 2005

LOCARNINI SA (guest ed): The control of hepatitis B: The role for chemoprevention. Semin Liver Dis 26:1, 2006

NATIONAL INSTITUTES OF HEALTH CONSENSUS DEVELOPMENT CONFERENCE: Management of hepatitis C. Hepatology 36(Suppl 1):1S, 2002

PAWLOTSKY J-M: Therapy of hepatitis C: From empiricism to eradication. Hepatology 43:S207, 2006

PEARLMAN BL: Chronic hepatitis C therapy: Changing the rules of duration. Clin Gastroenterol Hepatol 4:963, 2006

STRADER DB et al: AASLD practice guideline: Diagnosis, management, and treatment of hepatitis C. Hepatology 39:1147, 2004

301 Alcoholic Liver Disease
Mark E. Mailliard, Michael F. Sorrell

Chronic and excessive alcohol ingestion is one of the major causes of liver disease. The pathology of alcoholic liver disease comprises three major lesions, with the injury rarely existing in a pure form: (1) fatty liver, (2) alcoholic hepatitis, and (3) cirrhosis. Fatty liver is present in >90% of binge and chronic drinkers. A much smaller percentage of heavy drinkers will progress to alcoholic hepatitis, thought to be a precursor to cirrhosis. The prognosis of severe alcoholic liver disease is dismal; the mortality of patients with alcoholic hepatitis concurrent with cirrhosis is nearly 60% at 4 years. Although alcohol is considered a direct hepatotoxin, only between 10 and 20% of alcoholics will develop alcoholic hepatitis. The explanation for this apparent paradox is unclear but involves the complex interaction of facilitating and comorbid factors such as gender, heredity, and immunity.

ETIOLOGY AND PATHOGENESIS

Quantity and duration of alcohol intake are the most important risk factors involved in the development of alcoholic liver disease (Table 301-1). The roles of beverage type(s), i.e. wine, beer, or spirits, and pattern of drinking are less clear. Progress of the hepatic injury beyond the fatty liver stage seems to require additional risk factors that remain incompletely defined. Women are more susceptible to alcoholic liver injury when compared to men. They develop advanced liver disease with substantially less alcohol intake. Hispanic men have a much higher age-adjusted death rate in the United States from alcoholic cirrhosis than do non-Hispanic whites and blacks. In general, the time it takes to develop liver disease is directly related to the amount of alcohol consumed. It is useful in estimating alcohol consumption to understand that one beer, four ounces of wine, or one ounce of 80% spirits all contain ~12 g of alcohol. The threshold for developing alcoholic liver disease in men is an intake of >60–80 g/d of alcohol for 10 years, while women are at increased risk for developing similar degrees of liver injury by consuming 20–40 g/d. Ingestion of 160 g/d is associated with 25–fold increased risk of developing alcoholic cirrhosis. Gender-

TABLE 301-1 RISK FACTORS FOR ALCOHOLIC LIVER DISEASE

Risk Factor	Comment
Quantity	In men, 40–80 g/d of ethanol produces fatty liver; 160 g/d for 10–20 years causes hepatitis or cirrhosis. Only 15% of alcoholics develop alcoholic liver disease.
Gender	Women exhibit increased susceptibility to alcoholic liver disease at amounts >20 g/d; two drinks per day probably safe.
Hepatitis C	HCV infection concurrent with alcoholic liver disease is associated with younger age for severity, more advanced histology, decreased survival.
Genetics	Gene polymorphisms may include alcohol dehydrogenase, cytochrome P4502E1, and those associated with alcoholism (twin studies).
Malnutrition	Alcohol injury does not require malnutrition, but obesity and fatty liver from the effect of carbohydrate on the transcriptional control of lipid synthesis and transport may be factors. Patients should receive vigorous attention to nutritional support.

dependent differences result from poorly understood effects of estrogen and the metabolism of alcohol. Social, immunologic, and heritable factors have all been postulated to play a part in the development of the pathogenic process.

Chronic infection with hepatitis C (HCV) (Chap. 300) is an important comorbidity in the progression of alcoholic liver disease to cirrhosis in chronic and excessive drinkers. Even moderate alcohol intake of 20–50 g/d increases the risk of cirrhosis and hepatocellular cancer in HCV-infected individuals. Patients with both alcoholic liver injury and HCV infection develop decompensated liver disease at a younger age and have poorer overall survival. Increased liver iron stores and, rarely, porphyria cutanea tarda can occur as a consequence of the overlapping injurious processes secondary to alcohol abuse and HCV infection. In addition, alcohol intake of >50 g/d by HCV-infected patients decreases the efficacy of interferon-based antiviral therapy.

Our understanding of the pathogenesis of alcoholic liver injury is incomplete. Alcohol is a direct hepatotoxin, but ingestion of alcohol initiates a variety of metabolic responses that influence the final hepa-

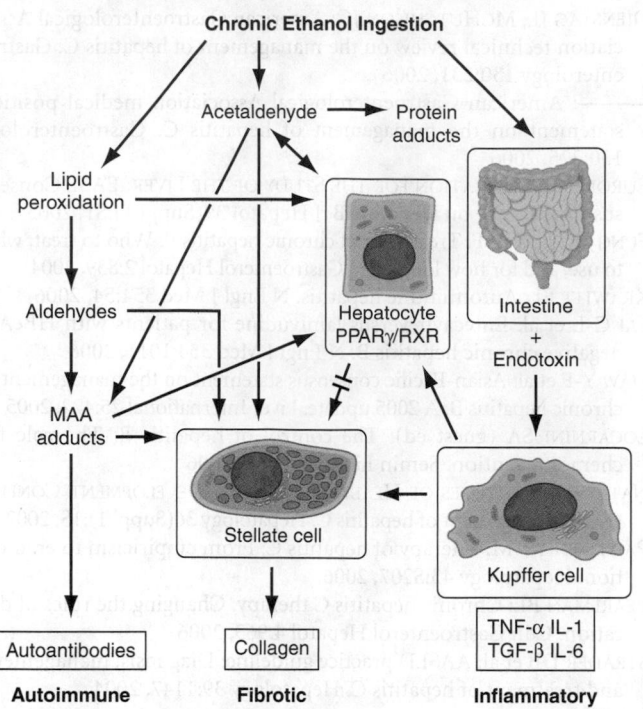

FIGURE 301-1 Biomedical and cellular pathogenesis of liver injury secondary to chronic ethanol ingestion. MAA, malondialdehyde-acetaldehyde; TNF, tumor necrosis factor; TGF, transforming growth factor; IL, interleukin; PPAR, peroxisome proliferator-activated receptor; RXR, retinoid X receptor.

totoxic response. The initial concept of malnutrition as the major pathogenic mechanism has been replaced by the understanding that the hepatic metabolism of alcohol initiates a pathogenic process involving production of toxic protein-aldehyde adducts, endotoxins, oxidative stress, immunologic activity, and pro-inflammatory cytokine release (Fig. 301-1). The complex interaction of intestinal and hepatic cells is crucial to alcohol-mediated liver injury. Tumor necrosis factor α (TNF-α) and intestine-derived endotoxemia facilitate hepatocyte apoptosis and necrosis. Stellate cell activation and collagen production are key events in hepatic fibrogenesis. The resulting fibrosis determines the architectural derangement of the liver following chronic alcohol ingestion.

PATHOLOGY

The liver has a limited repertoire in response to injury. Fatty liver is the initial and most common histologic response to hepatotoxic stimuli, including excessive alcohol ingestion. The accumulation of fat within the perivenular hepatocytes coincides with the location of alcohol dehydrogenase, the major enzyme responsible for alcohol metabolism. Continuing alcohol ingestion results in fat accumulation throughout the entire hepatic lobule. Despite extensive fatty change and distortion of the hepatocytes with macrovesicular fat, the cessation of drinking results in normalization of hepatic architecture and fat content within the liver. Alcoholic fatty liver has traditionally been regarded as entirely benign, but similar to the spectrum of nonalcoholic fatty liver disease (Chap. 303), the appearance of steatohepatitis and certain pathologic features such as giant mitochondria, perivenular fibrosis, and macrovesicular fat may be associated with progressive liver injury.

The transition between fatty liver and the development of alcoholic hepatitis is blurred. The hallmark of alcoholic hepatitis is hepatocyte injury characterized by ballooning degeneration, spotty necrosis, polymorphonuclear infiltrate, and fibrosis in the perivenular and perisinusoidal space of Disse. Mallory bodies are often present in florid cases but are neither specific nor necessary to establishing the diagnosis. Alcoholic hepatitis is thought to be a precursor to the devel-

opment of cirrhosis. However, like fatty liver, it is potentially reversible with cessation of drinking. Cirrhosis is present in up to 50% of patients with biopsy-proven alcoholic hepatitis and its regression is uncertain, even with abstention.

CLINICAL FEATURES

The clinical manifestations of alcoholic fatty liver are subtle and characteristically detected as a consequence of the patient's visit for a seemingly unrelated matter. Previously unsuspected hepatomegaly is often the only clinical finding. Occasionally, patients with fatty liver will present with right upper quadrant discomfort, tender hepatomegaly, nausea, and jaundice. Differentiation of alcoholic fatty liver from nonalcoholic fatty liver is difficult unless an accurate drinking history is ascertained. In every instance where liver disease is present, a thoughtful and sensitive drinking history should be obtained. Standard, validated questions accurately detect alcohol-related problems. Alcoholic hepatitis is associated with a wide gamut of clinical features. Cytokine production is thought to be responsible for the systemic manifestations of alcoholic hepatitis. Fever, spider nevi, jaundice, and abdominal pain simulating an acute abdomen represent the extreme end of the spectrum, while many patients will be entirely asymptomatic. Portal hypertension, ascites, or variceal bleeding can occur in the absence of cirrhosis. Recognition of the clinical features of alcoholic hepatitis is central to the initiation of an effective and appropriate diagnostic and therapeutic strategy. It is important to recognize that patients with alcoholic cirrhosis often exhibit clinical features identical to other causes of cirrhosis.

LABORATORY FEATURES

Patients with alcoholic liver disease are often identified through routine screening tests. The typical laboratory abnormalities seen in fatty liver are nonspecific and include modest elevations of the aspartate aminotransferase (AST), alanine aminotransferase (ALT), and γ-glutamyl transpeptidase (GGTP), accompanied by hypertriglyceridemia, hypercholesterolemia, and occasionally hyperbilirubinemia. In alcoholic hepatitis and in contrast to other causes of fatty liver, the AST and ALT are usually elevated two- to sevenfold. They are rarely >400 IU, and the AST/ALT ratio >1 (Table 301-2). Hyperbilirubinemia is common and is accompanied by modest increases in the alkaline phosphatase level. Derangement in hepatocyte synthetic function indicates more serious disease. Hypoalbuminemia and coagulopathy are common in advanced liver injury. Ultrasonography is useful in detecting fatty infiltration of the liver and determining liver size. The demonstration by ultrasound of portal vein flow reversal, ascites, and intraabdominal collaterals indicates serious liver injury with less potential for complete reversal of liver disease.

PROGNOSIS

Critically ill patients with alcoholic hepatitis have short-term (30 day) mortality rates >50%. Severe alcoholic hepatitis is heralded by coagulopathy (prothrombin time > 5 s), anemia, serum albumin concentrations <25 g/L (2.5 mg/dL), serum bilirubin levels > 137 μmol/L (8 mg/

TABLE 301-2	LABORATORY DIAGNOSIS OF ALCOHOLIC FATTY LIVER AND ALCOHOLIC HEPATITIS
Test	**Comment**
AST	Increased two- to sevenfold, <400 U/L, greater than ALT
ALT	Increased two- to sevenfold, <400 U/L
AST/ALT	Usually >1
GGTP	Not specific to alcohol, easily inducible, elevated in all forms of fatty liver
Bilirubin	May be markedly increased in alcoholic hepatitis despite modest elevation in alkaline phosphatase
PMN	If >5500/μL, predicts severe alcoholic hepatitis when discriminant function > 32

Note: AST, aspartate aminotransferase; ALT, alanine aminotransferase; GGTP, gamma-glutamyl transpeptidase; PMN, polymorphonuclear cells.

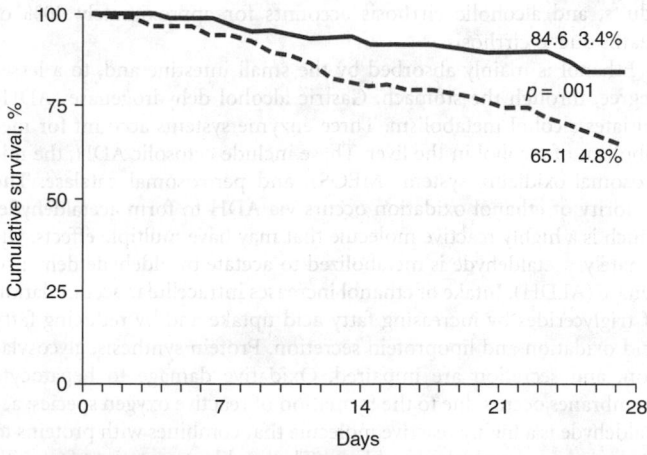

FIGURE 301-2 Effect of glucocorticoid therapy of severe alcoholic hepatitis on short-term survival: the result of a meta-analysis of individual data from three studies. Prednisolone, solid line; placebo, dotted line. (*Adapted from Mathurin et al., with permission from Elsevier Science.*)

dL), renal failure, and ascites. A discriminant function calculated as 4.6 × [prothrombin time control (seconds)] + serum bilirubin (mg/dL) can identify patients with a poor prognosis (discriminant function > 32). The presence of ascites, variceal hemorrhage, deep encephalopathy, or hepatorenal syndrome predicts a dismal prognosis. The pathologic stage of the injury can be helpful in predicting prognosis. Liver biopsy should be performed whenever possible to confirm the diagnosis, to establish potential reversibility of the liver disease, and to guide the therapeutic decisions.

Rx ALCOHOLIC LIVER DISEASE

Complete abstinence from alcohol is the cornerstone in the treatment of alcoholic liver disease. Improved survival and the potential for reversal of histologic injury regardless of the initial clinical presentation are associated with total avoidance of alcohol ingestion. Referral of patients to experienced alcohol counselors and/or alcohol treatment programs should be routine in the management of patients with alcoholic liver disease. Attention should be directed to the nutritional and psychosocial states during the evaluation and treatment periods. Because of data suggesting that the pathogenic mechanisms in alcoholic hepatitis involve cytokine release and the perpetuation of injury by immunologic processes, glucocorticoids have been extensively evaluated in the treatment of alcoholic hepatitis. Patients with severe alcoholic hepatitis, defined as a discriminant function > 32, were given prednisone, 40 mg/d, or prednisolone, 32 mg/d, for 4 weeks followed by a steroid taper (**Fig. 301-2**). Exclusion criteria included active gastrointestinal bleeding, sepsis, renal failure, or pancreatitis. Women with encephalopathy from severe alcoholic hepatitis may be particularly good candidates for glucocorticoids.

Newer understanding of the role of TNF-α expression and receptor activity in alcoholic liver injury has led to an examination of TNF inhibition as an alternative to glucocorticoids for severe alcoholic hepatitis. The nonspecific TNF inhibitor, pentoxifylline, recently demonstrated improved survival in the therapy of severe alcoholic hepatitis (**Fig. 301-3**). Preliminary trials of neutralizing monoclonal antibody specific for TNF have been disap-

TREATMENT FOR ALCOHOLIC HEPATITIS

Alcoholic Hepatitis
↓
Alcohol abstinence
Nutritional support
↓
Discriminant function ≥ 32
(with absence of comorbidity)
↓
Treatment options
↓   ↓
Preferred   Alternative
↓   ↓
Prednisolone 32 mg   Pentoxifylline 400 mg
PO daily for 4 weeks, PO tid for 4 weeks
then taper for 4 weeks

FIGURE 301-3 Treatment algorithm for alcoholic hepatitis. As identified by a calculated discriminant function > 32 (see text), patients with severe alcoholic hepatitis, without the presence of gastrointestinal bleeding or infection, would be candidates for either glucocorticoids or pentoxifylline administration.

pointing because of increased deaths secondary to infection. Because of inordinate surgical mortality and the high rates of recidivism following transplantation, patients with alcoholic hepatitis are not candidates for immediate liver transplantation. The transplant candidacy of these patients should be reevaluated after a defined period of sobriety.

FURTHER READINGS

AKRIVIADIS E et al: Pentoxifylline improves short-term survival in severe acute alcoholic hepatitis: A double blind placebo controlled trial. Gastroenterology 119:1637, 2000

BELL H et al: Long-term prognosis of patients with alcoholic liver cirrhosis: A 15-year follow-up study of 100 Norwegian patients admitted to one unit. Scand J Gastroenterol 9: 858, 2004

LEVITSKY J, MAILLIARD ME: Diagnosis and therapy of alcoholic liver disease. Semin Liver Dis 24: 233, 2004

MATHURIN P et al: Corticosteroids improve short-term survival in patients with severe alcoholic hepatitis (AH): Individual data analysis of the last three randomized placebo controlled double blind trials of corticosteroids in severe AH. J Hepatol 36:480, 2002

SAFDAR K, SCHIFF ER: Alcohol and hepatitis C. Semin Liver Dis 24: 305, 2004

302 Cirrhosis and Its Complications
Bruce R. Bacon

Cirrhosis is a condition that is defined histopathologically and has a variety of clinical manifestations and complications, some of which can be life-threatening. In the past, it has been thought that cirrhosis was never

reversible; however, it has become apparent that when the underlying insult that has caused the cirrhosis has been removed, there can be reversal of fibrosis. This is most apparent with the successful treatment of chronic hepatitis C; however, reversal of fibrosis is also seen in patients with hemochromatosis who have been successfully treated and in patients with alcoholic liver disease who have discontinued alcohol use.

Regardless of the cause of cirrhosis, the pathologic features consist of the development of fibrosis to the point that there is architectural

TABLE 302-1 CAUSES OF CIRRHOSIS

Alcoholism	Cardiac cirrhosis
Chronic viral hepatitis	Inherited metabolic liver disease
Hepatitis B	Hemochromatosis
Hepatitis C	Wilson's disease
Autoimmune hepatitis	α_1 Antitrypsin deficiency
Nonalcoholic steatohepatitis	Cystic fibrosis
Biliary cirrhosis	Cryptogenic cirrhosis
Primary biliary cirrhosis	
Primary sclerosing cholangitis	
Autoimmune cholangiopathy	

distortion with the formation of regenerative nodules. This results in a decrease in hepatocellular mass, and thus function, and an alteration of blood flow. The induction of fibrosis occurs with activation of hepatic stellate cells, resulting in the formation of increased amounts of collagen and other components of the extracellular matrix.

Clinical features of cirrhosis are the result of pathologic changes and mirror the severity of the liver disease. Most hepatic pathologists provide an assessment of grading and staging when evaluating liver biopsy samples. These grading and staging schemes vary between disease states and have been developed for most conditions, including chronic viral hepatitis, nonalcoholic fatty liver disease, and primary biliary cirrhosis. Advanced fibrosis usually includes bridging fibrosis with nodularity designated as stage 3 and cirrhosis designated as stage 4. Patients who have cirrhosis have varying degrees of compensated liver function, and clinicians need to differentiate between those who have stable, compensated cirrhosis and those who have decompensated cirrhosis. Patients who have developed complications of their liver disease and have become decompensated should be considered for liver transplantation. Many of the complications of cirrhosis will require specific therapy. *Portal hypertension* is a significant complicating feature of decompensated cirrhosis and is responsible for the development of ascites and bleeding from esophagogastric varices, two complications that signify decompensated cirrhosis. Loss of hepatocellular function results in jaundice, coagulation disorders, and hypoalbuminemia and contributes to the causes of portosystemic encephalopathy. The complications of cirrhosis are basically the same regardless of the etiology. Nonetheless, it is useful to classify patients by the cause of their liver disease (Table 302-1); patients can be divided into broad groups with alcoholic cirrhosis, cirrhosis due to chronic viral hepatitis, biliary cirrhosis, and other less-common causes such as cardiac cirrhosis, cryptogenic cirrhosis, and other miscellaneous causes.

ALCOHOLIC CIRRHOSIS

Excessive chronic alcohol use can cause several different types of chronic liver disease, including alcoholic fatty liver, alcoholic hepatitis, and alcoholic cirrhosis. Furthermore, use of excessive alcohol can contribute to liver damage in patients with other liver diseases, such as hepatitis C, hemochromatosis, and those patients who have fatty liver disease related to obesity. Chronic alcohol use can produce fibrosis in the absence of accompanying inflammation and/or necrosis. Fibrosis can be centrilobular, pericellular, or periportal. When fibrosis reaches a certain degree, there is disruption of the normal liver architecture and replacement of liver cells by regenerative nodules. In alcoholic cirrhosis, the nodules are usually <3 mm in diameter; this form of cirrhosis is referred to as *micronodular*. With cessation of alcohol use, larger nodules may form, resulting in a mixed micronodular and macronodular cirrhosis.

Pathogenesis Alcohol is the most commonly used drug in the United States, and more than two-thirds of adults drink alcohol each year. Thirty percent have had a binge within the past month, and over 7% of adults regularly consume more than two drinks per day. Unfortunately, more than 14 million adults in the United States meet the diagnostic criteria for alcohol abuse or dependence. In the United States, chronic liver disease is the 10th most common cause of death in

adults, and alcoholic cirrhosis accounts for approximately 40% of deaths due to cirrhosis.

Ethanol is mainly absorbed by the small intestine and, to a lesser degree, through the stomach. Gastric alcohol dehydrogenase (ADH) initiates alcohol metabolism. Three enzyme systems account for metabolism of alcohol in the liver. These include cytosolic ADH, the microsomal-oxidizing system (MEOS), and peroxisomal catalase. The majority of ethanol oxidation occurs via ADH to form acetaldehyde, which is a highly reactive molecule that may have multiple effects. Ultimately, acetaldehyde is metabolized to acetate by aldehyde dehydrogenase (ALDH). Intake of ethanol increases intracellular accumulation of triglycerides by increasing fatty acid uptake and by reducing fatty acid oxidation and lipoprotein secretion. Protein synthesis, glycosylation, and secretion are impaired. Oxidative damage to hepatocyte membranes occurs due to the formation of reactive oxygen species; acetaldehyde is a highly reactive molecule that combines with proteins to form protein-acetaldehyde adducts. These adducts may interfere with specific enzyme activities, including microtubular formation and hepatic protein trafficking. With acetaldehyde-mediated hepatocyte damage, certain reactive oxygen species can result in Kupffer cell activation. As a result, profibrogenic cytokines are produced that initiate and perpetuate stellate cell activation, with the resultant production of excess collagen and extracellular matrix. Connective tissue appears in both periportal and pericentral zones and eventually connects portal triads with central veins forming regenerative nodules. Hepatocyte loss occurs, and with increased collagen production and deposition, together with continuing hepatocyte destruction, the liver contracts and shrinks in size. This process generally takes from years to decades to occur and requires repeated insults.

Clinical Features The diagnosis of alcoholic liver disease requires an accurate history regarding both amount and duration of alcohol consumption. Patients with alcoholic liver disease can present with nonspecific symptoms such as vague right upper quadrant pain, fever, nausea and vomiting, diarrhea, anorexia, and malaise. Alternatively, they may present with more specific complications of chronic liver disease, including ascites, edema, or upper gastrointestinal (GI) hemorrhage. Many cases present incidentally at the time of autopsy or elective surgery. Other clinical manifestations include the development of jaundice or encephalopathy. The abrupt onset of any of these complications may be the first event prompting the patient to seek medical attention. Other patients may be identified in the course of an evaluation of routine laboratory studies that are found to be abnormal. On physical examination, the liver and spleen may be enlarged, with the liver edge being firm and nodular. Other frequent findings include scleral icterus, palmar erythema, spider angiomas, parotid gland enlargement, digital clubbing, muscle wasting, or the development of edema and ascites. Men may have decreased body hair and gynecomastia as well as testicular atrophy, which may be a consequence of hormonal abnormalities or a direct toxic effect of alcohol on the testes. In women with advanced alcoholic cirrhosis, menstrual irregularities usually occur, and some women may be amenorrheic. These changes are often reversible following cessation of alcohol.

Laboratory tests may be completely normal in patients with early compensated alcoholic cirrhosis. Alternatively, in advanced liver disease, many abnormalities usually are present. Patients may be anemic either from chronic GI blood loss, nutritional deficiencies, or hypersplenism related to portal hypertension, or as a direct suppressive effect of alcohol on the bone marrow. A unique form of hemolytic anemia (with spur cells and acanthocytes) called *Zieve's syndrome* can occur in patients with severe alcoholic hepatitis. Platelet counts are often reduced early in the disease, reflective of portal hypertension with hypersplenism. Serum total bilirubin can be normal or elevated with advanced disease. Direct bilirubin is frequently mildly elevated in patients with a normal total bilirubin, but the abnormality typically progresses as the disease worsens. Prothrombin times are often prolonged and usually do not respond to administration of parenteral vitamin K. Serum sodium levels are usually normal unless patients have ascites and then can be depressed, largely due to ingestion of excess free water. Serum aminotransferases (ALT, AST) are typically elevated, particularly in patients who continue to drink, with AST levels being higher than ALT levels, usually by a 2:1 ratio.

Diagnosis Patients who have any of the above-mentioned clinical features, physical examination findings, or laboratory studies should be considered to have alcoholic liver disease. The diagnosis, however, requires accurate knowledge that the patient is continuing to use and abuse alcohol. Furthermore, other forms of chronic liver disease (e.g., chronic viral hepatitis, metabolic or autoimmune liver diseases) must be considered or ruled out or, if present, an estimate of relative causality along with the alcohol use should be determined. Liver biopsy can be helpful to confirm a diagnosis, but generally when patients present with alcoholic hepatitis and are still drinking, liver biopsy is withheld until abstinence has been maintained for at least 6 months in order to determine residual, nonreversible disease.

In patients who have had complications of cirrhosis and who continue to drink, there is a <50% 5-year survival. In contrast, in those patients who are able to remain abstinent, the prognosis is significantly improved. In patients with advanced liver disease, the prognosis remains poor; however, in those individuals who are able to remain abstinent, liver transplantation is a viable option.

℞ ALCOHOLIC CIRRHOSIS

Abstinence is the cornerstone of therapy for patients with alcoholic liver disease. In addition, patients require good nutrition and long-term medical supervision in order to manage underlying complications that may develop. Complications such as the development of ascites and edema, variceal hemorrhage, or portosystemic encephalopathy all require specific management and treatment. Glucocorticoids are occasionally used in patients with severe alcoholic hepatitis in the absence of infection. Survival has been shown to improve in certain studies. Treatment is restricted to patients with a discriminant function (DF) value of >32. The DF is calculated as the serum total bilirubin plus the difference in the patient's prothrombin time compared to control (in seconds) multiplied by 4.6. In patients for whom this value is >32, there is improved survival at 28 days with the use of glucocorticoids.

Other therapies that have been used include oral pentoxifylline, which decreases the production of tumor necrosis factor α (TNF-α) and other proinflammatory cytokines. In contrast to glucocorticoids, with which complications can occur, pentoxifylline is relatively easy to administer and has few if any side effects. A variety of nutritional therapies have been tried with either parenteral or enteral feedings; however, it is unclear whether any of these modalities have significantly improved survival.

Recent studies have used parenterally administered inhibitors of TNF-α such as infliximab or etanercept. Early results have shown no adverse events; however, there was no clear-cut improvement in survival. Anabolic steroids, propylthiouracil, antioxidants, colchicine, and penicillamine have all been used but do not show clear-cut benefit and are not recommended.

As mentioned above, the cornerstone to treatment is cessation of alcohol use. Recent experience with medications that reduce craving for alcohol such as acamprosate calcium has been favorable. Patients may take other necessary medications even in the presence of cirrhosis. Acetaminophen use is often discouraged in patients with liver disease; however, if no more than 2 g of acetaminophen per day are consumed, there generally are no problems.

CIRRHOSIS DUE TO CHRONIC VIRAL HEPATITIS B OR C

Of patients exposed to the hepatitis C virus (HCV), approximately 80% develop chronic hepatitis C, and of those, about 20–30% will develop cirrhosis over 20–30 years. Many of these patients have had concomitant alcohol use, and the true incidence of cirrhosis due to hepatitis C alone is unknown. Nonetheless, this represents a significant number of patients. It is expected that an even higher percentage will go on to develop cirrhosis over longer periods of time. In the United States, approximately 5 million people have been exposed to the hepatitis C virus, with about 3^1/$_2$–4 million who are chronically

viremic. Worldwide, about 170 million individuals have hepatitis C, with some areas of the world (e.g., Egypt) having up to 15% of the population infected. HCV is a noncytopathic virus, and liver damage is probably immune-mediated. Progression of liver disease due to chronic hepatitis C is characterized by portal-based fibrosis with bridging fibrosis and nodularity developing, ultimately culminating in the development of cirrhosis. In cirrhosis due to chronic hepatitis C, the liver is small and shrunken with characteristic features of a mixed micro- and macronodular cirrhosis seen on liver biopsy. In addition to the increased fibrosis that is seen in cirrhosis due to hepatitis C, an inflammatory infiltrate is found in portal areas with interface hepatitis and occasionally some lobular hepatocellular injury and inflammation. In patients with HCV genotype 3, steatosis is often present.

Similar findings are seen in patients with cirrhosis due to chronic hepatitis B. Of patients exposed to hepatitis B, about 5% develop chronic hepatitis B, and about 20% of those patients will go on to develop cirrhosis. Special stains for HBc (hepatitis B core) and HBs (hepatitis B surface) antigen will be positive, and ground glass hepatocytes signifying HBsAg (hepatitis B surface antigen) may be present. In the United States, there are about 1.25 million carriers of hepatitis B, whereas in other parts of the world where hepatitis B virus (HBV) is endemic (i.e., Southeast Asia, sub-Saharan Africa), up to 15% of the population may be infected having acquired the infection vertically at the time of birth. Thus, over 300–400 million individuals are thought to have hepatitis B worldwide. Approximately 25% of these individuals may ultimately develop cirrhosis.

Clinical Features and Diagnosis Patients with cirrhosis due to either chronic hepatitis C or B can present with the usual symptoms and signs of chronic liver disease. Fatigue, malaise, vague right upper quadrant pain, and laboratory abnormalities are frequent presenting features. Diagnosis requires a thorough laboratory evaluation, including quantitative HCV RNA testing and analysis for HCV genotype, or hepatitis B serologies to include HBsAg, anti-HBs, HBeAg (hepatitis B e antigen), anti-HBe, and quantitative HBV DNA levels.

℞ CIRRHOSIS DUE TO CHRONIC VIRAL HEPATITIS B OR C

Management of complications of cirrhosis revolves around specific therapy for treatment of whatever complications occur, whether they be esophageal variceal hemorrhage, development of ascites and edema, or encephalopathy. In patients with chronic hepatitis B, numerous studies have shown beneficial effects of antiviral therapy, which is effective at viral suppression, as evidenced by reducing aminotransferase levels and HBV DNA levels, and improving histology by reducing inflammation and fibrosis. Several clinical trials and case series have demonstrated that patients with decompensated liver disease can become compensated with the use of antiviral therapy directed against hepatitis B. Currently available therapy includes lamivudine, adefovir, entecavir, and tenofovir. Interferon α can also be used for treating hepatitis B, but it should not be used in cirrhotics.

Treatment of patients with cirrhosis due to hepatitis C is a little more difficult because the side effects of pegylated interferon and ribavirin therapy are oftentimes difficult to manage in patients with cirrhosis. Dose-limiting cytopenias (platelets, white blood cells, red blood cells) or severe side effects can result in discontinuation of treatment. Nonetheless, if patients can tolerate treatment, and if it is successful, the benefit is great and disease progression is reduced.

CIRRHOSIS FROM AUTOIMMUNE HEPATITIS AND NONALCOHOLIC FATTY LIVER DISEASE

Other causes of posthepatitic cirrhosis include autoimmune hepatitis and cirrhosis due to nonalcoholic steatohepatitis. Many patients with autoimmune hepatitis (AIH) present with cirrhosis that is already established. Typically, these patients will not benefit from immunosuppressive therapy with glucocorticoids or azathioprine since the AIH is "burned out." In this situation, liver biopsy does not show a significant inflammatory infiltrate. Diagnosis in this setting requires positive autoimmune markers such as antinuclear antibody (ANA) or anti-smooth-muscle antibody (ASMA). When patients with AIH present with cirrhosis and active inflammation accompanied by elevated liver enzymes, there can be considerable benefit from the use of immunosuppressive therapy.

Patients with nonalcoholic steatohepatitis are increasingly being found to have progressed to cirrhosis. With the epidemic of obesity that continues in Western countries, more and more patients are identified with nonalcoholic fatty liver disease. Of these, a significant subset have nonalcoholic steatohepatitis and can progress to increased fibrosis and cirrhosis. Over the past several years, it has been increasingly recognized that many patients who were thought to have cryptogenic cirrhosis in fact have nonalcoholic steatohepatitis. As their cirrhosis progresses, they become catabolic and then lose the telltale signs of steatosis seen on biopsy. Management of complications of cirrhosis due to either AIH or nonalcoholic steatohepatitis is similar to that for other forms of cirrhosis.

BILIARY CIRRHOSIS

Biliary cirrhosis has pathologic features that are different from either alcoholic cirrhosis or posthepatitic cirrhosis, yet the manifestations of end-stage liver disease are the same. Cholestatic liver disease may result from necroinflammatory lesions, congenital or metabolic processes, or external bile duct compression. Thus, two broad categories reflect the anatomic sites of abnormal bile retention: *intrahepatic* and *extrahepatic*. The distinction is important for obvious therapeutic reasons. Extrahepatic obstruction may benefit from surgical or endoscopic biliary tract decompression, whereas intrahepatic cholestatic processes will not improve with such interventions and require a different approach.

The major causes of chronic cholestatic syndromes are primary biliary cirrhosis (PBC), autoimmune cholangitis, primary sclerosing cholangitis (PSC), and idiopathic adulthood ductopenia. These syndromes are usually clinically distinguished from each other by antibody testing, cholangiographic findings, and clinical presentation. However, they all share the histopathologic features of chronic cholestasis, such as cholate stasis, copper deposition, xanthomatous transformation of hepatocytes, and irregular so-called biliary fibrosis. In addition, there may be chronic portal inflammation, interface activity, and chronic lobular inflammation. Ductopenia is a result of this progressive disease as patients develop cirrhosis.

PRIMARY BILIARY CIRRHOSIS

PBC is seen in about 100–200 individuals per million, with a strong female preponderance and a median age of around 50 years at the time of diagnosis. The cause of PBC is unknown; it is characterized by portal inflammation and necrosis of cholangiocytes in small and medium-sized bile ducts. Cholestatic features prevail, and biliary cirrhosis is characterized by an elevated bilirubin level and progressive liver failure. Liver transplantation is the treatment of choice for patients with decompensated cirrhosis due to PBC. A variety of therapies have been proposed, but ursodeoxycholic acid (UDCA) is the only approved treatment that has some degree of efficacy by slowing the rate of progression of the disease.

Antimitochondrial antibodies (AMA) are present in about 90% of patients with PBC. These autoantibodies recognize intermitochondrial membrane proteins that are enzymes of the pyruvate dehydrogenase complex (PDC), the branched chain–2-oxoacid dehydrogenase complex, and the 2-oxogluterate dehydrogenase complex. Most relate to pyruvate dehydrogenase. These autoantibodies are not pathogenic but rather are useful markers for making a diagnosis of PBC.

Pathology Histopathologic analyses of liver biopsies of patients with PBC have resulted in identifying four distinct stages of the disease as it progresses. The earliest lesion is termed *chronic nonsuppurative destructive cholangitis* and is a necrotizing inflammatory process of the portal tracts. Medium and small bile ducts are infiltrated with lymphocytes and undergo duct destruction. Mild fibrosis and sometimes bile stasis can occur. With progression, the inflammatory infiltrate becomes less prominent, but the number of bile ducts is reduced and there is proliferation of smaller bile ductules. Increased fibrosis ensues with the expansion of periportal fibrosis to bridging fibrosis. Finally, cirrhosis, which may be micronodular or macronodular, develops.

Clinical Features Currently most patients with PBC are diagnosed well before the end-stage manifestations of the disease are present, and, as such, most patients are actually asymptomatic. When symptoms are present, they most prominently include a significant degree of fatigue out of proportion to what would be expected for either the severity of the liver disease or the age of the patient. Pruritus is seen in approximately 50% of patients at the time of diagnosis and can be debilitating. It may be intermittent and usually is most bothersome in the evening. In some patients, pruritus can develop toward the end of pregnancy, and there are examples of patients having been diagnosed with cholestasis of pregnancy rather than PBC. Pruritus that presents prior to the development of jaundice indicates severe disease and a poor prognosis.

Physical examination can show jaundice and other complications of chronic liver disease including hepatomegaly, splenomegaly, ascites, and edema. Other features that are unique to PBC include hyperpigmentation, xanthelasma, and xanthomata, which are related to the altered cholesterol metabolism seen in this disease. Hyperpigmentation is evident on the trunk and the arms and is seen in areas of exfoliation and lichenification associated with progressive scratching related to the pruritus. Bone pain resulting from osteopenia or osteoporosis is occasionally seen at the time of diagnosis.

Laboratory Findings Laboratory findings in PBC show cholestatic liver enzyme abnormalities with an elevation in γ-glutamyl transpeptidase and alkaline phosphatase (ALP) along with mild elevations in aminotransferases (ALT and AST). Immunoglobulins, particularly IgM, are typically increased. Hyperbilirubinemia usually is seen once cirrhosis has developed. Thrombocytopenia, leukopenia, and anemia may be seen in patients with portal hypertension and hypersplenism. Liver biopsy shows characteristic features as described above and should be evident to any experienced hepatopathologist. Up to 10% of patients with characteristic PBC will have features of AIH as well and are defined as having "overlap" syndrome. These patients are treated as PBC patients and may progress to cirrhosis with the same frequency as typical PBC patients.

Diagnosis PBC should be considered in patients with chronic cholestatic liver enzyme abnormalities. It is most often seen in middle-aged women. AMA testing may be negative, and it should be remembered that as many as 10% of patients with PBC may be AMA-negative. Liver biopsy is most important in this setting of AMA-negative PBC. In patients who are AMA-negative with cholestatic liver enzymes, PSC should be ruled out by way of cholangiography.

℞ PRIMARY BILIARY CIRRHOSIS

Treatment of the typical manifestations of cirrhosis are no different for PBC than for other forms of cirrhosis. UDCA has been shown to improve both biochemical and histologic features of the disease. Improvement is greatest when therapy is initiated early; the likelihood of significant improvement with UDCA is low in patients with PBC who present with manifestations of cirrhosis. UDCA is given in doses of 13–15 mg/kg per day; the medication is usually well-tolerated, although some patients have worsening pruritus with initiation of therapy. A small proportion of patients may have diarrhea or headache as a side effect of the drug. UDCA has been shown to slow the rate of progression of PBC, but it does not reverse or cure the disease. Patients with PBC require long-term follow-up by a physician experienced with the disease. Certain patients may need to be considered for liver transplantation should their liver disease decompensate.

The main symptoms of PBC are fatigue and pruritus, and symptom management is important. Several therapies have been tried for treatment of fatigue, but none of them have been successful; frequent naps should be encouraged. Pruritus is treated with antihistamines, narcotic receptor antagonists (naltrexone), and rifampin. Cholestyramine, a bile salt sequestering agent, has been helpful in some patients but is somewhat tedious and difficult to take. Plasmapheresis has been utilized rarely in patients with severe intractable pruritus. There is an increased incidence of osteopenia and osteoporosis in patients with cholestatic liver disease, and bone density testing should be performed. Treatment with a bisphosphonate should be instituted when bone disease is identified.

PRIMARY SCLEROSING CHOLANGITIS

As in PBC, the cause of PSC remains unknown. PSC is a chronic cholestatic syndrome that is characterized by diffuse inflammation and fibrosis involving the entire biliary tree, resulting in chronic cholestasis. This pathologic process ultimately results in obliteration of both the intra- and extrahepatic biliary tree, leading to biliary cirrhosis, portal hypertension, and liver failure. The cause of PSC remains unknown despite extensive investigation into various mechanisms related to bacterial and viral infections, toxins, genetic predisposition, and immunologic mechanisms, all of which have been postulated to contribute to the pathogenesis and progression of this syndrome.

Pathologic changes that can occur in PSC show bile duct proliferation as well as ductopenia and fibrous cholangitis (pericholangitis). Oftentimes, liver biopsy changes in PSC are not pathognomonic, and establishing the diagnosis of PSC must involve imaging of the biliary tree. Periductal fibrosis is occasionally seen on biopsy specimens and can be quite helpful in making the diagnosis. As the disease progresses, biliary cirrhosis is the final end-stage manifestation of PSC.

Clinical Features The usual clinical features of PSC are those found in cholestatic liver disease, with fatigue, pruritus, steatorrhea, deficiencies of fat-soluble vitamins, and the associated consequences. As in PBC, the fatigue is profound and nonspecific. Pruritus can oftentimes be debilitating and is related to the cholestasis. The severity of pruritus does not correlate with the severity of the disease. Metabolic bone disease, as seen in PBC, can occur with PSC and should be treated (see above).

Laboratory Findings Patients with PSC typically are identified in the course of an evaluation of abnormal liver enzymes. Most patients have at least a twofold increase in ALP and may have elevated aminotransferases as well. Albumin levels may be decreased, and prothrombin times are prolonged in a substantial proportion of patients at the time of diagnosis. Some degree of correction of a prolonged prothrombin time may occur with parenteral vitamin K. A small subset of patients have aminotransferase elevations greater than five times the upper limit of normal and may have features of AIH on biopsy. These individuals are thought to have an overlap syndrome between PSC and AIH. Autoantibodies are frequently positive in patients with the overlap syndrome but are typically negative in patients who only have PSC. One autoantibody, the perinuclear antineutrophil cytoplasmic antibody (P-ANCA) is positive in about 65% of patients with PSC. Over 50% of patients with PSC also have ulcerative colitis (UC); accordingly, once a diagnosis of PSC is established, colonoscopy should be performed looking for evidence of UC.

Diagnosis The definitive diagnosis of PSC requires cholangiographic imaging. Over the last several years, MRI with magnetic resonance cholangiopancreatography (MRCP) has been utilized as the imaging technique of choice for initial evaluation. Once patients are screened in this manner, some investigators feel that endoscopic retrograde cholangiopancreatography (ERCP) should also be performed to be certain whether or not a dominant stricture is present. Typical cholangiographic findings in PSC are multifocal stricturing and beading involving both the intrahepatic and extrahepatic biliary tree. However, though involvement may be of the intrahepatic bile ducts alone or of the extrahepatic bile ducts alone, more commonly both are involved. These strictures are typically short and with intervening segments of normal or slightly dilated bile ducts that are distributed diffusely, producing the classic beaded appearance. The gallbladder and cystic duct can be involved in up to 15% of cases. Patients with high-grade, diffuse stricturing of the intrahepatic bile ducts have an overall poor

prognosis. Gradually, biliary cirrhosis develops, and patients will progress to decompensated liver disease with all the manifestations of ascites, esophageal variceal hemorrhage, and encephalopathy.

PRIMARY SCLEROSING CHOLANGITIS

There is no specific proven treatment for PSC, although studies are currently ongoing using high-dose (20 mg/kg per day) UDCA to determine its benefit. Endoscopic dilatation of dominant strictures can be helpful, but the ultimate treatment is liver transplantation. A dreaded complication of PSC is the development of cholangiocarcinoma, which is a relative contraindication to liver transplantation. Symptoms of pruritus are common, and the approach is as mentioned previously for this problem in patients with PBC (see above).

CARDIAC CIRRHOSIS

Definition Patients with long-standing right-sided congestive heart failure may develop chronic liver injury and cardiac cirrhosis. This is an increasingly uncommon, if not rare, cause of chronic liver disease given the advances made in the care of patients with heart failure.

Etiology and Pathology In the case of long-term right-sided heart failure, there is an elevated venous pressure transmitted via the inferior vena cava and hepatic veins to the sinusoids of the liver, which become dilated and engorged with blood. The liver becomes enlarged and swollen, and with long-term passive congestion and relative ischemia due to poor circulation, centrilobular hepatocytes can become necrotic, leading to pericentral fibrosis. This fibrotic pattern can extend to the periphery of the lobule outward until a unique pattern of fibrosis causing cirrhosis can occur.

Clinical Features Patients typically have signs of congestive heart failure and will manifest an enlarged firm liver on physical examination. ALP levels are characteristically elevated, and aminotransferases may be normal or slightly increased with AST usually higher than ALT. It is unlikely that patients will develop variceal hemorrhage or encephalopathy.

Diagnosis The diagnosis is usually made in someone with clear-cut cardiac disease who has an elevated ALP and an enlarged liver. Liver biopsy shows a pattern of fibrosis that can be recognized by an experience hepatopathologist. Differentiation from Budd-Chiari syndrome (BCS) can be made by seeing extravasation of red blood cells in BCS, but not in cardiac hepatopathy. Venoocclusive disease can also affect hepatic outflow and has characteristic features on liver biopsy. Venoocclusive disease can be seen under the circumstances of conditioning for bone marrow transplant with radiation and chemotherapy; it can also be seen with the ingestion of certain herbal teas as well as pyrrolizidine alkaloids. This is typically seen in Caribbean countries and rarely in the United States. Treatment is based on management of the underlying cardiac disease.

OTHER TYPES OF CIRRHOSIS

There are several other less common causes of chronic liver disease that can progress to cirrhosis. These include inherited metabolic liver diseases such as hemochromatosis, Wilson's disease, α_1 antitrypsin (α_1 AT) deficiency, and cystic fibrosis. For all of these disorders, the manifestations of cirrhosis are similar, with some minor variations, to those seen in other patients with other causes of cirrhosis.

Hemochromatosis is an inherited disorder of iron metabolism that results in a progressive increase in hepatic iron deposition which, over time, can lead to a portal-based fibrosis progressing to cirrhosis, liver failure, and hepatocellular cancer. While the frequency of hemochromatosis is relatively common, with genetic susceptibility occurring in 1 in 250 individuals, the frequency of end-stage manifestations due to the disease is relatively low, and fewer than 5% of those patients who are genotypically susceptible will go on to develop severe liver disease from hemochromatosis. Diagnosis is made with serum iron studies showing an elevated transferrin saturation and an elevated ferritin level, along with abnormalities identified by *HFE* mutation analysis. Treatment is straightforward, with regular therapeutic phlebotomy.

Wilson's disease is an inherited disorder of copper homeostasis with failure to excrete excess amounts of copper, leading to an accumulation in the liver. This disorder is relatively uncommon, affecting 1 in 30,000 individuals. Wilson's disease typically affects adolescents and young adults. Prompt diagnosis before end-stage manifestations become irreversible can lead to significant clinical improvement. Diagnosis requires determination of ceruloplasmin levels, which are low; 24-hour urine copper levels, which are elevated; typical physical examination findings, including Kayser-Fleischer corneal rings, and characteristic liver biopsy findings. Treatment consists of copper chelating medications.

$\alpha_1 AT$ *deficiency* results from an inherited disorder that causes abnormal folding of the $\alpha_1 AT$ protein, resulting in failure of secretion of that protein from the liver. It is unknown how the retained protein leads to liver disease. Patients with $\alpha_1 AT$ deficiency at greatest risk for developing chronic liver disease have the ZZ genotype, but only about 10–20% of such individuals will develop chronic liver disease. Diagnosis is made by determining $\alpha_1 AT$ levels and genotype. Characteristic PAS-positive, diastase-resistant globules are seen on liver biopsy. The only effective treatment is liver transplantation, which is curative.

Cystic fibrosis is an uncommon inherited disorder affecting Caucasians of Northern European descent. A biliary-type cirrhosis can occur, and some patients derive benefit from the chronic use of UDCA.

MAJOR COMPLICATIONS OF CIRRHOSIS

The clinical course of patients with advanced cirrhosis is often complicated by a number of important sequelae that can occur regardless of the underlying cause of the liver disease. These include portal hypertension and its consequences of gastroesophageal variceal hemorrhage, splenomegaly, ascites, hepatic encephalopathy, spontaneous bacterial peritonitis (SBP), hepatorenal syndrome, and hepatocellular carcinoma (Table 302-2).

PORTAL HYPERTENSION

Portal hypertension is defined as the elevation of the hepatic venous pressure gradient (HVPG) to >5 mmHg. Portal hypertension is caused by a combination of two simultaneously occurring hemodynamic processes: (1) increased intrahepatic resistance to the passage of blood flow through the liver due to cirrhosis and regenerative nodules, and (2) increased splanchnic blood flow secondary to vasodilatation within the splanchnic vascular bed. Portal hypertension is directly responsible for the two major complications of cirrhosis, variceal hemorrhage and ascites. *Variceal hemorrhage* is an immediate life-threatening problem with a 20–30% mortality associated with each episode of bleeding. The portal venous system normally drains blood from the stomach, intestines, spleen, pancreas, and gallbladder, and the portal vein is formed by the confluence of the superior mesenteric and splenic veins. Deoxygenated blood from the small bowel drains into the superior mesenteric vein along with blood from the head of the pancreas, the ascending colon, and part of the transverse colon. Conversely, the splenic vein drains the spleen and the pancreas and is joined by the in-

TABLE 302-2 COMPLICATIONS OF CIRRHOSIS

Portal hypertension	Coagulopathy
Gastroesophageal varices	Factor deficiency
Portal hypertensive gastropathy	Fibrinolysis
Splenomegaly, hypersplenism	Thrombocytopenia
Ascites	Bone disease
Spontaneous bacterial peritonitis	Osteopenia
Hepatorenal syndrome	Osteoporosis
Type 1	Osteomalacia
Type 2	Hematologic abnormalities
Hepatic encephalopathy	Anemia
Hepatopulmonary syndrome	Hemolysis
Portopulmonary hypertension	Thrombocytopenia
Malnutrition	Neutropenia

TABLE 302-3 CLASSIFICATION OF PORTAL HYPERTENSION

Prehepatic
  Portal vein thrombosis
  Splenic vein thrombosis
  Massive splenomegaly (Banti's syndrome)
Hepatic
  Presinusoidal
    Schistosomiasis
    Congenital hepatic fibrosis
  Sinusoidal
    Cirrhosis—many causes
    Alcoholic hepatitis
  Postsinusoidal
    Hepatic sinusoidal obstruction (venoocclusive syndrome)
Posthepatic
  Budd-Chiari syndrome
  Inferior vena caval webs
  Cardiac causes
    Restrictive cardiomyopathy
    Constrictive pericarditis
    Severe congestive heart failure

ferior mesenteric vein, which brings blood from the transverse and descending colon as well as from the superior two-thirds of the rectum. Thus, the portal vein normally receives blood from almost the entire GI tract.

The causes of portal hypertension are usually subcategorized as prehepatic, intrahepatic, and posthepatic (Table 302-3). Prehepatic causes of portal hypertension are those affecting the portal venous system before it enters the liver; they include portal vein thrombosis and splenic vein thrombosis. Posthepatic causes encompass those affecting the hepatic veins and venous drainage to the heart; they include BCS, venoocclusive disease, and chronic right-sided cardiac congestion. Intrahepatic causes account for over 95% of cases of portal hypertension and are represented by the major forms of cirrhosis. Intrahepatic causes of portal hypertension can be further subdivided into presinusoidal, sinusoidal, and postsinusoidal causes. Postsinusoidal causes include venoocclusive disease, while presinusoidal causes include congenital hepatic fibrosis and schistosomiasis. Sinusoidal causes are related to cirrhosis from various causes.

Cirrhosis is the most common cause of portal hypertension in the United States, and clinically significant portal hypertension is present in >60% of patients with cirrhosis. Portal vein obstruction may be idiopathic or can occur in association with cirrhosis or with infection, pancreatitis, or abdominal trauma.

Coagulation disorders that can lead to the development of portal vein thrombosis include polycythemia vera; essential thrombocytosis; deficiencies in protein C, protein S, antithrombin 3, and factor V Leiden; and abnormalities in the gene regulating prothrombin production. Some patients may have a subclinical myeloproliferative disorder.

Clinical Features　The three primary complications of portal hypertension are gastroesophageal varices with hemorrhage, ascites, and hypersplenism. Thus, patients may present with upper GI bleeding, which on endoscopy is found to be due to esophageal or gastric varices, with the development of ascites along with peripheral edema, or with an enlarged spleen with associated reduction in platelets and white blood cells on routine laboratory testing.

ESOPHAGEAL VARICES　Over the last decade, it has become common practice to screen known cirrhotics with endoscopy to look for esophageal varices. Such screening studies have shown that approximately one-third of patients with histologically confirmed cirrhosis have varices. Approximately 5–15% of cirrhotics per year develop varices, and it is estimated that the majority of patients with cirrhosis will develop varices over their lifetime. Furthermore, it is anticipated that roughly one-third of patients with varices will develop bleeding. Several factors predict the risk of bleeding, including the severity of cirrhosis (Child's class); the height of wedged-hepatic vein pressure; the size of the varix; the location of the varix; and certain endoscopic stigmata, including red wale signs, hematocystic spots, diffuse erythema, bluish color, cherry-red spots, or white-nipple spots. Patients with tense ascites are also at increased risk for bleeding from varices.

Diagnosis In patients with cirrhosis who are being followed chronically, the development of portal hypertension is usually revealed by the presence of thrombocytopenia; the appearance of an enlarged spleen; or the development of ascites, encephalopathy and/or esophageal varices with or without bleeding. In previously undiagnosed patients, any of these features should prompt further evaluation to determine the presence of portal hypertension and liver disease. Varices should be identified by endoscopy. Abdominal imaging, either by CT or MRI, can be helpful in demonstrating a nodular liver and in finding changes of portal hypertension with intraabdominal collateral circulation. If necessary, interventional radiologic procedures can be performed to determine wedged and free hepatic vein pressures that will allow for the calculation of a wedged-to-free gradient, which is equivalent to the portal pressure. The average normal wedged-to-free gradient is 5 mmHg, and patients with a gradient >12 mmHg are at risk for variceal hemorrhage.

℞ VARICEAL HEMORRHAGE

Treatment for variceal hemorrhage as a complication of portal hypertension is divided into two main categories: (1) primary prophylaxis and (2) prevention of re-bleeding once there has been an initial variceal hemorrhage. Primary prophylaxis requires routine screening by endoscopy of all patients with cirrhosis. Once varices that are at increased risk for bleeding are identified, then primary prophylaxis can be achieved either through nonselective beta blockade or by variceal band ligation. Numerous placebo-controlled clinical trials of either propranolol or nadolol have been reported in the literature. The most rigorous studies were those that only included patients with significantly enlarged varices or with hepatic vein pressure gradients >12 mmHg. Patients treated with beta blockers have a lower risk of variceal hemorrhage than those treated with placebo over 1 and 2 years of follow-up. There is also a decrease in mortality related to variceal hemorrhage. Unfortunately, overall survival was improved in only one study. Further studies have demonstrated that the degree of reduction of portal pressure is a significant feature to determine success of therapy. Therefore, it is has been suggested that repeat measurements of hepatic vein pressure gradients may be used to guide pharmacologic therapy; however, this may be cost prohibitive. Several studies have evaluated variceal band ligation and variceal sclerotherapy as methods for providing primary prophylaxis.

Endoscopic variceal ligation (EVL) has achieved a level of success and comfort with most gastroenterologists who see patients with these complications of portal hypertension. Thus, in patients with cirrhosis who are screened for portal hypertension and are found to have large varices, it is recommended that they receive either beta blockade or primary prophylaxis with EVL.

The approach to patients once they have had a variceal bleed is first to treat the acute bleed, which can be life-threatening, and then to prevent further bleeding. Prevention of further bleeding is usually accomplished with repeated variceal band ligation until varices are obliterated. Treatment of acute bleeding requires both fluid and blood product replacement as well as prevention of subsequent bleeding with EVL.

The medical management of acute variceal hemorrhage includes the use of vasoconstricting agents, usually somatostatin or Octreotide. Vasopressin was used in the past but is no longer commonly used. Balloon tamponade (Sengstaken-Blakemore tube or Minnesota tube) can be used in patients who cannot get endoscopic therapy immediately or who need stabilization prior to endoscopic therapy. Control of bleeding can be achieved in the vast majority of cases; however, bleeding recurs in the majority of patients if definitive endoscopic therapy has not been instituted. Octreotide, a direct splanchnic vasoconstrictor, is given at dosages of 50–100 μg/h by continuous infusion. Endoscopic intervention is employed as first-line treatment to control bleeding acutely. Some endoscopists will use variceal injection therapy (sclerotherapy) as initial therapy, particularly when bleeding is vigorous. Variceal band ligation is used to control acute bleeding in over 90% of cases and should be repeated until obliteration of all varices is accomplished. When esophageal varices extend into the proximal stomach, band ligation is less successful. In these situations, when

bleeding continues from gastric varices, consideration for transjugular intrahepatic portosystemic shunt (TIPS) should be made. This technique creates a portosystemic shunt by a percutaneous approach using an expandable metal stent, which is advanced under angiographic guidance to the hepatic veins and then through the substance of the liver to create a direct portocaval shunt. This offers an alternative to surgery for acute decompression of portal hypertension. Encephalopathy can occur in as many as 20% of patients after TIPS and is particularly problematic in elderly patients and in those patients with preexisting encephalopathy. TIPS should be reserved for those individuals who fail endoscopic or medical management or who are poor surgical risks. TIPS can sometimes be used as a bridge to transplantation. Surgical esophageal transsection is a procedure that is rarely used and generally is associated with a poor outcome.

PREVENTION OF RECURRENT BLEEDING (Fig. 302-1) Once patients have had an acute bleed and have been managed successfully, attention should be paid to preventing recurrent bleeding. This usually requires repeated variceal band ligation until varices are obliterated. Beta blockade may be of adjunctive benefit in patients who are having recurrent variceal band ligation; however, once varices have been obliterated, the need for beta blockade is lessened. Despite successful variceal obliteration, many patients will still have portal hypertensive gastropathy from which bleeding can occur. Nonselective beta blockade may be helpful to prevent further bleeding from portal hypertensive gastropathy once varices have been obliterated.

Portosystemic shunt surgery is less commonly performed with the advent of TIPS; nonetheless, this procedure should be considered for patients with good hepatic synthetic function who could benefit by having portal decompressive surgery.

SPLENOMEGALY AND HYPERSPLENISM

Congestive splenomegaly is common in patients with portal hypertension. Clinical features include the presence of an enlarged spleen on

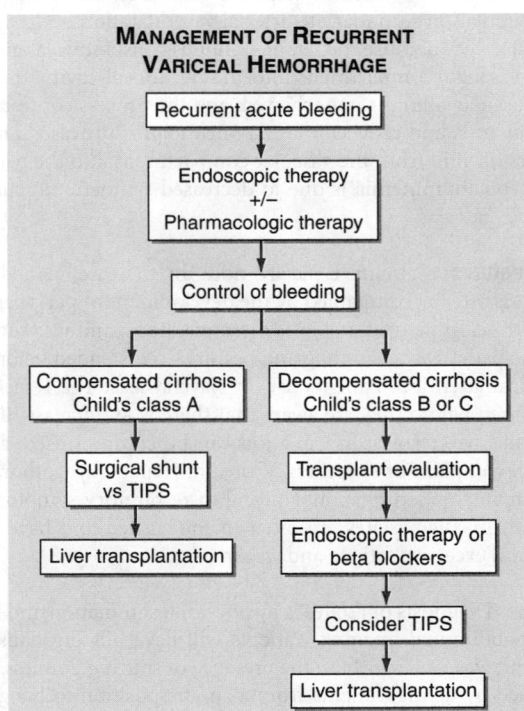

FIGURE 302-1 Management of recurrent variceal hemorrhage. This algorithm describes an approach to management of patients who have recurrent bleeding from esophageal varices. Initial therapy is generally with endoscopic therapy often supplemented by pharmacologic therapy. With control of bleeding, a decision needs to be made as to whether patients should go on to a surgical shunt or TIPS (if they are Child's class A) and be considered for transplant, or if they should have TIPS and be considered for transplant (if they are Child's class B or C). TIPS, transjugular intrahepatic portosystemic shunt.

physical examination and the development of thrombocytopenia and leukopenia in patients who have cirrhosis. Some patients will have fairly significant left-sided and left upper quadrant abdominal pain related to an enlarged and engorged spleen. Splenomegaly itself usually requires no specific treatment, although splenectomy can be successfully performed under very special circumstances.

Hypersplenism with the development of thrombocytopenia is a common feature of patients with cirrhosis and is usually the first indication of portal hypertension.

ASCITES

Definition   Ascites is the accumulation of fluid within the peritoneal cavity. Overwhelmingly, the most common cause of ascites is portal hypertension related to cirrhosis; however, clinicians should remember that malignant or infectious causes of ascites can be present as well, and careful differentiation of these other causes are obviously important for patient care.

Pathogenesis   The presence of portal hypertension contributes to the development of ascites in patients who have cirrhosis (Fig. 302-2). There is an increase in intrahepatic resistance, causing increased portal pressure, but there is also vasodilatation of the splanchnic arterial system, which in turn results in an increase in portal venous inflow. Both of these abnormalities result in increased production of splanchnic lymph. Vasodilating factors such as nitric oxide are responsible for the vasodilatory effect. These hemodynamic changes result in sodium retention by causing activation of the renin-angiotensin-aldosterone system with the development of hyperaldosteronism. The renal effects of increased aldosterone leading to sodium retention also contribute to the development of ascites. Sodium retention causes fluid accumulation and expansion of the extracellular fluid volume, which results in the formation of peripheral edema and ascites. Sodium retention is the consequence of a homeostatic response caused by underfilling of the arterial circulation secondary to arterial vasodilatation in the splanchnic vascular bed. Because the retained fluid is constantly leaking out of the intravascular compartment into the peritoneal cavity, the sensation of vascular filling is not achieved, and the process continues. Hypoalbuminemia and reduced plasma oncotic pressure also contribute to the loss of fluid from the vascular compartment into the peritoneal cavity. Hypoalbuminemia is due to decreased synthetic function in a cirrhotic liver.

Clinical Features   Patients typically note an increase in abdominal girth that is often accompanied by the development of peripheral edema. The development of ascites is often insidious, and it is surprising that some patients wait so long and become so distended before seeking medical attention. Patients usually have at least 1–2 L of fluid in the abdomen before they are aware that there is an increase. If ascitic fluid is massive, respiratory function can be compromised, and patients will complain of shortness of breath. Hepatic hydrothorax may also occur in this setting, contributing to respiratory symptoms. Patients with massive ascites are often malnourished and have muscle wasting and excessive fatigue and weakness.

Diagnosis   Diagnosis of ascites is by physical examination and is often aided by abdominal imaging. Patients will have bulging flanks, may have a fluid wave, or may have the presence of shifting dullness. This is determined by taking patients from a supine position to lying on either their left or right side and noting the movement of the dullness to percussion. Subtle amounts of ascites can be detected by ultrasound or CT scanning. Hepatic hydrothorax is more common on the right side and implicates a rent in the diaphragm with free flow of ascitic fluid into the thoracic cavity.

When patients present with ascites for the first time, it is recommended that a diagnostic paracentesis be performed to characterize the fluid. This should include the determination of total protein and albumin content, blood cell counts with differential, and cultures. In the appropriate setting, amylase may be measured and cytology per-

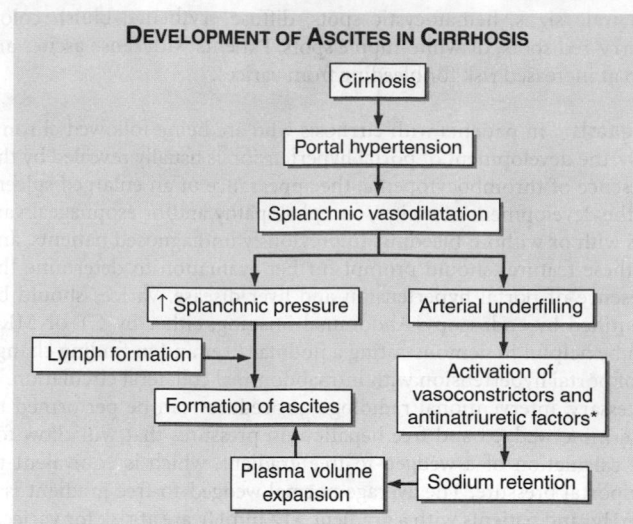

FIGURE 302-2 Development of ascites in cirrhosis. This flow diagram illustrates the importance of portal hypertension with splanchnic vasodilatation in the development of ascites. *Antinatriuretic factors include the renin-angiotensin-aldosterone system and the sympathetic nervous system.

formed. In patients with cirrhosis, the protein concentration of the ascitic fluid is quite low, with the majority of patients having an ascitic fluid protein concentration <1 g/dL. The development of the serum ascites-to-albumin gradient (SAAG) has replaced the description of exudative or transudative fluid. When the gradient between the serum albumin level and the ascitic fluid albumin level is >1.1 g/dL, then the cause of the ascites is most likely due to portal hypertension; this is most often in the setting of cirrhosis. When the gradient is <1.1 g/dL, infectious or malignant causes of ascites should be considered. When levels of ascitic fluid proteins are very low, patients are at increased risk for developing SBP. A high level of red blood cells in the ascitic fluid signifies a traumatic tap, or perhaps a hepatocellular cancer, or a ruptured omental varix. When the absolute level of polymorphonuclear leukocytes is >250 mm^3, then the question of ascitic fluid infection should be strongly considered. Ascitic fluid cultures should be obtained using bedside inoculation of culture media.

℞ ASCITES

Patients with small amounts of ascites can usually be managed with dietary sodium restriction alone. Most average diets in the United States contain 6 to 8 g of sodium per day and if patients eat at restaurants or fast food outlets, the amount of sodium in their diet can exceed this amount. Thus, it is often extremely difficult to get patients to change their dietary habits to ingest < 2 g of sodium per day, which is the amount that is recommended. Patients are frequently surprised to realize how much sodium is in the standard US diet and thus it is important to make educational pamphlets available to the patient. Often, a simple recommendation is to eat fresh or frozen foods, avoiding canned or processed foods, which are usually preserved with sodium. When a moderate amount of ascites is present, diuretic therapy is usually necessary. Traditionally, spironolactone at 100–200 mg/d as a single dose is started, and furosemide may be added at 40–80 mg/d, particularly in patients who have peripheral edema. In patients who have never received diuretics before, the failure of the above-mentioned dosages suggests that they are not being compliant with a low-sodium diet. If compliance is confirmed and ascitic fluid is not being mobilized, spironolactone can be increased to 400–600 mg/d and furosemide increased to 120–160 mg/d. If ascites is still present with these dosages of diuretics in patients who are compliant with a low-sodium diet, then they are defined as having *refractory ascites*, and alternative treatment modalities including repeated large-volume paracentesis, or a TIPS procedure should be considered (Fig. 302-3). Recent studies have shown that TIPS, while managing the ascites, does not improve survival in these patients. Unfortunately, TIPS is often associated with an increased frequency

FIGURE 302-3 Treatment of refractory ascites. In patients who develop azotemia in the course of receiving diuretics in the management of their ascites, some will require repeated large-volume paracentesis (LVP), some may be considered for transjugular intrahepatic portosystemic shunt (TIPS), and some would be good candidates for liver transplantation. These decisions are all individualized.

of hepatic encephalopathy and must be considered carefully on a case-by-case basis. The prognosis for patients with cirrhosis with ascites is poor, and some studies have shown that <50% of patients survive 2 years after the onset of ascites. Thus, there should be consideration for liver transplantation in patients with the onset of ascites.

SPONTANEOUS BACTERIAL PERITONITIS

SBP is a common and severe complication of ascites characterized by spontaneous infection of the ascitic fluid without an intraabdominal source. In patients with cirrhosis and ascites severe enough for hospitalization, SBP can occur in up to 30% of individuals and can have a 25% in-hospital mortality rate. Bacterial translocation is the presumed mechanism for development of SBP, with gut flora traversing the intestine into mesenteric lymph nodes, leading to bacteremia and seeding of the ascitic fluid. The most common organisms are *Escherichia coli* and other gut bacteria; however, gram-positive bacteria, including *Streptococcus viridans, Staphococcus aureus,* and *Enterococcus* sp., can also be found. If more than two organisms are identified, secondary bacterial peritonitis due to a perforated viscus should be considered. The diagnosis of SBP is made when the fluid sample has an absolute neutrophil count >250/mm³. Bedside cultures should be obtained when ascitic fluid is tapped. Patients with ascites may present with fever, altered mental status, elevated white blood cell count, and abdominal pain or discomfort, or they may present without any of these features. Therefore, it is necessary to have a high degree of clinical suspicion, and peritoneal taps are important for making the diagnosis. Treatment is with a second-generation cephalosporin, with cefotaxime being the most commonly used antibiotic. In patients with variceal hemorrhage, the frequency of SBP is significantly increased, and prophylaxis against SBP is recommended when a patient presents with upper GI bleeding. Furthermore, in patients who have had an episode(s) of SBP and recovered, once-weekly administration of antibiotics is used as prophylaxis for recurrent SBP.

HEPATORENAL SYNDROME

The hepatorenal syndrome (HRS) is a form of functional renal failure without renal pathology that occurs in about 10% of patients with advanced cirrhosis or acute liver failure. There are marked disturbances in the arterial renal circulation in patients with HRS; these include an increase in vascular resistance accompanied by a reduction in systemic vascular resistance. The reason for renal vasoconstriction is most likely multifactorial and is poorly understood. The diagnosis is made usually in the presence of a large amount of ascites in patients who have a step-wise progressive increase in creatinine. Type 1 HRS is character-

ized by a progressive impairment in renal function and a significant reduction in creatinine clearance within 1–2 weeks of presentation. Type 2 HRS is characterized by a reduction in glomerular filtration rate with an elevation of serum creatinine level, but it is fairly stable and is associated with a better outcome than that of Type 1 HRS.

HRS is often seen in patients with refractory ascites and requires exclusion of other causes of acute renal failure. Treatment has unfortunately been difficult, and in the past, dopamine or prostaglandin analogs were used as renal vasodilating medications. Carefully performed studies have failed to show clear-cut benefit from these therapeutic approaches. Currently, patients are treated with midodrine, an α-agonist, along with octreotide and intravenous albumin. The best therapy for HRS is liver transplantation; recovery of renal function is typical in this setting. In patients with either type 1 or type 2 HRS, the prognosis is poor unless transplant can be achieved within a short period of time.

HEPATIC ENCEPHALOPATHY

Portosystemic encephalopathy is a serious complication of chronic liver disease and is broadly defined as an alteration in mental status and cognitive function occurring in the presence of liver failure. In acute liver injury with fulminant hepatic failure, the development of encephalopathy is a requirement for a diagnosis of fulminant failure. Encephalopathy is much more commonly seen in patients with chronic liver disease. Gut-derived neurotoxins that are not removed by the liver because of vascular shunting and decreased hepatic mass get to the brain and cause the symptoms that we know of as hepatic encephalopathy. Ammonia levels are typically elevated in patients with hepatic encephalopathy, but the correlation between severity of liver disease and height of ammonia levels is often poor, and most hepatologists do not rely on ammonia levels to make a diagnosis. Other compounds and metabolites that may contribute to the development of encephalopathy include certain false neurotransmitters and mercaptans.

Clinical Features   In acute liver failure, changes in mental status can occur within weeks to months. Brain edema can be seen in these patients, with severe encephalopathy associated with swelling of the gray matter. Cerebral herniation is a feared complication of brain edema in acute liver failure, and treatment is meant to decrease edema with mannitol and judicious use of intravenous fluids.

In patients with cirrhosis, encephalopathy is often found as a result of certain precipitating events such as hypokalemia, infection, an increased dietary protein load, or electrolyte disturbances. Patients may be confused or exhibit a change in personality. They may actually be quite violent and difficult to manage; alternatively, patients may be very sleepy and difficult to arouse. Because precipitating events are so commonly found, they should be sought carefully. If patients have ascites, this should be tapped to rule out infection. Evidence of GI bleeding should be sought, and patients should be appropriately hydrated. Electrolytes should be measured and abnormalities corrected. In patients presenting with encephalopathy, asterixis is often present. Asterixis can be elicited by having patients extend their arms and bend their wrists back. In this maneuver, patients who are encephalopathic have a "liver flap"—i.e., a sudden forward movement of the wrist. This requires patients to be able to cooperate with the examiner and obviously cannot be elicited in patients who are severely encephalopathic or in hepatic coma.

The diagnosis of hepatic encephalopathy is clinical and requires an experienced clinician to recognize and put together all of the various features. Often when patients have encephalopathy for the first time, they are unaware of what is transpiring, but once they have been through the experience for the first time, they can identify when this is developing in subsequent situations and can often self-medicate to impair the development or worsening of encephalopathy.

℞ HEPATIC ENCEPHALOPATHY

Treatment is multifactorial and includes management of the above-mentioned precipitating factors. Sometimes hydration and correction of electrolyte imbalance is all that is necessary. In the past, restriction of dietary protein was considered for patients with encephalopathy; however, the negative impact of that maneuver on overall nutrition is thought to outweigh the benefit when treating encephalopathy, and it is thus discouraged. There may be some benefit to replacing animal-based protein with vegetable-based protein in some patients with encephalopathy that is difficult to manage. The mainstay of treatment for encephalopathy, in addition to correcting precipitating factors, is to use lactulose, a nonabsorbable disaccharide, which results in colonic acidification. Catharsis ensues, contributing to the elimination of nitrogenous products in the gut that are responsible for the development of encephalopathy. The goal of lactulose therapy is to promote 2–3 soft stools per day. Patients are asked to titrate their amount of ingested lactulose to achieve the desired effect. Poorly absorbed antibiotics are often used as adjunctive therapies for patients who have had a difficult time with lactulose. The alternating administration of neomycin and metronidazole has commonly been employed to reduce the individual side effects of each: neomycin for renal insufficiency and ototoxicity and metronidazole for peripheral neuropathy. More recently, rifaximin has been very effective in treating encephalopathy without the known side effects of neomycin or metronidazole. Zinc supplementation is sometimes helpful in patients with encephalopathy and is relatively harmless. The development of encephalopathy in patients with chronic liver disease is a poor prognostic sign, but this complication can be managed in the vast majority of patients.

MALNUTRITION IN CIRRHOSIS

Because the liver is principally involved in the regulation of protein and energy metabolism in the body, it is not surprising that patients with advanced liver disease are commonly malnourished. Once patients become cirrhotic, they are more catabolic, and muscle protein is metabolized. There are multiple factors that contribute to the malnutrition of cirrhosis, including poor dietary intake, alterations in gut nutrient absorption, and alterations in protein metabolism. Dietary supplementation for patients with cirrhosis is helpful in preventing patients from becoming catabolic.

ABNORMALITIES IN COAGULATION

Coagulopathy is almost universal in patients with cirrhosis. There is decreased synthesis of clotting factors and impaired clearance of anticoagulants. In addition, patients may have thrombocytopenia from hypersplenism due to portal hypertension. Vitamin K–dependent clotting factors are Factors II, VII, IX, and X. Vitamin K requires biliary excretion for its subsequent absorption; thus, in patients with chronic cholestatic syndromes, vitamin K absorption is frequently diminished. Intravenous or intramuscular vitamin K can quickly correct this abnormality. More commonly, the synthesis of vitamin K–dependent clotting factors is diminished because of a decrease in hepatic mass, and under these circumstances administration of parenteral vitamin K does not

improve the clotting factors or the prothrombin time. Platelet function is often abnormal in patients with chronic liver disease, in addition to decreases in platelet levels due to hypersplenism.

BONE DISEASE IN CIRRHOSIS

Osteoporosis is common in patients with chronic cholestatic liver disease because of malabsorption of vitamin D and decreased calcium ingestion. The rate of bone resorption exceeds that of new bone formation in patients with cirrhosis resulting in bone loss. Dual x-ray absorptiometry (DEXA) is a useful method for determining osteoporosis or osteopenia in patients with chronic liver disease. When a DEXA scan shows decreased bone mass, treatment should be administered with bisphosphonates that are effective at inhibiting resorption of bone and efficacious in the treatment of osteoporosis.

HEMATOLOGIC ABNORMALITIES IN CIRRHOSIS

Numerous hematologic manifestations of cirrhosis are present, including anemia from a variety of causes including hypersplenism, hemolysis, iron deficiency, and perhaps folate deficiency from malnutrition. Macrocytosis is a common abnormality in red blood cell morphology seen in patients with chronic liver disease, and neutropenia may be seen as a result of hypersplenism.

FURTHER READINGS

ARROYO V, COLMENERO J: Ascites and hepatorenal syndrome in cirrhosis: Pathophysiological basis of therapy and current management. J Hepatol 38:S69, 2003

BLEI AT, CORDOBA J: Hepatic encephalopathy. Am J Gastroenterol 96:1968, 2001

CÁRDENAS A, ARROYO V: Mechanisms of water and sodium retention in cirrhosis and the pathogenesis of ascites. Best Pract Res Clin Endocrinol Metab 17:607, 2003

DE FRANCHIS R: Updating consensus in portal hypertension: Report of the Baveno III Consensus Workshop on definitions, methodology, and therapeutic strategies in portal hypertension. J Hepatol 33:846, 2000

FERNANDEZ J et al: Diagnosis, treatment, and prevention of spontaneous bacterial peritonitis. Baillieres Best Pract Res Clin Gastroenterol 14:975, 2000

GINES P et al: Management of cirrhosis and ascites. N Engl J Med 350:1646, 2004

———— et al: Hyponatremia in cirrhosis: From pathogenesis to treatment. Hepatology 28:851, 1998

HALSTED CH: Nutrition and alcoholic liver disease. Semin Liver Dis 24:289, 2004

KROWKA MJ et al: Hepatopulmonary syndrome and portopulmonary hypertension: A report of the multicenter liver transplant database. Liver Transpl 10:174, 2004

303 Genetic, Metabolic, and Infiltrative Diseases Affecting the Liver
Bruce R. Bacon

There are a number of disorders of the liver that fit within the categories of genetic, metabolic, and infiltrative disorders. Inherited disorders include hemochromatosis, Wilson disease, α_1 antitrypsin (α_1AT) deficiency, and cystic fibrosis. Hemochromatosis is the most common disorder affecting Caucasian populations, with the genetic susceptibility for the disease being identified in 1 in 250 individuals. Over the past 10 years, it has become increasingly apparent that nonalcoholic fatty liver disease

(NAFLD) is the most common cause of elevated liver enzymes found in the U.S. population. With the obesity epidemic in the United States, it is estimated that 20% of the population may have abnormal liver enzymes on the basis of NAFLD and 3% may have nonalcoholic steatohepatitis (NASH). Infiltrative disorders of the liver are relatively rare.

GENETIC LIVER DISEASES

Hereditary Hemochromatosis Hereditary hemochromatosis (HH) is a common inherited disorder of iron metabolism (Chap. 351). Our knowledge of the disease and its phenotypic expression has changed since 1996 when the gene for HH, called *HFE*, was identified allowing for genetic testing for the two major mutations (C282Y, H63D) that are responsible for *HFE*-related HH. Subsequently, several additional genes/proteins involved in the regulation of iron homeostasis have been identified, contributing to a better understanding of cellular iron uptake and release and the characterization of additional causes of in-

TABLE 303-1 CLASSIFICATION OF IRON OVERLOAD SYNDROMES

Hereditary hemochromatosis (HH)
  HFE-related (type 1)
    C282Y/C282Y
    C282Y/H63D
    Other *HFE* mutations
  Non-*HFE*-related
    Juvenile HH
      HJV—hemojuvelin (type 2a)
      HAMP—hepcidin (type 2b)
    TfR2-related HH (type 3)
    Ferroportin-related HH (type 4)
    African iron overload

Secondary iron overload
  Iron-loading anemias
  Parenteral iron overload
  Chronic liver disease

Miscellaneous
  Neonatal iron overload
  Aceruloplasminemia
  Congenital atransferrinemia

Note: HJV, hemojuvelin; HAMP, hepcidin; TfR2, transferrin receptor 2.

herited iron overload (Table 303-1). All of these inherited syndromes result in the inappropriately high absorption of iron by the gastrointestinal mucosa, leading to the pathologic deposition of excess iron in the parenchymal cells of the liver, heart, pancreas, and other organs. Ultimately, parenchymal iron deposition leads to cell and tissue damage with the development of fibrosis and functional insufficiency. The liver is always the principal site of deposition of the majority of the excess absorbed iron, and the liver is always involved in symptomatic hemochromatosis. Recent studies have shown a central role for hepcidin, a 25-amino-acid peptide that is involved in the regulation of iron uptake by enterocytes and iron released by reticuloendothelial cells.

Most patients with HH are asymptomatic; however, when patients present with symptoms, they are frequently nonspecific and include weakness, fatigue, lethargy, and weight loss. Specific organ-related symptoms include abdominal pain, arthralgias, and symptoms and signs of chronic liver disease. Increasingly, most patients are now identified before they have symptoms, either through family studies or from the performance of screening iron studies. Several prospective population studies have shown that C282Y homozygosity is found in about 1 in 250 individuals of northern European descent, with the heterozygote frequency seen in approximately 1 in 10 individuals (Table 303-2). When systematic studies of either arthritis or diabetes clinics have looked specifically for HH, previously undiagnosed cases have been identified, often to the surprise of the clinician. These studies illustrate the need to consider HH in patients who present with the symptoms and signs known to occur in established HH. In older series of patients with HH, when patients were identified by symptoms or objective findings of the disease, women typically presented about 10 years later than men and there were about 10 times the number of men presenting as women, presumably because of the "protective" effect of menstrual blood loss and iron loss during pregnancy. More recently, when greater proportions of patients have been identified by screening blood tests or by family screening studies, the age of diagnosis for women was found to be approximately equivalent to that for men and the number of men identified was roughly equivalent to that of women.

When confronted with abnormal serum iron studies, clinicians should not wait for typical symptoms or findings of HH to appear before considering the diagnosis. However, once the diagnosis of HH is considered, either by an evaluation of abnormal screening iron studies, in the context of family studies, in a patient with an abnormal genetic test, or in the evaluation of a patient with any of the typical symptoms or clinical findings, definitive diagnosis is relatively straightforward. Fasting transferrin saturation [serum iron divided by total iron-binding capacity (TIBC) or transferrin, times 100%] and ferritin levels should be obtained. Both of these will be elevated in a symptomatic patient. It must be remembered that ferritin is an acute-phase reactant and can be elevated in a number of other inflammatory disorders, such as rheumatoid arthritis, or in various neoplastic diseases, such as lymphoma or other cancers. Also, serum ferritin is elevated in a majority of patients with NASH, in the absence of iron overload.

At present, if patients have an elevated transferrin saturation or ferritin level, then genetic testing should be performed; if they are a C282Y homozygote or a compound heterozygote (C282Y/H63D), the diagnosis is confirmed. If the ferritin is >1000 μg/L, the patient should be considered for liver biopsy since there is an increased frequency of advanced fibrosis in these individuals. If liver biopsy is performed, iron deposition is found in a periportal distribution with a periportal to pericentral gradient; iron is found predominantly in parenchymal cells, and Kupffer cells are spared.

℞ HEREDITARY HEMOCHROMATOSIS

Treatment of HH is relatively straightforward with weekly phlebotomy aimed to reduce iron stores, recognizing that each unit of blood contains 250 mg of iron. If patients are diagnosed and treated before the development of hepatic fibrosis, all complications of the disease can be avoided. Maintenance phlebotomy is required in most patients and usually can be achieved with 1 unit of blood removed every 2–3 months. Family studies should be performed with transferrin saturation, ferritin, and genetic testing offered to all first-degree relatives.

Wilson's Disease Wilson's disease is an inherited disorder of copper homeostasis first described in 1912 (Chap. 354). The Wilson's disease gene was identified in 1993 with the identification of *ATP7B*. This P-type ATPase is involved in copper transport and is necessary for the export of copper from the hepatocyte. Thus, in patients with mutations in *ATP7B*, copper is retained in the liver, leading to increased copper storage and ultimately liver disease as a result. Whereas hemochromatosis is found in 1 in 250 individuals, Wilson's disease is much less common, being seen in 1 in 30,000 individuals.

The clinical presentation of Wilson's disease is variable and includes chronic hepatitis, hepatic steatosis, and cirrhosis in adolescents and young adults. Neurologic manifestations indicate that liver disease is present and include speech disorders and various movement disorders. Diagnosis includes the demonstration of a reduced ceruloplasmin level, increased urinary excretion of copper, the presence of Kayser-Fleischer rings in the cornea of the eyes, and an elevated hepatic copper level, in the appropriate clinical setting. Whereas genetic testing is valuable in establishing the diagnosis of hemochromatosis, the genetic diagnosis of Wilson's disease is difficult because >200 mu-

TABLE 303-2 PREVALENCE OF C282Y HOMOZYGOTES WITHOUT IRON OVERLOAD IN POPULATION SCREENING STUDIES

Population Sample	Country	n	Prevalence of Homozygotes	C282Y Homozygotes with a Normal Ferritin, %
Electoral roll	New Zealand	1064	1 in 213	40
Primary care	United States	1653	1 in 276	50
Epidemiologic survey	Australia	3011	1 in 188	25
Blood donors	Canada	4211	1 in 327	81
General public	United States	41,038	1 in 270	33
Primary care	North America	44,082	1 in 227	25
	Total:	95,059	**Average:** 1 in 250	42

tations in *ATP7B* have been described with different degrees of frequency and penetration in certain populations.

℞ WILSON'S DISEASE

Treatment consists of copper chelating medications such as D-penicillamine and trientine. A role for zinc has also been established; zinc competes with copper absorption in the gut and induces metallothionein in the intestine, which then sequesters copper. Medical treatment is lifelong, and severe relapses leading to liver failure and death can occur with cessation of therapy. Liver transplantation is curative with respect to the underlying metabolic defect and restores the normal phenotype with respect to copper homeostasis.

α_1 Antitrypsin Deficiency α_1AT deficiency was first described in the late 1960s in patients with severe pulmonary disease. Shortly thereafter it was discovered to be a cause of neonatal liver disease, and now it is known to be a cause of liver disease in infancy, early childhood, adolescence, and in adults. The natural history of liver disease in α_1AT deficiency is quite variable. Many individuals with the ZZ genotype never develop disease throughout their entire lives. α_1AT deficiency becomes apparent in adults because of screening for liver disease in individuals who have liver function test abnormalities. The only hint to diagnosis may be coexistent lung disease at a relatively young age or a family history of liver and/or lung disease. Diagnosis is established by determining a reduced serum level of α_1AT as well as the performance of α_1AT genotyping. The ZZ genotype is found in about 1 in 2000 individuals; however, it should be remembered that liver disease can be found in individuals with the SZ genotype and occasionally in those with the MZ genotype. Liver biopsy in α_1AT disease shows characteristic PAS-positive diastase-resistant globules in the periphery of the hepatic lobule.

℞ α_1 ANTITRYPSIN DEFICIENCY

Treatment of α_1AT is nonspecific and supportive. Liver transplantation is curative. Recombinant AT administered IV has been used in patients with chronic lung disease due to α_1AT deficiency but is of no benefit in patients with α_1AT liver disease.

Cystic Fibrosis   Cystic fibrosis (CF) should also be considered as an inherited form of chronic liver disease, although the principal manifestations of CF include chronic lung disease and pancreatic insufficiency (Chap. 253). A small percentage of patients with CF who survive to adulthood have a form of biliary cirrhosis characterized by cholestatic liver enzyme abnormalities and the development of chronic liver disease. Ursodeoxycholic acid is occasionally helpful in improving liver test abnormalities and in reducing symptoms. The disease is slowly progressive.

METABOLIC LIVER DISEASES

Nonalcoholic Fatty Liver Disease   NAFLD was first described in the 1950s when fatty liver was characterized in a group of obese patients. In 1980, Ludwig and colleagues at the Mayo Clinic described 20 obese, diabetic, nonalcoholic patients who had similar findings on liver biopsy to patients with alcoholic liver disease, and the term nonalcoholic steatohepatitis was introduced. The prevalence of NAFLD in the United States and Europe ranges from 14–20%. This increased prevalence relates directly to the obesity epidemic seen in these populations. In the United States, NASH is thought to occur in ~3% of the general population, with fibrosis due to NASH being seen in >40% of significantly obese patients. The spectrum of NAFLD includes simple hepatic steatosis, which over time can progress to NASH, with the subsequent development of fibrosis and cirrhosis. Causes of macrovesicular steatosis are listed in Table 303-3. It is now known that many patients with hitherto identified "cryptogenic" cirrhosis in fact have liver disease on the basis of NASH, with the resolution of the steatosis once patients become catabolic due to cirrhosis.

Most patients who come to medical attention with NAFLD are identified as a result of incidentally discovered elevated liver enzymes

TABLE 303-3   CAUSES OF MACROVESICULAR STEATOSIS

Insulin resistance, hyperinsulinemia
   Centripetal obesity
   Type 2 diabetes

Medications
   Glucocorticoids
   Estrogens
   Tamoxifen
   Amiodarone

Nutritional
   Starvation
   Protein deficiency (Kwashiorkor)
   Choline deficiency

Liver disease
   Wilson disease
   Chronic hepatitis C—genotype 3
   Indian childhood cirrhosis
   Jejunoileal bypass

(ALT, AST). When patients are symptomatic, symptoms include fatigue or a vague right upper quadrant discomfort. ALT is generally higher than AST, and aminotransferases are only mildly (1.5–2 times the upper limit of normal) elevated. Recent studies have shown that many patients can have advanced NASH and even cirrhosis due to NASH with normal liver enzymes indicating that the prevalence of the disease may be even greater than was previously suspected. NASH is frequently seen in conjunction with other components of the metabolic syndrome (hypertension, diabetes mellitus, elevated lipids, and obesity), with NAFLD being considered the hepatic manifestation of this syndrome (Chap. 236). Insulin resistance is the underlying link between these various disorders and numerous studies have shown that virtually all patients with NASH have insulin resistance. Abnormal ferritin values are seen in ~50% of patients with NASH, and an elevated ferritin level may be a marker of insulin resistance in NASH.

The diagnosis of NAFLD requires a careful history to determine the amount of alcohol used. Most investigators in the field of fatty liver disease require that <20 g/d of alcohol be consumed to exclude alcoholic liver disease. Laboratory testing for hepatitis B and C, iron studies, and autoimmune serologies should also be determined. Imaging studies can show characteristic features of a fatty liver, but the ultimate diagnosis of either hepatic steatosis or NASH requires liver biopsy. Liver biopsy shows characteristic macrovesicular steatosis with occasional microvesicular fat being identified. A mixed inflammatory infiltrate is found in a lobular distribution. The histologic features of NASH are very similar to those seen in alcoholic liver disease; Mallory's hyaline can be seen in both disorders, although the number of hepatocytes containing Mallory's hyaline is frequently greater in alcoholic liver disease than in NASH. The fibrosis that occurs in NASH has a characteristic perivenular and perisinusoidal distribution. Most studies show that up to 30–40% of NASH patients can develop advanced fibrosis, with cirrhosis being identified in 10–15% of individuals. Increasingly, patients are being identified with cryptogenic cirrhosis who have most likely had NASH for decades. These patients can develop liver failure and require liver transplantation, and some patients can progress to the development of hepatocellular cancer.

℞ NONALCOHOLIC FATTY LIVER DISEASE

The mainstay of treatment of fatty liver disease is weight loss and exercise, which is often difficult to achieve in this population. As an aid to weight loss, orlistat, which is a reversible inhibitor of gastric and pancreatic lipase, has been shown to result in a small decrease in body weight and is usually fairly well tolerated. Bariatric surgery has been utilized and shows striking success, but is obviously a fairly drastic maneuver for induction of weight loss. Recent studies have focused on the presence of insulin resistance at the center of the pathophysiologic mechanisms of NAFLD. The thiazolidinedione medications are PPAR gamma inhibitors, which improve insulin sensitivity within the adipocyte and skeletal muscle by upregulating specific protein kinases involved in decreasing fatty acid synthesis. Two drugs—pioglitizone and rosiglitizone—are currently available and are being evaluated as potential therapeutic options in the treatment of NASH. Antioxidants have also been utilized, and small studies have shown benefit from vitamin E supplementation. Treatment of hyperlipidemia with statin-type agents has shown improvement in liver enzymes, but they have not been assessed for effects on histology. Ursodeoxycholic acid has been utilized and improves liver enzymes in patients with many liver diseases, but it has not been definitely helpful for fatty liver disease. At present, efforts should be directed to encouraging patients with NAFLD to lose weight.

Lipid Storage Diseases There are a number of rare lipid storage diseases that involve the liver, including the inherited disorders of Gaucher's and Niemann-Pick disease (Chap. 356). Other rare disorders include abetalipoproteinemia, Tangier disease, Fabray's disease, and types I and V hyperlipoproteinemia. Hepatomegaly is present due to increased fat deposition and increased glycogen found in the liver.

Porphyrias The porphyrias are a group of metabolic disorders in which there are defects in the biosynthesis of heme necessary for incorporation into numerous hemoproteins such as hemoglobin, myoglobin, catalase, and the cytochromes (Chap. 352). Porphyrias can present as either acute or chronic diseases, with the acute disorder causing recurring bouts of abdominal pain, and the chronic disorders characterized by painful skin lesions. Porphyria cutanea tarda (PCT) is the most commonly encountered porphyria. Patients present with characteristic vesicular lesions on sun-exposed areas of the skin, principally the dorsum of the hands, the tips of the ears, or the cheeks. About 40% of patients with PCT have mutations in the gene for hemochromatosis (*HFE*), and ~50% have hepatitis C; thus, iron studies and *HFE* mutation analysis as well as hepatitis C testing should be considered in all patients who present with PCT. PCT is also associated with excess alcohol use and some medications, most notably estrogens.

R₂ PORPHYRIAS

The mainstay of treatment of PCT is iron reduction by therapeutic phlebotomy, which is successful in reversing the skin lesions in the majority of patients. If hepatitis C is present, this should be treated as well. Acute intermittent porphyria presents with abdominal pain, with the diagnosis made by avoidance of certain precipitating factors such as starvation or certain diets. Intravenous heme as hematin has been used for treatment.

INFILTRATIVE DISORDERS

Amyloidosis Amyloidosis is a metabolic storage disease that results from deposition of insoluble proteins that are aberrantly folded and assembled and then deposited in a variety of tissues (Chap. 324). Amyloidosis is divided into two types, primary and secondary, based on the broad concepts of association with myeloma (primary) or chronic inflammatory illnesses (secondary). The disease is generally considered rare, although in certain disease states or in certain populations, it can be more common. For example, when associated with familial Mediterranean fever, it is seen in high frequency in Sephardic Jews and Ar-

menians living in Armenia and less frequently in Ashkenazi Jews, Turks, and Arabs. Amyloidosis frequently affects patients suffering from tuberculosis and leprosy and can be seen in upwards of 10–15% of patients with ankylosing spondylitis, rheumatoid arthritis, or Crohn's disease. In one surgical pathology series, amyloid was found in <1% of cases. The liver is commonly involved in cases of systemic amyloidosis, but it is frequently inapparent clinically and only documented at autopsy. Pathologic findings in the liver include positive staining with the Congo red histochemical stain where there is an apple-green birefringence noted under polarizing light.

Granulomas Granulomas are frequently found in the liver when patients are being evaluated for cholestatic liver enzyme abnormalities. Granulomas can be seen in primary biliary cirrhosis, but there are other characteristic clinical and laboratory findings that allow for a definitive diagnosis of that disorder. Granulomatous infiltration can also be seen as the principal hepatic manifestation of sarcoidosis, and this is the most common presentation of hepatic granulomas (Chap. 322). The vast majority of these patients do not require any specific treatment, other than what would normally be used for treatment of their sarcoidosis. A small subset, however, can develop a particularly bothersome desmoplastic reaction with a significant increase in fibrosis, which can progress to cirrhosis and liver failure. These patients may require treatment with immunosuppressive therapy and may require liver transplantation. In patients who have granulomas in the liver not associated with sarcoidosis, treatment is rarely needed.

Diagnosis requires liver biopsy, and it is important to establish a diagnosis so that a cause for the elevated liver enzymes is carefully identified. Some medications can cause granulomatous infiltration of the liver, the most notable of which is allopurinol.

Lymphoma Involvement of the liver with lymphoma can sometimes be with bulky mass lesions but can also be as a difficult-to-diagnose infiltrative disorder that does not show any characteristic findings on abdominal imaging studies (Chap. 105). Patients may present with severe liver disease, jaundice, hypoalbuminemia, mild to moderately elevated aminotransferases, and an elevated alkaline phosphatase.

A liver biopsy is required for diagnosis and should be considered when routine blood testing does not lead to a diagnosis of the liver dysfunction.

FURTHER READINGS

ALA A, SCHILSKY ML: Wilson disease: Pathophysiology, diagnosis, treatment, and screening. Clin Liver Dis 8:787, 2004

FLEMING R, BACON BR: Orchestration of iron homeostasis. N Eng J Med 352:1741, 2005

HARRISON SA, NEUSCHWANDER-TETRI BA: Nonalcoholic fatty liver disease and nonalcoholic steatohepatitis. Clin Liver Dis 8:861, 2004

O'NEILL J, POWELL L: Clinical aspects of hemochromatosis. Semin Liver Dis 25:381, 2005

PERLMUTTER DH: Alpha-1-antitrypsin deficiency: Diagnosis and treatment. Clin Liver Dis 8:839, 2004

304 Liver Transplantation
Jules L. Dienstag, Raymond T. Chung

Liver transplantation—the replacement of the native, diseased liver by a normal organ (allograft)—has matured from an experimental procedure reserved for desperately ill patients to an accepted, lifesaving operation applied more optimally in the natural history of end-stage liver disease. The preferred and technically most advanced approach is *orthotopic*

transplantation, in which the native organ is removed and the donor organ is inserted in the same anatomic location. Pioneered in the 1960s by Starzl at the University of Colorado and, later, at the University of Pittsburgh and by Calne in Cambridge, England, liver transplantation is now performed routinely worldwide. Success measured as 1-year survival has improved from ~30% in the 1970s to about 90% today. These improved prospects for prolonged survival, dating back to the early 1980s, resulted from refinements in operative technique, improvements in organ procurement and preservation, advances in immunosuppressive therapy, and, perhaps most influentially, more enlightened patient selection and timing. Despite the perioperative morbidity and mortality, the technical and management challenges of the procedure, and its costs, liver transplantation has become the approach of choice for selected patients whose chronic or acute liver disease is progressive, life-threatening, and unresponsive to medical therapy. Based on the current level of success, the number of liver transplants has continued to grow each year; in 2005, approximately 6000 patients received liver allografts in the United States. Still, the demand for new livers continues to outpace availability; in the same period, >17,000 patients in the United States were on a waiting list for a donor liver. In response to this drastic shortage of donor organs, many transplantation centers have begun to supplement cadaver-organ liver transplantation with living-donor transplantation.

INDICATIONS

Potential candidates for liver transplantation are children and adults who, in the absence of contraindications (see below), suffer from severe, irreversible liver disease for which alternative medical or surgical treatments have been exhausted or are unavailable. *Timing of the operation is of critical importance.* Indeed, improved timing and better patient selection are felt to have contributed more to the increased success of liver transplantation in the 1980s and beyond than all the impressive technical and immunologic advances combined. Although the disease should be advanced, and although opportunities for spontaneous or medically induced stabilization or recovery should be allowed, the procedure should be done sufficiently early to give the surgical procedure a fair chance for success. Ideally, transplantation should be considered in patients with end-stage liver disease who are experiencing or have experienced a life-threatening complication of hepatic decompensation or whose quality of life has deteriorated to unacceptable levels. Although patients with well-compensated cirrhosis can survive for many years, many patients with quasi-stable chronic liver disease have much more advanced disease than may be apparent. As discussed below, the better the status of the patient prior to transplantation, the higher will be the anticipated success rate of transplantation. The decision about *when* to transplant is complex and requires the combined judgment of an experienced team of hepatologists, transplant surgeons, anesthesiologists, and specialists in support services, not to mention the well-informed consent of the patient and the patient's family.

TRANSPLANTATION IN CHILDREN

Indications for transplantation in children are listed in Table 304-1. The most common is *biliary atresia. Inherited or genetic disorders of metabolism* associated with liver failure constitute another major indication for transplantation in children and adolescents. In Crigler-Naj-

TABLE 304-1 INDICATIONS FOR LIVER TRANSPLANTATION

Children	Adults
Biliary atresia	Primary biliary cirrhosis
Neonatal hepatitis	Secondary biliary cirrhosis
Congenital hepatic fibrosis	Primary sclerosing cholangitis
Alagille's disease[a]	Autoimmune hepatitis
Byler's disease[b]	Caroli's disease[c]
α_1-Antitrypsin deficiency	Cryptogenic cirrhosis
Inherited disorders of metabolism	Chronic hepatitis with cirrhosis
Wilson's disease	Hepatic vein thrombosis
Tyrosinemia	Fulminant hepatitis
Glycogen storage diseases	Alcoholic cirrhosis
Lysosomal storage diseases	Chronic viral hepatitis
Protoporphyria	Primary hepatocellular malignancies
Crigler-Najjar disease type I	Hepatic adenomas
Familial hypercholesterolemia	Nonalcoholic steatohepatitis
Primary hyperoxaluria type I	Familial amyloid polyneuropathy
Hemophilia	

[a]Arteriohepatic dysplasia, with paucity of bile ducts, and congenital malformations, including pulmonary stenosis.
[b]Intrahepatic cholestasis, progressive liver failure, mental and growth retardation.
[c]Multiple cystic dilatations of the intrahepatic biliary tree.

jar disease type I and in certain hereditary disorders of the urea cycle and of amino acid or lactate-pyruvate metabolism, transplantation may be the only way to prevent impending deterioration of CNS function, despite the fact that the native liver is structurally normal. Combined heart and liver transplantation has yielded dramatic improvement in cardiac function and in cholesterol levels in children with homozygous familial hypercholesterolemia; combined liver and kidney transplantation has been successful in patients with primary hyperoxaluria type I. In hemophiliacs with transfusion-associated hepatitis and liver failure, liver transplantation has been associated with recovery of normal Factor VIII synthesis.

TRANSPLANTATION IN ADULTS

Liver transplantation is indicated for end-stage *cirrhosis* of all causes (Table 304-1). In *sclerosing cholangitis* and *Caroli's disease* (multiple cystic dilatations of the intrahepatic biliary tree), recurrent infections and sepsis associated with inflammatory and fibrotic obstruction of the biliary tree may be an indication for transplantation. Because prior biliary surgery complicates, and is a relative contraindication for, liver transplantation, surgical diversion of the biliary tree has been all but abandoned for patients with sclerosing cholangitis. In patients who undergo transplantation for *hepatic vein thrombosis (Budd-Chiari syndrome)*, postoperative anticoagulation is essential; underlying myeloproliferative disorders may have to be treated but are not a contraindication to liver transplantation. If a donor organ can be located quickly, before life-threatening complications—including cerebral edema—set in, patients with acute liver failure are candidates for liver transplantation. Routine candidates for liver transplantation are patients with *alcoholic cirrhosis, chronic viral hepatitis,* and *primary hepatocellular malignancies.* Although all three of these categories are considered to be high risk, liver transplantation can be offered to carefully selected patients. Currently, chronic hepatitis C and alcoholic liver disease are the most common indications for liver transplantation, accounting for over 40% of all adult candidates who undergo the procedure. Patients with alcoholic cirrhosis can be considered as candidates for transplantation if they meet strict criteria for abstinence and reform; however, these criteria still do not prevent recidivism in up to a quarter of cases. Patients with chronic hepatitis C have early allograft and patient survival comparable to those of other subsets of patients after transplantation; however, reinfection in the donor organ is universal, recurrent hepatitis C is insidiously progressive, the impact of antiviral therapy is limited, allograft cirrhosis develops in 20–30% at 5 years, and cirrhosis and late organ failure are being recognized with increasing frequency beyond 5 years. In patients with chronic hepatitis B, in the absence of measures to prevent recurrent hepatitis B, survival after transplantation is reduced by approximately 10–20%; however, prophylactic use of hepatitis B immune globulin (HBIg) during and after transplantation increases the success of transplantation to a level comparable to that seen in patients with nonviral causes of liver decompensation. The specific oral antiviral drugs lamivudine, adefovir dipivoxil, and entecavir (Chap. 300) can be used both for prophylaxis against and for treatment of recurrent hepatitis B, facilitating further the management of patients undergoing liver transplantation for end-stage hepatitis B; most transplantation centers rely on a combination of HBIg and antiviral drugs to manage patients with hepatitis B. Issues of disease recurrence are discussed in more detail below. Patients with nonmetastatic primary hepatobiliary tumors—primary hepatocellular carcinoma (HCC), cholangiocarcinoma, hepatoblastoma, angiosarcoma, epithelioid hemangioendothelioma, and multiple or massive hepatic adenomata—have undergone liver transplantation; however, for some hepatobiliary malignancies, overall survival is significantly lower than that for other categories of liver disease. Most transplantation centers have reported 5-year recurrence-free survival rates in patients with unresectable HCC for single tumors <5 cm in diameter or for three or fewer lesions all <3 cm comparable to those seen in patients undergoing transplantation for nonmalignant indications. Consequently, liver transplantation is currently restricted to patients whose hepatic malignancies meet these criteria. Expanded criteria for patients with HCC are being evaluated. Because the likelihood of recurrent cholangiocarcino-

TABLE 304-2	CONTRAINDICATIONS TO LIVER TRANSPLANTATION
Absolute	**Relative**
Uncontrolled extrahepatobiliary infection	Age >70
Active, untreated sepsis	Prior extensive hepatobiliary surgery
Uncorrectable, life-limiting congenital anomalies	Portal vein thrombosis
Active substance or alcohol abuse	Renal failure
Advanced cardiopulmonary disease	Previous extrahepatic malignancy (not including nonmelanoma skin cancer)
Extrahepatobiliary malignancy (not including nonmelanoma skin cancer)	Severe obesity
Metastatic malignancy to the liver	Severe malnutrition/wasting
Cholangiocarcinoma	Medical noncompliance
AIDS	HIV seropositivity
Life-threatening systemic diseases	Intrahepatic sepsis
	Severe hypoxemia secondary to right-to-left intrapulmonary shunts (P_{O_2} < 50 mmHg)
	Severe pulmonary hypertension (mean PA pressure >35 mmHg)
	Uncontrolled psychiatric disorder

ma is very high, only highly selected patients with limited disease are being evaluated for transplantation after intensive chemotherapy and radiation.

CONTRAINDICATIONS

Absolute contraindications for transplantation include life-threatening systemic diseases, uncontrolled extrahepatic bacterial or fungal infections, preexisting advanced cardiovascular or pulmonary disease, multiple uncorrectable life-threatening congenital anomalies, metastatic malignancy, active drug or alcohol abuse (Table 304-2). Because carefully selected patients in their sixties and even seventies have undergone transplantation successfully, advanced age per se is no longer considered an absolute contraindication; however, in older patients a more thorough preoperative evaluation should be undertaken to exclude ischemic cardiac disease and other comorbid conditions. Advanced age (>70 years), however, should be considered a *relative contraindication*—that is, a factor to be taken into account with other relative contraindications. Other relative contraindications include portal vein thrombosis, HIV infection, preexisting renal disease not associated with liver disease, intrahepatic or biliary sepsis, severe hypoxemia (P_{O_2} <50 mmHg) resulting from right-to-left intrapulmonary shunts, portopulmonary hypertension with high mean pulmonary artery pressures (>35 mmHg), previous extensive hepatobiliary surgery, any uncontrolled serious psychiatric disorder, and lack of sufficient social supports. Any one of these relative contraindications is insufficient in and of itself to preclude transplantation. For example, the problem of portal vein thrombosis can be overcome by constructing a graft from the donor liver portal vein to the recipient's superior mesenteric vein. Now that highly active antiretroviral therapy has dramatically improved the survival of persons with HIV infection (Chap. 182), and because end-stage liver disease caused by chronic hepatitis C and B has emerged as a serious source of morbidity and mortality in the HIV-infected population, liver transplantation has now been performed successfully in selected HIV-positive persons who have excellent control of HIV infection. A multicenter National Institutes of Health (NIH) consortium is currently studying outcomes of liver transplantation in HIV-infected recipients.

TECHNICAL CONSIDERATIONS

CADAVER DONOR SELECTION

Cadaver donor livers for transplantation are procured primarily from victims of head trauma. Organs from brain-dead donors up to age 60 are acceptable if the following criteria are met: hemodynamic stability, adequate oxygenation, absence of bacterial or fungal infection, absence of abdominal trauma, absence of hepatic dysfunction, and serologic exclusion of hepatitis B and C viruses and HIV. Occasionally, organs from donors with hepatitis B and C are used, e.g., for recipients with prior

hepatitis B and C, respectively. Donor organs with antibody to hepatitis B core antigen (anti-HBc) can also be used when the need is especially urgent, and recipients of these organs are treated prophylactically with HBIg and other antiviral drugs. Cardiovascular and respiratory functions are maintained artificially until the liver can be removed. Transplantation of organs procured from deceased donors who have succumbed to cardiac death can be performed successfully under selected circumstances, when ischemic time is minimized and liver histology preserved. Compatibility in ABO blood group and organ size between donor and recipient are important considerations in donor selection; however, ABO-incompatible, split liver, or reduced-donor-organ transplants can be performed in emergency or marked donor-scarcity situations. Tissue typing for HLA matching is not required, and preformed cytotoxic HLA antibodies do not preclude liver transplantation. Following perfusion with cold electrolyte solution, the donor liver is removed and packed in ice. The use of University of Wisconsin (UW) solution, rich in lactobionate and raffinose, has permitted the extension of cold ischemic time up to 20 h; however, 12 h may be a more reasonable limit. Improved techniques for harvesting multiple organs from the same donor have increased the availability of donor livers, but the availability of donor livers is far outstripped by the demand. Currently in the United States, all donor livers are distributed through a nationwide organ-sharing network [United Network of Organ Sharing (UNOS)] designed to allocate available organs based on regional considerations and recipient acuity. Recipients who have the highest disease severity generally have the highest priority, but allocation strategies that balance highest urgency against best outcomes continue to evolve to distribute cadaver organs most effectively. Allocation based on the Child-Turcotte-Pugh (CTP) score, which uses five clinical variables (encephalopathy stage, ascites, bilirubin, albumin, and prothrombin time) and waiting time, has been replaced by allocation based upon urgency alone, calculated by the Model for End-Stage Liver Disease (MELD) score. The MELD score is based upon a mathematical model that includes bilirubin, creatinine, and prothrombin time expressed as international normalized ratio (INR) (Table 304-3). Neither waiting time (except as a tie breaker between two potential recipients with the same MELD scores) nor posttransplantation outcome is taken into account, but the MELD score has been shown to be the best predictor of pretransplantation mortality, satisfies the prevailing view that medical need should be the decisive determinant, and eliminates both the subjectivity inherent in the CTP scoring system (presence and degree of ascites and hepatic encephalopathy) and the

TABLE 304-3	UNITED NETWORK FOR ORGAN SHARING (UNOS) LIVER TRANSPLANTATION WAITING LIST CRITERIA

Status 1   Fulminant hepatic failure (including primary graft nonfunction and hepatic artery thrombosis within 7 days after transplantation as well as acute decompensated Wilson's disease)[a]

The Model for End-Stage Liver Disease (MELD) score, on a continuous scale,[b] determines allocation of the remainder of donor organs. This model is based upon the following calculation:

$3.78 \times \log_e$ bilirubin (mg/100 mL) + $11.2 \times \log_e$ international normalized ratio (INR) + $9.57 \times \log_e$ creatinine (mg/100 mL) + 6.43 (× 0 for alcoholic and cholestatic liver disease, × 1 for all other types of liver disease).[c,d,e]

Online calculators to determine MELD scores are available, such as the following: *www.unos.org/resources/meldPeldCalculator.asp*.

[a]For children <18 years of age, Status 1 includes acute or chronic liver failure plus hospitalization in an intensive care unit or inborn errors of metabolism. Status 1 is retained for those persons with fulminant hepatic failure and supersedes the MELD score.

[b]The MELD scale is continuous, with 34 levels ranging between 6 and 40. Donor organs usually do not become available unless the MELD score exceeds 20.

[c]Patients with stage T2 hepatocellular carcinoma receive 22 disease-specific points. An αfetoprotein level = 500 ng/mL is considered as stage I hepatocellular carcinoma even without evidence for a tumor on imaging.

[d]Creatinine is included because renal function is a validated predictor of survival in patients with liver disease. For adults undergoing dialysis twice a week, the creatinine in the equation is set to 4 mg/100 mL.

[e]For children <18 years of age, the Pediatric End-Stage Liver Disease (PELD) scale is used. This scale is based on albumin, bilirubin, INR, growth failure, and age. Status 1 is retained, but the PELD replaces Status 2 and 3.

differences in waiting times among different regions of the country. Under the CTP or the MELD system, highest priority (status 1) continues to be reserved for those patients with fulminant hepatic failure. Because candidates for liver transplantation who have HCC may not be sufficiently decompensated to compete for donor organs based upon urgency criteria alone, and because protracted waiting for cadaver donor organs results often in tumor growth beyond acceptable limits for transplantation, such patients are assigned disease-specific MELD points (Table 304-3).

LIVING-DONOR TRANSPLANTATION

Occasionally, especially for liver transplantation in children, one cadaver organ can be split between two (one adult and one child) recipients. A more viable alternative, transplantation of the right lobe of the liver from a healthy adult into an adult recipient, has gained increased popularity. Living-donor transplantation of the left lobe (left lateral segment), introduced in the early 1990s to alleviate the extreme shortage of donor organs for small children, accounts currently for approximately a third of all liver transplantation procedures in children. Driven by the shortage of cadaver organs, living-donor transplantation involving the more sizable right lobe is being considered with increasing frequency in adults; however, living-donor liver transplantation cannot be expected to solve the donor organ shortage. About 300 such procedures were done in 2005, representing only about 5% of all liver transplant operations done in the United States.

Living-donor transplantation can reduce waiting time and cold-ischemia time; is done under elective, rather than emergency, circumstances; and may be lifesaving in recipients who cannot afford to wait for a cadaver donor. The downside, of course, is the risk to the healthy donor (a mean of 10 weeks of medical disability; biliary complications in ~5%; postoperative complications such as wound infection, small-bowel obstruction, and incisional hernias in 9–19%; and, even, in 0.2–0.4%, death) as well as the increased frequency of biliary (15–32%) and vascular (10%) complications in the recipient. Potential donors must participate voluntarily without coercion, and transplantation teams should go to great lengths to exclude subtle coercive or inappropriate psychological factors as well as outline carefully to both donor and recipient the potential benefits and risks of the procedure. Donors for the procedure should be 18–60 years old; have a compatible blood type with the recipient; have no chronic medical problems or history of major abdominal surgery; be related genetically or emotionally to the recipient; and pass an exhaustive series of clinical, biochemical, and serologic evaluations to unearth disqualifying medical disorders. The recipient should meet the same UNOS criteria for liver transplantation as recipients of a cadaver donor allograft. The multicenter NIH A2ALL Study is collecting comprehensive data regarding outcomes of adult-to-adult living-donor liver transplantation (*http://www.nih-a2all.org/*).

SURGICAL TECHNIQUE

Removal of the recipient's native liver is technically difficult, particularly in the presence of portal hypertension with its associated collateral circulation and extensive varices. Further complicating removal is the presence of scarring from previous abdominal operations. The combination of portal hypertension and coagulopathy (elevated prothrombin time and thrombocytopenia) may translate into large blood product transfusion requirements. After the portal vein and infrahepatic and suprahepatic inferior venae cavae are dissected, the hepatic artery and common bile duct are dissected. Then the native liver is removed and the donor organ inserted. During the anhepatic phase, coagulopathy, hypoglycemia, hypocalcemia, and hypothermia are encountered and must be managed by the anesthesiology team. Caval, portal vein, hepatic artery, and bile duct anastomoses are performed in succession, the last by end-to-end suturing of the donor and recipient common bile ducts or by choledochojejunostomy to a Roux-en-Y loop if the recipient common bile duct cannot be used for reconstruction (e.g., in sclerosing cholangitis). A typical transplant operation lasts 8 h, with a range of 6–18 h. Because of excessive bleeding, large

volumes of blood, blood products, and volume expanders may be required during surgery; however, blood requirements have fallen sharply with improvements in surgical technique and experience.

As noted above, emerging alternatives to orthotopic liver transplantation include split-liver grafts, in which one donor organ is divided and inserted into two recipients; and living-donor procedures, in which the left (for children) or the right (for adults) lobe of the liver is harvested from a living donor for transplantation into the recipient. In the adult procedure, once the right lobe is removed from the donor, the donor right hepatic vein is anastomosed to the recipient right hepatic vein remnant, followed by donor-to-recipient anastomoses of the portal vein and then the hepatic artery. Finally, the biliary anastomosis is performed, duct-to-duct if practical or via Roux-en-Y anastomosis. Heterotopic liver transplantation, in which the donor liver is inserted without removal of the native liver, has met with very limited success and acceptance, except in a very small number of centers. In attempts to support desperately ill patients until a suitable donor organ can be identified, several transplantation centers are studying extracorporeal perfusion with bioartificial liver cartridges constructed from hepatocytes bound to hollow fiber systems and used as temporary hepatic-assist devices, but their efficacy remains to be established. Areas of research with the potential to overcome the shortage of donor organs include hepatocyte transplantation and xenotransplantation with genetically modified organs of nonhuman origin (e.g., swine).

POSTOPERATIVE COURSE AND MANAGEMENT

IMMUNOSUPPRESSIVE THERAPY

The introduction in 1980 of cyclosporine as an immunosuppressive agent contributed substantially to the improvement in survival after liver transplantation. Cyclosporine, a calcineurin inhibitor, blocks early activation of T cells and is specific for T cell functions that result from the interaction of the T cell with its receptor and that involve the calcium-dependent signal transduction pathway. As a result, the activity of cyclosporine leads to inhibition of lymphokine gene activation, blocking interleukins 2, 3, and 4, tumor necrosis factor α, and other lymphokines. Cyclosporine also inhibits B cell functions. This process occurs without affecting rapidly dividing cells in the bone marrow, which may account for the reduced frequency of posttransplantation systemic infections. The most common and important side effect of cyclosporine therapy is nephrotoxicity. Cyclosporine causes dose-dependent renal tubular injury and direct renal artery vasospasm. Following renal function, therefore, is important in monitoring cyclosporine therapy, perhaps even a more reliable indicator than blood levels of the drug. Nephrotoxicity is reversible and can be managed by dose reduction. Other adverse effects of cyclosporine therapy include hypertension, hyperkalemia, tremor, hirsutism, glucose intolerance, and gum hyperplasia.

Tacrolimus (originally labeled *FK 506*) is a macrolide lactone antibiotic isolated from a Japanese soil fungus, *Streptomyces tsukubaensis*. It has the same mechanism of action as cyclosporine but is 10–100 times more potent. Initially applied as "rescue" therapy for patients in whom rejection occurred despite the use of cyclosporine, tacrolimus was shown in two large, multicenter, randomized trials to be associated with a reduced frequency of acute rejection, refractory rejection, and chronic rejection. Although patient and graft survival are the same with these two drugs, the advantage of tacrolimus in minimizing episodes of rejection, reducing the need for additional glucocorticoid doses, and reducing the likelihood of bacterial and cytomegalovirus (CMV) infection has simplified the management of patients undergoing liver transplantation. In addition, the oral absorption of tacrolimus is more predictable than that of cyclosporine, especially during the early postoperative period when T-tube drainage interferes with the enterohepatic circulation of cyclosporine. As a result, in most transplantation centers tacrolimus has now supplanted cyclosporine for primary immunosuppression, and many centers rely on oral rather than intravenous administration from the outset. For transplantation centers that prefer cyclosporine, a new, better-absorbed microemulsion preparation is now available.

Although tacrolimus is more potent than cyclosporine, it is also more toxic and more likely to be discontinued for adverse events. The toxicity of tacrolimus is similar to that of cyclosporine; nephrotoxicity and neurotoxicity are the most commonly encountered adverse effects, and neurotoxicity (tremor, seizures, hallucinations, psychoses, coma) is more likely and more severe in tacrolimus-treated patients. Both drugs can cause diabetes mellitus, but tacrolimus does not cause hirsutism or gingival hyperplasia. Because of overlapping toxicity between cyclosporine and tacrolimus, especially nephrotoxicity, and because tacrolimus reduces cyclosporine clearance, these two drugs should not be used together. Since 99% of tacrolimus is metabolized by the liver, hepatic dysfunction reduces its clearance; in primary graft nonfunction (when, for technical reasons or because of ischemic damage prior to its insertion, the allograft is defective and does not function normally from the outset), tacrolimus doses have to be reduced substantially, especially in children. Both cyclosporine and tacrolimus are metabolized by the cytochrome P450 IIIA system, and therefore drugs that induce cytochrome P450 (e.g., phenytoin, phenobarbital, carbamazepine, rifampin) reduce available levels of cyclosporine and tacrolimus; drugs that inhibit cytochrome P450 (e.g., erythromycin, fluconazole, ketoconazole, clotrimazole, itraconazole, verapamil, diltiazem, nicardipine, cimetidine, danazol, metoclopramide, bromocriptine, and the HIV protease inhibitor ritonavir) increase cyclosporine and tacrolimus blood levels. Indeed, itraconazole is commonly used to help boost tacrolimus levels. Like azathioprine, cyclosporine and tacrolimus appear to be associated with a risk of lymphoproliferative malignancies (see below), which may occur earlier after cyclosporine or tacrolimus than after azathioprine therapy. Because of these side effects, combinations of cyclosporine or tacrolimus with prednisone and azathioprine—all at reduced doses—are preferable regimens for immunosuppressive therapy.

In patients with pretransplantation renal dysfunction or renal deterioration that occurs intraoperatively or immediately postoperatively, tacrolimus or cyclosporine therapy may not be practical; under these circumstances, induction or maintenance of immunosuppression with monoclonal antibodies to T cells, OKT3, may be appropriate. Therapy with OKT3 has been especially effective in reversing acute rejection in the posttransplant period and is the standard treatment for acute rejection that fails to respond to methylprednisolone boluses. Intravenous infusions of OKT3 may be complicated by transient fever, chills, and diarrhea, or by pulmonary edema, which can be fatal. When this drug is used to induce immunosuppression initially or to provide "rescue" in those who reject despite "conventional" therapy, the incidence of bacterial, fungal, and especially CMV infections is increased during and after such therapy. In some centers, ganciclovir antiviral therapy is initiated prophylactically as a routine along with OKT3. Because OKT3 is such a potent immunosuppressive agent, its use is more likely to be complicated by opportunistic infection or lymphoproliferative disorders; therefore, and because of the availability of alternative immunosuppressive drugs, OKT3 is used less often nowadays. Another immunosuppressive drug being used for patients undergoing liver transplantation is mycophenolic acid, a nonnucleoside purine metabolism inhibitor derived as a fermentation product from several *Penicillium* species. Mycophenolate has been shown to be better than azathioprine, when used with other standard immunosuppressive drugs, in preventing rejection after renal transplantation and has been adopted as well for use in liver transplantation. The most common adverse effects of mycophenolate are leukopenia and gastrointestinal complaints. Rapamycin, an inhibitor of later events in T cell activation, is approved for use in kidney transplantation but is not approved for use in liver transplant recipients because of the association with an increased frequency of hepatic artery thrombosis in the first month posttransplantation. Studies to examine the safety and efficacy of conversion to rapamycin from calcineurin inhibitors are ongoing. Because of its profound antiproliferative effects, rapamycin has also been suggested to be a useful immunosuppressive agent in patients with a prior or current history of malignancy, such as HCC. Further evaluation is underway.

The most important principle of immunosuppression is that the ideal approach strikes a balance between immunosuppression and immunologic competence. In general, given sufficient immunosuppres-

sion, acute liver allograft rejection is nearly always reversible. On the one hand, incompletely treated acute rejection predisposes to the development of chronic rejection, which can threaten graft survival. On the other hand, if the cumulative dose of immunosuppressive therapy is too large, the patient may succumb to opportunistic infection. In hepatitis C, pulse glucocorticoids or OKT3 use accelerate recurrent allograft hepatitis. Further complicating matters, acute rejection can be difficult to distinguish histologically from recurrent hepatitis C. Therefore, immunosuppressive drugs must be used judiciously, with strict attention to the infectious consequences of such therapy and careful confirmation of the diagnosis of acute rejection. In this vein, efforts have been made to minimize the use of glucocorticoids, a mainstay of immunosuppressive regimens, and steroid-free immunosuppression can be achieved in some instances. In this regard, patients who undergo liver transplantation for autoimmune diseases such as primary biliary cirrhosis, autoimmune hepatitis, and primary sclerosing cholangitis, are less likely to achieve freedom from steroids.

POSTOPERATIVE COMPLICATIONS

Complications of liver transplantation can be divided into hepatic and nonhepatic categories (Tables 304-4 and 304-5). In addition, both immediately postoperative and late complications are encountered. Patients who undergo liver transplantation as a rule have been chronically ill for protracted periods and may be malnourished and wasted. The impact of such chronic illness and the multisystem failure that accompanies liver failure continue to require attention in the postoperative period. Because of the massive fluid losses and fluid shifts that occur during the operation, patients may remain fluid-overloaded during the immediate postoperative period, straining cardiovascular reserve; this effect can be amplified in the face of transient renal dysfunction and pulmonary capillary vascular permeability. Continuous monitoring of cardiovascular and pulmonary function, measures to maintain the integrity of the intravascular compartment and to treat extravascular volume overload, and scrupulous attention to potential sources and sites of infection are of paramount importance. Cardiovascular instability may also result from the electrolyte imbalance that may accompany reperfusion of the donor liver as well as from restoration of systemic vascular resistance following implantation. Pulmonary function may be

TABLE 304-4	NONHEPATIC COMPLICATIONS OF LIVER TRANSPLANTATION
Fluid overload	
Cardiovascular instability	Arrhythmias
	Congestive heart failure
	Cardiomyopathy
Pulmonary compromise	Pneumonia
	Pulmonary capillary vascular permeability
	Fluid overload
Renal dysfunction	Prerenal azotemia
	Hypoperfusion injury (acute tubular necrosis)
	Drug nephrotoxicity
	↓ Renal blood flow secondary to ↑ intraabdominal pressure
Hematologic	Anemia 2° to gastrointestinal and/or intraabdominal bleeding
	Hemolytic anemia, aplastic anemia
	Thrombocytopenia
Infection	Bacterial: early, common postoperative infections
	Fungal/parasitic: late, opportunistic infections
	Viral: late, opportunistic infections, recurrent hepatitis
Neuropsychiatric	Seizures
	Metabolic encephalopathy
	Depression
	Difficult psychosocial adjustment
Diseases of donor	Infectious
	Malignant
Malignancy	B-cell lymphoma (posttransplantation lymphoproliferative disorders)
	De novo neoplasms (particularly squamous cell skin carcinoma)

TABLE 304-5 HEPATIC COMPLICATIONS OF LIVER TRANSPLANTATION

Hepatic Dysfunction Common after Major Surgery

Prehepatic	Pigment load
	Hemolysis
	Blood collections (hematomas, abdominal collections)
Intrahepatic	
Early	Hepatotoxic drugs and anesthesia
	Hypoperfusion (hypotension, shock, sepsis)
	Benign postoperative cholestasis
Late	Transfusion-associated hepatitis
	Exacerbation of primary hepatic disease
Posthepatic	Biliary obstruction
	↓ Renal clearance of conjugated bilirubin (renal dysfunction)

Hepatic Dysfunction Unique to Liver Transplantation

Primary graft nonfunction	
Vascular compromise	Portal vein obstruction
	Hepatic artery thrombosis
	Anastomotic leak with intraabdominal bleeding
Bile duct disorder	Stenosis, obstruction, leak
Rejection	
Recurrent primary hepatic disease	

compromised further by paralysis of the right hemidiaphragm associated with phrenic nerve injury. The hyperdynamic state with increased cardiac output that is characteristic of patients with liver failure reverses rapidly after successful liver transplantation.

Other immediate management issues include renal dysfunction. Prerenal azotemia, acute kidney injury associated with hypoperfusion (acute tubular necrosis), and renal toxicity caused by antibiotics, tacrolimus, or cyclosporine are encountered frequently in the postoperative period, sometimes necessitating dialysis. Hemolytic uremic syndrome can be associated with cyclosporine, tacrolimus, or OKT3. Occasionally, postoperative intraperitoneal bleeding may be sufficient to increase intraabdominal pressure, which, in turn, may reduce renal blood flow; this effect is rapidly reversible when abdominal distention is relieved by exploratory laparotomy to identify and ligate the bleeding site and to remove intraperitoneal clot.

Anemia may also result from acute upper gastrointestinal bleeding or from transient hemolytic anemia, which may be autoimmune, especially when blood group O livers are transplanted into blood group A or B recipients. This autoimmune hemolytic anemia is mediated by donor intrahepatic lymphocytes that recognize red blood cell A or B antigens on recipient erythrocytes. Transient in nature, this process resolves once the donor liver is repopulated by recipient bone marrow–derived lymphocytes; the hemolysis can be treated by transfusing blood group O red blood cells and/or by administering higher doses of glucocorticoids. Transient thrombocytopenia is also commonly encountered. Aplastic anemia, a late occurrence, is rare but has been reported in almost 30% of patients who underwent liver transplantation for acute, severe hepatitis of unknown cause.

Bacterial, fungal, or viral infections are common and may be life-threatening postoperatively. Early after transplant surgery, common postoperative infections predominate—pneumonia, wound infections, infected intraabdominal collections, urinary tract infections, and intravenous line infections—rather than opportunistic infections; these infections may involve the biliary tree and liver as well. Beyond the first postoperative month, the toll of immunosuppression becomes evident, and opportunistic infections—CMV, herpes viruses, fungal infections (*Aspergillus*, *Candida*, cryptococcal disease), mycobacterial infections, parasitic infections (*Pneumocystis*, *Toxoplasma*), bacterial infections (*Nocardia*, *Legionella*, and *Listeria*)—predominate. Rarely, early infections represent those transmitted with the donor liver, either infections present in the donor or infections acquired during procurement processing. De novo viral hepatitis infections acquired from the donor organ or, almost unheard of nowadays, from transfused blood products occur after typical incubation periods for these agents (well beyond the

first month). Obviously, infections in an immunosuppressed host demand early recognition and prompt management; prophylactic antibiotic therapy is administered routinely in the immediate postoperative period. Use of sulfamethoxazole with trimethoprim reduces the incidence of postoperative *Pneumocystis carinii* pneumonia. Antiviral prophylaxis for CMV with ganciclovir should be administered in patients at high risk (e.g., when a CMV-seropositive donor organ is implanted into a CMV-seronegative recipient).

Neuropsychiatric complications include seizures (commonly associated with cyclosporine and tacrolimus toxicity), metabolic encephalopathy, depression, and difficult psychosocial adjustment. Rarely, diseases are transmitted by the allograft from the donor to the recipient. In addition to viral and bacterial infections, malignancies of donor origin have occurred. Posttransplantation lymphoproliferative disorders, especially B cell lymphoma, are a recognized complication associated with immunosuppressive drugs such as azathioprine, tacrolimus, and cyclosporine (see above). Epstein-Barr virus has been shown to play a contributory role in some of these tumors, which may regress when immunosuppressive therapy is reduced. De novo neoplasms appear at increased frequency after liver transplantation, particularly squamous cell carcinomas of the skin. Routine screening should be performed.

Long-term complications after liver transplantation attributable primarily to immunosuppressive medications include diabetes mellitus (associated with glucocorticoids) as well as hypertension, hyperlipidemia, and chronic renal insufficiency (associated with cyclosporine and tacrolimus). Monitoring and treating these disorders is a routine component of posttransplantation care; in some cases, they respond to changes in immunosuppressive regimen, while in others, specific treatment of the disorder is introduced.

HEPATIC COMPLICATIONS

Hepatic dysfunction after liver transplantation is similar to the hepatic complications encountered after major abdominal and cardiothoracic surgery; however, in addition, there may be complications such as primary graft failure, vascular compromise, failure or stricture of the biliary anastomoses, and rejection. As in nontransplant surgery, postoperative jaundice may result from prehepatic, intrahepatic, and posthepatic sources. *Prehepatic* sources represent the massive hemoglobin pigment load from transfusions, hemolysis, hematomas, ecchymoses, and other collections of blood. *Early intrahepatic* liver injury includes effects of hepatotoxic drugs and anesthesia; hypoperfusion injury associated with hypotension, sepsis, and shock; and benign postoperative cholestasis. *Late intrahepatic* sources of liver injury include posttransfusion hepatitis and exacerbation of primary disease. *Posthepatic* sources of hepatic dysfunction include biliary obstruction and reduced renal clearance of conjugated bilirubin. Hepatic complications unique to liver transplantation include primary graft failure associated with ischemic injury to the organ during harvesting; vascular compromise associated with thrombosis or stenosis of the portal vein or hepatic artery anastomoses; vascular anastomotic leak; stenosis, obstruction, or leakage of the anastomosed common bile duct; recurrence of primary hepatic disorder (see below); and rejection.

TRANSPLANT REJECTION

Despite the use of immunosuppressive drugs, rejection of the transplanted liver still occurs in a proportion of patients, beginning 1–2 weeks after surgery. Clinical signs suggesting rejection are fever, right upper quadrant pain, and reduced bile pigment and volume. Leukocytosis may occur, but the most reliable indicators are increases in serum bilirubin and aminotransferase levels. Because these tests lack specificity, distinguishing among rejection and biliary obstruction, primary graft nonfunction, vascular compromise, viral hepatitis, CMV infection, drug hepatotoxicity, and recurrent primary disease may be difficult. Radiographic visualization of the biliary tree and/or percutaneous liver biopsy often helps to establish the correct diagnosis. Morphologic features of acute rejection include a mixed portal cellular infiltrate, bile duct injury, and/or endothelial inflammation ("endothelialitis"); some of these findings are reminiscent of graft-versus-host disease, primary biliary cirrhosis, or recurrent allograft hepatitis C. As soon as transplant rejection is suspected, treatment consists of intravenous methylprednisolone in repeated boluses; if this fails to abort rejection, many centers use antibodies to lymphocytes, such as OKT3, or polyclonal antilymphocyte globulin. Caution should be exercised when managing acute rejection with pulse glucocorticoids in patients with hepatitis C virus (HCV) infection, because of the high risk of triggering recurrent allograft hepatitis C.

Chronic rejection is a relatively rare outcome that can follow repeated bouts of acute rejection or that occurs unrelated to preceding rejection episodes. Morphologically, chronic rejection is characterized by progressive cholestasis, focal parenchymal necrosis, mononuclear infiltration, vascular lesions (intimal fibrosis, subintimal foam cells, fibrinoid necrosis), and fibrosis. This process may be reflected as ductopenia—the vanishing bile duct syndrome. Reversibility of chronic rejection is limited; in patients with therapy-resistant chronic rejection, retransplantation has yielded encouraging results.

OUTCOME

SURVIVAL
The survival rate for patients undergoing liver transplantation has improved steadily since 1983. One-year survival rates have increased from ~70% in the early 1980s to 85–90% from 2000 to 2006. Currently the 5-year survival rate exceeds 60%. An important observation is the relationship between clinical status before transplantation and outcome. For patients who undergo liver transplantation when their level of compensation is high (e.g., still working or only partially disabled), a 1-year survival rate of >85% is common. For those whose level of decompensation mandates continuous in-hospital care prior to transplantation, the 1-year survival rate is about 70%, while for those who are so decompensated that they require life support in an intensive care unit, the 1-year survival rate is ~50%. Since UNOS's adoption in 2002 of the MELD system for organ allocation, posttransplantation survival has been found to be affected adversely for candidates with MELD scores >25, considered high disease severity. Thus, irrespective of allocation scheme, high disease severity pretransplantation corresponds to diminished posttransplantation survival. Another important distinction in survival has been drawn between high-risk and low-risk patient categories. For patients who do not fit any "high-risk" designations, 1-year and 5-year survival rates of 85 and 80%, respectively, have been recorded. In contrast, among patients in high-risk categories—cancer, fulminant hepatitis, age >65, concurrent renal failure, respirator dependence, portal vein thrombosis, and history of a portacaval shunt or multiple right upper quadrant operations—survival statistics fall into the range of 60% at 1 year and 35% at 5 years. Survival after retransplantation for primary graft nonfunction is ~50%. Causes of failure of liver transplantation vary with time. Failures within the first 3 months result primarily from technical complications, postoperative infections, and hemorrhage. Transplant failures after the first 3 months are more likely to result from infection, rejection, or recurrent disease (such as malignancy or viral hepatitis).

RECURRENCE OF PRIMARY DISEASE
Features of autoimmune hepatitis, primary sclerosing cholangitis, and primary biliary cirrhosis overlap with those of rejection or posttransplantation bile-duct injury. Whether autoimmune hepatitis and sclerosing cholangitis recur after liver transplantation is controversial; data supporting recurrent autoimmune hepatitis (in up to a third of patients in some series) are more convincing than those supporting recurrent sclerosing cholangitis. Similarly, reports of recurrent primary biliary cirrhosis after liver transplantation have appeared; however, the histologic features of primary biliary cirrhosis and chronic rejection are virtually indistinguishable and occur as frequently in patients with primary biliary cirrhosis as in patients undergoing transplantation for other reasons. The presence of a florid inflammatory bile duct lesion is highly suggestive of the recurrence of primary biliary cirrhosis, but even this lesion can be observed in acute rejection. Hereditary disorders such as Wilson's disease and α_1 antitrypsin deficiency have not recurred after liver transplantation; however, recurrence of disordered iron metabolism has been observed in some patients with hemochromatosis. Hepatic vein thrombosis (Budd-Chiari syndrome) may recur; this can be minimized by treating underlying myeloproliferative disorders and by anticoagulation. Because cholangiocarcinoma recurs almost invariably, few centers now offer transplantation to such patients; however, a few highly selected patients with operatively confirmed stage I or II cholangiocarcinoma who undergo liver transplantation combined with neoadjuvant chemoradiation may experience excellent outcomes. In patients with intrahepatic hepatocellular carcinoma who meet criteria for transplantation, 1- and 5-year survivals are similar to those observed in patients undergoing liver transplantation for nonmalignant disease. Finally, metabolic disorders such as nonalcoholic steatohepatitis recur frequently, especially if the underlying metabolic predisposition is not altered.

Hepatitis A can recur after transplantation for fulminant hepatitis A, but such acute reinfection has no serious clinical sequelae. In fulminant hepatitis B, recurrence is not the rule; however, in the absence of any prophylactic measures, hepatitis B usually recurs after transplantation for end-stage chronic hepatitis B. Before the introduction of prophylactic antiviral therapy, immunosuppressive therapy sufficient to prevent allograft rejection led inevitably to marked increases in hepatitis B viremia, regardless of pretransplantation values. Overall graft and patient survival were poor, and some patients experienced a rapid recapitulation of severe injury—severe chronic hepatitis or even fulminant hepatitis—after transplantation. Also recognized in the era before availability of antiviral regimens was *fibrosing cholestatic hepatitis*, rapidly progressive liver injury associated with marked hyperbilirubinemia, substantial prolongation of the prothrombin time (both out of proportion to relatively modest elevations of aminotransferase activity), and rapidly progressive liver failure. This lesion has been suggested to represent a "choking off" of the hepatocyte by an overwhelming density of hepatitis B virus (HBV) proteins. Complications such as sepsis and pancreatitis were also observed more frequently in patients undergoing liver transplantation for hepatitis B prior to the introduction of antiviral therapy. The introduction of long-term prophylaxis with HBIg revolutionized liver transplantation for chronic hepatitis B. Neither preoperative hepatitis B vaccination, preoperative or postoperative interferon therapy, nor short-term (≤2 months) HBIg prophylaxis has been shown to be effective, but a retrospective analysis of data from several hundred European patients followed for 3 years after transplantation has shown that long-term (≥6 months) prophylaxis with HBIg is associated with a lowering of the risk of HBV reinfection from ~75% to 35% and a reduction in mortality from ~50% to 20%.

As a result of long-term HBIg use following liver transplantation for chronic hepatitis B, similar improvements in outcome have been observed in the United States, with 1-year survival rates between 75 and 90%. Currently, with HBIg prophylaxis, the outcome of liver transplantation for chronic hepatitis B is indistinguishable from that for chronic liver disease unassociated with chronic hepatitis B; essentially, medical concerns regarding liver transplantation for chronic hepatitis B have been eliminated. Passive immunoprophylaxis with HBIg is begun during the anhepatic stage of surgery, repeated daily for the first 6 postoperative days, then continued with infusions that are given either at regular intervals of 4–6 weeks or, alternatively, when anti-HBs levels fall below a threshold of 100 mIU/mL. The current approach in most centers is to continue HBIg indefinitely, which can add approximately $20,000 per year to the cost of care; some centers are evaluating regimens that shift to less frequent administration or to intramuscular administration in the late posttransplantation period. Still, occasionally "breakthrough" HBV infection occurs.

Further improving the outcome of liver transplantation for chronic hepatitis B is the current availability of such antiviral drugs as lamivudine, adefovir dipivoxil, and entecavir (Chap. 300). When these drugs are administered to patients with decompensated liver disease, a proportion improve sufficiently to postpone imminent liver transplantation. In addition, lamivudine can be used to prevent recurrence of HBV infection when administered *prior* to transplantation; to treat hepatitis B that recurs *after* transplantation, including in patients who break through HBIg prophylaxis; and to reverse the course of otherwise fatal fibrosing cholestatic hepatitis. Clinical trials have shown that lamivudine antiviral therapy reduces the level of HBV replication substantially, sometimes even resulting in clearance of hepatitis B surface antigen (HBsAg); reduces alanine aminotransferase (ALT) levels; and improves histologic features of necrosis and inflammation. Long-term use of lamivudine is safe and effective, but after several months a proportion of patients become resistant to lamivudine, resulting from YMDD (tyrosine-methionine-aspartate-aspartate) mutations in the HBV polymerase motif (Chap. 300). In approximately half of such resistant patients, hepatic deterioration may ensue. Fortunately, adefovir dipivoxil is available as well and can be used to treat lamivudine-associated YMDD variants, effectively "rescuing" patients experiencing hepatic decompensation after lamivudine breakthrough. Currently, most liver transplantation centers combine HBIg plus lamivudine or adefovir, and additional antivirals such as the more recently approved entecavir are being introduced as well. Clinical trials are underway to define the optimal application of these antiviral agents in the management of patients undergoing liver transplantation for chronic hepatitis B; conceivably, in the future, combinations of oral antiviral drugs may even supplant HBIg.

Prophylactic approaches applied to patients undergoing liver transplantation for chronic hepatitis B are being used as well for patients without hepatitis B who receive organs from donors with anti-HBc. Patients who undergo liver transplantation for chronic hepatitis B plus D are less likely to experience recurrent liver injury than patients undergoing liver transplantation for hepatitis B alone; still, such co-infected patients would also be offered standard posttransplantation prophylactic therapy for hepatitis B.

Accounting for up to 40% of all liver transplantation procedures, the most common indication for liver transplantation is end-stage liver disease resulting from chronic hepatitis C. Recurrence of HCV infection after liver transplantation can be documented in almost every patient if sufficiently sensitive virus markers are used. The clinical consequences of recurrent hepatitis C are limited during the first 5 years after transplantation. Nonetheless, despite the relative clinical benignity of recurrent hepatitis C in the early years after liver transplantation, and despite the negligible impact on patient survival during these early years, histologic studies have documented the presence of moderate to severe chronic hepatitis in more than half of all patients and bridging fibrosis or cirrhosis in ~10%. Moreover, progression to cirrhosis within 5 years is even more common, occurring in up to two-thirds of patients if moderate hepatitis is detected in a 1-year biopsy. Not surprisingly, then, for patients undergoing transplantation for hepatitis C, allograft and patient survival are diminished substantially between 5 and 10 years after transplantation. In a proportion of patients, even during the early posttransplantation period, recurrent hepatitis C may be sufficiently severe biochemically and histologically to merit antiviral therapy. Treatment with pegylated interferon can *suppress* HCV-associated liver injury but rarely leads to *sustained* benefit. Sustained virologic responses are the exception, and reduced tolerability is often dose-limiting. Preemptive combination antiviral therapy with pegylated interferon and the nucleoside analogue ribavirin immediately after transplantation does not appear to provide any advantage over therapy introduced after clinical hepatitis has occurred. Similarly, although interferon-based antiviral therapy is not recommended for patients with decompensated liver disease, some centers have experimented with pretransplantation antiviral therapy in an attempt to eradicate HCV replication prior to transplantation; preliminary results are promising, but interferon treatment of patients with end-stage liver disease can lead to worsening of hepatic decompensation, and HCV infection has recurred after transplantation in some of these recipients. Initial trials

of hepatitis C immune globulin preparations to prevent recurrent hepatitis C after liver transplantation have not been successful.

A small number succumb to early HCV-associated liver injury, and a syndrome reminiscent of fibrosing cholestatic hepatitis (see above) has been observed rarely. Because patients with more episodes of rejection receive more immunosuppressive therapy, and because immunosuppressive therapy enhances HCV replication, patients with severe or multiple episodes of rejection are more likely to experience early recurrence of hepatitis C after transplantation. Both high viral load and older donor age have been linked to recurrent HCV-induced liver disease and to earlier disease recurrence after transplantation.

Patients who undergo liver transplantation for end-stage alcoholic cirrhosis are at risk of resorting to drinking again after transplantation, a potential source of recurrent alcoholic liver injury. Currently, alcoholic liver disease is one of the more common indications for liver transplantation, accounting for 20–25% of all liver transplantation procedures, and most transplantation centers screen candidates carefully for predictors of continued abstinence. Recidivism is more likely in patients whose sobriety prior to transplantation was <6 months. For abstinent patients with alcoholic cirrhosis, liver transplantation can be undertaken successfully, with outcomes comparable to those for other categories of patients with chronic liver disease, when coordinated by a team approach that includes substance abuse counseling.

POSTTRANSPLANTATION QUALITY OF LIFE

Full rehabilitation is achieved in the majority of patients who survive the early postoperative months and escape chronic rejection or unmanageable infection. Psychosocial maladjustment interferes with medical compliance in a small number of patients, but most manage to adhere to immunosuppressive regimens, which must be continued indefinitely. In one study, 85% of patients who survived their transplant operations returned to gainful activities. In fact, some women have conceived and carried pregnancies to term after transplantation without demonstrable injury to their infants.

FURTHER READINGS

BERENGUER M: Treatment of hepatitis C after liver transplantation. Clin Liver Dis 9:579, 2005

BROWN RS JR et al: A survey of liver transplantation from living adult donors in the United States. N Engl J Med 348:818, 2003

CARITHERS RL JR: Liver transplantation. Liver Transpl 6:122, 2000

FISHMAN JA, RUBIN RH: Infection in organ-transplant recipients. N Engl J Med 338:1741, 1998

KEEFFE EB et al: Liver transplantation: Current status and novel approaches to liver replacement. Gastroenterology 120:749, 2001

KULKARNI S et al: Living donor liver transplantation for pediatric and adult recipients. Nat Clin Prac Gastro Hep 3:149, 2006

POST DJ et al: Immunosuppression in liver transplantation. Liver Transplant 11:1307, 2005

SCHREIBMAN IR, SCHIFF ER: Prevention and treatment of recurrent hepatitis B after liver transplantation: The current role of nucleoside and nucleotide analogues. *Ann Clin Microbiol Antimicrob* 5:8, 2006

SORRELL MF (ed): Liver transplantation in the new millennium. Semin Liver Dis 20:409, 2000

VARGAS HE et al: A concise update on the status of liver transplantation for hepatitis B virus: The challenges in 2002. Liver Transpl 8:2, 2002

WEBB K et al: Transplantation for alcoholic liver disease: Report of a consensus meeting. Liver Transplant 12:301, 2006

WIESNER R: Patient selection in an era of donor liver shortage: Current US policy. Nat Clin Prac Gastro Hep 2:24, 2005

305 Diseases of the Gallbladder and Bile Ducts

Norton J. Greenberger, Gustav Paumgartner

PHYSIOLOGY OF BILE PRODUCTION AND FLOW

BILE SECRETION AND COMPOSITION

Bile formed in the hepatic lobules is secreted into a complex network of canaliculi, small bile ductules, and larger bile ducts that run with lymphatics and branches of the portal vein and hepatic artery in portal tracts situated between hepatic lobules. These interlobular bile ducts coalesce to form larger septal bile ducts that join to form the right and left hepatic ducts, which in turn unite to form the common hepatic duct. The common hepatic duct is joined by the cystic duct of the gallbladder to form the common bile duct (CBD), which enters the duodenum (often after joining the main pancreatic duct) through the ampulla of Vater.

Hepatic bile is an isotonic fluid with an electrolyte composition resembling blood plasma. The electrolyte composition of gallbladder bile differs from that of hepatic bile because most of the inorganic anions, chloride and bicarbonate, have been removed by reabsorption across the gallbladder epithelium. As a result of water reabsorption, total solute concentration of bile increases from 3–4 g/dL in hepatic bile and 10–15 g/dL in gallbladder bile.

Major solute components of bile by moles percent include bile acids (80%), lecithin and traces of other phospholipids (16%), and unesterified cholesterol (4.0%). In the lithogenic state the cholesterol value can be as high as 8–10%. Other constituents include conjugated bilirubin, proteins (all immunoglobulins, albumin, metabolites of hormones, and other proteins metabolized in the liver), electrolytes, mucus, and, often, drugs and their metabolites.

The total daily basal secretion of hepatic bile is ~500–600 mL. Many substances taken up or synthesized by the hepatocyte are secreted into the bile canaliculi. The canalicular membrane forms microvilli and is associated with microfilaments of actin, microtubules, and other contractile elements. Prior to their secretion into the bile, many substances are taken up into the hepatocyte, while others such as phospholipids, a portion of primary bile acids, and some cholesterol are synthesized de novo in the hepatocyte. Three mechanisms are important in regulating bile flow: (1) active transport of bile acids from hepatocytes into the bile canaliculi, (2) active transport of other organic anions, and (3) cholangiocellular secretion. The last is a secretin-mediated and cyclic AMP–dependent mechanism that results in the secretion of a sodium- and bicarbonate-rich fluid into the bile ducts.

Active vectorial secretion of biliary constituents from the portal blood into the bile canaliculi is driven by a distinct set of polarized transport systems at the basolateral (sinusoidal) and the canalicular apical plasma membrane domains of the hepatocyte. Two sinusoidal bile salt uptake systems have been cloned in humans, the Na^+/taurocholate cotransporter (NTCP) and the organic anion transporting proteins (OATPs), which also transport a large variety of non-bile salt organic anions. Several ATP-dependent canalicular transport systems ("export pumps") have been identified, the most important of which are: the bile salt export pump (BSEP); the anionic conjugate export pump (MRP2), which mediates the canalicular excretion of various amphiphilic conjugates formed by phase II conjugation (e.g., bilirubin mono- and diglucuronides and drugs); the multidrug export pump (MDR1) for hydrophobic cationic compounds; and the phospholipid export pump (MDR3). Two hemitransporters ABCG5/G8, functioning as a couple, constitute the principal canalicular cholesterol and phytosterol transporter. F1C1 (ATP8B1) is an aminophospholipid transferase ("flippase") essential for maintaining the lipid asymmetry of the canalicular membrane. The canalicular membrane also contains ATP-independent transport systems such as the Cl/HCO_3 anion exchanger isoform 2 for canalicular bicarbonate secretion. For most of these transporters, genetic defects have been identified that are associated with various forms of cholestasis or defects of biliary excretion. F1C1 is defective in Byler's disease and results in ablation of all other ATP-dependent transporter functions. BSEP is defective in progressive familial intrahepatic cholestasis (PFIC) and benign recurrent intrahepatic cholestasis (BRIC) type 2 which can also be secondary to minor F1C1 (ATP8B1) mutations. Mutations of MRP2 cause the Dubin-Johnson syndrome, an inherited form of conjugated hyperbilirubinemia (Chap. 297). A defective MDR3 results in PFIC-3. ABCG5/G8, the canalicular half transporters for cholesterol and other neutral sterols, are defective in sitosterolemia. The cystic fibrosis transmembrane regulator (CFTR) located on bile duct epithelial cells but not on canalicular membranes is defective in cystic fibrosis, which is associated with impaired cholangiocellular pH regulation during ductular bile formation and chronic cholestatic liver disease, occasionally resulting in biliary cirrhosis.

THE BILE ACIDS

The primary bile acids, cholic acid and chenodeoxycholic acid (CDCA), are synthesized from cholesterol in the liver, conjugated with glycine or taurine, and secreted into the bile. Secondary bile acids, including deoxycholate and lithocholate, are formed in the colon as bacterial metabolites of the primary bile acids. However, lithocholic acid is much less efficiently absorbed from the colon than deoxycholic acid. Another secondary bile acid, found in low concentration, is ursodeoxycholic acid (UDCA), a stereoisomer of CDCA. In healthy subjects, the ratio of glycine to taurine conjugates in bile is ~3:1.

Bile acids are detergent-like molecules that in aqueous solutions and above a critical concentration of about 2 mM form molecular aggregates called *micelles*. Cholesterol alone is sparingly soluble in aqueous environments, and its solubility in bile depends on both the total lipid concentration and the relative molar percentages of bile acids and lecithin. Normal ratios of these constituents favor the formation of solubilizing *mixed micelles*, while abnormal ratios promote the precipitation of cholesterol crystals in bile via an intermediate liquid crystal phase.

In addition to facilitating the biliary excretion of cholesterol, bile acids facilitate the normal intestinal absorption of dietary fats, mainly cholesterol and fat-soluble vitamins, via a micellar transport mechanism (Chap. 288). Bile acids also serve as a major physiologic driving force for hepatic bile flow and aid in water and electrolyte transport in the small bowel and colon.

ENTEROHEPATIC CIRCULATION

Bile acids are efficiently conserved under normal conditions. Unconjugated, and to a lesser degree also conjugated, bile acids are absorbed by *passive diffusion* along the entire gut. Quantitatively much more important for bile salt recirculation, however, is the *active transport* mechanism for conjugated bile acids in the distal ileum (Chap. 288). The reabsorbed bile acids enter the portal bloodstream and are taken up rapidly by hepatocytes, reconjugated, and resecreted into bile (enterohepatic circulation).

The normal bile acid pool size is approximately 2–4 g. During digestion of a meal, the bile acid pool undergoes at least one or more enterohepatic cycles, depending on the size and composition of the meal. Normally, the bile acid pool circulates ~5–10 times daily. Intestinal absorption of the pool is about 95% efficient; therefore, fecal loss of bile acids is in the range of 0.2–0.4 g/d. In the steady state this fecal loss is compensated by an equal daily synthesis of bile acids by the liver, and thus the size of the bile acid pool is maintained. Bile acids returning to the liver suppress de novo hepatic synthesis of primary bile acids from cholesterol by inhibiting the rate-limiting enzyme cholesterol 7-hydroxylase. While the loss of bile salts in stool is usually matched by increased hepatic synthesis, the maximum rate of synthesis is ~5 g/d, which may be insufficient to replete the bile acid pool size when there is pronounced impairment of intestinal bile salt reabsorption.

GALLBLADDER AND SPHINCTERIC FUNCTIONS

In the fasting state, the sphincter of Oddi offers a high-pressure zone of resistance to bile flow from the CBD into the duodenum. This tonic contraction serves to (1) prevent reflux of duodenal contents into the pancreatic and bile ducts and (2) promote filling of the gallbladder. The major factor controlling the evacuation of the gallbladder is the peptide hormone cholecystokinin (CCK), which is released from the duodenal mucosa in response to the ingestion of fats and amino acids. CCK produces (1) powerful contraction of the gallbladder, (2) decreased resistance of the sphincter of Oddi, and (3) enhanced flow of biliary contents into the duodenum.

Hepatic bile is "concentrated" within the gallbladder by energy-dependent transmucosal absorption of water and electrolytes. Almost the entire bile acid pool may be sequestered in the gallbladder following an overnight fast for delivery into the duodenum with the first meal of the day. The normal capacity of the gallbladder is ~30 mL of bile.

DISEASES OF THE GALLBLADDER

CONGENITAL ANOMALIES

Anomalies of the biliary tract are not uncommon and include abnormalities in number, size, and shape (e.g., agenesis of the gallbladder, duplications, rudimentary or oversized "giant" gallbladders, and diverticula). *Phrygian cap* is a clinically innocuous entity in which a partial or complete septum (or fold) separates the fundus from the body. Anomalies of position or suspension are not uncommon and include left-sided gallbladder, intrahepatic gallbladder, retrodisplacement of the gallbladder, and "floating" gallbladder. The latter condition predisposes to acute torsion, volvulus, or herniation of the gallbladder.

GALLSTONES

Pathogenesis Gallstones are quite prevalent in most western countries. In the United States, several series have shown gallstones in at least 20% of women and in 8% of men over the age of 40 and in up to 40% of women over the age of 65 years. It is estimated that at least 25 million persons in the United States have gallstones and that ~1 million new cases of cholelithiasis develop each year.

Gallstones are formed because of abnormal bile constituents. They are divided into two major types: cholesterol stones account for 80% of the total, with pigment stones comprising the remaining 20%. Cholesterol gallstones usually contain >50% cholesterol monohydrate plus an admixture of calcium salts, bile pigments, proteins, and fatty acids, the latter in "brown" pigment stones. Pigment stones are composed primarily of calcium bilirubinate; they contain <20% cholesterol and are classified into "black" and "brown" types, the latter forming secondary to chronic biliary infection.

CHOLESTEROL STONES AND BILIARY SLUDGE Cholesterol is essentially water insoluble and requires aqueous dispersion into either micelles or vesicles, both of which require the presence of a second lipid to solubilize the cholesterol. Cholesterol and phospholipids are secreted into bile as unilamellar bilayered vesicles, which are converted into mixed micelles consisting of bile acids, phospholipids, and cholesterol by the action of bile acids. If there is an excess of cholesterol in relation to phospholipids and bile acids, unstable cholesterol-rich vesicles remain, which aggregate into large multilamellar vesicles from which cholesterol crystals precipitate (Fig. 305-1).

There are several important mechanisms in the formation of lithogenic (stone-forming) bile. The most important is increased biliary secretion of cholesterol. This may occur in association with obesity, high-caloric and cholesterol-rich diets, or drugs (e.g., clofibrate) and may result from increased activity of HMG-CoA reductase, the rate-limiting enzyme of hepatic cholesterol synthesis, and increased hepatic uptake of cholesterol from blood. In patients with gallstones, dietary cholesterol *increases* biliary cholesterol secretion. This does not occur in non-gallstone patients on high-cholesterol diets. In addition to environmental factors such as high-caloric and cholesterol-rich diets, genetic factors play an important role in gallstone disease. A large study of symptomatic gallstones in Swedish twins provided strong evidence for a role of genetic factors in gallstone pathogenesis. Genetic factors accounted for 25%, shared environmental factors for 13%, and indi-

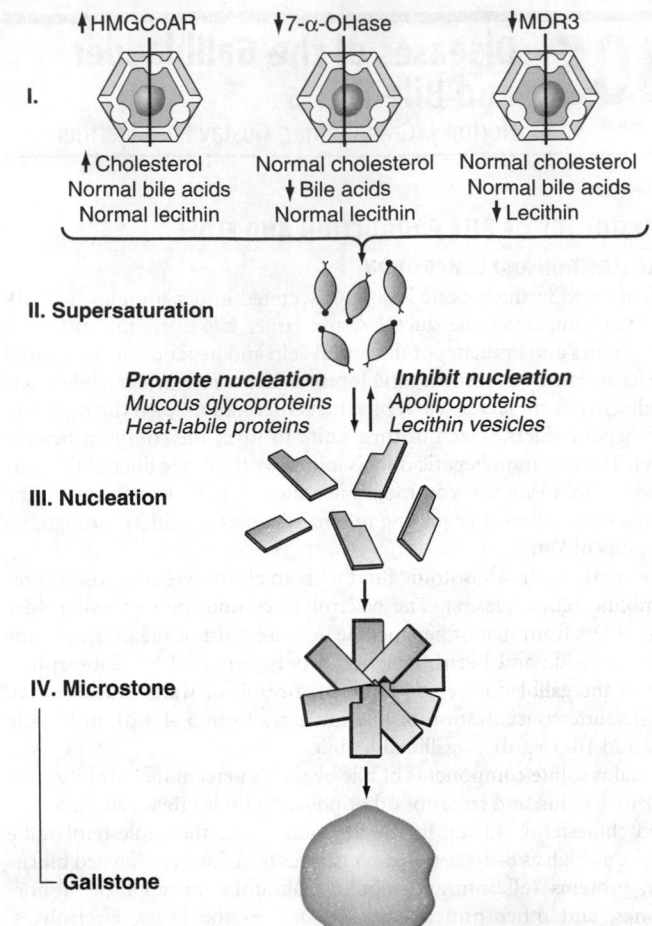

FIGURE 305-1 Scheme showing pathogenesis of cholesterol gallstone formation. Conditions or factors that increase the ratio of cholesterol to bile acids and phospholipids (lecithin) favor gallstone formation. HMG-CoAR, hydroxymethylglutaryl–coenzyme A reductase; 7-α-OHase, cholesterol, 7α-hydroxylase; MDR3, multidrug resistance–associated protein 3, also called phospholipid export pump.

vidual environmental factors for 62% of the phenotypic variation among monozygotic twins. A high prevalence of gallstones is found among first-degree relatives of gallstone carriers and in certain ethnic populations such as American Indians as well as Chilean Indians and Chilean Hispanics. A common genetic trait has been identified for some of these populations by mitochondrial DNA analysis. In some patients, impaired hepatic conversion of cholesterol to bile acids may also occur, resulting in an increase of the lithogenic cholesterol/bile acid ratio. Although most cholesterol stones have a polygenic basis, there are rare monogenic (mendelian) causes. Recently, a mutation in the *CYP7A1* gene has been described that results in a deficiency of the enzyme cholesterol 7-hydroxylase, which catalyzes the initial step in cholesterol catabolism and bile acid synthesis. The homozygous state is associated with hypercholesterolemia and gallstones. Because the phenotype is expressed in the heterozygote state, mutations in the *CYP7A1* gene may contribute to the susceptibility to cholesterol gallstone disease in the population. Mutations in the *MDR3* gene, which encodes the phospholipid export pump in the canalicular membrane of the hepatocyte, may cause defective phospholipid secretion into bile, resulting in cholesterol supersaturation of bile and formation of cholesterol gallstones in the gallbladder and in the bile ducts. Thus an excess of biliary cholesterol in relation to bile acids and phospholipids is primarily due to hypersecretion of cholesterol, but hyposecretion of bile acids or phospholipids may contribute. An additional disturbance of bile acid metabolism that is likely to contribute to supersaturation of bile with cholesterol is enhanced conversion of cholic acid to deoxycholic acid, with replacement of the cholic acid pool by an expanded deoxycholic acid pool. It may result from enhanced dehydroxylation of cholic acid and increased absorption of newly formed deoxycholic acid. An increased deoxycholate secretion is associated with hypersecretion of cholesterol into bile.

While supersaturation of bile with cholesterol is an important prerequisite for gallstone formation, it is generally not sufficient by itself to produce cholesterol precipitation in vivo. Most individuals with supersaturated bile do not develop stones because the time required for cholesterol crystals to nucleate and grow is longer than the time bile spends in the gallbladder.

An important mechanism is *nucleation* of cholesterol monohydrate crystals, which is greatly accelerated in human lithogenic bile. Accelerated nucleation of cholesterol monohydrate in bile may be due to either an *excess of pronucleating factors* or a *deficiency of antinucleating factors*. Mucin and certain non-mucin glycoproteins, principally immunoglobulins, appear to be pronucleating factors, while apolipoproteins AI and AII and other glycoproteins appear to be antinucleating factors. Cholesterol monohydrate crystal nucleation and crystal growth probably occur within the mucin gel layer. Vesicle fusion leads to liquid crystals, which, in turn, nucleate into solid cholesterol monohydrate crystals. Continued growth of the crystals occurs by direct nucleation of cholesterol molecules from supersaturated unilamellar or multilamellar biliary vesicles.

A third important mechanism in cholesterol gallstone formation is *gallbladder hypomotility*. If the gallbladder emptied all supersaturated or crystal-containing bile completely, stones would not be able to grow. A high percentage of patients with gallstones exhibits abnormalities of gallbladder emptying. Ultrasonographic studies show that gallstone patients display an increased gallbladder volume during fasting and also after a test meal (residual volume) and that fractional emptying after gallbladder stimulation is decreased. Gallbladder emptying is a major determinant of gallstone recurrence in patients who underwent biliary lithotripsy.

Biliary sludge is a thick mucous material that upon microscopic examination reveals lecithin-cholesterol crystals, cholesterol monohydrate crystals, calcium bilirubinate, and mucin gels. Biliary sludge typically forms a crescent-like layer in the most dependent portion of the gallbladder and is recognized by characteristic echoes on ultrasonography (see below). The presence of biliary sludge implies two abnormalities: (1) the normal balance between gallbladder mucin secretion and elimination has become deranged and (2) nucleation of biliary solutes has occurred. That biliary sludge may be a precursor form of gallstone disease is evident from several observations. In one study, 96 patients with gallbladder sludge were followed prospectively by serial ultrasound studies. In 18%, biliary sludge disappeared and did not recur for at least 2 years. In 60%, biliary sludge disappeared and reappeared; in 14%, gallstones (8% asymptomatic, 6% symptomatic) developed, and in 6%, severe biliary pain with or without acute pancreatitis occurred. In 12 patients, cholecystectomies were performed, 6 for gallstone-associated biliary pain and 3 in symptomatic patients with sludge but without gallstones who had prior attacks of pancreatitis; the latter did not recur after cholecystectomy. It should be emphasized that biliary sludge can develop with disorders that cause gallbladder hypomotility, i.e., surgery, burns, total parenteral nutrition, pregnancy, and oral contraceptives—all of which are associated with gallstone formation. However, the presence of biliary sludge implies supersaturation of bile with either cholesterol or calcium bilirubinate.

Two other conditions are associated with cholesterol stone or biliary sludge formation: pregnancy and very low calorie diet. There appear to be two key changes during pregnancy that contribute to a "cholelithogenic state": (1) a marked increase in cholesterol saturation during the third trimester and (2) sluggish gallbladder contraction in response to a standard meal, resulting in impaired gallbladder emptying. That these changes are related to pregnancy per se is supported by several studies that show reversal of these abnormalities quite rapidly after delivery. During pregnancy, gallbladder sludge develops in 20–0% of women and gallstones in 5–12%. Although biliary sludge is a

Cholesterol Stones

1. Demographic/genetic factors: Prevalence highest in North American Indians, Chilean Indians, and Chilean Hispanics, greater in Northern Europe and North America than in Asia, lowest in Japan; familial disposition; hereditary aspects
2. Obesity: Normal bile acid pool and secretion but increased biliary secretion of cholesterol
3. Weight loss: Mobilization of tissue cholesterol leads to increased biliary cholesterol secretion while enterohepatic circulation of bile acids is decreased
4. Female sex hormones
   a. Estrogens stimulate hepatic lipoprotein receptors, increase uptake of dietary cholesterol, and increase biliary cholesterol secretion
   b. Natural estrogens, other estrogens, and oral contraceptives lead to decreased bile salt secretion and decreased conversion of cholesterol to cholesteryl esters
5. Increasing age: Increased biliary secretion of cholesterol, decreased size of bile acid pool, decreased secretion of bile salts
6. Gallbladder hypomotility leading to stasis and formation of sludge
   a. Prolonged parenteral nutrition
   b. Fasting
   c. Pregnancy
   d. Drugs such as octreotide
7. Clofibrate therapy: Increased biliary secretion of cholesterol
8. Decreased bile acid secretion
   a. Primary biliary cirrhosis
   b. Genetic defect of the *CYP7A1* gene
9. Decreased phospholipid secretion: Genetic defect of the *MDR3* gene
10. Miscellaneous
    a. High-calorie, high-fat diet
    b. Spinal cord injury

Pigment Stones

1. Demographic/genetic factors: Asia, rural setting
2. Chronic hemolysis
3. Alcoholic cirrhosis
4. Pernicious anemia
5. Cystic fibrosis
6. Chronic biliary tract infection, parasite infections
7. Increasing age
8. Ileal disease, ileal resection or bypass

common finding during pregnancy, it is usually asymptomatic and often resolves spontaneously after delivery. Gallstones, which are less common than sludge and frequently associated with biliary colic, may also disappear after delivery because of spontaneous dissolution related to bile becoming unsaturated with cholesterol post partum.

Approximately 10–20% of persons with rapid weight reduction achieved through very low calorie dieting develop gallstones. In a study involving 600 patients who completed a 16-week, 520-kcal/d diet, UDCA in a dosage of 600 mg/d proved highly effective in preventing gallstone formation; gallstones developed in only 3% of UDCA recipients, compared to 28% of placebo-treated patients.

To summarize, cholesterol gallstone disease occurs because of several defects, which include (1) bile supersaturation with cholesterol, (2) nucleation of cholesterol monohydrate with subsequent crystal retention and stone growth, and (3) abnormal gallbladder motor function with delayed emptying and stasis. Other important factors known to predispose to cholesterol stone formation are summarized in Table 305-1.

PIGMENT STONES Black pigment stones are composed of either pure calcium bilirubinate or polymer-like complexes with calcium and mucin glycoproteins. They are more common in patients who have chronic hemolytic states (with increased conjugated bilirubin in bile), liver cirrhosis, Gilbert's syndrome, or cystic fibrosis. Gallbladder stones in patients with ileal diseases, ileal resection, or ileal bypass generally are also black pigment stones. Enterohepatic recycling of bilirubin in ileal disease states contributes to their pathogenesis. Brown pigment stones are composed of calcium salts of unconjugated biliru-

TABLE 305-2 DIAGNOSTIC EVALUATION OF THE GALLBLADDER

Diagnostic Advantages	Diagnostic Limitations	Comment
Gallbladder Ultrasound		
Rapid Accurate identification of gallstones (>95%) Simultaneous scanning of GB, liver, bile ducts, pancreas "Real-time" scanning allows assessment of GB volume, contractility Not limited by jaundice, pregnancy May detect very small stones	Bowel gas Massive obesity Ascites	Procedure of choice for detection of stones
Plain Abdominal X-Ray		
Low cost Readily available	Relatively low yield ? Contraindicated in pregnancy	Pathognomonic findings in: calcified gallstones Limey bile, porcelain GB Emphysematous cholecystitis Gallstone ileus
Oral Cholecystogram: Replaced by GBUS		
Radioisotope Scans (HIDA, DIDA, etc.)		
Accurate identification of cystic duct obstruction Simultaneous assessment of bile ducts	? Contraindicated in pregnancy Serum bilirubin >103–205 μmol/L (6–12 mg/dL) Cholecystogram of low resolution	Indicated for confirmation of suspected acute cholecystitis; less sensitive and less specific in chronic cholecystitis; useful in diagnosis of acalculous cholecystopathy, especially if given with CCK to assess gallbladder emptying

Note: GB, gallbladder; CCK, cholecystokinin; GBUS, gallbladder ultrasound.

bin with varying amounts of cholesterol and protein. They are caused by the presence of increased amounts of unconjugated, insoluble bilirubin in bile that precipitates to form stones. Deconjugation of an excess of soluble bilirubin mono- and diglucuronides may be mediated by endogenous β-glucuronidase but may also occur by spontaneous hydrolysis. Sometimes, the enzyme is also produced when bile is chronically infected by bacteria, and such stones are brown. Pigment stone formation is especially prominent in Asians and is often associated with infections in the gallbladder and biliary tree (Table 305-1).

Diagnosis Procedures of potential use in the diagnosis of cholelithiasis and other diseases of the gallbladder are detailed in Table 305-2. Ultrasonography of the gallbladder is very accurate in the identification of cholelithiasis and has replaced oral cholecystography (Fig. 305-2A). Stones as small as 2 mm in diameter may be confidently identified provided that firm criteria are used [e.g., acoustic "shadowing" of opacities that are within the gallbladder lumen and that change with the patient's position (by gravity)]. In major medical centers, the false-negative and false-positive rates for ultrasound in gallstone patients are ~2–4%. Biliary sludge is material of low echogenic activity that typically forms a layer in the most dependent position of the gallbladder. This layer shifts with postural changes but fails to produce acoustic shadowing; these two characteristics distinguish sludges from gallstones. Ultrasound can also be used to assess the emptying function of the gallbladder.

The plain abdominal film may detect gallstones containing sufficient calcium to be radiopaque (10–15% of cholesterol and ~50% of pigment stones). Plain radiography may also be of use in the diagnosis of emphysematous cholecystitis, porcelain gallbladder, limey bile, and gallstone ileus.

Oral cholecystography (OCG) has historically been a useful procedure for the diagnosis of gallstones but has been replaced by ultrasound. It may be used to assess the patency of the cystic duct and gallbladder emptying function. Further, OCG can also delineate the size and number of gallstones and determine whether they are calcified.

Radiopharmaceuticals such as ^{99m}Tc-labeled N-substituted iminodiacetic acids (HIDA, DIDA, DISIDA, etc.) are rapidly extracted from the blood and are excreted into the biliary tree in high concentration

FIGURE 305-2 Examples of ultrasound and radiologic studies of the biliary tract. A. An ultrasound study showing a distended gallbladder containing a single large stone (*arrow*) which casts an acoustic shadow. **B.** Endoscopic retrograde cholangiopancreatogram (ERCP) showing normal biliary tract anatomy. In addition to the endoscope and large vertical gallbladder filled with contrast dye, the common hepatic duct (chd), common bile duct (cbd), and pancreatic duct (pd) are shown. The arrow points to the ampulla of Vater. **C.** Endoscopic retrograde cholangiogram (ERC) showing choledocholithiasis. The biliary tract is dilatated and contains multiple radiolucent calculi. **D.** ERCP showing sclerosing cholangitis. The common bile duct shows areas that are strictured and narrowed.

even in the presence of mild to moderate serum bilirubin elevations. Failure to image the gallbladder in the presence of biliary ductal visualization may indicate cystic duct obstruction, acute or chronic cholecystitis, or surgical absence of the organ. Such scans have some application in the diagnosis of acute cholecystitis.

Symptoms of Gallstone Disease   Gallstones usually produce symptoms by causing inflammation or obstruction following their migration into the cystic duct or CBD. The most specific and characteristic symptom of gallstone disease is biliary colic that is a constant and often long-lasting pain (see below). Obstruction of the cystic duct or CBD by a stone produces increased intraluminal pressure and distention of the viscus that cannot be relieved by repetitive biliary contractions. The resultant visceral pain is characteristically a severe, steady ache or fullness in the epigastrium or right upper quadrant (RUQ) of the abdomen with frequent radiation to the interscapular area, right scapula, or shoulder.

Biliary colic begins quite suddenly and may persist with severe intensity for 30 min to 5 h, subsiding gradually or rapidly. It is steady rather than intermittent as would be suggested by the word *colic*, which must be regarded as a misnomer, although in widespread use. An episode of biliary pain persisting beyond 5 h should raise the suspicion of acute cholecystitis (see below). Nausea and vomiting frequently accompany episodes of biliary pain. An elevated level of serum bilirubin and/or alkaline phosphatase suggests a common duct stone. Fever or chills (rigors) with biliary pain usually imply a complication, i.e., cholecystitis, pancreatitis, or cholangitis. Complaints of vague epigastric fullness, dyspepsia, eructation, or flatulence, especially following a fatty meal, should not be confused with biliary pain. Such symptoms are frequently elicited from patients with or without gallstone disease but are not specific for biliary calculi. Biliary colic may be precipitated by eating a fatty meal, by consumption of a large meal following a period of prolonged fasting, or by eating a normal meal; it is frequently nocturnal, occurring within a few hours of retiring.

Natural History   Gallstone disease discovered in an asymptomatic patient or in a patient whose symptoms are not referable to cholelithiasis is a common clinical problem. The natural history of "silent," or asymptomatic, gallstones has occasioned much debate. A study of predominantly male silent gallstone patients suggests that the cumulative risk for the development of symptoms or complications is relatively low—10% at 5 years, 15% at 10 years, and 18% at 15 years. Patients remaining asymptomatic for 15 years were found to be unlikely to develop symptoms during further follow-up, and most patients who did develop complications from their gallstones experienced *prior* warning symptoms. Similar conclusions apply to diabetic patients with silent gallstones. Decision analysis has suggested that (1) the cumulative risk of death due to gallstone disease while on expectant management is small, and (2) prophylactic cholecystectomy is not warranted.

Complications requiring cholecystectomy are much more common in gallstone patients who have developed symptoms of biliary pain. Patients found to have gallstones at a young age are more likely to develop symptoms from cholelithiasis than are patients >60 years at the time of initial diagnosis. Patients with diabetes mellitus and gallstones may be somewhat more susceptible to septic complications, but the magnitude of risk of septic biliary complications in diabetic patients is incompletely defined.

℞ **GALLSTONES**

SURGICAL THERAPY   In asymptomatic gallstone patients, the risk of developing symptoms or complications requiring surgery is quite small (in the range of 1–2% per year). Thus a recommendation for cholecystectomy in a patient with gallstones should probably be based on assessment of three factors: (1) the presence of symptoms that are frequent enough or severe enough to interfere with the patient's general routine; (2) the presence of a prior complication of gallstone disease, i.e., history of acute cholecystitis, pancreatitis, gallstone fistula, etc.; or (3) the presence of an

underlying condition predisposing the patient to increased risk of gallstone complications (e.g., calcified or porcelain gallbladder and/or a previous attack of acute cholecystitis regardless of current symptomatic status). Patients with very large gallstones (>3 cm in diameter) and patients having gallstones in a congenitally anomalous gallbladder might also be considered for prophylactic cholecystectomy. Although young age is a worrisome factor in asymptomatic gallstone patients, few authorities would now recommend routine cholecystectomy in all young patients with silent stones. Laparoscopic cholecystectomy is a minimal-access approach for the removal of the gallbladder together with its stones. Its advantages include a markedly shortened hospital stay, minimal disability, as well as decreased cost, and it is the procedure of choice for most patients referred for elective cholecystectomy.

From several studies involving >4000 patients undergoing laparoscopic cholecystectomy, the following key points emerge: (1) complications develop in ~4% of patients, (2) conversion to laparotomy occurs in 5%, (3) the death rate is remarkably low (i.e., <0.1%), and (4) bile duct injuries are unusual (i.e., 0.2–0.5%) but more frequent than with open cholecystectomy. These data indicate why laparoscopic cholecystectomy has become the "gold standard" for treating symptomatic cholelithiasis.

MEDICAL THERAPY—GALLSTONE DISSOLUTION   Ursodeoxycholic acid (UDCA) decreases cholesterol saturation of bile and also appears to produce a lamellar liquid crystalline phase in bile that allows a dispersion of cholesterol from stones by physical-chemical means. UDCA may also retard cholesterol crystal nucleation. In carefully selected patients with a functioning gallbladder and with radiolucent stones <10 mm in diameter, complete dissolution can be achieved in ~50% of patients within 6 months to 2 years with UDCA at a dose of 8–10 mg/kg per day. The highest success rate (i.e., >70%) occurs in patients with small (<5 mm) floating radiolucent gallstones. Probably ≤ 10% of patients with *symptomatic* cholelithiasis are candidates for such treatment. However, in addition to the vexing problem of recurrent stones (30–50% over 3–5 years of follow-up), there is also the factor of taking an expensive drug for up to 2 years. The advantages and success of laparoscopic cholecystectomy have largely reduced the role of gallstone dissolution to patients who wish to avoid or are not candidates for elective cholecystectomy. However, patients with cholesterol gallstone disease who develop recurrent choledocholithiasis after cholecystectomy should be on long-term treatment with ursodeoxycholic acid.

ACUTE AND CHRONIC CHOLECYSTITIS
Acute Cholecystitis   Acute inflammation of the gallbladder wall usually follows obstruction of the cystic duct by a stone. Inflammatory response can be evoked by three factors: (1) *mechanical inflammation* produced by increased intraluminal pressure and distention with resulting ischemia of the gallbladder mucosa and wall, (2) *chemical inflammation* caused by the release of lysolecithin (due to the action of phospholipase on lecithin in bile) and other local tissue factors, and (3) *bacterial inflammation*, which may play a role in 50–85% of patients with acute cholecystitis. The organisms most frequently isolated by culture of gallbladder bile in these patients include *Escherichia coli*, *Klebsiella* spp., *Streptococcus* spp., and *Clostridium* spp.

Acute cholecystitis often begins as an attack of biliary pain that progressively worsens. Approximately 60–70% of patients report having experienced prior attacks that resolved spontaneously. As the episode progresses, however, the pain of acute cholecystitis becomes more generalized in the right upper abdomen. As with biliary colic, the pain of cholecystitis may radiate to the interscapular area, right scapula, or shoulder. Peritoneal signs of inflammation such as increased pain with jarring or on deep respiration may be apparent. The patient is anorectic and often nauseated. Vomiting is relatively common and may produce symptoms and signs of vascular and extracellular volume depletion. Jaundice is unusual early in the course of acute cholecystitis but may occur when edematous inflammatory changes involve the bile ducts and surrounding lymph nodes.

A low-grade fever is characteristically present, but shaking chills or rigors are not uncommon. The RUQ of the abdomen is almost invariably tender to palpation. An enlarged, tense gallbladder is palpable in 25–50% of patients. Deep inspiration or cough during subcostal palpation of the RUQ usually produces increased pain and inspiratory arrest (Murphy's sign). Localized rebound tenderness in the RUQ is common, as are abdominal distention and hypoactive bowel sounds from paralytic ileus, but generalized peritoneal signs and abdominal rigidity are usually lacking, in the absence of perforation.

The diagnosis of acute cholecystitis is usually made on the basis of a characteristic history and physical examination. The triad of sudden onset of RUQ tenderness, fever, and leukocytosis is highly suggestive. Typically, leukocytosis in the range of 10,000–15,000 cells per microliter with a left shift on differential count is found. The serum bilirubin is mildly elevated [<85.5 μmol/L (5 mg/dL)] in fewer than half of patients, while about one-fourth have modest elevations in serum aminotransferases (usually less than a fivefold elevation). Ultrasound will demonstrate calculi in 90–95% of cases and is useful for detection of signs of gallbladder inflammation including thickening of the wall, pericholecystic fluid, and dilation of the bile duct. The radionuclide (e.g., HIDA) biliary scan may be confirmatory if bile duct imaging is seen without visualization of the gallbladder.

Approximately 75% of patients treated medically have remission of acute symptoms within 2–7 days following hospitalization. In 25%, however, a complication of acute cholecystitis will occur despite conservative treatment (see below). In this setting, prompt surgical intervention is required. Of the 75% of patients with acute cholecystitis who undergo remission of symptoms, ~25% will experience a recurrence of cholecystitis within 1 year, and 60% will have at least one recurrent bout within 6 years. In view of the natural history of the disease, acute cholecystitis is best treated by early surgery whenever possible.

Mirizzi's syndrome is a rare complication in which a gallstone becomes impacted in the cystic duct or neck of the gallbladder causing compression of the CBD, resulting in CBD obstruction and jaundice. Ultrasound shows gallstone(s) lying outside the hepatic duct. Endoscopic retrograde cholangiopancreatography (ERCP) or percutaneous transhepatic cholangiography (PTC) or MRCP will usually demonstrate the characteristic extrinsic compression of the CBD. Surgery consists of removing the cystic duct, diseased gallbladder, and the impacted stone. The preoperative diagnosis of Mirizzi's syndrome is important to avoid CBD injury.

ACALCULOUS CHOLECYSTITIS In 5–10% of patients with acute cholecystitis, calculi obstructing the cystic duct are not found at surgery. In >50% of such cases, an underlying explanation for acalculous inflammation is not found. An increased risk for the development of acalculous cholecystitis is especially associated with serious trauma or burns, with the postpartum period following prolonged labor, and with orthopedic and other nonbiliary major surgical operations in the postoperative period. It may possibly complicate periods of prolonged parenteral hyperalimentation. For some of these cases, biliary sludge in the cystic duct may be responsible. Other precipitating factors include vasculitis, obstructing adenocarcinoma of the gallbladder, diabetes mellitus, torsion of the gallbladder, "unusual" bacterial infections of the gallbladder (e.g., *Leptospira*, *Streptococcus*, *Salmonella*, or *Vibrio cholerae*), and parasitic infestation of the gallbladder. Acalculous cholecystitis may also be seen with a variety of other systemic disease processes (sarcoidosis, cardiovascular disease, tuberculosis, syphilis, actinomycosis, etc.).

Although the clinical manifestations of acalculous cholecystitis are indistinguishable from those of calculous cholecystitis, the setting of acute gallbladder inflammation complicating severe underlying illness is characteristic of acalculous disease. Ultrasound, CT, or radionuclide examinations demonstrating a large, tense, static gallbladder without stones and with evidence of poor emptying over a prolonged period may be diagnostically useful in some cases. The complication rate for acalculous cholecystitis exceeds that for calculous cholecystitis. Successful management of acute acalculous cholecystitis appears to depend primarily on early diagnosis and surgical intervention, with meticulous attention to postoperative care.

ACALCULOUS CHOLECYSTOPATHY Disordered motility of the gallbladder can produce recurrent biliary pain in patients without gallstones. Infu-

sion of an octapeptide of CCK can be used to measure the gallbladder ejection fraction during cholescintigraphy. The surgical findings have included abnormalities such as chronic cholecystitis, gallbladder muscle hypertrophy, and/or a markedly narrowed cystic duct. Some of these patients may well have had antecedent gallbladder disease. The following criteria can be used to identify patients with acalculous cholecystopathy: (1) recurrent episodes of typical RUQ pain characteristic of biliary tract pain, (2) abnormal CCK cholescintigraphy demonstrating a gallbladder ejection fraction of <40%, and (3) infusion of CCK reproduces the patient's pain. An additional clue would be the identification of a large gallbladder on ultrasound examination. Finally, it should be noted that sphincter of Oddi dysfunction can also give rise to recurrent RUQ pain and CCK-scintigraphic abnormalities.

EMPHYSEMATOUS CHOLECYSTITIS So-called emphysematous cholecystitis is thought to begin with acute cholecystitis (calculous or acalculous) followed by ischemia or gangrene of the gallbladder wall and infection by gas-producing organisms. Bacteria most frequently cultured in this setting include anaerobes, such as *C. welchii* or *C. perfringens*, and aerobes, such as *E. coli*. This condition occurs most frequently in elderly men and in patients with diabetes mellitus. The clinical manifestations are essentially indistinguishable from those of nongaseous cholecystitis. The diagnosis is usually made on plain abdominal film by finding gas within the gallbladder lumen, dissecting within the gallbladder wall to form a gaseous ring, or in the pericholecystic tissues. The morbidity and mortality rates with emphysematous cholecystitis are considerable. Prompt surgical intervention coupled with appropriate antibiotics is mandatory.

Chronic Cholecystitis Chronic inflammation of the gallbladder wall is almost always associated with the presence of gallstones and is thought to result from repeated bouts of subacute or acute cholecystitis or from persistent mechanical irritation of the gallbladder wall by gallstones. The presence of bacteria in the bile occurs in >25% of patients with chronic cholecystitis. The presence of infected bile in a patient with *chronic* cholecystitis undergoing elective cholecystectomy probably adds little to the operative risk. Chronic cholecystitis may be asymptomatic for years, may progress to symptomatic gallbladder disease or to acute cholecystitis, or may present with complications (see below).

Complications of Cholecystitis · *EMPYEMA AND HYDROPS* Empyema of the gallbladder usually results from progression of acute cholecystitis with persistent cystic duct obstruction to superinfection of the stagnant bile with a pus-forming bacterial organism. The clinical picture resembles that of cholangitis with high fever, severe RUQ pain, marked leukocytosis, and often, prostration. Empyema of the gallbladder carries a high risk of gram-negative sepsis and/or perforation. Emergency surgical intervention with proper antibiotic coverage is required as soon as the diagnosis is suspected.

Hydrops or mucocele of the gallbladder may also result from prolonged obstruction of the cystic duct, usually by a large solitary calculus. In this instance, the obstructed gallbladder lumen is progressively distended, over a period of time, by mucus (mucocele) or by a clear transudate (hydrops) produced by mucosal epithelial cells. A visible, easily palpable, nontender mass sometimes extending from the RUQ into the right iliac fossa may be found on physical examination. The patient with hydrops of the gallbladder frequently remains asymptomatic, although chronic RUQ pain may also occur. Cholecystectomy is indicated, since empyema, perforation, or gangrene may complicate the condition.

GANGRENE AND PERFORATION Gangrene of the gallbladder results from ischemia of the wall and patchy or complete tissue necrosis. Underlying conditions often include marked distention of the gallbladder, vasculitis, diabetes mellitus, empyema, or torsion resulting in arterial occlusion. Gangrene usually predisposes to perforation of the gallbladder, but perforation may also occur in chronic cholecystitis without premonitory warning symptoms. *Localized perforations* are usually contained by the omentum or by adhesions produced by recurrent inflammation of the gallbladder. Bacterial superinfection of the walled-off gallbladder contents results in abscess formation. Most patients are best treated with cholecystectomy, but some seriously ill patients may be managed with cholecystostomy and drainage of the abscess. *Free perforation* is less common but is associated with a mortality rate of ~30%. Such patients may experience a sudden transient relief of RUQ pain as the distended gallbladder decompresses; this is followed by signs of generalized peritonitis.

FISTULA FORMATION AND GALLSTONE ILEUS *Fistulization* into an adjacent organ adherent to the gallbladder wall may result from inflammation and adhesion formation. Fistulas into the duodenum are most common, followed in frequency by those involving the hepatic flexure of the colon, stomach or jejunum, abdominal wall, and renal pelvis. Clinically "silent" biliary-enteric fistulas occurring as a complication of acute cholecystitis have been found in up to 5% of patients undergoing cholecystectomy. Asymptomatic cholecystoenteric fistulas may sometimes be diagnosed by finding gas in the biliary tree on plain abdominal films. Barium contrast studies or endoscopy of the upper gastrointestinal tract or colon may demonstrate the fistula. Treatment in the symptomatic patient usually consists of cholecystectomy, CBD exploration, and closure of the fistulous tract.

Gallstone ileus refers to mechanical intestinal obstruction resulting from the passage of a large gallstone into the bowel lumen. The stone customarily enters the duodenum through a cholecystoenteric fistula at that level. The site of obstruction by the impacted gallstone is usually at the ileocecal valve, provided that the more proximal small bowel is of normal caliber. The majority of patients do not give a history of either prior biliary tract symptoms or complaints suggestive of acute cholecystitis or fistulization. Large stones, >2.5 cm in diameter, are thought to predispose to fistula formation by gradual erosion through the gallbladder fundus. Diagnostic confirmation may occasionally be found on the plain abdominal film (e.g., small-intestinal obstruction with gas in the biliary tree and a calcified, ectopic gallstone) or following an upper gastrointestinal series (cholecystoduodenal fistula with small-bowel obstruction at the ileocecal valve). Laparotomy with stone extraction (or propulsion into the colon) remains the procedure of choice to relieve obstruction. Evacuation of large stones within the gallbladder should also be performed. In general, the gallbladder and its attachment to the intestines should be left alone.

LIMEY (MILK OF CALCIUM) BILE AND PORCELAIN GALLBLADDER Calcium salts may be secreted into the lumen of the gallbladder in sufficient concentration to produce calcium precipitation and diffuse, hazy opacification of bile or a layering effect on plain abdominal roentgenography. This so-called limey bile, or milk of calcium bile, is usually clinically innocuous, but cholecystectomy is recommended, especially when it occurs in a hydropic gallbladder. In the entity called *porcelain gallbladder*, calcium salt deposition within the wall of a chronically inflamed gallbladder may be detected on the plain abdominal film. Cholecystectomy is advised in all patients with porcelain gallbladder because in a high percentage of cases this finding appears to be associated with the development of carcinoma of the gallbladder.

℞ ACUTE CHOLECYSTITIS

MEDICAL THERAPY Although surgical intervention remains the mainstay of therapy for acute cholecystitis and its complications, a period of in-hospital stabilization may be required before cholecystectomy. Oral intake is eliminated, nasogastric suction may be indicated, and extracellular volume depletion and electrolyte abnormalities are repaired. Meperidine or nonsteroidal anti-inflammatory drugs (NSAIDs) are usually employed for analgesia because they may produce less spasm of the sphincter of Oddi than drugs such as morphine. Intravenous antibiotic therapy is usually indicated in patients with severe acute cholecystitis, even though bacterial superinfection of bile may not have occurred in the early stages of the inflammatory process. Antibiotic therapy is guided by

the most common organisms likely to be present, which are *E. coli, Klebsiella* spp., and *Streptococcus* spp. Effective antibiotics include ureidopenicillins such as piperacillin or mezlocillin, ampicillin sulbactam, ciprofloxacin, moxifloxacin, and third-generation cephalosporins. Anaerobic coverage by a drug such as metronidazole should be added if gangrenous or emphysematous cholecystitis is suspected. Imipenem/meropenem represent potent parenteral antibiotics that cover the whole spectrum of bacteria causing ascending cholangitis. They should, however, be reserved for the most severe, life-threatening infections when other regimens have failed (Chap. 143). Postoperative complications of wound infection, abscess formation, or sepsis are reduced in antibiotic-treated patients.

SURGICAL THERAPY The optimal timing of surgical intervention in patients with acute cholecystitis depends on stabilization of the patient. The clear trend is toward earlier surgery, and this is due in part to requirements for shorter hospital stays. Urgent (emergency) cholecystectomy or cholecystostomy is probably appropriate in most patients in whom a complication of acute cholecystitis such as empyema, emphysematous cholecystitis, or perforation is suspected or confirmed. In uncomplicated cases of acute cholecystitis, up to 30% of patients fail to resolve their symptoms on appropriate medical therapy, and progression of the attack or a supervening complication leads to the performance of early operation (within 24–72 h). The technical complications of surgery are not increased in patients undergoing early as opposed to delayed cholecystectomy. Delayed surgical intervention is probably best reserved for (1) patients in whom the overall medical condition imposes an unacceptable risk for early surgery and (2) patients in whom the diagnosis of acute cholecystitis is in doubt. Early cholecystectomy is the treatment of choice for most patients with acute cholecystitis. Mortality figures for emergency cholecystectomy in most centers approach 3%, while the mortality risk for elective or early cholecystectomy ~0.5% in patients under age 60. Of course, the operative risks increase with age-related diseases of other organ systems and with the presence of long- or short-term complications of gallbladder disease. Seriously ill or debilitated patients with cholecystitis may be managed with cholecystostomy and tube drainage of the gallbladder. Elective cholecystectomy may then be done at a later date.

Postcholecystectomy Complications Early complications following cholecystectomy include atelectasis and other pulmonary disorders, abscess formation (often subphrenic), external or internal hemorrhage, biliary-enteric fistula, and bile leaks. Jaundice may indicate absorption of bile from an intraabdominal collection following a biliary leak or mechanical obstruction of the CBD by retained calculi, intraductal blood clots, or extrinsic compression. Routine performance of intraoperative cholangiography during cholecystectomy has helped to reduce the incidence of these early complications.

Overall, cholecystectomy is a very successful operation that provides total or near-total relief of preoperative symptoms in 75–90% of patients. The most common cause of persistent postcholecystectomy symptoms is an overlooked symptomatic nonbiliary disorder (e.g., reflux esophagitis, peptic ulceration, pancreatitis, or—most often—irritable bowel syndrome). In a small percentage of patients, however, a disorder of the extrahepatic bile ducts may result in persistent symptomatology. These so-called postcholecystectomy syndromes may be due to (1) biliary strictures, (2) retained biliary calculi, (3) cystic duct stump syndrome, (4) stenosis or dyskinesia of the sphincter of Oddi, or (5) bile salt–induced diarrhea or gastritis.

CYSTIC DUCT STUMP SYNDROME In the absence of cholangiographically demonstrable retained stones, symptoms resembling biliary pain or cholecystitis in the postcholecystectomy patient have frequently been attributed to disease in a long (>1 cm) cystic duct remnant (cystic duct stump syndrome). Careful analysis, however, reveals that postcholecystectomy complaints are attributable to other causes in almost all patients in whom the symptom complex was originally thought to result from the existence of a long cystic duct stump. Accordingly, considerable care should be taken to investigate the possible role of other factors in the production of postcholecystectomy symptoms before attributing them to cystic duct stump syndrome.

PAPILLARY DYSFUNCTION, PAPILLARY STENOSIS, SPASM OF THE SPHINCTER OF ODDI, AND BILIARY DYSKINESIA Symptoms of biliary colic accompanied by signs of recurrent, intermittent biliary obstruction may be produced by papillary stenosis, papillary dysfunction, spasm of the sphincter of Oddi, and biliary dyskinesia. Papillary stenosis is thought to result from acute or chronic inflammation of the papilla of Vater or from glandular hyperplasia of the papillary segment. Five criteria have been used to define papillary stenosis: (1) upper abdominal pain, usually RUQ or epigastric; (2) abnormal liver tests; (3) dilatation of the common bile duct upon ERCP examination; (4) delayed (>45 min) drainage of contrast material from the duct; and (5) increased basal pressure of the sphincter of Oddi, a finding that may be of only minor significance. An alternative to ERCP is magnetic resonance cholangiography (MRC) if ERCP and/or biliary manometry are either unavailable or not feasible. In patients with papillary stenosis, quantitative hepatobiliary scintigraphy has revealed delayed transit from the common bile duct to the bowel, ductal dilatation, and abnormal time-activity dynamics. This technique can also be used before and after sphincterotomy to document improvement in biliary emptying. Treatment consists of endoscopic or surgical sphincteroplasty to ensure wide patency of the distal portions of both the bile and pancreatic ducts. The greater the number of the preceding criteria present, the greater the likelihood that a patient does have a degree of papillary stenosis sufficient to justify correction. The factors usually considered as indications for sphincterotomy include (1) prolonged duration of symptoms, (2) lack of response to symptomatic treatment, (3) presence of severe disability, and (4) the patient's choice of sphincterotomy over surgery (given a clear understanding on his or her part of the risks involved in both procedures).

Criteria for diagnosing dyskinesia of the sphincter of Oddi are even more controversial than those for papillary stenosis. Proposed mechanisms include spasm of the sphincter, denervation sensitivity resulting in hypertonicity, and abnormalities of the sequencing or frequency rates of sphincteric contraction waves. When thorough evaluation has failed to demonstrate another cause for the pain, and when cholangiographic and manometric criteria suggest a diagnosis of biliary dyskinesia, medical treatment with nitrites or anticholinergics to attempt pharmacologic relaxation of the sphincter has been proposed. Endoscopic biliary sphincterotomy (EBS) or surgical sphincteroplasty may be indicated in patients who fail to respond to a 2- to 3-month trial of medical therapy, especially if basal sphincter of Oddi pressures are elevated. EBS has become the procedure of choice for removing bile duct stones and for other biliary and pancreatic problems.

Bile Salt–Induced Diarrhea and Gastritis Postcholecystectomy patients may develop symptoms of dyspepsia, which have been attributed to duodenogastric reflux of bile. However, firm data linking these symptoms to bile gastritis after surgical removal of the gallbladder are lacking. Cholecystectomy induces persistent changes in gut transit, and these changes effect a noticeable modification of bowel habits. Cholecystectomy shortens gut transit time by accelerating passage of the fecal bolus through the colon with marked acceleration in the right colon, thus causing an increase in colonic bile acid output and a shift in bile acid composition toward the more diarrheagenic secondary bile acids. Diarrhea that is severe enough, i.e., three or more watery movements per day, can be classified as postcholecystectomy diarrhea, and this occurs in 5–10% of patients undergoing elective cholecystectomy. Treatment with bile acid sequestering agents such as cholestyramine or colestipol is often effective in ameliorating troublesome diarrhea.

THE HYPERPLASTIC CHOLECYSTOSES
The term *hyperplastic cholecystoses* is used to denote a group of disorders of the gallbladder characterized by excessive proliferation of normal tissue components.

Adenomyomatosis is characterized by a benign proliferation of gallbladder surface epithelium with glandlike formations, extramural sinuses, transverse strictures, and/or fundal nodule ("adenoma" or "adenomyoma") formation. Outpouchings of mucosa termed *Rokitansky-Aschoff sinuses* may be seen on oral cholecystography in conjunction with hyperconcentration of contrast medium. Characteristic dimpled filling defects also may be seen.

Cholesterolosis is characterized by abnormal deposition of lipid, especially cholesteryl esters within macrophages in the lamina propria of the gallbladder wall. In its diffuse form ("strawberry gallbladder"), the gallbladder mucosa is brick red and speckled with bright yellow flecks of lipid. The localized form shows solitary or multiple "cholesterol polyps" studding the gallbladder wall. Cholesterol stones of the gallbladder are found in nearly half the cases. Cholecystectomy is indicated in both adenomyomatosis and cholesterolosis when symptomatic or when cholelithiasis is present.

The prevalence of gallbladder polyps in the adult population is ~5%, with a marked male predominance. Few significant changes have been found over a 5-year period in asymptomatic patients with gallbladder polyps <10 mm in diameter. Cholecystectomy is recommended in symptomatic patients, as well as in asymptomatic patients >50 years of age, or in those whose polyps are >10 mm in diameter or associated with gallstones or polyp growth on serial ultrasonography.

DISEASES OF THE BILE DUCTS

CONGENITAL ANOMALIES
Biliary Atresia and Hypoplasia Atretic and hypoplastic lesions of the extrahepatic and large intrahepatic bile ducts are the most common biliary anomalies of clinical relevance encountered in infancy. The clinical picture is one of severe obstructive jaundice during the first month of life, with pale stools. When biliary atresia is suspected on the basis of clinical, laboratory, and imaging findings the diagnosis is confirmed by surgical exploration and operative cholangiography. Approximately 10% of cases of biliary atresia are treatable with roux-en-Y choledochojejunostomy, with the Kasai procedure (hepatic portoenterostomy) being attempted in the remainder in an effort to restore some bile flow. Most patients, even those having successful biliary-enteric anastomoses, eventually develop chronic cholangitis, extensive hepatic fibrosis, and portal hypertension.

Choledochal Cysts Cystic dilatation may involve the free portion of the CBD, i.e., choledochal cyst, or may present as diverticulum formation in the intraduodenal segment. In the latter situation, chronic reflux of pancreatic juice into the biliary tree can produce inflammation and stenosis of the extrahepatic bile ducts leading to cholangitis or biliary obstruction. Because the process may be gradual, ~50% of patients present with onset of symptoms after age 10. The diagnosis may be made by ultrasound, abdominal CT, MRC, or cholangiography. Only one-third of patients show the classic triad of abdominal pain, jaundice, and an abdominal mass. Ultrasonographic detection of a cyst separate from the gallbladder should suggest the diagnosis of choledochal cyst, which can be confirmed by demonstrating the entrance of extrahepatic bile ducts into the cyst. Surgical treatment involves excision of the "cyst" and biliary-enteric anastomosis. Patients with choledochal cysts are at increased risk for the subsequent development of cholangiocarcinoma.

Congenital Biliary Ectasia Dilatation of intrahepatic bile ducts may involve either the major intrahepatic radicles (Caroli's disease), the inter- and intralobular ducts (congenital hepatic fibrosis), or both. In Caroli's disease, clinical manifestations include recurrent cholangitis, abscess formation in and around the affected ducts, and, often, gallstone formation within portions of ectatic intrahepatic biliary radicles. Ultrasound, MRC, and CT are of great diagnostic value in demonstrating cystic dilatation of the intrahepatic bile ducts. Treatment with ongoing antibiotic therapy is usually undertaken in an effort to limit the frequency and severity of recurrent bouts of cholangitis. Progression to secondary biliary cirrhosis with portal hypertension, extrahepatic biliary obstruction, cholangiocarcinoma, or recurrent episodes of sepsis with hepatic abscess formation is common.

CHOLEDOCHOLITHIASIS

Pathophysiology and Clinical Manifestations Passage of gallstones into the CBD occurs in ~10–15% of patients with cholelithiasis. The incidence of common duct stones increases with increasing age of the patient, so that up to 25% of elderly patients may have calculi in the common duct at the time of cholecystectomy. Undetected duct stones are left behind in ~1–5% of cholecystectomy patients. The overwhelming majority of bile duct stones are cholesterol stones formed in the gallbladder, which then migrate into the extrahepatic biliary tree through the cystic duct. Primary calculi arising de novo in the ducts are usually pigment stones developing in patients with (1) hepatobiliary parasitism or chronic, recurrent cholangitis; (2) congenital anomalies of the bile ducts (especially Caroli's disease); (3) dilated, sclerosed, or strictured ducts; or (4) an *MDR3* gene defect leading to impaired biliary phospholipids secretion. Common duct stones may remain asymptomatic for years, may pass spontaneously into the duodenum, or (most often) may present with biliary colic or a complication.

Complications · CHOLANGITIS Cholangitis may be acute or chronic, and symptoms result from inflammation, which usually is caused by at least partial obstruction to the flow of bile. Bacteria are present on bile culture in ~75% of patients with acute cholangitis early in the symptomatic course. The characteristic presentation of acute cholangitis involves biliary pain, jaundice, and spiking fevers with chills (Charcot's triad). Blood cultures are frequently positive, and leukocytosis is typical. *Nonsuppurative acute cholangitis* is most common and may respond relatively rapidly to supportive measures and to treatment with antibiotics. In *suppurative acute cholangitis*, however, the presence of pus under pressure in a completely obstructed ductal system leads to symptoms of severe toxicity—mental confusion, bacteremia, and septic shock. Response to antibiotics alone in this setting is relatively poor, multiple hepatic abscesses are often present, and the mortality rate approaches 100% unless prompt endoscopic or surgical relief of the obstruction and drainage of infected bile are carried out. Endoscopic management of bacterial cholangitis is as effective as surgical intervention. ERCP with endoscopic sphincterotomy is safe and the preferred initial procedure for both establishing a definitive diagnosis and providing effective therapy.

OBSTRUCTIVE JAUNDICE Gradual obstruction of the CBD over a period of weeks or months usually leads to initial manifestations of jaundice or pruritus without associated symptoms of biliary colic or cholangitis. Painless jaundice may occur in patients with choledocholithiasis, but is much more characteristic of biliary obstruction secondary to malignancy of the head of the pancreas, bile ducts, or ampulla of Vater.

In patients whose obstruction is secondary to choledocholithiasis, associated chronic calculous cholecystitis is very common, and the gallbladder in this setting may be relatively indistensible. The absence of a palpable gallbladder in most patients with biliary obstruction from duct stones is the basis for *Courvoisier's law*, i.e., that the presence of a palpably enlarged gallbladder suggests that the biliary obstruction is secondary to an underlying malignancy rather than to calculous disease. Biliary obstruction causes progressive dilatation of the intrahepatic bile ducts as intrabiliary pressures rise. Hepatic bile flow is suppressed, and reabsorption and regurgitation of conjugated bilirubin into the bloodstream lead to jaundice accompanied by dark urine (bilirubinuria) and light-colored (acholic) stools.

CBD stones should be suspected in any patient with cholecystitis whose serum bilirubin level is >85.5 μmol/L (5 mg/dL). The maximum bilirubin level is seldom >256.5 μmol/L (15.0 mg/dL) in patients with choledocholithiasis unless concomitant hepatic disease or another factor leading to marked hyperbilirubinemia exists. Serum bilirubin levels ≥ 342.0 μmol/L (20 mg/dL) should suggest the possibility of neoplastic obstruction. The serum alkaline phosphatase level is almost always elevated in biliary obstruction. A rise in alkaline phosphatase often precedes clinical jaundice and may be the only abnormality in routine liver function tests. There may be a two- to tenfold elevation of serum aminotransferases, especially in association with acute obstruction. Follow-ing relief of the obstructing process, serum aminotransferase elevations usually return rapidly to normal, while the serum bilirubin level may take 1–2 weeks to return to normal. The alkaline phosphatase level usually falls slowly, lagging behind the decrease in serum bilirubin.

PANCREATITIS The most common associated entity discovered in patients with nonalcoholic acute pancreatitis is biliary tract disease. Biochemical evidence of pancreatic inflammation complicates acute cholecystitis in 15% of cases and choledocholithiasis in >30%, and the common factor appears to be the passage of gallstones through the common duct. Coexisting pancreatitis should be suspected in patients with symptoms of cholecystitis who develop (1) back pain or pain to the left of the abdominal midline, (2) prolonged vomiting with paralytic ileus, or (3) a pleural effusion, especially on the left side. Surgical treatment of gallstone disease is usually associated with resolution of the pancreatitis.

SECONDARY BILIARY CIRRHOSIS Secondary biliary cirrhosis may complicate prolonged or intermittent duct obstruction with or without recurrent cholangitis. Although this complication may be seen in patients with choledocholithiasis, it is more common in cases of prolonged obstruction from stricture or neoplasm. Once established, secondary biliary cirrhosis may be progressive even after correction of the obstructing process, and increasingly severe hepatic cirrhosis may lead to portal hypertension or to hepatic failure and death. Prolonged biliary obstruction may also be associated with clinically relevant deficiencies of the fat-soluble vitamins A, D, E, and K.

Diagnosis and Treatment The diagnosis of choledocholithiasis is usually made by cholangiography (Table 305-3), either preoperatively by ERCP or intraoperatively at the time of cholecystectomy. As many as 15% of patients undergoing cholecystectomy will prove to have CBD stones. When CBD stones are suspected prior to laparoscopic cholecystectomy, preoperative ERCP with endoscopic papillotomy and stone extraction is the preferred approach. It not only provides stone clearance but also defines the anatomy of the biliary tree in relationship to the cystic duct. CBD stones should be suspected in gallstone patients who have any of the following risk factors: (1) a history of jaundice or pancreatitis, (2) abnormal tests of liver function, and (3) ultrasonographic evidence of a dilated CBD or stones in the duct. Alternatively, if intraoperative cholangiography reveals retained stones, postoperative ERCP can be carried out. The need for preoperative ERCP is expected to decrease further as laparoscopic techniques for bile duct exploration improve.

The widespread use of laparoscopic cholecystectomy and ERCP has decreased the incidence of complicated biliary tract disease and the need for choledocholithotomy and T-tube drainage of the bile ducts. EBS followed by spontaneous passage or stone extraction is the treatment of choice in the management of patients with common duct stones, especially in elderly or poor-risk patients.

TRAUMA, STRICTURES, AND HEMOBILIA

Most benign strictures of the extrahepatic bile ducts result from surgical trauma and occur in about 1 in 500 cholecystectomies. Strictures may present with bile leak or abscess formation in the immediate postoperative period or with biliary obstruction or cholangitis as long as 2 years or more following the inciting trauma. The diagnosis is established by percutaneous or endoscopic cholangiography. Endoscopic brushing of biliary strictures may be helpful in establishing the nature of the lesion and is more accurate than bile cytology alone. When positive exfoliative cytology is obtained, the diagnosis of a neoplastic stricture is established. This procedure is especially important in patients with primary sclerosing cholangitis (PSC) who are predisposed to the development of cholangiocarcinomas. Successful operative correction of non-PSC bile duct strictures by a skillful surgeon with duct-to-bowel anastomosis is usually possible, although mortality rates from surgical complications, recurrent cholangitis, or secondary biliary cirrhosis are high.

TABLE 305-3 DIAGNOSTIC EVALUATION OF THE BILE DUCTS

Diagnostic Advantages	Diagnostic Limitations	Contraindications	Complications	Comment
Hepatobiliary Ultrasound				
Rapid Simultaneous scanning of GB, liver, bile ducts, pancreas Accurate identification of dilated bile ducts Not limited by jaundice, pregnancy Guidance for fine-needle biopsy	Bowel gas Massive obesity Ascites Barium Partial bile duct obstruction Poor visualization of distal CBD	None	None	Initial procedure of choice in investigating possible biliary tract obstruction
Computed Tomography				
Simultaneous scanning of GB, liver, bile ducts, pancreas Accurate identification of dilated bile ducts, masses Not limited by jaundice, gas, obesity, ascites High-resolution image Guidance for fine-needle biopsy	Extreme cachexia Movement artifact Ileus Partial bile duct obstruction	Pregnancy	Reaction to iodinated contrast, if used	Indicated for evaluation of hepatic or pancreatic masses Procedure of choice in investigating possible biliary obstruction if diagnostic limitations prevent HBUS
Magnetic Resonance Cholangiopancreatography				
Useful modality for visualizing pancreatic and biliary ducts Has excellent sensitivity for bile duct dilatation, biliary stricture, and intraductal abnormalities Can identify pancreatic duct dilatation or stricture, pancreatic duct stenosis, and pancreas divisum	Cannot offer therapeutic intervention High cost	Claustrophobia Certain metals (iron)	None	
Endoscopic Retrograde Cholangiopancreatography				
Simultaneous pancreatography Best visualization of distal biliary tract Bile or pancreatic cytology Endoscopic sphincterotomy and stone removal Biliary manometry	Gastroduodenal obstruction ? Roux en Y biliary-enteric anastomosis	Pregnancy ? Acute pancreatitis ? Severe cardiopulmonary disease	Pancreatitis Cholangitis, sepsis Infected pancreatic pseudocyst Perforation (rare) Hypoxemia, aspiration	Cholangiogram of choice in: Absence of dilated ducts ? Pancreatic, ampullary or gastroduodenal disease Prior biliary surgery Endoscopic sphincterotomy a treatment possibility
Percutaneous Transhepatic Cholangiogram				
Extremely successful when bile ducts dilated Best visualization of proximal biliary tract Bile cytology/culture Percutaneous transhepatic drainage	Nondilated or sclerosed ducts	Pregnancy Uncorrectable coagulopathy Massive ascites ? Hepatic abscess	Bleeding Hemobilia Bile peritonitis Bacteremia, sepsis	Indicated when ERCP is contraindicated or failed
Endoscopic Ultrasound				
Most sensitive method to detect ampullary stones				

Hemobilia may follow traumatic or operative injury to the liver or bile ducts, intraductal rupture of a hepatic abscess or aneurysm of the hepatic artery, biliary or hepatic tumor hemorrhage, or mechanical complications of choledocholithiasis or hepatobiliary parasitism. Diagnostic procedures such as liver biopsy, PTC, and transhepatic biliary drainage catheter placement may also be complicated by hemobilia. Patients often present with a classic triad of biliary pain, obstructive jaundice, and melena or occult blood in the stools. The diagnosis is sometimes made by cholangiographic evidence of blood clot in the biliary tree, but selective angiographic verification may be required. Although minor episodes of hemobilia may resolve without operative intervention, surgical ligation of the bleeding vessel is frequently required.

EXTRINSIC COMPRESSION OF THE BILE DUCTS

Partial or complete biliary obstruction may be produced by extrinsic compression of the ducts. The most common cause of this form of obstructive jaundice is carcinoma of the head of the pancreas. Biliary obstruction may also occur as a complication of either acute or chronic pancreatitis or involvement of lymph nodes in the porta hepatis by lymphoma or metastatic carcinoma. The latter should be distinguished from cholestasis resulting from massive replacement of the liver by tumor.

HEPATOBILIARY PARASITISM

Infestation of the biliary tract by adult helminths or their ova may produce a chronic, recurrent pyogenic cholangitis with or without multiple hepatic abscesses, ductal stones, or biliary obstruction. This condition is relatively rare but does occur in inhabitants of southern China and elsewhere in Southeast Asia. The organisms most commonly involved are trematodes or flukes, including *Clonorchis sinensis*, *Opisthorchis viverrini* or *O. felineus*, and *Fasciola hepatica*. The biliary tract also may be involved by intraductal migration of adult *Ascaris lumbricoides* from the duodenum or by intrabiliary rupture of hydatid cysts of the liver produced by *Echinococcus* spp. The diagnosis is made by cholangiography and the presence of characteristic ova on stool examination. When obstruction is present, the treatment of choice is laparotomy under antibiotic coverage, with common duct exploration and a biliary drainage procedure.

SCLEROSING CHOLANGITIS

Primary or idiopathic sclerosing cholangitis is characterized by a progressive, inflammatory, sclerosing, and obliterative process affecting the extrahepatic and/or the intrahepatic bile ducts. The disorder occurs up to 75% in association with inflammatory bowel disease, especially ulcerative colitis. It may also be associated with autoimmune pancreatitis; multifocal fibrosclerosis syndromes such as retroperitoneal, mediastinal, and/or periureteral fibrosis; Riedel's struma; or pseudotumor of the orbit.

Patients with primary sclerosing cholangitis often present with signs and symptoms of chronic or intermittent biliary obstruction: RUQ abdominal pain, pruritus, jaundice, or acute cholangitis. Late in the course, complete biliary obstruction, secondary biliary cirrhosis, hepatic failure, or portal hypertension with bleeding varices may occur. The diagnosis is usually established by finding multifocal, diffusely distributed strictures with intervening segments of normal or dilated ducts, producing a beaded appearance on cholangiography (Fig. 305-2D). The cholangiographic technique of choice in suspected cases is ERCP. When a diagnosis of sclerosing cholangitis has been established, a search for associated diseases, especially for chronic inflammatory bowel disease, should be carried out.

A recent study describes the natural history and outcome for 305 patients of Swedish descent with primary sclerosing cholangitis; 134 (44%) of the patients were asymptomatic at the time of diagnosis and, not surprisingly, had a significantly higher survival rate. The independent predictors of a bad prognosis were age, serum bilirubin concentration, and liver histologic changes. Cholangiocarcinoma was found in 24 patients (8%). Inflammatory bowel disease was closely associated with primary sclerosing cholangitis and had a prevalence of 81% in this study population.

Small duct PSC is defined by the presence of chronic cholestasis and hepatic histology consistent with PSC but with normal findings on cholangiography. Small duct PSC is found in ~5% of patients with PSC and may represent an earlier stage of PSC associated with a significantly better long-term prognosis. However, such patients may progress to classic PSC and/or end-stage liver disease with consequent necessity of liver transplantation.

In patients with AIDS, cholangiopancreatography may demonstrate a broad range of biliary tract changes as well as pancreatic duct obstruction and occasionally pancreatitis (Chap. 182). Further, biliary tract lesions in AIDS include infection and cholangiopancreatographic changes similar to those of PSC. Changes noted include: (1) diffuse involvement of intrahepatic bile ducts alone, (2) involvement of both intra- and extrahepatic bile ducts, (3) ampullary stenosis, (4) stricture of the intrapancreatic portion of the common bile duct, and (5) pancreatic duct involvement. Associated infectious organisms include *Cryptosporidium*, *Mycobacterium avium-intracellulare*, cytomegalovirus, *Microsporidia*, and *Isospora*. In addition, acalculous cholecystitis occurs in up to 10% of patients. ERCP sphincterotomy, while not without risk, provides significant pain reduction in patients with AIDS-associated papillary stenosis. Secondary sclerosing cholangitis may occur as a long-term complication of choledocholithiasis, cholangiocarcinoma, operative or traumatic biliary injury, or contiguous inflammatory processes.

Rx SCLEROSING CHOLANGITIS

Therapy with cholestyramine may help control symptoms of pruritus, and antibiotics are useful when cholangitis complicates the clinical picture. Vitamin D and calcium supplementation may help prevent the loss of bone mass frequently seen in patients with chronic cholestasis. Glucocorticoids, methotrexate, and cyclosporine have not been shown to be efficacious in PSC. UDCA in high dosage (20 mg/kg) improves serum liver tests, but an effect on survival has not been documented. In cases where high-grade biliary obstruction (dominant strictures) has occurred, balloon dilatation or stenting may be appropriate. Only rarely is surgical intervention indicated. Efforts at biliary-enteric anastomosis or stent placement may, however, be complicated by recurrent cholangitis and further progression of the stenosing process. The prognosis is unfavorable, with a median survival of 9 to 12 years following the diagnosis, regardless of therapy. Four variables (age, serum bilirubin level, histologic stage, and splenomegaly) predict survival in patients with PSC and serve as the basis for a risk score. PSC is one of the most common indications for liver transplantation.

FURTHER READINGS

APSTEIN MD, CAREY MC: Pathogenesis of cholesterol gallstones: A parsimonious hypothesis. Eur J Clin Invest 26:343, 1996

BROOME U et al: Natural history and outcome in 32 Swedish patients with small duct primary sclerosing cholangitis (PSC). J Hepatol 36:586, 2002

LAMMERT F, SAUERBRUCH T: Mechanisms of disease: The genetic epidemiology of gallbladder stones. Nat Clin Pract Gastroenterol Hepatol 2: 423, 2005

PAUMPARTNER G: Nonsurgical management of gallstone disease, in *Sleisenger and Fordtran's Gastrointestinal and Liver Disease*, 7th ed, M Feldman et al (eds). Philadelphia, Saunders, 2002, pp 1107–1115

PORTINCASA P et al: Cholesterol gallstone disease. Lancet 368:230, 2006

RANSOHOFF DF, GRACIE WA: Treatment of gallstones. Ann Intern Med 119:606, 1993

ZACKS SL et al: A population-based cohort study comparing laparoscopic cholecystectomy and open cholecystectomy. Ann J Gastroenterol 97:334, 2002

SECTION 3 — DISORDERS OF THE PANCREAS

306 Approach to the Patient with Pancreatic Disease

Phillip P. Toskes, Norton J. Greenberger

GENERAL CONSIDERATIONS

The clinical manifestations of acute and chronic pancreatitis and pancreatic insufficiency are protean. Thus, patients may present with hypertriglyceridemia, vitamin B_{12} malabsorption, hypercalcemia, hypocalcemia, hyperglycemia, ascites, pleural effusions, and chronic abdominal pain with normal blood amylase levels. Indeed, if the clinician considers pancreatitis as a possible diagnosis only when presented with a patient having classic symptoms (i.e., severe, constant epigastric pain that radiates through to the back, along with an elevated blood amylase or lipase level), only a minority of patients with pancreatitis will be diagnosed correctly.

As emphasized in Chap. 307, the etiologies as well as the clinical manifestations of pancreatitis are quite varied. Although it is well appreciated that pancreatitis is frequently secondary to alcohol abuse and biliary tract disease, it can also be caused by drugs, trauma, and viral infections and is associated with metabolic and connective tissue disorders. In ~30% of patients with acute pancreatitis and 25–40% of patients with chronic pancreatitis, the etiology is obscure.

Although good data exist concerning the frequency of acute pancreatitis (about 5000 new cases per year in the United States, with a mortality rate of about 10%), the number of patients who suffer with recurrent acute pancreatitis or chronic pancreatitis is largely undefined. These statistics have not changed over the past 25 years. Only one prospective study on the incidence of chronic pancreatitis is available; it showed an incidence of 8.2 new cases per 100,000 per year and a prevalence of 26.4 cases per 100,000. These numbers probably underestimate considerably the true incidence and prevalence, because non-alcohol-induced pancreatitis was largely ignored. At autopsy, the prevalence of chronic pancreatitis ranges from 0.04 to 5%. The relative inaccessibility of the pancreas to direct examination and the non-specificity of the abdominal pain associated with pancreatitis make the diagnosis of pancreatitis difficult and usually dependent on elevation of blood amylase and/or lipase levels. Many patients with chronic pancreatitis do not have elevated blood amylase or lipase levels. Some patients with chronic pancreatitis develop signs and symptoms of pancreatic exocrine insufficiency, and thus objective evidence for pancreatic disease can be demonstrated. However, there is a very large reservoir of pancreatic exocrine function. More than 90% of the pancreas must be damaged before maldigestion of fat and protein is manifested. Even the secretin stimulation test, which is the most sensitive method of assessing pancreatic exocrine function, is probably abnormal only when >60% of exocrine function has been lost. Noninvasive, indirect tests of pancreatic exocrine function (fecal elastase, serum trypsinogen) are much more likely to give abnormal results in patients with obvious pancreatic disease, i.e., pancreatic calcification, steatorrhea, or diabetes mellitus, than in patients with occult disease. Thus, the number of patients who have subclinical exocrine dysfunction (<90% loss of function) is unknown.

TESTS USEFUL IN THE DIAGNOSIS OF PANCREATIC DISEASE

Several tests have proved of value in the evaluation of pancreatic exocrine function. Examples of specific tests and their usefulness in the diagnosis of acute and chronic pancreatitis are summarized in Table 306-1 and Fig. 306-1. At most institutions, pancreatic function tests are performed if the diagnosis of pancreatic disease remains a possibility after noninvasive tests (ultrasound, CT) and invasive tests [endoscopic retrograde cholangiopancreatography (ERCP), endoscopic ultrasonography (EUS)] have given normal or inconclusive results. In this regard, tests employing *direct* stimulation of the pancreas are the most sensitive.

Pancreatic Enzymes in Body Fluids   The serum amylase and lipase levels are widely used as screening tests for acute pancreatitis in the patient with acute abdominal pain or back pain. Values greater than three times the upper limit of normal virtually clinch the diagnosis if gut perforation or infarction is excluded. In the absence of objective evidence of pancreatitis by abdominal ultrasound, CT scan, ERCP, or EUS, mild to moderate elevations of amylase and/or lipase are problematic in making a diagnosis of pancreatitis. In acute pancreatitis, the serum amylase is usually elevated within 24 h of onset and remains so for 1–3 days. Levels return to normal within 3–5 days unless there is extensive pancreatic necrosis, incomplete ductal obstruction, or pseudocyst formation. Approximately 85% of patients with acute pancreatitis have an elevated serum amylase level. This index may be normal, however, if (1) there is a delay (of 2–5 days) before blood samples are obtained, (2) the underlying disorder is chronic pancreatitis rather than acute pancreatitis, or (3) hypertriglyceridemia is present. Patients with hypertriglyceridemia and proven pancreatitis have been found to have spuriously low levels of amylase and perhaps lipase activity.

The serum amylase is often elevated in other conditions (Table 306-2), in part because the enzyme is found in many organs in addition to the pancreas (salivary glands, liver, small intestine, kidney, fallopian tube) and can be produced by various tumors (carcinomas of the lung, esophagus, breast, and ovary). An assay of serum trypsinogen (performed by several commercial laboratories) is quite helpful in this regard. Since this enzyme is secreted specifically by the pancreas, a normal serum trypsinogen level in a patient with minimal elevation of

serum amylase essentially rules out acute pancreatitis. Urinary amylase measurements, including the amylase/creatinine clearance ratio, are no more sensitive or specific than blood amylase levels. Isoamylase determinations do not accurately distinguish elevated blood amylase levels due to bona fide pancreatitis from elevated blood amylase levels due to a nonpancreatic source of amylase, especially when the blood amylase level is only moderately elevated.

Elevation of ascitic fluid amylase occurs in acute pancreatitis as well as in (1) pancreatogenous ascites due to disruption of the main pancreatic duct or a leaking pseudocyst and (2) other abdominal disorders that simulate pancreatitis (e.g., intestinal obstruction, intestinal infarction, and perforated peptic ulcer). Elevation of pleural fluid amylase occurs in acute pancreatitis, chronic pancreatitis, carcinoma of the lung, and esophageal perforation.

Lipase may now be the single best enzyme to measure for the diagnosis of acute pancreatitis. Improvements in substrates and technology offer clinicians improved options, especially when a turbidimetric assay is used. The newer lipase assays have colipase as a cofactor and are fully automated.

An assay for trypsinogen (or for trypsin-like immunoreactivity) has a theoretical advantage over amylase and lipase determinations in that the pancreas is the only organ that contains this enzyme. The test appears to be useful in the diagnosis of both acute and chronic pancreatitis. Sensitivity and specificity are comparable to those of amylase and lipase determinations. Since trypsinogen is also excreted by the kidney, elevated serum values are found in renal failure, as is the case with serum amylase and lipase levels. *No single blood test is reliable for the diagnosis of acute pancreatitis in patients with renal failure.* Determining whether a patient with renal failure and abdominal pain has pancreatitis remains a difficult clinical problem. A recent study found that serum amylase levels were elevated in patients with renal dysfunction only when creatinine clearance was <0.8 mL/s (<50 mL/min). In such patients, the serum amylase level was invariably <8.3 μkat/L (<500 IU/L) in the absence of objective evidence of acute pancreatitis. In that study, serum lipase and trypsin levels paralleled serum amylase values.

A recent study evaluated the sensitivity and specificity of five assays used to diagnose acute pancreatitis: two for amylase, one for lipase, one for trypsin-like immunoreactivity (TLI), and one for pancreatic isoamylase. The data obtained (1) show that, if the best cutoff level is used, all these assays have similar specificities and (2) suggest that total serum amylase is as good an indicator of acute pancreatitis as any of the alternatives. However, inherent in many such studies is the problem that the recognition and diagnosis of acute pancreatitis hinge on the finding of an elevated serum amylase level. The question arises as to whether any diagnostic test result can be proved superior to the total serum amylase level if hyperamylasemia is required for the diagnosis. In other studies, when "objective" confirmation of the clinical diagnosis of pancreatitis was required (ultrasonography, CT, laparotomy), the sensitivity of the serum amylase has been found to be as low as 68%. With these limitations in mind, the recommended screening tests for acute pancreatitis are *total serum amylase* and *serum lipase activities*. Serum amylase values greater than three times normal are highly specific.

Studies Pertaining to Pancreatic Structure • *RADIOLOGIC TESTS*   Plain films of the abdomen may provide useful information in patients with acute pancreatitis. The most frequent abnormalities include (1) a localized ileus, usually involving the jejunum ("sentinel loop"); (2) a generalized ileus with air-fluid levels; (3) the "colon cutoff sign," which results from isolated distention of the transverse colon; (4) duodenal distention with air-fluid levels; and (5) a mass, which is frequently a pseudocyst. In chronic pancreatitis, an important radiographic finding is pancreatic calcification, which characteristically is localized adjacent to and superimposed on the second lumbar vertebra (Fig. 307-3A).

Upper gastrointestinal x-rays may reveal displacement of the stomach by the retroperitoneal mass (Fig. 307-2A) or widening and effacement of the duodenal C loop, which also suggest the presence of a pancreatic mass, which could be inflammatory, cystic, or neoplastic. However, the use of x-ray films has been largely superseded by ultrasound.

TABLE 306-1 TESTS USEFUL IN THE DIAGNOSIS OF ACUTE AND CHRONIC PANCREATITIS AND PANCREATIC TUMORS

Test	Principle	Comment
Pancreatic Enzymes in Body Fluids		
Amylase		
1. Serum	Pancreatic inflammation leads to increased enzyme levels	Simple; 20–40% false negatives and positives; reliable if test results are three times the upper limit of normal
2. Urine	Renal clearance of amylase is increased in acute pancreatitis	May be abnormal when serum levels normal; false negatives and positives
3. Ascitic fluid	Disruption of gland or main pancreatic duct leads to increased amylase concentration	Can establish diagnosis of pancreatitis; false positives occur with intestinal obstruction and perforated ulcer
4. Pleural fluid	Exudative pleural effusion with pancreatitis	False positives occur with carcinoma of the lung and esophageal perforation
5. Isoenzymes	P isoamylases arise from the pancreas; S isoamylases are from other sources	More specific than total serum amylase in diagnosis of acute pancreatitis; useful in identifying nonpancreatic causes of hyperamylasemia
Serum lipase	Pancreatic inflammation leads to increased enzyme levels	New methods have greatly simplified determination; positive in 70–85% of cases
Serum trypsinogen	Pancreatic inflammation leads to increased levels	*Elevated* in acute pancreatitis; *decreased* in chronic pancreatitis *with* steatorrhea; normal in chronic pancreatitis *without* steatorrhea and in steatorrhea with normal pancreatic function
Studies Pertaining to Pancreatic Structure		
Radiologic and radionuclide tests		
1. Plain film of the abdomen	Abnormal in acute and chronic pancreatitis	Simple; normal in >50% of cases of both acute and chronic pancreatitis
2. Upper gastrointestinal x-rays	Abnormally thickened duodenal folds; displacement of stomach or widening of duodenal loop suggests a pancreatic mass (inflammatory, neoplastic, cystic)	Simple; frequently normal; largely superseded by US and CT scanning
3. Ultrasonography (US)	Can provide information on edema, inflammation, calcification, pseudocysts, and mass lesions	Simple, noninvasive; sequential studies quite feasible; useful in diagnosis of pseudocyst
4. CT scan	Permits detailed visualization of pancreas and surrounding structures	Useful in the diagnosis of pancreatic calcification, dilated pancreatic ducts, and pancreatic tumors; may not be able to distinguish between inflammatory and neoplastic mass lesions
5. Selective angiography	Can identify pancreatic neoplasms (1) by sheathing of celiac or superior mesenteric branches by tumor or (2) by tumor staining; displacement of vessels by tumor	Indicated (1) in suspected islet cell tumors and (2) before pancreatic or duodenal resection; most reliable features reflect nonresectable pancreatic cancer
6. Endoscopic retrograde cholangiopancreatography (ERCP)	Cannulation of pancreatic and common bile duct permits visualization of pancreatic-biliary ductal system	Provides diagnostic data in 60–85% of cases; differentiation of chronic pancreatitis from pancreatic carcinoma may be difficult
7. Endoscopic ultrasonography (EUS)	High-frequency transducer employed with EUS can produce very high resolution images and depict changes in the pancreatic duct and parenchyma with better detail	Exact role of EUS versus ERCP and CT not yet fully defined; sensitivity and specificity under study
8. Magnetic resonance cholangiopancreatography	Three-dimensional rendering has been used to produce very good images of the pancreatic duct by a noninvasive technique	May be used to evaluate patients judged to be at high risk for ERCP, such as the elderly; may replace ERCP as a diagnostic test, although large controlled studies need to be done
Pancreatic biopsy with US or CT guidance	Percutaneous biopsy with skinny needle and localization of lesion by US	High diagnostic yield; laparotomy avoided; requires special technical skills
Tests of Exocrine Pancreatic Function		
Direct stimulation of the pancreas with analysis of duodenal contents		
1. Secretin-pancreozymin (CCK) test	Secretin leads to increased output of pancreatic juice and HCO_3^-; CCK leads to increased output of pancreatic enzymes; pancreatic secretory response is related to the functional mass of pancreatic tissue	Sensitive enough to detect occult disease; involves duodenal intubation and fluoroscopy; poorly defined normal enzyme response; overlap in chronic pancreatitis; large secretory reserve capacity of the pancreas
Measurement of intraluminal digestion products		
1. Microscopic examination of stool for undigested meat fibers and fat	Lack of proteolytic and lipolytic enzymes causes decreased digestion of meat fibers and triglycerides	Simple, reliable; not sensitive enough to detect milder cases of pancreatic insufficiency
2. Quantitative stool fat determination	Lack of lipolytic enzymes brings about impaired fat digestion	Reliable, reference standard for defining severity of malabsorption; does not distinguish between maldigestion and malabsorption
3. Fecal nitrogen	Lack of proteolytic enzymes leads to impaired protein digestion, resulting in an increase in stool nitrogen	Does not distinguish between maldigestion and malabsorption; low sensitivity
Measurement of pancreatic enzymes in feces		
1. Elastase	Pancreatic secretion of proteolytic enzymes	Excellent specificity; sensitivity similar to that of serum trypsinogen
Miscellaneous tests		
1. Dual-labeled Schilling test	Intrinsic factor [^{57}Co]cobalamin and Hog R protein [^{58}Co]cobalamin are given together. Since proteases are necessary to cleave R protein, the ratio of labeled cobalamin excreted in urine is an index of exocrine dysfunction.	Time-consuming and expensive

FIGURE 306-1 An approach to the patient with suspected chronic pancreatitis. Endoscopic ultrasonography and magnetic resonance cholangiopancreatography are appropriate diagnostic alternatives. ERCP, endoscopic retrograde cholangiopancreatography.

Ultrasonography can provide important information in patients with acute pancreatitis, chronic pancreatitis, pancreatic calcification, pseudocyst, and pancreatic carcinoma. Echographic appearances can indicate the presence of edema, inflammation, and calcification (not obvious on plain films of the abdomen), as well as pseudocysts, mass lesions, and gallstones (Figs. 307-2*B* and 307-3*B*). In acute pancreatitis, the pancreas is characteristically enlarged. In pancreatic pseudocyst, the usual appearance is that of an echo-free, smooth, round fluid collection. Pancreatic carcinoma distorts the usual landmarks, and mass lesions >3.0 cm are usually detected as localized, echo-free solid lesions. Ultrasound is often the initial investigation for most patients with sus-

pected pancreatic disease. However, obesity, excess small- and large-bowel gas, and recently performed barium contrast examinations can interfere with ultrasound studies.

CT is the best imaging study for initial evaluation of a suspected chronic pancreatic disorder and for the complications of acute and chronic pancreatitis. It is especially useful in the detection of pancreatic tumors, fluid-containing lesions such as pseudocysts and abscesses, and calcium deposits (Figs. 307-3*C* and 307-4*A*). Most lesions are characterized by (1) enlargement of the pancreatic outline, (2) distortion of the pancreatic contour, and/or (3) a fluid filling that has a different attenuation coefficient than normal pancreas. However, it is difficult to distinguish between inflammatory and neoplastic lesions. Oral water-soluble contrast agents may be used to opacify the stomach and duodenum during CT scans; this strategy permits more precise delineation of various organs as well as mass lesions. Dynamic CT (using rapid IV administration of contrast) is useful in estimating the degree of pancreatic necrosis and in predicting morbidity and mortality. Spiral (helical) CT provides clear images much more rapidly and essentially negates artifact caused by patient movement (Fig. 307-2*D*).

Endoscopic ultrasonography (EUS) produces high-resolution images of the pancreatic parenchyma and pancreatic duct with a transducer fixed to an endoscope that can be directed onto the surface of the pancreas through the stomach or duodenum. EUS is replacing ERCP for diagnostic purposes in many centers. EUS allows one to obtain information about the pancreatic duct as well as the parenchyma and has no complications associated with it, in contrast to the 5–20% of post-ERCP pancreatitis observed. EUS is also very good in detecting common bile duct stones. Pancreatic masses can be biopsied via EUS and one can deliver nerve blocks through EUS. Although criteria for abnormalities on EUS in severe pancreatic disease have been developed, the true sensitivity and specificity of this procedure has yet to be determined. Currently chronic pancreatitis is diagnosed by EUS if three or more criteria listed in Table 306-3 are present. That concept has now been vigorously challenged since normal subjects and patients with nonulcer dyspepsia may have an abnormal EUS based on just three abnormalities. Many EUS experts are now requiring five or more abnormalities before chronic pancreatitis is diagnosed. Recent studies comparing EUS to the secretin test in patients with unexplained abdominal pain suspected of having chronic pancreatitis show a significantly better sensitivity and specificity for the secretin test over EUS in detecting early changes of chronic pancreatitis. The exact role of EUS versus CT, ERCP, or function testing has yet to be defined.

Magnetic resonance cholangiopancreatography (MRCP) is now being used to view both the bile duct and the pancreatic duct. Non-breath-holding and three-dimensional turbo spin-echo techniques are being utilized to produce superb MRCP images. The main pancreatic duct and common bile duct can be seen well, but there is still a question as to whether changes can be detected consistently in the secondary ducts. MRCP may be particularly useful to evaluate the pancreatic duct in high-risk patients such as the elderly because this is a noninvasive procedure.

Both EUS and MRCP may replace ERCP in some patients. As these techniques become more refined, they may well be the diagnostic tests of choice to evaluate the pancreatic duct. ERCP is still needed to perform therapy of bile duct and pancreatic duct lesions.

Selective catheterization of the celiac and superior mesenteric arteries combined with superselective catheterization of others arteries, such as

TABLE 306-2 CAUSES OF HYPERAMYLASEMIA AND HYPERAMYLASURIA

Pancreatic Disease

I. Pancreatitis	II. Pancreatic trauma
A. Acute	III. Pancreatic carcinoma
B. Chronic: ductal obstruction	
C. Complications of pancreatitis	
1. Pancreatic pseudocyst	
2. Pancreatogenous ascites	
3. Pancreatic abscess	
4. Pancreatic necrosis	

Nonpancreatic Disorders

I. Renal insufficiency	IV. Macroamylasemia
II. Salivary gland lesions	V. Burns
A. Mumps	VI. Diabetic ketoacidosis
B. Calculus	VII. Pregnancy
C. Irradiation sialadenitis	VIII. Renal transplantation
D. Maxillofacial surgery	IX. Cerebral trauma
III. "Tumor" hyperamylasemia	X. Drugs: morphine
A. Carcinoma of the lung	
B. Carcinoma of the esophagus	
C. Breast carcinoma, ovarian carcinoma	

Other Abdominal Disorders

I. Biliary tract disease: cholecystitis, choledocholithiasis
II. Intraabdominal disease
  A. Perforated or penetrating peptic ulcer
  B. Intestinal obstruction or infarction
  C. Ruptured ectopic pregnancy
  D. Peritonitis
  E. Aortic aneurysm
  F. Chronic liver disease
  G. Postoperative hyperamylasemia

TABLE 306-3 ENDOSCOPIC ULTRASONOGRAPHIC CRITERIA FOR CHRONIC PANCREATITIS

Ductal	Parenchymal
Stones	Echogenic strands
Echogenic ductal walls	Echogenic foci
Irregular ductal walls	Calcifications
Stricture	Lobular contour
Visible side branches	Cyst
Ductular dilatation	

the hepatic, splenic, and gastroduodenal arteries, permits visualization of the pancreas and detection of pancreatic neoplasms and pseudocysts. Pancreatic neoplasms can be identified by the sheathing of blood vessels by a mass lesion (Fig. 307-1D). Hormone-producing pancreatic tumors are especially likely to exhibit increased vascularity and tumor staining. Angiographic abnormalities are noted in many patients with pancreatic carcinoma but are uncommon in patients without pancreatic disease. Angiography complements ultrasonography and ERCP in the study of patients with a suspected pancreatic lesion and may be carried out if ERCP is either unsuccessful or nondiagnostic.

ERCP may provide useful information on the status of the pancreatic ductal system and thus aid in the differential diagnosis of pancreatic disease (Figs. 307-1C, 307-3D, and 307-4B). Pancreatic carcinoma is characterized by stenosis or obstruction of either the pancreatic duct or the common bile duct; both ductal systems are often abnormal. In chronic pancreatitis, ERCP abnormalities include (1) luminal narrowing; (2) irregularities in the ductal system with stenosis, dilation, sacculation, and ectasia; and (3) blockage of the pancreatic duct by calcium deposits. The presence of ductal stenosis and irregularity can make it difficult to distinguish chronic pancreatitis from carcinoma. It is important to be aware that ERCP changes interpreted as indicating chronic pancreatitis actually may be due to the effects of aging on the pancreatic duct or to the fact that the procedure was performed within several weeks of an attack of acute pancreatitis. Although aging may cause impressive ductal alterations, it does not affect the results of pancreatic function tests (i.e., the secretin test). Elevated serum and/or urine amylase levels after ERCP have been reported in 25–75% of patients, and clinical pancreatitis in 5–20% of patients. There are no satisfactory means to pharmacologically prevent ERCP-induced pancreatitis, despite many agents having been suggested and evaluated. The best way to prevent ERCP-induced pancreatitis is to not perform this procedure for diagnostic purposes in high-risk patients, who include women with acute relapsing pancreatitis in whom there is no evidence of biliary obstruction and patients with unexplained abdominal pain but no other abnormalities. If no lesion is found in the biliary and/or pancreatic ducts in a patient with repeated attacks of acute pancreatitis, manometric studies of the sphincter of Oddi may be indicated. Such studies, however, do increase the risk of post-ERCP/manometry acute pancreatitis. Such pancreatitis appears to be more common in patients with a nondilated pancreatic duct.

PANCREATIC BIOPSY WITH RADIOLOGIC GUIDANCE Percutaneous aspiration biopsy of a pancreatic mass often distinguishes a pancreatic inflammatory mass from a pancreatic neoplasm.

307 Acute and Chronic Pancreatitis
Norton J. Greenberger, Phillip P. Toskes

BIOCHEMISTRY AND PHYSIOLOGY OF PANCREATIC EXOCRINE SECRETION

GENERAL CONSIDERATIONS

The pancreas secretes 1500–3000 mL of isosmotic alkaline (pH > 8.0) fluid per day containing about 20 enzymes and zymogens. The pancreatic secretions provide the enzymes needed to effect the major digestive activity of the gastrointestinal tract and provide an optimal pH for the function of these enzymes.

REGULATION OF PANCREATIC SECRETION

The exocrine pancreas is influenced by intimately interacting hormonal and neural systems. *Gastric acid* is the stimulus for the release of secretin, which stimulates the secretion of pancreatic juice rich in water and electrolytes. Release of cholecystokinin (CCK) from the duodenum and

TESTS OF EXOCRINE PANCREATIC FUNCTION

Pancreatic function tests (Table 306-1) can be divided into the following:

1. *Direct stimulation of the pancreas* by IV infusion of secretin or secretin plus cholecystokinin (CCK) followed by collection and measurement of duodenal contents
2. Study of *intraluminal digestion products*, such as undigested meat fibers, stool fat, and fecal nitrogen
3. *Measurement of fecal pancreatic enzymes* such as elastase

The secretin test, used to detect diffuse pancreatic disease, is based on the physiologic principle that the pancreatic secretory response is directly related to the functional mass of pancreatic tissue. In the standard assay, secretin is given IV in a dose of 0.2 μg/kg of synthetic human or synthetic porcine secretin as either a bolus or a continuous infusion. Normal values for the standard secretin test are (1) volume output > 2.0 mL/kg per hour, (2) bicarbonate (HCO_3^-) concentration > 80 mmol/L, and (3) HCO_3^- output > 10 mmol/L in 1 h. The most reproducible measurement, giving the highest level of discrimination between normal subjects and patients with chronic pancreatitis, appears to be the maximal bicarbonate concentration.

There may be a dissociation between the results of the secretin test and those of tests of absorptive function. For example, patients with chronic pancreatitis often have abnormally low outputs of HCO_3^- after secretin but have normal fecal fat excretion. Thus the secretin test measures the secretory capacity of ductular epithelium, while fecal fat excretion indirectly reflects intraluminal lipolytic activity. Steatorrhea does not occur until intraluminal levels of lipase are markedly reduced, underscoring the fact that only small amounts of enzymes are necessary for intraluminal digestive activities. An abnormal secretin test result suggests only that chronic pancreatic damage is present; it will not consistently distinguish between chronic pancreatitis and pancreatic carcinoma.

The *serum trypsinogen level*, which is determined by radioimmunoassay, also has excellent specificity but is not very sensitive. It is a simple blood test that can detect severe damage to the exocrine pancreas. The normal values are 28–58 ng/mL, and any value <20 ng/mL reflects pancreatic steatorrhea.

Measurement of *intraluminal digestion products*, i.e., undigested muscle fibers, stool fat, and fecal nitrogen, is discussed in Chap. 288. The amount of human elastase in stool reflects the pancreatic output of this proteolytic enzyme. Decreased elastase activity in stool is an excellent test to detect severe pancreatic exocrine insufficiency in patients with chronic pancreatitis and cystic fibrosis. Tests useful in the diagnosis of exocrine pancreatic insufficiency and the differential diagnosis of malabsorption are also discussed in Chaps. 288 and 307.

jejunum is largely triggered by long-chain fatty acids, certain essential amino acids (tryptophan, phenylalanine, valine, methionine), and gastric acid itself. CCK evokes an enzyme-rich secretion from the pancreas. The *parasympathetic nervous system* (via the vagus nerve) exerts significant control over pancreatic secretion. Secretion evoked by secretin and CCK depends on permissive roles of vagal afferent and efferent pathways. This is particularly true for enzyme secretion, whereas water and bicarbonate secretions are heavily dependent on the hormonal effects of secretin and CCK. Also, vagal stimulation effects the release of vasoactive intestinal peptide (VIP), a secretin agonist. Bile salts also stimulate pancreatic secretion, thereby integrating the functions of the biliary tract, pancreas, and small intestine.

Pancreatic exocrine secretion is influenced by inhibitory neuropeptides such as somatostatin, pancreatic polypeptide, peptide YY, neuropeptide Y, enkephalin, pancreastatin, calcitonin gene–related peptides, glucagon, and galanin. Although pancreatic polypeptide and peptide YY may act primarily on nerves outside the pancreas, somatostatin acts at multiple sites. Nitric oxide is also an important neurotransmitter. The mechanism of action of these various factors has not been fully defined.

WATER AND ELECTROLYTE SECRETION

Bicarbonate is the ion of primary physiologic importance within pancreatic secretion. The ductal cells secrete bicarbonate predominantly derived from plasma (93%) rather than intracellular metabolism (7%). Bicarbonate enters through the sodium bicarbonate co-transporter with depolarization caused by chloride efflux through the cystic fibrosis transmembrane conductance regulator (CFTR). Secretin and VIP, both of which increase intracellular cyclic AMP, act on the ductal cells opening the CFTR in promoting secretion. CCK, acting as a neuromodulator, markedly potentiates the stimulatory effects of secretin. Acetylcholine also plays an important role in ductal cell secretion. Bicarbonate helps neutralize gastric acid and creates the appropriate pH for the activity of pancreatic enzymes.

ENZYME SECRETION

The acinar cell is highly compartmentalized and is concerned with the secretion of pancreatic enzymes. Proteins synthesized by the rough endoplasmic reticulum are processed in the Golgi and then targeted to the appropriate site, whether that be zymogen granules, lysosomes, or other cell compartments. The pancreas secretes amylolytic, lipolytic, and proteolytic enzymes. *Amylolytic enzymes*, such as amylase, hydrolyze starch to oligosaccharides and to the disaccharide maltose. The *lipolytic enzymes* include lipase, phospholipase A, and cholesterol esterase. Bile salts inhibit lipase in isolation; but colipase, another constituent of pancreatic secretion, binds to lipase and prevents this inhibition. Bile salts activate phospholipase A and cholesterol esterase. *Proteolytic enzymes* include endopeptidases (trypsin, chymotrypsin), which act on internal peptide bonds of proteins and polypeptides; exopeptidases (carboxypeptidases, aminopeptidases), which act on the free carboxyl- and amino-terminal ends of peptides, respectively; and elastase. The proteolytic enzymes are secreted as inactive precursors (zymogens). Ribonucleases (deoxyribonucleases, ribonuclease) are also secreted. *Enterokinase*, an enzyme found in the duodenal mucosa, cleaves the lysine-isoleucine bond of trypsinogen to form trypsin. Trypsin then activates the other proteolytic zymogens in a cascade phenomenon. All pancreatic enzymes have pH optima in the alkaline range. The nervous system initiates pancreatic enzyme secretion. The neurologic stimulation is cholinergic, involving extrinsic innervation by the vagus nerve and subsequent innervation by intrapancreatic cholinergic nerves. The stimulatory neurotransmitters are acetylcholine and gastrin-releasing peptides. These neurotransmitters activate calcium-dependent second messenger systems resulting in the release of zymogen granules. VIP is present in intrapancreatic nerves and potentiates the effect of acetylcholine. In contrast to other species, there are no CCK receptors on acinar cells in humans. CCK in physiologic concentrations stimulates pancreatic secretion by stimulating central vagal and intrapancreatic nerves.

AUTOPROTECTION OF THE PANCREAS

Autodigestion of the pancreas is prevented by the packaging of proteases in precursor form and by the synthesis of protease inhibitors, i.e., pancreatic secretory trypsin inhibitor (PSTI) and serine protease inhibitor, kazal type 1 (SPINK1). These protease inhibitors are found in the acinar cell, the pancreatic secretions, and the α_1- and α_2-globulin fractions of plasma. In addition, low calcium concentrations within the pancreas decrease trypsin activity. Loss of any of these protective mechanisms leads to zymogen activation, autodigestion, and acute pancreatitis.

EXOCRINE-ENDOCRINE RELATIONSHIPS

Insulin appears to be needed locally for secretin and CCK to promote exocrine secretion; thus, it acts in a permissive role for these two hormones.

ENTEROPANCREATIC AXIS AND FEEDBACK INHIBITION

Pancreatic enzyme secretion is controlled, at least in part, by a negative feedback mechanism induced by the presence of active serine proteases in the duodenum. To illustrate, perfusion of the duodenal lumen with phenylalanine causes a prompt increase in plasma CCK levels as well as increased secretion of chymotrypsin. However, simultaneous perfusion with trypsin blunts both responses. Conversely, perfusion of the duodenal lumen with protease inhibitors actually leads to enzyme hypersecretion. The available evidence supports the concept that the duodenum contains a peptide called *CCK-releasing factor* (CCK-RF) that is involved in stimulating CCK release. It appears that serine proteases inhibit pancreatic secretion by acting on a CCK-releasing peptide in the lumen of the small intestine. Thus the integrative result of both bicarbonate and enzyme secretion depends on a feedback process for both bicarbonate and pancreatic enzymes. Acidification of the duodenum releases secretin, which stimulates vagal-vagal and other neural pathways to activate pancreatic duct cells, which secrete bicarbonate. This bicarbonate then neutralizes the duodenal acid, and the feedback loop is completed. Duodenal proteins lead to a reduction in free proteases, thereby leading to an increase in free CCK-RF. CCK-RF is then released into the blood in physiologic concentrations, acting primarily through the neural pathways (vagal-vagal). This leads to acetylcholine-mediated pancreatic enzyme secretion. Proteases continue to be secreted from the pancreas until the protein within the duodenum and CCK-RF are digested. At this point, the free duodenal proteases rise again, thus completing this step in the feedback process.

ACUTE PANCREATITIS

GENERAL CONSIDERATIONS

Pancreatic inflammatory disease may be classified as (1) acute pancreatitis or (2) chronic pancreatitis. The pathologic spectrum of acute pancreatitis varies from *interstitial pancreatitis*, which is usually a mild and self-limited disorder, to *necrotizing pancreatitis*, in which the degree of pancreatic necrosis correlates with the severity of the attack and its systemic manifestations.

The incidence of pancreatitis varies in different countries and depends on cause, e.g., alcohol, gallstones, metabolic factors, and drugs (Table 307-1). The estimated incidence in England is 5.4/100,000 per year; in the United States it is 79.8/100,000 per year, thus resulting in >200,000 new cases of acute pancreatitis annually.

ETIOLOGY AND PATHOGENESIS

There are many causes of acute pancreatitis (Table 307-1), but the mechanisms by which these conditions trigger pancreatic inflammation have not been identified. Gallstones continue to be the leading cause of acute pancreatitis in most series (30–60%). Alcohol is the second most common cause, responsible for 15–30% of cases in the United States. The incidence of pancreatitis in alcoholics is surprisingly low (5/100,000), indicating that in addition to the amount of alcohol ingested unknown factors affect a person's susceptibility to pancreatic injury. The mechanism of injury is not well understood. Hypertriglyceridemia is the cause of acute pancreatitis in 1.3–3.8% of cases; serum triglyceride levels are usually >11.3 mmol/L (>1000 mg/dL). Most patients with hypertriglyceridemia, when subsequently examined, show evidence of an underlying derangement in lipid metabolism, probably unrelated to pancreatitis. Patients with diabetes mellitus who have developed ketoacidosis or who are on certain medications may also develop high triglyceride levels. Acute pancreatitis occurs in 5–20% of patients following endoscopic retrograde cholangiopancreatography (ERCP). Approximately 2–5% of cases of acute pancreatitis are drug-related. Drugs cause pancreatitis either by a hypersensitivity reaction or by the generation of a toxic metabolite, although in some cases it is not clear which of these mechanisms is operative (Table 307-1).

Autodigestion is one pathogenic theory, according to which pancreatitis results when proteolytic enzymes (e.g., trypsinogen, chymotrypsinogen, proelastase, and phospholipase A) are activated in the pancreas rather than in the intestinal lumen. A number of factors (e.g., endotoxins, exotoxins, viral infections, ischemia, anoxia, and direct trauma) are believed to activate these proenzymes. Activated proteolytic enzymes, especially trypsin, not only digest pancreatic and peripancreatic tissues but also can activate other enzymes, such as elastase and phospholipase.

TABLE 307-1 CAUSES OF ACUTE PANCREATITIS

Common Causes

Gallstones (including microlithiasis)
Alcohol (acute and chronic alcoholism)
Hypertriglyceridemia
Endoscopic retrograde cholangiopancreatography (ERCP), especially after
  biliary manometry
Trauma (especially blunt abdominal trauma)
Postoperative (abdominal and nonabdominal operations)
Drugs (azathioprine, 6-mercaptopurine, sulfonamides, estrogens,
  tetracycline, valproic acid, anti-HIV medications)
Sphincter of Oddi dysfunction

Uncommon Causes

Vascular causes and vasculitis (ischemic-hypoperfusion states after cardiac
  surgery)
Connective tissue disorders and thrombotic thrombocytopenic purpura (TTP)
Cancer of the pancreas
Hypercalcemia
Periampullary diverticulum
Pancreas divisum
Hereditary pancreatitis
Cystic fibrosis
Renal failure

Rare Causes

Infections (mumps, coxsackievirus, cytomegalovirus, echovirus, parasites)
Autoimmune (e.g., Sjögren's syndrome)

**Causes to Consider in Patients with Recurrent Bouts of Acute
Pancreatitis without an Obvious Etiology**

Occult disease of the biliary tree or pancreatic ducts, especially microlithiasis,
  sludge
Drugs
Hypertriglyceridemia
Pancreas divisum
Pancreatic cancer
Sphincter of Oddi dysfunction
Cystic fibrosis
Idiopathic

ACTIVATION OF PANCREATIC ENZYMES IN THE PATHOGENESIS OF ACUTE PANCREATITIS

Several recent studies have suggested that pancreatitis is a disease that evolves in three phases. The initial phase is characterized by intrapancreatic digestive enzyme activation and acinar cell injury. Zymogen activation appears to be mediated by lysosomal hydrolases such as cathepsin B which become co-localized with digestive enzymes in intracellular organelles; it is currently believed that acinar cell injury is the consequence of zymogen activation. The second phase of pancreatitis involves the activation, chemoattraction, and sequestration of neutrophils in the pancreas, resulting in an intrapancreatic inflammatory reaction of variable severity. Neutrophil depletion induced by prior administration of an antineutrophil serum has been shown to reduce the severity of experimentally induced pancreatitis. There is also evidence to support the concept that neutrophil sequestration can activate trypsinogen. Thus, intrapancreatic acinar cell activation of trypsinogen could be a two-step process, i.e., with a neutrophil-independent and a neutrophil-dependent phase. The third phase of pancreatitis is due to the effects of activated proteolytic enzymes and cytokines, released by the inflamed pancreas, on distant organs. Activated proteolytic enzymes, especially trypsin, not only digest pancreatic and peripancreatic tissues but also activate other enzymes such as elastase and phospholipase. The active enzymes then digest cellular membranes and cause proteolysis, edema, interstitial hemorrhage, vascular damage, coagulation necrosis, fat necrosis, and parenchymal cell necrosis. Cellular injury and death result in the liberation of bradykinin peptides, vasoactive substances, and histamine that can produce vasodilation, increased vascular permeability, and edema with profound effects on many organs, most notably the lung. The

systemic inflammatory response syndrome (SIRS) and acute respiratory distress syndrome (ARDS) as well as multiorgan failure may occur as result of this cascade of local as well as distant effects.

The course of acute pancreatitis appears to be modified by genetic factors that can increase the susceptibility and/or modify the severity of pancreatic injury. Four susceptibility genes have been identified: (1) cationic trypsinogen mutations (PRSS1m, R122Hm, and N291), (2) pancreatic secretory trypsin inhibitor (SPINK1), (3) cystic fibrosis transmembrane conductance regulator (CFTR), and (4) monocyte chemotactic protein (MCP-1). Experimental and clinical data indicate that MCP-1 may be an important inflammatory mediator in the early pathologic process of acute pancreatitis, a determinant of the severity of the inflammatory response, and a promoter of organ failure. MCP-1 helps drive the inflammatory response after pancreatic injury. The MCP-1 2518 G allele polymorphism is a gain-of-function promoter that increases MCP-1 expression. In a recent study, 14 patients with severe pancreatitis all had elevated MCP-1 levels, with the mean value being eightfold greater than 116 controls and also eightfold greater than 63 patients with mild pancreatitis; 5 of the 14 died. The MCP-1 2518 G allele is a risk factor for severe acute pancreatitis. MCP-1 levels measured early in the course of acute pancreatitis appear to be an accurate predictor of severity and death.

APPROACH TO THE PATIENT:
Abdominal Pain

Abdominal pain is the major symptom of acute pancreatitis. Pain may vary from a mild and tolerable discomfort to severe, constant, and incapacitating distress. Characteristically, the pain, which is steady and boring in character, is located in the epigastrium and periumbilical region and often radiates to the back as well as to the chest, flanks, and lower abdomen. The pain is frequently more intense when the patient is supine, and patients often obtain relief by sitting with the trunk flexed and knees drawn up. Nausea, vomiting, and abdominal distention due to gastric and intestinal hypomotility and chemical peritonitis are also frequent complaints.

Physical examination frequently reveals a distressed and anxious patient. Low-grade fever, tachycardia, and hypotension are fairly common. Shock is not unusual and may result from (1) hypovolemia secondary to exudation of blood and plasma proteins into the retroperitoneal space (a "retroperitoneal burn"); (2) increased formation and release of kinin peptides, which cause vasodilation and increased vascular permeability; and (3) systemic effects of proteolytic and lipolytic enzymes released into the circulation. Jaundice occurs infrequently; when present, it usually is due to edema of the head of the pancreas with compression of the intrapancreatic portion of the common bile duct. Erythematous skin nodules due to subcutaneous fat necrosis may occur. In 10–20% of patients, there are pulmonary findings, including basilar rales, atelectasis, and pleural effusion, the latter most frequently left-sided. Abdominal tenderness and muscle rigidity are present to a variable degree, but, compared with the intense pain, these signs may be unimpressive. Bowel sounds are usually diminished or absent. An enlarged pancreas with organized necrosis or a pseudocyst may be palpable in the upper abdomen. A faint blue discoloration around the umbilicus (Cullen's sign) may occur as the result of hemoperitoneum, and a blue-red-purple or green-brown discoloration of the flanks (Turner's sign) reflects tissue catabolism of hemoglobin. The latter two findings, which are uncommon, indicate the presence of a severe necrotizing pancreatitis.

LABORATORY DATA

The diagnosis of acute pancreatitis is usually established by the detection of an increased level of serum amylase. Values threefold or more above normal virtually clinch the diagnosis if overt salivary gland disease and gut perforation or infarction are excluded. However, there appears to be no definite correlation between the severity of pancreatitis and the degree of serum amylase elevation. After 48–72 h, even with continuing evidence of pancreatitis, total serum amylase values tend to return to normal. However, pancreatic isoamylase and lipase levels

TABLE 307-2	RISK FACTORS THAT ADVERSELY AFFECT SURVIVAL IN ACUTE PANCREATITIS

Severe Acute Pancreatitis

1. Associated with organ failure and/or local complications such as necrosis
2. Clinical manifestations
   a. Obesity BMI > 30
   b. Hemoconcentration (hematocrit > 44%)
   c. Age > 70
3. Organ failure[a]
   a. Shock
   b. Pulmonary insufficiency (P_{O_2} < 60)
   c. Renal failure (CR > 2.0 mg%)
   d. GI bleeding
4. ≥ 3 Ransom criteria (not fully utilizable until 48 h)
5. Apache II score > 8 (cumbersome)

[a]Usually declares itself shortly after onset.

may remain elevated for 7–14 days. It will be recalled that amylase elevations in serum and urine occur in many conditions other than pancreatitis (Table 306-2). Importantly, patients with *acidemia* (arterial pH ≤ 7.32) may have spurious elevations in serum amylase. In one study, 12 of 33 patients with acidemia had elevated serum amylase, but only 1 had an elevated lipase value; in 9, salivary-type amylase was the predominant serum isoamylase. This finding explains why patients with diabetic ketoacidosis may have marked elevations in serum amylase without any other evidence of acute pancreatitis. Serum lipase activity increases in parallel with amylase activity. Measurement of both enzymes is important as serum amylase tends to be higher in gallstone pancreatitis and serum lipase higher in alcohol-associated pancreatitis. A threefold elevated serum lipase value is usually diagnostic of acute pancreatitis; these tests are especially helpful in patients with nonpancreatic causes of hyperamylasemia (Table 307-2). Markedly increased levels of peritoneal or pleural fluid amylase [>1500 nmol/L (>5000 U/dL)] are also helpful, if present, in establishing the diagnosis.

Leukocytosis (15,000–20,000 leukocytes per μL) occurs frequently. Patients with more severe disease may show hemoconcentration with hematocrit values >44% because of loss of plasma into the retroperitoneal space and peritoneal cavity. Hemoconcentration may be the harbinger of more severe disease, i.e., pancreatic necrosis. *Hyperglycemia* is common and is due to multiple factors, including decreased insulin release, increased glucagon release, and an increased output of adrenal glucocorticoids and catecholamines. *Hypocalcemia* occurs in ~25% of patients, and its pathogenesis is incompletely understood. Although earlier studies suggested that the response of the parathyroid gland to a decrease in serum calcium is impaired, subsequent observations have failed to confirm this idea. Intraperitoneal saponification of calcium by fatty acids in areas of fat necrosis occurs occasionally, with large amounts (up to 6.0 g) dissolved or suspended in ascitic fluid. Such "soap formation" may also be significant in patients with pancreatitis, mild hypocalcemia, and little or no obvious ascites. *Hyperbilirubinemia* [serum bilirubin > 68 μmol/L (>4.0 mg/dL)] occurs in ~10% of patients. However, jaundice is transient, and serum bilirubin levels return to normal in 4–7 days. Serum alkaline phosphatase and aspartate aminotransferase (AST) levels are also transiently elevated and parallel serum bilirubin values. Markedly elevated serum lactic dehydrogenase (LDH) levels [>8.5 μmol/L (>500 U/dL)] suggest a poor prognosis. Serum albumin is decreased to 30 g/L (3.0 g/dL) in ~10% of patients; this finding is associated with more severe pancreatitis and a higher mortality rate (Table 307-2). *Hypertriglyceridemia* occurs in 15 to 20% of patients, and serum amylase and lipase levels in these individuals are often spuriously normal (Chap. 306). Approximately 25% of patients have *hypoxemia* (arterial P_{O_2} ≤ 60 mmHg), which may herald the onset of ARDS. Finally, the electrocardiogram is occasionally abnormal in acute pancreatitis with ST-segment and T-wave abnormalities simulating myocardial ischemia.

A CT scan can confirm the clinical impression of acute pancreatitis even in the face of normal serum amylase levels. Importantly, CT is quite helpful in indicating the severity of acute pancreatitis and the risk of morbidity and mortality and in evaluating the complications of acute pancreatitis (see below). Sonography is useful in acute pancreatitis to evaluate the gallbladder. Radiologic studies useful in the diagnosis of acute pancreatitis are discussed in Chap. 306 and listed in Table 306-1.

DIAGNOSIS

Any severe acute pain in the abdomen or back should suggest acute pancreatitis. The diagnosis is usually entertained when a patient with a possible predisposition to pancreatitis presents with severe and constant abdominal pain, nausea, emesis, fever, tachycardia, and abnormal findings on abdominal examination. Laboratory studies frequently reveal leukocytosis, hypocalcemia, and hyperglycemia. The diagnosis is usually confirmed by the finding of a threefold or greater elevated level of serum amylase and/or lipase. Not all the above features have to be present for the diagnosis to be established. Strong indicators include hemoconcentration (hematocrit > 44%) and signs of organ failure (Table 307-2).

The *differential diagnosis* should include the following disorders: (1) perforated viscus, especially peptic ulcer; (2) acute cholecystitis and biliary colic; (3) acute intestinal obstruction; (4) mesenteric vascular occlusion; (5) renal colic; (6) myocardial infarction; (7) dissecting aortic aneurysm; (8) connective tissue disorders with vasculitis; (9) pneumonia; and (10) diabetic ketoacidosis. A penetrating duodenal ulcer can usually be identified by imaging studies or endoscopy. A perforated duodenal ulcer is readily diagnosed by the presence of free intraperitoneal air. It may be difficult to differentiate acute cholecystitis from acute pancreatitis, since an elevated serum amylase may be found in both disorders. Pain of biliary tract origin is more right-sided or epigastric than periumbilical and is gradual in onset; ileus is usually absent. Sonography and radionuclide scanning are helpful in establishing the diagnosis of cholelithiasis and cholecystitis. Intestinal obstruction due to mechanical factors can be differentiated from pancreatitis by the history of colicky pain, findings on abdominal examination, and x-rays of the abdomen showing changes characteristic of mechanical obstruction. Acute mesenteric vascular occlusion is usually evident in elderly debilitated patients with brisk leukocytosis, abdominal distention, and bloody diarrhea, in whom paracentesis shows sanguineous fluid and angiography shows vascular occlusion. Serum as well as peritoneal fluid amylase levels are increased, however, in patients with intestinal infarction. Systemic lupus erythematosus and polyarteritis nodosa may be confused with pancreatitis, especially since pancreatitis may develop as a complication of these diseases. Diabetic ketoacidosis is often accompanied by abdominal pain and elevated total serum amylase levels, thus closely mimicking acute pancreatitis. However, the serum lipase level is not elevated in diabetic ketoacidosis.

COURSE OF THE DISEASE AND COMPLICATIONS

It is important to identify patients with acute pancreatitis who have an increased risk of dying. Multiple factor scoring systems (Ranson, Imrie, Apache II) are difficult to use, show poor predictive powers, and have not been uniformly embraced by clinicians. The key indicators of a severe attack of pancreatitis are listed in Table 307-2 and include age > 70 years, body mass index (BMI) > 30, hematocrit > 44%, and admission C-reactive protein > 150 mg/L. However, it is organ failure, in which respiratory failure (P_{O_2} < 60 mmHg) dominates, that determines outcome in the majority of difficult to manage cases. The presence of shock (systolic blood pressure < 90 mmHg or tachycardia > 130), renal failure [serum creatinine > 177 μmol/L (>2.0 mg/dL)], and gastrointestinal bleeding (>500 mL/24 h) are also key factors. The high mortality rate of such severely ill patients is due in large part to multiorgan failure, especially during the first week, and warrants intensive monitoring and/or a combination of radiologic and surgical means, as discussed in detail below.

The local and systemic complications of acute pancreatitis are listed in Table 307-3. In the first 2–3 weeks after pancreatitis, patients frequently develop an inflammatory mass, which may be due to organized pancreatic necrosis (with or without infection) or a pseudocyst. Pancreatic abscess develops later, i.e., usually after 6 weeks. Systemic

TABLE 307-3 COMPLICATIONS OF ACUTE PANCREATITIS

Local

Necrosis	Pancreatic ascites
Sterile	Disruption of main pancreatic
Infected	duct
Organized	Leaking pseudocyst
Pancreatic fluid collections	Involvement of contiguous organs
Pancreatic abscess	by necrotizing pancreatitis
Pancreatic pseudocyst	Massive intraperitoneal
Pain	hemorrhage
Rupture	Thrombosis of blood vessels
Hemorrhage	(splenic vein, portal vein)
Infection	Bowel infarction
Obstruction of gastrointestinal	Obstructive jaundice
tract (stomach, duodenum,	
colon)	

Systemic

Pulmonary	Renal
Pleural effusion	Oliguria
Atelectasis	Azotemia
Mediastinal abscess	Renal artery and/or renal vein
Pneumonitis	thrombosis
Adult respiratory distress syndrome	Acute tubular necrosis
Cardiovascular	Metabolic
Hypotension	Hyperglycemia
Hypovolemia	Hypertriglyceridemia
Sudden death	Hypocalcemia
Nonspecific ST-T changes in elec-	Encephalopathy
trocardiogram simulating myo-	Sudden blindness (Purtscher's
cardial infarction	retinopathy)
Pericardial effusion	Central nervous system
Hematologic	Psychosis
Disseminated intravascular	Fat emboli
coagulation	Fat necrosis
Gastrointestinal hemorrhage	Subcutaneous tissues
Peptic ulcer disease	(erythematous nodules)
Erosive gastritis	Bone
Hemorrhagic pancreatic necrosis	Miscellaneous (mediastinum,
with erosion into major blood	pleura, nervous system)
vessels	
Portal vein thrombosis, variceal	
hemorrhage	

complications include pulmonary, cardiovascular, hematologic, renal, metabolic, and central nervous system abnormalities. Pancreatitis and hypertriglyceridemia constitute an association in which cause and effect remain incompletely understood. However, several reasonable conclusions can be drawn. First, hypertriglyceridemia can precede and apparently cause pancreatitis. Second, the vast majority (>80%) of patients with acute pancreatitis do not have hypertriglyceridemia. Third, almost all patients with pancreatitis and hypertriglyceridemia have preexisting abnormalities in lipoprotein metabolism. Fourth, many of the patients with this association have persistent hypertriglyceridemia after recovery from pancreatitis and are prone to recurrent episodes of pancreatitis. Fifth, any factor (e.g., drugs or alcohol) that causes an abrupt increase in serum triglycerides to levels >11 mmol/L (1000 mg/dL) can precipitate a bout of pancreatitis that can be associated with significant complications and even become fulminant. To avert the risk of triggering pancreatitis, a fasting serum triglyceride measurement should be obtained before estrogen replacement therapy is begun in postmenopausal women. Fasting levels < 3.4 mmol/L (300 mg/dL) pose no risk, whereas levels > 8.5 mmol/L (750 mg/dL) are associated with a high probability of developing pancreatitis. Finally, patients with a deficiency of apolipoprotein CII have an increased incidence of pancreatitis; apolipoprotein CII activates lipoprotein lipase, which is important in clearing chylomicrons from the bloodstream.

Purtscher's retinopathy, a relatively unusual complication, is manifested by a sudden and severe loss of vision in a patient with acute pancreatitis. It is characterized by a peculiar funduscopic appearance with cotton-wool spots and hemorrhages confined to an area limited by the optic disk and macula; it is believed to be due to occlusion of the posterior retinal artery with aggregated granulocytes.

The two most common causes of acute pancreatitis are biliary tract disease and alcoholism; other causes are listed in Table 307-1. The risk of acute pancreatitis in patients with at least one gallstone <5 mm in diameter is fourfold greater than that in patients with larger stones. However, after a conventional workup, a specific cause is not identified in ~30% of patients.

In one series of 31 patients diagnosed initially as having idiopathic acute pancreatitis, 23 were found to have occult gallstone disease. Thus, approximately two-thirds of patients with recurrent acute pancreatitis without an obvious cause actually have occult gallstone disease due to microlithiasis. Other diseases of the biliary tree and pancreatic ducts that can cause acute pancreatitis include choledochocele; ampullary tumors; pancreas divisum; and pancreatic duct stones, stricture, and tumor. Approximately 2–4% of patients with pancreatic carcinoma present with acute pancreatitis.

Recurrent Pancreatitis Approximately 25% of patients who have had an attack of acute pancreatitis have a recurrence. The two most common etiologic factors are alcohol and cholelithiasis. In patients with recurrent pancreatitis without an obvious cause the differential diagnosis should encompass occult biliary tract disease including microlithiasis, hypertriglyceridemia, drugs, pancreatic cancer, sphincter of Oddi dysfunction, pancreas divisum, cystic fibrosis, and pancreatic cancer (Table 307-1).

Pancreatitis in Patients with AIDS The incidence of acute pancreatitis is increased in patients with AIDS for two reasons: (1) the high incidence of infections involving the pancreas, such as infections with cytomegalovirus, *Cryptosporidium*, and the *Mycobacterium avium* complex; and (2) the frequent use by patients with AIDS of medications such as didanosine, pentamidine, trimethoprim-sulfamethoxazole, and protease inhibitors (Chap. 182).

℞ ACUTE PANCREATITIS

In most patients (85–90%) with acute pancreatitis, the disease is self-limited and subsides spontaneously, usually within 3–7 days after treatment is instituted. Conventional measures include (1) analgesics for pain, (2) IV fluids and colloids to maintain normal intravascular volume, and (3) no oral alimentation. Controlled trials have shown that nasogastric suction offers no clear-cut advantages in the treatment of mild to moderately severe acute pancreatitis. Its use, therefore, must be considered elective rather than mandatory.

It has been demonstrated that CCK-stimulated pancreatic secretion is almost abolished in four different experimental models of acute pancreatitis. This finding probably explains why drugs to block pancreatic secretion in acute pancreatitis have failed to have any therapeutic benefit. For this and other reasons, anticholinergic drugs are not indicated in acute pancreatitis. In addition to nasogastric suction and anticholinergic drugs, other therapies designed to "rest the pancreas" by inhibiting pancreatic secretion have not changed the course of the disease.

ROLE OF ANTIBIOTICS The benefit of antibiotic prophylaxis in the treatment of necrotizing acute pancreatitis remains controversial. A Cochrane database review of four randomized controlled trials (218 patients) compared antibiotic therapy with supportive medical treatment. Antibiotic prophylaxis reduced all-cause mortality from 17% to 6% and pancreatic sepsis from 32% to 21%, but did not differ from supportive therapy for rates of extrapancreatic infection, operative treatment, fungal infection, or length of hospital stay. However, none of the four studies were double blind and they varied in case mix and in choice and duration of antibiotic treatment.

A recent double-blind placebo-controlled trial investigated the effect of ciprofloxacin and metronidazole on the course and outcome of 114 patients with predicted severe acute pancreatitis. Although there were fewer multiorgan failure and extrapancreatic infections in the antibiotic treated group, this study detected no benefit of antibiotic prophylaxis with regard to the risk of developing infected pancreatic necrosis. However, the high crossover rate to antibiotic therapy in 21 of 56 patients in the placebo group may have contributed to the negative results.

Although the optimal drugs and duration of therapy remain incompletely defined, the current recommendation in patients with necrotizing acute pancreatitis is the use of a systemic antibiotic such as imipenem cilastin, 500 mg thrice daily for 7 days.

Intraabdominal *Candida* infection during acute necrotizing pancreatitis is increasing in frequency and is associated with increased use of antibiotics. In one representative trial, intraabdominal *Candida* infection was found in 13 of 37 cases and was associated with a mortality rate fourfold greater than that associated with intraabdominal bacterial infection alone. Given the impact of *Candida* infection on the mortality rate in acute necrotizing pancreatitis and the apparent benefit of prophylactic antibiotics, these data suggest earlier use of fungicides.

Several other drugs have been evaluated by prospective controlled trials and found ineffective in the treatment of acute pancreatitis. The list, by no means complete, includes glucagon, H_2 blockers, protease inhibitors such as aprotinin, glucocorticoids, calcitonin, nonsteroidal anti-inflammatory drugs (NSAIDs), and lexipafant, a platelet-activating factor inhibitor. A recent meta-analysis of somatostatin, octreotide, and the antiprotease gabexate mesylate in therapy of acute pancreatitis suggested (1) a reduced mortality rate but no change in complications with octreotide, and (2) no effect on the mortality rate but reduced pancreatic damage with gabexate.

A CT scan, especially a dynamic contrast-enhanced CT (CECT) scan, provides valuable information on the severity and prognosis of acute pancreatitis **(Fig. 307-1)**. In particular, a CECT scan allows estimation of the presence and extent of pancreatic necrosis. Recent studies suggest that the likelihood of prolonged pancreatitis or a serious complication is negligible when the CT severity index is 1 or 2 and low with scores of 3–6. However, patients with scores of 7–10 had a 92% morbidity rate and a 17% mortality rate. Necrosis is present in 12–20% of patients with acute pancreatitis. Those with necrosis have a morbidity rate of 50% and mortality rate of 20%, whereas those without necrosis have a morbidity rate <10% and a negligible mortality rate. A few retrospective studies have raised concern that the use of IV contrast early in the course of acute pancreatitis might intensify pancreatic necrosis. However, since prospective human studies are not available, it is reasonable to reserve CECT scans for patients with severe pancreatitis or suspected local septic complications.

The patient with mild to moderate pancreatitis usually requires treatment with IV fluids and fasting. A clear liquid diet is frequently started on the third to sixth day and a regular diet by the fifth to seventh day. The decision to reintroduce oral intake is usually based on the following criteria: (1) a decrease in or resolution of abdominal pain; (2) the patient is hungry;

and (3) organ dysfunction, if present, has resolved. Elevation of serum amylase/lipase or persistent inflammatory changes seen on CT scans should not discourage feeding a hungry asymptomatic patient. In this regard, persistence of inflammatory changes on CT scans or persistent elevations in serum amylase/lipase may not resolve for weeks to months. The patient with unremitting *fulminant pancreatitis* usually requires inordinate amounts of fluid and close attention to complications such as cardiovascular collapse, respiratory insufficiency, and pancreatic infection. The latter should be managed by a combination of radiologic and surgical means (see below). While earlier uncontrolled studies suggested that *peritoneal lavage* through a percutaneous dialysis catheter was helpful in severe pancreatitis, subsequent studies indicate that this treatment does not influence the outcome of such attacks. Aggressive surgical pancreatic debridement (necrosectomy) should be undertaken soon after confirmation of the presence of infected necrosis, and multiple operations may be required. Since the mortality rate from sterile acute necrotizing pancreatitis is ~10%, laparotomy with adequate drainage and removal of necrotic tissue should be considered if conventional therapy does not halt the patient's deterioration. The use of total parenteral nutrition (TPN) makes it possible to give nutritional support to patients with severe, acute, or protracted pancreatitis who are unable to eat normally. It has been suggested that enteral feeding with a nasojejunal tube may be preferred over TPN because of decreased infection. Less expensive enteral feeds meet approximately only 50% of nutritional needs, whereas TPN meets 90% of those needs. There are no large, well-controlled trials comparing enteral feeds to TPN in patients with severe acute pancreatitis. Only a small percentage of patients with acute pancreatitis need hyperalimentation.

Patients with severe gallstone-induced pancreatitis may improve dramatically if papillotomy is carried out within the first 36–72 h of the attack. Studies indicate that only those patients with gallstone pancreatitis who are in the very severe group should be considered for urgent ERCP. Finally, the treatment for patients with hypertriglyceridemia-associated pancreatitis includes (1) weight loss to ideal weight, (2) a lipid-restricted diet, (3) exercise, (4) avoidance of alcohol and of drugs that can elevate serum triglycerides (i.e., estrogens, vitamin A, thiazides, and propanolol), and (5) control of diabetes.

INFECTED PANCREATIC NECROSIS, ABSCESS, AND PSEUDOCYST

Infected pancreatic necrosis should be differentiated from pancreatic abscess. The former is a diffuse infection of an acutely inflamed, ne-

A

B

FIGURE 307-1 Acute pancreatitis: CT evolution. *A.* Contrast-enhanced CT scan of the abdomen performed on admission of a patient with clinical evidence of acute pancreatitis. Note the mildly decreased density of the body of the pancreas to the left of the midline (*arrow*). There are a few linear strands in the peripancreatic fat, suggesting inflammation (*open arrows*). A small amount of fluid is seen in the anterior pararenal space (*arrowhead*). ***B.*** Nine days after admission, there is a marked worsening with severe inflammation of the pancreas evidenced by anterior displacement of the posterior gastric wall (*arrows*), increased inflammation of the peripancreatic fat, and increased pancreatic effusion in the anterior perirenal space and around the splenic vein (*open arrows*). (*Courtesy of Dr. PR Ros, University of Florida College of Medicine; with permission.*)

crotic pancreas occurring most often in the first 2–4 weeks after the onset of pancreatitis. In contrast, a pancreatic abscess is an ill-defined, liquid collection of pus that evolves over a longer period, often 4–6 weeks. It tends to be less life-threatening and is associated with a lower rate of surgical mortality. Infected pancreatic necrosis should be treated by surgical debridement because the solid component of the infected pancreas is not amenable to effective radiologically guided percutaneous evacuation. Pancreatic abscess can be treated surgically or, in selected cases, by percutaneous drainage. The necrotic pancreas becomes secondarily infected in 20–35% of patients, most frequently with gram-negative bacteria of alimentary origin. Whether infection occurs depends on several factors, including the extent of pancreatic and peripancreatic necrosis, the degree of pancreatic ischemia and hypoperfusion, and the presence of organ or multiorgan failure.

The early diagnosis of pancreatic infection can be accomplished by CT-guided needle aspiration. In one study, 60 patients, representing 5% of all admissions for acute pancreatitis, were suspected of harboring a pancreatic infection on the basis of fever, leukocytosis, and an abnormal CT scan (pseudocyst or extrapancreatic fluid collection). Importantly, 60% of these patients had a pancreatic infection, and 55% of these infections developed in the first 3 weeks. These findings suggest that only guided aspiration can reliably distinguish sterile from infected pancreatic necrosis. The following are guidelines for patients meeting the above selection criteria: (1) Pseudocysts should be aspirated promptly in seriously ill patients because more than half may be infected, whereas asymptomatic pseudocysts need not be; (2) extrapancreatic fluid collections need not be aspirated promptly, because most are sterile; (3) if a necrotic pancreas is found initially to be sterile but fever and leukocytosis persist, 5–7 days of observation should be allowed to pass before reaspiration is considered, as clinical improvement frequently occurs; and (4) if fever and leukocytosis recur after an interval of well-being, reaspiration should be considered.

Severe pancreatitis with the presence of key risk factors, postoperative pancreatitis, early oral feeding, early laparotomy, and perhaps injudicious use of antibiotics predispose to the development of pancreatic abscess, which occurs in 3–4% of patients with acute pancreatitis. Pancreatic abscess may also develop because of a communication between a pseudocyst and the colon, inadequate surgical drainage of a pseudocyst, or needling of a pseudocyst. The characteristic signs of abscess are fever, leukocytosis, ileus, and rapid deterioration in a patient previously recovering from pancreatitis. Sometimes, however, the only manifestations are persistent fever and signs of continuing pancreatic inflammation. Drainage of pancreatic abscesses (now seen less frequently) by percutaneous techniques, using CT guidance, has been frequently successful with resolution in 50–60% of patients. Laparotomy with radical sump drainage and possibly resection of necrotic tissue are occasionally required.

Pseudocysts of the pancreas are collections of tissue, fluid, debris, pancreatic enzymes, and blood that develop over a period of 4–6 weeks after the onset of acute pancreatitis; they form in ~15% of patients with acute pancreatitis. In contrast to true cysts, pseudocysts do not have an epithelial lining; their walls consist of necrotic tissue, granulation tissue, and fibrous tissue. Many lesions that have the imaging appearance of a pseudocyst are actually organized necrosis. Disruption of the pancreatic ductal system is common. However, the subsequent course of this disruption varies widely, ranging from spontaneous healing to continuous leakage of pancreatic juice, which results in tense ascites. Pseudocysts are preceded by pancreatitis in 90% of cases and by trauma in 10%. Approximately 85% are located in the body or tail of the pancreas and 15% in the head. Some patients have two or more pseudocysts. Abdominal pain, with or without radiation to the back, is the usual presenting complaint. A palpable, tender mass may be found in the middle or left upper abdomen. The serum amylase level is elevated in 75% of patients at some point during their illness and may fluctuate markedly.

On x-ray examination, 75% of pseudocysts can be seen to displace some portion of the gastrointestinal tract (Fig. 307-2). Sonography, however, is reliable in detecting pseudocysts. Sonography also permits differentiation between an edematous, inflamed pancreas, which can give rise to a palpable mass, and an actual pseudocyst. Furthermore, se-

rial ultrasound studies will indicate whether a pseudocyst has resolved. CT complements ultrasonography in the diagnosis of pancreatic pseudocyst (Fig. 307-2), especially when the pseudocyst is infected.

In earlier studies with sonography, pseudocysts were seen to resolve in 25–40% of patients. Pseudocysts that are >5 cm in diameter may persist for >6 weeks. Recent natural history studies have suggested that noninterventional, expectant management is the best course in selected patients with minimal symptoms and no evidence of active alcohol use in whom the pseudocyst appears mature by radiography and does not resemble a cystic neoplasm. A significant number of these pseudocysts resolve spontaneously >6 weeks after their formation. Also, these studies demonstrate that large pseudocyst size is not an absolute indication for interventional therapy and that many peripancreatic fluid collections detected on CT in cases of acute pancreatitis resolve spontaneously. A pseudocyst that does not resolve spontaneously may lead to serious complications, such as (1) pain caused by expansion of the lesion and pressure on other viscera, (2) rupture, (3) hemorrhage, and (4) abscess. Rupture of a pancreatic pseudocyst is a particularly serious complication. Shock almost always supervenes, and mortality rates range from 14% if the rupture is not associated with hemorrhage to >60% if hemorrhage has occurred. Rupture and hemorrhage are the prime causes of death from pancreatic pseudocyst. A triad of findings—an increase in the size of the mass, a localized bruit over the mass, and a sudden decrease in hemoglobin level and hematocrit without obvious external blood loss—should alert one to the possibility of hemorrhage from a pseudocyst. Thus, in patients who are stable and free of complications and in whom serial ultrasound studies show that the pseudocyst is shrinking, conservative therapy is indicated. Conversely, if the pseudocyst is expanding and is complicated by rupture, hemorrhage, or abscess, the patient should be operated on. With ultrasound or CT guidance, sterile chronic pseudocysts can be treated safely with single or repeated needle aspiration or more prolonged catheter drainage with a success rate of 45–75%. The success rate of these techniques for infected pseudocysts is considerably less (40–50%). Patients who do not respond to drainage require surgical therapy for internal or external drainage of the cyst.

Pseudoaneurysms develop in up to 10% of patients with acute pancreatitis at sites reflecting the distribution of pseudocysts and fluid collections (Fig. 307-2D). The splenic artery is most frequently involved, followed by the inferior and superior pancreatic duodenal arteries. This diagnosis should be suspected in patients with pancreatitis who develop upper gastrointestinal bleeding without an obvious cause or in whom thin-cut CT scanning reveals a contrast-enhanced lesion within or adjacent to a suspected pseudocyst. Arteriography is necessary to confirm the diagnosis and allow treatment.

PANCREATIC ASCITES AND PANCREATIC PLEURAL EFFUSIONS

Pancreatic ascites is usually due to disruption of the main pancreatic duct, often by an internal fistula between the duct and the peritoneal cavity or a leaking pseudocyst (Chap. 44). This diagnosis is suggested in a patient with an elevated serum amylase level in whom the ascites fluid has both increased levels of albumin [>30 g/L (>3.0 g/dL)] and a markedly elevated level of amylase. The fluid in true pancreatic ascites usually has an amylase concentration of >20,000 U/L as a result of the ruptured duct or leaking pseudocyst. Lower amylase elevations may be found in the peritoneal fluid of patients with acute pancreatitis. In addition, ERCP often demonstrates passage of contrast material from a major pancreatic duct or a pseudocyst into the peritoneal cavity. As many as 15% of patients with pseudocysts have concurrent pancreatic ascites. The differential diagnosis should include intraperitoneal carcinomatosis, tuberculous peritonitis, constrictive pericarditis, and Budd-Chiari syndrome.

℞ PANCREATIC ASCITES AND PANCREATIC PLEURAL EFFUSIONS

If the pancreatic duct disruption is posterior, an internal fistula may develop between the pancreatic duct and the pleural space, producing a pleu-

A

B

C

D

FIGURE 307-2 Pseudocyst of pancreas. A. Upper gastrointestinal x-ray showing displacement of stomach by pseudocyst. **B.** Sonogram showing pseudocyst (*cyst*). GB, gallbladder; MPV, portal vein. Behind the large pseudocyst is seen the calcified head of the pancreas. A dilated common bile duct (*asterisk*) is noted. **C.** CT scan showing pseudocyst. Note the large, lobulated fluid collection (*arrows*) surrounding the tail of the pancreas (*arrowheads*). Note also the dense, thin rim in the periphery representing the fibrous capsule of the pseudocyst. **D.** Spiral CT showing a pseudocyst (*small arrow*) with a pseudoaneurysm (light area in pseudocyst). Note the demonstration of the main pancreatic duct (*big arrow*), even though this duct is minimally dilated by ERCP. (*A, B, courtesy of Dr. CE Forsmark, University of Florida College of Medicine; C, D, courtesy of Dr. PR Ros, University of Florida College of Medicine; with permission.*)

ral effusion, which is usually left-sided and often massive. This complication is best treated by ERCP and stent placement and infrequently requires thoracentesis or chest tube drainage. If the pancreatic duct disruption is anterior, amylase- and lipase-rich peritoneal fluid accumulate. ERCP and stenting are the preferred initial approach.

Treatment may require nasogastric suction and parenteral alimentation to decrease pancreatic secretion. In addition, paracentesis may be necessary to keep the peritoneal cavity free of fluid and, it is hoped, to effect sealing of the leak. The long-acting somatostatin analogue octreotide, which inhibits pancreatic secretion, is useful in cases of pancreatic ascites and pleural effusion. If ascites continues to recur after 2–3 weeks of medical management, the patient should be operated on after pancreatography to define the anatomy of the abnormal duct. Patients in whom ERCP identifies two or more sites of extravasation are unlikely to respond to conservative management and/or stenting.

CHRONIC PANCREATITIS AND PANCREATIC EXOCRINE INSUFFICIENCY

PATHOPHYSIOLOGY

Chronic pancreatitis is a disease process characterized by irreversible damage to the pancreas as distinct from the reversible changes noted in acute pancreatitis. The condition is best defined by the presence of histologic abnormalities, including chronic inflammation, fibrosis, and progressive destruction of both exocrine and eventually endocrine tissue. A number of etiologies may result in chronic pancreatitis, but all may ultimately lead to irreversible morphologic damage to the pancreas, and these etiologies may produce the cardinal complications of chronic pancreatitis such as abdominal pain, steatorrhea, and diabetes mellitus.

The events that initiate the inflammatory process in the pancreas are still not well understood. Current experimental and clinical observations have shown that alcohol has a direct toxic effect on the pancreas. While patients with alcohol-induced pancreatitis generally consume large amounts of alcohol, some consume very little, as little as ≤ 50 g/d. Prolonged consumption of socially acceptable amounts of alcohol is compatible with the development of chronic pancreatitis. Findings of extensive pancreatic fibrosis in patients who died during their first attack of clinical acute alcohol-induced pancreatitis support the concept that such patients already have chronic pancreatitis.

The biochemical and molecular mechanisms that may be important to the pathogenesis of chronic pancreatitis continue to be explored. Overexpression of fibroblasts and growth factors in tissue in patients with chronic pancreatitis has been reported. High levels of transforming growth factor α and its receptor protein epidermal growth factor have been documented in patients with chronic pancreatitis. It is yet to be determined whether these observations are truly relevant in the pathogenesis of chronic pancreatitis.

ETIOLOGIC CONSIDERATIONS

Among adults in the United States, alcoholism is the most common cause of clinically apparent chronic pancreatitis, while cystic fibrosis is the most frequent cause in children. In up to 25% of adults in the United States with chronic pancreatitis, the cause is not known. That is, they are labeled as *idiopathic chronic pancreatitis*. Recent investigations have indicated that up to 15% of patients with idiopathic pancreatitis may have pancreatitis due to genetic defects (Table 307-4).

Whitcomb and associates studied several large families with hereditary chronic pancreatitis and were able to identify a genetic defect that affects the gene encoding for trypsinogen. Several additional defects of this gene have also been described. The defect allows trypsinogen to be resistant to the effect of trypsin inhibitor, become spontaneously activated, and to remain activated. It is hypothesized that this continual activation of digestive enzymes within the gland leads to acute injury and, finally, chronic pancreatitis. This group of investigators has also reported that a second form of hereditary chronic pancreatitis tends to present later, has a female predominance, and frequently leads to chronic pancreatitis.

Several other groups of investigators have documented mutations of *CFTR*. This gene functions as a cyclic AMP–regulated chloride channel. In patients with cystic fibrosis, the high concentration of macromolecules can block the pancreatic ducts. It must be appreciated, however, that there is a great deal of heterogeneity in relationship to the *CFTR* gene defect. More than 1000 putative mutations of the *CFTR* gene have been identified. Attempts to elucidate the relationship between the genotype and pancreatic manifestations have been hampered by the number of mutations. The ability to detect *CFTR* mutations has led to the recognition that the clinical spectrum of the disease is broader than previously thought. Two recent studies have clarified the association between mutations of the *CFTR* gene and another monosymptomatic form of cystic fibrosis, i.e., chronic pancreatitis. It is estimated that in patients with idiopathic pancreatitis, the frequency of a single *CFTR* mutation is 11 times the expected frequency and the frequency of two mutant alleles is 80 times the expected frequency. In these studies, the patients were adults when the diagnosis of pancreatitis was made; none had any clinical evidence of pulmonary disease, and sweat test results were not diagnostic of cystic fibrosis. The prevalence of such mutations is unclear, and further studies are certainly needed. In addition, the therapeutic and prognostic implication of these findings with respect to managing pancreatitis remains to be determined. Long-term follow-up of affected patients is needed. *CFTR* mutations are common in the general population. It is unclear whether the *CFTR* mutation alone can lead to pancreatitis as an autosomal recessive disease. A recent study evaluated 39 patients with idiopathic chronic pancreatitis to assess the risk associated with these mutations. Patients with two *CFTR* mutations (compound heterozygotes) demonstrated *CFTR* function at a level between that seen in typical cystic fibrosis and cystic fibrosis carriers and had a 40-fold increased risk of pancreatitis. The presence of an *N34S SPINK1* mutation increased the risk 20-fold. A combination of two *CFTR* mutations and an *N34S SPINK1* mutation increased the risk of pancreatitis 900-fold. Table 307-4 lists recognized causes of chronic pancreatitis and pancreatic exocrine insufficiency.

AUTOIMMUNE PANCREATITIS

Autoimmune pancreatitis (AIP) is an increasingly recognized disorder of presumed autoimmune etiology that is associated with characteristic clinical, histologic, and morphologic findings (Table 307-5). It has been referred to by a variety of names including *sclerosing pancreatitis*, *tumefactive pancreatitis*, and *nonalcoholic destructive pancreatitis* depending, in part, upon the specific pathologic findings and the presence of extrapancreatic manifestations. However, it is generally believed that the pathologic heterogeneity may reflect different stages or manifestations of the same disease.

Clinical Features of Chronic Pancreatitis   Patients with chronic pancreatitis seek medical attention predominantly because of two symptoms:

TABLE 307-4	CHRONIC PANCREATITIS AND PANCREATIC EXOCRINE INSUFFICIENCY: TIGAR-O CLASSIFICATION SYSTEM
Toxic-metabolic	**Autoimmune**
Alcoholic	Isolated autoimmune CP
Tobacco smoking	Autoimmune CP associated with
Hypercalcemia	Sjögren's syndrome
Hyperlipidemia	Inflammatory bowel disease
Chronic renal failure	Primary biliary cirrhosis
Medications—phenacetin	
abuse	**Recurrent and severe acute**
Toxins—organotin	**pancreatitis**
compounds	Postnecrotic (severe acute pancreatitis)
(e.g., DBTC)	Recurrent acute pancreatitis
	Vascular diseases/ischemia
Idiopathic	Postirradiation
Early onset	
Late onset	**Obstructive**
Tropical	Pancreas divisum
	Sphincter of Oddi disorders
Genetic	(controversial)
Hereditary pancreatitis	Duct obstruction (e.g., tumor)
Cationic trypsinogen	Preampullary duodenal wall cysts
CFTR mutations	Posttraumatic pancreatic duct scars
SPINK1 mutations	

CP, chronic pancreatitis; TIGAR-O, toxic-metabolic, idiopathic, genetic, autoimmune, recurrent and severe acute pancreatitis, obstructive.

TABLE 307-5	CLINICAL FEATURES OF AUTOIMMUNE PANCREATITIS (AIP)

- Mild symptoms usually abdominal pain, but without frequent attacks of pancreatitis, which are unusual
- Presentation with obstructive jaundice
- Diffuse swelling and enlargement of the pancreas, especially the head, the latter mimicking carcinoma of the pancreas
- Diffuse irregular narrowing of the pancreatic duct in ERCP
- Increased levels of serum gamma globulins especially IgG₄
- Presence of other auto-antibodies (ANA), rheumatoid factor (RF)
- Can occur with other autoimmune diseases Sjögren's syndrome, PSC, UC, rheumatoid arthritis
- Extra pancreatic bile duct changes such as stricture of the common bile duct and intrahepatic ducts
- Absence of pancreatic calcifications or cysts
- Pancreatic biopsies reveal extensive fibrosis and lymphoplasmacytic infiltration
- Glucocorticoids are effective in alleviating symptoms, decreasing size of the pancreas, and reversing histopathologic changes
- ⅔ of patients present with either obstructive jaundice or a "mass" in the head of the pancreas mimicking carcinoma

TABLE 307-6 LARGE DUCT VERSUS SMALL DUCT CHRONIC PANCREATITIS

	Large Duct	Small Duct
Sex Predominance	Male	Female
Diagnostic Tests		
Secretin test	Abnormal	Abnormal
Serum trypsinogen	Often abnormal	Usually normal
Fecal elastase	Often abnormal	Usually normal
Pancreatic calcification on plain film of the abdomen	Frequent	Infrequent
ERCP	Often markedly abnormal	Minimally abnormal to normal
Natural History		
Progression to steatorrhea	Frequent	Rare
Therapy of pain		
Pancreatic enzymes	Poor response	Good to excellent response
Surgical procedures	Sometimes helpful	Not usually indicated

abdominal pain or maldigestion. The abdominal pain may be quite variable in location, severity, and frequency. The pain can be constant or intermittent with frequent pain-free intervals. Eating may exacerbate the pain, leading to a fear of eating with consequent weight loss. The spectrum of abdominal pain ranges from mild to quite severe with narcotic dependence as a frequent consequence. Maldigestion is manifested as chronic diarrhea, steatorrhea, weight loss, and fatigue. Patients with abdominal pain may or may not progress to maldigestion, and ~20% of patients will present with symptoms of maldigestion without a history of abdominal pain. Patients with chronic pancreatitis have significant morbidity and mortality and utilize appreciable amounts of societal resources. Despite the steatorrhea, clinically apparent deficiencies of fat-soluble vitamins are surprisingly uncommon. Physical findings in these patients are usually unimpressive so that there is a disparity between the severity of abdominal pain and the physical signs, which usually consist of some mild tenderness and mild temperature elevation.

It is helpful to differentiate chronic pancreatitis into its different forms. One obvious demarcation is whether the patient has small-duct or large-duct disease. Table 307-6 describes features that distinguish between these two kinds of pancreatitis. The pathogenesis, diagnostic approach, clinical course, and treatment results vary greatly between these two forms of chronic pancreatitis. In contrast to acute pancreatitis, the serum amylase and lipase levels are usually not elevated in chronic pancreatitis. Elevation of serum bilirubin and alkaline phosphatase may indicate cholestasis secondary to chronic inflammation and/or stricture around the common bile duct. Many patients have impaired glucose tolerance with elevated fasting blood glucose levels. The diagnostic test with the best sensitivity and specificity is the hormone stimulation test utilizing secretin. It becomes abnormal when ≥ 60% of the pancreatic exocrine function has been lost. This usually correlates well with the onset of chronic abdominal pain. Approximately 40% of patients with chronic pancreatitis have cobalamin (vitamin B_{12}) malabsorption. This can be corrected by the administration of oral pancreatic enzymes. The serum trypsinogen and D-xylose excretion tests are useful in patients with pancreatic steatorrhea. The trypsinogen level will be abnormal and the D-xylose excretion usually normal in such patients. A decrease of serum trypsinogen level to <20 mg/mL strongly suggests severe pancreatic exocrine insufficiency, as does a fecal elastase of <100 µg per gram of stool.

Utilizing radiographic techniques (Figs. 307-3 and 307-4), it can be shown that diffuse calcifications noted on plain film of the abdomen usually indicate ~80% damage to the pancreas. While alcohol is by far the most common cause of pancreatic calcification, such calcification may also be noted in severe protein-calorie malnutrition, hereditary pancreatitis, posttraumatic pancreatitis, hypercalcemic pancreatitis, islet cell tumors, and idiopathic chronic pancreatitis. Abdominal ultrasonography, CT scanning, and ERCP greatly aid in the diagnosis of pancreatic disease (Fig. 307-3). In addition to excluding a pseudocyst and pancreatic cancer, sonography and CT may show calcification, dilated ducts, or an atrophic pancreas. ERCP or magnetic resonance cholangiopancreatography (MRCP) provides a direct view of the pancreatic duct and

may show a pseudocyst missed by sonography or CT. The role of endoscopic ultrasonography (EUS) in diagnosing early chronic pancreatitis is still being defined. EUS complements pancreatic function tests, and a combination of a hormone-stimulation function test and EUS is the most complete way to evaluate the presence or extent of chronic pancreatitis (Chap. 306). Whether EUS can detect early chronic pancreatitis, i.e., small-duct disease, with the same degree of accuracy as the hormone-stimulation test is controversial. Recent data comparing these modalities head-to-head would indicate that EUS is not a sensitive test for detecting early chronic pancreatitis (Chap. 306) and may lead to false-positive tests in patients who have dyspepsia or even in normal controls.

Complications of Chronic Pancreatitis The complications of chronic pancreatitis are protean and are listed in Table 307-7. Although most patients have impaired glucose tolerance, diabetic ketoacidosis and coma are uncommon. Likewise, end-organ damage (retinopathy, neuropathy, nephropathy) is also uncommon. A nondiabetic retinopathy may be due to either vitamin A and/or zinc deficiency. Gastrointestinal bleeding may occur from peptic ulceration, gastritis, a pseudocyst eroding into the duodenum, or ruptured varices secondary to splenic vein thrombosis due to inflammation of the tail of the pancreas. Jaundice, cholestasis, and biliary cirrhosis may occur from the chronic inflammatory reaction around the intrapancreatic portion of the common bile duct. Twenty years after the diagnosis of chronic pancreatitis, the cumulative risk of pancreatic carcinoma is 4%. Patients with hereditary pancreatitis are at a tenfold higher risk for pancreatic cancer.

℞ CHRONIC PANCREATITIS

The treatment of steatorrhea with pancreatic enzymes is straightforward even though complete correction of steatorrhea is unusual. Enzyme therapy usually brings diarrhea under control and restores absorption of fat to an acceptable level. Thus, pancreatic enzymes, largely from porcine sources, have been the cornerstone of pancreatic therapy. In treating steatorrhea, it is important to use a potent pancreatic formulation that will deliver sufficient lipase into the duodenum to correct maldigestion and decrease steatorrhea (Table 307-8).

The management of pain in patients with chronic pancreatitis is problematic. In patients with large-duct disease usually from alcohol-induced chronic pancreatitis, ductal decompression has been the therapy of choice. Among such patients, 80% seem to obtain immediate relief; however, at the end of 3 years, half the patients have recurrence of pain. Preliminary data suggest that large doses of octreotide may decrease the pain in patients with large-duct disease.

Octreotide was initially selected and evaluated for the treatment of abdominal pain associated with large-duct chronic pancreatitis. It is a somatostatin analogue that inhibits pancreatic secretion and lowers blood CCK levels. A multicenter, double-blinded, placebo-controlled, dose-ranging study showed that 200 µg of octreotide given SC three times daily was superior to placebo and decreased the abdominal pain of patients. Octreotide significantly relieves pain in some patients with severe chronic pancreatitis refractory to other forms of therapy, including surgery.

In patients with small-duct disease, conventional nonenteric coated enzyme preparations containing high concentrations of serine proteases relieve pain. The patients who respond best to these proteases are those with an abnormal hormone stimulation test or minimal changes on ERCP and normal fat absorption. It appears that these serum proteases relieve pain by catabolizing a CCK-releasing peptide that ultimately leads to a lower CCK level in the blood and, thus, less stimulation to the pancreas. This feedback inhibition mechanism appears to be operative in the upper small intestine. Nonenteric coated enzymes are preferable because when given with a proton pump inhibitor, those enzymes that escape acid destruction within the stomach are delivered directly into the duodenum, where the

FIGURE 307-3 Radiologic abnormalities in chronic pancreatitis. A. Pancreatic calcification (*arrows*) and stenosis (tapering) of the intrahepatic portion of the common bile duct demonstrated by percutaneous transhepatic cholangiography. **B.** Pancreatic calcification (*large white arrow*) demonstrated by sonography. Note dilated pancreatic duct (*thin white arrow*) and splenic vein (*open arrow*). **C.** Pancreatic calcification (*vertical arrows*) and dilated pancreatic duct (*horizontal arrow*) demonstrated by CT scan. **D.** Endoscopic retrograde cholangiogram shows grossly dilated pancreatic ducts (*arrows*) in a patient with long-standing pancreatitis.

feedback principle is operative. Enteric-coated enzymes, although appropriate for treating steatorrhea, are not the enzymes of choice for treating abdominal pain because the enteric-coated compounds have been demonstrated to open their enteric coat when they pass beyond the duodenum and into the mid small intestine. This feedback principle is not operative in that part of the intestine. The ideal pancreatic enzyme preparation will be one that has enteric-coated lipase and free proteases. The free proteases would enter into the duodenum and evoke a positive feedback control mechanism, and the enteric-coated lipase would open beyond the duodenum and enhance fat absorption. Table 307-8 lists the frequently utilized pancreatic enzyme preparations in the United States.

Gastroparesis is also quite common in patients with chronic pancreatitis, particularly those who have small-duct painful chronic pancreatitis. It is important to recognize this because treatment with enzymes may fail simply because gastroparesis is preventing the appropriate delivery of enzymes into the upper intestine where the enzymes can then act via a feedback inhibition process. In patients with small-duct disease and painful chronic pancreatitis, it is important to evaluate gastric emptying and if gastric emptying is impaired, to effect proper emptying with prokinetic agents. In this setting enzyme therapy is more apt to be successful.

Endoscopic treatment of chronic pancreatitis pain may involve sphincterotomy, stenting, stone extraction, and drainage of a pancreatic pseudocyst. Therapy directed to the pancreatic duct would seem to be most appropriate in the setting of a dominant stricture, if a ductal stone has led to obstruction. The use of endoscopic stenting for patients with chronic pain, but without a dominant stricture, has not been proven in any controlled trials. It is now appreciated that significant complications can occur from stenting, i.e., bleeding, cholangitis, stent migration, and stent clogging. All of these may lead to pancreatitis. Importantly, damage to the pancreatic duct and the pancreatic parenchyma can occur following stenting.

Total pancreatectomy and autologous islet cell transplantation have been used in selected patients with chronic pancreatitis and abdominal pain refractory to conventional therapy. The patients who have benefited the most to date have chronic pancreatitis without prior pancreatic surgery or evidence of islet cell insufficiency. The role of this procedure remains to be fully defined but may be an option in lieu of ductal decompression surgery or pancreatic resection in patients with intractable, painful small-duct disease, particularly as the standard surgical procedures tend to decrease islet cell yield.

HEREDITARY PANCREATITIS

Hereditary pancreatitis is a rare disease that is similar to chronic pancreatitis except for an early age of onset and evidence of hereditary factors

FIGURE 307-4 Chronic pancreatitis and pancreatic calculi: CT scan and ERCP appearance. **A.** In this contrast-enhanced CT scan of the abdomen, there is evidence of an atrophic pancreas with multiple calcifications (*arrows*). Note the markedly dilated pancreatic duct seen in this section through the body and tail (*open arrows*). **B.** ERCP in the same patient demonstrates the dilated pancreatic duct as well as an intrapancreatic duct calculus (*arrows*). These findings correlate nicely with the CT scan appearance.

(involving an autosomal dominant gene with incomplete penetrance). A genome-wide search using genetic linkage analysis identified the hereditary pancreatitis gene on chromosome 7. Mutations in ion codons 29 (exon 2) and 122 (exon 3) of the cationic trypsinogen gene cause autosomal dominant forms of hereditary pancreatitis. The codon 122 mutations lead to a substitution of the corresponding arginine with another amino acid, usually histidine. This substitution, when it occurs, eliminates a fail-safe trypsin self-destruction site necessary to eliminate trypsin that is prematurely activated within the acinar cell. These patients have recurring attacks of severe abdominal pain that may last from a few days to a few weeks. The serum amylase and lipase levels may be elevated during acute attacks but are usually normal. Patients frequently develop pancreatic calcification, diabetes mellitus, and steatorrhea; in addition, they have an increased incidence of pancreatic carcinoma, with the cumulative incidence being as high as 40% by age 70. Such patients often require ductal decompression for pain relief. Abdominal complaints in relatives of patients with hereditary pancreatitis should raise the question of pancreatic disease.

Pancreatic Secretory Trypsin Inhibitor (PSTI) Gene Mutations PSTI, or SPINK1, is a 56-amino-acid peptide that specifically inhibits trypsin by physically blocking its active site. SPINK1 acts as the first line of defense against prematurely activated trypsinogen in the acinar cell. Recently, it has been shown that the frequency of SPINK1 mutations in patients with idiopathic chronic pancreatitis is markedly increased, suggesting that these mutations may be associated with pancreatitis.

PANCREATIC ENDOCRINE TUMORS

Pancreatic endocrine tumors are discussed in Chap. 344.

OTHER CONDITIONS

ANNULAR PANCREAS

When the ventral pancreatic anlage fails to migrate correctly to make contact with the dorsal anlage, the result may be a ring of pancreatic tissue encircling the duodenum. Such an annular pancreas may cause intestinal obstruction in the neonate or the adult. Symptoms of post-prandial fullness, epigastric pain, nausea, and vomiting may be present for years before the diagnosis is entertained. The radiographic findings are symmetric dilation of the proximal duodenum with bulging of the recesses on either side of the annular band, effacement but not destruction of the duodenal mucosa, accentuation of the findings in the right anterior oblique position, and lack of change on repeated examinations. The differential diagnosis should include duodenal webs, tumors of the pancreas or duodenum, postbulbar peptic ulcer, regional enteritis, and adhesions. Patients with annular pancreas have an increased incidence of pancreatitis and peptic ulcer. Because of these and other potential complications, the treatment is surgical even if the condition has been present for years. Retrocolic duodenojejunostomy is the procedure of choice, although some surgeons advocate Billroth II gastrectomy, gastroenterostomy, and vagotomy.

PANCREAS DIVISUM

Pancreas divisum occurs when the embryologic ventral and dorsal pancreatic anlagen fail to fuse, so that pancreatic drainage is accom-

---

TABLE 307-7 COMPLICATIONS OF CHRONIC PANCREATITIS

Narcotic addiction	Gastrointestinal bleeding
Impaired glucose tolerance	Jaundice
Gastroparesis	Cholangitis and/or biliary cirrhosis
Cobalamin malabsorption	Subcutaneous fat necrosis
Nondiabetic retinopathy	Bone pain
Effusions with high amylase content	Pancreatic cancer

TABLE 307-8 FREQUENTLY UTILIZED PANCREATIC ENZYME PREPARATIONS

	Protease[a] (× 1000)	Lipase[a] (× 1000)
Nonenteric Coated		
Viokase 8 (Axcan Scandipharm, Birmingham, AL)	30	8
Viokase 16 (Axcan Scandipharm)	60	16
Kuzyme HP (Schwartz, Milwaukee, WI)	30	8
Cotazym (Organon, East Orange, NJ)	30	8
Enteric Coated		
Creon 5 (Solvay, Marietta, GA)	18.75	5
Creon 10 (Solvay)	37.5	10
Creon 20 (Solvay)	75	20
Pancrease MT4 (McNeil Pharmaceuticals, Ft. Washington, PA)	12	4
Pancrease MT10 (McNeil Pharmaceuticals)	30	10
Pancrease MT16 (McNeil Pharmaceuticals)	48	16
Ultrase 12 (Scandipharm, Birmingham, AL)	39	12
Ultrase 18 (Scandipharm)	58.5	18
Ultrase 20 (Scandipharm)	65	20
Cotazym-S (Organon)	20	5

[a]United States Pharmacopea units per tablet or capsule.
Manufacturers and their locations follow names of drugs.
For pain 4 to 8 nonenteric coated tablets four times daily.
For maldigestion 1–2 enteric coated capsules with each meal.

plished mainly through the accessory papilla. Pancreas divisum is the most common congenital anatomic variant of the human pancreas. Current evidence indicates that this anomaly does not predispose to the development of pancreatitis in the great majority of patients who harbor it. However, the combination of pancreas divisum and a small accessory orifice could result in dorsal duct obstruction. The challenge is to identify this subset of patients with dorsal duct pathology. Cannulation of the dorsal duct by ERCP is not as easily done as is cannulation of the ventral duct. Patients with pancreatitis and pancreas divisum demonstrated by ERCP should be treated with conservative measures. In many of these patients, pancreatitis is idiopathic and unrelated to the pancreas divisum. Endoscopic or surgical intervention is indicated only when the above methods fail. If marked dilation of the dorsal duct can be demonstrated, surgical ductal decompression should be performed. The appropriate therapy for patients without dilation of the dorsal duct is not yet defined. It should be stressed that the ERCP appearance of pancreas divisum—i.e., a small-caliber ventral duct with an arborizing pattern—may be mistaken as representing an obstructed main pancreatic duct secondary to a mass lesion.

MACROAMYLASEMIA

In macroamylasemia, amylase circulates in the blood in a polymer form too large to be easily excreted by the kidney. Patients with this condition demonstrate an elevated serum amylase value, a low urinary amylase value, and a C_{am}/C_{cr} ratio of <1%. The presence of macroamylase can be documented by chromatography of the serum. The prevalence of macroamylasemia is 1.5% of the nonalcoholic general adult hospital population. Usually macroamylasemia is an incidental finding and is not related to disease of the pancreas or other organs.

Macrolipasemia has now been documented in a few patients with cirrhosis or non-Hodgkin's lymphoma. In these patients, the pancreas appeared normal on ultrasound and CT examination. Lipase was shown to be complexed with immunoglobulin A. Thus, the possibility of *both* macroamylasemia and macrolipasemia should be considered in patients with elevated blood levels of these enzymes.

ACKNOWLEDGMENTS
This chapter represents a revised version of the chapter by Dr. Norton J. Greenberger, Dr. Phillip P. Toskes, and Dr. Kurt J. Isselbacher that was in the previous editions of Harrison's.

FURTHER READINGS

GUPTA V, TOSKES PP: Diagnosis and management of chronic pancreatitis. Postgrad Med J 81:491, 2005

ISENMAN R et al: Prophylactic antibiotic treatment in patients with predicted severe acute pancreatitis: A placebo controlled, double-blinded trial. Gastroenterology 126:997, 2004

SOMOGYI L et al: Recurrent acute pancreatitis: An algorithmic approach to identification and elimination of inciting factors. Gastroenterology 120:708, 2001

THOMSON A: Enteral versus parenteral nutritional support in acute pancreatitis: A clinical review. J Gastroenterol Hepatol 21:22, 2006

YADAY Y et al: A critical evaluation of laboratory tests in acute pancreatitis. Am J Gastroenterol 97:1309, 2002

308   Introduction to the Immune System

Barton F. Haynes, Kelly A. Soderberg, Anthony S. Fauci

DEFINITIONS

- *Adaptive immune system*—recently evolved system of immune responses mediated by T and B lymphocytes. Immune responses by these cells are based on specific antigen recognition by clonotypic receptors that are products of genes that rearrange during development and throughout the life of the organism. Additional cells of the adaptive immune system include various types of antigen-presenting cells.
- *Antibody*—B cell–produced molecules encoded by genes that rearrange during B cell development consisting of immunoglobulin heavy and light chains that together form the central component of the B cell receptor for antigen. Antibody can exist as B cell surface antigen-recognition molecules or as secreted molecules in plasma and other body fluids (Table 308-11).
- *Antigens*—foreign or self-molecules that are recognized by the adaptive and innate immune systems resulting in immune cell triggering, T cell activation, and/or B cell antibody production.
- *Antimicrobial peptides*—small peptides <100 amino acids in length that are produced by cells of the innate immune system and have anti-infectious agent activity (Table 308-2).
- *Apoptosis*—the process of *programmed cell death* whereby signaling through various "death receptors" on the surface of cells [e.g., tumor necrosis factor (TNF) receptors, CD95] leads to a signaling cascade that involves activation of the caspase family of molecules and leads to DNA cleavage and cell death. Apoptosis, which does not lead to induction of inordinate inflammation, is to be contrasted with *cell necrosis*, which does lead to induction of inflammatory responses.
- *B lymphocytes*—bone marrow–derived or bursal-equivalent lymphocytes that express surface immunoglobulin (the B cell receptor for antigen) and secrete specific antibody after interaction with antigen (Figs. 308-2, 308-6).
- *B cell receptor for antigen*—complex of surface molecules that rearrange during postnatal B cell development, made up of surface immunoglobulin (Ig) and associated Ig αβ chain molecules that recognize nominal antigen via Ig heavy and light chain variable regions, and signal the B cell to terminally differentiate to make antigen-specific antibody (Fig. 308-8).
- *CD classification of human lymphocyte differentiation antigens*—the development of monoclonal antibody technology led to the discovery of a large number of new leukocyte surface molecules. In 1982, the First International Workshop on Leukocyte Differentiation Antigens was held to establish a nomenclature for cell-surface molecules of human leukocytes. From this and subsequent leukocyte differentiation workshops has come the *cluster of differentiation (CD) classification* of leukocyte antigens (Table 308-1).
- *Chemokines*—soluble molecules that direct and determine immune cell movement and circulation pathways.
- *Complement*—cascading series of plasma enzymes and effector proteins whose function is to lyse pathogens and/or target them to be phagocytized by neutrophils and monocyte/macrophage lineage cells of the reticuloendothelial system (Fig. 308-5).
- *Co-stimulatory molecules*—molecules of antigen-presenting cells (such as B7-1 and B7-2 or CD40) that lead to T cell activation when bound by ligands on activated T cells (such as CD28 or CD40 ligand) (Fig. 308-7).
- *Cytokines*—soluble proteins that interact with specific cellular receptors that are involved in the regulation of the growth and activation of immune cells and mediate normal and pathologic inflammatory and immune responses (Tables 308-6, 308-8, 308-9).
- *Dendritic cells*—myeloid and/or lymphoid lineage antigen-presenting cells of the adaptive immune system. Immature dendritic cells, or dendritic cell precursors, are key components of the innate immune system by responding to infections with production of high levels of cytokines. Dendritic cells are key initiators both of innate immune responses via cytokine production and of adaptive immune responses via presentation of antigen to T lymphocytes (Figs. 308-2, 308-3, Table 308-5).
- *Innate immune system*—ancient immune recognition system of host cells bearing germ line–encoded pattern recognition receptors (PRRs) that recognize pathogens and trigger a variety of mechanisms of pathogen elimination. Cells of the innate immune system include natural killer (NK) cell lymphocytes, monocytes/macrophages, dendritic cells, neutrophils, basophils, eosinophils, tissue mast cells, and epithelial cells (Tables 308-2, 308-3, 308-4, 308-5, 308-10).
- *Large granular lymphocytes*—lymphocytes of the innate immune system with azurophilic cytotoxic granules that have NK cell activity capable of killing foreign and host cells with few or no self–major histocompatibility complex (MHC) class I molecules (Fig. 308-4).
- *Natural killer cells*—large granular lymphocytes that kill target cells expressing few or no human leukocyte antigen (HLA) class I molecules, such as malignantly transformed cells and virally infected cells. NK cells express receptors that inhibit killer cell function when self–MHC class I is present (Fig. 308-4).
- *Pathogen-associated molecular patterns* (PAMPs)—Invariant molecular structures expressed by large groups of microorganisms that are recognized by host cellular pattern recognition receptors in the mediation of innate immunity (Fig. 308-1).
- *Pattern recognition receptors* (PRRs)—germ line–encoded receptors expressed by cells of the innate immune system that recognize pathogen-associated molecular patterns (Table 308-3).
- *T cells*—thymus-derived lymphocytes that mediate adaptive cellular immune responses including T helper, T regulatory, and cytotoxic T lymphocyte effector cell functions (Figs. 308-2, 308-3, 308-6).
- *T cell receptor for antigen*—complex of surface molecules that rearrange during postnatal T cell development made up of clonotypic T cell receptor (TCR) α and β chains that are associated with the CD3 complex composed of invariant γ, δ, ε, ζ, and η chains. TCR-α and -β chains recognize peptide fragments of protein antigen physically bound in antigen-presenting cell MHC class I or II molecules, leading to signaling via the CD3 complex to mediate effector functions (Fig. 308-7).
- *Tolerance*—B and T cell nonresponsiveness to antigens that results from encounter with foreign or self-antigens by B and T lymphocytes in the absence of expression of antigen-presenting cell co-stimulatory molecules. Tolerance to antigens may be induced and maintained by multiple mechanisms either centrally (in the thymus for T cells or bone marrow for B cells) or peripherally at sites throughout the peripheral immune system.

INTRODUCTION

The human immune system has evolved over millions of years from both invertebrate and vertebrate organisms to develop sophisticated defense mechanisms to protect the host from microbes and their virulence factors. The normal immune system has three key properties: a highly diverse repertoire of antigen receptors that enables recognition of a nearly infinite range of pathogens; immune memory, to mount rapid recall immune responses; and immunologic tolerance, to avoid immune damage to normal self-tissues. From invertebrates, humans have inherited the innate immune system, an ancient defense system that uses germ line–encoded proteins to recognize pathogens. Cells of the innate immune system, such as macrophages, dendritic cells, and natural killer (NK) lymphocytes, recognize pathogen-associated molecular patterns (PAMPs) that are highly conserved among many microbes and use a diverse set of pattern recognition receptor molecules (PRRs). Important components of the recognition of microbes by the innate immune system include (1) recognition by germ line–encoded host molecules, (2) recognition of key microbe virulence factors but not recognition of self-molecules, and (3) nonrecognition of benign foreign molecules or microbes. Upon contact with pathogens, macrophages and NK cells may kill pathogens directly or, in concert with dendritic cells, may activate a series of events that both slow the infection and recruit the more recently evolved arm of the human immune system, the adaptive immune system.

Adaptive immunity is found only in vertebrates and is based on the generation of antigen receptors on T and B lymphocytes by gene rearrangements, such that individual T or B cells express unique antigen receptors on their surface capable of specifically recognizing diverse antigens of the myriad infectious agents in the environment. Coupled with finely tuned specific recognition mechanisms that maintain tolerance (nonreactivity) to self-antigens, T and B lymphocytes bring both *specificity* and *immune memory* to vertebrate host defenses.

This chapter describes the cellular components, key molecules (Table 308-1), and mechanisms that make up the innate and adaptive immune systems, and describes how adaptive immunity is recruited to the defense of the host by innate immune responses. An appreciation of the cellular and molecular bases of innate and adaptive immune responses is critical to understanding the pathogenesis of inflammatory, autoimmune, infectious, and immunodeficiency diseases.

TABLE 308-1 HUMAN LEUKOCYTE SURFACE ANTIGENS—THE CD CLASSIFICATION OF LEUKOCYTE DIFFERENTIATION ANTIGENS

Surface Antigen (Other Names)	Family	Molecular Mass, kDa	Distribution	Ligand(s)	Function
CD1a (T6, HTA-1)	Ig	49	CD, cortical thymocytes, Langerhans type of dendritic cells	TCRγδ T cells	CD1 molecules present lipid antigens of intracellular bacteria such as *M. leprae* and *M. tuberculosis* to TCRγδ T cells.
CD1b	Ig	45	CD, cortical thymocytes, Langerhans type of dendritic cells	TCRγδ T cells	
CD1c	Ig	43	DC, cortical thymocytes, subset of B cells, Langerhans type of dendritic cells	TCRγδ T cells	
CD1d	Ig	?	Cortical thymocytes, intestinal epithelium, Langerhans type of dendritic cells	TCRγδ T cells	
CD2 (T12, LFA-2)	Ig	50	T, NK	CD58, CD48, CD59, CD15	Alternative T cell activation, T cell anergy, T cell cytokine production, T- or NK-mediated cytolysis, T cell apoptosis, cell adhesion
CD3 (T3, Leu-4)	Ig	γ:25–28, δ:21–28, ε:20–25, η:21–22, ζ:16	T	Associates with the TCR	T cell activation and function; ζ is the signal transduction components of the CD3 complex
CD4 (T4, Leu-3)	Ig	55	T, myeloid	MHC-II, HIV, gp120, IL-16, SABP	T cell selection, T cell activation, signal transduction with p56*lck*, primary receptor for HIV
CD7 (3A1, Leu-9)	Ig	40	T, NK	K-12 (CD7L)	T and NK cell signal transduction and regulation of IFN-γ, TNF-α production
CD8 (T8, Leu-2)	Ig	34	T	MHC-I	T cell selection, T cell activation, signal transduction with p56*lck*
CD14 (LPS-receptor)	LRG	53–55	M, G (weak), not by myeloid progenitors	Endotoxin (lipopolysaccharide), lipoteichoic acid, PI	TLR4 mediates with LPS and other PAMP activation of innate immunity
CD19 B4	Ig	95	B (except plasma cells), FDC	Not known	Associates with CD21 and CD81 to form a complex involved in signal transduction in B cell development, activation, and differentiation
CD20 (B1)	Unassigned	33–37	B (except plasma cells)	Not known	Cell signaling, may be important for B cell activation and proliferation
CD21 (B2, CR2, EBV-R, C3dR)	RCA	145	Mature B, FDC, subset of thymocytes	C3d, C3dg, iC3b, CD23, EBV	Associates with CD19 and CD81 to form a complex involved in signal transduction in B cell development, activation, and differentiation; Epstein-Barr virus receptor
CD22 (BL-CAM)	Ig	130–140	Mature B	CDw75	Cell adhesion, signaling through association with p72*sky*, p53/56*lyn*, PI3 kinase, SHP1, fLCγ
CD23 (FcεRII, B6, Leu-20, BLAST-2)	C-type lectin	45	B, M, FDC	IgE, CD21, CD11b, CD11c	Regulates IgE synthesis, cytokine release by monocytes

(continued)

Surface Antigen (Other Names)	Family	Molecular Mass, kDa	Distribution	Ligand(s)	Function
CD28	Ig	44	T, plasma cells	CD80, CD86	Co-stimulatory for T cell activation; involved in the decision between T cell activation and anergy
CD40	TNFR	48–50	B, DC, EC, thymic epithelium, MP, cancers	CD154	B cell activation, proliferation, and differentiation, formation of GCs, isotype switching, rescue from apoptosis
CD45 (LCA, T200, B220)	PTP	180, 200, 210, 220	All leukocytes	Galectin-1, CD2, CD3, CD4	T and B activation, thymocyte development, signal transduction, apoptosis
CD45RA	PTP	210, 220	Subset T, medullary thymocytes, "naive" T	Galectin-1, CD2, CD3, CD4	Isoforms of CD45 containing exon 4 (A), restricted to a subset of T cells
CD45RB	PTP	200, 210, 220	All leukocytes	Galectin-1, CD2, CD3, CD4	Isoforms of CD45 containing exon 5 (B)
CD45RC	PTP	210, 220	Subset T, medullary thymocytes, "naive" T	Galectin-1, CD2, CD3, CD4	Isoforms of CD45 containing exon 6 (C), restricted to a subset of T cells
CD45RO	PTP	180	Subset T, cortical thymocytes, "memory" T	Galectin-1, CD2, CD3, CD4	Isoforms of CD45 containing no differentially spliced exons, restricted to a subset of T cells
CD80 (B7-1, BB1)	Ig	60	Activated B and T, MP, DC	CD28, CD152	Co-regulator of T cell activation; signaling through CD28 stimulates and through CD152 inhibits T cell activation
CD86 (B7-2, B70)	Ig	80	Subset B, DC, EC, activated T, thymic epithelium	CD28, CD152	Co-regulator of T cell activation; signaling through CD28 stimulates and through CD152 inhibits T cell activation
CD95 (APO-1, Fas)	TNFR	135	Activated T and B	Fas ligand	Mediates apoptosis
CD152 (CTLA-4)	Ig	30–33	Activated T	CD80, CD86	Inhibits T cell proliferation
CD154 (CD40L)	TNF	33	Activated CD4+ T, subset CD8+ T, NK, M, basophil	CD40	Co-stimulatory for T cell activation, B cell proliferation and differentiation

Note: CTLA, cytotoxic T lymphocyte–associated protein; DC, dendritic cells; EBV, Epstein-Barr virus; EC, endothelial cells; ECM, extracellular matrix; Fcγ RIIIA, low-affinity IgG receptor isoform A; FDC, follicular dendritic cells; G, granulocytes; GC, germinal center; GPI, glycosyl phosphotidylinositol; HTA, human thymocyte antigen; IgG, immunoglobulin G; LCA, leukocyte common antigen; LPS, lipopolysaccharide; MHC-I, major histocompatibility complex class I; MP, macrophages; Mr, relative molecular mass; NK, natural killer cells; P, platelets; PBT, peripheral blood T cells; PI, phosphotidylinositol; PI3K, phosphotidyl-inositol 3-kinase; PLC, phospholipase C; PTP, protein tyrosine phosphatase; TCR, T cell receptor; TNF, tumor necrosis factor; TNFR, tumor necrosis factor receptor. For an expanded list of cluster of differentiation (CD) human antigens, see Harrison's Online at http://harrisons.accessmedicine.com; and for a full list of CD human antigens from the most recent Human Workshop on Leukocyte Differentiation Antigens (VII), see http://www.ncbi.nlm.nih.gov/prow/guide.

Source: Compiled from T Kishimoto et al (eds): *Leukocyte Typing VI,* New York, Garland Publishing 1997; R Brines et al: Immunology Today 18S:1, 1997; and S Shaw (ed): *Protein Reviews on the Web* http://www.ncbi.nlm.nih.gov/prow/guide.

THE INNATE IMMUNE SYSTEM

All multicellular organisms, including humans, have developed the use of a limited number of germ line–encoded molecules that recognize large groups of pathogens. Because of the myriad human pathogens, host molecules of the human innate immune system sense "danger signals" and either recognize PAMPs, the common molecular structures shared by many pathogens, or recognize host cell molecules produced in response to infection such as heat shock proteins and fragments of the extracellular matrix. PAMPs must be conserved structures vital to pathogen virulence and survival, such as bacterial endotoxin, so that pathogens cannot mutate molecules of PAMPs to evade human innate immune responses. PRRs are host proteins of the innate immune system that recognize PAMPs or host danger signal molecules (Tables 308-2, 308-3). Thus, recognition of pathogen molecules by hematopoietic and nonhematopoietic cell types leads to activation/production of the complement cascade, cytokines, and antimicrobial peptides as effector molecules. In addition, pathogen PAMPs and host danger signal molecules activate dendritic cells to mature and to express molecules on the dendritic cell surface that optimize antigen presentation to respond to foreign antigens.

PATTERN RECOGNITION

Major PRR families of proteins include C-type lectins, leucine-rich proteins, macrophage scavenger receptor proteins, plasma pentraxins, lipid transferases, and integrins (Table 308-3). A major group of PRR collagenous glycoproteins with C-type lectin domains are termed *collectins* and include the serum protein mannose-binding lectin (MBL). MBL and other collectins, as well as two other protein families—the pentraxins (such as C-reactive protein and serum amyloid P) and macrophage scavenger receptors—all have the property of opsonizing (coating) bacteria for phagocytosis by macrophages and can also activate the complement cascade to lyse bacteria. Integrins are cell-surface adhesion molecules that signal cells after cells bind bacterial lipopolysaccharide (LPS) and activate phagocytic cells to ingest pathogens.

A series of recent discoveries has revealed the mechanisms of connection between the innate and adaptive immune systems; these include (1) a plasma protein, LPS-binding protein, which binds and transfers LPS to the macrophage LPS receptor, CD14; and (2) a human family of proteins called *Toll-like receptor proteins* (TLR), some of which are associated with CD14, bind LPS, and signal epithelial cells, dendritic cells, and macrophages to produce cytokines and upregulate cell-surface molecules that signal the initiation of adaptive immune responses (Fig. 308-1, Tables 308-3, 308-4). Proteins in the Toll family

TABLE 308-2 **MAJOR COMPONENTS OF THE INNATE IMMUNE SYSTEM**

Pattern recognition receptors (PRR)	C type lectins, leucine-rich proteins, scavenger receptors, pentraxins, lipid transferases, integrins
Antimicrobial peptides	α-Defensins, β-defensins, cathelin, protegrin, granulsyin, histatin, secretory leukoprotease inhibitor, and probiotics
Cells	Macrophages, dendritic cells, NK cells, NK-T cells, neutrophils, eosinophils, mast cells, basophils, and epithelial cells
Complement components	Classic and alternative complement pathway, and proteins that bind complement components
Cytokines	Autocrine, paracrine, endocrine cytokines that mediate host defense and inflammation, as well as recruit, direct, and regulate adaptive immune responses

Note: NK cells, natural killer cells.

TABLE 308-3   MAJOR PATTERN RECOGNITION RECEPTORS (PRR) OF THE INNATE IMMUNE SYSTEM

PRR Protein Family	Sites of Expression	Examples	Ligands (PAMPs)	Functions of PRR
Toll-like receptors	Multiple cell types	TLR2-10	(see Fig. 308-1 and Table 308-4) Bacterial and viral carbohydrates	Activate innate immune cells to respond to multiple pathogens and initiate adaptive immune responses.
C-type Lectins	Plasma proteins	Collectins		Opsonization of bacteria and virus, activation of complement
Humoral			Terminal mannose	
Cellular	Macrophages, dendritic cell	Macrophage mannose receptor	Carbohydrate on HLA molecules	Phagocytosis of pathogens
	Natural killer (NK) cells	NKG2-A		Inhibits killing of host cells expressing HLA+ self peptides
Leucine-rich proteins	Macrophages, dendritic cells, epithelial cells	CD14	Lipopolysaccharide (LPS)	Binds LPS and Toll proteins
Scavenger receptors	Macrophage	Macrophage scavenger receptors	Bacterial cell walls	Phagocytosis of bacteria
Pentraxins	Plasma protein	C-creative proteins	Phosphatidyl choline	Opsonization of bacteria, activation of complement
	Plasma protein	Serum amyloid P	Bacterial cell walls	Opsonization of bacteria, activation of complement
Lipid transferases	Plasma protein	LPS binding protein	LPS	Binds LPS, transfers LPS to CD14
Integrins	Macrophages, dendritic cells, NK cells	CD11b,c; CD18	LPS	Signals cells, activates phagocytosis

Note: PAMPs, pathogen-associated molecular patterns.
Source: Adapted with permission from R Medzhitov, CA Janeway, Innate immunity: Impact on the adaptive immune response. Curr Opin Immunol 9:4, 1997.

(TLR 1–10) can be expressed on macrophages, dendritic cells, and B cells as well as on a variety of nonhematopoietic cell types, including respiratory epithelial cells (Tables 308-4, 308-5). Upon ligation, these receptors activate a series of intracellular events that lead to the killing of bacteria- and viral-infected cells as well as to the recruitment and ultimate activation of antigen-specific T and B lymphocytes (Fig. 308-1). Importantly, signaling by massive amounts of LPS through TLR4 leads to the release of large amounts of cytokines that mediate LPS-induced shock. Mutations in TLR4 proteins in mice protect from LPS shock, and TLR mutations in humans protect from LPS-induced inflammatory diseases such as LPS-induced asthma (Fig. 308-1).

Cells of invertebrates and vertebrates produce antimicrobial small peptides (<100 amino acids) that can act as endogenous antibodies (Table 308-2). Some of these peptides are produced by epithelia that line various organs, while others are found in macrophages or neutrophils that ingest pathogens. Antimicrobial peptides have been identified that kill bacteria such as *Pseudomonas* spp., *Escherichia coli*, and *Mycobacterium tuberculosis*.

EFFECTOR CELLS OF INNATE IMMUNITY

Cells of the innate immune system and their roles in the first line of host defense are listed in Table 308-5. Equally important as their roles in the mediation of innate immune responses are the roles that each cell type plays in recruiting T and B lymphocytes of the adaptive immune system to engage in specific antipathogen responses.

Monocytes-Macrophages Monocytes arise from precursor cells within bone marrow (Fig. 308-2) and circulate with a half-life ranging from 1 to 3 days. Monocytes leave the peripheral circulation by marginating in capillaries and migrating into a vast extravascular pool. Tissue macrophages arise from monocytes that have migrated out of the circulation and by in situ proliferation of macrophage precursors in tissue. Common locations where tissue macrophages (and certain of their specialized forms) are found are lymph node, spleen, bone marrow, perivascular connective tissue, serous cavities such as the peritoneum, pleura, skin connective tissue, lung (alveolar macrophages), liver (Kupffer cells), bone (osteoclasts), central nervous system (microglia cells), and synovium (type A lining cells).

In general, monocytes-macrophages are on the first line of defense associated with innate immunity and ingest and destroy microorganisms through the release of toxic products such as hydrogen peroxide (H_2O_2) and nitric oxide (NO). Inflammatory mediators produced by

FIGURE 308-1 Overview of major TLR signaling pathways. All TLRs signal through MyD88, with the exception of TLR3. TLR4 and the TLR2 subfamily (TLR1, TLR2, TLR6) also engage TIRAP. TLR3 signals through TRIF. TRIF is also used in conjunction with TRAM in the TLR4–MyD88-independent pathway. Dashed arrrows indicate translocation into the nucleus. LPS, lipopolysaccharide; dsRNA, double-strand RNA; ssRNA, single-strand RNA; MAPK, mitogen-activated protein kinases; NF-κB, nuclear factor-κB; IRF3, interferon regulatory factor 3. (*Adapted from D van Duin, R Medzhitov, AC Shaw, 2005, with permission.*)

TABLE 308-4 THE ROLE OF PRRS IN MODULATION OF T CELL RESPONSES

2023

PRR Family	PRRs	Ligand	DC or Macrophage Cytokine Response	Adaptive Immune Response
TLRs	TLR2 (heterodimer with TLR1 or 6)	Lipopeptides Pam-3-cys (TLR 2/1) MALP (TLR 2/6)	Low IL-12p70 High IL-10 IL-6	T_H1 T_H2 T regulatory
	TLR3	dsRNA	IL-12p70 IFN-α IL-6	T_H1
	TLR4	E. coli LPS	High IL-12p70 Intermediate IL-10 IL-6	T_H1
	TLR5	Flagellin	High IL-12p70 Low IL-12p70	T_H1 T_H2
	TLR7/8	ssRNA Imidazoquinolines	High IL-12p70 IFN-α IL-6	T_H1
	TLR9	CpG DNA	High IL-12p70 Low IL-10 IL-6 IFN-α	T_H1
	TLR10	?	?	?
C-type lectins	DC-SIGN	Env of HIV; core protein of HCV; components of M. tuberculosis; H. pylori, Lewis Ag	H. pylori, Lewis Ag Suppresses IL-12p70 Suppression of TLR signaling in DCs	T_H2 T regulatory
NOD	NOD2	Muramyl dipeptide of peptidoglycan	Induces IL-10 in DCs	Weak T cell response (tolerogenic?)
Mannose receptor	Mannose receptor	Mannosylated lipoarabinomannans from bacillus Calmette-Guerin and M. tuberculosis	Suppression of IL-12 and TLR signaling in DCs	Weak T cell response? (tolerogenic?)

Note: dsRNA, double-strand RNA; ssRNA, single-strand RNA; LPS, lipopolysaccharide; T_H2, helper T cell; T_H1, helper T cell; CpG, sequences in DNA recognized by TLR-9; MALP, macrophage-activating lipopeptide; DC-SIGN, DC-specific C-type lectin; NOD, NOTCH protein domain; TLR, toll-like receptor; HIV, human immunodeficiency virus; HCV, hepatitis C.
Source: B Pulendran, J Immunol 174:2457, 2005. Copyright 2005 The American Association of Immunologists, Inc.; with permission.

TABLE 308-5 CELLS OF THE INNATE IMMUNE SYSTEM AND THEIR MAJOR ROLES IN TRIGGERING ADAPTIVE IMMUNITY

Cell Type	Major Role in Innate Immunity	Major Role in Adaptive Immunity
Macrophages	Phagocytose and kill bacteria; produce antimicrobial peptides; bind (LPS); produce inflammatory cytokines	Produce IL-1 and TNFα to upregulate lymphocyte adhesion molecules and chemokines to attract antigen-specific lymphocyte. Produce IL-12 to recruit T_H1 T helper cell responses; upregulate co-stimulatory and MHC molecules to facilitate T and B lymphocyte recognition and activation. Macrophages and dendritic cells, after LPS signaling, upregulate co-stimulatory molecules B7-1 (CD80) and B7-2 (CD86) that are required for activation of antigen-specific anti-pathogen T cells. There are also Toll-like proteins on B cells and dendritic cells that after LPS ligation, induce CD80 and CD86 on these cells for T cell antigen presentation.
Plasmacytoid f dendritic cells (DCs) of lymphoid lineage	Produce large amounts of interferon-α (IFN-α) which has antitumor and antiviral activity, and are found in T cell zones of lymphoid organs; they circulate in blood.	IFN-α is a potent activator of macrophage and mature DCs to phagocytose invading pathogens and present pathogen antigens to T and B cells
Myeloid dendritic cells are of two types; interstitial and Langerhans-derived	Interstitial DCs are strong producers of IL-12 and IL-10 and are located in T cell zones of lymphoid organs, circulate in blood, and are present in the interstices of the lung, heart, and kidney; Langerhans DCs are strong producers of IL-12; are located in T cell zones of lymph nodes, skin epithelia, and the thymic medulla; and circulate in blood	Interstitial DCs are potent activator of macrophage and mature DCs to phagocytose invading pathogens and present pathogen antigens to T and B cells
Natural killer (NK) cells	Kill foreign and host cells that have low levels of MHC+ self peptides. Express NK receptors that inhibit NK function in the presence of high expression of self-MHC.	Produce TNF-α and IFN-γ that recruit T_H1 helper T cell responses
NK-T cells	Lymphocytes with both T cell and NK surface markers that recognize lipid antigens of intracellular bacteria such as M. tuberculosis by CD1 molecules and kill host cells infected with intracellular bacteria.	Produce IL-4 to recruit T_H2 helper T cell responses, IgG1 and IgE production
Neutrophils	Phagocytose and kill bacteria, produce antimicrobial peptides	Produce nitric oxide synthase and nitric oxide that inhibit apoptosis in lymphocytes and can prolong adaptive immune responses
Eosinophils	Kill invading parasites	Produce IL-5 that recruits Ig-specific antibody responses
Mast cells and basophils	Release TNF-α, IL-6, IFN-γ in response to a variety of bacterial PAMPs	Produce IL-4 that recruits T_H2 helper T cell responses and recruit IgG1- and IgE-specific antibody responses
Epithelial cells	Produce anti-microbial peptides; tissue specific epithelia produce mediator of local innate immunity, e.g. lung epithelial cells produce surfactant proteins (proteins within the collectin family) that bind and promote clearance of lung invading microbes	Produces TGF-β that triggers IgA-specific antibody responses.

Note: LPS, lipopolysaccharide; PAMP, pathogen-associated molecular patterns; TNF-α, tumor necrosis factor-alpha; IL-4, IL-5, IL-6, IL-10 and IL-12, interleukin 4, 5, 6, 10 or 12, respectively.
Source: Adapted with permission from R Medzhitov, CA Janeway: Innate immunity: Impact on the adaptive immune response. Curr Opinion Immunol 9:4–9, 1997a.

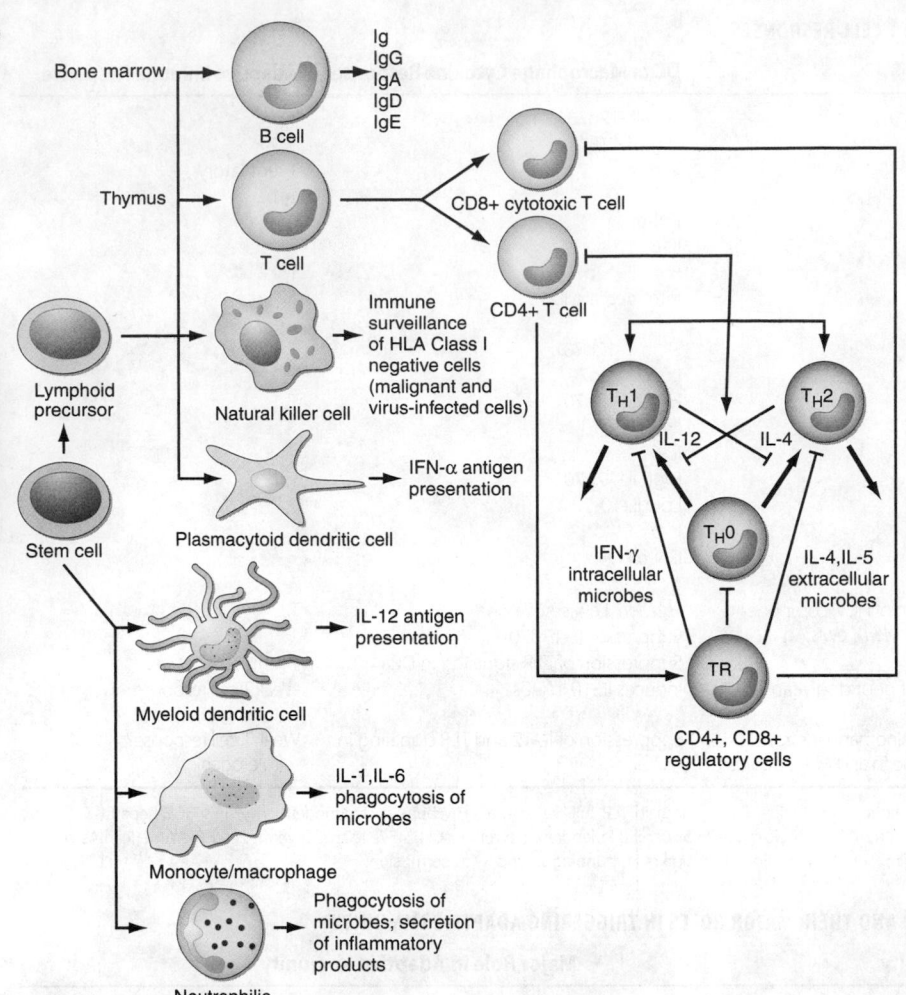

FIGURE 308-2 Schematic model of intercellular interactions of adaptive immune system cells. In this figure the arrows denote that cells develop from precursor cells or produce cytokines or antibodies; lines ending with bars indicate suppressive intercellular interactions. Stem cells differentiate into either T cells, antigen-presenting dendritic cells, natural killer cells, macrophages, granulocytes, or B cells. Foreign antigen is processed by dendritic cells, and peptide fragments of foreign antigen are presented to CD4+ and/or CD8+ T cells. CD8+ T cell activation leads to induction of cytotoxic T lymphocyte (CTL) or killer T cell generation, as well as induction of cytokine-producing CD8+ cytotoxic T cells. For antibody production against the same antigen, active antigen is bound to sIg within the B cell receptor complex and drives B cell maturation into plasma cells that secrete Ig. T_H1 or T_H2 CD4+ T cells producing interleukin (IL) 4, IL-5, or interferon (IFN)γ regulate the Ig class switching and determine the type of antibody produced. CD4+, CD25+ T regulatory cells produce IL-10 and downregulate T and B cell responses once the microbe has been eliminated. GM-CSF, granulocyte-macrophage colony stimulating factor; TNF, tumor necrosis factor.

manner, dendritic cells "cross-present" infectious agent antigens of macrophages to T cells. Activated macrophages can also mediate antigen-nonspecific lytic activity and eliminate cell types such as tumor cells in the absence of antibody. This activity is largely mediated by cytokines (i.e., TNF-α and IL-1). Monocytes-macrophages express lineage-specific molecules (e.g., the cell-surface LPS receptor, CD14) as well as surface receptors for a number of molecules, including the Fc region of IgG, activated complement components, and various cytokines (Table 308-6).

Dendritic Cells Human dendritic cells (DCs) are heterogenous and contain two subsets, myeloid DCs and plasmacytoid DCs. Myeloid DCs can differentiate into either macrophages/monocytes or tissue-specific DCs such as Langerhans cells in skin. Plasmacytoid DCs are inefficient antigen-presenting cells but are potent producers of type I interferon (IFN) (e.g., IFN-α) in response to viral infections. The maturation of DCs is regulated through cell-to-cell contact and soluble factors, and DCs attract immune effectors through secretion of chemokines.

When dendritic cells come in contact with bacterial products, viral proteins, or host proteins released as danger signals from distressed host cells (Figs. 308-2, 308-3), infectious agent molecules bind to various TLRs and activate dendritic cells to release cytokines and chemokines that drive cells of the innate immune system to become activated to respond to the invading organism, and recruit T and B cells of the adaptive immune system to respond. Plasmacytoid DCs produce IFN-α that is antiviral and activates NK cell killing of pathogen-infected cells; it also activates T cells to mature into antipathogen killer T cells. Following contact with pathogens, both plasmacytoid and myeloid DCs produce chemokines that attract T helper cells, B cells, polymorphonuclear cells, and naïve and memory T cells as well as regulatory T cells to ultimately dampen the immune response once the pathogen is controlled. TLR engagement on dendritic cells upregulates dendritic cell MHC class II, B7-1 (CD80), and B7-2 (CD86), which enhance specific antigen presentation and induce dendritic cell cytokine production (Table 308-1). Thus, dendritic cells are important bridges between early (innate) and later (adaptive) immunity. DCs modulate and determine the types of immune responses induced by pathogens via the TLRs expressed on DCs (TLR7-9 on plasmacytoid DCs, TLR4 on monocytoid DCs) and via the TLR adapter proteins that are induced to associate with TLRs (Fig. 308-1, Table 308-4). In addition, other PRRs, such as C-type lectins, NOD, and mannose receptors, upon ligation by pathogen products, activate cells of the adaptive immune system and, like TLR stimulation, by a variety of factors, determine the type and quality of the adaptive immune response that is triggered (Table 308-4).

Large Granular Lymphocytes/Natural Killer Cells Large granular lymphocytes (LGLs) or NK cells account for ~5–10% of peripheral blood lymphocytes. NKs cells are nonadherent, nonphagocytic cells with large azurophilic cytoplasmic granules. NKs cells express surface receptors for the Fc portion of IgG (CD16) and for NCAM-I (CD56), and many NK cells express some T lineage markers, particularly CD8,

macrophages attract additional effector cells such as neutrophils to the site of infection. Macrophage mediators include prostaglandins; leukotrienes; platelet activating factor; cytokines such as interleukin (IL) 1, tumor necrosis factor (TNF) α, IL-6, and IL-12; and chemokines (Tables 308-6 to 308-9).

Although monocytes-macrophages were originally thought to be the major antigen-presenting cells (APCs) of the immune system, it is now clear that cell types called dendritic cells are the most potent and effective APCs in the body (see below). Monocytes-macrophages mediate innate immune effector functions such as destruction of antibody-coated bacteria, tumor cells, or even normal hematopoietic cells in certain types of autoimmune cytopenias. Monocytes-macrophages ingest bacteria or are infected by viruses, and in doing so, they frequently undergo apoptosis. Macrophages that are "stressed" by intracellular infectious agents are recognized by dendritic cells as infected and apoptotic cells and are phagocytosed by dendritic cells. In this

TABLE 308-6 **CYTOKINES AND CYTOKINE RECEPTORS**   **2025**

Cytokine	Receptor	Cell Source	Cell Target	Biologic Activity
IL-1α,β	Type I IL-1r, Type II IL-1r	Monocytes/macrophages, B cells, fibroblasts, most epithelial cells including thymic epithelium, endothelial cells	All cells	Upregulated adhesion molecule expression, neutrophil and macrophage emigration, mimics shock, fever, upregulated hepatic acute phase protein production, facilitates hematopoiesis.
IL-2	IL-2r α,β, common γ	T cells	T cells, B cells NK cells, monocytes/macrophages	T cell activation and proliferation, B cell growth, NK cell proliferation and activation, enhanced monocyte/macrophage cytolytic activity.
IL-3	IL-3r, common β	T cells, NK cells, mast cells	Monocytes/macrophages, mast cells, eosinophils, bone marrow progenitors	Stimulation of hematopoietic progenitors.
IL-4	IL-4r α, common γ	T cells, mast cells, basophils	T cells, B cells, NK cells, monocytes/macrophages, neutrophils, eosinophils, endothelial cells, fibroblasts	Stimulates T$_H$2 helper T cell differentiation and proliferation. Stimulates B cell Ig class switch to IgG1 and IgE anti-inflammatory action on T cells, monocytes.
IL-5	IL-5r α, common γ	T cells, mast cells and eosinophils	Eosinophils, basophils, murine B cells	Regulates eosinophil migration and activation.
IL-6	IL-6r, gp130	Monocytes/macrophages, B cells, fibroblasts, most epithelium including thymic epithelium, endothelial cells	T cells, B cells, epithelial cells, hepatocytes, monocytes/macrophages	Induction of acute phase protein production, T and B cell differentiation and growth, myeloma cell growth, osteoclast growth and activation.
IL-7	IL-7r α, common γ	Bone marrow, thymic epithelial cells	T cells, B cells, bone marrow cells	Differentiation of B, T and NK cell precursors, activation of T and NK cells.
IL-8	CXCR1, CXCR2	Monocytes/macrophages, T cells, neutrophils, fibroblasts, endothelial cells, epithelial cells	Neutrophils, T cells, monocytes/macrophages, endothelial cells, basophils	Induces neutrophil, monocyte and T cell migration, induces neutrophil adherence to endothelial cells, histamine release from basophils, stimulates angiogenesis. Suppresses proliferations of hepatic precursors.
IL-9	IL-9r α, common γ	T cells	Bone marrow progenitors, B cells, T cells, mast cells	Induces mast cell proliferation and function, synergizes with IL-4 in IgG and IgE production, T cell growth, activation and differentiation.
IL-10	IL-10r	Monocytes/macrophages, T cells, B cells, keratinocytes, mast cells	Monocytes/macrophages, T cells, B cells, NK cells, mast cells	Inhibits macrophage proinflammatory cytokine production, downregulates cytokine class II antigen and B7-1 and B7-2 expression, inhibits differentiation of T$_H$1, helper T cells, inhibits NK cell function, stimulates mast cell proliferation and function, B cell activation and differentiation.
IL-11	IL-11, gp130	Bone marrow stromal cells	Megakaryocytes, B cells, hepatocytes	Induces megakaryocyte colony formation and maturation, enhances antibody responses, stimulates acute-phase protein production
IL-12 (35 kD and 40 kD subunits)	IL-12r	Activated macrophages, dendritic cells, neutrophils	T cells, NK cells	Induces T$_H$1 T helper cell formation and lymphokine-activated killer cell formation. Increases CD8+ CTL cytolytic activity; ↓IL-17, ↑γ-IFN.
IL-13	IL-13/IL-4	T cells (T$_H$2)	Monocytes/macrophages, B cells, endothelial cells, keratinocytes	Upregulation of VCAM-1 and C-C chemokine expression on endothelial cells, B cell activation and differentiation, inhibits macrophage proinflammatory cytokine production.
IL-14	Unknown	T cells	Normal and malignant B cells	Induces B cell proliferation
IL-15	IL-15r α, common γ, IL2r β	Monocytes/macrophages, epithelial cells, fibroblasts	T cells, NK cells	T cell activation and proliferation. Promotes angiogenesis, and NK cells.
IL-16	CD4	Mast cells, eosinophils, CD8+ T cells, respiratory epithelium	CD4+ T cells, monocytes/macrophages, eosinophils	Chemoattraction of CD4+ T cells, monocytes, and eosinophils. Inhibits HIV replication. Inhibits T cell activation through CD3/T cell receptor
IL-17	IL17r	CD4+ T cells	Fibroblasts, endothelium, epithelium	Enhanced cytokine secretion.
IL-18	IL-18r (IL-1R related protein)	Keratinocytes, macrophages	T cells, B cells, NK cells	Upregulated IFNγ production, enhanced NK cell cytotoxicity.
IL-21	IL-δγ chain/IL-21R	CD4 T cells	NK cells	Down-regulates NK cell activating molecules, NKG2D/DAP10
IL-23	IL-12Rb1/IL23R	Macrophages, other cell types	T cells	Opposite effects of IL-12 (↓IL-17, ↑γ-IFN)
IFNα	Type I interferon receptor	All cells	All cells	Anti-viral activity. Stimulates T cell, macrophage, and NK cell activity. Direct anti-tumor effects. Upregulates MHC class I antigen expression. Used therapeutically in viral and autoimmune conditions.
IFNβ	Type I interferon receptor	All cells	All cells	Anti-viral activity. Stimulates T cell, macrophage, and NK cell activity. Direct anti-tumor effects. Upregulates MHC class I antigen expression. Used therapeutically in viral and autoimmune conditions

(continued)

CHAPTER 308 Introduction to the Immune System

Cytokine	Receptor	Cell Source	Cell Target	Biologic Activity
IFNγ	Type II interferon receptor	T cells, NK cells	All cells	Regulates macrophage and NK cell activations. Stimulates immunoglobulin secretion by B cells. Induction of class II histocompatibility antigens. T_H1 T cell differentiation.
TNFα	TNFrI, TNFrII	Monocytes/macrophages, mast cells, basophils, eosinophils, NK cells, B cells, T cells, keratinocytes, fibroblasts, thymic epithelial cells	All cells except erythrocytes	Fever, anorexia, shock, capillary leak syndrome, enhanced leukocyte cytotoxicity, enhanced NK cell function, acute phase protein synthesis, pro-inflammatory cytokine induction.
TNFβ	TNFrI, TNFrII	T cells, B cells	All cells except erythrocytes	Cell cytotoxicity, lymph node and spleen development.
LTβ	LTβR	T cells	All cells except erythrocytes	Cell cytotoxicity, normal lymph node development
G-CSF	G-CSFr; gp130	Monocytes/macrophages, fibroblasts, endothelial cells, thymic epithelial cells, stromal cells	Myeloid cells, endothelial cells	Regulates myelopoiesis. Enhances survival and function of neutrophils. Clinical use in reversing neutropenia after cytotoxic chemotherapy.
GM-CSF	GM-CSFr, common β	T cells, monocytes/macrophages, fibroblasts, endothelial cells, thymic epithelial cells	Monocytes/macrophages, neutrophils, eosinophils, fibroblasts, endothelial cells	Regulates myelopoiesis. Enhances macrophage bactericidal and tumoricidal activity. Mediator of dendritic cell maturation and function. Upregulates NK cell function. Clinical use in reversing neutropenia after cytotoxic chemotherapy.
M-CSF	M-CSFr (c-fms protooncogene)	Fibroblasts, endothelial cells, monocytes/macrophages, T cells, B cells, epithelial cells including thymic epithelium	Monocytes/macrophages	Regulates monocyte/macrophage production and function.
LIF	LIFr; gp130	Activated T cells, bone marrow stromal cells, thymic epithelium	Megakaryocytes, monocytes, hepatocytes, possibly lymphocyte subpopulations	Induces hepatic acute phase protein production. Stimulates macrophage differentiation. Promotes growth of myeloma cells and hematopoietic progenitors. Stimulates thromboiesis.
OSM	OSMr; LIFr; gp130	Activated monocytes/macrophages and T cells, bone marrow stromal cells, some breast carcinoma cell lines, myeloma cells	Neurons, hepatocytes, monocytes/macrophages, adipocytes, alveolar epithelial cells, embryonic stem cells, melanocytes, endothelial cells, fibroblasts, myeloma cells	Induces hepatic acute phase protein production. Stimulates macrophage differentiation. Promotes growth of myeloma cells and hematopoietic progenitors. Stimulates thromboiesis. Stimulates growth of Kaposi's sarcoma cells.
SCF	SCFr (c-kit protooncogene)	Bone marrow stromal cells and fibroblasts	Embryonic stem cells, myeloid and lymphoid precursors, mast cells.	Stimulates hematopoietic progenitor cell growth, mast cell growth, promotes embryonic stem cell migration.
TGFβ (3 isoforms)	Type I, II, III TGFβ receptor	Most cell types	Most cell types	Down-regulates T cell, macrophage and granulocyte responses. Stimulates synthesis of matrix proteins. Stimulates angiogenesis.
Lymphotactin/ SCM-1	Unknown	NK cells, mast cells, double negative thymocytes, activated CD8+ T cells	T cells, NK cells	Chemoattractant for lymphocytes. Only known chemokine of C class.
MCP-1	CCR2	Fibroblasts, smooth muscle cells, activated PBMCs	Monocytes/macrophages, NK cells, memory T cells, basophils	Chemoattractant for monocytes, activated memory T cells, and NK cells. Induces granule release from CD8+ T cells and NK cells. Potent histamine releasing factor for basophiles. Suppresses proliferation of hematopoietic precursors. Regulates monocyte protease production.
MCP-2	CCR1, CCR2	Fibroblasts, activated PBMCs	Monocytes/macrophages, T cells, eosinophils, basophils, NK cells	Chemoattractant for monocytes, memory and naïve T cells, eosinophils, ?NK cells. Activates basophils and eosinophils. Regulates monocyte protease production.
MCP-3	CCR1, CCR2	Fibroblasts, activated PBMCs	Monocytes/macrophages, T cells, eosinophils, basophils, NK cells, dendritic cells	Chemoattractant for monocytes, memory and naïve T cells, dendritic cells, eosinophils, ?NK cells. Activates basophils and eosinophils. Regulates monocyte protease production.
MCP-4	CCR2, CCR3	Lung, colon, small intestinal epithelial cells, activated endothelial cells	Monocytes/macrophages, T cells eosinophils, basophils	Chemoattractant for monocytes, T cells, eosinophils and basophils
Eotaxin	CCR3	Pulmonary epithelial cells, heart	Eosinophils, basophils	Potent chemoattractant for eosinophils and basophils. Induces allergic airways disease. Acts in concert with IL-5 to activate eosinophils. Antibodies to eotaxin inhibit airway inflammation.

(continued)

TABLE 308-6 CYTOKINES AND CYTOKINE RECEPTORS (CONTINUED)

Cytokine	Receptor	Cell Source	Cell Target	Biologic Activity
TARC	CCR4	Thymus, dendritic cells, activated T cells	T cells, NK cells	Chemoattractant for T and NK cells.
MDC	CCR4	Monocytes/macrophages, dendritic cells, thymus	Activated T cells	Chemoattractant for activated T cells. Inhibits infection with T cell tropic HIV.
MIP-1α	CCR1, CCR5	Monocytes/macrophages, T cells	Monocytes/macrophages, T cells, dendritic cells, NK cells, eosinophils, basophils	Chemoattractant for monocytes, T cells, dendritic cells, NK cells, and weak chemoattractant for eosinophils and basophils. Activates NK cell function. Suppresses proliferation of hematopoietic precursors. Necessary for myocarditis associated with Coxsackie virus infection. Inhibits infection with monocytotropic HIV.
MIP-1β	CCR5	Monocytes/macrophages, T cells	Monocytes/macrophages, T cells, NK cells, dendritic cells	Chemoattractant for monocytes, T cells, and NK cells. Activates NK cell function. Inhibits infection with monocytotropic HIV.
RANTES	CCR1, CCR2, CCR5	Monocytes/macrophages, T cells, fibroblasts, eosinophils	Monocytes/macrophages, T cells, NK cells, dendritic cells, eosinophils, basophils	Chemoattractant for monocytes/macrophages, CD4+ CD45Ro+T cells, CD8+ T cells, NK cells, eosinophils, and basophils. Induces histamine release from basophils. Inhibits infections with monocytotropic HIV.
LARC/MIP-3α/ Exodus-1	CCR6	Dendritic cells, fetal liver cells, activated T cells	T cells, B cells	Chemoattractant for lymphocytes.
ELC/MIP-3β	CCR7	Thymus, lymph node, appendix	Activated T cells and B cells	Chemoattractant for B and T cells. Receptor upregulated on EBV infected B cells and HSV infected T cells.
I-309/TCA-3	CCR8	Activated T cells	Monocytes/macrophages, T cells	Chemoattractant for monocytes. Prevents glucocorticoid-induced apoptosis in some T cell lines.
SLC/TCA-4/ Exodus-2	Unknown	Thymic epithelial cells, lymph node, appendix and spleen	T cells	Chemoattractant for T lymphocytes. Inhibits hematopoiesis.
DC-CK1/PARC	Unknown	Dendritic cells in secondary lymphoid tissues	Naïve T cells	May have a role in induction of immune responses.
TECK	Unknown	Dendritic cells, thymus, liver, small intestine	T cells, monocytes/macrophages, dendritic cells	Thymic dendritic cell-derived cytokine, possibly involved in T cell development
GROα/MGSA	CXCR2	Activated granulocytes, monocyte/macrophages, and epithelial cells.	Neutrophils, epithelial cells, ?endothelial cells	Neutrophil chemoattractant and activator. Mitogenic for some melanoma cell lines. Suppresses proliferation of hematopoietic precursors. Angiogenic activity.
GROβ/MIP-2α	CXCR2	Activated granulocytes and monocyte/macrophages	Neutrophils and ?endothelial cells.	Neutrophil chemoattractant and activator. Angiogenic activity.
NAP-2	CXCR2	Platelets	Neutrophils, basophils	Derived from platelet basic protein. Neutrophil chemoattractant and activator.
IP-10	CXCR3	Monocytes/macrophages, T cells, fibroblasts, endothelial cells, epithelial cells	Activated T cells, tumor infiltrating lymphocytes, ?endothelial cells, ?NK cells	IFNγ-inducible protein that is a chemoattractant for T cells. Suppresses proliferation of hematopoietic precursors.
MIG	CXCR3	Monocytes/macrophages, T cells, fibroblasts	Activated T cells, tumor infiltrating lymphocytes	IFNγ-inducible protein that is a chemoattractant for T cells. Suppresses proliferation of hematopoietic precursors.
SDF-1	CXCR4	Fibroblasts	T cells, dendritic cells, ?basophils, ?endothelial cells	Low potency, high efficacy T cell chemoattractant. Required for B-lymphocyte development. Prevents infection of CD4+, CXCR4+ cells by T cell tropic HIV.
Fractalkine	CX3CR1	Activated endothelial cells	NK cells, T cells, monocytes/macrophages	Cell surface chemokine/mucin hybrid molecule that functions as a chemoattractant, leukocyte activator and cell adhesion molecule.
PF-4	Unknown	Platelets, megakaryocytes	Fibroblasts, endothelial cells	Chemoattractant for fibroblasts. Suppresses proliferation of hematopoietic precursors. Inhibits endothelial cell proliferation and angiogenesis.

Note: IL, interleukin; NK, natural killer; T$_H$1 and T$_H$2 helper T cell subsets; Ig, immunoglobulin; CXCR, CXC-type chemokine receptor; B7-1, CD80, B7-2, CD86; PBMC, peripheral blood mononuclear cells; VCAM, vascular cell adhesion molecule; IFN, interferon; MHC, major histocompatibility complex; TNF, tumor necrosis factor; G-CSF, granulocyte colony-stimulating factor; GM-CSF, granulocyte-macrophage CSF; M-CSF, macrophage CSF; HIV, human immunodeficiency virus; LIF, leukemia inhibitory factor; OSM, oncostatin M; SCF, stem cell factor; TGF, transforming growth factor; MCP, monocyte chemotactic protein; CCR, CC-type chemokine receptor; TARC, thymus and activation-regulated chemokine; MDC, macrophage-derived chemokine; MIP, macrophage inflammatory protein; RANTES, regulated on activation, normally T-cell expressed and secreted; LARC, liver and activation-regulated chemokine; EBV, Epstein-Barr virus; ELC, EB11 ligand chemokine (MIP-1β); HSV, herpes simplex virus; TCA, T-cell activation protein; DC-CK, dendritic cell chemokine; PARC, pulmonary and activation-regulated chemokine; SLC, secondary lymphoid tissue chemokine; TECK, thymus expressed chemokine; GRP, growth-related peptide; MGSA, melanoma growth-stimulating activity; NAP, neutrophil-activating protein; IP-10, IFN-γ-inducible protein-10; MIG, monoteine induced by IFN-γ; SDF, stromal cell-derived factor; PF, platelet factor.

Source: Used with permission from Sundy JS, Patel DD, and Haynes BF: Appendix B, in *Inflammation, Basic Principles and Clinical Correlates*, 3rd ed, J Gallin and R Snyderman (eds). Philadelphia, Lippincott Williams and Wilkins, 1999.

TABLE 308-7 CC, CXC$_1$, CX$_3$, C$_1$ AND XC FAMILIES OF CHEMOKINES AND CHEMOKINE RECEPTORS[a]

Chemokine Receptor	Chemokine Ligands	Cell Types	Disease Connection
CCR1	CCL3 (MIP-1α), CCL5 (RANTES), CCL7 (MCP-3), CCL14 (HCC1)	T cells, monocytes, eosinophils, basophils	Rheumatoid arthritis, multiple sclerosis
CCR2	CCL2 (MCP-1), CCL8 (MCP-2), CCL7 (MCP-3), CCL13 (MCP-4), CCL16 (HCC4)	Monocytes, dendritic cells (immature), memory T cells	Atherosclerosis, rheumatoid arthritis, multiple sclerosis, resistance to intracellular pathogens, type 2 diabetes mellitus
CCR3	CCL11 (eotaxin), CCL13 (eotaxin-2), CCL7 (MCP-3), CCL5 (RANTES), CCL8 (MCP-2), CCL13 (MCP-4)	Eosinophils, basophils, mast cells, T$_H$2, platelets	Allergic asthma and rhinitis
CCR4	CCL17 (TARC), CCL22 (MDC)	T cells (T$_H$2) dendritic cells (mature), basophils, macrophages, platelets	Parasitic infection, graft rejection, T-cell homing to skin
CCR5	CCL3 (MIP-1α), CCL4 (MIP-1β), CCL5 (RANTES), CCL11 (eotaxin), CCL14 (HCC1), CCL16 (HCC4)	T cells, monocytes	HIV-1 coreceptor (T-tropic strains), transplant rejection
CCR6	CCL20 (MIP-3β, LARC)	T cells (T regulatory and memory), B cells, dendritic cells	Mucosal humoral immunity, allergic asthma, intestinal T-cell homing
CCR7	CCL19 (ELC), CCL21 (SLC)	T cells, dendritic cells (mature)	Transport of T cells and dendritic cells to lymph nodes, antigen presentation, and cellular immunity
CCR8	CCL1 (1309)	T cells (T$_H$2), monocytes, dendritic cells	Dendritic-cell migration to lymph node, type 2 cellular immunity, granuloma formation
CCR9	CCL25 (TECK)	T cells, IgA+ plasma cells	Homing of T cells and IgA+ plasma cells to the intestine, inflammatory bowel disease
CCR10	CCL27 (CTACK, CCL28 (MEC)	T cells	T-cell homing to intestine and skin
CXCR1	CXCL8 (interleukin-8), CXCL6 (GCP2)	Neutrophils, monocytes	Inflammatory lung disease, COPD
CXCR2	CXCL8, CXCL1 (GROα), CXCL2 (GROβ), CXCL3 (GROγ), CXCL5 (ENA-78), CXCL6	Neutrophils, monocytes, microvascular endothelial cells	Inflammatory lung disease, COPD, angiogenic for tumor growth
CXCR3-A	CXCL9 (MIG), CXCL10 (IP-10), CXCL11 (I-TAC)	Type 1 helper cells, mast cells, mesangial cells	Inflammatory skin disease, multiple sclerosis, transplant rejection
CXCR3-B	CXCL4 (PF4), CXCL9 (MIG), CXCL10 (IP-10), CXCL11 (I-TAC)	Microvascular endothelial cells, neoplastic cells	Angiostatic for tumor growth
CXCR4	CXCL12 (SDF-1)	Widely expressed	HIV-1 coreceptor (T-cell–tropic), tumor metastases, hematopoiesis
CXCR5	CXCL13 (BCA-1)	B cells, follicular helper T cells	Formation of B-cell follicles
CXCR6	CXCL16 (SR-PSOX)	CD8+ T cells, natural killer cells, and memory CD4+ T cells	Inflammatory liver disease, atherosclerosis (CXCL16)
CX$_3$CR1	CX3CL1 (fractalkine)	Macrophages, endothelial cells, smooth-muscle cells	Atherosclerosis
XCR1	XCL1 (lymphotactin), XCL2	T cells, natural killer cells	Rheumatoid arthritis, IgA nephropathy, tumor response

[a]MIP denotes macrophage inflammatory protein, MCP monocyte chemoattractant protein, HCC hemofiltrate chemokine, T$_H$2 type 2 helper T cells, TARC thymus and activation-regulated chemokine, MDC macrophage-derived chemokine, LARC liver and activation-regulated chemokine, ELC Epstein-Barr I1-ligand chemokine, SLC secondary lymphoid-tissue chemokine, TECK thymus-expressed chemokine, CTACK cutaneous T-cell–attracting chemokine, and MEC mammary-enriched chemokine.
GCP denotes granulocyte chemotactic protein, COPD chronic obstructive pulmonary disease, GRO growth-regulated oncogene, ENA epithelial-cell–derived neutrophil-activating peptide, MIG monokine induced by interferon-γ, IP-10 interferon inducible 10, I-TAC interferon-inducible T-cell alpha chemoattractant, PF platelet factor, SDF stromal-cell–derived factor, HIV human immunodeficiency virus, BCA-1 B-cell chemoattractant 1, and SR-PSOX scavenger receptor for phosphatidylserine-containing oxidized lipids

Source: From Charo and Ramsohoff, 2006 with permission.

and proliferate in response to IL-2. NK cells arise in both bone marrow and thymic microenvironments.

Functionally, NK cells share features with both monocytes-macrophages and neutrophils in that they mediate both antibody-dependent cellular cytotoxicity (ADCC) and NK cell activity. ADCC is the binding of an opsonized (antibody-coated) target cell to an Fc receptor–bearing effector cell via the Fc region of antibody, resulting in lysis of the target by the effector cell. NK cell activity is the nonimmune (i.e., effector cell never having had previous contact with the target), MHC-unrestricted, non-antibody-mediated killing of target cells, which are usually malignant cell types, transplanted foreign cells, or virus-infected cells. Thus, NK cell activity may play an important role in immune surveillance and destruction of malignant and virally infected host cells. NK cell hyporesponsiveness is also observed in patients with *Chédiak-Higashi syndrome*, an autosomal recessive disease associated with fusion of cytoplasmic granules and defective degranulation of neutrophil lysosomes.

The ability of NK cells to kill target cells is inversely related to target cell expression of MHC class I molecules. Thus, NK cells kill target cells with low or no levels of MHC class I expression and are prevented from killing target cells with high levels of class I expression. NK cells have surface-inhibiting killer immunoglobulin-like receptors (KIRs) that bind to classic MHC class I molecules in a polymorphic way and inhibit NK cell killing of human leukocyte antigen (HLA) positive cells. NK cell inactivation by KIRs is a central mechanism to prevent damage to normal host cells. However, to eliminate malignant and virally infected cells, NK cells also require activation through recognition of NK activation molecules on the surface of target cells (Fig. 308-4). Three molecules on NK cells—NKp46, NKp30, and NKp44—are collectively referred to as *natural cytotoxicity receptors (NCRs)* and mediate NK cell activation against target cells; the ligands to which they bind on target cells remain unknown. In addition, two coreceptors on NK cells, 2B4 and NTB-A, can serve as either activators or inhibitors of NK cells, depending on the ligand and signaling pathways that become activated. Thus, NK cell signaling is a highly coordinated series of inhibiting and activating signals that are coordinated to all NK cells such that they do not respond to uninfected, nonmalignant self-cells, but they are activated to attack malignant and virally infected cells. Recent evidence suggests that NK cells, though not possessing rearranging immune recognition genes, may be able to mediate recall responses for certain immune reactions such as contact hypersensitivity.

Some NK cells express CD3 and are termed *NK/T cells*. NK/T cells can also express oligoclonal forms of the TCR for antigen that can recognize lipid molecules of intracellular bacteria when presented in the

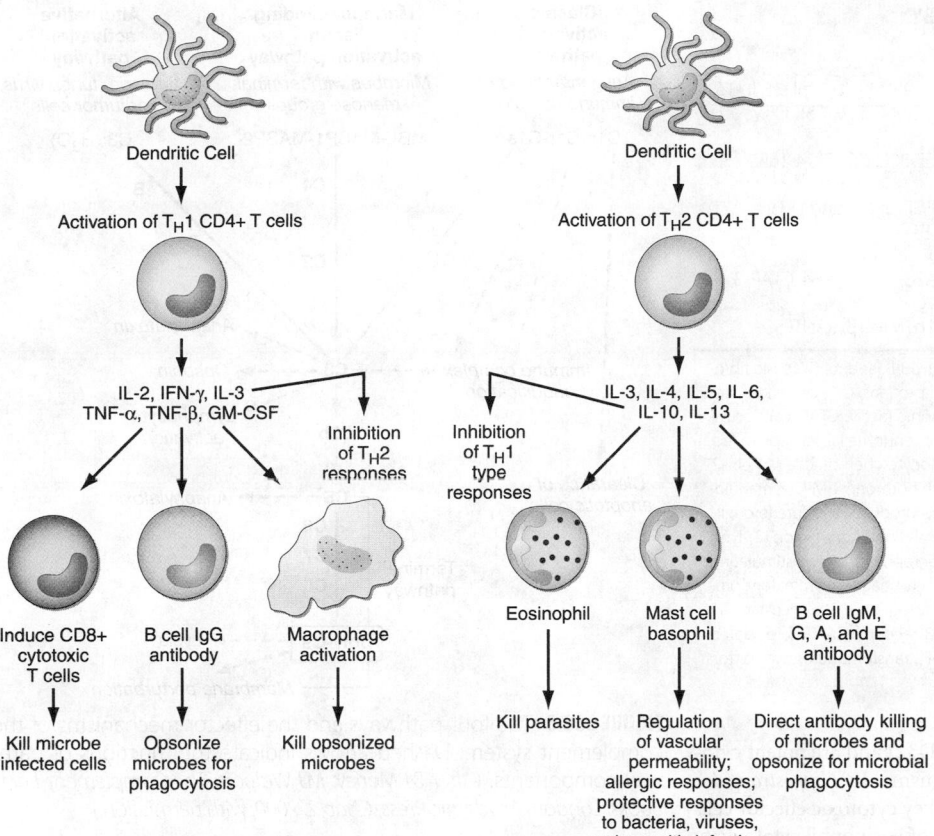

FIGURE 308-3 CD4+ helper T1 (T$_H$1) cells and T$_H$2 T cells secrete distinct but overlapping sets of cytokines. T$_H$1 CD4+ cells are frequently activated in immune and inflammatory reactions against intracellular bacteria or viruses, while T$_H$2 CD4+ cells are frequently activated for certain types of antibody production against parasites and extracellular encapsulated bacteria; they are also activated in allergic diseases. GM-CSF, granulocyte-macrophage colony stimulating factor; IFN, interferon; IL, interleukin; TNF, tumor necrosis factor. *(Adapted from S Romagnani: CD4 effector cells, in J Gallin, R Snyderman (eds): Inflammation: Basic Principles and Clinical Correlates, 3d ed. Philadelphia, Lippincott Williams & Wilkins, 1999; with permission.)*

context of CD1 molecules on APCs. This mode of recognition of intracellular bacteria such as *Listeria monocytogenes* and *M. tuberculosis* by NK/T cells leads to induction of activation of DCs and is thought to be an important defense mechanism against these organisms.

Neutrophils, Eosinophils, and Basophils

Granulocytes are present in nearly all forms of inflammation and are amplifiers and effectors of innate immune responses (Fig. 308-3). Unchecked accumulation and activation of granulocytes can lead to host tissue damage, as seen in neutrophil- and eosinophil-mediated *systemic necrotizing vasculitis*. Granulocytes are derived from stem cells in bone marrow. Each type of granulocyte (neutrophil, eosinophil, or basophil) is derived from a different subclass of progenitor cell, which is stimulated to proliferate by colony-stimulating factors (Table 308-6). During terminal maturation of granulocytes, class-specific nuclear morphology and cytoplasmic granules appear that allow for histologic identification of granulocyte type.

Neutrophils express Fc receptors for IgG (CD16) and receptors for activated complement components (C3b or CD35). Upon interaction of neutrophils with opsonized bacteria or immune complexes, azurophilic granules (containing myeloperoxidase, lysozyme, elastase, and other enzymes) and specific granules (containing lactoferrin, lysozyme, collagenase, and other enzymes) are released, and microbicidal superoxide radicals (O_2^-) are generated at the neutrophil surface. The generation of superoxide leads to inflammation by direct injury to tissue and by alteration of macromolecules such as collagen and DNA.

FIGURE 308-4 Receptors and ligands involved in human NK cell-mediated cytotoxicity. NK cell activation is the final result of the engagement of a number of receptors that have opposite functions. A simplified model of the surface receptors and their ligands involved in NK cell activation (green) or inactivation (red) is shown. KIRS are killer immunoglobulin-like receptors. In the absence of inhibitory signals, activating NK cell receptor ligation with molecules on the target cell results in NK cell triggering and target cell lysis. This event occurs in MHC class I HLA-defective cells, such as tumors or virus-infected cells. In the case of normal cells that express MHC class I, the interaction between inhibitory receptors and MHC class I delivers signals that overcome NK cell triggering, thus preventing target cell lysis. Although the cellular natural cytotoxic receptor (NCR) ligands have not yet been identified, the ligands for NG2D are represented by stress-inducible MICA, MICB, and ULBPs. The ligand for 2B4 is CD48, which is expressed by hematopoietic cells, whereas the ligand for NTB-A is itself on target cells. The + and − symbols denote activating or inhibitory signals, respectively. *(From Moretta A. et al. Nature Immunol., vol. 3, 2002; with permission.)*

TABLE 308-8	MAJOR STRUCTURAL FAMILIES OF CYTOKINES
Four α-helix-bundle family interleukins	Interleukin-2 (IL-2) Subfamily: Interleukins: IL-2, IL-3, IL-4, IL-5, IL-6, IL-7, IL-9, IL-11, IL-12, IL-13, IL-15, IL-21, IL-23 Not called interleukins: Colony-stimulating factor-1 (CSF1), granulocyte–macrophage colony-stimulating factor (CSF2), Flt-3 ligand, erythropoietin (EPO), thrombopoietin (THPO), leukocyte inhibitory factor (LIF) Not interleukins: Growth hormone (GH1), prolactin (PRL), leptin (LEP), cardiotrophin (CTF1), ciliary neurotrophic factor (CNTF), cytokine receptor-like factor 1 (CLC or CLF) Interferon (IFN) subfamily: IFN-β, IFN-α IL-10 subfamily: IL-10, IL-19, IL-20, IL-22, IL-24 and IL-26
IL-1 family	IL-1α, (IL1A), IL-1β, (IL1B), IL-18 (IL18) and paralogues, IL-17A, IL-17B, IL-17C, IL-17D, IL-17E, IL-17F
Chemokines	IL-8, MCP-1, MCP-2, MCP-3, MCP-4, eotaxin, TARC, LARC/MIP-3α, MDC, MIP-1α, MIP-1β, RANTES, MIP-3β, I-309, SLC, PARC, TECK, GROα, GROβ, NAP-2, IP-19, MIG, SDF-1, PF4

Note: GRO, growth-related peptide; IL interleukin; IP, INFg-inducible protein; LARC, liver and activation-regulated chemokine; MCP, monocyte chemotactic protein; MDC, macrophage-derived chemokine; MIG monotenine-induced by IFNg; MIP, macrophage inflammatory protein; NAP, neutrophil-activating protein; PARC, pulmonary and activation-regulated chemokine; PF4, platelet factor; RANTES, regulated on activation normally T cell expressed and secreted; SDF, stromal-cell derived factor; SLC, secondary lymphoid tissue.

Source: Adapted with permission from JW Schrader, Trends Immunology 23:573, 2002.

TABLE 308-9   CYTOKINES FAMILIES GROUPED BY STRUCTURAL SIMILARITY

Hematopoietins	IL-2, IL-3, IL-4, IL-5, IL-6, IL-7, IL-9, IL-11, IL-12, IL-15, IL-16, IL-17, IL-21, IL-23, EPO, LIF, GM-CSF, G-CSF, OSM, CNTF, GH, and TPO
	TNF-α, LT-α, LT-β, CD40L, CD30L, CD27L, 4-1BBL, OX40, OPG, and FasL
IL-1	IL-1α, IL-1β, IL-1ra, IL-18, bFGF, aFGF, and ECGF
PDGF	PDGF A, PDGF B, and M-CSF
TGF-β	TGF-β and BMPs (1,2,4 etc.)
C-X-C chemokines	IL-8, Gro-α/β/γ, NAP-2, ENA78, GCP-2, PF4, CTAP-3, Mig, and IP-10
C-C chemokines	MCP-1, MCP-2, MCP-3, MIP-1α, MIP-1β, RANTES

Note: aFGF, acidic fibroblast growth factor; 4-1 BBL, 401 BB ligand; bFGF, basic fibroblast growth factor; BMP, bone marrow morphogenetic proteins; C-C, cysteine-cysteine; CD, cluster of differentiation; CNTF, ciliary neurotrophic factor; CTAP, connective tissue activating peptide; C-X-C, cysteine-x-cysteine; ECGF, endothelial cell growth factor; EPO, erythropoietin; FasL, Fas ligand; GCP-2, granulocyte chemotactic protein-2; G-CSF, granulocyte colony-stimulating factor; GH, growth hormone; Gro, growth-related gene products; IFN, interferon; IL, interleukin; IP, interferon-γ inducible protein; LIF, leukemia inhibitory factor; LT, lymphotoxin; MCP, monocyte chemoattractant; M-CSF, macrophage colony-stimulating factor; Mig, monokine induced by interferon-γ; MIP, macrophage inflammatory protein; NAP-2, neutrophil activating protein-2; OPG, osteoprotegerin; OSM, oncostatin M; PDGF, platelet-derived growth factor; PF, platelet factor; R, receptor; RANTES, regulated on activation, normal T cell-expressed and –secreted; TGF, transforming growth factor; TNF, tumor necrosis factor; TPO, thyroperoxidase.

FIGURE 308-5 The four pathways and the effector mechanisms of the complement system. Dashed arrows indicate the functions of pathway components. (*After BJ Morley, MJ Walport: The Complement Facts Books. London, Academic Press, Chap 2, 2000; with permission.*)

Eosinophils express Fc receptors for IgG (CD32) and are potent cytotoxic effector cells for various parasitic organisms. In *Nippostrongylus brasiliensis* helminth infection, eosinophils are key cytotoxic effector cells in removal of these parasites. Key to regulation of eosinophil cytotoxicity to *N. brasiliensis* worms are antigen-specific T helper cells that produce IL-4, thus providing an example of regulation of innate immune responses by adaptive immunity antigen-specific T cells. Intracytoplasmic contents of eosinophils, such as major basic protein, eosinophil cationic protein, and eosinophil-derived neurotoxin, are capable of directly damaging tissues and may be responsible in part for the organ system dysfunction in the *hypereosinophilic syndromes* (Chap. 61). Since the eosinophil granule contains anti-inflammatory types of enzymes (histaminase, arylsulfatase, phospholipase D), eosinophils may homeostatically downregulate or terminate ongoing inflammatory responses.

Basophils and tissue mast cells are potent reservoirs of cytokines such as IL-4 and can respond to bacteria and viruses with antipathogen cytokine production through multiple TLRs expressed on their surface. Mast cells and basophils can also mediate immunity through the binding of antipathogen antibodies. This is a particularly important host defense mechanism against parasitic diseases. Basophils express high-affinity surface receptors for IgE (FcRI) and, upon cross-

linking of basophil-bound IgE by antigen, can release histamine, eosinophil chemotactic factor of anaphylaxis, and neutral protease—all mediators of allergic immediate (anaphylaxis) hypersensitivity responses (Table 308-10). In addition, basophils express surface receptors for activated complement components (C3a, C5a), through which mediator release can be directly effected. Thus, basophils, like most cells of the immune system, can be activated in the service of host defense against pathogens, or they can be activated for mediation release and cause pathogenic responses in allergic and inflammatory diseases. For further discussion of tissue mast cells, see Chap. 311.

The Complement System   The complement system, an important soluble component of the innate immune system, is a series of plasma enzymes, regulatory proteins, and proteins that are activated in a cascading fashion, resulting in cell lysis. There are four pathways of the complement system: the classic activation pathway activated by antigen/antibody immune complexes, the MBL (a serum collectin; Table 308-3) activation pathway activated by microbes with terminal mannose groups, the alternative activation pathway activated by microbes or tumor cells, and the terminal pathway that is common to the first three pathways and leads to the membrane attack complex that lyses cells (Fig. 308-5). The series of enzymes of the complement system are serine proteases.

Activation of the classic complement pathway via immune complex binding to C1q links the innate and adaptive immune systems via specific antibody in the immune complex. The alternative complement activation pathway is antibody-independent and is activated by binding of C3 directly to pathogens and "altered self" such as tumor cells. In the renal glomerular inflammatory disease *IgA nephropathy*, IgA activates the alternative complement pathway and causes glomerular damage and decreased renal function. Activation of the classic complement pathway via C1, C4, and C2 and activation of the alternative pathway via factor D, C3, and factor B both lead to cleavage and activation of C3. C3 activation fragments, when bound to target surfaces such as bacteria and other foreign antigens, are critical for opsonization (coating by antibody and complement) in preparation for phagocytosis. The MBL pathway substitutes MBL-associated serine proteases (MASPs) 1 and 2 for C1q, C1r, and C1s to activate C4. The MBL activation pathway is activated by mannose on the surface of bacteria and viruses.

TABLE 308-10   EXAMPLES OF MEDIATORS RELEASED FROM HUMAN CELLS AND BASOPHILS

Mediator	Actions
Histamine	Smooth-muscle contraction, increased vascular permeability
Slow reacting substance of anaphylaxis (SRSA) (leukotriene C4, D4, E4)	Smooth-muscle contraction
Eosinophil chemotactic factor of anaphylaxis (ECF-A)	Chemotactic attraction of eosinophils
Platelet-activating factor	Activates platelets to secrete serotonin and other mediators: smooth-muscle contraction; induces vascular permeability
Neutrophil chemotactic factor (NCF)	Chemotactic attraction of neutrophils
Leukotactic activity (leukotriene B4)	Chemotactic attraction of neutrophils
Heparin	Anticoagulant
Basophil kallikrein of anaphylaxis (BK-A)	Cleaves kininogen to form bradykinin

The three pathways of complement activation all converge on the final common terminal pathway. C3 cleavage by each pathway results in activation of C5, C6, C7, C8, and C9, resulting in the membrane attack complex that physically inserts into the membranes of target cells or bacteria and lyses them.

Thus, complement activation is a critical component of innate immunity for responding to microbial infection. The functional consequences of complement activation by the three initiating pathways and the terminal pathway are shown in Fig. 308-5. In general the cleavage products of complement components facilitate microbe or damaged cell clearance (C1q, C4, C3), promote activation and enhancement of inflammation (anaphylatoxins, C3a, C5a), and promote microbe or opsonized cell lysis (membrane attack complex).

CYTOKINES

Cytokines are soluble proteins produced by a wide variety of hematopoietic and nonhematopoietic cell types (Tables 308-6 to 308-9). They are critical for both normal innate and adaptive immune responses, and their expression may be perturbed in most immune, inflammatory, and infectious disease states.

Cytokines are involved in the regulation of the growth, development, and activation of immune system cells and in the mediation of the inflammatory response. In general, cytokines are characterized by considerable redundancy; different cytokines have similar functions. In addition, many cytokines are pleiotropic in that they are capable of acting on many different cell types. This pleiotropism results from the expression on multiple cell types of receptors for the same cytokine (see below), leading to the formation of "cytokine networks." The action of cytokines may be (1) autocrine when the target cell is the same cell that secretes the cytokine, (2) paracrine when the target cell is nearby, and (3) endocrine when the cytokine is secreted into the circulation and acts distal to the source.

Cytokines have been named based on presumed targets or based on presumed functions. Those cytokines that are thought to primarily target leukocytes have been named interleukins (IL-1, -2, -3, etc.). Many cytokines that were originally described as having a certain function have retained those names (granulocyte colony-stimulating factor or G-CSF, etc.). Cytokines belong in general to three major structural families: the hemopoietin family; the TNF, IL-1, platelet-derived growth factor (PDGF), and transforming growth factor (TGF) β families; and the CXC and c-c chemokine families (Table 308-8). Chemokines are cytokines that regulate cell movement and trafficking; they act through G protein–coupled receptors and have a distinctive three-dimensional structure. IL-8 is the only chemokine that early on was named an interleukin (Table 308-6).

In general, cytokines exert their effects by influencing gene activation that results in cellular activation, growth, differentiation, functional cell-surface molecule expression, and cellular effector function. In this regard, cytokines can have dramatic effects on the regulation of immune responses and the pathogenesis of a variety of diseases. Indeed, T cells have been categorized on the basis of the pattern of cytokines that they secrete, which results in either humoral immune response (T_H2) or cell-mediated immune response (T_H1) (Fig. 308-3).

Cytokine receptors can be grouped into five general families based on similarities in their extracellular amino acid sequences and conserved structural domains. The immunoglobulin (Ig) superfamily represents a large number of cell-surface and secreted proteins. The IL-1 receptors (type 1, type 2) are examples of cytokine receptors with extracellular Ig domains.

The hallmark of the hematopoietic growth factor (type 1) receptor family is that the extracellular regions of each receptor contain two conserved motifs. One motif, located at the N terminus, is rich in cysteine residues. The other motif is located at the C terminus proximal to the transmembrane region and comprises five amino acid residues, tryptophan-serine-X-tryptophan-serine (WSXWS). This family can be grouped on the basis of the number of receptor subunits they have and on the utilization of shared subunits. A number of cytokine receptors, i.e., IL-6, IL-11, IL-12, and leukemia inhibitory factor, are paired

with gp130. There is also a common 150-kDa subunit shared by IL-3, IL-5, and granulocyte-macrophage colony-stimulating factor (GM-CSF) receptors. The gamma chain (γ_c) of the IL-2 receptor is common to the IL-2, IL-4, IL-7, IL-9, and IL-15 receptors. Thus, the specific cytokine receptor is responsible for ligand-specific binding, while the subunits such as gp130, the 150-kDa subunit, and γ_c are important in signal transduction. The γ_c gene is on the X chromosome, and mutations in the γ_c protein result in the X-linked form of severe combined immune deficiency syndrome (X-SCID) (Chap. 310).

The members of the interferon (type II) receptor family include the receptors for IFN-γ and -β, which share a similar 210-amino-acid binding domain with conserved cysteine pairs at both the amino and carboxy termini. The members of the TNF (type III) receptor family share a common binding domain composed of repeated cysteine-rich regions. Members of this family include the p55 and p75 receptors for TNF (TNFR1 and TNFR2, respectively); CD40 antigen, which is an important B cell–surface marker involved in immunoglobulin isotype switching; fas/Apo-1, whose triggering induces apoptosis; CD27 and CD30, which are found on activated T cells and B cells; and nerve growth factor receptor.

The common motif for the seven transmembrane helix family was originally found in receptors linked to GTP-binding proteins. This family includes receptors for chemokines (Table 308-7), β-adrenergic receptors, and retinal rhodopsin. It is important to note that two members of the chemokine receptor family, CXC chemokine receptor type 4 (CXCR4) and β chemokine receptor type 5 (CCR5), have been found to serve as the two major coreceptors for binding and entry of HIV into CD4-expressing host cells (Chap. 182).

Significant advances have been made in defining the signaling pathways through which cytokines exert their effects intracellularly. The Janus family of protein tyrosine kinases (JAK) is a critical element involved in signaling via the hematopoietin receptors. Four JAK kinases, JAK1, JAK2, JAK3, and Tyk2, preferentially bind different cytokine receptor subunits. Cytokine binding to its receptor brings the cytokine receptor subunits into apposition and allows a pair of JAKs to transphosphorylate and activate one another. The JAKs then phosphorylate the receptor on the tyrosine residues and allow signaling molecules to bind to the receptor, where these molecules become phosphorylated. Signaling molecules bind the receptor because they have domains (SH2, or src homology 2 domains) that can bind phosphorylated tyrosine residues. There are a number of these important signaling molecules that bind the receptor, such as the adapter molecule SHC, which can couple the receptor to the activation of the mitogen-activated protein kinase pathway. In addition, an important class of substrate of the JAKs is the signal transducers and activators of transcription (STAT) family of transcription factors. STATs have SH2 domains that enable them to bind to phosphorylated receptors, where they are then phosphorylated by the JAKs. It appears that different STATs have specificity for different receptor subunits. The STATs then dissociate from the receptor and translocate to the nucleus, bind to DNA motifs that they recognize, and regulate gene expression. The STATs preferentially bind DNA motifs that are slightly different from one another and thereby control transcription of specific genes. The importance of this pathway is particularly relevant to lymphoid development. Mutations of JAK3 itself also result in a disorder identical to X-SCID; however, since JAK3 is found on chromosome 19 and not on the X chromosome, JAK3 deficiency occurs in boys and girls (Chap. 310).

THE ADAPTIVE IMMUNE SYSTEM

Adaptive immunity is characterized by antigen-specific responses to a foreign antigen or pathogen. A key feature of adaptive immunity is that following the initial contact with antigen (immunologic priming), subsequent antigen exposure leads to more rapid and vigorous immune responses (immunologic memory). The adaptive immune system consists of dual limbs of cellular and humoral immunity. The principal effectors of cellular immunity are T lymphocytes, while the principal effectors of humoral immunity are B lymphocytes. Both B and T lymphocytes derive from a common stem cell (Fig. 308-6).

FIGURE 308-6 Development stages of T and B cells. Elements of the developing T and B cell receptor for antigen are shown schematically. The classification into the various stages of B cell development is primarily defined by rearrangement of the immunoglobulin (Ig), heavy (H), and light (L) chain genes and by the absence or presence of specific surface markers. *[Adapted from CA Janeway et al, (eds): Immunobiology. The Immune Systemic Health and Disease, 4th ed, New York, Garland, 1999; with permission.]* The classification of stages of T cell development is primarily defined by cell surface marker protein expression (sCD3, surface CD3 expression; cCD3, cytoplasmic CD3 expression; TCR, T cell receptor).

The proportion and distribution of immunocompetent cells in various tissues reflect cell traffic, homing patterns, and functional capabilities. Bone marrow is the major site of maturation of B cells, monocytes-macrophages, dendritic cells, and granulocytes and contains pluripotent stem cells that, under the influence of various colony-stimulating factors, are capable of giving rise to all hematopoietic cell types. T cell precursors also arise from hematopoietic stem cells and home to the thymus for maturation. Mature T lymphocytes, B lymphocytes, monocytes, and dendritic cells enter the circulation and home to peripheral lymphoid organs (lymph nodes, spleen) and mucosal surface–associated lymphoid tissue (gut, genitourinary, and respiratory tracts) as well as the skin and mucous membranes and await activation by foreign antigen.

T Cells The pool of effector T cells is established in the thymus early in life and is maintained throughout life both by new T cell production in the thymus and by antigen-driven expansion of virgin peripheral T cells into "memory" T cells that reside in peripheral lymphoid organs. The thymus exports ~2% of the total number of thymocytes

per day throughout life, with the total number of daily thymic emigrants decreasing by ~3% per year during the first four decades of life.

Mature T lymphocytes constitute 70–80% of normal peripheral blood lymphocytes (only 2% of the total-body lymphocytes are contained in peripheral blood), 90% of thoracic duct lymphocytes, 30–40% of lymph node cells, and 20–30% of spleen lymphoid cells. In lymph nodes, T cells occupy deep paracortical areas around B cell germinal centers, and in the spleen, they are located in periarteriolar areas of white pulp (Chap. 60). T cells are the primary effectors of cell-mediated immunity, with subsets of T cells maturing into CD8+ cytotoxic T cells capable of lysis of virus-infected or foreign cells (short-lived effector T cells). Two populations of long-lived memory T cells are triggered by infections: effector memory and central memory T cells. Effector memory T cells reside in nonlymphoid organs and respond rapidly to repeated pathogenic infections with cytokine production and cytotoxic functions to kill virus-infected cells. Central memory T cells home to lymphoid organs where they replenish long- and short-lived and effector memory T cells as needed.

In general, CD4+ T cells are also the primary regulatory cells of T and B lymphocyte and monocyte function by the production of cytokines and by direct cell contact (Fig. 308-2). In addition, T cells regulate erythroid cell maturation in bone marrow, and through cell contact (CD40 ligand) have an important role in activation of B cells and induction of Ig isotype switching.

Human T cells express cell-surface proteins that mark stages of intrathymic T cell maturation or identify specific functional subpopulations of mature T cells. Many of these molecules mediate or participate in important T cell functions (Table 308-1, Fig. 308-6).

The earliest identifiable T cell precursors in bone marrow are CD34+ pro-T cells (i.e., cells in which TCR genes are neither rearranged nor expressed). In the thymus, CD34+ T cell precursors begin cytoplasmic (c) synthesis of components of the CD3 complex of TCR-associated molecules (Fig. 308-6). Within T cell precursors, TCR for antigen gene rearrangement yields two T cell lineages, expressing either TCRαβ chains or TCRγδ chains. T cells expressing the TCRαβ chains constitute the majority of peripheral T cells in blood, lymph node, and spleen and terminally differentiate into either CD4+ or CD8+ cells. Cells expressing TCRγδ chains circulate as a minor population in blood; their functions, although not fully understood, have been postulated to be those of immune surveillance at epithelial surfaces and cellular defenses against mycobacterial organisms and other intracellular bacteria through recognition of bacterial lipids.

In the thymus, the recognition of self-peptides on thymic epithelial cells, thymic macrophages, and dendritic cells plays an important role in shaping the T cell repertoire to recognize foreign antigen (*positive selection*) and in eliminating highly autoreactive T cells (*negative selection*). As immature cortical thymocytes begin to express surface TCR for antigen, autoreactive thymocytes are destroyed (negative selection), thymocytes with TCRs capable of interacting with foreign antigen peptides in the context of self-MHC antigens are activated and develop to maturity (positive selection), and thymocytes with TCR that are incapable of binding to self-MHC antigens die of attrition (*no selection*). Mature thymocytes that are positively selected are either CD4+ helper T cells or MHC class II–restricted cytotoxic (killer) T cells, or they are CD8+ T cells destined to become MHC class I–restricted cytotoxic T cells. *MHC class I– or class II–restricted* means that T cells recognize antigen peptide fragments only when they are presented in the antigen-recognition site of a class I or class II MHC molecule, respectively (Chap. 309).

After thymocyte maturation and selection, CD4 and CD8 thymocytes leave the thymus and migrate to the peripheral immune system. The thymus continues to be a contributor to the peripheral immune system, well into adult life, both normally and when the peripheral T cell pool is damaged, such as occurs in AIDS and cancer chemotherapy.

MOLECULAR BASIS OF T CELL RECOGNITION OF ANTIGEN The TCR for antigen is a complex of molecules consisting of an antigen-binding heterodimer of either αβ or γδ chains noncovalently linked with five CD3 subunits (γ, δ, ε, ζ, and η) (Fig. 308-7). The CD3 ζ chains are either disulfide-linked homodimers (CD3-ζ$_2$) or disulfide-linked heterodimers composed of one ζ chain and one η chain. TCRαβ or TCRγδ molecules must be associated with CD3 molecules to be inserted into the T cell surface membrane, TCRα being paired with TCRβ and TCRγ being paired with TCRδ. Molecules of the CD3 complex mediate transduction of T cell activation signals via TCRs, while TCRα and -β or -γ and -δ molecules combine to form the TCR antigen-binding site.

The α, β, γ, and δ TCR for antigen molecules have amino acid sequence homology and structural similarities to immunoglobulin heavy and light chains and are members of the *immunoglobulin gene superfamily* of molecules. The genes encoding TCR molecules are encoded as clusters of gene segments that rearrange during the course of T cell maturation. This creates an efficient and compact mechanism for housing the diversity requirements of antigen receptor molecules. The TCRα chain is on chromosome 14 and consists of a series of V (variable), J (joining), and C (constant) regions. The TCRβ chain is on chromosome 7 and consists of multiple V, D (diversity), J, and C TCRβ loci. The TCRγ chain is on chromosome 7, and the TCRδ chain is in the middle of the TCRα locus on chromosome 14. Thus, molecules of the TCR for antigen have constant (framework) and variable regions, and the gene segments encoding the α, β, γ, and δ chains of these molecules are recombined and selected in the thymus, culminating in synthesis of the completed molecule. In both T and B cell precursors (see below), DNA rearrangements of antigen receptor genes involve the same enzymes, recombinase activating gene (RAG)1 and RAG2, both DNA-dependent protein kinases.

TCR diversity is created by the different V, (D), and J segments that are possible for each receptor chain by the many permutations of V, D, and J segment combinations, by "N-region diversification" due to the addition of nucleotides at the junction of rearranged gene segments,

FIGURE 308-7 Signaling through the T cell receptor. Activation signals are mediated via immunoreceptor tyrosine-based activation (ITAM) sequences in LAT and CD3 chains (blue bars) that bind to enzymes and transduce activation signals to the nucleus via the indicated intracellular activation pathways. Ligation of the T-cell receptor (TCR) by MHC complexed with antigen results in sequential activation of LCK and g-chain–associated protein kinase of 70 kDa (ZAP70). ZAP70 phosphorylates several downstream targets, including LAT (linker for activation of T cells) and SLP76 [SCR homology 2 (SH2) domain-containing leukocyte protein of 76 kDa]. SLP76 is recruited to membrane-bound LAT through its constitutive interaction with GADS (GRB2-related adaptor protein). Together, SLP76 and LAT nucleate a multimolecular signaling complex, which induces a host of downstream responses, including calcium flux, mitogen-activated protein kinase (MAPK) activation, integrin activation, and cytoskeletal reorganization. [*Adapted from GA Koretzky, F Abtahaian, MA Silverman, Nature 6(1):67–78, 2006; with permission.*]

and by the pairing of individual chains to form a TCR dimer. As T cells mature in the thymus, the repertoire of antigen-reactive T cells is modified by selection processes that eliminate many autoreactive T cells, enhance the proliferation of cells that function appropriately with self-MHC molecules and antigen, and allow T cells with nonproductive TCR rearrangements to die.

TCRαβ cells do not recognize native protein or carbohydrate antigens. Instead, T cells recognize only short (~9–13 amino acids) peptide fragments derived from protein antigens taken up or produced in APCs. Foreign antigens may be taken up by endocytosis into acidified intracellular vesicles or by phagocytosis and degraded into small peptides that associate with MHC class II molecules (exogenous antigen-presentation pathway). Other foreign antigens arise endogenously in the cytosol (such as from replicating viruses) and are broken down into small peptides that associate with MHC class I molecules (endogenous antigen-presenting pathway). Thus, APCs proteolytically degrade foreign proteins and display peptide fragments embedded in the MHC class I or II antigen-recognition site on the MHC molecule surface, where foreign peptide fragments are available to bind to TCRαβ or TCRγδ chains of reactive T cells. CD4 molecules act as adhesives and, by direct binding to MHC class II (DR, DQ, or DP) molecules, stabilize the interaction of TCR with peptide antigen (Fig. 308-7). Similarly, CD8 molecules also act as adhesives to stabilize the TCR-antigen interaction by direct CD8 molecule binding to MHC class I (A, B, or C) molecules.

Antigens that arise in the cytosol and are processed via the endogenous antigen-presentation pathway are cleaved into small peptides by a complex of proteases called the *proteasome*. From the proteasome, antigen peptide fragments are transported from the cytosol into the lumen of the endoplasmic reticulum by a heterodimeric complex termed *transporters associated with antigen processing*, or TAP proteins. There, MHC class I molecules in the endoplasmic reticulum membrane physically associate with processed cytosolic peptides. Following peptide association with class I molecules, peptide–class I complexes are exported to the Golgi apparatus, and then to the cell surface, for recognition by CD8+ T cells.

Antigens taken up from the extracellular space via endocytosis into intracellular acidified vesicles are degraded by vesicle proteases into peptide fragments. Intracellular vesicles containing MHC class II molecules fuse with peptide-containing vesicles, thus allowing peptide fragments to physically bind to MHC class II molecules. Peptide–MHC class II complexes are then transported to the cell surface for recognition by CD4+ T cells (Chap. 309).

Whereas it is generally agreed that the TCRαβ receptor recognizes peptide antigens in the context of MHC class I or class II molecules, lipids in the cell wall of intracellular bacteria such as *M. tuberculosis* can also be presented to a wide variety of T cells, including subsets of CD4, CD8 TCRαβ T cells, TCRγδ T cells, and a subset of CD8+ TCRαβ T cells. Importantly, bacterial lipid antigens are not presented in the context of MHC class I or II molecules, but rather are presented in the context of MHC-related CD1 molecules. Some γδ T cells that recognize lipid antigens via CD1 molecules have very restricted TCR usage, do not need antigen priming to respond to bacterial lipids, and may actually be a form of innate rather than acquired immunity to intracellular bacteria.

Just as foreign antigens are degraded and their peptide fragments presented in the context of MHC class I or class II molecules on APCs, endogenous self-proteins also are degraded and self-peptide fragments are presented to T cells in the context of MHC class I or class II molecules on APCs. In peripheral lymphoid organs, there are T cells that are capable of recognizing self-protein fragments but normally are *anergic* or *tolerant*, i.e., nonresponsive to self-antigenic stimulation, due to lack of self-antigen upregulating APC *co-stimulatory molecules* such as B7-1 (CD80) and B7-2 (CD86) (see below).

Once engagement of mature T cell TCR by foreign peptide occurs in the context of self–MHC class I or class II molecules, binding of non-antigen-specific adhesion ligand pairs such as CD54-CD11/CD18 and CD58-CD2 stabilizes MHC peptide–TCR binding, and the expression of these adhesion molecules is upregulated (Fig. 308-7). Once antigen ligation of the TCR occurs, the T cell membrane is partitioned into *lipid membrane microdomains*, or *lipid rafts*, that coalesce the key signaling molecules TCR/CD3 complex, CD28, CD2, LAT (linker for activation of T cells), intracellular activated (dephosphorylated) src family protein tyrosine kinases (PTKs), and the key CD3ζ-associated protein-70 (ZAP-70) PTK (Fig. 308-7). Importantly, during T cell activation, the CD45 molecule, with protein tyrosine phosphatase activity is partitioned away from the TCR complex to allow activating phosphorylation events to occur. The coalescence of signaling molecules of activated T lymphocytes in *microdomains* has suggested that T cell–APC interactions can be considered *immunologic synapses*, analogous in function to neuronal synapses.

After TCR-MHC binding is stabilized, activation signals are transmitted through the cell to the nucleus and lead to the expression of gene products important in mediating the wide diversity of T cell functions such as the secretion of IL-2. The TCR does not have intrinsic signaling activity but is linked to a variety of signaling pathways via immunoreceptor tyrosine-based activation motifs (ITAMs) expressed on the various CD3 chains that bind to proteins that mediate signal transduction. Each of the pathways results in the activation of particular transcription factors that control the expression of cytokine and cytokine receptor genes. Thus, antigen-MHC binding to the TCR induces the activation of the src family of PTKs, fyn and lck (lck is associated with CD4 or CD8 co-stimulatory molecules); phosphorylation of CD3ζ chain; activation of the related tyrosine kinases ZAP-70 and syk; and downstream activation of the calcium-dependent calcineurin pathway, the ras pathway, and the protein kinase C pathway. Each of

these pathways leads to activation of specific families of transcription factors (including NF-AT, fos and jun, and rel/NF-κB) that form heteromultimers capable of inducing expression of IL-2, IL-2 receptor, IL-4, TNF-α, and other T cell mediators.

In addition to the signals delivered to the T cell from the TCR complex and CD4 and CD8, molecules on the T cell such as CD28 and inducible co-stimulator (ICOS) and molecules on dendritic cells such as B7-1 (CD80) and B7-2 (CD86) also deliver important co-stimulatory signals that upregulate T cell cytokine production and are essential for T cell activation. If signaling through CD28 or ICOS does not occur, or if CD28 is blocked, the T cell becomes anergic rather than activated (see "Immune Tolerance and Autoimmunity," below).

T CELL SUPERANTIGENS Conventional antigens bind to MHC class I or II molecules in the groove of the αβ heterodimer and bind to T cells via the V regions of the TCRα and -β chains. In contrast, superantigens bind directly to the lateral portion of the TCRβ chain and MHC class II β chain and stimulate T cells based solely on the Vβ gene segment utilized independent of the D, J, and Vα sequences present. *Superantigens* are protein molecules capable of activating up to 20% of the peripheral T cell pool, whereas conventional antigens activate <1 in 10,000 T cells. T cell superantigens include staphylococcal enterotoxins and other bacterial products. Superantigen stimulation of human peripheral T cells occurs in the clinical setting of *staphylococcal toxic shock syndrome*, leading to massive overproduction of T cell cytokines that leads to hypotension and shock (Chap. 129).

B Cells Mature B cells constitute 10–15% of human peripheral blood lymphocytes, 20–30% of lymph node cells, 50% of splenic lymphocytes, and ~10% of bone marrow lymphocytes. B cells express on their surface intramembrane immunoglobulin (Ig) molecules that function as B cell receptors (BCRs) for antigen in a complex of Ig-associated α and β signaling molecules with properties similar to those described in T cells (Fig. 308-8). Unlike T cells, which recognize only processed peptide fragments of conventional antigens embedded in the notches of MHC class I and class II antigens of APCs, B cells are capable of recognizing and proliferating to whole unprocessed native antigens via antigen binding to B cell surface Ig (sIg) receptors. B cells also express surface receptors for the Fc region of IgG molecules (CD32) as well as receptors for activated complement components (C3d or CD21, C3b or CD35). The primary function of B cells is to produce antibodies. B cells also serve as APCs and are highly efficient at antigen processing. Their antigen-presenting function is enhanced by a variety of cytokines. Mature B cells are derived from bone marrow precursor cells that arise continuously throughout life (Fig. 308-6).

B lymphocyte development can be separated into antigen-independent and antigen-dependent phases. Antigen-independent B cell development occurs in primary lymphoid organs and includes all stages of B cell maturation up to the sIg+ mature B cell. Antigen-dependent B cell maturation is driven by the interaction of antigen with the mature B cell sIg, leading to memory B cell induction, Ig class switching, and plasma cell formation. Antigen-dependent stages of B cell maturation occur in secondary lymphoid organs, including lymph node, spleen, and gut Peyer's patches. In contrast to the T cell repertoire that is generated intrathymically before contact with foreign antigen, the repertoire of B cells expressing diverse antigen-reactive sites is modified by further alteration of Ig genes after stimulation by antigen—a process called *somatic mutation*—which occurs in lymph node germinal centers.

During B cell development, diversity of the antigen-binding variable region of Ig is generated by an ordered set of Ig gene rearrangements that are similar to the rearrangements undergone by TCR α, β, γ, and δ genes. For the heavy chain, there is first a rearrangement of D segments to J segments, followed by a second rearrangement between a V gene segment and the newly formed D-J sequence; the C segment is aligned to the V-D-J complex to yield a functional Ig heavy chain gene (V-D-J-C). During later stages, a functional κ or λ light chain gene is generated by rearrangement of a V segment to a J segment, ultimately yielding an intact Ig molecule composed of heavy and light chains.

FIGURE 308-8 B-cell-receptor (BCR) activation results in the sequential activation of protein tyrosine kinases, which results in the formation of a signaling complex and activation of downstream pathways as shown. Whereas SLP76 is recruited to the membrane through GADS and LAT, the mechanism of SLP65 recruitment is unclear. Studies have indicated two mechanisms: (a) direct binding by the SH2 domain of SLP65 to immunoglobulin (Ig) of the BCR complex or (b) membrane recruitment through a leucine zipper in the amino terminus of SLP65 and an unknown binding partner. ADAP, adhesion- and degranulation-promoting adaptor protein; AP1, activator protein 1; BTK, Bruton's tyrosine kinase; DAG, diacylglycerol; GRB2, growth-factor-receptor-bound protein 2; HPK1, haematopoietic progenitor kinase 1; InsP₃, inositol-1,4,5-trisphosphate; ITK , interleukin-2-inducible T-cell kinase; NCK, non-catalytic region of tyrosine kinase; NF-B, nuclear factor B; PKC, protein kinase C; PLC, phospholipase C; PtdIns(4,5)P₂, phosphatidylinositol-4,5-bisphosphate; RASGRP, RAS guanyl-releasing protein; SOS, son of sevenless homologue; SYK, spleen tyrosine kinase. [*Adapted from GA Koretzky, F Abtahian, MA Silverman, Nat Rev Immunol 6(1):67–78, 2006; with permission.*]

The process of Ig gene rearrangement is regulated and results in a single antibody specificity produced by each B cell, with each Ig molecule comprising one type of heavy chain and one type of light chain. Although each B cell contains two copies of Ig light and heavy chain genes, only one gene of each type is productively rearranged and expressed in each B cell, a process termed *allelic exclusion.*

There are ~300 V_κ genes and 5 J_κ genes, resulting in the pairing of V_κ and J_κ genes to create >1500 different light chain combinations. The number of distinct κ light chains that can be generated is increased by somatic mutations within the V_κ and J_κ genes, thus creating large numbers of possible specificities from a limited amount of germ-line genetic information. As noted above, in heavy chain Ig gene rearrangement, the VH domain is created by the joining of three types of germ-line genes called V_H, D_H, and J_H, thus allowing for even greater diversity in the variable region of heavy chains than of light chains.

The most immature B cell precursors (early pro-B cells) lack cytoplasmic Ig (cIg) and sIg (Fig. 308-6). The large pre-B cell is marked by the acquisition of the surface pre-BCR composed of μ heavy (H) chains and a pre-B light chain, termed ψLC. ψLC is a surrogate light chain receptor encoded by the nonrearranged V pre-B and the λ5 light chain locus (the pre-BCR). Pro- and pre-B cells are driven to proliferate and mature by signals from bone marrow stroma—in particular, IL-7. Light chain rearrangement occurs in the small pre-B cell stage such that the full BCR is expressed at the immature B cell stage. Imma-

ture B cells have rearranged Ig light chain genes and express sIgM. As immature B cells develop into mature B cells, sIgD is expressed as well as sIgM. At this point, B lineage development in bone marrow is complete, and B cells exit into the peripheral circulation and migrate to secondary lymphoid organs to encounter specific antigens.

Random rearrangements of Ig genes occasionally generate self-reactive antibodies, and mechanisms must be in place to correct these mistakes. One such mechanism is BCR editing, whereby autoreactive BCRs are mutated to not react with self-antigens. If receptor editing is unsuccessful in eliminating autoreactive B cells, then autoreactive B cells undergo negative selection in the bone marrow through induction of apoptosis after BCR engagement of self-antigen.

After leaving the bone marrow, B cells populate peripheral B cell sites, such as lymph node and spleen, and await contact with foreign antigens that react with each B cell's clonotypic receptor. Antigen-driven B cell activation occurs through the BCR, and a process known as *somatic hypermutation* takes place whereby point mutations in rearranged H- and L-genes give rise to mutant sIg molecules, some of which bind antigen better than the original sIg molecules. Somatic hypermutation, therefore, is a process whereby memory B cells in peripheral lymph organs have the best binding, or the highest-affinity antibodies. This overall process of generating the best antibodies is called *affinity maturation of antibody.*

Lymphocytes that synthesize IgG, IgA, and IgE are derived from sIgM+, sIgD+ mature B cells. Ig class switching occurs in lymph node and other peripheral lymphoid tissue germinal centers. CD40 on B cells and CD40 ligand on T cells constitute a critical co-stimulatory receptor-ligand pair of immune-stimulatory molecules. Pairs of CD40+ B cells and CD40 ligand+ T cells bind and drive B cell Ig switching via T cell–produced cytokines such as IL-4 and TGF-β. IL-1, -2, -4, -5, and -6 synergize to drive mature B cells to proliferate and differentiate into Ig-secreting cells.

Humoral Mediators of Adaptive Immunity: Immunoglobulins Immunoglobulins are the products of differentiated B cells and mediate the humoral arm of the immune response. The primary functions of antibodies are to bind specifically to antigen and bring about the inactivation or removal of the offending toxin, microbe, parasite, or other foreign substance from the body. The structural basis of Ig molecule function and Ig gene organization has provided insight into the role of antibodies in normal protective immunity, pathologic immune-mediated damage by immune complexes, and autoantibody formation against host determinants.

All immunoglobulins have the basic structure of two heavy and two light chains (Fig. 308-8). Immunoglobulin isotype (i.e., G, M, A, D, E) is determined by the type of Ig heavy chain present. IgG and IgA isotypes can be divided further into subclasses (G1, G2, G3, G4, and A1, A2) based on specific antigenic determinants on Ig heavy chains. The characteristics of human immunoglobulins are outlined in **Table 308-11.** The four chains are covalently linked by disulfide bonds. Each

TABLE 308-11 PHYSICAL, CHEMICAL, AND BIOLOGIC PROPERTIES OF HUMAN IMMUNOGLOBULINS

Property	IgG	IgA	IgM	IgD	IgE
Usual molecular form	Monomer	Monomer, dimer	Pentamer, hexamer	Monomer	Monomer
Other chains	None	J chain, SC	J chain	None	None
Subclasses	G1, G2, G3, G4	A1, A2	None	None	None
Heavy chain allotypes	Gm (=30)	No A1, A2m (2)	None	None	None
Molecular mass, kDa	150	160, 400	950, 1150	175	190
Sedimentation constant, Sw20	6.6S	7S, 11S	19S	7S	8S
Carbohydrate content, %	3	7	10	9	13
Serum level in average adult, mg/mL	9.5–12.5	1.5–2.6	0.7–1.7	0.04	0.0003
Percentage of total serum Ig	75–85	7–15	5–10	0.3	0.019
Serum half-life, days	23	6	5	3	2.5
Synthesis rate, mg/kg per day	33	65	7	0.4	0.016
Antibody valence	2	2,4	10, 12	2	2
Classical complement activation	+(G1, 2?, 3)	–	++	–	–
Alternate complement activation	+(G4)	+	–	+	–
Binding cells via Fc	Macrophages, neutrophils, large granular lymphocytes	Lymphocytes	Lymphocytes	None	Mast cells, basophils, B cells
Biologic properties	Placental transfer, secondary Ab for most antipathogen responses	Secretory immunoglobulin	Primary Ab responses	Marker for mature B cells	Allergy, antiparasite responses

Source: After L Carayannopoulos and JD Capra, in WE Paul (ed): *Fundamental Immunology*, 3d ed. New York, Raven, 1993; with permission.

chain is made up of a V region and C regions (also called *domains*), themselves made up of units of ~110 amino acids. Light chains have one variable (V_L) and one constant (C_L) unit; heavy chains have one variable unit (V_H) and three or four constant (C_H) units, depending on isotype. As the name suggests, the constant, or C, regions of Ig molecules are made up of homologous sequences and share the same primary structure as all other Ig chains of the same isotype and subclass. Constant regions are involved in biologic functions of Ig molecules. The C_{H2} domain of IgG and the C_{H4} units of IgM are involved with the binding of the C1q portion of C1 during complement activation. The C_H region at the carboxy-terminal end of the IgG molecule, the Fc region, binds to surface Fc receptors (CD16, CD32, CD64) of macrophages, dendritic cells, NK cells, B cells, neutrophils, and eosinophils.

Variable regions (V_L and V_H) constitute the antibody-binding (Fab) region of the molecule. Within the V_L and V_H regions are hypervariable regions (extreme sequence variability) that constitute the antigen-binding site unique to each Ig molecule. The idiotype is defined as the specific region of the Fab portion of the Ig molecule to which antigen binds. Antibodies against the idiotype portion of an antibody molecule are called *anti-idiotype antibodies*. The formation of such antibodies in vivo during a normal B cell antibody response may generate a negative (or "off") signal to B cells to terminate antibody production.

IgG constitutes ~75–85% of total serum immunoglobulin. The four IgG subclasses are numbered in order of their level in serum, IgG1 being found in greatest amounts and IgG4 the least. IgG subclasses have clinical relevance in their varying ability to bind macrophage and neutrophil Fc receptors and to activate complement (Table 308-11). Moreover, selective deficiencies of certain IgG subclasses give rise to clinical syndromes in which the patient is inordinately susceptible to bacterial infections. IgG antibodies are frequently the predominant antibody made after rechallenge of the host with antigen (secondary antibody response).

IgM antibodies normally circulate as a 950-kDa pentamer with 160-kDa bivalent monomers joined by a molecule called the *J chain*, a 15-kDa nonimmunoglobulin molecule that also effects polymerization of IgA molecules. IgM is the first immunoglobulin to appear in the immune response (primary antibody response) and is the initial type of antibody made by neonates. Membrane IgM in the monomeric form also functions as a major antigen receptor on the surface of mature B cells (Fig. 308-8). IgM is an important component of immune complexes in autoimmune diseases. For example, IgM antibodies against IgG molecules (rheumatoid factors) are present in high titers in *rheumatoid arthritis*, other collagen diseases, and some infectious diseases (*subacute bacterial endocarditis*).

IgA constitutes only 7–15% of total serum immunoglobulin but is the predominant class of immunoglobulin in secretions. IgA in secre-

tions (tears, saliva, nasal secretions, gastrointestinal tract fluid, and human milk) is in the form of secretory IgA (sIgA), a polymer consisting of two IgA monomers, a joining molecule, again called the J chain, and a glycoprotein called the *secretory protein*. Of the two IgA subclasses, IgA1 is primarily found in serum, whereas IgA2 is more prevalent in secretions. IgA fixes complement via the alternative complement pathway and has potent antiviral activity in humans by prevention of virus binding to respiratory and gastrointestinal epithelial cells.

IgD is found in minute quantities in serum and, together with IgM, is a major receptor for antigen on the B cell surface. IgE, which is present in serum in very low concentrations, is the major class of immunoglobulin involved in arming mast cells and basophils by binding to these cells via the Fc region. Antigen cross-linking of IgE molecules on basophil and mast cell surfaces results in release of mediators of the immediate hypersensitivity response (Table 308-11).

CELLULAR INTERACTIONS IN REGULATION OF NORMAL IMMUNE RESPONSES

The net result of activation of the humoral (B cell) and cellular (T cell) arms of the adaptive immune system by foreign antigen is the elimination of antigen directly by specific effector T cells or in concert with specific antibody. Figure 308-2 is a simplified schematic diagram of the T and B cell responses indicating some of these cellular interactions.

The expression of adaptive immune cell function is the result of a complex series of immunoregulatory events that occur in phases. Both T and B lymphocytes mediate immune functions, and each of these cell types, when given appropriate signals, passes through stages, from activation and induction through proliferation, differentiation, and ultimately effector functions. The effector function expressed may be at the end point of a response, such as secretion of antibody by a differentiated plasma cell, or it might serve a regulatory function that modulates other functions, such as is seen with CD4+ and CD8+ T lymphocytes that modulate both differentiation of B cells and activation of CD8+ cytotoxic T cells.

CD4 helper T cells can be subdivided on the basis of cytokines produced (Fig. 308-2). Activated T_H1-type helper T cells secrete IL-2, IFN-γ, IL-3, TNF-α, GM-CSF, and TNF-β, while activated T_H2-type helper T cells secrete IL-3, -4, -5, -6, -10, and -13. T_H1 CD4+ T cells, through elaboration of IFN-γ, have a central role in mediating intracellular killing by a variety of pathogens. T_H1 CD4+ T cells also provide T cell help for generation of cytotoxic T cells and some types of opsonizing antibody, and they generally respond to antigens that lead to delayed hypersensitivity types of immune responses for many intracellular viruses and bacteria (such as HIV or *M. tuberculosis*). In contrast, T_H2 cells have a primary role in regulatory humoral immunity and isotype switching. T_H2 cells, through production of IL-4 and IL-

10, have a regulatory role in limiting proinflammatory responses mediated by T_H1 cells (Fig. 308-2). In addition, T_H2 CD4+ T cells provide help to B cells for specific Ig production and respond to antigens that require high antibody levels for foreign antigen elimination (extracellular encapsulated bacteria such as *Streptococcus pneumoniae* and certain parasite infections). The type of T cell response generated in an immune response is determined by the microbe PAMPs presented to the dendritic cells, the TLRs on the dendritic cells that become activated, the types of dendritic cells that are activated, and the cytokines that are produced (Table 308-4). Commonly, myeloid dendritic cells produce IL-12 and activate T_H1 T cell responses that result in IFN-γ and cytotoxic T cell induction, and plasmacytoid dendritic cells produce IFN-α and lead to T_H2 responses that result in IL-4 production and enhanced antibody responses.

As shown in Figs. 308-2 and 308-3, upon activation by dendritic cells, T cell subsets that produce IL-2, IL-3, IFN-γ, and/or IL-4, -5, -6, -10, and -13 are generated and exert positive and negative influences on effector T and B cells. For B cells, trophic effects are mediated by a variety of cytokines, particularly T cell–derived IL-3, -4, -5, and -6, that act at sequential stages of B cell maturation, resulting in B cell proliferation, differentiation, and ultimately antibody secretion. For cytotoxic T cells, trophic factors include inducer T cell secretion of IL-2, IFN-γ, and IL-12.

An important type of immunomodulatory T cell that controls immune responses is *CD4+ and CD8+ T regulatory cells*. These cells constitutively express the α chain of the IL-2 receptor (CD25), produce large amounts of IL-10, and can suppress both T and B cell responses. T regulatory cells are induced by immature dendritic cells and play key roles in maintaining tolerance to self-antigens in the periphery. Loss of T regulatory cells is the cause of organ-specific autoimmune disease in mice such as autoimmune thyroiditis, adrenalitis, and oophoritis (see "Immune Tolerance and Autoimmunity," below). T regulatory cells also play key roles in controlling the magnitude and duration of immune responses to microbes. Normally, after the initial immune response to a microbe has eliminated the invader, T regulatory cells are activated to suppress the antimicrobe response and prevent host injury. Some microbes have adapted to induce T regulatory cell activation at the site of infection to promote parasite infection and survival. In *Leishmania* infection, the parasite locally induces T regulatory cell accumulation at skin infection sites that dampens anti-*Leishmania* T cell responses and prevents elimination of the parasite. It is thought that many chronic infections such as by *M. tuberculosis* are associated with abnormal T regulatory cell activation that prevents elimination of the microbe.

Although B cells recognize native antigen via B cell surface Ig receptors, B cells require T cell help to produce high-affinity antibody of multiple isotypes that are the most effective in eliminating foreign antigen. This T cell dependence likely functions in the regulation of B cell responses and in protection against excessive autoantibody production. T cell–B cell interactions that lead to high-affinity antibody production require (1) processing of native antigen by B cells and expression of peptide fragments on the B cell surface for presentation to T_H cells, (2) the ligation of B cells by both the TCR complex and the CD40 ligand, (3) induction of the process termed *antibody isotype switching* in antigen-specific B cell clones, and (4) induction of the process of affinity maturation of antibody in the germinal centers of B cell follicles of lymph node and spleen.

Naïve B cells express cell-surface IgD and IgM, and initial contact of naïve B cells with antigen is via binding of native antigen to B cell–surface IgM. T cell cytokines, released following T_H2 cell contact with B cells or by a "bystander" effect, induce changes in Ig gene conformation that promote recombination of Ig genes. These events then result in the "switching" of expression of heavy chain exons in a triggered B cell, leading to the secretion of IgG, IgA, or, in some cases, IgE antibody with the same V region antigen specificity as the original IgM antibody, for response to a wide variety of extracellular bacteria, protozoa, and helminths. CD40 ligand expression by activated T cells is critical for induction of B cell antibody isotype switching and for B cell responsiveness to cytokines. Patients with mutations in T cell

CD40 ligand have B cells that are unable to undergo isotype switching, resulting in lack of memory B cell generation and the immunodeficiency syndrome of *X-linked hyper-IgM syndrome* (Chap. 310).

IMMUNE TOLERANCE AND AUTOIMMUNITY

Immune tolerance is defined as the absence of activation of pathogenic autoreactivity. *Autoimmune diseases* are syndromes caused by the activation of T or B cells or both, with no evidence of other causes such as infections or malignancies (Chap. 312). Once thought to be mutually exclusive, immune tolerance and autoimmunity are now both recognized to be present normally in health; when abnormal, they represent extremes from the normal state. For example, it is now known that low levels of autoreactivity of T and B cells with self-antigens in the periphery are critical to their survival. Similarly, low levels of autoreactivity and thymocyte recognition of self-antigens in the thymus are the mechanisms whereby (1) normal T cells are positively selected to survive and leave the thymus to respond to foreign microbes in the periphery, and (2) T cells highly reactive to self-antigens are negatively selected and die to prevent overly self-reactive T cells from getting into the periphery (central tolerance). However, not all self-antigens are expressed in the thymus to delete highly self-reactive T cells, and there are mechanisms for peripheral tolerance induction of T cells as well. Unlike the presentation of microbial antigens by mature dendritic cells, the presentation of self-antigens by immature dendritic cells neither activates nor matures the dendritic cells to express high levels of co-stimulatory molecules such as B7-1 (CD80) or B7-2 (CD86). When peripheral T cells are stimulated by dendritic cells expressing self-antigens in the context of HLA molecules, sufficient stimulation of T cells occurs to keep them alive, but otherwise they remain anergic, or nonresponsive, until they contact a dendritic cell with high levels of co-stimulatory molecules expressing microbial antigens. In the latter setting, normal T cells then become activated to respond to the microbe. If B cells have high-self-reactivity BCRs, they normally undergo receptor editing to express a less autoreactive receptor or are induced to die. Although many autoimmune diseases are characterized by abnormal or pathogenic autoantibody production (Table 308-12), most autoimmune diseases are caused by a combination of excess T and B cell reactivity.

Multiple factors contribute to the genesis of clinical autoimmune disease syndromes, including genetic susceptibility (Table 308-13), environmental immune stimulants such as drugs (e.g., procainamide and dilantin with drug-induced systemic lupus erythematosus), infectious agent triggers (such as Epstein-Barr virus and autoantibody production against red blood cells and platelets), and loss of T regulatory cells (leading to thyroiditis, adrenalitis, and oophoritis).

Immunity at Mucosal Surfaces Mucosa covering the respiratory, digestive, and urogenital tracts, the eye conjunctiva, the inner ear, and the ducts of all exocrine glands contain cells of the innate and adaptive mucosal immune system that protect these surfaces against pathogens. In the healthy adult, mucosa-associated lymphoid tissue (MALT) contains 80% of all immune cells within the body and constitutes the largest mammalian lymphoid organ system.

MALT has three main functions: (1) to protect the mucous membranes from invasive pathogens, (2) to prevent uptake of foreign antigens from food, commensal organisms, and airborne pathogens and particulate matter, and (3) to prevent pathologic immune responses from foreign antigens if they do cross the mucosal barriers of the body.

MALT is a compartmentalized system of immune cells that functions independently from systemic immune organs. Whereas the systemic immune organs are essentially sterile under normal conditions and respond vigorously to pathogens, MALT immune cells are continuously bathed in foreign proteins and commensal bacteria, and they must select those pathogenic antigens that must be eliminated. MALT contains anatomically defined foci of immune cells in the intestine, tonsil, appendix, and peribronchial areas that are inductive sites for mucosal immune responses. From these sites immune T and B cells migrate to effector sites in mucosal parenchyma and exocrine glands where mucosal immune cells eliminate pathogen-infected cells. In addition to mucosal immune

TABLE 308-12 RECOMBINANT OR PURIFIED AUTOANTIGENS RECOGNIZED BY AUTOANTIBODIES ASSOCIATED WITH HUMAN AUTOIMMUNE DISORDERS

Autoantigen	Autoimmune Diseases	Autoantigen	Autoimmune Diseases
Cell- or Organ-Specific Autoimmunity			
Acetylcholine receptor	Myasthenia gravis	Insulin receptor	Type B insulin resistance, acanthosis, systemic lupus erythematosus (SLE)
Actin	Chronic active hepatitis, primary bilary cirrhosis	Intrinsic factor type 1	Pernicious anemia
Adenine nucleotide translator (ANT)	Dilated cardiomyopathy, myocarditis	Leukocyte function-associated antigen (LFA-1)	Treatment-resistant Lyme arthritis
β-Adrenoreceptor	Dilated cardiomyopathy	Myelin-associated glycoprotein (MAG)	Polyneuropathy
Aromatic L-amino acid decarboxylase	Autoimmune polyendocrine syndrome type 1 (APS-1)	Myelin-basic protein	Multiple sclerosis, demyelinating diseases
Asialoglycoprotein receptor	Autoimmune hepatitis	Myelin oligodendrocyte glycoprotein (MOG)	Multiple sclerosis
Bactericidal/permeability-increasing protein (Bpi)	Cystic fibrosis vasculitides	Myosin	Rheumatic fever
Calcium-sensing receptor	Acquired hypoparathyroidism	p-80-Collin	Atopic dermatitis
Cholesterol side-chain cleavage enzyme (CYPIIa)	Autoimmune polyglandular syndrome-1	Pyruvate dehydrogenase complex-E2 (PDC-E2)	Primary biliary cirrhosis
Collagen type IV-α3-chain	Goodpasture syndrome	Sodium iodide symporter (NIS)	Graves' disease, autoimmune hypothyroidism
Cytochrome P450 2D6 (CYP2D6)	Autoimmune hepatitis		
Desmin	Crohn disease, coronary artery disease	SOX-10	Vitiligo
Desmoglein 1	Pemphigus foliaceus	Thyroid and eye muscle shared protein	Thyroid-associated ophthalmopathy
Desmoglein 3	Pemphigus vulgaris		
F-actin	Autoimmune hepatitis	Thyroglobulin	Autoimmune thyroiditis
GM gangliosides	Guillain-Barré syndrome	Thyroid peroxidase	Autoimmune Hashimoto thyroiditis
Glutamate decarboxylase (GAD65)	Type 1 diabetes, stiff man syndrome	Throtropin receptor	Graves' disease
Glutamate receptor (GLUR)	Rasmussen encephalitis	Tissue transglutaminase	Celiac disease
H/K ATPase	Autoimmune gastritis	Transcription coactivator p75	Atopic dermatitis
17-α-Hydroxylase (CYP17)	Autoimmune polyglandular syndrome-1	Tryptophan hydroxylase	Autoimmune polyglandular syndrome-1
21-Hydroxylase (CYP21)	Addison disease	Tyrosinase	Vitiligo, metastatic melanoma
IA-2 (ICA512)	Type 1 diabetes	Tyrosine hydroxylase	Autoimmune polyglandular syndrome-1
Insulin	Type 1 diabetes, insulin hypoglycemic syndrome (Hirata disease)		
Systemic Autoimmunity			
ACTH	ACTH deficiency	Histone H2A-H2B-DNA	SLE
Aminoacyl-tRAN histidyl synthetase	Myositis, dermatomyositis	IgE receptor	Chronic idiopathic urticaria
Aminoacyl-tRNA synthetase (several)	Polymyositis, dermatomyositis	Keratin	RA
Cardiolipin	SLE, anti-phospholipid syndrome	Ku-DNA-protein kinase	SLE
Carbonic anhydrase II	SLE, Sjögren syndrome, systemic sclerosis	Ku-nucleoprotein	Connective tissue syndrome
		La phosphoprotein (La 55-B)	Sjögren syndrome
Collagen (multiple types)	Rheumatoid arthritis (RA), SLE, progressive systemic sclerosis	Myeloperoxidase	Necrotizing and crescentic glomerulonephritis (NCGN), systemic vasculitis
Centromere-associated proteins	Systemic sclerosis	Proteinase 3 (PR3)	Wegener granulomatosis, Churg-Strauss syndrome
DNA-dependent nucleosine-stimulated ATPase	Dermatomyositis		
Fibrillarin	Scleroderma	RNA polymerase I–III (RNP)	Systemic sclerosis, SLE
Fibronectin	SLE, RA, morphea	Signal recognition protein (SRP54)	Polymyositis
Glucose-6-phosphate isomerase	RA	Topoisomerase-1 (Scl-70)	Scleroderma, Raynaud syndrome
β2-Glycoprotein I (B2-GPI)	Primary antiphospholipid syndrome	Tublin	Chronic liver disease, visceral leishmaniasis
Golgin (95, 97, 160, 180)	Sjögren syndrome, SLE, RA	Vimentin	Systemic autoimmune disease
Heat shock protein	Various immune-related disorders		
Hemidesmosomal protein 180	Bullous pemphigoid, herpes gestationis, cicatricial pemphigoid		
Plasma Protein and Cytokine Autoimmunity			
C1 inhibitor	Autoimmune C1 deficiency	Glycoprotein IIb/IIIg and Ib/IX	Autoimmune thrombocytopenia purpura
C1q	SLE, membrane proliferative glomerulonephritis (MPGN)	IgA	Immunodeficiency associated with SLE, pernicious anemia, thyroiditis, Sjögren's syndrome and chronic active hepatitis
Cytokines (IL-1α, IL-1β, IL-6, IL-10, LIF)	RA, systemic sclerosis, normal subjects		
Factor II, factor V, factor VII, factor VIII, factor IX, factor X, factor XI, thrombin vWF	Prolonged coagulation time		
		Oxidized LDL (OxLDL)	Atherosclerosis
Cancer and Paraneoplastic Autoimmunity			
Amphiphysin	Neuropathy, small-cell lung cancer	p62 (IGF-II mRNA-binding protein)	Hepatocellular carcinoma (China)
Cyclin B1	Hepatocellular carcinoma	Recoverin	Cancer-associated retinopathy
DNA topoisomerase II	Liver cancer	Ri protein	Paraneoplastic opsoclonus myoclonus ataxia
Desmoplakin	Paraneoplastic pemphigus		
Gephyrin	Paraneoplastic stiff man syndrome	βIV spectrin	Lower motor neuron syndrome
Hu proteins	Paraneoplastic encephalomyelitis	Synaptotagmin	Lambert-Eaton myasthenic syndrome
Neuronal nicotinic acetylcholine receptor	Subacute autonomic neuropathy, cancer	Voltage-gated calcium channels	Lambert-Eaton myasthenic syndrome
p53	Cancer, SLE	Yo protein	Paraneoplastic cerebellar degeneration

Source: From A Lernmark et al: J Clin Invest 108:1091, 2001; with permission.

Protein	Defect	Disease or Syndrome	Observation in Animal Models or Humans
Cytokines and Signaling Proteins			
Tumor necrosis factor (TNF) α	Overexpression	Inflammatory bowel disease (IBD), arthritis, vasculitis	Mice
TNF-α	Underexpression	Systemic lupus erythematosus (SLE)	Mice
Interleukin-1-receptor antagonist	Underexpression	Arthritis	Mice
IL-2	Overexpression	IBD	Mice
IL-7	Overexpression	IBD	Mice
IL-10	Overexpression	IBD	Mice
IL-2 receptor	Overexpression	IBD	Mice
IL-10 receptor	Overexpression	IBD	Mice
IL-3	Overexpression	Demyelinating syndrome	Mice
Interferon-δ	Overexpression in skin	SLE	Mice
STAT-3	Underexpression	IBD	Mice
STAT-4	Overexpression	IBD	Mice
Transforming growth factor (TGF) β	Underexpression	Systemic wasting syndrome and IBD	Mice
TGF-β receptor in T cells	Underexpression	SLE	Mice
Programmed death (PD-1)	Underexpression	SLE-like syndrome	Mice
Cytotoxic T lymphocyte, antigen-4 (CTLA-4)	Underexpression	Systemic lymphoproliferative disease	Mice
IL-10	Underexpression	IBD (mouse)	Mice and humans
		Type 1 diabetes, thyroid disease, primary (human)	
Major Histocompatibility Locus Molecules[a]			
HLA B27	Allele expression or over-expression	Inflammatory bowel disease	Rats and humans
Complement deficiency of C1, 2, 3 or 4	Underexpression		Humans
LIGHT (TNF superfamily 14)	Overexpression	Systemic lymphoproliferative (mouse) and autoimmunity	Mice
HLA class II DQB10301, DQB10302	Allele expression	Juvenile-onset diabetes	Human
HLA class II DQB10401, DQB10402	Allele expression	Rheumatoid arthritis	Humans
HLA class I B27	Allele expression	Ankylosing spondylitis, IBD	Rats and humans
Apoptosis Proteins			
TNFactor receptor 1 (TNF-R1)	Underexpression	Familial periodic fever syndrome	Humans
Fas (CD95; Apo-1)	Underexpression	Autoimmune lymphoproliferative syndrome type 1 (ALPS 1); malignant lymphoma; bladder cancer	Humans
Fas ligand	Underexpression	SLE (only one case identified)	Humans
Perforin	Underexpression	Familial hemophagocytic lymphohistiocytosis (FHL)	Humans
Caspase 10	Underexpression	Autoimmune lymphoproliferative syndrome type II (ALPS II)	Humans
bcl-10	Underexpression	Non-Hodgkin's lymphoma	Humans
P53	Underexpression	Various malignant neoplasms	Humans
Bax	Underexpression	Colon cancer; hematopoietic malignancies	Humans
bcl-2	Underexpression	Non-Hodgkin's lymphoma	Humans
c-IAP2	Underexpression	Low-grade MALT lymphoma	Humans
NAIP1	Underexpression	Spinal muscular atrophy	Humans

[a]Many autoimmune diseases are associated with a myriad of major compatibility complex gene allele (HLA) types. They are presented here as examples.
Note: MALT, mucosa-associated lymphoid tissue.

Source: Adopted from L Mullauer et al: Mutat Res 488:211, 2001; A Davidson, B Diamond: N Engl J Med 345:340, 2001; with permission.

responses, all mucosal sites have strong mechanical and chemical barriers and cleansing functions to repel pathogens.

Key components of MALT include specialized epithelial cells called "membrane" or "M" cells that take up antigens and deliver them to dendritic cells or other APCs. Effector cells in MALT include B cells producing antipathogen neutralizing antibodies of secretory IgA as well as IgG isotype, T cells producing similar cytokines as in systemic immune system response, and T helper and cytotoxic T cells that respond to pathogen infected cells.

Secretory IgA is produced in amounts of >50 mg/kg of body weight per 24 h and functions to inhibit bacterial adhesion, inhibit macromolecule absorption in the gut, neutralize viruses, and enhance antigen elimination in tissue through binding to IgA and receptor-mediated transport of immune complexes through epithelial cells.

Recent studies have demonstrated the importance of commensal gut and other mucosal bacteria to the health of the human immune system. Normal commensal flora induces anti-inflammatory events in the gut and protects epithelial cells from pathogens through TLRs and other PRR signaling. When the gut is depleted of normal commensal flora, the immune system becomes abnormal, with loss of T_H1 T cell

function. Restoration of the normal gut flora can reestablish the balance in T helper cell ratios characteristic of the normal immune system. When the gut barrier is intact, either antigens do not transverse the gut epithelium or, when pathogens are present, a self-limited, protective MALT immune response eliminates the pathogen (Fig. 308-9). However, when the gut barrier breaks down, immune responses to commensal flora antigens can cause inflammatory bowel diseases such as *Crohn's disease* and, perhaps, *ulcerative colitis* (Fig. 308-9) (Chap. 289). Uncontrolled MALT immune responses to food antigens, such as gluten, can cause *celiac disease* (Chap. 289).

THE CELLULAR AND MOLECULAR CONTROL OF PROGRAMMED CELL DEATH

The process of apoptosis (programmed cell death) plays a crucial role in regulating normal immune responses to antigen. In general, a wide variety of stimuli trigger one of several apoptotic pathways to eliminate microbe-infected cells, eliminate cells with damaged DNA, or eliminate activated immune cells that are no longer needed (Fig. 308-10). The largest known family of "death receptors" is the tumor necrosis factor receptor (TNF-R) family [TNF-R1, TNF-R2, Fas (CD95), death receptor 3 (DR3), death receptor 4 (DR4, TRAIL-R1), and death receptor 5 (DR5,

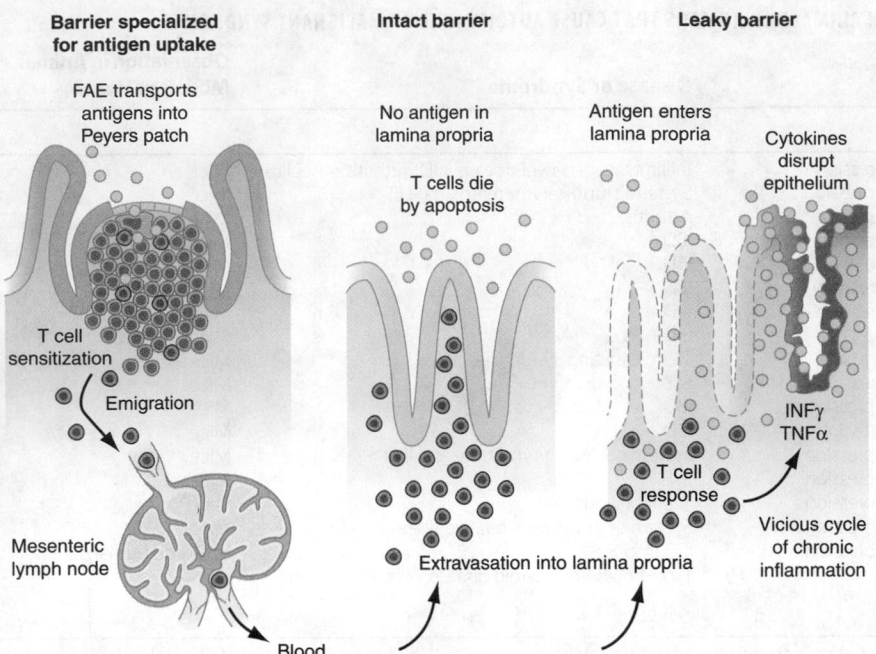

Barrier specialized for antigen uptake

FAE transports antigens into Peyers patch

T cell sensitization

Emigration

Mesenteric lymph node

Blood

Intact barrier

No antigen in lamina propria

T cells die by apoptosis

Extravasation into lamina propria

Leaky barrier

Antigen enters lamina propria

Cytokines disrupt epithelium

INFγ TNFα

T cell response

Vicious cycle of chronic inflammation

FIGURE 308-9 Increased epithelial permeability may be important in the development of chronic gut T cell–mediated inflammation. CD4 T cells activated by gut antigens in Peyer's patches migrate to the LP. In healthy individuals, these cells die by apoptosis. Increased epithelial permeability may allow sufficient antigen to enter the LP to trigger T cell activation, breaking tolerance mediated by immunosuppressive cytokines and perhaps T regulatory cells. Pro-inflammatory cytokines then further increase epithelial permeability, setting up a vicious cycle of chronic inflammation. *(From T MacDonald, G Monteleone: Science 307:1924, 2005; with permission.)*

sites of antigen localization; (2) antigen-nonspecific recognition of pathogens by macrophages and other cells and systems of the innate immune system; (3) specific recognition of foreign antigens mediated by T and B lymphocytes; (4) amplification of the inflammatory response with recruitment of specific and nonspecific effector cells by complement components, cytokines, kinins, arachidonic acid metabolites, and mast cell–basophil products; and (5) macrophage, neutrophil, and lymphocyte participation in destruction of antigen with ultimate removal of antigen particles by phagocytosis (by macrophages or neutrophils) or by direct cytotoxic mechanisms (involving macrophages, neutrophils, DCs, and lymphocytes). Under normal circumstances, orderly progression of host defenses through these phases results in a well-controlled immune and inflammatory response that protects the host from the offending antigen. However, dysfunction of any of the host defense systems can damage host tissue and produce clinical disease. Furthermore, for certain pathogens or antigens, the normal immune response itself might contribute substantially to the tissue damage. For example, the immune and inflammatory response in the brain to certain pathogens such as *M. tuberculosis* may be responsible for much of the morbidity of this disease in that organ system (Chap. 158). In addition, the morbidity associated with certain pneumonias such as that caused by *Pneumocystis carinii* may be associated more with inflammatory infiltrates than with the tissue destructive effects of the microorganism itself (Chap. 200).

TRAIL-R2)]; their ligands are all in the TNF-α family. Binding of ligands to these death receptors leads to a signaling cascade that involves activation of the *caspase* family of molecules that leads to DNA cleavage and cell death. Two other pathways of programmed cell death involve nuclear *p53* in the elimination of cells with abnormal DNA and *mitochondrial cytochrome c* to induce cell death in damaged cells (Fig. 308-10). A number of human diseases have now been described that result from, or are associated with, mutated apoptosis genes (Table 308-13). These include mutations in the TNF-R1 in *hereditary periodic fever (familial Mediterranean fever)* (Chap. 291), Fas and Fas ligand in autoimmune and lymphoproliferation syndromes, and multiple associations of mutations in genes in the apoptotic pathway with malignant syndromes.

MECHANISMS OF IMMUNE-MEDIATED DAMAGE TO MICROBES OR HOST TISSUES

Several responses by the host innate and adaptive immune systems to foreign microbes culminate in rapid and efficient elimination of microbes. In these scenarios, the classic weapons of the adaptive immune system (T cells, B cells) interface with cells (macrophages, dendritic cells, NK cells, neutrophils, eosinophils, basophils) and soluble products (microbial peptides, pentraxins, complement and coagulation systems) of the innate immune system (Chaps. 61 and 311).

There are five general phases of host defenses: (1) migration of leukocytes to

FIGURE 308-10 Scheme of major apoptosis pathways. DD, death domain; DED, death effector domain. *(From L Mullauer et al: Mutat Res 488:211, 2001; with permission.)*

The Molecular Basis of Lymphocyte–Endothelial Cell Interactions

The control of lymphocyte circulatory patterns between the bloodstream and peripheral lymphoid organs operates at the level of lymphocyte–endothelial cell interactions to control the specificity of lymphocyte subset entry into organs. Similarly, lymphocyte–endothelial cell interactions regulate the entry of lymphocytes into inflamed tissue. Adhesion molecule expression on lymphocytes and endothelial cells regulates the retention and subsequent egress of lymphocytes within tissue sites of antigenic stimulation, delaying cell exit from tissue and preventing reentry into the circulating lymphocyte pool (Fig. 308-11). All types of lymphocyte migration begin with lymphocyte attachment to specialized regions of vessels, termed *high endothelial venules* (HEVs). An important concept is that adhesion molecules do not generally bind their ligand until a conformational change (ligand activation) occurs in the adhesion molecule that allows ligand binding. Induction of a conformation-dependent determinant on an adhesion molecule can be accomplished by cytokines or via ligation of other adhesion molecules on the cell.

The first stage of lymphocyte–endothelial cell interactions, *attachment and rolling*, occurs when lymphocytes leave the stream of flowing blood cells in a postcapillary venule and roll along venule endothelial cells (Fig. 308-11). Lymphocyte rolling is mediated by the L-selectin molecule (LECAM-1, LAM-1, CD62L) and slows cell transit time through venules, allowing time for activation of adherent cells.

The second stage of lymphocyte–endothelial cell interactions, *firm adhesion with activation-dependent stable arrest*, requires stimulation of lymphocytes by chemoattractants or by endothelial cell–derived cytokines. Cytokines thought to participate in adherent cell activation include members of the IL-8 family, platelet-activation factor, leukotriene B$_4$, and C5a. In addition, HEVs express chemokines, SLC (CCL21) and ELC (CCL19), which participate in this process. Following activation by chemoattractants, lymphocytes shed L-selectin from the cell surface and upregulate cell CD11b/18 (MAC-1) or CD11a/18 (LFA-1) molecules, resulting in firm attachment of lymphocytes to HEVs.

Lymphocyte homing to peripheral lymph nodes involves adhesion of L-selectin to glycoprotein HEV ligands collectively referred to as *peripheral node addressin (PNAd)*, whereas homing of lymphocytes to intestine Peyer's patches primarily involves adhesion of the α4,β7 integrin to mucosal addressin cell adhesion molecule-1 (MAdCAM-1) on the Peyer's patch HEVs. However, for migration to mucosal Peyer's patch lymphoid aggregates, naïve lymphocytes primarily use L-selectin, whereas memory lymphocytes use α4,β7 integrin. α4,β1 integrin (CD49d/CD29, VLA-4)–VCAM-1 interactions are important in the initial interaction of memory lymphocytes with HEVs of multiple organs in sites of inflammation (Table 308-14).

The third stage of leukocyte emigration in HEVs is *sticking and arrest*. Sticking of the lymphocyte to endothelial cells and arrest at the site of sticking are mediated predominantly by ligation of αL,β2 integrin LFA-1 to the integrin ligand ICAM-1 on HEVs. While the first three stages of lymphocyte attachment to HEVs take only a few seconds, the fourth stage of lymphocyte emigration, *transendothelial migration*, takes ~10 min. Although the molecular mechanisms that control lymphocyte transendothelial migration are not fully characterized, the HEV CD44 molecule and molecules of the HEV glycocalyx (extracellular matrix) are thought to play important regulatory roles

FIGURE 308-11 Key migration steps of immune cells at sites of inflammation. Inflammation due to tissue damage or infection induces the release of cytokines (not shown) and inflammatory chemoattractants (red arrowheads) from distressed stromal cells and "professional" sentinels, such as mast cells and macrophages (not shown). The inflammatory signals induce upregulation of endothelial selectins and immunoglobulin "superfamily" members, particularly ICAM-1 and/or VCAM-1. Chemoattractants, particularly chemokines, are produced by or translocated across venular endothelial cells (red arrow) and are displayed in the lumen to rolling leukocytes. Those leukocytes that express the appropriate set of trafficking molecules undergo a multistep adhesion cascade (steps 1–3) and then polarize and move by diapedesis across the venular wall (steps 4 and 5). Diapedesis involves transient disassembly of endothelial junctions and penetration through the underlying basement membrane (step 6). Once in the extravascular (interstitial) space, the migrating cell uses different integrins to gain "footholds" on collagen fibers and other ECM molecules, such as laminin and fibronectin, and on inflammation-induced ICAM-1 on the surface of parenchymal cells (step 7). The migrating cell receives guidance cues from distinct sets of chemoattractants, particularly chemokines, which may be immobilized on glycosaminoglycans (GAG) that "decorate" many ECM molecules and stromal cells. Inflammatory signals also induce tissue-resident DCs to undergo maturation. Once DCs process material from damaged tissues and invading pathogens, they upregulate CCR7, which allows them to enter draining lymph vessels that express the CCR7 ligancd CCL21 (and CCL19). In lymph nodes (LN), these antigen-loaded mature DCs activate naïve T cells and expand pools of effector lymphocytes, which enter the blood and migrate back to the site of inflammation. T cells in tissue also use this CCR7-dependent route to migrate from peripheral sites to draining lymph nodes through afferent lymphatics. [*Adapted from AD Luster, R Alon, UH von Andrian, Nat Immunol 6(12):1182–1190, 2005; with permission.*]

TABLE 308-14 TRAFFICKING MOLECULES INVOLVED IN INFLAMMATORY DISEASE PROCESSES

Disease	Key Effector Cell	Proposed Leukocyte Receptors for Endothelial Traffic Signals		
		L-Selectin, Ligand	GPCR	Integrin[a]
Acute Inflammation				
Myocardial infarction	Neutrophil	PSGL-1	CXCR1, CXCR2, PAFR, BLT1	LFA-1, Mac-1
Stroke	Neutrophil	L-selectin, PSGL-1	CXCR1, CXCR2, PAFR, BLT1	LFA-1, Mac-1
Ischemia-reperfusion	Neutrophil	PSGL-1	CXCR1, CXCR2, PAFR, BLT1	LFA-1, Mac-1
T$_H$1 Inflammation				
Atherosclerosis	Monocyte	PSGL-1	CCR1, CCR2, BLT1, CXCR2, CX3CR1	VLA-4
	T$_H$1	PSGL-1	CXCR3, CCR5	VLA-4
Multiple sclerosis	T$_H$1	PSGL-1 (?)	CXCR3, CXCR6	VLA-4, LFA-1
	Monocyte	PSGL-1 (?)	CCR2, CCR1	VLA-4, LFA-1
Rheumatoid arthritis	Monocyte	PSGL-1	CCR1, CCR2	VLA-1, VLA-2, VLA-4, LFA-1
	T$_H$1	PSGL-1	CXCR3, CXCR6	VLA-1, VLA-2, VLA-4, LFA-1
	Neutrophil	L-selectin, PSGL-1	CXCR2, BLT1	LFA-1[b]
Psoriasis	Skin-homing T$_H$1	CLA	CCR4, CCR10, CXCR3	VLA-4[c], LFA-1
Crohn disease	Gut-homing T$_H$1	PSGL-1	CCR9, CXCR3	$\alpha_4\beta_7$, LFA-1
Type I diabetes	T$_H$1	PSGL-1 (?)	CCR4, CCR5	VLA-4, LFA-1
	CD8	L-selectin (?), PSGL-1 (?)	CXCR3	VLA-4, LFA-1
Allograft rejection	CD8	PSGL-1	CXCR3, CX3CR1, BLT1	VLA-4, LFA-1
	B cell	L-selectin, PSGL-1	CXCR5, CXCR4	VLA-4, LFA-1
Hepatitis	CD8	PSGL-1	CXCR3, CCR5, CXCR6	VLA-4
Lupus	T$_H$1	None	CXCR6	VLA-4[d]
	Plasmacytoid DC	L-selectin, CLA	CCR7, CXCR3, ChemR23	LFA-1, Mac-1
	B cell	CLA (?)	CXCR5, CXCR4	LFA-1
T$_H$2 Inflammation				
Asthma	T$_H$2	PSGL-1	CCR4, CCR8, BLT1	LFA-1
	Eosinophil	PSGL-1	CCR3, PAFR, BLT1	VLA-4, LFA-1
	Mast cells	PSGL-1	CCR2, CCR3, BLT1	VLA-4, LFA-1
Atopic dermatitis	Skin-homing T$_H$2	CLA	CCR4, CCR10	VLA-4, LFA-1

[a]Various β_1 integrins have been linked in different ways in basal lamina and interstitial migration of distinct cell types and inflammatory settings.
[b]In some settings, Mac-1 has been linked to transmigration.
[c]CD44 can act in concert with VLA-4 in particular models of leukocyte arrest.
[d]T$_H$2 cells require VAP-1 to traffic to inflamed liver.
Source: From AD Luster, UH von Adrian: *Nature Immunol* vol.6, 2005, with permission.

in this process (Fig. 308-11). Finally, expression of matrix metalloproteases capable of digesting the subendothelial basement membrane, rich in nonfibrillar collagen, appears to be required for the penetration of lymphoid cells into the extravascular sites.

Abnormal induction of HEV formation and use of the molecules discussed above have been implicated in the induction and maintenance of inflammation in a number of chronic inflammatory diseases. In animal models of type 1 diabetes mellitus, MAdCAM-1 and Gly-CAM-1 have been shown to be highly expressed on HEVs in inflamed pancreatic islets, and treatment of these animals with inhibitors of L-selectin and α4 integrin function blocked the development of type 1 diabetes mellitus (Chap. 338). A similar role for abnormal induction of the adhesion molecules of lymphocyte emigration has been suggested in *rheumatoid arthritis* (Chap. 314), *Hashimoto's thyroiditis* (Chap. 335), *Graves' disease* (Chap. 335), *multiple sclerosis* (Chap. 375), *Crohn's disease* (Chap. 289), and *ulcerative colitis* (Chap. 289).

Immune-Complex Formation Clearance of antigen by immune-complex formation between antigen and antibody is a highly effective mechanism of host defense. However, depending on the level of immune complexes formed and their physicochemical properties, immune complexes may or may not result in host and foreign cell

damage. After antigen exposure, certain types of soluble antigen-antibody complexes freely circulate and, if not cleared by the reticuloendothelial system, can be deposited in blood vessel walls and in other tissues such as renal glomeruli and cause *vasculitis* or *glomerulonephritis* syndromes (Chaps. 277 and 319).

Immediate-Type Hypersensitivity Helper T cells that drive antiallergen IgE responses are usually T$_H$2-type inducer T cells that secrete IL-4, IL-5, IL-6, and IL-10. Mast cells and basophils have high-affinity receptors for the Fc portion of IgE (FcRI), and cell-bound antiallergen IgE effectively "arms" basophils and mast cells. Mediator release is triggered by antigen (allergen) interaction with Fc receptor–bound IgE, the mediators released are responsible for the pathophysiologic changes of *allergic diseases* (Table 308-10). Mediators released from mast cells and basophils can be divided into three broad functional types: (1) those that increase vascular permeability and contract smooth muscle (histamine, platelet-activating factor, SRS-A, BK-A), (2) those that are chemotactic for or activate other inflammatory cells (ECF-A, NCF, leukotriene B$_4$), and (3) those that modulate the release of other mediators (BK-A, platelet-activating factor) (Chap. 311).

Cytotoxic Reactions of Antibody In this type of immunologic injury, complement-fixing (C1-binding) antibodies against normal or foreign cells or tissues (IgM, IgG1, IgG2, IgG3) bind complement via the classic pathway and initiate a sequence of events similar to that initiated by immune-complex deposition, resulting in cell lysis or tissue injury. Examples of antibody-mediated cytotoxic reactions include red cell lysis in *transfusion reactions, Goodpasture's syndrome* with anti–glomerular basement membrane antibody formation, and *pemphigus vulgaris* with antiepidermal antibodies inducing blistering skin disease.

Classic Delayed-Type Hypersensitivity Reactions Inflammatory reactions initiated by mononuclear leukocytes and not by antibody alone have been termed *delayed-type hypersensitivity reactions*. The term *delayed* has been used to contrast a secondary cellular response that appears 48–72 h after antigen exposure with an *immediate* hypersensitivity response generally seen within 12 h of antigen challenge and initiated by basophil mediator release or preformed antibody. For example, in an individual previously infected with *M. tuberculosis* organisms, intradermal placement of tuberculin purified-protein derivative as a skin test challenge results in an indurated area of skin at 48–72 h, indicating previous exposure to tuberculosis.

The cellular events that result in classic delayed-type hypersensitivity responses are centered around T cells (predominantly, though not exclusively, IFN-γ, IL-2, and TNF-α-secreting T$_H$1-type helper T cells) and macrophages. Recently NK cells have been suggested to play a major role in the form of delayed hypersensitivity that occurs following skin contact with immunogens. First, local immune and inflammatory responses at the site of foreign antigen upregulate endothelial cell adhesion molecule expression, promoting the accumulation of lymphocytes at the tissue site. In the general schemes outlined in Figs. 308-2 and 308-3, antigen is processed by dendritic cells and presented to small numbers of CD4+ T cells expressing a TCR specific for the antigen. IL-12 produced by APCs induces T cells to produce IFN-γ (T$_H$1 response). Macrophages frequently undergo epithelioid cell transformation and fuse to form multinucleated giant cells in response to IFN-γ. This type of mononuclear cell infiltrate is termed *granulomatous inflammation*. Examples of diseases in which delayed-type hypersensitivity plays a major role are fungal infections (*histoplasmosis*; Chap. 192), mycobacterial infections (*tuberculosis, leprosy*; Chaps. 158 and 159), chlamydial infections (*lymphogranuloma venereum*; Chap. 169), helminth infections (*schistosomiasis*; Chap. 212), reactions to toxins (*berylliosis*; Chap. 250), and hypersensitivity reactions to organic dusts (*hypersensitivity pneumonitis*; Chap. 249). In addition, delayed-type hypersensitivity responses play important roles in tissue damage in autoimmune diseases such as *rheumatoid arthritis, temporal arteritis,* and *Wegener's granulomatosis* (Chaps. 314 and 319).

CLINICAL EVALUATION OF IMMUNE FUNCTION

Clinical assessment of immunity requires investigation of the four major components of the immune system that participate in host defense and in the pathogenesis of autoimmune diseases: (1) humoral immunity (B cells); (2) cell-mediated immunity (T cells, monocytes); (3) phagocytic cells of the reticuloendothelial system (macrophages), as well as polymorphonuclear leukocytes; and (4) complement. Clinical problems that require an evaluation of immunity include chronic infections, recurrent infections, unusual infecting agents, and certain autoimmune syndromes. The type of clinical syndrome under evaluation can provide information regarding possible immune defects (Chap. 310). Defects in cellular immunity generally result in viral, mycobacterial, and fungal infections. An extreme example of deficiency in cellular immunity is AIDS (Chap. 182). Antibody deficiencies result in recurrent bacterial infections, frequently with organisms such as *S. pneumoniae* and *Haemophilus influenzae* (Chap. 310). Disorders of phagocyte function are frequently manifested by recurrent skin infections, often due to *Staphylococcus aureus* (Chap. 61). Finally, deficiencies of early and late complement components are associated with autoimmune phenomena and recurrent *Neisseria* infections (Table 308-15). For further discussion of useful initial screening tests of immune function, see Chap. 310.

IMMUNOTHERAPY

Most current therapies for autoimmune and inflammatory diseases involve the use of nonspecific immune-modulating or immunosuppressive agents such as glucocorticoids or cytotoxic drugs. The goal of development of new treatments for immune-mediated diseases is to design ways to specifically interrupt pathologic immune responses, leaving nonpathologic immune responses intact. Novel ways to interrupt pathologic immune responses that are under investigation include the use of anti-inflammatory cytokines or specific cytokine inhibitors as anti-inflammatory agents; the use of monoclonal antibodies against T or B lymphocytes as therapeutic agents; the induction of anergy by administration of soluble CTLA-4 protein; the use of intravenous Ig for certain infections and immune complex–mediated diseases; the use of specific cytokines to reconstitute components of the immune system; and bone marrow transplantation to replace the pathogenic immune system with a more normal immune system (Table 308-16) (Chaps. 61, 310, and 182).

Cytokines and Cytokine Inhibitors Recently a humanized mouse anti-TNF-α monoclonal antibody (MAb) has been shown to be effective in both rheumatoid arthritis and ulcerative colitis. Use of anti-TNF-α antibody therapy has resulted in clinical improvement in patients with these diseases and has opened the way for targeting TNF-α to treat other severe forms of autoimmune and/or inflammatory disease. Blockage of TNF-α has been effective in *rheumatoid arthritis, psoriasis, Crohn's disease,* and *ankylosing spondylitis*. Anti-TNF-α MAb (infliximab) has been approved by the FDA for treatment of patients with rheumatoid arthritis.

Other cytokine inhibitors under investigation are recombinant soluble TNF-α receptor (R) fused to human Ig and soluble IL-1 receptor (termed *IL-1 receptor antagonist*, or IL-1 ra). Soluble TNF-αR (etanercept) and IL-1 ra act to inhibit the activity of pathogenic cytokines in rheumatoid arthritis, i.e., TNF-α and IL-1, respectively. Similarly, anti-IL-6, IFN-β, and IL-11 act to inhibit pathogenic proinflammatory cytokines. Anti-IL-6 inhibits IL-6 activity, while IFN-β and IL-11 decrease IL-1 and TNF- production.

Of particular note has been the successful use of IFN-γ in the treatment of the phagocytic cell defect in *chronic granulomatous disease* (Chap. 61). Intermittent infusions of IL-2 in HIV-infected individuals in the early or intermediate stages of disease have resulted in substantial and sustained increases in CD4+ T cells.

Monoclonal Antibodies to T and B Cells The OKT3 MAb against human T cells has been used for several years as a T cell–specific immunosuppressive agent that can substitute for horse anti-thymocyte globulin (ATG) in the treatment of solid organ transplant rejection. OKT3 produces fewer allergic reactions than ATG but does induce human anti-mouse Ig antibody—thus limiting its use. Anti-CD4 MAb therapy has been used in trials to treat patients with rheumatoid arthritis. While inducing profound immunosuppression, anti-CD4 MAb treatment also induces susceptibility to severe infections. Treatment of patients with a MAb against the T cell molecule CD40 ligand (CD154) is under investigation to induce tolerance to organ transplants, with promising results reported in animal studies. Monoclonal antibodies to the CD25 (IL-2α) receptor are being used for treatment of graft-versus-host disease in bone marrow transplantation, and anti-CD20 MAb (rituximab) is being tested for anti–B cell therapy for *antineutrophil cytoplasmic antibody–associated vasculitis* (Chap. 319). Anti-IgE monoclonal antibody (omalizumab) is being tested for blocking antigen-specific IgE that causes *hay fever* and *allergic rhinitis* (Chap. 311).

Tolerance Induction Specific immunotherapy has moved into a new era with the introduction of soluble CTLA-4 protein into clinical trials. Use of this molecule to block T cell activation via TCR/CD28 ligation during organ or bone marrow transplantation has showed promising results in animals and in early human clinical trials. Specifically, treatment of bone marrow with CTLA-4 protein reduces rejection of the graft in HLA-mismatched bone marrow transplantation. In addition, promising results with soluble CTLA-4 have been reported in the downmodulation of autoimmune T cell responses in the treatment of psoriasis; new trials of the drug are ongoing for treatment of systemic lupus erythematosus (Chap. 313).

TABLE 308-15	COMPLEMENT DEFICIENCIES AND ASSOCIATED DISEASES
Component	**Associated Diseases**
Classic Pathway	
Clq, Clr, Cls, C4	Immune-complex syndromes,[a] pyogenic infections
C2	Immune-complex syndromes,[a] few with pyogenic infections
C1 Inhibitor	Rare immune-complex disease, few with pyogenic infections
C3 and Alternative Pathway C3	
C3	Immune-complex syndromes,[a] pyogenic infections
D	Pyogenic infections
Properdin	*Neisseria* infections
I	Pyogenic infections
H	Hemolytic uremic syndrome
Membrane Attack Complex	
C5, C6, C7, C8	Recurrent *Neisseria* infections, immune-complex disease
C9	Rare *Neisseria* infections

[a]Immune-complex syndromes include systemic lupus erythematosus (SLE) and SLE-like syndromes, glomerulonephritis, and vasculitis syndromes.
Source: After JA Schifferli, DK Peters: Lancet 88:957, 1983, with permission.

PART 14

Disorders of the Immune System, Connective Tissue, and Joints

TABLE 308-16 CURRENT STATUS OF DEVELOPMENT OF IMMUNOMODULATORY AGENTS

Agents	Rationale	Status
Cytokines and Cytokine Inhibitors to Inhibit Immune Responses and Inflammation		
Anti-TNF-α monoclonal antibody; humanized mouse chimeric MAb, infliximab, fully humanized MAb, adalimumab	Inhibit TNF-α	FDA approved for rheumatoid arthritis, Crohn's colitis (infliximab); FDA approved for rheumatoid arthritis (adalimumab)
Recombinant TNF-receptor-Ig fusion protein (etanercept)	Inhibit TNF-α	FDA approved for rheumatoid arthritis, juvenile rheumatoid arthritis, psoriasis
Recombinant IL-1 receptor antagonist (IL-1Ra) (anakinra)	Inhibit IL-1α and -β	FDA approved for rheumatoid arthritis
Monoclonal Antibodies or Toxins Against T or B Cells		
Anti-CD3 and T cell murine monoclonal antibody (OKT3)	Inhibit T cell function; induce T cell lymphopenia	FDA approved for treatment of cardiac and renal allograft rejection
Diphtheria toxin-IL2 fusion protein	Kills activated T cells	FDA approved for GVHD and transplant repertoire; understudy to kill T regulatory cell to embrace tumor vaccine efficacy
Humanized anti-CD3 monoclonal antibody (hOKT3 gamma-1)	Eliminates auto-reactive T cells	Human study underway in Type I diabetes, psoriasis
Humanized anti-CD25 (IL-2R) monoclonal antibody (daclizumab)	Eliminates activated T cells	FDA approved for graft versus host disease; studies underway in ulcerative colitis
Anti-CD40 ligand (CD154) monoclonal antibody	Inhibit CD40-CD40 ligand interaction; induces T cell tolerance	In primate trials for prevention of renal allograft rejection
Humanized anti-CD20 (anti-B cell) monoclonal antibody (rituximab)	Eliminates autoreactive B cells	Human study underway for treatment of ANCA+ vasculitis
Humanized anti-IgE monoclonal antibody (omalizumab)	Block allergy causing IgE	Human study underway for allergy (Hay fever, allergic rhinitis)
Soluble T Cell Molecule		
Soluble CTLA-4 protein	Inhibit CD28-B7-1 and B7-2 interactions; induces tolerance to organ grafts; inhibit autoimmune T cell reactivity in autoimmune diseases	In trials for preventing GVHD in bone marrow transplantation and for treatment of psoriasis and systemic lupus erythematosus
Intravenous Immunoglobin		
IVIg	Reticuloendothelial cell blockage; complement inhibition; regulation of idiotype/anti-idiotype antibodies; modulation of cytokine production; modulation of lymphocyte production	FDA approved for Kawasaki's disease and immune thrombocytopenia purpura; treatment of GVHD, multiple sclerosis, myasthenia gravis, Guillain-Barré syndrome, and chronic inflammatory demyelinating polyneuropathy supported by clinical trials
Cytokines for Immune Reconstitution		
IL-2	Induce proliferation of peripheral memory CD4+ and CD8+ T cells	In trial for treatment of HIV infection
IL-7	Induce renewed thymopoiesis	Under consideration for treatment of disease associated with T cell deficiency
Hematopoietic Stem Cell Transplantation		
Hematopoietic stem transplantation for immune reconstitution	Remove pathologic autoreactive immune system and replace with less autoreactive immunity	In clinical trials for systemic lupus erythematosus, multiple sclerosis, and scleroderma

Note: FDA, Food and Drug Administration; GVHD, graft-versus-host disease; ANCA, anti-neutrophil cytoplasmic antibody.

Intravenous Immunoglobulin (IVIg) IVIg has been used successfully to block reticuloendothelial cell function and immune complex clearance in various immune cytopenias such as immune thrombocytopenia (Chap. 109). In addition, IVIg is useful for prevention of tissue damage in certain inflammatory syndromes such as Kawasaki disease (Chap. 319) and as Ig replacement therapy for certain types of immunoglobulin deficiencies (Chap. 310). In addition, controlled clinical trials support the use of IVIg in selected patients with graft-versus-host disease, multiple sclerosis, myasthenia gravis, Guillain-Barré syndrome, and chronic demyelinating polyneuropathy (Table 308-16).

Stem Cell Transplantation Hematopoietic stem cell transplantation (SCT) is now being comprehensively studied to treat several autoimmune diseases, including systemic lupus erythematosus, multiple sclerosis, and scleroderma. The goal of immune reconstitution in autoimmune disease syndromes is to replace a dysfunctional immune system with a normally reactive immune cell repertoire. Preliminary results in patients with scleroderma and lupus have showed encouraging results. Controlled clinical trials in these three diseases are now being launched in the United States and Europe to compare the toxicity and efficacy of conventional immunosuppression therapy with that of myeloablative autologous SCT.

Thus, a number of recent insights into immune system function have spawned a new field of interventional immunotherapy and have enhanced the prospect for development of specific and nontoxic therapies for immune and inflammatory diseases.

FURTHER READINGS

ANDREAKOS ETH et al: Role of cytokines, in *Rheumatoid Arthritis*, EW St. Clair et al (eds). Philadelphia, Lippincott Williams & Wilkins, 2004, pp 134–149

BACKHED F et al: Host-bacterial mutualism in the human intestine. Science 307:1915, 2005

BLANDER JM et al: Toll-dependent selection of microbial antigens for presentation by dendritic cells. Nature 440:808, 2006

COLONNA M et al: Dendritic cells at the host-pathogen interface. Nat Immunol 7:117, 2006

DAVIDSON A, DIAMOND B: Autoimmune diseases. N Engl J Med 345:340, 2001

DIAMOND B et al: The immune tolerance network and rheumatic disease: Immune tolerance comes to the clinic. Arthritis Rheum 44:1730, 2001

DRAYTON DL et al: Lymphoid organ development: From ontogeny to neogenesis. Nat Immunol 7:344, 2006

HAYNES BF et al: The role of the thymus in immune reconstitution in aging bone marrow transplantation and AIDS. Annu Rev Immunol 18:529, 2000

HOLMGREN J et al: Mucosal immunity and vaccines. Nat Med 11(4 Suppl):S45, 2005

JANEWAY CA et al (eds): *Immunobiology. The Immune System in Health and Disease*, 5th ed. New York, Garland, 1999

KELLEY WN et al (eds): *Textbook of Rheumatology*, 4th ed. Philadelphia, Saunders, 1993, chaps. 6, 7, 10, 13, 15, 16

KORETZKY GA et al: SLP76 and SLP65: Complex regulation of signalling in lymphocytes and beyond. Nat Rev Immunol 6:67, 2006

LERNMARK A: Autoimmune diseases: Are markers ready for prediction? J Clin Invest 108:1091, 2001

LUSTER AD et al: Immune cell migration in inflammation: Present and future therapeutic targets. Nat Immunol 6:1182, 2005

MACDONALD TT et al: Immunity, inflammation, and allergy in the gut. Science 307:1920, 2005

MORETTA A et al: Major histocompatibility complex class I–specific receptors on human natural killer and T lymphocytes. Immunol Rev 155:105, 1997

———— et al: What is a natural killer cell? Nat Immunol 3:6, 2002

MORETTA L et al: Human natural killer cells: Molecular mechanisms controlling NK cell activation and tumor cell lysis. Immunol Lett 100:7, 2005

MORLEY BJ, WALPORT MJ: *The Complement Facts Books.* London, Academic Press, 2000, chap. 2

MULLAUER L et al: Mutations in apoptosis genes: A pathogenetic factor for human disease. Mutat Res 488:211, 2001

RIVERA J et al: Molecular regulation of mast cell activation. J Allergy Clin Immunol 6:1214, 2006

ROMAGNANI S: CD4 effector cells, in *Inflammation: Basic Principles and Clinical Correlates*, 3d ed, J Gallin, R Snyderman (eds). Philadelphia, Lippincott Williams & Wilkins, 1999, pp 177–184

SAKAGUCHI S: Regulatory T cells: Mediating compromises between host and parasite. Nat Immunol 4:10, 2003

SCHRADER JW: Interleukin is as interleukin does. Trends Immunol 23:573, 2002

SHEVACH EM: Regulatory T cells in autoimmunity. Annu Rev Immunol 18:423, 2000

SHINKAI K et al: Helper T cells regulate type-2 innate immunity in vivo. Nature 420:825, 2002

SARTOR RB: Therapeutic manipulation of the enteric microflora in inflammatory bowel diseases: Antibiotics, probiotics, and prebiotics. Gastroenterology 6:1620, 2004

VAN DUIN D et al: Triggering TLR signaling in vaccination. Trends Immunol 27:49, 2006

YOKOYAMA WM: Contact hypersensitivity: Not just T cells! Nat Immunol 7:437, 2006

309 The Major Histocompatibility Complex

Gerald T. Nepom

THE HLA COMPLEX AND ITS PRODUCTS

The human major histocompatibility complex (MHC), commonly called the human leukocyte antigen (HLA) complex, is a 4-megabase (Mb) region on chromosome 6 (6p21.3) that is densely packed with expressed genes. The best known of these genes are the HLA class I and class II genes, whose products are critical for immunologic specificity and transplantation histocompatibility, and they play a major role in susceptibility to a number of autoimmune diseases. Many other genes in the HLA region are also essential to the innate and antigen-specific functioning of the immune system. The HLA region shows extensive conservation with the MHC of other mammals in terms of genomic organization, gene sequence, and protein structure and function. Much of our understanding of the MHC has come from investigation of the MHC in mice, which is termed the *H-2 complex*, and to a lesser degree from other species as well. Nonetheless, in this chapter discussion will be confined to information applicable to the MHC in humans.

The *HLA class I genes* are located in a 2-Mb stretch of DNA at the telomeric end of the HLA region (Fig. 309-1). The classic (MHC class Ia) HLA-A, -B, and -C loci, the products of which are integral participants in the immune response to intracellular infections, tumors, and allografts, are expressed in all nucleated cells and are highly polymorphic in the population. *Polymorphism* refers to a high degree of allelic variation within a genetic locus that leads to extensive variation between different individuals expressing different alleles. Over 450 alleles at HLA-A, 780 at HLA-B, and 230 at HLA-C have been identified in different human populations, making this the most highly polymorphic segment known within the human genome. Each of the alleles at these loci encodes a

heavy chain (also called an α *chain*) that associates noncovalently with the nonpolymorphic light chain β$_2$-*microglobulin*, encoded on chromosome 15.

The nomenclature of HLA genes and their products reflects the grafting of newer DNA sequence information on an older system based on serology. Among class I genes, alleles of the HLA-A, -B, and -C loci were originally identified in the 1950s, 1960s, and 1970s by alloantisera, derived primarily from multiparous women, who in the course of normal pregnancy produce antibodies against paternal antigens expressed on fetal cells. The serologic allotypes were designated by consecutive numbers, e.g., HLA-A1, HLA-B8. Currently, under World Health Organization (WHO) nomenclature, class I alleles are given a single designation that indicates locus, serologic specificity, and sequence-based subtype. For example, HLA-A*0201 indicates subtype 1 of the serologically defined allele HLA-A2. Subtypes that differ from each other at the nucleotide but not the amino acid sequence level are designated by an extra numeral, e.g., HLA-B*07021 and HLA-B*07022 are two variants of the HLA-B702 subtype of HLA-B*07. The nomenclature of class II genes, discussed below, is made more complicated by the fact that both chains of a class II molecule are encoded by closely linked HLA-encoded loci, both of which may be polymorphic, and by the presence of differing numbers of isotypic DRB loci in different individuals. It has become clear that accurate

FIGURE 309-1 Physical map of the HLA region, showing the class I and class II loci, other immunologically important loci, and a sampling of other genes mapped to this region. Gene orientation is indicated by arrowheads. Scale is in kilobase (kb). The approximate genetic distance from DP to A is 3.2 cM. This includes 0.8 cM between A and B (including 0.2 cM between C and B), 0.4–0.8 cM between B and DR-DQ, and 1.6–2.0 cM between DR-DQ and DP.

FIGURE 309-2 A. The trimolecular complex of TCR (*top*), MHC molecule (*bottom*) and a bound peptide form the structural determinants of specific antigen recognition. Other panels (*B* and *C*) show the domain structure of MHC class I (B) and class II (C) molecules. The α_1 and α_2 domains of class I and the α_1 and β_1 domains of class II form a β-sheet platform that forms the floor of the peptide-binding groove, and α helices that form the sides of the groove. The α_3 (A) and β_2 domains (B) project from the cell surface and form the contact sites for CD8 and CD4, respectively. *(Adapted from EL Reinhertz et al: Science 286:1913, 1999; and C Janeway et al: Immunobiology Bookshelf, 2d ed, Garland Publishing, New York, 1997; with permission.)*

HLA genotyping requires DNA sequence analysis, and the identification of alleles at the DNA sequence level has contributed greatly to the understanding of the role of HLA molecules as peptide-binding ligands, to the analysis of associations of HLA alleles with certain diseases, to the study of the populations genetics of HLA, and to a clearer understanding of the contribution of HLA differences to allograft rejection and graft-vs-host disease. Current databases of HLA class I and class II sequences can be accessed by internet (e.g., from the IMGT/HLA Database, *http://www.ebi.ac.uk/imgt/hla*), and frequent updates of HLA gene lists are published in several journals.

The biologic significance of this MHC genetic diversity, resulting in extreme variation in the human population, is evident from the perspective of the structure of MHC molecules. As shown in Fig. 309-2, the MHC class I and class II genes encode MHC molecules that bind small peptides, and together this complex (pMHC; peptide-MHC) forms the ligand for recognition by T lymphocytes, through the antigen-specific T cell receptor. There is a direct link between the genetic variation and this structural interaction: The allelic changes in genetic sequence result in diversification of the peptide-binding capabilities of each MHC molecule and in differences for specific TCR binding. Thus, different pMHC complexes bind different antigens and are targets for recognition by different T cells.

The class I MHC and class II MHC structures, shown in Figs. 309-2B and 309-2C, are structurally closely related, although there are a few key differences. While both bind peptides and present them to T cells, the binding pockets have different shapes, which influences the types of immune responses that result (discussed below). In addition, there are structural contact sites for T cell molecules known as CD8 and CD4, expressed on the class I or class II membrane-proximal domains, respectively. This ensures that when peptide antigens are presented by class I molecules, the responding T cells are predominantly of the CD8 class, and similarly, that T cells responding to class II pMHC complexes are predominantly CD4.

The nonclassic, or class Ib, MHC molecules, HLA-E, -F, and -G, are much less polymorphic than MHC Ia and appear to have distinct functions. The HLA-E molecule, which has a peptide repertoire restricted to signal peptides cleaved from classic MHC class I molecules, is the major self-recognition target for the natural killer (NK) cell inhibitory receptors NKG2A or NKG2C paired with CD94 (see below and Chap. 308); four HLA-E alleles are known. HLA-G is expressed selectively in extravillous trophoblasts, the fetal cell population directly

in contact with maternal tissues. It binds a wide array of peptides, is expressed in six different alternatively spliced forms, and provides inhibitory signals to both NK cells and T cells, presumably in the service of maintaining maternofetal tolerance. The function of HLA-F remains largely unknown.

Additional class I–like genes have been identified, some HLA-linked and some encoded on other chromosomes, that show only distant homology to the class Ia and Ib molecules but share the three-dimensional class I structure. Those on chromosome 6p21 include MIC-A and MIC-B, which are encoded centromeric to HLA-B, and HLA-HFE, located 3 to 4 cM (centi-Morgan) telomeric of HLA-F. MIC-A and MIC-B do not bind peptide but are expressed on gut and other epithelium in a stress-inducible manner and serve as activation signals for certain γδ T cells, NK cells, CD8 T cells, and activated macrophages, acting through the activating NKG2D receptors. Sixty-one MIC-A and twenty-five MIC-B alleles are known, and additional diversification comes from variable alanine repeat sequences in the transmembrane domain. HLA-HFE encodes the gene defective in hereditary hemochromatosis (Chap. 351). Among the non-HLA, class I–like genes, CD1 refers to a family of molecules that present glycolipids or other nonpeptide ligands to certain T cells, including T cells with NK activity; FcRn binds IgG within lysosomes and protects it from catabolism (Chap. 308); and Zn-α_2-glycoprotein 1 binds a nonpeptide ligand and promotes catabolism of triglycerides in adipose tissue. Like the HLA-A, -B, -C, -E, -F, and -G heavy chains, each of which forms a heterodimer with β_2-microglobulin (Fig. 309-2), the class I–like molecules, HLA-HFE, FcRn, and CD1 also bind to β_2-microglobulin, but MIC-A, MIC-B, and Zn-α_2-glycoprotein 1 do not.

The *HLA class II region* is also illustrated in Fig. 309-1. Multiple class II genes are arrayed within the centromeric 1 Mb of the HLA region, forming distinct haplotypes. A *haplotype* refers to an array of alleles at polymorphic loci along a chromosomal segment. Multiple class II genes are present on a single haplotype, clustered into three major subregions: HLA-DR, -DQ, and -DP. Each of these subregions contains at least one functional alpha (A) locus and one functional beta (B) locus. Together these encode proteins that form the α and β polypeptide chains of a mature class II HLA molecule. Thus, the DRA and DRB genes encode an HLA-DR molecule; products of the DQAl and DQBl genes form an HLA-DQ molecule; and the DPAl and DPBl genes encode an HLA-DP molecule. There are several DRB genes (DRB1, DRB2, DRB3, etc.), so that two expressed DR molecules are encoded on most haplotypes by combining the α-chain product of the DRA gene with separate β chains. More than 438 alleles have been identified at the HLA-DRB1 locus, with most of the variation occurring within limited segments encoding residues that interact with antigens. Detailed analysis of sequences and population distribution of these alleles strongly suggests that this diversity is actively selected by environmental pressures associated with pathogen diversity.

The class II region was originally termed the *D-region*. The allelic gene products were first detected by their ability to stimulate lymphocyte proliferation by *mixed lymphocyte reaction* and were named Dw1, Dw2, etc. Subsequently, serology was used to identify gene products on peripheral blood B cells, and the antigens were termed *DR* (D-related). After additional class II loci were identified, these came to be known as DQ and DP. In the DQ region, both DQA1 and DQB1 are polymorphic, with 34 DQA1 alleles and 71 DQB1 alleles. The current nomenclature is largely analogous to that discussed above for class I, using the convention "locus * allele." Thus, for example, subtypes of the serologically defined specificity DR4, encoded by the DRB1 locus, are termed DRB1*0401, -0402, etc. In addition to allelic polymorphism, products of different DQA1 alleles can, with some limitations, pair with products of different DQB1 alleles through both *cis* and *trans* pairing to create combinatorial complexity and expand the number of expressed class II molecules. Because of the enormous allelic diversity in the general population, most individuals are heterozygous at all of the class I and class II loci. Thus, most individuals express six classic class I molecules (two each of HLA-A, -B, and -C) and around eight class II molecules—two DP, two DR (more in the case of haplotypes with additional functional DRB genes), and up to four DQ (two *cis* and two *trans*).

OTHER GENES IN THE MHC

In addition to the class I and class II genes themselves, there are numerous genes interspersed among the HLA loci that have interesting and important immunologic functions. Our current concept of the function of MHC genes now encompasses many of these additional genes, some of which are also highly polymorphic. Indeed, direct comparison of the complete DNA sequences for two of the entire 4-Mb MHC regions from different haplotypes show >18,000 variations, encoding an extremely high potential for biologic diversity. Specific examples include the TAP and LMP genes, as discussed in more detail below, which encode molecules that participate in intermediate steps in the HLA class I biosynthetic pathway. Another set of HLA genes, DMA and DMB, perform an analogous function for the class II pathway. These genes encode an intracellular molecule that facilitates the proper complexing of HLA class II molecules with antigen (see below). The *HLA class III region* is a name given to a cluster of genes between the class I and class II complexes, which includes genes for the two closely related cytokines tumor necrosis factor (TNF)-α and lymphotoxin (TNF-β); the complement components C2, C4, and Bf; heat shock protein (HSP)70; and the enzyme 21-hydroxylase.

The class I genes HLA-A, -B, and -C are expressed in all nucleated cells, although generally to a higher degree on leukocytes than on nonleukocytes. In contrast, the class II genes show a more restricted distribution: HLA-DR and HLA-DP genes are constitutively expressed on most cells of the myeloid cell lineage, whereas all three class II gene families (HLA-DR, -DQ, and -DP) are inducible by certain stimuli provided by inflammatory cytokines such as interferon γ. Within the lymphoid lineage, expression of these class II genes is constitutive on B cells and inducible on human T cells. Most endothelial and epithelial cells in the body, including the vascular endothelium and the intestinal epithelium, are also inducible for class II gene expression. Thus, while these somatic tissues normally express only class I and not class II genes, during times of local inflammation they are recruited by cytokine stimuli to express class II genes as well, thereby becoming active participants in ongoing immune responses. Class II expression is controlled largely at the transcriptional level through a conserved set of promoter elements that interact with a protein known as *CIITA*. Cytokine-mediated induction of CIITA is a principal method by which tissue-specific expression of HLA gene expression is controlled. Other HLA genes involved in the immune response, such as TAP and LMP, are also susceptible to upregulation by signals such as interferon γ. Sequence data for the entire HLA region can be accessed on the internet (e.g., *http://www.sanger.ac.uk/HGP/Chr6/MHC*). Many new genes have been discovered, the functions of which remain to be determined, as well as numerous microsatellite regions and other genetic elements. The gene density of the class II region is high, with approximately one protein encoded every 30 kb, and that of the class I and class III regions is even higher, with approximately one protein encoded every 15 kb.

LINKAGE DISEQUILIBRIUM

In addition to extensive polymorphism at the class I and class II loci, another characteristic feature of the HLA complex is *linkage disequilibrium*. This is formally defined as a deviation from Hardy-Weinberg equilibrium for alleles at linked loci. This is reflected in the very low recombination rates between certain loci within the HLA complex. For example, recombination between DR and DQ loci is almost never observed in family studies, and characteristic haplotypes with particular arrays of DR and DQ alleles are found in every population. Similarly, the complement components C2, C4, and Bf are almost invariably inherited together, and the alleles at these loci are found in characteristic haplotypes. In contrast, there is a recombinational hotspot between DQ and DP, which are separated by 1–2 cM of genetic distance, despite their close physical proximity. Certain extended haplotypes encompassing the interval from DQ into the class I region are commonly found, the most notable being the haplotype DR3-B8-A1, which is found, in whole or in part, in 10–30% of northern European Caucasians. It has been hypothesized that selective pressures may maintain linkage disequilibrium in HLA, but this remains to be determined. As discussed below under HLA and immunologic disease, one consequence of the phenomenon of linkage disequilibrium has been the resulting difficulty in assigning HLA-disease associations to a single allele at a single locus.

MHC STRUCTURE AND FUNCTION

Class I and class II molecules display a distinctive structural architecture, which contains specialized functional domains responsible for the unique genetic and immunologic properties of the HLA complex. The principal known function of both class I and class II HLA molecules is to bind antigenic peptides in order to present antigen to an appropriate T cell. The ability of a particular peptide to satisfactorily bind to an individual HLA molecule is a direct function of the molecular fit between the amino acid residues on the peptide with respect to the amino acid residues of the HLA molecule. The bound peptide forms a tertiary structure called the *MHC-peptide complex*, which communicates with T lymphocytes through binding to the T cell receptor (TCR) molecule. The first site of TCR-MHC-peptide interaction in the life of a T cell occurs in the thymus, where self-peptides are presented to developing thymocytes by MHC molecules expressed on thymic epithelium and hematopoietically derived antigen-presenting cells, which are primarily responsible for positive and negative selection, respectively (Chap. 308). Thus, the population of MHC–T cell complexes expressed in the thymus shapes the TCR repertoire. Mature T cells encounter MHC molecules in the periphery both in the maintenance of tolerance (Chap. 312) and in the initiation of immune responses. The MHC-peptide-TCR interaction is the central event in the initiation of most antigen-specific immune responses, since it is the structural determinant of the specificity. For potentially immunogenetic peptides, the ability of a given peptide to be generated and bound by an HLA molecule is a primary feature of whether or not an immune response to that peptide can be generated, and the repertoire of peptides that a particular individual's HLA molecules can bind exerts a major influence over the specificity of that individual's immune response.

When a TCR molecule binds to an HLA-peptide complex, it forms intermolecular contacts with both the antigenic peptide and with the HLA molecule itself. The outcome of this recognition event depends on the density and duration of the binding interaction, accounting for a dual specificity requirement for activation of the T cell. That is, the

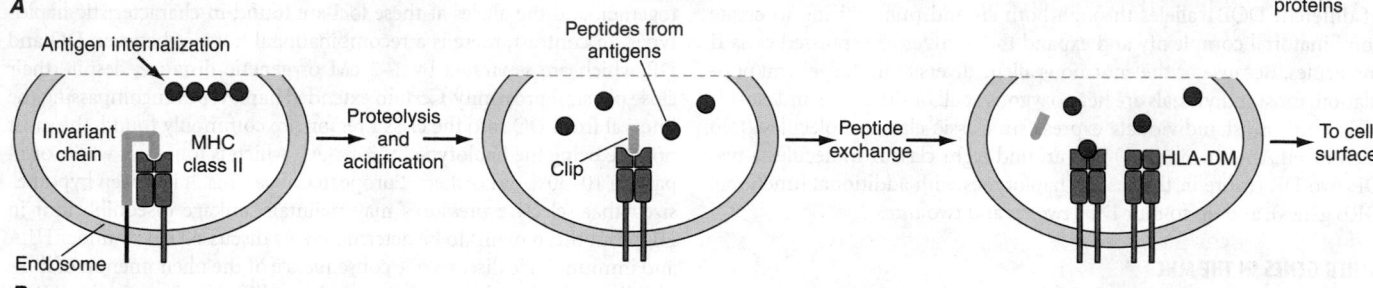

FIGURE 309-3 Biosynthesis of class I (A) and class II (B) molecules.
A. Nascent heavy chain (HC) becomes associated with β_2-microglobulin (β2m) and peptide through interactions with a series of chaperones. Peptides generated by the proteasome are transported into the endoplasmic reticulum (ER) by TAP. Peptides undergo N-terminal trimming in the ER and become associated with chaperones, including gp96 and PDI. Once peptide binds to HC-β2m, the HC-β2m-peptide trimeric complex exits the ER and is transported by the secretory pathway to the cell surface. In the Golgi, the N-linked oligosaccharide undergoes maturation, with addition of sialic acid residues. Molecules are not necessarily drawn to scale. **B.** Pathway of HLA class II molecule assembly and antigen processing. After transport through the Golgi and post-Golgi compartment, the class II–invariant chain complex moves to an acidic endosome, where the invariant chain is proteolytically cleaved into fragments and displaced by antigenic peptides, facilitated by interactions with the DMA-DMB chaperone protein. This class II molecule–peptide complex is then transported to the cell surface.

TCR must be specific both for the antigenic peptide and for the HLA molecule. The polymorphic nature of the presenting molecules, and the influence that this exerts on the peptide repertoire of each molecule, results in the phenomenon of *MHC restriction* of the T cell specificity for a given peptide. The binding of CD8 or CD4 molecules to the class I or class II molecule, respectively, also contributes to the interaction between T cell and the HLA-peptide complex, by providing for the selective activation of the appropriate T cell.

CLASS I STRUCTURE

(Fig. 309-2*B*) As noted above, MHC class I molecules provide a cell-surface display of peptides derived from intracellular proteins, and they also provide the signal for self-recognition by NK cells. Surface-expressed class I molecules consist of an MHC-encoded 44-kD glycoprotein heavy chain, a non-MHC-encoded 12-kD light chain β_2-microglobulin, and an antigenic peptide, typically 8–11 amino acids in length and derived from intracellularly produced protein. The heavy chain displays a prominent peptide-binding groove. In HLA-A and -B molecules, the groove is ~3 nm in length by 1.2 nm in maximum width (30 Å × 12 Å), whereas it is apparently somewhat wider in HLA-C. Antigenic peptides are noncovalently bound in an extended conformation within the peptide-binding groove, with both N- and C-terminal ends anchored in pockets within the groove (A and F pockets, respectively) and, in many cases, with a prominent kink, or arch, approximately one-third of the way from the N-terminus that elevates the peptide main chain off the floor of the groove.

A remarkable property of peptide binding by MHC molecules is the ability to form highly stable complexes with a wide array of peptide sequences. This is accomplished by a combination of peptide sequence–independent and peptide sequence–dependent bonding. The former consists of hydrogen bond and van der Waals interactions between conserved residues in the peptide-binding groove and charged or polar atoms along the peptide backbone. The latter is dependent upon the six side pockets that are formed by the irregular surface produced by protrusion of amino acid side chains from within the binding groove. The side chains lining the pockets interact with some of the peptide side chains. The sequence polymorphism among different class I alleles and isotypes predominantly affects the residues that line these pockets, and the interactions of these residues with peptide residues constitute the sequence-dependent bonding that confers a particular sequence "motif" on the range of peptides that can bind any given MHC molecule.

CLASS I BIOSYNTHESIS

(Fig. 309-3*A*) The biosynthesis of the classic MHC class I molecules reflects their role in presenting endogenous peptides. The heavy chain is cotranslationally inserted into the membrane of the endoplasmic reticulum (ER), where it becomes glycosylated and associates sequentially with the chaperone proteins calnexin and ERp57. It then forms a complex with β_2-microglobulin, and this complex associates with the chaperone calreticulin and the MHC-encoded molecule tapasin, which physically links the class I complex to TAP, the MHC-encoded transporter associated with antigen processing. Meanwhile, peptides generated within the cytosol from intracellular proteins by the multi-subunit, multicatalytic proteasome complex are actively transported into the ER by TAP, where they are trimmed by a peptidase known as *ERAAP* (ER aminopeptidase associated with antigen processing). At this point, peptides with appropriate sequence complementarity bind specific class I molecules to form complete, folded heavy chain–β_2-microglobulin–peptide trimer complexes. These are transported rapidly from the ER, through the *cis*- and *trans*-Golgi where the N-linked oligosaccharide is further processed, and thence to the cell surface.

Most of the peptides transported by TAP are produced in the cytosol by proteolytic cleavage of intracellular proteins by the multisubunit, multicatalytic proteasome, and inhibitors of the proteasome dramatically reduce expression of class I–presented antigenic peptides. A thiol-dependent oxidoreductase Erp57, which mediates disulfide bond rearrangements, also appears to play an important role in folding the class I–peptide complex into a stable multicomponent molecule. The MHC-encoded proteasome subunits LMP2 and LMP7 may influence the spectrum of peptides produced but are not essential for proteasome function.

CLASS I FUNCTION

Peptide Antigen Presentation On any given cell, a class I molecule occurs in 100,000–200,000 copies and binds several hundred to several thousand distinct peptide species. The vast majority of these peptides are self-peptides to which the host immune system is tolerant by one or more of the mechanisms that maintain tolerance, e.g., clonal deletion in the thymus or clonal anergy or clonal ignorance in the periphery (Chaps. 308 and 312). However, class I molecules bearing foreign peptides expressed in a permissive immunologic context activate CD8 T cells, which, if naïve, will then differentiate into cytolytic T lymphocytes (CTLs). These T cells and their progeny, through their $\alpha\beta$ TCRs, are then capable of Fas/CD95- and/or perforin-mediated cytotoxicity and/or cytokine secretion (Chap. 308) upon further encounter with the class I–peptide combination that originally activated it, and also with other combinations of class I molecule plus peptide that present a similar immunochemical stimulus to the TCR. As alluded to above, this phenomenon by which T cells recognize foreign antigens in the context of specific MHC alleles is termed *MHC restriction*, and the specific MHC molecule is termed the *restriction element*. The most common source of foreign peptides presented by class I molecules is viral infection, in the course of which peptides from viral proteins enter the class I pathway. The generation of a strong CTL response that destroys virally infected cells represents an important antigen-specific defense against many viral infections (Chap. 308). In the case of some viral infections—hepatitis B, for example—CTL-induced target cell apoptosis is thought to be a more important mechanism of tissue damage than any direct cytopathic effect of the virus itself. The importance of the class I pathway in the defense against viral infection is underscored by the identification of a number of viral products that interfere with the normal class I biosynthetic pathway and thus block the immunogenetic expression of viral antigens.

Other examples of intracellularly generated peptides that can be presented by class I molecules in an immunogenic manner include peptides derived from nonviral intracellular infectious agents (e.g., *Listeria*, *Plasmodium*), tumor antigens, minor histocompatibility antigens, and certain autoantigens. There are also situations in which cell surface–expressed class I molecules are thought to acquire and present exogenously derived peptides.

HLA Class I Receptors and NK Cell Recognition (Chap. 308) NK cells, which play an important role in innate immune responses, are activated to cytotoxicity and cytokine secretion by contact with cells that lack MHC class I expression, and NK cell activation is inhibited by cells that express MHC class I. In humans, the recognition of class I molecules by NK cells is carried out by three classes of receptor families, the killer cell–inhibitory cell receptor (KIR) family, the leukocyte Ig-like receptor (LIR) family, and the CD94/NKG2 family. The KIR family, also called CD158, is encoded on chromosome 19q13.4. KIR gene no-

menclature is based on the number of domains (2D or 3D) and the presence of long (L) or short (S) cytoplasmic domains. The KIR2DL1 and S1 molecules primarily recognize alleles of HLA-C, which possess a lysine at position 80 (HLA-Cw2, -4, -5 and -6), while the KIR2DL2/S2 and KIR2DL3/S3 families primarily recognize alleles of HLA-C with asparagine at this position (HLA-Cw1,-3, -7 and -8). The KIR3DL1 and S1 molecules predominantly recognize HLA-B alleles that fall into the HLA-Bw4 class determined by residues 77–83 in the α_1 domain of the heavy chain, while the KIR3DL2 molecule is an inhibitory receptor for HLA-A*03. One of the KIR products, KIR2DL4, is known to be an activating receptor for HLA-G. The most common KIR haplotype in Caucasians contains one activating KIR and six inhibitory KIR genes, although there is a great deal of diversity in the population, with >100 different combinations. It appears that most individuals have at least one inhibitory KIR for a self-HLA class I molecule, providing a structural basis for NK cell target specificity, which helps prevent NK cells from attacking normal cells.

The LIR gene family (CD85, also called ILT) is encoded centromeric of the KIR locus on 19q13.4, and it encodes a variety of inhibitory immunoglobulin-like receptors expressed on many lymphocyte and other hematopoietic lineages. Interaction of LIR-1 (ILT2) with NK or T cells inhibits activation and cytotoxicity, mediated by many different HLA class I molecules, including HLA-G. HLA-F also appears to interact with LIR molecules, although the functional context for this is not understood.

The third family of NK receptors for HLA is encoded in the NK complex on chromosome 12p12.3-13.1 and consists of CD94 and five NKG2 genes, A/B, C, E/H, D, and F. These molecules are C-type (calcium-binding) lectins, and most function as disulfide-bonded heterodimers between CD94 and one of the NKG2 glycoproteins. The principle ligand of CD94/NKG2A receptors is the HLA-E molecule, complexed to a peptide derived from the signal sequence of classic HLA class I molecules and HLA-G. Thus, analogous to the way in which KIR receptors recognize HLA-C, the NKG2 receptor monitors self–class I expression, albeit indirectly through peptide recognition in the context of HLA-E. NKG2C, -E, and -H appear to have similar specificities but act as activating receptors. NKG2D is expressed as a homodimer and functions as an activating receptor expressed on NK cells, $\gamma\delta$ TCR T cells, and activated CD8 T cells. When complexed with an adaptor called DAP10, NKG2D recognizes MIC-A and MIC-B molecules and activates the cytolytic response. NKG2D also binds a class of molecules known as *ULBP*, structurally related to class I molecules but not encoded in the MHC. The function of NK cells in immune responses is discussed in Chap. 308.

CLASS II STRUCTURE

(Fig. 309-2C) A specialized functional architecture similar to that of the class I molecules can be seen in the example of a class II molecule depicted in Fig. 309-2C, with an antigen-binding cleft arrayed above a supporting scaffold that extends the cleft toward the external cellular environment. However, in contrast to the HLA class I molecular structure, β_2-microglobulin is not associated with class II molecules. Rather, the class II molecule is a heterodimer, composed of a 29-kD α chain and a 34-kD β chain. The amino-terminal domains of each chain form the antigen-binding elements which, like the class I molecule, cradle a bound peptide in a groove bounded by extended α-helical loops, one encoded by the A (α chain) gene and one by the B (β chain) gene. Like the class I groove, the class II antigen-binding groove is punctuated by pockets that contact the side chains of amino acid residues of the bound peptide, but unlike the class I groove, it is open at both ends. Therefore, peptides bound by class II molecules vary greatly in length, since both the N- and C-terminal ends of the peptides can extend through the open ends of this groove. Approximately 11 amino acids within the bound peptide form intimate contacts with the class II molecule itself, with backbone hydrogen bonds and specific side chain interactions combining to provide, respectively, stability and specificity to the binding (Fig. 309-4).

The genetic polymorphisms that distinguish different class II genes correspond to changes in the amino acid composition of the class II

FIGURE 309-4 Specific intermolecular interactions determine peptide binding to MHC class II molecules. A short peptide sequence derived from alpha-gliadin (*A*) is accommodated within the MHC class II binding groove by specific interactions between peptide side chains (the P1–P9 residues illustrated in *B*) and corresponding pockets in the MHC class II structure. The latter are determined by the genetic polymorphisms of the MHC gene, in this case encoding an HLA-DQ2 molecule. *C.* This shows the extensive hydrogen bond and salt bridge network which tightly constrains the pMHC complex and presents the complex of antigen and restriction element for CD4 T cell recognition. (*From C Kim et al.*)

molecule, and these variable sites are clustered predominantly around the pocket structures within the antigen-binding groove. As with class I, this is a critically important feature of the class II molecule, which explains how genetically different individuals have functionally different HLA molecules.

BIOSYNTHESIS AND FUNCTION OF CLASS II MOLECULES

(Fig. 309-3*B*) The intracellular assembly of class II molecules occurs within a specialized compartmentalized pathway that differs dramatically from the class I pathway described above. As illustrated in Fig. 309-3*B*, the class II molecule assembles in the ER in association with a chaperone molecule, known as the *invariant chain*. The invariant chain performs at least two roles. First, it binds to the class II molecule and blocks the peptide-binding groove, thus preventing antigenic peptides from binding. This role of the invariant chain appears to account for one of the important differences between class I and class II MHC pathways, since it can

explain why class I molecules present endogenous peptides from proteins newly synthesized in the ER but class II molecules generally do not. Second, the invariant chain contains molecular localization signals that direct the class II molecule to traffic into post-Golgi compartments known as *endosomes*, which develop into specialized acidic compartments where proteases cleave the invariant chain, and antigenic peptides can now occupy the class II groove. The specificity and tissue distribution of these proteases appear to be an important way in which the immune system regulates access to the peptide-binding groove and T cells become exposed to specific self-antigens. Differences in protease expression in the thymus and in the periphery may in part determine which specific peptide sequences comprise the peripheral repertoire for T cell recognition. It is at this stage in the intracellular pathway, after cleavage of the invariant chain, that the MHC-encoded DM molecule catalytically facilitates the exchange of peptides within the class II groove to help optimize the specificity and stability of the MHC-peptide complex.

Once this MHC-peptide complex is deposited in the outer cell membrane it becomes the target for T cell recognition via a specific TCR expressed on lymphocytes. Because the endosome environment contains internalized proteins retrieved from the extracellular environment, the class II–peptide complex often contains bound antigens that were originally derived from extracellular proteins. In this way, the class II peptide–loading pathway provides a mechanism for immune surveillance of the extracellular space. This appears to be an important feature that permits the class II molecule to bind foreign peptides, distinct from the endogenous pathway of class I–mediated presentation.

ROLE OF HLA IN TRANSPLANTATION

The development of modern clinical transplantation in the decades since the 1950s provided a major impetus for elucidation of the HLA system, as allograft survival is highest when donor and recipient are HLA-identical. Although many molecular events participate in transplantation rejection, allogeneic differences at class I and class II loci play a major role. Class I molecules can promote T cell responses in several different ways. In the cases of allografts in which the host and donor are mismatched at one or more class I loci, host T cells can be activated by classic *direct alloreactivity*, in which the antigen receptors on the host T cells react with the foreign class I molecule expressed on the allograft. In this situation, the response of any given TCR may be dominated by the allogeneic MHC molecule, the peptide bound to it, or some combination of the two. Another type of host antigraft T cell response involves the uptake and processing of donor MHC antigens by host antigen-presenting cells and the subsequent presentation of the resulting peptides by host MHC molecules. This mechanism is termed *indirect alloreactivity*.

In the case of class I molecules on allografts that are shared by the host and the donor, a host T cell response may still be triggered because of peptides that are presented by the class I molecules of the graft but not of the host. The most common basis for the existence of these endogenous antigen peptides, called *minor histocompatibility antigens*, is a genetic difference between donor and host at a non-MHC locus encoding the structural gene for the protein from which the peptide is derived. These loci are termed *minor histocompatibility loci*, and non-identical individuals typically differ at many such loci. CD4 T cells react to analogous class II variation, both direct and indirect, and class II differences alone are sufficient to drive allograft rejection.

ASSOCIATION OF HLA ALLELES WITH SUSCEPTIBILITY TO DISEASE

It has long been postulated that infectious agents provide the driving force for the allelic diversification seen in the HLA system. An important corollary of this hypothesis is that resistance to specific pathogens may differ between individuals, based on HLA genotype. Observations of specific HLA genes associated with resistance to malaria or dengue fever, persistence of hepatitis B, and to disease progression in HIV infection are consistent with this model. For example, failure to clear persistent hepatitis B or C viral infection may reflect the inability of particular HLA molecules to present viral antigens effectively to T cells. Similarly, both protective and susceptible HLA allelic associations have been described for human papilloma virus–associated cervical neoplasia, implicating the MHC as an influence in mediating viral clearance in this form of cancer.

Pathogen diversity is probably also the major selective pressure favoring HLA heterozygosity. The extraordinary scope of HLA allelic diversity increases the likelihood that most new pathogens will be recognized by some HLA molecules, helping to assure immune fitness to the host. However, another consequence of diversification is that some alleles may become preferentially selective for recognition of self-antigens as well. Indeed, particular HLA alleles are strongly associated with certain disease states, particularly for some common autoimmune diseases (Chap. 312). By comparing allele frequencies in patients with any particular disease and in control populations, >100 such associations have been identified, some of which are listed in Table 309-1. The strength of genetic association is reflected in the term *relative risk*, which is a statistical odds ratio representing the risk of disease for an individual carrying a particular genetic marker compared with the risk for individuals in that population without that marker. The nomenclature shown in Table 309-1 reflects both the HLA serotype (e.g., DR3, DR4) and the HLA genotype (e.g., DRB1*0301, DRB1*0401). It very likely the class I and class II alleles themselves are the true susceptibility alleles for most of these associations. However, because of the extremely strong linkage disequilibrium between the DR and DQ loci, in some cases it has been difficult to determine the specific locus or combination of class II loci involved. In some cases, the susceptibility gene may be one of the HLA-linked genes located near the class I or class II region, but not the HLA gene itself, and in other cases the susceptibility gene may be a non-HLA gene, such as TNF-α, which is nearby. Indeed, since linkage disequilibrium of some haplotypes extends across large segments of the MHC region, it is quite possible that combinations of genes may account for the particular associations of HLA haplotypes with disease. For example, on some haplotypes associated with rheumatoid arthritis, both HLA-

DRB1 alleles and a particular polymorphism associated with the TNF locus may be contributory to disease risk. Other candidates for similar epistatic effects include the IKBL gene and the MICA locus, potentially in combination with classic HLA class II risk alleles.

As might be predicted from the known function of the class I and class II gene products, almost all of the diseases associated with specific HLA alleles have an immunologic component to their pathogenesis. It should be stressed that even the strong HLA associations with disease (those associations with relative risk of ≥10) implicate normal, rather than defective, alleles. Most individuals who carry these susceptibility genes do not express the associated disease; in this way the particular HLA gene is permissive for disease but requires other environmental (e.g., the presence of specific antigens) or genetic factors for full penetrance. In each case studied, even in diseases with very strong HLA associations, the concordance of disease in monozygotic twins is higher than in HLA-identical dizygotic twins or other sibling pairs, indicating that non-HLA genes contribute to susceptibility and can significantly modify the risk attributable to HLA.

Another group of diseases is genetically linked to HLA, not because of the immunologic function of HLA alleles, but rather because they

TABLE 309-1	SIGNIFICANT HLA CLASS I AND CLASS II ASSOCIATIONS WITH DISEASE		
	Marker	**Gene**	**Strength of Association**
Spondyloarthropathies			
Ankylosing spondylitis	B27	B*2702, -04, -05	++++
Reiter's syndrome	B27		++++
Acute anterior uveitis	B27		+++
Reactive arthritis (*Yersinia, Salmonella, Shigella, Chlamydia*)	B27		+++
Psoriatic spondylitis	B27		+++
Collagen-vascular diseases			
Juvenile arthritis, pauciarticular	DR8		++
	DR5		++
Rheumatoid arthritis	DR4	DRB1*0401, -04, -05	+++
Sjögren's syndrome	DR3		++
Systemic lupus erythematosus			
Caucasian	DR3		+
Japanese	DR2		++
Autoimmune gut & skin			
Gluten-sensitive enteropathy (celiac disease)	DQ2	DQA1*0501 DQB1*0201	+++
Chronic active hepatitis	DR3		++
Dermatitis herpetiformis	DR3		+++
Psoriasis vulgaris	Cw6		++
Pemphigus vulgaris	DR4	DRB1*0402	+++
	DQ1	DQB1*0503	
Bullous pemphigoid variant	DQ7	DQB1*0301	+
Autoimmune endocrine			
Type 1 diabetes mellitus	DR4	DQB1*0302	+++
	DQ8	DRB1*0401, -04	
	DR3		++
	DR2	DQB1*0602	—[a]
Hyperthyroidism (Graves')	B8		+
	DR3		+
Hyperthyroidism (Japanese)	B35		+
Adrenal insufficiency	DR3		++
Autoimmune neurologic			
Myasthenia gravis	B8		+
	DR3		+
Multiple sclerosis	DR2	DRB1*1501 DRB5*0101	++
Other			
Behçet's disease	B51		++
Congenital adrenal hyperplasia	B47	21-OH (Cyp21B)	+++
Narcolepsy	DR2	DQB1*0602	++++
Goodpasture's syndrome (anti-GBM)	DR2		++

[a]Strong negative association; i.e., genetic association with protection from diabetes.

are caused by autosomal dominant or recessive abnormal alleles at loci that happen to reside in or near the HLA region. Examples of these are 21-hydroxylase deficiency (Chap. 336), hemochromatosis (Chap. 351), and spinocerebellar ataxia (Chap. 369).

CLASS I ASSOCIATIONS WITH DISEASE

Although the associations of human disease with particular HLA alleles or haplotypes predominantly involve the class II region, there are also several prominent disease associations with class I alleles. These include the association of Behçet's disease (Chap. 320) with HLA-B51, psoriasis vulgaris (Chap. 53) with HLA-Cw6, and, most notably, the spondyloarthropathies (Chap. 318) with HLA-B27. Twenty-five HLA-B locus alleles, designated HLA-B*2701–B*2725, encode the family of B27 class I molecules. All of the subtypes share a common B pocket in the peptide-binding groove, a deep, negatively charged pocket that shows a strong preference for binding the arginine side chain. In addition, B27 is among the most negatively charged of HLA class I heavy chains, and the overall preference is for positively charged peptides. HLA-B*2705 is the predominant subtype in Caucasians and most other non-Oriental populations, and this subtype is very highly associated with ankylosing spondylitis (AS) (Chap. 318), both in its idiopathic form and in association with chronic inflammatory bowel disease or psoriasis vulgaris. It is also associated with reactive arthritis (ReA) (Chap. 318), with other idiopathic forms of peripheral arthritis (undifferentiated spondyloarthropathy), and with recurrent acute anterior uveitis. B27 is found in 50–90% of individuals with these conditions, compared with a prevalence of ~7% in North American Caucasians. The prevalence of B27 in patients with idiopathic AS is 90%, and in AS complicated by iritis or aortic insufficiency it is close to 100%. The absolute risk of spondyloarthropathy in unselected B27+ individuals has been variously estimated at 2–13% and >20% if a B27+ first-degree relative is affected. The concordance rate of AS in identical twins is very high, at least 65%. It can be concluded that the B27 molecule itself is involved in disease pathogenesis, based on strong evidence from clinical epidemiology and on the occurrence of a spondyloarthropathy-like disease in HLA-B27 transgenic rats. Both AS and ReA are associated with the B27 subtypes B*2702, -04, and -05, and anecdotal association has been reported for subtypes B*2701, -03, -07, -08, -10, and -11.

The association of B27 with these diseases may derive from the specificity of a particular peptide or family of peptides bound to B27 or through another mechanism that is independent of the peptide specificity of B27. The first alternative can be further subdivided into mechanisms that involve T cell recognition of B27-peptide complexes and those that do not. A variety of other roles for B27 in disease pathogenesis have been postulated, including molecular or antigenic mimicry between B27 and certain bacteria and reduced killing of intracellular bacteria in cells expressing B27. HLA-B27 has been shown to form heavy chain homodimers, utilizing the cysteine residue at position 67 of the B57 α chain. These homodimers are expressed on the surface of lymphocytes and monocytes from patients with AS, and receptors including KIR3DL1, KIR3DL2, and ILT4 are capable of binding to them. Whether these interactions contribute to disease susceptibility or pathogenesis is currently unknown.

CLASS II DISEASE ASSOCIATIONS

As can be seen in Table 309-1, the majority of associations of HLA and disease are with class II alleles. Several diseases have complex HLA genetic associations.

Celiac Disease In the case of celiac disease (Chap. 288), it is probable that the HLA-DQ genes are the primary basis for the disease association. HLA-DQ genes present on both the celiac-associated DR3 and DR7 haplotypes include the DQB1*0201 gene, and further detailed studies have documented a specific class II αβ dimer encoded by the DQA1*0501 and DQB1*0201 genes, which appears to account for the HLA genetic contribution to celiac disease susceptibility. This specific HLA association with celiac disease may have a straightforward expla-

nation: peptides derived from the wheat gluten component gliaden are bound to the molecule encoded by DQA1*0501 and DQB1*0201 and presented to T cells. A gliaden-derived peptide that has been implicated in this immune activation binds the DQ class II dimer best when the peptide contains a glutamine to glutamic acid substitution. It has been proposed that tissue transglutaminase, an enzyme present at increased levels in the intestinal cells of celiac patients, converts glutamine to glutamic acid in gliadin, creating peptides that are capable of being bound by the DQ2 molecule and presented to T cells.

Pemphigus Vulgaris In the case of pemphigus vulgaris (Chap. 55), there are two HLA genes associated with disease, DRB1*0402- and -DQB1*0503. Peptides derived from desmoglien3, an epidermal autoantigen, bind to the DRB1*0402- and DQB1*0503-encoded HLA molecules, and this combination of specific peptide binding and disease-associated class II molecule is sufficient to stimulate desmoglien-specific T cells. A bullous pemphigoid clinical variant, not involving desmoglien recognition, has been found to be associated with HLA-DQB1*0301.

Juvenile Arthritis Pauciarticular juvenile arthritis (Chap. 314) is an autoimmune disease associated with genes at the DRB1 locus and also with genes at the DPB1 locus. Patients with both DPB1*0201 and a DRB1 susceptibility allele (usually DRB1*08 or -*05) have a higher relative risk than expected from the additive effect of those genes alone. In juvenile patients with rheumatoid factor–positive polyarticular disease, heterozygotes carrying both DRB1*0401 and -*0404 have a relative risk > 100, reflecting an apparent synergy in individuals inheriting both of these susceptibility genes.

Type 1 Diabetes Mellitus Type 1 (autoimmune) diabetes mellitus (Chap. 338) is associated with MHC genes on more than one haplotype. The presence of both the DR3 and DR4 haplotypes in one individual confers a 20-fold increased risk for type 1 diabetes; the strongest single association is with DQB1*0302, and all haplotypes that carry a DQB1*0302 gene are associated with type 1 diabetes, whereas related haplotypes that carry a different DQB1 gene are not. However, the relative risk associated with inheritance of this gene can be modified, depending on other HLA genes present either on the same or a second haplotype. For example, the presence of a DR2-positive haplotype containing a DQB1*0602 gene is associated with decreased risk. This gene, DQB1*0602, is considered "protective" for type 1 diabetes. Even some DRB1 genes that can occur on the same haplotype as DQB1*0302 may modulate risk, so that individuals with the DR4 haplotype that contains DRB1*0403 are less susceptible to type 1 diabetes than individuals with other DR4-DQB1*0302 haplotypes.

Although the presence of a DR3 haplotype in combination with the DR4-DQB1*0302 haplotype is a very high risk combination for diabetes susceptibility, the specific gene on the DR3 haplotype that is responsible for this synergy is not yet identified. There are some characteristic structural features of the diabetes-associated DQ molecule encoded by DQB1*0302, particularly the capability for binding peptides that have negatively charged amino acids near their C-termini. This may indicate a role for specific antigenic peptides or T cell interactions in the immune response to islet-associated proteins.

HLA and Rheumatoid Arthritis The HLA genes associated with rheumatoid arthritis (RA) (Chap. 314) encode a distinctive sequence of amino acids from codons 67–74 of the DRβ molecule: RA-associated class II molecules carry the sequence LeuLeuGluGlnArgArgAlaAla or LeuLeuGluGlnLysArgAlaAla in this region, while non-RA-associated genes carry one or more differences in this region. These residues form a portion of the molecule that lies in the middle of the α-helical portion of the DRB1-encoded class II molecule, termed the *shared epitope*.

The highest risk for susceptibility to RA comes in individuals who carry both a DRB1*0401 and DRB1*0404 gene. These DR4-positive RA-associated alleles are most frequent among patients with more severe, erosive disease. Several mechanisms have been proposed that link the shared epitope to immune reactivity in RA. This portion of the class II molecule may allow preferential binding of an arthritogenic peptide, it may favor the expansion of a type of self-reactive T lymphocyte, or it may itself form part of the pMHC ligand recognized by TCR that initiates synovial tissue recognition.

MOLECULAR MECHANISMS FOR HLA-DISEASE ASSOCIATIONS

As noted above, HLA molecules play a key role in the selection and establishment of the antigen-specific T cell repertoire and a major role in the subsequent activation of those T cells during the initiation of an immune response. Precise genetic polymorphisms characteristic of individual alleles dictate the specificity of these interactions and thereby instruct and guide antigen-specific immune events. These same genetically determined pathways are therefore implicated in disease pathogenesis when specific HLA genes are responsible for autoimmune disease susceptibility.

The fate of developing T cells within the thymus is determined by the affinity of interaction between T cell receptor and HLA molecules bearing self-peptides, and thus the particular HLA types of each individual control the precise specificity of the T cell repertoire (Chap. 308). The primary basis for HLA-associated disease susceptibility may well lie within this thymic maturation pathway. The positive selection of potentially autoreactive T cells, based on the presence of specific HLA susceptibility genes, may establish the threshold for disease risk in a particular individual.

At the time of onset of a subsequent immune response, the primary role of the HLA molecule is to bind peptide and present it to antigen-specific T cells. The HLA complex can therefore be viewed as encoding genetic determinants of precise immunologic activation events. Antigenic peptides that bind particular HLA molecules are capable of stimulating T cell immune responses; peptides that do not bind are not presented to T cells and are not immunogenic. This genetic control of the immune response is mediated by the polymorphic sites within the HLA antigen–binding groove that interact with the bound peptides. In autoimmune and immune-mediated diseases, it is likely that specific tissue antigens that are targets for pathogenic lymphocytes are complexed with the HLA molecules encoded by specific susceptibility alleles. In autoimmune diseases with an infectious etiology, it is likely that immune responses to peptides derived from the initiating pathogen are bound and presented by particular HLA molecules to activate T lymphocytes that play a triggering or contributory role in disease pathogenesis. The concept that early events in disease initiation are triggered by specific HLA-peptide complexes offers some prospects for therapeutic intervention, since it may be possible to design compounds that interfere with the formation or function of specific HLA-peptide–T cell receptor interactions.

When considering mechanisms of HLA associations with immune response and disease, it is well to remember that just as HLA genetics are complex, so are the mechanisms likely to be heterogeneous. Immune-mediated disease is a multistep process in which one of the HLA-associated functions is to establish a repertoire of potentially reactive T cells, while another HLA-associated function is to provide the essential peptide-binding specificity for T cell recognition. For diseases with multiple HLA genetic associations, it is possible that both of these interactions occur and synergize to advance an accelerated pathway of disease.

FURTHER READINGS

COLBERT RA: The immunobiology of HLA-B27: Variations on a theme. Curr Mol Med 4:21, 2004

HERTL M et al: T cell control in autoimmune bullous skin disorders. J Clin Invest 116:1159, 2006

JONES EY et al: MHC class II proteins and disease: A structural perspective. Nat Rev Immunol 6:271, 2006

KIM C et al: Structural basis for HLA-DQ2-mediated presentation of gluten epitopes in celiac disease. Proc Natl Acad Sci USA 101:4175, 2004

MARTIN M, CARRINGTON M: Immunogenetics of viral infections. Curr Opin Immunol 17:510, 2005

NEPOM GT: Major histocompatibility complex-directed susceptibility to rheumatoid arthritis. Adv Immunol 68:315, 1998

———, KWOK WW: Molecular basis for HLA-DQ associations with IDDM. Diabetes 47:1177, 1998

SHIINA T et al: An update of the HLA genomic region, locus information and disease associations: 2004. Tissue Antigens 64:631, 2004

TROWSDALE J: HLA genomics in the third millennium. Curr Opin Immunol 17:498, 2005

310 Primary Immune Deficiency Diseases

Max D. Cooper, Harry W. Schroeder, Jr.

Specific adaptive immune responses are mediated by developmentally independent, but functionally interacting, families of lymphocytes. T lymphocytes mediate cellular immunity, while B lymphocytes and their plasma cell progeny produce antibodies to provide humoral immunity. The activities of B and T cells and their products in host defense are closely integrated with innate immune functions of other cells of the reticuloendothelial system. Dendritic cells, Langerhans cells in the skin, and macrophages play an important role in the trapping and presentation of antigens to T and B cells to initiate the immune response. Macrophages also become effector cells, especially when activated by cytokine products of lymphocytes. The scavenger activity of macrophages and polymorphonuclear leukocytes is directed and made specific by antibodies in concert with cytokines and the complement system. Natural killer (NK) cells, a population of granular lymphocytes with receptors specific for major histocompatibility complex (MHC) class I molecules, may spontaneously kill tumor and virus-infected cells, activities that are enhanced by the cytokine products of immune and inflammatory cells. Killing by NK cells can also be targeted by IgG antibodies for which NK cells have cell-surface receptors. The interaction of basophils and tissue mast cells with IgE antibodies in causation of immediate-type hypersensitivity is discussed in Chap. 311. Consideration of these interrelationships is an important part of the analysis of patients with suspected immune deficiency.

DIFFERENTIATION OF T AND B CELLS

The functional deficits that occur in both congenital and acquired immunodeficiencies are usefully viewed as being caused by defects at various points along the differentiation pathways of immunocompetent cells. Lymphoid progenitors derived from hematopoietic stem cells may migrate to the thymus to begin T cell development or remain in the fetal liver or bone marrow where they enter the B and NK cell pathways of development (Fig. 310-1). Immature T and B cells then migrate through the circulation to the spleen, lymph nodes, intestine, and other peripheral lymphoid organs. In these sites, they may encounter antigens presented by dendritic cells or macrophages and respond with proliferation, differentiation, and mediation of immune responses. Chapter 308 provides a general account of their roles in cellular and humoral immunity.

Differentiation of T or B cells may be arrested at either the primary or secondary stages. Reflecting the complex cellular interactions involved in immune responses and the pivotal role played by T lymphocytes, immune deficiencies primarily involving T cells are also associated with abnormal B cell function.

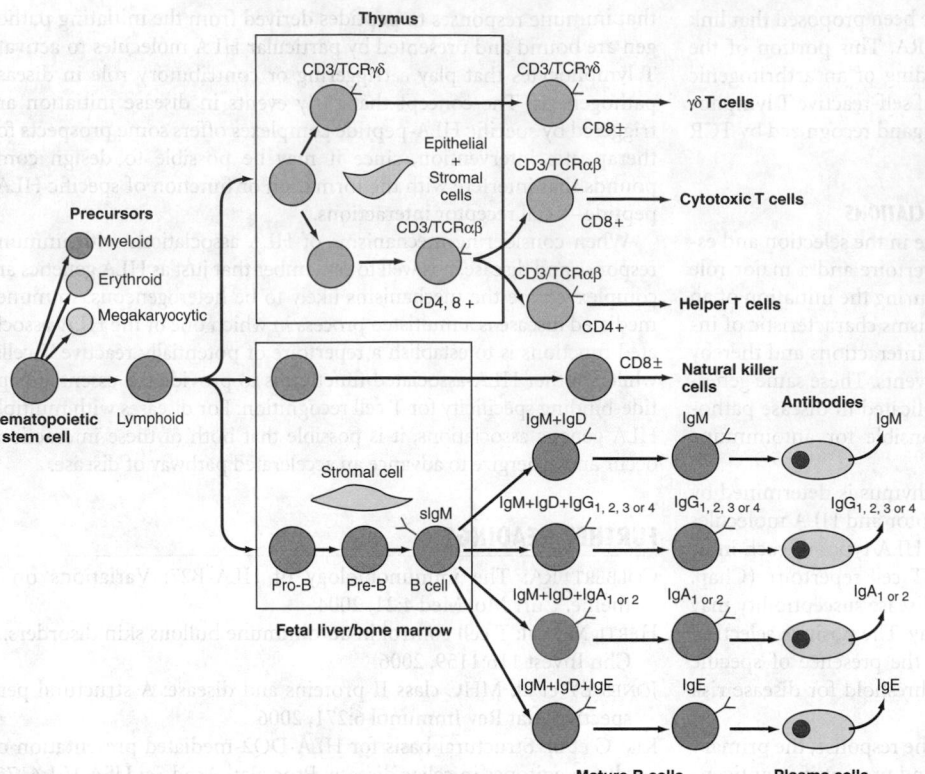

FIGURE 310-1 **Hypothetical model outlining the differentiation of hematopoietic stem cells along T, B, and NK cell lineages.** The antigen-presenting dendritic cells, not shown here, are derived from both lymphoid and myeloid progenitors. Failure to develop T and B cells may result from defective stem cells or from inborn metabolic errors affecting both cell types. Rarely, other hematopoietic cell lines are also absent. Absence of either T or B cells suggests malfunction of central lymphoid tissues, including the thymus and the fetal liver–bone marrow complex. B cell deficiency may result from failure to generate pre-B cells from their stem cell precursors or from failure of pre-B cells to give rise to their B lymphocyte progeny. Similarly, differentiation may be arrested at several levels within the T cell lineage; arrests at the thymocyte level and failure to develop the helper subset have been observed in immunodeficient patients. Agammaglobulinemia and deficiencies of some T cell functions may occur despite the presence of normal numbers of B or T cells in the circulation. Failure of B lymphocytes to differentiate to plasma cells can be due to intrinsic cellular abnormalities or to faulty T cell regulation.

CLINICAL DISEASE FEATURES COMMON TO IMMUNE DEFICIENCY

Immunodeficiency syndromes, whether congenital, spontaneously acquired, or iatrogenic, are characterized by unusual susceptibility to infection and not infrequently associated with autoimmune disease and lymphoreticular malignancies. The types of infection often provide the first clue to the nature of the immunologic defect.

Patients with *defects in humoral immunity* have recurrent or chronic sinopulmonary infection, meningitis, and bacteremia, most commonly caused by pyogenic bacteria such as *Haemophilus influenzae, Streptococcus pneumoniae,* and *Staphylococcus aureus.* These and other pyogenic organisms also cause frequent infections in individuals who have either neutropenia or a deficiency of the pivotal third component of complement (C3). The tripartite collaboration of antibody, complement, and phagocytes in host defense against pyogenic organisms makes it important to assess all three systems in individuals with unusual susceptibility to bacterial infections.

Antibody-deficient patients in whom cell-mediated immunity is intact have an interesting response to viral infections. The clinical course of primary infection with viruses such as varicella zoster or rubeola, unless complicated by bacterial infection, does not differ significantly from that of the normal host. However, multiple bouts of chickenpox and measles may occur. Such observations suggest that intact T cells may be sufficient for control of established viral infections, while antibodies play an important role in limiting the initial dissemination of virus and

in providing long-lasting protection. Exceptions to this generalization are becoming more widely recognized. Agammaglobulinemic patients fail to clear hepatitis B virus from their circulation and have a progressive, and often fatal, course. Poliomyelitis has occurred following live-virus vaccination in some patients. Notably, antibody-deficient patients may become chronically infected and continue to excrete large amounts of virus for years. Chronic encephalitis, which may progress over a period of months to years, is a particular threat in congenitally agammaglobulinemic boys. Echoviruses and adenoviruses have been isolated from brain, spinal fluid, or other sites in such patients.

The occurrence of an unusually serious infection—for example, *H. influenzae* meningitis in an older child or adult—warrants consideration of humoral immune deficiency. Recurrent bacterial pneumonias also suggest this possibility. Chronic otitis media occurs frequently in patients with hypogammaglobulinemia and is significant because of its relative rarity in normal adults. Pansinusitis, although almost invariably present in immunoglobulin deficiency, is a less helpful finding because it is not rare in apparently normal people. Bacterial infections of the skin or urinary tract are less frequent problems in hypogammaglobulinemic patients. Infestation with the intestinal parasite *Giardia lamblia* is a frequent cause of diarrhea in antibody-deficient patients.

Abnormalities of T cell-mediated immunity predispose to disseminated virus infections, particularly with latent viruses such as *Herpes simplex* (Chap. 172), *Varicella zoster* (Chap. 173), and cytomegalovirus (Chap. 175). In addition, patients so affected almost invariably develop mucocutaneous candidiasis and frequently acquire systemic fungal infections. Pneumonia caused by *Pneumocystis carinii* is also common (Chap. 200). Severe enteritis caused by *Cryptosporidium* infection may extend to the biliary tract to result in sclerosing cholangitis.

T cell deficiency is always accompanied by some abnormality of antibody responses (Fig. 310-1), although this may or may not be reflected by hypogammaglobulinemia. This explains in part why patients with primary T cell defects are also subject to overwhelming bacterial infection.

The most severe form of immune deficiency occurs in individuals who lack both cell-mediated and humoral immune functions. Individuals with severe combined immunodeficiency (SCID) are susceptible to the whole range of infectious agents including organisms not ordinarily considered pathogenic. Multiple infections with viruses, bacteria, and fungi occur, often simultaneously. Because donor lymphocytes cannot be rejected by these recipients, blood transfusions can produce fatal graft-versus-host disease.

EVALUATION OF IMMUNODEFICIENT PATIENTS

A careful history and physical examination will usually indicate whether the major problem involves the antibody-complement-phagocyte system or cell-mediated immunity. A history of contact dermatitis due to poison ivy suggests intact cellular immunity. Persistent mucocutaneous candidiasis suggests deficient cell-mediated immunity. Lymphopenia and the absence of palpable lymph nodes may be important findings. However, patients with profound immunodeficiency may

TABLE 310-1 LABORATORY EVALUATION OF HOST DEFENSE STATUS

Initial Screening Assays[a]

Complete blood count with differential smear
Serum immunoglobulin levels: IgM, IgG, IgA, IgD, IgE

Other Readily Available Assays

Quantification of blood mononuclear cell populations by immunofluorescence assays employing monoclonal antibody markers[b]
  T cells: CD3, CD4, CD8, TCRαβ, TCRγδ
  B cells: CD19, CD20, CD21, Ig(μ, δ, γ, α, κ, λ), Ig-associated molecules (α, β)
  Activation markers: HLA-DR, CD25, CD80 (B cells), CD154 (T cells)
  NK cells: CD16/CD56
  Monocytes: CD15
T cell functional evaluation
  1. Delayed hypersensitivity skin tests (PPD, *Candida*, histoplasmin, tetanus toxoid)
  2. Proliferative response to mitogens (anti-CD3 antibody, phytohemagglutinin, concanavalin A) and allogeneic cells (mixed lymphocyte response)
  3. Cytokine production
B cell functional evaluation
  1. Natural or commonly acquired antibodies: isohemagglutinins; antibodies to common viruses (influenza, rubella, rubeola) and bacterial toxins (diphtheria, tetanus)
  2. Response to immunization with protein (tetanus toxoid) and carbohydrate (pneumococcal vaccine, *H. influenzae B* vaccine) antigens
  3. Quantitative IgG subclass determinations
Complement
  1. CH$_{50}$ assays (classic and alternative pathways)
  2. C3, C4, and other components
Phagocyte function
  1. Reduction of nitroblue tetrazolium
  2. Chemotaxis assays
  3. Bactericidal activity

[a]Together with a history and physical examination, these tests will identify more than 95% of patients with primary immunodeficiencies.
[b]The menu of monoclonal antibody markers may be expanded or contracted to focus on particular clinical questions.

---

have diffuse lymphoid hyperplasia. Most immunodeficiencies may be diagnosed by thoughtful use of tests available in local or regional clinical laboratories. More precise evaluation of immunologic functions and treatment may require referral to specialized centers. Table 310-1 presents a résumé of widely available laboratory investigations.

HUMORAL IMMUNITY

With rare exceptions, deficiency of humoral immunity is accompanied by diminished serum concentration of one or more classes of immunoglobulin. Normal values vary with age, and adult concentrations of IgM (1.0±0.4 g/L) are reached at about 1 year, of IgG (10.0±3.0 g/L) at 5–6 years, and of IgA (2.5±1.0 g/L) by puberty (Chap. 308). The wide range of values among normal adults creates difficulty in defining the lower limits of normal. Reasonable estimates for low values are below 0.4 g/L for IgM, 5 g/L for IgG, and 0.5 g/L for IgA. In the presence of borderline hypogammaglobulinemia, assessing the patient's capacity to produce specific antibodies becomes particularly important. Isohemagglutinins are valuable standard assays, and measurements of pre- and postimmunization titers to tetanus toxoid, diphtheria toxoid, *H. influenzae* capsular polysaccharide, and *S. pneumoniae* serotypes provide a comprehensive assessment of humoral responsiveness.

Estimation of numbers of circulating B and T lymphocytes is of value in determining the pathogenesis of certain types of immune deficiency. B lymphocytes are identified by the presence of membrane-bound immunoglobulins, their associated α- and β-chain units, and other lineage-specific molecules on the B cell surface (Table 310-1), which can be identified and enumerated by specific monoclonal antibodies.

Since antibody deficiency may be mimicked clinically by deficiency of complement components, measurement of total hemolytic complement (CH$_{50}$) should be a part of the evaluation of host defense. Mea-

surement of C3 alone is inadequate for screening, since deficiencies of both early and late complement components may predispose to bacterial infection (Chap. 308).

CELLULAR IMMUNITY

T lymphocytes may be enumerated by their expression of the TCR/CD3 complex of surface molecules (TCR, T cell receptor). The CD4 molecule serves as a marker for helper T cells, although macrophages also express this molecule in relatively low levels. Conversely, CD8α/β heterodimers are expressed by cytotoxic T cells. CD8 is also expressed by some γδ T cells and by NK cells as CD8αα homodimeric molecules.

Normal levels of serum immunoglobulins and antibody responsiveness are reliable indices of intact helper T cell function. T lymphocyte function can be measured directly by delayed hypersensitivity skin testing using a variety of antigens to which the majority of older children and adults have been sensitized. A generally useful skin test antigen is a 1:5 dilution of tetanus toxoid injected intradermally, since almost all individuals will have been sensitized. Purified protein derivative (PPD), histoplasmin, mumps antigen, and extracts of *Candida* or *Trichophyton* also may be used.

T lymphocyte function may be estimated in vitro by the capacity of cells to proliferate in response to antigens to which the patient has been sensitized, to lymphocytes from an unrelated donor, to antibodies that cross-link the CD3/TCR complex, or to the T cell mitogens, such as phytohemagglutinin and concanavalin A. The response is usually quantified 3 days later by measurement of incorporation of radioactive thymidine into newly synthesized DNA. The production of cytokines (or interleukins) by activated T cells can be measured, as can the ability of T cells activated in mixed lymphocyte culture to lyse target cells. Finally, assays exist for detection of defects in T cell surface receptors and specific elements of their signal transduction pathways.

CLASSIFICATION

Primary immunodeficiencies may be either congenital or manifested later in life and are currently classified according to mode of inheritance and whether the genetic defect affects T cells, B cells, or both (Table 310-2). The following discussion emphasizes three related concepts: (1) that immunodeficiencies are logically viewed as defects of cellular differentiation; (2) that these defects may involve either primary development of T or B cells or the antigen-dependent phase of their differentiation; and (3) that defects of B cell formation may in some instances reflect faulty T-B collaboration.

Secondary immunodeficiencies are those not caused by intrinsic abnormalities in development or function of T and B cells. The best known of these is AIDS, which may follow infection with the human immunodeficiency virus (Chap. 182). Other examples are immune deficiency associated with malnutrition, protein-losing enteropathy, and intestinal lymphangiectasia. Also considered secondary are immunodeficiencies resulting from hypercatabolic states such as occur in myotonic dystrophy; immunodeficiency associated with lymphoreticular malignancy; and immunodeficiency resulting from treatment with x-rays, antilymphocyte antibodies, or immunosuppressive drugs.

INCIDENCE

As a group, the primary immunodeficiencies are relatively common. The most frequent, isolated IgA deficiency, occurs in approximately 1 in 600 individuals in Europe and North America. Common variable immunodeficiency, a related disorder characterized by panhypogammaglobulinemia, is the next most common disorder. Both of these immunodeficiency states often become clinically evident in young adults.

The more severe forms of primary immunodeficiency are relatively rare, have their onset early in life, and all too frequently result in death during childhood. However, patients with congenital hypogammaglobulinemia may lead relatively healthy lives with adequate antibody-replacement therapy. In a referral center for patients with immunodeficiency diseases, approximately two-thirds of the immunodeficient patients will be adults.

TABLE 310-2 PRIMARY IMMUNODEFICIENCIES—LABORATORY AND CLINICAL FEATURES

| | Lymphocytes | | | Cellular Immunity | Humoral Immunity | | | | Antibody Responses | Common Infections |
| | | | | | Serum Immunoglobulins | | | | | |
	B	T	NK		M	G	A	E		
Severe Combined Immunodeficiency (SCID)										
Adenosine deaminse (ADA) deficiency	−	−	+	−	↓	↓	↓	↓	−	Bacteria, viruses, fungi
Artemis deficiency (SCIDA)	−	−	+	−	↓	↓	↓	↓	−	Bacteria, viruses, fungi
CD45 deficiency	+	−	−	−	↓	↓	↓	↓	−	Bacteria, viruses, fungi
Cernunnos deficiency	−	−	+	−	↓	↓	↓	↓	−	Bacteria, viruses, fungi
DNA ligase IV (LIG4) deficiency	−	−	+	−	↓	↓	↓	↓	−	Bacteria, viruses, fungi
Interleukin receptor γ chain deficiency (X-linked SCID)	+	−	−	−	N	↓	↓	↓	−	Bacteria, viruses, fungi
Janus-associated kinase 3 (JAK3) deficiency	+	−	−	−	N	↓	↓	↓	−	Bacteria, viruses, fungi
Recombinase activating gene (RAG 1/2) deficiency	−	−	+	−	↓	↓	↓	↓	−	Bacteria, viruses, fungi
Reticular dysgenesis	−	−	−	−	↓	↓	↓	↓	−	Bacteria, viruses, fungi
TAP-1 or TAP-2 deficiency (MHC class I deficiency)	+	±	+	−	N	N	N	N	+	Bacteria, viruses, fungi
Primary T Cell Deficiency										
CD8 deficiency	+	±	+	±	N	N	N	N	+	Bacteria
diGeorge syndrome	+	−	+	−	N	N	N	N	±	Bacteria, viruses, fungi
Interleukin 7 receptor α (IL7RA) deficiency	+	−	+	−	N	N	N	N	±	Bacteria, viruses, fungi
MHC class II deficiency	+	±	+	+	N	↓	↓	↓	±	Bacteria, viruses, fungi
LCK deficiency	+	±	+	+	N	↓	↓	↓	±	Bacteria, viruses, fungi
Orai1 deficiency	+	+	±	−	↑	N/↑	↑	−	±	Bacteria, viruses, fungi
Nude syndrome (wing helix nude deficiency)	+	−	+	−	N	N/↓	N/↓	N/↓	±	Bacteria, viruses, fungi
Purine nucleotide phosphorylase (PNP) deficiency	+	−	+	−	N	↓	↓	↓	±	Bacteria, viruses, fungi
T cell receptor deficiency (CD3γ, δ, ε, and ζ deficiencies)	+	±	+	−	N	N	N	N	±	Bacteria, viruses, fungi
Zap70 tyrosine kinase deficiency	+	±	+	−	N	N/↓	N/↓	N/↓	±	Bacteria, viruses, fungi
Predominantly Antibody Deficiency										
IgG subclass deficiency	+	+	+	+	N	N/↓	N/↓	N	±	Bacteria
Autosomal agammaglobulinemia (recessive: λ5, Igβ, or BLNK deficiency; dominant: LRRC8)	−	+	+	+	↓	↓	↓	↓	−	Bacteria, *Giardia lamblia*
Common variable immune deficiency (MHC-associated, ICOS, TACI, BAFFR, CD19)	+	+	+	+	N/↓	↓	↓	↓	−	Bacteria, *Giardia lamblia*
Selective IgA deficiency (MHC-associated, TACI)	+	+	+	+	N	N	↓	N	±	Bacteria, *Giardia lamblia*
X-linked agammaglobulinemia	−	+	+	+	↓	↓	↓	↓	−	Bacteria, *Giardia lamblia*
Hyper-IgM syndrome										
Activation-induced cytidine deaminase (AID) deficiency	+	+	+	+	N/↑	↓	↓	↓	±	Bacteria
Uracil-DNA Glycosylase (UNG) deficiency	+	+	+	+	N/↑	↓	↓	↓	±	Bacteria
X-linked CD40 ligand deficiency	+	+	+	+	N/↑	↓	N/↓	↓	±	Bacteria, viruses, fungi
X-linked IKK-γ (NEMO) deficiency	+	+	+	+	N/↑	↓	↓	↓	±	Bacteria, viruses, fungi
CD40 deficiency	+	+	+	+	N/↑	↓	N/↓	↓	±	Bacteria, viruses, fungi
Other Well-Defined Immunodeficiency Syndromes										
Hyper IgE syndrome	+	+	+	+	N	N	N	↑↑↑	+	Bacteria
Wiskott-Aldrich syndrome	+	±	+	±	↓	N	↑	↑	±	Bacteria
Interferon γ receptor deficiency	+	+	+	+	N	N	N	N	+	Mycobacteria, viruses
Interleukin 1 receptor–associated kinase 4 deficiency	+	+	+	+	N	N	N	N	±	Bacteria, fungi
Interleukin 12 and interleukin 12 receptor deficiency	+	+	+	+	N	N	N	N	+	Mycobacteria, *Salmonella*
Whim Syndrome	+	+	+	+	N/↓	↓	N/↓	−	+	Bacteria, Warts
X-linked lymphoproliferative syndrome	+	+	+	+	N	N/↓	N/↓	N/↓	±	Epstein-Barr virus

Note: B, B cells; N, normal; NK, natural killer lymphocytes; T, T cells, +, normal levels; −, reduced or absent levels.

SEVERE COMBINED IMMUNODEFICIENCY

The SCID syndrome is characterized by gross functional impairment of both humoral and cell-mediated immunity and by susceptibility to devastating fungal, bacterial, and viral infections. The syndrome is inherited either as an X-linked or autosomal recessive defect, and affected infants rarely survive beyond 1 year without treatment.

The overall incidence of SCID is 1 in 100,000 to 1 in 1,000,000. The syndrome has been associated with mutations in one of several genes whose products are necessary for the normal differentiation of T, B, and, sometimes, NK cells. Genetic deficiencies in Orai1, a vital calcium channel component in T cells, and CD45, a tyrosine phosphatase that is essential for TCR signaling and development, may lead to a T⁻B⁺NK⁺ SCID phenotype. A T⁻B⁺NK⁺ SCID phenotype may result from a function-loss mutation in the *IL-7 receptor α chain (IL7RA)* gene, since T cell production and survival is dependent on IL-7 stimulation.

In one autosomal recessive form of SCID characterized by severe lymphopenia, the failure in both T and B cell development is due to mutations in the *RAG-1* or *RAG-2* genes, the combined activities of which are needed for V(D)J recombination. A function-loss mutation in either the *DNA-dependent tyrosine kinase, Artemis, ligase IV (LIG4)* or the *Cernunnos* genes may cause SCID, since they also encode essential enzymes for the V(D)J gene rearrangement process. About half of patients with autosomal recessive SCID are deficient in an enzyme involved in purine metabolism, adenosine deaminase (ADA), due to mutations in the *ADA* gene. The abortive lymphoid differentiation associated with ADA deficiency is due to intracellular accumulation of adenosine and deoxyadenosine nucleotides that trigger apoptosis of immature T and B lineage cells.

SCID may also occur with an X-linked inheritance pattern. Aborted thymocyte differentiation and an absence of peripheral T cells and NK cells are seen in X-linked SCID. B lymphocytes are present in normal numbers but are functionally defective. The defective gene encodes a common γ chain of the receptors for interleukin (IL) 2, -4, -7, -9, and -15, thus disrupting the action of this important set of lymphokines. The same T⁻NK⁻B⁺ SCID phenotype seen in X-linked SCID can be inherited as an autosomal recessive disease due to mutations in the gene for JAK3 protein kinase deficiency. This enzyme associates with the common γ chain of the receptors for IL-2, -4, -7, -9, and -15 to serve as a key element in their signal transduction pathways.

℞ SEVERE COMBINED IMMUNODEFICIENCY

The cellular defects in SCID patients logically rest with the pluripotent hematopoietic stem cells or their lymphoid progenitor progeny. Accordingly, the immunologic deficits in all of the different types of SCID patients may be repaired by transplantation of histocompatible bone marrow as a source of stem cells in that the stromal microenvironments of these individuals are intact and capable of supporting T and B cell development. However, antibody deficiency requiring immunoglobulin replacement therapy may persist for years in the recipient γc-, JAK3-, IL-7Rα-, Orai1-, and CD45-deficient patients, unless their defective B cells are eliminated prior to bone marrow transplantation to allow replacement with normal B cells of donor origin. Ex vivo insertion of a γc transgene into bone marrow progenitors has successfully corrected the immune deficiency of X-linked SCID patients. Notably, however, chance insertion of the γc transgene near a tumor-suppressor gene has been associated with development of a T cell lymphoproliferative disorder in several treated patients. In ADA-deficient patients without histocompatible bone marrow donors, the administration of exogenous ADA (conjugated to polyethylene glycol to prolong its half-life) may improve immunologic function and clinical status. Hematopoietic stem cell gene therapy has also been used successfully in treating ADA-deficient SCID patients; myeloablative conditioning was required to clear a space in the bone marrow for the ADA transduced cells. Treatment of SCID patients should be performed in centers with a strong research interest in this problem. It is crucial that these patients be recognized and treated early. Live viral vaccines or blood transfusions must be avoided because they cause fatal infections and graft-versus-host disease in SCID patients.

PRIMARY T CELL IMMUNODEFICIENCY

Reflecting the diversity of T cell functions, abnormalities of T cell development may be responsible for a wide spectrum of immune deficiencies, including combined immunodeficiency, selective defects in cell-mediated immunity, and syndromes presenting as antibody deficiency. These defects may be acquired (Chap. 182) as well as congenital.

The diGeorge Syndrome
This classic example of isolated T cell deficiency results from maldevelopment of thymic epithelial elements derived from the third and fourth pharyngeal pouches. The gene defect has been mapped to chromosomal position 22q11 in most patients with the diGeorge syndrome, and to 10p in others. Defective development of organs dependent on cells of embryonic neural crest origin includes congenital cardiac defects, particularly those involving the great vessels; hypocalcemic tetany, due to failure of parathyroid development; and absence of a normal thymus. Facial abnormalities may include abnormal ears, shortened philtrum, micrognathia, and hypertelorism. Serum immunoglobulin concentrations are frequently normal, but antibody responses, particularly of IgG and IgA isotypes, are usually impaired. T cell levels are reduced, whereas B cell levels are normal. Affected individuals often have a small, histologically normal thymus located near the base of the tongue or in the neck, allowing most patients to develop functional T cells in numbers that may or may not be adequate for host defense.

The Nude Syndrome
The human disease counterpart to the *nude* mouse is caused by mutations of the *whn* (winged-helix-nude) gene that result in impairment of hair follicle and epithelial thymic development. The human *nude* phenotype is characterized by congenital baldness, nail dystrophy, and severe T cell immunodeficiency.

T Cell Receptor Deficiency
Since the expression and function of antigen-specific TCRs is dependent on their signal-transducing CD3γ, δ, ε, and ζ chains, defective genes for any of these receptor components can impair T cell development and function. CD3γ mutations result in a selective deficit in CD8 T cells, whereas CD3ε mutations lead to a preferential reduction in CD4 T cells, thus implying differences in the signal transduction roles for each CD3 component. CD3δ and CD3ζ deficiencies may result in complete absence of T cell development.

MHC Class II Deficiency
Because T cells are required for B cell responses to most antigens, any gene defect (or acquired disorder) that interferes with T cell development and cell-mediated immunity will also compromise antibody production and humoral immunity. MHC class II deficiency results in one such immunodeficiency in that the TCRαβ must see protein antigens as peptide fragments held within the α helical grooves of class II and class I molecules encoded by the MHC. Antigen-presenting cells in individuals with this relatively rare disorder fail to express the class II molecules DP, DQ, and DR on their surface. Although some affected individuals produce CD4-bearing T lymphocytes in their thymus, these cannot recognize antigen properly to function as normal helper T cells. The defective T cell function leads to recurrent bronchopulmonary infections, chronic diarrhea, and severe viral infections that usually prove fatal before 4 years of age. This immunodeficiency disease is caused by mutations in genes that encode essential transcriptional factors that bind to promoter elements for the *MHC class II* genes. The *class II transactivator (CIITA)* gene is mutated in one subgroup of MHC class II–deficient patients, whereas mutations in *RFX* genes encoding additional transcriptional factors for *MHC class II* genes are responsible for the defective development and function of CD4 T cells in other families: *RFXANK* in subgroup B, *RFX5* in subgroup C, and *RFXAP* in subgroup D.

ZAP70 Tyrosine Kinase Deficiency
Recurrent and opportunistic infections begin within the first year of life in individuals with a deficiency in ZAP70 tyrosine kinase, a pivotal component in the TCR/CD3 signal transduction cascade. The rare inheritance of mutations in both alleles of the *ZAP70* gene results in a selective deficiency of CD8 T cells and dysfunction of CD4 T cells, which are present in normal numbers. Severe immunodeficiency is the inevitable consequence.

Purine Nucleoside Phosphorylation Deficiency
Function-loss mutations of the *purine nucleoside phosphorylase (PNP)* gene are associated with a severe and selective deficiency of T lymphocyte function. This enzyme functions in the same purine salvage pathway as ADA; toxic effects of the PNP deficiency are thought to result from the intracellular accumulation of deoxyguanosine triphosphate.

Ataxia-Telangiectasia
Ataxia-telangiectasia (AT) is an autosomal recessive genetic disorder characterized by cerebellar ataxia, oculocutaneous telangiectasia, and immunodeficiency. The mutant *ATM* gene has sequence similarity to the phosphatidyl-inositol-3 kinases that are

involved in signal transduction. The *ATM* gene belongs to a conserved family of genes that monitor DNA repair and coordinate DNA synthesis with cell division. The deleterious effects of the *ATM* gene are widespread. Truncal ataxia may become evident when walking begins and is progressive. Telangiectasia, primarily represented by dilated blood vessels in the ocular sclera, in a butterfly area of the face, and on the ears, is an early diagnostic feature. Immunodeficiency may be clinically manifest by recurrent and chronic sinopulmonary infection leading to bronchiectasis, although not all patients have overt immunodeficiency. Ovarian agenesis is a frequent occurrence. Persistence of very high serum levels of oncofetal proteins, including α-fetoprotein and carcinoembryonic antigen, may be of diagnostic value. Frequent causes of death are chronic pulmonary disease and malignancy. Lymphomas are most common, although carcinomas also occur.

The immunologic abnormalities seem to be related to maldevelopment of the thymus. The markedly hypoplastic thymus is similar in appearance to an embryonic thymus. The peripheral T cell pool is reduced in size, especially in lymphoid tissue compartments. Cutaneous anergy and delayed rejection of skin allografts are common. Although B lymphocyte development is normal, most patients are deficient in serum IgE and IgA, and a smaller number have reduced serum levels of IgG, particularly of the IgG2, IgG4 subclasses.

The defect in DNA repair mechanisms in AT patients renders their cells highly susceptible to radiation-induced chromosomal damage and resultant tumor development. AT is a rare disorder, with an incidence of 1 in 10,000 to 1 in 100,000, but 1% of the population is heterozygous for an AT mutation. This is important because the heterozygous state also predisposes to enhanced cellular radiosensitivity and cancer, especially breast cancer in females (Chap. 368).

℞ PRIMARY T CELL IMMUNODEFICIENCY

Therapeutic options other than symptomatic treatment are limited for this group of patients. Live vaccines and blood transfusions containing viable T cells should be assiduously avoided. Exposure to x-irradiation also should be avoided in patients with AT. Therapeutic intervention in the form of an epithelial thymic transplant can repair the T cell deficiency in patients with the nude syndrome and in the most severe cases of the diGeorge syndrome where T cells are absent. Treatment by bone marrow transplantation is sometimes successful after myeloablative conditioning in patients with PNP and MHC class II deficiencies. Preventive therapy for *P. carinii* in the form of trimethoprim/sulfamethoxazole should be considered. Immunoglobulin infusions are also recommended for those T cell–deficient individuals with severe antibody deficiency reflected by low serum levels of IgG.

IMMUNOGLOBULIN DEFICIENCY SYNDROMES

X-Linked Agammaglobulinemia   Males with this syndrome often begin to have recurrent bacterial infections in the first year of life when maternally derived immunoglobulins have disappeared. Although B cell progenitors are found in the bone marrow, affected individuals have very few immunoglobulin-bearing B lymphocytes in their circulation and typically lack primary and secondary lymphoid follicles. Mutations of *Bruton's tyrosine kinase (Btk)* gene are responsible for X-linked agammaglobulinemia. The developmental block due to the deficiency of this pre-BCR and BCR signaling enzyme is evident at the pre-B cell level (Fig. 310-1). B cells in heterozygous female carriers exclusively utilize the X chromosome with the normal *Btk* gene, while random X chromosome usage occurs in T cells and myeloid cells. A variant disorder, *X-linked agammaglobulinemia with growth hormone deficiency*, has been associated with *Btk* mutations that result in a truncated message.

Agammaglobulinemia is a misnomer, since most of these patients synthesize some immunoglobulins. Within the same family, some affected males may have substantial levels of IgM, IgG, and IgA, while others are nearly agammaglobulinemic. Btk-deficient patients typically are very deficient in circulating B lymphocytes. The few B lymphocytes that escape the block in pre-B cell differentiation are hyporesponsive, making antibody replacement therapy essential in these patients.

Sinopulmonary bacterial infections constitute the most frequent clinical problem. Mycoplasma infections may cause arthritis in some of these patients. Chronic encephalitis of viral etiology, sometimes associated with dermatomyositis, can be a fatal complication. All of these complications are reduced by treatment with intravenous immunoglobulins.

Autosomal Agammaglobulinemia   This syndrome can result from mutations in a variety of genes whose products are required for B lineage differentiation. Homozygous function-loss mutations in any of the genes coding pre-B receptor components—μ *heavy chain, surrogate light chain (VpreB and VLL1)*, Igα, and Igβ—can block pre-B cell differentiation, thereby leading to the absence of B cells, agammaglobulinemia, and recurrent bacterial infections. Disruption of B cell development may also occur as a consequence of mutations in genes coding for key elements in the pre-B receptor signaling pathway such as the adaptor B-cell linker protein (BLNK). Truncation of *LRRC8*, a gene of unknown function that is expressed in progenitor B cells, also leads to an absence of mature B cells in heterozygous individuals.

Transient Hypogammaglobulinemia of Infancy   This diagnosis is reserved for those rare instances in which normal physiologic hypogammaglobulinemia of infancy is unusually prolonged and severe. IgG levels normally drop to 3.0–4.0 g/L between 3 and 6 months of age as maternally derived IgG is catabolized. The IgG levels subsequently rise, reflecting the infant's own antibody production. Periodic immunologic assessment is needed to differentiate transient hypogammaglobulinemia from other forms of antibody deficiency. Antibody replacement therapy is recommended only in the face of severe or recurrent infections.

IgA Deficiency   IgA deficiency and common variable immunodeficiency (CVID) represent polar ends of a clinical spectrum due to the same underlying gene defect(s) in a large subset of these patients. The two disorders feature similar B cell differentiation arrests, differing only in the extent of the immunoglobulin class deficiencies. Over a period of years, IgA-deficient patients may progress to the panhypogammaglobulinemia phenotype characteristic of CVID, and vice versa. Both immunoglobulin deficiency phenotypes are found in the same family.

An inability to produce antibodies of the IgA1 and IgA2 subclasses occurs in approximately 1 in 600 individuals of European origin, a much higher incidence than is seen for other primary immunodeficiencies. IgA deficiency and CVID are frequently associated with MHC haplotypes that are more common in Caucasians. Accordingly, IgA deficiency is much less common in people of Sub-Saharan African and East Asian origin. In Japan, for example, the incidence is approximately 1 in 18,500. Function-loss mutations in a variety of non-MHC genes have been defined in families with IgA-deficient/CVID members. These include the genes for ICOS, an immune co-stimulator molecule used by T cells to activate B cells in germinal centers, BAFFR and TACI, the receptors for B cell–activating factor (BAFF), and CD19, the B cell co-stimulatory receptor.

Individuals with isolated IgA deficiency may appear healthy or present with an increased number of acute and chronic respiratory infections that may lead to bronchiectasis. Chronic diarrheal diseases also occur. Associated reductions in the IgG2 and IgG4 subclasses are associated with the increased infections in some IgA-deficient individuals. The incidence of asthma and other atopic diseases among IgA-deficient patients is high. Conversely, the incidence of IgA deficiency among atopic children has been found to be more than 20 times that in the normal population. IgA deficiency can also be associated with arthritis (Chap. 314) and systemic lupus erythematosus (Chap. 313). IgA-deficient patients frequently produce autoantibodies. They may produce antibodies to IgA that make them vulnerable to severe anaphylactic reactions when transfused with normal blood or blood products containing IgA.

The clinical consequences of IgA deficiency are best appreciated by lifelong study of affected individuals. Among 204 healthy young adults whose IgA deficiency was identified when they served as blood donors,

80% experienced episodes of infections, drug allergy, autoimmune disorders, or atopic disease during the next 20 years of their life. They had an increased susceptibility to pneumonia, recurrent episodes of respiratory infections, and a higher incidence of autoimmune diseases, including vitiligo, autoimmune thyroiditis, and rheumatoid arthritis.

Although IgA deficiency is often familial, it can also occur in association with congenital intrauterine infections, such as toxoplasmosis, rubella, and cytomegalovirus infection. It may follow treatment with phenytoin, penicillamine, or other medications in genetically susceptible individuals.

Treatment of IgA deficiency is essentially symptomatic. IgA cannot be effectively replaced by exogenous immunoglobulin or plasma, and use of either can increase the risk of development of antibodies to IgA. However, immunoglobulin infusions may benefit IgA-deficient individuals in whom IgG2 and IgG4 subclass deficiencies are associated with severe infections. IgA-deficient patients in need of transfusion should be screened for the presence of antibodies to IgA and ideally should be given blood only from IgA-deficient donors.

Common Variable Immunodeficiency This diagnostic category includes a heterogeneous group, mostly adults, who have in common the clinical manifestations of deficient production of all the different classes of antibodies. These hypogammaglobulinemic patients usually have normal numbers of B lymphocytes that are clonally diverse but phenotypically immature. B lymphocytes in these patients are able to recognize antigens and respond with proliferation, but they are impaired in their ability to become memory B cells and mature plasma cells. This abortive differentiation pattern leads to the frequent occurrence of nodular B lymphocyte hyperplasia that may result in splenomegaly and intestinal lymphoid hyperplasia of massive proportion.

It is important to consider the diagnosis of common variable immunodeficiency in adults with chronic pulmonary infections, some of whom will present with bronchiectasis. Intestinal diseases—including chronic giardiasis, intestinal malabsorption, and atrophic gastritis with pernicious anemia—are common in this group of patients. Patients with common variable immunodeficiency may also present with signs and symptoms highly suggestive of lymphoid malignancy, including fever, weight loss, anemia, thrombocytopenia, splenomegaly, generalized lymphadenopathy, and lymphocytosis. Histologic examination of lymphoid tissues usually reveals germinal center hyperplasia that may be difficult to distinguish from nodular lymphoma (Chap. 105). Demonstration of a normal κ/λ light chain ratio and other evidence for polyclonality of circulating and tissue B lymphocytes can serve to distinguish these patients from those having a monoclonal B cell malignancy with secondary hypogammaglobulinemia. The administration of intravenous immunoglobulin in adequate doses (see below) is an essential part of the prevention and treatment of all these complications.

IgG Subclass Deficiencies Selective deficiencies in one or more of the four IgG subclasses are seen in some patients with repeated infections. The IgG subclass deficiency may easily go undetected when the total serum IgG level is measured, because IgG2, IgG3, and IgG4 together account for only 30–40% of the IgG antibodies. However, the availability of subclass-specific monoclonal antibodies allows precise measurement of IgG subclass levels.

Homozygous deletions of genes encoding the constant region of the different γ chains are the basis for the IgG subclass deficiency in some individuals. For example, deletion of the $C\alpha1$, $C\gamma2$, $C\gamma4$, and $C\varepsilon$ genes in the heavy chain locus on both chromosomes 14 was responsible for one individual's inability to make IgA1, IgG2, IgG4, and IgE. Because other components of their immune system are intact, individuals with this and other patterns of C_H gene deletions may not have unusual infections.

Most of the IgG subclass–deficient individuals with repeated infections appear to have regulatory defects that prevent normal B cell differentiation. The defect may extend to other isotypes. IgA deficiency may accompany IgG2 and IgG4 subclass deficiencies (see "IgA Deficiency," above); an inability to produce IgM antibodies to polysaccharide antigens often reflects a broader defect in antibody responsiveness. While

patients with IgG subclass deficiency may benefit from administration of immunoglobulin, a thorough assessment of humoral immunity is needed to identify the relatively few who need this therapy.

X-Linked Immunodeficiency with Hyper IgM In this syndrome, IgG and IgA levels typically are very low, while IgM levels may be very high, normal, or even low. The development of B lymphocytes bearing IgM and IgD and the absence of IgG and IgA B lymphocytes indicate a defect in isotype switching. The defective CD40L (CD154) gene in these patients encodes a transiently expressed molecule on activated T cells that is the ligand for the CD40 molecule on dendritic (D) cells and B cells. Gene mutations that preclude normal CD40 ligand expression prevent normal T and B cell cooperation, germinal center formation, V-region diversification by somatic hypermutation, and isotype switching. T cell responses are also compromised in these CD40 ligand–deficient patients because their T cells are deprived of an important activation stimulus as a consequence of the defective T, D, and B cell interactions (Chap. 308). Consequently, these patients experience more severe infections than those occurring with other hypogammaglobulinemic states. In addition to recurrent bacterial infections, pneumonia may be caused by *P. carinii*, cytomegalovirus, *Aspergillus*, *Cryptosporidium*, and other unusual organisms. Enteritis due to cryptosporidial infection may extend into the biliary tract to result in a sclerosing cholangitis and hepatic cirrhosis. Neutropenia is frequent in affected males and increases their vulnerability to infections. Immunodeficiency with hyper-IgM is also seen in patients of both sexes who have function-loss mutations of the CD40 gene or genes coding for components of CD40/CD40L signaling pathways. Impaired signaling through the nuclear factor–kappa B (NF-κB) pathway due to NF-κB essential modulator (NEMO) mutations can cause an X-linked hyper-IgM and anhidrotic ectodermal dysplasia (XHM-ED) syndrome with or without osteopetrosis and lymphedema.

Hyper-IgM syndrome also results from function-loss mutations of the *activation-induced cytidine deaminase (AID)* or *uracil-DNA glycosylase (UNG)* genes. Both AID, which is expressed solely in B cells, and UNG, which removes uracil in DNA resulting from deamination of cytosine, are directly involved in somatic hypermutation of the immunoglobulin variable region and class switch recombination, but they do not contribute to T cell immune function. The IgM antibodies made by patients with AID deficiency are of relatively low affinity due to the defective somatic hypermutation. The immune deficiency in AID- and UNG-deficient patients is similar to that observed in other pure hypogammaglobulinemic states.

Rx IMMUNOGLOBULIN DEFICIENCY SYNDROMES

Replacement therapy with human immunoglobulin is the therapeutic cornerstone for antibody-deficient patients who have recurrent infections and who are deficient in IgG. Maintenance of serum IgG levels above 6.0 g/L will prevent most systemic infections in these patients. These serum levels can usually be achieved by intravenous administration of immunoglobulin, 400–500 mg/kg, at 3- to 4-week intervals. Subcutaneous administration of immunoglobulin is a viable alternative means of therapy, especially for patients at risk for adverse events during intravenous administration or in situations where access to medical personnel is difficult. In patients with mild to moderate IgG deficiency (3.0–5.0 g/L) or isolated IgG subclass deficiencies, the decision to treat should be based on evaluation of clinical symptoms and antibody responses to antigenic challenge. Since immunoglobulin preparations are composed almost entirely of IgG antibodies, they are of no value for repairing deficiencies of immunoglobulins other than IgG. Infusions of immunoglobulin are also not benign. Previous outbreaks of hepatitis C virus infections in hypogammaglobulinemic patients receiving contaminated immunoglobulin preparations have led to improved safety measures for current commercial preparations. Some antibody-deficient patients develop symptoms of diaphoresis, tachycardia, flank pain, and hypotension during immunoglobulin infusion. This reaction may be resolved by slowing the rate of immunoglobulin infusion. Thrombotic complications, including stroke, myocardial infarction, and pulmonary emboli, have also been reported to be associated with rapid immunoglobulin infusion. Serious anaphylactic reactions may occur as a consequence of antibodies produced by the patient against donor immunoglobulins, particularly IgA (Chap. 107). The potential for severe adverse reactions merits administration of the initial immunoglobulin infusion under medical supervision in a hospital or clinic setting.

A heightened index of suspicion of infection is essential for antibody-deficient patients. Identification of infectious agents in order to select appropriate antibiotic, antiparasitic, or antiviral therapy is also very important. Because immunoglobulin infusions do not suffice to eliminate chronic sinopulmonary infections with *H. influenzae* and other microorganisms, prolonged antibiotic therapy may be required to treat these infections effectively and to prevent progression to pulmonary fibrosis and bronchiectasis. Regular postural drainage with chest percussion can be especially important in management of these patients. Infestation with *G. lamblia*, a common cause of chronic diarrhea in antibody-deficient patients, usually responds to therapy with metronidazole.

Cryptosporidial infections in CD40 ligand–deficient patients may respond to long-term treatment with amphotericin B and flucytosine. The neutropenia frequently associated with infections in these patients may resolve with successful treatment of infections and with antibody replacement therapy. Bone marrow transplantation following myeloablative pretransplantation therapy can be curative for boys with this devastating immunodeficiency. This treatment has a much greater chance of success when performed during childhood.

MISCELLANEOUS IMMUNODEFICIENCY SYNDROMES

Infection with *Candida albicans* is the almost universal accompaniment of severe deficiencies in T cell–mediated immunity. *Chronic mucocutaneous candidiasis* is different because superficial candidiasis is usually the only manifestation of immunodeficiency in this syndrome. These patients rarely develop systemic infection with *Candida* or other fungal agents and are not unusually susceptible to virus or bacterial disease. No uniformity of immunologic defects has been identified in these patients. Humoral immunity, including ability to make specific anti-*Candida* antibodies, is usually normal. Some patients are anergic to a variety of antigens and others only to *Candida*. The syndrome is often congenital and may be associated with single or multiple endocrinopathies as well as iron deficiency. Treatment of associated conditions may lead to improvement or even cure of *Candida* infection. In other patients, intensive treatment with amphotericin B coupled with surgical removal of infected nails has led to sustained improvement. Oral antifungal agents, such as fluconazole and itraconazole, may also be effective.

One well-defined genetic disorder, *autoimmune polyendocrinopathy-candidiasis-ectodermal dystrophy* (APECED), is caused by autoimmune regulator (*AIRE*) gene mutations. The AIRE transcription factor upregulates thymic expression of many extrathymic tissue-specific proteins, such as insulin, for the purpose of inducing T cell tolerance to self-antigens. Patients experiencing all three major symptoms of APECED commonly develop candidiasis, hypoparathyroidism, and Addison's disease in chronologic order during childhood, although only two of these manifestations are required for diagnosis. Less common symptoms, such as insulin-dependent diabetes mellitus, autoimmune thyroid diseases, chronic atrophic gastritis, chronic active hepatitis, vitiligo, and cholelithiasis, may appear as late as the fifth or sixth decades of life.

Interferon γ Receptor Deficiency This immunodeficiency is characterized by serious infections caused by bacille Calmette-Guérin (BCG) vaccine and environmental nontuberculous mycobacteria. Associated salmonella infections occur in a minority of the cases. This syndrome can be caused by mutations in genes for the *interferon γ receptor signal-transducing chain* (IFNGR2) gene or the *ligand binding chain of the interferon γ receptor* (IFNGR1) gene. Null mutations in both *IFNGR1* alleles are responsible for a more severe autosomal recessive form. A less severe form, inherited in an autosomal dominant pattern, is caused by *IFNGR1* mutations in a small deletional hotspot that result in a receptor chain lacking the cytoplasmic tail. Accumulation of the truncated receptor on the surface of macrophages compromises their response to interferon (IFN) γ and the killing of ingested mycobacterium.

Interleukin 12 Receptor Deficiency Mutations in the gene coding the β1 subunit of the IL-12 receptor can also result in disseminated mycobacterial infections attributable to BCG and nontuberculous mycobacteria, and in some cases non-typhi salmonella infections. Although the clinical manifestations are usually less severe than in patients with complete IFNGR1 deficiency, IL-12 receptor deficiency may predispose individuals to clinical tuberculosis as well. The IL-12 receptor–deficient patients suffer from the deficient production of IFN-γ by their otherwise normal NK and T cells, but the therapeutic use of IFN-γ may cure their mycobacterial infection.

Immunodeficiency with Thymoma Hypogammaglobulinemia in association with spindle cell thymoma is usually seen relatively late in adult life. Bacterial infections and severe diarrhea often reflect the antibody deficiency, whereas fungal and viral infections are infrequent complications. T cell numbers and cell-mediated immunity are usually normal, but these patients are very deficient in circulating B lymphocytes and pre-B cells in the bone marrow. They frequently have eosinopenia and may also develop erythroid aplasia. Complete bone marrow failure is less common. The relationship between the benign spindle cell thymoma and abnormalities of variable hematopoietic cell lineages remains conjectural, and treatment is limited to immunoglobulin administration and symptomatic therapy.

Wiskott-Aldrich Syndrome This X-linked disease characterized by eczema, thrombocytopenia, and repeated infections is caused by mutations in the *WASP* gene. The WASP protein is expressed in cells of all hematopoietic lineages, although it serves a cytoskeletal organizing role for signaling elements that are particularly important in platelets and T cells. WASP deficient platelets are small and have a shortened half-life. Affected male infants often present with bleeding, and most do not survive childhood, dying of complications of bleeding, infection, or lymphoreticular malignancy. The immunologic defects include low serum concentrations of IgM, while IgA and IgG are normal and IgE is frequently increased. Although the number and class distribution of B lymphocytes are usually normal, these patients fail to make antibodies to polysaccharide antigens normally, and responses to protein antigens may be impaired late in the course of the disease. Most patients eventually acquire severe T cell deficiency, rendering them vulnerable to overwhelming infections with herpes simplex virus and other infectious agents.

Transplantation of histocompatible bone marrow from a sibling donor following myeloablative therapy can correct both the hematologic and immunologic abnormalities. In patients lacking a suitable donor, intravenous immunoglobulin infusions or splenectomy may improve platelet counts and reduce the risk of serious hemorrhage. Because of the increased risk of pneumococcal bacteremia, splenectomized patients should receive prophylactic penicillin.

X-Linked Lymphoproliferative Syndrome This disease involves a selective impairment in immune elimination of Epstein-Barr virus (EBV). A fulminant and fatal outcome is the consequence of EBV infection in approximately half of the affected males. Hypogammaglobulinemia is the outcome in 30%, and B cell malignancies are acquired in approximately 25% of EBV-infected patients. The disease may be manifested from early childhood onward, depending on the time of EBV infection. Carrier females handle EBV infections normally. Cytotoxic T cells and NK cells are primarily responsible for control of EBV infection in normal persons. In males with the X-linked lymphoproliferative syndrome, this process is impaired as a consequence of mutations in a gene coding a T cell and NK cell signaling element called SH2D1A or SAP. Intravenous immunoglobulins should be administered to affected males who develop hypogammaglobulinemia. Bone marrow transplantation from an HLA-matched donor may be curative, especially in younger children with this syndrome. Myeloablative chemotherapy is a necessary prerequisite to successful bone marrow transplantation, thereby increasing the risk of this procedure.

Hyper-IgE Syndrome The hyper IgE syndrome (Chap. 61) is characterized by recurrent abscesses involving skin, lungs, and other organs and very high IgE levels. IgE levels may decline with time to reach normal levels in approximately 20% of affected adults. Staphylococcal infection is common to all patients, but most have infections with other pyogenic organisms as well. Abnormal neutrophil chemotaxis is an inconsistent finding, and diminished antibody responses to secondary immunization have been noted. Nonimmunologic features include impaired shedding of the primary teeth, recurrent bone fractures, hyperextensible joints, and scoliosis. Males and females are affected in an inheritance pattern suggesting an autosomal dominant defect with variable penetrance, but the gene defect has not been identified. Prophylaxis with penicillinase-resistant penicillins or cephalosporins is highly recommended to prevent staphylococcal infections. Pneumatoceles, a frequent complication of pneumonias, may require surgical excision.

METABOLIC ABNORMALITIES ASSOCIATED WITH IMMUNODEFICIENCY

The relation of deficiencies of the purine salvage enzymes adenosine deaminase and purine nucleoside phosphorylase to immunodeficiency was discussed earlier. The syndrome of *acrodermatitis enteropathica* includes severe desquamating skin lesions, intractable diarrhea, bizarre neurologic symptoms, variable combined immunodeficiency, and an often fatal outcome. This disease is apparently caused by an inborn error of metabolism resulting in malabsorption of dietary zinc and can be treated effectively by parenteral or large oral doses of zinc. Zinc deficiency might in part account for the immunodeficiency that accompanies severe malnutrition. Inherited deficiency of transcobalamin II, the serum carrier molecule responsible for transport of vitamin B_{12} to tissues, is associated with failure of immunoglobulin production as well as megaloblastic anemia, leukopenia, thrombocytopenia, and severe malabsorption. All abnormalities of this rare disorder are reversed by administration of vitamin B_{12}. Finally, primary immunodeficiencies are associated with or are secondary to a number of diverse diseases (**Chap. e26**).

CONCLUSION

Defective genes have been identified for most of the primary immunodeficiency diseases that are currently recognized (**Chap. e26**). It can be anticipated that different gene mutations will be identified in other individuals with increased susceptibility to infection. Identification of the mutant genes is the first step toward a better understanding of the pathogenesis of immunodeficiency disease and improved therapeutic strategies. The ultimate goal for these individuals is successful gene repair.

FURTHER READINGS

BONILLA FA, GEHA RS: Update on primary immunodeficiency diseases. J Allergy Clin Immunol 117:S435, 2006

BUCKLEY RH: Molecular defects in human severe combined immunodeficiency and approaches to immune reconstitution. Ann Rev Immunol 22:625, 2004

CHINEN J, PUCK JM: Successes and risks of gene therapy in primary immunodeficiencies. J Allergy Clin Immunol 113:595, 2004

OCHS HD et al (eds): *Primary Immunodeficiency Diseases: A Molecular and Cellular Approach*, 2d ed. New York, Oxford University Press, 2006

ORANGE JS: Use of intravenous immunoglobulin in human disease: A review of evidence by members of the Primary Immunodeficiency Committee of the American Academy of Allergy, Asthma, and Immunology. J Allergy Clin Immunol 117:S525, 2006

SALZER U, GRIMBACHER B: TACItly changing tunes: Farewell to a yin and yang of BAFF receptor and TACI in humoral immunity? New genetic defects in common variable immunodeficiency. Curr Opin Allergy Clin Immunol 5:496, 2005

SHEARER WT, FISCHER A: The last 80 years in primary immunodeficiency: How far have we come, how far need we go? J Allergy Clin Immunol 117:748, 2006

SECTION 2 ▸ DISORDERS OF IMMUNE-MEDIATED INJURY

---

311 Allergies, Anaphylaxis, and Systemic Mastocytosis
K. Frank Austen

The term *atopic allergy* implies a familial tendency to manifest such conditions as asthma, rhinitis, urticaria, and eczematous dermatitis (atopic dermatitis) alone or in combination. However, individuals without an atopic background may also develop hypersensitivity reactions, particularly urticaria and anaphylaxis, associated with the same class of antibody, IgE, found in atopic individuals. Inasmuch as the mast cell is the key effector cell of the biologic response in allergic rhinitis, urticaria, anaphylaxis, and systemic mastocytosis, the introduction to these clinical problems will consider the developmental biology, activation pathway, product profile, and target tissues for this cell type.

The binding of IgE to human mast cells and basophils, a process termed *sensitization*, prepares these cells for subsequent antigen-specific activation. The sensitization of the high-affinity Fc receptor for IgE, designated FcεRI, also stabilizes the cellular expression of the receptor. FcεRI is composed of one α, one β, and two disulfide-linked γ chains, which together cross the plasma membrane seven times. The α chain is responsible for IgE binding, and the β and γ chains provide for signal transduction that follows the aggregation of the sensitized tetrameric receptors by polymeric antigen. Signal transduction is initiated through the action of an Src family–related tyrosine kinase, termed *Lyn*, that is constitutively associated with the β chain. Lyn transphosphorylates the canonical immunoreceptor tyrosine-based activation motifs (ITAMs) of the β and γ chains of the receptor, resulting in recruitment of more active Lyn to the β chain and of Syk tyrosine kinase. The phosphorylated tyrosines in the ITAMs function as binding sites for the tandem *src* homology two (SH2) domains within Syk. Syk activates not only phospholipase Cγ, which associates with the Linker of Activated T Cells at the plasma membrane, but also phosphatidylinositol 3-kinase to provide phosphatidylinositol-3,4,5-trisphosphate, which allows membrane targeting of the Tec family kinase Btk and its activation by Lyn. In addition, the Src family tyrosine kinase Fyn becomes activated after aggregation of IgE receptors and phosphorylates the adapter protein Gab2 that enhances activation of phosphatidylinositol 3-kinase. Indeed, this additional input is essential for mast cell activation, but it can be partially inhibited by Lyn, indicating that the extent of mast cell activation is in part regulated by the interplay between these src family kinases. Activated phospholipase Cγ cleaves phospholipid membrane substrates to provide inositol-1,4,5-trisphosphate (IP_3) and 1,2-diacylglycerols (1,2-DAGs) so as to mobilize intracellular calcium and activate protein kinase C, respectively. The subsequent opening of calcium-regulated activated channels provides the sustained elevations of intracellular calcium required to recruit the mitogen-activated protein kinases, ERK, JNK, and p38 (serine/threonine kinases), which provide cascades to augment arachidonic acid release and to mediate nuclear translocation of transcription factors for various cytokines. The calcium ion–dependent activation of phospholipases cleaves membrane phospholipids to generate lysophospholipids, which, like 1,2-DAG, may facilitate the fusion of the secretory granule perigranular membrane with the cell membrane, a step that releases the membrane-free granules containing the preformed mediators of mast cell effects.

The secretory granule of the human mast cell has a crystalline structure, unlike mast cells of lower species. IgE-dependent cell activation results in solubilization and swelling of the granule contents within the first minute of receptor perturbation; this reaction is followed by the ordering of intermediate filaments about the swollen granule, movement of the granule toward the cell surface, and fusion of the perigranular membrane with that of other granules and with the plasmalemma to form extracellular channels for mediator release while maintaining cell viability.

In addition to exocytosis, aggregation of FcεRI initiates two other pathways for generation of bioactive products, namely, lipid mediators and cytokines. The biochemical steps involved in expression of such cytokines as tumor necrosis factor α (TNF-α), interleukin (IL) 1, IL-6, IL-4, IL-5, IL-13, granulocyte-macrophage colony-stimulating factor (GM-CSF), and others including an array of chemokines, have not been specifically defined for mast cells. Inhibition studies of cytokine production (IL-1β, TNF-α, and IL-6) in mouse mast cells with cyclosporine or FK506 reveal binding to the ligand-specific immunophilin and attenuation of the calcium ion– and calmodulin-dependent serine/threonine phosphatase, calcineurin.

Lipid mediator generation (Fig. 311-1) involves translocation of calcium ion–dependent cytosolic phospholipase A_2 to the outer nuclear membrane, with subsequent release of arachidonic acid for metabolic processing by the distinct prostanoid and leukotriene pathways. The constitutive prostaglandin endoperoxide synthase-1 (PGHS-1/cyclooxygenase-1) and the de novo inducible PGHS-2 (cyclooxygenase-2) convert released arachidonic acid to the sequential intermediates, prostaglandins G_2 and H_2. The glutathione-dependent hematopoietic prostaglandin D_2 (PGD$_2$) synthase then converts PGH$_2$ to PGD$_2$, the predominant mast cell prostanoid. The PGD$_2$ receptors, DP$_1$ and DP$_2$, are distributed to smooth muscle as well as to T$_H$2 lymphocytes, eosinophils, and basophils implicated in allergic inflammation.

For the leukotriene biosynthetic pathway, the released arachidonic acid is metabolized by 5-lipoxygenase (5-LO) in the presence of an integral nuclear membrane protein, the 5-LO activating protein (FLAP). The calcium ion–dependent translocation of 5-LO to the nuclear membrane converts the arachidonic acid to the sequential intermediates, 5-hydroperoxyeicosatetraenoic acid and leukotriene (LT) A$_4$. LTA$_4$ is conjugated with reduced glutathione by LTC$_4$ synthase, an integral nuclear membrane protein homologous to FLAP. Intracellular LTC$_4$ is released by a carrier-specific export step for extracellular conversion to LTD$_4$ and LTE$_4$ by sequential removal of glutamic acid and glycine. Alternatively, cytosolic LTA$_4$ hydrolase converts some LTA$_4$ to the dihydroxy leukotriene LTB$_4$, which also undergoes specific export. Two receptors for LTB$_4$, BLT$_1$ and BLT$_2$, mediate chemotaxis of human neutrophils. Two receptors for the cysteinyl leukotrienes, CysLT$_1$ and CysLT$_2$, are present on smooth muscle of the airways and the microvasculature and on hematopoietic cells such as macrophages, eosinophils, and mast cells. Whereas CysLT$_1$ has a preference for LTD$_4$ and is blocked by the receptor antagonists in clinical use, CysLT$_2$ is equally responsive to LTC$_4$ and is unaffected by these antagonists. The lysophospholipid formed during release of arachidonic acid from 1-O-alkyl-2-acyl-sn-glyceryl-3-phosphorylcholine can be acetylated in the second position to form platelet-activating factor (PAF).

Unlike most other cells of bone marrow origin, mast cells leave the marrow and circulate as committed progenitors lacking their definitive secretory granules and characteristic FcεRI. These committed progeni-

FIGURE 311-1 Pathways for biosynthesis and release of membrane-derived lipid mediators from mast cells. In the 5-lipoxygenase pathway leukotriene A$_4$ (LTA$_4$) is the intermediate from which the terminal-pathway enzymes generate the distinct final products, leukotriene C$_4$ (LTC$_4$) and leukotriene B$_4$ (LTB$_4$), which leave the cell by separate saturable transport systems. Gamma glutamyl transpeptidase and a dipeptidase then cleave glutamic acid and glycine from LTC$_4$ to form LTD$_4$ and LTE$_4$, respectively. The major mast cell product of the cyclooxygenase system is PGD$_2$.

tors express the receptor, c-*kit*, for stem cell factor (SCF), and unlike other lineages, they retain and increase its expression with maturation. The SCF interaction with c-*kit* is an absolute requirement for the development of constitutive tissue mast cells residing in skin and connective tissue sites and for the T$_H$2 cell–dependent comitogenesis providing mast cells to mucosal surfaces. Indeed, in clinical T cell deficiencies, mast cells are absent from the intestinal mucosa but are present in the submucosa. Based on the immunodetection of secretory granule neutral proteases, mast cells in the lung parenchyma and intestinal mucosa selectively express tryptase, and those in the intestinal and airway submucosa, skin, lymph nodes, and breast parenchyma express tryptase, chymase, and carboxypeptidase A (CPA). The secretory granules of mast cells selectively positive for tryptase exhibit closed scrolls with a periodicity suggestive of a crystalline structure by electron microscopy; whereas the secretory granules of mast cells with multiple proteases are scroll-poor, with an amorphous or lattice-like appearance.

Mast cells are distributed at cutaneous and mucosal surfaces and in submucosal tissues about venules and could influence the entry of foreign substances by their rapid response capability (Fig. 311-2). Upon stimulus-specific activation and secretory granule exocytosis, histamine and acid hydrolases are solubilized, whereas the neutral proteases, which are cationic, remain largely complexed to the anionic proteoglycans, heparin and chrondroitin sulfate E, so as to function in concert. Histamine and the various lipid mediators (PGD$_2$, LTC$_4$/D$_4$/E$_4$, PAF) alter venular permeability, thereby allowing influx of plasma proteins such as complement and immunoglobulins, whereas LTB$_4$ mediates leukocyte–endothelial cell adhesion and subsequent directed migration (chemotaxis). The accumulation of leukocytes and plasma opsonins would facilitate defense of the microenvironment. The inflammatory response can also be detrimental, as in bronchial asthma, where the smooth-muscle constrictor activity of the cysteinyl leukotrienes is evident and much more potent than that of histamine.

The cellular component of the mast cell–mediated inflammatory response would be augmented and sustained by cytokines and chemo-

Lipid mediators
- LTB$_4$
- LTC$_4$
- PAF
- PGD$_2$

Secretory granule preformed mediators
- Histamine
- Proteoglycans
- Tryptase and chymase
- Carboxypeptidase A

Cytokines
- IL-3
- IL-4
- IL-5
- IL-6
- GM-CSF
- IL-13
- IL-1
- INF–γ
- TNF–α
- Chemokines

Activated mast cell

Leukocyte responses
- Adherence
- Chemotaxis
- IgE production
- Mast cell proliferation
- Eosinophil activation

Fibroblast responses
- Proliferation
- Vacuolation
- Globopentaosylceramide production
- Collagen production

Substrate responses
- Activation of matrix metalloproteases
- Activation of coagulation cascade

Microvascular responses
- Augmented venular permeability
- Leukocyte adherence
- Constriction
- Dilatation

FIGURE 311-2 Bioactive mediators of three categories generated by IgE-dependent activation of murine mast cells can elicit common but sequential target cell effects leading to acute and sustained inflammatory responses. LT, leukotriene; PAF, platelet-activating factor; PGD$_2$, prostaglandin D$_2$; IL, interleukin; GM-CSF, granulocyte-macrophage colony-stimulating factor; INF, interferon; TNF, tumor necrosis factor.

kines of mast cell origin. IgE-dependent activation of human skin mast cells in situ elicits TNF-α production and release, which in turn induces endothelial cell responses favoring leukocyte adhesion. Similarly, activation of purified human lung mast cells or cord blood–derived cultured mast cells in vitro results in substantial production of proinflammatory (TNF-α) and immunomodulatory cytokines (IL-4, IL-5, IL-13) and chemokines. Bronchial biopsies of patients with bronchial asthma reveal that mast cells are immunohistochemically positive for IL-4 and IL-5, but that the predominant localization of IL-4, IL-5, and GM-CSF is to T cells, defined as T$_H$2 by this profile. IL-4 modulates the T cell phenotype to the T$_H$2 subtype, determines the isotype switch to IgE (as does IL-13), and upregulates FcεRI-mediated expression of cytokines by mast cells.

An immediate and late cellular phase of allergic inflammation can be induced in the skin, nose, or lung of some allergic humans with local allergen challenge. In the immediate phase of a local challenge, there is pruritus and watery discharge from the nose, bronchospasm and mucus secretion in the lungs, and a wheal-and-flare response with pruritus in the skin. The reduced nasal patency, reduced pulmonary function, or evident erythema with swelling at the skin site in a late-phase response at 6 to 8 h is associated with biopsy findings of infiltrating and activated T$_H$2 cells, eosinophils, basophils, and even some neutrophils. This allergic inflammation proceeding from early mast cell activation to late cellular infiltration has been used as an experimental surrogate of perennial rhinitis or bronchial asthma. However, in bronchial asthma there is a separate variable, intrinsic hyperreactivity of the airways.

Consideration of the mechanism of immediate-type hypersensitivity diseases in the human has focused largely on the IgE-dependent recognition of otherwise nontoxic substances. A region of chromosome 5 (5q23-31) contains genes implicated in the control of IgE levels including IL-4 and IL-13, as well as IL-3 and IL-9 involved in reactive mast cell hyperplasia and IL-5 and GM-CSF central to eosinophil development and their enhanced tissue viability. Genes with linkage to the specific IgE response to particular allergens include those encoding the major histocompatibility complex (MHC) and certain chains of the T cell receptor (TCR-αδ). The complexity of atopy and the associated diseases includes susceptibility, severity, and therapeutic responses, each of which is among the separate variables modulated by both innate and adaptive immune stimuli.

The induction of allergic disease requires sensitization of a predisposed individual to a specific allergen. The greatest propensity for the development of atopic allergy occurs in childhood and early adoles-

cence. The allergen is processed by antigen-presenting cells of the monocytic lineage located throughout the body at surfaces that contact the outside environment, such as the nose, lungs, eyes, skin, and intestine. These antigen-presenting cells present the epitope-bearing peptides via their MHC to particular T helper cell subsets. The T cell response depends both on cognate recognition through various ligand/receptor interactions and on the cytokine microenvironment, with IL-4 directing a T$_H$2 response and interferon (IFN)γ a T$_H$1 profile. The T$_H$2 response is associated with activation of specific B cells that can also present allergens or that transform into plasma cells for antibody production. Synthesis and release into the plasma of allergen-specific IgE results in sensitization of FcεR1-bearing cells such as mast cells and basophils, which become activated upon exposure to the specific allergen. In certain diseases, including those associated with atopy, the monocyte and eosinophil populations can express a trimeric FcεR1 which lacks the β chain, and yet respond to its aggregation.

ANAPHYLAXIS

DEFINITION

The life-threatening anaphylactic response of a sensitized human appears within minutes after administration of specific antigen and is manifested by respiratory distress, laryngeal edema, and/or intense bronchospasm, often followed by vascular collapse or by shock without antecedent respiratory difficulty. Cutaneous manifestations exemplified by pruritus and urticaria with or without angioedema are characteristic of such systemic anaphylactic reactions. Gastrointestinal manifestations include nausea, vomiting, crampy abdominal pain, and diarrhea.

PREDISPOSING FACTORS AND ETIOLOGY

There is no convincing evidence that age, sex, race, or geographic location predisposes a human to anaphylaxis except through exposure to some immunogen. According to most studies, atopy does not predispose individuals to anaphylaxis from penicillin therapy or venom of a stinging insect but is a risk factor for allergens in food or latex.

The materials capable of eliciting the systemic anaphylactic reaction in humans include the following: heterologous proteins in the form of hormones (insulin, vasopressin, parathormone); enzymes (trypsin, chymotrypsin, penicillinase, streptokinase); pollen extracts (ragweed, grass, trees); nonpollen extracts (dust mites, dander of cats, dogs, horses, and laboratory animals); food (peanuts, milk, eggs, seafood, nuts, grains, beans, gelatin in capsules); monoclonal antibodies; occupation-related products (latex rubber products); and Hymenoptera venom (yellow jacket, yellow and baldfaced hornets, paper wasp, honey bee, imported fire ants); polysaccharides such as dextran and thiomersal as a vaccine preservative; drugs such as protamine; antibiotics (penicillins, cephalosporins, amphotericin B, nitrofurantoin, quinolones); chemotherapy agents (carboplatin, paclitaxel, doxorubicin); local anesthetics (procaine, lidocaine); muscle relaxants (suxamethonium, gallamine, pancuronium); vitamins (thiamine, folic acid); diagnostic agents (sodium dehydrocholate, sulfobromophthalein); and occupation-related chemicals (ethylene oxide), which are considered to function as haptens that form immunogenic conjugates with host proteins. The conjugating hapten may be the parent compound, a nonenzymatically derived storage product, or a metabolite formed in the host.

PATHOPHYSIOLOGY AND MANIFESTATIONS

Individuals differ in the time of appearance of symptoms and signs, but the hallmark of the anaphylactic reaction is the onset of some manifestation within seconds to minutes after introduction of the antigen, generally by injection or less commonly by ingestion. There may be upper or lower airway obstruction or both. Laryngeal edema may be experienced as a "lump" in the throat, hoarseness, or stridor, while bronchial obstruction is associated with a feeling of tightness in the chest and/or audible wheezing. Patients with bronchial asthma are predisposed to severe involvement of the lower airways. Flushing with diffuse erythema and a feeling of warmth may occur. A characteristic feature is the eruption of well-circumscribed, discrete cutaneous wheals with erythematous, raised, serpiginous borders and blanched centers. These urticarial eruptions are intensely pruritic and may be localized or disseminated. They may coalesce to form giant hives, and they seldom persist beyond 48 h. A localized, nonpitting, deeper edematous cutaneous process, angioedema, may also be present. It may be asymptomatic or cause a burning or stinging sensation.

In fatal cases with clinical bronchial obstruction, the lungs show marked hyperinflation on gross and microscopic examination. The microscopic findings in the bronchi, however, are limited to luminal secretions, peribronchial congestion, submucosal edema, and eosinophilic infiltration, and the acute emphysema is attributed to intractable bronchospasm that subsides with death. The angioedema resulting in death by mechanical obstruction occurs in the epiglottis and larynx, but the process is also evident in the hypopharynx and to some extent in the trachea; on microscopic examination there is wide separation of the collagen fibers and the glandular elements; vascular congestion and eosinophilic infiltration are also present. Patients dying of vascular collapse without antecedent hypoxia from respiratory insufficiency have visceral congestion with a presumptive loss of intravascular blood volume. The associated electrocardiographic abnormalities, with or without infarction, noted in some patients may reflect a primary cardiac event mediated by mast cells or be secondary to a critical reduction in blood volume.

The angioedematous and urticarial manifestations of the anaphylactic syndrome have been attributed to release of endogenous histamine. A role for the cysteinyl leukotrienes in causing marked bronchiolar constriction seems likely. Vascular collapse without respiratory distress in response to experimental challenge with the sting of a hymenopteran was associated with marked and prolonged elevations in blood histamine and intravascular coagulation and kinin generation. The finding that patients with systemic mastocytosis and episodic vascular collapse excrete large amounts of PGD_2 metabolites in addition to histamine suggests that PGD_2 is also of importance in the hypotensive anaphylactic reactions. The actions of the array of mast cell–derived mediators are likely additive or synergistic at the target tissues.

DIAGNOSIS

The diagnosis of an anaphylactic reaction depends on a history revealing the onset of the symptoms and signs within minutes after the responsible material is encountered. It is appropriate to rule out a complement-mediated immune complex reaction, an idiosyncratic response to a nonsteroidal anti-inflammatory drug (NSAID), or the direct effect of certain drugs or diagnostic agents on mast cells. Intravenous administration of a chemical mast cell–degranulating agent, including opiate derivatives and radiographic contrast media, may elicit generalized urticaria, angioedema, and a sensation of retrosternal oppression with or without clinically detectable bronchoconstriction or hypotension. Aspirin and other NSAIDs such as indomethacin, aminopyrine, and mefenamic acid may precipitate a life-threatening episode of obstruction of upper or lower airways, especially in patients with asthma, that is clinically indistinguishable from anaphylaxis but is not associated with the presence of specific IgE or elevation of blood tryptase. This syndrome, which is commonly associated with nasal polyposis, is due to inhibition of PGHS-1 with corresponding unregulated, amplified generation of the cysteinyl leukotrienes via the 5-LO/LTC$_4$ synthase pathway. In the transfusion anaphylactic reaction that occurs in patients with IgA deficiency, the responsible specificity resides in IgG or IgE anti-IgA; the mechanism of the reaction mediated by IgG anti-IgA is presumed to be complement activation with secondary mast cell participation.

The presence of specific IgE in the blood of patients with systemic anaphylaxis has been demonstrated by passive transfer of the serum intradermally into a normal recipient, followed in 24 h by antigen challenge into the same site, with subsequent development of a wheal and flare, the *Prausnitz-Küstner reaction*. To avoid the hazards of transferring hepatitis or other infections, it is preferable to use the serum to seek passive sensitization of a human leukocyte suspension enriched with basophils for subsequent antigen-induced histamine release. Furthermore, radioimmunoassays using purified antigens can demonstrate specific IgE in serum of patients with anaphylactic reactions. Elevations of tryptase levels in serum implicate mast cell activation in an adverse systemic reaction and are particularly informative with episodes of hypotension during general anesthesia or when there has been a fatal outcome.

℞ ANAPHYLAXIS

Early recognition of an anaphylactic reaction is mandatory, since death occurs within minutes to hours after the first symptoms. Mild symptoms such as pruritus and urticaria can be controlled by administration of 0.3 to 0.5 mL of 1:1000 (1.0 mg/mL) epinephrine SC or IM, with repeated doses as required at 5- to 20-min intervals for a severe reaction. If the antigenic material was injected into an extremity, the rate of absorption may be reduced by prompt application of a tourniquet proximal to the reaction site, administration of 0.2 mL of 1:1000 epinephrine into the site, and removal without compression of an insect stinger, if present. An IV infusion should be initiated to provide a route for administration of 2.5 mL epinephrine, diluted 1:10,000, at 5- to 10-min intervals, volume expanders such as normal saline, and vasopressor agents such as dopamine if intractable hypotension occurs. Replacement of intravascular volume due to postcapillary venular leakage may require several liters of saline. Epinephrine provides both α- and β-adrenergic effects, resulting in vasoconstriction, bronchial smooth-muscle relaxation, and attenuation of enhanced venular permeability. When epinephrine fails to control the anaphylactic reaction, hypoxia due to airway obstruction or related to a cardiac arrhythmia, or both, must be considered. Oxygen alone via a nasal catheter or with nebulized albuterol may be helpful, but either endotracheal intubation or a tracheostomy is mandatory for oxygen delivery if progressive hypoxia develops. Ancillary agents such as the antihistamine diphenhydramine, 50 to 100 mg IM or IV, and aminophylline, 0.25 to 0.5 g IV, are appropriate for urticaria-angioedema and bronchospasm, respectively. Intravenous glucocorticoids, 0.5–1.0 mg/kg of medrol, are not effective for the acute event but may alleviate later recurrence of bronchospasm, hypotension, or urticaria.

PREVENTION

Prevention of anaphylaxis must take into account the sensitivity of the recipient, the dose and character of the diagnostic or therapeutic agent, and the effect of the route of administration on the rate of absorption. Beta blockers are relatively contraindicated in persons at risk for anaphylactic reactions, especially those sensitive to Hymenoptera venom or those undergoing immunotherapy for respiratory system allergy. If there is a definite history of a past anaphylactic reaction, even though mild, it is advisable to select a structurally unrelated agent. A knowledge of cross-reactivity among agents is critical since, for example, cephalosporins have a cross-reactive ring structure with the penicillins. A prick or scratch skin test should precede an intradermal skin test, since the latter has a higher risk of causing anaphylaxis. These tests should be performed before the administration of certain materials that are likely to elicit anaphylactic reactions, such as allergenic extracts. Skin testing for antibiotics or chemotherapeutic agents should be performed only on patients with a positive clinical history consistent with an IgE-mediated reaction and in imminent need of the antibiotic in question; skin testing is of no value for non-IgE-mediated eruptions. With regard to penicillin, two-thirds of patients with a positive reaction history and positive skin tests to benzylpenicilloyl-polylysine (BPL) and/or the minor determinant mixture (MDM) of benzylpenicillin products experience allergic reactions with treatment, and these are almost uniformly of the anaphylactic type in those patients with minor determinant reactivity. Even patients without a history of previous clinical reactions have a 2–6% incidence of positive skin tests to the two test materials, and about 3 per 1000 with a negative history experience anaphylaxis with therapy, with a mortality of about 1 per 100,000.

Desensitization with most antibiotics and other classes of therapeutic agents can proceed by the IV, SC, or oral route. Typically, graded quantities of the drug are given by the selected route using double doses until a therapeutic dosage is achieved. Due to the risk of systemic anaphylaxis during the course of desensitization, such a procedure should be performed only in a setting in which resuscitation equipment is at hand and an IV line is in place. It is critical to give the therapeutic agent at regular intervals throughout the treatment period to prevent the reestablishment of a significant pool of sensitized cells.

A different form of protection involves the development of blocking antibody of the IgG class, which is protective against Hymenoptera venom–induced anaphylaxis by interacting with antigen so that less reaches the sensitized tissue mast cells. The maximal risk for systemic anaphylactic reactions in persons with Hymenoptera sensitivity occurs in association with a currently positive skin test. Although there is only low-grade cross-reactivity between honey bee and yellow jacket venoms, there is a high degree of cross-reactivity between yellow jacket venom and the rest of the vespid venoms (yellow or baldfaced hornets and wasps). Prevention involves modification of outdoor activities to exclude bare feet, wearing perfumed toiletries, eating in areas attractive to insects, clipping hedges or grass, and hauling away trash or fallen fruit. As with each anaphylactic sensitivity, the individual should wear an informational bracelet and have immediate access to an unexpired auto-injectable epinephrine kit. The limitations of lifestyle and the psychological duress can be addressed by venom immunotherapy. Although it has been recommended that venom therapy be continued indefinitely or until the skin and specific serum IgE tests are unremarkable, there is evidence that 5 years of treatment induces a state of resistance to sting reactions that is independent of serum levels of specific IgG or IgE. For children with a systemic reaction limited to skin, the likelihood of progression to more serious respiratory or vascular manifestations is low, and thus immunotherapy is not recommended.

URTICARIA AND ANGIOEDEMA

DEFINITION

Urticaria and angioedema may appear separately or together as cutaneous manifestations of localized nonpitting edema; a similar process may occur at mucosal surfaces of the upper respiratory or gastrointestinal tract. *Urticaria* involves only the superficial portion of the dermis, presenting as well-circumscribed wheals with erythematous raised serpiginous borders with blanched centers that may coalesce to become giant wheals. *Angioedema* is a well-demarcated localized edema involving the deeper layers of the skin, including the subcutaneous tissue. Recurrent episodes of urticaria and/or angioedema of less than 6 weeks' duration are considered acute, whereas attacks persisting beyond this period are designated chronic.

PREDISPOSING FACTORS AND ETIOLOGY

The occurrence of urticaria and angioedema is probably more frequent than usually described because of the evanescent, self-limited nature of such eruptions, which seldom require medical attention when limited to the skin. Although persons in any age group may experience acute or chronic urticaria and/or angioedema, these lesions increase in frequency after adolescence, with the highest incidence occurring in persons in the third decade of life; indeed, one survey of college students indicated that 15–20% had experienced a pruritic wheal reaction.

The classification of urticaria-angioedema presented in Table 311-1 focuses on the different mechanisms for eliciting clinical disease and can be useful for differential diagnosis; nonetheless, most cases of chronic urticaria are idiopathic. Urticaria and/or angioedema occurring during the appropriate season in patients with seasonal respiratory allergy or as a result of exposure to animals or molds is attributed to inhalation or physical contact with pollens, animal dander, and mold spores, respectively. However, urticaria and angioedema secondary to inhalation are relatively uncommon compared to urticaria and angioedema elicited by ingestion of fresh fruits, shellfish, fish, milk products, chocolate, legumes including peanuts, and various drugs that may elicit not only the anaphylactic syndrome with prominent gastrointestinal complaints but also chronic urticaria.

Additional etiologies include physical stimuli such as cold, heat, solar rays, exercise, and mechanical irritation. The physical urticarias can be distinguished by the precipitating event and other aspects of the clinical presentation. *Dermographism*, which occurs in 1–4% of the population, is defined by the appearance of a linear wheal at the site of a brisk stroke with a firm object or by any configuration appropriate to the eliciting event. Dermographism has a prevalence that peaks in the second to third decades. It is not influenced by an atopic diathesis and has a duration generally of <5 years. *Pressure urticaria*, which often accompanies chronic idiopathic urticaria, presents in response to a sustained stimulus such as a shoulder strap or belt, running (feet), or manual labor (hands). *Cholinergic urticaria* is distinctive in that the pruritic wheals are of small size (1–2 mm) and are surrounded by a large area of erythema; attacks are precipitated by fever, a hot bath or shower, or exercise and are presumptively attributed to a rise in core body temperature. *Exercise-related anaphylaxis* can be precipitated by exertion alone or can be dependent on prior food ingestion. The clinical presentation can be limited to flushing, erythema, and pruritic urticaria but may progress to angioedema of the face, oropharynx, larynx, or intestine or to vascular collapse; it is distinguished from cholinergic urticaria by presenting with wheals of conventional size and by not occurring with fever or a hot bath. *Cold urticaria* is local at body areas exposed to low ambient temperature or cold objects (ice cube) but can progress to vascular collapse with immersion in cold water (swimming). *Solar urticaria* is subdivided into six groups by the response to specific portions of the light spectrum. *Vibratory angioedema* may occur after years of occupational exposure or can be idiopathic; it may be accompanied by cholinergic urticaria. Other rare forms of physical allergy, always defined by stimulus-specific elicitation, include *local heat urticaria*, *aquagenic urticaria* from contact with water of any temperature (sometimes associated with polycythemia vera), and *contact urticaria* from direct interaction with some chemical substance.

Angioedema without urticaria due to generation of bradykinin occurs with C1 inhibitor (C1INH) deficiency that may be inborn as an autosomal dominant characteristic or may be acquired through appearance of an autoantibody. The angiotensin-converting enzyme (ACE) inhibitors can provoke a similar clinical presentation in 0.1–0.5% of hypertensive patients due to attenuated degradation of brady-

TABLE 311-1 CLASSIFICATION OF URTICARIA AND/OR ANGIOEDEMA

1. IgE-dependent
   a. Specific antigen sensitivity (pollens, foods, drugs, fungi, molds, Hymenoptera venom, helminths)
   b. Physical: dermographism, cold, solar
   c. Autoimmune
2. Bradykinin-mediated
   a. Hereditary angioedema: C1 inhibitor deficiency: null (type 1) and dysfunctional (type 2)
   b. Acquired angioedema: C1 inhibitor deficiency: anti-idiotype and anti-C1 inhibitor
   c. Angiotensin-converting enzyme inhibitors
3. Complement-mediated
   a. Necrotizing vasculitis
   b. Serum sickness
   c. Reactions to blood products
4. Nonimmunologic
   a. Direct mast cell–releasing agents (opiates, antibiotics, curare, D-tubocurarine, radiocontrast media)
   b. Agents that alter arachidonic acid metabolism (aspirin and nonsteroidal anti-inflammatory agents, azo dyes, and benzoates)
5. Idiopathic

kinin. The urticaria and angioedema associated with classic serum sickness or with hypocomplementemic cutaneous necrotizing angiitis are believed to be immune-complex diseases. The drug reactions to mast cell granule–releasing agents and to NSAIDs may be systemic, resembling anaphylaxis, or limited to cutaneous sites.

PATHOPHYSIOLOGY AND MANIFESTATIONS

Urticarial eruptions are distinctly pruritic, involve any area of the body from the scalp to the soles of the feet, and appear in crops of 12- to 36-h duration, with old lesions fading as new ones appear. Most of the physical urticarias (cold, cholinergic, dermatographism) are an exception with individual lesions lasting less than 2 h. The most common sites for urticaria are the extremities and face, with angioedema often being periorbital and in the lips. Although self-limited in duration, angioedema of the upper respiratory tract may be life-threatening due to laryngeal obstruction, while gastrointestinal involvement may present with abdominal colic, with or without nausea and vomiting, and may precipitate unnecessary surgical intervention. No residual discoloration occurs with either urticaria or angioedema unless there is an underlying process leading to superimposed extravasation of erythrocytes.

The pathology is characterized by edema of the superficial dermis in urticaria and of the subcutaneous tissue and deep dermis in angioedema. Collagen bundles in affected areas are widely separated, and the venules are sometimes dilated. Any perivenular infiltrate consists of lymphocytes, eosinophils, and neutrophils that are present in varying combination and numbers.

Perhaps the best-studied example of IgE- and mast cell–mediated urticaria and angioedema is *cold urticaria*. Cryoglobulins or cold agglutinins may be recognized, but not in the majority of patients. Immersion of an extremity in an ice bath precipitates angioedema of the distal portion with urticaria at the air interface within minutes of the challenge. Histologic studies reveal marked mast cell degranulation with associated edema of the dermis and subcutaneous tissues. The venous effluent of the cold-challenged and angioedematous extremity shows a marked rise in plasma content of histamine, whereas the venous effluent of the contralateral normal extremity contains no increment of this mediator. Elevated levels of histamine have been found in the plasma of venous effluent and in the fluid of suction blisters at experimentally induced lesional sites in patients with dermographism, pressure urticaria, vibratory angioedema, light urticaria, and heat urticaria. By ultrastructural analysis, the pattern of mast cell degranulation in cold urticaria resembles an IgE-mediated response with solubilization of granule contents, fusion of the perigranular and cell membranes, and discharge of granule contents, whereas in a dermographic lesion there is an additional superimposed zonal (piecemeal) degranulation. Elevations of plasma histamine levels with biopsy-proven mast cell degranulation have also been demonstrated with generalized attacks of *cholinergic urticaria* and *exercise-related anaphylaxis* precipitated experimentally in subjects exercising on a treadmill while wearing a wet suit; however, only in cholinergic urticaria is there a concomitant decrease in pulmonary function.

Up to 40% of patients with chronic urticaria have autoantibodies to IgE or more commonly to the α chain of FcεRI. In these patients, autologous serum injected into their own skin can induce a wheal and flare involving mast cell activation. An association with antibodies to microsomal peroxidase and/or thyroglobulin has been observed often with clinically significant Hashimoto's thyroiditis. In vitro studies reveal that these autoantibodies can mediate basophil degranulation with enhancement by serum as a source of the anaphylatoxic fragment, C5a.

Hereditary angioedema is an autosomal dominant disease due to a deficiency of C1INH (type 1) in about 85% of patients and to a dysfunctional protein (type 2) in the remainder. In the acquired form there is excessive consumption of C1INH due either to immune complexes formed between anti-idiotypic antibody and monoclonal IgG presented by B cell lymphomas or to an autoantibody directed to C1INH. C1INH blocks the catalytic function of activated factor XII (Hageman factor) and of kallikrein, as well as the C1r/C1s components of C1. During clinical attacks of angioedema, C1INH-deficient patients have elevated plasma levels of bradykinin, particularly in the venous effluent of an involved extremity, and reduced levels of prekallikrein and high-molecular-weight kininogen, from which bradykinin is cleaved. The parallel decline in the complement substrates C4 and C2 reflects the action of activated C1 during such attacks. Mice with targeted disruption of the gene for C1INH exhibit a chronic increase in vascular permeability. The pathobiology is aggravated by administration of an ACE inhibitor (captopril) and is attenuated by breeding the C1INH null strain to a bradykinin 2 receptor (Bk2R) null strain. As ACE is also described as kininase II, the use of blockers results in impaired bradykinin degradation and explains the angioedema occurring idiosyncratically in hypertensive patients with a normal C1INH.

DIAGNOSIS

The rapid onset and self-limited nature of urticarial and angioedematous eruptions are distinguishing features. Additional characteristics are the occurrence of the urticarial crops in various stages of evolution and the asymmetric distribution of the angioedema. Urticaria and/or angioedema involving IgE-dependent mechanisms are often appreciated by historic considerations implicating specific allergens or physical stimuli, by seasonal incidence, and by exposure to certain environments. Direct reproduction of the lesion with physical stimuli is particularly valuable because it so often establishes the cause of the lesion. The diagnosis of an environmental allergen based on the clinical history can be confirmed by skin testing or assay for allergen-specific IgE in serum. IgE-mediated urticaria and/or angioedema may or may not be associated with an elevation of total IgE or with peripheral eosinophilia. Fever, leukocytosis, and an elevated sedimentation rate are absent.

The classification of urticarial and angioedematous states noted in Table 311-1 in terms of possible mechanisms necessarily includes some differential diagnostic points. Hypocomplementemia is not observed in IgE-mediated mast cell disease and may reflect either an acquired abnormality generally attributed to the formation of immune complexes or a genetic deficiency of C1INH. Chronic recurrent urticaria, generally in females, associated with arthralgias, an elevated sedimentation rate, and normo- or hypocomplementemia suggests an underlying cutaneous necrotizing angiitis. Vasculitic urticaria typically persists longer than 72 h, whereas conventional urticaria often has a duration of <24–48 h. Confirmation depends on a biopsy that reveals cellular infiltration, nuclear debris, and fibrinoid necrosis of the venules. The same pathobiologic process accounts for the urticaria in association with such diseases as systemic lupus erythematosus or viral hepatitis with or without an associated arteritis. Serum sickness per se or a similar clinical entity due to drugs includes not only urticaria but also pyrexia, lymphadenopathy, myalgia, and arthralgia or arthritis. Urticarial reactions to blood products or intravenous administration of immunoglobulin are defined by the event and generally are not progressive unless the recipient is IgA-deficient in the former case or the reagent is aggregated in the latter.

The diagnosis of hereditary angioedema is suggested not only by family history but also by the lack of pruritus and of urticarial lesions, the prominence of recurrent gastrointestinal attacks of colic, and episodes of laryngeal edema. Laboratory diagnosis depends on demonstrating a deficiency of C1INH antigen (type 1) or a nonfunctional protein (type 2) by a catalytic inhibition assay. While levels of C1 are normal, its substrates, C4 and C2, are chronically depleted and fall further during attacks due to the activation of additional C1. The acquired forms of C1INH deficiency have the same clinical manifestations but differ in the lack of a familial element and exhibit a reduction of C1 function and C1q protein as well as C1INH, C4, and C2. Inborn and acquired C1INH deficiency and ACE inhibitor–elicited angioedema are associated with elevated levels of bradykinin.

Urticaria and angioedema can be differentiated from contact sensitivity, a vesicular eruption that progresses to chronic thickening of the skin with continued allergenic exposure. They can also be differentiated from atopic dermatitis, a condition that may present as erythema, edema, papules, vesiculation, and oozing proceeding to a subacute and chronic stage in which vesiculation is less marked or absent and scaling, fissuring, and lichenification predominate in a distribution that characteristically involves the flexor surfaces. In cutaneous mastocytosis, the reddish brown macules and papules, characteristic of urticaria pigmentosa, urticate with pruritus upon trauma; and in systemic mastocytosis, without or with urticaria pigmentosa, there is an episodic systemic flushing with or without urtication but no angioedema.

℞ URTICARIA AND ANGIOEDEMA

Identification of the etiologic factor(s) and its elimination provide the most satisfactory therapeutic program; this approach is feasible to varying degrees with IgE-mediated reactions to allergens or physical stimuli. For most forms of urticaria, H_1 antihistamines such as chlorpheniramine or diphenhydramine, and including the nonsedating class such as loratadine, desloratadine, fexofenadine, or cetirizine, are effective in attenuating both urtication and pruritus. Cyproheptadine in dosages beginning at 8 mg and ranging up to 32 mg daily and especially hydroxyzine in dosages beginning at 40 mg and ranging up to 200 mg daily have proven effective when H_1 antihistamines have been inadequate. Addition of an H_2 antagonist such as cimetidine, ranitidine, or famotidine in conventional dosages may add benefit when H_1 antihistamines are inadequate. Doxepin, a dibenzoxepin tricyclic compound with both H_1 and H_2 receptor antagonist activity, is yet another alternative. A CysLT$_1$ antagonist such as montelukast, 10 mg/d, or zafirlukast, 20 mg twice a day, can be add-on therapy. Topical glucocorticoids are of no value, and systemic glucocorticoids are generally avoided in idiopathic, allergen-induced, or physical urticarias due to their long-term toxicity. Systemic glucocorticoids are useful in the management of patients with pressure urticaria, with vasculitic urticaria (especially with eosinophil prominence), with idiopathic angioedema with or without urticaria, or with chronic urticaria that responds poorly to conventional treatment. With persistent vasculitic urticaria, hydroxychloroquine or colchicine may be added to the regimen after hydroxyzine and before or along with systemic glucocorticoids. Cyclosporine can be efficacious for patients with chronic idiopathic or chronic autoimmune urticaria that is severe and poorly responsive to other modalities and/or where a glucocorticoid requirement is excessive.

The therapy of inborn C1INH deficiency has been simplified by the finding that attenuated androgens correct the biochemical defect and afford prophylactic protection; their efficacy is attributed to production by the normal gene of an amount of functional C1INH sufficient to control the spontaneous activation of C1. The antifibrinolytic agent ε-aminocaproic acid may be used for preoperative prophylaxis but is contraindicated in patients with thrombotic tendencies or ischemia due to arterial atherosclerosis. Infusion of isolated C1INH protein and SC administration of a bradykinin 2 receptor antagonist are each being assessed for amelioration of attacks.

SYSTEMIC MASTOCYTOSIS

DEFINITION

Systemic mastocytosis is defined by a clonal expansion of mast cells that in most instances is indolent and nonneoplastic. The mast cell expansion is generally recognized only in bone marrow and in the normal peripheral distribution sites of the cells, such as skin, gastrointestinal mucosa, liver, and spleen. Mastocytosis occurs at any age and has a slight preponderance in males. The prevalence of systemic mastocytosis is not known, a familial occurrence is rare, and atopy is not increased.

CLASSIFICATION AND PATHOPHYSIOLOGY

A recent consensus classification for mastocytosis recognizes cutaneous mastocytosis with variants and four systemic forms (Table 311-2). The form designated as *indolent systemic mastocytosis* (ISM) accounts for the majority of patients; it implies that there is no evidence of an associated hematologic disorder, liver disease, or lymphadenopathy and is not known to alter life expectancy. In *systemic mastocytosis associated with clonal hematologic non-mast cell lineage disease* (SM-AHNMD), the prognosis is determined by the nature of the associated disorder, which

TABLE 311-2   CLASSIFICATION OF MASTOCYTOSIS
Cutaneous mastocytosis (CM)
Urticaria pigmentosa (UP)/maculopapular cutaneous mastocytosis (MPCM)
Variants: plaque form, nodular form; telangiectasia macularis eruptiva perstans (TMEP); diffuse cutaneous mastocytosis (DCM)
Solitary mastocytoma of skin
Indolent systemic mastocytosis (ISM)
Systemic mastocytosis with an associated clonal hematologic non-mast cell lineage disease (SM-AHNMD)
Aggressive systemic mastocytosis (ASM)
Variant: lymphadenopathic mastocytosis with eosinophilia
Mast cell leukemia (MCL)
Mast cell sarcoma (MCS)

Source: Modified from P Valent et al, in ES Jaffe et al (eds): *World Health Organization Classification of Tumors: Pathology and Genetics in Tumors of Hematopoietic and Lymphoid Tissues*, Lyon, IARC Press, 2001.

can range from dysmyelopoiesis to leukemia. In *aggressive systemic mastocytosis* (ASM), mast cell infiltration/proliferation in multiple organs such as liver, spleen, gut, CNS, and/or bone, results in a poor prognosis; a subset of these patients has prominent eosinophilia with hepatosplenomegaly and lymphadenopathy. *Mast cell leukemia* is the rarest form of the disease and is invariably fatal at present; the peripheral blood contains circulating, metachromatically staining, atypical mast cells.

A point mutation of A to T at codon 816 of *c-kit* that causes an aspartic acid to valine substitution is found in multiple cell lineages in patients with mastocytosis, indicating a somatic gain-in-function mutation. This substitution, as well as other rare mutations of *c-kit*, is characteristic of adults with SM-AHNMD but is also detected in patients with ISM or cutaneous mastocytosis, as might be anticipated because mast cells at any site are of bone marrow lineage. In infants and children with cutaneous manifestations, namely, urticaria pigmentosa or bullous lesions, visceral involvement is usually lacking, and resolution is common because gain-in-function mutations are infrequent.

CLINICAL MANIFESTATIONS

The clinical manifestations of systemic mastocytosis, distinct from a leukemic complication, are due to tissue occupancy by the mast cell mass, the tissue response to that mass, and the release of bioactive substances acting at both local and distal sites. The pharmacologically induced manifestations are pruritus, flushing, palpitations and vascular collapse, gastric distress, lower abdominal crampy pain, and recurrent headache. The increase in cell burden is evidenced by the lesions of urticaria pigmentosa at skin sites, and directly causes bone pain and malabsorption. Mast cell–mediated fibrotic changes occur in liver, spleen, and bone marrow but not in gastrointestinal tissue or skin. Immunofluorescent analysis of bone marrow and skin lesions in ISM and of spleen, lymph node, and skin in ASM has revealed only one mast cell phenotype, namely, scroll-poor cells expressing tryptase, chymase, and CPA.

The cutaneous lesions of urticaria pigmentosa are reddish-brown macules or papules that respond to trauma with urtication and erythema (Darier's sign). The apparent incidence of these lesions is ≥90% in patients with ISM and <50% in those with SM-AHNMD or ASM. Approximately 1% of patients with ISM have skin lesions that appear as tan-brown macules with striking patchy erythema and associated telangiectasia (telangiectasia macularis eruptiva perstans). In the upper gastrointestinal tract, gastritis and peptic ulcer are a significant problem. In the lower intestinal tract, the occurrence of diarrhea and abdominal pain is attributed to increased motility due to mast cell mediators, and this can be aggravated by malabsorption, which can also cause secondary nutritional insufficiency and osteomalacia. The periportal fibrosis associated with mast cell infiltration and a prominence of eosinophils may lead to portal hypertension and ascites. In some patients, flushing and recurrent vascular collapse are markedly aggravated by an idiosyncratic response to a minimal dosage of NSAIDs. The neuropsychiatric disturbances are clinically most evident as impaired recent memory, decreased attention span, and "migraine-like" headaches. Patients may ex-

TABLE 311-3   DIAGNOSTIC CRITERIA FOR SYSTEMIC MASTOCYTOSIS*

Major: Multifocal dense infiltrates of mast cells in bone marrow or other extracutaneous tissues with confirmation by immunodetection of tryptase or metachromasia

Minor: Abnormal mast cell morphology with a spindle shape and/or multilobed or eccentric nucleus

  Aberrant mast cell surface phenotype with expression of CD25 and CD2 (IL-2 receptor) in addition to C117 (c-kit)

  Detection of codon 816 mutation in peripheral blood cells, bone marrow cells, or lesional tissue

  Total serum tryptase (mostly alpha) greater than 20 ng/mL

*Diagnosis requires either major and one minor or three minor criteria.

perience exacerbation of a specific clinical sign or symptom with alcohol ingestion, use of mast cell–interactive narcotics, or ingestion of NSAIDs.

DIAGNOSIS

Although the diagnosis of mastocytosis is generally suspected on the basis of the clinical history and physical findings, and can be supported by laboratory procedures, it can be established only by a tissue diagnosis. By recent convention, the diagnosis of systemic mastocytosis depends heavily on bone marrow biopsy to meet the criteria of one major plus one minor or three minor findings (Table 311-3). The bone marrow provides the major criterion by revealing aggregates of mast cells, often in paratrabecular and perivascular locations with lymphocytes and eosinophils, as well as the minor criteria of an abnormal mast cell morphology, an aberrant mast cell membrane immunophenotype, or a codon 816 mutation in any cell type. A serum total tryptase level and/or a 24-h urine collection for measurement of histamine, histamine metabolites, or metabolites of PGD_2 are noninvasive approaches to consider before bone marrow biopsy. The α form of tryptase is elevated in more than one-half of patients with systemic mastocytosis and provides a minor criterion; the β form is increased in patients undergoing an anaphylactic reaction. Additional studies directed by the presentation include a bone scan or skeletal survey; contrast studies of the upper gastrointestinal tract with small-bowel follow-through, computed tomography scan, or endoscopy; and a neuropsychiatric evaluation, including an electroencephalogram.

The differential diagnosis requires the exclusion of other flushing disorders. The 24-h urine assessment of 5-hydroxy-indoleacetic acid and metanephrines should exclude a carcinoid tumor or a pheochromocytoma. Most patients with recurrent anaphylaxis, including the idiopathic group, present with angioedema and/or wheezing, which are not manifestations of systemic mastocytosis.

℞ SYSTEMIC MASTOCYTOSIS

The management of systemic mastocytosis uses a stepwise and symptom/sign–directed approach that includes an H_1 antihistamine for flushing and pruritus, an H_2 antihistamine or proton pump inhibitor for gastric acid hypersecretion, oral cromolyn sodium for diarrhea and abdominal pain, and aspirin for severe flushing with or without associated vascular collapse, despite use of H_1 and H_2 antihistamines, to block biosynthesis of PGD_2. Systemic glucocorticoids appear to alleviate the malabsorption. Headaches are generally managed with tricyclic antidepressants and other neurotransmitter-modifying agents. Ketotifen has been used to alleviate flushing in patients with gastric intolerance to NSAIDs and in patients with bone pain or intractable headaches. The efficacy of IFN-α in ASM is controversial, and this may relate to dosage limitations due to side effects. Treatment with hydroxyurea to reduce the mast cell lineage progenitors may have merit in ASM. Chemotherapy is appropriate for the frank leukemias. Although c-kit is a receptor tyrosine kinase, the gain-in-function mutation of codon 816 is not susceptible to inhibition by imatinib mesylate.

ALLERGIC RHINITIS

DEFINITION

Allergic rhinitis is characterized by sneezing; rhinorrhea; obstruction of the nasal passages; conjunctival, nasal, and pharyngeal itching; and lacrimation, all occurring in a temporal relationship to allergen exposure. Although commonly seasonal due to elicitation by airborne pollens, it can be perennial in an environment of chronic exposure. The incidence of allergic rhinitis in North America is about 7%, with the peak occurring in childhood and adolescence. The prevalence in North America is nearly 20%.

PREDISPOSING FACTORS AND ETIOLOGY

Allergic rhinitis generally presents in atopic individuals, i.e., in persons with a family history of a similar or related symptom complex and a personal history of collateral allergy expressed as eczematous dermatitis, urticaria, and/or asthma (Chap. 248). Up to 40% of patients with rhinitis manifest asthma, whereas ~70% of individuals with asthma experience rhinitis. Symptoms generally appear before the fourth decade of life and tend to diminish gradually with aging, although complete spontaneous remissions are uncommon. A relatively small number of weeds that depend on wind rather than insects for cross-pollination, as well as grasses and some trees, produce sufficient quantities of pollen suitable for wide distribution by air currents to elicit seasonal allergic rhinitis. The dates of pollination of these species generally vary little from year to year in a particular locale but may be quite different in another climate. In the temperate areas of North America, trees typically pollinate from March through May, grasses in June and early July, and ragweed from mid-August to early October. Molds, which are widespread in nature because they occur in soil or decaying organic matter, may propagate spores in a pattern dependent on climatic conditions. Perennial allergic rhinitis occurs in response to allergens that are present throughout the year, including desquamating epithelium in animal dander, cockroach-derived proteins, mold spores, or dust, which has mites such as *Dermatophagoides farinae* and *D. pteronyssinus*. Dust mites are scavengers of flecks of human skin and coat the digestate with mite-specific protein for excretion. In up to one-half of patients with perennial rhinitis, no clear-cut allergen can be demonstrated as causative. The ability of allergens to cause rhinitis rather than lower respiratory symptoms may be attributed to their large size, 10 to 100 μm, and retention within the nose.

PATHOPHYSIOLOGY AND MANIFESTATIONS

Episodic rhinorrhea, sneezing, obstruction of the nasal passages with lacrimation, and pruritus of the conjunctiva, nasal mucosa, and oropharynx are the hallmarks of allergic rhinitis. The nasal mucosa is pale and boggy, the conjunctiva congested and edematous, and the pharynx is generally unremarkable. Swelling of the turbinates and mucous membranes with obstruction of the sinus ostia and eustachian tubes precipitates secondary infections of the sinuses and middle ear, respectively. Nasal polyps, representing mucosal protrusions containing edema fluid with variable numbers of eosinophils, can increase obstructive symptoms and can concurrently arise within the nasopharynx or sinuses. Nasal polyps may occur independent of allergic rhinitis in patients with the aspirin-intolerant triad of rhinosinusitis and asthma.

The nose presents a large mucosal surface area through the folds of the turbinates and serves to adjust the temperature and moisture content of inhaled air and to filter out particulate materials >10 μm in size by impingement in a mucous blanket; ciliary action moves the entrapped particles toward the pharynx. Entrapment of pollen and digestion of the outer coat by mucosal enzymes such as lysozymes release protein allergens generally of 10,000 to 40,000 molecular weight. The initial interaction occurs between the allergen and intraepithelial mast cells and then proceeds to involve deeper perivenular mast cells, both of which are sensitized with specific IgE. During the symptomatic season when the mucosae are already swollen and hyperemic, there is enhanced adverse reactivity to the seasonal pollen as well as to antigenically unrelated pollens for which there is underlying hypersensitivity due to improved penetration of the allergens. Biopsy specimens of nasal mucosa during seasonal rhinitis show submucosal edema with infiltration by eosinophils, along with some basophils and neutrophils.

The mucosal surface fluid contains IgA that is present because of its secretory piece and also IgE, which apparently arrives by diffusion from plasma cells in proximity to mucosal surfaces. IgE fixes to mucosal and submucosal mast cells, and the intensity of the clinical response to inhaled allergens is quantitatively related to the naturally occurring pollen dose. In sensitive individuals, the introduction of allergen into the nose is associated with sneezing, "stuffiness," and discharge, and the fluid contains histamine, PGD_2, and leukotrienes. Thus the mast cells of the nasal mucosa and submucosa generate and release mediators through IgE-dependent reactions that are capable of producing tissue edema and eosinophilic infiltration.

DIAGNOSIS

The diagnosis of seasonal allergic rhinitis depends largely on an accurate history of occurrence coincident with the pollination of the offending weeds, grasses, or trees. The continuous character of perennial allergic rhinitis due to contamination of the home or place of work makes historic analysis difficult, but there may be a variability in symptoms that can be related to exposure to animal dander, dust mite and/or cockroach allergens, fungal spores, or work-related allergens such as latex. Patients with perennial rhinitis commonly develop the problem in adult life, and manifest nasal congestion and a postnasal discharge, often associated with thickening of the sinus membranes demonstrated by radiography. Perennial nonallergic rhinitis associated with nasal eosinophils (NARES) occurs in the middle decades of life and is characterized by nasal obstruction, anosmia, chronic sinusitis, and frequent aspirin intolerance. The term *vasomotor rhinitis* designates a condition of enhanced reactivity of the nasopharynx in which a symptom complex resembling perennial allergic rhinitis occurs with nonspecific stimuli and without tissue eosinophilia or an allergic etiology. Other entities to be excluded are structural abnormalities of the nasopharynx; exposure to irritants; gustatory or ethanol-induced rhinitis; hypothyroidism; upper respiratory infection; pregnancy with prominent nasal mucosal edema; prolonged topical use of α-adrenergic agents in the form of nose drops (rhinitis medicamentosa); and the use of certain therapeutic agents such as rauwolfia, β-adrenergic antagonists, estrogens, progesterone, ACE inhibitors, aspirin and NSAIDS, and drugs for erectile dysfunction (phosphodiesterase-5 inhibitors).

The nasal secretions of allergic patients are rich in eosinophils, and a modest peripheral eosinophilia is a common feature. Local or systemic neutrophilia implies infection. Total serum IgE is frequently elevated, but the demonstration of immunologic specificity for IgE is critical to an etiologic diagnosis. A skin test by the intracutaneous route (puncture or prick) with the allergens of interest provides a rapid and reliable approach to identifying allergen-specific IgE that has sensitized cutaneous mast cells. A positive intracutaneous skin test with 1:10–1:20 weight/volume of extract has a high predictive value for the presence of allergy. An intradermal test with a 1:500–1:1000 dilution of 0.05 mL may follow if indicated by history when the intracutaneous test is negative; but while more sensitive, it is less reliable due to the reactivity of some asymptomatic individuals at the test dose. Skin testing by the intracutaneous route for food allergens can be supportive of the clinical history. A double-blind, placebo-controlled challenge may document a food allergy, but such a procedure does bear the risk of an anaphylactic reaction. An elimination diet is safer but is tedious and less definitive. Food allergy is uncommon as a cause of allergic rhinitis.

Newer methodology for detecting total IgE, including the development of enzyme-linked immunosorbent assays (ELISA) employing anti-IgE bound to either a solid-phase or a liquid-phase particle, provides rapid and cost-effective determinations. Measurements of specific anti-IgE in serum are obtained by its binding to an allergen and quantitation by subsequent uptake of labeled anti-IgE. As compared to the skin test, the assay of specific IgE in serum is less sensitive but has high specificity.

PREVENTION

Avoidance of exposure to the offending allergen is the most effective means of controlling allergic diseases; removal of pets from the home to avoid animal danders, utilization of air-filtration devices to minimize

the concentrations of airborne pollens, elimination of cockroach-derived proteins by chemical destruction of the pest and careful food storage, travel to nonpollinating areas during the critical periods, and even a change of domicile to eliminate a mold spore problem may be necessary. Control of dust mites by allergen avoidance includes use of plastic-lined covers for mattresses, pillows, and comforters; using a filter-equipped vacuum cleaner; washing bedding and clothes at temperatures >54.5°C (above 130°F); and elimination of carpets and drapes.

℞ ALLERGIC RHINITIS

Although allergen avoidance is the most cost-effective means of managing allergic rhinitis, treatment with pharmacologic agents represents the standard approach to seasonal or perennial allergic rhinitis. Oral antihistamines of the H_1 class are effective for nasopharyngeal itching, sneezing, and watery rhinorrhea and for such ocular manifestations as itching, tearing, and erythema, but they are not efficacious for the nasal congestion. The older antihistamines are sedating, and they induce psychomotor impairment, including reduced eye-hand coordination and impaired automobile driving skills. Their anticholinergic (muscarinic) effects include visual disturbance, urinary retention, and constipation. Because the newer H_1 antihistamines such as fexofenadine, loratadine, desloratadine, cetirizine, and azelastine are less lipophilic and more H_1 selective, their ability to cross the blood-brain barrier is reduced, and thus their sedating and anticholinergic side effects are minimized. These newer antihistamines do not differ appreciably in efficacy for relief of rhinitis and/or sneezing. Oral antihistamines have little benefit on congestion. Azelastine nasal spray may benefit individuals with nonallergic vasomotor rhinitis, but it has an adverse effect of dysgeusia (taste perversion) in some patients. Because antihistamines have little effect on congestion, α-adrenergic agents such as phenylephrine or oximetazoline are generally used topically to alleviate nasal congestion and obstruction. However, the duration of their efficacy is limited because of rebound rhinitis (i.e., 7- to 14-day use can lead to rhinitis medicamentosa) and such systemic responses as hypertension. Oral α-adrenergic agonist decongestants containing pseudoephedrine are standard for the management of nasal congestion, generally in combination with an antihistamine. These pseudoephedrine combination products can cause insomnia and are precluded in patients with narrow angle glaucoma, urinary retention, severe hypertension, marked coronary artery disease, or a first trimester pregnancy. The CysLT1 blocker, montelukast, is approved for both seasonal and perennial rhinitis. Cromolyn sodium, a nasal spray, is essentially without side effects and is used prophylactically on a continuous basis during the season. The clinical efficacy of cromolyn sodium used prophylactically is less than that of second-generation oral antihistamines. Intranasal high-potency glucocorticoids are the most potent drugs available for the relief of established rhinitis, seasonal or perennial, and are effective in relieving nasal congestion. They provide efficacy with substantially reduced side effects as compared with this same class of agent administered orally. Their most frequent side effect is local irritation, with *Candida* overgrowth being a rare occurrence. The currently available intranasal glucocorticoids—beclomethasone, flunisolide, budesonide, fluticasone, and mometasone—are equally effective clinically, achieving up to 70% overall symptom relief with some variation in the time period for onset of benefit. Topical ipratropium is an anticholinergic agent effective in reducing rhinorrhea, including that in patients with perennial symptoms, and it can be additionally efficacious when combined with intranasal steroids. Local treatment with cromolyn sodium may be effective in mild allergic conjunctivitis. Topical antihistamines such as olopatadine, azelastine, or epinastine provide rapid relief of itching and redness and are more effective than oral antihistamines.

Immunotherapy, often termed *hyposensitization*, consists of repeated subcutaneous injections of gradually increasing concentrations of the allergen(s) considered to be specifically responsible for the symptom complex. Controlled studies of ragweed, grass, dust mite, and cat dander allergens administered for treatment of allergic rhinitis have demonstrated at least partial relief of symptoms and signs. The duration of such immunotherapy is 3–5 years, with discontinuation being based on minimal symptoms over two consecutive seasons of exposure. Clinical benefit appears related to the administration of a high dose of relevant allergen advancing from weekly to monthly intervals. Patients should remain at the treatment site for at least 20 min after allergen administration so that any anaphylactic consequence can be managed. Local reactions with erythema and induration are not uncom-

MANAGEMENT OF RHINITIS

FIGURE 311-3 Algorithm for the diagnosis and management of rhinitis. ENT, ear, nose, and throat surgeon.

mon and may persist for 1 to 3 days. Immunotherapy is contraindicated in patients with significant cardiovascular disease or unstable asthma and should be conducted with particular caution in any patient requiring β-adrenergic blocking therapy because of the difficulty in managing an anaphylactic complication. The response to immunotherapy is derived from a complex of cellular and humoral effects that likely includes a modulation in T cell cytokine production. Immunotherapy should be reserved for clearly documented seasonal or perennial rhinitis, clinically related to defined allergen exposure with confirmation by the presence of allergen-specific IgE. Early studies suggest that systemic treatment with a monoclonal antibody

to IgE (omalizumab) that blocks mast cell sensitization has efficacy for allergic rhinitis and can be used with immunotherapy to enhance safety and efficacy. However, current approval is only to treat patients with persistent allergic asthma not controlled by inhaled glucocorticoid therapy. A sequence for the management of allergic or perennial rhinitis based on an allergen-specific diagnosis and stepwise management as required for symptom control would include the following: (1) identification of the offending allergen(s) by history with confirmation of the presence of allergen-specific IgE by skin test and/or serum assay; (2) avoidance of the offending allergen; and (3) medical management in a stepwise fashion (**Fig. 311-3**). Mild intermittent symptoms of allergic rhinitis are treated with oral antihistamines, oral CysLT1 antagonists, intranasal antihistamines, or intranasal cromolyn prophylaxis. Moderate to more severe allergic rhinitis is managed with intranasal glucocorticoids plus oral antihistamines, oral CysLT1 antagonists, or antihistamine-decongestant combinations. Persistent allergic rhinitis requiring the daily use of intranasal glucocorticoids with add-on interventions such as oral antihistamines, decongestant combinations, or topical ipratropium merits consideration of allergen-specific immunotherapy. Even a brief course of oral prednisone can be indicated.

FURTHER READINGS

AUSTEN KF, KANAOKA Y: *Lipids*, in SHE Kaufmann, R Medzhitov, S Gordon (eds): *The Innate Immune Response to Infection*. Washington, DC, ASM Press, 2004, pp 417–431

BENOIST C, MATHIS D: Mast cells in autoimmune disease. Nature 420:875, 2002

GALLI SJ et al: Mast cells in the development of adaptive immune responses. Nat Immunol 6:135, 2005

SOTER NA, KAPLAN AP: Urticaria and angioedema, in IM Freedberg et al (eds): *Fitzpatrick's Dermatology in General Medicine*, 6th ed. New York, McGraw-Hill, 2003, pp 1129–1139

VALENTINE MD: Insect venom allergy, in KF Austen et al (eds): *Immunologic Diseases*, 6th ed. Philadelphia, Lippincott Williams & Wilkins, 2001

WOROBEC A, METCALFE DD: Anaphylactic syndrome, in KF Austen et al (eds): *Immunologic Diseases*, 6th ed. Philadelphia, Lippincott Williams & Wilkins, 2001

TABLE 312-1 **MECHANISMS PREVENTING AUTOIMMUNITY** 2071

312 Autoimmunity and Autoimmune Diseases

Peter E. Lipsky, Betty Diamond

TABLE 312-1 **MECHANISMS PREVENTING AUTOIMMUNITY**

1. Sequestration of self-antigen
2. Generation and maintenance of tolerance
   a. Central deletion of autoreactive lymphocytes
   b. Peripheral anergy of autoreactive lymphocytes
   c. Receptor replacement by autoreactive lymphocytes
3. Regulatory mechanisms

One of the classically accepted features of the immune system is the capacity to distinguish self from nonself. Although they are able to recognize and generate reactions to a vast array of foreign materials, most animals do not mount immune responses to self-antigens under ordinary circumstances and thus are tolerant to self. Whereas recognition of self plays an important role in shaping both the T cell and B cell repertoires of immune receptors and plays an essential role in the recognition of nominal antigen by T cells, the development of potentially harmful immune responses to self-antigens is, in general, precluded. Autoimmunity therefore represents the end result of the breakdown of one or more of the basic mechanisms regulating immune tolerance.

The essential feature of an autoimmune disease is that tissue injury is caused by the immunologic reaction of the organism with its own tissues. Autoimmunity, on the other hand, refers merely to the presence of antibodies or T lymphocytes that react with self-antigens and does not necessarily imply that the development of self-reactivity has pathogenic consequences.

Autoimmunity may be seen in normal individuals and in higher frequency in normal older people. In addition, autoreactivity may develop during various infectious conditions. The expression of autoimmunity may be self-limited, as occurs with many infectious processes, or persistent. When autoimmunity is induced by an inciting event, such as infection or tissue damage from trauma or infarction, there may or may not be ensuing pathology. Even in the presence of organ pathology, it may be difficult to determine whether the damage is mediated by autoreactivity. Thus, the presence of self-reactivity may be either the cause or a consequence of an ongoing pathologic process.

MECHANISMS OF AUTOIMMUNITY

Since Ehrlich first postulated the existence of mechanisms to prevent the generation of self-reactivity in 1900, ideas concerning the nature of this inhibition have developed in parallel with the progressive increase in understanding of the immune system. Burnet's clonal selection theory included the idea that interaction of lymphoid cells with their specific antigens during fetal or early postnatal life would lead to elimination of such "forbidden clones." This idea became untenable, however, when it was shown by a number of investigators that autoimmune diseases could be induced by simple immunization procedures that autoantigen-binding cells could be demonstrated easily in the circulation of normal individuals, and that self-limited autoimmune phenomena frequently developed during infections. These observations indicated that clones of cells capable of responding to autoantigens were present in the repertoire of antigen-reactive cells in normal adults and suggested that mechanisms in addition to clonal deletion were responsible for preventing their activation.

Currently, three general processes are thought to be involved in the maintenance of selective unresponsiveness to autoantigens (Table 312-1): (1) sequestration of self-antigens, rendering them inaccessible to the immune system; (2) specific unresponsiveness (tolerance or anergy) of relevant T or B cells; and (3) limitation of potential reactivity by regulatory mechanisms.

Derangements of these normal processes may predispose to the development of autoimmunity (Table 312-2). In general, these abnormal responses relate to stimulation by exogenous agents, usually bacterial or viral, or endogenous abnormalities in the cells of the immune system. Microbial superantigens, such as staphylococcal protein A and staphylococcal enterotoxins, are substances that can stimulate a broad range of T and B cells based upon specific interactions with selected families of immune receptors, irrespective of their antigen specificity. If autoantigen-reactive T and/or B cells express these receptors, au-

toimmunity might develop. Alternatively, molecular mimicry or cross-reactivity between a microbial product and a self-antigen might lead to activation of autoreactive lymphocytes. One of the best examples of autoreactivity and autoimmune disease resulting from molecular mimicry is rheumatic fever, in which antibodies to the M protein of streptococci cross-react with myosin, laminin, and other matrix proteins. Deposition of these autoantibodies in the heart initiates an inflammatory response. Molecular mimicry between microbial proteins and host tissues has been reported in type 1 diabetes mellitus, rheumatoid arthritis, and multiple sclerosis. The capacity of nonspecific stimulation of the immune system to predispose to the development of autoimmunity has been explored in a number of models; one is provided by the effect of adjuvants on the production of autoimmunity. Autoantigens become much more immunogenic when administered with adjuvant. It is presumed that infectious agents may be able to overcome self-tolerance because they possess molecules, such as bacterial endotoxin, that have adjuvant-like effects on the immune system by stimulating cells through Toll-like receptors.

Endogenous derangements of the immune system may also contribute to the loss of immunologic tolerance to self-antigens and the development of autoimmunity (Table 312-2). Many autoantigens reside in immunologically privileged sites, such as the brain or the anterior chamber of the eye. These sites are characterized by the inability of engrafted tissue to elicit immune responses. Immunologic privilege results from a number of events, including the limited entry of proteins from those sites into lymphatics, the local production of immunosuppressive cytokines such as transforming growth factor β, and the local expression of molecules such as Fas ligand that can induce apoptosis of activated T cells. Lymphoid cells remain in a state of immunologic ignorance (neither activated nor anergized) to proteins expressed uniquely in immunologically privileged sites. If the privileged site is damaged by trauma or inflammation, or if T cells are activated elsewhere, proteins expressed at this site can become the targets of immunologic assault. Such an event may occur in multiple sclerosis and sympathetic ophthalmia, in which antigens uniquely expressed in the brain and eye, respectively, become the target of activated T cells.

Alterations in antigen presentation may also contribute to autoimmunity. This may occur by epitope spreading, in which protein determinants (*epitopes*) not routinely seen by lymphocytes (*cryptic epitopes*)

TABLE 312-2 **MECHANISMS OF AUTOIMMUNITY**

I. Exogenous
   A. Molecular mimicry
   B. Superantigenic stimulation
   C. Microbial adjuvanticity
II. Endogenous
   A. Altered antigen presentation
      1. Loss of immunologic privilege
      2. Presentation of novel or crytic epitopes (epitope spreading)
      3. Alteration of self-antigen
      4. Enhanced function of antigen-presenting cells
         a. Costimulatory molecule expression
         b. Cytokine production
   B. Increased T cell help
      1. Cytokine production
      2. Costimulatory molecules
   C. Increased B cell function
   D. Apoptotic defects
   E. Cytokine imbalance
   F. Altered immunoregulation

are recognized as a result of immunologic reactivity to associated molecules. For example, animals immunized with one protein component of a multimolecular complex may be induced to produce antibodies to the other components of the complex. Finally, inflammation, drug exposure, or normal senescence may cause a primary chemical alteration in proteins, resulting in the generation of immune responses that cross-react with normal self-proteins. Alterations in the availability and presentation of autoantigens may be important components of immunoreactivity in certain models of organ-specific autoimmune diseases. In addition, these factors may be relevant in understanding the pathogenesis of various drug-induced autoimmune conditions. However, the diversity of autoreactivity manifest in non-organ-specific systemic autoimmune diseases suggests that these conditions might result from a more general activation of the immune system rather than from an alteration in individual self-antigens.

A number of experimental models have suggested that intense stimulation of T lymphocytes can produce nonspecific signals that bypass the need for antigen-specific helper T cells and lead to polyclonal B cell activation with the formation of multiple autoantibodies. For example, antinuclear, antierythrocyte, and antilymphocyte antibodies are produced during the chronic graft-versus-host reaction. In addition, true autoimmune diseases, including autoimmune hemolytic anemia and immune complex–mediated glomerulonephritis, can also be induced in this manner. While it is clear that such diffuse activation of helper T cell activity can cause autoimmunity, nonspecific stimulation of B lymphocytes can also lead to the production of autoantibodies. Thus, the administration of polyclonal B cell activators, such as bacterial endotoxin, to normal mice leads to the production of a number of autoantibodies, including those directed to DNA and IgG (rheumatoid factor).

Aberrant selection of the B or T cell repertoire at the time of antigen receptor expression can also predispose to autoimmunity. For example, B cell immunodeficiency caused by an absence of the B cell receptor–associated kinase, Bruton's tyrosine kinase, leads to X-linked agammaglobulinemia. This syndrome is characterized by reduced B cell activation, but also by diminished negative selection of autoreactive B cells, resulting in increased autoreactivity within a deficient B cell repertoire. Likewise, negative selection of autoreactive T cells in the thymus requires expression of the autoimmune regulator (AIRE) gene that enables the expression of tissue-specific proteins in thymic medullary epithelial cells. Peptides from these proteins are expressed in the context of MHC molecules and mediate the elimination of autoreactive T cells. The absence of AIRE gene expression leads to a failure of negative selection of autoreactive cells, autoantibody production, and severe inflammatory destruction of multiple organs. Individuals deficient in AIRE gene expression develop autoimmune polyendocrinopathy-candidiasis-ectodermal dystrophy (APECED).

Primary alterations in the activity of T and/or B cells, cytokine imbalances, or defective immunoregulatory circuits may also contribute to the emergence of autoimmunity. For example, decreased apoptosis, as can be seen in animals with defects in Fas (CD95) or Fas ligand or in patients with related abnormalities, can be associated with the development of autoimmunity. Similarly, diminished production of tumor necrosis factor (TNF) and interleukin (IL) 10 has been reported to be associated with the development of autoimmunity.

Autoimmunity may also result from an abnormality of immunoregulatory mechanisms. Observations made in both human autoimmune disease and animal models suggest that defects in the generation and expression of regulatory T cell activity may allow for the production of autoimmunity. It has recently been appreciated that the IPEX (immunodysregulation, polyendocrinopathy, enteropathy X-linked) syndrome results from the failure to express the FOXP3 gene, which encodes a molecule critical in the differentiation of regulatory T cells. Administration of normal regulatory T cells or factors derived from them can prevent the development of autoimmune disease in rodent models of autoimmunity.

It should be apparent that no single mechanism can explain all the varied manifestations of autoimmunity. Furthermore, genetic evaluation has shown that a number of abnormalities often need to converge to induce an autoimmune disease. Additional factors that appear to be important determinants in the induction of autoimmunity include age, sex (many autoimmune diseases are far more common in women), genetic background, exposure to infectious agents, and environmental contacts. How all of these disparate factors affect the capacity to develop self-reactivity is currently being intensively investigated.

GENETIC CONSIDERATIONS Evidence in humans that there are susceptibility genes for autoimmunity comes from family studies and especially from studies of twins. Studies in type 1 diabetes mellitus, rheumatoid arthritis, multiple sclerosis, and systemic lupus erythematosus (SLE) have shown that approximately 15–30% of pairs of monozygotic twins show disease concordance, compared with <5% of dizygotic twins. The occurrence of different autoimmune diseases within the same family has suggested that certain susceptibility genes may predispose to a variety of autoimmune diseases. Genetic mapping has begun to identify chromosomal regions that predispose to specific autoimmune diseases. One gene is a phosphatase expressed by a variety of hematopoietic cells that downregulates antigen receptor–mediated stimulation, PTPN22. A loss-of-function polymorphism of this gene is associated with both type 1 diabetes mellitus and rheumatoid arthritis in some populations. In addition to this evidence from humans, certain inbred mouse strains reproducibly develop specific spontaneous or experimentally induced autoimmune diseases, whereas others do not. These findings have led to an extensive search for genes that determine susceptibility to autoimmune disease.

The most consistent association for susceptibility to autoimmune disease has been with particular alleles of the major histocompatibility complex (MHC). It has been suggested that the association of MHC genotype with autoimmune disease relates to differences in the ability of different allelic variations of MHC molecules to present autoantigenic peptides to autoreactive T cells. An alternative hypothesis involves the role of MHC alleles in shaping the T cell receptor repertoire during T cell ontogeny in the thymus. Additionally, specific MHC gene products may be themselves the source of peptides that can be recognized by T cells. Cross-reactivity between such MHC peptides and peptides derived from proteins produced by common microbes may trigger autoimmunity by molecular mimicry. However, MHC genotype alone does not determine the development of autoimmunity. Identical twins are far more likely to develop the same autoimmune disease than MHC-identical nontwin siblings, suggesting that genetic factors other than the MHC also affect disease susceptibility. Recent studies of the genetics of type 1 diabetes mellitus, SLE, rheumatoid arthritis, and multiple sclerosis in humans and mice have shown that there are several independently segregating disease susceptibility loci in addition to the MHC.

There is evidence that several other genes are important in increasing susceptibility to autoimmune disease. In humans, inherited homozygous deficiency of the early proteins of the classic pathway of complement (C1, C4, or C2) is very strongly associated with the development of SLE. In mice and humans, abnormalities in the genes encoding proteins involved in the regulation of apoptosis, including Fas (CD95, tumor necrosis factor receptor superfamily 6) and Fas ligand (CD95 ligand; CD178, tumor necrosis factor ligand superfamily 6), are strongly associated with the development of autoimmunity. There is also evidence that inherited variation in the level of expression of certain cytokines, such as TNF or IL-10, may also increase susceptibility to autoimmune disease.

A further important factor in disease susceptibility is the hormonal status of the patient. Many autoimmune diseases show a strong sex bias, which appears in most cases to relate to the hormonal status of women.

IMMUNOPATHOGENIC MECHANISMS IN AUTOIMMUNE DISEASES

The mechanisms of tissue injury in autoimmune diseases can be divided into antibody-mediated and cell-mediated processes. Representative examples are listed in Table 312-3.

TABLE 312-3	MECHANISMS OF TISSUE DAMAGE IN AUTOIMMUNE DISEASE		
Effector	**Mechanism**	**Target**	**Disease**
Autoantibody	Blocking or inactivation	α Chain of the nicotinic acetylcholine receptor	Myasthenia gravis
		Phospholipid–β_2-glyco-protein 1 complex	Antiphospholipid syndrome
		Insulin receptor	Insulin-resistant diabetes mellitus
		Intrinsic factor	Pernicious anemia
	Stimulation	TSH receptor (LATS)	Graves' disease
		Proteinase-3 (ANCA)	Wegener's granulomatosis
		Epidermal cadherin$_1$ Desmoglein 3	Pemphigus vulgaris
	Complement activation	α_3 Chain of collagen IV	Goodpasture's syndrome
	Immune-complex formation	Double-strand DNA	Systemic lupus erythematosus
		Ig	Rheumatoid arthritis
	Opsonization	Platelet GpIIb:IIIa	Autoimmune thrombocytopenic purpura
		Rh antigens, I antigen	Autoimmune hemolytic anemia
	Antibody-dependent cellular cytotoxicity	Thyroid peroxidase, thyroglobulin	Hashimoto's thyroiditis
T cells	Cytokine production	?	Rheumatoid arthritis, multiple sclerosis, type 1 diabetes mellitus
	Cellular cytotoxicity	?	Type 1 diabetes mellitus

Note: ANCA, antineutrophil cytoplasmic antibody; LATS, long-acting thyroid stimulator; TSH, thyroid-stimulating hormone.

The pathogenicity of autoantibodies can be mediated through several mechanisms, including opsonization of soluble factors or cells, activation of an inflammatory cascade via the complement system, and interference with the physiologic function of soluble molecules or cells.

In autoimmune thrombocytopenic purpura, opsonization of platelets targets them for elimination by phagocytes. Likewise, in autoimmune hemolytic anemia, binding of immunoglobulin to red cell membranes leads to phagocytosis and lysis of the opsonized cell. Goodpasture's syndrome, a disease characterized by lung hemorrhage and severe glomerulonephritis, represents an example of antibody binding leading to local activation of complement and neutrophil accumulation and activation. The autoantibody in this disease binds to the α_3 chain of type IV collagen in the basement membrane. In SLE, activation of the complement cascade at sites of immunoglobulin deposition in renal glomeruli is considered to be a major mechanism of renal damage.

Autoantibodies can also interfere with normal physiologic functions of cells or soluble factors. Autoantibodies against hormone receptors can lead to stimulation of cells or to inhibition of cell function through interference with receptor signaling. For example, long-acting thyroid stimulators, which are autoantibodies that bind to the receptor for thyroid-stimulating hormone (TSH), are present in Graves' disease and function as agonists, causing the thyroid to respond as if there were an excess of TSH. Alternatively, antibodies to the insulin receptor can cause insulin-resistant diabetes mellitus through receptor blockade. In myasthenia gravis, autoantibodies to the acetylcholine receptor can be detected in 85–90% of patients and are responsible for muscle weakness. The exact location of the antigenic epitope, the valence and affinity of the antibody, and perhaps other characteristics determine whether activation or blockade results from antibody binding.

Antiphospholipid antibodies are associated with thromboembolic events in primary and secondary antiphospholipid syndrome and have also been associated with fetal wastage. The major antibody is directed to the phospholipid–β_2-glycoprotein I complex and appears to exert a procoagulant effect. In pemphigus vulgaris, autoantibodies bind to a component of the epidermal cell desmosome, desmoglein 3, and play a role in the induction of the disease. They exert their pathologic effect by disrupting cell-cell junctions through stimulation of the production of epithelial proteases, leading to blister formation. Cytoplasmic antineutrophil cytoplasmic antibody (c-ANCA), found in Wegener's granulomatosis, is an antibody to an intracellular antigen, the 29-kDa serine protease (proteinase-3). In vitro experiments have shown that IgG anti-c-ANCA causes cellular activation and degranulation of primed neutrophils.

It is important to note that autoantibodies of a given specificity may cause disease only in genetically susceptible hosts, as has been shown in experimental models of myasthenia gravis. Finally, some autoantibodies seem to be markers for disease but have as yet no known pathogenic potential.

AUTOIMMUNE DISEASES

Manifestations of autoimmunity are found in a large number of pathologic conditions. However, their presence does not necessarily imply that the pathologic process is an autoimmune disease. A number of attempts to establish formal criteria for the diagnosis of autoimmune diseases have been made, but none is universally accepted. One set of criteria is shown in Table 312-4; however, this should be viewed merely as a guide in consideration of the problem.

To classify a disease as autoimmune, it is necessary to demonstrate that the immune response to a self-antigen causes the observed pathology. Initially, the demonstration that antibodies against the affected tissue could be detected in the serum of patients suffering from various diseases was taken as evidence that these diseases had an autoimmune basis. However, such autoantibodies are also found when tissue damage is caused by trauma or infection, and the autoantibody is secondary to tissue damage. Thus, it is necessary to show that autoimmunity is pathogenic before classifying a disease as autoimmune.

If the autoantibodies are pathogenic, it may be possible to transfer disease to experimental animals by the administration of autoantibodies, with the subsequent development of pathology in the recipient similar to that seen in the patient from whom the antibodies were obtained. This has been shown, for example, in Graves' disease. Some autoimmune diseases can be transferred from mother to fetus and are observed in the newborn babies of diseased mothers. The symptoms of the disease in the newborn usually disappear as the levels of the maternal antibody decrease. An exception is congenital heart block, in which damage to the developing conducting system of the heart as a result of transfer of anti-Ro antibody from the mother results in permanent heart block.

In most situations, the critical factors that determine when the development of autoimmunity results in autoimmune disease have not been delineated. The relationship of autoimmunity to the development of autoimmune disease may relate to the fine specificity of the

TABLE 312-4	HUMAN AUTOIMMUNE DISEASE: PRESUMPTIVE EVIDENCE FOR AN IMMUNOLOGIC PATHOGENESIS

Major Criteria
1. Presence of autoantibodies or evidence of cellular reactivity to self
2. Documentation of relevant autoantibody or lymphocytic infiltrate in the pathologic lesion
3. Demonstration that relevant autoantibody or T cells can cause tissue pathology
   a. Transplacental transmission
   b. Adaptive transfer into animals
   c. In vitro impact on cellular function

Supportive Evidence
1. Reasonable animal model
2. Beneficial effect from immunosuppressive agents
3. Association with other evidence of autoimmunity
4. No evidence of infection or other obvious cause

TABLE 312-5 **SOME AUTOIMMUNE DISEASES**

Organ Specific

Graves' disease	Vitiligo
Hashimoto's thyroiditis	Autoimmune hemolytic anemia
Autoimmune polyglandular syndrome	Autoimmune thrombocytopenic purpura
Type 1 diabetes mellitus	Pernicious anemia
Insulin-resistant diabetes mellitus	Myasthenia gravis
Immune-mediated infertility	Multiple sclerosis
Autoimmune Addison's disease	Guillain-Barré syndrome
Pemphigus vulgaris	Stiff-man syndrome
Pemphigus foliaceus	Acute rheumatic fever
Dermatitis herpetiformis	Sympathetic ophthalmia
Autoimmune alopecia	Goodpasture's syndrome

Organ Nonspecific (Systemic)

Systemic lupus erythematosus	Wegener's granulomatosis
Rheumatoid arthritis	Antiphospholipid syndrome
Systemic necrotizing vasculitis	Sjögren's syndrome

antibodies or T cells or their specific effector capabilities. In many circumstances, a mechanistic understanding of the pathogenic potential of autoantibodies has not been established. In some autoimmune diseases, biased production of cytokines by helper T (T_H) cells may play a role in pathogenesis. In this regard, T cells can differentiate into specialized effector cells that predominantly produce interferon γ (T_H1) or IL-4 (T_H2) (Chap. 308). The former facilitate macrophage activation and classic cell-mediated immunity, whereas the latter are thought to have regulatory functions and are involved in the resolution of normal immune responses and also the development of responses to a variety of parasites. In a number of autoimmune diseases, such as rheumatoid arthritis, multiple sclerosis, type 1 diabetes mellitus, and Crohn's disease, there appears to be biased differentiation of T_H1 cells, with resultant organ damage.

ORGAN-SPECIFIC VERSUS SYSTEMIC AUTOIMMUNE DISEASES

Autoimmune diseases form a spectrum, from those specifically affecting a single organ to systemic disorders with involvement of many organs (Table 312-5). Hashimoto's autoimmune thyroiditis is an example of an organ-specific autoimmune disease (Chap. 335). In this disorder, there is a specific lesion in the thyroid associated with infiltration of mononuclear cells and damage to follicular cells. Antibody to thyroid constituents can be demonstrated in nearly all cases. Other organ- or tissue-specific autoimmune disorders include pemphigus vulgaris, autoimmune hemolytic anemia, idiopathic thrombocytopenic purpura, Goodpasture's syndrome, myasthenia gravis, and sympathetic ophthalmia. One important feature of some organ-specific autoimmune diseases is the tendency for overlap, such that an individual with one specific syndrome is more likely to develop a second syndrome. For example, there is a high incidence of pernicious anemia in individuals with autoimmune thyroiditis. More striking is the tendency for individuals with an organ-specific autoimmune disease to develop multiple other manifestations of autoimmunity without the development of associated organ pathology. Thus, as many as 50% of individuals with pernicious anemia have non-cross-reacting antibodies to thyroid constituents, whereas patients with myasthenia gravis may develop antinuclear antibodies, antithyroid antibodies, rheumatoid factor, antilymphocyte antibodies, and polyclonal hypergammaglobulinemia. Part of the explanation for this may relate to the genetic elements shared by individuals with these different diseases.

Systemic autoimmune diseases differ from organ-specific diseases in that pathologic lesions are found in multiple diverse organs and tissues. The hallmark of these conditions is the demonstration of associated relevant autoimmune manifestations that are likely to be etiologic in the organ pathology. SLE represents the prototype of these disorders because of its abundance of autoimmune manifestations.

SLE is a disease of protean manifestations that characteristically involves the kidneys, joints, skin, serosal surfaces, blood vessels, and central nervous system (Chap. 313). The disease is associated with a vast array of autoantibodies whose production appears to be a part of a generalized hyperreactivity of the humoral immune system. Other features of SLE include generalized B cell hyperresponsiveness, polyclonal hypergammaglobulinemia, and increased titers of antibodies to commonly encountered viral antigens.

℞ AUTOIMMUNE DISEASES

Treatment of autoimmune diseases can focus on either suppressing the induction of autoimmunity, restoring normal regulatory mechanisms, or inhibiting the effector mechanisms. To eliminate autoreactive cells, immunosuppressive or ablative therapies are most commonly used. In recent years, cytokine blockade has been demonstrated to be effective in preventing immune activation in some diseases. New therapies are currently in clinical trials to target lymphoid cells more specifically, either by blocking a costimulatory signal needed for T or B cell activation, by eliminating the effector T cells or B cells, or by using autoantigen itself to induce tolerance. One major advance in inhibiting effector mechanisms has been the introduction of cytokine blockade, targeting TNF or IL-1, that appears to limit organ damage in some diseases. Biologicals that interface with T cell activation (abatacept) or delete B cells (rituximab) have also recently been approved for the treatment of rheumatoid arthritis. Therapies that prevent target organ damage or support target organ function remain an important therapeutic approach to autoimmune disease.

FURTHER READINGS

BECHLER EC et al: Gene Expression profiling in human autoimmunity. Immunol Rev 210:120, 2006

FIJINAMI RS et al: Molecular mimicry, bystander activation, or viral persistence: Infections and autoimmune disease. Clin Microbiol Rev 19:80, 2006

GEULD SB et al: Silencing of autoreactive B cells by anergy: A fresh perspective. Curr Opin Immunol 18:292, 2006

KANG HK, DATTA SK: Regulatory T cells in lupus. Int Rev Immunol 25(1–2):5, 2006

KIROU KA et al: Soluble mediators as therapeutic targets in systemic lupus erythematosus: Cytokines, immunoglobulin receptors, and the complement system. Rheum Dis Clin North Am 32:103, 2006

NOTARANGELO LD et al: Immunodeficiencies with autoimmune consequences. Adv Immunol 89:321, 2006

SEELEN MA et al: Role of complement in innate and autoimmunity. J Nephrol 18:642, 2005

SHEPAHELOVICH D, SHOENFELD Y: Prediction and prevention of autoimmune diseases: Additional aspects of the mosaic of autoimmunity. Lupus 15:183, 2006

SIGAL LH: Protecting against autoimmunity-tolerance: Mechanisms of negative selection in the thymus. J Clin Rheumatol 12:99, 2006

YOUINOU P et al: B lymphocytes on the front line of autoimmunity. Autoimmun Rev 5:215, 2006

313 Systemic Lupus Erythematosus

Bevra Hannahs Hahn

DEFINITION AND PREVALENCE

Systemic lupus erythematosus (SLE) is an autoimmune disease in which organs and cells undergo damage mediated by tissue-binding autoantibodies and immune complexes. Ninety percent of patients are women of child-bearing years; people of both sexes, all ages, and all ethnic groups are susceptible. Prevalence of SLE in the United States is 15–50 per 100,000; the highest prevalence among ethnic groups studied is in African Americans.

PATHOGENESIS AND ETIOLOGY

The proposed pathogenic mechanisms of SLE are illustrated in Fig. 313-1. Interactions between susceptibility genes and environmental factors result in abnormal immune responses. Those responses include (1) activation of innate immunity (dendritic cells) by CpG DNA, DNA in immune complexes, and RNA in RNA/protein self-antigens; (2) lowered activation thresholds of adaptive immunity cells (antigen-specific T and B lymphocytes); (3) ineffective regulatory and inhibitory CD4+ and CD8+ T cells; and (4) reduced clearance of apoptotic cells and of immune complexes. Self-antigens (nucleosomal DNA/protein; RNA/protein in Sm, Ro, and La; phospholipids) are available for recognition by the immune system in surface blebs of apoptotic cells; thus antigens, autoantibodies, and immune complexes persist for prolonged periods of time, allowing inflammation and disease to develop. Immune activation of circulating and tissue-bound cells is accompanied by increased secretion of proinflammatory tumor necrosis factor (TNF) α and type 1 and 2 interferons (IFNs), and the B cell–driving cytokines B lymphocyte stimulator (BLyS) and interleukin (IL) 10. Upregulation of genes induced by interferons is a genetic "signature" of SLE. However, lupus T and natural killer (NK) cells fail to produce enough IL-2 and transforming growth factor (TGF) to induce regulatory CD4+ and inhibitory CD8+ T cells. The result of these abnormalities is sustained production of pathogenic autoantibodies (referred to in Fig. 313-1 and described in Table 313-1) and immune complexes, which bind to target tissues, with activation of complement and phagocytic cells that recognize Ig-coated circulating blood cells. Activation of complement and immune cells leads to release of chemotaxins, cytokines, chemokines, vasoactive peptides, and destructive enzymes. In the setting of chronic inflammation, accumulation of growth factors and products of chronic oxidation contribute to irreversible tissue damage in glomeruli, arteries, lungs, and other tissues.

SLE is a multigenic disease. In most genetically susceptible individuals, normal alleles of multiple normal genes each contribute a small amount to abnormal immune responses; if enough variations accumulate, disease results. Some predisposing genes confirmed in at least two independent cohorts are listed in Fig. 313-1. Homozygous deficiencies of early components of complement (C1q,r,s; C2; C4) confer strong predisposition to SLE, but such deficiencies are rare. Each of the other genes listed

increases risk for SLE by only 1.5- to 3-fold. Some gene alleles probably contribute to disease susceptibility by influencing clearance of apoptotic cells (C1q, MBL) or immune complexes (FcR 2A and 3A), antigen presentation (HLA-DR2,3,8), B cell maturation (IL-10), T cell activation (PTPN22), or chemotaxis (MCP-1). None of these hypotheses is proven. In addition to influencing disease susceptibility in various ethnic groups, some genes influence clinical manifestations of disease (e.g., FcR2A/3A, MBL, PDCD1 for nephritis; MCP-1 for arthritis and vasculitis). A region on chromosome 16 contains genes that predispose to SLE, rheumatoid arthritis, psoriasis, and Crohn's disease, suggesting the presence of "autoimmunity genes" that, when interacting with other genes, predispose to different autoimmune diseases. There are likely to be protective gene alleles as well. All these gene combinations influence immune responses to the external and internal environment; when such responses are too high and/or too prolonged, autoimmune disease results.

Female sex is permissive for SLE; females of many mammalian species make higher antibody responses than males. Women exposed to estrogen-containing oral contraceptives or hormone replacement have an increased risk of developing SLE (1.2- to 2-fold). Estradiol binds to receptors on T and B lymphocytes, increasing activation and survival of those cells, thus favoring prolonged immune responses.

Several environmental stimuli may influence SLE (Fig. 313-1). Exposure to ultraviolet light causes flares of SLE in approximately 70% of patients, possibly by increasing apoptosis in skin cells or by altering DNA and intracellular proteins to make them antigenic. It is likely that some infections induce a normal immune response that matures to contain some T and B cells that recognize self-antigens; such cells are not appropriately regulated, and autoantibody production occurs. Most SLE patients have autoantibodies for 3 years or more before the first symptoms of disease, suggesting that regulation controls the degree of autoimmunity for years before quantities and qualities of autoantibodies and pathogenic B and T cells actually cause clinical disease. Epstein-Barr virus (EBV) may be one infectious agent that can trigger SLE in susceptible individuals. Children and adults with SLE are more

1. Genes

C1q,C2,C4
HLA-D2,3,8
MBL
FcR 2A,3A,2B
IL-10
MCP-1
PTPN22

Environment

UV light
Gender
?Infection
?EBV
Others

2. Abnormal Immune Response

DC
Ag
T cell
B cell

Defective suppressive networks

3. Autoantibodies Immune Complexes

C3
C3a

4. Inflammation

Rash
Nephritis
Arthritis
Leukopenia
CNS dz
Carditis
Clotting
Etc.

Chr. inflam.
Chr. oxid.

5. Damage

Renal Failure
Artherosclerosis
Pulm fibrosis
Stroke
Damage from Rx
Etc.

FIGURE 313-1 Pathogenesis of SLE. Genes confirmed in more than one independent cohort as increasing susceptibility to SLE or lupus nephritis are listed. Gene-environment interactions result in abnormal immune responses that generate pathogenic autoantibodies and immune complexes that deposit in tissue, activate complement, cause inflammation, and over time lead to irreversible organ damage. Ag, antigen; C1q, complement system; C3, complement component; CNS, central nervous system; DC, dendritic cell; EBV, Epstein-Barr virus; HLA, human leukocyte antigen; FcR, immunoglobulin Fc-binding receptor; IL, interleukin; MBL, mannose-binding ligand; MCP, monocyte chemotactic protein; PTPN, phosphotyrosine phosphatase; UV, ultraviolet.

TABLE 313-1 AUTOANTIBODIES IN SYSTEMIC LUPUS ERYTHEMATOSUS (SLE)

Antibody	Prevalence, %	Antigen Recognized	Clinical Utility
Antinuclear antibodies	98	Multiple nuclear	Best screening test; repeated negative tests make SLE unlikely
Anti-dsDNA	70	DNA (double-stranded)	High titers are SLE-specific and in some patients correlate with disease activity, nephritis, vasculitis
Anti-Sm	25	Protein complexed to 6 species of nuclear U1 RNA	Specific for SLE; no definite clinical correlations; most patients also have anti-RNP; more common in African Americans and Asians than Caucasians
Anti-RNP	40	Protein complexed to U1 RNAγ	Not specific for SLE; high titers associated with syndromes that have overlap features of several rheumatic syndromes including SLE; more common in African Americans than Caucasians
Anti-Ro (SS-A)	30	Protein complexed to hY RNA, primarily 60 kDa and 52 kDa	Not specific for SLE; associated with sicca syndrome, subacute cutaneous lupus, and neonatal lupus with congenital heart block; associated with decreased risk for nephritis
Anti-La (SS-B)	10	47-kDa protein complexed to hY RNA	Usually associated with anti-Ro; associated with decreased risk for nephritis
Antihistone	70	Histones associated with DNA (in nucleosome, chromatin)	More frequent in drug-induced lupus than in SLE
Antiphospholipid	50	Phospholipids, β2 glycoprotein 1 cofactor, prothrombin	Three tests available—ELISAs for cardiolipin and β2G1, sensitive prothrombin time (DRVVT); predisposes to clotting, fetal loss, thrombocytopenia
Antierythrocyte	60	Erythrocyte membrane	Measured as direct Coombs' test; a small proportion develops overt hemolysis
Antiplatelet	30	Surface and altered cytoplasmic antigens in platelets	Associated with thrombocytopenia but sensitivity and specificity are not good; this is not a useful clinical test
Antineuronal (includes anti-glutamate receptor)	60	Neuronal and lymphocyte surface antigens	In some series a positive test in CSF correlates with active CNS lupus
Antiribosomal P	20	Protein in ribosomes	In some series a positive test in serum correlates with depression or psychosis due to CNS lupus

Note: CNS, central nervous system; CSF, cerebrospinal fluid; DRVVT, dilute Russell viper venom time; ELISA, enzyme-linked immunosorbent assay.

likely to be infected by EBV than age-, sex-, and ethnicity-matched controls—an observation confirmed in African-American adults in another population. EBV activates and infects B lymphocytes and survives in those cells for decades; it also contains amino acid sequences that mimic sequences on human spliceosomes (RNA/protein antigens often recognized by autoantibodies in people with SLE). Thus, interplay between genetic susceptibility, environment, sex, and abnormal immune responses results in autoimmunity (Chap. 312).

PATHOLOGY

In SLE, biopsies of affected skin show deposition of Ig at the dermal-epidermal junction (DEJ), injury to basal keratinocytes, and inflammation dominated by T lymphocytes in the DEJ and around blood vessels and dermal appendages. Clinically unaffected skin may also show Ig deposition at the DEJ.

In renal biopsies, the pattern and severity of injury are important in diagnosis and in selecting the best therapy. Most published clinical studies of lupus nephritis have used the World Health Organization (WHO) classification of lupus nephritis. However, the International Society of Nephrology (ISN) and the Renal Pathology Society (RPS) have published a new, similar classification (Table 313-2) that will probably replace the WHO standards. An advantage of the ISN/RPS classification is the addition of "a" for active and "c" for chronic changes, giving the physician information regarding the potential reversibility of disease. All the classification systems focus on glomerular disease, although the presence of tubular interstitial and vascular disease is important to clinical outcomes. In general, class III and IV disease, as well as class V accompanied by III or IV disease, should be treated with aggressive immunosuppression if possible, because there is a high risk for end-stage renal disease (ESRD) if patients are untreated or undertreated. Treatment for lupus nephritis is not recommended in patients with class I or II disease or with extensive irreversible changes. In children, a diagnosis of SLE can be established on the basis of renal histology without meeting additional diagnostic criteria (Table 313-3).

Histologic abnormalities in blood vessels may also determine therapy. Patterns of vasculitis are not specific for SLE but may indicate active disease: leukocytoclastic vasculitis is most common (Chap. 319).

Lymph node biopsies are usually performed to rule out infection or malignancies. In SLE, they show nonspecific diffuse chronic inflammation.

DIAGNOSIS

The diagnosis of SLE is based on characteristic clinical features and autoantibodies. Current criteria (2006) for classification are listed in Table 313-3 (new criteria are being developed), and an algorithm for diagnosis and initial therapy is shown in Fig. 313-2. The criteria are intended for confirming the diagnosis of SLE in patients included in studies; the author uses them in individual patients for estimating the probability that a disease is SLE. Any combination of ≥4 of 11 criteria, well documented at any time during an individual's history, makes it likely that the patient has SLE. (Specificity and sensitivity are ~95% and ~75%, respectively.) In many patients, criteria accrue over time. Antinuclear antibodies (ANA) are positive in >98% of patients during the course of disease; repeated negative tests suggest that the diagnosis is not SLE, unless other autoantibodies are present (Fig. 313-2). High-titer IgG antibodies to double-stranded DNA and antibodies to the Sm antigen are both specific for SLE and, therefore, favor the diagnosis in the presence of compatible clinical manifestations. The presence in an individual of multiple autoantibodies without clinical symptoms should not be considered diagnostic for SLE, although such persons are at increased risk since clinical SLE begins in most patients years after autoantibodies appear.

INTERPRETATION OF CLINICAL MANIFESTATIONS

When a diagnosis of SLE is made, it is important to establish the severity and potential reversibility of the illness and to estimate the possible consequences of various therapeutic interventions. In the following paragraphs, descriptions of some disease manifestations begin with relatively mild problems and progress to those more life-threatening.

Overview and Systemic Manifestations At its onset, SLE may involve one or several organ systems; over time, additional manifestations may occur (Tables 313-3 and 313-4). Most of the autoantibodies characteristic of each person are present at the time clinical manifestations appear (Tables 313-1 and 313-3). Severity of SLE varies from mild and intermittent to severe and fulminant. Most patients experience exacer-

TABLE 313-2 CLASSIFICATION OF LUPUS NEPHRITIS (INTERNATIONAL SOCIETY OF NEPHROLOGY AND RENAL PATHOLOGY SOCIETY)

Class I: Minimal Mesangial Lupus Nephritis
Normal glomeruli by light microscopy, but mesangial immune deposits by immunofluorescence.

Class II: Mesangial Proliferative Lupus Nephritis
Purely mesangial hypercellularity of any degree or mesangial matrix expansion by light microscopy, with mesangial immune deposits. A few isolated subepithelial or subendothelial deposits may be visible by immunofluorescence or electron microscopy, but not by light microscopy.

Class III: Focal Lupus Nephritis
Active or inactive focal, segmental or global endo- or extracapillary glomerulonephritis involving <50% of all glomeruli, typically with focal subendothelial immune deposits, with or without mesangial alterations.
  Class III (A): Active lesions—focal proliferative lupus nephritis
  Class III (A/C): Active and chronic lesions—focal proliferative and sclerosing lupus nephritis
  Class III (C): Chronic inactive lesions with glomerular scars—focal sclerosing lupus nephritis

Class IV: Diffuse Lupus Nephritis
Active or inactive diffuse, segmental or global endo- or extracapillary glomerulonephritis involving 50% of all glomeruli, typically with diffuse subendothelial immune deposits, with or without mesangial alterations. This class is divided into diffuse segmental (IV-S) lupus nephritis when 50% of the involved glomeruli have segmental lesions, and diffuse global (IV-G) lupus nephritis when 50% of the involved glomeruli have global lesions. *Segmental* is defined as a glomerular lesion that involves less than half of the glomerular tuft. This class includes cases with diffuse wire loop deposits but with little or no glomerular proliferation.
  Class IV-S (A): Active lesions—diffuse segmental proliferative lupus nephritis
  Class IV-G (A): Active lesions—diffuse global proliferative lupus nephritis
  Class IV-S (A/C): Active and chronic lesions—diffuse segmental proliferative and sclerosing lupus nephritis
  Class IV-G (A/C): Active and chronic lesions—diffuse global proliferative and sclerosing lupus nephritis
  Class IV-S (C): Chronic inactive lesions with scars—diffuse segmental sclerosing lupus nephritis
  Class IV-G (C): Chronic inactive lesions with scars—diffuse global sclerosing lupus nephritis

Class V: Membranous Lupus Nephritis
Global or segmental subepithelial immune deposits or their morphologic sequelae by light microscopy and by immunofluorescence or electron microscopy, with or without mesangial alterations. Class V lupus nephritis may occur in combination with class III or IV, in which case both will be diagnosed. Class V lupus nephritis may show advanced sclerosis.

Class VI: Advanced Sclerotic Lupus Nephritis
≥90% of glomeruli globally sclerosed without residual activity.

Indicate and grade (mild, moderate, severe) tubular atrophy, interstitial inflammation and fibrosis, severity of arteriosclerosis or other vascular lesions.
Source: JJ Weening et al: Kidney Int 65:521, 2004. Reprinted by permission from Macmillan Publishers Ltd., Copyright 2004.

bations interspersed with periods of relative quiescence; permanent complete remissions (absence of symptoms with no treatment) are rare. Systemic symptoms, particularly fatigue and myalgias/arthralgias, are present most of the time. Severe systemic illness requiring glucocorticoid therapy can occur with fever, prostration, weight loss, and anemia with or without other organ-targeted manifestations.

Musculoskeletal Manifestations   Most people with SLE have intermittent polyarthritis, varying from mild to disabling, characterized by soft tissue swelling and tenderness in joints, most commonly in hands, wrists, and knees. Joint deformities (hands and feet) develop in only 10%. Erosions on joint x-rays are rare; their presence suggests a non-lupus inflammatory arthropathy such as rheumatoid arthritis (Chap. 314); some experts think that erosions can occur in SLE. If pain persists in a single joint, such as knee, shoulder, or hip, a diagnosis of ischemic necrosis of bone should be considered, particularly if there are no other manifestations of active SLE. The prevalence of ischemic necrosis of bone is increased in SLE, especially in patients treated with systemic glucocorticoids. Myositis with clinical muscle weakness, elevated creatine kinase levels, positive MRI scan, and muscle necrosis and inflammation on biopsy can occur, although most patients have myalgias without frank myositis. Glucocorticoid thera-

pies (commonly) and antimalarial therapies (rarely) can also cause muscle weakness; these adverse effects must be distinguished from active disease.

Cutaneous Manifestations   Lupus dermatitis can be classified as discoid lupus erythematosus (DLE), systemic rash, subacute cutaneous lupus erythematosus (SCLE), or "other." Discoid lesions are roughly circular with slightly raised, scaly hyperpigmented erythematous rims and depigmented, atrophic centers in which all dermal appendages are permanently destroyed. Lesions can be disfiguring, particularly on the face and scalp. Treatment consists primarily of topical or locally injected glucocorticoids and systemic antimalarials. Only 5% of people with DLE have SLE (although half have positive ANA); however, among individuals with SLE, as many as 20% have DLE. The most common SCLE rash is a photosensitive, slightly raised erythema, occasionally scaly, on the face (particularly the cheeks and nose—the "butterfly" rash), ears, chin, V region of the neck, upper back, and extensor surfaces of the arms. Worsening of this rash often accompanies flare of systemic disease. SCLE consists of scaly red patches similar to psoriasis or circular flat red-rimmed lesions. Patients with these manifestations are exquisitely photosensitive; most have antibodies to Ro (SS-A). Other SLE rashes include recurring urticaria, lichen planus–like dermatitis, bullae, and panniculitis ("lupus profundus"). Rashes can be minor or severe; they may be the major disease manifestation. Small, painful ulcerations on the oral or nasal mucosa are common in SLE; the lesions resemble aphthous ulcers.

Renal Manifestations   Nephritis is usually the most serious manifestation of SLE, particularly since nephritis and infection are the leading causes of mortality in the first decade of disease. Since nephritis is asymptomatic in most lupus patients, urinalysis should be ordered in any person suspected of having SLE. The classification of lupus nephritis is primarily histologic (see "Pathology," above, and Table 313-2). Renal biopsy is useful in planning current and near-future therapies. Patients with dangerous proliferative forms of glomerular damage (ISN III and IV) usually have microscopic hematuria and proteinuria (>500 mg per 24 h); approximately one-half develop nephrotic syndrome, and most develop hypertension. If diffuse proliferative glomerulonephritis (DPGN) is untreated, virtually all patients develop ESRD within 2 years of diagnosis. Therefore, aggressive immunosup-

TABLE 313-3 DIAGNOSTIC CRITERIA FOR SYSTEMIC LUPUS ERYTHEMATOSUS

Malar rash	Fixed erythema, flat or raised, over the malar eminences
Discoid rash	Erythematous circular raised patches with adherent keratotic scaling and follicular plugging; atrophic scarring may occur
Photosensitivity	Exposure to ultraviolet light causes rash
Oral ulcers	Includes oral and nasopharyngeal ulcers, observed by physician
Arthritis	Nonerosive arthritis of two or more peripheral joints, with tenderness, swelling, or effusion
Serositis	Pleuritis or pericarditis documented by ECG or rub or evidence of effusion
Renal disorder	Proteinuria >0.5 g/d or ≥3+, or cellular casts
Neurologic disorder	Seizures or psychosis without other causes
Hematologic disorder	Hemolytic anemia or leukopenia (<4000/μL) or lymphopenia (<1500/μL) or thrombocytopenia (<100,000/μL) in the absence of offending drugs
Immunologic disorder	Anti-dsDNA, anti-Sm, and/or anti-phospholipid
Antinuclear antibodies	An abnormal titer of ANA by immunofluorescence or an equivalent assay at any point in time in the absence of drugs known to induce ANAs

If ≥4 of these criteria, well documented, are present at any time in a patient's history, the diagnosis is likely to be SLE. Specificity is ~95%; sensitivity is ~75%.
Note: ANA, antinuclear antibodies; dsDNA, double-strand DNA; ECG, electrocardiography.
Source: Criteria published by EM Tan et al: Arthritis Rheum 25:1271, 1982; update by MC Hochberg, Arthritis Rheum 40:1725, 1997.

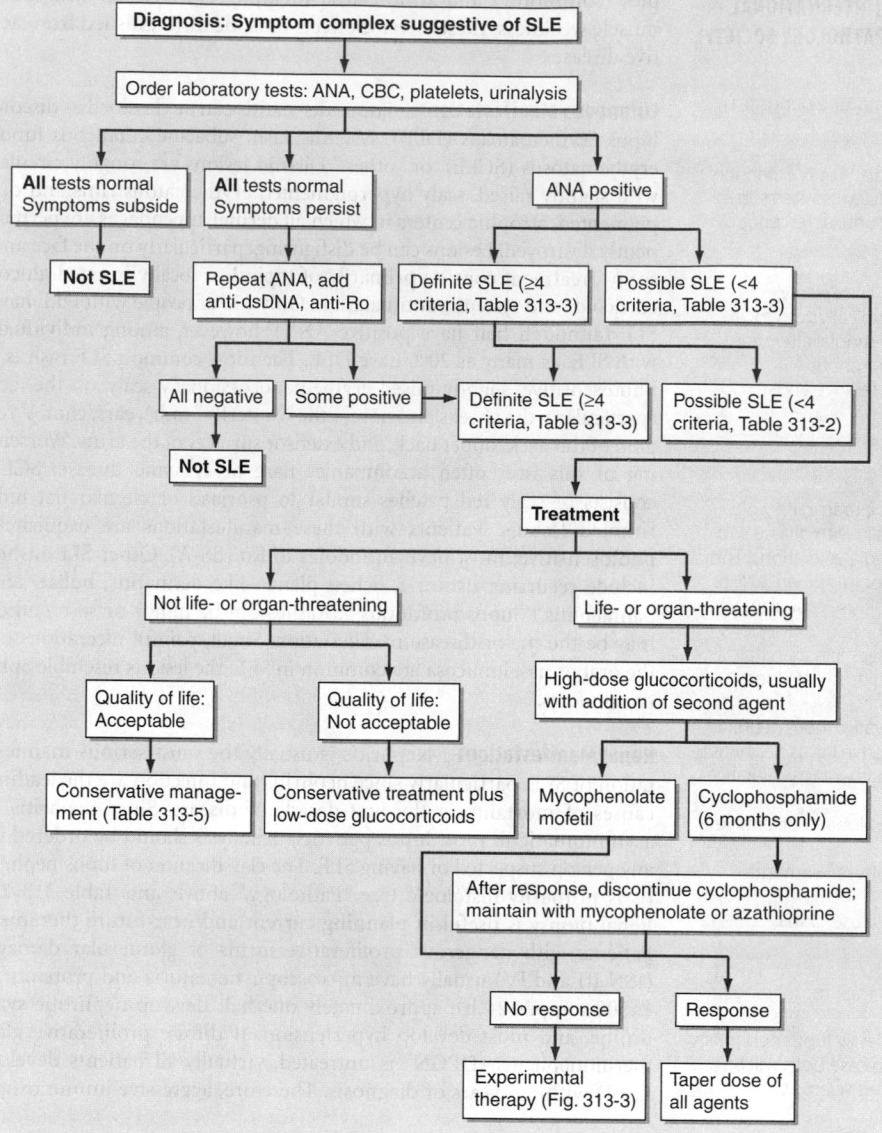

FIGURE 313-2 Algorithm for diagnosis and initial therapy of SLE. ANA, antinuclear antibodies; CBC, complete blood count.

pression is indicated (usually systemic glucocorticoids plus a cytotoxic drug), unless damage is irreversible (Fig. 313-2, Table 313-5). African Americans are more likely to develop ESRD than are Caucasians, even with the most current therapies. Overall in the United States, ~20% of individuals with lupus DPGN die or develop ESRD within 10 years of diagnosis. Such individuals require aggressive control of SLE and of the complications of renal disease and of therapy. A small proportion of SLE patients with proteinuria (usually nephrotic) have membranous glomerular changes without proliferation on renal biopsy. Their outcome is better than for those with DPGN, but proteinuria is less likely to improve on lupus nephritis immunosuppressive therapies. Lupus nephritis tends to be an ongoing disease, with flares requiring re-treatment over many years. For most people with lupus nephritis, accelerated atherosclerosis becomes important after several years of disease; attention must be given to control of blood pressure, hyperlipidemia, and hyperglycemia.

Nervous System Manifestations   There are many central nervous system (CNS) and peripheral nervous system manifestations of SLE; in some patients these are the major cause of morbidity and mortality. It is useful to approach this diagnostically by asking first whether the symptoms result from SLE or another condition (such as infection in immunosuppressed individuals). If symptoms are related to SLE, it

should be determined whether they are caused by a diffuse process or vascular occlusive disease. The most common manifestation of diffuse CNS lupus is cognitive dysfunction, including difficulties with memory and reasoning. Headaches are also common. When excruciating, they often indicate SLE flare; when milder, they are difficult to distinguish from migraine or tension headaches. Seizures of any type may be caused by lupus; treatment often requires both antiseizure and immunosuppressive therapies. Psychosis can be the dominant manifestation of SLE; it must be distinguished from glucocorticoid-induced psychosis. The latter usually occurs in the first weeks of glucocorticoid therapy, at daily doses of ≥40 mg of prednisone or equivalent; psychosis resolves over several days after glucocorticoids are decreased or stopped. Myelopathy is not rare and is often disabling; rapid immunosuppressive therapy starting with glucocorticoids is standard of care.

Vascular Occlusions   The prevalence of transient ischemic attacks, strokes, and myocardial infarctions is increased in patients with SLE. These vascular events are increased in, but not exclusive to, SLE patients with antibodies to phospholipids (aPL). It is likely that antiphospholipid antibodies are associated with hypercoagulability and acute thrombotic events, whereas chronic disease is associated with accelerated atherosclerosis. Ischemia in the brain can be caused by focal occlusion (either noninflammatory or associated with vasculitis) or by embolization from carotid artery plaque or from fibrinous vegetations of Libman-Sacks endocarditis. Appropriate tests for aPL (see below) and for sources of emboli should be ordered in such patients to estimate the need for, intensity of, and duration of anti-inflammatory and/or anticoagulant therapies. In SLE, myocardial infarctions are primarily manifestations of accelerated atherosclerosis. The increased risk for vascular events is seven- to tenfold overall, and higher in women <45 years old with SLE. Characteristics associated with increased risk for atherosclerosis include older age, hypertension, dyslipidemia, dysfunctional proinflammatory high-density lipoproteins, repeated high scores for disease activity, high cumulative or daily doses of glucocorticoids, and high levels of homocysteine. When it is most likely that an event results from clotting, long-term anticoagulation is the therapy of choice. Two processes can occur at once—vasculitis plus bland vascular occlusions—in which case it is appropriate to treat with anticoagulation plus immunosuppression. The role of statin therapies in SLE is being investigated.

Pulmonary Manifestations   The most common pulmonary manifestation of SLE is pleuritis with or without pleural effusion. This manifestation, when mild, may respond to treatment with nonsteroidal anti-inflammatory drugs (NSAIDs); when more severe, patients require a brief course of glucocorticoid therapy. Pulmonary infiltrates also occur as a manifestation of active SLE and are difficult to distinguish from infection on imaging studies. Life-threatening pulmonary manifestations include interstitial inflammation leading to fibrosis, shrinking lung syndrome, and intraalveolar hemorrhage; all of these probably require early aggressive immunosuppressive therapy as well as supportive care.

TABLE 313-4	CLINICAL MANIFESTATIONS OF SLE AND PREVALENCE OVER THE ENTIRE COURSE OF DISEASE[a]

Manifestation	Prevalence, %
Systemic: Fatigue, malaise, fever, anorexia, weight loss	95
Musculoskeletal	95
Arthralgias/myalgias	95
Nonerosive polyarthritis	60
Hand deformities	10
Myopathy/myositis	25/5
Ischemic necrosis of bone	15
Cutaneous	80
Photosensitivity	70
Malar rash	50
Oral ulcers	40
Alopecia	40
Discoid rash	20
Vasculitis rash	20
Other (e.g., urticaria, subacute cutaneous lupus)	15
Hematologic	85
Anemia (chronic disease)	70
Leukopenia (<4000/μL)	65
Lymphopenia (<1500/μL)	50
Thrombocytopenia (<100,000/μL)	15
Lymphadenopathy	15
Splenomegaly	15
Hemolytic anemia	10
Neurologic	60
Cognitive disorder	50
Mood disorder	40
Headache	25
Seizures	20
Mono-, polyneuropathy	15
Stroke, TIA	10
Acute confusional state or movement disorder	2–5
Aseptic meningitis, myelopathy	<1
Cardiopulmonary	60
Pleurisy, pericarditis, effusions	30–50
Myocarditis, endocarditis	10
Lupus pneumonitis	10
Coronary artery disease	10
Interstitial fibrosis	5
Pulmonary hypertension, ARDS, hemorrhage	<5
Shrinking lung syndrome	<5
Renal	30–50
Proteinuria >500 mg/24 h, cellular casts	30–50
Nephrotic syndrome	25
End-stage renal disease	5–10
Gastrointestinal	40
Nonspecific (nausea, mild pain, diarrhea)	30
Abnormal liver enzymes	40
Vasculitis	5
Thrombosis	15
Venous	10
Arterial	5
Ocular	15
Sicca syndrome	15
Conjunctivitis, episcleritis	10
Vasculitis	5

[a]Numbers indicate percent of patients who have the manifestation at some time during the course of illness.

Note: ARDS, acute respiratory distress syndrome; TIA, transient ischemic attack.

Cardiac Manifestations Pericarditis is the most frequent cardiac manifestation; it usually responds to anti-inflammatory therapy and infrequently leads to tamponade. More serious cardiac manifestations are myocarditis and fibrinous endocarditis of Libman-Sacks. The endocardial involvement can lead to valvular insufficiencies, most commonly of the mitral or aortic valves, or to embolic events. It has not been proven that glucocorticoid or other immunosuppressive therapies lead to improvement of lupus myocarditis or endocarditis, but it is usual practice to administer a trial of high-dose steroids along with appropriate supportive therapy for heart failure, arrhythmia, or embolic events. As discussed above, patients with SLE are at increased risk for myocardial infarction, usually due to accelerated atherosclerosis,

which probably results from chronic inflammation and/or chronic oxidative damage to lipids and to organs.

Hematologic Manifestations The most frequent hematologic manifestation of SLE is anemia, usually normochromic normocytic, reflecting chronic illness. Hemolysis can be rapid in onset and severe, requiring high-dose glucocorticoid therapy, which is effective in most patients. Leukopenia is also common and almost always consists of lymphopenia, not granulocytopenia; this rarely predisposes to infections and by itself usually does not require therapy. Thrombocytopenia may be a recurring problem. If platelet counts are >40,000/μL and abnormal bleeding is absent, therapy may not be required. High-dose glucocorticoid therapy (e.g., 1 mg/kg per day of prednisone or equivalent) is usually effective for the first few episodes of severe thrombocytopenia. Recurring or prolonged hemolytic anemia or thrombocytopenia, or disease requiring an unacceptably high dose of daily glucocorticoids, should be treated with an additional strategy (see "Treatment," below).

Gastrointestinal Manifestations Nausea, sometimes with vomiting, and diarrhea can be manifestations of an SLE flare, as can diffuse abdominal pain caused by autoimmune peritonitis and/or intestinal vasculitis. Increases in serum aspartate aminotransferase (AST) and alanine aminotransferase (ALT) are common when SLE is active. These manifestations usually improve promptly during systemic glucocorticoid therapy. Vasculitis involving the intestine may be life-threatening; perforations, ischemia, bleeding, and sepsis are frequent complications. Aggressive immunosuppressive therapy with high-dose glucocorticoids is recommended for short-term control; evidence of recurrence is an indication for additional therapies.

Ocular Manifestations Sicca syndrome (Sjögren's syndrome; Chap. 317) and nonspecific conjunctivitis are common in SLE and rarely threaten vision. In contrast, retinal vasculitis and optic neuritis are serious manifestations: blindness can develop over days to weeks. Aggressive immunosuppression is recommended, although there are no controlled trials to prove effectiveness. Complications of glucocorticoid therapy include cataracts (common) and glaucoma.

LABORATORY TESTS

Laboratory tests serve (1) to establish or rule out the diagnosis; (2) to follow the course of disease, particularly to suggest that a flare is occurring or organ damage is developing; and (3) to identify adverse effects of therapies.

Tests for Autoantibodies (Tables 313-1 and 313-3) Diagnostically, the most important autoantibodies to detect are ANA since the test is positive in >95% of patients, usually at the onset of symptoms. A few patients develop ANA within 1 year of symptom onset; repeated testing may thus be useful. ANA-negative lupus exists but is very rare in adults and is usually associated with other autoantibodies (anti-Ro or anti-DNA). High-titer IgG antibodies to double-stranded DNA (dsDNA) (but not to single-stranded DNA) are specific for SLE. There is no international standardized test for ANA; variability between different service laboratories is high. Enzyme-linked immunosorbent assays (ELISA) and immunofluorescent reactions of sera with the dsDNA in the flagellate *Crithidia luciliae* have ~60% sensitivity for SLE; identification of high-avidity anti-dsDNA in the Farr assay is not as sensitive but may correlate better with risk for nephritis. Titers of anti-dsDNA vary over time. In some patients, increases in quantities of anti-dsDNA herald a flare, particularly of nephritis or vasculitis. Antibodies to Sm are also specific for SLE and assist in diagnosis; anti-Sm antibodies do not usually correlate with disease activity or clinical manifestations. aPL are not specific for SLE, but their presence fulfills one classification criterion and they identify patients at increased risk for venous or arterial clotting, thrombocytopenia, and fetal loss. There are two widely accepted tests that measure different antibodies (anticardiolipin and the lupus anticoagulant): (1) ELISA for anticardiolipin (internationally standardized with good reproducibility) and (2) a sensitive phospholipid-based activated prothrombin time such as the dilute Russell venom viper test. Some centers also recommend measurement of anti-

TABLE 313-5 MEDICATIONS FOR THE MANAGEMENT OF SLE

Medication	Dose Range	Drug Interactions	Serious or Common Adverse Effects
NSAIDs, salicylates (Ecotrin[a] and St. Joseph's aspirin[a] approved by FDA for use in SLE)	Doses toward upper limit of recommended range usually required	A2R/ACE inhibitors, glucocorticoids, fluconazole, methotrexate, thiazides	NSAIDs: Higher incidence of aseptic meningitis, transaminitis, decreased renal function, vasculitis of skin; entire class, especially COX-2-specific inhibitors, may increase risk for myocardial infarction Salicylates: ototoxicity, tinnitus Both: GI events and symptoms, allergic reactions, dermatitis, dizziness, acute renal failure, edema, hypertension
Topical glucocorticoids	Mid-potency for face; mid to high potency other areas	None known	Atrophy of skin, contact dermatitis, folliculitis, hypopigmentation, infection
Topical sunscreens	SPF 15 at least; 30+ preferred	None known	Contact dermatitis
Hydroxychloroquine[a] (quinacrine can be added or substituted)	200–400 mg qd (100 mg qd)	None known	Retinal damage, agranulocytosis, aplastic anemia, ataxia, cardiomyopathy, dizziness, myopathy, ototoxicity, peripheral neuropathy, pigmentation of skin, seizures, thrombocytopenia Quinacrine usually causes diffuse yellow skin coloration
DHEA (dehydroepiandrosterone)	200 mg qd	Unclear	Acne, menstrual irregularities, high serum levels of testosterone
Methotrexate b (for dermatitis, arthritis)	10–25 mg once a week, PO or SC, with folic acid; decrease dose if CrCl < 60 mL/min	Acitretin, leflunomide, NSAIDs and salicylates, penicillins, probenecid, sulfonamides, trimethoprim	Anemia, bone marrow suppression, leucopenia, thrombocytopenia, hepatotoxicity, nephrotoxicity, infections, neurotoxicity, pulmonary fibrosis, pneumonitis, severe dermatitis, seizures
Glucocorticoids, oral[a] (several specific brands are approved by FDA for use in SLE)	Prednisone, prednisolone: 0.5–1 mg/kg per day for severe SLE 0.07–0.3 mg/kg per day or qod for milder disease	A2R/ACE antagonists, antiarrhythmics class III, β2, cyclosporine, NSAIDs and salicylates, phenothiazines, phenytoins, quinolones, rifampin, risperidone, thiazides, sulfonylureas, warfarin	Infection, VZV infection, hypertension, hyperglycemia, hypokalemia, acne, allergic reactions, anxiety, aseptic necrosis of bone, cushingoid changes, CHF, fragile skin, insomnia, menstrual irregularities, mood swings, osteoporosis, psychosis
Methylprednisolone sodium succinate, IV[a] (approved for lupus nephritis)	For severe disease, 1 g IV qd × 3 days	As for oral glucocorticoids	As for oral glucocorticoids (if used repeatedly); anaphylaxis
Cyclophosphamide[b] IV Oral	7–25 mg/kg q month × 6; consider mesna administration with dose 1.5–3 mg/kg per day Decrease dose for CrCl < 25 mL/min	Allopurinol, bone marrow suppressants, colony-stimulating factors, doxorubicin, rituximab, succinylcholine, zidovudine	Infection, VZV infection, bone marrow suppression, leukopenia, anemia, thrombocytopenia, hemorrhagic cystitis (less with IV), carcinoma of the bladder, alopecia, nausea, diarrhea, malaise, malignancy, ovarian and testicular failure
Mycophenolate mofetil[b]	2–3 g/d PO; decrease dose if CrCl <25 mL/min	Acyclovir, antacids, azathioprine, bile acid–binding resins, ganciclovir, iron, salts, probenecid, oral contraceptives	Infection, leukopenia, anemia, thrombocytopenia, lymphoma, lymphoproliferative disorders, malignancy, alopecia, cough, diarrhea, fever, GI symptoms, headache, hypertension, hypercholesterolemia, hypokalemia, insomnia, peripheral edema, transaminitis, tremor, rash
Azathioprine[b]	2–3 mg/kg per day PO; decrease frequency of dose if CrCl < 50 mL/min	ACE inhibitors, allopurinol, bone marrow suppressants, interferons, mycophenolate mofetil, rituximab, warfarin, zidovudine	Infection, VZV infection, bone marrow suppression, leukopenia, anemia, thrombocytopenia, pancreatitis, hepatotoxicity, malignancy, alopecia, fever, flulike illness, GI symptoms

[a]Indicates medication is approved for use in SLE by the U.S. Food and Drug Administration.

[b]Indicates the medication has been used with glucocorticoids in the trials showing efficacy.

Note: A2R, angiotensin 2 receptor; ACE, angiotensin-converting enzyme; CHF, congestive heart failure; CrCl, creatinine clearance; FDA, U.S. Food and Drug Administration; GI, gastrointestinal; NSAIDs, nonsteroidal anti-inflammatory drugs; SPF, sun protection factor; VZV, varicella-zoster virus.

bodies to β2 glycoprotein 1, a serum protein cofactor that is the target of most antibodies to cardiolipin and some lupus anticoagulants. High titers of IgG anticardiolipin (>50 IU) indicate high risk for a clinical episode of clotting. Quantities of aPL may vary markedly over time; repeated testing is justified if clinical manifestations of the antiphospholipid antibody syndrome (APS) appear. To make a diagnosis of APS, with or without SLE, requires the presence of clotting and/or repeated fetal losses plus at least two positive tests for aPL, at least 12 weeks apart.

An additional autoantibody test with predictive value (not used for diagnosis) detects anti-Ro, which indicates increased risk for neonatal lupus, sicca syndrome, and SCLE. Women with child-bearing potential and SLE should be screened for aPL and anti-Ro.

Standard Tests for Diagnosis Screening tests for complete blood count, platelet count, and urinalysis may detect abnormalities that contribute to the diagnosis and influence management decisions.

Tests for Following Disease Course It is useful to follow tests that indicate the status of organ involvement known to be present during SLE flares. These might include hemoglobin levels, platelet counts, urinalysis,

and serum levels of creatinine or albumin. There is great interest in identification of additional markers of disease activity. Candidates include levels of anti-DNA antibodies, several components of complement (C3 is most widely available), activated complement products (including those that bind to the C4d receptor on erythrocytes), IFN-inducible genes, soluble IL-2, and urinary adiponectin or monocyte chemotactic protein 1. None is uniformly agreed upon as a reliable indicator of flare or of response to therapeutic interventions. The physician should determine for each patient whether certain laboratory test changes predict flare. If so, altering therapy in response to these changes has been shown to prevent flares. In addition, given the increased prevalence of atherosclerosis in SLE, it is advisable to follow the recommendations of the National Cholesterol Education Program for testing and treatment, including scoring of SLE as an independent risk factor, similar to diabetes mellitus.

℞ SYSTEMIC LUPUS ERYTHEMATOSUS

There is no cure for SLE, and complete sustained remissions are rare. Therefore, the physician should plan to control acute, severe flares and then develop maintenance strategies that suppress symptoms to an acceptable level and prevent organ damage. Usually patients will endure some adverse effects of medications. Therapeutic choices depend on (1) whether disease manifestations are life-threatening or likely to cause organ damage, justifying aggressive therapies; (2) whether manifestations are potentially reversible; and (3) the best approaches to preventing complications of disease and its treatments. Therapies, doses, and adverse effects are listed in Table 313-5.

CONSERVATIVE THERAPIES FOR MANAGEMENT OF NON-LIFE-THREATENING DISEASE
Among patients with fatigue, pain, and autoantibodies of SLE, but without major organ involvement, management can be directed to suppression of symptoms. Analgesics and antimalarials are mainstays. NSAIDs are useful analgesics/anti-inflammatories, particularly for arthritis/arthralgias. However, two major issues currently indicate caution in using NSAIDs. First, SLE patients compared with the general population are at increased risk for NSAID-induced aseptic meningitis, elevated serum transaminases, hypertension, and renal dysfunction. Second, all NSAIDs, particularly those that inhibit cyclooxygenase-2 specifically, may increase risk for myocardial infarction. Acetaminophen to control pain may be a good strategy, but NSAIDs may be more effective in some patients, and the relative hazards of NSAIDs compared with low-dose glucocorticoid therapy have not been established. Antimalarials (hydroxychloroquine, chloroquine, and quinacrine) often reduce dermatitis, arthritis, and fatigue. A randomized, placebo-controlled, prospective trial has shown that hydroxychloroquine reduces the number of disease flares; it may also reduce accrual of tissue damage over time. Because of potential retinal toxicity, patients receiving antimalarials should undergo ophthalmologic examinations at least annually. A placebo-controlled prospective trial suggests that administration of dehydroepiandrosterone may reduce disease activity. If quality of life is inadequate in spite of these conservative measures, treatment with low doses of systemic glucocorticoids may be necessary.

LIFE-THREATENING SLE: PROLIFERATIVE FORMS OF LUPUS NEPHRITIS
The mainstay of treatment for any inflammatory life-threatening or organ-threatening manifestations of SLE is systemic glucocorticoids (0.5–2 mg/kg per day PO or 1000 mg of methylprednisolone sodium succinate IV daily for 3 days followed by 0.5–1 mg/kg of daily prednisone or equivalent). Evidence that glucocorticoid therapy is life-saving comes from retrospective studies from the predialysis era; survival is significantly better in people with DPGN treated with high-dose daily glucocorticoids (40–60 mg of prednisone daily for 4–6 months) versus lower doses. Currently, high doses are recommended for much shorter periods; recent trials of interventions for severe SLE employ 4–6 weeks of these doses. Thereafter, doses are tapered as rapidly as the clinical situation permits, usually to a maintenance dose varying from 5 to 10 mg of prednisone or equivalent per day or from 10 to 20 mg every other day. Most patients with an episode of severe lupus require many years of maintenance therapy with low-dose glucocorticoids, which can be increased to prevent or treat disease flares. Frequent attempts to gradually reduce the glucocorticoid requirement are recommended since virtually everyone develops important adverse effects (Table 313-5). Prospective controlled trials in active lupus nephritis show that administration of high doses of glucocorticoids (1000 mg of methylprednisolone daily for 3 days) by intravenous routes compared with daily oral routes shortens the time to maximal improvement by a few weeks but does not result in better renal function. It has become standard practice to initiate therapy for active, potentially life-threatening SLE with high-dose IV glucocorticoid pulses, based on studies in lupus nephritis. This approach must be tempered by safety considerations, such as the presence of conditions adversely affected by glucocorticoids (infection, hyperglycemia, hypertension, osteoporosis, etc.).

Cytotoxic/immunosuppressive agents added to glucocorticoids are recommended to treat serious SLE. Almost all prospective controlled trials in SLE involving cytotoxic agents have been conducted in patients with lupus nephritis, and always in combination with glucocorticoids. Therefore, the following recommendations apply to treatment of nephritis; there is little information regarding the efficacy of mycophenolate mofetil in other forms of SLE. Either cyclophosphamide (an alkylating agent) or mycophenolate mofetil (a relatively lymphocyte-specific inhibitor of inosine monophosphatase and therefore of purine synthesis) is an acceptable choice for induction of improvement in severely ill patients; azathioprine (a purine analogue and cycle-specific antimetabolite) may be effective but is slower to influence response. In patients whose renal biopsies show ISN grade III or IV disease, early treatment with combinations of glucocorticoids and cyclophospha-

mide reduces progression to ESRD and improves survival. Short-term studies with glucocorticoids plus mycophenolate mofetil show that this regimen is safer than and not inferior to cyclophosphamide in inducing improvement, and that mycophenolate (or azathioprine) is safer than cyclophosphamide in maintaining improvement after a 6-month induction phase. If cyclophosphamide is used, the recommended dose is 500–750 mg/m^2 intravenously, monthly for 3–6 months, then discontinuation with introduction of mycophenolate or azathioprine. The incidence of ovarian failure, a common effect of cyclophosphamide therapy, can be reduced by treatment with a gonadotropin-releasing hormone agonist prior to each cyclophosphamide dose. European studies have suggested that cyclophosphamide at doses of 500 mg total every 2 weeks for six doses is as effective as the higher dose and longer duration recommended above, over a period of 5–7 years. The great majority of those patients were Caucasian; it is not clear that the data apply to all U.S. populations. Cyclophosphamide and mycophenolate responses begin 3–16 weeks after treatment is initiated, whereas glucocorticoid responses may begin within 24 h. Patients with high serum creatinine levels [e.g., ≥265 μmol/L (>3.0 mg/dL)] many months in duration and high chronicity scores on renal biopsy are not likely to respond. Regarding the efficacy of mycophenolate compared with cyclophosphamide, most studies of the former are short-term (<5 years). Such data are useful but may not adequately describe the overall utility of that approach, since cyclophosphamide compared with glucocorticoids alone reduces ESRD—a change that can be detected in study cohorts ~5 years after therapy is introduced. The recommended duration of cyclophosphamide therapy is controversial. There are data to support treatment (1) once monthly IV for 6 months followed by 2 more years of quarterly doses, (2) for 12 weeks followed by azathioprine, and (3) for 6 months followed by azathioprine or mycophenolate. In general, cyclophosphamide may be discontinued when it is clear that a patient is improving; possibility of disease flare is reduced by continuing therapy with one of the cytotoxic/immunosuppressive drugs discussed above. Response of lupus nephritis to cyclophosphamide and glucocorticoids is better in Caucasian groups than in African Americans. Mycophenolate may be a better choice for African Americans, but results of long-term studies are needed before this recommendation can be validated. The adverse effects most likely to influence patient choice against the use of cyclophosphamide are a high rate of irreversible ovarian or testicular failure with increasing cumulative doses, nausea and malaise that often accompany each IV dose, alopecia, and frequent infections.

Since glucocorticoid-plus-cyclophosphamide therapy has many adverse effects and is often disliked by patients, there has been a search for different therapies that are less toxic; this led to the recent study and use of mycophenolate. Azathioprine (a purine antagonist) added to glucocorticoids probably reduces the number of SLE flares and the maintenance glucocorticoid requirement; it can also help sustain improvement induced by faster-acting treatments (glucocorticoids plus mycophenolate or cyclophosphamide). Patients who have homozygous deficiency of the TMPT enzyme, which is required to metabolize the 6-mercaptopurine product of azathioprine, should not receive azathioprine because they are at increased risk for bone marrow suppression. Daily oral azathioprine has fewer adverse effects than cyclophosphamide. Good improvement occurs in ~80% of lupus nephritis patients receiving either cyclophosphamide or mycophenolate at 1–2 years of follow-up. However, at least 50% of these individuals have flares of nephritis over the next 5 years, and re-treatment is required. Chlorambucil is an alkylating agent that can be substituted for cyclophosphamide; the risk of irreversible bone marrow suppression may be greater with this agent. Methotrexate (a folinic acid antagonist) may have a role in the treatment of arthritis and dermatitis but probably not in life-threatening disease. The role of leflunomide, a relatively lymphocyte-specific pyrimidine antagonist licensed for use in rheumatoid arthritis, is being studied in patients with SLE. Cyclosporine, which inhibits production of IL-2 and inhibits T lymphocyte functions, has not been studied in prospective controlled trials in SLE but is nonetheless used by some clinicians. Since it has potential nephrotoxicity, but no bone marrow toxicity, the author uses it (in doses of 3–5 mg/kg per day PO) in patients with steroid-resistant cytopenias of SLE or in steroid-resistant patients who have developed bone marrow suppression from standard cytotoxic agents.

It is important to note that there are few if any randomized, controlled, prospective studies of any agents in life-threatening SLE that does not include nephritis. Therefore, use of glucocorticoids plus cyclophosphamide or mycophenolate in other life-threatening conditions is based on studies in nephritis.

SPECIAL CONDITIONS IN SLE THAT MAY REQUIRE ADDITIONAL OR DIFFERENT THERAPIES   Pregnancy and Lupus

Fertility rates for men and women with SLE are probably normal. However, rate of fetal loss is increased (approximately two- to threefold) in women with SLE. Fetal demise is higher in mothers with high disease activity, antiphospholipid antibodies, and/or nephritis. Suppression of disease activity can be achieved by administration of systemic glucocorticoids. A placental enzyme, 11-β-dehydrogenase 2, deactivates glucocorticoids; it is more effective in deactivating prednisone and prednisolone than the fluorinated glucocorticoids dexamethasone and betamethasone. Therefore, maternal SLE should be controlled with prednisone/prednisolone at the lowest effective doses for the shortest time required. Adverse effects of prenatal glucocorticoid exposure (primarily betamethasone) on offspring may include low birth weight, developmental abnormalities in the CNS, and predilection toward adult metabolic syndrome. In SLE patients with aPL (on at least two occasions) and prior fetal losses, treatment with heparin (standard or low-molecular-weight) plus low-dose aspirin has been shown in prospective controlled trials to increase significantly the proportion of live births. An additional potential problem for the fetus is the presence of antibodies to Ro, sometimes associated with neonatal lupus consisting of rash and congenital heart block. The latter can be life-threatening; therefore the presence of anti-Ro requires vigilant monitoring of fetal heart rates with prompt intervention (delivery if possible) if distress occurs. Women with SLE usually tolerate pregnancy without disease flares. However, a small proportion develops severe flares requiring aggressive glucocorticoid therapy or early delivery. Poor maternal outcomes are highest in women with active nephritis or irreversible organ damage in kidneys, brain, or heart.

Lupus and Antiphospholipid Antibody Syndrome   Patients with SLE who have venous or arterial clotting, and/or repeated fetal losses, and at least two positive tests for aPL have APS and should be managed with long-term anticoagulation. A target international normalized ratio (INR) of 2.0–2.5 is recommended for patients with one episode of venous clotting; an INR of 3.0–3.5 is recommended for patients with recurring clots or arterial clotting, particularly in the central nervous system. Recommendations are based on both retrospective and prospective studies of posttreatment clotting events and adverse effects from anticoagulation.

Microvascular Thrombotic Crisis (Thrombotic Thrombocytopenic Purpura, Hemolytic Uremic Syndrome)   This syndrome of hemolysis, thrombocytopenia, and microvascular thrombosis in kidneys, brain, and other tissues carries a high mortality rate and occurs most commonly in young individuals with lupus nephritis. The most useful laboratory tests are identification of schistocytes on peripheral blood smears and elevated serum levels of lactate dehydrogenase. Plasma exchange or extensive plasmapheresis is usually life-saving; there is no evidence that cytotoxic drugs are effective.

Lupus Dermatitis   Patients with any form of lupus dermatitis should minimize exposure to ultraviolet light, employing appropriate clothing and sunscreens with a sun protection factor of at least 15. Topical glucocorticoids and antimalarials (such as hydroxychloroquine) are effective in reducing lesion severity in most patients and are relatively safe. Systemic treatment with retinoic acid is a useful strategy in patients with inadequate improvement on topical glucocorticoids and antimalarials; adverse effects are potentially severe (particularly fetal abnormalities), and there are stringent reporting requirements for its use in the United States. Extensive, pruritic, bullous, or ulcerating dermatitides usually improve promptly after institution of systemic glucocorticoids; tapering may be accompanied by flare of lesions, thus necessitating use of a second medication such as hydroxychloroquine, ret-

inoids, or cytotoxic medications such as methotrexate or azathioprine. In therapy-resistant lupus dermatitis there are reports of success with topical tacrolimus (caution must be exerted because of the possible increased risk for malignancies) or with systemic dapsone or thalidomide (the extreme danger of fetal deformities from thalidomide requires permission from and supervision by the supplier).

PREVENTIVE THERAPIES   Prevention of complications of SLE and its therapy include providing appropriate vaccinations (the administration of influenza and pneumococcal vaccines has been studied in patients with SLE; flare rates are similar to those receiving placebo) and suppressing recurrent urinary tract infections. In addition, strategies to prevent osteoporosis should be initiated in most patients likely to require long-term glucocorticoid therapy and/or with other predisposing factors. Control of hypertension and appropriate prevention strategies for atherosclerosis, including monitoring and treatment of dyslipidemias, management of hyperglycemia, and obesity, are recommended.

EXPERIMENTAL THERAPIES   Figure 313-3 shows the targets of several new biologicals, and mycophenolate, all of which are currently in clinical trials. Most strategies target T or B lymphocytes, particularly those undergoing activation, rather than entire cell populations. Some therapies, as indicated by bold boxes, are licensed by the U.S. Food and Drug Administration for use in diseases other than SLE. Several studies have employed vigorous immunosuppression with high-dose cyclophosphamide plus anti-T cell strategies, with rescue by transplantation of autologous hematopoietic stem cells for the treatment of severe and refractory SLE. A recent report showed an estimated mortality rate over 5 years of 15% and sustained remission in 50%. It is hoped that the next edition of this text will recommend more effective and less toxic approaches to treatment of SLE based on some of these strategies.

PATIENT OUTCOMES, PROGNOSIS, AND SURVIVAL

Survival in patients with SLE in the United States, Canada, Europe, and China is approximately 95% at 5 years, 90% at 10 years, and 78% at 20 years. In the United States, African Americans and Hispanic Americans with a mestizo heritage have a worse progno-

FIGURE 313-3 Experimental therapies for SLE in clinical trials in 2006. Green boxes surround interventions that are licensed for use by the U.S. Food and Drug Administration in diseases other than SLE. Blue boxes surround experimental products that are not licensed for use in any disease. APRIL, a proliferation-inducing ligand; BCMA, B cell maturation antigen; BCR, B cell receptor; BLyS, B lymphocyte stimulator; CTLA4, cytotoxic T cell lymphocyte antigen; DR, human leukocyte antigen molecule; IMPDH, inosine monophosphate dehydrogenase; MP/DC, macrophage/dendritic cell; TCR, T cell receptor.

sis than Caucasians, whereas Africans in Africa and Hispanic Americans with a Puerto Rican origin do not. The relative importance of gene mixtures and environmental differences accounting for ethnic differences is not known. In societies where modern medical care (and organ transplantation) is available only to those who can pay, glucocorticoid therapies are usually the sole therapy for severe lupus; prognosis is worse than in the developed world. Poor prognosis (~50% mortality in 10 years) in most series is associated with (at the time of diagnosis) high serum creatinine levels [>124 μmol/L (>1.4 mg/dL)], hypertension, nephrotic syndrome (24-h urine protein excretion >2.6 g), anemia [hemoglobin <124 g/L (<12.4 g/dL)], hypoalbuminemia, hypocomplementemia, aPL, male sex, and ethnicity (African American, Hispanic, and mestizo heritage). Data regarding outcomes in SLE patients with renal transplants show mixed results: some series have a twofold increase in graft rejection compared to patients with other causes of ESRD, whereas others show no differences. Overall patient survival is comparable (85% at 2 years). Lupus nephritis occurs in approximately 10% of transplanted kidneys. Disability in patients with SLE is common due primarily to chronic fatigue, arthritis, and pain, as well as renal disease. As many as 25% of patients may experience remissions, sometimes for a few years, but these are rarely permanent. The leading causes of death in the first decade of disease are systemic disease activity, renal failure, and infections; subsequently, thromboembolic events become increasingly frequent causes of mortality.

DRUG-INDUCED LUPUS

This is a syndrome of positive ANA associated with symptoms such as fever, malaise, arthritis or intense arthralgias/myalgias, serositis, and/or rash. The syndrome appears during therapy with certain medications and biologic agents, is predominant in Caucasians, has less female predilection than SLE, rarely involves kidneys or brain, is rarely associated with anti-dsDNA, is commonly associated with antibodies to histones, and usually resolves over several weeks after discontinuation of the offending medication. The list of substances that can induce lupus-like disease is long. Among the most frequent are the antiarrhythmics procainamide, disopyramide, and propafenone; the antihypertensive hydralazine; several angiotensin-converting enzyme inhibitors and beta blockers; the antithyroid propylthiouracil; the antipsychotics chlorpromazine and lithium; the anticonvulsants carbamazepine and phenytoin; the antibiotics isoniazid, minocycline, and macrodantin; the antirheumatic sulfasalazine; the diuretic hydrochlorothiazide; the antihyperlipidemics lovastatin and simvastatin; and interferons and TNF inhibitors. ANA usually appears before symptoms; however, many of the medications mentioned above induce ANA in patients who never develop symptoms of drug-induced lupus. It is appropriate to test for ANA at the first hint of relevant symptoms and to use test results to help decide whether to withdraw the suspect agent.

FURTHER READINGS

DOOLEY MA, GINZLER EM: Newer therapeutic approaches for SLE: Immunosuppressive agents. Rheum Dis Clin North Am 32:91, 2006

KASITANON N et al: Predictors of survival in systemic lupus erythematosus. Medicine (Baltimore) 85:147, 2006

KRISHNAN S et al: Autoimmunity in systemic lupus erythematosus: Integrating genes and biology. Semin Immunol 18:230, 2006

WALLACE DJ, HAHN BH (eds): *Dubois' Lupus Erythematosus*, 7th ed. Philadelphia, Lippincott Williams & Wilkins, 2006

314 Rheumatoid Arthritis
Peter E. Lipsky

Rheumatoid arthritis (RA) is a chronic multisystem disease of unknown cause. Although there are a variety of systemic manifestations, the characteristic feature of established RA is persistent inflammatory synovitis, usually involving peripheral joints in a symmetric distribution. The potential of the synovial inflammation to cause cartilage damage and bone erosions and subsequent changes in joint integrity is the hallmark of the disease. Despite its destructive potential, the course of RA can be quite variable. Some patients may experience only a mild oligoarticular illness of brief duration with minimal joint damage, but most will have a relentless progressive polyarthritis with marked functional impairment.

EPIDEMIOLOGY AND GENETICS

The prevalence of RA is ~0.8% of the population (range 0.3–2.1%); women are affected approximately three times more often than men. The prevalence increases with age, and sex differences diminish in the older age group. RA is seen throughout the world and affects all races. However, the incidence and severity seem to be less in rural sub-Saharan Africa and in Caribbean blacks. The onset is most frequent during the fourth and fifth decades of life, with 80% of all patients developing the disease between the ages of 35 and 50. The incidence of RA is more than six times greater in 60- to 64-year-old women compared to 18- to 29-year-old women. Recent data indicate that the incidence of RA may be diminishing. Moreover, disease severity appears to be declining, although it is uncertain whether this reflects more aggressive therapeutic interventions.

Family studies indicate a genetic predisposition. For example, severe RA is found at approximately four times the expected rate in first-degree relatives of individuals with disease associated with the presence of the autoantibody, rheumatoid factor; ~10% of patients with RA will have an affected first-degree relative. Moreover, monozygotic twins are at least four times more likely to be concordant for RA than dizygotic twins, who have a similar risk of developing RA as nontwin siblings. Only 15–20% of monozygotic twins are concordant for RA, however, implying that factors other than genetics play an important etiopathogenic role. Despite this, genetic factors are thought to explain ~60% of the disease susceptibility of RA. Of note, the highest risk for concordance of RA is noted in twins who have two HLA-DRB1 alleles known to be associated with RA. The class II major histocompatibility complex allele HLA-DR4 (DRβ1*0401) and related alleles are known to be major genetic risk factors for RA. Early studies showed that as many as 70% of patients with RA express HLA-DR4 compared with 28% of control individuals. This association is particularly strong for individuals who develop RA associated with antibodies to cyclic citrullinated polypeptides (CCP). An association with HLA-DR4 has been noted in many populations, but not all. In some populations, including Israeli Jews, Asian Indians, and Yakima Indians of North America, however, there is no association between the development of RA and HLA-DR4. In these individuals, there is an association between RA and the closely related HLA-DR1 (DRβ1*0101). The term *shared epitope* has been used to denote the HLA-β1 alleles that appear to convey increased risk for RA because they have similar amino acids in the third hypervariable region of the peptide binding cleft of the molecule. It has been estimated that the risk of developing RA in a person with DRβ1*0401 or the closely related DRβ1*0404 is 1 in 35 and 1 in 20, respectively, whereas the presence of both alleles puts persons at an even greater risk. In certain groups of patients, there does not appear to be a clear association between HLA-DR4–related epitopes and RA. Thus, nearly 75% of African-American RA patients do not have this genetic element. Moreover, there is an association with HLA-DR10 (DRβ1*1001) in Spanish and Italian patients, with HLA-DR9 (DRβ1*0901) in Chileans, and with HLA-DR3 (DRβ1*0301) in Arab populations.

Additional genes in the HLA-D complex may also convey altered susceptibility to RA. These include portions of the HLA region outside of the coding regions of HLA-DR molecules that increase risk. In addition, certain HLA-DR alleles, including HLA-DR5 (DRβ1*1101), HLA-DR2 (DRβ1*1501), HLA-DR3 (DRβ1*0301), and HLA-DR7

(DRβ1*0701), may protect against the development of RA in that they tend to be found at lower frequency in RA patients than in controls. A recent classification of HLA-β1 alleles based on the sequence of the third hypervariable region, encoding a portion of the peptide binding cleft, has established a hierarchy of disease susceptibility. Alleles of a group that contained a lysine at position 71 conveyed the highest risk, whereas alleles of a group that contained an arginine at position 71 also conveyed increased risk compared to all other HLF-β1 alleles. It has been estimated that HLA genes contribute about one-third of the genetic susceptibility to RA. Thus, genes outside the HLA complex also contribute. Recent analyses have identified PTPN22, a phosphatase involved in antigen receptor signaling in lymphocytes, FcRL3, a molecule involved in regulating B cell activation, PADI4, an enzyme involved in conversion of citrulline to arginine in proteins, and CTLA4, a molecule involved in regulation of T cell activation, as susceptibility genes for RA, in at least some populations. Except for PADI4, these genes also appear to convey risk for other autoimmune diseases.

Genetic risk factors do not fully account for the incidence of RA, suggesting that environmental factors also play a role in the etiology of the disease. This is emphasized by epidemiologic studies in Africa that have indicated that climate and urbanization have a major impact on the incidence and severity of RA in groups of similar genetic background. Smoking has clearly been identified as a risk for RA in persons expressing an HLA-β1 susceptibility allele. Such persons have an increased risk to develop severe RA associated with antibodies to CCP.

ETIOLOGY

The cause of RA remains unknown. It has been suggested that RA might be a manifestation of the response to an infectious agent in a genetically susceptible host. Because of the worldwide distribution of RA, it has been hypothesized that if an infectious agent is involved, the organism must be ubiquitous. A number of possible causative agents have been suggested, including *Mycoplasma*, Epstein-Barr virus (EBV), cytomegalovirus, parvovirus, and rubella virus, but convincing evidence that these or other infectious agents cause RA has not emerged. The process by which an infectious agent might cause chronic inflammatory arthritis with a characteristic distribution also remains unknown.

PATHOLOGY AND PATHOGENESIS

Microvascular injury and an increase in the number of synovial lining cells appear to be the earliest lesions in rheumatoid synovitis. The nature of the insult causing this response is not known. Subsequently, an increased number of synovial lining cells is seen along with perivascular infiltration with mononuclear cells. Before the onset of clinical symptoms, the perivascular infiltrate is predominantly composed of myeloid cells, whereas in symptomatic arthritis, T cells can also be found, although their number does not appear to correlate with symptoms. As the process continues, the synovium becomes edematous and protrudes into the joint cavity as villous projections.

Light-microscopic examination discloses a characteristic constellation of features, which include hyperplasia and hypertrophy of the synovial lining cells; focal or segmental vascular changes, including microvascular injury, thrombosis, and neovascularization; edema; and infiltration with mononuclear cells, often collected into aggregates around small blood vessels (Fig. 314-1). The endothelial cells of the rheumatoid synovium have the appearance of high endothelial venules of lymphoid organs that have been altered by cytokine exposure to facilitate entry of cells into tissue. Rheumatoid synovial endothelial cells express increased amounts of various adhesion molecules involved in this process. Although this pathologic picture is typical of RA, it can also be seen in a variety of other chronic inflammatory arthritides. The mononuclear cell collections are variable in composition and size. The predominant infiltrating cell is the T lymphocyte. CD4+ T cells predominate over CD8+ T cells and are frequently found in close proximity to HLA-DR+ macrophages and dendritic cells. Increased numbers of a separate population of T cells expressing the γδ form of the T cell receptor have also been found in the synovium, although they remain a minor population there and their role in RA has not been delineated.

FIGURE 314-1 Histology of rheumatoid synovitis. A. The characteristic features of rheumatoid inflammation with hyperplasia of the lining layer (*arrow*) and mononuclear infiltrates in the sublining layer (*double arrow*). **B.** A higher magnification of the largely CD4+ T cell infiltrate around postcapillary venules (*arrow*).

The major population of T cells in the rheumatoid synovium is composed of CD4+ memory T cells that form the majority of cells aggregated around postcapillary venules. Scattered throughout the tissue are CD8+ T cells. Both populations express the early activation antigen, CD69. Besides the accumulation of T cells, rheumatoid synovitis is also characterized by the infiltration of variable numbers of B cells and antibody-producing plasma cells. In advanced disease, structures similar to germinal centers of secondary lymphoid organs may be observed in the synovium, but these are observed only in a small fraction of patients. Both polyclonal immunoglobulin and the autoantibody rheumatoid factor are produced within the synovial tissue, which leads to the local formation of immune complexes. Antibodies to synovial tissue components may also contribute to inflammation. Recent evidence suggests that antibodies to CCP, which are generated within the synovium, may contribute to RA synovitis. Increased numbers of activated mast cells are also found in the rheumatoid synovium. Local release of the contents of their granules may contribute to inflammation. Finally, the synovial fibroblasts in RA manifest evidence of activation in that they produce a number of enzymes such as collagenase and cathepsins that can degrade components of the articular matrix. These activated fibroblasts are particularly prominent in the lining layer and at the interface with bone and cartilage. Osteoclasts are also prominent at sites of bone erosion. Activated mesenchymal stromal cells, similar to those found in normal bone marrow, can also be found in the rheumatoid synovium.

The rheumatoid synovium is characterized by the presence of a number of secreted products of activated lymphocytes, macrophages, and fibroblasts. The local production of these cytokines and chemokines appears to account for many of the pathologic and clinical manifestations of RA. These effector molecules include those that are derived from T lymphocytes, those originating from activated myeloid cells, and those secreted by other cell types in the synovium, such as fibroblasts and endothelial cells. The activity of these chemokines and cytokines appears to account for many of the features of rheumatoid synovitis, including the synovial tissue inflammation, synovial fluid inflammation, synovial proliferation, and cartilage and bone damage, as well as the systemic manifestations of RA. In addition to the production of effector molecules that propagate the inflammatory process, local factors are produced that tend to slow the inflammation, including specific inhibitors of cytokine action and additional cytokines, such as transforming growth factor β (TGF-β), which inhibits many of the features of rheumatoid synovitis including T cell activation and proliferation, B cell differentiation, and migration of cells into the inflammatory site, and may be involved in generating a population of regulatory T cells, as a means to control inflammation.

These findings have suggested that the propagation of RA is an immunologically mediated event, although the original initiating stimulus has not been characterized. One view is that the inflammatory process in the tissue is driven by the CD4+ T cells infiltrating the synovium. Evidence for this includes (1) the predominance of CD4+ T cells in the synovium; (2) the increase in soluble interleukin (IL) 2 receptors, a product of activated T cells, in blood and synovial fluid of patients with active RA; and (3) amelioration of the disease by removal of T cells by thoracic duct drainage or peripheral lymphapheresis or suppression of their proliferation or function by drugs, such as cyclosporine, leflunomide, or nondepleting monoclonal antibodies to CD4, or inhibitors of T cell activation, such as the T cell co-stimulation competitor, CTLA-4·Ig (abatacept). In addition, the association of RA with certain HLA-DR alleles, whose only known functions are to shape the repertoire of CD4+ T cells during ontogeny in the thymus and bind and present antigenic peptides to CD4+ T cells in the periphery, strongly implies a role for CD4+ T cells in the pathogenesis of the disease. Within the rheumatoid synovium, the CD4+ T cells differentiate predominantly into T_H1-like effector cells producing the proinflammatory cytokine interferon (IFN)γ and appear to be deficient in differentiation into T_H2-like effector cells capable of producing the anti-inflammatory cytokine IL-4. As a result of the ongoing secretion of IFN-γ without the regulatory influences of IL-4, macrophages are activated to produce the proinflammatory cytokines IL-1 and tumor necrosis factor (TNF) and also increase expression of HLA molecules. Direct contact between activated T cells and myeloid cells may also lead to the production of proinflammatory cytokines by the latter. Moreover, T lymphocytes express surface molecules such as CD154 (CD40 ligand) and also produce a variety of cytokines that promote B cell proliferation and differentiation into antibody-forming cells and therefore may also promote local B cell stimulation. The resultant production of immunoglobulin and rheumatoid factor can lead to immune-complex formation with consequent complement activation and exacerbation of the inflammatory process by the production of the anaphylatoxins, C3a and C5a, and the chemotactic factor C5a. In addition, antibodies may be produced to other self-antigens, such as CCP, that can contribute to disease pathogenesis. The tissue inflammation is reminiscent of chronic inflammatory responses to persistent microorganisms, although it has become clear that the number of T cells producing cytokines such as IFN-γ is less than is found in typical delayed-type hypersensitivity reactions, perhaps owing to the large amount of reactive oxygen species produced locally in the synovium that can dampen T cell function or the action of local regulatory cells. It remains unclear whether the persistent T cell activity represents a response to a persistent exogenous antigen or to altered autoantigens such as collagen, immunoglobulin, one of the heat shock proteins, or CCP. Alternatively, it could represent persistent responsiveness to activated autologous cells such as might occur as a result of EBV infection or persistent response to a foreign antigen or superantigen in the synovial tissue. Finally, rheumatoid inflammation could reflect persistent stimulation of T cells by synovial-derived antigens that cross-react with determinants introduced during antecedent exposure to foreign antigens or infectious microorganisms. The important contribution of B lymphocytes to the chronic inflammatory process has been emphasized by the observation that treatment with a monoclonal antibody to the B cell marker, CD20 (rituximab), caused prompt depletion of B lymphocytes, a decline in serum rheumatoid factor titers, and a partial amelioration of signs and symptoms of inflammation.

Overriding the chronic inflammation in the synovial tissue is an acute inflammatory process in the synovial fluid. The exudative synovial fluid contains more polymorphonuclear leukocytes (PMNLs) than mononuclear cells. A number of mechanisms play a role in stimulating the exudation of synovial fluid. Locally produced antibodies to tissue components and immune complexes can activate complement and generate anaphylatoxins and chemotactic factors. Local production of chemokines and cytokines with chemotactic activity as well as inflammatory mediators such as leukotriene B_4 and products of complement activation can attract neutrophils. Moreover, many of these same agents can also stimulate the endothelial cells of postcapillary venules to become more efficient at binding circulating cells. The net result is the enhanced migration of PMNLs into the synovial site. In addition, vasoactive mediators such as histamine produced by the mast cells that infiltrate the rheumatoid synovium may also facilitate the exudation of inflammatory cells into the synovial fluid. Finally, the vasodilatory effects of locally produced prostaglandin E_2 may also facilitate entry of inflammatory cells into the inflammatory site. Once in the synovial fluid, the PMNLs can ingest immune complexes, with the resultant production of reactive oxygen metabolites and other inflammatory mediators, further adding to the inflammatory milieu. Locally produced cytokines and chemokines can additionally stimulate PMNLs. The production of large amounts of cyclooxygenase and lipoxygenase pathway products of arachidonic acid metabolism by cells in the synovial fluid and tissue further accentuates the signs and symptoms of inflammation.

The precise mechanism by which bone and cartilage destruction occurs has not been completely resolved. Although the synovial fluid contains a number of enzymes potentially able to degrade cartilage, the majority of destruction occurs in juxtaposition to the inflamed synovium, or pannus, that spreads to cover the articular cartilage. This vascular granulation tissue is composed of proliferating fibroblasts, small blood vessels, and a variable number of mononuclear cells and produces a large amount of degradative enzymes, including collagenase and stromelysin, that may facilitate tissue damage. The cytokines IL-1 and TNF play an important role by stimulating the cells of the pannus to produce collagenase and other neutral proteases. These same two cytokines also activate chondrocytes in situ, stimulating them to produce proteolytic enzymes that can degrade cartilage locally and also inhibiting synthesis of new matrix molecules. Finally, these two cytokines, along with IL-6, may contribute to the local demineralization of bone by contributing to the activation of osteoclasts that accumulate at the site of local bone resorption. Prostaglandin E_2 produced by fibroblasts and macrophages may also contribute to bone demineralization. The common final pathway of bone erosion is likely to involve the activation of osteoclasts that are present in large numbers at these sites. Systemic manifestations of RA can be accounted for by release of inflammatory effector molecules from the synovium. These include IL-1, TNF, and IL-6, which account for many of the manifestations of active RA, including malaise, fatigue, and elevated levels of serum acute-phase reactants. The importance of TNF in producing these manifestations is emphasized by the prompt amelioration of symptoms following administration of a monoclonal antibody to TNF or a soluble TNF receptor Ig construct to patients with RA. This is associated with a decrease in production of other proinflammatory cytokines, including IL-1 and IL-6. Other cytokines may also contribute to the inflammatory milieu, including IL-17. In addition, immune complexes produced within the synovium and entering the circulation may account for other features of the disease, such as systemic vasculitis.

As shown in Fig. 314-2, the pathology of RA evolves over the duration of this chronic disease. The earliest event appears to be a nonspecific inflammatory response initiated by an unknown stimulus and characterized by accumulation of macrophages and other mononuclear cells within the sublining layer of the synovium. The activity of these cells is demonstrated by the increased appearance of macrophage-derived cytokines, including TNF, IL-1β, and IL-6. Subsequently, activation and differentiation of memory CD4+ T cells is induced, presumably in response to antigenic peptides displayed by a variety of antigen-presenting cells in the synovial tissue. The activated memory T cells are capable of producing cytokines, especially IFN-γ, which amplify and perpetuate the inflammation. The presence of activated T cells expressing CD154 (CD40 ligand) can induce polyclonal B cell stimulation and differentiation of memory B cells and plasma cells that produce autoantibodies locally. The cascade of cytokines produced in the synovium activates a variety of cells in the synovium, bone, and cartilage to produce effector molecules that can cause tissue damage characteristic of chronic inflammation. It is important to em-

Nonspecific Inflammation
Initiation

T Cell Activation
Amplification

Tissue Injury
Chronic inflammation

FIGURE 314-2 The progression of rheumatoid synovitis. This figure depicts the evolution of the pathogenic mechanisms and ultimate pathologic changes involved in the development of rheumatoid synovitis. The stages of rheumatoid arthritis are proposed to be an initiation phase of nonspecific inflammation, followed by an amplification phase resulting from T cell activation, and finally a stage of chronic inflammation with tissue injury. A variety of stimuli may initiate the initial phase of nonspecific inflammation, which may last for a protracted period of time with no or moderate symptoms. When activation of memory T cells in response to a variety of peptides presented by antigen-presenting cells occurs in genetically susceptible individuals, amplification of inflammation occurs with the promotion of local rheumatoid factor and other autoantibody production and enhanced capacity to mediate tissue damage.

phasize that there is no current way to predict the progress from one stage of inflammation to the next, and once established, each can influence the other. Important features of this model include the following: (1) the major pathologic events vary with time in this chronic disease; (2) the time required to progress from one step to the next may vary in different patients, and the events, once established, may persist simultaneously; (3) once established, the major pathogenic events operative in an individual patient may vary at different times; (4) the process is chronic and reiterative, with successive events stimulating progressive amplification of inflammation; and (5) once memory T cells and B cells have been generated, anti-inflammatory and anticytokine therapy may be capable of suppressing disease manifestations but not preventing recrudescence of disease activity once therapy is discontinued. These considerations have important implications with regard to appropriate treatment.

CLINICAL MANIFESTATIONS

Onset Characteristically, RA is a chronic polyarthritis. In approximately two-thirds of patients, it begins insidiously with fatigue, anorexia, generalized weakness, and vague musculoskeletal symptoms until the appearance of synovitis becomes apparent. This prodrome may persist for weeks or months and defy diagnosis. Specific symptoms usually appear gradually as several joints, especially those of the hands, wrists, knees, and feet, become affected in a symmetric fashion. In ~10% of individuals, the onset is more acute, with a rapid development of polyarthritis, often accompanied by constitutional symptoms, including fever, lymphadenopathy, and splenomegaly. In approximately one-third of patients, symptoms may initially be confined to one or a few joints. Although the pattern of joint involvement may remain asymmetric in some patients, a symmetric pattern is more typical.

Signs and Symptoms of Articular Disease Pain, swelling, and tenderness may initially be poorly localized to the joints. Pain in affected joints, aggravated by movement, is the most common manifestation of established RA. It corresponds in pattern to the joint involvement but does not always correlate with the degree of apparent inflammation.

Generalized stiffness is frequent and is usually greatest after periods of inactivity. Morning stiffness of >1-h duration is an almost invariable feature of inflammatory arthritis. Notably, however, the presence of morning stiffness may not reliably distinguish between chronic inflammatory and noninflammatory arthritides, as it is also found frequently in the latter. The majority of patients will experience constitutional symptoms such as weakness, easy fatigability, anorexia, and weight loss. Although fever to 40°C occurs on occasion, temperature elevation in >38°C is unusual and suggests the presence of an intercurrent problem such as infection.

Clinically, synovial inflammation causes swelling, tenderness, and limitation of motion. Initially, impairment in physical function is caused by pain and inflammation, and disability owing to this is a frequent early feature of aggressive RA. Warmth is usually evident on examination, especially of large joints such as the knee, but erythema is infrequent. Pain originates predominantly from the joint capsule, which is abundantly supplied with pain fibers and is markedly sensitive to stretching or distention. Joint swelling results from accumulation of synovial fluid, hypertrophy of the synovium, and thickening of the joint capsule. Initially, motion is limited by pain. The inflamed joint is usually held in flexion to maximize joint volume and minimize distention of the capsule. Later, fibrous or bony ankylosis or soft tissue contractures lead to fixed deformities.

Although inflammation can affect any diarthrodial joint, RA most often causes symmetric arthritis with characteristic involvement of certain specific joints such as the proximal interphalangeal and metacarpophalangeal joints. The distal interphalangeal joints are rarely involved. Synovitis of the wrist joints is a nearly uniform feature of RA and may lead to limitation of motion, deformity, and median nerve entrapment (carpal tunnel syndrome). Synovitis of the elbow joint often leads to flexion contractures that may develop early in the disease. The knee joint is commonly involved with synovial hypertrophy, chronic effusion, and frequently ligamentous laxity. Pain and swelling behind the knee may be caused by extension of inflamed synovium into the popliteal space (Baker's cyst). Arthritis in the forefoot, ankles, and subtalar joints can produce severe pain with ambulation as well as a number of deformities. Axial involvement is usually limited to the upper cervical spine. Involvement of the lumbar spine is not seen, and lower back pain cannot be ascribed to rheumatoid inflammation. On occasion, inflammation from the synovial joints and bursae of the upper cervical spine leads to atlantoaxial subluxation. This usually presents as pain in the occiput but on rare occasions may lead to compression of the spinal cord.

With persistent inflammation, a variety of characteristic joint changes develop. These can be attributed to a number of pathologic events, including laxity of supporting soft tissue structures; damage or weakening of ligaments, tendons, and the joint capsule; cartilage degradation; muscle imbalance; and unopposed physical forces associated with the use of affected joints. Characteristic changes of the hand include (1) radial deviation at the wrist with ulnar deviation of the digits, often with palmar subluxation of the proximal phalanges ("Z" deformity); (2) hyperextension of the proximal interphalangeal joints, with compensatory flexion of the distal interphalangeal joints (swan-neck deformity); (3) flexion contracture of the proximal interphalangeal joints and extension of the distal interphalangeal joints (boutonnière deformity); and (4) hyperextension of the first interphalangeal joint and flexion of the first metacarpophalangeal joint with a consequent loss of thumb mobility and pinch. Typical joint changes may also develop in the feet, including eversion at the hindfoot (subtalar joint), plantar subluxation of the metatarsal heads, widening of the forefoot, hallux valgus, and lateral deviation and dorsal subluxation of the toes. Later in the disease, disability is more related to structural damage to articular structures.

Extraarticular Manifestations RA is a systemic disease with a variety of extraarticular manifestations. It is estimated that as many as 40% of patients may have extraarticular manifestations, and in ~15% these are severe. On occasion, extraarticular manifestations may be the major evidence of disease activity and source of morbidity and require management per se. As a rule, these manifestations occur in individuals with high titers of autoantibodies to the Fc component of immunoglobulin G (rheumatoid factors) or with antibodies to CCP. Although the frequency of patients with severe extraarticular manifestations appears to be declining, these patients have an increased mortality compared to other persons with RA or age-matched normal controls.

Rheumatoid nodules may develop in 20–30% of persons with RA. They are usually found on periarticular structures, extensor surfaces, or other areas subjected to mechanical pressure, but they can develop elsewhere, including the pleura and meninges. Common locations include the olecranon bursa, the proximal ulna, the Achilles tendon, and the occiput. Nodules vary in size and consistency and are rarely symptomatic, but on occasion they break down as a result of trauma or become infected. They are found almost invariably in individuals with circulating rheumatoid factor. Histologically, rheumatoid nodules consist of a central zone of necrotic material including collagen fibrils, noncollagenous filaments, and cellular debris; a midzone of palisading macrophages that express HLA-DR antigens; and an outer zone of granulation tissue. Examination of early nodules has suggested that the initial event may be a focal vasculitis. In some patients, treatment with methotrexate can increase the number of nodules dramatically.

Clinical weakness and atrophy of skeletal muscle are common. Muscle atrophy may be evident within weeks of the onset of RA and is usually most apparent in musculature approximating affected joints. Muscle biopsy may show type II fiber atrophy and muscle fiber necrosis with or without a mononuclear cell infiltrate.

Rheumatoid vasculitis (Chap. 319), which can affect nearly any organ system, is seen in patients with severe RA and high titers of circulating rheumatoid factor. Rheumatoid vasculitis is very uncommon in African Americans. In its most aggressive form, rheumatoid vasculitis can cause polyneuropathy and mononeuritis multiplex, cutaneous ulceration and dermal necrosis, digital gangrene, and visceral infarction. While such widespread vasculitis is very rare, more limited forms are not uncommon, especially in white patients with high titers of rheumatoid factor. Neurovascular disease presenting either as a mild distal sensory neuropathy or as mononeuritis multiplex may be the only sign of vasculitis. Cutaneous vasculitis usually presents as crops of small brown spots in the nail beds, nail folds, and digital pulp. Larger ischemic ulcers, especially in the lower extremity, may also develop. Myocardial infarction secondary to rheumatoid vasculitis has been reported, as has vasculitic involvement of lungs, bowel, liver, spleen, pancreas, lymph nodes, and testes. Renal vasculitis is rare.

Pleuropulmonary manifestations, which are more commonly observed in men, include pleural disease, interstitial fibrosis, pleuropulmonary nodules, pneumonitis, and arteritis. Evidence of pleuritis is found commonly at autopsy, but symptomatic disease during life is infrequent. Typically, the pleural fluid contains very low levels of glucose in the absence of infection. Pleural fluid complement is also low compared with the serum level when these are related to the total protein concentration. Pulmonary fibrosis can produce impairment of the diffusing capacity of the lung. Pulmonary nodules may appear singly or in clusters. When they appear in individuals with pneumoconiosis, a diffuse nodular fibrotic process (Caplan's syndrome) may develop. On occasion, pulmonary nodules may cavitate and produce a pneumothorax or bronchopleural fistula. Rarely, pulmonary hypertension secondary to obliteration of the pulmonary vasculature occurs. In addition to pleuropulmonary disease, upper airway obstruction from cricoarytenoid arthritis or laryngeal nodules may develop.

Clinically apparent heart disease attributed to the rheumatoid process was thought previously to be rare, but evidence of asymptomatic pericarditis is found at autopsy in 50% of cases. Pericardial fluid has a low glucose level and is frequently associated with the occurrence of pleural effusion. Although pericarditis is usually asymptomatic, on rare occasions death has occurred from tamponade. Chronic constrictive pericarditis may also occur. More recently, an increased incidence of congestive heart failure and death from cardiovascular disease has been associated with RA. This relates to the level of disease activity and can be mitigated with appropriate anti-inflammatory therapy.

RA tends to spare the central nervous system directly, although vasculitis can cause peripheral neuropathy. *Neurologic manifestations* may also result from atlantoaxial or midcervical spine subluxations. Nerve entrapment secondary to proliferative synovitis or joint deformities may produce neuropathies of median, ulnar, radial (interosseous branch), or anterior tibial nerves.

The rheumatoid process involves the *eye* in <1% of patients. Affected individuals usually have long-standing disease and nodules. The two principal manifestations are episcleritis, which is usually mild and transient, and scleritis, which involves the deeper layers of the eye and is a more serious inflammatory condition. Histologically, the lesion is similar to a rheumatoid nodule and may result in thinning and perforation of the globe (scleromalacia perforans). From 15–20% of persons with RA may develop Sjögren's syndrome with attendant keratoconjunctivitis sicca.

Felty's syndrome consists of chronic RA, splenomegaly, neutropenia, and, on occasion, anemia and thrombocytopenia. It is most common in individuals with long-standing disease. These patients frequently have high titers of rheumatoid factor, subcutaneous nodules, and other manifestations of systemic rheumatoid disease. Felty's syndrome is very uncommon in African Americans. It may develop after joint inflammation has regressed. Circulating immune complexes are often present, and evidence of complement consumption may be seen. The leukopenia is a selective neutropenia with polymorphonuclear leukocyte counts of <1500 cells/μL and sometimes <1000 cell/μL. Bone marrow examination usually reveals moderate hypercellularity with a paucity of mature neutrophils. However, the bone marrow may be normal, hyperactive, or hypoactive; maturation arrest may be seen. Hypersplenism has been proposed as one of the causes of leukopenia, but splenomegaly is not invariably found and splenectomy does not always correct the abnormality. Excessive margination of granulocytes caused by antibodies to these cells, complement activation, or binding of immune complexes may contribute to granulocytopenia. Patients with Felty's syndrome have increased frequency of infections usually associated with neutropenia. The cause of the increased susceptibility to infection is related to the defective function of PMNLs as well as the decreased number of cells.

Osteoporosis secondary to rheumatoid involvement is common and may be aggravated by glucocorticoid therapy. Glucocorticoid treatment may cause significant loss of bone mass, especially early in the course of therapy, even when low doses are employed. Osteopenia in RA involves both juxtaarticular bone and long bones distant from involved joints. RA is associated with a modest decrease in mean bone mass and a moderate increase in the risk of fracture. Bone mass appears to be adversely affected by functional impairment and active inflammation, especially early in the course of the disease.

RA is associated with an increased incidence of lymphoma, especially large B cell lymphoma. Notably, this is particularly observed in those with persistent inflammatory disease.

RA in the Elderly The incidence of RA continues to increase past age 60. It has been suggested that elderly-onset RA might have a poorer prognosis, as manifested by more persistent disease activity, more frequent radiographically evident deterioration, more frequent systemic involvement, and more rapid functional decline. Aggressive disease is largely restricted to those patients with high titers of rheumatoid factor. By contrast, elderly patients who develop RA without elevated titers of rheumatoid factor (seronegative disease) generally have less severe, often self-limited disease.

LABORATORY FINDINGS

No tests are specific for diagnosing RA. However, rheumatoid factors, which are autoantibodies reactive with the Fc portion of IgG, are found in more than two-thirds of adults with the disease and have classically been used to evaluate patients with RA. Widely utilized tests largely detect IgM rheumatoid factors. The presence of rheumatoid factor is not specific for RA, as rheumatoid factor is found in 5% of healthy persons. The frequency of rheumatoid factor in the general population increases with age, and 10–20% of individuals >65 years have a positive test. In addition, a number of conditions besides RA are associated with the presence of rheumatoid factor. These include systemic lupus erythematosus, Sjögren's syndrome, chronic liver disease, sarcoidosis, interstitial pulmonary fibrosis, infectious mononucleosis, hepatitis B, tuberculosis, leprosy, syphilis, subacute bacterial endocarditis, visceral leishmaniasis, schistosomiasis, and malaria. In addition, rheumatoid factor may appear transiently in normal individuals after vaccination or transfusion and may also be found in relatives of individuals with RA.

The presence of rheumatoid factor does not establish the diagnosis of RA as the predictive value of the presence of rheumatoid factor in determining a diagnosis of RA is poor. Thus fewer than one-third of unselected patients with a positive test for rheumatoid factor will be found to have RA. Therefore, the rheumatoid factor test is not useful as a screening procedure. However, the presence of rheumatoid factor can be of prognostic significance because patients with high titers tend to have more severe and progressive disease with extraarticular manifestations. Rheumatoid factor is uniformly found in patients with nodules or vasculitis. In summary, a test for the presence of rheumatoid factor can be employed to confirm a diagnosis in individuals with a suggestive clinical presentation and, if present in high titer, to designate patients at risk for severe systemic disease.

Antibodies to CCP (designated anti-CCP) can also be used to evaluate patients with RA. Although these antibodies are most commonly found in rheumatoid factor–positive patients, on occasion they can be detected in the absence of rheumatoid factor. In addition, the anti-CCP test has a similar sensitivity and a better specificity for RA than does rheumatoid factor, and, therefore, some have advocated its use to evaluate RA patients instead of rheumatoid factor. This is particularly the case in individuals with early RA, in whom assessment of anti-CCP may be the most useful to confirm the diagnosis and establish a likely prognosis. The presence of anti-CCP is most common in persons with aggressive disease, with a tendency for developing bone erosions. The development of anti-CCP is most frequent in individuals with an RA associated HLA-β1 allele and in those who smoke cigarettes, and may occur before the development of clinical manifestations of RA. However, as with rheumatoid factor, the presence of anti-CCP is not useful to predict the future development of RA because it can be found in ~1.5% of normal individuals, most of whom will not develop RA, and occasionally in persons with other rheumatic diseases. However, it is a useful test to confirm a diagnosis of RA and to estimate prognosis.

Normochromic, normocytic anemia is frequently present in active RA. It is thought to reflect ineffective erythropoiesis; large stores of iron are found in the bone marrow. In general, anemia and thrombocytosis correlate with disease activity. The white blood cell count is usually normal, but a mild leukocytosis may be present. Leukopenia may also exist without the full-blown picture of Felty's syndrome. Eosinophilia, when present, usually reflects severe systemic disease.

The erythrocyte sedimentation rate (ESR) is increased in nearly all patients with active RA. The levels of a variety of other acute-phase reactants including ceruloplasmin and C-reactive protein are also elevated, and generally such elevations correlate with disease activity and the likelihood of progressive joint damage.

Synovial fluid analysis confirms the presence of inflammatory arthritis, although none of the findings is specific. The fluid is usually turbid, with reduced viscosity, increased protein content, and a slightly decreased or normal glucose concentration. The white cell count varies between 5 and 50,000/μL; PMNLs predominate. A synovial fluid white blood cell count >2000/μL with >75% polymorphonuclear leukocytes is highly characteristic of inflammatory arthritis, although not diagnostic of RA. Total hemolytic complement, C3, and C4 are markedly diminished in synovial fluid relative to total protein concentration as a result of activation of the classic complement pathway by locally produced immune complexes.

RADIOGRAPHIC EVALUATION

Early in the disease, radiographic evaluations of the affected joints are usually not helpful in establishing a diagnosis. They reveal only that which is apparent from physical examination, namely, evidence of soft tissue swelling and joint effusion. As the disease progresses, abnormalities become more pronounced, but none of the radiographic findings is diagnostic of RA. The diagnosis, however, is supported by a characteristic pattern of abnormalities, including the tendency toward symmetric involvement. Juxtaarticular osteopenia may become apparent within weeks of onset. Loss of articular cartilage and bone erosions develop after months of sustained activity. The primary value of radiography is to determine the extent of cartilage destruction and bone erosion produced by the disease, particularly when one is attempting to estimate the aggressive nature of the disease, monitoring the impact of therapy with disease-modifying drugs, or determining the need for surgical intervention. Other means of imaging bones and joints, including ^{99m}Tc bisphosphonate bone scanning and MRI, may be capable of detecting early inflammatory changes that are not apparent from standard radiography but are rarely necessary in the routine evaluation of patients with RA.

CLINICAL COURSE AND PROGNOSIS

The course of RA is quite variable and difficult to predict in an individual patient. The current therapeutic approach of early aggressive intervention appears to have mitigated the clinical course of RA, resulting in less persistent inflammation, disability, joint damage, and mortality. Classically, most patients had experienced persistent but fluctuating disease activity, accompanied by a variable degree of joint abnormalities and functional impairment. After 10–12 years, <20% of patients had no evidence of disability or joint abnormalities. Moreover, within 10 years, ~50% of patients had work disability. All of these outcomes are thought to be positively influenced by early aggressive intervention. A number of features are correlated with a greater likelihood of developing joint abnormalities or disabilities. These include the presence of >20 inflamed joints, a markedly elevated ESR, radiographic evidence of bone erosions, the presence of rheumatoid nodules, high titers of serum rheumatoid factor or anti-CCP antibodies, the presence of functional disability, persistent inflammation, advanced age at onset, the presence of comorbid conditions, low socioeconomic status or educational level, or the presence of HLA-DRβ1*0401 or -DRβ*0404. The presence of one or more of these implies the presence of more aggressive disease with a greater likelihood of developing progressive joint abnormalities and disability. Persistent elevation of the ESR, disability, and pain on longitudinal follow-up are good predictors of work disability, whereas persistent synovitis of >12 weeks is associated with an increased likelihood of developing bone erosions. Patients who lack these features have more indolent disease with a slower progression to joint abnormalities and disability. The pattern of disease onset does not appear to predict the development of disabilities. Approximately 15% of patients with RA will have a short-lived inflammatory process that remits without major disability. These individuals tend to lack the aforementioned features associated with more aggressive disease.

Several features of patients with RA appear to have prognostic significance. Remissions of disease activity are most likely to occur during the first year. White females tend to have more persistent synovitis and more progressively erosive disease than males. Persons who present with high titers of rheumatoid factor, anti-CCP antibodies, C-reactive protein, and haptoglobin also have a worse prognosis, as do individuals with subcutaneous nodules or radiographic evidence of erosions at the time of initial evaluation. Sustained disease activity of >1 year's duration portends a poor outcome, and persistent elevation of acute-phase reactants appears to correlate strongly with radiographic progression. Before the use of early aggressive therapy, a large proportion of inflamed joints manifested erosions within 2 years, whereas the subsequent course of erosions was highly variable; however, in general, radiographic damage appears to progress at a constant rate in patients with RA. Foot joints are affected more frequently than hand joints. Despite the decrease in the rate of progressive joint damage with time, functional disability, which develops early in the course of the disease, continues to worsen at the same rate, although the most rapid rate of functional loss occurs within the first 2 years of disease. Early in the course of RA, disability is more associated with pain and inflammation, whereas later in the course of the disease, damage to articular structures makes a greater contribution.

The median life expectancy of persons with RA is shortened by 3–7 years. Of the 2.5-fold increase in mortality rate, RA itself is a contributing feature in 15–30%. The increased mortality rate seems to be limited to patients with more severe articular disease and can be attributed largely to infection and gastrointestinal bleeding and an increased risk of cardiovascular disease. Recent evidence has emphasized the important role of cardiovascular disease in the increased mortality of RA patients, and this appears to diminish with effective anti-inflammatory therapy. Drug therapy may also play a role in the increased mortality rate seen in individuals with RA. Factors correlated with early death include disability, disease duration or severity, persistent inflammation, glucocorticoid use, age at onset, and low socioeconomic or educational status.

DIAGNOSIS

The diagnosis of RA can be delayed because of the nonspecific nature of initial symptoms. The diagnosis of RA is easily made in persons with typical established disease. The typical picture of bilateral symmetric inflammatory polyarthritis involving small and large joints in both the upper and lower extremities with sparing of the axial skeleton except the cervical spine suggests the diagnosis. Constitutional features indicative of the inflammatory nature of the disease, such as morning stiffness, support the diagnosis. Demonstration of subcutaneous nodules is a helpful diagnostic feature. Additionally, the presence of rheumatoid factor, anti-CCP antibodies, inflammatory synovial fluid with increased numbers of PMNLs, and radiographic findings of juxtaarticular bone demineralization and erosions of the affected joints substantiate the diagnosis.

The diagnosis is somewhat more difficult early in the course when only constitutional symptoms or intermittent arthralgias or arthritis in an asymmetric distribution may be present. A period of observation may be necessary before the diagnosis can be established. A definitive diagnosis of RA depends predominantly on characteristic clinical features and the exclusion of other inflammatory processes. The isolated finding of a positive test for rheumatoid factor, anti-CCP antibody, or an elevated ESR or CRP, especially in an older person with joint pains, should not itself be used as evidence of RA.

In 1987, the American College of Rheumatology developed revised criteria for the classification of RA (Table 314-1). These criteria demonstrate a sensitivity of 91–94% and a specificity of 89% when used to classify patients with RA compared with control subjects with rheumatic diseases other than RA. Although these criteria were developed as a means of disease classification for investigational purposes, they can be useful as guidelines for establishing the diagnosis. Failure to meet these criteria, however, especially during the early stages of the disease, does not exclude the diagnosis. Indeed, these criteria do not effectively differentiate patients with new-onset RA from those with a variety of other forms of early inflammatory arthritis. Moreover, in patients with early arthritis, the criteria do not discriminate effectively between patients who subsequently develop persistent, disabling, or erosive disease and those who do not.

TABLE 314-1 THE 1987 REVISED CRITERIA FOR THE CLASSIFICATION OF RA

1. Guidelines for classification
  a. Four of seven criteria are required to classify a patient as having rheumatoid arthritis (RA).
  b. Patients with two or more clinical diagnoses are not excluded.
2. Criteria^a
  a. Morning stiffness: Stiffness in and around the joints lasting 1 h before maximal improvement.
  b. Arthritis of three or more joint areas: At least three joint areas, observed by a physician simultaneously, have soft tissue swelling or joint effusions, not just bony overgrowth. The 14 possible joint areas involved are right or left proximal interphalangeal, metacarpophalangeal, wrist, elbow, knee, ankle, and metatarsophalangeal joints.
  c. Arthritis of hand joints: Arthritis of wrist, metacarpophalangeal joint, or proximal interphalangeal joint.
  d. Symmetric arthritis: Simultaneous involvement of the same joint areas on both sides of the body.
  e. Rheumatoid nodules: Subcutaneous nodules over bony prominences, extensor surfaces, or juxtaarticular regions observed by a physician.
  f. Serum rheumatoid factor: Demonstration of abnormal amounts of serum rheumatoid factor by any method for which the result has been positive in less than 5% of normal control subjects.
  g. Radiographic changes: Typical changes of RA on posteroanterior hand and wrist radiographs that must include erosions or unequivocal bony decalcification localized in or most marked adjacent to the involved joints.

^aCriteria a–d must be present for at least 6 weeks. Criteria b–e must be observed by a physician.
Source: From Arnett et al.

℞ RHEUMATOID ARTHRITIS

GENERAL PRINCIPLES The goals of therapy of RA are (1) relief of pain, (2) reduction of inflammation, (3) protection of articular structures, (4) maintenance of function, and (5) control of systemic involvement. Since the etiology of RA is unknown, the pathogenesis is not completely delineated, and the mechanisms of action of some of the therapeutic agents employed are uncertain, therapy remains somewhat empirical. None of the therapeutic interventions is curative, and therefore all must be viewed as palliative, aimed at relieving the signs and symptoms of the disease. The various therapies employed are directed at nonspecific suppression of the inflammatory or immunologic process with the expectation of ameliorating symptoms and preventing progressive damage to articular structures.

Management of patients with RA involves an interdisciplinary approach, which attempts to deal with the various problems that these individuals encounter with functional as well as psychosocial interactions. A variety of physical therapy modalities may be useful in decreasing the symptoms of RA. Rest ameliorates symptoms and can be an important component of the total therapeutic program. In addition, splinting to reduce unwanted motion of inflamed joints may be useful. Exercise directed at maintaining muscle strength and joint mobility without exacerbating joint inflammation is also an important aspect of the therapeutic regimen. A variety of orthotic and assistive devices can be helpful in supporting and aligning deformed joints to reduce pain and improve function. Education of the patient and family is an important component of the therapeutic plan to help those involved become aware of the potential impact of the disease and make appropriate accommodations in lifestyle to maximize satisfaction and minimize stress on joints.

Medical management of RA involves five general approaches. The first is the use of nonsteroidal anti-inflammatory drugs (NSAIDs) and simple analgesics to control the symptoms and signs of the local inflammatory process. These agents are rapidly effective at mitigating signs and symptoms, but they appear to exert minimal effect on the progression of the disease. Recently, specific inhibitors of the isoform of cyclooxygenase (COX) that is upregulated at inflammatory sites (COX-2) have been developed. COX inhibitors (known as Coxibs), which selectively inhibit COX-2 and not COX-1, have been shown to be as effective as classic NSAIDs, which inhibit both isoforms of COX, but to cause significantly less gastroduodenal ulceration. However, these agents are associated with an increased risk of cardiovascular events, and therefore their use must be guided by a careful assessment of risk/benefit ratio. An important additional second line of therapy involves use of low-dose oral glucocorticoids. Although low-dose glucocorticoids have been widely used to suppress signs and symptoms of inflammation, recent evidence indicates that they may also retard the development and progression of bone erosions. In addition, the use of low-dose glucocorticoids increases the anti-inflammatory effects of agents such as methotrexate as well as the protective effect of these agents on bone damage. An initial course of low-dose glucocorticoids should be considered in patients either alone or when therapy with disease modifying anti-rheumatic drugs (DMARDs) is considered. Intraarticular glucocorticoids can often provide transient symptomatic relief when systemic medical therapy has failed to resolve inflammation. The third line of agents includes the DMARDs just mentioned. These agents appear to have the capacity to decrease elevated levels of acute-phase reactants in treated patients and, therefore, are thought to modify the inflammatory component of RA and thus its destructive capacity. These agents include methotrexate, sulfasalazine, hydroxychloroquine, gold salts, or D-penicillamine, although the latter two are now used infrequently. Combinations of DMARDs appear to be more effective than single agents in controlling the signs and symptoms of RA. A fourth group of agents are the biologics, which include TNG-neutralizing agents (infliximab, etanercept, and adalimumab), IL-1-neutralizing agents (anakinra), those that deplete B cells (rituximab), and those that interfere with T cell activation (abatacept). These agents have been shown to have a major impact on the signs and symptoms of RA and also to slow progressive damage to articular structures. A fifth group of agents are the immunosuppressive and cytotoxic drugs, including leflunomide, cyclosporine, azathioprine, and cyclophosphamide, that have been shown to ameliorate the disease process in some patients. Additional approaches have been employed in an attempt to control the signs and symptoms of RA. Substituting omega-3 fatty acids such as eicosapentaenoic acid found in certain fish oils for dietary omega-6 essential fatty acids found in meat has also been shown to provide symptomatic improvement in patients with RA. A variety of nontraditional approaches have also been claimed to be effective in treating RA, including diets, plant and animal extracts, vaccines, hormones, and topical preparations of various sorts. Many of these are costly, and none has been shown to be effective. However, belief in their efficacy ensures their continued use by some patients.

DRUGS   Disease-Modifying Anti-Rheumatic Drugs   Clinical experience has delineated a number of agents—the DMARDs—that appear to have the capacity to alter the course of RA. Despite having no chemical or pharmacologic similarities, in practice these agents share a number of characteristics. They exert minimal direct nonspecific anti-inflammatory or analgesic effects, and therefore NSAIDs must be continued during their administration, except in a few cases when true remissions are induced with them. The appearance of benefit from DMARD therapy is usually delayed for weeks or months. As many as two-thirds of patients develop some clinical improvement as a result of therapy with any of these agents, although the induction of true remissions is unusual. In addition to clinical improvement, there is frequently an improvement in serologic evidence of disease activity, and titers of rheumatoid factor and C-reactive protein and the ESR frequently decline. Moreover, DMARD therapy, especially early in the disease course, retards the development of bone erosions.

No characteristic features of patients have emerged that predict responsiveness to a DMARD. Moreover, the indications for the initiation of therapy with one of these agents are not well defined. Recently, evidence has emerged that the initiation of DMARD therapy early in the course of RA clearly has a major impact on the development of bone erosions and the progression to disability. It is now felt that DMARD therapy should be begun as soon as the diagnosis of RA is established, especially in those with any evidence of aggressive disease with a poor prognosis.

Which DMARD should be the drug of first choice remains controversial, and trials have failed to demonstrate a consistent advantage of one over the other. Despite this, methotrexate has emerged as the DMARD of choice especially in individuals with risk factors for development of bone erosions or persistent synovitis of >3 months' duration, because of its relatively rapid onset of action, its capacity to effect sustained improvement with ongoing therapy, and the higher level of patient retention on therapy. Methotrexate is usually employed on a weekly schedule of 7.5–25 mg given either orally in divided doses or, if necessary, SC or IM to avoid gastrointestinal toxicity. Recent trials have documented the efficacy of methotrexate and have indicated that its onset of action is more rapid than other DMARDs, and patients tend to remain on therapy with methotrexate longer than they remain on other DMARDs because of better clinical responses and less toxicity. Long-term trials have indicated that methotrexate does not induce remission but rather suppresses symptoms while it is being administered. Maximal improvement is observed after 6 months of therapy, with little additional improvement thereafter. Major toxicity includes gastrointestinal upset, oral ulceration, and liver function abnormalities that appear to be dose-related and reversible and hepatic fibrosis that can be quite insidious, requiring liver biopsy for detection in its early stages. Drug-induced pneumonitis has also been reported. Liver biopsy is recommended for individuals with persistent or repetitive liver function abnormalities. Concurrent administration of folic acid or folinic acid may diminish the frequency of some side effects, although efficacy may be diminished somewhat. In this regard, each of the DMARDs is associated with toxicity, and therefore careful patient monitoring is necessary. Toxicity of the various agents also becomes important in determining the drug of first choice. Of note, failure to respond or development of toxicity to one DMARD does not preclude responsiveness to another. Thus, a similar percentage of RA patients who have failed to respond to one DMARD will respond to another when it is given as the second disease-modifying drug.

GLUCOCORTICOID THERAPY   Systemic glucocorticoid therapy can provide effective symptomatic therapy in patients with RA. Low-dose (<7.5 mg/d) prednisone is a useful additive therapy to control symptoms. Moreover, recent evidence suggests that low-dose glucocorticoid therapy may retard the progression of bone erosions and that an initial course of low-dose glucocorticoids may have a long-term protective effect against bone damage. Monthly pulses with high-dose glucocorticoids may be useful in some patients and may hasten the response when therapy with a DMARD is initiated. Finally, a course of low-dose oral glucocorticoids combined with DMARD therapy can be beneficial in controlling signs and symptoms rapidly and affording long-term retardation of bone erosion.

BIOLOGICS   Recently, biologic agents that bind and neutralize TNF have become available. One of these is a TNF type II receptor fused to IgG1 (etanercept), the second is a chimeric mouse/human monoclonal antibody to TNF (infliximab), and the third is a fully human antibody to TNF (adalimumab). Clinical trials have shown that parenteral administration of any of these TNF-neutralizing agents is remarkably effective at controlling signs and symptoms of RA in patients who have failed DMARD therapy, as well as in DMARD-naïve patients. Repetitive therapy with these agents is effective with or without concomitant methotrexate, although combination therapy with methotrexate or another DMARD appears to provide the greatest benefit. These agents not only are effective in persistently controlling signs and symptoms of RA in a majority of patients, but they have also been shown to slow the rate of progression of joint damage assessed radiographically and to improve disability. Side effects include the potential for an increased risk of serious infections. Particularly notable is the capacity of TNF blockade to increase the risk of developing reactivation of dormant tuberculosis. It is prudent to carry out tuberculin skin testing and, if necessary, further evaluation with chest radiographs before beginning therapy with an anti-TNF agent to limit the chance of inciting reactivation of tuberculosis. Anti-TNF therapy also has the potential to increase the risk of lymphoma and possibly other malignancies in treated patients. TNF-neutralizing therapy can also induce the development of anti-DNA antibodies, but rarely is there associated evidence of signs and symptoms of systemic lupus erythematosus. Other side effects include infusion or injection site reactions and rarely the development of demyelinating central nervous system disease. Although these side effects are uncommon, their occurrence mandates that TNF-neutralizing therapy be supervised by physicians with experience in their use.

Anakinra is a recombinant IL-1 receptor antagonist that competitively blocks the binding of IL-1β and IL-1α to the IL-1 receptor and thereby inhibits the activity of these two related proinflammatory cytokines. Anakinra has been shown to improve the signs and symptoms of RA, to decrease disability, and to slow progression of articular damage assessed radiographically. It can be given as monotherapy or in combination with methotrexate. The major side effects are injection site reactions. In general, the clinical impact of anakinra appears to be less than that of TNF-neutralizing therapy, but it may be used in those in whom TNF-neutralizing therapy is precluded. It is rarely effective in those who have failed TNF-neutralizing therapy.

Combining anakinra with a TNF-blocking agent does not increase efficacy and is associated with an increased frequency of infection, and, therefore, is not recommended. Rituximab, a chimeric antibody directed to CD20 that depletes mature B cells, has been approved for treatment of RA patients who have failed anti-TNF therapy. In combination with methotrexate, this therapy can improve signs and symptoms in these patients and also retard the progress of bone damage. The major adverse events relate to transfusion reactions that can be controlled with glucocorticoids. Although the optimal regimen has not been established, therapy can be repeated usually at 6-month intervals when circulating B cells return.

Abatacept is a fusion protein consisting of CTLA4 and the Fc portion of IgG1. It inhibits T cell activation by competitively inhibiting the co-stimulation of T cells that results from interaction of T cell–expressed CD28 and CD80/86 expressed by antigen-presenting cells. It can be used with or without methotrexate, although its efficacy is greater as co-therapy with methotrexate. It has a positive effect on signs and symptoms of RA and also retards progressive bone damage. It is usually reserved for patients who have failed TNF-neutralizing therapy or in those who have contraindications to TNF blockade. Abatacept is tolerated quite well. Combining abatacept with a TNF-blocking agent does not increase efficacy, and is associated with more adverse events, including serious infections, and, therefore, is not recommended.

DIAGNOSIS OF RHEUMATOID ARTHRITIS

Risk factors for disability/erosions?
Rheumatoid factor
Anti-CCP antibody
Multiple swollen joints
Elevated acute-phase reactants
DR4+ (Shared epitope)
Erosions on x-ray
Disability

FIGURE 314-3 Algorithm for the medical management of rheumatoid arthritis. Coxib, COX-2 inhibitors; DMARD, disease-modifying anti-rheumatic drug; CCP, cyclic citrullinated polypeptide; MTX, methotrexate; SSA, sulfasalazine; TNF, tumor necrosis factor.

IMMUNOSUPPRESSIVE THERAPY   The immunosuppressive drugs azathioprine, leflunomide, cyclosporine, and cyclophosphamide have been shown to be effective in the treatment of RA and to exert therapeutic effects similar to those of the DMARDs. However, these agents appear to be no more effective than the DMARDs. Moreover, they cause a variety of toxic side effects, and cyclophosphamide appears to predispose the patient to the development of malignant neoplasms. Therefore, these drugs have been reserved for patients who have clearly failed therapy with DMARDs and biologics. On occasion, extraarticular disease such as rheumatoid vasculitis may require cytotoxic immunosuppressive therapy.

Leflunomide is metabolized to an active metabolite that acts to inhibit dihydroorotate dehydrogenase, an essential enzyme in the pyrimidine biosynthetic pathway. Its predominant action is to inhibit the proliferation of T lymphocytes. Leflunomide has been shown to control the signs and symptoms of RA and to slow the progression of joint damage as effectively as methotrexate. Leflunomide can be given alone or with methotrexate and is the most frequently employed immunosuppressive agent used to treat patients with RA. It is used as monotherapy in patients who have had adverse reactions to methotrexate or inadequate responses to it. The major side effect is the associated increase in liver function enzymes that occurs in 5% of patients receiving leflunomide alone and in >50% of individuals taking leflunomide with methotrexate.

SURGERY   Surgery plays a role in the management of patients with severely damaged joints. Although arthroplasties and total joint replacements can be done on a number of joints, the most successful procedures are carried out on hips, knees, and shoulders. Realistic goals of these procedures are relief of pain and reduction of disability. Reconstructive hand surgery may lead to cosmetic improvement and some functional benefit. Open or arthroscopic synovectomy may be useful in some patients with persistent monarthritis, especially of the knee. Although synovectomy may offer short-term relief of symptoms, it does not appear to retard bone destruction or alter the natural history of the disease. In addition, early tenosynovectomy of the wrist may prevent tendon rupture.

APPROACH TO THE PATIENT:
Rheumatoid Arthritis

An approach to the medical management of patients with RA is depicted in Fig. 314-3. The principles underlying care of these patients reflect the value of early appropriately aggressive intervention, the variability of the disease, the frequent persistent nature of the inflammation and its potential to cause disability, the relationship between sustained inflammation and bone erosions and mortality, and the need to reevaluate the patient frequently for symptomatic response to therapy, progression of disability and joint damage, and side effects of treatment. At the onset of disease it is difficult to predict the natural history of an individual patient's illness. Therefore, the classic approach was to attempt to alleviate the patient's symptoms with NSAIDs or Coxibs. Some patients may have mild disease that requires no additional therapy. However, most patients will require additional therapy, and the treating physician must be vigilant and prepared to institute appropriate therapy as soon as indicated. Nearly all patients will benefit from a course of low-dose glucocorticoids, and this should be considered routinely. If the patient has any evidence of aggressive disease, as described above, or persistent synovitis for >3 months, initiation of DMARD therapy should be considered as early as feasible. In RA patients there appears to be a window of opportunity early in the course of the disease, during which initiation of aggressive therapy can have a major impact on subsequent damage to articular structures and disability.

At some time during most patients' course, the possibility of initiating DMARD therapy is entertained. The presence of risk factors for bone damage or disability or persistent synovitis of >3 months' duration are usual indications to initiate DMARD therapy. The decision to begin use of a DMARD and/or low-dose oral glucocorticoids requires experience and clinical judgment as well as the ability to assess joint swelling and functional activity and the patient's pain tolerance and expectation of therapy accurately. In this setting, the fully informed patient must play an active role in the decision to begin DMARD and/or low-dose oral glucocorticoid therapy, after careful review of the therapeutic and toxic potential of the various drugs. If DMARD therapy, usually methotrexate, fails to control signs and symptoms of RA, a decision to add or switch to a biologic agent is considered. These are quite potent at controlling signs and symptoms of RA, slowing damage to articular structures, and limiting disability but are very expensive and associated with serious adverse events. The decision to employ these agents requires considerable experience, judgment, and the agreement of a fully informed patient.

If a patient responds to a DMARD, therapy is continued with careful monitoring to avoid toxicity. All DMARDs provide a suppressive effect and therefore require prolonged administration. Even with successful therapy, local injection of glucocorticoids may be necessary to diminish inflammation that may persist in a limited number of joints. In addition, NSAIDs or Coxibs may be necessary to mitigate symptoms. Even after inflammation has totally resolved, symptoms from loss of cartilage and supervening degenerative joint disease or altered joint function may require additional treatment. Surgery may also be necessary to relieve pain or diminish the functional impairment secondary to alterations in joint function.

FURTHER READINGS

ARNETT FC et al: The American Rheumatism Association 1987 Revised Criteria for the Classification of Rheumatoid Arthritis. Arthritis Rheum 31:315, 1988

BERGLIN E et al: Radiological outcome in rheumatoid arthritis is predicted by presence of antibodies against cyclic citrullinated peptide before and at disease onset, and by IgA-RF at disease onset. Ann Rheum Dis 65(4):453, 2006

BONGARTZ T et al: Anti-TNF antibody therapy in rheumatoid arthritis and the risk of serious infections and malignancies: Systematic review and meta-analysis of rare harmful effects in randomized controlled trials. JAMA 295(19):2275, 2006

BREEDVELD FC et al: The PREMIER study: A multicenter, randomized, double-blind clinical trial of combination therapy with adalimumab plus methotrexate versus methotrexate alone or adalimumab alone in patients with early, aggressive rheumatoid arthritis who had not had previous methotrexate treatment. Arthritis Rheum 54(1):26, 2006

COHEN SB et al: A multicentre, double-blind, randomised, placebo-controlled trial of anakinra (Kineret), a recombinant interleukin 1 receptor antagonist, in patients with rheumatoid arthritis treated with background methotrexate. Ann Rheum Dis 63(9):1062, 2004 Epub 2004 Apr 13

COSTENBADER KH et al: Smoking intensity, duration, and cessation, and the risk of rheumatoid arthritis in women. Am J Med 119(6):503, 2006

DA SILVA JA et al: Safety of low-dose glucocorticoid treatment in rheumatoid arthritis: Published evidence and prospective trial data. Ann Rheum Dis 65(3):285, 2006 Epub 2005 Aug 17. Review

EMERY P et al: The efficacy and safety of rituximab in patients with active rheumatoid arthritis despite methotrexate treatment. Arthritis Rheum 54(5):1390, 2006

FINCKH A et al: The effectiveness of anti-tumor necrosis factor therapy in preventing progressive radiographic joint damage in rheumatoid arthritis: a population-based study. Arthritis Rheum 54(1):54, 2006

GOLDBACH-MANSKY R, LIPSKY PE: New concepts in the treatment of rheumatoid arthritis. Annu Rev Med 54:197, 2003 Epub 2001 Dec 3. Review

KUHN KA et al: Antibodies against citrullinated proteins enhance tissue injury in experimental autoimmune arthritis. J Clin Invest 116(4):961, 2006

LIPSKY PE et al: Infliximab and methotrexate in the treatment of rheumatoid arthritis. Anti-Tumor Necrosis Factor Trial in Rheumatoid Arthritis with Concomitant Therapy Study Group. N Engl J Med 343(22):1594, 2000

MESSORI A et al: New drugs for rheumatoid arthritis. N Engl J Med 351(9):937, 2004

SMOLEN JS et al and the ACTIVE-CONTROLLED STUDY OF PATIENTS RECEIVING INFLIXIMAB FOR THE TREATMENT OF RHEUMATOID ARTHRITIS OF EARLY ONSET (ASPIRE) STUDY GROUP: Predictors of joint damage in patients with early rheumatoid arthritis treated with high-dose methotrexate with or without concomitant infliximab: results from the ASPIRE trial. Arthritis Rheum 54(3):702, 2006

TURESSON C, MATTESON EL: Genetics of rheumatoid arthritis. Mayo Clin Proc 81(1):94, 2006

315 Acute Rheumatic Fever
Jonathan R. Carapetis

Acute rheumatic fever (ARF) is a multisystem disease resulting from an autoimmune reaction to infection with group A streptococci. Although many parts of the body may be affected, almost all of the manifestations resolve completely. The exception is cardiac valvular damage [rheumatic heart disease (RHD)], which may persist after the other features have disappeared.

ARF and RHD are diseases of poverty. They were common in all countries until the early twentieth century, when their incidence began to decline in industrialized nations. This decline was largely attributable to improved living conditions—particularly less crowded housing and better hygiene—which resulted in reduced transmission of group A streptococci. The introduction of antibiotics and improved systems of medical care had a supplemental effect. Recurrent outbreaks of ARF began in the 1980s in the Rocky Mountain states of the United States, where elevated rates persist.

The virtual disappearance of ARF and reduction in the incidence of RHD in industrialized countries during the twentieth century unfortunately was not replicated in developing countries, where these diseases continue unabated. RHD is the most common cause of heart disease in children in developing countries and is a major cause of mortality and morbidity in adults as well. It was recently estimated that between 15 and 19 million people worldwide are affected by RHD, with approximately one-quarter of a million deaths occurring each year. Some 95% of ARF cases and RHD deaths now occur in developing countries.

Although ARF and RHD are relatively common in all developing countries, they occur at particularly elevated rates in certain regions. These "hot spots" are sub-Saharan Africa, Pacific nations, Australasia, and the Indian subcontinent (Fig. 315-1).

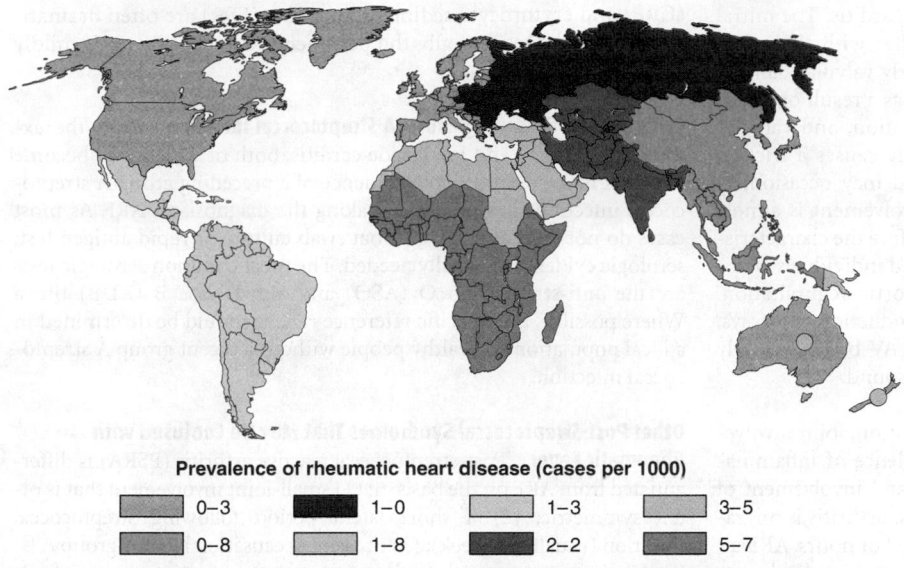

FIGURE 315-1 Prevalence of rheumatic heart disease in children aged 5–14 years. *Circles within Australia and New Zealand represent indigenous populations, and also Pacific Islanders in New Zealand. (Reprinted with permission from JR Carapetis et al: Lancet Infect Dis.)*

Prevalence of rheumatic heart disease (cases per 1000)

0–3	1–0
0–8	1–8
	1–3
	2–2
3–5	
5–7	

Epitopes present in the cell wall, cell membrane, and the A, B, and C repeat regions of the streptococcal M protein are immunologically similar to molecules in human myosin, tropomyosin, keratin, actin, laminin, vimentin, and N-acetylglucosamine. This molecular mimicry is the basis for the autoimmune response that leads to ARF. It has been hypothesized that human molecules—particularly epitopes in cardiac myosin—result in T cell sensitization. These T cells are then recalled following subsequent exposure to group A streptococci bearing immunologically similar epitopes.

However, myosin cross-reactivity with M protein does not explain the valvular damage that is the hallmark of rheumatic carditis, given that myosin is not present in valvular tissue. The link may be laminin, another α-helical coiled-coil protein like myosin and M protein, which is found in cardiac endothelium and is recognized by anti-myosin, anti-M protein T cells. Moreover, antibodies to cardiac valve tissue cross-react with the N-acetylglucosamine of group A streptococcal carbohydrate, and there is some evidence that these antibodies may be responsible for valvular damage.

EPIDEMIOLOGY

ARF is mainly a disease of children aged 5–14 years. Initial episodes become less common in older adolescents and young adults and are rare in persons aged >30 years. By contrast, recurrent episodes of ARF remain relatively common in adolescents and young adults. This pattern contrasts with the prevalence of RHD, which peaks between 25 and 40 years. There is no clear gender association for ARF, but RHD more commonly affects females, sometimes up to twice as frequently as males.

PATHOGENESIS

Organism Factors Based on currently available evidence, ARF is exclusively caused by infection of the upper respiratory tract with group A streptococci. It is now thought that any strain of group A streptococcus has the potential to cause ARF. Potential role of skin infection and of groups C and G streptococci are currently being investigated. It has been postulated that a series of preceding streptococcal infections is needed to "prime" the immune system prior to the final infection that directly causes disease.

Host Factors Approximately 3–6% of any population may be susceptible to ARF, and this proportion does not vary dramatically between populations. Findings of familial clustering of cases and concordance in monozygotic twins—particularly for chorea—confirm that susceptibility to ARF is an inherited characteristic. Particular HLA class II alleles appear to be strongly associated with susceptibility. Associations have also been described with high levels of circulating mannose-binding lectin and polymorphisms of transforming growth factor β_1 gene and immunoglobulin genes. High-level expression of a particular alloantigen present on B cells, D8-17, has been found in patients with a history of ARF in many populations, with intermediate-level expression in first-degree family members, suggesting that this may be a marker of inherited susceptibility.

The Immune Response When a susceptible host encounters a group A streptococcus, an autoimmune reaction results, which leads to damage to human tissues as a result of cross-reactivity between epitopes on the organism and the host (Fig. 315-2).

CLINICAL FEATURES

There is a latent period of ~3 weeks (1–5 weeks) between the precipitating group A streptococcal infection and the appearance of the clinical features of ARF. The exceptions are chorea and indolent carditis, which may follow prolonged latent periods lasting up to 6 months. Although many patients report a prior sore throat, the preceding group A streptococcal infection is commonly subclinical; in these cases it can only be confirmed using streptococcal antibody testing. The most common clinical presentation of ARF is polyarthritis and fever. Polyarthritis is present in 60–75% of cases and carditis in 50–60%. The prevalence of chorea in ARF varies substantially between populations, ranging from <2% to 30%. Erythema marginatum and subcutaneous nodules are now rare, being found in <5% of cases.

Heart Involvement Up to 60% of patients with ARF progress to RHD. The endocardium, pericardium, or myocardium may be affect-

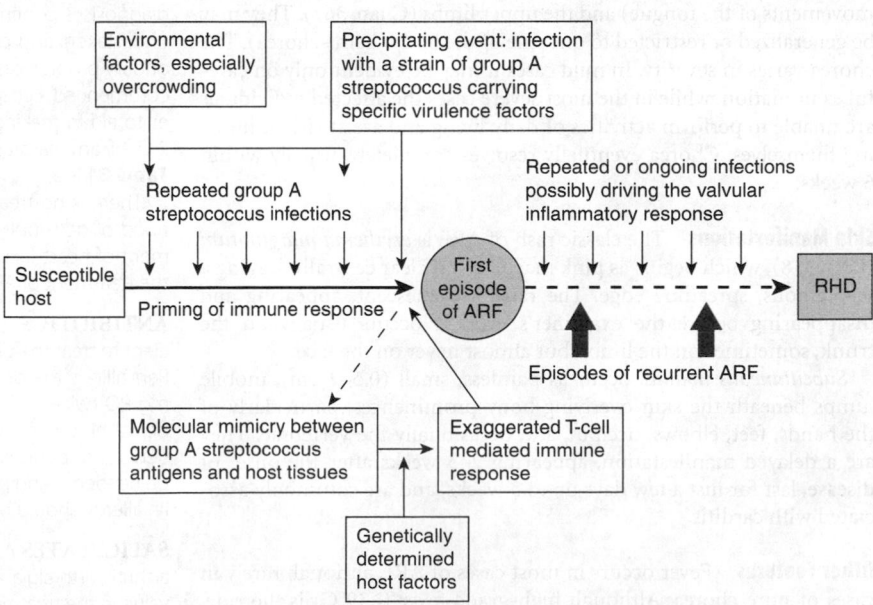

FIGURE 315-2 Pathogenetic pathway for acute rheumatic fever and rheumatic heart disease. *(Reprinted with permission from Lancet 366:155, 2005.)*

ed. Valvular damage is the hallmark of rheumatic carditis. The mitral valve is almost always affected, sometimes together with the aortic valve; isolated aortic valve involvement is rare. Early valvular damage leads to regurgitation. Over ensuing years, usually as a result of recurrent episodes, leaflet thickening, scarring, calcification, and valvular stenosis may develop. Pericarditis most commonly causes a friction rub or a small effusion on echocardiography and may occasionally cause pleuritic central chest pain. Myocardial involvement is almost never responsible in itself for cardiac failure. Therefore the characteristic manifestation of carditis in previously unaffected individuals is mitral regurgitation, sometimes accompanied by aortic regurgitation. Myocardial inflammation may affect electrical conduction pathways, leading to P-R interval prolongation (first-degree AV block or rarely higher-level block) and softening of the first heart sound.

Joint Involvement To qualify as a major manifestation, joint involvement in ARF must be arthritic, i.e., objective evidence of inflammation, with hot, swollen, red and/or tender joints and involvement of more than one joint (i.e., polyarthritis). The typical arthritis is migratory, moving from one joint to another over a period of hours. ARF almost always affects the large joints—most commonly the knees, ankles, hips, and elbows—and is asymmetric. The pain is severe and usually disabling until anti-inflammatory medication is commenced.

Less severe joint involvement is also relatively common but qualifies only as a minor manifestation. Arthralgia without objective joint inflammation usually affects large joints in the same migratory pattern as polyarthritis. In some populations, aseptic monoarthritis may be a presenting feature of ARF. This may occur because of early commencement of anti-inflammatory medication before the typical migratory pattern is established.

The joint manifestations of ARF are highly responsive to salicylates and other nonsteroidal anti-inflammatory drugs (NSAIDs). Indeed, joint involvement that persists more than 1 or 2 days after starting salicylates is unlikely to be due to ARF. Conversely, if salicylates are commenced early in the illness, before fever and migratory polyarthritis have become manifest, it may be difficult to make a diagnosis of ARF. For this reason, salicylates and other NSAIDs should be withheld—and pain managed with acetaminophen or codeine—until the diagnosis is confirmed.

Chorea Sydenham's chorea commonly occurs in the absence of other manifestations, follows a prolonged latent period after group A streptococcal infection, and is found mainly in females. The choreiform movements affect particularly the head (causing characteristic darting movements of the tongue) and the upper limbs (Chap. 367). They may be generalized or restricted to one side of the body (hemi-chorea). The chorea varies in severity. In mild cases it may be evident only on careful examination, while in the most severe cases the affected individuals are unable to perform activities of daily living and are at risk of injuring themselves. Chorea eventually resolves completely, usually within 6 weeks.

Skin Manifestations The classic rash of ARF is *erythema marginatum* (Chap. 18), which begins as pink macules that clear centrally, leaving a serpiginous, spreading edge. The rash is evanescent, appearing and disappearing before the examiner's eyes. It occurs usually on the trunk, sometimes on the limbs, but almost never on the face.

Subcutaneous nodules occur as painless, small (0.5–2 cm), mobile lumps beneath the skin overlying bony prominences, particularly of the hands, feet, elbows, occiput, and occasionally the vertebrae. They are a delayed manifestation, appearing 2–3 weeks after the onset of disease, last for just a few days up to 3 weeks, and are commonly associated with carditis.

Other Features Fever occurs in most cases of ARF, although rarely in cases of pure chorea. Although high-grade fever (≥39°C) is the rule, lower grade temperature elevations are not uncommon. Elevated acute-phase reactants are also present in most cases. C-reactive protein

(CRP) and erythrocyte sedimentation rate (ESR) are often dramatically elevated. Occasionally the peripheral leukocyte count is mildly elevated.

Evidence of a Preceding Group A Streptococcal Infection With the exception of chorea and low-grade carditis, both of which may become manifest many months later, evidence of a preceding group A streptococcal infection is essential in making the diagnosis of ARF. As most cases do not have a positive throat swab culture or rapid antigen test, serologic evidence is usually needed. The most common serologic tests are the anti-streptolysin O (ASO) and anti-DNase B (ADB) titers. Where possible, age-specific reference ranges should be determined in a local population of healthy people without a recent group A streptococcal infection.

Other Post-Streptococcal Syndromes That May Be Confused with Rheumatic Fever Post-streptococcal reactive arthritis (PSRA) is differentiated from ARF on the basis of: (1) small-joint involvement that is often symmetric; (2) a short latent period following streptococcal infection (usually <1 week); (3) occasional causation by non-group A β-hemolytic streptococcal infection; (4) slower responsiveness to salicylates; and (5) the absence of other features of ARF, particularly carditis.

Pediatric Autoimmune Neuropsychiatric Disorders Associated with Streptococcal infection (PANDAS) is a term that links a range of tic disorders and obsessive-compulsive symptoms with group A streptococcal infections. People with PANDAS are said not to be at risk of carditis, unlike patients with Sydenham's chorea. The diagnoses of PANDAS and PSRA should rarely be made in populations with a high incidence of ARF.

Confirming the Diagnosis Because there is no definitive test, the diagnosis of ARF relies on the presence of a combination of typical clinical features together with evidence of the precipitating group A streptococcal infection, and the exclusion of other diagnoses. This uncertainty led Dr. T. Duckett Jones in 1944 to develop a set of criteria (subsequently known as the *Jones criteria*) to aid in the diagnosis. An expert panel convened by the World Health Organization (WHO) clarified the use of the Jones criteria in ARF recurrences (Table 315-1). These criteria include a preceding streptococcal type A infection as well as some combination of major and minor manifestations.

℞ ACUTE RHEUMATIC FEVER

Patients with possible ARF should be followed closely to ensure that the diagnosis is confirmed, treatment of heart failure and other symptoms is undertaken, and preventive measures including commencement of secondary prophylaxis, inclusion on an ARF registry, and health education are commenced. Echocardiography should be performed on all possible cases to aid in making the diagnosis and to determine the severity at baseline of any carditis. Other tests that should be performed are listed in **Table 315-2**.

There is no treatment for ARF that has been proven to alter the likelihood of developing, or the severity of, RHD. With the exception of treatment of heart failure, which may be life-saving in cases of severe carditis, the treatment of ARF is symptomatic.

ANTIBIOTICS All patients with ARF should receive antibiotics sufficient to treat the precipitating group A streptococcal infection (Chap. 130). Penicillin is the drug of choice and can be given orally (as penicillin, 500 mg PO twice daily for 10 days) or as a single dose of 1.2 million units IM benzathine penicillin G. Erythromycin, 250 mg bid, may be used for patients with penicillin allergy. Because long-term secondary prophylaxis will be needed—and penicillin is the drug of choice for this—reported penicillin allergy should be confirmed, preferably in consultation with an allergist.

SALICYLATES AND NSAIDS These may be used for the treatment of arthritis, arthralgia, and fever, once the diagnosis is confirmed. They are of no value in the treatment of carditis or chorea. Aspirin is the drug of choice. An initial dose of 80–100 mg/kg per day in children (4–8 g/d in adults) in 4–5 divided doses is often needed for the first few days up to 2 weeks. A lower dose

TABLE 315-1 2002–2003 WORLD HEALTH ORGANIZATION CRITERIA FOR THE DIAGNOSIS OF RHEUMATIC FEVER AND RHEUMATIC HEART DISEASE (BASED ON THE 1992 REVISED JONES CRITERIA)

Diagnostic Categories	Criteria
Primary episode of rheumatic fever[a]	Two major or one major and two minor manifestations plus evidence of preceding group A streptococcal infection
Recurrent attack of rheumatic fever in a patient without established rheumatic heart disease	Two major or one major and two minor manifestations plus evidence of preceding group A streptococcal infection
Recurrent attack of rheumatic fever in a patient with established rheumatic heart disease[b]	Two minor manifestations plus evidence of preceding group A streptococcal infection[c]
Rheumatic chorea	Other major manifestations or evidence of group A streptococcal infection not required
Insidious onset rheumatic carditis[b]	
Chronic valve lesions of rheumatic heart disease (patients presenting for the first time with pure mitral stenosis or mixed mitral valve disease and/or aortic valve disease)[d]	Do not require any other criteria to be diagnosed as having rheumatic heart disease
Major manifestations	Carditis
	Polyarthritis
	Chorea
	Erythema marginatum
	Subcutaneous nodules
Minor manifestations	Clinical: fever, polyarthralgia
	Laboratory: elevated erythrocyte sedimentation rate or leukocyte count[e]
	Electrocardiogram: prolonged P-R interval
Supporting evidence of a preceding streptococcal infection within the last 45 days	Elevated or rising anti-streptolysin O or other streptococcal antibody, or
	A positive throat culture, or
	Rapid antigen test for group A streptococcus, or
	Recent scarlet fever[e]

[a]Patients may present with polyarthritis (or with only polyarthralgia or monoarthritis) and with several (3 or more) other minor manifestations, together with evidence of recent group A streptococcal infection. Some of these cases may later turn out to be rheumatic fever. It is prudent to consider them as cases of "probable rheumatic fever" (once other diagnoses are excluded) and advise regular secondary prophylaxis. Such patients require close follow up and regular examination of the heart. This cautious approach is particularly suitable for patients in vulnerable age groups in high incidence settings.
[b]Infective endocarditis should be excluded.
[c]Some patients with recurrent attacks may not fulfil these criteria.
[d]Congenital heart disease should be excluded.
[e]1992 Revised Jones criteria do not include elevated leukocyte count as a laboratory minor manifestation (but do include elevated C-reactive protein), and do not include recent scarlet fever as supporting evidence of a recent streptococcal infection.

Source: Reprinted with permission from WHO Expert Consultation on Rheumatic Fever and Rheumatic Heart Disease (2001: Geneva, Switzerland): *Rheumatic Fever and Rheumatic Heart Disease: Report of a WHO Expert Consultation* (WHO Tech Rep Ser, 923). Geneva, World Health Organization, 2004.

should be used if symptoms of salicylate toxicity emerge, such as nausea, vomiting, or tinnitus. When the acute symptoms are substantially resolved, the dose can be reduced to 60–70 mg/kg per day for a further 2–4 weeks. Fever, joint manifestations, and elevated acute-phase reactants sometimes recur up to 3 weeks after the medication is discontinued. This does not indicate a recurrence and can be managed by recommencing salicylates for a brief period. Although less well studied, naproxen at a dose of 10–20 mg/kg per day has been reported to lead to good symptomatic response.

CONGESTIVE HEART FAILURE Glucocorticoids The use of glucocorticoids in ARF remains controversial. Two meta-analyses have failed to demonstrate a benefit of glucocorticoids compared to placebo or salicylates in improving the short- or longer term outcome of carditis. However, the studies included in these meta-analyses all took place >40 years ago and did not use medications in common usage today. Many clinicians treat cases of severe carditis (causing heart failure) with glucocorticoids in the belief that they may reduce the acute inflammation and result in more rapid resolution of failure. However, the potential benefits of this treatment should be balanced against the possible adverse effects, including gastrointestinal bleeding and fluid retention. If used, prednisone or prednisolone are recommended at doses of 1–2 mg/kg per day (maximum, 80 mg). Intravenous methylprednisolone may be used in very severe carditis. Glucocorticoids are often only required for a few days or up to a maximum of 3 weeks.

MANAGEMENT OF HEART FAILURE See Chap. 227.

BED REST Traditional recommendations for long-term bed rest, once the cornerstone of management, are no longer widely practiced. Instead, bed rest should be prescribed as needed while arthritis and arthralgia are present, and for patients with heart failure. Once symptoms are well controlled, gradual mobilization can commence as tolerated.

CHOREA Medications to control the abnormal movements do not alter the duration or outcome of chorea. Milder cases can usually be managed by providing a calm environment. In patients with severe chorea, carbamazepine or sodium valproate are preferred to haloperidol. A response may not be seen for 1–2 weeks, and a successful response may only be to reduce rather than resolve the abnormal movements. Medication should be continued for 1–2 weeks after symptoms subside.

INTRAVENOUS IMMUNOGLOBULIN (IVIG) Small studies have suggested that IVIg may lead to more rapid resolution of chorea but has shown no benefit on the short- or long-term outcome of carditis in ARF without chorea. In the absence of better data, IVIg is *not* recommended except in cases of severe chorea refractory to other treatments.

PROGNOSIS

Untreated, ARF lasts on average 12 weeks. With treatment, patients are usually discharged from hospital within 1–2 weeks. Inflammatory markers should be monitored every 1–2 weeks until they have normalized (usually within 4–6 weeks), and an echocardiogram should be performed after 1 month to determine if there has been progression of carditis. Cases with more severe carditis need close clinical and echocardiographic monitoring in the longer term.

Once the acute episode has resolved, the priority in management is to ensure long-term clinical follow-up and adherence to a regimen of secondary prophylaxis. Patients should be entered onto the local

TABLE 315-2 RECOMMENDED TESTS IN CASES OF POSSIBLE ACUTE RHEUMATIC FEVER

Recommended for all cases
White blood cell count
Erythrocyte sedimentation rate
C-reactive protein
Blood cultures if febrile
Electrocardiogram (repeat in 2 weeks and 2 months if prolonged P-R interval or other rhythm abnormality)
Chest x-ray if clinical or echocardiographic evidence of carditis
Echocardiogram (consider repeating after 1 month if negative)
Throat swab (preferably before giving antibiotics)—culture for group A streptococcus
Anti-streptococcal serology: both anti-streptolysin O and anti-DNase B titres, if available (repeat 10–14 days later if 1st test not confirmatory)

Tests for alternative diagnoses, depending on clinical features
Repeated blood cultures if possible endocarditis
Joint aspirate (microscopy and culture) for possible septic arthritis
Copper, ceruloplasmin, anti-nuclear antibody, drug screen for choreiform movements
Serology and auto-immune markers for arboviral, auto-immune or reactive arthritis

Source: Reprinted with permission from National Heart Foundation of Australia.

TABLE 315-3 SUGGESTED DURATION OF SECONDARY PROPHYLAXIS[a]

Category of Patient	Duration of Prophylaxis
Patient without proven carditis	For 5 years after the last attack or 18 years of age (whichever is longer)
Patient with carditis (mild mitral regurgitation or healed carditis)	For 10 years after the last attack, or 25 years of age (whichever is longer)
More severe valvular disease	Lifelong
Valvular surgery	Lifelong

[a]These are only recommendations and must be modified by individual circumstances as warranted.

Source: Reprinted with permission from WHO Expert Consultation on Rheumatic Fever and Rheumatic Heart Disease (2001: Geneva, Switzerland): *Rheumatic Fever and Rheumatic Heart Disease: Report of a WHO Expert Consultation* (WHO Tech Rep Ser, 923). Geneva, World Health Organization, 2004.

ARF registry (if present) and contact made with primary care practitioners to ensure a plan for follow-up and administration of secondary prophylaxis before the patient is discharged. Patients and their families should also be educated about their disease, emphasizing the importance of adherence to secondary prophylaxis. If carditis is present, they should also be informed of the need for antibiotic prophylaxis against endocarditis for dental and surgical procedures.

PREVENTION

Primary Prevention Ideally, primary prevention would entail elimination of the major risk factors for streptococcal infection, particularly overcrowded housing and inadequate hygiene infrastructure. This is difficult to achieve in most places where ARF is common.

Therefore, the mainstay of primary prevention for ARF remains primary prophylaxis, i.e., the timely and complete treatment of group A streptococcal sore throat with antibiotics. If commenced within 9 days of sore throat onset, a course of 10 days of penicillin V (500 mg bid PO in adults) or a single IM injection of 1.2 million units of benzathine penicillin G will prevent almost all cases of ARF that would otherwise have developed. This important strategy relies on individuals presenting for medical care when they have a sore throat, the availability of trained health and microbiology staff along with the materials and infrastructure to take throat swabs, and a reliable supply of penicillin. Unfortunately, many of these elements are not available in developing countries. Moreover, the majority of cases of ARF do not follow a sore throat sufficiently severe for the patient to seek medical attention.

Secondary Prevention The mainstay of controlling ARF and RHD is secondary prevention. Because patients with ARF are at dramatically higher risk than the general population of developing a further episode of ARF after a group A streptococcal infection, they should receive long-term penicillin prophylaxis to prevent recurrences. The best antibiotic for secondary prophylaxis is benzathine penicillin G (1.2 million units, or 600,000 units if <30 kg) delivered every 4 weeks or more frequently (e.g., every 3 weeks or even every 2 weeks) to persons considered to be at particularly high risk. Oral penicillin V (250 mg) can be given twice-daily instead but is somewhat less effective than benzathine penicillin G. Penicillin allergic patients can receive erythromycin (250 mg) twice daily.

The duration of secondary prophylaxis is determined by many factors, in particular the duration since the last episode of ARF (recurrences become less likely with increasing time), age (recurrences are less likely with increasing age), and the severity of RHD (if severe, it may be prudent to avoid even a very small risk of recurrence because of the potentially serious consequences) (Table 315-3). Secondary prophylaxis is best delivered as part of a coordinated RHD control program, based around a registry of patients. Registries improve the ability to follow patients and identify those who default from prophylaxis and institute strategies to improve adherence.

FURTHER READINGS

CARAPETIS JR et al: Acute rheumatic fever. Lancet 366:155, 2005

CARAPETIS JR et al: The global burden of group A streptococcal diseases. Lancet Infect Dis 5:685, 2005

CILLIERS AM: Rheumatic fever and its management. BMJ 333:1153, 2006

GUILHERME L et al: Molecular mimicry in the autoimmune pathogenesis of rheumatic heart disease. Autoimmunity 39:31, 2006

NATIONAL HEART FOUNDATION OF AUSTRALIA: *Diagnosis and Management of Acute Rheumatic Fever and Rheumatic Heart Disease in Australia: Complete Evidence-Based Review and Guideline.* Melbourne, National Heart Foundation of Australia, 2006

SPECIAL WRITING GROUP OF THE COMMITTEE ON RHEUMATIC FEVER, ENDOCARDITIS AND KAWASAKI DISEASE OF THE AMERICAN HEART ASSOCIATION: Guidelines for the diagnosis of acute rheumatic fever: Jones criteria, 1992 update. JAMA 268:2069, 1992

316 Systemic Sclerosis (Scleroderma) and Related Disorders
John Varga

DEFINITION

Systemic sclerosis (SSc) is a chronic systemic disorder of unknown etiology. SSc is characterized by thickening of the skin (scleroderma) and distinctive involvement of multiple internal organs, most notably the lungs, gastrointestinal tract, heart, and kidneys. The early stage of the disease, associated with prominent inflammatory features, is followed by the development of widespread functional and structural alterations in multiple vascular beds and progressive visceral organ dysfunction due to fibrosis. The presence of thickened skin (scleroderma) distinguishes SSc from other connective tissue diseases. Scleroderma-like skin induration can occur in various disorders in addition to localized forms of scleroderma (Table 316-1), and it is important to accurately differentiate these conditions from SSc. The disease is highly heterogeneous. Patients with SSc can be classified into two distinct subsets defined by the distribution pattern and extent of skin involvement, as well as other clinical and laboratory manifestations (Table 316-2). Diffuse cutaneous SSc (dcSSc) presents with progressive skin induration, starting in the fingers and ascending from distal to proximal extremities, the face, and the trunk. These patients are at risk for early pulmonary fibrosis and acute renal involvement. In limited cutaneous SSc (lcSSc), patients generally have long-standing Raynaud's phenomenon before other manifestations of SSc appear. Skin induration is limited to the fingers (sclerodactyly), distal extremities, and face, and the trunk is not affected. A subset of patients with lcSSc have prominent calcinosis cutis, Raynaud's phenomenon, esophageal dysmotility, sclerodactyly, and telangiectasia, a constellation termed *CREST syndrome*. However, these features may also be seen in patients with dcSSc. Visceral organ involvement in lcSSc tends to show insidious progression. Although the long-term prognosis of lcSSc is better than that of dcSSc, pulmonary arterial hypertension (PAH), hypothyroidism, and primary biliary cirrhosis may occur in the late stage of the former. In some patients, Raynaud's phenomenon and other typical features of SSc occur in the absence of detectable skin thickening. This syndrome has been termed *SSc sine scleroderma*.

EPIDEMIOLOGY

 SSc is an acquired sporadic disease with a worldwide distribution and affecting all races. In the United States, the incidence is 9–19 cases per million per year. The only community-based survey of SSc yielded a prevalence of 286 cases per million population. There are an estimated 100,000 cases of SSc in the United States, although this number may be significantly higher if patients who do not

TABLE 316-1 CONDITIONS ASSOCIATED WITH SCLERODERMA-LIKE INDURATION

Systemic sclerosis
    Limited cutaneous SSc
    Diffuse cutaneous SSc
Localized scleroderma
    Guttate morphea, diffuse morphea
    Linear scleroderma, coup de sabre, hemifacial atrophy
Overlap syndromes
    Mixed connective tissue disease
    SSc/polymyositis
Undifferentiated connective tissue disease
Scleredema and diabetic scleredema
Scleromyxedema (papular mucinosis)
Nephrogenic fibrosing syndrome (nephrogenic fibrosing dermatopathy)
Chronic graft-versus-host disease
Diffuse fasciitis with eosinophilia (Shulman disease, eosinophilic fasciitis)
Eosinophilia-myalgia syndrome
Chemically induced scleroderma-like conditions
    Vinyl chloride–induced disease
    Pentazocine-induced skin fibrosis
Paraneoplastic syndrome

meet strict classification criteria are also included. Studies from England, Australia, and Japan showed rates of SSc that were lower than in the United States. Age, gender, and ethnicity are important factors determining disease susceptibility. Like other connective tissue diseases, SSc shows a female predominance, greatest in the childbearing years and declining after menopause. While SSc can present at any age, the most common age of onset is in the range of 30–50 years. African Americans have a higher incidence than whites, and disease onset occurs at an earlier age. Furthermore, African Americans are more likely to have the diffuse cutaneous form of SSc with interstitial lung involvement as well as a worse prognosis.

GENETIC CONSIDERATIONS SSc shows a non-Mendelian pattern of inheritance. The concordance rate for SSc among twins is low (4.7%), although concordance for the presence of antinuclear antibodies is significantly greater. A genetic contribution to disease susceptibility is indicated by the fact that 1.6% of SSc patients have a first-degree relative with SSc. The risk of other autoimmune diseases, including systemic lupus erythematosus (Chap. 313) and rheumatoid arthritis (Chap. 314), is also increased. Among Choctaw Native Americans, SSc prevalence as high as 4690 per million has been reported. Genetic investigations in SSc to date have focused on polymorphisms of candidate genes, particularly those involved in immunity and inflammation, vascular function, and connective tissue homeostasis. Associations of single nucleotide polymorphism (SNP) with SSc have been reported in the genes encoding angiotensin-converting enzyme (ACE); endothelin-1 and nitric oxide synthase; B cell markers (CD19); chemokines (monocyte chemoattractant protein-1) and chemokine receptors; cytokines [interleukin 1α, IL-4, and tumor necrosis factor α (TNF-α)]; growth factors and their receptors [connective tissue growth factor (CTGF) and transforming growth factor β (TGF-β)]; and extracellular matrix proteins [fibronectin, fibrillin, and secreted protein acidic-rich in cysteine (SPARC)].

ENVIRONMENTAL FACTORS

Patients with SSc have increased serum antibodies to human cytomegalovirus (hCMV), and antitopoisomerase-I (Scl-70) autoantibodies recognize antigenic epitopes present on the hCMV-derived proteins, suggesting molecular mimicry as a possible mechanistic link between hCMV infection and SSc. Evidence of human parvovirus B19 infection in SSc patients has also been presented; however, the etiologic role of viruses remains unproven. Reports of apparent geographic clustering of SSc

cases suggesting shared environmental exposures have not been substantiated by careful investigation. An epidemic of a novel syndrome with features suggestive of SSc occurred in Spain in the 1980s. The outbreak, termed *toxic oil syndrome* and affecting over 20,000 individuals, was linked to consumption of contaminated rapeseed oils used for cooking. A similar epidemic outbreak, termed *eosinophilia-myalgia syndrome* (EMS), occurred a decade later in the United States. Affected individuals presented with marked peripheral blood eosinophilia and severe myalgia, followed by the development of scleroderma-like chronic skin lesions. The epidemic was linked to the consumption of imported batches of L-tryptophan used as dietary supplements. The incidence rate of new cases of EMS showed a dramatic decline following the nationwide recall of L-tryptophan products. While both of these apparently novel toxic-epidemic syndromes were characterized by scleroderma-like chronic skin changes and variable visceral organ involvement, their clinical, pathological, and laboratory features clearly distinguished them from SSc. The incidence of SSc is increased among miners exposed to silica. Other occupational exposures tentatively linked with SSc include polyvinyl chloride, epoxy resins, and aromatic hydrocarbons including toluene and trichloroethylene. Drugs implicated in SSc-like illnesses include bleomycin, pentazocine and cocaine, and appetite suppressants linked with pulmonary hypertension. Case reports and series describing SSc in women with silicone breast implants had raised concern regarding a possible etiologic role of silicone in SSc. However, large-scale epidemiologic investigations found no evidence of increased risk of SSc.

PATHOGENESIS

A comprehensive view of the pathogenesis of SSc must take into account the three cardinal features of the disease: (1) vasculopathy, (2) cellular and humoral immunity, and (3) progressive visceral and vascular fibrosis in multiple organs (Fig. 316-1). Autoimmunity and altered endothelial cell function and vascular reactivity may be the earliest manifestations of SSc. Complex interplay between these processes is thought to initiate and then amplify and sustain the fibrotic process.

Animal Models of Disease There is no single animal model that reproduces all three cardinal processes that underlie the pathogenesis of SSc, but some models recapitulate selected disease characteristics. The tight-skin mouse is a naturally occurring fibrosis model characterized by spontaneous skin thickening. The mutation responsible for the phenotype, a duplication in the fibrillin-1 gene, results in defective extracellular matrix assembly and aberrant activation of TGF-β. Mutations in the fibrillin-1 gene have not been described in patients with SSc. Chronic fibrosis in the skin and lungs can be induced in mice by bleomycin injections or by transplantation of HLA-mismatched bone marrow or spleen cells. Increasingly, manipulation of mice via mutagenesis or targeted genetic modification such as knock-out or transgenesis are utilized to create new models for SSc and to dissect the roles of individual molecules in the underlying processes. For instance, genetic targeting of Smad3, an intracellular TGF-β signal transducer, or of the chemokine monocyte chemoattractant protein-1 (MCP-1) yielded mice that were resistant to bleomycin-induced scleroderma.

TABLE 316-2 SUBSETS OF SYSTEMIC SCLEROSIS (SSC): LIMITED CUTANEOUS SSC VERSUS DIFFUSE CUTANEOUS SSC

Features	Limited Cutaneous SSc	Diffuse Cutaneous SSc
Skin involvement	Limited to fingers, distal to elbows, face; slow progression	Diffuse: fingers, extremities, face, trunk; rapid progression
Raynaud's phenomenon	Precedes skin involvement; associated with critical ischemia	Onset contemporaneous with skin involvement
Pulmonary fibrosis	May occur, moderate	Frequent, early and severe
Pulmonary arterial hypertension	Frequent, late, may be isolated	May occur, associated with pulmonary fibrosis
Scleroderma renal crisis	Very rare	Occurs in 15%; early
Calcinosis cutis	Frequent, prominent	May occur, mild
Characteristic autoantibodies	Anticentromere	Antitopoisomerase I (Scl-70)

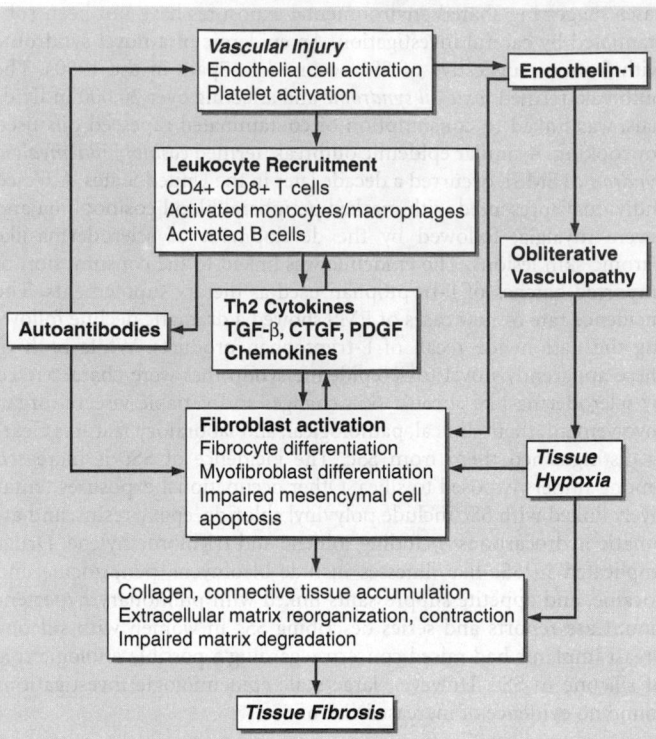

FIGURE 316-1 The pathogenesis of systemic sclerosis. Initial vascular injury in genetically susceptible individuals leads to functional and structural vascular alterations, inflammation, and autoimmunity. The inflammatory and immune responses initiate and sustain fibroblast activation and differentiation, resulting in pathological fibrogenesis and irreversible tissue damage.

Vasculopathy Vascular involvement in SSc is extensive and has important clinical consequences. Raynaud's phenomenon, an early manifestation, is characterized by an altered blood-flow response to cold challenge. This initially reversible vascular abnormality is associated with alterations in the autonomic and peripheral nervous systems, with impaired production of neuropeptides such as calcitonin gene-related peptide from sensory afferent nerves and heightened sensitivity of α_2-adrenergic receptors on vascular smooth-muscle cells. While isolated Raynaud's phenomenon is relatively benign and nonprogressive, in patients with SSc it is associated with irreversible morphological and functional changes. Viruses, superoxide radicals, and vascular cytotoxic factors such as serum proteases, complement, and circulating antiendothelial cell autoantibodies may each contribute to endothelial cell injury in early SSc. Endothelial injury results in dysregulated production of endothelium-derived vasodilatory (nitric oxide and prostacyclin) and vasoconstricting (endothelin-1) substances, as well as increased expression of intercellular adhesion molecule 1 (ICAM-1) and other surface adhesion molecules. Microvessels show enhanced permeability and transendothelial leukocyte diapedesis, activation of coagulation and fibrinolytic cascades, and platelet aggregation. Smooth-muscle cell-like myointimal cells proliferate, the basement membrane is thickened and reduplicated, and fibrosis of the adventitial layers develops. The vasculopathic process affects capillaries, arterioles, and even large vessels in many organs, resulting in reduced blood flow and impaired tissue oxygenation.

Progressive luminal occlusion due to intimal and medial hypertrophy and adventitial fibrosis, combined with persistent endothelial cell damage and apoptosis, establish a vicious cycle culminating in the striking absence of blood vessels seen on angiograms of the hands and kidneys of patients with late-stage disease. Damaged endothelium promotes platelet aggregation with release of platelet alpha granules including thromboxane, a potent vasoconstrictor, and of platelet-derived growth factor (PDGF). Vascular compromise is further aggravated by defective fibrinolysis. Oxidative stress due to ischemia-reperfusion is associated with generation of free radicals that further damage the endothelium through peroxidation of membrane lipids. Paradoxically, the process of revascularization that normally reestablishes blood flow to ischemic tissue is defective in SSc. Failure of vasculogenesis occurs in the setting of elevated serum levels of vascular endothelial growth factor (VEGF) and other angiogenic factors. The number of bone marrow–derived CD34+ CD133+ endothelial progenitor cells is markedly reduced in the circulation, and their differentiation in vitro into mature endothelial cells is impaired. Thus, widespread obliterative vasculopathy and failure to repair damaged vessels are hallmarks of SSc.

Cellular and Humoral Autoimmunity In the early stages of SSc, activated T cells and monocytes/macrophages accumulate in lesional skin, lungs, and other effected organs. Infiltrating T cells express CD45 and HLA-DR activation markers and display restricted receptor signatures indicative of oligoclonal expansion in response to (unknown) antigen. Circulating CD4+ T cells have elevated levels of chemokine receptors and α_1 integrin adhesion molecules accounting for their enhanced ability to bind to endothelium and to fibroblasts. Endothelial cells express ICAM-1 and other adhesion molecules that facilitate leukocyte diapedesis. Activated macrophages and T cells show a T_H2-polarized immune response and secrete IL-4 and IL-13. T_H2 cytokines induce the production of TGF-β and promote collagen synthesis and other profibrotic responses, whereas the T_H1 cytokine interferon γ (IFN-γ) inhibits collagen synthesis and blocks cytokine-mediated fibroblast activation. Because TGF-β stimulates its own synthesis, as well as that of CTGF (also termed CCN2) and other cytokines, TGF-β establishes an autocrine/paracrine stimulatory loop that sustains activation of fibroblasts and other effector cells (Chaps. 308 and 312).

Circulating autoantibodies occur in virtually all patients with SSc. These mutually exclusive autoantibodies are highly specific for SSc and show strong association with individual disease phenotypes and genetically determined HLA haplotypes. Autoantibody levels correlate with disease severity, and titers fluctuate with disease activity. Some SSc-specific autoantibodies are antinuclear and directed against proteins involved in mitosis, such as topoisomerase-I, centromere, and the RNA polymerases; others are directed against cell-surface antigens or secreted proteins. While autoantibodies have well-established clinical utility as diagnostic and prognostic markers, their pathogenetic role in the clinical manifestations of SSc remains uncertain. Topoisomerase-I autoantibodies can directly bind to fibroblasts, and autoantibodies to fibroblasts, endothelial cells, PDGF cell-surface receptors, fibrillin-1, and matrix metalloproteinase enzymes have been described in SSc patients. Some of these autoantibodies may play a direct role in tissue damage.

Multiple potential mechanisms have been proposed to account for the generation of autoantibodies in SSc. According to one theory, in patients with SSc, certain proteins undergo modifications such as proteolytic cleavage, increased expression, or altered subcellular localization, resulting in their recognition by the immune system. For example, the protease granzyme B is released from cytotoxic T cells, cleaves peptides, and generates potential neo-epitopes that can break immune tolerance. Recent studies implicate B cells in both the autoimmune and fibrotic responses in SSc. In addition to their well-recognized role in antibody production, B cells can also present antigen, produce IL-6 and TGF-β, and modulate T cell and dendritic cell function. In patients with SSc, B cells show elevated expression of the CD19 membrane receptor, the naive B cell compartment is expanded, and numbers of memory B cells and early plasma cells are reduced. Gene expression profiling of lesional skin has identified mRNA expression signatures characteristic of activated B cells.

Fibrosis Fibrosis affecting multiple organs distinguishes SSc from other connective tissue diseases. Fibrosis characteristically follows and is thought to be a consequence of autoimmunity and vascular damage. The process, characterized by progressive replacement of normal tissue architecture with dense connective tissue, accounts for substantial morbidity and mortality in SSc. Fibroblasts are mesenchymal cells responsible for maintaining the functional and structural integrity of connective tissue. When activated by TGF-β and related factors, fibroblasts proliferate, migrate, elaborate collagen and extracellular matrix, secrete growth factors and cytokines and express surface receptors for them, and transdifferentiate into myofibroblasts. Together, these responses allow fibroblasts to repair tissue injury under normal circumstances. While the fibroblast repair program is rapid and self-limited under physiologic conditions, the activation of fibroblasts in pathological fibrosis is sustained and amplified, resulting in exaggerated matrix remodeling and scar formation.

In addition to resident connective tissue fibroblasts, circulating mesenchymal progenitor cells of bone marrow origin also contribute to fibrosis. The factors that regulate the production of mesenchymal progenitor cells in the bone marrow and their trafficking from the circulation into lesional tissue, and promote their differentiation in situ into matrix-producing adhesive and contractile fibrocytes, are unknown. Fibroblasts can undergo transdifferentiation into smooth-muscle–like myofibroblasts. While myofibroblasts can be transiently detected during normal wound healing, they persist in tissue during pathological fibrogenesis, possibly due to abnormal resistance to apoptosis. Myofibroblasts contribute to scar formation via their ability to produce collagen and TGF-β and to contract the surrounding extracellular matrix, converting it into dense scar.

Fibroblasts explanted from SSc lesional tissues display an abnormal phenotype in culture indicative of autonomous activation. Compared to normal fibroblasts, SSc fibroblasts are characterized by variably increased rates of collagen gene transcription. Furthermore, they display smooth-muscle actin stress fibers; enhanced synthesis and secretion of extracellular matrix molecules, cytokines, and growth factors; expression of chemokine receptors and cell surface adhesion molecules; resistance to apoptosis; and constitutive autocrine TGF-β signaling. The abnormal "scleroderma phenotype" persists during serial passage of these cells in vitro. The mechanisms underlying the autonomously activated phenotype are unknown; persistent fibroblast activation via autocrine stimulatory loops involving TGF-β, selection of activated fibroblast subpopulations driven by hypoxia or immune factors, intrinsic abnormalities in SSc fibroblasts, and altered cell-matrix interaction may be involved. Recent studies indicate that intracellular blockade of TGF-β signaling can partially "normalize" the activated phenotype in SSc lesional fibroblasts, suggesting that autocrine TGF-β signaling contributes to the persistent fibrogenic phenotype of SSc fibroblasts. Results from global transcriptome analyses of SSc fibroblasts show differential expression of many extracellular matrix genes, including collagens, fibronectin, and fibrillins. A majority of the abnormally expressed genes could be mechanistically linked to TGF-β responses, but other fibrogenic signaling pathways also operate in SSc.

PATHOLOGY

The distinguishing pathologic hallmark of SSc is the combination of widespread obliterative vasculopathy of small arteries and arterioles and fibrosis in the skin and internal organs. Whereas in established SSc these lesions occur in the absence of inflammation, in relatively early-stage disease, perivascular cellular infiltrates may be detected in multiple organs prior to the appearance of fibrosis. In the skin, infiltrates are located in the reticular dermis and are composed primarily of CD4+ T lymphocytes. In addition, CD8+ T cells, monocytes/macrophages, plasma cells, mast cells, and occasionally B cells may be detected. In the lungs the majority of infiltrating T cells are CD8+. Evidence of eosinophil degranulation in the absence of intact eosinophils may be found. The vascular lesion is characterized by intimal proliferation in the small and medium-sized arteries, resulting in luminal narrowing. Obliterative vasculopathy is a late finding most prominent in the heart, lungs, kidneys, and intestinal tract. Tissue fibrosis is found in the skin, lungs, gastrointestinal tract, heart, tendon sheath, perifascicular tissue surrounding skeletal muscle, and some endocrine organs. In these tissues, accumulation of connective tissue composed of collagens, fibronectin, proteoglycans, and other structural macromolecules leads to progressive replacement of normal tissue architecture, resulting in functional impairment of affected organs.

Skin In the skin, fibrosis causes massive dermal expansion and obliteration of the hair follicles, sweat glands, and other appendages (Fig. 316-2A). Collagen fiber accumulation is prominent in the reticular dermis, and the fibrotic process invades the subjacent adipose layer with entrapment of fat cells. The epidermis is atrophic, and the rete pegs are effaced.

FIGURE 316-2 Pathologic findings in systemic sclerosis. A. Dermal sclerosis. The skin is thickened due to marked expansion of the dermis. Thick bundles of densely packed collagen replaces skin appendages. **B.** Early interstitial lung disease. Diffuse fibrosis of the alveolar septae and a chronic inflammatory cell infiltrate. Trichrome stain. **C.** Pulmonary arterial obliterative vasculopathy. Striking intimal hyperplasia and narrowing of the lumen of a small pulmonary artery, with minimal interstitial fibrosis, in a patient with limited cutaneous SSc.

Lungs Patchy infiltration of the alveolar walls with CD8+ lymphocytes, macrophages, and eosinophils occurs in early disease. With progression, interstitial fibrosis and vascular damage dominate the pathological picture, often coexisting within the same lesions in patients with dcSSc. Pulmonary fibrosis is characterized by expansion of the alveolar interstitium, with accumulation of collagen and other connective tissue proteins. The most common histologic pattern is nonspecific interstitial pneumonitis (Fig. 316-2B). Progressive thickening of the alveolar septae results in obliteration of the airspaces and honeycombing, as well as loss of pulmonary blood vessels. This process impairs gas exchange and contributes to worsening of pulmonary hypertension. Intimal thickening of the pulmonary arteries, best seen with elastin stain, underlies pulmonary hypertension (Fig. 316-2C) and, at autopsy, is often associated with multiple pulmonary emboli and evidence of myocardial fibrosis.

Gastrointestinal Tract Pathologic changes can be found at any level from the mouth to the rectum. The lower esophagus is frequently involved, with prominent fibrosis of the lamina propria and submucosa and atrophy of the muscular layers; striated muscle in the upper third of the esophagus is generally spared. Characteristic vascular lesions are often present. Replacement of the normal intestinal tract architecture results in disordered peristaltic activity, with gastroesophageal reflux, dysmotility, and small-bowel obstruction. Chronic reflux is associated with esophageal inflammation, ulcerations, and stricture formation and may lead to premalignant Barrett's metaplasia.

Kidneys In the kidneys, lesions in the interlobular arteries predominate, whereas glomerulonephritis is rare. Chronic renal ischemia is associated with shrunken glomeruli. Patients with scleroderma renal crisis show dramatic changes in small renal arteries with reduplication of elastic lamina, marked intimal proliferation, and narrowing of the lumen, often accompanied by thrombosis and microangiopathic hemolysis.

Heart The heart is frequently affected, with prominent involvement of the myocardium and pericardium. The characteristic arteriolar lesions of intimal proliferation and luminal narrowing are accompanied by contraction band necrosis, reflecting ischemia-reperfusion injury, and patchy myocardial fibrosis that may also involve the conduction system.

Other Organs Synovitis may be found in early SSc; however, with progression of the disease, the synovium becomes fibrotic. Fibrosis of tendon sheaths and fascia produces palpable and sometimes audible tendon friction rubs. Inflammatory myositis and, in later stages, muscle atrophy and fibrosis are common findings. Fibrosis of the thyroid gland and of the minor salivary glands may be seen.

CLINICAL FEATURES

Overview Systemic sclerosis can affect virtually every organ (Table 316-3). The disease shows a great deal of variability in its clinical expression from one patient to the next. Patients can be classified into one of two major subsets defined by the degree of clinically involved skin (Table 316-2). In dcSSc, internal organ involvement occurs early and is often progressive. In contrast, lcSSc presents with long-standing Raynaud's phenomenon, is associated with indolent skin and limited internal organ involvement, and carries a better prognosis. While classification of SSc into diffuse and limited cutaneous subsets is useful, disease expression is far more complex, and several distinct phenotypes are recognized within each subset. For example, 10–15% of patients with lcSSc develop severe pulmonary artery hypertension without significant interstitial lung disease (ILD). Other patients have systemic features of SSc without appreciable skin involvement (SSc sine scleroderma). Unique clinical phenotypes of SSc associate with specific autoantibodies (Table 316-4). Patients with "overlap" have typical SSc features coexisting with clinical and laboratory evidence of another autoimmune disease such as polymyositis, autoimmune thyroid disease, Sjögren's syndrome, polyarthritis, autoimmune liver disease, or systemic lupus erythematosus.

The term *scleroderma* refers to localized scleroderma and is used to describe a group of localized fibrosing skin disorders that primarily affect children (Table 316-1). In contrast to SSc, localized scleroderma is rarely associated with internal organ involvement. Morphea presents as solitary or multiple circular patches of thickened skin and, less commonly, widespread induration (generalized morphea); the fingers are spared. Linear scleroderma—streaks of thickened skin, typically in one or both lower extremities—may affect the subcutaneous tissues with fibrosis and atrophy of supporting structures, muscle, and bone. In children, the growth of affected long bones can be retarded. When linear scleroderma lesions cross joints, significant contractures can develop.

Initial Clinical Presentation The initial clinical presentation is quite different in the diffuse and the limited cutaneous forms of the disease. In dcSSc, the interval between Raynaud's phenomenon and appearance of other manifestations is generally brief (weeks to months). Soft tissue swelling and intense pruritus are signs of the early inflammatory "edematous" phase of dcSSc. The skin on the fingers, hands, distal limbs, and face is usually affected first. Patients may note diffuse hyperpigmentation. Carpal tunnel syndrome can occur. Arthralgias are common and may be associated with muscle weakness and decreased joint mobility. During the ensuing weeks to months, the inflammatory edematous phase evolves into the "fibrotic" phase. Fibrosis starts in the dermis and is associated with loss of body hair, reduced production of skin oils, and a decline in sweating capacity. The subcutaneous tissue becomes affected, with fat atrophy and fibrosis of underlying fascia, muscle, and other soft tissue structures. Progressive flexion contractures of the fingers ensue. The wrists, elbows, shoulders, hip girdles, knees, and ankles are also affected due to fibrosis of the supporting joint structures. While advancing skin involvement is the most visible manifestation of early active dcSSc, progressive internal organ involvement occurs during this stage. The initial 4 years of the disease is the period of rapidly evolving systemic involvement; if organ failure does not occur during this period, the systemic process may then stabilize without further progression.

The course of the disease in lcSSc is more indolent and relatively benign. The period between the onset of Raynaud's phenomenon and

TABLE 316-4 AUTOANTIBODIES IN SYSTEMIC SCLEROSIS (SSC)

Target Antigen	SSc Subset	Characteristic Clinical Association
Topoisomerase-I	dcSSc	ILD, cardiac involvement, scleroderma renal crisis
Centromere proteins	lcSSc	Digital ischemia, calcinosis, isolated PAH
U3-RNP	dcSSc	PAH, ILD, scleroderma renal crisis, myositis
Th/T0	lcSSc	ILD, PAH
PM/Scl	lcSSc	Calcinosis, myositis
U1-RNP	MCTD	PAH
RNA polymerase III	dcSSc	Extensive skin, scleroderma renal crisis

Note: dcSSc, diffuse cutaneous SSc; lcSSc, limited cutaneous SSc; ILD, interstitial lung disease; PAH, pulmonary arterial hypertension.

TABLE 316-3 INTERNAL ORGAN INVOLVEMENT: LIMITED CUTANEOUS AND DIFFUSE CUTANEOUS FORMS OF SYSTEMIC SCLEROSIS

Features	Limited Cutaneous SSc (%)	Diffuse Cutaneous SSc (%)
Skin involvement	90[a]	100
Raynaud's phenomenon	99	98
Esophageal involvement	90	80
Pulmonary fibrosis	35	65
Pulmonary arterial hypertension	25	15
Myopathy	11	23
Cardiac involvement	9	12
Scleroderma renal crisis	2	15

[a]10% of lcSSc patients have SSc sine scleroderma.

additional manifestations such as gastroesophageal reflux, telangiectasia, or calcinosis is commonly several years. Raynaud's phenomenon tends to be more severe in lcSSc and is frequently associated with critical digital ischemia, ulcerations, and autoamputation. Although significant renal involvement or pulmonary fibrosis is uncommon, isolated pulmonary artery hypertension develops in 10–15% of patients with lcSSc. Overlap of SSc with other autoimmune syndromes, including the sicca complex, polyarthritis, cutaneous vasculitis, and biliary cirrhosis, occurs primarily in the lcSSc subset.

ORGAN INVOLVEMENT

Raynaud's Phenomenon Raynaud's phenomenon, defined as episodic vasoconstriction in the fingers and toes, develops in virtually every patient with SSc. In some, episodes may also affect the tip of the nose and earlobes. Attacks are triggered by exposure to cold, a decrease in temperature, emotional stress, and vibration. In colder climates, patients commonly experience an increase in the frequency and severity of episodes during the winter months. Typical attacks start with pallor, followed by cyanosis of variable duration. Eventually erythema develops spontaneously or with rewarming of the digit. The progression of the three color phases reflects the underlying pathogenic mechanisms of vasoconstriction, ischemia, and reperfusion. Some patients with Raynaud's phenomenon may experience only pallor or cyanosis.

As much as 3–5% of the general population has Raynaud's phenomenon, and it is more frequent in women. In the absence of associated signs or symptoms of an underlying condition, Raynaud's phenomenon is classified as primary, and represents an exaggerated physiological response to cold. Secondary Raynaud's phenomenon occurs as a complication of SSc and other connective tissue diseases, hematological and endocrine conditions, and occupational disorders, as well as in association with the use of beta blockers such as atenolol, anticancer drugs such as cisplatin and bleomycin, and a variety of other medications. Distinguishing primary versus secondary Raynaud's phenomenon can present a diagnostic challenge. The lack of an underlying cause for Raynaud's phenomenon on the basis of the history and physical examination; a positive family history of Raynaud's phenomenon; absence of digital tissue necrosis, ulceration, or gangrene; and a negative test for antinuclear antibodies support the diagnosis of primary Raynaud's phenomenon. Secondary Raynaud's phenomenon tends to develop at an older age (>30 years), is clinically more severe (episodes more frequent, prolonged, and painful), and is frequently associated with ischemic lesions and infarction in the digits (Fig. 316-3). The cutaneous capillaries at the nailbed can be viewed under a drop of grade B immersion oil using a low-power stereoscopic microscope. Nailfold microscopy may be helpful in Raynaud's phenomenon; patients with primary Raynaud's phenomenon have normal capillaries

FIGURE 316-3 Digital necrosis. Sharply demarcated necrosis of the fingertip in a patient with limited cutaneous SSc.

FIGURE 316-4 Sclerodactyly. Note skin induration and fixed flexion contractures at the proximal interphalangeal joints in a patient with limited cutaneous SSc.

that appear as regularly spaced parallel vascular loops, whereas in SSc and other connective tissue diseases, nailfold capillaries are distorted with widened and irregular loops, dilated lumen, and areas of vascular "dropout." In patients with SSc, Raynaud's-like abnormal vascular reactivity may involve multiple vascular beds, and cold-induced episodic vasospasm has been documented in the pulmonary, renal, gastrointestinal, and coronary circulations.

Skin Features Clinically evident skin thickening is the hallmark of SSc that distinguishes it from other connective tissue diseases. The distribution of skin thickening is invariably symmetrical and bilateral. In the early stages of dcSSc, edema is gradually replaced by skin thickening that characteristically advances from distal to proximal extremities in an ascending centripetal fashion. In the affected areas, the skin is firm, coarse, and thickened. The extremities and trunk may be darkly pigmented. In some patients, diffuse tanning in the absence of sun exposure is a very early manifestation of skin involvement. In dark-skinned patients, vitiligo-like hypopigmentation may occur. Because pigment loss spares the perifollicular areas, a "salt-and-pepper" appearance of the skin may be seen; this pattern is most common on the scalp, upper back, and chest. Dermal sclerosis due to collagen accumulation causes obliteration of hair follicles, sweat glands, and sebaceous glands, resulting in hair loss, decreased sweating, and dry skin. Transverse creases on the dorsum of the fingers disappear (Fig. 316-4). The fingers develop fixed flexion contractures, causing reduced hand mobility and muscle atrophy. Skin thickening in combination with fibrosis of the subjacent tendons accounts for contractures of the wrists, elbows, and knees. Thick ridges at the neck due to firm adherence of skin to the underlying platysma muscle interfere with neck extension. The face assumes a characteristic "mauskopf" appearance with taut and shiny skin, loss of wrinkles, and occasionally an expressionless facies due to reduced mobility of the eyelids, cheeks, and mouth. Thinning of the lips with accentuation of the central incisor teeth and fine wrinkles (radial furrowing) around the mouth complete the picture. The oral aperture may be dramatically reduced; microstomia interferes with eating and oral hygiene. The nose assumes a pinched, beak-like appearance.

In established SSc of long duration, the affected skin is firmly bound to the subcutaneous fat (tethering) and undergoes thinning and atrophy. Macular telangiectasia 2–20 mm in diameter occur frequently, particularly in lcSSc. These skin lesions, which resemble the telangiectasia seen in hereditary hemorrhagic telangiectasia, are prominent on the face, hands, lips, and oral cavity. Breakdown of atrophic skin leads to slow-healing ulcerations that are most common at the extensor surfaces of the proximal interphalangeal joints. Other sites for skin ulcerations include the volar pads of the fingertips and bony prominences such as the elbows and malleoli. Chronic ulcers are painful and may become secondarily infected, resulting in osteomyelitis. Healing of ischemic fingertip ulcerations leaves characteristic digital "pits." Soft tissue loss at the fingertips due to ischemia is frequent and may be associated with striking resorption of the terminal phalanges (acro-osteolysis) (Fig. 316-5).

Calcium deposits occur in the skin and soft tissues, particularly in patients with lcSSc who are positive for anticentromere antibodies.

FIGURE 316-5 Acro-osteolysis. Note dissolution of terminal phalanges in a patient with long-standing limited cutaneous SSc.

The deposits, varying in size from tiny punctate lesions to large conglomerate masses, are composed of calcium hydroxyapatite crystals and can be readily visualized on plain x-rays. Frequent locations include the finger pads, palms, extensor surfaces of the forearms, and the olecranon and prepatellar bursae (Fig. 316-6). Paraspinal calcifications may cause neurological complications. Calcific deposits are generally noted as persistent firm, nontender subcutaneous lumps and may occasionally ulcerate through the overlying skin, producing drainage of chalky white material, pain, and local inflammation.

Pulmonary Features   Pulmonary involvement can be documented in most patients with SSc and is now the leading cause of death. The two main types of significant pulmonary involvement are ILD and PAH; many patients develop some degree of both complications. Less frequent pulmonary manifestations include aspiration pneumonitis complicating gastroesophageal reflux, pulmonary hemorrhage due to endobronchial telangiectasia, obliterative bronchiolitis, pleural reactions, restrictive ventilatory defect due to chest wall fibrosis, and spontaneous pneumothorax. The incidence of lung cancer, particularly bronchoalveolar carcinoma, may be increased in patients with SSc.

Pulmonary involvement may remain asymptomatic until it is advanced. The most frequent presenting symptoms of pulmonary involvement—exertional dyspnea, fatigue, and reduced exercise tolerance—are often subtle and slowly progressive. A chronic dry cough may be present. Physical examination may reveal "Velcro" crackles at the lung bases. Pulmonary function testing (PFT) is a sensitive method for detecting early pulmonary involvement in asymptomatic patients. The most common abnormalities are reductions in forced vital capacity (FVC) or single breath diffusing capacity (DLCO). A reduction in DLCO that is significantly out of proportion to the reduction

FIGURE 316-6 Calcinosis cutis. Note large calcific deposit breaking through the skin in a patient with limited cutaneous SSc.

in FVC suggests pulmonary vascular disease, but may also be due to anemia. With exercise, patients show a decrease in PO_2.

INTERSTITIAL LUNG DISEASE (ILD)   Some evidence of ILD can be found at autopsy in up to 90% of patients with SSc and by thin-section high-resolution computed tomography (HRCT) in 85%. ILD and pulmonary fibrosis cause restrictive lung disease with impaired gas exchange, characterized on PFT by decreased FVC and DLCO but unaffected flow rates. Clinically significant ILD develops in 16–43% of patients with SSc, the frequency depending on the detection method used and the characteristics of the patient population. Risk factors include male gender, African-American race, diffuse skin involvement, severe gastroesophageal reflux, and the presence of topoisomerase-I autoantibodies, as well as a low FVC or DLCO at initial presentation. In patients who develop significant ILD, the most rapid progression in lung disease occurs early in the course of the disease (within the first 3 years), when the FVC declines by an average of 32% per year.

Chest radiography is useful for ruling out infection and other causes of pulmonary involvement, but it is relatively insensitive for detection of early ILD. HRCT of the chest is more sensitive and may show reticular linear opacities predominantly in the lower lobes, even in asymptomatic patients (Fig. 316-7). Additional findings include mediastinal lymphadenopathy, nodules, and honeycombing. Ground-glass opacification, seen in 50% of patients, is not specific for identifying alveolitis or predicting rapidly progressing lung disease. Bronchoalveolar lavage (BAL) may be useful for identifying inflammation in the lower respiratory tract and ruling out infection. In some studies, an elevated proportion of neutrophils (>2%) and/or eosinophils (>3%) in the BAL fluid was associated with more extensive lung disease, more rapid decline in FVC, and reduced survival. Lung biopsy is indicated only in patients with atypical findings on chest radiographs and should be thoracoscopically guided. The histologic pattern on lung biopsy may be helpful in predicting the risk of progression of ILD. The most common pattern in SSc, nonspecific interstitial pneumonitis, carries a better prognosis than usual interstitial pneumonitis. Recent studies suggest that measurement of serum markers such as KL-6, a glycoprotein found in type II pneumocytes and alveolar macrophages, may have utility in the detection and serial monitoring of ILD in patients with SSc.

FIGURE 316-7 High-resolution CT scan of the lungs. Note peripheral bilateral reticulonodular opacifications in the lower lobes of the lungs in a patient with diffuse cutaneous SSc.

PULMONARY ARTERIAL HYPERTENSION (PAH) PAH, defined as a mean pulmonary arterial pressure >25 mm Hg at rest, as determined by right heart catheterization, is increasingly recognized as a major complication of SSc. Approximately 12–25% of SSc patients have evidence of PAH. In these patients, PAH may occur in association with ILD or as an isolated pulmonary abnormality. The natural history of SSc-associated PAH is variable, but in many patients it follows a relentlessly downhill course with development of right heart failure and significant mortality. Risk factors for PAH include limited cutaneous disease with anticentromere antibodies, late age at disease onset, severe Raynaud's phenomenon, and the presence of U1-RNP, U3-RNP (fibrillarin), and B23 antibodies.

Patients with early PAH are generally asymptomatic. The initial symptom is typically exertional dyspnea and reduced exercise capacity. With progression, angina, exertional near-syncope, and symptoms and signs of right-sided heart failure appear. Physical examination shows tachypnea, a prominent pulmonic S2 heart sound, palpable right ventricular heave, elevated jugular venous pressure, and dependent edema. Doppler echocardiography provides an estimate of pulmonary arterial systolic pressures and also indicates the presence of valvular abnormalities or left ventricular systolic or diastolic dysfunction that could cause pulmonary hypertension due to elevated pulmonary venous pressures. Echocardiogram-derived estimates of pulmonary arterial systolic pressures exceeding 40 mm Hg at rest suggest PAH. Pulmonary function testing may show a reduced DLCO in isolation or combined with a restrictive pattern. Right heart catheterization is required to confirm the presence of PAH and accurately assess its severity. Recent studies indicate that elevated serum levels of brain natriuretic peptide (BNP) and N-terminal BNP correlate with the presence and severity of PAH, suggesting a potential role for BNP measurements in screening SSc patients for PAH and in monitoring response to treatment. The prognosis of PAH is determined by the degree of pulmonary arterial pressure elevation.

Gastrointestinal Involvement The gastrointestinal tract is affected in up to 90% of patients with SSc and may be asymptomatic or present with unexplained weight loss. Gastrointestinal involvement is characterized by abnormal motility of the esophagus, stomach, and small and large intestines. The pathological features are similar throughout the length of the gastrointestinal tract, with prominent atrophy and fibrosis of smooth muscle, intact mucosa, and obliterative small-vessel vasculopathy. Oropharyngeal manifestations are frequent and are due to a combination of xerostomia, reduced oral aperture, and periodontal disease. Symptoms of gastroesophageal reflux disease (GERD) develop early. Most patients have heartburn, regurgitation, and dysphagia. A combination of reduced lower esophageal sphincter pressure, impaired esophageal clearance of refluxed gastric contents due to diminished motility in the distal two-thirds of the esophagus, and delayed gastric emptying accounts for GERD. Severe erosive esophagitis may be found on endoscopy in patients with minimal symptoms. Endoscopy may be necessary to rule out opportunistic infections with Candida, herpes virus, and cytomegalovirus. Esophageal strictures and Barrett's esophagus may complicate chronic GERD. Because Barrett's esophagus is associated with adenocarcinoma, SSc patients with this lesion need to undergo periodic endoscopy and biopsy. Extra-esophageal manifestations of GERD, such as hoarseness and chronic cough, and aspiration pneumonitis aggravating ILD may occur.

Gastroparesis is common and may cause early satiety, abdominal pain and distension, and aggravated reflux symptoms. The presence and severity of gastroparesis can be assessed by radionuclide gastric emptying studies. Gastric vascular ectasia may occur in the antrum. These subepithelial lesions, part of the diffuse small-vessel vasculopathy of SSc, give a watermelon appearance on endoscopy. Patients with watermelon stomach may have recurrent episodes of occult gastrointestinal bleeding, resulting in unexplained anemia. Manometric testing shows abnormalities in the upper small intestines of most patients with SSc. Impaired motility may result in malabsorption and chronic diarrhea secondary to bacterial overgrowth. Fat and protein malabsorption and B12 and vita-

min D deficiency ensue, sometimes culminating in severe malnutrition. Disturbed intestinal motor function can also cause intestinal pseudoobstruction. Patients present with recurrent episodes of acute abdominal pain, nausea, and vomiting. Radiographic studies show acute intestinal obstruction, and the major diagnostic challenge is to differentiate pseudoobstruction, which responds to supportive care and intravenous nutritional supplementation, from mechanical obstruction. Colonic involvement may cause constipation, fecal incontinence, and rectal prolapse. In late-stage SSc, wide-mouth sacculations in the colon may occur, causing perforation and bleeding. An occasional radiologic finding is pneumatosis cystoides intestinalis due to air trapping in the bowel wall that may rupture and cause benign pneumoperitoneum. Primary biliary cirrhosis may coexist with SSc.

Renal Involvement Hypertension and chronic nonprogressive proteinuria are frequent in SSc. Scleroderma renal crisis, which is the most dreaded complication of SSc, occurs in 20–25% of patients, most commonly within 4 years of the onset of the disease. Until the advent of ACE inhibitor drugs, short-term survival of patients with scleroderma renal crisis was <10%. The pathogenesis of scleroderma renal crisis involves obliterative vasculopathy of the renal cortical arteries. Progressive reduction in renal blood flow, aggravated by vasospasm, leads to juxtaglomerular apparatus hyperplasia, renin secretion, and activation of the renin-angiotensin axis, with further renal vasoconstriction resulting in a vicious cycle that culminates in malignant hypertension. Factors that further compromise already impaired renal blood flow, such as dehydration and hypotension, play a role in precipitating scleroderma renal crisis. Risk factors include African-American race, male gender, diffuse and rapidly progressive skin involvement, and autoantibodies to RNA polymerase III. The presence of palpable tendon friction rubs, pericardial effusion, new unexplained anemia, and thrombocytopenia may predict impending scleroderma renal crisis. High-risk patients should be monitored closely and counseled to check their blood pressure daily. Patients with lcSSc only infrequently develop scleroderma renal crisis. Because there is a significant association between glucocorticoid use and the onset of scleroderma renal crisis, prednisone should be avoided in high-risk SSc patients.

Patients characteristically present with abrupt onset of malignant hypertension. They may complain of severe headache, blurred vision, and chest pain and have striking elevation of blood pressure. In approximately 10% of patients, blood pressure remains normal (normotensive renal crisis). Urinalysis shows proteinuria and microscopic hematuria; thrombocytopenia and evidence of a microangiopathic hemolysis with fragmented red blood cells is seen. Rapidly progressive oliguric renal failure generally follows. In some patients, scleroderma renal crisis is misdiagnosed as thrombotic thrombocytopenic purpura. A creatinine >3 mg/dl at presentation predicts poor outcome, with permanent hemodialysis and high mortality. Prompt aggressive intervention with ACE inhibitors to achieve blood pressure control before renal failure results in significantly improved prognosis.

Cardiac Involvement Cardiac involvement is manifested by myocardial and pericardial disease and conduction system abnormalities. Cardiac involvement can also occur secondary to PAH and scleroderma renal crisis. Despite the presence of widespread obliterative vasculopathy in SSc, the frequency of clinical or pathological coronary artery disease is not elevated. Most patients with cardiac involvement remain asymptomatic until heart failure or serious arrhythmias occur. Overt signs of cardiac involvement in SSc are associated with increased mortality. Thallium perfusion studies document abnormal cardiac perfusion in a majority of patients. Raynaud's-like episodic vasospasm of the coronary arteries has been described. Echocardiographic evidence of left ventricular diastolic dysfunction is frequent. Diastolic dysfunction may be due to hypertension or myocardial fibrosis, but its clinical significance is unclear. Myocarditis can develop in association with inflammatory polymyositis. Conduction defects and arrhythmias due to fibrosis or ischemia of the conduction system are frequent. Pericardial effusions may occur, causing symptoms and, rarely, tamponade.

Musculoskeletal Complications Carpal tunnel syndrome occurs frequently and may be a presenting manifestation of SSc. Generalized arthralgia and stiffness are prominent in early disease. Joint mobility is progressively impaired, especially in patients with dcSSc. Most commonly affected are the hands, where contractures at the proximal interphalangeal joints and wrists develop, sometimes accompanied by tendon friction rubs characterized by leathery crepitation that can be heard or palpated upon passive movement. Tendon rubs are due to extensive fibrosis and adhesion of the tendon sheaths and fascial planes at the affected joint. Movement at the elbows, shoulders, and knees is frequently reduced. True joint inflammation is uncommon; however, occasional patients develop features of rheumatoid arthritis and, rarely, severe erosive asymmetrical polyarthritis of the joints in the hands. Muscle weakness may reflect deconditioning, disuse atrophy, and malnutrition. Less commonly, inflammatory myositis indistinguishable from idiopathic polymyositis may occur. A chronic noninflammatory myopathy characterized by atrophy and fibrosis in the absence of elevated muscle enzyme levels is seen in some patients with late-stage SSc. Bone resorption , a frequent late complication, occurs most commonly in the terminal phalanges, where it causes loss of the distal tufts (acro-osteolysis) (Fig. 316-5). Acro-osteolysis of the mandibular condyles can lead to bite difficulties. Osteolysis can also affect the ribs and distal clavicles.

Other Disease Manifestations Many SSc patients develop dry eyes and dry mouth (sicca complex). Biopsy of the minor salivary glands shows fibrosis rather than focal lymphocytic infiltration characteristic of primary Sjögren's syndrome (Chap. 317). Hypothyroidism is common and generally due to fibrosis of the thyroid gland. Whereas the central nervous system is generally spared in SSc, sensory trigeminal neuropathy due to fibrosis or vasculopathy can occur, presenting with gradual onset of pain and numbness. Pregnancy in women with SSc is associated with an increased rate of adverse fetal outcomes. Furthermore, worsening cardiopulmonary involvement may occur during pregnancy, and new onset of scleroderma renal crisis has been described. Erectile dysfunction is frequent in men with SSc and may be the initial disease manifestation. Inability to attain or maintain penile erection is due to vascular insufficiency and fibrosis.

LABORATORY FEATURES

Anemia is frequent in patients with SSc and may have different etiologies. Most common is a mild normocytic or microcytic anemia due to chronic inflammation. Serum iron is low or normal, whereas ferritin levels are elevated. Iron deficiency anemia may indicate gastrointestinal bleeding caused by watermelon stomach or chronic esophagitis. Macrocytic anemia, indicating a maturation disorder, may be caused by folate and vitamin B_{12} deficiency due to small bowel bacterial overgrowth and malabsorption, or by drugs that interfere with cellular DNA metabolism, such as methotrexate or alkylating agents. Acute microangiopathic hemolytic anemia, caused by mechanical trauma and fragmentation of red blood cells during their passage through microvessels coated with fibrin or platelet thrombi, frequently accompanies scleroderma renal crisis. Thrombocytopenia and leukopenia occur rarely and generally indicate drug toxicity. In contrast to other connective tissue diseases, the erythrocyte sedimentation rate (ESR) is generally normal; an elevation may indicate coexisting myositis or malignancy.

Antinuclear autoantibodies can be detected in almost all patients with SSc and are present at disease onset. Some of these autoantibodies, such as those directed against topoisomerase-I (Scl-70) and centromere, are very highly specific for SSc and are mutually exclusive. Furthermore, a patient's specific autoantibody profile remains stable over time. Each of the eight distinct autoantibodies described in SSc shows a strong association with a particular disease phenotype (Table 316-4). Topoisomerase-I antibodies are detected in 31% of patients with dcSSc, but in only 13% of patients with lcSSc; conversely, anticentromere antibodies are detected in 38% of patients with lcSSc, but in only 2% of patients with dcSSc. Topoisomerase-I antibodies generally occur in patients with dcSSc and early-onset ILD. Anticentromere antibodies occur in patients

with lcSSc with PAH, whereas cardiac and renal involvement and significant ILD are rare in these patients. Patients with topoisomerase-I antibody have reduced survival compared to those without this antibody; whereas patients with anticentromere antibody have improved survival compared to those without this antibody. The characteristic nucleolar immunofluorescene pattern of SSc detected on serological testing is due to antibody recognition of U3-RNP (fibrillarin), Th/To, and PM/Scl. No direct pathogenic role has been established for SSc-associated autoantibodies; however, recent studies indicate that antibody titers correlate with disease severity and fluctuate with disease activity.

Diagnosis The diagnosis of SSc is made primarily on clinical grounds and is generally straightforward in patients with established disease. The presence of skin induration, with a characteristic symmetrical distribution pattern associated with typical visceral organ manifestations, establishes the diagnosis with a high degree of certainty. While the conditions listed in Table 316-1 may be associated with variable skin induration, the distribution pattern of these lesions, absence of Raynaud's phenomenon, and lack of typical visceral organ manifestations or SSc-specific autoantibodies help to differentiate these conditions from SSc. Occasionally, full-thickness biopsy of the skin may be indicated to establish the diagnosis of scleredema, scleromyxedema, or nephrogenic systemic fibrosis. In lcSSc a history of antecedent Raynaud's phenomenon and gastroesophageal reflux symptoms, coupled with the presence of sclerodactyly, often in combinations with telangiectasia and calcinosis cutis, helps to establish the diagnosis. The finding of digital tip pitting scars and radiological evidence of pulmonary fibrosis in the lower lobes are particularly helpful diagnostically. Primary Raynaud's phenomenon is a common disorder that must be differentiated from early or limited SSc. Nailfold microscopy is particularly helpful in this situation, because in primary Raynaud's phenomenon the nailfold capillaries are normal, whereas in SSc capillary abnormalities can be detected even before other disease manifestations.

Establishing the diagnosis of SSc in early disease may be a challenge. In patients with dcSSc, initial symptoms are often nonspecific and relate to inflammation. Raynaud's phenomenon may be absent at this stage, and patients complain of fatigue, swelling, aching, and stiffness; muscle weakness and weight loss may be prominent. Physical examination may reveal diffuse edema and swelling of the fingers. Patients are sometimes diagnosed as early rheumatoid arthritis, systemic lupus erythematosus, myositis, or, most commonly, undifferentiated connective tissue disease. Within weeks to months, Raynaud's phenomenon develops, and the disease assumes its characteristic clinical features with advancing induration of the skin. The presence of antinuclear and SSc-specific autoantibodies, most commonly anticentromere or antitopoisomerase-I, provides a high degree of diagnostic specificity. Raynaud's phenomenon with fingertip ulcerations or other evidence of digital ischemia, coupled with telangiectasia, distal esophageal dysmotility, unexplained ILD, or PAH, or malignant hypertension with renal failure in the absence of skin induration, suggests the diagnosis of SSc sine scleroderma. These patients generally have anticentromere antibodies.

℞ SYSTEMIC SCLEROSIS

OVERVIEW To date, no therapy has been shown to significantly alter the natural history of SSc. In contrast, multiple interventions are highly effective in alleviating the symptoms and in slowing the progression of the cumulative organ damage. A significant reduction in disease-related mortality has been noted during the past 25 years. Because of the marked heterogeneity in clinical presentations, patients with SSc need careful investigation, and evaluation and treatment approaches must be individually tailored according to each patient's unique needs. Optimal management incorporates the following principles: prompt and accurate diagnosis; classification and risk stratification based on clinical and laboratory evaluation; early recognition of organ-based complications and assessment of their extent, severity, and likelihood of deterioration; ongoing regular monitoring for progression, disease activity, and response to therapy; and continuing patient education. In order to minimize irreversible organ damage, the approach to the management of life-threatening complications must be proactive, with regular screening and initiation of appropriate intervention at the earliest possible opportunity. In light of the highly complex and multisystemic nature of SSc, a holistic approach that integrates care by specialists from multiple disciplines is best. Most patients are treated with combinations of drugs that act upon different aspects of the disease. It is important that patients become familiar with the full spectrum of potential complications, have a thorough understanding of the therapeutic options and natural history of the disease, and be encouraged to partner with their physicians in its management. This typically requires a long-term relationship between patient and physician, with ongoing counseling and encouragement.

Disease-Modifying Treatments Immunosuppressive agents that are effective in controlling other connective tissue diseases have generally shown modest or no benefit in the treatment of SSc. Glucocorticoids may decrease stiffness and aching in patients with early-stage dcSSc but do not influence the progression of skin or internal organ involvement. Furthermore, use of glucocorticoids in high doses is associated with an increased risk of scleroderma renal crisis. Therefore glucocorticoids should be avoided if possible; when absolutely necessary, they should be given at the lowest dose possible and for brief periods only. Cyclophosphamide has been extensively studied, in light of its efficacy in the treatment of vasculitis (Chap. 319), systemic lupus erythematosus (Chap. 313) and other autoimmune diseases (Chap. 312). A number of retrospective uncontrolled clinical trials evaluated the efficacy of daily oral and intermittent intravenous cyclophosphamide in SSc-related ILD. These studies, as well as a recent placebo-controlled multicenter clinical trial, showed that cyclophosphamide reduced the progression of ILD in patients with early symptomatic disease, with stabilization, and, rarely, modest improvement in abnormalities of pulmonary function and HRCT. Improvement in the extent of skin induration has also been noted. Patients with early-stage SSc and evidence of progressive pulmonary involvement appear to be candidates for cyclophosphamide therapy. Cyclophosphamide is generally given for 6–12 months, but the optimal duration of therapy has not been established. The benefits of cyclophosphamide need to be balanced by its potential toxicity. Well-recognized adverse effects include bone marrow suppression, opportunistic infections, hemorrhagic cystitis and bladder cancer, premature ovarian failure, and late secondary malignancies.

In small clinical trials, methotrexate, an antimetabolite used extensively in the treatment of rheumatoid arthritis, showed a modest therapeutic benefit. The potential profibrotic effects of methotrexate, manifested as infrequent liver cirrhosis and ILD, raise concern regarding its use in a fibrotic disorder. Mycophenolate mofetil treatment was associated with improved skin induration in uncontrolled studies and was generally well tolerated. Therapeutic immunomodulation using cyclosporine, azathioprine, extracorporeal photophoresis, thalidomide, or rapamycin is currently not well-supported by the literature. Immune ablation using high-dose chemotherapy, followed by autologous peripheral stem cell reconstitution, has been performed in SSc. Because uncontrolled studies have shown that stem cell transplantation in patients with extensive SSc and poor prognosis was associated with variable clinical response, this form of intervention is currently undergoing evaluation in randomized prospective clinical trials. In light of its substantial morbidity and mortality, autologous stem cell transplantation in SSc is still considered experimental.

Because widespread tissue fibrosis causes progressive organ damage in dcSSc, drugs that interfere with the fibrotic process represent a rational approach to therapy. D-penicillamine has been extensively used in SSc as an antifibrotic agent. Retrospective studies indicated that, by virtue of its immunosuppressive activity and ability to prevent cross-linking of extracellular collagen fibers, D-penicillamine stabilized and improved skin induration, prevented new internal organ involvement, and improved survival. However, a randomized controlled clinical trial in early active SSc found no difference in the extent of skin involvement between patients treated with standard-dose (750 mg/d) or very low-dose (125 mg every other d) D-penicillamine. Minocycline, recombinant relaxin, and INF-γ have failed to show meaningful clinical benefit in small studies.

The goal of vascular therapy is to control episodes of Raynaud's phenomenon, prevent the development and enhance the healing of ischemic complications, and slow the progression of obliterative vasculopathy. Patients with Raynaud's phenomenon should be instructed to dress warmly, minimize cold exposure or stress, and avoid drugs that could precipitate or exacerbate vasospastic episodes. Some patients may respond to biofeedback therapy. Calcium channel blockers such as nifedepine or diltiazem are commonly used but show only moderate benefit, and their use is often limited by side effects (palpitations, dependent edema, light-headedness). While ACE inhibitors are not effective for reducing the frequency or severity of episodes, angiotensin II receptor blockers such as losartan are effective and generally well tolerated. Additional vasoactive therapies for Raynaud's phenomenon include α_1-adrenergic receptor blockers (e.g., prazosine), 5-phosphodiesterase inhibitors (e.g., sildenafil), serotonin reuptake inhibitors (e.g., fluoxetine), topical nitroglycerine, and intravenous prostaglandins. Low-dose aspirin and dipyridamole prevent platelet aggregation and may have a role as adjunctive agents. In patients with ischemic ulcerations on the fingers, the endothelin-1 receptor antagonist bosentan reduces the development of new ulcers. Digital sympathectomy may be effective in some patients with severe Raynaud's phenomenon associated with ischemia. Empiric long-term therapy with statins and antioxidants may delay the progression of vascular damage and obliteration.

Treatment of Gastrointestinal Complications Because gastroesophageal reflux is very common, all patients with SSc should be treated for this complication. Significant reflux may occur in the absence of symptoms. Patients should be instructed to elevate the head of the bed and eat frequent small meals. Proton pump inhibitors and H2 blockers are effective and may need to be given in relatively high doses. Recurrent bleeding from vascular ectasia in the gastric antrum (watermelon stomach) is amenable to treatment with laser photocoagulation. Bacterial overgrowth due to small-bowel dysmotility causes bloating and diarrhea and may lead to malabsorption and severe malnutrition. Aggressive treatment with short courses of rotating broad-spectrum antibiotics such as metronidazole, erythromycin, and tetracycline can eradicate bacterial overgrowth. Parenteral hyperalimentation is indicated if malnutrition develops. Chronic hypomotility of the small bowel may respond to octreotide injections.

Treatment of Pulmonary Arterial Hypertension Patients with SSc should be screened for the presence of PAH on a regular basis. When PAH is symptomatic, treatment should be started with an oral endothelin-1 receptor antagonist. Most patients should also receive diuretics, oral anticoagulation, and digoxin when appropriate. Endothelin-1 receptor antagonists such as bosentan have been shown to improve exercise tolerance and slow the rate of clinical deterioration in pulmonary arterial hypertension. If hypoxemia is documented, supplemental oxygen should be given by nasal cannula in order to avoid hypoxia-induced secondary pulmonary vasoconstriction. Inhibitors of phosphodiesterase type 5 (e.g., sildenafil) have been shown to have short-term efficacy in PAH and may be used in combination with bosentan. If inadequate clinical response or progression of disease is seen, parenteral prostacyclin analogues may be used. Epoprostenol or treprostinil are administered intravenously or by continuous subcutaneous infusion, and iloprost by frequent inhalations. Lung transplantation remains an option for some SSc patients who fail therapy.

Treatment of Renal Crisis Scleroderma renal crisis is a medical emergency because its outcome is largely determined by the extent of renal damage present at the time when aggressive therapy is initiated. Prompt recognition of impending or early scleroderma renal crisis is therefore essential, and efforts should be made to avoid its occurrence. High-risk patients with early SSc and extensive and progressive skin involvement should be instructed to monitor their blood pressure daily and report significant alterations to their physician immediately. They should avoid nonsteroidal anti-inflammatory drugs (NSAIDs) and glucocorticoids. When scleroderma renal crisis occurs, treatment should be started promptly with ACE inhibitors. Kidney biopsy is rarely indicated in this setting. Short-term dialysis may be appropriate, particularly because substantial renal recovery can occur following renal crisis, and patients may be able to discontinue dialysis. Kidney transplantation is considered for patients who are unable to discontinue dialysis after 1–2 years.

Skin Care Because skin involvement in SSc is never life-threatening, stabilizes, and may even regress spontaneously over time, the overall management of the disease should not be dictated by its cutaneous manifestations. The inflammatory symptoms of early skin involvement can be effectively controlled with systemic antihistamines and cautious use of low-dose glucocorticoids (less than 5 mg/d of prednisone) for brief periods. Retrospective studies have shown that D-penicillamine reduced the extent and progression of skin induration; however, these benefits could not be substantiated in a controlled prospective trial. Cyclophosphamide and methotrexate have also been shown to have modest effects on skin induration. Because induration is associated with dryness, patients should use hydrophilic ointments and bath oils. Regular skin massage is helpful. Telangiectasia may present a cosmetic problem, especially when they occur on the face. Treatment with pulsed dye laser may be effective. Fingertip ulcerations should be protected by occlusive dressing to promote healing and prevent infection. Infected skin ulcers are treated with topical antibiotics. Surgical debridement may be indicated. No therapy has been shown to be effective in preventing the formation of calcific soft tissue deposits or in promoting their dissolution.

COURSE AND PROGNOSIS

The natural history of SSc is highly variable and difficult to predict, especially in early stages when the specific disease subset—diffuse or limited cutaneous form—is not clear. Patient with dcSSc have a more rapidly progressive disease and worse prognosis than those with lcSSc.

In dcSSc, early inflammatory symptoms such as fatigue, edema, arthralgia, and pruritus tend to subside 2–4 years after the onset of disease, and the extent of skin thickening reaches a plateau after which it generally shows slow regression. It is during the early edematous stage, generally lasting <3 years, that visceral organ involvement develops and progresses. While existing visceral organ involvement, such as pulmonary fibrosis, may continue to progress, new organ involvement is rare after the skin involvement reaches its peak. Scleroderma renal crisis almost invariably occurs within the first 4 years of disease. In dcSSc patients with late-stage disease (>6 years), the skin is usually soft and atrophic. Skin regression characteristically occurs in an order that is the reverse of initial involvement, with softening on the trunks followed by proximal and then distal extremities. Sclerodactyly and finger contractures generally persist. Cutaneous telangiectasia and calcinosis are common, making it difficult to differentiate late-stage dcSSc from lcSSc. Relapse or recurrence of skin thickening after the peak of skin involvement has been reached is rare. Patients with lcSSc follow a clinical course that is markedly different than that of dcSSc, and lcSSc carries a better prognosis. In this subset of SSc, Raynaud's phenomenon typically precedes other disease manifestations by years or even decades. Visceral organ complications such as PAH generally develop late and tend to be slowly progressive.

SSc confers a substantial increase in the risk of premature death, with five–eightfold higher age- and gender-adjusted mortality rates compared to the general population. In one population-based study of SSc patients with all forms of the disease, the median survival was 11 years. In patients with dcSSc, 5- and 10-year survivals are 70 and 55%, respectively, whereas in patients with lcSSc, 5- and 10-year survivals are 90 and 75%, respectively. The prognosis of SSc correlates with the extent of skin involvement, which itself is a surrogate for visceral organ involvement. Major causes of death in SSc are PAH, pulmonary fibrosis, gastrointestinal involvement, cardiac involvement, and scleroderma renal crisis. Lung cancer and excess cardiovascular deaths also contribute to increased mortality. Markers of worse prognosis include male gender, older age of disease onset, African-American race, extensive skin thickening with truncal involvement, evidence of significant or progressive visceral organ involvement, and the presence of topoisomerase-I antibodies. Additional findings demonstrable at initial evaluation that are associated with increased mortality include an elevated ESR, anemia, and proteinuria. In one study, SSc patients with extensive skin involvement, lung vital capacity <55% predicted, significant gastrointestinal involvement (pseudoobstruction or malabsorption), evidence of cardiac involvement (arrhythmias or congestive heart failure), or scleroderma renal crisis had a cumulative 9-year survival <40%. The severity of PAH is itself strongly associated with mortality, and SSc patients who had a mean pulmonary arterial pressure ≥45 mmHg had a 33% 3-year survival. The introduction of ACE inhibitors in the early 1980s had a dramatic impact on survival of patients with scleroderma renal crisis, from a <20% 1-year survival in the pretreatment era to a >70% 1-year survival currently.

MIXED CONNECTIVE TISSUE DISEASE

Patients with features of lcSSc coexisting with features of systemic lupus erythematosus, polymyositis, and rheumatoid arthritis may have mixed connective tissue disease (MCTD). This overlap syndrome is generally associated with the presence of high titers of autoantibodies to U1-RNP. The characteristic initial presentation is Raynaud's phenomenon associated with puffy fingers and myalgia. Gradually, lcSSc features of sclerodactyly, calcinosis, and cutaneous telangiectasia develop. Skin rashes suggestive of systemic lupus erythematosus (malar rash, photosensitivity) or of dermatomyositis (heliotrope rash on the eyelids, erythematous rash on the knuckles) occur. While arthralgia is common, some patients develop erosive polyarthritis. Pulmonary fibrosis and isolated or secondary PAH may develop. Other manifestations include esophageal dysmotility, pericarditis, Sjögren's syndrome, and renal disease, especially membranous glomerulonephritis. Laboratory evaluation indicates features of inflammation with elevated ESR and hypergammaglobulinemia. While anti-U1RNP antibodies are detected in the serum in high titers, SSc-specific autoantibodies are not found. In contrast to SSc, patients with MCTD often show a good response to treatment with glucocorticoids, and the long-term prognosis is better than that of SSc. Whether MCTD is a truly distinct entity or is, rather, a subset of systemic lupus erythematosus or SSc remains controversial.

EOSINOPHILIC FASCIITIS

Eosinophilic fasciitis is a rare idiopathic disorder associated with scleroderma-like induration of the skin that generally develops rapidly and involves the upper extremities. Adults are primarily affected. The skin has a coarse cobblestone "peau d'orange" appearance. In contrast to SSc, internal organ involvement is rare in eosinophilic fasciitis, and Raynaud's phenomenon is absent. Furthermore, skin involvement spares the fingers. Full-thickness biopsy of the lesional skin reveals marked subcutaneous fibrosis and thickening of the subcutaneous fascial layers. Inflammation and eosinophil infiltration in the fascia are variably present. In the acute phase of the illness, peripheral blood eosinophilia is generally present but may be transient. Autoantibodies do not occur. Treatment with glucocorticoids leads to prompt resolution of the eosinophilia, but skin changes show only slow and variable improvement. The prognosis of patients with eosinophilic fasciitis is good.

FURTHER READINGS

ABRAHAM DJ, VARGA J: Scleroderma: From cell and molecular mechanisms to disease models. Trends Immunol 26:587, 2005

FEGHALI-BOSTWICK C et al: Analysis of systemic sclerosis in twins reveals low concordance for disease and high concordance for the presence of antinuclear antibodies. Arthritis Rheum 48:1956, 2003

KUWANA M et al: Defective vasculogenesis in systemic sclerosis. Lancet 364:603, 2004

MAYES MD et al: Prevalence, incidence, survival, and disease characteristics of systemic sclerosis in a large US population. Arthritis Rheum 48:2246, 2003

SATO S et al: Altered blood B lymphocyte homeostasis in systemic sclerosis: Expanded naive B cells and diminished but activated memory B cells. Arthritis Rheum 50:1918, 2004

SCUSSEL-LONZETTI L et al: Predicting mortality in systemic sclerosis: Analysis of a cohort of 309 French Canadian patients with emphasis on features at diagnosis as predictive factors for survival. Medicine (Baltimore) 81:154, 2002

TASHKIN DP et al: Cyclophosphamide versus placebo in scleroderma lung disease. N Engl J Med 354:2655, 2006

WHITFIELD ML et al: Systemic and cell type-specific gene expression patterns in SSc skin. Proc Natl Acad Sci U S A 100:12319, 2003

317 Sjögren's Syndrome
Haralampos M. Moutsopoulos

DEFINITION, INCIDENCE, AND PREVALENCE

Sjögren's syndrome is a chronic, slowly progressive autoimmune disease characterized by lymphocytic infiltration of the exocrine glands resulting in xerostomia and dry eyes. Approximately one-third of patients present with systemic manifestations; a small but significant number of patients may develop malignant lymphoma. The disease presents alone (primary Sjögren's syndrome) or in association with other autoimmune rheumatic diseases (secondary Sjögren's syndrome) (Table 317-1).

Middle-aged women (female-to-male ratio, 9:1) are primarily affected, although it may occur in all ages, including childhood. The prevalence of primary Sjögren's syndrome is approximately 0.5–1.0%, while 30% of patients with autoimmune rheumatic diseases suffer from secondary Sjögren's syndrome.

PATHOGENESIS

Sjögren's syndrome is characterized by both T cell lymphocytic infiltration of the exocrine glands and B lymphocyte hyperreactivity. An oligomonoclonal B cell process, which is characterized by cryoprecipitable monoclonal immunoglobulins with rheumatoid factor activity, is evident in up to 25% of patients.

Sera of patients with Sjögren's syndrome often contain autoantibodies directed against non-organ-specific antigens such as immunoglobulins (rheumatoid factors) and extractable nuclear and cytoplasmic antigens (Ro/SS-A, La/SS-B). Ro/SS-A autoantigen consists of two polypeptides (52 and 60 kDa) in conjunction with cytoplasmic RNAs, whereas the 48-kDa La/SS-B protein is bound to RNA III polymerase transcripts. Autoantibodies to Ro/SS-A and La/SS-B antigens are usually detected at the time of diagnosis and are associated with earlier disease onset, longer disease duration, salivary gland enlargement, more severe lymphocytic infiltration of minor salivary glands, and certain extraglandular manifestations. Antibodies to α-fodrin (120 kDa), a salivary gland–specific protein, have been found in sera of patients with Sjögren's syndrome. The major infiltrating cells in the affected exocrine glands are activated T and B lymphocytes. Macrophages and natural killer cells are rarely detected. In chronic lesions, a small but persistent number of dendritic cells are apparent in lymphoid follicle–like formations resembling germinal centers. Glandular epithelial cells undergo apoptotic death prompted by both extracellular (Fas/FasLigand and Perforin/granzymes) and intracellular (increased apoptotic vs. antiapoptotic molecules, e.g., Bax vs. Bcl-2) mechanisms. Infiltrating lymphocytes not only provide apoptotic messages to epithelial cells but also tend to be resistant to apoptosis. Ductal and acinar epithelial cells appear to play a significant role in the initiation and perpetuation of the autoimmune injury. They express class II major histocompatibility complex (MHC) and co-stimulatory molecules and thus are able to provide signals essential for lymphocytic activation. Autoantigens that are normally intracellular are disclosed on the surface of the cells, probably through the aforementioned apoptotic mechanisms. Finally, they inappropriately produce proinflammatory cytokines and lymphoattractant chemokines necessary for sustaining the autoimmune lesion and progressing to more sophisticated ectopic germinal center formation. Recent studies have shown that, similar to T cells, CD40+ B cells also have a tendency to be resistant to apoptosis. B cell activating factor (BAFF) has been found to be elevated in patients with Sjögren's syndrome, especially those with hypergammaglobulinemia, and probably accounts for this antiapoptotic effect. Interestingly, glandular epithelial cells seem to have an active role in the production of BAFF. The triggering factor for epithelial activation appears to be a persistent enteroviral infection (possibly by Coxsackie virus strains).

A defect in cholinergic activity mediated through the M3 receptor, which leads to neuroepithelial dysfunction and diminished glandular secretions, has been proposed. Finally, the observation that the water-channel protein aquaporin-5 redistributes from the apical membranes to the cytoplasm of acinar epithelial cells offers another alternative theory for Sjögren's syndrome pathogenesis.

Immunogenetic studies have demonstrated that HLA-B8, -DR3, and -DRw52 are prevalent in patients with primary Sjögren's syndrome. Molecular analysis of HLA class II genes has revealed that patients with Sjögren's syndrome, regardless of their ethnic origin, are highly associated with the HLA DQA1*0501 allele, pointing out that genetic predisposition may play an important role.

CLINICAL MANIFESTATIONS

The majority of Sjögren's syndrome patients have symptoms related to diminished lacrimal and salivary gland function. In most patients, the primary syndrome runs a slow and benign course. The initial manifestations can be mucosal or nonspecific dryness, and 8–10 years may elapse from the initial symptoms to full-blown development of the disease.

The principal oral symptom of Sjögren's syndrome is dryness (xerostomia). Patients complain of difficulty in swallowing dry food, inability to speak continuously, a burning sensation, increase in dental caries, and problems in wearing complete dentures. Physical examination shows a dry, erythematous, sticky oral mucosa. There is atrophy of the filiform papillae on the dorsum of the tongue, and saliva from the major glands is either not expressible or cloudy. Enlargement of the parotid or other major salivary glands occurs in two-thirds of patients with primary Sjögren's syndrome but is uncommon in those with the secondary syndrome. Diagnostic tests include sialometry, sialography, and scintigraphy. The labial minor salivary gland biopsy permits histopathologic confirmation of the focal lymphocytic infiltrates.

Ocular involvement is the other major manifestation of Sjögren's syndrome. Patients usually complain of a sandy or gritty feeling under the eyelids. Other symptoms include burning, accumulation of thick strands at the inner canthi, decreased tearing, redness, itching, eye fatigue, and increased photosensitivity. These symptoms are attributed to the destruction of corneal and bulbar conjunctival epithelium, defined as *keratoconjunctivitis sicca*. Diagnostic evaluation of keratoconjunctivitis sicca includes measurement of tear flow by Schirmer's I test and tear composition as assessed by the tear breakup time or tear lysozyme content. Slit-lamp examination of the cornea and conjunctiva after rose Bengal staining reveals punctuate corneal ulcerations and attached filaments of corneal epithelium.

Involvement of other exocrine glands occurs less frequently and includes a decrease in mucous gland secretions of the upper and lower respiratory tree, resulting in dry nose, throat, and trachea (xerotrachea), and diminished secretion of the exocrine glands of the gastrointestinal tract, leading to esophageal mucosal atrophy, atrophic gastritis, and subclinical pancreatitis. Dyspareunia due to dryness of the external genitalia and dry skin also may occur.

Extraglandular (systemic) manifestations are seen in one-third of patients with Sjögren's syndrome (Table 317-2), while they are very rare in patients with Sjögren's syndrome associated with rheumatoid arthritis. These patients complain more often of easy fatigability, low-grade fever, Raynaud's phenomenon, myalgias, and arthralgias. Most patients with primary Sjögren's syndrome experience at least one episode of nonerosive arthritis during the course of their disease. Manifestations of pulmonary involvement are frequently evident histologically but rarely clinically important. Dry cough is the major manifestation

TABLE 317-1	ASSOCIATION OF SJÖGREN'S SYNDROME WITH OTHER AUTOIMMUNE DISEASES

Rheumatoid arthritis
Systemic lupus erythematosus
Scleroderma
Mixed connective tissue disease
Primary biliary cirrhosis
Vasculitis
Chronic active hepatitis

TABLE 317-2	INCIDENCE OF EXTRAGLANDULAR MANIFESTATIONS IN PRIMARY SJÖGREN'S SYNDROME

Clinical Manifestation	Percent
Arthralgias/arthritis	60
Raynaud's phenomenon	37
Lymphadenopathy	14
Lung involvement	14
Vasculitis	11
Kidney involvement	9
Liver involvement	6
Lymphoma	6
Splenomegaly	3
Peripheral neuropathy	2
Myositis	1

that is attributed to small airway disease. Renal involvement includes interstitial nephritis, clinically manifested by hyposthenuria and renal tubular dysfunction with or without acidosis. Untreated acidosis may lead to nephrocalcinosis. Glomerulonephritis is a rare finding that occurs in patients with mixed cryoglobulinemia, or systemic lupus erythematosus overlapping with Sjögren's syndrome. Vasculitis affects small and medium-sized vessels. The most common clinical features are purpura, recurrent urticaria, skin ulcerations, glomerulonephritis, and mononeuritis multiplex. Sensorineural hearing loss was found in one-half of patients with Sjögren's syndrome and correlated with the presence of anticardiolipin antibodies, while anti-Ro/SSA positivity is associated with congenital heart block.

It has been suggested that primary Sjögren's syndrome with vasculitis may also present with multifocal, recurrent, and progressive nervous system disease, such as hemiparesis, transverse myelopathy, hemisensory deficits, seizures, and movement disorders. Aseptic meningitis and multiple sclerosis also have been reported in these patients.

Lymphoma is a well-known manifestation of Sjögren's syndrome that usually presents later in the illness. Persistent parotid gland enlargement, purpura, leukopenia, cryoglobulinemia, and low C4 complement levels are manifestations suggesting the development of lymphoma. Interestingly, the same risk factors account for glomerulonephritis and are those that confer increased mortality. Most lymphomas are extranodal, low-grade marginal zone B cell lymphomas and are usually detected incidentally upon evaluating the labial biopsy. The affected lymph nodes are usually peripheral. Survival is decreased in patients with B symptoms, lymph node mass >7 cm in diameter, and high or intermediate histologic grade.

TABLE 317-3	DIFFERENTIAL DIAGNOSIS OF SICCA SYMPTOMS

Xerostomia	Dry Eye	Bilateral Parotid Gland Enlargement
Viral infections	Inflammation	Viral infections
Drugs	Stevens-Johnson	Mumps
Psychotherapeutic	syndrome	Influenza
Parasympatholytic	Pemphigoid	Epstein-Barr
Antihypertensive	Chronic conjunctivitis	Coxsackievirus A
Psychogenic	Chronic blepharitis	Cytomegalovirus
Irradiation	Sjögren's syndrome	HIV
Diabetes mellitus	Toxicity	Sarcoidosis
Trauma	Burns	Amyloidosis
Sjögren's syndrome	Drugs	Sjögren's syndrome
	Neurologic conditions	Metabolic
	Impaired lacrimal	Diabetes mellitus
	gland function	Hyperlipoprotein-
	Impaired eyelid	emias
	function	Chronic pancreatitis
	Miscellaneous	Hepatic cirrhosis
	Trauma	Endocrine
	Hypovitaminosis A	Acromegaly
	Blink abnormality	Gonadal
	Lid scarring	hypofunction
	Anesthetic cornea	
	Epithelial irregularity	

TABLE 317-4	DIFFERENTIAL DIAGNOSIS OF SJÖGREN'S SYNDROME

HIV Infection and Sicca Syndrome	Sjögren's Syndrome	Sarcoidosis
Predominant in young males	Predominant in middle-aged women	Invariable
Lack of autoantibodies to Ro/SS-A and/or La/SS-B	Presence of autoantibodies	Lack of autoantibodies to Ro/SS-A and/or La/SS-B
Lymphoid infiltrates of salivary glands by CD8+ lymphocytes	Lymphoid infiltrates of salivary glands by CD4+ lymphocytes	Granulomas in salivary glands
Association with HLA-DR5	Association with HLA-DR3 and -DRw52	Unknown
Positive serologic tests for HIV	Negative serologic tests for HIV	Negative serologic tests for HIV

Routine laboratory tests reveal mild normochromic, normocytic anemia. An elevated erythrocyte sedimentation rate is found in approximately 70% of patients.

DIAGNOSIS AND DIFFERENTIAL DIAGNOSIS

The diagnosis of primary Sjögren's syndrome is obtained if the patient presents with eye and/or mouth dryness, the eye tests disclose keratoconjunctivitis sicca, the mouth evaluation reveals the classic manifestations of the syndrome, and the patient's serum reacts with Ro/SS-A and/or La/SS-B autoantigens. Labial biopsy is needed when the diagnosis is uncertain or to rule out other conditions that may cause dry mouth or eyes or parotid gland enlargement (Tables 317-3, 317-4). Validated diagnostic criteria have been established by a European study and have now been further improved by a European-American study group (Table 317-5). Hepatitis C virus infection should be ruled out since, apart from serologic tests, the remainder of the clinicopathologic picture is almost identical to that of Sjögren's syndrome.

TABLE 317-5	REVISED INTERNATIONAL CLASSIFICATION CRITERIA FOR SJÖGREN'S SYNDROME[a,b,c]

I. Ocular symptoms: a positive response to at least one of three validated questions.
  1. Have you had daily, persistent, troublesome dry eyes for more than 3 months?
  2. Do you have a recurrent sensation of sand or gravel in the eyes?
  3. Do you use tear substitutes more than three times a day?
II. Oral symptoms: a positive response to at least one of three validated questions.
  1. Have you had a daily feeling of dry mouth for more than 3 months?
  2. Have you had recurrent or persistently swollen salivary glands as an adult?
  3. Do you frequently drink liquids to aid in swallowing dry foods?
III. Ocular signs: objective evidence of ocular involvement defined as a positive result to at least one of the following two tests:
  1. Shirmer's I test, performed without anesthesia ($\leq$5 mm in 5 min)
  2. Rose Bengal score or other ocular dye score ($\geq$4 according to van Bijsterveld's scoring system)
IV. Histopathology: In minor salivary glands focal lymphocytic sialoadenitis, with a focus score $\geq$1.
V. Salivary gland involvement: objective evidence of salivary gland involvement defined by a positive result to at least one of the following diagnostic tests:
  1. Unstimulated whole salivary flow ($\leq$1.5 mL in 15 min)
  2. Parotid sialography
  3. Salivary scintigraphy
VI. Antibodies in the serum to Ro/SS-A or La/SS-B antigens, or both

[a]Exclusion criteria: Past head and neck radiation treatment, hepatitis C infection, AIDS, preexisting lymphoma, sarcoidosis, graft versus host disease, use of anticholinergic drugs.
[b]Primary Sjögren's syndrome: any four of the six items, as long as item IV (histopathology) or VI (serology) is positive, or any three of the four objective criteria items (items III, IV, V, VI).
[c]In patients with a potentially associated disease (e.g., another well-defined connective tissue disease), the presence of item I or item II plus any two from among items III, IV, and V may be considered as indicative of secondary Sjögren's syndrome.
Source: From Vitali C et al.

TREATMENT ALGORITHM FOR SJÖGREN'S SYNDROME

FIGURE 317-1 Treatment algorithm for Sjögren's syndrome.

recommended. Certain drugs that may decrease lacrimal and salivary secretion such as diuretics, antihypertensive drugs, anticholinergics, and antidepressants should be avoided.

For xerostomia the best replacement is water. Propionic acid gels may be used to treat vaginal dryness. To stimulate secretions, pilocarpine (5 mg thrice daily) or cevimeline (30 mg thrice daily) administered orally appears to improve sicca manifestations, and both are well tolerated. Hydroxychloroquine (200 mg) is helpful for arthralgias.

Patients with renal tubular acidosis should receive sodium bicarbonate orally (0.5–2.0 mmol/kg in four divided doses). Glucocorticoids (1 mg/kg per day) and/or immunosuppressive agents (e.g., cyclophosphamide) are indicated only for the treatment of systemic vasculitis. Anti–tumor necrosis factor agents appear ineffective, while anti-CD20 monoclonal antibody therapy in combination with a classic CHOP regimen leads to increased survival in patients with lymphoma.

FURTHER READINGS

KASSAN S, MOUTSOPOULOS HM: Clinical manifestations and early diagnosis of Sjögren syndrome. Arch Intern Med 164:1275, 2004

MAVRAGANI CP et al: The management of Sjögren's syndrome. Nat Clin Pract Rheum 2:252, 2006

MITSIAS DI et al: The role of epithelial cells in the initiation and perpetuation of autoimmune lesion: Lessons from Sjögren's syndrome (autoimmune epithelitis). Lupus 15:255, 2006

PIJPE J et al: Rituximab treatment in patients with primary Sjögren's syndrome: An open-label phase II study. Arthritis Rheum 52:2740, 2005

TRIANTAFYLLOPOULOU A et al: Evidence for coxsackievirus infection in primary Sjögren's syndrome. Arthritis Rheum 50:2897, 2004

VITALI C et al: Classification criteria for Sjögren's syndrome: A revised version of the European criteria proposed by the American-European Consensus Group. Ann Rheum Dis 61:554, 2002

℞ SJÖGREN'S SYNDROME

Treatment of Sjögren's syndrome is aimed at symptomatic relief and limiting the damaging local effects of chronic xerostomia and keratoconjunctivitis sicca by substituting or simulating the missing secretions (**Fig. 317-1**).

To replace deficient tears, there are several readily available ophthalmic preparations (Tearisol; Liquifilm; 0.5% methylcellulose; Hypo Tears). If corneal ulcerations are present, eye patching and boric acid ointments are

318 The Spondyloarthritides
Joel D. Taurog

The spondyloarthritides are a group of disorders that share certain clinical features and genetic associations. These disorders include ankylosing spondylitis, reactive arthritis, psoriatic arthritis and spondylitis, enteropathic arthritis and spondylitis, juvenile-onset spondyloarthritis, and undifferentiated spondyloarthritis. The similarities in clinical manifestations and genetic predisposition suggest that these disorders share pathogenic mechanisms.

ANKYLOSING SPONDYLITIS

Ankylosing spondylitis (AS) is an inflammatory disorder of unknown cause that primarily affects the axial skeleton; peripheral joints and extraarticular structures are also frequently involved. The disease usually begins in the second or third decade; male to female prevalence is between 2:1 and 3:1. Older names include *Marie-Strümpell disease* or *Bechterew's disease*.

EPIDEMIOLOGY

AS shows a striking correlation with the histocompatibility antigen HLA-B27 and occurs worldwide roughly in proportion to the prevalence of this antigen (Chap. 309). In North American Caucasians, the prevalence of B27 is 7%, whereas it is 90% in patients with AS, independent of disease severity.

In population surveys, AS is present in 1–6% of adults inheriting B27, whereas the prevalence is 10–30% among B27+ adult first-degree relatives of AS probands. The concordance rate in identical twins is approximately 65%. It appears that susceptibility to AS is determined largely by genetic factors, with B27 comprising about one-third of the genetic component. Probable linkage has been found to the interleukin 1 (IL-1) gene cluster on chromosome 2 and to several other genomic regions.

PATHOLOGY

The sites of axial inflammation in AS are inaccessible to routine biopsy and are rarely approached surgically. Knowledge of the axial histopathology is therefore based on a limited number of mostly advanced cases. Sacroiliitis is often the earliest manifestations of AS. Synovitis, pannus, myxoid marrow, subchondral granulation tissue and marrow edema, enthesitis, and chondroid differentiation are found. Macrophages, T cells, and osteoclasts are prevalent. Eventually the eroded joint margins are gradually replaced by fibrocartilage regeneration and then by ossification. The joint may become totally obliterated.

In the spine, early in the process there is inflammatory granulation tissue at the junction of annulus fibrosus and vertebral bone. The outer annular fibers are eroded and eventually replaced by bone, forming the beginning of a bony syndesmophyte, which then grows by continued enchondral ossification, ultimately bridging the adjacent vertebral bodies. Ascending progression of this process leads to the "bamboo spine." Other lesions in the spine include diffuse osteoporosis, erosion of vertebral bodies at the disk margin, "squaring" of vertebrae, and inflammation and destruction of the disk-bone border. Inflammatory arthritis of the apophyseal joints is common, with erosion of cartilage by pannus, often followed by bony ankylosis.

Bone mineral density is diminished in the spine and proximal femur early in the course of the disease, before the advent of significant immobilization.

Peripheral synovitis in AS shows marked vascularity, lining layer hyperplasia, lymphoid infiltration, and pannus formation. Central cartilaginous erosions caused by proliferation of subchondral granulation tissue are common.

Inflammation in the fibrocartilaginous enthesis, the region where a tendon, ligament, or joint capsule attaches to bone, is a characteristic lesion in AS and other SpA, both at axial and peripheral sites. Enthesitis is associated with prominent edema of the adjacent bone marrow and is often characterized by erosive lesions that eventually undergo ossification.

PATHOGENESIS

The pathogenesis of AS is incompletely understood but is almost certainly immune-mediated. There is lively controversy regarding the primary site of disease initiation. A unifying concept is that the AS disease process begins at sites where articular cartilage, ligaments, and other structures attach to bone. The dramatic response of the disease to therapeutic blockade of tumor necrosis factor α (TNF-α) indicates that this cytokine plays a central role in the immunopathogenesis of AS. The inflamed sacroiliac joint is infiltrated with CD4+ and CD8+ T cells and macrophages and shows high levels of TNF-α, particularly early in the disease course. Abundant TGF-β has been found in more advanced lesions. Peripheral synovitis in AS and the other spondyloarthritides is characterized by neutrophils, macrophages expressing CD68 and CD163, CD4+ and CD8+ T cells, and B cells. There is prominent staining for ICAM-1, VCAM-1, matrix metalloproteinase-3 (MMP-3), and myeloid-related proteins 8 and 14 (MRP-8 and MRP-14). Unlike rheumatoid arthritis (RA) synovium, citrullinated proteins and cartilage gp39 peptide-MHC complexes are absent.

No specific event or exogenous agent that triggers the onset of disease has been identified, although overlapping features with reactive arthritis and inflammatory bowel disease (IBD) suggest that enteric bacteria may play a role. Elevated serum titers of antibodies to certain enteric bacteria are common in AS patients, but no role for these antibodies in the pathogenesis of AS has been identified. Strong evidence that B27 plays a direct role is provided by genetic epidemiology studies and by the finding that rats transgenic for B27 spontaneously develop dramatic arthritis and spondylitis. It has yet to be determined whether the role of B27 involves classical peptide antigen presentation to CD8+ T cells or some other mechanism, or both. More generally, the relative degree of participation of innate and adaptive immunity remains to be determined.

CLINICAL MANIFESTATIONS

The symptoms of the disease are usually first noticed in late adolescence or early adulthood; the median age in western countries is 23. In 5% of patients, symptoms begin after age 40. The initial symptom is usually dull pain, insidious in onset, felt deep in the lower lumbar or gluteal region, accompanied by low-back morning stiffness of up to a few hours' duration that improves with activity and returns following periods of inactivity. Within a few months of onset, the pain has usually become persistent and bilateral. Nocturnal exacerbation of pain that forces the patient to rise and move around may be frequent.

In some patients, bony tenderness (presumably reflecting enthesitis) may accompany back pain or stiffness, while in others it may be the predominant complaint. Common sites include the costosternal junctions, spinous processes, iliac crests, greater trochanters, ischial tuberosities, tibial tubercles, and heels. Occasionally, bony chest pain is the presenting complaint. Arthritis in the hips and shoulders ("root" joints) occurs in 25–35% of patients, in many cases early in the disease course. Arthritis of peripheral joints other than the hips and shoulders, usually asymmetric, occurs in up to 30% of patients and can occur at any stage of the disease. Neck pain and stiffness from involvement of the cervical spine are usually relatively late manifestations. Occasional patients, particularly in the older age group, present with predominantly constitutional symptoms.

AS often has a juvenile onset in developing countries. Peripheral arthritis and enthesitis usually predominate, with axial symptoms supervening in late adolescence.

Initially, physical findings mirror the inflammatory process. The most specific findings involve loss of spinal mobility, with limitation of anterior and lateral flexion and extension of the lumbar spine and of chest expansion. Limitation of motion is usually out of proportion to the degree of bony ankylosis, reflecting muscle spasm secondary to pain and inflammation. Pain in the sacroiliac joints may be elicited either with direct pressure or with maneuvers that stress the joints. In addition, there is commonly tenderness upon palpation at the sites of symptomatic bony tenderness and paraspinous muscle spasm.

The Schober test is a useful measure of lumbar spine flexion. The patient stands erect, with heels together, and marks are made directly over the spine 5 cm below and 10 cm above the lumbosacral junction (identified by a horizontal line between the posterosuperior iliac spines). The patient then bends forward maximally, and the distance between the two marks is measured. The distance between the two marks increases by ≥5 cm in the case of normal mobility and by <4 cm in the case of decreased mobility. Chest expansion is measured as the difference between maximal inspiration and maximal forced expiration in the fourth intercostal space in males or just below the breasts in females. Normal chest expansion is ≥5 cm.

Limitation or pain with motion of the hips or shoulders is usually present if either of these joints is involved. It should be emphasized that early in the course of mild cases, symptoms may be subtle and nonspecific, and the physical examination may be completely normal.

The course of the disease is extremely variable, ranging from the individual with mild stiffness and radiographically equivocal sacroiliitis to the patient with a totally fused spine and severe bilateral hip arthritis, accompanied by severe peripheral arthritis and extraarticular manifestations. Pain tends to be persistent early in the disease and then becomes intermittent, with alternating exacerbations and quiescent periods. In a typical severe untreated case with progression of the spondylitis to syndesmophyte formation, the patient's posture undergoes characteristic changes, with obliterated lumbar lordosis, buttock atrophy, and accentuated thoracic kyphosis. There may be a forward stoop of the neck or flexion contractures at the hips, compensated by flexion at the knees. Disease progression can be estimated clinically from loss of height, limitation of chest expansion and spinal flexion, and occiput-to-wall distance. Occasional individuals are encountered with advanced physical findings who report having never had significant symptoms.

For a given patient, the rate of progression of radiographically demonstrable damage is linear over decades. In some but not all studies, onset of the disease in adolescence and early hip involvement correlate with a worse prognosis. The disease in women tends to progress less frequently to total spinal ankylosis, although there is some evidence for an increased prevalence of isolated cervical ankylosis and peripheral arthritis in women. In industrialized countries, peripheral arthritis (distal to hips and shoulders) occurs overall in less than half of patients with AS, usually as a late manifestation, whereas in developing countries, the prevalence is much higher, with onset typically early in the disease course. Pregnancy has no consistent effect on AS, with symptoms improving, remaining the same, or deteriorating in about one-third of pregnant patients, respectively.

The most serious complication of the spinal disease is spinal fracture, which can occur with even minor trauma to the rigid, osteoporotic spine. The lower cervical spine is most commonly involved. These fractures are often displaced and cause spinal cord injury. A recent survey suggested a >10% lifetime risk of fracture. Occasionally, fracture through a diskovertebral junction and adjacent neural arch, termed *pseudoarthrosis* and occurring most commonly in the thoracolumbar spine, can be an unrecognized source of persistent localized pain and/or neurologic dysfunction. Wedging of thoracic vertebrae is common and correlates with accentuated kyphosis.

The most common extraarticular manifestation is acute anterior uveitis, which occurs in 40% of patients and can antedate the spondylitis. Attacks are typically unilateral, causing pain, photophobia, and increased lacrimation. These tend to recur, often in the opposite eye. Cataracts and secondary glaucoma are not uncommon sequelae. Up to 60% of patients have inflammation in the colon or ileum. This is usually asymptomatic, but frank inflammatory bowel disease (IBD) occurs in 5–10% of patients with AS (see "Enteropathic Arthritis," below). About 10% of patients meeting criteria for AS have psoriasis (see "Psoriatic Arthritis," below). Aortic insufficiency, sometimes producing symptoms of congestive heart failure, occurs in a few percent of patients, occasionally early in the course of the spinal disease but usually after prolonged disease. Third-degree heart block may occur alone or together with aortic insufficiency. Subclinical pulmonary lesions and cardiac dysfunction may be relatively common. Cauda equina syndrome and upper pulmonary lobe fibrosis are rare late complications. Retroperitoneal fibrosis is a rare associated condition. Prostatitis has been reported to have an increased prevalence. Amyloidosis is rare (Chap. 324).

Several validated measures of disease activity and functional outcome have recently been developed for AS. Despite the persistence of the disease, most patients remain gainfully employed. Some but not all studies of survival in AS have suggested that AS shortens life span, compared with the general population. Mortality attributable to AS is largely the result of spinal trauma, aortic insufficiency, respiratory failure, amyloid nephropathy, or complications of therapy such as upper gastrointestinal hemorrhage.

LABORATORY FINDINGS

No laboratory test is diagnostic of AS. In most ethnic groups, B27 is present in approximately 90% of patients. Erythrocyte sedimentation rate (ESR) and C-reactive protein (CRP) are often, but not always, elevated. Mild anemia may be present. Patients with severe disease may show an elevated alkaline phosphatase level. Elevated serum IgA levels are common. Rheumatoid factor, anti-CCP, and antinuclear antibodies are largely absent unless caused by a coexistent disease, although the latter may appear with anti-TNF therapy. Synovial fluid from peripheral joints in AS is nonspecifically inflammatory. In cases with restriction of chest wall motion, decreased vital capacity and increased functional residual capacity are common, but airflow measurements are normal and ventilatory function is usually well maintained.

RADIOGRAPHIC FINDINGS

Radiographically demonstrable sacroiliitis is usually present in AS. The earliest changes by standard radiography are blurring of the cortical margins of the subchondral bone, followed by erosions and sclerosis. Progression of the erosions leads to "pseudowidening" of the joint space; as fibrous and then bony ankylosis supervene, the joints may become obliterated. The changes and progression of the lesions are usually symmetric.

In the lumbar spine, progression of the disease leads to straightening, caused by loss of lordosis, and reactive sclerosis, caused by osteitis of the anterior corners of the vertebral bodies with subsequent erosion, leading to "squaring" of the vertebral bodies. Progressive ossification leads to eventual formation of marginal syndesmophytes, visible on plain films as bony bridges connecting successive vertebral bodies anteriorly and laterally.

In mild cases, years may elapse before unequivocal sacroiliac abnormalities are evident on plain radiographs. Computed tomography (CT) and magnetic resonance imaging (MRI) can detect abnormalities reliably at an earlier stage than plain radiography. Dynamic MRI with fat saturation, either short tau inversion recovery (STIR) sequence or T1-weighted images with contrast enhancement, is highly sensitive and specific for identifying early intraarticular inflammation, cartilage changes, and underlying bone marrow edema in sacroiliitis (Fig. 318-1). These techniques are also highly sensitive for evaluation of acute and chronic spinal changes (Fig. 318-2).

Reduced bone mineral density can be detected by dual-energy x-ray absorptiometry of the femoral neck and the lumbar spine. Falsely elevated readings related to spinal ossification can be avoided by using a lateral projection of the L3 vertebral body.

DIAGNOSIS

It is important to establish the diagnosis of early AS before the development of irreversible deformity. This goal presents a challenge for several reasons: (1) back pain is very common, but AS is much less common; (2) an early presumptive diagnosis often relies on clinical grounds requiring considerable expertise; (3) young individuals with early AS are often reluctant to seek medical care. The widely used modified New York criteria (1984) are classification rather than diagnostic criteria, and they are insensitive in early or mild cases. These consist of the following: (1) a history of inflammatory back pain (see below), (2) limitation of motion of the lumbar spine in both the sagittal and frontal planes, (3) limited chest ex-

FIGURE 318-1 Early sacroiliitis in a patient with AS, indicated by prominent sacral bone marrow edema (asterisks) on a coronal oblique STIR (short tau inversion recovery) magnetic resonance image. (*From DS Levine et al: Clin Radiol 59:400, 2004.*)

Baseline   **Week 24**

FIGURE 318-2 Spinal inflammation (spondylodiscitis) in a patient with AS and its dramatic response to treatment with infliximab. Gadolinium-enhanced T1-weighted magnetic resonance images, with fat saturation, at baseline and after 24 weeks of infliximab therapy. (*From J Braun et al.*)

pansion, and (4) definite radiographic sacroiliitis. Criterion 4 plus any one of the other three criteria is sufficient for a diagnosis of definite AS. Dynamic MRI is definitely more sensitive than plain radiography. Although its exact sensitivity and specificity remain to be defined, it is recommended in suspected cases in which plain radiography either fails to show definite changes or is undesirable (e.g., in young women or children).

The presence of B27 is neither necessary nor sufficient for the diagnosis. However, in accord with Bayes' theorem, the presence or absence of B27 greatly increases or decreases, respectively, the probability of AS in patients with equivocal clinical findings lacking radiographic abnormalities. Moreover, the absence of B27 in a typical case of AS significantly increases the probability of coexistent IBD.

AS must be differentiated from numerous other causes of low-back pain, some far more common than AS. For several decades, the following five features have been used to distinguish the inflammatory back pain of AS: (1) age of onset below 40, (2) insidious onset, (3) duration >3 months before medical attention is sought, (4) morning stiffness, and (5) improvement with exercise or activity. The most common causes of back pain other than AS are primarily mechanical or degenerative rather than primarily inflammatory and do not show clustering of these features. A recent reassessment has led to the following proposed criteria for inflammatory back pain in adults ≤50 years old: (1) morning stiffness >30 min, (2) improvement with exercise but not with rest, (3) awakening from back pain during only the second half of the night, and (4) alternating buttock pain.

Less-common metabolic, infectious, and malignant causes of back pain must also be differentiated from AS, including infectious spondylitis, spondylodiscitis, and sacroiliitis. Ochronosis can produce a phenotype that is clinically and radiographically similar to AS. Calcification and ossification of paraspinous ligaments occur in *diffuse idiopathic skeletal hyperostosis* (DISH), which occurs in the middle-aged and elderly and is usually not symptomatic. Ligamentous calcification gives the appearance of "flowing wax" on the anterior bodies of the vertebrae. Intervertebral disk spaces are preserved, and sacroiliac and apophyseal joints appear normal, helping to differentiate DISH from spondylosis and from AS, respectively.

℞ ANKYLOSING SPONDYLITIS

Any management of AS should include an exercise program designed to maintain posture and range of motion. Until recently, nonsteroidal anti-in-

flammatory drugs (NSAIDs) have been the mainstay of pharmacologic therapy for AS. These agents reduce pain and tenderness and increase mobility in many patients with AS. Moreover, in a recent 2–year randomized controlled study, radiographic progression of AS was significantly slower in patients taking daily NSAIDs than in those taking them only as needed for severe pain or stiffness. However, many patients with AS have continued symptoms and develop deformity despite NSAID therapy. Beginning in 2000, dramatic responses to anti-TNF-α therapy were reported in patients with AS and other spondyloarthritides. Patients with AS treated with either infliximab (chimeric human/mouse anti-TNF-α monoclonal antibody), etanercept (soluble p75 TNF-α receptor–IgG fusion protein), or adalimumab (human anti-TNF-α monoclonal antibody) have shown rapid, profound, and sustained reductions in all clinical and laboratory measures of disease activity. Patients with long-standing disease and even some with complete spinal ankylosis have shown striking improvement in both objective and subjective indicators of disease activity and function, including morning stiffness, pain, spinal mobility, peripheral joint swelling, CRP, and ESR. MRI studies indicate substantial resolution of bone marrow edema, enthesitis, and joint effusions in the sacroiliac joints, spine, and peripheral joints (Fig. 318-2). Similar results have been obtained in large randomized controlled trials of all three agents and many open label studies. About half of the patients achieve a ≥50% reduction in the Bath Ankylosing Spondylitis Disease Activity Index (BASDAI), the most commonly used measure of disease activity. Increased bone mineral density is found as early as 24 weeks after onset of therapy. Whether radiographic disease progression is slowed has not yet been determined definitively.

The dosages of these agents used in AS patients have usually been similar to those in RA. Infliximab is given as an intravenous infusion, typically at a dose of 3–5 mg/kg body weight, and then repeated 2 weeks later, again 6 weeks later, and then at 8-week intervals. Some success has been achieved with longer intervals, including infusion only upon recurrence of symptoms. Etanercept is given by subcutaneous injection in a dose of 25 mg twice weekly or 50 mg once weekly. Adalimumab is given by subcutaneous injection in a dose of 40 mg biweekly.

Although these potent immunosuppressive agents have so far been relatively safe, seven types of side effects are not rare: (1) serious infections, including disseminated tuberculosis; (2) hematologic disorders, such as pancytopenia; (3) demyelinating disorders; (4) exacerbation of congestive heart failure; (5) systemic lupus erythematosus–related autoantibodies and clinical features; (6) hypersensitivity infusion or injection site reactions; and (7) severe liver disease. Increased incidence of malignancy is of theoretical concern but has not been observed in AS patients treated for up to 5 years.

Because of the expense, potentially serious side effects, and unknown long-term effects of these agents, their use should be restricted to patients with a definite diagnosis and active disease (BASDAI ≥ 4 out of 10 and expert opinion) that is inadequately responsive to therapy with at least two different NSAIDs. Before initiation of anti-TNF therapy, all patients should be tested for tuberculin reactivity, and reactors (≥5 mm) should be treated with anti-TB agents. Contraindications include active infection or high risk of infection; malignancy or premalignancy; and history of systemic lupus erythematosus, multiple sclerosis, or related autoimmunity. Pregnancy and breast-feeding are relative contraindications. Continuation beyond 12 weeks of therapy requires a 50% reduction in BASDAI (or absolute reduction of 2 out of 10) and favorable expert opinion. Sulfasalazine, in doses of 2–3 g/d, has been shown to be of modest benefit, primarily for peripheral arthritis. A therapeutic trial of this agent should precede any use of anti-TNF agents in patients with predominantly peripheral arthritis. Methotrexate, although widely used, has not been shown to be of benefit in AS, nor has any therapeutic role for gold or oral glucocorticoids been documented. Potential benefit in AS has been reported for thalidomide, 200 mg/d, perhaps acting through inhibition of TNF-α.

The most common indication for surgery in patients with AS is severe hip joint arthritis, the pain and stiffness of which are usually dramatically relieved by total hip arthroplasty. A small number of patients may benefit from surgical correction of extreme flexion deformities of the spine or of atlantoaxial subluxation.

Attacks of uveitis are usually managed effectively with local glucocorticoid administration in conjunction with mydriatic agents, although systemic glucocorticoids or even immunosuppressive drugs and rarely infliximab may be required in some cases. TNF inhibitors reduce the frequency of attacks of uveitis in patients with AS. A few individuals have developed new or recurrent uveitis subsequent to the use of a TNF inhibitor, especially etanercept.

Coexistent cardiac disease may require pacemaker implantation and/or aortic valve replacement. Management of osteoporosis of the axial skeleton is at present similar to that used for primary osteoporosis, since data specific for AS are not available.

REACTIVE ARTHRITIS

Reactive arthritis (ReA) refers to acute nonpurulent arthritis complicating an infection elsewhere in the body. In recent years, the term has been used primarily to refer to spondyloarthritis following enteric or urogenital infections. Other forms of reactive and infection-related arthritis not associated with B27 and showing a spectrum of clinical features different from spondyloarthritis, such as rheumatic fever or Lyme disease, are discussed in Chaps. 315 and 166.

HISTORIC BACKGROUND

The association of acute arthritis with episodes of diarrhea or urethritis has been recognized for centuries. A large number of cases during World Wars I and II focused attention on the triad of arthritis, urethritis, and conjunctivitis, which became known as *Fiessenger-Leroy-Reiter syndrome*, often with additional mucocutaneous lesions. These eponyms are now of historic interest only.

The identification of bacterial species capable of triggering the clinical syndrome and the finding that many patients possess the B27 antigen have led to the unifying concept of ReA as a clinical syndrome triggered by specific etiologic agents in a genetically susceptible host. A similar spectrum of clinical manifestations can be triggered by enteric infection with any of several *Shigella*, *Salmonella*, *Yersinia*, and *Campylobacter* species; by genital infection with *Chlamydia trachomatis*; and by other agents as well. The triad of arthritis, urethritis, and conjunctivitis represents part of the spectrum of the clinical manifestations of ReA. For the purposes of this chapter, the use of the term *ReA* will be restricted to those cases of spondyloarthritis in which there is at least presumptive evidence for a related antecedent infection. Patients with clinical features of ReA who lack evidence of an antecedent infection will be considered to have *undifferentiated spondyloarthritis*, discussed below.

EPIDEMIOLOGY

Following the first reports of association of ReA with HLA-B27, in most hospital-based series in which *Shigella*, *Yersinia*, or *Chlamydia* were the triggering infectious agents, 60–85% of patients were found to be B27 positive, with a lower prevalence in ReA triggered by *Salmonella* and *Campylobacter*. In more recent community-based or common source epidemic studies, the prevalence of B27 has often been below 50%, and in some instances not elevated at all. The most common age range is 18–40 years, but ReA can occur both in children over 5 years of age and in older adults.

The gender ratio in ReA following enteric infection is nearly 1:1, whereas venereally acquired ReA occurs predominantly in men. The overall prevalence and incidence of ReA are difficult to assess because of the variable prevalence of the triggering infections and genetic susceptibility factors in different populations. In Scandinavian countries, an annual incidence of 10–28/100,000 has been reported. The spondyloarthritides were formerly almost unknown in sub-Saharan Africa. However, ReA and other peripheral spondyloarthritides have now become the most common rheumatic diseases in Africans in the wake of the AIDS epidemic, without association to B27, which is very rare in these populations. Spondyloarthritis in Africans with HIV infection usually occurs in individuals with stage I disease (as classified by the World Health Organization). It is often the first manifestation of infection and often remits with disease progression. In contrast, western Caucasian patients with HIV and spondyloarthritis are predominantly B27 positive, and the arthritis flares as AIDS advances.

PATHOLOGY

Synovial histology is similar to that of other spondyloarthritides. Enthesitis shows increased vascularity and macrophage infiltration of fibrocartilage. Microscopic histopathologic evidence of inflammation has occasionally been noted in the colon and ileum of patients with postvenereal ReA, but much less commonly than in postenteric ReA. The skin lesions of keratoderma blenorrhagica, which is associated mainly with venereally acquired ReA, are histologically indistinguishable from psoriatic lesions.

ETIOLOGY AND PATHOGENESIS

Of the four *Shigella* species *S. sonnei*, *S. boydii*, *S. flexneri*, and *S. dysenteriae*, *S. flexneri* has most often been implicated in cases of ReA, both sporadic and epidemic. Recent data suggest that *S. sonnei* and *S. dysenteriae* trigger some cases of ReA.

Other bacteria identified definitively as triggers of ReA include several *Salmonella* spp., *Yersinia enterocolitica*, *Y. pseudotuberculosis*, *Campylobacter jejuni*, and *Chlamydia trachomatis*. There is also increasing evidence implicating *Clostridium difficile*, *Campylobacter coli*, certain toxigenic *E. coli*, and possibly *Ureaplasma urealyticum and Mycoplasma genitalium*. Respiratory infection with *Chlamydia pneumoniae* has also been implicated. There are numerous isolated reports of acute arthritis preceded by other bacterial, viral, or parasitic infections, but whether the microorganisms involved are actual triggers of ReA remains to be determined.

It has not been determined whether ReA occurs by the same pathogenic mechanism following infection with each of these microorganisms, nor has the mechanism been fully elucidated in the case of any one of the known bacterial triggers. Most, if not all, of the triggering organisms produce lipopolysaccharide (LPS) and share a capacity to attack mucosal surfaces, to invade host cells, and to survive intracellularly. Antigens from *Chlamydia*, *Yersinia*, *Salmonella*, and *Shigella* have been shown to be present in the synovium and/or synovial fluid leukocytes of patients with ReA for long periods following the acute attack. In ReA triggered by *Y. enterocolitica*, bacterial LPS and heat shock protein antigens have been found in peripheral blood cells years after the triggering infection. *Yersinia* DNA and *C. trachomatis* DNA and RNA have been detected in synovial tissue from ReA patients, suggesting the presence of viable organisms despite uniform failure to culture the organism from these specimens. The dormant form of *C. trachomatis* that persists in synovium transcriptionally upregulates many genes orthologous to genes upregulated in persistent *M. tuberculosis* infection.

T cells that specifically respond to antigens of the inciting organism have been found in inflamed synovium but not in peripheral blood of patients with ReA. These T cells are predominantly CD4+, but CD8+ B27-restricted bacteria-specific cytolytic T cells have also been isolated in *Yersinia*- and *C. trachomatis*-induced ReA. A unique conserved T cell antigen receptor sequence has been identified in B27-restricted synovial T cells in ReA. Unlike the synovial CD4 T cells in RA, which are predominantly of the T_H1 phenotype, those in ReA also show a T_H2 phenotype. A T regulatory 1 (Tr1) phenotype with elevated IL-10 and TGF-beta in T, B, and macrophage lineages has also been found in ReA synovium. IL-10 promoter haplotypes have been found to be significantly different in ReA patients than in B27+ controls.

HLA-B27 seems to be associated with more severe and chronic forms of ReA, but its pathogenic role remains to be determined. HLA-B27 significantly prolongs the intracellular survival of *Y. enterocolitica* and *S. enteritidis* in human and mouse cell lines. Prolonged intracellular bacterial survival, promoted by B27, other factors, or both, may permit trafficking of infected leukocytes from the site of primary infection to joints, where a T cell response to persistent bacterial antigens may then promote arthritis.

CLINICAL FEATURES

The clinical manifestations of ReA constitute a spectrum that ranges from an isolated, transient monarthritis to severe multisystem disease. A careful history will usually elicit evidence of an antecedent infection 1–4 weeks before onset of symptoms of the reactive disease. However, in a sizable minority, no clinical or laboratory evidence of an antecedent infection can be found. In many cases of presumed venereally acquired reactive disease, there is a history of a recent new sexual partner, even in the absence of laboratory evidence of infection.

Constitutional symptoms are common, including fatigue, malaise, fever, and weight loss. The musculoskeletal symptoms are usually acute in onset. Arthritis is usually asymmetric and additive, with involvement of new joints occurring over a period of a few days to 1–2 weeks. The joints of the lower extremities, especially the knee, ankle, and subtalar, metatarsophalangeal, and toe interphalangeal joints, are the most common sites of involvement, but the wrist and fingers can be involved as well. The arthritis is usually quite painful, and tense joint effusions are not uncommon, especially in the knee. Patients often cannot walk without support. Dactylitis, or "sausage digit," a diffuse swelling of a solitary finger or toe, is a distinctive feature of ReA and other peripheral spondyloarthritides but can be seen in polyarticular gout and sarcoidosis. Tendinitis and fasciitis are particularly characteristic lesions, producing pain at multiple insertion sites (entheses), especially the Achilles insertion, the plantar fascia, and sites along the axial skeleton. Spinal and low-back pain are quite common and may be caused by insertional inflammation, muscle spasm, acute sacroiliitis, or, presumably, arthritis in intervertebral articulations.

Urogenital lesions may occur throughout the course of the disease. In males, urethritis may be marked or relatively asymptomatic and may be either an accompaniment of the triggering infection or a result of the reactive phase of the disease. Prostatitis is also common. Similarly, in females, cervicitis or salpingitis may be caused either by the infectious trigger or by the sterile reactive process.

Ocular disease is common, ranging from transient, asymptomatic conjunctivitis to an aggressive anterior uveitis that occasionally proves refractory to treatment and may result in blindness.

Mucocutaneous lesions are frequent. Oral ulcers tend to be superficial, transient, and often asymptomatic. The characteristic skin lesions, *keratoderma blennorrhagica*, consist of vesicles that become hyperkeratotic, ultimately forming a crust before disappearing. They are most common on the palms and soles but may occur elsewhere as well. In patients with HIV infection, these lesions are often extremely severe and extensive, sometimes dominating the clinical picture (Chap. 182). Lesions on the glans penis, termed *circinate balanitis*, are common; these consist of vesicles that quickly rupture to form painless superficial erosions, which in circumcised individuals can form crusts similar to those of keratoderma blennorrhagica. Nail changes are common and consist of onycholysis, distal yellowish discoloration, and/or heaped-up hyperkeratosis.

Less-frequent or rare manifestations of ReA include cardiac conduction defects, aortic insufficiency, central or peripheral nervous system lesions, and pleuropulmonary infiltrates.

Arthritis typically persists 3–5 months, but courses up to 1 year can occur. Chronic joint symptoms persist in about 15% of patients and in up to 60% in hospital-based series. Recurrences of the acute syndrome are also common. Work disability or forced change in occupation are common in those with persistent joint symptoms. Chronic heel pain is often particularly distressing. Low-back pain, sacroiliitis, and frank AS are also common sequelae. In most studies, HLA-B27–positive patients have shown a worse outcome than B27-negative patients. Patients with *Yersinia*-induced arthritis have less chronic disease than those whose initial episode follows epidemic shigellosis.

LABORATORY AND RADIOGRAPHIC FINDINGS

The ESR is usually elevated during the acute phase of the disease. Mild anemia may be present, and acute-phase reactants tend to be increased. Synovial fluid is nonspecifically inflammatory. In most ethnic groups, about half the patients are B27 positive. It is unusual for the triggering infection to persist at the site of primary mucosal infection through the time of onset of the reactive disease, but it may occasionally be possible to culture the organism, e.g., in the case of *Yersinia*- or *Chlamydia*-induced disease. Serologic evidence of a recent infection may be present, such as a marked elevation of antibodies to *Yersinia*, *Salmonella*, or

Chlamydia. Polymerase chain reaction (PCR) of first-voided urine specimens for chlamydial DNA is said to have high sensitivity.

In early or mild disease, radiographic changes may be absent or confined to juxtaarticular osteoporosis. With long-standing persistent disease, marginal erosions and loss of joint space can be seen in affected joints. Periostitis with reactive new bone formation is characteristic of the disease, as it is with all the spondyloarthritides. Spurs at the insertion of the plantar fascia are common.

Sacroiliitis and spondylitis may be seen as late sequelae. The sacroiliitis is more commonly asymmetric than in AS, and the spondylitis, rather than ascending symmetrically from the lower lumbar segments, can begin anywhere along the lumbar spine. The syndesmophytes may be coarse and nonmarginal, arising from the middle of a vertebral body, a pattern rarely seen in primary AS. Progression to spinal fusion is uncommon.

DIAGNOSIS

ReA is a clinical diagnosis with no definitively diagnostic laboratory test or radiographic finding. The diagnosis should be entertained in any patient with an acute inflammatory, asymmetric, additive arthritis or tendinitis. The evaluation should include questioning regarding possible triggering events such as an episode of diarrhea or dysuria. On physical examination, attention must be paid to the distribution of the joint and tendon involvement and to possible sites of extraarticular involvement, such as the eyes, mucous membranes, skin, nails, and genitalia. Synovial fluid analysis may be helpful in excluding septic or crystal-induced arthritis. Culture, serology, or molecular methods may help to identify a triggering infection.

Although typing for B27 is not needed to secure the diagnosis in clear-cut cases, it may have prognostic significance in terms of severity, chronicity, and the propensity for spondylitis and uveitis. Furthermore, if positive, it can be helpful diagnostically in atypical cases, but a negative test is of little diagnostic value. HIV testing is often indicated and may be necessary in order to select appropriate therapy.

It is important to differentiate ReA from disseminated gonococcal disease (Chap. 137), both of which can be venereally acquired and associated with urethritis. Unlike ReA, gonococcal arthritis and tenosynovitis tend to involve both upper and lower extremities equally, to lack back symptoms, and to be associated with characteristic vesicular skin lesions. A positive gonococcal culture from the urethra or cervix does not exclude a diagnosis of ReA; however, culturing gonococci from blood, skin lesion, or synovium establishes the diagnosis of disseminated gonococcal disease. PCR assay for *Neisseria gonorrhoeae* and *C. trachomatis* may be helpful. Occasionally, only a therapeutic trial of antibiotics can distinguish the two.

ReA shares many features in common with psoriatic arthropathy. However, psoriatic arthritis is usually gradual in onset; the arthritis tends to affect primarily the upper extremities; there is less associated periarthritis; and there are usually no associated mouth ulcers, urethritis, or bowel symptoms.

℞ REACTIVE ARTHRITIS

Most patients with ReA benefit to some degree from NSAIDs, although acute symptoms are rarely completely ameliorated, and some patients fail to respond at all. Indomethacin, 75–150 mg/d in divided doses, is the initial treatment of choice, but other NSAIDs may be tried.

Prompt, appropriate antibiotic treatment of acute chlamydial urethritis or enteric infection may prevent the emergence of ReA. However, several controlled trials have failed to demonstrate any benefit for antibiotic therapy that is initiated after onset of arthritis. One long-term follow-up study suggested that although antibiotic therapy had no effect on the acute episode of ReA, it helped prevent subsequent chronic spondyloarthritis. Another such study failed to demonstrate any long-term benefit.

Multicenter trials have suggested that sulfasalazine, up to 3 g/d in divided doses, may be beneficial to patients with persistent ReA.* Patients with persistent disease may respond to azathioprine, 1–2 mg/kg per day, or to methotrexate, up to 20 mg per week. Although no trials of anti-TNF-α in ReA have been reported, anecdotal evidence supports the use of these agents in severe chronic cases, although lack of response has also been observed.*

Tendinitis and other enthesitic lesions may benefit from intralesional glucocorticoids. Uveitis may require aggressive treatment with glucocorticoids to prevent serious sequelae. Skin lesions ordinarily require only symptomatic treatment. In patients with HIV infection and ReA, many of whom have severe skin lesions, the skin lesions in particular respond to antiretroviral therapy. Cardiac complications are managed conventionally; management of neurologic complications is symptomatic.

Comprehensive management includes counseling of patients in the avoidance of sexually transmitted disease and exposure to enteropathogens, as well as appropriate use of physical therapy, vocational counseling, and continued surveillance for long-term complications such as ankylosing spondylitis.

PSORIATIC ARTHRITIS

Psoriatic arthritis (PsA) refers to an inflammatory arthritis that characteristically occurs in individuals with psoriasis.

HISTORIC BACKGROUND

The association between arthritis and psoriasis was noted in the nineteenth century. In the 1960s, on the basis of epidemiologic and clinical studies, it became clear that unlike RA the arthritis associated with psoriasis was usually seronegative, often involved the distal interphalangeal (DIP) joints of the fingers and the spine and sacroiliac joints, had distinctive radiographic features, and showed considerable familial aggregation. In the 1970s, PsA was included in the broader category of the spondyloarthritides because of features similar to those of AS and ReA.

EPIDEMIOLOGY

Estimates of the prevalence of PsA among individuals with psoriasis range from 5 to 30%. In Caucasian populations, psoriasis is estimated to have a prevalence of 1–3%. Psoriasis and PsA are less common in other races in the absence of HIV infection. First-degree relatives of PsA patients have an elevated risk for psoriasis, for PsA itself, and for other forms of spondyloarthritis. Of patients with psoriasis, 30% have an affected first-degree relative. In monozygotic twins, the concordance for psoriasis is ≥65%, and for PsA ≥30%. A variety of HLA associations have been found. The HLA-Cw6 gene is directly associated with psoriasis, particularly familial juvenile onset (type I) psoriasis. HLA-B27 is associated with psoriatic spondylitis (see below). HLA-DR7, -DQ3, and -B57 are associated with PsA because of linkage disequilibrium with Cw6. Other associations include HLA-B13, -B37, -B38, -B39, and DR4. The MIC-A-A9 allele at the HLA-B-linked MIC-A locus has also recently been reported associated with PsA, as have certain killer immunoglobulin-like receptor (KIR) alleles. The complex inheritance patterns of psoriasis and PsA suggest that several unlinked allelic loci are required for susceptibility. However, only the MHC has shown consistent linkage from study to study.

PATHOLOGY

The inflamed synovium in PsA resembles that of RA, although with somewhat less hyperplasia and cellularity than in RA, and somewhat greater vascularity. Some studies have indicated a higher tendency to synovial fibrosis in PsA. Unlike RA, PsA shows prominent enthesitis, with histology similar to that of the other spondyloarthritides.

PATHOGENESIS

PsA is almost certainly immune-mediated and probably shares pathogenic mechanisms with psoriasis. PsA synovium shows infiltration with T cells, B cells, macrophages, and NK receptor–expressing cells, with upregulation of leukocyte homing receptors. Clonally expanded CD8+ T cells are frequent in PsA. Cytokine production in the synovium in PsA resembles that in psoriatic skin lesions and in RA synovium, having predominantly a T_H1 pattern. Interleukin (IL) 2, interferon γ, TNF-α, and IL-1β, -6, -8, -10, -12, -13, and -15 are found in PsA synovium or synovial fluid. Consistent with the extensive bone lesions in PsA, patients with PsA have been found to have a marked increase in osteoclastic precursors in peripheral blood and upregulation of RANKL (receptor activator of NF-κβ ligand) in the synovial lining layer.

CLINICAL FEATURES

In 60–70% of cases, psoriasis precedes joint disease. In 15–20%, the two manifestations appear within 1 year of each other. In about 15–20% of cases, the arthritis precedes the onset of psoriasis and can present a diagnostic challenge. The frequency in men and women is almost equal, although the frequency of disease patterns differs somewhat in the two sexes. The disease can begin in childhood or late in life but typically begins in the fourth or fifth decade, at an average age of 37 years.

The spectrum of arthropathy associated with psoriasis is quite broad. Many classification schemes have been proposed. In the original scheme of Wright and Moll, five patterns are described: (1) arthritis of the DIP joints; (2) asymmetric oligoarthritis; (3) symmetric polyarthritis similar to RA; (4) axial involvement (spine and sacroiliac joints); and (5) arthritis mutilans, a highly destructive form of disease. These patterns are not fixed, and the pattern that persists chronically often differs from that of the initial presentation. A simpler scheme in recent use contains three patterns: oligoarthritis, polyarthritis, and axial arthritis.

Nail changes in the fingers or toes occur in 90% of patients with PsA, compared with 40% of psoriatic patients without arthritis, and pustular psoriasis is said to be associated with more severe arthritis. Several articular features distinguish PsA from other joint disorders. Dactylitis occurs in >30%; enthesitis and tenosynovitis are also common and are probably present in most patients although often not appreciated on physical examination. Shortening of digits because of underlying osteolysis is particularly characteristic of PsA, and there is a much greater tendency than in RA for both fibrous and bony ankylosis of small joints. Rapid ankylosis of one or more proximal interphalangeal (PIP) joints early in the course of disease is not uncommon. Back and neck pain and stiffness are also common in PsA.

Arthropathy confined to the DIP joints predominates in about 15% of cases. Accompanying nail changes in the affected digits are almost always present. These joints are also often affected in the other patterns of PsA. Approximately 30% of patients have asymmetric oligoarthritis. This pattern commonly involves a knee or another large joint with a few small joints in the fingers or toes, often with dactylitis. Symmetric polyarthritis occurs in about 40% of PsA patients at presentation. It may be indistinguishable from RA in terms of the joints involved, but other features characteristic of PsA are usually also present. In general, peripheral joints in PsA tend to be somewhat less tender than in RA, although signs of inflammation are usually present. Almost any peripheral joint can be involved. Axial arthropathy without peripheral involvement is found in about 5% of PsA patients. It may be indistinguishable from idiopathic AS, although more neck involvement and less thoracolumbar spinal involvement is characteristic, and nail changes are not found in idiopathic AS. About 5% of PsA patients have arthritis mutilans, in which there can be widespread shortening of digits ("telescoping"), sometimes coexisting with ankylosis and contractures in other digits.

Six patterns of nail involvement are identified: pitting, horizontal ridging, onycholysis, yellowish discoloration of the nail margins, dystrophic hyperkeratosis, and combinations of these findings. Other extraarticular manifestations of the spondyloarthritides are common. Eye involvement, either conjunctivitis or uveitis, is reported in 7–33% of PsA patients. Unlike the uveitis associated with AS, the uveitis in PsA is more often bilateral, chronic, and/or posterior. Aortic valve insufficiency has been found in <4% of patients, usually after long-standing disease.

Widely varying estimates of clinical outcome have been reported in PsA. At its worst, severe PsA with arthritis mutilans is at least as crippling and ultimately fatal as severe RA. Unlike RA, however, many pa-

---

*Azathioprine, methotrexate, sulfasalazine, pamidronate, and thalidomide have not been approved for this purpose by the U.S. Food and Drug Administration at the time of publication.

tients with PsA experience temporary remissions. Overall, erosive disease develops in the majority of patients, progressive disease with deformity and disability is common, and in some large published series, mortality was found to be significantly increased compared with the general population.

The psoriasis and associated arthropathy seen with HIV infection both tend to be severe and can occur in populations with very little psoriasis in noninfected individuals. Severe enthesopathy, dactylitis, and rapidly progressive joint destruction are seen, but axial involvement is very rare. This condition is prevented by or responds well to antiretroviral therapy.

LABORATORY AND RADIOGRAPHIC FINDINGS

There are no diagnostic laboratory tests for PsA. ESR and CRP are often elevated. A small percentage of patients may have low titers of rheumatoid factor or antinuclear antibodies. Uric acid may be elevated in the presence of extensive psoriasis. HLA-B27 is found in 50–70% of patients with axial disease, but ≤15–20% in patients with only peripheral joint involvement.

The peripheral and axial arthropathies in PsA show a number of radiographic features that distinguish them from RA and AS, respectively. Characteristics of peripheral PsA include DIP involvement, including the classic "pencil-in-cup" deformity; marginal erosions with adjacent bony proliferation ("whiskering"); small-joint ankylosis; osteolysis of phalangeal and metacarpal bone, with telescoping of digits; and periostitis and proliferative new bone at sites of enthesitis (Fig. 318-3). Characteristics of axial PsA include asymmetric sacroiliitis; compared with idiopathic AS, less zygoapophyseal joint arthritis, fewer and less symmetric and delicate syndesmophytes; fluffy hyperperiostosis on anterior vertebral bodies; severe cervical spine involvement, with a tendency to atlantoaxial subluxation but relative sparing of the thoracolumbar spine; and paravertebral ossification. Ultrasound and MRI both readily demonstrate enthesitis and tendon sheath effusions that can be difficult to assess on physical examination. A recent MRI study of 68 PsA patients found sacroiliitis in 35%, unrelated to B27 but correlated with restricted spinal movement.

DIAGNOSIS

The diagnosis of PsA is primarily clinical, based on the presence of psoriasis and characteristic peripheral or spinal joint symptoms, signs, and imaging. Diagnosis can be challenging when the arthritis precedes psoriasis, the psoriasis is undiagnosed or obscure, or the joint involvement closely resembles another form of arthritis. A high index of sus-

picion is needed in any patient with an undiagnosed inflammatory arthropathy. The history should include inquiry about psoriasis in the patient and family members. Patients should be asked to disrobe for the physical examination, and psoriasiform lesions should be sought in the scalp, ears, umbilicus, and gluteal folds in addition to more accessible sites; the finger and toe nails should also be carefully examined. Axial symptoms or signs, dactylitis, enthesitis, ankylosis, the pattern of joint involvement, and characteristic radiographic changes can be helpful clues. The differential diagnosis of isolated DIP involvement is short. Osteoarthritis (Heberden's nodes) is usually not inflammatory; gout involving more than one DIP joint often involves other sites and is accompanied by tophi; the very rare entity multicentric reticulohistiocytosis involves other joints and has characteristic small pearly periungual skin nodules; and the uncommon entity inflammatory osteoarthritis, like the others, lacks the nail changes of PsA. Radiography can be helpful in all of these cases and in distinguishing between psoriatic spondylitis and idiopathic AS. A history of trauma to an affected joint preceding the onset of arthritis is said to occur more frequently in PsA than in other types of arthritis, perhaps reflecting the Koebner phenomenon in which psoriatic skin lesions can arise at sites of the skin trauma.

℞ PSORIATIC ARTHRITIS

Ideally, coordinated therapy is directed at both the skin and joints in PsA. As described above for AS, use of the anti-TNF-α agents has revolutionized the treatment of PsA. Prompt and dramatic resolution of both arthritis and skin lesions has been observed in large, randomized controlled trials of etanercept, infliximab, and adalimumab. Many of the responding patients had long-standing disease that was resistant to all previous therapy, as well as extensive skin disease. The clinical response is more dramatic than in RA, and delay of disease progression has been demonstrated radiographically The anti-T cell biologic agent Alefacept, in combination with methotrexate, has also been proven effective in both psoriatic arthritis and psoriasis.

Other treatment for PsA has been based on drugs that have efficacy in RA and/or in psoriasis. Although methotrexate in doses of 15–25 mg/week and sulfasalazine (usually given in doses of 2–3 g/d) have each been found to have clinical efficacy in controlled trials, neither effectively halts progression of erosive joint disease. Other agents with efficacy in psoriasis reported to benefit PsA are cyclosporine, retinoic acid derivatives, and psoralen plus ultraviolet light (PUVA). There is controversy regarding the efficacy in PsA of gold and antimalarials, which have been widely used in RA. The pyrimidine synthetase inhibitor leflunomide has been shown in a randomized controlled trial to be beneficial in both psoriasis and psoriatic arthritis.

All of these treatments require careful monitoring. Immunosuppressive therapy may be used cautiously in HIV-associated PsA if the HIV infection is well controlled.

In one large prospective series, 7% of patients with PsA required musculoskeletal surgery beginning at a mean of 13 years' disease duration. Indications for surgery are similar to those in RA, although there is an impression that outcomes in PsA may be less satisfactory.

UNDIFFERENTIATED AND JUVENILE-ONSET SPONDYLOARTHRITIS

Many patients, usually young adults, present with some features of one or more of the spondyloarthritides discussed above but lack criteria for these diagnoses. For example, a patient may present with inflammatory synovitis of one knee, Achilles tendinitis, and dactylitis of one digit, or sacroiliitis in the absence of other criteria for AS. Such patients are said to have undifferentiated spondyloarthritis, or simply spondyloarthritis, as defined by the European Spondyloarthropathy Study Group (ESSG criteria, Fig. 318-4). Some of these patients may have ReA in which the triggering infection remains clinically silent. In some other cases, the patient subsequently develops IBD or psoriasis or the process eventually meets criteria for AS. Approximately half the patients with undifferentiated spondyloarthritis are HLA-B27 positive, and thus the absence of B27 is not useful in establishing or excluding

FIGURE 318-3 Characteristic lesions of psoriatic arthritis. Inflammation is prominent in the DIP joints (left 5th, 4th, 2nd; right 3rd and 5th) and PIP joints (left 2nd, right 2nd, 4th, and 5th). There is dactylitis in the left 2nd finger and thumb, with pronounced telescoping of the left 2nd finger. Nail dystrophy (hyperkeratosis and onycholysis) affects each of the fingers except the left 3rd finger, the only finger without arthritis. (*Courtesy of Donald Raddatz, MD; with permission.*)

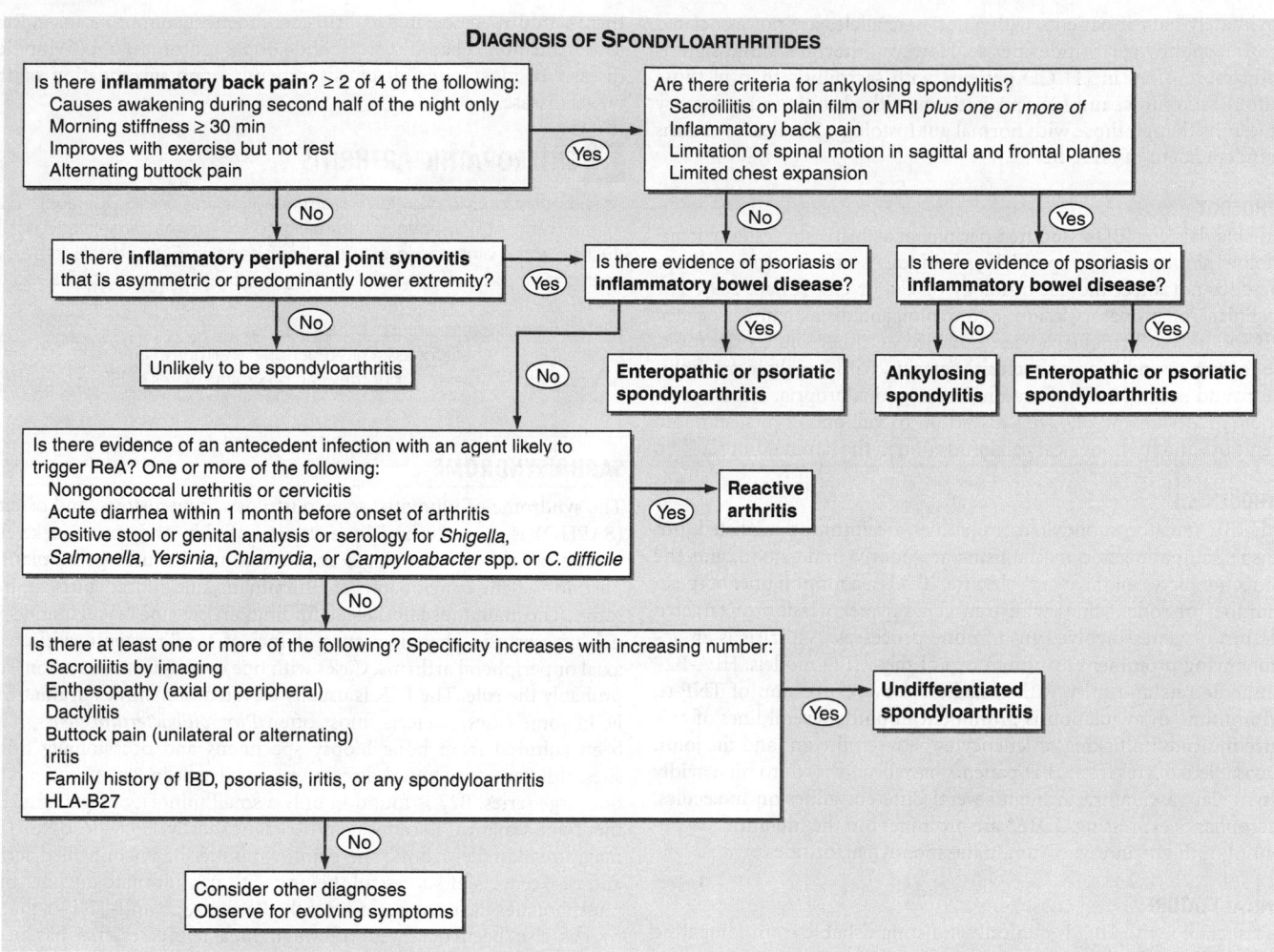

FIGURE 318-4 Algorithm for diagnosis of the spondyloarthritides, adapted from the European Spondyloarthropathy Study Group criteria and the Amor criteria *(M Dougados et al: Arthritis Rheum 34:1218, 1991; B Amor: Rev Rhum Mal Ostéoartic 57:85, 1990).* Sensitivity and specificity for any given decision arm are approximately 80%. If a diagnosis of psoriatic arthropathy, reactive arthritis, or undifferentiated spondyloarthritis is made on the basis of peripheral arthropathy, then HIV infection needs to be considered.

the diagnosis. In familial cases, which are much more frequently B27 positive, there is often eventual progression to AS.

In juvenile-onset spondyloarthritis, which begins between ages 7 and 16, most commonly in boys (60–80%), an asymmetric, predominantly lower-extremity oligoarthritis and enthesitis without extraarticular features is the typical mode of presentation. The prevalence of B27 in this condition, which has been termed the seronegative, enthesopathy, arthropathy (SEA) syndrome, is approximately 80%. Many, but not all, of these patients go on to develop AS in late adolescence or adulthood.

Management of undifferentiated spondyloarthritis is similar to that of the other spondyloarthritides. Response to anti-TNF-α therapy has been documented, and this therapy is indicated in severe, persistent cases not responsive to other treatment. One recent study reported significant benefit in patients with long-standing undifferentiated spondyloarthropathy treated for 9 months with doxycycline and rifampin. These data await confirmation.

Current pediatric textbooks and journals should be consulted for information on management of juvenile-onset spondyloarthritis. An algorithm for the diagnosis of the spondyloarthritides in adults is presented in Fig. 318-4.

ENTEROPATHIC ARTHRITIS

HISTORIC BACKGROUND

A relationship between arthritis and IBD was observed in the 1930s. The relationship was further defined by the epidemiologic studies in the 1950s and 1960s and included in the concept of the spondyloarthritides in the 1970s.

EPIDEMIOLOGY

Both of the common forms of IBD, ulcerative colitis (UC) and Crohn's disease (CD) (Chap. 289), are associated with spondyloarthritis. UC and CD both have an estimated prevalence of 0.05–0.1%, and the incidence of each is thought to have increased in recent decades. AS and peripheral arthritis are both associated with UC and with CD. Wide variations have been reported in the estimated frequencies of these associations. In recent series, AS was diagnosed in 1–10%, and peripheral arthritis in 10–50%, of patients with IBD. Inflammatory back pain and enthesopathy are common, and many patients have sacroiliitis on imaging studies.

The prevalence of UC or CD in patients with AS is thought to be 5–10%. However, investigation of unselected spondyloarthritis patients by ileocolonoscopy has revealed that from one-third to two-thirds of patients with AS have subclinical intestinal inflammation that is evident either macroscopically or histologically. These lesions have also been found in patients with undifferentiated spondyloarthritis or ReA (both enterically and urogenitally acquired).

Both UC and CD have a tendency to familial aggregation, more so for CD. HLA associations have been weak and inconsistent. HLA-B27 is found in up to 70% of patients with IBD and AS, but in ≤15% of patients with IBD and peripheral arthritis or IBD alone. Three alleles of the *NOD2/CARD15* gene on chromosome 16 have been found in approximately half of patients with CD. These alleles are not associated with the spondyloarthritides per se. However, they are found significantly more often in (1) CD patients with sacroiliitis than in those without sacroiliitis, and (2) SpA patients with chronic inflammatory gut lesions than in those with normal gut histology. These associations are independent of HLA-B27.

PATHOLOGY

Available data for IBD-associated peripheral arthritis suggest a synovial histology similar to other spondyloarthritides. Association with arthropathy does not affect the gut histology of UC or CD (Chap. 289). The subclinical inflammatory lesions in the colon and distal ileum associated with spondyloarthritis have been classified as either acute or chronic. The former resemble acute bacterial enteritis, with largely intact architecture and neutrophilic infiltration in the lamina propria. The latter resemble the lesions of CD, with distortion of villi and crypts, aphthoid ulceration, and mononuclear cell infiltration in the lamina propria.

PATHOGENESIS

Both IBD and the spondyloarthropathies are immune-mediated, but the specific pathogenic mechanisms are poorly understood, and the connection between the two is obscure. IBD is a common phenotype in a number of rodent lines with transgenic overexpression or targeted deletion of genes involved in immune processes. Arthritis is an accompanying prominent feature in two of these IBD models, HLA-B27 transgenic rats and mice with constitutive overexpression of TNF-α, and immune dysregulation is prominent in both. Several lines of evidence indicate trafficking of leukocytes between the gut and the joint. Mucosal leukocytes from IBD patients have been shown to bind avidly to synovial vasculature through several different adhesion molecules. Macrophages expressing CD163 are prominent in the inflammatory lesions of both gut and synovium in the spondyloarthritides.

CLINICAL FEATURES

AS associated with IBD is clinically indistinguishable from idiopathic AS. It runs a course independent of the bowel disease, and in many patients it precedes the onset of IBD, sometimes by many years. Peripheral arthritis not infrequently begins before onset of overt bowel disease. The spectrum of peripheral arthritis includes acute self-limited attacks of oligoarthritis that often coincide with relapses of IBD, and more chronic and symmetric polyarticular arthritis that runs a course independent of IBD activity. The patterns of joint involvement are similar in UC and CD. In general, erosions and deformities are infrequent in IBD-associated peripheral arthritis, and joint surgery is rarely required. Dactylitis and enthesopathy are occasionally found. In addition to the ~20% of IBD patients with spondyloarthritis, a comparable percentage have arthralgias or fibromyalgia symptoms.

Other extraintestinal manifestations of IBD are seen in addition to arthropathy, including uveitis, pyoderma gangrenosum, erythema nodosum, and finger clubbing, all somewhat more common in CD than UC. The uveitis shares the features described above for PsA-associated uveitis.

LABORATORY AND RADIOGRAPHIC FINDINGS

Laboratory findings reflect the inflammatory and metabolic manifestations of IBD. Joint fluid is usually at least mildly inflammatory. Of patients with AS and IBD, 30–70% carry the HLA-B27 gene, compared with >90% of patients with AS alone and 50–70% of those with AS and psoriasis. Hence, definite or probable AS in a B27-negative individual in the absence of psoriasis should prompt a search for occult IBD. Radiographic changes in the axial skeleton are the same as in uncomplicated AS. Erosions are uncommon in peripheral arthritis but may occur, particularly in the metatarsophalangeal joints. Isolated destructive hip disease has been described.

DIAGNOSIS

Diarrhea and arthritis are both common conditions that can coexist for a variety of reasons. When etiopathogenically related, reactive arthritis and IBD-associated arthritis are the most common causes. Rare causes include celiac disease, blind loop syndromes, and Whipple's disease. In most cases, diagnosis depends upon investigation of the bowel disease.

℞ ENTEROPATHIC ARTHRITIS

As with the spondyloarthritides, treatment of CD has been revolutionized by therapy with anti-TNF agents. Infliximab and adalimumab are effective for induction and maintenance of clinical remission in CD, and infliximab has been shown to be effective in fistulizing CD. IBD-associated arthritis also responds to these agents. Other treatment for IBD, including sulfasalazine and related drugs, systemic glucocorticoids, and immunosuppressive drugs, are also usually of benefit for associated peripheral arthritis. NSAIDs are generally helpful and well tolerated, but they can precipitate flares of IBD.

SAPHO SYNDROME

The syndrome of synovitis, acne, pustulosis, hyperostosis, and osteitis (SAPHO) is characterized by a variety of skin and musculoskeletal manifestations. Dermatologic manifestations include palmoplantar pustulosis, acne conglobata, acne fulminans, and hidradenitis suppurativa. The main musculoskeletal findings are sternoclavicular and spinal hyperostosis, chronic recurrent foci of sterile osteomyelitis, and axial or peripheral arthritis. Cases with one or a few manifestations are probably the rule. The ESR is usually elevated, sometimes dramatically. In some cases, bacteria, most often *Propionibacterium acnes*, have been cultured from bone biopsy specimens and occasionally other sites. Inflammatory bowel disease was coexistent in 8% of patients in one large series. B27 is found in only a small minority of patients. Either bone scan or CT scan is helpful diagnostically. High-dose NSAIDs may provide relief from bone pain. A number of uncontrolled series and case reports of successful therapy with pamidronate or other bisphosphonates have appeared recently. Response to anti-TNF-α therapy has also been observed, although in a few cases this has been associated with a flare of skin manifestations. Successful prolonged antibiotic therapy has also been reported.

WHIPPLE'S DISEASE

Whipple's disease (see also Chap. 288) is a rare chronic bacterial infection, mostly of middle-aged Caucasian men, caused by *Tropheryma whippelii*. At least 75% of affected individuals develop an oligo- or polyarthritis. The joint manifestations usually precede other symptoms of the disease by 5 years or more; they are thus particularly important because antibiotic therapy is curative, whereas the untreated disease is fatal. Large and small peripheral joints and sacroiliac joints may be involved. The arthritis is abrupt in onset, migratory, usually lasts hours to a few days, and then resolves completely. Chronic polyarthritis and joint space loss, visible on x-ray, can occur but are not typical. Eventually prolonged diarrhea, malabsorption, and weight loss occur. Other manifestations of systemic disease include fever, edema, serositis, endocarditis, pneumonia, hypotension, lymphadenopathy, hyperpigmentation, subcutaneous nodules, clubbing, and uveitis. Central nervous system involvement eventually develops in 80% of untreated patients, with cognitive changes, headache, diplopia, and papilledema, and may be appreciated by abnormalities on MRI. Oculomasticatory and oculofacial-skeletal myorhythmia, accompanied by supranuclear vertical gaze palsy, are said to be pathognomonic. Laboratory abnormalities include anemia and changes from malabsorption. There is at most a weak association with HLA-B27. Synovial fluid is usually inflammatory. Radiography rarely shows joint erosions but may show sacroiliitis. Abdominal CT may reveal lymphadenopathy. Foamy macrophages containing PAS-staining bacterial remnants can be seen in biopsies of small intestine, synovium, lymph node, and other tissues.

The complete genome sequence of *T. whippelii* was published in 2003. Diagnosis is established by PCR amplification of sequences of the 16S ribosomal gene or other genes of *T. whippelii* in biopsied tissue. In the future, this may be supplanted or complemented by serologic tests. The syndrome responds best to therapy with penicillin (or ceftriaxone) and streptomycin for 2 weeks followed by trimethoprim-sulfamethoxazole for 1–2 years. Monitoring for central nervous system relapse is critical.

FURTHER READINGS

BORENSTEIN D: Inflammatory arthritides of the spine: Surgical versus nonsurgical treatment. Clin Orthop Relat Res 443:208, 2006

BRAUN J et al: Major reduction in spinal inflammation in patients with ankylosing spondylitis after treatment with infliximab: Results of a multicenter, randomized, double-blind, placebo-controlled magnetic resonance imaging study. Arthritis Rheum 54:1646, 2006

FELDTKELLER E et al: Prevalence and annual incidence of vertebral fractures in patients with ankylosing spondylitis. Rheumatol Int 26:234, 2006

KIM TH et al: Pathogenesis of ankylosing spondylitis and reactive arthritis. Curr Opin Rheumatol 17:400, 2005

LEIRISALO-REPO M: Reactive arthritis. Scand J Rheumatol 34:251, 2005

MEASE PJ et al: Alefacept in combination with methotrexate for the treatment of psoriatic arthritis: Results of a randomized, double-blind, placebo-controlled study. Arthritis Rheum 54:1638, 2006

REVEILLE JD, ARNETT FC: Spondyloarthritis: Update on pathogenesis and management. Am J Med 118:592, 2005

RUDWALEIT M et al: Inflammatory back pain in ankylosing spondylitis: A reassessment of the clinical history for application as classification and diagnostic criteria. Arthritis Rheum 54:569, 2006

TAYLOR W et al: Classification criteria for psoriatic arthritis. Development of new criteria from a large international study. Arthritis Rheum, 54:2665, 2006

ZOCHLING J et al: ASAS/EULAR recommendations for the management of ankylosing spondylitis. Ann Rheum Dis 65:442, 2006

319 The Vasculitis Syndromes
Carol A. Langford, Anthony S. Fauci

DEFINITION

Vasculitis is a clinicopathologic process characterized by inflammation of and damage to blood vessels. The vessel lumen is usually compromised, and this is associated with ischemia of the tissues supplied by the involved vessel. A broad and heterogeneous group of syndromes may result from this process, since any type, size, and location of blood vessel may be involved. Vasculitis and its consequences may be the primary or sole manifestation of a disease; alternatively, vasculitis may be a secondary component of another primary disease. Vasculitis may be confined to a single organ, such as the skin, or it may simultaneously involve several organ systems.

CLASSIFICATION

A major feature of the vasculitic syndromes as a group is the fact that there is a great deal of heterogeneity at the same time as there is considerable overlap among them. This heterogeneity and overlap in addition to a lack of understanding of the pathogenesis of these syndromes have been major impediments to the development of a coherent classification system for these diseases. Table 319-1 lists the major vasculitis syndromes. The distinguishing and overlapping features of these syndromes are discussed below.

PATHOPHYSIOLOGY AND PATHOGENESIS

Generally, most of the vasculitic syndromes are assumed to be mediated at least in part by immunopathogenic mechanisms that occur in response to certain antigenic stimuli (Table 319-2). However, evidence

TABLE 319-1 VASCULITIS SYNDROMES

Primary Vasculitis Syndromes	Secondary Vasculitis Syndromes
Wegener's granulomatosis	Drug-induced vasculitis
Churg-Strauss syndrome	Serum sickness
Polyarteritis nodosa	Vasculitis associated with other
Microscopic polyangiitis	primary diseases
Giant cell arteritis	Infection
Takayasu's arteritis	Malignancy
Henoch-Schönlein purpura	Rheumatic disease
Idiopathic cutaneous vasculitis	
Essential mixed cryoglobulinemia	
Behçet's syndrome	
Isolated vasculitis of the central nervous system	
Cogan's syndrome	
Kawasaki disease	

TABLE 319-2 POTENTIAL MECHANISMS OF VESSEL DAMAGE IN VASCULITIS SYNDROMES

Pathogenic immune complex formation and/or deposition
  Henoch-Schönlein purpura
  Vasculitis associated with collagen vascular diseases
  Serum sickness and cutaneous vasculitis syndromes
  Hepatitis C–associated essential mixed cryoglobulinemia
  Hepatitis B–associated polyarteritis nodosa
Production of antineutrophilic cytoplasmic antibodies
  Wegener's granulomatosis
  Churg-Strauss syndrome
  Microscopic polyangiitis
Pathogenic T lymphocyte responses and granuloma formation
  Giant cell arteritis
  Takayasu's arteritis
  Wegener's granulomatosis
  Churg-Strauss syndrome

Source: Adapted from Sneller and Fauci.

supporting this hypothesis is for the most part indirect and may reflect epiphenomena as opposed to true causality. Furthermore, it is unknown why some individuals might develop vasculitis in response to certain antigenic stimuli, whereas others do not. It is likely that a number of factors are involved in the ultimate expression of a vasculitic syndrome. These include the genetic predisposition, environmental exposures, and the regulatory mechanisms associated with immune response to certain antigens.

Pathogenic Immune-Complex Formation Vasculitis is generally considered within the broader category of *immune-complex diseases* that include serum sickness and certain of the connective tissue diseases, of which systemic lupus erythematosus (Chap. 313) is the prototype. Although deposition of immune complexes in vessel walls is the most widely accepted pathogenic mechanism of vasculitis, the causal role of immune complexes has not been clearly established in most of the vasculitic syndromes. Circulating immune complexes need not result in deposition of the complexes in blood vessels with ensuing vasculitis, and many patients with active vasculitis do not have demonstrable circulating or deposited immune complexes. The actual antigen contained in the immune complex has only rarely been identified in vasculitic syndromes. In this regard, hepatitis B antigen has been identified in both the circulating and deposited immune complexes in a subset of patients with systemic vasculitis, most notably in polyarteritis nodosa (PAN; see below). The syndrome of essential mixed cryoglobulinemia is strongly associated with hepatitis C virus infection; hepatitis C virions and hepatitis C virus antigen-antibody complexes have been identified in the cryoprecipitates of these patients (see below).

The mechanisms of tissue damage in immune complex–mediated vasculitis resemble those described for serum sickness. In this model, antigen-antibody complexes are formed in antigen excess and are deposited in vessel walls whose permeability has been increased by vasoactive amines such as histamine, bradykinin, and leukotrienes released from platelets or from mast cells as a result of IgE-triggered mechanisms. The deposition of complexes results in activation of complement components, particularly C5a, which is strongly chemotactic for neutrophils. These cells then infiltrate the vessel wall, phagocytose the immune complexes, and release their intracytoplasmic enzymes, which damage the vessel wall. As the process becomes subacute or chronic, mononuclear cells infiltrate the vessel wall. The common denominator of the resulting syndrome is compromise of the vessel lumen with ischemic changes in the tissues supplied by the involved vessel. Several variables may explain why only certain types of immune complexes cause vasculitis and why only certain vessels are affected in individual patients. These include the ability of the reticuloendothelial system to clear circulating complexes from the blood, the size and physicochemical properties of immune complexes, the relative degree of turbulence of blood flow, the intravascular hydrostatic pressure in different vessels, and the preexisting integrity of the vessel endothelium.

Antineutrophil Cytoplasmic Antibodies (ANCA)   ANCA are antibodies directed against certain proteins in the cytoplasmic granules of neutrophils and monocytes. These autoantibodies are present in a high percentage of patients with certain systemic vasculitis syndromes, particularly Wegener's granulomatosis and microscopic polyangiitis, and in patients with necrotizing and crescentic glomerulonephritis. There are two major categories of ANCA based on different targets for the antibodies. The terminology of *cytoplasmic ANCA* (c-ANCA) refers to the diffuse, granular cytoplasmic staining pattern observed by immunofluorescence microscopy when serum antibodies bind to indicator neutrophils. Proteinase-3, the 29-kDa neutral serine proteinase present in neutrophil azurophilic granules, is the major c-ANCA antigen. More than 90% of patients with typical active Wegener's granulomatosis have detectable antibodies to proteinase-3 (see below). The terminology of *perinuclear ANCA* (p-ANCA) refers to the more localized perinuclear or nuclear staining pattern of the indicator neutrophils. The major target for p-ANCA is the enzyme myeloperoxidase; other targets that can produce a p-ANCA pattern of staining include elastase, cathepsin G, lactoferrin, lysozyme, and bactericidal/permeability-increasing protein. However, only antibodies to myeloperoxidase have been convincingly associated with vasculitis. Antimyeloperoxidase antibodies have been reported to occur in variable percentages of patients with microscopic polyangiitis, Churg-Strauss syndrome, crescentic glomerulonephritis, Goodpasture's syndrome, and Wegener's granulomatosis (see below). A p-ANCA pattern of staining that is not due to antimyeloperoxidase antibodies has been associated with nonvasculitic entities such as rheumatic and nonrheumatic autoimmune diseases, inflammatory bowel disease, certain drugs, and infections such as endocarditis and bacterial airway infections in patients with cystic fibrosis.

It is unclear why patients with these vasculitis syndromes develop antibodies to myeloperoxidase or proteinase-3, whereas such antibodies are rare in other inflammatory diseases and autoimmune diseases. There are a number of in vitro observations that suggest possible mechanisms whereby these antibodies can contribute to the pathogenesis of the vasculitis syndromes. Proteinase-3 and myeloperoxidase reside in the azurophilic granules and lysosomes of resting neutrophils and monocytes, where they are apparently inaccessible to serum antibodies. However, when neutrophils or monocytes are primed by tumor necrosis factor (TNF) α or interleukin (IL) 1, proteinase-3 and myeloperoxidase translocate to the cell membrane where they can interact with extracellular ANCA. The neutrophils then degranulate and produce reactive oxygen species that can cause tissue damage. Furthermore, ANCA-activated neutrophils can adhere to and kill endothelial cells in vitro. Activation of neutrophils and monocytes by ANCA also induces the release of proinflammatory cytokines such as IL-1 and IL-8. Recent adoptive transfer experiments in genetically engineered mice provide further evidence for a direct pathogenic role of ANCA in vivo. In contradiction, however, a number of clinical and laboratory observations argue against a primary pathogenic role for ANCA. Patients may have active Wegener's granulomatosis in the absence of ANCA; the absolute height of the antibody titers does not correlate well with disease activity; and patients with Wegener's granulomatosis in remission may continue to have high antiproteinase-3 (c-ANCA) titers for years (see below). Thus, the role of these autoantibodies in the pathogenesis of systemic vasculitis remains unclear.

Pathogenic T Lymphocyte Responses and Granuloma Formation   In addition to the classic immune complex–mediated mechanisms of vasculitis as well as ANCA, other immunopathogenic mechanisms may be involved in damage to vessels. The most prominent of these are delayed hypersensitivity and cell-mediated immune injury as reflected in the histopathologic feature of granulomatous vasculitis. However, immune complexes themselves may induce granulomatous responses. Vascular endothelial cells can express HLA class II molecules following activation by cytokines such as interferon (IFN) γ. This allows these cells to participate in immunologic reactions such as interaction with CD4+ T lymphocytes in a manner similar to antigen-presenting macrophages. Endothelial cells can secrete IL-1, which may activate T lymphocytes and initiate or propagate in situ immunologic processes within the blood vessel. In addition, IL-1 and TNF-α are potent inducers of endothelial-leukocyte adhesion molecule 1 (ELAM-1) and vascular cell adhesion molecule 1 (VCAM-1), which may enhance the adhesion of leukocytes to endothelial cells in the blood vessel wall. Other mechanisms such as direct cellular cytotoxicity, antibody directed against vessel components, or antibody-dependent cellular cytotoxicity have been suggested in certain types of vessel damage. However, there is no convincing evidence to support their causal contribution to the pathogenesis of any of the recognized vasculitic syndromes.

APPROACH TO THE PATIENT:
Vasculitis

The diagnosis of vasculitis is often considered in any patient with an unexplained systemic illness. However, there are certain clinical abnormalities that when present alone or in combination should suggest a diagnosis of vasculitis. These include palpable purpura, pulmonary infiltrates and microscopic hematuria, chronic inflammatory sinusitis, mononeuritis multiplex, unexplained ischemic events, and glomerulonephritis with evidence of multisystem disease. A number of nonvasculitic diseases may also produce some or all of these abnormalities. Thus, the first step in the workup of a patient with suspected vasculitis is to exclude other diseases that produce clinical manifestations that can mimic vasculitis (Table 319-3). It is particularly important to exclude infectious diseases with features that overlap those of vasculitis, especially if the patient's clinical condition is deteriorating rapidly and empirical immunosuppressive treatment is being contemplated.

Once diseases that mimic vasculitis have been excluded, the workup should follow a series of progressive steps that establish the diagnosis of vasculitis and determine, where possible, the category of the vasculitis syndrome (Fig. 319-1). This approach is of considerable importance since several of the vasculitis syndromes require aggressive therapy with glucocorticoids and cytotoxic agents, while other syndromes usually resolve spontaneously and require symptomatic treatment only. The definitive diagnosis of vasculitis is made upon biopsy of involved tissue. The yield of "blind" biopsies of organs with no subjective or objective evidence of involvement is very low and should be avoided. When syndromes such as PAN, Takayasu's arteritis, or isolated central nervous system (CNS) vasculitis are suspected, angiogram of organs with suspected involvement should be performed. However, angiograms should not be

TABLE 319-3	CONDITIONS THAT CAN MIMIC VASCULITIS

Infectious diseases
    Bacterial endocarditis
    Disseminated gonococcal infection
    Pulmonary histoplasmosis
    Coccidioidomycosis
    Syphilis
    Lyme disease
    Rocky Mountain spotted fever
    Whipple's disease
Coagulopathies/thrombotic microangiopathies
    Antiphospholipid antibody syndrome
    Thrombotic thrombocytopenic purpura
Neoplasms
    Atrial myxoma
    Lymphoma
    Carcinomatosis
Drug toxicity
    Cocaine
    Amphetamines
    Ergot alkaloids
    Methysergide
    Arsenic
Sarcoidosis
Atheroembolic disease
Goodpasture's syndrome
Amyloidosis
Migraine
Cryofibrinogenemia

performed routinely when patients present with localized cutaneous vasculitis with no clinical indication of visceral involvement.

The constellation of clinical, laboratory, biopsy, and radiographic findings usually allows proper categorization to a specific syndrome, and therapy where appropriate should be initiated according to this information (see individual syndromes below). If an offending antigen that precipitates the vasculitis is recognized, the antigen should be removed where possible. If the vasculitis is associated with an underlying disease such as an infection, neoplasm, or connective tissue disease, the underlying disease should be treated. If the syndrome does not resolve following removal of an offending antigen or treatment of an underlying disease, or if there is no recognizable underlying disease, treatment should be initiated according to the category of the vasculitis syndrome. Treatment options will be considered under the individual syndromes (see below), and general principles of therapy will be considered at the end of the chapter.

WEGENER'S GRANULOMATOSIS

Definition *Wegener's granulomatosis* is a distinct clinicopathologic entity characterized by granulomatous vasculitis of the upper and lower respiratory tracts together with glomerulonephritis. In addition, variable degrees of disseminated vasculitis involving both small arteries and veins may occur.

Incidence and Prevalence Wegener's granulomatosis is an uncommon disease with an estimated prevalence of 3 per 100,000. It is extremely rare in blacks compared with whites; the male-to-female ratio is 1:1. The disease can be seen at any age; ~15% of patients are <19 years of age, but only rarely does the disease occur before adolescence; the mean age of onset is ~40 years.

Pathology and Pathogenesis The histopathologic hallmarks of Wegener's granulomatosis are necrotizing vasculitis of small arteries and veins together with granuloma formation, which may be either intravascular or extravascular (Fig. 319-2). Lung involvement typically appears as multiple, bilateral, nodular cavitary infiltrates (Fig. 319-3), which on biopsy almost invariably reveal the typical necrotizing granulomatous vasculitis. Upper airway lesions, particularly those in the si-

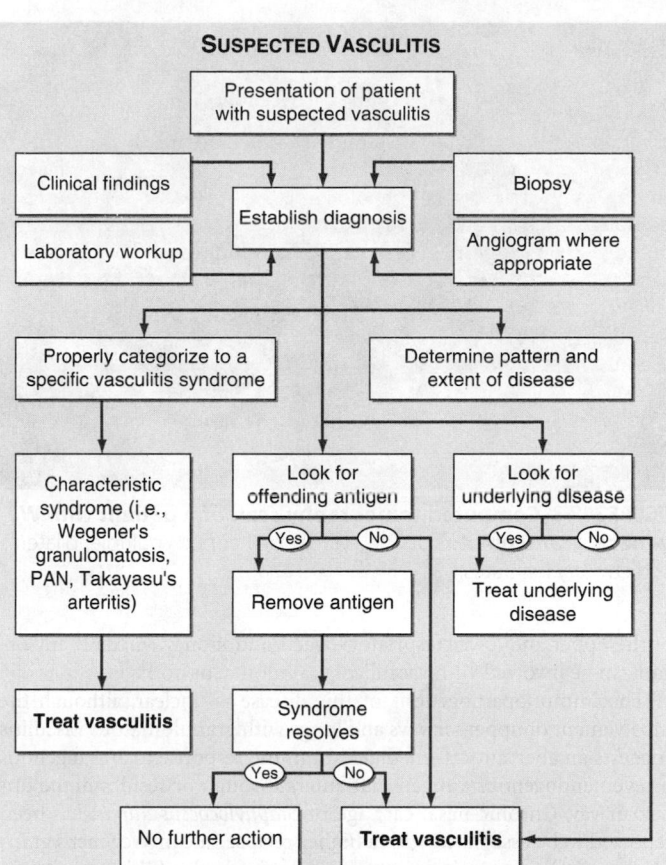

FIGURE 319-1 Algorithm for the approach to a patient with suspected diagnosis of vasculitis. PAN, polyarteritis nodosa.

nuses and nasopharynx, typically reveal inflammation, necrosis, and granuloma formation, with or without vasculitis.

In its earliest form, renal involvement is characterized by a focal and segmental glomerulitis that may evolve into a rapidly progressive crescentic glomerulonephritis. Granuloma formation is only rarely seen on renal biopsy. In contrast to other forms of glomerulonephritis, evidence of immune complex deposition is not found in the renal lesion of Wegener's granulomatosis. In addition to the classic triad of disease

FIGURE 319-2 Lung histology in Wegener's granulomatosis. This area of geographic necrosis has a serpiginous border of histiocytes and giant cells surrounding a central necrotic zone. Vasculitis is also present with neutrophils and lymphocytes infiltrating the wall of a small arteriole (upper right). *(Courtesy of William D. Travis, MD; with permission.)*

FIGURE 319-3 Computed tomography scan of a patient with Wegener's granulomatosis. The patient developed multiple, bilateral, and cavitary infiltrates.

of the upper and lower respiratory tracts and kidney, virtually any organ can be involved with vasculitis, granuloma, or both.

The immunopathogenesis of this disease is unclear, although the involvement of upper airways and lungs with granulomatous vasculitis suggests an aberrant cell-mediated immune response to an exogenous or even endogenous antigen that enters through or resides in the upper airway. Chronic nasal carriage of *Staphylococcus aureus* has been reported to be associated with a higher relapse rate of Wegener's granulomatosis; however, there is no evidence for a role of this organism in the pathogenesis of the disease.

Peripheral blood mononuclear cells obtained from patients with Wegener's granulomatosis manifest increased secretion of IFN-γ but not of IL-4, IL-5, or IL-10 compared to normal controls. In addition, TNF-α production from peripheral blood mononuclear cells and CD4+ T cells is elevated. Furthermore, monocytes from patients with Wegener's granulomatosis produce increased amounts of IL-12. These findings indicate an unbalanced T_H1-type T cell cytokine pattern in this disease that may have pathogenic and perhaps ultimately therapeutic implications.

A high percentage of patients with Wegener's granulomatosis develop ANCA, and these autoantibodies may play a role in the pathogenesis of this disease (see above).

Clinical and Laboratory Manifestations Involvement of the upper airways occurs in 95% of patients with Wegener's granulomatosis. Patients often present with severe upper respiratory tract findings such as paranasal sinus pain and drainage and purulent or bloody nasal discharge, with or without nasal mucosal ulceration (Table 319-4). Nasal septal perforation may follow, leading to saddle nose deformity. Serous otitis media may occur as a result of eustachian tube blockage. Subglottic tracheal stenosis resulting from active disease or scarring occurs in ~16% of patients and may result in severe airway obstruction.

Pulmonary involvement may be manifested as asymptomatic infiltrates or may be clinically expressed as cough, hemoptysis, dyspnea, and chest discomfort. It is present in 85–90% of patients. Endobronchial disease, either in its active form or as a result of fibrous scarring, may lead to obstruction with atelectasis.

Eye involvement (52% of patients) may range from a mild conjunctivitis to dacryocystitis, episcleritis, scleritis, granulomatous sclerouveitis, ciliary vessel vasculitis, and retroorbital mass lesions leading to proptosis.

Skin lesions (46% of patients) appear as papules, vesicles, palpable purpura, ulcers, or subcutaneous nodules; biopsy reveals vasculitis, granuloma, or both. Cardiac involvement (8% of patients) manifests as pericarditis, coronary vasculitis, or, rarely, cardiomyopathy. Nervous

TABLE 319-4 WEGENER'S GRANULOMATOSIS: FREQUENCY OF CLINICAL MANIFESTATIONS IN 158 PATIENTS STUDIED AT THE NATIONAL INSTITUTES OF HEALTH

Manifestation	Percent at Disease Onset	Percent Throughout Course of Disease
Kidney		
Glomerulonephritis	18	77
Ear/nose/throat	73	92
Sinusitis	51	85
Nasal disease	36	68
Otitis media	25	44
Hearing loss	14	42
Subglottic stenosis	1	16
Ear pain	9	14
Oral lesions	3	10
Lung	45	85
Pulmonary infiltrates	25	66
Pulmonary nodules	24	58
Hemoptysis	12	30
Pleuritis	10	28
Eyes		
Conjunctivitis	5	18
Dacryocystitis	1	18
Scleritis	6	16
Proptosis	2	15
Eye pain	3	11
Visual loss	0	8
Retinal lesions	0	4
Corneal lesions	0	1
Iritis	0	2
Other[a]		
Arthralgias/arthritis	32	67
Fever	23	50
Cough	19	46
Skin abnormalities	13	46
Weight loss (>10% body weight)	15	35
Peripheral neuropathy	1	15
Central nervous system disease	1	8
Pericarditis	2	6
Hyperthyroidism	1	3

[a]Fewer than 1% had parotid, pulmonary artery, breast, or lower genitourinary (urethra, cervix, vagina, testicular) involvement.
Source: Hoffman et al.

system manifestations (23% of patients) include cranial neuritis, mononeuritis multiplex, or, rarely, cerebral vasculitis and/or granuloma.

Renal disease (77% of patients) generally dominates the clinical picture and, if left untreated, accounts directly or indirectly for most of the mortality in this disease. Although it may smolder in some cases as a mild glomerulitis with proteinuria, hematuria, and red blood cell casts, it is clear that once clinically detectable renal functional impairment occurs, rapidly progressive renal failure usually ensues unless appropriate treatment is instituted.

While the disease is active, most patients have nonspecific symptoms and signs such as malaise, weakness, arthralgias, anorexia, and weight loss. Fever may indicate activity of the underlying disease but more often reflects secondary infection, usually of the upper airway.

Characteristic laboratory findings include a markedly elevated erythrocyte sedimentation rate (ESR), mild anemia and leukocytosis, mild hypergammaglobulinemia (particularly of the IgA class), and mildly elevated rheumatoid factor. Thrombocytosis may be seen as an acute-phase reactant. Approximately 90% of patients with active Wegener's granulomatosis have a positive antiproteinase-3 ANCA. However, in the absence of active disease, the sensitivity drops to ~60–70%. A small percentage of patients with Wegener's granulomatosis may have antimyeloperoxidase rather than antiproteinase-3 antibodies.

Patients with Wegener's granulomatosis have been found to have an increased incidence of venous thrombotic events. Although routine anticoagulation for all patients is not recommended, a heightened awareness for any clinical features suggestive of deep venous thrombosis or pulmonary emboli is warranted.

Diagnosis The diagnosis of Wegener's granulomatosis is made by the demonstration of necrotizing granulomatous vasculitis on tissue biopsy in a patient with compatible clinical features. Pulmonary tissue offers the highest diagnostic yield, almost invariably revealing granulomatous vasculitis. Biopsy of upper airway tissue usually reveals granulomatous inflammation with necrosis but may not show vasculitis. Renal biopsy can confirm the presence of pauci-immune glomerulonephritis.

The specificity of a positive antiproteinase-3 ANCA for Wegener's granulomatosis is very high, especially if active glomerulonephritis is present. However, the presence of ANCA should be adjunctive and, with very rare exceptions, should not substitute for a tissue diagnosis. False-positive ANCA titers have been reported in certain infectious and neoplastic diseases.

In its typical presentation, the clinicopathologic complex of Wegener's granulomatosis usually provides ready differentiation from other disorders. However, if all the typical features are not present at once, it needs to be differentiated from the other vasculitides, Goodpasture's syndrome (Chap. 277), relapsing polychondritis (Chap. 321), tumors of the upper airway or lung, and infectious diseases such as histoplasmosis (Chap. 192), mucocutaneous leishmaniasis (Chap. 205), and rhinoscleroma (Chap. 31) as well as noninfectious granulomatous diseases.

Of particular note is the differentiation from *midline granuloma* and *upper airway neoplasms*, which are part of the spectrum of *midline destructive diseases*. These diseases lead to extreme tissue destruction and mutilation localized to the midline upper airway structures including the sinuses; erosion through the skin of the face commonly occurs, a feature that is extremely rare in Wegener's granulomatosis. Although blood vessels may be involved in the intense inflammatory reaction and necrosis, primary vasculitis is seen rarely. When systemic involvement occurs, it usually declares itself as a neoplastic process. In this regard, it is likely that midline granuloma is part of the spectrum of *angiocentric immunoproliferative lesions*. The latter are considered to represent a spectrum of postthymic T cell proliferative lesions and should be treated as such (Chap. 105). The term *idiopathic* has been applied to midline granuloma when extensive diagnostic workup including multiple biopsies has failed to reveal anything other than inflammation and necrosis. Under these circumstances, it is possible that the tumor cells were masked by the intensive inflammatory response. Such cases have responded to local irradiation with 50 Gy (5000 rad). Upper airway lesions should never be irradiated in Wegener's granulomatosis. Cocaine-induced tissue injury can be another important mimic of Wegener's granulomatosis in patients who present with isolated midline destructive disease. ANCA that target human neutrophil elastase can be found in patients with cocaine-induced midline destructive lesions and can confound the differentiation from Wegener's granulomatosis.

Wegener's granulomatosis must also be differentiated from *lymphomatoid granulomatosis*, which is an Epstein-Barr virus–positive B cell proliferation that is associated with an exuberant T cell reaction. Lymphomatoid granulomatosis is characterized by lung, skin, CNS, and kidney involvement in which atypical lymphocytoid and plasmacytoid cells infiltrate nonlymphoid tissue in an angioinvasive manner. In this regard, it clearly differs from Wegener's granulomatosis in that it is not an inflammatory vasculitis in the classic sense but an infiltration of vessels with atypical mononuclear cells; granuloma may be present in involved tissues. Up to 50% of patients may develop a true malignant lymphoma.

℞ WEGENER'S GRANULOMATOSIS

CYCLOPHOSPHAMIDE INDUCTION FOR SEVERE DISEASE

Wegener's granulomatosis was formerly universally fatal, usually within a few months after the onset of clinically apparent renal disease. Glucocorticoids alone led to some symptomatic improvement, with little effect on the ultimate course of the disease. It has been well established that the most effective therapy in this disease is cyclophosphamide given in doses of 2 mg/kg per day orally together with glucocorticoids. The leukocyte count should be monitored closely during therapy, and the dosage of cyclophosphamide should be adjusted in order to maintain the count above 3000/μL, which generally maintains the neutrophil count at ~1500/μL. With this approach, clinical remission can usually be induced and maintained without causing severe leukopenia with its associated risk of infection. As it was originally studied, cyclophosphamide was continued for 1 year following the induction of complete remission and gradually tapered and discontinued thereafter.

At the initiation of therapy, glucocorticoids should be administered together with cyclophosphamide. This can be given as prednisone, 1 mg/kg per day initially (for the first month of therapy) as a daily regimen, with gradual conversion to an alternate-day schedule followed by tapering and discontinuation after ~6 months.

Using the above regimen, the prognosis of this disease is excellent; marked improvement is seen in >90% of patients, and complete remissions are achieved in 75% of patients. A number of patients who developed irreversible renal failure but who achieved subsequent remission on appropriate therapy have undergone successful renal transplantation.

Despite the dramatic remissions induced by the therapeutic regimen described above, long-term follow-up of patients has revealed that ~50% of remissions are later associated with one or more relapses. Reinduction of remission is almost always achieved; however, a high percentage of patients ultimately have some degree of morbidity from irreversible features of their disease, such as varying degrees of renal insufficiency, hearing loss, tracheal stenosis, saddle nose deformity, and chronically impaired sinus function. The determination of relapse should be based on objective evidence of disease activity, taking care to rule out other features that may have a similar appearance such as infection, medication toxicity, or chronic disease sequelae. The ANCA titer can be misleading. Many patients who achieve remission continue to have elevated titers for years. In addition, one study found that >40% of patients who were in remission and had a fourfold increase in ANCA titer did not have a relapse in disease. Patients who relapse may not do so until many months or years after the rise in ANCA titer. Thus, a rise in ANCA titer by itself is not a harbinger of immediate disease relapse and should not lead to reinstitution or increase in immunosuppressive therapy. However, such a finding should prompt the clinician to examine the patient carefully for any objective evidence of active disease and to monitor that patient closely.

Certain types of morbidity are related to toxic side effects of treatment. Glucocorticoid-related side effects can include diabetes mellitus, cataracts, life-threatening infectious disease complications, serious osteoporosis, and severe cushingoid features. The risk of such toxicities can be reduced with the use of an alternate-day glucocorticoid regimen as outlined in the preceding regimen. Cyclophosphamide-related toxicities are more frequent and severe. Cystitis to varying degrees occurs in at least 30% of patients, bladder cancer in 6%, myelodysplasia in 2%, and there is a high risk of permanent infertility in both men and women.

Some reports have indicated therapeutic success with less frequent and severe toxic side effects using intermittent boluses of IV cyclophosphamide (1 g/m² per month) in place of daily administration. However, we and others have found an increased rate of relapse with bolus IV cyclophosphamide. We therefore strongly recommend that the drug be given as daily oral therapy.

In patients with immediately life-threatening disease, such as rapidly progressive glomerulonephritis, a regimen of daily cyclophosphamide and glucocorticoids is clearly the treatment of choice to induce remission. However, after patients have achieved remission, which typically occurs within 3–6 months, consideration should be given to stopping cyclophosphamide and beginning methotrexate or azathioprine for remission maintenance. This approach is aimed at lessening the toxicity associated with chronic cyclophosphamide therapy. Methotrexate is administered orally starting at a dosage of 0.3 mg/kg as a single weekly dose, not to exceed 15 mg/week. If the treatment is well tolerated after 1–2 weeks, the dosage should be increased by 2.5 mg weekly up to a dosage of 20–25 mg/week and maintained at that level. This regimen is given for 2 years past remission, after which time it is tapered by 2.5 mg each month until discontinuation. To lessen toxicity, methotrexate is often given together with folic acid, 1 mg daily, or folinic acid, 5–10 mg once a week 24 h following methotrexate. Azathioprine, 2 mg/kg per day, has also proven effective in maintaining remission following induction with daily cyclophosphamide. There have been no studies to date comparing methotrexate to azathioprine for remission maintenance. In the absence of such data, the choice of agent is often based on toxicity profile, as methotrexate cannot be given to patients with renal insufficiency or chronic liver disease. In patients who are unable to receive methotrexate or azathioprine or who have relapsed through such treatment, emerging data suggest that mycophenolate mofetil, 1000 mg twice a day, may also sustain remission following cyclophosphamide induction in selected patients.

METHOTREXATE INDUCTION FOR NONSEVERE DISEASE For selected patients whose disease is not immediately life threatening or in those patients who have experienced significant cyclophosphamide toxicity, methotrexate together with glucocorticoids given at the dosages described above may be considered as an alternative for initial therapy.

BIOLOGIC THERAPIES Biologic therapies have increasingly been investigated in Wegener's granulomatosis. Etanercept, a dimeric fusion protein containing the 75-kDa TNF receptor bound to human IgG1, was not found to sustain remission when used adjunctively to standard therapy and should not be used in the treatment of Wegener's granulomatosis. Favorable preliminary results with the use of rituximab (anti-CD20) in Wegener's granulomatosis have been reported. However, pending further investigation of this agent through rigorous prospective trials, rituximab should not be used in place of standard treatments that are of proven efficacy.

TRIMETHOPRIM-SULFAMETHOXAZOLE Although certain reports have indicated that trimethoprim-sulfamethoxazole (TMP-SMX) may be of benefit in the treatment of Wegener's granulomatosis, there are no firm data to substantiate this, particularly in patients with serious renal and pulmonary disease. In a study examining the effect of TMP-SMX on relapse, decreased relapses were shown only with regard to upper airway disease, and no differences in major organ relapses were observed. TMP-SMX alone should never be used to treat active Wegener's granulomatosis outside of the upper airway.

ORGAN-SPECIFIC TREATMENT Not all manifestations of Wegener's granulomatosis require or respond to cytotoxic therapy. In managing non-major organ disease, such as that isolated to the sinus, joints, or skin, the risks of treatment should be carefully weighed against the benefits. Given the potential toxicities of this agent, treatment with cyclophosphamide is rarely if ever justified for the treatment of isolated sinus disease in Wegener's granulomatosis. Although patients with non-major organ disease may be effectively treated without cytotoxic therapy, these individuals must be monitored closely for the development of disease activity affecting the lungs, kidneys, or other major organs. Subglottic tracheal stenosis and endobronchial stenosis are examples of disease manifestations that do not typically respond to systemic immunosuppressive treatment.

CHURG-STRAUSS SYNDROME

Definition Churg-Strauss syndrome, also referred to as *allergic angiitis and granulomatosis*, was described in 1951 by Churg and Strauss and is characterized by asthma, peripheral and tissue eosinophilia, extravascular granuloma formation, and vasculitis of multiple organ systems.

Incidence and Prevalence Churg-Strauss syndrome is an uncommon disease with an estimated annual incidence of 1–3 per million. The disease can occur at any age with the possible exception of infants. The mean age of onset is 48 years, with a female-to-male ratio of 1.2:1.

Pathology and Pathogenesis The necrotizing vasculitis of Churg-Strauss syndrome involves small and medium-sized muscular arteries, capillaries, veins, and venules. A characteristic histopathologic feature of Churg-Strauss syndrome is granulomatous reactions that may be present in the tissues or even within the walls of the vessels themselves. These are usually associated with infiltration of the tissues with eosinophils. This process can occur in any organ in the body; lung involvement is predominant, with skin, cardiovascular system, kidney,

peripheral nervous system, and gastrointestinal tract also commonly involved. Although the precise pathogenesis of this disease is uncertain, its strong association with asthma and its clinicopathologic manifestations, including eosinophilia, granuloma, and vasculitis, point to aberrant immunologic phenomena.

Clinical and Laboratory Manifestations Patients with Churg-Strauss syndrome often exhibit nonspecific manifestations such as fever, malaise, anorexia, and weight loss, which are characteristic of a multisystem disease. The pulmonary findings in Churg-Strauss syndrome clearly dominate the clinical picture with severe asthmatic attacks and the presence of pulmonary infiltrates. Mononeuritis multiplex is the second most common manifestation and occurs in up to 72% of patients. Allergic rhinitis and sinusitis develop in up to 61% of patients and are often observed early in the course of disease. Clinically recognizable heart disease occurs in ~14% of patients and is an important cause of mortality. Skin lesions occur in ~51% of patients and include purpura in addition to cutaneous and subcutaneous nodules. The renal disease in Churg-Strauss syndrome is less common and generally less severe than that of Wegener's granulomatosis and microscopic polyangiitis.

The characteristic laboratory finding in virtually all patients with Churg-Strauss syndrome is a striking eosinophilia, which reaches levels >1000 cells/μL in >80% of patients. Evidence of inflammation as evidenced by elevated ESR, fibrinogen, or α_2-globulins can be found in 81% of patients. The other laboratory findings reflect the organ systems involved. Approximately 48% of patients with Churg-Strauss syndrome have circulating ANCA that is usually antimyeloperoxidase.

Diagnosis Although the diagnosis of Churg-Strauss syndrome is optimally made by biopsy in a patient with the characteristic clinical manifestations (see above), histologic confirmation can be challenging as the pathognomonic features often do not occur simultaneously. In order to be diagnosed with Churg-Strauss syndrome, a patient should have evidence of asthma, peripheral blood eosinophilia, and clinical features consistent with vasculitis.

℞ CHURG-STRAUSS SYNDROME

The prognosis of untreated Churg-Strauss syndrome is poor, with a reported 5-year survival of 25%. With treatment, prognosis is favorable, with one study finding a 78-month actuarial survival rate of 72%. Myocardial involvement is the most frequent cause of death and is responsible for 39% of patient mortality. Glucocorticoids alone appear to be effective in many patients. Dosage tapering is often limited by asthma, and many patients require low-dose prednisone for persistent asthma many years after clinical recovery from vasculitis. In glucocorticoid failure or in patients who present with fulminant multisystem disease, the treatment of choice is a combined regimen of daily cyclophosphamide and prednisone (see "Wegener's Granulomatosis" for a detailed description of this therapeutic regimen).

POLYARTERITIS NODOSA

Definition PAN, also referred to as *classic PAN*, was described in 1866 by Kussmaul and Maier. It is a multisystem, necrotizing vasculitis of small and medium-sized muscular arteries in which involvement of the renal and visceral arteries is characteristic. PAN does not involve pulmonary arteries, although bronchial vessels may be involved; granulomas, significant eosinophilia, and an allergic diathesis are not observed.

Incidence and Prevalence It is difficult to establish an accurate incidence of PAN because previous reports have included PAN and microscopic polyangiitis as well as other related vasculitides. PAN, as currently defined, is felt to be a very uncommon disease.

Pathology and Pathogenesis The vascular lesion in PAN is a necrotizing inflammation of small and medium-sized muscular arteries.

The lesions are segmental and tend to involve bifurcations and branchings of arteries. They may spread circumferentially to involve adjacent veins. However, involvement of venules is not seen in PAN and, if present, suggests microscopic polyangiitis (see below). In the acute stages of disease, polymorphonuclear neutrophils infiltrate all layers of the vessel wall and perivascular areas, which results in intimal proliferation and degeneration of the vessel wall. Mononuclear cells infiltrate the area as the lesions progress to the subacute and chronic stages. Fibrinoid necrosis of the vessels ensues with compromise of the lumen, thrombosis, infarction of the tissues supplied by the involved vessel, and, in some cases, hemorrhage. As the lesions heal, there is collagen deposition, which may lead to further occlusion of the vessel lumen. Aneurysmal dilatations up to 1 cm in size along the involved arteries are characteristic of PAN. Granulomas and substantial eosinophilia with eosinophilic tissue infiltrations are not characteristically found and suggest Churg-Strauss syndrome (see above).

Multiple organ systems are involved, and the clinicopathologic findings reflect the degree and location of vessel involvement and the resulting ischemic changes. As mentioned above, pulmonary arteries are not involved in PAN, and bronchial artery involvement is uncommon. The pathology in the kidney in classic PAN is that of arteritis without glomerulonephritis. In patients with significant hypertension, typical pathologic features of glomerulosclerosis may be seen. In addition, pathologic sequelae of hypertension may be found elsewhere in the body.

The presence of hepatitis B antigenemia in ~10–30% of patients with systemic vasculitis, particularly of the PAN type, together with the isolation of circulating immune complexes composed of hepatitis B antigen and immunoglobulin, and the demonstration by immunofluorescence of hepatitis B antigen, IgM, and complement in the blood vessel walls, strongly suggest the role of immunologic phenomena in the pathogenesis of this disease. Hairy cell leukemia can be associated with PAN; the pathogenic mechanisms of this association are unclear.

Clinical and Laboratory Manifestations Nonspecific signs and symptoms are the hallmarks of PAN. Fever, weight loss, and malaise are present in over one-half of cases. Patients usually present with vague symptoms such as weakness, malaise, headache, abdominal pain, and myalgias that can rapidly progress to a fulminant illness. Specific complaints related to the vascular involvement within a particular organ system may also dominate the presenting clinical picture as well as the entire course of the illness (Table 319-5). In PAN, renal involvement most commonly manifests as hypertension, renal insufficiency, or hemorrhage due to microaneurysms.

TABLE 319-5	**CLINICAL MANIFESTATIONS RELATED TO ORGAN SYSTEM INVOLVEMENT IN CLASSIC POLYARTERITIS NODOSA**

Organ System	Percent Incidence	Clinical Manifestations
Renal	60	Renal failure, hypertension
Musculoskeletal	64	Arthritis, arthralgia, myalgia
Peripheral nervous system	51	Peripheral neuropathy, mononeuritis multiplex
Gastrointestinal tract	44	Abdominal pain, nausea and vomiting, bleeding, bowel infarction and perforation, cholecystitis, hepatic infarction, pancreatic infarction
Skin	43	Rash, purpura, nodules, cutaneous infarcts, livedo reticularis, Raynaud's phenomenon
Cardiac	36	Congestive heart failure, myocardial infarction, pericarditis
Genitourinary	25	Testicular, ovarian, or epididymal pain
Central nervous system	23	Cerebral vascular accident, altered mental status, seizure

Source: From TR Cupps, AS Fauci: *The Vasculitides.* Philadelphia, Saunders, 1981.

There are no diagnostic serologic tests for PAN. In >75% of patients, the leukocyte count is elevated with a predominance of neutrophils. Eosinophilia is seen only rarely and, when present at high levels, suggests the diagnosis of Churg-Strauss syndrome. The anemia of chronic disease may be seen, and an elevated ESR is almost always present. Other common laboratory findings reflect the particular organ involved. Hypergammaglobulinemia may be present, and up to 30% of patients have a positive test for hepatitis B surface antigen. Antibodies against myeloperoxidase or proteinase-3 (ANCA) are rarely found in patients with PAN.

Diagnosis The diagnosis of PAN is based on the demonstration of characteristic findings of vasculitis on biopsy material of involved organs. In the absence of easily accessible tissue for biopsy, the angiographic demonstration of involved vessels, particularly in the form of aneurysms of small and medium-sized arteries in the renal, hepatic, and visceral vasculature, is sufficient to make the diagnosis. Aneurysms of vessels are not pathognomonic of PAN; furthermore, aneurysms need not always be present, and angiographic findings may be limited to stenotic segments and obliteration of vessels. Biopsy of symptomatic organs such as nodular skin lesions, painful testes, and nerve/muscle provides the highest diagnostic yields.

℞ POLYARTERITIS NODOSA

The prognosis of untreated PAN is extremely poor, with a reported 5-year survival rate between 10 and 20%. Death usually results from gastrointestinal complications, particularly bowel infarcts and perforation, and cardiovascular causes. Intractable hypertension often compounds dysfunction in other organ systems, such as the kidneys, heart, and CNS, leading to additional late morbidity and mortality in PAN. With the introduction of treatment, survival rate has increased substantially. Favorable therapeutic results have been reported in PAN with the combination of prednisone and cyclophosphamide (see "Wegener's Granulomatosis" for a detailed description of this therapeutic regimen). In less severe cases of PAN, glucocorticoids alone have resulted in disease remission. Favorable results have also been reported in the treatment of PAN related to hepatitis B virus with antiviral therapy in combination with glucocorticoids and plasma exchange. Careful attention to the treatment of hypertension can lessen the acute and late morbidity and mortality associated with renal, cardiac, and CNS complications of PAN. Following successful treatment, relapse of PAN has been estimated to occur in only 10% of patients.

MICROSCOPIC POLYANGIITIS

Definition The term *microscopic polyarteritis* was introduced into the literature by Davson in 1948 in recognition of the presence of glomerulonephritis in patients with PAN. In 1992, the Chapel Hill Consensus Conference on the Nomenclature of Systemic Vasculitis adopted the term *microscopic polyangiitis* to connote a necrotizing vasculitis with few or no immune complexes affecting small vessels (capillaries, venules, or arterioles). Glomerulonephritis is very common in microscopic polyangiitis, and pulmonary capillaritis often occurs. The absence of granulomatous inflammation in microscopic polyangiitis is said to differentiate it from Wegener's granulomatosis.

Incidence and Prevalence The incidence of microscopic polyangiitis has not yet been reliably established due to its previous inclusion as part of PAN. The mean age of onset is ~57 years of age, and males are slightly more frequently affected than females.

Pathology and Pathogenesis The vascular lesion in microscopic polyangiitis is histologically similar to that in PAN. Unlike PAN, the vasculitis seen in microscopic polyangiitis has a predilection to involve capillaries and venules in addition to small and medium-sized arteries. Immunohistochemical staining reveals a paucity of immunoglobulin deposition in the vascular lesion of microscopic polyangiitis, suggesting that immune complex formation does not play a role in the pathogenesis of this syndrome. The renal lesion seen in microscopic polyangiitis is identical to that of Wegener's granulomatosis. Like Wegener's granulomatosis, microscopic polyangiitis is highly associated with the presence of ANCA, which may play a role in pathogenesis of this syndrome (see above).

Clinical and Laboratory Manifestations   Because of its predilection to involve the small vessels, microscopic polyangiitis and Wegener's granulomatosis share similar clinical features. Disease onset may be gradual with initial symptoms of fever, weight loss, and musculoskeletal pain; however, it is often acute. Glomerulonephritis occurs in at least 79% of patients and can be rapidly progressive, leading to renal failure. Hemoptysis may be the first symptom of alveolar hemorrhage, which occurs in 12% of patients. Other manifestations include mononeuritis multiplex and gastrointestinal tract and cutaneous vasculitis. Upper airways disease and pulmonary nodules are not typically found in microscopic polyangiitis and, if present, suggest Wegener's granulomatosis.

Features of inflammation may be seen, including an elevated ESR, anemia, leukocytosis, and thrombocytosis. ANCA are present in 75% of patients with microscopic polyangiitis, with antimyeloperoxidase antibodies being the predominant ANCA associated with this disease.

Diagnosis   The diagnosis is based on histologic evidence of vasculitis or pauci-immune glomerulonephritis in a patient with compatible clinical features of multisystem disease. Although microscopic polyangiitis is strongly ANCA-associated, no studies have as yet established the sensitivity and specificity of ANCA in this disease.

℞ MICROSCOPIC POLYANGIITIS

The 5-year survival rate for patients with treated microscopic polyangiitis is 74%, with disease-related mortality occurring from alveolar hemorrhage or gastrointestinal, cardiac, or renal disease. To date there has been limited disease-specific information on the treatment of microscopic polyangiitis. Available data together with a predilection for this disease to affect the small vessels support a therapeutic approach similar to that used in Wegener's granulomatosis. Patients with immediately life-threatening disease should be treated with the combination of prednisone and daily cyclophosphamide (see "Wegener's Granulomatosis" for a detailed description of this therapeutic regimen). Disease relapse has been observed in at least 34% of patients. Treatment for such relapses would be similar to that used at the time of initial presentation and based upon site and severity of disease.

GIANT CELL ARTERITIS AND POLYMYALGIA RHEUMATICA

Definition   *Giant cell arteritis*, also referred to as *cranial arteritis* or *temporal arteritis*, is an inflammation of medium- and large-sized arteries. It characteristically involves one or more branches of the carotid artery, particularly the temporal artery. However, it is a systemic disease that can involve arteries in multiple locations, particularly the aorta and its main branches.

Giant cell arteritis is closely associated with *polymyalgia rheumatica*, which is characterized by stiffness, aching, and pain in the muscles of the neck, shoulders, lower back, hips, and thighs. Most commonly, polymyalgia rheumatica occurs in isolation, but it may be seen in 40–50% of patients with giant cell arteritis. In addition, ~10–20% of patients who initially present with features of isolated polymyalgia rheumatica later go on to develop giant cell arteritis. This strong clinical association together with data from pathophysiologic studies has increasingly supported that giant cell arteritis and polymyalgia rheumatica represent differing clinical spectrums of a single disease process.

Incidence and Prevalence   Giant cell arteritis occurs almost exclusively in individuals >50 years. It is more common in women than in men and is rare in blacks. The incidence of giant cell arteritis varies widely in different studies and in different geographic regions. A high incidence has been found in Scandinavia and in regions of the United States with large Scandinavian populations, compared to a lower inci-

dence in southern Europe. The annual incidence rates in individuals ≥50 years range from 6.9–32.8 per 100,000 population. Familial aggregation has been reported, as has an association with HLA-DR4. In addition, genetic linkage studies have demonstrated an association of giant cell arteritis with alleles at the HLA-DRB1 locus, particularly HLA-DRB1*04 variants. In Olmsted County, Minnesota, the annual incidence of polymyalgia rheumatica in individuals ≥50 years is 58.7 per 100,000 population.

Pathology and Pathogenesis   Although the temporal artery is most frequently involved in giant cell arteritis, patients often have a systemic vasculitis of multiple medium- and large-sized arteries, which may go undetected. Histopathologically, the disease is a panarteritis with inflammatory mononuclear cell infiltrates within the vessel wall with frequent giant cell formation. There is proliferation of the intima and fragmentation of the internal elastic lamina. Pathophysiologic findings in organs result from the ischemia related to the involved vessels.

Experimental data support that giant cell arteritis is an antigen-driven disease in which activated T lymphocytes, macrophages, and dendritic cells play a critical role in the disease pathogenesis. Sequence analysis of the T cell receptor of tissue-infiltrating T cells in lesions of giant cell arteritis indicates restricted clonal expansion, suggesting the presence of an antigen residing in the arterial wall. Giant cell arteritis is believed to be initiated in the adventitia where CD4+ T cells become activated and orchestrate macrophage differentiation. T cells recruited to vasculitic lesions in patients with giant cell arteritis produce predominantly IL-2 and IFN-γ, and the latter has been suggested to be involved in the progression to overt arteritis.

Clinical and Laboratory Manifestations   Giant cell arteritis is characterized clinically by the complex of fever, anemia, high ESR, and headaches in a patient over the age of 50 years. Other manifestations include malaise, fatigue, anorexia, weight loss, sweats, arthralgias, and associated polymyalgia rheumatica.

In patients with involvement of the temporal artery, headache is the predominant symptom and may be associated with a tender, thickened, or nodular artery, which may pulsate early in the disease but may become occluded later. Scalp pain and claudication of the jaw and tongue may occur. A well-recognized and dreaded complication of giant cell arteritis, particularly in untreated patients, is ischemic optic neuropathy, which may lead to serious visual symptoms, even sudden blindness in some patients. However, most patients have complaints relating to the head or eyes before visual loss. Attention to such symptoms with institution of appropriate therapy (see below) will usually avoid this complication. Claudication of the extremities, strokes, myocardial infarctions, and infarctions of visceral organs have been reported. Of note, giant cell arteritis is associated with an increased risk of aortic aneurysm, which is usually a late complication and may lead to dissection and death.

Characteristic laboratory findings in addition to the elevated ESR include a normochromic or slightly hypochromic anemia. Liver function abnormalities are common, particularly increased alkaline phosphatase levels. Increased levels of IgG and complement have been reported. Levels of enzymes indicative of muscle damage such as serum creatine kinase are not elevated.

Diagnosis   The diagnosis of giant cell arteritis and its associated clinicopathologic syndrome can often be suggested clinically by the demonstration of the complex of fever, anemia, and high ESR with or without symptoms of polymyalgia rheumatica in a patient >50 years. The diagnosis is confirmed by biopsy of the temporal artery. Since involvement of the vessel may be segmental, positive yield is increased by obtaining a biopsy segment of 3–5 cm together with serial sectioning of biopsy specimens. Ultrasonography of the temporal artery has been reported to be helpful in diagnosis. A temporal artery biopsy should be obtained as quickly as possible in the setting of ocular signs and symptoms, and under these circumstances therapy should not be delayed pending a biopsy. In this regard, it has been reported that temporal artery biopsies may show vasculitis even after ~14 days of glucocorticoid therapy. A dramatic clinical response to a trial of glucocorticoid therapy can further support the diagnosis.

Isolated polymyalgia rheumatica is a clinical diagnosis made by the presence of typical symptoms of stiffness, aching, and pain in the muscles of the hip and shoulder girdle, an increased ESR, the absence of clinical features suggestive of giant cell arteritis, and a prompt therapeutic response to low dose prednisone.

℞ GIANT CELL ARTERITIS AND POLYMYALGIA RHEUMATICA

Disease-related mortality from giant cell arteritis is very uncommon with fatalities occurring from cerebrovascular events, myocardial infarction, or aortic aneurysm rupture.

The goals of treatment in giant cell arteritis are to reduce symptoms and, most importantly, to prevent visual loss. Giant cell arteritis and its associated symptoms are exquisitely sensitive to glucocorticoid therapy. Treatment should begin with prednisone, 40–60 mg/d for ~1 month, followed by a gradual tapering. When ocular signs and symptoms occur, it is important that therapy be initiated or adjusted to control them. Although the optimal duration of glucocorticoid therapy has not been established, most series have found that patients require treatment for ≥2 years. Symptom recurrence during prednisone tapering develops in 60–85% of patients with giant cell arteritis, requiring a dosage increase. The ESR can serve as a useful indicator of inflammatory disease activity in monitoring and tapering therapy and can be used to judge the pace of the tapering schedule. However, minor increases in the ESR can occur as glucocorticoids are being tapered and do not necessarily reflect an exacerbation of arteritis, particularly if the patient remains symptom-free. Under these circumstances, the tapering should continue with caution. Glucocorticoid toxicity occurs in 35–65% of patients and represents an important cause of patient morbidity. Aspirin has been found to reduce the occurrence of cranial ischemic complications in giant cell arteritis and should be given in addition to glucocorticoids in patients who do not have contraindications. The use of weekly methotrexate as a glucocorticoid-sparing agent has been examined in two randomized placebo-controlled trials that reached conflicting conclusions.

Patients with isolated polymyalgia rheumatica respond promptly to prednisone, which can be started at a lower dose of 10–20 mg/d. Similar to giant cell arteritis, the ESR can serve as a useful indicator in monitoring and prednisone reduction. Recurrent polymyalgia symptoms develop in the majority of patients during prednisone tapering. One study of weekly methotrexate found that the use of this drug reduced the prednisone dose on average by only 1 mg and did not decrease prednisone-related side effects.

TAKAYASU'S ARTERITIS

Definition *Takayasu's arteritis* is an inflammatory and stenotic disease of medium- and large-sized arteries characterized by a strong predilection for the aortic arch and its branches. For this reason, it is often referred to as the *aortic arch syndrome*.

Incidence and Prevalence Takayasu's arteritis is an uncommon disease with an estimated annual incidence rate of 1.2–2.6 cases per million. It is most prevalent in adolescent girls and young women. Although it is more common in Asia, it is neither racially nor geographically restricted.

Pathology and Pathogenesis The disease involves medium- and large-sized arteries, with a strong predilection for the aortic arch and its branches; the pulmonary artery may also be involved. The most commonly affected arteries seen by angiography are listed in Table 319-6. The involvement of the major branches of the aorta is much more marked at their origin than distally. The disease is a panarteritis with inflammatory mononuclear cell infiltrates and occasionally giant cells. There are marked intimal proliferation and fibrosis, scarring and vascularization of the media, and disruption and degeneration of the elastic lamina. Narrowing of the lumen occurs with or without thrombosis. The vasa vasorum are frequently involved. Pathologic changes in

| | **TABLE 319-6** | **FREQUENCY OF ARTERIOGRAPHIC ABNORMALITIES AND POTENTIAL CLINICAL MANIFESTATIONS OF ARTERIAL INVOLVEMENT IN TAKAYASU'S ARTERITIS** |

Artery	Percent of Arteriographic Abnormalities	Potential Clinical Manifestations
Subclavian	93	Arm claudication, Raynaud's phenomenon
Common carotid	58	Visual changes, syncope, transient ischemic attacks, stroke
Abdominal aorta[a]	47	Abdominal pain, nausea, vomiting
Renal	38	Hypertension, renal failure
Aortic arch or root	35	Aortic insufficiency, congestive heart failure
Vertebral	35	Visual changes, dizziness
Coeliac axis[a]	18	Abdominal pain, nausea, vomiting
Superior mesenteric[a]	18	Abdominal pain, nausea, vomiting
Iliac	17	Leg claudication
Pulmonary	10–40	Atypical chest pain, dyspnea
Coronary	<10	Chest pain, myocardial infarction

[a]Arteriographic lesions at these locations are usually asymptomatic but may potentially cause these symptoms.
Source: Kerr et al.

various organs reflect the compromise of blood flow through the involved vessels.

Immunopathogenic mechanisms, the precise nature of which is uncertain, are suspected in this disease. As with several of the vasculitis syndromes, circulating immune complexes have been demonstrated, but their pathogenic significance is unclear.

Clinical and Laboratory Manifestations Takayasu's arteritis is a systemic disease with generalized as well as vascular symptoms. The generalized symptoms include malaise, fever, night sweats, arthralgias, anorexia, and weight loss, which may occur months before vessel involvement is apparent. These symptoms may merge into those related to vascular compromise and organ ischemia. Pulses are commonly absent in the involved vessels, particularly the subclavian artery. The frequency of arteriographic abnormalities and the potentially associated clinical manifestations are listed in Table 319-6. Hypertension occurs in 32 to 93% of patients and contributes to renal, cardiac, and cerebral injury.

Characteristic laboratory findings include an elevated ESR, mild anemia, and elevated immunoglobulin levels.

Diagnosis The diagnosis of Takayasu's arteritis should be suspected strongly in a young woman who develops a decrease or absence of peripheral pulses, discrepancies in blood pressure, and arterial bruits. The diagnosis is confirmed by the characteristic pattern on arteriography, which includes irregular vessel walls, stenosis, poststenotic dilatation, aneurysm formation, occlusion, and evidence of increased collateral circulation. Complete aortic arteriography by catheter-directed dye arteriography or magnetic resonance arteriography should be obtained, in order to fully delineate the distribution and degree of arterial disease. Histopathologic demonstration of inflamed vessels adds confirmatory data; however, tissue is rarely readily available for examination.

℞ TAKAYASU'S ARTERITIS

The long-term outcome of patients with Takayasu's arteritis has varied widely between studies. Although two North American reports found overall survival to be ≥94%, the 5-year mortality rate from other studies has ranged from 0–35%. Disease-related mortality most often occurs from congestive heart failure, cerebrovascular events, myocardial infarction, aneurysm rupture, or renal failure. Even in the absence of life-threatening disease Takayasu's arteritis can be associated with significant morbidity. The course of the disease is variable, and although spontaneous remissions may occur, Takayasu's arteritis is most often chronic and relapsing. Although glucocorticoid therapy in doses of 40–60 mg prednisone per day alleviates symptoms, there are no convincing studies that indicate that they increase survival. The combination of glucocorticoid therapy for acute signs and symptoms and an aggressive surgical and/or angioplastic approach to stenosed vessels has markedly improved outcome and decreased morbidity by lessening the risk of stroke, correcting hypertension due to renal artery stenosis, and improving blood flow to ischemic viscera and limbs. Unless it is urgently required, surgical correction of stenosed arteries should be undertaken only when the vascular inflammatory process is well controlled with medical therapy. In individuals who are refractory to or unable to taper glucocorticoids, methotrexate in doses up to 25 mg per week has yielded encouraging results.

HENOCH-SCHÖNLEIN PURPURA

Definition   *Henoch-Schönlein purpura*, also referred to as *anaphylactoid purpura*, is a distinct systemic vasculitis syndrome that is characterized by palpable purpura (most commonly distributed over the buttocks and lower extremities), arthralgias, gastrointestinal signs and symptoms, and glomerulonephritis. It is a small-vessel vasculitis.

Incidence and Prevalence   Henoch-Schönlein purpura is usually seen in children; most patients range in age from 4–7 years; however, the disease may also be seen in infants and adults. It is not a rare disease; in one series it accounted for between 5 and 24 admissions per year at a pediatric hospital. The male-to-female ratio is 1.5:1. A seasonal variation with a peak incidence in spring has been noted.

Pathology and Pathogenesis   The presumptive pathogenic mechanism for Henoch-Schönlein purpura is immune-complex deposition. A number of inciting antigens have been suggested including upper respiratory tract infections, various drugs, foods, insect bites, and immunizations. IgA is the antibody class most often seen in the immune complexes and has been demonstrated in the renal biopsies of these patients.

Clinical and Laboratory Manifestations   In pediatric patients, palpable purpura is seen in virtually all patients; most patients develop polyarthralgias in the absence of frank arthritis. Gastrointestinal involvement, which is seen in almost 70% of pediatric patients, is characterized by colicky abdominal pain usually associated with nausea, vomiting, diarrhea, or constipation and is frequently accompanied by the passage of blood and mucus per rectum; bowel intussusception may occur. Renal involvement occurs in 10–50% of patients and is usually characterized by mild glomerulonephritis leading to proteinuria and microscopic hematuria, with red blood cell casts in the majority of patients (Chap. 277); it usually resolves spontaneously without therapy. Rarely, a progressive glomerulonephritis will develop. In adults, presenting symptoms are most frequently related to the skin and joints, while initial complaints related to the gut are less common. Although certain studies have found that renal disease is more frequent and more severe in adults, this has not been a consistent finding. However, the course of renal disease in adults may be more insidious and thus requires close follow-up. Myocardial involvement can occur in adults but is rare in children.

Laboratory studies generally show a mild leukocytosis, a normal platelet count, and occasionally eosinophilia. Serum complement components are normal, and IgA levels are elevated in about one-half of patients.

Diagnosis   The diagnosis of Henoch-Schönlein purpura is based on clinical signs and symptoms. Skin biopsy specimen can be useful in confirming leukocytoclastic vasculitis with IgA and C3 deposition by immunofluorescence. Renal biopsy is rarely needed for diagnosis but may provide prognostic information in some patients.

℞ HENOCH-SCHÖNLEIN PURPURA

The prognosis of Henoch-Schönlein purpura is excellent. Mortality is exceedingly rare, and 1–5% of children progress to end-stage renal disease. Most patients recover completely, and some do not require therapy. Treatment is similar for adults and children. When glucocorticoid therapy is required, prednisone, in doses of 1 mg/kg per day and tapered according to clinical response, has been shown to be useful in decreasing tissue edema, arthralgias, and abdominal discomfort; however, it has not proven beneficial in the treatment of skin or renal disease and does not appear to shorten the duration of active disease or lessen the chance of recurrence. Patients with rapidly progressive glomerulonephritis have been anecdotally reported to benefit from intensive plasma exchange combined with cytotoxic drugs. Disease recurrences have been reported in 10–40% of patients.

IDIOPATHIC CUTANEOUS VASCULITIS

Definition   The term *cutaneous vasculitis* is defined broadly as inflammation of the blood vessels of the dermis. Due to its heterogeneity, cutaneous vasculitis has been described by a variety of terms including *hypersensitivity vasculitis* and *cutaneous leukocytoclastic angiitis*. However, cutaneous vasculitis is not one specific disease but a manifestation that can be seen in a variety of settings. In >70% of cases, cutaneous vasculitis occurs either as part of a primary systemic vasculitis or as a secondary vasculitis related to an inciting agent or an underlying disease (see "Secondary Vasculitis," below). In the remaining 30% of cases, cutaneous vasculitis occurs idiopathically.

Incidence and Prevalence   Cutaneous vasculitis represents the most commonly encountered vasculitis in clinical practice. The exact incidence of idiopathic cutaneous vasculitis has not been determined due to the predilection for cutaneous vasculitis to be associated with an underlying process and the variability of its clinical course.

Pathology and Pathogenesis   The typical histopathologic feature of cutaneous vasculitis is the presence of vasculitis of small vessels. Postcapillary venules are the most commonly involved vessels; capillaries and arterioles may be involved less frequently. This vasculitis is characterized by a *leukocytoclasis*, a term that refers to the nuclear debris remaining from the neutrophils that have infiltrated in and around the vessels during the acute stages. In the subacute or chronic stages, mononuclear cells predominate; in certain subgroups, eosinophilic infiltration is seen. Erythrocytes often extravasate from the involved vessels, leading to palpable purpura.

Clinical and Laboratory Manifestations   The hallmark of idiopathic cutaneous vasculitis is the predominance of skin involvement. Skin lesions may appear typically as palpable purpura; however, other cutaneous manifestations of the vasculitis may occur, including macules, papules, vesicles, bullae, subcutaneous nodules, ulcers, and recurrent or chronic urticaria. The skin lesions may be pruritic or even quite painful, with a burning or stinging sensation. Lesions most commonly occur in the lower extremities in ambulatory patients or in the sacral area in bedridden patients due to the effects of hydrostatic forces on the postcapillary venules. Edema may accompany certain lesions, and hyperpigmentation often occurs in areas of recurrent or chronic lesions.

There are no specific laboratory tests diagnostic of idiopathic cutaneous vasculitis. A mild leukocytosis with or without eosinophilia is characteristic, as is an elevated ESR. Laboratory studies should be aimed towards ruling out features to suggest an underlying disease or a systemic vasculitis.

Diagnosis   The diagnosis of cutaneous vasculitis is made by the demonstration of vasculitis on biopsy. An important diagnostic principle in patients with cutaneous vasculitis is to search for an etiology of the vasculitis—be it an exogenous agent, such as a drug or an infection, or an endogenous condition, such as an underlying disease (Fig. 319-1).

In addition, a careful physical and laboratory examination should be performed to rule out the possibility of systemic vasculitis. This should start with the least invasive diagnostic approach and proceed to the more invasive only if clinically indicated.

Rx IDIOPATHIC CUTANEOUS VASCULITIS

When an antigenic stimulus is recognized as the precipitating factor in the cutaneous vasculitis, it should be removed; if this is a microbe, appropriate antimicrobial therapy should be instituted. If the vasculitis is associated with another underlying disease, treatment of the latter often results in resolution of the former. In situations where disease is apparently self-limited, no therapy, except possibly symptomatic therapy, is indicated. When cutaneous vasculitis persists and when there is no evidence of an inciting agent, an associated disease, or an underlying systemic vasculitis, the decision to treat should be based on weighing the balance between the degree of symptoms and the risk of treatment. Some cases of idiopathic cutaneous vasculitis resolve spontaneously, while others remit and relapse. In those patients with persistent vasculitis, a variety of therapeutic regimens have been tried with variable results. In general, the treatment of idiopathic cutaneous vasculitis has not been satisfactory. Fortunately, since the disease is generally limited to the skin, this lack of consistent response to therapy usually does not lead to a life-threatening situation. Glucocorticoids are often used in the treatment of idiopathic cutaneous vasculitis. Therapy is usually instituted as prednisone, 1 mg/kg per day, with rapid tapering where possible, either directly to discontinuation or by conversion to an alternate-day regimen followed by ultimate discontinuation. In cases that prove refractory to glucocorticoids, a trial of a cytotoxic agent may be indicated. Patients with chronic vasculitis isolated to cutaneous venules rarely respond dramatically to any therapeutic regimen, and cytotoxic agents should be used only as a last resort in these patients. Methotrexate and azathioprine have been used in such situations in anecdotal reports. Although cyclophosphamide is the most effective therapy for the systemic vasculitides, it should almost never be used for idiopathic cutaneous vasculitis because of the potential toxicity. Other agents with which there have been anecdotal reports of success include dapsone, colchicine, and nonsteroidal anti-inflammatory agents.

ESSENTIAL MIXED CRYOGLOBULINEMIA

Definition Cryoglobulins are cold-precipitable monoclonal or polyclonal immunoglobulins. Cryoglobulinemia may be associated with a systemic vasculitis characterized by palpable purpura, arthralgias, weakness, neuropathy, and glomerulonephritis. Although this can be observed in association with a variety of underlying disorders including multiple myeloma, lymphoproliferative disorders, connective tissue diseases, infection, and liver disease, in many instances it appeared to be idiopathic. Because of the apparent absence of an underlying disease and the presence of cryoprecipitate containing oligoclonal/polyclonal immunoglobulins, this entity was referred to as *essential mixed cryoglobulinemia*. Since the discovery of hepatitis C, it has been established that in the vast majority of patients, essential mixed cryoglobulinemia is related to an aberrant immune response to chronic hepatitis C infection.

Incidence and Prevalence The incidence of essential mixed cryoglobulinemia has not been established. It has been estimated, however, that 5% of patients with chronic hepatitis C will develop the syndrome of essential mixed cryoglobulinemia.

Pathology and Pathogenesis Skin biopsies in essential mixed cryoglobulinemia reveal an inflammatory infiltrate surrounding and involving blood vessel walls, with fibrinoid necrosis, endothelial cell hyperplasia, and hemorrhage. Deposition of immunoglobulin and complement is common. Abnormalities of uninvolved skin including basement membrane alterations and deposits in vessel walls may be found. Membranoproliferative glomerulonephritis is responsible for 80% of all renal lesions in essential mixed cryoglobulinemia.

The association between hepatitis C and essential mixed cryoglobulinemia has been supported by the high frequency of documented

hepatitis C infection, the presence of hepatitis C RNA and anti–hepatitis C antibodies in serum cryoprecipitates, evidence of hepatitis C antigens in vasculitic skin lesions, and the effectiveness of antiviral therapy (see below). Current evidence suggest that in the majority of cases, essential mixed cryoglobulinemia occurs when an aberrant immune response to hepatitis C infection leads to the formation of immune complexes consisting of hepatitis C antigens, polyclonal hepatitis C–specific IgG, and monoclonal IgM rheumatoid factor. The deposition of these immune complexes in blood vessel walls triggers an inflammatory cascade that results in the clinical syndrome of essential mixed cryoglobulinemia.

Clinical and Laboratory Manifestations The most common clinical manifestations of essential mixed cryoglobulinemia are cutaneous vasculitis, arthritis, peripheral neuropathy, and glomerulonephritis. Renal disease develops in 10–30% of patients. Life-threatening rapidly progressive glomerulonephritis or vasculitis of the CNS, gastrointestinal tract, or heart occurs infrequently.

The presence of circulating cryoprecipitates is the fundamental finding in essential mixed cryoglobulinemia. Rheumatoid factor is almost always found and may be a useful clue to the disease when cryoglobulins are not detected. Hypocomplementemia occurs in 90% of patients. An elevated ESR and anemia occur frequently. Evidence for hepatitis C infection must be sought in all patients by testing for hepatitis C antibodies and hepatitis C RNA.

Rx ESSENTIAL MIXED CRYOGLOBULINEMIA

Acute mortality from essential mixed cryoglobulinemia is uncommon, but the presence of glomerulonephritis is a poor prognostic sign for overall outcome. In such patients, 15% progress to end-stage renal disease, with 40% later experiencing fatal cardiovascular disease, infection, or liver failure. As indicated above, the majority of cases are associated with hepatitis C infection. In such patients, treatment with IFN-α and ribavirin (Chap. 298) can prove beneficial. Clinical improvement with antiviral therapy is dependent on the virologic response. Patients who clear hepatitis C from the blood have objective improvement in their vasculitis along with significant reductions in levels of circulating cryoglobulins, IgM, and rheumatoid factor. However, substantial portions of patients with hepatitis C do not have a sustained virologic response to such therapy, and the vasculitis typically relapses with the return of viremia. While transient improvement can be observed with glucocorticoids, a complete response is seen in only 7% of patients. Plasmapheresis and cytotoxic agents have been used in anecdotal reports. These observations have not been confirmed, and such therapies carry significant risks.

BEHÇET'S SYNDROME

Behçet's syndrome is a clinicopathologic entity characterized by recurrent episodes of oral and genital ulcers, iritis, and cutaneous lesions. The underlying pathologic process is a leukocytoclastic venulitis, although vessels of any size and in any organ can be involved. This disorder is described in detail in Chap. 320.

ISOLATED VASCULITIS OF THE CENTRAL NERVOUS SYSTEM

Isolated vasculitis of the CNS which is also called *primary angiitis of the CNS* (PACNS) is an uncommon clinicopathologic entity characterized by vasculitis restricted to the vessels of the CNS without other apparent systemic vasculitis. Although the arteriole is most commonly affected, vessels of any size can be involved. The inflammatory process is usually composed of mononuclear cell infiltrates with or without granuloma formation.

Patients may present with severe headaches, altered mental function, and focal neurologic defects. Systemic symptoms are generally absent. Devastating neurologic abnormalities may occur depending on the extent of vessel involvement. The diagnosis can be suggested by abnormal MRI of the brain, an abnormal lumbar puncture, and/or

FIGURE 319-4 Cerebral angiogram from a 32-year-old male with central nervous system vasculitis. Dramatic beading (*arrow*) typical of vasculitis is seen.

demonstration of characteristic vessel abnormalities on arteriography (Fig. 319-4) but it is confirmed by biopsy of the brain parenchyma and leptomeninges. In the absence of a brain biopsy, care should be taken not to misinterpret as true primary vasculitis angiographic abnormalities that might actually be related to another cause. The differential diagnosis includes infection, atherosclerosis, emboli, connective tissue disease, sarcoidosis, malignancy, vasospasm, and drug-associated causes. The prognosis of this disease is poor; however, some reports indicate that glucocorticoid therapy, alone or together with cyclophosphamide administered as described above, has induced sustained clinical remissions in a small number of patients.

COGAN'S SYNDROME

Cogan's syndrome is characterized by interstitial keratitis together with vestibuloauditory symptoms. It may be associated with a systemic vasculitis, particularly aortitis with involvement of the aortic valve. Glucocorticoids are the mainstay of treatment. Initiation of treatment as early as possible after the onset of hearing loss improves the likelihood of a favorable outcome.

KAWASAKI DISEASE

Kawasaki disease, also referred to as *mucocutaneous lymph node syndrome,* is an acute, febrile, multisystem disease of children. Some 80% of cases occur prior to the age of 5, with the peak incidence occurring at ≤2 years. It is characterized by nonsuppurative cervical adenitis and changes in the skin and mucous membranes such as edema; congested conjunctivae; erythema of the oral cavity, lips, and palms; and desquamation of the skin of the fingertips. Although the disease is generally benign and self-limited, it is associated with coronary artery aneurysms in ~25% of cases, with an overall case-fatality rate of 0.5–2.8%. These complications usually occur between the third and fourth weeks of illness during the convalescent stage. Vasculitis of the coronary arteries is seen in almost all the fatal cases that have been autopsied. There is typical intimal proliferation and infiltration of the vessel wall with mononuclear cells. Beadlike aneurysms and thromboses may be seen along the artery. Other manifestations include pericarditis, myocarditis, myocardial ischemia and infarction, and cardiomegaly.

Apart from the up to 2.8% of patients who develop fatal complications, the prognosis of this disease for uneventful recovery is excellent. High-dose IV γ globulin (2 g/kg as a single infusion over 10 h) together with aspirin (100 mg/kg per day for 14 days followed by 3–5 mg/kg per day for several weeks) have been shown to be effective in reducing the prevalence of coronary artery abnormalities when administered early in the course of the disease.

POLYANGIITIS OVERLAP SYNDROMES

Some patients with systemic vasculitis manifest clinicopathologic characteristics that do not fit precisely into any specific disease but have overlapping features of different vasculitides. Active systemic vasculitis in such settings has the same potential for causing irreversible organ system damage as when it occurs in one of the defined syndromes listed in Table 319-1. The diagnostic and therapeutic considerations as well as the prognosis for these patients depend on the sites and severity of active vasculitis. Patients with vasculitis that could potentially cause irreversible damage to a major organ system should be treated as described under "Wegener's granulomatosis."

SECONDARY VASCULITIS

DRUG-INDUCED VASCULITIS

Vasculitis associated with drug reactions usually presents as palpable purpura that may be generalized or limited to the lower extremities or other dependent areas; however, urticarial lesions, ulcers, and hemorrhagic blisters may also occur (Chap. 56). Signs and symptoms may be limited to the skin, although systemic manifestations such as fever, malaise, and polyarthralgias may occur. Although the skin is the predominant organ involved, systemic vasculitis may result from drug reactions. Drugs that have been implicated in vasculitis include allopurinol, thiazides, gold, sulfonamides, phenytoin, and penicillin (Chap. 56).

An increasing number of drugs have been reported to cause vasculitis associated with antimyeloperoxidase ANCA. Of these, the best evidence of causality exists for hydralazine and propylthiouracil. The clinical manifestations in ANCA-positive drug-induced vasculitis can range from cutaneous lesions to glomerulonephritis and pulmonary hemorrhage. Outside of drug discontinuation, treatment should be based on the severity of the vasculitis. Patients with immediately life-threatening small-vessel vasculitis should initially be treated with glucocorticoids and cyclophosphamide as described for Wegener's granulomatosis. Following clinical improvement, consideration may be given for tapering such agents along a more rapid schedule.

SERUM SICKNESS AND SERUM SICKNESS–LIKE REACTIONS

These reactions are characterized by the occurrence of fever, urticaria, polyarthralgias, and lymphadenopathy 7–10 days after primary exposure and 2–4 days after secondary exposure to a heterologous protein (classic serum sickness) or a nonprotein drug such as penicillin or sulfa (serum sickness–like reaction). Most of the manifestations are not due to a vasculitis; however, occasional patients will have typical cutaneous venulitis that may progress rarely to a systemic vasculitis.

VASCULITIS ASSOCIATED WITH OTHER UNDERLYING PRIMARY DISEASES

Certain *infections* may directly trigger an inflammatory vasculitic process. For example, rickettsias can invade and proliferate in the endothelial cells of small blood vessels causing a vasculitis (Chap. 167). In addition, the inflammatory response around blood vessels associated with certain systemic fungal diseases such as histoplasmosis (Chap. 192) may mimic a primary vasculitic process. A leukocytoclastic vasculitis predominantly involving the skin with occasional involvement of other organ systems may be a minor component of many other infections. These include *subacute bacterial endocarditis, Epstein-Barr virus infection, HIV infection,* as well as a number of other infections.

Vasculitis can be associated with certain *malignancies,* particularly lymphoid or reticuloendothelial neoplasms. Leukocytoclastic venulitis confined to the skin is the most common finding; however, widespread systemic vasculitis may occur. Of particular note is the association of *hairy cell leukemia* (Chap. 105) with PAN.

| TABLE 319-7 | MAJOR TOXIC SIDE EFFECTS OF DRUGS COMMONLY USED IN THE TREATMENT OF SYSTEMIC VASCULITIS |

Glucocorticoids

Osteoporosis	Growth suppression in children
Cataracts	Hypertension
Glaucoma	Avascular necrosis of bone
Diabetes mellitus	Myopathy
Electrolyte abnormalities	Alterations in mood
Metabolic abnormalities	Psychosis
Suppression of inflammatory and	Pseudotumor cerebri
immune responses leading to	Peptic ulcer diathesis
opportunistic infections	Pancreatitis
Cushingoid features	

Cyclophosphamide

Bone marrow suppression	Hypogammaglobulinemia
Cystitis	Pulmonary fibrosis
Bladder carcinoma	Myelodysplasia
Gonadal suppression	Oncogenesis
Gastrointestinal intolerance	Teratogenicity
	Opportunistic infections

Methotrexate

Gastrointestinal intolerance	Pneumonitis
Stomatitis	Teratogenicity
Bone marrow suppression	Opportunistic infections
Hepatotoxicity (may lead to fibrosis or cirrhosis)	

A number of *connective tissue diseases* have vasculitis as a secondary manifestation of the underlying primary process. Foremost among these are *systemic lupus erythematosus* (Chap. 313), *rheumatoid arthritis* (Chap. 314), *inflammatory myositis* (Chap. 383), *relapsing polychondritis* (Chap. 321), and *Sjögren's syndrome* (Chap. 317). The most common form of vasculitis in these conditions is the small-vessel venulitis isolated to the skin. However, certain patients may develop a fulminant systemic necrotizing vasculitis.

Secondary vasculitis has also been observed in association with *ulcerative colitis, congenital deficiencies of various complement components, retroperitoneal fibrosis, primary biliary cirrhosis, α_1-antitrypsin deficiency,* and *intestinal bypass surgery.*

PRINCIPLES OF TREATMENT

Once a diagnosis of vasculitis has been established, a decision regarding therapeutic strategy must be made (Fig. 319-1). The vasculitis syndromes represent a wide spectrum of diseases with varying degrees of severity. Since the potential toxic side effects of certain therapeutic regimens may be substantial, the risk-versus-benefit ratio of any therapeutic approach should be weighed carefully. Specific therapeutic regimens are discussed above for the individual vasculitis syndromes; however, certain general principles regarding therapy should be considered. On the one hand, glucocorticoids and/or cytotoxic therapy should be instituted immediately in diseases where irreversible organ system dysfunction and high morbidity and mortality have been clearly established. Wegener's granulomatosis is the prototype of a severe systemic vasculitis requiring such a therapeutic approach (see above). On the other hand, when feasible, aggressive therapy should be avoided for vasculitic manifestations that rarely result in irreversible organ system dysfunction and that usually do not respond to such therapy. For example, idiopathic cutaneous vasculitis usually resolves with symptomatic treatment, and prolonged courses of glucocorticoids uncommonly result in clinical benefit. Cytotoxic agents have not proved to be beneficial in idiopathic cutaneous vasculitis, and their toxic side effects generally outweigh any potential beneficial effects. Glucocorticoids should be initiated in those systemic vasculitides that cannot be specifically categorized or for which there is no established standard therapy; cytotoxic therapy should be added in these diseases only if an adequate response does not result or if remission can only be achieved

and maintained with an unacceptably toxic regimen of glucocorticoids. When remission is achieved, one should continually attempt to taper glucocorticoids to an alternate-day regimen and discontinue when possible. When using cytotoxic regimens, one should base the choice of agent upon the available therapeutic data supporting efficacy in that disease, the site and severity of organ involvement, and the toxicity profile of the drug.

Physicians should be thoroughly aware of the toxic side effects of therapeutic agents employed (Table 319-7). Many of the side effects of glucocorticoid therapy are markedly decreased in frequency and duration in patients on alternate-day regimens compared to daily regimens. When cyclophosphamide is administered chronically in doses of 2 mg/kg per day for substantial periods of time (one to several years), the incidence of cystitis is at least 30% and the incidence of bladder cancer is at least 6%. Bladder cancer can occur several years after discontinuation of cyclophosphamide therapy; therefore, monitoring for bladder cancer should continue indefinitely in patients who have received prolonged courses of daily cyclophosphamide. Instructing the patient to take cyclophosphamide all at once in the morning with a large amount of fluid throughout the day in order to maintain a dilute urine can reduce the risk of bladder injury. Significant alopecia is unusual in the chronically administered, low-dose regimen. Permanent infertility can occur in both men and women. Bone marrow suppression is an important toxicity of cyclophosphamide and can be observed during glucocorticoid tapering or over time, even after periods of stable measurements. Monitoring of the complete blood count every 1–2 weeks for as long as the patient receives cyclophosphamide can effectively prevent cytopenias. When the white blood count (WBC) is maintained at >3000/μL, and the patient is not receiving daily glucocorticoids, the incidence of life-threatening opportunistic infections is low. However, the WBC is not an accurate predictor of risk of all opportunistic infections; and infections with *Pneumocystis jiroveci* and certain fungi can be seen in the face of WBCs that are within normal limits, particularly in patients receiving glucocorticoids. All vasculitis patients who are not allergic to sulfa and who are receiving daily glucocorticoids in combination with a cytotoxic drug should receive TMP-SMX as prophylaxis against *P. jiroveci* infection.

Finally, it should be emphasized that each patient is unique and requires individual decision-making. The above outline should serve as a framework to guide therapeutic approaches; however, flexibility should be practiced in order to provide maximal therapeutic efficacy with minimal toxic side effects in each patient.

FURTHER READINGS

GUILLEVIN L et al: Microscopic polyangiitis. Clinical and laboratory findings in eighty-five patients. Arthritis Rheum 42:421, 1999

HOFFMAN GS, SPECKS U: Antineutrophil cytoplasmic antibodies. Arthritis Rheum 41:1521, 1998

—— et al: Wegener's granulomatosis: An analysis of 158 patients. Ann Intern Med 116:488, 1992

JENNETTE JC et al: Nomenclature of systemic vasculitis. Proposal of an international consensus conference. Arthritis Rheum 37:187, 1994

KERR G et al: Takayasu arteritis. Ann Intern Med 120:919, 1994

LANGFORD CA et al: Use of cytotoxic agents and cyclosporine in the treatment of autoimmune disease. Part 2: Inflammatory bowel disease, systemic vasculitis, and therapeutic toxicity. Ann Intern Med 129:49, 1998

—— et al: Use of a cyclophosphamide-induction methotrexate-maintenance regimen for the treatment of Wegener's granulomatosis: extended follow-up and rate of relapse. Am J Med 114:463, 2003

LUDVIKSSON BR et al: Active Wegener's granulomatosis is associated with HLA-DR+ CD4+ T cells exhibiting an unbalanced Th-1 type T cell cytokine pattern: Reversal with IL-10. J Immunol 160:3602, 1998

SNELLER MC, FAUCI AS: Pathogenesis of vasculitis syndromes. Med Clin North Am 81:221, 1997

320 Behçet's Syndrome
Haralampos M. Moutsopoulos

DEFINITION, INCIDENCE, AND PREVALENCE

Behçet's syndrome is a multisystem disorder presenting with recurrent oral and genital ulcerations as well as ocular involvement. The diagnosis is clinical and based on internationally agreed diagnostic criteria (Table 320-1).

The syndrome affects young males and females from the Mediterranean region, the Middle East, and the Far East, suggesting a link with the ancient Silk Route. Males and females are affected equally, but males often have more severe disease. Blacks are very infrequently affected.

PATHOGENESIS

The etiology and pathogenesis of this syndrome remain obscure. The main pathologic lesion is systemic perivasculitis with early neutrophil infiltration, endothelial swelling, and fibrinoid necrosis. Apart from neutrophils, increased numbers of infiltrating Tγδ cells are observed. Circulating autoantibodies against α-enolase of endothelial cells and *anti–Saccharomyces cerevisiae antibodies* (ASCA—characteristic of Crohn's disease) are found to be present in the later stages of the disease. A tendency toward venous thrombus formation accounts for many of the consequences of Behçet's syndrome, though it is not clear whether it is due to additional thrombophilic factors (e.g., factor V–Leiden mutation, reduced activated protein C levels) or to the inflammatory vasculitis per se. Finally, the strong association with HLA-B5 (B51) alloantigen (present almost exclusively on areas of the aforementioned Silk Route) and the fact that ~1 in 10 patients has an affected relative underscore the genetic basis of Behçet's syndrome.

CLINICAL FEATURES

The recurrent aphthous ulcerations are a sine qua non for the diagnosis. The ulcers are usually painful, are shallow or deep with a central yellowish necrotic base, appear singly or in crops, and are located anywhere in the oral cavity. The ulcers persist for 1–2 weeks and subside without leaving scars. The genital ulcers are less common but more specific, do not affect the glans penis or urethra, and produce scrotal scars.

Skin involvement includes folliculitis, erythema nodosum, an acne-like exanthem, and, infrequently, vasculitis. Nonspecific skin inflammatory reactivity to any scratches or intradermal saline injection (pathergy test) is a common and specific manifestation.

Eye involvement with scarring and bilateral panuveitis is the most dreaded complication, since it occasionally progresses rapidly to blindness. The eye disease is usually present at the onset but may also develop within the first few years. In addition to iritis, posterior uveitis, retinal vessel occlusions, and optic neuritis can be seen in some patients with the syndrome. Hypopyon uveitis, a specific but rare manifestation, is a layer of pus visible on the anterior chamber; it usually indicates severe retinal vascular disease.

The arthritis of Behçet's syndrome is not deforming and affects the knees and ankles.

Superficial or deep peripheral vein thrombosis is seen in one-fourth of patients. Pulmonary emboli are a rare complication. The superior vena cava is obstructed occasionally, producing a dramatic clinical picture. Arterial involvement occurs infrequently and presents with aortitis or peripheral arterial aneurysm and arterial thrombosis. Pul-

TABLE 320-1	DIAGNOSTIC CRITERIA OF BEHÇET'S DISEASE

Recurrent oral ulceration plus two of the following:
    Recurrent genital ulceration
    Eye lesions
    Skin lesions
    Pathergy test

monary artery vasculitis presenting with dyspnea, cough, chest pain, hemoptysis, and infiltrates on chest roentgenograms has been reported recently in 5% of patients and should be differentiated from thromboembolic disease since it warrants anti-inflammatory and not thrombolytic therapy.

Neurologic involvement (5–10%) appears mainly in the parenchymal form (80%); it is associated with brainstem involvement and has a serious prognosis (*CNS-Behçet's syndrome*). Dural sinus thrombi (20%) are associated with headache and increased intracranial pressure. MRI and/or proton magnetic resonance spectroscopy (MRS) are very sensitive and should be employed if CNS-Behçet's syndrome is suspected.

Gastrointestinal involvement consists of mucosal ulcerations of the gut, resembling Crohn's disease.

Laboratory findings are mainly nonspecific indices of inflammation, such as leukocytosis and elevated erythrocyte sedimentation rate, as well as C-reactive protein levels; autoantibodies (see above) may be found.

℞ BEHÇET'S SYNDROME

The severity of the syndrome usually abates with time. Apart from the patients with CNS-Behçet's syndrome and major vessel disease, the life expectancy seems to be normal, and the only serious complication is blindness.

Mucous membrane involvement may respond to topical glucocorticoids in the form of mouthwash or paste. In more serious cases, thalidomide (100 mg/d) is effective. Thrombophlebitis is treated with aspirin, 325 mg/d. Colchicine can be beneficial for the mucocutaneous manifestations of the syndrome. Uveitis and CNS-Behçet's syndrome require systemic glucocorticoid therapy (prednisone, 1 mg/kg per day) and azathioprine, 2–3 mg/kg per day. Interferon has proved to be very effective not only for CNS-Behçet's syndrome but also for refractory uveitis. Preliminary data suggest that anti–tumor necrosis factor therapy may be an alternative treatment modality for panuveitis. Early initiation of azathioprine tends to favorably affect the long-term prognosis of Behçet's syndrome.

FURTHER READINGS

INTERNATIONAL STUDY GROUP FOR BEHÇET'S DISEASE: Criteria for diagnosis of Behçet's disease. Lancet 335:1078, 1990

KURAL-SEYAHI E et al: The long-term mortality and morbidity of Behçet syndrome: A 2-decade outcome survey of 387 patients followed at a dedicated center. Medicine (Baltimore) 82:60, 2003

LEE KH et al: Human alpha-enolase from endothelial cells as a target antigen of anti-endothelial cell antibody in Behçet's disease. Arthritis Rheum 48:2025, 2003

MELIKOGLU M et al: Short-term trial of etanercept in Behçet's disease: A double blind, placebo controlled study. J Rheumatol 32:98, 2005

VERITY DH et al: Behçet's disease: From Hippocrates to the third millennium. Br J Ophthalmol 87:1175, 2003

YURDAKUL S et al: Behçet syndrome. Curr Opin Rheumatol 16:38, 2004

321 Relapsing Polychondritis
Carol A. Langford, Bruce C. Gilliland†

Relapsing polychondritis is an uncommon inflammatory disorder of unknown cause characterized by an episodic and generally progressive course affecting predominantly the cartilage of the ears, nose, and laryngotracheobronchial tree. Other manifestations include scleritis, neurosensory hearing loss, polyarthritis, cardiac abnormalities, skin lesions, and glomerulonephritis. The peak age of onset is between the ages of 40–50 years, but relapsing polychondritis may affect children and the elderly. It is found in all races, and both sexes are equally affected. No familial tendency is apparent. A significantly higher frequency of HLA-DR4 has been found in patients with relapsing polychondritis than in normal individuals. A predominant subtype allele(s) of HLA-DR4 was not found. Approximately 30% of patients with relapsing polychondritis will have another rheumatologic disorder, the most frequent being systemic vasculitis, followed by rheumatoid arthritis, systemic lupus erythematosus (SLE), Sjögren's syndrome, or ankylosing spondylitis. Nonrheumatic disorders associated with relapsing polychondritis include inflammatory bowel disease, primary biliary cirrhosis, and myelodysplastic syndrome (Table 321-1).

Diagnostic criteria were suggested over 20 years ago by McAdam et al. and modified by Damiani and Levine a few years later. These criteria continue to be generally used in clinical practice. McAdam et al. proposed the following: (1) recurrent chondritis of both auricles; (2) nonerosive inflammatory arthritis; (3) chondritis of nasal cartilage; (4) inflammation of ocular structures, including conjunctivitis, keratitis, scleritis/episcleritis, and/or uveitis; (5) chondritis of the laryngeal and/or tracheal cartilages; and (6) cochlear and/or vestibular damage manifested by neurosensory hearing loss, tinnitus, and/or vertigo. The diagnosis is certain when three or more of these features are present along with a positive biopsy from the ear, nasal, or respiratory cartilage. Damiani and Levine later suggested that the diagnosis could be made when one or more of the above features and a positive biopsy were present, when two or more separate sites of cartilage inflammation were present that responded to glucocorticoids or dapsone, or when three or more of the above features were present. A biopsy is not necessary in most patients with clinically evident disease.

PATHOLOGY AND PATHOPHYSIOLOGY
The earliest abnormality of hyaline and elastic cartilage noted histologically is a focal or diffuse loss of basophilic staining indicating depletion of proteoglycan from the cartilage matrix. Inflammatory infiltrates are found adjacent to involved cartilage and consist predominantly of mononuclear cells and occasional plasma cells. In acute disease, polymorphonuclear white cells may also be present. Destruction of cartilage begins at the outer edges and advances centrally. There is lacunar breakdown and loss of chondrocytes. Degenerating cartilage is replaced by granulation tissue and later by fibrosis and focal areas of calcification. Small loci of cartilage regeneration may be present. Immunofluorescence studies have shown immunoglobulins and complement at sites of involvement. Extracellular granular material observed in the degenerating cartilage matrix by electron microscopy has been interpreted to be enzymes, immunoglobulins, or proteoglycans.

Immunologic mechanisms play a role in the pathogenesis of relapsing polychondritis. Immunoglobulin and complement deposits are found at sites of inflammation. In addition, antibodies to type II collagen and to matrilin-1 and immune complexes are detected in the sera of some patients. The possibility that an immune response to type II collagen may be important in the pathogenesis is supported experimentally by the occurrence of auricular chondritis in rats immunized with type II collagen. Antibodies to type II collagen are found in the sera of these animals, and immune deposits are detected at sites of ear inflammation.

†Deceased. A contributor to HPIM since the 11th edition, Dr. Gilliland passed away on February 17, 2007.

Humoral immune responses to type IX and type XI collagen, matrilin-1, and cartilage oligomeric matrix protein have been demonstrated in some patients. In a study, rats immunized with matrilin-1 were found to develop severe inspiratory stridor and swelling of the nasal septum. The rats had severe inflammation with erosions of the involved cartilage, which was characterized by increased numbers of CD4+ and CD8+ T cells in the lesions. The cartilage of the joints and ear pinna was not involved. All had IgG antibodies to matrilin-1. Matrilin-1 is a noncollagenous protein present in the extracellular matrix in cartilage. It is present in high concentrations in the trachea and is also present in the nasal septum but not in articular cartilage. A subsequent study demonstrated serum anti-matrilin-1 antibodies in approximately 13% of patients with relapsing polychondritis; approximately 70% of these patients had respiratory symptoms. Cell-mediated immunity may also be operative in causing tissue injury, since lymphocyte transformation can be demonstrated when lymphocytes of patients are exposed to cartilage extracts. T cells specific for type II collagen have been found in some patients, and CD4+ T cells have been observed at sites of cartilage inflammation. The accumulating data strongly suggest that both humoral and cell-mediated immunity play an important role in the pathogenesis of relapsing polychondritis.

Dissolution of cartilage matrix can be induced by the intravenous injection of crude papain, a proteolytic enzyme, into young rabbits, which results in collapse of their normally rigid ears within 4 h. Reconstitution of the matrix occurs in about 7 days. In relapsing polychondritis, loss of cartilage matrix also most likely results from action of proteolytic enzymes released from chondrocytes, polymorphonuclear white cells, and monocytes that have been activated by inflammatory mediators.

CLINICAL MANIFESTATIONS
The onset of relapsing polychondritis is frequently abrupt with the appearance of one or two sites of cartilaginous inflammation. Fever, fatigue, and weight loss occur and may precede the clinical signs of relapsing polychondritis by several weeks. Relapsing polychondritis may go unrecognized for several months or even years in patients who only initially manifest intermittent joint pain and/or swelling, or who have unexplained eye inflammation, hearing loss, valvular heart disease, or pulmonary symptoms. The pattern of cartilaginous involvement and the frequency of episodes vary widely among patients.

Auricular chondritis is the most frequent presenting manifestation of relapsing polychondritis in 40% of patients and eventually affects about 85% of patients (Table 321-2). One or both ears are involved, either sequentially or simultaneously. Patients experience the sudden onset of pain, tenderness, and swelling of the cartilaginous portion of the ear (Fig. 321-1). Earlobes are spared because they do not contain cartilage. The overlying skin has a beefy red or violaceous color. Prolonged or recurrent episodes result in a flabby or droopy ear as a sequela of cartilage destruction. Swelling may close off the eustachian tube (causing otitis media) or the external auditory meatus, either of which can impair hearing. Inflammation of the internal auditory artery or its cochlear branch produces hearing loss, vertigo, ataxia, nausea, and vomiting. Vertigo is almost always accompanied by hearing loss. The

TABLE 321-1 DISORDERS ASSOCIATED WITH RELAPSING POLYCHONDRITIS[a]

Systemic vasculitis
Rheumatoid arthritis
Systemic lupus erythematosus
Sjögren's syndrome
Spondyloarthritides
Behçet's syndrome
Inflammatory bowel disease
Primary biliary cirrhosis
Myelodysplastic syndrome

[a]Systemic vasculitis is the most common association followed by rheumatoid arthritis, systemic lupus erythematosus, and Sjögren's syndrome.
Source: Modified from Michet.

TABLE 321-2 **CLINICAL MANIFESTATIONS OF RELAPSING POLYCHONDRITIS**

Clinical Feature	Frequency, %	
	Presenting	Cumulative
Auricular chondritis	43	89
Arthritis	32	72
Nasal chondritis	21	61
Ocular inflammation	18	59
Laryngotracheal symptoms	23	55
Reduced hearing	7	40
Saddle nose deformity	11	25
Cutaneous	4	25
Laryngotracheal stricture	15	23
Vasculitis	2	14
Elevated creatinine	7	13
Aortic or mitral regurgitation	0	12

Source: Modified from Kent et al.

cartilage of the nose becomes inflamed during the first or subsequent attacks. Approximately 50% of patients will eventually have nose involvement. Patients may experience nasal stuffiness, rhinorrhea, and epistaxis. The bridge of the nose becomes red, swollen, and tender and may collapse, producing a saddle deformity (Fig. 321-2). In some patients, the saddle deformity develops insidiously without overt inflammation. Saddle nose is observed more frequently in younger patients, especially in women.

Arthritis is the presenting manifestation in relapsing polychondritis in approximately one-third of patients and may be present for several months before other features appear. Eventually, more than half the patients will have arthritis. The arthritis is usually asymmetric and oligo- or polyarticular, and it involves both large and small peripheral joints. An episode of arthritis lasts from a few days to several weeks and resolves spontaneously without residual joint deformity. Attacks of arthritis may not be temporally related to other manifestations of relapsing polychondritis. The joints are warm, tender, and swollen. Joint fluid has been reported to be noninflammatory. In addition to peripheral joints, inflammation may involve the costochondral, sternomanubrial, and sternoclavicular cartilages. Destruction of these cartilages may result in a pectus excavatum deformity or even a flail anterior chest wall. Relapsing polychondritis may occur in patients with preexisting rheumatoid arthritis, Reiter's syndrome, psoriatic arthritis, or ankylosing spondylitis.

FIGURE 321-1 ***Left.*** The pinna is erythematous, swollen, and tender. Not shown is the ear lobule that is spared as there is no underlying cartilage. ***Right.*** The pinna is thickened and deformed. The destruction of the underlying cartilage results in a floppy ear. *(Reprinted from the Clinical Slide Collection on the Rheumatic Diseases, ©1991, 1995, 1997, 1998, 1999. Used by permission of the American College of Rheumatology.)*

FIGURE 321-2 Saddle nose results from destruction and collapse of the nasal cartilage. *(Reprinted from the Clinical Slide Collection on the Rheumatic Diseases, ©1991, 1995, 1997, 1998, 1999. Used by permission of the American College of Rheumatology.)*

Eye manifestations occur in more than half of patients and include conjunctivitis, episcleritis, scleritis, iritis, and keratitis. Eye involvement is seldom the presenting feature. Ulceration and perforation of the cornea may occur and cause blindness. Other manifestations include eyelid and periorbital edema, proptosis, cataracts, optic neuritis, extraocular muscle palsies, retinal vasculitis, and renal vein occlusion.

Laryngotracheobronchial involvement occurs in ~50% of patients. Symptoms include hoarseness, a nonproductive cough, and tenderness over the larynx and proximal trachea. Mucosal edema, strictures, and/or collapse of laryngeal or tracheal cartilage may cause stridor and life-threatening airway obstruction necessitating tracheostomy. Collapse of cartilage in bronchi leads to pneumonia and, when extensive, to respiratory insufficiency.

Aortic regurgitation occurs in about 5% of patients and is due to progressive dilation of the aortic ring or to destruction of the valve cusps. Mitral and other heart valves are affected less often. Other cardiac manifestations include pericarditis, myocarditis, and conduction abnormalities. Aneurysms of the proximal, thoracic, or abdominal aorta may occur even in the absence of active chondritis and occasionally rupture.

Systemic vasculitis may occur in association with relapsing polychondritis. Vasculitides include isolated cutaneous vasculitis, polyarteritis nodosa, giant cell arteritis, and Takayasu's arteritis (Chap. 319). Neurologic abnormalities usually occur as a result of underlying vasculitis, manifesting as seizures, strokes, ataxia, and peripheral and cranial nerve neuropathies. Cranial nerves II, III, VI, and VII are most often involved. Approximately 25% of patients have skin lesions, none of which is characteristic for relapsing polychondritis but can reflect an associated vasculitis. These include purpura, erythema nodosum, erythema multiforme, angioedema/urticaria, livedo reticularis, and panniculitis. Segmental necrotizing glomerulonephritis with crescent formation has been noted in some patients, usually in association with microscopic polyangiitis, but may occur in the absence of systemic vasculitis.

The course of disease is highly variable, with episodes lasting from a few days to several weeks and then subsiding spontaneously. Attacks may recur at intervals varying from weeks to months. In other patients, the disease has a chronic, smoldering course. In a few patients, the disease may be limited to one or two episodes of cartilage inflammation. In one study, the 5-year estimated survival rate was 74% and the 10-year survival rate 55%. In contrast to earlier series, only about half the deaths could be attributed to relapsing polychondritis or complications of treatment. Pulmonary complications accounted for only 10% of all fatalities. In general, patients with more widespread disease have a worse prognosis.

LABORATORY FINDINGS

Mild leukocytosis and normocytic, normochromic anemia are often present. Eosinophilia is observed in 10% of patients. The erythrocyte sedimentation rate and C-reactive protein are usually elevated. Rheumatoid factor and antinuclear antibody tests are occasionally positive in low titers. Antibodies to type II collagen are present in fewer than half the patients and are not specific. Circulating immune complexes may be detected, especially in patients with early active disease. Elevated levels of γ globulin may be present. Antineutrophil cytoplasmic antibodies (ANCA), either cytoplasmic (C-ANCA) or perinuclear (P-ANCA), are found in some patients with active disease. The upper and lower airways can be evaluated by imaging techniques such as linear tomography, laryngotracheography, and CT, and by bronchoscopy. MRI is helpful in evaluation of the larynx and trachea. Bronchography is performed to demonstrate bronchial narrowing. Intrathoracic airway obstruction can also be evaluated by inspiratory-expiratory flow studies. The chest film may show narrowing of the trachea and/or the main bronchi, widening of the ascending or descending aorta due to an aneurysm, and cardiomegaly when aortic insufficiency is present. MRI can be used in assessing aortic aneurysmal dilatation. Radiographs may show calcification at previous sites of cartilage damage involving ear, nose, larynx, or trachea.

DIAGNOSIS

Diagnosis is based on recognition of the typical clinical features. Biopsies of the involved cartilage from the ear, nose, or respiratory tract will confirm the diagnosis but are only necessary when clinical features are not typical. Patients with Wegener's granulomatosis may have a saddle nose and pulmonary involvement but can be distinguished by the absence of auricular involvement and the presence of granulomatous lesions in the tracheobronchial tree. Patients with Cogan's syndrome have interstitial keratitis and vestibular and auditory abnormalities, but this syndrome does not involve the respiratory tract or ears. Reiter's syndrome may initially resemble relapsing polychondritis because of oligoarticular arthritis and eye involvement, but it is distinguished in time by the appearance of urethritis and typical mucocutaneous lesions and the absence of nose or ear cartilage involvement. Rheumatoid arthritis may initially suggest relapsing polychondritis because of arthritis and eye inflammation. The arthritis in rheumatoid arthritis, however, is erosive and symmetric. In addition, rheumatoid factor titers are usually high compared with those in relapsing polychondritis. Bacterial infection of the pinna may be mistaken for relapsing polychondritis but differs by usually involving only one ear, including the earlobe. Auricular cartilage may also be damaged by trauma or frostbite.

Relapsing polychondritis may develop in patients with a variety of autoimmune disorders, including SLE, rheumatoid arthritis, Sjögren's syndrome, and vasculitis. In most cases, these disorders antedate the appearance of polychondritis, usually by months or years. It is likely that these patients have an immunologic abnormality that predisposes them to development of this group of autoimmune disorders.

℞ **RELAPSING POLYCHONDRITIS**

In patients with active chondritis, prednisone, 40–60 mg/d, is often effective in suppressing disease activity; it is tapered gradually once disease is controlled. In some patients, prednisone can be stopped, while in others low doses in the range of 10–15 mg/d are required for continued suppression of disease. Dapsone instead of prednisone has been effective in suppressing inflammation in some patients. Immunosuppressive drugs such as methotrexate, cyclophosphamide, azathioprine, or cyclosporine should be reserved for patients who fail to respond to prednisone or who require high doses for control of disease activity. Patients with significant ocular inflammation often require intraocular steroids as well as high doses of prednisone. Heart valve replacement or repair of an aortic aneurysm may be necessary. When obstruction is severe, tracheostomy is required. Stents may be necessary in patients with tracheobronchial collapse.

FURTHER READINGS

KENT PD et al: Relapsing polychondritis. Curr Opin Rheumatol 16:56, 2004

LETKO E et al: Relapsing polychondritis: A clinical review. Semin Arthritis Rheum 31:384, 2002

MICHET CJ et al: Relapsing polychondritis. Survival and predictive role of early disease manifestations. Ann Intern Med 104:74, 1986

STAATS BA et al: Relapsing polychondritis. Semin Respir Crit Care Med 23:145, 2002

TRENTHAM DE, LE CH: Relapsing polychondritis. Ann Intern Med 129:114, 1998

322 Sarcoidosis
Robert P. Baughman, Elyse E. Lower

DEFINITION

Sarcoidosis is an inflammatory disease characterized by the presence of noncaseating granulomas. The disease is often multisystem and requires the presence of involvement in two or more organs for a specific diagnosis. The finding of granulomas is not specific for sarcoidosis, and other conditions known to cause granulomas must be ruled out. These conditions include mycobacterial and fungal infections, malignancy, and environmental agents such as beryllium. While sarcoidosis can affect virtually every organ of the body, the lung is most commonly affected. Other organs commonly affected are the liver, skin, and eye. The clinical outcome of sarcoidosis varies, with remission occurring in over half the patients within a few years of diagnosis; however, the remaining patients develop a chronic disease that lasts for decades.

ETIOLOGY

Despite multiple investigations, the cause of sarcoidosis remains unknown. Currently, the most likely etiology is an infectious or noninfectious environmental agent that triggers an inflammatory response in a genetically susceptible host. Among the possible infectious agents, careful studies have shown a much higher incidence of *Propionibacter acnes* in the lymph nodes of sarcoidosis patients compared to controls. An animal model has shown that *P. acnes* can induce a granulomatous response in mice similar to sarcoidosis. Other studies support the possibility of an atypical mycobacterium, although these have yet to be confirmed by blinded studies with adequate controls. Recent studies have demonstrated the presence of a mycobacterial protein [*Mycobacterium tuberculosis* catalase-peroxidase (mKatG)] in the granulomas of some sarcoidosis patients. This protein is very resistant to degradation and may represent the persistent antigen in sarcoidosis. Environmental exposures to insecticides and mold have been associated with an increased risk for disease. In addition, health care workers appear to have an increased risk. Some authors have suggested that sarcoidosis is not due to a single agent but represents a particular host response to multiple agents. An interesting approach to finding the etiology of sarcoidosis is to correlate the environmental exposures to genetic markers. These studies have supported the hypothesis that a genetically susceptible host is a key factor in the disease.

INCIDENCE AND PREVALENCE

Sarcoidosis is seen worldwide, with the highest prevalence reported in the Nordic population. In the United States, the disease has been reported more commonly in blacks than whites, with the ratio of blacks to whites ranging from 3:1 to 17:0. Women appear to be slightly more susceptible than men. The lower estimate is the result of a recent study from a large health maintenance organization in Detroit. The earlier American studies finding the higher incidence in blacks may have been influenced by the fact that blacks seem to develop more extensive and chronic pulmonary disease. Since most sarcoidosis clinics are run by pulmonologists, a selection bias may have occurred. Worldwide, the prevalence of the disease varies from 20–60 per 100,000 for many groups such as Japanese, Italians, and American whites. Higher rate occurs in Ireland and Nordic countries. In one closely observed community in Sweden, the lifetime risk for developing sarcoidosis was 3%.

Sarcoidosis often occurs in young, otherwise healthy adults. It is uncommon to diagnose the disease in someone under age 18. However, it has become clear that a second peak in incidence develops around age 60. In a study of >700 newly diagnosed sarcoidosis patients in the United States, half the patients were ≥40 years at the time of diagnosis.

Although most cases of sarcoidosis are sporadic, a familial form of the disease exists. At least 5% of patients with sarcoidosis will have a family member with sarcoidosis. Sarcoidosis patients who are Irish or American blacks seem to have a two to three times higher rate of familial disease.

PATHOPHYSIOLOGY AND IMMUNOPATHOGENESIS

The granuloma is the pathologic hallmark of sarcoidosis. A distinct feature of sarcoidosis is the local accumulation of inflammatory cells. Extensive studies in the lung using bronchoalveolar lavage (BAL) have demonstrated that the initial inflammatory response is an influx of T helper cells. In addition, there is an accumulation of activated monocytes. Figure 322-1 is a proposed model for sarcoidosis. Using the HLA-CD4 complex, antigen-presenting cells present an unknown antigen to the helper T cell. Studies have clarified that specific HLA haplotypes such as HLA-DRB1*1101 are associated with an increased risk for developing sarcoidosis. In addition, different HLA haplotypes are associated with different clinical outcomes.

The macrophage/helper T cell cluster leads to activation with the increased release of several cytokines. These include interleukin (IL) 2 released from the T cell and interferon γ and tumor necrosis factor (TNF) released by the macrophage. The T cell is a necessary part of the initial inflammatory response. In advanced, untreated HIV infection, patients who lack helper T cells rarely develop sarcoidosis. In contrast, several reports confirm that sarcoidosis becomes unmasked as HIV-infected individuals receive antiretroviral therapy, with subsequent restoration of their immune system. In contrast, treatment of established pulmonary sarcoidosis with cyclosporine, a drug that downregulates helper T cell responses, seems to have little impact on sarcoidosis.

The granulomatous response of sarcoidosis can resolve with or without therapy. However, in at least 20% of patients with sarcoidosis, a chronic form of the disease develops. This persistent form of the disease is associated with the secretion of high levels of IL-8. Also, studies have reported that in patients with this chronic form of disease excessive amounts of TNF are released in the areas of inflammation.

It is sometimes difficult to determine early on the ultimate clinical outcome of sarcoidosis. One form of the disease, *Löfgren's syndrome*, consists of erythema nodosum, hilar adenopathy on chest roentgenogram, and uveitis. Löfgren's syndrome is associated with a good prognosis, with >90% of patients experiencing disease resolution within 2 years. Recent studies have demonstrated that the HLA-DQB1*0201 is highly associated with Löfgren's syndrome. In contrast, patients with the disfiguring skin condition lupus pernio or cardiac or neurologic involvement rarely experience disease remission.

CLINICAL MANIFESTATIONS

The presentation of sarcoidosis ranges from patients who are asymptomatic to those with organ failure. It is unclear how often sarcoidosis is asymptomatic. In countries where routine chest roentgenogram screening is performed, 20–30% of pulmonary cases are detected in asymptomatic individuals. The inability to screen for other asymptomatic forms of the disease would suggest that as many as a third of sarcoidosis patients are asymptomatic.

Respiratory complaints including cough and dyspnea are the most common presenting symptoms. In many cases, the patient presents with a 2–4 week history of these symptoms. Unfortunately, due to the nonspecific nature of pulmonary symptoms, the patient may see physicians for up to a year before a diagnosis is confirmed. The diagnosis of sarcoidosis is usually only suggested when a chest roentgenogram is performed.

Symptoms related to cutaneous and ocular disease are the next two most common complaints. Skin lesions are often nonspecific. However, since these lesions are readily observed, the patient and treating physician are often led to a diagnosis. In contrast to patients with pulmonary disease, patients with cutaneous lesions are more likely to be diagnosed within 6 months of symptoms.

Nonspecific constitutional symptoms include fatigue, fever, night sweats, and weight loss. Fatigue is perhaps the most common constitutional symptom that affects these patients. Given its insidious nature, patients are usually not aware of the association with their sarcoidosis until their disease resolves.

The overall incidence of sarcoidosis at the time of diagnosis and eventual common organ involvement are summarized in Table 322-1. Over time, skin, eye, and neurologic involvement seem more apparent. In the United States, the frequency of specific organ involvement appears to be affected by age, race, and gender. For example, eye disease

FIGURE 322-1 Schematic representation of initial events of sarcoidosis. The antigen-presenting cell and helper T cell complex leads to the release of multiple cytokines. This forms a granuloma. Over time, the granuloma may resolve or lead to chronic disease, including fibrosis.

TABLE 322-1 FREQUENCY OF COMMON ORGAN INVOLVEMENT AND LIFETIME RISK[a]

	Presentation, %[b]	Follow-up, %[c]
Lung	95	94
Skin	24	43
Eye	12	29
Extrathoracic lymph node	15	16
Liver	12	14
Spleen	7	8
Neurologic	5	16
Cardiac	2	3

[a]Patients could have more than one organ involved.
[b]From ACCESS study of 736 patients evaluated within 6 months of diagnosis.
[c]From follow-up of 1024 sarcoidosis patients seen at the University of Cincinnati Interstitial Lung Disease and Sarcoidosis Clinic from 2002–2006.

FIGURE 322-2 Posterior-anterior chest roentgenogram demonstrating bilateral hilar adenopathy, stage 1 disease.

FIGURE 322-3 High-resolution CT scan of chest demonstrating patchy reticular nodularity, including areas of confluence.

is more common among blacks. Under the age of 40, it occurs more frequently in women. However, in those diagnosed over the age of 40, eye disease is more common in men.

LUNG

Lung involvement occurs in >90% of sarcoidosis patients. The most commonly used method for detecting lung disease is still the chest roentgenogram. Figure 322-2 illustrates the chest roentgenogram from a sarcoidosis patient with bilateral hilar adenopathy. Although the CT scan has changed the diagnostic approach to interstitial lung disease, the CT scan is not usually considered a monitoring tool for patients with sarcoidosis. Figure 322-3 demonstrates some of the characteristic CT features, including peribronchial thickening and reticular nodular changes, which are predominantly subpleural. The peribronchial thickening seen on CT scan seems to explain the high yield of granulomas from bronchial biopsies performed for diagnosis.

While the CT scan is more sensitive, the standard scoring system described by Scadding in 1961 for chest roentgenograms remains the preferred method of characterizing the chest involvement. Stage 1 is hilar adenopathy alone (Fig. 322-2), often with right paratracheal involvement. Stage 2 is a combination of adenopathy plus infiltrates, whereas stage 3 reveals infiltrates alone. Stage 4 consists of fibrosis. Usually the infiltrates in sarcoidosis are predominantly an upper lobe process. Only in a few noninfectious diseases is an upper lobe predominance noted. In addition to sarcoidosis, the differential diagnosis of upper lobe disease includes hypersensitivity pneumonitis, silicosis, and Langerhans cell histiocytosis. For infectious diseases, tuberculosis and *Pneumocystis* pneumonia can often present as upper lobe diseases.

Lung volumes, mechanics, and diffusion all are useful in evaluating interstitial lung diseases such as sarcoidosis. The diffusion of carbon monoxide (DL_{CO}) is the most sensitive test for an interstitial lung disease. Reduced lung volumes are a reflection of the restrictive lung disease seen in sarcoidosis. However, a third of the patients presenting with sarcoidosis still have lung volumes within the normal range, despite abnormal chest roentgenograms and dyspnea.

Approximately half of sarcoidosis patients present with obstructive disease, reflected by a reduced ratio of forced vital capacity expired in time interval t (FEV_t/FVC). Cough is a very common symptom. Airway involvement causing varying degrees of obstruction underlies the cough in most sarcoidosis patients. However, airway hyperreactivity as determined by methacholine challenge will be positive in some of these patients. A few patients with cough will respond to traditional bronchodilators as the only form of treatment. In some cases, high-dose inhaled glucocorticoids alone are useful.

Pulmonary arterial hypertension is reported in at least 5% of sarcoidosis patients. Either direct vascular involvement or the consequence of fibrotic changes in the lung can lead to pulmonary arterial hypertension. In sarcoidosis patients with end-stage fibrosis awaiting lung transplant, 70% will have pulmonary arterial hypertension. This is a much higher incidence than that reported for other fibrotic lung diseases. In less advanced, but still symptomatic, patients pulmonary arterial hypertension has been noted in up to 50% of the cases. Because sarcoidosis-associated pulmonary arterial hypertension may respond to therapy, evaluation for this should be considered in persistently symptomatic patients.

SKIN

Skin involvement is eventually identified in over a third of patients with sarcoidosis. The classic cutaneous lesions include erythema nodosum, maculopapular lesions, hyper- and hypopigmentation, keloid formation, and subcutaneous nodules. A specific complex of involvement of the bridge of the nose, the area beneath the eyes, and the cheeks is referred to as *lupus pernio* (Fig. 322-4) and is diagnostic for a chronic form of sarcoidosis.

In contrast, erythema nodosum is a transient rash that can be seen in association with hilar adenopathy and uveitis (Löfgren's syndrome). Erythema nodosum is more common in women and in certain self-described demographic groups including Caucasians and Puerto

FIGURE 322-4 Chronic inflammatory lesions around nose, eyes, and cheeks, referred to as lupus pernio.

FIGURE 322-5 Maculopapular lesions on the trunk of a sarcoidosis patient.

Ricans. In the United States, the other manifestations of skin sarcoidosis, especially lupus pernio, are more common in blacks than whites.

The maculopapular lesions from sarcoidosis are the most common chronic form of the disease (Fig. 322-5). These are often overlooked by the patient and physician, since they are chronic and not painful. Initially, these lesions are usually purplish papules elevated up to 1 cm and <3 cm in diameter. They can become confluent and infiltrate large areas of the skin. With treatment, the color and induration may fade. Because these lesions are caused by noncaseating granulomas, the diagnosis of sarcoidosis can be readily made by a skin biopsy.

EYE

The frequency of ocular manifestations for sarcoidosis varies depending on race. In Japan, >70% of sarcoidosis patients develop ocular disease, while in the United States only 30% have eye disease, with problems more common in blacks than whites. Although the most common manifestation is an anterior uveitis, over a quarter of patients will have inflammation at the posterior of the eye, including retinitis and pars planitis. While symptoms such as photophobia, blurred vision, and increased tearing can occur, some asymptomatic patients still have active inflammation. Initially asymptomatic patients with ocular sarcoidosis can eventually develop blindness. Therefore, it is recommended that all patients with sarcoidosis receive a dedicated ophthalmologic examination. Sicca is seen in over half of the chronic sarcoidosis patients. Dry eyes appear to be a reflection of prior lacrimal gland disease. Although the patient may no longer have active inflammation, the dry eyes may require natural tears or other lubricants.

LIVER

Using biopsies to detect granulomatous disease, liver involvement can be identified in over half of sarcoidosis patients. However, using liver function studies, only 20–30% of patients will have evidence of liver involvement. The most common abnormality of liver function is an elevation of the alkaline phosphatase level, consistent with an obstructive pattern. In addition, elevated transaminase levels can occur. An elevated bilirubin level is a marker for more advanced liver disease. Overall, only 5% of sarcoidosis patients have sufficient symptoms from their liver disease to require specific therapy. Although symptoms can be due to hepatomegaly, more frequently symptoms result from extensive intrahepatic cholestasis leading to portal hypertension. In this case, ascites and esophageal varices can occur. It is rare that a sarcoidosis patient will require a liver transplant, because even the patient with cirrhosis due to sarcoidosis can respond to systemic therapy. On a cautionary note, patients with both sarcoidosis and hepatitis C should avoid therapy with interferon α because of its association with the development or worsening of granulomatous disease.

BONE MARROW AND SPLEEN

One or more bone marrow manifestations can be identified in many sarcoidosis patients. The most common hematologic problem is lymphopenia, which is a reflection of sequestration of the lymphocytes into the areas of inflammation. Anemia occurs in 20% of patients and leukopenia is less common. Bone marrow examination will reveal granulomas in about a third of patients. Splenomegaly can be detected in 5–10% of patients, but splenic biopsy reveals granulomas in 60% of patients. The CT scan can be relatively specific for sarcoidosis involvement of the spleen (Fig. 322-6). Both bone marrow and spleen involvement are more common in blacks than whites. These manifestations alone are rarely an indication for therapy. On occasion, splenectomy may be indicated for massive symptomatic splenomegaly or profound pancytopenia.

CALCIUM METABOLISM

Hypercalcemia and/or hypercalciuria occurs in about 10% of sarcoidosis patients. It is more common in whites than blacks and in men. The mechanism of abnormal calcium metabolism is increased production of 1,25-dihydroxyvitamin D by the granuloma itself. The 1,25-dihydroxyvitamin D causes increased intestinal absorption of calcium, leading to hypercalcemia with a suppressed parathyroid hormone (PTH) level (Chap. 347). Increased exogenous vitamin D from diet or sunlight exposure may exacerbate this problem. Serum calcium should be determined as part of the initial evaluation of all sarcoidosis patients, and a repeat determination may be useful during the summer months with increased sun exposure. In patients with a history of renal calculi, a 24-h urine calcium measurement should be obtained. If a sarcoidosis patient with a history of renal calculi is to be placed on calcium supplements, a follow-up 24-h urine calcium level should be measured.

RENAL DISEASE

Direct kidney involvement occurs in <5% of sarcoidosis patients. It is associated with granulomas in the kidney itself and can lead to nephritis. However, hypercalcemia is the most likely cause of sarcoidosis-associated renal disease. In 1–2% of sarcoidosis patients, acute renal failure has been encountered as a result of hypercalcemia. Treatment of the hypercalcemia with glucocorticoids and other therapies often improves, but does not totally resolve, the renal dysfunction.

NERVOUS SYSTEM

Neurologic disease is reported in 5–10% of sarcoidosis patients and appears to be of equal frequency across all ethnic groups. Any part of the central or peripheral nervous system can be affected. The presence of granulomatous inflammation is often visible on MRI studies. The MRI with gadolinium enhancement may demonstrate space-occupy-

FIGURE 322-6 CT scan of the abdomen after oral and intravenous contrast. The stomach is compressed by the enlarged spleen. Within the spleen, areas of hypo- and hyperdensity are identified.

ing lesions, but the MRI can be negative due to small lesions or the effect of systemic therapy in reducing the inflammation. The cerebral spinal fluid (CSF) findings include a lymphocytic meningitis with a mild increase in protein. The CSF glucose is usually normal but can be low. Certain areas of the nervous system are more commonly affected in neurosarcoidosis. These include cranial nerve involvement, basilar meningitis, myelopathy, and anterior hypothalamic disease with associated diabetes insipidus (Chap. 334). Seizures and cognitive changes also occur. Of the cranial nerves, seventh nerve paralysis can be transient and can be mistaken for Bell's palsy (idiopathic seventh nerve paralysis). Since this form of neurosarcoidosis often resolves within weeks and does not recur, it may have occurred prior to a definitive diagnosis of sarcoidosis. Optic neuritis is another cranial nerve manifestation of sarcoidosis. This manifestation is more chronic and usually requires long-term systemic therapy. It can be associated with both anterior and posterior uveitis. Differentiating between neurosarcoidosis and multiple sclerosis can be difficult at times. Optic neuritis can occur in both diseases. In some patients with sarcoidosis, multiple enhancing white matter abnormalities may be detected by MRI, suggesting multiple sclerosis. In such cases, the presence of meningeal enhancement or hypothalamic involvement suggests neurosarcoidosis, as does evidence of extraneurologic disease such as pulmonary or skin involvement, which also suggests sarcoidosis. Since the response of neurosarcoidosis to glucocorticoids and cytotoxic therapy is different from that of multiple sclerosis, differentiating between these disease entities is important.

CARDIAC

The presence of cardiac involvement is influenced by race. Over a quarter of Japanese sarcoidosis patients develop cardiac disease, whereas only 5% of sarcoidosis patients in the United States and Europe develop cardiac disease. However, there is no apparent difference between whites and blacks. Cardiac disease usually presents as either congestive heart failure or cardiac arrhythmias. Both manifestations result from infiltration of the heart muscle by granulomas. Diffuse granulomatous involvement of the heart muscle can lead to ejection fractions below 10%. Even in this situation, improvement in the ejection fraction can occur with systemic therapy. Arrhythmias can also occur with diffuse infiltration or with more patchy cardiac involvement. If the AV node is infiltrated, heart block can occur. This can be detected by routine electrocardiography. Ventricular arrhythmias and sudden death due to ventricular tachycardia are common causes of death. Arrhythmias are best detected using 24-h ambulatory monitoring. Because ventricular arrhythmias are usually multifocal due to patchy multiple granulomas in the heart, ablation therapy is not useful. Patients with significant ventricular arrhythmias should be considered for an implanted defibrillator, which appears to have reduced the rate of death in cardiac sarcoidosis. While systemic therapy can be useful in treating the arrhythmias, patients may still have malignant arrhythmias up to 6 months after starting successful treatment, and the risk for recurrent arrhythmias occurs whenever medications are tapered.

MUSCULOSKELETAL SYSTEM

Direct granulomatous bone and muscle involvement as documented by x-ray, MRI (**Fig. 322-7**), gallium scan, or biopsy can be seen in about 10% of sarcoidosis patients. However, a larger percentage of sarcoidosis patients complain of myalgias and arthralgias. These complaints are similar to those reported by patients with other inflammatory diseases, including chronic infections such as mononucleosis. Fatigue associated with sarcoidosis may be overwhelming for many patients. Recent studies have demonstrated a link between fatigue and small peripheral nerve fiber disease in sarcoidosis.

OTHER ORGAN INVOLVEMENT

Although sarcoidosis can affect any organ of the body, rarely does it involve the breast, testes, ovary, or stomach. Because of the rarity of involvement, a mass in one of these areas requires a biopsy to rule out other diseases including cancer. For example, in a study of breast prob-

FIGURE 322-7 MRI of wrist demonstrating large cyst in a sarcoidosis patient (*line*).

lems in female sarcoidosis patients, a breast lesion was more likely to be granulomas from sarcoidosis than from breast cancer. However, findings on the physical examination or mammogram cannot reliably differentiate between these lesions. More importantly, as women with sarcoidosis age, breast cancer becomes more common. Therefore, it is recommended that routine screening including mammography be performed along with other imaging studies (ultrasound, MRI) or biopsy as clinically indicated.

COMPLICATIONS

Sarcoidosis is usually a self-limited, non-life-threatening disease. However, organ-threatening disease can occur. These complications can include blindness, paraplegia, or renal failure. Death from sarcoidosis occurs in about 5% of patients seen in sarcoidosis referral clinics. The usual causes of death related to sarcoidosis are from lung, cardiac, neurologic, or liver involvement. In respiratory failure, an elevation of the right atrial pressure is a poor prognostic finding. Lung complications can also include infections such as mycetoma, which can subsequently lead to massive bleeding. In addition, the use of immunosuppressive agents can increase the incidence of serious infections.

LABORATORY FINDINGS

The chest roentgenogram remains the most commonly used tool to assess lung involvement in sarcoidosis. As noted above, the chest roentgenogram classifies involvement into four stages, with stages 1 and 2 having hilar and paratracheal adenopathy. The CT scan has been used increasingly in evaluating interstitial lung disease. In sarcoidosis, the presence of adenopathy and a nodular infiltrate is not specific for sarcoidosis. Adenopathy up to 2 cm can be seen in other inflammatory lung diseases such as idiopathic pulmonary fibrosis. However, adenopathy >2 cm in the short axis supports the diagnosis of sarcoidosis over other interstitial lung diseases.

Gallium 67 scanning has been used over the years to detect inflammatory activity in various parts of the body. A negative scan can be easily misinterpreted as the scan will quickly revert to normal during glucocorticoid therapy. In addition, the test requires that the patient return 2–4 days later. More recently, the positive emission tomography (PET) scan, using radiolabeled fluorodeoxy glucose as the marker, has provided information similar to that of the gallium scan. While the sensitivity of PET scanning has not been fully evaluated in sarcoidosis, it is important to recognize that a positive PET scan may be due to the granulomas from sarcoidosis and not to disseminated malignancy.

Serum levels of angiotensin-converting enzyme (ACE) can be helpful in the diagnosis of sarcoidosis. However, the test has somewhat low sensitivity and specificity. Elevated levels of ACE are reported in 60% of patients with acute disease and only 20% of patients with chronic disease. Although there are several causes for mild elevation of ACE, including diabetes, elevations of >50% of the upper limit of normal are seen in only a few conditions including sarcoidosis, leprosy, Gaucher's disease, hyperthyroidism, and disseminated granulomatous infections such as miliary tuberculosis. The ACE level in lymphoma is usually lower than normal, which may provide a useful distinction from sarcoidosis. There is an insertion/deletion (I/D) polymorphism of the *ACE* gene on what is felt to be in the noncritical part of the gene. There is a phenotypic difference for ACE levels, with II polymorphism having the lowest and DD polymorphism the highest levels of ACE for both sarcoidosis patients and healthy controls. There is no clear-cut association between ACE phenotype and clinical manifestation of disease. Because the ACE level is determined by a biologic assay, the concurrent use of an ACE inhibitor such as lisinopril will lead to a very low ACE level.

DIAGNOSIS

The diagnosis of sarcoidosis requires both compatible clinical features and pathologic findings. Since the cause of sarcoidosis remains elusive, the diagnosis cannot be made with 100% certainty. Nevertheless, the diagnosis can be made with reasonable certainty based on history and physical features along with laboratory and pathologic findings.

Patients are usually evaluated for possible sarcoidosis based on two scenarios (Fig. 322-8). In the first scenario, a patient may undergo a biopsy revealing a noncaseating granuloma in either a pulmonary or an extrapulmonary organ. If the clinical presentation is consistent with sarcoidosis and there is no alternative cause for the granulomas identified, then the patient is felt to have sarcoidosis.

In the second scenario, signs or symptoms suggesting sarcoidosis such as the presence of bilateral adenopathy may be present in an otherwise asymptomatic patient or a patient with uveitis or a rash consistent with sarcoidosis. At this point, a diagnostic procedure should be performed. For the patient with a compatible skin lesion, a skin biopsy should be considered. Other biopsies to consider could include liver, extrathoracic lymph node, or muscle. In some cases, a biopsy of the affected organ may not be easy to perform (such as a brain or spinal cord lesion). In other cases, such as an endomyocardial biopsy, the likelihood of a positive biopsy is low. Because of the high rate of pulmonary involvement in these cases, the lung may be easier to approach by bronchoscopy. During the bronchoscopy, a transbronchial biopsy, bronchial biopsy, or transbronchial needle aspirate of an enlarged mediastinal lymph node can be performed.

If the biopsy reveals granulomas, an alternative diagnosis such as infection or malignancy must be excluded. Bronchoscopic washings can be sent for cultures for fungi and tuberculosis. For the pathologist, the more tissue that is provided, the more comfortable is the diagnosis of sarcoidosis. A needle aspirate may be adequate in an otherwise classic case of sarcoidosis, but may be insufficient in a patient in whom lymphoma or fungal infection is a likely alternative diagnosis. Since granulomas can be seen on the edge of a lymphoma, the presence of a few granulomas from a needle aspirate may not be sufficient to clarify the diagnosis. Mediastinoscopy remains the procedure of choice to confirm the presence or absence of lymphoma in the mediastinum. Alternatively, for most patients, evidence of extrathoracic disease (e.g., eye involvement) may further support the diagnosis of sarcoidosis.

For patients with negative pathology, positive supportive tests may increase the likelihood of the diagnosis of sarcoidosis. These tests include an elevated ACE level, which can also be elevated in other granulomatous diseases but not in malignancy. A positive gallium scan can support the diagnosis if increased activity is noted in the parotids and lacrimal glands (*Panda sign*) or in the right paratracheal and left hilar

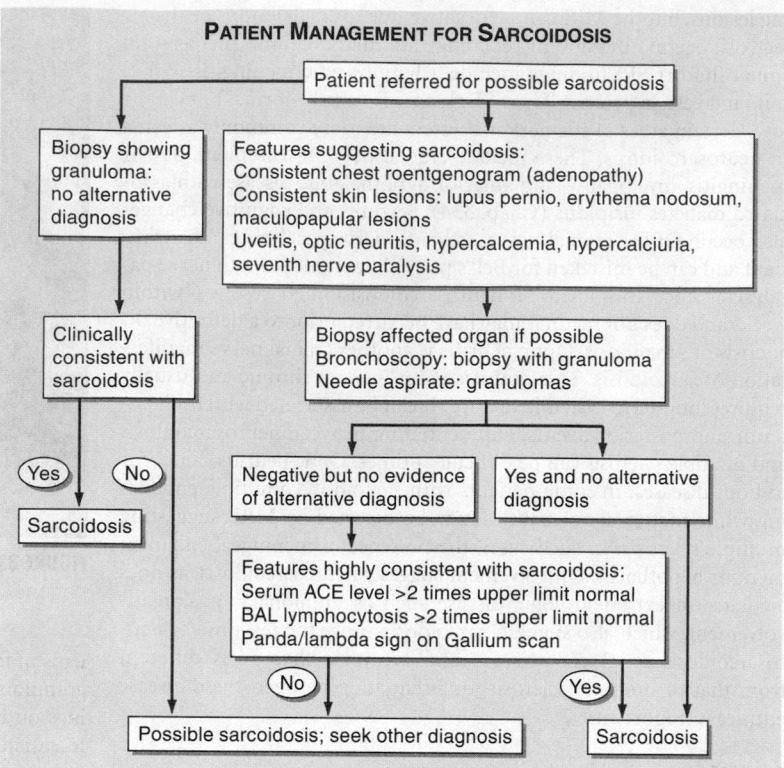

PATIENT MANAGEMENT FOR SARCOIDOSIS

FIGURE 322-8 Proposed approach to management of patient with possible sarcoidosis. Presence of one or more of these features supports the diagnosis of sarcoidosis: uveitis, optic neuritis, hypercalcemia, hypercalciuria, seventh cranial nerve paralysis, diabetes insipidus.

area (*lambda sign*). A BAL is often performed during the bronchoscopy. An increase in the percentage of lymphocytes supports the diagnosis of sarcoidosis. The use of the lymphocyte markers CD4 and CD8 can be used to determine the CD4/CD8 ratio of these increased lymphocytes in the BAL fluid. A ratio of > 3.5 is strongly supportive of sarcoidosis but is less sensitive than an increase in lymphocytes alone. Although in general, an increase in BAL lymphocytes is supportive of the diagnosis, other conditions must be considered.

These supportive tests when combined with commonly associated clinical features of the disease, which are not diagnostic of sarcoidosis, can enhance the diagnostic probability. These nondiagnostic features include uveitis, renal stones, hypercalcemia, seventh cranial nerve paralysis, or erythema nodosum.

The *Kveim-Siltzbach procedure* is a specific diagnostic test for sarcoidosis. An intradermal injection of specially prepared tissue derived from the spleen of a known sarcoidosis patient is biopsied 4–6 weeks after injection. If noncaseating granulomas are seen, this is highly specific for the diagnosis of sarcoidosis. Unfortunately, there is no commercially available Kviem-Siltzbach reagent, and some locally prepared batches have lower specificity. Thus, this test is of historic interest and is rarely used in current clinical practice.

Because the diagnosis of sarcoidosis can never be certain, over time other features may arise that lead to an alternative diagnosis. On the other hand, evidence for new organ involvement may eventually confirm the diagnosis of sarcoidosis.

PROGNOSIS

The risk of death or loss of organ function remains low in sarcoidosis. Poor outcomes usually occur in patients who present with advanced disease in whom treatment seems to have little impact. In these cases, irreversible fibrotic changes have frequently occurred.

For the majority of patients, initial presentation occurs during the granulomatous phase of the disease as depicted in Fig. 322-1. It is

ALGORITHM FOR MANAGEMENT OF SARCOIDOSIS

FIGURE 322-9 The management of acute sarcoidosis is based on level of symptoms and extent of organ involvement. In patients with mild symptoms, no therapy may be needed unless specified manifestations are noted.

clear that many patients resolve their disease within 2–5 years. These patients are felt to have acute, self-limiting sarcoidosis. On the other hand, there is a form of the disease that does not resolve within the first 2–5 years. These chronic patients can be identified at presentation by certain risk factors at presentation such as fibrosis on chest roentgenogram, presence of lupus pernio, bone cysts, cardiac or neurologic disease (except isolated seventh nerve paralysis), and presence of renal calculi due to hypercalciuria. Recent studies also indicate that patients who require glucocorticoids for any manifestation of their disease in the first 6 months of presentation have a >50% chance of having chronic disease. In contrast, <10% of patients who require systemic therapy in the first 6 months will require chronic therapy.

℞ SARCOIDOSIS

The indications for therapy should be based on symptoms. The patient with elevated liver function tests or an abnormal chest roentgenogram probably does not benefit from treatment. However, these patients should be monitored for evidence of progressive, symptomatic disease.

One approach to therapy is summarized in **Figs. 322-9** and **322-10**. We have divided the approach into treating acute versus chronic disease. For acute disease, no therapy remains a viable option for patients with no or mild symptoms. For symptoms confined to only one organ, topical therapy is preferable. For multiorgan disease or disease too extensive for topical therapy, an approach to systemic therapy is outlined. Glucocorticoids remain the drugs of choice for this disease. However, the decision to continue to treat with glucocorticoids or to add steroid-sparing agents depends on the tolerability, duration, and dosage of glucocorticoids. **Table 322-2** summarizes the dosage and monitoring of several commonly used drugs. According to the available trials, evidence-based recommendations are made. Most of these recommendations are for pulmonary disease because most of the trials were performed only in pulmonary disease. Treatment recommendations for extrapulmonary disease are usually similar with a few modifications. For example, the dosage of glucocorticoids is usually higher for neurosarcoidosis and lower for cutaneous disease. There was some suggestion that higher doses would be beneficial for cardiac sarcoidosis, but one study found

that initial doses >40 mg/d prednisone were associated with a worse outcome.

While most patients receive glucocorticoids as their initial systemic therapy, toxicity associated with prolonged therapy often leads to steroid-sparing alternatives. The antimalarial drugs such as hydroxychloroquine are more effective for skin than pulmonary disease. Minocycline may also be useful for cutaneous sarcoidosis. For pulmonary and other extrapulmonary disease, cytotoxic agents are often employed. These include methotrexate, azathioprine, chlorambucil, and cyclophosphamide. The most widely studied cytotoxic agent has been methotrexate. This agent works in approximately two-thirds of sarcoidosis patients, regardless of the disease manifestation. As noted in Table 322-2, specific guidelines for monitoring therapy have been recommended. Cytokine modulators such as thalidomide and pentoxifylline have also been used in a limited number of cases.

The anti-TNF agents have recently been studied in sarcoidosis, with prospective randomized trials of both etanercept and infliximab completed. Etanercept has a limited role as a steroid-sparing agent. On the other hand, infliximab significantly improves lung function when given to patients with chronic disease already on glucocorticoids and cytotoxic agents. The difference in response for these two agents is similar to that observed in Crohn's disease, where infliximab is effective and etanercept is not. In addition, increased risks for reactivation of tuberculosis are reported for infliximab compared to etanercept. The differential response rate could be explained by differences in mechanism of action since etanercept is a TNF receptor antagonist and infliximab is a monoclonal antibody against TNF. The peak dosage of the drug may also be different, since etanercept is given SC whereas infliximab is given IV. A higher peak dose may lead to better intracellular penetration and therefore affect the transmembrane TNF. In contrast to etanercept, infliximab binds to TNF on the surface of some cells that are releasing TNF and this can lead to cell lysis. This effect has been documented in Crohn's disease.

The role of the newer therapeutic agents for sarcoidosis is still evolving. However, these targeted therapies confirm that TNF may be an important target, especially in the treatment of chronic disease. However, the majority of cases either do not require therapy or can be controlled with glucocorticoids and cytotoxic agents.

MANAGEMENT ALGORITHM OF CHRONIC DISEASE

FIGURE 322-10 Approach to chronic disease is based on whether glucocorticoid therapy is tolerated or not.

TABLE 322-2   COMMONLY USED DRUGS TO TREAT SARCOIDOSIS

Drug	Initial Dose	Maintenance Dose	Monitoring	Toxicity	Support Therapy[a]	Support Monitoring[a]
Prednisone	20–40 mg qd	Taper to 5–10 mg	Glucose, blood pressure, bone density	Diabetes, osteoporosis	A: Acute pulmonary D: Extrapulmonary	
Hydroxychloroquine	200–400 mg qd	400 mg qd	Eye exam q6–12 mo	Ocular	B: Some forms of disease	D: Routine eye exam
Methotrexate	10 mg qw	2.5–15 mg qw	CBC, renal, hepatic q2mo	Hematologic, nausea, hepatic, pulmonary	B: Steroid sparing C: Some forms chronic disease	D: Routine hematologic, renal, and hepatic monitoring
Azathioprine	50–150 mg qd	50–200 mg qd	CBC, renal q2mo	Hematologic, nausea	C: Some forms chronic disease	D: Routine hematologic monitoring
Infliximab	3–5 mg/kg q2wk for 2 doses	3–10 mg/kg q4–8 wk	Initial PPD	Infections, allergic reaction, carcinogen	B: Chronic pulmonary disease	C: Caution in patients with latent tuberculosis or advanced congestive heart failure

[a]Grade A: supported by at least two double-blind randomized control trials; grade B: supported by prospective cohort studies; grade C: supported primarily by two or more retrospective studies; grade D: only one retrospective study or based on experience in other diseases.

Note: CBC, complete blood count; PPD, purified protein derivative test for tuberculosis.
Source: Adapted from Baughman and Selroos.

FURTHER READINGS

BAUGHMAN RP, SELROOS O: Evidence-based approach to treatment of sarcoidosis, in PG Gibson et al (eds): *Evidence-Based Respiratory Medicine*. Oxford, BMJ Books Blackwell, 2005, pp 491–508

——— et al: Clinical characteristics of patients in a case control study of sarcoidosis. Am J Respir Crit Care Med 164:1885, 2001

HUNNINGHAKE GW et al: ATS/ERS/WASOG statement on sarcoidosis. American Thoracic Society/European Respiratory Society/World Association of Sarcoidosis and other Granulomatous Disorders. Sarcoidosis Vasc Diffuse Lung Dis 16:149, 1999

JUDSON MA and the ACCESS Research group: Defining organ involvement in sarcoidosis: The ACCESS proposed instrument. Sarcoidosis Vasc Diffuse Lung Dis 16:75, 1999

NEWMAN LS et al: A case control etiologic study of sarcoidosis: Environmental and occupational risk factors. Am J Respir Crit Care Med 170:1324, 2004

ROSSMAN MD et al: HLA-DRB1*1101: A significant risk factor for sarcoidosis in blacks and whites. Am J Hum Genet 73:720, 2003

SATO H et al: HLA-DQB1*0201: A marker for good prognosis in British and Dutch patients with sarcoidosis. Am J Respir Cell Mol Biol 27:406, 2002

SONG Z et al: Mycobacterial catalase-peroxidase is a tissue antigen and target of the adaptive immune response in systemic sarcoidosis. J Exp Med 201:755, 2005

YEAGER H et al: Pulmonary and psychosocial findings at enrollment in the ACCESS study. Sarcoidosis Vasc Diffuse Lung Dis 22:147, 2005

ZIEGENHAGEN MW et al: Exaggerated TNF-alpha release of alveolar macrophages in corticosteroid resistant sarcoidosis. Sarcoidosis Vasc Diffuse Lung Dis 19:185, 2002

323 Familial Mediterranean Fever
Daniel L. Kastner

Familial Mediterranean fever (FMF) is the prototype of a group of inherited diseases (Table 323-1) that are characterized by recurrent episodes of fever with serosal, synovial, or cutaneous inflammation and, in some individuals, the eventual development of systemic AA amyloidosis (Chap. 324). Because of the relative infrequency of high-titer autoantibodies or antigen-specific T cells, the term *autoinflammatory* has been proposed to describe these disorders, rather than autoimmune.

BACKGROUND AND PATHOPHYSIOLOGY

FMF was first recognized among Armenians, Arabs, Turks, and non-Ashkenazi (primarily North African and Iraqi) Jews. With the advent of genetic testing, FMF has been documented with increasing frequency among Ashkenazi Jews and Italians, and occasional cases have been confirmed even in the absence of known Mediterranean ancestry. FMF is recessively inherited, but, particularly in countries where families are small, a positive family history can only be elicited in ~50% of cases. DNA testing demonstrates carrier frequencies as high as 1:3 among affected populations, suggesting a heterozygote advantage.

The FMF gene encodes a 781-amino acid, ~95 kDa protein denoted *pyrin* (or *marenostrin*) that is expressed in granulocytes, eosinophils, monocytes, dendritic cells, and synovial and peritoneal fibroblasts.

The N-terminal 92 amino acids of pyrin define a motif, the PYRIN domain, that is similar in structure to death domains, death effector domains, and caspase recruitment domains. PYRIN domains mediate homotypic protein-protein interactions and have been found in several other proteins, including cryopyrin, which is mutated in three other recurrent fever syndromes. Through a number of mechanisms, including the interaction of the PYRIN domain with an intermediary adaptor protein, pyrin regulates caspase-1 [interleukin (IL) 1β-converting enzyme], and thereby IL-1β secretion. Pyrin-deficient mice exhibit heightened sensitivity to endotoxin, excessive IL-1β production, and impaired monocyte apoptosis.

ACUTE ATTACKS

Febrile episodes in FMF may begin even in early infancy; 90% of patients have had their first attack by age 20. Typical FMF episodes generally last 24–72 h, with arthritic attacks tending to last somewhat longer. In some patients the episodes occur with great regularity, but more often the frequency of attacks varies over time, ranging from as often as once every few days to remissions lasting several years. Attacks are often unpredictable, although some patients relate them to physical exertion, emotional stress, or menses; pregnancy may be associated with remission.

If measured, fever is nearly always present throughout FMF attacks. Severe hyperpyrexia and even febrile seizures may be seen in infants, and fever is sometimes the only manifestation of FMF in young children.

Over 90% of FMF patients experience abdominal attacks at some time. Episodes range in severity from dull, aching pain and distention

TABLE 323-1 THE HEREDITARY PERIODIC FEVER SYNDROMES

	FMF	TRAPS	HIDS	MWS	FCAS	NOMID
Ethnicity	Jewish, Arab, Turkish, Armenian, Italian	Any ethnic group	Predominantly Dutch, northern European	Any ethnic group	Any ethnic group	Any ethnic group
Inheritance	Recessive	Dominant	Recessive	Dominant	Dominant	Usually de novo mutations
Gene/chromosome	MEFV/16p13.3	TNFRSF1A/12p13	MVK/12q24	CIAS1/1q44	CIAS1/1q44	CIAS1/1q44
Protein	Pyrin	p55 TNF receptor	Mevalonate kinase	Cryopyrin	Cryopyrin	Cryopyrin
Attack length	1–3 days	Often > 7 days	3–7 days	1–2 days	Minutes–3 days	Continuous, with flares
Serosa	Pleurisy, peritonitis; asymptomatic pericardial effusions	Pleurisy, peritonitis, pericarditis	Abd pain, but seldom peritonitis; pleurisy, pericarditis uncommon	Abd pain common; pleurisy, pericarditis rare	Rare	Rare
Skin	Erysipeloid erythema	Centrifugally migrating erythema	Diffuse maculopapular rash; oral ulcers	Diffuse urticaria-like rash	Cold-induced urticaria-like rash	Diffuse urticaria-like rash
Joints	Acute monoarthritis; chronic hip arthritis (rare)	Acute monoarthritis, arthralgia	Arthralgia, oligoarthritis	Arthralgia, large joint oligoarthritis	Polyarthralgia	Epiphyseal, patellar overgrowth, clubbing
Muscle	Exercise-induced myalgia common; protracted febrile myalgia rare	Migratory myalgia	Uncommon	Myalgia common	Sometimes myalgia	Sometimes myalgia
Eyes, ears	Uncommon	Periorbital edema, conjunctivitis, rarely uveitis	Uncommon	Conjunctivitis, episcleritis, optic disc edema; sensorineural hearing loss	Conjunctivitis	Conjunctivitis, uveitis, optic disc edema, blindness, sensorineural hearing loss
CNS	Aseptic meningitis rare	Headache	Headache	Headache	Headache	Aseptic meningitis, seizures
Amyloidosis	Most common in M694V homozygotes	~15% of cases	Not described	~25% of cases	Uncommon	Late complication
Treatment	Oral colchicine prophylaxis	Glucocorticoids, etanercept	NSAIDs for fever; IL-1β and TNF inhibitors investigational	Anakinra (IL-1 receptor antagonist)	Anakinra	Anakinra

Abbreviations: FMF, familial Mediterranean fever; TNF, tumor necrosis factor; TRAPS, TNF receptor–associated periodic syndrome; HIDS, hyperimmunoglobulin D with periodic fever syndrome; MWS, Muckle-Wells syndrome; FCAS, familial cold autoinflammatory syndrome; NOMID, neonatal-onset multisystem inflammatory disease; Abd, abdominal; CNS, central nervous system; NSAIDs, nonsteroidal anti-inflammatory drugs.

with mild tenderness on direct palpation to severe generalized pain with absent bowel sounds, rigidity, rebound tenderness, and air-fluid levels on upright radiographs. CT scanning may demonstrate a small amount of fluid in the abdominal cavity. If such patients undergo exploratory laparotomy, a sterile, neutrophil-rich peritoneal exudate is present, sometimes with adhesions from previous episodes. Ascites is rare.

Pleural attacks are usually manifested by unilateral, sharp, stabbing chest pain. Radiographs may show atelectasis and sometimes an effusion. If performed, thoracentesis demonstrates an exudative fluid rich in neutrophils. After repeated attacks, pleural thickening may develop.

FMF arthritis is most frequent among individuals homozygous for the M694V mutation, which is especially common in the non-Ashkenazi Jewish population. Acute arthritis in FMF is usually monoarticular, affecting the knee, ankle, or hip, although other patterns can be seen, particularly in children. Large sterile effusions rich in neutrophils are frequent, without commensurate erythema or warmth. Even after repeated arthritic attacks, radiographic changes are rare. Before the advent of colchicine prophylaxis, chronic arthritis of the knee or hip were seen in ~5% of FMF patients with arthritis. Chronic sacroiliitis can occur in FMF irrespective of the HLA-B27 antigen, even in the face of colchicine therapy. In the United States, FMF patients are much more likely to have arthralgia than arthritis.

The most characteristic cutaneous manifestation of FMF is erysipelas-like erythema, a raised erythematous rash that most commonly occurs on the dorsum of the foot, ankle, or lower leg, alone or in combination with abdominal pain, pleurisy, or arthritis. Biopsy demonstrates perivascular infiltrates of granulocytes and monocytes. This rash is seen most often in M694V homozygotes and is relatively rare in the United States.

Exercise-induced (nonfebrile) myalgia is common in FMF, and a small percentage of patients develop a protracted febrile myalgia that can last several weeks. Symptomatic pericardial disease is rare, although some patients have small pericardial effusions as an incidental echocardiographic finding. Unilateral acute scrotal inflammation may occur in prepubertal boys. Aseptic meningitis has been reported in FMF but the causal connection is controversial. Vasculitis, including Henoch-Schönlein purpura and polyarteritis nodosum (Chap. 319) may be seen at increased frequency in FMF.

Laboratory features of FMF attacks are consistent with acute inflammation and include an elevated erythrocyte sedimentation rate, leukocytosis, thrombocytosis (in children), and elevations in C-reactive protein, fibrinogen, haptoglobin, and serum immunoglobulins. Transient albuminuria and hematuria may also be seen.

AMYLOIDOSIS

Before the advent of colchicine prophylaxis, systemic amyloidosis was a common complication of FMF. It is caused by deposition of a fragment of serum amyloid A, an acute-phase reactant, in the kidneys, adrenals, intestine, spleen, lung, and testes (Chap. 324). Amyloidosis should be suspected in patients who have proteinuria between attacks; renal or rectal biopsy are used most often to establish the diagnosis. Risk factors include the M694V homozygous genotype, positive family history (independent of FMF mutational status), the SAA 1 genotype, male gender, noncompliance with colchicine therapy, and having grown up in the Middle East.

DIAGNOSIS

For typical cases, physicians experienced with FMF can often make the diagnosis on clinical grounds alone. Clinical criteria sets for FMF have

CHAPTER 323 Familial Mediterranean Fever

been shown to have high sensitivity and specificity in parts of the world where the pretest probability of FMF is high. Genetic testing can provide a useful adjunct in ambiguous cases or for physicians not experienced in FMF. Most of the disease-associated FMF mutations are in exon 10 of the gene, with a smaller group of mutations in exon 2. An updated list of mutations for FMF and other hereditary periodic fevers can be found online at *http://fmf.igh.cnrs.fr/infevers/*.

Genetic testing has permitted a broadening of the clinical spectrum and geographic distribution of FMF and may be of prognostic value. Most studies indicate that M694V homozygotes have an earlier age of onset and a higher frequency of arthritis, rash, and amyloidosis. In contrast, the E148Q mutation is usually associated with milder disease. E148Q is sometimes found in *cis* with exon 10 mutations, which complicates the interpretation of genetic test results. Only ~70% of patients with clinically typical FMF have two identifiable mutations in *trans*, suggesting either that current screening methods do not detect all of the relevant mutations or that one mutation may be sufficient to cause disease under some circumstances. In these cases clinical judgment is very important, and sometimes a therapeutic trial of colchicine may help to confirm the diagnosis. Genetic testing of unaffected individuals is usually inadvisable, because of the possibility of nonpenetrance and the potential impact of a positive test on future insurability.

If a patient is seen during his or her first attack, the differential diagnosis may be broad, although delimited by the specific organ involvement. After several attacks the differential diagnosis may include the other hereditary periodic fever syndromes (Table 323-1); the syndrome of periodic fever with aphthous ulcers, pharyngitis, and cervical adenopathy (PFAPA); systemic-onset juvenile rheumatoid arthritis or adult Still's disease; porphyria; hereditary angioedema; inflammatory bowel disease; and, in women, gynecologic disorders.

℞ FAMILIAL MEDITERRANEAN FEVER

The treatment of choice for FMF is daily oral colchicine, which decreases the frequency and intensity of attacks and prevents the development of amyloidosis in compliant patients. Intermittent dosing at the onset of attacks is not as effective as daily prophylaxis and is of unproven value in preventing amyloidosis. The usual adult dose of colchicine is 1.2–1.8 mg/d, which causes substantial reduction in symptoms in two-thirds of patients and some improvement in >90%. Children may require lower doses, although not proportionately to body weight.

Common side effects of colchicine include bloating, abdominal cramps, lactose intolerance, and diarrhea. They can be minimized by starting at a low dose and gradually advancing as tolerated, splitting the dose, use of simethecone for flatulence, and avoidance of dairy products. If taken by either parent at the time of conception, colchicine may cause a small increase in the risk of trisomy 21 (Down syndrome). In elderly patients with renal insufficiency, colchicine can cause a myoneuropathy characterized by proximal muscle weakness and elevation of the creatine kinase. Cyclosporine inhibits hepatic excretion of colchicine by its effects on the MDR-1 transport system, sometimes leading to colchicine toxicity in patients who have undergone renal transplantation for amyloidosis. Intravenous colchicine should generally not be administered to patients already taking oral colchicine, because severe, sometimes fatal, toxicity can occur in this setting.

There are no established alternatives for the small number of patients who do not respond to colchicine or cannot tolerate therapeutic dosages, although the IL-1 receptor antagonist and inhibitors of interferon-α and tumor necrosis factor (TNF) are investigational. Bone marrow transplantation has been suggested for refractory FMF, but the risk-benefit ratio is currently regarded as unacceptable.

OTHER HEREDITARY RECURRENT FEVERS

Within 5 years of the discovery of the FMF gene, three additional genes causing five other hereditary periodic fever syndromes were identified, catalyzing a paradigm shift in diagnosis and treatment of these disorders.

TNF RECEPTOR–ASSOCIATED PERIODIC SYNDROME (TRAPS) TRAPS is caused by dominantly inherited mutations in the extracellular domains of the 55-kDa TNF receptor (TNFRSF1A, p55). Although originally described in a large Irish family (and hence the name *familial Hibernian fever*), TRAPS has a broad ethnic distribution. TRAPS episodes often begin in childhood. The duration of attacks ranges from 1–2 days to as long as several weeks, and in severe cases symptoms may be nearly continuous. In addition to peritoneal, pleural, and synovial attacks similar to FMF, TRAPS patients frequently have ocular inflammation (most often conjunctivitis and/or periorbital edema), and a distinctive migratory myalgia with overlying painful erythema may be present. TRAPS patients generally respond better to glucocorticoids than to prophylactic colchicine. About 15% develop amyloidosis. The diagnosis of TRAPS is based on the demonstration of *TNFRSF1A* mutations in the presence of characteristic symptoms. Leukocytes from patients with certain TRAPS mutations exhibit a defect in TNF receptor-shedding, possibly impairing normal homeostasis. However, a more complex picture is emerging, with a number of functional abnormalities, some of which are ligand-independent, contributing to the autoinflammatory phenotype. Etanercept, a TNF inhibitor, ameliorates TRAPS attacks, although its effect on amyloidosis is unproven.

Hyperimmunoglobulinemia D with Periodic Fever Syndrome (HIDS)

HIDS is a recessively inherited recurrent fever syndrome found primarily in individuals of northern European ancestry. It is caused by mutations in mevalonate kinase (*MVK*), encoding an enzyme involved in the synthesis of cholesterol and nonsterol isoprenoids. Attacks usually begin in infancy, and last 3–5 days. Clinically distinctive features include painful cervical adenopathy, a diffuse maculopapular rash sometimes affecting the palms and soles, and aphthous ulcers; pleurisy is rare, as is amyloidosis. Although originally defined by the persistent elevation of serum IgD, disease activity is not related to IgD levels, and some patients with FMF or TRAPS may have modestly increased serum IgD. Moreover, occasional patients with *MVK* mutations and periodic fever have normal IgD levels. All patients with mutations have markedly elevated urinary mevalonate levels during their febrile attacks, although the inflammatory manifestations are likely to be due to a deficiency of isoprenoids rather than an excess of mevalonate. There is currently no established treatment for HIDS.

The Cryopyrinopathies Three hereditary febrile syndromes, familial cold autoinflammatory syndrome (FCAS), Muckle-Wells syndrome (MWS), and neonatal-onset multisystem inflammatory disease (NOMID), are all caused by mutations in *CIAS1*, the gene encoding cryopyrin (or NALP3), and represent a clinical spectrum of disease. FCAS patients develop chills, fever, headache, arthralgia, conjunctivitis, and an urticaria-like rash in response to generalized cold exposure. In MWS, an urticarial rash is noted, but it is not usually induced by cold; MWS patients also develop fevers, abdominal pain, limb pain, arthritis, conjunctivitis, and, over time, sensorineural hearing loss. NOMID is the most severe of the three disorders, with chronic aseptic meningitis, a characteristic arthropathy, and rash. Like the FMF protein, pyrin, cryopyrin has an N-terminal PYRIN domain. Cryopyrin regulates IL-1β production through the formation of a macromolecular complex termed the *inflammasome*. Macrophages from cryopyrin-deficient mice exhibit decreased IL-1β production in response to certain Gram-positive bacteria, bacterial RNA, and monosodium urate crystals. Patients with all three cryopyrinopathies show a dramatic response to daily injections of anakinra, the IL-1 receptor antagonist.

FURTHER READINGS

HOFFMAN HM et al: Prevention of cold-associated acute inflammation in familial cold autoinflammatory syndrome by interleukin-1 receptor antagonist. Lancet 364:1779, 2004

HULL KM et al: The TNF receptor–associated periodic syndrome (TRAPS). Emerging concepts of an autoinflammatory disorder. Medicine (Baltimore) 81:349, 2002

LOBITO AA et al: Abnormal disulfide-linked oligomerization results in ER retention and altered signaling by TNFR1 mutants in

TNFR1-associated periodic fever syndrome (TRAPS). Blood 108:1320, 2006

MANDEY SH et al: A role for geranylgeranylation in interleukin-1β secretion. Arthritis Rheum 54:3690, 2006

MARIATHASAN S, MONACK DM: Inflammasome adaptors and sensors: Intracellular regulators of infection and inflammation. Nat Rev Immunol 7:31, 2007

MASTERS SL et al: Recent advances in the molecular pathogenesis of hereditary recurrent fevers. Curr Opin Allergy Clin Immunol 6:428, 2006

324 Amyloidosis
David C. Seldin, Martha Skinner

GENERAL PRINCIPLES

Amyloidosis is a term for diseases that are due to the extracellular deposition of insoluble polymeric protein fibrils in tissues and organs. These diseases are a subset of a growing group of disorders caused by misfolding of proteins. Among these are Alzheimer's disease and other neurodegenerative diseases, transmissible prion diseases, and some genetic diseases caused by mutations that lead to misfolding and protein loss of function, such as certain of the cystic fibrosis mutations. Amyloid fibrils share a common β-pleated sheet structural conformation that confers unique staining properties. The name *amyloid* is attributed to the pathologist Virchow, who in 1854 thought such deposits were cellulose-like.

Amyloid diseases are defined by the biochemical nature of the protein in the fibril deposits and are classified according to whether they are systemic or localized, acquired or inherited, and by their clinical patterns (Table 324-1). The accepted nomenclature is *AX*, where *A* indicates amyloidosis and *X* represents the protein in the fibril. *AL* is amyloid composed of immunoglobulin (Ig) light chains (LCs), and is called *primary systemic amyloidosis*; it arises from a clonal B cell disorder, usually myeloma. *AF* groups the familial amyloidoses, most commonly due to transthyretin, the transport protein for thyroid hormone and retinol binding protein. *AA* amyloid is composed of the acute phase reactant serum amyloid A protein and occurs in the setting of chronic inflammatory or infectious diseases. The disease associated with AA amyloid is called *secondary amyloidosis*. *Aβ₂M* is amyloid composed of β₂-microglobulin and occurs in individuals with end-stage renal disease (ESRD) of long duration. *Aβ* is the most common form of localized amyloidosis. Aβ is in the brain in Alzheimer's disease and is derived from abnormal proteolytic processing of the amyloid precursor protein (APP).

Diagnosis and treatment of the amyloidoses rests upon the pathologic diagnosis of amyloid deposits and immunohistochemical or biochemical identification of amyloid type (Fig. 324-1). In the systemic amyloidoses, the involved organs can be biopsied, but amyloid deposits may be found in any tissue of the body. Historically, blood vessels of the gingiva or rectal mucosa were examined, but the most easily accessible tissue, positive in more than 80% of patients with systemic amyloid, is fat. After local anesthesia, needle aspiration of fat from the abdominal wall can be expelled onto a slide and stained, avoiding even a minor surgical procedure. If this material is negative, kidney biopsy, endomyocardial biopsy, liver biopsy, or an endoscopic biopsy can be consid-

ered. The regular β sheet structure of amyloid deposits exhibit a unique green birefringence by polarized light microscopy when stained with Congo red dye; the 10-nm diameter fibrils can be seen by electron microscopy. Once amyloid is found, the protein type must be determined, usually by immunohistochemistry or immunoelectron microscopy. Careful evaluation of the patient profile and clinical presentation, including age and ethnic origin, organ system involvement, underlying diseases, and family history should provide a clue to the type of amyloid.

The mechanisms of fibril formation and tissue toxicity remain controversial. A common underlying mechanism involves formation of intermolecular dimers by trans β sheet interactions of partially unfolded APP, leading to the formation of multimers and higher-order polymers. Factors that contribute to fibrillogenesis include variant or unstable protein structure; extensive β-sheet conformation of the precursor protein; proteolytic processing of the precursor protein; association with components of the serum or extracellular matrix (e.g., amyloid P-component, "amyloid enhancing factor" in spleen extracts,

TABLE 324-1 AMYLOID FIBRIL PROTEINS AND THEIR PRECURSORS

Amyloid Protein	Precursor	Systemic (S) or Localized (L)	Syndrome or Involved Tissues
AL	Immunoglobulin light chain	S, L	Primary Myeloma-associated
AH	Immunoglobulin heavy chain	S, L	Primary Myeloma-associated
ATTR	Transthyretin	S	Familial Senile systemic
		L?	Tenosynovium
Aβ₂M	β₂-microglobulin	S	Hemodialysis
		L?	Joints
AA	(Apo)serum AA	S	Secondary, reactive
AApoAI	Apolipoprotein AI	S	Familial
		L	Aortic
AApoAII	Apolipoprotein AII	S	Familial
AGel	Gelsolin	S	Familial
ALys	Lysozyme	S	Familial
AFib	Fibrinogen α-chain	S	Familial
ACys	Cystatin C	S	Familial
ABri[a]	ABriPP	L, S?	Familial dementia, British
ADan[a]	*ADanPP*	*L*	*Familial dementia, Danish*
Aβ	Aβ protein precursor (AβPP)	L	Alzheimer's disease, aging
APrP	Prion protein	L	Spongiform encephalopathies
ACal	(Pro)calcitonin	L	C-cell thyroid tumors
AIAPP	Islet amyloid polypeptide	L	Islets of Langerhans Insulinomas
AANF	Atrial natriuretic factor	L	Cardiac atria
APro	Prolactin	L	Aging pituitary Prolactinomas
AIns	Insulin	L	Iatrogenic
AMed	Lactadherin	L	Senile aortic, media
AKer	Kerato-epithelin	L	Cornea; familial
A(tbn)[b]	*tbn[b]*	*L*	*Pindborg tumors*
ALac	*Lactoferrin*	*L*	*Cornea; familial*

[a]ADan is coming from the same gene as ABri and has identical N-terminal sequence. It will be a matter of further discussion whether ADan should be included in the nomenclature as a separate protein (see text).
[b]To be named.

Note: Proteins in italics are preliminary.

Source: Reprinted from P Westermark et al: A primer of amyloid nomenclature. Amyloid 14(3):179–183, 2007. With permission from Taylor & Francis Ltd. (*http://www.tandf.co.uk/journals*).

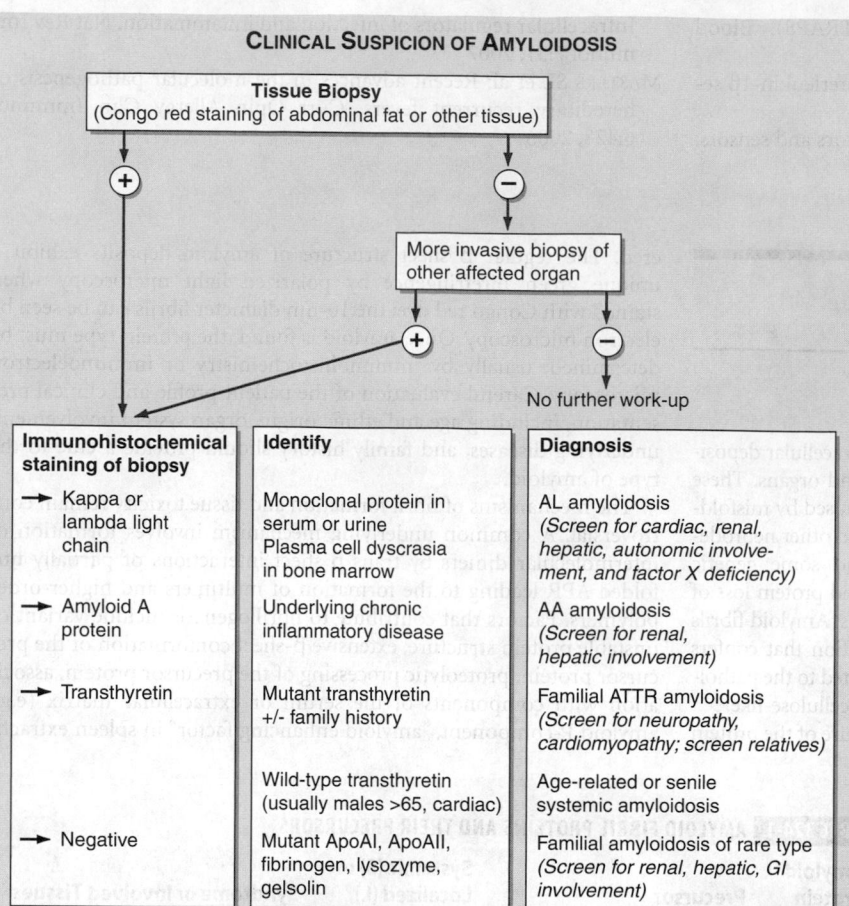

CLINICAL SUSPICION OF AMYLOIDOSIS

Tissue Biopsy
(Congo red staining of abdominal fat or other tissue)

(+) (−)

More invasive biopsy of other affected organ

(+) (−)

No further work-up

Immunohistochemical staining of biopsy	Identify	Diagnosis
→ Kappa or lambda light chain	Monoclonal protein in serum or urine Plasma cell dyscrasia in bone marrow	AL amyloidosis *(Screen for cardiac, renal, hepatic, autonomic involvement, and factor X deficiency)*
→ Amyloid A protein	Underlying chronic inflammatory disease	AA amyloidosis *(Screen for renal, hepatic involvement)*
→ Transthyretin	Mutant transthyretin +/- family history	Familial ATTR amyloidosis *(Screen for neuropathy, cardiomyopathy; screen relatives)*
	Wild-type transthyretin (usually males >65, cardiac)	Age-related or senile systemic amyloidosis
→ Negative	Mutant ApoAl, ApoAll, fibrinogen, lysozyme, gelsolin	Familial amyloidosis of rare type *(Screen for renal, hepatic, GI involvement)*

FIGURE 324-1 Algorithm for the diagnosis of amyloidosis and determination of type: Clinical suspicion: unexplained nephropathy, cardiomyopathy, neuropathy, enteropathy, arthropathy, and macroglossia. ApoAl, apolipoprotein Al; ApoAll, apolipoprotein All; GI, gastrointestinal.

apolipoprotein E, or glycosaminoglycans); and local physical properties, including pH of the tissue. Once the fibrils reach a critical size, they become insoluble and deposit in extracellular tissue sites. These macromolecular deposits interfere with organ function, at least in part due to cellular uptake of oligomeric amyloid precursors producing toxicity to target cells.

The clinical syndromes of the amyloidoses are associated with relatively nonspecific alterations in routine laboratory tests. Blood counts are usually normal, although the erythrocyte sedimentation rate is frequently elevated. Patients with renal involvement will usually have proteinuria, which can be as much as 30 g/d, producing hypoalbuminemia lower than 1 g/dL. Patients with cardiac involvement will often have elevation of brain naturietic peptide (BNP), pro-BNP, and troponin. These can be useful for monitoring disease activity and have been proposed as prognostic factors; they can be falsely elevated in the presence of renal insufficiency. Patients with liver involvement, even when it is advanced, usually develop cholestasis with an elevated alkaline phosphatase but minimal elevation of the transaminases and preservation of synthetic function. In AL amyloidosis, endocrinopathies can occur, with laboratory testing demonstrating hypothyroidism, hypoadrenalism, or even hypopituitarism. These findings are not specific for amyloidosis. Diagnosis of amyloidosis rests upon two pillars: the identification of fibrillar deposits in tissues and the typing of the amyloid.

AL AMYLOIDOSIS

ETIOLOGY AND INCIDENCE

AL amyloidosis is most frequently caused by a clonal expansion of plasma cells in the bone marrow that secrete a clonal Ig LC that deposits as

amyloid fibrils in tissues. It may be purely serendipitous whether the clonal plasma cells produce an LC that misfolds and produces AL amyloidosis, or folds properly allowing the cells to inexorably expand over time and develop into multiple myeloma (Chap. 106). It is also possible that the two processes have differing molecular etiologies. AL amyloidosis can occur in multiple myeloma and other B lymphoproliferative diseases, including non-Hodgkin's lymphoma (Chap. 105) and Waldenstrom's macroglobulinemia (Chap. 106). AL amyloidosis is the most common type of systemic amyloidosis in North America. Its incidence has been estimated at 4.5 per 100,000; however, ascertainment continues to be inadequate, and the true incidence may be much higher. AL amyloidosis, like other plasma cell diseases, usually occurs after age 40 and is often rapidly progressive and fatal if untreated. It occurs in about 15% of myelomas. About 20% of all patients with AL amyloidosis have myeloma; the rest have other B cell disorders.

DIAGNOSIS

Identification of a clonal plasma cell dyscrasia distinguishes AL from other types of amyloidosis. More than 90% of patients have a serum or urine monoclonal Ig protein that can be detected by immunofixation electrophoresis (Fig. 324-2A) or free light chain assay. The standard serum protein electrophoresis (SPEP) and urine protein electrophoresis (UPEP) are not useful screening tests because the clonal Ig in AL amyloidosis, unlike in multiple myeloma, is often not present in sufficient quantity in the serum to produce a monoclonal "M-spike" by these tests. A commercially available nephelometric assay accurately quantifies abnormal LCs that circulate free of heavy chains in both multiple myeloma and AL amyloidosis. In AL, elevated levels of free LCs with a shift in the normal ratio of free kappa to lambda is seen in 75% of patients. Lambda LCs are more common than kappa LCs in AL amyloidosis. Examining the ratio is essential because in renal failure free light chain clearance is reduced, and both types of LCs will be elevated. In addition, an increased percentage of plasma cells in the bone marrow is noted in about 90% of patients; those cells are monoclonal by immunohistochemical staining for kappa and lambda (Fig. 324-2B), or by fluorescence-activated cell sorter. However, a monoclonal serum protein by itself is not diagnostic of amyloidosis, since monoclonal gammopathy of uncertain significance (MGUS) is common in older patients (Chap. 106). However, when MGUS is present in a patient with biopsy-proven amyloidosis, the AL type is strongly suspected. Immunohistochemical staining of the amyloid deposits is useful if they bind one light chain antibody in preference to the other; some AL deposits bind many antisera nonspecifically. Immunoelectron microscopy can be more reliable but is not widely available. Mass spectrometry-based microsequencing of small amounts of protein extracted from fibril deposits may ultimately be the most reliable way to identify the components of the fibrils. In ambiguous cases, other forms of amyloidosis should be thoroughly excluded.

PATHOLOGY AND CLINICAL FEATURES

Amyloid deposits are usually widespread in AL amyloidosis and can be present in the interstitium of any organ except the central nervous system. The amyloid fibril deposits are composed of intact 23 kDa monoclonal Ig LCs or smaller fragments, 11–18 kDa in size, representing the variable (V) region alone, or the V region and a portion of the constant (C) region. Although all kappa and lambda LC subtypes have been identified in AL amyloid fibrils, lambda subtypes predominate,

FIGURE 324-2 Laboratory features of AL amyloidosis. A. Serum immunofixation electrophoresis reveals an IgGκ monoclonal protein; the serum protein electrophoresis is often normal. **B.** Bone marrow biopsy specimen in another patient, stained with antibody to λ light chain and developed with horseradish peroxidase, exhibits clonotypic λ-positive plasma cells (400x); antibody staining for κ would reveal few or no κ-positive cells. *(Photomicrograph courtesy of C. O'Hara; with permission.)*

and the lambda VI subtype appears to have unique structural properties that predispose it to fibril formation, often in the kidney.

AL amyloidosis is usually a rapidly progressive disease that presents with characteristic clinical syndromes, recognition of which is key to making the diagnosis. Initial symptoms of fatigue and weight loss are common, but the diagnosis is rarely made until symptoms referable to a specific organ appear. The kidneys are the most frequently affected organ (80%). Renal amyloidosis is usually manifested by proteinuria,

which is often in the nephrotic range and associated with significant hypoalbuminemia and edema or anasarca; rarely, tubular rather than glomerular deposition of amyloid can produce azotemia without significant proteinuria. Cardiac symptoms are the second most common presentation (40%), but cardiac dysfunction is associated with death in 75% of patients. The electrocardiogram may show low voltage with a pseudo-infarct pattern. With significant cardiac involvement, the echocardiogram will display concentrically thickened ventricles (the interventricular septal thickness is a useful parameter to monitor) and diastolic dysfunction; however, systolic function is preserved until late in the disease. Nervous system features include a peripheral sensory neuropathy (18%), carpal tunnel syndrome (25%), and/or autonomic dysfunction with gastrointestinal motility disturbances (early satiety, diarrhea, constipation) and orthostatic hypotension (16%). Macroglossia, with an enlarged, indented, or immobile tongue, is pathognomonic of AL amyloidosis and is seen in 10% of patients. Hepatomegaly, seen in 34% of patients, may be massive with cholestatic liver function abnormalities, although liver failure is uncommon. The spleen is frequently involved, and there may be functional hyposplenism in the absence of significant splenomegaly. Many patients report "easy bruising" due to amyloid deposits in capillaries and deficiency of clotting factor X; cutaneous ecchymoses appear, particularly around the eyes, giving the "raccoon-eyes" sign. Other findings include nail dystrophy, alopecia, and amyloid arthropathy with thickening of synovial membranes (**Fig. 324-3**).

℞ AL AMYLOIDOSIS

Extensive multisystem involvement typifies AL amyloidosis, and median survival with no treatment is usually about one year from the time of diagnosis. Current therapies target the clonal bone marrow plasma cells using approaches employed for multiple myeloma. Treatment with cyclic oral melphalan and prednisone can decrease the plasma cell burden but produces complete hematologic remission in only a few percent of patients and minimal organ responses and improvement in survival (median 2 years). The substitution of pulses of high-dose dexamethasone for prednisone produces a higher response rate and more durable remissions, although dexamethasone is not always well tolerated by patients with significant edema or cardiac disease. High-dose intravenous melphalan followed by autologous stem cell transplantation is far more effective than oral melphalan and prednisone. Complete hematologic response rates are about 40%, as measured by complete loss of clonal plasma cells in the bone marrow and disappearance of the monoclonal LC by immunofixation electrophoresis. In patients without a complete hematologic response, a significant improvement is often seen in hematologic parameters. Similar rates of improvement are seen in organ function and quality of life, with an extended survival exceeding that previously seen in this disease. The complete hematologic responses appear to be more durable than those seen in multiple myeloma and may even signal cure, as remissions of more than 10 years are documented. Unfortunately, only about half of AL amyloidosis patients are eligible for such aggressive treatment, and even at specialized treatment centers, peritransplant mortality is higher than for other hematologic diseases because of impaired organ function. Amy-

FIGURE 324-3 Clinical signs of AL amyloidosis. A. Macroglossia. **B.** Periorbital ecchymoses. **C.** Fingernail dystrophy.

loid cardiomyopathy, poor nutritional status, impaired performance status, and multiple-organ disease contribute to excess morbidity and mortality. The bleeding diathesis due to adsorption of clotting factor X to amyloid fibrils also confers high mortality during myelosuppressive therapy; however, this syndrome occurs in only a few percent of patients. Age alone, or renal insufficiency, does not have a major impact on morbidity or outcome, and these factors alone should not exclude patients from such treatment. In selected patients, tandem transplantation may offer an even higher rate of hematologic response.

For patients with impaired cardiac function or arrhythmias due to amyloid involvement of the myocardium, median survival is only about 6 months without treatment, and stem cell mobilization and high-dose chemotherapy are dangerous. In these patients, cardiac transplantation can be performed, followed by treatment with high-dose melphalan and stem cell rescue to prevent amyloid deposition in the transplanted heart or other organs. Thalidomide and lenalidomide have activity; lenalidomide is reasonably well-tolerated and, particularly in combination with dexamethasone, produces complete hematologic remissions and improvement in organ function. Novel agents such as the proteasome inhibitor bortezomib are also under investigation for AL amyloidosis.

Supportive care is important for patients with any type of amyloidosis. For nephrotic syndrome, diuretics and supportive stockings can ameliorate edema; angiotensin-converting enzyme inhibitors should be used with caution and have not been shown to slow renal disease progression. Congestive heart failure due to amyloid cardiomyopathy is also best treated with diuretics; it is important to note that digitalis, calcium channel blockers, and beta blockers are relatively contraindicated as they can interact with amyloid fibrils and produce heart block and worsening heart failure. Amiodarone has been used for atrial and ventricular arrhythmias. Automatic implantable defibrillators have reduced effectiveness due to the thickened myocardium. Atrial ablation is another effective approach for atrial fibrillation. For conduction abnormalities, ventricular pacing may be indicated. Atrial contractile dysfunction is common in amyloid cardiomyopathy, and is an indication for anticoagulation. Autonomic neuropathy can be treated with α agonists such as midodrine to support the blood pressure; gastrointestinal dysfunction may respond to motility or bulk agents. Nutritional supplementation, either orally or parenterally, is also important.

In localized AL, amyloid deposits can be produced by clonal plasma cells infiltrating local sites in the airways, bladder, skin, or lymph nodes (Table 324-1). Deposits may respond to surgical intervention or radiation therapy; systemic treatment is generally not appropriate. Patients should be referred to a center familiar with management of these rare manifestations of amyloidosis.

AA AMYLOIDOSIS

ETIOLOGY AND INCIDENCE

AA amyloidosis can occur in association with almost any of the chronic inflammatory states (e.g., rheumatoid arthritis, lupus, Crohn's disease) or chronic infections such as tuberculosis or subacute bacterial endocarditis. In the United States and Europe, AA amyloidosis has become uncommon, occurring in <1% of patients with these diseases, perhaps because of advances in anti-inflammatory and antimicrobial therapies. Nonetheless, in Finland AA amyloidosis was reported to be the most common cause of nephrotic syndrome in patients with rheumatoid arthritis. AA amyloidosis is more common in Turkey and the Middle East, where it occurs in association with familial Mediterranean fever (Chap. 323). It is the only type of systemic amyloidosis that occurs in children.

PATHOLOGY AND CLINICAL FEATURES

Deposits are more limited in AA amyloidosis than in AL amyloidosis; they usually begin in the kidneys. Hepatomegaly, splenomegaly, and autonomic neuropathy can occur as the disease progresses; cardiomyopathy occurs rarely. The symptoms and signs are similar to those described for AL amyloidosis. The AA amyloid fibrils are usually composed of an 8-kDa, 76 amino acid N-terminal portion of a 12-kDa precursor protein, serum amyloid A (SAA). SAA is an acute-phase apoprotein synthesized in the liver and transported by high-density li-

poprotein, HDL3, in the plasma. Several years of an underlying inflammatory disease causing chronic elevation of SAA usually precedes fibril formation, although infections can produce AA deposition more quickly. In mouse models and perhaps in people, AA fibril formation can be accelerated by an amyloid enhancing factor present in high concentration in the spleen (which may be early SAA aggregates or deposits), by basement membrane heparan sulfate proteoglycan, or by seeding with AA or heterologous fibrils.

℞ AA AMYLOIDOSIS

The primary therapy in AA amyloidosis is treatment of the underlying inflammatory or infectious disease. Treatment that suppresses or eliminates the inflammation or infection also decreases the SAA protein concentration. For familial Mediterranean fever, colchicine in a dose of 1.2–1.8 mg/d is the appropriate treatment. Colchicine has not been helpful for AA amyloidosis of other causes or for other amyloidoses. A multicenter randomized phase III trial has recently been completed using eprodisate, designed to interfere with the interaction of AA amyloid protein with glycosaminoglycans in tissues and thus prevent or disrupt fibril formation. This drug is well tolerated and appears to markedly delay progression of AA renal disease, regardless of the underlying inflammatory process. Eprodisate is the first targeted inhibitor for diseases of protein misfolding and deposition to become available to patients.

AF AMYLOIDOSIS

The inherited AF amyloidoses are autosomal dominant diseases in which a variant plasma protein forms amyloid deposits, beginning in midlife. These diseases are rare, with an estimated incidence of <1 per 100,000. The most common form of AF is caused by mutation of the abundant plasma protein transthyretin (TTR, also known as *prealbumin*). More than 100 TTR mutations are known, and most are associated with ATTR amyloidosis. One variant, Ile122, has a carrier frequency that may be as high as 4% in the African-American population and is associated with late-onset cardiac amyloidosis. The actual incidence of disease in the African-American population is the subject of ongoing clinical research, but it would be wise to consider this in the differential diagnosis of African-American patients who present with concentric cardiac hypertrophy and evidence of diastolic dysfunction, whether or not they have a history of hypertension. Even wild-type TTR can form fibrils, leading to so-called senile systemic amyloidosis (SSA) in older patients. It can be found in up to 25% of autopsies in patients over age 80, and it can produce a clinical syndrome of amyloid cardiomyopathy that is similar to that occurring in younger patients with mutant TTR. Other familial amyloidoses, caused by variant apolipoproteins AI or AII, gelsolin, fibrinogen Aα, or lysozyme, are reported in only a few families worldwide.

In ATTR and in other forms of familial amyloidosis, the variant structure of the precursor protein is the key factor in fibril formation. The role of aging is intriguing, since patients born with the variant proteins do not have clinically apparent disease until middle age, despite the lifelong presence of the abnormal protein. Further evidence of an age-related "trigger" is the occurrence of SSA in the elderly, caused by the deposition of fibrils derived from normal TTR.

CLINICAL FEATURES

AF amyloidosis has a variable presentation but is usually consistent within affected kindreds with the same mutant protein. A family history makes AF more likely, but many patients present sporadically with new mutations. ATTR usually presents as a syndrome of familial amyloidotic polyneuropathy or familial amyloidotic cardiomyopathy; within a family, the age of disease onset is usually consistent. Peripheral neuropathy begins as a lower-extremity sensory and motor neuropathy and progresses to the upper extremities. Autonomic neuropathy is manifest by gastrointestinal symptoms of diarrhea with weight loss and orthostatic hypotension. Patients with TTR Met-30, the commonest mutation, have normal echocardiograms but may have conduction defects and require a pacemaker. Patients with TTR Ala-60 and several other mutations have myocardial thickening similar to that caused by AL amyloidosis, although heart failure is less common and the prognosis is better. Vitreous opacities caused by amyloid deposits are pathognomonic of ATTR amyloidosis.

Other AF syndromes include those associated with inherited mutations in apolipoprotein AI (AApoAI), apolipoprotein AII (AApoAII), fibrinogen (AFib), lysozyme (ALys), and gelsolin (AGel) that cause amyloid fibril deposition. These are very rare disorders with slowly progressing dysfunction of kidneys, liver, gastrointestinal tract, and, in the case of gelsolin, abnormalities of the cranial nerves and cornea.

Patients with AF amyloidosis can present with clinical syndromes that mimic those of patients with AL. Patients who do not have a plasma cell disorder should be screened for AF. This is particularly important in ethnic populations with a high carrier frequency of AF alleles (e.g., patients of Portuguese decent, African Americans). Variant TTR proteins can usually be detected by isoelectric focusing, but DNA sequencing is the gold standard for diagnosis for ATTR and the other AF mutations.

℞ ATTR AMYLOIDOSIS

Without intervention, survival after ATTR disease onset is 5–15 years. Orthotopic liver transplantation removes the major source of variant TTR production and replaces it with a source of normal TTR; it also arrests disease progression and leads to improvement in autonomic and peripheral neuropathy in some patients. Cardiomyopathy often does not improve, and in some patients it can worsen after liver transplantation, perhaps due to deposition of wild-type TTR as seen in SSA. Compounds have been identified that stabilize TTR in a non-pathogenic tetrameric conformation. The first of these, diflunisal, is being studied in a multicenter phase III trial, and screens for other agents are ongoing.

Aβ_2M AMYLOIDOSIS

Aβ_2M amyloidosis is composed of β_2-microglobulin, the invariant chain of class I human leukocyte antigens, and produces rheumatologic manifestations in patients on long-term hemodialysis. β_2-microglobulin is excreted by the kidney, and levels become elevated in ESRD. The molecular mass of β_2M is 11.8 kDa, above the molecular mass cutoff of some dialysis membranes. The incidence of this disease appears to be declining with newer dialysis techniques.

Aβ_2M amyloidosis usually presents with carpal tunnel syndrome, persistent joint effusions, spondyloarthropathy, and cystic bone lesions. Carpal tunnel syndrome is often the first symptom of disease. In the past, persistent joint effusions accompanied by mild discomfort had been seen in up to 50% of patients on dialysis for more than 12

years. Involvement is bilateral, and large joints (shoulders, knees, wrists, and hips) are more frequently affected. The synovial fluid is non-inflammatory, and β_2M amyloid deposits can be found if the sediment is stained with Congo red. Although less common, visceral β_2M amyloid deposits do occasionally occur in the gastrointestinal tract, heart, tendons, and subcutaneous tissues of the buttocks. There is no specific therapy for Aβ_2M amyloidosis, but cessation of dialysis after renal allograft may lead to symptomatic improvement.

SUMMARY

A diagnosis of amyloidosis should be considered in patients with unexplained nephropathy, cardiomyopathy (particularly with diastolic dysfunction), neuropathy (either peripheral or autonomic), enteropathy, or the pathognomonic soft tissue findings of macroglossia and periorbital ecchymoses. Pathologic identification of amyloid fibrils can be made; Congo red staining of aspirated abdominal fat is the initial test of choice in most cases. Accurate typing using a combination of immunologic, biochemical, and genetic testing is essential to choosing the appropriate therapy (see algorithm for workup, Fig. 324-1). For difficult cases, referral centers can provide specialized diagnostic techniques and access to clinical trials.

FURTHER READINGS

AKAR H et al: Quantitative serum free light-chain assay in the diagnostic evaluation of AL amyloidosis. Amyloid J Protein Folding Disorders 12:210, 2005

BENSON M: Amyloidosis, in *The Metabolic and Molecular Bases of Inherited Disease*, 8th ed, CR Scriver et al (eds). New York, McGraw-Hill, 2001, pp 5345–5378

DEMBER LM et al: Effect of intravenous melphalan and autologous blood stem cell transplant on AL amyloidosis–associated renal disease. Ann Intern Med 134:746, 2001

MERLINI G, BELLOTTI V: Molecular mechanisms of amyloidosis. N Engl J Med 349:583, 2003

RAJKUMAR SV, GERTZ MA: Advances in the treatment of amyloidosis. N Engl J Med 356:2413, 2007

SELDIN DC et al: Improvement in quality of life of patients with AL amyloidosis treated with high-dose melphalan and autologous stem cell transplantation. Blood 104:1888, 2004

——— et al: Successful treatment of AL amyloidosis with high-dose melphalan and autologous stem cell transplantation in patients over age 65. Blood 108:3945, 2006

SKINNER M et al: High-dose melphalan and autologous stem-cell transplantation in patients with AL amyloidosis: An 8-year study. Ann Intern Med 140:85, 2004

SECTION 3 ▸ DISORDERS OF THE JOINTS AND ADJACENT TISSUES

325 Approach to Articular and Musculoskeletal Disorders

John J. Cush, Peter E. Lipsky

Musculoskeletal complaints account for >315 million outpatient visits per year. Recent surveys by the Centers for Disease Control and Prevention suggest that 33% (69.9 million) of the U.S. population is affected by arthritis or joint disorders. Many of these are self-limited conditions requiring minimal evaluation and only symptomatic therapy and reassurance. However, in some patients, specific musculoskele-

tal symptoms or their persistence may herald a more serious condition that requires further evaluation or laboratory testing to establish a diagnosis or document the extent and nature of the pathologic process. The goal of the musculoskeletal evaluation is to formulate a differential diagnosis that leads to an accurate diagnosis and timely therapy, while avoiding excessive diagnostic testing and unnecessary treatment (Table 325-1). There are several urgent conditions that must be diagnosed promptly to avoid significant morbid or mortal sequelae. These "red flag" diagnoses include septic arthritis, acute crystal-induced arthritis (e.g., gout), and fracture. Each may be suspected by its acute onset and monarticular or focal presentation (see below).

Individuals with musculoskeletal complaints should be evaluated with a thorough history, a comprehensive physical examination, and,

TABLE 325-1	EVALUATION OF PATIENTS WITH MUSCULOSKELETAL COMPLAINTS

Goals
  Accurate diagnosis
  Timely provision of therapy
  Avoidance of unnecessary diagnostic testing
Approach
  Anatomic localization of complaint (articular vs. nonarticular)
  Determination of the nature of the pathologic process (inflammatory vs. noninflammatory)
  Determination of the extent of involvement (monarticular, polyarticular, focal, widespread)
  Determination of chronology (acute vs. chronic)
  Consider the most common disorders first
  Formulation of a differential diagnosis

if appropriate, laboratory testing. The initial encounter should determine whether the musculoskeletal complaint is (1) *articular* or *nonarticular* in origin, (2) *inflammatory* or *noninflammatory* in nature, (3) *acute* or *chronic* in duration, and (4) *localized* or *widespread* (*systemic*) in distribution.

With such an approach and an understanding of the pathophysiologic processes that underlie musculoskeletal complaints, a diagnosis can be made in the vast majority of individuals. However, some patients will not fit immediately into an established diagnostic category. Many musculoskeletal disorders resemble each other at the outset, and some may take weeks or months to evolve into a readily recognizable diagnostic entity. This consideration should temper the desire to establish a definitive diagnosis at the first encounter.

ARTICULAR VERSUS NONARTICULAR

The musculoskeletal evaluation must discriminate the anatomic origin(s) of the patient's complaint. For example, ankle pain can result from a variety of pathologic conditions involving disparate anatomic structures, including gonococcal arthritis, calcaneal fracture, Achilles tendinitis, cellulitis, and peripheral neuropathy. Distinguishing between articular and nonarticular conditions requires a careful and detailed examination. Articular structures include the synovium, synovial fluid, articular cartilage, intraarticular ligaments, joint capsule, and juxtaarticular bone. Nonarticular (or periarticular) structures, such as supportive extraarticular ligaments, tendons, bursae, muscle, fascia, bone, nerve, and overlying skin, may be involved in the pathologic process. Although musculoskeletal complaints are often ascribed to the joints, nonarticular disorders (rather than articular) more frequently underlie such complaints. Distinguishing between these potential sources of pain may be challenging to the unskilled examiner. Articular disorders may be characterized by deep or diffuse pain, pain or limited range of motion on active and passive movement, and swelling (caused by synovial proliferation, effusion, or bony enlargement), crepitation, instability, "locking," or deformity. By contrast, nonarticular disorders tend to be painful on active, but not passive (or assisted), range of motion, demonstrate point or focal tenderness in regions adjacent to articular structures, and have physical findings remote from the joint capsule. Moreover, nonarticular disorders seldom demonstrate swelling, crepitus, instability, or deformity.

INFLAMMATORY VERSUS NONINFLAMMATORY DISORDERS

In the course of a musculoskeletal evaluation, the examiner should determine the nature of the underlying pathologic process and whether inflammatory or noninflammatory findings exist. Inflammatory disorders may be infectious (infection with *Neisseria gonorrhoea* or *Mycobacterium tuberculosis*), crystal-induced (gout, pseudogout), immune-related [rheumatoid arthritis (RA), systemic lupus erythematosus (SLE)], reactive (rheumatic fever, Reiter's syndrome), or idiopathic. Inflammatory disorders may be identified by any of the four cardinal signs of inflammation (erythema, warmth, pain, or swelling), systemic symptoms (fatigue, fever, rash, weight loss), or laboratory evidence of inflammation

[elevated erythrocyte sedimentation rate (ESR) or C-reactive protein (CRP), thrombocytosis, anemia of chronic disease, or hypoalbuminemia]. Articular stiffness commonly accompanies chronic musculoskeletal disorders. However, the severity and duration of stiffness may be diagnostically important. Morning stiffness related to inflammatory disorders (such as RA or polymyalgia rheumatica) is precipitated by prolonged rest, is described as severe, lasts for hours, and may improve with activity and anti-inflammatory medications. By contrast, intermittent stiffness (also known as gel phenomenon), associated with noninflammatory conditions [such as osteoarthritis (OA)], is precipitated by brief periods of rest, usually lasts <60 min, and is exacerbated by activity. Fatigue may accompany inflammation (as seen in RA and polymyalgia rheumatica) but may also be prominent in fibromyalgia (a noninflammatory disorder), anemia, cardiac failure, endocrinopathy, poor nutrition, poor sleep, or depression. Noninflammatory disorders may be related to trauma (rotator cuff tear), repetitive use (bursitis, tendonitis), degeneration or ineffective repair (OA), neoplasm (pigmented villonodular synovitis), or pain amplification (fibromyalgia). Noninflammatory disorders are often characterized by pain without synovial swelling or warmth, absence of inflammatory or systemic features, daytime gel phenomena rather than morning stiffness, and normal (for age) or negative laboratory investigations.

Identification of the nature of the underlying process and the site of the complaint will enable the examiner to narrow the diagnostic considerations and to assess the need for immediate diagnostic or therapeutic intervention, or for continued observation. **Figure 325-1** presents a logical approach to the evaluation of patients with musculoskeletal complaints.

In the formulation of a differential diagnosis, the examiner should be mindful of the most common causes of musculoskeletal complaints (**Fig. 325-2**). Thus, the prevalence of these disorders in the general population may facilitate an early diagnosis. As trauma, fracture, and fibromyalgia are among the most common causes of presentation, these should be considered during the initial encounter. The frequency of these disorders is best clarified by dividing patients according to their age. Hence, those <60 years are commonly affected by repetitive use/strain disorders, gout (men only), RA, spondyloarthritis, and infectious arthritis. Patients >60 years are frequently affected by OA, crystal (gout and pseudogout) arthritis, polymyalgia rheumatica, osteoporotic fracture, and septic arthritis.

CLINICAL HISTORY

Additional historic features may reveal important clues to the diagnosis. Aspects of the patient profile, complaint chronology, extent of joint involvement, and precipitating factors can provide important information. Certain diagnoses are more frequent in different *age* groups (Fig. 325-2). SLE and reactive arthritis occur more frequently in the young, whereas fibromyalgia and RA are frequent in middle age and OA and polymyalgia rheumatica are more prevalent among the elderly. Diagnostic clustering is also evident when *sex* and *race* are considered. Gout and the spondyloarthropathies (e.g., ankylosing spondylitis) are more common in men, whereas RA, fibromyalgia, and lupus are more frequent in women. *Racial predilections* may be influential. Thus, polymyalgia rheumatica, giant cell arteritis, and Wegener's granulomatosis commonly affect whites, whereas sarcoidosis and SLE more commonly affect African Americans. *Familial aggregation* may be seen in disorders such as ankylosing spondylitis, gout, and Heberden's nodes of OA.

The chronology of the complaint is an important diagnostic feature and can be divided into the *onset*, *evolution*, and *duration*. The onset of disorders such as septic arthritis or gout tends to be abrupt, whereas OA, RA, and fibromyalgia may have more indolent presentations. The patients' complaints may evolve differently and be classified as chronic (OA), intermittent (crystal or Lyme arthritis), migratory (rheumatic fever, gonococcal or viral arthritis), or additive (RA, psoriatic arthritis). Musculoskeletal disorders are typically classified as acute or chronic based upon a symptom duration that is either less than or greater than 6 weeks, respectively. Acute arthropathies tend to be infectious, crystal-induced, or reactive. Chronic conditions include non-

FIGURE 325-1 Algorithm for the diagnosis of musculoskeletal complaints. An approach to formulating a differential diagnosis (shown in italics). (ESR, erythrocyte sedimentation rate; CRP, C-reactive protein; DIP, distal interphalangeal; CMC, carpometacarpal; PIP, proximal interphalangeal; MCP, metacarpophalangeal; MTP, metatarsophalangeal; PMR, polymyalgia rheumatica; SLE, systemic lupus erythematosus; JA, juvenile arthritis.)

whereas lower extremity arthritis is characteristic of reactive arthritis and gout at their onset. Involvement of the axial skeleton is common in OA and ankylosing spondylitis but is infrequent in RA, with the notable exception of the cervical spine.

The clinical history should also identify *precipitating events*, such as trauma, drug administration (Table 325-2), or antecedent or intercurrent illnesses, that may have contributed to the patient's complaint. Certain comorbidities may predispose to musculoskeletal consequences. This is especially so for diabetes mellitus (carpal tunnel syndrome), renal insufficiency (gout), psoriasis (psoriatic arthritis), myeloma (low back pain), cancer (myositis), and osteoporosis (fracture) or when using certain drugs such as glucocorticoids (osteonecrosis, septic arthritis) and diuretics or chemotherapy (gout). Lastly, a thorough *rheumatic review of systems* may disclose useful diagnostic information. A variety of musculoskeletal disorders may be associated with systemic features such as fever (SLE, infection), rash (SLE, psoriatic arthritis), nail abnormalities (psoriatic or reactive arthritis), myalgias (fibromyalgia, myopathy), or weakness (polymyositis, neuropathy). In addition, some conditions are associated with involvement of other organ systems including the eyes (Behçet's disease, sarcoidosis, spondyloarthritis), gastrointestinal tract (scleroderma, inflammatory bowel disease), genitourinary tract (reactive arthritis, gonococcemia), or the nervous system (Lyme disease, vasculitis).

Lastly, the examiner should assess the level of pain and physical limitation that accompanies the complaint. The intensity of the patient's pain, stiffness, or weakness can be quantified (0–10) verbally or with the use of a 10-cm visual analogue scale (0 = no pain and 10 = the worst possible pain). Functional limitation and disability should be identified and recorded for future comparisons. There are several validated functional measures that are easily incorporated into the musculoskeletal evaluation, such as the modified Health Assessment Questionnaire (Fig. 325-3).

RHEUMATOLOGIC EVALUATION OF THE ELDERLY

The incidence of rheumatic diseases rises with age, such that 58% of those >65 years will have joint complaints. Musculoskeletal disorders in elderly patients are often not diagnosed because the signs and symptoms may be insidious, overlooked, or overshadowed by comorbidities. These difficulties are compounded by the diminished reliability of laboratory testing in the elderly, who often manifest nonpathologic abnormal results. For example, the ESR may be misleadingly elevated, and low-titer positive tests for rheumatoid factor and antinuclear antibodies (ANAs) may be seen in up to 15% of elderly pa-

inflammatory or immunologic arthritides (e.g., OA, RA) and nonarticular disorders (e.g., fibromyalgia).

The *extent* of articular involvement is often diagnostic. Articular disorders are classified based on the number of joints involved, as either *monarticular* (one joint), *oligoarticular* or *pauciarticular* (two or three joints), or *polyarticular* (more than three joints). Although crystal and infectious arthritis are often mono- or oligoarticular, OA and RA are polyarticular disorders. Nonarticular disorders may be classified as either focal or widespread. Complaints secondary to tendinitis or carpal tunnel syndrome are typically focal, whereas weakness and myalgia, due to polymyositis or fibromyalgia, are more diffuse in their presentation. Joint involvement in RA tends to be symmetric, whereas the spondyloarthropathies and gout are often asymmetric and oligoarticular. The upper extremities are frequently involved in RA and OA,

MOST COMMON MUSCULOSKELETAL CONDITIONS

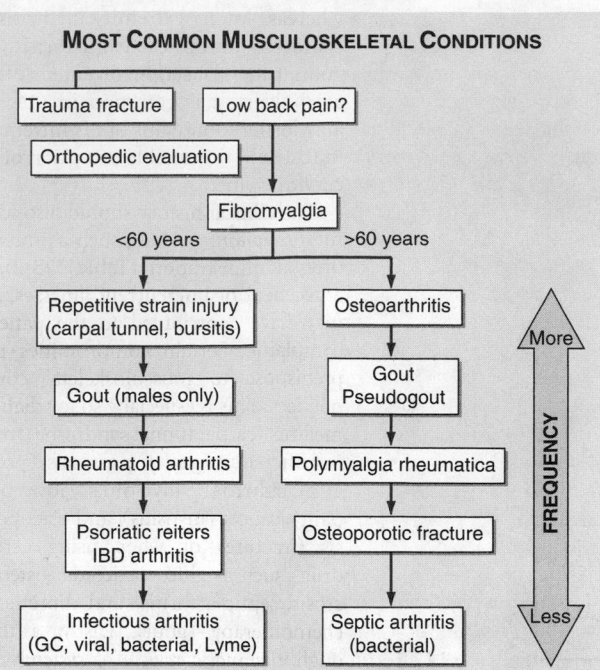

FIGURE 325-2 Algorithm for consideration of the most common musculoskeletal conditions. (IBD, inflammatory bowel disease; GC, gonococcal.)

tients. Although nearly all rheumatic disorders afflict the elderly, certain diseases and drug-induced disorders (Table 325-2) are more common in this age group. The elderly should be approached in the same manner as other patients with musculoskeletal complaints, but with an emphasis on identifying the potential rheumatic consequences of medical comorbidities and therapies. OA, osteoporosis, gout, pseudogout, polymyalgia rheumatica, vasculitis, drug-induced SLE, and chronic salicylate toxicity are all more common in the elderly than in other individuals. The physical examination should identify the nature of the musculoskeletal complaint as well as coexisting diseases that may influence diagnosis and choice of treatment.

TABLE 325-2 DRUG-INDUCED MUSCULOSKELETAL CONDITIONS

Arthralgias
Quinidine, cimetidine, quinolones, chronic acyclovir, interferon, IL-2, nicardipine, vaccines, rifabutin, aromatase and HIV protease inhibitors
Myalgias/myopathy
Glucocorticoids, penicillamine, hydroxychloroquine, AZT, lovastatin, simvastatin, pravastatin, clofibrate, interferon, IL-2, alcohol, cocaine, taxol, docetaxel, colchicine, quinolones, cyclosporine
Tendon rupture
Quinolones, glucocorticoids
Gout
Diuretics, aspirin, cytotoxics, cyclosporine, alcohol, moonshine, ethambutol
Drug-induced lupus
Hydralazine, procainamide, quinidine, phenytoin, carbemazepine, methyldopa, isoniazid, chlorpromazine, lithium, penicillamine, tetracyclines, TNF inhibitors, ACE inhibitors, ticlopidine
Osteonecrosis
Glucocorticoids, alcohol, radiation, bisphosphonates
Osteopenia
Glucocorticoids, chronic heparin, phenytoin, methotrexate
Scleroderma
Vinyl chloride, bleomycin, pentazocine, organic solvents, carbidopa, tryptophan, rapeseed oil
Vasculitis
Allopurinol, amphetamines, cocaine, thiazides, penicillamine, propylthiouracil, montelukast, TNF inhibitors, hepatitis B vaccine, trimethoprim/sulfamethoxazole

Note: IL-2, interleukin 2; TNF, tumor necrosis factor; ACE, angiotensin-converting enzyme.

Modified Health Assessment Questionnaire

Today are you able to (check box)	No difficulty	Some difficulty	Much difficulty	Cannot do
Dress yourself; including laces & buttons?				
Get in and out of bed?				
Lift a full cup or glass to your mouth?				
Walk outdoors on flat ground?				
Wash and dry your entire body?				
Bend down & pick up clothing from floor?				
Turn regular faucets on and off?				
Get in and out of a car?				

FIGURE 325-3 Modified Health Assessment Questionnaire. (From T Pincus et al: Arthritis Rheum 26:1346, 1983; with permission.)

PHYSICAL EXAMINATION

The goal of the physical examination is to ascertain the structures involved, the nature of the underlying pathology, the functional consequences of the process, and the presence of systemic or extraarticular manifestations. A knowledge of topographic anatomy is necessary to identify the primary site(s) of involvement and differentiate articular from nonarticular disorders. The musculoskeletal examination depends largely on careful inspection, palpation, and a variety of specific physical maneuvers to elicit diagnostic signs (Table 325-3). Although most articulations of the appendicular skeleton can be examined in this manner, adequate inspection and palpation are not possible for many axial (e.g., zygapophyseal) and inaccessible (e.g., sacroiliac or hip) joints. For such joints, there is a greater reliance upon specific maneuvers and imaging for assessment.

Examination of involved and uninvolved joints will determine whether *pain, warmth, erythema,* or *swelling* is present. The locale and level of pain elicited by palpation or movement should be quantified. One example would be to count the number of tender joints on palpation of 28 easily examined joints [proximal interphalangeals (PIPs), metacarpophalangeals (MCPs), wrists, elbows, shoulders, and knees]

TABLE 325-3 GLOSSARY OF MUSCULOSKELETAL TERMS

Crepitus
A palpable (less commonly audible) vibratory or crackling sensation elicited with joint motion; fine joint crepitus is common and often insignificant in large joints; coarse joint crepitus indicates advanced cartilaginous and degenerative changes (as in osteoarthritis)
Subluxation
Alteration of joint alignment such that articulating surfaces incompletely approximate each other
Dislocation
Abnormal displacement of articulating surfaces such that the surfaces are not in contact
Range of motion
For diarthrodial joints, the arc of measurable movement through which the joint moves in a single plane
Contracture
Loss of full movement resulting from a fixed resistance caused either by tonic spasm of muscle (reversible) or to fibrosis of periarticular structures (permanent)
Deformity
Abnormal shape or size of a structure; may result from bony hypertrophy, malalignment of articulating structures, or damage to periarticular supportive structures
Enthesitis
Inflammation of the entheses (tendinous or ligamentous insertions on bone)
Epicondylitis
Infection or inflammation involving an epicondyle

(with a range of 0–28). Similarly, the number of swollen joints (0–28) can be counted and recorded. Careful examination should distinguish between true articular swelling (caused by synovial effusion or synovial proliferation) and nonarticular (or periarticular) involvement, which usually extends beyond the normal joint margins. Synovial effusion can be distinguished from synovial hypertrophy or bony hypertrophy by palpation or specific maneuvers. For example, small to moderate knee effusions may be identified by the "bulge sign" or "ballottement of the patellae." Bursal effusions (e.g., effusions of the olecranon or prepatellar bursa) are often focal, periarticular, overlie bony prominences, and are fluctuant with sharply defined borders. Joint *stability* can be assessed by palpation and by the application of manual stress. *Subluxation* or *dislocation*, which may be secondary to traumatic, mechanical, or inflammatory causes, can be assessed by inspection and palpation. Joint *swelling or volume* can be assessed by palpation. Distention of the articular capsule usually causes pain and evident swelling. The patient will attempt to minimize the pain by maintaining the joint in the position of least intraarticular pressure and greatest volume, usually partial flexion. For this reason, inflammatory effusions may give rise to flexion contractures. Clinically, this may be detected as fluctuant or "squishy" swelling, voluntary or fixed flexion deformities, or diminished range of motion—especially on extension, when joint volumes are decreased. Active and passive *range of motion* should be assessed in all planes, with contralateral comparison. Serial evaluations of the joints should record the number of tender and swollen joints and the range of motion, using a goniometer to quantify the arc of movement. Each joint should be passively manipulated through its full range of motion (including, as appropriate, flexion, extension, rotation, abduction, adduction, lateral bending, inversion, eversion, supination, pronation, medial/lateral deviation, plantar- or dorsiflexion). Limitation of motion is frequently caused by effusion, pain, deformity, or contracture. If passive motion exceeds active motion, a periarticular process (e.g., tendon rupture or myopathy) should be considered. *Contractures* may reflect antecedent synovial inflammation or trauma. Joint *crepitus* may be felt during palpation or maneuvers and may be especially coarse in OA. Joint *deformity* usually indicates a long-standing or aggressive pathologic process. Deformities may result from ligamentous destruction, soft tissue contracture, bony enlargement, ankylosis, erosive disease, or subluxation. Examination of the musculature will document strength, atrophy, pain, or spasm. Appendicular muscle weakness should be characterized as proximal or distal. Muscle strength should be assessed by observing the patient's performance (e.g., walking, rising from a chair, grasping, writing). Strength may also be graded on a 5-point scale: 0 for no movement; 1 for trace movement or twitch; 2 for movement with gravity eliminated; 3 for movement against gravity only; 4 for movement against gravity and resistance; and 5 for normal strength. The examiner should assess for often-overlooked nonarticular or periarticular involvement, especially when articular complaints are not supported by objective findings referable to the joint capsule. The identification of soft tissue/nonarticular pain will prevent unwarranted and often expensive additional evaluations. Specific maneuvers may reveal common nonarticular abnormalities, such as a carpal tunnel syndrome (which can be identified by Tinel's or Phalen's sign). Other examples of soft tissue abnormalities include olecranon bursitis, epicondylitis (e.g., tennis elbow), enthesitis (e.g., Achilles tendinitis), and trigger points associated with fibromyalgia.

APPROACH TO REGIONAL RHEUMATIC COMPLAINTS

Although all patients should be evaluated in a logical and thorough manner, many cases with focal musculoskeletal complaints are caused by commonly encountered disorders that exhibit a predictable pattern of onset, evolution, and localization; they can often be diagnosed immediately on the basis of limited historic information and selected maneuvers or tests. Although nearly every joint could be approached in this manner, the evaluation of four common involved anatomic regions—the hand, shoulder, hip, and knee—are reviewed here.

HAND PAIN

Focal or unilateral hand pain may result from trauma, overuse, infection, or a reactive or crystal-induced arthritis. By contrast, bilateral hand complaints commonly suggest a degenerative (e.g., OA), systemic, or inflammatory/immune (e.g., RA) etiology. The distribution or pattern of joint involvement is highly suggestive of certain disorders (Fig. 325-4). Thus, OA (or degenerative arthritis) may manifest as distal interphalangeal (DIP) and PIP joint pain with bony hypertrophy sufficient to produce Heberden's and Bouchard's nodes, respectively. Pain, with or without bony swelling, involving the base of the thumb (first carpometacarpal joint) is also highly suggestive of OA. By contrast, RA tends to involve the PIP, MCP, intercarpal, and carpometacarpal joints (wrist) with pain, prolonged stiffness, and palpable synovial tissue hypertrophy. Psoriatic arthritis may mimic the pattern of joint involvement seen in OA (DIP and PIP joints), but can be distinguished by the presence of inflammatory signs (erythema, warmth, synovial swelling), with or without carpal involvement, nail pitting or onycholysis. Hemochromatosis should be considered when degenerative changes (bony hypertrophy) are seen at the second and third MCP joints with associated chondrocalcinosis or episodic, inflammatory wrist arthritis.

Soft tissue swelling over the dorsum of the hand and wrist may suggest an inflammatory extensor tendon tenosynovitis possibly caused by gonococcal infection, gout, or inflammatory arthritis (e.g., RA). The diagnosis is suggested by local warmth, swelling, or pitting edema and may be confirmed when pain is induced by maintaining the wrist in a fixed, neutral position and flexing the digits distal to the MCP joints to stretch the extensor tendon sheaths.

Focal wrist pain localized to the radial aspect may be caused by De Quervain's tenosynovitis resulting from inflammation of the tendon sheath(s) involving the abductor pollicis longus or extensor pollicis brevis (Fig. 325-4). This commonly results from overuse or follows pregnancy and may be diagnosed with Finkelstein's test. A positive result is present when radial wrist pain is induced after the thumb is flexed and placed inside a clenched fist and the patient actively deviates the hand downward with ulnar deviation at the wrist. Carpal tun-

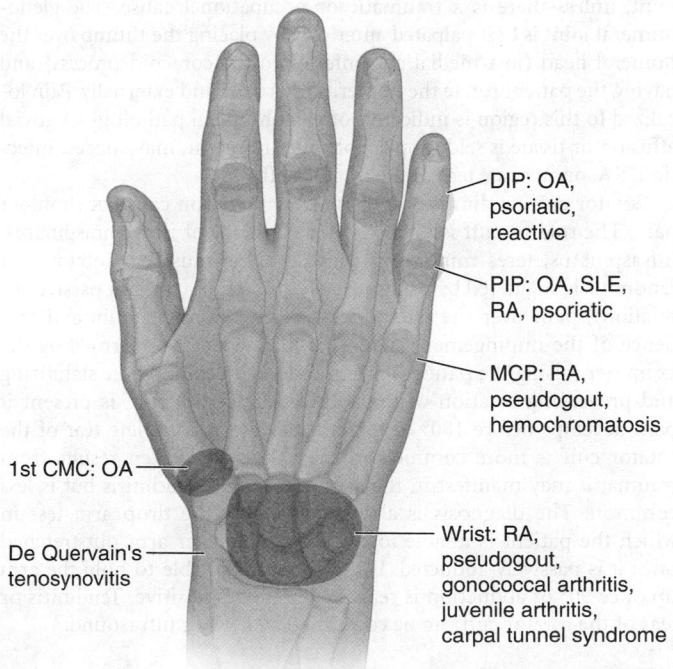

FIGURE 325-4 Sites of hand or wrist involvement and their potential disease associations. (DIP, distal interphalangeal; OA, osteoarthritis; PIP, proximal interphalangeal; SLE, systemic lupus erythematosus; RA, rheumatoid arthritis; MCP, metacarpophalangeal; CMC, carpometacarpal.) (*From Cush et al, with permission.*)

DIP: OA, psoriatic, reactive

PIP: OA, SLE, RA, psoriatic

MCP: RA, pseudogout, hemochromatosis

1st CMC: OA

De Quervain's tenosynovitis

Wrist: RA, pseudogout, gonococcal arthritis, juvenile arthritis, carpal tunnel syndrome nel syndrome is another common disorder of the upper extremity and results from compression of the median nerve within the carpal tunnel. Manifestations include paresthesia in the thumb, second and third fingers, and radial half of the fourth finger and, at times, atrophy of thenar musculature. Carpal tunnel syndrome is commonly associated with pregnancy, edema, trauma, OA, inflammatory arthritis, and infiltrative disorders (e.g., amyloidosis). The diagnosis is suggested by a positive Tinel's or Phalen's sign. With each test, paresthesia in a median nerve distribution is induced or increased by either "thumping" the volar aspect of the wrist (Tinel's sign) or pressing the extensor surfaces of both flexed wrists against each other (Phalen's sign).

SHOULDER PAIN

During the evaluation of shoulder disorders, the examiner should carefully note any history of trauma, fibromyalgia, infection, inflammatory disease, occupational hazards, or previous cervical disease. In addition, the patient should be questioned as to the activities or movement(s) that elicit shoulder pain. Shoulder pain is referred frequently from the cervical spine but may also be referred from intrathoracic lesions (e.g., a Pancoast tumor) or from gall bladder, hepatic, or diaphragmatic disease. Fibromyalgia should be suspected when glenohumeral pain is accompanied by diffuse periarticular (i.e., subacromial, bicipital) pain and tender points (i.e., trapezius or supraspinatus). The shoulder should be put through its full range of motion both actively and passively (with examiner assistance): forward flexion, extension, abduction, adduction, and rotation. Manual inspection of the periarticular structures will often provide important diagnostic information. The examiner should apply direct manual pressure over the subacromial bursa that lies lateral to and immediately beneath the acromion. Subacromial bursitis is a frequent cause of shoulder pain. Anterior to the subacromial bursa, the bicipital tendon traverses the bicipital groove. This tendon is best identified by palpating it in its groove as the patient rotates the humerus internally and externally. Direct pressure over the tendon may reveal pain indicative of bicipital tendinitis. Palpation of the acromioclavicular joint may disclose local pain, bony hypertrophy, or, uncommonly, synovial swelling. Whereas OA and RA commonly affect the acromioclavicular joint, OA seldom involves the glenohumeral joint, unless there is a traumatic or occupational cause. The glenohumeral joint is best palpated anteriorly by placing the thumb over the humeral head (just medial and inferior to the coracoid process) and having the patient rotate the humerus internally and externally. Pain localized to this region is indicative of glenohumeral pathology. Synovial effusion or tissue is seldom palpable but, if present, may suggest infection, RA, or an acute tear of the rotator cuff.

Rotator cuff tendinitis or tear is a very common cause of shoulder pain. The rotator cuff is formed by the tendons of the supraspinatus, infraspinatus, teres minor, and subscapularis muscles. Rotator cuff tendinitis is suggested by pain on active abduction (but not passive abduction), pain over the lateral deltoid muscle, night pain, and evidence of the impingement sign. This maneuver is performed by the examiner raising the patient's arm into forced flexion while stabilizing and preventing rotation of the scapula. A positive sign is present if pain develops before 180° of forward flexion. A complete tear of the rotator cuff is more common in the elderly and often results from trauma; it may manifest in the same manner as tendinitis but is less common. The diagnosis is also suggested by the drop arm test in which the patient is unable to maintain his or her arm outstretched once it is passively abducted. If the patient is unable to hold the arm up once 90° of abduction is reached, the test is positive. Tendinitis or tear of the rotator cuff can be confirmed by MRI or ultrasound.

KNEE PAIN

A careful history should delineate the chronology of the knee complaint and whether there are predisposing conditions, trauma, or medications that might underlie the complaint. For example, patellofemoral disease (e.g., OA) may cause anterior knee pain that worsens with climbing stairs. Observation of the patient's gait is also important. The knee should be carefully inspected in the upright (weight-bear-

ing) and prone positions for swelling, erythema, contusion, laceration, or malalignment. The most common form of malalignment in the knee is *genu varum* (bowlegs) or *genu valgum* (knock knees). Bony swelling of the knee joint commonly results from hypertrophic osseous changes seen with disorders such as OA and neuropathic arthropathy. Swelling caused by hypertrophy of the synovium or synovial effusion may manifest as a fluctuant, ballotable, or soft tissue enlargement in the suprapatellar pouch (suprapatellar reflection of the synovial cavity) or regions lateral and medial to the patella. Synovial effusions may also be detected by balloting the patella downward toward the femoral groove or by eliciting a "bulge sign." With the knee extended the examiner should manually compress, or "milk," synovial fluid down from the suprapatellar pouch and lateral to the patellae. The application of manual pressure lateral to the patella may cause an observable shift in synovial fluid (bulge) to the medial aspect. The examiner should note that this maneuver is only effective in detecting small to moderate effusions (<100 mL). Inflammatory disorders such as RA, gout, pseudogout, and reactive arthritis may involve the knee joint and produce significant pain, stiffness, swelling, or warmth. A popliteal or *Baker's cyst* is best palpated with the knee partially flexed and is best viewed posteriorly with the patient standing and knees fully extended to visualize popliteal swelling or fullness.

Anserine bursitis is an often missed periarticular cause of knee pain in adults. The pes anserine bursa underlies the semimembranosus tendon and may become inflamed and painful following trauma, overuse, or inflammation. It is often tender in patients with fibromyalgia. Anserine bursitis manifests primarily as point tenderness inferior and medial to the patella and overlies the medial tibial plateau. Swelling and erythema may not be present. Other forms of bursitis may also present as knee pain. The prepatellar bursa is superficial and is located over the inferior portion of the patella. The infrapatellar bursa is deeper and lies beneath the patellar ligament before its insertion on the tibial tubercle.

Internal derangement of the knee may result from trauma or degenerative processes. Damage to the meniscal cartilage (medial or lateral) frequently presents as chronic or intermittent knee pain. Such an injury should be suspected when there is a history of trauma or athletic activity and when the patient relates symptoms of "locking," clicking, or "giving way" of the joint. Pain may be elicited during palpation over the ipsilateral joint line or when the knee is stressed laterally or medially. A positive McMurray test may indicate a meniscal tear. To perform this test, the knee is first flexed at 90°, and the leg is then extended while the lower extremity is simultaneously torqued medially or laterally. A painful click during inward rotation may indicate a lateral meniscus tear, and pain during outward rotation may indicate a tear in the medial meniscus. Lastly, damage to the cruciate ligaments should be suspected with acute onset of pain, possibly with swelling, a history of trauma, or a synovial fluid aspirate that is grossly bloody. Examination of the cruciate ligaments is best accomplished by eliciting a drawer sign. With the patient recumbent, the knee should be partially flexed and the foot stabilized on the examining surface. The examiner should manually attempt to displace the tibia anteriorly or posteriorly with respect to the femur. If anterior movement is detected, then anterior cruciate ligament damage is likely. Conversely, significant posterior movement may indicate posterior cruciate damage. Contralateral comparison will assist the examiner in detecting significant anterior or posterior movement.

HIP PAIN

The hip is best evaluated by observing the patient's gait and assessing range of motion. The vast majority of patients reporting "hip pain" localize their pain unilaterally to the posterior or gluteal musculature (Fig. 325-5). Such pain may or may not be associated with low back pain and tends to radiate down the posterolateral aspect of the thigh. This presentation frequently results from degenerative arthritis of the lumbosacral spine and commonly follows a dermatomal distribution with involvement of nerve roots between L5 and S1. Some individuals instead localize their "hip pain" laterally to the area overlying the tro-

Anterior　　　Posterior/lateral

Enthesitis
(anterior superior
iliac crest)

True hip pain
Iliopsoasbursitis

Meralgia
paresthetica

Sacroiliac pain

Buttock pain
referred from
lumbosacral
spine

Trochanteric
bursitis

Ischiogluteal
bursitis

Sciatica

FIGURE 325-5 Origins of hip pain and dysesthesias. *(From Cush et al, with permission.)*

women are caused by the uricosuric effects of estrogen. Urinary uric acid levels are normally <750 mg per 24 h. Although hyperuricemia [especially levels >535 μmol/L (9 mg/dL)] is associated with an increased incidence of gout and nephrolithiasis, levels do not correlate with the severity of disease. Uric acid levels (and the risk of gout) may be increased by inborn errors of metabolism (Lesch-Nyhan syndrome), disease states (renal insufficiency, myeloproliferative disease, psoriasis), or drugs (alcohol, cytotoxic therapy, thiazides). Although nearly all patients with gout will demonstrate hyperuricemia at some time during their illness, up to 40% of patients with an acute gouty attack will have normal serum uric acid levels. Monitoring serum uric acid may be useful in assessing the response to hypouricemic therapy or chemotherapy.

Serologic tests for rheumatoid factor, cyclic citrullinated peptide (CCP) antibodies, ANAs, complement levels, Lyme and antineutrophil cytoplasmic antibodies (ANCA), or antistreptolysin O (ASO) titer should be carried out only when there is clinical evidence to suggest an associated diagnosis, as these have poor predictive value when used for screening, especially when the pretest probability is low. Although 4–5% of a healthy population will have positive tests for rheumatoid factor and ANAs, only 1% and <0.4% of the population will have RA or SLE, respectively. IgM rheumatoid factor (autoantibodies against the Fc portion of IgG) is found in 80% of patients with RA and may also be seen in low titers in patients with chronic infections (*tuberculosis*, leprosy); other autoimmune diseases (SLE, Sjögren's syndrome); and chronic pulmonary, hepatic, or renal diseases. When considering RA, anti-CCP antibodies are comparably sensitive but more specific than rheumatoid factor. In RA, the presence of anti-CCP and rheumatoid factor antibodies may indicate a greater risk for more severe, erosive polyarthritis. ANAs are found in nearly all patients with SLE and may also be seen in patients with other autoimmune diseases (polymyositis, scleroderma, antiphospholipid syndrome), drug-induced lupus (resulting from hydralazine, procainamide, quinidine, tetracyclines, tumor necrosis factor inhibitors), chronic liver or renal disorders, and advanced age. Positive ANAs are found in 5% of adults and in up to 14% of elderly or chronically ill individuals. The ANA test is very sensitive but poorly specific for lupus, as <5% of all positive results will be caused by lupus alone. The interpretation of a positive ANA test may depend on the magnitude of the titer and the pattern observed by immunofluorescence microscopy (Table 325-4). Diffuse and speckled patterns are least specific, whereas a peripheral, or rim, pattern [related to autoantibodies against double-stranded (native) DNA] is highly specific and suggestive of lupus. Centromeric patterns are seen in patients with limited scleroderma (CREST syndrome) or primary biliary sclerosis, and nucleolar patterns may be seen in patients with diffuse systemic sclerosis or inflammatory myositis.

Aspiration and analysis of synovial fluid are always indicated in acute monarthritis or when an infectious or crystal-induced arthropathy is suspected. Synovial fluid may distinguish between noninflammatory and inflammatory processes by analysis of the appearance, viscosity, and cell count. Tests for synovial fluid glucose, protein, lactate dehydrogenase, lactic acid, or autoantibodies are not recommended as they have no diagnostic value. Normal synovial fluid is clear or a pale straw color and is viscous, primarily because of the high levels of hyaluronate. Noninflammatory synovial fluid is clear, viscous, and amber-colored, with a white blood cell count of <2000/μL and a predominance of mononuclear cells. The viscosity of synovial fluid is assessed by expressing fluid from the syringe one drop at a time. Normally, there is a stringing effect, with a long tail behind each synovial drop. Effusions caused by OA or trauma will have normal viscosity. Inflammatory fluid is turbid and yellow, with an increased white

chanteric bursa. Because of the depth of this bursa, swelling and warmth are usually absent. Diagnosis of trochanteric bursitis can be confirmed by inducing point tenderness over the trochanteric bursa. Gluteal and trochanteric pain may also indicate underlying fibromyalgia. Range of movement may be limited by pain. Pain in the hip joint is less common and tends to be located anteriorly, over the inguinal ligament; it may radiate medially to the groin or along the anteromedial thigh. Uncommonly, iliopsoas bursitis may mimic true hip joint pain. Diagnosis of iliopsoas bursitis may be suggested by a history of trauma or inflammatory arthritis. Pain associated with iliopsoas bursitis is localized to the groin or anterior thigh and tends to worsen with hyperextension of the hip; many patients prefer to flex and externally rotate the hip to reduce the pain from a distended bursa.

LABORATORY INVESTIGATIONS

The vast majority of musculoskeletal disorders can be easily diagnosed by a complete history and physical examination. An additional objective of the initial encounter is to determine whether additional investigations or immediate therapy are required. A number of features indicate the need for additional evaluation. Monarticular conditions require additional evaluation, as do traumatic or inflammatory conditions and conditions accompanied by neurologic changes or systemic manifestations of serious disease. Finally, individuals with chronic symptoms (>6 weeks), especially when there has been a lack of response to symptomatic measures, are candidates for additional evaluation. The extent and nature of the additional investigation should be dictated by the clinical features and suspected pathologic process. Laboratory tests should be used to confirm a specific clinical diagnosis and not be used to screen or evaluate patients with vague rheumatic complaints. Indiscriminate use of broad batteries of diagnostic tests and radiographic procedures is rarely a useful or cost-effective means to establish a diagnosis.

Besides a complete blood count, including a white blood cell (WBC) and differential count, the routine evaluation should include a determination of an acute-phase reactant such as the ESR or CRP, which can be useful in discriminating inflammatory from noninflammatory disorders. Both are inexpensive and easily obtained and may be elevated with infection, inflammation, autoimmune disorders, neoplasia, pregnancy, renal insufficiency, and advanced age.

Serum uric acid determinations are useful only when gout has been diagnosed and therapy contemplated. Uric acid, the end product of purine metabolism, is primarily excreted in the urine. Serum values range from 238–516 μmol/L (4.0–8.6 mg/dL) in men; the lower values

TABLE 325-4 ANTINUCLEAR ANTIBODY (ANA) PATTERNS AND CLINICAL ASSOCIATIONS

ANA Pattern	Antigen Identified	Clinical Correlate
Diffuse	Deoxyribonucleo-protein	Nonspecific
	Histones	Drug-induced lupus, lupus
Peripheral (rim)	ds-DNA	50% of SLE (specific)
Speckled	U1-RNP	>90% of MCTD
	Sm	30% of SLE (specific)
	Ro (SS-A)	Sjögrens 60%, SCLE, neonatal lupus, ANA(–) lupus
	La (SS-B)	50% of Sjögrens, 15% lupus
	Scl-70	40% of diffuse scleroderma
	PM-1	Polymyositis (PM), dermatomyositis
	Jo-1	PM w/ pneumonitis + arthritis
Nucleolar	RNA polymerase I, others	40% of PSS
Centromere	Kinetochore	75% CREST (limited scleroderma)

Note: SLE, systemic lupus erythematosus; MCTD, mixed connective tissue disease; SCLE, subacute cutaneous lupus erythematosus; PSS, progressive systemic sclerosis; CREST, calcinosis, *R*aynaud phenomenon, *e*sophageal involvement; *s*clerodactyly; and *t*elangiectasia.

cell count (2000–50,000/μL) and a polymorphonuclear leukocyte predominance. Inflammatory fluid has reduced viscosity, diminished hyaluronate, and little or no tail following each drop of synovial fluid. Such effusions are found in RA, gout, and other inflammatory arthritides. Septic fluid is opaque and purulent, with a WBC count usually >50,000/μL, a predominance of polymorphonuclear leukocytes (>75%), and low viscosity. Such effusions are typical of septic arthritis but may occur with RA or gout. In addition, hemorrhagic synovial fluid may be seen with trauma, hemarthrosis, or neuropathic arthritis. An algorithm for synovial fluid aspiration and analysis is shown in Fig. 325-6. Synovial fluid should be analyzed immediately for appearance, viscosity, and cell count. Monosodium urate crystals (observed in gout) are seen by polarized microscopy and are long, needle-shaped, negatively birefringent, and usually intracellular. In chondrocalcinosis and pseudogout, calcium pyrophosphate dihydrate crystals are usually short, rhomboid-shaped, and positively birefringent. Whenever infection is suspected, synovial fluid should be Gram-stained and cultured appropriately. If gonococcal arthritis is suspected, immediate plating of the fluid on appropriate culture medium is indicated. Synovial fluid from patients with chronic monarthritis should also be cultured for *M. tuberculosis* and fungi. Last, it should be noted that crystal-induced and septic arthritis occasionally occur together in the same joint.

DIAGNOSTIC IMAGING IN JOINT DISEASES

Conventional radiography has been a valuable tool in the diagnosis and staging of articular disorders. Plain x-rays are most appropriate when there is a history of trauma, suspected chronic infection, progressive disability, or monarticular involvement; when therapeutic alterations are considered; or when a baseline assessment is desired for what appears to be a chronic process. However, in acute inflammatory arthritis, early radiography is rarely helpful in establishing a diagnosis and may only reveal soft tissue swelling or juxtaarticular demineralization. As the disease progresses, calcification (of soft tissues, cartilage, or bone), joint space narrowing, erosions, bony ankylosis, new bone formation (sclerosis, osteophytes, or periostitis), or subchondral cysts may develop and suggest specific clinical entities. Consultation with a radiologist will help define the optimal imaging modality, technique, or positioning and prevent the need for further studies.

Additional imaging techniques may possess greater diagnostic sensitivity and facilitate early diagnosis in a limited number of articular disorders and in selected circumstances and are indicated when conventional radiography is inadequate or nondiagnostic (Table 325-5). *Ultrasonography* is useful in the detection of soft tissue abnormalities

INTERPRETATION OF SYNOVIAL FLUID ASPIRATION

Strongly consider synovial fluid aspiration and analysis if there is
• Monarthritis (acute or chronic)
• Trauma with joint effusion
• Monarthritis in a patient with chronic polyarthritis
• Suspicion of joint infection, crystal-induced arthritis, or hemarthrosis

Analyze fluid for
• Appearance, viscosity
• WBC count, differential
• Gram stain, culture, and sensitivity (if indicated)
• Crystal identification by polarized microscopy

Is the effusion hemorrhagic?

No / Yes

Inflammatory or noninflammatory articular condition

Consider
• Trauma or mechanical derangement
• Coagulopathy
• Neuropathic arthropathy
• Other

Is the WBC > 2000/μL?

No / Yes

Consider noninflammatory articular conditions
• Osteoarthritis
• Trauma
• Other

Consider inflammatory or septic arthritis

Is the % PMNs > 75%?

No

Yes

Consider other inflammatory or septic arthritides
• Gram stain, culture mandatory

Are crystals present?

No

Yes

Crystal identification for specific diagnosis
• Gout
• Pseudogout

Is the WBC > 50,000/μL?

No / Yes

Probable inflammatory arthritis

Possible septic arthritis

FIGURE 325-6 Algorithmic approach to the use and interpretation of synovial fluid aspiration and analysis. [WBC, white blood cell (count); PMNs, polymorphonuclear (leukocytes).]

that cannot be fully appreciated by clinical examination. Although inexpensive, it is seldom the preferred method of evaluation. The foremost application of ultrasound is in the diagnosis of synovial (Baker's) cysts, although rotator cuff tears and various tendon injuries may be evaluated with ultrasound by an experienced operator. *Radionuclide scintigraphy* provides useful information regarding the metabolic status of bone and, along with radiography, is well suited for total-body assessment of the extent and distribution of skeletal involvement. Radionuclide imaging is a very sensitive, but poorly specific, means of detecting inflammatory or metabolic alterations in bone or periarticular soft tissue structures. The limited tissue contrast resolution of scintigraphy may obscure the distinction between a bony or periarticular process and may necessitate the additional use of MRI. Scintigraphy, using ^{99m}Tc, ^{67}Ga, or ^{111}In-labeled WBCs has been applied to a variety of articular disorders with variable success (Table 325-5). Although [^{99m}Tc] pertechnate or diphosphate scintigraphy (Fig. 325-7) may be useful in identifying osseous infection, neoplasia, inflammation, increased blood flow, bone remodeling, heterotopic bone formation, or avascular necrosis, MRI is preferred in most instances. The poor specificity of ^{99m}Tc scanning has largely limited its use to surveys for bone

TABLE 325-5 DIAGNOSTIC IMAGING TECHNIQUES FOR MUSCULOSKELETAL DISORDERS

Method	Imaging Time, h	Cost[a]	Current Indications
Ultrasound[b]	<1	+	Synovial cysts Rotator cuff tears Tendon injury
Radionuclide scintigraphy			
^{99m}Tc	1–4	++	Metastatic bone survey Evaluation of Paget's disease Acute and chronic osteomyelitis
^{111}In-WBC	24	+++	Acute infection Prosthetic infection Acute osteomyelitis
^{67}Ga	24–48	++++	Acute and chronic infection Acute osteomyelitis
Computed tomography	<1	+++	Herniated intervertebral disk Sacroiliitis Spinal stenosis Spinal trauma Osteoid osteoma Stress fracture
Magnetic resonance imaging	1/2–2	+++++	Avascular necrosis Osteomyelitis Intraarticular derangement and soft tissue injury Derangements of axial skeleton and spinal cord Herniated intervertebral disk Pigmented villonodular synovitis Inflammatory and metabolic muscle pathology

[a]Relative cost for imaging study.
[b]Results depend on operator.

disc), sacroiliitis, osteoid osteoma, and stress fractures. Helical or spiral CT (with or without contrast angiography) is a novel technique that is rapid, cost effective, and sensitive in diagnosing pulmonary embolism or obscure fractures, often in the setting of initially equivocal findings. High-resolution CT can be advocated in the evaluation of suspected or established infiltrative lung disease (e.g., scleroderma or rheumatoid lung). The recent use of hybrid [positron emission tomography (PET)/CT or single photon emission CT (SPECT/CT)] scans in metastatic evaluations have incorporated CT to provide better anatomic localization of scintigraphic abnormalities.

MRI has significantly advanced the ability to image musculoskeletal structures. MRI has the advantages of providing multiplanar images with fine anatomic detail and contrast resolution (Fig. 325-8) that allows for the superior ability to visualize bone marrow and soft tissue periarticular structures. Although more costly with a longer procedural time than CT, the MRI has become the preferred technique when evaluating complex musculoskeletal disorders.

MRI can image fascia, vessels, nerve, muscle, cartilage, ligaments, tendons, pannus, synovial effusions, and bone marrow. Visualization of particular structures can be enhanced by alter-

metastases and Paget's disease of bone. Gallium scanning utilizes ^{67}Ga, which binds serum and cellular transferrin and lactoferrin, and is preferentially taken up by neutrophils, macrophages, bacteria, and tumor tissue (e.g., lymphoma). As such, it is primarily used in the identification of occult infection or malignancy. Scanning with ^{111}In-labeled WBCs has been used to detect osteomyelitis and infectious and inflammatory arthritis. Nevertheless, the use of ^{111}In-labeled WBC or ^{67}Ga scanning has largely been replaced by MRI, except when there is a suspicion of prosthetic joint infections.

CT provides detailed visualization of the axial skeleton. Articulations previously considered difficult to visualize by radiography (e.g., zygapophyseal, sacroiliac, sternoclavicular, hip joints) can be effectively evaluated using CT. CT has been demonstrated to be useful in the diagnosis of low back pain syndromes (e.g., spinal stenosis vs. herniated

FIGURE 325-7 **[^{99m}Tc]diphosphonate scintigraphy of the feet of a 33-year-old black male with reactive arthritis,** manifested by sacroiliitis, urethritis, uveitis, asymmetric oligoarthritis, and enthesitis. This bone scan demonstrates increased uptake indicative of enthesitis involving the insertions of the left Achilles tendon, plantar aponeurosis, and right tibialis posterior tendon as well as arthritis of the right first interphalangeal joint.

FIGURE 325-8 **Superior sensitivity of MRI in the diagnosis of osteonecrosis of the femoral head.** A 45-year-old woman receiving high-dose glucocorticoids developed right hip pain. Conventional x-rays (*top*) demonstrated only mild sclerosis of the right femoral head. T1-weighted MRI (*bottom*) demonstrated low-density signal in the right femoral head, diagnostic of osteonecrosis.

ing the pulse sequence to produce either T1- or T2-weighted spin echo, gradient echo, or inversion recovery [including short tau inversion recovery (STIR)] images. Because of its sensitivity to changes in marrow fat, MRI is a sensitive but nonspecific means of detecting osteonecrosis, osteomyelitis, and marrow inflammation indicating overlying synovitis or osteitis (Fig. 325-8). Because of its enhanced soft tissue resolution, MRI is more sensitive than arthrography or CT in the diagnosis of soft tissue injuries (e.g., meniscal and rotator cuff tears); intraarticular derangements; marrow abnormalities (osteonecrosis, myeloma); and spinal cord or nerve root damage or synovitis.

FURTHER READINGS

AVOUAC J et al: Diagnostic and predictive value of anti-cyclic citrullinated protein antibodies in rheumatoid arthritis: A systematic literature review. Ann Rheum Dis 65(7):845, 2006

CUSH JJ et al: Evaluation of musculoskeletal complaints, in *Rheumatology: Diagnosis and Therapeutics,* 2d ed, JJ Cush, A Kavanaugh, CM Stein (eds). Philadelphia, Lippincott Williams & Wilkins, 2005, pp 3–20

HOOTMAN JM, HELMICK CG: Projections of US prevalence of arthritis and associated activity limitations. Arthritis Rheum 54(1):226, 2006

KAVANAUGH A: The utility of immunologic laboratory tests in patients with rheumatic diseases. Arthritis Rheum 44:2221, 2001

ORY PA: Radiography in the assessment of musculoskeletal conditions. Best Pract Res Clin Rheumatol 17(3):495, 2003

RUDWALEIT M et al: How to diagnose axial spondyloarthritis early. Ann Rheum Dis 63(5):535, 2004

SHMERLING RH et al: Synovial fluid tests: What should be ordered? JAMA 264:1009, 1990

SIVA C et al: Diagnosing acute monoarthritis in adults: A practical approach for the family physician. Am Fam Physician 68(1):83, 2003

326 Osteoarthritis
David T. Felson

Osteoarthritis (OA) is the most common type of arthritis. Its high prevalence, especially in the elderly, and the high rate of disability related to disease make it a leading cause of disability in the elderly. Because of the aging of Western populations and because obesity, a major risk factor, are increasing in prevalence, the occurrence of osteoarthritis is on the rise. In the United States, osteoarthritis prevalence will increase from 66–100% by the year 2020.

OA affects certain joints, yet spares others (Fig. 326-1). Commonly affected joints include the cervical and lumbosacral spine, hip, knee, and first metatarsal phalangeal joint (MTP). In the hands, the distal and proximal interphalangeal joints and the base of the thumb are often affected. Usually spared are the wrist, elbow, and ankle. Our joints were designed in an evolutionary sense, when humans were still brachiating apes. We thus develop OA in joints that were ill designed for these tasks, i.e., joints involved in pincer grip in the hands and lower extremity weight-bearing joints. Some joints, like the ankles, may be spared because their articular cartilage may be uniquely resistant to loading stresses.

OA can be diagnosed based on structural abnormalities or on the symptoms these abnormalities evoke. Based on cadaveric studies, structural changes of OA are nearly universal by the elderly years. These include cartilage loss (seen as joint space loss on x-rays) and osteophytes. Many persons with x-ray evidence of OA have no joint symptoms and, while the prevalence of structural abnormalities is of interest in understanding disease pathogenesis, what matters more from a clinical and public health perspective is the prevalence of symptomatic OA. Symptoms, usually joint pain, determine disability, visits to clinicians, and disease costs.

Symptomatic OA of the knee (pain on most days of a recent month in a knee plus x-ray evidence of OA in that knee) occurs in ~12% of persons age ≥60 in the United States and 6% of all adults age ≥30. Symptomatic hip OA is roughly one-third as common as disease in the knee. While radiographically evident hand OA and the appearance of bony enlargement in affected hand joints (Fig. 326-2) are extremely common in older persons, most cases are often not symptomatic. Even so, recent studies suggest that symptomatic hand OA occurs in ~10% of elderly individuals and often produces measurable physical functional limitation.

The prevalence of OA correlates strikingly with age. Regardless of how it is defined, OA is uncommon in adults under age 40 and highly prevalent in those over age 60. It is also a disease that, at least in middle-aged and elderly persons, is much more common in women than in men, and sex differences in prevalence increase with age.

FIGURE 326-1 Joints affected by osteoarthritis.

First carpometacarpal

Distal and proximal interphalangeal

Cervical vertebrae

Lower lumbar vertebrae

Hip

Knee

First metatarsophalangeal

FIGURE 326-2 Severe osteoarthritis of the hands affecting the distal interphalangeal joints (Heberden's nodes) and the proximal interphalangeal joints (Bouchard's nodes). There is no clear bony enlargement of the other common site in the hands, the thumb base.

X-ray evidence of OA is common in the lower back and neck, but back pain and neck pain have not been tied to findings of OA on x-ray. Thus, back pain and neck pain are treated separately (Chap. 16).

DEFINITION

OA is joint failure, a disease in which all structures of the joint have undergone pathologic change, often in concert. The pathologic sine qua non of disease is hyaline articular cartilage loss, present in a focal and, initially, nonuniform manner. This is accompanied by increasing thickness and sclerosis of the subchondral bony plate, by outgrowth of osteophytes at the joint margin, by stretching of the articular capsule, by mild synovitis in many affected joints, and by weakness of muscles bridging the joint. In knees, meniscal degeneration is part of the disease. There are numerous pathways that lead to joint failure, but the initial step is often joint injury in the setting of a failure of protective mechanisms.

JOINT PROTECTIVE MECHANISMS AND THEIR FAILURE

Joint protectors include: joint capsule and ligaments, muscle, sensory afferents, and underlying bone. Joint capsule and ligaments serve as joint protectors by providing a limit to excursion, thereby fixing the range of joint motion.

Synovial fluid reduces friction between articulating cartilage surfaces, thereby serving as a major protector against friction-induced cartilage wear. This lubrication function depends on the molecule *lubricin*, a mucinous glycoprotein secreted by synovial fibroblasts whose concentration diminishes after joint injury and in the face of synovial inflammation.

The ligaments, along with overlying skin and tendons, contain mechanoreceptor sensory afferent nerves. These mechanoreceptors fire at different frequencies throughout a joint's range of motion, providing feedback by way of the spinal cord to muscles and tendons. As a consequence, these muscles and tendons can assume the right tension at appropriate points in joint excursion to act as optimal joint protectors, anticipating joint loading.

Muscles and tendons that bridge the joint are key joint protectors. Their co-contractions at the appropriate time in joint movement provide the appropriate power and acceleration for the limb to accomplish its tasks. Focal stress across the joint is minimized by muscle contraction that decelerates the joint before impact and assures that when joint impact arrives, it is distributed broadly across the joint surface.

The bone underneath the cartilage may also provide a shock-absorbing function, as it may give way subtly to an oncoming impulse load.

Failure of these joint protectors increases the risk of joint injury and OA. For example, in animals, OA develops rapidly when a sensory nerve to the joint is sectioned and joint injury induced. Similarly, in humans, Charcot arthropathy, which is a severe and rapidly progressive OA, develops when minor joint injury occurs in the presence of posterior column peripheral neuropathy. Another example of joint protector failure is rupture of ligaments, a well-known cause of the early development of OA.

Cartilage and Its Role in Joint Failure In addition to being a primary target tissue for disease, cartilage also functions as a joint protector. A thin rim of tissue at the ends of two opposing bones, cartilage is lubricated by synovial fluid to provides an almost frictionless surface across which these two bones move. The compressible stiffness of cartilage compared to bone provides the joint with impact-absorbing capacity. Both the smooth frictionless surface and the compressive stiffness of cartilage serve as protective mechanisms preventing joint injury.

Since the earliest changes of OA may occur in cartilage and abnormalities there can accelerate disease development, understanding the structure and physiology of cartilage is critical to an appreciation of disease pathogenesis. The two major macromolecules in cartilage are type 2 collagen, which provides cartilage its tensile strength, and aggrecan, a proteoglycan macromolecule linked with hyaluronic acid, which consists of highly negatively charged glycosaminoglycans. In normal cartilage, type 2 collagen is woven tightly, constraining the aggrecan

molecules in the interstices between collagen strands, forcing these highly negatively charged molecules into close proximity with one another. The aggrecan molecule, through electrostatic repulsion of its negative charges, gives cartilage its compressive stiffness. Chondrocytes, the cells within this avascular tissue, synthesize all elements of the matrix. In addition, they produce enzymes that break down the matrix and cytokines and growth factors, which in turn provide autocrine/paracrine feedback that modulates synthesis of matrix molecules (Fig. 326-3). Cartilage matrix synthesis and catabolism are in a dynamic equilibrium influenced by the cytokine and growth factor environment and by mechanical stress. While chondrocytes synthesize numerous enzymes, especially matrix metalloproteinases (MMP), there are only a few that are critical in regulating cartilage breakdown. Type 2 cartilage is degraded primarily by MMP-13 (collagenase 3), with other collagenases playing a minor role. Aggrecan degradation is complex but appears to be a consequence, in part, of activation of aggrecanase 1 (ADAMTS-4) and perhaps of MMPs. Both collagenase and aggrecanase act primarily in the territorial matrix surrounding chondrocytes; however, as the osteoarthritic process develops, their activities and effects spread throughout the matrix, especially in the superficial layers of cartilage.

The synovium and chondrocytes synthesize numerous growth factors and cytokines. Chief among them is interleukin (IL) 1, which exerts transcriptional effects on chondrocytes, stimulating production of proteinases and suppressing cartilage matrix synthesis. In animal models of OA, IL-1 blockade prevents cartilage loss. Tumor necrosis factor (TNF) α may play a similar role to that of IL-1. These cytokines also induce chondrocytes to synthesize prostaglandin E_2, nitric oxide, and bone morphogenic protein 2 (BMP-2), which together have complex effects on matrix synthesis and degradation. Nitric oxide inhibits aggrecan synthesis and enhances proteinase activity, whereas BMP-2 is a potent stimulator of anabolic activity. At early stages in the matrix response to injury and in the healthy response to loading, the net effect of cytokine stimulation may be matrix turnover but, ultimately, excess IL-1 triggers a process of matrix degradation. Enzymes in the matrix are held in check by activation inhibitors, including tissue inhibitor of metalloproteinase (TIMP). Growth factors are also part of this complex network, with insulin-like growth factor type 1 and transforming growth factor β playing prominent roles in stimulating anabolism by chondrocytes.

While healthy cartilage is metabolically sluggish, with slow matrix turnover and a net balance of synthesis and degradation, cartilage in early OA or after an injury is highly metabolically active. In the latter situation, stimulated chondrocytes synthesize enzymes and new matrix molecules, with those enzymes becoming activated in the matrix, causing release of degraded aggrecan and type 2 collagen into cartilage and into the synovial fluid. OA cartilage is characterized by gradual depletion of aggrecan, an unfurling of the tightly woven collagen matrix, and loss of type 2 collagen. With these changes comes increasing vulnerability of cartilage, which no longer has compressive stiffness.

RISK FACTORS

Joint vulnerability and joint loading are the two major factors contributing to the development of OA. On the one hand, a vulnerable joint whose protectors are dysfunctional can develop OA with minimal levels of loading, perhaps even levels encountered during ever day activities. On the other hand, in a young joint with competent protectors, a major acute injury or long-term overloading is necessary to precipitate disease. Risk factors for OA can be understood in terms of their effect either on joint vulnerability or on loading (Fig. 326-4).

Systemic Risk Factors Age is the most potent risk factor for OA, with prevalence and incidence of disease rising dramatically with age. Radiographic evidence of OA is rare in individuals under age 40; however, in some joints, such as the hands, OA occurs in >50% of persons over age 70. Aging increases joint vulnerability through several mechanisms. Whereas dynamic loading of joints stimulates cartilage matrix by chondrocytes in young cartilage, aged cartilage is less responsive to these stimuli. Indeed, because of the poor responsiveness of older cartilage to such stimulation, cartilage transplant operations are far more

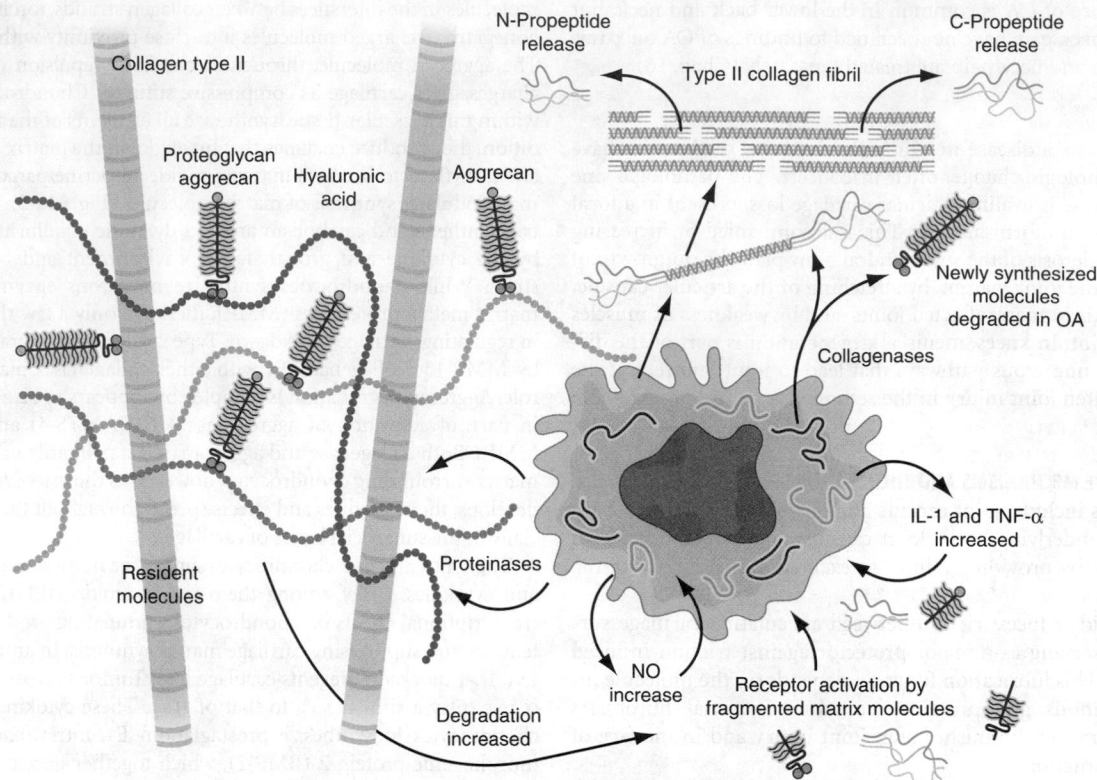

FIGURE 326-3 The chondrocyte and its products, type II collagen, aggrecan and enzymes which degrade these structures along with molecules stimulating chondrocytes. [*From AR Poole et al: Ann Rheum Dis 61 (S): ii78, 2002.*]

challenging in older than in younger persons. Partly because of this failure to synthesize matrix with loading, cartilage thins with age, and thinner cartilage experiences higher shear stress at basal layers and is at greater risk of cartilage damage. Aging also increases the likelihood of failure of major joint protectors. Muscles that bridge the joint become weaker with age and also respond less quickly to oncoming impulses. Sensory nerve input slows with age, retarding the feedback loop of mechanoreceptors to muscles and tendons related to their tension and position. Ligaments stretch with age, making them less able to absorb

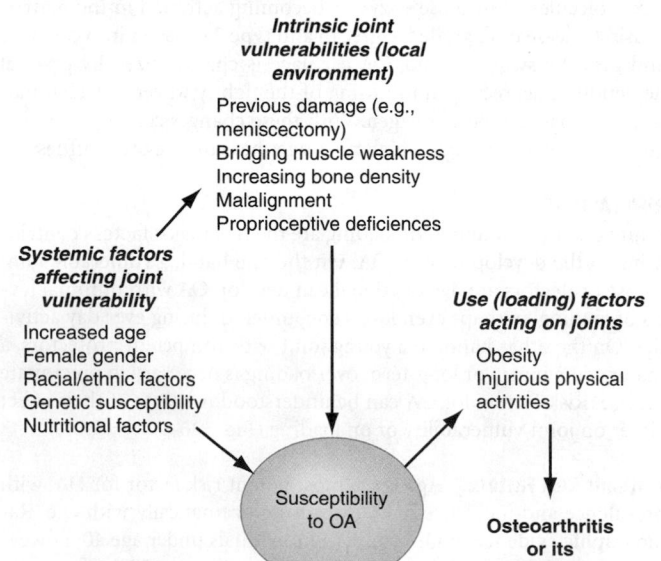

FIGURE 326-4 Risk factors for osteoarthritis either contribute to the susceptibility of the joint (systemic factors or factors in the local joint environment) or they increase risk by the load they put on the joint. Usually a combination of loading and susceptibility factors is required to cause disease or its progression.

impulses. A combination of all of these factors work in concert to increase the vulnerability of older joints to OA.

Older women are at high risk of OA in all joints, a risk that emerges as women reach their sixth decade. While hormone loss with menopause may contribute to this risk, there is little understanding of the vulnerability of older women's joints to OA.

Heritability and Genetics OA is a highly heritable disease, but its heritability varies by joint. Fifty percent of the hand and hip OA in the community is attributable to inheritance, i.e., to disease present in other members of the family. However, the heritable proportion of knee OA is at most 30%, with some studies suggesting no heritability at all. Whereas many people with OA have disease in multiple joints, this "generalized OA" phenotype is rarely inherited and is more often a consequence of aging.

Emerging evidence suggests that persons with genetic mutations in proteins that regulate the transcription of major cartilage molecules are at high risk of OA. One gene implicated is *FRZB*, in which a mutation may put a woman at high risk of hip OA. *FRZB* is a gene for a Frizzle protein that antagonizes an extracellular Wnt ligand, and the Wnt signaling pathway plays a critical role in matrix synthesis and joint development.

Global Considerations Hip OA is rare in China and in immigrants from China to the United States. However, OA in the knees, is at least as common, if not more so, in Chinese than in Caucasians from the United States, and knee OA represents a major cause of disability in China. Anatomic differences between Chinese and Caucasian hips may account for much of the difference in prevalence, with Caucasian hips having a higher prevalence of anatomic predispositions to the development of OA. Persons from Africa, but not African Americans, may also have a very low rate of hip OA.

Risk Factors in the Joint Environment Some risk factors increase vulnerability of the joint through local effects on the joint environment. With changes in joint anatomy, for example, load across the joint is no longer distributed evenly across the joint surface, but rather shows an increase in focal stress. In the hip, three uncommon developmental abnormalities occurring in utero or childhood, congenital dysplasia, Legg-Perthes disease, and slipped femoral capital epiphysis, leave a child with distortions of hip joint anatomy that often lead to OA later in life. Girls are predominantly affected by acetabular dysplasia, a mild form of congenital dislocation, whereas the other abnormalities more often affect boys. Depending on the severity of the anatomic abnormalities, hip OA occurs either in young adulthood (severe abnormalities) or middle age (mild abnormalities).

Major injuries to a joint also can produce anatomic abnormalities that leave the joint susceptible to OA. For example, a fracture through the joint surface often causes OA in joints in which the disease is otherwise rare such as the ankle and the wrist. Avascular necrosis can lead to collapse of dead bone at the articular surface, producing anatomic irregularities and subsequent OA.

Tears of ligaments that protect the joints, such as the anterior cruciate ligament in the knee and the labrum in the hip, can increase joint susceptibility and lead to premature OA. While meniscal tears may increase the risk of OA, meniscectomy operations, including selective ones, increase the risk of later disease, perhaps independent of the tear that led to the operation. Even injuries that do not produce diagnosed joint injuries may increase risk of OA, perhaps because the structural injury was not detected at the time. For example, in the Framingham study subjects, men with a history of major knee injury, but no surgery, had a 3.5-fold increased risk for subsequent knee OA.

Another source of anatomic abnormality is malalignment across the joint (Fig. 326-5). This factor has been best studied in the knee, which is the fulcrum of the longest lever arm in the body. Varus (bow-legged) knees with OA are at exceedingly high risk of cartilage loss in the medial or inner compartment of the knee, whereas valgus (knock-kneed) malalignment predisposes to rapid cartilage loss in the lateral compartment. Malalignment causes this effect by decreasing contact area during loading, increasing stress on a focal area or cartilage, which then breaks down. There is evidence that malalignment in the knee not only causes cartilage loss but leads to underlying bone damage, producing bone marrow lesions seen on MRI.

While it is likely that the weakness in muscles bridging a joint increase the risk of OA in that joint, there is no definitive evidence in this regard.

Patients with knee OA have impaired proprioception across their knees, and this may predispose them to further disease progression. The role of bone in serving as a shock absorber for impact load is not well understood, but persons with increased bone density are at high risk of OA, suggesting that the resistance of bone to impact during joint use may play a role in disease development.

Loading Factors · *OBESITY* Three to six times body weight is exerted across the knee during single leg stance. Any increase in weight may be multiplied by this factor to reveal the excess force across the knee in overweight persons during walking. Obesity is a well-recognized and potent risk factor for the development of knee OA and, less so, for hip OA. Obesity precedes the development of disease and is not just a consequence of the inactivity present in those with disease. Obesity is a stronger risk factor for disease in women than in men, and in women, the relationship of weight to the risk of disease is linear, so that with each increase in weight, there is a commensurate increase in risk. Weight loss in women lowers the risk of developing symptomatic disease. Not only is obesity a risk factor for OA in weight-bearing joints, but obese persons have more severe symptoms from the disease.

Obesity's effect on the development and progression of disease is mediated mostly through the increased loading in weight-bearing joints that occurs in overweight persons. However, a modest association of obesity with an increased risk of hand OA suggests that there may be a systemic metabolic factor circulating in obese persons that affects disease risk also.

REPEATED USE OF JOINT There are two categories of repetitive joint use, occupational use and leisure time physical activities. Workers performing repetitive tasks as part of their occupations for many years are at high risk of developing OA in the joints they use repeatedly. For example, farmers are at high risk for hip OA, miners have high rates of OA in knees and spine, and shipyard and dockyard workers have a higher prevalence of disease in knees and fingers than do office workers. Even within a textile mill, women whose jobs required fine pincer grip [increasing the stress across the interphalangeal (IP) joints] had much more distal IP (DIP) joint OA than women of the same age whose jobs required repeated power grip, a motion that does not stress the DIP joints. Workers whose jobs require regular knee bending or lifting or carrying heavy loads have a high rate of knee OA. One reason why workers may get disease is that during long days at work, their muscles may gradually become exhausted, no longer serving as effective joint protectors.

While exercise is a major element of the treatment of OA, certain types of exercise may paradoxically increase the risk of disease. While recreational runners are not at increased risk of knee OA, studies suggest that they do have a modest increased risk of disease in the hip. However, persons who have already sustained major knee injuries are at increased risk of progressive knee OA as a consequence of running. Compared to nonrunners, elite runners (professional runners and those on Olympic teams) have high risks of both knee and hip OA. Given the widespread recommendation to adopt a healthier, more exercise-filled lifestyle; longitudinal epidemiologic studies of exercise contain cautionary notes. For example, women with increased levels of physical activity, either as teenagers or at age 50, had a higher risk of developing symptomatic hip disease later in life than women who were sedentary. Other athletic activities that pose high risks of joint injury, such as football, may thereby predispose to OA.

PATHOLOGY

The pathology of OA provides evidence of the panarticular involvement of disease. Cartilage initially shows surface fibrillation and irregularity. As disease progresses, focal erosions develop there, and these eventually extend down to the subjacent bone. With further progression, cartilage erosion down to bone expands to involve a larger proportion of the joint surface, even though OA remains a focal disease with nonuniform loss of cartilage (Fig. 326-6).

After an injury to cartilage, chondrocytes undergo mitosis and clustering. While the metabolic activity of these chondrocyte clusters is high, the net effect of this activity is to promote proteoglycan depletion in the matrix surrounding the chondrocytes. This is because the catabolic activity is greater than the synthetic. As disease develops, collagen matrix becomes damaged, the negative charges of proteoglycans get exposed, and cartilage swells from ionic attraction to water molecules. Because in damaged cartilage proteoglycans are no longer forced into close proximity, cartilage does not bounce back after loading as it did when healthy, and cartilage becomes vulnerable to further injury. Chondrocytes at the basal level of cartilage undergo apoptosis.

Normal   Varus   Knock knees (valgus)

FIGURE 326-5 The two types of limb malalignment in the frontal plane: *varus,* in which the stress is placed across the medial compartment of the knee joint, and *valgus,* which places excess stress across the lateral compartment of the knee.

FIGURE 326-6 Pathologic changes of osteoarthritis in a toe joint. Note the nonuniform loss of cartilage (arrowhead vs. solid arrow), the increased thickness of the subchondral bone envelope (solid arrow), and the osteophyte (open arrow). (*From the American College of Rheumatology slide collection.*)

With loss of cartilage come alterations in subchondral bone. Stimulated by growth factors and cytokines, osteoclasts and osteoblasts in the subchondral bony plate, just underneath cartilage, become activated. Bone formation produces a thickening and stiffness of the subchondral plate that occurs even before cartilage ulcerates. Trauma to bone during joint loading may be the primary factor driving this bone response, with healing from injury (including microcracks) producing stiffness. Small areas of osteonecrosis usually exist in joints with advanced disease. Bone death may also be caused by bone trauma with shearing of microvasculature, leading to a cutoff of vascular supply to some bone areas.

At the margin of the joint, near areas of cartilage loss, osteophytes form. These start as outgrowths of new cartilage and, with neurovascular invasion from the bone, this cartilage ossifies. Osteophytes are an important radiographic hallmark of OA. In malaligned joints, osteophytes grow larger on the side of the joint subject to most loading stress (e.g., in varus knees, osteophytes grow larger on the medial side).

The synovium produces lubricating fluids that minimize shear stress during motion. In healthy joints, the synovium consists of a single discontinuous layer filled with fat and containing two types of cells, macrophages and fibroblasts, but, in OA, it can sometimes become edematous and inflamed. There is a migration of macrophages from the periphery into the tissue, and cells lining the synovium proliferate. Enzymes secreted by the synovium digest cartilage matrix that has been sheared from the surface of the cartilage.

Additional pathologic changes occur in the capsule, which stretches, becomes edematous, and can become fibrotic.

The pathology of OA is not identical across joints. In hand joints with severe OA, for example, there are often cartilage erosions in the center of the joint probably produced by bony pressure from the opposite side of the joint. Bone remodeling is a prominent feature of hand OA, in part because of the thin cartilage in each hand joint. In hand OA, pathology has also been noted in ligament site insertions, which may help propagate disease.

Basic calcium phosphate and calcium pyrophosphate dihydrate crystals are present microscopically in most joints with end-stage OA. Their role in osteoarthritic cartilage is unclear, but their release from cartilage into the joint space and joint fluid likely triggers synovial inflammation, which can, in turn, produce release of enzymes and trigger nociceptive stimulation.

SOURCES OF PAIN

Because cartilage is aneural, cartilage loss in a joint is not accompanied by pain. Thus, pain in OA likely arises from structures outside the car-

tilage. Innervated structures in the joint include the synovium, ligaments, joint capsule, muscles, and subchondral bone. Most of these are not visualized by the x-ray, and the severity of x-ray changes in OA correlates poorly with pain severity.

Based on MRI studies in osteoarthritic knees comparing those with and without pain and on studies mapping tenderness in unanesthetized joints, likely sources of pain include synovial inflammation, joint effusions, and bone marrow edema. Modest synovitis develops in many but not all osteoarthritic joints. Some diseased joints have no synovitis, whereas others have synovial inflammation that approaches the severity of joints with rheumatoid arthritis (Chap. 314). The presence of synovitis on MRI is correlated with the presence and severity of knee pain. Capsular stretching from fluid in the joint stimulates nociceptive fibers there, inducing pain. Increased focal loading as part of the disease not only damages cartilage but probably also injures the underlying bone. As a consequence, bone marrow edema appears on the MRI; histologically, this edema may signal the presence of microcracks and scar, which are the consequences of trauma. These lesions may stimulate bone nociceptive fibers. Also, hemostatic pressure within bone rises in OA, and the increased pressure itself may stimulate nociceptive fibers, causing pain. Lastly, osteophytes themselves may be a source of pain. When osteophytes grow, neurovascular innervation penetrates through the base of the bone into the cartilage and into the developing osteophyte.

Pain may arise from outside the joint also, including bursae near the joints. Common sources of pain near the knee are anserine bursitis and iliotibial band syndrome.

CLINICAL FEATURES

Joint pain from OA is activity-related. Pain comes on either during or just after joint use and then gradually resolves. Examples include knee or hip pain with going up or down stairs, pain in weight-bearing joints when walking, and, for hand OA, pain after cooking. Early in disease, pain is episodic, triggered often by a day or two of overactive use of a diseased joint, such as a person with knee OA taking a long run and noticing a few days of pain thereafter. As disease progresses, the pain becomes continuous and even begins to be bothersome at night. Stiffness of the affected joint may be prominent, but morning stiffness is usually brief (<30 min).

In knees, buckling may occur, in part, due to weakness of muscles crossing the joint. Mechanical symptoms, such as buckling, catching, or locking, could also signify internal derangement, such as meniscal tears, and need to be evaluated. In the knee, pain with activities requiring knee flexion, such as stair climbing and arising from a chair, often emanates from the patellofemoral compartment of the knee, which does not actively articulate until the knee is bent ~35°.

OA is the most common cause of chronic knee pain in persons over age 45, but the differential diagnosis is long. Inflammatory arthritis is likely if there is prominent morning stiffness and many other joints are affected. Bursitis occurs commonly around knees and hips. A physical examination should focus on whether tenderness is over the joint line (at the junction of the two bones around which the joint is articulating) or is outside of it. Anserine bursitis, medial and distal to the knee, is an extremely common cause of chronic knee pain that may respond to a glucocorticoid injection. Prominent nocturnal pain in the absence of end-stage OA merits a distinct workup. For hip pain, OA can be detected by loss of internal rotation on passive movement, and pain isolated to an area lateral to the hip joint usually reflects the presence of trochanteric bursitis.

No blood tests are routinely indicated for workup of patients with OA unless less symptoms and signs suggest inflammatory arthritis. Examination of the synovial fluid is often more helpful diagnostically than an x-ray. If the synovial fluid white count is >1000 per μL, inflammatory arthritis or gout or pseudogout are likely, the latter two being also identified by the presence of crystals.

X-rays are indicated to evaluate chronic hand pain and hip pain thought to be due to OA, as the diagnosis is often unclear without confirming radiographs. For knee pain, x-rays should be obtained if

FIGURE 326-7 X-ray of knee with medial osteoarthritis. Note the narrowed joint space on medial side of the joint only (*white arrow*), the sclerosis of the bone in the medial compartment providing evidence of cortical thickening (*black arrow*), and the osteophytes in the medial femur (*white wedge*).

symptoms or signs are not typical of OA or if knee pain persists after effective treatment. In OA, radiographic findings (Fig. 326-7) correlate poorly with the presence and severity of pain. Further, radiographs may be normal in early disease as they are insensitive to cartilage loss and other early findings.

While MRI may reveal the extent of pathology in an osteoarthritic joint, it is not indicated as part of the diagnostic workup. Findings such as meniscal tears in cartilage and bone lesions occur in most patients with OA in the knee, but almost never warrant a change in therapy.

℞ OSTEOARTHRITIS

The goals of the treatment of OA are to alleviate pain and minimize loss of physical function. To the extent that pain and loss of function are consequences of inflammation, of weakness across the joint, and of laxity and instability, the treatment of OA involves addressing each of these impairments. Comprehensive therapy consists of a multimodality approach including nonpharmacologic and pharmacologic elements.

Patients with mild and intermittent symptoms may need only reassurance or nonpharmacologic treatments. Patients with ongoing, disabling pain are likely to need both nonpharmaco- and pharmacotherapy.

Treatments for knee OA have been more completely evaluated than those for hip and hand OA or for disease in other joints. Thus, while the principles of treatment are identical for OA in all joints, we shall focus below on the treatment of knee OA, noting specific recommendations for disease in other joints, especially when they differ from those for disease in the knee.

NONPHARMACOTHERAPY   Since OA is a mechanically driven disease, the mainstay of treatment involves altering loading across the painful joint and improving the function of joint protectors, so they can better distribute load across the joint. Ways of lessening focal load across the joint include

(1) avoiding activities that overload the joint, as evidenced by their causing pain;
(2) improving the strength and conditioning of muscles that bridge the joint, so as to optimize their function; and
(3) unloading the joint, either by redistributing load within the joint with a brace or a splint or by unloading the joint during weight bearing with a cane or a crutch.

The simplest effective treatment for many patients is to avoid activities that precipitate pain. For example, for the middle-aged patient whose long-distance running brings on symptoms of knee OA, a less demanding form of weight-bearing activity may alleviate all symptoms. For an older person whose daily constitutionals up and down hills bring on knee pain, routing the constitutional away from hills might eliminate symptoms.

Each pound of weight increases the loading across the knee three- to sixfold. Weight loss may have a commensurate multiplier effect, unloading

both knees and hips. Thus, weight loss, especially if substantial, may lessen symptoms of knee and hip OA.

In hand joints affected by OA, splinting, by limiting motion, often minimizes pain for patients with involvement either in the base of the thumb or in the DIP or proximal IP joints. With an appropriate splint, function can often be preserved. Weight-bearing joints such as knees and hips can be unloaded by using a cane in the hand opposite to the affected joint for partial weight bearing. A physical therapist can help teach the patient how to use the cane optimally, including ensuring that its height is optimal for unloading. Crutches or walkers can serve a similar beneficial function.

Exercise   Osteoarthritic pain in knees or hips during weight bearing results in lack of activity and poor mobility and, because OA is so common, the inactivity that results represent a public health concern, increasing the risk of cardiovascular disease and of obesity. Aerobic capacity is poor in most elders with symptomatic knee OA, worse than others of the same age.

The development of weakness in muscles that bridge osteoarthritic joints is multifactorial in etiology. First, there is a decline in strength with age. Second, with limited mobility comes disuse muscle atrophy. Third, patients with painful knee or hip OA alter their gait so as to lessen loading across the affected joint, and this further diminishes muscle use. Fourth, "arthrogenous inhibition" may occur, whereby contraction of muscles bridging the joint is inhibited by a nerve afferent feedback loop emanating in a swollen and stretched joint capsule; this prevents maximal attainment of voluntary maximal strength. Since adequate muscle strength and conditioning are critical to joint protection, weakness in a muscle that bridges a diseased joint makes the joint more susceptible to further damage and pain. The degree of weakness correlates strongly with the severity of joint pain and the degree of physical limitation. One of the cardinal elements of the treatment of OA is to improve the functioning of muscles surrounding the joint.

At least for knee OA, trials have shown that exercise lessens pain and improves physical function. Most effective exercise regimens consist of aerobic and/or resistance training, the latter of which focuses on strengthening muscles across the joint. Exercises are likely to be effective, especially if they train muscles for the activities a person performs daily. Some exercises may actually increase pain in the joint; these should be avoided, and the regimen needs to be individualized to optimize effectiveness and minimize discomfort. Range-of-motion exercises, which do not strengthen muscles, and isometric exercises that strengthen muscles, but not through range of motion, are unlikely to be effective by themselves. Isokinetic and isotonic strengthening (strengthening that occurs when a person flexes or extends the knees against resistance) have been shown consistently to be efficacious. Low-impact exercises, including water aerobics and water resistance training, are often better tolerated by patients than exercises involving impact loading, such as running or treadmill exercises. A patient should be referred to an exercise class or to a therapist who can create an individualized regimen, and then an individualized home-based regimen can be crafted.

There is no strong evidence that patients with hip or hand OA benefit from therapeutic exercise, although for any patient with OA, individualized exercise programs should be tried. Adherence to exercise over the long term is the major challenge to an exercise prescription. In trials involving patients with knee OA who are interested in exercise treatment, a third to over a half of patients stopped exercising by 6 months. Less than 50% continued regular exercise at 1 year. The strongest predictor of continued exercise in a patient is a previous personal history of successful exercise. Physicians should reinforce the exercise prescription at each clinic visit, help the patient recognize barriers to ongoing exercise, and identify convenient times for exercise to be done routinely. The combination of exercise with calorie restriction is especially effective in lessening pain.

One clinical trial has suggested that, among those with very early OA, participating in a strengthening and multimodality exercise program led to improvement in cartilage biochemistry, as evidenced by MRI imaging. There is little other evidence, however, that strengthening or other exercise has an effect on joint structure.

Correction of Malalignment   Malalignment in the frontal plane (varus-valgus) markedly increases the stress across the joint, which can lead to progression of disease and to pain and disability (Fig. 326-5). Correcting malalignment, either surgically or with bracing, can relieve pain in persons whose knees are maligned. Malalignment develops over years as a consequence of gradual anatomic alterations of the joint and bone, and correcting it is often very challenging. One way is with a fitted brace, which takes an often varus osteoarthritic knee and straightens it by putting valgus stress across the knee. Unfortunately, many patients are unwilling to wear a realigning knee brace, plus in patients with obese legs, braces may slip with usage and lose their realigning effect. They are indicated for willing patients who can learn to put them on correctly and on whom they do not slip.

Other ways of correcting malalignment across the knee include the use of orthotics in footwear. Unfortunately, while they may have modest effects on knee alignment, trials have heretofore not demonstrated efficacy of a lateral wedge orthotic vs. placebo wedges.

Pain from the patellofemoral compartment of the knee can be caused by tilting of the patella or patellar malalignment with the patella riding laterally (or less often, medially) in the femoral trochlear groove. Using a brace to realign the patella, or tape to pull the patella back into the trochlear sulcus or reduce its tilt, has been shown, when compared to placebo taping in clinical trials, to lessen patellofemoral pain. However, patients may find it difficult to apply tape, and skin irritation from the tape is common. Commercial patellar braces may be a solution, but they have not been tested.

While their effect on malalignment is questionable, neoprene sleeves pulled to cover the knee lessen pain and are easy to use and popular among patients. The explanation for their therapeutic effect on pain is unclear.

In patients with knee OA, acupuncture produces modest pain relief compared to placebo needles and may be an adjunctive treatment.

PHARMACOTHERAPY While nonpharmacologic approaches to therapy constitute its mainstay, pharmacotherapy serves an important adjunctive role in OA treatment. Available drugs are administered using oral, topical, and intraarticular routes.

Acetaminophen, Nonsteroidal Anti-inflammatory Drugs (NSAIDs), and COX-2 Inhibitors

Acetaminophen (paracetamol) is the initial analgesic of choice for patients with OA in knee, hip, or hands. For some patients, it is adequate to control symptoms, in which case more toxic drugs such as NSAIDs can be avoided. Doses up to 1 g 4 times daily can be used **(Table 326-1)**.

NSAIDs are the most popular drugs to treat osteoarthritic pain. In clinical trials, NSAIDs produce ~30% greater improvement in pain than high-dose acetaminophen. Occasional patients treated with NSAIDs experience dramatic pain relief, whereas others experience little improvement. Initially, NSAIDs should be taken on an "as needed" basis because side effects are less frequent with low intermittent doses, which may be highly efficacious. If occasional medication use is insufficiently effective, then daily treatment with NSAIDs is indicated, with an anti-inflammatory dose selected (Table 326-1). Patients should be reminded to take low-dose aspirin and NSAIDs at different times to eliminate drug interactions.

NSAIDs have substantial and frequent side effects, the most common of which is upper gastrointestinal toxicity, including dyspepsia, nausea, bloating, gastrointestinal bleeding, and ulcer disease. Some 30–40% of patients experience upper gastrointestinal (GI) side effects so severe as to require discontinuation of medication. Strategies to avoid or minimize the risk of nonsteroidal related GI side effects include:

- Take medications after food.
- Avoid use of two NSAIDs.
- Use a relatively safe NSAID. In terms of GI toxicity, meta-analyses have suggested that nonacetylated salicylates, ibuprofen and nabumetone, are among the safer NSAIDs; more dangerous ones include piroxicam, ketorolac, and ketoprofen.
- For persons at high risk of GI bleeding and/or complications, prescribe a gastroprotective agent (Table 326-1).

Major NSAID-related GI side effects can occur in patients who do not complain of upper GI symptoms. In one study of patients hospitalized for GI bleeding, 81% had no premonitory symptoms.

TABLE 326-1 PHARMACOLOGIC TREATMENT FOR OSTEOARTHRITIS

Treatment	Dosage	Comments
Acetaminophen	Up to 1 g qid	Prolongs half-life of warfarin
NSAIDs[a]		Take with food. High rates of gastrointestinal side effects, including ulcers and bleeding, occur. Patients at high risk for gastrointestinal side effects should also take either a proton-pump inhibitor or misoprostol.[b] There is an increased concern about side effects (gastrointestinal or bleeding) when taken with acetylsalicylic acid. Can also cause edema and renal insufficiency.
Naproxen	375–500 mg bid	
Salsalate	1500 mg bid	
Ibuprofen	600–800 mg 3–4 times a day	
Cyclooxygenase-2 inhibitors Celecoxib	100–200 mg/d	High doses are associated with an increased risk of myocardial infarction and stroke. Can cause edema and renal insufficiency.
Opiates	Various	Common side effects include dizziness, sedation, nausea or vomiting, dry mouth, constipation, urinary retention, and pruritis. Respiratory and central nervous system depression can occur.
Capsaicin	0.025–0.075% cream 3–4 times a day	Can irritate mucous membranes.
Intraarticular injections Hyaluronans Steroids	Varies from 3 to 5 weekly injections depending on preparation	Mild to moderate pain at injection site. Controversy exists re: efficacy.

[a]NSAIDs denotes nonsteroidal anti-inflammatory drugs.
[b]Patients at high risk include those with previous gastrointestinal events, persons ≥60 years, and persons taking glucocorticoids. Trials have shown the efficacy of proton-pump inhibitors and misoprostol in the prevention of ulcers and bleeding. Misoprostol is associated with a high rate of diarrhea and cramping; therefore, proton-pump inhibitors are more widely used to reduce NSAID-related gastrointestinal symptoms.
Source: Adapted from Felson.

There are other common side effects of NSAIDs, including the tendency to develop edema, because of prostaglandin inhibition of afferent blood supply to glomeruli in the kidneys and, for similar reasons, a predilection toward reversible renal insufficiency. Blood pressure may increase modestly in some NSAID-treated patients.

Alternative anti-inflammatory medications are cyclooxygenase-2 (COX-2) inhibitors. While their rate of GI side effects may be less than for conventional NSAIDs, their risk of causing edema and renal insufficiency is similar. In addition, COX-2 inhibitors, especially at high dose, increase the risk of myocardial infarction and of stroke. This is because selective COX-2 inhibitors reduce prostaglandin I_2 production by vascular endothelium, but do not inhibit platelet thromboxane A_2 production, leading to an increased risk of intravascular thrombosis.

Intraarticular Injections: Glucocorticoids and Hyaluronic Acid

Since synovial Inflammation is likely to be a major cause of pain in patients with OA, local anti-inflammatory treatments administered intraarticularly may be effective in ameliorating pain, at least temporarily. Glucocorticoid injections provide such efficacy, but work better than placebo injections for only 1 or 2 weeks. This may be because the disease remains mechanically driven and, when a person begins to use the joint, the loading factors that induce pain return. Glucocorticoid injections are useful to get patients over acute flares of pain and may be especially indicated if the patient has coexistent OA and crystal deposition disease, especially from calcium pyrophosphate dihydrate crystals (Chap. 327). There is no evidence that repeated glucocorticoid injections into the joint are dangerous.

Hyaluronic acid injections can be given for treatment of symptoms in knee and hip OA, but there is controversy as to whether they have efficacy vs. placebo (Table 326-1).

Optimal therapy for OA is often achieved by trial and error, with each patient having idiosyncratic responses to specific treatments. When medical therapies have failed and the patient has an unacceptable reduction in their quality of life and ongoing pain and disability, then at least for knee and hip OA, total joint arthroplasty is indicated.

SURGERY For knee OA, several operations are available. Among the most popular surgeries, at least in the United States, is arthroscopic debridement and lavage. A well done randomized trial evaluating this operation showed that its efficacy was no greater than that of sham surgery for relief of pain or disability. There is controversy as to whether mechanical symptoms such as buckling, which are extremely common in patients with knee OA, respond to arthroscopic debridement. While buckling is usually due to muscle weakness, a history of a recent injury, along with knee catching or locking, may suggest a meniscal tear is contributing to this symptom. In such cases arthroscopic debridement with partial meniscal resection might be warranted.

For patients with knee OA isolated to the medial compartment, operations to realign the knee to lessen medial loading can relieve pain. These include a high tibial osteotomy, in which the tibia is broken just below the tibial plateau and realigned so as to load the lateral, nondiseased compartment, or a unicompartmental replacement with realignment. Each surgery may provide the patient with years of pain relief before they require a total knee replacement.

Ultimately, when the patient with knee or hip OA has failed medical treatment modalities and remains in pain, with limitations of physical function that compromise the quality of life, the patient should be referred for total knee or hip arthroplasty. These are highly efficacious operations that relieve pain and improve function in the vast majority of patients. Currently failure rates are ~1% per year, although these rates are higher in obese patients. The chance of surgical success is greater in centers where at least 50 such operations are performed yearly or with surgeons who perform a similar number annually. The timing of knee or hip replacement is critical. If the patient suffers for many years until their functional status has declined substantially, with considerable muscle weakness, postoperative functional status may not improve to a level achieved by others who underwent operation earlier in their disease course.

Cartilage Regeneration   Chondrocyte transplantation has not been found to be efficacious in OA, perhaps because OA includes pathology of joint mechanics, which is not corrected by chondrocyte transplants. Similarly, abrasion arthroplasty (chondroplasty) has not been well studied for efficacy in OA, but it produces fibrocartilage in place of damaged hyaline cartilage. Both of these surgical attempts to regenerate and reconstitute articular cartilage may be more likely to be efficacious early in disease when joint malalignment and many of the other noncartilage abnormalities that characterize OA have not yet developed.

FURTHER READINGS

BENNELL K, HINMAN R: Exercise as a treatment for osteoarthritis. Curr Opin Rheumatol 17: 634, 2005

BRANDT K et al (eds): *Osteoarthritis*, 2d ed. Oxford, Oxford University Press, 2003

FELSON DT: Osteoarthritis of the knee. N Engl J Med 354: 841, 2006

KROHN K: Footwear alterations and bracing as treatments for knee osteoarthritis. Curr Opin Rheumatol 17: 653, 2005

LO G et al: Intraarticular hyaluronic acid in treatment of knee osteoarthritis. A meta-analysis. JAMA 290:3115, 2003

327 Gout and Other Crystal-Associated Arthropathies
H. Ralph Schumacher, Lan X. Chen

The use of polarizing light microscopy during synovial fluid analysis in 1961 by McCarty and Hollander and the subsequent application of other crystallographic techniques, such as electron microscopy, energy-dispersive elemental analysis, and x-ray diffraction, have allowed investigators to identify the roles of different microcrystals, including monosodium urate (MSU), calcium pyrophosphate dihydrate (CPPD), calcium apatite (apatite), and calcium oxalate (CaOx), in inducing acute or chronic arthritis or periarthritis. The clinical events that result from deposition of MSU, CPPD, apatite, and CaOx have many similarities but also important differences. Prior to the use of crystallographic techniques in rheumatology, much of what was considered to be gouty arthritis in fact was not. Because of often similar clinical presentations, the need to perform synovial fluid analysis to distinguish the type of crystal involved must be emphasized. Polarized light microscopy alone can identify most typical crystals; apatite, however, is an exception. Aspiration and analysis of effusions are also important to assess the possibility of infection. Apart from the identification of specific microcrystalline materials or organisms, synovial fluid characteristics in crystal-associated diseases are nonspecific, and synovial fluid can be inflammatory or noninflammatory. A list of possible musculoskeletal manifestations of crystal-associated arthritis is shown in Table 327-1.

GOUT

Gout is a metabolic disease most often affecting middle-aged to elderly men and postmenopausal women. It is the result of an increased body pool of urate with hyperuricemia. It is typically characterized by episodic acute and chronic arthritis, due to deposition of MSU crystals in joints and connective tissue tophi, and the risk for deposition in kidney interstitium or uric acid nephrolithiasis (Chap. 353).

ACUTE AND CHRONIC ARTHRITIS

Acute arthritis is the most frequent early clinical manifestation of gout. Usually, only one joint is affected initially, but polyarticular acute gout

TABLE 327-1	MUSCULOSKELETAL MANIFESTATIONS OF CRYSTAL-INDUCED ARTHRITIS
Acute mono- or polyarthritis	Destructive arthropathies
Bursitis	Pseudo-rheumatoid arthritis
Tendinitis	Pseudo-ankylosing spondylitis
Enthesitis	Spinal stenosis
Tophaceous deposits	Crown dens syndrome
Peculiar type of osteoarthritis	Carpal tunnel syndrome
Synovial osteochondromatosis	Tendon rupture

can occur in subsequent episodes. The metatarsophalangeal joint of the first toe is often involved, but tarsal joints, ankles, and knees are also commonly affected. Especially in elderly patients or in advanced disease, finger joints may be involved. Inflamed Heberden's or Bouchard's nodes may be a first manifestation of gouty arthritis. The first episode of acute gouty arthritis frequently begins at night with dramatic joint pain and swelling. Joints rapidly become warm, red, and tender, with a clinical appearance that often mimics cellulitis. Early attacks tend to subside spontaneously within 3–10 days, and most patients have intervals of varying length with no residual symptoms until the next episode. Several events may precipitate acute gouty arthritis: dietary excess, trauma, surgery, excessive ethanol ingestion, hypouricemic therapy, and serious medical illnesses such as myocardial infarction and stroke.

After many acute mono- or oligoarticular attacks, a proportion of gouty patients may present with a chronic nonsymmetric synovitis, causing potential confusion with rheumatoid arthritis (Chap. 314). Less commonly, chronic gouty arthritis will be the only manifestation and, more rarely, the disease will manifest only as periarticular tophaceous deposits in the absence of synovitis. Women represent only 5–20% of all patients with gout. Premenopausal gout is rare; it is seen mostly in individuals with a strong family history of gout. Kindreds of precocious gout in young females caused by decreased renal urate clearance and renal insufficiency have been described. Most women with gouty arthritis are postmenopausal and elderly, have osteoarthritis and arterial hypertension causing mild renal insufficiency, and are usually receiving diuretics.

Laboratory Diagnosis   Even if the clinical appearance strongly suggests gout, the diagnosis should be confirmed by needle aspiration of acutely or chronically involved joints or tophaceous deposits. Acute septic arthritis, several of the other crystalline-associated arthropathies, pal-

FIGURE 327-1 Extracellular and intracellular monosodium urate crystals, as seen in a fresh preparation of synovial fluid, illustrate needle- and rod-shaped strongly negative birefringent crystals (compensated polarized light microscopy; 400×).

indromic rheumatism, and psoriatic arthritis may present with similar clinical features. During acute gouty attacks, strongly birefringent needle-shaped MSU crystals with negative elongation are typically seen both intracellularly and extracellularly (Fig. 327-1). Synovial fluid cell counts are elevated from 2000 to 60,000/µL. Effusions appear cloudy due to the increased numbers of leukocytes. Large amounts of crystals occasionally produce a thick pasty or chalky joint fluid. Bacterial infection can coexist with urate crystals in synovial fluid; if there is any suspicion of septic arthritis, joint fluid must also be cultured.

MSU crystals can also often be demonstrated in the first metatarsophalangeal joint and in knees not acutely involved with gout. Arthrocentesis of these joints is a useful technique to establish the diagnosis of gout between attacks.

Serum uric acid levels can be normal or low at the time of the acute attack, as inflammatory cytokines can be uricosuric and effective initiation of hypouricemic therapy can precipitate attacks. This limits the value of serum uric acid determinations for the diagnosis of gout. Nevertheless, serum urate levels are almost always elevated at some time and are important to use to follow the course of hypouricemic therapy. A 24-h urine collection for uric acid can, in some cases, be useful in assessing the risk of stones, in elucidating overproduction or underexcretion of uric acid, and in deciding if it might be appropriate to use a uricosuric therapy (Chap. 353). Excretion of >800 mg of uric acid per 24 h on a regular diet suggests that causes of overproduction of purine should be considered. Urinalysis, serum creatinine, hemoglobin, white blood cell (WBC) count, liver function tests, and serum lipids should be obtained because of possible pathologic sequelae of gout and other associated diseases requiring treatment, and as baselines because of possible adverse effects of gout treatment.

Radiographic Features Early in the disease radiographic studies may only confirm clinically evident swelling. Cystic changes, well-defined erosions with sclerotic margins (often with overhanging bony edges), and soft tissue masses are characteristic radiographic features of advanced chronic tophaceous gout.

℞ GOUT

ACUTE GOUTY ARTHRITIS The mainstay of treatment during an acute attack is the administration of anti-inflammatory drugs such as nonsteroidal anti-inflammatory drugs (NSAIDs), colchicine, or glucocorticoids. NSAIDs are most often used in individuals without complicating comorbid conditions. Both colchicine and NSAIDs may be poorly tolerated and dangerous in the elderly and in the presence of renal insufficiency and gastrointestinal disorders. In attacks involving one or two joints, intraarticular glucocorticoid injections may be preferable and effective. Ice pack applications and rest of the involved joints can be helpful. Colchicine given orally

is a traditional and effective treatment, if used early in the attack. One to two 0.6-mg tablets can be given every 6–8 h over several days with subsequent tapering. This is generally better tolerated than the formerly advised hourly regimen. The drug must be stopped promptly at the first sign of loose stools, and symptomatic treatment must be given for the diarrhea. Intravenous colchicine is occasionally used, e.g., as pre- or postoperative prophylaxis in 1- to 2-mg doses when patients cannot take medications orally. Life-threatening colchicine toxicity and sudden death have been described with the administration of >4 mg/d IV. The IV colchicine should be given slowly through an established venous line over 10 min in a soluset. The total dose should never exceed 4 mg.

NSAIDs given in full anti-inflammatory doses are effective in ~90% of patients, and the resolution of signs and symptoms usually occurs in 5–8 days. The most effective drugs are any of those with a short half-life and include indomethacin, 25–50 mg tid; ibuprofen, 800 mg tid; or diclofenac, 50 mg tid. Oral glucocorticoids such as prednisone, 30–50 mg/d as the initial dose and gradually tapered with the resolution of the attack can be effective in polyarticular gout. For single or few involved joints intraarticular triamcinolone acetonide, 20–40 mg, or methylprednisolone, 25–50 mg, have been effective and well tolerated. Adrenocorticotropic hormone (ACTH) as an intramuscular injection of 40–80 IU in a single dose or every 12 h for 1–2 days can be effective in patients with acute polyarticular refractory gout or in those with a contraindication for using colchicine or NSAIDs.

HYPOURICEMIC THERAPY Ultimate control of gout requires correction of the basic underlying defect, the hyperuricemia. Attempts to normalize serum uric acid to <300–360 µmol/L (5.0–6.0 mg/dL) to prevent recurrent gouty attacks and eliminate tophaceous deposits entail a commitment to long-term hypouricemic regimens and medications that generally are required for life. Hypouricemic therapy should be considered when, as in most patients, the hyperuricemia cannot be corrected by simple means (control of body weight, low-purine diet, increase in liquid intake, limitation of ethanol use, and avoidance of diuretics). The decision to initiate hypouricemic therapy is usually made taking into consideration the number of acute attacks (urate lowering may be cost effective after two attacks), serum uric acid levels [progression is more rapid in patients with serum uric acid >535 µmol/L (>9.0 mg/dL)], patient's willingness to commit to lifelong therapy, or presence of uric acid stones. Urate-lowering therapy should be initiated in any patient who already has tophi or chronic gouty arthritis. Uricosuric agents, such as probenecid, can be used in patients with good renal function who underexcrete uric acid, with <600 mg in a 24-h urine sample. Urine volume must be maintained by ingestion of 1500 mL of water every day. Probenecid can be started at a dosage of 250 mg twice daily and increased gradually as needed up to 3 g in order to maintain a serum uric acid level <300 µmol/L (5 mg/dL). Probenecid is generally not effective in patients with serum creatinine levels of >177 µmol/L (2.0 mg/dL). These patients may require allopurinol or benzbromarone (not available in the United States). The latter is another uricosuric drug that is more effective in patients with renal failure. Recent reports have identified that losartan, fenofibrate, and amlodipine have some mild uricosuric effects.

The xanthine oxidase inhibitor allopurinol is by far the most commonly used hypouricemic agent and is the best drug to lower serum urate in overproducers, urate stone formers, and patients with renal disease. It can be given in a single morning dose, 100–300 mg initially and increasing up to 800 mg if needed. In patients with chronic renal disease, the initial allopurinol dosage should be lower and adjusted depending on the serum creatinine concentration; for example, with a creatinine clearance of 10 mL/min, one would generally use 100 mg every other day. Doses can gradually be increased to reach the target urate level; however, more studies are needed to provide exact guidance. Patients with frequent acute attacks may also require lower initial doses to prevent exacerbations. Toxicity of allopurinol has been recognized increasingly in patients with renal failure who use thiazide diuretics and in those patients allergic to penicillin and ampicillin. The most serious side effects include skin rash with progression to life-threatening toxic epidermal necrolysis, systemic vasculitis, bone marrow suppression, granulomatous hepatitis, and renal failure. Patients with mild cutaneous reactions to allopurinol can reconsider the use of a uricosuric agent or undergo an attempt at desensitization to allopurinol. They can also pay increased attention to diet and should be aware of new alternative agents under investigation (see below). Urate-lowering drugs are generally not initiated during acute attacks but after the patient is stable and low-dose colchicine has been initiated to decrease the risk of flares that often occur with urate lowering. Colchicine prophylaxis in doses of 0.6 mg one to two times daily is usually continued, along with the hypouricemic therapy, until the patient is normouricemic and without gouty attacks for 6 months or as long as tophi are present. New urate-lowering drugs undergoing investigation include a PEGylated uricase and a new specific xanthine oxidase inhibitor, febuxostat.

CPPD DEPOSITION DISEASE

PATHOGENESIS

The deposition of CPPD crystals in articular tissues is most common in the elderly, occurring in 10–15% of persons aged 65–75 years and 30–50% of those >85 years. In most cases this process is asymptomatic, and the cause of CPPD deposition is uncertain. Because >80% of patients are >60 years and 70% have preexisting joint damage from other conditions, it is likely that biochemical changes in aging or diseased cartilage favor crystal nucleation. In patients with CPPD arthritis there is an increased production of inorganic pyrophosphate and decreased levels of pyrophosphatases in cartilage extracts. Mutations in the *ANKH* gene described in both familial and sporadic cases can increase elaboration and extracellular transport of pyrophosphate. The increase in pyrophosphate production appears to be related to enhanced activity of ATP pyrophosphohydrolase and 5′-nucleotidase, which catalyze the reaction of ATP to adenosine and pyrophosphate. This pyrophosphate could combine with calcium to form CPPD crystals in matrix vesicles or on collagen fibers. There are decreased levels of cartilage glycosaminoglycans that normally inhibit and regulate crystal nucleation. In vitro studies have demonstrated that transforming growth factor β_1 and epidermal growth factor both stimulate the production of pyrophosphate by articular cartilage and thus may contribute to the deposition of CPPD crystals.

Release of CPPD crystals into the joint space is followed by the phagocytosis of these crystals by monocyte-macrophages and neutrophils, which respond by releasing chemotactic and inflammatory substances.

A minority of patients with CPPD arthropathy have metabolic abnormalities or hereditary CPPD disease (Table 327-2). These associations suggest that a variety of different metabolic products may enhance CPPD deposition either by directly altering cartilage or inhibiting inorganic pyrophosphatases. Included among these conditions are hyperparathyroidism, hemochromatosis, hypophosphatasia, and hypomagnesemia. The presence of CPPD arthritis in individuals <50 years old should lead to consideration of these metabolic disorders and inherited forms of disease, including those identified in a variety of ethnic groups (Table 327-2). Genomic DNA studies performed on different kindreds have shown a possible location of genetic defects on chromosome 8q or on chromosome 5p in a region that expresses the gene of the membrane pyrophosphate channel (*ANKH* gene). Mutations as noted above described in the *ANKH* gene in kindreds with CPPD arthritis can increase extracellular pyrophosphate and induce CPPD crystal formation. Investigation of younger patients with CPPD

TABLE 327-2 CONDITIONS ASSOCIATED WITH CALCIUM PYROPHOSPHATE DIHYDRATE DISEASE

Aging
Disease-associated
  Primary hyperparathyroidism
  Hemochromatosis
  Hypophosphatasia
  Hypomagnesemia
  Chronic gout
  Postmeniscectomy
Epiphyseal dysplasias
Hereditary: Slovakian-Hungarian, Spanish, Spanish-American (Argentinian,[a] Colombian, and Chilean), French,[a] Swedish, Dutch, Canadian, Mexican-American, Italian-American,[a] German-American, Japanese, Tunisian, Jewish, English[a]

[a]Mutations in the *ANKH* gene.

---

deposition should include inquiry for evidence of familial aggregation and evaluation of serum calcium, phosphorus, alkaline phosphatase, magnesium, serum iron, and transferrin.

CLINICAL MANIFESTATIONS

CPPD arthropathy may be asymptomatic, acute, subacute, or chronic or cause acute synovitis superimposed on chronically involved joints. Acute CPPD arthritis was originally termed *pseudogout* by McCarty and coworkers because of its striking similarity to gout. Other clinical manifestations of CPPD deposition include (1) induction or enhancement of peculiar forms of osteoarthritis; (2) induction of severe destructive disease that may radiographically mimic neuropathic arthritis; (3) production of symmetric proliferative synovitis, clinically similar to rheumatoid arthritis and frequently seen in familial forms with early onset; (4) intervertebral disk and ligament calcification with restriction of spine mobility, mimicking ankylosing spondylitis (also seen in hereditary forms); and (5) rarely spinal stenosis (most commonly seen in the elderly) (Table 327-1).

The knee is the joint most frequently affected in CPPD arthropathy. Other sites include the wrist, shoulder, ankle, elbow, and hands. Rarely, the temporomandibular joint and ligamentum flavum of the spinal canal are involved. Clinical and radiographic evidence indicates that CPPD deposition is polyarticular in at least two-thirds of patients. When the clinical picture resembles that of slowly progressive osteoarthritis, diagnosis may be difficult. Joint distribution may provide important clues suggesting CPPD disease. For example, primary osteoarthritis rarely involves a metacarpophalangeal, wrist, elbow, shoulder, or ankle joint. If radiographs reveal punctate and/or linear radiodense deposits in fibrocartilaginous joint menisci or articular hyaline cartilage (*chondrocalcinosis*), the diagnostic likelihood of CPPD disease is further enhanced. *Definitive diagnosis* requires demonstration of typical crystals in synovial fluid or articular tissue (Fig. 327-2). In the absence of joint effusion or indications to obtain a synovial biopsy, chondrocalcinosis is presumptive of CPPD deposition. One exception is chondrocalcinosis due to CaOx in some patients with chronic renal failure.

Acute attacks of CPPD arthritis may be precipitated by trauma. Rapid diminution of serum calcium concentration, as may occur in severe medical illness or after surgery (especially parathyroidectomy), can also lead to pseudogout attacks.

In as many as 50% of cases, episodes of CPPD-induced inflammation are associated with low-grade fever and, on occasion, temperatures as high as 40°C. Whether or not radiographic proof of chondrocalcino-

FIGURE 327-2 Intracellular and extracellular calcium pyrophosphate dihydrate crystals, as seen in a fresh preparation of synovial fluid, illustrate rectangular, rod-shaped, and rhomboid weakly positive birefringent crystals (compensated polarized light microscopy; 400×).

sis is evident in the involved joint(s), synovial fluid analysis with microbial cultures is essential to rule out the possibility of infection. In fact, infection in a joint with any microcrystalline deposition process can lead to crystal shedding and subsequent synovitis from both crystals and microorganisms. Synovial fluid in acute CPPD disease has inflammatory characteristics. The leukocyte count can range from several thousand cells to 100,000 cells/μL, the mean being about 24,000 cells/μL and the predominant cell being the neutrophil. Polarized light microscopy usually reveals rhomboid, square, or rod-like crystals with weak positive birefringence inside tissue fragments and fibrin clots and in neutrophils (Fig. 327-2). CPPD crystals may coexist with MSU and apatite in some cases.

℞ CPPD DEPOSITION DISEASE

Untreated acute attacks may last a few days to as long as a month. Treatment by joint aspiration and NSAIDs or by intraarticular glucocorticoid injection may result in return to prior status in ≤10 days. For patients with frequent recurrent attacks of pseudogout, daily prophylactic treatment with low doses of colchicine may be helpful in decreasing the frequency of the attacks. Severe polyarticular attacks usually require short courses of glucocorticoids. Unfortunately, there is no effective way to remove CPPD deposits from cartilage and synovium. Uncontrolled studies suggest that the administration of antimalarial agents or even methotrexate may be helpful in controlling persistent synovitis. Patients with progressive destructive large-joint arthropathy may require joint replacement.

CALCIUM APATITE DEPOSITION DISEASE

PATHOGENESIS

Apatite is the primary mineral of normal bone and teeth. Abnormal accumulation can occur in areas of tissue damage (dystrophic calcification), in hypercalcemic or hyperparathyroid states (metastatic calcification), and in certain conditions of unknown cause (Table 327-3). In chronic renal failure, hyperphosphatemia can contribute to extensive apatite deposition both in and around joints. Familial aggregation is rarely seen; no association with *ANKH* mutations has been described thus far. Apatite crystals are deposited primarily on matrix vessels. Incompletely understood alterations in matrix proteoglycans, phosphatases, hormones, and cytokines can probably influence crystal formation.

Apatite aggregates are commonly present in synovial fluid in an extremely destructive chronic arthropathy of the elderly that occurs most often in shoulders (Milwaukee shoulder) and in a similar process in hips, knees, and erosive osteoarthritis of fingers. Joint destruction is associated with damage to cartilage and supporting structures, leading to instability and deformity. Progression tends to be indolent, and synovial fluid leukocyte counts are usually <2000/μL. Symptoms range from minimal to severe pain and disability that may lead to joint replacement

TABLE 327-3	CONDITIONS ASSOCIATED WITH APATITE DEPOSITION DISEASE

Aging
Osteoarthritis
Hemorrhagic shoulder effusions in the elderly (Milwaukee shoulder)
Destructive arthropathy
Tendinitis, bursitis
Tumoral calcinosis (sporadic cases)
Disease-associated
  Hyperparathyroidism
  Milk-alkali syndrome
  Renal failure/long-term dialysis
  Connective tissue diseases (e.g., systemic sclerosis, idiopathic myositis, SLE)
  Heterotopic calcification following neurologic catastrophes (e.g., stroke, spinal cord injury)
Heredity
  Bursitis, arthritis
  Tumoral calcinosis
  Fibrodysplasia ossificans progressiva

Note: SLE, systemic lupus erythematosus.

surgery. Whether severely affected patients merely represent an extreme synovial tissue response to the apatite crystals that are so common in osteoarthritis is uncertain. Synovial lining cell cultures exposed to apatite (or CPPD) crystals markedly increase the release of collagenases and neutral proteases, underscoring the destructive potential of abnormally stimulated synovial lining cells.

CLINICAL MANIFESTATIONS

Periarticular or articular deposits may occur and may be associated with acute reversible inflammation and/or chronic damage to the joint capsule, tendons, bursa, or articular surfaces. The most common sites of apatite deposition include bursae and tendons in and/or around the knees, shoulders, hips, and fingers. Clinical manifestations include asymptomatic radiographic abnormalities, acute synovitis, bursitis, tendinitis, and chronic destructive arthropathy. Although the true incidence of apatite arthritis is not known, 30–50% of patients with osteoarthritis have apatite microcrystals in their synovial fluid. Such crystals can frequently be identified in clinically stable osteoarthritic joints, but they are more likely to come to attention in persons experiencing acute or subacute worsening of joint pain and swelling. The synovial fluid leukocyte count in apatite arthritis is usually low (<2000/μL), despite dramatic symptoms, with predominance of mononuclear cells.

DIAGNOSIS

Intra- and/or periarticular calcifications with or without erosive, destructive, or hypertrophic changes may be seen on radiographs (Fig. 327-3). These should be distinguished from the linear calcifications typical of CPPD deposition disease.

Definitive diagnosis of apatite arthropathy depends on identification of crystals from synovial fluid or tissue (Fig. 327-3). Individual crystals, which generally contain mostly carbonate substituted apatite, are very small and can be seen only by electron microscopy. Clumps of crystals may appear as 1- to 20-μm shiny intra- or extracellular non-birefringent globules or aggregates that stain purplish with Wright's stain and bright red with alizarin red S. Absolute identification depends on electron microscopy with energy-dispersive elemental analysis, x-ray diffraction, or infrared spectroscopy, but these are usually not required in clinical diagnosis.

℞ CALCIUM APATITE DEPOSITION DISEASE

Treatment of apatite arthritis or periarthritis is nonspecific. Acute attacks of bursitis or synovitis may be self-limiting, resolving in days to several weeks. Aspiration of effusions and the use of either NSAIDs or oral colchicine for 2 weeks or intra- or periarticular injection of a depot glucocorticoid appear to shorten the duration and intensity of symptoms. Periarticular apatite deposits may be resorbed with resolution of attacks. Agents to lower serum phosphate levels may lead to resorption of deposits in renal failure patients receiving hemodialysis. In patients with underlying severe destructive articular changes, response to medical therapy is usually less rewarding.

CaOx DEPOSITION DISEASE

PATHOGENESIS

Primary oxalosis is a rare hereditary metabolic disorder (Chap. 358). Enhanced production of oxalic acid may result from at least two different enzyme defects, leading to hyperoxalemia and deposition of calcium oxalate crystals in tissues. Nephrocalcinosis, renal failure, and death usually occur before age 20. Acute and/or chronic CaOx arthritis and periarthritis may complicate primary oxalosis during later years of illness.

Secondary oxalosis is more common than the primary disorder. It is one of the many metabolic abnormalities that complicate end-stage renal disease. In chronic renal disease, calcium oxalate deposits have long been recognized in visceral organs, blood vessels, bones, and even cartilage. However, it was not until 1982 that such deposits were demonstrated to be one of the causes of arthritis in chronic renal failure. Thus far, reported patients have been dependent on long-term hemodialysis or peritoneal dialysis (Chap. 275), and many had received ascorbic acid supplements. Ascorbic acid is metabolized to oxalate,

A

B

FIGURE 327-3 A. Radiograph showing calcification due to apatite crystals surrounding an eroded joint. **B.** An electron micrograph demonstrates dark needle-shaped apatite crystals within a vacuole of a synovial fluid mononuclear cell (30,000×).

which is inadequately cleared in uremia and by dialysis. Such supplements are now usually avoided in dialysis programs because of the risk of enhancing hyperoxalosis and its sequelae.

CLINICAL MANIFESTATIONS AND DIAGNOSIS
CaOx aggregates can be found in bone, articular cartilage, synovium, and periarticular tissues. From these sites, crystals may be shed, causing acute synovitis. Persistent aggregates of CaOx can, like apatite and CPPD, stimulate synovial cell proliferation and enzyme release, result-

FIGURE 327-4 Bipyramidal and small polymorphic calcium oxalate crystals from synovial fluid are classical finding in CaOx arthropathy (ordinary light microscopy; 400×).

ing in progressive articular destruction. Deposits have been documented in fingers, wrists, elbows, knees, ankles, and feet.

Clinical features of acute CaOx arthritis may not be distinguishable from those due to sodium urate, CPPD, or apatite. Radiographs may reveal chondrocalcinosis or soft tissue calcifications. CaOx-induced synovial effusions are usually noninflammatory, with <2000 leukocytes/μL, or mildly inflammatory. Neutrophils or mononuclear cells can predominate. CaOx crystals have a variable shape and variable birefringence to polarized light. The most easily recognized forms are bipyramidal, have strong birefringence (Fig. 327-4), and stain with alizarin red S.

Rx CALCIUM OXALATE DEPOSITION DISEASE

Treatment of CaOx arthropathy with NSAIDs, colchicine, intraarticular glucocorticoids, and/or an increased frequency of dialysis has produced only slight improvement. In primary oxalosis, liver transplantation has induced a significant reduction in crystal deposits (Chap. 358).

ACKNOWLEDGMENT
This chapter has been revised from an original version written by Antonio Reginato, MD, in previous editions of Harrison's Principles of Internal Medicine.

FURTHER READINGS

CHOI HK et al: Pathogenesis of gout. Ann Intern Med 143:499-516, 2005
MALDONADO I et al: Oxalate crystal deposition disease. Curr Rheumatol Rep 4:257, 2002
MOLLOY ES, MCCARTHY GM: Hydroxyapatite deposition disease of the joint. Curr Rheumatol Rep 5:215, 2003
SCHUMACHER HR, CHEN LX: Newer therapeutic approaches: Gout. Rheum Dis Clin North Am 32:235, 2006
WORTMANN RL et al (eds): *Crystal-Induced Arthropathies: Gout, Pseudogout and Apatite-Associated Syndromes.* New York, Taylor & Francis, 427 pp, 2006
ZAKA R, WILLIAMS CJ: Genetics of chondrocalcinosis. Osteoarthritis Cartilage, 13:745, 2005

328 Infectious Arthritis
Lawrence C. Madoff

INTRODUCTION
Although *Staphylococcus aureus, Neisseria gonorrhoeae,* and other bacteria are the most common causes of infectious arthritis, various mycobacteria, spirochetes, fungi, and viruses also infect joints (Table 328-1).

Since acute bacterial infection can rapidly destroy articular cartilage, all inflamed joints must be evaluated without delay to exclude noninfectious processes and to determine appropriate antimicrobial therapy and drainage procedures. For more detailed information on infectious arthritis due to specific organisms, the reader is referred to the chapters on those organisms.

Acute bacterial infection typically involves a single joint or a few joints. Subacute or chronic monarthritis or oligoarthritis suggests mycobacterial or fungal infection; episodic inflammation is seen in syph-

TABLE 328-1 DIFFERENTIAL DIAGNOSIS OF ARTHRITIS SYNDROMES

Acute Monarticular Arthritis	Chronic Monarticular Arthritis	Polyarticular Arthritis
Staphylococcus aureus	*Mycobacterium tuberculosis*	*Neisseria meningitidis*
Streptococcus pneumoniae	Nontuberculous mycobacteria	*N. gonorrhoeae*
β-Hemolytic streptococci	*Borrelia burgdorferi*	Nongonococcal bacterial arthritis
Gram-negative bacilli	*Treponema pallidum*	Bacterial endocarditis
Neisseria gonorrhoeae	*Candida* species	*Candida* species
Candida species	*Sporothrix schenckii*	Poncet's disease (tuberculous
Crystal-induced arthritis	*Coccidioides immitis*	rheumatism)
Fracture	*Blastomyces dermatitidis*	Hepatitis B virus
Hemarthrosis	*Aspergillus* species	Parvovirus B19
Foreign body	*Cryptococcus neoformans*	HIV
Osteoarthritis	*Nocardia* species	Human T-lymphotropic virus
Ischemic necrosis	*Brucella* species	type I
Monarticular rheumatoid arthritis	Legg-Calvé-Perthes disease	Rubella virus
	Osteoarthritis	Arthropod-borne viruses
		Sickle cell disease flare
		Reactive arthritis
		Serum sickness
		Acute rheumatic fever
		Inflammatory bowel disease
		Systemic lupus erythematosus
		Rheumatoid arthritis/Still's
		disease
		Other vasculitides
		Sarcoidosis

ilis, Lyme disease, and the reactive arthritis that follows enteric infections and chlamydial urethritis. Acute polyarticular inflammation occurs as an immunologic reaction during the course of endocarditis, rheumatic fever, disseminated neisserial infection, and acute hepatitis B. Bacteria and viruses occasionally infect multiple joints, the former most commonly in persons with rheumatoid arthritis.

APPROACH TO THE PATIENT:
Infectious Arthritis

Aspiration of synovial fluid—an essential element in the evaluation of potentially infected joints—can be performed without difficulty in most cases by the insertion of a large-bore needle into the site of maximal fluctuance or tenderness or by the route of easiest access. Ultrasonography or fluoroscopy may be used to guide aspiration of difficult-to-localize effusions of the hip and, occasionally, the shoulder and other joints. Normal synovial fluid contains <180 cells (predominantly mononuclear cells) per microliter. Synovial cell counts averaging 100,000/μL (range, 25,000–250,000/μL), with >90% neutrophils, are characteristic of acute bacterial infections. Crystal-induced, rheumatoid, and other noninfectious inflammatory arthritides are usually associated with <30,000–50,000 cells/μL; cell counts of 10,000–30,000/μL, with 50–70% neutrophils and the remainder lymphocytes, are common in mycobacterial and fungal infections. Definitive diagnosis of an infectious process relies on identification of the pathogen in stained smears of synovial fluid, isolation of the pathogen from cultures of synovial fluid and blood, or detection of microbial nucleic acids and proteins by polymerase chain reaction (PCR)–based assays and immunologic techniques.

ACUTE BACTERIAL ARTHRITIS

Pathogenesis Bacteria enter the joint from the bloodstream; from a contiguous site of infection in bone or soft tissue; or by direct inoculation during surgery, injection, animal or human bite, or trauma. In hematogenous infection, bacteria escape from synovial capillaries, which have no limiting basement membrane, and within hours provoke neutrophilic infiltration of the synovium. Neutrophils and bacteria enter the joint space; later, bacteria adhere to articular cartilage. Degradation of cartilage begins within 48 h as a result of increased intraarticular pressure, release of pro-

teases and cytokines from chondrocytes and synovial macrophages, and invasion of the cartilage by bacteria and inflammatory cells. Histologic studies reveal bacteria lining the synovium and cartilage as well as abscesses extending into the synovium, cartilage, and—in severe cases—subchondral bone. Synovial proliferation results in the formation of a pannus over the cartilage, and thrombosis of inflamed synovial vessels develops. Bacterial factors that appear important in the pathogenesis of infective arthritis include various surface-associated adhesins in *S. aureus* that permit adherence to cartilage and endotoxins that promote chondrocyte-mediated breakdown of cartilage.

Microbiology The hematogenous route of infection is the most common route in all age groups, and nearly every bacterial pathogen is capable of causing septic arthritis. In infants, group B streptococci, gram-negative enteric bacilli, and *S. aureus* are the usual pathogens. Since the advent of the *Haemophilus influenzae* vaccine, *S. aureus*, *Streptococcus pyogenes* (group A *Streptococcus*), and (in some centers) *Kingella kingae* have predominated among children <5 years of age. Among young adults and adolescents, *N. gonorrhoeae* is the most commonly implicated organism. *S. aureus* accounts for most nongonococcal isolates in adults of all ages; gram-negative bacilli, pneumococci, and β-hemolytic streptococci—particularly groups A and B, but also groups C, G, and F—are involved in up to one-third of cases in older adults, especially those with underlying comorbid illnesses.

Infections after surgical procedures or penetrating injuries are due most often to *S. aureus* and occasionally to other gram-positive bacteria or gram-negative bacilli. Infections with coagulase-negative staphylococci are unusual except after the implantation of prosthetic joints or arthroscopy. Anaerobic organisms, often in association with aerobic or facultative bacteria, are found after human bites and when decubitus ulcers or intraabdominal abscesses spread into adjacent joints. Polymicrobial infections complicate traumatic injuries with extensive contamination. Bites and scratches from cats and other animals may introduce *Pasteurella multocida* into joints, and bites from humans may introduce *Eikenella corrodens* or other components of the oral flora.

Nongonococcal Bacterial Arthritis · EPIDEMIOLOGY Although hematogenous infections with virulent organisms such as *S. aureus*, *H. influenzae*, and pyogenic streptococci occur in healthy persons, there is an underlying host predisposition in many cases of septic arthritis. Patients with rheumatoid arthritis have the highest incidence of infective arthritis (most often secondary to *S. aureus*) because of chronically inflamed joints; glucocorticoid therapy; and frequent breakdown of rheumatoid nodules, vasculitic ulcers, and skin overlying deformed joints. Diabetes mellitus, glucocorticoid therapy, hemodialysis, and malignancy all carry an increased risk of infection with *S. aureus* and gram-negative bacilli. Tumor necrosis factor (TNF) inhibitors (etanercept and infliximab), increasingly used for the treatment of rheumatoid arthritis, predispose to mycobacterial infections and possibly to other pyogenic bacterial infections and could be associated with septic arthritis in this population. Pneumococcal infections complicate alcoholism, deficiencies of humoral immunity, and hemoglobinopathies. Pneumococci, *Salmonella*, and *H. influenzae* cause septic arthritis in persons infected with HIV. Persons with primary immunoglobulin deficiency are at risk for mycoplasmal arthritis, which results in permanent joint damage if treatment with tetracycline and IV immunoglobulin (IVIg) replacement is not administered promptly. IV drug users acquire staphylococcal and streptococcal infections from their own flora and acquire pseudomonal and other gram-negative infections from drugs and injection paraphernalia.

clinically, and infection and crystal-induced disease occasionally occur together. Organisms are seen on synovial fluid smears in nearly three-quarters of infections with *S. aureus* and streptococci and in 30–50% of infections due to gram-negative and other bacteria. Cultures of synovial fluid are positive in >90% of cases. Inoculation of synovial fluid into bottles containing liquid media for blood cultures increases the yield of culture, especially if the pathogen is a fastidious organism or the patient is taking an antibiotic. Although not yet widely available, PCR-based assays for bacterial DNA will also be useful for the diagnosis of partially treated or culture-negative bacterial arthritis.

Rx NONGONOCOCCAL BACTERIAL ARTHRITIS

Prompt administration of systemic antibiotics and drainage of the involved joint can prevent destruction of cartilage, postinfectious degenerative arthritis, joint instability, or deformity. Once samples of blood and synovial fluid have been obtained for culture, empirical antibiotics should be given that are directed against bacteria visualized on smears or against the pathogens that are likely, given the patient's age and risk factors. Initial therapy should consist of the IV administration of bactericidal agents; direct instillation of antibiotics into the joint is not necessary to achieve adequate levels in synovial fluid and tissue. An IV third-generation cephalosporin such as cefotaxime (1 g every 8 h) or ceftriaxone (1–2 g every 24 h) provides adequate empirical coverage for most community-acquired infections in adults when smears show no organisms. Either oxacillin or nafcillin (2 g every 4 h) is used if there are gram-positive cocci on the smear. If methicillin-resistant *S. aureus* is a possible pathogen (e.g., when it is widespread in the community or in hospitalized patients), IV vancomycin (1 g every 12 h) should be given. In addition, an aminoglycoside or third-generation cephalosporin should be given to IV drug users or other patients in whom *Pseudomonas aeruginosa* may be the responsible agent.

Definitive therapy is based on the identity and antibiotic susceptibility of the bacteria isolated in culture. Infections due to staphylococci are treated with oxacillin, nafcillin, or vancomycin for 4 weeks. Pneumococcal and streptococcal infections due to penicillin-susceptible organisms respond to 2 weeks of therapy with penicillin G (2 million units IV every 4 h); infections caused by *H. influenzae* and by strains of *S. pneumoniae* that are resistant to penicillin are treated with cefotaxime or ceftriaxone for 2 weeks. Most enteric gram-negative infections can be cured in 3–4 weeks by a second- or third-generation cephalosporin given IV or by a fluoroquinolone, such as levofloxacin (500 mg IV or PO every 24 h). *P. aeruginosa* infection should be treated for at least 2 weeks with a combination regimen of an aminoglycoside plus either an extended-spectrum penicillin, such as mezlocillin (3 g IV every 4 h), or an antipseudomonal cephalosporin, such as ceftazidime (1 g IV every 8 h). If tolerated, this regimen is continued for an additional 2 weeks; alternatively, a fluoroquinolone, such as ciprofloxacin (750 mg PO twice daily), is given by itself or with the penicillin or cephalosporin in place of the aminoglycoside.

Timely drainage of pus and necrotic debris from the infected joint is required for a favorable outcome. Needle aspiration of readily accessible joints such as the knee may be adequate if loculations or particulate matter in the joint does not prevent its thorough decompression. Arthroscopic drainage and lavage may be employed initially or within several days if repeated needle aspiration fails to relieve symptoms, decrease the volume of the effusion and the synovial white cell count, and clear bacteria from smears and cultures. In some cases, arthrotomy is necessary to remove loculations and debride infected synovium, cartilage, or bone. Septic arthritis of the hip is best managed with arthrotomy, particularly in young children, in whom infection threatens the viability of the femoral head. Septic joints do not require immobilization except for pain control before symptoms are alleviated by treatment. Weight bearing should be avoided until signs of inflammation have subsided, but frequent passive motion of the joint is indicated to maintain full mobility. While addition of glucocorticoids to antibiotic treatment improves the outcome of *S. aureus* arthritis in experimental animals, no clinical trials have yet evaluated this approach in humans.

FIGURE 328-1 Acute septic arthritis of the sternoclavicular joint.
A man in his 40s with a history of cirrhosis presented with a new onset of fever and lower neck pain. He had no history of IV drug use or previous catheter placement. Jaundice and a painful swollen area over his left sternoclavicular joint were evident on physical exam. Cultures of blood drawn at admission grew group B *Streptococcus*. The patient recovered after treatment with IV penicillin. *(Courtesy of Francisco M. Marty, MD, Brigham & Women's Hospital, Boston; with permission.)*

CLINICAL MANIFESTATIONS Some 90% of patients present with involvement of a single joint—most commonly the knee; less frequently the hip; and still less often the shoulder, wrist, or elbow. Small joints of the hands and feet are more likely to be affected after direct inoculation or a bite. Among IV drug users, infections of the spine, sacroiliac joints, or sternoclavicular joints (Fig. 328-1) are more common than infections of the appendicular skeleton. Polyarticular infection is most common among patients with rheumatoid arthritis and may resemble a flare of the underlying disease.

The usual presentation consists of moderate to severe pain that is uniform around the joint, effusion, muscle spasm, and decreased range of motion. Fever in the range of 38.3°–38.9°C (101°–102°F) and sometimes higher is common but may be lacking, especially in persons with rheumatoid arthritis, renal or hepatic insufficiency, or conditions requiring immunosuppressive therapy. The inflamed, swollen joint is usually evident on examination except in the case of a deeply situated joint, such as the hip, shoulder, or sacroiliac joint. Cellulitis, bursitis, and acute osteomyelitis, which may produce a similar clinical picture, should be distinguished from septic arthritis by their greater range of motion and less-than-circumferential swelling. A focus of extraarticular infection, such as a boil or pneumonia, should be sought. Peripheral-blood leukocytosis with a left shift and elevation of the erythrocyte sedimentation rate (ESR) or C-reactive protein level are common.

Plain radiographs show evidence of soft tissue swelling, joint-space widening, and displacement of tissue planes by the distended capsule. Narrowing of the joint space and bony erosions indicate advanced infection and a poor prognosis. Ultrasound is useful for detecting effusions in the hip, and CT or MRI can demonstrate infections of the sacroiliac joint, the sternoclavicular joint, and the spine very well.

LABORATORY FINDINGS Specimens of peripheral blood and synovial fluid should be obtained before antibiotics are administered. Blood cultures are positive in up to 50–70% of *S. aureus* infections but are less frequently positive in infections due to other organisms. The synovial fluid is turbid, serosanguineous, or frankly purulent. Gram-stained smears confirm the presence of large numbers of neutrophils. Levels of total protein and lactate dehydrogenase in synovial fluid are elevated, and the glucose level is depressed; however, these findings are not specific for infection, and measurement of these levels is not necessary to make the diagnosis. The synovial fluid should be examined for crystals, because gout and pseudogout can resemble septic arthritis

Gonococcal Arthritis • *EPIDEMIOLOGY* Although its incidence has declined in recent years, gonococcal arthritis (Chap. 137) has accounted for up to 70% of episodes of infectious arthritis in persons <40 years of age in the United States. Arthritis due to *N. gonorrhoeae* is a consequence of bacteremia arising from gonococcal infection or, more frequently, from asymptomatic gonococcal mucosal colonization of the urethra, cervix, or pharynx. Women are at greatest risk during menses and during pregnancy and overall are two to three times more likely than men to develop disseminated gonococcal infection (DGI) and arthritis. Persons with complement deficiencies, especially of the terminal components, are prone to recurrent episodes of gonococcemia. Strains of gonococci that are most likely to cause DGI include those that produce transparent colonies in culture, have the type IA outer-membrane protein, or are of the AUH-auxotroph type.

CLINICAL MANIFESTATIONS AND LABORATORY FINDINGS   The most common manifestation of DGI is a syndrome of fever, chills, rash, and articular symptoms. Small numbers of papules that progress to hemorrhagic pustules develop on the trunk and the extensor surfaces of the distal extremities. Migratory arthritis and tenosynovitis of the knees, hands, wrists, feet, and ankles are prominent. The cutaneous lesions and articular findings are believed to be the consequence of an immune reaction to circulating gonococci and immune-complex deposition in tissues. Thus, cultures of synovial fluid are consistently negative, and blood cultures are positive in <45% of patients. Synovial fluid may be difficult to obtain from inflamed joints and usually contains only 10,000–20,000 leukocytes/μL.

True gonococcal septic arthritis is less common than the DGI syndrome and always follows DGI, which is unrecognized in one-third of patients. A single joint, such as the hip, knee, ankle, or wrist, is usually involved. Synovial fluid, which contains >50,000 leukocytes/μL, can be obtained with ease; the gonococcus is only occasionally evident in gram-stained smears, and cultures of synovial fluid are positive in <40% of cases. Blood cultures are almost always negative.

Because it is difficult to isolate gonococci from synovial fluid and blood, specimens for culture should be obtained from potentially infected mucosal sites. Cultures and gram-stained smears of skin lesions are occasionally positive. All specimens for culture should be plated onto Thayer-Martin agar directly or in special transport media at the bedside and transferred promptly to the microbiology laboratory in an atmosphere of 5% CO_2, as generated in a candle jar. PCR-based assays are extremely sensitive in detecting gonococcal DNA in synovial fluid. A dramatic alleviation of symptoms within 12–24 h after the initiation of appropriate antibiotic therapy supports a clinical diagnosis of the DGI syndrome if cultures are negative.

Rx GONOCOCCAL ARTHRITIS

Initial treatment consists of ceftriaxone (1 g IV or IM every 24 h) to cover possible penicillin-resistant organisms. Once local and systemic signs are clearly resolving and if the sensitivity of the isolate permits, the 7-day course of therapy can be completed with an oral agent such as ciprofloxacin (500 mg twice daily) if sensitivity allows. If penicillin-susceptible organisms are isolated, amoxicillin (500 mg three times daily) may be used. Suppurative arthritis usually responds to needle aspiration of involved joints and 7–14 days of antibiotic treatment. Arthroscopic lavage or arthrotomy is rarely required. Patients with DGI should be treated for *Chlamydia trachomatis* infection unless this infection is ruled out by appropriate testing.

It is noteworthy that arthritis symptoms similar to those seen in DGI occur in meningococcemia. A dermatitis-arthritis syndrome, purulent monarthritis, and reactive polyarthritis have been described. All respond to treatment with IV penicillin.

SPIROCHETAL ARTHRITIS

Lyme Disease   Lyme disease (Chap. 166) due to infection with the spirochete *Borrelia burgdorferi* causes arthritis in up to 70% of persons who are not treated. Intermittent arthralgias and myalgias—but not arthritis—occur within days or weeks of inoculation of the spirochete by the *Ixodes* tick. Later, there are three patterns of joint disease: (1) Fifty percent of untreated persons experience intermittent episodes of monarthritis or oligoarthritis involving the knee and/or other large joints. The

symptoms wax and wane without treatment over months, and each year 10–20% of patients report loss of joint symptoms. (2) Twenty percent of untreated persons develop a pattern of waxing and waning arthralgias. (3) Ten percent of untreated patients develop chronic inflammatory synovitis resulting in erosive lesions and destruction of the joint. Serologic tests for IgG antibodies to *B. burgdorferi* are positive in >90% of persons with Lyme arthritis, and a PCR-based assay detects *Borrelia* DNA in 85%.

Rx LYME ARTHRITIS

Lyme arthritis generally responds well to therapy. A regimen of oral doxycycline (100 mg twice daily for 30 days), oral amoxicillin (500 mg four times daily for 30 days), or parenteral ceftriaxone (2 g/d for 2–4 weeks) is recommended. Patients who do not respond to a total of 2 months of oral therapy or 1 month of parenteral therapy are unlikely to benefit from additional antibiotic therapy and are treated with anti-inflammatory agents or synovectomy. Failure of therapy is associated with host features such as the HLA-DR4 genotype, persistent reactivity to OspA (outer-surface protein A), and the presence of hLFA-1 (human leukocyte function–associated antigen 1), which cross-reacts with OspA.

Syphilitic Arthritis   Articular manifestations occur in different stages of syphilis (Chap. 162). In early congenital syphilis, periarticular swelling and immobilization of the involved limbs (Parrot's pseudoparalysis) complicate osteochondritis of long bones. Clutton's joint, a late manifestation of congenital syphilis that typically develops between the ages of 8 and 15 years, is caused by chronic painless synovitis with effusions of large joints, particularly the knees and elbows. Secondary syphilis may be associated with arthralgias; with symmetric arthritis of the knees and ankles and occasionally of the shoulders and wrists; and with sacroiliitis. The arthritis follows a subacute to chronic course with a mixed mononuclear and neutrophilic synovial-fluid pleocytosis (typical cell counts, 5000–15,000/μL). Immunologic mechanisms may contribute to the arthritis, and symptoms usually improve rapidly with penicillin therapy. In tertiary syphilis, Charcot's joint is a result of sensory loss due to tabes dorsalis. Penicillin is not helpful in this setting.

MYCOBACTERIAL ARTHRITIS

Tuberculous arthritis (Chap. 158) accounts for ~1% of all cases of tuberculosis and for 10% of extrapulmonary cases. The most common presentation is chronic granulomatous monarthritis. An unusual syndrome, Poncet's disease, is a reactive symmetric form of polyarthritis that affects persons with visceral or disseminated tuberculosis. No mycobacteria are found in the joints, and symptoms resolve with antituberculous therapy.

Unlike tuberculous osteomyelitis (Chap. 120), which typically involves the thoracic and lumbar spine (50% of cases), tuberculous arthritis primarily involves the large weight-bearing joints, in particular the hips, knees, and ankles, and only occasionally involves smaller non-weight-bearing joints. Progressive monarticular swelling and pain develop over months or years, and systemic symptoms are seen in only half of all cases. Tuberculous arthritis occurs as part of a disseminated primary infection or through late reactivation, often in persons with HIV infection or other immunocompromised hosts. Coexistent active pulmonary tuberculosis is unusual.

Aspiration of the involved joint yields fluid with an average cell count of 20,000/μL, with ~50% neutrophils. Acid-fast staining of the fluid yields positive results in fewer than one-third of cases, and cultures are positive in 80%. Culture of synovial tissue taken at biopsy is positive in ~90% of cases and shows granulomatous inflammation in most. DNA amplification methods such as PCR can shorten the time to diagnosis to 1 or 2 days. Radiographs reveal peripheral erosions at the points of synovial attachment, periarticular osteopenia, and eventually joint-space narrowing. Therapy for tuberculous arthritis is the same as that for tuberculous pulmonary disease, requiring the administration of multiple agents for 6–9 months. Therapy is more prolonged in immunosuppressed individuals, such as those infected with HIV.

A   **B**   **C**

FIGURE 328-2 Chronic arthritis caused by ***Histoplasma capsulatum*** in the left knee. **A.** A man in his 60s from El Salvador presented with a history of progressive knee pain and difficulty walking for several years. He had undergone arthroscopy for a meniscal tear 7 years before presentation (without relief) and had received several intraarticular glucocorticoid injections. The patient developed significant deformity of the knee over time, including a large effusion in the lateral aspect. **B.** An x-ray of the knee showed multiple abnormalities, including severe medial femorotibial joint-space narrowing, several large subchondral cysts within the tibia and the patellofemoral compartment, a large su-prapatellar joint effusion, and a large soft-tissue mass projecting laterally over the knee. **C.** MRI further defined these abnormalities and demonstrated the cystic nature of the lateral knee abnormality. Synovial biopsies demonstrated chronic inflammation with giant cells, and cultures grew *H. capsulatum* after 3 weeks of incubation. All clinical cystic lesions and the effusion resolved after 1 year of treatment with itraconazole. The patient underwent a left total knee replacement for definitive treatment. *(Courtesy of Francisco M. Marty, MD, Brigham & Women's Hospital, Boston; with permission.)*

Various atypical mycobacteria (Chap. 160) found in water and soil may cause chronic indolent arthritis. Such disease results from trauma and direct inoculation associated with farming, gardening, or aquatic activities. Smaller joints, such as the digits, wrists, and knees, are usually involved. Involvement of tendon sheaths and bursae is typical. The mycobacterial species involved include *Mycobacterium marinum*, *M. avium-intracellulare*, *M. terrae*, *M. kansasii*, *M. fortuitum*, and *M. chelonae*. In persons who have HIV infection or are receiving immunosuppressive therapy, hematogenous spread to the joints has been reported for *M. kansasii*, *M. avium-intracellulare*, and *M. haemophilum*. Diagnosis usually requires biopsy and culture, and therapy is based on antimicrobial susceptibility patterns.

FUNGAL ARTHRITIS

Fungi are an unusual cause of chronic monarticular arthritis. Granulomatous articular infection with the endemic dimorphic fungi *Coccidioides immitis*, *Blastomyces dermatitidis*, and (less commonly) *Histoplasma capsulatum* (Fig. 328-2) results from hematogenous seeding or direct extension from bony lesions in persons with disseminated disease. Joint involvement is an unusual complication of sporotrichosis (infection with *Sporothrix schenckii*) among gardeners and other persons who work with soil or sphagnum moss. Articular sporotrichosis is six times more common among men than among women, and alcoholics and other debilitated hosts are at risk for polyarticular infection.

Candida infection involving a single joint—usually the knee, hip, or shoulder—results from surgical procedures, intraarticular injections, or (among critically ill patients with debilitating illnesses, such as diabetes mellitus or hepatic or renal insufficiency, and patients receiving immunosuppressive therapy) hematogenous spread. *Candida* infections in IV drug users typically involve the spine, sacroiliac joints, or other fibrocartilaginous joints. Unusual cases of arthritis due to *Aspergillus* species, *Cryptococcus neoformans*, *Pseudallescheria boydii*, and the dematiaceous fungi have also resulted from direct inoculation or disseminated hematogenous infection in immunocompromised persons.

The synovial fluid in fungal arthritis usually contains 10,000–40,000 cells/μL, with ~70% neutrophils. Stained specimens and cultures of synovial tissue often confirm the diagnosis of fungal arthritis when studies of synovial fluid give negative results. Treatment consists of drainage and lavage of the joint and systemic administration of an antifungal agent directed at a specific pathogen. The doses and dura-tion of therapy are the same as for disseminated disease (see Part 7, Section 16). Intraarticular instillation of amphotericin B has been used in addition to IV therapy.

VIRAL ARTHRITIS

Viruses produce arthritis by infecting synovial tissue during systemic infection or by provoking an immunologic reaction that involves joints. As many as 50% of women report persistent arthralgias and 10% report frank arthritis within 3 days of the rash that follows natural infection with rubella virus and within 2–6 weeks after receipt of live-virus vaccine. Episodes of symmetric inflammation of fingers, wrists, and knees uncommonly recur for >1 year, but a syndrome of chronic fatigue, low-grade fever, headaches, and myalgias can persist for months or years. IVIg has been helpful in selected cases. Self-limited monarticular or migratory polyarthritis may develop within 2 weeks of the parotitis of mumps; this sequela is more common among men than among women. Approximately 10% of children and 60% of women develop arthritis after infection with parvovirus B19. In adults, arthropathy sometimes occurs without fever or rash. Pain and stiffness, with less prominent swelling (primarily of the hands but also of the knees, wrists, and ankles), usually resolve within weeks, although a small proportion of patients develop chronic arthropathy.

About 2 weeks before the onset of jaundice, up to 10% of persons with acute hepatitis B develop an immune complex–mediated, serum sickness–like reaction with maculopapular rash, urticaria, fever, and arthralgias. Less common developments include symmetric arthritis involving the hands, wrists, elbows, or ankles and morning stiffness that resembles a flare of rheumatoid arthritis. Symptoms resolve at the time jaundice develops. Many persons with chronic hepatitis C infection report persistent arthralgia or arthritis, both in the presence and in the absence of cryoglobulinemia. Painful arthritis involving larger joints often accompanies the fever and rash of several arthropod-borne viral infections, including those caused by chikungunya, O'nyong-nyong, Ross River, Mayaro, and Barmah Forest viruses. Symmetric arthritis involving the hands and wrists may occur during the convalescent phase of infection with lymphocytic choriomeningitis virus. Patients infected with an enterovirus frequently report arthralgias, and echovirus has been isolated from patients with acute polyarthritis.

Several arthritis syndromes are associated with HIV infection. Reiter's syndrome with painful lower-extremity oligoarthritis often follows an episode of urethritis in HIV-infected persons. HIV-associated Reiter's syndrome appears to be extremely common among persons with the HLA-B27 haplotype, but sacroiliac joint disease is unusual and is seen mostly in the absence of HLA-B27. Up to one-third of HIV-infected persons with psoriasis develop psoriatic arthritis. Painless monarthropathy and persistent symmetric polyarthropaty occasionally complicate HIV infection. Chronic persistent oligoarthritis of the shoulders, wrists, hands, and knees occurs in women infected with human T cell lymphotropic virus type I. Synovial thickening, destruction of articular cartilage, and leukemic-appearing atypical lymphocytes in synovial fluid are characteristic, but progression to T cell leukemia is unusual.

PARASITIC ARTHRITIS

Arthritis due to parasitic infection is rare. The guinea worm *Dracunculus medinensis* may cause destructive joint lesions in the lower extremities as migrating gravid female worms invade joints or cause ulcers in adjacent soft tissues that become secondarily infected. Hydatid cysts infect bones in 1–2% of cases of infection with *Echinococcus granulosus*. The expanding destructive cystic lesions may spread to and destroy adjacent joints, particularly the hip and pelvis. In rare cases, chronic synovitis has been associated with the presence of schistosomal eggs in synovial biopsies. Monarticular arthritis in children with lymphatic filariasis appears to respond to therapy with diethylcarbamazine, even in the absence of microfilariae in synovial fluid. Reactive arthritis has been attributed to hookworm, *Strongyloides*, *Cryptosporidium*, and *Giardia* infection in case reports, but confirmation is required.

POSTINFECTIOUS OR REACTIVE ARTHRITIS

Reiter's syndrome, a reactive polyarthritis, develops several weeks after ~1% of cases of nongonococcal urethritis and 2% of enteric infections, particularly those due to *Yersinia enterocolitica*, *Shigella flexneri*, *Campylobacter jejuni*, and *Salmonella* species. Only a minority of these patients have the other findings of classic Reiter's syndrome, including urethritis, conjunctivitis, uveitis, oral ulcers, and rash. Studies have identified microbial DNA or antigen in synovial fluid or blood, but the pathogenesis of this condition is poorly understood.

Reiter's syndrome is most common among young men (except after *Yersinia* infection) and has been linked to the HLA-B27 locus as a potential genetic predisposing factor. Patients report painful, asymmetric oligoarthritis affecting mainly the knees, ankles, and feet. Low-back pain is common, and radiographic evidence of sacroiliitis is found in patients with long-standing disease. Most patients recover within 6 months, but prolonged recurrent disease is more common in cases following chlamydial urethritis. Anti-inflammatory agents help to relieve symptoms, but the role of prolonged antibiotic therapy in eliminating microbial antigen from the synovium is controversial.

Migratory polyarthritis and fever constitute the usual presentation of acute rheumatic fever in adults (Chap. 315). This presentation is distinct from that of poststreptococcal reactive arthritis, which also follows infections with group A *Streptococcus* but is not migratory, lasts beyond the typical 3-week maximum of acute rheumatic fever, and responds poorly to aspirin.

INFECTIONS IN PROSTHETIC JOINTS

Infection complicates 1–4% of total joint replacements. The majority of infections are acquired intraoperatively or immediately postoperatively as a result of wound breakdown or infection; less commonly, these joint infections develop later after joint replacement and are the result of hematogenous spread or direct inoculation. The presentation may be acute, with fever, pain, and local signs of inflammation, especially in infections due to *S. aureus*, pyogenic streptococci, and enteric bacilli. Alternatively, infection may persist for months or years without causing constitutional symptoms when less virulent organisms, such as coagulase-negative staphylococci or diphtheroids, are involved. Such indolent infections are usually acquired during joint implanta-

tion and are discovered during evaluation of chronic unexplained pain or after a radiograph shows loosening of the prosthesis; the ESR and C-reactive protein level are usually elevated in such cases.

The diagnosis is best made by needle aspiration of the joint; accidental introduction of organisms during aspiration must be meticulously avoided. Synovial fluid pleocytosis with a predominance of polymorphonuclear leukocytes is highly suggestive of infection, since other inflammatory processes uncommonly affect prosthetic joints. Culture and Gram's stain usually yield the responsible pathogen. Use of special media for unusual pathogens such as fungi, atypical mycobacteria, and *Mycoplasma* may be necessary if routine and anaerobic cultures are negative.

℞ PROSTHETIC JOINT INFECTIONS

Treatment includes surgery and high doses of parenteral antibiotics, which are given for 4–6 weeks because bone is usually involved. In most cases, the prosthesis must be replaced to cure the infection. Implantation of a new prosthesis is best delayed for several weeks or months because relapses of infection occur most commonly within this time frame. In some cases, reimplantation is not possible, and the patient must manage without a joint, with a fused joint, or even with amputation. Cure of infection without removal of the prosthesis is occasionally possible in cases that are due to streptococci or pneumococci and that lack radiologic evidence of loosening of the prosthesis. In these cases, antibiotic therapy must be initiated within several days of the onset of infection, and the joint should be drained vigorously either by open arthrotomy or arthroscopically. In selected patients who prefer to avoid the high morbidity associated with joint removal and reimplantation, suppression of the infection with antibiotics may be a reasonable goal. A high cure rate with retention of the prosthesis has been reported when the combination of oral rifampin and ciprofloxacin is given for 3–6 months to persons with staphylococcal prosthetic joint infection of short duration. This approach, which is based on the ability of rifampin to kill organisms adherent to foreign material and in the stationary growth phase, requires confirmation in prospective trials.

Prevention   To avoid the disastrous consequences of infection, candidates for joint replacement should be selected with care. Rates of infection are particularly high among patients with rheumatoid arthritis, persons who have undergone previous surgery on the joint, and persons with medical conditions requiring immunosuppressive therapy. Perioperative antibiotic prophylaxis, usually with cefazolin, and measures to decrease intraoperative contamination, such as laminar flow, have lowered the rates of perioperative infection to <1% in many centers. After implantation, measures should be taken to prevent or rapidly treat extraarticular infections that might give rise to hematogenous spread to the prosthesis. The effectiveness of prophylactic antibiotics for the prevention of hematogenous infection following dental procedures has not been demonstrated; in fact, viridans streptococci and other components of the oral flora are extremely unusual causes of prosthetic joint infection. Accordingly, the American Dental Association and the American Academy of Orthopaedic Surgeons do not recommend antibiotic prophylaxis for most dental patients with total joint replacements. They do, however, recommend prophylaxis for patients who may be at high risk of hematogenous infection, including those with inflammatory arthropathies, immunosuppression, type 1 diabetes mellitus, joint replacement within 2 years, previous prosthetic joint infection, malnourishment, or hemophilia. The recommended regimen is amoxicillin (2 g PO) 1 h before dental procedures associated with a high incidence of bacteremia. Clindamycin (600 mg PO) is suggested for patients allergic to penicillin.

ACKNOWLEDGMENTS
The contributions of James H. Maguire and the late Scott J. Thaler to this chapter in earlier editions are gratefully acknowledged.

FURTHER READINGS

BARDIN T: Gonococcal arthritis. Best Pract Res Clin Rheumatol 17:201, 2003

Donatto KC: Orthopedic management of septic arthritis. Rheum Dis Clin North Am 24:275, 1998

Franssila R, Hedman K: Infection and musculoskeletal conditions: Viral causes of arthritis. Best Pract Res Clin Rheumatol 20:1139, 2006

Harrington JT: Mycobacterial and fungal arthritis. Curr Opin Rheumatol 10:335, 1998

Medina Rodriguez F: Rheumatic manifestations of human immunodeficiency virus infection. Rheum Dis Clin North Am 29:145, 2003

Meehan AM et al: Outcome of penicillin-susceptible streptococcal prosthetic joint infection treated with debridement and retention of the prosthesis. Clin Infect Dis 36:845, 2003

Shirtliff ME, Mader JT: Acute septic arthritis. Clin Microbiol Rev 15:527, 2002

Stengel D et al: Systematic review and meta-analysis of antibiotic therapy for bone and joint infections. Lancet Infect Dis 1:175, 2001

Tarkowski A: Infection and musculoskeletal conditions: Infectious arthritis. Best Pract Res Clin Rheumatol 20:1029, 2006

Zimmerli W et al: Prosthetic-joint infections. N Engl J Med 351:145, 2004

329 Fibromyalgia
Carol A. Langford, Bruce C. Gilliland†

Fibromyalgia is a commonly encountered disorder characterized by chronic widespread musculoskeletal pain, stiffness, paresthesia, disturbed sleep, and easy fatigability along with multiple painful tender points, which are widely and symmetrically distributed. Fibromyalgia affects predominantly women in a ratio of 9:1 compared to men. This disorder is found in most countries, in most ethnic groups, and in all types of climates. The prevalence of fibromyalgia in the general population of a community in the United States using the 1990 American College of Rheumatology (ACR) classification criteria (see below) was reported to be 3.4% in women and 0.5% in men. Contrary to some previous reports, fibromyalgia was not found to be present mainly in young women but, rather, to be most prevalent in women ≥50 years. The prevalence increased with age, being 7.4% in women between the ages of 70 and 79. Although not common, fibromyalgia also occurs in children. The reported prevalence of fibromyalgia in some rheumatology clinics has been as high as 20%. Most patients present with fibromyalgia between the ages of 30–50 years.

PATHOGENESIS

Several causative mechanisms for fibromyalgia have been postulated to explain abnormal pain perception. Several abnormalities of the central nervous system have been suggested. Disturbed sleep has been implicated as a factor in the pathogenesis. Nonrestorative sleep or awakening unrefreshed has been observed in most patients with fibromyalgia. Sleep electroencephalographic studies in patients with fibromyalgia have shown disruption of normal stage 4 sleep [non–rapid eye movement (NREM) sleep] by many repeated α-wave intrusions. The idea that stage 4 sleep deprivation has a role in causing this disorder was supported by the observation that symptoms of fibromyalgia developed in normal subjects whose stage 4 sleep was disrupted artificially by induced α-wave intrusions. This sleep disturbance, however, has been demonstrated in healthy individuals; in emotionally distressed individuals; and in patients with sleep apnea, fever, osteoarthritis, or rheumatoid arthritis. Low levels of serotonin metabolites have been reported in the cerebrospinal fluid (CSF) of patients with fibromyalgia, suggesting that a deficiency of serotonin, a neurotransmitter that regulates pain and NREM sleep, might also be involved in the pathogenesis of fibromyalgia. Fibromyalgia patients as a group have been reported by some investigators to have reduced levels of growth hormone, which is important for muscle repair and strength. Growth hormone is secreted normally during stage 4 sleep, which is disturbed in patients with fibromyalgia. The reduction of growth hormone may explain the extended periods of muscle pain following exertion in these patients. The level of the neurotransmitter substance P has been reported to be increased in the CSF of fibromyalgia patients and may play a role in spreading muscle pain. Patients with fibromyalgia have a decreased cortisol response to stress. Low urinary free cortisol and a diminished cortisol response to corticotropin-releasing hormone suggest an abnormal hypothalamic-pituitary-adrenal axis. Autonomic dysfunction has also been suggested to play a role in the pathogenesis of fibromyalgia. Some patients experience orthostatic hypotension on tilt-table testing and may have increased resting supine heart rates. Disturbances of the autonomic and peripheral nervous system may also account for the dry eyes and mouth and the cold sensitivity and Raynaud's-like symptoms seen in patients with fibromyalgia. Single photon emission computed tomography (SPECT) imaging has demonstrated reduced blood flow to the thalamus, caudate nucleus, and pontine tectum, which are areas in the brain involved in the signaling, integration, and modulation of pain. Patients with fibromyalgia have been shown to perceive stimuli such as heat or pressure as painful with less degree of stimulation than normal individuals. The actual threshold for detecting stimuli appears to be similar in both patients and normal subjects. Studies have also suggested that patients with fibromyalgia may have psychophysiologic abnormalities in their ability to inhibit irrelevant somatosensory stimulation.

Many patients with fibromyalgia have psychological abnormalities; there has been disagreement as to whether some of these abnormalities represent reactions to the chronic pain or whether the symptoms of fibromyalgia are a reflection of psychiatric disturbance. Approximately 30% of patients fit a psychiatric diagnosis, the most common being depression, anxiety, somatization, and hypochondriasis. Studies have also shown a high prevalence of sexual and physical abuse and eating disorders. However, fibromyalgia also occurs in patients without significant psychiatric problems.

Since patients experience pain from muscle and musculotendinous sites, many studies have been done to examine muscle, both structurally and physiologically. Inflammation or diagnostic muscle abnormalities have not been found. Evidence indicates deconditioning of muscles, and patients experience a greater degree of postexertional pain than do unaffected persons. A better understanding of fibromyalgia awaits further studies.

CLINICAL MANIFESTATIONS

Symptoms are generalized musculoskeletal aching and stiffness and fatigue. Patients may complain of low back pain, which may radiate into the buttocks and legs. Others complain of pain and tightness in the neck and across the upper posterior shoulders. Patients complain of muscle pain after even mild exertion, and some degree of pain is always present. The pain has been described as a burning or gnawing pain or as soreness, stiffness, or aching. Pain may begin in one region, such as the shoulders, neck, or lower back (Chap. 330) before it eventually becomes widespread. Patients may complain of joint pain and perceive that their joints are swollen; however, joint examination yields normal findings. Stiffness is generally present on arising in the morning; usually it improves during the day, but in some patients it lasts all day. Patients may complain of numbness of their hands and feet. They may also feel colder overall than others in the home, and some may experience Raynaud's-like phenomena or actual Raynaud's phenomenon. Patients complain of feeling fatigued and exhausted and wake up tired. They also awaken frequently at night and have trouble falling back to sleep. Patients may experience cognitive impairment with difficulty thinking and loss of short-term memory. Headaches, including migraine type, are also common symptoms. Others experience episodes of light-headedness, dizziness, anxiety, or depression. Symptoms are made worse by stress or anxiety, cold, damp weather, and overexertion. Patients often feel better during warmer weather and vacations.

---

†Deceased. A contributor to HPIM since the 11th edition, Dr. Gilliland passed away on February 17, 2007.

FIGURE 329-1 Tender points in fibromyalgia. Suboccipital muscle insertion at base of skull; anterior aspect of intertransverse process spaces at C5–7; midpoint of upper border of trapezius muscle; above scapular spine near medial border of scapula; second costochondral junction; lateral epicondyle; upper outer quadrant of buttocks; posterior aspect of trochanteric prominence; medial fat pad of knee (all bilateral). *(From the brochure "Fibromyalgia," Arthritis Information, Advice and Guidance, Disease Series. Used by permission of the Arthritis Foundation.)*

The characteristic feature on physical examination is the demonstration of specific sites or points, which are more tender or painful than the same sites in normal individuals. The ACR Criteria for Fibromyalgia defines 18 tender points (Fig. 329-1). These points of tenderness are remarkably constant in location. A moderate and consistent degree of pressure should be used in digital palpation of these tender points. As a guideline to reduce variability in the interpretation of point tenderness, the amount of force applied should be 4 kg (~9 lb), which is the degree of force required to just blanch the examiner's thumbnail. This amount of pressure does not produce significant tenderness or pain in normal subjects. Some workers recommend that the tender site be palpated using a rolling motion, which may be more effective in eliciting the tenderness. The tender sites can also be examined using a dolorimeter, which is a spring-loaded pressure gauge; however, digital palpation appears to be as effective and accurate. Some investigators have quantitated the degree of tenderness or pain, but the number of tender point sites is more diagnostic. Some patients are tender all over although still more tender or painful at the specific tender point sites.

Skinfold tenderness may be present, particularly over the upper scapular region. Subcutaneous nodules may be felt at sites of tenderness. Nodules in similar locations are present in normal persons but are not tender.

Fibromyalgia may be triggered by emotional stress, infections and other medical illness, surgery, hypothyroidism, and trauma. It has appeared in some patients with hepatitis C infection, HIV infection, parvovirus B19 infection, or Lyme disease. In the latter situation, fibromyalgia may persist despite adequate antibiotic treatment for Lyme disease, and especially anxious patients may believe that they still have Lyme disease. Disorders commonly associated with fibromyalgia include irritable bowel syndrome, irritable bladder, headaches (including migraine headaches), dysmenorrhea, premenstrual syndrome, restless leg syndrome, temporomandibular joint pain, noncardiac chest pain, Raynaud's phenomenon, and sicca syndrome.

The course of fibromyalgia is variable. Symptoms wax and wane in some patients, while in others pain and fatigue are persistent regardless of therapy. Studies from tertiary medical centers indicate a poor

prognosis for most patients. The prognosis may be better in community-treated patients. In a community-based study reported after 2 years of treatment, 24% of patients were in remission, and 47% no longer fulfilled the ACR criteria for fibromyalgia.

DIAGNOSIS

Fibromyalgia is diagnosed by a history of widespread musculoskeletal pain present for at least 3 months and the demonstration of significant tenderness or pain in at least 11 of the 18 tender point sites on digital palpation (Fig. 329-1). The ACR criteria are useful for standardizing the diagnosis; however, not all patients with fibromyalgia meet these criteria (Table 329-1). Some patients have fewer tender sites and more regional pain and may be considered to have fibromyalgia.

The musculoskeletal and neurologic examinations are normal in fibromyalgia patients, and there are no laboratory abnormalities. Fibromyalgia may occur in patients with rheumatoid arthritis, systemic lupus erythematosus (SLE), other connective tissue diseases, or other medical illness. A distinction is no longer made between primary and secondary fibromyalgia (concomitant with other disease), as the signs and symptoms are similar. Fibromyalgia and chronic fatigue syndrome have many similarities (Chap. 384). Both are associated with fatigue, abnormal sleep, musculoskeletal pain, impaired memory and concentration, and psychiatric conditions such as less severe forms of depression and anxiety. Patients with chronic fatigue syndrome, however, are more likely to have symptoms suggesting a viral illness. These include mild fever, sore throat, and pain in the axillary and anterior and posterior cervical lymph nodes. The onset of chronic fatigue syndrome is usually sudden; patients are usually able to date the onset. While many patients with chronic fatigue syndrome have tender or painful points, the diagnosis does not require their presence. Patients with fibromyalgia may be misdiagnosed with SLE or Sjögren's syndrome as these disorders have in common symptoms of musculoskeletal pain, dry eyes, cold hands, and fatigue. The antinuclear antibody (ANA) test may also be positive. The frequency of a positive ANA test in fibromyalgia patients, however, is the same as sex- and aged-matched normal controls. The predictive value of a positive ANA test in patients without characteristic symptoms and objective features of a connective tissue disease is quite low. Discretion is advised before or-

TABLE 329-1	THE AMERICAN COLLEGE OF RHEUMATOLOGY 1990 CRITERIA FOR THE CLASSIFICATION OF FIBROMYALGIA[a]

1. History of widespread pain. Pain is considered widespread when all of the following are present:
   a. Pain in the left side of the body
   b. Pain in the right side of the body
   c. Pain above the waist
   d. Pain below the waist
   e. Axial skeletal pain (cervical spine or anterior chest or thoracic spine or low back)
2. Pain on digital palpation in at least 11 of the following 18 tender point sites (see Fig. 329-1):
   a. Occiput: bilateral, at the suboccipital muscle insertion
   b. Low cervical: bilateral, at the anterior aspect of the intertransverse spaces at C5–7
   c. Trapezius: bilateral, at the midpoint of the upper border
   d. Supraspinatus: bilateral, at the origin, above the scapular spine near the medial border
   e. Second rib: bilateral, at the second costochondral junction, just lateral to the junction on the upper surface
   f. Lateral epicondyle: bilateral, 2 cm distal to the epicondyle
   g. Gluteal: bilateral, in the upper outer quadrant of the buttock
   h. Greater trochanter: bilateral, posterior to the trochanteric prominence
   i. Knee: bilateral, at the medial fat pad proximal to the joint line

Digital palpation should be performed with a moderate degree of pressure. For a tender point to be considered positive, the subject must state that the palpation was painful. "Tender" is not to be considered painful.

---

[a]For purposes of classification, patients will be said to have fibromyalgia if both criteria are satisfied. Widespread pain must have been present for at least 3 months. The presence of a second clinical disorder does not exclude the diagnosis of fibromyalgia.

Source: Modified from F Wolfe et al: Arthritis Rheum 33:171, 1990.

dering an ANA test. Patients with fibromyalgia may complain of muscle weakness, but on muscle strength testing, they have "giveaway" weakness secondary to pain. Proximal muscle weakness and elevated muscle enzymes distinguish patients with polymyositis. Polymyalgia rheumatica is distinguished from fibromyalgia in an elderly patient by the presence of more proximal muscle stiffness and pain and an elevated erythrocyte sedimentation rate. Patients should be evaluated for hypothyroidism, which may have symptoms similar to fibromyalgia or may accompany fibromyalgia. Disturbed sleep, musculoskeletal pain, and fatigue occur in patients with sleep apnea and restless leg syndrome. A distinguishing feature of sleep apnea is the presence of significant daytime somnolence. These patients should be referred to a sleep laboratory for evaluation and treatment. Myofascial pain syndrome, which involves an area such as the shoulder or neck, may represent a localized form of fibromyalgia (Chap. 330). Some patients with this syndrome progress to fibromyalgia.

The diagnosis of fibromyalgia has taken on a more complex significance in regard to labor and industry issues. This has become a significant issue since it has been reported that 10–25% of patients are not able to work in any capacity, while others require modification of their work. Disability evaluation in fibromyalgia is controversial. The diagnosis of fibromyalgia is not accepted by all. It is hard to evaluate patients' perceptions of their inability to function. The determination of tender points can also be subjective, on the part of both the physician and the patient, particularly when issues of compensation are pending. Patients also encounter difficulty in having their illness recognized as a disability. Physicians have been placed in the inappropriate role of assessing the patient's disability. Physicians are not in a position to quantitate disability at the workplace; that is better done by a work evaluation specialist. Better instruments are clearly needed for measuring disability, particularly in patients with fibromyalgia.

℞ FIBROMYALGIA

Patients should be informed that they have a condition that is not crippling, deforming, or degenerative, and that treatment is available. The initial step in treatment is to improve the quality of sleep. The use of tricyclics such as amitriptyline (10–50 mg), nortriptyline (10–75 mg), and doxepin (10–25 mg) or a pharmacologically similar drug, cyclobenzaprine (10–40 mg), 1–2 h before bedtime will give the patient restorative sleep (stage 4 sleep), resulting in clinical improvement. Patients should be started on a low dose, which is increased gradually as needed. Side effects of these tricyclics and cyclobenzaprine limit their use; these include constipation, dry mouth, weight gain, drowsiness, and difficulty thinking. Trazodone or zol-

pidem also improves sleep quality. In patients with restless leg syndrome, clonazepam may be effective. Depression and anxiety should next be treated with appropriate drugs and, when indicated, with psychiatric counseling. Duloxetine, a serotonin/norepinephrine reuptake inhibitor, has shown benefit for the management of symptoms associated with fibromyalgia in patients with or without major depressive disorder.

Fluoxetine, sertraline, paroxetine, citalopram, or other newer selective serotonin reuptake inhibitors can be used as antidepressants. Other useful antidepressants are trazodone and venlafaxine. Alprazolam and lorazepam are effective for anxiety. Patients may also benefit by regular aerobic exercises, which are started after patients begin to have improved sleep and less pain and fatigue. Exercise should be of a low-impact type and begun at a low level. Eventually the patient should be exercising 20–30 min, 3–4 days a week. Regular stretching exercises are also very important. Salicylates or other nonsteroidal anti-inflammatory drugs (NSAIDs) only partially improve symptoms. Glucocorticoids have been of little benefit and should not be used in these patients. Opiate analgesics should be avoided. For pain, acetaminophen or tramadol may be useful. Also, gabapentin (300–1200 mg/d in divided doses) may reduce pain. Local measures such as heat, massage, injection of tender sites with steroids or lidocaine, and acupuncture provide only temporary relief of symptoms. Other therapies that may help to varying degrees include biofeedback, behavioral modification, hypnotherapy, and stress management and relaxation response training. Life stresses should be identified and discussed with the patient, and the patient should be provided with help on how to cope with these stresses. Patients may benefit from a multidisciplinary team approach involving a mental health professional, a physical therapist, and a physical medicine and rehabilitation specialist. Group therapy may be beneficial. Patients should be well educated about their disorder and taught the importance of self-help. There are patient support groups in many communities. While treatment of fibromyalgia is effective in some patients, others continue to have chronic disease, which is relieved only partially if at all.

FURTHER READINGS

BRADLEY LA, ALARCON GS: Fibromyalgia, in *Arthritis and Allied Conditions*, 15th ed, WJ Koopman (ed). Philadelphia, Lippincott Williams & Wilkins, 2005, pp 1869–1910

BURKHAM J: Fibromyalgia, in *Kelley's Textbook of Rheumatology*, 7th ed, ED Harris et al (eds). Philadelphia, Saunders, 2005, pp 522–536

GOLDENBERG DL: Fibromyalgia syndrome a decade later: What have we learned? Arch Intern Med 159:777, 1999

WOLFE F et al: The prevalence and characteristics of fibromyalgia in the general population. Arthritis Rheum 38:19, 1995

330 Arthritis Associated with Systemic Disease, and Other Arthritides

Carol A. Langford, Bruce C. Gilliland†

ARTHRITIS ASSOCIATED WITH SYSTEMIC DISEASE

ARTHROPATHY OF ACROMEGALY

Acromegaly is the result of excessive production of growth hormone by an adenoma in the anterior pituitary gland (Chap. 333). Middle-aged persons are most often affected. The excessive secretion of growth hormone along with insulin-like growth factor I stimulates proliferation of cartilage, periarticular connective tissue, and bone, resulting in several musculoskeletal abnormalities, including osteoarthritis, back pain, muscle weakness, and carpal tunnel syndrome.

---

†Deceased. A contributor to HPIM since the 11th edition, Dr. Gilliland passed away on February 17, 2007.

An arthropathy resembling osteoarthritis is a common feature, affecting most often the knees, shoulders, hips, and hands. Single or multiple joints may be affected. The overgrowth of cartilage initially produces widening of the joint space. The newly synthesized cartilage is not developed in an organized manner, making it susceptible to fissuring, ulceration, and destruction. Ligamental laxity of the joint resulting from the growth of connective tissue also contributes to the development of osteoarthritis. With breakdown and loss of cartilage, the joint space narrows, and subchondral sclerosis and osteophytes appear on radiographs. Joint examination reveals marked crepitus and hypermobility. Joint fluid is noninflammatory. Calcium pyrophosphate dihydrate crystals are found in the cartilage in some cases of acromegaly arthropathy and, when shed into the joint, can produce attacks of pseudogout. Chondrocalcinosis may also be observed radiographically. Approximately half of the patients with acromegaly experience back pain, which is predominantly lumbosacral. Hypermobility of the spine may be a contributing factor in back pain. Radiograph of the spine shows normal or increased intervertebral disk spaces, hypertrophic anterior osteophytes, and ligamental calcification. These changes are similar to those observed in patients with diffuse idiopathic skeletal hyperostosis. Dorsal kyphosis in conjunction with elongation of the ribs contributes to the development of the barrel chest seen in acromegalic patients. The hands and feet become enlarged owing to soft tissue proliferation. The fingers are thickened and have spadelike distal tufts. One-third of patients have a thickened heel pad. Approximately 25% of patients have Raynaud's phenomenon.

Carpal tunnel syndrome occurs in about half of patients. The median nerve is compressed by the excessive growth of connective tissue in the carpal tunnel. The median nerve also becomes enlarged. Patients with acromegaly also develop proximal muscle weakness, which is thought to be caused by the effect of growth hormone on muscle. Results of muscle enzyme assays and electromyography are normal. Muscle biopsy specimens show muscle fibers of varying size and no inflammatory changes.

ARTHROPATHY OF HEMOCHROMATOSIS

Hemochromatosis is a disorder of iron storage. Excessive amounts of iron are absorbed from the intestine, leading to iron deposition in parenchymal cells, which results in tissue damage and impairment of organ function (Chap. 351). Symptoms of hemochromatosis usually begin between the ages of 40 and 60 but can occur earlier. Arthritis, which occurs in 20–40% of patients, usually begins after the age of 50 and may be the first clinical feature of hemochromatosis. The arthropathy is an osteoarthritis-like disorder affecting the small joints of the hands, followed later by larger joints such as knees, ankles, shoulders, and hips. The second and third metacarpophalangeal joints of both hands are often the first joints affected; they can provide an important clue to the possibility of hemochromatosis. Patients experience stiffness and pain. Morning stiffness usually lasts less than half an hour. The affected joints are enlarged and mildly tender. Synovial tissue is not appreciably increased. Radiographs show irregular narrowing of the joint space, subchondral sclerosis, and subchondral cysts. There is juxtaarticular proliferation of bone, with frequent hooklike osteophytes. The synovial fluid is noninflammatory. The synovium shows mild to moderate proliferation of lining cells, fibrosis, and a low number of inflammatory cells, which are mononuclear. In approximately half of patients, there is evidence of calcium pyrophosphate deposition disease (CPPD), and patients may experience episodes of pseudogout. Iron can be demonstrated in the lining cells of the synovium and also in chondrocytes.

Iron may damage the articular cartilage in several ways. Iron catalyzes superoxide-dependent lipid peroxidation, which may play a role in joint damage. In animal models, ferric iron has been shown to interfere with collagen formation. Iron has also been shown to increase the release of lysosomal enzymes from cells in the synovial membrane. Iron may also play a role in the development of chondrocalcinosis. Iron inhibits synovial tissue pyrophosphatase in vitro and, therefore, may inhibit pyrophosphatase in vivo, resulting in chondrocalcinosis. Iron in synovial cells may also inhibit the clearance of calcium pyrophosphate from the joint.

℞ ARTHROPATHY OF HEMOCHROMATOSIS

The treatment of hemochromatosis is repeated phlebotomy. Unfortunately, this treatment has little effect on the arthritis, which, along with chondrocalcinosis, usually continues to progress. Treatment of the arthritis consists of administration of acetaminophen and nonsteroidal anti-inflammatory drugs (NSAIDs). Acute pseudogout attacks are treated with higher doses of an NSAID or a short course of glucocorticoids. Placement of a hip or knee prosthesis has been successful in advanced disease.

HEMOPHILIC ARTHROPATHY

Hemophilia is a sex-linked recessive genetic disorder characterized by the absence or deficiency of factor VIII (hemophilia A, or classic hemophilia) or factor IX (hemophilia B, or Christmas disease) (Chap. 110). Hemophilia A is by far the more common type, constituting 85% of cases. Spontaneous hemarthrosis is a common problem with both types of hemophilia and can lead to a chronic deforming arthritis. The frequency and severity of hemarthrosis are related to the degree of clotting factor deficiency. Hemarthrosis is not common in other inherited disorders of coagulation, such as von Willebrand disease or factor V deficiency.

Hemarthrosis becomes evident after 1 year of age, when the child begins to walk and run. In order of frequency, the joints most commonly affected are the knees, ankles, elbows, shoulders, and hips. Small joints of the hands and feet are occasionally involved.

In the initial stage of arthropathy, hemarthrosis produces a warm, tensely swollen, and painful joint. The patient holds the affected joint in flexion and guards against any movement. Blood in the joint remains liquid because of the absence of intrinsic clotting factors and the absence of tissue thromboplastin in the synovium. The blood in the joint space is resorbed over a period of a week or longer, depending on the size of the hemarthrosis. Joint function usually returns to normal or baseline in about 2 weeks.

Recurrent hemarthrosis leads to the development of a chronic arthritis. The involved joints remain swollen, and flexion deformities develop. In the later stages of arthropathy, joint motion is restricted and function is severely limited. Joint ankylosis, subluxation, and laxity are features of end-stage disease.

Bleeding into muscle and soft tissue also causes musculoskeletal disorders. When bleeding into the iliopsoas muscle occurs, the hip is held in flexion because of the pain, resulting in a hip flexion contracture. Rotation of the hip is preserved, which distinguishes this problem from intraarticular hemorrhage. Expansion of the hematoma may place pressure on the femoral nerve, resulting in a femoral neuropathy. Another problem is shortening of the heel cord secondary to bleeding into the gastrocnemius. Hemorrhage into a closed compartment space, such as the volar compartment in the forearm, can result in muscle necrosis, neuropathy, and flexion deformities of the wrist and fingers. When bleeding involves periosteum or bone, a pseudotumor forms. These occur distal to the elbows or knees in children and improve with treatment of the hemophilia. Surgical removal is indicated if the pseudotumor continues to enlarge. In adults, they occur in the femur and pelvis and are usually refractory to treatment. When bleeding occurs in muscle, cysts may develop within the muscle. Needle aspiration of a cyst is contraindicated because it can induce bleeding.

Septic arthritis can occur in hemophilia and is difficult at times to distinguish from acute hemarthrosis on physical examination. Whenever there is suspicion of an infected joint, the joint should be aspirated immediately, the fluid cultured, and the patient started on antibiotics that provide broad coverage until the results of the culture are known. The patient should be infused with the deficient clotting factor before the joint is tapped to decrease the risk of further bleeding.

Radiographs of joints reflect the stage of disease. In early stages there is only capsule distention; later, juxtaarticular osteopenia, marginal erosions, and subchondral cysts develop. In late disease, the joint space is narrowed and there is bony overgrowth. The changes are similar to those observed in osteoarthritis. Unique features of hemophilic arthropathy are widening of the femoral intercondylar notch, enlargement of the proximal radius, and squaring of the distal end of the patella.

Recurrent hemarthrosis produces synovial hyperplasia and hypertrophy. A pannus covers the cartilage. Cartilage is damaged by collagenase and other degradative enzymes released by mononuclear cells in the overlying synovium. Hemosiderin is found in synovial lining cells, the subsynovium, and chondrocytes and may also play a role in cartilage destruction.

℞ HEMARTHROSIS

The treatment of hemarthrosis is initiated with the immediate infusion of factor VIII or IX at the first sign of joint or muscle hemorrhage. The patient is placed at bed rest, with the involved joint in as much extension as the patient can tolerate. Analgesic doses of an NSAID and local icing may help with the pain. NSAIDs can be given safely for short periods even though they have a stabilizing effect on platelets. Studies have shown no significant abnormalities in platelet function or bleeding time in hemophiliacs receiving ibuprofen. The cyclooxygenase-2 inhibitors do not interfere with platelet function and can be safely given for pain where their use is felt to be safe and indicated based upon the risks versus benefits. Synovectomy, open or arthroscopic, may be indicated in patients with chronic synovial proliferation and recurrent hemarthrosis. Hypertrophied synovium is very vascular and subject to bleeding. Both types of synovectomy reduce the number of hemarthroses and slow the roentgenographic progression of hemophilic arthropathy. Open surgical synovectomy, however, is associated with some loss of range of motion. Radiosynovectomy with either yttrium 90 silicate or phosphorus 31 colloid also has been effective and may be a useful alternative when surgical synovectomy is not practical. Total joint replacement is indicated for severe joint destruction and incapacitating pain. Because of the young age of hemophilic patients, total-joint prostheses may need to be replaced more than once during their lives.

ARTHROPATHIES ASSOCIATED WITH HEMOGLOBINOPATHIES

Sickle Cell Disease
Sickle cell disease (Chap. 99) is associated with several musculoskeletal abnormalities (Table 330-1). Children under the age of 5 may develop diffuse swelling, tenderness, and warmth of the hands and feet lasting from 1 to 3 weeks. The condition, referred to as *sickle cell dactylitis* or *hand-foot syndrome*, has also been observed in sickle cell disease and sickle cell thalassemia. Dactylitis is believed to result from infarction of the bone marrow and cortical bone leading to periostitis and soft tissue swelling. Radiographs show periosteal elevation, subperiosteal new bone formation, and areas of radiolucency and increased density involving the metacarpals, metatarsals, and proximal phalanges. These bone changes disappear after several months. The syndrome leaves little or no residual damage. Because hematopoiesis ceases in the small bones of hands and feet with age, the syndrome is rarely seen after age 4 or 5 and does not occur in adults.

Sickle cell crisis is often associated with periarticular pain and joint effusions. The joint and periarticular area are warm and tender. Knees and elbows are most often affected, but other joints can be involved. Joint effusions are noninflammatory, with white cell counts <1000/μL; mononuclear cells predominate. There have been a few reports of sterile inflammatory effusion with high cell counts consisting of mostly polymorphonuclear white cells. Synovial biopsies have shown mild lining cell proliferation and microvascular thrombosis. Scintigraphic studies have shown decreased marrow uptake adjacent to the involved joint. The joint effusion and periarticular pain are considered to be the result of ischemia and infarction of the synovium and adjacent bone and bone marrow. The treatment is that for sickle cell crisis (Chap. 99).

Patients with sickle cell disease may also develop osteomyelitis, which commonly involves the long tubular bones (Chap. 120). These patients are particularly susceptible to bacterial infections, especially *Salmonella* infections, which are found in more than half of cases. The most common isolate is *S. typhimurium* (Chap. 146). Radiographs of the involved site show periosteal elevation initially, followed by disruption of the cortex. Treatment of the infection results in healing of the bone lesion. Sickle cell disease is also associated with bone infarction resulting from thrombosis secondary to the sickling of red cells. Bone infarction also occurs in hemoglobin sickle cell disease and sickle cell thalassemia (Chap. 99). The bone pain in sickle cell crisis is due to bone and bone marrow infarction. In children, infarction of the epiphyseal growth plate interferes with normal growth of the affected extremity. Radiographically, infarction of the bone cortex results in periosteal elevation and irregular thickening of the bone cortex. Infarction in the bone marrow leads to lysis, fibrosis, and new bone formation.

Avascular necrosis of the head of the femur is seen in ~5% of patients. It also occurs in the humeral head and less commonly in the distal femur, tibial condyles, distal radius, vertebral bodies, and other juxtaarticular sites. The mechanism for avascular necrosis is most likely the same as for bone infarction. Subchondral hemorrhage may play a role in the deterioration of articular cartilage. Irregularity of the femoral head or of other bone surfaces affected by avascular necrosis eventually results in degenerative joint disease. Radiograph of the affected joint may show patchy radiolucency and density followed by flattening of the bone. MRI is a sensitive technique for detecting early avascular necrosis as well as bone infarction elsewhere. Total hip replacement and placement of prostheses in other joints may improve function and relieve pain in those patients with severe joint destruction.

Septic arthritis is occasionally encountered in sickle cell disease (Chap. 328). Multiple joints may be infected. Joint infection may re-

TABLE 330-1	MUSCULOSKELETAL ABNORMALITIES IN SICKLE CELL DISEASE	
Sickle cell dactylitis	Avascular necrosis
Joint effusions in sickle cell crises	Bone changes secondary to marrow hyperplasia
Osteomyelitis	
Infarction of bone	Septic arthritis
Infarction of bone marrow	Gouty arthritis

sult from hematogenous spread or from spread of contiguous osteomyelitis. Microorganisms identified include *Staphylococcus aureus*, *Streptococcus*, *Escherichia coli*, and *Salmonella*. The latter is not seen as frequently in septic arthritis as it is in osteomyelitis. Acute gouty arthritis is uncommon in sickle cell disease, even though 40% of patients are hyperuricemic. Hyperuricemia is due to overproduction of uric acid secondary to increased red cell turnover. Attacks may be polyarticular.

The bone marrow hyperplasia in sickle cell disease results in widening of the medullary cavities, thinning of the cortices, and coarse trabeculations and central cupping of the vertebral bodies. These changes are also seen to a lesser degree in hemoglobin sickle cell disease and sickle cell thalassemia. In normal individuals, red marrow is located mostly in the axial skeletal, but in sickle cell disease, red marrow is found in the bones of the extremities and even in the tarsal and carpal bones. Vertebral compression may lead to dorsal kyphosis, and softening of the bone in the acetabulum may result in protrusio acetabuli.

Thalassemia
β-Thalassemia is a congenital disorder of hemoglobin synthesis characterized by impaired production of β chains (Chap. 99). Bone and joint abnormalities occur in β-thalassemia, being most common in the major and intermedia groups. In one study, ~50% of patients with β-thalassemia had evidence of symmetric ankle arthropathy, characterized by a dull aching pain aggravated by weight bearing. The onset was most often in the second or third decade of life. The degree of ankle pain in these patients varied. Some patients experienced self-limited ankle pain, which occurred only after strenuous physical activity and lasted several days to weeks. Other patients had chronic ankle pain, which became worse with walking. Symptoms eventually abated in a few patients. Compression of the ankle, calcaneus, or forefoot was painful in some patients. Synovial fluid from two patients was noninflammatory. Radiographs of ankle showed osteopenia, widened medullary spaces, thin cortices, and coarse trabeculations. These findings were largely the result of bone marrow expansion. The joint space was preserved. Specimens of bone from three patients revealed osteomalacia, osteopenia, and microfractures. Increased osteoblasts as well as increased foci of bone resorption were present on the bone surface. Iron staining was found in the bone trabeculae, in osteoid, and in the cement line. Synovium showed hyperplasia of lining cells, which contained deposits of hemosiderin. This arthropathy was considered to be related to the underlying bone pathology. The role of iron overload or abnormal bone metabolism in the pathogenesis of this arthropathy is not known. The arthropathy was treated with analgesics and splints. Patients were also transfused to decrease hematopoiesis and bone marrow expansion.

Patients with β-thalassemia major and intermedia also have involvement of other joints, including the knees, hips, and shoulders. Acquired hemochromatosis with arthropathy has been described in a patient with thalassemia. Gouty arthritis and septic arthritis can occur. Avascular necrosis is not a feature of thalassemia because there is no sickling of red cells leading to thrombosis and infarction.

β-Thalassemia minor (trait) is also associated with joint manifestations. Chronic seronegative oligoarthritis affecting predominantly ankles, wrists, and elbows has been described. These patients had mild persistent synovitis without large effusions. Joint erosions were not seen. Recurrent episodes of an acute asymmetric arthritis have also been reported; episodes last less than a week and may affect knees, ankles, shoulders, elbows, wrists, and metacarpal phalangeal joints. The mechanism for this arthropathy is unknown. Treatment with nonsteroidal drugs was not particularly effective.

(See also Chap. 350) Musculoskeletal manifestations may be the first indication of a hereditary disorder of lipoprotein metabolism. Patients with familial hypercholesterolemia (previously referred to as *type II hyperlipoproteinemia*) may have recurrent migratory polyarthritis involving knees and other large peripheral joints and, to a lesser degree, peripheral small joints. In a few patients, the arthritis is monarticular. Fever may accompany the arthritis. Pain ranges from moderate to very severe to incapacitating. The involved joints can be warm, erythematous, swollen, and tender. Arthritis usually has a sudden onset, lasts from a few days to 2 weeks, and does not cause joint damage. Episodes may suggest acute gout attacks. Several attacks occur per year. Synovial fluid from involved joints is not inflammatory and contains few white cells and no crystals. Joint involvement may actually represent inflammatory periarthritis or peritendinitis and not intraarticular disease. The recurrent, transient nature of the arthritis may suggest rheumatic fever, especially since patients with hyperlipoproteinemia have an elevated erythrocyte sedimentation rate and a falsely elevated antistreptolysin O titer. Patients may also experience Achilles tendinitis, which can be very painful. Attacks of tendinitis come on gradually and last only a few days. Fever is not present. Patients may be asymptomatic between attacks. During an attack the Achilles tendon is warm, erythematous, swollen, and tender to palpation. Achilles tendinitis and other joint manifestations often precede the appearance of xanthomas and may be the first clinical indication of hyperlipoproteinemia. Attacks of tendinitis may occur following treatment with a lipid-lowering drug. Patients can also have tendinous xanthomas in the Achilles, patellar, and extensor tendons of the hands and feet. Xanthomas have also been reported in the peroneal tendon, the plantar aponeurosis, and the periosteum overlying the distal tibia. These xanthomas are located within tendon fibers. Tuberous xanthomas are soft subcutaneous masses located over the extensor surfaces of the elbows, knees, and hands, as well as on the buttocks. They appear in childhood in homozygous patients and after the age of 30 in heterozygous patients. Patients with elevated plasma levels of very low-density lipoprotein (VLDL) and triglyceride (previously referred to as *type IV hyperlipoproteinemia*) may also have a mild inflammatory arthritis affecting large and small peripheral joints, usually in an asymmetric pattern with only a few joints involved at a time. The onset of arthritis is usually in middle age. Arthritis may be persistent or recurrent, with episodes lasting a few days to weeks. Joint pain is severe in some patients. Patients may experience morning stiffness. Joint tenderness and periarticular hyperesthesia may also be present, as may synovial thickening. Joint fluid is usually noninflammatory and without crystals but may have increased white blood cell counts with predominantly mononuclear cells. The fluid is occasionally lactescent. Radiographs may show juxtaarticular osteopenia and cystic lesions. Large bone cysts have been noted in a few patients. Xanthoma and bone cysts are also observed in other lipoprotein disorders. The pathogenesis of arthritis in patients with familial hypercholesterolemia or with elevated levels of VLDL and triglyceride is not well understood. Salicylates, other NSAIDs, or analgesics usually provide relief of symptoms. Clinical improvement may also occur in patients treated with lipid-lowering agents; however, patients treated with an HMG-CoA reductase inhibitor may experience myalgias, and a few patients may develop polymyositis or even rhabdomyolysis. Myositis has also been reported with the use of niacin (Chap. 384).

OTHER ARTHRITIDES

NEUROPATHIC JOINT DISEASE

Neuropathic joint disease (Charcot's joint) is a progressive destructive arthritis associated with loss of pain sensation, proprioception, or both. In addition, normal muscular reflexes that modulate joint movement are decreased. Without these protective mechanisms, joints are subjected to repeated trauma, resulting in progressive cartilage and bone damage. Neuropathic arthropathy was first described by Jean-Martin Charcot in 1868 in patients with tabes dorsalis. The term *Char-*

FIGURE 330-1 Charcot arthropathy associated with diabetes mellitus. Lateral foot radiograph demonstrating complete loss of the arch due to bony fragmentation and dislocation in the midfoot. (*Courtesy of Andrew Neckers, MD, and Jean Schils, MD; with permission.*)

cot joint is commonly used interchangeably with *neuropathic joint*. Today, diabetes mellitus is the most frequent cause of neuropathic joint disease (Fig. 330-1). A variety of other disorders are associated with neuropathic arthritis including leprosy, yaws, syringomyelia, meningomyelocele, congenital indifference to pain, peroneal muscular atrophy (Charcot-Marie-Tooth disease), and amyloidosis. An arthritis resembling neuropathic joint disease is seen in patients who have received frequent intraarticular glucocorticoid injections into a weight-bearing joint and in patients with CPPD. The distribution of joint involvement depends on the underlying neurologic disorder (Table 330-2). In tabes dorsalis, knees, hips, and ankles are most commonly affected; in syringomyelia, the glenohumeral joint, elbow, and wrist; and in diabetes mellitus, the tarsal and tarsometatarsal joints.

Pathology and Pathophysiology The pathologic changes in the neuropathic joint are similar to those found in the severe osteoarthritic joint. There is fragmentation and eventual loss of articular cartilage with eburnation of the underlying bone. Osteophytes are found at the joint margins. With more advanced disease, erosions are present on the joint surface. Fractures, devitalized bone, and intraarticular loose bodies may be present. Microscopic fragments of cartilage and bone are seen in the synovial tissue.

At least two underlying mechanisms are believed to be involved in the pathogenesis of neuropathic arthritis. An abnormal autonomic nervous system is thought to be responsible for the increased blood flow to the joint and subsequent resorption of bone. Loss of bone, particularly in the diabetic foot, may be the initial manifestation. With the loss of deep pain, proprioception, and protective neuromuscular reflexes, the joint is subjected to repeated injuries including ligamental tears and bone fractures. The mechanism of injury that occurs following frequent intraarticular glucocorticoid injections is thought to be due to the analgesic effect of glucocorticoids leading to overuse of an already damaged joint, which results in accelerated cartilage damage. It is not understood why only a few patients with neuropathies develop neuropathic arthritis.

Clinical Manifestations Neuropathic joint disease usually begins in a single joint and then progresses to involve other joints, depending on the underlying neurologic disorder. The involved joint progressively becomes enlarged from bony overgrowth and synovial effusion. Loose bodies may be palpated in the joint cavity. Joint instability, subluxation,

TABLE 330-2	DISORDERS ASSOCIATED WITH NEUROPATHIC JOINT DISEASE
Diabetes mellitus	Amyloidosis
Tabes dorsalis	Leprosy
Meningomyelocele	Congenital indifference to pain
Syringomyelia	Peroneal muscular atrophy

and crepitus occur as the disease progresses. Neuropathic joints may develop rapidly, and a totally disorganized joint with multiple bony fragments may evolve in a patient within weeks or months. The amount of pain experienced by the patient is less than would be anticipated based on the degree of joint involvement. Patients may experience sudden joint pain from intraarticular fractures of osteophytes or condyles.

Neuropathic arthritis is encountered most often in patients with diabetes mellitus, with the incidence estimated in the range of 0.5%. The usual age of onset is ≥50 years following several years of diabetes, but exceptions occur. The tarsal and tarsometatarsal joints are most often affected, followed by the metatarsophalangeal and talotibial joints. The knees and spine are occasionally involved. In about 20%, neuropathic arthritis may be present in both feet. Patients often attribute the onset of foot pain to antecedent trauma such as twisting their foot. Neuropathic changes may develop rapidly following a foot fracture or dislocation. Swelling of the foot and ankle are often present. Downward collapse of the tarsal bones leads to convexity of the sole, referred to as a "rocker foot." Large osteophytes may protrude from the top of the foot. Calluses frequently form over the metatarsal heads and may lead to infected ulcers and osteomyelitis. Radiographs may show resorption and tapering of the distal metatarsal bones. The term *Lisfranc fracture-dislocation* is sometimes used to describe the destructive changes at the tarsometatarsal joints.

Diagnosis The diagnosis of neuropathic arthritis is based on the clinical features and characteristic radiographic findings in a patient with an underlying sensory neuropathy. The differential diagnosis of neuropathic arthritis includes osteomyelitis, osteonecrosis, advanced osteoarthritis, stress fractures, and CPPD. Radiographs in neuropathic arthritis initially show changes of osteoarthritis with joint space narrowing, subchondral bone sclerosis, osteophytes, and joint effusions followed later by marked destructive and hypertrophic changes. Soft tissue swelling, bone resorption, fractures, large osteophytes, extraarticular bone fragments, and subluxation are present with advanced arthropathy. The radiographic findings of neuropathic arthritis may be difficult to differentiate from those of osteomyelitis, especially in the diabetic foot. The joint margins in a neuropathic joint tend to be distinct, while in osteomyelitis, they are blurred. Imaging studies and cultures of fluid and tissue from the joint are often required to exclude osteomyelitis. MRI is helpful in differentiating these disorders. Another useful study is a bone scan using indium 111–labeled white blood cells or indium 111–labeled immunoglobulin G, which will show an increased uptake in osteomyelitis but not in a neuropathic joint. A technetium bone scan will not distinguish osteomyelitis from neuropathic arthritis, as increased uptake is observed in both. The joint fluid in neuropathic arthritis is noninflammatory; may be xanthochromic or even bloody; and may contain fragments of synovium, cartilage, and bone. The finding of calcium pyrophosphate dihydrate crystals suggests the diagnosis of a crystal-associated neuropathic-like arthropathy. In the absence of such crystals, the presence of increased number of leukocytes may indicate osteomyelitis.

℞ NEUROPATHIC JOINT DISEASE

The primary focus of treatment is to provide stabilization of the joint. Treatment of the underlying disorder, even if successful, does not usually alter the joint disease. Braces and splints are helpful. Their use requires close surveillance, since patients may be unable to appreciate pressure from a poorly adjusted brace. In the diabetic patient, early recognition and treatment of a Charcot's foot by prohibiting weight-bearing of the foot for at least 8 weeks may possibly prevent severe disease from developing. Fusion of a very unstable joint may improve function, but nonunion is frequent, especially when immobilization of the joint is inadequate.

HYPERTROPHIC OSTEOARTHROPATHY AND CLUBBING

Hypertrophic osteoarthropathy (HOA) is characterized by clubbing of digits and, in more advanced stages, by periosteal new bone formation and synovial effusions. HOA occurs in primary or familial form and usually begins in childhood. The secondary form of HOA is associated

FIGURE 330-2 Clubbing of fingers. *(Reprinted from the Clinical Slide Collection on the Rheumatic Diseases, Copyright 1991, 1995. Used by permission of the American College of Rheumatology.)*

with intrathoracic malignancies, suppurative lung disease, congenital heart disease, and a variety of other disorders and is more common in adults. Clubbing is almost always a feature of HOA but can occur as an isolated manifestation (Fig. 330-2). The presence of clubbing in isolation is generally considered to represent either an early stage or an element in the spectrum of HOA. The presence of only clubbing in a patient usually has the same clinical significance as HOA.

Pathology and Pathophysiology In HOA, the bone changes in the distal extremities begin as periostitis followed by new bone formation. At this stage, a radiolucent area may be observed between the new periosteal bone and subjacent cortex. As the process progresses, multiple layers of new bone are deposited, which become contiguous with the cortex and result in cortical thickening. The outer portion of bone is laminated in appearance, with an irregular surface. Initially, the process of periosteal new bone formation involves the proximal and distal diaphyses of the tibia, fibula, radius, and ulna and, less frequently, the femur, humerus, metacarpals, metatarsals, and phalanges. Occasionally, scapulae, clavicles, ribs, and pelvic bones are also affected. In long-standing disease, these changes extend to involve metaphyses and musculotendinous insertions. The adjacent interosseous membranes may become ossified. The distribution of the bone manifestations is usually bilateral and symmetric. The soft tissue overlying the distal third of the arms and legs may be thickened. Mononuclear cell infiltration may be present in the adjacent soft tissue. Proliferation of connective tissue occurs in the nail bed and volar pad of digits, giving the distal phalanges a clubbed appearance. Small blood vessels in the clubbed digits are dilated and have thickened walls. In addition, the number of arteriovenous anastomoses is increased. The synovia of involved joints show edema, varying degrees of synovial cell proliferation, thickening of the subsynovium, vascular congestion, vascular obliteration with thrombi, and small numbers of lymphocyte infiltrates.

Several theories have been suggested for the pathogenesis of HOA. Most have been disproved or have not explained the development in all clinical disorders associated with HOA. Previously proposed neurogenic and humoral theories are no longer considered likely explanations for HOA. The neurogenic theory was based on the observation that vagotomy resulted in symptomatic improvement in a small number of patients with lung tumors and HOA. It was postulated that vagal stimuli from the tumor site led via a neural reflex to efferent nerve impulses to the distal extremities, resulting in HOA. This theory, however, did not explain HOA in conditions where vagal stimulation did not occur, as in cyanotic congenital heart disease or arterial aneurysms. The humoral theory postulated that soluble substances that are normally inactivated or removed during passage through the lung reached the systemic circulation in an active form and stimulated the changes of HOA. Substances proposed included prostaglandins, ferritin, bradykinin, estrogen, and growth hormone. These substances seemed unlikely candidates, since their blood levels in HOA patients overlapped those in individuals without HOA. Furthermore, these substances did not explain the development of localized HOA associated with arterial aneurysms or infected arterial grafts.

Recent studies have suggested a role for platelets in the development of HOA. It has been observed that megakaryocytes and large platelet particles, present in venous circulation, were fragmented in their passage through normal lung. In patients with cyanotic congenital heart disease and in other disorders associated with right-to-left shunts, these large platelet particles bypass the lung and reach the distal extremities, where they can interact with endothelial cells. Platelet clumps have been demonstrated to form on an infected heart valve in bacterial endocarditis, in the wall of arterial aneurysms, and on infected arterial grafts. These platelet particles may also reach the distal extremities and interact with endothelial cells. Platelet-endothelial activation in the distal portion of extremities would then result in the release of platelet-derived growth factor (PDGF) and other factors leading to the proliferation of connective tissue and periosteum. Stimulation of fibroblasts by PDGF and transforming growth factor β results in cell growth and collagen synthesis. Elevated plasma levels of von Willebrand factor antigen have been found in patients with both primary and secondary forms of HOA, indicating endothelial activation or damage. Abnormalities of collagen synthesis have been demonstrated in the involved skin of patients with primary HOA. Fibroblasts from affected skin were shown to have increased collagen synthesis, increased $\alpha1(I)$ procollagen mRNA, and evidence for upregulation of collagen transcription. Other factors are undoubtedly involved in the pathogenesis of HOA, and further studies are needed to better understand this disorder.

Clinical Manifestations Primary or familial HOA, also referred to as *pachydermoperiostitis* or *Touraine-Solente-Golé syndrome*, usually begins insidiously at puberty. In a smaller number of patients, the onset is in the first year of life. The disorder is inherited as an autosomal dominant trait with variable expression and is nine times more common in boys than in girls. Approximately one-third of patients have a family history of primary HOA.

Primary HOA is characterized by clubbing, periostitis, and unusual skin features. A small number of patients with this syndrome do not express clubbing. The skin changes and periostitis are prominent features of this syndrome. The skin becomes thickened and coarse. Deep nasolabial folds develop, and the forehead may become furrowed. Patients may have heavy-appearing eyelids and ptosis. The skin is often greasy, and there may be excessive sweating of the hands and feet. Patients may also experience acne vulgaris, seborrhea, and folliculitis. In a few patients, the skin over the scalp becomes very thick and corrugated, a feature that has been descriptively termed *cutis verticis gyrata*. The distal extremities, particularly the legs, become thickened owing to proliferation of new bone and soft tissue; when the process is extensive, the distal lower extremities resemble those of an elephant. The periostitis is usually not painful, as it may be in secondary HOA. Clubbing of the fingers may be extensive, producing large, bulbous deformities and clumsiness. Clubbing also affects the toes. Patients may experience articular and periarticular pain, especially in the ankles and knees, and joint motion may be mildly restricted owing to periarticular bone overgrowth. Noninflammatory effusions occur in the wrists, knees, and ankles. Synovial hypertrophy is not found. Associated abnormalities observed in patients with primary HOA include hypertrophic gastropathy, bone marrow failure, female escutcheon, gynecomastia, and cranial suture defects. In patients with primary HOA, the symptoms disappear when adulthood is reached.

HOA secondary to an underlying disease occurs more frequently than primary HOA. It accompanies a variety of disorders and may precede clinical features of the associated disorder by months. Clubbing is more frequent than the full syndrome of HOA in patients with associated illnesses. Because clubbing evolves over months and is usually asymptomatic, it is often recognized first by the physician and not the patient. Patients may experience a burning sensation in their fingertips. Clubbing is characterized by widening of the fingertips, enlargement of the distal volar pad, convexity of the nail contour, and the loss of the normal 15° angle between the proximal nail and cuticle. The thickness of the digit at the base of the nail is greater than the thickness at the distal interphalangeal joint. An objective measurement of finger clubbing can be made by determining the diameter at the base of the nail and at the distal interphalangeal joint of all 10 digits. Clubbing is present when the sum of the individual digit ratios is >10. At the bedside, clubbing can be appreciated by having the patient place the dorsal surface of the distal phalanges of the fourth fingers together with the nails of the fourth fingers opposing each other. Normally, an open area is visible between the bases of the opposing fingernails; when clubbing is present, this open space is no longer visible. The base of the nail feels spongy when compressed, and the nail can be easily rocked on its bed. Marked periungual erythema is usually present. When clubbing is advanced, the finger may have a drumstick appearance, and the distal interphalangeal joint can be hyperextended. Periosteal involvement in the distal extremities may produce a burning or deep-seated aching pain. The pain can be quite incapacitating and is aggravated by dependency and relieved by elevation of the affected limbs. The overlying soft tissue may be swollen, and the skin slightly erythematous. Pressure applied over the distal forearms and legs may be quite painful.

Patients may also experience joint pain, most often in the ankles, wrists, and knees. Joint effusions may be present; usually they are small and noninflammatory. The small joints of the hands are rarely affected. Severe joint or bone pain may be the presenting symptom of an underlying lung malignancy and may precede the appearance of clubbing. In addition, the progression of HOA tends to be more rapid when associated with malignancies, most notably bronchogenic carcinoma. Unlike primary HOA, excessive sweating and oiliness of the skin and thickening of the facial skin are uncommon in secondary HOA.

HOA occurs in 5–10% of patients with intrathoracic malignancies, the most common being bronchogenic carcinoma and pleural tumors (Table 330-3). Lung metastases infrequently cause HOA. HOA is also seen in patients with intrathoracic infections, including lung abscesses, empyema, bronchiectasis, chronic obstructive lung disease, and, uncommonly, pulmonary tuberculosis. HOA may also accompany chronic interstitial pneumonitis, sarcoidosis, and cystic fibrosis. In the latter, clubbing is more common than the full syndrome of HOA. Other causes of clubbing include congenital heart disease with right-to-left shunts, bacterial endocarditis, Crohn's disease, ulcerative colitis, sprue, and neoplasms of the esophagus, liver, and small and large bowel. In patients with congenital heart disease with right-to-left shunts, clubbing alone occurs more often than the full syndrome of HOA.

Unilateral clubbing has been found in association with aneurysms of major extremity arteries, with infected arterial grafts, and with arteriovenous fistulas of brachial vessels. Clubbing of the toes but not fingers has been associated with an infected abdominal aortic aneurysm and patent ductus arteriosus. Clubbing of a single digit may follow trauma and has been reported in tophaceous gout and sarcoidosis.

TABLE 330-3 DISORDERS ASSOCIATED WITH HYPERTROPHIC OSTEOARTHROPATHY

Pulmonary	Cardiovascular
Bronchogenic carcinoma and other neoplasms	Cyanotic congenital heart disease
Lung abscesses, empyema, bronchiectasis	Subacute bacterial endocarditis
Chronic interstitial pneumonitis	Infected arterial grafts[a]
Cystic fibrosis	Aortic aneurysm[b]
Chronic obstructive lung disease	Aneurysm of major extremity artery[a]
Sarcoidosis	Patent ductus arteriosus[b]
Gastrointestinal	Arteriovenous fistula of major extremity vessel[a]
Inflammatory bowel disease	Thyroid (thyroid acropachy)
Sprue	Hyperthyroidism (Graves' disease)
Neoplasms: esophagus, liver, bowel	

[a]Unilateral involvement.
[b]Bilateral lower extremity involvement.

While clubbing occurs more commonly than the full syndrome in most diseases, periostitis in the absence of clubbing has been observed in the affected limb of patients with infected arterial grafts.

Hyperthyroidism (Graves' disease), treated or untreated, is occasionally associated with clubbing and periostitis of the bones of the hands and feet. This condition is referred to as *thyroid acropachy*. Periostitis is asymptomatic and occurs in the midshaft and diaphyseal portion of the metacarpal and phalangeal bones. The long bones of the extremities are seldom affected. Elevated levels of long-acting thyroid stimulator are found in the serum of these patients.

Laboratory Findings The laboratory abnormalities reflect the underlying disorder. The synovial fluid of involved joints has <500 white cells per microliter, and the cells are predominantly mononuclear. Radiographs show a faint radiolucent line beneath the new periosteal bone along the shaft of long bones at their distal end. These changes are observed most frequently at the ankles, wrists, and knees. The ends of the distal phalanges may show osseous resorption. Radionuclide studies show pericortical linear uptake along the cortical margins of long bones that may be present before any radiographic changes.

℞ HYPERTROPHIC OSTEOARTHROPATHY

The treatment of HOA is to identify the associated disorder and treat it appropriately. The symptoms and signs of HOA may disappear completely with removal or effective chemotherapy of a tumor or with antibiotic therapy and drainage of a chronic pulmonary infection. Vagotomy or percutaneous block of the vagus nerve leads to symptomatic relief in some patients. Aspirin, NSAIDs, or analgesics may help control symptoms of HOA.

REFLEX SYMPATHETIC DYSTROPHY SYNDROME

The reflex sympathetic dystrophy syndrome is now referred to as *complex regional pain syndrome, type 1*, by the new Classification of the International Association for the Study of Pain. It is characterized by pain and swelling, usually of a distal extremity, accompanied by vasomotor instability, trophic skin changes, and the rapid development of bony demineralization. Reflex sympathetic dystrophy syndrome, including its treatment, is covered in greater detail in Chap. 371.

TIETZE SYNDROME AND COSTOCHONDRITIS

Tietze syndrome is manifested by painful swelling of one or more costochondral articulations. The age of onset is usually before 40, and both sexes are affected equally. In most patients only one joint is involved, usually the second or third costochondral joint. The onset of anterior chest pain may be sudden or gradual. The pain may radiate to the arms or shoulders and is aggravated by sneezing, coughing, deep inspirations, or twisting motions of the chest. The term *costochondritis* is often used interchangeably with *Tietze syndrome*, but some workers restrict the former term to pain of the costochondral articulations without swelling. Costochondritis is observed in patients over age 40; tends to affect the third, fourth, and fifth costochondral joints; and occurs more often in women. Both syndromes may mimic cardiac or upper abdominal causes of pain. Rheumatoid arthritis, ankylosing spondylitis, and Reiter's syndrome may involve costochondral joints but are distinguished easily by their other clinical features. Other skeletal causes of anterior chest wall pain are xiphoidalgia and the slipping rib syndrome, which usually involves the tenth rib. Malignancies such as breast cancer, prostate cancer, plasma cell cytoma, and sarcoma can invade the ribs, thoracic spine, or chest wall and produce symptoms suggesting Tietze syndrome. They should be easily distinguishable by radiographs and biopsy. Analgesics, anti-inflammatory drugs, and local glucocorticoid injections usually relieve symptoms.

MYOFASCIAL PAIN SYNDROME

Myofascial pain syndrome is characterized by localized musculoskeletal pain and tenderness in association with trigger points. The pain is deep and aching and may be accompanied by a burning sensation. Myofascial pain may follow trauma, overuse, or prolonged static contraction of a muscle or muscle group, which may occur when reading or writing at a desk or working at a computer. In addition, this syndrome may be associated with underlying osteoarthritis of the neck or low back. Trigger points are a diagnostic feature of this syndrome. Pain is referred from trigger points to defined areas distant from the original tender points. Palpation of the trigger point reproduces or accentuates the pain. The trigger points are usually located in the center of a muscle belly, but they can occur at other sites, such as costosternal junctions, the xiphoid process, ligamentous and tendinous insertions, fascia, and fatty areas. Trigger point sites in muscle have been described as feeling indurated and taut, and palpation may cause the muscle to twitch. These findings, however, have been shown not to be unique for myofascial pain syndrome, since in a controlled study they were also present in fibromyalgia patients and normal subjects. Myofascial pain most often involves the posterior neck, low back, shoulders, and chest. Chronic pain in the muscles of the posterior neck may involve referral of pain from the trigger point in the erector neck muscle or upper trapezius to the head, leading to persistent headaches, which may last for days. Trigger points in the paraspinal muscles of the low back may refer pain to the buttock. Pain may be referred down the leg from a trigger point in the gluteus medius and can mimic sciatica. A trigger point in the infraspinatus muscle may produce local and referred pain over the lateral deltoid and down the outside of the arm into the hand. Injection of a local anesthetic such as 1% lidocaine into the trigger point site often results in pain relief. Another useful technique is first to spray from the trigger point toward the area of referred pain with an agent such as ethyl chloride and then to stretch the muscle. This maneuver may need to be repeated several times. Massage and application of ultrasound to the affected area also may be beneficial. Patients should be instructed in methods to prevent muscle stresses related to work and recreation. Posture and resting positions are important in preventing muscle tension. The prognosis in most patients is good. In some patients, myofascial pain syndrome may evolve into fibromyalgia (Chap. 329). Patients at risk for developing fibromyalgia are thought to be those with anxiety, depression, nonrestorative sleep, and fatigue.

TUMORS OF JOINTS

Primary tumors and tumor-like disorders of synovium are uncommon but should be considered in the differential diagnosis of monarticular joint disease. In addition, metastases to bone and primary bone tumors adjacent to a joint may produce joint symptoms. **For further discussion, see Chap. 94.**

Pigmented villonodular synovitis is characterized by the slowly progressive, exuberant, benign proliferation of synovial tissue, usually involving a single joint. The most common age of onset is in the third decade, and women are affected slightly more often than men. The cause of this disorder is unknown.

The synovium has a brownish color and numerous large, finger-like villi that fuse to form pedunculated nodules. There is marked hyperplasia of synovial cells in the stroma of the villi. Hemosiderin granules and lipids are found in the cytoplasm of macrophages and in the interstitial tissue. Multinucleated giant cells may be present. The proliferative synovium grows into the subsynovial tissue and invades adjacent cartilage and bone.

The clinical picture of pigmented villonodular synovitis is characterized by the insidious onset of swelling and pain in one joint, most commonly the knee. Other joints affected include the hips, ankles, calcaneocuboid joints, elbows, and small joints of the fingers or toes. The disease may also involve the common flexor sheath of the hands or fingers. Less commonly, tendon sheaths in the wrist, ankle, or foot may be involved. Symptoms may be mild and intermittent and may be present for years before the patient seeks medical attention. Radiographs may show joint space narrowing, erosions, and subchondral cysts. The joint fluid contains blood and is dark red or almost black in color. Lipid-containing macrophages may be present in the fluid. The joint fluid may be clear if hemorrhages have not occurred.

The treatment of pigmented villonodular synovitis is complete synovectomy. With incomplete synovectomy, the villonodular synovitis recurs, and the rate of tissue growth may be faster than it was originally. Irradiation of the involved joint has been successful in some patients.

Synovial chondromatosis is a disorder characterized by multiple focal metaplastic growths of normal-appearing cartilage in the synovium or tendon sheath. Segments of cartilage break loose and continue to grow as loose bodies. When calcification and ossification of loose bodies occur, the disorder is referred to as *synovial osteochondromatosis*. The disorder is usually monarticular and affects young to middle-aged individuals. The knee is most often involved, followed by hip, elbow, and shoulder. Symptoms are pain, swelling, and decreased motion of the joint. Radiographs may show several rounded calcifications within the joint cavity. Treatment is synovectomy; however, the tumor may recur.

Hemangiomas occur in synovium and in tendon sheaths. The knee is affected most commonly. Recurrent episodes of joint swelling and pain usually begin in childhood. The joint fluid is bloody. Treatment is excision of the lesion. *Lipomas* occur most often in the knee, originating in the subsynovial fat on either side of the patellar tendon. Lipomas also appear in tendon sheaths of the hands, wrists, feet, and ankles. In some instances, surgical removal is necessary.

Synovial sarcoma is a malignant neoplasm often found near a large joint of both upper and lower extremities, being more common in the lower extremity. It seldom arises within the joint itself. Synovial sarcomas constitute 10% of soft tissue sarcomas. The tumor is believed to arise from primitive mesenchymal tissue that differentiates into epithelial cells and/or spindle cells. Small foci of calcification may be present in the tumor mass. It occurs most often in young adults and is more common in men. The tumor presents as a slowly growing deep seated mass near a joint, without much pain. The area of the knee is the most common site, followed by the foot, ankle, elbow, and shoulder. Other primary sites include the buttocks, abdominal wall, retroperitoneum, and mediastinum. The tumor spreads along tissue planes. The most common site of visceral metastasis is lung. The diagnosis is made by biopsy. Treatment is wide resection of the tumor including adjacent muscle and regional lymph nodes, followed by chemotherapy and radiation therapy. Currently used chemotherapeutic agents are doxorubicin, ifosfamide, and cisplatin. Amputation of the involved distal extremity may be required. Chemotherapy may be beneficial in some patients with metastatic disease. Isolated pulmonary metastasis can be surgically removed. The 5-year survival with treatment is variable depending on the staging of the tumor, ranging from approximately 25% to 60% or higher. Synovial sarcomas tend to recur locally and eventually metastasize to regional lymph nodes, lungs, and skeleton.

FURTHER READINGS

ALTMAN RD, TENENBAUM J: Hypertrophic osteoarthropathy, in *Kelley's Textbook of Rheumatology*, 7th ed, ED Harris et al (eds). Philadelphia, Saunders, 2005, pp 1748–1753

CRONIN ME: Rheumatic aspects of endocrinopathies, in *Arthritis and Allied Conditions*, 15th ed, WJ Koopman (ed). Philadelphia, Lippincott Williams & Wilkins, 2005, pp 2559–2576

HECK LW JR: Arthritis associated with hematologic disorders, storage diseases, disorders of lipid metabolism, and dysproteinemias, in *Arthritis and Allied Conditions*, 15th ed, WJ Koopman (ed). Philadelphia, Lippincott Williams & Wilkins, 2005, pp 1969–1990

331 Periarticular Disorders of the Extremities
Carol A. Langford, Bruce C. Gilliland†

A number of periarticular disorders have become increasingly common over the past two to three decades, due in part to greater participation in recreational sports by individuals of a wide range of ages. This chapter discusses some of the more common periarticular disorders of the extremities.

BURSITIS

Bursitis is inflammation of a bursa, which is a thin-walled sac lined with synovial tissue. The function of the bursa is to facilitate movement of tendons and muscles over bony prominences. Excessive frictional forces from overuse, trauma, systemic disease (e.g., rheumatoid arthritis, gout), or infection may cause bursitis. *Subacromial bursitis* (subdeltoid bursitis) is the most common form of bursitis. The subacromial bursa, which is contiguous with the subdeltoid bursa, is located between the undersurface of the acromion and the humeral head and is covered by the deltoid muscle. Bursitis is caused by repetitive overhead motion and often accompanies rotator cuff tendinitis. Another frequently encountered form is *trochanteric bursitis*, which involves the bursa around the insertion of the gluteus medius onto the greater trochanter of the femur. Patients experience pain over the lateral aspect of the hip and upper thigh and have tenderness over the posterior aspect of the greater trochanter. External rotation and resisted abduction of the hip elicit pain. *Olecranon bursitis* occurs over the posterior elbow, and when the area is acutely inflamed, infection or gout should be excluded by aspirating the bursa and performing a Gram stain and culture on the fluid as well as examining the fluid for urate crystals. *Achilles bursitis* involves the bursa located above the insertion of the tendon to the calcaneus and results from overuse and wearing tight shoes. *Retrocalcaneal bursitis* involves the bursa that is located between the calcaneus and posterior surface of the Achilles tendon. The pain is experienced at the back of the heel, and swelling appears on the medial and/or lateral side of the tendon. It occurs in association with spondyloarthropathies, rheumatoid arthritis, gout, or trauma. *Ischial bursitis* (weaver's bottom) affects the bursa separating the gluteus medius from the ischial tuberosity and develops from prolonged sitting and pivoting on hard surfaces. *Iliopsoas bursitis* affects the bursa that lies between the iliopsoas muscle and hip joint and is lateral to the femoral vessels. Pain is experienced over this area and is made worse by hip extension and flexion. *Anserine bursitis* is an inflammation of the sartorius bursa located over the medial side of the tibia just below the knee and under the conjoint tendon and is manifested by pain on climbing stairs. Tenderness is present over the insertion of the conjoint tendon of the sartorius, gracilis, and semitendinosus. *Prepatellar bursitis* (housemaid's knee) occurs in the bursa situated between the patella and overlying skin and is caused by kneeling on hard surfaces. Gout or infection may also occur at this site. Treatment of bursitis consists of prevention of the aggravating situation, rest of the involved part, administration of a nonsteroidal anti-inflammatory drug (NSAID) where appropriate for an individual patient, or local glucocorticoid injection.

ROTATOR CUFF TENDINITIS AND IMPINGEMENT SYNDROME

Tendinitis of the rotator cuff is the major cause of a painful shoulder and is currently thought to be caused by inflammation of the tendon(s). The rotator cuff consists of the tendons of the supraspinatus, infraspinatus, subscapularis, and teres minor muscles, and inserts on the humeral tuberosities. Of the tendons forming the rotator cuff, the supraspinatus tendon is the most often affected, probably because of its repeated impingement (*impingement syndrome*) between the humeral head and the undersurface of the anterior third of the acromion and coracoacromial ligament above as well as the reduction in its blood supply that occurs with abduction of the arm (Fig. 331-1). The tendon of the infraspinatus and that of the long

---

†Deceased. A contributor to HPIM since the 11th edition, Dr. Gilliland passed away on February 17, 2007.

FIGURE 331-1 Coronal section of the shoulder illustrating the relationships of the glenohumeral joint, the joint capsule, the subacromial bursa, and the rotator cuff (supraspinatus tendon). *[From F Kozin, in Arthritis and Allied Conditions, 13th ed, WJ Koopman (ed). Baltimore, Williams & Wilkins, 1997, with permission.]*

head of the biceps are less commonly involved. The process begins with edema and hemorrhage of the rotator cuff, which evolves to fibrotic thickening and eventually to rotator cuff degeneration with tendon tears and bone spurs. Subacromial bursitis also accompanies this syndrome. Symptoms usually appear after injury or overuse, especially with activities involving elevation of the arm with some degree of forward flexion. Impingement syndrome occurs in persons participating in baseball, tennis, swimming, or occupations that require repeated elevation of the arm. Those over age 40 are particularly susceptible. Patients complain of a dull aching in the shoulder, which may interfere with sleep. Severe pain is experienced when the arm is actively abducted into an overhead position. The arc between 60° and 120° is especially painful. Tenderness is present over the lateral aspect of the humeral head just below the acromion. NSAIDs, local glucocorticoid injection, and physical therapy may relieve symptoms. Surgical decompression of the subacromial space may be necessary in patients refractory to conservative treatment.

Patients may tear the supraspinatus tendon acutely by falling on an outstretched arm or lifting a heavy object. Symptoms are pain along with weakness of abduction and external rotation of the shoulder. Atrophy of the supraspinatus muscles develops. The diagnosis is established by arthrogram, ultrasound, or MRI. Surgical repair may be necessary in patients who fail to respond to conservative measures. In patients with moderate-to-severe tears and functional loss, surgery is indicated.

CALCIFIC TENDINITIS

This condition is characterized by deposition of calcium salts, primarily hydroxyapatite, within a tendon. The exact mechanism of calcification is not known but may be initiated by ischemia or degeneration of the tendon. The supraspinatus tendon is most often affected because it is frequently impinged on and has a reduced blood supply when the arm is abducted. The condition usually develops after age 40. Calcification within the tendon may evoke acute inflammation, producing sudden and severe pain in the shoulder. However, it may be asymptomatic or not related to the patient's symptoms.

BICIPITAL TENDINITIS AND RUPTURE

Bicipital tendinitis, or tenosynovitis, is produced by friction on the tendon of the long head of the biceps as it passes through the bicipital groove. When the inflammation is acute, patients experience anterior shoulder pain that radiates down the biceps into the forearm. Abduction and external rotation of the arm are painful and limited. The bicipital groove is very tender to palpation. Pain may be elicited along

the course of the tendon by resisting supination of the forearm with the elbow at 90° (Yergason's supination sign). Acute rupture of the tendon may occur with vigorous exercise of the arm and is often painful. In a young patient, it should be repaired surgically. Rupture of the tendon in an older person may be associated with little or no pain and is recognized by the presence of persistent swelling of the biceps ("Popeye" muscle) produced by the retraction of the long head of the biceps. Surgery is usually not necessary in this setting.

DE QUERVAIN'S TENOSYNOVITIS

In this condition, inflammation involves the abductor pollicis longus and the extensor pollicis brevis as these tendons pass through a fibrous sheath at the radial styloid process. The usual cause is repetitive twisting of the wrist. It may occur in pregnancy, and it also occurs in mothers who hold their babies with the thumb outstretched. Patients experience pain on grasping with their thumb, such as with pinching. Swelling and tenderness are often present over the radial styloid process. The Finkelstein sign is positive, which is elicited by having the patient place the thumb in the palm and close the fingers over it. The wrist is then ulnarly deviated, resulting in pain over the involved tendon sheath in the area of the radial styloid. Treatment consists initially of splinting the wrist and an NSAID. When severe or refractory to conservative treatment, glucocorticoid injections can be very effective.

PATELLAR TENDINITIS (JUMPER'S KNEE)

Tendinitis involves the patellar tendon at its attachment to the lower pole of the patella. Patients may experience pain when jumping during basketball or volleyball, going up stairs, or doing deep knee squats. Tenderness is noted on examination over the lower pole of the patella. Treatment consists of rest, icing, and NSAIDs, followed by strengthening and increasing flexibility.

ADHESIVE CAPSULITIS

Often referred to as "frozen shoulder," adhesive capsulitis is characterized by pain and restricted movement of the shoulder, usually in the absence of intrinsic shoulder disease. Night pain is often present in the affected shoulder. Adhesive capsulitis, however, may follow bursitis or tendinitis of the shoulder or be associated with systemic disorders such as chronic pulmonary disease, myocardial infarction, and diabetes mellitus. Prolonged immobility of the arm contributes to the development of adhesive capsulitis, and reflex sympathetic dystrophy is thought to be a pathogenic factor. The capsule of the shoulder is thickened, and a mild chronic inflammatory infiltrate and fibrosis may be present.

Adhesive capsulitis occurs more commonly in women after age 50. Pain and stiffness usually develop gradually over several months to a year but progress rapidly in some patients. Pain may interfere with sleep. The shoulder is tender to palpation, and both active and passive movement are restricted. Radiographs of the shoulder show osteopenia. The diagnosis is confirmed by arthrography, in that only a limited amount of contrast material, usually <15 mL, can be injected under pressure into the shoulder joint.

In most patients, the condition improves spontaneously 1–3 years after onset. While pain usually improves, most patients are left with some limitation of shoulder motion. Early mobilization of the arm following an injury to the shoulder may prevent the development of this disease. Slow but forceful injection of contrast material into the joint may lyse adhesions and stretch the capsule, resulting in improvement of shoulder motion. Manipulation under anesthesia may be helpful in some patients. Once the disease is established, therapy may have little effect on its natural course. Local injections of glucocorticoids, NSAIDs, and physical therapy may provide relief of symptoms.

LATERAL EPICONDYLITIS (TENNIS ELBOW)

Lateral epicondylitis, or tennis elbow, is a painful condition involving the soft tissue over the lateral aspect of the elbow. The pain originates at or near the site of attachment of the common extensors to the lateral epicondyle and may radiate into the forearm and dorsum of the wrist. This painful condition is thought to be caused by small tears of the extensor aponeurosis resulting from repeated resisted contractions of the extensor muscles. The pain usually appears after work or recreational activities involving repeated motions of wrist extension and supination against resistance. Most patients with this disorder injure themselves in activities other than tennis, such as pulling weeds, carrying suitcases or briefcases, or using a screwdriver. The injury in tennis usually occurs when hitting a backhand with the elbow flexed. Shaking hands and opening doors can reproduce the pain. Striking the lateral elbow against a solid object may also induce pain.

The treatment is usually rest along with administration of an NSAID. Ultrasound, icing, and friction massage may also help relieve pain. When pain is severe, the elbow is placed in a sling or splinted at 90° of flexion. When the pain is acute and well localized, injection of a glucocorticoid using a small-gauge needle may be effective. Following injection, the patient should be advised to rest the arm for at least 1 month and avoid activities that would aggravate the elbow. Once symptoms have subsided, the patient should begin rehabilitation to strengthen and increase flexibility of the extensor muscles before resuming physical activity involving the arm. A forearm band placed 2.5–5.0 cm (1–2 in.) below the elbow may help to reduce tension on the extensor muscles at their attachment to the lateral epicondyle. The patient should be advised to restrict activities requiring forcible extension and supination of the wrist. Improvement may take several months. The patient may continue to experience mild pain but, with care, can usually avoid the return of debilitating pain. In an occasional patient, surgical release of the extensor aponeurosis may be necessary.

MEDIAL EPICONDYLITIS

Medial epicondylitis is an overuse syndrome resulting in pain over the medial side of the elbow with radiation into the forearm. The cause of this syndrome is considered to be repetitive resisted motions of wrist flexion and pronation, which lead to microtears and granulation tissue at the origin of the pronator teres and forearm flexors, particularly the flexor carpi radialis. This overuse syndrome is usually seen in patients >35 years and is much less common than lateral epicondylitis. It occurs most often in work-related repetitive activities but also occurs with recreational activities such as swinging a golf club (golfer's elbow) or throwing a baseball. On physical examination, there is tenderness just distal to the medial epicondyle over the origin of the forearm flexors. Pain can be reproduced by resisting wrist flexion and pronation with the elbow extended. Radiographs are usually normal. The differential diagnosis of patients with medial elbow symptoms include tears of the pronator teres, acute medial collateral ligament tear, and medial collateral ligament instability. Ulnar neuritis has been found in 25–50% of patients with medial epicondylitis and is associated with tenderness over the ulnar nerve at the elbow as well as hypesthesia and paresthesia on the ulnar side of the hand.

The initial treatment of medial epicondylitis is conservative, involving rest, NSAIDs, friction massage, ultrasound, and icing. Some patients may require splinting. Injections of glucocorticoids at the painful site may also be effective. Patients should be instructed to rest at least 1 month. Also, patients should be started on physical therapy once the pain has subsided. In patients with chronic debilitating medial epicondylitis that remains unresponsive after at least a year of treatment, surgical release of the flexor muscle at its origin may be necessary and is often successful.

PLANTAR FASCIITIS

Plantar fasciitis is a common cause of foot pain in adults, with the peak incidence occurring in people between the ages of 40–60 years. It is also seen more frequently in a younger population consisting of runners, aerobic exercise dancers, and ballet dancers. The pain originates at or near the site of the plantar fascia attachment to the medial tuberosity of the calcaneus. The plantar fascia is a thick fibrous band that extends distally, dividing into five slips that insert into each metatarsal head. Its function is to tighten and elevate the longitudinal arch as well as to invert the hind foot during the push-off phase of gait.

Plantar fasciitis is thought to be the result of repetitive microtrauma to the tissue. Pathology of involved fascia reveals degeneration of fibrous tissue with or without fibroblast proliferation and chronic inflammation. Several factors that increase the risk of developing plantar fasciitis include obesity, pes planus (excessive pronation of the foot), pes cavus (high-arched foot), limited dorsiflexion of the ankle, prolonged standing, walking on hard surfaces, and faulty shoes. In runners, excessive running and a change to a harder running surface may precipitate plantar fasciitis.

The diagnosis of plantar fasciitis can usually be made on the basis of history and physical examination alone. The onset of inferior heel pain of plantar fasciitis is typically gradual, but in some individuals it can be abrupt. Patients experience severe pain with the first steps on arising in the morning or following inactivity during the day. The pain usually lessens with weight-bearing activity during the day, only to worsen with continued activity. Pain is made worse on walking barefoot or up stairs. On examination, maximal tenderness is elicited on palpation over the inferior heel corresponding to the site of attachment of the plantar fascia.

Imaging studies may be indicated when the diagnosis is not clear. Plain radiographs may show heel spurs, which are of little diagnostic significance as they may be present in patients with or without plantar fasciitis. A calcaneal stress fracture may be detected on plain radiographs; however, a bone scan is more sensitive. Bone scan in plantar fasciitis demonstrates increased uptake at the attachment of the plantar fascia to the calcaneus. Ultrasonography in plantar fasciitis can demonstrate thickening of the fascia and diffuse hypoechogenicity, indicating edema at the attachment of the plantar fascia to the calcaneus. MRI is a sensitive method for detecting plantar fasciitis, but it is usually not required for establishing the diagnosis.

The differential diagnosis of inferior heel pain includes calcaneal stress fractures, the spondyloarthritides, rheumatoid arthritis, gout, neoplastic or infiltrative bone processes, and nerve compression/entrapment syndromes. The diagnosis of these disorders is made on clinical features, imaging studies, and laboratory findings, which distinguish them from plantar fasciitis.

Long-term studies have found that resolution of symptoms occurs within 12 months in more than 80% of patients with plantar fasciitis. Treatment should begin immediately with the diagnosis of plantar fasciitis. The patient is advised to reduce or discontinue activities that can exacerbate plantar fasciitis. Initial treatment consists of ice, heat, massage, and stretching. Stretching of the plantar fascia and calf muscles are commonly employed and can be beneficial. Orthotics provide medial arch support and can be effective in relieving symptoms. Foot strapping or taping are commonly performed, and some patients may benefit by wearing a night splint designed to keep the ankle in a neutral position. A short course of NSAIDs can be given to alleviate symptoms in patients where the benefits outweigh the risks. Local glucocorticoid injections have also been shown to be efficacious but may carry an increased risk for plantar fascia rupture. Plantar fasciotomy is reserved for those patients who have failed to improve after at least 6–12 months of conservative treatment.

FURTHER READINGS

BUCHBINDER R: Plantar fasciitis. N Engl J Med 350:2159, 2004

FRIEMAN BG et al: Rotator cuff disease: A review of diagnosis, pathophysiology, and current trends in treatment. Arch Phys Med Rehabil 75:604, 1994

HUSNI EM, DONOHUE JP: Painful shoulder and reflex sympathetic dystrophy syndrome, in *Arthritis and Allied Conditions*, 15th ed, WJ Koopman (ed). Philadelphia, Lippincott Williams & Wilkins, 2005, pp 2133–2152

MARTIN SD, THORNHILL TS: Shoulder pain, in *Kelley's Textbook of Rheumatology*, 7th ed, ED Harris et al (eds). Philadelphia, Saunders, 2005, pp 557–587

NEER CS II: Impingement lesions. Clin Orthop 173:70, 1983

332 Principles of Endocrinology
J. Larry Jameson

The management of endocrine disorders requires a broad understanding of intermediary metabolism, reproductive physiology, bone metabolism, and growth. Accordingly, the practice of endocrinology is intimately linked to a conceptual framework for understanding hormone secretion, hormone action, and principles of feedback control. The endocrine system is evaluated primarily by measuring hormone concentrations, thereby arming the clinician with valuable diagnostic information. Most disorders of the endocrine system are amenable to effective treatment, once the correct diagnosis is determined. Endocrine deficiency disorders are treated with physiologic hormone replacement; hormone excess conditions, usually due to benign glandular adenomas, are managed by removing tumors surgically or by reducing hormone levels medically.

SCOPE OF ENDOCRINOLOGY

The specialty of endocrinology encompasses the study of glands and the hormones they produce. The term *endocrine* was coined by Starling to contrast the actions of hormones secreted internally (endocrine) with those secreted externally (*exocrine*) or into a lumen, such as the gastrointestinal tract. The term *hormone*, derived from a Greek phrase meaning "to set in motion," aptly describes the dynamic actions of hormones as they elicit cellular responses and regulate physiologic processes through feedback mechanisms.

Unlike many other specialties in medicine, it is not possible to define endocrinology strictly along anatomic lines. The classic endocrine glands—pituitary, thyroid, parathyroid, pancreatic islets, adrenal, and gonads—communicate broadly with other organs through the nervous system, hormones, cytokines, and growth factors. In addition to its traditional synaptic functions, the brain produces a vast array of peptide hormones, spawning the discipline of neuroendocrinology. Through the production of hypothalamic releasing factors, the central nervous system (CNS) exerts a major regulatory influence over pituitary hormone secretion (Chap. 333). The peripheral nervous system stimulates the adrenal medulla. The immune and endocrine systems are also intimately intertwined. The adrenal glucocorticoid, cortisol, is a powerful immunosuppressant. Cytokines and interleukins (ILs) have profound effects on the functions of the pituitary, adrenal, thyroid, and gonads. Common endocrine diseases, such as autoimmune thyroid disease and type 1 diabetes mellitus, are caused by dysregulation of immune surveillance and tolerance. Less common diseases such as polyglandular failure, Addison's disease, and lymphocytic hypophysitis also have an immunologic basis.

The interdigitation of endocrinology with physiologic processes in other specialties sometimes blurs the role of hormones. For example, hormones play an important role in maintenance of blood pressure, intravascular volume, and peripheral resistance in the cardiovascular system. Vasoactive substances such as catecholamines, angiotensin II, endothelin, and nitric oxide are involved in dynamic changes of vascular tone, in addition to their multiple roles in other tissues. The heart is the principal source of atrial natriuretic peptide, which acts in classic endocrine fashion to induce natriuresis at a distant target organ (the kidney). Erythropoietin, a traditional circulating hormone, is made in the kidney and stimulates erythropoiesis in the bone marrow (Chap. 58). The kidney is also integrally involved in the renin-angiotensin axis (Chap. 336) and is a primary target of several hormones, including parathyroid hormone (PTH), mineralocorticoids, and vasopressin. The gastrointestinal tract produces a surprising number of peptide hormones such as cholecystokinin, ghrelin, gastrin, secretin, and vasoactive intestinal peptide, among many others. Carcinoid and islet tumors can secrete excessive amounts of these hormones, leading to specific clinical syndromes (Chap. 344). Many of these gastrointestinal hormones are also produced in the CNS, where their functions remain poorly understood. As new hormones such as inhibin, ghrelin, and leptin are discovered, they become integrated into the science and practice of medicine on the basis of their functional roles rather than their tissues of origin.

Characterization of hormone receptors frequently reveals unexpected relationships to factors in nonendocrine disciplines. The growth hormone (GH) and leptin receptors, for example, are members of the cytokine receptor family. The G protein–coupled receptors (GPCRs), which mediate the actions of many peptide hormones, are used in numerous physiologic processes, including vision, smell, and neurotransmission.

NATURE OF HORMONES

Hormones can be divided into five major classes: (1) *amino acid derivatives* such as dopamine, catecholamine, and thyroid hormone (TH); (2) *small neuropeptides* such as gonadotropin-releasing hormone (GnRH), thyrotropin-releasing hormone (TRH), somatostatin, and vasopressin; (3) *large proteins* such as insulin, luteinizing hormone (LH), and PTH produced by classic endocrine glands; (4) *steroid hormones* such as cortisol and estrogen that are synthesized from cholesterol-based precursors; and (5) *vitamin derivatives* such as retinoids (vitamin A) and vitamin D. A variety of *peptide growth factors*, most of which act locally, share actions with hormones. As a rule, amino acid derivatives and peptide hormones interact with cell-surface membrane receptors. Steroids, thyroid hormones, vitamin D, and retinoids are lipid-soluble and interact with intracellular nuclear receptors.

HORMONE AND RECEPTOR FAMILIES

Many hormones and receptors can be grouped into families, reflecting their structural similarities (Table 332-1). The evolution of these families generates diverse but highly selective pathways of hormone action. Recognizing these relationships allows extrapolation of information gleaned from one hormone or receptor to other family members.

The glycoprotein hormone family, consisting of thyroid-stimulating hormone (TSH), follicle-stimulating hormone (FSH), LH, and human chorionic gonadotropin (hCG), illustrates many features of related hormones. The glycoprotein hormones are heterodimers that have the α subunit in common; the β subunits are distinct and confer specific biologic actions. The overall three-dimensional architecture of the β subunits is similar, reflecting the locations of conserved disulfide bonds that restrain protein conformation. The cloning of the β-subunit genes from multiple species suggests that this family arose from a common ancestral gene, probably by gene duplication and subsequent divergence to evolve new biologic functions.

As the hormone families enlarge and diverge, their receptors must co-evolve, if new biologic functions are to be derived. Related GPCRs, for example, have evolved for each of the glycoprotein hormones. These receptors are structurally similar, and each is coupled to the $G_s\alpha$ signaling pathway. However, there is minimal overlap of hormone

TABLE 332-1 MEMBRANE RECEPTOR FAMILIES AND SIGNALING PATHWAYS

Receptors	Effectors	Signaling Pathways
G Protein–Coupled Seven-Transmembrane (GPCR)		
β-Adrenergic LH, FSH, TSH Glucagon	$G_s\alpha$, adenylate cyclase	Stimulation of cyclic AMP production, protein kinase A
PTH, PTHrP ACTH, MSH GHRH, CRH	Ca^{2+} channels	Calmodulin, Ca^{2+}-dependent kinases
α-Adrenergic Somatostatin	$G_i\alpha$	Inhibition of cyclic AMP production Activation of K^+, Ca^{2+} channels
TRH, GnRH	G_q, G_{11}	Phospholipase C, diacylglycerol, IP_3, protein kinase C, voltage-dependent Ca^{2+} channels
Receptor Tyrosine Kinase		
Insulin, IGF-I	Tyrosine kinases, IRS	MAP kinases, PI 3-kinase; AKT, also known as protein kinase B, PKB
EGF, NGF	Tyrosine kinases, ras	Raf, MAP kinases, RSK
Cytokine Receptor–Linked Kinase		
GH, PRL	JAK, tyrosine kinases	STAT, MAP kinase, PI 3-kinase, IRS-1
Serine Kinase		
Activin, TGF-β, MIS	Serine kinase	Smads

Note: IP_3, inositol triphosphate; IRS, insulin receptor substrates; MAP, mitogen-activated protein; MSH, melanocyte-stimulating hormone; NGF, nerve growth factor; PI, phosphatylinositol; RSK, ribosomal S6 kinase; TGF-β, transforming growth factor β. For all other abbreviations, see text.

binding. For example, TSH binds with high specificity to the TSH receptor but interacts minimally with the LH or the FSH receptor. Nonetheless, there can be subtle physiologic consequences of hormone cross-reactivity with other receptors. Very high levels of hCG during pregnancy stimulate the TSH receptor and increase TH levels, resulting in a compensatory decrease in TSH.

Insulin, insulin-like growth factor (IGF) I, and IGF-II share structural similarities that are most apparent when precursor forms of the proteins are compared. In contrast to the high degree of specificity seen with the glycoprotein hormones, there is moderate cross-talk among the members of the insulin/IGF family. High concentrations of an IGF-II precursor produced by certain tumors (e.g., sarcomas) can cause hypoglycemia, partly because of binding to insulin and IGF-I receptors (Chap. 96). High concentrations of insulin also bind to the IGF-I receptor, perhaps accounting for some of the clinical manifestations seen in severe insulin resistance.

Another important example of receptor cross-talk is seen with PTH and parathyroid hormone–related peptide (PTHrP) (Chap. 347). PTH is produced by the parathyroid glands, whereas PTHrP is expressed at high levels during development and by a variety of tumors (Chap. 96). These hormones share amino acid sequence similarity, particularly in their amino-terminal regions. Both hormones bind to a single PTH receptor that is expressed in bone and kidney. Hypercalcemia and hypophosphatemia may therefore result from excessive production of either hormone, making it difficult to distinguish hyperparathyroidism from hypercalcemia of malignancy solely on the basis of serum chemistries. However, sensitive and specific assays for PTH and PTHrP now allow these disorders to be separated more readily.

Based on their specificities for DNA binding sites, the nuclear receptor family can be subdivided into type 1 receptors (GR, MR, AR, ER, PR) that bind steroids and type 2 receptors (TR, VDR, RAR, PPAR) that bind TH, vitamin D, retinoic acid, or lipid derivatives. Certain functional domains in nuclear receptors, such as the zinc finger DNA-binding domains, are highly conserved. However, selective

amino acid differences within this domain confer DNA sequence specificity. The hormone-binding domains are more variable, providing great diversity in the array of small molecules that bind to different nuclear receptors. With few exceptions, hormone binding is highly specific for a single type of nuclear receptor. One exception involves the glucocorticoid and mineralocorticoid receptors. Because the mineralocorticoid receptor also binds glucocorticoids with high affinity, an enzyme (11β-hydroxysteroid dehydrogenase) located in renal tubular cells inactivates glucocorticoids, allowing selective responses to mineralocorticoids such as aldosterone. However, when very high glucocorticoid concentrations occur, as in Cushing's syndrome, the glucocorticoid degradation pathway becomes saturated, allowing excessive cortisol levels to exert mineralocorticoid effects (sodium retention, potassium wasting). This phenomenon is particularly pronounced in ectopic adrenocorticotropic hormone (ACTH) syndromes (Chap. 336). Another example of relaxed nuclear receptor specificity involves the estrogen receptor, which can bind an array of compounds, some of which share little structural similarity to the high-affinity ligand estradiol. This feature of the estrogen receptor makes it susceptible to activation by "environmental estrogens" such as resveratrol, octylphenol, and many other aromatic hydrocarbons. On the other hand, this lack of specificity provides an opportunity to synthesize a remarkable series of clinically useful antagonists (e.g., tamoxifen) and selective estrogen response modulators (SERMs) such as raloxifene. These compounds generate distinct conformations that alter receptor interactions with components of the transcription machinery (see below), thereby conferring their unique actions.

HORMONE SYNTHESIS AND PROCESSING

The synthesis of peptide hormones and their receptors occurs through a classic pathway of gene expression: transcription → mRNA → protein → posttranslational protein processing → intracellular sorting, membrane integration, or secretion (Chap. 62).

Many hormones are embedded within larger precursor polypeptides that are proteolytically processed to yield the biologically active hormone. Examples include: proopiomelanocortin (POMC) → ACTH; proglucagon → glucagon; proinsulin → insulin; pro-PTH → PTH, among others. In many cases, such as POMC and proglucagon, these precursors generate multiple biologically active peptides. It is provocative that hormone precursors are typically inactive, presumably adding an additional level of regulatory control. This is true not only for peptide hormones but also for certain steroids (testosterone → dihydrotestosterone) and thyroid hormone ($T_4 → T_3$).

Hormone precursor processing is intimately linked to intracellular sorting pathways that transport proteins to appropriate vesicles and enzymes, resulting in specific cleavage steps, followed by protein folding and translocation to secretory vesicles. Hormones destined for secretion are translocated across the endoplasmic reticulum under the guidance of an amino-terminal signal sequence that is subsequently cleaved. Cell-surface receptors are inserted into the membrane via short segments of hydrophobic amino acids that remain embedded within the lipid bilayer. During translocation through the Golgi and endoplasmic reticulum, hormones and receptors are also subject to a variety of posttranslational modifications, such as glycosylation and phosphorylation, which can alter protein conformation, modify circulating half-life, and alter biologic activity.

Synthesis of most steroid hormones is based on modifications of the precursor, cholesterol. Multiple regulated enzymatic steps are required for the synthesis of testosterone (Chap. 340), estradiol (Chap. 341), cortisol (Chap. 336), and vitamin D (Chap. 346). This large number of synthetic steps predisposes to multiple genetic and acquired disorders of steroidogenesis.

Although endocrine genes contain regulatory DNA elements similar to those found in many other genes, their exquisite control by other hormones also necessitates the presence of specific hormone response elements. For example, the TSH genes are repressed directly by thyroid hormones acting through the thyroid hormone receptor (TR), a member of the nuclear receptor family. Steroidogenic enzyme gene expression requires specific transcription factors, such as steroidogenic factor-1 (SF-1), acting in conjunction with signals transmitted by trophic hormones (e.g., ACTH or LH). For some hormones, substantial regulation occurs at the level of translational efficiency. Insulin biosynthesis, while requiring ongoing gene transcription, is regulated primarily at the translational level in response to elevated levels of glucose or amino acids.

HORMONE SECRETION, TRANSPORT, AND DEGRADATION

The circulating level of a hormone is determined by its rate of secretion and its circulating half-life. After protein processing, peptide hormones (GnRH, insulin, GH) are stored in secretory granules. As these granules mature, they are poised beneath the plasma membrane for imminent release into the circulation. In most instances, the stimulus for hormone secretion is a releasing factor or neural signal that induces rapid changes in intracellular calcium concentrations, leading to secretory granule fusion with the plasma membrane and release of its contents into the extracellular environment and bloodstream. Steroid hormones, in contrast, diffuse into the circulation as they are synthesized. Thus, their secretory rates are closely aligned with rates of synthesis. For example, ACTH and LH induce steroidogenesis by stimulating the activity of *steroidogenic acute regulatory* (StAR) protein (transports cholesterol into the mitochondrion) along with other rate-limiting steps (e.g., cholesterol side-chain cleavage enzyme, CYP11A1) in the steroidogenic pathway.

Hormone transport and degradation dictate the rapidity with which a hormonal signal decays. Some hormonal signals are evanescent (e.g., somatostatin), whereas others are longer-lived (e.g., TSH). Because somatostatin exerts effects in virtually every tissue, a short half-life allows its concentrations and actions to be controlled locally. Structural modifications that impair somatostatin degradation have been useful for generating long-acting therapeutic analogues, such as octreotide (Chap. 333). On the other hand, the actions of TSH are highly specific for the thyroid gland. Its prolonged half-life accounts for relatively constant serum levels, even though TSH is secreted in discrete pulses.

An understanding of circulating hormone half-life is important for achieving physiologic hormone replacement, as the frequency of dosing and the time required to reach steady state are intimately linked to rates of hormone decay. T_4, for example, has a circulating half-life of 7 days. Consequently, >1 month is required to reach a new steady state, but single daily doses are sufficient to achieve constant hormone levels. T_3, in contrast, has a half-life of 1 day. Its administration is associated with more dynamic serum levels and it must be administered two to three times per day. Similarly, synthetic glucocorticoids vary widely in their half-lives; those with longer half-lives (e.g., dexamethasone) are associated with greater suppression of the hypothalamic-pituitary-adrenal (HPA) axis. Most protein hormones [e.g., ACTH, GH, prolactin (PRL); PTH, LH] have relatively short half-lives (<20 min), leading to sharp peaks of secretion and decay. The only accurate way to profile the pulse frequency and amplitude of these hormones is to measure levels in frequently sampled blood (every 10 min or less) over long durations (8–24 h). Because this is not practical in a clinical setting, an alternative strategy is to pool three to four samples drawn at about 30-min intervals, recognizing that pulsatile secretion makes it difficult to establish a narrow normal range. Rapid hormone decay is useful in certain clinical settings. For example, the short half-life of PTH allows the use of intraoperative PTH determinations to confirm successful removal of an adenoma. This is particularly valuable diagnostically when there is a possibility of multicentric disease or parathyroid hyperplasia, as occurs with multiple endocrine neoplasia (MEN) or renal insufficiency.

Many hormones circulate in association with serum-binding proteins. Examples include: (1) T_4 and T_3 binding to thyroxine-binding globulin (TBG), albumin, and thyroxine-binding prealbumin (TBPA); (2) cortisol binding to cortisol-binding globulin (CBG); (3) androgen and estrogen binding to sex hormone–binding globulin (SHBG) (also called testosterone-binding globulin, TeBG); (4) IGF-I and -II binding to multiple IGF-binding proteins (IGFBPs); (5) GH interactions with

GH-binding protein (GHBP), a circulating fragment of the GH receptor extracellular domain; and (6) activin binding to follistatin. These interactions provide a hormonal reservoir, prevent otherwise rapid degradation of unbound hormones, restrict hormone access to certain sites (e.g., IGFBPs), and modulate the unbound, or "free," hormone concentrations. Although a variety of binding protein abnormalities have been identified, most have little clinical consequence, aside from creating diagnostic problems. For example, TBG deficiency can greatly reduce total TH levels, but the free concentrations of T_4 and T_3 remain normal. Liver disease and certain medications can also influence binding protein levels (e.g., estrogen increases TBG) or cause displacement of hormones from binding proteins (e.g., salsalate displaces T_4 from TBG). In general, only unbound hormone is available to interact with receptors and thereby elicit a biologic response. Short-term perturbations in binding proteins change the free hormone concentration, which in turn induces compensatory adaptations through feedback loops. SHBG changes in women are an exception to this self-correcting mechanism. When SHBG decreases because of insulin resistance or androgen excess, the unbound testosterone concentration is increased, potentially leading to hirsutism (Chap. 50). The increased unbound testosterone level does not result in an adequate compensatory feedback correction because estrogen, and not testosterone, is the primary regulator of the reproductive axis.

An additional exception to the unbound hormone hypothesis involves megalin, a member of the LDL receptor family that serves as an endocytotic receptor for carrier-bound vitamins A and D, and SHBG-bound androgens and estrogens. Following internalization, the carrier proteins are degraded in lysosomes and release their bound ligands within the cells. Megalin deficiency in mice impairs androgen-dependent testis descent and estrogen-mediated vaginal opening, confirming a functional role in these steroid-dependent events.

HORMONE ACTION THROUGH RECEPTORS

Receptors for hormones are divided into two major classes—membrane and nuclear. *Membrane receptors* primarily bind peptide hormones and catecholamines. *Nuclear receptors* bind small molecules that can diffuse across the cell membrane, such as TH, steroids, and vitamin D. Certain general principles apply to hormone-receptor interactions, regardless of the class of receptor. Hormones bind to receptors with specificity and an affinity that generally coincides with the dynamic range of circulating hormone concentrations. Low concentrations of free hormone (usually 10^{-12} to 10^{-9} M) rapidly associate and dissociate from receptors in a bimolecular reaction, such that the occupancy of the receptor at any given moment is a function of hormone concentration and the receptor's affinity for the hormone. Receptor numbers vary greatly in different target tissues, providing one of the major determinants of specific cellular responses to circulating hormones. For example, ACTH receptors are located almost exclusively in the adrenal cortex, and FSH receptors are found only in the gonads. In contrast, insulin and TRs are widely distributed, reflecting the need for metabolic responses in all tissues.

MEMBRANE RECEPTORS

Membrane receptors for hormones can be divided into several major groups: (1) seven transmembrane GPCRs, (2) tyrosine kinase receptors, (3) cytokine receptors, and (4) serine kinase receptors (Fig. 332-1). The *seven transmembrane GPCR family* binds a remarkable array of hormones, including large proteins (e.g., LH, PTH), small peptides (e.g., TRH, somatostatin), catecholamines (epinephrine, dopamine), and even minerals (e.g., calcium). The extracellular domains of GPCRs vary widely in size and are the major binding site for large hormones. The transmembrane-spanning regions are composed of hydrophobic α-helical domains that traverse the lipid bilayer. Like some channels, these domains are thought to circularize and form a hydrophobic pocket into which certain small ligands fit. Hormone binding induces conformational changes in these domains, transducing structural changes to the intracellular domain, which is a docking site for G proteins.

FIGURE 332-1 Membrane receptor signaling. MAPK, mitogen-activated protein kinase; PKA, -C, protein kinase A, C; TGF, transforming growth factor. For other abbreviations, see text.

The large family of *G proteins*, so named because they bind guanine nucleotides (GTP, GDP), provides great diversity for coupling receptors to different signaling pathways. G proteins form a heterotrimeric complex that is composed of various α and βγ subunits. The α subunit contains the guanine nucleotide–binding site and hydrolyzes GTP → GDP. The βγ subunits are tightly associated and modulate the activity of the α subunit, as well as mediating their own effector signaling pathways. G protein activity is regulated by a cycle that involves GTP hydrolysis and dynamic interactions between the α and βγ subunits. Hormone binding to the receptor induces GDP dissociation, allowing Gα to bind GTP and dissociate from the βγ complex. Under these conditions, the Gα subunit is activated and mediates signal transduction through various enzymes such as adenylate cyclase or phospholipase C. GTP hydrolysis to GDP allows reassociation with the βγ subunits and restores the inactive state. As described below, a variety of endocrinopathies result from G protein mutations or from mutations in receptors that modify their interactions with G proteins.

There are more than a dozen isoforms of the Gα subunit. $G_s\alpha$ stimulates, whereas $G_i\alpha$ inhibits, adenylate cyclase, an enzyme that generates the second messenger, cyclic AMP, leading to activation of protein kinase A (Table 332-1). G_q subunits couple to phospholipase C, generating diacylglycerol and inositol triphosphate, leading to activation of protein kinase C and the release of intracellular calcium.

The *tyrosine kinase receptors* transduce signals for insulin and a variety of growth factors, such as IGF-I, epidermal growth factor (EGF), nerve growth factor, platelet-derived growth factor, and fibroblast growth factor. The cysteine-rich extracellular ligand-binding domains contain growth factor binding sites. After ligand binding, this class of receptors undergoes autophosphorylation, inducing interactions with intracellular adaptor proteins such as Shc and insulin receptor substrates. In the case of the insulin receptor, multiple kinases are activated, including the Raf-Ras-MAPK and the Akt/protein kinase B pathways. The tyrosine kinase receptors play a prominent role in cell growth and differentiation as well as in intermediary metabolism.

The GH and PRL receptors belong to the *cytokine receptor* family (Chap. 308). Analogous to the tyrosine kinase receptors, ligand binding induces receptor interaction with intracellular kinases—the Janus kinases (JAKs), which phosphorylate members of the signal transduction and activators of transcription (STAT) family—as well as with other signaling pathways (Ras, PI3-K, MAPK). The activated STAT proteins translocate to the nucleus and stimulate expression of target genes.

The *serine kinase receptors* mediate the actions of activins, transforming growth factor β, müllerian-inhibiting substance (MIS, also known as anti-müllerian hormone, AMH), and bone morphogenic proteins (BMPs). This family of receptors (consisting of type I and II subunits) signal through proteins termed *smads* (fusion of terms for *Caenorhabditis elegans* sma + mammalian mad). Like the STAT proteins, the smads serve a dual role of transducing the receptor signal and acting as transcription factors. The pleomorphic actions of these growth factors dictate that they act primarily in a local (paracrine or autocrine) manner. Binding proteins, such as follistatin (which binds activin and other members of this family), function to inactivate the growth factors and restrict their distribution.

NUCLEAR RECEPTORS

The family of nuclear receptors has grown to nearly 100 members, many of which are still classified as orphan receptors because their ligands, if they exist, remain to be identified (Fig. 332-2). Otherwise, most nuclear receptors are classified based on the nature of their ligands. Though all nuclear receptors ultimately act to increase or decrease gene transcription, some (e.g., glucocorticoid receptor) reside primarily in the cytoplasm, whereas others (e.g., thyroid hormone receptor) are always located in the nucleus. After ligand binding, the cytoplasmically localized receptors translocate to the nucleus. There is growing evidence that certain nuclear receptors (e.g., glucocorticoid, estrogen) can also act at the membrane or in the cytoplasm to activate or repress signal transduction pathways, providing a mechanism for cross-talk between membrane and nuclear receptors.

The structures of nuclear receptors have been extensively studied, including by x-ray crystallography. The DNA binding domain, consisting of two zinc fingers, contacts specific DNA recognition sequences in target genes. Most nuclear receptors bind to DNA as dimers. Consequently, each monomer recognizes an individual DNA motif, referred to as a "half-site." The steroid receptors, including the glucocorticoid, estrogen, progesterone, and androgen receptors, bind to DNA as homodimers. Consistent with this twofold symmetry, their DNA recognition half-sites are palindromic. The thyroid, retinoid, peroxisome proliferator activated, and vitamin D receptors bind to DNA preferentially as heterodimers in combination with retinoid X receptors (RXRs). Their DNA half-sites are arranged as direct repeats. Receptor specificity for DNA sequences is determined by (1) the sequence of the half-site, (2) the orientation of the half-sites (palindromic, direct repeat), and (3) the spacing between the half-sites. For example, vitamin D, thyroid, and retinoid receptors recognize similar tandemly repeated half-sites (TAAGTCA), but these DNA repeats are spaced by three, four, and five nucleotides, respectively.

The carboxy-terminal hormone-binding domain mediates transcriptional control. For type II receptors, such as thyroid hormone receptor (TR) and retinoic acid receptor (RAR), co-repressor proteins bind to the receptor in the absence of ligand and silence gene transcription. Hormone binding induces conformational changes, triggering the release of co-repressors and inducing the recruitment of coactivators that stimulate transcription. Thus, these receptors are capable of mediating dramatic changes in the level of gene activity. Certain disease states are associated with defective regulation of these events. For example, mutations in the TR prevent co-repressor dissociation, resulting in a dominant form of hormone resistance (Chap. 335). In promyelocytic leukemia, fusion of RARα to other nuclear proteins causes aberrant gene silencing and prevents normal cellular differentiation. Treatment with retinoic acid reverses this repression and allows cellular differentiation and apoptosis to occur. Most type 1 steroid receptors interact weakly with co-repressors, but ligand binding still induces interactions with an

Homodimer Steroid Receptors	Heterodimer Receptors	Orphan Receptors
ER, AR, PR, GR	TR, VDR, RAR, PPAR	SF-1, DAX-1, HNF4α

Ligands

DNA response elements

| Ligand induces coactivator binding | Ligand dissociates corepressors and induces coactivator binding | Constitutive activator or repressor binding |

Gene Expression

— Hormone + : Activated

Basal — Hormone + : Silenced, Activated

— Receptor + : Activated

FIGURE 332-2 Nuclear receptor signaling. ER, estrogen receptor; AR, androgen receptor; PR, progesterone receptor; GR, glucocorticoid receptor; TR, thyroid hormone receptor; VDR, vitamin D receptor; RAR, retinoic acid receptor; PPAR, peroxisome proliferator activated receptor; SF-1, steroidogenic factor-1; DAX, dosage sensitive sex-reversal, adrenal hypoplasia congenita, X-chromosome; HNF4α, hepatic nuclear factor 4α.

array of coactivators. X-ray crystallography shows that various SERMs induce distinct estrogen receptor conformations. The tissue-specific responses caused by these agents in breast, bone, and uterus appear to reflect distinct interactions with coactivators. The receptor-coactivator complex stimulates gene transcription by several pathways, including (1) recruitment of enzymes (histone acetyl transferases) that modify chromatin structure, (2) interactions with additional transcription factors on the target gene, and (3) direct interactions with components of the general transcription apparatus to enhance the rate of RNA polymerase II–mediated transcription. Studies of nuclear receptor-mediated transcription show that these are dynamic events involving relatively rapid (e.g., 30–60 min) cycling of transcription complexes on any given target gene.

FUNCTIONS OF HORMONES

The functions of individual hormones are described in detail in subsequent chapters. Nevertheless, it is useful to illustrate how most biologic responses require integration of several different hormone pathways. The physiologic functions of hormones can be divided into three general areas: (1) growth and differentiation, (2) maintenance of homeostasis, and (3) reproduction.

GROWTH

Multiple hormones and nutritional factors mediate the complex phenomenon of growth (Chap. 333). Short stature may be caused by GH deficiency, hypothyroidism, Cushing's syndrome, precocious puberty, malnutrition, chronic illness, or genetic abnormalities that affect the epiphyseal growth plates (e.g., *FGFR3* or *SHOX* mutations). Many factors (GH, IGF-I, TH) stimulate growth, whereas others (sex steroids) lead to epiphyseal closure. Understanding these hormonal interactions is important in the diagnosis and management of growth disorders. For example, delaying exposure to high levels of sex steroids may enhance the efficacy of GH treatment.

MAINTENANCE OF HOMEOSTASIS

Though virtually all hormones affect homeostasis, the most important among these are the following:

1. TH—controls about 25% of basal metabolism in most tissues

2. Cortisol—exerts a permissive action for many hormones in addition to its own direct effects
3. PTH—regulates calcium and phosphorus levels
4. Vasopressin—regulates serum osmolality by controlling renal free water clearance
5. Mineralocorticoids—control vascular volume and serum electrolyte (Na⁺, K⁺) concentrations
6. Insulin—maintains euglycemia in the fed and fasted states

The defense against hypoglycemia is an impressive example of integrated hormone action (Chap. 339). In response to the fasted state and falling blood glucose, insulin secretion is suppressed, resulting in decreased glucose uptake and enhanced glycogenolysis, lipolysis, proteolysis, and gluconeogenesis to mobilize fuel sources. If hypoglycemia develops (usually from insulin administration or sulfonylureas), an orchestrated counterregulatory response occurs—glucagon and epinephrine rapidly stimulate glycogenolysis and gluconeogenesis, whereas GH and cortisol act over several hours to raise glucose levels and antagonize insulin action.

Although free-water clearance is primarily controlled by vasopressin, cortisol and TH are also important for facilitating renal tubular responses to vasopressin (Chap. 334). PTH and vitamin D function in an interdependent manner to control calcium metabolism (Chap. 346). PTH stimulates renal synthesis of 1,25-dihydroxyvitamin D, which increases calcium absorption in the gastrointestinal tract and enhances PTH action in bone. Increased calcium, along with vitamin D, feeds back to suppress PTH, thereby maintaining calcium balance.

Depending on the severity of a given stress and whether it is acute or chronic, multiple endocrine and cytokine pathways are activated to mount an appropriate physiologic response. In severe acute stress such as trauma or shock, the sympathetic nervous system is activated and catecholamines are released, leading to increased cardiac output and a primed musculoskeletal system. Catecholamines also increase mean blood pressure and stimulate glucose production. Multiple stress-induced pathways converge on the hypothalamus, stimulating several hormones including vasopressin and corticotropin-releasing hormone (CRH). These hormones, in addition to cytokines (tumor necrosis factor α, IL-2, IL-6), increase ACTH and GH production. ACTH stimulates the adrenal gland, increasing cortisol, which in turn helps to sustain blood pressure and dampen the inflammatory response. Increased vasopressin acts to conserve free water.

REPRODUCTION

The stages of reproduction include: (1) sex determination during fetal development (Chap. 343); (2) sexual maturation during puberty (Chaps. 340 and 341); (3) conception, pregnancy, lactation, and childrearing (Chap. 341); and (4) cessation of reproductive capability at menopause (Chap. 342). Each of these stages involves an orchestrated interplay of multiple hormones, a phenomenon well illustrated by the dynamic hormonal changes that occur during each 28-day menstrual cycle. In the early follicular phase, pulsatile secretion of LH and FSH stimulates the progressive maturation of the ovarian follicle. This results in gradually increasing estrogen and progesterone levels, leading to enhanced pituitary sensitivity to GnRH, which, when combined with accelerated GnRH secretion, triggers the LH surge and rupture of the mature follicle. Inhibin, a protein produced by the granulosa cells, enhances follicular growth and feeds back to the pituitary to selectively suppress FSH, without affecting LH. Growth factors such as EGF and

IGF-I modulate follicular responsiveness to gonadotropins. Vascular endothelial growth factor and prostaglandins play a role in follicle vascularization and rupture.

During pregnancy, the increased production of prolactin, in combination with placentally derived steroids (e.g., estrogen and progesterone), prepares the breast for lactation. Estrogens induce the production of progesterone receptors, allowing for increased responsiveness to progesterone. In addition to these and other hormones involved in lactation, the nervous system and oxytocin mediate the suckling response and milk release.

HORMONAL FEEDBACK REGULATORY SYSTEMS

Feedback control, both negative and positive, is a fundamental feature of endocrine systems. Each of the major hypothalamic-pituitary-hormone axes is governed by negative feedback, a process that maintains hormone levels within a relatively narrow range (Chap. 333). Examples of hypothalamic-pituitary negative feedback include (1) thyroid hormones on the TRH-TSH axis, (2) cortisol on the CRH-ACTH axis, (3) gonadal steroids on the GnRH-LH/FSH axis, and (4) IGF-I on the growth hormone–releasing hormone (GHRH)-GH axis (Fig. 332-3). These regulatory loops include both positive (e.g., TRH, TSH) and negative components (e.g., T_4, T_3), allowing for exquisite control of hormone levels. As an example, a small reduction of TH triggers a rapid increase of TRH and TSH secretion, resulting in thyroid gland stimulation and increased TH production. When the TH reaches a normal level, it feeds back to suppress TRH and TSH, and a new steady state is attained. Feedback regulation also occurs for endocrine systems that do not involve the pituitary gland, such as calcium feedback on PTH, glucose inhibition of insulin secretion, and leptin feedback on the hypothalamus. An understanding of feedback regulation provides important insights into endocrine testing paradigms (see below).

Positive feedback control also occurs but is not well understood. The primary example is estrogen-mediated stimulation of the mid-cycle LH surge. Though chronic low levels of estrogen are inhibitory, gradually rising estrogen levels stimulate LH secretion.

This effect, which is illustrative of an endocrine rhythm (see below), involves activation of the hypothalamic GnRH pulse generator. In addition, estrogen-primed gonadotropes are extraordinarily sensitive to GnRH, leading to a ten- to twentyfold amplification of LH release.

PARACRINE AND AUTOCRINE CONTROL

The aforementioned examples of feedback control involve classic endocrine pathways in which hormones are released by one gland and act on a distant target gland. However, local regulatory systems, often involving growth factors, are increasingly recognized. *Paracrine regulation* refers to factors released by one cell that act on an adjacent cell in the same tissue. For example, somatostatin secretion by pancreatic islet δ cells inhibits insulin secretion from nearby β cells. *Autocrine regulation* describes the action of a factor on the same cell from which it is produced. IGF-I acts on many cells that produce it, including chondrocytes, breast epithelium, and gonadal cells. Unlike endocrine actions, paracrine and autocrine control are difficult to document because local growth factor concentrations cannot be readily measured.

Anatomic relationships of glandular systems also greatly influence hormonal exposure—the physical organization of islet cells enhances their intercellular communication; the portal vasculature of the hypothalamic-pituitary system exposes the pituitary to high concentrations of hypothalamic releasing factors; testicular seminiferous tubules gain exposure to high testosterone levels produced by the interdigitated Leydig cells; the pancreas receives nutrient information from the gastrointestinal tract; and the liver is the proximal target of insulin action because of portal drainage from the pancreas.

HORMONAL RHYTHMS

The feedback regulatory systems described above are superimposed on hormonal rhythms that are used for adaptation to the environment. Seasonal changes, the daily occurrence of the light-dark cycle, sleep, meals, and stress are examples of the many environmental events that affect hormonal rhythms. The *menstrual cycle* is repeated on average every 28 days, reflecting the time required to follicular maturation and ovulation (Chap. 341). Essentially all pituitary hormone rhythms are entrained to sleep and to the *circadian cycle*, generating reproducible patterns that are repeated approximately every 24 h. The HPA axis, for example, exhibits characteristic peaks of ACTH and cortisol production in the early morning, with a nadir during the night. Recognition of these rhythms is important for endocrine testing and treatment. Patients with Cushing's syndrome characteristically exhibit increased midnight cortisol levels when compared to normal individuals (Chap. 336). In contrast, morning cortisol levels are similar in these groups, as cortisol is normally high at this time of day in normal individuals. The HPA axis is more susceptible to suppression by glucocorticoids administered at night as they blunt the early morning rise of ACTH. Understanding these rhythms allows glucocorticoid replacement that mimics diurnal production by administering larger doses in the morning than in the afternoon. Disrupted sleep rhythms can alter hormonal regulation. For example, sleep deprivation causes mild insulin resistance and hypertension, which are reversible at least in the short term.

Other endocrine rhythms occur on a more rapid time scale. Many peptide hormones are secreted in discrete bursts every few hours. LH and FSH secretion are exquisitely sensitive to GnRH pulse frequency. Intermittent pulses of GnRH are required to maintain pituitary sensitivity, whereas continuous exposure to GnRH causes pituitary gonadotrope desensitization. This feature of the hypothalamic-pituitary-gonadotrope axis forms the basis for using long-acting GnRH agonists to treat central precocious puberty or to decrease testosterone levels in the management of prostate cancer.

It is important to be aware of the pulsatile nature of hormone secretion and the rhythmic patterns of hormone production when relating serum hormone measurements to normal values. For some hormones,

FIGURE 332-3 Feedback regulation of endocrine axes. CNS, central nervous system.

TABLE 332-2 CAUSES OF ENDOCRINE DYSFUNCTION

Type of Endocrine Disorder	Examples
Hyperfunction	
Neoplastic	
Benign	Pituitary adenomas, hyperparathyroidism, autonomous thyroid or adrenal nodules, pheochromocytoma
Malignant	Adrenal cancer, medullary thyroid cancer, carcinoid
Ectopic	Ectopic ACTH, SIADH secretion
Multiple endocrine neoplasia	MEN 1, MEN 2
Autoimmune	Graves' disease
Iatrogenic	Cushing's syndrome, hypoglycemia
Infectious/inflammatory	Subacute thyroiditis
Activating receptor mutations	LH, TSH, Ca^{2+} and PTH receptors, G$_s\alpha$
Hypofunction	
Autoimmune	Hashimoto's thyroiditis, type 1 diabetes mellitus, Addison's disease, polyglandular failure
Iatrogenic	Radiation-induced hypopituitarism, hypothyroidism, surgical
Infectious/inflammatory	Adrenal insufficiency, hypothalamic sarcoidosis
Hormone mutations	GH, LHβ, FSHβ, vasopressin
Enzyme defects	21-Hydroxylase deficiency
Developmental defects	Kallmann syndrome, Turner syndrome, transcription factors
Nutritional/vitamin deficiency	Vitamin D deficiency, iodine deficiency
Hemorrhage/infarction	Sheehan's syndrome, adrenal insufficiency
Hormone resistance	
Receptor mutations	
Membrane	GH, vasopressin, LH, FSH, ACTH, GnRH, GHRH, PTH, leptin, Ca^{2+}
Nuclear	AR, TR, VDR, ER, GR, PPAR$_\gamma$
Signaling pathway mutations	Albright's hereditary osteodystrophy
Postreceptor	Type 2 diabetes mellitus, leptin resistance

Note: AR, androgen receptor; ER, estrogen receptor; GR, glucocorticoid receptor; PPAR, peroxisome proliferator activated receptor; SIADH, syndrome of inappropriate antidiuretic hormone; TR, thyroid hormone receptor; VDR, vitamin D receptor. For all other abbreviations, see text.

integrated markers have been developed to circumvent hormonal fluctuations. Examples include 24-h urine collections for cortisol, IGF-I as a biologic marker of GH action, and HbA1c as an index of long-term (weeks to months) blood glucose control.

Often, one must interpret endocrine data only in the context of other hormones. For example, PTH levels are typically assessed in combination with serum calcium concentrations. A high serum calcium level in association with elevated PTH is suggestive of hyperparathyroidism, whereas a suppressed PTH in this situation is more likely to be caused by hypercalcemia of malignancy or other causes of hypercalcemia. Similarly, TSH should be elevated when T$_4$ and T$_3$ concentrations are low, reflecting reduced feedback inhibition. When this is not the case, it is important to consider secondary hypothyroidism, which is caused by a defect at the level of the pituitary.

PATHOLOGIC MECHANISMS OF ENDOCRINE DISEASE

Endocrine diseases can be divided into three major types of conditions: (1) hormone excess, (2) hormone deficiency, and (3) hormone resistance (Table 332-2).

CAUSES OF HORMONE EXCESS

Syndromes of hormone excess can be caused by neoplastic growth of endocrine cells, autoimmune disorders, and excess hormone administration. Benign endocrine tumors, including parathyroid, pituitary, and adrenal adenomas, often retain the capacity to produce hormones, perhaps reflecting the fact that they are relatively well differentiated.

Many endocrine tumors exhibit subtle defects in their "set points" for feedback regulation. For example, in Cushing's disease, impaired feedback inhibition of ACTH secretion is associated with autonomous function. However, the tumor cells are not completely resistant to feedback, as evidenced by ACTH suppression by higher doses of dexamethasone (e.g., high-dose dexamethasone test) (Chap. 336). Similar set point defects are also typical of parathyroid adenomas and autonomously functioning thyroid nodules.

The molecular basis of some endocrine tumors, such as the MEN syndromes (MEN 1, 2A, 2B), have provided important insights into tumorigenesis (Chap. 345). MEN 1 is characterized primarily by the triad of parathyroid, pancreatic islet, and pituitary tumors. MEN 2 predisposes to medullary thyroid carcinoma, pheochromocytoma, and hyperparathyroidism. The *MEN1* gene, located on chromosome 11q13, encodes a putative tumor-suppressor gene, menin. Analogous to the paradigm first described for retinoblastoma, the affected individual inherits a mutant copy of the *MEN1* gene, and tumorigenesis ensues after a somatic "second hit" leads to loss of function of the normal *MEN1* gene (through deletion or point mutations).

In contrast to inactivation of a tumor-suppressor gene, as occurs in MEN 1 and most other inherited cancer syndromes, MEN 2 is caused by activating mutations in a single allele. In this case, activating mutations of the *RET* protooncogene, which encodes a receptor tyrosine kinase, leads to thyroid C cell hyperplasia in childhood before the development of medullary thyroid carcinoma. Elucidation of this pathogenic mechanism has allowed early genetic screening for *RET* mutations in individuals at risk for MEN 2, permitting identification of those who may benefit from prophylactic thyroidectomy and biochemical screening for pheochromocytoma and hyperparathyroidism.

Mutations that activate hormone receptor signaling have been identified in several GPCRs. For example, activating mutations of the LH receptor cause a dominantly transmitted form of male-limited precocious puberty, reflecting premature stimulation of testosterone synthesis in Leydig cells (Chap. 340). Activating mutations in these GPCRs are predominantly located in the transmembrane domains and induce receptor coupling to G$_s\alpha$, even in the absence of hormone. Consequently, adenylate cyclase is activated, and cyclic AMP levels increase in a manner that mimics hormone action. A similar phenomenon results from activating mutations in G$_s\alpha$. When these occur early in development, they cause McCune-Albright syndrome. When they occur only in somatotropes, the activating G$_s\alpha$ mutations cause GH-secreting tumors and acromegaly (Chap. 333).

In autoimmune Graves' disease, antibody interactions with the TSH receptor mimic TSH action, leading to hormone overproduction (Chap. 335). Analogous to the effects of activating mutations of the TSH receptor, these stimulating autoantibodies induce conformational changes that release the receptor from a constrained state, thereby triggering receptor coupling to G proteins.

CAUSES OF HORMONE DEFICIENCY

Most examples of hormone deficiency states can be attributed to glandular destruction caused by autoimmunity, surgery, infection, inflammation, infarction, hemorrhage, or tumor infiltration (Table 332-2). Autoimmune damage to the thyroid gland (Hashimoto's thyroiditis) and pancreatic islet β cells (type 1 diabetes mellitus) is a prevalent cause of endocrine disease. Mutations in a number of hormones, hormone receptors, transcription factors, enzymes, and channels can also lead to hormone deficiencies.

HORMONE RESISTANCE

Most severe hormone resistance syndromes are due to inherited defects in membrane receptors, nuclear receptors, or the pathways that transduce receptor signals. These disorders are characterized by defective hormone action, despite the presence of increased hormone levels. In complete androgen resistance, for example, mutations in the androgen receptor a female phenotypic appearance in genetic (XY) males, even though LH and testosterone levels are increased (Chap. 343). In addition to these relatively rare genetic disorders, more common acquired forms of functional hormone resistance include insulin resistance in type 2 diabetes mellitus, leptin resistance in obesity, and GH resistance in catabolic states. The pathogenesis of functional resistance involves receptor downregulation and postreceptor desensitization of signaling pathways; functional forms of resistance are generally reversible.

APPROACH TO THE PATIENT:
Endocrine Disease

Because endocrinology interfaces with numerous physiologic systems, there is no standard endocrine history and examination. Moreover, because most glands are relatively inaccessible, the examination usually focuses on the manifestations of hormone excess or deficiency, as well as direct examination of palpable glands, such as the thyroid and gonads. For these reasons, it is important to evaluate patients in the context of their presenting symptoms, review of systems, family and social history, and exposure to medications that may affect the endocrine system. Astute clinical skills are required to detect subtle symptoms and signs suggestive of underlying endocrine disease. For example, a patient with Cushing's syndrome may manifest specific findings, such as central fat redistribution, striae, and proximal muscle weakness, in addition to features seen commonly in the general population, such as obesity, plethora, hypertension, and glucose intolerance. Similarly, the insidious onset of hypothyroidism—with mental slowing, fatigue, dry skin, and other features—can be difficult to distinguish from similar, nonspecific findings in the general population. Clinical judgment, based on knowledge of disease prevalence and pathophysiology, is required to decide when to embark on more extensive evaluation of these disorders. Laboratory testing plays an essential role in endocrinology by allowing quantitative assessment of hormone levels and dynamics. Radiologic imaging tests, such as CT scan, MRI, thyroid scan, and ultrasound, are also used for the diagnosis of endocrine disorders. However, these tests are generally employed only after a hormonal abnormality has been established by biochemical testing.

HORMONE MEASUREMENTS AND ENDOCRINE TESTING Radioimmunoassays are the most important diagnostic tool in endocrinology, as they allow sensitive, specific, and quantitative determination of steady-state and dynamic changes in hormone concentrations. Radioimmunoassays use antibodies to detect specific hormones. For many peptide hormones, these measurements are now configured to use two different antibodies to increase binding affinity and specificity. There are many variations of these assays; a common format involves using one antibody to capture the antigen (hormone) onto an immobilized surface and a second antibody, coupled to a chemilumenescent (ICMA) or radioactive (IRMA) signal to detect the antigen. These assays are sensitive enough to detect plasma hormone concentrations in the picomolar to nanomolar range, and they can readily distinguish structurally related proteins, such as PTH from PTHrP. A variety of other techniques are used to measure specific hormones, including mass spectroscopy, various forms of chromatography, and enzymatic methods; bioassays are now rarely used.

Most hormone measurements are based on plasma or serum samples. However, urinary hormone determinations remain useful for the evaluation of some conditions. Urinary collections over 24 h provide an integrated assessment of the production of a hormone or metabolite, many of which vary during the day. It is important to assure complete collections of 24-h urine samples; simultaneous measurement of creatinine provides an internal control for the adequacy of collection and can be used to normalize some hormone measurements. A 24-h urine free cortisol measurement largely reflects the amount of unbound cortisol, thus providing a reasonable index of biologically available hormone. Other commonly used urine determinations include 17-hydroxycorticosteroids, 17-ketosteroids, vanillylmandelic acid, metanephrine, catecholamines, 5-hydroxyindoleacetic acid, and calcium.

The value of quantitative hormone measurements lies in their correct interpretation in a clinical context. The normal range for most hormones is relatively broad, often varying by a factor of two- to tenfold. The normal ranges for many hormones are gender- and age-specific. Thus, using the correct normative database is an essential part of interpreting hormone tests. The pulsatile nature of hormones and factors that can affect their secretion, such as sleep, meals, and medications, must also be considered. Cortisol values increase fivefold between midnight and dawn; reproductive hormone levels vary dramatically during the female menstrual cycle.

For many endocrine systems, much information can be gained from basal hormone testing, particularly when different components of an endocrine axis are assessed simultaneously. For example, low testosterone and elevated LH levels suggest a primary gonadal problem, whereas a hypothalamic-pituitary disorder is likely if both LH and testosterone are low. Because TSH is a sensitive indicator of thyroid function, it is generally recommended as a first-line test for thyroid disorders. An elevated TSH level is almost always the result of primary hypothyroidism, whereas a low TSH is most often caused by thyrotoxicosis. These predictions can be confirmed by determining the free thyroxine level. Elevated calcium and PTH levels suggest hyperparathyroidism, whereas PTH is suppressed in hypercalcemia caused by malignancy or granulomatous diseases. A suppressed ACTH in the setting of hypercortisolemia, or increased urine free cortisol, is seen with hyperfunctioning adrenal adenomas.

It is not uncommon, however, for baseline hormone levels associated with pathologic endocrine conditions to overlap with the normal range. In this circumstance, dynamic testing is useful to further separate the two groups. There are a multitude of dynamic endocrine tests, but all are based on principles of feedback regulation, and most responses can be remembered based on the pathways that govern endocrine axes. *Suppression tests* are used in the setting of suspected endocrine hyperfunction. An example is the dexamethasone suppression test used to evaluate Cushing's syndrome (Chaps. 333 and 336). *Stimulation tests* are generally used to assess endocrine hypofunction. The ACTH stimulation test, for example, is used to assess the adrenal gland response in patients with suspected adrenal insufficiency. Other stimulation tests use hypothalamic-releasing factors such as TRH, GnRH, CRH, and GHRH to evaluate pituitary hormone reserve (Chap. 333). Insulin-induced hypoglycemia evokes pituitary ACTH and GH responses. Stimulation tests based on reduction or inhibition of endogenous hormones are now used infrequently. Examples include metyrapone inhibition of cortisol synthesis and clomiphene inhibition of estrogen feedback.

SCREENING AND ASSESSMENT OF COMMON ENDOCRINE DISORDERS Many endocrine disorders are prevalent in the adult population (Table 332-3) and can be diagnosed and managed by general internists, family practitioners, or other primary health care providers. The high prevalence and clinical impact of certain endocrine diseases justifies vigilance for features of these disorders during routine physical examinations; laboratory screening is indicated in selected high-risk populations.

TABLE 332-3 EXAMPLES OF PREVALENT ENDOCRINE AND METABOLIC DISORDERS IN THE ADULT

Disorder	Approx. Prevalence in Adults[a]	Screening/Testing Recommendations[b]	Chapter
Obesity	31% BMI ≥30 65% BMI ≥25	Calculate BMI Measure waist circumference Exclude secondary causes Consider comorbid complications	75

Type 2 diabetes mellitus	>7%	Beginning at age 45, screen every 3 years, or earlier in high-risk groups:
		   Fasting plasma glucose (FPG) > 126 mg/dL
		   Random plasma glucose > 200 mg/dL
		An elevated HbA1c
		Consider comorbid complications
			338

Hyperlipidemia	20–25%	Cholesterol screening at least every 5 years; more often in high-risk groups Lipoprotein analysis (LDL, HDL) for increased cholesterol, CAD, diabetes Consider secondary causes	350
Hypothyroidism	5–10%, women 0.5–2%, men	TSH; confirm with free T$_4$ Screen women after age 35 and every 5 years thereafter	335
Graves' disease	1–3%, women 0.1%, men	TSH, free T$_4$	335
Thyroid nodules and neoplasia	5% palpable >25% by ultrasound	Physical examination of thyroid Fine-needle aspiration biopsy	335
Osteoporosis	5–10%, women 2–4%, men	Bone mineral density measurements in women >65 years or in postmenopausal women or men at risk Exclude secondary causes	348
Hyperparathyroidism	0.1–0.5%, women > men	Serum calcium PTH, if calcium is elevated Assess comorbid conditions	347
Infertility	10%, couples	Investigate both members of couple Semen analysis in male Assess ovulatory cycles in female Specific tests as indicated	340, 341
Polycystic ovarian syndrome	5–10%, women	Free testosterone, DHEAS Consider comorbid conditions	341
Hirsutism	5–10%	Free testosterone, DHEAS Exclude secondary causes Additional tests as indicated	50
Menopause	Median age, 51	FSH	342
Hyperprolactinemia	15% in women with amenorrhea or galactorrhea	PRL level MRI, if not medication-related	333
Erectile dysfunction	20–30%	Careful history, PRL, testosterone Consider secondary causes (e.g., diabetes)	49
Gynecomastia	15%	Often, no tests are indicated Consider Klinefelter syndrome Consider medications, hypogonadism, liver disease	340
Klinefelter syndrome	0.2%, men	Karyotype Testosterone	343
Turner syndrome	0.03%, women	Karyotype Consider comorbid conditions	343

[a]The prevalence of most disorders varies among ethnic groups and with aging. Data based primarily on U.S. population.

[b]See individual chapters for additional information on evaluation and treatment. Early test-ing is indicated in patients with signs and symptoms of disease or in those at increased risk.

Note: BMI, body mass index; CAD, coronary artery disease; DHEAS, dehydroepiandrosterone; HDL, high-density lipoprotein; LDL, low-density lipoprotein. For other abbreviations, see text.

FURTHER READINGS

DeGroot LJ, Jameson JL (eds): *Endocrinology*, 5th ed. Philadelphia, Elsevier, 2006

Hammes A et al: Role of endocytosis in cellular uptake of sex steroids. Cell 122:751, 2005

Leo CP et al: Hormonal genomics. Endocr Rev 23:369, 2002

Marx SJ, Simonds WF: Hereditary hormone excess: Genes, molecular pathways, and syndromes. Endocr Rev 26:615, 2005

Smith CL et al: Coregulator function: A key to understanding tissue specificity of selective receptor modulators. Endocr Rev 25:45, 2004

Weinstein LS et al: Minireview: GNAS: Normal and abnormal functions. Endocrinology 145:5459, 2004

333 Disorders of the Anterior Pituitary and Hypothalamus

Shlomo Melmed, J. Larry Jameson

The anterior pituitary is often referred to as the "master gland" because, together with the hypothalamus, it orchestrates the complex regulatory functions of multiple other endocrine glands. The anterior pituitary gland produces six major hormones: (1) prolactin (PRL), (2) growth hormone (GH), (3) adrenocorticotropin hormone (ACTH), (4) luteinizing hormone (LH), (5) follicle-stimulating hormone (FSH), and (6) thyroid-stimulating hormone (TSH) (Table 333-1). Pituitary hormones are secreted in a pulsatile manner, reflecting stimulation by an array of specific hypothalamic releasing factors. Each of these pituitary hormones elicits specific responses in peripheral target tissues. The hormonal products of these peripheral glands, in turn, exert feedback control at the level of the hypothalamus and pituitary to modulate pituitary function (Fig. 333-1). Pituitary tumors cause char-

TABLE 333-1   ANTERIOR PITUITARY HORMONE EXPRESSION AND REGULATION

Cell	Corticotrope	Somatotrope	Lactotrope	Thyrotrope	Gonadotrope
Tissue-specific transcription factor	T-Pit	Prop-1, Pit-1	Prop-1, Pit-1	Prop-1, Pit-1, TEF	SF-1, DAX-1
Fetal appearance	6 weeks	8 weeks	12 weeks	12 weeks	12 weeks
Hormone	POMC	GH	PRL	TSH	FSH LH
Chromosomal locus	2p	17q	6	α–6q; β-1p	β-11p; β-19q
Protein	Polypeptide	Polypeptide	Polypeptide	Glycoprotein α, β subunits	Glycoprotein α, β subunits
Amino acids	266 (ACTH 1–39)	191	199	211	210 204
Stimulators	CRH, AVP, gp-130 cytokines	GHRH, Ghrelin	Estrogen, TRH, VIP	TRH	GnRH, activins, estrogen
Inhibitors	Glucocorticoids	Somatostatin, IGF-I	Dopamine	T_3, T_4, dopamine, somatostatin, glucocorticoids	Sex steroids, inhibin
Target gland	Adrenal	Liver, other tissues	Breast, other tissues	Thyroid	Ovary, testis
Trophic effect	Steroid production	IGF-I production, growth induction, insulin antagonism	Milk production	T_4 synthesis and secretion	Sex steroid production, follicle growth, germ cell maturation
Normal range	ACTH, 4–22 pg/L	<0.5 µg/L[a]	M < 15; F <20 µg/L	0.1–5 mU/L	M, 5–20 IU/L, F (basal), 5–20 IU/L

[a]Hormone secretion integrated over 24 h.

Note: M, male; F, female. For other abbreviations, see text.

Source: Adapted from I Shimon, S Melmed, in S Melmed, P Conn (eds): *Endocrinology: Basic and Clinical Principles*. Totowa, NJ, Humana, 2005.

PART 15
Endocrinology and Metabolism

acteristic hormone excess syndromes. Hormone deficiency may be inherited or acquired. Fortunately, efficacious treatments exist for the various pituitary hormone excess and deficiency syndromes. Nonetheless, these diagnoses are often elusive, emphasizing the importance of recognizing subtle clinical manifestations and performing the correct laboratory diagnostic tests. For discussion of disorders of the posterior pituitary, or neurohypophysis, see Chap. 334.

ANATOMY AND DEVELOPMENT

ANATOMY

The pituitary gland weighs ~600 mg and is located within the sella turcica ventral to the diaphragma sella; it comprises anatomically and functionally distinct anterior and posterior lobes. The sella is contiguous to vascular and neurologic structures, including the cavernous sinuses, cranial nerves, and optic chiasm. Thus, expanding intrasellar pathologic processes may have significant central mass effects in addition to their endocrinologic impact.

Hypothalamic neural cells synthesize specific releasing and inhibiting hormones that are secreted directly into the portal vessels of the pituitary stalk. Blood supply of the pituitary gland is derived from the superior and inferior hypophyseal arteries (Fig. 333-2). The hypothalamic-pituitary portal plexus provides the major blood source for the anterior pituitary, allowing reliable transmission of hypothalamic peptide pulses without significant systemic dilution; consequently, pituitary cells are exposed to releasing or inhibiting factors and in turn release their hormones as discrete pulses (Fig. 333-3).

The posterior pituitary is supplied by the inferior hypophyseal arteries. In contrast to the anterior pituitary, the posterior lobe is directly innervated by hypothalamic neurons (supraopticohypophyseal and tuberohypophyseal nerve tracts) via the pituitary stalk (Chap. 334). Thus, posterior pituitary production of vasopressin [antidiuretic hormone (ADH)] and oxytocin is particularly sensitive to neuronal damage by lesions that affect the pituitary stalk or hypothalamus.

PITUITARY DEVELOPMENT

The embryonic differentiation and maturation of anterior pituitary cells have been elucidated in considerable detail. Pituitary development from Rathke's pouch involves a complex interplay of lineage-specific transcription factors expressed in pluripotent stem cells and gradients of locally produced growth factors (Table 333-1). The transcription factor Pit-1 determines cell-specific expression of GH, PRL, and TSH in somatotropes, lactotropes, and thyrotropes. Expression of high levels of estrogen receptors in cells that contain Pit-1 favors PRL expression, whereas thyrotrope embryonic factor (TEF) induces TSH expression. Pit-1 binds to GH, PRL, and TSH gene regulatory ele-

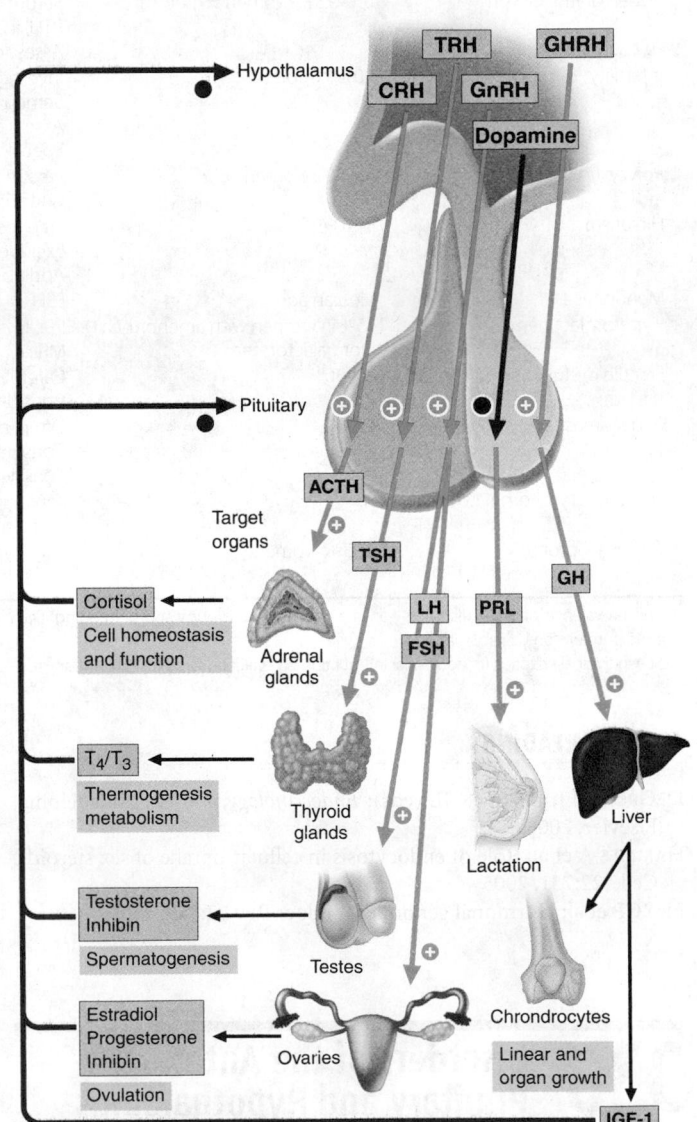

FIGURE 333-1 Diagram of pituitary axes. Hypothalamic hormones regulate anterior pituitary trophic hormones that, in turn, determine target gland secretion. Peripheral hormones feed back to regulate hypothalamic and pituitary hormones. For abbreviations, see text.

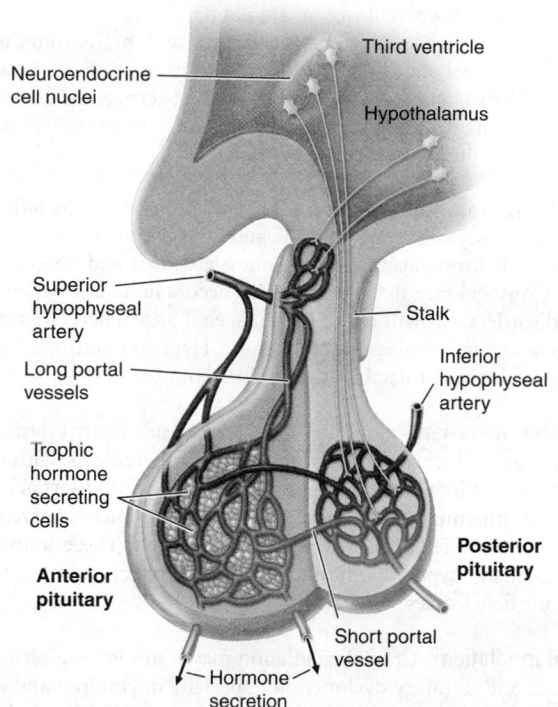

FIGURE 333-2 Diagram of hypothalamic-pituitary vasculature. The hypothalamic nuclei produce hormones that traverse the portal system and impinge on anterior pituitary cells to regulate pituitary hormone secretion. Posterior pituitary hormones are derived from direct neural extensions.

ments, as well as to recognition sites on its own promoter, providing a mechanism for perpetuating selective pituitary phenotypic stability. The transcription factor Prop-1 induces the pituitary development of Pit-1-specific lineages, as well as gonadotropes. Gonadotrope cell development is further defined by the cell-specific expression of the nuclear receptors, steroidogenic factor (SF-1) and DAX-1. Development of corticotrope cells, which express the proopiomelanocortin (POMC) gene, requires the T-Pit transcription factor. Abnormalities of pituitary development caused by mutations of Pit-1, Prop-1, SF-1, DAX-1, and T-Pit result in a series of rare, selective or combined, pituitary hormone deficits.

HYPOTHALAMIC AND ANTERIOR PITUITARY INSUFFICIENCY

Hypopituitarism results from impaired production of one or more of the anterior pituitary trophic hormones. Reduced pituitary function can result from inherited disorders; more commonly, it is acquired and reflects the mass effects of tumors or the consequences of inflammation or vascular damage. These processes may also impair synthesis or secretion of hypothalamic hormones, with resultant pituitary failure (Table 333-2).

FIGURE 333-3 Hypothalamic gonadotropin-releasing hormone (GnRH) pulses induce secretory pulses of luteinizing hormone (LH).

TABLE 333-2	ETIOLOGY OF HYPOPITUITARISM^a

Development/structural
  Transcription factor defect
  Pituitary dysplasia/aplasia
  Congenital CNS mass, encephalocele
  Primary empty sella
  Congenital hypothalamic disorders (septo-optic dysplasia, Prader-Willi syndrome, Laurence-Moon-Biedl syndrome, Kallmann syndrome)
Traumatic
  Surgical resection
  Radiation damage
  Head injuries
Neoplastic
  Pituitary adenoma
  Parasellar mass (meningioma, germinoma, ependymoma, glioma)
  Rathke's cyst
  Craniopharyngioma
  Hypothalamic hamartoma, gangliocytoma
  Pituitary metastases (breast, lung, colon carcinoma)
  Lymphoma and leukemia
  Meningioma
Infiltrative/inflammatory
  Lymphocytic hypophysitis
  Hemochromatosis
  Sarcoidosis
  Histiocytosis X
  Granulomatous hypophysitis
Vascular
  Pituitary apoplexy
  Pregnancy-related (infarction with diabetes; postpartum necrosis)
  Sickle cell disease
  Arteritis
Infections
  Fungal (histoplasmosis)
  Parasitic (toxoplasmosis)
  Tuberculosis
  Pneumocystis carinii

^{a}Trophic hormone failure associated with pituitary compression or destruction usually occurs sequentially GH > FSH > LH > TSH > ACTH. During childhood, growth retardation is often the presenting feature, and in adults hypogonadism is the earliest symptom.

DEVELOPMENTAL AND GENETIC CAUSES OF HYPOPITUITARISM

Pituitary Dysplasia Pituitary dysplasia may result in aplastic, hypoplastic, or ectopic pituitary gland development. Because pituitary development requires midline cell migration from the nasopharyngeal Rathke's pouch, midline craniofacial disorders may be associated with pituitary dysplasia. Acquired pituitary failure in the newborn can also be caused by birth trauma, including cranial hemorrhage, asphyxia, and breech delivery.

SEPTO-OPTIC DYSPLASIA Hypothalamic dysfunction and hypopituitarism may result from dysgenesis of the septum pellucidum or corpus callosum. Affected children have mutations in the *HESX1* gene, which is involved in early development of the ventral prosencephalon. These children exhibit variable combinations of cleft palate, syndactyly, ear deformities, hypertelorism, optic atrophy, micropenis, and anosmia. Pituitary dysfunction leads to diabetes insipidus, GH deficiency and short stature, and, occasionally, TSH deficiency.

Tissue-Specific Factor Mutations Several pituitary cell–specific transcription factors, such as Pit-1 and Prop-1, are critical for determining the development and function of specific anterior pituitary cell lineages. Autosomal dominant or recessive Pit-1 mutations cause combined GH, PRL, and TSH deficiencies. These patients present with growth failure and varying degrees of hypothyroidism. The pituitary may appear hypoplastic on magnetic resonance imaging (MRI).

Prop-1 is expressed early in pituitary development and appears to be required for Pit-1 function. Familial and sporadic *PROP1* mutations result in combined GH, PRL, TSH, and gonadotropin deficiency. Over 80% of these patients have growth retardation; by adulthood, all are deficient in TSH and gonadotropins, and a small minority later develop ACTH deficiency. Because of gonadotropin deficiency, they do not enter puberty spontaneously. In some cases, the pituitary gland is enlarged. *TPIT* mutations result in ACTH deficiency associated with hypocortisolism.

Developmental Hypothalamic Dysfunction • *KALLMANN SYNDROME* This syndrome results from defective hypothalamic gonadotropin-releasing hormone (GnRH) synthesis and is associated with anosmia or hyposmia due to olfactory bulb agenesis or hypoplasia (Chap. 340). The syndrome may also be associated with color blindness, optic atrophy, nerve deafness, cleft palate, renal abnormalities, cryptorchidism, and neurologic abnormalities such as mirror movements. Defects in the *KAL* gene, which maps to chromosome Xp22.3, prevent embryonic migration of GnRH neurons from the hypothalamic olfactory placode to the hypothalamus. Genetic abnormalities, in addition to *KAL* mutations, can also cause isolated GnRH deficiency, as autosomal recessive (i.e., *GPR54*) and dominant (i.e., *FGFR1*) modes of transmission have been described. GnRH deficiency prevents progression through puberty. Males present with delayed puberty and pronounced hypogonadal features, including micropenis, probably the result of low testosterone levels during infancy. Female patients present with primary amenorrhea and failure of secondary sexual development.

Kallmann syndrome and other causes of congenital GnRH deficiency are characterized by low LH and FSH levels and low concentrations of sex steroids (testosterone or estradiol). In sporadic cases of isolated gonadotropin deficiency, the diagnosis is often one of exclusion after eliminating other causes of hypothalamic-pituitary dysfunction. Repetitive GnRH administration restores normal pituitary gonadotropin responses, pointing to a hypothalamic defect.

Long-term treatment of men with human chorionic gonadotropin (hCG) or testosterone restores pubertal development and secondary sex characteristics; women can be treated with cyclic estrogen and progestin. Fertility may also be restored by the administration of gonadotropins or by using a portable infusion pump to deliver subcutaneous, pulsatile GnRH.

BARDET-BIEDL SYNDROME This is a rare genetically heterogeneous disorder characterized by mental retardation, renal abnormalities, obesity, and hexadactyly, brachydactyly, or syndactyly. Central diabetes insipidus may or may not be associated. GnRH deficiency occurs in 75% of males and half of affected females. Retinal degeneration begins in early childhood, and most patients are blind by age 30. Ten subtypes of Bardet-Biedl syndrome (BBS) have been identified with genetic linkage to nine different loci. Several of the loci encode genes involved in basal body cilia function, which may account for the diverse clinical manifestations.

LEPTIN AND LEPTIN RECEPTOR MUTATIONS Deficiencies of leptin, or its receptor, cause a broad spectrum of hypothalamic abnormalities including hyperphagia, obesity, and central hypogonadism (Chap. 74). Decreased GnRH production in these patients results in attenuated pituitary FSH and LH synthesis and release.

Prader-Willi Syndrome This is a contiguous gene syndrome resulting from deletion of the paternal copies of the imprinted *SNRPN* gene, the *NECDIN* gene, and possibly other genes on chromosome 15q. Prader-Willi Syndrome is associated with hypogonadotropic hypogonadism, hyperphagia-obesity, chronic muscle hypotonia, mental retardation, and adult-onset diabetes mellitus (Chap. 63). Multiple somatic defects also involve the skull, eyes, ears, hands, and feet. Diminished hypothalamic oxytocin- and vasopressin-producing nuclei have been reported. Deficient GnRH synthesis is suggested by the observation that chronic GnRH treatment restores pituitary LH and FSH release.

ACQUIRED HYPOPITUITARISM
Hypopituitarism may be caused by accidental or neurosurgical trauma; vascular events such as apoplexy; pituitary or hypothalamic neoplasms such as pituitary adenomas, craniopharyngiomas, lymphoma, or metastatic tumors; inflammatory disease such as lymphocytic hy-

pophysitis; infiltrative disorders such as sarcoidosis, hemochromatosis (Chap. 351), and tuberculosis; or irradiation.

Increasing evidence suggests that patients with brain injury including trauma, subarachnoid hemorrhage, and irradiation have transient hypopituitarism and require intermittent long-term endocrine follow-up, as permanent hypothalamic or pituitary dysfunction will develop in 25–40% of these patients.

Hypothalamic Infiltration Disorders These disorders—including sarcoidosis, histiocytosis X, amyloidosis, and hemochromatosis—frequently involve both hypothalamic and pituitary neuronal and neurochemical tracts. Consequently, diabetes insipidus occurs in half of patients with these disorders. Growth retardation is seen if attenuated GH secretion occurs before pubertal epiphyseal closure. Hypogonadotropic hypogonadism and hyperprolactinemia are also common.

Inflammatory Lesions Pituitary damage and subsequent dysfunction can be seen with chronic infections such as tuberculosis, with opportunistic fungal infections associated with AIDS, and in tertiary syphilis. Other inflammatory processes, such as granulomas or sarcoidosis, may mimic the features of a pituitary adenoma. These lesions may cause extensive hypothalamic and pituitary damage, leading to trophic hormone deficiencies.

Cranial Irradiation Cranial irradiation may result in long-term hypothalamic and pituitary dysfunction, especially in children and adolescents, as they are more susceptible to damage following whole-brain or head and neck therapeutic irradiation. The development of hormonal abnormalities correlates strongly with irradiation dosage and the time interval after completion of radiotherapy. Up to two-thirds of patients ultimately develop hormone insufficiency after a median dose of 50 Gy (5000 rad) directed at the skull base. The development of hypopituitarism occurs over 5–15 years and usually reflects hypothalamic damage rather than primary destruction of pituitary cells. Although the pattern of hormone loss is variable, GH deficiency is most common, followed by gonadotropin and ACTH deficiency. When deficiency of one or more hormones is documented, the possibility of diminished reserve of other hormones is likely. Accordingly, anterior pituitary function should be evaluated over the long term in previously irradiated patients, and replacement therapy instituted when appropriate (see below).

Lymphocytic Hypophysitis This often occurs in postpartum women; it usually presents with hyperprolactinemia and MRI evidence of a prominent pituitary mass often resembling an adenoma, with mildly elevated PRL levels. Pituitary failure caused by diffuse lymphocytic infiltration may be transient or permanent but requires immediate evaluation and treatment. Rarely, isolated pituitary hormone deficiencies have been described, suggesting a selective autoimmune process targeted to specific cell types. Most patients manifest symptoms of progressive mass effects with headache and visual disturbance. The erythrocyte sedimentation rate is often elevated. As the MRI image may be indistinguishable from that of a pituitary adenoma, hypophysitis should be considered in a postpartum woman with a newly diagnosed pituitary mass before embarking on unnecessary surgical intervention. The inflammatory process often resolves after several months of glucocorticoid treatment, and pituitary function may be restored, depending on the extent of damage.

Pituitary Apoplexy Acute intrapituitary hemorrhagic vascular events can cause substantial damage to the pituitary and surrounding sellar structures. Pituitary apoplexy may occur spontaneously in a preexisting adenoma; post-partum (Sheehan's syndrome); or in association with diabetes, hypertension, sickle cell anemia, or acute shock. The hyperplastic enlargement of the pituitary during pregnancy increases the risk for hemorrhage and infarction. Apoplexy is an endocrine emergency that may result in severe hypoglycemia, hypotension, central nervous system (CNS) hemorrhage, and death. Acute symptoms may include

TABLE 333-3 TESTS OF PITUITARY SUFFICIENCY

Hormone	Test	Blood Samples	Interpretation
Growth hormone	Insulin tolerance test: Regular insulin (0.05–0.15 U/kg IV)	–30, 0, 30, 60, 120 min for glucose and GH	Glucose < 40 mg/dL; GH should be >3 µg/L
	GHRH test: 1 µg/kg IV	0, 15, 30, 45, 60, 120 min for GH	Normal response is GH >3 µg/L
	L-Arginine test: 30 g IV over 30 min	0, 30, 60, 120 min for GH	Normal response is GH >3 µg/L
	L-dopa test: 500 mg PO	0, 30, 60, 120 min for GH	Normal response is GH >3 µg/L
Prolactin	TRH test: 200–500 µg IV	0, 20, and 60 min for TSH and PRL	Normal prolactin is >2 µg/L and increase >200% of baseline
ACTH	Insulin tolerance test: Regular insulin (0.05–0.15 U/kg IV)	–30, 0, 30, 60, 90 min for glucose and cortisol	Glucose <40 mg/dL Cortisol should increase by >7 µg/dL or to >20 µg/dL
	CRH test: 1 µg/kg ovine CRH IV at 0800 h	0, 15, 30, 60, 90, 120 min for ACTH and cortisol	Basal ACTH increases 2- to 4-fold and peaks at 20–100 pg/mL Cortisol levels >20–25 µg/dL
	Metyrapone test: Metyrapone (30 mg/kg) at midnight	Plasma 11-deoxycortisol and cortisol at 8 A.M.; ACTH can also be measured	Plasma cortisol should be <4 µg/dL to assure an adequate response Normal response is 11 deoxycortisol >7.5 µg/dL or ACTH >75 pg/mL
	Standard ACTH stimulation test: ACTH 1-24 (Cosyntropin), 0.25 mg IM or IV	0, 30, 60 min for cortisol and aldosterone	Normal response is cortisol >21 µg/dL and aldosterone response of >4 ng/dL above baseline
	Low-dose ACTH test: ACTH 1-24 (Cosyntropin), 1 µg IV	0, 30, 60 min for cortisol	Cortisol should be >21 µg/dL
	3-day ACTH stimulation test consists of 0.25 mg ACTH 1-24 given IV over 8 h each day		Cortisol >21 µg/dL
TSH	Basal thyroid function tests: T₄, T₃, TSH	Basal tests	Low free thyroid hormone levels in the setting of TSH levels that are not appropriately increased
	TRH test: 200–500 µg IV	0, 20, 60 min for TSH and PRL[a]	TSH should increase by >5 mU/L unless thyroid hormone levels are increased
LH, FSH	LH, FSH, testosterone, estrogen	Basal tests	Basal LH and FSH should be increased in postmenopausal women Low testosterone levels in the setting of low LH and FSH
	GnRH test: GnRH (100 µg) IV	0, 30, 60 min for LH and FSH	In most adults, LH should increase by 10 IU/L and FSH by 2 IU/L Normal responses are variable
Multiple hormones	Combined anterior pituitary test: GHRH (1 µg/kg), CRH (1 µg/kg), GnRH (100 µg), TRH (200 µg) are given IV	–30, 0, 15, 30, 60, 90, 120 min for GH, ACTH, cortisol, LH, FSH, and TSH	Combined or individual releasing hormone responses must be elevated in the context of basal target gland hormone values and may not be uniformly diagnostic (see text)

[a]Evoked PRL response indicates lactotrope integrity.

Note: For abbreviations, see text.

severe headache with signs of meningeal irritation, bilateral visual changes, ophthalmoplegia, and, in severe cases, cardiovascular collapse and loss of consciousness. Pituitary computed tomography (CT) or MRI may reveal signs of intratumoral or sellar hemorrhage, with deviation of the pituitary stalk and compression of pituitary tissue.

Patients with no evident visual loss or impaired consciousness can be observed and managed conservatively with high-dose glucocorticoids. Those with significant or progressive visual loss or loss of consciousness require urgent surgical decompression. Visual recovery after surgery is inversely correlated with the length of time after the acute event. Therefore, severe ophthalmoplegia or visual deficits are indications for early surgery. Hypopituitarism is very common after apoplexy.

Empty Sella A partial or apparently totally empty sella is often an incidental MRI finding. These patients usually have normal pituitary function, implying that the surrounding rim of pituitary tissue is fully functional. Hypopituitarism, however, may develop insidiously. Pituitary masses may undergo clinically silent infarction with development of a partial or totally empty sella by cerebrospinal fluid (CSF) filling the dural herniation. Rarely, small but functional pituitary adenomas may arise within the rim of pituitary tissue, and these are not always visible on MRI.

PRESENTATION AND DIAGNOSIS

The clinical manifestations of hypopituitarism depend on which hormones are lost and the extent of the hormone deficiency. GH deficien-

cy causes growth disorders in children and leads to abnormal body composition in adults (see below). Gonadotropin deficiency causes menstrual disorders and infertility in women and decreased sexual function, infertility, and loss of secondary sexual characteristics in men. TSH and ACTH deficiency usually develop later in the course of pituitary failure. TSH deficiency causes growth retardation in children and features of hypothyroidism in children and in adults. The secondary form of adrenal insufficiency caused by ACTH deficiency leads to hypocortisolism with relative preservation of mineralocorticoid production. PRL deficiency causes failure of lactation. When lesions involve the posterior pituitary, polyuria and polydipsia reflect loss of vasopressin secretion. Epidemiologic studies have documented an increased mortality rate in patients with longstanding pituitary damage, primarily from increased cardiovascular and cerebrovascular disease.

LABORATORY INVESTIGATION

Biochemical diagnosis of pituitary insufficiency is made by demonstrating low levels of trophic hormones in the setting of low target hormone levels. For example, low free thyroxine in the setting of a low or inappropriately normal TSH level suggests secondary hypothyroidism. Similarly, a low testosterone level without elevation of gonadotropins suggests hypogonadotropic hypogonadism. Provocative tests may be required to assess pituitary reserve (Table 333-3). GH responses to insulin-induced hypoglycemia, arginine, L-dopa, growth hormone–releasing hormone (GHRH), or growth hormone–releasing peptides (GHRPs) can be used to assess GH reserve. Corticotropin-releasing

TABLE 333-4 HORMONE REPLACEMENT THERAPY FOR ADULT HYPOPITUITARISM[a]

Trophic Hormone Deficit	Hormone Replacement
ACTH	Hydrocortisone (10–20 mg A.M.; 5–10 mg P.M.)
	Cortisone acetate (25 mg A.M.; 12.5 mg P.M.)
	Prednisone (5 mg A.M.; 2.5 mg P.M.)
TSH	L-Thyroxine (0.075–0.15 mg daily)
FSH/LH	Males
	Testosterone enanthate (200 mg IM every 2 weeks)
	Testosterone skin patch (5 mg/d)
	Females
	Conjugated estrogen (0.65–1.25 mg qd for 25 days)
	Progesterone (5–10 mg qd) on days 16–25
	Estradiol skin patch (0.5 mg, every other day)
	For fertility: Menopausal gonadotropins, human chorionic gonadotropins
GH	Adults: Somatotropin (0.1–1.25 mg SC qd)
	Children: Somatotropin [0.02–0.05 (mg/kg per day)]
Vasopressin	Intranasal desmopressin (5–20 μg twice daily)
	Oral 300–600 μg qd

[a]All doses shown should be individualized for specific patients and should be reassessed during stress, surgery, or pregnancy. Male and female fertility requirements should be managed as discussed in Chap. 45.

Note: For abbreviations, see text.

hormone (CRH) administration induces ACTH release, and administration of synthetic ACTH (cortrosyn) evokes adrenal cortisol release as an indirect indicator of pituitary ACTH reserve (Chap. 336). ACTH reserve is most reliably assessed during insulin-induced hypoglycemia. However, this test should be performed cautiously in patients with suspected adrenal insufficiency because of enhanced susceptibility to hypoglycemia and hypotension. Insulin-induced hypoglycemia is contraindicated in patients with active coronary artery disease or seizure disorders.

℞ **HYPOPITUITARISM**

Hormone replacement therapy, including glucocorticoids, thyroid hormone, sex steroids, growth hormone, and vasopressin, is usually safe and free of complications. Treatment regimens that mimic physiologic hormone production allow for maintenance of satisfactory clinical homeostasis. Effective dosage schedules are outlined in **Table 333-4**. Patients in need of glucocorticoid replacement require careful dose adjustments during stressful events such as acute illness, dental procedures, trauma, and acute hospitalization (Chap. 336).

HYPOTHALAMIC, PITUITARY, AND OTHER SELLAR MASSES

PITUITARY TUMORS

Pituitary adenomas are the most common cause of pituitary hormone hypersecretion and hyposecretion syndromes in adults. They account for ~15% of all intracranial neoplasms. At autopsy, up to one-quarter of all pituitary glands harbor an unsuspected microadenoma (<10 mm diameter). Similarly, pituitary imaging detects small clinically inapparent pituitary lesions in at least 10% of individuals.

Pathogenesis Pituitary adenomas are benign neoplasms that arise from one of the five anterior pituitary cell types. The clinical and biochemical phenotype of pituitary adenomas depend on the cell type from which they are derived. Thus, tumors arising from lactotrope (PRL), somatotrope (GH), corticotrope (ACTH), thyrotrope (TSH), or gonadotrope (LH, FSH) cells hypersecrete their respective hormones (Table 333-5). Plurihormonal tumors that express combinations of GH, PRL, TSH, ACTH, and the glycoprotein hormone α subunit may be diagnosed by careful immunocytochemistry or may manifest as clinical syndromes that combine features of these hormonal hypersecretory syndromes. Morphologically, these tumors may

arise from a single polysecreting cell type or comprise cells with mixed function within the same tumor.

Hormonally active tumors are characterized by autonomous hormone secretion with diminished responsiveness to physiologic inhibitory pathways. Hormone production does not always correlate with tumor size. Small hormone-secreting adenomas may cause significant clinical perturbations, whereas larger adenomas that produce less hormone may be clinically silent and remain undiagnosed (if no central compressive effects occur). About one-third of all adenomas are clinically nonfunctioning and produce no distinct clinical hypersecretory syndrome. Most of these arise from gonadotrope cells and may secrete small amounts of α- and β-glycoprotein hormone subunits or, very rarely, intact circulating gonadotropins. True pituitary carcinomas with documented extracranial metastases are exceedingly rare.

Almost all pituitary adenomas are monoclonal in origin, implying the acquisition of one or more somatic mutations that confer a selective growth advantage. In addition to direct studies of oncogene mutations, this model is supported by X-chromosomal inactivation analyses of tumors in female patients heterozygous for X-linked genes. Consistent with their clonal origin, complete surgical resection of small pituitary adenomas usually cures hormone hypersecretion. Nevertheless, hypothalamic hormones, such as GHRH or CRH, also enhance mitotic activity of their respective pituitary target cells, in addition to their role in pituitary hormone regulation. Thus, patients harboring rare abdominal or chest tumors elaborating ectopic GHRH or CRH may present with somatotrope or corticotrope hyperplasia.

Several etiologic genetic events have been implicated in the development of pituitary tumors. The pathogenesis of sporadic forms of acromegaly has been particularly informative as a model of tumorigenesis. GHRH, after binding to its G protein–coupled somatotrope receptor, utilizes cyclic AMP as a second messenger to stimulate GH secretion and somatotrope proliferation. A subset (~35%) of GH-secreting pituitary tumors contain sporadic mutations in Gsα (Arg 201 → Cys or His; Gln 227 → Arg). These mutations inhibit intrinsic GTPase activity, resulting in constitutive elevation of cyclic AMP, Pit-1 induction, and activation of cyclic AMP response element binding protein (CREB), thereby promoting somatotrope cell proliferation and GH secretion.

Characteristic loss of heterozygosity (LOH) in various chromosomes has been documented in large or invasive macroadenomas, suggesting the presence of putative tumor suppressor genes at these loci. LOH of chromosome regions on 11q13, 13, and 9 is present in up to 20% of sporadic pituitary tumors including GH-, PRL-, and ACTH-producing adenomas and in some nonfunctioning tumors.

TABLE 333-5 CLASSIFICATION OF PITUITARY ADENOMAS[a]

Adenoma Cell Origin	Hormone Product	Clinical Syndrome
Lactotrope	PRL	Hypogonadism, galactorrhea
Gonadotrope	FSH, LH, subunits	Silent or hypogonadism
Somatotrope	GH	Acromegaly/gigantism
Corticotrope	ACTH	Cushing's disease
Mixed growth hormone and prolactin cell	GH, PRL	Acromegaly, hypogonadism, galactorrhea
Other plurihormonal cell	Any	Mixed
Acidophil stem cell	PRL, GH	Hypogonadism, galactorrhea, acromegaly
Mammosomatotrope	PRL, GH	Hypogonadism, galactorrhea, acromegaly
Thyrotrope	TSH	Thyrotoxicosis
Null cell	None	Pituitary failure
Oncocytoma	None	Pituitary failure

[a]Hormone-secreting tumors are listed in decreasing order of frequency. All tumors may cause local pressure effects, including visual disturbances, cranial nerve palsy, and headache.

Note: For abbreviations, see text.

Source: Adapted from S Melmed, in JL Jameson (ed): *Principles of Molecular Medicine*, Totowa, Humana Press, 1998.

Compelling evidence also favors growth factor promotion of pituitary tumor proliferation. Basic fibroblast growth factor (bFGF) is abundant in the pituitary and has been shown to stimulate pituitary cell mitogenesis. Other factors involved in initiation and promotion of pituitary tumors include loss of negative-feedback inhibition (as seen with primary hypothyroidism or hypogonadism) and estrogen-mediated or paracrine angiogenesis. Growth characteristics and neoplastic behavior may also be influenced by several activated oncogenes, including *RAS* and pituitary tumor transforming gene (*PTTG*).

Genetic Syndromes Associated with Pituitary Tumors Several familial syndromes are associated with pituitary tumors, and the genetic mechanisms for some of these have been unraveled.

Multiple endocrine neoplasia (MEN) 1 is an autosomal dominant syndrome characterized primarily by a genetic predisposition to parathyroid, pancreatic islet, and pituitary adenomas (Chap. 345). MEN1 is caused by inactivating germline mutations in *MENIN*, a constitutively expressed tumor-suppressor gene located on chromosome 11q13. Loss of heterozygosity, or a somatic mutation of the remaining normal *MENIN* allele, leads to tumorigenesis. About half of affected patients develop prolactinomas; acromegaly and Cushing's syndrome are less commonly encountered.

Carney syndrome is characterized by spotty skin pigmentation, myxomas, and endocrine tumors including testicular, adrenal, and pituitary adenomas. Acromegaly occurs in about 20% of patients. A subset of patients have mutations in the R1α regulatory subunit of protein kinase A (*PRKAR1A*).

McCune-Albright syndrome consists of polyostotic fibrous dysplasia, pigmented skin patches, and a variety of endocrine disorders, including GH-secreting pituitary tumors, adrenal adenomas, and autonomous ovarian function (Chap. 341). Hormonal hypersecretion is the result of constitutive cyclic AMP production caused by inactivation of the GTPase activity of Gsα. The Gsα mutations occur postzygotically, leading to a mosaic pattern of mutant expression.

Familial acromegaly is a rare disorder in which family members may manifest either acromegaly or gigantism. The disorder is associated with LOH at a chromosome 11q13 locus distinct from that of *MENIN*.

OTHER SELLAR MASSES

Craniopharyngiomas are benign, suprasellar cystic masses that present with headaches, visual field deficits, and variable degrees of hypopituitarism. They are derived from Rathke's pouch and arise near the pituitary stalk, commonly extending into the suprasellar cistern. Craniopharyngiomas are often large, cystic, and locally invasive. Many are partially calcified, providing a characteristic appearance on skull x-ray and CT images. More than half of all patients present before age 20, usually with signs of increased intracranial pressure, including headache, vomiting, papilledema, and hydrocephalus. Associated symptoms include visual field abnormalities, personality changes and cognitive deterioration, cranial nerve damage, sleep difficulties, and weight gain. Hypopituitarism can be documented in about 90% and diabetes insipidus occurs in about 10%. About half of affected children present with growth retardation. MRI is generally superior to CT to evaluate cystic structure and tissue components of craniopharyngiomas. CT is useful to define calcifications and to evaluate invasion into surrounding bony structures and sinuses.

Treatment usually involves transcranial or transsphenoidal surgical resection followed by postoperative radiation of residual tumor. Surgery alone is curative in less than half of patients because of adherence to vital structures or because of small tumor deposits in the hypothalamus or brain parenchyma. The goal of surgery is to remove as much tumor as possible without risking complications associated with efforts to remove firmly adherent or inaccessible tissue. In the absence of radiotherapy, about 75% of tumors recur, and 10-year survival is less than 50%. In patients with incomplete resection, radiotherapy improves 10-year survival to 70–90% but is associated with increased risk of secondary malignancies. Most patients require lifelong pituitary hormone replacement.

Developmental failure of Rathke's pouch obliteration may lead to *Rathke's cysts*, which are small (<5 mm) cysts entrapped by squamous epithelium, and are found in about 20% of individuals at autopsy. Although Rathke's cleft cysts do not usually grow and are often diagnosed incidentally, about a third present in adulthood with compressive symptoms, diabetes insipidus, and hyperprolactinemia due to stalk compression. Rarely, internal hydrocephalus develops. The diagnosis is suggested preoperatively by visualizing the cyst wall on MRI, which distinguishes these lesions from craniopharyngiomas. Cyst contents range from CSF-like fluid to mucoid material. *Arachnoid cysts* are rare and generate an MRI image isointense with cerebrospinal fluid.

Sella chordomas usually present with bony clival erosion, local invasiveness, and, on occasion, calcification. Normal pituitary tissue may be visible on MRI, distinguishing chordomas from aggressive pituitary adenomas. Mucinous material may be obtained by fine-needle aspiration.

Meningiomas arising in the sellar region may be difficult to distinguish from nonfunctioning pituitary adenomas. Meningiomas typically enhance on MRI and may show evidence of calcification or bony erosion. Meningiomas may cause compressive symptoms.

Histiocytosis X comprises a variety of syndromes associated with foci of eosinophilic granulomas. Diabetes insipidus, exophthalmos, and punched-out lytic bone lesions (*Hand-Schüller-Christian disease*) are associated with granulomatous lesions visible on MRI, as well as a characteristic axillary skin rash. Rarely, the pituitary stalk may be involved.

Pituitary metastases occur in ~3% of cancer patients. Blood-borne metastatic deposits are found almost exclusively in the posterior pituitary. Accordingly, diabetes insipidus can be a presenting feature of lung, gastrointestinal, breast, and other pituitary metastases. About half of pituitary metastases originate from breast cancer; about 25% of patients with metastatic breast cancer have such deposits. Rarely, pituitary stalk involvement results in anterior pituitary insufficiency. The MRI diagnosis of a metastatic lesion may be difficult to distinguish from an aggressive pituitary adenoma; the diagnosis may require histologic examination of excised tumor tissue. Primary or metastatic lymphoma, leukemias, and plasmacytomas also occur within the sella.

Hypothalamic hamartomas and *gangliocytomas* may arise from astrocytes, oligodendrocytes, and neurons with varying degrees of differentiation. These tumors may overexpress hypothalamic neuropeptides including GnRH, GHRH, or CRH. In GnRH-producing tumors, children present with precocious puberty, psychomotor delay, and laughing-associated seizures. Medical treatment of GnRH-producing hamartomas with long-acting GnRH analogues effectively suppresses gonadotropin secretion and controls premature pubertal development. Rarely, hamartomas are also associated with craniofacial abnormalities; imperforate anus; cardiac, renal, and lung disorders; and pituitary failure as features of *Pallister-Hall syndrome*, which is caused by mutations in the carboxyterminus of the *GLI3* gene. Hypothalamic hamartomas are often contiguous with the pituitary, and preoperative MRI diagnosis may not be possible. Histologic evidence of hypothalamic neurons in tissue resected at transsphenoidal surgery may be the first indication of a primary hypothalamic lesion.

Hypothalamic gliomas and *optic gliomas* occur mainly in childhood and usually present with visual loss. Adults have more aggressive tumors; about a third are associated with neurofibromatosis.

Brain germ-cell tumors may arise within the sellar region. These include *dysgerminomas*, which are frequently associated with diabetes insipidus and visual loss. They rarely metastasize. *Germinomas*, *embryonal carcinomas*, *teratomas*, and *choriocarcinomas* may arise in the parasellar region and produce hCG. These germ-cell tumors present with precocious puberty, diabetes insipidus, visual field defects, and thirst disorders. Many patients are GH-deficient with short stature.

METABOLIC EFFECTS OF HYPOTHALAMIC LESIONS
Lesions involving the anterior and preoptic hypothalamic regions cause paradoxical vasoconstriction, tachycardia, and hyperthermia. Acute hyperthermia is usually due to a hemorrhagic insult, but poikilothermia may also occur. Central disorders of thermoregulation result from posterior hypothalamic damage. The *periodic hypothermia*

syndrome comprises episodic attacks of rectal temperatures <30°C, sweating, vasodilation, vomiting, and bradycardia (Chap. 20). Damage to the ventromedial hypothalamic nuclei by craniopharyngiomas, hypothalamic trauma, or inflammatory disorders may be associated with *hyperphagia* and *obesity*. This region appears to contain an energy-satiety center where melanocortin receptors are influenced by leptin, insulin, POMC products, and gastrointestinal peptides (Chap. 74). Polydipsia and hypodipsia are associated with damage to central osmoreceptors located in preoptic nuclei (Chap. 334). Slow-growing hypothalamic lesions can cause increased somnolence and disturbed sleep cycles as well as obesity, hypothermia, and emotional outbursts. Lesions of the central hypothalamus may stimulate sympathetic neurons, leading to elevated serum catecholamine and cortisol levels. These patients are predisposed to cardiac arrhythmias, hypertension, and gastric erosions.

EVALUATION

Local Mass Effects Clinical manifestations of sellar lesions vary, depending on the anatomic location of the mass and direction of its extension (Table 333-6). The dorsal sellar diaphragm presents the least resistance to soft tissue expansion from the sella; consequently, pituitary adenomas frequently extend in a suprasellar direction. Bony invasion may occur as well.

Headaches are common features of small intrasellar tumors, even with no demonstrable suprasellar extension. Because of the confined nature of the pituitary, small changes in intrasellar pressure stretch the dural plate; however, headache severity correlates poorly with adenoma size or extension.

Suprasellar extension can lead to visual loss by several mechanisms, the most common being compression of the optic chiasm, but direct invasion of the optic nerves or obstruction of CSF flow leading to secondary visual disturbances also occurs. Pituitary stalk compression by a hormonally active or inactive intrasellar mass may compress the portal vessels, disrupting pituitary access to hypothalamic hormones and dopamine; this results in hyperprolactinemia and concurrent loss of other pituitary hormones. This "stalk section" phenomenon may also be caused by trauma, whiplash injury with posterior clinoid stalk compression, or skull base fractures. Lateral mass invasion may impinge on

TABLE 333-6 FEATURES OF SELLAR MASS LESIONS[a]

Impacted Structure	Clinical Impact
Pituitary	Hypogonadism
	Hypothyroidism
	Growth failure and adult hyposomatotropism
	Hypoadrenalism
Optic chiasm	Loss of red perception
	Bitemporal hemianopia
	Superior or bitemporal field defect
	Scotoma
	Blindness
Hypothalamus	Temperature dysregulation
	Appetite and thirst disorders
	Obesity
	Diabetes insipidus
	Sleep disorders
	Behavioral dysfunction
	Autonomic dysfunction
Cavernous sinus	Opthalmoplegia with or without ptosis or diplopia
	Facial numbness
Frontal lobe	Personality disorder
	Anosmia
Brain	Headache
	Hydrocephalus
	Psychosis
	Dementia
	Laughing seizures

[a]As the intrasellar mass expands, it first compresses intrasellar pituitary tissue, then usually invades dorsally through the dura to lift the optic chiasm or laterally to the cavernous sinuses. Bony erosion is rare, as is direct brain compression. Microadenomas may present with headache.

the cavernous sinus and compress its neural contents, leading to cranial nerve III, IV, and VI palsies as well as effects on the ophthalmic and maxillary branches of the fifth cranial nerve (Chap. 371). Patients may present with diplopia, ptosis, ophthalmoplegia, and decreased facial sensation, depending on the extent of neural damage. Extension into the sphenoid sinus indicates that the pituitary mass has eroded through the sellar floor. Aggressive tumors rarely invade the palate roof and cause nasopharyngeal obstruction, infection, and CSF leakage. Temporal and frontal lobe involvement may lead to uncinate seizures, personality disorders, and anosmia. Direct hypothalamic encroachment by an invasive pituitary mass may cause important metabolic sequelae, including precocious puberty or hypogonadism, diabetes insipidus, sleep disturbances, dysthermia, and appetite disorders.

MRI Sagittal and coronal T1-weighted MRI imaging, before and after administration of gadolinium, allow precise visualization of the pituitary gland with clear delineation of the hypothalamus, pituitary stalk, pituitary tissue and surrounding suprasellar cisterns, cavernous sinuses, sphenoid sinus, and optic chiasm. Pituitary gland height ranges from 6 mm in children to 8 mm in adults; during pregnancy and puberty, the height may reach 10–12 mm. The upper aspect of the adult pituitary is flat or slightly concave, but in adolescent and pregnant individuals, this surface may be convex, reflecting physiologic pituitary enlargement. The stalk should be midline and vertical. CT scan is indicated to define the extent of bony erosion or the presence of calcification.

Anterior pituitary gland soft tissue consistency is slightly heterogeneous on MRI, and signal intensity resembles that of brain matter on T1-weighted imaging (Fig. 333-4). Adenoma density is usually lower than that of surrounding normal tissue on T1-weighted imaging, and the signal intensity increases with T2-weighted images. The high phospholipid content of the posterior pituitary results in a "pituitary bright spot."

Sellar masses are commonly encountered as incidental findings on MRI, and most of these are pituitary adenomas (incidentalomas). In the absence of hormone hypersecretion, these small lesions can be safely monitored by MRI, which is performed annually and then less often if there is no evidence of growth. Resection should be considered for incidentally discovered macroadenomas, as about one-third become invasive or cause local pressure effects. If hormone hypersecretion is evident, specific therapies are indicated. When larger masses (>1 cm) are encountered, they should also be distinguished from nonadenomatous lesions. Meningiomas are often associated with bony hyperostosis; craniopharyngiomas may be calcified and are usually hypodense, whereas gliomas are hyperdense on T2-weighted images.

FIGURE 333-4 Pituitary adenoma. Coronal T1-weighted postcontrast MR image shows a homogeneously enhancing mass (*arrowheads*) in the sella turcica and suprasellar region compatible with a pituitary adenoma; the small arrows outline the carotid arteries.

TABLE 333-7	SCREENING TESTS FOR FUNCTIONAL PITUITARY ADENOMAS	
	Test	**Comments**
Acromegaly	Serum IGF-I	Interpret IGF-I relative to age- and gender-matched controls
	Oral glucose tolerance test with GH obtained at 0, 30, and 60 min	Normal subjects should suppress growth hormone to <1 µg/L
Prolactinoma	Serum PRL	Exclude medications
		MRI of the sella should be ordered if prolactin is elevated
Cushing's disease	24-h urinary free cortisol	Ensure urine collection is total and accurate
	Dexamethasone (1 mg) at 11 P.M. and fasting plasma cortisol measured at 8 A.M.	Normal subjects suppress to <5 µg/dL
	ACTH assay	Distinguishes adrenal adenoma (ACTH suppressed) from ectopic ACTH or Cushing's disease (ACTH normal or elevated)

Note: For abbreviations, see text.

Ophthalmologic Evaluation

Because optic tracts may be contiguous to an expanding pituitary mass, reproducible visual field assessment that uses perimetry techniques should be performed on all patients with sellar mass lesions that abut the optic chiasm (Chap. 29). Bitemporal hemianopia or superior bitemporal defects are classically observed, reflecting the location of these tracts within the inferior and posterior part of the chiasm. Homonymous cuts reflect postchiasmal and monocular field cuts prechiasmal lesions. Loss of red perception is an early sign of optic tract pressure. Early diagnosis reduces the risk of blindness, scotomas, or other visual disturbances.

Laboratory Investigation

The presenting clinical features of functional pituitary adenomas (e.g., acromegaly, prolactinomas, or Cushing's syndrome) should guide the laboratory studies (Table 333-7). However, for a sellar mass with no obvious clinical features of hormone excess, laboratory studies are geared towards determining the nature of the tumor and assessing the possible presence of hypopituitarism. When a pituitary adenoma is suspected based on MRI, initial hormonal evaluation usually includes (1) basal PRL; (2) insulin-like growth factor (IGF) I; (3) 24-h urinary free cortisol (UFC) and/or overnight oral dexamethasone (1 mg) suppression test; (4) α subunit, FSH, and LH; and (5) thyroid function tests. Additional hormonal evaluation may be indicated based on the results of these tests. Pending more detailed assessment of hypopituitarism, a menstrual history, testosterone and 8 A.M. cortisol levels, and thyroid function tests usually identify patients with pituitary hormone deficiencies that require hormone replacement before further testing or surgery.

Histologic Evaluation

Immunohistochemical staining of pituitary tumor specimens obtained at transsphenoidal surgery confirms clinical and laboratory studies and provides a histologic diagnosis when hormone studies are equivocal and in cases of clinically nonfunctioning tumors. Occasionally, ultrastructural assessment by electron microscopy is required for diagnosis.

℞ HYPOTHALAMIC, PITUITARY, AND OTHER SELLAR MASSES

OVERVIEW Successful management of sellar masses requires accurate diagnosis as well as selection of optimal therapeutic modalities. Most pituitary tumors are benign and slow-growing. Clinical features result from local mass effects and hormonal hypo- or hypersecretion syndromes caused directly by the adenoma or as a consequence of treatment. Thus, lifelong management and follow-up are necessary for these patients.

MRI technology with gadolinium enhancement for pituitary visualization, new advances in transsphenoidal surgery and in stereotactic radio-

therapy (including gamma-knife radiotherapy), and novel therapeutic agents have improved pituitary tumor management. The goals of pituitary tumor treatment include normalization of excess pituitary secretion, amelioration of symptoms and signs of hormonal hypersecretion syndromes, and shrinkage or ablation of large tumor masses with relief of adjacent structure compression. Residual anterior pituitary function should be preserved and can sometimes be restored by removing the tumor mass. Ideally, adenoma recurrence should be prevented.

TRANSSPHENOIDAL SURGERY Transsphenoidal rather than transfrontal resection is the desired surgical approach for pituitary tumors, except for the rare invasive suprasellar mass surrounding the frontal or middle fossa, the optic nerves, or invading posteriorly behind the clivus. Intraoperative microscopy facilitates visual distinction between adenomatous and normal pituitary tissue, as well as microdissection of small tumors that may not be visible by MRI (**Fig. 333-5**). Transsphenoidal surgery also avoids the cranial invasion and manipulation of brain tissue required by subfrontal surgical approaches. Endoscopic techniques with three-dimensional intraoperative localization have improved visualization and access to tumor tissue.

In addition to correction of hormonal hypersecretion, pituitary surgery is indicated for mass lesions that impinge on surrounding structures. Surgical decompression and resection are required for an expanding pituitary mass accompanied by persistent headache, progressive visual field defects, cranial nerve palsies, internal hydrocephalus, and, occasionally, intrapituitary hemorrhage and apoplexy. Transsphenoidal surgery is sometimes used for pituitary tissue biopsy to establish a histologic diagnosis.

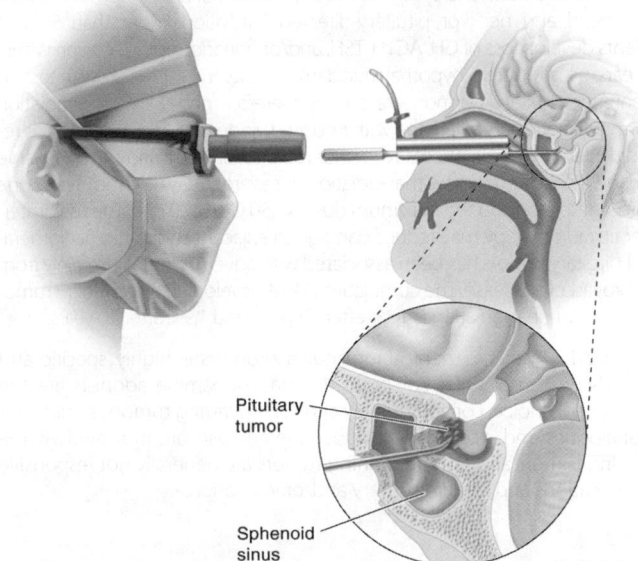

FIGURE 333-5 Transsphenoidal resection of pituitary mass via the endonasal approach. *(Adapted from Fahlbusch R: Endocrinol Metab Clin 21:669, 1992.)*

Whenever possible, the pituitary mass lesion should be selectively excised; normal tissue should be manipulated or resected only when critical for effective mass dissection. Nonselective hemihypophysectomy or total hypophysectomy may be indicated if no mass lesion is clearly discernible, multifocal lesions are present, or the remaining nontumorous pituitary tissue is obviously necrotic. This strategy, however, increases the likelihood of hypopituitarism and the need for lifelong hormonal replacement.

Preoperative mass effects, including visual field defects or compromised pituitary function, may be reversed by surgery, particularly when these deficits are not long-standing. For large and invasive tumors, it is necessary to determine the optimal balance between maximal tumor resection and preservation of anterior pituitary function, especially for preserving growth and reproductive function in younger patients. Similarly, tumor invasion outside of the sella is rarely amenable to surgical cure; the surgeon must judge the risk-benefit ratio of extensive tumor resection.

Side Effects Tumor size, the degree of invasiveness, and experience of the surgeon largely determine the incidence of surgical complications. Operative mortality is about 1%. Transient diabetes insipidus and hypopituitarism occur in up to 20% of patients. Permanent diabetes insipidus, cranial nerve damage, nasal septal perforation, or visual disturbances may be encountered in up to 10% of patients. CSF leaks occur in 4% of patients. Less common complications include carotid artery injury, loss of vision, hypothalamic damage, and meningitis. Permanent side effects are rare after surgery for microadenomas.

RADIATION Radiation is used either as a primary therapy for pituitary or parasellar masses or, more commonly, as an adjunct to surgery or medical therapy. Focused megavoltage irradiation is achieved by precise MRI localization, using a high-voltage linear accelerator and accurate isocentric rotational arcing. A major determinant of accurate irradiation is reproduction of the patient's head position during multiple visits and maintenance of absolute head immobility. A total of <50 Gy (5000 rad) is given as 180-cGy (180-rad) fractions split over about 6 weeks. Stereotactic radiosurgery delivers a large single high-energy dose from a cobalt 60 source (gamma knife), linear accelerator, or cyclotron. Long-term effects of gamma-knife surgery are as yet unknown.

The role of radiation therapy in pituitary tumor management depends on multiple factors including the nature of the tumor, age of the patient, and the availability of surgical and radiation expertise. Because of its relatively slow onset of action, radiation therapy is usually reserved for postsurgical management. As an adjuvant to surgery, radiation is used to treat residual tumor and in an attempt to prevent regrowth. Irradiation offers the only effective means for ablating significant postoperative residual nonfunctioning tumor tissue. In contrast, PRL-, GH-, and sometimes ACTH-secreting tumor tissues are amenable to medical therapy.

Side Effects In the short term, radiation may cause transient nausea and weakness. Alopecia and loss of taste and smell may be more long-lasting. Failure of pituitary hormone synthesis is common in patients who have undergone head and neck or pituitary-directed irradiation. More than 50% of patients develop loss of GH, ACTH, TSH, and/or gonadotropin secretion within 10 years, usually due to hypothalamic damage. Lifelong follow-up with testing of anterior pituitary hormone reserve is therefore necessary after radiation treatment. Optic nerve damage with impaired vision due to optic neuritis is reported in about 2% of patients who undergo pituitary irradiation. Cranial nerve damage is uncommon now that radiation doses are ≤2 Gy (200 rad) at any one treatment session and the maximum dose is <50 Gy (5000 rad). The use of stereotactic radiotherapy may reduce damage to adjacent structures. Radiotherapy of pituitary tumors has been associated with adverse mortality, mainly from cerebrovascular disease. The cumulative risk of developing a secondary tumor after conventional radiation is 1.3% after 10 years and 1.9% after 20 years.

MEDICAL Medical therapy for pituitary tumors is highly specific and depends on tumor type. For prolactinomas, dopamine agonists are the treatment of choice. For acromegaly and TSH-secreting tumors, somatostatin analogues and, occasionally, dopamine agonists are indicated. ACTH-secreting tumors and nonfunctioning tumors are generally not responsive to medications and require surgery and/or irradiation.

PROLACTIN

SYNTHESIS

PRL consists of 198 amino acids and has a molecular mass of 21,500 kDa; it is weakly homologous to GH and human placental lactogen

(hPL), reflecting the duplication and divergence of a common GH-PRL-hPL precursor gene on chromosome 6. PRL is synthesized in lactotropes, which constitute about 20% of anterior pituitary cells. Lactotropes and somatotropes are derived from a common precursor cell that may give rise to a tumor secreting both PRL and GH. Marked lactotrope cell hyperplasia develops during the last two trimesters of pregnancy and the first few months of lactation. These transient functional changes in the lactotrope population are induced by estrogen.

SECRETION

Normal adult serum PRL levels are about 10–25 μg/L in women and 10–20 μg/L in men. PRL secretion is pulsatile, with the highest secretory peaks occurring during rapid eye movement sleep. Peak serum PRL levels (up to 30 μg/L) occur between 4:00 and 6:00 A.M. The circulating half-life of PRL is about 50 min.

PRL is unique among the pituitary hormones in that the predominant central control mechanism is inhibitory, reflecting dopamine-mediated suppression of PRL release. This regulatory pathway accounts for the spontaneous PRL hypersecretion that occurs after pituitary stalk section, often a consequence of compressive mass lesions at the skull base. Pituitary, dopamine type 2 (D_2) receptors mediate PRL inhibition. Targeted disruption (gene knockout) of the murine D_2 receptor in mice results in hyperprolactinemia and lactotrope proliferation. As discussed below, dopamine agonists play a central role in the management of hyperprolactinemic disorders.

Thyrotropin-releasing hormone (TRH) (pyro Glu-His-Pro-NH2) is a hypothalamic tripeptide that releases prolactin within 15–30 min after intravenous injection. The physiologic relevance of TRH for PRL regulation is unclear, and it appears primarily to regulate TSH (Chap. 335). *Vasoactive intestinal peptide* (VIP) also induces PRL release, whereas glucocorticoids and thyroid hormone weakly suppress PRL secretion.

Serum PRL levels rise transiently after exercise, meals, sexual intercourse, minor surgical procedures, general anesthesia, acute myocardial infarction, and other forms of acute stress. PRL levels increase significantly (about tenfold) during pregnancy and decline rapidly within 2 weeks of parturition. If breastfeeding is initiated, basal PRL levels remain elevated; suckling stimulates reflex increases in PRL levels that last for about 30–45 min. Breast suckling activates neural afferent pathways in the hypothalamus that induce PRL release. With time, the suckling-induced responses diminish and interfeeding PRL levels return to normal.

ACTION

The PRL receptor is a member of the type I cytokine receptor family that also includes GH and interleukin (IL) 6 receptors. Ligand binding induces receptor dimerization and intracellular signaling by Janus kinase (JAK), which stimulates translocation of the signal transduction and activators of transcription (STAT) family to activate target genes. In the breast, the lobuloalveolar epithelium proliferates in response to PRL, placental lactogens, estrogen, progesterone, and local paracrine growth factors, including IGF-I.

PRL acts to induce and maintain lactation, decrease reproductive function, and suppress sexual drive. These functions are geared toward ensuring that maternal lactation is sustained and not interrupted by pregnancy. PRL inhibits reproductive function by suppressing hypothalamic GnRH and pituitary gonadotropin secretion and by impairing gonadal steroidogenesis in both women and men. In the ovary, PRL blocks folliculogenesis and inhibits granulosa cell aromatase activity, leading to hypoestrogenism and anovulation. PRL also has a luteolytic effect, generating a shortened, or inadequate, luteal phase of the menstrual cycle. In men, attenuated LH secretion leads to low testosterone levels and decreased spermatogenesis. These hormonal changes decrease libido and reduce fertility in patients with hyperprolactinemia.

HYPERPROLACTINEMIA

Etiology Hyperprolactinemia is the most common pituitary hormone hypersecretion syndrome in both men and women. PRL-secreting pitu-

TABLE 333-8 ETIOLOGY OF HYPERPROLACTINEMIA[a]

I. Physiologic hypersecretion
Pregnancy
Lactation
Chest wall stimulation
Sleep
Stress

II. Hypothalamic–pituitary stalk damage
Tumors
　Craniopharyngioma
　Suprasellar pituitary mass
　　extension
　Meningioma
　Dysgerminoma
　Metastases
Empty sella
Lymphocytic hypophysitis
Adenoma with stalk
　compression
Granulomas
Rathke's cyst
Irradiation
Trauma
　Pituitary stalk section
　Suprasellar surgery

III. Pituitary hypersecretion
Prolactinoma
Acromegaly

IV. Systemic disorders
Chronic renal failure
Hypothyroidism
Cirrhosis
Pseudocyesis
Epileptic seizures

V. Drug-induced hypersecretion
Dopamine receptor blockers
　Phenothiazines: chlorpromazine,
　　perphenazine
　Butyrophenones: haloperidol
　Thioxanthenes
　Metoclopramide
Dopamine synthesis inhibitors
　α-Methyldopa
Catecholamine depletors
　Reserpine
Opiates
H_2 antagonists
　Cimetidine, ranitidine
Imipramines
　Amitriptyline, amoxapine
Serotonin-reuptake inhibitors
　Fluoxetine
Calcium channel blockers
　Verapamil
Hormones
　Estrogens
　Antiandrogens
　TRH

Note: Hyperprolactinemia >100 μg/L almost invariably is indicative of a prolactin-secreting pituitary adenoma. Physiologic causes, hypothyroidism, and drug-induced hyperprolactinemia should be excluded before extensive evaluation.

itary adenomas (prolactinomas) are the most common cause of PRL levels >100 μg/L (see below). Less pronounced PRL elevation can also be seen with microprolactinomas but is more commonly caused by drugs, pituitary stalk compression, hypothyroidism, or renal failure (Table 333-8).

Pregnancy and lactation are the important physiologic causes of hyperprolactinemia. Sleep-associated hyperprolactinemia reverts to normal within an hour of awakening. Nipple stimulation and sexual orgasm may also increase PRL. Chest wall stimulation or trauma (including chest surgery and herpes zoster) invoke the reflex suckling arc with resultant hyperprolactinemia. Chronic renal failure elevates PRL by decreasing peripheral clearance. Primary hypothyroidism is associated with mild hyperprolactinemia, probably because of compensatory TRH secretion.

Lesions of the hypothalamic-pituitary region that disrupt hypothalamic dopamine synthesis, portal vessel delivery, or lactotrope responses are associated with hyperprolactinemia. Thus, hypothalamic tumors, cysts, infiltrative disorders, and radiation-induced damage cause elevated PRL levels, usually in the range of 30–100 μg/L. Plurihormonal adenomas (including GH and ACTH tumors) may directly hypersecrete PRL. Pituitary masses, including clinically nonfunctioning pituitary tumors, may compress the pituitary stalk to cause hyperprolactinemia.

Drug-induced inhibition or disruption of dopaminergic receptor function is a common cause of hyperprolactinemia (Table 333-8). Thus, antipsychotics and antidepressants are a relatively common cause of mild hyperprolactinemia. Methyldopa inhibits dopamine synthesis and verapamil blocks dopamine release, also leading to hyperprolactinemia. Hormonal agents that induce PRL include estrogens, antiandrogens, and TRH.

Presentation and Diagnosis Amenorrhea, galactorrhea, and infertility are the hallmarks of hyperprolactinemia in women. If hyperprolactinemia develops prior to menarche, primary amenorrhea results. More commonly, hyperprolactinemia develops later in life and leads to oligomenorrhea and, ultimately, to amenorrhea. If hyperprolactine-

mia is sustained, vertebral bone mineral density can be reduced compared with age-matched controls, particularly when associated with pronounced hypoestrogenemia. Galactorrhea is present in up to 80% of hyperprolactinemic women. Although usually bilateral and spontaneous, it may be unilateral or only expressed manually. Patients may also complain of decreased libido, weight gain, and mild hirsutism.

In men with hyperprolactinemia, diminished libido, infertility, or visual loss (from optic nerve compression) are the usual presenting symptoms. Gonadotropin suppression leads to reduced testosterone, impotence, and oligospermia. True galactorrhea is uncommon in men with hyperprolactinemia. If the disorder is longstanding, secondary effects of hypogonadism are evident, including osteopenia, reduced muscle mass, and decreased beard growth.

The diagnosis of idiopathic hyperprolactinemia is made by exclusion of known causes of hyperprolactinemia in the setting of a normal pituitary MRI. Some of these patients may harbor small microadenomas below MRI sensitivity (~2 mm).

GALACTORRHEA

Galactorrhea, the inappropriate discharge of milk-containing fluid from the breast, is considered abnormal if it persists for longer than 6 months after childbirth or discontinuation of breastfeeding. Postpartum galactorrhea associated with amenorrhea is a self-limiting disorder usually associated with moderately elevated PRL levels. Galactorrhea may occur spontaneously, or it may be elicited by nipple pressure. In both men and women, galactorrhea may vary in color and consistency (transparent, milky, or bloody) and arise either unilaterally or bilaterally. Mammography or ultrasound is indicated for bloody discharges (particularly from a single duct), which may be caused by breast cancer. Galactorrhea is commonly associated with hyperprolactinemia caused by any of the conditions listed in Table 333-8. Acromegaly is associated with galactorrhea in about one-third of patients. Treatment of galactorrhea usually involves managing the underlying disorder (e.g., replacing T_4 for hypothyroidism; discontinuing a medication; treating prolactinoma).

Laboratory Investigation Basal, fasting morning PRL levels (normally <20 μg/L) should be measured to assess hypersecretion. Because hormone secretion is pulsatile and levels vary widely in some individuals with hyperprolactinemia, it may be necessary to measure levels on several different occasions when clinical suspicion is high. Both false-positive and false-negative results may be encountered. In patients with markedly elevated PRL levels (>1000 μg/L), results may be falsely lowered because of assay artifacts; sample dilution is required to measure these high values accurately. Falsely elevated values may be caused by aggregated forms of circulating PRL, which are biologically inactive (macroprolactinemia). Hypothyroidism should be excluded by measuring TSH and T_4 levels.

℞ HYPERPROLACTINEMIA

Treatment of hyperprolactinemia depends on the cause of elevated PRL levels. Regardless of the etiology, however, treatment should be aimed at normalizing PRL levels to alleviate suppressive effects on gonadal function, halt galactorrhea, and preserve bone mineral density. Dopamine agonists are effective for many different causes of hyperprolactinemia (see Treatment for "Prolactinoma," below).

If the patient is taking a medication known to cause hyperprolactinemia, the drug should be withdrawn, if possible. For psychiatric patients who require neuroleptic agents, dose titration or the addition of a dopamine agonist can help restore normoprolactinemia and alleviate reproductive symptoms. However, dopamine agonists sometimes worsen the underlying psychiatric condition, especially at high doses. Hyperprolactinemia usually resolves after adequate thyroid hormone replacement in hypothyroid patients or after renal transplantation in patients undergoing dialysis. Resection of hypothalamic or sellar mass lesions can reverse hyperprolactinemia caused by reduced dopamine tone. Granulomatous infiltrates occasionally respond to glucocorticoid administration. In patients with irreversible hypothalamic damage, no treatment may be warranted. In up to 30% of patients with hyperprolactinemia—with or without a visible pituitary microadenoma—the condition resolves spontaneously.

PROLACTINOMA

Etiology and Prevalence

Tumors arising from lactotrope cells account for about half of all functioning pituitary tumors, with an annual incidence of ~3/100,000 population. Mixed tumors secreting combinations of GH and PRL, ACTH and PRL, and rarely TSH and PRL, are also seen. These plurihormonal tumors are usually recognized by immunohistochemistry, often without apparent clinical manifestations from the production of additional hormones. Microadenomas are classified as <1 cm in diameter and do not usually invade the parasellar region. Macroadenomas are >1 cm in diameter and may be locally invasive and impinge on adjacent structures. The female:male ratio for microprolactinomas is 20:1, whereas the gender ratio is near 1:1 for macroadenomas. Tumor size generally correlates directly with PRL concentrations; values >100 μg/L are usually associated with macroadenomas. Men tend to present with larger tumors than women, possibly because the features of hypogonadism are less readily evident. PRL levels remain stable in most patients, reflecting the slow growth of these tumors. About 5% of microadenomas progress in the long term to macroadenomas. Hyperprolactinemia resolves spontaneously in about 30% of microadenomas.

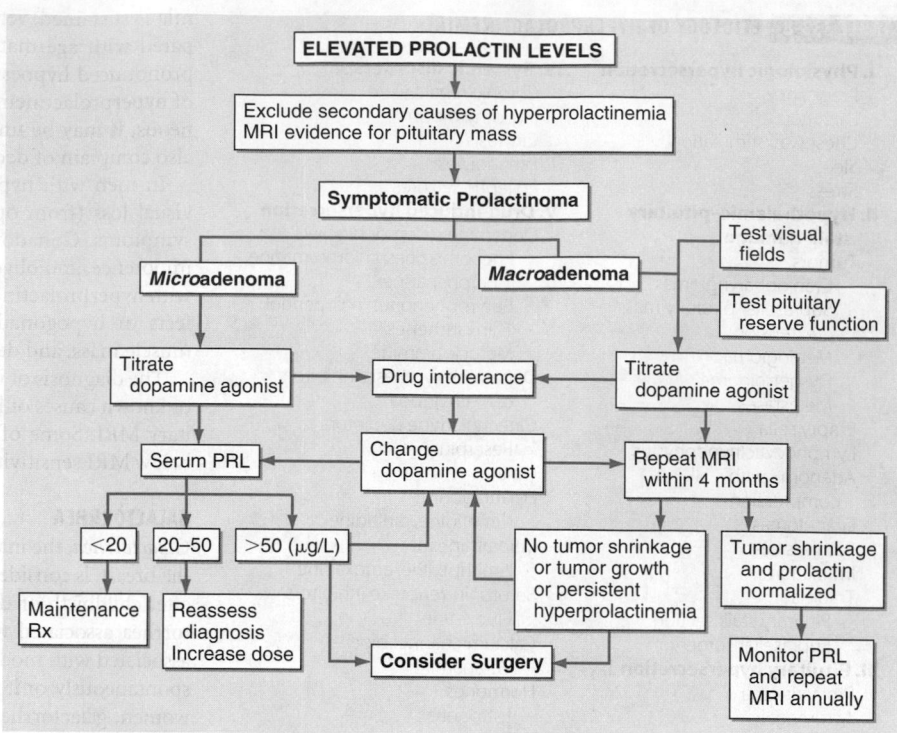

FIGURE 333-6 Management of prolactinoma. MRI, magnetic resonance imaging; PRL, prolactin.

Presentation and Diagnosis

Women usually present with amenorrhea, infertility, and galactorrhea. If the tumor extends outside of the sella, visual field defects or other mass effects may be seen. Men often present with impotence, loss of libido, infertility, or signs of central CNS compression including headaches and visual defects. Assuming that physiologic and medication-induced causes of hyperprolactinemia are excluded (Table 333-8), the diagnosis of prolactinoma is likely with a PRL level >100 μg/L. PRL levels <100 μg/L may be caused by microadenomas, other sellar lesions that decrease dopamine inhibition, or nonneoplastic causes of hyperprolactinemia. For this reason, an MRI should be performed in all patients with hyperprolactinemia. It is important to remember that hyperprolactinemia caused secondarily by the mass effects of nonlactotrope lesions is also corrected by treatment with dopamine agonists, despite failure to shrink the underlying mass. Consequently, PRL suppression by dopamine agonists does not necessarily indicate that the lesion is a prolactinoma.

℞ PROLACTINOMA

As microadenomas rarely progress to become macroadenomas, no treatment may be needed if fertility is not desired. Estrogen replacement is indicated to prevent bone loss and other consequences of hypoestrogenemia and does not appear to increase the risk of tumor enlargement. These patients should be monitored by regular serial PRL and MRI measurements.

For symptomatic microadenomas, therapeutic goals include control of hyperprolactinemia, reduction of tumor size, restoration of menses and fertility, and resolution of galactorrhea. Dopamine agonist doses should be titrated to achieve maximal PRL suppression and restoration of reproductive function (Fig. 333-6). A normalized PRL level does not ensure reduced tumor size. However, tumor shrinkage is not usually seen in those who do not respond with lowered PRL levels. For macroadenomas, formal visual field testing should be performed before initiating dopamine agonists. MRI and visual fields should be assessed at 6- to 12-month intervals until the mass shrinks and annually thereafter until maximum size reduction has occurred.

MEDICAL Oral dopamine agonists (cabergoline or bromocriptine) are the mainstay of therapy for patients with micro- or macroprolactinomas. Dopamine agonists suppress PRL secretion and synthesis as well as lacto-

trope cell proliferation. About 20% of patients are resistant to dopaminergic treatment; these adenomas may exhibit decreased D_2 dopamine receptor numbers or a postreceptor defect. D_2 receptor gene mutations in the pituitary have not been reported.

Cabergoline An ergoline derivative, cabergoline is a long-acting dopamine agonist with high D_2 receptor affinity. The drug effectively suppresses PRL for >14 days after a single oral dose and induces prolactinoma shrinkage in most patients. Cabergoline (0.5 to 1.0 mg twice weekly) achieves normoprolactinemia and resumption of normal gonadal function in ~80% of patients with microadenomas; galactorrhea improves or resolves in 90% of patients. Cabergoline normalizes PRL and shrinks ~70% of macroprolactinomas. Mass effect symptoms, including headaches and visual disorders, usually improve dramatically within days after cabergoline initiation; improvement of sexual function requires several weeks of treatment but may occur before complete normalization of prolactin levels. After initial control of PRL levels has been achieved, cabergoline should be reduced to the lowest effective maintenance dose. In ~5% of treated patients, hyperprolactinemia may resolve and not recur when dopamine agonists are discontinued after long-term treatment. Cabergoline may also be effective in patients resistant to bromocriptine. Adverse effects and drug intolerance are encountered less commonly than with bromocriptine.

Bromocriptine The ergot alkaloid bromocriptine mesylate is a dopamine receptor agonist that suppresses prolactin secretion. Because it is short-acting, the drug is preferred when pregnancy is desired. In microadenomas bromocriptine rapidly lowers serum prolactin levels to normal in up to 70% of patients, decreases tumor size, and restores gonadal function. In patients with macroadenomas, prolactin levels are also normalized in 70% of patients and tumor mass shrinkage (≥50%) is achieved in up to 40% of patients.

Therapy is initiated by administering a low bromocriptine dose (0.625–1.25 mg) at bedtime with a snack, followed by gradually increasing the dose. Most patients are successfully controlled with a daily dose of ≤7.5 mg (2.5 mg tid).

Other Dopamine Agonists These include *pergolide mesylate*, an ergot derivative with dopaminergic properties; *lisuride*, an ergot derivative; and *quinagolide* (CV 205-502, Norprolac), a nonergot oral dopamine agonist with specific D_2 receptor activity.

Side Effects Side effects of dopamine agonists include constipation, nasal stuffiness, dry mouth, nightmares, insomnia, and vertigo; decreasing the dose usually alleviates these problems. Nausea, vomiting, and postural hypotension with faintness may occur in ~25% of patients after the initial dose. These symptoms may persist in some patients. In general, fewer side effects are reported with cabergoline. For the approximately 15% of patients who are intolerant of oral bromocriptine, cabergoline may be better tolerated. Intravaginal administration of bromocriptine is often efficacious in patients with intractable gastrointestinal side effects. Auditory hallucinations, delusions, and mood swings have been reported in up to 5% of patients and may be due to the dopamine agonist properties or to the lysergic acid derivative of the compounds. Rare reports of leukopenia, thrombocytopenia, pleural fibrosis, cardiac arrhythmias, and hepatitis have been described.

Surgery Indications for surgical adenoma debulking include dopamine resistance or intolerance, or the presence of an invasive macroadenoma with compromised vision that fails to improve after drug treatment. Initial PRL normalization is achieved in about 70% of microprolactinomas after surgical resection, but only 30% of macroadenomas can be successfully resected. Follow-up studies have shown that hyperprolactinemia recurs in up to 20% of patients within the first year after surgery; long-term recurrence rates exceed 50% for macroadenomas. Radiotherapy for prolactinomas is reserved for patients with aggressive tumors that do not respond to maximally tolerated dopamine agonists and/or surgery.

PREGNANCY The pituitary increases in size during pregnancy, reflecting the stimulatory effects of estrogen and perhaps other growth factors. About 5% of microadenomas significantly increase in size, but 15–30% of macroadenomas grow during pregnancy. Bromocriptine has been used for more than 30 years to restore fertility in women with hyperprolactinemia, without evidence of teratogenic effects. Nonetheless, most authorities recommend strategies to minimize fetal exposure to the drug. For women taking bromocriptine who desire pregnancy, mechanical contraception should be used through three regular menstrual cycles to allow for conception timing. When pregnancy is confirmed, bromocriptine should be discontinued and PRL levels followed serially, especially if headaches or visual symptoms occur. For women harboring macroadenomas, regular visual field testing is recommended, and the drug should be reinstituted if tumor growth is apparent. Although pituitary MRI may be safe during pregnancy, this procedure should be reserved for symptomatic patients with severe headache and/or visual field defects. Surgical decompression may be indicated if vision is threatened. Although comprehensive data support the efficacy and relative safety of bromocriptine-facilitated fertility, patients should be advised of potential unknown deleterious effects and the risk of tumor growth during pregnancy. As cabergoline is long-acting with a high D_2-receptor affinity, it is not approved for use in women when fertility is desired.

GROWTH HORMONE

SYNTHESIS

GH is the most abundant anterior pituitary hormone, and GH-secreting somatotrope cells constitute up to 50% of the total anterior pituitary cell population. Mammosomatotrope cells, which co-express PRL with GH, can be identified using double immunostaining techniques. Somatotrope development and GH transcription are determined by expression of the cell-specific Pit-1 nuclear transcription factor. Five distinct genes on chromosome 17q22 encode GH and related proteins. The pituitary GH gene (*hGH-N*) produces two alternatively spliced products that give rise to 22-kDa GH (191 amino acids) and a less abundant 20-kDa GH molecule, with similar biologic activity. Placental syncytiotrophoblast cells express a GH variant (*hGH-V*) gene; the related hormone human chorionic somatotropin (HCS) is expressed by distinct members of the gene cluster.

SECRETION

GH secretion is controlled by complex hypothalamic and peripheral factors. *GHRH* is a 44-amino-acid hypothalamic peptide that stimulates GH synthesis and release. Ghrelin, an octanoylated gastric-derived peptide, as well as synthetic agonists of the *GHRP* receptor, induce GHRH and also directly stimulate GH release. *Somatostatin* [somatotropin-release inhibiting factor (SRIF)] is synthesized in the medial preoptic area of the hypothalamus and inhibits GH secretion. GHRH is secreted in discrete spikes that elicit GH pulses, whereas

SRIF sets basal GH tone. SRIF is also expressed in many extrahypothalamic tissues, including the CNS, gastrointestinal tract, and pancreas, where it also acts to inhibit islet hormone secretion. *IGF-I*, the peripheral target hormone for GH, feeds back to inhibit GH; estrogen induces GH, whereas chronic glucocorticoid excess suppresses GH release.

Surface receptors on the somatotrope regulate GH synthesis and secretion. The GHRH receptor is a G protein–coupled receptor (GPCR) that signals through intracellular cyclic AMP pathway to stimulate somatotrope cell proliferation as well as GH production. Inactivating mutations of the GHRH receptor cause profound dwarfism (see below). A distinct surface receptor for ghrelin, a gastric-derived GH secretagogue, is expressed in the hypothalamus and pituitary. Somatostatin binds to five distinct receptor subtypes (SSTR1 to SSTR5); SSTR2 and SSTR5 subtypes preferentially suppress GH (and TSH) secretion.

GH secretion is pulsatile, with highest peak levels occurring at night, generally correlating with sleep onset. GH secretory rates decline markedly with age so that hormone levels in middle age are about 15% of pubertal levels. These changes are paralleled by an age-related decline in lean muscle mass. GH secretion is also reduced in obese individuals, though IGF-I levels may not be suppressed, suggesting a change in the setpoint for feedback control. Elevated GH levels occur within an hour of deep sleep onset as well as after exercise, physical stress, trauma, and during sepsis. Integrated 24-h GH secretion is higher in women and is also enhanced by estrogen replacement. Using standard assays, random GH measurements are undetectable in ~50% of daytime samples obtained from healthy subjects and are also undetectable in most obese and elderly subjects. Thus, single random GH measurements do not distinguish patients with adult GH deficiency from normal persons.

GH secretion is profoundly influenced by nutritional factors. Using newer ultrasensitive chemiluminescence-based GH assays with a sensitivity of 0.002 µg/L, a glucose load can be shown to suppress GH to <0.7 µg/L in women and to <0.07 µg/L in men. Increased GH pulse frequency and peak amplitudes occur with chronic malnutrition or prolonged fasting. GH is stimulated by intravenous L-arginine, dopamine, and apomorphine (a dopamine receptor agonist), as well as by α-adrenergic pathways. β-Adrenergic blockage induces basal GH and enhances GHRH- and insulin-evoked GH release.

ACTION

The pattern of GH secretion may affect tissue responses. The higher GH pulsatility observed in men, as compared to the relatively continuous GH secretion in women, may be an important biologic determinant of linear growth patterns and liver enzyme induction.

The 70-kDa peripheral GH receptor protein shares structural homology with the cytokine/hematopoietic superfamily. A fragment of the receptor extracellular domain generates a soluble GH binding protein (GHBP) that interacts with GH in the circulation. The liver and cartilage contain the greatest number of GH receptors. GH binding to receptor dimers is followed by signaling through the JAK/STAT pathway. The activated STAT proteins translocate to the nucleus, where they modulate expression of GH-regulated target genes. GH analogues that bind to the receptor, but are incapable of mediating receptor signaling, are potent antagonists of GH action. A GH receptor antagonist (pegvisomant) has been approved for treatment of acromegaly.

GH induces protein synthesis and nitrogen retention and impairs glucose tolerance by antagonizing insulin action. GH also stimulates lipolysis, leading to increased circulating fatty acid levels, reduced omental fat mass, and enhanced lean body mass. GH promotes sodium, potassium, and water retention and elevates serum levels of inorganic phosphate. Linear bone growth occurs as a result of complex hormonal and growth factor actions, including those of IGF-I. GH stimulates epiphyseal prechondrocyte differentiation. These precursor cells produce IGF-I locally and are also responsive to the growth factor.

INSULIN-LIKE GROWTH FACTORS

Although GH exerts direct effects in target tissues, many of its physiologic effects are mediated indirectly through IGF-I, a potent growth and differentiation factor. The liver is the major source of circulating IGF-I. In peripheral tissues, IGF-I exerts local paracrine actions that appear to be both dependent on and independent of GH. Thus, GH administration induces circulating IGF-I as well as stimulating IGF-I production in multiple tissues.

Both IGF-I and -II are bound to high-affinity circulating IGF-binding proteins (IGFBPs) that regulate IGF bioactivity. Levels of IGFBP3 are GH-dependent, and it serves as the major carrier protein for circulating IGF-I. GH deficiency and malnutrition are usually associated with low IGFBP3 levels. IGFBP1 and -2 regulate local tissue IGF action but do not bind appreciable amounts of circulating IGF-I.

Serum IGF-I concentrations are profoundly affected by physiologic factors. Levels increase during puberty, peak at 16 years, and subsequently decline by >80% during the aging process. IGF-I concentrations are higher in women than in men. Because GH is the major determinant of hepatic IGF-I synthesis, abnormalities of GH synthesis or action (e.g., pituitary failure, GHRH receptor defect, or GH receptor defect) reduce IGF-I levels. Hypocaloric states are associated with GH resistance; IGF-I levels are therefore low with cachexia, malnutrition, and sepsis. In acromegaly, IGF-I levels are invariably high and reflect a log-linear relationship with GH concentrations.

IGF-I Physiology IGF-I has been approved for use in patients with GH-resistance syndromes. Injected IGF-I (100 μg/kg) induces hypoglycemia, and lower doses improve insulin sensitivity in patients with severe insulin resistance and diabetes. In cachectic subjects, IGF-I infusion (12 μg/kg per hour) enhances nitrogen retention and lowers cholesterol levels. Longer-term subcutaneous IGF-I injections enhance protein synthesis and are anabolic. Although bone formation markers are induced, bone turnover may also be stimulated by IGF-I.

IGF-I side effects are dose-dependent, and overdose may result in hypoglycemia, hypotension, fluid retention, temporomandibular jaw pain, and increased intracranial pressure, all of which are reversible. Avascular femoral head necrosis has been reported. Chronic excess IGF-I would presumably result in features of acromegaly.

DISORDERS OF GROWTH AND DEVELOPMENT

Skeletal Maturation and Somatic Growth The growth plate is dependent on a variety of hormonal stimuli including GH, IGF-I, sex steroids, thyroid hormones, paracrine growth factors, and cytokines. The growth-promoting process also requires caloric energy, amino acids, vitamins, and trace metals and consumes about 10% of normal energy production. Malnutrition impairs chondrocyte activity and reduces circulating IGF-I and IGFBP3 levels.

Linear bone growth rates are very high in infancy and are pituitary-dependent. Mean growth velocity is ~6 cm/year in later childhood and is usually maintained within a given range on a standardized percentile chart. Peak growth rates occur during midpuberty when bone age is 12 (girls) or 13 (boys). Secondary sexual development is associated with elevated sex steroids that cause progressive epiphyseal growth plate closure. *Bone age* is delayed in patients with all forms of true GH deficiency or GH receptor defects that result in attenuated GH action.

Short stature may occur as a result of constitutive intrinsic growth defects or because of acquired extrinsic factors that impair growth. In general, delayed bone age in a child with short stature is suggestive of a hormonal or systemic disorder, whereas normal bone age in a short child is more likely to be caused by a genetic cartilage dysplasia or growth plate disorder (Chap. 357).

GH Deficiency in Children • *GH DEFICIENCY* Isolated GH deficiency is characterized by short stature, micropenis, increased fat, high-pitched voice, and a propensity to hypoglycemia due to relatively unopposed insulin action. Familial modes of inheritance are seen in one-third of these individuals and may be autosomal dominant, recessive, or X-linked. About 10% of children with GH deficiency have mutations in the *GH-N* gene, including gene deletions and a wide range of point mutations. Mutations in transcription factors Pit-1 and Prop-1, which control somatotrope development, cause GH deficiency in combination with oth-

er pituitary hormone deficiencies, which may become manifest only in adulthood. The diagnosis of *idiopathic GH deficiency* (IGHD) should be made only after known molecular defects have been excluded.

GHRH RECEPTOR MUTATIONS Recessive mutations of the GHRH receptor gene in subjects with severe proportionate dwarfism are associated with low basal GH levels that cannot be stimulated by exogenous GHRH, GHRP, or insulin-induced hypoglycemia. The syndrome exemplifies the importance of the GHRH receptor for somatotrope cell proliferation and hormonal responsiveness.

GROWTH HORMONE INSENSITIVITY This is caused by defects of GH receptor structure or signaling. Homozygous or heterozygous mutations of the GH receptor are associated with partial or complete GH insensitivity and growth failure (*Laron syndrome*). The diagnosis is based on normal or high GH levels, with decreased circulating GHBP, and low IGF-I levels. Very rarely, defective IGF-I, IGF-I receptor, or IGF-I signaling defects are also encountered. *STAT5B* mutations result in immunodeficiency with abrogated GH signaling, leading to short stature with normal or elevated GH levels and low IGF-I levels.

NUTRITIONAL SHORT STATURE Caloric deprivation and malnutrition, uncontrolled diabetes, and chronic renal failure represent secondary causes of abrogated GH receptor function. These conditions also stimulate production of proinflammatory cytokines, which act to further exacerbate the block of GH-mediated signal transduction. Children with these conditions typically exhibit features of acquired short stature with elevated GH and low IGF-I levels. Circulating GH receptor antibodies may rarely cause peripheral GH insensitivity.

PSYCHOSOCIAL SHORT STATURE Emotional and social deprivation lead to growth retardation accompanied by delayed speech, discordant hyperphagia, and attenuated response to administered GH. A nurturing environment restores growth rates.

Presentation and Diagnosis Short stature is commonly encountered in clinical practice, and the decision to evaluate these children requires clinical judgment in association with auxologic data and family history. Short stature should be comprehensively evaluated if a patient's height is >3 SD below the mean for age or if the growth rate has decelerated. Skeletal maturation is best evaluated by measuring a radiologic bone age, which is based mainly on the degree of growth plate fusion. Final height can be predicted using standardized scales (Bayley-Pinneau or Tanner-Whitehouse) or estimated by adding 6.5 cm (boys) or subtracting 6.5 cm (girls) from the midparental height.

Laboratory Investigation Because GH secretion is pulsatile, GH deficiency is best assessed by examining the response to provocative stimuli including exercise, insulin-induced hypoglycemia, and other pharmacologic tests that normally increase GH to >7 μg/L in children. Random GH measurements do not distinguish normal children from those with true GH deficiency. Adequate adrenal and thyroid hormone replacement should be assured before testing. Age- and gender-matched IGF-I levels are not sufficiently sensitive or specific to make the diagnosis but can be useful to confirm GH deficiency. Pituitary MRI may reveal pituitary mass lesions or structural defects.

℞ DISORDERS OF GROWTH AND DEVELOPMENT

Replacement therapy with recombinant GH (0.02–0.05 mg/kg per day subcutaneously) restores growth velocity in GH-deficient children to ~10 cm/year. If pituitary insufficiency is documented, other associated hormone deficits should be corrected—especially adrenal steroids. GH treatment is also moderately effective for accelerating growth rates in children with Turner syndrome and chronic renal failure.

In patients with GH insensitivity and growth retardation due to mutations of the GH receptor, treatment with IGF-I bypasses the dysfunctional GH receptor.

TABLE 333-9	FEATURES OF ADULT GROWTH HORMONE DEFICIENCY	
Clinical		**Imaging**

Clinical
Impaired quality of life
  Decreased energy and drive
  Poor concentration
  Low self-esteem
  Social isolation
Body composition changes
  Increased body fat mass
  Central fat deposition
  Increased waist-hip ratio
  Decreased lean body mass
Reduced exercise capacity
  Reduced maximum O₂ uptake
  Impaired cardiac function
  Reduced muscle mass
Cardiovascular risk factors
  Impaired cardiac structure
    and function
  Abnormal lipid profile
  Decreased fibrinolytic activity
  Atherosclerosis
  Omental obesity

Imaging
Pituitary: Mass or structural damage
Bone: Reduced bone mineral density
Abdomen: Excess omental adiposity
Laboratory
Evoked GH <3 ng/mL
IGF-I and IGFBP3 low or normal
Increased LDL-cholesterol
Concomitant gonadotropin, TSH,
  and/or ACTH reserve deficits may
  be present

Note: LDL, low-density lipoprotein; for other abbreviations, see text.

ADULT GH DEFICIENCY (AGHD)

This disorder is usually caused by hypothalamic or pituitary somatotrope damage. Acquired pituitary hormone deficiency follows a typical pattern whereby loss of adequate GH reserve foreshadows subsequent hormone deficits. The sequential order of hormone loss is usually GH → FSH/LH → TSH → ACTH.

Presentation and Diagnosis The clinical features of AGHD include changes in body composition, lipid metabolism, and quality of life and cardiovascular dysfunction (Table 333-9). Body composition changes are common and include reduced lean body mass, increased fat mass with selective deposition of intraabdominal visceral fat, and increased waist-to-hip ratio. Hyperlipidemia, left ventricular dysfunction, hypertension, and increased plasma fibrinogen levels may also be present. Bone mineral content is reduced, with resultant increased fracture rates. Patients may experience social isolation, depression, and difficulty in maintaining gainful employment. Adult hypopituitarism is associated with a threefold increased cardiovascular mortality rate in comparison to age- and sex-matched controls, and this may be due to GH deficiency.

Laboratory Investigation AGHD is rare, and in light of the nonspecific nature of associated clinical symptoms, patients appropriate for testing should be carefully selected on the basis of well-defined criteria. With few exceptions, testing should be restricted to patients with the following predisposing factors: (1) pituitary surgery, (2) pituitary or hypothalamic tumor or granulomas, (3) history of cranial irradiation, (4) radiologic evidence of a pituitary lesion, (5) childhood requirement for GH replacement therapy, or, rarely, (6) unexplained low age- and sex-matched IGF-I levels. The transition of the GH-deficient adolescent to adulthood requires retesting to document adult GH deficiency. Up to 20% of patients previously treated for childhood-onset GH deficiency are found to be GH-sufficient on repeat testing as adults.

A significant proportion (~25%) of truly GH-deficient adults have low-normal IGF-I levels. Thus, as in the evaluation of GH deficiency in children, valid age- and gender-matched IGF-I measurements provide a useful index of therapeutic responses but are not sufficiently sensitive for diagnostic purposes. The most validated test to distinguish pituitary-sufficient patients from those with AGHD is insulin-induced (0.05–0.1 U/kg) hypoglycemia. After glucose reduction to ~40 mg/dL, most individuals experience neuroglycopenic symptoms (Chap. 339), and peak GH release occurs at 60 min and remains elevated for up to 2 h. About 90% of healthy adults exhibit GH responses >5 μg/L; AGHD is defined by a peak GH response to hypoglycemia of <3 μg/L. Although insulin-induced hypoglycemia is safe when per-

formed under appropriate supervision, it is contraindicated in patients with diabetes, ischemic heart disease, cerebrovascular disease, or epilepsy, and in elderly patients. Alternative stimulatory tests include intravenous arginine (30 g), GHRH (1 μg/kg), and GHRP-6 (90 μg). Combinations of these tests may evoke GH secretion in subjects not responsive to a single test.

℞ ADULT GH DEFICIENCY

Once the diagnosis of AGHD is unequivocally established, replacement of GH may be indicated. Contraindications to therapy include the presence of an active neoplasm, intracranial hypertension, or uncontrolled diabetes and retinopathy. The starting dose of 0.1–0.2 mg/d should be titrated (up to a maximum of 1.25 mg/d) to maintain IGF-I levels in the mid-normal range for age- and gender-matched controls **(Fig. 333-7)**. Women require higher doses than men, and elderly patients require less GH. Long-term GH maintenance sustains normal IGF-I levels and is associated with persistent body composition changes (e.g., enhanced lean body mass and lower body fat). High-density lipoprotein cholesterol increases, but total cholesterol and insulin levels do not change significantly. Lumbar spine bone mineral density increases, but this response is gradual (>1 year). Many patients note significant improvement in quality of life when evaluated by standardized questionnaires. The effect of GH replacement on mortality rates in GH-deficient patients is currently the subject of long-term prospective investigation.

About 30% of patients exhibit reversible dose-related fluid retention, joint pain, and carpal tunnel syndrome, and up to 40% exhibit myalgias and paresthesia. Patients receiving insulin require careful monitoring for dosing adjustments, as GH is a potent counterregulatory hormone for insulin action. Patients with type 2 diabetes mellitus initially develop further insulin resistance. However, glycemic control improves with the sustained loss of abdominal fat associated with long-term GH replacement. Headache, increased intracranial pressure, hypertension, atrial fibrillation, and tinnitus occur rarely. Prevalence of pituitary tumor regrowth and potential progression of skin lesions are currently being assessed in long-term surveillance programs. To date, development of these potential side effects does not appear significant.

ACROMEGALY

Etiology GH hypersecretion is usually the result of a somatotrope adenoma but may rarely be caused by extrapituitary lesions (Table 333-10). In addition to more common GH-secreting somatotrope adenomas, mixed mammosomatotrope tumors and acidophilic stem-cell adenomas secrete both GH and PRL. In patients with acidophilic stem-cell adenomas, features of hyperprolactinemia (hypogonadism

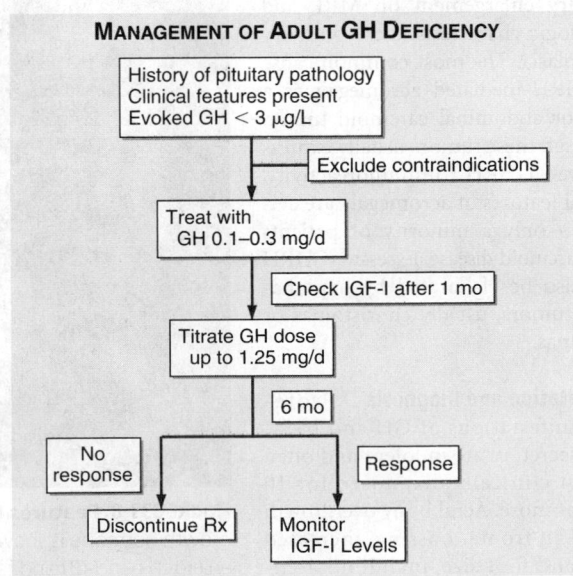

FIGURE 333-7 Management of adult growth hormone (GH) deficiency. IGF, insulin-like growth factor.

TABLE 333-10 CAUSES OF ACROMEGALY	
	Prevalence, %
Excess Growth Hormone Secretion	
Pituitary	98
Densely or sparsely granulated GH cell adenoma	60
Mixed GH cell and PRL cell adenoma	25
Mammosomatrope cell adenoma	10
Plurihormonal adenoma	
GH cell carcinoma or metastases	
Multiple endocrine neoplasia-1 (GH cell adenoma)	
McCune-Albright syndrome	
Ectopic sphenoid or parapharyngeal sinus pituitary adenoma	
Extrapituitary tumor	
Pancreatic islet cell tumor	<1
Lymphoma	
Excess Growth Hormone–Releasing Hormone Secretion	
Central	<1
Hypothalamic hamartoma, choristoma, ganglioneuroma	<1
Peripheral	<1
Bronchial carcinoid, pancreatic islet cell tumor, small cell lung cancer, adrenal adenoma, medullary thyroid carcinoma, pheochromocytoma	

Source: Adapted from S Melmed: N Engl J Med 322:966, 1990.

and galactorrhea) predominate over the less clinically evident signs of acromegaly. Occasionally, mixed plurihormonal tumors are encountered that secrete ACTH, the glycoprotein hormone subunit, or TSH, in addition to GH. Patients with partially empty sellae may present with GH hypersecretion due to a small GH-secreting adenoma within the compressed rim of pituitary tissue; some of these may reflect the spontaneous necrosis of tumors that were previously larger. GH-secreting tumors rarely arise from ectopic pituitary tissue remnants in the nasopharynx or midline sinuses.

There are case reports of ectopic GH secretion by tumors of pancreatic, ovarian, lung, or hematopoietic origin. Excess GHRH production may cause acromegaly because of chronic stimulation of somatotropes. These patients present with classic features of acromegaly, elevated GH levels, pituitary enlargement on MRI, and pathologic characteristics of pituitary hyperplasia. The most common cause of GHRH-mediated acromegaly is a chest or abdominal carcinoid tumor. Although these tumors usually express positive GHRH immunoreactivity, clinical features of acromegaly are evident in only a minority of patients with carcinoid disease. Excessive GHRH may also be elaborated by hypothalamic tumors, usually choristomas or neuromas.

Presentation and Diagnosis Protean manifestations of GH and IGF-I hypersecretion are indolent and often are not clinically diagnosed for 10 years or more. Acral bony overgrowth results in frontal bossing, increased hand and foot size, mandibular enlargement with prognathism, and widened space between the lower inci-

sor teeth. In children and adolescents, initiation of GH hypersecretion prior to epiphyseal long bone closure is associated with development of pituitary gigantism (Fig. 333-8). Soft tissue swelling results in increased heel pad thickness, increased shoe or glove size, ring tightening, characteristic coarse facial features, and a large fleshy nose. Other commonly encountered clinical features include hyperhidrosis, deep and hollow-sounding voice, oily skin, arthropathy, kyphosis, carpal tunnel syndrome, proximal muscle weakness and fatigue, acanthosis nigricans, and skin tags. Generalized visceromegaly occurs, including cardiomegaly, macroglossia, and thyroid gland enlargement.

The most significant clinical impact of GH excess occurs with respect to the cardiovascular system. Coronary heart disease, cardiomyopathy with arrhythmias, left ventricular hypertrophy, decreased diastolic function, and hypertension occur in about 30% of patients. Upper airway obstruction with sleep apnea occurs in more than 60% of patients and is associated with both soft tissue laryngeal airway obstruction and central sleep dysfunction. Diabetes mellitus develops in 25% of patients with acromegaly, and most patients are intolerant of a glucose load (as GH counteracts the action of insulin). Acromegaly is associated with an increased risk of colon polyps and mortality from colonic malignancy; polyps are diagnosed in up to one-third of patients. Overall mortality is increased about threefold and is due primarily to cardiovascular and cerebrovascular disorders and respiratory disease. Unless GH levels are controlled, survival is reduced by an average of 10 years compared with an age-matched control population.

Laboratory Investigation Age- and gender-matched serum IGF-I levels are elevated in acromegaly. Consequently, an IGF-I level provides a useful laboratory screening measure when clinical features raise the possibility of acromegaly. Due to the pulsatility of GH secretion, measurement of a single random GH level is not useful for the diagnosis or exclusion of acromegaly and does not correlate with disease severity. The diagnosis of acromegaly is confirmed by demonstrating the failure of GH suppression to <1 μg/L within 1–2 h of an oral glucose load (75 g). Using newer ultrasensitive GH assays, normal nadir GH levels are even lower (<0.05 μg/L). About 20% of patients exhibit a paradoxical

FIGURE 333-8 Features of acromegaly/gigantism. A 22-year-old man with gigantism due to excess growth hormone is shown to the left of his identical twin. The increased height and prognathism **(A)** and enlarged hand **(B)** and foot **(C)** of the affected twin are apparent. Their clinical features began to diverge at the age of approximately 13 years. (*Reproduced from R Gagel, IE McCutcheon: N Engl J Med 324:524, 1999; with permission.*)

GH rise after glucose. PRL should be measured, as it is elevated in ~25% of patients with acromegaly. Thyroid function, gonadotropins, and sex steroids may be attenuated because of tumor mass effects. Because most patients will undergo surgery with glucocorticoid coverage, tests of ACTH reserve in asymptomatic patients are more efficiently deferred until after surgery.

Rx ACROMEGALY

Surgical resection of GH-secreting adenomas is the initial treatment for most patients (**Fig. 333-9**). Somatostatin analogues are used as adjuvant treatment for preoperative shrinkage of large invasive macroadenomas, immediate relief of debilitating symptoms, and reduction of GH hypersecretion, in frail patients experiencing morbidity, in patients who decline surgery, or, when surgery fails, to achieve biochemical control. Irradiation or repeat surgery may be required for patients who cannot tolerate or do not respond to adjunctive medical therapy. The high rate of late hypopituitarism and the slow rate (5–15 years) of biochemical response are the main disadvantages of radiotherapy. Irradiation is relatively ineffective in normalizing IGF-I levels. Stereotactic ablation of GH-secreting adenomas by gamma-knife radiotherapy is promising, but long-term results are not available and the side effects have not been clearly delineated. Somatostatin analogues may be given while awaiting the full benefits of radiotherapy. Systemic sequelae of acromegaly, including cardiovascular disease, diabetes, and arthritis, should also be managed aggressively. Maxillofacial surgery for mandibular repair may be indicated.

SURGERY Transsphenoidal surgical resection by an experienced surgeon is the preferred primary treatment for both microadenomas (cure rate ~70%) and macroadenomas (<50% cured). Soft tissue swelling improves immediately after tumor resection. GH levels return to normal within an hour, and IGF-I levels are normalized within 3–4 days. In ~10% of patients, acromegaly may recur several years after apparently successful surgery; hypopituitarism develops in up to 15% of patients.

SOMATOSTATIN ANALOGUES Somatostatin analogues exert their therapeutic effects through SSTR2 and -5 receptors, both of which are invariably expressed by GH-secreting tumors. Octreotide acetate is an eight-amino-acid synthetic somatostatin analogue. In contrast to native somatostatin, the analogue is relatively resistant to plasma degradation. It has a 2-h serum half-life and possesses fortyfold greater potency than native somatostatin to suppress GH. Octreotide is administered by subcutaneous injection, beginning with 50 µg tid; the dose can be gradually increased up to 1500 µg/d. Fewer than 10% of patients do not respond to the analogue. Octreotide suppresses integrated GH levels to <5 µg/L in ~70% of patients and to <2 µg/L in up to 60% of patients. It normalizes IGF-I levels in ~75% of treated patients. Prolonged use of the analogue is not associated with desensitization, even after ≥20 years of treatment. Rapid relief of headache and soft tissue swelling occurs in ~75% of patients within days to weeks of treatment initiation. Subjective clinical benefits of octreotide therapy occur more frequently than biochemical remission, and most patients report symptomatic improvement, including amelioration of headache, perspiration, obstructive apnea, and cardiac failure. Modest pituitary tumor size reduction occurs in about 40% of patients, but this effect is reversed when treatment is stopped.

The long-acting somatostatin depot formulations, octreotide and lanreotide, are the preferred medical treatment for patients with acromegaly. *Sandostatin-LAR* is a sustained-release, long-acting formulation of octreotide incorporated into microspheres that sustain drug levels for several weeks after intramuscular injection. GH suppression occurs for as long as 6 weeks after a 30-mg injection; long-term monthly treatment sustains GH and IGF-I suppression and also reduces pituitary tumor size in ~50% of patients. *Lanreotide*, a slow-release depot somatostatin preparation, is a cyclic somatostatin octapeptide analogue that suppresses GH and IGF-I hypersecretion for 10–14 days after a 30-mg intramuscular injection. Long-term administration controls GH hypersecretion in two-thirds of treated patients and improves patient compliance because of the long interval required between drug injections. A subcutaneous long-acting gel formulation is also available. Lanreotide is not currently approved in the USA.

Side Effects Somatostatin analogues are well tolerated in most patients. Adverse effects are short-lived and mostly relate to drug-induced suppression of gastrointestinal motility and secretion. Nausea, abdominal discomfort, fat malabsorption, diarrhea, and flatulence occur in one-third of patients, and these symptoms usually remit within 2 weeks. Octreotide suppresses postprandial gallbladder contractility and delays gallbladder emptying; up to 30% of patients develop long-term echogenic sludge or asymptomatic cholesterol gallstones. Other side effects include mild glucose intolerance due to transient insulin suppression, asymptomatic bradycardia, hypothyroxinemia, and local injection site discomfort.

GH RECEPTOR ANTAGONISTS Pegvisomant antagonizes endogenous GH action by blocking peripheral GH binding to its receptor. Consequently, serum IGF-I levels are suppressed, reducing the deleterious effects of excess endogenous GH. Pegvisomant is administered by daily subcutaneous injection (10–20 mg), and normalizes IGF-I in >90% of patients. GH levels, however, remain elevated as the drug does not have antitumor actions. Side effects include reversible liver enzyme elevation, lipodystrophy, and injection site pain. Tumor size should be monitored by MRI.

Combined treatment with monthly octreotide-LAR and weekly or biweekly pegvisomant injections has been effectively used for resistant patients.

DOPAMINE AGONISTS Bromocriptine and cabergoline may suppress GH secretion in some patients, particularly those with cosecretion of PRL. High bromocriptine doses (≥20 mg/d) are usually required to achieve modest GH therapeutic efficacy. Cabergoline also modestly suppresses GH when given at a relatively high dose of 0.5 mg/d. Combined treatment with octreotide and cabergoline may induce additive biochemical control compared to either drug alone.

RADIATION External radiation therapy or high-energy stereotactic techniques are used as adjuvant therapy for acromegaly. An advantage of radiation is that patient compliance with long-term treatment is not required. Tumor mass is reduced, and GH levels are attenuated over time. However, 50% of patients require at least 8 years for GH levels to be suppressed to <5 µg/L; this level of GH reduction is achieved in about 90% of patients after 18 years but represents suboptimal GH suppression. Patients may require interim medical therapy for several years prior to attaining

FIGURE 333-9 Management of acromegaly. GH, growth hormone; CNS, central nervous system; IGF, insulin-like growth factor. (*Adapted from S. Melmed et al: J Clin Endocrinol Metab 83:2646, 1998; © The Endocrine Society.*)

MANAGEMENT OF ACROMEGALY

GH-Secreting Adenoma → Assess likelihood of surgical cure

- Likely → Debulking required for CNS pressure effects → Surgery → Measure GH/IGF-I
  - controlled → Monitor
  - elevated → Somatostatin analogue → Measure GH/IGF-I → controlled → Monitor
- Unlikely → Somatostatin analogue → Measure GH/IGF-I → controlled → Monitor

Measure GH/IGF-I → Improve somatostatin analogue efficacy: increase dose/frequency; add dopamine agonist or GH receptor antagonist

uncontrolled → Measure GH/IGF-I
- controlled → Monitor
- uncontrolled → • GH receptor antagonist • Radiation therapy • Reoperation

maximal radiation benefits. Most patients also experience hypothalamic-pituitary damage, leading to gonadotropin, ACTH, and/or TSH deficiency within 10 years of therapy.

In summary, surgery is the preferred primary treatment for GH-secreting microadenomas (Fig. 333-9). The high frequency of GH hypersecretion after macroadenoma resection usually necessitates adjuvant or primary medical therapy for these larger tumors. Patients unable to receive or respond to unimodal medical treatment may benefit from combined treatments, or can be offered radiation.

ADRENOCORTICOTROPIN HORMONE (See also Chap. 336)

SYNTHESIS

ACTH-secreting corticotrope cells constitute about 20% of the pituitary cell population. ACTH (39 amino acids) is derived from the POMC precursor protein (266 amino acids) that also generates several other peptides, including β-lipotropin, β-endorphin, met-enkephalin, α melanocyte-stimulating hormone (MSH), and corticotropin-like intermediate lobe protein (CLIP). The POMC gene is potently suppressed by glucocorticoids and induced by CRH, arginine vasopressin (AVP), and proinflammatory cytokines, including IL-6, as well as leukemia inhibitory factor.

CRH, a 41-amino-acid hypothalamic peptide synthesized in the paraventricular nucleus as well as in higher brain centers, is the predominant stimulator of ACTH synthesis and release. The CRH receptor is a GPCR that is expressed on the corticotrope and induces POMC transcription.

SECRETION

ACTH secretion is pulsatile and exhibits a characteristic circadian rhythm, peaking at 6 A.M. and reaching a nadir about midnight. Adrenal glucocorticoid secretion, which is driven by ACTH, follows a parallel diurnal pattern. ACTH circadian rhythmicity is determined by variations in secretory pulse amplitude rather than changes in pulse frequency. Superimposed on this endogenous rhythm, ACTH levels are increased by AVP, physical stress, exercise, acute illness, and insulin-induced hypoglycemia.

Loss of cortisol feedback inhibition, as occurs in primary adrenal failure, results in extremely high ACTH levels. Glucocorticoid-mediated negative regulation of the hypothalamo-pituitary-adrenal (HPA) axis occurs as a consequence of both hypothalamic CRH suppression and direct attenuation of pituitary POMC gene expression and ACTH release.

Acute inflammatory or septic insults activate the HPA axis through the integrated actions of proinflammatory cytokines, bacterial toxins, and neural signals. The overlapping cascade of ACTH-inducing cytokines [tumor necrosis factor (TNF); IL-1, -2, and -6; and leukemia inhibitory factor] activates hypothalamic CRH and AVP secretion, pituitary POMC gene expression, and local paracrine pituitary cytokine networks. The resulting cortisol elevation restrains the inflammatory response and enables host protection. Concomitantly, cytokine-mediated central glucocorticoid receptor resistance impairs glucocorticoid suppression of the HPA. Thus, the neuroendocrine stress response reflects the net result of highly integrated hypothalamic, intrapituitary, and peripheral hormone and cytokine signals.

ACTION

The major function of the HPA axis is to maintain metabolic homeostasis and to mediate the neuroendocrine stress response. ACTH induces adrenocortical steroidogenesis by maintaining adrenal cell proliferation and function. The receptor for ACTH, designated *melanocortin-2 receptor*, is a GPCR that induces steroidogenesis by stimulating a cascade of steroidogenic enzymes (Chap. 336).

ACTH DEFICIENCY

Presentation and Diagnosis Secondary adrenal insufficiency occurs as a result of pituitary ACTH deficiency. It is characterized by fatigue,

weakness, anorexia, nausea, vomiting, and, occasionally, hypoglycemia. In contrast to primary adrenal failure, hypocortisolism associated with pituitary failure is not usually accompanied by pigmentation changes or mineralocorticoid deficiency. *TPIT* mutations result in primary ACTH deficiency.

ACTH deficiency is commonly due to glucocorticoid withdrawal following treatment-associated suppression of the HPA axis. Isolated ACTH deficiency may occur after surgical resection of an ACTH-secreting pituitary adenoma that has suppressed the HPA axis; this phenomenon is suggestive of a surgical cure. The mass effects of other pituitary adenomas or sellar lesions may lead to ACTH deficiency, but usually in combination with other pituitary hormone deficiencies. Partial ACTH deficiency may be unmasked in the presence of an acute medical or surgical illness, when clinically significant hypocortisolism reflects diminished ACTH reserve.

Laboratory Diagnosis Inappropriately low ACTH levels in the setting of low cortisol levels are characteristic of diminished ACTH reserve. Low basal serum cortisol levels are associated with blunted cortisol responses to ACTH stimulation and impaired cortisol response to insulin-induced hypoglycemia, or testing with metyrapone or CRH. For description of provocative ACTH tests, see "Tests of Pituitary-Adrenal Responsiveness" in Chap. 336.

℞ ACTH DEFICIENCY

Glucocorticoid replacement therapy improves most features of ACTH deficiency. The total daily dose of hydrocortisone replacement should not exceed 30 mg daily, divided into two or three doses. Prednisone (5 mg each morning; 2.5 mg each evening) is longer-acting and has fewer mineralocorticoid effects than hydrocortisone. Some authorities advocate lower maintenance doses in an effort to avoid cushingoid side effects. Doses should be increased several-fold during periods of acute illness or stress.

CUSHING'S SYNDROME (ACTH-PRODUCING ADENOMA)
(See also Chap. 336)

Etiology and Prevalence Pituitary corticotrope adenomas account for 70% of patients with endogenous causes of Cushing's syndrome. However, it should be emphasized that iatrogenic hypercortisolism is the most common cause of cushingoid features. Ectopic tumor ACTH production, cortisol-producing adrenal adenomas, adrenal carcinoma, and adrenal hyperplasia account for the other causes; rarely, ectopic tumor CRH production is encountered.

ACTH-producing adenomas account for about 10–15% of all pituitary tumors. Because the clinical features of Cushing's syndrome often lead to early diagnosis, most ACTH-producing pituitary tumors are relatively small microadenomas. However, macroadenomas are also seen, and some ACTH-secreting adenomas are clinically silent. Cushing's disease is 5–10 times more common in women than in men. These pituitary adenomas exhibit unrestrained ACTH secretion, with resultant hypercortisolemia. However, they retain partial suppressibility in the presence of high doses of administered glucocorticoids, providing the basis for dynamic testing to distinguish pituitary and nonpituitary causes of Cushing's syndrome.

Presentation and Diagnosis The diagnosis of Cushing's syndrome presents two great challenges: (1) to distinguish patients with pathologic cortisol excess from those with physiologic or other disturbances of cortisol production; and (2) to determine the etiology of cortisol excess.

Typical features of chronic cortisol excess include thin, fragile skin, central obesity, hypertension, plethoric moon facies, purple striae and easy bruisability, glucose intolerance or diabetes mellitus, gonadal dysfunction, osteoporosis, proximal muscle weakness, signs of hyperandrogenism (acne, hirsutism), and psychological disturbances (depression, mania, and psychoses) (Table 333-11). Hematopoietic features of hypercortisolism include leukocytosis, lymphopenia, and eosinopenia. Immune suppression includes delayed hypersensitivity. The protean manifesta-

TABLE 333-11 CLINICAL FEATURES OF CUSHING'S SYNDROME (ALL AGES)

Symptoms/Signs	Frequency, %
Obesity or weight gain (>115% ideal body weight)	80
Thin skin	80
Moon facies	75
Hypertension	75
Purple skin striae	65
Hirsutism	65
Abnormal glucose tolerance	55
Impotence	55
Menstrual disorders (usually amenorrhea)	60
Plethora	60
Proximal muscle weakness	50
Truncal obesity	50
Acne	45
Bruising	45
Mental changes	45
Osteoporosis	40
Edema of lower extremities	30
Hyperpigmentation	20
Hypokalemic alkalosis	15
Diabetes mellitus	15

Source: Adapted from MA Magiokou et al, in ME Wierman (ed), *Diseases of the Pituitary.* Totowa, NJ, Humana, 1997.

tions of hypercortisolism make it challenging to decide which patients mandate formal laboratory evaluation. Certain features make pathologic causes of hypercortisolism more likely—these include characteristic central redistribution of fat, thin skin with striae and bruising, and proximal muscle weakness. In children and in young females, early osteoporosis may be particularly prominent. The primary cause of death is cardiovascular disease, but infections and risk of suicide are also increased.

Rapid development of features of hypercortisolism associated with skin hyperpigmentation and severe myopathy suggests an ectopic source of ACTH. Hypertension, hypokalemic alkalosis, glucose intolerance, and edema are also more pronounced in these patients. Serum potassium levels <3.3 mmol/L are evident in ~70% of patients with ectopic ACTH secretion but are seen in <10% of patients with pituitary-dependent Cushing's syndrome.

Laboratory Investigation The diagnosis of Cushing's syndrome is based on laboratory documentation of endogenous hypercortisolism. Measurements of 24-h urine free cortisol (UFC) is a precise and cost-effective screening test. Alternatively, the failure to suppress plasma cortisol after an overnight 1-mg dexamethasone suppression test can be used to identify patients with hypercortisolism. As nadir levels of cortisol occur at night, elevated midnight samples of cortisol are suggestive of Cushing's syndrome. Basal plasma ACTH levels often distinguish patients with ACTH-independent (adrenal or exogenous glucocorticoid) from those with ACTH-dependent (pituitary, ectopic ACTH) Cushing's syndrome. Mean basal ACTH levels are about eightfold higher in patients with ectopic ACTH secretion compared to those with pituitary ACTH-secreting adenomas. However, extensive overlap of ACTH levels in these two disorders precludes using ACTH to make the distinction. Instead, dynamic testing, based on differential sensitivity to glucocorticoid feedback, or ACTH stimulation in response to CRH or cortisol reduction is used to discriminate ectopic versus pituitary sources of excess ACTH (Table 333-12). Very rarely, circulating CRH levels are elevated, reflecting ectopic tumor-derived secretion of CRH and often ACTH. For further discussion of dynamic testing for Cushing's syndrome, see Chap. 336.

Most ACTH-secreting pituitary tumors are <5 mm in diameter, and about half are undetectable by sensitive MRI. The high prevalence of incidental pituitary microadenomas diminishes the ability to distinguish ACTH-secreting pituitary tumors accurately by MRI.

Inferior Petrosal Venous Sampling Because pituitary MRI with gadolinium enhancement is insufficiently sensitive to detect small (<2 mm)

pituitary ACTH-secreting adenomas, bilateral inferior petrosal sinus ACTH sampling before and after CRH administration may be required to distinguish these lesions from ectopic ACTH-secreting tumors that may have similar clinical and biochemical characteristics. Simultaneous assessment of ACTH concentrations in each inferior petrosal vein and in the peripheral circulation provides a strategy for confirming and localizing pituitary ACTH production. Sampling is performed at baseline and 2, 5, and 10 min after intravenous ovine CRH (1 μg/kg) injection. An increased ratio (>2) of inferior petrosal: peripheral vein ACTH confirms pituitary Cushing's syndrome. After CRH injection, peak petrosal:peripheral ACTH ratios of ≥3 confirm the presence of a pituitary ACTH-secreting tumor. The sensitivity of this test is >95%, with very rare false-positive results. False-negative results may be encountered in patients with aberrant venous drainage. Petrosal sinus catheterizations are technically difficult, and about 0.05% of patients develop neurovascular complications. The procedure should not be performed in patients with hypertension or in the presence of a well-visualized pituitary adenoma on MRI.

Rx CUSHING'S SYNDROME

Selective transsphenoidal resection is the treatment of choice for Cushing's syndrome **(Fig. 333-10)**. The remission rate for this procedure is ~80% for microadenomas but <50% for macroadenomas. After successful tumor resection, most patients experience a postoperative period of symptomatic ACTH deficiency that lasts for up to 12 months. This usually requires low-dose cortisol replacement, as patients experience steroid withdrawal symptoms as well as having a suppressed HPA axis. Biochemical recurrence occurs in approximately 5% of patients in whom surgery was initially successful.

When initial surgery is unsuccessful, repeat surgery is sometimes indicated, particularly when a pituitary source for ACTH is well documented. In older patients, in whom issues of growth and fertility are less important, hemi- or total hypophysectomy may be necessary if a discrete adenoma is

TABLE 333-12 DIFFERENTIAL DIAGNOSIS OF ACTH-DEPENDENT CUSHING'S SYNDROME[a]

	ACTH-Secreting Pituitary Tumor	Ectopic ACTH Secretion
Etiology	Pituitary corticotrope adenoma Plurihormonal adenoma	Bronchial, abdominal carcinoid Small cell lung cancer Thymoma
Gender	F > M	M > F
Clinical features	Slow onset	Rapid onset Pigmentation Severe myopathy
Serum potassium <3.3 μg/L	<10%	75%
24-h urinary free cortisol (UFC)	High	High
Basal ACTH level	Inappropriately high	Very high
Dexamethasone suppression 1 mg overnight		
Low dose (0.5 mg q6h)	Cortisol >5 μg/dL	Cortisol >5 μg/dL
High dose (2 mg q6h)	Cortisol <5 μg/dL	Cortisol >5 μg/dL
UFC > 80% suppressed	Microadenomas: 90% Macroadenomas: 50%	10%
Inferior petrosal sinus sampling (IPSS) Basal		
IPSS: peripheral	>2	<2
CRH-induced IPSS: peripheral	>3	<3

[a]ACTH-independent causes of Cushing's syndrome are diagnosed by suppressed ACTH levels and an adrenal mass in the setting of hypercortisolism. Iatrogenic Cushing's syndrome is excluded by history.

Note: ACTH, adrenocorticotropin hormone; F, female; M, male; CRH, corticotropin-releasing hormone.

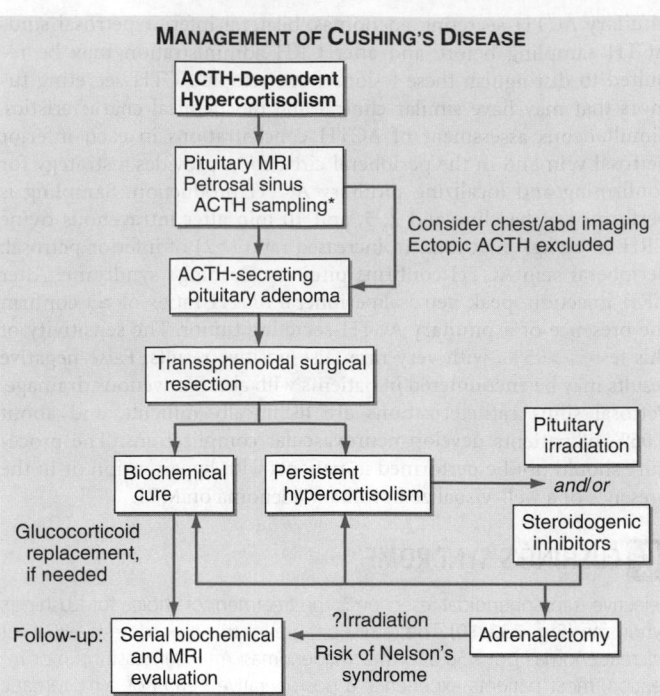

FIGURE 333-10 Management of Cushing's syndrome. ACTH, adrenocorticotropin hormone; MRI, magnetic resonance imaging. *, Not usually required.

not recognized. Pituitary irradiation may be used after unsuccessful surgery, but it cures only about 15% of patients. Because radiation is slow and only partially effective in adults, steroidogenic inhibitors are used in combination with pituitary irradiation to block the adrenal effects of persistently high ACTH levels.

Ketoconazole, an imidazole derivative antimycotic agent, inhibits several P450 enzymes and effectively lowers cortisol in most patients with Cushing's disease when administered twice daily (600–1200 mg/d). Elevated hepatic transaminases, gynecomastia, impotence, gastrointestinal upset, and edema are common side effects. *Metyrapone* (2–4 g/d) inhibits 11β-hydroxylase activity and normalizes plasma cortisol in up to 75% of patients. Side effects include nausea and vomiting, rash, and exacerbation of acne or hirsutism. *Mitotane* (o,p′-DDD; 3–6 g/d orally in four divided doses) suppresses cortisol hypersecretion by inhibiting 11β-hydroxylase and cholesterol side-chain cleavage enzymes and by destroying adrenocortical cells. Side effects of mitotane include gastrointestinal symptoms, dizziness, gynecomastia, hyperlipidemia, skin rash, and hepatic enzyme elevation. It may also lead to hypoaldosteronism. Other agents include *aminoglutethimide* (250 mg tid), *trilostane* (200–1000 mg/d), *cyproheptadine* (24 mg/d), and IV *etomidate* (0.3 mg/kg per hour). Glucocorticoid insufficiency is a potential side effect of agents used to block steroidogenesis.

The use of steroidogenic inhibitors has decreased the need for bilateral adrenalectomy. Removal of both adrenal glands corrects hypercortisolism but may be associated with significant morbidity and necessitates permanent glucocorticoid and mineralocorticoid replacement. Adrenalectomy in the setting of residual corticotrope adenoma tissue predisposes to the development of *Nelson's syndrome*, a disorder characterized by rapid pituitary tumor enlargement and increased pigmentation secondary to high ACTH levels. Radiation therapy may be indicated to prevent the development of Nelson's syndrome after adrenalectomy.

GONADOTROPINS: FSH AND LH

SYNTHESIS AND SECRETION
Gonadotrope cells constitute about 10% of anterior pituitary cells and produce two gonadotropins—LH and FSH. Like TSH and hCG, LH and FSH are glycoprotein hormones consisting of α and β subunits. The α subunit is common to these glycoprotein hormones; specificity is conferred by the β subunits, which are expressed by separate genes.

Gonadotropin synthesis and release are dynamically regulated. This is particularly true in women, in whom the rapidly fluctuating gonadal steroid levels vary throughout the menstrual cycle. Hypothalamic GnRH, a 10-amino-acid peptide, regulates the synthesis and secretion of both LH and FSH. GnRH is secreted in discrete pulses every 60–120 min, which in turn elicit LH and FSH pulses (Fig. 333-3). The pulsatile mode of GnRH input is essential to its action; pulses prime gonadotrope responsiveness, whereas continuous GnRH exposure induces desensitization. Based on this phenomenon, long-acting GnRH agonists are used to suppress gonadotropin levels in children with precocious puberty and in men with prostate cancer (Chap. 91) and are used in some ovulation-induction protocols to reduce endogenous gonadotropins (Chap. 341). Estrogens act at the hypothalamic and pituitary levels to control gonadotropin secretion. Chronic estrogen exposure is inhibitory, whereas rising estrogen levels, as occur during the preovulatory surge, exert positive feedback to increase gonadotropin pulse frequency and amplitude. Progesterone slows GnRH pulse frequency but enhances gonadotropin responses to GnRH. Testosterone feedback in men also occurs at the hypothalamic and pituitary levels and is mediated in part by its conversion to estrogens.

Although GnRH is the main regulator of LH and FSH secretion, FSH synthesis is also under separate control by the gonadal peptides inhibin and activin, which are members of the transforming growth factor β (TGF-β) family. Inhibin selectively suppresses FSH, whereas activin stimulates FSH synthesis (Chap. 341).

ACTION
The gonadotropin hormones interact with their respective GPCRs expressed in the ovary and testis, evoking germ-cell development and maturation and steroid hormone biosynthesis. In women, FSH regulates ovarian follicle development and stimulates ovarian estrogen production. LH mediates ovulation and maintenance of the corpus luteum. In men, LH induces Leydig cell testosterone synthesis and secretion and FSH stimulates seminiferous tubule development and regulates spermatogenesis.

GONADOTROPIN DEFICIENCY
Hypogonadism is the most common presenting feature of adult hypopituitarism, even when other pituitary hormones are also deficient. It is often a harbinger of hypothalamic or pituitary lesions that impair GnRH production or delivery through the pituitary stalk. As noted above, hypogonadotropic hypogonadism is a common presenting feature of hyperprolactinemia.

A variety of inherited and acquired disorders are associated with *isolated hypogonadotropic hypogonadism* (IHH) (Chap. 340). Hypothalamic defects associated with GnRH deficiency include two X-linked disorders, Kallmann syndrome (see above) and mutations in the *DAX1* gene, as well as dominant mutations in *FGFR1*. Mutations in GPR54, the GnRH receptor, and the LH β or FSH β subunit genes are additional causes of selective gonadotropin deficiency. Acquired forms of GnRH deficiency leading to hypogonadotropism are seen in association with anorexia nervosa (Chap. 76), stress, starvation, and extreme exercise, but may also be idiopathic. Hypogonadotropic hypogonadism in these disorders is reversed by removal of the stressful stimulus, or caloric replenishment.

Presentation and Diagnosis In premenopausal women, hypogonadotropic hypogonadism presents as diminished ovarian function leading to oligomenorrhea or amenorrhea, infertility, decreased vaginal secretions, decreased libido, and breast atrophy. In hypogonadal adult men, secondary testicular failure is associated with decreased libido and potency, infertility, decreased muscle mass with weakness, reduced beard and body hair growth, soft testes, and characteristic fine facial wrinkles. Osteoporosis occurs in both untreated hypogonadal women and men.

Laboratory Investigation Central hypogonadism is associated with low or inappropriately normal serum gonadotropin levels in the setting of low sex hormone concentrations (testosterone in men, estradiol in women). Because gonadotropin secretion is pulsatile, valid assessments may require repeated measurements or using pooled serum samples. Men have abnormal semen analysis.

Intravenous GnRH (100 µg) stimulates gonadotropes to secrete LH (which peaks within 30 min) and FSH (which plateaus during the ensuing 60 min). Normal responses vary according to menstrual cycle stage, age, and sex of the patient. Generally, LH levels increase about threefold, whereas FSH responses are less pronounced. In the setting of gonadotropin deficiency, a normal gonadotropin response to GnRH indicates intact gonadotrope function and suggests a hypothalamic abnormality. An absent response, however, cannot reliably distinguish pituitary from hypothalamic causes of hypogonadism. For this reason, GnRH testing usually adds little to the information gained from baseline evaluation of the hypothalamic-pituitary-gonadotrope axis, except in cases of isolated GnRH deficiency (e.g., Kallmann syndrome).

MRI examination of the sellar region and assessment of other pituitary functions are usually indicated in patients with documented central hypogonadism.

℞ GONADOTROPIN DEFICIENCY

In males, testosterone replacement is necessary to achieve and maintain normal growth and development of the external genitalia, secondary sex characteristics, male sexual behavior, and androgenic anabolic effects including maintenance of muscle function and bone mass. Testosterone may be administered by intramuscular injections every 1–4 weeks or using patches that are replaced daily (Chap. 340). Testosterone gels are also available. Gonadotropin injections [hCG or human menopausal gonadotropin (hMG)] over 12–18 months are used to restore fertility. Pulsatile GnRH therapy (25–150 ng/kg every 2 h), administered by a subcutaneous infusion pump, is also effective for treatment of hypothalamic hypogonadism when fertility is desired.

In premenopausal women, cyclical replacement of estrogen and progesterone maintains secondary sexual characteristics and integrity of genitourinary tract mucosa and prevents premature osteoporosis (Chap. 341). Gonadotropin therapy is used for ovulation induction. Follicular growth and maturation are initiated using hMG or recombinant FSH; hCG is subsequently injected to induce ovulation. As in men, pulsatile GnRH therapy can be used to treat hypothalamic causes of gonadotropin deficiency.

NONFUNCTIONING AND GONADOTROPIN-PRODUCING PITUITARY ADENOMAS
Etiology and Prevalence   Nonfunctioning pituitary adenomas include those that secrete little or no pituitary hormones, as well as tumors that produce too little hormone to result in recognizable clinical features. They are the most common type of pituitary adenoma and are usually macroadenomas at the time of diagnosis because clinical features are inapparent until tumor mass effects occur. Based on immunohistochemistry, most clinically nonfunctioning adenomas can be shown to originate from gonadotrope cells. These tumors typically produce small amounts of intact gonadotropins (usually FSH) as well as uncombined α, LH β, and FSH β subunits. Tumor secretion may lead to elevated α and FSH β subunits and, rarely, to increased LH β subunit levels. Some adenomas express α subunits without FSH or LH. TRH administration often induces an atypical increase of tumor-derived gonadotropins or subunits.

Presentation and Diagnosis   Clinically nonfunctioning tumors often present with optic chiasm pressure and other symptoms of local expansion or may be incidentally discovered on an MRI performed for another indication (incidentaloma). Menstrual disturbances or ovarian hyperstimulation rarely occur in women with large tumors that produce FSH and LH. More commonly, adenoma compression of the pituitary stalk or surrounding pituitary tissue leads to attenuated LH and features of hypogonadism. PRL levels are usually slightly increased, also because of stalk compression. It is important to distinguish this circumstance from true prolactinomas, as most nonfunctioning tumors respond poorly to treatment with dopamine agonists.

Laboratory Investigation   The goal of laboratory testing in clinically nonfunctioning tumors is to classify the type of the tumor, to identify hormonal markers of tumor activity, and to detect possible hypopituitarism. Free α subunit levels may be elevated in 10–15% of patients with nonfunctioning tumors. In female patients, peri- or postmenopausal basal FSH concentrations are difficult to distinguish from tumor-derived FSH elevation. Premenopausal women have cycling FSH levels, also preventing clear-cut diagnostic distinction from tumor-derived FSH. In men, gonadotropin-secreting tumors may be diagnosed because of slightly increased gonadotropins (FSH > LH) in the setting of a pituitary mass. Testosterone levels are usually low, despite the normal or increased LH level, perhaps reflecting reduced LH bioactivity or the loss of normal LH pulsatility. Because this pattern of hormone tests is also seen in primary gonadal failure and, to some extent, with aging (Chap. 340), the finding of increased gonadotropins alone are insufficient for the diagnosis of a gonadotropin-secreting tumor. In the majority of patients with gonadotrope adenomas, TRH administration stimulates LH β subunit secretion; this response is not seen in normal individuals. GnRH testing, however, is not helpful for making the diagnosis. For nonfunctioning and gonadotropin-secreting tumors, the diagnosis usually rests on immunohistochemical analyses of resected tumor tissue, as the mass effects of these tumors usually necessitate resection.

Although acromegaly or Cushing's syndrome usually presents with unique clinical features, clinically inapparent somatotrope or corticotrope adenomas can be excluded by a normal IGF-I value and normal 24-h urinary free cortisol levels. If PRL levels are <100 µg/L in a patient harboring a pituitary mass, a nonfunctioning adenoma causing pituitary stalk compression should be considered.

℞ NONFUNCTIONING AND GONADOTROPIN-PRODUCING PITUITARY ADENOMAS

Asymptomatic small nonfunctioning adenomas with no threat to vision may be followed with regular MRI and visual field testing without immediate intervention. However, for larger macroadenomas, transsphenoidal surgery reduces tumor size and relieves mass effects (**Fig. 333-11**). Although it is not usually possible to remove all adenoma tissue surgically, vision improves in 70% of patients with preoperative visual field defects. Preexisting hypopituitarism that results from tumor mass effects commonly improves or may resolve completely. Beginning about 6 months postoperatively, MRI scans should be performed yearly to detect tumor regrowth. Within 5–6 years following successful surgical resection, ~15% of nonfunctioning tumors recur. When substantial tumor remains after transsphenoidal surgery, adjuvant radiotherapy may be indicated to prevent tumor regrowth. Radiotherapy may be deferred if no postoperative residual mass is evident.

Nonfunctioning pituitary tumors respond poorly to dopamine agonist treatment, with modest tumor shrinkage occurring in <10% of patients. Although SSTR subtypes 2 and 5 have been identified on nonfunctioning pituitary adenomas, octreotide is largely ineffective for shrinking these tumors. The selective GnRH antagonist, Nal-Glu GnRH, suppresses FSH hypersecretion but has no effect on adenoma size.

THYROID-STIMULATING HORMONE

SYNTHESIS AND SECRETION
TSH-secreting thyrotrope cells constitute 5% of the anterior pituitary cell population. TSH is structurally related to LH and FSH. It shares a common α subunit with these hormones but contains a specific TSH β subunit. TRH is a hypothalamic tripeptide (pyroglutamyl histidyl-prolinamide) that acts through a GPCR to stimulate TSH synthesis and secretion; it also stimulates the lactotrope cell to secrete PRL. TSH secretion is stimulated by TRH, whereas thyroid hormones, dopamine, somatostatin, and glucocorticoids suppress TSH by overriding TRH induction.

Thyrotrope growth and TSH secretion are both induced when negative feedback inhibition by thyroid hormones is removed. Thus, thyroid damage (including surgical thyroidectomy), radiation-induced hypothyroidism, chronic thyroiditis, or prolonged goitrogen exposure are associated with increased TSH. Long-standing untreated hypothyroidism can lead to thyrotrope hyperplasia and pituitary enlargement, which may be evident on MRI.

ACTION

TSH is secreted in pulses, though the excursions are modest in comparison to other pituitary hormones because of the low amplitude of the pulses and the relatively long half-life of TSH. Consequently, single determinations of TSH suffice to assess its circulating levels. TSH binds to a GPCR on thyroid follicular cells to stimulate thyroid hormone synthesis and release (Chap. 335).

TSH DEFICIENCY

Features of central hypothyroidism due to TSH deficiency mimic those seen with primary hypothyroidism but are generally less severe. Pituitary hypothyroidism is characterized by low basal TSH levels in the setting of low free thyroid hormone. In contrast, patients with hypothyroidism of hypothalamic origin (presumably due to a lack of endogenous TRH) may exhibit normal or even slightly elevated TSH levels. The TSH produced in this circumstance appears to have reduced biologic activity because of altered glycosylation.

TRH (200 μg) injected intravenously causes a two- to threefold increase in TSH (and PRL) levels within 30 min. Although TRH testing can be used to assess TSH reserve, abnormalities of the thyroid axis can usually be detected based on basal free T$_4$ and TSH levels, and TRH testing is rarely indicated.

Thyroid-replacement therapy should be initiated after establishing adequate adrenal function. Dose adjustment is based on thyroid hormone levels and clinical parameters rather than the TSH level.

TSH-SECRETING ADENOMAS

TSH-producing macroadenomas are rare but are often large and locally invasive when they occur. Patients usually present with thyroid goiter and hyperthyroidism, reflecting overproduction of TSH. Diagnosis is based on demonstrating elevated serum free T$_4$ levels, inappropriately normal or high TSH secretion, and MRI evidence of a pituitary adenoma.

It is important to exclude other causes of inappropriate TSH secretion, such as resistance to thyroid hormone, an autosomal dominant disorder caused by mutations in the thyroid hormone β receptor (Chap. 335). The presence of a pituitary mass and elevated α subunit levels are suggestive of a TSH-secreting tumor. Dysalbuminemic hyperthyroxinemia syndromes, caused by mutations in serum thyroid hormone binding proteins, are also characterized by elevated thyroid hormone levels, but with normal rather than suppressed TSH levels. Moreover, free thyroid hormone levels are normal in these disorders, most of which are familial.

℞ TSH-SECRETING ADENOMAS

The initial therapeutic approach is to remove or debulk the tumor mass surgically, using either a transsphenoidal or subfrontal approach. Total resection is not often achieved as most of these adenomas are large and locally invasive. Normal circulating thyroid hormone levels are achieved in about two-thirds of patients after surgery. Thyroid ablation or antithyroid drugs (methimazole or propylthiouracil) can be used to reduce thyroid hormone levels. Somatostatin analogue treatment effectively normalizes TSH and α subunit hypersecretion, shrinks the tumor mass in 50% of patients, and improves visual fields in 75% of patients; euthyroidism is re-

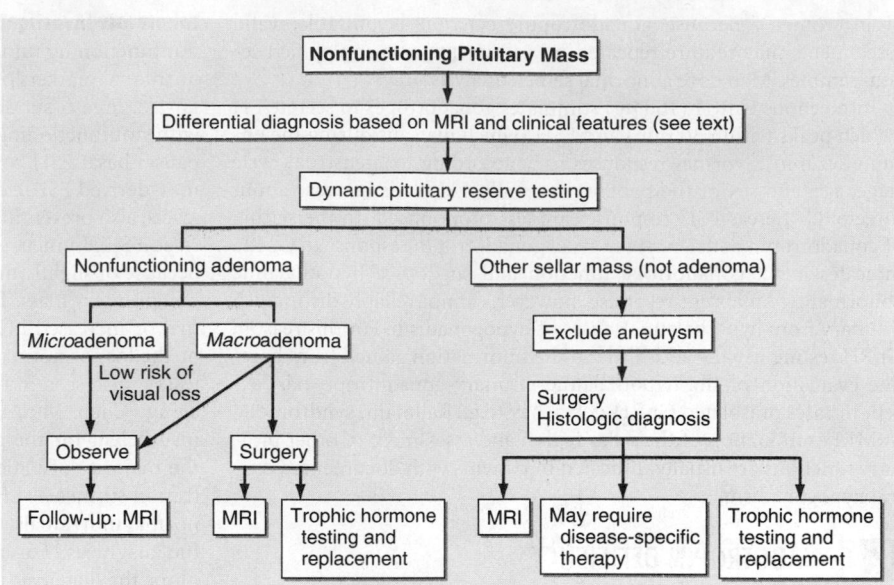

FIGURE 333-11 Management of a nonfunctioning pituitary mass.

stored in most patients. In some patients, octreotide markedly suppresses TSH, causing biochemical hypothyroidism that requires concomitant thyroid hormone replacement. Lanreotide (30 mg intramuscularly), a long-acting somatostatin analogue (see above), effectively suppresses TSH and thyroid hormone in patients treated every 14 days.

DIABETES INSIPIDUS

See Chap. 334 for diagnosis and treatment of diabetes insipidus.

FURTHER READINGS

AIMARETTI G et al: Residual pituitary function after brain injury-induced hypopituitarism: A prospective 12-month study. J Clin Endocrinol Metab 90:6085, 2005

CATUREGLI P et al: Autoimmune hypophysitis. Endocr Rev 26:599, 2005

COLAO A et al: Predictors of remission of hyperprolactinaemia after long-term withdrawal of cabergoline therapy. Clin Endocrinol (Oxf) Sep;67(3):426, 2007

COZZI R et al: Primary treatment of acromegaly with octreotide LAR: A long-term (up to nine years) prospective study of its efficacy in the control of disease activity and tumor shrinkage. J Clin Endocrinol Metab 91:1397, 2006

GILLAM MP et al: Advances in the treatment of prolactinomas. Endocr Rev 27:485, 2006

ILIAS I et al: Cushing's syndrome due to ectopic corticotropin secretion: Twenty years' experience at the National Institutes of Health. J Clin Endocrinol Metab 90:4955, 2005

JALLAD RS et al: Does partial surgical tumour removal influence the response to octreotide-LAR in acromegalic patients previously resistant to the somatostatin analogue? Clin Endocrinol (Oxf) 67:310, 2007

LIU H et al: Systematic review: The safety and efficacy of growth hormone in the healthy elderly. Ann Intern Med 146:104, 2007

MELMED S: Acromegaly. N Engl J Med 355(24):2558, 2006

——— et al: A critical analysis of pituitary tumor shrinkage during primary therapy of acromegaly. J Clin Endocrinol Metab 90:4405, 2005

MINNITI G et al: Risk of second brain tumor after conservative surgery and radiotherapy for pituitary adenomas: Update after an additional 10 years. J Clin Endocrinol Metab 90:800, 2005

MOLITCH ME: Evaluation and treatment of adult growth hormone deficiency: An Endocrine Society Clinical Practice Guideline. J Clin Endocrinol Metab 91:1621, 2006

334 Disorders of the Neurohypophysis

Gary L. Robertson

The neurohypophysis, or posterior pituitary gland, is formed by axons that originate in large cell bodies in the supraoptic and paraventricular nuclei of the hypothalamus. It produces two hormones: (1) arginine vasopressin (AVP), also known as antidiuretic hormone; and (2) oxytocin. AVP acts on the renal tubules to reduce water loss by concentrating the urine. Oxytocin stimulates postpartum milk letdown in response to suckling. AVP deficiency causes diabetes insipidus (DI), characterized by the production of large amounts of dilute urine. Excessive or inappropriate AVP production predisposes to hyponatremia if water intake is not reduced in parallel with urine output.

VASOPRESSIN

ACTION

AVP is a nonapeptide composed of a six-membered disulfide ring and a tripeptide tail (Fig. 334-1). The most important, if not the only, physiologic action of AVP is to reduce water excretion by promoting concentration of urine. This antidiuretic effect is achieved by increasing the hydroosmotic permeability of cells that line the distal tubule and medullary collecting ducts of the kidney (Fig. 334-2). In the absence of AVP, these cells are impermeable to water and reabsorb little, if any, of the relatively large volume of dilute filtrate that enters from the proximal nephron. This results in the excretion of very large volumes (as much as 0.2 mL/kg per min) of maximally dilute urine (specific gravity and osmolarity ~1.000 and 50 mosmol/L, respectively), a condition known as a *water diuresis*. In the presence of AVP, these cells become selectively permeable to water, allowing it to diffuse back down the osmotic gradient created by the hypertonic renal medulla. As a result, the dilute fluid passing through the tubules is concentrated and the rate of urine flow decreases. The magnitude of this effect varies in direct proportion to the plasma AVP concentration and, at maximum levels, approximates a urine flow rate as low as 0.35 mL/min and a urine osmolarity as high as 1200 mosmol/L. AVP action is mediated via binding to G protein–coupled V_2 receptors on the serosal surface of the cell, activation of adenyl cyclase, and insertion into the luminal surface of water channels composed of a protein known as *aquaporin 2*.

At high concentrations, AVP also causes contraction of smooth muscle in blood vessels and in the gastrointestinal tract, induces glycogenolysis in the liver, and potentiates adrenocorticotropic hormone (ACTH) release by corticotropin-releasing factor. These effects are mediated by V_{1a} or V_{1b} receptors that are coupled to phospholipase C. Their role, if any, in human physiology/pathophysiology is still uncertain.

SYNTHESIS AND SECRETION

AVP secretion is synthesized via a polypeptide precursor that includes AVP, neurophysin, and copeptin. After preliminary processing and folding, the precursor is packaged in neurosecretory vesicles where it is transported down the axon, further processed to AVP, and stored until the hormone and other components are released by exocytosis into peripheral blood.

FIGURE 334-1 Primary structures of arginine vasopressin (AVP), oxytocin, and desmopressin.

AVP secretion is regulated primarily by the "effective" osmotic pressure of body fluids. This control is mediated by specialized hypothalamic cells, known as *osmoreceptors*, which are extremely sensitive to small changes in the plasma concentration of sodium and certain other solutes but are insensitive to other solutes such as urea or glucose. The osmoreceptors appear to include inhibitory as well as stimulatory components that function in concert to form a threshold, or set point, control system for AVP release. Below this threshold, plasma AVP is suppressed to levels that permit the development of a maximum water diuresis. Above it, plasma AVP rises steeply in direct proportion to plasma osmolarity, quickly reaching levels sufficient to effect a maximum antidiuresis. The absolute levels of plasma osmolarity/sodium at which minimally and maximally effective levels of plasma AVP occur vary appreciably from person to person, owing apparently to genetic influences on the set and sensitivity of the system. However, the average threshold, or set point, for AVP release corresponds to a plasma os-

FIGURE 334-2 Antidiuretic effect of arginine vasopressin (AVP) in the regulation of urine volume. In a typical 70-kg adult, the kidney filters ~180 L/d of plasma. Of this, ~144 L (80%) is reabsorbed isosmotically in the proximal tubule and another 8 L (4–5%) is reabsorbed without solute in the descending limb of Henle's loop. The remainder is diluted to an osmolarity of ~60 mmol/kg by selective reabsorption of sodium and chloride in the ascending limb. In the absence of AVP, the urine issuing from the loop passes largely unmodified through the distal tubules and collecting ducts, resulting in a maximum water diuresis. In the presence of AVP, solute-free water is reabsorbed osmotically through the principal cells of the collecting ducts, resulting in the excretion of a much smaller volume of concentrated urine. This antidiuretic effect is mediated via a G protein–coupled V_2 receptor that increases intracellular cyclic AMP, thereby inducing translocation of aquaporin 2 (AQP 2) water channels into the apical membrane. The resultant increase in permeability permits an influx of water that diffuses out of the cell through AQP 3 and AQP 4 water channels on the basal-lateral surface. The net rate of flux across the cell is determined by the number of AQP 2 water channels in the apical membrane and the strength of the osmotic gradient between tubular fluid and the renal medulla. Tight junctions on the lateral surface of the cells serve to prevent unregulated water flow.

molarity or sodium of about 280 mosmol/L or 135 meq/L, respectively; levels only 2–4% higher normally result in maximum antidiuresis. Though relatively stable in a healthy adult, the set of the osmoregulatory system can also be lowered by pregnancy, the menstrual cycle, estrogen, and relatively large, acute reductions in blood pressure or volume.

The effects of acute changes in blood volume or pressure are mediated largely by neuronal afferents that originate in transmural pressure receptors of the heart and large arteries and project via the vagus and glossopharyngeal nerves to the brain stem, from whence postsynaptic projections ascend to the hypothalamus. These pathways maintain a tonic inhibitory tone that decreases when blood volume or pressure falls by >10–20%. This baroregulatory system is probably of minor importance in the physiology of AVP secretion because the hemodynamic changes required to affect it do not usually occur during normal activities. However, the baroregulatory system undoubtedly plays an important role in AVP secretion in patients with large, acute disturbances of hemodynamic function.

AVP secretion can also be stimulated by nausea, acute hypoglycemia, glucocorticoid deficiency, smoking, and, possibly, hyperangiotensinemia. The emetic stimuli are extremely potent since they typically elicit immediate, 50- to 100-fold increases in plasma AVP, even when the nausea is transient and unassociated with vomiting or other symptoms. They appear to act via the emetic center in the medulla and can be completely blocked by treatment with antiemetics such as fluphenazine. There is no evidence that pain or other noxious stresses have any affect on AVP unless they elicit a vasovagal reaction with its associated nausea and hypotension.

METABOLISM

AVP distributes rapidly into a space roughly equal to the extracellular fluid volume. It is cleared irreversibly with a $t_{1/2}$ of 10–30 min. Most AVP clearance is due to degradation in the liver and kidneys. During pregnancy, the metabolic clearance of AVP is increased three- to fourfold due to placental production of an N-terminal peptidase.

THIRST

Because AVP cannot reduce water loss below a certain minimum level obligated by urinary solute load and evaporation from skin and lungs, a mechanism for ensuring adequate intake is essential for preventing dehydration. This vital function is performed by the thirst mechanism. Like AVP, thirst is regulated primarily by an osmostat that is located in the anteromedial hypothalamus and is able to detect very small changes in the plasma concentration of sodium and certain other effective solutes. The thirst osmostat appears to be "set" about 5% higher than the AVP osmostat. This arrangement ensures that thirst, polydipsia, and dilution of body fluids do not occur until plasma osmolarity/sodium start to exceed the defensive capacity of the antidiuretic mechanism.

OXYTOCIN

Oxytocin is also a nonapeptide and differs from AVP only at positions 3 and 8 (Fig. 334-1). However, it has relatively little antidiuretic effect and seems to act mainly on mammary ducts to facilitate milk letdown during nurs-

ing. It may also help to initiate or facilitate labor by stimulating contraction of uterine smooth muscle, but it is not yet clear if this action is physiologic or necessary for normal delivery.

DEFICIENCIES OF VASOPRESSIN SECRETION AND ACTION

DIABETES INSIPIDUS

Clinical Characteristics Decreased secretion or action of AVP usually manifests as DI, a syndrome characterized by the production of abnormally large volumes of dilute urine. The 24-h urine volume is >50 mL/kg body weight and the osmolarity is <300 mosmol/L. The polyuria produces symptoms of urinary frequency, enuresis, and/or nocturia, which may disturb sleep and cause mild daytime fatigue or somnolence. It is also associated with thirst and a commensurate increase in fluid intake (polydipsia). Clinical signs of dehydration are uncommon unless fluid intake is impaired.

Etiology Deficient secretion of AVP can be primary or secondary. The primary form usually results from agenesis or irreversible destruction of the neurohypophysis and is variously referred to as *neurohypophyseal DI*, *pituitary DI*, or *central DI*. It can be caused by a variety of congenital, acquired, or genetic disorders but almost half the time it is idiopathic (Table 334-1). The genetic form of neurohypophyseal DI is

TABLE 334-1   CAUSES OF DIABETES INSIPIDUS

Pituitary diabetes insipidus	Nephrogenic diabetes insipidus
Acquired	Acquired
Head trauma (closed and penetrating)	Drugs
Neoplasms	Lithium
Primary	Demeclocycline
Craniopharyngioma	Methoxyflurane
Pituitary adenoma (suprasellar)	Amphotericin B
Dysgerminoma	Aminoglycosides
Meningioma	Cisplatin
Metastatic (lung, breast)	Rifampin
Hematologic (lymphoma, leukemia)	Foscarnet
Granulomas	Metabolic
Neurosarcoid	Hypercalcemia, hypercalciuria
Histiocytosis	Hypokalemia
Xanthoma disseminatum	Obstruction (ureter or urethra)
Infectious	Vascular
Chronic meningitis	Sickle cell disease and trait
Viral encephalitis	Ischemia (acute tubular necrosis)
Toxoplasmosis	Granulomas
Inflammatory	Neurosarcoid
Lymphocytic infundibuloneurohypophysitis	Neoplasms
Wegener's granulomatosis	Sarcoma
Lupus erythematosus	Infiltration
Scleroderma	Amyloidosis
Chemical toxins	Pregnancy
Tetrodotoxin	Idiopathic
Snake venom	Genetic
Vascular	X-linked recessive (AVP receptor-2 gene)
Sheehan's syndrome	Autosomal recessive (aquaporin-2 gene)
Aneurysm (internal carotid)	Autosomal dominant (aquaporin-2 gene)
Aortocoronary bypass	**Primary polydipsia**
Hypoxic encephalopathy	Acquired
Pregnancy (vasopressinase)	Psychogenic
Idiopathic	Schizophrenia
Congenital malformations	Obsessive-compulsive disorder
Septooptic dysplasia	Dipsogenic (abnormal thirst)
Midline craniofacial defects	Granulomas
Holoprosencephaly	Neurosarcoid
Hypogenesis, ectopia of pituitary	Infectious
Genetic	Tuberculous meningitis
Autosomal dominant (*AVP-neurophysin gene*)	Head trauma (closed and penetrating)
Autosomal recessive (*AVP-neurophysin gene*)	Demyelination
Autosomal recessive-Wolfram-(4p – *WFS 1 gene*)	Multiple sclerosis
X-linked recessive (Xq28)	Drugs
Deletion chromosome 7q	Lithium
	Carbamazepine
	Idiopathic
	Iatrogenic

usually transmitted in an autosomal dominant mode and is caused by diverse mutations in the coding region of the AVP–neurophysin II (or *AVP-NPII*) gene. All of the mutations alter one or more amino acids known to be critical for correct folding of the prohormone, thus interfering with its processing and trafficking through the endoplasmic reticulum. The AVP deficiency and DI develop several months to several years after birth and appear to result from selective degeneration of AVP-producing magnocellular neurons, probably caused by accumulation of misfolded precursor. An autosomal recessive form due to an inactivating mutation in the AVP portion of the gene, an X-linked recessive form due to an unidentified gene on Xq28, and an autosomal recessive form due to mutations of the *WFS 1* gene responsible for Wolfram's syndrome (diabetes insipidus, diabetes mellitus, optic atrophy, and neural deafness; DIDMOAD), have also been described. A primary deficiency of plasma AVP can also result from increased metabolism by an N-terminal aminopeptidase produced by the placenta. It is referred to as *gestational DI* since the signs and symptoms manifest during pregnancy and usually remit several weeks after delivery. However, a subclinical deficiency in AVP secretion can often be demonstrated in the nonpregnant state, indicating that damage to the neurohypophysis may also contribute to the AVP deficiency.

Secondary deficiencies of AVP result from inhibition of secretion by excessive intake of fluids. They are referred to as *primary polydipsia* and can be divided into three subcategories. One of them, called *dipsogenic DI*, is characterized by inappropriate thirst caused by a reduction in the "set" of the osmoregulatory mechanism. It sometimes occurs in association with multifocal diseases of the brain such as neurosarcoid, tuberculous meningitis, or multiple sclerosis but is often idiopathic. The second subtype, called *psychogenic polydipsia*, is not associated with thirst, and the polydipsia seems to be a feature of psychosis. The third subtype, which may be referred to as *iatrogenic polydipsia*, results from recommendations to increase fluid intake for its presumed health benefits.

Primary deficiencies in the antidiuretic action of AVP result in *nephrogenic DI* (Table 334-1). They can be genetic, acquired, or caused by exposure to various drugs. The genetic form is usually transmitted in an X-linked mode and is caused by mutations in the coding region of the V_2 receptor gene. Autosomal recessive or dominant forms result from mutations in the gene encoding the aquaporin protein that forms the water channels in the distal nephron.

Secondary deficiencies in the antidiuretic response to AVP result from polyuria per se. They are caused by washout of the medullary concentration gradient and/or suppression of aquaporin function. They usually resolve 24–48 h after the polyuria is corrected but often complicate interpretation of acute tests commonly used for differential diagnosis.

Pathophysiology When the secretion or action of AVP is reduced below 80–85% of normal, urine concentration ceases and the rate of output increases to symptomatic levels. If the defect is primary (e.g., the patient has pituitary, gestational, or nephrogenic DI), the polyuria results in a small (1–2%) decrease in body water and a commensurate increase in plasma osmolarity and sodium concentration that stimulate thirst and a compensatory increase in water intake. As a result, *overt physical or laboratory signs of dehydration do not develop unless the patient also has a defect in thirst* (see below) *or fails to drink for some other reason.*

The severity of the antidiuretic defect varies markedly among patients with pituitary, gestational, or nephrogenic DI. In some, the deficiencies in AVP secretion or action are so severe that basal urine output approximates the maximum (10–15 mL/min); even an intense stimulus such as nausea or severe dehydration does not raise plasma AVP enough to concentrate the urine. In others, however, the deficiency in AVP secretion or action is incomplete, and a modest stimulus such as a few hours of fluid deprivation, smoking, or a vasovagal reaction increases plasma AVP sufficiently to produce a profound antidiuresis. The maximum urine osmolarity achieved in these patients is usually less than normal, largely because their maximal concentrating

capacity is temporarily impaired by chronic polyuria. However, in a few patients with partial pituitary or nephrogenic DI, it can reach levels as high as 800 mosmol/L.

In primary polydipsia, the pathogenesis of the polydipsia and polyuria is the reverse of that in pituitary, nephrogenic, and gestational DI. Thus, the excessive intake of fluids slightly increases body water, thereby reducing plasma osmolarity, AVP secretion, and urinary concentration. The latter results in a compensatory increase in urinary free-water excretion that varies in direct proportion to intake. Therefore, clinically appreciable overhydration is uncommon unless the compensatory water diuresis is impaired by a drug or disease that stimulates or mimics endogenous AVP.

In the dipsogenic form of primary polydipsia, fluid intake is excessive because the osmotic threshold for thirst appears to be reset to the left, often well below that for AVP release. When deprived of fluids or subjected to some other acute osmotic or nonosmotic stimulus, these individuals invariably increase plasma AVP normally, but the resultant increase in urine concentration is usually subnormal because their renal capacity to concentrate the urine is also blunted by chronic polyuria. Thus, their antidiuretic response to these stimuli may be indistinguishable from that in patients with partial pituitary, partial gestational, or partial nephrogenic DI. Patients with psychogenic or iatrogenic polydipsia respond similarly to fluid restriction but do not complain of thirst and usually offer other explanations for their high fluid intake.

Differential Diagnosis When symptoms of urinary frequency, enuresis, nocturia, and/or persistent thirst are present, a 24-h urine should be collected on an ad libitum fluid intake. If the volume exceeds 50 mL/kg per day (3500 mL in a 70-kg man), polyuria is present. If the osmolarity is >300 mosmol/L, the polyuria is due to a solute diuresis and the patient should be evaluated for glucosuria or other less common causes of excessive solute excretion. However, if the 24-h urine osmolarity is <300 mosmol/L, the patient has a water diuresis and should be evaluated further to determine which type of DI is present.

In differentiating between the various types of DI, the history, physical examination, and routine laboratory tests may be helpful but are rarely sufficient because few, if any, of the findings are pathognomonic. Except in the rare patient who is clearly dehydrated under basal conditions of ad libitum fluid intake, this evaluation should begin with a *fluid deprivation test*. To minimize patient discomfort, avoid excessive dehydration, and maximize the information obtained, the test should be started in the morning and water balance should be monitored closely with hourly measurements of body weight, plasma osmolarity and/or sodium concentration, and urine volume and osmolarity.

If fluid deprivation does not result in urine concentration (osmolarity > 300 mosmol/L, specific gravity > 1.010) before body weight decreases by 5% or plasma osmolarity/sodium exceed the upper limit of normal, the patient has severe pituitary or severe nephrogenic DI. These disorders can usually be distinguished by administering desmopressin (DDAVP, 0.03 μg/kg SC or IV) and repeating the measurement of urine osmolarity 1–2 h later. An increase of >50% indicates severe pituitary DI, whereas a smaller or absent response is strongly suggestive of nephrogenic DI.

If fluid deprivation results in concentration of the urine, the differential diagnosis is more difficult because the patient can have either partial pituitary DI, partial nephrogenic DI, or a form of primary polydipsia. In this situation, the change in urine osmolarity after the administration of desmopressin does not differentiate the possible disorders because the responses are variable and overlap in the three types of DI. The best way to differentiate between them is to measure plasma or urine AVP before and during the fluid deprivation test and analyze the results in relation to the concurrent plasma or urine osmolarity (Fig. 334-3). This approach invariably differentiates partial nephrogenic DI from partial pituitary DI and primary polydipsia. It also differentiates partial pituitary DI from primary polydipsia if the hormone is measured when plasma osmolarity or sodium is clearly above the normal range. The requisite level of hypertonic dehydration

FIGURE 334-3 Relationship of plasma AVP to urine osmolarity (*left*) and plasma osmolarity (*right*) before and during fluid deprivation–hypertonic saline infusion test in patients who are normal (blue zones) or have primary polydipsia (blue zones), pituitary diabetes insipidus (green zones), or nephrogenic diabetes insipidus (pink zones).

may be difficult to produce by fluid deprivation alone when the urine is concentrated. Therefore, it is usually necessary to infuse hypertonic (3%) saline at a rate of 0.1 mL/kg per min while continuing the fluid deprivation and repeat the AVP measurements as soon as plasma osmolarity rises to >300 mosmol/L (Na^+ > 145 mmol/L). This endpoint is usually reached within 30–120 min.

The differential diagnosis of DI may also be facilitated by MRI of the pituitary and hypothalamus. In most healthy adults and children, the posterior pituitary emits a hyperintense signal in T1-weighted mid-sagittal images. This "bright spot" is almost always present in patients with primary polydipsia but is invariably absent or abnormally small in patients with pituitary DI. It is usually also small or absent in nephrogenic DI presumably because of high secretion and turnover of vasopressin. Thus, a normal bright spot virtually excludes pituitary DI, is against nephrogenic DI, and strongly suggests primary polydipsia. Lack of the bright spot is less helpful, however, because it is absent not only in pituitary and nephrogenic DI but also in some normal persons and in patients with empty sella who do not have DI.

The other way to distinguish between the three basic types of DI is to closely monitor the effects of antidiuretic therapy on changes in water balance.

R_x DIABETES INSIPIDUS

The signs and symptoms of uncomplicated pituitary DI can be eliminated completely by treatment with desmopressin (DDAVP), a synthetic analogue of AVP (Fig. 334-1). It acts selectively at V_2 receptors to increase urine concentration and decrease urine flow in a dose-dependent manner (**Fig. 334-4**). It is also more resistant to degradation than AVP and has a three- to fourfold longer duration of action. Desmopressin (DDAVP) can be given by IV or SC injection, nasal inhalation, or oral tablet. The doses required to completely control pituitary DI vary widely, depending on the patient and the route of administration. However, they usually range from 1–2 μg qd or bid by injection, 10–20 μg bid or tid by nasal spray, or 100–400 μg bid or tid orally. The onset of action is rapid, ranging from as little as 15 min after injection to 60 min after oral administration. When given in doses sufficient to completely normalize urinary osmolarity and flow, desmopressin produces a slight (1–3%) increase in total-body water and a commensurate decrease in plasma osmolarity and sodium concentration that rapidly eliminate thirst and polydipsia. Consequently, water balance is maintained and hyponatremia does not develop unless the patient has an associated abnormality in the osmoregulation of thirst or ingests/receives excessive amounts of fluid for some other reason. Fortunately, thirst is usually normal in patients with pituitary DI, and the other causes of excessive intake can usually be eliminated by educating the patient about the risks of drinking for reasons other than thirst. Therefore, desmopressin can usually be given safely in doses sufficient to maintain a completely normal urine output without subjecting the patient to the

inconvenience and discomfort of allowing intermittent escape to prevent water intoxication.

Primary polydipsia cannot be treated safely with desmopressin. It inhibits the polyuria but, unlike pituitary DI, does not eliminate the urge to drink. Therefore, it almost always produces water intoxication within 24–48 h. Iatrogenic polydipsia can often be corrected by patient counseling, but there is no effective treatment for either psychogenic or dipsogenic DI.

The symptoms and signs of nephrogenic DI are not affected by treatment with desmopressin but may be reduced by treatment with a thiazide diuretic and/or amiloride in conjunction with a low-sodium diet. Inhibitors of prostaglandin synthesis (e.g., indomethacin) are also very effective in some patients.

ADIPSIC HYPERNATREMIA

Clinical Characteristics Adipsic hypernatremia is a syndrome characterized by chronic or recurrent hypertonic dehydration caused by a deficiency in the osmoregulation of thirst. The hypernatremia varies widely in severity and is usually associated with signs of hypovolemia such as tachycardia, postural hypotension, azotemia, hyperuricemia, and hypokalemia. Muscle weakness, pain, rhabdomyolysis, hyperglycemia, hyperlipidemia, and acute renal failure may also occur. DI is usually not present at least at presentation.

Pathophysiology Adipsic hypernatremia is caused by agenesis or destruction of the hypothalamic osmoreceptors that normally regulate thirst and AVP secretion (Fig. 334-5). The deficiency of osmoregulation is usually due to a congenital or acquired disease in the hypothal-

FIGURE 334-4 Effect of desmopressin therapy on water balance in patient with uncomplicated pituitary diabetes insipidus. Note that treatment rapidly reduces thirst and fluid intake as well as urine output to normal, with only a slight increase in body water (weight) and decrease in plasma osmolarity/sodium. [*From Endocrinology and Metabolism, 4th ed, P Felig, L Frohman (eds). New York, McGraw-Hill, 2001, with permission.*]

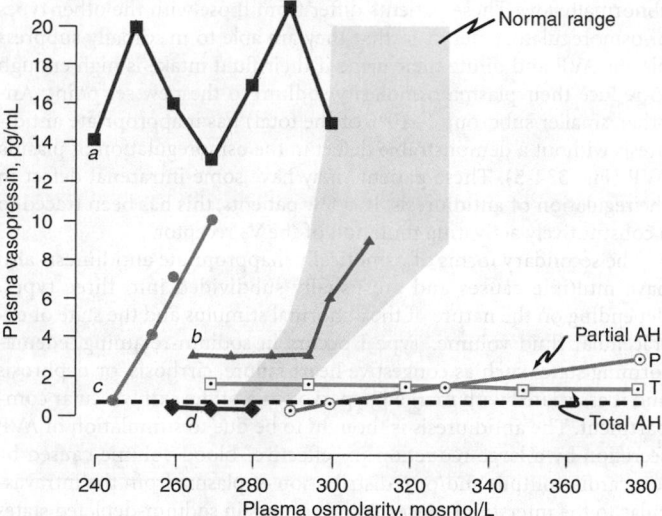

FIGURE 334-5 Heterogeneity of osmoregulatory dysfunction in adipsic hypernatremia (AH) and the syndrome of inappropriate antidiuresis (SIAD). Each line depicts schematically the relationship of plasma arginine vasopressin (AVP) to plasma osmolarity during water loading and/or infusion of 3% saline in a patient with either AH (open symbols) or SIAD (closed symbols). The shaded area indicates the normal range of the relationship. The horizontal broken line indicates the plasma AVP level below which the hormone is undetectable and urinary concentration usually does not occur. Lines P and T represent patients with a selective deficiency in the osmoregulation of thirst and AVP that is either partial (○) or total (□). In the latter, plasma AVP does not change in response to increases or decreases in plasma osmolarity but remains within a range sufficient to concentrate the urine even if overhydration produces hypotonic hyponatremia. In contrast, if the osmoregulatory deficiency is partial (○), rehydration of the patient suppresses plasma AVP to levels that result in urinary dilution and polyuria before plasma osmolarity and sodium are reduced to normal. Lines a–d represent different defects in the osmoregulation of plasma AVP observed in patients with SIAD. In a (■), plasma AVP is markedly elevated and fluctuates widely without relation to changes in plasma osmolarity, indicating complete loss of osmoregulation. In b (▲), plasma AVP remains fixed at a slightly elevated level until plasma osmolarity reaches the normal range at which point it begins to rise appropriately, indicating a selective defect in the inhibitory component of the osmoregulatory mechanism. In c (●), plasma AVP rises in close correlation with plasma osmolarity before the latter reaches the normal range, indicating downward resetting of the osmostat. In d (◆), plasma AVP appears to be osmoregulated normally, suggesting that the inappropriate antidiuresis is caused by some other abnormality.

amus (Table 334-2). Whatever the cause, the lack of thirst results in a failure to drink enough water to replenish renal and extrarenal losses resulting in hypernatremic, hypertonic dehydration. In most patients, the osmoregulation of AVP secretion is also impaired partially or completely (Fig. 334-5). If the deficiency is partial, severe dehydration stimulates the release of enough AVP to concentrate the urine. However, as rehydration decreases the hypertonicity and hypovolemia, plasma AVP falls and polyuria develops. Patients with a complete lack of osmoregulation do not develop DI at any level of hydration because they cannot osmotically suppress or stimulate AVP secretion. Therefore, they have permanent inappropriate antidiuresis and develop hyponatremia if overhydrated during treatment. In most patients, the neurohypophysis as well as the AVP response to hemodynamic or emetic stimuli are normal. Consequently, hypovolemia and/or hypotension become the dominant influence on AVP release, especially when the dehydration is severe. In some, however, the neurohypophysis is also deficient, resulting in a combination of chronic pituitary DI and hypodipsia that is particularly difficult to manage.

TABLE 334-2	CAUSES OF ADIPSIC HYPERNATREMIA

Acquired
  Vascular: Occlusion anterior communicating artery
  Tumors
    Primary
      Craniopharyngioma
      Pinealoma, germinoma
      Meningioma
      Glioma
    Metastatic (lung, breast)
  Granulomas: Neurosarcoid
              Histiocytosis
  Trauma: Closed
          Penetrating (pituitary-hypothalamic surgery)
  Psychogenic: Psychotic depression
  Other: Hydrocephalus
         Neurodegenerative
         AIDS, cytomegalovirus encephalitis
  Idiopathic
Congenital
  Midline malformation (septum and corpus callosum)
  Microcephaly
Genetic: Autosomal recessive (Schinzel-Giedion syndrome)

Differential Diagnosis Adipsic hypernatremia should be distinguished from hypernatremia caused by physical restrictions to drinking (e.g., coma, paralysis, restraints, absence of fresh water) or intake of large amounts of sodium. This distinction can usually be made from the history, physical examination, and routine laboratory tests. If a conscious patient denies thirst and/or does not drink vigorously when hypernatremic, the diagnosis of hypodipsia or adipsia can be made with confidence irrespective of the volume status. If the patient is obtunded at the time of presentation, the possibility of adipsic hypernatremia can be evaluated after rehydration by assessing the thirst and plasma AVP response to a controlled fluid deprivation–hypertonic saline infusion test similar to that described for evaluation of DI. A history of one or more previous episodes of hypernatremia is also virtually diagnostic.

℞ ADIPSIC HYPERNATREMIA

Severe dehydration in adipsic hypernatremia should be corrected by administering water by mouth, if the patient is alert, or 0.45% saline IV, if the patient is obtunded or uncooperative. The number of liters of free water required to correct the deficit (ΔFW) can be estimated from body weight in kg (BW) and the serum sodium concentration in mmol/L (S_{Na}) by the formula $\Delta FW = 0.5BW \times [(S_{Na} - 140)/140]$. If serum glucose ($S_{Glu}$) is elevated, the measured S_{Na} should be corrected (S_{Na}^*) by the formula $S_{Na}^* = S_{Na} + [(S_{Glu} - 90)/36]$. This amount plus an allowance for continuing insensible and urinary losses should be given over a 24- to 48-h period. Close monitoring of serum sodium as well as fluid intake and urinary output is essential because, depending on the extent of osmoreceptor deficiency (Fig. 334-5), some patients will develop AVP-deficient DI requiring desmopressin therapy to complete rehydration; others will develop hyponatremia and a syndrome of inappropriate antidiuresis (SIAD)-like picture if overhydrated. If hyperglycemia and/or hypokalemia are present, insulin and/or potassium supplements should be given with the expectation that both can be discontinued soon after rehydration is complete. Plasma urea/creatinine should be monitored closely for signs of acute renal failure.

Once the patient has been rehydrated, an MRI of the brain and tests of anterior pituitary function should be performed to look for the cause and collateral defects in other hypothalamic functions. A long-term management plan to prevent or minimize recurrence of the fluid and electrolyte imbalance should also be developed. This should include a practical method that the patient can use to regulate fluid intake in accordance with day-to-day variations in water balance. The most effective way to do this is to prescribe desmopressin to control DI, if it is present, and teach the patient how to use day-to-day changes in body weight as a guide for adjusting fluid intake. It may also be possible to adjust fluid intake by monitoring day-to-day changes in serum sodium using equipment recently developed for home use. Prescribing a constant fluid intake is ineffective and potentially dangerous because it does not take into account the large, uncontrolled variations in insensible loss that inevitably result from changes in ambient temperature and physical activity.

EXCESS VASOPRESSIN SECRETION AND ACTION

HYPONATREMIA (See also Chap. 46)

Clinical Characteristics Excessive secretion or action of AVP results in the production of decreased volumes of more highly concentrated urine. If not accompanied by a commensurate reduction in fluid intake or an increase in insensible loss, the reduction in urine output results in excess water retention with expansion and dilution of all body fluids. In some patients, excessive intake results from inappropriate thirst. If the hyponatremia develops gradually or has been present for more than a few days, it may be largely asymptomatic. However, if it develops acutely, it is almost always accompanied by symptoms and signs of water intoxication that may include mild headache, confusion, anorexia, nausea, vomiting, coma, and convulsions. Severe hyponatremia may be lethal.

Etiology Hyponatremia and impaired urinary dilution can be caused by a primary defect in the regulation of AVP secretion or action or can be secondary to a recognized nonosmotic stimulus such as hypovolemia, hypotension, nausea, or glucocorticoid deficiency. The primary forms are generally referred to as SIAD. They have many different causes, including ectopic production of AVP by lung cancer or other neoplasms; eutopic release by various diseases or drugs; and exogenous administration of AVP, desmopressin, or large doses of oxytocin (Table 334-3). The ectopic forms result from abnormal expression of the AVP-NPII gene by primary or metastatic malignancies. The eutopic forms occur most often in patients with acute infections or strokes but have also been associated with many other diseases and injuries. The mechanisms by which these diseases disrupt osmoregulation are not known. The defect in osmoregulation can take any of four distinct forms (Fig. 334-5). In one of the most common (reset osmostat), AVP secretion remains fully responsive to changes in plasma osmolarity/sodium, but the threshold, or set point, of the osmoregulatory system is

abnormally low. These patients differ from those with the other types of osmoregulatory defect in that they are able to maximally suppress plasma AVP and dilute their urine if their fluid intake is high enough to reduce their plasma osmolarity/sodium to the new set point. Another, smaller subgroup (~10% of the total) has inappropriate antidiuresis without a demonstrable defect in the osmoregulation of plasma AVP (Fig. 334-5). These patients may have some intrarenal defect in the regulation of antidiuresis. In a few patients, this has been traced to a constitutively activating mutation of the V_2 receptor.

The secondary forms of osmotically inappropriate antidiuresis also have multiple causes and are usually subdivided into three types, depending on the nature of the abnormal stimulus and the state of extracellular fluid volume. Type I occurs in sodium-retaining, edema-forming states such as congestive heart failure, cirrhosis, or nephrosis and is associated with marked hypervolemia of the extravascular compartment. The antidiuresis is thought to be due to stimulation of AVP secretion by a large reduction in "effective" blood volume caused by low cardiac output and/or redistribution of plasma from the intravascular to the interstitial space. Type II occurs in sodium-depleted states such as severe gastroenteritis, diuretic abuse, or mineralocorticoid deficiency and is due to stimulation of AVP by a large reduction in blood volume and/or pressure. In both types, the abnormal AVP secretion appears to be due to resetting of the osmostat similar to that in some patients with SIAD. Type IIIA results from stimulation of AVP secretion by nausea or isolated glucocorticoid deficiency. In this case, the hyponatremia is not associated with overt hyper- or hypovolemia and can closely resemble SIAD (type IIIB) in which extracellular volume also appears to be normal (Table 334-4). However, they must be distinguished because their treatments differ. In type IIIA, the excess AVP secretion can be corrected quickly and completely by treatments (antiemetics or glucocorticoids) that are not useful in type IIIB (SIAD).

Pathophysiology When osmotic suppression of antidiuresis is impaired for any reason, significant expansion and dilution of body fluids occurs only if water intake exceeds the rate of insensible and urinary losses. The excess water intake is sometimes due to an associated defect in the osmoregulation of thirst but can also be psychogenic or iatrogenic, including the administration of IV fluids.

In SIAD, the excessive retention of water has two other effects. First, by increasing extracellular volume, it increases glomerular filtration and atrial natriuretic hormone, suppresses plasma renin activity, and increases urinary sodium excretion. This natriuresis serves to counteract the extracellular hypervolemia but aggravates the hyponatremia. Second, by producing hyponatremia, it increases intracellular volume in all organs including the brain. This swelling increases intracranial pressure, which is probably responsible for the symptoms of acute water intoxication. Within a few days, this swelling may be counteracted by inactivation or elimination of intracellular solutes, resulting in the remission of symptoms even though the hyponatremia persists. The pathophysiology of type IIIA (euvolemic) hyponatremia is probably similar to SIAD.

In type I (edematous) or type II (hypovolemic) hyponatremia, the antidiuretic effect of hemodynamically induced AVP release is enhanced by decreased distal delivery of glomerular filtrate that results from increased reabsorption of sodium in proximal nephrons. Again, if the marked reduction in urine output that ensues is not associated with a commensurate reduction in water intake or an increase in insensible loss, body fluids are expanded and diluted, resulting in hyponatremia. Unlike SIAD, however, glomerular filtration is reduced and plasma renin activity and aldosterone are elevated due to the hypovolemic stimulus. Thus, urinary sodium is low (unless sodium reabsorption is impaired by a diuretic) and the hyponatremia is usually accompanied by hypokalemia, azotemia, and hyperuricemia. The sodium retention is an appropriate compensatory response to severe volume and sodium depletion present in type II but is inappropriate and deleterious in type I since body sodium and extracellular volume are already markedly increased.

Differential Diagnosis SIAD is a diagnosis of exclusion that can usually be accomplished with routine historic, physical, and laboratory infor-

TABLE 334-3	CAUSES OF SYNDROME OF INAPPROPRIATE ANTIDIURESIS (SIAD)

Neoplasms	Neurologic
Carcinomas	Guillain-Barré syndrome
Lung	Multiple sclerosis
Duodenum	Delirium tremens
Pancreas	Amyotrophic lateral sclerosis
Ovary	Hydrocephalus
Bladder, ureter	Psychosis
Other neoplasms	Peripheral neuropathy
Thymoma	Congenital malformations
Mesothelioma	Agenesis corpus callosum
Bronchial adenoma	Cleft lip/palate
Carcinoid	Other midline defects
Gangliocytoma	Metabolic
Ewing's sarcoma	Acute intermittent porphyria
Head trauma (closed and penetrating)	Pulmonary
Infections	Asthma
Pneumonia, bacterial or viral	Pneumothorax
Abscess, lung or brain	Positive-pressure respiration
Cavitation (aspergillosis)	Drugs
Tuberculosis, lung or brain	Vasopressin or desmopressin
Meningitis, bacterial or viral	Chlorpropamide
Encephalitis	Oxytocin, high dose
AIDS	Vincristine
Vascular	Carbamazepine
Cerebrovascular occlusions, hemorrhage	Nicotine
Cavernous sinus thrombosis	Phenothiazines
	Cyclophosphamide
	Tricyclic antidepressants
	Monoamine oxidase inhibitors
	Serotonin reuptake inhibitors

TABLE 334-4 **DIFFERENTIAL DIAGNOSIS OF HYPONATREMIA BASED ON CLINICAL ASSESSMENT OF EXTRACELLULAR FLUID VOLUME (ECFV)**

Clinical Findings	Type I, Hypervolemic	Type II, Hypovolemic	Type IIIA, Euvolemic	Type IIIB, Euvolemic (SIAD)
History				
CHF, cirrhosis, or nephrosis	Yes	No	No	No
Salt and water loss	No	Yes	No	No
ACTH–cortisol deficiency and/or nausea and vomiting	No	No	Yes	No
Physical examination				
Generalized edema, ascites	Yes	No	No	No
Postural hypotension	Maybe	Maybe	Maybe[a]	No
Laboratory				
BUN, creatinine	High-normal	High-normal	Low-normal	Low-normal
Uric acid	High-normal	High-normal	Low-normal	Low-normal
Serum potassium	Low-normal	Low-normal[b]	Normal[c]	Normal
Serum albumin	Low-normal	High-normal	Normal	Normal
Serum cortisol	Normal-high	Normal-high[d]	Low[e]	Normal
Plasma renin activity	High	High	Low[f]	Low
Urinary sodium (meq unit of time)[g]	Low	Low[h]	High[i]	High[i]

[a]Postural hypotension may occur in secondary (ACTH-dependent) adrenal insufficiency even though ECFV and aldosterone are usually normal.

[b]Serum potassium may be high if hypovolemia is due to aldosterone deficiency.

[c]Serum potassium may be low if vomiting causes alkalosis.

[d]Serum cortisol is low if hypovolemia is due to primary adrenal insufficiency (Addison's disease).

[e]Serum cortisol will be normal or high if the cause is nausea and vomiting rather than secondary (ACTH-dependent) adrenal insufficiency.

[f]Plasma renin activity may be high if the cause is secondary (ACTH) adrenal insufficiency.

[g]Urinary sodium should be expressed as the *rate of excretion* rather than the concentration. In a hyponatremic adult, an excretion rate > 25 meq/day (or 25 μeq/mg of creatinine) could be considered high.

[h]The rate of urinary sodium excretion may be high if the hypovolemia is due to diuretic abuse, primary adrenal insufficiency, or other causes of renal sodium wasting.

[i]The rate of urinary sodium excretion may be low if intake is curtailed by symptoms or treatment.

Note: SIAD, syndrome of inappropriate antidiuresis; CHF, congestive heart failure; ACTH, adrenocorticotropic hormone; BUN, blood urea nitrogen.

mation. In a patient with hyponatremia, the possibility of simple dilution caused by an osmotically driven shift of water from the intracellular to the extracellular space should be excluded by measuring plasma glucose and/or plasma osmolarity. If the glucose is not elevated enough to account for the hyponatremia [serum sodium decreases ~1 meq/L for each rise in glucose of 2.0 mmol/L (36 mg/dL)] and/or plasma osmolarity is reduced in proportion to sodium (each decrease in serum sodium of 1 meq/L should reduce plasma osmolarity by ~2 mosmol/L), the hyponatremia is "true" and can be typed or classified by standard clinical indicators of the extracellular fluid volume (Table 334-4). If these findings are ambiguous or contradictory, measuring the rate of urinary sodium excretion or plasma renin activity may be helpful. These measurements can be misleading, however, if SIAD is stable or resolving or if the patient has type II hyponatremia due to a primary defect in renal conservation of sodium, surreptitious diuretic abuse, or hyporeninemic hypoaldosteronism. The latter may be suspected if serum potassium is elevated instead of low as is usually seen in types I and II hyponatremia. Measurements of plasma AVP are currently of no diagnostic value since the abnormalities are similar in all three types of hyponatremia. In patients who fulfill the clinical criteria for type III (euvolemic) hyponatremia, plasma cortisol should also be measured to rule out secondary adrenal insufficiency. If cortisol is normal and there is no history of nausea/vomiting or other obvious cause for type III hyponatremia, a careful search for occult lung cancer should also be undertaken.

Rx HYPONATREMIA

The management of patients with hyponatremia differs depending not only on the type but also on the severity and duration of symptoms. In a patient with SIAD (type IIIB) and few symptoms, the objective is to gradually reduce body water by restricting total fluid intake to less than the sum of urinary and insensible losses. Because the water derived from food (300–700 mL/d) usually approximates basal insensible losses in adults, total discretionary intake (all liq-

uids) should be at least 500 mL less than urinary output. If achieved, this deficit usually reduces body water and increases serum sodium by about 1–2% per day. If more rapid correction of the hyponatremia is desired to eliminate severe symptoms or signs, the fluid restriction can be supplemented by IV infusion of hypertonic (3%) saline. This treatment has the advantage of correcting the sodium deficiency that is partly responsible for the hyponatremia and also produces a solute diuresis that serves to remove some of the excess water. However, if hypertonic saline is given too rapidly in a patient in whom hyponatremia has been present for >24–48 h, it also has the potential to produce central pontine myelinolysis, an acute, potentially fatal neurologic syndrome characterized by quadriparesis, ataxia, and abnormal extraocular movements. The risk of this complication can be minimized by observing several precautions: 3% saline should be infused at a rate ≤0.05 mL/kg body weight per min; the effect should be monitored continuously by STAT measurements of serum sodium at least once every 2 h; and the infusion should be stopped as soon as serum sodium increases by 12 mmol/L or to 130 mmol/L, whichever comes first. Urinary output should also be monitored continuously since SIAD can remit spontaneously at any time, resulting in an acute water diuresis that greatly accelerates the rate of rise in serum sodium produced by fluid restriction and 3% saline infusion.

In chronic, persistent SIAD, the hyponatremia can be corrected by treatment with demeclocycline, 150–300 mg PO three or four times a day, or fludrocortisone, 0.05–0.2 mg PO twice a day. The effect of the demeclocycline manifests in 7–14 days and is due to production of a reversible form of nephrogenic DI. Potential side effects include phototoxicity and azotemia. The effect of fludrocortisone also requires 1–2 weeks and is partly due to increased retention of sodium and possibly inhibition of thirst. It also increases urinary potassium excretion, which may require replacement through dietary adjustments or supplements. Fludrocortisone may induce hypertension, occasionally necessitating discontinuation of the treatment.

Nonpeptide AVP antagonists that block the antidiuretic effect of AVP have also been used experimentally in acute and chronic SIAD. They produce a dose-dependent increase in urinary free-water excretion, which, if combined with a modest restriction of fluid intake, gradually reduce body water and correct the hyponatremia. These studies have shown no adverse effect but, like hypertonic saline, the antagonists probably carry the risk of inducing osmotic demyelination if the hyponatremia is corrected too rapidly. One of them, a combined V_2/V_{1a} antagonist (Conivaptan), has recently been approved for short term in-hospital treatment of SIAD, and other antagonists are currently in phase III trials.

In euvolemic hyponatremia due to protracted nausea and vomiting or isolated glucocorticoid deficiency (type IIIA), all abnormalities can be corrected quickly and completely by giving an antiemetic or hydrocortisone. As with other treatments, care must be taken to ensure that serum sodium does not rise too quickly or too far.

In type I hyponatremia, fluid restriction is also appropriate and somewhat effective, if it can be maintained. However, infusion of hypertonic saline is contraindicated because it further increases total body sodium and edema and may precipitate cardiovascular decompensation. Preliminary studies with antagonists of V_2 receptors indicate that they are almost as effective in type I hyponatremia as they are in SIAD, but they have not yet been approved for this indication.

In type II hyponatremia, the defect in AVP secretion and water balance can usually be corrected easily and quickly by stopping the loss of sodium and water and/or replacing the deficits by mouth or IV infusion of normal or hypertonic saline. As with the treatment of other forms of hyponatremia, care must be taken to ensure that plasma sodium does not increase too rapidly. Fluid restriction and administration of AVP antagonists are contraindicated in type II as they would only aggravate the underlying volume depletion and could result in hemodynamic collapse.

FURTHER READINGS

BICHET DG: Hereditary polyuric disorders: New concepts and differential diagnosis. Semin Nephrol 26:224, 2006

CHRISTENSEN JH, RITTIG S: Familial neurohypophyseal diabetes insipidus—an update. Semin Nephrol 26:209, 2006

FELDMAN BJ et al: Nephrogenic syndrome of inappropriate antidiuresis. N Engl J Med 352:1884, 2005

ROBERTSON GL: Antidiuretic hormone: Normal and disordered function. Endocrinol Metab Clin North Am 30:671, 2001

VERBALIS JG: Vasopressin V2 receptor antagonists. J Mol Endocrinol 29:1, 2002

——— (ed): Hyponatremia: New understanding, new therapy. Am J Med 119(Suppl 1): 1, 2006

335 Disorders of the Thyroid Gland

J. Larry Jameson, Anthony P. Weetman

The thyroid gland produces two related hormones, thyroxine (T_4) and triiodothyronine (T_3) (Fig. 335-1). Acting through nuclear receptors, these hormones play a critical role in cell differentiation during development and help maintain thermogenic and metabolic homeostasis in the adult. Autoimmune disorders of the thyroid gland can either stimulate the overproduction of thyroid hormones (*thyrotoxicosis*) or cause glandular destruction and hormone deficiency (*hypothyroidism*). In addition, benign nodules and various forms of thyroid cancer are relatively common and amenable to detection by physical examination.

ANATOMY AND DEVELOPMENT

The thyroid (Greek *thyreos*, shield, plus *eidos*, form) consists of two lobes that are connected by an isthmus. It is located anterior to the trachea between the cricoid cartilage and the suprasternal notch. The normal thyroid is 12–20 g in size, highly vascular, and soft in consistency. Four parathyroid glands, which produce parathyroid hormone (Chap. 347), are located posterior to each pole of the thyroid. The recurrent laryngeal nerves traverse the lateral borders of the thyroid gland and must be identified during thyroid surgery to avoid vocal cord paralysis.

The thyroid gland develops from the floor of the primitive pharynx during the third week of gestation. The developing gland migrates along the thyroglossal duct to reach its final location in the neck. This feature accounts for the rare ectopic location of thyroid tissue at the base of the tongue (lingual thyroid) as well as the occurrence of thyroglossal duct cysts along this developmental tract. Thyroid hormone synthesis normally begins at about 11 weeks' gestation.

Neural crest derivatives from the ultimobranchial body give rise to thyroid medullary C cells that produce calcitonin, a calcium-lowering hormone. The C cells are interspersed throughout the thyroid gland, although their density is greatest in the juncture of the upper one-third and lower two-thirds of the gland.

Thyroid gland development is orchestrated by the coordinated expression of several developmental transcription factors. Thyroid transcription factor (TTF) 1, TTF-2, and paired homeobox-8 (PAX-8) are expressed selectively, but not exclusively, in the thyroid gland. In combination, they dictate thyroid cell development and the induction of thyroid-specific genes such as thyroglobulin (Tg), thyroid peroxidase (TPO), the sodium iodide symporter (NIS), and the thyroid-stimulating hormone receptor (TSH-R). Mutations in these developmental transcription factors or their downstream target genes are rare causes of thyroid agenesis or dyshormonogenesis, though the causes of most forms of congenital hypothyroidism remain unknown (Table 335-1). Because congenital hypothyroidism occurs in approximately 1 in 4000 newborns, neonatal screening is now performed in most industrialized countries (see below). Transplacental passage of maternal thyroid hormone occurs before the fetal thyroid gland begins to function and provides partial support to a fetus with congenital hypothyroidism. Early thyroid hormone replacement in newborns with congenital hypothyroidism prevents potentially severe developmental abnormalities.

The thyroid gland consists of numerous spherical follicles composed of thyroid follicular cells that surround secreted colloid, a proteinaceous fluid containing large amounts of thyroglobulin, the protein precursor of thyroid hormones (Fig. 335-2). The thyroid follicular cells are polarized—the basolateral surface is apposed to the bloodstream and an apical surface faces the follicular lumen. Increased demand for thyroid hormone is regulated by thyroid-stimulating hormone (TSH), which binds to its receptor on the basolateral surface of the follicular cells, leading to Tg reabsorption from the follicular lumen and proteolysis within the cell to yield thyroid hormones for secretion into the bloodstream.

REGULATION OF THE THYROID AXIS

TSH, secreted by the thyrotrope cells of the anterior pituitary, plays a pivotal role in control of the thyroid axis and serves as the most useful physiologic marker of thyroid hormone action. TSH is a 31-kDa hormone composed of α and β subunits; the α subunit is common to the other glycoprotein hormones [luteinizing hormone, follicle-stimulating hormone, human chorionic gonadotropin (hCG)], whereas the TSH β subunit is unique to TSH. The extent and nature of carbohydrate modification are modulated by thyrotropin-releasing hormone (TRH) stimulation and influence the biologic activity of the hormone.

The thyroid axis is a classic example of an endocrine feedback loop. Hypothalamic TRH stimulates pituitary production of TSH, which, in turn, stimulates thyroid hormone synthesis and secretion. Thyroid hormones feed back to inhibit TRH and TSH production (Fig. 335-2). The "set-point" in this axis is established by TSH. TRH is the major positive regulator of TSH synthesis and secre-

FIGURE 335-1 Structures of thyroid hormones. Thyroxine (T_4) contains four iodine atoms. Deiodination leads to production of the potent hormone triiodothyronine (T_3), or the inactive hormone reverse T_3.

Thyroxine (T_4)
3,5,3',5'-Tetraiodothyronine

Deiodinase 1 or 2
(5'-Deiodination)

Deiodinase 3>2
(5-Deiodination)

Tri-iodothyronine (T_3)
3,5,3'-Triiodothyronine

Reverse T_3 (rT_3)
3,3',5'-Triiodothyronine

TABLE 335-1	GENETIC CAUSES OF CONGENITAL HYPOTHYROIDISM	
Defective Gene Protein	**Inheritance**	**Consequences**
PROP-1	Autosomal recessive	Combined pituitary hormone deficiencies with preservation of adrenocorticotropic hormone
PIT-1	Autosomal recessive Autosomal dominant	Combined deficiencies of growth hormone, prolactin, thyroid-stimulating hormone (TSH)
TSHβ	Autosomal recessive	TSH deficiency
TTF-1 (TITF-1)	Autosomal dominant	Variable thyroid hypoplasia, choreoathetosis, pulmonary problems
TTF-2 (FOXE-1)	Autosomal recessive	Thyroid agenesis, choanal atresia, spiky hair
PAX-8	Autosomal dominant	Thyroid dysgenesis
TSH-receptor	Autosomal recessive	Resistance to TSH
$G_{s\alpha}$ (Albright hereditary osteodystrophy)	Autosomal dominant	Resistance to TSH
Na^+/I^- symporter	Autosomal recessive	Inability to transport iodide
THOX2	Autosomal dominant	Organification defect
Thyroid peroxidase	Autosomal recessive	Defective organification of iodide
Thyroglobulin	Autosomal recessive	Defective synthesis of thyroid hormone
Pendrin	Autosomal recessive	Pendred's syndrome: sensorineural deafness and partial organification defect in thyroid
Dehalogenase	Autosomal recessive	Loss of iodide reutilization

thyroid hormone increase basal TSH production and enhance TRH-mediated stimulation of TSH. High thyroid hormone levels rapidly and directly suppress TSH gene expression secretion and inhibit TRH stimulation of TSH, indicating that thyroid hormones are the dominant regulator of TSH production. Like other pituitary hormones, TSH is released in a pulsatile manner and exhibits a diurnal rhythm; its highest levels occur at night. However, these TSH excursions are modest in comparison to those of other pituitary hormones, in part because TSH has a relatively long plasma half-life (50 min). Consequently, single measurements of TSH are adequate for assessing its circulating level. TSH is measured using immunoradiometric assays that are highly sensitive and specific. These assays readily distinguish between normal and suppressed TSH values; thus, TSH can be used for the diagnosis of hyperthyroidism (low TSH) as well as hypothyroidism (high TSH).

tion. Peak TSH secretion occurs ~15 min after administration of exogenous TRH. Dopamine, glucocorticoids, and somatostatin suppress TSH but are not of major physiologic importance except when these agents are administered in pharmacologic doses. Reduced levels of

FIGURE 335-2 Regulation of thyroid hormone synthesis. *Left.* Thyroid hormones T_4 and T_3 feed back to inhibit hypothalamic production of thyrotropin-releasing hormone (TRH) and pituitary production of thyroid-stimulating hormone (TSH). TSH stimulates thyroid gland production of T_4 and T_3. ***Right.*** Thyroid follicles are formed by thyroid epithelial cells surrounding proteinaceous colloid, which contains thyroglobulin. Follicular cells, which are polarized, synthesize thyroglobulin and carry out thyroid hormone biosynthesis (see text for details). TSH-R, thyroid-stimulating hormone receptor; Tg, thyroglobulin; NIS, sodium-iodide symporter; TPO, thyroid peroxidase; DIT, diiodotyrosine; MIT, monoiodotyrosine.

THYROID HORMONE SYNTHESIS, METABOLISM, AND ACTION

THYROID HORMONE SYNTHESIS

Thyroid hormones are derived from Tg, a large iodinated glycoprotein. After secretion into the thyroid follicle, Tg is iodinated on tyrosine residues that are subsequently coupled via an ether linkage. Reuptake of Tg into the thyroid follicular cell allows proteolysis and the release of newly synthesized T_4 and T_3.

Iodine Metabolism and Transport Iodide uptake is a critical first step in thyroid hormone synthesis. Ingested iodine is bound to serum proteins, particularly albumin. Unbound iodine is excreted in the urine. The thyroid gland extracts iodine from the circulation in a highly efficient manner. For example, 10–25% of radioactive tracer (e.g., ^{123}I) is taken up by the normal thyroid gland over 24 h; this value can rise to 70–90% in Graves' disease. Iodide uptake is mediated by the Na^+/I^- symporter (NIS), which is expressed at the basolateral membrane of thyroid follicular cells. NIS is most highly expressed in the thyroid gland, but low levels are present in the salivary glands, lactating breast, and placenta. The iodide transport mechanism is highly regulated, allowing adaptation to variations in dietary supply. Low iodine levels increase the amount of NIS and stimulate uptake, whereas high iodine levels suppress NIS expression and uptake. The selective expression of NIS in the thyroid allows isotopic scanning, treatment of hyperthyroidism, and ablation of thyroid cancer with radioisotopes of iodine, without significant effects on other organs. Mutation of the *NIS* gene is a rare cause of congenital hypothyroidism, underscoring its importance in thyroid hormone synthesis. Another iodine transporter, pendrin, is located on the apical surface of thyroid cells and mediates iodine efflux into the lumen. Mutation of the *PENDRIN* gene causes *Pendred syndrome*, a disorder characterized by defective organification of iodine, goiter, and sensorineural deafness.

Iodine deficiency is prevalent in many mountainous regions and in central Africa, central South America, and northern Asia (Fig. 335-3). The World Health Organization (WHO) estimates that about 2 billion people are iodine-deficient, based on urinary excretion data. In areas of relative iodine deficiency, there is an increased prevalence of goiter and, when deficiency is severe, hypothyroidism and cretinism. *Cretinism* is characterized by mental and growth retardation and occurs when children who live in iodine-deficient regions are not treated with iodine or thyroid hormone to restore normal thyroid hormone levels during early life. These children are often born to mothers with iodine deficiency, and it is likely that maternal thyroid hormone deficiency worsens the condition. Concomitant selenium deficiency may also contribute to the neurologic manifesta-

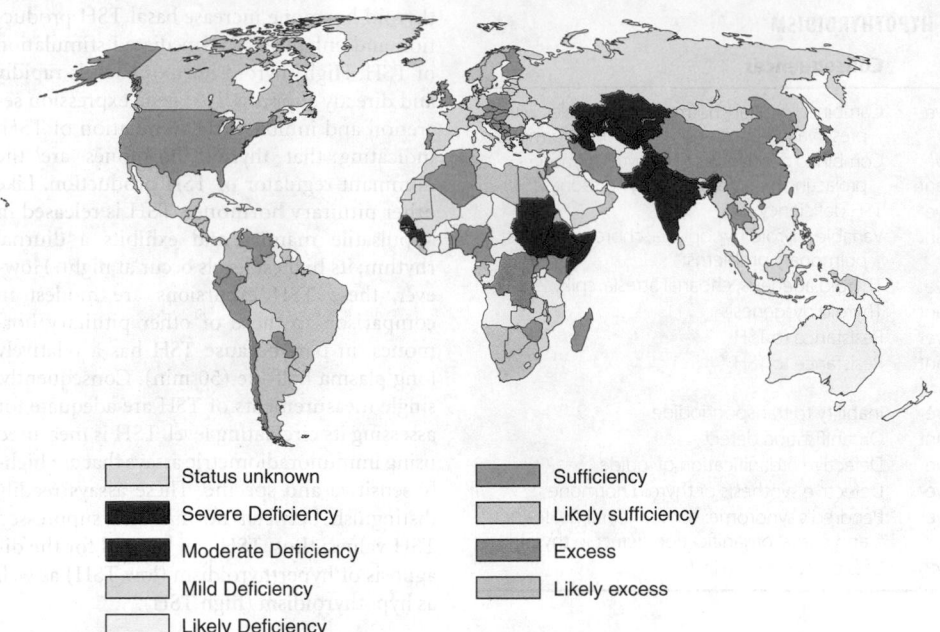

Status unknown

Severe Deficiency

Moderate Deficiency

Mild Deficiency

Likely Deficiency

Sufficiency

Likely sufficiency

Excess

Likely excess

FIGURE 335-3 Worldwide iodine nutrition. Data are from the WHO and the International Council for the Control of Iodine Deficiency Disorders (*http://indorgs.virginia.edu/iccidd/mi/cidds.html*).

tions of cretinism. Iodine supplementation of salt, bread, and other food substances has markedly reduced the prevalence of cretinism. Unfortunately, however, iodine deficiency remains the most common cause of preventable mental deficiency, often because of societal resistance to food additives or the cost of supplementation. In addition to overt cretinism, mild iodine deficiency can lead to subtle reduction of IQ. Oversupply of iodine, through supplements or foods enriched in iodine (e.g., shellfish, kelp), is associated with an increased incidence of autoimmune thyroid disease. The recommended average daily intake of iodine is 150 μg/d for adults, 90–120 μg/d for children, and 200 μg/d for pregnant women. Urinary iodine is >10 μg/dL in iodine-sufficient populations.

Organification, Coupling, Storage, Release After iodide enters the thyroid, it is trapped and transported to the apical membrane of thyroid follicular cells, where it is oxidized in an organification reaction that involves TPO and hydrogen peroxide. The reactive iodine atom is added to selected tyrosyl residues within Tg, a large (660 kDa) dimeric protein that consists of 2769 amino acids. The iodotyrosines in Tg are then coupled via an ether linkage in a reaction that is also catalyzed by TPO. Either T_4 or T_3 can be produced by this reaction, depending on the number of iodine atoms present in the iodotyrosines. After coupling, Tg is taken back into the thyroid cell, where it is processed in lysosomes to release T_4 and T_3. Uncoupled mono- and diiodotyrosines (MIT, DIT) are deiodinated by the enzyme dehalogenase, thereby recycling any iodide that is not converted into thyroid hormones.

Disorders of thyroid hormone synthesis are rare causes of congenital hypothyroidism. The vast majority of these disorders are due to recessive mutations in TPO or Tg, but defects have also been identified in the TSH-R, NIS, pendrin, hydrogen peroxide generation, and dehalogenase. Because of the biosynthetic defect, the gland is incapable of synthesizing adequate amounts of hormone, leading to increased TSH and a large goiter.

TSH Action TSH regulates thyroid gland function through the TSH-R, a seven-transmembrane G protein–coupled receptor (GPCR). The TSH-R is coupled to the α subunit of stimulatory G protein ($G_{s\alpha}$), which activates adenylyl cyclase, leading to increased production of cyclic AMP. TSH also stimulates phosphatidylinositol turnover by activating phospholipase C. The functional role of the TSH-R is exemplified by the consequences of naturally occurring mutations. Recessive loss-of-function mutations cause thyroid hypoplasia and congenital hypothyroidism. Dominant gain-of-function mutations cause sporadic or familial hyperthyroidism that is characterized by goiter, thyroid cell hyperplasia, and autonomous function. Most of these activating mutations occur in the transmembrane domain of the receptor. They are thought to mimic the conformational changes induced by TSH binding or the interactions of thyroid-stimulating immunoglobulins (TSI) in Graves' disease. Activating TSH-R mutations also occur as somatic events and lead to clonal selection and expansion of the affected thyroid follicular cell (see below).

Other Factors that Influence Hormone Synthesis and Release Although TSH is the dominant hormonal regulator of thyroid gland growth and function, a variety of growth factors, most produced locally in the thyroid gland, also influence thyroid hormone synthesis. These include insulin-like growth factor I (IGF-I), epidermal growth factor, transforming growth factor β (TGF-β), endothelins, and various cytokines. The quantitative roles of these factors are not well understood, but they are important in selected disease states. In acromegaly, for example, increased levels of growth hormone and IGF-I are associated with goiter and predisposition to multinodular goiter (MNG). Certain cytokines and interleukins (ILs) produced in association with autoimmune thyroid disease induce thyroid growth, whereas others lead to apoptosis. Iodine deficiency increases thyroid blood flow and upregulates the NIS, stimulating more efficient uptake. Excess iodide transiently inhibits thyroid iodide organification, a phenomenon known as the *Wolff-Chaikoff effect*. In individuals with a normal thyroid, the gland escapes from this inhibitory effect and iodide organification resumes; the suppressive action of high iodide may persist, however, in patients with underlying autoimmune thyroid disease.

THYROID HORMONE TRANSPORT AND METABOLISM

Serum Binding Proteins T_4 is secreted from the thyroid gland in about twentyfold excess over T_3 (Table 335-2). Both hormones are bound to plasma proteins, including thyroxine-binding globulin (TBG); transthyretin (TTR, formerly known as thyroxine-binding prealbumin, or TBPA); and albumin. The plasma-binding proteins increase the pool of circulating hormone, delay hormone clearance, and may modulate hormone delivery to selected tissue sites. The concentration of TBG is relatively low (1–2 mg/dL), but because of its high affinity for thyroid hormones ($T_4 > T_3$), it carries about 80% of the bound hormones. Albumin has relatively low affinity for thyroid hormones but has a high plasma concentration (~3.5 g/dL), and it binds up to 10% of T_4 and 30% of T_3. TTR carries about 10% of T_4 but little T_3.

TABLE 335-2	CHARACTERISTICS OF CIRCULATING T_4 AND T_3	
Hormone Property	**T_4**	**T_3**
Serum concentrations		
Total hormone	8 μg/dL	0.14 μg/dL
Fraction of total hormone in the free form	0.02%	0.3%
Free (unbound) hormone	$21 \times 10^{-12} M$	$6 \times 10^{-12} M$
Serum half-life	7 d	0.75 d
Fraction directly from the thyroid	100%	20%
Production rate, including peripheral conversion	90 μg/d	32 μg/d
Intracellular hormone fraction	~20%	~70%
Relative metabolic potency	0.3	1
Receptor binding	$10^{-10} M$	$10^{-11} M$

When the effects of the various binding proteins are combined, approximately 99.98% of T_4 and 99.7% of T_3 are protein-bound. Because T_3 is less tightly bound than T_4, the amount of unbound T_3 is greater than unbound T_4, even though there is less total T_3 in the circulation. The unbound, or free, concentrations of the hormones are $\sim 2 \times 10^{-11}\ M$ for T_4 and $\sim 6 \times 10^{-12}\ M$ for T_3, which roughly correspond to the thyroid hormone receptor binding constants for these hormones (see below). The unbound hormone is thought to be biologically available to tissues, although the discovery of megalin as a cellular transporter of protein-bound steroids raises the possibility of distinct transport systems for bound and unbound hormones. Nonetheless, the homeostatic mechanisms that regulate the thyroid axis are directed toward maintenance of normal concentrations of unbound hormones.

Abnormalities of Thyroid Hormone Binding Proteins

A number of inherited and acquired abnormalities affect thyroid hormone binding proteins. X-linked TBG deficiency is associated with very low levels of total T_4 and T_3. However, because unbound hormone levels are normal, patients are euthyroid and TSH levels are normal. It is important to recognize this disorder to avoid efforts to normalize total T_4 levels, as this leads to thyrotoxicosis and is futile because of rapid hormone clearance in the absence of TBG. TBG levels are elevated by estrogen, which increases sialylation and delays TBG clearance. Consequently, in women who are pregnant or taking estrogen-containing contraceptives, elevated TBG increases total T_4 and T_3 levels; however, unbound T_4 and T_3 levels are normal. These features explain why women with hypothyroidism require increased amounts of l-thyroxine replacement when TBG levels are increased by pregnancy or estrogen treatment. Mutations in TBG, TTR, and albumin may increase the binding affinity for T_4 and/or T_3 and cause disorders known as *euthyroid hyperthyroxinemia* or *familial dysalbuminemic hyperthyroxinemia* (FDH) (Table 335-3). These disorders result in increased total T_4 and/or T_3, but unbound hormone levels are normal. The familial nature of the disorders, and the fact that TSH levels are normal rather than suppressed, should suggest this diagnosis. Unbound hormone levels (ideally measured by dialysis) are normal in FDH. The diagnosis can be confirmed by using tests that measure the affinities of radiolabeled hormone binding to specific transport proteins or by performing DNA sequence analyses of the abnormal transport protein genes.

Certain medications, such as salicylates and salsalate, can displace thyroid hormones from circulating binding proteins. Although these drugs transiently perturb the thyroid axis by increasing free thyroid hormone levels, TSH is suppressed until a new steady state is reached, thereby restoring euthyroidism. Circulating factors associated with acute illness may also displace thyroid hormone from binding proteins (see "Sick Euthyroid Syndrome," below).

Deiodinases

T_4 may be thought of as a precursor for the more potent T_3. T_4 is converted to T_3 by the deiodinase enzymes (Fig. 335-1). Type I deiodinase, which is located primarily in thyroid, liver, and kidney, has a relatively low affinity for T_4. Type II deiodinase has a higher affinity for T_4 and is found primarily in the pituitary gland, brain, brown fat, and thyroid gland. Expression of type II deiodinase allows it to regulate T_3 concentrations locally, a property that may be important in the context of levothyroxine (T_4) replacement. Type II deiodinase is also regulated by thyroid hormone; hypothyroidism induces the enzyme, resulting in enhanced $T_4 \rightarrow T_3$ conversion in tissues such as brain and pituitary. $T_4 \rightarrow T_3$ conversion is impaired by fasting, systemic illness or acute trauma, oral contrast agents, and a variety of medications (e.g., propylthiouracil, propranolol, amiodarone, glucocorticoids). Type III deiodinase inactivates T_4 and T_3 and is the most important source of reverse T_3 (rT_3). Massive hemangiomas that express type III deiodinase are a rare cause of hypothyroidism in infants.

THYROID HORMONE ACTION

Thyroid Hormone Transport

Circulating thyroid hormones enter cells by passive diffusion and via the monocarboxylate 8 (MCT8) transporter that was identified in patients with multiple neurologic deficits and thyroid function abnormalities (low T4, high T3, and high TSH). After entering cells, thyroid hormones act primarily through nuclear receptors, although they also stimulate plasma membrane and mitochondrial enzymatic responses.

Nuclear Thyroid Hormone Receptors

Thyroid hormones bind with high affinity to nuclear *thyroid hormone receptors* (TRs) α and β. Both TRα and TRβ are expressed in most tissues, but their relative expression levels vary among organs; TRα is particularly abundant in brain, kidney, gonads, muscle, and heart, whereas TRβ expression is relatively high in the pituitary and liver. Both receptors are variably spliced to form unique isoforms. The TR$\beta2$ isoform, which has a unique amino terminus, is selectively expressed in the hypothalamus and pituitary, where it plays a role in feedback control of the thyroid axis. The TR$\alpha2$ isoform contains a unique carboxy terminus that precludes thyroid hormone binding; it may function to block the action of other TR isoforms.

The TRs contain a central DNA-binding domain and a C-terminal ligand-binding domain. They bind to specific DNA sequences, termed *thyroid response elements* (TREs), in the promoter regions of target genes (Fig. 335-4). The receptors bind as homodimers or, more commonly, as heterodimers with retinoic acid X receptors (RXRs) (Chap. 332). The activated receptor can either stimulate gene transcription (e.g., myosin heavy chain α) or inhibit transcription (e.g., TSH β-subunit gene), depending on the nature of the regulatory elements in the target gene.

Thyroid hormones (T_3 and T_4) bind with similar affinities to TRα and TRβ. However, structural differences in the ligand binding domains provide the potential for developing receptor-selective agonists

TABLE 335-3	CONDITIONS ASSOCIATED WITH EUTHYROID HYPERTHYROXINEMIA		
Disorder	**Cause**	**Transmission**	**Characteristics**
Familial dysalbuminemic hyperthyroxinemia (FDH)	Albumin mutations, usually R218H	AD	Increased T_4 Normal unbound T_4 Rarely increased T_3
TBG			
Familial excess	Increased TBG production	XL	Increased total T_4, T_3 Normal unbound T_4, T_3
Acquired excess	Medications (estrogen), pregnancy, cirrhosis, hepatitis	Acquired	Increased total T_4, T_3 Normal unbound T_4, T_3
Transthyretin[a]			
Excess	Islet tumors	Acquired	Usually normal T_4, T_3
Mutations	Increased affinity for T_4 or T_3	AD	Increased total T_4, T_3 Normal unbound T_4, T_3
Medications: propranolol, ipodate, iopanoic acid, amiodarone	Decreased $T_4 \rightarrow T_3$ conversion	Acquired	Increased T_4 Decreased T_3 Normal or increased TSH
Sick-euthyroid syndrome	Acute illness, especially psychiatric disorders	Acquired	Transiently increased unbound T_4 Decreased TSH T_4 and T_3 may also be decreased (see text)
Resistance to thyroid hormone (RTH)	Thyroid hormone receptor β mutations	AD	Increased unbound T_4, T_3 Normal or increased TSH Some patients clinically thyrotoxic

[a]Also known as thyroxine-binding prealbumin, TBPA.

Note: AD, autosomal dominant; TBG, thyroxine-binding globulin; TSH, thyroid-stimulating hormone; XL, X-linked.

FIGURE 335-4 Mechanism of thyroid hormone receptor action. The thyroid hormone receptor (TR) and retinoid X receptor (RXR) form heterodimers that bind specifically to thyroid hormone response elements (TRE) in the promoter regions of target genes. In the absence of hormone, TR binds co-repressor (CoR) proteins that silence gene expression. The numbers refer to a series of ordered reactions that occur in response to thyroid hormone: (1) T_4 or T_3 enters the nucleus; (2) T_3 binding dissociates CoR from TR; (3) Coactivators (CoA) are recruited to the T_3-bound receptor; (4) gene expression is altered.

or antagonists. T_3 is bound with 10–15 times greater affinity than T_4, which explains its increased hormonal potency. Though T_4 is produced in excess of T_3, receptors are occupied mainly by T_3, reflecting $T_4 \rightarrow T_3$ conversion by peripheral tissues, greater T_3 bioavailability in the plasma, and receptors' greater affinity for T_3. After binding to TRs, thyroid hormone induces conformational changes in the receptors that modify its interactions with accessory transcription factors. In the absence of thyroid hormone binding, the aporeceptors bind to co-repressor proteins that inhibit gene transcription. Hormone binding dissociates the co-repressors and allows the recruitment of coactivators that enhance transcription. The discovery of TR interactions with co-repressors explains the fact that TR silences gene expression in the absence of hormone binding. Consequently, hormone deficiency has a profound effect on gene expression because it causes gene repression as well as loss of hormone-induced stimulation. This concept has been corroborated by the finding that targeted deletion of the TR genes in mice has a less-pronounced phenotypic effect than hormone deficiency.

Thyroid Hormone Resistance Resistance to thyroid hormone (RTH) is an autosomal dominant disorder characterized by elevated thyroid hormone levels and inappropriately normal or elevated TSH. Individuals with RTH do not, in general, exhibit signs and symptoms that are typical of hypothyroidism because hormone resistance is partial and is compensated by increased levels of thyroid hormone. The clinical features of RTH can include goiter, attention deficit disorder, mild reduction in IQ, delayed skeletal maturation, tachycardia, and impaired metabolic responses to thyroid hormone.

RTH is caused by mutations in the TRβ receptor gene. These mutations, located in restricted regions of the ligand-binding domain, cause loss of receptor function. However, because the mutant receptors retain the capacity to dimerize with RXRs, bind to DNA, and recruit co-repressor proteins, they function as antagonists of the remaining normal TRβ and TRα receptors. This property, referred to as "dominant negative" activity, explains the autosomal dominant mode of transmission. The diagnosis is suspected when unbound thyroid hormone levels are increased without suppression of TSH. Similar hormonal abnormalities are found in other affected family members, although the TRβ mutation arises de novo in about 20% of patients. DNA sequence analysis of the TRβ gene provides a definitive diagnosis. RTH must be distinguished from other causes of euthyroid hyper-

thyroxinemia (e.g., FDH) and inappropriate secretion of TSH by TSH-secreting pituitary adenomas (Chap. 333). In most patients, no treatment is indicated; the importance of making the diagnosis is to avoid inappropriate treatment of mistaken hyperthyroidism and to provide genetic counseling.

PHYSICAL EXAMINATION

In addition to the examination of the thyroid itself, the physical examination should include a search for signs of abnormal thyroid function and the extrathyroidal features of ophthalmopathy and dermopathy (see below). Examination of the neck begins by inspecting the seated patient from the front and side and noting any surgical scars, obvious masses, or distended veins. The thyroid can be palpated with both hands from behind or while facing the patient, using the thumbs to palpate each lobe. It is best to use a combination of these methods, especially when nodules are small. The patient's neck should be slightly flexed to relax the neck muscles. After locating the cricoid cartilage, the isthmus can be identified and followed laterally to locate either lobe (normally the right lobe is slightly larger than the left). By asking the patient to swallow sips of water, thyroid consistency can be better appreciated as the gland moves beneath the examiner's fingers.

Features to be noted include thyroid size, consistency, nodularity, and any tenderness or fixation. An estimate of thyroid size (normally 12–20 g) should be made, and a drawing is often the best way to record findings. However, ultrasound is the method of choice when it is important to determine thyroid size accurately. The size, location, and consistency of any nodules should also be defined. A bruit over the gland indicates increased vascularity, as occurs in hyperthyroidism. If the lower borders of the thyroid lobes are not clearly felt, a goiter may be retrosternal. Large retrosternal goiters can cause venous distention over the neck and difficulty breathing, especially when the arms are raised (Pemberton's sign). With any central mass above the thyroid, the tongue should be extended, as thyroglossal cysts then move upward. The thyroid examination is not complete without assessment for lymphadenopathy in the supraclavicular and cervical regions of the neck.

LABORATORY EVALUATION

Measurement of Thyroid Hormones The enhanced sensitivity and specificity of *TSH assays* have greatly improved laboratory assessment of thyroid function. Because TSH levels change dynamically in response to alterations of T_4 and T_3, a logical approach to thyroid testing is to first determine whether TSH is suppressed, normal, or elevated. With rare exceptions (see below), a normal TSH level excludes a primary abnormality of thyroid function. This strategy depends on the use of immunochemiluminometric assays (ICMAs) for TSH that are sensitive enough to discriminate between the lower limit of the reference range and the suppressed values that occur with thyrotoxicosis. Extremely sensitive (fourth generation) assays can detect TSH levels ≤0.004 mU/L, but for practical purposes assays sensitive to ≤0.1 mU/L are sufficient. The widespread availability of the TSH ICMA has rendered the TRH stimulation test obsolete, as the failure of TSH to rise after an intravenous bolus of 200–400 μg TRH has the same implications as a suppressed basal TSH measured by ICMA.

The finding of an abnormal TSH level must be followed by measurements of circulating thyroid hormone levels to confirm the diagnosis of hyperthyroidism (suppressed TSH) or hypothyroidism (elevated TSH). Radioimmunoassays are widely available for serum *total T_4* and *total T_3*. T_4 and T_3 are highly protein-bound, and numerous factors (illness, medications, genetic factors) can influence protein binding. It is useful, therefore, to measure the free, or unbound, hormone levels, which correspond to the biologically available hormone pool. Two direct methods are used to measure *unbound thyroid hormones*: (1) unbound thyroid hormone competition with radiolabeled T_4 (or an analogue) for binding to a solid-phase antibody, and (2) physical separation of the unbound hormone fraction by ultracentrifugation or equilibrium dialysis. Though early unbound hormone immunoassays suffered from artifacts, newer assays correlate well with the results of the more technically demanding and expensive physical separation methods. An indirect method to estimate unbound thyroid hormone levels is to calculate the free T_3 or free T_4 index from the total T_4 or T_3 concentration and the *thyroid hormone binding ratio* (THBR). The latter is derived from the *T_3-resin uptake test*, which determines the distribution of radiolabeled T_3 between an absorbent resin and the unoccupied thyroid hormone binding proteins in the sample. The binding of the labeled T_3 to the resin is increased when there is reduced unoccupied protein binding sites (e.g., TBG deficiency) or increased total thyroid hormone in the sample; it is decreased under the opposite circumstances. The product of THBR and total T_3 or T_4 provides the *free T_3 or T_4 index*. In effect, the index corrects for anomalous total hormone values caused by abnormalities in hormone-protein binding.

Total thyroid hormone levels are *elevated* when TBG is increased due to estrogens (pregnancy, oral contraceptives, hormone therapy, tamoxifen), and *decreased* when TBG binding is reduced (androgens, nephrotic syndrome). Genetic disorders and acute illness can also cause abnormalities in thyroid hormone binding proteins, and various drugs [phenytoin, carbamazepine, salicylates, and nonsteroidal anti-inflammatory drugs (NSAIDs)] can interfere with thyroid hormone binding. Because unbound thyroid hormone levels are normal and the patient is euthyroid in all of these circumstances, assays that measure unbound hormone are preferable to those for total thyroid hormones.

For most purposes, the unbound T_4 level is sufficient to confirm thyrotoxicosis, but 2–5% of patients have only an elevated T_3 level (T_3 toxicosis). Thus, unbound T_3 levels should be measured in patients with a suppressed TSH but normal unbound T_4 levels.

There are several clinical conditions in which the use of TSH as a screening test may be misleading, particularly without simultaneous unbound T_4 determinations. Any severe nonthyroidal illness can cause abnormal TSH levels (see below). Although hypothyroidism is the most common cause of an elevated TSH level, rare causes include a TSH-secreting pituitary tumor (Chap. 333), thyroid hormone resistance, and assay artifact. Conversely, a suppressed TSH level, particularly <0.1 mU/L, usually indicates thyrotoxicosis but may also be seen during the first trimester of pregnancy (due to hCG secretion), after treatment of hyperthyroidism (because TSH can remain suppressed for several months), and in response to certain medications (e.g., high doses of glucocorticoids or dopamine). Importantly, secondary hypothyroidism, caused by hypothalamic-pituitary disease, is associated with a variable (low to high-normal) TSH level, which is inappropriate for the low T_4 level. Thus, *TSH should not be used to assess thyroid function in patients with suspected or known pituitary disease.*

Tests for the end-organ effects of thyroid hormone excess or depletion, such as estimation of basal metabolic rate, tendon reflex relaxation rates, or serum cholesterol, are not useful as clinical determinants of thyroid function.

Tests to Determine the Etiology of Thyroid Dysfunction Autoimmune thyroid disease is detected most easily by measuring circulating antibodies against TPO and Tg. As antibodies to Tg alone are uncommon, it is reasonable to measure only TPO antibodies. About 5–15% of euthyroid women and up to 2% of euthyroid men have thyroid antibodies; such individuals are at increased risk of developing thyroid dysfunction. Almost all patients with autoimmune hypothyroidism, and up to 80% of those with Graves' disease, have TPO antibodies, usually at high levels.

TSI are antibodies that stimulate the TSH-R in Graves' disease. They can be measured in bioassays or indirectly in assays that detect antibody binding to the receptor. The main use of these assays is to predict neonatal thyrotoxicosis caused by high maternal levels of TSI in the last trimester of pregnancy.

Serum Tg levels are increased in all types of thyrotoxicosis except *thyrotoxicosis factitia* caused by self-administration of thyroid hormone. Tg levels are particularly increased in thyroiditis, reflecting thyroid tissue destruction and release of Tg. The main role for Tg measurement, however, is in the follow-up of thyroid cancer patients. After total thyroidectomy and radioablation, Tg levels should be undetectable; measurable levels indicate incomplete ablation or recurrent cancer.

Radioiodine Uptake and Thyroid Scanning The thyroid gland selectively transports radioisotopes of iodine (^{123}I, ^{125}I, ^{131}I) and ^{99m}Tc pertechnetate, allowing thyroid imaging and quantitation of radioactive tracer fractional uptake.

Nuclear imaging of Graves' disease is characterized by an enlarged gland and increased tracer uptake that is distributed homogeneously. Toxic adenomas appear as focal areas of increased uptake, with suppressed tracer uptake in the remainder of the gland. In toxic MNG, the gland is enlarged—often with distorted architecture—and there are multiple areas of relatively increased or decreased tracer uptake. Subacute thyroiditis is associated with very low uptake because of follicular cell damage and TSH suppression. Thyrotoxicosis factitia is also associated with low uptake.

Although the use of fine-needle aspiration (FNA) biopsy has diminished the use of thyroid scans in the evaluation of solitary thyroid nodules, the functional features of thyroid nodules have some prognostic significance. So-called cold nodules, which have diminished tracer uptake, are usually benign. However, these nodules are more likely to be malignant (~5–10%) than so-called hot nodules, which are almost never malignant.

Thyroid scanning is also used in the follow-up of thyroid cancer. After thyroidectomy and ablation using ^{131}I, there is diminished radioiodine uptake in the thyroid bed, allowing the detection of metastatic thyroid cancer deposits that retain the ability to transport iodine. Whole-body scans using 111–185 MBq (3–5 mCi) ^{131}I are typically performed after thyroid hormone withdrawal to raise the TSH level or after the administration of recombinant human TSH.

Thyroid Ultrasound Ultrasonography is used increasingly to assist in the diagnosis of nodular thyroid disease, a reflection of the limitations of the physical examination and improvements in ultrasound technology. Using 10-MHz instruments, spatial resolution and image quality are excellent, allowing the detection of nodules and cysts >3 mm. In addition to detecting thyroid nodules, ultrasound is useful for monitoring nodule size and for the aspiration of cystic lesions. Ultrasound-guided FNA biopsy of thyroid lesions lowers the rate of inadequate sampling. Ultrasonography is also used in the evaluation of recurrent thyroid cancer, including possible spread to cervical lymph nodes.

HYPOTHYROIDISM

Iodine deficiency remains the most common cause of hypothyroidism worldwide. In areas of iodine sufficiency, autoimmune disease (Hashimoto's thyroiditis) and iatrogenic causes (treatment of hyperthyroidism) are most common (Table 335-4).

CONGENITAL HYPOTHYROIDISM

Prevalence Hypothyroidism occurs in about 1 in 4000 newborns. It may be transient, especially if the mother has TSH-R blocking antibodies or has received antithyroid drugs, but permanent hypothyroidism occurs in the majority. Neonatal hypothyroidism is due to thyroid gland dysgenesis in 80–85%, to inborn errors of thyroid hormone synthesis in 10–15%, and is TSH-R antibody-mediated in 5% of affected newborns. The developmental abnormalities are twice as common in girls. Mutations that cause congenital hypothyroidism are being increasingly recognized, but the vast majority remain idiopathic (Table 335-1).

Clinical Manifestations The majority of infants appear normal at birth, and <10% are diagnosed based on clinical features, which include prolonged jaundice, feeding problems, hypotonia, enlarged tongue, delayed bone maturation, and umbilical hernia. Importantly, permanent neurologic damage results if treatment is delayed. Typical features of adult hypothyroidism may also be present (Table 335-5). Other congenital malformations, especially cardiac, are four times more common in congenital hypothyroidism.

Diagnosis and Treatment Because of the severe neurologic consequences of untreated congenital hypothyroidism, neonatal screening

TABLE 335-4 **CAUSES OF HYPOTHYROIDISM**

Primary

Autoimmune hypothyroidism: Hashimoto's thyroiditis, atrophic thyroiditis

Iatrogenic: ^{131}I treatment, subtotal or total thyroidectomy, external irradiation of neck for lymphoma or cancer

Drugs: iodine excess (including iodine-containing contrast media and amiodarone), lithium, antithyroid drugs, p-aminosalicylic acid, interferon-α and other cytokines, aminoglutethimide

Congenital hypothyroidism: absent or ectopic thyroid gland, dyshormonogenesis, TSH-R mutation

Iodine deficiency

Infiltrative disorders: amyloidosis, sarcoidosis, hemochromatosis, scleroderma, cystinosis, Riedel's thyroiditis

Overexpression of type 3 deoiodinase in infantile hemangioma

Transient

Silent thyroiditis, including postpartum thyroiditis

Subacute thyroiditis

Withdrawal of thyroxine treatment in individuals with an intact thyroid

After ^{131}I treatment or subtotal thyroidectomy for Graves' disease

Secondary

Hypopituitarism: tumors, pituitary surgery or irradiation, infiltrative disorders, Sheehan's syndrome, trauma, genetic forms of combined pituitary hormone deficiencies

Isolated TSH deficiency or inactivity

Bexarotene treatment

Hypothalamic disease: tumors, trauma, infiltrative disorders, idiopathic

Note: TSH, thyroid-stimulating hormone; TSH-R, TSH receptor.

programs have been established. These are generally based on measurement of TSH or T_4 levels in heel-prick blood specimens. When the diagnosis is confirmed, T_4 is instituted at a dose of 10–15 μg/kg per day, and the dose is adjusted by close monitoring of TSH levels. T_4 requirements are relatively great during the first year of life, and a high circulating T_4 level is usually needed to normalize TSH. Early treatment with T_4 results in normal IQ levels, but subtle neurodevelopmental abnormalities may occur in those with the most severe hypothyroidism at diagnosis or when treatment is suboptimal.

AUTOIMMUNE HYPOTHYROIDISM

Classification Autoimmune hypothyroidism may be associated with a goiter (Hashimoto's, or *goitrous thyroiditis*) or, at the later stages of the disease, minimal residual thyroid tissue (*atrophic thyroiditis*). Because the autoimmune process gradually reduces thyroid function, there is a phase of compensation when normal thyroid hormone levels are maintained by a rise in TSH. Though some patients may have minor symptoms, this state is called *subclinical hypothyroidism*. Later, unbound T_4 levels fall and TSH levels rise further; symptoms become more readily apparent at this stage (usually TSH >10 mU/L), which is referred to as *clinical hypothyroidism* or *overt hypothyroidism*.

Prevalence The mean annual incidence rate of autoimmune hypothyroidism is up to 4 per 1000 women and 1 per 1000 men. It is more common in certain populations, such as the Japanese, probably because of genetic factors and chronic exposure to a high-iodine diet.

TABLE 335-5 **SIGNS AND SYMPTOMS OF HYPOTHYROIDISM (DESCENDING ORDER OF FREQUENCY)**

Symptoms	Signs
Tiredness, weakness	Dry coarse skin; cool peripheral extremities
Dry skin	
Feeling cold	Puffy face, hands, and feet (myxedema)
Hair loss	
Difficulty concentrating and poor memory	Diffuse alopecia
	Bradycardia
Constipation	Peripheral edema
Weight gain with poor appetite	Delayed tendon reflex relaxation
Dyspnea	Carpal tunnel syndrome
Hoarse voice	Serous cavity effusions
Menorrhagia (later oligomenorrhea or amenorrhea)	
Paresthesia	
Impaired hearing	

The mean age at diagnosis is 60 years, and the prevalence of overt hypothyroidism increases with age. Subclinical hypothyroidism is found in 6–8% of women (10% over the age of 60) and 3% of men. The annual risk of developing clinical hypothyroidism is about 4% when subclinical hypothyroidism is associated with positive TPO antibodies.

Pathogenesis In Hashimoto's thyroiditis, there is a marked lymphocytic infiltration of the thyroid with germinal center formation, atrophy of the thyroid follicles accompanied by oxyphil metaplasia, absence of colloid, and mild to moderate fibrosis. In atrophic thyroiditis, the fibrosis is much more extensive, lymphocyte infiltration is less pronounced, and thyroid follicles are almost completely absent. Atrophic thyroiditis likely represents the end stage of Hashimoto's thyroiditis rather than a distinct disorder.

As with most autoimmune disorders, susceptibility to autoimmune hypothyroidism is determined by a combination of genetic and environmental factors, and the risk of either autoimmune hypothyroidism or Graves' disease is increased among siblings. HLA-DR polymorphisms are the best documented genetic risk factors for autoimmune hypothyroidism, especially HLA-DR3, -DR4, and -DR5 in Caucasians. A weak association also exists between polymorphisms in *CTLA-4*, a T cell–regulatory gene, and autoimmune hypothyroidism. Both of these genetic associations are shared by other autoimmune diseases, which may explain the relationship between autoimmune hypothyroidism and other autoimmune diseases, especially type 1 diabetes mellitus, Addison's disease, pernicious anemia, and vitiligo (Chap. 345). HLA-DR and *CTLA*-4 polymorphisms account for approximately half of the genetic susceptibility to autoimmune hypothyroidism. The other contributory loci remain to be identified. A gene on chromosome 21 may be responsible for the association between autoimmune hypothyroidism and Down syndrome. The female preponderance of thyroid autoimmunity is most likely due to sex steroid effects on the immune response, but an X chromosome–related genetic factor is also possible, which may account for the high frequency of autoimmune hypothyroidism in Turner syndrome. Environmental susceptibility factors are poorly defined at present. A high iodine intake may increase the risk of autoimmune hypothyroidism by immunologic effects or direct thyroid toxicity. There is no convincing evidence for a role of infection except for the congenital rubella syndrome, in which there is a high frequency of autoimmune hypothyroidism. Viral thyroiditis does not induce subsequent autoimmune thyroid disease.

The thyroid lymphocytic infiltrate in autoimmune hypothyroidism is composed of activated CD4+ and CD8+ T cells, as well as B cells. Thyroid cell destruction is primarily mediated by the CD8+ cytotoxic T cells, which destroy their targets by either perforin-induced cell necrosis or granzyme B–induced apoptosis. In addition, local T cell production of cytokines, such as tumor necrosis factor (TNF), IL-1, and interferon γ (IFN-γ), may render thyroid cells more susceptible to apoptosis mediated by death receptors, such as Fas, which are activated by their respective ligands on T cells. These cytokines also impair thyroid cell function directly and induce the expression of other proinflammatory molecules by the thyroid cells themselves, such as cytokines, HLA class I and class II molecules, adhesion molecules, CD40, and nitric oxide. Administration of high concentrations of cytokines for therapeutic purposes (especially IFN-α) is associated with increased autoimmune thyroid disease, possibly through mechanisms similar to those in sporadic disease.

Antibodies to Tg and TPO are clinically useful markers of thyroid autoimmunity, but any pathogenic effect is restricted to a secondary role in amplifying an ongoing autoimmune response. TPO antibodies fix complement, and complement membrane attack complexes are present in the thyroid in autoimmune hypothyroidism. However, transplacental passage of Tg or TPO antibodies has no effect on the fetal thyroid, which suggests that T cell–mediated injury is required to initiate autoimmune damage to the thyroid.

Up to 20% of patients with autoimmune hypothyroidism have antibodies against the TSH-R, which, in contrast to TSI, do not stimulate the receptor but prevent the binding of TSH. These TSH-R-blocking antibodies therefore cause hypothyroidism and, especially in Asian patients, thyroid atrophy. Their transplacental passage may induce transient neonatal hypothyroidism. Rarely, patients have a mixture of TSI- and TSH-R-blocking antibodies, and thyroid function can oscillate between hyperthyroidism and hypothyroidism as one or the other antibody becomes dominant. Predicting the course of disease in such individuals is difficult, and they require close monitoring of thyroid function. Bioassays can be used to document that TSH-R-blocking antibodies reduce the cyclic AMP–inducing effect of TSH on cultured TSH-R-expressing cells, but these assays are difficult to perform. Assays that measure the binding of antibodies to the receptor by competition with radiolabeled TSH [TSH-binding inhibiting immunoglobulins (TBII)] do not distinguish between TSI- and TSH-R-blocking antibodies, but a positive result in a patient with spontaneous hypothyroidism is strong evidence for the presence of blocking antibodies. The use of these assays does not generally alter clinical management, although they may be useful to confirm the cause of transient neonatal hypothyroidism.

Clinical Manifestations   The main clinical features of hypothyroidism are summarized in Table 335-5. The onset is usually insidious, and the patient may become aware of symptoms only when euthyroidism is restored. Patients with Hashimoto's thyroiditis may present because of goiter rather than symptoms of hypothyroidism. The goiter may not be large but is usually irregular and firm in consistency. It is often possible to palpate a pyramidal lobe, normally a vestigial remnant of the thyroglossal duct. Rarely, uncomplicated Hashimoto's thyroiditis is associated with pain.

Patients with atrophic thyroiditis or the late stage of Hashimoto's thyroiditis present with symptoms and signs of hypothyroidism. The skin is dry, and there is decreased sweating, thinning of the epidermis, and hyperkeratosis of the stratum corneum. Increased dermal glycosaminoglycan content traps water, giving rise to skin thickening without pitting (*myxedema*). Typical features include a puffy face with edematous eyelids and nonpitting pretibial edema (Fig. 335-5). There is pallor, often with a yellow tinge to the skin due to carotene accumulation. Nail growth is retarded, and hair is dry, brittle, difficult to manage, and falls out easily. In addition to diffuse alopecia, there is thinning of the outer third of the eyebrows, although this is not a specific sign of hypothyroidism.

Other common features include constipation and weight gain (despite a poor appetite). In contrast to popular perception, the weight gain is usually modest and due mainly to fluid retention in the myxedematous tissues. Libido is decreased in both sexes, and there may be oligomenorrhea or amenorrhea in long-standing disease, but menorrhagia is also common. Fertility is reduced and the incidence of miscarriage is increased. Prolactin levels are often modestly increased (Chap. 333) and may contribute to alterations in libido and fertility and cause galactorrhea.

Myocardial contractility and pulse rate are reduced, leading to a reduced stroke volume and bradycardia. Increased peripheral resistance may be accompanied by hypertension, particularly diastolic. Blood flow is diverted from the skin, producing cool extremities. Pericardial effusions occur in up to 30% of patients but rarely compromise cardiac function. Though alterations in myosin heavy chain isoform expression have been documented, cardiomyopathy is unusual. Fluid may also accumulate in other serous cavities and in the middle ear, giving rise to conductive deafness. Pulmonary function is generally normal, but dyspnea may be caused by pleural effusion, impaired respiratory muscle function, diminished ventilatory drive, or sleep apnea.

FIGURE 335-5 Facial appearance in hypothyroidism. Note puffy eyes and thickened, pale skin.

Carpal tunnel and other entrapment syndromes are common, as is impairment of muscle function with stiffness, cramps, and pain. On examination, there may be slow relaxation of tendon reflexes and pseudomyotonia. Memory and concentration are impaired. Rare neurologic problems include reversible cerebellar ataxia, dementia, psychosis, and myxedema coma. *Hashimoto's encephalopathy* has been defined as a steroid-responsive syndrome associated with TPO antibodies, myoclonus, and slow-wave activity on electroencephalography, but the relationship with thyroid autoimmunity or hypothyroidism is not established. The hoarse voice and occasionally clumsy speech of hypothyroidism reflect fluid accumulation in the vocal cords and tongue.

The features described above are the consequence of thyroid hormone deficiency. However, autoimmune hypothyroidism may be associated with signs or symptoms of other autoimmune diseases, particularly vitiligo, pernicious anemia, Addison's disease, alopecia areata, and type 1 diabetes mellitus. Less-common associations include celiac disease, dermatitis herpetiformis, chronic active hepatitis, rheumatoid arthritis, systemic lupus erythematosus (SLE), and Sjögren's syndrome. Thyroid-associated ophthalmopathy, which usually occurs in Graves' disease (see below), occurs in about 5% of patients with autoimmune hypothyroidism.

Autoimmune hypothyroidism is uncommon in children and usually presents with slow growth and delayed facial maturation. The appearance of permanent teeth is also delayed. Myopathy, with muscle swelling, is more common in children than in adults. In most cases, puberty is delayed, but precocious puberty sometimes occurs. There may be intellectual impairment if the onset is before 3 years and the hormone deficiency is severe.

Laboratory Evaluation   A summary of the investigations used to determine the existence and cause of hypothyroidism is provided in Fig. 335-6. A normal TSH level excludes primary (but not secondary) hypothyroidism. If the TSH is elevated, an unbound T_4 level is needed to confirm the presence of clinical hypothyroidism, but T_4 is inferior to TSH when used as a screening test, as it will not detect subclinical hypothyroidism. Circulating unbound T_3 levels are normal in about 25% of patients, reflecting adaptive deiodinase responses to hypothyroidism. T_3 measurements are therefore not indicated.

EVALUATION OF HYPOTHYROIDISM

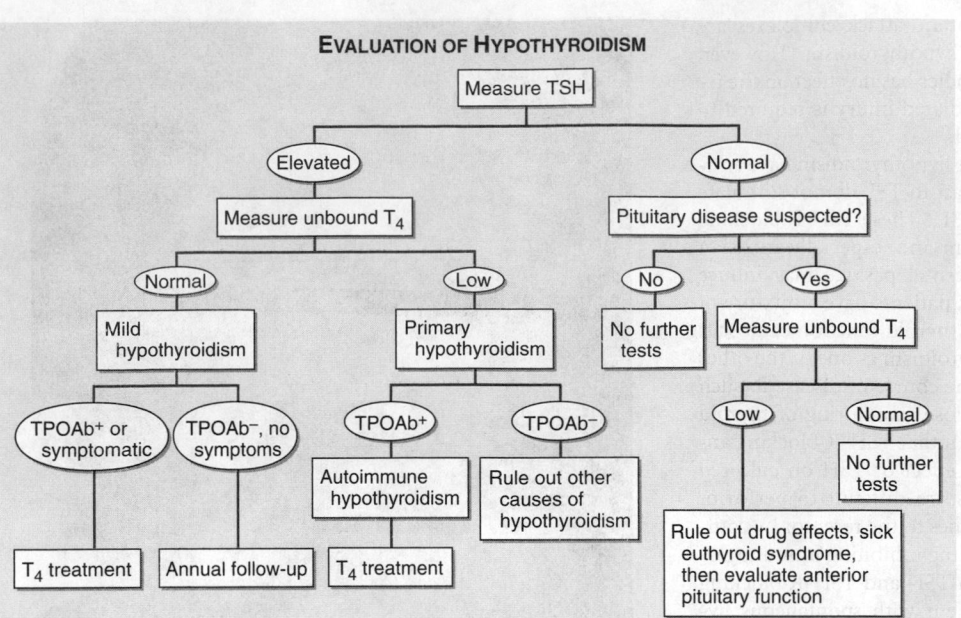

FIGURE 335-6 Evaluation of hypothyroidism. TPOAb⁺, thyroid peroxidase antibodies present; TPOAb⁻, thyroid peroxidase antibodies not present; TSH, thyroid-stimulating hormone.

Once clinical or subclinical hypothyroidism is confirmed, the etiology is usually easily established by demonstrating the presence of TPO antibodies, which are present in >90% of patients with autoimmune hypothyroidism. TBII can be found in 10–20% of patients, but these determinations are not needed routinely. If there is any doubt about the cause of a goiter associated with hypothyroidism, FNA biopsy can be used to confirm the presence of autoimmune thyroiditis. Other abnormal laboratory findings in hypothyroidism may include increased creatine phosphokinase, elevated cholesterol and triglycerides, and anemia (usually normocytic or macrocytic). Except when accompanied by iron deficiency, the anemia and other abnormalities gradually resolve with thyroxine replacement.

Differential Diagnosis An asymmetric goiter in Hashimoto's thyroiditis may be confused with a multinodular goiter or thyroid carcinoma, in which thyroid antibodies may also be present. Ultrasound can be used to show the presence of a solitary lesion or a multinodular goiter rather than the heterogeneous thyroid enlargement typical of Hashimoto's thyroiditis. FNA biopsy is useful in the investigation of focal nodules. Other causes of hypothyroidism are discussed below but rarely cause diagnostic confusion (Table 335-4).

OTHER CAUSES OF HYPOTHYROIDISM

Iatrogenic hypothyroidism is a common cause of hypothyroidism and can often be detected by screening before symptoms develop. In the first 3–4 months after radioiodine treatment, transient hypothyroidism may occur due to reversible radiation damage. Low-dose thyroxine treatment can be withdrawn if recovery occurs. Because TSH levels are suppressed by hyperthyroidism, unbound T_4 levels are a better measure of thyroid function than TSH in the months following radioiodine treatment. Mild hypothyroidism after subtotal thyroidectomy may also resolve after several months, as the gland remnant is stimulated by increased TSH levels.

Iodine deficiency is responsible for endemic goiter and cretinism but is an uncommon cause of adult hypothyroidism unless the iodine intake is very low or there are complicating factors, such as the consumption of thiocyanates in cassava or selenium deficiency. Though hypothyroidism due to iodine deficiency can be treated with thyroxine, public health measures to improve iodine intake should be advocated to eliminate this problem. Iodized salt or bread or a single bolus of oral or intramuscular iodized oil have all been used successfully.

Paradoxically, chronic iodine excess can also induce goiter and hypothyroidism. The intracellular events that account for this effect are unclear, but individuals with autoimmune thyroiditis are especially susceptible. Iodine excess is responsible for the hypothyroidism that occurs in up to 13% of patients treated with amiodarone (see below). Other drugs, particularly lithium, may also cause hypothyroidism. Transient hypothyroidism caused by thyroiditis is discussed below.

Secondary hypothyroidism is usually diagnosed in the context of other anterior pituitary hormone deficiencies; isolated TSH deficiency is very rare (Chap. 333). TSH levels may be low, normal, or even slightly increased in secondary hypothyroidism; the latter is due to secretion of immunoactive but bioinactive forms of TSH. The diagnosis is confirmed by detecting a low unbound T_4 level. The goal of treatment is to maintain T_4 levels in the upper half of the reference range, as TSH levels cannot be used to monitor therapy.

℞ HYPOTHYROIDISM

CLINICAL HYPOTHYROIDISM If there is no residual thyroid function, the daily replacement dose of levothyroxine is usually 1.6 μg/kg body weight (typically 100–150 μg). In many patients, however, lower doses suffice until residual thyroid tissue is destroyed. In patients who develop hypothyroidism after the treatment of Graves' disease, there is often underlying autonomous function, necessitating lower replacement doses (typically 75–125 μg/d).

Adult patients under 60 without evidence of heart disease may be started on 50–100 μg levothyroxine (T_4) daily. The dose is adjusted on the basis of TSH levels, with the goal of treatment being a normal TSH, ideally in the lower half of the reference range. TSH responses are gradual and should be measured about 2 months after instituting treatment or after any subsequent change in levothyroxine dosage. The clinical effects of levothyroxine replacement are often slow to appear. Patients may not experience full relief from symptoms until 3–6 months after normal TSH levels are restored. Adjustment of levothyroxine dosage is made in 12.5- or 25-μg increments if the TSH is high; decrements of the same magnitude should be made if the TSH is suppressed. Patients with a suppressed TSH of any cause, including T_4 overtreatment, have an increased risk of atrial fibrillation and reduced bone density.

Although dessicated animal thyroid preparations (thyroid extract USP) are available, they are not recommended as the ratio of T3 to T4 is nonphysiologic. The use of levothyroxine combined with liothyronine (triiodothyronine, T_3) has been advocated, but benefit has not been confirmed in several prospective studies. There is no place for liothyronine alone as long-term replacement, because the short half-life necessitates three or four daily doses and is associated with fluctuating T_3 levels.

Once full replacement is achieved and TSH levels are stable, follow-up measurement of TSH is recommended at annual intervals and may be extended to every 2–3 years if a normal TSH is maintained over several years. It is important to ensure ongoing adherence, however, as patients do not feel any symptomatic difference after missing a few doses of levothyroxine, and this sometimes leads to self-discontinuation.

In patients of normal body weight who are taking ≥200 μg of levothyroxine per day, an elevated TSH level is often a sign of poor adherence to treatment. This is also the likely explanation for fluctuating TSH levels, despite a constant levothyroxine dosage. Such patients often have normal or high unbound T_4 levels, despite an elevated TSH, because they remember to take medication for a few days before testing; this is sufficient to normalize T_4, but not TSH, levels. It is important to consider variable adherence, as this pattern of thyroid function tests is otherwise suggestive of disorders associated with inappropriate TSH secretion (Table 335-3). Because T_4 has a long half-life (7 days), patients who miss doses can be advised to take two or three doses of the skipped tablets at once. Other causes of increased levothyroxine requirements must be excluded, particularly malabsorption (e.g., celiac disease, small-bowel surgery), estrogen therapy, and drugs that interfere with T_4 absorption or clearance such as cholestyramine, ferrous sulfate, calcium supplements, lovastatin, aluminum hydroxide, rifampicin, amiodarone, carbamazepine, and phenytoin.

SUBCLINICAL HYPOTHYROIDISM By definition, subclinical hypothyroidism refers to biochemical evidence of thyroid hormone deficiency in patients who have few or no apparent clinical features of hypothyroidism. There are no universally accepted recommendations for the management of subclinical hypothyroidism, but the most recently published guidelines do not recommend treatment when TSH levels are below 10 mU/L. It is important to confirm that any elevation of TSH is sustained over a 3-month period before treatment is given. As long as excessive treatment is avoided, there is no risk in correcting a slightly increased TSH. Moreover, there is a risk that patients will progress to overt hypothyroidism, particularly when the TSH level is elevated and TPO antibodies are present. Treatment is administered by starting with a low dose of levothyroxine (25–50 μg/d) with the goal of normalizing TSH. If thyroxine is not given, thyroid function should be evaluated annually.

SPECIAL TREATMENT CONSIDERATIONS Rarely, levothyroxine replacement is associated with pseudotumor cerebri in children. Presentation appears to be idiosyncratic and occurs months after treatment has begun. Women with a history or high risk of hypothyroidism should ensure that they are euthyroid prior to conception and during early pregnancy as maternal hypothyroidism may adversely affect fetal neural development. Thyroid function should be evaluated immediately after pregnancy is confirmed and at the beginning of the second and third trimesters. The dose of levothyroxine may need to be increased by ≥50% during pregnancy and returned to previous levels after delivery. Elderly patients may require up to 20% less thyroxine than younger patients. In the elderly, especially patients with known coronary artery disease, the starting dose of levothyroxine is 12.5–25 μg/d with similar increments every 2–3 months until TSH is normalized. In some patients it may be impossible to achieve full replacement, despite optimal antianginal treatment. *Emergency surgery* is generally safe in patients with untreated hypothyroidism, although routine surgery in a hypothyroid patient should be deferred until euthyroidism is achieved.

Myxedema coma still has a high mortality rate, despite intensive treatment. Clinical manifestations include reduced level of consciousness, sometimes associated with seizures, as well as the other features of hypothyroidism (Table 335-5). Hypothermia can reach 23°C (74°F). There may be a history of treated hypothyroidism with poor compliance, or the patient may be previously undiagnosed. Myxedema coma almost always occurs in the elderly and is usually precipitated by factors that impair respiration, such as drugs (especially sedatives, anesthetics, antidepressants), pneumonia, congestive heart failure, myocardial infarction, gastrointestinal bleeding, or cerebrovascular accidents. Sepsis should also be suspected. Exposure to cold may also be a risk factor. Hypoventilation, leading to hypoxia and hypercapnia, plays a major role in pathogenesis; hypoglycemia and dilutional hyponatremia also contribute to the development of myxedema coma.

Levothyroxine can initially be administered as a single intravenous bolus of 500 μg, which serves as a loading dose. Although further levothyroxine is not strictly necessary for several days, it is usually continued at a dose of 50–100 μg/d. If suitable intravenous preparation is not available, the same initial dose of levothyroxine can be given by nasogastric tube (though absorption may be impaired in myxedema). An alternative is to give liothyronine (T_3) intravenously or via nasogastric tube, in doses ranging from 10 to 25 μg every 8–12 h. This treatment has been advocated because $T_4 \rightarrow T_3$ conversion is impaired in myxedema coma. However, excess liothyronine has the potential to provoke arrhythmias. Another option is to combine levothyroxine (200 μg) and liothyronine (25 μg) as a single, initial intravenous bolus followed by daily treatment with levothyroxine (50–100 μg/d) and liothyronine (10 μg every 8 h).

Supportive therapy should be provided to correct any associated metabolic disturbances. External warming is indicated only if the temperature is <30°C, as it can result in cardiovascular collapse (Chap. 20). Space blankets should be used to prevent further heat loss. Parenteral hydrocortisone (50 mg every 6 h) should be administered, as there is impaired adrenal reserve in profound hypothyroidism. Any precipitating factors should be treated, including the early use of broad-spectrum antibiotics, pending the exclusion of infection. Ventilatory support with regular blood gas analysis is usually needed during the first 48 h. Hypertonic saline or intravenous glucose may be needed if there is severe hyponatremia or hypoglycemia; hypotonic intravenous fluids should be avoided because they may exacerbate water retention secondary to reduced renal perfusion and inappropriate vasopressin secretion. The metabolism of most medications is impaired, and sedatives should be avoided if possible or used in reduced doses. Medication blood levels should be monitored, when available, to guide dosage.

THYROTOXICOSIS

Thyrotoxicosis is defined as the state of thyroid hormone excess and is not synonymous with *hyperthyroidism*, which is the result of excessive thyroid function. However, the major etiologies of thyrotoxicosis are hyperthyroidism caused by Graves' disease, toxic MNG, and toxic adenomas. Other causes are listed in Table 335-6.

GRAVES' DISEASE

Epidemiology Graves' disease accounts for 60–80% of thyrotoxicosis. The prevalence varies among populations, depending mainly on iodine intake (high iodine intake is associated with an increased prevalence of Graves' disease). Graves' disease occurs in up to 2% of women but is one-tenth as frequent in men. The disorder rarely begins before adolescence and typically occurs between 20 and 50 years of age, but it also occurs in the elderly.

Pathogenesis As in autoimmune hypothyroidism, a combination of environmental and genetic factors, including polymorphisms in HLA-DR, *CTLA-4*, and *PTPN22* (a T cell regulatory gene), contribute to Graves' disease susceptibility. The concordance for Graves' disease in monozygotic twins is 20–30%, compared to <5% in dizygotic twins. Indirect evidence suggests that stress is an important environmental factor, presumably operating through neuroendocrine effects on the immune system. Smoking is a minor risk factor for Graves' disease and a major risk factor for the development of ophthalmopathy. Sudden increases in iodine intake may precipitate Graves' disease, and there is a threefold increase in the occurrence of Graves' disease in the postpartum period.

TABLE 335-6 **CAUSES OF THYROTOXICOSIS**

Primary hyperthyroidism
Graves' disease
Toxic multinodular goiter
Toxic adenoma
Functioning thyroid carcinoma metastases
Activating mutation of the TSH receptor
Activating mutation of $G_{s\alpha}$ (McCune-Albright syndrome)
Struma ovarii
Drugs: iodine excess (Jod-Basedow phenomenon)

Thyrotoxicosis without hyperthyroidism
Subacute thyroiditis
Silent thyroiditis
Other causes of thyroid destruction: amiodarone, radiation, infarction of adenoma
Ingestion of excess thyroid hormone (thyrotoxicosis factitia) or thyroid tissue

Secondary hyperthyroidism
TSH-secreting pituitary adenoma
Thyroid hormone resistance syndrome: occasional patients may have features of thyrotoxicosis
Chorionic gonadotropin-secreting tumors[a]
Gestational thyrotoxicosis[a]

[a]Circulating TSH levels are low in these forms of secondary hyperthyroidism.
Note: TSH, thyroid-stimulating hormone.

The hyperthyroidism of Graves' disease is caused by TSI that are synthesized in the thyroid gland as well as in bone marrow and lymph nodes. Such antibodies can be detected by bioassays or by using the more widely available TBII assays. The presence of TBII in a patient with thyrotoxicosis implies the existence of TSI, and these assays are useful in monitoring pregnant Graves' patients in whom high levels of TSI can cross the placenta and cause neonatal thyrotoxicosis. Other thyroid autoimmune responses, similar to those in autoimmune hypothyroidism (see above), occur concurrently in patients with Graves' disease. In particular, TPO antibodies occur in up to 80% of cases and serve as a readily measurable marker of autoimmunity. Because the coexisting thyroiditis can also affect thyroid function, there is no direct correlation between the level of TSI and thyroid hormone levels in Graves' disease. In the long term, spontaneous autoimmune hypothyroidism may develop in up to 15% of Graves' patients.

Cytokines appear to play a major role in thyroid-associated ophthalmopathy. There is infiltration of the extraocular muscles by activated T cells; the release of cytokines such as IFN-γ, TNF, and IL-1 results in fibroblast activation and increased synthesis of glycosaminoglycans that trap water, thereby leading to characteristic muscle swelling. Late in the disease, there is irreversible fibrosis of the muscles. Orbital fibroblasts may be particularly sensitive to cytokines, perhaps explaining the anatomic localization of the immune response. Though the pathogenesis of thyroid-associated ophthalmopathy remains unclear, there is mounting evidence that the TSH-R may be a shared autoantigen that is expressed in the orbit and this would explain the close association with autoimmune thyroid disease. Increased fat is an additional cause of retrobulbar tissue expansion. The increase in intraorbital pressure can lead to proptosis, diplopia, and optic neuropathy

Clinical Manifestations   Signs and symptoms include features that are common to any cause of thyrotoxicosis (Table 335-7) as well as those specific for Graves' disease. The clinical presentation depends on the severity of thyrotoxicosis, the duration of disease, individual susceptibility to excess thyroid hormone, and the patient's age. In the elderly, features of thyrotoxicosis may be subtle or masked, and patients may present mainly with fatigue and weight loss, a condition known as *apathetic thyrotoxicosis*.

Thyrotoxicosis may cause unexplained weight loss, despite an enhanced appetite, due to the increased metabolic rate. Weight gain occurs in 5% of patients, however, because of increased food intake. Other prominent features include hyperactivity, nervousness, and irritability, ultimately leading to a sense of easy fatigability in some patients. Insomnia and impaired concentration are common; apathetic thyrotoxicosis may be mistaken for depression in the elderly. Fine tremor is a frequent finding, best elicited by having patients stretch out their fingers while feeling the fingertips with the palm. Common neurologic manifestations include hyperreflexia, muscle wasting, and proximal myopathy without fasciculation. Chorea is a rare feature. Thyrotoxicosis is sometimes associated with a form of hypokalemic periodic paralysis; this disorder is particularly common in Asian males with thyrotoxicosis.

The most common cardiovascular manifestation is sinus tachycardia, often associated with palpitations, occasionally caused by supraventricular tachycardia. The high cardiac output produces a bounding pulse, widened pulse pressure, and an aortic systolic murmur and can lead to worsening of angina or heart failure in the elderly or those with preexisting heart disease. Atrial fibrillation is more common in patients >50 years. Treatment of the thyrotoxic state alone converts atrial fibrillation to normal sinus rhythm in about half of patients, suggesting the existence of an underlying cardiac problem in the remainder.

The skin is usually warm and moist, and the patient may complain of sweating and heat intolerance, particularly during warm weather. Palmar erythema, onycholysis, and, less commonly, pruritus, urticaria, and diffuse hyperpigmentation may be evident. Hair texture may become fine, and a diffuse alopecia occurs in up to 40% of patients, persisting for months after restoration of euthyroidism. Gastrointestinal transit time is decreased, leading to increased stool frequency, often with diarrhea and occasionally mild steatorrhea. Women frequently experience oligomenorrhea or amenorrhea; in men there may be impaired sexual function and, rarely, gynecomastia. The direct effect of thyroid hormones on bone resorption leads to osteopenia in longstanding thyrotoxicosis; mild hypercalcemia occurs in up to 20% of patients, but hypercalciuria is more common. There is a small increase in fracture rate in patients with a previous history of thyrotoxicosis.

In Graves' disease the thyroid is usually diffusely enlarged to two–three times its normal size. The consistency is firm, but less so than in MNG. There may be a thrill or bruit due to the increased vascularity of the gland and the hyperdynamic circulation.

Lid retraction, causing a staring appearance, can occur in any form of thyrotoxicosis and is the result of sympathetic overactivity. However, Graves' disease is associated with specific eye signs that comprise *Graves' ophthalmopathy* (Fig. 335-7A). This condition is also called *thyroid-associated ophthalmopathy*, as it occurs in the absence of Graves' disease in 10% of patients. Most of these individuals have autoimmune hypothyroidism or thyroid antibodies. The onset of Graves' ophthalmopathy occurs within the year before or after the diagnosis of thyrotoxicosis in 75% of patients but can sometimes precede or follow thyrotoxicosis by several years, accounting for some cases of euthyroid ophthalmopathy.

Some patients with Graves' disease have little clinical evidence of ophthalmopathy. However, the enlarged extraocular muscles typical of the disease, and other subtle features, can be detected in almost all patients when investigated by ultrasound or CT imaging of the orbits. Unilateral signs are found in up to 10% of patients. The earliest manifestations of ophthalmopathy are usually a sensation of grittiness, eye discomfort, and excess tearing. About a third of patients have proptosis, best detected by visualization of the sclera between the lower border of the iris and the lower eyelid, with the eyes in the primary position. Proptosis can be measured using an exophthalmometer. In severe cases, proptosis may cause corneal exposure and damage, especially if the lids fail to close during sleep. Periorbital edema, scleral injection, and chemosis are also frequent. In 5–10% of patients, the muscle swelling is so severe that diplopia results, typically but not exclusively when the patient looks up and laterally. The most serious manifestation is compression of the optic nerve at the apex of the orbit, leading to papilledema, peripheral field defects, and, if left untreated, permanent loss of vision.

Many scoring systems have been used to gauge the extent and activity of the orbital changes in Graves' disease. The "NO SPECS" scheme is an acronym derived from the following eye changes:

0 = **N**o signs or symptoms
1 = **O**nly signs (lid retraction or lag), no symptoms
2 = **S**oft tissue involvement (periorbital edema)
3 = **P**roptosis (>22 mm)
4 = **E**xtraocular muscle involvement (diplopia)
5 = **C**orneal involvement
6 = **S**ight loss

TABLE 335-7	SIGNS AND SYMPTOMS OF THYROTOXICOSIS (DESCENDING ORDER OF FREQUENCY)

Symptoms	Signs[a]
Hyperactivity, irritability, dysphoria	Tachycardia; atrial fibrillation in the elderly
Heat intolerance and sweating	Tremor
Palpitations	Goiter
Fatigue and weakness	Warm, moist skin
Weight loss with increased appetite	Muscle weakness, proximal myopathy
Diarrhea	Lid retraction or lag
Polyuria	Gynecomastia
Oligomenorrhea, loss of libido	

[a]Excludes the signs of ophthalmopathy and dermopathy specific for Graves' disease.

TSH level is suppressed and total and unbound thyroid hormone levels are increased. In 2–5% of patients (and more in areas of borderline iodine intake), only T_3 is increased (T_3 toxicosis). The converse state of T_4 toxicosis, with elevated total and unbound T_4 and normal T_3 levels, is occasionally seen when hyperthyroidism is induced by excess iodine, providing surplus substrate for thyroid hormone synthesis. Measurement of TPO antibodies is useful in differential diagnosis. Measurement of TBII or TSI will confirm the diagnosis but is not needed routinely. Associated abnormalities that may cause diagnostic confusion in thyrotoxicosis include elevation of bilirubin, liver enzymes, and ferritin. Microcytic anemia and thrombocytopenia may occur.

Differential Diagnosis Diagnosis of Graves' disease is straightforward in a patient with biochemically confirmed thyrotoxicosis, diffuse goiter on palpation, ophthalmopathy, positive TPO or TSH-R antibodies, and often a personal or family history of autoimmune disorders. For patients with thyrotoxicosis who lack these features, the most reliable diagnostic method is a radionuclide (^{99m}Tc, ^{123}I, or ^{131}I) scan of the thyroid, which will distinguish the diffuse, high uptake of Graves' disease from nodular thyroid disease, destructive thyroiditis, ectopic thyroid tissue, and factitious thyrotoxicosis. In secondary hyperthyroidism due to a TSH-secreting pituitary tumor, there is also a diffuse goiter. The presence of a nonsuppressed TSH level and the finding of a pituitary tumor on CT or MRI scan readily identify such patients.

Clinical features of thyrotoxicosis can mimic certain aspects of other disorders, including panic attacks, mania, pheochromocytoma, and weight loss associated with malignancy. The diagnosis of thyrotoxicosis can be easily excluded if the TSH and unbound T_3 levels are normal. A normal TSH also excludes Graves' disease as a cause of diffuse goiter.

Clinical Course Clinical features generally worsen without treatment; mortality was 10–30% before the introduction of satisfactory therapy. Some patients with mild Graves' disease experience spontaneous re-

FIGURE 335-7 Features of Graves' disease. A. Ophthalmopathy in Graves' disease; lid retraction, periorbital edema, conjunctival injection, and proptosis are marked. **B.** Thyroid dermopathy over the lateral aspects of the shins. **C.** Thyroid acropachy.

Although useful as a mnemonic, the NO SPECS scheme is inadequate to describe the eye disease fully, and patients do not necessarily progress from one class to another. When Graves' eye disease is active and severe, referral to an ophthalmologist is indicated and objective measurements are needed, such as lid fissure width; corneal staining with fluorescein; and evaluation of extraocular muscle function (e.g., Hess chart), intraocular pressure and visual fields, acuity, and color vision.

Thyroid dermopathy occurs in <5% of patients with Graves' disease (Fig. 335-7*B*), almost always in the presence of moderate or severe ophthalmopathy. Although most frequent over the anterior and lateral aspects of the lower leg (hence the term *pretibial myxedema*), skin changes can occur at other sites, particularly after trauma. The typical lesion is a noninflamed, indurated plaque with a deep pink or purple color and an "orange-skin" appearance. Nodular involvement can occur, and the condition can rarely extend over the whole lower leg and foot, mimicking elephantiasis. *Thyroid acropachy* refers to a form of clubbing found in <1% of patients with Graves' disease (Fig. 335-7*C*). It is so strongly associated with thyroid dermopathy that an alternative cause of clubbing should be sought in a Graves' patient without coincident skin and orbital involvement.

Laboratory Evaluation Investigations used to determine the existence and cause of thyrotoxicosis are summarized in Fig. 335-8. In Graves' disease, the

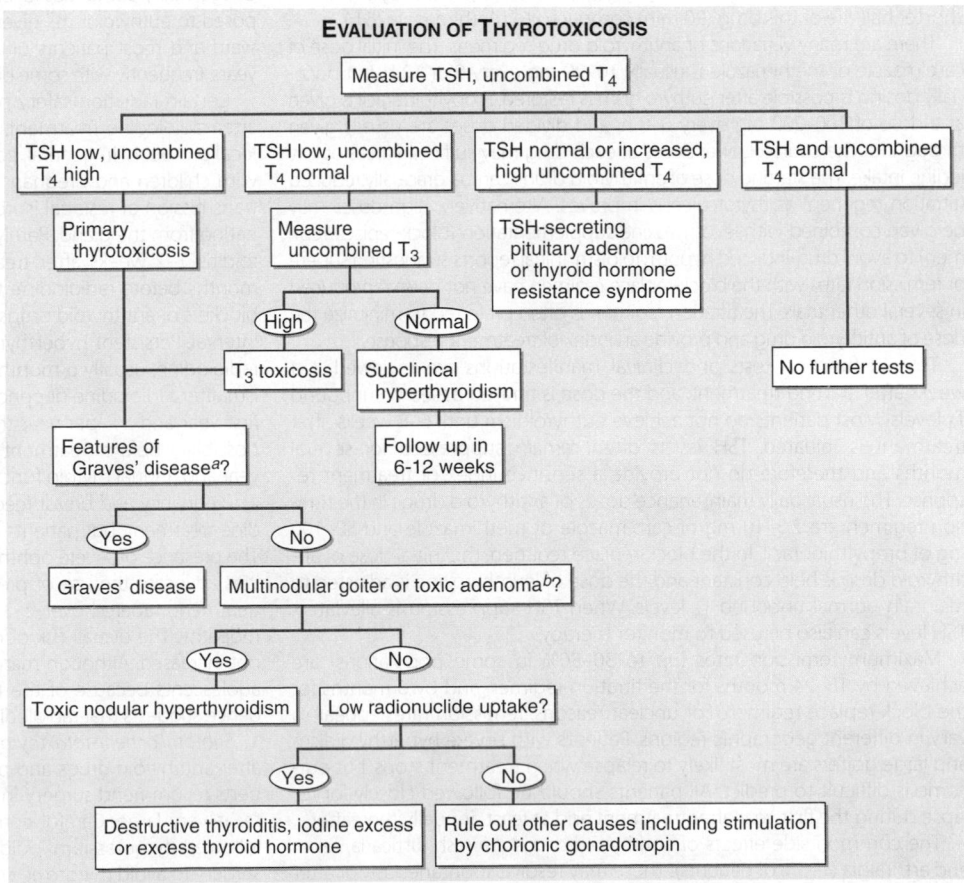

EVALUATION OF THYROTOXICOSIS

Measure TSH, uncombined T_4

- TSH low, uncombined T_4 high → Primary thyrotoxicosis → Features of Graves' disease^a? → Yes → Graves' disease / No → Multinodular goiter or toxic adenoma^b? → Yes → Toxic nodular hyperthyroidism / No → Low radionuclide uptake? → Yes → Destructive thyroiditis, iodine excess or excess thyroid hormone / No → Rule out other causes including stimulation by chorionic gonadotropin
- TSH low, uncombined T_4 normal → Measure uncombined T_3 → High → T_3 toxicosis / Normal → Subclinical hyperthyroidism → Follow up in 6-12 weeks
- TSH normal or increased, high uncombined T_4 → TSH-secreting pituitary adenoma or thyroid hormone resistance syndrome
- TSH and uncombined T_4 normal → No further tests

FIGURE 335-8 Evaluation of thyrotoxicosis. ^{a}Diffuse goiter, positive TPO antibodies, ophthalmopathy, dermopathy; ^{b}can be confirmed by radionuclide scan. TSH, thyroid-stimulating hormone.

lapses and remissions. Rarely, there may be fluctuation between hypo- and hyperthyroidism due to changes in the functional activity of TSH-R antibodies. About 15% of patients who enter remission after treatment with antithyroid drugs develop hypothyroidism 10–15 years later as a result of the destructive autoimmune process.

The clinical course of ophthalmopathy does not follow that of the thyroid disease. Ophthalmopathy typically worsens over the initial 3–6 months, followed by a plateau phase over the next 12–18 months, with spontaneous improvement, particularly in the soft tissue changes. However, the course is more fulminant in up to 5% of patients, requiring intervention in the acute phase if there is optic nerve compression or corneal ulceration. Diplopia may appear late in the disease due to fibrosis of the extraocular muscles. Some studies suggest that radioiodine treatment for hyperthyroidism worsens the eye disease in a small proportion of patients (especially smokers). Antithyroid drugs or surgery have no adverse effects on the clinical course of ophthalmopathy. Thyroid dermopathy, when it occurs, usually appears 1–2 years after the development of Graves' hyperthyroidism; it may improve spontaneously.

℞ GRAVES' DISEASE

The *hyperthyroidism* of Graves' disease is treated by reducing thyroid hormone synthesis, using antithyroid drugs, or reducing the amount of thyroid tissue with radioiodine (^{131}I) treatment or by thyroidectomy. Antithyroid drugs are the predominant therapy in many centers in Europe and Japan, whereas radioiodine is more often the first line of treatment in North America. These differences reflect the fact that no single approach is optimal and that patients may require multiple treatments to achieve remission.

The main *antithyroid drugs* are the thionamides, such as propylthiouracil, carbimazole, and the active metabolite of the latter, methimazole. All inhibit the function of TPO, reducing oxidation and organification of iodide. These drugs also reduce thyroid antibody levels by mechanisms that remain unclear, and they appear to enhance rates of remission. Propylthiouracil inhibits deiodination of $T_4 \rightarrow T_3$. However, this effect is of minor benefit, except in the most severe thyrotoxicosis, and is offset by the much shorter half-life of this drug (90 min) compared to methimazole (6 h).

There are many variations of antithyroid drug regimens. The initial dose of carbimazole or methimazole is usually 10–20 mg every 8 or 12 h, but once-daily dosing is possible after euthyroidism is restored. Propylthiouracil is given at a dose of 100–200 mg every 6–8 h, and divided doses are usually given throughout the course. Lower doses of each drug may suffice in areas of low iodine intake. The starting dose of antithyroid drugs can be gradually reduced (titration regimen) as thyrotoxicosis improves. Alternatively, high doses may be given combined with levothyroxine supplementation (block-replace regimen) to avoid drug-induced hypothyroidism. Initial reports suggesting superior remission rates with the block-replace regimen have not been reproduced in several other trials. The titration regimen is often preferred to minimize the dose of antithyroid drug and provide an index of treatment response.

Thyroid function tests and clinical manifestations are reviewed 3–4 weeks after starting treatment, and the dose is titrated based on unbound T_4 levels. Most patients do not achieve euthyroidism until 6–8 weeks after treatment is initiated. TSH levels often remain suppressed for several months and therefore do not provide a sensitive index of treatment response. The usual daily maintenance doses of antithyroid drugs in the titration regimen are 2.5–10 mg of carbimazole or methimazole and 50–100 mg of propylthiouracil. In the block-replace regimen, the initial dose of antithyroid drug is held constant and the dose of levothyroxine is adjusted to maintain normal unbound T_4 levels. When TSH suppression is alleviated, TSH levels can also be used to monitor therapy.

Maximum remission rates (up to 30–50% in some populations) are achieved by 18–24 months for the titration regimen and by 6 months for the block-replace regimen. For unclear reasons, remission rates appear to vary in different geographic regions. Patients with severe hyperthyroidism and large goiters are most likely to relapse when treatment stops, but outcome is difficult to predict. All patients should be followed closely for relapse during the first year after treatment and at least annually thereafter.

The common side effects of antithyroid drugs are rash, urticaria, fever, and arthralgia (1–5% of patients). These may resolve spontaneously or after substituting an alternative antithyroid drug. Rare but major side effects include hepatitis, an SLE-like syndrome, and, most importantly, agranulocy-tosis (<1%). It is essential that antithyroid drugs are stopped and not restarted if a patient develops major side effects. Written instructions should be provided regarding the symptoms of possible agranulocytosis (e.g., sore throat, fever, mouth ulcers) and the need to stop treatment pending a complete blood count to confirm that agranulocytosis is not present. Management of agranulocytosis is described in Chap. 102. It is not useful to monitor blood counts prospectively, as the onset of agranulocytosis is idiosyncratic and abrupt.

Propranolol (20–40 mg every 6 h) or longer-acting beta blockers such as atenolol, may be helpful to control adrenergic symptoms, especially in the early stages before antithyroid drugs take effect. The need for anticoagulation with coumadin should be considered in all patients with atrial fibrillation. If digoxin is used, increased doses are often needed in the thyrotoxic state.

Radioiodine causes progressive destruction of thyroid cells and can be used as initial treatment or for relapses after a trial of antithyroid drugs. There is a small risk of thyrotoxic crisis (see below) after radioiodine, which can be minimized by pretreatment with antithyroid drugs for at least a month before treatment. Antecedent treatment with antithyroid drugs should be considered for all elderly patients or for those with cardiac problems, to deplete thyroid hormone stores before administration of radioiodine. Carbimazole or methimazole must be stopped at least 3 days before radioiodine administration to achieve optimum iodine uptake. Propylthiouracil has a prolonged radioprotective effect and should be stopped several weeks before radioiodine is given, or a larger dose of radioiodine will be necessary.

Efforts to calculate an optimal dose of radioiodine that achieves euthyroidism without a high incidence of relapse or progression to hypothyroidism have not been successful. Some patients inevitably relapse after a single dose because the biologic effects of radiation vary between individuals, and hypothyroidism cannot be uniformly avoided even using accurate dosimetry. A practical strategy is to give a fixed dose based on clinical features, such as the severity of thyrotoxicosis, the size of the goiter (increases the dose needed), and the level of radioiodine uptake (decreases the dose needed). ^{131}I dosage generally ranges between 185 MBq (5 mCi) to 555 MBq (15 mCi). Incomplete treatment or early relapse is more common in males and in patients <40 years of age. Many authorities favor an approach aimed at thyroid ablation (as opposed to euthyroidism), given that levothyroxine replacement is straightforward and most patients ultimately progress to hypothyroidism over 5–10 years, frequently with some delay in the diagnosis of hypothyroidism.

Certain radiation safety precautions are necessary in the first few days after radioiodine treatment, but the exact guidelines vary depending on local protocols. In general, patients need to avoid close, prolonged contact with children and pregnant women for several days because of possible transmission of residual isotope and excessive exposure to radiation emanating from the gland. Rarely there may be mild pain due to radiation thyroiditis 1–2 weeks after treatment. Hyperthyroidism can persist for 2–3 months before radioiodine takes full effect. For this reason, β-adrenergic blockers or antithyroid drugs can be used to control symptoms during this interval. Persistent hyperthyroidism can be treated with a second dose of radioiodine, usually 6 months after the first dose. The risk of hypothyroidism after radioiodine depends on the dosage but is at least 10–20% in the first year and 5% per year thereafter. Patients should be informed of this possibility before treatment and require close follow-up during the first year and annual thyroid function testing.

Pregnancy and breast feeding are absolute contraindications to radioiodine treatment, but patients can conceive safely 6 months after treatment. The presence of severe ophthalmopathy requires caution, and some authorities advocate the use of prednisone, 40 mg/d, at the time of radioiodine treatment, tapered over 2–3 months to prevent exacerbation of ophthalmopathy. The overall risk of cancer after radioiodine treatment in adults is not increased. Although many physicians avoid radioiodine in children and adolescents because of the theoretical risks of malignancy, emerging evidence suggests that radioiodine can be used safely in older children.

Subtotal or near-total thyroidectomy is an option for patients who relapse after antithyroid drugs and prefer this treatment to radioiodine. Some experts recommend surgery in young individuals, particularly when the goiter is very large. Careful control of thyrotoxicosis with antithyroid drugs, followed by potassium iodide (3 drops SSKI orally tid), is needed prior to surgery to avoid thyrotoxic crisis and to reduce the vascularity of the gland. The major complications of surgery—bleeding, laryngeal edema, hypoparathyroidism, and damage to the recurrent laryngeal nerves—are unusual when the procedure is performed by highly experienced surgeons. Recurrence rates in the best series are <2%, but the rate of hypothyroidism is only slightly less than that following radioiodine treatment.

The titration regimen of antithyroid drugs should be used to manage Graves' disease in *pregnancy*, as blocking doses of these drugs produce fetal hypothyroidism. Propylthiouracil is usually used because of relatively low transplacental transfer and its ability to block $T_4 \rightarrow T_3$ conversion. Also, carbimazole and methimazole have been associated with rare cases of fetal *aplasia cutis* and other defects, such as choanal atresia. The lowest effective dose of propylthiouracil should be given, and it is often possible to stop treatment in the last trimester since TSI tend to decline in pregnancy. Nonetheless, the transplacental transfer of these antibodies rarely causes *fetal* or *neonatal thyrotoxicosis*. Poor intrauterine growth, a fetal heart rate of >160 beats/min, and high levels of maternal TSI in the last trimester may herald this complication. Antithyroid drugs given to the mother can be used to treat the fetus and may be needed for 1–3 months after delivery, until the maternal antibodies disappear from the baby's circulation. The postpartum period is a time of major risk for relapse of Graves' disease. Breast-feeding is safe with low doses of antithyroid drugs. Graves' disease in *children* is usually managed with antithyroid drugs, often given as a prolonged course of the titration regimen. Surgery or radioiodine may be indicated for severe disease.

Thyrotoxic crisis, or *thyroid storm*, is rare and presents as a life-threatening exacerbation of hyperthyroidism, accompanied by fever, delirium, seizures, coma, vomiting, diarrhea, and jaundice. The mortality rate due to cardiac failure, arrhythmia, or hyperthermia is as high as 30%, even with treatment. Thyrotoxic crisis is usually precipitated by acute illness (e.g., stroke, infection, trauma, diabetic ketoacidosis), surgery (especially on the thyroid), or radioiodine treatment of a patient with partially treated or untreated hyperthyroidism. Management requires intensive monitoring and supportive care, identification and treatment of the precipitating cause, and measures that reduce thyroid hormone synthesis. Large doses of propylthiouracil (600 mg loading dose and 200–300 mg every 6 h) should be given orally or by nasogastric tube or per rectum; the drug's inhibitory action on $T_4 \rightarrow T_3$ conversion makes it the antithyroid drug of choice. One hour after the first dose of propylthiouracil, stable iodide is given to block thyroid hormone synthesis via the Wolff-Chaikoff effect (the delay allows the antithyroid drug to prevent the excess iodine from being incorporated into new hormone). A saturated solution of potassium iodide (5 drops SSKI every 6 h), or ipodate or iopanoic acid (0.5 mg every 12 h), may be given orally. (Sodium iodide, 0.25 g intravenously every 6 h is an alternative but is not generally available.) Propranolol should also be given to reduce tachycardia and other adrenergic manifestations (40–60 mg orally every 4 h; or 2 mg intravenously every 4 h). Although other β-adrenergic blockers can be used, high doses of propranolol decrease $T_4 \rightarrow T_3$ conversion, and the doses can be easily adjusted. Caution is needed to avoid acute negative inotropic effects, but controlling the heart rate is important, as some patients develop a form of high-output heart failure. Additional therapeutic measures include glucocorticoids (e.g., dexamethasone, 2 mg every 6 h), antibiotics if infection is present, cooling, oxygen, and intravenous fluids.

Ophthalmopathy requires no active treatment when it is mild or moderate, as there is usually spontaneous improvement. General measures include meticulous control of thyroid hormone levels, cessation of smoking, and an explanation of the natural history of ophthalmopathy. Discomfort can be relieved with artificial tears (e.g., 1% methylcellulose), eye ointment, and the use of dark glasses with side frames. Periorbital edema may respond to a more upright sleeping position or a diuretic. Corneal exposure during sleep can be avoided by using patches or taping the eyelids shut. Minor degrees of diplopia improve with prisms fitted to spectacles. Severe ophthalmopathy, with optic nerve involvement or chemosis resulting in corneal damage, is an emergency requiring joint management with an ophthalmologist. Short-term benefit can be gained in about two-thirds of patients by the use of high-dose glucocorticoids (e.g., prednisone, 40–80 mg daily), sometimes combined with cyclosporine. Glucocorticoid doses are tapered by 5 mg every 2 weeks, but the taper often results in reemergence of congestive symptoms. Pulse therapy with intravenous methylprednisolone (e.g., 1 g of methylprednisolone in 250 mL of saline infused over 2 h daily for 1 week) followed by an oral regimen is also used. When glucocorticoids are ineffective, orbital decompression can be achieved by removing bone from any wall of the orbit, thereby allowing displacement of fat and swollen extraocular muscles. The transantral route is used most often, as it requires no external incision. Proptosis recedes an average of 5 mm, but there may be residual or even worsened diplopia. Once the eye disease has stabilized, surgery may be indicated for relief of diplopia and correction of the appearance. External beam radiotherapy of the orbits has been used for many years, especially for ophthalmopathy of recent onset, but the objective evidence that this therapy is beneficial remains equivocal.

Thyroid dermopathy does not usually require treatment but can cause cosmetic problems or interfere with the fit of shoes. Surgical removal is not indicated. If necessary, treatment consists of topical, high-potency glucocorticoid ointment under an occlusive dressing. Octreotide may be beneficial in some cases.

OTHER CAUSES OF THYROTOXICOSIS

Destructive thyroiditis (subacute or silent thyroiditis) typically presents with a short thyrotoxic phase due to the release of preformed thyroid hormones and catabolism of Tg (see "Subacute Thyroiditis," below). True hyperthyroidism is absent, as demonstrated by a low radionuclide uptake. Circulating Tg levels are usually increased. Other causes of thyrotoxicosis with low or absent thyroid radionuclide uptake include *thyrotoxicosis factitia*; iodine excess and, rarely, ectopic thyroid tissue, particularly teratomas of the ovary (*struma ovarii*); and functional metastatic follicular carcinoma. Whole-body radionuclide studies can demonstrate ectopic thyroid tissue, and thyrotoxicosis factitia can be distinguished from destructive thyroiditis by the clinical features and low levels of Tg. Amiodarone treatment is associated with thyrotoxicosis in up to 10% of patients, particularly in areas of low iodine intake (see below).

TSH-secreting pituitary adenoma is a rare cause of thyrotoxicosis. It can be identified by the presence of an inappropriately normal or increased TSH level in a patient with hyperthyroidism, diffuse goiter, and elevated T_4 and T_3 levels (Chap. 333). Elevated levels of the subunit of TSH, released by the TSH-secreting adenoma, support this diagnosis, which can be confirmed by demonstrating the pituitary tumor on MRI or CT scan. A combination of transsphenoidal surgery, sella irradiation, and octreotide may be required to normalize TSH, as many of these tumors are large and locally invasive at the time of diagnosis. Radioiodine or antithyroid drugs can be used to control thyrotoxicosis.

Thyrotoxicosis caused by *toxic MNG* and *hyperfunctioning solitary nodules* is discussed below.

THYROIDITIS

A clinically useful classification of thyroiditis is based on the onset and duration of disease (Table 335-8).

ACUTE THYROIDITIS

Acute thyroiditis is rare and due to suppurative infection of the thyroid. In children and young adults, the most common cause is the presence of a piriform sinus, a remnant of the fourth branchial pouch that connects the oropharynx with the thyroid. Such sinuses are predominantly left-sided. A long-standing goiter and degeneration in a thyroid malignancy are risk factors in the elderly. The patient presents

TABLE 335-8	**CAUSES OF THYROIDITIS**

Acute
  Bacterial infection: especially *Staphylococcus*, *Streptococcus*, and *Enterobacter*
  Fungal infection: *Aspergillus*, *Candida*, *Coccidioides*, *Histoplasma*, and *Pneumocystis*
  Radiation thyroiditis after ^{131}I treatment
  Amiodarone (may also be subacute or chronic)
Subacute
  Viral (or granulomatous) thyroiditis
  Silent thyroiditis (including postpartum thyroiditis)
  Mycobacterial infection
Chronic
  Autoimmunity: focal thyroiditis, Hashimoto's thyroiditis, atrophic thyroiditis
  Riedel's thyroiditis
  Parasitic thyroiditis: echinococcosis, strongyloidiasis, cysticercosis
  Traumatic: after palpation

with thyroid pain, often referred to the throat or ears, and a small, tender goiter that may be asymmetric. Fever, dysphagia, and erythema over the thyroid are common, as are systemic symptoms of a febrile illness and lymphadenopathy.

The differential diagnosis of *thyroid pain* includes subacute or, rarely, chronic thyroiditis, hemorrhage into a cyst, malignancy including lymphoma, and, rarely, amiodarone-induced thyroiditis or amyloidosis. However, the abrupt presentation and clinical features of acute thyroiditis rarely cause confusion. The erythrocyte sedimentation rate (ESR) and white cell count are usually increased, but thyroid function is normal. FNA biopsy shows infiltration by polymorphonuclear leukocytes; culture of the sample can identify the organism. Caution is needed in immunocompromised patients as fungal, mycobacterial, or *Pneumocystis* thyroiditis can occur in this setting. Antibiotic treatment is guided initially by Gram stain and subsequently by cultures of the FNA biopsy. Surgery may be needed to drain an abscess, which can be localized by CT scan or ultrasound. Tracheal obstruction, septicemia, retropharyngeal abscess, mediastinitis, and jugular venous thrombosis may complicate acute thyroiditis but are uncommon with prompt use of antibiotics.

SUBACUTE THYROIDITIS

This is also termed *de Quervain's thyroiditis, granulomatous thyroiditis,* or *viral thyroiditis.* Many viruses have been implicated, including mumps, coxsackie, influenza, adenoviruses, and echoviruses, but attempts to identify the virus in an individual patient are often unsuccessful and do not influence management. The diagnosis of subacute thyroiditis is often overlooked because the symptoms can mimic pharyngitis. The peak incidence occurs at 30–50 years, and women are affected three times more frequently than men.

Pathophysiology   The thyroid shows a characteristic patchy inflammatory infiltrate with disruption of the thyroid follicles and multinucleated giant cells within some follicles. The follicular changes progress to granulomas accompanied by fibrosis. Finally, the thyroid returns to normal, usually several months after onset. During the initial phase of follicular destruction, there is release of Tg and thyroid hormones, leading to increased circulating T_4 and T_3 and suppression of TSH (Fig. 335-9). During this destructive phase, radioactive iodine uptake is low or undetectable. After several weeks, the thyroid is depleted of stored thyroid hormone and a phase of hypothyroidism typically occurs, with low unbound T_4 (and sometimes T_3) and moderately increased TSH levels. Radioactive iodine uptake returns to normal or is even increased as a result of the rise in TSH. Finally, thyroid hormone and TSH levels return to normal as the disease subsides.

Clinical Manifestations   The patient usually presents with a painful and enlarged thyroid, sometimes accompanied by fever. There may be features of thyrotoxicosis or hypothyroidism, depending on the phase of the illness. Malaise and symptoms of an upper respiratory tract infection may precede the thyroid-related features by several weeks. In other patients, the onset is acute, severe, and without obvious antecedent. The patient typically complains of a sore throat, and examination reveals a small goiter that is exquisitely tender. Pain is often referred to the jaw or ear. Complete resolution is the usual outcome, but permanent hypothyroidism can occur, particularly in those with coincidental thyroid autoimmunity. A prolonged course over many months, with one or more relapses, occurs in a small percentage of patients.

Laboratory Evaluation   As depicted in Fig. 335-9, thyroid function tests characteristically evolve through three distinct phases over about 6 months: (1) thyrotoxic phase, (2) hypothyroid phase, and (3) recovery phase. In the thyrotoxic phase, T_4 and T_3 levels are increased, reflecting their discharge from the damaged thyroid cells, and TSH is suppressed. The T_4/T_3 ratio is greater than in Graves' disease or thyroid autonomy, in which T_3 is often disproportionately increased. The diagnosis is confirmed by a high ESR and low radioiodine uptake. The white blood cell count may be increased, and thyroid antibodies are

FIGURE 335-9 Clinical course of subacute thyroiditis. The release of thyroid hormones is initially associated with a thyrotoxic phase and suppressed thyroid-stimulating hormone (TSH). A hypothyroid phase then ensues, with low T_4 and TSH levels that are initially low but gradually increase. During the recovery phase, increased TSH levels combined with resolution of thyroid follicular injury leads to normalization of thyroid function, often several months after the beginning of the illness. ESR, erythrocyte sedimentation rate; UT$_4$, unbound T$_4$.

negative. If the diagnosis is in doubt, FNA biopsy may be useful, particularly to distinguish unilateral involvement from bleeding into a cyst or neoplasm.

℞ SUBACUTE THYROIDITIS

Relatively large doses of aspirin (e.g., 600 mg every 4–6 h) or NSAIDs are sufficient to control symptoms in many cases. If this treatment is inadequate, or if the patient has marked local or systemic symptoms, glucocorticoids should be given. The usual starting dose is 40–60 mg prednisone, depending on severity. The dose is gradually tapered over 6–8 weeks, in response to improvement in symptoms and the ESR. If a relapse occurs during glucocorticoid withdrawal, treatment should be started again and withdrawn more gradually. In these patients, it is useful to wait until the radioactive iodine uptake normalizes before stopping treatment. Thyroid function should be monitored every 2–4 weeks using TSH and unbound T$_4$ levels. Symptoms of thyrotoxicosis improve spontaneously but may be ameliorated by β-adrenergic blockers; antithyroid drugs play no role in treatment of the thyrotoxic phase. Levothyroxine replacement may be needed if the hypothyroid phase is prolonged, but doses should be low enough (50 to 100 μg daily) to allow TSH-mediated recovery.

SILENT THYROIDITIS

Painless thyroiditis, or *"silent" thyroiditis,* occurs in patients with underlying autoimmune thyroid disease. It has a clinical course similar to that of subacute thyroiditis, except that there is little or no thyroid tenderness. The condition occurs in up to 5% of women 3–6 months after pregnancy and is then termed *postpartum thyroiditis.* Typically, patients have a brief phase of thyrotoxicosis lasting 2–4 weeks, followed by hypothyroidism for 4–12 weeks, and then resolution; often, however, only one phase is apparent. The condition is associated with the presence of TPO antibodies antepartum, and it is three times more common in women with type 1 diabetes mellitus. As in subacute thyroiditis, the radioactive iodine uptake is initially suppressed. In addition to the painless goiter, silent thyroiditis can be distinguished from subacute thyroiditis by a normal ESR and the presence of TPO antibodies. Glucocorticoid treatment is not indicated for silent thyroiditis. Severe thyrotoxic symptoms can be managed with a brief course of propranolol, 20–40 mg three or four times daily. Thyroxine replacement may be needed for the hypothyroid phase but should be withdrawn after 6–9 months, as recovery is the rule. Annual follow-up thereafter is recommended, as a proportion of these individuals develop permanent hypothyroidism.

DRUG-INDUCED THYROIDITIS

Patients receiving cytokines such as IFN-α or IL-2 may develop painless thyroiditis. IFN-α, which is used to treat chronic hepatitis B or C and hematological and skin malignancies, causes thyroid dysfunction in up to 5% of treated patients. It has been associated with painless thyroiditis, hypothyroidism, and Graves' disease, and is most common in women with TPO antibodies prior to treatment. For discussion of amiodarone, see "Amiodarone Effects on Thyroid Function," below.

CHRONIC THYROIDITIS

Focal thyroiditis is present in 20–40% of euthyroid autopsy cases and is associated with serologic evidence of autoimmunity, particularly the presence of TPO antibodies. These antibodies are 4–10 times more common in otherwise healthy women than men. The most common clinically apparent cause of chronic thyroiditis is *Hashimoto's thyroiditis*, an autoimmune disorder that often presents as a firm or hard goiter of variable size (see above). *Riedel's thyroiditis* is a rare disorder that typically occurs in middle-aged women. It presents with an insidious, painless goiter with local symptoms due to compression of the esophagus, trachea, neck veins, or recurrent laryngeal nerves. Dense fibrosis disrupts normal gland architecture and can extend outside the thyroid capsule. Despite these extensive histologic changes, thyroid dysfunction is uncommon. The goiter is hard, nontender, often asymmetric, and fixed, leading to suspicion of a malignancy. Diagnosis requires open biopsy as FNA biopsy is usually inadequate. Treatment is directed to surgical relief of compressive symptoms. Tamoxifen may also be beneficial. There is an association between Riedel's thyroiditis and idiopathic fibrosis at other sites (retroperitoneum, mediastinum, biliary tree, lung, and orbit).

SICK EUTHYROID SYNDROME

Any acute, severe illness can cause abnormalities of circulating TSH or thyroid hormone levels in the absence of underlying thyroid disease, making these measurements potentially misleading. The major cause of these hormonal changes is the release of cytokines such as IL-6. Unless a thyroid disorder is strongly suspected, the routine testing of thyroid function should be avoided in acutely ill patients.

The most common hormone pattern in sick euthyroid syndrome (SES) is a decrease in total and unbound T_3 levels (low T_3 syndrome) with normal levels of T_4 and TSH. The magnitude of the fall in T_3 correlates with the severity of the illness. T_4 conversion to T_3 via peripheral deiodination is impaired, leading to increased reverse T_3 (rT_3). Despite this effect, decreased clearance rather than increased production is the major basis for increased rT_3. Also, T_4 is alternately metabolized to the hormonally inactive T_3 sulfate. It is generally assumed that this low T_3 state is adaptive, as it can be induced in normal individuals by fasting. Teleologically, the fall in T_3 may limit catabolism in starved or ill patients.

Very sick patients may exhibit a dramatic fall in total T_4 and T_3 levels (low T_4 syndrome). This state has a poor prognosis. A key factor in the fall in T_4 levels is altered binding to TBG. T_4 assays usually demonstrate a normal unbound T_4 level in such patients, depending on the assay method used. Fluctuation in TSH levels also creates challenges in the interpretation of thyroid function in sick patients. TSH levels may range from <0.1 to >20 mU/L; these alterations reverse after recovery, confirming the absence of underlying thyroid disease. A rise in cortisol or administration of glucocorticoids may provide a partial explanation for decreased TSH levels. The exact mechanisms underlying the subnormal TSH seen in 10% of sick patients and the increased TSH seen in 5% remain unclear but may be mediated by cytokines including IL-12 and IL-18.

Any severe illness can induce changes in thyroid hormone levels, but certain disorders exhibit a distinctive pattern of abnormalities. Acute liver disease is associated with an initial rise in total (but not unbound) T_3 and T_4 levels, due to TBG release; these levels become subnormal with progression to liver failure. A transient increase in total and unbound T_4 levels, usually with a normal T_3 level, is seen in 5–30% of acutely ill psychiatric patients. TSH values may be transiently low, normal, or high in these patients. In the early stage of HIV infection, T_3 and T_4 levels rise, even if there is weight loss. T_3 levels fall with progression to AIDS, but TSH usually remains normal. Renal disease is often accompanied by low T_3 concentrations, but with normal rather than increased rT_3 levels, due to an unknown factor that increases uptake of rT_3 into the liver.

The diagnosis of SES is challenging. Historic information may be limited, and patients often have multiple metabolic derangements. Useful features to consider include previous history of thyroid disease and thyroid function tests, evaluation of the severity and time course of the patient's acute illness, documentation of medications that may affect thyroid function or thyroid hormone levels, and measurements of rT_3 together with unbound thyroid hormones and TSH. The diagnosis of SES is frequently presumptive, given the clinical context and pattern of laboratory values; only resolution of the test results with clinical recovery can clearly establish this disorder. Treatment of SES with thyroid hormone (T_4 and/or T_3) is controversial, but most authorities recommend monitoring the patient's thyroid function tests during recovery, without administering thyroid hormone, unless there is historic or clinical evidence suggestive of hypothyroidism. Sufficiently large randomized controlled trials using thyroid hormone are unlikely to resolve this therapeutic controversy in the near future, because clinical presentations and outcomes are highly variable.

AMIODARONE EFFECTS ON THYROID FUNCTION

Amiodarone is a commonly used type III antiarrhythmic agent (Chap. 226). It is structurally related to thyroid hormone and contains 39% iodine by weight. Thus, typical doses of amiodarone (200 mg/d) are associated with very high iodine intake, leading to >fortyfold increases in plasma and urinary iodine levels. Moreover, because amiodarone is stored in adipose tissue, high iodine levels persist for >6 months after discontinuation of the drug. Amiodarone inhibits deiodinase activity, and its metabolites function as weak antagonists of thyroid hormone action. Amiodarone has the following effects on thyroid function: (1) acute, transient suppression of thyroid function; (2) hypothyroidism in patients susceptible to the inhibitory effects of a high iodine load; and (3) thyrotoxicosis that may be caused by a Jod-Basedow effect from the iodine load in the setting of MNG, a thyroiditis-like condition, or possibly induction of autoimmune Graves' disease.

The initiation of amiodarone treatment is associated with a transient decrease of T_4 levels, reflecting the inhibitory effect of iodine on T_4 release. Soon thereafter, most individuals escape from iodide-dependent suppression of the thyroid (Wolff-Chaikoff effect), and the inhibitory effects on deiodinase activity and thyroid hormone receptor action become predominant. These events lead to the following pattern of thyroid function tests: increased T_4, decreased T_3, increased rT_3, and a transient increase of TSH (up to 20 mU/L). TSH levels normalize or are slightly suppressed by 1–3 months.

The incidence of hypothyroidism from amiodarone varies geographically, apparently correlating with iodine intake. Hypothyroidism occurs in up to 13% of amiodarone-treated patients in iodine-replete countries, such as the United States, but is less common (<6% incidence) in areas of lower iodine intake, such as Italy or Spain. The pathogenesis appears to involve an inability of the thyroid gland to escape from the Wolff-Chaikoff effect in autoimmune thyroiditis. Consequently, amiodarone-associated hypothyroidism is more common in women and individuals with positive TPO antibodies. It is usually unnecessary to discontinue amiodarone for this side effect, as levothyroxine can be used to normalize thyroid function. TSH levels should be monitored, because T_4 levels are often increased for the reasons described above.

The management of amiodarone-induced thyrotoxicosis (AIT) is complicated by the fact that there are several causes of thyrotoxicosis and because the increased thyroid hormone levels exacerbate underlying arrhythmias and coronary artery disease. Amiodarone treatment causes thyrotoxicosis in 10% of patients living in areas of low iodine intake and in 2% of patients in regions of high iodine intake. There are two major forms of AIT, although some patients have features of both. Type 1 AIT is associated with an underlying thyroid abnormality (preclinical Graves' disease or nodular goiter). Thyroid hormone synthesis becomes excessive as a result of increased iodine exposure (Jod-Basedow phenomenon). Type 2 AIT occurs in individuals with no intrinsic thyroid abnormalities and is the result of drug-induced lysosomal activation leading to destructive thyroiditis with histiocyte accumulation in the thyroid. Mild forms of type 2 AIT can resolve spontaneously or can occasionally lead to hypothyroidism. Color-flow doppler thyroid scanning shows increased vascularity in type 1 AIT but decreased vascularity in type 2 AIT. Thyroid scintiscans are difficult to interpret in this setting, because the high endogenous iodine levels diminish tracer uptake. However, the presence of normal or increased uptake favors type 1 AIT.

In AIT the drug should be stopped, if possible, although this is often impractical because of the underlying cardiac disorder. Discontinuation of amiodarone will not have an acute effect because of its storage and prolonged half-life. High doses of antithyroid drugs can be used in type 1 AIT but are often ineffective. In type 2 AIT, oral contrast agents, such as sodium ipodate (500 mg/d) or sodium tyropanoate (500 mg, 1–2 doses/d), rapidly reduce T_4 and T_3 levels, decrease $T_4 \rightarrow T_3$ conversion, and may block tissue uptake of thyroid hormones. Potassium perchlorate, 200 mg every 6 h, has been used to reduce thyroidal iodide content. Perchlorate treatment has been associated with agranulocytosis, though the risk appears relatively low with short-term use. Glucocorticoids, administered as for subacute thyroiditis, are of variable benefit in type 2 AIT. Lithium blocks thyroid hormone release and can provide modest benefit. Near-total thyroidectomy rapidly decreases thyroid hormone levels and may be the most effective long-term solution, if the patient can undergo the procedure safely.

THYROID FUNCTION IN PREGNANCY

Five factors alter thyroid function in pregnancy: (1) the transient increase in hCG during the first trimester, which stimulates the TSH-R; (2) the estrogen-induced rise in TBG during the first trimester, which is sustained during pregnancy; (3) alterations in the immune system, leading to the onset, exacerbation, or amelioration of an underlying autoimmune thyroid disease (see above); (4) increased thyroid hormone metabolism by the placenta; and (5) increased urinary iodide excretion, which can cause impaired thyroid hormone production in areas of marginal iodine sufficiency. Women with a precarious iodine intake (<50 μg/d) are most at risk of developing a goiter during pregnancy, and iodine supplementation should be considered to prevent maternal and fetal hypothyroidism and the development of neonatal goiter.

The rise in circulating hCG levels during the first trimester is accompanied by a reciprocal fall in TSH that persists into the middle of pregnancy. This appears to reflect weak binding of hCG, which is present at very high levels, to the TSH-R. Rare individuals have been described with variant TSH-R sequences that enhance hCG binding and TSH-R activation. hCG-induced changes in thyroid function can result in transient gestational hyperthyroidism and/or *hyperemesis gravidarum*, a condition characterized by severe nausea and vomiting and risk of volume depletion. Antithyroid drugs are rarely needed, and parenteral fluid replacement usually suffices until the condition resolves.

Maternal hypothyroidism occurs in 2–3% of women of child-bearing age and is associated with increased risk of developmental delay in the offspring. Consequently, TSH screening for hypothyroidism is indicated in early pregnancy and should be considered in women who are planning pregnancy, particularly if they have a goiter or strong family history of autoimmune thyroid disease. Thyroid hormone requirements are increased by 25–50 μg/d during pregnancy.

GOITER AND NODULAR THYROID DISEASE

Goiter refers to an enlarged thyroid gland. Biosynthetic defects, iodine deficiency, autoimmune disease, and nodular diseases can each lead to goiter, though by different mechanisms. Biosynthetic defects and io-

dine deficiency are associated with reduced efficiency of thyroid hormone synthesis, leading to increased TSH, which stimulates thyroid growth as a compensatory mechanism to overcome the block in hormone synthesis. Graves' disease and Hashimoto's thyroiditis are also associated with goiter. In Graves' disease, the goiter results mainly from the TSH-R–mediated effects of TSI. The goitrous form of Hashimoto's thyroiditis occurs because of acquired defects in hormone synthesis, leading to elevated levels of TSH and its consequent growth effects. Lymphocytic infiltration and immune system–induced growth factors also contribute to thyroid enlargement in Hashimoto's thyroiditis. Nodular disease is characterized by the disordered growth of thyroid cells, often combined with the gradual development of fibrosis. Because the management of goiter depends on the etiology, the detection of thyroid enlargement on physical examination should prompt further evaluation to identify its cause.

Nodular thyroid disease is common, occurring in about 3–7% of adults when assessed by physical examination. Using more sensitive techniques, such as ultrasound, it is present in >25% of adults. Thyroid nodules may be solitary or multiple, and they may be functional or nonfunctional.

DIFFUSE NONTOXIC (SIMPLE) GOITER

Etiology and Pathogenesis When diffuse enlargement of the thyroid occurs in the absence of nodules and hyperthyroidism, it is referred to as a *diffuse nontoxic goiter*. This is sometimes called *simple goiter*, because of the absence of nodules, or *colloid goiter*, because of the presence of uniform follicles that are filled with colloid. Worldwide, diffuse goiter is most commonly caused by iodine deficiency and is termed *endemic goiter* when it affects >5% of the population. In nonendemic regions, *sporadic goiter* occurs, and the cause is usually unknown. Thyroid enlargement in teenagers is sometimes referred to as *juvenile goiter*. In general, goiter is more common in women than men, probably because of the greater prevalence of underlying autoimmune disease and the increased iodine demands associated with pregnancy.

In *iodine-deficient areas*, thyroid enlargement reflects a compensatory effort to trap iodide and produce sufficient hormone under conditions in which hormone synthesis is relatively inefficient. Somewhat surprisingly, TSH levels are usually normal or only slightly increased, suggesting increased sensitivity to TSH or activation of other pathways that lead to thyroid growth. Iodide appears to have direct actions on thyroid vasculature and may indirectly affect growth through vasoactive substances such as endothelins and nitric oxide. Endemic goiter is also caused by exposure to environmental *goitrogens* such as cassava root, which contains a thiocyanate; vegetables of the Cruciferae family (e.g., brussels sprouts, cabbage, and cauliflower); and milk from regions where goitrogens are present in grass. Though relatively rare, inherited defects in thyroid hormone synthesis lead to a diffuse nontoxic goiter. Abnormalities at each step in hormone synthesis, including iodide transport (NIS), Tg synthesis, organification and coupling (TPO), and the regeneration of iodide (dehalogenase), have been described.

CLINICAL MANIFESTATIONS AND DIAGNOSIS

If thyroid function is preserved, most goiters are asymptomatic. Spontaneous hemorrhage into a cyst or nodule may cause the sudden onset of localized pain and swelling. Examination of a diffuse goiter reveals a symmetrically enlarged, nontender, generally soft gland without palpable nodules. Goiter is defined, somewhat arbitrarily, as a lateral lobe with a volume greater than the thumb of the individual being examined. If the thyroid is markedly enlarged, it can cause tracheal or esophageal compression. These features are unusual, however, in the absence of nodular disease and fibrosis. *Substernal goiter* may obstruct the thoracic inlet. *Pemberton's sign* refers to symptoms of faintness with evidence of facial congestion and external jugular venous obstruction when the arms are raised above the head, a maneuver that draws the thyroid into the thoracic inlet. Respiratory flow measurements and CT or MRI should be used to evaluate substernal goiter in patients with obstructive signs or symptoms.

Thyroid function tests should be performed in all patients with goiter to exclude thyrotoxicosis or hypothyroidism. It is not unusual, particularly in iodine deficiency, to find a low total T_4, with normal T_3 and TSH, reflecting enhanced $T_4 \rightarrow T_3$ conversion. A low TSH, particularly in older patients, suggests the possibility of thyroid autonomy or undiagnosed Graves' disease, causing subclinical thyrotoxicosis. TPO antibodies may be useful to identify patients at increased risk of autoimmune thyroid disease. Low urinary iodine levels (<10 μg/dL) support a diagnosis of iodine deficiency. Thyroid scanning is not generally necessary but will reveal increased uptake in iodine deficiency and most cases of dyshormonogenesis. Ultrasound is not generally indicated in the evaluation of diffuse goiter unless a nodule is palpable on physical examination.

℞ DIFFUSE NONTOXIC (SIMPLE) GOITER

Iodine or thyroid hormone replacement induces variable regression of goiter in iodine deficiency, depending on how long it has been present and the degree of fibrosis that has developed. Because of the possibility of underlying thyroid autonomy, caution should be exercised when instituting suppressive thyroxine therapy in patients with goiter, particularly if the baseline TSH is in the low–normal range. In younger patients, the dose of levothyroxine can be started at 100 μg/d and adjusted to suppress the TSH into the low–normal but detectable range. Treatment of elderly patients should be initiated at 50 μg/d. The efficacy of suppressive treatment is greater in younger patients and for those with soft goiters. Significant regression is usually seen within 3–6 months of treatment; after this time it is unlikely to occur. In older patients, and in those with some degree of nodular disease or fibrosis, fewer than one-third demonstrate significant shrinkage of the goiter. Surgery is rarely indicated for diffuse goiter. Exceptions include documented evidence of tracheal compression or obstruction of the thoracic inlet, which are more likely to be associated with substernal multinodular goiters (see below). Subtotal or near-total thyroidectomy for these or cosmetic reasons should be performed by an experienced surgeon to minimize complication rates, which occur in up to 10% of cases. Surgery should be followed by mild suppressive treatment with levothyroxine to prevent regrowth of the goiter. Radioiodine reduces goiter size by about 50% in the majority of patients. It is rarely associated with transient acute swelling of the thyroid, which is usually inconsequential unless there is severe tracheal narrowing. If not treated with levothyroxine, patients should be followed after radioiodine treatment for the possible development of hypothyroidism.

NONTOXIC MULTINODULAR GOITER

Etiology and Pathogenesis Depending on the population studied, MNG occurs in up to 12% of adults. MNG is more common in women than men and increases in prevalence with age. It is more common in iodine-deficient regions but also occurs in regions of iodine sufficiency, reflecting multiple genetic, autoimmune, and environmental influences on the pathogenesis.

There is typically wide variation in nodule size. Histology reveals a spectrum of morphologies ranging from hypercellular regions to cystic areas filled with colloid. Fibrosis is often extensive, and areas of hemorrhage or lymphocytic infiltration may be seen. Using molecular techniques, most nodules within a MNG are polyclonal in origin, suggesting a hyperplastic response to locally produced growth factors and cytokines. TSH, which is usually not elevated, may play a permissive or contributory role. Monoclonal lesions also occur within a MNG, reflecting mutations in genes that confer a selective growth advantage to the progenitor cell.

Clinical Manifestations Most patients with nontoxic MNG are asymptomic and, by definition, euthyroid. MNG typically develops over many years and is detected on routine physical examination or when an individual notices an enlargement in the neck. If the goiter is large enough, it can ultimately lead to compressive symptoms including difficulty swallowing, respiratory distress (tracheal compression), or plethora (venous congestion), but these symptoms are uncommon. Symptomatic MNGs are usually extraordinarily large and/or develop

fibrotic areas that cause compression. Sudden pain in a MNG is usually caused by hemorrhage into a nodule but should raise the possibility of invasive malignancy. Hoarseness, reflecting laryngeal nerve involvement, also suggests malignancy.

Diagnosis On examination, thyroid architecture is distorted, and multiple nodules of varying size can be appreciated. Because many nodules are deeply embedded in thyroid tissue or reside in posterior or substernal locations, it is not possible to palpate all nodules. A TSH level should be measured to exclude subclinical hyper- or hypothyroidism, but thyroid function is usually normal. Tracheal deviation is common, but compression must usually exceed 70% of the tracheal diameter before there is significant airway compromise. Pulmonary function testing can be used to assess the functional effects of compression and to detect tracheomalacia, which characteristically causes inspiratory stridor. CT or MRI can be used to evaluate the anatomy of the goiter and the extent of substernal extension, which is often much greater than is apparent on physical examination. A barium swallow may reveal the extent of esophageal compression. The risk of malignancy in MNG is similar to that in solitary nodules. Ultrasonography can be used to identify which nodules should be biopsied, including large, dominant nodules or those with sonographic characteristics suggestive of malignancy (e.g., microcalcifications, hypoechogenicity, increased vascularity).

℞ NONTOXIC MULTINODULAR GOITER

Most nontoxic MNGs can be managed conservatively. T_4 suppression is rarely effective for reducing goiter size and introduces the risk of thyrotoxicosis, particularly if there is underlying autonomy or if it develops during treatment. If levothyroxine is used, it should be started at low doses (50 μg) and advanced gradually while monitoring the TSH level to avoid excessive suppression. Contrast agents and other iodine-containing substances should be avoided because of the risk of inducing the *Jod-Basedow effect*, characterized by enhanced thyroid hormone production by autonomous nodules. Radioiodine is being used with increasing frequency because it often decreases goiter size and may selectively ablate regions of autonomy. Dosage of ^{131}I depends on the size of the goiter and radioiodine uptake but is usually about 3.7 MBq (0.1 mCi) per gram of tissue, corrected for uptake [typical dose 370–1070 Mbq (10 to 29 mCi)]. Repeat treatment may be needed. It is possible to achieve a 40–50% reduction in goiter size in most patients. Earlier concerns about radiation-induced thyroid swelling and tracheal compression have diminished as recent studies have shown this complication to be rare. When acute compression occurs, glucocorticoid treatment or surgery may be needed. Radiation-induced hypothyroidism is less common than after treatment for Graves' disease. However, posttreatment autoimmune thyrotoxicosis may occur in up to 5% of patients treated for nontoxic MNG. Surgery remains highly effective but is not without risk, particularly in older patients with underlying cardiopulmonary disease.

TOXIC MULTINODULAR GOITER

The pathogenesis of toxic MNG appears to be similar to that of nontoxic MNG; the major difference is the presence of functional autonomy in toxic MNG. The molecular basis for autonomy in toxic MNG remains unknown. As in nontoxic goiters, many nodules are polyclonal, while others are monoclonal and vary in their clonal origins. Genetic abnormalities known to confer functional autonomy, such as activating TSH-R or $G_{s\alpha}$ mutations (see below), are not usually found in the autonomous regions of toxic MNG goiter.

In addition to features of goiter, the clinical presentation of toxic MNG includes subclinical hyperthyroidism or mild thyrotoxicosis. The patient is usually elderly and may present with atrial fibrillation or palpitations, tachycardia, nervousness, tremor, or weight loss. Recent exposure to iodine, from contrast dyes or other sources, may precipitate or exacerbate thyrotoxicosis. The TSH level is low. The T_4 level may be normal or minimally increased; T_3 is often elevated to a greater degree than T_4. Thyroid scan shows heterogeneous uptake with multiple regions of increased and decreased uptake; 24-h uptake of radioiodine may not be increased.

Rx TOXIC MULTINODULAR GOITER

The management of toxic MNG is challenging. Antithyroid drugs, often in combination with beta blockers, can normalize thyroid function and address clinical features of thyrotoxicosis. This treatment, however, often stimulates the growth of the goiter, and in contrast to Graves' disease, spontaneous remission does not occur. Radioiodine can be used to treat areas of autonomy as well as to decrease the mass of the goiter. Usually, however, some degree of autonomy remains, presumably because multiple autonomous regions emerge as soon as others are treated. Nonetheless, a trial of radioiodine should be considered before subjecting patients, many of whom are elderly, to surgery. Surgery provides definitive treatment of underlying thyrotoxicosis as well as goiter. Patients should be rendered euthyroid using antithyroid drugs before operation.

HYPERFUNCTIONING SOLITARY NODULE

A solitary, autonomously functioning thyroid nodule is referred to as *toxic adenoma*. The pathogenesis of this disorder has been unraveled by demonstrating the functional effects of mutations that stimulate the TSH-R signaling pathway. Most patients with solitary hyperfunctioning nodules have acquired somatic, activating mutations in the TSH-R (**Fig. 335-10**). These mutations, located primarily in the receptor transmembrane domain, induce constitutive receptor coupling to $G_{s\alpha}$, increasing cyclic AMP levels and leading to enhanced thyroid follicular cell proliferation and function. Less commonly, somatic mutations are identified in $G_{s\alpha}$. These mutations, which are similar to those seen in McCune-Albright syndrome (Chap. 341) or in a subset of somatotrope adenomas (Chap. 333), impair GTP hydrolysis, also causing constitutive activation of the cyclic AMP signaling pathway. In most series, activating mutations in either the TSH-R or the $G_{s\alpha}$ subunit genes are identified in >90% of patients with solitary hyperfunctioning nodules.

FIGURE 335-10 Activating mutations of the TSH-R. Mutations (*) that activate the thyroid-stimulating hormone receptor (TSH-R) reside mainly in transmembrane 5 and intracellular loop 3, though mutations have occurred in a variety of different locations. The effect of these mutations is to induce conformational changes that mimic TSH binding, thereby leading to coupling to stimulatory G protein ($G_{s\alpha}$) and activation of adenylate cyclase (AC), an enzyme that generates cyclic AMP.

Thyrotoxicosis is usually mild. The disorder is suggested by the presence of the thyroid nodule, which is generally large enough to be palpable, and by the absence of clinical features suggestive of Graves' disease or other causes of thyrotoxicosis. A thyroid scan provides a definitive diagnostic test, demonstrating focal uptake in the hyperfunctioning nodule and diminished uptake in the remainder of the gland, as activity of the normal thyroid is suppressed.

Rx HYPERFUNCTIONING SOLITARY NODULE

Radioiodine ablation is usually the treatment of choice. Because normal thyroid function is suppressed, ^{131}I is concentrated in the hyperfunctioning nodule with minimal uptake and damage to normal thyroid tissue. Relatively large radioiodine doses [e.g., 370–1110 MBq (10–29.9 mCi) ^{131}I] have been shown to correct thyrotoxicosis in about 75% of patients within 3 months. Hypothyroidism occurs in <10% of patients over the next 5 years. Surgical resection is also effective and is usually limited to enucleation of the adenoma or lobectomy, thereby preserving thyroid function and minimizing risk of hypoparathyroidism or damage to the recurrent laryngeal nerves. Medical therapy using antithyroid drugs and beta blockers can normalize thyroid function but is not an optimal long-term treatment. Ethanol injection under ultrasound guidance has been used successfully in some centers to ablate hyperfunctioning nodules. Repeated injections (often more than 5 sessions) are required to reduce nodule size. Normal thyroid function can be achieved in most patients using this technique.

BENIGN NEOPLASMS

The various types of benign thyroid nodules are listed in **Table 335-9**. These lesions are common (5–10% adults), particularly when assessed by sensitive techniques such as ultrasound. The risk of malignancy is very low for *macrofollicular adenomas* and *normofollicular adenomas*. *Microfollicular, trabecular, and Hürthle cell variants* raise greater concern, and the histology is more difficult to interpret. About one-third of palpable nodules are *thyroid cysts*. These may be recognized by their

TABLE 335-9 CLASSIFICATION OF THYROID NEOPLASMS

	Approximate Prevalence, %
Benign	
Follicular epithelial cell adenomas	
Macrofollicular (colloid)	
Normofollicular (simple)	
Microfollicular (fetal)	
Trabecular (embryonal)	
Hürtle cell variant (oncocytic)	
Malignant	
Follicular epithelial cell	
Well-differentiated carcinomas	
Papillary carcinomas	80–90
Pure papillary	
Follicular variant	
Diffuse sclerosing variant	
Tall cell, columnar cell variants	
Follicular carcinomas	5–10
Minimally invasive	
Widely invasive	
Hürthle cell carcinoma (oncocytic)	
Insular carcinoma	
Undifferentiated (anaplastic) carcinomas	
C cell (calcitonin-producing)	
Medullary thyroid cancer	10
Sporadic	
Familial	
MEN 2	
Other malignancies	
Lymphomas	1–2
Sarcomas	
Metastases	
Others	

Note: MEN, multiple endocrine neoplasia.

ultrasound appearance or based on aspiration of large amounts of pink or straw-colored fluid (colloid). Many are mixed cystic/solid lesions, in which case it is desirable to aspirate cellular components under ultrasound or harvest cells after cytospin of cyst fluid. Cysts frequently recur, even after repeated aspiration, and may require surgical excision if they are large or if the cytology is suspicious. Sclerosis has been used with variable success but is often painful and may be complicated by infiltration of the sclerosing agent.

The treatment approach for benign nodules is similar to that for MNG. TSH suppression with levothyroxine decreases the size of about 30% of nodules and may prevent further growth. The TSH level should be suppressed into the low–normal range, assuming there are no contraindications; alternatively, nodule size can be monitored without suppression. If a nodule has not decreased in size after 6–12 months of suppressive therapy, treatment should be discontinued since little benefit is likely to accrue from long-term treatment.

THYROID CANCER

Thyroid carcinoma is the most common malignancy of the endocrine system. Malignant tumors derived from the follicular epithelium are classified according to histologic features. Differentiated tumors, such as papillary thyroid cancer (PTC) or follicular thyroid cancer (FTC), are often curable, and the prognosis is good for patients identified with early-stage disease. In contrast, anaplastic thyroid cancer (ATC) is aggressive, responds poorly to treatment, and is associated with a bleak prognosis.

The incidence of thyroid cancer (~9/100,000 per year) increases with age, plateauing after about age 50 (Fig. 335-11). Age is also an important prognostic factor—thyroid cancer at a young age (<20) or in older persons (>45) is associated with a worse prognosis. Thyroid cancer is twice as common in women as men, but male sex is associated with a worse prognosis. Additional important risk factors include a history of childhood head or neck irradiation, large nodule size (≥4 cm), evidence for local tumor fixation or invasion into lymph nodes, and the presence of metastases (Table 335-10).

Several unique features of thyroid cancer facilitate its management: (1) thyroid nodules are readily palpable, allowing early detection and biopsy by FNA; (2) iodine radioisotopes can be used to diagnose (^{123}I) and treat (^{131}I) differentiated thyroid cancer, reflecting the unique uptake of this anion by the thyroid gland; and (3) serum markers allow the detection of residual or recurrent disease, including the use of Tg levels for PTC and FTC and calcitonin for medullary thyroid cancer (MTC).

CLASSIFICATION

Thyroid neoplasms can arise in each of the cell types that populate the gland, including thyroid follicular cells, calcitonin-producing C cells,

FIGURE 335-11 Age-associated incidence (——◆——) and mortality (——●——) rates for invasive thyroid cancer. [*Adapted from LAG Ries et al (eds): SEER Cancer Statistics Review, 1973–1996, Bethesda, National Cancer Institute, 1999.*]

TABLE 335-10 RISK FACTORS FOR THYROID CARCINOMA IN PATIENTS WITH THYROID NODULE

History of head and neck irradiation	Family history of thyroid cancer or MEN 2
Age <20 or >45 years	Vocal cord paralysis, hoarse voice
Bilateral disease	Nodule fixed to adjacent structures
Increased nodule size (>4 cm)	Extrathyroidal extension
New or enlarging neck mass	Suspected lymph node involvement
Male sex	Iodine deficiency (follicular cancer)

Note: MEN, multiple endocrine neoplasia.

lymphocytes, and stromal and vascular elements, as well as metastases from other sites (Table 335-9). The American Joint Committee on Cancer (AJCC) has designated a staging system using the TNM classification (Table 335-11). Several other classification and staging systems are also widely used, some of which place greater emphasis on histologic features or risk factors such as age or gender.

PATHOGENESIS AND GENETIC BASIS

Radiation Early studies of the pathogenesis of thyroid cancer focused on the role of external radiation, which predisposes to chromosomal breaks, presumably leading to genetic rearrangements and loss of tumor-suppressor genes. External radiation of the mediastinum, face, head, and neck region was administered in the past to treat an array of conditions, including acne and enlargement of the thymus, tonsils, and adenoids. Radiation exposure increases the risk of benign and malignant thyroid nodules, is associated with multicentric cancers, and shifts the incidence of thyroid cancer to an earlier age group. Radiation from nuclear fallout also increases the risk of thyroid cancer. Children seem more predisposed to the effects of radiation than adults. Of note, radiation derived from ^{131}I therapy appears to contribute minimal increased risk of thyroid cancer.

TSH and Growth Factors Many differentiated thyroid cancers express TSH receptors and, therefore, remain responsive to TSH. This observation provides the rationale for T_4 suppression of TSH in patients with thyroid cancer. Residual expression of TSH receptors also allows TSH-stimulated uptake of ^{131}I therapy (see below).

Oncogenes and Tumor-Suppressor Genes Thyroid cancers are monoclonal in origin, consistent with the idea that they originate as a consequence of mutations that confer a growth advantage to a single cell. In addition to increased rates of proliferation, some thyroid cancers exhibit impaired apoptosis and features that enhance invasion, angiogenesis, and metastasis. By analogy with the model of multi-step carcinogenesis proposed for colon cancer (Chap. 79), thyroid neoplasms have been analyzed for a variety of genetic alterations, but

TABLE 335-11 THYROID CANCER CLASSIFICATION^a

Papillary or follicular thyroid cancers		
	<45 years	**>45 years**
Stage I	Any T, any N, M0	T1, N0, M0
Stage II	Any T, any N, M1	T2 or T3, N0, M0
Stage III	—	T4, N0, M0
		Any T, N1, M0
Stage IV	—	Any T, any N, M1
Anaplastic thyroid cancer		
Stage IV	All cases are stage IV	
Medullary thyroid cancer		
Stage I	T1, N0, M0	
Stage II	T2–T4, N0, M0	
Stage III	Any T, N1, M0	
Stage IV	Any T, any N, M1	

^{a}Criteria include: T, the size and extent of the primary tumor (T1 ≤ 1 cm; 1 cm < T2 ≤ 4 cm; T3 > 4 cm; T4 direct invasion through the thyroid capsule); N, the absence (N0) or presence (N1) of regional node involvement; M, the absence (M0) or presence (M1) of metastases.

Source: American Joint Committee on Cancer staging system for thyroid cancers using the TNM classification.

TABLE 335-12 GENETIC ALTERATIONS IN THYROID NEOPLASIA

Gene/Protein	Type of Gene	Chromosomal Location	Genetic Abnormality	Tumor
TSH receptor	GPCR receptor	14q31	Point mutations	Toxic adenoma, differentiated carcinomas
$G_{s\alpha}$	G protein	20q13.2	Point mutations	Toxic adenoma, differentiated carcinomas
RET/PTC	Receptor tyrosine kinase	10q11.2	Rearrangements PTC1: (inv(10)q11.2q21) PTC2: (t(10;17)(q11.2;q23)) PTC3: ELE1/TK	PTC
RET	Receptor tyrosine kinase	10q11.2	Point mutations	MEN 2, medullary thyroid cancer
BRAF	MEK kinase	7q24	Point mutations, rearrangements	PTC
TRK	Receptor tyrosine kinase	1q23-24	Rearrangements	Multinodular goiter, papillary thyroid cancer
RAS	Signal transducing p21	Hras 11p15.5 Kras 12p12.1; Nras 1p13.2	Point mutations	Differentiated thyroid carcinoma, adenomas
p53	Tumor suppressor, cell cycle control, apoptosis	17p13	Point mutations Deletion, insertion	Anaplastic cancer
APC	Tumor suppressor, adenomatous polyposis coli gene	5q21-q22	Point mutations	Anaplastic cancer, also associated with familial polyposis coli
p16 (MTS1, CDKN2A)	Tumor suppressor, cell cycle control	9p21	Deletions	Differentiated carcinomas
p21/WAF	Tumor suppressor, cell cycle control	6p21.2	Overexpression	Anaplastic cancer
MET	Receptor tyrosine kinase	7q31	Overexpression	Follicular thyroid cancer
c-MYC	Receptor tyrosine kinase	8q24.12.-13	Overexpression	Differentiated carcinoma
PTEN	Phosphatase	10q23	Point mutations	PTC in Cowden's syndrome (multiple hamartomas, breast tumors, gastrointestinal polyps, thyroid tumors)
CTNNB1	β-Catenin	3p22	Point mutations	Anaplastic cancer
Loss of heterozygosity (LOH)	?Tumor suppressors	3p; 11q13 Other loci	Deletions	Differentiated thyroid carcinomas, anaplastic cancer
PAX8-PPARγ1	Transcription factor Nuclear receptor fusion	t(2;3)(q13;p25)	Translocation	Follicular adenoma or carcinoma

Note: TSH, thyroid-stimulating hormone; $G_{s\alpha}$, G-protein stimulating α-subunit; RET, rearranged during transfection proto-oncogene; PTC, papillary thyroid cancer; TRK, tyrosine kinase receptor; RAS, rat sarcoma proto-oncogene; p53, p53 tumor suppressor gene; MET, met proto-oncogene (hepatocyte growth factor receptor); c-MYC, cellular homologue of myelocytomatosis virus proto-oncogene; PTEN, phosphatase and tensin homologue; APC, adenomatous polyposis coli; MTS, multiple tumor suppressor; CDKN2A, cyclin-dependent kinase inhibitor 2A; P21, p21 tumor suppressor; WAF, wild-type p53 activated fragment; GPCR, G protein–coupled receptor; ELE1/TK, ret-activating gene ele1/tyrosine kinase; MEN 2, multiple endocrine neoplasia-2; PAX8, Paired domain transcription factor; PPARγ1, peroxisome-proliferator activated receptor γ1; BRAF, v-raf homologue, B1; MEK, mitogen extracellular signal-regulated kinase.

Source: Adapted with permission from P Kopp, JL Jameson, in JL Jameson (ed): *Principles of Molecular Medicine*. Totowa, NJ, Humana Press, 1998.

without clear evidence of an ordered acquisition of somatic mutations as they progress from the benign to the malignant state. On the other hand, certain mutations are relatively specific for thyroid neoplasia, some of which correlate with histologic classification (Table 335-12).

Activating mutations of the TSH-R and the $G_{s\alpha}$ subunit are associated with autonomously functioning nodules. Though these mutations induce thyroid cell growth, this type of nodule is almost always benign.

Activation of the RET-RAS-BRAF signaling pathway is seen in most PTCs, though the types of mutations are heterogeneous. A variety of rearrangements involving the *RET* gene on chromosome 10 brings this receptor tyrosine kinase under the control of other promoters, leading to receptor overexpression. *RET* rearrangements occur in 20–40% of PTCs in different series and were observed with increased frequency in tumors developing after the Chernobyl radiation accident. Rearrangements in PTC have also been observed for another tyrosine kinase gene, *TRK1*, which is located on chromosome 1. To date, the identification of PTC with *RET* or *TRK1* rearrangements has not proven useful for predicting prognosis or treatment responses. *BRAF* mutations appear to be the most common genetic alteration in PTC. These mutations activate the kinase, which stimulates the mitogen-activated protein MAP kinase (MAPK) cascade. *RAS* mutations, which also stimulate the MAPK cascade, are found in about 20–30% of thyroid neoplasms, including both PTC and FTC. Of note, simultaneous *RET*, *BRAF*, and *RAS* mutations do not occur in the same tumor, suggesting that activation of the MAPK cascade is critical for tumor development, independent of the step that initiates the cascade.

As noted above, *RAS* mutations also occur in FTCs. In addition, a rearrangement of the thyroid developmental transcription factor PAX8 with the nuclear receptor PPARγ is identified in a significant fraction of FTCs. Loss of heterozygosity of 3p or 11q, consistent with deletions of tumor-suppressor genes, is also common in FTCs.

Most of the mutations seen in differentiated thyroid cancers have also been detected in ATCs. Mutations in CTNNB1, which encodes β-catenin, occur in about two-thirds of ATCs, but not in PTC or FTC. Mutations of the tumor suppressor p53 also play an important role in the development of ATC. Because p53 plays a role in cell cycle surveillance, DNA repair, and apoptosis, its loss may contribute to the rapid acquisition of genetic instability as well as poor treatment responses (Chap. 80) (Table 335-12).

MTC, when associated with multiple endocrine neoplasia (MEN) type 2, harbors an inherited mutation of the *RET* gene. Unlike the rearrangements of *RET* seen in PTC, the mutations in MEN2 are point mutations that induce constitutive activity of the tyrosine kinase (Chap. 345). MTC is preceded by hyperplasia of the C cells, raising the likelihood that as-yet-unidentified "second hits" lead to cellular transformation. A subset of sporadic MTC contain somatic mutations that activate *RET*.

WELL-DIFFERENTIATED THYROID CANCER

Papillary PTC is the most common type of thyroid cancer, accounting for 70–90% of well-differentiated thyroid malignancies. Microscopic PTC is present in up to 25% of thyroid glands at autopsy, but most of these lesions are very small (several millimeters) and are not clinically significant. Characteristic cytologic features of PTC help make the diagnosis by FNA or after surgical resection; these include psammoma bodies, cleaved nuclei with an "orphan-Annie" appearance caused by large nucleoli, and the formation of papillary structures.

PTC tends to be multifocal and to invade locally within the thyroid gland as well as through the thyroid capsule and into adjacent structures in the neck. It has a propensity to spread via the lymphatic system but can metastasize hematogenously as well, particularly to bone and lung. Because of the relatively slow growth of the tumor, a significant burden of pulmonary metastases may accumulate, sometimes with remarkably few symptoms. The prognostic implication of lymph node spread is debated. Lymph node involvement by thyroid cancer can be remarkably well tolerated but appears to increase the risk of recurrence and mortality, particularly in older patients. The staging of PTC by the TNM system is outlined in Table 335-11. Most papillary cancers are identified in the early stages (>80% stages I or II) and have an excellent prognosis, with survival curves similar to expected survival (Fig. 335-12A). Mortality is markedly increased in stage IV disease (distant metastases), but this group comprises only about 1% of patients. The treatment of PTC is described below.

Follicular The incidence of FTC varies widely in different parts of the world; it is more common in iodine-deficient regions. FTC is difficult to diagnose by FNA because the distinction between benign and malignant follicular neoplasms rests largely on evidence of invasion into vessels, nerves, or adjacent structures. FTC tends to spread by hematogenous routes leading to bone, lung, and central nervous system metastases. Mortality rates associated with FTC are less favorable than for PTC, in part because a larger proportion of patients present with stage IV disease (Fig. 335-12B). Poor prognostic features include distant metastases, age >50 years, primary tumor size >4 cm, Hürthle cell histology, and the presence of marked vascular invasion.

℞ WELL-DIFFERENTIATED THYROID CANCER

SURGERY All well-differentiated thyroid cancers should be surgically excised. In addition to removing the primary lesion, surgery allows accurate histologic diagnosis and staging, and multicentric disease is commonly found in the contralateral thyroid lobe. Lymph node spread can also be assessed at the time of surgery, and involved nodes can be removed. Recommendations about the extent of surgery vary for stage I disease, as survival rates are similar for lobectomy and near-total thyroidectomy. Lobectomy is associated with a lower incidence of hypoparathyroidism and injury to the recurrent laryngeal nerves. However, it is not possible to monitor Tg levels or to perform whole-body ^{131}I scans in the presence of the residual lobe. Moreover, if final staging or subsequent follow-up indicates the need for radioiodine scanning or treatment, repeat surgery is necessary to remove the remaining thyroid tissue. Therefore, near-total thyroidectomy is preferable in almost all patients; complication rates are acceptably low if the surgeon is highly experienced in the procedure. Postsurgical radioablation of the remnant thyroid tissue is increasingly being used as it may destroy remaining or multifocal thyroid carcinoma, and it facilitates the use of Tg determinations and radioiodine scanning for long-term follow-up by eliminating residual normal or neoplastic tissue.

TSH SUPPRESSION THERAPY As most tumors are still TSH-responsive, levothyroxine suppression of TSH is a mainstay of thyroid cancer treatment. Though TSH suppression clearly provides therapeutic benefit, there are no prospective studies that identify the optimal level of TSH suppression. A reasonable goal is to suppress TSH as much as possible without subjecting the patient to unnecessary side effects from excess thyroid hormone, such as atrial fibrillation, osteopenia, anxiety, and other manifestations of thyrotoxicosis. For patients at low risk of recurrence, TSH should be suppressed into the low but detectable range (0.1–0.5 IU/L). For patients at high risk of recurrence or with known metastatic disease, complete TSH suppression is indicated if there are no strong contraindications to mild thyrotoxicosis. In this instance, unbound T_4 must also be monitored to avoid excessive treatment.

RADIOIODINE TREATMENT Well-differentiated thyroid cancer still incorporates radioiodine, though less efficiently than normal thyroid follicular cells. Radioiodine uptake is determined primarily by expression of the NIS and is stimulated by TSH, requiring expression of the TSH-R. The retention time for radioactivity is influenced by the extent to which the tumor retains differentiated functions such as iodide trapping and organification. After near-total thyroidectomy, substantial thyroid tissue often remains, particularly in the thyroid bed and surrounding the parathyroid glands. Consequently, ^{131}I ablation is necessary to eliminate remaining normal thyroid tissue and to treat residual tumor cells.

Indications The use of therapeutic doses of radioiodine remains an area of controversy in thyroid cancer management. However, postoperative thyroid ablation and radioiodine treatment of known residual PTC or FTC clearly reduces recurrence rates but has a smaller impact on mortality, particularly in patients at relatively low risk. This low-risk group includes most patients with stage 1 PTC with primary tumors <1.5 cm in size. For patients with larger papillary tumors, spread to the adjacent lymph nodes, FTC, or evidence of metastases, thyroid ablation and radioiodine treatment are generally indicated.

^{131}I Thyroid Ablation and Treatment As noted above, the decision to use ^{131}I for thyroid ablation should be coordinated with the surgical approach, as radioablation is much more effective when there is minimal remaining normal thyroid tissue. A typical strategy is to treat the patient for several weeks postoperatively with liothyronine (25 μg bid or tid), followed by thyroid hormone withdrawal. Ideally, the TSH level should increase to >50 IU/L over 3–4 weeks. The level to which TSH rises is dictated largely by the amount of normal thyroid tissue remaining postoperatively. Recombinant human TSH (rhTSH) has also been used to enhance ^{131}I uptake for postsurgical ablation. It appears to be at least as effective as thyroid hor-

FIGURE 335-12 Survival rates in patients with differentiated thyroid cancer. A. Papillary cancer, cohort of 1851 patients. I, 1107 (60%); II, 408 (22%); III, 312 (17%); IV, 24 (1%); n = 1185. **B.** Follicular cancer, cohort of 153 patients. I, 42 (27%); II, 82 (54%); III, 6 (4%); IV, 23 (15%); n = 153. [*Adapted from PR Larsen et al: William's Textbook of Endocrinology, 9th ed, JD Wilson et al (eds). Philadelphia, Saunders, 1998, pp 389–575, with permission.*]

PART 15

Endocrinology and Metabolism

mone withdrawal and should be particularly useful as residual thyroid tissue prevents an adequate endogenous TSH rise. rhTSH is currently approved for postoperative ablation in Europe but not in the United States.

A pretreatment scanning dose of ^{131}I [usually 111–185 MBq (3–5 mCi)] can reveal the amount of residual tissue and provides guidance about the dose needed to accomplish ablation. However, because of concerns about radioactive "stunning" that impairs subsequent treatment, there is a trend to avoid pretreatment scanning and to proceed directly to ablation, unless there is suspicion that the amount of residual tissue will alter therapy. A maximum outpatient ^{131}I dose is 1110 MBq (29.9 mCi) in the United States, though ablation is often more complete using greater doses [1850–3700 MBq (50–100 mCi)]. Patients should be placed on a low-iodine diet (<50 µg/d urinary iodine) to increase radioiodine uptake. In patients with known residual cancer, the larger doses ensure thyroid ablation and may destroy remaining tumor cells. A whole-body scan following the high-dose radioiodine treatment is useful to identify possible metastatic disease.

Follow-Up Whole-Body Thyroid Scanning and Thyroglobulin Determinations An initial whole-body scan should be performed about 6 months after thyroid ablation. The strategy for follow-up management of thyroid cancer has been altered by the availability of rhTSH to stimulate ^{131}I uptake and by the improved sensitivity of Tg assays to detect residual or recurrent disease. A scheme for using either rhTSH or thyroid hormone withdrawal for thyroid scanning is summarized in **Fig. 335-13**. After thyroid ablation, rhTSH can be used in follow-up to stimulate Tg and ^{131}I uptake without subjecting patients to thyroid hormone withdrawal and its associated symptoms of hypothyroidism as well as the risk of tumor growth after prolonged TSH stimulation. Alternatively, in patients who are likely to require ^{131}I treatment, the traditional approach of thyroid hormone withdrawal can be used to increase TSH. This involves switching patients from levothyroxine (T_4) to the more rapidly cleared hormone liothyronine (T_3), thereby allowing TSH to increase more quickly. Because TSH stimulates Tg levels, Tg measurements should be obtained after administration of rhTSH or when TSH levels have risen after thyroid hormone withdrawal.

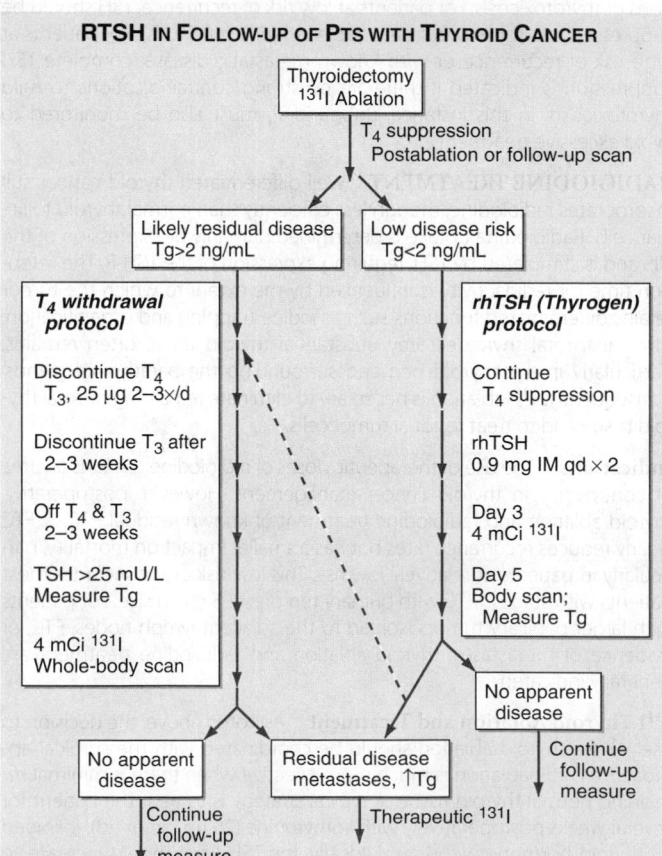

FIGURE 335-13 Use of recombinant thyroid-stimulating hormone (TSH) in the follow-up of patients with thyroid cancer. Tg, thyroglobulin; rhTSH, recombinant human TSH.

In low-risk patients who have no clinical evidence of residual disease after ablation and a basal Tg <1 ng/ml, increasing evidence supports the use of rhTSH-stimulated Tg levels 1 year after ablation, without the need for radioiodine scanning. If stimulated Tg levels are low (<2 ng/ml) and, ideally, undetectable, these patients can be managed with suppressive therapy and measurements of unstimulated Tg every 6–12 months. The absence of Tg antibodies should be confirmed in these patients. On the other hand, patients with residual disease on whole-body scanning or those with elevated Tg levels require additional ^{131}I therapy. In addition, most authorities advocate radioiodine treatment for scan-negative, Tg-positive (Tg >5–10 ng/mL) patients, as many derive therapeutic benefit from a large dose of ^{131}I.

In addition to radioiodine, external beam radiotherapy is also used to treat specific metastatic lesions, particularly when they cause bone pain or threaten neurologic injury (e.g., vertebral metastases).

ANAPLASTIC AND OTHER FORMS OF THYROID CANCER
Anaplastic Thyroid Cancer As noted above, ATC is a poorly differentiated and aggressive cancer. The prognosis is poor, and most patients die within 6 months of diagnosis. Because of the undifferentiated state of these tumors, the uptake of radioiodine is usually negligible, but it can be used therapeutically if there is residual uptake. Chemotherapy has been attempted with multiple agents, including anthracyclines and paclitaxel, but it is usually ineffective. External beam radiation therapy can be attempted and continued if tumors are responsive.

Thyroid Lymphoma Lymphoma in the thyroid gland often arises in the background of Hashimoto's thyroiditis. A rapidly expanding thyroid mass suggests the possibility of this diagnosis. Diffuse large-cell lymphoma is the most common type in the thyroid. Biopsies reveal sheets of lymphoid cells that can be difficult to distinguish from small-cell lung cancer or ATC. These tumors are often highly sensitive to external radiation. Surgical resection should be avoided as initial therapy because it may spread disease that is otherwise localized to the thyroid. If staging indicates disease outside of the thyroid, treatment should follow guidelines used for other forms of lymphoma (Chap. 105).

MEDULLARY THYROID CARCINOMA
MTC can be sporadic or familial and accounts for about 5–10% of thyroid cancers. There are three familial forms of MTC: MEN 2A, MEN 2B, and familial MTC without other features of MEN (Chap. 345). In general, MTC is more aggressive in MEN 2B than in MEN 2A, and familial MTC is more aggressive than sporadic MTC. Elevated serum calcitonin provides a marker of residual or recurrent disease. It is reasonable to test all patients with MTC for *RET* mutations, as genetic counseling and testing of family members can be offered to those individuals who test positive for mutations.

The management of MTC is primarily surgical. Unlike tumors derived from thyroid follicular cells, these tumors do not take up radioiodine. External radiation treatment and chemotherapy may provide palliation in patients with advanced disease (Chap. 345).

APPROACH TO THE PATIENT:
A Thyroid Nodule

Palpable thyroid nodules are found in about 5% of adults, but the prevalence varies considerably worldwide. Given this high prevalence rate, it is common for the practitioner to identify thyroid nodules. The main goal of this evaluation is to identify, in a cost-effective manner, the small subgroup of individuals with malignant lesions.

As described above, nodules are more common in iodine-deficient areas, in women, and with aging. Most palpable nodules are >1 cm in diameter, but the ability to feel a nodule is influenced by its location within the gland (superficial versus deeply embedded), the anatomy of the patient's neck, and the experience of the examiner. More sensitive methods of detection, such as CT, thyroid ultrasound, and pathologic studies, reveal thyroid nodules in >20% of glands. The presence of these thyroid incidentalomas has led to

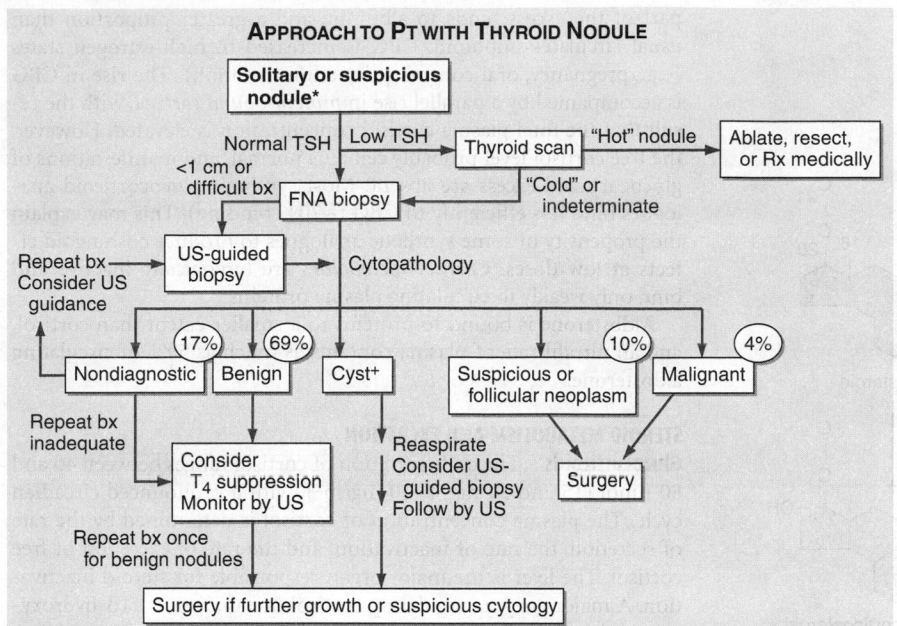

APPROACH TO PT WITH THYROID NODULE

FIGURE 335-14 Approach to the patient with a thyroid nodule. See text and references for details. †About one-third of nodules are cystic or mixed solid-cystic. US, ultrasound; TSH, thyroid-stimulating hormone; FNA, fine-needle aspiration.

should be performed within 2–5 years to confirm the benign status of the nodule.

Nondiagnostic biopsies occur for many reasons, including a fibrotic reaction with relatively few cells available for aspiration, a cystic lesion in which cellular components reside along the cyst margin, or a nodule that may be too small for accurate aspiration. For these reasons, ultrasound-guided FNA is indicated when the FNA is repeated. Ultrasound is also increasingly used for initial biopsies in an effort to enhance nodule localization and the accuracy of sampling. Ultrasound characteristics are also useful for deciding which nodules to biopsy when multiple nodules are present. Sonographic characteristics suggestive of malignancy include microcalcifications, increased vascularity, and hypoechogenicity within the nodule.

The evaluation of a thyroid nodule is stressful for most patients. They are concerned about the possibility of thyroid cancer, whether verbalized or not. It is constructive, therefore, to review the diagnostic approach and to reassure patients when no malignancy is found. When a suspicious lesion or thyroid cancer is identified, an explanation of the generally favorable prognosis and available treatment options should be provided.

FURTHER READINGS

ABALOVICH M et al: Management of thyroid dysfunction during pregnancy and postpartum: An Endocrine Society Clinical Practice Guideline. J Clin Endocrinol Metab 92(Suppl):S1, 2007

COOPER DS: Antithyroid drugs. N Engl J Med 352:905, 2005

——— et al: Management guidelines for patients with thyroid nodules and differentiated thyroid cancer. Thyroid 16:1, 2006

DE FELICE M, DI LAURO R: Thyroid development and its disorders: Genetics and molecular mechanisms. Endo Rev 25:722, 2004

DEGROOT LJ et al: Thyroid gland (Part 10, Vol 2), in *Endocrinology*, 5th ed, LJ DeGroot, JL Jameson (eds). Philadelphia, Elsevier Saunders, 2006

ESCOBAR-MORREALE HF et al: Treatment of hypothyroidism with combinations of levothyroxine plus liothyronine. J Clin Endocrinol Metab 90:4946, 2005

GHARIB H et al: Subclinical thyroid dysfunction: a joint statement on management from the American Association of Clinical Endocrinologists, the American Thyroid Association, and the Endocrine Society. J Clin Endocrinol Metab 90:581, 2005

GRUTERS A ET AL: Molecular genetic defects in congenital hypothyroidism. Eur J Endocrinol 151(Suppl 3):U39, 2004

KONDO T et al: Pathogenetic mechanisms in thyroid follicular cell neoplasia. Nat Rev Cancer 6:292, 2006

PEARCE EN: Diagnosis and management of thyrotoxicosis. BMJ 332(7554):1369, 2006

ROBERTS CGP, LADENSON PW: Hypothyroidism. Lancet 363:793, 2004

WEETMAN AP: Cellular immune responses in autoimmune thyroid disease. Clin Endocrinol 61:405, 2004

much debate about how to detect nodules and which nodules to investigate further. Most authorities still rely on physical examination to detect thyroid nodules, reserving ultrasound for monitoring nodule size or as an aid in thyroid biopsy.

An approach to the evaluation of a solitary nodule is outlined in Fig. 335-14. Most patients with thyroid nodules have normal thyroid function tests. Nonetheless, thyroid function should be assessed by measuring a TSH level, which may be suppressed by one or more autonomously functioning nodules. If the TSH is suppressed, a radionuclide scan is indicated to determine if the identified nodule is "hot," as lesions with increased uptake are almost never malignant and FNA is unnecessary. Otherwise, FNA biopsy should be the first step in the evaluation of a thyroid nodule. FNA has good sensitivity and specificity when performed by physicians familiar with the procedure and when the results are interpreted by experienced cytopathologists. The technique is particularly good for detecting PTC. The distinction of benign and malignant follicular lesions is often not possible using cytology alone.

In several large studies, FNA biopsies yielded the following findings: 70% benign, 10% malignant or suspicious for malignancy, and 20% nondiagnostic or yielding insufficient material for diagnosis. Characteristic features of malignancy mandate surgery. A diagnosis of follicular neoplasm also warrants surgery, as benign and malignant lesions cannot be distinguished based on cytopathology or frozen section. The management of patients with benign lesions is more variable. Many authorities advocate TSH suppression, whereas others monitor nodule size without suppression. With either approach, thyroid nodule size should be monitored, ideally using ultrasound. Repeat FNA is indicated if a nodule enlarges, and a second biopsy should be performed within 2–5 years to confirm the benign status of the nodule.

336 Disorders of the Adrenal Cortex
Gordon H. Williams, Robert G. Dluhy

BIOCHEMISTRY AND PHYSIOLOGY

The adrenal cortex produces three major classes of steroids: (1) glucocorticoids, (2) mineralocorticoids, and (3) adrenal androgens. Consequently, normal adrenal function is important for modulating intermediary metabolism and immune responses through glucocorticoids; blood pressure, vascular volume, and electrolytes through mineralocorticoids; and secondary sexual characteristics (in females) through androgens. The adrenal axis plays an important role in the stress response by rapidly increasing cortisol levels. Adrenal disorders include hyperfunction (Cushing's syndrome) and hypofunction (adrenal insufficiency), as well as a variety of genetic abnormalities of steroidogenesis.

FIGURE 336-1 Basic steroid structure and nomenclature.

STEROID NOMENCLATURE

The basic structure of steroids is built upon a five-ring nucleus (Fig. 336-1). The carbon atoms are numbered in a sequence beginning with ring A. Adrenal steroids contain either 19 or 21 carbon atoms. The C_{19} steroids have methyl groups at C-18 and C-19. C_{19} steroids with a ketone group at C-17 are termed *17-ketosteroids*; C_{19} steroids have predominantly androgenic activity. The C_{21} steroids have a 2-carbon side chain (C-20 and C-21) attached at position 17 and methyl groups at C-18 and C-19; C_{21} steroids with a hydroxyl group at position 17 are termed *17-hydroxycorticosteroids*. The C_{21} steroids have either glucocorticoid or mineralocorticoid properties.

BIOSYNTHESIS OF ADRENAL STEROIDS

Cholesterol, derived from the diet and from endogenous synthesis, is the substrate for steroidogenesis. Uptake of cholesterol by the adrenal cortex is mediated by the low-density lipoprotein (LDL) receptor. With long-term stimulation of the adrenal cortex by adrenocorticotropic hormone (ACTH), the number of LDL receptors increases. The three major adrenal biosynthetic pathways lead to the production of glucocorticoids (cortisol), mineralocorticoids (aldosterone), and adrenal androgens (dehydroepiandrosterone). Separate zones of the adrenal cortex synthesize specific hormones (Fig. 336-2). This zonation is accompanied by the selective expression of the genes encoding the enzymes unique to the formation of each type of steroid: aldosterone synthase is normally expressed only in the outer (glomerulosa) cell layer, whereas 21- and 17-hydroxylase are expressed in the (inner) fasciculata-reticularis cell layers, which are the sites of cortisol and androgen biosynthesis, respectively.

STEROID TRANSPORT

Cortisol circulates in the plasma as free cortisol, protein-bound cortisol, and cortisol metabolites. *Free cortisol* is a physiologically active hormone that is not protein-bound and therefore can act directly on tissue sites. Normally, <5% of circulating cortisol is free. Only the unbound cortisol and its metabolites are filterable at the glomerulus. Increased quantities of free steroid are excreted in the urine in states characterized by hypersecretion of cortisol, because the unbound fraction of plasma cortisol rises. Plasma has two cortisol-binding systems. One is a high-affinity, low-capacity α_2-globulin termed *transcortin* or *cortisol-binding globulin* (CBG), and the other is a low-affinity, high-capacity protein, *albumin*. Cortisol binding to CBG is reduced in areas of inflammation, thus increasing the local concentration of free cortisol. When the concentration of cortisol is >700 nmol/L (25 µg/dL),

part of the excess binds to albumin, and a greater proportion than usual circulates unbound. CBG is increased in high-estrogen states (e.g., pregnancy, oral contraceptive administration). The rise in CBG is accompanied by a parallel rise in *protein-bound cortisol*, with the result that the total plasma cortisol concentration is elevated. However, the free cortisol level probably remains normal, and manifestations of glucocorticoid excess are absent. Most synthetic glucocorticoid analogues bind less efficiently to CBG (~70% binding). This may explain the propensity of some synthetic analogues to produce cushingoid effects at low doses. *Cortisol metabolites* are biologically inactive and bind only weakly to circulating plasma proteins.

Aldosterone is bound to proteins to a smaller extent than cortisol, and an ultrafiltrate of plasma contains as much as 50% of circulating aldosterone.

STEROID METABOLISM AND EXCRETION

Glucocorticoids The daily secretion of cortisol ranges between 40 and 80 µmol (15 and 30 mg; 8–10 mg/m²), with a pronounced circadian cycle. The plasma concentration of cortisol is determined by the rate of secretion, the rate of inactivation, and the rate of excretion of free cortisol. The liver is the major organ responsible for steroid inactivation. A major enzyme regulating cortisol metabolism is 11β-hydroxysteroid dehydrogenase (11β-HSD). There are two isoforms: 11β-HSD 1 is primarily expressed in the liver and acts as a reductase, converting the inactive cortisone to the active glucocorticoid, cortisol; the 11β-HSD 2 isoform is expressed in a number of tissues and converts cortisol to the inactive metabolite, cortisone. Mutations in the *HSD11β1* gene are associated with rapid cortisol turnover, leading to activation of the hypothalamic-pituitary-adrenal (HPA) axis and excessive adrenal androgen production in women. In animal models, excess omental expression of 11β-HSD 1 increases local glucocorticoid production and is associated with central obesity and insulin resistance. The oxidative reaction of 11β-HSD 1 is increased in hypothyroidism. Mutations in the *HSD11β2* gene cause the syndrome of *apparent mineralocorticoid excess*, reflecting insufficient inactivation of cortisol in the kidney, allowing inappropriate cortisol activation of the mineralocorticoid receptor (see below).

Mineralocorticoids In individuals with normal salt intake, the average daily secretion of aldosterone ranges between 0.1 and 0.7 µmol (50 and 250 µg). During a single passage through the liver, >75% of circulating aldosterone is normally inactivated by conjugation with glucuronic acid. However, under certain conditions, such as congestive failure, this rate of inactivation is reduced.

Adrenal Androgens The major androgen secreted by the adrenal is dehydroepiandrosterone (DHEA) and its sulfuric acid ester (DHEAS). Approximately 15–30 mg of these compounds is secreted daily. Smaller amounts of androstenedione, 11β-hydroxyandrostenedione, and testosterone are secreted. DHEA is the major precursor of the urinary 17-ketosteroids. Two-thirds of the urine 17-ketosteroids in the male are derived from adrenal metabolites, and the remaining one-third comes from testicular androgens. In the female, almost all urine 17-ketosteroids are derived from the adrenal.

Steroids diffuse passively through the cell membrane and bind to intracellular receptors (Chap. 332). Glucocorticoids and mineralocorticoids bind with nearly equal affinity to the mineralocorticoid receptor (MR). However, only glucocorticoids bind to the glucocorticoid receptor (GR). After the steroid binds to the receptor, the steroid-receptor complex is transported to the nucleus, where it binds to specific sites on steroid-regulated genes, altering levels of transcription. Some actions of glucocorticoids (e.g., anti-inflammatory effects) are mediated by GR-mediated inhibition of other transcription factors, such as activating protein-1 (AP-1) or nuclear factor kappa B (NFκB), which normally stimulate the activity of various cytokine genes. Because cortisol binds to the MR with the same affinity as aldosterone, mineralocorticoid specificity is achieved by local metabolism of cortisol to the inactive compound cortisone by 11β-HSD 2. The glucocorticoid effects of other

FIGURE 336-2 Biosynthetic pathways for adrenal steroid production; major pathways to mineralocorticoids, glucocorticoids, and androgens. 3β-HSD, 3β-hydroxysteroid dehydrogenase.

steroids, such as high-dose progesterone, correlate with their relative binding affinities for the GR. Inherited defects in the GR cause glucocorticoid resistance states. Individuals with GR defects have high levels of cortisol but do not have manifestations of hypercortisolism.

ACTH PHYSIOLOGY

ACTH and a number of other peptides (lipotropins, endorphins, and melanocyte-stimulating hormones) are processed from a larger precursor molecule of 31,000 mol wt—proopiomelanocortin (POMC) (Chap. 333). POMC is made in a variety of tissues, including brain, anterior and posterior pituitary, and lymphocytes. The constellation of POMC-derived peptides secreted depends on the tissue. ACTH, a 39-amino-acid peptide, is synthesized and stored in basophilic cells of the anterior pituitary. The N-terminal 18-amino-acid fragment of ACTH has full biologic potency, and shorter N-terminal fragments have partial biologic activity. Release of ACTH and related peptides from the anterior pituitary gland is stimulated by corticotropin-releasing hormone (CRH), a 41-amino-acid peptide produced in the median eminence of the hypothalamus (Fig. 336-3). Urocortin, a neuropeptide related to CRH, mimics many of the central effects of CRH (e.g., appetite suppression, anxiety), but its role in ACTH regulation is unclear. Some related peptides such as β-lipotropin (β-LPT) are released in equimolar concentrations with ACTH, suggesting that they are cleaved enzymatically from the parent POMC before or during the secretory process. However, β-endorphin levels may or may not correlate with circulating levels of ACTH, depending on the nature of the stimulus.

The major factors controlling ACTH release include CRH, the free cortisol concentration in plasma, stress, and the sleep-wake cycle (Fig. 336-3). Plasma ACTH varies during the day as a result of its pulsatile secretion and follows a circadian pattern, with a peak just prior to wak-

FIGURE 336-3 The hypothalamic-pituitary-adrenal axis. The main sites for feedback control by plasma cortisol are the pituitary gland (1) and the hypothalamic corticotropin-releasing center (2). Feedback control by plasma cortisol also occurs at the locus coeruleus/sympathetic system (3) and may involve higher nerve centers (4) as well. There may also be a short feedback loop involving inhibition of corticotropin-releasing hormone (CRH) by adrenocorticotropic hormone (ACTH) (5). Hypothalamic neurotransmitters influence CRH release; serotoninergic and cholinergic systems stimulate the secretion of CRH and ACTH; adrenergic agonists and γ-aminobutyric acid (GABA) probably inhibit CRH release. The opioid peptides β-endorphin and enkephalin inhibit, and vasopressin and angiotensin II augment, the secretion of CRH and ACTH. β-LPT, β-lipotropin; POMC, pro-opiomelanocortin; LC, locus coeruleus; NE, norepinephrine.

ing and a nadir before sleeping. If a new sleep-wake cycle is adopted, the pattern changes over several days to conform to it. ACTH and cortisol levels also increase in response to eating. Stress (e.g., pyrogens, surgery, hypoglycemia, exercise, and severe emotional trauma) causes the release of CRH and arginine vasopressin (AVP) and activation of the sympathetic nervous system. These changes in turn enhance ACTH release, acting individually or in concert. For example, AVP release acts synergistically with CRH to amplify ACTH secretion; CRH also stimulates the locus coeruleus/sympathetic system. Stress-related secretion of ACTH abolishes the circadian periodicity of ACTH levels but is, in turn, suppressed by prior high-dose glucocorticoid administration. The normal pulsatile, circadian pattern of ACTH release is regulated by CRH; this mechanism is the so-called open feedback loop. CRH secretion, in turn, is influenced by hypothalamic neurotransmitters including the serotoninergic and cholinergic pathways. The immune system also influences the HPA axis (Fig. 336-4). For example, inflammatory cytokines [tumor necrosis factor (TNF)α, interleukin (IL) 1α, IL-1β, and IL-6] produced by monocytes increase ACTH release by stimulating secretion of CRH and/or AVP. Finally, ACTH release is regulated by the level of free cortisol in plasma. Cortisol decreases the responsive-

ness of pituitary corticotropic cells to CRH; the response of the POMC mRNA to CRH is also inhibited by glucocorticoids. In addition, glucocorticoids inhibit the locus coeruleus/sympathetic system and CRH release. The latter servomechanism establishes the primacy of cortisol in the control of ACTH secretion. The suppression of ACTH secretion that results in adrenal atrophy following *prolonged* glucocorticoid therapy is caused primarily by suppression of hypothalamic CRH release, as exogenous CRH administration in this circumstance produces a rise in plasma ACTH. Cortisol also exerts feedback effects on higher brain centers (hippocampus, reticular system, and septum) and perhaps on the adrenal cortex.

The biologic half-life of ACTH in the circulation is <10 min. The action of ACTH is also rapid; within minutes of its release, the concentration of steroids in the adrenal venous blood increases. ACTH stimulates steroidogenesis via activation of adenyl cyclase. Adenosine-3', 5'-monophosphate (cyclic AMP), in turn, stimulates the synthesis of protein kinase enzymes, thereby resulting in the phosphorylation of proteins that activate steroid biosynthesis.

RENIN-ANGIOTENSIN PHYSIOLOGY

Renin is a proteolytic enzyme that is produced and stored in the granules of the juxtaglomerular cells surrounding the afferent arterioles of glomeruli in the kidney. Renin acts on the basic substrate angiotensinogen (a circulating α$_2$-globulin made in the liver) to form the decapeptide angiotensin I (Fig. 336-5). Angiotensin I is then enzymatically transformed by angiotensin-converting enzyme (ACE), which is present in many tissues (particularly the pulmonary vascular endothelium), to the octapeptide angiotensin II by the removal of the two C-terminal amino acids. Angiotensin II is a potent pressor agent and exerts its action by a direct effect on arteriolar smooth muscle. In addition, angiotensin II stimulates production of aldosterone by the zona glomerulosa of the adrenal cortex; the heptapeptide angiotensin III may also stimulate aldosterone production. The two major classes of angiotensin receptors are termed *AT1* and *AT2*; AT1 may exist as two subtypes α and β. Most of the effects of angiotensins II and III are mediated by the AT1 receptor. Angiotensinases rapidly destroy angiotensin II (half-life, 1 min), while the half-life of renin is more prolonged (10–20 min). In addition

FIGURE 336-4 The immune-adrenal axis. Cortisol has anti-inflammatory properties that include effects on the microvasculature, cellular actions, and the suppression of inflammatory cytokines (the so-called immune-adrenal axis). A stress such as sepsis increases adrenal secretion, and cortisol in turn suppresses the immune response via this system. −, suppression; +, stimulation; CRH, corticotropin-releasing hormone; ACTH, adrenocorticotropic hormone; IL, interleukin; TNF, tumor necrosis factor; PAF, platelet activating factor.

FIGURE 336-5 The interrelationship of the volume and potassium feedback loops on aldosterone secretion. Integration of signals from each loop determines the level of aldosterone secretion.

to circulating renin-angiotensin, many tissues have a local renin-angiotensin system and the ability to produce angiotensin II. These tissues include the uterus, placenta, vascular tissue, heart, brain, and, particularly, the adrenal cortex and kidney. Although the role of locally generated angiotensin II is not established, it may modulate the growth and function of the adrenal cortex and vascular smooth muscle.

The amount of renin released reflects the combined effects of four interdependent factors. The *juxtaglomerular cells*, which are specialized myoepithelial cells that cuff the afferent arterioles, act as miniature pressure transducers, sensing renal perfusion pressure and corresponding changes in afferent arteriolar perfusion pressures. For example, a reduction in circulating blood volume leads to a corresponding reduction in renal perfusion pressure and afferent arteriolar pressure (Fig. 336-5). This change is perceived by the juxtaglomerular cells as a decreased stretch exerted on the afferent arteriolar walls, and the juxtaglomerular cells release more renin into the renal circulation. This results in the formation of angiotensin I, which is converted in the kidney and peripherally to angiotensin II by ACE. Angiotensin II influences sodium homeostasis via two major mechanisms: it changes renal blood flow so as to maintain a constant glomerular filtration rate, thereby changing the filtration fraction of sodium, and it stimulates the adrenal cortex to release aldosterone. Increasing plasma levels of aldosterone enhance renal sodium retention and thus result in expansion of the extracellular fluid volume (ECFV), which, in turn, dampens the stimulus for renin release. In this context, the renin-angiotensin-aldosterone system regulates volume by modifying renal hemodynamics and tubular sodium transport.

A second control mechanism for renin release is centered in the *macula densa cells*, a group of distal convoluted tubular epithelial cells directly opposed to the juxtaglomerular cells. They may function as chemoreceptors, monitoring the sodium (or chloride) load presented to the distal tubule. Under conditions of increased delivery of filtered sodium to the macula densa, a signal is conveyed to decrease juxtaglomerular cell release of renin, thereby modulating the glomerular filtration rate and the filtered load of sodium.

The *sympathetic nervous system* regulates the release of renin in response to assumption of the upright posture. The mechanism is either a direct effect on the juxtaglomerular cell to increase adenyl cyclase activity or an indirect effect on either the juxtaglomerular or the macula densa cells via vasoconstriction of the afferent arteriole.

Finally, circulating factors influence renin release. Increased dietary intake of potassium decreases renin release, whereas decreased potassium intake increases it. The significance of these effects is unclear. *Angiotensin II* exerts negative feedback control on renin release that is independent of alterations in renal blood flow, blood pressure, or aldosterone secretion. *Atrial natriuretic peptides* also inhibit renin release. Thus, the control of renin release involves both *intrarenal* (pressor receptor and macula densa) and *extrarenal* (sympathetic nervous system, potassium, angiotensin, etc.) mechanisms. Steady-state

renin levels reflect all these factors, with the intrarenal mechanism predominating.

GLUCOCORTICOID PHYSIOLOGY

The division of adrenal steroids into glucocorticoids and mineralocorticoids is arbitrary in that most glucocorticoids have some mineralocorticoid-like properties. The descriptive term *glucocorticoid* is used for adrenal steroids whose predominant action is on intermediary metabolism. Their overall actions are directed at enhancing the production of the high-energy fuel, glucose, and reducing all other metabolic activity not directly involved in that process. Sustained activation, however, results in a pathophysiologic state, e.g., Cushing's syndrome. The principal glucocorticoid is cortisol (hydrocortisone). The effect of glucocorticoids on intermediary metabolism is mediated by the GR. Physiologic effects of glucocorticoids include the regulation of protein, carbohydrate, lipid, and nucleic acid metabolism. Glucocorticoids raise the blood glucose level by antagonizing the secretion and actions of insulin, thereby inhibiting peripheral glucose uptake, which promotes hepatic glucose synthesis (gluconeogenesis) and hepatic glycogen content. The actions on protein metabolism are mainly catabolic, resulting in an increase in protein breakdown and nitrogen excretion. In large part, these actions reflect a mobilization of glycogenic amino acid precursors from peripheral supporting structures, such as bone, skin, muscle, and connective tissue, due to protein breakdown and inhibition of protein synthesis and amino acid uptake. Hyperaminoacidemia also facilitates gluconeogenesis by stimulating glucagon secretion. Glucocorticoids act directly on the liver to stimulate the synthesis of certain enzymes, such as tyrosine aminotransferase and tryptophan pyrrolase. Glucocorticoids regulate fatty acid mobilization by enhancing the activation of cellular lipase by lipid-mobilizing hormones (e.g., catecholamines and pituitary peptides).

The actions of cortisol on protein and adipose tissue vary in different parts of the body. For example, pharmacologic doses of cortisol can deplete the protein matrix of the vertebral column (trabecular bone), whereas long bones (which are primarily compact bone) are affected only minimally; similarly, peripheral adipose tissue mass decreases, whereas abdominal and interscapular fat expand.

Glucocorticoids have anti-inflammatory properties, which are probably related to effects on the microvasculature and to suppression of inflammatory cytokines. In this sense, glucocorticoids modulate the immune response via the so-called immune-adrenal axis (Fig. 336-4). This "loop" is one mechanism by which a stress, such as sepsis, increases adrenal hormone secretion, and the elevated cortisol level in turn suppresses the immune response. For example, cortisol maintains vascular responsiveness to circulating vasoconstrictors and opposes the increase in capillary permeability during acute inflammation. Glucocorticoids cause a leukocytosis that reflects release from the bone marrow of mature cells as well as inhibition of their egress through the capillary wall. Glucocorticoids produce a depletion of circulating eosinophils and lymphoid tissue, specifically T cells, by causing a redistribution from the circulation into other compartments. Thus, cortisol impairs cell-mediated immunity. Glucocorticoids also inhibit the production and action of the mediators of inflammation, such as the lymphokines and prostaglandins. Glucocorticoids inhibit the production and action of interferon by T lymphocytes and the production of IL-1 and IL-6 by macrophages. The antipyretic action of glucocorticoids may be explained by an effect on IL-1, which appears to be an endogenous pyrogen (Chap. 17). Glucocorticoids also inhibit the production of T cell growth factor (IL-2) by T lymphocytes. Glucocorticoids reverse macrophage activation and antagonize the action of migration-inhibiting factor (MIF), leading to reduced adherence of macrophages to vascular endothelium. Glucocorticoids reduce prostaglandin and leukotriene production by inhibiting the activity of phospholipase A_2, thus blocking release of arachidonic acid from phospholipids. Finally, glucocorticoids inhibit the production and inflammatory effects of bradykinin, platelet-activating factor, and seroto-nin. It is probably only at pharmacologic dosages that antibody production is reduced and lysosomal membranes are stabilized, the latter effect suppressing the release of acid hydrolases.

Cortisol levels respond within minutes to stress, whether physical (trauma, surgery, exercise), psychological (anxiety, depression), or physiologic (hypoglycemia, fever). The reasons why elevated glucocorticoid levels protect the organism under stress are not understood, but in conditions of glucocorticoid deficiency, such stresses may cause hypotension, shock, and death. Consequently, in individuals with adrenal insufficiency, glucocorticoid administration should be increased during stress.

Cortisol has major effects on body water. It helps regulate the ECFV by retarding the migration of water into cells and by promoting renal water excretion, the latter effect mediated by suppression of vasopressin secretion, by an increase in the rate of glomerular filtration, and by a direct action on the renal tubule. The consequence is to prevent water intoxication by increasing solute-free water clearance. Glucocorticoids also have weak mineralocorticoid-like properties, and high doses promote renal tubular sodium reabsorption and increased urine potassium excretion. Glucocorticoids can also influence behavior; emotional disorders may occur with either an excess or a deficit of cortisol. Finally, cortisol suppresses the secretion of pituitary POMC and its derivative peptides (ACTH, β-endorphin, and β-LPT) and the secretion of hypothalamic CRH and vasopressin.

MINERALOCORTICOID PHYSIOLOGY
Mineralocorticoids modify function in two classes of cells—epithelial and nonepithelial.

Effects on Epithelia   Classically, mineralocorticoids are considered major regulators of ECFV and are the major determinants of potassium metabolism. These effects are mediated by the binding of aldosterone to the MR in epithelial cells, primarily the principal cells in the renal cortical collecting duct. Because of its electrochemical gradient, sodium passively enters these cells from the urine via epithelial sodium channels located on the luminal membrane and is actively extruded from the cell via the Na/K-activated ATPase ("sodium pump") located on the basolateral membrane. The sodium pump also provides the driving force of potassium loss into the urine through potassium-selective luminal channels, again assisted by the electrochemical gradient for potassium in these cells. Aldosterone stimulates all three of these processes by increasing gene expression directly (for the sodium pump and the potassium channels) or via a complex process (for epithelial sodium channels) to increase both the number and activity of the sodium channels. Water passively follows the transported sodium, thus expanding intra- and extravascular volume.

Because the concentration of hydrogen ion is greater in the lumen than in the cell, hydrogen ion is also actively secreted. Mineralocorticoids also act on the epithelium of the salivary ducts, sweat glands, and gastrointestinal tract to cause reabsorption of sodium in exchange for potassium.

When normal individuals are given aldosterone, an initial period of sodium retention is followed by natriuresis, and sodium balance is reestablished after 3–5 days. As a result, edema does not develop. This process is referred to as the *escape phenomenon*, signifying an "escape" by the renal tubules from the sodium-retaining action of aldosterone. While renal hemodynamic factors may play a role in the escape, the level of atrial natriuretic peptide also increases. However, it is important to realize that there is no escape from the potassium-losing effects of mineralocorticoids.

Effect on Nonepithelial Cells   The MR has been identified in a number of nonepithelial cells, e.g., neurons in the brain, myocytes, endothelial cells, and vascular smooth-muscle cells. In these cells, the actions of aldosterone differ from those in epithelial cells in several ways:

1. They do not modify sodium-potassium homeostasis.
2. The groups of regulated genes differ, although only a few are known; for example, in nonepithelial cells, aldosterone modifies the expression of several collagen genes controlling tissue growth

factors, e.g., transforming growth factor (TGF) β, plasminogen activator inhibitor, type 1 (PAI-1), adiponectin, and leptin.

3. In some of these tissues (e.g., myocardium and brain), the MR is not protected by the 11-HSD 2 enzyme. Thus, cortisol rather than aldosterone may be activating the MR. In other tissues (e.g., the vasculature), 11-HSD 2 is expressed in a manner similar to that of the kidney. Therefore, aldosterone is activating the MR.
4. Some effects on nonepithelial cells may be via nongenomic mechanisms. These actions are too rapid—occurring within 1–2 min and peaking within 5–10 min—to be considered genomic, suggesting that they are secondary to activation of a cell-surface receptor. However, no cell-surface MR has been identified, raising the possibility that the same MR is mediating both genomic and nongenomic effects. In the vasculature, the nongenomic effects mediated by aldosterone include an increase in the phosphorylation of protein kinase C and extracellular regulated kinase (ERK), and a reduction in the phosphorylation of epithelial nitric oxide synthase. In the intact organism, some, if not all, of both nongenomic and genomic effects are mediated via an interaction between the MR, aldosterone, and proteins in specialized areas in the target cell's surface membrane termed *caveolae*. However, caveolin proteins are not always required as aldosterone still produces adverse cardiovascular effects in caveolin-knockout animals. Rapid, nongenomic effects have also been described for other steroids including estradiol, progesterone, thyroxine, and vitamin D.
5. Some of these tissues—the myocardium and vasculature—may also produce aldosterone, although this theory is controversial and may be both species- and condition-specific.

Regulation of Aldosterone Secretion   Three primary mechanisms control adrenal aldosterone secretion: the renin-angiotensin system, potassium, and ACTH (Table 336-1). Whether these are also the primary regulatory mechanisms modifying nonadrenal production is uncertain. The renin-angiotensin system controls ECFV via regulation of aldosterone secretion (Fig. 336-5). In effect, the renin-angiotensin system maintains the circulating blood volume constant by causing aldosterone-induced sodium retention during volume deficiency and by decreasing aldosterone-dependent sodium retention when volume is ample. There is an increasing body of evidence indicating that some tissues, in addition to the kidney, produce angiotensin II and may participate in the regulation of aldosterone secretion either from the adrenal or extraadrenal sources. Intriguingly, the adrenal itself is capable of synthesizing angiotensin II. What role(s) the extrarenal production of angiotensin II plays in normal physiology is still largely unknown. However, the tissue renin-angiotensin system is activated in utero in response to growth and development and/or later in life in response to injury.

Potassium ion directly stimulates aldosterone secretion, independent of the circulating renin-angiotensin system, which it suppresses (Fig. 336-5). In addition to a direct effect, potassium also modifies al-

TABLE 336-1   FACTORS REGULATING ALDOSTERONE BIOSYNTHESIS

Factor	Effect
Renin-angiotensin system	Stimulation
Sodium ion	Inhibition (?physiologic)
Potassium ion	Stimulation
Neurotransmitters	
Dopamine	Inhibition
Serotonin	Stimulation
Pituitary hormones	
ACTH	Stimulation
Non-ACTH pituitary hormones (e.g., growth hormone)	Permissive (for optimal response to sodium restriction)
β-Endorphin	Stimulation
γ-Melanocyte-stimulating hormone	Permissive
Atrial natriuretic peptide	Inhibition
Ouabain-like factors	Inhibition
Endothelin	Stimulation

Note: ACTH, adrenocorticotropic hormone.

dosterone secretion indirectly by activating the local renin-angiotensin system in the zona glomerulosa. This effect can be blocked by the administration of ACE inhibitors that reduce the local production of angiotensin II and thereby reduce the acute aldosterone response to potassium. An increase in serum potassium of as little as 0.1 mmol/L increases plasma aldosterone levels under certain circumstances. Oral potassium loading therefore increases aldosterone secretion, plasma levels, and excretion.

Physiologic amounts of ACTH stimulate aldosterone secretion acutely, but this action is not sustained unless ACTH is administered in a pulsatile fashion. Most studies relegate ACTH to a minor role in the control of aldosterone. For example, subjects receiving high-dose glucocorticoid therapy, and with presumed complete suppression of ACTH, have normal aldosterone secretion in response to sodium restriction.

Prior dietary intake of both potassium and sodium can alter the magnitude of the aldosterone response to acute stimulation. This effect results from a change in the expression and activity of aldosterone synthase. Increasing potassium intake or decreasing sodium intake sensitizes the response of the glomerulosa cells to acute stimulation by ACTH, angiotensin II, and/or potassium.

Neurotransmitters (dopamine and serotonin) and some peptides, such as atrial natriuretic peptide, γ-melanocyte-stimulating hormone (γ-MSH), and β-endorphin, also participate in the regulation of aldosterone secretion (Table 336-1). Thus, the control of aldosterone secretion involves both stimulatory and inhibitory factors.

ANDROGEN PHYSIOLOGY

Androgens regulate male secondary sexual characteristics and can cause virilizing symptoms in women (Chap. 50). Adrenal androgens have a minimal effect in males whose sexual characteristics are predominately determined by gonadal steroids (testosterone). In females, however, several androgen-like effects, e.g., sexual hair, are largely mediated by adrenal androgens. The principal adrenal androgens are DHEA, androstenedione, and 11-hydroxyandrostenedione. DHEA and androstenedione are weak androgens and exert their effects via conversion to the potent androgen testosterone in extraglandular tissues. DHEA also has poorly understood effects on the immune and cardiovascular systems. Adrenal androgen formation is regulated by ACTH, not by gonadotropins. Adrenal androgens are suppressed by exogenous glucocorticoid administration.

LABORATORY EVALUATION OF ADRENOCORTICAL FUNCTION

A basic assumption is that measurements of the plasma or urinary level of a given steroid reflect the rate of adrenal *secretion* of that steroid. However, urine *excretion* values may not truly reflect the secretion rate because of improper collection or altered metabolism. Plasma levels reflect the level of secretion only at the time of measurement. The plasma level (PL) depends on two factors: the secretion rate (SR) of the hormone and the rate at which it is metabolized, i.e., its metabolic clearance rate (MCR). These three factors can be related as follows:

$$PL = \frac{SR}{MCR} \quad \text{or} \quad SR = MCR \times PL$$

BLOOD LEVELS

Peptides The plasma levels of ACTH and angiotensin II can be measured by immunoassay techniques. Basal ACTH secretion shows a circadian rhythm, with lower levels in the early evening than in the morning. However, ACTH is secreted in a pulsatile manner, leading to rapid fluctuations superimposed on this circadian rhythm. Angiotensin II levels also vary diurnally and are influenced by dietary sodium and potassium intakes and posture. Both upright posture and sodium restriction elevate angiotensin II levels.

Most clinical determinations of the renin-angiotensin system, however, involve measurements of peripheral *plasma renin activity* (PRA) in which the renin activity is gauged by the generation of angiotensin I during a standardized incubation period. This method depends on the presence of sufficient angiotensinogen in the plasma as substrate. The

generated angiotensin I is measured by radioimmunoassay. The PRA depends on the dietary sodium intake and on whether the patient is ambulatory. In normal humans, the PRA shows a diurnal rhythm characterized by peak values in the morning and a nadir in the afternoon. An alternative approach is to measure plasma active renin, which is easier and not dependent on endogenous substrate concentration. PRA and active renin correlate very well on low-sodium diets but less well on high-sodium diets.

Steroids Cortisol and aldosterone are both secreted episodically, and levels vary during the day, with peak values in the morning and low levels in the evening. In addition, the plasma level of aldosterone, but not of cortisol, is increased by dietary potassium loading, by sodium restriction, or by assumption of the upright posture. Measurement of the sulfate conjugate of DHEA may be a useful index of adrenal androgen secretion, as little DHEA sulfate is formed in the gonads and because the half-life of DHEA sulfate is 7–9 h. However, DHEA sulfate levels reflect both DHEA production and sulfatase activity.

URINE LEVELS

For the assessment of glucocorticoid secretion, the urine 17-hydroxycorticosteroid assay has been replaced by measurement of urinary free cortisol. Elevated levels of urinary free cortisol correlate with states of hypercortisolism, reflecting changes in the levels of unbound, physiologically active circulating cortisol. Normally, the rate of excretion is higher in the daytime (7 A.M.–7 P.M.) than at night (7 P.M.–7 A.M.).

Urinary 17-ketosteroids originate in either the adrenal gland or the gonad. In normal women, 90% of urinary 17-ketosteroids is derived from the adrenal, and in men 60–70% is of adrenal origin. Urine 17-ketosteroid values are highest in young adults and decline with age.

A carefully timed urine collection is a prerequisite for all excretory determinations. Urinary creatinine should be measured simultaneously to determine the accuracy and adequacy of the collection procedure.

STIMULATION TESTS

Stimulation tests are useful in the diagnosis of hormone deficiency states.

Tests of Glucocorticoid Reserve Within minutes after administration of ACTH, cortisol levels increase. This responsiveness can be used as an index of the functional reserve of the adrenal gland for production of cortisol. Under maximal ACTH stimulation, cortisol secretion increases tenfold, to 800 μmol/d (300 mg/d), but maximal stimulation can be achieved only with prolonged ACTH infusions.

A screening test (the so-called rapid ACTH stimulation test) involves the administration of 25 units (0.25 mg) of cosyntropin IV or IM and measurement of plasma cortisol levels before administration and 30 and 60 min after administration; the test can be performed at any time of the day. The most clear-cut criterion for a normal response is a stimulated cortisol level of >500 nmol/L (>18 μg/dL), and the minimal stimulated normal increment of cortisol is >200 nmol/L (>7 μg/dL) above baseline. Severely ill patients with elevated basal cortisol levels may show no further increases following acute ACTH administration.

Tests of Mineralocorticoid Reserve and Stimulation of the Renin-Angiotensin System Stimulation tests use protocols designed to create a programmed volume depletion, such as sodium restriction, diuretic administration, or upright posture. A simple, potent test consists of severe sodium restriction and upright posture. After 3–5 days of a 10-mmol/d sodium intake, rates of aldosterone secretion or excretion should increase two- to threefold over the control values. Supine morning plasma aldosterone levels are usually increased three- to sixfold, and they increase a further two- to fourfold in response to 2–3 h of upright posture.

When the dietary sodium intake is normal, stimulation testing requires the administration of a potent diuretic, such as 40–80 mg furosemide, followed by 2–3 h of upright posture. The normal response is a two- to fourfold rise in plasma aldosterone levels.

SUPPRESSION TESTS

Suppression tests to document hypersecretion of adrenal hormones involve measurement of the target hormone response after standardized suppression of its tropic hormone.

Tests of Pituitary-Adrenal Suppressibility The ACTH release mechanism is sensitive to the circulating glucocorticoid level. When blood levels of glucocorticoid are increased in normal individuals, less ACTH is released from the anterior pituitary and less steroid is produced by the adrenal gland. The integrity of this feedback mechanism can be tested clinically by giving a glucocorticoid and judging the suppression of ACTH secretion by analysis of urine steroid levels and/or plasma cortisol and ACTH levels. A potent glucocorticoid such as dexamethasone is used, so that the agent can be given in an amount small enough not to contribute significantly to the pool of steroids to be analyzed.

The best *screening* procedure is the overnight dexamethasone suppression test. This involves the measurement of plasma cortisol levels at 8 A.M. following the oral administration of 1 mg dexamethasone the previous midnight. The 8 A.M. value for plasma cortisol in normal individuals should be <140 nmol/L (5 μg/dL).

The definitive test of adrenal suppressibility involves administering 0.5 mg dexamethasone every 6 h for two successive days while collecting urine over a 24-h period for determination of creatinine and free cortisol and/or measuring plasma cortisol levels. In a patient with a normal hypothalamic-pituitary ACTH release mechanism, a fall in the urine free cortisol to <25 nmol/d (10 μg/d) or of plasma cortisol to <140 nmol/L (5 μg/dL) is seen on the second day of administration.

A normal response to either suppression test implies that the glucocorticoid regulation of ACTH and its control of the adrenal glands is physiologically normal. However, an isolated abnormal result, particularly to the overnight suppression test, does not in itself demonstrate pituitary and/or adrenal disease.

Tests of Mineralocorticoid Suppressibility These tests rely on an expansion of ECFV, which should decrease circulating plasma renin activity and decrease the secretion and/or excretion of aldosterone. Various tests differ in the rate at which ECFV is expanded. One convenient suppression test involves the IV infusion of 500 mL/h of normal saline solution for 4 h, which normally suppresses plasma aldosterone levels to <220 pmol/L (<8 ng/dL) from a sodium-restricted diet or to <140 pmol/L (<5 ng/dL) from a normal sodium intake. Alternatively, a high-sodium diet can be administered for 3 days with 0.2 mg fludrocortisone twice daily. Aldosterone excretion is measured on the third day and should be <28 nmol/d (10 μg/d). These tests should not be performed in potassium-depleted individuals since they carry a risk of precipitating hypokalemia.

TESTS OF PITUITARY-ADRENAL RESPONSIVENESS

Stimuli such as insulin-induced hypoglycemia, AVP, and pyrogens induce the release of ACTH from the pituitary by an action on higher neural centers or on the pituitary itself. Insulin-induced hypoglycemia is particularly useful, because it stimulates the release of both growth hormone and ACTH. In this test, regular insulin (0.05–0.1 U/kg body weight) is given intravenously as a bolus to reduce the fasting glucose level to at least 50% below basal. The normal cortisol response is a rise to >500 nmol/L (18 μg/dL). Glucose levels must be monitored during insulin-induced hypoglycemia, and it should be terminated by feeding or IV glucose, if subjects develop symptoms of hypoglycemia. This test is contraindicated in individuals with coronary artery disease or a seizure disorder.

Metyrapone inhibits 11β-hydroxylase in the adrenal. As a result, the conversion of 11-deoxycortisol (compound S) to cortisol is impaired, causing 11-deoxycortisol to accumulate in the blood and the blood level of cortisol to decrease (Fig. 336-2). The hypothalamic-pituitary axis responds to the declining cortisol blood levels by releasing more ACTH. Note that assessment of the response depends on both an intact hypothalamic-pituitary axis and an intact adrenal gland.

Although modifications of the original metyrapone test have been described, a commonly used protocol involves administering 750 mg of the drug by mouth every 4 h over a 24-h period and comparing the control and postmetyrapone plasma levels of 11-deoxycortisol, cortisol, and ACTH. In normal individuals, plasma 11-deoxycortisol levels should be >210 nmol/L (7 μg/dL) and ACTH levels should be >17 pmol/L (75 pg/mL) following metyrapone administration. The metyrapone test does not accurately reflect ACTH reserve if subjects are ingesting exogenous glucocorticoids or drugs that accelerate the metabolism of metyrapone (e.g., phenytoin).

A direct and selective test of the pituitary corticotrophs can be achieved with CRH. The bolus injection of ovine CRH (corticorelin ovine triflutate; 1 μg/kg body weight) stimulates secretion of ACTH and β-LPT in normal human subjects within 15–60 min. In normal individuals, the mean increment in ACTH is 9 pmol/L (40 pg/mL). However, the magnitude of the ACTH response is less than that produced by insulin-induced hypoglycemia, implying that additional factors (such as vasopressin) augment stress-induced increases in ACTH secretion.

The rapid ACTH test can often distinguish between primary and secondary adrenal insufficiency, because aldosterone secretion is preserved in secondary adrenal failure by the renin-angiotensin system and potassium. Cosyntropin (25 units) is given IV or IM, and plasma cortisol and aldosterone levels are measured before and at 30 and 60 min after administration. The cortisol response is abnormal in both groups, but patients with secondary insufficiency show an increase in aldosterone levels of at least 140 pmol/L (5 ng/dL). No aldosterone response is seen in patients in whom the adrenal cortex is destroyed. Alternatively, ACTH at a physiologic dose (1 μg), the so-called low-dose ACTH test, may be used to detect secondary adrenal insufficiency. An abnormal response is similar to that in the rapid ACTH test. However, levels need to be measured at 30 min, and the ACTH needs to be directly injected IV because it can be absorbed by plastic tubing. Because the use of a bolus of exogenous ACTH does not invariably exclude a diagnosis of secondary adrenocortical insufficiency, direct tests of pituitary ACTH reserve (metyrapone test, insulin-induced hypoglycemia) may be required in the appropriate clinical setting.

HYPERFUNCTION OF THE ADRENAL CORTEX

Excess cortisol is associated with Cushing's syndrome; excess aldosterone causes aldosteronism; and excess adrenal androgens cause adrenal virilism. These syndromes do not always occur in the "pure" form but may have overlapping features.

CUSHING'S SYNDROME

Etiology Cushing described a syndrome characterized by truncal obesity, hypertension, fatigability and weakness, amenorrhea, hirsutism, purplish abdominal striae, edema, glucosuria, osteoporosis, and a basophilic tumor of the pituitary. As awareness of this syndrome has increased, the diagnosis of Cushing's syndrome has been broadened into the classification shown in Table 336-2. Regardless of etiology, all

---

TABLE 336-2 CAUSES OF CUSHING'S SYNDROME

Adrenal hyperplasia
  Secondary to pituitary ACTH overproduction
    Pituitary-hypothalamic dysfunction
    Pituitary ACTH-producing micro- or macroadenomas
  Secondary to ACTH or CRH-producing nonendocrine tumors
    (bronchogenic carcinoma, carcinoid of the thymus, pancreatic
    carcinoma, bronchial adenoma)
Adrenal macronodular hyperplasia (including ectopic expression of GIP
  receptors in the adrenal cortex)
Adrenal micronodular dysplasia
  Sporadic
  Familial (Carney's syndrome)
Adrenal neoplasia
  Adenoma
  Carcinoma
Exogenous, iatrogenic causes
  Prolonged use of glucocorticoids
  Prolonged use of ACTH

Note: ACTH, adrenocorticotropic hormone; CRH, corticotropin-releasing hormone; GIP, gastric inhibitory peptide.

cases of endogenous Cushing's syndrome are due to increased production of cortisol by the adrenal. In most cases, the cause is *bilateral adrenal hyperplasia* due to hypersecretion of pituitary ACTH or ectopic production of ACTH by a nonpituitary source. The incidence of pituitary-dependent adrenal hyperplasia is three times greater in women than in men, and the most frequent age of onset is the third or fourth decade. Most evidence indicates that the primary defect is the de novo development of a pituitary adenoma, as tumors are found in >90% of patients with pituitary-dependent adrenal hyperplasia. Alternatively, the defect may occasionally reside in the hypothalamus or in higher neural centers, leading to release of CRH inappropriate to the level of circulating cortisol. This primary defect leads to hyperstimulation of the pituitary, resulting in hyperplasia or tumor formation. In surgical series, most individuals with hypersecretion of pituitary ACTH are found to have a microadenoma (<10 mm in diameter; 50% are ≤5 mm in diameter), but a pituitary macroadenoma (>10 mm) or diffuse hyperplasia of the corticotrope cells may be found. Traditionally, only an individual who has an ACTH-producing pituitary tumor is defined as having Cushing's *disease*, whereas Cushing's *syndrome* refers to all causes of excess cortisol: exogenous ACTH tumor, adrenal tumor, pituitary ACTH-secreting tumor, or excessive glucocorticoid treatment.

The *ectopic ACTH syndrome* is caused by nonpituitary tumors that secrete either ACTH and/or CRH and cause bilateral adrenal hyperplasia (Chap. 96). The ectopic production of CRH results in clinical, biochemical, and radiologic features indistinguishable from those caused by hypersecretion of pituitary ACTH. The typical signs and symptoms of Cushing's syndrome may be absent or minimal with ectopic ACTH production, and hypokalemic alkalosis is a prominent manifestation. Most of these cases are associated with the primitive small cell (oat cell) type of bronchogenic carcinoma or with carcinoid tumors of the thymus, pancreas, or ovary; medullary carcinoma of the thyroid; or bronchial adenomas. The onset of Cushing's syndrome may be sudden, particularly in patients with carcinoma of the lung, and this feature accounts in part for the failure of these patients to exhibit the classic manifestations. On the other hand, patients with carcinoid tumors or pheochromocytomas have longer clinical courses and usually exhibit the typical cushingoid features. The ectopic secretion of ACTH is also accompanied by the accumulation of ACTH fragments in plasma and by elevated plasma levels of ACTH precursor molecules. Because such tumors may produce large amounts of ACTH, baseline steroid values are usually very high and increased skin pigmentation may be present.

Approximately 20–25% of patients with Cushing's syndrome have an adrenal neoplasm. These tumors are usually unilateral, and about half are malignant. Occasionally, patients have biochemical features both of pituitary ACTH excess and of an adrenal adenoma. These individuals may have *nodular hyperplasia* of both adrenal glands, often the result of prolonged ACTH stimulation in the absence of a pituitary adenoma. Two additional entities cause nodular hyperplasia: a familial disorder in children or young adults (so-called pigmented micronodular dysplasia; see below) and an abnormal cortisol response to gastric inhibitory polypeptide or luteinizing hormone, secondary to ectopic expression of receptors for these hormones in the adrenal cortex.

The most common cause of Cushing's syndrome is *iatrogenic* administration of steroids for a variety of reasons. Although the clinical features bear some resemblance to those seen with adrenal tumors, these patients are usually distinguishable on the basis of history and laboratory studies.

Clinical Signs, Symptoms, and Laboratory Findings Many of the signs and symptoms of Cushing's syndrome follow logically from the known action of glucocorticoids (Table 336-3). Catabolic responses in peripheral supportive tissue causes muscle weakness and fatigability, osteoporosis, broad violaceous cutaneous striae (Fig. 336-6), and easy bruisability. The latter signs are secondary to weakening and rupture of collagen fibers in the dermis. Osteoporosis may cause collapse of vertebral bodies and pathologic fractures of other bones. Decreased bone mineralization is particularly pronounced in children. Increased hepatic gluconeogene-

TABLE 336-3 FREQUENCY OF SIGNS AND SYMPTOMS IN CUSHING'S SYNDROME

Sign or Symptom	Percent of Patients
Typical habitus (centripetal obesity)[a]	97
Increased body weight	94
Fatigability and weakness	87
Hypertension (blood pressure > 150/90)	82
Hirsutism[a]	80
Amenorrhea	77
Broad violaceous cutaneous striae[a]	67
Personality changes	66
Ecchymoses[a]	65
Proximal myopathy[a]	62
Edema	62
Polyuria, polydipsia	23
Hypertrophy of clitoris	19

[a]Features more specific for Cushing's syndrome.

sis and insulin resistance can cause impaired glucose tolerance. Overt diabetes mellitus occurs in <20% of patients, who probably are individuals with a predisposition to this disorder. Hypercortisolism promotes the deposition of adipose tissue in characteristic sites, notably the upper face (producing the typical "moon" facies), the interscapular area (producing the "buffalo hump"), supraclavicular fat pads, and the mesenteric bed (producing "truncal" obesity) (Fig. 336-6). Rarely, episternal fatty tumors and mediastinal widening secondary to fat accumulation occur. The reason for this peculiar distribution of adipose tissue is not known, but it is associated with insulin resistance and/or elevated insulin levels. The face appears plethoric, even in the absence of any increase in red blood cell concentration. Hypertension is common, and emotional changes may be profound, ranging from irritability and emotional lability to severe depression, confusion, or even frank psychosis. In women, increased levels of adrenal androgens can cause acne, hirsutism, and oligomenorrhea or amenorrhea. Some signs and symptoms in patients with hypercortisolism—i.e., obesity, hypertension, osteoporosis, and diabetes—are nonspecific and therefore are less helpful in diagnosing the condition. On the other hand, easy bruising, typical striae, myopathy, and virilizing signs (although less frequent) are, if present, more suggestive of Cushing's syndrome (Table 336-3).

Except in iatrogenic Cushing's syndrome, plasma and urine cortisol levels are elevated. Occasionally, hypokalemia, hypochloremia, and metabolic alkalosis are present, particularly with ectopic production of ACTH.

Diagnosis The diagnosis of Cushing's syndrome depends on the demonstration of increased cortisol production and failure to suppress

FIGURE 336-6 Clinical features of Cushing's syndrome. Note the central obesity and wide, violaceous striae.

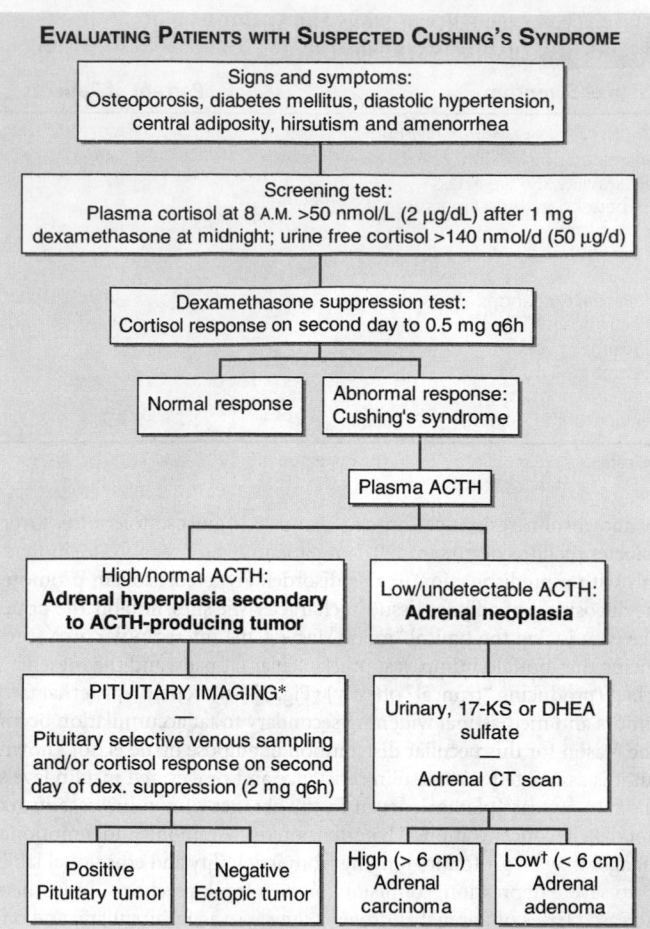

EVALUATING PATIENTS WITH SUSPECTED CUSHING'S SYNDROME

Signs and symptoms:
Osteoporosis, diabetes mellitus, diastolic hypertension, central adiposity, hirsutism and amenorrhea

Screening test:
Plasma cortisol at 8 A.M. >50 nmol/L (2 μg/dL) after 1 mg dexamethasone at midnight; urine free cortisol >140 nmol/d (50 μg/d)

Dexamethasone suppression test:
Cortisol response on second day to 0.5 mg q6h

Normal response

Abnormal response:
Cushing's syndrome

Plasma ACTH

High/normal ACTH:
Adrenal hyperplasia secondary to ACTH-producing tumor

Low/undetectable ACTH:
Adrenal neoplasia

PITUITARY IMAGING*
—
Pituitary selective venous sampling and/or cortisol response on second day of dex. suppression (2 mg q6h)

Urinary, 17-KS or DHEA sulfate
—
Adrenal CT scan

Positive Pituitary tumor

Negative Ectopic tumor

High (> 6 cm) Adrenal carcinoma

Low† (< 6 cm) Adrenal adenoma

FIGURE 336-7 Evaluating patients suspected of having Cushing's syndrome. *A microadenoma or macroadenoma may be visualized by pituitary magnetic resonance scanning. †Risk of carcinoma in adrenal tumors 4–6 cm is 6%. Radiographic clues include tumor heterogeneity and irregular borders (see Fig. 336-8). 17-KS, 17-ketosteroids; DHEA, dehydroepiandrosterone; ACTH, adrenocorticotropic hormone; CT, computed tomography.

cortisol secretion normally when dexamethasone is administered (Chap. 333). Once the diagnosis is established, further testing is designed to determine the etiology (Fig. 336-7 and Table 336-4).

For initial screening, the overnight dexamethasone suppression test is recommended (see above). In difficult cases (e.g., in obese or depressed patients), measurement of a 24-h urine free cortisol can also be used as a screening test. A level >140 nmol/d (50 μg/d) is suggestive of Cushing's syndrome. The definitive diagnosis is then established by failure of urinary cortisol to fall to <25 nmol/d (10 μg/d) or of plasma cortisol to fall to <140 nmol/L (5 μg/dL) after a standard low-dose dexamethasone suppression test (0.5 mg every 6 h for 48 h). Owing to circadian variability, plasma cortisol and, to a certain extent, ACTH determinations are not meaningful when performed in isolation, but the absence of the normal fall of plasma cortisol at midnight is consis-

tent with Cushing's syndrome because there is loss of the diurnal cortisol rhythm.

The task of determining the etiology of Cushing's syndrome is complicated by the fact that all the available tests lack specificity and by the fact that the tumors producing this syndrome are prone to spontaneous and often dramatic changes in hormone secretion (periodic hormonogenesis). No test has a specificity >95%, and it may be necessary to use a combination of tests to arrive at the correct diagnosis.

Plasma ACTH levels can be useful in distinguishing the various causes of Cushing's syndrome, particularly in separating ACTH-dependent from ACTH-independent causes. In general, measurement of plasma ACTH is useful in the diagnosis of ACTH-independent etiologies of the syndrome, since most adrenal tumors cause low or undetectable ACTH levels [<2 pmol/L (10 pg/mL)]. Furthermore, ACTH-secreting pituitary macroadenomas and ACTH-producing nonendocrine tumors usually result in elevated ACTH levels. In the ectopic ACTH syndrome, ACTH levels may be elevated to >110 pmol/L (500 pg/mL), and in most patients the level is >40 pmol/L (200 pg/mL). In Cushing's syndrome as the result of a microadenoma or pituitary-hypothalamic dysfunction, ACTH levels range from 6–30 pmol/L (30–150 pg/mL) [normal, <14 pmol/L (<60 pg/mL)], with half of values falling in the normal range. However, the main problem with the use of ACTH levels in the differential diagnosis of Cushing's syndrome is that ACTH levels may be similar in individuals with hypothalamic-pituitary dysfunction, pituitary microadenomas, ectopic CRH production, and ectopic ACTH production (especially carcinoid tumors) (Table 336-4).

A useful step to distinguish patients with an ACTH-secreting pituitary microadenoma or hypothalamic-pituitary dysfunction from those with other forms of Cushing's syndrome is to determine the response of cortisol output to administration of high-dose dexamethasone (2 mg every 6 h for 2 days). An alternative 8-mg, overnight high-dose dexamethasone test has been developed; however, this test has a lower sensitivity and specificity than the standard test. When the diagnosis of Cushing's syndrome is clear-cut on the basis of baseline urinary and plasma assays, the high-dose dexamethasone suppression test may be used without performing the preliminary low-dose suppression test. The high-dose suppression test provides close to 100% specificity if the criterion used is suppression of urinary free cortisol by >90%. Occasionally, in individuals with bilateral nodular hyperplasia and/or ectopic CRH production, steroid output is also suppressed. Failure of low- and high-dose dexamethasone administration to suppress cortisol production (Table 336-4) can occur in patients with adrenal hyperplasia secondary to an ACTH-secreting pituitary macroadenoma or an ACTH-producing tumor of nonendocrine origin and in those with adrenal neoplasms.

Because of these difficulties, several additional tests have been advocated, such as the metyrapone and CRH infusion tests. The rationale underlying these tests is that steroid hypersecretion by an adrenal tumor or the ectopic production of ACTH will suppress the hypothalamic-pituitary axis so that inhibition of pituitary ACTH release can be demonstrated by either test. Thus, most patients with pituitary-hypothalamic dysfunction and/or a microadenoma have an increase in steroid or ACTH secretion in response to metyrapone or CRH administration, whereas most patients with ectopic ACTH-producing tumors do not. Most pituitary macroadenomas also respond to CRH, but their response to metyrapone is variable. However, false-positive and false-negative CRH tests can occur in patients with ectopic ACTH and pituitary tumors.

The main diagnostic dilemma in Cushing's syndrome is to distinguish those instances due to microadenomas of the pituitary from those due to ectopic sources (e.g., carcinoids or pheochromocytoma) that produce CRH and/or ACTH. The clinical manifestations are

TABLE 336-4 DIAGNOSTIC TESTS TO DETERMINE THE TYPE OF CUSHING'S SYNDROME

Test	Pituitary Macroadenoma	Pituitary Microadenoma	Ectopic ACTH or CRH Production	Adrenal Tumor
Plasma ACTH level	↑ to ↑↑	N to ↑	↑ to ↑↑↑	↓
Percent who respond to high-dose dexamethasone	<10	95	<10	<10
Percent who respond to CRH	>90	>90	<10	<10

Note: ACTH, adrenocorticotropic hormone; CRH, corticotropin-releasing hormone; N, normal; ↑, elevated; ↓, decreased. See text for definition of a response.

similar unless the ectopic tumor produces other symptoms, such as diarrhea and flushing from a carcinoid tumor or episodic hypertension from a pheochromocytoma. Sometimes, one can distinguish between ectopic and pituitary ACTH production by using metyrapone or CRH tests, as noted above. In these situations, CT of the pituitary gland is usually normal. MRI with the enhancing agent gadolinium may be better than CT for this purpose but demonstrates pituitary microadenomas in only half of patients with Cushing's disease. Because microadenomas can be detected in up to 10–20% of individuals without known pituitary disease, a positive imaging study does not prove that the pituitary is the source of ACTH excess. In those with negative imaging studies, selective petrosal sinus venous sampling for ACTH is now used in many referral centers. ACTH levels are measured at baseline, 2, 5, and 10 min after ovine CRH (1 μ/kg IV) injections. Peak petrosal:peripheral ACTH ratios of >3:1 confirm the presence of a pituitary ACTH-secreting tumor. In centers where petrosal sinus sampling is performed frequently, it has proved highly sensitive for distinguishing pituitary and nonpituitary sources of ACTH excess. However, the catheterization procedure is technically difficult, and complications have occurred.

The diagnosis of a *cortisol-producing adrenal adenoma* is suggested by low ACTH and disproportionate elevations in baseline urine free cortisol levels with only modest changes in urinary 17-ketosteroids or plasma DHEA sulfate. Adrenal androgen secretion is usually reduced in these patients owing to the cortisol-induced suppression of ACTH and subsequent involution of the androgen-producing zona reticularis.

The diagnosis of *adrenal carcinoma* is suggested by a palpable abdominal mass and by markedly elevated baseline values of both urine 17-ketosteroids and plasma DHEA sulfate. Plasma and urine cortisol levels are variably elevated. Adrenal carcinoma is usually resistant to both ACTH stimulation and dexamethasone suppression. Elevated adrenal androgen secretion often leads to virilization in the female. Estrogen-producing adrenocortical carcinoma usually presents with gynecomastia in men and dysfunctional uterine bleeding in women. These adrenal tumors secrete increased amounts of androstenedione, which is converted peripherally to the estrogens estrone and estradiol. Adrenal carcinomas that produce Cushing's syndrome are often associated with elevated levels of the intermediates of steroid biosynthesis (especially 11-deoxycortisol), suggesting inefficient conversion of the intermediates to the final product. This feature also accounts for the characteristic increase in 17-ketosteroids. Approximately 20% of adrenal carcinomas are not associated with endocrine syndromes and are presumed to be nonfunctioning or to produce biologically inactive steroid precursors. In addition, the excessive production of steroids is not always clinically evident (e.g., androgens in adult men).

Differential Diagnosis • PSEUDO-CUSHING'S SYNDROME Problems in diagnosis include patients with obesity, chronic alcoholism, depression, and acute illness of any type. Extreme *obesity* is uncommon in Cushing's syndrome; furthermore, with exogenous obesity, the adiposity is generalized, not truncal. On adrenocortical testing, abnormalities in patients with exogenous obesity are usually modest. Basal urine steroid excretion levels in obese patients are also either normal or slightly elevated, and the diurnal pattern in blood and urine levels is normal. Patients with *chronic alcoholism* and those with *depression* share similar abnormalities in steroid output: modestly elevated urine cortisol, blunted circadian rhythm of cortisol levels, and resistance to suppression using the overnight dexamethasone test. In contrast to alcoholic subjects, depressed patients do not have signs and symptoms of Cushing's syndrome. Following discontinuation of alcohol and/or improvement in the emotional status, results of steroid testing usually return to normal. One or more of three tests have been used to differentiate mild Cushing's syndrome and pseudo-Cushing's syndrome. The serum cortisol level following the standard 2-day low-dose dexamethasone test has very high sensitivity and specificity. Although the CRH test alone is less useful, in combination with the low-dose dexamethasone test, there is nearly complete discrimination between these two conditions. Finally, a midnight cortisol level obtained in awake patients may have similar predictive value as the low-dose dexametha-

sone test if a cut-off of 210 nmol/L (7.5 μg/dL) is used. Patients with *acute illness* often have abnormal results on laboratory tests and fail to exhibit pituitary-adrenal suppression in response to dexamethasone, since major stress (such as pain or fever) interrupts the normal regulation of ACTH secretion. *Iatrogenic Cushing's syndrome*, induced by the administration of glucocorticoids or other steroids such as megestrol that bind to the glucocorticoid receptor, is indistinguishable by physical findings from endogenous adrenocortical hyperfunction. The distinction can be made, however, by measuring blood or urine cortisol levels in a basal state; in the iatrogenic syndrome these levels are low secondary to suppression of the pituitary-adrenal axis. The severity of iatrogenic Cushing's syndrome is related to the total steroid dose, the biologic half-life of the steroid, and the duration of therapy. Also, individuals taking afternoon and evening doses of glucocorticoids develop Cushing's syndrome more readily and with a smaller total daily dose than do patients taking morning doses only.

Radiologic Evaluation for Cushing's Syndrome The preferred radiologic study for visualizing the adrenals is a CT scan of the abdomen (Fig. 336-8). CT is of value both for localizing adrenal tumors and for diagnosing bilateral hyperplasia. All patients believed to have hypersecretion of pituitary ACTH should have a pituitary MRI scan with gadolinium contrast. Even with this technique, small microadenomas may be undetectable; alternatively, false-positive masses due to cysts or nonsecretory lesions of the normal pituitary may be imaged. In patients with ectopic ACTH production, high-resolution chest CT is a useful first step.

Evaluation of Asymptomatic Adrenal Masses Many incidental masses (so-called incidentalomas) are discovered during radiographic testing for another condition, rather than testing performed because of a suspected adrenal disorder. This is not surprising since ~6% of adult/elderly subjects at autopsy have adrenocortical adenomas. However, the prevalence of incidental adenomas is age-dependent, i.e., cortical adenomas are very uncommon in individuals <30 years of age.

An important early step in the evaluation of adrenal incidentalomas is to determine whether the patient has a history of prior malignancy. In this circumstance, the adrenal mass will be a metastasis in about one-half of the patients. If the primary tumor is being treated and there are no other metastases, it may be prudent to obtain a biopsy of the mass. A CT-guided fine-needle aspiration (FNA) can usually identify nonadrenal or metastatic tissue. However, pheochromocytoma should always be excluded before a FNA is performed.

The next step is to determine whether the tumor is functioning, although the great majority (70–80%) are nonsecretory. Overt clinical symptoms are usually absent in incidentally discovered adrenal masses, but the clinician should search for subtle signs and symptoms of hormonal overproduction, such as Cushingoid features and paroxysmal symptomatology. All patients with incidentally discovered masses should be screened for pheochromocytoma (Chap. 337), regardless of radiographic features that are considered typical for cortical adenomas (see below). Measurement of plasma free metanephrines is the recommended test due its high sensitivity, and a negative test essentially rules out this disorder. All patients should also be screened with an overnight dexamethasone-suppression test since autonomous cortisol production in patients without typical features of hypercortisolism (so-called preclinical or subclinical Cushing's syndrome) is the most common hypersecretory syndrome in incidentally discovered adrenal masses (Fig. 336-9). Such patients may experience side effects of mild overproduction of cortisol (such as hypertension, glucose intolerance, and osteoporosis) and may benefit from excision of the mass. Patients with hypertension should also be screened for primary aldosteronism by measurement of plasma aldosterone and plasma renin activity. Finally, females with signs of androgen excess or males with feminization should be tested for the overproduction of the appropriate sex steroids.

A major consideration is whether the incidentally discovered mass is an adrenocortical carcinoma (ACC). Although the probability of

FIGURE 336-8 CT and MRI of the adrenal glands. A. Normal adrenal on CT. **B.** Normal adrenal on T1-weighted MRI. **C.** CT of benign adrenal adenoma. Right adrenal mass with 1.5 cm homogeneous attenuation (–5 Hounsfield units). **D.** Right adrenal mass (2 cm) showing homogeneous intermediate signal intensity on MRI in-phase gradient echo sequence. **E.** There is homogeneous loss of signal on the corresponding out-of-phase sequence, consistent with a diagnosis of adrenal adenoma.

ACC is very low (<0.01%), and the vast majority of adrenal masses are benign adenomas, ACC is associated with a poor prognosis, especially if discovered at a late stage. Radiographic characterization of the adrenal mass has been crucial in this decision-making process; size and imaging phenotype are the best predictors of possible malignancy. Features suggestive of malignancy include: large size (>4–6 cm), irregular margins and tumor inhomogeneity, soft tissue calcifications visible on CT, and high unenhanced CT attenuation values (>10 HU). Similar findings characteristic of malignancy are seen on chemical-shift MRI. In contrast, the common benign adrenocortical adenoma is characterized by diameter < 4 cm and tumor homogeneity with sharp margins and low unenhanced CT values (<10 HU). FNA is not useful to distinguish between benign and malignant primary adrenal tumors. If the radiographic criteria favor a benign adrenocortical neoplasm, reassurance is gained if the mass remains unchanged in size at follow-up scanning in 3–6 months. On the other hand, benign cortical adenomas may increase in size (up to 1–2 cm) over several years of follow-up.

℞ CUSHING'S SYNDROME

ADRENAL NEOPLASM   Adrenal adenomas may be resected using laparoscopic techniques. Because of the possibility of atrophy of the contralateral adrenal, the patient should be treated with glucocorticoids and mineralocorticoids pre- and postoperatively as if for total adrenalectomy, even when a unilateral lesion is suspected, the routine being similar to that for an Addisonian patient undergoing elective surgery (see below).

Despite operative intervention, most patients with adrenal carcinoma die within 3 years of diagnosis. Metastases occur most often to liver and lung. The principal drug for the treatment of adrenocortical carcinoma is mitotane (o,p'-DDD), an isomer of the insecticide DDT. Mitotane suppresses cortisol production and decreases plasma and urine steroid levels. Al-

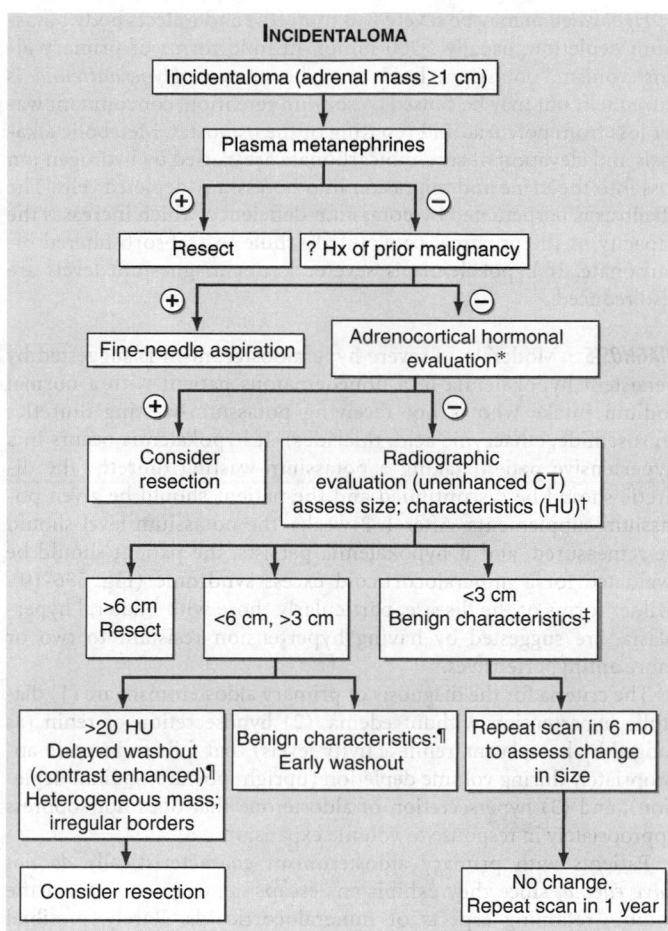

FIGURE 336-9 Incidentaloma. *Adrenocortical hormonal evaluation: Dexamethasone suppression test in all patients; plasma renin activity/aldosterone ratio for hypertensives; sex steroid (DHEA sulfate, estradiol) for clinical signs in females and males, respectively. †Hounsfield units (HU): a measurement of x-ray attenuation or lipid content of neoplasms. A lipid-rich mass (< 10 HU) is diagnostic of a benign cortical adenoma. ‡Benign characteristics: homogeneous mass, smooth borders, HU <10. ¶Benign adrenal adenomas are also characterized by earlier washout of contrast enhancement than other neoplasms.

though its cytotoxic action is relatively selective for the glucocorticoid-secreting zone of the adrenal cortex, the zona glomerulosa may also be inhibited. Because mitotane also alters the extraadrenal metabolism of cortisol, plasma and urinary cortisol levels must be assessed to titrate the effect. The drug is usually given in divided doses three to four times a day, with the dose increased gradually to tolerability (usually <6 g daily). At higher doses, almost all patients experience side effects, which may be gastrointestinal (anorexia, diarrhea, vomiting) or neuromuscular (lethargy, somnolence, dizziness). All patients treated with mitotane should receive long-term glucocorticoid maintenance therapy, and, in some, mineralocorticoid replacement is appropriate. In approximately one-third of patients, both tumor and metastases regress, but long-term survival is not altered. In many patients, mitotane only inhibits steroidogenesis and does not cause regression of tumor metastases. Osseous metastases are usually refractory to the drug and should be treated with radiation therapy. Mitotane can also be given as adjunctive therapy after surgical resection of an adrenal carcinoma, although there is no evidence that this improves survival. Because of the absence of a long-term benefit with mitotane, alternative chemotherapeutic approaches based on platinum therapy have been used. However, there are no data presently available indicating a prolongation of life.

BILATERAL HYPERPLASIA Patients with hyperplasia usually have a relative or absolute increase in ACTH levels. Since therapy would logi-

cally be directed at reducing ACTH levels, the ideal primary treatment for ACTH- or CRH-producing tumors, whether pituitary or ectopic, is surgical removal. Occasionally (particularly with ectopic ACTH production) surgical excision is not possible because the disease is far advanced. In this situation, "medical" or surgical adrenalectomy may correct the hypercortisolism.

Controversy exists as to the proper treatment for bilateral adrenal hyperplasia when the source of the ACTH overproduction is not apparent. In some centers, these patients (especially those who suppress after the administration of a high-dose dexamethasone test) undergo surgical exploration of the pituitary via a transsphenoidal approach in the expectation that a microadenoma will be found (Chap. 333). However, in most circumstances selective petrosal sinus venous sampling is recommended, and the patient is referred to an appropriate center if the procedure is not available locally. If a microadenoma is not found at the time of exploration, total hypophysectomy may be needed. Complications of transsphenoidal surgery include cerebrospinal fluid rhinorrhea, diabetes insipidus, panhypopituitarism, and optic or cranial nerve injuries.

In other centers, total adrenalectomy is the treatment of choice. The cure rate with this procedure is close to 100%. The adverse effects include the certain need for lifelong mineralocorticoid and glucocorticoid replacement and a 10–20% probability of a pituitary tumor developing over the next 10 years (Nelson's syndrome; Chap. 333). It is uncertain whether these tumors arise de novo or if they were present prior to adrenalectomy but were too small to be detected. Periodic radiologic evaluation of the pituitary gland by MRI as well as serial ACTH measurements should be performed in all individuals after bilateral adrenalectomy for Cushing's disease. Such pituitary tumors may become locally invasive and impinge on the optic chiasm or extend into the cavernous or sphenoid sinuses.

Except in children, pituitary irradiation is rarely used as primary treatment, being reserved rather for postoperative tumor recurrences. In some centers, high levels of gamma radiation can be focused on the desired site with less scattering to surrounding tissues by using stereotactic techniques. Side effects of radiation include ocular motor palsy and hypopituitarism. There is a long lag time between treatment and remission, and the remission rate is usually <50%.

Finally, in occasional patients in whom a surgical approach is not feasible, "medical" adrenalectomy may be indicated **(Table 336-5)**. Inhibition of steroidogenesis may also be indicated in severely cushingoid patients prior to surgical intervention. Chemical adrenalectomy may be accomplished by the administration of the inhibitor of steroidogenesis ketoconazole (600–1200 mg/d). In addition, mitotane (2 or 3 g/d) and/or the blockers of steroid synthesis aminoglutethimide (1 g/d) and metyrapone (2 or 3 g/d) may be effective either alone or in combination. Mitotane is slow to take effect (weeks). Mifepristone, a competitive inhibitor of the binding of glucocorticoid to its receptor, may be a treatment option. Adrenal insufficiency is a risk with all these agents, and replacement steroids may be required.

ALDOSTERONISM

Aldosteronism is a syndrome associated with hypersecretion of the mineralocorticoid aldosterone. In *primary* aldosteronism the cause for the excessive aldosterone production resides within the adrenal gland; in *secondary* aldosteronism the stimulus is extraadrenal.

TABLE 336-5 **TREATMENT MODALITIES FOR PATIENTS WITH ADRENAL HYPERPLASIA SECONDARY TO PITUITARY ACTH HYPERSECRETION**

Treatments to reduce pituitary ACTH production
   Transsphenoidal resection of microadenoma
   Radiation therapy
Treatments to reduce or eliminate adrenocortical cortisol secretion
   Bilateral adrenalectomy
   Medical adrenalectomy (metyrapone, mitotane, aminoglutethimide, ketoconazole)[a]

[a]Not curative but effective as long as chronically administered in selected patients.
Note: ACTH, adrenocorticotropic hormone.

Primary Aldosteronism with an Adrenal Tumor In the original descriptions of excessive and inappropriate aldosterone production, the disease was the result of an *aldosterone-producing adrenal adenoma* (Conn's syndrome). Most cases involve a unilateral adenoma, which is usually small and may occur on either side. Rarely, primary aldosteronism is due to an adrenal carcinoma. Aldosteronism is twice as common in women as in men, usually occurs between the ages of 30 and 50, and is present in ~1% of unselected hypertensive patients.

Primary Aldosteronism without an Adrenal Tumor In many patients with clinical and biochemical features of primary aldosteronism, a solitary adenoma is not found at surgery. Instead, these patients have *bilateral cortical nodular hyperplasia*. In the literature, this disease is also termed *idiopathic hyperaldosteronism*, and/or *nodular hyperplasia*. The cause is unknown. Often it is difficult to distinguish these patients from those with low renin essential hypertension. In contrast to patients with an aldosteronoma, those with bilateral hyperplasia are unlikely to have hypokalemia and usually have lower levels of aldosterone and less radiologic evidence for adrenal pathology. They constitute perhaps as many as 80% of patients with primary aldosteronism and largely contribute to the increased prevalence of primary aldosteronism reported during the past few years. Although the prevalence of the tumor form of primary aldosteronism in the general hypertension population remains in the ≤1% range, the prevalence of the bilateral hyperplasia form has been reported to range as high as 10%, depending on the criteria used and the study population.

SIGNS AND SYMPTOMS Hypersecretion of aldosterone increases the renal distal tubular exchange of intratubular sodium for secreted potassium and hydrogen ions, with progressive depletion of body potassium and development of hypokalemia. Most patients have diastolic hypertension, which may be very severe, and headaches. The hypertension is probably due to the increased sodium reabsorption and extracellular volume expansion. *Potassium depletion* is responsible for the muscle weakness and fatigue and is due to the effect of potassium depletion on the muscle cell membrane. The polyuria results from impairment of urinary concentrating ability and is often associated with polydipsia. However, some individuals with mild disease, particularly most with the bilateral hyperplasia type, may have potassium levels in the low normal range and therefore have no symptoms associated with hypokalemia.

Electrocardiographic and roentgenographic signs of left ventricular enlargement are, in part, secondary to the hypertension. However, the left ventricular hypertrophy is disproportionate to the level of blood pressure when compared to individuals with essential hypertension, and regression of the hypertrophy occurs even if blood pressure is not reduced after removal of an aldosteronoma. If potassium depletion is present, there may be electrocardiographic signs of hypokalemia including prominent U waves, cardiac arrhythmias, and premature contractions. In the absence of associated congestive heart failure, renal disease, or preexisting abnormalities (such as thrombophlebitis), edema is characteristically absent. However, structural damage to the cerebral circulation, retinal vasculature, and kidney occurs more frequently than would be predicted based on the level and duration of the hypertension. Proteinuria may occur in as many as 50% of patients with primary aldosteronism, and renal failure occurs in up to 15%. Thus, it is probable that excess aldosterone production induces cardiovascular damage independent of its effect on blood pressure.

LABORATORY FINDINGS Laboratory findings depend on both the duration and the severity of potassium depletion. An overnight concentration test often reveals impaired ability to concentrate the urine, probably secondary to the hypokalemia. Urine pH is neutral to alkaline because of excessive secretion of ammonium and bicarbonate ions to compensate for the metabolic alkalosis. Again these findings are infrequent in patients with bilateral hyperplasia.

Hypokalemia may be severe (<3 mmol/L) and reflects body potassium depletion, usually >300 mmol. In mild forms of primary aldosteronism, potassium levels may be normal. *Hypernatremia* is infrequent but may be caused by sodium retention, concomitant water loss from polyuria, and resetting of the osmostat. Metabolic alkalosis and elevation of serum bicarbonate are caused by hydrogen ion loss into the urine and migration into potassium-depleted cells. The alkalosis is perpetuated by potassium deficiency, which increases the capacity of the proximal convoluted tubule to reabsorb filtered bicarbonate. If hypokalemia is severe, serum magnesium levels are also reduced.

DIAGNOSIS Moderate to severe hyperaldosteronism is suggested by persistent hypokalemia in a nonedematous patient with a normal sodium intake who is not receiving potassium-wasting diuretics (furosemide, ethacrynic acid, thiazides). If hypokalemia occurs in a hypertensive patient taking a potassium-wasting diuretic, the diuretic should be discontinued and the patient should be given potassium supplements. After 1–2 weeks, the potassium level should be remeasured, and if hypokalemia persists, the patient should be evaluated for a mineralocorticoid excess syndrome (Fig. 336-10). Milder forms of the disease, particularly those with bilateral hyperplasia, are suggested by having hypertension resistant to two or more antihypertensives.

The criteria for the diagnosis of primary aldosteronism are (1) diastolic hypertension without edema, (2) hyposecretion of renin (as judged by low plasma renin activity levels) that fails to increase appropriately during volume depletion (upright posture, sodium depletion), and (3) hypersecretion of aldosterone that does not suppress appropriately in response to volume expansion.

Patients with primary aldosteronism characteristically *do not have edema*, since they exhibit an "escape" phenomenon from the sodium-retaining aspects of mineralocorticoids. Rarely, pretibial edema is present in patients with associated nephropathy and azotemia.

The estimation of plasma renin activity is of limited value in separating patients with primary aldosteronism from those with hypertension of other causes. Although failure of plasma renin activity to rise normally during volume-depletion maneuvers is a criterion for the diagnosis of primary aldosteronism, suppressed renin activity also occurs in 25% of patients with essential hypertension.

Although a renin measurement alone lacks specificity, the ratio of serum aldosterone to plasma renin activity is a very useful screening test. A high ratio (>30), when aldosterone is expressed as ng/dL and plasma renin activity as ng/mL per hour, strongly suggests autonomy of aldosterone secretion. Aldosterone levels need to be >500 pmol/L (>15 ng/dL) when salt intake is not restricted. In some centers, the aldosterone/plasma renin activity ratio is used as a primary screen test in all normokalemic, difficult-to-control hypertensive patients, in addition to those with hypokalemia. Ultimately, it is necessary to demonstrate a lack of aldosterone suppression to diagnose primary aldosteronism (Fig. 336-10). The autonomy exhibited in these patients refers only to the resistance to suppression of secretion during volume expansion; aldosterone can and does respond in a normal or above-normal fashion to the stimulus of potassium loading or ACTH infusion.

Once hyposecretion of renin and failure of aldosterone secretion suppression are demonstrated, aldosterone-producing adenomas should be localized by abdominal CT scan, using a high-resolution scanner as many aldosteronomas are <1 cm in size. If the CT scan is negative, percutaneous transfemoral bilateral adrenal vein catheterization with adrenal vein sampling may demonstrate a two- to threefold increase in plasma aldosterone concentration on the involved side. In cases of hyperaldosteronism secondary to cortical nodular hyperplasia, no lateralization is found. It is important for samples to be obtained simultaneously, if possible, and for cortisol levels to be measured to ensure that false localization does not reflect dilution or an ACTH- or stress-induced rise in aldosterone levels. In a patient

EVALUATING HYPERTENSIVE PATIENTS WITH SUSPECTED MINERALOCORTICOID EXCESS STATES

FIGURE 336-10 Diagnostic flowchart for evaluating patients with possible mineralocorticoid excess states, including primary aldosteronism (PA). *Serum K+ may be normal in some patients with mild mineralocorticoid excess states or those who are taking potassium-sparing diuretics (spironolactone, triamterene) or those who ingest low sodium and high potassium intakes. †Inadequate control of hypertension (HTN) on three antihypertensives (including a diuretic). ‡This step should not be taken if hypertension is severe (diastolic pressure > 115 mmHg) or if cardiac failure is present. Also, serum potassium levels should be corrected before the infusion of a saline solution. Alternative methods that produce comparable suppression of aldosterone secretion include oral sodium loading (200 mmol/d) and the administration of fludrocortisone, 0.2 mg bid, for 3–4 days. ¶For example, Liddle's syndrome, apparent mineralocorticoid excess syndrome, or a deoxycorticosterone-secreting tumor. §Consider diagnosis of glucocorticoid-remediable aldosteronism (GRA) in patients with early-onset HTN (< 20 years old) or those with a positive family history of early-onset HTN or primary aldosteronism. See text. AVS, bilateral adrenal vein sampling, to lateralize aldosterone production in APA or confirm bilateral secretion in IH; CT, computed tomography; MRA, mineralocorticoid receptor antagonist.

with an adenoma, the aldosterone/cortisol ratio lateralizes to the side of the lesion.

DIFFERENTIAL DIAGNOSIS   Patients with hypertension and hypokalemia may have either primary or secondary hyperaldosteronism (Fig. 336-11). A useful maneuver to distinguish between these conditions is the measurement of plasma renin activity. Secondary hyperaldosteronism in patients with accelerated hypertension is due to elevated plasma renin levels; in contrast, patients with primary aldosteronism have suppressed plasma renin levels. Indeed, in patients with a serum potassium concentration < 2.5 mmol/L, a high ratio of plasma aldosterone to plasma renin activity in a random sample is usually sufficient to establish the diagnosis of primary aldosteronism without additional testing. Ectopic ACTH production should also be considered in patients with hypertension and severe hypokalemia.

The most common problem is to distinguish between hyperaldosteronism due to an adenoma and that due to idiopathic bilateral nodular hyperplasia. This distinction is important because hypertension associated with idiopathic hyperplasia does not usually benefit from bilateral adrenalectomy, whereas hypertension associated with aldosterone-producing tumors is usually improved or cured by removal of the adenoma. Although patients with idiopathic bilateral nodular hyperplasia tend to have higher potassium levels (many in the normal range), lower aldosterone secretion, and higher plasma renin activity than do patients with primary aldosteronism, differentiation is impossible solely on clinical and/or biochemical grounds. An anomalous postural decrease in plasma aldosterone and elevated plasma 18-hydroxycorticosterone levels are present in most patients with a unilateral lesion. However, these tests are also of limited diagnostic value in the individual patient, because some adenoma patients have an increase in plasma aldosterone with upright posture, so-called renin-responsive aldosteronoma. A definitive diagnosis is best made by radiographic studies, including bilateral adrenal vein catheterization, as noted above.

Primary aldosteronism must also be distinguished from other *hypermineralocorticoid states*. In a few instances, hypertensive patients with hypokalemic alkalosis have adenomas that secrete deoxycorticosterone. Such patients have reduced plasma renin activity levels, but aldosterone levels are either normal or reduced, suggesting the diagnosis of mineralocorticoid excess due to a hormone other than aldosterone. Several inherited disorders have clinical features similar to those of primary aldosteronism (see below).

℞ PRIMARY ALDOSTERONISM

Primary aldosteronism due to an adenoma is usually treated by surgical excision of the adenoma. Where possible, a laparoscopic approach is favored. However, dietary sodium restriction and the administration of an aldosterone antagonist—e.g., spironolactone—are effective in many cases. Hypertension and hypokalemia are usually controlled by doses of 25–100 mg of spironolactone every 8 h. In some patients, medical man-

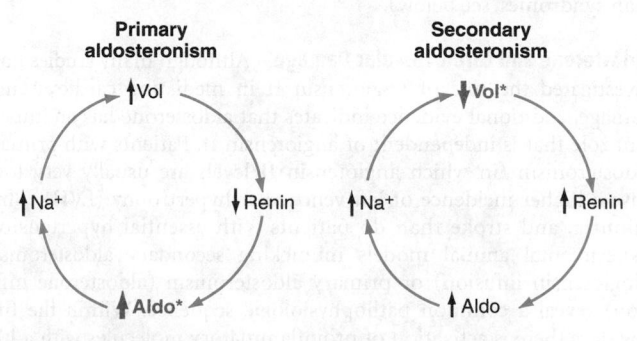

FIGURE 336-11 Responses of the renin-aldosterone volume control loop in primary versus secondary aldosteronism.

CHAPTER 336 Disorders of the Adrenal Cortex

agement has been successful for years, but chronic therapy in men is usually limited by side effects of spironolactone such as gynecomastia, decreased libido, and impotence. Eplerenone, a less potent but more specific MR antagonist with minimal, if any, antiandrogen effect is also useful in doses of 50–150 mg every 8 h.

When idiopathic bilateral hyperplasia is suspected, surgery is indicated only when significant, symptomatic hypokalemia cannot be controlled with medical therapy, i.e., by spironolactone, eplerenone, triamterene, or amiloride. Hypertension associated with idiopathic hyperplasia is usually not benefited by bilateral adrenalectomy.

Secondary Aldosteronism *Secondary aldosteronism* refers to an appropriately increased production of aldosterone in response to activation of the renin-angiotensin system (Fig. 336-11). The production rate of aldosterone is often higher in patients with secondary aldosteronism than in those with primary aldosteronism. Secondary aldosteronism usually occurs in association with the accelerated phase of hypertension or on the basis of an underlying edema disorder. Secondary aldosteronism in pregnancy is a normal physiologic response to estrogen-induced increases in circulating levels of renin substrate and plasma renin activity and to the antialdosterone actions of progestogens.

Secondary aldosteronism in hypertensive states is due either to a primary overproduction of renin (primary reninism) or to an overproduction of renin secondary to a decrease in renal blood flow and/or perfusion pressure (Fig. 336-11). Secondary hypersecretion of renin can be due to a narrowing of one or both of the major renal arteries by atherosclerosis or by fibromuscular hyperplasia. Overproduction of renin from both kidneys also occurs in severe arteriolar nephrosclerosis (malignant hypertension) or with profound renal vasoconstriction (the accelerated phase of hypertension). The secondary aldosteronism is characterized by hypokalemic alkalosis, moderate to severe increases in plasma renin activity, and moderate to marked increases in aldosterone levels.

Secondary aldosteronism with hypertension can also be caused by rare renin-producing tumors (primary reninism). In these patients, the biochemical characteristics are of renal vascular hypertension, but the primary defect is renin secretion by a juxtaglomerular cell tumor. The diagnosis can be made by demonstration of normal renal vasculature and/or demonstration of a space-occupying lesion in the kidney by radiographic techniques and documentation of a unilateral increase in renal vein renin activity. Rarely, these tumors arise in tissues such as the ovary.

Secondary aldosteronism is present in many forms of *edema*. The rate of aldosterone secretion is usually increased in patients with edema caused by either cirrhosis or the nephrotic syndrome. In congestive heart failure, elevated aldosterone secretion varies depending on the severity of cardiac failure. The stimulus for aldosterone release in these conditions appears to be *arterial hypovolemia* and/or hypotension. Thiazides and furosemide often exaggerate secondary aldosteronism via volume depletion; hypokalemia and, on occasion, alkalosis can then become prominent features. On occasion, secondary hyperaldosteronism occurs without edema or hypertension (Bartter and Gitelman syndromes, see below).

Aldosterone and Cardiovascular Damage Although many studies have investigated the role of angiotensin II in mediating cardiovascular damage, additional evidence indicates that aldosterone has an important role that is independent of angiotensin II. Patients with primary aldosteronism (in which angiotensin II levels are usually very low) have a higher incidence of left ventricular hypertrophy (LVH), albuminuria, and stroke than do patients with essential hypertension. Experimental animal models mimicking secondary aldosteronism (angiotensin infusion) or primary aldosteronism (aldosterone infusion) reveal a common pathophysiologic sequence. Within the first few days there is activation of proinflammatory molecules with a histologic picture of perivascular macrophage infiltrate and inflammation, followed by cellular death, fibrosis, and ventricular hypertrophy. These events are prevented if a MR antagonist is used or if adrenalec-

tomy is performed initially. The same pathophysiologic sequence is seen in animals with average aldosterone levels and cardiovascular damage, i.e., diabetes mellitus, or genetic hypertensive rats. There are two important additional observations. First, the level of sodium intake is a critical co-factor. If salt intake is severely restricted, no damage occurs even though the aldosterone levels are markedly elevated. Thus, it is not the level of aldosterone per se that is responsible for the damage, but its level relative to the volume or sodium status of the individual. Second, the dose of an MR antagonist required to prevent cardiovascular damage in these experimental models is much lower than that required to induce substantial volume depletion.

Several clinical trials support these experimental results. In the RALES trial, patients with class II/IV heart failure were randomized to standard care or a low dose of the MR antagonist, spironolactone. There was a 30% reduction in all-cause mortality and cardiovascular mortality and hospitalizations after 36 months. Two studies in hypertensive subjects addressed the question of the relative importance of a reduction of angiotensin II formation versus blockade of the MR in mediating cardiovascular damage. Subjects were randomized to eplerenone (an MR antagonist), enalapril (an ACE inhibitor), or both agents. In the first study, the subjects had LVH, with the endpoint being a reduction in LVH. In the second, the subjects had diabetes mellitus and proteinuria, with the endpoint being a reduction in proteinuria. In both studies, all three treatment arms substantially reduced the primary endpoint; however, the most potent effect occurred in the combination arms of the studies. In the monotherapy LVH arms, the reduction in LVH was similar, while in the proteinuria study, eplerenone produced a greater reduction than did enalapril. A follow-up study in diabetics with proteinuria provided insight into the maximally effective therapeutic dose. In this study, all subjects were treated with enalapril and randomized to treatment with placebo or 50 mg or 100 mg of eplerenone. The two doses reduced proteinuria to the same extent. These results, coupled with the low dose of spironolactone that was highly effective in the RALES trial, suggest that the maximally effective dose necessary to reduce cardiovascular damage is much lower than that required to reduce blood pressure maximally. The final study was the EPHESUS trial, where individuals who developed congestive heart failure after an acute myocardial infarction were randomized to standard-of-care treatment with or without a small dose of eplerenone. Eplerenone administration produced a significantly greater reduction in mortality (15–17%) and in cardiovascular-related hospitalizations than the placebo arm. These clinical studies provide strong support to the hypothesis that MR blockade has a significant added advantage over standard-of-care therapy in reducing cardiovascular mortality and surrogate adverse cardiovascular endpoints.

SYNDROMES OF ADRENAL ANDROGEN EXCESS

Adrenal androgen excess results from excess production of DHEA and androstenedione, which are converted to testosterone in extraglandular tissues; elevated testosterone levels account for most of the virilization. Adrenal androgen excess may be associated with the secretion of greater or smaller amounts of other adrenal hormones and may, therefore, present as "pure" syndromes of virilization or as "mixed" syndromes associated with excessive glucocorticoids and Cushing's syndrome. For further discussion of hirsutism and virilization, see Chap. 50.

HYPOFUNCTION OF THE ADRENAL CORTEX

Cases of adrenal insufficiency can be divided into two general categories: (1) those associated with primary inability of the adrenal to elaborate sufficient quantities of hormone, and (2) those associated with a secondary failure due to inadequate ACTH formation or release (Table 336-6).

PRIMARY ADRENOCORTICAL DEFICIENCY (ADDISON'S DISEASE)

The original description of Addison's disease—"general languor and debility, feebleness of the heart's action, irritability of the stomach, and

TABLE 336-6 CLASSIFICATION OF ADRENAL INSUFFICIENCY

Primary Adrenal Insuffiency

Anatomic destruction of gland (chronic or acute)
  "Idiopathic" atrophy (autoimmune, adrenoleukodystrophy)
  Surgical removal
  Infection (tuberculous, fungal, viral—especially in AIDS patients)
  Hemorrhage
  Invasion: metastatic
Metabolic failure in hormone production
  Congenital adrenal hyperplasia
  Enzyme inhibitors (metyrapone, ketoconazole, aminoglutethimide)
  Cytotoxic agents (mitotane)
ACTH-blocking antibodies
Mutation in ACTH receptor gene
Adrenal hypoplasia congenita

Secondary Adrenal Insufficiency

Hypopituitarism due to hypothalamic-pituitary disease
Suppression of hypothalamic-pituitary axis
  By exogenous steroid
  By endogenous steroid from tumor

Note: ACTH, adrenocorticotropic hormone.

a peculiar change of the color of the skin"—summarizes the dominant clinical features. Advanced cases are usually easy to diagnose, but recognition of the early phases can be challenging.

Incidence Acquired forms of primary insufficiency are relatively rare, may occur at any age, and affect both sexes equally. Because of the common therapeutic use of steroids, secondary adrenal insufficiency is relatively common.

Etiology and Pathogenesis Addison's disease results from progressive destruction of the adrenals, which must involve >90% of the glands before adrenal insufficiency appears. The adrenal is a frequent site for chronic granulomatous diseases, predominantly tuberculosis but also histoplasmosis, coccidioidomycosis, and cryptococcosis. In early series, tuberculosis was responsible for 70–90% of cases, but the most frequent cause now is *idiopathic* atrophy, and an autoimmune mechanism is probably responsible. Rarely, other lesions are encountered, such as adrenoleukodystrophy, bilateral hemorrhage, tumor metastases, HIV, cytomegalovirus (CMV), amyloidosis, adrenomyeloneuropathy, familial adrenal insufficiency, or sarcoidosis.

Although half of patients with idiopathic atrophy have circulating adrenal antibodies, autoimmune destruction is probably secondary to cytotoxic T lymphocytes. Specific adrenal antigens to which autoantibodies may be directed include 21-hydroxylase (CYP21A2) and side chain cleavage enzyme, but the significance of these antibodies in the pathogenesis of adrenal insufficiency is unknown. Some antibodies cause adrenal insufficiency by blocking the binding of ACTH to its receptors. Some patients also have antibodies to thyroid, parathyroid, and/or gonadal tissue (Chap. 345). There is also an increased incidence of chronic lymphocytic thyroiditis, premature ovarian failure, type 1 diabetes mellitus, and hypo- or hyperthyroidism. The presence of two or more of these autoimmune endocrine disorders in the same person defines the polyglandular autoimmune syndrome type II. Additional features include pernicious anemia, vitiligo, alopecia, nontropical sprue, and myasthenia gravis. Within families, multiple generations are affected by one or more of the above diseases. Type II polyglandular syndrome is associated with a mutant gene on chromosome 6 as well as with HLA alleles B8 and DR3.

The combination of parathyroid and adrenal insufficiency and chronic mucocutaneous candidiasis constitutes type I polyglandular autoimmune syndrome. Other autoimmune diseases in this disorder include pernicious anemia, chronic active hepatitis, alopecia, primary hypothyroidism, and premature gonadal failure. There is no HLA association; this syndrome is inherited as an autosomal recessive trait. It is caused by mutations in the *a*utoimmune *p*olyendocrinopathy candi-

diasis *e*ctodermal *d*ystrophy (APECED) gene located on chromosome 21q22.3. The gene encodes a transcription factor thought to be involved in lymphocyte function. The type I syndrome usually presents during childhood, whereas the type II syndrome is usually manifested in adulthood.

Clinical suspicion of adrenal insufficiency should be high in patients with AIDS (Chap. 182). CMV regularly involves the adrenal glands (so-called CMV necrotizing adrenalitis), and involvement with *Mycobacterium avium-intracellulare*, *Cryptococcus*, and Kaposi's sarcoma has been reported. Adrenal insufficiency in AIDS patients may not be manifest clinically, but tests of adrenal reserve frequently give abnormal results. When interpreting tests of adrenocortical function, it is important to remember that medications such as rifampin, phenytoin, ketoconazole, megestrol, and opiates may cause or potentiate adrenal insufficiency. Adrenal hemorrhage and infarction occur in patients on anticoagulants and in those with circulating anticoagulants and hypercoagulable states, such as the antiphospholipid syndrome.

There are several rare genetic causes of adrenal insufficiency that present primarily in infancy and childhood (see below).

Clinical Signs and Symptoms Adrenocortical insufficiency caused by gradual adrenal destruction is characterized by an insidious onset of fatigability, weakness, anorexia, nausea and vomiting, weight loss, cutaneous and mucosal pigmentation, hypotension, and occasionally hypoglycemia (Table 336-7). Depending on the duration and degree of adrenal hypofunction, the manifestations vary from mild chronic fatigue to fulminating shock associated with acute destruction of the glands, as described by Waterhouse and Friderichsen.

Asthenia is the cardinal symptom. Early it may be sporadic, usually most evident at times of stress; as adrenal function becomes more impaired, the patient is continuously fatigued, and bed rest is necessary.

Hyperpigmentation may be striking or absent. It commonly appears as a diffuse brown, tan, or bronze darkening of parts such as the elbows or creases of the hand and of areas that normally are pigmented such as the areolae about the nipples. Bluish-black patches may appear on the mucous membranes. Some patients develop dark freckles, and irregular areas of vitiligo may paradoxically be present. As an early sign, tanning following sun exposure may be persistent.

Arterial hypotension with postural accentuation is frequent, and blood pressure may be in the range of 80/50 or less.

Abnormalities of gastrointestinal function are often the presenting complaint. Symptoms vary from mild anorexia with weight loss to fulminating nausea, vomiting, diarrhea, and ill-defined abdominal pain, which may be so severe as to be confused with an acute abdomen. Patients may have personality changes, usually consisting of excessive irritability and restlessness. Enhancement of the sensory modalities of taste, olfaction, and hearing is reversible with therapy. Axillary and pubic hair may be decreased in women due to loss of adrenal androgens.

Laboratory Findings In the early phase of gradual adrenal destruction, there may be no demonstrable abnormalities in the routine laboratory parameters, but adrenal reserve is decreased—i.e., while basal steroid

TABLE 336-7 FREQUENCY OF SYMPTOMS AND SIGNS IN ADRENAL INSUFFICIENCY

Sign or Symptom	Percent of Patients
Weakness	99
Pigmentation of skin	98
Weight loss	97
Anorexia, nausea, and vomiting	90
Hypotension (<110/70)	87
Pigmentation of mucous membranes	82
Abdominal pain	34
Salt craving	22
Diarrhea	20
Constipation	19
Syncope	16
Vitiligo	9

output may be normal, a subnormal increase occurs after stress. Adrenal stimulation with ACTH uncovers abnormalities in this stage of the disease, eliciting a subnormal increase of cortisol levels or no increase at all. In more advanced stages of adrenal destruction, serum sodium, chloride, and bicarbonate levels are reduced, and the serum potassium level is elevated. The hyponatremia is due both to loss of sodium into the urine (due to aldosterone deficiency) and to movement into the intracellular compartment. This extravascular sodium loss depletes ECFV and accentuates hypotension. Elevated plasma vasopressin and angiotensin II levels may contribute to the hyponatremia by impairing free water clearance. Hyperkalemia is due to a combination of aldosterone deficiency, impaired glomerular filtration, and acidosis. Basal levels of cortisol and aldosterone are subnormal and fail to increase following ACTH administration. Mild to moderate hypercalcemia occurs in 10–20% of patients for unclear reasons. The electrocardiogram may show nonspecific changes, and the electroencephalogram exhibits a generalized reduction and slowing. There may be a normocytic anemia, a relative lymphocytosis, and a moderate eosinophilia.

Diagnosis The diagnosis of adrenal insufficiency should be made only with ACTH stimulation testing to assess adrenal reserve capacity for steroid production (see above for ACTH test protocols). In brief, the best screening test is the cortisol response 60 min after 250 μg of cosyntropin given IM or IV. Cortisol levels should be >495 nmol/L (18 μg/dL). If the response is abnormal, then primary and secondary adrenal insufficiency can be distinguished by measuring aldosterone levels from the same blood samples. In secondary, but not primary, adrenal insufficiency, the aldosterone increment will be normal [≥150 pmol/L (5 ng/dL)]. Furthermore, in primary adrenal insufficiency, plasma ACTH and associated peptides (β-LPT) are elevated because of loss of the usual cortisol-hypothalamic-pituitary feedback relationship, whereas in secondary adrenal insufficiency, plasma ACTH values are low or "inappropriately" normal (Fig. 336-12).

Differential Diagnosis Because weakness and fatigue are common, diagnosis of early adrenocortical insufficiency may be difficult. However, the combination of mild gastrointestinal distress, weight loss, anorexia, and a suggestion of increased pigmentation makes it mandatory to perform ACTH stimulation testing to rule out adrenal insufficiency, particularly before steroid treatment is begun. Weight loss is useful in evaluating the significance of weakness and malaise. Racial pigmentation may be a confounding feature, but a *recent* and progressive *increase* in pigmentation is usually reported by the patient with gradual adrenal destruction. Hyperpigmentation is usually absent when adrenal destruction is rapid, as in bilateral adrenal hemorrhage. The fact that hyperpigmentation occurs with other diseases may also present a problem, but the appearance and distribution of pigment in adrenal insufficiency are usually characteristic. When doubt exists, measurement of ACTH levels and testing of adrenal reserve with the infusion of ACTH provide clear-cut differentiation.

℞ ADRENAL INSUFFICIENCY

All patients with adrenal insufficiency should receive specific hormone replacement. These patients require careful education about the disease. Replacement therapy should correct both glucocorticoid and mineralocorticoid deficiencies. Hydrocortisone (cortisol) is the mainstay of treatment. The dose for most adults (depending on size) is 20–30 mg/d. Patients are advised to take glucocorticoids with meals or, if that is impractical, with milk or an antacid, because the drugs may increase gastric acidity and exert direct toxic effects on the gastric mucosa. To simulate the normal diurnal adrenal rhythm, two-thirds of the dose is taken in the morning, and the remaining one-third is taken in the late afternoon. Some patients exhibit insomnia, irritability, and mental excitement after initiation of therapy; in these, the dosage should be reduced. Other situations that may necessitate smaller doses are hypertension and diabetes mellitus. Obese individuals and those on anticonvulsive medications may require increased dosages. Measurements of plasma ACTH or cortisol or of urine cortisol levels do not appear to be useful in determining optimal glucocorticoid dosages.

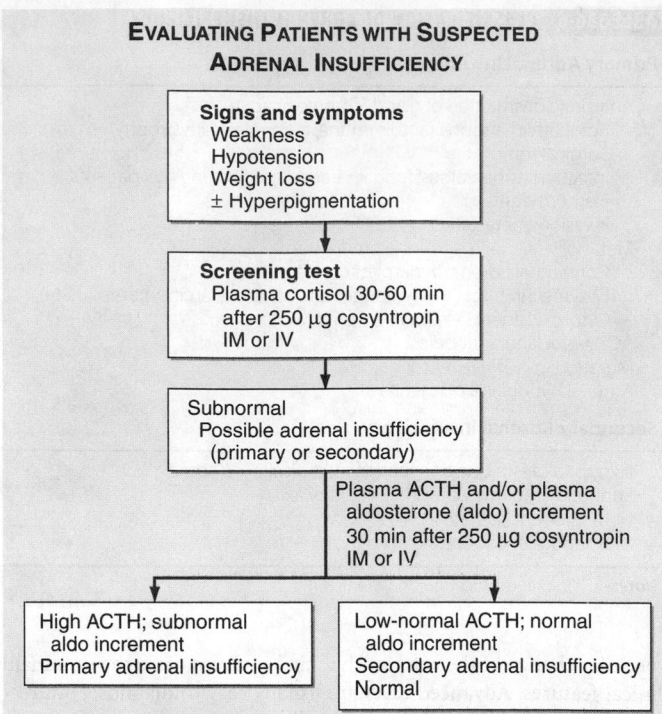

EVALUATING PATIENTS WITH SUSPECTED ADRENAL INSUFFICIENCY

Signs and symptoms
Weakness
Hypotension
Weight loss
± Hyperpigmentation

↓

Screening test
Plasma cortisol 30-60 min after 250 μg cosyntropin IM or IV

↓

Subnormal
Possible adrenal insufficiency (primary or secondary)

↓

Plasma ACTH and/or plasma aldosterone (aldo) increment 30 min after 250 μg cosyntropin IM or IV

High ACTH; subnormal aldo increment
Primary adrenal insufficiency

Low-normal ACTH; normal aldo increment
Secondary adrenal insufficiency
Normal

FIGURE 336-12 Diagnostic flowchart for evaluating patients with suspected adrenal insufficiency. Plasma adrenocorticotropic hormone (ACTH) levels are low in secondary adrenal insufficiency. In adrenal insufficiency secondary to pituitary tumors or idiopathic panhypopituitarism, other pituitary hormone deficiencies are present. On the other hand, ACTH deficiency may be isolated, as seen following prolonged use of exogenous glucocorticoids. Because the isolated blood levels obtained in these screening tests may not be definitive, the diagnosis may need to be confirmed by a continuous 24-h ACTH infusion. Normal subjects and patients with secondary adrenal insufficiency may be distinguished by insulin tolerance or metyrapone testing.

Since the replacement dosage of hydrocortisone does not replace the mineralocorticoid component of the adrenal hormones, mineralocorticoid supplementation is usually needed. This is accomplished by the administration of 0.05–0.1 mg fludrocortisone per day PO. Patients should also be instructed to maintain an ample intake of sodium (3–4 g/d).

The adequacy of mineralocorticoid therapy can be assessed by measurement of blood pressure and serum electrolytes. Blood pressure should be normal and without postural changes; serum sodium, potassium, creatinine, and urea nitrogen levels should also be normal. Measurement of plasma renin levels may also be useful in titrating the dose.

In female patients with adrenal insufficiency, androgen levels are also low. Thus, some physicians believe that daily replacement with 25–50 mg of DHEA PO may improve quality of life and bone mineral density.

Complications of glucocorticoid therapy, with the exception of gastritis, are *rare* at the dosages recommended for treatment of adrenal insufficiency. Complications of mineralocorticoid therapy include hypokalemia, hypertension, cardiac enlargement, and even congestive heart failure due to sodium retention. Periodic measurements of body weight, serum potassium level, and blood pressure are useful. All patients with adrenal insufficiency should carry medical identification, should be instructed in the parenteral self-administration of steroids, and should be registered with a medical alerting system.

Special Therapeutic Problems During periods of intercurrent illness, especially in the setting of fever, the dose of hydrocortisone should be doubled. With severe illness it should be increased to 75–150 mg/d. When oral administration is not possible, parenteral routes should be employed. Likewise, before surgery or dental extractions, supplemental glucocorticoids should be administered. Patients should also be advised to increase the dose of fludrocortisone and to add salt to their otherwise normal diet during periods of strenuous exercise with sweating, during extremely hot weather, and with gastrointestinal upsets such as diarrhea. A simple strate-

TABLE 336-8	STEROID THERAPY SCHEDULE FOR A PATIENT WITH ADRENAL INSUFFICIENCY UNDERGOING SURGERY[a]				
	Hydrocortisone Infusion, Continuous, mg/h		Hydrocortisone (Orally)		Fludrocortisone (Orally), 8 A.M.
			8 A.M.	4 P.M.	
Routine daily medication			20	10	0.1
Day before operation			20	10	0.1
Day of operation	10				
Day 1	5–7.5				
Day 2	2.5–5				
Day 3	2.5–5	or	40	20	0.1
Day 4	2.5–5	or	40	20	0.1
Day 5			40	20	0.1
Day 6			20	20	0.1
Day 7			20	10	0.1

[a]All steroid doses are given in milligrams. An alternative approach is to give 100 mg hydrocortisone as an IV bolus injection every 8 h on the day of the operation (see text).

gy is to supplement the diet one to three times daily with salty broth [250 mL (1 cup) of beef or chicken bouillon contains 35 mmol of sodium]. For a representative program of steroid therapy for the patient with adrenal insufficiency who is undergoing major surgery, see **Table 336-8**. This schedule is designed so that on the day of surgery it will mimic the output of cortisol in normal individuals undergoing prolonged major stress (10 mg/h, 250–300 mg/d). Thereafter, if the patient is improving and is afebrile, the dose of hydrocortisone is tapered by 20–30% daily. Mineralocorticoid administration is unnecessary at hydrocortisone doses >100 mg/d because of the mineralocorticoid effects of hydrocortisone at such dosages.

SECONDARY ADRENOCORTICAL INSUFFICIENCY

ACTH deficiency causes *secondary* adrenocortical insufficiency; it may be a selective deficiency, as is seen following prolonged administration of excess glucocorticoids, or it may occur in association with deficiencies of multiple pituitary hormones (panhypopituitarism) (Chap. 333). Patients with secondary adrenocortical hypofunction have many symptoms and signs in common with those having primary disease but are *not hyperpigmented*, since ACTH and related peptide levels are low. In fact, plasma ACTH levels distinguish between primary and secondary adrenal insufficiency, since they are elevated in the former and decreased to absent in the latter. Patients with total pituitary insufficiency have manifestations of multiple hormone deficiencies. An additional feature distinguishing primary adrenocortical insufficiency is the *near-normal level of aldosterone secretion* seen in pituitary and/or isolated ACTH deficiencies (Fig. 336-12). Patients with pituitary insufficiency may have hyponatremia, which can be dilutional or secondary to a subnormal increase in aldosterone secretion in response to severe sodium restriction. However, severe *dehydration, hyponatremia*, and *hyperkalemia* are characteristic of severe mineralocorticoid insufficiency and favor a diagnosis of primary adrenocortical insufficiency.

Patients receiving long-term steroid therapy, despite physical findings of Cushing's syndrome, may develop adrenal insufficiency because of prolonged pituitary-hypothalamic suppression and adrenal atrophy secondary to the loss of endogenous ACTH. These patients have two deficits, a loss of adrenal responsiveness to ACTH and a failure of pituitary ACTH release. They are characterized by low blood cortisol and ACTH levels, a low baseline rate of steroid excretion, and abnormal ACTH and metyrapone responses. Most patients with steroid-induced adrenal insufficiency eventually recover normal HPA responsiveness, but recovery time varies from days to months. The rapid ACTH test provides a convenient assessment of recovery of HPA function. Because the plasma cortisol concentrations after injection of cosyntropin and during insulin-induced hypoglycemia are usually similar, the rapid ACTH test assesses the integrated HPA function (see "Tests of Pituitary-Adrenal Responsiveness," above). Some investigators suggest using the low-dose (1 μg) ACTH test for suspected secondary ACTH deficiency. Additional tests to assess pituitary ACTH reserve include the standard metyrapone and insulin-induced hypoglycemia tests.

Glucocorticoid therapy in patients with secondary adrenocortical insufficiency does not differ from that for the primary disorder. Mineralocorticoid therapy is usually not necessary, as aldosterone secretion is preserved.

ACUTE ADRENOCORTICAL INSUFFICIENCY

Acute adrenocortical insufficiency may result from several processes. On the one hand, *adrenal crisis* may be a rapid and overwhelming intensification of chronic adrenal insufficiency, usually precipitated by sepsis or surgical stress. Alternatively, acute hemorrhagic destruction of both adrenal glands can occur in previously well individuals. In children, this event is usually associated with septicemia with *Pseudomonas* or meningococcemia (Waterhouse-Friderichsen syndrome). In adults, anticoagulant therapy or a coagulation disorder may result in bilateral adrenal hemorrhage. Occasionally, bilateral adrenal hemorrhage in the newborn results from birth trauma. Hemorrhage has been observed during pregnancy, following idiopathic adrenal vein thrombosis, and as a complication of venography (e.g., infarction of an adenoma). The third and most frequent cause of acute insufficiency is the rapid withdrawal of steroids from patients with adrenal atrophy owing to chronic steroid administration. Acute adrenocortical insufficiency may also occur in patients with congenital adrenal hyperplasia or those with decreased adrenocortical reserve when they are given drugs capable of inhibiting steroid synthesis (mitotane, ketoconazole) or of increasing steroid metabolism (phenytoin, rifampin).

Adrenal Crisis The long-term survival of patients with adrenocortical insufficiency depends largely on the prevention and treatment of adrenal crisis. Consequently, the occurrence of infection, trauma (including surgery), gastrointestinal upsets, or other stresses necessitates an immediate increase in hormone. In untreated patients, preexisting symptoms are intensified. Nausea, vomiting, and abdominal pain may become intractable. Fever may be severe or absent. Lethargy deepens into somnolence, and hypovolemic vascular collapse ensues. In contrast, patients previously maintained on chronic glucocorticoid therapy may not exhibit dehydration or hypotension until they are in a preterminal state, since mineralocorticoid secretion is usually preserved. In all patients in crisis, a precipitating cause should be sought.

℞ ADRENAL CRISIS

Treatment is directed primarily toward repletion of circulating glucocorticoids and replacement of the sodium and water deficits. Hence an IV infusion of 5% glucose in normal saline solution should be started with a bolus IV infusion of 100 mg hydrocortisone followed by a continuous infusion of hydrocortisone at a rate of 10 mg/h. An alternative approach is to administer a 100-mg bolus of hydrocortisone IV every 6 h. However, only continuous infusion maintains the plasma cortisol constantly at stress levels [>830 nmol/L (30 μg/dL)]. Effective treatment of hypotension requires glucocorticoid replacement and repletion of sodium and water deficits. If the crisis was preceded by prolonged nausea, vomiting, and dehydration, several liters of saline solution may be required in the first few hours. Vasoconstrictive agents (such as dopamine) may be indicated in extreme conditions as adjuncts to volume replacement. With large doses of steroid, i.e., 100–200 mg hydrocortisone, the patient receives a maximal mineralocorticoid effect, and supplementary mineralocorticoid is superfluous. Following improvement, the steroid dosage is tapered over the next few days to maintenance levels, and mineralocorticoid therapy is reinstituted if needed (Table 336-8).

ADRENAL CORTICOL INSUFFICIENCY IN ACUTELY ILL PATIENTS

The physiology of the HPA axis is dramatically altered during critical illnesses such as trauma, surgery, sepsis, and shock. In such situations cortisol levels rise four- to sixfold, diurnal variation is abolished, and the unbound fractions of cortisol rise in the circulation and in target tissues. Inadequate cortisol production during critical illness can result in hypotension, reduced systemic vascular resistance, shock, and death.

A major area of controversy in presumably normal individuals is the correlation of clinical outcomes with the cortisol levels measured during critical illness. Subnormal cortisol production during acute severe illness has been termed "functional" or "relative" adrenal insufficiency. Conceptually, the elevated cortisol levels that are observed are viewed as insufficient to control the inflammatory response and maintain blood pressure. Observational and experimental data in acute illness support this concept since routine stress doses of hydrocortisone reduce inflammatory markers and improve blood pressure and blood flow without impairing immune responses. Thus, if such patients can be identified, treatment with supplementary cortisol could be beneficial.

Clinical trial data support the concept that most patients with septic shock have relative adrenal insufficiency, defined as a <255-μmol/L (<9-μg/dL) increment between peak and baseline cortisol levels following administration of 250 μg of cosystropin as an IV bolus. If patients with relative adrenal insufficiency are treated for 7 days with standard stress doses of hydrocortisone, 50 mg every 6 h and 50 μg of 9-alpha fludrocortisone, 28-day survival is increased and steroid-treated subjects are more likely to have pressor agents withdrawn than placebo-treated subjects. No differences in adverse events have been reported between placebo- and steroid-treated subjects, and responders to cosyntropin receive no benefit from steroid treatment.

Thus, experimental and clinical trial data strongly support treating patients with relative adrenal insufficiency for a week. However, it has been difficult to establish a level of cortisol in a critically ill patient below which replacement glucocorticoids may improve prognosis. In most circumstances the cortisol level obtained, either randomly or following a cosyntropin test, needs to be interpreted in the context of the clinical picture. Many have accepted that a random cortisol level of ≤441 nmol/L (15 μg/dL) is indicative of relative adrenal insufficiency and a random cortisol level >938 nmol/L (34 μg/dL) usually excludes that diagnosis. In patients who have random cortisol levels between 441 and 938 nmol/L (15 and 34 μg/dL), a cosyntropin stimulation test may identify patients with diminished adrenal reserve [increment < 255 nmol/L (9 μg/dL)] who may benefit from supplementary cortisol treatment. However, many acutely ill subjects who are hemodynamically stable without pressor treatment have values below this level. Thus, the clinical state is still an important factor to be considered before initiating steroid therapy.

One approach is to assume that an acutely ill patient with hemodynamic instability not secondary to blood loss, particularly if septic shock is present, has relative adrenal insufficiency until proven otherwise. Treatment with supplementary cortisol should be initiated promptly following the measurement of a random cortisol level and/or performing a cosyntropin stimulation test. Such patients should be treated with 50–75 mg of hydrocortisone IV every 6 h as bolus treatment or the same amount as a continuous infusion. This dose of hydrocortisone is sufficient to saturate the MR, and additional treatment with 9-alpha fludrocortisone is not necessary. Treatment can be terminated if the cortisol levels obtained at the outset are appropriately elevated. On the other hand, those patients with abnormal testing should be treated for 1 week and then tapered. In surviving patients, pituitary-adrenal function should be reevaluated after resolution of the critical illness.

HYPOALDOSTERONISM

Isolated aldosterone deficiency accompanied by normal cortisol production occurs in association with hyporeninism, as an inherited biosynthetic defect, postoperatively following removal of aldosterone-secreting adenomas, during protracted heparin administration, in pretectal disease of the nervous system, and in severe postural hypotension.

The feature common to all forms of hypoaldosteronism is the inability to increase aldosterone secretion appropriately in response to salt re-striction. Most patients have unexplained hyperkalemia, which is often exacerbated by restriction of dietary sodium intake. In severe cases, urine sodium wastage occurs at a normal salt intake, whereas in milder forms, excessive loss of urine sodium occurs only with salt restriction.

Most cases of isolated hypoaldosteronism occur in patients with a deficiency in renin production (so-called hyporeninemic hypoaldosteronism), most commonly in adults with diabetes mellitus and mild renal failure and in whom hyperkalemia and metabolic acidosis are out of proportion to the degree of renal impairment. Plasma renin levels fail to rise normally following sodium restriction and postural changes. The pathogenesis is uncertain. Possibilities include renal disease (the most likely), autonomic neuropathy, ECFV expansion, and defective conversion of renin precursors to active renin. Aldosterone levels also fail to rise normally after salt restriction and volume contraction; this effect is probably related to the hyporeninism, since biosynthetic defects in aldosterone secretion usually cannot be demonstrated. In these patients, aldosterone secretion increases promptly after ACTH stimulation, but it is uncertain whether the magnitude of the response is normal. On the other hand, the level of aldosterone appears to be subnormal in relationship to the hyperkalemia.

Hypoaldosteronism can also be associated with high renin levels and low or elevated levels of aldosterone (see below). Severely ill patients may also have hyperreninemic hypoaldosteronism; such patients have a high mortality rate (80%). Hyperkalemia is not present. Possible explanations for the hypoaldosteronism include adrenal necrosis (uncommon) or a shift in steroidogenesis from mineralocorticoids to glucocorticoids, possibly related to prolonged ACTH stimulation.

Before the diagnosis of isolated hypoaldosteronism is considered for a patient with hyperkalemia, "pseudohyperkalemia" (e.g., hemolysis, thrombocytosis) should be excluded by measuring the *plasma* potassium level. The next step is to demonstrate a normal cortisol response to ACTH stimulation. Then, the response of renin and aldosterone levels to stimulation (upright posture, sodium restriction) should be measured. Low renin and aldosterone levels establish the diagnosis of hyporeninemic hypoaldosteronism. A combination of high renin levels and low aldosterone levels is consistent with an aldosterone biosynthetic defect or a selective unresponsiveness to angiotensin II. Finally, there is a condition that clinically and biochemically mimics hypoaldosteronism with elevated renin levels. However, the aldosterone levels are not low but high—so-called pseudohypoaldosteronism. This inherited condition is caused by a mutation in the epithelial sodium channel (see below).

℞ HYPOALDOSTERONISM

The treatment is to replace the mineralocorticoid deficiency. For practical purposes, the administration of 0.05–0.15 mg fludrocortisone PO daily should restore electrolyte balance if salt intake is adequate (e.g., 150–200 mmol/d). However, patients with hyporeninemic hypoaldosteronism may require higher doses of mineralocorticoid to correct hyperkalemia. This need poses a potential risk in patients with hypertension, mild renal insufficiency, or congestive heart failure. An alternative approach is to reduce salt intake and to administer furosemide, which can ameliorate acidosis and hyperkalemia. Occasionally, a combination of these two approaches is efficacious.

GENETIC CONSIDERATIONS — Glucocorticoid Diseases

Congenital Adrenal Hyperplasia Congenital adrenal hyperplasia (CAH) is the consequence of recessive mutations that cause one of several distinct enzymatic defects (see below). Because cortisol is the principal adrenal steroid regulating ACTH elaboration and because ACTH stimulates adrenal growth and function, a block in cortisol synthesis may result in the enhanced secretion of adrenal androgens and/or mineralocorticoids depending on the site of the enzyme block. In severe congenital virilizing hyperplasia, the adrenal output of cortisol may be so compromised as to cause adrenal deficiency despite adrenal hyperplasia.

CAH is the most common adrenal disorder of infancy and childhood (Chap. 343). Partial enzyme deficiencies can be expressed after adolescence, predominantly in women with hirsutism and oligomenorrhea but minimal virilization. Late-onset adrenal hyperplasia may account for 5–25% of cases of hirsutism and oligomenorrhea in women, depending on the population.

Etiology Enzymatic defects have been described in 21-hydroxylase (CYP21A2), 17α-hydroxylase/17,20-lyase (CYP17), 11β-hydroxylase (CYP11B1), and in (3β-HSD2) (Fig. 336-2). Although the genes encoding these enzymes have been cloned, the diagnosis of specific enzyme deficiencies with genetic techniques is not practical because of the large number of different deletions and missense mutations. CYP21A2 deficiency is closely linked to the HLA-B locus of chromosome 6 so that HLA typing and/or DNA polymorphism can be used to detect the heterozygous carriers and to diagnose affected individuals in some families. The clinical expression in the different disorders is variable, ranging from virilization of the female (CYP2/A2) to feminization of the male (3β-HSD2) (Chap. 343).

Adrenal virilization in the female at birth is associated with ambiguous external genitalia (*female pseudohermaphroditism*). Virilization begins after the fifth month of intrauterine development. At birth there may be enlargement of the clitoris, partial or complete fusion of the labia, and sometimes a urogenital sinus in the female. If the labial fusion is nearly complete, the female infant has external genitalia resembling a penis with hypospadias. In the *postnatal* period, CAH is associated with virilization in the female and isosexual precocity in the male. The excessive androgen levels result in accelerated growth, so that bone age exceeds chronologic age. Because epiphyseal closure occurs early, growth stops, but truncal development continues, the characteristic appearance being a short child with a well-developed trunk.

The most common form of CAH (95% of cases) is a result of impairment of CYP21A2. In addition to cortisol deficiency, aldosterone secretion is decreased in approximately one-third of the patients. Thus, with CYP21A2 deficiency, adrenal virilization occurs with or without a salt-losing tendency due to aldosterone deficiency (Fig. 336-2).

CYP11B1 deficiency causes a "hypertensive" variant of CAH. Hypertension and hypokalemia occur because of the impaired conversion of 11-deoxycorticosterone to corticosterone, resulting in the accumulation of 11-deoxycorticosterone, a potent mineralocorticoid. The degree of hypertension is variable. Steroid precursors are shunted into the androgen pathway.

CYP17 deficiency is characterized by hypogonadism, hypokalemia, and hypertension. This rare disorder causes decreased production of cortisol and shunting of precursors into the mineralocorticoid pathway with hypokalemic alkalosis, hypertension, and suppressed plasma renin activity. Usually, 11-deoxycorticosterone production is elevated. Because CYP17 hydroxylation is required for biosynthesis of both adrenal androgens and gonadal testosterone and estrogen, this defect is associated with sexual immaturity, high gonadotropin levels, and low urinary 17-ketosteroid excretion. Female patients have primary amenorrhea and lack of development of secondary sexual characteristics. Because of deficient androgen production, male patients have either ambiguous external genitalia or a female phenotype (*underandrogenization*). Exogenous glucocorticoids can correct the hypertensive syndrome, and treatment with appropriate gonadal steroids results in sexual maturation.

With 3β-HSD2 deficiency, conversion of pregnenolone to progesterone is impaired, so that the synthesis of both cortisol and aldosterone is blocked, with shunting into the adrenal androgen pathway via 17α-hydroxypregnenolone and DHEA. Because DHEA is a weak androgen, and because this enzyme deficiency is also present in the gonad, the genitalia of the male fetus may be incompletely virilized or feminized. Conversely, in the female, overproduction of DHEA may produce partial virilization.

Diagnosis The diagnosis of CAH should be considered in infants having episodes of acute adrenal insufficiency or salt-wasting or hypertension. The diagnosis is further suggested by the finding of hypertrophy of the clitoris, fused labia, or a urogenital sinus in the female or of isosexual precocity in the male. In infants and children with a CYP21A2 defect, increased urine 17-ketosteroid excretion and increased plasma DHEA sulfate levels are typically associated with an increase in the blood levels of 17-hydroxyprogesterone and the excretion of its urinary metabolite pregnanetriol. Demonstration of elevated levels of 17-hydroxyprogesterone in amniotic fluid at 14–16 weeks of gestation allows prenatal detection of affected female infants. Prenatal genetic testing is also possible in families in whom the specific genetic defect is known.

The diagnosis of a *salt-losing form* of CAH due to defects in CYP21A2 is suggested by episodes of acute adrenal insufficiency with hyponatremia, hyperkalemia, dehydration, and vomiting. These infants and children often crave salt and have laboratory findings indicating deficits in both cortisol and aldosterone secretion.

With the *hypertensive form* of CAH due to CYP11B1 deficiency, 11-deoxycorticosterone and 11-deoxycortisol accumulate. The diagnosis is confirmed by demonstrating increased levels of 11-deoxycortisol in the blood or increased amounts of tetrahydro-11-deoxycortisol in the urine. Elevation of 17-hydroxyprogesterone levels does not imply a coexisting CYP21A2 deficiency.

Very high levels of urine DHEA with low levels of pregnanetriol and of cortisol metabolites in urine are characteristic of children with 3β-HSD2 deficiency. Marked salt-wasting may also occur.

Adults with *late-onset adrenal hyperplasia* (partial deficiency of CYP21A2, CYP11B1, or 3β-HSD2) are characterized by normal or moderately elevated levels of urinary 17-ketosteroids and plasma DHEA sulfate. A high basal level of a precursor of cortisol biosynthesis (such as 17-hydroxyprogesterone, 17-hydroxypregnenolone, or 11-deoxycortisol), or elevation of such a precursor after ACTH stimulation, confirms the diagnosis of a partial deficiency. Measurement of steroid precursors 60 min after bolus administration of ACTH is usually sufficient. Adrenal androgen output is easily suppressed by the standard low-dose (2 mg) dexamethasone test.

℞ CONGENITAL ADRENAL HYPERPLASIA

Therapy in CAH patients consists of daily administration of glucocorticoids to suppress pituitary ACTH secretion. Because of its low cost and intermediate half-life, prednisone is the drug of choice except in infants, in whom hydrocortisone is usually used. In adults with late-onset adrenal hyperplasia, the smallest single bedtime dose of a long- or intermediate-acting glucocorticoid that suppresses pituitary ACTH secretion should be administered. The amount of steroid required by children with CAH is ~1–1.5 times the normal cortisol production rate of 27–35 μmol (10–13 mg) of cortisol per square meter of body surface per day and is given in divided doses two or three times per day. The dosage schedule is governed by repetitive analysis of the urinary 17-ketosteroids, plasma DHEA sulfate, and/or precursors of cortisol biosynthesis. Skeletal growth and maturation must also be monitored closely, as overtreatment with glucocorticoid replacement therapy retards linear growth.

Receptor Mutations *Isolated glucocorticoid deficiency* is a rare autosomal recessive disease secondary to a mutation in the ACTH receptor. Usually mineralocorticoid function is normal. Adrenal insufficiency is manifest within the first 2 years of life as hyperpigmentation, convulsions, and/or frequent episodes of hypoglycemia. In some patients the adrenal insufficiency is associated with achalasia and alacrima—Allgrove's, or triple A, syndrome. However, in some triple A syndrome patients, no mutation in the ACTH receptor has been identified, suggesting that a distinct genetic abnormality causes this syndrome. *Adrenal hypoplasia congenita* is a rare X-linked disorder caused by a mutation in the *DAX1* gene. This gene encodes an orphan nuclear receptor that plays an important role in the development of the adrenal cortex and also the hypothalamic-pituitary-gonadal axis. Thus, patients present with signs and symptoms secondary to deficiencies of all three major adrenal steroids—cortisol, aldosterone, and adrenal androgens—as well as gonadotropin deficiency. Finally a rare cause of hypercortisolism without cushingoid stigmata is *primary cortisol resistance* due to mutations in the glucocorticoid receptor. The resistance is incomplete because patients do not exhibit signs of adrenal insufficiency.

Miscellaneous Conditions Adrenoleukodystrophy causes severe demyelination and early death in children, and adrenomyeloneuropathy is associated with a mixed motor and sensory neuropathy with spastic paraplegia in adults; both disorders are associated with elevated circulating levels of very long chain fatty acids and cause adrenal insufficiency. Autosomal recessive mutations in the s*teroidogenic* a*cute* r*egulatory* (STAR) protein gene cause congenital lipoid adrenal hyperplasia (Chap. 343), which is characterized by adrenal insufficiency and defective gonadal steroidogenesis. In genetic males, this leads to female phenotype. In genetic females, sexual differentiation is normal but there is premature ovarian failure. Because STAR mediates cholesterol transport into the mitochondrion, mutations in the protein cause massive lipid accumulation in steroidogenic cells, ultimately leading to cell toxicity.

MINERALOCORTICOID DISEASES

Some forms of CAH have a mineralocorticoid component (see above). Others are caused by a mutation in other enzymes or ion channels important in mediating or mimicking aldosterone's action.

Hypermineralocorticoidism • *LOW PLASMA RENIN ACTIVITY* Rarely, hypermineralocorticoidism is due to a defect in cortisol biosynthesis, specifically 11- or 17-hydroxylation. ACTH levels are increased, with a resultant increase in the production of the mineralocorticoid 11-deoxy-corticosterone. Hypertension and hypokalemia can be corrected by glucocorticoid administration. The definitive diagnosis is made by demonstrating an elevation of precursors of cortisol biosynthesis in the blood or urine or by direct demonstration of the genetic defect.

Glucocorticoid administration can also ameliorate hypertension or produce normotension even though a hydroxylase deficiency cannot be identified. These patients have normal to slightly elevated aldosterone levels that do not suppress in response to saline but do suppress in response to 2 days of dexamethasone (2 mg/d). The condition is inherited as an autosomal dominant trait and is termed *glucocorticoid-remediable aldosteronism* (GRA). This entity is secondary to a chimeric gene duplication whereby the 11-β hydroxylase gene promoter (which is under the control of ACTH) is fused to the aldosterone synthase coding sequence. Thus, aldosterone synthase activity is ectopically expressed in the zona fasciculata and is regulated by ACTH, in a fashion similar to the regulation of cortisol secretion. Screening for this defect is best performed by assessing the presence or absence of the chimeric gene. Because the abnormal gene may be present in the absence of hypokalemia, its frequency as a cause of hypertension is unknown. Individuals with suppressed plasma renin levels and juvenile-onset hypertension or a history of early-onset hypertension in first-degree relatives should be screened for this disorder. Early hemorrhagic stroke also occurs in GRA-affected individuals.

GRA documented by genetic analysis may be treated with glucocorticoid administration or antimineralocorticoids, i.e., spironolactone, triamterene, or amiloride. Glucocorticoids should be used only in small doses to avoid inducing iatrogenic Cushing's syndrome. A combination approach is often necessary.

HIGH PLASMA RENIN ACTIVITY *Bartter syndrome* is characterized by severe hyperaldosteronism (hypokalemic alkalosis) with moderate to marked increases in renin activity and hypercalciuria, but normal blood pressure and no edema; this disorder usually begins in childhood. Renal biopsy shows juxtaglomerular hyperplasia. Bartter syndrome is caused by a mutation in the renal Na-K-2Cl co-transporter gene. The pathogenesis involves a defect in the renal conservation of sodium or chloride. The renal loss of sodium is thought to stimulate renin secretion and aldosterone production. Hyperaldosteronism produces potassium depletion, and hypokalemia further elevates prostaglandin production and plasma renin activity. In some cases, the hypokalemia may be potentiated by a defect in renal conservation of potassium.

Gitelman syndrome is an autosomal recessive trait characterized by renal salt wasting and as a result, as in Bartter syndrome, activation of the renin-angiotensin-aldosterone system. As a consequence affected individuals have low blood pressure, low serum potassium, low serum magnesium, and high serum bicarbonate. In contrast to Bartter syndrome, urinary calcium excretion is reduced. Gitelman syndrome results from loss-of-function mutations of the renal thiazide-sensitive Na-Cl co-transporter.

Increased Mineralocorticoid Action *Liddle syndrome* is a rare autosomal dominant disorder that mimics hyperaldosteronism. The defect is in the genes encoding the β or η subunits of the epithelial sodium channel. Both renin and aldosterone levels are low, owing to the constitutively activated sodium channel and the resulting excess sodium reabsorption in the renal tubule.

A rare autosomal recessive cause of hypokalemia and hypertension is 11β-HSD 2 deficiency, in which cortisol cannot be converted to cortisone and hence binds to the MR and acts as a mineralocorticoid. This condition, also termed *apparent mineralocorticoid excess syndrome*, is caused by a defect in the gene encoding the renal isoform of this enzyme, 11β-HSD 2. Patients can be identified either by documenting an increased ratio of cortisol to cortisone in the urine or by genetic analysis. Patients with the 11β-HSD deficiency syndrome can be treated with small doses of dexamethasone, which suppresses ACTH and endogenous cortisol production but binds less well to the mineralocorticoid receptor than does cortisol.

The ingestion of candies or chewing tobacco containing certain forms of licorice produces a syndrome that mimics primary aldosteronism. The component of such agents that causes sodium retention is glycyrrhizinic acid, which inhibits 11β-HSD 2 and hence allows cortisol to act as a mineralocorticoid. The diagnosis is established or excluded by a careful history.

Decreased Mineralocorticoid Production or Action In patients with a deficiency in aldosterone biosynthesis, the transformation of corticosterone into aldosterone is impaired, owing to a mutation in the aldosterone synthase (CYP11B2) gene. These patients have low to absent aldosterone secretion, elevated plasma renin levels, and elevated levels of the intermediates of aldosterone biosynthesis (corticosterone and 18-hydroxycorticosterone).

Pseudohypoaldosteronism type I (PHA-I) is an autosomal recessive disorder that is seen in the neonatal period and is characterized by salt wasting, hypotension, hyperkalemia, and high renin and aldosterone levels. In contrast to the gain-of-function mutations in the epithelial sodium channel in Liddle syndrome, mutations in PHA-I result in loss of epithelial sodium channel function.

PHARMACOLOGIC CLINICAL USES OF ADRENAL STEROIDS

The widespread use of glucocorticoids emphasizes the need for a thorough understanding of the metabolic effects of these agents. Before adrenal hormone therapy is instituted, the expected gains should be weighed against undesirable effects. Several important questions should be addressed before initiating therapy. First, how serious is the disorder (the more serious, the greater the likelihood that the risk/benefit ratio will be positive)? Second, how long will therapy be required (the longer the therapy, the greater the risk of adverse side effects)? Third, does the individual have preexisting conditions that glucocorticoids may exacerbate (Table 336-9)? If so, then a careful risk/benefit assessment is required to ensure that the ratio is favorable given the increased likelihood of harm by steroids in these patients. Supplementary measures to minimize undesirable metabolic effects are shown in Table 336-10. Fourth, which preparation is best?

The following considerations should be taken into account in deciding which steroid preparation to use:

1. *The biologic half-life.* The rationale behind alternate-day therapy is to decrease the metabolic effects of the steroids for a significant part of each 48-h period while still producing a pharmacologic effect durable enough to be effective. Too long a half-life would defeat the first

TABLE 336-9	A CHECKLIST PRIOR TO THE ADMINISTRATION OF GLUCOCORTICOIDS IN PHARMACOLOGIC DOSES

Presence of tuberculosis or other chronic infection (chest x-ray, tuberculin test)
Evidence of impaired glucose intolerance, history of gestational diabetes, or strong family history of type 2 diabetes mellitus in first-degree relative
Evidence of preexisting (or high risk for) osteoporosis (bone density assessment in organ transplant recipients or postmenopausal patients)
History of peptic ulcer, gastritis, or esophagitis (stool guaiac test)
Evidence of hypertension, cardiovascular disease, or hyperlipidemia (triglyceride level)
History of psychological disorders

TABLE 336-10 SUPPLEMENTARY MEASURES TO MINIMIZE UNDESIRABLE METABOLIC EFFECTS OF GLUCOCORTICOIDS

Diet
  Monitor caloric intake to prevent weight gain.
  Diabetic diet if glucose intolerant.
  Restrict sodium intake to prevent edema and minimize hypertension.
  Provide supplementary potassium if necessary.
Consider antacid, H$_2$ receptor antagonist, and/or H+, K+,-ATPase inhibitor therapy
Institute all-day steroid schedule, if possible
  Patients receiving steroid therapy over a prolonged period (months) should have an appropriate increase in hormone level during periods of acute stress. A rule of thumb is to *double* the maintenance dose.
Minimize loss of bone mineral density
  Consider administering gonadal hormone replacement therapy in post-menopausal women:
    0.625–1.25 mg conjugated estrogens given cyclically with progesterone, unless the uterus is absent (testosterone replacement in hypogonadal men)
  Ensure adequate calcium intake (should be ~1200 mg/d elemental calcium).
  Administer a minimum of 800–1000 IU/d supplemental vitamin D.
  Measure blood levels of calciferol and 1,25(OH)$_2$ vitamin D. Supplement as needed.
  Consider administering bisphosphonate prophylactically, orally, or parenterally in high-risk patients.

TABLE 336-11 GLUCOCORTICOID PREPARATIONS

Commonly Used Name[a]	Estimated Potency[b]	
	Glucocorticoid	Mineralocorticoid
Short-Acting		
Hydrocortisone	1	1
Cortisone	0.8	0.8
Intermediate-Acting		
Prednisone	4	0.25
Prednisolone	4	0.25
Methylprednisolone	5	<0.01
Triamcinolone	5	<0.01
Long-Acting		
Paramethasone	10	<0.01
Betamethasone	25	<0.01
Dexamethasone	30–40	<0.01

[a]The steroids are divided into three groups according to the duration of biologic activity. Short-acting preparations have a biologic half-life <12 h; long-acting, >48 h; and intermediate, between 12 and 36 h. Triamcinolone has the longest half-life of the intermediate-acting preparations.

[b]Relative milligram comparisons with hydrocortisone, setting the glucocorticoid and mineralocorticoid properties of hydrocortisone as 1. Sodium retention is insignificant for commonly employed doses of methylprednisolone, triamcinolone, paramethasone, betamethasone, and dexamethasone.

purpose, and too short a half-life would defeat the second. In general, the more potent the steroid, the longer its biologic half-life.

2. *The mineralocorticoid effects of the steroid.* Most synthetic steroids have less mineralocorticoid effect than hydrocortisone (Table 336-11).

3. *The biologically active form of the steroid.* Cortisone and prednisone have to be converted to biologically active metabolites before anti-inflammatory effects can occur. Because of this, in a condition for which steroids are known to be effective and when an adequate dose has been given without response, one should consider substituting hydrocortisone or prednisolone for cortisone or prednisone.

4. *The cost of the medication.* This is a serious consideration if chronic administration is planned. Prednisone is the least expensive of available steroid preparations.

5. *The type of formulation.* Topical steroids have the distinct advantage over oral steroids in reducing the likelihood of systemic side effects. In addition, some inhaled steroids have been designed to minimize side effects by increasing their hepatic inactivation if they are swallowed. However, all topical steroids can be absorbed into the systemic circulation.

FURTHER READINGS

ALLEN DB: Effects of inhaled steroids on growth, bone metabolism, and adrenal function. Adv Periatr 53:101, 2006

BERNINI GP et al: Unique association of non-functioning pheochromocytoma, ganglioneuroma, adrenal cortical adenoma, hepatic and vertebral hemangiomas in a patient with a new intronic variant in the VHL gene. J Endocrinol Invest 28:1032, 2005

DLUHY RG, WILLIAMS GH: Aldosterone: Villain or bystander? N Engl J Med 351:8, 2004

EPSTEIN M et al: Selective aldosterone blockade with eplerenone produces albuminuria in patients with Type 2 diabetes. Clin J Am Soc Nephrol 1:940, 2006

FINDLING JW, RAFF H: Cushing's syndrome: Important issues in diagnosis and management. J Clin Endocrinol Metab 91:3746, 2006

GANNON TA et al: Adrenal insufficiency in the critically ill trauma population. Am Surg 72: 373, 2006

HOOD SJ et al: The spironolactone, amiloride, losartan, and thiazide (SALT) double-blind crossover trial in patients with low-renin hypertension and elevated aldosterone-renin ratio. Circulation 116:268, 2007

MATTSSON C, YOUNG WF JR: Primary aldosteronism: Diagnostic and treatment strategies. Nat Clin Pract Nephrol 2:198, 2006

MOTTA-RAMIREZ GA et al: Comparison of CT findings in symptomatic and incidentally discovered pheochromocytomas. Am J Roentgenol 185:684, 2005

NAIR KS et al: DHEA in elderly women and DHEA or testosterone in elderly men. N Engl J Med 355:1647, 2006

NIEMAN LK, ILIAS I: Evaluation and treatment of Cushing's syndrome. Am J Med 118:1340, 2005

TORRESANI T, BIASON-LAUBER A: Congenital adrenal hyperplasia: Diagnostic advances. J Inherit Metab Dis 30:563, 2007

YOUNG WF, JR: Clinical practice: The incidentally discovered adrenal mass. N Engl J Med 356:601, 2007

337 Pheochromocytoma
Hartmut P.H. Neumann

Pheochromocytomas and paragangliomas are catecholamine-producing tumors derived from the sympathetic or parasympathetic nervous system. These tumors may arise sporadically or be inherited as features of multiple endocrine neoplasia type 2 or several other pheochromocytoma-associated syndromes. The diagnosis of pheochromocytomas provides a potentially correctable cause of hypertension, and their removal can prevent hypertensive crises that can be lethal. The clinical presentation is variable, ranging from an adrenal incidentaloma to a patient in hypertensive crisis with associated cerebrovascular or cardiac complications.

EPIDEMIOLOGY

Pheochromocytoma is estimated to occur in 2–8 out of 1 million persons per year, and about 0.1% of hypertensive patients harbor a pheochromocytoma. Autopsy series reveal prevalence figures of 0.2%. The mean age at diagnosis is about 40 years, although the tumors can occur from early childhood until late in life. The "rule of tens" for pheochromocytomas states that about 10% are bilateral, 10% are extraadrenal, and 10% are malignant. However, these percentages are higher in the inherited syndromes.

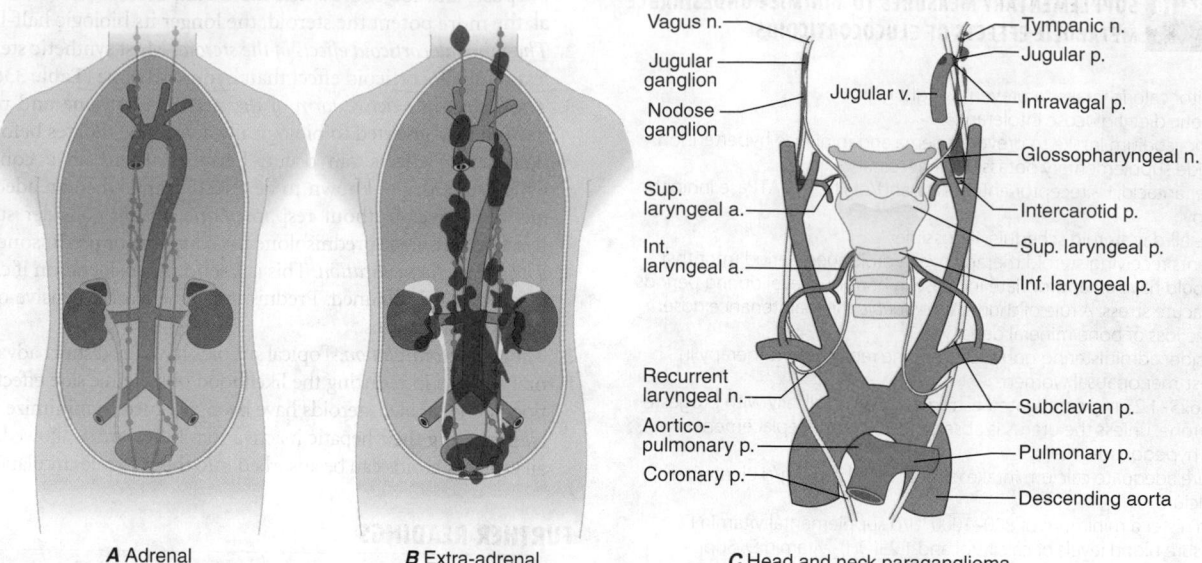

A Adrenal pheochromocytoma

B Extra-adrenal pheochromocytoma

C Head and neck paraganglioma

FIGURE 337-1 The paraganglial system and topographic sites (in red) of pheochromocytomas and paragangliomas. [**A,B,** from WM Manger, RW Gifford RW, Clinical and experimental pheochromocytoma. Cambridge, Blackwell Science, 1996 and **C,** from GG Glenner, PM Grimley, Tumors of the extra-adrenal paraganglion system (including chemoreceptors), Atlas of Tumor Pathology, 2d Series, Fascicle 9. Washington, DC, AFIP, 1974.]

ETIOLOGY AND PATHOGENESIS

Pheochromocytomas and paragangliomas are well-vascularized tumors that arise from cells derived from the sympathetic (e.g., adrenal medulla) or parasympathetic (e.g., carotid body, glomus vagale) paraganglia (Fig. 337-1). The name *pheochromocytoma* reflects the black-colored staining caused by chromaffin oxidation of catecholamines. Although a variety of nomenclatures have been used to describe these tumors, most clinicians use the term *pheochromocytoma* to describe symptomatic catecholamine-producing tumors, including those located in extraadrenal retroperitoneal, pelvic, and thoracic sites. The term *paraganglioma* is used to describe catecholamine-producing tumors in the head and neck, as well as tumors that arise from the parasympathetic nervous system, which may secrete little or no catecholamines.

The etiology of most sporadic pheochromocytomas and paragangliomas is unknown. However, about 25% of patients have an inherited condition, including germ-line mutations in the *RET, VHL, NF1, SDHB, SDHC,* or *SDHD* genes. Biallelic gene inactivation has been demonstrated for the *VHL, NF1,* and *SDH* genes, whereas *RET* mutations activate the receptor tyrosine kinase activity. SDH is an enzyme of the Krebs cycle and the mitochondrial respiratory chain. The VHL protein is a component of a ubiquitin E3 ligase. *VHL* mutations reduce protein degradation, resulting in upregulation of components involved in cell cycle progression, glucose metabolism, and oxygen sensing.

CLINICAL FEATURES

The clinical presentation is so variable that pheochromocytoma has been termed "the great masquerader" (Table 337-1). Among the presenting symptoms, episodes of palpitations, headaches, and profuse sweating are typical and constitute a classic triad. The presence of all the three symptoms, in association with hypertension, makes pheochromocytoma a likely diagnosis. On the other hand, a pheochromocytoma can be asymptomatic for years, and some tumors have grown to a considerable size before patients noted symptoms.

The dominant sign is hypertension. Classically, patients have episodic hypertension, but sustained hypertension is also frequent. Catecholamine crises can lead to heart failure, pulmonary edema, arrhythmias, and intracranial hemorrhage. During episodes of hormone release, which can occur at very divergent intervals, patients are anxious and pale, and they experience tachycardia and palpitations. These paroxysms generally last less than an hour and may be precipitated by surgery, positional changes, exercise, pregnancy, urination (particularly bladder pheochromocytomas), and various medications (e.g., tricyclic antidepressants, opiates, metoclopramide).

DIAGNOSIS

The diagnosis is based on documentation of catecholamine excess by biochemical testing and localization of the tumor by imaging. Both are of equal importance, although measurement of catecholamines is traditionally the first step.

Biochemical Testing Pheochromocytomas and paragangliomas synthesize and store catecholamines, which include norepinephrine (noradrenaline), epinephrine (adrenaline), and dopamine. Elevated plasma and urinary levels of catecholamines and the methylated metabolites, metanephrines, are the cornerstone for the diagnosis. The hormonal activity of tumors fluctuates, resulting in considerable variation in serial catecholamine measurements. Thus, there is some value in obtaining tests during or soon after a symptomatic crisis. On the other hand, most tumors continuously leak O-methylated metabolites, which are detected by metanephrine measurements.

Catecholamines and metanephrines can be measured using many different methods (e.g., high-performance liquid chromatography, enzyme-linked immunosorbent assay, other immunoassays). In a clinical context suspicious for pheochromocytoma, when values are increased two to three times the upper limit of normal, a pheochromocytoma is highly likely, regardless of the assay used, assuming an appropriate

TABLE 337-1	CLINICAL FEATURES ASSOCIATED WITH PHEOCHROMOCYTOMA
Headaches	Weight loss
Sweating attacks	Paradoxical response to antihypertensive drugs
Palpitation and tachycardia	
Hypertension, sustained or paroxysmal	Polyuria and polydipsia
	Constipation
Anxiety and panic attacks	Orthostatic hypotension
Pallor	Dilated cardiomyopathy
Nausea	Erythrocytosis
Abdominal pain	Elevated blood sugar
Weakness	Hypercalcemia

TABLE 337-2	BIOCHEMICAL AND IMAGING METHODS USED FOR PHEOCHROMOCYTOMA AND PARAGANGLIOMA DIAGNOSIS		
Diagnostic Method		**Sensitivity**	**Specificity**
24-h urinary tests			
Vanillylmandelic acid		++	++++
Catecholamines		+++	+++
Fractionated metanephrines		++++	++
Total metanephrines		+++	++++
Plasma tests			
Catecholamines		+++	++
Free metanephrines		++++	+++
Chromogranin A		+++	++
CT		++++	+++
MRI		++++	+++
MIBG scintigraphy		+++	++++
Somatostatin receptor scintigraphy[a]		++	++
Dopa (dopamine) PET (preliminary data)		++++	++++

[a]Particularly high in head and neck paragangliomas.

Note: MIBG, metaiodobenzylguanidine; PET, positron-emission tomography.

clinical context. However, as summarized in Table 337-2, the sensitivity and specificity of available biochemical tests varies greatly, and these differences are important when assessing patients with borderline catecholamine elevation. Urinary tests for VMA, metanephrines (total or fractionated), and catecholamines are widely available and commonly used for initial testing. Among these tests, the fractionated metanephrines and catecholamines are the most sensitive. Plasma tests are more convenient and include measurements of catecholamines, metanephrines, and chromagranin A, a secretory product of endocrine cells. Plasma metanephrine measurements are most sensitive and are less susceptible to false-positive elevations from stress, including venipuncture. Although the incidence of false-positive test results has been reduced by the introduction of newer assays, physiologic stress responses and medications (e.g., levodopa, labetalol, sympathomimetics) that increase catecholamines can still confound testing. Because the tumors are relatively rare, borderline elevations are likely to be false positives. In this circumstance, repeated testing, often using different assays, may clarify the diagnosis. If possible, physiologic (e.g., heart failure, shock, hypertension) or pharmacologic (clonidine withdrawal, tricyclic antidepressants) factors that might cause false positives should be eliminated. The pattern of catecholamines can help in localizing the tumor, as epinephrine is virtually never increased in extraadrenal pheochromocytomas.

Pharmacologic tests, such as the phentolamine test, the glucagon provocation test, and the clonidine suppression test, are of relatively low sensitivity and are rarely used.

Diagnostic Imaging A variety of methods have been used to localize pheochromocytomas and paragangliomas (Table 337-2). CT and MRI are similar in sensitivity. CT should be performed with contrast. T2-weighted MRI with gadolinium contrast is optimal for detecting pheochromocytomas and is somewhat better than CT for imaging extraadrenal pheochromocytomas and paragangliomas. About 5% of adrenal incidentalomas, usually detected by CT or MRI, prove to be pheochromocytomas after endocrinologic evaluation.

Tumors can also be localized using radioactive tracers including ^{131}I- or ^{123}I-metaiodobenzylguanidine (MIBG), ^{111}In-somatostatin analogues, or ^{18}F-dopa (or dopamine) positron-emission tomography (PET). Because these agents exhibit selective uptake in paragangliomas, nuclear imaging is particularly useful in the hereditary syndromes.

Differential Diagnosis When entertaining the possibility of a pheochromocytoma, other disorders to consider include essential hypertension, anxiety attacks, use of cocaine or amphetamines, mastocytosis or carcinoid syndrome (usually lacking hypertension), intracranial lesions, clonidine withdrawal, autonomic epilepsy, and factitious crises (usually from sympathomimetic amines). When an asymptomatic adrenal mass is identified, likely diagnoses other than pheochromocyto-

ma include a nonfunctioning adrenal adenoma, aldosteronoma, and cortisol-producing adenoma (Cushing's syndrome).

℞ PHEOCHROMOCYTOMA

Complete tumor removal is the ultimate therapeutic goal. Preoperative patient preparation is essential for safe surgery. α-Adrenergic blockers (phenoxybenzamine) should be initiated at relatively low doses (e.g., 5–10 mg orally three times per day) and increased as tolerated every few days. Because patients are volume constricted, liberal salt intake and hydration are necessary to avoid orthostasis. Adequate alpha blockade generally requires 10–14 days, with a typical final dose of 20–30 mg phenoxybenzamine three times per day. Oral prazosin or intravenous phentolamine can be used to manage paroxysms while awaiting adequate alpha blockade. Before surgery, the blood pressure should be consistently below 160/90 mmHg, with moderate orthostasis. Beta blockers (e.g., 10 mg propranolol three to four times per day) can be added after starting alpha blockers, and increased as needed, if tachycardia persists. Because beta blockers can induce a paradoxical increase in blood pressure in the absence of alpha blockade, they should be administered only after effective alpha blockade. Other antihypertensives, such as calcium-channel blockers or angiotensin-converting enzyme inhibitors, have also been used when blood pressure is difficult to control with phenoxybenzamine alone.

Surgery should be performed by teams of anesthesiologists and surgeons with experience in the management of pheochromocytomas. Blood pressure can be labile during surgery, particularly at the onset of intubation or when manipulating the tumor. Nitroprusside infusion is useful for intraoperative hypertensive crises, and hypotension usually responds to volume infusion. Although laparotomy was the traditional surgical approach, laparoscopy, using either a transperitoneal or retroperitoneal (for bilateral adrenalectomy) approach, is associated with fewer complications and a faster recovery. Atraumatic endoscopic surgery was introduced in the early 1990s and has now become the method of choice. It may be possible to preserve the normal adrenal cortex, particularly in hereditary disorders in which bilateral pheochromocytomas are more likely. Extraadrenal abdominal pheochromocytomas can also be removed endoscopically. Postoperatively, catecholamine normalization should be documented. An adrenocorticotropic hormone test should be used to exclude cortisol deficiency when bilateral adrenal cortex–sparing surgery is performed.

MALIGNANT PHEOCHROMOCYTOMA

About 5–10% of pheochromocytomas and paragangliomas are malignant. The diagnosis of malignant pheochromocytoma is problematic. Typical histologic criteria of cellular atypia, presence of mitoses, and invasion of vessels or adjacent tissues do not reliably identify which tumors have the capacity to metastasize. Thus, the term *malignant pheochromocytoma* is generally restricted to tumors with distant metastases, most commonly found in lungs, bone, or liver, suggesting a vascular pathway of spread. Because hereditary syndromes are associated with multifocal tumor sites, these features should be anticipated in patients with germ-line mutations of *RET*, *VHL*, *SDHD*, or *SDHB*. However, distant metastases also occur in these syndromes, especially carriers of *SDHB* mutations.

Treatment of malignant pheochromocytoma or paraganglioma is challenging. Options include tumor mass reduction; alpha blockers for symptoms; chemotherapy; and nuclear medicine radiotherapy. Averbuch's chemotherapy protocol includes dacarbazine (600 mg/m² days 1 and 2), cyclophosphamide (750 mg/m² day 1), and vincristine (1.4 mg/m² day 1), repeated every 21 days for three to six cycles. Palliation (stable disease to shrinkage) is achieved in about half of patients. An alternative is ^{131}I-MIBG treatment using 200-mCi doses at monthly intervals, over three to six cycles. The prognosis of metastatic pheochromocytoma or paraganglioma is variable, with a 5-year survival of 30–60%.

PHEOCHROMOCYTOMA IN PREGNANCY

Pheochromocytomas are occasionally diagnosed in pregnancy. Endoscopic removal, preferably in the forth to sixth month of gestation, is possible and can be followed by uneventful childbirth. Regular screening in families with inherited pheochromocytomas provides an oppor-

TABLE 337-3 PHEOCHROMOCYTOMA- AND PARAGANGLIOMA-ASSOCIATED SYNDROMES

	MEN 2	VHL	PGL4	PGL3	PGL1	NF 1
Mean age at diagnosis	34	16	34	41	26	43
Multifocal	65%	55%	12%	11%	48%	20%
Adrenal/abdominal extraadrenal	97%/3%	92%/17%	42%/58%	0	86%/57%	94%/6%
Thoracic	0	5%	12%	0	29%	0
Head and neck paraganglioma	0	0	6%	100%	48%	0
Malignancy	3%	4%	24%	0	0	12%
Associated tumors	Medullary thyroid carcinoma, primary hyperparathyroidism	Eye hemangiomas, hemangioblastomas of the CNS, clear cell renal carcinoma, pancreatic islet cell tumors, endolymphatic sac tumors of the inner ear	Renal cell carcinoma in a minority	No regular association with other tumors		Neurofibromas, café au lait spots, axillary freckling, optic pathway tumors, iris hamartomas
Inheritance	Autosomal dominant	Autosomal dominant	Autosomal dominant	Autosomal dominant, no manifestation in offspring of mothers	Autosomal dominant	Autosomal dominant
Gene name	*RET*	*VHL*	*SDHB*	*SDHC*	*SDHD*	*NF1*
Gene location	10q11.2	3p25–26	1p36	1q23	11q23	17q11.2
No. of exons	21	3	8	6	4	57

Note: CNS, central nervous system; MEN 2, multiple endocrine neoplasia type 2; NF 1, neurofibromatosis type 1; PGL, paraganglioma syndrome; VHL, von Hippel-Lindau syndrome.

Source: Adapted from the Freiburg International Pheochromocytoma and Paraganglioma Registry.

tunity to identify and remove asymptomatic tumors in women of reproductive age.

PHEOCHROMOCYTOMA-ASSOCIATED SYNDROMES

About 25–33% of patients with pheochromocytoma or paraganglioma have an inherited syndrome (Table 337-3). The mean age at diagnosis is about 15 years lower in patients with inherited syndromes compared to those with sporadic tumors.

Neurofibromatosis type 1 (NF 1) was the first described pheochromocytoma-associated syndrome (Chap. 374). The *NF1* gene functions as a tumor suppressor by regulating the ras signaling cascade. Classic features of neurofibromatosis include multiple neurofibromas, café au lait spots, axillary freckling of the skin, and Lisch nodules of the iris (Fig. 337-2). Pheochromocytomas occur in only about 1% of these patients and are located predominantly in the adrenals. Malignant pheochromocytoma is not infrequent.

The most well-known pheochromocytoma-associated syndrome is the autosomal dominant disorder *multiple endocrine neoplasia type 2A and type 2B (MEN 2A, MEN 2B)* (Chap. 345). Both types of MEN 2 are caused by mutations in *RET* (*rearranged in transfection*), which en-

FIGURE 337-2 Neurofibromatosis. A. MRI of bilateral adrenal pheochromocytoma. **B.** Cutaneous neurofibromas. **C.** Lisch nodules of the iris. **D.** Axillary freckling. [**A,** *from HPH Neumann et al: The Keio J Med 54(1):15, 2005; with permission.*]

FIGURE 337-3 Multiple endocrine neoplasia type 2. Multifocal medullary thyroid carcinoma shown by (**A**) MIBG scintigraphy and (**B**) operative specimen; arrows demonstrate the tumors; arrowheads show the tissue bridge of the cut specimen. Bilateral adrenal pheochromocytoma shown by (**C**) MIBG scintigraphy, (**D**) CT imaging, and (**E**) operative specimens. [*From HPH Neumann et al: The Keio J Med 54(1):15, 2005; with permission.*]

codes a tyrosine kinase. The locations of *RET* mutations correlate with the severity of disease and the type of MEN 2 (Chap. 345). MEN 2A is characterized by medullary thyroid carcinoma (MTC), pheochromocytoma, and hyperparathyroidism; MEN 2B also includes MTC and pheochromocytoma, as well as multiple mucosal neuromas, though it typically lacks hyperparathyroidism. Although MTC is seen in virtually all patients with MEN 2, pheochromocytoma occurs in only about 50% of patients. Most pheochromocytomas are benign, located in the adrenals, and bilateral (Fig. 337-3). Pheochromocytoma may be symptomatic before MTC. Prophylactic thyroidectomy is being performed in many carriers of *RET* mutations; pheochromocytomas should be excluded before surgery in these patients.

Von Hippel-Lindau syndrome (VHL) is an autosomal dominant disorder that predisposes to retinal and cerebellar hemangioblastomas, which also occur in the brain stem and spinal cord (Fig. 337-4). Other important features of VHL are clear cell renal carcinomas, pancreatic islet cell tumors, endolymphatic sac tumors (ELSTs) of the inner ear, cystadenomas of the epididymis and broad ligament, and multiple pancreatic or renal cysts.

The *VHL* gene encodes an E3 ubiquitin ligase that regulates expression of hypoxia-inducible factor-1 (HIF-1), among other genes. Loss of *VHL* is associated with increased expression of vascular endothelial growth factor (VEGF), which induces angiogenesis. Although the *VHL* gene can be inactivated by all types of mutations, patients with pheochromocytoma predominantly have missense mutations. About 20–30% of patients with VHL have pheochromocytomas, but in some families, the incidence can reach 90%. The recognition of pheochromocytoma as a VHL-associated feature provides an opportunity to diagnose retinal, renal, and central nervous system tumors at an earlier stage.

The *paraganglioma syndromes (PGL)* have been classified by genetic analyses of families with head and neck paragangliomas. The susceptibility genes encode subunits of the enzyme succinate dehydrogenase (SDH), a component in the Kreb's cycle and the mitochondrial electron transport chain. SDH is formed by four subunits (A–D). Mutations of *SDHB* (PGL4), *SDHC* (PGL3), and *SDHD* (PGL1) predispose to three of the paraganglioma syndromes (Table 337-3). The gene for PGL2 has not been identified yet. Mutations of SDHA do not predispose to paraganglioma tumors but instead cause Leigh disease, a form of encephalopathy. The transmission of *SDHC* and *SDHB* mutations is autosomal dominant. In contrast, SDHD families exhibit a gene imprinting effect: only the offspring of affected fathers develop tumors. In a small number of patients with familial pheochromocytoma, a mutation has not yet been identified.

PGL1 is most frequent, followed by PGL4, and PGL3 is rare. Adrenal, extraadrenal abdominal, and thoracic pheochromocytomas are components of PGL1 and PGL4, but not of PGL3 (Fig. 337-5). About one-third of the patients develop metastases.

GUIDELINES FOR GENETIC SCREENING IN PATIENTS WITH PHEOCHROMOCYTOMA OR PARAGANGLIOMA

In addition to family history, general features suggesting an inherited syndrome include young age, multifocal tumors, extraadrenal tumors, or malignant tumors (Fig. 337-6). Given the relatively high prevalence of familial syndromes among patients who present with pheochromocytoma or paraganglioma, it is useful to identify germline mutations, even in patients without a known family history. A first step is to search for clinical features of inherited syndromes and to perform an in-depth, multigenerational family history. Each of these syndromes exhibits autosomal dominant transmission with variable penetrance (Table 337-3). Cutaneous neurofibromas, café au

FIGURE 337-4 Von Hippel-Lindau disease with extraparaganglial features. Retinal angioma (**A**); hemangioblastomas of cerebellum are shown by MRI in (**B**) brain stem; (**C** and **D**) spinal cord; (**E**) carcinoma of the right kidney, cysts of the left kidney; and (**F**) multiple pancreatic cysts. [*A,D, from HPH Neumann et al: Adv Nephrol Necker Hosp 27:361, 1997. Copyright Elsevier. B, from Inherited Disorders of the Kidney, SH Morgan, J-P Grunfeld (eds). Oxford, Oxford Univ Press, 1998. E,F, from HPH Neumann et al: Contrib Nephrol 136:193, 2001. Copyright S. Karger AG, Basel.*]

lait spots, and axillary freckling suggest neurofibromatosis. Germ-line mutations in *NF1* have not been reported in patients with sporadic pheochromocytomas. Thus, *NF1* testing does not need to be performed in the absence of other clinical features of neurofibromatosis. A personal or family history of medullary thyroid cancer or parathyroid tumors strongly suggests MEN 2 and should prompt testing for *RET* mutations. A history of visual impairment, or tumors of the cerebellum, kidney, brain stem or spinal cord, suggests the possibility of VHL.

A single adrenal pheochromocytoma in a patient with an otherwise unremarkable history may still be associated with mutations of *VHL*, *RET*, *SDHB*, or *SDHD* (in decreasing order of frequency). Two-thirds of extraadrenal tumors are associated with one of these syndromes, and multifocal tumors occur with decreasing frequency in carriers of *RET*, *SDHD*, *VHL*, and *SDHB* mutations. About 25% of head and neck paragangliomas are associated with germ-line mutations of one of the SDH subunit genes (particularly *SDHD*) and are rare in carriers of *VHL* or *RET* mutations.

FIGURE 337-5 Paraganglioma syndrome. PGL1, a patient with incomplete resection of a left carotid body tumor and the *SDHD* W5X mutation. **A.** ^{18}F-dopa positron-emission tomography demonstrating tumor uptake in the right jugular glomus, the right carotid body, the left carotid body, the left coronary glomus, and the right adrenal gland. Note the physiologic accumulation of the radiopharmaceutical agent in the kidneys, liver, gallbladder, renal pelvis, and the urinary bladder. **B** and **C.** CT angiography with 3D reconstruction. Arrows point to the paraganglial tumors. [*From S Hoegerle et al: Eur J Nucl Med Mol Imaging 30(5):689, 2003; with permission.*]

FIGURE 337-6 Mutation distribution in the *RET*, *VHL*, *NF1*, *SDHB*, *SDHC*, and *SDHD* genes. The bars depict the frequency of sporadic or various inherited forms of pheochromocytoma in different age groups. The inherited disorders are much more common among younger individuals presenting with pheochromocytoma. *(Data from the Freiburg International Pheochromocytoma and Paraganglioma Registry.)*

Once the underlying syndrome is diagnosed, the benefit of genetic testing can be extended to relatives. For this purpose, it is necessary to identify the germ-line mutation in the proband and, after genetic counseling, perform DNA sequence analyses of the responsible gene in relatives to determine if they are affected (Chap. 64). Other family members may benefit from biochemical screening for tumors in individuals who carry a germ-line mutation.

FURTHER READINGS

BAUSCH B et al: Clinical and genetic characteristics of patients with neurofibromatosis type 1 and pheochromocytoma. N Engl J Med 354:2729, 2006

——— et al: Germline NF1 mutational spectra and loss-of-heterozygosity analyses in patients with pheochromocytoma and neurofibromatosis type 1. J Clin Endocrinol Metab 92:2784, 2007

LENDERS JW et al: Phaeochromocytoma. Lancet 366:665, 2005

NEUMANN HP et al: Distinct clinical features of paraganglioma syndromes associated with *SDHB* and *SDHD* gene mutations. JAMA 292:943, 2004

——— et al: Evidence of MEN-2 in the original description of classic pheochromocytoma. N Engl J Med 357:1311, 2007

——— et al: Germ-line mutations in nonsyndromic pheochromocytoma. N Engl J Med 346:1459, 2002

SCHOLZ T et al: Clinical review: Current treatment of malignant pheochromocytoma. J Clin Endocrinol Metab 92:1217, 2007

WALZ MK et al: Laparoscopic and retroperitoneoscopic treatment of pheochromocytomas and retroperitoneal paragangliomas: Results of 161 tumors in 126 patients. World J Surg 30:899, 2006

338 Diabetes Mellitus
Alvin C. Powers

Diabetes mellitus (DM) refers to a group of common metabolic disorders that share the phenotype of hyperglycemia. Several distinct types of DM exist and are caused by a complex interaction of genetics and environmental factors. Depending on the etiology of the DM, factors contributing to hyperglycemia include reduced insulin secretion, decreased glucose utilization, and increased glucose production. The metabolic dysregulation associated with DM causes secondary pathophysiologic changes in multiple organ systems that impose a tremendous burden on the individual with diabetes and on the health care system. In the United States, DM is the leading cause of end-stage renal disease (ESRD), nontraumatic lower extremity amputations, and adult blindness. It also predisposes to cardiovascular diseases. With an increasing incidence worldwide, DM will be a leading cause of morbidity and mortality for the foreseeable future.

CLASSIFICATION

DM is classified on the basis of the pathogenic process that leads to hyperglycemia, as opposed to earlier criteria such as age of onset or type of therapy (Fig. 338-1). The two broad categories of DM are designated type 1 and type 2 (Table 338-1). Both types of diabetes are preceded by a phase of abnormal glucose homeostasis as the pathogenic processes progresses. Type 1 diabetes is the result of complete or near-total insulin deficiency. Type 2 DM is a heterogeneous group of disorders characterized by variable degrees of insulin resistance, impaired insulin secretion, and increased glucose production. Distinct genetic and metabolic defects in insulin action and/or secretion give rise to the common phenotype of hyperglycemia in type 2 DM and have important potential

Type of Diabetes	Normal glucose tolerance	Hyperglycemia		
		Pre-diabetes	Diabetes Mellitus	
		Impaired fasting glucose or impaired glucose tolerance	Not insulin requiring	Insulin required for control / Insulin required for survival
Type 1				
Type 2				
Other specific types				
Gestational Diabetes				
Time (years)				
FPG	<5.6 mmol/L (100 mg/dL)	5.6–6.9 mmol/L (100–125 mg/dL)	≥7.0 mmol/L (126 mg/dL)	
2-h PG	<7.8 mmol/L (140 mg/dL)	7.8–11.1 mmol/L (140–199 mg/dL)	≥11.1 mmol/L (200 mg/dL)	

FIGURE 338-1 Spectrum of glucose homeostasis and diabetes mellitus (DM). The spectrum from normal glucose tolerance to diabetes in type 1 DM, type 2 DM, other specific types of diabetes, and gestational DM is shown from left to right. In most types of DM, the individual traverses from normal glucose tolerance to impaired glucose tolerance to overt diabetes. Arrows indicate that changes in glucose tolerance may be bi-directional in some types of diabetes. For example, individuals with type 2 DM may return to the impaired glucose tolerance category with weight loss; in gestational DM diabetes may revert to impaired glucose tolerance or even normal glucose tolerance after delivery. The fasting plasma glucose (FPG) and 2-h plasma glucose (PG), after a glucose challenge for the different categories of glucose tolerance, are shown at the lower part of the figure. These values do not apply to the diagnosis of gestational DM. Some types of DM may or may not require insulin for survival, hence the dotted line. (Conventional units are used in the figure.) *(Adapted from the American Diabetes Association, 2007.)*

TABLE 338-1 **ETIOLOGIC CLASSIFICATION OF DIABETES MELLITUS**

I. Type 1 diabetes (β-cell destruction, usually leading to absolute insulin deficiency)
   A. Immune-mediated
   B. Idiopathic
II. Type 2 diabetes (may range from predominantly insulin resistance with relative insulin deficiency to a predominantly insulin secretory defect with insulin resistance)
III. Other specific types of diabetes
   A. Genetic defects of β cell function characterized by mutations in:
     1. Hepatocyte nuclear transcription factor (HNF) 4α (MODY 1)
     2. Glucokinase (MODY 2)
     3. HNF-1α (MODY 3)
     4. Insulin promoter factor-1 (IPF-1; MODY 4)
     5. HNF-1β (MODY 5)
     6. NeuroD1 (MODY 6)
     7. Mitochondrial DNA
     8. Subunits of ATP-sensitive potassium channel
     9. Proinsulin or insulin conversion
   B. Genetic defects in insulin action
     1. Type A insulin resistance
     2. Leprechaunism
     3. Rabson-Mendenhall syndrome
     4. Lipodystrophy syndromes
   C. Diseases of the exocrine pancreas—pancreatitis, pancreatectomy, neoplasia, cystic fibrosis, hemochromatosis, fibrocalculous pancreatopathy, mutations in carboxyl ester lipase
   D. Endocrinopathies—acromegaly, Cushing's syndrome, glucagonoma, pheochromocytoma, hyperthyroidism, somatostatinoma, aldosteronoma
   E. Drug- or chemical-induced—Vacor, pentamidine, nicotinic acid, glucocorticoids, thyroid hormone, diazoxide, β-adrenergic agonists, thiazides, phenytoin, α-interferon, protease inhibitors, clozapine
   F. Infections—congenital rubella, cytomegalovirus, coxsackie
   G. Uncommon forms of immune-mediated diabetes—"stiff-person" syndrome, anti-insulin receptor antibodies
   H. Other genetic syndromes sometimes associated with diabetes—Down's syndrome, Klinefelter's syndrome, Turner's syndrome, Wolfram's syndrome, Friedreich's ataxia, Huntington's chorea, Laurence-Moon-Biedl syndrome, myotonic dystrophy, porphyria, Prader-Willi syndrome
IV. Gestational diabetes mellitus (GDM)

Note: MODY, maturity onset of diabetes of the young.
Source: Adapted from American Diabetes Association, 2007.

therapeutic implications now that pharmacologic agents are available to target specific metabolic derangements. Type 2 DM is preceded by a period of abnormal glucose homeostasis classified as impaired fasting glucose (IFG) or impaired glucose tolerance (IGT).

Two features of the current classification of DM diverge from previous classifications. First, the terms *insulin-dependent diabetes mellitus* (IDDM) and *noninsulin-dependent diabetes mellitus* (NIDDM) are obsolete. Since many individuals with type 2 DM eventually require insulin treatment for control of glycemia, the use of the term NIDDM generated considerable confusion. A second difference is that age is not a criterion in the classification system. Although type 1 DM most commonly develops before the age of 30, an autoimmune beta cell destructive process can develop at any age. It is estimated that between 5 and 10% of individuals who develop DM after age 30 have type 1 DM. Likewise, type 2 DM more typically develops with increasing age but is now being diagnosed more frequently in children and young adults, particularly in obese adolescents.

OTHER TYPES OF DM

Other etiologies for DM include specific genetic defects in insulin secretion or action, metabolic abnormalities that impair insulin secretion, mitochondrial abnormalities, and a host of conditions that impair glucose tolerance (Table 338-1). *Maturity onset diabetes of the young* (MODY) is a subtype of DM characterized by autosomal dominant inheritance, early onset of hyperglycemia (usually <25 years), and impairment in insulin secretion (discussed below). Mutations in the insulin receptor cause a group of rare disorders characterized by severe insulin resistance.

DM can result from pancreatic exocrine disease when the majority of pancreatic islets are destroyed. Hormones that antagonize insulin action can also lead to DM. Thus, DM is often a feature of endocrinopathies such as acromegaly and Cushing's disease. Viral infections have been implicated in pancreatic islet destruction but are an extremely rare cause of DM. A form of acute onset of type 1 diabetes, termed *fulminant diabetes*, has been noted in Japan and may be related to viral infection of islets.

GESTATIONAL DIABETES MELLITUS (GDM)

Glucose intolerance may develop during pregnancy. Insulin resistance is related to the metabolic changes of late pregnancy, and the increased insulin requirements may lead to IGT. GDM occurs in ~4% of pregnancies in the United States; most women revert to normal glucose tolerance post-partum but have a substantial risk (30–60%) of developing DM later in life.

EPIDEMIOLOGY

The worldwide prevalence of DM has risen dramatically over the past two decades, from an estimated 30 million cases in 1985 to 177 million in 2000. Based on current trends, >360 million individuals will have diabetes by the year 2030 (Fig. 338-2). Although the prevalence of both type 1 and type 2 DM is increasing worldwide, the prevalence of type 2 DM is rising much more rapidly because of increasing obesity and reduced activity levels as countries become more industrialized. This is true in most countries, and 6 of the top 10 countries with the highest rates are in Asia. In the United States, the Centers for Disease Control and Prevention (CDC) estimated that 20.8 million persons, or 7% of the population, had diabetes in 2005 (~30% of individuals with diabetes were undiagnosed). Approximately 1.5

FIGURE 338-2 Worldwide prevalence of diabetes mellitus. The prevalence of diabetes in 2000 and the projected prevalence in 2030 are shown by geographical region. *(Used with permission from Diabetes Action Now: An Initiative of the World Health Organization and the International Diabetes Federation, 2004, as adapted from S Wild et al: Diabetes Care 27:1047, 2004.)*

million individuals (>20 years) were newly diagnosed with diabetes in 2005. DM increases with aging. In 2005, the prevalence of DM in the United Sates was estimated to be 0.22% in those <20 years and 9.6% in those >20 years. In individuals >60 years, the prevalence of DM was 20.9%. The prevalence is similar in men and women throughout most age ranges (10.5% and 8.8% in individuals >20 years) but is slightly greater in men >60 years. Worldwide estimates project that in 2030 the greatest number of individuals with diabetes will be 45–64 years of age.

There is considerable geographic variation in the incidence of both type 1 and type 2 DM. Scandinavia has the highest incidence of type 1 DM (e.g., in Finland, the incidence is 35/100,000 per year). The Pacific Rim has a much lower rate (in Japan and China, the incidence is 1–3/100,000 per year) of type 1 DM; Northern Europe and the United States have an intermediate rate (8–17/100,000 per year). Much of the increased risk of type 1 DM is believed to reflect the frequency of high-risk HLA alleles among ethnic groups in different geographic locations. The prevalence of type 2 DM and its harbinger, IGT, is highest in certain Pacific islands, intermediate in countries such as India and the United States, and relatively low in Russia. This variability is likely due to genetic, behavioral, and environmental factors. DM prevalence also varies among different ethnic populations within a given country. In 2005, the CDC estimated that the prevalence of DM in the United States (age > 20 years) was 13.3% in African Americans, 9.5% in Latinos, 15.1% in Native Americans (American Indians and Alaska natives), and 8.7% in non-Hispanic whites. Individuals belonging to Asian-American or Pacific-Islander ethnic groups in Hawaii are twice as likely to have diabetes compared to non-Hispanic whites. The onset of type 2 DM occurs, on average, at an earlier age in ethnic groups other than non-Hispanic whites.

Diabetes is a major cause of mortality, but several studies indicate that diabetes is likely underreported as a cause of death. In the United States, diabetes was listed as the sixth-leading cause of death in 2002; a recent estimate suggested that diabetes was the fifth leading cause of death worldwide and was responsible for almost 3 million deaths annually (1.7–5.2% of deaths worldwide).

DIAGNOSIS

The National Diabetes Data Group and World Health Organization have issued diagnostic criteria for DM (Table 338-2) based on the following premises: (1) the spectrum of fasting plasma glucose (FPG) and the response to an oral glucose load (OGTT—oral glucose tolerance test) varies among normal individuals, and (2) DM is defined as the level of glycemia at which diabetes-specific complications occur rather than on deviations from a population-based mean. For example, the prevalence of retinopathy in Native Americans (Pima Indian population) begins to increase at a FPG > 6.4 mmol/L (116 mg/dL) (Fig. 338-3).

Glucose tolerance is classified into three categories based on the FPG (Fig. 338-1): (1) FPG < 5.6 mmol/L (100 mg/dL) is considered normal; (2) FPG = 5.6–6.9 mmol/L (100–125 mg/dL) is defined as IFG; and (3) FPG ≥7.0 mmol/L (126 mg/dL) warrants the diagnosis of DM. Based on the OGTT, IGT is defined as plasma glucose levels between 7.8 and 11.1 mmol/L (140 and 199 mg/dL) and diabetes is de-

FPG (mg/dL)	70-	89-	93-	97-	100-	105-	109-	116-	136-	226-
2-h PG (mg/dL)	38-	94-	106-	116-	126-	138-	156-	185-	244-	364-
HbA1c (%)	3.4-	4.8-	5.0-	5.2-	5.3-	5.5-	5.7-	6.0-	6.7-	9.5-

FIGURE 338-3 Relationship of diabetes-specific complication and glucose tolerance. This figure shows the incidence of retinopathy in Pima Indians as a function of the fasting plasma glucose (FPG), the 2-h plasma glucose after a 75-g oral glucose challenge (2-h PG), or glycated hemoglobin (A1C). Note that the incidence of retinopathy greatly increases at a fasting plasma glucose >116 mg/dL, or a 2-h plasma glucose of 185 mg/dL, or a A1C >6.0%. (Blood glucose values are shown in mg/dL; to convert to mmol/L, divide value by 18.) (*Copyright 2002, American Diabetes Association. From Diabetes Care 25(Suppl 1): S5–S20, 2002.*)

fined as a glucose > 11.1 mmol/L (200 mg/dL) 2 h after a 75-g oral glucose load (Table 338-2). Some individuals have both IFG and IGT. Individuals with IFG and/or IGT, recently designated *pre-diabetes* by the American Diabetes Association (ADA), are at substantial risk for developing type 2 DM (25–40% risk over the next 5 years) and have an increased risk of cardiovascular disease.

The current criteria for the diagnosis of DM emphasize that the FPG is the most reliable and convenient test for identifying DM in asymptomatic individuals. A random plasma glucose concentration ≥11.1 mmol/L (200 mg/dL) accompanied by classic symptoms of DM (polyuria, polydipsia, weight loss) is sufficient for the diagnosis of DM (Table 338-2). Oral glucose tolerance testing, although still a valid means for diagnosing DM, is not recommended as part of routine care.

Some investigators have advocated the hemoglobin A1C (A1C) as a diagnostic test for DM. Though there is a strong correlation between elevations in the plasma glucose and the A1C (discussed below), the relationship between the FPG and the A1C in individuals with normal glucose tolerance or mild glucose intolerance is less clear, and thus the use of the A1C is not currently recommended to diagnose diabetes.

The diagnosis of DM has profound implications for an individual from both a medical and financial standpoint. Thus, these diagnostic criteria must be satisfied before assigning the diagnosis of DM. Abnormalities on screening tests for diabetes should be repeated before making a definitive diagnosis of DM, unless acute metabolic derangements or a markedly elevated plasma glucose are present (Table 338-2). The revised criteria also allow for the diagnosis of DM to be withdrawn in situations where the FPG reverts to normal.

SCREENING

Widespread use of the FPG as a screening test for type 2 DM is recommended because: (1) a large number of individuals who meet the current criteria for DM are asymptomatic and unaware that they have the disorder, (2) epidemiologic studies suggest that type 2 DM may be present for up to a decade before diagnosis, (3) as many as 50% of individuals with type 2 DM have one or more diabetes-specific complications at the time of their diagnosis, and (4) treatment of type 2 DM may favorably alter the natural history of DM. The ADA recommends screening all individuals >45 years every 3 years and screening individuals at an earlier age if they are overweight [body mass index (BMI) > 25 km/m²] and have one additional risk factor for diabetes

---

TABLE 338-2 CRITERIA FOR THE DIAGNOSIS OF DIABETES MELLITUS

- Symptoms of diabetes plus random blood glucose concentration ≥11.1 mmol/L (200 mg/dL)[a] *or*
- Fasting plasma glucose ≥7.0 mmol/L (126 mg/dL)[b] *or*
- Two-hour plasma glucose ≥11.1 mmol/L (200 mg/dL) during an oral glucose tolerance test[c]

[a]Random is defined as without regard to time since the last meal.
[b]Fasting is defined as no caloric intake for at least 8 h.
[c]The test should be performed using a glucose load containing the equivalent of 75 g anhydrous glucose dissolved in water; not recommended for routine clinical use.
Note: In the absence of unequivocal hyperglycemia and acute metabolic decompensation, these criteria should be confirmed by repeat testing on a different day.
Source: Adapted from American Diabetes Association, 2007.

TABLE 338-3 **RISK FACTORS FOR TYPE 2 DIABETES MELLITUS**

Family history of diabetes (i.e., parent or sibling with type 2 diabetes)
Obesity (BMI ≥25 kg/m²)
Habitual physical inactivity
Race/ethnicity (e.g., African American, Latino, Native American, Asian
   American, Pacific Islander)
Previously identified IFG or IGT
History of GDM or delivery of baby >4 kg (>9 lb)
Hypertension (blood pressure ≥140/90 mmHg)
HDL cholesterol level <35 mg/dL (0.90 mmol/L) and/or a triglyceride level
   >250 mg/dL (2.82 mmol/L)
Polycystic ovary syndrome or acanthosis nigricans
History of vascular disease

Note: BMI, body mass index; IFG, impaired fasting glucose; IGT, impaired glucose tolerance; GDM, gestational diabetes mellitus; HDL, high-density lipoprotein.
Source: Adapted from American Diabetes Association, 2007.

(Table 338-3). In contrast to type 2 DM, a long asymptomatic period of hyperglycemia is rare prior to the diagnosis of type 1 DM. A number of immunologic markers for type 1 DM are becoming available (discussed below), but their routine use is discouraged pending the identification of clinically beneficial interventions for individuals at high risk for developing type 1 DM.

INSULIN BIOSYNTHESIS, SECRETION, AND ACTION

BIOSYNTHESIS

Insulin is produced in the beta cells of the pancreatic islets. It is initially synthesized as a single-chain 86-amino-acid precursor polypeptide, preproinsulin. Subsequent proteolytic processing removes the amino-terminal signal peptide, giving rise to proinsulin. Proinsulin is structurally related to insulin-like growth factors I and II, which bind weakly to the insulin receptor. Cleavage of an internal 31-residue fragment from proinsulin generates the C peptide and the A (21 amino acids) and B (30 amino acids) chains of insulin, which are connected by disulfide bonds. The mature insulin molecule and C peptide are stored together and cosecreted from secretory granules in the beta cells. Because the C peptide is cleared more slowly than insulin, it is a useful marker of insulin secretion and allows discrimination of endogenous and exogenous sources of insulin in the evaluation of hypoglycemia (Chaps. 339 and 344). Pancreatic beta cells cosecrete islet amyloid polypeptide (IAPP) or amylin, a 37-amino-acid peptide, along with insulin. The role of IAPP in normal physiology is unclear, but it is the major component of the amyloid fibrils found in the islets of patients with type 2 diabetes, and an analogue is sometimes used in treating both type 1 and type 2 DM. Human insulin is now produced by recombinant DNA technology; structural alterations at one or more residues are useful for modifying its physical and pharmacologic characteristics (see below).

SECRETION

Glucose is the key regulator of insulin secretion by the pancreatic beta cell, although amino acids, ketones, various nutrients, gastrointestinal peptides, and neurotransmitters also influence insulin secretion. Glucose levels > 3.9 mmol/L (70 mg/dL) stimulate insulin synthesis, primarily by enhancing protein translation and processing. Glucose stimulation of insulin secretion begins with its transport into the beta cell by the GLUT2 glucose transporter (Fig. 338-4). Glucose phosphorylation by glucokinase is the rate-limiting step that controls glucose-regulated insulin secretion. Further metabolism of glucose-6-phosphate via glycolysis generates ATP, which inhibits the activity of an ATP-sensitive K⁺ channel. This channel consists of two separate proteins: one is the binding site for certain oral hypoglycemics (e.g., sulfonylureas, meglitinides); the other is an inwardly rectifying K⁺ channel protein (Kir6.2). Inhibition of this K⁺ channel induces beta cell membrane depolarization, which opens voltage-dependent calcium channels (leading to an influx of calcium), and stimulates insulin secretion. Insulin secretory profiles reveal a pulsatile pattern of hormone release, with small secreto-

FIGURE 338-4 **Diabetes and abnormalities in glucose-stimulated insulin secretion.** Glucose and other nutrients regulate insulin secretion by the pancreatic beta cell. Glucose is transported by the GLUT2 glucose transporter; subsequent glucose metabolism by the beta cell alters ion channel activity, leading to insulin secretion. The SUR receptor is the binding site for drugs that act as insulin secretagogues. Mutations in the events or proteins underlined are a cause of maturity onset diabetes of the young (MODY) or other forms of diabetes. SUR, sulfonylurea receptor; ATP, adenosine triphosphate; ADP, adenosine diphosphate; cAMP, cyclic adenosine monophosphate. (Adapted from WL Lowe, in JL Jameson (ed): Principles of Molecular Medicine. Totowa, NJ, Humana, 1998.)

ry bursts occurring about every 10 min, superimposed upon greater amplitude oscillations of about 80–150 min. Incretins are released from neuroendocrine cells of the gastrointestinal tract following food ingestion and amplify glucose-stimulated insulin secretion and suppress glucagon secretion. Glucagon-like peptide 1 (GLP-1), the most potent incretin, is released from L cells in the small intestine and stimulates insulin secretion only when the blood glucose is above the fasting level. Incretin analogues, such as exena-tide, are being used to enhance endogenous insulin secretion (see below).

ACTION

Once insulin is secreted into the portal venous system, ~50% is degraded by the liver. Unextracted insulin enters the systemic circulation where it binds to receptors in target sites. Insulin binding to its receptor stimulates intrinsic tyrosine kinase activity, leading to receptor autophosphorylation and the recruitment of intracellular signaling molecules, such as insulin receptor substrates (IRS) (Fig. 338-5). IRS and other adaptor proteins initiate a complex cascade of phosphorylation and dephosphorylation reactions, resulting in the widespread metabolic and mitogenic effects of insulin. As an example, activation of the phosphatidylinositol-3'-kinase (PI-3-kinase) pathway stimulates translocation of glucose transporters (e.g., GLUT4) to the cell surface, an event that is crucial for glucose uptake by skeletal muscle and fat. Activation of other insulin receptor signaling pathways induces glycogen synthesis, protein synthesis, lipogenesis, and regulation of various genes in insulin-responsive cells.

Glucose homeostasis reflects a balance between hepatic glucose production and peripheral glucose uptake and utilization. Insulin is the most important regulator of this metabolic equilibrium, but neural input, metabolic signals, and other hormones (e.g., glucagon) result in integrated control of glucose supply and utilization (Chap. 339; see Fig. 339-1). In the fasting state, low insulin levels increase glucose production by promoting hepatic gluconeogenesis and glycogenolysis and reduce glucose uptake in insulin-sensitive tissues (skeletal muscle and fat),

FIGURE 338-5 Insulin signal transduction pathway in skeletal muscle. The insulin receptor has intrinsic tyrosine kinase activity and interacts with insulin receptor substrates (IRS and Shc) proteins. A number of "docking" proteins bind to these cellular proteins and initiate the metabolic actions of insulin [GrB-2, SOS, SHP-2, p65, p110, and phosphatidylinositol-3′-kinase (PI-3-kinase)]. Insulin increases glucose transport through PI-3-kinase and the Cbl pathway, which promotes the translocation of intracellular vesicles containing GLUT4 glucose transporter to the plasma membrane. *(Adapted from WL Lowe, in Principles of Molecular Medicine, JL Jameson (ed). Totowa, NJ, Humana, 1998; A Virkamaki et al: J Clin Invest 103:931, 1999. For additional details see AR Saltiel, CR Kahn: Nature 414:799, 2001.)*

thereby promoting mobilization of stored precursors such as amino acids and free fatty acids (lipolysis). Glucagon, secreted by pancreatic alpha cells when blood glucose or insulin levels are low, stimulates glycogenolysis and gluconeogenesis by the liver and renal medulla. Postprandially, the glucose load elicits a rise in insulin and fall in glucagon, leading to a reversal of these processes. Insulin, an anabolic hormone, promotes the storage of carbohydrate and fat and protein synthesis. The major portion of postprandial glucose is utilized by skeletal muscle, an effect of insulin-stimulated glucose uptake. Other tissues, most notably the brain, utilize glucose in an insulin-independent fashion.

PATHOGENESIS

TYPE 1 DM

Type 1 DM is the result of interactions of genetic, environmental, and immunologic factors that ultimately lead to the destruction of the pancreatic beta cells and insulin deficiency. Type 1 DM results from autoimmune beta cell destruction and most, but not all, individuals have evidence of islet-directed autoimmunity. Some individuals who have the clinical phenotype of type 1 DM lack immunologic markers indicative of an autoimmune process involving the beta cells. These individuals are thought to develop insulin deficiency by unknown, nonimmune mechanisms and are ketosis prone; many are African American or Asian in heritage. The temporal development of type 1 DM is shown schematically as a function of beta cell mass in Fig. 338-6. Individuals with a genetic susceptibility have normal beta cell mass at birth but begin to lose beta cells secondary to autoimmune destruction that occurs over months to years. This autoimmune process is thought to be triggered by an infectious or environmental stimulus and to be sustained by a beta cell–specific molecule. In the majority, immunologic markers appear after the triggering event but before diabetes becomes clinically overt. Beta cell mass then begins to decline, and insulin secretion becomes progressively impaired, although normal glucose tolerance is maintained. The rate of decline in beta cell mass varies widely among individuals, with some patients progressing rapidly to clinical diabetes and others evolving more slowly. Features of diabetes do not become evident until a majority of beta cells are destroyed (~80%). At this point, residual functional beta cells still exist but are insufficient in number to maintain glucose tolerance. The events that trigger the transition from glucose intolerance to frank dia-

betes are often associated with increased insulin requirements, as might occur during infections or puberty. After the initial clinical presentation of type 1 DM, a "honeymoon" phase may ensue during which time glycemic control is achieved with modest doses of insulin or, rarely, insulin is not needed. However, this fleeting phase of endogenous insulin production from residual beta cells disappears as the autoimmune process destroys the remaining beta cells, and the individual becomes completely insulin deficient.

GENETIC CONSIDERATIONS Susceptibility to type 1 DM involves multiple genes. The concordance of type 1 DM in identical twins ranges between 30 and 70%, indicating that additional modifying factors are likely involved in determining whether diabetes develops. The major susceptibility gene for type 1 DM is located in the HLA region on chromosome 6. Polymorphisms in the HLA complex account for 40–50% of the genetic risk of developing type 1 DM. This region contains genes that encode the class II MHC molecules, which present antigen to helper T cells and thus are involved in initiating the immune response (Chap. 309). The ability of class II MHC molecules to present antigen is dependent on the amino acid composition of their antigen-binding sites. Amino acid substitutions may influence the specificity of the immune response by altering the binding affinity of different antigens for class II molecules.

Most individuals with type 1 DM have the HLA DR3 and/or DR4 haplotype. Refinements in genotyping of HLA loci have shown that the haplotypes DQA1*0301, DQB1*0302, and DQB1*0201 are most strongly associated with type 1 DM. These haplotypes are present in 40% of chil-

FIGURE 338-6 Temporal model for development of type 1 diabetes. Individuals with a genetic predisposition are exposed to an immunologic trigger that initiates an autoimmune process, resulting in a gradual decline in beta cell mass. The downward slope of the beta cell mass varies among individuals and may not be continuous. This progressive impairment in insulin release results in diabetes when ~80% of the beta cell mass is destroyed. A "honeymoon" phase may be seen in the first 1 or 2 years after the onset of diabetes and is associated with reduced insulin requirements. *[Adapted from Medical Management of Type 1 Diabetes, 3d ed, JS Skyler (ed). American Diabetes Association, Alexandria, VA, 1998.]*

dren with type 1 DM as compared to 2% of the normal U.S. population. However, most individuals with predisposing haplotypes do not develop diabetes.

In addition to MHC class II associations, at least 10 different genetic loci contribute susceptibility to type 1 DM (loci recently identified include polymorphisms in the promoter region of the insulin gene, the CTLA-4 gene, interleukin-2 receptor, *IFIH1*, and PTPN22). Genes that confer protection against the development of the disease also exist. The haplotype DQA1*0102, DQB1*0602 is extremely rare in individuals with type 1 DM (<1%) and appears to provide protection from type 1 DM.

Although the risk of developing type 1 DM is increased tenfold in relatives of individuals with the disease, the risk is relatively low: 3–4% if the parent has type 1 diabetes and 5–15% in a sibling (depending on which HLA haplotypes are shared). Hence, most individuals with type 1 DM do not have a first-degree relative with this disorder.

Pathophysiology Although other islet cell types [alpha cells (glucagon-producing), delta cells (somatostatin-producing), or PP cells (pancreatic polypeptide-producing)] are functionally and embryologically similar to beta cells and express most of the same proteins as beta cells, they are inexplicably spared from the autoimmune process. Pathologically, the pancreatic islets are infiltrated with lymphocytes (in a process termed *insulitis*). After all beta cells are destroyed, the inflammatory process abates, the islets become atrophic, and most immunologic markers disappear. Studies of the autoimmune process in humans and in animal models of type 1 DM (NOD mouse and BB rat) have identified the following abnormalities in the humoral and cellular arms of the immune system: (1) islet cell autoantibodies; (2) activated lymphocytes in the islets, peripancreatic lymph nodes, and systemic circulation; (3) T lymphocytes that proliferate when stimulated with islet proteins; and (4) release of cytokines within the insulitis. Beta cells seem to be particularly susceptible to the toxic effect of some cytokines [tumor necrosis factor α (TNF-α), interferon γ, and interleukin 1 (IL-1)]. The precise mechanisms of beta cell death are not known but may involve formation of nitric oxide metabolites, apoptosis, and direct CD8+ T cell cytotoxicity. The islet destruction is mediated by T lymphocytes rather than islet autoantibodies, as these antibodies do not generally react with the cell surface of islet cells and are not capable of transferring DM to animals. Suppression of the autoimmune process (cyclosporine, T lymphocyte antibodies) at the time of diagnosis of diabetes slows the decline in beta cell destruction, but the safety of such interventions is unknown.

Pancreatic islet molecules targeted by the autoimmune process include insulin, glutamic acid decarboxylase (GAD, the biosynthetic enzyme for the neurotransmitter GABA), ICA-512/IA-2 (homology with tyrosine phosphatases), and phogrin (insulin secretory granule protein). With the exception of insulin, none of the autoantigens are beta cell specific, which raises the question of how the beta cells are selectively destroyed. Current theories favor initiation of an autoimmune process directed at one beta cell molecule, which then spreads to other islet molecules as the immune process destroys beta cells and creates a series of secondary autoantigens. The beta cells of individuals who develop type 1 DM do not differ from beta cells of normal individuals, since islets transplanted from a genetically identical twin are destroyed by a recurrence of the autoimmune process of type 1 DM.

Immunologic Markers Islet cell autoantibodies (ICAs) are a composite of several different antibodies directed at pancreatic islet molecules such as GAD, insulin, and IA-2/ICA-512 and serve as a marker of the autoimmune process of type 1 DM. Assays for autoantibodies to GAD-65 are commercially available. Testing for ICAs can be useful in classifying the type of DM as type 1 and in identifying nondiabetic individuals at risk for developing type 1 DM. ICAs are present in the majority of individuals (>75%) diagnosed with new-onset type 1 DM, in a significant minority of individuals with newly diagnosed type 2 DM (5–10%), and occasionally in individuals with GDM (<5%). ICAs

are present in 3–4% of first-degree relatives of individuals with type 1 DM. In combination with impaired insulin secretion after IV glucose tolerance testing, they predict a >50% risk of developing type 1 DM within 5 years. Without this impairment in insulin secretion, the presence of ICAs predicts a 5-year risk of <25%. Based on these data, the risk of a first-degree relative developing type 1 DM is relatively low. At present, the measurement of ICAs in nondiabetic individuals is a research tool because no treatments have been approved to prevent the occurrence or progression to type 1 DM.

Environmental Factors Numerous environmental events have been proposed to trigger the autoimmune process in genetically susceptible individuals; however, none have been conclusively linked to diabetes. Identification of an environmental trigger has been difficult because the event may precede the onset of DM by several years (Fig. 338-6). Putative environmental triggers include viruses (coxsackie and rubella most prominently), bovine milk proteins, and nitrosourea compounds.

Prevention of Type 1 DM A number of interventions have successfully delayed or prevented diabetes in animal models. Some interventions have targeted the immune system directly (immunosuppression, selective T cell subset deletion, induction of immunologic tolerance to islet proteins), whereas others have prevented islet cell death by blocking cytotoxic cytokines or increasing islet resistance to the destructive process. Though results in animal models are promising, these interventions have not been successful in preventing type 1 DM in humans. The Diabetes Prevention Trial—type 1 concluded that administering insulin (IV or PO) to individuals at high risk for developing type 1 DM did not prevent type 1 DM. In patients with new-onset type 1 diabetes, treatment with anti-CD3 monoclonal antibodies has recently been shown to slow the decline in C-peptide levels.

TYPE 2 DM
Insulin resistance and abnormal insulin secretion are central to the development of type 2 DM. Although the primary defect is controversial, most studies support the view that insulin resistance precedes an insulin secretory defect but that diabetes develops only when insulin secretion becomes inadequate.

GENETIC CONSIDERATIONS Type 2 DM has a strong genetic component. The concordance of type 2 DM in identical twins is between 70 and 90%. Individuals with a parent with type 2 DM have an increased risk of diabetes; if both parents have type 2 DM, the risk approaches 40%. Insulin resistance, as demonstrated by reduced glucose utilization in skeletal muscle, is present in many nondiabetic, first-degree relatives of individuals with type 2 DM. The disease is polygenic and multifactorial since in addition to genetic susceptibility, environmental factors (such as obesity, nutrition, and physical activity) modulate the phenotype. The genes that predispose to type 2 DM are incompletely identified, but recent genome-wide association studies have identified several genes that convey a relatively small risk for type 2 DM (relative risk of 1.1-1.5). Most prominent is a variant of the transcription factor 7-like 2 gene that has been associated with type 2 diabetes in several populations and with impaired glucose tolerance in one population at high risk for diabetes. Genetic polymorphisms associated with type 2 diabetes have also been found in the genes encoding the peroxisome proliferators-activated receptor-γ, inward rectifying potassium channel expressed in beta cells, zinc transporter expressed in beta cells, IRS, and calpain 10. The mechanisms by which these genetic alterations increase the susceptibility to type 2 diabetes are not clear, but several are predicted to alter insulin secretion. Investigation using genome-wide scanning for polymorphisms associated with type 2 DM is ongoing.

Pathophysiology Type 2 DM is characterized by impaired insulin secretion, insulin resistance, excessive hepatic glucose production, and abnormal fat metabolism. Obesity, particularly visceral or central (as

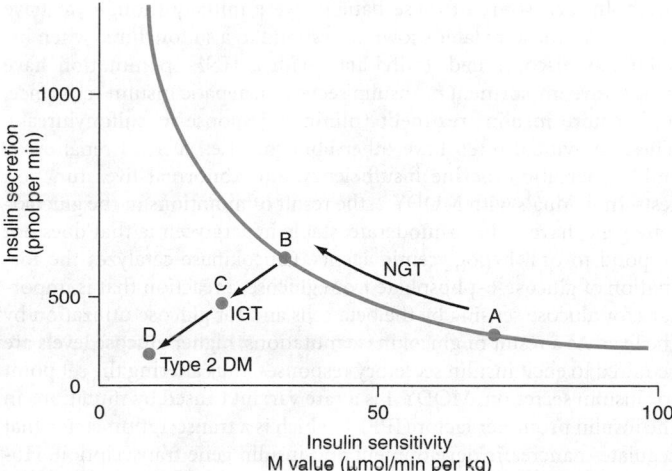

FIGURE 338-7 Metabolic changes during the development of type 2 diabetes mellitus (DM). Insulin secretion and insulin sensitivity are related, and as an individual becomes more insulin resistant (by moving from point A to point B), insulin secretion increases. A failure to compensate by increasing the insulin secretion results initially in impaired glucose tolerance (IGT; point C) and ultimately in type 2 DM (point D). (Adapted from SE Kahn: J Clin Endocrinol Metab 86:4047, 2001; RN Bergman, M Ader: Trends Endocrinol Metab 11:351, 2000.)

evidenced by the hip-waist ratio), is very common in type 2 DM. In the early stages of the disorder, glucose tolerance remains near-normal, despite insulin resistance, because the pancreatic beta cells compensate by increasing insulin output (Fig. 338-7). As insulin resistance and compensatory hyperinsulinemia progress, the pancreatic islets in certain individuals are unable to sustain the hyperinsulinemic state. IGT, characterized by elevations in postprandial glucose, then develops. A further decline in insulin secretion and an increase in hepatic glucose production lead to overt diabetes with fasting hyperglycemia. Ultimately, beta cell failure may ensue.

Metabolic Abnormalities • ABNORMAL MUSCLE AND FAT METABOLISM Insulin resistance, the decreased ability of insulin to act effectively on target tissues (especially muscle, liver, and fat), is a prominent feature of type 2 DM and results from a combination of genetic susceptibility and obesity. Insulin resistance is relative, however, since supernormal levels of circulating insulin will normalize the plasma glucose. Insulin dose-response curves exhibit a rightward shift, indicating reduced sensitivity, and a reduced maximal response, indicating an overall decrease in maximum glucose utilization (30–60% lower than in normal individuals). Insulin resistance impairs glucose utilization by insulin-sensitive tissues and increases hepatic glucose output; both effects contribute to the hyperglycemia. Increased hepatic glucose output predominantly accounts for increased FPG levels, whereas decreased peripheral glucose usage results in postprandial hyperglycemia. In skeletal muscle, there is a greater impairment in nonoxidative glucose usage (glycogen formation) than in oxidative glucose metabolism through glycolysis. Glucose metabolism in insulin-independent tissues is not altered in type 2 DM.

The precise molecular mechanism leading to insulin resistance in type 2 DM has not been elucidated. Insulin receptor levels and tyrosine kinase activity in skeletal muscle are reduced, but these alterations are most likely secondary to hyperinsulinemia and are not a primary defect. Therefore, "postreceptor" defects in insulin-regulated phosphorylation/dephosphorylation may play the predominant role in insulin resistance (Fig. 338-5). For example, a PI-3-kinase signaling defect may reduce translocation of GLUT4 to the plasma membrane. Other abnormalities include the accumulation of lipid within skeletal myocytes, which may impair mitochondrial oxidative phosphorylation and reduce insulin-stimulated mitochondrial ATP production. Impaired fatty acid oxidation and lipid accumulation within skeletal myocytes may generate reactive

oxygen species such as lipid peroxides. Of note, not all insulin signal transduction pathways are resistant to the effects of insulin (e.g., those controlling cell growth and differentiation using the mitogenic-activated protein kinase pathway). Consequently, hyperinsulinemia may increase the insulin action through these pathways, potentially accelerating diabetes-related conditions such as atherosclerosis.

The obesity accompanying type 2 DM, particularly in a central or visceral location, is thought to be part of the pathogenic process. The increased adipocyte mass leads to increased levels of circulating free fatty acids and other fat cell products (Chap. 74). For example, adipocytes secrete a number of biologic products (nonesterified free fatty acids, retinol-binding protein 4, leptin, TNF-α, resistin, and adiponectin). In addition to regulating body weight, appetite, and energy expenditure, adipokines also modulate insulin sensitivity. The increased production of free fatty acids and some adipokines may cause insulin resistance in skeletal muscle and liver. For example, free fatty acids impair glucose utilization in skeletal muscle, promote glucose production by the liver, and impair beta cell function. In contrast, the production by adipocytes of adiponectin, an insulin-sensitizing peptide, is reduced in obesity and this may contribute to hepatic insulin resistance. Adipocyte products and adipokines also produce an inflammatory state and may explain why markers of inflammation such as IL-6 and C-reactive protein are often elevated in type 2 DM. Inhibition of inflammatory signaling pathways such as the nuclear factor κB (NFκB) pathway appears to reduce insulin resistance and improve hyperglycemia in animal models.

IMPAIRED INSULIN SECRETION Insulin secretion and sensitivity are interrelated (Fig. 338-7). In type 2 DM, insulin secretion initially increases in response to insulin resistance to maintain normal glucose tolerance. Initially, the insulin secretory defect is mild and selectively involves glucose-stimulated insulin secretion. The response to other nonglucose secretagogues, such as arginine, is preserved. Eventually, the insulin secretory defect progresses to a state of grossly inadequate insulin secretion.

The reason(s) for the decline in insulin secretory capacity in type 2 DM is unclear. The assumption is that a second genetic defect—superimposed upon insulin resistance—leads to beta cell failure. Islet amyloid polypeptide or amylin is cosecreted by the beta cell and forms the amyloid fibrillar deposit found in the islets of individuals with long-standing type 2 DM. Whether such islet amyloid deposits are a primary or secondary event is not known. The metabolic environment of diabetes may also negatively impact islet function. For example, chronic hyperglycemia paradoxically impairs islet function ("glucose toxicity") and leads to a worsening of hyperglycemia. Improvement in glycemic control is often associated with improved islet function. In addition, elevation of free fatty acid levels ("lipotoxicity") and dietary fat may also worsen islet function. Beta cell mass is decreased in individuals with long-standing type 2 diabetes.

INCREASED HEPATIC GLUCOSE AND LIPID PRODUCTION In type 2 DM, insulin resistance in the liver reflects the failure of hyperinsulinemia to suppress gluconeogenesis, which results in fasting hyperglycemia and decreased glycogen storage by the liver in the postprandial state. Increased hepatic glucose production occurs early in the course of diabetes, though likely after the onset of insulin secretory abnormalities and insulin resistance in skeletal muscle. As a result of insulin resistance in adipose tissue and obesity, free fatty acid (FFA) flux from adipocytes is increased, leading to increased lipid [very low density lipoprotein (VLDL) and triglyceride] synthesis in hepatocytes. This lipid storage or steatosis in the liver may lead to nonalcoholic fatty liver disease (Chap. 303) and abnormal liver function tests. This is also responsible for the dyslipidemia found in type 2 DM [elevated triglycerides, reduced high-density lipoprotein (HDL), and increased small dense low-density lipoprotein (LDL) particles].

Insulin Resistance Syndromes The insulin resistance condition comprises a spectrum of disorders, with hyperglycemia representing one of the most readily diagnosed features. The *metabolic syndrome*, the *insulin resistance syndrome*, or *syndrome X* are terms used to describe a constellation of metabolic derangements that includes insulin resistance, hypertension, dyslipidemia (low HDL and elevated triglycerides), central or visceral obesity, type 2 diabetes or IGT/IFG, and accelerated cardiovascular disease. This syndrome is discussed in Chap. 236.

A number of relatively rare forms of severe insulin resistance include features of type 2 DM or IGT (Table 338-1). Acanthosis nigricans and signs of hyperandrogenism (hirsutism, acne, and oligomenorrhea in women) are also common physical features. Two distinct syndromes of severe insulin resistance have been described in adults: (1) type A, which affects young women and is characterized by severe hyperinsulinemia, obesity, and features of hyperandrogenism; and (2) type B, which affects middle-aged women and is characterized by severe hyperinsulinemia, features of hyperandrogenism, and autoimmune disorders. Individuals with the type A insulin resistance syndrome have an undefined defect in the insulin-signaling pathway; individuals with the type B insulin resistance syndrome have autoantibodies directed at the insulin receptor. These receptor autoantibodies may block insulin binding or may stimulate the insulin receptor, leading to intermittent hypoglycemia.

Polycystic ovary syndrome (PCOS) is a common disorder that affects premenopausal women and is characterized by chronic anovulation and hyperandrogenism (Chap. 341). Insulin resistance is seen in a significant subset of women with PCOS, and the disorder substantially increases the risk for type 2 DM, independent of the effects of obesity.

Prevention Type 2 DM is preceded by a period of IGT, and a number of lifestyle modifications and pharmacologic agents prevent or delay the onset of DM. The Diabetes Prevention Program (DPP) demonstrated that intensive changes in lifestyle (diet and exercise for 30 min/day five times/week) in individuals with IGT prevented or delayed the development of type 2 DM by 58% compared to placebo. This effect was seen in individuals regardless of age, sex, or ethnic group. In the same study, metformin prevented or delayed diabetes by 31% compared to placebo. The lifestyle intervention group lost 5–7% of their body weight during the 3 years of the study. Studies in Finnish and Chinese populations noted similar efficacy of diet and exercise in preventing or delaying type 2 DM; acarbose, metformin, thiazolidinediones, and orlistat prevent or delay type 2 DM but are not approved for this purpose. When administered to nondiabetic individuals for other reasons (cardiac, cholesterol lowering, etc.), pravastatin reduced the number of new cases of diabetes. Individuals with a strong family history of type 2 DM and individuals with IFG or IGT should be strongly encouraged to maintain a normal BMI and engage in regular physical activity. Pharmacologic therapy for individuals with prediabetes is currently controversial because its cost-effectiveness and safety profile are not known. A recent ADA Consensus panel concluded that metformin, but not other medications, could be considered in individuals with both IFG and IGT who are at very high risk for progression to diabetes (age < 60 years, BMI ≥ 35 kg/m^2, family history of diabetes in first-degree relative, elevated triglycerides, reduced HDL, hypertension, or A1C > 6.0%).

GENETICALLY DEFINED, MONOGENIC FORMS OF DIABETES MELLITUS

Several monogenic forms of DM have been identified. Six different variants of MODY, caused by mutations in genes encoding islet-enriched transcription factors or glucokinase (Fig. 338-4), are transmitted as autosomal dominant disorders. MODY 1, MODY 3, and MODY 5 are caused by mutations in the hepatocyte nuclear transcription factor (HNF) 4α, HNF-1α, and HNF-1β, respectively. As their names imply, these transcription factors are expressed in the liver but also in other tissues, including the pancreatic islets and kidney. These factors most likely affect islet development or the expression of genes important in glucose-stimulated insulin secretion or the maintenance of beta cell mass. For example, individuals with an HNF-1α mutation have a progressive decline in glycemic control but respond to sulfonyl-

ureas. In fact, some of these patients were initially thought to have type 1 DM but were later shown to respond to a sulfonylurea when insulin was discontinued. Individuals with a HNF-1β mutation have progressive impairment of insulin secretion, hepatic insulin resistance, and require insulin treatment (minimal response to sulfonylureas). These individual often have other abnormalities such as renal cysts, mild pancreatic exocrine insufficiency, and abnormal liver function tests. Individuals with MODY 2, the result of mutations in the glucokinase gene, have mild-to-moderate, stable hyperglycemia that does not respond to oral hypoglycemic agents. Glucokinase catalyzes the formation of glucose-6-phosphate from glucose, a reaction that is important for glucose sensing by the beta cells and for glucose utilization by the liver. As a result of glucokinase mutations, higher glucose levels are required to elicit insulin secretory responses, thus altering the set point for insulin secretion. MODY 4 is a rare variant caused by mutations in the insulin promoter factor (IPF) 1, which is a transcription factor that regulates pancreatic development and insulin gene transcription. Homozygous inactivating mutations cause pancreatic agenesis, whereas heterozygous mutations result in DM. Studies of populations with type 2 DM suggest that mutations in MODY-associated genes are rare (<5%) causes of type 2 DM.

Transient or permanent neonatal diabetes (onset < 6 months of age) may be caused by several genetic mutations and requires treatment with insulin. Mutations in subunits of the ATP-sensitive potassium channel subunits (Kir6.2 and ABCC8) (Fig. 338-4) are the major causes of permanent neonatal diabetes. Although these activating mutations impair glucose-stimulated insulin secretion, these individuals may respond to sulfonylureas and improve their glycemic control and can be treated with these agents. Homozygous glucokinase mutations cause a severe form of neonatal diabetes.

ACUTE COMPLICATIONS OF DM

Diabetic ketoacidosis (DKA) and hyperglycemic hyperosmolar state (HHS) are acute complications of diabetes. DKA was formerly considered a hallmark of type 1 DM, but it also occurs in individuals who lack immunologic features of type 1 DM and who can subsequently be treated with oral glucose-lowering agents (these obese individuals with type 2 DM are often of Hispanic or African-American descent). HHS is primarily seen in individuals with type 2 DM. Both disorders are associated with absolute or relative insulin deficiency, volume depletion, and acid-base abnormalities. DKA and HHS exist along a continuum of hyperglycemia, with or without ketosis. The metabolic similarities and differences in DKA and HHS are highlighted in Table 338-4. Both disor-

TABLE 338-4 LABORATORY VALUES IN DIABETIC KETOACIDOSIS (DKA) AND HYPERGLYCEMIC HYPEROSMOLAR STATE (HHS) (REPRESENTATIVE RANGES AT PRESENTATION)

	DKA	HHS
Glucose,^{a} mmol/L (mg/dL)	13.9–33.3 (250–600)	33.3–66.6 (600–1200)
Sodium, meq/L	125–135	135–145
Potassium^a	Normal to ↑	Normal
Magnesium^a	Normal^b	Normal
Chloride^a	Normal	Normal
Phosphate^a	↓	Normal
Creatinine	Slightly ↑	Moderately ↑
Osmolality (mOsm/mL)	300–320	330–380
Plasma ketones^a	++++	+/–
Serum bicarbonate,^{a} meq/L	<15 meq/L	Normal to slightly ↓
Arterial pH	6.8–7.3	>7.3
Arterial P_{CO_2},^{a} mmHg	20–30	Normal
Anion gap^a [Na – (Cl + HCO$_3$)]	↑	Normal to slightly ↑

^{a}Large changes occur during treatment of DKA.
^{b}Although plasma levels may be normal or high at presentation, total-body stores are usually depleted.

TABLE 338-5	MANIFESTATIONS OF DIABETIC KETOACIDOSIS

Symptoms
    Nausea/vomiting
    Thirst/polyuria
    Abdominal pain
    Shortness of breath
Precipitating events
    Inadequate insulin administration
    Infection (pneumonia/UTI/
        gastroenteritis/sepsis)
    Infarction (cerebral, coronary,
        mesenteric, peripheral)
    Drugs (cocaine)
    Pregnancy
	Physical findings
	    Tachycardia
	    Dehydration/hypotension
	    Tachypnea/Kussmaul respirations/
	        respiratory distress
	    Abdominal tenderness (may
	        resemble acute pancreatitis or
	        surgical abdomen)
	    Lethargy/obtundation/cerebral
	        edema/possibly coma

Note: UTI, urinary tract infection.

ders are associated with potentially serious complications if not promptly diagnosed and treated.

DIABETIC KETOACIDOSIS

Clinical Features   The symptoms and physical signs of DKA are listed in Table 338-5 and usually develop over 24 h. DKA may be the initial symptom complex that leads to a diagnosis of type 1 DM, but more frequently it occurs in individuals with established diabetes. Nausea and vomiting are often prominent, and their presence in an individual with diabetes warrants laboratory evaluation for DKA. Abdominal pain may be severe and can resemble acute pancreatitis or ruptured viscus. Hyperglycemia leads to glucosuria, volume depletion, and tachycardia. Hypotension can occur because of volume depletion in combination with peripheral vasodilatation. Kussmaul respirations and a fruity odor on the patient's breath (secondary to metabolic acidosis and increased acetone) are classic signs of the disorder. Lethargy and central nervous system depression may evolve into coma with severe DKA but should also prompt evaluation for other reasons for altered mental status (infection, hypoxia, etc.). Cerebral edema, an extremely serious complication of DKA, is seen most frequently in children. Signs of infection, which may precipitate DKA, should be sought on physical examination, even in the absence of fever. Tissue ischemia (heart, brain) can also be a precipitating factor.

Pathophysiology   DKA results from relative or absolute insulin deficiency combined with counterregulatory hormone excess (glucagon, catecholamines, cortisol, and growth hormone). Both insulin deficiency and glucagon excess, in particular, are necessary for DKA to develop. The decreased ratio of insulin to glucagon promotes gluconeogenesis, glycogenolysis, and ketone body formation in the liver, as well as increases in substrate delivery from fat and muscle (free fatty acids, amino acids) to the liver.

The combination of insulin deficiency and hyperglycemia reduces the hepatic level of fructose-2,6-phosphate, which alters the activity of phosphofructokinase and fructose-1,6-bisphosphatase. Glucagon excess decreases the activity of pyruvate kinase, whereas insulin deficiency increases the activity of phosphoenolpyruvate carboxykinase. These changes shift the handling of pyruvate toward glucose synthesis and away from glycolysis. The increased levels of glucagon and catecholamines in the face of low insulin levels promote glycogenolysis. Insulin deficiency also reduces levels of the GLUT4 glucose transporter, which impairs glucose uptake into skeletal muscle and fat and reduces intracellular glucose metabolism (Fig. 338-5).

Ketosis results from a marked increase in free fatty acid release from adipocytes, with a resulting shift toward ketone body synthesis in the liver. Reduced insulin levels, in combination with elevations in catecholamines and growth hormone, increase lipolysis and the release of free fatty acids. Normally, these free fatty acids are converted to triglycerides or VLDL in the liver. However, in DKA, hyperglucagonemia alters hepatic metabolism to favor ketone body formation, through activation of the enzyme carnitine palmitoyltransferase I. This enzyme is crucial for regulating fatty acid transport into the mitochondria,

where beta oxidation and conversion to ketone bodies occur. At physiologic pH, ketone bodies exist as ketoacids, which are neutralized by bicarbonate. As bicarbonate stores are depleted, metabolic acidosis ensues. Increased lactic acid production also contributes to the acidosis. The increased free fatty acids increase triglyceride and VLDL production. VLDL clearance is also reduced because the activity of insulin-sensitive lipoprotein lipase in muscle and fat is decreased. Hypertriglyceridemia may be severe enough to cause pancreatitis.

DKA is initiated by inadequate levels of plasma insulin (Table 338-5). Most commonly, DKA is precipitated by increased insulin requirements, as might occur during a concurrent illness. Failure to augment insulin therapy often compounds the problem. Occasionally, complete omission of insulin by the patient or health care team (in a hospitalized patient with type 1 DM) precipitates DKA. Patients using insulin infusion devices with short-acting insulin are at increased risk of DKA, since even a brief interruption in insulin delivery (e.g., mechanical malfunction) quickly leads to insulin deficiency.

Laboratory Abnormalities and Diagnosis   The timely diagnosis of DKA is crucial and allows for prompt initiation of therapy. DKA is characterized by hyperglycemia, ketosis, and metabolic acidosis (increased anion gap) along with a number of secondary metabolic derangements (Table 338-4). Occasionally, the serum glucose is only minimally elevated. Serum bicarbonate is frequently <10 mmol/L, and arterial pH ranges between 6.8 and 7.3, depending on the severity of the acidosis. Despite a total-body potassium deficit, the serum potassium at presentation may be mildly elevated, secondary to the acidosis. Total-body stores of sodium, chloride, phosphorous, and magnesium are also reduced in DKA but are not accurately reflected by their levels in the serum because of dehydration and hyperglycemia. Elevated blood urea nitrogen (BUN) and serum creatinine levels reflect intravascular volume depletion. Interference from acetoacetate may falsely elevate the serum creatinine measurement. Leukocytosis, hypertriglyceridemia, and hyperlipoproteinemia are commonly found as well. Hyperamylasemia may suggest a diagnosis of pancreatitis, especially when accompanied by abdominal pain. However, in DKA the amylase is usually of salivary origin and thus is not diagnostic of pancreatitis. Serum lipase should be obtained if pancreatitis is suspected.

The measured serum sodium is reduced as a consequence of the hyperglycemia [1.6-mmol/L (1.6 meq) reduction in serum sodium for each 5.6-mmol/L (100 mg/dL) rise in the serum glucose]. A normal serum sodium in the setting of DKA indicates a more profound water deficit. In "conventional" units, the calculated serum osmolality [2 × (serum sodium + serum potassium) + plasma glucose (mg/dL)/18 + BUN/2.8] is mildly to moderately elevated, though to a lesser degree than that found in HHS (see below).

In DKA, the ketone body, β-hydroxybutyrate, is synthesized at a threefold greater rate than acetoacetate; however, acetoacetate is preferentially detected by a commonly used ketosis detection reagent (nitroprusside). Serum ketones are present at significant levels (usually positive at serum dilution of ≥1:8). The nitroprusside tablet, or stick, is often used to detect urine ketones; certain medications such as captopril or penicillamine may cause false-positive reactions. Serum or plasma assays for β-hydroxybutyrate more accurately reflect the true ketone body level.

The metabolic derangements of DKA exist along a spectrum, beginning with mild acidosis with moderate hyperglycemia evolving into more severe findings. The degree of acidosis and hyperglycemia do not necessarily correlate closely since a variety of factors determine the level of hyperglycemia (oral intake, urinary glucose loss). Ketonemia is a consistent finding in DKA and distinguishes it from simple hyperglycemia. The differential diagnosis of DKA includes starvation ketosis, alcoholic ketoacidosis (bicarbonate usually > 15 meq/L) and other increased anion gap acidosis (Chap. 48).

℞ DIABETIC KETOACIDOSIS

The management of DKA is outlined in **Table 338-6**. After initiating IV fluid replacement and insulin therapy, the agent or event that precipitated the

TABLE 338-6 **MANAGEMENT OF DIABETIC KETOACIDOSIS**

1. Confirm diagnosis (↑plasma glucose, positive serum ketones, metabolic acidosis).
2. Admit to hospital; intensive-care setting may be necessary for frequent monitoring or if pH < 7.00 or unconscious.
3. Assess:
    Serum electrolytes (K+, Na+, Mg2+, Cl−, bicarbonate, phosphate)
    Acid-base status—pH, HCO3−, PCO2, β-hydroxybutyrate
    Renal function (creatinine, urine output)
4. Replace fluids: 2–3 L of 0.9% saline over first 1–3 h (10–15 mL/kg per hour); subsequently, 0.45% saline at 150–300 mL/h; change to 5% glucose and 0.45% saline at 100–200 mL/h when plasma glucose reaches 250 mg/dL (14 mmol/L).
5. Administer short-acting insulin: IV (0.1 units/kg) or IM (0.3 units/kg), then 0.1 units/kg per hour by continuous IV infusion; increase 2- to 3-fold if no response by 2–4 h. If initial serum potassium is < 3.3 mmol/L (3.3 meq/L), do not administer insulin until the potassium is corrected to > 3.3 mmol/L (3.3.meq/L).
6. Assess patient: What precipitated the episode (noncompliance, infection, trauma, infarction, cocaine)? Initiate appropriate workup for precipitating event (cultures, CXR, ECG).
7. Measure capillary glucose every 1–2 h; measure electrolytes (especially K+, bicarbonate, phosphate) and anion gap every 4 h for first 24 h.
8. Monitor blood pressure, pulse, respirations, mental status, fluid intake and output every 1–4 h.
9. Replace K+: 10 meq/h when plasma K+ < 5.5 meq/L, ECG normal, urine flow and normal creatinine documented; administer 40–80 meq/h when plasma K+ < 3.5 meq/L or if bicarbonate is given.
10. Continue above until patient is stable, glucose goal is 150–250 mg/dL, and acidosis is resolved. Insulin infusion may be decreased to 0.05–0.1 units/kg per hour.
11. Administer intermediate or long-acting insulin as soon as patient is eating. Allow for overlap in insulin infusion and subcutaneous insulin injection.

Note: CXR, chest x-ray; ECG, electrocardiogram.
Source: Adapted from M Sperling, in *Therapy for Diabetes Mellitus and Related Disorders*, American Diabetes Association, Alexandria, VA, 1998; and AE Kitabchi et al: Diabetes Care 29:2739, 2006.

episode of DKA should be sought and aggressively treated. If the patient is vomiting or has altered mental status, a nasogastric tube should be inserted to prevent aspiration of gastric contents. Central to successful treatment of DKA is careful monitoring and frequent reassessment to ensure that the patient and the metabolic derangements are improving. A comprehensive flow sheet should record chronologic changes in vital signs, fluid intake and output, and laboratory values as a function of insulin administered.

After the initial bolus of normal saline, replacement of the sodium and free water deficit is carried out over the next 24 h (fluid deficit is often 3–5 L). When hemodynamic stability and adequate urine output are achieved, IV fluids should be switched to 0.45% saline at a rate of 200–300 mL/h, depending on the calculated volume deficit. The change to 0.45% saline helps to reduce the trend toward hyperchloremia later in the course of DKA. Alternatively, initial use of lactated Ringer's IV solution may reduce the hyperchloremia that commonly occurs with normal saline.

A bolus of IV (0.1 units/kg) or IM (0.3 units/kg) short-acting insulin should be administered immediately (Table 338-6), and subsequent treatment should provide continuous and adequate levels of circulating insulin. Intravenous administration is preferred (0.1 units/kg per hour), because it assures rapid distribution and allows adjustment of the infusion rate as the patient responds to therapy. In mild episodes of DKA, short-acting insulin analogues can be used subcutaneously. Intravenous regular insulin should be continued until the acidosis resolves and the patient is metabolically stable. As the acidosis and insulin resistance associated with DKA resolve, the insulin infusion rate can be decreased (to 0.05–0.1 units/kg per hour). Intermediate or long-acting insulin, in combination with SC short-acting insulin, should be administered as soon as the patient resumes eating, as this facilitates transition to an outpatient insulin regimen and reduces length of hospital stay. It is crucial to continue the insulin infusion until adequate insulin levels are achieved by the SC route. Even relatively brief periods of inadequate insulin administration in this transition phase may result in DKA relapse.

Hyperglycemia usually improves at a rate of 4.2–5.6 mmol/L (75–100 mg/dL) per hour as a result of insulin-mediated glucose disposal, reduced hepatic glucose release, and rehydration. The latter reduces catecholamines, increases urinary glucose loss, and expands the intravascular volume. The decline in the plasma glucose within the first 1–2 h may be more rapid and is mostly related to volume expansion. When the plasma glucose reaches 13.9 mmol/L (250 mg/dL), glucose should be added to the 0.45% saline infusion to maintain the plasma glucose in the 11.1–13.9 mmol/L (200–250 mg/dL) range, and the insulin infusion should be continued. Ketoacidosis begins to resolve as insulin reduces lipolysis, increases peripheral ketone body use, suppresses hepatic ketone body formation, and promotes bicarbonate regeneration. However, the acidosis and ketosis resolve more slowly than hyperglycemia. As ketoacidosis improves, β-hydroxybutyrate is converted to acetoacetate. Ketone body levels may appear to increase if measured by laboratory assays that use the nitroprusside reaction, which only detects acetoacetate and acetone. The improvement in acidosis and anion gap, a result of bicarbonate regeneration and decline in ketone bodies, is reflected by a rise in the serum bicarbonate level and the arterial pH. Depending on the rise of serum chloride, the anion gap (but not bicarbonate) will normalize. A hyperchloremic acidosis [serum bicarbonate of 15–18 mmol/L (15–18 meq/L)] often follows successful treatment and gradually resolves as the kidneys regenerate bicarbonate and excretes chloride.

Potassium stores are depleted in DKA [estimated deficit 3–5 mmol/kg (3–5 meq/kg)]. During treatment with insulin and fluids, various factors contribute to the development of hypokalemia. These include insulin-mediated potassium transport into cells, resolution of the acidosis (which also promotes potassium entry into cells), and urinary loss of potassium salts of organic acids. Thus, potassium repletion should commence as soon as adequate urine output and a normal serum potassium are documented. If the initial serum potassium level is elevated, then potassium repletion should be delayed until the potassium falls into the normal range. Inclusion of 20–40 meq of potassium in each liter of IV fluid is reasonable, but additional potassium supplements may also be required. To reduce the amount of chloride administered, potassium phosphate or acetate can be substituted for the chloride salt. The goal is to maintain the serum potassium >3.5 mmol/L (3.5 meq/L). If the initial serum potassium is <3.3 mmol/L (3.3 meq/L), do not administer insulin until the potassium is supplemented to >3.3 mmol/L (3.3 meq/L).

Despite a bicarbonate deficit, bicarbonate replacement is not usually necessary. In fact, theoretical arguments suggest that bicarbonate administration and rapid reversal of acidosis may impair cardiac function, reduce tissue oxygenation, and promote hypokalemia. The results of most clinical trials do not support the routine use of bicarbonate replacement, and one study in children found that bicarbonate use was associated with an increased risk of cerebral edema. However, in the presence of severe acidosis (arterial pH < 7.0 after initial hydration), the ADA advises bicarbonate [50 mmol/L (meq/L) of sodium bicarbonate in 200 mL of sterile water with 10 meq/L KCl over 1 h if pH = 6.9–7.0; or 100 mmol/L (meq/L) of sodium bicarbonate in 400 mL of sterile water with 20 meq/L KCl over 2 h if pH < 6.9]. Repeat the dose of bicarbonate every 2 h until the arterial pH is >7.0. Hypophosphatemia may result from increased glucose usage, but randomized clinical trials have not demonstrated that phosphate replacement is beneficial in DKA. If the serum phosphate < 0.32 mmol/L (1.0 mg/dL), then phosphate supplement should be considered and the serum calcium monitored. Hypomagnesemia may develop during DKA therapy and may also require supplementation.

With appropriate therapy, the mortality of DKA is low (<5%) and is related more to the underlying or precipitating event, such as infection or myocardial infarction. The major nonmetabolic complication of DKA therapy is cerebral edema, which most often develops in children as DKA is resolving. The etiology of and optimal therapy for cerebral edema are not well established, but overreplacement of free water should be avoided. Venous thrombosis, upper gastrointestinal bleeding, and acute respiratory distress syndrome occasionally complicate DKA.

Following treatment, the physician and patient should review the sequence of events that led to DKA to prevent future recurrences. Foremost is patient education about the symptoms of DKA, its precipitating factors, and the management of diabetes during a concurrent illness. During illness or when oral intake is compromised, patients should: (1) frequently measure the capillary blood glucose; (2) measure urinary ketones when the serum glucose > 16.5 mmol/L (300 mg/dL); (3) drink fluids to maintain hydration; (4) continue or increase insulin; and (5) seek medical attention if dehydration, persistent vomiting, or uncontrolled hyperglycemia develop. Using these strategies, early DKA can be prevented or detected and treated appropriately on an outpatient basis.

HYPERGLYCEMIC HYPEROSMOLAR STATE

Clinical Features The prototypical patient with HHS is an elderly individual with type 2 DM, with a several week history of polyuria, weight loss, and diminished oral intake that culminates in mental confusion, lethargy, or coma. The physical examination reflects profound dehydration and hyperosmolality and reveals hypotension, tachycardia, and altered mental status. Notably absent are symptoms of nausea, vomiting, and abdominal pain and the Kussmaul respirations characteristic of DKA. HHS is often precipitated by a serious, concurrent illness such as myocardial infarction or stroke. Sepsis, pneumonia, and other serious infections are frequent precipitants and should be sought. In addition, a debilitating condition (prior stroke or dementia) or social situation that compromises water intake usually contributes to the development of the disorder.

Pathophysiology Relative insulin deficiency and inadequate fluid intake are the underlying causes of HHS. Insulin deficiency increases hepatic glucose production (through glycogenolysis and gluconeogenesis) and impairs glucose utilization in skeletal muscle (see above discussion of DKA). Hyperglycemia induces an osmotic diuresis that leads to intravascular volume depletion, which is exacerbated by inadequate fluid replacement. The absence of ketosis in HHS is not completely understood. Presumably, the insulin deficiency is only relative and less severe than in DKA. Lower levels of counterregulatory hormones and free fatty acids have been found in HHS than in DKA in some studies. It is also possible that the liver is less capable of ketone body synthesis or that the insulin/glucagon ratio does not favor ketogenesis.

Laboratory Abnormalities and Diagnosis The laboratory features in HHS are summarized in Table 338-4. Most notable are the marked hyperglycemia [plasma glucose may be >55.5 mmol/L (1000 mg/dL)], hyperosmolality (>350 mosmol/L), and prerenal azotemia. The measured serum sodium may be normal or slightly low despite the marked hyperglycemia. The corrected serum sodium is usually increased [add 1.6 meq to measured sodium for each 5.6-mmol/L (100 mg/dL) rise in the serum glucose]. In contrast to DKA, acidosis and ketonemia are absent or mild. A small anion gap metabolic acidosis may be present secondary to increased lactic acid. Moderate ketonuria, if present, is secondary to starvation.

℞ HYPERGLYCEMIC HYPEROSMOLAR STATE

Volume depletion and hyperglycemia are prominent features of both HHS and DKA. Consequently, therapy of these disorders shares several elements (Table 338-6). In both disorders, careful monitoring of the patient's fluid status, laboratory values, and insulin infusion rate is crucial. Underlying or precipitating problems should be aggressively sought and treated. In HHS, fluid losses and dehydration are usually more pronounced than in DKA due to the longer duration of the illness. The patient with HHS is usually older, more likely to have mental status changes, and more likely to have a life-threatening precipitating event with accompanying comorbidities. Even with proper treatment, HHS has a substantially higher mortality than DKA (up to 15% in some clinical series).

Fluid replacement should initially stabilize the hemodynamic status of the patient (1–3 L of 0.9% normal saline over the first 2–3 h). Because the fluid deficit in HHS is accumulated over a period of days to weeks, the rapidity of reversal of the hyperosmolar state must balance the need for free water repletion with the risk that too rapid a reversal may worsen neurologic function. If the serum sodium > 150 mmol/L (150 meq/L), 0.45% saline should be used. After hemodynamic stability is achieved, the IV fluid administration is directed at reversing the free water deficit using hypotonic fluids (0.45% saline initially then 5% dextrose in water, D_5W). The calculated free water deficit (which averages 9–10 L) should be reversed over the next 1–2 days (infusion rates of 200–300 mL/h of hypotonic solution).

Potassium repletion is usually necessary and should be dictated by repeated measurements of the serum potassium. In patients taking diuretics, the potassium deficit can be quite large and may be accompanied by magnesium deficiency. Hypophosphatemia may occur during therapy and can be improved by using KPO_4 and beginning nutrition.

As in DKA, rehydration and volume expansion lower the plasma glucose initially, but insulin is also required. A reasonable regimen for HHS begins with an IV insulin bolus of 0.1 units/kg followed by IV insulin at a constant infusion rate of 0.1 units/kg per hour. If the serum glucose does not fall, increase the insulin infusion rate by twofold. As in DKA, glucose should be added to IV fluid when the plasma glucose falls to 13.9 mmol/L (250 mg/dL), and the insulin infusion rate should be decreased to 0.05–0.1 units/kg per hour. The insulin infusion should be continued until the patient has resumed eating and can be transferred to a SC insulin regimen. The patient should be discharged from the hospital on insulin, though some patients can later switch to oral glucose-lowering agents.

CHRONIC COMPLICATIONS OF DM

The chronic complications of DM affect many organ systems and are responsible for the majority of morbidity and mortality associated with the disease. Chronic complications can be divided into vascular and nonvascular complications (Table 338-7). The vascular complications of DM are further subdivided into microvascular (retinopathy, neuropathy, nephropathy) and macrovascular complications [coronary artery disease (CAD), peripheral arterial disease (PAD), cerebrovascular disease]. Nonvascular complications include problems such as gastroparesis, infections, and skin changes. Long-standing diabetes may be associated with hearing loss. Whether type 2 DM in elderly individuals is associated with impaired mental function is not clear.

The risk of chronic complications increases as a function of the duration of hyperglycemia; they usually become apparent in the second decade of hyperglycemia. Since type 2 DM often has a long asymptomatic period of hyperglycemia, many individuals with type 2 DM have complications at the time of diagnosis.

The microvascular complications of both type 1 and type 2 DM result from chronic hyperglycemia. Large, randomized clinical trials of individuals with type 1 or type 2 DM have conclusively demonstrated that a reduction in chronic hyperglycemia prevents or delays retinopathy, neuropathy, and nephropathy. Other incompletely defined factors may modulate the development of complications. For example, despite long-standing DM, some individuals never develop nephropathy or retinopathy. Many of these patients have glycemic control that is indistinguishable from those who develop microvascular complications, suggesting that there is a genetic susceptibility for developing particular complications.

Evidence implicating a causative role for chronic hyperglycemia in the development of macrovascular complications is less conclusive.

TABLE 338-7	CHRONIC COMPLICATIONS OF DIABETES MELLITUS

Microvascular
  Eye disease
    Retinopathy (nonproliferative/proliferative)
    Macular edema
  Neuropathy
    Sensory and motor (mono- and polyneuropathy)
    Autonomic
  Nephropathy
Macrovascular
  Coronary artery disease
  Peripheral arterial disease
  Cerebrovascular disease
Other
  Gastrointestinal (gastroparesis, diarrhea)
  Genitourinary (uropathy/sexual dysfunction)
  Dermatologic
  Infectious
  Cataracts
  Glaucoma
  Periodontal disease

However, coronary heart disease events and mortality are two to four times greater in patients with type 2 DM. These events correlate with fasting and postprandial plasma glucose levels as well as with the A1C. Other factors (dyslipidemia and hypertension) also play important roles in macrovascular complications.

MECHANISMS OF COMPLICATIONS

Although chronic hyperglycemia is an important etiologic factor leading to complications of DM, the mechanism(s) by which it leads to such diverse cellular and organ dysfunction is unknown. Four prominent theories, which are not mutually exclusive, have been proposed to explain how hyperglycemia might lead to the chronic complications of DM.

One theory is that increased intracellular glucose leads to the formation of advanced glycosylation end products (AGEs) via the nonenzymatic glycosylation of intra- and extracellular proteins. Nonenzymatic glycosylation results from the interaction of glucose with amino groups on proteins. AGEs have been shown to cross-link proteins (e.g., collagen, extracellular matrix proteins), accelerate atherosclerosis, promote glomerular dysfunction, reduce nitric oxide synthesis, induce endothelial dysfunction, and alter extracellular matrix composition and structure. The serum level of AGEs correlates with the level of glycemia, and these products accumulate as glomerular filtration rate declines.

A second theory is based on the observation that hyperglycemia increases glucose metabolism via the sorbitol pathway. Intracellular glucose is predominantly metabolized by phosphorylation and subsequent glycolysis, but when increased, some glucose is converted to sorbitol by the enzyme aldose reductase. Increased sorbitol concentration alters redox potential, increases cellular osmolality, generates reactive oxygen species, and likely leads to other types of cellular dysfunction. However, testing of this theory in humans, using aldose reductase inhibitors, has not demonstrated significant beneficial effects on clinical endpoints of retinopathy, neuropathy, or nephropathy.

A third hypothesis proposes that hyperglycemia increases the formation of diacylglycerol leading to activation of protein kinase C (PKC). Among other actions, PKC alters the transcription of genes for fibronectin, type IV collagen, contractile proteins, and extracellular matrix proteins in endothelial cells and neurons. Inhibitors of PKC are being studied in clinical trials.

A fourth theory proposes that hyperglycemia increases the flux through the hexosamine pathway, which generates fructose-6-phosphate, a substrate for O-linked glycosylation and proteoglycan production. The hexosamine pathway may alter function by glycosylation of proteins such as endothelial nitric oxide synthase or by changes in gene expression of transforming growth factor β (TGF-β) or plasminogen activator inhibitor-1 (PAI-1).

Growth factors appear to play an important role in DM-related complications, and their production is increased by most of these proposed pathways. Vascular endothelial growth factor A (VEGF-A) is increased locally in diabetic proliferative retinopathy and decreases after laser photocoagulation. TGF-β is increased in diabetic nephropathy and stimulates basement membrane production of collagen and fibronectin by mesangial cells. Other growth factors, such as platelet-derived growth factor, epidermal growth factor, insulin-like growth factor I, growth hormone, basic fibroblast growth factor, and even insulin, have been suggested to play a role in DM-related complications. A possible unifying mechanism is that hyperglycemia leads to increased production of reactive oxygen species or superoxide in the mitochondria; these compounds may activate all four of the pathways described above. Although hyperglycemia serves as the initial trigger for complications of diabetes, it is still unknown whether the same pathophysiologic processes are operative in all complications or whether some pathways predominate in certain organs.

GLYCEMIC CONTROL AND COMPLICATIONS

The Diabetes Control and Complications Trial (DCCT) provided definitive proof that reduction in chronic hyperglycemia can prevent many of the early complications of type 1 DM. This large multicenter clinical trial randomized over 1400 individuals with type 1 DM to either intensive or conventional diabetes management, and prospectively evaluated the development of retinopathy, nephropathy, and neuropathy. Individuals in the intensive diabetes management group received multiple administrations of insulin each day along with extensive educational, psychological, and medical support. Individuals in the conventional diabetes management group received twice-daily insulin injections and quarterly nutritional, educational, and clinical evaluation. The goal in the former group was normoglycemia; the goal in the latter group was prevention of symptoms of diabetes. Individuals in the intensive diabetes management group achieved a substantially lower hemoglobin A1C (7.3%) than individuals in the conventional diabetes management group (9.1%).

The DCCT demonstrated that improvement of glycemic control reduced nonproliferative and proliferative retinopathy (47% reduction), microalbuminuria (39% reduction), clinical nephropathy (54% reduction), and neuropathy (60% reduction). Improved glycemic control also slowed the progression of early diabetic complications. There was a nonsignificant trend in reduction of macrovascular events during the trial (most individuals were young and had a low risk of cardiovascular disease). The results of the DCCT predicted that individuals in the intensive diabetes management group would gain 7.7 additional years of vision, 5.8 additional years free from ESRD, and 5.6 years free from lower extremity amputations. If all complications of DM were combined, individuals in the intensive diabetes management group would experience 15.3 more years of life without significant microvascular or neurologic complications of DM, compared to individuals who received standard therapy. This translates into an additional 5.1 years of life expectancy for individuals in the intensive diabetes management group. The benefit of the improved glycemic control during the DCCT persisted even after the study concluded and glycemic control worsened. For example, individuals in the intensive diabetes management group for a mean of 6.5 years had a 42–57% reduction in cardiovascular events [nonfatal myocardial infarction (MI), stroke, or death from a cardiovascular event] at a mean follow-up of 17 years, even though their subsequent glycemic control was the same as those in the conventional diabetes management group.

The benefits of an improvement in glycemic control occurred over the entire range of A1C values (Fig. 338-8), suggesting that at any A1C level, an improvement in glycemic control is beneficial. The goal of therapy is to achieve an A1C level as close to normal as possible, without subjecting the patient to excessive risk of hypoglycemia.

The United Kingdom Prospective Diabetes Study (UKPDS) studied the course of >5000 individuals with type 2 DM for >10 years. This study utilized multiple treatment regimens and monitored the effect

FIGURE 338-8 Relationship of glycemic control and diabetes duration to diabetic retinopathy. The progression of retinopathy in individuals in the Diabetes Control and Complications Trial is graphed as a function of the length of follow-up with different curves for different A1C values. (*Adapted from The Diabetes Control and Complications Trial Research Group: Diabetes 44:968, 1995.*)

of intensive glycemic control and risk factor treatment on the development of diabetic complications. Newly diagnosed individuals with type 2 DM were randomized to (1) intensive management using various combinations of insulin, a sulfonylurea, or metformin; or (2) conventional therapy using dietary modification and pharmacotherapy with the goal of symptom prevention. In addition, individuals were randomly assigned to different antihypertensive regimens. Individuals in the intensive treatment arm achieved an A1C of 7.0%, compared to a 7.9% A1C in the standard treatment group. The UKPDS demonstrated that each percentage point reduction in A1C was associated with a 35% reduction in microvascular complications. As in the DCCT, there was a continuous relationship between glycemic control and development of complications. Improved glycemic control did not conclusively reduce (nor worsen) cardiovascular mortality but was associated with improvement with lipoprotein risk profiles, such as reduced triglycerides and increased HDL.

One of the major findings of the UKPDS was that strict blood pressure control significantly reduced both macro- and microvascular complications. In fact, the beneficial effects of blood pressure control were greater than the beneficial effects of glycemic control. Lowering blood pressure to moderate goals (144/82 mmHg) reduced the risk of DM-related death, stroke, microvascular end points, retinopathy, and heart failure (risk reductions between 32 and 56%).

Similar reductions in the risks of retinopathy and nephropathy were also seen in a small trial of lean Japanese individuals with type 2 DM randomized to either intensive glycemic control or standard therapy with insulin (Kumamoto study). These results demonstrate the effectiveness of improved glycemic control in individuals of different ethnicity and, presumably, a different etiology of DM (i.e., phenotypically different from those in the DCCT and UKPDS).

The findings of the DCCT, UKPDS, and Kumamoto study support the idea that chronic hyperglycemia plays a causative role in the pathogenesis of diabetic microvascular complications. These landmark studies prove the value of metabolic control and emphasize the importance of (1) intensive glycemic control in all forms of DM, and (2) early diagnosis and strict blood pressure control in type 2 DM.

OPHTHALMOLOGIC COMPLICATIONS OF DIABETES MELLITUS

DM is the leading cause of blindness between the ages of 20 and 74 in the United States. The gravity of this problem is highlighted by the finding that individuals with DM are 25 times more likely to become legally blind than individuals without DM. Blindness is primarily the result of progressive diabetic retinopathy and clinically significant macular edema. Diabetic retinopathy is classified into two stages: nonproliferative and proliferative. Nonproliferative diabetic retinopathy usually appears late in the first decade or early in the second decade of the disease and is marked by retinal vascular microaneurysms, blot hemorrhages, and cotton wool spots (Fig. 338-9). Mild nonproliferative retinopathy progresses to more extensive disease, characterized by changes in venous vessel caliber, intraretinal microvascular abnormalities, and more numerous microaneurysms and hemorrhages. The pathophysiologic mechanisms invoked in nonproliferative retinopathy include loss of retinal pericytes, increased retinal vascular permeability, alterations in retinal blood flow, and abnormal retinal microvasculature, all of which lead to retinal ischemia.

The appearance of neovascularization in response to retinal hypoxia is the hallmark of proliferative diabetic retinopathy (Fig. 338-9). These newly formed vessels appear near the optic nerve and/or macula and rupture easily, leading to vitreous hemorrhage, fibrosis, and ultimately retinal detachment. Not all individuals with nonproliferative retinopathy develop proliferative retinopathy, but the more severe the nonproliferative disease, the greater the chance of evolution to proliferative retinopathy within 5 years. This creates an important opportunity for early detection and treatment of diabetic retinopathy. Clinically significant macular edema can occur when only nonproliferative retinopathy is present. Fluorescein angiography is useful to detect macular edema, which is associated with a 25% chance of moderate visual loss over the next 3 years.

FIGURE 338-9 Diabetic retinopathy results in scattered hemorrhages, yellow exudates, and neovascularization. This patient has neovascular vessels proliferating from the optic disc, requiring urgent pan retinal laser photocoagulation.

Duration of DM and degree of glycemic control are the best predictors of the development of retinopathy; hypertension is also a risk factor. Nonproliferative retinopathy is found in almost all individuals who have had DM for >20 years (25% incidence with 5 years, and 80% incidence with 15 years of type 1 DM). Although there is genetic susceptibility for retinopathy, it confers less influence than either the duration of DM or the degree of glycemic control.

℞ DIABETIC RETINOPATHY

The most effective therapy for diabetic retinopathy is prevention. Intensive glycemic and blood pressure control will delay the development or slow the progression of retinopathy in individuals with either type 1 or type 2 DM. Paradoxically, during the first 6–12 months of improved glycemic control, established diabetic retinopathy may transiently worsen. Fortunately, this progression is temporary, and in the long term, improved glycemic control is associated with less diabetic retinopathy. Individuals with known retinopathy are candidates for prophylactic photocoagulation when initiating intensive therapy. Once advanced retinopathy is present, improved glycemic control imparts less benefit, though adequate ophthalmologic care can prevent most blindness.

Regular, comprehensive eye examinations are essential for all individuals with DM. Most diabetic eye disease can be successfully treated if detected early. Routine, nondilated eye examinations by the primary care provider or diabetes specialist are inadequate to detect diabetic eye disease, which requires an ophthalmologist for optimal care of these disorders. Laser photocoagulation is very successful in preserving vision. Proliferative retinopathy is usually treated with panretinal laser photocoagulation, whereas macular edema is treated with focal laser photocoagulation. Although exercise has not been conclusively shown to worsen proliferative diabetic retinopathy, most ophthalmologists advise individuals with advanced diabetic eye disease to limit physical activities associated with repeated Valsalva maneuvers. Aspirin therapy (650 mg/d) does not appear to influence the natural history of diabetic retinopathy.

RENAL COMPLICATIONS OF DIABETES MELLITUS

Diabetic nephropathy is the leading cause of ESRD in the United States and a leading cause of DM-related morbidity and mortality. Both microalbuminuria and macroalbuminuria in individuals with DM are associated with increased risk of cardiovascular disease. Individuals with diabetic nephropathy commonly have diabetic retinopathy.

Like other microvascular complications, the pathogenesis of diabetic nephropathy is related to chronic hyperglycemia. The mechanisms by which chronic hyperglycemia leads to ESRD, though incompletely defined, involve the effects of soluble factors (growth factors, angiotensin II, endothelin, AGEs), hemodynamic alterations in the renal microcirculation (glomerular hyperfiltration or hyperper-

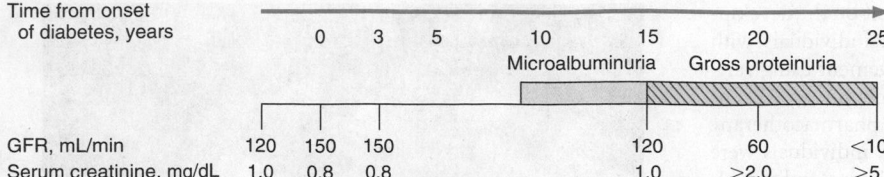

	0	3	5	10	15	20	25
				Microalbuminuria	Gross proteinuria		
GFR, mL/min	120	150	150		120	60	<10
Serum creatinine, mg/dL	1.0	0.8	0.8		1.0	>2.0	>5

FIGURE 338-10 Time course of development of diabetic nephropathy. The relationship of time from onset of diabetes, the glomerular filtration rate (GFR), and the serum creatinine are shown. *(Adapted from RA DeFranzo, in Therapy for Diabetes Mellitus and Related Disorders, 3d ed. American Diabetes Association, Alexandria, VA, 1998.)*

fusion, increased glomerular capillary pressure), and structural changes in the glomerulus (increased extracellular matrix, basement membrane thickening, mesangial expansion, fibrosis). Some of these effects may be mediated through angiotensin II receptors. Smoking accelerates the decline in renal function. Because only 20–40% of patients with diabetes develop diabetic nephropathy, additional susceptibility factors remain unidentified. One known risk factor is a family history of diabetic nephropathy.

The natural history of diabetic nephropathy is characterized by a fairly predictable sequence of events that was initially defined for individuals with type 1 DM but appears to be similar in type 2 DM (Fig. 338-10). Glomerular hyperperfusion and renal hypertrophy occur in the first years after the onset of DM and are associated with an increase of the glomerular filtration rate (GFR). During the first 5 years of DM, thickening of the glomerular basement membrane, glomerular hypertrophy, and mesangial volume expansion occur as the GFR returns to normal. After 5–10 years of type 1 DM, ~40% of individuals begin to excrete small amounts of albumin in the urine. Microalbuminuria is defined as 30–300 mg/d in a 24-h collection or 30–300 µg/mg creatinine in a spot collection (preferred method). Although the appearance of microalbuminuria in type 1 DM is an important risk factor for progression to overt proteinuria (>300 mg/d), only ~50% of individuals progress to macroalbuminuria over the next 10 years. In some individuals with type 1 diabetes and microalbuminuria of short duration, the microalbuminuria regresses. Once macroalbuminuria is present, there is a steady decline in GFR, and ~50% of individuals reach ESRD in 7–10 years. Once macroalbuminuria develops, blood pressure rises slightly and the pathologic changes are likely irreversible. Some individuals with type 1 or type 2 DM have a decline in GFR in the absence of micro- or macroalbuminuria and this is the basis for assessing the GFR on an annual basis using serum creatinine.

The nephropathy that develops in type 2 DM differs from that of type 1 DM in the following respects: (1) microalbuminuria or macroalbuminuria may be present when type 2 DM is diagnosed, reflecting its long asymptomatic period; (2) hypertension more commonly accompanies microalbuminuria or macroalbuminuria in type 2 DM; and (3) microalbuminuria may be less predictive of diabetic nephropathy and progression to macroalbuminuria in type 2 DM. Finally, it should be noted that albuminuria in type 2 DM may be secondary to factors unrelated to DM, such as hypertension, congestive heart failure (CHF), prostate disease, or infection. Diabetic nephropathy and ESRD secondary to DM develop more commonly in African Americans, Native Americans, and Hispanic individuals than in Caucasians with type 2 DM.

Type IV renal tubular acidosis (hyporeninemic hypoaldosteronism) may occur in type 1 or 2 DM. These individuals develop a propensity to hyperkalemia, which may be exacerbated by medications [especially angiotensin-converting enzyme (ACE) inhibitors and angiotensin receptor blockers (ARBs)]. Patients with DM are predisposed to radiocontrast-induced nephrotoxicity. Risk factors for radiocontrast-induced nephrotoxicity are preexisting nephropathy and volume depletion. Individuals with DM undergoing radiographic procedures with contrast dye should be well hydrated before and after dye exposure, and the serum creatinine should be monitored for 24 h following the procedure.

Rx DIABETIC NEPHROPATHY

The optimal therapy for diabetic nephropathy is prevention by control of glycemia. As part of comprehensive diabetes care, microalbuminuria should be detected at an early stage when effective therapies can be instituted. The recommended strategy for detecting microalbuminuria is outlined in **Fig. 338-11** and includes annual measurement of the serum creatinine to estimate GFR. Interventions effective in slowing progression from microalbuminuria to macroalbuminuria include: (1) normalization of glycemia, (2) strict blood pressure control, and (3) administration of ACE inhibitors or ARBs. Dyslipidemia should also be treated.

Improved glycemic control reduces the rate at which microalbuminuria appears and progresses in type 1 and type 2 DM. However, once macroalbuminuria exists, it is unclear whether improved glycemic control will slow progression of renal disease. During the phase of declining renal function, insulin requirements may fall as the kidney is a site of insulin degradation. Furthermore, many glucose-lowering medications (sulfonylureas and metformin) are contraindicated in advanced renal insufficiency.

Many individuals with type 1 or type 2 DM develop hypertension. Numerous studies in both type 1 and type 2 DM demonstrate the effectiveness of strict blood pressure control in reducing albumin excretion and slowing the decline in renal function. Blood pressure should be maintained at <130/80 mmHg in diabetic individuals without proteinuria. A slightly lower blood pressure (125/75) should be considered for individuals with microalbuminuria or macroalbuminuria (see "Hypertension," below).

Either ACE inhibitors or ARBs should be used to reduce the progression from microalbuminuria to macroalbuminuria and the associated decline in GFR that accompanies macroalbuminuria in individuals with type 1 or type 2 DM (see "Hypertension," below). Although direct comparisons of ACE inhibitors and ARBs are lacking, most experts believe that the two classes of drugs are equivalent in the patient with diabetes. ARBs can be used as an alternative in patients who develop ACE inhibitor–associated cough or angioedema. After 2–3 months of therapy in patients with microalbuminuria, the drug dose is increased until either the microalbuminuria disappears or the maximum dose is reached. If use of either ACE inhibitors or ARBs is not possible, then calcium channel blockers (non-dihydropyridine class), beta blockers, or diuretics should be used. However, their efficacy in slowing the fall in the GFR is not

FIGURE 338-11 Screening for microalbuminuria should be performed in patients with type 1 diabetes for ≥ 5 years, in patients with type 2 diabetes, and during pregnancy. Non-diabetes-related conditions that might increase microalbuminuria are urinary tract infection, hematuria, heart failure, febrile illness, severe hyperglycemia, severe hypertension, and vigorous exercise. *(Adapted from RA DeFronzo, in Therapy for Diabetes Mellitus and Related Disorders, 3d ed. American Diabetes Association, Alexandria, VA, 1998.)*

proven. Blood pressure control with any agent is extremely important, but a drug-specific benefit in diabetic nephropathy, independent of blood pressure control, has been shown only for ACE inhibitors and ARBs in patients with DM.

The ADA suggests modest restriction of protein intake in diabetic individuals with microalbuminuria (0.8 g/kg per day) or macroalbuminuria (<0.8 g/kg per day, which is the adult Recommended Daily Allowance, or ~10% of the daily caloric intake).

Nephrology consultation should be considered when the estimated GFR < 60 mL/min per 1.743 m². Once macroalbuminuria ensues, the likelihood of ESRD is very high. As compared to nondiabetic individuals, hemodialysis in patients with DM is associated with more frequent complications, such as hypotension (due to autonomic neuropathy or loss of reflex tachycardia), more difficult vascular access, and accelerated progression of retinopathy. Survival after the onset of ESRD is shorter in the diabetic population compared to nondiabetics with similar clinical features. Atherosclerosis is the leading cause of death in diabetic individuals on dialysis, and hyperlipidemia should be treated aggressively. Renal transplantation from a living-related donor is the preferred therapy but requires chronic immunosuppression. Combined pancreas-kidney transplant offers the promise of normoglycemia and freedom from dialysis.

NEUROPATHY AND DIABETES MELLITUS

Diabetic neuropathy occurs in ~50% of individuals with long-standing type 1 and type 2 DM. It may manifest as polyneuropathy, mononeuropathy, and/or autonomic neuropathy. As with other complications of DM, the development of neuropathy correlates with the duration of diabetes and glycemic control. Additional risk factors are BMI (the greater the BMI, the greater the risk of neuropathy) and smoking. The presence of cardiovascular disease, elevated triglycerides, and hypertension is also associated with diabetic peripheral neuropathy. Both myelinated and unmyelinated nerve fibers are lost. Because the clinical features of diabetic neuropathy are similar to those of other neuropathies, the diagnosis of diabetic neuropathy should be made only after other possible etiologies are excluded (Chap. 379). The ADA recommends screening for distal symmetric neuropathy beginning with the initial diagnosis of diabetes and screening for autonomic neuropathy 5 years after diagnosis of type 1 DM and at the time of diagnosis of type 2 DM. All individuals with diabetes should then be screened annually for both forms of neuropathy.

Polyneuropathy/Mononeuropathy The most common form of diabetic neuropathy is distal symmetric polyneuropathy. It most frequently presents with distal sensory loss, but up to 50% of patients do not have symptoms of neuropathy. Hyperesthesia, paresthesia, and dysesthesia also may occur. Any combination of these symptoms may develop as neuropathy progresses. Symptoms may include a sensation of numbness, tingling, sharpness, or burning that begins in the feet and spreads proximally. Neuropathic pain develops in some of these individuals, occasionally preceded by improvement in their glycemic control. Pain typically involves the lower extremities, is usually present at rest, and worsens at night. Both an acute (lasting <12 months) and a chronic form of painful diabetic neuropathy have been described. As diabetic neuropathy progresses, the pain subsides and eventually disappears, but a sensory deficit in the lower extremities persists. Physical examination reveals sensory loss, loss of ankle reflexes, and abnormal position sense.

Diabetic polyradiculopathy is a syndrome characterized by severe disabling pain in the distribution of one or more nerve roots. It may be accompanied by motor weakness. Intercostal or truncal radiculopathy causes pain over the thorax or abdomen. Involvement of the lumbar plexus or femoral nerve may cause severe pain in the thigh or hip and may be associated with muscle weakness in the hip flexors or extensors (diabetic amyotrophy). Fortunately, diabetic polyradiculopathies are usually self-limited and resolve over 6–12 months.

Mononeuropathy (dysfunction of isolated cranial or peripheral nerves) is less common than polyneuropathy in DM and presents with pain and motor weakness in the distribution of a single nerve. A vascular etiology has been suggested, but the pathogenesis is unknown.

Involvement of the third cranial nerve is most common and is heralded by diplopia. Physical examination reveals ptosis and ophthalmoplegia with normal pupillary constriction to light. Sometimes other cranial nerves IV, VI, or VII (Bell's palsy) are affected. Peripheral mononeuropathies or simultaneous involvement of more than one nerve (mononeuropathy multiplex) may also occur.

Autonomic Neuropathy Individuals with long-standing type 1 or 2 DM may develop signs of autonomic dysfunction involving the cholinergic, noradrenergic, and peptidergic (peptides such as pancreatic polypeptide, substance P, etc.) systems. DM-related autonomic neuropathy can involve multiple systems, including the cardiovascular, gastrointestinal, genitourinary, sudomotor, and metabolic systems. Autonomic neuropathies affecting the cardiovascular system cause a resting tachycardia and orthostatic hypotension. Reports of sudden death have also been attributed to autonomic neuropathy. Gastroparesis and bladder-emptying abnormalities are often caused by the autonomic neuropathy seen in DM (discussed below). Hyperhidrosis of the upper extremities and anhidrosis of the lower extremities result from sympathetic nervous system dysfunction. Anhidrosis of the feet can promote dry skin with cracking, which increases the risk of foot ulcers. Autonomic neuropathy may reduce counterregulatory hormone release, leading to an inability to sense hypoglycemia appropriately (hypoglycemia unawareness; Chap. 339), thereby subjecting the patient to the risk of severe hypoglycemia and complicating efforts to improve glycemic control.

℞ DIABETIC NEUROPATHY

Treatment of diabetic neuropathy is less than satisfactory. Improved glycemic control should be aggressively pursued and will improve nerve conduction velocity, but symptoms of diabetic neuropathy may not necessarily improve. Efforts to improve glycemic control may be confounded by autonomic neuropathy and hypoglycemia unawareness. Risk factors for neuropathy such as hypertension and hypertriglyceridemia should be treated. Avoidance of neurotoxins (alcohol) and smoking, supplementation with vitamins for possible deficiencies (B₁₂, folate; Chap. 71), and symptomatic treatment are the mainstays of therapy. Loss of sensation in the foot places the patient at risk for ulceration and its sequelae; consequently, prevention of such problems is of paramount importance. Patients with symptoms or signs of neuropathy (see "Physical Examination," below) should check their feet daily and take precautions (footwear) aimed at preventing calluses or ulcerations. If foot deformities are present, a podiatrist should be involved.

Chronic, painful diabetic neuropathy is difficult to treat but may respond to antidepressants (tricyclic antidepressants such as amitriptyline, desipramine, nortriptyline, imipramine or selective serotonin norepinephrine reuptake inhibitors such as duloxetine) or anticonvulsants (gabapentin, pregabalin, carbamazepine, lamotrigine). Two agents, duloxetine and pregabalin, have been approved by the U.S. Food and Drug Administration (FDA) for pain associated with diabetic neuropathy. However, pending further study, most recommend beginning with other agents such as a tricyclic antidepressant and switching if there is no response or if side effects develop. Aldose reductase inhibitors do not offer significant symptomatic relief. Referral to a pain management center may be necessary. Since the pain of acute diabetic neuropathy may resolve over time, medications may be discontinued as progressive neuronal damage from DM occurs.

Therapy of orthostatic hypotension secondary to autonomic neuropathy is also challenging. A variety of agents have limited success (fludrocortisone, midodrine, clonidine, octreotide, and yohimbine) but each has significant side effects. Nonpharmacologic maneuvers (adequate salt intake, avoidance of dehydration and diuretics, and lower extremity support hose) may offer some benefit.

GASTROINTESTINAL/GENITOURINARY DYSFUNCTION

Long-standing type 1 and 2 DM may affect the motility and function of gastrointestinal (GI) and genitourinary systems. The most prominent GI symptoms are delayed gastric emptying (gastroparesis) and altered small- and large-bowel motility (constipation or diarrhea). Gastroparesis may present with symptoms of anorexia, nausea, vomiting, early satiety, and abdominal bloating. Microvascular complications (retinopathy and neuropathy) are usually present. Nuclear medicine scintigraphy after ingestion of a radiolabeled meal is the best study to document delayed gastric emptying, but may not correlate well with symptoms. Noninvasive "breath tests" following ingestion of a radiolabeled meal are under development. Though parasympathetic dysfunction secondary to chronic hyperglycemia is important in the development of gastroparesis, hyperglycemia itself also impairs gastric emptying. Nocturnal diarrhea, alternating with constipation, is a feature of DM-related GI autonomic neuropathy. In type 1 DM, these symptoms should also prompt evaluation for celiac sprue because of its increased frequency. Esophageal dysfunction in long-standing DM may occur but is usually asymptomatic.

Diabetic autonomic neuropathy may lead to genitourinary dysfunction including cystopathy, erectile dysfunction, and female sexual dysfunction (reduced sexual desire, dyspareunia, reduced vaginal lubrication). Symptoms of diabetic cystopathy begin with an inability to sense a full bladder and a failure to void completely. As bladder contractility worsens, bladder capacity and the post-void residual increase, leading to symptoms of urinary hesitancy, decreased voiding frequency, incontinence, and recurrent urinary tract infections. Diagnostic evaluation includes cystometry and urodynamic studies.

Erectile dysfunction and retrograde ejaculation are very common in DM and may be one of the earliest signs of diabetic neuropathy (Chap. 49). Erectile dysfunction, which increases in frequency with the age of the patient and the duration of diabetes, may occur in the absence of other signs of diabetic autonomic neuropathy.

Rx GASTROINTESTINAL/GENITOURINARY DYSFUNCTION

Current treatments for these complications of DM are inadequate. Improved glycemic control should be a primary goal, as some aspects (neuropathy, gastric function) may improve. Smaller, more frequent meals that are easier to digest (liquid) and low in fat and fiber may minimize symptoms of gastroparesis. Agents with some efficacy include dopamine agonists metoclopramide, 5–10 mg, and domperidone, 10–20 mg, before each meal. Erythromycin interacts with the motilin receptor and may promote gastric emptying. Diabetic diarrhea in the absence of bacterial overgrowth is treated symptomatically with loperamide and may respond to octreotide (50–75 μg three times daily, SC). Treatment of bacterial overgrowth with antibiotics is sometimes useful (Chap. 288).

Diabetic cystopathy should be treated with timed voiding or self-catheterization, possibly with the addition of bethanechol. Drugs that inhibit type 5 phosphodiesterase are effective for erectile dysfunction, but their efficacy in individuals with DM is slightly lower than in the nondiabetic population (Chap. 49). Sexual dysfunction in women may be improved with use of vaginal lubricants, treatment of vaginal infections, and systemic or local estrogen replacement.

CARDIOVASCULAR MORBIDITY AND MORTALITY

Cardiovascular disease is increased in individuals with type 1 or type 2 DM. The Framingham Heart Study revealed a marked increase in PAD, CHF, CAD, MI, and sudden death (risk increase from one- to fivefold) in DM. The American Heart Association has designated DM as a major risk factor for cardiovascular disease (same category as smoking, hypertension, and hyperlipidemia). Type 2 diabetes patients without a prior MI have a similar risk for coronary artery–related events as nondiabetic individuals who have had a prior MI. Because of the extremely high prevalence of underlying cardiovascular disease in individuals with diabetes (especially in type 2 DM), evidence of atherosclerotic vascular disease (e.g., cardiac stress test) should be sought in an individual with diabetes who has symptoms suggestive of cardiac ischemia, peripheral or carotid arterial disease, a resting electrocardiogram indicative of prior infarction, plans to initiate an exercise program, proteinuria, or two other cardiac risk factors (ADA recommendations). Whether and how to screen asymptomatic individuals with diabetes for CAD is controversial. The absence of chest pain ("silent ischemia") is common in individuals with diabetes, and a thorough cardiac evalu-

ation is indicated in individuals undergoing major surgical procedures. The prognosis for individuals with diabetes who have CAD or MI is worse than for nondiabetics. CAD is more likely to involve multiple vessels in individuals with DM.

The increase in cardiovascular morbidity and mortality appears to relate to the synergism of hyperglycemia with other cardiovascular risk factors. For example, after controlling for all known cardiovascular risk factors, type 2 DM increases the cardiovascular death rate twofold in men and fourfold in women. Risk factors for macrovascular disease in diabetic individuals include dyslipidemia, hypertension, obesity, reduced physical activity, and cigarette smoking. Additional risk factors more prevalent in the diabetic population include microalbuminuria, macroalbuminuria, an elevation of serum creatinine, and abnormal platelet function. Insulin resistance, as reflected by elevated serum insulin levels, is associated with an increased risk of cardiovascular complications in individuals with and without DM. Individuals with insulin resistance and type 2 DM have elevated levels of plasminogen activator inhibitors (especially PAI-1) and fibrinogen, which enhances the coagulation process and impairs fibrinolysis, thus favoring the development of thrombosis. Diabetes is also associated with endothelial, vascular smooth-muscle, and platelet dysfunction.

Evidence that improved glycemic control reduces cardiovascular complications in DM is inconclusive. In the DCCT, the number of cardiovascular events in patients with type 1 diabetes did not differ between the standard and intensively treated groups during the trial but were reduced at follow-up 17 years later (see above). An improvement in the lipid profile of individuals in the intensive group (lower total and LDL cholesterol, lower triglycerides) during intensive diabetes management was noted. Trials to examine whether improved glycemic control reduces cardiovascular events in type 2 diabetes are underway. Concerns about the atherogenic potential of insulin remain, since in nondiabetic individuals, higher serum insulin levels (indicative of insulin resistance) are associated with a greater risk of cardiovascular morbidity and mortality. In the UKPDS, improved glycemic control did not conclusively reduce cardiovascular mortality. Importantly, treatment with insulin and the sulfonylureas did not appear to increase the risk of cardiovascular disease in individuals with type 2 DM, refuting prior claims about the atherogenic potential of these agents.

In addition to CAD, cerebrovascular disease is increased in individuals with DM (threefold increase in stroke). Individuals with DM have an increased incidence of CHF. The etiology of this abnormality is probably multifactorial and includes factors such as myocardial ischemia from atherosclerosis, hypertension, and myocardial cell dysfunction secondary to chronic hyperglycemia.

Rx CARDIOVASCULAR DISEASE

In general, the treatment of coronary disease is not different in the diabetic individual (Chap. 237). Revascularization procedures for CAD, including percutaneous coronary interventions (PCI) and coronary artery bypass grafting (CABG), may be less efficacious in the diabetic individual. Initial success rates of PCI in diabetic individuals are similar to those in the nondiabetic population, but diabetic patients have higher rates of restenosis and lower long-term patency and survival rates in older studies. More recently, the use of drug-eluting stents and a GPIIb/IIIa platelet inhibitor has improved the outcomes in diabetic patients, and whether there is a difference in efficacy of PCI in diabetic individuals is not clear. Although CABG may be preferred over PCI in diabetic individuals with multivessel CAD or recent Q-wave MI, PCI is preferred in patients with single-vessel CAD or two-vessel disease (no involvement of left anterior descending).

The ADA has emphasized the importance of glycemic control and aggressive cardiovascular risk modification in all individuals with DM (see below). Past trepidation about using beta blockers in individuals who have diabetes should not prevent use of these agents since they clearly benefit diabetic patients after MI. ACE inhibitors (or ARBs) may also be particularly beneficial and should be considered in individuals with type 2 DM and other risk factors (smoking, dyslipidemia, history of cardiovascular disease, microalbuminuria). Patients with atypical chest pain or an abnormal resting EKG should be screened for CHD. Screening of asymptomatic individuals with diabetes is controversial.

Antiplatelet therapy reduces cardiovascular events in individuals with DM who have CAD. Current recommendations by the ADA include the use of aspirin for secondary prevention of coronary events. Although data demonstrating efficacy in primary prevention of coronary events in DM are lacking, antiplatelet therapy should be strongly considered, especially in diabetic individuals >30 years of age with other coronary risk factors such as hypertension, smoking, family history, or dyslipidemia. The aspirin dose (75–162 mg) is the same as that in nondiabetic individuals. Aspirin therapy does not have detrimental effects on renal function or hypertension, nor does it influence the course of diabetic retinopathy.

Cardiovascular Risk Factors · *DYSLIPIDEMIA* Individuals with DM may have several forms of dyslipidemia (Chap. 350). Because of the additive cardiovascular risk of hyperglycemia and hyperlipidemia, lipid abnormalities should be assessed aggressively and treated as part of comprehensive diabetes care (Fig. 338-12). The most common pattern of dyslipidemia is hypertriglyceridemia and reduced HDL cholesterol levels. DM itself does not increase levels of LDL, but the small dense LDL particles found in type 2 DM are more atherogenic because they are more easily glycated and susceptible to oxidation.

Almost all treatment studies of diabetic dyslipidemia have been performed in individuals with type 2 DM because of the greater frequency of dyslipidemia in this form of diabetes. Interventional studies have shown that the beneficial effects of LDL reduction are similar in the diabetic and nondiabetic populations. Large prospective trials of primary and secondary intervention for CHD have included some individuals with type 2 DM, and subset analyses have consistently found that reductions in LDL reduce cardiovascular events and morbidity in individuals with DM. Most clinical trials used HMG CoA reductase inhibitors, although gemfibrozil is also beneficial. No prospective studies have addressed similar questions in individuals with type 1 DM. Since the frequency of cardiovascular disease is low in children and young adults with diabetes, assessment of CV risk should be incorporated into the guidelines discussed below.

Based on the guidelines provided by the ADA and the American Heart Association, priorities in the treatment of hyperlipidemia are: (1) lower the LDL cholesterol, (2) raise the HDL cholesterol, and (3) decrease the triglycerides. A treatment strategy depends on the pattern of lipoprotein abnormalities (Fig. 338-12). Initial therapy for all forms of dyslipidemia should include dietary changes, as well as the same life-style modifications recommended in the nondiabetic population (smoking cessation, blood pressure control, weight loss, increased physical activity). The dietary recommendations for individuals with DM are similar to those advocated by the National Cholesterol Education Program (Chap. 350) and include increased monounsaturated fat and carbohydrates and reduced saturated fats and cholesterol. Though viewed as important, the response to dietary alterations is often modest (<10% reduction in the LDL). Improvement in glycemic control will lower triglycerides and have a modest beneficial effect by raising HDL. HMG CoA reductase inhibitors are the agents of choice for lowering the LDL. According to guidelines of the ADA and the American Heart Association, the target lipid values in diabetic individuals (age >40 years) without cardiovascular disease should be: LDL < 2.6 mmol/L (100 mg/dL); HDL > 1.1 mmol/L (40 mg/dL) in men and >1.38 mmol/L (50 mg/dL) in women; and triglycerides < 1.7 mmol/L (150 mg/dL). The rationale for these goals is that the risk of CHD is similar to that in patients without diabetes who have had a prior MI. In patients >40 years, the ADA recommends addition of statin, regardless of the LDL, to reduce LDL by 30–40%. If the patient is known to have cardiovascular disease, the ADA recommends an LDL goal of <1.8 mmol/L (70 mg/dL) as an "option" [in keeping with evidence that such a goal is beneficial in non-diabetic individuals with CAD (Chap. 350)]. Fibrates have some efficacy and should be considered when the HDL is low in the setting of a mild elevation of the LDL. Combination therapy with an HMG CoA reductase inhibitor and a fibrate or another lipid-lowering agent (ezetimibe, niacin) may be needed to reach LDL or HDL goals, but statin/fibrate combinations increase the possibility of side effects such as myositis. Nicotinic acid effectively raises HDL and can be used

FIGURE 338-12 Dyslipidemia management in diabetes. *Second-line treatment: fibric acid derivative, ezetimibe, niacin, or bile acid–binding resin. †See text for pharmacologic treatment based on age and risk profile. LDL, low-density lipoprotein; HDL, high-density lipoprotein.

in patients with diabetes, but high doses (>2 g/d) may worsen glycemic control and increase insulin resistance. Bile acid–binding resins should not be used if hypertriglyceridemia is present. Pharmacologic therapy of dyslipidemia to achieve a LDL < 2.6 mmol/L (100 mg/dL) should be considered in diabetic individuals <40 years of age without cardiovascular disease if the individual also has other risk factors.

HYPERTENSION Hypertension can accelerate other complications of DM, particularly cardiovascular disease and nephropathy. In targeting the goal of BP < 130/80, therapy should first emphasize life-style modifications such as weight loss, exercise, stress management, and sodium restriction. Realizing that more than one agent is usually required to reach a blood pressure goal, the ADA recommends that all patients with diabetes and hypertension be treated with an ACE inhibitor or an ARB. Subsequently, agents that reduce cardiovascular risk (beta blockers, thiazide diuretics, and calcium channel blockers) should be incorporated into the regimen. While ACE inhibitors and ARBs are likely equivalent in most patients with diabetes and renal disease, the ADA recommends: (1) in patients with type 1 diabetes, hypertension, and micro- or macroalbuminuria, an ACE inhibitor slowed progression of nephropathy; (2) in patients with type 2 diabetes, hypertension, and microalbuminuria, an ACE inhibitor or an ARB slowed the progression to macroalbuminuria; and (3) in patients with type 2 diabetes, hypertension, macroalbuminuria, and renal insufficiency, an ARB slowed the decline in GFR. Additional points of emphasis include:

1. ACE inhibitors are either glucose- and lipid-neutral or glucose- and lipid-beneficial and thus positively impact the cardiovascular risk profile. Calcium channel blockers, central adrenergic antagonists, and vasodilators are lipid- and glucose-neutral.
2. Beta blockers and thiazide diuretics can increase insulin resistance and negatively impact the lipid profile; beta blockers may slightly increase the risk of developing type 2 DM. Although often questioned because of the potential masking of hypoglycemic symptoms, beta blockers are safe in most patients with diabetes and reduce cardiovascular events.
3. Sympathetic inhibitors and α-adrenergic blockers may worsen orthostatic hypotension in the diabetic individual with autonomic neuropathy.
4. Equivalent reduction in blood pressure by different classes of agents may not translate into equivalent protection from cardiovascular and renal endpoints. Thiazides, beta blockers, ACE inhibitors, and ARBs positively impact cardiovascular endpoints (MI or stroke).
5. Non-dihydropyridine calcium channel blockers (verapamil and diltiazem), rather than dihydropyridine agents (amlodipine and nifedipine), are preferred in diabetics.

CHAPTER 338

Diabetes Mellitus

6. A blood pressure goal of <125/75 is suggested for individuals with macroalbuminuria, hypertension, and diabetes.

7. Serum potassium and renal function should be monitored.

Because of the high prevalence of atherosclerotic disease in individuals with DM, the possibility of renovascular hypertension should be considered when the blood pressure is not readily controlled.

LOWER EXTREMITY COMPLICATIONS

DM is the leading cause of nontraumatic lower extremity amputation in the United States. Foot ulcers and infections are also a major source of morbidity in individuals with DM. The reasons for the increased incidence of these disorders in DM involve the interaction of several pathogenic factors: neuropathy, abnormal foot biomechanics, PAD, and poor wound healing. The peripheral sensory neuropathy interferes with normal protective mechanisms and allows the patient to sustain major or repeated minor trauma to the foot, often without knowledge of the injury. Disordered proprioception causes abnormal weight bearing while walking and subsequent formation of callus or ulceration. Motor and sensory neuropathy lead to abnormal foot muscle mechanics and to structural changes in the foot (hammer toe, claw toe deformity, prominent metatarsal heads, Charcot joint). Autonomic neuropathy results in anhidrosis and altered superficial blood flow in the foot, which promote drying of the skin and fissure formation. PAD and poor wound healing impede resolution of minor breaks in the skin, allowing them to enlarge and to become infected.

Approximately 15% of individuals with DM develop a foot ulcer (great toe or MTP areas are most common), and a significant subset will ultimately undergo amputation (14–24% risk with that ulcer or subsequent ulceration). Risk factors for foot ulcers or amputation include: male sex, diabetes >10 years' duration, peripheral neuropathy, abnormal structure of foot (bony abnormalities, callus, thickened nails), peripheral arterial disease, smoking, history of previous ulcer or amputation, and poor glycemic control. Large callouses are often precursors to or overlie ulcerations.

℞ LOWER EXTREMITY COMPLICATIONS

The optimal therapy for foot ulcers and amputations is prevention through identification of high-risk patients, education of the patient, and institution of measures to prevent ulceration. High-risk patients should be identified during the routine foot examination performed on all patients with DM (see "Ongoing Aspects of Comprehensive Diabetes Care," below). Patient education should emphasize: (1) careful selection of footwear, (2) daily inspection of the feet to detect early signs of poor-fitting footwear or minor trauma, (3) daily foot hygiene to keep the skin clean and moist, (4) avoidance of self-treatment of foot abnormalities and high-risk behavior (e.g., walking barefoot), and (5) prompt consultation with a health care provider if an abnormality arises. Patients at high risk for ulceration or amputation may benefit from evaluation by a foot care specialist. Interventions directed at risk factor modification include orthotic shoes and devices, callus management, nail care, and prophylactic measures to reduce increased skin pressure from abnormal bony architecture. Attention to other risk factors for vascular disease (smoking, dyslipidemia, hypertension) and improved glycemic control are also important.

Despite preventive measures, foot ulceration and infection are common and represent a serious problem. Due to the multifactorial pathogenesis of lower extremity ulcers, management of these lesions is multidisciplinary and often demands expertise in orthopedics, vascular surgery, endocrinology, podiatry, and infectious diseases. The plantar surface of the foot is the most common site of ulceration. Ulcers may be primarily neuropathic (no accompanying infection) or may have surrounding cellulitis or osteomyelitis. Cellulitis without ulceration is also frequent and should be treated with antibiotics that provide broad-spectrum coverage, including anaerobes (see below).

An infected ulcer is a clinical diagnosis, since superficial culture of any ulceration will likely find multiple possible bacterial pathogens. The infection surrounding the foot ulcer is often the result of multiple organisms (gram-positive and -negative organisms and anaerobes), and gas gangrene may develop in the absence of clostridial infection. Cultures taken from the surface of the ulcer are not helpful; a culture from the debrided ulcer base or from purulent drainage or aspiration of the wound is the most helpful. Wound depth should be determined by inspection and probing with a blunt-tipped sterile instrument. Plain radiographs of the foot should be performed to assess the possibility of osteomyelitis in chronic ulcers that have not responded to therapy. Nuclear medicine bone scans may be helpful, but overlying subcutaneous infection is often difficult to distinguish from osteomyelitis. Indium-labeled white cell studies are more useful in determining if the infection involves bony structures or only soft tissue, but they are technically demanding. MRI of the foot may be the most specific modality, although distinguishing bony destruction due to osteomyelitis from destruction secondary to Charcot arthropathy is difficult. If surgical debridement is necessary, bone biopsy and culture may provide the answer.

Osteomyelitis is best treated by a combination of prolonged antibiotics (IV then oral) and possibly debridement of infected bone. The possible contribution of vascular insufficiency should be considered in all patients. Noninvasive blood-flow studies are often unreliable in DM, and angiography may be required, recognizing the risk of contrast-induced nephrotoxicity. Peripheral arterial bypass procedures are often effective in promoting wound healing and in decreasing the need for amputation of the ischemic limb.

A growing number of possible treatments for diabetic foot ulcers exist, but they have yet to demonstrate clear efficacy in prospective, controlled trials. A consensus statement from the ADA identified six interventions with demonstrated efficacy in diabetic foot wounds: (1) off-loading, (2) debridement, (3) wound dressings, (4) appropriate use of antibiotics, (5) revascularization, and (6) limited amputation. Off-loading is the complete avoidance of weight bearing on the ulcer, which removes the mechanical trauma that retards wound healing. Bed rest and a variety of orthotic devices or contact casting limit weight bearing on wounds or pressure points. Surgical debridement is important and effective, but clear efficacy of other modalities for wound cleaning (enzymes, soaking, whirlpools) is lacking. Dressings such as hydrocolloid dressings promote wound healing by creating a moist environment and protecting the wound. Antiseptic agents should be avoided. Topical antibiotics are of limited value. Referral for physical therapy, orthotic evaluation, and rehabilitation should occur once the infection is controlled.

Mild or non-limb-threatening infections can be treated with oral antibiotics (cephalosporin, clindamycin, amoxicillin/clavulanate, and fluoroquinolones), surgical debridement of necrotic tissue, local wound care (avoidance of weight bearing over the ulcer), and close surveillance for progression of infection. More severe ulcers may require IV antibiotics as well as bed rest and local wound care. Urgent surgical debridement may be required. Strict control of glycemia should be a goal (see below). Intravenous antibiotics should provide broad-spectrum coverage directed toward *Staphylococcus aureus*, streptococci, gram-negative aerobes, and anaerobic bacteria. Initial antimicrobial regimens include ertapenem, piperacillin/tazobactam, cefotetan, ampicillin/sulbactam, linezolid, or the combination of clindamycin and a fluoroquinolone. Severe infections, or infections that do not improve after 48 h of antibiotic therapy, require expansion of antimicrobial therapy to treat methicillin-resistant *S. aureus* (e.g., vancomycin) and *Pseudomonas aeruginosa*. If the infection surrounding the ulcer is not improving with IV antibiotics, reassessment of antibiotic coverage and reconsideration of the need for surgical debridement or revascularization are indicated. With clinical improvement, oral antibiotics and local wound care can be continued on an outpatient basis with close follow-up.

New information about wound biology has led to a number of new technologies (e.g., living skin equivalents and growth factors such as basic fibroblast growth factor) that may prove useful, especially in neuropathic ulcers. Recombinant platelet-derived growth factor has some benefit and complements the therapies of off-loading, debridement, and antibiotics. Hyperbaric oxygen has been used, but rigorous proof of efficacy is lacking. Negative wound pressure has been shown to accelerate wound healing of plantar wounds.

INFECTIONS

Individuals with DM have a greater frequency and severity of infection. The reasons for this include incompletely defined abnormalities in cell-mediated immunity and phagocyte function associated with hyperglycemia, as well as diminished vascularization. Hyperglycemia aids the colonization and growth of a variety of organisms (*Candida* and other fungal species). Many common infections are more frequent and severe in the diabetic population, whereas several rare infections are seen almost exclusively in the diabetic population. Examples of this latter category include rhinocerebral mucormycosis, emphysematous infections of the gall bladder and urinary tract, and "malignant" or invasive otitis externa. Invasive otitis externa is usually secondary to *P. aeruginosa* infection in the soft tissue surrounding the external auditory canal, usually begins with pain and discharge, and may rapidly progress to osteomyelitis and meningitis. These infections should be sought, in particular, in patients presenting with HHS.

Pneumonia, urinary tract infections, and skin and soft tissue infections are all more common in the diabetic population. In general, the organisms that cause pulmonary infections are similar to those found in the nondiabetic population; however, gram-negative organisms, *S. aureus*, and *Mycobacterium tuberculosis* are more frequent pathogens. Urinary tract infections (either lower tract or pyelonephritis) are the result of common bacterial agents such as *Escherichia coli*, though several yeast species (*Candida* and *Torulopsis glabrata*) are commonly observed. Complications of urinary tract infections include emphysematous pyelonephritis and emphysematous cystitis. Bacteriuria occurs frequently in individuals with diabetic cystopathy. Susceptibility to furunculosis, superficial candidal infections, and vulvovaginitis are increased. Poor glycemic control is a common denominator in individuals with these infections. Diabetic individuals have an increased rate of colonization of *S. aureus* in the skin folds and nares. Diabetic patients also have a greater risk of postoperative wound infections. Strict glycemic control reduces postoperative infections in diabetic individuals undergoing CABG and should be the goal in all diabetic patients with an infection.

DERMATOLOGIC MANIFESTATIONS

The most common skin manifestations of DM are protracted wound healing and skin ulcerations. Diabetic dermopathy, sometimes termed *pigmented pretibial papules*, or "diabetic skin spots," begins as an erythematous area and evolves into an area of circular hyperpigmentation. These lesions result from minor mechanical trauma in the pretibial region and are more common in elderly men with DM. Bullous diseases, bullosa diabeticorum (shallow ulcerations or erosions in the pretibial region), are also seen. *Necrobiosis lipoidica diabeticorum* is a rare disorder of DM that predominantly affects young women with type 1 DM, neuropathy, and retinopathy. It usually begins in the pretibial region as an erythematous plaque or papules that gradually enlarge, darken, and develop irregular margins, with atrophic centers and central ulceration. They may be painful. Vitiligo occurs at increased frequency in individuals with type 1 diabetes. *Acanthosis nigricans* (hyperpigmented velvety plaques seen on the neck, axilla, or extensor surfaces) is sometimes a feature of severe insulin resistance and accompanying diabetes. Generalized or localized *granuloma annulare* (erythematous plaques on the extremities or trunk) and *scleredema* (areas of skin thickening on the back or neck at the site of previous superficial infections) are more common in the diabetic population. *Lipoatrophy* and *lipohypertrophy* can occur at insulin injection sites but are unusual with the use of human insulin. Xerosis and pruritus are common and are relieved by skin moisturizers.

APPROACH TO THE PATIENT:
Diabetes Mellitus

DM and its complications produce a wide range of symptoms and signs; those secondary to acute hyperglycemia may occur at any stage of the disease, whereas those related to chronic complications begin to appear during the second decade of hyperglycemia. Individuals with previously undetected type 2 DM may present with chronic complications of DM at the time of diagnosis. The history and physical examination should assess for symptoms or signs of acute hyperglycemia and should screen for the chronic complications and conditions associated with DM.

HISTORY A complete medical history should be obtained with special emphasis on DM-relevant aspects such as weight, family history of DM and its complications, risk factors for cardiovascular

disease, exercise, smoking, and ethanol use. Symptoms of hyperglycemia include polyuria, polydipsia, weight loss, fatigue, weakness, blurry vision, frequent superficial infections (vaginitis, fungal skin infections), and slow healing of skin lesions after minor trauma. Metabolic derangements relate mostly to hyperglycemia (osmotic diuresis, reduced glucose entry into muscle) and to the catabolic state of the patient (urinary loss of glucose and calories, muscle breakdown due to protein degradation and decreased protein synthesis). Blurred vision results from changes in the water content of the lens and resolves as the hyperglycemia is controlled.

In a patient with established DM, the initial assessment should also include special emphasis on prior diabetes care, including the type of therapy, prior hemoglobin A1C levels, self-monitoring blood glucose results, frequency of hypoglycemia, presence of DM-specific complications, assessment of the patient's knowledge about diabetes, exercise, and nutrition. The chronic complications may afflict several organ systems, and an individual patient may exhibit some, all, or none of the symptoms related to the complications of DM (see above). In addition, the presence of DM-related comorbidities should be sought (cardiovascular disease, hypertension, dyslipidemia).

PHYSICAL EXAMINATION In addition to a complete physical examination, special attention should be given to DM-relevant aspects such as weight or BMI, retinal examination, orthostatic blood pressure, foot examination, peripheral pulses, and insulin injection sites. Blood pressure > 130/80 mmHg is considered hypertension in individuals with diabetes. Careful examination of the lower extremities should seek evidence of peripheral neuropathy, calluses, superficial fungal infections, nail disease, ankle reflexes, and foot deformities (such as hammer or claw toes and Charcot foot) in order to identify sites of potential skin ulceration. Vibratory sensation (128-MHz tuning fork at the base of the great toe), the ability to sense touch with a monofilament (5.07, 10-g monofilament), and pinprick sensation are useful to detect moderately advanced diabetic neuropathy. Since periodontal disease is more frequent in DM, the teeth and gums should also be examined.

CLASSIFICATION OF DM IN AN INDIVIDUAL PATIENT The etiology of diabetes in an individual with new-onset disease can usually be assigned on the basis of clinical criteria. Individuals with type 1 DM tend to have the following characteristics: (1) onset of disease prior to age 30; (2) lean body habitus; (3) requirement of insulin as the initial therapy; (4) propensity to develop ketoacidosis; and (5) an increased risk of other autoimmune disorders such as autoimmune thyroid disease, adrenal insufficiency, pernicious anemia, celiac disease, and vitiligo. In contrast, individuals with type 2 DM often exhibit the following features: (1) develop diabetes after the age of 30; (2) are usually obese (80% are obese, but elderly individuals may be lean); (3) may not require insulin therapy initially; and (4) may have associated conditions such as insulin resistance, hypertension, cardiovascular disease, dyslipidemia, or PCOS. In type 2 DM, insulin resistance is often associated with abdominal obesity (as opposed to hip and thigh obesity) and hypertriglyceridemia. Although most individuals diagnosed with type 2 DM are older, the age of diagnosis is declining, and there is a marked increase among overweight children and adolescents. Some individuals with phenotypic type 2 DM present with DKA but lack autoimmune markers and may be later treated with oral glucose-lowering agents rather than insulin (have been termed *ketosis-prone type 2 DM*). On the other hand, some individuals (5–10%) with the phenotypic appearance of type 2 DM do not have absolute insulin deficiency but have autoimmune markers (ICA, GAD antibodies) suggestive of type 1 DM (termed *latent autoimmune diabetes of the adult*). Such individuals are more likely to be <50 years of age, have a normal BMI, and have a personal or family history of other autoimmune disease. They are much more likely to require insulin treatment within 5 years. However, it is remains difficult to categorize some patients unequivocally. Individuals who deviate from the clinical profile of type 1 and type 2 DM, or who have other associated defects such as deafness, pancreatic exocrine disease, and other endocrine disorders, should be classified accordingly (Table 338-1).

LABORATORY ASSESSMENT The laboratory assessment should first determine whether the patient meets the diagnostic criteria for DM (Table 338-2) and then assess the degree of glycemic control (A1C, discussed below). In addition to the standard laboratory evaluation, the patient should be screened for DM-associated conditions (e.g., microalbuminuria, dyslipidemia, thyroid dysfunction). Individuals at high risk for cardiovascular disease should be screened for asymptomatic CAD by appropriate cardiac stress testing, when indicated.

The classification of the type of DM may be facilitated by laboratory assessments. Serum insulin or C-peptide measurements do not always distinguish type 1 from type 2 DM, but a low C-peptide level confirms a patient's need for insulin. Many individuals with new-onset type 1 DM retain some C-peptide production. Measurement of islet cell antibodies at the time of diabetes onset may be useful if the type of DM is not clear based on the characteristics described above.

LONG-TERM TREATMENT

OVERALL PRINCIPLES

The goals of therapy for type 1 or type 2 DM are to: (1) eliminate symptoms related to hyperglycemia, (2) reduce or eliminate the long-term microvascular and macrovascular complications of DM, and (3) allow the patient to achieve as normal a lifestyle as possible. To reach these goals, the physician should identify a target level of glycemic control for each patient, provide the patient with the educational and pharmacologic resources necessary to reach this level, and monitor/treat DM-related complications. Symptoms of diabetes usually resolve when the plasma glucose is <11.1 mmol/L (200 mg/dL), and thus most DM treatment focuses on achieving the second and third goals. The treatment goals for patients with diabetes are summarized in Table 338-8.

The care of an individual with either type 1 or type 2 DM requires a multidisciplinary team. Central to the success of this team are the patient's participation, input, and enthusiasm, all of which are essential for optimal diabetes management. Members of the health care team include the primary care provider and/or the endocrinologist or diabetologist, a certified diabetes educator, and a nutritionist. In addition, when the complications of DM arise, subspecialists (including neurol-ogists, nephrologists, vascular surgeons, cardiologists, ophthalmologists, and podiatrists) with experience in DM-related complications are essential.

A number of names are sometimes applied to different approaches to diabetes care, such as intensive insulin therapy, intensive glycemic control, and "tight control." The current chapter, however, will use the term *comprehensive diabetes care* to emphasize the fact that optimal diabetes therapy involves more than plasma glucose management. Though glycemic control is central to optimal diabetes therapy, comprehensive diabetes care of both type 1 and type 2 DM should also detect and manage DM-specific complications and modify risk factors for DM-associated diseases. In addition to the physical aspects of DM, social, family, financial, cultural, and employment-related issues may impact diabetes care. The International Diabetes Federation (IDF), recognizing that resources available for diabetes care varies widely throughout the world, has issued guidelines for standard care (a well-developed service base and with health care funding systems consuming a significant part of their national wealth), minimal care (health care settings with very limited resources), and comprehensive care (health care settings with considerable resources). This chapter provides guidance for this comprehensive level of diabetes care.

PATIENT EDUCATION ABOUT DM, NUTRITION, AND EXERCISE

The patient with type 1 or type 2 DM should receive education about nutrition, exercise, care of diabetes during illness, and medications to lower the plasma glucose. Along with improved compliance, patient education allows individuals with DM to assume greater responsibility for their care. Patient education should be viewed as a continuing process with regular visits for reinforcement; it should not be a process that is completed after one or two visits to a nurse educator or nutritionist. The ADA refers to education about the individualized management plan for the patient as diabetes self-management education (DSME). More frequent contact between the patient and the diabetes management team (electronic, telephone, etc.) improves glycemic control.

Diabetes Education The diabetes educator is a health care professional (nurse, dietician, or pharmacist) with specialized patient education skills who is certified in diabetes education (e.g., American Association of Diabetes Educators). Education topics important for optimal diabetes care include self-monitoring of blood glucose; urine ketone monitoring (type 1 DM); insulin administration; guidelines for diabetes management during illnesses; management of hypoglycemia; foot and skin care; diabetes management before, during, and after exercise; and risk factor–modifying activities.

Nutrition *Medical nutrition therapy* (MNT) is a term used by the ADA to describe the optimal coordination of caloric intake with other aspects of diabetes therapy (insulin, exercise, weight loss). The ADA has issued recommendations for three types of MNT. Primary prevention measures of MNT are directed at preventing or delaying the onset of type 2 DM in high-risk individuals (obese or with pre-diabetes) by promoting weight reduction. Medical treatment of obesity is a rapidly evolving area and is discussed in Chap. 75. Secondary prevention measures of MNT are directed at preventing or delaying diabetes-related complications in diabetic individuals by improving glycemic control. Tertiary prevention measures of MNT are directed at managing diabetes-related complications (cardiovascular disease, nephropathy) in diabetic individuals. For example, in individuals with diabetes and chronic kidney disease, protein intake should be limited to 0.8 g/kg of body weight per day. MNT in patients with diabetes and cardiovascular disease should incorporate dietary principles used in non-diabetic patients with cardiovascular disease. While the recommendations for all three types of MNT overlap; this chapter emphasizes secondary prevention measures of MNT. Pharmacologic approaches that facilitate weight loss and bariatric surgery should be considered in selected patients (Chap. 75).

As for the general population, a diet that includes fruits, vegetables, fiber-containing foods, and low-fat milk is advised. Like other aspects of DM therapy, MNT must be adjusted to meet the goals of the indi-

TABLE 338-8	TREATMENT GOALS FOR ADULTS WITH DIABETES[a]	
Index	**Goal**
Glycemic control[b]	
A1C	<7.0[c]
Preprandial capillary plasma glucose	5.0–7.2 mmol/L (90–130 mg/dL)
Peak postprandial capillary plasma glucose	<10.0 mmol/L (<180 mg/dL)[d]
Blood pressure	<130/80[e]
Lipids[f]	
Low-density lipoprotein	<2.6 mmol/L (<100 mg/dL)
High-density lipoprotein	>1.1 mmol/L (>40 mg/dL)[g]
Triglycerides	<1.7 mmol/L (<150 mg/dL)

[a]As recommended by the ADA; Goals should be developed for each patient (see text). Goals may be different for certain patient populations.
[b]A1C is primary goal.
[c]While the ADA recommends an A1C < 7.0% in general, in the individual patient it recommends an ". . . A1C as close to normal (<6.0%) as possible without significant hypoglycemia. . . ." Normal range for A1C—4.0–6.0 (DCCT-based assay).
[d]One-two hours after beginning of a meal.
[e]In patients with reduced GFR and macroalbuminuria, the goal is <125/75.
[f]In decreasing order of priority.
[g]For women, some suggest a goal that is 0.25 mmol/L (10 mg/dL) higher.
Source: Adapted from American Diabetes Association, 2007.

TABLE 338-9	NUTRITIONAL RECOMMENDATIONS FOR ADULTS WITH DIABETES[a]

Fat
- 20–35% of total caloric intake
- Saturated fat < 7% of total calories
- <200 mg/day of dietary cholesterol
- Two or more servings of fish/week provide ω-3 polyunsaturated fatty acids
- Minimal trans fat consumption

Carbohydrate
- 45–65% of total caloric intake (low-carbohydrate diets are not recommended)
- Amount and type of carbohydrate important[b]
- Sucrose-containing foods may be consumed with adjustments in insulin dose

Protein
- 10–35% of total caloric intake (high-protein diets are not recommended)

Other components
- Fiber-containing foods may reduce postprandial glucose excursions
- Nonnutrient sweeteners

[a]See text for differences for patients with type 1 or type 2 diabetes. As for the general population, a healthy diet includes fruits, vegetables, and fiber-containing foods.
[b]Amount of carbohydrate determined by estimating grams of carbohydrate in diet; glycemic index reflects how consumption of a particular food affects the blood glucose.
Source: Adapted from American Diabetes Association, 2007.

vidual patient. Furthermore, MNT education is an important component of comprehensive diabetes care and should be reinforced by regular patient education. In general, the components of optimal MNT are similar for individuals with type 1 or type 2 DM (Table 338-9). Historically, nutrition education imposed restrictive, complicated regimens on the patient. Current practices have greatly changed, though many patients and health care providers still view the diabetic diet as monolithic and static. For example, MNT now includes foods with sucrose and seeks to modify other risk factors such as hyperlipidemia and hypertension rather than focusing exclusively on weight loss in individuals with type 2 DM. The *glycemic index* is an estimate of the postprandial rise in the blood glucose when a certain amount of that food is consumed. Consumption of foods with a low glycemic index appears to reduce postprandial glucose excursions and improve glycemic control. Reduced calorie and nonnutritive sweeteners are useful. Currently, evidence does not support supplementation of the diet with vitamins, antioxidants (vitamin C and E), or micronutrients (chromium) in patients with diabetes. The goal of MNT in the individual with type 1 DM is to coordinate and match the caloric intake, both temporally and quantitatively, with the appropriate amount of insulin. MNT in type 1 DM and self-monitoring of blood glucose must be integrated to define the optimal insulin regimen. The ADA encourages patients and providers to utilize carbohydrate counting or exchange systems to estimate the nutrient content of a meal or snack. Based on the patient's estimate of the carbohydrate content of meal, an insulin-to-carbohydrate ratio determines the bolus insulin dose for a meal or snack. MNT must be flexible enough to allow for exercise, and the insulin regimen must allow for deviations in caloric intake. An important component of MNT in type 1 DM is to minimize the weight gain often associated with intensive diabetes management.

The goals of MNT in type 2 DM are slightly different and address the greatly increased prevalence of cardiovascular risk factors (hypertension, dyslipidemia, obesity) and disease in this population. The majority of these individuals are obese, and weight loss is strongly encouraged and should remain an important goal. Hypocaloric diets and modest weight loss (5–7%) often result in rapid and dramatic glucose lowering in individuals with new-onset type 2 DM. Nevertheless, numerous studies document that long-term weight loss is uncommon. MNT for type 2 DM should emphasize modest caloric reduction, reduced fat intake, increased physical activity, and reduction of hyperlipidemia and hypertension. Increased consumption of soluble, dietary fiber may improve glycemic control in individuals with type 2 DM. Weight loss and exercise improve insulin resistance.

Exercise Exercise has multiple positive benefits including cardiovascular risk reduction, reduced blood pressure, maintenance of muscle mass, reduction in body fat, and weight loss. For individuals with type 1 or type 2 DM, exercise is also useful for lowering plasma glucose (during and following exercise) and increasing insulin sensitivity. In patients with diabetes, the ADA recommends 150 min/week (distributed over at least 3 days) of aerobic physical activity. In patients with type 2 DM, the exercise regimen should also include resistance training.

Despite its benefits, exercise presents challenges for individuals with DM because they lack the normal glucoregulatory mechanisms (normally, insulin falls and glucagon rises during exercise). Skeletal muscle is a major site for metabolic fuel consumption in the resting state, and the increased muscle activity during vigorous, aerobic exercise greatly increases fuel requirements. Individuals with type 1 DM are prone to either hyperglycemia or hypoglycemia during exercise, depending on the preexercise plasma glucose, the circulating insulin level, and the level of exercise-induced catecholamines. If the insulin level is too low, the rise in catecholamines may increase the plasma glucose excessively, promote ketone body formation, and possibly lead to ketoacidosis. Conversely, if the circulating insulin level is excessive, this relative hyperinsulinemia may reduce hepatic glucose production (decreased glycogenolysis, decreased gluconeogenesis) and increase glucose entry into muscle, leading to hypoglycemia.

To avoid exercise-related hyper- or hypoglycemia, individuals with type 1 DM should: (1) monitor blood glucose before, during, and after exercise; (2) delay exercise if blood glucose is >14 mmol/L (250 mg/dL) and ketones are present; (3) if the blood glucose is <5.6 mmol/L (100 mg/dL), ingest carbohydrate before exercising; (3) monitor glucose during exercise and ingest carbohydrate to prevent hypoglycemia; (4) decrease insulin doses (based on previous experience) before exercise and inject insulin into a nonexercising area; and (5) learn individual glucose responses to different types of exercise and increase food intake for up to 24 h after exercise, depending on intensity and duration of exercise. In individuals with type 2 DM, exercise-related hypoglycemia is less common but can occur in individuals taking either insulin or insulin secretagogues.

Because asymptomatic cardiovascular disease appears at a younger age in both type 1 and type 2 DM, formal exercise tolerance testing may be warranted in diabetic individuals with any of the following: age >35 years, diabetes duration >15 years (type 1 DM) or >10 years (type 2 DM), microvascular complications of DM (retinopathy, microalbuminuria, or nephropathy), PAD, other risk factors of CAD, or autonomic neuropathy. Untreated proliferative retinopathy is a relative contraindication to vigorous exercise, as this may lead to vitreous hemorrhage or retinal detachment.

MONITORING THE LEVEL OF GLYCEMIC CONTROL

Optimal monitoring of glycemic control involves plasma glucose measurements by the patient and an assessment of long-term control by the physician (measurement of hemoglobin A1C and review of the patient's self-measurements of plasma glucose). These measurements are complementary: the patient's measurements provide a picture of short-term glycemic control, whereas the A1C reflects average glycemic control over the previous 2–3 months.

Self-Monitoring of Blood Glucose Self-monitoring of blood glucose (SMBG) is the standard of care in diabetes management and allows the patient to monitor his or her blood glucose at any time. In SMBG, a small drop of blood and an easily detectable enzymatic reaction allow measurement of the capillary plasma glucose. Many glucose monitors can rapidly and accurately measure glucose (calibrated to provide plasma glucose value even though blood glucose is measured) in small amounts of blood (3–10 μl) obtained from the fingertip; alternative testing sites (e.g., forearm) are less reliable, especially when the blood glucose is changing rapidly (postprandially). A large number of blood glucose monitors are available, and the certified diabetes educator is critical in helping the patient select the optimal device and learn to use it properly. By combining glucose measurements with diet history, medication changes, and exercise history, the physician and patient can improve the treatment program.

The frequency of SMBG measurements must be individualized and adapted to address the goals of diabetes care. Individuals with type 1 DM or individuals with type 2 DM taking multiple insulin injections each day should routinely measure their plasma glucose three or more times per day to estimate and select mealtime boluses of short-acting insulin and to modify long-acting insulin doses. Most individuals with type 2 DM require less frequent monitoring, though the optimal frequency of SMBG has not been clearly defined. Individuals with type 2 DM who are taking insulin should utilize SMBG more frequently than those on oral agents. Individuals with type 2 DM who are on oral medications should utilize SMBG as a means of assessing the efficacy of their medication and the impact of diet. Since plasma glucose levels fluctuate less in these individuals, one to two SMBG measurements per day (or fewer in patients who are on oral agents or are diet-controlled) may be sufficient. Most measurements in individuals with type 1 or type 2 DM should be performed prior to a meal and supplemented with postprandial measurements to assist in reaching postprandial glucose targets (Table 338-8). Urine glucose testing does not provide an accurate assessment of glycemic control.

Devices for continuous blood glucose monitoring are the subject of intense investigation, as some systems have been approved by the FDA and others are in various stages of development. Currently, the use of these devices in routine diabetes management is limited, and they do not replace the need for a traditional glucose meter. This rapidly evolving technology requires substantial expertise on the part of the diabetes management team and the patient. Current continuous glucose monitoring systems (CGMS) measure the glucose in interstitial fluid that is in equilibrium with the blood glucose. Alarms notify the patient if the blood glucose falls into the hypoglycemic range. The FDA refers to these as "minimally invasive" or "noninvasive" depending on how the interstitial fluid is obtained. Several devices use an indwelling subcutaneous catheter to monitor interstitial fluid glucose and provide either real time or retrospective glucose values. Although clinical experience with these devices is limited, they appear to provide useful short-term information about the patterns of glucose changes as well as an enhanced ability to detect hypoglycemic episodes.

Ketones are an indicator of early diabetic ketoacidosis and should be measured in individuals with type 1 DM when the plasma glucose is consistently >16.7 mmol/L (300 mg/dL); during a concurrent illness; or with symptoms such as nausea, vomiting, or abdominal pain. Blood measurement of β-hydroxybutyrate is preferred over urine testing with nitroprusside-based assays that measure only acetoacetate and acetone.

Assessment of Long-Term Glycemic Control   Measurement of glycated hemoglobin is the standard method for assessing long-term glycemic control. When plasma glucose is consistently elevated, there is an increase in nonenzymatic glycation of hemoglobin; this alteration reflects the glycemic history over the previous 2–3 months, since erythrocytes have an average life span of 120 days (glycemic level in the preceding month contributes about 50% to the A1C value). There are numerous laboratory methods for measuring the various forms of glycated hemoglobin, and these have significant interassay variations. Since glycated hemoglobin measurements are usually compared to prior measurements, it is essential for the assay results to be comparable. Depending on the assay methodology, hemoglobinopathies, anemias, reticulocytosis, transfusions, and uremia may interfere with the A1C result. Measurement of A1C at the "point of care" allows for more rapid feedback and may therefore assist in adjustment of therapy.

Glycated hemoglobin or A1C should be measured in all individuals with DM during their initial evaluation and as part of their comprehensive diabetes care. As the primary predictor of long-term complications of DM, the A1C should mirror, to a certain extent, the short-term measurements of SMBG. These two measurements are complementary in that recent intercurrent illnesses may impact the SMBG measurements but not the A1C. Likewise, postprandial and nocturnal hyperglycemia may not be detected by the SMBG of fasting and preprandial

capillary plasma glucose but will be reflected in the A1C. In standardized assays, the A1C approximates the following mean plasma glucose values: an A1C of 6% is 7.5 mmol/L (135 mg/dL), 7% is 9.5 mmol/L (170 mg/dL), 8% is 11.5 mmol/L (205 mg/dL), etc. [A 1% rise in the A1C translates into a 2.0-mmol/L (35 mg/dL) increase in the mean glucose.] In patients achieving their glycemic goal, the ADA recommends measurement of the A1C at least twice per year. More frequent testing (every 3 months) is warranted when glycemic control is inadequate, when therapy has changed, or in most patients with type 1 DM. The degree of glycation of other proteins, such as albumin, can be used as an alternative indicator of glycemic control when the A1C is inaccurate (hemolytic anemia, hemoglobinopathies). The fructosamine assay (measuring glycated albumin) reflects the glycemic status over the prior 2 weeks. Alternative assays of glycemic control (including the 1,5 anhydroglucitol assay) should not be routinely used since studies demonstrating that it accurately predicts the complications of DM are lacking.

℞ TYPE 1 AND TYPE 2 DIABETES MELLITUS

ESTABLISHMENT OF TARGET LEVEL OF GLYCEMIC CONTROL Because the complications of DM are related to glycemic control, normoglycemia or near normoglycemia is the desired, but often elusive, goal for most patients. However, normalization of the plasma glucose for long periods of time is extremely difficult, as demonstrated by the DCCT. Regardless of the level of hyperglycemia, improvement in glycemic control will lower the risk of diabetes complications (Fig. 338-8).

The target for glycemic control (as reflected by the A1C) must be individualized, and the goals of therapy should be developed in consultation with the patient after considering a number of medical, social, and lifestyle issues. Some important factors to consider include the patient's age, ability to understand and implement a complex treatment regimen, presence and severity of complications of diabetes, ability to recognize hypoglycemic symptoms, presence of other medical conditions or treatments that might alter the response to therapy, lifestyle and occupation (e.g., possible consequences of experiencing hypoglycemia on the job), and level of support available from family and friends.

The ADA suggests that the glycemic goal is to achieve an A1C as close to normal as possible without significant hypoglycemia. In general, the target A1C should be <7.0% (Table 338-8) with a more stringent target (<6%) for many patients. A higher A1C goal may be appropriate for the very young or old or in individuals with limited life span or comorbid conditions. The major consideration is the frequency and severity of hypoglycemia, since this becomes more common with a more stringent A1C goal. Other groups (International Diabetes Federation and American Association of Clinical Endocrinology) have suggested that the A1C goal should be ≤6.5% in most individuals, based primarily on the observation that there is no lower limit of A1C in terms of reducing diabetes-specific complications.

TYPE 1 DIABETES MELLITUS   **General Aspects**   The ADA recommendations for fasting and bedtime glycemic goals and A1C targets are summarized in Table 338-8. The goal is to design and implement insulin regimens that mimic physiologic insulin secretion. Because individuals with type 1 DM partially or completely lack endogenous insulin production, administration of basal, exogenous insulin is essential for regulating glycogen breakdown, gluconeogenesis, lipolysis, and ketogenesis. Likewise, insulin replacement for meals should be appropriate for the carbohydrate intake and promote normal glucose utilization and storage.

Intensive Management   Intensive diabetes management has the goal of achieving euglycemia or near-normal glycemia. This approach requires multiple resources including thorough and continuing patient education, comprehensive recording of plasma glucose measurements and nutrition intake by the patient, and a variable insulin regimen that matches glucose intake and insulin dose. Insulin regimens usually include multiple-component insulin regimens, multiple daily injections (MDI), or insulin infusion devices (each discussed below).

The benefits of intensive diabetes management and improved glycemic control include a reduction in the microvascular complications of DM and a reduction in the macrovascular complications of DM, which persists after a period of near-normoglycemia. From a psychological standpoint, the patient experiences greater control over his or her diabetes and often notes an improved sense of well-being, greater flexibility in the timing and content of meals, and the capability to alter insulin dosing with exercise. In addition, intensive diabetes management in pregnancy reduces the risk of fetal malformations and morbidity. Intensive diabetes management is strongly encouraged in newly diagnosed patients with type 1 DM because it may prolong the period of C-peptide production, which may result in better glycemic control and a reduced risk of serious hypoglycemia.

Although intensive management confers impressive benefits, it is also accompanied by significant personal and financial costs and is therefore not appropriate for all individuals.

Insulin Preparations Current insulin preparations are generated by recombinant DNA technology and consist of the amino acid sequence of human insulin or variations thereof. Animal insulin (beef or pork) is no longer used. In the United States, most insulin is formulated as U-100 (100 units/mL), whereas in some other countries it is available in other concentrations (e.g., U-40 = 40 units/mL). Human insulin has been formulated with distinctive pharmacokinetics or genetically modified to more closely mimic physiologic insulin secretion. Insulins can be classified as short-acting or long-acting **(Table 338-10)**. For example, one short-acting insulin formulation, insulin lispro, is an insulin analogue in which the 28th and 29th amino acids (lysine and proline) on the insulin B chain have been reversed by recombinant DNA technology. Insulin aspart and insulin glulisine are other genetically modified insulin analogues with properties similar to lispro. These insulin analogues have full biologic activity but less tendency for self aggregation, resulting in more rapid absorption and onset of action and a shorter duration of action. These characteristics are particularly advantageous for allowing entrainment of insulin injection and action to rising plasma glucose levels following meals. The shorter duration of action also appears to be associated with a decreased number of hypoglycemic episodes, primarily because the decay of insulin action corresponds to the decline in plasma glucose after a meal. Thus, insulin aspart, lispro, or glulisine is preferred over regular insulin for prandial coverage. Insulin glargine is a long-acting biosynthetic human insulin that differs from normal insulin in that asparagine is replaced by glycine at amino acid 21, and two arginine residues are added to the C-terminus of the B chain. Compared to NPH insulin, the onset of insulin glargine action is later, the duration of action is longer (~24 h), and there is no pronounced peak. A lower incidence of hypoglycemia, especially at night, has been reported with insulin glargine when compared to NPH insulin. Insulin detemir has a fatty acid side chain that prolongs its action by slowing absorption and catabolism. Regular and NPH insulin have the native insulin amino acid sequence. Regular insulin formulated as U-500 (500 units/mL) is available and sometimes useful in severely insulin resistant patients.

Basal insulin requirements are provided by long-acting (NPH insulin, insulin glargine, or insulin detemir) insulin formulations. These are usually prescribed with short-acting insulin in an attempt to mimic physiologic insulin release with meals. Although mixing of NPH and short-acting insulin formulations is common practice, this mixing may alter the insulin absorption profile (especially the short-acting insulins). For example, lispro absorption is delayed by mixing with NPH. The alteration in insulin absorption when the patient mixes different insulin formulations should not discourage mixing insulins. However, the following guidelines should be followed: (1) mix the different insulin formulations in the syringe immediately before injection (inject within 2 min after mixing); (2) do not store insulin as a mixture; (3) follow the same routine in terms of insulin mixing and administration to standardize the physiologic response to injected insulin; and (4) do not mix insulin glargine or detemir with other insulins. The miscibility of human regular and NPH insulin allows for the production of combination insulins that contain 70% NPH and 30% regular (70/30), or equal mixtures of NPH and regular (50/50). Other combination insulin formulations are insulin aspart (70/30) and insulin lispro (75/25 and 50/50). By including some insulin analogue mixed with protamine, these combina-

TABLE 338-10 PHARMACOKINETICS OF INSULIN PREPARATIONS

Preparation	Time of Action		
	Onset, h	Peak, h	Effective Duration, h
Short-acting, subcutaneous			
Lispro	<0.25	0.5–1.5	3–4
Aspart	<0.25	0.5–1.5	3–4
Glulisine	<0.25	0.5–1.5	3–4
Regular	0.5–1.0	2–3	4–6
Short-acting, inhaled			
Inhaled regular insulin	<0.25	0.5–1.5	4–6
Long-acting			
NPH	1–4	6–10	10–16
Detemir	1–4	—[a]	12–20
Glargine	1–4	—[a]	24
Insulin Combinations			
75/25–75% protamine lispro, 25% lispro	<0.25	1.5 h[b]	Up to 10–16
70/30–70% protamine aspart, 30% aspart	<0.25	1.5 h[b]	Up to 10–16
50/50–50% protamine lispro, 50% lispro	<0.25	1.5 h[b]	Up to 10–16
70/30–70% NPH, 30% regular insulin	0.5–1	Dual	10–16
50/50–50% NPH, 50% regular insulin	0.5–1	Dual	10–16

[a]Glargine has minimal peak activity; detemir has some peak activity at 6–14 h.
[b]Dual: two peaks; one at 2–3 h; the second several hours later.
Source: Adapted from JS Skyler, *Therapy for Diabetes Mellitus and Related Disorders*, American Diabetes Association, Alexandria, VA, 2004.

tions have a short-acting and long-acting profile (Table 338-10). While more convenient for the patient (only two injections/day), combination insulin formulations do not allow independent adjustment of short-acting and long-acting activity. Several insulin formulations are available as insulin "pens," which may be more convenient for some patients.

Insulin can also be delivered by inhalation by using a powder formulation of regular insulin and a delivery device. For insulin delivery, the patient uses a powdered formulation of insulin (a "blister") and a specialized inhaler to release a cloud of insulin into a reservoir from which the aerosolized insulin is inhaled. Inhaled insulin is short-acting, with an onset of action similar to insulin analogues but with a duration of action similar to regular insulin. It is therefore used for prandial coverage. Inhaled insulin must either be combined with an injected long-acting insulin to provide basal insulin coverage in type 1 or type 2 DM (Table 338-10) or used in combination with oral agents in patients with type 2 DM. Inhaled insulin appears to be similar to injected regular insulin in terms of glycemic control. It is available in 1- and 3-mg "blisters," which are equivalent to 3 and 8 units of injected regular insulin. To deliver a larger dose requires the use of more than one blister. Inhaled insulin is not approved for use in patients who smoke or have chronic lung diseases. Pulmonary function testing should be performed before starting inhaled insulin and repeated after 6 months of treatment and then annually. Side effects include cough, which improves with continued use, and hypoglycemia in a frequency similar to that seen with injected regular insulin. Long-term safety of inhaled insulin is not known. Proper use of the inhalation device requires patient education. Inhaled insulin has no physiologic advantage over injected short-acting insulin but may be considered in selected patients with type 2 DM who are unwilling to use injected insulin. Other inhaled insulin formulations are under development.

Insulin Regimens Representations of the various insulin regimens that may be utilized in type 1 DM are illustrated in **Fig. 338-13**. Although the insulin profiles are depicted as "smooth," symmetric curves, there is considerable patient-to-patient variation in the peak and duration. In all regimens, long-acting insulins (NPH, glargine, or detemir) supply basal insulin, whereas regular, insulin aspart, glulisine, or lispro insulin provides prandial insulin. Short-acting insulin analogues should be injected just before (<20 min) or just after a meal; regular insulin is given 30–45 min prior to a meal.

A shortcoming of current insulin regimens is that injected insulin immediately enters the systemic circulation, whereas endogenous insulin is secreted into the portal venous system. Thus, exogenous insulin administration exposes the liver to subphysiologic insulin levels. No insulin regimen reproduces the precise insulin secretory pattern of the pancreatic islet. However, the most physiologic regimens entail more frequent insulin injections, greater reliance on short-acting insulin, and more frequent capillary plas-

FIGURE 338-13 Representative insulin regimens for the treatment of diabetes. For each panel, the *y*-axis shows the amount of insulin effect and the *x*-axis shows the time of day. B, breakfast; L, lunch; S, supper; HS, bedtime; CSII, continuous subcutaneous insulin infusion. *Lispro, glulisine, or insulin aspart can be used. The time of insulin injection is shown with a vertical arrow. The type of insulin is noted above each insulin curve. **A.** A multiple-component insulin regimen consisting of long-acting insulin (^, one shot of glargine or two shots of detemir) to provide basal insulin coverage and three shots of glulisine, lispro, or insulin aspart to provide glycemic coverage for each meal. **B.** The injection of two shots of long-acting insulin (^, NPH or detemir) and short-acting insulin [glulisine, lispro, insulin aspart (solid red line), or regular (green dashed line)]. Only one formulation of short-acting insulin is used. **C.** Insulin administration by insulin infusion device is shown with the basal insulin and a bolus injection at each meal. The basal insulin rate is decreased during the evening and increased slightly prior to the patient awakening in the morning. Glulisine, lispro, or insulin aspart is used in the insulin pump. [*Adapted from H Lebovitz (ed): Therapy for Diabetes Mellitus. American Diabetes Association, Alexandria, VA, 2004.*]

ma glucose measurements. In general, individuals with type 1 DM require 0.5–1.0 U/kg per day of insulin divided into multiple doses, with ~50% of the insulin given as basal insulin.

Multiple-component insulin regimens refer to the combination of basal insulin and bolus insulin (preprandial short-acting insulin). The timing and dose of short-acting, preprandial insulin are altered to accommodate the SMBG results, anticipated food intake, and physical activity. Such regimens offer the patient with type 1 diabetes more flexibility in terms of lifestyle and the best chance for achieving near normoglycemia. One such regimen, shown in Fig. 338-13*B*, consists of basal insulin with glargine or detemir and preprandial lispro, glulisine, or insulin aspart. The insulin aspart, glulisine, or lispro dose is based on individualized algorithms that integrate the preprandial glucose and the anticipated carbohydrate intake. To determine the meal component of the preprandial insulin dose, the patient uses an insulin:carbohydrate ratio (a common ratio is 1–1.5 units/10 g of carbohydrate, but this must be determined for each individual). To this insulin dose is added the supplemental or correcting insulin based on the preprandial blood glucose [one formula uses 1 unit of insulin for every 2.7 mmol/L (50 mg/dL) over the preprandial glucose target; another formula uses (body weight in kg) × (blood glucose – desired glucose in mg/dL)/1500]. An alternative multiple-component insulin regimen consists of bedtime NPH insulin, a small dose of NPH insulin at breakfast (20–30% of bedtime dose), and preprandial short-acting insulin. Other variations of this regimen are in use but have the disadvantage that NPH has a significant peak, making hypoglycemia more common. Frequent SMBG (>3 times per day) is absolutely essential for all types of insulin regimens.

One commonly used regimen consists of twice-daily injections of a long-acting insulin like NPH (detemir could be used instead) mixed with a short-acting insulin before the morning and evening meal (Fig. 338-13*A*). Such regimens usually prescribe two-thirds of the total daily insulin dose in the morning (with about two-thirds given as long-acting insulin and one-third as short-acting) and one-third before the evening meal (with approximately one-half given as long-acting insulin and one-half as short-acting). The drawback to such a regimen is that it enforces a rigid schedule on the patient, in terms of daily activity and the content and timing of meals. Although it is simple and effective at avoiding severe hyperglycemia, it does not generate near-normal glycemic control in most individuals with type 1 DM. Moreover, if the patient's meal pattern or content varies or if physical activity is increased, hyperglycemia or hypoglycemia may result. Moving the long-acting insulin from before the evening meal to bedtime may avoid nocturnal hypoglycemia and provide more insulin as glucose levels rise in the early morning (so-called dawn phenomenon). The insulin dose in such regimens should be adjusted based on SMBG results with the following general assumptions: (1) the fasting glucose is primarily determined by the prior evening long-acting insulin; (2) the pre-lunch glucose is a function of the morning short-acting insulin; (3) the pre-supper glucose is a function of the morning long-acting insulin; and (4) the bedtime glucose is a function of the pre-supper, short-acting insulin. This is not an optimal regimen for the patient with type 1 DM, but is sometimes used for patients with type 2 diabetes.

Continuous subcutaneous insulin infusion (CSII) is a very effective insulin regimen for the patient with type 1 diabetes (Fig. 338-13*C*). To the basal insulin infusion, a preprandial insulin ("bolus") is delivered by the insulin infusion device based on instructions from the patient, who uses an individualized algorithm incorporating the preprandial plasma glucose and anticipated carbohydrate intake (see above). These sophisticated insulin infusion devices can accurately deliver small doses of insulin (microliters per hour) and have several advantages: (1) multiple basal infusion rates can be programmed to accommodate nocturnal versus daytime basal insulin requirement, (2) basal infusion rates can be altered during periods of exercise, (3) different waveforms of insulin infusion with meal-related bolus allow better matching of insulin depending on meal composition, and (4) programmed algorithms consider prior insulin administration and blood glucose values in calculating the insulin dose. These devices require a health professional with considerable experience with insulin infusion devices and very frequent patient interactions with the diabetes management team. Insulin infusion devices present unique challenges, such as infection at the infusion site, unexplained hyperglycemia because the infusion set becomes obstructed, or diabetic ketoacidosis if the pump becomes disconnected. Since most physicians use lispro, glulisine, or insulin aspart in CSII, the extremely short half-life of these insulins quickly lead to insulin deficiency if the delivery system is interrupted. Essential to the safe use of infusion devices is thorough patient education about pump function and frequent SMBG. Efforts to create a closed loop system in which data from continuous glucose measurement regulates the insulin infusion rate continue.

Other Agents That Improve Glucose Control The role of amylin, a 37-amino-acid peptide cosecreted with insulin from pancreatic beta cells, in normal glucose homeostasis is uncertain. However, based on the rationale that patients who are insulin deficient are also amylin deficient, an analogue of amylin (pramlintide) was created and found to reduce postprandial glycemic excursions in type 1 and type 2 diabetic patients taking insulin. Pramlintide injected just before a meal slows gastric emptying and suppresses glucagon but does not alter insulin levels. Pramlintide is approved for insulin-treated patients with type 1 and type 2 DM. Addition of pramlintide produces a modest reduction in the A1C and seems to dampen meal-related glucose excursions. In type 1 diabetes, pramlintide is started as a 15-µg SC injection before each meal and titrated up to a maximum of 30–60 µg as tolerated. In type 2 DM, pramlintide is started as a 60-µg SC injection before each meal and may be titrated up to a maximum of 120 µg. The major side effects are nausea and vomiting, and dose escalations should be slow to limit these side effects. Because pramlintide slows gastric emptying, it may influence absorption of other medications and should not be used in combination with other drugs that slow GI motility. The short-acting insulin given before the meal should initially be reduced to avoid hypoglycemia and then titrated as the effects of the pramlintide

FIGURE 338-14 Essential elements in comprehensive diabetes care of type 2 diabetes.

become evident. α-Glucosidase inhibitors are another type of agent that may be used in patients with type 1 DM (see below).

TYPE 2 DIABETES MELLITUS **General Aspects** The goals of therapy for type 2 DM are similar to those in type 1. While glycemic control tends to dominate the management of type 1 DM, the care of individuals with type 2 DM must also include attention to the treatment of conditions associated with type 2 DM (obesity, hypertension, dyslipidemia, cardiovascular disease) and detection/management of DM-related complications **(Fig. 338-14)**. DM-specific complications may be present in up to 20–50% of individuals with newly diagnosed type 2 DM. Reduction in cardiovascu-

lar risk is of paramount importance as this is the leading cause of mortality in these individuals. Efforts to achieve blood pressure and lipid goals (Table 338-8) should begin in concert with glucose-lowering interventions.

Type 2 diabetes management should begin with MNT (discussed above). An exercise regimen to increase insulin sensitivity and promote weight loss should also be instituted. Pharmacologic approaches to the management of type 2 DM include oral glucose-lowering agents, insulin, and other agents that improve glucose control; most physicians and patients prefer oral glucose-lowering agents as the initial choice (discussed below after review of various medications). Any therapy that improves glycemic control reduces "glucose toxicity" to the islet cells and improves endogenous insulin secretion. However, type 2 DM is a progressive disorder and ultimately requires multiple therapeutic agents and often insulin.

Glucose-Lowering Agents Advances in the therapy of type 2 DM have generated considerable enthusiasm for oral glucose-lowering agents that target different pathophysiologic processes in type 2 DM. Based on their mechanisms of action, glucose-lowering agents are subdivided into agents that increase insulin secretion, reduce glucose production, increase insulin sensitivity, and enhance GLP-1 action **(Table 338-11)**. Glucose-lowering agents (with the exception of α-glucosidase inhibitors and an amylin analogue) are ineffective in type 1 DM and should not be used for glucose management of severely ill individuals with type 2 DM. Insulin is sometimes the initial glucose-lowering agent.

Insulin Secretagogues Insulin secretagogues stimulate insulin secretion by interacting with the ATP-sensitive potassium channel on the beta cell (Fig. 338-4). These drugs are most effective in individuals with type 2 DM of relatively recent onset (<5 years), who have residual endogenous insulin production. At maximum doses, first-generation sulfonylureas are similar in potency to second-generation agents but have a longer half-life,

TABLE 383-11 GLUCOSE-LOWERING THERAPIES FOR TYPE 2 DIABETES

	Mechanism of Action	Examples	A1C Reduction (%)[a]	Agent-Specific Advantages	Agent-Specific Disadvantages	Contraindications/ Relative Contraindications
Oral						
Biguanides	↓ Hepatic glucose production, weight loss, glucose, utilization, insulin resistance	Metformin	1–2	Weight loss	Lactic acidosis, diarrhea, nausea	Serum creatinine >1.5 mg/dL (men) >1.4 mg/dL (women), CHF, radiographic contrast studies, seriously ill patients, acidosis
α–Glucosidase inhibitors	↓ Glucose absorption	Acarbose, Miglitol	0.5–0.8	Reduce postprandial glycemia	GI flatulence, liver function tests	Renal/liver disease
Dipeptidyl peptidase IV inhibitors	Prolong endogenous GLP-1 action	Sitagliptin	0.5–1.0	Does not cause hypoglycemia		Reduce dose with renal disease
Insulin secretagogues—sulfonylureas	↑ Insulin secretion	Table 338-12	1–2	Lower fasting blood glucose	Hypoglycemia, weight gain	Renal/liver disease
Insulin secretagogues—non-sulfonylureas	↑ Insulin secretion	Table 338-12	1–2	Short onset of action, lowers postprandial glucose	Hypoglycemia	Renal/liver disease
Thiazolidinediones	↓ Insulin resistance, ↑ glucose utilization	Rosiglitazone, Pioglitazone	0.5–1.4	Lower insulin requirements	Peripheral edema, CHF, weight gain, fractures, macular edema; rosiglitazone may increase risk of MI	Congestive heart failure, liver disease
Parenteral						
Insulin	↑ Glucose utilization and other anabolic actions	Table 323-11	No limit	Known safety profile	Injection, weight gain, hypoglycemia	
GLP-1 agonist	↑ Insulin, ↓ Glucagon, slow gastric emptying	Exenatide	0.5–1.0	Weight loss	Injection, nausea, ↑ risk of hypoglycemia with insulin secretagogues	Renal disease, agents that also slow GI motility
Amylin agonist[b]	Slow gastric emptying, ↓ Glucagon	Pramlintide	0.25–0.5	Reduce postprandial glycemia, weight loss	Injection, nausea, ↑ risk of hypoglycemia with insulin	Agents that also slow GI motility
Medical nutrition therapy and physical activity	↓ Insulin, resistance, ↑ insulin secretion	Low-calorie, low-fat diet, exercise	1–2	Other health benefits	Compliance difficult, long-term success low	

[a]A1C reduction depends partly on starting A1C.
[b]Amylin agonist is approved for use in type 1 and type 2 diabetes.

TABLE 338-12 CHARACTERISTICS OF ORAL AGENTS THAT INCREASE INSULIN SECRETION

Generic Name	Approved Daily Dosage Range, mg	Duration of Action, h
Sulfonylurea—first generation		
Chlorpropamide	100–500	>48
Tolazamide	100–1000	12–24
Tolbutamide	500–3000	6–12
Sulfonylurea—second generation		
Glimepiride	1–8	24
Glipizide	2.5–40	12–18
Glipizide (extended release)	5–10	24
Glyburide	1.25–20	12–24
Glyburide (micronized)	0.75–12	12–24
Nonsulfonylureas		
Repaglinide	0.5–16	2–6
Nateglinide	180–360	2–4

Source: Adapted from BR Zimmerman (ed): *Medical Management of Type 2 Diabetes,* 4th ed. American Diabetes Association, Alexandria, VA, 1998.

a greater incidence of hypoglycemia, and more frequent drug interactions **(Table 338-12).** Thus, second-generation sulfonylureas are generally preferred. An advantage to a more rapid onset of action is better coverage of the postprandial glucose rise, but the shorter half-life of such agents requires more than once-a-day dosing. Sulfonylureas reduce both fasting and postprandial glucose and should be initiated at low doses and increased at 1- to 2-week intervals based on SMBG. In general, sulfonylureas increase insulin acutely and thus should be taken shortly before a meal; with chronic therapy, though, the insulin release is more sustained. Glimepiride and glipizide can be given in a single daily dose and are preferred over glyburide. Repaglinide and nateglinide are not sulfonylureas but also interact with the ATP-sensitive potassium channel. Because of their short half-life, these agents are given with each meal or immediately before to reduce meal-related glucose excursions.

Insulin secretagogues are generally well tolerated. All of these agents, however, have the potential to cause profound and persistent hypoglycemia, especially in elderly individuals. Hypoglycemia is usually related to delayed meals, increased physical activity, alcohol intake, or renal insufficiency. Individuals who ingest an overdose of some agents develop prolonged and serious hypoglycemia and should be monitored closely in the hospital (Chap. 339). Most sulfonylureas are metabolized in the liver to compounds (some of which are active) that are cleared by the kidney. Thus, their use in individuals with significant hepatic or renal dysfunction is not advisable. Weight gain, a common side effect of sulfonylurea therapy, results from the increased insulin levels and improvement in glycemic control. Some sulfonylureas have significant drug interactions with alcohol and some medications including warfarin, aspirin, ketoconazole, α-glucosidase inhibitors, and fluconazole. A related isoform of ATP-sensitive potassium channels is present in the myocardium and the brain. All of these agents except glyburide have a low affinity for this isoform. Despite concerns that this agent might affect the myocardial response to ischemia and observational studies suggesting that sulfonylureas increase cardiovascular risk, the UKPDS did not show an increased cardiac mortality with glyburide.

Biguanides Metformin is representative of this class of agents. It reduces hepatic glucose production through an undefined mechanism and improves peripheral glucose utilization slightly (Table 338-11). Metformin reduces fasting plasma glucose and insulin levels, improves the lipid profile, and promotes modest weight loss. The initial starting dose of 500 mg once or twice a day can be increased to 1000 mg bid. An extended-release form is available and may have fewer gastrointestinal side effects (diarrhea, anorexia, nausea, metallic taste). Because of its relatively slow onset of action and gastrointestinal symptoms with higher doses, the dose should be escalated every 2–3 weeks based on SMBG measurements. The major toxicity of metformin, lactic acidosis, can be prevented by careful patient selection. Metformin should not be used in patients with renal insufficiency [serum creatinine > 133 μmol/L (1.5 mg/dL) in men or > 124 μmol/L (1.4 mg/dL) in women, with adjustments for age], any form of acidosis, CHF, liver disease, or severe hypoxia. Metformin should be discontinued in patients who are seriously ill, in patients who can take nothing orally, and in

those receiving radiographic contrast material. Insulin should be used until metformin can be restarted.

α-Glucosidase Inhibitors α-Glucosidase inhibitors (acarbose and miglitol) reduce postprandial hyperglycemia by delaying glucose absorption; they do not affect glucose utilization or insulin secretion (Table 338-11). Postprandial hyperglycemia, secondary to impaired hepatic and peripheral glucose disposal, contributes significantly to the hyperglycemic state in type 2 DM. These drugs, taken just before each meal, reduce glucose absorption by inhibiting the enzyme that cleaves oligosaccharides into simple sugars in the intestinal lumen. Therapy should be initiated at a low dose (25 mg of acarbose or miglitol) with the evening meal and may be increased to a maximal dose over weeks to months (50–100 mg for acarbose or 50 mg for miglitol with each meal). The major side effects (diarrhea, flatulence, abdominal distention) are related to increased delivery of oligosaccharides to the large bowel and can be reduced somewhat by gradual upward dose titration. α-Glucosidase inhibitors may increase levels of sulfonylureas and increase the incidence of hypoglycemia. Simultaneous treatment with bile acid resins and antacids should be avoided. These agents should not be used in individuals with inflammatory bowel disease, gastroparesis, or a serum creatinine >177 μmol/L (2.0 mg/dL). This class of agents is not as potent as other oral agents in lowering the hemoglobin A1C but is unique because it reduces the postprandial glucose rise even in individuals with type 1 DM. If hypoglycemia from other diabetes treatments occurs while taking these agents, the patient should consume glucose since the degradation and absorption of complex carbohydrates will be retarded.

Thiazolidinediones Thiazolidinediones reduce insulin resistance. These drugs bind to the PPAR-γ (peroxisome proliferator-activated receptor-γ) nuclear receptor. The PPAR-γ receptor is found at highest levels in adipocytes but is expressed at lower levels in many other tissues. Agonists of this receptor regulate a large number of genes, promote adipocyte differentiation, reduce hepatic fat accumulation, and appear to reduce insulin resistance indirectly by enhancing fatty acid storage and possibly by increasing adiponectin levels (Table 338-11). Thiazolidinediones promote a redistribution of fat from central to peripheral locations. Circulating insulin levels decrease with use of the thiazolidinediones, indicating a reduction in insulin resistance. Although direct comparisons are not available, the two currently available thiazolidinediones appear to have similar efficacy; the therapeutic range for pioglitazone is 15–45 mg/d in a single daily dose, and for rosiglitazone the total daily dose is 2–8 mg/d administered either once daily or twice daily in divided doses. The ability of thiazolidinediones to influence cardiovascular disease or other features of the metabolic syndrome is under investigation.

The prototype of this class of drugs, troglitazone, was withdrawn from the U.S. market after reports of hepatotoxicity and an association with an idiosyncratic liver reaction that sometimes led to hepatic failure. Although rosiglitazone and pioglitazone do not appear to induce the liver abnormalities seen with troglitazone, the FDA recommends measurement of liver function tests prior to initiating therapy with a thiazolidinedione and at regular intervals (every 2 months for the first year and then periodically). Rosiglitazone raises LDL, HDL, and triglycerides slightly. Pioglitazone raises HDL to a greater degree and LDL a lesser degree but lowers triglycerides. The clinical significance of the lipid changes with these agents is not known and may be difficult to ascertain since most patients with type 2 diabetes are also treated with a statin. Emphasis should be placed on reaching lipid, blood pressure, and glycemic targets rather than the type of therapy needed to reach those goals. Thiazolidinediones are associated with weight gain (2–3 kg), a small reduction in the hematocrit, and a mild increase in plasma volume. Peripheral edema and CHF may occur and is more common in individuals also treated with insulin. These agents are contraindicated in patients with liver disease or CHF (class III or IV). Recent metanalyses have suggested that rosiglitazone is associated with an increased risk of myocardial infarction. The FDA has issued an alert that rare patients taking these agents may experience a worsening of diabetic macular edema. An increased risk of fractures has been noted in women taking these agents. Thiazolidinediones have been shown to induce ovulation in premenopausal women with PCOS. Women should be warned about the risk of pregnancy, since the safety of thiazolidinediones in pregnancy is not established.

Insulin Therapy in Type 2 DM Insulin should be considered as the initial therapy in type 2 DM, particularly in lean individuals or those with severe weight loss, in individuals with underlying renal or hepatic disease that precludes oral glucose-lowering agents, or in individuals who are hospitalized or acutely ill. Insulin therapy is ultimately required by a substantial number of individuals with type 2 DM because of the progressive nature of the disorder and the relative insulin deficiency that develops in patients with long-standing diabetes. Both physician and patient reluctance often delay the initiation of insulin therapy, but glucose control and patient well-being are improved by insulin therapy in patients who have not reached the glycemic target.

Because endogenous insulin secretion continues and is capable of providing some coverage of mealtime caloric intake, insulin is usually initiated in a single dose of long-acting insulin (0.3–0.4 U/kg per day), given either before breakfast and in the evening (NPH) or just before bedtime (NPH, glargine, detemir). Since fasting hyperglycemia and increased hepatic glucose production are prominent features of type 2 DM, bedtime insulin is more effective in clinical trials than a single dose of morning insulin. Glargine given at bedtime has less nocturnal hypoglycemia than NPH insulin. Some physicians prefer a relatively low, fixed starting dose of intermediate-acting insulin (15–20 units in the morning and 5–10 units at bedtime) to avoid hypoglycemia. The insulin dose may then be adjusted in 10% increments as dictated by SMBG results. Both morning and bedtime long-acting insulin may be used in combination with oral glucose-lowering agents (biguanides, α-glucosidase inhibitors, or thiazolidinediones). The combination of insulin and a thiazolidinedione promotes weight gain and edema and is a less desirable combination. Initially, basal insulin may be sufficient, but often prandial insulin coverage is needed as diabetes progresses. Other insulin formulations that have a combination of short-acting and long-acting insulin (Table 338-10) are sometimes used in patients with type 2 DM because of convenience but do not allow independent adjustment of short-acting and long-acting insulin dose. In selected patients with type 2 DM (usually insulin deficient as defined by C-peptide level), insulin infusion devices may be considered.

Agents That Enhance GLP-1 Receptor Signaling   "Incretins" amplify glucose-stimulated insulin secretion. Agents that either act as a GLP-1 agonist or enhance endogenous GLP-1 activity have become available and are under development. Exenatide, a synthetic version of a peptide originally found in the saliva of the Gila monster (exendin-4), is an analogue of GLP-1. Unlike native GLP-1 which has a half-life of <5 min, differences in the exenatide amino acid sequence render it resistant to the enzyme that degrades GLP-1 (dipeptidyl peptidase IV, or DPP-IV). Thus, exenatide has prolonged GLP-1-like action by binding to GLP-1 receptors found in islets, the gastrointestinal tract, and the brain. Exenatide increases glucose-stimulated insulin secretion, suppresses glucagon, and slows gastric emptying. Exenatide does not promote weight gain; in fact, most patients experience modest weight loss. It appears that GLP-1 agonists also suppress appetite. Exenatide, approved for combination with other oral agents for type 2 DM, should be started as a 5-μg SC injection before the morning and evening meal and increased to 10 μg twice daily, depending on the response and side effects (nausea being the limiting factor). The A1C reductions with exenatide are modest compared to those with some oral agents. Exenatide is approved only for use as adjunct or combination therapy with metformin or sulfonylureas; studies of its efficacy in combination with other oral agents are underway. Exenatide should not be used in patients taking insulin. The major side effects are nausea, vomiting, and diarrhea; some patients taking insulin secretagogues may require a reduction in those agents to prevent hypoglycemia. Because it slows gastric emptying and may influence the absorption of other drugs, the timing of administration should be coordinated. Whether exenatide enhances beta cell survival, promotes beta cell proliferation, or alters the natural history of type 2 DM is not known. Other GLP-1 receptor agonists and formulations are under development. DPP-IV inhibitors represent a new class of oral agents that inhibit degradation of native GLP-1 and thus enhance incretin effect. These agents promote insulin secretion in the absence of hypoglycemia or weight gain, and appear to have a preferential effect on postprandial blood glucose. The FDA has approved the first DPP-IV inhibitor, sitagliptin, for use with diet and exercise to improve glycemic control in adult individuals with type 2 DM. It can also be used in combination with metformin or a thiazolidinedione. Sitagliptin is administered at a dose of 100 mg orally once daily. Reduced doses should be given to patients with moderate (creatinine clearance 30–50 mL/min, 50 mg once daily) or severe (creatinine clearance < 30 mL/min, 25 mg once daily) renal insufficiency. Renal function should be assessed prior to initiation of

sitagliptin therapy and periodically thereafter. Clinical experience with this agent is limited.

Choice of Initial Glucose-Lowering Agent   The level of hyperglycemia should influence the initial choice of therapy. Assuming maximal benefit of MNT and increased physical activity has been realized, patients with mild to moderate hyperglycemia [FPG < 11.1–13.9 mmol/L (200–250 mg/dL)] often respond well to a single, oral glucose-lowering agent. Patients with more severe hyperglycemia [FPG > 13.9 mmol/L (250 mg/dL)] may respond partially but are unlikely to achieve normoglycemia with oral monotherapy. A stepwise approach that starts with a single agent and adds a second agent to achieve the glycemic target can be used (see "Combination Therapy," below). Insulin can be used as initial therapy in individuals with severe hyperglycemia [FPG > 13.9–16.7 mmol/L (250–300 mg/dL)] or in those who are symptomatic from the hyperglycemia. This approach is based on the rationale that more rapid glycemic control will reduce "glucose toxicity" to the islet cells, improve endogenous insulin secretion, and possibly allow oral glucose-lowering agents to be more effective. If this occurs, the insulin may be discontinued.

Insulin secretagogues, biguanides, α-glucosidase inhibitors, thiazolidinediones, and insulin are approved for monotherapy of type 2 DM. Although each class of oral glucose-lowering agents has unique advantages and disadvantages, certain generalizations apply: (1) insulin secretagogues, biguanides, DPP-IV inhibitors, and thiazolidinediones improve glycemic control to a similar degree (1–2% reduction in A1C) and are more effective than α-glucosidase inhibitors; (2) assuming a similar degree of glycemic improvement, no clinical advantage to one class of drugs has been demonstrated, and any therapy that improves glycemic control is likely beneficial; (3) insulin secretagogues and α-glucosidase inhibitors begin to lower the plasma glucose immediately, whereas the glucose-lowering effects of the biguanides and thiazolidinediones are delayed by several weeks to months; (4) not all agents are effective in all individuals with type 2 DM (primary failure); (5) biguanides, α-glucosidase inhibitors, DPP-IV inhibitors, and thiazolidinediones do not directly cause hypoglycemia; and (6) most individuals will eventually require treatment with more than one class of oral glucose-lowering agents or insulin, reflecting the progressive nature of type 2 DM.

Considerable clinical experience exists with metformin and sulfonylureas because they have been available for several decades. It is assumed that the α-glucosidase inhibitors, DPP-IV inhibitors, and thiazolidinediones, which are newer classes of oral glucose-lowering drugs, will reduce DM-related complications by improving glycemic control, although long-term data are not yet available. The thiazolidinediones are theoretically attractive because they target a fundamental abnormality in type 2 DM, namely insulin resistance. However, all of these agents are currently more costly than metformin and sulfonylureas.

A reasonable treatment algorithm for initial therapy uses metformin as initial therapy because of its efficacy, known side-effect profile, and relatively low cost **(Fig. 338-15)**. Metformin has the advantage that it promotes mild weight loss, lowers insulin levels, and improves the lipid profile slightly. Based on SMBG results and the A1C, the dose of metformin should be increased until the glycemic target is achieved or maximum dose is reached.

Approximately one-third of individuals will reach their target glycemic goal using metformin as monotherapy.

Combination Therapy with Glucose-Lowering Agents   A number of combinations of therapeutic agents are successful in type 2 DM, and the dosing of agents in combination is the same as when the agents are used alone. Because mechanisms of action of the first and second agents are different, the effect on glycemic control is usually additive. Several fixed dose combinations of oral agents are available, but evidence that they are superior to titration of single agent to a maximum dose and then addition of a second agent is lacking. If adequate control is not achieved with the combination of two agents (based on reassessment of the A1C every 3 months), a third oral agent or basal insulin should be added (Fig. 338-15).

Treatment with insulin becomes necessary as type 2 DM enters the phase of relative insulin deficiency (as seen in long-standing DM) and is signaled by inadequate glycemic control with one or two oral glucose-lowering agents. Insulin alone or in combination should be used in patients who fail to reach the glycemic target. For example, a single dose of long-acting insulin at bedtime is effective in combination with metformin. As endogenous insulin production falls further, multiple injections of long-acting and short-acting insulin regimens are necessary to control postprandial glucose excursions. These insulin regimens are identical to the long-acting and short-acting combination regimens discussed above for type 1 DM. Since the hyperglycemia of type 2 DM tends to be more "stable," these regimens can be increased in 10% increments every 2–3 days using the fasting blood glucose results. The daily insulin dose required can become quite large (1–2 units/kg per day) as endogenous insulin production falls and insulin resistance persists. Individuals who require >1 unit/kg per day of long-acting insulin should be considered for combination therapy with metformin or a thiazolidinedione. The addition of metformin or a thiazolidinedione can reduce insulin requirements in some individuals with type 2 DM, while maintaining or even improving glycemic control. Insulin plus a thiazolidinedione promotes weight gain and is associated with peripheral edema. Addition of a thiazolidinedione to a patient's insulin regimen may necessitate a reduction in the insulin dose to avoid hypoglycemia.

EMERGING THERAPIES Whole pancreas transplantation (performed concomitantly with a renal transplant) may normalize glucose tolerance and is an important therapeutic option in type 1 DM, though it requires substantial expertise and is associated with the side effects of immunosuppression. Pancreatic islet transplantation has been plagued by limitations in pancreatic islet isolation and graft survival and remains an area of clinical investigation. Many individuals with long-standing type 1 DM still produce very small amounts of insulin or have insulin-positive cells within the pancreas. This suggests that beta cells are slowly regenerating but are quickly destroyed by the autoimmune process. Thus, efforts to suppress the autoimmune process and to stimulate beta cell regeneration are underway both at the time of diagnosis and in years after the diagnosis of type 1 DM. Closed-loop pumps that infuse the appropriate amount of insulin in response to changing glucose levels are potentially feasible now that continuous glucose-monitoring technology has been developed.

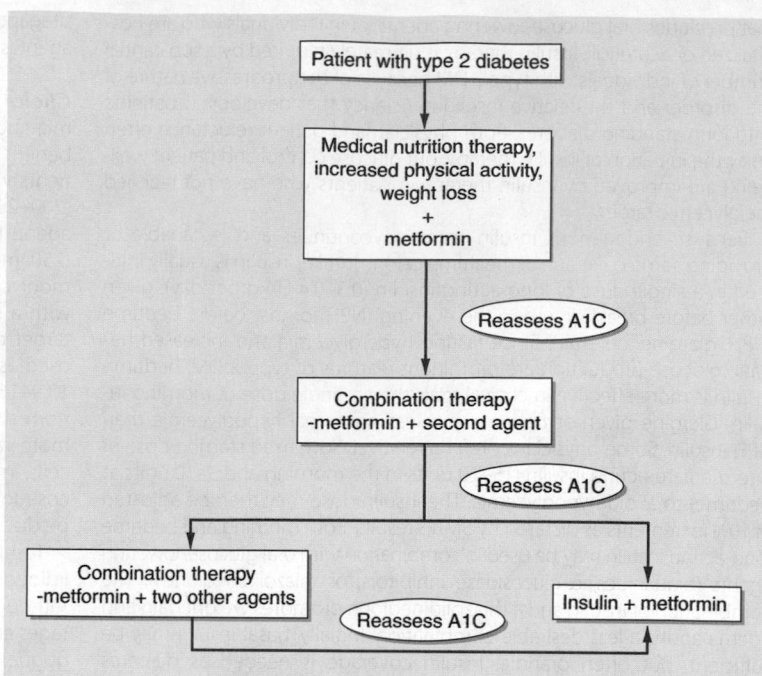

FIGURE 338-15 Glycemic management of type 2 diabetes. See text for discussion of treatment of severe hyperglycemia or symptomatic hyperglycemia. Agents that can be combined with metformin include insulin secretagogues, thiazolidinediones, α-glucosidase inhibitors, DPP-IV inhibitors, and exenatide. A1C, hemoglobin A1C.

COMPLICATIONS OF THERAPY FOR DIABETES MELLITUS

As with any therapy, the benefits of efforts directed towards glycemic control must be weighed against the risks of treatment. Side effects of intensive treatment include an increased frequency of serious hypoglycemia, weight gain, increased economic costs, and greater demands on the patient. In the DCCT, quality of life was very similar in the intensive and standard therapy groups. The most serious complication of therapy for DM is hypoglycemia, and its treatment with oral glucose or glucagon injection is discussed in Chap. 339. Severe, recurrent hypoglycemia warrants examination of treatment regimen and glycemic goal for the individual patient. Weight gain occurs with most (insulin, insulin secretagogues, thiazolidinediones) but not all (metformin, α-glucosidase inhibitors, exenatide) therapies that improve glycemic control. It is partially due to the anabolic effects of insulin and the reduction in glucosuria. In the DCCT, individuals with the greatest weight gain exhibited increases in LDL cholesterol and triglycerides as well as increases in blood pressure (both systolic and diastolic) similar to those seen in individuals with type 2 DM and insulin resistance. These effects could increase the risk of cardiovascular disease. As discussed previously, transient worsening of diabetic retinopathy or neuropathy sometimes accompanies improved glycemic control.

ONGOING ASPECTS OF COMPREHENSIVE DIABETES CARE

The morbidity and mortality of DM-related complications can be greatly reduced by timely and consistent surveillance procedures (Table 338-13). These screening procedures are indicated for all individuals with DM, but numerous studies have documented that most individuals with diabetes do not receive comprehensive diabetes care. Screening for dyslipidemia and hypertension should be performed annually. In addition to routine health maintenance, individuals with diabetes should also receive the pneumococcal and tetanus vaccines (at recommended intervals) and the influenza vaccine (annually). As discussed above, aspirin therapy should be considered in many patients with diabetes.

An annual comprehensive eye examination should be performed by a qualified optometrist or ophthalmologist. If abnormalities are detected, further evaluation and treatment require an ophthalmologist skilled in diabetes-related eye disease. Because many individuals with type 2 DM have had asymptomatic diabetes for several years before diagnosis, the ADA recommends the following ophthalmologic examination schedule: (1) individuals with type 1 DM should have an initial eye examination within 3–5 years of diagnosis, (2) individuals with type 2 DM should have an initial eye examination at the time of diabetes diagnosis, (3) women with DM who are pregnant or contemplating pregnancy should have an eye examination prior to conception and during the first trimester, and (4) individuals whose eye examination is normal can have a repeat examination in 2–3 years rather than annually.

An annual foot examination should: (1) assess blood flow, sensation (monofilament testing, pin prick, or tuning fork), ankle reflexes, and nail care; (2) look for the presence of foot deformities such as hammer or claw toes and Charcot foot; and (3) identify sites of poten-

TABLE 338-13	GUIDELINES FOR ONGOING MEDICAL CARE FOR PATIENTS WITH DIABETES

- Self-monitoring of blood glucose (individualized frequency)
- A1C testing (2–4 times/year)
- Patient education in diabetes management (annual)
- Medical nutrition therapy and education (annual)
- Eye examination (annual)
- Foot examination (1–2 times/year by physician; daily by patient)
- Screening for diabetic nephropathy (annual; see Fig. 338-11)
- Blood pressure measurement (quarterly)
- Lipid profile and serum creatinine (estimate GFR) (annual)
- Influenza/pneumococcal immunizations
- Consider antiplatelet therapy (see text)

Note: A1C, hemoglobin A1C.

tial ulceration. Calluses and nail deformities should be treated by a podiatrist; the patient should be discouraged from self-care of even minor foot problems, but should be strongly encouraged to check his/her feet daily for any early lesions. The ADA advises a visual foot inspection in patients with symptoms or signs of diabetic neuropathy at 3- or 6-month intervals.

An annual microalbuminuria measurement (albumin-to-creatinine ratio in spot urine) is advised in individuals with type 1 or type 2 DM and no protein on a routine urinalysis (Fig. 338-10). If the urinalysis detects proteinuria, the amount of protein should be quantified by standard urine protein measurements. If the urinalysis was negative for protein in the past, microalbuminuria should be the annual screening examination. Routine urine protein measurements do not detect low levels of albumin excretion. Screening should commence 5 years after the onset of type 1 DM and at the time of diagnosis of type 2 DM. Regardless of protein excretion results, the GFR should be estimated using the serum creatinine in all patients on an annual basis.

SPECIAL CONSIDERATIONS IN DIABETES MELLITUS

PSYCHOSOCIAL ASPECTS

As with any chronic, debilitating disease, the individual with DM faces a series of challenges that affect all aspects of daily life. The individual with DM must accept that he or she may develop complications related to DM. Even with considerable effort, normoglycemia can be an elusive goal, and solutions to worsening glycemic control may not be easily identifiable. The patient should view him- or herself as an essential member of the diabetes care team and not as someone who is cared for by the diabetes team. Emotional stress may provoke a change in behavior so that individuals no longer adhere to a dietary, exercise, or therapeutic regimen. This can lead to the appearance of either hyper- or hypoglycemia. Eating disorders, including binge eating disorders, bulimia, and anorexia nervosa, appear to occur more frequently individuals with type 1 or type 2 DM (Chap. 76).

MANAGEMENT IN THE HOSPITALIZED PATIENT

Virtually all medical and surgical subspecialties are involved in the care of hospitalized patients with diabetes. Hyperglycemia, whether in a patient with known diabetes or in someone without known diabetes, appears to be a predictor of poor outcome in hospitalized patients. General anesthesia, surgery, infection, or concurrent illness raises the levels of counterregulatory hormones (cortisol, growth hormone, catecholamines, and glucagon) and cytokines that may lead to transient insulin resistance and hyperglycemia. These factors increase insulin requirements by increasing glucose production and impairing glucose utilization and thus may worsen glycemic control. The concurrent illness or surgical procedure may lead to variable insulin absorption and also prevent the patient with DM from eating normally and may promote hypoglycemia. Glycemic control should be assessed (with A1C) and, if feasible, should be optimized prior to surgery. Electrolytes, renal function, and intravascular volume status should be assessed as well. The high prevalence of cardiovascular disease in individuals with DM (especially in type 2 DM) may require preoperative cardiovascular evaluation.

Glycemic control appears to improve the clinical outcomes in a variety of settings. In fact, many patients who do not have preexisting diabetes but who develop modest blood glucose elevations during their hospitalization appear to benefit from achieving near-normoglycemia using insulin treatment. For example, maintenance of a near-normal glucose with a continuous insulin infusion reduced the risk of postoperative infection after CABG and reduced the morbidity and mortality in patients in a surgical intensive care unit. In a number of cross-sectional studies of patients with diabetes, a greater degree of hyperglycemia was associated with worse cardiac, neurologic, and infectious outcomes. The goals of diabetes management during hospitalization are near-normoglycemia, avoidance of hypoglycemia, and transition back to the outpatient diabetes treatment regimen. The ADA suggests

these glycemic goals for critically ill patients: ". . .as close to 6.1 mmol/L (110 mg/dL) and generally <10 mmol/L (180 mg/dL, postprandial)." In noncritically ill patients, the suggested glycemic goals are as close as possible to 5.0–7.2 mmol/L (90–130 mg/dL) preprandially and <10 mmol/L (180 mg/dL) postprandially. This process requires integrating information regarding the plasma glucose, diabetes treatment regimen, and clinical status of the patient.

The physician caring for an individual with diabetes in the perioperative period, during times of infection or serious physical illness, or simply when fasting for a diagnostic procedure must monitor the plasma glucose vigilantly, adjust the diabetes treatment regimen, and provide glucose infusion as needed. Depending on the severity of the patient's illness and the hospital setting, the physician can use either an insulin infusion or subcutaneous insulin. A "consistent carbohydrate diabetes meal plan" for hospitalized patients provides a predictable amount of carbohydrate for a particular meal each day (but not necessarily the same amount for breakfast, lunch, and supper). The hospital diet should be determined by a nutritionist; terms such as "ADA diet" or "low-sugar diet" are no longer used. Several different treatment regimens (IV or SC insulin regimens) can be employed successfully.

Insulin infusions can effectively control plasma glucose in the perioperative period and when the patient is unable to take anything by mouth. The absorption of subcutaneous insulin may be variable in such situations. Regular insulin is preferred over insulin analogues for IV insulin infusion since it is less expensive and equally effective. The physician must consider carefully the clinical setting in which an insulin infusion will be utilized, including whether adequate ancillary personnel are available to monitor the plasma glucose frequently and whether they can adjust the insulin infusion rate to maintain the plasma glucose within the optimal range.

Because of the short half-life of IV regular insulin, it is necessary to administer long-acting insulin prior to discontinuation of the insulin infusion to avoid a period of insulin deficiency. An alternative to an insulin infusion is basal or "scheduled" insulin provided by SC, long-acting insulin supplemented by prandial or "corrective" insulin using a short-acting insulin (insulin analogues preferred). The use of "sliding scale" insulin alone, where no insulin is given unless the blood glucose is elevated, is inadequate for in-patient glucose management and should not be used. The short-acting, pre-prandial insulin dose should include coverage for food consumption (based on anticipated carbohydrate intake) plus a corrective or supplemental insulin based on the patient's insulin sensitivity and the blood glucose. For example, if the patient is thin (and likely insulin sensitive), a corrective insulin supplement might be 1 unit for each 2.7 mmol/L (50 mg/dL) over the glucose target. If the patient is obese and insulin resistant, then the insulin supplement might be 2 units for each 2.7 mmol/L (50 mg/dL) over the glucose target. It is critical to individualize the regimen and adjust the basal or "scheduled" insulin dose frequently, based on the corrective insulin required.

Individuals with type 1 DM who are undergoing general anesthesia and surgery, or who are seriously ill, should receive continuous insulin, either through an IV insulin infusion or by SC administration of a reduced dose of long-acting insulin. Short-acting insulin alone is insufficient. Prolongation of a surgical procedure or delay in the recovery room is not uncommon and may result in periods of insulin deficiency leading to DKA. Insulin infusion is the preferred method for managing patients with type 1 DM in the perioperative period or when serious concurrent illness is present (0.5–1.0 units/h of regular insulin). Insulin-infusion algorithms jointly developed and implemented by nursing and physician staff are advised. If the diagnostic or surgical procedure is brief and performed under local or regional anesthesia, a reduced dose of SC, long-acting insulin may suffice (30–50% reduction, with short-acting insulin held or reduced). This approach facilitates the transition back to long-acting insulin after the procedure. Glucose may be infused to prevent hypoglycemia. The blood glucose should be monitored frequently during the illness or in the perioperative period.

Individuals with type 2 DM can be managed with either regular insulin infusion, or a reduced dose of SC long-acting insulin (25–50% reduction) plus preprandial, short-acting insulin. Oral glucose-lowering agents should be discontinued upon admission and are not useful in regulating the plasma glucose in clinical situations where the insulin requirements and glucose intake are changing rapidly. Moreover, these oral agents may be dangerous if the patient is fasting (e.g., hypoglycemia with sulfonylureas). Metformin should be withheld when radiographic contrast media will be given or if severe CHF, acidosis, or declining renal function is present.

Total Parenteral Nutrition (See also Chap. 73.) Total parenteral nutrition (TPN) greatly increases insulin requirements. In addition, individuals not previously known to have DM may become hyperglycemic during TPN and require insulin treatment. Intravenous insulin infusion is the preferred treatment for hyperglycemia, and rapid titration to the required insulin dose is done most efficiently using a separate insulin infusion. After the total insulin dose has been determined, insulin may be added directly to the TPN solution or, preferably, given as a separate infusion. Often, individuals receiving either TPN or enteral nutrition receive their caloric loads continuously and not at "meal times"; consequently, SC insulin regimens must be adjusted.

Glucocorticoids Glucocorticoids increase insulin resistance, decrease glucose utilization, increase hepatic glucose production, and impair insulin secretion. These changes lead to a worsening of glycemic control in individuals with DM and may precipitate diabetes in other individuals ("steroid-induced diabetes"). The effects of glucocorticoids on glucose homeostasis are dose-related, usually reversible, and most pronounced in the postprandial period. If the FPG is near the normal range, oral diabetes agents (e.g., sulfonylureas, metformin) may be sufficient to reduce hyperglycemia. If the FPG > 11.1 mmol/L (200 mg/dL), oral agents are usually not efficacious and insulin therapy is required. Short-acting insulin may be required to supplement long-acting insulin in order to control postprandial glucose excursions.

Reproductive Issues Reproductive capacity in either men or women with DM appears to be normal. Menstrual cycles may be associated with alterations in glycemic control in women with DM. Pregnancy is associated with marked insulin resistance; the increased insulin requirements often precipitate DM and lead to the diagnosis of GDM. Glucose, which at high levels is a teratogen to the developing fetus, readily crosses the placenta, but insulin does not. Thus, hyperglycemia from the maternal circulation may stimulate insulin secretion in the fetus. The anabolic and growth effects of insulin may result in macrosomia. GDM complicates ~4% of pregnancies in the United States. The incidence of GDM is greatly increased in certain ethnic groups, including African Americans and Latinos, consistent with a similar increased risk of type 2 DM. Current recommendations advise screening for glucose intolerance between weeks 24 and 28 of pregnancy in women with high risk for GDM (≥25 years; obesity; family history of DM; member of an ethnic group such as Latino, Native American, Asian American, African American, or Pacific Islander). Therapy for GDM is similar to that for individuals with pregnancy-associated diabetes and involves MNT and insulin, if hyperglycemia persists. Oral glucose-lowering agents have not been approved for use during pregnancy. With current practices, the morbidity and mortality of the mother with GDM and the fetus are not different from those in the nondiabetic population. Individuals who develop GDM are at marked increased risk for developing type 2 DM in the future and should be screened periodically for DM. Most individuals with GDM revert to normal glucose tolerance after delivery, but some will continue to have overt diabetes or impairment of glucose tolerance. In addition, children of women with GDM appear to be at risk for obesity and glucose intolerance and have an increased risk of diabetes beginning in the later stages of adolescence.

Pregnancy in individuals with known DM requires meticulous planning and adherence to strict treatment regimens. Intensive diabetes management and normalization of the A1C are essential for individuals with existing DM who are planning pregnancy. The most crucial period of glycemic control is soon after fertilization. The risk of fetal malformations is increased 4–10 times in individuals with uncontrolled DM at the time of conception, and normal plasma glucose during the preconception period and throughout the periods of organ development in the fetus should be the goal.

LIPODYSTROPHIC DM

Lipodystrophy, or the loss of subcutaneous fat tissue, may be generalized in certain genetic conditions such as leprechaunism. Generalized lipodystrophy is associated with severe insulin resistance and is often accompanied by acanthosis nigricans and dyslipidemia. Localized lipodystrophy associated with insulin injections has been reduced considerably by the use of human insulin.

Protease Inhibitors and Lipodystrophy Protease inhibitors used in the treatment of HIV disease (Chap. 182) have been associated with a centripetal accumulation of fat (visceral and abdominal area), accumulation of fat in the dorsocervical region, loss of extremity fat, decreased insulin sensitivity (elevations of the fasting insulin level and reduced glucose tolerance on IV glucose tolerance testing), and dyslipidemia. Although many aspects of the physical appearance of these individuals resemble Cushing's syndrome, increased cortisol levels do not account for this appearance. The possibility remains that this is related to HIV infection by some undefined mechanism, since some features of the syndrome were observed before the introduction of protease inhibitors. Therapy for HIV-related lipodystrophy is not well established.

FURTHER READINGS

AMERICAN DIABETES ASSOCIATION: Clinical practice recommendations 2007. Diabetes Care 30:S4, 2007

———: Nutrition recommendations and interventions for diabetes—2006. Diabetes Care 29:2140, 2006

BAX JJ et al: Screening for coronary artery disease in patients with diabetes. Diabetes Care 30:2729, 2007

BOLEN S et al: Systematic review: Comparative effectiveness and safety of oral medications for type 2 diabetes mellitus. Ann Intern Med 147:386, 2007

EISENBARTH GS: Update in type 1 diabetes. J Clin Endocrinol Metab 92:2403, 2007

GROSS JL et al: Diabetic nephropathy: Diagnosis, prevention, and treatment. Diabetes Care 28:164, 2005

INZUCCHI SE: Management of hyperglycemia in the hospital setting. N Engl J Med 355:1903, 2006

NATHAN DM et al: Intensive diabetes treatment and cardiovascular disease in patients with type 1 diabetes. N Engl J Med 353:2643, 2005

SAUDEK CD et al: Assessing glycemia in diabetes using self-monitoring blood glucose and hemoglobin A1c. JAMA 295:1688, 2006

STUMVOLL M et al: Type 2 diabetes: Principles of pathogenesis and therapy. Lancet 365:1333, 2005

VINIK A et al: Diabetic neuropathies: Clinical manifestations and current treatment options. Nat Clin Pract Endocrinol Metab 2:269, 2006

ZIMMET P et al: Global and societal implications of the diabetes epidemic. Nature 414:782, 2001

339 Hypoglycemia
Philip E. Cryer

Hypoglycemia is most commonly caused by drugs used to treat diabetes mellitus or by exposure to other drugs, including alcohol. However, a number of other disorders, including insulinoma, critical organ failure, sepsis and inanition, hormone deficiencies, non-β-cell tumors, inherited metabolic disorders, and prior gastric surgery, may cause hypoglycemia (Table 339-1). Hypoglycemia is most convincingly documented by *Whipple's triad:* (1) symptoms consistent with hypoglycemia, (2) a low plasma glucose concentration measured with a precise method (not a glucose monitor), and (3) relief of those symptoms after the plasma glucose level is raised. The lower limit of the fasting plasma glucose concentration is normally approximately 70 mg/dL (3.9 mmol/L), but substantially lower venous glucose levels occur normally, late after a meal. Glucose levels <55 mg/dL (3.0 mmol/L) with symptoms that are relieved promptly after the glucose level is raised document hypoglycemia. Hypoglycemia can cause serious morbidity; if severe and prolonged, it can be fatal. It should be considered in any patient with episodes of confusion, an altered level of consciousness, or a seizure.

SYSTEMIC GLUCOSE BALANCE AND GLUCOSE COUNTERREGULATION

Glucose is an obligate metabolic fuel for the brain under physiologic conditions. The brain cannot synthesize glucose or store more than a few minutes' supply as glycogen and therefore requires a continuous supply of glucose from the arterial circulation. As the arterial plasma glucose concentration falls below the physiologic range, blood-to-brain glucose transport becomes insufficient to support brain energy metabolism and function. However, redundant glucose counterregulatory mechanisms normally prevent or rapidly correct hypoglycemia.

Plasma glucose concentrations are normally maintained within a relatively narrow range, roughly 70–110 mg/dL (3.9–6.1 mmol/L) in the fasting state with transient higher excursions after a meal, despite wide variations in exogenous glucose delivery from meals and in endogenous glucose utilization by, for example, exercising muscle. Between meals and during fasting, plasma glucose levels are maintained by endogenous glucose production, hepatic glycogenolysis, and hepatic (and renal) gluconeogenesis (Fig. 339-1). Although hepatic glycogen stores are usually sufficient to maintain plasma glucose levels for approximately 8 h, this time period can be shorter if glucose demand is increased by exercise or if glycogen stores are depleted by illness or starvation.

Gluconeogenesis requires a coordinated supply of precursors from muscle and adipose tissue to the liver (and kidneys). Muscle provides lactate, pyruvate, alanine, glutamine, and other amino acids. Triglycerides in adipose tissue are broken down into fatty acids and glycerol, which is a gluconeogenic precursor. Fatty acids provide an alternative oxidative fuel to tissues other than the brain (which requires glucose).

Systemic glucose balance—maintenance of the normal plasma glucose concentration—is accomplished by a network of hormones, neural signals, and substrate effects that regulate endogenous glucose production and glu-

cose utilization by tissues other than the brain (Chap. 338). Among the regulatory factors, insulin plays a dominant role (Table 339-2; Fig. 339-1). As plasma glucose levels decline within the physiologic range in the fasting state, pancreatic β cell insulin secretion decreases, thereby increasing hepatic glycogenolysis and hepatic (and renal) gluconeogenesis. Low insulin levels also reduce glucose utilization in peripheral

TABLE 339-1 CAUSES OF HYPOGLYCEMIA

Fasting (Postabsorptive) Hypoglycemia

Drugs
   Especially insulin, sulfonylureas, ethanol
   Sometimes quinine, pentamidine
   Rarely salicylates, sulfonamides, others
Critical illnesses
   Hepatic, renal, or cardiac failure
   Sepsis
   Inanition
Hormone deficiencies
   Cortisol, growth hormone, or both
   Glucagon and epinephrine (in insulin-deficient diabetes)
Non-β-cell tumors
Endogenous hyperinsulinism
   Insulinoma
   Other β cell disorders
   Insulin secretagogue (sulfonylurea, other)
   Autoimmune (autoantibodies to insulin or the insulin receptor)
   Ectopic insulin secretion
Disorders of infancy or childhood
   Transient intolerance of fasting
   Congenital hyperinsulinism
   Inherited enzyme deficiencies

Reactive (Postprandial) Hypoglycemia

Alimentary (postgastrectomy)
Noninsulinoma pancreatogenous hypoglycemia syndrome
   In the absence of prior surgery
   Following Roux-en-Y-gastric bypass
Other causes of endogenous hyperinsulinism
Hereditary fructose intolerance, galactosemia
Idiopathic

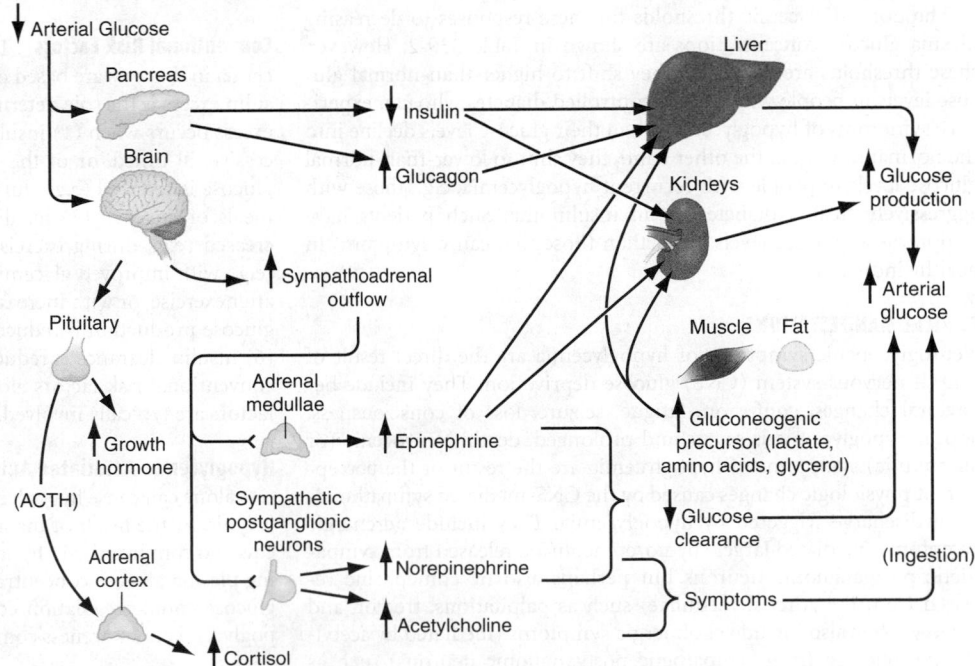

FIGURE 339-1 Physiology of glucose counterregulation—the mechanisms that normally prevent or rapidly correct hypoglycemia. In insulin-deficient diabetes, the key counterregulatory responses—suppression of insulin and increases of glucagon—are lost, and the stimulation of sympathoadrenal outflow is attenuated.

TABLE 339-2 PHYSIOLOGIC RESPONSES TO DECREASING PLASMA GLUCOSE CONCENTRATIONS

Response	Glycemic Threshold, mmol/L (mg/dL)	Physiologic Effects	Role in the Prevention or Correction of Hypoglycemia (Glucose Counterregulation)
↓ Insulin	4.4–4.7 (80–85)	↑ R_a (↓R_d)	Primary glucose regulatory factor/first defense against hypoglycemia
↑ Glucagon	3.6–3.9 (65–70)	↑ R_a	Primary glucose counterregulatory factor/second defense against hypoglycemia
↑ Epinephrine	3.6–3.9 (65–70)	↑ R_a, ↓ R_c	Third defense against hypoglycemia, critical when glucagon is deficient
↑ Cortisol and growth hormone	3.6–3.9 (65–70)	↑ R_a, ↓ R_c	Involved in defense against prolonged hypoglycemia, not critical
Symptoms	2.8–3.1 (50–55)	Recognition of hypoglycemia	Prompt behavioral defense against hypoglycemia (food ingestion)
↓ Cognition	<2.8 (<50)	—	(Compromises behavioral defense against hypoglycemia)

Note: R_a, rate of glucose appearance, glucose production by the liver and kidneys; R_c, rate of glucose clearance, glucose utilization relative to the ambient plasma glucose concentration; R_d, rate of glucose disappearance, glucose utilization by the brain (which is unaltered by the glucoregulatory hormones) and by insulin-sensitive tissues such as skeletal muscle (which is regulated by insulin, epinephrine, cortisol, and growth hormone).

tissues, inducing lipolysis and proteolysis, thereby releasing gluconeogenic precursors. Thus, a decrease in insulin secretion is the first defense against hypoglycemia.

As plasma glucose levels decline just below the physiologic range, glucose counterregulatory (plasma glucose–raising) hormones are released (Table 339-2; Fig. 339-1). Among these, pancreatic α cell glucagon, which stimulates hepatic glycogenolysis, plays a primary role. Glucagon is the second defense against hypoglycemia. Adrenomedullary epinephrine, which stimulates hepatic glycogenolysis and gluconeogenesis (and renal gluconeogenesis), is not normally critical. However, it becomes critical when glucagon is deficient. Epinephrine is the third defense against hypoglycemia. When hypoglycemia is prolonged, cortisol and growth hormone also support glucose production and limit glucose utilization.

As plasma glucose levels fall to lower levels, symptoms prompt the behavioral defense against hypoglycemia, including the ingestion of food (Table 339-2; Fig. 339-1).

The normal glycemic thresholds for these responses to decreasing plasma glucose concentrations are shown in Table 339-2. However, these thresholds are dynamic. They shift to higher-than-normal glucose levels in people with poorly controlled diabetes who can experience symptoms of hypoglycemia when their glucose levels decline into the normal range. On the other hand, they shift to lower-than-normal glucose levels in people with recurrent hypoglycemia, e.g., those with aggressively treated diabetes or an insulinoma. Such patients have symptoms at glucose levels lower than those that cause symptoms in healthy individuals.

CLINICAL MANIFESTATIONS

Neuroglycopenic symptoms of hypoglycemia are the direct result of central nervous system (CNS) glucose deprivation. They include behavioral changes, confusion, fatigue, seizure, loss of consciousness, and, if hypoglycemia is severe and prolonged, death. Neurogenic (or autonomic) symptoms of hypoglycemia are the result of the perception of physiologic changes caused by the CNS-mediated sympathoadrenal discharge triggered by hypoglycemia. They include adrenergic symptoms (mediated largely by norepinephrine released from sympathetic postganglionic neurons but perhaps also by epinephrine released from the adrenal medullae) such as palpitations, tremor, and anxiety. They also include cholinergic symptoms (mediated by acetylcholine released from sympathetic postganglionic neurons) such as sweating, hunger, and paresthesias. Clearly, these are nonspecific symptoms. Their attribution to hypoglycemia requires a corresponding low plasma glucose concentration and their resolution after the glucose level is raised (Whipple's triad).

Common signs of hypoglycemia include diaphoresis and pallor. Heart rate and systolic blood pressure are typically raised, but these findings may not be prominent. Neuroglycopenic manifestations are often observable. Transient focal neurologic deficits occur occasionally. Permanent neurologic deficits are rare.

ETIOLOGY AND PATHOPHYSIOLOGY

Hypoglycemia is most commonly a result of the treatment of diabetes. This topic is therefore addressed before considering other causes of hypoglycemia.

HYPOGLYCEMIA IN DIABETES
Impact and Frequency Hypoglycemia is the limiting factor in the glycemic management of diabetes. First, it causes recurrent morbidity in most people with type 1 diabetes (T1DM) and many with type 2 diabetes (T2DM) and is sometimes fatal. Second, it precludes maintenance of euglycemia over a lifetime of diabetes and thus full realization of the well-established benefits of glycemic control. Third, it causes a vicious cycle of recurrent hypoglycemia by producing hypoglycemia-associated autonomic failure—the clinical syndromes of defective glucose counterregulation and of hypoglycemia unawareness.

Hypoglycemia is a fact of life for people with T1DM. They suffer an average of two episodes of symptomatic hypoglycemia per week and at least one episode of severe, at least temporarily disabling, hypoglycemia each year. An estimated 2–4% of people with T1DM die as a result of hypoglycemia. Overall, hypoglycemia is less frequent in T2DM. Metformin, thiazolidinediones, α-glucosidase inhibitors, glucagon-like peptide-1 (GLP-1) receptor agonists or analogues, and dipeptidyl peptidase-IV (DPP-IV) inhibitors should not cause hypoglycemia. However, they increase the risk when combined with an insulin secretagogue, such as one of the sulfonylureas, or with insulin. Notably, the frequency of hypoglycemia approaches that in T1DM as persons with T2DM develop insulin deficiency and require treatment with insulin.

Conventional Risk Factors The conventional risk factors for hypoglycemia in diabetes are based on the premise that relative or absolute insulin excess is the sole determinant of risk. Relative or absolute insulin excess occurs when (1) insulin (or insulin secretagogue) doses are excessive, ill-timed, or of the wrong type; (2) the influx of exogenous glucose is reduced (e.g., during an overnight fast or following missed meals or snacks); (3) insulin-independent glucose utilization is increased (e.g., during exercise); (4) sensitivity to insulin is increased (e.g., with improved glycemic control, in the middle of the night, late after exercise, or with increased fitness or weight loss); (5) endogenous glucose production is reduced (e.g., following alcohol ingestion); and (6) insulin clearance is reduced (e.g., in renal failure). However, these conventional risk factors alone explain a minority of episodes; other factors are typically involved.

Hypoglycemia-Associated Autonomic Failure While marked insulin excess alone can cause hypoglycemia, iatrogenic hypoglycemia in diabetes is typically the result of the interplay of relative or absolute insulin excess and compromised physiologic and behavioral defenses against falling plasma glucose concentrations (Table 339-2; Fig. 339-2). Defective glucose counterregulation compromises physiologic defense, and hypoglycemia unawareness compromises behavioral defense.

DEFECTIVE GLUCOSE COUNTERREGULATION In the setting of endogenous insulin deficiency, insulin levels do not decrease as plasma glucose levels fall; the first defense against hypoglycemia is lost. Furthermore, because the decrement in intraislet insulin is normally a signal to stim-

FIGURE 339-2 Hypoglycemia-associated autonomic failure in insulin-deficient diabetes. *(Adapted from Cryer PE: N Engl J Med 350:2272, 2004. Copyright Massachusetts Medical Society, 2004.)*

ulate glucagon secretion, glucagon levels do not increase as plasma glucose levels fall further; the second defense against hypoglycemia is lost. Finally, the increase in epinephrine levels, the third defense against hypoglycemia, in response to a given level of hypoglycemia is typically attenuated. The glycemic threshold for the sympathoadrenal (adrenomedullary epinephrine and sympathetic neural norepinephrine) response is shifted to lower plasma glucose concentrations. That is typically the result of recent antecedent iatrogenic hypoglycemia. In the setting of absent decrements in insulin and of absent increments in glucagon, the attenuated increment in epinephrine causes the clinical syndrome of defective glucose counterregulation. Affected patients are at 25-fold or greater increased risk of severe iatrogenic hypoglycemia during aggressive glycemic therapy of their diabetes compared with those with normal epinephrine responses.

HYPOGLYCEMIA UNAWARENESS The attenuated sympathoadrenal response (largely the reduced sympathetic neural response) to hypoglycemia causes the clinical syndrome of hypoglycemia unawareness, i.e., loss of the warning adrenergic and cholinergic symptoms that previously allowed the patient to recognize developing hypoglycemia and therefore abort the episode by ingesting carbohydrates. Affected patients are at a sixfold increased risk of severe iatrogenic hypoglycemia during aggressive glycemic therapy of their diabetes.

HYPOGLYCEMIA-ASSOCIATED AUTONOMIC FAILURE The concept of hypoglycemia-associated autonomic failure (HAAF) in diabetes posits that recent antecedent iatrogenic hypoglycemia (or sleep or prior exercise) causes both defective glucose counterregulation (by reducing the epinephrine response to a given level of subsequent hypoglycemia in the setting of absent insulin and glucagon responses) and hypoglycemia unawareness (by reducing the sympathoadrenal response to a given level of subsequent hypoglycemia). These impaired responses create a vicious cycle of recurrent iatrogenic hypoglycemia (Fig. 339-2). Hypoglycemia unawareness, and to some extent the reduced epinephrine component of defective glucose counterregulation, is reversible by as little as 2–3 weeks of scrupulous avoidance of hypoglycemia in most affected patients.

Based on this pathophysiology, additional risk factors for hypoglycemia in diabetes include (1) insulin deficiency that indicates that insulin levels will not decrease and glucagon levels will not increase as plasma glucose levels fall; (2) a history of severe hypoglycemia or of hypoglycemia unawareness, implying recent antecedent hypoglycemia, that indicates that the sympathoadrenal response will be attenuated; and (3) lower HbA$_{1C}$ levels or lower glycemic goals that, all other factors being equal, increase the probability of recent antecedent hypoglycemia.

Hypoglycemia Risk Factor Reduction It is possible to reduce the risk of hypoglycemia while maintaining a degree of glycemic control in patients with diabetes. This involves application of the principles of aggressive glycemic therapy (Chap. 338)—patient education and empowerment, frequent self-monitoring of blood glucose, flexible insulin (and other drug) regimens including the use of insulin analogues, individualized glycemic goals, and ongoing professional guidance and support—and consideration of both the conventional risk factors and those indicative of compromised glucose counterregulation. Given a history of hypoglycemia unawareness, a 2- to 3-week period of scrupulous avoidance of hypoglycemia is indicated.

FASTING HYPOGLYCEMIA

There are many causes of fasting (postabsorptive) hypoglycemia (Table 339-1). However, drugs are the most common cause by far. Those used to treat diabetes mellitus (see above) are frequent offenders, as is alcohol. Of the critical illnesses that cause hypoglycemia, sepsis is the most common. Relevant hormone deficiencies, non-β-cell tumors, and endogenous hyperinsulinism, as well as hypoglycemic disorders with their onset in infancy and childhood, are rare.

Drugs Insulin and insulin secretagogues suppress glucose production and stimulate glucose utilization. Ethanol blocks gluconeogenesis but not glycogenolysis. Thus, alcohol-induced hypoglycemia typically occurs after a several-day ethanol binge during which the person eats little food, thereby causing glycogen depletion. Ethanol is usually measurable in blood at the time of presentation, but its levels correlate poorly with plasma glucose concentrations. Because gluconeogenesis becomes the predominant route of glucose production during prolonged hypoglycemia, alcohol can contribute to the progression of hypoglycemia in patients with insulin-treated diabetes.

Salicylates in large doses can cause hypoglycemia by inhibiting glucose production. Sulfonamides also rarely cause hypoglycemia by stimulating insulin secretion.

Pentamidine is toxic to pancreatic β cells. It causes insulin release initially, with hypoglycemia in about 10% of treated patients, and can cause diabetes later. Quinine also stimulates insulin secretion. However, the relative contribution of hyperinsulinemia to the pathogenesis of hypoglycemia in critically ill patients with malaria treated with quinine is debated. Quinolone antibiotics, particularly gatifloxacin, have been reported to cause hypoglycemia, often in the setting of drug-treated diabetes. Among the antiarrhythmic drugs, quinidine, disopyramide, and cibenzoline have been reported to cause hypoglycemia.

Hypoglycemia has been attributed to many other drugs, including the nonselective β-adrenergic antagonist propanolol. Since the glycemic actions of epinephrine and the adrenergic symptoms of hypoglycemia (but not the cholinergic symptoms such as sweating) are mediated by β$_2$-adrenergic receptors, it is reasonable to use a relatively selective β$_1$-adrenergic antagonist (e.g., atenolol or metoprolol) in a setting in which hypoglycemia might occur.

Critical Illness Among hospitalized patients, serious illnesses such as renal, hepatic, or cardiac failure, sepsis, and inanition are second only to drugs as causes of hypoglycemia.

Rapid and extensive hepatic destruction (e.g., toxic hepatitis) causes fasting hypoglycemia because the liver is the major site of endogenous glucose production. The mechanism of hypoglycemia in patients with cardiac failure is unknown. It may involve hepatic congestion and hypoxia. Although the kidneys are a source of glucose production, hypoglycemia in patients with renal failure is also caused by the reduced clearance of insulin and reduced mobilization of gluconeogenic precursors in renal failure.

Sepsis is a relatively common cause of hypoglycemia. Increased glucose utilization is induced by cytokine production in macrophage-rich tissues such as the liver, spleen, and lung. Hypoglycemia develops if glucose production fails to keep pace. Cytokine-induced inhibition of gluconeogenesis in the setting of nutritional glycogen depletion, in combination with hepatic and renal hypoperfusion, may also contribute to hypoglycemia.

Hypoglycemia can be seen with starvation, perhaps because of loss of whole-body fat stores and subsequent depletion of gluconeogenic precursors (e.g., amino acids), necessitating increased glucose utilization.

Hormone Deficiencies Neither cortisol nor growth hormone is critical to the prevention of hypoglycemia, at least in adults. Nonetheless, hypoglycemia can occur with prolonged fasting in patients with primary adrenocortical failure (Addison's disease) or hypopituitarism. Anorexia and weight loss are typical features of chronic cortisol deficiency and likely result in glycogen depletion. Cortisol deficiency is associated with impaired gluconeogenesis and low levels of gluconeogenic precursors, suggesting that substrate-limited gluconeogenesis, in the setting of glycogen depletion, is the cause of hypoglycemia. Growth hormone deficiency can cause hypoglycemia in young children. In addition to extended fasting, high rates of glucose utilization (e.g., during exercise or in pregnancy) or low rates of glucose production (e.g., following alcohol ingestion) can precipitate hypoglycemia in adults with previously unrecognized hypopituitarism.

Hypoglycemia is not a feature of the epinephrine-deficient state that results from bilateral adrenalectomy, when glucocorticoid replacement is adequate, nor does it occur during pharmacologic adrenergic blockade when other glucoregulatory systems are intact. Combined deficiencies of glucagon and epinephrine play a key role in the pathogenesis of iatrogenic hypoglycemia in people with insulin-deficient diabetes. Otherwise, deficiencies of these hormones are not usually considered in the differential diagnosis of a hypoglycemic disorder.

Non-β-Cell Tumors Fasting hypoglycemia, often termed non-islet cell tumor hypoglycemia, occurs occasionally in patients with large mesenchymal or epithelial tumors (e.g., hepatomas, adrenocortical carcinomas, carcinoids). The glucose kinetic patterns resemble those of hyperinsulinism (see below), but insulin secretion is suppressed appropriately during hypoglycemia. In most instances, hypoglycemia is due to overproduction of an incompletely processed form of insulin-like growth factor II ("big IGF-II") that does not complex normally with circulating binding proteins and thus more readily gains access to target tissues. The tumors are usually apparent clinically, and free IGF-II levels [and levels of pro-IGF-II (E1-21)] are elevated. Curative surgery is seldom possible, but reduction of tumor bulk may ameliorate hypoglycemia. Therapy with a glucocorticoid, growth hormone, or both has also been reported to alleviate hypoglycemia.

Endogenous Hyperinsulinism Hypoglycemia due to endogenous hyperinsulinism can be caused by (1) a primary β cell disorder, typically a β cell tumor (insulinoma), sometimes multiple insulinomas, or, especially in infants and young children, a functional β cell disorder with β cell hypertrophy or hyperplasia; (2) a β cell secretagogue such as a sulfonylurea; (3) an autoantibody to insulin; or (4) rarely, ectopic insulin secretion. None of these causes is common. Endogenous hyperinsulinism is more likely in an overtly healthy individual without clues to other potential causes of hypoglycemia. Accidental, surreptitious, or even malicious administration of an insulin secretagogue or insulin also should be considered in such an individual.

The fundamental pathophysiologic feature of endogenous hyperinsulinism caused by a primary β cell disorder or an insulin secretagogue is the failure of insulin secretion to fall to very low levels during hypoglycemia. This is assessed by measuring plasma insulin, C-peptide (the connecting peptide that is cleaved from proinsulin to produce insulin), and glucose concentrations during hypoglycemia; proinsulin levels also can be measured. Insulin, C-peptide, and proinsulin levels need not be high relative to normal, euglycemic values; they are often inappropriately high in the setting of a low plasma glucose concentration. Critical diagnostic findings are a plasma insulin concentration ≥3 μU/mL (≥18 pmol/L) and a plasma C-peptide concentration ≥0.6 ng/mL (≥0.2 nmol/L) (with a plasma proinsulin concentration ≥5.0 pmol/L) when the plasma glucose concentration is <55 mg/dL (<3.0 mmol/L) with symptoms of hypoglycemia.

Most primary β cell disorders, such as an insulinoma, cause fasting hypoglycemia. The diagnostic strategy is to make the above measurements during spontaneous, symptomatic hypoglycemia, i.e., after an overnight fast, an extended outpatient fast, or, if necessary, an inpatient prolonged (48- or 72-h) fast. It is necessary to screen the plasma for sulfonylureas and other insulin secretagogues (repaglinide, nateglinide) at the time of hypoglycemia since these produce an insulin, C-peptide, proinsulin, and glucose pattern indistinguishable from that produced by an insulinoma. Autoantibodies to insulin also should be sought but need not be measured at the time of hypoglycemia. The noninsulinoma pancreatogenous hypoglycemia syndrome, which also causes postprandial hyperinsulinemic hypoglycemia, is discussed later. The rare autoantibodies to the insulin receptor are sometimes agonists; insulin secretion is suppressed during hypoglycemia but insulin levels tend to be inappropriately high, perhaps because of decreased clearance of insulin via the receptor. Ectopic insulin secretion has been reported, but it must be quite rare and is usually not considered in the differential diagnosis of a hypoglycemic disorder. Finally, the finding of inappropriately high insulin levels but low C-peptide levels during hypoglycemia indicates exogenous insulin administration. A diagnostic algorithm for a patient with suspected endogenous hyperinsulinism is shown in **Fig. 339-3.**

Insulinomas are uncommon—the yearly incidence is estimated to be 1 in 250,000—but because more than 90% are benign, they are a treatable cause of potentially fatal hypoglycemia. The median age at presentation is 50 years in sporadic cases, but it usually presents in the third decade when it is a component of multiple endocrine neoplasia type 1 (Chap. 345). More than 99% of insulinomas are within the substance of the pancreas and they are usually small (90% <2.0 cm). Therefore, they come to clinical attention because of hypoglycemia rather than mass effects. Computed tomography detects approximately 70–80% of insulinomas, and magnetic resonance imaging detects about 85%. These methods detect metastases in the roughly 10% of patients with a malignant insulinoma. Transabdominal ultrasound will often identify insulinomas, and endoscopic ultrasound has a sensitivity of about 90%. Somatostatin receptor scintigraphy is thought to detect insulinomas in about half of patients. Selective pancreatic arterial calcium injections, with the endpoint of a sharp increase in hepatic venous insulin levels, regionalizes insulinomas with high sensitivity, but this invasive procedure is seldom necessary. The same is true of transhepatic portal venous sampling. Intraoperative pancreatic ultrasonography almost invariably localizes insulinomas that are not readily palpable by the surgeon. Surgical resection of a solitary insulinoma is generally curative. Diazoxide, which inhibits insulin secretion, or the somatostatin analogue octreotide can be used to treat hypoglycemia in patients with unresectable tumors.

DISORDERS OF INFANCY AND CHILDHOOD

Discussion of the various disorders that cause hypoglycemia in infancy and childhood, including multiple causes of transient intolerance of fasting, congenital hyperinsulinism, and inherited enzyme deficiencies, is beyond the scope of this chapter.

REACTIVE HYPOGLYCEMIA

Reactive (postprandial) hypoglycemia occurs exclusively after meals. Its diagnosis requires documentation of Whipple's triad after a mixed meal. The diagnosis should not be made on the basis of seemingly low venous plasma glucose concentrations after an oral glucose load. It can occur following gastrectomy. Termed *alimentary hypoglycemia*, this is thought to be the result of early hyperinsulinemia caused by rapid increments in plasma glucose and enhanced secretion of the gut incretin GLP-1 coupled with suppression of glucagon secretion by GLP-1. Administration of an α-glucosidase inhibitor (e.g., acarbose or miglitol)

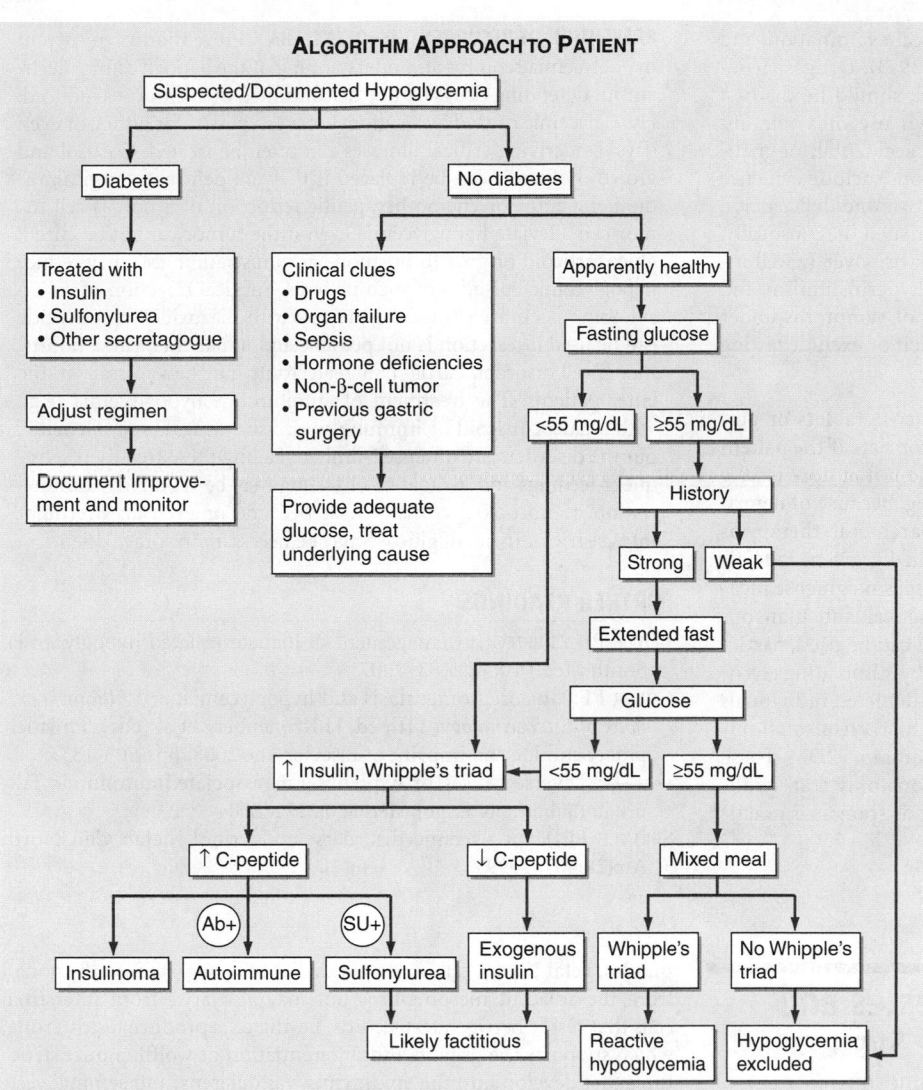

ALGORITHM APPROACH TO PATIENT

Suspected/Documented Hypoglycemia

→ Diabetes
→ No diabetes

Diabetes:
Treated with
- Insulin
- Sulfonylurea
- Other secretagogue

→ Adjust regimen

→ Document Improvement and monitor

No diabetes:
Clinical clues
- Drugs
- Organ failure
- Sepsis
- Hormone deficiencies
- Non-β-cell tumor
- Previous gastric surgery

→ Provide adequate glucose, treat underlying cause

Apparently healthy
→ Fasting glucose
→ <55 mg/dL | ≥55 mg/dL

≥55 mg/dL → History → Strong / Weak

Strong → Extended fast → Glucose → <55 mg/dL | ≥55 mg/dL

<55 mg/dL → ↑ Insulin, Whipple's triad

↑ Insulin, Whipple's triad → ↑ C-peptide / ↓ C-peptide

≥55 mg/dL → Mixed meal

↑ C-peptide → (Ab+) → Autoimmune ; (SU+) → Sulfonylurea ; Insulinoma

↓ C-peptide → Exogenous insulin → Likely factitious

Mixed meal → Whipple's triad → Reactive hypoglycemia ; No Whipple's triad → Hypoglycemia excluded

FIGURE 339-3 Diagnostic approach to a patient with documented hypoglycemia or suspected hypoglycemia based on a history of suggestive symptoms, a low plasma glucose concentration, or both. Ab+, positive for antibody to insulin; SU+, positive for sulfonylurea (or other secretagogue).

and laboratory features with insulinoma. It is most common among health care workers, patients with diabetes or their relatives, and people with a history of other factitious illnesses. However, it should be considered in all patients being evaluated for hypoglycemia of obscure cause. Accidental ingestion of an insulin secretagogue (e.g., the result of a pharmacy error) also occurs.

Analytical error in the measurement of plasma glucose concentrations is rare. On the other hand, glucose monitors used to guide treatment of diabetes are not quantitative instruments, particularly at low glucose levels, and these should not be used for the definitive diagnosis of hypoglycemia. Even with a quantitative method, low measured glucose concentrations can be artifactual, e.g., the result of continued glucose metabolism by the formed elements of the blood ex vivo, particularly in the presence of leukocytosis, erythrocytosis, or thrombocytosis, or if separation of the serum from the formed elements is delayed (pseudohypoglycemia).

APPROACH TO THE PATIENT:
Hypoglycemia

In addition to recognition and documentation of hypoglycemia, and often urgent treatment, diagnosis of the hypoglycemic mechanism is critical for choosing a treatment that prevents, or at least minimizes, recurrent hypoglycemia. A diagnostic algorithm is shown in Fig. 339-3.

RECOGNITION AND DOCUMENTATION
Hypoglycemia is suspected in patients with typical symptoms; in the presence of confusion, an altered level of consciousness, or a seizure; or in a clinical setting in which hypoglycemia is known to occur. Urgent treatment is often necessary in patients with suspected hypoglycemia. Blood should be drawn, whenever possible, before the administration of glucose to allow documentation of a low plasma glucose concentration. Convincing documentation of hypoglycemia requires the fulfillment of Whipple's triad. Thus, the ideal time to measure the plasma glucose level is during a symptomatic episode. A normal glucose level excludes hypoglycemia as the cause of the symptoms. A low glucose level confirms that hypoglycemia is the cause of the symptoms, provided the latter resolve after the glucose level is raised. When the cause of the hypoglycemic episode is obscure, additional measurements, while the glucose level is low and before treatment, should include plasma insulin, C-peptide, and ethanol concentrations, as well as levels of insulin secretagogues.

When the history suggests prior hypoglycemia, and a potential mechanism is not apparent, the diagnostic strategy is to measure the plasma glucose, insulin, and C-peptide levels under conditions when hypoglycemia would be expected, typically during fasting. On the other hand, while it cannot be ignored, a distinctly low plasma glucose concentration measured in a patient without corresponding symptoms raises the possibility of an artifact (pseudohypoglycemia).

DIAGNOSIS OF THE HYPOGLYCEMIC MECHANISM In a patient with documented hypoglycemia, a plausible hypoglycemic mechanism

is a conceptually attractive treatment, although controlled clinical trials documenting its efficacy are lacking.

Reactive hypoglycemia also occurs in patients with autoantibodies to insulin and in the noninsulinoma pancreatogenous hypoglycemia syndrome. Affected patients have symptomatic hyperinsulinemic postprandial hypoglycemia (but negative 72-h fasts) that remits following partial pancreatectomy. Histologic findings include β cell hypertrophy with or without hyperplasia. A similar syndrome following Roux-en-Y gastric bypass surgery for obesity has been described.

The existence of a clinically relevant idiopathic reactive hypoglycemia syndrome is debated. The issue is whether symptoms are caused by hypoglycemia, an exaggerated sympathoadrenal response to declining glucose levels late after a meal, or some glucose-independent mechanism. In any event, caution should be exercised before labeling a person with a diagnosis of hypoglycemia. Frequent feedings, avoidance of simple sugars, and high-protein diets are commonly recommended to patients thought to have idiopathic reactive hypoglycemia. The efficacy of these approaches has not been established by controlled clinical trials.

FACTITIOUS AND ARTIFACTUAL HYPOGLYCEMIA
Factitious hypoglycemia, caused by surreptitious or even malicious administration of insulin or an insulin secretagogue, shares many clinical

can often be deduced from the history, physical examination, and available laboratory data (Table 339-1; Fig. 339-3). Drugs, particularly those used to treat diabetes or alcohol, should be the first consideration, even in the absence of known use of a relevant drug, given the possibility of surreptitious, accidental, or malicious drug administration. Other considerations include evidence of a relevant critical illness, less commonly hormone deficiencies, and rarely a non–β-cell tumor that can be pursued diagnostically. Absent one of these mechanisms, in an otherwise overtly well individual, one should consider endogenous hyperinsulinism and proceed with measurements and assessment of symptoms under fasting conditions of sufficient duration to elicit or exclude fasting hypoglycemia.

URGENT TREATMENT   Oral treatment with glucose tablets or glucose-containing fluids, candy, or food is appropriate if the patient is able and willing to take these. A reasonable initial dose is 20 g of glucose. If the patient is unable or unwilling, because of neuroglycopenia, to take carbohydrates orally, parenteral therapy is necessary. Intravenous glucose (25 g) should be given and followed by a glucose infusion guided by serial plasma glucose measurements. If intravenous therapy is not practical, subcutaneous or intramuscular glucagon (1.0 mg in adults) can be used, particularly in patients with T1DM. Because it acts by stimulating glycogenolysis, glucagon is ineffective in glycogen-depleted individuals (e.g., those with alcohol-induced hypoglycemia). It also stimulates insulin secretion and is therefore less useful in T2DM. These treatments raise plasma glucose concentrations only transiently, and patients should therefore be urged to eat as soon as is practical to replete glycogen stores.

PREVENTION OF RECURRENT HYPOGLYCEMIA   Prevention of recurrent hypoglycemia requires an understanding of the hypoglycemic mechanism. Offending drugs can be discontinued or their doses reduced. Hypoglycemia caused by a sulfonylurea can persist for hours, or even days. Underlying critical illnesses can often be treated. Cortisol and growth hormone can be replaced if they are deficient. Surgical, radiotherapeutic, or chemotherapeutic reduction of a non–β-cell tumor can alleviate hypoglycemia even if the tumor cannot be cured; glucocorticoid or growth hormone administration also may reduce hypoglycemic episodes in such patients. Surgical resection of an insulinoma is curative; medical therapy with diazoxide or octreotide can be used if resection is not possible and in patients with a nontumor β cell disorder. Partial pancreatectomy may be necessary in the latter patients. The treatment of autoimmune hypoglycemia (e.g., with a glucocorticoid or immunosuppressive drugs) is problematic, but the disorders are often self-limited. Failing these treatments, frequent feedings and avoidance of fasting may be required. Administration of uncooked cornstarch at bedtime or even an overnight intragastric infusion of glucose may be necessary in some patients.

FURTHER READINGS

Boyle PJ, Zrebiec J: Management of diabetes-related hypoglycemia. South Med J 100(2):183, 2007

Cryer PE: Glucose homeostasis and hypoglycemia, in *Williams Textbook of Endocrinology*, 11th ed, H Kronenberg et al (eds). Philadelphia, Saunders, an imprint of Elsevier, Inc 2008, pp 1503-1533

———: Diverse causes of hypoglycemia-associated autonomic failure in diabetes. N Engl J Med 350:2272, 2004

Service FJ: Hypoglycemic disorders. Endocrinol Metab Clin North Am 28:467, 1999

340   Disorders of the Testes and Male Reproductive System
Shalender Bhasin, J. Larry Jameson

The male reproductive system regulates sex differentiation, virilization, and the hormonal changes that accompany puberty, ultimately leading to spermatogenesis and fertility. Under the control of the pituitary hormones—luteinizing hormone (LH) and follicle-stimulating hormone (FSH)—the Leydig cells of the testes produce testosterone and germ cells are nurtured by Sertoli cells to divide, differentiate, and mature into sperm. During embryonic development, testosterone and dihydrotestosterone (DHT) induce the wolffian duct and virilization of the external genitalia. During puberty, testosterone promotes somatic growth and the development of secondary sex characteristics. In the adult, testosterone is necessary for spermatogenesis and stimulation of libido and normal sexual function. This chapter focuses on the physiology of the testes and disorders associated with decreased androgen production, which may be caused by gonadotropin deficiency or by primary testis dysfunction. A variety of testosterone formulations now allow more physiologic androgen replacement. Infertility occurs in ~5% of men and is increasingly amenable to treatment by hormone replacement or by using sperm transfer techniques. For further discussion of sexual dysfunction, disorders of the prostate, and testicular cancer, see Chaps. 49, 91, 92, respectively.

DEVELOPMENT AND STRUCTURE OF THE TESTIS

The fetal testis develops from the undifferentiated gonad after expression of a genetic cascade that is initiated by the SRY (sex-related gene on the Y chromosome) (Chap. 343). SRY induces differentiation of Sertoli cells, which surround germ cells and, together with peritubular myoid cells, form testis cords that will later develop into seminiferous tubules. Fetal Leydig cells and endothelial cells migrate into the gonad from the adjacent mesonephros but may also arise from interstitial cells that reside between testis cords. Leydig cells produce testosterone, which supports the growth and differentiation of wolffian duct structures that develop into the epididymis, vas deferens, and seminal vesicles. Testosterone is also converted to DHT (see below), which induces formation of the prostate and the external male genitalia, including the penis, urethra, and scrotum. Testicular descent through the inguinal canal is controlled in part by Leydig cell production of insulin-like factor 3 (INSL3), which acts via a receptor termed *Great* (*G* protein–coupled *receptor affecting testis* descent). Sertoli cells produce müllerian inhibiting substance (MIS), which causes regression of the müllerian structures, including the fallopian tube, uterus, and upper segment of the vagina.

NORMAL MALE PUBERTAL DEVELOPMENT

Although *puberty* commonly refers to the maturation of the reproductive axis and the development of secondary sex characteristics, it involves a coordinated response of multiple hormonal systems including the adrenal gland and the growth hormone (GH) axis (Fig. 340-1). The development of secondary sex characteristics is initiated by *adrenarche*, which usually occurs between 6 and 8 years of age when the adrenal gland begins to produce greater amounts of androgens from the zona reticularis, the principal site of dehydroepiandrosterone (DHEA) production. The sex maturation process is greatly accelerated by the activation of the hypothalamic-pituitary axis and the production of gonadotropin-releasing hormone (GnRH). The GnRH pulse generator in the hypothalamus is active during fetal life and early infancy but is quiescent until the early stages of puberty, when the sensitivity to steroid inhibition is gradually lost, causing reactivation of GnRH secretion. Although the pathways that initiate reactivation of the GnRH pulse generator have been elusive, mounting evidence supports involvement of GPR54, a G protein–coupled receptor that binds an endogenous ligand, metastin. Individuals with mutations of GPR54 fail to enter puberty,

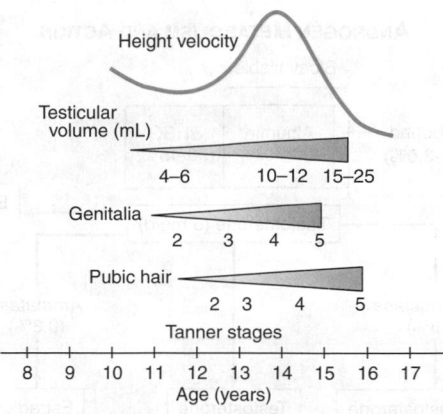

FIGURE 340-1 Pubertal events in males. Sexual maturity ratings for genitalia and pubic hair and divided into five stages. *(From WA Marshall, JM Tanner: Variations in the pattern of pubertal changes in boys. Arch Dis Child 45:13, 1970.)*

and experiments in primates demonstrate that infusion of the ligand is sufficient to induce premature puberty. Leptin, a hormone produced by adipose cells, may play a permissive role in the onset of puberty, as leptin-deficient individuals also fail to enter puberty (Chap. 74).

The early stages of puberty are characterized by nocturnal surges of LH and FSH. Growth of the testes is usually the first sign of puberty, reflecting an increase in seminiferous tubule volume. Increasing levels of testosterone deepen the voice and increase muscle growth. Conversion of testosterone to DHT leads to growth of the external genitalia and pubic hair. DHT also stimulates prostate and facial hair growth and initiates recession of the temporal hairline. The growth spurt occurs at a testicular volume of about 10–12 mL. GH increases early in puberty and is stimulated in part by the rise in gonadal steroids. GH increases the level of insulin-like growth factor 1 (IGF-1), which enhances linear bone growth. The prolonged pubertal exposure to gonadal steroids (mainly estradiol) ultimately causes epiphyseal closure and limits further bone growth.

REGULATION OF TESTICULAR FUNCTION

REGULATION OF THE HYPOTHALAMIC-PITUITARY-TESTIS AXIS IN ADULT MAN

Hypothalamic GnRH regulates the production of the pituitary gonadotropins, LH and FSH (Fig. 340-2). GnRH is released in discrete pulses approximately every 2 h, resulting in corresponding pulses of LH and FSH. These dynamic hormone pulses account in part for the wide variations in LH and testosterone, even within the same individual. LH acts primarily on the Leydig cell to stimulate testosterone synthesis. The regulatory control of androgen synthesis is mediated by testosterone and estrogen feedback on both the hypothalamus and the pituitary. FSH acts on the Sertoli cell to regulate spermatogenesis and the production of Sertoli products such as inhibin B, which acts to selectively suppress pituitary FSH. Despite these somewhat distinct Leydig and Sertoli cell–regulated pathways, testis function is integrated at several levels: GnRH regulates both gonadotropins; spermatogenesis requires high levels of testosterone; numerous paracrine interactions between Leydig and Sertoli cells are necessary for normal testis function.

THE LEYDIG CELL: ANDROGEN SYNTHESIS

LH binds to its seven transmembrane, G protein–coupled receptor to activate the cyclic AMP pathway. Stimulation of the LH receptor induces *s*teroid *a*cute *r*egulatory (StAR) protein, along with several steroidogenic enzymes involved in androgen synthesis. LH receptor mutations cause Leydig cell hypoplasia or agenesis, underscoring the importance of this pathway for Leydig cell development and function. The rate-limiting process in testosterone synthesis is the delivery of cholesterol by the StAR protein to the inner mitochondrial membrane. Peripheral benzodiazepine receptor, a mitochondrial cholesterol-binding protein, is also an acute regulator of Leydig cell steroidogenesis.

FIGURE 340-2 Human pituitary gonadotropin axis, structure of testis, seminiferous tubule. E$_2$, 17β estradiol; DHT, dihydrotestosterone.

The five major enzymatic steps involved in testosterone synthesis are summarized in Fig. 340-3. After cholesterol transport into the mitochondrion, the formation of pregnenolone by CYP11A1 (side chain cleavage enzyme) is a limiting enzymatic step. The 17α-hydroxylase and the 17,20-lyase reactions are catalyzed by a single enzyme, CYP17; posttranslational modification (phosphorylation) of this enzyme and the presence of specific enzyme cofactors confer 17,20-lyase activity selectively in the testis and zona reticularis of the adrenal gland. Testosterone can be converted to the more potent DHT by 5α-reductase, or it can be aromatized to estradiol by CYP19 (aromatase).

Testosterone Transport and Metabolism In males, 95% of circulating testosterone is derived from testicular production (3–10 mg/d). Direct secretion of testosterone by the adrenal and the peripheral conversion of androstenedione to testosterone collectively account for another 0.5 mg/d of testosterone. Only a small amount of DHT (70 μg/d) is secreted directly by the testis; most circulating DHT is derived from peripheral conversion of testosterone. Most of the daily production of estradiol (approximately 45 μg/d) in men is derived from aromatase-mediated peripheral conversion of testosterone and androstenedione.

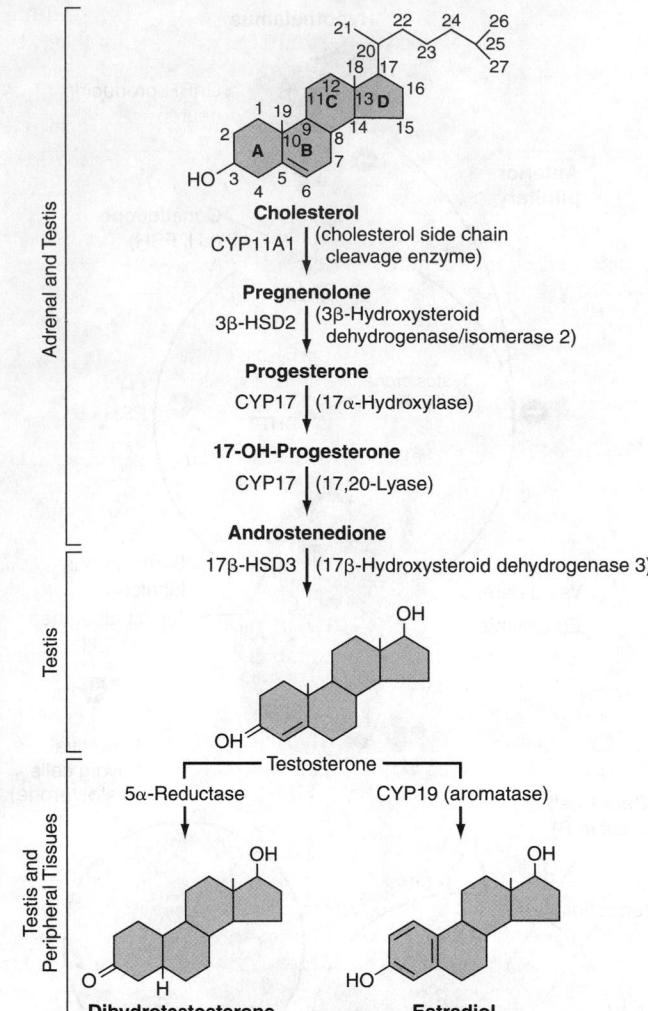

FIGURE 340-3 The biochemical pathway in the conversion of 27-carbon sterol cholesterol to androgens and estrogens.

FIGURE 340-4 Androgen metabolism and actions. SHBG, sex hormone–binding globulin.

Circulating testosterone is bound to two plasma proteins: sex hormone–binding globulin (SHBG) and albumin (Fig. 340-4). SHBG binds testosterone with much greater affinity than albumin. Only 0.5–3% of testosterone is unbound. According to the "free hormone" hypothesis, only the unbound fraction is biologically active; however, albumin-bound hormone dissociates readily in the capillaries and may be bioavailable. The finding that SHBG-bound testosterone may be internalized through endocytic pits by binding to a protein called megalin have challenged the "free hormone" hypothesis. SHBG concentrations are decreased by androgens, obesity, insulin, and nephrotic syndrome. Conversely, estrogen administration, hyperthyroidism, many chronic inflammatory illnesses, and aging are associated with high SHBG concentrations.

Testosterone is metabolized predominantly in the liver, although some degradation occurs in peripheral tissues, particularly the prostate and the skin. In the liver, testosterone is converted by a series of enzymatic steps that involve 5α- and 5β-reductases, 3α- and 3β-hydroxysteroid dehydrogenases, and 17β-hydroxysteroid dehydrogenase into androsterone, etiocholanolone, DHT, and 3-α-androstanediol. These compounds undergo glucuronidation or sulfation before being excreted by the kidneys.

Mechanism of Androgen Action The androgen receptor (AR) is structurally related to the nuclear receptors for estrogen, glucocorticoids, and progesterone (Chap. 332). The AR is encoded by a gene on the long arm of the X chromosome and has a molecular mass of about 110 kDa. A polymorphic region in the amino terminus of the receptor, which contains a variable number of glutamine repeats, modifies the transcriptional activity of the receptor. The AR protein is distributed in both the cytoplasm and

the nucleus. Androgen binding to the AR causes it to translocate into the nucleus, where it binds to DNA or other transcription factors already bound to DNA. The ligand also induces conformational changes that allow the recruitment and assembly of tissue-specific cofactors. Thus, the AR is a ligand-regulated transcription factor. Some androgen effects may be mediated by nongenomic AR signal transduction pathways. Testosterone binds to AR with half the affinity of DHT. The DHT-AR complex also has greater thermostability and a slower dissociation rate than the testosterone-AR complex. However, the molecular basis for selective testosterone versus DHT actions remains incompletely explained.

THE SEMINIFEROUS TUBULES: SPERMATOGENESIS
The seminiferous tubules are convoluted, closed loops with both ends emptying into the rete testis, a network of progressively larger efferent ducts that ultimately form the epididymis (Fig. 340-2). The seminiferous tubules total about 600 m in length and comprise about two-thirds of testis volume. The walls of the tubules are formed by polarized Sertoli cells that are apposed to peritubular myoid cells. Tight junctions between Sertoli cells create a blood-testis barrier. Germ cells comprise the majority of the seminiferous epithelium (~60%) and are intimately embedded within the cytoplasmic extensions of the Sertoli cells, which function as "nurse cells." Germ cells progress through characteristic stages of mitotic and meiotic divisions. A pool of type A spermatogonia serve as stem cells capable of self-renewal. Primary spermatocytes are derived from type B spermatogonia and undergo meiosis before progressing to spermatids that undergo spermiogenesis (a differentiation process involving chromatin condensation, acquisition of an acrosome, elongation of cytoplasm, and formation of a tail) and are released from Sertoli cells as mature spermatozoa. The complete differentiation process into mature sperm requires 74 days. Peristaltic-type action by peritubular myoid cells transports sperm into the efferent ducts. The spermatozoa spend an additional 21 days in the epididymis, where they undergo further maturation and capacitation. The normal adult testes produce >100 million sperm per day.

Naturally occurring mutations in the *FSHβ* gene and in the FSH receptor confirm an important, but not essential, role for this pathway in spermatogenesis. Females with these mutations are hypogonadal and infertile because ovarian follicles do not mature; males exhibit variable degrees of reduced spermatogenesis, presumably because of impaired Sertoli cell function. Because Sertoli cells produce inhibin B, an inhibitor of FSH, seminiferous tubule damage (e.g., by radiation) causes a selective increase of FSH. Testosterone reaches very high concentrations locally in the testis and is essential for spermatogenesis. Several cytokines and growth factors are also involved in the regulation of spermatogenesis by paracrine and autocrine mechanisms. A number of knockout mouse models exhibit impaired germ cell development or spermatogenesis, presaging possible mutations associated with male infertility. The human Y chromosome contains a small pseudoautosomal region that can recombine with homologous regions of the X chromosome. Most of the Y chromosome does not recombine with the X chromosome and is referred to as the male-specific region of the Y (MSY). The MSY contains 156 transcription units that encode for 26 proteins, including nine families of Y-specific multicopy genes; many of these Y-specific genes are also testis-specific and necessary for spermatogenesis. Microdeletions of several Y chromosome azoospermia factor (*AZF*) genes (e.g., RNA-binding motif, *RBM*; deleted in azoospermia, *DAZ*) are associated with oligospermia or azoospermia.

℞ MALE FACTOR INFERTILITY

Treatment options for male factor infertility have expanded greatly in recent years. Secondary hypogonadism is highly amenable to treatment with pulsatile GnRH or gonadotropins (see below). In vitro techniques have provided new opportunities for patients with primary testicular failure and disorders of sperm transport. Choice of initial treatment options depends on sperm concentration and motility. Expectant management should be attempted initially in men with mild male factor infertility (sperm count of $15-20 \times 10^6/\text{mL}$ and normal motility). Moderate male factor infertility ($10-15 \times 10^6/\text{mL}$ and 20–40% motility) should begin with intrauterine insemination alone or in combination with treatment of the female partner with clomiphene or gonadotropins, but it may require in vitro fertilization (IVF) with or without intracytoplasmic sperm injection (ICSI). For men with a severe defect (sperm count of $<10 \times 10^6/\text{mL}$, 10% motility), IVF with ICSI or donor sperm should be used.

CLINICAL AND LABORATORY EVALUATION OF MALE REPRODUCTIVE FUNCTION

HISTORY AND PHYSICAL EXAMINATION

The history should focus on developmental stages such as puberty and growth spurts, as well as androgen-dependent events such as early morning erections, frequency and intensity of sexual thoughts, and frequency of masturbation or intercourse. Although libido and the overall frequency of sexual acts are decreased in androgen-deficient men, young hypogonadal men may achieve erections in response to visual erotic stimuli. Men with acquired androgen deficiency often report decreased energy and increased irritability.

The physical examination should focus on secondary sex characteristics such as hair growth, gynecomastia, testicular volume, prostate, and height and body proportions. *Eunuchoid proportions* are defined as an arm span >2 cm greater than height and suggest that androgen deficiency occurred before epiphyseal fusion. Hair growth in the face, axilla, chest, and pubic regions is androgen-dependent; however, changes may not be noticeable unless androgen deficiency is severe and prolonged. Ethnicity also influences the intensity of hair growth (Chap. 50). Testicular volume is best assessed by using a Prader orchidometer. Testes range from 3.5 to 5.5 cm in length, which corresponds to a volume of 12–25 mL. Advanced age does not influence testicular size, although the consistency becomes less firm. Asian men generally have smaller testes than western Europeans, independent of differences in body size. Because of its possible role in infertility, the presence of varicocele should be sought by palpation while the patient is standing; it is more common on the left side. Patients with Klinefelter syndrome have markedly reduced testicular volumes (1–2 mL). In congenital hypogonadotropic hypogonadism, testicular volumes provide a good index for the degree of gonadotropin deficiency and the likelihood of response to therapy.

GONADOTROPIN AND INHIBIN MEASUREMENTS

LH and FSH are measured using two-site immunoradiometric, immunofluorometric, or chemiluminescent assays, which have very low cross-reactivity with other pituitary glycoprotein hormones and human chorionic gonadotropin (hCG) and have sufficient sensitivity to measure the low levels present in patients with hypogonadotropic hypogonadism. In men with a low testosterone level, an LH level can distinguish primary (high LH) versus secondary (low or inappropriately normal LH) hypogonadism. An elevated LH level indicates a primary defect at the testicular level, whereas a low or inappropriately normal LH level suggests a defect at the hypothalamic-pituitary level. LH pulses occur about every 1–3 h in normal men. Thus, gonadotropin levels fluctuate, and samples should be pooled or repeated when results are equivocal. FSH is less pulsatile than LH because it has a longer half-life. Increased FSH suggests damage to the seminiferous tubules. Inhibin B, a Sertoli cell product that suppresses FSH, is reduced with seminiferous tubule damage. Inhibin B is a dimer with α-β_B subunits and is measured by two-site immunoassays.

GnRH Stimulation Testing   The GnRH test is performed by measuring LH and FSH concentrations at baseline and at 30 and 60 min after intravenous administration of 100 μg of GnRH. A minimally acceptable response is a twofold LH increase and a 50% FSH increase. In the prepubertal period or with severe GnRH deficiency, the gonadotrope may not respond to a single bolus of GnRH because it has not been primed by endogenous hypothalamic GnRH; in these patients, GnRH responsiveness may be restored by chronic, pulsatile GnRH administration. With the availability of sensitive and specific LH assays, GnRH stimulation testing is used rarely except to evaluate gonadotrope function in patients who have undergone pituitary surgery or have a space-occupying lesion in the hypothalamic-pituitary region.

TESTOSTERONE ASSAYS

Total Testosterone   Total testosterone includes both unbound and protein-bound testosterone and is measured by radioimmunoassays, immunometric assays, or liquid chromatography tandem mass spectrometry (LC-MS/MS). LC-MS/MS involves extraction of serum by organic solvents, separation of testosterone from other steroids by high-performance liquid chromatography and mass spectrometry, and quantitation of unique testosterone fragments by mass spectrometry. LC-MS/MS provides accurate and sensitive measurements of testosterone levels even in the low range and is emerging as the method of choice for testosterone measurement. A single random sample provides a good approximation of the average testosterone concentration with the realization that testosterone levels fluctuate in response to pulsatile LH. Testosterone is generally lower in the late afternoon and is reduced by acute illness. The testosterone concentration in healthy young men ranges from 300 to 1000 ng/dL in most laboratories, although these reference ranges are not derived from population-based random samples. Alterations in SHBG levels due to aging, obesity, some types of medications, or chronic illness, or on a congenital basis, can affect total testosterone levels.

Measurement of Unbound Testosterone Levels   Most circulating testosterone is bound to SHBG and to albumin; only 0.5–3% of circulating testosterone is unbound, or "free." The unbound testosterone concentration can be measured by equilibrium dialysis or calculated from total testosterone, SHBG, and albumin concentrations by using published mass-action equations. Tracer analogue methods are relatively inexpensive and convenient, but they are inaccurate. *Bioavailable testosterone* refers to unbound testosterone plus testosterone that is loosely bound to albumin; it can be estimated by the ammonium sulfate precipitation method.

hCG Stimulation Test   The hCG stimulation test is performed by administering a single injection of 1500–4000 IU of hCG intramuscularly and measuring testosterone levels at baseline and 24, 48, 72, and 120 h after hCG injection. An alternative regimen involves three injections of 1500 units of hCG on successive days and measuring testosterone levels 24 h after the last dose. An acceptable response to hCG is a doubling of the testosterone concentration in adult men. In prepubertal boys, an increase in testosterone to >150 ng/dL indicates the presence of testicular tissue. No response may indicate an absence of testicular tissue or marked impairment of Leydig cell function. Measurement of MIS, a Sertoli cell product, is also used to detect the presence of testes in prepubertal boys with cryptorchidism.

SEMEN ANALYSIS

Semen analysis is the most important step in the evaluation of male infertility. Samples are collected by masturbation following a period of abstinence for 2–3 days. Semen volumes and sperm concentrations vary considerably among fertile men, and several samples may be needed before concluding that the results are abnormal. Analysis should be performed within an hour of collection. The normal ejaculate volume is 2–6 mL and contains sperm counts of >20 million/mL, with a motility of >50% and >15% normal morphology. Some men with low sperm counts are nevertheless fertile. A variety of tests for sperm function can be performed in specialized laboratories, but these add relatively little to the treatment options.

TESTICULAR BIOPSY

Testicular biopsy is useful in some patients with oligospermia or azoospermia as an aid in diagnosis and indication for the feasibility of treatment. Using local anesthesia, fine-needle aspiration biopsy is performed to aspirate tissue for histology. Alternatively, open biopsies can be performed under local or general anesthesia when more tissue is required. A normal biopsy in an azoospermic man with a normal FSH level suggests obstruction of the vas deferens, which may be correctable surgically. Biopsies are also used to harvest sperm for ICSI and to classify disorders such as hypospermatogenesis (all stages present but in reduced numbers), germ cell arrest (usually at primary spermatocyte stage), and Sertoli cell–only syndrome (absent germ cells) or hyalinization (sclerosis with absent cellular elements).

DISORDERS OF SEXUAL DIFFERENTIATION

See Chap. 343.

DISORDERS OF PUBERTY

PRECOCIOUS PUBERTY

Puberty in boys before age 9 is considered precocious. *Isosexual precocity* refers to premature sexual development consistent with phenotypic sex and includes features such as the development of facial hair and phallic growth. Isosexual precocity is divided into gonadotropin-dependent and gonadotropin-independent causes of androgen excess (Table 340-1). *Heterosexual precocity* refers to the premature development of estrogenic features in boys, such as breast development.

Gonadotropin-Dependent Precocious Puberty
This disorder, called *central precocious puberty* (CPP), is less common in boys than in girls. It is caused by premature activation of the GnRH pulse generator, sometimes because of central nervous system (CNS) lesions such as hypothalamic hamartomas, but it is often idiopathic. CPP is characterized by gonadotropin levels that are inappropriately elevated for age. Because pituitary priming has occurred, GnRH elicits LH and FSH responses typical of those seen in puberty or in adults. MRI should be performed to exclude a mass, structural defect, infection, or inflammatory process.

Gonadotropin-Independent Precocious Puberty
Androgens from the testis or the adrenal are increased but gonadotropins are low. This group of disorders includes hCG-secreting tumors; congenital adrenal hyperplasia; sex steroid–producing tumors of the testis, adrenal, and ovary; accidental or deliberate exogenous sex steroid administration; hypothyroidism; and activating mutations of the LH receptor or $G_s\alpha$ subunit.

FAMILIAL MALE-LIMITED PRECOCIOUS PUBERTY
Also called *testotoxicosis*, familial male-limited precocious puberty is an autosomal dominant

---

TABLE 340-1 CAUSES OF PRECOCIOUS OR DELAYED PUBERTY IN BOYS

I. Precocious puberty
  A. Gonadotropin-dependent
    1. Idiopathic
    2. Hypothalamic hamartoma or other lesions
    3. CNS tumor or inflammatory state
  B. Gonadotropin-independent
    1. Congenital adrenal hyperplasia
    2. hCG-secreting tumor
    3. McCune-Albright syndrome
    4. Activating LH receptor mutation
    5. Exogenous androgens

II. Delayed puberty
  A. Constitutional delay of growth and puberty
  B. Systemic disorders
    1. Chronic disease
    2. Malnutrition
    3. Anorexia nervosa
  C. CNS tumors and their treatment (radiotherapy and surgery)
  D. Hypothalamic-pituitary causes of pubertal failure (low gonadotropins)
    1. Congenital disorders (Table 340-2)
      a. Hypothalamic syndromes (e.g., Prader-Willi)
      b. Idiopathic hypogonadotropic hypogonadism
      c. Kallmann syndrome
      d. GnRH receptor mutations
      e. Adrenal hypoplasia congenita
      f. PROP1 mutations
      g. Other mutations affecting pituitary development/function
    2. Acquired disorders
      a. Pituitary tumors
      b. Hyperprolactinemia
  E. Gonadal causes of pubertal failure (elevated gonadotropins)
    1. Klinefelter syndrome
    2. Bilateral undescended testes or anorchia
    3. Orchitis
    4. Chemotherapy or radiotherapy
  F. Androgen insensitivity

Note: CNS, central nervous system; hCG, human chronic gonadotropin; LH, luteinizing hormone; GnRH, gonadotropin-releasing hormone.

---

disorder caused by activating mutations in the LH receptor, leading to constitutive stimulation of the cyclic AMP pathway and testosterone production. Clinical features include premature androgenization in boys, growth acceleration in early childhood, and advanced bone age followed by premature epiphyseal fusion. Testosterone is elevated, and LH is suppressed. Treatment options include inhibitors of testosterone synthesis (e.g., ketoconazole), androgen receptor antagonists (e.g., flutamide), and aromatase inhibitors (e.g., anastrazole).

MCCUNE-ALBRIGHT SYNDROME This is a sporadic disorder caused by somatic (postzygotic) activating mutations in the $G_s\alpha$ subunit that links G protein–coupled receptors to intracellular signaling pathways (Chap. 349). The mutations impair the guanosine triphosphatase activity of the $G_s\alpha$ protein, leading to constitutive activation of adenylyl cyclase. Like activating LH receptor mutations, this stimulates testosterone production and causes gonadotropin-independent precocious puberty. In addition to sexual precocity, affected individuals may have autonomy in the adrenals, pituitary, and thyroid glands. Café au lait spots are characteristic skin lesions that reflect the onset of the somatic mutations in melanocytes during embryonic development. Polyostotic fibrous dysplasia is caused by activation of the parathyroid hormone receptor pathway in bone. Treatment is similar to that in patients with activating LH receptor mutations. Bisphosphonates have been used to treat bone lesions.

CONGENITAL ADRENAL HYPERPLASIA Boys with congenital adrenal hyperplasia (CAH) who are not well controlled with glucocorticoid suppression of adrenocorticotropic hormone (ACTH) can develop premature virilization because of excessive androgen production by the adrenal gland (Chaps. 336 and 343). LH is low, and the testes are small. Rarely, adrenal rests may develop within the testis because of chronic ACTH stimulation.

Heterosexual Sexual Precocity Breast enlargement in prepubertal boys can result from familial aromatase excess, estrogen-producing tumors in the adrenal gland, Sertoli cell tumors in the testis, marijuana smoking, or exogenous estrogens or androgens. Occasionally, germ cell tumors that secrete hCG can be associated with breast enlargement due to excessive stimulation of estrogen production (see "Gynecomastia," below).

APPROACH TO THE PATIENT:
Precocious Puberty

After verification of precocious development, serum LH and FSH levels should be measured to determine whether gonadotropins are increased in relation to chronologic age (gonadotropin-dependent) or whether sex steroid secretion is occurring independent of LH and FSH (gonadotropin-independent). In children with gonadotropin-dependent precocious puberty, CNS lesions should be excluded by history, neurologic examination, and MRI scan of the head. If organic causes are not found, one is left with the diagnosis of idiopathic central precocity. Patients with high testosterone but suppressed LH concentrations have gonadotropin-independent sexual precocity; in these patients, DHEA sulfate (DHEAS) and 17α-hydroxyprogesterone should be measured. High levels of testosterone and 17α-hydroxyprogesterone suggest the possibility of CAH due to 21α-hydroxylase or 11β-hydroxylase deficiency. If testosterone and DHEAS are elevated, adrenal tumors should be excluded by obtaining a CT scan of the adrenal glands. Patients with elevated testosterone but without increased 17α-hydroxyprogesterone or DHEAS should undergo careful evaluation of the testis by palpation and ultrasound to exclude a Leydig cell neoplasm. Activating mutations of the LH receptor should be considered in children with gonadotropin-independent precocious puberty in whom CAH, androgen abuse, and adrenal and testicular neoplasms have been excluded.

℞ PRECOCIOUS PUBERTY

In patients with a known cause (e.g., a CNS lesion or a testicular tumor), therapy should be directed towards the underlying disorder. In patients with idiopathic CPP, long-acting GnRH analogues can be used to suppress gonadotropins and decrease testosterone, halt early pubertal development, delay accelerated bone maturation, and prevent early epiphyseal closure, without causing osteoporosis. The treatment is most effective for increasing final adult height if it is initiated before age 6. Puberty resumes after discontinuation of the GnRH analogue. Counseling is an important aspect of the overall treatment strategy.

In children with gonadotropin-independent precocious puberty, inhibitors of steroidogenesis, such as ketoconazole, and AR antagonists have been used empirically. Long-term treatment with spironolactone (a weak androgen antagonist), testolactone (aromatase inhibitor), and ketoconazole has been reported to normalize growth rate and bone maturation and to improve predicted height in small, nonrandomized trials in boys with familial male-limited precocious puberty.

DELAYED PUBERTY

Puberty is delayed in boys if it has not ensued by age 14, an age that is 2–2.5 standard deviations above the mean for healthy children. Delayed puberty is more common in boys than in girls. There are four main categories of delayed puberty: (1) constitutional delay of growth and puberty (~60% of cases); (2) functional hypogonadotropic hypogonadism caused by systemic illness or malnutrition (~20% of cases); (3) hypogonadotropic hypogonadism caused by genetic or acquired defects in the hypothalamic-pituitary region (~10% of cases); and (4) hypergonadotropic hypogonadism secondary to primary gonadal failure (~15% of cases) (Table 340-1). Functional hypogonadotropic hypogonadism is more common in girls than in boys. Permanent causes of hypogonadotropic or hypergonadotropic hypogonadism are identified in <25% of boys with delayed puberty.

APPROACH TO THE PATIENT:
Delayed Puberty

Any history of systemic illness, eating disorders, excessive exercise, social and psychological problems, and abnormal patterns of linear growth during childhood should be verified. Boys with pubertal delay may have accompanying emotional and physical immaturity relative to their peers, which can be a source of anxiety. Physical examination should focus on height; arm span; weight; visual fields; and secondary sex characteristics, including hair growth, testicular volume, phallic size, and scrotal reddening and thinning. Testicular size >2.5 cm generally indicates that the child has entered puberty.

The main diagnostic challenge is to distinguish those with constitutional delay, who will progress through puberty at a later age, from those with an underlying pathologic process. Constitutional delay should be suspected when there is a family history and when there are delayed bone age and short stature. Pituitary priming by pulsatile GnRH is required before LH and FSH are synthesized and secreted normally. Thus, blunted responses to exogenous GnRH can be seen in patients with constitutional delay, GnRH deficiency, or pituitary disorders (see "GnRH Stimulation Testing," above). On the other hand, low-normal basal gonadotropin levels or a normal response to exogenous GnRH is consistent with an early stage of puberty, which is often heralded by nocturnal GnRH secretion. Thus, constitutional delay is a diagnosis of exclusion that requires ongoing evaluation until the onset of puberty and the growth spurt.

℞ DELAYED PUBERTY

If therapy is considered appropriate, it can begin with 25–50 mg testosterone enanthate or testosterone cypionate every 2 weeks, or by using a 2.5-mg testosterone patch or 25-mg testosterone gel. Because aromatization of testosterone to estrogen is obligatory for mediating androgen effects on epiphyseal fusion, concomitant treatment with aromatase inhibitors may allow attainment of greater final adult height. Testosterone treatment should be interrupted after 6 months to determine if endogenous LH and FSH secretion have ensued. Other causes of delayed puberty should be considered when there are associated clinical features or when boys do not enter puberty spontaneously after a year of observation or treatment.

Reassurance without hormonal treatment is appropriate for many individuals with presumed constitutional delay of puberty. However, the impact of delayed growth and pubertal progression on a child's social relationships and school performance should be weighed. Also, boys with constitutional delay of puberty are less likely to achieve their full genetic height potential and have reduced total body bone mass as adults, mainly due to narrow limb bones and vertebrae as a result of impaired periosteal expansion during puberty. Administration of androgen therapy to boys with constitutional delay does not affect final height, and when administered with an aromatase inhibitor, it may improve final height.

DISORDERS OF THE MALE REPRODUCTIVE AXIS DURING ADULTHOOD

HYPOGONADOTROPIC HYPOGONADISM

Because LH and FSH are trophic hormones for the testes, impaired secretion of these pituitary gonadotropins results in secondary hypogonadism, which is characterized by low testosterone in the setting of low LH and FSH. Those with the most severe deficiency have complete absence of pubertal development, sexual infantilism, and, in some cases, hypospadias and undescended testes. Patients with partial gonadotropin deficiency have delayed or arrested sex development. The 24-h LH secretory profiles are heterogeneous in patients with hypogonadotropic hypogonadism, reflecting variable abnormalities of LH pulse frequency or amplitude. In severe cases, basal LH is low and there are no LH pulses. A smaller subset of patients has low-amplitude LH pulses or markedly reduced pulse frequency. Occasionally, only sleep-entrained LH pulses occur, reminiscent of the pattern seen in the early stages of puberty. Hypogonadotropic hypogonadism can be classified

TABLE 340-2 **CAUSES OF CONGENITAL HYPOGONADOTROPIC HYPOGONADISM**

Gene	Locus	Inheritance	Associated Features
KAL1	Xp22	X-linked	Anosmia, renal agenesis, synkinesia, cleft lip/palate, oculomotor/visuospatial defects, gut malrotations
NELF	9q34.3	AR	Anosmia, hypogonadotropic hypogonadism
FGFR1	8p11-p12	AD	Anosmia, cleft lip/palate, synkinesia, syndactyly
PROK2	20p13	AR	Anosmia, hypogonadotropic hypogonadism
LEP	7q31	AR	Obesity
LEPR	1p31	AR	Obesity
PC1	5q15-21	AR	Obesity, diabetes mellitus, ACTH deficiency
HESX1	3p21	AR	Septooptic dysplasia, CPHD
		AD	Isolated GH insufficiency
LHX3	9q34	AR	CPHD (ACTH spared), cervical spine rigidity
PROP1	5q35	AR	CPHD (ACTH usually spared)
GPR54	19p13	AR	None
GNRHR	4q21	AR	None
FSHβ	11p13	AR	↑ LH
LHβ	19q13	AR	↑ FSH
SF1 (NR5A1)	9p33	AD/AR	Primary adrenal failure, XY sex reversal
DAX1 (NR0B1)	Xp21	X-linked	Primary adrenal failure, impaired spermatogenesis

Abbreviations: ACTH, adrenocorticotropic hormone; AD, autosomal dominant; AR, autosomal recessive; CPHD, combined pituitary hormone deficiency; KAL1, Interval-1 gene; NELF, nasal embryonic LHRH factor; FGFR1, fibroblast growth factor receptor 1; PROK2, prokineticin 2; LEP, leptin; LEPR, leptin receptor; PC1, prohormone convertase 1; HESX1, homeo box gene expressed in embryonic stem cells 1; LHX3, LIM homeobox gene 3; PROP1, Prophet of Pit 1; GPR54, G protein–coupled receptor 54; GNRHR, gonadotropin-releasing hormone receptor; FSHβ, follicle-stimulating hormone β-subunit; LHβ, luteinizing hormone β-subunit; SF1, steroidogenic factor 1; DAX1, dosage-sensitive sex-reversal, adrenal hypoplasia congenita, X-chromosome.

into congenital and acquired disorders. Congenital disorders most commonly involve GnRH deficiency, which leads to gonadotropin deficiency. Acquired disorders are much more common than congenital disorders and may result from a variety of sellar mass lesions or infiltrative diseases of the hypothalamus or pituitary.

Congenital Disorders Associated with Gonadotropin Deficiency

Most cases of congenital hypogonadotropic hypogonadism are idiopathic, despite extensive endocrine testing and imaging studies of the sellar region. Among known causes, familial hypogonadotropic hypogonadism can be transmitted as an X-linked (20%), autosomal recessive (30%), or autosomal dominant (50%) trait. Some individuals with idiopathic hypogonadotropic hypogonadism (IHH) have sporadic mutations in the same genes that cause inherited forms of the disorder. *Kallmann syndrome* is an X-linked disorder caused by mutations in the *KAL1* gene, which encodes anosmin, a protein that mediates the migration of neural progenitors of the olfactory bulb and GnRH-producing neurons. These individuals have GnRH deficiency and variable combinations of anosmia or hyposmia, renal defects, and neurologic abnormalities including mirror movements. Gonadotropin secretion and fertility can be restored by administration of pulsatile GnRH or by gonadotropin replacement. Mutations in the *FGFR1* gene cause an autosomal dominant form of hypogonadotropic hypogonadism that clinically resembles Kallmann syndrome. Prokineticin 2 (PROK2) also encodes a protein involved in migration and development of olfactory and GnRH neurons. Recessive mutations in PROK2 cause anosmia and hypogonadotropic hypogonadism. The *FGFR1* gene product may be the receptor for the *KAL1* gene product, anosmin, thereby explaining the similarity in clinical features. Other autosomal dominant causes remain unexplained. X-linked hypogonadotropic hypogonadism also occurs in *adrenal hypoplasia congenita*, a disorder caused by mutations in the *DAX1* gene, which encodes a nuclear receptor in the adrenal gland and reproductive axis. Adrenal hypoplasia congenita is characterized by absent development of the adult zone of the adrenal cortex, leading to neonatal adrenal insufficiency. Puberty usually does not occur or is arrested, reflecting variable degrees of gonadotropin deficiency. Although sexual differentiation is normal, some patients have testicular dysgenesis and impaired spermatogenesis despite gonadotropin replacement. Less commonly, adrenal hypoplasia congenita, sex reversal, and hypogonadotropic hypogonadism can be caused by mutations of steroidogenic factor 1 (SF1). *GnRH receptor mutations*

account for ~40% of autosomal recessive and 10% of sporadic cases of hypogonadotropic hypogonadism. These patients have decreased LH response to exogenous GnRH. Some receptor mutations alter GnRH binding affinity, allowing apparently normal responses to pharmacologic doses of exogenous GnRH, whereas other mutations may alter signal transduction downstream of hormone binding. Recessive mutations in the G protein–coupled receptor GPR54 cause gonadotropin deficiency without anosmia. Patients retain responsiveness to exogenous GnRH, suggesting an abnormality in the neural pathways controlling GnRH release. Rarely, recessive mutations in the *LHβ* or *FSHβ* genes have been described in patients with selective deficiencies of these gonadotropins. Deletions or mutations of the *GnRH* gene have not been found in patients with hypogonadotropic hypogonadism.

A number of homeodomain transcription factors are involved in the development and differentiation of the specialized hormone-producing cells within the pituitary gland (Table 340-2). Patients with mutations of *PROP1* have combined pituitary hormone deficiency that includes GH, prolactin (PRL) thyroid-stimulating hormone (TSH), LH, and FSH, but not ACTH. *LHX3* mutations cause combined pituitary hormone deficiency in association with cervical spine rigidity. *HESX1* mutations cause septooptic dysplasia and combined pituitary hormone deficiency.

Prader-Willi syndrome is characterized by obesity, hypotonic musculature, mental retardation, hypogonadism, short stature, and small hands and feet. Prader-Willi syndrome is a genomic imprinting disorder caused by deletions of the proximal portion of paternally derived chromosome 15q, uniparental disomy of the maternal alleles, or mutations of the genes/loci involved in imprinting (Chap. 63). *Laurence-Moon syndrome* is an autosomal recessive disorder characterized by obesity, hypogonadism, mental retardation, polydactyly, and retinitis pigmentosa. Recessive mutations of leptin, or its receptor, cause severe obesity and pubertal arrest, apparently because of hypothalamic GnRH deficiency (Chap. 74).

Acquired Hypogonadotropic Disorders • SEVERE ILLNESS, STRESS, MALNUTRITION, AND EXERCISE

These may cause reversible gonadotropin deficiency. Although gonadotropin deficiency and reproductive dysfunction are well documented in these conditions in women, men exhibit similar but less-pronounced responses. Unlike women, most male runners and other endurance athletes have normal gonadotropin and sex steroid levels, despite low body fat and frequent intensive exercise. Testosterone levels fall at the onset of illness and recover during recuperation. The magnitude of gonadotropin suppression generally correlates with the severity of illness. Although hypogonadotropic hypogonadism is the most common cause of androgen deficiency in patients with acute illness, some have elevated levels of LH and FSH, which suggest primary gonadal dysfunction. The pathophysiology of reproductive dysfunction during acute illness is unknown but likely involves a combination of cytokine and/or glucocorticoid effects. There is a high frequency of low testosterone levels in patients with chronic illnesses such as HIV infection, end-stage renal disease, chronic obstructive lung disease, and many types of cancer and in patients receiving glucocorticoids. About 20% of HIV-infected men with low testosterone levels have elevated LH and FSH levels; these patients presumably have primary testicular dysfunction. The remaining 80% have either normal or low LH and FSH levels; these men have a central hypothalamic-pituitary defect or a dual defect involving both the testis and the hypothalamic-pituitary centers. Muscle wasting is common in chronic diseases associated with hypogonadism, which also leads to debility, poor quality of life, and adverse outcome of disease. There is great interest in exploring strategies that can reverse androgen deficiency or attenuate the sarcopenia associated with chronic illness.

Men using opioids for relief of cancer or noncancerous pain or because of addiction often have suppressed testosterone and LH levels; the degree of suppression is dose-related. Opioids suppress GnRH secretion and alter the sensitivity to feedback inhibition by gonadal steroids. Men who are heavy users of marijuana have decreased testosterone secretion and sperm production. The mechanism of marijuana-induced hypogonadism is decreased GnRH secretion. Gynecomastia observed in marijuana users can also be caused by plant estrogens in crude preparations.

OBESITY   In men with mild to moderate obesity, SHBG levels decrease in proportion to the degree of obesity, resulting in lower total testosterone levels. However, free testosterone levels usually remain within the normal range. The decrease in SHBG levels is caused by increased circulating insulin, which inhibits SHBG production. Estradiol levels are higher in obese men compared to healthy, nonobese controls, because of aromatization of testosterone to estradiol in adipose tissue. Weight loss is associated with reversal of these abnormalities including an increase in total and free testosterone levels and a decrease in estradiol levels. A subset of massively obese men may have a defect in the hypothalamic-pituitary axis as suggested by low free testosterone in the absence of elevated gonadotropins. Weight gain in adult men can accelerate the rate of age-related decline in testosterone levels.

HYPERPROLACTINEMIA   (See also Chap. 333.) Elevated PRL levels are associated with hypogonadotropic hypogonadism. PRL inhibits hypothalamic GnRH secretion either directly or through modulation of tuberoinfundibular dopaminergic pathways. A PRL-secreting tumor may also destroy the surrounding gonadotropes by invasion or compression of the pituitary stalk. Treatment with dopamine agonists reverses gonadotropin deficiency, although there may be a delay relative to PRL suppression.

SELLAR MASS LESIONS   Neoplastic and nonneoplastic lesions in the hypothalamus or pituitary can directly or indirectly affect gonadotrope function. In adults, pituitary adenomas constitute the largest category of space-occupying lesions affecting gonadotropin and other pituitary hormone production. Pituitary adenomas that extend into the suprasellar region can impair GnRH secretion and mildly increase PRL secretion (usually <50 μg/L) because of impaired tonic inhibition by dopaminergic pathways. These tumors should be distinguished from prolactinomas, which typically secrete higher PRL levels. The presence of diabetes insipidus suggests the possibility of a craniopharyngioma, infiltrative disorder, or other hypothalamic lesions (Chap. 334).

HEMOCHROMATOSIS   (See also Chap. 351.) Both the pituitary and testis can be affected by excessive iron deposition. However, the pituitary defect is the predominant lesion in most patients with hemochromatosis and hypogonadism. The diagnosis of hemochromatosis is suggested by the association of characteristic skin discoloration, hepatic enlargement or dysfunction, diabetes mellitus, arthritis, cardiac conduction defects, and hypogonadism.

PRIMARY TESTICULAR CAUSES OF HYPOGONADISM

Common causes of primary testicular dysfunction include Klinefelter syndrome, uncorrected cryptorchidism, cancer chemotherapy, radiation to the testes, trauma, torsion, infectious orchitis, HIV infection, anorchia syndrome, and myotonic dystrophy. Primary testicular disorders may be associated with impaired spermatogenesis, decreased androgen production, or both. See Chap. 343 for disorders of testis development, androgen synthesis, and androgen action.

Klinefelter Syndrome   (See also Chap. 343.) Klinefelter syndrome is the most common chromosomal disorder associated with testicular dysfunction and male infertility. It occurs in about 1 in 1000 live-born males. Azoospermia is the rule in men with Klinefelter syndrome who

have the 47,XXY karyotype; however, men with mosaicism may have germ cells, especially at a younger age. Testicular histology shows hyalinization of seminiferous tubules and absence of spermatogenesis. Although their function is impaired, the number of Leydig cells appears to increase. Testosterone is decreased and estradiol is increased, leading to clinical features of undervirilization and gynecomastia. Men with Klinefelter syndrome are at increased risk of breast cancer, non-Hodgkin's lymphoma, and lung cancer, and reduced risk of prostate cancer. Periodic mammography for breast cancer surveillance is recommended for men with Klinefelter syndrome.

Cryptorchidism   Cryptorchidism occurs when there is incomplete descent of the testis from the abdominal cavity into the scrotum. About 3% of full-term and 30% of premature male infants have at least one cryptorchid testis at birth, but descent is usually complete by the first few weeks of life. The incidence of cryptorchidism is <1% by 9 months of age. Cryptorchidism is associated with increased risk of malignancy and infertility. Unilateral cryptorchidism, even when corrected before puberty, is associated with decreased sperm count, possibly reflecting unrecognized damage to the fully descended testis or other genetic factors. Epidemiologic, clinical, and molecular evidence supports the idea that cryptorchidism, hypospadias, impaired spermatogenesis, and testicular cancer may be causally related to common genetic and environment perturbations, and are components of the testicular dysgenesis syndrome.

Acquired Testicular Defects   *Viral orchitis* may be caused by the mumps virus, echovirus, lymphocytic choriomeningitis virus, and group B arboviruses. Orchitis occurs in as many as one-fourth of adult men with mumps; the orchitis is unilateral in about two-thirds and bilateral in the remainder. Orchitis usually develops a few days after the onset of parotitis but may precede it. The testis may return to normal size and function or undergo atrophy. Semen analysis returns to normal for three-fourths of men with unilateral involvement but normal for only one-third of men with bilateral orchitis. *Trauma*, including testicular torsion, can also cause secondary atrophy of the testes. The exposed position of the testes in the scrotum renders them susceptible to both thermal and physical trauma, particularly in men with hazardous occupations.

The testes are sensitive to *radiation damage*. Doses >200 mGy (20 rad) are associated with increased FSH and LH levels and damage to the spermatogonia. After ~800 mGy (80 rad), oligospermia or azoospermia develops, and higher doses may obliterate the germinal epithelium. Permanent androgen deficiency in adult men is uncommon after therapeutic radiation; however, most boys given direct testicular radiation therapy for acute lymphoblastic leukemia have permanently low testosterone levels. Sperm banking should be considered before patients undergo radiation treatment or chemotherapy.

Drugs interfere with testicular function by several mechanisms, including inhibition of testosterone synthesis (e.g., ketoconazole), blockade of androgen action (e.g., spironolactone), increased estrogen (e.g., marijuana), or direct inhibition of spermatogenesis (e.g., chemotherapy).

Combination chemotherapy for acute leukemia, Hodgkin's disease, and testicular and other cancers may impair Leydig cell function and cause infertility. The degree of gonadal dysfunction depends on the type of chemotherapeutic agent and the dose and duration of therapy. Because of high response rates and the young age of these men, infertility and androgen deficiency have emerged as important long-term complications of cancer chemotherapy. Cyclophosphamide and combination regimens containing procarbazine are particularly toxic to germ cells. Thus, 90% of men with Hodgkin's lymphoma receiving MOPP (mechlorethamine, oncovin, procarbazine, prednisone) therapy develop azoospermia or extreme oligozoospermia; newer regimens that do not include procarbazine, such as ABVD (adriamycin, bleomycin, vinblastine, dacarbazine), are less toxic to germ cells.

Alcohol, when consumed in excess for prolonged periods, decreases testosterone, independent of liver disease or malnutrition. Elevated estradiol and decreased testosterone levels may occur in men taking digitalis.

The occupational and recreational history should be carefully evaluated in all men with infertility because of the toxic effects of many *chemical agents* on spermatogenesis. Known environmental hazards include microwaves and ultrasound and chemicals such as nematocide dibromochloropropane, cadmium, phthalates, and lead. In some populations, sperm density is said to have declined by as much as 40% in the past 50 years. Environmental estrogens or antiandrogens may be partly responsible.

Testicular failure also occurs as a part of *polyglandular autoimmune insufficiency* (Chap. 345). Sperm antibodies can cause isolated male infertility. In some instances, these antibodies are secondary phenomena resulting from duct obstruction or vasectomy. Granulomatous diseases can affect the testes, and testicular atrophy occurs in 10–20% of men with lepromatous leprosy because of direct tissue invasion by the mycobacteria. The tubules are involved initially, followed by endarteritis and destruction of Leydig cells.

Systemic disease can cause primary testis dysfunction in addition to suppressing gonadotropin production. In cirrhosis, a combined testicular and pituitary abnormality leads to decreased testosterone production independent of the direct toxic effects of ethanol. Impaired hepatic extraction of adrenal androstenedione leads to extraglandular conversion to estrone and estradiol, which partially suppresses LH. Testicular atrophy and gynecomastia are present in approximately one-half of men with cirrhosis. In chronic renal failure, androgen synthesis and sperm production decrease despite elevated gonadotropins. The elevated LH level is due to reduced clearance, but it does not restore normal testosterone production. About one-fourth of men with renal failure have hyperprolactinemia. Improvement in testosterone production with hemodialysis is incomplete, but successful renal transplantation may return testicular function to normal. Testicular atrophy is present in one-third of men with sickle cell anemia. The defect may be at either the testicular or the hypothalamic-pituitary level. Sperm density can decrease temporarily after acute febrile illness in the absence of a change in testosterone production. Infertility in men with celiac disease is associated with a hormonal pattern typical of androgen resistance, namely elevated testosterone and LH levels.

Neurologic diseases associated with altered testicular function include myotonic dystrophy, spinobulbar muscular atrophy, and paraplegia. In myotonic dystrophy, small testes may be associated with impairment of both spermatogenesis and Leydig cell function. Spinobulbar muscular atrophy is caused by an expansion of the glutamine repeat sequences in the amino-terminal region of the AR; this expansion impairs function of the AR, but it is unclear how the alteration is related to the neurologic manifestations. Men with spinobulbar muscular atrophy often have undervirilization and infertility as a late manifestation. Spinal cord lesions that cause paraplegia can lead to a temporary decrease in testosterone levels and may cause persistent defects in spermatogenesis; some patients retain the capacity for penile erection and ejaculation.

ANDROGEN INSENSITIVITY SYNDROMES

Mutations in the AR cause resistance to the action of testosterone and DHT. These X-linked mutations are associated with variable degrees of defective male phenotypic development and undervirilization (Chap. 343). Although not technically hormone-insensitivity syndromes, two genetic disorders impair testosterone conversion to active sex steroids. Mutations in the *SRD5A2* gene, which encodes 5α-reductase type 2, prevent the conversion of testosterone to DHT, which is necessary for the normal development of the male external genitalia. Mutations in the *CYP19* gene, which encodes aromatase, prevent testosterone conversion to estradiol. Males with *CYP19* mutations have delayed epiphyseal fusion, tall stature, eunuchoid proportions, and osteoporosis, consistent with evidence from an estrogen receptor–deficient individual that these testosterone actions are mediated indirectly via estrogen.

GYNECOMASTIA

Gynecomastia refers to enlargement of the male breast. It is caused by excess estrogen action and is usually the result of an increased estrogen/androgen ratio. True gynecomastia is associated with glandular breast tissue that is >4 cm in diameter and often tender. Glandular tissue enlargement should be distinguished from excess adipose tissue: glandular tissue is firmer and contains fibrous-like cords. Gynecomastia occurs as a normal physiologic phenomenon in the newborn (due to transplacental transfer of maternal and placental estrogens), during puberty (high estrogen to androgen ratio in early stages of puberty), and with aging (increased fat tissue and increased aromatase activity), but it can also result from pathologic conditions associated with androgen deficiency or estrogen excess. The prevalence of gynecomastia increases with age and body mass index (BMI), likely because of increased aromatase activity in adipose tissue. Medications that alter androgen metabolism or action may also cause gynecomastia. The relative risk of breast cancer is increased in men with gynecomastia, although the absolute risk is relatively small.

PATHOLOGIC GYNECOMASTIA

Any cause of *androgen deficiency* can lead to gynecomastia, reflecting an increased estrogen/androgen ratio, as estrogen synthesis still occurs by aromatization of residual adrenal and gonadal androgens. Gynecomastia is a characteristic feature of Klinefelter syndrome (Chap. 343). *Androgen insensitivity* disorders also cause gynecomastia. *Excess estrogen production* may be caused by tumors, including Sertoli cell tumors in isolation or in association with Peutz-Jegher syndrome or Carney complex. Tumors that produce hCG, including some testicular tumors, stimulate Leydig cell estrogen synthesis. *Increased conversion of androgens to estrogens* can be a result of increased availability of substrate (androstenedione) for extraglandular estrogen formation (CAH, hyperthyroidism, and most feminizing adrenal tumors) or to diminished catabolism of androstenedione (liver disease) so that estrogen precursors are shunted to aromatase in peripheral sites. Obesity is associated with increased aromatization of androgen precursors to estrogens. Extraglandular aromatase activity can also be increased in tumors of the liver or adrenal gland or rarely as an inherited disorder. Several families with *increased peripheral aromatase activity* inherited as an autosomal dominant or as an X-linked disorder have been described. In some families with this disorder, an inversion in chromosome 15q21.2-3 causes the CYP19 gene to be activated by the regulatory elements of contiguous genes resulting in excessive estrogen production in the fat and other extragonadal tissues. *Drugs* can cause gynecomastia by acting directly as estrogenic substances (e.g., oral contraceptives, phytoestrogens, digitalis), inhibiting androgen synthesis (e.g., ketoconazole), or action (e.g., spironolactone).

Because up to two-thirds of pubertal boys and half of hospitalized men have palpable glandular tissue that is benign, detailed investigation or intervention is not indicated in all men presenting with gynecomastia (Fig. 340-5). In addition to the extent of gynecomastia, recent onset, rapid growth, tender tissue, and occurrence in a lean subject should prompt more extensive evaluation. This should include a careful drug history, measurement and examination of the testes, assessment of virilization, evaluation of liver function, and hormonal measurements including testosterone, estradiol, and androstenedione, LH, and hCG. A karyotype should be obtained in men with very small testes to exclude Klinefelter syndrome. In spite of extensive evaluation, the etiology is established in fewer than one-half of patients.

℞ GYNECOMASTIA

When the primary cause can be identified and corrected, breast enlargement usually subsides over several months. However, if gynecomastia is of long duration, surgery is the most effective therapy. Indications for surgery include severe psychological and/or cosmetic problems, continued growth or tenderness, or suspected malignancy. In patients who have painful gynecomastia and in whom surgery cannot be performed, treatment with antiestrogens such as tamoxifen (20 mg/d) can reduce pain and breast tissue size in over half the patients. Aromatase inhibitors can be effective in the early proliferative phase of the disorder, although the experience is largely based on the use of testolactone, a relatively weak aromatase inhibitor; placebo-controlled trials with more potent aromatase inhibitors such

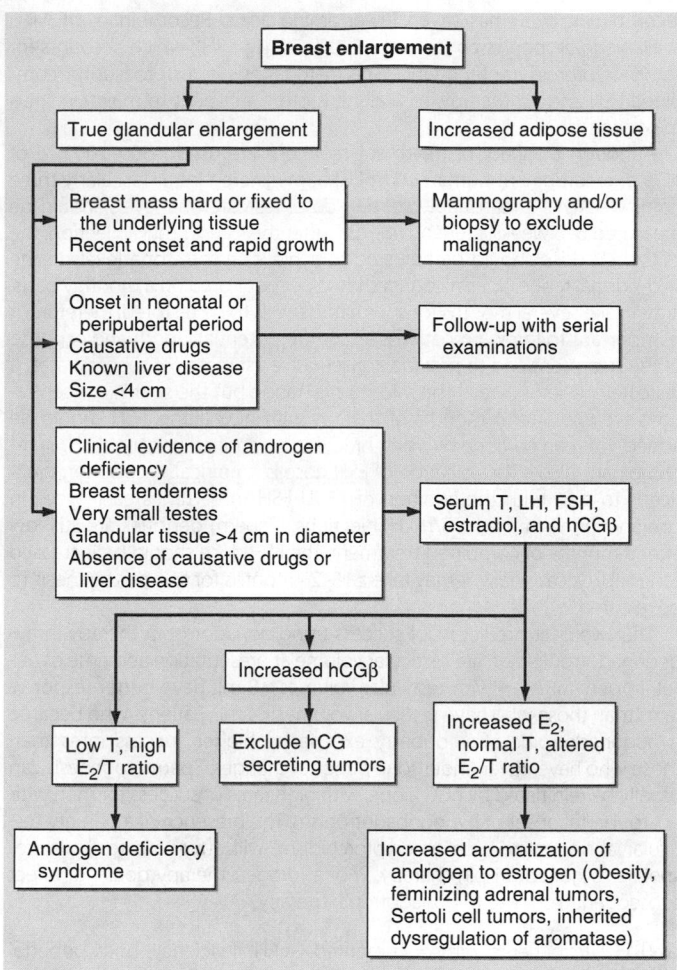

FIGURE 340-5 Evaluation of gynecomastia. T, testosterone; LH, lute-inizing hormone; FSH, follicle-stimulating hormones; hCGβ, human chorionic gonadotropin β; E$_2$, 17β-estradiol.

as anastrozole, fadrozole, letrozole, or formestane are needed. In a random-ized trial in men with established gynecomastia, anastrozole proved no more effective than placebo in reducing breast size.

AGING-RELATED CHANGES IN MALE REPRODUCTIVE FUNCTION

A number of cross-sectional and longitudinal studies (e.g., The Balti-more Longitudinal Study of Aging and the Massachusetts Male Aging Study) have established that testosterone concentrations decrease with advancing age. This age-related decline starts in the third decade of life and progresses slowly; the rate of decline in testosterone concentra-tions is greater for men with chronic illness and for those taking medi-cations than in healthy older men. Because SHBG concentrations are higher in older men than in younger men, free or bioavailable testoste-rone concentrations decline with aging to a greater extent than total testosterone concentrations. The age-related decline in testosterone is due to defects at all levels of the hypothalamic-pituitary-testicular axis: pulsatile GnRH secretion is attenuated, LH response to GnRH is re-duced, and testicular response to LH is impaired. However, the gradu-al rise of LH with aging suggests that testis dysfunction is the main cause of declining androgen levels. The term *andropause* has been used to denote age-related decline in testosterone concentrations; this term is a misnomer because there is no discrete time when testosterone con-centrations decline abruptly.

In epidemiologic surveys, low total and bioavailable testosterone concentrations have been associated with decreased appendicular skel-etal muscle mass and strength, decreased self-reported physical func-tion, higher visceral fat mass, insulin resistance, and increased risk of coronary artery disease and mortality. In systematic reviews of ran-domized controlled trials, testosterone therapy of healthy older men with low or low-normal testosterone levels was associated with greater increments in lean body mass, grip strength, and self-reported physi-cal function than that associated with placebo. Testosterone therapy also induced greater improvement in vertebral but not femoral bone mineral density. Testosterone therapy of older men with sexual dys-function and unequivocally low testosterone levels improves libido, but testosterone effects on erectile function and response to selective phosphodiesterase inhibitors have been inconsistent. Testosterone ther-apy has not been shown to improve depression scores, fracture risk, cognitive function, or clinical outcomes in older men. Furthermore, the long-term risks of testosterone supplementation in older men remain largely unknown. In particular, physiologic testosterone replacement might increase the risk of prostate cancer or exacerbate cardiovascular disease. Population screening of all older men for low testosterone lev-els is not recommended, and testing should be restricted to men who have symptoms or physical features attributable to androgen deficien-cy. Testosterone therapy is not recommended for all older men with low testosterone levels. In older men with significant symptoms of an-drogen deficiency who have testosterone levels below 200 ng/dL, tes-tosterone therapy may be considered on an individualized basis and should be instituted after careful discussion of the risks and benefits (see "Testosterone Replacement," below).

Testicular morphology, semen production, and fertility are main-tained up to a very old age in men. Although concern has been expressed about age-related increases in germ cell mutations and impairment of DNA repair mechanisms, the frequency of chromosomal aneuploidy or structural abnormalities does not increase in the sperm of older men. However, the incidence of autosomal dominant diseases, such as achon-droplasia, polyposis coli, Marfan syndrome, and Apert's syndrome, in-creases in the offspring of men who are advanced in age, consistent with transmission of sporadic missense mutations.

APPROACH TO THE PATIENT:
Androgen Deficiency

Hypogonadism is often heralded by decreased sex drive, reduced frequency of sexual intercourse or inability to maintain erections, reduced beard growth, loss of muscle mass, decreased testicular size, and gynecomastia. Less than 10% of patients with erectile dys-function alone have testosterone deficiency. Thus, it is useful to look for a constellation of symptoms and signs suggestive of andro-gen deficiency. Except when extreme, these clinical features may be difficult to distinguish from changes that occur with normal aging. Moreover, androgen deficiency may develop gradually. Population studies, such as the Massachusetts Male Aging Study, suggest that about 4% of men between the ages of 40 and 70 have testosterone levels <150 ng/dL. Thus, androgen deficiency is not uncommon.

When symptoms or clinical features suggest possible androgen deficiency, the laboratory evaluation is initiated by the measure-ment of total testosterone, preferably in the morning (Fig. 340-6). A total testosterone level <200 ng/dL measured by a reliable assay, in association with symptoms, is evidence of testosterone deficien-cy. An early-morning testosterone level >350 ng/dL makes the di-agnosis of androgen deficiency unlikely. In men with testosterone levels between 200 and 350 ng/dL, the total testosterone level should be repeated and a free testosterone level should be measured. In older men and in patients with other clinical states that are associ-ated with alterations in SHBG levels, a direct measurement of free testosterone level by equilibrium dialysis can be useful in unmask-ing testosterone deficiency.

When androgen deficiency has been confirmed by low testoste-rone concentrations, LH should be measured to classify the patient as having primary (high LH) or secondary (low or inappropriately normal LH) hypogonadism. An elevated LH level indicates that the defect is at the testicular level. Common causes of primary testicu-lar failure include Klinefelter syndrome, HIV infection, uncorrected

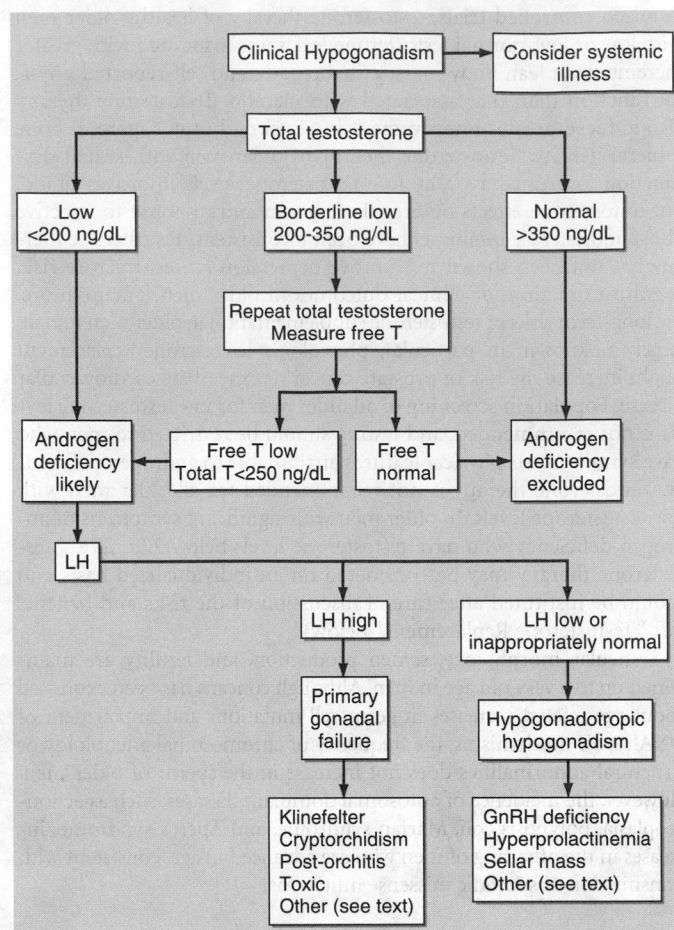

FIGURE 340-6 Evaluation of hypogonadism. T, testosterone; LH, luteinizing hormone; GnRH, gonadotropin-releasing hormone.

cryptorchidism, cancer chemotherapeutic agents, radiation, surgical orchiectomy, or prior infectious orchitis. Unless causes of primary testicular failure are known, a karyotype should be performed in men with low testosterone and elevated LH to exclude Klinefelter syndrome. Men who have a low testosterone but "inappropriately normal" or low LH levels have secondary hypogonadism; their defect resides at the hypothalamic-pituitary level. Common causes of acquired secondary hypogonadism include space-occupying lesions of the sella, hyperprolactinemia, chronic illness, hemochromatosis, excessive exercise, and substance abuse. Measurement of PRL and MRI scan of the hypothalamic-pituitary region can help exclude the presence of a space-occupying lesion. Patients in whom known causes of hypogonadotropic hypogonadism have been excluded are classified as having IHH. It is not unusual for congenital causes of hypogonadotropic hypogonadism, such as Kallmann syndrome, to be diagnosed in young adults.

℞ AGE-RELATED REPRODUCTIVE DYSFUNCTION

GONADOTROPINS Gonadotropin therapy is used to establish or restore fertility in patients with gonadotropin deficiency of any cause. Several gonadotropin preparations are available. Human menopausal gonadotropin (hMG; purified from the urine of postmenopausal women) contains 75 IU FSH and 75 IU LH per vial. hCG (purified from the urine of pregnant women) has little FSH activity and resembles LH in its ability to stimulate testosterone production by Leydig cells. Recombinant hCG is now available. Because of the expense of hMG, treatment is usually begun with hCG alone, and hMG is added later to promote the FSH-dependent stages of spermatid development. Recombinant human FSH (hFSH) is now available and is indistinguishable from purified urinary hFSH in its biologic activity and pharmacokinetics in vitro and in vivo, although the mature β subunit of

recombinant hFSH has seven fewer amino acids. Recombinant hFSH is available in ampoules containing 75 IU (~7.5 μg FSH), which accounts for >99% of protein content. Once spermatogenesis is restored using combined FSH and LH therapy, hCG alone is often sufficient to maintain spermatogenesis.

Although a variety of treatment regimens are used, 1500–2000 IU of hCG or recombinant human LH (rhLH) administered intramuscularly three times weekly is a reasonable starting dose. Testosterone levels should be measured 6–8 weeks later and 48–72 h after the hCG or rhLH injection; the hCG/rhLH dose should be adjusted to achieve testosterone levels in the mid-normal range. Sperm counts should be monitored on a monthly basis. It may take several months for spermatogenesis to be restored; therefore, it is important to forewarn patients about the potential length and expense of the treatment and to provide conservative estimates of success rates. If testosterone levels are in the mid-normal range but the sperm concentrations are low after 6 months of therapy with hCG alone, FSH should be added. This can be done by using hMG, highly purified urinary hFSH, or recombinant hFSH. The selection of FSH dose is empirical. A common practice is to start with the addition of 75 IU FSH three times each week in conjunction with the hCG/rhLH injections. If sperm densities are still low after 3 months of combined treatment, the FSH dose should be increased to 150 IU. Occasionally, it may take ≥18–24 months for spermatogenesis to be restored.

The two best predictors of success using gonadotropin therapy in hypogonadotropic men are testicular volume at presentation and time of onset. In general, men with testicular volumes >8 mL have better response rates than those who have testicular volumes <4 mL. Patients who became hypogonadotropic after puberty experience higher success rates than those who have never undergone pubertal changes. Spermatogenesis can usually be reinitiated by hCG alone, with high rates of success for men with postpubertal onset of hypogonadotropism. The presence of a primary testicular abnormality, such as cryptorchidism, will attenuate testicular response to gonadotropin therapy. Prior androgen therapy does not affect subsequent response to gonadotropin therapy.

GNRH In patients with documented GnRH deficiency, both pubertal development and spermatogenesis can be successfully induced by pulsatile administration of low doses of GnRH. This response requires normal pituitary and testicular function. Therapy usually begins with an initial dose of 25 ng/kg per pulse administered subcutaneously every 2 h by a portable infusion pump. Testosterone, LH, and FSH levels should be monitored. The dose of GnRH is increased until testosterone levels reach the mid-normal range. Doses ranging from 25 to 200 ng/kg may be required to induce virilization. Once pubertal changes have been initiated, the dose of GnRH can often be reduced. Increased sperm counts and testicular volume have been reported in >70% of treated men, and improvements in sexual function and virilization can be induced in >90% of patients. Cutaneous infections occur but are infrequent and minor. Carrying a portable infusion device can be cumbersome, and follow-up of these patients requires physician supervision and laboratory monitoring. Some patients with IHH have cryptorchidism; men with this additional testicular defect may not respond to GnRH or gonadotropin therapy.

Comparative studies of gonadotropin therapy and pulsatile GnRH administration demonstrate that these two therapies are similar in terms of the time to first appearance of sperm or pregnancy rates; both approaches are equally effective in inducing spermatogenesis in men with hypogonadotropic hypogonadism caused by GnRH deficiency. However, most patients find intermittent gonadotropin injections preferable to wearing a continuous infusion pump.

TESTOSTERONE REPLACEMENT Androgen therapy is indicated to restore testosterone levels to normal to correct features of androgen deficiency. Testosterone replacement improves libido and overall sexual activity; increases energy, lean muscle mass, and bone density; and gives the patient a better sense of well-being. The benefits of testosterone replacement therapy have only been proven in men who have documented androgen deficiency, as demonstrated by testosterone levels that are well below the lower limit of normal (<250 ng/dL).

Testosterone is available in a variety of formulations with distinct pharmacokinetics **(Table 340-3)**. Testosterone serves as a prohormone and is converted to 17β-estradiol by aromatase and to 5α-dihydrotestosterone by 5α-reductase. Therefore, when evaluating testosterone formulations, it

Formulation	Regimen	Pharmacokinetic Profile	DHT and Estradiol	Advantages	Disadvantages
Testosterone enanthate or cypionate	100 mg IM weekly or 200 mg IM every 2 weeks	After a single IM injection, serum testosterone levels rise into the supraphysiologic range and then decline gradually into the hypogonadal range by the end of the dosing interval	DHT and estradiol levels rise in proportion to the increase in testosterone levels; T:DHT and T:E$_2$ ratios do not change	Corrects symptoms of androgen deficiency Relatively inexpensive, if self-administered Flexibility of dosing	Requires IM injection Peaks and troughs in serum testosterone levels
Scrotal testosterone patch[a]	One scrotal patch designed to nominally deliver 6 mg over 24 h applied daily	Normalizes serum testosterone levels in many but not all androgen-deficient men	Serum estradiol levels are in the physiologic male range, but DHT levels rise into the supraphysiologic range; T:DHT ratio is significantly lower than in healthy men	Corrects symptoms of androgen deficiency	To promote optimum adherence of the patch, scrotal skin needs to be shaved High DHT levels
Nongenital transdermal system	1 or 2 patches, designed to nominally deliver 5–10 mg testosterone over 24 h applied daily on nonpressure areas	Restores serum testosterone, DHT, and estradiol levels into the physiologic male range	T:DHT and T:estradiol levels are in the physiologic male range	Ease of application, corrects symptoms of androgen deficiency, and mimics the normal diurnal rhythm of testosterone secretion Lesser increase in hemoglobin than injectable esters	Serum testosterone levels in some androgen-deficient men maybe in the low-normal range; these men may need application of 2 patches daily Skin irritation at the application site may be a problem for some patients
Testosterone gel	5–10 g testosterone gel containing 50–100 mg testosterone applied daily	Restores serum testosterone and estradiol levels into the physiologic male range	Serum DHT levels are higher and T:DHT ratios are lower in hypogonadal men treated with the testosterone gel than in healthy eugonadal men	Corrects symptoms of androgen deficiency, provides flexibility of dosing, ease of application, good skin tolerability	Potential of transfer to a female partner or child by direct skin-to-skin contact; moderately high DHT levels
17-α methyl testosterone	17-α alkylated compound that should not be used because of potential for liver toxicity	Orally active			Clinical responses are variable; potential for liver toxicity; should not be used for treatment of androgen deficiency
Buccal, bioadhesive, testosterone tablets	30 mg controlled release, bioadhesive tablets used twice daily	Absorbed from the buccal mucosa	Normalizes serum testosterone and DHT levels in hypogonadal men	Corrects symptoms of androgen deficiency in healthy, hypogonadal men	Gum-related adverse events in 16% of treated men
Oral testosterone undecanoate[b]	40–80 mg orally 2 or 3 times daily with meals	When administered in oleic acid, testosterone undecanoate is absorbed through the lymphatics, bypassing the portal system; considerable variability in the same individual on different days and among individuals	High DHT:T ratio	Convenience of oral administration	Not approved in the USA Variable clinical responses, variable serum testosterone levels, high DHT:T ratio
Injectable long-acting testosterone undecanoate in oil[b]	1000 mg injected IM followed by 1000 mg at 6 weeks, then 1000 mg every 12 weeks	When administered at a dose of 1000 mg IM, serum testosterone levels are maintained in the normal range in a majority of treated men	DHT and estradiol levels rise in proportion to the increase in testosterone levels; T:DHT and T:E$_2$ ratios do not change	Corrects symptoms of androgen deficiency Requires infrequent administration	Requires IM injection of a large volume (4 mL)
Testosterone pellets	4–6 200-mg pellets implanted SC	Serum testosterone peaks at 1 month and then sustained in normal range for 4–6 months	T:DHT and T:E$_2$ ratios do not change	Corrects symptoms of androgen deficiency	Requires surgical incision for insertions; pellets may extrude spontaneously

[a]Not currently available in the United States.
[b]Formulation available outside the United States but not currently approved by the U.S. Food and Drug Administration.
Abbreviations: IM, intramuscular; DHT, dihydrotestosterone; T, testosterone; E$_2$, 17β-estradiol; SC, subcutaneously.
Source: Reproduced from the Endocrine Society Guideline for Testosterone Therapy of Androgen Deficiency Syndromes in Adult Men (Bhasin et al).

is important to consider whether the formulation being used can achieve physiologic estradiol and DHT concentrations, in addition to normal testosterone concentrations. Although testosterone concentrations at the lower end of the normal male range can restore sexual function, it is not clear whether low-normal testosterone levels can maintain bone mineral density and muscle mass. The current recommendation is to restore testosterone levels to the mid-normal range.

Oral Derivatives of Testosterone Testosterone is well-absorbed after oral administration but quickly degrades during the first pass through the liver. Therefore, it is not possible to achieve sustained blood levels of testosterone after oral administration of crystalline testosterone. 17α-Alkylated derivatives of testosterone (e.g., 17α-methyl testosterone, oxandrolone, fluoxymesterone) are relatively resistant to hepatic degradation and can be administered orally; however, because of the potential for hepatotoxicity, including cholestatic jaundice, peliosis, and hepatoma, these formulations should not be used for testosterone replacement. Hereditary angioedema due to C1 esterase deficiency is the only exception to this general recommendation; in this condition, oral 17α-alkylated androgens are useful because they stimulate hepatic synthesis of the C1 esterase inhibitor.

Injectable Forms of Testosterone The esterification of testosterone at the 17β-hydroxy position makes the molecule hydrophobic and extends its duration of action. The slow release of testosterone ester from an oily depot in the muscle accounts for its extended duration of action. The longer the side chain, the greater the hydrophobicity of the ester and longer the duration of action. Thus, testosterone enanthate and cypionate with longer side chains have longer duration of action than testosterone propionate. Within 24 h after intramuscular administration of 200 mg testosterone enanthate or cypionate, testosterone levels rise into the high-normal or supraphysiologic range and then gradually decline into the hypogonadal range over the next 2 weeks. A bimonthly regimen of testosterone enanthate or cypionate therefore results in peaks and troughs in testosterone levels that are accompanied by changes in a patient's mood, sexual desire, and energy level. The kinetics of testosterone enanthate and cypionate are similar. Estradiol and DHT levels are normal if testosterone replacement is physiologic.

Transdermal Testosterone Patch The nongenital testosterone patch, when applied in an appropriate dose, can normalize testosterone, DHT, and estradiol levels 4–12 h after application. Sexual function and a sense of well-being are restored in androgen-deficient men treated with the nongenital patch. One 5-mg patch may not be sufficient to increase testosterone into the mid-normal male range in all hypogonadal men; some patients may need daily administration of two 5-mg patches to achieve the targeted testosterone concentrations. The transdermal patches are more expensive than testosterone esters. The use of testosterone patches may be associated with skin irritation in some individuals.

Testosterone Gel Two testosterone gels, Androgel and Testim, are available in 2.5- and 5-g unit doses that nominally deliver 25 and 50 mg of testosterone to the application site. Initial pharmacokinetic studies have demonstrated that 5-, 7.5-, and 10-g doses applied daily to the skin can maintain total and free testosterone concentrations in the mid- to high-normal range in hypogonadal men. Total and free testosterone concentrations are uniform throughout the 24-h period. The current recommendations are to begin with a 50-mg dose and adjust the dose based on testosterone levels. The advantages of the testosterone gel include the ease of application, its invisibility after application, and its flexibility of dosing. A major concern is the potential for inadvertent transfer of the gel to a sexual partner or to children who may come in close contact with the patient. The ratio of DHT to testosterone concentrations is higher in men treated with the testosterone gel.

A buccal adhesive testosterone tablet, which adheres to the buccal mucosa and releases testosterone as it is slowly dissolved, has been approved. After twice-daily application of 30-mg tablets, serum testosterone levels are maintained within the normal male range in a majority of treated hypogonadal men. The adverse effects include buccal ulceration and gum problems in a few subjects. The clinical experience with this formulation is limited, and the effects of food and brushing on absorption have not been studied in detail.

Testosterone Formulations Not Available in the United States Testosterone undecanoate, when administered orally in oleic acid, is absorbed preferentially through the lymphatics into the systemic circulation and is spared the first-pass degradation in the liver. Doses of 40–80 mg orally, two or three times daily, are typically used. However, the clinical responses are variable and suboptimal. DHT-to-testosterone ratios are higher in hypogonadal men treated with oral testosterone undecanoate, as compared to eugonadal men.

Implants of crystalline testosterone can be inserted in the subcutaneous tissue by means of a trocar through a small skin incision. Testosterone is released by surface erosion of the implant and absorbed into the systemic circulation. Four to six 200-mg implants can maintain testosterone in the mid- to high-normal range for up to 6 months. Potential drawbacks include incising the skin for insertion and removal, and spontaneous extrusions and fibrosis at the site of the implant.

After initial priming, long-acting testosterone undecanoate in oil, when administered intramuscularly every 12 weeks, maintains serum testosterone, estradiol, and DHT in the normal male range and corrects symptoms of androgen deficiency in a majority of treated men. However, large injection volume (4 mL) is its relative drawback.

Novel Androgen Formulations A number of androgen formulations with better pharmacokinetics or more selective activity profiles are under development. A biodegradable testosterone microsphere formulation provides physiologic testosterone levels for 10–11 weeks. Two long-acting esters, testosterone buciclate and testosterone undecanoate, when injected intramuscularly, can maintain circulating testosterone concentrations in the male range for 7–12 weeks. Initial clinical trials have demonstrated the feasibility of administering testosterone by the sublingual or buccal routes. 7α-Methyl-19-nortestosterone is an androgen that cannot be 5α-reduced; therefore, compared to testosterone, it has relatively greater agonist activity in muscle and gonadotropin suppression but lesser activity on the prostate.

Analogous to the selective estrogen receptor modulators, such as raloxifene, it may be possible to develop selective androgen receptor modulators (SARMs) that exert the desired physiologic effects on muscle, bone, or sexual function but without adversely affecting the prostate and the cardiovascular system.

Pharmacologic Uses of Androgens Androgens and selective androgen receptor modulators are being evaluated as anabolic therapies for functional limitations associated with aging and chronic illness. Testosterone supplementation increases skeletal muscle mass, maximal voluntary strength, and muscle power in healthy men, hypogonadal men, older men with low testosterone levels, HIV-infected men with weight loss, and men receiving glucocorticoids. These anabolic effects of testosterone are related to testosterone dose and circulating concentrations. Systematic reviews have confirmed that testosterone therapy of HIV-infected men with weight loss promotes improvements in body weight, lean body mass, muscle strength, and depression indices, leading to recommendations that testosterone be considered as an adjunctive therapy in HIV-infected men who are experiencing unexplained weight loss and who have low testosterone levels. Similarly, in glucocorticoid-treated men, testosterone therapy should be considered to maintain muscle mass and strength, and vertebral bone mineral density. It is unknown whether testosterone therapy of older men with functional limitations can improve physical function, reduce disability, and improve health-related quality of life. Concerns about potential adverse effects of testosterone on prostate and cardiovascular event rates have encouraged the development of selective androgen receptor modulators that are preferentially anabolic and spare the prostate.

Testosterone administration induces hypertrophy of both type 1 and 2 fibers and increases satellite cell (muscle progenitor cells) and myonuclear number. Androgens promote the differentiation of mesenchymal, multipotent progenitor cells into the myogenic lineage and inhibit their differentiation into the adipogenic lineage. Testosterone may have additional effects on satellite cell replication and muscle protein synthesis, which may contribute to an increase in muscle mass.

Other indications for androgen therapy are in selected patients with anemia due to bone marrow failure (an indication largely supplanted by erythropoietin) or for hereditary angioedema.

Male Hormonal Contraception Based on Combined Administration of Testosterone and Gonadotropin Inhibitors Supraphysiologic doses of testosterone (200 mg testosterone enanthate weekly) act by suppressing LH and FSH secretion and induce azoospermia in 50% of Caucasian men and >95% of Chinese men. Because of concern about long-term adverse effects of supraphysiologic testosterone doses, regimens that combine other gonadotropin inhibitors, such as GnRH antagonists and progestins with replacement doses of testosterone, are being investigated. Oral etonogestrel daily in combination with intramuscular testosterone decanoate every 4–6 weeks induced azoospermia or severe oligozoospermia (sperm density <1 million/mL) in 99% of treated men over a 1-year period. This regimen was associated with weight gain, decreased testicular volume, and decreased plasma high-density lipoprotein (HDL) cholesterol; the long-term safety has not been demonstrated. Selective androgen receptor modulators that are more potent inhibitors of gonadotropins than testosterone and spare the prostate hold promise for their contraceptive potential.

Recommended Regimens for Androgen Replacement Testosterone esters are administered weekly at doses of 75–100 mg intramuscularly, or 150–200 mg every 2 weeks. One or two 5-mg nongenital testosterone patches can be applied daily over the skin of the back, thigh, or upper arm away from pressure areas. Testosterone gel is typically applied over a covered area of skin at a dose of 5–10 g daily; patients should wash their hands after gel application. Bioadhesive buccal testosterone tablets at a dose of 30 mg are typically applied twice daily on the buccal mucosa.

Establishing Efficacy of Testosterone Replacement Therapy Because a clinically useful marker of androgen action is not available, restoration of testosterone levels into the mid-normal range remains the goal of therapy. Measurements of LH and FSH are not useful in assessing the adequacy of testosterone replacement. Testosterone should be measured 3 months after initiating therapy to assess adequacy of therapy. In patients who are treated with testosterone enanthate or cypionate, testosterone levels should be 350–600 ng/dL 1 week after the injection. If testosterone levels are outside this range, adjustments should be made to either the dose or the interval between injections. In men on transdermal patch or gel, or buccal testosterone therapy, testosterone levels should be in the mid-normal range (500–700 ng/dL) 4–12 h after application. If testosterone levels are outside this range, the dose should be adjusted.

Restoration of sexual function, secondary sex characteristics, and energy level and sense of well-being are important objectives of testosterone replacement therapy. The patient should also be asked about sexual desire and activity, the presence of early morning erections, and the ability to achieve and maintain erections adequate for sexual intercourse. Some hypogonadal men continue to complain about sexual dysfunction even after testosterone replacement has been instituted; these patients may benefit from counseling. The hair growth in response to androgen replacement is variable and depends on ethnicity. Hypogonadal men with prepubertal onset of androgen deficiency who begin testosterone therapy in their late 20s or 30s may find it difficult to adjust to their newly found sexuality and may benefit from counseling. If the patient has a sexual partner, the partner should be included in counseling because of the dramatic physical and sexual changes that occur with androgen treatment.

Contraindications for Androgen Administration Testosterone administration is contraindicated in men with a history of prostate or breast cancer **(Table 340-4)**. Testosterone should not be prescribed to men with severe symptoms of benign prostatic hypertrophy (American Urological Association symptom score >19) or with baseline prostate-specific antigen (PSA) >3 ng/mL without a urologic evaluation. Testosterone replacement should not be administered to men with baseline hematocrit ≥50%. Testosterone can induce and exacerbate sleep apnea because of its neuromuscular effects on the upper airway. Testosterone should not be administered to men with congestive heart failure with class III or IV symptoms.

Monitoring Potential Adverse Experiences The clinical effectiveness and safety of testosterone replacement therapy should be performed 3

TABLE 340-4 CONDITIONS IN WHICH TESTOSTERONE ADMINISTRATION IS ASSOCIATED WITH A RISK OF ADVERSE OUTCOME

Conditions in which testosterone administration is associated with very high risk of serious adverse outcomes:
  Metastatic prostate cancer
  Breast cancer
Conditions in which testosterone administration is associated with moderate to high risk of adverse outcomes
  Undiagnosed prostate nodule or induration
  Unexplained PSA elevation
  Erythrocytosis (hematocrit >50%)
  Severe lower urinary tract symptoms associated with benign prostatic hypertrophy as indicated by American Urological Association/International prostate symptom score >19
  Unstable severe congestive heart failure (class III or IV)

Note: PSA, prostate-specific antigen.
Source: Reproduced from the Endocrine Society Guideline for Testosterone Therapy of Androgen Deficiency Syndromes in Adult Men (Bhasin et al).

TABLE 340-5 MONITORING OF MEN RECEIVING TESTOSTERONE THERAPY

1. Evaluate the patient 3 months after treatment starts and then annually to assess whether symptoms have responded to treatment and whether the patient is suffering from any adverse effects.
2. Monitor testosterone levels 2 or 3 months after initiation of testosterone therapy.
  The therapy should aim to raise serum testosterone levels into the mid-normal range.
  Injectable testosterone enanthate or cypionate: Measure serum testosterone levels midway between injections. If testosterone is >700 ng/dL (24.5 nmol/L) or <350 ng/dL (12.3 nmol/L), adjust dose or frequency.
  Transdermal patch: Assess testosterone levels 3–12 hours after application of the patch; adjust dose to achieve testosterone levels in the mid-normal range.
  Buccal testosterone bioadhesive tablet: Assess levels immediately before or after application of fresh system.
  Transdermal gel: Assess testosterone level any time after patient has been on treatment for at least 1 week; adjust dose to achieve serum testosterone levels in the mid-normal range.
  Oral testosterone undecanoate[a]: Monitor serum testosterone levels 3–5 h after ingestion.
  Injectable testosterone undecanoate[a]: Measure serum testosterone level just prior to each subsequent injection and adjust the dosing interval to maintain serum testosterone in mid-normal range.
3. Check hematocrit at baseline, at 3 months, and then annually. If hematocrit is >54%, stop therapy until hematocrit decreases to a safe level; evaluate the patient for hypoxia and sleep apnea; reinitiate therapy with a reduced dose.
4. Measure bone mineral density of lumbar spine and/or femoral neck after 1–2 years of testosterone therapy in hypogonadal men with osteoporosis or low trauma fracture, consistent with regional standard of care.
5. Perform digital rectal examination and check PSA level before initiating treatment, at 3 months, and then in accordance with guidelines for prostate cancer screening depending on the age and race of the patient.
6. Obtain urological consultation if there is:
  Verified serum PSA concentration >4.0 ng/mL
  An increase in serum PSA concentration >1.4 ng/mL within any 12-month period of testosterone treatment
  A PSA velocity of >0.4 ng/mL/year using the PSA level after 6 months of testosterone administration as the reference (only applicable if PSA data are available for a period exceeding 2 years)
  Detection of a prostatic abnormality on digital rectal examination
  An AUA/IPSS of >19
7. Evaluate formulation-specific adverse effects at each visit.
  Buccal testosterone tablets: Inquire about alterations in taste and examine the gums and oral mucosa for irritation.
  Injectable testosterone esters (enanthate and cypionate): Ask about fluctuations in mood or libido.
  Testosterone patches: Look for skin reaction at the application site.
  Testosterone gels: Advise patients to cover the application sites with a shirt and to wash the skin with soap and water before having skin-to-skin contact, as testosterone gels leave a testosterone residue on the skin that can be transferred to a woman or child who might come in close contact. Serum testosterone levels are maintained when the application site is washed 4–6 hours after application of the testosterone gel.

[a]Not approved for clinical use in the United States.
Note: PSA, prostate-specific antigen; AUA, American Urological Association; IPSS, international prostate symptom score.
Source: Reproduced from the Endocrine Society Guideline for Testosterone Therapy of Androgen Deficiency Syndromes in Adult Men (Bhasin et al).

and 6 months after initiating testosterone therapy and annually thereafter **(Table 340-5)**. Potential adverse effects include acne, oiliness of skin, erythrocytosis, breast tenderness and enlargement, leg edema, induction and exacerbation of obstructive sleep apnea, and increased risk of prostate cancer, though it may increase the incidence of detection rather than the actual occurrence rate. In addition, there may be formulation-specific adverse effects such as skin irritation with transdermal patch, risk of gel transfer to a sexual partner with testosterone gels, buccal ulceration and gum problems with buccal testosterone, and pain and mood fluctuation with injectable testosterone esters.

Hemoglobin Levels Administration of testosterone to androgen-deficient men is typically associated with a 3–5% increase in hemoglobin levels, but the magnitude of hemoglobin increase may be greater in men who have sleep apnea, a significant smoking history, or chronic obstructive lung disease. Erythrocytosis is the most frequent adverse event reported in testosterone trials in middle-aged and older men and is also the most frequent cause of treatment discontinuation in these trials. The frequency of erythrocytosis is higher in older men than younger men and higher in hypogonadal men treated with injectable testosterone esters than in those treated with transdermal formulations, presumably due to the higher testosterone dose delivered by the typical regimens of testosterone esters. If hematocrit rises above 54%, testosterone therapy should be stopped until hematocrit has fallen to <50%. After evaluation of the patient for hypoxia and sleep apnea, testosterone therapy may be reinitiated at a lower dose.

Digital Examination of the Prostate and Serum PSA Levels Testosterone replacement therapy increases prostate volume to the size seen in age-matched controls but should not increase prostate volume beyond that expected for age. There is no evidence that testosterone replacement causes prostate cancer. However, androgen administration can exacerbate preexisting prostate cancer. Many older men harbor microscopic foci of cancer in their prostates. It is not known whether long-term testosterone administration will induce these microscopic foci to grow into clinically significant cancers.

PSA levels are lower in testosterone-deficient men and are restored to normal after testosterone replacement. There is considerable test-retest variability in PSA measurements; the average interassay coefficient of variation of PSA assays is 15%. The 95% confidence interval for the change in PSA values, measured 3–6 months apart, is 1.4 ng/mL. Increments in PSA levels after testosterone supplementation in androgen-deficient men are generally <0.5 ng/mL, and increments >1.0 ng/mL over a 3–6-month period are unusual. Nevertheless, administration of testosterone to men with baseline PSA levels between 2.5 and 4.0 ng/mL will cause PSA levels to exceed 4.0 ng/mL for some, and many of these men may undergo prostate biopsies. PSA velocity criterion can be used for patients who have sequential PSA measurements for >2 years; a change of >0.40 ng/mL per year merits closer urologic follow-up.

Cardiovascular Risk Assessment The long-term effects of testosterone supplementation on cardiovascular risk are unknown. Testosterone effects on lipids depend on the dose (physiologic or supraphysiologic), the route of administration (oral or parenteral), and the formulation (whether aromatizable or not). Physiologic testosterone replacement by an aromatizable androgen has a modest effect on HDL or no effect at all. In middle-aged men with low testosterone levels, physiologic testosterone replacement has been shown to improve insulin sensitivity and reduce visceral obesity. In epidemiologic studies, testosterone concentrations are inversely related to waist-to-hip ratio and directly correlated with HDL cholesterol levels. These data suggest that physiologic testosterone concentration is correlated with factors associated with reduced cardiovascular risk. However, no prospective studies have examined the effect on testosterone replacement on cardiovascular risk.

Androgen Abuse by Athletes and Recreational Bodybuilders The illicit use of androgenic steroids to enhance athletic performance is widespread among professional and high school athletes and recreational bodybuilders. Although androgen supplementation increases skeletal muscle mass and strength, whether and how androgens improve athletic performance is unknown. The most commonly used androgenic steroids include testosterone esters, nandrolone, stanozolol, methandienone, and methenolol. Athletes generally use increasing doses of multiple steroids in a practice known as stacking. A majority of athletes who abuse androgenic steroids also use other drugs that are perceived to be muscle-building or performance-enhancing, such as growth hormone; IGF-1; insulin; stimulants such as amphetamine, clenbuterol, ephedrine, and thyroxine; and drugs perceived to reduce adverse effects such as hCG, aromatase inhibitors, or estrogen antagonists.

The adverse effects of androgen abuse include a marked decrease in plasma HDL cholesterol and an increase in LDL cholesterol, changes in clotting factors, suppression of spermatogenesis resulting in reduced fertility, and increase in liver enzymes. Elevations of liver enzymes, hepatic neoplasms, and peliosis hepatis have been reported, mostly with the use of oral, 17-α alkylated androgenic steroids but not with parenterally administered testosterone or its esters. There are anecdotal reports of the association of androgenic steroid use with "rage reactions." Breast tenderness and enlargement are not uncommon among athletes abusing aromatizable androgens. Oral 17-α alkylated androgens also can induce insulin resistance and glucose intolerance. A serious, underappreciated adverse effect of androgen use is the suppression of the hypothalamic-pituitary-testicular axis. Upon discontinuation of exogenous androgen use, the suppressed hypothalamic-pituitary axis may take weeks to months to recover. During this period when testosterone levels are low, the athletes may experience sexual dysfunction, hot flushes, fatigue, and depressed mood, causing some athletes to resume androgen use and thus perpetuating the cycle of abuse, withdrawal symptoms, and dependence. Also, the use of nonsterile needles confers the risk of local infection, sepsis, hepatitis, and HIV infection. Disproportionate gains in muscle mass and strength without commensurate adaptations in tendons and other connective tissues may predispose to the risk of tendon injuries.

Accredited laboratories use gas chromatography-mass spectrometry or liquid chromatography-mass spectrometry to detect anabolic steroid abuse. In recent years, the availability of high-resolution mass spectrometry and tandem mass spectrometry has further improved the sensitivity of detecting androgen abuse. Illicit testosterone use is detected generally by the application of the measurement of urinary testosterone to epitestosterone ratio and further confirmed by the use of the $^{13}C:^{12}C$ ratio in testosterone by the use of isotope ratio combustion mass spectrometry. Exogenous testosterone administration increases urinary testosterone glucuronide excretion and consequently the testosterone to epitestosterone ratio. Ratios above 6 suggest exogenous testosterone use but can also reflect genetic variation. Synthetic testosterone has a lower $^{13}C:^{12}C$ ratio than endogenously produced testosterone and these differences in $^{13}C:^{12}C$ ratio can be detected by isotope ratio combustion mass spectrometry, which is used to confirm exogenous testosterone use in individuals with a high testosterone to epitestosterone ratio.

FURTHER READINGS

ACHERMANN JC et al: Inherited disorders of the gonadotropin hormones. Mol Cell Endocrinol 179:89, 2001

BHASIN S: An approach to infertile men. J Clin Endocrinol Metab 92:1995, 2007

——— et al: Testosterone therapy in adult men with androgen deficiency syndromes: An endocrine society clinical practice guideline. J Clin Endocrinol Metab 91:1995, 2006

BOLONA ER et al: Testosterone use in men with sexual dysfunction: A systematic review and meta-analysis of randomized placebo-controlled trials. Mayo Clin Proc 82:20, 2007

FELDMAN HA et al: Age trends in the level of serum testosterone and other hormones in middle-aged men: Longitudinal results from the Massachusetts male aging study. J Clin Endocrinol Metab 87:589, 2002

FERLIN A et al: Molecular and clinical characterizations of Y chromosome microdeletions in infertile men: A 10-year experience in Italy. J Clin Endocrinol Metab 92:762, 2007

SEDLMEYER IL, PALMERT MR: Delayed puberty: Analysis of a large case series from an academic center. J Clin Endocrinol Metab 87:1613, 2002

341 The Female Reproductive System: Infertility and Contraception
Janet E. Hall

The female reproductive system regulates the hormonal changes responsible for puberty and adult reproductive function. Normal reproductive function in women requires the dynamic integration of hormonal signals from the hypothalamus, pituitary, and ovary, resulting in repetitive cycles of follicle development, ovulation, and preparation of the endometrial lining of the uterus for implantation should conception occur.

For further discussion of related topics, see the following chapters: menstrual cycle disorders (Chap. 51), hyperandrogenic disorders (Chap. 50), sexually transmitted diseases (Chap. 124), sexual differentiation (Chap. 343), menopause (Chap. 342), gynecologic malignancies (Chap. 93), and male hormonal contraception (Chap. 340).

FIGURE 341-1 Ovarian germ cell number is maximal at mid-gestation, then decreases precipitously.

DEVELOPMENT OF THE OVARY AND EARLY FOLLICULAR GROWTH

The ovary orchestrates the development and release of a mature oocyte and also elaborates hormones (e.g., estrogen, progesterone, inhibin) that are critical for pubertal development and preparation of the uterus for conception, implantation, and the early stages of pregnancy. To achieve these functions in repeated monthly cycles, the ovary undergoes some of the most dynamic changes of any organ in the body.

Primordial germ cells can be identified by the third week of gestation and their migration to the genital ridge is complete by 6 weeks' gestation. Germ cells can only persist within the genital ridge and are then referred to as *oogonia*. In contrast to testis development, germ cells are essential for induction of normal ovarian development, reflecting a key role of oogonia in the formation of primordial follicles. Although one X chromosome undergoes X inactivation in somatic cells, it is reactivated in oogonia and genes on both X chromosomes are required for normal ovarian development. A streak ovary containing only stromal cells is found in patients with 45, X Turner syndrome (Chap. 343).

Starting at ~8 weeks' gestation, oogonia begin to enter prophase of the first meiotic division and become primary oocytes. This allows the oocyte to be surrounded by a single layer of flattened granulosa cells to form a primordial follicle. Granulosa cells are derived from mesonephric cells that invade the ovary early in its development, pushing the germ cells to the periphery or ovarian cortex. Although recent studies have reopened the debate, the weight of evidence supports the concept that the ovary contains a nonrenewable pool of germ cells. Through the combined processes of mitosis, meiosis, and atresia, the population of oogonia reaches its maximum of 6–7 million by 20 weeks' gestation after which there is inexorable loss of both oogonia and primordial follicles through the process of atresia. At birth, oogonia are no longer present in the ovary, and only 1–2 million germ cells remain (Fig. 341-1).

The oocyte persists in prophase of the first meiotic division until just before ovulation, when meiosis resumes. The quiescent primordial follicles are recruited to further growth and differentiation through a highly regulated process that limits the size of the developing cohort to ensure that folliculogenesis can continue throughout the reproductive life span. This initial recruitment of primordial follicles to form primary follicles is characterized by growth of the oocyte and the transition from squamous to cuboidal granulosa cells (Fig. 341-2). The theca interna cells that surround the developing follicle begin to form as the primary follicle grows. Acquisition of a zona pellucida by the oocyte and the presence of several layers of surrounding cuboidal granulosa cells mark the development of secondary

FIGURE 341-2 The primordial to primary follicle transition involves somatic cell differentiation to cuboidal granulosa cells and the formation of a theca cell layer from the surrounding stromal cells. These steps require the cooperative interaction of signals from the oocyte and the somatic cells. AMH, anti-müllerian hormone; bFGF, basic fibroblast growth factor; KL, kit ligand; BMP, bone morphogenic protein. (*From Knight and Glister, 2006; with permission.*)

follicles. It is at this stage that granulosa cells develop follicle-stimulating hormone (FSH), estradiol, and androgen receptors and communicate with one another through the development of gap junctions.

In murine models, genes that regulate ovarian development and follicle formation have been identified (Fig. 341-3). Bidirectional signals between the oocyte and its surrounding somatic cells are essential for normal follicular development. For example, the oocyte-derived factor in the germline α (FIGα) is required for initial follicle formation. Anti-müllerian hormone (AMH) and activins derived from somatic cells induce the development of primary follicles from primordial follicles. Oocyte-derived growth differentiation factor 9 (GDF-9) is required for migration of pre-theca cells to the outer surface of the developing follicle (Fig. 341-2). GDF-9 is also required for formation of secondary follicles, as are granulosa cell–derived KIT ligand (KITL) and the forkhead transcription factor (Foxl2). All of these genes are potential candidates for premature ovarian failure in women, and mutations in the human *FOXL2* gene have already been shown to cause

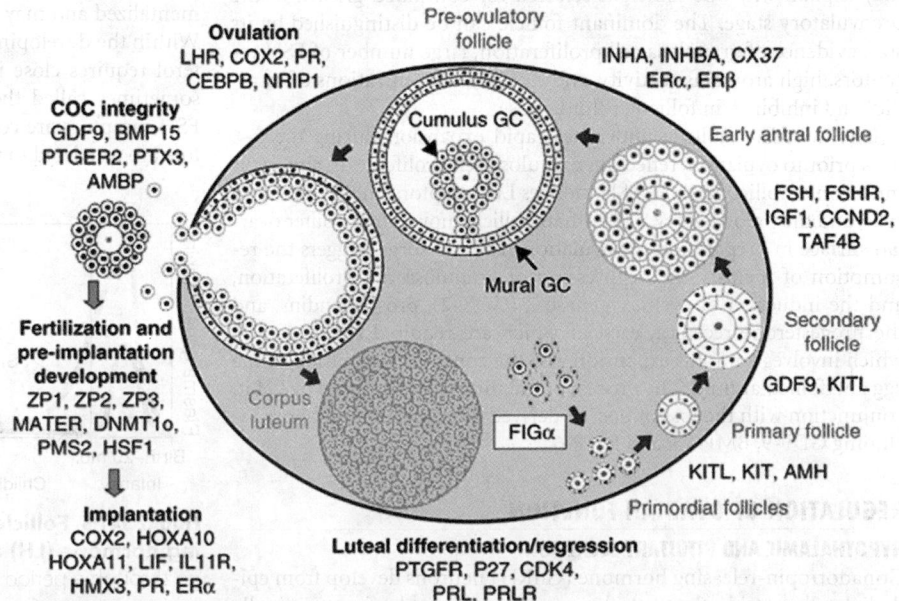

FIGURE 341-3 Specific genes control the orderly development of ovarian development and follicle formation. (*From MM Matzuk, DJ Lamb: Nat Cell Biol 4:Suppl S41–9, 2002; with permission.*)

Primordial follicles

Primary follicles

Graffian follicle

Corpus luteum

FIGURE 341-4 Development of ovarian follicles. *(Courtesy of JH Eichhorn and D Roberts, Massachusetts General Hospital; with permission.)*

the syndrome of blepharophimosis/ptosis/epicanthus inversus, which is associated with ovarian failure.

DEVELOPMENT OF A MATURE FOLLICLE

The early stages of follicle growth are primarily driven by intraovarian factors, whereas maturation to the state required for ovulation, including the resumption of meiosis in the oocyte, requires the combined stimulus of FSH and luteinizing hormone (LH). Recruitment of secondary follicles from the resting follicle pool requires the direct action of FSH. Accumulation of follicular fluid between the layers of granulosa cells creates an antrum that divides the granulosa cells into two functionally distinct groups: mural cells that line the follicle wall and cumulus cells that surround the oocyte (Fig. 341-4). A single dominant follicle emerges from the growing follicle pool within the first 5–7 days after the onset of menses, and the majority of follicles fall off their growth trajectory and become atretic. Autocrine actions of activin and bone morphogenic protein 6 (BMP-6), derived from the granulosa cells, and paracrine actions of GDF-9, BMP-15, and BMP-6, derived from the oocyte, are involved in granulosa cell proliferation and modulation of FSH responsiveness. Differential exposure to these factors may explain why one follicle is selected for continued growth to the preovulatory stage. The dominant follicle can be distinguished by its size, evidence of granulosa cell proliferation, large number of FSH receptors, high aromatase activity, and elevated concentrations of estradiol and inhibin A in follicular fluid.

The dominant follicle undergoes rapid expansion during the 5–6 days prior to ovulation, reflecting granulosa cell proliferation and accumulation of follicular fluid. FSH induces LH receptors on the granulosa cells, and the preovulatory, or Graffian, follicle moves to the outer ovarian surface in preparation for ovulation. The LH surge triggers the resumption of meiosis, the suppression of granulosa cell proliferation, and the induction of cyclooxygenase 2 (COX-2), prostaglandins, and the progesterone receptor, each of which are required for ovulation, which involves cumulus expansion and the controlled expulsion of the egg and follicular fluid. The process of luteinization is induced by LH in conjunction with the loss of oocyte-derived luteinization inhibitors including GDF-9, BMP-15, and BMP-6.

REGULATION OF OVARIAN FUNCTION

HYPOTHALAMIC AND PITUITARY SECRETION

Gonadotropin-releasing hormone (GnRH) neurons develop from epithelial cells outside the central nervous system and migrate, initially alongside the olfactory neurons, to the medial basal hypothalamus. Approximately 7000 GnRH neurons, scattered throughout the medial basal hypothalamus, establish contacts with capillaries of the pituitary portal system in the median eminence. GnRH is secreted into the pituitary portal system in discrete pulses to stimulate synthesis and secretion of LH and FSH from pituitary gonadotropes, which comprise ~10% of cells in the pituitary (Chap. 333). Functional connections of GnRH neurons with the portal system are established by the end of the first trimester, coinciding with the production of pituitary gonadotropins. Thus, like the ovary, the hypothalamic and pituitary components of the reproductive system are present before birth. However, the high levels of estradiol and progesterone produced by the placenta suppress hormonal secretion in the fetus.

After birth, and the removal of placental steroids, gonadotropin levels rise. FSH levels are much higher in girls than in boys. This rise in FSH is associated with ovarian activation (evident on ultrasound) and increased inhibin B and estradiol levels. By 12–20 months of age, the reproductive axis is again suppressed, and a period of relative quiescence persists until puberty (Fig. 341-5). At the onset of puberty, pulsatile GnRH secretion induces pituitary gonadotropin production. In the early stages of puberty, LH and FSH secretion are apparent only during sleep, but as puberty develops, pulsatile gonadotropin secretion occurs throughout the day and night.

The mechanisms responsible for the childhood quiescence and pubertal reactivation of the reproductive axis remain incompletely understood. GnRH neurons in the hypothalamus respond to both excitatory and inhibitory factors. Increased sensitivity to the inhibitory influence of gonadal steroids has long been implicated in the inhibition of GnRH secretion during childhood. Metabolic signals, such as adipocyte-derived leptin, also play a permissive role in reproductive function (Chap. 74). Studies of patients with isolated GnRH deficiency reveal that mutations in the G protein–coupled receptor 54 (*GPR54*) gene preclude the onset of puberty. The ligand for this receptor, metastin, is derived from the parent peptide, kisspeptin-1 (KISS1), and is a powerful stimulant for GnRH release. A potential role for metastin in the onset of puberty has been suggested by upregulation of KISS1 and GPR54 transcripts in the hypothalamus at the time of puberty. The KISS/GPR54 system may also be involved in estrogen feedback regulation of GnRH secretion.

OVARIAN STEROIDS

Ovarian steroid–producing cells do not store hormones but produce them in response to LH and FSH during the normal menstrual cycle. The sequence of steps and the enzymes involved in the synthesis of steroid hormones are similar in the ovary, adrenal, and testes. However, the specific enzymes required to catalyze specific steps are compartmentalized and may not be abundant or even present in all cell types. Within the developing ovarian follicle, estrogen synthesis from cholesterol requires close integration between theca and granulosa cells— sometimes called the *two-cell model for steroidogenesis* (Fig. 341-6). FSH receptors are confined to the granulosa cells, whereas LH receptors are restricted to the theca cells until the late stages of follicular de-

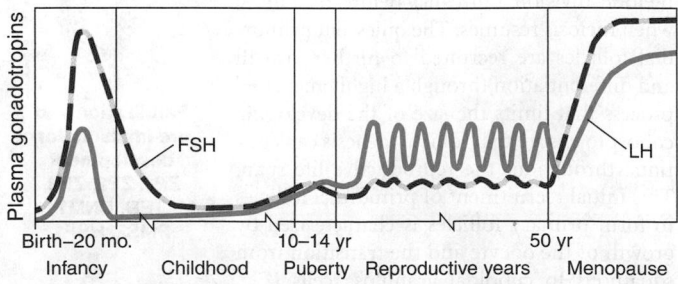

FIGURE 341-5 Follicle-stimulating hormone (FSH) and luteinizing hormone (LH) are increased during the neonatal years but go through a period of childhood quiescence before increasing again during puberty. Gonadotropin levels are cyclic during the reproductive years and increase dramatically with the loss of negative feedback that accompanies menopause.

FIGURE 341-6 Estrogen production in the ovary requires the cooperative function of the theca and granulosa cells under the control of luteinizing hormone (LH) and follicle-stimulating hormone (FSH). HSD, hydroxysteroid dehydrogenase; OHP, hydroxyprogesterone.

velopment, when they are also found on granulosa cells. The theca cells surrounding the follicle are highly vascularized and use cholesterol, derived primarily from circulating lipoproteins, as the starting point for the synthesis of androstenedione and testosterone under the control of LH. Androstenedione and testosterone are transferred across the basal lamina to the granulosa cells, which receive no direct blood supply. The mural granulosa cells are particularly rich in aromatase and, under the control of FSH, produce estradiol, the primary steroid secreted from the follicular phase ovary and the most potent estrogen. Theca cell–produced androstenedione and, to a lesser extent, testosterone are also secreted into peripheral blood, where they can be converted to dihydrotestosterone in skin and to estrogens in adipose tissue. The hilar interstitial cells of the ovary are functionally similar to Leydig cells and are also capable of secreting androgens. Although stromal cells proliferate in response to androgens [as in polycystic ovarian syndrome (PCOS)], they do not secrete androgens.

Rupture of the follicle at the time of ovulation is accompanied by the development of a rich capillary network induced by angiogenic factors such as granulosa-cell derived vascular endothelial growth factor (VEGF), making it possible for large molecules such as low-density lipoprotein (LDL) to reach the luteinized granulosa and theca lutein cells. Luteinized granulosa cells express genes involved in progestin synthesis. Theca lutein cells produce 17-hydroxyprogesterone, a substrate for aromatization by the luteinized granulosa cells. While the major secretory product of the corpus luteum is progesterone, estradiol and 17-hydroxyprogesterone are also produced. LH is critical for normal structure and function of the corpus luteum. Because LH and human chorionic gonadotropin (hCG) bind to a common receptor, the role of LH in support of the corpus luteum can be replaced by hCG in the first 10 weeks after conception, and hCG is commonly used for luteal phase support in the treatment of infertility.

Steroid Hormone Actions (See Chap. 332) Both estrogen and progesterone play critical roles in the expression of secondary sexual characteristics in women. Estrogen promotes development of the ductule system in the breast, whereas progesterone is responsible for glandular development. In the reproductive tract, estrogens create a receptive environment for fertilization and support pregnancy and parturition through carefully coordinated changes in the endometrium, thickening of the vaginal mucosa, thinning of the cervical mucus, and uterine growth and contractions. Progesterone induces secretory activity in the estrogen-primed endometrium, increases the viscosity of cervical mucus, and inhibits uterine contractions. Both gonadal steroids play critical roles in the negative and positive feedback controls of gonado-

tropin secretion. Progesterone also increases basal body temperature and has therefore been used clinically as a marker of ovulation.

The vast majority of circulating estrogens and androgens are carried in the blood bound to carrier proteins, which restrain their free diffusion into cells and prolong their clearance, serving as a reservoir. High-affinity binding proteins include sex hormone–binding globulin (SHBG), which binds androgens with somewhat greater affinity than estrogens, and corticosteroid-binding globulin (CBG), which also binds progesterone. Modulations in binding protein levels by insulin, androgens, and estrogens contribute to high bioavailable testosterone levels in PCOS and to high circulating estrogen and progesterone levels during pregnancy.

Estrogens act primarily through binding to the nuclear receptors, estrogen receptor (ER) α and β. Transcriptional coactivators and co-repressors modulate ER action (Chap. 332). Both ER subtypes are present in the hypothalamus, pituitary, ovary, and reproductive tract. Although ERα and -β exhibit some functional redundancy, there is also a high degree of specificity, particularly in cell type expression. For example, ERα functions in the ovarian theca cells, whereas ERβ is critical for granulosa cell function. There is also evidence for membrane-initiated signaling by estrogen. Similar signaling mechanisms pertain for progesterone with evidence of transcriptional regulation through progesterone receptor (PR) A and B protein isoforms, as well as rapid membrane signaling.

OVARIAN PEPTIDES

Inhibin was initially isolated from gonadal fluids based on its ability to selectively inhibit FSH secretion from pituitary cells. Inhibin is a heterodimer composed of an α-subunit and a βA- or βB-subunit to form inhibin A or inhibin B, both of which are secreted from the ovary. Activin is a homodimer of inhibin β subunits with the capacity to stimulate the synthesis and secretion of FSH. Inhibins and activins are members of the transforming growth factor β (TGF-β) superfamily of growth and differentiation factors. During the purification of inhibin, follistatin, an unrelated monomeric protein that inhibits FSH secretion, was discovered. Follistatin inhibits FSH secretion indirectly through binding and neutralizing activin.

Inhibin B is secreted from the granulosa cells of small antral follicles, whereas inhibin A is present in both granulosa and theca cells and is secreted by dominant follicles. Inhibin A is also present in luteinized granulosa cells and is a major secretory product of the corpus luteum. Inhibin B increases in serum in response to FSH and is used clinically as a marker of ovarian reserve. Inhibin B also plays an important negative feedback role on FSH, independent of estradiol, during the menstrual cycle. Although activin is also secreted from the ovary, the excess of follistatin in serum, combined with its nearly irreversible binding of activin, make it unlikely that ovarian activin plays an endocrine role in FSH regulation. However, as indicated above, there is evidence that activin plays an autocrine/paracrine role in the ovary, and it may also act locally in the pituitary to modulate FSH production.

Müllerian-inhibiting substance (MIS) (also known as anti-müllerian hormone, AMH) plays an important role in ovarian biology in addition to its traditional role in the degeneration of the müllerian ducts in the male. MIS is produced by granulosa cells and, like inhibin B, is a marker of ovarian reserve. MIS may also inhibit the recruitment of primordial follicles into the follicle pool by inhibiting aromatase expression.

HORMONAL INTEGRATION OF THE NORMAL MENSTRUAL CYCLE

The sequence of changes responsible for mature reproductive function is coordinated through a series of negative and positive feedback loops that alter pulsatile GnRH secretion, the pituitary response to GnRH, and the relative secretion of LH and FSH from the gonadotrope. The frequency and amplitude of pulsatile GnRH secretion influence the differential synthesis and secretion of LH and FSH, with slow frequencies favoring FSH synthesis and increased amplitudes favoring LH synthesis. Activin is produced in both pituitary gonadotropes and folliculostellate cells and stimulates the synthesis and secretion of FSH. Inhibins function as potent antagonists of activins through sequestration of the ac-

FIGURE 341-7 The reproductive system in women is critically dependent on both negative feedback of gonadal steroids and inhibin to modulate follicle-stimulating hormone (FSH) secretion and on estrogen positive feedback to generate the preovulatory luteinizing hormone (LH) surge. GnRH, gonadotropin-releasing hormone.

tivin receptors. Although inhibin is expressed in the pituitary, gonadal inhibin is the principal source of feedback inhibition of FSH.

For the majority of the cycle, the reproductive system functions in a classic endocrine negative feedback mode. Estradiol and progesterone inhibit GnRH secretion, and the inhibins act at the pituitary to selectively inhibit FSH synthesis and secretion (Fig. 341-7). This negative feedback control of FSH is critical to development of the single mature oocyte that characterizes normal reproductive function in women. In addition to these negative feedback controls, the menstrual cycle is uniquely dependent on estrogen-induced positive feedback to produce an LH surge that is essential for ovulation of a mature follicle. The neural signaling pathways that distinguish estrogen negative versus positive feedback are incompletely understood.

THE FOLLICULAR PHASE

This phase is characterized by recruitment of a cohort of secondary follicles and the ultimate selection of a dominant preovulatory follicle (Fig. 341-8). The follicular phase begins, by convention, on the first day of menses. However, follicular recruitment is initiated by the rise in FSH that begins in the late luteal phase in conjunction with the loss of negative feedback of gonadal steroids and likely inhibin A. The fact that a 20–30% increase in FSH is adequate for follicular recruitment speaks to the marked sensitivity of the resting follicle pool to FSH. The resultant granulosa cell proliferation is responsible for stimulating early follicular phase levels of inhibin B. Inhibin B in conjunction with rising levels of estradi-

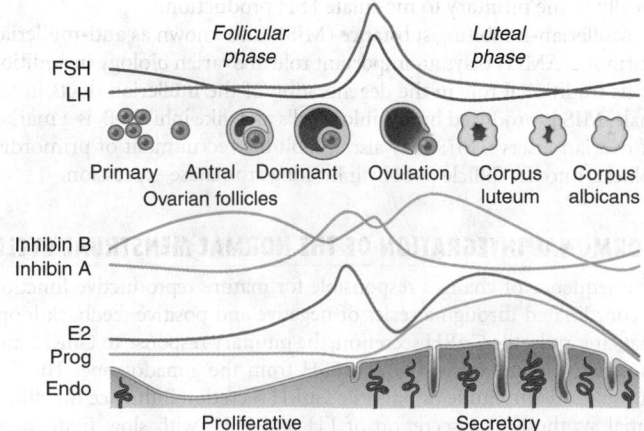

FIGURE 341-8 Relationship between gonadotropins, follicle development, gonadal secretion, and endometrial changes during the normal menstrual cycle. FSH, follicle-stimulating hormone; LH, luteinizing hormone; E₂, estradiol; Prog, progesterone; Endo, endometrium.

ol, and probably inhibin A, restrain FSH secretion during this critical period such that only a single follicle matures in the vast majority of cycles. The increased risk of multiple gestation associated with the increased levels of FSH characteristic of advanced maternal age, or with exogenous gonadotropin administration in the treatment of infertility, attest to the importance of the negative feedback regulation of FSH. With further growth of the dominant follicle, estradiol and inhibin A increase exponentially and the follicle acquires LH receptors. Increasing levels of estradiol are responsible for proliferative changes in the endometrium. The exponential rise in estradiol results in positive feedback on the pituitary, leading to the generation of an LH surge (and a smaller FSH surge), thereby triggering ovulation and luteinization of the granulosa cells.

THE LUTEAL PHASE

This phase begins with the formation of the corpus luteum from the ruptured follicle in response to ovulation signals. Progesterone and inhibin A are produced from the luteinized granulosa cells, which continue to aromatize theca-derived androgen precursors, producing estradiol. The combined actions of estrogen and progesterone are responsible for the secretory changes in the endometrium that are necessary for implantation. The corpus luteum is supported by LH but has a finite life span because of diminished sensitivity to LH. The demise of the corpus luteum results in a progressive decline in hormonal support of the endometrium. Inflammation or local hypoxia and ischemia result in vascular changes in the endometrium leading to the release of cytokines, cell death, and shedding of the endometrium.

If conception occurs, hCG produced by the trophoblast binds to LH receptors on the corpus luteum, maintaining steroid hormone production and preventing involution of the corpus luteum. The corpus luteum is essential for the hormonal maintenance of the endometrium during the first 6–10 weeks of pregnancy until this function is taken over by the placenta.

CLINICAL ASSESSMENT OF OVARIAN FUNCTION

Menstrual bleeding should become regular within 2 to 4 years of menarche, although anovulatory and irregular cycles are common before that. For the remainder of adult reproductive life, the cycle length counted from the first day of menses to the first day of subsequent menses, is ~28 days, with a range of 25–35 days. However, cycle-to-cycle variability for an individual woman is ± 2 days. Luteal phase length is relatively constant between 12 and 14 days in normal cycles; thus, the major variability in cycle length is due to variations in the follicular phase. The duration of menstrual bleeding in ovulatory cycles varies between 4 and 6 days. There is a gradual shortening of cycle length with age such that women over the age of 35 have cycles that are shorter than during their younger reproductive years. Anovulatory cycles increase as women approach the menopause, and bleeding patterns may be erratic.

Women who report regular monthly bleeding with cycles that do not vary by >4 days generally have ovulatory cycles, but several other clinical signs can be used to assess the likelihood of ovulation. Some women experience *mittelschmerz*, described as mid-cycle pelvic discomfort that is thought to be caused by the rapid expansion of the dominant follicle at the time of ovulation. A constellation of premenstrual moliminal symptoms such as bloating, breast tenderness, and food cravings often occur several days before menses in ovulatory cycles, but their absence cannot be used as evidence of anovulation. Methods that can be used to determine whether ovulation is likely include a serum progesterone level >5 ng/mL ~7 days before expected menses, an increase in basal body temperature of >0.5°F (0.24°C) in the second half of the cycle due to the thermoregulatory effect of progesterone, or the detection of the urinary LH surge using ovulation predictor kits. Because ovulation occurs ~36 h after the LH surge, urinary LH can be helpful in timing intercourse to coincide with ovulation.

Ultrasound can be used to detect the growth of the fluid-filled antrum of the developing follicle and to assess endometrial proliferation in response to increasing estradiol levels in the follicular phase, as well as the characteristic echogenicity of the secretory endometrium of the luteal phase.

TABLE 341-1	MEAN AGE (YEARS) OF PUBERTAL MILESTONES IN GIRLS, WITH 95% CONFIDENCE INTERVALS				
	Onset of Breast/Pubic Hair Development	Age of Peak Height Velocity	Menarche	Final Breast/Pubic Hair Development	Adult Height
Caucasian	10.2	11.9	12.6	14.3	17.1
African Amercan	9.6	11.5	12	13.6	16.5

Source: From FM Biro et al: J Pediatr 148:234, 2006.

PUBERTY

NORMAL PUBERTAL DEVELOPMENT IN GIRLS

The first menstrual period (*menarche*) occurs relatively late in the series of developmental milestones that characterize normal pubertal development (Table 341-1). Menarche is preceded by the appearance of pubic and then axillary hair as a result of maturation of the zona reticularis in the adrenal gland and increased adrenal androgen secretion, particularly dehydroepiandrosterone (DHEA). The triggers for adrenarche remain unknown but may involve increases in body mass index as well as in utero and neonatal factors. Menarche is also preceded by breast development (*thelarche*), which is exquisitely sensitive to the very low levels of estrogens that result from peripheral conversion of adrenal androgens and the low levels of estrogen secreted from the ovary early in pubertal maturation. Breast development precedes the appearance of pubic and axillary hair in ~60% of girls. The interval between the onset of breast development and menarche is ~2 years. There has been a gradual decline in the age of menarche over the past century, attributed in large part to improvement in nutrition, and there is a relationship between adiposity and earlier sexual maturation in girls. In the United States, menarche occurs at an average age of 12.5 years (Table 341-1). Much of the variation in the timing of puberty is due to genetic factors, with heritability estimates of 50–80%. Both adrenarche and breast development occur ~1 year earlier in African-American compared with Caucasian girls, although the timing of menarche differs by only 6 months between these ethnic groups.

Other important hormonal changes also occur in conjunction with puberty. Growth hormone (GH) levels increase early in puberty, stimulated in part by the pubertal increases in estrogen secretion. GH increases IGF-I, which enhances linear growth. The growth spurt is generally less pronounced in girls than in boys, with a peak growth velocity of ~7 cm/year. Linear growth is ultimately limited by closure of epiphyses in the long bones as a result of prolonged exposure to estrogen. Puberty is also associated with mild insulin resistance.

DISORDERS OF PUBERTY

The differential diagnosis of precocious and delayed puberty is similar in boys and girls. However, there are differences in the timing of normal puberty and differences in the relative frequency of specific disorders in girls compared with boys.

Precocious Puberty Traditionally, precocious puberty has been defined as the development of secondary sexual characteristics before the age of 8 in girls based on data from Marshall and Tanner in British girls studied in the 1960s. More recent studies led to recommendations that girls be evaluated for precocious puberty if breast development or pubic hair were present at <7 years of age for Caucasian girls or <6 years for African-American girls.

Precocious puberty is most often centrally mediated (Table 341-2), resulting from early activation of the hypothalamic-pituitary-ovarian axis. It is characterized by pulsatile LH secretion and an enhanced LH and FSH response to exogenous GnRH (two- to threefold stimulation) (Table 341-3). True precocity is marked by advancement in bone age of >2 SD, a recent history of growth acceleration, and progression of secondary sexual characteristics. In girls, centrally mediated precocious puberty is idiopathic in ~85% of cases; however, neurogenic causes must also be considered. GnRH agonists that induce pituitary desensitization are the mainstay of treatment to prevent premature epiphyseal closure and preserve adult height, as well to manage psychosocial repercussions of precocious puberty.

Peripherally mediated precocious puberty does not involve activation of the hypothalamic-pituitary-ovarian axis and is characterized by suppressed gonadotropins in the presence of elevated estradiol. Management of peripheral precocious puberty involves treating the underlying disorder (Table 341-2) and limiting the effects of gonadal steroids using aromatase inhibitors, inhibitors of steroidogenesis, and

TABLE 341-3	EVALUATION OF PRECOCIOUS AND DELAYED PUBERTY		
		Precocious	Delayed
Initial screening tests			
History and physical		x	x
Assessment of growth velocity		x	x
Bone age		x	x
LH, FSH		x	x
Estradiol, testosterone		x	x
DHEAS		x	x
17-Hydroxyprogesterone		x	
TSH, T₄		x	x
Complete blood count			x
Sedimentation rate, C-reactive protein			x
Electrolytes, renal function			x
Liver enzymes			x
IGF-I, IGFBP-3			x
Urinalysis			x
Secondary tests			
Pelvic ultrasound		x	
Cranial MRI		x	x
β-hCG		x	
GnRH/agonist stimulation test		x	x
ACTH stimulation test		x	
Inflammatory bowel disease panel		x	x
Celiac disease panel			x
Prolactin			x
Karyotype			x

Note: LH, luteinizing hormone; FSH, follicle-stimulating hormone; DHEAS, dehydroepiandrosterone sulfate; TSH, thyroid-stimulating hormone; T₄, thyroxine; IGF, insulin-like growth factor; IGFBP-3, IGF-binding protein 3; hCG, human chorionic gonadotropin; ACTH, adrenocorticotropic hormone.

TABLE 341-2	DIFFERENTIAL DIAGNOSIS OF PRECOCIOUS PUBERTY	
Central (GnRH dependent)	**Peripheral (GnRH independent)**
Idiopathic	Congenital adrenal hyperplasia
CNS tumors	Estrogen-producing tumors
Hamartomas	Adrenal tumors
Astrocytomas	Ovarian tumors
Adenomyomas	Gonadotropin/hCG-producing
Gliomas	tumors
Germinomas	Exogenous exposure to estro-
CNS infection	gen or androgen
Head trauma	McCune-Albright syndrome
Iatrogenic	Aromatase excess syndrome
Radiation	
Chemotherapy	
Surgical	
CNS malformation	
Arachnoid or suprasellar cysts	
Septo-optic dysplasia	
Hydrocephalus	

Note: GnRH, gonadotropin-releasing hormone; CNS, central nervous system; hCG, human chorionic gonadotropin.

estrogen receptor blockers. It is important to be aware that central precocious puberty can also develop in girls whose precocity was initially peripherally mediated, as in McCune-Albright syndrome and congenital adrenal hyperplasia.

Incomplete and intermittent forms of precocious puberty may also occur. For example, premature breast development may occur in girls before the age of 2 years, with no further progression and without significant advancement in bone age, androgen production, or compromised height. Premature adrenarche can also occur in the absence of progressive pubertal development, but it must be distinguished from late-onset congenital adrenal hyperplasia and androgen-secreting tumors, in which case it may be termed *heterosexual precocity*. Premature adrenarche may be associated with obesity, hyperinsulinemia, and subsequent predisposition to PCOS.

Delayed Puberty Delayed puberty (Table 341-4) is defined as the absence of secondary sexual characteristics by age 13 in girls. The diagnostic considerations are very similar to those for primary amenorrhea (Chap. 51). Between 25 and 40% of delayed puberty in girls is of ovarian origin, with Turner syndrome constituting a majority of such patients. Functional hypogonadotropic hypogonadism encompasses diverse etiologies such as systemic illnesses, including celiac disease and chronic renal disease, and endocrinopathies, such as diabetes and hypothyroidism. In addition, girls appear to be particularly susceptible to the adverse effects of abnormalities in energy balance that result from exercise, dieting, and/or eating disorders. Together these reversible conditions account for ~25% of delayed puberty in girls. Congenital hypogonadotropic hypogonadism in girls or boys can be caused by mutations in several different

TABLE 341-4 DIFFERENTIAL DIAGNOSIS OF DELAYED PUBERTY

Hypergonadotropic
- Ovarian
  - Turner syndrome
  - Gonadal dysgenesis
  - Chemotherapy/radiation therapy
  - Galactosemia
  - Autoimmune oophoritis
  - Congenital lipoid hyperplasia
- Steroidogenic enzyme abnormalities
  - 17α-hydroxylase deficiency
  - Aromatase deficiency
- Gonadotropin/receptor mutations
  - FSHβ, LHR, FSHR
- Androgen resistance syndrome

Hypogonadotropic
- Genetic
  - Hypothalamic syndromes
    - Letpin/leptin receptor
    - HESX1 (septooptic dysplasia)
    - PC1 (prohormone convertase)
  - IHH and Kallmann syndrome
    - KAL, FGFR1
    - GnRHR, GPR54
  - Abnormalities of pituitary development/function
    - PROP1
- CNS tumors/infiltrative disorders
  - Craniopharyngioma
  - Astrocytoma, germinoma, glioma
  - Prolactinomas, other pituitary tumors
  - Histiocytosis X
- Chemotherapy/radiation
- Functional
  - Chronic diseases
  - Malnutrition
  - Excessive exercise
  - Eating disorders

Note: FSHβ, follicle-stimulating hormone β chain; FSHR, FSH receptor; LHR, luteinizing hormone receptor; HESX1, homeobox, embryonic stem cell expressed 1; IHH, idiopathic hypogonadotropic hypogonadism; KAL, Kallmann; FGFR1, fibroblast growth factor 1; GnRHR, gonadotropin-releasing hormone receptor; GPR54, G protein-coupled receptor 54; PROP1, prophet of Pit1, paired-like homeodomain transcription factor; CNS, central nervous system.

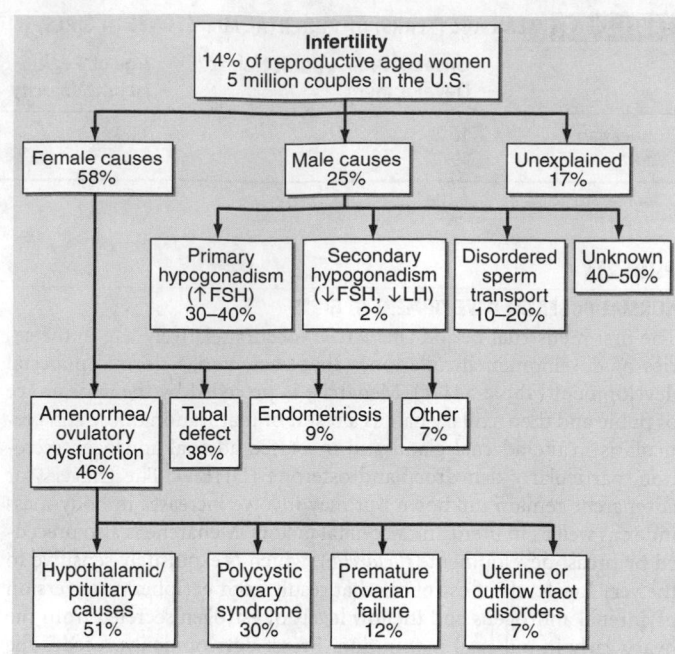

FIGURE 341-9 Causes of infertility. FSH, follicle-stimulating hormone; LH, luteinizing hormone.

genes or combinations of genes (Chap. 340, Table 340-2). Family studies suggest that genes identified in association with absent puberty may cause delayed puberty and that there may be a genetic susceptibility to environmental stresses such as diet and exercise. Although neuroanatomic causes of delayed puberty are considerably less common in girls than in boys, it is always important to rule these out in the setting of hypogonadotropic hypogonadism.

INFERTILITY

DEFINITION AND PREVALENCE
Infertility is defined as the inability to conceive after 12 months of unprotected sexual intercourse. In a study of 5574 English and American women who ultimately conceived, pregnancy occurred in 50% within 3 months, 72% within 6 months, and 85% within 12 months. These findings are consistent with predictions based on *fecundability*, the probability of achieving pregnancy in one menstrual cycle (approximately 20–25% in healthy young couples). Assuming a fecundability of 0.25, 98% of couples should conceive within 13 months. Based on this definition, the National Survey of Family Growth reports a 14% rate of infertility in the United States in married women aged 15–44. The infertility rate has remained relatively stable over the past 30 years, although the proportion of couples without children has risen, reflecting a trend to delay childbearing. This trend has important implications because of an age-related decrease in fecundability, which begins at age 35 and decreases markedly after age 40.

CAUSES OF INFERTILITY
The spectrum of infertility ranges from reduced conception rates or the need for medical intervention to irreversible causes of infertility. Infertility can be attributed primarily to male factors in 25%, female factors in 58%, and is unexplained in about 17% of couples (Fig. 341-9). Not uncommonly, both male and female factors contribute to infertility.

APPROACH TO THE PATIENT:
Infertility

INITIAL EVALUATION In all couples presenting with infertility, the initial evaluation includes discussion of the appropriate timing of intercourse and discussion of modifiable risk factors such as smoking, alcohol, caffeine, and obesity. A description of the range of investigations that may be required and a brief description of infertility treatment options, including adoption, should be reviewed. Initial investigations are focused on determining whether the primary cause of the infertility is male, female, or both. These investigations include a semen analysis in the male, confirmation of ovulation in the female, and, in the majority of situations, documentation of tubal patency in the female. In some cases, after an extensive workup excluding all male and female factors, a specific cause cannot be identified and infertility may ultimately be classified as unexplained.

PSYCHOLOGICAL ASPECTS OF INFERTILITY Infertility is invariably associated with psychological stress related not only to the diagnostic and therapeutic procedures themselves but also to repeated cycles of hope and loss associated with each new procedure or cycle of treatment that does not result in the birth of a child. These feelings are often combined with a sense of isolation from friends and family. Counseling and stress-management techniques should be introduced early in the evaluation of infertility. Infertility and its treatment do not appear to be associated with long-term psychological sequelae.

FEMALE CAUSES Abnormalities in menstrual function constitute the most common cause of female infertility. These disorders, which include ovulatory dysfunction and abnormalities of the uterus or outflow tract, may present as amenorrhea or as irregular or short menstrual cycles. A careful history and physical examination and a limited number of laboratory tests will help to determine whether the abnormality is: (1) hypothalamic or pituitary (low FSH, LH, and estradiol with or without an increase in prolactin), (2) PCOS (irregular cycles and hyperandrogenism in the absence of other causes of androgen excess), (3) ovarian (low estradiol with increased FSH), or (4) uterine or outflow tract abnormality. The frequency of these diagnoses depends on whether the amenorrhea is primary or occurs after normal puberty and menarche (see Fig. 51-2). The approach to further evaluation of these disorders is described in detail in Chap. 51.

Ovulatory Dysfunction In women with a history of regular menstrual cycles, *evidence of ovulation* should be sought as described above. An endometrial biopsy to exclude luteal phase insufficiency is no longer considered an essential part of the infertility workup for most patients. Even in the presence of ovulatory cycles, evaluation of *ovarian reserve* is recommended for women over 35 by measurement of FSH on day 3 of the cycle or in response to clomiphene, an estrogen antagonist (see below). An FSH level < 10 IU/mL on cycle day 3 predicts adequate ovarian oocyte reserve. Antral follicle count, inhibin B, and MIS are also being investigated as indicators of ovarian reserve.

Tubal Disease This may result from pelvic inflammatory disease (PID), appendicitis, endometriosis, pelvic adhesions, tubal surgery, and previous use of an intrauterine device (IUD). However, a cause is not identified in up to 50% of patients with documented tubal factor infertility. Because of the high prevalence of tubal disease, evaluation of tubal patency by hysterosalpingogram (HSG) or laparoscopy should occur early in the majority of couples with infertility. Subclinical infections with *Chlamydia trachomatis* may be an underdiagnosed cause of tubal infertility and requires the treatment of both partners.

Endometriosis *Endometriosis* is defined as the presence of endometrial glands or stroma outside the endometrial cavity and uterine musculature. Its presence is suggested by a history of dyspareunia (painful intercourse), worsening dysmenorrhea that often begins before menses, or by a thickened rectovaginal septum or deviation of the cervix on pelvic examination. The pathogenesis of the infertility associated with endometriosis is unclear but may involve effects on the normal endometrium as well as adhesions. Endometriosis is often clinically silent, however, and can only be excluded definitively by laparoscopy.

MALE CAUSES (See also Chap. 340) Known causes of male infertility include primary testicular disease, disorders of sperm transport, and hypothalamic-pituitary disease resulting in secondary hypogonadism. However, the etiology is not ascertained in up to half of men with suspected male factor infertility. The key initial diagnostic test is a *semen analysis*. Testosterone levels should be measured if the sperm count is low on repeated examination or if there is clinical evidence of hypogonadism.

℞ INFERTILITY

The treatment of infertility should be tailored to the problems unique to each couple. In many situations, including unexplained infertility, mild to moderate endometriosis, and/or borderline semen parameters, a stepwise approach to infertility is optimal, beginning with low-risk interventions and moving to more invasive, higher risk interventions only if necessary. After determination of all infertility factors and their correction, if possible, this approach might include, in increasing order of complexity: (1) expectant management, (2) clomiphene citrate (see below) with or without intrauterine insemination (IUI), (3) gonadotropins with or without IUI, and (4) in vitro fertilization (IVF). The time used to complete the evaluation, correction, and expectant management can be longer in women <30 years of age, but this process should be advanced rapidly in women >35. In some situations expectant management will not be appropriate.

OVULATORY DYSFUNCTION Treatment of ovulatory dysfunction should first be directed at identification of the etiology of the disorder to allow specific management when possible. Dopamine agonists, for example, may be indicated in patients with hyperprolactinemia (Chap. 333); lifestyle modification may be successful in women with low body weight or a history of intensive exercise (Chap. 76).

Medications used for ovulation induction include clomiphene citrate, gonadotropins, and pulsatile GnRH. *Clomiphene citrate* is a nonsteroidal estrogen antagonist that increases FSH and LH levels by blocking estrogen negative feedback at the hypothalamus. The efficacy of clomiphene for ovulation induction is highly dependent on patient selection. It induces ovulation in ~60% of women with PCOS and is the initial treatment of choice. It may be combined with agents that modify insulin levels, such as metformin. Clomiphene citrate is less successful in patients with hypogonadotropic hypogonadism. *Aromatase inhibitors* have also been investigated for the treatment of infertility. Initial studies are promising, but these medications have not been approved for this indication.

Gonadotropins are highly effective for ovulation induction in women with hypogonadotropic hypogonadism and PCOS and are used to induce multiple follicular recruitment in unexplained infertility and in older reproductive-aged women. Disadvantages include a significant risk of multiple gestation and the risk of ovarian hyperstimulation, but careful monitoring and a conservative approach to ovarian stimulation reduce these risks. Currently available gonadotropins include urinary preparations of LH and FSH, highly purified FSH, and recombinant FSH. Though FSH is the key component, there is growing data that the addition of some LH (or hCG) may improve results, particularly in hypogonadotropic patients.

Pulsatile GnRH is highly effective for restoring ovulation in patients with hypothalamic amenorrhea. Pregnancy rates are similar to those following the use of gonadotropins, but rates of multiple gestation are lower and there is virtually no risk of ovarian hyperstimulation. Unfortunately, pulsatile GnRH is not widely available in the United States.

None of these methods are effective in women with premature ovarian failure in whom donor oocyte or adoption are the methods of choice.

TUBAL DISEASE If hysterosalpingography suggests a tubal or uterine cavity abnormality, or if a patient is ≥35 at the time of initial evaluation, laparoscopy with tubal lavage is recommended, often with a hysteroscopy. Although tubal reconstruction may be attempted if tubal disease is identified, it is generally being replaced by the use of IVF. These patients are at increased risk of developing an ectopic pregnancy.

ENDOMETRIOSIS Though 60% of women with minimal or mild endometriosis may conceive within 1 year without treatment, laparoscopic resection or ablation appears to improve conception rates. Medical management of advanced stages of endometriosis is widely used for symptom control but has not been shown to enhance fertility. In moderate to severe endometriosis, conservative surgery is associated with pregnancy rates of 50 and 39%, respectively, compared with rates of 25 and 5% with expectant management alone. In some patients, IVF may be the treatment of choice.

MALE FACTOR INFERTILITY The treatment options for male factor infertility have expanded greatly in recent years (Chap. 340). Secondary hypogonadism is highly amenable to treatment with pulsatile GnRH or gonadotropins. In vitro techniques have provided new opportunities for patients with primary testicular failure and disorders of sperm transport. Choice of initial treatment options depends on sperm concentration and motility. Expectant management should be attempted initially in men with mild male factor infertility (sperm count of 15 to 20 × 10^6/mL and normal motility). Moderate male factor infertility (10 to 15 × 10^6/mL and 20–40% motility) should begin with IUI alone or in combination with treatment of the female partner with clomiphene or gonadotropins, but it may require IVF with or without intracytoplasmic sperm injection (ICSI). For men with a severe defect (sperm count of <10 × 10^6/mL; 10% motility), IVF with ICSI or donor sperm should be used. If ICSI is performed because of azoospermia due to congenital bilateral absence of the vas deferens, genetic testing and counseling should be provided because of the risk of cystic fibrosis.

ASSISTED REPRODUCTIVE TECHNOLOGIES The development of assisted reproductive technologies (ART) has dramatically altered the treatment of male and female infertility. IVF is indicated for patients with many causes of infertility that have not been successfully managed with more conservative approaches. IVF or ICSI is often the treatment of choice in couples with a significant male factor or tubal disease, whereas IVF using donor oocytes is used in patients with premature ovarian failure and in women of advanced reproductive age. Success rates depend on the age of the woman and the cause of the infertility and are generally 18–24% per cycle when initiated in women <40. In women >40, there is a marked decrease in both the number of oocytes retrieved and their ability to be fertilized. Though often effective, IVF is expensive and requires careful monitoring of ovulation induction and invasive techniques including the aspiration of multiple follicles. IVF is associated with a significant risk of multiple gestation (31% twins, 6% triplets, and 0.2% higher order multiples).

CONTRACEPTION

Though various forms of contraception are widely available, ~30% of births in the United States are the result of unintended pregnancy. Teenage pregnancies continue to represent a serious public health problem in the United States, with >1 million unintended pregnancies each year—a significantly greater incidence than in other industrialized nations.

Contraceptive methods are widely used (Table 341-5). Only 15% of couples report having unprotected sexual intercourse in the past 3 months. A reversible form of contraception is used by >50% of couples, while sterilization (in either the male or female) has been employed as a permanent form of contraception by over a third of couples. Pregnancy termination is relatively safe when directed by health care professionals but is rarely the option of choice.

No single contraceptive method is ideal, although all are safer than carrying a pregnancy to term. The effectiveness of a given method of contraception depends not only on the efficacy of the method itself. Discrepancies between theoretical and actual effectiveness emphasize the importance of patient education and compliance when considering various forms of contraception (Table 341-5). Knowledge of the advantages and disadvantages of each contraceptive is essential for counseling an individual

about the methods that are safest and most consistent with his or her lifestyle. The World Health Organization (WHO) has extensive family planning resources for the physician and patient that can be accessed on line.

BARRIER METHODS

Barrier contraceptives (such as condoms, diaphragms, and cervical caps) and spermicides are easily available, reversible, and have fewer side effects than hormonal methods. However, their effectiveness is highly dependent on adherence and proper use (Table 341-5). A major advantage of barrier contraceptives is the protection provided against sexually transmitted diseases (STIs) (Chap. 124). Consistent use is associated with a decreased risk of HIV, gonorrhea, nongonococcal urethritis, and genital herpes, probably due in part to the concomitant use of spermicides. Natural membrane condoms may be less effective than latex condoms, and petroleum-based lubricants can degrade condoms and decrease their efficacy for preventing HIV infection. A highly effective female condom, which also provides protection against STIs, was approved in 1994 but has not achieved widespread use.

STERILIZATION

Sterilization is the method of birth control most frequently chosen by fertile men and multiparous women >30 (Table 341-5). Sterilization refers to a procedure that prevents fertilization by surgical interruption of the fallopian tubes in women or the vas deferens in men. Although tubal ligation and vasectomy are potentially reversible, these procedures should be considered permanent and should not be undertaken without patient counseling.

Several methods of *tubal ligation* have been developed, all of which are highly effective with a 10-year cumulative pregnancy rate of 1.85 per 100 women. However, when pregnancy does occur, the risk of ectopic pregnancy may be as high as 30%. The success rate of tubal reanastomosis depends on the method used, but even after successful reversal, the risk of ectopic pregnancy remains high. In addition to prevention of pregnancy, tubal ligation reduces the risk of ovarian cancer, possibly by limiting the upward migration of potential carcinogens.

Vasectomy is a highly effective outpatient surgical procedure that has little risk. The development of azoospermia may be delayed for 2–6 months, and other forms of contraception must be used until two

TABLE 341-5 EFFECTIVENESS OF DIFFERENT FORMS OF CONTRACEPTION

Method of Contraception	Theoretical[a] Effectiveness, %	Actual[a] Effectiveness, %	Percent Continuing Use at 1 Year[b]	Contraceptive Methods Used by U.S. Women[c]
Barrier methods				
Condoms	98	88	63	20
Diaphragm	94	82	58	2
Cervical cap	94	82	50	<1
Spermicides	97	79	43	1
Sterilization				
Male	99.9	99.9	100	11
Female	99.8	99.6	100	28
Intrauterine device				1
Copper T380	99	97	78	
Progestasert	98	97	81	
Mirena	99.9	99.8		
Oral contraceptive pill			72	27
Combination	99.9	97		
Progestin only	99.5	97		
Long-acting progestins				
Depo-Provera	99.7	99.7	70	<1

[a]Adapted from J Trussel et al: Obstet Gynecol 76:558, 1990.
[b]Adapted from Contraceptive Technology Update. Contraceptive Technology, Feb. 1996, Vol 17, No 1, pp 13–24.
[c]Adapted from LJ Piccinino and WD Mosher: Fam Plan Perspective 30:4, 1998.

sperm-free ejaculations provide proof of sterility. Reanastomosis may restore fertility in 30–50% of men, but the success rate declines with time after vasectomy and may be influenced by factors such as the development of anti-sperm antibodies.

INTRAUTERINE DEVICES

IUDs inhibit pregnancy primarily through a spermicidal effect caused by a sterile inflammatory reaction produced by the presence of a foreign body in the uterine cavity (copper IUDs) or by the release of progestins (Progestasert, Mirena). IUDs provide a high level of efficacy in the absence of systemic metabolic effects, and ongoing motivation is not required to ensure efficacy once the device has been placed. However, only 1% of women in the United States use this method compared to a utilization rate of 15–30% in much of Europe and Canada, despite evidence that the newer devices are not associated with increased rates of pelvic infection and infertility, as occurred with earlier devices. An IUD should not be used in women at high risk for development of STI or in women at high risk for bacterial endocarditis. The IUD may not be effective in women with uterine leiomyomas because they alter the size or shape of the uterine cavity. IUD use is associated with increased menstrual blood flow, although this is less pronounced with the progesterone-releasing IUD than the copper-containing device.

HORMONAL METHODS

Oral Contraceptive Pills Because of their ease of use and efficacy, oral contraceptive pills are the most widely used form of hormonal contraception. They act by suppressing ovulation, changing cervical mucus, and altering the endometrium. The current formulations are made from synthetic estrogens and progestins. The estrogen component of the pill consists of ethinyl estradiol or mestranol, which is metabolized to ethinyl estradiol. Multiple synthetic progestins are used. Norethindrone and its derivatives are used in many formulations. Low-dose norgestimate and the more recently developed progestins (desogestrel, gestodene, drospirenone) have a less androgenic profile; levonorgestrel appears to be the most androgenic of the progestins and should be avoided in patients with hyperandrogenic symptoms. The three major formulations of oral contraceptives are (1) fixed-dose estrogen-progestin combination, (2) phasic estrogen-progestin combination, and (3) progestin only. Each of these formulations is administered daily for 3 weeks followed by a week of no medication during which menstrual bleeding generally occurs. Two extended oral contraceptives have recently been approved for use in the United States; Seasonale is a 3-month preparation with 84 days of active drug and 7 day of placebo, Lybrel is a continuous preparation containing 90 μg of levonorgestrel and 20 μg of ethinyl estradiol. Current doses of ethinyl estradiol range from 20–50 μg. However, indications for the 50-μg dose are rare, and the majority of formulations contain 35 μg of ethinyl estradiol. The reduced estrogen and progesterone content in the second- and third-generation pills has decreased both side effects and risks associated with oral contraceptive use (Table 341-6). At the currently used doses, patients must be cautioned not to miss pills due to the potential for ovulation. Side effects, including break-through bleeding, amenorrhea, breast tenderness, and weight gain, are often responsive to a change in formulation.

The microdose progestin-only minipill is less effective as a contraceptive, having a pregnancy rate of 2–7 per 100 women-years. However, it may be appropriate for women with cardiovascular disease or for women who cannot tolerate synthetic estrogens.

New Methods A *weekly contraceptive patch* (Ortho Evra) is available and has similar efficacy to oral contraceptives but may be associated with less breakthrough bleeding. Approximately 2% of patches fail to adhere, and a similar percentage of women have skin reactions. Efficacy is lower in women >90 kg. The amount of estrogen delivered may be comparable to that of a 40-μg ethinyl estradiol oral contraceptive, raising the possibility of increased risk of venous thromboembolism, which must be balanced against potential benefits for women not able

TABLE 341-6 ORAL CONTRACEPTIVES: CONTRAINDICATIONS AND DISEASE RISK

Contraindications
Absolute
  Previous thromboembolic event or stroke
  History of an estrogen-dependent tumor
  Active liver disease
  Pregnancy
  Undiagnosed abnormal uterine bleeding
  Hypertriglyceridemia
  Women over age 35 who smoke heavily (>15 cigarettes per day)
Relative
  Hypertension
  Women receiving anticonvulsant drug therapy

Disease Risks
Increased
  Coronary heart disease—increased only in smokers > 35; no relation to progestin type
  Hypertension—relative risk 1.8 (current users) and 1.2 (previous users)
  Venous thrombosis—relative risk ~4; markedly increased with factor V Leiden or prothrombin-gene mutations (see Chap. 110)
  Stroke—increased only in combination with hypertension; unclear relation to migraine headache
  Cerebral vein thrombosis—relative risk ~13–15; synergistic with prothrombin-gene mutation
  Cervical cancer—relative risk 2–4
Decreased
  Ovarian cancer—50% reduction in risk
  Endometrial cancer—40% reduction in risk

to successfully use other methods. A *monthly contraceptive estrogen/progestin injection* (Lunelle) is highly effective, with a first-year failure rate of <0.2%, but it may be less effective in obese women. Its use is associated with bleeding irregularities that diminish over time. Fertility returns rapidly after discontinuation. A *monthly vaginal ring* (NuvaRing) that is intended to be left in place during intercourse is also available for contraceptive use. It is highly effective, with a 12-month failure rate of 0.7%. Ovulation returns within the first recovery cycle after discontinuation.

Long-Term Contraceptives Long-term progestin administration in the form of Depo-Provera acts primarily by inhibiting ovulation and causing changes in the endometrium and cervical mucus that result in decreased implantation and sperm transport. Depo-Provera requires an IM injection and is effective for 3 months, but return of fertility after discontinuation may be delayed for up to 12–18 months. Although highly effective, Norplant is no longer being manufactured. Amenorrhea, irregular bleeding, and weight gain are the most common adverse effects associated with both injectable forms of contraception. A major advantage of the injectable progestin-based contraceptives is the apparent lack of increased arterial and venous thromboembolic events, but increased gallbladder disease and decreased bone density may result.

POSTCOITAL CONTRACEPTION

Postcoital contraceptive methods prevent implantation or cause regression of the corpus luteum and are highly efficacious if used appropriately. Unprotected intercourse without regard to the time of the month carries an 8% incidence of pregnancy, an incidence that can be reduced to 2% by the use of emergency contraceptives within 72 h of unprotected intercourse. A notice published in 1997 by the U.S. Food and Drug Administration indicated that certain oral contraceptive pills could be used within 72 h of unprotected intercourse [Ovral (2 tablets, 12 h apart) and Lo/Ovral (4 tablets, 12 h apart)]. Preven (50 mg ethinyl estradiol and 0.25 mg levonorgestrel) and Plan B (0.75 mg Levonorgestrel) are now approved for postcoital contraception. Side effects are common with these high doses of hormones and include nausea, vomiting, and breast soreness. Recent studies suggest that 600 mg mifepristone (RU486), a progesterone receptor antagonist, may be equally as effective as or more effective than hormonal regimens, with fewer side effects. Mifepristone is now available in the United States as

Mifeprex, to be used with or without misoprostol (synthetic prostaglandin E$_1$, an off-label indication for this use of misoprostol).

FURTHER READINGS

BOIVIN J et al: International estimates of infertility prevalence and treatment-seeking: Potential need and demand for infertility medical care. Hum Reprod 22:1506, 2007

FISHER WA, BLACK A: Contraception in Canada: A review of method choices, characteristics, adherence and approaches to counseling. CMAJ 176:953, 2007

KNIGHT PG, GLISTER C: TGF-β superfamily members and ovarian follicle development. Reproduction 132:191, 2006

PRACTICE COMMITTEE OF THE AMERICAN SOCIETY OF REPRODUCTIVE MEDICINE: Hormonal contraception: Recent advances and controversies. Fertil Steril 86:S229, 2006

ROY A, MATZUK MM: Deconstructing mammalian reproduction: Using knockouts to define fertility pathways. Reproduction 131:207, 2006

SEMINARA SB: Mechanisms of disease: The first kiss—a crucial role for kisspeptin-1 and its receptor, G-protein-coupled receptor 54, in puberty and reproduction. Nat Clin Pract Endocrinol Metab 2:328, 2006

342 The Menopause Transition and Postmenopausal Hormone Therapy

JoAnn E. Manson, Shari S. Bassuk

Menopause is the permanent cessation of menstruation due to loss of ovarian follicular function. It is diagnosed retrospectively after 12 months of amenorrhea. The average age at menopause is 51 years among U.S. women. *Perimenopause* refers to the time period preceding menopause, when fertility wanes and menstrual cycle irregularity increases, until the first year after cessation of menses. The onset of perimenopause precedes the final menses by 2–8 years, with a mean duration of 4 years. Smoking accelerates the menopausal transition by 2 years.

Although the peri- and postmenopausal transitions share many symptoms, the physiology and clinical management differ. Low-dose oral contraceptives have become a therapeutic mainstay in perimenopause, whereas postmenopausal hormone therapy (HT) has been a common method of symptom alleviation after menstruation ceases.

PERIMENOPAUSE

PHYSIOLOGY

Ovarian mass and fertility decline sharply after age 35 and even more precipitously during perimenopause; depletion of primary follicles, a process that begins before birth, occurs steadily until menopause (Chap. 341). In perimenopause, intermenstrual intervals shorten significantly (typically by 3 days) due to an accelerated follicular phase. Follicle-stimulating hormone (FSH) levels rise, due to altered folliculogenesis and reduced inhibin secretion. In contrast to the consistently high FSH and low estradiol levels seen in menopause, perimenopause is characterized by "irregularly irregular" hormone levels. The propensity for anovulatory cycles can produce a hyperestrogenic, hypoprogestagenic environment that may account for the increased incidence of endometrial hyperplasia or carcinoma, uterine polyps, and leiomyoma observed among women of perimenopausal age. Mean serum levels of selected ovarian and pituitary hormones during the menopausal transition are shown in **Fig. 342-1**. With transition into menopause, estradiol levels fall markedly, whereas estrone levels are relatively preserved, reflecting peripheral aromatization of adrenal and ovarian androgens. FSH levels increase more than those of luteinizing hormone (LH), presumably because of the loss of inhibin, as well as estrogen feedback.

DIAGNOSTIC TESTS

Because of their extreme intraindividual variability, FSH and estradiol levels are imperfect diagnostic indicators of perimenopause in menstruating women. However, a low FSH in the early follicular phase (days 2–5) of the menstrual cycle is inconsistent with a diagnosis of perimenopause. FSH measurement can also aid in assessing fertility; levels of <20 mIU/mL, 20 to <30 mIU/ mL, and ≥30 mIU/mL measured on day 3 of the cycle indicate a good, fair, and poor likelihood of achieving pregnancy, respectively.

SYMPTOMS

Determining whether symptoms that develop in midlife are due to ovarian senescence or to other age-related changes is difficult. There is strong evidence that the menopausal transition can cause hot flashes, night sweats, irregular bleeding, and vaginal dryness, and moderate evidence that it can cause sleep disturbances in some women. There is inconclusive or insufficient evidence that ovarian aging is a major cause of mood swings, depression, impaired memory or concentration, somatic symptoms, urinary incontinence, or sexual dysfunction. In one U.S. study, nearly 60% of women reported hot flashes in the 2 years before their final menses. Symptom intensity, duration, frequency, and effects on quality of life are highly variable.

℞ PERIMENOPAUSE

For women with irregular or heavy menses or hormonally related symptoms that impair quality of life, low-dose combined oral contraceptives are a staple of therapy. Static doses of estrogen and progestin (e.g., 20 μg of ethinyl estradiol and 1 mg of norethindrone acetate daily for 21 days each month) can eliminate vasomotor symptoms and restore regular cyclicity. Oral contraceptives provide other benefits, including protection against ovarian and endometrial cancers and increased bone density, although it is not clear whether use during perimenopause decreases fracture risk later in life. Moreover, the contraceptive benefit is important, given that the unintentional pregnancy rate among women in their forties rivals that of adolescents. Contraindications to oral contraceptive use include cigarette smoking, liver disease, a history of thromboembolism or cardiovascular disease, breast cancer, or unexplained vaginal bleeding. Progestin-only formulations (e.g., 0.35 mg norethindrone daily) or medroxyprogesterone (Depo-Provera) injections (e.g., 150 mg IM every 3 months) may provide an alternative for the treatment of perimenopausal menorrhagia in women who smoke or have cardiovascular risk factors. Although progestins neither regularize cycles nor reduce the number of bleeding days, they reduce the volume of menstrual flow.

FIGURE 342-1 Mean serum levels of ovarian and pituitary hormones during the menopausal transition. FSH, follicle-stimulating hormone; LH, luteinizing hormone. *(From JL Shifren, I Schiff: The aging ovary. J Womens Health Gend Based Med 9:S-3, 2000, with permission.)*

Nonhormonal strategies to reduce menstrual flow include use of non-steroidal anti-inflammatory agents such as mefenamic acid (initial dose of 500 mg at start of menses, then 250 mg qid for 2–3 days) or, when medical approaches fail, endometrial ablation. It should be noted that menorrhagia requires an evaluation to rule out uterine disorders. Transvaginal ultrasound with saline enhancement is useful for detecting leiomyomata or polyps, and endometrial aspiration can identify hyperplastic changes.

TRANSITION TO MENOPAUSE For sexually active women using contraceptive hormones to alleviate perimenopausal symptoms, the question of when and if to switch to HT must be individualized. Doses of estrogen and progestogen (either synthetic progestins or natural forms of progesterone) in HT are lower than those in oral contraceptives and have not been documented to prevent pregnancy. Although a 1-year absence of spontaneous menses reliably indicates ovulation cessation, it is not possible to assess the natural menstrual pattern while a woman is taking an oral contraceptive. Women willing to switch to a barrier method of contraception should do so; if menses occur spontaneously, oral contraceptive use can be resumed. The average age of final menses among relatives can serve as a guide for when to initiate this process, which can be repeated yearly until menopause has occurred.

MENOPAUSE AND POSTMENOPAUSAL HORMONE THERAPY

One of the most complex health care decisions facing women is whether to use postmenopausal HT. Once prescribed primarily to relieve vasomotor symptoms, HT has been promoted as a strategy to forestall various disorders that accelerate after menopause, including osteoporosis and cardiovascular disease. In 2000, nearly 40% of postmenopausal women age 50–74 in the United States had used HT. This widespread use occurred despite the paucity of conclusive data, until recently, on the health consequences of such therapy. Although many women rely on their health care providers for a definitive answer to the question of whether to use postmenopausal hormones, balancing the benefits and risks for an individual patient is challenging.

Although observational studies suggest that HT prevents cardiovascular and other chronic diseases, the apparent benefits may result at least in part from differences between women who opt to take postmenopausal hormones and women who do not. Those choosing HT tend to be healthier, have greater access to medical care, are more compliant with prescribed treatments, and maintain a more health-promoting lifestyle. Randomized trials, which eliminate these confounding factors, have not consistently confirmed the benefits found in observational studies. Indeed, the largest HT trial to date, the Women's Health Initiative (WHI), which examined more than 27,000 postmenopausal women age 50–79 (mean age, 63) for an average of 5–7 years, was stopped early because of an overall unfavorable risk-benefit ratio in the estrogen-progestin arm and an excess risk of stroke that was not offset by a reduced risk of coronary heart disease (CHD) in the estrogen-only arm.

The following summary offers a decision-making guide based on a synthesis of currently available evidence. Prevention of cardiovascular disease is eliminated from the equation due to lack of evidence for such benefits in recent randomized clinical trials.

BENEFITS AND RISKS OF POSTMENOPAUSAL HORMONE THERAPY
(Table 342-1)

Definite Benefits • **SYMPTOMS OF MENOPAUSE** Compelling evidence, including data from randomized clinical trials, indicates that estrogen therapy is highly effective for controlling vasomotor and genitourinary symptoms. Alternative approaches, including the use of antidepressants (such as venlafaxine, 75–150 mg/d), gabapentin (300–900 mg/d), clonidine (0.1–0.2 mg/d), or vitamin E (400–800 IU/d), or the consumption of soy-based products or other phytoestrogens, may also alleviate vasomotor symptoms, although they are less effective than HT. For genitourinary symptoms, the efficacy of vaginal estrogen is similar to that of oral or transdermal estrogen.

OSTEOPOROSIS (See also Chap. 348)

Bone Density By reducing bone turnover and resorption rates, estrogen slows the aging-related bone loss experienced by most postmenopausal women. More than 50 randomized trials have demonstrated that postmenopausal estrogen therapy, with or without a progestogen, rapidly increases bone mineral density at the spine by 4–6% and at the hip by 2–3%, and maintains those increases during treatment.

Fractures Data from observational studies indicate a 50–80% lower risk of vertebral fracture and a 25–30% lower risk of hip, wrist, and other peripheral fractures among current estrogen users; addition of a progestogen does not appear to modify this benefit. Discontinuation of estrogen therapy leads to a diminution of protection. In the WHI, 5–7 years of either combined estrogen-progestin or estrogen-only therapy was associated with a 30–40% reduction in hip fracture and 20–30% fewer total fractures among a population unselected for osteoporosis. Bisphosphonates (such as alendronate, 10 mg/d or 70 mg once per week; risedronate, 5 mg/d or 35 mg once per week; or ibandronate, 2.5 mg/d or 150 mg once per month or 3 mg every 3 months IV) and raloxifene (60 mg/d), a selective estrogen receptor modulator (SERM), have been shown in randomized trials to increase bone mass density and decrease fracture rates. A recently available option for treatment of osteoporosis is parathyroid hormone (teriparatide, 20 μg/d SC). These agents, unlike estrogen, do not appear to have adverse effects on the endometrium or breast. Increased physical activity and adequate calcium (1000–1500 mg/d through diet or supplements in two to three divided doses) and vitamin D (400–800 IU/d) intakes may also reduce the risk of osteoporosis-related fractures.

Definite Risks • **ENDOMETRIAL CANCER (WITH ESTROGEN ALONE)** A combined analysis of 30 observational studies found a tripling of endometrial cancer risk among short-term (1–5 years) users of unopposed estrogen and a nearly tenfold increased risk among users for 10 or more years. These findings are supported by results from the randomized Postmenopausal Estrogen/Progestin Interventions (PEPI) trial, in which 24% of women assigned to unopposed estrogen for 3 years developed atypical endometrial hyperplasia, a premalignant lesion, compared with only 1% of women assigned to placebo. Use of a progestogen, which opposes the effects of estrogen on the endometrium, eliminates these risks.

VENOUS THROMBOEMBOLISM A meta-analysis of 12 studies—8 case-control, 1 cohort, and 3 randomized trials—found that current estrogen use was associated with a doubling of venous thromboembolism risk in postmenopausal women. Relative risks of thromboembolic events were even greater (2.7–5.1) in the three trials included in the meta-analysis. Results from the WHI indicate a twofold increase in risk of venous and pulmonary thromboembolism associated with estrogen-progestin and a one-third increase in this risk with estrogen-only therapy.

BREAST CANCER (WITH ESTROGEN-PROGESTIN) An increased risk of breast cancer has been found among current or recent estrogen users in observational studies; this risk is directly related to duration of use. In a meta-analysis of 51 case-control and cohort studies, short-term use (<5 years) of postmenopausal HT did not appreciably elevate breast cancer incidence, whereas long-term use (≥5 years) was associated with a 35% increase in risk. In contrast to findings for endometrial cancer, combined estrogen-progestin regimens appear to increase breast cancer risk more than estrogen alone. Data from randomized trials also indicate that estrogen-progestin raises breast cancer risk. In the WHI, women assigned to receive combination hormones for an average of 5.6 years were 24% more likely to develop breast cancer than women assigned to placebo, but 7.1 years of estrogen-only therapy did not increase risk. Indeed, the WHI showed a trend toward a reduction in breast cancer risk with estrogen alone, although it is unclear whether this finding would pertain to formulations of estrogen other than conjugated equine estrogens or to treatment durations longer than 7 years. In the Heart and Estrogen/progestin Replacement Study (HERS), 4 years of combination therapy was associated with a 27% increase in breast cancer risk. Although the latter finding was not

TABLE 342-1 BENEFITS AND RISKS OF POSTMENOPAUSAL HORMONE THERAPY (HT) IN PRIMARY PREVENTION SETTINGS[a]

		Benefit or Risk		
		Relative		Absolute
Outcome	Effect	Observational Studies	WHI[b], Except Where Noted	WHI[b], Except Where Noted
Definite Benefits				
Symptoms of menopause	Definite improvement	↓ 70–80% decreased risk	↓65–90% decreased risk[c]	
Osteoporosis	Definite increase in bone mineral density and decrease in fracture risk	↓ 20–50% decreased risk for fracture	E+P: ↓ 33% decreased risk for hip fracture E: ↓ 39% decreased risk for hip fracture	E+P: 50 fewer hip fractures (110 vs 160) per 100,000 woman-years E: 60 fewer hip fractures (110 vs 170) per 100,000 woman-years
Definite Risks				
Endometrial cancer	Definite increase in risk with estrogen alone; no increase in risk with estrogen-progestin	E+P: No increase in risk E: ↑ >300% increased risk (1–5 years); >600% increased risk (≥5 years)	E+P: No increase in risk E: Not applicable	E+P: No difference in risk E: 46 excess cases per 100,000 woman-years with unopposed estrogen (observational studies)[d]
Venous thromboembolism	Definite increase in risk	↑ 110% increased risk	E+P: ↑ 106% increased risk E: ↑ 32% increased risk	E+P: 180 excess cases (350 vs 170) per 100,000 woman-years E: 80 excess cases (300 vs 220) per 100,000 woman-years
Breast cancer	Increase in risk with long-term use (≥5 years) of estrogen-progestin	E+P: ↑ 63% increased risk (≥5 years) E: ↑ 20% increased risk (≥5 years)	E+P: ↑ 24% increased risk E: No increase in risk	10–30 excess cases per 10,000 women using HT for 5 years; 30–90 excess cases per 10,000 women after 10 years use; 50–200 excess cases per 10,000 women after 15 years use (estimate derived from observational data and WHI E+P findings)
Gallbladder disease	Definite increase in risk	↑ 110% increased risk	E+P: ↑ 67% increased risk E: ↑ 93% increased risk	E+P: 180 excess cases (460 vs 280) per 100,000 woman-years E: 310 excess cases (650 vs 340) per 100,000 woman-years
Probable or Uncertain Risks and Benefits				
Coronary heart disease	Probable increase in risk among older women and women many years past menopause; possible decrease in risk or no effect in younger or recently menopausal women	E+P: ↓ 36% decreased risk E: ↓ 45% decreased risk	E+P: ↑ 24% increased risk E: No increase or decrease in risk	E+P: 60 excess cases (390 vs 330) per 100,000 woman-years E: No difference in risk
Stroke	Probable increase in risk	↑ 12% increased risk	E+P: ↑ 31% increased risk E: ↑ 39% increased risk	E+P: 70 excess cases (310 vs 240) per 100,000 woman-years E: 120 excess cases (440 vs 320) per 100,000 woman-years
Ovarian cancer	Probable increase in risk with long-term use (≥5 years)	E+P: No effect (<4 years use) E: ↑ 80% increased risk (≥10 years)	E+P: ↑ 58% increased risk[e] E: Not yet available	E+P: 10 excess cases (40 vs 30) per 100,000 woman-years[e]
Colorectal cancer	Probable decrease in risk with estrogen-progestin	↓ 34% decreased risk	E+P: ↓ 37% decreased risk E: No increase or decrease in risk	E+P: 70 fewer cases (90 vs 160) per 100,000 woman-years E: No difference in risk
Diabetes mellitus	Probable decrease in risk	↓ 20% decreased risk	E+P: ↓ 21% decreased risk E: ↓ 12% decreased risk[e]	E+P: 150 fewer cases (610 vs 760) per 100,000 woman-years E: 140 fewer cases (1160 vs 1300) per 100,000 woman-years[e]
Cognitive dysfunction	Unproven decrease in risk (inconsistent data from observational studies and randomized trials)	↓ 34% decreased risk	↑ 76% increased risk for dementia at age ≥65	120–230 excess cases of dementia per 100,000 woman-years

[a]E, estrogen alone; E+P, estrogen plus progestin. Most studies have assessed conjugated equine estrogen alone or in combination with medroxyprogesterone acetate.
[b]WHI, Women's Health Initiative. The estrogen-plus-progestin arm of the WHI assessed 5.6 years of conjugated equine estrogen (0.625 mg/d) plus medroxyprogesterone acetate (2.5 mg/d) versus placebo. The estrogen-alone arm of the WHI assessed 7.1 years of conjugated equine estrogen (0.625 mg/d) versus placebo.
[c]Data are from other randomized trials. The WHI was not designed to assess effect of HT on menopausal symptoms.
[d]JE Manson, KA Martin: N Engl J Med 345:34, 2001.
[e]Not statistically significant.

statistically significant, the totality of evidence strongly implicates estrogen-progestin therapy in breast carcinogenesis.

GALLBLADDER DISEASE Large observational studies report a two- to three-fold increased risk of gallstones or cholecystectomy among postmenopaus-al women taking oral estrogen. In the WHI, women randomized to estrogen-progestin or estrogen alone had a 67% and 93% greater risk, respectively, of undergoing cholecystectomy than those assigned to placebo. Increased risks were also observed in HERS. Transdermal HT may not increase the risk of gallbladder disease, but further research is needed.

STROKE Until recently, HT had been enthusiastically recommended as a possible cardioprotective agent. In the past three decades, multiple observational studies suggested, in the aggregate, that estrogen use leads to a 35–50% reduction in CHD incidence among postmenopausal women. The biologic plausibility of such an association is supported by data from randomized trials demonstrating that exogenous estrogen lowers plasma low-density lipoprotein (LDL) cholesterol and raises high-density lipoprotein (HDL) cholesterol levels by 10–15%. Administration of estrogen also favorably affects lipoprotein(a) levels, LDL oxidation, endothelial vascular function, fibrinogen, and plasminogen activator inhibitor-1. However, estrogen therapy also has unfavorable effects on other biomarkers of cardiovascular risk: it boosts triglyceride levels; promotes coagulation via factor VII, prothrombin fragments 1 and 2, and fibrinopeptide A elevations; and raises levels of the inflammatory marker C-reactive protein.

Randomized trials of estrogen or combined estrogen-progestin in women with preexisting cardiovascular disease have not confirmed the benefits reported in observational studies. In HERS, a secondary prevention trial designed to test the efficacy and safety of estrogen-progestin therapy on clinical cardiovascular outcomes, the 4-year incidence of coronary mortality and nonfatal myocardial infarction was similar in the active treatment and placebo groups, and a 50% increase in risk of coronary events was noted during the first year of the study among participants assigned to the active treatment group. Although it is possible that progestin may mitigate estrogen's benefits, the Estrogen Replacement and Atherosclerosis (ERA) trial indicated that angiographically determined progression of coronary atherosclerosis was unaffected by either opposed or unopposed estrogen treatment. Moreover, the Papworth Hormone Replacement Therapy Atherosclerosis Study, a trial of transdermal estradiol with and without norethindrone; the Women's Estrogen for Stroke Trial (WEST), a trial of oral 17β-estradiol; and the EStrogen in the Prevention of ReInfarction Trial (ESPRIT), a trial of oral estradiol valerate, found no cardiovascular benefits of the regimens studied. Thus, in clinical trials, HT has not proved effective for the secondary prevention of cardiovascular disease in postmenopausal women.

Primary prevention trials also suggest an early increase in cardiovascular risk and absence of cardioprotection with postmenopausal HT. Results from the WHI suggest a deleterious cardiovascular effect of HT. Women assigned to 5.6 years of estrogen-progestin therapy were 24% more likely to develop CHD and 31% more likely to suffer a stroke than those assigned to placebo. In the estrogen-only arm of the WHI, a similar increase in stroke and no effect on CHD were observed.

However, a closer look at available data suggests that timing of initiation of HT may critically influence the association between such therapy and CHD. Estrogen may slow early stages of atherosclerosis but have adverse effects on advanced atherosclerotic lesions. It has been hypothesized that the prothrombotic and proinflammatory effects of estrogen manifest themselves predominantly among women with subclinical lesions who initiate HT well after the menopausal transition, whereas women with less arterial damage who start HT early in menopause may derive cardiovascular benefit because they have not yet developed advanced lesions. Nonhuman primate data support this concept. Conjugated estrogens had no effect on the extent of coronary artery plaque in cynomolgus monkeys assigned to estrogen alone or combined with progestin starting 2 years (approximately 6 human years) after oophorectomy and well after the establishment of atherosclerosis. However, administration of exogenous hormones immediately after oophorectomy, during the early stages of atherosclerosis, reduced the extent of plaque by 70%.

Lending further credence to this hypothesis are results of subgroup analyses of observational and clinical trial data. For example, although there was no association between estrogen-only therapy and CHD in the WHI study cohort as a whole, such therapy was associated with a CHD risk reduction of 37% among participants age 50–59. By contrast, a risk reduction of only 8% was observed among those age 60–69, and a risk increase of 11% was found among those age 70–79. Due to the relatively small number of cases of myocardial infarction or coronary death (the primary definition of CHD in the WHI), especially in the younger women, these intra- and inter-age group differences were not statistically significant. However, when the definition of CHD was widened to include coronary bypass surgery or percutaneous coronary interventions, estrogen-only therapy was associated with a significant 45% reduction in CHD among women in the youngest age group. Moreover, estrogen was associated with lower levels of coronary artery calcified plaque.

Although age did not have a similar effect in the estrogen-progestin arm of the WHI, CHD risks steadily increased with years since menopause. Estrogen-progestin was associated with an 11% risk reduction for women less than 10 years beyond menopause but was associated with a 22% increase in risk for women 10–19 years from menopause, and a 71% increase in risk for women 20 years or more from menopause (only the latter was statistically significant). In the large observational Nurses' Health Study, women who chose to start HT within 4 years of menopause experienced a lower risk of CHD than did nonusers, whereas those who began therapy 10 or more years after menopause appeared to receive little coronary benefit. Because observational studies include a high proportion of women who begin HT within 3–4 years of menopause and clinical trials include a high proportion of women 12 or more years past menopause, these findings help to reconcile some of the apparent discrepancies between the two types of studies.

Whether age at initiation of HT influences stroke risk is not well understood. Further research is needed on age, time since menopause, and other clinical characteristics as well as on biomarkers that predict increases or decreases in cardiovascular risk associated with exogenous HT. Furthermore, it remains uncertain whether different doses, formulations, or routes of administration of HT will produce different cardiovascular effects.

COLORECTAL CANCER Observational studies have suggested that HT reduces risks of colon and rectal cancer, although the estimated magnitudes of the relative benefits ranged from 8 to 34% in various meta-analyses. In the WHI, the sole trial to examine the issue, estrogen-progestin was associated with a significant 44% reduction in colorectal cancer over a 5.6-year period, although no benefit was seen with 7 years of estrogen–only therapy.

COGNITIVE DECLINE AND DEMENTIA A meta-analysis of 10 case-control and 2 cohort studies suggested that postmenopausal HT is associated with a 34% decreased risk of dementia. Subsequent randomized trials, including the WHI, however, have failed to demonstrate any benefit of estrogen or estrogen-progestin therapy on the progression of mild to moderate Alzheimer's disease and/or have indicated a potential adverse effect of HT on the incidence of dementia, at least in women age 65 and older. Determining whether timing of initiation of HT influences cognitive outcomes will require further study.

OVARIAN CANCER AND OTHER DISORDERS On the basis of limited observational and randomized data, it has been hypothesized that HT increases the risk of ovarian cancer and reduces the risk of type 2 diabetes mellitus. Results from the WHI support these hypotheses.

APPROACH TO THE PATIENT:
Postmenopausal Hormone Therapy

The rational use of postmenopausal HT requires balancing the potential benefits and risks. Figure 342-2 provides one approach to decision making. The clinician should first determine whether the patient has moderate to severe menopausal symptoms, the only indication for initiating systemic HT (urogenital symptoms in the absence of vasomotor symptoms may be treated with vaginal estrogen). The benefits and risks of such therapy should then be reviewed with the patient, giving more emphasis to absolute than to relative measures of effect, and pointing out uncertainties in clinical knowledge where relevant. (Because chronic disease rates generally increase with age, absolute risks tend to be greater in older women, even when relative risks remain similar.) Potential side effects—es-

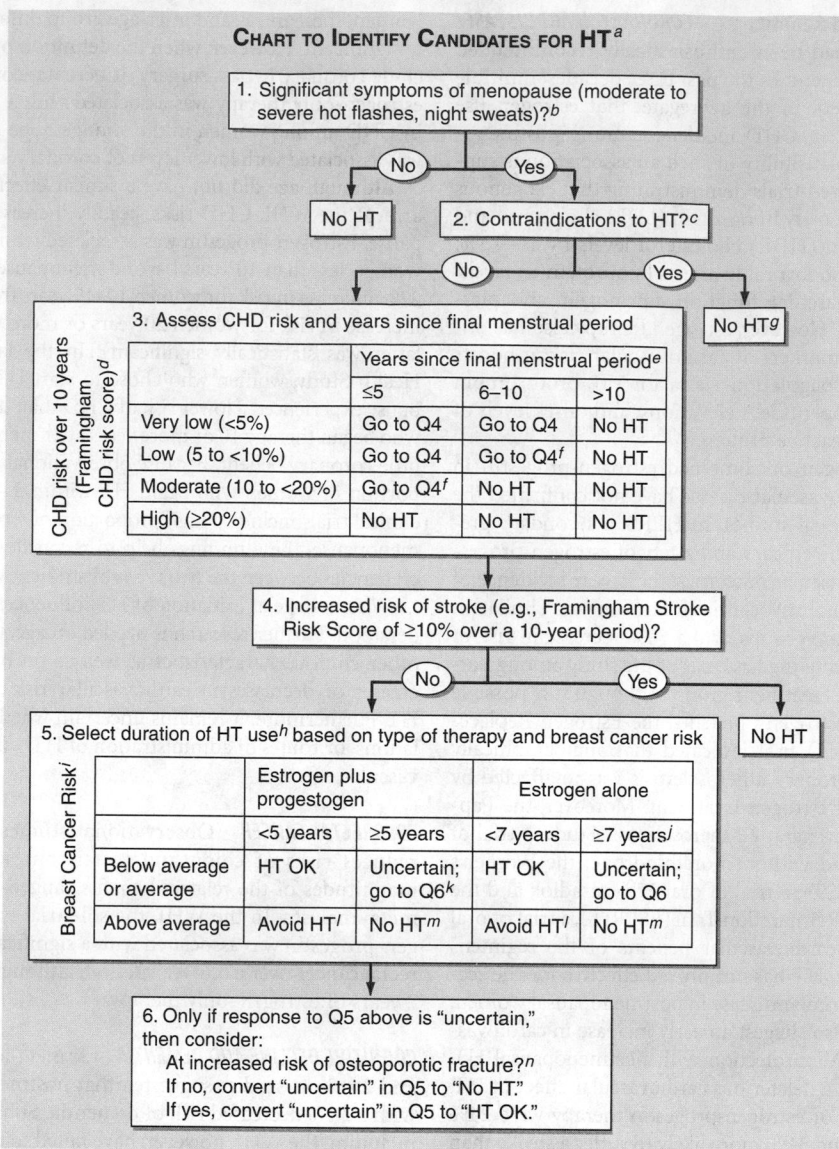

CHART TO IDENTIFY CANDIDATES FOR HT[a]

1. Significant symptoms of menopause (moderate to severe hot flashes, night sweats)?[b]

No → No HT

Yes → 2. Contraindications to HT?[c]

No → 3. Assess CHD risk and years since final menstrual period

Yes → No HT[g]

CHD risk over 10 years (Framingham CHD risk score)[d]	Years since final menstrual period[e]		
	≤5	6–10	>10
Very low (<5%)	Go to Q4	Go to Q4	No HT
Low (5 to <10%)	Go to Q4	Go to Q4[f]	No HT
Moderate (10 to <20%)	Go to Q4[f]	No HT	No HT
High (≥20%)	No HT	No HT	No HT

4. Increased risk of stroke (e.g., Framingham Stroke Risk Score of ≥10% over a 10-year period)?

No → 5. Select duration of HT use[h] based on type of therapy and breast cancer risk

Yes → No HT

Breast Cancer Risk[i]	Estrogen plus progestogen		Estrogen alone	
	<5 years	≥5 years	<7 years	≥7 years[j]
Below average or average	HT OK	Uncertain; go to Q6[k]	HT OK	Uncertain; go to Q6
Above average	Avoid HT[l]	No HT[m]	Avoid HT[l]	No HT[m]

6. Only if response to Q5 above is "uncertain," then consider:
   At increased risk of osteoporotic fracture?[n]
   If no, convert "uncertain" in Q5 to "No HT."
   If yes, convert "uncertain" in Q5 to "HT OK."

FIGURE 342-2 Flowchart for identifying appropriate candidates for postmenopausal hormone therapy (HT). CHD, coronary heart disease.
[a]Reassess each step at least once every 6–12 months (assuming patient's continued preference for HT).
[b]Women who have vaginal dryness without moderate to severe vasomotor symptoms may be candidates for vaginal estrogen.
[c]Traditional contraindications: unexplained vaginal bleeding; active liver disease; history of venous thromboembolism due to pregnancy, oral contraceptive use, or unknown etiology; blood clotting disorder; history of breast or endometrial cancer; history of CHD, stroke, transient ischemic attack, or diabetes. For other contraindications, including high triglycerides (>400 mg/dL); active gallbladder disease; and history of venous thromboembolism due to past immobility, surgery, or bone fracture; oral HT should be avoided but transdermal HT may be an option (see f below).
[d]10-Year risk of CHD, based on Framingham Coronary Heart Disease Risk Score (Expert Panel on Detection, Evaluation, and Treatment of High Blood Cholesterol in Adults: JAMA 285:2486, 2001), as modified by JE Manson, with SS Bassuk: Hot Flashes, Hormones & Your Health. New York, McGraw-Hill, 2007.
[e]Women >10 years past menopause are not good candidates for starting (first use of) HT.
[f]Avoid oral HT. Transdermal HT may be an option because it has a less adverse effect on clotting factors, triglyceride levels, and inflammation factors than oral HT.

[g]Consider selective serotonin or serotonin-norepinephrine reuptake inhibitor, gabapentin, clonidine, soy, or alternative.
[h]HT should be continued only if moderate to severe menopausal symptoms persist. The recommended cutpoints for duration are based on results of the Women's Health Initiative estrogen-progestin and estrogen-alone trials, which lasted 5.6 and 7.1 years, respectively. For longer durations of HT use, balance of benefits and risks is not known.
[i]Above-average risk of breast cancer: one or more first-degree relatives with breast cancer; susceptibility genes such as BRCA1 or BRCA2; or a personal history of breast biopsy demonstrating atypia.
[j]Women with premature surgical menopause may take HT until average age at menopause (age 51 in the United States) and then follow flowchart for subsequent decision making.
[k]If progestogen is taken daily, avoid extending duration. If progestogen is cyclical or infrequent, avoid extending duration more than 1–2 years.
[l]If menopausal symptoms are severe, estrogen plus progestin can be taken for 2–3 years maximum and estrogen alone for 4–5 years maximum.
[m]If at high risk of osteoporotic fracture (see Q6), consider bisphosphonate, raloxifene, or alternative.
[n]Increased risk of osteoporotic fracture: documented osteopenia, personal or family history of nontraumatic fracture, current smoking, or weight <125 lb.

Source: Adapted from JE Manson with SS Bassuk: Hot Flashes, Hormones & Your Health. New York, McGraw-Hill, 2007.

pecially vaginal bleeding that may result from use of combined estrogen-progestogen formulations recommended for women with an intact uterus—should be noted. The patient's own preference regarding therapy should be elicited and factored into the decision. Contraindications to HT should be assessed routinely and include unexplained vaginal bleeding; active liver disease; venous thromboembolism; history of endometrial cancer (except stage 1 without deep invasion) or breast cancer; and history of CHD, stroke, transient ischemic attack, or diabetes. Relative contraindications include hypertriglyceridemia (>400 mg/dL) and active gallbladder disease; in such cases, transdermal estrogen may be an option. Primary prevention of heart disease should not be viewed as an expected benefit of HT, and an increase in stroke and a small early increase in coronary artery disease risk should be considered. Nevertheless, such therapy may be appropriate if the noncoronary benefits of treatment clearly outweigh risks. A woman who suffers an acute coronary event or stroke while on HT should stop therapy immediately.

Short-term use (<5 years) of HT is appropriate for relief of menopausal symptoms among women without contraindications to such use. However, such therapy should be avoided among women with an elevated baseline risk of future cardiovascular events. Women who have contraindications, or are opposed to HT, may derive benefit from the use of certain antidepressants (including venlafaxine, fluoxetine, or paroxetine), gabapentin, clonidine, soy, or black cohosh, and, for genitourinary symptoms, intravaginal estrogen creams or devices.

Long-term use (≥5 years) of HT, especially estrogen-progestogen, is more problematic because a heightened risk of breast cancer must be factored into the decision. Reasonable candidates for such use include a small percentage of postmenopausal women and comprise those who have persistent severe vasomotor symptoms along with an increased risk of osteoporosis (e.g., those with osteopenia, a personal or family history of nontraumatic fracture, or a weight below 125 lb), who also have no personal or family history of breast cancer in a first-degree relative or other contraindications, and who have a strong personal preference for therapy. Poor candidates are women with elevated cardiovascular risk, those at increased risk of breast cancer (e.g., women who have a first-degree relative with breast cancer, susceptibility genes such as *BRCA1* or *BRCA2*, or a personal history of cellular atypia detected by breast biopsy), and those at low risk of osteoporosis. Even in reasonable candidates, strategies to minimize dose and duration of use should be employed. For example, women using HT to relieve intense vasomotor symptoms in early postmenopause should consider discontinuing therapy before 5 years, resuming it only if such symptoms persist. Because of the role

of progestogens in increasing breast cancer risk, regimens that employ cyclic rather than continuous progestogen exposure should be considered if treatment is extended. For prevention of osteoporosis, alternative therapies such as bisphosphonates or SERMs should be considered. Research on androgen-containing preparations has been limited, particularly in terms of long-term safety. Additional research on the effects of these agents on cardiovascular disease, glucose tolerance, and breast cancer will be of particular interest.

In addition to HT, control of symptoms and prevention of chronic disease can be accomplished by lifestyle choices, including smoking abstention, adequate physical activity, and a healthy diet. An expanding array of pharmacologic options—e.g., bisphosphonates, SERMs, and other agents for osteoporosis, and cholesterol-lowering or antihypertensive agents for cardiovascular disease—should also reduce the widespread reliance on hormone use. However, short-term HT may still benefit some women.

FURTHER READINGS

ADVISORY PANEL OF THE NORTH AMERICAN MENOPAUSE SOCIETY: Estrogen and progestin use in peri- and postmenopausal women: March 2007 Position Statement of the North American Menopause Society. Menopause 14:168, 2007

AMERICAN COLLEGE OF OBSTETRICIANS AND GYNECOLOGISTS TASK FORCE ON HORMONE THERAPY: Hormone therapy. Obstet Gynecol 104:S1, 2004

HSIA J et al: Conjugated equine estrogens and coronary heart disease. Arch Intern Med 166:357, 2006

MANSON JE et al: Estrogen plus progestin and the risk of coronary heart disease. N Engl J Med 349:523, 2003

——— et al: Estrogen therapy and coronary-artery calcification. N Engl J Med 356:2591, 2007

MANSON JE, WITH BASSUK SS: *Hot Flashes, Hormones & Your Health.* New York: McGraw-Hill, 2007

ROBERTS H: Managing the menopause. BMJ 334(7596):736, 2007

ROSSOUW JE et al: Postmenopausal hormone therapy and risk of cardiovascular disease by age and years since menopause. JAMA 297:1465, 2007

STEERING COMMITTEE FOR THE WOMEN'S HEALTH INITIATIVE: Effects of conjugated equine estrogen in postmenopausal women with hysterectomy: Principal results from the Women's Health Initiative randomized controlled trial. JAMA 291:1701, 2004

WARREN MP: Historical perspectives in postmenopausal hormone therapy: Defining the right dose and duration. Mayo Clin Proc 82(2):219, 2007

343 Disorders of Sex Development
John C. Achermann, J. Larry Jameson

Sex development begins in utero but continues into young adulthood with the achievement of sexual maturity and reproductive capability. The early stages of sex development can be divided into three major components: chromosomal sex, gonadal sex (sex determination), and phenotypic sex (sex differentiation) (Fig. 343-1). Abnormalities at each of these stages can result in disorders of sex development (DSD). The child born with ambiguous genitalia requires urgent assessment, as some causes, such as congenital adrenal hyperplasia (CAH), can be associated with life-threatening adrenal crises. Early gender assignment and clear communication with parents about the diagnosis and treatment options are essential. The involvement of an experienced multidisciplinary team is crucial for planning surgical intervention (if needed), medical management, and counseling. DSD can also manifest later in life due to subtler forms of gonadal dysfunction [e.g., Klinefelter syndrome (KS)] and

are often diagnosed by internists. Because DSD are associated with a variety of psychological, reproductive, and metabolic consequences, an open dialogue must be established between patient and health care providers to ensure continuity and attention to these issues.

NORMAL SEX DEVELOPMENT

Chromosomal sex describes the X and/or Y chromosome complement (46,XY male; 46,XX female) that is established at the time of fertilization. The presence of a normal Y chromosome determines that testis development will occur, even in the presence of multiple X chromosomes (e.g., 47,XXY or 48,XXXY). The loss of an X chromosome impairs gonad development (45,X or 45,X/46,XY mosaicism). Fetuses with no X chromosome (45,Y) are not viable.

Gonadal sex refers to the assignment of gonadal tissue as testis or ovary. The embryonic gonad is bipotential and can develop (from ~40 days gestation) into either a testis or ovary, depending on which genes are expressed (Fig. 343-2). Testis development is initiated by expression of the Y chromosome gene *SRY* (sex-determining region on the Y chromosome), which encodes an HMG box transcription factor. *SRY*

FIGURE 343-1 Sex development can be divided into three major components: chromosomal sex, gonadal sex, and phenotypic sex. T, testosterone; DHT, dihydrotestosterone; MIS, müllerian-inhibiting substance.

is transiently expressed in cells destined to become Sertoli cells and serves as a pivotal switch to establish the testis lineage. Mutation of *SRY* prevents testis development in chromosomal 46,XY males, whereas translocation of *SRY* in 46,XX females is sufficient to induce testis development and a male phenotype. Other genes are necessary to continue testis development. *SOX9* (*SRY*-related HMG-box gene 9) is upregulated in the developing male gonad but is suppressed in the female gonad. Transgenic expression of *SOX9* is sufficient to initiate testis formation in mice, and mutations that disrupt *SOX9* impair testis development. *WT1* (Wilms' tumor–related gene 1) acts early in the genetic pathway and regulates the transcription of several genes including *SF1*, *DAX1*, and *AMH* (encoding *MIS*, müllerian-inhibiting substance). *SF1* (steroidogenic factor 1) encodes a nuclear receptor that functions in cooperation with other transcription factors to regulate a large array of adrenal and gonadal genes, including many genes involved in steroidogenesis. Heterozygous *SF1* mutations account for ~10% of XY

FIGURE 343-2 The genetic regulation of gonadal development. *WT1*, Wilms' tumor–related gene 1; *SF1*, steroidogenic factor 1; *SRY*, sex-determining region on the Y chromosome; *SOX9*, SRY-related HMG-box gene 9; *DHH*, desert hedgehog; *ATRX*, (α-thalassemia, mental retardation on the X); *DAX1*, dosage sensitive sex-reversal, adrenal hypoplasia congenita on the X chromosome, gene 1; DMRT 1/2, doublesex MAB3-related transcription factor 1/2; *WNT4*, wingless-type MMTV integration site 4; *FST*, follistatin; *BMP2* and 15, bone morpho factors 2 and 15; *FOXL2*, forkhead transcription factor L2; *GDF9*, growth differentiation factor 9; *AMH*, anti-müllerian hormone (müllerian-inhibiting substance); *DHT*, dihydrotestosterone; *RSPO1*, R-spondin 1.

patients with gonadal dysgenesis and impaired androgenization, indicating the sensitivity of the testis to *SF1* gene dosage. The early expression pattern of *SF1* in the gonad parallels that of another orphan nuclear receptor, *DAX1* (dosage sensitive sex-reversal, adrenal hypoplasia congenita on the X chromosome, gene 1). *DAX1* is downregulated as the testis develops. Duplication of *DAX1* impairs testis development, possibly by antagonizing the function of SRY and SF1. Deletions or mutations of *DAX1*, on the other hand, lead to disordered formation of testis cords, again revealing the exquisite sensitivity of the male sex-determining pathway to gene dosage effects. In addition to the genes mentioned above, studies of human and murine mutations indicate that at least 15 other genes are also involved in gonadal differentiation, development, and final positioning of the gonad (Fig. 343-2). These genes encode an array of signaling molecules and paracrine growth factors, in addition to transcription factors.

Although ovarian development was once considered to be a "default" process, it is now clear that specific genes are expressed during the earliest stages of ovary development (e.g., follistatin) (Fig. 343-2). Once the ovary has formed, additional genes are required for normal follicular development [e.g., follicle-stimulating hormone (FSH) receptor, GDF9]. Steroidogenesis in the ovary requires the development of follicles containing granulosa cells and theca cells surrounding the oocytes (Chap. 341). Thus, there is relatively limited ovarian steroidogenesis until gonadotropins are produced at puberty.

Germ cells also develop in a sex dimorphic manner. In the developing ovary, primordial germ cells (PGCs) enter meiosis, whereas they proliferate and then undergo mitotic arrest in the developing testis. PGC entry into meiosis is initiated by retinoic acid, which activates *STRA8* (*stimulated by retinoic acid 8*) and other genes involved in meiosis. The developing testis produces high levels of CYP26B1, an enzyme that degrades retinoic acid, thereby preventing PGC entry into meiosis.

Phenotypic sex refers to the structures of the external and internal genitalia and secondary sex characteristics. The male phenotype requires the secretion of anti-müllerian hormone (AMH, müllerian-inhibiting substance) from Sertoli cells and testosterone from testicular Leydig cells. AMH is a member of the transforming growth factor (TGF) β family and acts through specific receptors to cause regression of the müllerian structures (60–80 days gestation). At ~60–140 days gestation, testosterone supports the development of wolffian structures, including the epididymides, vasa deferentia, and seminal vesicles. Testosterone is the precursor for dihydrotestosterone (DHT), a potent androgen that promotes development of the external genitalia, including the penis and scrotum (65–100 days, and thereafter) (Fig. 343-3). The urogenital sinus develops into the prostate and prostatic urethra in the male and into the urethra and lower portion of the vagina in the female. The genital tubercle becomes the glans penis in the male and the clitoris in the female. The urogenital swellings form the scrotum or the labia majora, and the urethral folds fuse to form the shaft of the penis and the male urethra or the labia minora. In the female, wolffian ducts regress and the müllerian ducts form the fallopian tubes, uterus, and upper segment of the vagina. A normal female phenotype will develop in the absence of the gonad, but estrogen is needed for maturation of the uterus and breast at puberty.

DISORDERS OF CHROMOSOMAL SEX

Disorders of chromosomal sex result from abnormalities in the number or structure of the X or Y chromosomes (Table 343-1).

KLINEFELTER SYNDROME (47,XXY)

Pathophysiology The classic form of KS (47,XXY) occurs following meiotic nondisjunction of the sex chromosomes during gametogenesis (40% during spermatogenesis, 60% during oogenesis) (Chap. 63). Mosaic forms of KS (46,XY/47,XXY) are thought to result from chromosomal mitotic nondisjunction within the zygote, and occur in at least 10% of individuals with this condition. Other chromosomal variants of KS (e.g., 48,XXYY; 48,XXXY) have been reported but are less common.

FIGURE 343-3 Normal sex development. A. Internal urogenital tract. **B.** External genitalia. *[After JD Wilson, JE Griffin, in E Braunwald et al (eds): Harrison's Principles of Internal Medicine, 15th ed. New York, McGraw-Hill, 2001.]*

ing in vitro fertilization in men with oligospermia or with intracytoplasmic sperm injection (ICSI) following retrieval of spermatozoa by testicular sperm extraction techniques. In specialized centers, successful spermatozoa retrieval using this technique is possible in >50% of men with non-mosaic KS. Following ICSI and embryo transfer, successful pregnancies can be achieved in ~50% of these cases. The risk of transmission of this chromosomal abnormality needs to be considered, and preimplantation screening may be desired.

TURNER SYNDROME (GONADAL DYSGENESIS; 45,X)

Pathophysiology Approximately one-half of individuals with Turner syndrome (TS) have a 45,X karyotype, about 20% have 45,X/46,XX mosaicism, and the remainder have structural abnormalities of the X chromosome such as X fragments, isochromosomes, or rings. The clinical features of TS result from haploinsufficiency of multiple X chromosomal genes (e.g., short stature homeobox, *SHOX*). However, imprinted genes may also be affected when the inherited X has different parental origins.

Clinical Features TS is characterized by bilateral streak gonads, primary amenorrhea, short stature, and multiple congenital anomalies in phenotypic females. It affects ~1 in 2500 women and is diagnosed at different ages depending on the dominant clinical features (Table 343-1). Prenatally, a diagnosis of TS is usually made incidentally after chorionic villous sampling or amniocentesis for unrelated reasons, such as advanced maternal age. Prenatal ultrasound findings include increased nuchal translucency and reduced fetal growth in some cases. The postnatal diagnosis of TS should be considered in female neonates or infants with lymphedema, nuchal folds, low hairline, or left-sided cardiac defects, and in girls with unexplained growth failure or pubertal delay. Although limited spontaneous pubertal development occurs in up to 30% of girls with TS (10%, 45,X; 30–40%, 45,X/46,XX), and ~2% reach menarche, the vast majority of women with TS develop complete ovarian failure. This diagnosis should be considered, therefore, in all women who present with primary or secondary amenorrhea and elevated gonadotropin levels.

℞ TURNER SYNDROME

The management of girls and women with TS requires a multidisciplinary approach because of the number of potentially involved organ systems. Detailed cardiac and renal evaluation should be performed at the time of diagnosis. Individuals with congenital heart defects (CHD) (30%) (bicuspid aortic valve, 30–50%; coarctation of the aorta, 30%; aortic root dilatation, 5%) require long-term follow-up by an experienced cardiologist, antibiotic prophylaxis for dental or surgical procedures, and serial imaging of aortic root dimensions, as progressive aortic root dilatation is associated with increased risk of aortic dissection. Individuals found to have congenital renal and urinary tract malformations (30%) are at risk for urinary tract infections, hypertension, and nephrocalcinosis. Hypertension can occur independent of cardiac and renal malformations and should be monitored and treated as in other patients with essential hypertension. Clitoral enlargement or other evidence of virilization suggests the presence of covert, translocated Y chromosomal material and is associated with increased risk of gonado-

Clinical Features KS is characterized by small testes, infertility, gynecomastia, eunuchoid proportions, and poor virilization in phenotypic males. It has an incidence of at least 1 in 1000 men, but many are not diagnosed. In severe cases, individuals present prepubertally with small testes, or with impaired androgenization and gynecomastia at the time of puberty. Developmental delay and learning disabilities may be a feature. Later in life, eunuchoid features or infertility lead to the diagnosis. Testes are small and firm [median length 2.5 cm (4 mL volume); almost always <3.5 cm (12 mL)], and typically seem inappropriately small for the degree of androgenization. Biopsies are not usually necessary but reveal seminiferous tubule hyalinization and azoospermia. Other clinical features of KS are listed in Table 343-1. Plasma concentrations of FSH and luteinizing hormone (LH) are increased in most patients with 47,XXY (90 and 80%, respectively) and plasma testosterone is decreased (50–75%), reflecting primary gonadal failure. Estradiol is often increased because of chronic Leydig cell stimulation by LH and because of aromatization of androstenedione by adipose tissue; the increased ratio of estradiol/testosterone results in gynecomastia. Patients with mosaic forms of KS have less severe clinical features, larger testes, and sometimes achieve spontaneous fertility.

℞ KLINEFELTER SYNDROME

Gynecomastia should be treated by surgical reduction if it causes concern (Chap. 340). Androgen supplementation improves virilization, libido, energy, hypofibrinolysis, and bone mineralization in underandrogenized men but may occasionally worsen gynecomastia (Chap. 340). Fertility has been achieved us-

TABLE 343-1 CLINICAL FEATURES OF CHROMOSOMAL DISORDERS OF SEX DEVELOPMENT (DSD)

Disorder	Common Chromosomal Complement	Gonad	Genitalia		Breast Development	Clinical Features
			External	Internal		
Klinefelter syndrome	47,XXY or 46,XY/ 47,XXY	Hyalinized testes	Male	Male	Gynecomastia	Small testes, azoospermia, decreased facial and axillary hair, decreased libido, tall stature & increased leg length, decreased penile length, increased risk of breast tumors, thromboembolic disease, learning difficulties, obesity, diabetes mellitus, varicose veins
Turner syndrome	45,X or 45,X/ 46,XX	Streak gonad or immature ovary	Female	Hypoplastic female	Immature female	Infancy: lymphedema, web neck, shield chest, low set hair line, cardiac defects and coarctation of the aorta, urinary tract malformations & horseshoe kidney Childhood: short stature, cubitus valgus, short neck, short 4th metacarpals, hypoplastic nails, micrognathia, scoliosis, otitis media & sensorineural hearing loss, ptosis & amblyopia, multiple nevi & keloid formation, autoimmune thyroid disease, visuo-spatial learning difficulties Adulthood: pubertal failure & primary amenorrhea, hypertension, obesity, dyslipidemia, impaired glucose tolerance & insulin resistance, autoimmune thyroid disease, cardiovascular disease, aortic root dilatation, osteoporosis, inflammatory bowel disease, chronic hepatic dysfunction, increased risk of colon cancer, hearing loss
Mixed gonadal dysgenesis	45,X/46,XY	Testis or streak gonad	Variable	Variable	Usually male	Short stature, increased risk of gonadal tumors, some Turner syndrome features
True hermaphroditism (ovotesticular DSD)	46,XX/46,XY	Testis & ovary or ovotestis	Variable	Variable	Gynecomastia	Possible increased risk of gonadal tumors

blastoma, apparently the consequence of Y chromosomal genes distinct from *SRY*. Regular assessment of thyroid function, weight, dentition, hearing, speech, vision, and educational issues should be performed during childhood. Otitis media and middle ear disease are prevalent in childhood (50–85%), and sensorineural hearing loss becomes progressively frequent with age (70–90%). Autoimmune hypothyroidism (15–30%) can occur in childhood but has a mean age of onset in the third decade. Counseling about long-term growth and fertility issues should be provided. Patient support groups are active throughout the world.

The treatment of short stature in children with TS remains a challenge, as untreated final height rarely exceeds 150 cm. High-dose recombinant growth hormone stimulates growth rate in children with TS and may be used alone or in combination with low doses of the nonaromatizable anabolic steroid oxandrolone (up to 0.05 mg/kg per day) in the older child (>8 years). However, final height increments are often modest (5–10 cm), and individualization of treatment regimens to response may be beneficial. Girls with evidence of gonadal failure require estrogen replacement to induce breast and uterine development, to support growth, and to maintain bone mineralization. Most physicians now choose to initiate low-dose estrogen therapy (one-tenth to one-eighth of the adult replacement dose) to induce puberty at an age-appropriate time (~12 years). Doses of estrogen are increased gradually to allow feminization over a 2–3 year period. Progestins are later added to regulate withdrawal bleeds, and some women with TS have now achieved successful pregnancy after ovum donation and in vitro fertilization. Long-term follow-up of women with TS involves careful surveillance of sex hormone replacement and reproductive function, bone mineralization, cardiac function and aortic root dimensions, blood pressure, weight and glucose tolerance, hepatic and lipid profiles, thyroid function, and hearing.

MIXED GONADAL DYSGENESIS (45,X/46,XY)

Mixed gonadal dysgenesis typically results from 45,X/46,XY mosaicism. The phenotype of patients with this condition varies considerably. Although some patients have a predominantly female phenotype with somatic features of TS, streak gonads, and müllerian structures, most 45,X/46,XY individuals have a male phenotype and testes, and the diagnosis is made incidentally after amniocentesis or during investigation of infertility. In practice, most children referred for assessment

have ambiguous genitalia and variable somatic features. A female sex-of-rearing is often chosen (60%) if phallic development is poor and uterine structures are present. However, gonadectomy is indicated to prevent further androgen secretion and to prevent development of gonadoblastoma (up to 25%). Individuals raised as males may require reconstructive surgery for hypospadias and removal of dysgenetic gonads. Scrotal testes can be preserved but need regular examination for tumor development. Biopsy for carcinoma in situ is recommended in adolescence, and testosterone supplementation may be required for virilization in puberty. Height potential is usually limited.

OVOTESTICULAR DSD

Ovotesticular DSD (formerly called *true hermaphroditism*) occurs when both an ovary and testis, or when an ovotestis, are found in one individual. For unclear reasons, gonadal asymmetry most often occurs with a testis on the right and an ovary on the left. Most individuals with this diagnosis have a 46,XX karyotype, especially in Sub-Sahara Africa. A 46,XX/46,XY chimeric karyotype is less common and has a variable phenotype depending on the proportion of each cell line. Fluorescence in situ hybridization (FISH) or polymerase chain reaction (PCR) for *SRY* may detect translocations of this region of the Y chromosome in a subset of patients.

DISORDERS OF GONADAL AND PHENOTYPIC SEX

The clinical features of patients with disorders of gonadal and phenotypic sex are divided into the underandrogenization of 46,XY males (46,XY DSD) or excess androgenization of 46,XX females (46,XX DSD). These disorders comprise a spectrum of phenotypes ranging from "46,XY phenotypic females" or "46,XX males" to individuals with ambiguous genitalia.

46,XY DSD (UNDERANDROGENIZED MALES)

Underandrogenization of the 46,XY fetus (formerly called *male pseudohermaphroditism*) reflects defects in androgen production or action. It can result from disorders of testis development, defects of androgen synthesis, or resistance to testosterone and DHT (Table 343-2).

TABLE 343-2 DISORDERS CAUSING UNDERANDROGENIZATION IN KARYOTYPIC MALES (46,XY DSD)

Disorders of testis development
  True hermaphroditism (46,XY)
  Gonadal dysgenesis
  Absent testis syndrome
Disorders of androgen synthesis
  LH receptor mutations
  Smith-Lemli-Opitz syndrome
  Steroidogenic acute regulatory protein mutations
  Cholesterol side chain cleavage (CYP11A1) deficiency
  3β-Hydroxysteroid dehydrogenase 2 (HSD3B2) deficiency
  17α-Hydroxylase/17,20-lyase (CYP17) deficiency
  P450 oxidoreductase deficiency (POR)
  17β-Hydroxysteroid dehydrogenase 3 (HSD17B3) deficiency
  5α-Reductase 2 deficiency (SRD5A2)
Disorders of androgen action
  Androgen insensitivity syndrome
  Androgen receptor cofactor defects
Other disorders of male reproductive tract
  Persistent müllerian duct syndrome
  Isolated hypospadias
  Cryptorchidism or undescended testes

Note: DSD, disorders of sex development.

Disorders of Testis Development • *TESTICULAR DYSGENESIS* Patients with *pure* (or *complete*) *gonadal dysgenesis* (*Swyer syndrome*) have streak gonads, müllerian structures [due to insufficient AMH/müllerian inhibiting substance (MIS) secretion], and a complete absence of androgenization. Patients with *partial gonadal dysgenesis* (*dysgenetic testes*) produce enough MIS to regress the uterus and, sometimes, sufficient testosterone for partial androgenization. Gonadal dysgenesis can result from mutations or deletions of testis-promoting genes (*WT1, SF1, SRY, SOX9, DHH, ATRX, ARX, DMRT*) or duplication of chromosomal loci containing *WNT4* or *DAX1* (Table 343-3). Among these, deletions or mutations of *SRY* and heterozygous mutations of *SF1* appear to be most common but still account for <25% of cases. Associated clinical features may be present, reflecting additional functional roles for these genes. For example, renal dysfunction occurs in patients with specific *WT1* mutations (Denys-Drash and Frasier syndromes), primary adrenal failure occurs with some patients with *SF1* mutations, and severe cartilage abnormalities (campomelic dysplasia) are the predominant clinical feature of *SOX9* mutations. Dysgenetic testes should be removed to prevent malignancy, and estrogens can be used to induce secondary sex characteristics in 46,XY individuals raised as females. *Absent (vanishing) testis syndrome* (*bilateral anorchia*) reflects regression of the testis during development. The etiology is unknown, but the absence of müllerian structures indicates adequate secretion of

CHAPTER 343 Disorders of Sex Development

TABLE 343-3 GENETIC CAUSES OF UNDERANDROGENIZATION OF KARYOTYPIC MALES (46,XY DSD)

Gene	Inheritance	Gonad	Uterus	External Genitalia	Associated Features
Disorders of Testis Development					
WT1	AD	Dysgenetic testis	+/−	Female or ambiguous	Wilms' tumor, renal abnormalities, gonadal tumors (WAGR, Denys-Drash & Frasier syndromes)
SF1	AR/AD	Dysgenetic testis	+/−	Female or ambiguous	Primary adrenal failure
SRY	Y	Dysgenetic testis or ovotestis	+/−	Female or ambiguous	
SOX9	AD	Dysgenetic testis or ovotestis	+/−	Female or ambiguous	Campomelic dysplasia
DHH	AR	Dysgenetic testis	+	Female	Minifascicular neuropathy
ATRX	X	Dysgenetic testis	−	Female or ambiguous	α-Thalassemia, developmental delay
ARX	X	Dysgenetic testis	−	Male or ambiguous	Mental retardation; X-linked lissencephaly
DAX1	dupXp21	Dysgenetic testis	+/−	Female or ambiguous	
WNT4	dup1p35	Dysgenetic testis	+	Ambiguous	
Disorders of Androgen Synthesis					
LHR	AR	Testis	−	Female, ambiguous or micropenis	Leydig cell hypoplasia
DHCR7	AR	Testis	−	Variable	Smith-Lemli-Opitz syndrome: coarse facies, second-third toe syndactyly, failure to thrive, developmental delay, cardiac & visceral abnormalities
StAR	AR	Testis	−	Female or ambiguous	Congenital lipoid adrenal hyperplasia (primary adrenal failure)
CYP11A1	AR	Testis	−	Ambiguous	Primary adrenal failure
HSD3B2	AR	Testis	−	Ambiguous	CAH, primary adrenal failure, partial androgenization due to ↑ DHEA
CYP17	AR	Testis	−	Female or ambiguous	CAH, hypertension due to ↑ corticosterone & 11-deoxycorticosterone, except in isolated 17,20 lyase deficiency
POR	AR	Testis	−	Ambiguous or male	Mixed features of 21-hydroxylase deficiency and 17α-hydroxylase/17,20 lyase deficiency, sometimes associated with Antley-Bixler craniosynostosis
HSD17B3	AR	Testis	−	Female or ambiguous	Partial androgenization at puberty, ↑ androstenedione:testosterone ratio
SRD5A2	AR	Testis	−	Ambiguous or micropenis	Partial androgenization at puberty, ↑ testosterone: dihydrotestosterone ratio
Disorders of Androgen Action					
Androgen receptor	X	Testis	−	Female, ambiguous, micropenis or normal male	Phenotypic spectrum from complete androgen insensitivity syndrome (female external genitalia) and partial androgen insensitivity (ambiguous) to normal male genitalia and infertility

Note: AR, autosomal recessive; AD, autosomal dominant; *WT1*, Wilms' tumor-related gene 1; WAGR, Wilms' tumor, aniridia, genitourinary anomalies, and mental retardation; *SF1*, steroidogenic factor 1; *SRY*, sex-related gene on the Y chromosome; *SOX9*, SRY-related HMG-box gene 9; *DHH*, desert hedgehog; *ATRX*, (α-thalassemia, mental retardation on the X); *ARX*, aristaless related homeobox, X-linked; *DAX1*, dosage sensitive sex-reversal, adrenal hypoplasia congenita on the X chromosome, gene 1; *WNT4*, wingless-type mouse mammary tumor virus integration site, 4; *LHR*, LH receptor; *DHCR7*, sterol 7δ reductase; *StAR*, steroidogenic acute regulatory protein; *CYP11A1*, P450 cholesterol side-chain cleavage; *HSD3B2*, 3β-hydroxysteroid dehydrogenase type 2; *CYP17*, 17α-hydroxylase and 17,20-lyase; *POR*, P450 oxidoreductase deficiency; *HSD17B3*, 17β-hydroxysteroid dehydrogenase type 3; *CYP19*, aromatase; *SRD5A2*, 5α-reductase type 2.

FIGURE 343-4 Simplified overview of glucocorticoid and androgen synthesis pathways. Defects in *CYP21A2* and *CYP11B1* shunt steroid precursors into the androgen pathway and cause androgenization of 46,XX females. Testosterone and dihydrotestosterone are synthesized in the testicular Leydig cells. Defects in enzymes involved in androgen synthesis result in underandrogenization of 46,XY males. *StAR*, steroidogenic acute regulatory protein. [*After JD Wilson, JE Griffin, in E Braunwald et al (eds): Harrison's Principles of Internal Medicine, 15th ed. New York, McGraw-Hill, 2001.*]

adrenal insufficiency in severe cases, but the accumulation of dehydroepiandrosterone (DHEA) has a mild androgenizing effect resulting in ambiguous genitalia or hypospadias. Patients with congenital adrenal hyperplasia due to *17α-hydroxylase (CYP17) deficiency* have variable underandrogenization and develop hypertension and hypokalemia due to the potent salt-retaining effects of corticosterone and 11-deoxycorticosterone. Patients with complete loss of *17α-hydroxylase* function often present as phenotypic females who fail to enter puberty and are found to have inguinal testes and hypertension in adolescence. Some mutations in *CYP17* selectively impair 17,20 lyase activity, without altering 17α-hydroxylase activity, leading to underandrogenization without mineralocorticoid excess and hypertension. Mutations in *P450 oxidoreductase (POR)* affect multiple steroidogenic enzymes leading to impaired androgenization and a biochemical pattern of apparent combined 21-hydroxylase and 17α-hydroxylase deficiency, sometimes with skeletal abnormalities (Antley-Bixler craniosynostosis). Defects in *17β-hydroxysteroid dehydrogenase type 3 (HSD17B3)* and *5α-reductase type 2 (SRD5A2)* interfere with the synthesis of testosterone and DHT, respectively. These conditions are characterized by minimal or absent androgenization in utero, but some phallic development can occur during adolescence due to the action of other enzyme isoforms. Individuals with *5α-reductase type 2* deficiency have normal wolffian structures and do not usually develop breast tissue. In some cultures, these individuals change gender role behavior from female to male at puberty, because the increase in testosterone induces muscle mass and other virilizing features. DHT cream can improve prepubertal phallic growth in patients raised as male. Individuals raised as female require gonadectomy before adolescence and estrogen replacement at puberty.

MIS in utero. Early testicular regression causes impaired androgenization in utero and, in most cases, androgenization of the external genitalia is either normal or slightly impaired (e.g., micropenis, hypospadias). These individuals can be offered testicular prostheses and should receive androgen replacement in adolescence.

Disorders of Androgen Synthesis Defects in the pathway that regulates androgen synthesis (Fig. 343-4) cause underandrogenization of the male fetus (Table 343-3). Müllerian regression is unaffected because Sertoli cell function is preserved.

LH RECEPTOR Mutations in the LH receptor cause Leydig cell hypoplasia and androgen deficiency. Defects of LH receptor synthesis or function preclude hCG (human chorionic gonadotropin) stimulation of Leydig cells in utero, as well as LH stimulation of Leydig cells late in gestation and during the neonatal period. As a result, testosterone and DHT synthesis are insufficient for normal androgenization of the internal and external genitalia, causing a spectrum of phenotypes that range from complete underandrogenization to micropenis, depending on the severity of the mutation.

STEROIDOGENIC ENZYME PATHWAYS Mutations in *steroidogenic acute regulatory protein (StAR)* and *CYP11A1* affect both adrenal and gonadal steroidogenesis (Chap. 336). Affected individuals (46,XY) usually have severe early-onset salt-losing adrenal failure and a female phenotype. Defects in *3β-hydroxysteroid dehydrogenase type 2 (HSD3B2)* also cause

Disorders of Androgen Action • *ANDROGEN INSENSITIVITY SYNDROME* Mutations in the androgen receptor (AR) cause resistance to androgen (testosterone, DHT) action or the *androgen insensitivity syndrome* (AIS). AIS is a spectrum of disorders that affects at least 1 in 100,000 chromosomal males. Because the androgen receptor is X-linked, only males are affected and maternal carriers are phenotypically normal. XY individuals with *complete AIS (formerly called testicular feminization syndrome)* have a female phenotype, normal breast development (due to aromatization of testosterone), a short vagina but no uterus (because MIS production is normal), scanty pubic and axillary hair, and female psychosexual orientation. Gonadotropins and testosterone levels can be low, normal, or elevated, depending on the degree of androgen resistance and the contribution of estradiol to feedback inhibition of the hypothalamic-pituitary gonadal axis. Most patients present with inguinal herniae (containing testes) in childhood or with primary amenorrhea in adulthood. Gonadectomy is usually performed, as there is a low risk of malignancy, and estrogen replacement is prescribed. Alternatively, the gonads can be left in situ until breast development is complete. The use of graded dilators in adolescence is usually sufficient to dilate the vagina and permit sexual intercourse.

Partial AIS (Reifenstein syndrome) results from less severe AR mutations. Patients often present in infancy with perineoscrotal hypospadias, small undescended testes, and with gynecomastia at the time of puberty. Those individuals raised as males require hypospadias repair in childhood and breast reduction in adolescence. Supplemental testosterone rarely enhances androgenization significantly, as endogenous testosterone is already increased. More severely underandrogenized patients present with clitoral enlargement and labial fusion and may be raised as females. The surgical and psychosexual management of these patients is complex and requires active involvement of the parents and the patient during the appropriate stages of development. *Azoospermia* and male-factor infertility has also been described in association with mild loss-of-function mutations in the androgen receptor. Trinucleotide (CAG) repeat expansion, from a mean of 22 repeats to >40 repeats, within a highly polymorphic region of the androgen receptor is associated with spinal and bulbar muscular atrophy (also known as Kennedy disease). These patients may show evidence of partial androgen insensitivity in adolescence or adulthood (e.g., gynecomastia).

OTHER DISORDERS AFFECTING 46,XY MALES

Persistent müllerian duct syndrome is the presence of a uterus in an otherwise normal male. This condition can result from mutations in AMH or its receptor (AMHR2). The uterus may be removed, but damage to vasa deferentia must be avoided. *Isolated hypospadias* occurs in ~1 in 200 males and is treated by surgical repair. Most cases are idiopathic, although evidence of penoscrotal hypospadias, poor phallic development, and/or bilateral cryptorchidism require investigation for an underlying disorder of sex development (e.g., defect in testosterone action). Unilateral undescended testes (cryptorchidism) affects more than 3% of boys at birth. Orchidopexy should be considered if the testis has not descended by 6–12 months of age. Bilateral cryptorchidism occurs less frequently and should raise suspicion of gonadotropin deficiency or DSD. A subset of patients with cryptorchidism have mutations in the insulin-like 3 (*INSL3*) gene or its receptor LGR8 (also known as *GREAT*), which mediates normal testicular descent. Ascending testis is being increasingly recognized as a distinct condition for which management is currently unclear. *Syndromic associations* and *intrauterine growth retardation* also occur relatively frequently in association with impaired testicular function or target-tissue responsiveness, but the underlying etiology of many of these conditions is unknown.

46,XX DSD (ANDROGENIZED FEMALES)

Inappropriate androgenization of females (formerly called *female pseudohermaphroditism*) occurs when the gonad (ovary) contains androgen-secreting testicular material or after increased androgen exposure (Table 343-4).

TABLE 343-4 DISORDERS CAUSING ANDROGENIZATION IN KARYOTYPIC FEMALES (46,XX DSD)

Ovarian transdifferentiation
   True hermaphroditism (46,XX)
   XX male (46,XX testicular DSD)
Increased androgen synthesis
   3β-Hydroxysteroid dehydrogenase 2 (*HSD3B2*) deficiency (mild)
   21-Hydroxylase (*CYP21A2*) deficiency
   P450 oxidoreductase (*POR*) deficiency
   11β-Hydroxylase (*CYP11B1*) deficiency
   Aromatase (*CYP19*) deficiency
   Glucocorticoid receptor mutations
Increased androgen exposure
   Maternal virilizing tumors (e.g., luteomas of pregnancy)
   Androgenic drugs
Nonvirilizing disorders of the female reproductive tract
   Ovarian dysgenesis
   Müllerian agenesis
   Vaginal agenesis

Note: DSD, disorders of sex development.

Gonadal Transdifferentiation Testicular tissue can develop in 46,XX testicular DSD (46,XX males) following translocation of *SRY* or duplication of *SOX9* or defects in *RSPO1* (Table 343-5).

Increased Androgen Exposure • *21-HYDROXYLASE DEFICIENCY (CONGENITAL ADRENAL HYPERPLASIA)* The *classic form* of 21-hydroxylase deficiency (21-OHD) is the most common cause of CAH (Chap. 336). It has an incidence of between 1 in 10,000 and 15,000 and is the most frequent cause of androgenization in chromosomal 46,XX females (Table 343-5). Affected individuals are homozygous or compound heterozygous for severe mutations in the enzyme 21-hydroxylase (*CYP21A2*). This mutation causes a block in adrenal glucocorticoid and mineralocorticoid synthesis, increasing 17-hydroxyprogesterone, and shunting steroid precursors into the androgen synthesis pathway (Fig. 343-4). Glucocorticoid insufficiency causes a compensatory elevation of adrenocorticotropin (ACTH), resulting in adrenal hyperplasia and additional synthesis of steroid precursors proximal to the enzymatic block. Increased androgen synthesis in utero causes androgenization of the female fetus in the first trimester. Ambiguous genitalia are seen at birth, with varying degrees of clitoral enlargement and labial fusion. Excess androgen production causes gonadotropin-independent precocious puberty in males with 21-OHD.

TABLE 343-5 GENETIC CAUSES OF ANDROGENIZATION OF KARYOTYPIC FEMALES (46,XX DSD)

Gene	Inheritance	Gonad	Uterus	External Genitalia	Associated Features
Ovarian Transdifferentiation					
SRY	Translocation	Testis or ovotestis	−	Male or ambiguous	
SOX9	dup17q24	Unknown	−	Male or ambiguous	
RSPO1	AR	Testis or ovotestis	±	Male or ambiguous	Palmarplantar hyperkeratosis, squamous cell skin carcinoma
Increased Androgen Synthesis					
HSD3B2	AR	Ovary	+	Clitoromegaly	CAH, primary adrenal failure, mild androgenization due to ↑ DHEA
CYP21A2	AR	Ovary	+	Ambiguous	CAH, phenotypic spectrum from severe salt-losing forms associated with adrenal failure to simple virilizing forms with compensated adrenal function, ↑ 17-hydroxyprogesterone
POR	AR	Ovary	+	Ambiguous or female	Mixed features of 21-hydroxylase deficiency and 17α-hydroxylase/17,20 lyase deficiency, sometimes associated with Antley-Bixler craniosynostosis
CYP11B1	AR	Ovary	+	Ambiguous	CAH, hypertension due to ↑ 11-deoxycortisol & 11-deoxycorticosterone
CYP19	AR	Ovary	+	Ambiguous	Maternal virilization during pregnancy, absent breast development at puberty
Glucocorticoid receptor	AR	Ovary	+	Ambiguous	↑ ACTH, 17-hydroxyprogesterone and cortisol; failure of dexamethasone suppression

Note: DSD, disorders of sex development; AR, autosomal recessive; *SRY*, sex-related gene on the Y chromosome; *SOX9*, SRY-related HMG-box gene 9; CAH, congenital adrenal hyperplasia; *HSD3B2*, 3β-hydroxysteroid dehydrogenase type 2; *CYP21A2*, 21-hydroxylase; POR, P450 oxidoreductase deficiency; *CYP11B1*, 11β-hydroxylase; *CYP19*, aromatase; ACTH, adrenocorticotropin; *RSPO1*, R-spondin 1.

The *salt-wasting* form of 21-OHD results from severe combined glucocorticoid and mineralocorticoid deficiency. A salt-wasting crisis usually manifests between 7 and 21 days of life and is a potentially life-threatening event requiring urgent fluid resuscitation and steroid treatment. Thus, a diagnosis of 21-OHD should be considered in any baby with ambiguous genitalia with bilateral non-palpable gonads. Males (46,XY) with 21-OHD have no genital abnormalities at birth but are equally susceptible to adrenal insufficiency and salt-losing crises.

Females with the *classic simple virilizing* form of 21-OHD also present with genital ambiguity. They have impaired cortisol biosynthesis but do not develop salt loss. Patients with *nonclassic 21-OHD* produce normal amounts of cortisol and aldosterone, but at the expense of producing excess androgens. Hirsutism (60%), oligomenorrhea (50%), and acne (30%) are the most frequent presenting features. This is one of the most frequent recessive disorders in humans, with an incidence as high as 1 in 100–500 in many populations and 1 in 27 in Ashkenazi Jews of Eastern European origin.

Biochemical features of acute salt-wasting 21-OHD are hypoglycemia, hyponatremia, hyperkalemia, low cortisol and aldosterone, and elevated 17-hydroxyprogesterone, ACTH, and plasma renin activity. Presymptomatic diagnosis of classic 21-OHD is now made by neonatal screening tests for increased 17-hydroxyprogesterone in many centers. In most cases, 17-hydroxyprogesterone is markedly increased. In adults, ACTH stimulation (0.25 mg cosyntropin IV) with assays for 17-hydroxyprogesterone at 0 and 30 min can be useful for detecting nonclassic 21-OHD and heterozygotes (Chap. 336).

℞ CONGENITAL ADRENAL HYPERPLASIA

Acute salt-wasting crises require fluid resuscitation, IV hydrocortisone, and correction of hypoglycemia. Once stabilized, glucocorticoids must be given to correct the cortisol insufficiency and to suppress ACTH stimulation, thereby preventing further virilization, rapid skeletal maturation, and the development of polycystic ovaries. Typically, hydrocortisone (10–20 mg/m^2 per d in three divided doses) is used with a goal of partially suppressing 17-hydroxyprogesterone (100–<1000 ng/dL). The aim of treatment is to use the lowest glucocorticoid dose that adequately suppresses adrenal androgen production without causing signs of glucocorticoid excess, such as impaired growth and obesity. Salt-wasting conditions are treated with mineralocorticoid replacement. Infants usually need salt supplements up to the first year of life. Plasma renin activity and electrolytes are used to monitor mineralocorticoid replacement. Some patients with simple-virilizing 21-OHD also benefit from mineralocorticoid supplements. Newer therapeutic approaches, such as anti-androgens and aromatase inhibitors (to block premature epiphyseal closure), are under evaluation. Parents and patients should be aware of the need for increased doses of steroids during sickness, and patients should carry medic alert systems.

Older adolescents and adults are often treated with prednisolone, or dexamethasone at night, to provide more complete ACTH suppression. Steroid doses should be adjusted to individual requirements as overtreatment results in weight gain and hypertension and can affect bone turnover. Androstenedione and testosterone may be useful measurements of long-term control with less fluctuation than 17-hydroxyprogesterone. Mineralocorticoid requirements often decrease in adulthood, and doses should be reduced to avoid hypertension. In very severe cases, adrenalectomy has been advocated but incurs the risks of major surgery and total adrenal insufficiency.

Girls with significant genital androgenization due to classic 21-OHD usually undergo vaginal reconstruction and clitoral reduction (maintaining the glans and nerve supply), but the optimal timing of these procedures is debated. There is a higher threshold for undertaking clitoral surgery in some centers as long-term sensation and ability to achieve orgasm can be affected, but the long-term results of newer techniques are not yet known. If surgery is performed in infancy, surgical revision or regular vaginal dilatation may be needed in adolescence or adulthood, and long-term psycho-

logical support and psychosexual counseling may be appropriate. Women with 21-OHD frequently develop polycystic ovaries and have reduced fertility, especially when control is poor. Fecundity is achieved in 50–90% of women, but ovulation induction (or even adrenalectomy) is frequently required. Dexamethasone should be avoided in pregnancy. Men with poorly controlled 21-OHD may develop testicular adrenal rests and are at risk for reduced fertility. Prenatal treatment of 21-OHD by the administration of dexamethasone to mothers has been shown to reduce the degree of androgenization in affected female fetuses. However, treatment of the mother and child must be started ideally before 6–7 weeks; long-term effects of prenatal dexamethasone exposure on fetal development are still under evaluation.

The treatment of other forms of CAH includes mineralocorticoid and glucocorticoid replacement for salt-losing conditions (e.g., *StAR, CYP11A1, HSD3B2*), suppression of ACTH drive with glucocorticoids in disorders associated with hypertension (e.g., *CYP17, CYP11B1*), and appropriate sex-hormone replacement in adolescence and adulthood, where necessary.

OTHER CAUSES Increased androgen synthesis can also occur in CAH due to defects in *POR*, *11β-hydroxylase (CYP11B1)* and *3β-hydroxysteroid dehydrogenase type 2 (HSD3B2)*, and with mutations in the genes encoding *aromatase (CYP19)* and the glucocorticoid receptor. Increased androgen exposure in utero can occur with maternal virilizing tumors and with ingestion of androgenic compounds.

OTHER DISORDERS AFFECTING 46,XX FEMALES

Congenital absence of the vagina occurs in association with *müllerian agenesis* or *hypoplasia* as part of the Mayer-Rokitansky-Kuster-Hauser syndrome (*WNT4* mutations). This diagnosis should be considered in otherwise phenotypically normal females with primary amenorrhea. Rarer associated features include renal (agenesis) and cervical spinal abnormalities.

GLOBAL CONSIDERATIONS

The approach to the child or adolescent with ambiguous genitalia or other DSD requires cultural sensitivity, as the concepts of sex and gender vary widely. Rare genetic DSD can occur more frequently in specific populations (e.g., *5β-reductase type 2* in the Dominican Republic). Different forms of CAH also show ethnic and geographic variability. In many countries, appropriate biochemical tests may not be readily available, and access to appropriate forms of surgery or treatment may be limited.

FURTHER READINGS

Bojesen A, Gravholt CH: Klinefelter syndrome in clinical practice. Nat Clin Pract Urol 4:192, 2007

Bondy CA for the Turner Syndrome Consensus Study Group: Care of girls and women with Turner syndrome: A guideline of the Turner Syndrome Study Group. J Clin Endocrinol Metab 92:10, 2007

Cools M et al: Germ cell tumors in the intersex gonad: Old paths, new directions, moving frontiers. Endocrinol Rev 27:468, 2006

Lee PA et al: Consensus statement of management of intersex disorders. Pediatrics 118:e488, 2006

MacLaughlin DT, Donahoe PK: Sex determination and differentiation. N Engl J Med 350:367, 2004

Ogilvie CM et al: Congenital adrenal hyperplasia in adults: A review of medical, surgical and psychological issues. Clin Endocrinol 64:2, 2006

Wilhelm D et al: Sex determination and gonadal development in mammals. Physiol Rev 87:1, 2007

Wilson CA, Davies DC: The control of sexual differentiation of the reproductive system and brain. Reproduction 133:331, 2007

344 Endocrine Tumors of the Gastrointestinal Tract and Pancreas

Robert T. Jensen

GENERAL FEATURES OF GASTROINTESTINAL (GI) NEUROENDOCRINE TUMORS

Gastrointestinal neuroendocrine tumors (NETs) are derived from the diffuse neuroendocrine system of the GI tract, which is composed of amine- and acid-producing cells with different hormonal profiles, depending on the site of origin. The tumors they produce can be divided into carcinoid tumors and pancreatic endocrine tumors (PETs). These tumors were originally classified as APUDomas (for *amine precursor uptake and decarboxylation*), as were pheochromocytomas, melanomas, and medullary thyroid carcinomas because they share certain cytochemical features as well as various pathologic, biologic, and molecular features (Table 344-1). It was originally proposed that APUDomas had a similar embryonic origin from neural crest cells, but it is now known the peptide-secreting cells are not of neuroectodermal origin. Nevertheless, the concept is useful because the tumors have important similarities as well as some differences (Table 344-1).

CLASSIFICATION/PATHOLOGY/TUMOR BIOLOGY OF NETS

NETs are generally composed of monotonous sheets of small round cells with uniform nuclei; mitoses are uncommon. They can be tenta-

---

TABLE 344-1 **GENERAL CHARACTERISTICS OF GI NEUROENDOCRINE TUMORS [CARCINOIDS, PANCREATIC ENDOCRINE TUMORS (PETS)]**

I. Share general neuroendocrine cell markers
  A. Chromogranins (A, B, C) are acidic monomeric soluble proteins found in the large secretory granules; chromogranin A is most widely used.
  B. Neuron-specific enolase (NSE) is the γ-γ dimer of the enzyme enolase and is a cytosolic marker of neuroendocrine differentiation.
  C. Synaptophysin is an integral membrane glycoprotein of 38,000 molecular weight found in small vesicles of neurons and neuroendocrine tumors.
II. Pathologic similarities
  A. All are APUDomas showing *amine precursor uptake and decarboxylation*
  B. Ultrastructurally they have dense-core secretory granules (>80 nm).
  C. Histologically appear similar with few mitoses and uniform nuclei
  D. Frequently synthesize multiple peptides/amines, which can be detected immunocytochemically but may not be secreted
  E. Presence or absence of clinical syndrome or type cannot be predicted by immunocytochemical studies
  F. Histologic classifications do not predict biologic behavior; only invasion or metastases establishes malignancy.
III. Similarities of biologic behavior
  A. Generally slow growing, but a proportion is aggressive.
  B. Secrete biologically active peptides/amines, which can cause clinical symptoms.
  C. Generally have high densities of somatostatin receptors, which are used for both localization and treatment.
IV. Similarities/differences in molecular abnormalities
  A. Similarities
    1. Uncommon—alterations in common oncogenes (*ras, jun, fos*, etc.).
    2. Uncommon—alterations in common tumor-suppressor genes (p53, retinoblastoma).
    3. Alterations at MEN-1 locus (11q13) and p16^{INK4a} (9p21) occur in a proportion (10–30%).
    4. Methylation of various genes occurs in 40–87% (*ras*-associated domain family I, p14, p16, O^6 methyl guanosine methyltransferase, retinoic acid receptor β)
  B. Differences
    1. PETs—loss of 3p (8–47%), 3q (8–41%), 11q (21–62%), 6q (18–68%). Gains at 17q (10–55%), 7q (16–68%).
    2. Carcinoids—loss of 18q (38–67%) > 18p (33–43%) > 9p, 16q21 (21–23%). Gains at 17q, 19p (57%).

---

tively identified on routine histology; however, these tumors are now principally recognized by their histologic staining patterns due to shared cellular proteins. Historically, silver staining was used and tumors were classified as showing an argentaffin reaction if they took up and reduced silver, or as being argyrophilic if they did not reduce it. More recently immunocytochemical localization of chromogranins (A, B, C), neuron-specific enolase, or synaptophysin, which are all neuroendocrine cell markers, are used (Table 344-1). Chromogranin A is currently the most widely used.

Ultrastructurally, these tumors possess electron-dense neurosecretory granules and frequently contain small clear vesicles that correspond to synaptic vesicles of neurons. NETs synthesize numerous peptides, growth factors, and bioactive amines that may be ectopically secreted, giving rise to a specific clinical syndrome (Table 344-2). The diagnosis of the specific syndrome requires the clinical features of the disease and cannot be made from the immunocytochemistry results alone. Furthermore, pathologists cannot distinguish between benign and malignant NETs unless metastases or invasion are present.

Carcinoid tumors are frequently classified according to their anatomic area of origin (i.e., foregut, midgut, hindgut) because tumors with similar embryonic origin share functional manifestations, histochemistry, and secretory products (Table 344-3). Foregut tumors generally have a low serotonin (5HT) content, are argentaffin-negative but argyrophilic, occasionally secrete adrenocorticotropic hormone (ACTH) or 5-hydroxytryptophan (5HTP) causing an atypical carcinoid syndrome (Fig. 344-1), are often multihormonal, and may metastasize to bone. They uncommonly produce a clinical syndrome due to the secreted products. Midgut carcinoids are argentaffin-positive, have a high 5HT content, most frequently cause the typical carcinoid syndrome when they metastasize (Table 344-3, Fig. 344-1), release 5HT and tachykinins (substance P, neuropeptide K, substance K), rarely secrete 5HTP or ACTH, and uncommonly metastasize to bone. Hindgut carcinoids (rectum, transverse and descending colon) are argentaffin-negative, often argyrophilic, rarely contain 5HT or cause the carcinoid syndrome (Fig. 344-1, Table 344-3), rarely secrete 5HTP or ACTH, contain numerous peptides, and may metastasize to bone.

PETs can be classified into nine well-established specific functional syndromes (Table 344-2), four possible specific functional syndromes (PETs secreting calcitonin, renin, luteinizing hormone, or erythropoietin), and nonfunctional PETs [pancreatic polypeptide (PP)-secreting tumors; PPomas]. Each of the functional syndromes is associated with symptoms due to the specific hormone released. In contrast, nonfunctional PETs release no products that cause a specific clinical syndrome. "Nonfunctional" is a misnomer in the strict sense because they frequently ectopically secrete a number of peptides (PP, chromogranin A, ghrelin, neurotensin, α subunits of human chorionic gonadotropin (hCG), neuron-specific enolase); however, they cause no specific clinical syndrome. The symptoms caused by nonfunctional PETs are entirely due to the tumor per se.

Carcinoid tumors can occur in almost any GI tissue (Table 344-3); however, at present most (70%) take origin from one of three sites: bronchus, jejunoileum, or colon/rectum. In the past, carcinoid tumors most frequently were reported in the appendix (i.e., 40%); however, the bronchus/lung and small intestine are now the most common sites. Overall, GI carcinoids are the most common site for these tumors, comprising 64%, with the respiratory tract second at 28%.

The term *pancreatic endocrine tumor*, although widely used and therefore retained here, is also a misnomer, strictly speaking, because these tumors can occur either almost entirely in the pancreas (insulinomas, glucagonomas, nonfunctional PETs, PETs causing hypercalcemia) or at both pancreatic and extrapancreatic sites [gastrinomas, VIPomas (VIP, vasoactive intestinal peptide), somatostatinomas, GRFomas (GRF, growth hormone–releasing factor)]. PETs are also called *islet cell tumors*; however, this term is discouraged because it is not established that they originate from the islets, and many can occur at extrapancreatic sites.

A uniform World Health Organization (WHO) classification for all GI NETs (including carcinoids and PETs) divides them into three general categories: (1a) well-differentiated NETs, (1b) well-differentiated

TABLE 344-2 GI NEUROENDOCRINE TUMOR SYNDROMES

Name	Biologically Active Peptide(s) Secreted	Incidence (New Cases/10⁶ Population/ Year)	Tumor Location	Malignant, %	Associated with MEN-1, %	Main Symptoms/ Signs
Established Specific Functional Syndrome						
Carcinoid tumor						
Carcinoid syndrome	Serotonin, possibly tachykinins, motilin, prostaglandins	0.5–2	Midgut (75–87%) Foregut (2–33%) Hindgut (1–8%) Unknown (2–15%)	95–100	Rare	Diarrhea (32–84%) Flushing (63–75%) Pain (10–34%) Asthma (4–18%) Heart disease (11–41%)
Pancreatic endocrine tumor						
Zollinger-Ellison syndrome	Gastrin	0.5–1.5	Duodenum (70%) Pancreas (25%) Other sites (5%)	60–90	20–25	Pain (79–100%) Diarrhea (30–75%) Esophageal symptoms (31–56%)
Insulinoma	Insulin	1–2	Pancreas (>99%)	<10	4–5	Hypoglycemic symptoms (100%)
VIPoma (Verner-Morrison syndrome, pancreatic cholera, WDHA)	Vasoactive intestinal peptide	0.05–0.2	Pancreas (90%, adult) Other (10%, neural, adrenal, periganglionic)	40–70	6	Diarrhea (90–100%) Hypokalemia (80–100%) Dehydration (83%)
Glucagonoma	Glucagon	0.01–0.1	Pancreas (100%)	50–80	1–20	Rash (67–90%) Glucose intolerance (38–87%) Weight loss (66–96%)
Somatostatinoma	Somatostatin	Rare	Pancreas (55%) Duodenum/jejunum (44%)	>70	45	Diabetes mellitus (63–90%) Cholelithiases (65–90%) Diarrhea (35–90%)
GRFoma	Growth hormone-releasing hormone	Unknown	Pancreas (30%) Lung (54%) Jejunum (7%) Other (13%)	>60	16	Acromegaly (100%)
ACTHoma	ACTH	Rare	Pancreas (4–16% all ectopic Cushing's)	>95	Rare	Cushing's syndrome (100%)
PET causing carcinoid syndrome	Serotonin, ? tachykinins	Rare (43 cases)	Pancreas (<1% all carcinoids)	60–88	Rare	Same as carcinoid syndrome above
PET causing hypercalcemia	PTHrP, others unknown	Rare	Pancreas (rare cause of hypercalcemia)	84	Rare	Abdominal pain due to hepatic metastases
Possible Specific Functional Syndrome						
PET secreting calcitonin	Calcitonin	Rare	Pancreas (rare cause of hypercalcitonemia)	>80	16	Diarrhea (50%)
PET secreting renin	Renin	Rare	Pancreas	Unknown	No	Hypertension
PET secreting luteinizing hormone	Luteinizing hormone	Rare	Pancreas	Unknown	No	Anovulation, virilization (female); reduced libido (male)
PET secreting erythropoietin	Erythropoietin	Rare	Pancreas	100	No	Polycythemia
No Functional Syndrome						
PPoma/nonfunctional	None	1–2	Pancreas (100%)	>60	18–44	Weight loss (30–90%) Abdominal mass (10–30%) Pain (30–95%)

Note: MEN, multiple endocrine neoplasia; VIPoma, tumor secreting vasoactive intestinal peptide; WDHA, watery diarrhea, hypokalemia, and achlorhydria syndrome; ACTH, adrenocorticotropic hormone; PET, pancreatic endocrine tumor; PTHrP, parathyroid hormone–related peptide; PPoma, tumor secreting pancreatic polypeptide.

neuroendocrine carcinomas of low-grade malignancy, and (2) poorly differentiated neuroendocrine carcinomas that are usually small cell neuroendocrine carcinomas of high-grade malignancy. The term *carcinoid* is synonymous with *well-differentiated NETs* (1a). This classification is further divided on the basis of tumor location and biology. Furthermore, for the first time a standard TNM classification has been proposed for the GI foregut NETs. The availability of this WHO classification and the TNM classification should greatly facilitate the comparison of clinical, pathological and prognostic features and results of treatment in GI NETs from different studies.

The exact incidence of carcinoid tumors or PETs varies according to whether only symptomatic or all tumors are considered. The incidence of clinically significant carcinoids is 7–13 cases/million population per year, whereas any malignant carcinoids at autopsy are reported in 21–84 cases/million population per year. Clinically significant PETs have a prevalence of 10 cases per million population with insulinomas, gastrinomas, and nonfunctional PETs having an incidence of 0.5–2 cases per million population per year (Table 344-2). VIPomas are 2- to 8-fold less common, glucagonomas are 17- to 30-fold less common, and somatostatinomas the least common. In autop-

TABLE 344-3 CARCINOID TUMOR LOCATION, FREQUENCY OF METASTASES, AND ASSOCIATION WITH THE CARCINOID SYNDROME

	Location (% of Total)	Incidence of Metastases	Incidence of Carcinoid Syndrome
Foregut			
Esophagus	<0.1	—	—
Stomach	4.6	10	9.5
Duodenum	2.0	—	3.4
Pancreas	0.7	71.9	20
Gallbladder	0.3	17.8	5
Bronchus, lung, trachea	27.9	5.7	13
Midgut			
Jejunum	1.8	⎰58.4	9
Ileum	14.9	⎱	9
Meckel's diverticulum	0.5		13
Appendix	4.8	38.8	<1
Colon	8.6	51	5
Liver	0.4	32.2	—
Ovary	1.0	32	50
Testis	<0.1	—	50
Hindgut			
Rectum	13.6	3.9	—

Source: Location is from the PAN-SEER data (1973–1999), and incidence of metastases from the SEER data (1992–1999), reported by IM Modlin et al: Cancer 97:934, 2003. Incidence of carcinoid syndrome is from 4349 cases studied from 1950–1971, reported by JD Godwin, Cancer 36:560, 1975.

sy studies 0.5–1.5% of all cases have a PET; however, in <1 in 1000 cases was a functional tumor thought to occur.

Both carcinoid tumors and PETs commonly show malignant behavior (Tables 344-2, -3). With PETs, except for insulinomas in which <10% are malignant, 50–100% in different series are malignant. With carcinoid tumors, the percentage showing malignant behavior varies in different locations. For the three most common sites of occurrence the incidence of metastases varies greatly from jejunoileum (58%) > lung/bronchus (6%) > rectum (4%). With both carcinoid tumors and PETs, a number of factors influence survival and the aggressiveness of the tumor (Table 344-4). The presence of liver metastases is the single most important prognostic factor in single and multivariate analyses for both carcinoid tumors and PETs. Particularly important in the development of liver metastases is the size of the primary tumor. For example, with small-intestinal carcinoids, the most frequent cause of the carcinoid syndrome due to metastatic disease in the liver (Table 344-2), metastases occur in 15–25% if the tumor diameter is <1 cm, 58–80% if it is 1–2 cm, and >75% if >2 cm. Similar data exist for gastrinomas and other PETs, where the size of the primary tumor has been shown to be an independent predictor of the development of liver metastases. The presence of lymph node metastases, the depth of invasion, various histologic features [differentiation, mitotic rates, growth indices, vessel density, vascular endothelial growth factor (VEGF), and CD10 metalloproteinase expression], elevated serum alkaline phosphatase levels, and flow cytometric results (such as the presence of aneuploidy) are all

TABLE 344-4 PROGNOSTIC FACTORS IN NEUROENDOCRINE TUMORS

Both carcinoid tumors and PETs
  Presence of liver metastases ($p < .001$)
  Extent of liver metastases ($p < .001$)
  Presence of lymph node metastases ($p < .001$)
  Depth of invasion ($p < .001$)
  Elevated serum alkaline phosphatase levels ($p = .003$)
  Primary tumor site ($p < .001$)
  Primary tumor size ($p < .005$)
  Various histologic features
    Tumor differentiation ($p < .001$)
    High growth indices (high Ki-67 index, PCNA expression)
    High mitotic counts ($p < .001$)
    Vascular or perineural invasion
    Vessel density (low microvessel density, increased lymphatic density)
    Low VEGF, high CD10 metalloproteinase expression
    Flow cytometric features (i.e., aneuploidy)
Carcinoid tumors
  Presence of carcinoid syndrome
  Laboratory results [urinary 5-HIAA level ($p < .01$), plasma neuropeptide K ($p < .05$), serum chromogranin A ($p < .01$)]
  Presence of a second malignancy
  Male sex ($p < .001$)
  Older age ($p < .01$)
  Mode of discovery (incidental > symptomatic)
  Molecular findings [TGF-α expression ($p < .05$), chr 16q LOH or gain chr 4p ($p < .05$)]
PETs
  Ha-Ras oncogene or p53 overexpression
  Female sex
  MEN-1 syndrome absent
  Laboratory findings (increased chromogranin A in some studies; gastrinomas—increased gastrin level)
  Molecular findings [increased HER2/*neu* expression ($p = .032$), chr 1q, 3p, 3q, or 6q LOH ($p = .0004$), EGF receptor overexpression ($p = .034$), gains in chr 7q, 17q, 17p, 20q]

Note: PET, pancreatic endocrine tumor; Ki-67, proliferation-associated nuclear antigen recognized by Ki-67 monoclonal antibody; PCNA, proliferating cell nuclear antigen; 5HIAA, 5-hydroxyindoleacetic acid; TGF-α, transforming growth factor α; chr, chromosome; LOH, loss of heterozygosity; MEN, multiple endocrine neoplasia; EGF, epidermal growth factor.

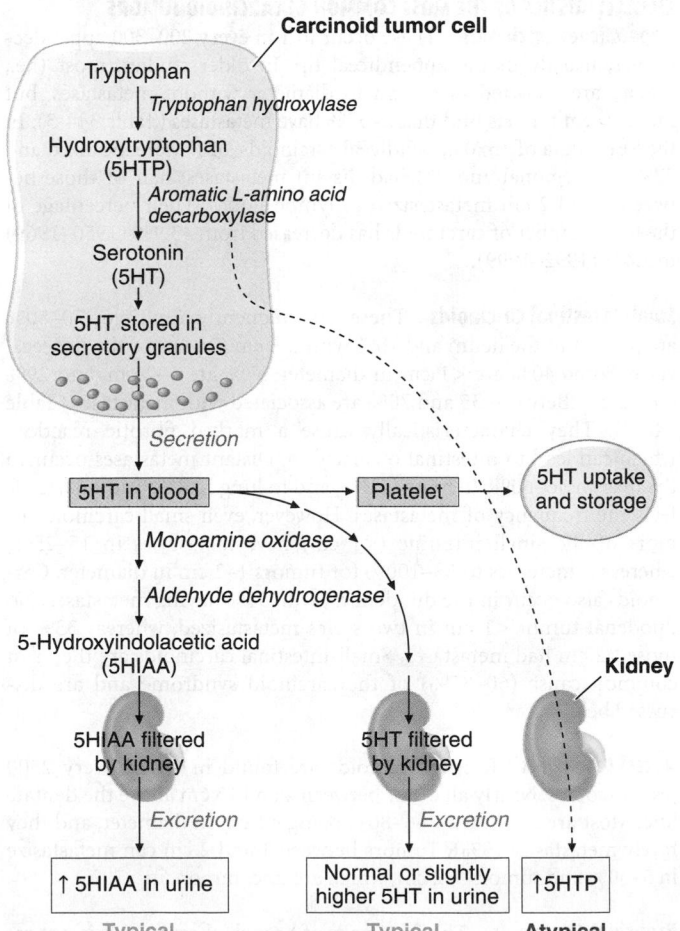

FIGURE 344-1 Synthesis, secretion, and metabolism of serotonin (5HT) in patients with typical and atypical carcinoid syndromes. Abbreviations: 5HIAA, 5-hydroxyindolacetic acid.

TABLE 344-5 GENETIC SYNDROMES ASSOCIATED WITH AN INCREASED INCIDENCE OF NEUROENDOCRINE TUMORS [NETS (CARCINOIDS OR PANCREATIC ENDOCRINE TUMORS) (PETS)]

Syndrome	Location of Gene Mutation and Gene Product	NETs Seen/Frequency
Multiple endocrine neoplasia type 1 (MEN-1)	11q13 (encodes 610-amino-acid protein, menin)	80–100% develop PETs: (nonfunctional > gastrinoma > insulinoma) Carcinoids: gastric (13–30%), bronchial/thymic (8%)
von Hippel–Lindau disease	3q25 (encodes 213-amino-acid protein)	12–17% develop PETs (almost always nonfunctional)
von Recklinghausen's disease [neurofibromatosis 1 (NF-1)]	17q11.2 (encodes 2485-amino-acid protein, neurofibromin)	Duodenal somatostatinomas (usually nonfunctional) Rarely insulinoma, gastrinoma
Tuberous sclerosis	9q34 (TSCI) encodes 1164-amino-acid protein, hamartin) 16p13 (TSC2) (encodes 1807-amino-acid protein, tuberin)	Uncommonly develop PETs [nonfunctional and functional (insulinoma, gastrinoma)]

important prognostic factors for the development of metastatic disease (Table 344-4). For patients with carcinoid tumors, additional poor prognostic factors include the development of the carcinoid syndrome, older age, male sex, the presence of a symptomatic tumor, or higher levels of a number of tumor markers [5-hydroxyindolacetic acid (5HIAA), neuropeptide K, chromogranin A]. With PETs or gastrinomas, the best studied PET, a worse prognosis is associated with female sex, overexpression of the ha-ras oncogene or p53, the absence of multiple endocrine neoplasia-type 1 (MEN-1), and higher levels of various tumor markers (i.e., chromogranin A, gastrin).

A number of genetic disorders are associated with an increased incidence of NETs (Table 344-5). Each one is caused by a loss of a possible tumor-suppressor gene. The most important is MEN-1, an autosomal dominant disorder due to a defect in a 10-exon gene on 11q13, which encodes for a 610-amino acid nuclear protein, menin (Chap. 345). Patients with MEN-1 develop hyperparathyroidism due to parathyroid hyperplasia in 95–100%, PETs in 80–100%, pituitary adenomas in 54–80%, bronchial carcinoids in 8%, thymic carcinoids in 8%, and gastric carcinoids in 13–30% of the patients with Zollinger-Ellison syndrome (ZES). In patients with MEN-1, 80–100% develop nonfunctional PETs; functional PETs occur in 80%, with 54% developing ZES, 21% insulinomas, 3% glucagonomas, and 1% VIPomas. MEN-1 is present in 20–25% of all patients with ZES, in 4% with insulinomas, and in a low percentage (<5%) of the other PETs.

Three phacomatoses associated with NETs are von Hippel–Lindau disease (VHL), von Recklinghausen's disease [neurofibromatosis (NF) type 1], and tuberous sclerosis (Bourneville's disease). VHL is an autosomal dominant disorder due to defects in a gene on chromosome 3p25, which encodes a 213-amino-acid protein that interacts with the elongin family of proteins as a transcriptional regulator (Chaps. 278, 337, 345, 374). In addition to cerebellar hemangioblastomas, renal cancer, and pheochromocytomas, 10–17% of these patients develop a PET. Most are nonfunctional although insulinomas and VIPomas are reported. Patients with NF-1 have defects in a gene on chromosome 17q11.2 encoding for a 2845-amino-acid protein, neurofibromin, which functions in normal cells as a suppressor of the ras signaling cascade (Chap. 374). Up to 12% of these patients develop an upper GI carcinoid tumor, characteristically in the periampullary region (54%). Many are classified as somatostatinomas because they contain somatostatin immunocytochemically; however, they uncommonly secrete somatostatin or produce a clinical somatostatinoma syndrome. NF-1 has rarely been associated with insulinomas and ZES. Tuberous sclerosis is caused by mutations that alter either the 1164-amino-acid protein, hamartin (TSC1), or the 1807-amino-acid protein, tuberin (TSC2) (Chap. 374). Both hamartin and tuberin interact in a pathway related to cytosolic G protein regulation. A few cases including nonfunctional and functional PETs (insulinomas and gastrinomas) have been reported in these patients (Table 344-5).

In contrast to most common nonendocrine tumors such as carcinoma of the breast, colon, lung, or stomach, alterations in common oncogenes (ras, myc, fos, src, jun) or tumor-suppressor genes (p53, retinoblastoma susceptibility gene) have not been found in PETs or carcinoid tumors. Alterations that may be important in their pathogenesis include changes in the MEN-1 gene, p16/MTS1 tumor-suppressor gene, and DPC 4/Smad 4 gene; amplification of the HER-2/neu protooncogene and growth factors and their receptors; methylation of a number of genes likely resulting in their inactivation; and deletions of unknown tumor-suppressor genes as well as gains in other unknown genes (Table 344-1). Comparative genomic hybridization and genome-wide allelotyping studies have shown differences in chromosomal losses and gains between PETs and carcinoids, some of which have prognostic significance (Table 344-4). Mutations in the MEN-1 gene are likely particularly important. Loss of heterozygosity at the MEN-1 locus on chromosome 11q13 is seen in 93% of sporadic PETs (i.e., in patients without MEN-1) and in 26–75% of sporadic carcinoid tumors. Mutations in the MEN-1 gene are reported in 31–34% of sporadic gastrinomas. The presence of a number of these molecular alterations (PET or carcinoid) correlates with tumor growth, tumor size, disease extent or invasiveness and may have prognostic significance.

CARCINOID TUMORS AND CARCINOID SYNDROME

CHARACTERISTICS OF THE MOST COMMON GI CARCINOID TUMORS

Appendiceal Carcinoids These occur in 1 in every 200–300 appendectomies, usually in the appendiceal tip. In older studies, most (i.e., >90%) are reported as <1 cm in diameter without metastases, but more recent reports find that 2–35% have metastases (Table 344-3). In the SEER data of 1570 appendiceal carcinoids, 62% were localized and 27% had regional and 8% had distant metastases; half of those between 1 and 2 cm metastasized to lymph nodes. Their percentage of the total number of carcinoids has decreased from 43.9% (1950–1969) to 2.4% (1992–1999).

Small Intestinal Carcinoids These are frequently multiple; 70–80% are present in the ileum and 70% within 6 cm (24 in.) of the ileocecal valve. Some 40% are <1 cm in diameter, 32% are 1–2 cm, and 29% are >2 cm. Between 35 and 70% are associated with metastases (Table 344-3). They characteristically cause a marked fibrotic reaction, which can lead to intestinal obstruction. Distant metastases occur to the liver in 36–60%, to bone in 3%, and to lung in 4%. Tumor size affects the frequency of metastases. However, even small carcinoid tumors of the small intestine (<1 cm) have metastases in 15–25%, whereas it increases to 58–100% for tumors 1–2 cm in diameter. Carcinoids also occur in the duodenum, with 31% having metastases. No duodenal tumor <1 cm in two series metastasized, whereas 33% of those >2 cm had metastases. Small-intestinal carcinoids are the most common cause (60–87%) of the carcinoid syndrome and are discussed below.

Rectal Carcinoids Rectal carcinoids are found in ~1 of every 2500 proctoscopies. Nearly all occur between 4 and 13 cm above the dentate line. Most are small, with 66–80% being <1 cm in diameter, and they rarely metastasize (5%). Tumors between 1 and 2 cm can metastasize in 5–30% and tumors > 2 cm, which are uncommon, in >70%.

Bronchial Carcinoids The frequency of bronchial carcinoids is not related to smoking. A number of different classifications of bronchial carcinoid tumors are proposed. In some studies, lung NETs are classified into four categories: typical carcinoid [also called bronchial carcinoid tumor, Kulchitsky cell carcinoma (KCC)-I]; atypical carcinoid (also called well-differentiated neuroendocrine carcinoma, KCC-II); intermediate small cell neuroendocrine carcinoma; and small cell neuroendocarcinoma (KCC-III). Another proposed classification includes three categories of lung NETs: benign or low-grade malignant (typical carcinoid), low-grade malignant (atypical carcinoid), and high-grade malignant (poorly differentiated carcinoma of the large cell or small cell type). These different categories of lung NETs have different prognoses, varying from excellent for typical carcinoid to poor for small cell neuroendocrine carcinomas.

Gastric Carcinoids These account for 3 of every 1000 gastric neoplasms. It is thought that three different subtypes of gastric carcinoids occur. Each originates from gastric enterochromaffin-like (ECL) cells in the gastric mucosa. Two subtypes are associated with hypergastrinemic states, either chronic atrophic gastritis (type I) (80% of all gastric carcinoids) or ZES, almost always as part of the MEN-1 syndrome (type II) (6% of all cases). These tumors generally pursue a benign course, with 9–30% associated with metastases. They are usually multiple, small, and infiltrate only to the submucosa. The third subtype of gastric carcinoid (type III) (sporadic) occurs without hypergastrinemia (14% of all carcinoids) and pursues an aggressive course, with 54–66% developing metastases. Sporadic carcinoids are usually single, large tumors, 50% have atypical histology, and they can be a cause of the carcinoid syndrome. Gastric carcinoids as a percentage of all carcinoids are increasing in frequency [1.96% (1969–71), 3.6% (1973–91), 5.8% (1991–99)].

CARCINOID TUMORS WITHOUT THE CARCINOID SYNDROME

The age of patients at diagnosis ranges from 10–93 years with a mean of 63 years for small intestine and 66 years for the rectum. The presentation is diverse and related to the site of origin and extent of malignant spread. In the appendix, carcinoid tumors are usually found incidentally during surgery for suspected appendicitis. Small-intestinal carcinoids in the jejunoileum present with periodic abdominal pain (51%), intestinal obstruction with ileus/invagination (31%), an abdominal tumor (17%), or GI bleeding (11%). Because of the vagueness of the symptoms, the diagnosis is usually delayed ~2 years from onset of the symptoms, ranging up to 20 years. Duodenal, gastric, and rectal carcinoids are most frequently found by chance at endoscopy. The most common symptoms of rectal carcinoids are melena/bleeding (39%), constipation (17%), and diarrhea (12%). Bronchial carcinoids are frequently discovered as a lesion on a chest radiograph, and 31% of the patients are asymptomatic. Thymic carcinoids present as anterior mediastinal masses on chest radiograph or CT scan. Ovarian and testicular carcinoids usually present as masses discovered on physical examination or ultrasound. Metastatic carcinoid tumor in the liver frequently presents as hepatomegaly in a patient who may have minimal symptoms and near-normal liver function tests.

CARCINOID TUMORS WITH SYSTEMIC SYMPTOMS DUE TO SECRETED PRODUCTS

Carcinoid tumors can contain numerous GI peptides: gastrin, insulin, somatostatin, motilin, neurotensin, tachykinins (substance K, substance P, neuropeptide K), glucagon, gastrin-releasing peptide, VIP, PP, other biologically active peptides (ACTH, calcitonin, growth hormone), prostaglandins and bioactive amines (5HT). These substances may or may not be released in sufficient amounts to cause symptoms. In various studies of patients with carcinoid tumors, elevated serum levels of PP were found in 43%, motilin in 14%, gastrin in 15%, and VIP in 6%. Foregut carcinoids are more likely to produce various GI peptides than midgut carcinoids. Ectopic ACTH production causing Cushing's syndrome is increasingly seen with foregut carcinoids (respiratory tract primarily) and in some series was the most common cause of the ectopic ACTH syndrome, accounting for 64% of all cases. Acromegaly due to GRF release occurs with foregut carcinoids, as does the somatostatinoma syndrome, but rarely occurs with duodenal carcinoids. The most common systemic syndrome with carcinoid tumors is the carcinoid syndrome.

TABLE 344-6 CLINICAL CHARACTERISTICS IN PATIENTS WITH CARCINOID SYNDROME

	At Presentation	During Course of Disease
Symptoms/signs		
Diarrhea	32–73%	68–84%
Flushing	23–65%	63–74%
Pain	10%	34%
Asthma/wheezing	4–8%	3–18%
Pellagra	2%	5%
None	12%	22%
Carcinoid heart disease present	11%	14–41%
Demographics		
Male	46–59%	46–61%
Age		
Mean	57 yrs	52–54 yrs
Range	25–79 yrs	9–91 yrs
Tumor location		
Foregut	5–9%	2–33%
Midgut	78–87%	60–87%
Hindgut	1–5%	1–8%
Unknown	2–11%	2–15%

CARCINOID SYNDROME

Clinical Features The cardinal features at presentation as well as during the disease course are shown in Table 344-6. Flushing and diarrhea are the two most common symptoms, occurring in up to 73% initially and in up to 89% during the course of the disease. The characteristic flush is of sudden onset; it is a deep red or violaceous erythema of the upper body, especially the neck and face, often associated with a feeling of warmth, and occasionally associated with pruritus, lacrimation, diarrhea, or facial edema. Flushes may be precipitated by stress, alcohol, exercise, certain foods such as cheese, or by certain agents such as catecholamines, pentagastrin, and serotonin reuptake inhibitors. Flushing episodes may be brief, lasting 2–5 min, especially initially, or may last hours, especially later in the disease course. Flushing is usually seen with midgut carcinoids but can also occur with foregut carcinoids. With bronchial carcinoids the flushes are frequently prolonged for hours to days, reddish in color, and associated with salivation, lacrimation, diaphoresis, diarrhea, and hypotension. The flush associated with gastric carcinoids is also reddish in color but patchy in distribution over the face and neck. It may be provoked by food and have accompanying pruritus.

Diarrhea is present in 32–73% initially and 68–84% at some time in their disease course. Diarrhea usually occurs with flushing (85% of cases). The diarrhea is usually described as watery with 60% having <1 L/day of diarrhea. Steatorrhea is present in 67%, and in 46% it is >15 g/d (normal <7 g). Abdominal pain may be present with the diarrhea or independently in 10–34% of cases.

Cardiac manifestations occur in 11% initially and in 14–41% at some time in the disease course. The cardiac disease is due to fibrosis involving the endocardium, primarily on the right side, although left side lesions can occur also. The dense fibrous deposits are most commonly on the ventricular aspect of the tricuspid valve and less commonly on the pulmonary valve cusps. They can result in constriction of the valves and pulmonic stenosis is usually predominant, whereas the tricuspid valve is often fixed open, resulting in regurgitation predominating. Up to 80% of patients with cardiac lesions develop heart failure. Lesions on the left side are much less extensive, occur in 30% at autopsy, and most frequently affect the mitral valve.

Other clinical manifestations include wheezing or asthma-like symptoms (8–18%) and pellagra-like skin lesions (2–25%). A variety of noncardiac problems due to increased fibrous tissue have been reported including retroperitoneal fibrosis causing urethral obstruction, Peyronie's disease of the penis, intraabdominal fibrosis, and occlusion of the mesenteric arteries or veins.

Pathobiology In different studies, carcinoid syndrome occurred in 8% of 8876 patients with carcinoid tumors with a rate of 1.4–18.4%. It only occurs when sufficient concentrations of secreted products by the tumor reach the systemic circulation. In 91% of cases this occurs after distant metastases to the liver. Rarely primary gut carcinoids with nodal metastases with extensive retroperitoneal invasion, pancreatic carcinoids with retroperitoneal lymph nodes, or carcinoids of the lung or ovary with direct access to the systemic circulation can cause the carcinoid syndrome without hepatic metastases. All carcinoid tumors do not have the same propensity to metastasize and cause the carcinoid syndrome. Midgut carcinoids account for 60–67% of the cases of carcinoid syndrome, foregut tumors for 2–33%, hindgut for 1–8%, and an unknown primary location for 2–15% (Tables 344-2, 344-3).

One of the main secretory products of carcinoid tumors involved in the carcinoid syndrome is 5HT (Fig. 344-1), which is synthesized from tryptophan. Up to 50% of dietary tryptophan can be used in this synthetic pathway by tumor cells, which can result in inadequate supplies for conversion to niacin; hence, some patients (2.5%) develop pellagra-like lesions. 5HT has numerous biologic effects including stimulating intestinal secretion with inhibition of absorption, stimulating increases in intestinal motility, and stimulating fibrogenesis. In various studies 56–88% of all carcinoid tumors were associated with 5HT overproduction; however, 12–26% of patients did not have the carcinoid syndrome. In one study, platelet 5HT was elevated in 96% of patients with midgut carcinoids, in 43% with foregut tumors, and in 0% with hindgut tumors. In 90–100% of patients with the carcinoid syndrome, evidence of 5HT overproduction is noted. 5HT is thought to be predominantly responsible for the diarrhea by its effects on gut motility and intestinal secretion, primarily through $5HT_3$ and, to a lesser degree, $5HT_4$ receptors. Serotonin receptor antagonists (especially $5HT_3$ antagonists) relieve the diarrhea in most patients. Additional studies suggest prostaglandin E_2 and tachykinins may be important mediators of the diarrhea in some patients. 5HT does not appear to be involved in the flushing because flushing is not relieved by serotonin receptor antagonists. In patients with gastric carcinoids the red, patchy pruritic flush is likely due to histamine release, because it can be prevented by H_1 and H_2 receptor antagonists. Numerous studies show tachykinins are stored in carcinoid tumors and released during flushing. However, octreotide can relieve the flushing induced by pentagastrin in these patients without altering the stimulated increase in plasma substance P, suggesting that other mediators must be involved in the flushing. Both histamine and 5HT may be responsible for the wheezing as well as the fibrotic reactions involving the heart, causing Peyronie's disease and intraabdominal fibrosis. The exact mechanism of the heart disease is unclear. The valvular heart disease caused by the appetite-suppressant drug dexfenfluramine is histologically indistinguishable from that observed in carcinoid disease. Furthermore, ergot-containing dopamine receptor agonists used for Parkinson's disease (pergolide, cabergoline) cause valvular heart disease that closely resembles that seen in the carcinoid syndrome. Metabolites of fenfluramine, as well as the dopamine receptor agonists, have high affinity for $5HT_{2B}$ receptors, activation of which is known to cause fibroblast mitogenesis. High levels of $5HT_{2B}$ receptors are known to occur in heart valves. Studies on cultured interstitial cells from human cardiac valves demonstrate that these valvulopathic drugs induce mitogenesis by activating $5HT_{2B}$ receptors and stimulating upregulation of transforming growth factor β and collagen biosynthesis. These observations support the conclusion that 5HT overproduction by carcinoid tumors is important in mediating the valvular changes, possibly by activating $5HT_{2B}$ receptors in the endocardium. Both the magnitude of serotonin overproduction and prior chemotherapy are important predictors of progression of the heart disease. Atrial naturetic peptide overproduction is also reported in patients with cardiac disease, but its role in the pathogenesis is unknown.

Patients may develop either a typical or atypical carcinoid syndrome. In patients with the typical form, characteristically caused by a midgut carcinoid tumor, the conversion of tryptophan to 5HTP is the rate-limiting step (Fig. 344-1). Once 5HTP is formed it is rapidly converted to 5HT and stored in secretory granules of the tumor or in platelets. A small amount remains in plasma that is converted to 5HIAA, which appears in large amounts in the urine. These patients have an expanded 5HT pool size, increased blood and platelet 5HT, and increased urinary 5HIAA. Some carcinoid tumors cause an atypical carcinoid syndrome thought due to a deficiency in the enzyme dopa decarboxylase, and thus, 5HTP cannot be converted to 5HT and instead is secreted into the bloodstream. In these patients, plasma 5HT levels are normal but urinary levels may be increased because some 5HTP is converted to 5HT in the kidney. Characteristically, urinary 5HTP and 5HT are increased, but urinary 5HIAA levels are only slightly elevated. Foregut carcinoids are the most likely to cause an atypical carcinoid syndrome.

One of the most immediate life-threatening complications of the carcinoid syndrome is the development of a carcinoid crisis. This is more frequent in patients who have intense symptoms or have greatly increased urinary 5HIAA levels (i.e., >200 mg/d). The crises may occur spontaneously or be provoked by stress, anesthesia, chemotherapy, or a biopsy. Patients develop intense flushing, diarrhea, abdominal pain, cardiac abnormalities including tachycardia, hypertension, or hypotension. If not adequately treated, it can be a terminal event.

DIAGNOSIS OF THE CARCINOID SYNDROME AND CARCINOID TUMORS

The diagnosis of carcinoid syndrome relies on measurement of urinary or plasma serotonin or its metabolites in the urine. The measurement of 5HIAA is most frequently used. False-positive elevations may occur if the patient is eating serotonin-rich foods such as bananas, pineapple, walnuts, pecans, avocados, or hickory nuts or is taking certain medications (cough syrup containing guaifenesin, acetaminophen, salicylates, or L-dopa). The normal range in daily urinary 5HIAA excretion is 2 to 8 mg/d. In one study, 92% of patients with carcinoid syndrome had 5HT overproduction; in another, 5HIAA had a 73% sensitivity and 100% specificity for carcinoid syndrome.

Most physicians use only the urinary 5HIAA excretion rate; however, plasma and platelet serotonin levels, if available, may give additional information. Platelet serotonin levels are more sensitive than urinary 5HIAA but are not generally available. Because patients with foregut carcinoids may produce an atypical carcinoid syndrome, if this syndrome is suspected and urinary 5HIAA is minimally elevated or normal, other urinary metabolites of tryptophan, such as 5HTP or 5HT, should be measured.

Flushing occurs in a number of other conditions, such as systemic mastocytosis, chronic myeloid leukemia with increased histamine release, and menopause; as a reaction to alcohol or glutamate; and as a side effect of chlorpropamide, calcium channel blockers, and nicotinic acid. None of these conditions cause an increased urinary 5HIAA.

The diagnosis of carcinoid tumor can be suggested by the carcinoid syndrome, by recurrent abdominal symptoms in a healthy-appearing individual, or by discovering hepatomegaly or hepatic metastases associated with minimal symptoms. Ileal carcinoids, which are 25% of all clinically detected carcinoids, should be suspected in patients with bowel obstruction, abdominal pain, flushing, or diarrhea.

Serum chromogranin A levels are elevated in 56–100% of patients with carcinoid tumors, and the level correlates with tumor bulk. Serum chromogranin A levels are not specific for carcinoid tumors because they are also elevated in patients with PETs and other NETs. Plasma neuron-specific enolase levels are also used as a marker of carcinoid tumors but are less sensitive than chromogranin A, being increased in only 17–47% of patients.

℞ CARCINOID SYNDROME AND NONMETASTATIC CARCINOID TUMORS

CARCINOID SYNDROME Treatment includes avoiding conditions that precipitate flushing, dietary supplementation with nicotinamide, treatment of heart failure with diuretics, treatment of wheezing with oral bronchodilators, and controlling the diarrhea with antidiarrheal agents such as loperamide or diphenoxylate. If patients still have symptoms, serotonin receptor antagonists or somatostatin analogues are the drugs of choice.

FIGURE 344-2 Structure of somatostatin and synthetic analogues used for diagnostic or therapeutic indications.

There are 14 subclasses of 5HT receptors, and antagonists for most are not available. The $5HT_1$ and $5HT_2$ receptor antagonists methysergide, cyproheptadine, and ketanserin have all been used to control the diarrhea but usually do not decrease flushing. Methysergide use is limited because it can cause retroperitoneal fibrosis. Ketanserin diminishes diarrhea in 30–100% of patients. $5HT_3$ receptor antagonists (ondansetron, tropisetron, alosetron) can control diarrhea and nausea in up to 100% of patients and occasionally ameliorate the flushing. A combination of histamine H_1 and H_2 receptor antagonists (i.e., diphenhydramine and cimetidine or ranitidine) may control flushing in patients with foregut carcinoids.

Synthetic analogues of somatostatin (octreotide, lanreotide) are the most widely used agents to control the symptoms of patients with carcinoid syndrome (**Fig. 344-2**). These drugs are effective at relieving symptoms and decreasing urinary 5HIAA levels in patients with carcinoid syndrome. Octreotide controls symptoms in >80% of patients, including the diarrhea and flushing, and 70% of patients have a >50% decrease in urinary 5HIAA excretion. Patients with mild to moderate symptoms should initially be treated with 100 μg SC every 8 h. Individual responses vary, and some patients have received as much as 3000 μg/d. Some 40% of patients escape control after a median of 4 months, and the dose may need to be increased. Similar results are reported with lanreotide.

In patients with carcinoid crises, somatostatin analogues are effective at both treating the condition as well as preventing symptoms during known precipitating events such as surgery, anesthesia, chemotherapy, or stress. It is recommended that octreotide, 150–250 μg SC every 6–8 h, be used 24–48 h before anesthesia and then continued throughout the procedure.

Sustained-release preparations of both octreotide [octreotide-LAR (long-acting release)] and lanreotide [lanreotide-PR (prolonged release, lanreotide autogel)] permit infrequent injections. Octreotide-LAR (30 mg/month) gives a plasma level ≥ 1 ng/mL for 25 days, whereas this requires 3–6 injections per day of the non-sustained-release form. Lanreotide-PR is given IM every 10–14 days, and the lanreotide autogel every 4–6 weeks. Each of the sustained-release forms is highly effective at controlling the symptoms of the carcinoid syndrome (61–85% of patients).

Short-term side effects occur in 40–60% of patients receiving SC somatostatin analogues. Pain at the injection site and side effects related to the GI tract (59% discomfort, 15% nausea, diarrhea) are the most common. They are usually short-lived and do not interrupt treatment. Important long-term side effects include gallstone formation, steatorrhea, and deterioration in glucose tolerance. The overall incidence of gallstones/biliary sludge in one study was 52%, with 7% having symptomatic disease requiring surgical treatment.

Interferon α (IFN-α) is effective in controlling symptoms of the carcinoid syndrome, either alone or combined with hepatic artery embolization. With IFN-α alone the response rate is 42%, and with IFN-α with hepatic artery embolization, diarrhea was controlled for 1 year in 43% and flushing in 86%.

Hepatic artery embolization alone or with chemotherapy (chemoembolization) has been used to control the symptoms of carcinoid syndrome. Embolization alone is reported to control symptoms in up to 76% of patients and chemoembolization (5-fluorouracil, doxorubicin, cisplatin, mitomycin) in 60–75% of patients. Hepatic artery embolization can have major side effects including nausea, vomiting, pain, and fever. In two studies, 5–7% of patients died from complications of hepatic artery occlusion.

Other drugs have been used successfully in small numbers of patients to control the symptoms of carcinoid syndrome. Parachlorophenylanine can inhibit tryptophan hydroxylase and the conversion of tryptophan to 5HTP. However, its severe side effects, including psychiatric disturbances, make it intolerable for long-term use. α-Methyldopa inhibits the conversion of 5HTP to 5HT; however, its effects are only partial.

CARCINOID TUMORS (NONMETASTATIC) Surgery is the only potentially curative therapy. The extent of surgical resection is determined by the size of the primary. With appendiceal carcinoids, appendectomy was curative in 103 patients followed for up to 35 years. With rectal carcinoids <1 cm, local resection is curative. With small-intestinal carcinoids <1 cm, consensus had not been reached. Because 15–69% of small-intestinal carcinoids this size have metastases, some recommend a wide resection with en bloc resection of the adjacent lymph-bearing mesentery. If the carcinoid tumor is >2 cm in rectal, appendiceal, or small-intestinal sites, a full cancer operation should be done. This includes a right hemicolectomy for appendiceal carcinoid, an abdominoperineal resection or low anterior resection for rectal carcinoids and an en bloc resection of adjacent lymph nodes for small-intestinal carcinoids. For carcinoids 1–2 cm in diameter, a simple appendectomy is proposed by some for appendiceal tumors, whereas others favor a formal right hemicolectomy. For 1- to 2-cm rectal carcinoids, a wide local full-thickness excision is performed.

With type I or II gastric carcinoids, which are usually <1 cm, endoscopic removal is recommended. In type I or II gastric carcinoids >2 cm or if there is local invasion, some recommend total gastrectomy, whereas others recommend antrectomy in type 1 to reduce the hypergastrinemia; antrectomy produced regression of the carcinoids in a number of studies. For types I and III gastric carcinoids of 1 to 2 cm, there is no agreement, with some recommending endoscopic treatment, others surgical treatment. With type III gastric carcinoids >2 cm, excision and regional lymph node clearance is recommended. Most tumors <1 cm are treated endoscopically. Resection of isolated or limited hepatic metastases may be beneficial (see below).

PANCREATIC ENDOCRINE TUMORS

Functional PETs usually present clinically with symptoms due to the hormone-excess state. Only late in the course of the disease does the tumor per se cause prominent symptoms such as abdominal pain. In contrast, all of the symptoms due to nonfunctional PETs are due to the tumor per se. The overall result of this is that some functional PETs may present with severe symptoms with a small or undetectable primary tumor, whereas nonfunctional tumors almost always present late in their disease course with large tumors, which are usually metastatic. The mean delay between onset of continuous symptoms and diagnosis of a functional PET syndrome is 4–7 years. Therefore, the diagnoses are frequently missed for extended periods of time.

Rx PANCREATIC ENDOCRINE TUMOR

Treatment of PETs requires two different strategies. (1) Treatment must be directed at the hormone excess state, such as the gastric acid hypersecretion in gastrinomas or hypoglycemia in insulinomas. Ectopic hormone secretion usually causes the presenting symptoms and can cause life-threatening complications. (2) With all of the tumors except insulinomas, >50% are malignant (Table 344-2); therefore, treatment must also be directed against the tumor itself. Because these tumors are frequently widespread, surgical resection for cure, which addresses both treatment aspects, is not possible.

GASTRINOMA (ZOLLINGER-ELLISON SYNDROME)

A gastrinoma is a NET that secretes gastrin; the resultant hypergastrinemia causes gastric acid hypersecretion (ZES). The chronic gastric acid hypersecretion leads to growth of the gastric mucosa with increased numbers of parietal cells and proliferation of gastric ECL cells. The gastric acid hypersecretion characteristically causes peptic ulcer disease (PUD), often refractory and severe, as well as diarrhea. The most common presenting symptoms are abdominal pain (70–100%), diarrhea (37–73%), and gastroesophageal reflux disease (GERD) (30–35%); 10–20% have diarrhea only. Although peptic ulcers may occur in unusual locations, most patients have a typical duodenal ulcer. Important observations that should suggest this diagnosis include PUD with diarrhea; PUD in an unusual location or with multiple ulcers; and PUD refractory to treatment, associated with prominent gastric folds, associated with findings suggestive of MEN-1 (endocrinopathy, family history of ulcer or endocrinopathy, nephrolithiases), or without *Helicobacter pylori* present. *H. pylori* is present in >90% of idiopathic peptic ulcers but is present in <50% of patients with gastrinomas. Chronic unexplained diarrhea should also suggest gastrinoma.

About 20–25% of patients have MEN-1, and in most cases hyperparathyroidism is present prior to the gastrinoma. These patients are treated differently from those without MEN-1; therefore, MEN-1 should be sought in all patients by family history, by measuring plasma ionized calcium and prolactin levels and plasma hormone levels (parathormone, growth hormone).

Most gastrinomas (50–70%) are present in the duodenum, followed by the pancreas (20–40%) and other intraabdominal sites (mesentery, lymph nodes, biliary tract, liver, stomach, ovary). Three cases with two extraabdominal sites have been described: gastrinomas of the left ventricular septum of the heart and non–small cell lung cancer. In MEN-1, the gastrinomas are also usually in the duodenum (70–90%) or the pancreas (10–30%), and they are almost always multiple. About 60–90% of gastrinomas are malignant (Table 344-2) with metastatic spread to lymph nodes and liver. Distant metastases to bone occur in 12–30% of patients with liver metastases.

Diagnosis The diagnosis of gastrinoma requires the demonstration of fasting hypergastrinemia and an increased basal gastric acid output (BAO) (hyperchlorhydria). Greater than 98% of patients with gastrinomas have fasting hypergastrinemia, although in 40–60% the level may be less than tenfold elevated. Therefore, when the diagnosis is suspected, a fasting gastrin level should be determined first. Potent gastric acid–suppressant drugs such as proton pump inhibitors (e.g., omeprazole, esomeprazole) can suppress acid secretion sufficiently to cause hypergastrinemia; because of their prolonged duration of action, the drugs need to be discontinued for a week before the gastrin determination. If the gastrin level is elevated, it is important to show it is increased when gastric pH ≤ 2.0; physiologic hypergastrinemia secondary to achlorhydria (atrophic gastritis, pernicious anemia) is one of the most common causes of hypergastrinemia. Nearly all gastrinoma patients have a fasting pH ≤ 2 when off antisecretory drugs. If the fasting

gastrin > 1000 ng/L (10 times increased) and the pH ≤ 2.0, which occurs in 40–60% of patients with gastrinoma, the diagnosis is established after ruling out the possibility of retained antrum syndrome by history. In patients with hypergastrinemia with fasting gastrin < 1000 ng/L and gastric pH ≤ 2.0, other conditions such as *H. pylori* infections, antral G cell hyperplasia/hyperfunction, gastric outlet obstruction, or rarely, renal failure can masquerade as a gastrinoma. To establish the diagnosis in this group, a determination of BAO and a secretin stimulation test should be done. In patients with gastrinomas without previous gastric acid–reducing surgery, the BAO is usually (>90%) elevated (i.e., >15 meq/h). The secretin stimulation test is usually positive, with the criterion of >120 ng/L increase over the basal level having the highest sensitivity (94%) and specificity (100%).

Rx GASTRINOMAS

Gastric acid hypersecretion in patients with gastrinomas can be controlled in almost every case by oral gastric antisecretory drugs. Because of their long duration of action and potency, allowing once or twice a day dosing, the proton pump inhibitors are the drugs of choice. Histamine H₂-receptor antagonists are also effective, although more frequent dosing (q 4–8 h) and high doses are frequently required. In patients with MEN-1 with hyperparathyroidism, correction of the hyperparathyroidism increases the sensitivity to gastric antisecretory drugs and decreases the basal acid output.

With the increased ability to control acid hypersecretion, >50% of the patients who are not cured (>60% of patients) will die from tumor-related causes. At presentation careful imaging studies are essential to localize the extent of the tumor. A third of patients present with hepatic metastases, and in <15% of those with hepatic metastases the disease is limited, so that surgical resection may be possible. Surgical cure is possible in 30% of patients without MEN-1 or liver metastases (40% of all patients). In patients with MEN-1, long-term surgical cure is rare because the tumors are multiple, frequently with lymph node metastases. Therefore, all patients with gastrinomas without MEN-1 or a medical condition limiting life expectancy should undergo surgery by an experienced surgeon.

INSULINOMAS

An insulinoma is an endocrine tumor of the pancreas derived from beta cells that ectopically secretes insulin, which results in hypoglycemia. The average age of occurrence is 40–50 years. The most common clinical symptoms are due to the effect of the hypoglycemia on the central nervous system (neuroglycemic symptoms) and include confusion, headache, disorientation, visual difficulties, irrational behavior, or even coma. Also, most patients have symptoms due to excess catecholamine release secondary to the hypoglycemia including sweating, tremor, and palpitations. Characteristically these attacks are associated with fasting.

Insulinomas are generally small (>90% < 2 cm), usually not multiple (90%), and only 5–15% are malignant; they almost invariably occur only in the pancreas, distributed equally in the pancreatic head, body, and tail.

Insulinomas should be suspected in all patients with hypoglycemia, especially with a history suggesting attacks provoked by fasting or with a family history of MEN-1. Insulin is synthesized as proinsulin, a 21-amino-acid α-chain and a 30-amino-acid β-chain connected by a 33-amino-acid connecting peptide (C peptide). In insulinomas, in addition to elevated plasma insulin levels, elevated plasma proinsulin levels are found and C-peptide levels can be elevated.

Diagnosis The diagnosis of insulinoma requires the demonstration of an elevated plasma insulin level at the time of hypoglycemia. A number of other conditions may cause fasting hypoglycemia, such as the inadvertent or surreptitious use of insulin or oral hypoglycemic agents, severe liver disease, alcoholism, poor nutrition, or other extrapancreatic tumors. The most reliable test to diagnose insulinoma is a fast up to 72 h with serum glucose, C-peptide, and insulin measurements every 4–8 h. If at any point the patient becomes symptomatic or glucose levels are persistently <2.2 mmol/L (40 mg/dL), the test should be terminated and repeat samples for the above studies obtained before glucose is given. Some 70–80% of patients will develop hypoglycemia during the first 24 h and 98% by 48 h. In nonobese normal subjects, serum insulin levels should decrease to <43 pmol/L (<6 μU/mL) when blood glucose decreases to ≤2.2 mmol/L (≤40 mg/dL) and the ratio of insulin to glucose is <0.3 (in mg/dL). In addition to having an insulin level >6 μU/mL when blood glucose is ≤40 mg/dL, some investigators also require an elevated C-peptide and serum proinsulin level, an insulin/glucose ratio >0.3, and a decreased plasma β-hydroxybutyrate level for the diagnosis of insulinomas. Surreptitious use of insulin or hypoglycemic agents may be difficult to distinguish from insulinomas. The combination of proinsulin levels (normal in exogenous insulin/hypoglycemic agent users), C-peptide levels (low in exogenous insulin users), antibodies to insulin (positive in exogenous insulin users), and measurement of sulfonylurea levels in serum or plasma will allow the correct diagnosis to be made. The diagnosis of insulinoma has been complicated by the introduction of specific insulin assays that do not also interact with proinsulin, as do many of the older radioimmunoassays (RIAs), and therefore give lower plasma insulin levels. The increased use of these specific insulin assays has resulted in increased numbers of patients with insulinomas having lower plasma insulin values than the 43 pmol/L (6 μU/mL) levels proposed to be characteristic of insulinomas by RIA. In these patients the assessment of proinsulin and C-peptide levels at the time of hypoglycemia are particularly helpful for establishing the correct diagnosis.

℞ INSULINOMAS

Only 5–15% of insulinomas are malignant; therefore, after appropriate imaging (see below), surgery should be performed. In different studies, 75–95% of patients are cured by surgery. Before surgery, the hypoglycemia can be controlled by frequent small meals and the use of diazoxide (150–800 mg/d). Diazoxide is a benzothiadiazide whose hyperglycemic effect is attributed to inhibition of insulin release. Its side effects are sodium retention and GI symptoms such as nausea. Approximately 50–60% of patients respond to diazoxide. Other agents effective in some patients to control the hypoglycemia include verapamil and diphenylhydantoin. Long-acting somatostatin analogues such as octreotide are acutely effective in 40% of patients. However, octreotide needs to be used with care because it inhibits growth hormone secretion and can alter plasma glucagon levels; therefore, in some patients it can worsen the hypoglycemia.

For the 5–15% of patients with malignant insulinomas, the above drugs or somatostatin analogues are used initially. If they are not effective, various anti-tumor treatments such as hepatic arterial embolization, chemoembolization, or chemotherapy have been used (see below).

GLUCAGONOMAS

A glucagonoma is an endocrine tumor of the pancreas that secretes excessive amounts of glucagon, which causes a distinct syndrome characterized by dermatitis, glucose intolerance or diabetes, and weight loss. Glucagonomas principally occur between 45 and 70 years of age. The tumor is clinically heralded by a characteristic dermatitis (migratory necrolytic erythema) (67–90%), accompanied by glucose intolerance (40–90%), weight loss (66–96%), anemia (33–85%), diarrhea (15–29%), and thromboembolism (11–24%). The rash starts usually as an annular erythema at intertriginous and periorificial sites, especially in the groin or buttock. It subsequently becomes raised and bullae form; when the bullae rupture, eroded areas form. The lesions can wax and wane. A characteristic laboratory finding is hypoaminoacidemia, which occurs in 26–100% of patients.

Glucagonomas are generally large tumors (5–10 cm) at diagnosis. Some 50–80% occur in the pancreatic tail. From 50–82% have evidence of metastatic spread at presentation, usually to the liver. Glucagonomas are rarely extrapancreatic and usually occur singly.

Diagnosis The diagnosis is confirmed by demonstrating an increased plasma glucagon level (normal is <150 ng/L). Plasma glucagon levels are >1000 ng/L in 90%, between 500 and 1000 ng/L in 7%, and <500

ng/L in 3%. A plasma glucagon level >1000 ng/L is considered diagnostic of glucagonoma. Other diseases causing increased plasma glucagon levels include renal insufficiency, acute pancreatitis, hypercorticism, hepatic insufficiency, prolonged fasting, or familial hyperglucagonomia. With the exception of cirrhosis, these disorders do not increase plasma glucagon to >500 ng/L.

℞ GLUCAGONOMAS

In 50–80% of patients, metastases are present, so curative surgical resection is not possible. Surgical debulking in patients with advanced disease or other anti-tumor treatments may be beneficial (see below). Long-acting somatostatin analogues such as octreotide or lanreotide improve the skin rash in 75% of patients and may improve the weight loss, pain, and diarrhea but usually do not improve the glucose intolerance.

SOMATOSTATINOMA SYNDROME

The somatostatinoma syndrome is due to a NET that secretes excessive amounts of somatostatin, which causes a distinct syndrome characterized by diabetes mellitus, gallbladder disease, diarrhea, and steatorrhea. There is no general distinction in the literature between a tumor that contains somatostatin-like immunoreactivity (somatostatinoma) and does (11–45%), or does not (55–89%) produce a clinical syndrome (somatostatinoma syndrome) by secreting somatostatin. In one review of 173 cases of somatostatinomas, only 11% were associated with the somatostatinoma syndrome. The mean age of patients is 51 years. Somatostatinomas occur primarily in the pancreas and small intestine, and the frequency of the symptoms differs in each. Each of the usual symptoms is more frequent in pancreatic than intestinal somatostatinomas: diabetes mellitus (95% vs. 21%), gallbladder disease (94% vs. 43%), diarrhea (92% vs. 38%), steatorrhea (83% vs. 12%), hypochlorhydria (86% vs. 12%), and weight loss (90% vs. 69%). Somatostatinomas occur in the pancreas in 56–74% of cases, with the primary location being in the pancreatic head. The tumors are usually solitary (90%) and large, with a mean size of 4.5 cm. Liver metastases are frequent, being present in 69–84% of patients.

Somatostatin is a tetradecapeptide that is widely distributed in the central nervous system and GI tract, where it functions as a neurotransmitter or has paracrine and autocrine actions. It is a potent inhibitor of many processes including release of almost all hormones, acid secretion, intestinal and pancreatic secretion, and intestinal absorption. Most of the clinical manifestations are directly related to these inhibitory actions.

Diagnosis In most cases somatostatinomas have been found by accident either at the time of cholecystectomy or during endoscopy. The presence of psammoma bodies in a duodenal tumor should particularly raise suspicion. Duodenal somatostatin-containing tumors are increasingly associated with von Recklinghausen's disease. Most of these do not cause the somatostatinoma syndrome. The diagnosis of the somatostatinoma syndrome requires the demonstration of elevated plasma somatostatin levels.

℞ SOMATOSTATINOMAS

Pancreatic tumors are frequently (70–92%) metastatic at presentation, whereas 30–69% of small-intestinal somatostatinomas have metastases. Surgery is the treatment of choice for those without widespread hepatic metastases. Symptoms in patients with the somatostatinoma syndrome are improved by octreotide treatment.

VIPOMAS

VIPomas are endocrine tumors that secrete excessive amounts of VIP, which causes a distinct syndrome characterized by large-volume diarrhea, hypokalemia, and dehydration. This syndrome is also called Verner-Morrison syndrome, pancreatic cholera, and WDHA syndrome for *w*atery *d*iarrhea, *h*ypokalemia, and *a*chlorhydria, which some patients develop. The mean age of patients with this syndrome is 49 years; however, it can occur in children and when it does, it is usually caused by a ganglioneuroma or ganglioneuroblastoma.

The principal symptoms are large-volume diarrhea (100%) severe enough to cause hypokalemia (80–100%), dehydration (83%), hypochlorhydria (54–76%), and flushing (20%). The diarrhea is secretory in nature, persisting during fasting, is almost always >1 L/d and >3 L/d in 70%. Most patients do not have accompanying steatorrhea (16%), and the increased stool volume is due to increased excretion of sodium and potassium, which, with the anions, account for the osmolality of the stool. Patients frequently have hyperglycemia (25–50%) and hypercalcemia (25–50%).

VIP is a 28-amino-acid peptide important as a neurotransmitter, ubiquitously present in the central nervous system and GI tract. Its known actions include stimulation of small-intestinal chloride secretion, effects on smooth-muscle contractility, inhibition of acid secretion, and vasodilatory effects, which explain most features of the clinical syndrome.

In adults 80–90% of VIPomas are pancreatic in location, with the rest due to VIP-secreting pheochromocytomas, intestinal carcinoids, and, rarely, ganglioneuromas. These tumors are usually solitary, 50–75% are in the pancreatic tail, and 37–68% have hepatic metastases at diagnosis. In children <10 years old, the syndrome is usually due to ganglioneuromas or ganglioblastomas and is less often malignant (10%).

Diagnosis The diagnosis requires the demonstration of an elevated plasma VIP level and the presence of large-volume diarrhea. A stool volume of <700 mL/day is proposed to exclude the diagnosis of VIPoma. By fasting the patient, a number of causes can be excluded that cause marked diarrhea. Other diseases that can give a secretory large-volume diarrhea include gastrinomas, chronic laxative abuse, carcinoid syndrome, systemic mastocytosis, rarely medullary thyroid cancer, diabetes, and AIDS. Of these conditions, only VIPomas cause a marked increase in plasma VIP.

℞ VASOACTIVE INTESTINAL PEPTIDOMAS

The most important initial treatment in these patients is to correct their dehydration, hypokalemia, and electrolyte losses with fluid and electrolyte replacement. These patients may require 5 L/d of fluid and >350 meq/day of potassium. Because 37–68% of adults with VIPomas have metastatic disease in the liver at presentation, a significant number of patients cannot be cured surgically. In these patients long-acting somatostatin analogues such as octreotide or lanreotide are the drugs of choice.

Octreotide will control the diarrhea in 87% of patients. In nonresponsive patients the combination of glucocorticoids and octreotide has proved helpful in a small number of patients. Other drugs reported to be helpful in small numbers of patients include prednisone (60–100 mg/d), clonidine, indomethacin, phenothiazines, loperamide, lidamidine, lithium, propanolol, and metoclopramide. Treatment of advanced disease with embolization, chemoembolization, and chemotherapy may also be helpful (see below).

NONFUNCTIONAL PANCREATIC ENDOCRINE TUMORS

Nonfunctional PETs are endocrine tumors that originate in the pancreas and either secrete no products or their products do not cause a specific clinical syndrome. The symptoms are due entirely to the tumor per se. Nonfunctional PETs secrete chromogranin A (90–100%), chromogranin B (90–100%), PP (58%), α-hCG (40%), and β-hCG (20%). Because the symptoms are due to the tumor alone, patients with nonfunctional PETs usually present late in their disease course with invasive tumors and hepatic metastases (64–92%), and the tumors are usually large (72% > 5 cm). The tumors are usually solitary except in patients with MEN-1, where they are multiple. They occur primarily in the pancreatic head. Even though these tumors do not cause a functional syndrome, immunocytochemical studies show they synthesize numerous peptides and cannot be distinguished from functional tumors by immunocytochemistry.

The most common symptoms are abdominal pain (30–80%); jaundice (20–35%); weight loss, fatigue, or bleeding; and 10–15% are found incidentally. The average time from the beginning of symptoms to diagnosis is 5 years.

Diagnosis The diagnosis is established by histologic confirmation in a patient without either clinical symptoms or elevated plasma hormone levels. Even though chromogranin A levels are elevated in almost every patient, this is not specific for this disease as it can be found in functional PETs, carcinoids, and other neuroendocrine disorders. Plasma PP is increased in 22–71% of patients and should strongly suggest the diagnosis in a patient with a pancreatic mass because it is usually normal in patients with pancreatic adenocarcinomas. Elevated plasma PP is not diagnostic of this tumor because it is elevated in a number of other conditions such as chronic renal failure, old age, inflammatory conditions, and diabetes.

℞ NONFUNCTIONAL PANCREATIC ENDOCRINE TUMORS

Unfortunately, surgical curative resection can be considered only in the minority of the patients because 64–92% present with metastatic disease. Treatment is directed against the tumor per se using chemotherapy, embolization, chemoembolization, or hormonal therapy (see below).

GRFOMAS

GRFomas are endocrine tumors that secrete excessive amounts of GRF that causes acromegaly. The true frequency of this syndrome is not known. GRF is a 44-amino-acid peptide, and 25–44% of PETs have GRF immunoreactivity, although it is uncommonly secreted. GRFomas are lung tumors in 47–54% of cases, PETs in 29–30%, and small-intestinal carcinoids in 8–10%; up to 12% occur at other sites. Patients have a mean age of 38 years, and the symptoms are usually due to either acromegaly or the tumor itself. The acromegaly caused by GRFomas is indistinguishable from classic acromegaly. The pancreatic tumors are usually large (>6 cm), and liver metastases are present in 39%. They should be suspected in any patient with acromegaly and an abdominal tumor, in a patient with MEN-1 with acromegaly, or in a patient without a pituitary adenoma with acromegaly or associated with hyperprolactinemia, which occurs in 70% of GRFomas. GRFomas are an uncommon cause of acromegaly. The diagnosis is established by performing plasma assays for GRF and growth hormone. The normal level for GRF is <5 μg/L in men and <10 μg/L in women. Most GRFomas have a plasma GRF level ≥ 300 μg/L. Patients with GRFomas also have increased plasma insulin-like growth factor 1 levels similar to those in classic acromegaly. Surgery is the treatment of choice if diffuse metastases are not present. Long-acting somatostatin analogues such as octreotide or lanreotide are the agents of choice, with 75–100% of patients responding.

OTHER RARE PANCREATIC ENDOCRINE TUMOR SYNDROMES

Cushing's syndrome (ACTHoma) due to a PET occurs in 4–16% of all ectopic Cushing's syndrome cases. It occurs in 5% of cases of sporadic gastrinomas, almost invariably in patients with hepatic metastases, and is an independent poor prognostic factor. Paraneoplastic hypercalcemia due to PETs releasing parathyroid hormone–related peptide (PTHrP), a PTH-like material, or unknown factor, is rarely reported. The tumors are usually large, and liver metastases are usually present. Most (88%) appear to be due to release of PTHrP. PETs can occasionally cause the carcinoid syndrome. PETs secreting calcitonin have been proposed as a specific clinical syndrome. Half of the patients have diarrhea, which disappears with resection of the tumor. The proposal that this could be a discrete syndrome is supported by finding that 25–42% of patients with medullary thyroid cancer with hypercalcitonemia develop diarrhea, likely secondary to a motility disorder. A renin-producing PET has been described in a patient presenting with hypertension; PETs secreting luteinizing hormone, resulting in masculinization or decreased libido, and a PET secreting erythropoietin, resulting in polycythemia have also been reported (Table 344-2). Ghrelin is a 28-amino-acid peptide with a number of metabolic and immunologic functions. Although it is detectable immunohistochemically in most PETs, only 1 in 24 patients (4%) with a PET had elevated plasma ghrelin levels in one study and the patient was asymptomatic. Release of ghrelin by a PET may be clinically silent.

TUMOR LOCALIZATION

Localization of the primary tumor and defining the extent of disease are essential to the proper management of all carcinoids and PETs. Numerous tumor localization methods are used in both types of NETs, including conventional imaging studies (CT, MRI, transabdominal ultrasound, selective angiography), somatostatin receptor scintigraphy (SRS), and positron emission tomographic scanning. In PETs, endoscopic ultrasound (EUS) and functional localization by measuring venous hormonal gradients are also reported useful. Bronchial carcinoids are usually detected by a standard chest radiography and assessed by CT. Rectal, duodenal, colonic, and gastric carcinoids are usually detected by GI endoscopy.

PETs, as well as carcinoid tumors, frequently overexpress high-affinity somatostatin receptors in both their primary tumors and their metastases. Of the five types of somatostatin receptors (sst_{1-5}), radiolabeled octreotide binds with high affinity to sst_2 and sst_5, lower for sst_3, and has a very low affinity for sst_1 and sst_4. Between 90 and 100% of carcinoid tumors and PETs possess sst_2, and many also have the other four sst subtypes. Interaction with these receptors can be used to localize NETs using [^{111}In-DTPA-D-Phe^1]octreotide and radionuclide scanning (SRS) as well as for treatment of the hormone excess state with octreotide or lanreotide, as discussed earlier. Because of its sensitivity and ability to localize tumor throughout the body, SRS is now the initial imaging modality of choice for localizing both primary and metastatic NETs. SRS localizes tumor in 73–89% of patients with carcinoids and in 56–100% of patients with PETs, except for insulinomas. Insulinomas are usually small and have low densities of sst receptors, resulting in SRS being positive in only 12–50% of patients with insulinomas. Figure 344-3 shows an example of the increased sensitivity of SRS in a patient with a carcinoid tumor. The CT scan (Fig. 344-3, *top*) shows a single liver metastasis, whereas the SRS demonstrates three metastases in the liver in multiple locations (Fig. 344-3, *bottom*). Occasional false-positive responses with SRS can occur (12% in one study) because numerous other normal tissues and diseases can have high densities of sst receptors, including granulomas (sarcoid, TB, etc.), thyroid diseases (goiter, thyroiditis), and activated lymphocytes (lymphomas, wound infections). For PETs located in the pancreas, EUS is highly sensitive, localizing 77–93% of insulinomas, which occur almost exclusively within the pancreas. EUS is less sensitive for extrapancreatic tumors. If liver metastases are identified by SRS, either a CT or MRI is then recommended to assess the size and exact location of the metastases because SRS does not give information on tumor size. Functional localization measuring hormone gradients after intra-arterial calcium injections in insulinomas (insulin) or gastrin gradients after secretin injections in gastrinoma is a sensitive method, being positive in 80–100% of patients. However, this method gives only regional localization and therefore is reserved for cases where other imaging modalities are negative. Positron emission tomographic scanning with ^{18}F-fluoro-DOPA in patients with carcinoids or with ^{11}C-5HTP in patients with PETs or carcinoids has greater sensitivity than conventional imaging studies or SRS and will likely be used increasingly in the future.

Rx ADVANCED DISEASE (DIFFUSE METASTATIC DISEASE)

The single most important prognostic factor for survival is the presence of liver metastases (**Fig. 344-4**). For patients with foregut carcinoids without hepatic metastases, the 5-year survival in one study was 95% and with distant metastases, 20%. With gastrinomas, the 5-year survival without liver metastases is 98%, with limited metastases in one hepatic

FIGURE 344-3 Ability of CT scanning (*top*) or somatostatin receptor scintigraphy (SRS) (*bottom*) to localize metastatic carcinoid in the liver.

lobe it is 78%, and with diffuse metastases, 16%. A number of different modalities are reported to be effective in advanced disease including cytoreductive surgery (removal of all visible tumor), treatment with chemotherapy, somatostatin analogues, IFN-α, hepatic embolization alone or with chemotherapy (chemoembolization), radiotherapy, and liver transplantation.

SPECIFIC ANTITUMOR TREATMENTS Cytoreductive surgery, unfortunately, is only possible in the 9–22% of patients who have limited hepatic metastases. Although no randomized studies have proven that hepatic resection extends life, results from a number of studies suggest it likely increases survival and therefore is recommended, if possible.

Chemotherapy for metastatic carcinoid tumors has generally been disappointing, with response rates of 0–40% with various two- or three-drug combinations. Chemotherapy for PETs has been more successful with tumor shrinkage reported in 30–70% of patients. The current regimen of choice is streptozotocin and doxorubicin.

Long-acting somatostatin analogues such as octreotide, lanreotide, and IFN-α rarely decrease tumor size (i.e., 0–17%); however, these drugs have tumoristatic effects, stopping additional growth in 26–95% of patients with NETs. How long tumor stabilization lasts or whether it prolongs survival has not been established.

Hepatic embolization and chemoembolization (with dacarbazine, cisplatin, doxorubicin, 5-fluorouracil, or streptozotocin) have been reported to decrease tumor bulk and to help control the symptoms of the hormone-excess state. These modalities are generally reserved for cases in which treatment with somatostatin analogues, IFN-α (carcinoids), or chemotherapy (PETs) fails. Embolization, when combined with treatment with octreotide and IFN-α, significantly reduces tumor progression ($p = .008$)

FIGURE 344-4 Effect of the presence and extent of liver metastases on survival in patients with gastrinomas (**A**) or carcinoid tumors (**B**). ZES, Zollinger-Ellison syndrome. *(A is drawn from data from 199 patients with gastrinomas modified from F Yu et al: J Clin Oncol 17:615, 1999. B is drawn from data from 71 patients with foregut carcinoid tumors from EW McDermott et al: Br J Surg 81:1007, 1994.)*

over treatment with embolization and octreotide alone in patients with advanced midgut carcinoids.

Radiotherapy with radiolabeled somatostatin analogues that are internalized by the tumors is an approach under investigation. Three different radionuclides are being used: (1) high doses of [^{111}In-DTPA-D-Phe^{1}]octreotide (Fig. 344-2), which emits γ-rays, internal conversion, and Auger electrons; yttrium-90, which emits high-energy β-particles coupled by a DOTA chelating group to octreotide or octreotate; and (3) ^{177}lutetium-coupled analogues, which emit both β- and γ-rays. All are being tested. Tumor stabilization is reported in 41–81%, 44–88%, and 23–40%, respectively, and a decrease in tumor size in 8–30%, 6–37%, and 38%, respectively, of patients with advanced metastatic NETs. These results suggest this novel therapy may be helpful, especially in patients with advanced metastatic disease.

The use of liver transplantation has been abandoned for treatment of most metastatic tumors to the liver. However, for metastatic NETs it is still a consideration. In a review of 103 cases of malignant NETs (48 PETs, 43 carcinoids), the 2- and 5-year survival rates were 60% and 47%, respectively. However, recurrence-free survival was low (<24%). It was concluded that for younger patients with metastatic NETs limited to the liver, liver transplantation may be justified.

FURTHER READINGS

FORRER F et al: Peptide receptor radiotherapy. Best Practice Res Clin Endocrinol Metab 21:111, 2007

JENSEN RT, DOHERTY GM: Carcinoid tumors and the carcinoid syndrome, in *Cancer: Principles and Practice of Oncology*, 7th ed, VT DeVita Jr, S Hellman, SA Rosenberg (eds). Philadelphia, Lippincott Williams and Wilkins, 2005, pp 1559–1574

MODLIN IM et al: Therapeutic options for gastrointestinal carcinoids. Clin Gastrointest Hepatol 4:526, 2006

OBERG K, ERIKSSON B: Neuroendocrine tumors. Best Pract Res Clin Endocrinol Metabol 21:1, 2007

RINDI G, BORDI C: Aetiology, molecular pathogenesis and genetics. Best Pract Res Clin Gastroenterol 19:519, 2005

——— et al (ed): Consensus guidelines on the management of patients with digestive neuroendocrine tumors. Neuroendocrinology 84:151, 2006

345 Disorders Affecting Multiple Endocrine Systems

Camilo Jimenez, Robert F. Gagel

NEOPLASTIC DISORDERS AFFECTING MULTIPLE ENDOCRINE ORGANS

Multiple endocrine neoplasia syndrome is defined as a disorder with neoplasms in two or more different hormonal tissues in several members of a family. Several distinct genetic disorders predispose to endocrine gland neoplasia and cause hormone excess syndromes (Table 345-1). DNA-based genetic testing is now available for these disorders, but effective management requires an understanding of endocrine neoplasia and the range of clinical features that may be manifested in an individual patient.

MULTIPLE ENDOCRINE NEOPLASIA (MEN) TYPE 1

MEN1, or Wermer's syndrome, is inherited as an autosomal dominant trait. This syndrome is characterized by neoplasia of the parathyroid glands, enteropancreatic tumors, anterior pituitary adenomas, and other neuroendocrine tumors with variable penetrance (Table 345-1). Although rare, MEN1 is the most common multiple endocrine neoplasia syndrome with an estimated prevalence of 2–20 per 100,000 in the gen-

eral population. This syndrome is caused by inactivating mutations of the tumor-suppressor gene *MEN1* located at chromosome 11q13. The *MEN1* gene codes for a nuclear protein called Menin. Menin interacts with JunD, suppressing the JunD-dependent transcriptional activation. It is unclear how this accounts for Menin growth regulatory activity, since JunD is associated with inhibition of cell growth. Each child born to an affected parent has a 50% probability of inheriting the gene. The variable penetrance of the several neoplastic components can make the differential diagnosis and treatment challenging.

Clinical Manifestations *Primary hyperparathyroidism* is the most common manifestation of MEN1, with an estimated penetrance of 95–100%. Hypercalcemia may develop during the teenage years, and most individuals are affected by age 40 (Fig. 345-1). Hyperparathyroidism is the earliest manifestation of the syndrome in most MEN1 patients. The neoplastic changes in hyperparathyroidism provide a specific example of one of the cardinal features of endocrine tumors in MEN1—multicentricity. The neoplastic changes inevitably affect multiple parathyroid glands, making surgical cure difficult. Screening for hyperparathyroidism involves measurement of either an albumin-adjusted or ionized serum calcium level. The diagnosis is established by demonstrating elevated levels of serum calcium and intact parathyroid hormone. Manifestations of hyperparathyroidism of MEN1 do not differ substantially from those in sporadic hyperparathyroidism and include calcium-containing kidney stones, kidney failure, nephrocalcinosis, bone abnormalities (i.e., osteoporosis, osteitis fibrosa cystica), and gastrointestinal and musculoskeletal complaints. Management is challenging because of early onset, significant recurrence rates, and the multiplicity of parathyroid gland involvement. Differentiation of hyperparathyroidism of MEN1 from other forms of familial primary hyperparathyroidism is usually based on family history, histologic features of resected parathyroid tissue, the presence of a *MEN1* mutation and, sometimes, long-term observation to determine whether other manifestations of MEN1 develop. Parathyroid hyperplasia is the most common cause of hyperparathyroidism in MEN1, although single and multiple adenomas have been described. Hyperplasia of one or more parathyroid glands is common in younger patients; adenomas are usually found in older patients or those with long-standing disease.

Enteropancreatic tumors are the second most common manifestation of MEN1, with an estimated penetrance of 50%. They tend to occur in parallel with hyperparathyroidism (Fig. 345-1); 30% are malignant. Most of these tumors secrete peptide hormones that cause specific clinical syndromes. These syndromes, however, may have an insidious onset and a slow progression, making their diagnosis difficult and in many cases delayed. Some enteropancreatic tumors do not secrete hormones. These "silent" tumors are usually found during radiographic screening. Metastasis, most commonly to the liver, is not uncommon.

Gastrinomas are the most common enteropancreatic tumors observed in MEN1 patients and result in the Zollinger-Ellison syndrome (ZES). ZES is caused by excessive gastrin production and occurs in more than one-half of MEN1 patients with small carcinoid-like tumors in the duodenal wall or, less often, by pancreatic islet cell tumors. There may be more than one gastrin-producing tumor, making localization difficult. The robust acid production may cause esophagitis, duodenal ulcers throughout the duodenum, ulcers involving the proximal jejunum, and diarrhea. The ulcer diathesis is commonly refractory to conservative therapy such as antacids. The diagnosis is made by finding increased gastric acid secretion, elevated basal gastrin levels in the serum [generally >115 pmol/L (200 pg/mL)], and an exaggerated response of serum gastrin to either secretin or calcium. Other causes of elevated serum gastrin levels, such as achlorhydria, treatment with H_2 receptor antagonists or proton pump inhibitors, retained gastric antrum, small-bowel resection, gastric outlet obstruction, and hypercalcemia, should be excluded (Fig. 345-1). High-resolution, early-phase CT scanning, abdominal MRI with contrast, octreotide scan, and/or endoscopic ultrasound provide the best preoperative techniques for identification of the primary and metastatic gastrinoma; intraoperative ultrasonography is the most sensitive method for detection of small tumors. Approximately one-fourth of all ZES occurs in the context of MEN1.

Insulinomas are the second most common enteropancreatic tumors in patients who suffer from MEN1. Unlike gastrinomas, most insuli-

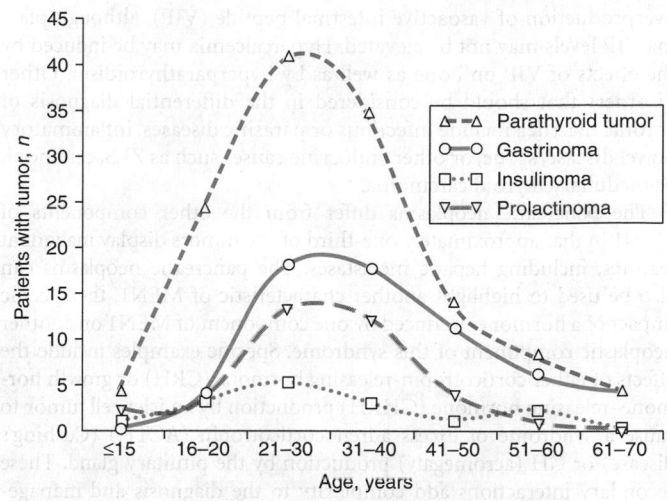

FIGURE 345-1 Age at onset of endocrine tumor expression in multiple endocrine neoplasia type 1 (MEN1). Data derived from retrospective analysis for each endocrine organ hyperfunction in 130 cases of MEN1. Age at onset is the age at first symptom or, with tumors not causing symptoms, age at the time of the first abnormal finding on a screening test. The rate of diagnosis of hyperparathyroidism increased sharply between ages 16 and 20 years. *(Reprinted with permission from S Marx et al: Ann Intern Med 129:484, 1998.)*

nomas originate in the pancreas bed, becoming the most common pancreatic tumor in MEN1. Hypoglycemia caused by insulinomas is observed in about one-third of MEN1 patients with pancreatic islet cell tumors (Fig. 345-1). The tumors may be benign or malignant (25%). The diagnosis can be suggested by documenting hypoglycemia during a short fast with simultaneous inappropriate elevation of serum insulin and C-peptide levels. More commonly, it is necessary to subject the patient to a supervised 12- to 72-h fast to provoke hypoglycemia (Chap. 339). Large insulinomas may be identified by CT or MRI scanning; small tumors not detected by conventional radiographic techniques may be localized by endoscopic ultrasound or by selective arteriographic injection of calcium into each of the arteries that supply the pancreas and sampling the hepatic vein for insulin to determine the anatomic region containing the tumor. Intraoperative ultrasonography is frequently used to localize these tumors. The trend to earlier diagnosis of, hence, smaller tumors has reduced the usefulness of octreotide scanning, which is positive in a minority of these patients.

Glucagonoma, seen occasionally in MEN1, causes a syndrome of hyperglycemia, skin rash (necrolytic migratory erythema), anorexia, glossitis, anemia, depression, diarrhea, and venous thrombosis. In about half of these patients the plasma glucagon level is high, leading to its designation as the *glucagonoma syndrome*, although elevation of the plasma glucagon level in MEN1 patients is not necessarily associated with these symptoms. Some patients with this syndrome also have elevated plasma ghrelin levels. The glucagonoma syndrome may represent a complex interaction between glucagon and ghrelin overproduction and the nutritional status of the patient.

The *Verner-Morrison*, or *watery diarrhea*, *syndrome* consists of watery diarrhea, hypokalemia, hypochlorhydria, and metabolic acidosis. The diarrhea can be voluminous and is almost always found in association with an islet cell tumor, prompting use of the term *pancreatic cholera*. However, the syndrome is not restricted to pancreatic islet tumors and has been observed with carcinoids or other tumors. This syndrome is believed to be due to

TABLE 345-1	DISEASE ASSOCIATIONS IN THE MULTIPLE ENDOCRINE NEOPLASIA (MEN) SYNDROMES

MEN1	MEN2	Mixed Syndromes
Parathyroid hyperplasia or adenoma	**MEN2A** MTC	**Von Hippel–Lindau syndrome** Pheochromocytoma
Islet cell hyperplasia, adenoma, or carcinoma	Pheochromocytoma Parathyroid hyperplasia or adenoma	Islet cell tumor Renal cell carcinoma
Pituitary hyperplasia or adenoma	**MEN2A with cutaneous lichen amyloidosis**	Hemangioblastoma of central nervous system
Other less common manifestations: foregut carcinoid, pheochromocytoma, subcutaneous or visceral lipomas	**MEN2A with Hirschsprung disease** **Familial MTC** **MEN2B** MTC Pheochromocytoma Mucosal and gastrointestinal neuromas Marfanoid features	Retinal angiomas **Neurofibromatosis with features of MEN1 or 2** **Carney complex** Myxomas of heart, skin, and breast Spotty cutaneous pigmentation Testicular, adrenal, and GH-producing pituitary tumors Peripheral nerve schwannomas

Abbreviations: GH, growth hormone; MTC, medullary thyroid carcinoma.

overproduction of vasoactive intestinal peptide (VIP), although plasma VIP levels may not be elevated. Hypercalcemia may be induced by the effects of VIP on bone as well as by hyperparathyroidism. Other disorders that should be considered in the differential diagnosis of chronic diarrhea include infectious or parasitic diseases, inflammatory bowel disease, sprue, or other endocrine causes such as ZES, carcinoid, or medullary thyroid carcinoma.

The pancreatic neoplasms differ from the other components of MEN1 in that approximately one-third of the tumors display malignant features, including hepatic metastases. The pancreatic neoplasms can also be used to highlight another characteristic of MEN1, the specific impact of a hormone produced by one component of MEN1 on another neoplastic component of this syndrome. Specific examples include the effects of either corticotropin-releasing hormone (CRH) or growth hormone–releasing hormone (GHRH) production by an islet cell tumor to cause a syndrome of excess adrenocorticotropin (ACTH) (Cushing's disease) or GH (acromegaly) production by the pituitary gland. These secondary interactions add complexity to the diagnosis and management of these tumor syndromes. Pancreatic islet cell tumors are diagnosed by identification of a characteristic clinical syndrome, hormonal assays with or without provocative stimuli, or radiographic techniques. One approach involves annual screening of individuals at risk with measurement of basal and meal-stimulated levels of pancreatic polypeptide to identify the tumors as early as possible; the rationale of this screening strategy is the concept that surgical removal of islet cell tumors at an early stage will be curative. Other approaches to screening include measurement of serum gastrin and pancreatic polypeptide levels every 2–3 years, with the rationale that pancreatic neoplasms will be detected at a later stage but can be managed medically, if possible, or by surgery. High-resolution, early-phase CT scanning or endoscopic ultrasound provides the best preoperative technique for identification of these tumors; intraoperative ultrasonography is the most sensitive method for detection of small tumors.

Pituitary tumors occur in 20–30% of patients with MEN1 and tend to be multicentric. These tumors can exhibit aggressive behavior and local invasiveness that makes them difficult to resect (Chap. 333). Prolactinomas are most common (Fig. 345-1) and are diagnosed by finding serum prolactin levels >200 μg/L, with or without a pituitary mass evident by MRI. Values <200 μg/L may be due to a prolactin-secreting neoplasm or to compression of the pituitary stalk by a different type of pituitary tumor. Acromegaly due to excessive GH production is the second most common syndrome caused by pituitary tumors in MEN1 and can rarely be due to production of GHRH by an islet cell tumor (see above). Cushing's disease can be caused by ACTH-producing pituitary tumors or by ectopic production of ACTH or CRH by other components of MEN1 syndrome including islet cell or carcinoid tumors or adrenal adenomas. Diagnosis of pituitary Cushing's disease is generally best accomplished by a high-dose dexamethasone suppression test or by petrosal venous sinus sampling for ACTH after IV injection of CRH. Differentiation of a primary pituitary tumor from an ectopic CRH-producing tumor may be difficult because the pituitary is the source of ACTH in both disorders; documentation of CRH production by a pancreatic islet or carcinoid tumor may be the only method of proving ectopic CRH production.

Adrenal cortical tumors are found in almost one-half of gene carriers but are rarely functional; malignancy in the cortical adenomas is uncommon. Rare cases of pheochromocytoma have been described in the context of MEN1. Due to its rarity, screening for these tumors is only indicated when there are suggestive symptoms.

Carcinoid tumors in MEN1 are of the foregut type and are derived from thymus, lung, stomach, or duodenum; they may metastasize or be locally invasive. These tumors usually produce serotonin, calcitonin, or CRH; the typical carcinoid syndrome with flushing, diarrhea, and bronchospasm is rare (Chap. 344). Mediastinal carcinoid tumors (an upper mediastinal mass) are more common in men; bronchial carcinoid tumors are more common in women. Carcinoid tumors are a late manifestation of MEN1; some reports have emphasized the importance of routine chest CT screening for mediastinal carcinoid tu-

FIGURE 345-2 Schematic depiction of the *MEN1* gene and the distribution of mutations. The shaded areas show coding sequence. The closed circles show the relative distribution of mutations, mostly inactivating, in each exon. Mutation data are derived from the Human Gene Mutation Database from which more detailed information can be obtained (*www.uwcm.ac.uk/uwcm/mg/hgmd0.html*). *(From M Krawczak, DN Cooper: Trends Genet 13:1321, 1998.)*

mors because of their high rate of malignant transformation and aggressive behavior.

UNUSUAL MANIFESTATIONS OF MEN1 Subcutaneous or visceral lipomas and cutaneous leiomyomas may also be present but rarely undergo malignant transformation. Skin angiofibromas or collagenomas are seen in most patients with MEN1 when carefully sought.

 GENETIC CONSIDERATIONS *MEN1* gene mutations are found in >90% of families with the syndrome (**Fig. 345-2**). Genetic testing can be performed in individuals at risk for the development of MEN1 and is now commercially available in the United States and Europe. The major value of genetic testing in a kindred with an identifiable mutation is the assignment or exclusion of gene carrier status. In those identified as carrying the mutant gene, routine screening for individual manifestations of MEN1 should be performed as outlined above. Those with negative genetic test results in a kindred with a known germline mutation can be excluded from further screening for MEN1. A significant percentage of sporadic parathyroid, islet cell, and carcinoid tumors also have loss or mutation of *MEN1*. It is presumed that these mutations are somatic and occur in a single cell, leading to subsequent transformation.

℞ MULTIPLE ENDOCRINE NEOPLASIA TYPE 1

Almost everyone who inherits a mutant *MEN1* gene develops at least one clinical manifestation of the syndrome. Most develop hyperparathyroidism, 80% develop pancreatic islet cell tumors, and more than half develop pituitary tumors. For most of these tumors, initial surgery is not curative and patients frequently require multiple surgical procedures and surgery on two or more endocrine glands during a lifetime. For this reason, it is essential to establish clear goals for management of these patients rather than to recommend surgery casually each time a tumor is discovered. Ranges for acceptable management are discussed below.

HYPERPARATHYROIDISM Individuals with serum calcium levels >3.0 mmol/L (12 mg/dL), evidence of calcium nephrolithiasis or renal dysfunction, neuropathic or muscular symptoms, or bone involvement (including osteopenia) or individuals <50 years of age should undergo parathyroid exploration. There is less agreement regarding the necessity for parathyroid exploration in individuals who do not meet these criteria, and observation may be appropriate in the MEN1 patient with asymptomatic hyperparathyroidism.

When parathyroid surgery is indicated in MEN1, there are two approaches. In the first, all parathyroid tissue is identified and removed at the time of primary operation, and parathyroid tissue is implanted in the nondominant forearm. Thymectomy should also be performed because of the potential for later development of malignant carcinoid tumors. If reoperation for hyperparathyroidism is necessary at a later date, transplanted parathyroid tissue can be resected from the forearm with titration of tissue removal to lower the intact parathyroid hormone (PTH) to <50% of basal.

Another approach is to remove 3–3.5 parathyroid glands from the neck (leaving ~50 mg of parathyroid tissue), carefully marking the location of residual tissue so that the remaining tissue can be located easily during subsequent surgery. If this approach is utilized, intraoperative PTH measurements should be utilized to monitor adequacy of removal of parathyroid tissue with a goal of reducing postoperative serum intact PTH to ≤50% of basal values.

The use of high-resolution CT scanning (1 mm) and imaging during three phases of contrast flow has substantially improved the ability to identify aberrantly located parathyroid tissue. As this issue arises with some frequency in the context of parathyroid disease in MEN1, this technique should be utilized to locate parathyroid tissue before reoperation for a failed exploration, and it may be useful prior to the initial operation.

PANCREATIC ISLET CELL TUMORS (See Chap. 344 for discussion of pancreatic islet cell tumors not associated with MEN1.) Two features of pancreatic islet cell tumors in MEN1 complicate the management. First, the pancreatic islet cell tumors are multicentric, malignant about a third of the time, and cause death in 10–20% of patients. Second, performance of a total pancreatectomy to prevent malignancy causes diabetes mellitus, a disease with significant long-term complications that include neuropathy, retinopathy, and nephropathy. These features make it difficult to formulate clear-cut guidelines, but some general concepts appear to be valid. (1) Islet cell tumors producing insulin, glucagon, VIP, GHRH, or CRH should be resected because medical therapy for the hormonal effects of these tumors are generally ineffective. (2) Gastrin-producing islet cell tumors that cause ZES are frequently multicentric. Recent experience suggests that a high percentage of ZES in MEN1 is caused by duodenal wall carcinoid tumors and that resection of these tumors improves the cure rate. Treatment with H2 receptor antagonists (cimetidine or ranitidine) or proton pump inhibitors (omeprazole, lansoprazole, esomeprazole, etc.) provides an alternative, and some think preferable, therapy to surgery for control of ulcer disease in patients with multicentric tumors or with hepatic metastases. (3) In families in which there is a high incidence of malignant islet cell tumors that cause death, total pancreatectomy at an early age may be considered to prevent malignancy.

Management of metastatic islet cell carcinoma is unsatisfactory. Hormonal abnormalities can sometimes be controlled. For example, ZES can be treated with H2 receptor antagonists or proton pump inhibitors; the somatostatin analogues, octreotide or lanreotide, are useful in the management of carcinoid, glucagonoma, and the watery diarrhea syndrome. Bilateral adrenalectomy may be required for ectopic ACTH syndrome if medical therapy is ineffective (Chap. 336). Islet cell carcinomas frequently metastasize to the liver but may grow slowly. Hepatic artery embolization, radiofrequency ablation, or chemotherapy (5-fluorouracil, streptozocin, chlorozotocin, doxorubicin, or dacarbazine) may reduce tumor mass, control symptoms of hormone excess, and prolong life; however, these treatments are never curative. Consideration should be given to participation in clinical trials of new agents that target specific molecular pathways.

PITUITARY TUMORS Treatment of prolactinomas with dopamine agonists (bromocriptine, cabergoline, or quinagolide) usually returns the serum prolactin level to normal and prevents further tumor growth (Chap. 333). Surgical resection of a prolactinoma is rarely curative but may relieve mass effects. Transsphenoidal resection is appropriate for neoplasms that secrete ACTH, GH, or the α-subunit of the pituitary glycoprotein hormones. Octreotide reduces tumor mass in one-third of GH-secreting tumors and reduces GH and insulin-like growth factor I levels in >75% of patients. Pegvisomant, a GH antagonist, rapidly lowers insulin-like growth factor levels in patients with acromegaly (Chap. 333). Radiation therapy may be useful for large or recurrent tumors.

Improvements in the management of MEN1, particularly the earlier recognition of islet cell and pituitary tumors, have improved outcomes in these patients. As a result, other neoplastic manifestations that develop later in the course of this disorder, such as carcinoid syndrome, are now seen with increased frequency.

MULTIPLE ENDOCRINE NEOPLASIA TYPE 2

Clinical Manifestations Medullary thyroid carcinoma (MTC) and pheochromocytoma are associated in two major syndromes: MEN type 2A and MEN type 2B (Table 345-1). MEN2A is the combination of MTC, hyperparathyroidism, and pheochromocytoma. Three subvariants of MEN2A are familial medullary thyroid carcinoma (FMTC), MEN2A with cutaneous lichen amyloidosis, and MEN2A with Hirschsprung disease. MEN2B is the combination of MTC, pheochromocytoma, mucosal neuromas, intestinal ganglioneuromatosis, and marfanoid features.

MULTIPLE ENDOCRINE NEOPLASIA TYPE 2A MTC is the most common manifestation. This tumor usually develops in childhood, beginning as hyperplasia of the calcitonin-producing cells (C cells) of the thyroid. MTC is typically located at the junction of the upper one-third and lower two-thirds of each lobe of the thyroid, reflecting the high density of C cells in this location; tumors >1 cm in size are frequently associated with local or distant metastases. Measurement of the serum calcitonin level after calcium or pentagastrin injection makes it possible to diagnose this disorder at an early stage in its development (see below).

Pheochromocytoma occurs in ~50% of patients with MEN2A and causes palpitations, nervousness, headaches, and sometimes sweating (Chap. 337). About half of the tumors are bilateral, and >50% of patients who have had unilateral adrenalectomy develop a pheochromocytoma in the contralateral gland within a decade. A second feature of these tumors is a disproportionate increase in the secretion of epinephrine relative to norepinephrine. This characteristic differentiates the MEN2 pheochromocytomas from sporadic pheochromocytoma and those associated with von Hippel–Lindau (VHL) syndrome, hereditary paraganglioma, or neurofibromatosis. Capsular invasion is common, but metastasis is uncommon. Finally, the pheochromocytomas are almost always found in the adrenal gland, differentiating the pheochromocytomas in MEN2 from the extraadrenal tumors more commonly found in hereditary paraganglioma syndromes.

Hyperparathyroidism occurs in 15–20% of patients, with the peak incidence in the third or fourth decade. The manifestations of hyperparathyroidism do not differ from those in other forms of primary hyperparathyroidism (Chap. 347). Diagnosis is established by finding hypercalcemia, hypophosphatemia, hypercalciuria, and an inappropriately high serum level of intact parathyroid hormone. Multiglandular parathyroid hyperplasia is the most common histologic finding, although with long-standing disease adenomatous changes may be superimposed on hyperplasia.

The most common subvariant of MEN2A is familial MTC, an autosomal dominant syndrome in which MTC is the only manifestation (Table 345-1). The clinical diagnosis of FMTC is established by the identification of MTC in multiple generations without a pheochromocytoma. Since the penetrance of pheochromocytoma is 50% in MEN2A, it is possible that MEN2A could masquerade as FMTC in small kindreds. It is important to consider this possibility carefully before classifying a kindred as having FMTC; failure to do so could lead to death or serious morbidity from pheochromocytoma in an affected kindred member. The difficulty of differentiating MEN2A and FMTC is discussed further below.

MULTIPLE ENDOCRINE NEOPLASIA TYPE 2B The association of MTC, pheochromocytoma, mucosal neuromas, and a marfanoid habitus is designated MEN2B. MTC in MEN2B develops earlier and is more aggressive than in MEN2A. Metastatic disease has been described prior to 1 year of age, and death may occur in the second or third decade of life. However, the prognosis is not invariably bad even in patients with metastatic disease, as evidenced by a number of multigenerational families with this disease.

Pheochromocytoma occurs in more than half of MEN2B patients and does not differ from that in MEN2A. Hypercalcemia is rare in MEN2B, and there are no well-documented examples of hyperparathyroidism.

The mucosal neuromas and marfanoid body habitus are the most distinctive features and are recognizable in childhood. Neuromas are present on the tip of the tongue, under the eyelids, and throughout the gastrointestinal tract and are true neuromas, distinct from neurofibromas. The most common presentation in children relates to gastrointestinal symptomatology including intermittent colic, pseudoobstruction, and diarrhea.

GENETIC CONSIDERATIONS Mutations of the *RET* proto-oncogene have been identified in most patients with MEN2 (**Fig. 345-3**). *RET* encodes a tyrosine kinase receptor, that in combination with a co-receptor, GFRα, is normally activated by glial cell–derived neurotrophic factor (GDNF) or other members of this transforming growth factor β–like family of peptides including artemin, persephin, and neurturin. In the C cell there is evidence that persephin normally activates the *RET*/GFRα-4 receptor complex and is partially responsible for migration of the C cells into the thyroid gland, whereas in the gastrointestinal tract, GDNF activates the *RET*/GFRα-1 complex. *RET* mutations induce constitutive activity of the receptor, explaining the autosomal dominant transmission of the disorder.

Naturally occurring mutations localize to two regions of the *RET* tyrosine kinase receptor. The first is a cysteine-rich extracellular domain; point mutations in the coding sequence for one of six cysteines (codons 609, 611, 618, 620, 630, or 634) cause amino acid substitutions that induce receptor dimerization and activation in the absence of its ligand. Codon 634 mutations occur in 80% of MEN2A kindreds and are most commonly associated with classic MEN2A features (Figs. 345-3 and 345-2); an arginine substitution at this codon accounts for half of all MEN2A mutations. All reported families with MEN2A and cutaneous lichen amyloidosis have a codon 634 mutation. Mutations of codons 609, 611, 618, or 620 occur in 10–15% of MEN2A kindreds and are more commonly associated with FMTC (Fig. 345-3). Mutations in codons 609, 618, and 620 have also been identified in a variant of MEN2A that includes Hirschsprung disease (Fig. 345-3). The second region of the *RET* tyrosine kinase that is mutated in MEN2 is in the substrate recognition pocket at codon 918 (Fig. 345-3). This activating mutation is present in ~95% of patients with MEN2B and accounts for 5% of all *RET* proto-oncogene mutations in MEN2. Mutations of codon 883 and 922 have also been identified in a few patients with MEN2B.

Uncommon mutations (<5% of the total) include those of codons 533 (exon 8), 666, 768, 777, 790, 791, 804, 891, and 912. Mutations associated with only FMTC include codons 533, 768, and 912. With greater experience, mutations that were once associated with FMTC only (666, 791, V804L, V804M, and 891) have since been found in MEN2A as there have been occasional descriptions of pheochromocytoma. At present it is reasonable to conclude that only kindreds with codon 533, 768, or 912 mutations are consistently associated with FMTC; in kindreds with all other *RET* mutations, pheochromocytoma is a possibility. The recognition that germline mutations occur in at least 6% of patients with apparently sporadic MTC has led to the firm recommendation that all patients with MTC should be screened for these mutations. The effort to screen patients with sporadic MTC when combined with the fact that new kindreds with classic MEN2A are being recognized less frequently has led to a shift in the mutation frequencies. These findings mirror results in other malignancies where germline mutations of cancer-causing genes contribute to a greater percentage of apparently sporadic cancer than previously considered. The recognition of new *RET* mutations suggests that more will be identified in the future.

Somatic mutations (found only in the tumor and not transmitted in the germline) of the *RET* proto-oncogene have been identified in sporadic MTC; 25–35% of sporadic tumors have codon 918 mutations, and somatic mutations in codons 630, 768, and 804 have also been identified (Fig. 345-3).

℞ MULTIPLE ENDOCRINE NEOPLASIA TYPE 2

SCREENING FOR MULTIPLE ENDOCRINE NEOPLASIA TYPE 2
Death from MTC can be prevented by early thyroidectomy. The identification of *RET* proto-oncogene mutations and the application of DNA-based molecular diagnostic techniques to identify these mutations has simplified the screening process. During the initial evaluation of a kindred, a *RET* proto-oncogene analysis should be performed on an individual with proven MEN2A. Establishment of the specific germline mutation facilitates the subsequent analysis of other family members. Each family member at risk should be tested twice for the presence of the specific mutation; the second analysis should be performed on a new DNA sample and, ideally, in a second laboratory to exclude sample mix-up or technical error (see www.genetests.org for an up-to-date list of laboratory testing sites). Both false-positive and false-negative analyses have been described; a false-negative test result is of the greatest concern because calcitonin testing is now rarely performed as a diagnostic backup study; if there is a genetic test error, a child may present in the second or third decade with metastatic MTC. Individuals in a kindred with a known mutation who have two normal analyses can be excluded from further screening.

There is general consensus that children with codon 883, 918, and 922 mutations, those associated with MEN2B, should have a total thyroidectomy and central lymph node dissection (level VI) performed during the first months of life or soon after identification of the syndrome. If local metastasis is discovered, a more extensive lymph node dissection (levels II to V) is generally indicated. In children with codon 611, 618, 620, 630, 634, and 891 mutations, thyroidectomy should be performed before the age of 6 years because of reports of local metastatic disease in children this age. Finally, there are kindreds with codon 609, 768, 790, 791, 804, and 912 mutations where the phenotype of MTC appears to be less aggressive. The clinician caring for children with one of these mutations faces a dilemma. In many kindreds there has never been a death from MTC caused by one of these mutations. However, in other kindreds there are examples of metastatic disease occurring early in life. For example, metastatic disease prior to the age of 6 years has been described with codon 609 and 804 mutations and before the age of 14 years in a patient with a codon 912 mutation. In kindreds with these mutations, two management approaches have been suggested: (1) perform a total thyroidectomy with or without central node dissection at some arbitrary age (perhaps 6–10 years of age), or (2) continue annual or biannual calcitonin provocative testing with performance of total thyroidectomy with or without central neck dissection when the test becomes abnormal. The pentagastrin test involves measurement of serum calcitonin basally and 2, 5, 10, and 15 min after a bolus injection of 5 μg pentagastrin per kilogram body weight. Patients should be

FIGURE 345-3 Schematic diagram of the *RET* proto-oncogene showing mutations found in MEN type 2 and sporadic medullary thyroid carcinoma (MTC). The *RET* proto-oncogene is located on the proximal arm of chromosome 10q (10q11.2). Activating mutations of two functional domains of RET tyrosine kinase receptor have been identified. The first affects a cysteine-rich (Cys-Rich) region in the extracellular portion of the receptor. Each germline mutation changes a cysteine at codons 609, 611, 618, 620, or 634 to another amino acid. The second region is the intracellular tyrosine kinase (TK) domain. Codon 634 mutations account for ~80% of all germline mutations. Mutations of codons 630, 768, 883, and 918 have been identified as somatic (nongermline) mutations that occur in a single parafollicular or C cell within the thyroid gland in sporadic MTC. A codon 918 mutation is the most common somatic mutation. Abbreviations: MEN2, multiple endocrine neoplasia type 2; CLA, cutaneous lichen amyloidosis; FMTC, familial medullary thyroid carcinoma; Signal, the signal peptide; Cadherin, a cadherin-like region in the extracellular domain; TM, transmembrane domain; TK, tyrosine kinase domain.

warned before pentagastrin injection of epigastric tightness, nausea, warmth, and tingling of extremities and reassured that the symptoms will last ~2 min. If pentagastrin is unavailable, an alternative is a short calcium infusion, performed by obtaining a baseline serum calcitonin and then infusing 150 mg calcium salt IV over 10 min with measurement of serum calcitonin at 5, 10, 15, 30 min after initiation of the infusion.

The *RET* proto-oncogene analysis should be performed in patients with suspected MEN2B to detect codon 883, 918, and 922 mutations, especially in newborn children where the diagnosis is suspected but the clinical phenotype is not fully developed. Other family members at risk for MEN2B should also be tested because the mucosal neuromas can be subtle. Most MEN2B mutations represent de novo mutations derived from the paternal allele. In the rare families with proven germline transmission of MTC but no identifiable *RET* proto-oncogene mutation (sequencing of the entire *RET* gene should be performed), annual pentagastrin or calcium testing should be performed on members at risk.

Annual screening for pheochromocytoma in patients with germline *RET* mutations should be performed by measuring basal plasma or 24-h urine catecholamines and metanephrines. The goal is to identify a pheochromocytoma before it causes significant symptoms or is likely to cause sudden death, an event most commonly associated with large tumors. Although there are kindreds with FMTC and specific *RET* mutations in which no pheochromocytomas have been identified (Fig. 345-3), clinical experience is insufficient to exclude pheochromocytoma screening in these individuals. Radiographic studies, such as MRI or CT scans, are generally reserved for individuals with abnormal screening tests or with symptoms suggestive of pheochromocytoma (Chap. 337). Women should be tested during pregnancy because undetected pheochromocytoma can cause maternal death during childbirth.

Measurement of serum calcium and parathyroid hormone levels every 2–3 years provides an adequate screen for hyperparathyroidism, except in those families in which hyperparathyroidism is a prominent component, where measurements should be made annually.

MEDULLARY THYROID CARCINOMA Hereditary MTC is a multicentric disorder. Total thyroidectomy with a central lymph node dissection should be performed in children who carry the mutant gene. Incomplete thyroidectomy leaves the possibility of later transformation of residual C cells. The goal of early therapy is cure, and a strategy that does not accomplish this goal is short-sighted. Long-term follow-up studies indicate an excellent outcome, with ~90% of children free of disease 15–20 years after surgery. In contrast, 15–25% of patients in whom the diagnosis is made on the basis of a palpable thyroid nodule die from the disease within 15–20 years.

In adults with MTC > 1 cm in size, metastases to regional lymph nodes are common (>75%). Total thyroidectomy with central lymph node dissection and selective dissection of other regional chains provide the best chance for cure. In patients with extensive local metastatic disease in the neck, external radiation may prevent local recurrence or reduce tumor mass but is not curative. Chemotherapy with combinations of adriamycin, vincristine, cyclophosphamide, and dacarbazine may provide palliation. Clinical trials with small compounds that interact with the ATP-binding pocket of the RET receptor and prevent phosphorylation of tyrosine (tyrosine kinase inhibitors) have shown promise for treatment of hereditary MTC. Some of these agents will be entering phase II and III trials and should be considered in patients with metastatic disease. Phase I and II studies of some of these agents have documented tumor regression and lowering of calcitonin and carcinoembryonic antigen in some patients.

PHEOCHROMOCYTOMA The long-term goal for management of pheochromocytoma is to prevent death and cardiovascular complications. Improvements in radiographic imaging of the adrenals make direct examination of the apparently normal contralateral gland during surgery less important, and the rapid evolution of laparoscopic abdominal or retroperitoneal surgery has simplified management of early pheochromocytoma. The major question is whether to remove both adrenal glands or to remove only the affected adrenal at the time of primary surgery. Issues to be considered in making this decision include the possibility of malignancy (<15 reported cases), the high probability of developing pheochromocytoma in the apparently unaffected gland over an 8- to 10-year period, and the risks of adrenal insufficiency caused by removal of both glands (at least two deaths related to adrenal insufficiency have occurred in MEN2 patients). Most clinicians recommend removing only the affected gland. If both adrenals are removed, glucocorticoid and min-

eralocorticoid replacement is mandatory. An alternative approach is to perform a cortical-sparing adrenalectomy, removing the pheochromocytoma and adrenal medulla, leaving the adrenal cortex behind. This approach is usually successful and eliminates the necessity for steroid hormone replacement in most patients, although the pheochromocytoma recurs in a small percentage.

HYPERPARATHYROIDISM Hyperparathyroidism has been managed by one of two approaches. Removal of 3.5 glands with maintenance of the remaining half gland in the neck is the usual procedure. In families in whom hyperparathyroidism is a prominent manifestation (almost always associated with a codon 634 *RET* mutation) and recurrence is common, total parathyroidectomy with transplantation of parathyroid tissue into the nondominant forearm is preferred. This approach is discussed above in the context of hyperparathyroidism associated with MEN 1.

OTHER GENETIC ENDOCRINE TUMOR SYNDROMES

A number of mixed syndromes exist in which the neoplastic associations differ from those in MEN 1 or 2 (Table 345-1).

The cause of VHL syndrome, the association of central nervous system tumors, renal cell carcinoma, pheochromocytoma, and islet cell neoplasms, is a mutation in the *VHL* tumor-suppressor gene. Germline-inactivating mutations of the *VHL* gene cause tumor formation when there is additional loss or somatic mutation of the normal *VHL* allele in brain, kidney, pancreatic islet, or adrenal medullary cells. Missense mutations been identified in >40% of VHL families with pheochromocytoma, suggesting that families with this type of mutation should be surveyed routinely for pheochromocytoma. A point that may be useful in differentiating VHL from MEN1 (overlapping features include islet cell tumor and rare pheochromocytoma) or MEN2 (overlapping feature is pheochromocytoma) is that hyperparathyroidism rarely occurs in VHL.

The molecular defect in type 1 neurofibromatosis inactivates neurofibromin, a cell membrane–associated protein that normally activates a GTPase. Inactivation of this protein impairs GTPase and causes continuous activation of p21 Ras and its downstream tyrosine kinase pathway. Endocrine tumors also form in less common neoplastic genetic syndromes. These include Cowden's disease, Carney complex, familial acromegaly, and familial carcinoid syndrome. Carney complex comprises myxomas of the heart, skin, and breast; peripheral nerve schwannomas; spotty skin pigmentation; and testicular, adrenal, and GH–secreting pituitary tumors. Linkage analysis has identified two loci: chromosome 2p in half of families and 17q in the others. The 17q gene has been identified as the regulatory subunit (type IA) of protein kinase A (*PRKA1A*).

IMMUNOLOGIC SYNDROMES AFFECTING MULTIPLE ENDOCRINE ORGANS

When immune dysfunction affects two or more endocrine glands and other nonendocrine immune disorders are present, the *polyglandular autoimmune* (PGA) *syndromes* should be considered. The PGA syndromes are classified as two main types: the type I syndrome starts in childhood and is characterized by mucocutaneous candidiasis, hypoparathyroidism, and adrenal insufficiency; the type II, or Schmidt, syndrome is more likely to present in adults and most commonly comprises adrenal insufficiency, thyroiditis, or type 1 diabetes mellitus. Some authors have attempted to subdivide PGA II on the basis of association with some autoimmune disorders but not others (i.e., type II and type III). The type III syndrome is heterogeneous and may consist of autoimmune thyroid disease along with a variety of other autoimmune endocrine disorders (Table 345-2). However, little information is gained by making this subdivision in terms of understanding pathogenesis or prevention of future endocrine complications in individual patients or in the affected families.

POLYGLANDULAR AUTOIMMUNE SYNDROME TYPE I

PGA type I is usually recognized in the first decade of life and requires two of three components for diagnosis: mucocutaneous candidiasis, hypoparathyroidism, and adrenal insufficiency. Mucocutaneous candidiasis and hypoparathyroidism present with similar high frequency (100% and 79–96%, respectively). Adrenal insufficiency is observed

TABLE 345-2 FEATURES OF POLYGLANDULAR AUTOIMMUNE (PGA) SYNDROMES

PGA I	PGA II
Epidemiology	
Autosomal recessive	Polygenic inheritance
Mutations in APECED gene	HLA-DR3 and HLA-DR4 associated
Childhood onset	Adult onset
Equal male:female ratio	Female predominance
Disease Associations	
Mucocutaneous candidiasis	Adrenal insufficiency
Hypoparathyroidism	Hypothyroidism
Adrenal insufficiency	Graves' disease
Hypogonadism	Type 1 diabetes
Alopecia	Hypogonadism
Hypothyroidism	Hypophysitis
Dental enamel hypoplasia	Myasthenia gravis
Malabsorption	Vitiligo
Chronic active hepatitis	Alopecia
Vitiligo	Pernicious anemia
Pernicious anemia	Celiac disease

Note: APECED, autoimmune polyendocrinopathy-candidiasis-ectodermal dystrophy.

in 60–72% of patients. Mineralocorticoids and glucocorticoids may be lost simultaneously or sequentially. PGA type 1 is also called *autoimmune polyendocrinopathy-candidiasis-ectodermal dystrophy* (APECED). Other endocrine defects can include gonadal failure (60% female, 14% male), hypothyroidism (5%), and destruction of the beta cells of the pancreatic islets and development of insulin-dependent (type 1) diabetes mellitus (14% lifetime risk). Additional features include hypoplasia of the dental enamel, nail dystrophy, tympanic membrane sclerosis, vitiligo, keratopathy, and gastric parietal cell dysfunction resulting in pernicious anemia (13%). Some patients develop autoimmune hepatitis (12%), malabsorption (variably attributed to intestinal lymphangiectasia, bacterial overgrowth, or hypoparathyroidism), asplenism, achalasia, and cholelithiasis (Table 345-2). At the outset, only one organ may be involved, but the number increases with time so that patients eventually manifest two to five components of the syndrome.

Most patients initially present with oral candidiasis in childhood; it is poorly responsive to treatment (Chap. 347) and relapses frequently. Chronic hypoparathyroidism usually occurs before adrenal insufficiency develops. More than 60% of postpubertal women develop premature hypogonadism. The endocrine components, including adrenal insufficiency and hypoparathyroidism, may not develop until the fourth decade, making continued surveillance necessary.

Type I PGA syndrome is not associated with a particular HLA type and is usually inherited as an autosomal recessive trait. It may occur sporadically. The responsible gene, designated as either *APECED* or *AIRE*, encodes a transcription factor that is expressed in thymus and lymph nodes; a variety of different mutations have been reported. The mechanism by which these mutations lead to the diverse manifestations of type I PGA is still unknown.

POLYGLANDULAR AUTOIMMUNE SYNDROME TYPE II

PGA type II is characterized by two or more of the endocrinopathies listed in Table 345-2. Most often these include primary adrenal insufficiency, Graves' disease or autoimmune hypothyroidism, type 1 diabetes mellitus, or primary hypogonadism. Because adrenal insufficiency is relatively rare, it is frequently used to define the presence of the syndrome. Among patients with adrenal insufficiency, type 1 diabetes mellitus coexists in 52% and autoimmune thyroid disease occurs in 69%. However, many patients with antimicrosomal and antithyroglobulin antibodies never develop abnormalities of thyroid function. Thus, increased antibody titers alone are poor predictors of future disease. Other associated conditions include hypophysitis, celiac disease (2–3%), atrophic gastritis, and pernicious anemia (13%). Vitiligo, caused by antibodies against the melanocyte, and alopecia are less common than in the type I syndrome. Mucocutaneous candidiasis does not occur. A few patients develop a late-onset, usually transient hypoparathyroidism caused by antibodies that compete with parathyroid hormone for binding to the parathyroid hormone receptor. Up to 25% of patients with myasthenia gravis, and an even higher percentage who have myasthenia and a thymoma, have PGA type II.

The type II syndrome is familial in nature, often transmitted as an autosomal dominant trait with incomplete penetrance. Like many of the individual autoimmune endocrinopathies, certain HL-DR3 and -DR4 alleles increase disease susceptibility; several different genes probably contribute to the expression of this syndrome.

A variety of autoantibodies are seen in PGA type II, including antibodies directed against: (1) thyroid antigens such as thyroid peroxidase, thyroglobulin, or the thyroid-stimulating hormone (TSH) receptor; (2) adrenal side chain cleavage enzyme, steroid 21-hydroxylase, or ACTH receptor; and (3) pancreatic islet glutamic acid decarboxylase or the insulin receptor, among others. The roles of cytokines such as interferon and cell-mediated immunity are unclear.

DIAGNOSIS

The clinical manifestations of adrenal insufficiency often develop slowly, may be difficult to detect, and can be fatal if not diagnosed and treated appropriately. Thus, prospective screening should be performed routinely in all patients and family members at risk for PGA types I and II. The most effective screening test for adrenal disease is a cosyntropin stimulation test (Chap. 336). A fasting blood glucose level can be obtained to screen for hyperglycemia. Additional screening tests should include measurements of TSH, luteinizing hormone, follicle-stimulating hormone, and, in men, testosterone levels. In families with suspected type I PGA syndrome, calcium and phosphorus levels should be measured. These screening studies should be performed every 1–2 years up to about age 50 in families with PGA type II syndrome and until about age 40 in patients with type I syndrome. Screening measurements of autoantibodies against potentially affected endocrine organs are of uncertain prognostic value. The differential diagnosis of PGA syndrome should include the DiGeorge syndrome (hypoparathyroidism due to glandular agenesis and mucocutaneous candidiasis), Kearns-Sayre syndrome (hypoparathyroidism, primary hypogonadism, type 1 diabetes mellitus, and panhypopituitarism), Wolfram's syndrome (congenital diabetes insipidus and diabetes mellitus), IPEX syndrome (*im*munodysregulation, *p*olyendocrinopathy, and *e*nteropathy, X-linked), and congenital rubella (type 1 diabetes mellitus and hypothyroidism).

℞ POLYGLANDULAR AUTOIMMUNE SYNDROME

With the exception of Graves' disease, the management of each of the endocrine components of the disease involves hormone replacement and is covered in detail in the chapters on adrenal, thyroid, gonadal, and parathyroid disease (Chaps. 335, 336, 340, 341, 347). Some aspects of therapy deserve special emphasis. Primary hypothyroidism can mask adrenal insufficiency by prolonging the half-life of cortisol; consequently, administration of thyroid hormone to a patient with unsuspected adrenal insufficiency can precipitate adrenal crisis. Thus, all patients with hypothyroidism in the context of PGA syndrome should be screened for adrenal disease and, if it is present, be treated with glucocorticoids prior to or concurrently with thyroid hormone therapy. Hypoglycemia or decreasing insulin requirements in a patient with diabetes mellitus type 1 may be the earliest symptom of adrenal insufficiency. Consequently, such patients should be screened for adrenal disease. Treatment of mucocutaneous candidiasis with ketoconazole may induce adrenal insufficiency. This drug may also elevate liver enzymes, making the diagnosis of autoimmune hepatitis more difficult. Hypocalcemia in PGA type II is more commonly due to malabsorption associated with celiac disease than to hypoparathyroidism.

OTHER AUTOIMMUNE ENDOCRINE SYNDROMES

Insulin Resistance Caused by Antibodies Rare insulin-resistance syndromes occur in patients who develop antibodies that block the interaction of insulin with its receptor. Conversely, other classes of anti-insulin receptor antibodies can activate the receptor and can cause hypoglycemia; this disorder should be considered in the differential diagnosis of fasting hypoglycemia (Chap. 339).

Patients with insulin receptor antibodies and acanthosis nigricans are often middle-aged women who acquire insulin resistance in association with other autoimmune disorders such as systemic lupus erythematosus or Sjögren's syndrome. Vitiligo, alopecia, Raynaud's phenomenon, and arthritis may also be seen. Other autoimmune endocrine disorders, including thyrotoxicosis, hypothyroidism, and hypogonadism, occur rarely. Acanthosis nigricans, a velvety, hyperpigmented, thickened skin lesion, is prominent on the dorsum of the neck and other skin fold areas in the axillae or groin and often heralds the diagnosis in these patients. However, acanthosis nigricans also occurs in patients with obesity or polycystic ovarian syndrome, in which insulin resistance appears to be due to a postreceptor defect; thus acanthosis nigricans itself is not diagnostic of the immunologic form of insulin resistance.

Some patients with acanthosis nigricans have mild glucose intolerance, with a compensatory increase in insulin secretion that is only detected when insulin levels are measured. Others have severe diabetes mellitus requiring massive doses of insulin (several thousand units per day) to lower the blood glucose levels. The nature of the antibodies determines the manifestations; though insulin resistance is more common, fasting hypoglycemia can result from insulinomimetic antibodies.

Insulin-resistant diabetes mellitus associated with anti-insulin antibodies occurs in patients with ataxia telangiectasia. This is an autosomal recessive disorder caused by mutations in *ATM*, a gene involved in cellular responses to ionizing radiation and oxidative damage. This disorder is characterized by ataxia, telangiectasia, immune abnormalities, and an increased incidence of malignancies.

Autoimmune Insulin Syndrome with Hypoglycemia   This disorder typically occurs in patients with other autoimmune disorders and is caused by polyclonal autoantibodies that bind to endogenously synthesized insulin. If the insulin dissociates from the antibodies several hours or more after a meal, hypoglycemia can result. Most cases of the syndrome have been described from Japan, and there may be a genetic component. In plasma cell dyscrasias such as multiple myeloma, the plasma cells may produce monoclonal antibodies against insulin and cause hypoglycemia by a similar mechanism.

Antithyroxine Antibodies and Hypothyroidism   Circulating autoantibodies against thyroid hormones in patients with both immune thyroid disease and plasma cell dyscrasias such as Waldenström's macroglobulinemia can bind thyroid hormones, decrease their biologic activity, and result in primary hypothyroidism. In other patients the antibodies simply interfere with thyroid hormone immunoassays and cause false elevations or decreases in measured hormone levels.

Crow-Fukase Syndrome   The features of this syndrome are highlighted by an acronym that emphasizes its important features: *p*olyneuropathy, *o*rganomegaly, *e*ndocrinopathy, *M*-proteins, and *s*kin changes (POEMS). The most important feature is a severe, progressive sensorimotor polyneuropathy associated with a plasma cell dyscrasia. Localized collections of plasma cells (plasmacytomas) can cause sclerotic bone lesions and produce monoclonal IgG or IgA proteins. Endocrine manifestations in men or women include hyperprolactinemia, diabetes mellitus type 2, primary hypothyroidism, and adrenal insufficiency. Additional findings include ovarian failure and amenorrhea in women and testicular failure, impotence, and gynecomastia in men. Skin changes include hyperpigmentation, thickening of the dermis, hirsutism, and hyperhidrosis. Hepatomegaly and lymphadenopathy occur in about two-thirds of patients, and splenomegaly is seen in about one-third. Other manifestations include increased cerebrospinal fluid pressure with papilledema, peripheral edema, ascites, pleural effusions, glomerulonephritis, and fever. Median survival may be >10 years, though shorter in patients with extravascular volume overload or clubbing.

The systemic nature of the disorder may cause confusion with other connective tissue diseases. The endocrine manifestations suggest an autoimmune basis of the disorder, but circulating antibodies against endocrine cells have not been demonstrated. Increased serum and tissue levels of interleukin 6, interleukin 1β, vascular endothelial growth factor, matrix metalloproteins, and tumor necrosis factor α are present, but the pathophysiologic basis for the POEMS syndrome is uncertain. Therapy directed against the plasma cell dyscrasia such as local radiation of bony lesions, chemotherapy, thalidomide, plasmapheresis, bone marrow or stem cell transplantation, and treatment with all-*trans* retinoic acid may improve the endocrine manifestations.

FURTHER READINGS

ASARI R et al: Estimated risk of pheochromocytoma recurrence after adrenal-sparing surgery in patients with multiple endocrine neoplasia type 2A. Arch Surg 141:1199, 2006

CLARKE JT: Narrative review: Fabry disease. Ann Intern Med 146:425, 2007

DEGROOT JW et al: RET as a diagnostic and therapeutic target in sporadic and hereditary endocrine tumors. Endocr Rev 27:535, 2006

DITTMAR M et al: Polyglandular autoimmune syndromes: Immunogenetics and long-term follow-up. J Clin Endocrinol Metab 88:2983, 2003

LINHART A, ELLIOTT PM: The heart in Anderson-Fabry disease and other lysosomal storage disorders. Heart 93:528, 2007

NAKAMURA E, KAELIN WG JR: Recent insights into the molecular pathogenesis of pheochromocytoma and paraganglioma. Endocr Pathol 17:97, 2006

OZAWA A et al: The parathyroid/pituitary variant of men1 usually has causes other than p27kip1 mutations. J Clin Endocrinol Metab 92(5):1948, 2007

PELLEGATA NS et al: Germ-line mutations in p27Kip1 cause a multiple endocrine neoplasia syndrome in rats and humans. Proc Natl Acad Sci USA 103:15558, 2006

PLAZA-MENACHO I et al: Current concepts in RET-related genetics, signaling and therapeutics. Trends Genet 22:627, 2006

SEVIN M et al: The adult form of Niemann-Pick disease type C. Brain 130:120, 2007

SECTION 2   DISORDERS OF BONE AND MINERAL METABOLISM

346   Bone and Mineral Metabolism in Health and Disease

F. Richard Bringhurst, Marie B. Demay, Stephen M. Krane, Henry M. Kronenberg

BONE STRUCTURE AND METABOLISM

Bone is a dynamic tissue that is remodeled constantly throughout life. The arrangement of compact and cancellous bone provides a strength and density suitable for both mobility and protection. In addition, bone provides a reservoir for calcium, magnesium, phosphorus, sodium, and other ions necessary for homeostatic functions. The skeleton is highly vascular and receives about 10% of the cardiac output. Remodeling of bone is accomplished by two distinct cell types: osteoblasts produce bone matrix and osteoclasts resorb the matrix.

The extracellular components of bone consist of a solid mineral phase in close association with an organic matrix, of which 90–95% is type I collagen (Chap. 357). The noncollagenous portion of the organic matrix is heterogeneous and contains serum proteins, such as albumin, as well as many locally produced proteins, whose functions are incompletely understood. These proteins include cell attachment/sig-

A

B

FIGURE 346-1 Pathways regulating development of (A) osteoblasts and (B) osteoclasts. Hormones, cytokines, and growth factors that control cell proliferation and differentiation are shown above the arrows. Transcription factors and other markers specific for various stages of development are depicted below the arrows. BMPs, bone morphogenic proteins; wnts, wingless-type, mouse mammary tumor virus integration site; PTH, parathyroid hormone; Vit D, vitamin D; IGFs,

insulin-like growth factors; Runx2, Runt-related transcription factor 2; M-CSF, macrophage colony-stimulating factor; PU-1, a monocyte- and B lymphocyte–specific ets family transcription factor; NFκB, nuclear factor κB; TRAF, tumor necrosis factor receptor–associated factors; RANK ligand, receptor activator of NFκB ligand; IL-1, interleukin-1; IL-6, interleukin-6. *(Modified from T Suda et al: Endocr Rev 20:345, 1999, with permission.)*

naling proteins, such as thrombospondin, osteopontin, and fibronectin; calcium-binding proteins such as matrix gla protein and osteocalcin; and proteoglycans such as biglycan and decorin. Some of these proteins organize collagen fibrils; others influence mineralization and binding of the mineral phase to the matrix.

The mineral phase is made up of calcium and phosphate and is best characterized as a poorly crystalline hydroxyapatite. The mineral phase of bone is deposited initially in intimate relation to the collagen fibrils and is found in specific locations in the "holes" between the collagen fibrils. This architectural arrangement of mineral and matrix results in a two-phase material well suited to withstand mechanical stresses. The organization of collagen influences the amount and type of mineral phase formed in bone. Although the primary structures of type I collagen in skin and bone tissues are similar, there are differences in posttranslational modifications and distribution of intermolecular cross-links. The holes in the packing structure of the collagen are larger in mineralized collagen of bone and dentin than in unmineralized collagens such as tendon. Single amino-acid substitutions in the helical portion of either the α1 (*COL1A1*) or α2 (*COL1A2*) chains of type I collagen disrupt the organization of bone in osteogenesis imperfecta. The severe skeletal fragility associated with these disorders highlights the importance of the fibrillar matrix in the structure of bone (Chap. 357).

Osteoblasts synthesize and secrete the organic matrix. They are derived from cells of mesenchymal origin (Fig. 346-1A). Active osteoblasts are found on the surface of newly forming bone. As an osteoblast secretes matrix, which is then mineralized, the cell becomes an *osteocyte*, still connected with its blood supply through a series of canaliculi. Osteocytes comprise the vast majority of the cells in bone. They are thought to be the mechanosensors in bone that communicate signals to surface osteoblasts and their progenitors through the canalic-

ular network. Mineralization of the matrix, both in trabecular bone and in osteones of compact cortical bone (*haversian systems*), begins soon after the matrix is secreted (primary mineralization) but is not completed for several weeks or even longer (secondary mineralization). While this mineralization takes advantage of the high concentrations of calcium and phosphate already near saturation in serum, mineralization is a carefully regulated process dependent on the activity of osteoblast-derived alkaline phosphatase, which probably works by hydrolyzing inhibitors of mineralization.

Genetic studies in humans and mice have identified several key genes that control osteoblast development. Core-binding factor A1 (*CBFA1*, also called *Runx2*), is a transcription factor expressed specifically in chondrocyte (cartilage cells) and osteoblast progenitors, as well as in hypertrophic chondrocytes and mature osteoblasts. *Runx2* regulates the expression of several important osteoblast proteins including osterix (another transcription factor needed for osteoblast maturation), osteopontin, bone sialoprotein, type I collagen, osteocalcin, and receptor-activator of NFκB (RANK) ligand. *Runx2* expression is regulated, in part, by bone morphogenic proteins (BMPs). *Runx2*-deficient mice are devoid of osteoblasts, whereas mice with a deletion of only one allele (*Runx2 +/−*) exhibit a delay in formation of the clavicles and some cranial bones. The latter abnormalities are similar to those in the human disorder *cleidocranial dysplasia*, which is also caused by heterozygous inactivating mutations in *Runx2*.

The paracrine signaling molecule, Indian hedgehog (Ihh), also plays a critical role in osteoblast development, as evidenced by Ihh-deficient mice that lack osteoblasts in bone formed on a cartilage mold (endochondral ossification). Signals originating from members of the wnt (wingless-type mouse mammary tumor virus integration site) family of paracrine factors are also important. Humans and mice missing a wnt-family co-receptor, LRP5 (lipoprotein receptor–related

FIGURE 346-2 Schematic representation of bone remodeling. The cycle of bone remodeling is carried out by the basic multicellular unit (BMU), comprising a group of osteoclasts and osteoblasts. In cortical bone, the BMUs tunnel through the tissue, whereas in cancellous bone, they move across the trabecular surface. The process of bone remodeling is initiated by contraction of the lining cells and the recruitment of osteoclast precursors. These precursors fuse to form multinucleated, active osteoclasts that mediate bone resorption. Osteoclasts adhere to bone and subsequently remove it by acidification and proteolytic digestion. As the BMU advances, osteoclasts leave the resorption site and osteoblasts move in to cover the excavated area and begin the process of new bone formation by secreting osteoid, which is eventually mineralized into new bone. After osteoid mineralization, osteoblasts flatten and form a layer of lining cells over new bone.

protein 5), have osteoporosis. Remarkably, humans with an overactive form of LPR5 have increased bone mass. Numerous other growth-regulatory factors affect osteoblast function, including the three closely related transforming growth factor βs, fibroblast growth factors (FGFs) 2 and 18, platelet-derived growth factor, and insulin-like growth factors (IGFs) I and II. Hormones such as parathyroid hormone (PTH) and 1,25-dihydroxyvitamin D [1,25(OH)₂D] activate receptors expressed by osteoblasts to assure mineral homeostasis and to influence a variety of bone cell functions.

Resorption of bone is carried out mainly by *osteoclasts*, multinucleated cells that are formed by fusion of cells derived from the common precursor of macrophages and osteoclasts. Multiple factors regulating osteoclast development have been identified (Fig. 346-1*B*). Factors produced by osteoblasts or marrow stromal cells allow osteoblasts to control osteoclast development and activity. Macrophage colony-stimulating factor (M-CSF) plays a critical role during several steps in the pathway and ultimately leads to fusion of osteoclast progenitor cells to form multinucleated, active osteoclasts. RANK ligand, a member of the tumor necrosis factor (TNF) family, is expressed on the surface of osteoblast progenitors and stromal fibroblasts. In a process involving cell-cell interactions, RANK ligand binds to the RANK receptor on osteoclast progenitors, stimulating osteoclast differentiation and activation. Alternatively, a soluble decoy receptor, referred to as osteoprotegerin, can bind RANK ligand and inhibit osteoclast differentiation. Several growth factors and cytokines (including interleukins 1, 6, and 11; TNF; and interferon γ) modulate osteoclast differentiation and function. Most hormones that influence osteoclast function do not directly target this cell but instead influence M-CSF and RANK ligand signaling by osteoblasts. Both PTH and 1,25(OH)₂D increase osteoclast number and activity, whereas estrogen decreases osteoclast number and activity by this indirect mechanism. Calcitonin, in contrast, binds to its receptor on the basal surface of osteoclasts and directly inhibits osteoclast function.

Osteoclast-mediated resorption of bone takes place in scalloped spaces (*Howship's lacunae*) where the osteoclasts are attached through a specific α$_v$β$_3$ integrin to components of the bone matrix such as osteopontin. The osteoclast forms a tight seal to the underlying matrix and secretes protons, chloride, and proteinases into a confined space likened to an extracellular lysosome. The active osteoclast surface forms a ruffled border that contains a specialized proton-pump ATPase, which secretes acid and solubilizes the mineral phase. Carbonic anhydrase (type II isoenzyme) within the osteoclast generates the needed protons. The bone matrix is resorbed in the acid environment adjacent to the ruffled border by proteases that act at low pH, such as cathepsin K.

In the embryo and in the growing child, bone develops by remodeling and replacing previously calcified cartilage (endochondral bone formation) or is formed without a cartilage matrix (intramembranous bone formation). Chondrocytes proliferate, secrete and mineralize a matrix, enlarge (hypertrophy), and then die, thereby enlarging bone and providing the matrix and factors that stimulate endochondral bone formation. This program is regulated by both local factors, such as IGF-I and -II, parathyroid hormone–related peptide (PTHrP), and FGFs, and by systemic hormones such as growth hormone, glucocorticoids, and estrogen.

New bone, whether formed in infants or in adults during repair, has a relatively high ratio of cells to matrix and is characterized by coarse fiber bundles of collagen that are interlaced and randomly dispersed (woven bone). In adults, the more mature bone is organized with fiber bundles regularly arranged in parallel or concentric sheets (lamellar bone). In long bones, deposition of lamellar bone in a concentric arrangement around blood vessels forms the haversian systems. Growth in length of bones is dependent on proliferation of cartilage cells and on the endochondral sequence at the growth plate. Growth in width and thickness is accomplished by formation of bone at the periosteal surface and by resorption at the endosteal surface, with the rate of formation exceeding that of resorption. In adults, after the growth plates close, growth in length and endochondral bone formation cease, except for some activity in the cartilage cells beneath the articular surface. Even in adults, however, remodeling of bone (within haversian systems as well as trabecular bone) continues throughout life. In adults, ~4% of the surface of trabecular bone (such as iliac crest) is involved in active resorption, whereas 10–15% of trabecular surfaces is covered with osteoid. Radioisotope studies indicate that as much as 18% of the total skeletal calcium is deposited and removed each year. Thus, bone is an active metabolizing tissue that requires an intact blood supply. The cycle of bone resorption and formation is a highly orchestrated process carried out by the basic multicellular unit, composed of a group of osteoclasts and osteoblasts (Fig. 346-2).

The response of bone to fractures, infection, and interruption of blood supply and to expanding lesions is relatively limited. Dead bone must be resorbed, and new bone must be formed, a process carried out in association with growth of new blood vessels into the involved area. In injuries that disrupt the organization of the tissue, such as a fracture in which apposition of fragments is poor or when motion exists at the fracture site, the progenitor stromal cells differentiate into cells with functional capacities different from those of osteoblasts, and varying amounts of fibrous tissue and cartilage are formed. When there is good apposition with fixation and little motion at the fracture site, repair occurs predominantly by formation of new bone without other scar tissue.

Remodeling of bone occurs along lines of force generated by mechanical stress. The signals from these mechanical stresses are sensed by osteocytes, which transmit signals to osteoclasts or osteoblasts, or their precursors. A bowing deformity increases new bone formation at the concave surface and resorption at the convex surface, seemingly designed to produce the strongest mechanical structure. Expanding lesions in bone, such as tumors, induce resorption at the surface in contact with the tumor, by producing ligands, such as PTHrP, that stimulate osteoclast differentiation and function. Even in a disorder as architecturally disruptive as Paget's disease, remodeling is dictated by mechanical forces. Thus, bone plasticity reflects the interaction of cells with each other and with the environment.

Measurement of the products of osteoblast and osteoclast activity can assist in the diagnosis and management of bone diseases. Osteoblast activity can be assessed by measuring serum bone-specific alkaline phosphatase. Similarly, osteocalcin, a protein secreted from osteoblasts, is made virtually only by osteoblasts. Osteoclast activity can be assessed by measurement of products of collagen degradation. Collagen molecules are covalently linked to each other in the extracellular matrix through the formation of hydroxypyridinium crosslinks (Chap. 357). These cross-linked peptides can be measured both in urine and in blood.

CALCIUM METABOLISM

Over 99% of the 1–2 kg of calcium present normally in the adult human body resides in the skeleton, where it provides mechanical stability and serves as a reservoir sometimes needed to maintain extracellular fluid (ECF) calcium concentration (Fig. 346-3). Skeletal calcium accretion first becomes significant during the third trimester of fetal life, accelerates throughout childhood and adolescence, reaches a peak in early adulthood, and gradually declines thereafter at rates that rarely exceed 1–2% per year. These slow changes in total skeletal calcium content contrast with relatively high daily rates of closely matched fluxes of calcium into and out of bone (~250–500 mg each), a process mediated by coupled osteoblastic and osteoclastic activity. Another 0.5–1% of skeletal calcium is freely exchangeable (e.g., in chemical equilibrium) with that in the ECF.

The concentration of ionized calcium in the ECF must be maintained within a narrow range because of the critical role it plays in a wide array of cellular functions, especially those involved in neuromuscular activity, secretion, and signal transduction. Intracellular cytosolic free calcium levels are ~100 nmol/L and are 10,000-fold lower than ionized calcium concentration in the blood and ECF (1.1–1.3 mmol/L). This steep chemical gradient promotes rapid calcium influx through various membrane calcium channels that can be activated by hormones, metabolites, or neurotransmitters, swiftly changing cellular function. In blood, total calcium concentration is normally 2.2–2.6 mM (8.5–10.5 mg/dL), of which ~50% is ionized. The remainder is bound ionically to negatively charged proteins (predominantly albumin and immunoglobulins) or loosely complexed with phosphate, citrate, sulfate, or other anions. Alterations in serum protein concentrations directly affect the total blood calcium concentration, even if the ionized calcium concentration remains normal. An algorithm to correct for protein changes adjusts the total serum calcium (in mg/dL) upward by 0.8 times the deficit in serum albumin (g/dL) or by 0.5 times the deficit in serum immunoglobulin (in g/dL). Such corrections provide only rough approximations of actual free calcium concentrations, however, and may be misleading, particularly during acute illness. Acidosis also alters ionized calcium by reducing its association with proteins. The best practice is to measure blood ionized calcium directly by a method that employs calcium-selective electrodes in acute settings during which calcium abnormalities might occur.

Control of the ionized calcium concentration in the ECF ordinarily is accomplished by adjusting the rates of calcium movement across intestinal and renal epithelia. These adjustments are mediated mainly via changes in blood levels of the hormones PTH and 1,25(OH)$_2$D. Blood ionized calcium directly suppresses PTH secretion by activating parathyroid calcium-sensing receptors (CaSRs). Also, ionized calcium indirectly affects PTH secretion via effects on 1,25(OH)$_2$D production. This active vitamin D metabolite inhibits PTH production by an incompletely understood mechanism of negative feedback (Chap. 347).

Normal dietary calcium intake in the United States varies widely, ranging from 10–37 mmol/d (400–1500 mg/d). Many individuals, in an effort to prevent osteoporosis, routinely supplement this further with oral calcium salts to a total intake of 37–50 mmol/d (1500–2000 mg/d). Intestinal absorption of ingested calcium involves both active (transcellular) and passive (paracellular) mechanisms. Passive calcium absorption is nonsaturable and approximates 5% of daily calcium intake, whereas the active mechanism, controlled principally by 1,25(OH)$_2$D, normally ranges from 20–70%. Active calcium transport occurs mainly in the proximal small bowel (duodenum and proximal jejunum), although some active calcium absorption occurs in most segments of the small intestine. Optimal rates of calcium absorption require gastric acid. This is especially true for weakly dissociable calcium supplements such as calcium carbonate. In fact, large boluses of calcium carbonate are poorly absorbed because of their neutralizing effect upon gastric acid. In achlorhydric subjects or for those taking drugs that inhibit gastric acid secretion, supplements should be taken with meals to optimize their absorption. Use of calcium citrate may be preferable in these circumstances. Calcium absorption may also be blunted in disease states such as pancreatic or biliary insufficiency, in which ingested calcium remains bound to unabsorbed fatty acids or other food constituents. At high levels of calcium intake, synthesis of 1,25(OH)$_2$D is reduced, which decreases the rate of active intestinal calcium absorption. The opposite occurs with dietary calcium restriction. Some calcium, ~2.5–5.0 mmol/d (100–200 mg/d), is excreted as an obligate component of intestinal secretions and is not regulated by calciotropic hormones.

The feedback-controlled hormonal regulation of intestinal absorptive efficiency results in a relatively constant daily net calcium absorption of ~5–7.5 mmol/d (200–400 mg/d), despite large changes in daily dietary calcium intake. This daily load of absorbed calcium is excreted by the kidneys in a manner that is also tightly regulated by the concentration of ionized calcium in the blood. Approximately 8–10 g/d of calcium are filtered by the glomeruli, of which only 2–3% appears in the urine. Most filtered calcium (65%) is reabsorbed in the proximal tubules via a passive, paracellular route that is coupled to concomitant NaCl reabsorption and not specifically regulated. The cortical thick ascending limb of Henle's loop (cTAL) reabsorbs roughly another 20% of filtered calcium, also via a paracellular mechanism. Calcium reabsorption in the cTAL requires a tight-junctional protein called paracellin-1 and is inhibited by increased blood concentrations of calcium or magnesium, acting via the CaSR, which is highly expressed on basolateral membranes in this nephron segment. Operation of the renal CaSR provides a mechanism, independent of those engaged directly by PTH or 1,25(OH)$_2$D, whereby serum ionized calcium can control renal calcium reabsorption. Finally, ~10% of filtered calcium is reabsorbed in the distal convoluted tubules (DCT) by a transcellular mechanism. Calcium enters the luminal surface of the cell through specific apical calcium channels, whose number is regulated. It then moves across the cell in association with a specific calcium-binding protein (calbindin-D28k) that buffers cytosolic calcium concentrations

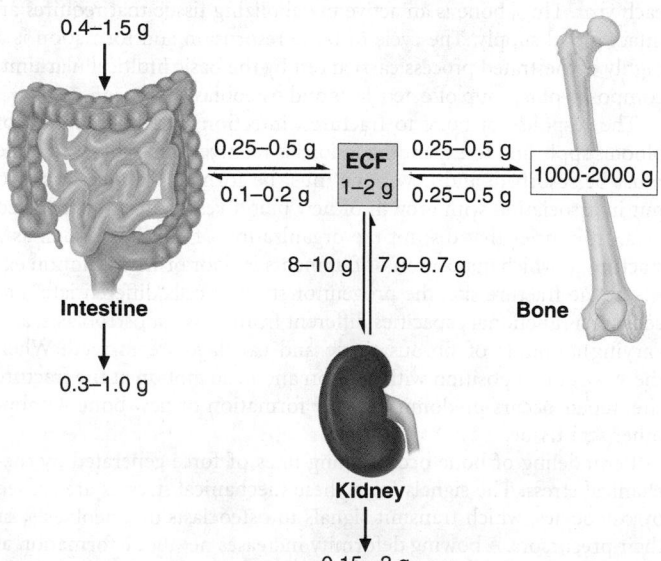

FIGURE 346-3 Calcium homeostasis. Schematic illustration of calcium content of extracellular fluid (ECF) and bone as well as of diet and feces; magnitude of calcium flux per day as calculated by various methods is shown at sites of transport in intestine, kidney, and bone. Ranges of values shown are approximate and chosen to illustrate certain points discussed in text. In conditions of calcium balance, rates of calcium release from and uptake into bone are equal.

from the large mass of transported calcium. Ca^{2+}-ATPases and Na^+/Ca^{2+} exchangers actively extrude calcium across the basolateral surface and thereby maintain the transcellular calcium gradient. All of these processes are stimulated, directly or indirectly, by PTH. The DCT is also the site of action of thiazide diuretics, which lower urinary calcium excretion. Conversely, dietary sodium loads, or increased distal sodium delivery caused by loop diuretics or saline infusion, reduce DCT calcium reabsorption.

The homeostatic mechanisms that normally maintain a constant serum ionized calcium concentration may fail at extremes of calcium intake or when the hormonal systems or organs involved are compromised. Thus, even with maximal activity of the vitamin D–dependent intestinal active transport system, sustained calcium intakes <5 mmol/d (<200 mg/d) cannot provide enough net calcium absorption to replace obligate losses via the intestine, kidney, sweat, or other secretions. In this case, increased blood levels of PTH and $1,25(OH)_2D$ activate osteoclastic bone resorption to obtain needed calcium from bone, which leads to progressive bone loss and negative calcium balance. Increased PTH and $1,25(OH)_2D$ also enhance renal calcium reabsorption, and $1,25(OH)_2D$ enhances calcium absorption in the gut. At very high calcium intakes [>100 mmol/d; >4 g/d], passive intestinal absorption continues to deliver calcium into the ECF, despite maximally downregulated intestinal active transport and renal tubular calcium reabsorption. This can cause severe hypercalciuria, nephrocalcinosis, progressive renal failure, and hypercalcemia (e.g., "milk alkali syndrome"). Deficiency or excess of PTH or vitamin D, intestinal disease, and renal failure represent other commonly encountered challenges to normal calcium homeostasis (Chap. 347).

PHOSPHORUS METABOLISM

Although 85% of the ~600 g of body phosphorus is present in bone mineral, phosphorus is also a major intracellular constituent, both as the free anion(s) and as a component of numerous organophosphate compounds including structural proteins, enzymes, transcription factors, carbohydrate and lipid intermediates, high-energy stores (ATP, creatine phosphate), and nucleic acids. Unlike calcium, phosphorus exists intracellularly at concentrations close to those present in ECF (e.g., 1–2 mmol/L). In cells and in the ECF, phosphorus exists in several forms, predominantly as $H_2PO_4^-$ or $NaHPO_4^-$, with perhaps 10% as HPO_4^{2-}. This mixture of anions will be referred to here as "phosphate." In serum, about 12% of phosphorus is bound to proteins. Concentrations of phosphates in blood and ECF are generally expressed in terms of elemental phosphorus, the normal range in adults being 0.75–1.45 mmol/L (2.5–4.5 mg/dL). Because the volume of the intracellular fluid compartment is twice that of the ECF, measurements of ECF phosphate may not accurately reflect phosphate availability within cells that follows even modest shifts of phosphate from one compartment to the other.

Phosphate is widely available in foods and is efficiently absorbed (65%) by the small intestine, even in the absence of vitamin D. On the other hand, phosphate absorptive efficiency may be further enhanced (to 85–90%) via active transport mechanisms that are stimulated by $1,25(OH)_2D$. These involve activation of Na^+/PO_4^{2-} co-transporters that move phosphate into intestinal cells against an unfavorable electrochemical gradient. Daily net intestinal phosphate absorption varies widely according to the composition of the diet but is generally in the range of 500–1000 mg/d. Phosphate absorption can be inhibited by large doses of calcium salts or by sevelamer hydrochloride (Renagel), strategies commonly used to control levels of serum phosphate in renal failure. Aluminum hydroxide antacids also reduce phosphate absorption but are less commonly used because of the potential for aluminum toxicity. Low serum phosphate directly stimulates renal proximal tubular synthesis of $1,25(OH)_2D$.

Serum phosphate levels vary by as much as 50% on a normal day. This reflects the effect of food intake but also an underlying circadian rhythm that produces a nadir between 7 and 10 A.M. Carbohydrate administration, especially as IV dextrose solutions in fasting subjects, can decrease serum phosphate by >0.7 mmol/L (2 mg/dL) due to rapid uptake into, and utilization by, cells. A similar response is observed in the treatment of diabetic ketoacidosis and during metabolic or respiratory alkalosis. Because of this wide variation in serum phosphate, it is best to perform measurements in the basal, fasting state.

Control of serum phosphate is determined mainly by the rate of renal tubular reabsorption of the filtered load, which is ~4–6 g/d. Because intestinal phosphate absorption is highly efficient, urinary excretion is not constant but varies directly with dietary intake. The fractional excretion of phosphate (ratio of phosphate to creatinine clearance) is generally in the range of 10–15%. The proximal tubule is the principal site at which renal phosphate reabsorption is regulated. This is accomplished by changes in the apical expression and activity of a specific Na^+/PO_4^{2-} co-transporter (NaPi-2) in the proximal tubule. Apical expression of NaPi-2 is rapidly reduced by PTH, the major known hormonal regulator of renal phosphate excretion. FGF23 can dramatically impair phosphate reabsorption (see below). Activating *FGF23* mutations cause the rare disorder autosomal dominant hypophosphatemic rickets. In contrast to PTH, this molecule also leads to reduced synthesis of $1,25(OH)_2D$, which may worsen the resulting hypophosphatemia by lowering intestinal phosphate absorption. Renal reabsorption of phosphate is responsive to changes in dietary intake, such that experimental dietary phosphate restriction leads to a dramatic lowering of urinary phosphate within hours, preceding any decline in serum phosphate (e.g., filtered load). This physiologic renal adaptation to changes in dietary phosphate availability occurs independently of PTH. Findings in *FGF23*-knockout mice suggest that FGF23 normally acts to lower blood phosphate and $1,25(OH)_2D$ levels. In turn, elevations of blood phosphate increases blood levels of FGF23.

Renal phosphate reabsorption is impaired by hypocalcemia, hypomagnesemia, and severe hypophosphatemia. Phosphate clearance is enhanced by ECF volume expansion and impaired by dehydration. Phosphate retention is an important pathophysiologic feature of renal insufficiency (Chap. 274).

HYPOPHOSPHATEMIA

Causes Hypophosphatemia can occur by one or more of three primary mechanisms: (1) inadequate intestinal phosphate absorption, (2) excessive renal phosphate excretion, or (3) rapid redistribution of phosphate from the ECF into bone or soft tissue (Table 346-1). Because phosphate is so abundant in foods, inadequate intestinal absorption is almost never observed now that aluminum hydroxide antacids, which bind phosphate in the gut, are no longer commonly used. Fasting or starvation, however, may result in depletion of body phosphate and predispose to subsequent hypophosphatemia during refeeding, especially if this is accomplished with IV glucose alone.

Chronic hypophosphatemia usually signifies a persistent renal tubular phosphate-wasting disorder. Excessive activation of PTH/PTHrP receptors in the proximal tubule, because of primary or secondary hyperparathyroidism or because of the PTHrP-mediated hypercalcemia syndrome in malignancy (Chap. 347), is among the more common causes of renal hypophosphatemia, especially because of the high prevalence of vitamin D deficiency in older Americans. Familial hypocalciuric hypercalcemia and Jansen's chondrodystrophy are rare examples of genetic disorders in this category (Chap. 347).

Several genetic and acquired diseases cause PTH/PTHrP-independent tubular phosphate wasting, with associated rickets and osteomalacia. All of these diseases manifest severe hypophosphatemia; renal phosphate wasting, sometimes accompanied by aminoaciduria; low blood levels of $1,25(OH)_2D$; low-normal serum levels of calcium; and evidence of impaired cartilage or bone mineralization. Analysis of these diseases has led to the discovery of a "new" hormone, FGF23, that is an important physiologic regulator of phosphate metabolism. FGF23 decreases phosphate reabsorption in the proximal tubule and also suppresses the 1-hydroxylase responsible for synthesis of $1,25(OH)_2D$. FGF23 is synthesized by cells of the osteoblast lineage. High-phosphate diets increase FGF23 levels, and low-phosphate diets decrease them. Autosomal dominant hypophosphatemic rickets (ADHR) was the first disease linked to abnormalities in FGF23. ADHR results from activating mutations in the gene encoding FGF23. The most common inherited cause of hypophosphatemia is X-linked hypophosphatemic rickets (XL-HR), which results from inactivating mutations in an endopeptidase

TABLE 346-1 **CAUSES OF HYPOPHOSPHATEMIA**

I. Reduced renal tubular phosphate reabsorption
  A. PTH/PTHrP-dependent
    1. Primary hyperparathyroidism
    2. Secondary hyperparathyroidism
      a. Vitamin D deficiency/resistance
      b. Calcium starvation/malabsorption
      c. Bartter syndrome
      d. Autosomal recessive renal hypercalciuria with hypomagnesemia
    3. PTHrP-dependent hypercalcemia of malignancy
    4. Familial hypocalciuric hypercalcemia
  B. PTH/PTHrP-independent
    1. Genetic hypophosphatemia
      a. X-linked hypophosphatemic rickets
      b. Dent disease
      c. Autosomal dominant hypophosphatemic rickets
      d. Fanconi syndrome(s)
      e. Cystinosis
      f. Wilson disease
      g. McCune-Albright syndrome (fibrous dysplasia)
      h. Idiopathic hypercalciuria (absorptive subtype)
      i. Hereditary hypophosphatemia with hypercalciuria (Bedouins)
    2. Tumor-induced osteomalacia
    3. Other systemic disorders
      a. Poorly controlled diabetes mellitus
      b. Alcoholism
      c. Hyperaldosteronism
      d. Hypomagnesemia
      e. Amyloidosis
      f. Hemolytic uremic syndrome
      g. Renal transplantation or partial liver resection
      h. Rewarming or induced hyperthermia
    4. Drugs or toxins
      a. Ethanol
      b. Acetazolamide, other diuretics
      c. High-dose estrogens or glucocorticoids
      d. Heavy metals (lead, cadmium)
      e. Toluene, N-methyl formamide
      f. Cisplatin, ifosfamide, foscarnet, rapamycin
      g. Calcitonin, pamidronate
II. Impaired intestinal phosphate absorption
  A. Aluminum-containing antacids
  B. Sevalamer
III. Shifts of extracellular phosphate into cells
  A. Intravenous glucose
  B. Insulin therapy of prolonged hyperglycemia or diabetic ketoacidosis
  C. Catecholamines (epinephrine, dopamine, albuterol)
  D. Acute respiratory alkalosis
  E. Gram-negative sepsis, toxic shock syndrome
  F. Recovery from starvation or acidosis
  G. Rapid cellular proliferation
    1. Leukemic blast crisis
    2. Intensive erythropoetin, other CSF therapy
IV. Accelerated net bone formation
  A. Following parathyroidectomy
  B. Treatment of vitamin D deficiency, Paget disease
  C. Osteoblastic metastases

Note: CSF, cerebrospinal fluid.

termed *PHEX* (*p*hosphate-regulating gene with *h*omologies to *e*ndopeptidases on the *X* chromosome) that is most abundantly expressed on the surface of mature osteoblasts. Patients with XLH usually have high FGF23 levels, and ablation of the FGF23 gene reverses the hypophosphatemia found in the mouse version of XLH. How inactivation of PHEX leads to increased levels of FGF23 has not yet been determined. A third hypophosphatemic disorder, tumor-induced osteomalacia (TIO), is an acquired disorder in which tumors, usually of mesenchymal origin and generally histologically benign, secrete molecules that induce renal phosphate wasting. The hypophosphatemic syndrome resolves completely within hours to days following successful resection of the responsible tumor. Such tumors express large amounts of FGF23 mRNA, and patients with TIO usually exhibit elevations of FGF23 in their blood.

Dent's disease is an X-linked recessive disorder caused by inactivating mutations in CLCN5, a chloride transporter expressed in endosomes of the proximal tubule; features include hypercalciuria, hypophosphatemia, and recurrent kidney stones. Renal phosphate wasting is common among poorly controlled diabetics and alcoholics, who therefore are at risk for iatrogenic hypophosphatemia when treated with insulin or IV glucose, respectively. Diuretics and certain other drugs and toxins can cause defective renal tubular phosphate reabsorption (Table 346-1).

In hospitalized patients, hypophosphatemia is often attributable to massive redistribution of phosphate from the ECF into cells. Insulin therapy of diabetic ketoacidosis is a paradigm for this phenomenon, in which the severity of the hypophosphatemia is related to the extent of antecedent depletion of phosphate and other electrolytes (Chap. 338). The hypophosphatemia is usually greatest at a point many hours after initiation of insulin therapy and is difficult to predict from baseline measurements of serum phosphate at the time of presentation, when prerenal azotemia can obscure significant phosphate depletion. Other factors that may contribute to such acute redistributive hypophosphatemia include antecedent starvation or malnutrition, administration of IV glucose without other nutrients, elevated blood catecholamines (endogenous or exogenous), respiratory alkalosis, and recovery from metabolic acidosis.

Hypophosphatemia can also occur transiently (over weeks to months) during the phase of accelerated net bone formation following parathyroidectomy for severe primary hyperparathyroidism or during treatment of vitamin D deficiency or lytic Paget's disease. This is usually most prominent in patients who preoperatively have evidence of high bone turnover (e.g., high serum levels of alkaline phosphatase). Osteoblastic metastases can also lead to this syndrome.

Clinical and Laboratory Findings The clinical manifestations of severe hypophosphatemia reflect a generalized defect in cellular energy metabolism because of ATP depletion, a shift from oxidative phosphorylation toward glycolysis, and associated tissue or organ dysfunction. Acute, severe hypophosphatemia occurs mainly or exclusively in hospitalized patients with underlying serious medical or surgical illness and preexisting phosphate depletion due to excessive urinary losses, severe malabsorption, or malnutrition. Chronic hypophosphatemia tends to be less severe, with a clinical presentation dominated by musculoskeletal complaints such as bone pain, pseudofractures, and proximal muscle weakness or, in children, rickets and short stature.

Neuromuscular manifestations of severe hypophosphatemia are variable but may include muscle weakness, lethargy, confusion, disorientation, hallucinations, dysarthria, dysphagia, oculomotor palsies, anisocoria, nystagmus, ataxia, cerebellar tremor, ballismus, hyporeflexia, impaired sphincter control, distal sensory deficits, paresthesia, hyperesthesia, generalized or Guillain Barré–like ascending paralysis, seizures, coma, and death. Serious sequelae such as paralysis, confusion, and seizures are likely only at phosphate concentrations <0.25 mmol/L (<0.8 mg/dL). Rhabdomyolysis may develop during rapidly progressive hypophosphatemia. The diagnosis of hypophosphatemia-induced rhabdomyolysis may be overlooked, as up to 30% of patients with acute hypophosphatemia (<0.7 mM) have creatine phosphokinase elevations that peak 1–2 days after the nadir in serum phosphate, when the release of phosphate from injured myocytes may have led to a near-normalization of circulating levels of phosphate.

Respiratory failure and cardiac dysfunction, reversible with phosphate treatment, may occur at serum phosphate levels of 0.5–0.8 mmol/L (1.5–2.5 mg/dL). Renal tubular defects, including tubular acidosis, glycosuria, and impaired reabsorption of sodium and calcium, may occur. Hematologic abnormalities correlate with reductions in intracellular ATP and 2,3-diphosphoglycerate and may include erythrocyte microspherocytosis and hemolysis; impaired oxyhemoglobin dissociation; defective leukocyte chemotaxis, phagocytosis, and bacterial killing; and platelet dysfunction with spontaneous gastrointestinal hemorrhage.

R̄x HYPOPHOSPHATEMIA

Severe hypophosphatemia [<0.75 mmol/L (<2 mg/dL)], particularly in the setting of underlying phosphate depletion, constitutes a dangerous electrolyte abnormality that should be corrected promptly. Unfortunately, the

TABLE 346-2 **INTRAVENOUS THERAPY OF HYPOPHOSPHATEMIA**

Consider

Likely severity of underlying phosphate depletion
Concurrent parenteral glucose administration
Presence of neuromuscular, cardiopulmonary, or hematologic complications of hypophosphatemia
Renal function [reduce dose by 50% if serum creatinine >220 μmol/L (>2.5 mg/dL)]
Serum calcium level (correct hypocalcemia first; reduce dose by 50% in hypercalcemia)

Guidelines

Serum Phosphorus, mM (mg/dL)	Rate of Infusion, mmol/h	Duration, h	Total Administered, mmol
<0.8 (<2.5)	2.0	6	12
<0.5 (<1.5)	4.0	6	24
<0.3 (<1.0)	8.0	6	48

Rates shown are calculated for a 70-kg person; levels of serum calcium and phosphorus must be measured every 6 to 12 h during therapy; infusions can be repeated to achieve stable serum phosphorus levels > 0.8 mmol/L (>2.5 mg/dL); most formulations available in the United States provide 3 mmol/mL of sodium or potassium phosphate.

cumulative deficit in body phosphate cannot be easily predicted from knowledge of the circulating level of phosphate, and therapy must be approached empirically. The threshold for IV phosphate therapy and the dose administered should reflect consideration of renal function, the likely severity and duration of the underlying phosphate depletion, and the presence and severity of symptoms consistent with those of hypophosphatemia. In adults, phosphate may be safely administered IV as neutral mixtures of sodium and potassium phosphate salts at initial doses of 0.2–0.8 mmol/kg of elemental phosphorus over 6 h (e.g., 10–50 mmol over 6 h), with doses >20 mmol/6 h reserved for those who have serum levels <0.5 mmol/L (1.5 mg/dL) and normal renal function. A suggested approach is presented in **Table 346-2**. Serum levels of phosphate and calcium must be monitored closely (every 6–12 h) throughout treatment. It is necessary to avoid a serum calcium-phosphorus product >50 to reduce the risk of heterotopic calcification. Hypocalcemia, if present, should be corrected before administering IV phosphate. Less severe hypophosphatemia, in the range of 0.5–0.8 mmol/L (1.5–2.5 mg/dL), can usually be treated with oral phosphate in divided doses of 750–2000 mg/d, as elemental phosphorus; higher doses can cause bloating and diarrhea.

Management of chronic hypophosphatemia requires knowing the cause(s) of the disorder. Hypophosphatemia related to the secondary hyperparathyroidism of vitamin D deficiency usually responds to treatment with vitamin D and calcium alone. XLHR, ADHR, TIO, and related renal tubular disorders are usually managed with divided oral doses of phosphate, often with calcium and 1,25(OH)$_2$D supplements to bypass the block in renal 1,25(OH)$_2$D synthesis and prevent secondary hyperparathyroidism caused by suppression of ECF calcium levels. Thiazide diuretics may be used to prevent nephrocalcinosis in patients who are managed this way. Complete normalization of hypophosphatemia is generally not possible in these conditions. Optimal therapy of TIO is extirpation of the responsible tumor, which may be localized by radiographic skeletal survey or bone scan (many are located in bone) or by radionuclide scanning using sestamibi or labeled octreotide. Successful treatment of TIO-induced hypophosphatemia with octreotide has been reported in a small number of patients.

HYPERPHOSPHATEMIA

Causes When the filtered load of phosphate and glomerular filtration rate (GFR) are normal, control of serum phosphate levels is achieved by adjusting the rate at which phosphate is reabsorbed by the proximal tubular NaPi-2 co-transporter. The principal hormonal regulator of NaPi-2 activity is PTH. Hyperphosphatemia, defined in adults as a fasting serum phosphate concentration >1.8 mmol/L (5.5 mg/dL), usually results from impaired glomerular filtration, hypoparathyroidism, excessive delivery of phosphate into the ECF (from bone, gut, or parenteral phosphate therapy), or some combination of these factors

TABLE 346-3 **CAUSES OF HYPERPHOSPHATEMIA**

I. Impaired renal phosphate excretion
  A. Renal insufficiency
  B. Hypoparathyroidism
    1. Developmental
    2. Autoimmune
    3. After neck surgery or radiation
    4. Activating mutations of the calcium-sensing receptor
  C. Parathyroid suppression
    1. Parathyroid-independent hypercalcemia
      a. Vitamin D or vitamin A intoxication
      b. Sarcoidosis, other granulomatous diseases
      c. Immobilization, osteolytic metastases
      d. Milk-alkali syndrome
    2. Severe hypermagnesemia or hypomagnesemia
  D. Pseudohypoparathyroidism
  E. Acromegaly
  F. Tumoral calcinosis
  G. Heparin therapy
II. Massive extracellular fluid phosphate loads
  A. Rapid administration of exogenous phosphate (intravenous, oral, rectal)
  B. Extensive cellular injury or necrosis
    1. Crush injuries
    2. Rhabdomyolysis
    3. Hyperthermia
    4. Fulminant hepatitis
    5. Cytotoxic therapy
    6. Severe hemolytic anemia
  C. Transcellular phosphate shifts
    1. Metabolic acidosis
    2. Respiratory acidosis

(Table 346-3). The upper limit of normal serum phosphate concentrations is higher in children and neonates [2.4 mmol/L (7 mg/dL)]. It is useful to distinguish hyperphosphatemia caused by impaired renal phosphate excretion from that which results from excessive delivery of phosphate into the ECF (Table 346-3).

In chronic renal insufficiency, reduced GFR leads to phosphate retention. Hyperphosphatemia, in turn, further impairs renal synthesis of 1,25(OH)$_2$D and stimulates PTH secretion and hypertrophy, both directly and indirectly (by lowering blood ionized calcium levels). Thus, hyperphosphatemia is a major cause of the secondary hyperparathyroidism of renal failure and must be addressed early in the course of the disease (Chaps. 274 and 347).

Hypoparathyroidism leads to hyperphosphatemia via increased expression of NaPi-2 co-transporters in the proximal tubule. Hypoparathyroidism, or parathyroid suppression, has multiple potential causes including autoimmune disease; developmental, surgical, or radiation-induced absence of functional parathyroid tissue; vitamin D intoxication or other causes of PTH-independent hypercalcemia; cellular PTH resistance (pseudohypoparathyroidism or hypomagnesemia); infiltrative disorders such as Wilson disease and hemochromatosis; and impaired PTH secretion caused by hypermagnesemia, severe hypomagnesemia, or activating mutations in the CaSR. Hypocalcemia may also contribute directly to impaired phosphate clearance, as calcium infusion can induce hyperphosphaturia in hypoparathyroid subjects. Increased tubular phosphate reabsorption also occurs in acromegaly, during heparin administration, and in tumoral calcinosis. Tumoral calcinosis is a caused by a rare group of genetic disorders in which the *FGF23* gene is either inactivated directly or in which FGF23 is processed in a way that leads to low levels of active FGF23 in the bloodstream. These abnormalities cause elevated serum 1,25(OH)$_2$D, parathyroid suppression, increased intestinal calcium absorption, and focal hyperostosis with large, lobulated periarticular heterotopic ossifications (especially at shoulders or hips) and are accompanied by hyperphosphatemia. In some forms of tumoral calcinosis serum phosphorus levels are normal.

When large amounts of phosphate are rapidly delivered into the ECF, hyperphosphatemia can occur despite normal renal function. Examples include overzealous IV phosphate therapy, oral or rectal administration of large amounts of phosphate-containing laxatives or enemas (especially in children), extensive soft tissue injury or necrosis (crush injuries, rhabdomyolysis, hyperthermia, fulminant hepatitis, cytotoxic chemotherapy), extensive hemolytic anemia, or transcellular phosphate shifts induced by severe metabolic or respiratory acidosis.

Clinical Findings   The clinical consequences of acute, severe hyperphosphatemia are due mainly to the formation of widespread calcium phosphate precipitates and resulting hypocalcemia. Thus, tetany, seizures, accelerated nephrocalcinosis (with renal failure, hyperkalemia, hyperuricemia, and metabolic acidosis), and pulmonary or cardiac calcifications (including development of acute heart block) may occur. The severity of these complications relates to the elevation of serum phosphate levels, which can reach concentrations as high as 7 mmol/L (20 mg/dL) in instances of massive soft tissue injury or tumor lysis syndrome.

℞ HYPERPHOSPHATEMIA

Therapeutic options for management of severe hyperphosphatemia are limited. Volume expansion may enhance renal phosphate clearance. Aluminum hydroxide antacids or sevalamer may be helpful in chelating and limiting absorption of offending phosphate salts present in the intestine. Hemodialysis is the most effective therapeutic strategy and should be considered early in the course of severe hyperphosphatemia, especially in the setting of renal failure and symptomatic hypocalcemia.

MAGNESIUM METABOLISM

Magnesium is the major intracellular divalent cation. Normal concentrations of extracellular magnesium and calcium are crucial for normal neuromuscular activity. Intracellular magnesium forms a key complex with ATP and is an important cofactor for a wide range of enzymes, transporters, and nucleic acids required for normal cellular function, replication, and energy metabolism. The concentration of magnesium in serum is closely regulated within the range of 0.7–1.0 mmol/L (1.5–2.0 meq/L; 1.7–2.4 mg/dL), of which 30% is protein-bound and another 15% is loosely complexed to phosphate and other anions. Half of the 25 g (1000 mmol) of total body magnesium is located in bone, only half of which is insoluble in the mineral phase. Almost all extraskeletal magnesium is present within cells, where the total concentration is 5 mM, 95% of which is bound to proteins and other macromolecules. Because only 1% of body magnesium resides in the ECF, measurements of serum magnesium levels may not accurately reflect the level of total body magnesium stores.

Dietary magnesium content normally ranges from 6–15 mmol/d (140–360 mg/d), of which 30–40% is absorbed, mainly in the jejunum and ileum. Intestinal magnesium absorptive efficiency is stimulated by 1,25(OH)$_2$D and can reach 70% during magnesium deprivation. Urinary magnesium excretion normally matches net intestinal absorption and is ~4 mmol/d (100 mg/d). Regulation of serum magnesium concentrations is achieved mainly by control of renal magnesium reabsorption. Only 20% of filtered magnesium is reabsorbed in the proximal tubule, whereas 60% is reclaimed in the cTAL and another 5–10% in the DCT. Magnesium reabsorption in the cTAL occurs via a paracellular route that requires both a lumen-negative potential, created by NaCl reabsorption, and the tight-junction protein, paracellin-1. Magnesium reabsorption in the cTAL is increased by PTH but inhibited by hypercalcemia or hypermagnesemia, both of which activate the CaSR in this nephron segment.

HYPOMAGNESEMIA

Causes   Hypomagnesemia usually signifies substantial depletion of body magnesium stores (0.5–1 mmol/kg). Hypomagnesemia can result from intestinal malabsorption; protracted vomiting, diarrhea, or intestinal drainage; defective renal tubular magnesium reabsorption; or rapid shifts of magnesium from the ECF into cells, bone, or third spaces (Table 346-4). Dietary magnesium deficiency is unlikely except possibly in the setting of alcoholism. A rare genetic disorder causing selective intestinal magnesium malabsorption has been described (primary infantile hypomagnesemia). Another rare inherited disor-

TABLE 346-4	CAUSES OF HYPOMAGNESEMIA

I. Impaired intestinal absorption
  A. Primary infantile hypomagnesemia
  B. Malabsorption syndromes
  C. Vitamin D deficiency
II. Increased intestinal losses
  A. Protracted vomiting/diarrhea
  B. Intestinal drainage, fistulae
III. Impaired renal tubular reabsorption
  A. Genetic magnesium-wasting syndromes
    1. Gitelman syndrome
    2. Bartter syndrome
    3. Paracellin-1 mutations
    4. Na$^+$,K$^+$-ATPase g-subunit mutations (FXYD2)
    5. Autosomal dominant, with low bone mass
  B. Acquired renal disease
    1. Tubulointerstitial disease
    2. Postobstruction, ATN (diuretic phase)
    3. Renal transplantation
  C. Drugs and toxins
    1. Ethanol
    2. Diuretics (loop, thiazide, osmotic)
    3. Cisplatin
    4. Pentamidine, foscarnet
    5. Cyclosporine
    6. Aminoglycosides, amphotericin B
  D. Other
IV. Extracellular fluid volume expansion
  A. Hyperaldosteronism
  B. SIADH
  C. Diabetes mellitus
  D. Hypercalcemia
  E. Phosphate depletion
  F. Metabolic acidosis
  G. Hyperthyroidism
V. Rapid shifts from extracellular fluid
  A. Intracellular redistribution
    1. Recovery from diabetic ketoacidosis
    2. Refeeding syndrome
    3. Correction of respiratory acidosis
    4. Catecholamines
  B. Accelerated bone formation
    1. Post parathyroidectomy
    2. Treatment of vitamin D deficiency
    3. Osteoblastic metastases
  C. Other
    1. Pancreatitis, burns, excessive sweating
    2. Pregnancy (3rd trimester) and lactation

Note: ATN, acute tubular necrosis; SIADH, syndrome of inappropriate anti-diuretic hormone.

der (hypomagnesemia with secondary hypocalcemia) is caused by mutations in the gene encoding TRPM6, a protein that, along with TRPM7, forms a channel important for both intestinal and renal magnesium transport. Malabsorptive states, often compounded by vitamin D deficiency, can critically limit magnesium absorption and produce hypomagnesemia, despite the compensatory effects of secondary hyperparathyroidism and of hypocalcemia and hypomagnesemia to enhance cTAL magnesium reabsorption. Diarrhea or surgical drainage fluid may contain ≥5 mmol/L of magnesium.

Several genetic magnesium-wasting syndromes are described, including inactivating mutations of genes encoding the DCT NaCl co-transporter (Gitelman syndrome), proteins required for cTAL Na-K-2Cl transport (Bartter syndrome), paracellin-1 (autosomal recessive renal hypomagnesemia with hypercalciuria), a DCT Na$^+$,K$^+$-ATPase γ-subunit (autosomal dominant renal hypomagnesemia with hypocalciuria), the FXYD2 γ-subunit of the distal tubular basolateral Na$^+$,K$^+$-ATPase, and a mitochondrial DNA gene encoding a mitochondrial tRNA. ECF expansion, hypercalcemia, and severe phosphate depletion may impair magnesium reabsorption, as can various forms of renal injury, including those caused by drugs such as cisplatin, cyclosporine, aminoglycosides, and pentamidine (Table 346-4). A rising blood concentration of ethanol directly impairs tubular magnesium reabsorption, and persistent glycosuria with osmotic diuresis leads to magnesium wasting and likely contributes to the high frequency of hypomagnesemia in poorly controlled diabetics. Magnesium depletion is aggravated by metabolic acidosis, which causes intracellular losses as well.

Hypomagnesemia due to rapid shifts of magnesium from ECF into the intracellular compartment can occur during recovery from diabetic ketoacidosis, from starvation, or from respiratory acidosis. Less acute shifts may be seen during rapid bone formation after parathyroidectomy, with treatment of vitamin D deficiency, or with osteoblastic metastases. Large amounts of magnesium may be lost with acute pancreatitis, extensive burns, protracted and severe sweating, and during pregnancy and lactation.

Clinical and Laboratory Findings Hypomagnesemia may cause generalized alterations in neuromuscular function, including tetany, tremor, seizures, muscle weakness, ataxia, nystagmus, vertigo, apathy, depression, irritability, delirium, and psychosis. Patients are usually asymptomatic when serum magnesium concentrations are >0.5 mmol/L (1 meq/L; 1.2 mg/dL), although the severity of symptoms may not correlate with serum magnesium levels. Cardiac arrhythmias may occur, including sinus tachycardia, other supraventricular tachycardias, and ventricular arrhythmias. Electrocardiographic abnormalities may include prolonged PR or QT intervals, T-wave flattening or inversion, and ST straightening. Sensitivity to digitalis toxicity may be enhanced.

Other electrolyte abnormalities often seen with hypomagnesemia, including hypocalcemia (with hypocalciuria) and hypokalemia, may not be easily corrected unless magnesium is administered as well. The hypocalcemia may be a result of concurrent vitamin D deficiency, although hypomagnesemia can cause impaired synthesis of $1,25(OH)_2D$, cellular resistance to PTH and, at very low serum magnesium [<0.4 mmol/L (<0.8 meq/L; <1 mg/dL)], a defect in PTH secretion; these abnormalities are reversible with therapy.

℞ HYPOMAGNESEMIA

Mild, asymptomatic hypomagnesemia may be treated with oral magnesium salts [$MgCl_2$, MgO, $Mg(OH)_2$] in divided doses totaling 20–30 mmol/d (40–60 meq/d). Diarrhea may occur with larger doses. More severe hypomagnesemia should be treated parenterally, preferably with IV $MgCl_2$, which can be administered safely as a continuous infusion of 50 mmol/d (100 meq Mg^{2+}/d) if renal function is normal. If GFR is reduced, the infusion rate should be lowered by 50–75%. Use of IM $MgSO_4$ is discouraged; the injections are painful and provide relatively little magnesium (2 mL of 50% $MgSO_4$ supplies only 4 mmol). $MgSO_4$ may be given IV instead of $MgCl_2$, although the sulfate anions may bind calcium in serum and urine and aggravate hypocalcemia. Serum magnesium should be monitored at intervals of 12–24 h during therapy, which may continue for several days because of impaired renal conservation of magnesium (only 50–70% of the daily IV magnesium dose is retained) and delayed repletion of intracellular deficits, which may be as high as 1–1.5 mmol/kg (2–3 meq/kg).

It is important to consider the need for calcium, potassium, and phosphate supplementation in patients with hypomagnesemia. Vitamin D deficiency frequently coexists and should be treated with oral or parenteral vitamin D or 25(OH)D [but not $1,25(OH)_2D$, which may impair tubular magnesium reabsorption, possibly via PTH suppression]. In severely hypomagnesemic patients with concomitant hypocalcemia and hypophosphatemia, administration of IV magnesium alone may worsen hypophosphatemia, provoking neuromuscular symptoms or rhabdomyolysis, due to rapid stimulation of PTH secretion. This is avoided by administering both calcium and magnesium.

HYPERMAGNESEMIA

Causes Hypermagnesemia is rarely seen in the absence of renal insufficiency, as normal kidneys can excrete large amounts (250 mmol/d) of magnesium. Mild hypermagnesemia due to excessive reabsorption in the cTAL occurs with calcium-sensing receptor mutations in familial hypocalciuric hypercalcemia and has been described in some patients with adrenal insufficiency, hypothyroidism, or hypothermia. Massive exogenous magnesium exposures, usually via the gastrointestinal

TABLE 346-5 CAUSES OF HYPERMAGNESEMIA

Impaired Mg excretion	Rapid Mg mobilization from soft
Renal failure	tissues
Familial hypocalciuric	Trauma
hypercalcemia	Extensive burns
Excessive Mg intake	Shock, sepsis
Cathartics	Post cardiac arrest
Intestinal obstruction/perforation	Other disorders
following magnesium ingestion	Adrenal insufficiency
Parenteral magnesium	Hypothyroidism
administration	Hypothermia
Magnesium-rich urologic irrigants	

tract, can overwhelm renal excretory capacity and cause life-threatening hypermagnesemia (Table 346-5). A notable example of this is prolonged retention of even normal amounts of magnesium-containing cathartics in patients with intestinal ileus, obstruction, or perforation. Extensive soft tissue injury or necrosis can also deliver large amounts of magnesium into the ECF in patients who have suffered trauma, shock, sepsis, cardiac arrest, or severe burns.

Clinical and Laboratory Findings The most prominent clinical manifestations of hypermagnesemia are vasodilation and neuromuscular blockade, which may appear at serum magnesium concentrations >2 mmol/L (>4 meq/L; >4.8 mg/dL). Hypotension, refractory to vasopressors or volume expansion, may be an early sign. Nausea, lethargy, and weakness may progress to respiratory failure, paralysis, and coma, with hypoactive tendon reflexes, at serum magnesium levels >4 mmol/L. Other findings may include gastrointestinal hypomotility or ileus; facial flushing; pupillary dilation; paradoxical bradycardia; prolongation of PR, QRS, and QT intervals; heart block; and, at serum magnesium levels approaching 10 mmol/L, asystole.

Hypermagnesemia, acting via the CaSR, causes hypocalcemia and hypercalciuria due to both parathyroid suppression and impaired cTAL calcium reabsorption.

℞ HYPERMAGNESEMIA

Successful treatment of hypermagnesemia generally involves identifying and interrupting the source of magnesium and employing measures to increase magnesium clearance from the ECF. Use of magnesium-free cathartics or enemas may be helpful in clearing ingested magnesium from the gastrointestinal tract. Vigorous IV hydration should be attempted, if appropriate. Hemodialysis is effective and may be required in patients with significant renal insufficiency. Calcium, administered IV in doses of 100–200 mg over 1–2 h, has been reported to provide temporary improvement in signs and symptoms of hypermagnesemia.

VITAMIN D

SYNTHESIS AND METABOLISM

$1,25$-dihydroxyvitamin D $[1,25(OH)_2D]$ is the major steroid hormone involved in mineral ion homeostasis regulation. Vitamin D and its metabolites are hormones and hormone precursors rather than vitamins, since in the proper biologic setting, they can be synthesized endogenously (Fig. 346-4). In response to ultraviolet radiation of the skin, a photochemical cleavage results in the formation of vitamin D from 7-dehydrocholesterol. Cutaneous production of vitamin D is decreased by melanin and high solar protection factor sunblocks, which effectively impair skin penetration of ultraviolet light. The increased use of sunblocks in North America and Western Europe and a reduction in the magnitude of solar exposure of the general population over the past several decades has led to an increased reliance on dietary sources of vitamin D. In the United States and Canada, these sources largely consist of fortified cereals and dairy products, in addition to fish oils and egg yolks. Vitamin D from plant sources is in the form of vitamin D_2, whereas that from animal sources is vitamin D_3. These two forms have equivalent biologic activity and are activated equally well by the

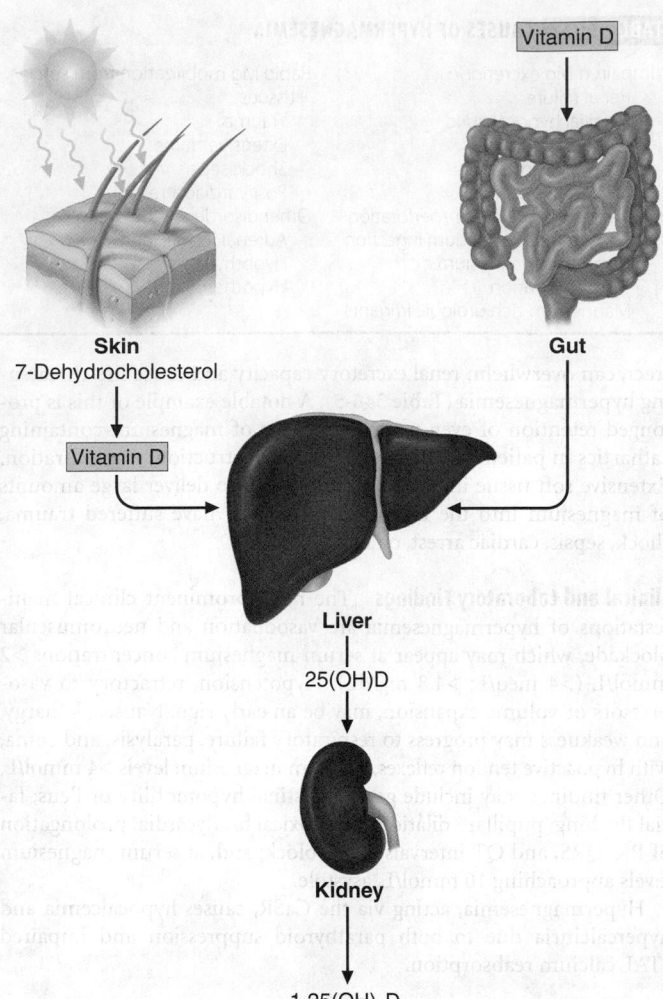

Skin
7-Dehydrocholesterol

Gut

Vitamin D

Liver

25(OH)D

Kidney

1,25(OH)₂D

FIGURE 346-4 Vitamin D synthesis and activation. Vitamin D is synthesized in the skin in response to ultraviolet radiation and is also absorbed from the diet. It is then transported to the liver, where it undergoes 25-hydroxylation. This metabolite is the major circulating form of vitamin D. The final step in hormone activation, 1α-hydroxylation, occurs in the kidney.

vitamin D hydroxylases in humans. Vitamin D enters the circulation, whether absorbed from the intestine or synthesized cutaneously, bound to vitamin D–binding protein, an α-globulin synthesized in the liver. Vitamin D is subsequently 25-hydroxylated in the liver by cytochrome P450–like enzymes in the mitochondria and microsomes. The activity of this hydroxylase is not tightly regulated, and the resultant metabolite, 25-hydroxyvitamin D [25(OH)D], is the major circulating and storage form of vitamin D. Approximately 88% of 25(OH)D circulates bound to the vitamin D–binding protein, 0.03% is free, and the rest circulates bound to albumin. The half-life of 25(OH)D is approximately 2–3 weeks; however, it is dramatically shortened when vitamin D–binding protein levels are reduced, as can occur with increased urinary losses in the nephrotic syndrome.

The second hydroxylation, required for the formation of the mature hormone, occurs in the kidney (Fig. 346-5). The 25-hydroxyvitamin D-1α-hydroxylase is a tightly regulated cytochrome P450–like mixed function oxidase expressed in the proximal convoluted tubule cells of the kidney. PTH and hypophosphatemia are the major inducers of this microsomal enzyme, whereas calcium, FGF23, and the enzyme's product, 1,25(OH)₂D, repress it. The 25-hydroxyvitamin D-1α-hydroxylase is also present in epidermal keratinocytes, but keratinocyte production of 1,25(OH)₂D is not thought to contribute to circulating levels of this hormone. In addition to being present in the trophoblastic layer of the placenta, the 1α-hydroxylase is produced by macrophages associated with granulomata and lymphomas. In these latter pathologic states, the

activity of the enzyme is induced by interferon γ and TNF-α but is not regulated by calcium or 1,25(OH)₂D; therefore, hypercalcemia, associated with elevated levels of 1,25(OH)₂D, may be observed. Treatment of sarcoidosis-associated hypercalcemia with glucocorticoids, ketoconazole, or chloroquine reduces 1,25(OH)₂D production and effectively lowers serum calcium. In contrast, chloroquine has not been shown to lower the elevated serum 1,25(OH)₂D levels in patients with lymphoma.

The major pathway for inactivation of vitamin D metabolites is an additional hydroxylation step by the vitamin D 24-hydroxylase, an enzyme that is expressed in most tissues. 1,25(OH)₂D is the major inducer of this enzyme; therefore, this hormone promotes its own inactivation, thereby limiting its biologic effects. Polar metabolites of 1,25(OH)₂D are secreted into the bile and reabsorbed via the enterohepatic circulation. Impairment of this recirculation, seen with diseases of the terminal ileum, leads to accelerated losses of vitamin D metabolites.

ACTIONS OF 1,25(OH)₂D

1,25(OH)₂D mediates its biologic effects by binding to a member of the nuclear receptor superfamily, the vitamin D receptor (VDR). This

Vitamin D₃

Vitamin D-
25 hydroxylase

Liver

25(OH)D₃

25(OH)D-1α-
hydroxylase

Pᵢ and
other factors

Kidney

1,25(OH)₂D₃

1,25(OH)₂D₃

PTH

Bone

PTH

**Parathyroid
glands**

Intestine

Ca²⁺ HPO₄²⁻

Calcification

Ca²⁺ HPO₄²⁻

**Blood
calcium**

FIGURE 346-5 Schematic representation of the hormonal control loop for vitamin D metabolism and function. A reduction in the serum calcium below ~2.2 mmol/L (8.8 mg/dL) prompts a proportional increase in the secretion of parathyroid hormone (PTH) and so mobilizes additional calcium from the bone. PTH promotes the synthesis of 1,25(OH)₂D in the kidney, which, in turn, stimulates the mobilization of calcium from bone and intestine and regulates the synthesis of PTH by negative feedback.

receptor belongs to the subfamily that includes the thyroid hormone receptors, the retinoid receptors and the peroxisome proliferator–activated receptors; however, in contrast to the other members of this subfamily, only one VDR isoform has been isolated. The VDR binds to target DNA sequences as a heterodimer with the retinoid X receptor, recruiting a series of coactivators that modify chromatin and approximate the VDR to the basal transcriptional apparatus, resulting in the induction of target gene expression. The mechanism of transcriptional repression by the VDR varies with different target genes but has been shown to involve either interference with the action of activating transcription factors or the recruitment of novel proteins to the VDR complex, resulting in transcriptional repression.

The affinity of the VDR for $1,25(OH)_2D$ is approximately three orders of magnitude higher than that for other vitamin D metabolites. Under normal physiologic circumstances, these other metabolites are not thought to stimulate receptor-dependent actions. However, in states of vitamin D toxicity, the markedly elevated levels of $25(OH)D$ may lead to hypercalcemia by interacting directly with the VDR and by displacing $1,25(OH)_2D$ from vitamin D–binding protein, resulting in increased bioavailability of the active hormone.

The VDR is expressed in a wide range of cells and tissues. The molecular actions of $1,25(OH)_2D$ have been most extensively studied in tissues involved in the regulation of mineral ion homeostasis. This hormone is a major inducer of calbindin 9K, a calcium-binding protein expressed in the intestine, which is thought to play an important role in the active transport of calcium across the enterocyte. The two major calcium transporters expressed by intestinal epithelia, TRPV5 and TRPV6 (transient receptor potential vanilloid), are also vitamin D responsive. By inducing the expression of these and other genes in the small intestine, $1,25(OH)_2D$ increases the efficiency of intestinal calcium absorption, and it has also been shown to have several important actions in the skeleton. The VDR is expressed in osteoblasts and regulates the expression of several genes in this cell. These genes include the bone matrix proteins, osteocalcin and osteopontin, which are upregulated by $1,25(OH)_2D$, in addition to type I collagen, which is transcriptionally repressed by $1,25(OH)_2D$. Both $1,25(OH)_2D$ and parathyroid hormone induce the expression of RANK ligand, which promotes osteoclast differentiation and increases osteoclast activity, by binding to RANK on osteoclast progenitors and mature osteoclasts. This is the mechanism by which $1,25(OH)_2D$ induces bone resorption. However, the skeletal features associated with VDR-knockout mice (rickets, osteomalacia) are largely corrected by increasing calcium and phosphorus intake, underscoring the importance of vitamin D action in the gut.

The VDR is expressed in the parathyroid gland, and $1,25(OH)_2D$ has been shown to have antiproliferative effects on parathyroid cells and to suppress the transcription of the parathyroid hormone gene. These effects of $1,25(OH)_2D$ on the parathyroid gland are an important part of the rationale for current therapies directed at preventing and treating hyperparathyroidism associated with renal insufficiency.

The VDR is also expressed in tissues and organs that do not play a role in mineral ion homeostasis. Notable in this respect is the observation that $1,25(OH)_2D$ has an antiproliferative effect on several cell types, including keratinocytes, breast cancer cells, and prostate cancer cells. The effects of $1,25(OH)_2D$ and the VDR on keratinocytes are particularly intriguing. Alopecia is seen in humans and mice with mutant VDRs but is not a feature of vitamin D deficiency; thus, the effects of the VDR on the hair follicle are ligand-independent.

VITAMIN D DEFICIENCY

The mounting concern about the relationship between solar exposure and the development of skin cancer has led to increased reliance on dietary sources of vitamin D. Although the prevalence of vitamin D deficiency varies, the third National Health and Nutrition Examination Survey (NHANES III) revealed that vitamin D deficiency is prevalent throughout the United States. The clinical syndrome of vitamin D deficiency can be a result of deficient production of vitamin D in the skin, lack of dietary intake, accelerated losses of vitamin D, impaired vitamin D activation or resistance to the biologic effects of $1,25(OH)_2D$ (Table

TABLE 346-6 CAUSES OF IMPAIRED VITAMIN D ACTION	
Vitamin D deficiency	Impaired 1α-hydroxylation
Impaired cutaneous production	Hypoparathyroidism
Dietary absence	Renal failure
Malabsorption	Ketoconazole
Accelerated loss of vitamin D	1α-hydroxylase mutation
Increased metabolism (barbiturates, phenytoin, rifampin)	Oncogenic osteomalacia
	X-linked hypophosphatemic
Impaired enterohepatic	rickets
circulation	Target organ resistance
Impaired 25-hydroxylation	Vitamin D receptor mutation
Liver disease	Phenytoin
Isoniazid	

346-6). The elderly and nursing home residents are particularly at risk for vitamin D deficiency, since both the efficiency of vitamin D synthesis in the skin and the absorption of vitamin D from the intestine decline with age. Similarly, intestinal malabsorption of dietary fats leads to vitamin D deficiency. This is further exacerbated in the presence of terminal ileal disease, which results in impaired enterohepatic circulation of vitamin D metabolites. In addition to intestinal diseases, accelerated inactivation of vitamin D metabolites can be seen with drugs that induce hepatic cytochrome P450 mixed function oxidases, such as barbiturates, phenytoin, and rifampin. Impaired 25-hydroxylation, associated with severe liver disease or isoniazid, is an infrequent cause of vitamin D deficiency. Impaired 1α-hydroxylation is prevalent in the population with profound renal dysfunction, due to an increase in circulating FGF23 levels and a decrease in functional renal mass. Thus, therapeutic interventions should be considered in patients whose creatinine clearance is <0.5 mL/s (30 mL/min). Mutations in the renal 1α-hydroxylase are the basis for the genetic disorder, pseudo-vitamin D–deficiency rickets. This autosomal recessive disorder presents with the syndrome of vitamin D deficiency in the first year of life. Patients present with growth retardation, rickets, and hypocalcemic seizures. Serum $1,25(OH)_2D$ levels are low, despite normal $25(OH)D$ levels and elevated PTH levels. Treatment with vitamin D metabolites that do not require 1α-hydroxylation results in disease remission, although lifelong therapy is required. A second autosomal recessive disorder, hereditary vitamin D–resistant rickets, a consequence of vitamin D receptor mutations, is a greater therapeutic challenge. These patients present in a similar fashion during the first year of life, but alopecia often accompanies the disorder, demonstrating a functional role of the VDR in postnatal hair regeneration. Serum levels of $1,25(OH)_2D$ are dramatically elevated in these individuals, both because of increased production due to stimulation of 1α-hydroxylase activity as a consequence of secondary hyperparathyroidism and because of impaired inactivation, since induction of the 24-hydroxylase by $1,25(OH)_2D$ requires an intact VDR. Since the receptor mutation results in hormone resistance, daily calcium and phosphorus infusions may be required to bypass the defect in intestinal mineral ion absorption.

Regardless of the cause, the clinical manifestations of vitamin D deficiency are largely a consequence of impaired intestinal calcium absorption. Mild to moderate vitamin D deficiency is asymptomatic, whereas long-standing vitamin D deficiency results in hypocalcemia accompanied by secondary hyperparathyroidism, impaired mineralization of the skeleton (osteopenia on x-ray or decreased bone mineral density), and proximal myopathy. In the absence of an intercurrent illness, the hypocalcemia associated with long-standing vitamin D deficiency rarely presents with acute symptoms of hypocalcemia, such as numbness, tingling, or seizures. However, the concurrent development of hypomagnesemia, which impairs parathyroid function, or the administration of potent bisphosphonates, which impair bone resorption, can lead to acute symptomatic hypocalcemia in vitamin D–deficient individuals.

RICKETS AND OSTEOMALACIA

In children, prior to epiphyseal fusion, vitamin D deficiency results in growth retardation associated with an expansion of the growth plate known as *rickets*. Three layers of chondrocytes are present in the normal growth plate: the reserve zone, the proliferating zone, and the hypertrophic zone. Rickets associated with impaired vitamin D action is characterized by expansion of the hypertrophic chondrocyte layer. The proliferation and differentiation of the chondrocytes in the rachitic growth plate are normal, and the expansion of the growth plate is a consequence of impaired apoptosis of the late hypertrophic chondrocytes, an event that precedes replacement of these cells by osteoblasts during endochondral bone formation. Investigations in murine models demonstrate that hypophosphatemia, which in vitamin D deficiency is a consequence of secondary hyperparathyroidism, is a key etiologic factor in the development of the rachitic growth plate.

The hypocalcemia and hypophosphatemia that accompany vitamin D deficiency result in impaired mineralization of bone matrix proteins, a condition known as *osteomalacia*. Osteomalacia is also a feature of long-standing hypophosphatemia, which may be a consequence of renal phosphate wasting or chronic use of etidronate or phosphate-binding antacids. This hypomineralized matrix is biomechanically inferior to normal bone; as a result, patients with vitamin D deficiency are prone to bowing of weight-bearing extremities and skeletal fractures. Vitamin D and calcium supplementation have been shown to decrease the incidence of hip fracture among ambulatory nursing home residents in France, suggesting that undermineralization of bone contributes significantly to morbidity in the elderly. Proximal myopathy is a striking feature of severe vitamin D deficiency, both in children and in adults. Rapid resolution of the myopathy is observed upon vitamin D treatment.

Though vitamin D deficiency is the most common cause of rickets and osteomalacia, many disorders lead to inadequate mineralization of the growth plate and bone. Calcium deficiency without vitamin D deficiency, the disorders of vitamin D metabolism previously discussed, and hypophosphatemia can all lead to inefficient mineralization. Even in the presence of normal calcium and phosphate levels, chronic acidosis and drugs such as bisphosphonates can lead to osteomalacia. The inorganic calcium/phosphate mineral phase of bone cannot form at low pH, and bisphosphonates bind to and prevent mineral crystal growth. Since alkaline phosphatase is necessary for normal mineral deposition, probably because the enzyme can hydrolyze inhibitors of mineralization such as inorganic pyrophosphate, genetic inactivation of the alkaline phosphatase gene (hereditary hypophosphatasia) can also lead to osteomalacia in the setting of normal calcium and phosphate levels.

DIAGNOSIS OF VITAMIN D DEFICIENCY, RICKETS, AND OSTEOMALACIA

The most specific screening test for vitamin D deficiency in otherwise healthy individuals is a serum 25(OH)D level. While the normal ranges vary, levels of 25(OH)D < 37 nmol/L (<15 ng/mL) are associated with increasing PTH levels and lower bone density; optimal vitamin D levels are >62 nmol/L (>25 ng/mL). Vitamin D deficiency leads to impaired intestinal absorption of calcium, resulting in decreased serum total and ionized calcium values. This hypocalcemia results in secondary hyperparathyroidism, a homeostatic response that initially maintains serum calcium levels at the expense of the skeleton. Due to the PTH-induced increase in bone turnover, alkaline phosphatase levels are often increased. In addition to increasing bone resorption, PTH decreases urinary calcium excretion, while promoting phosphaturia. This results in hypophosphatemia, which exacerbates the mineralization defect in the skeleton. With prolonged vitamin D deficiency resulting in osteomalacia, calcium stores in the skeleton become relatively inaccessible, since osteoclasts cannot resorb unmineralized osteoid, and frank hypocalcemia ensues. Since PTH is a major stimulus for the renal 25(OH)D 1α-hydroxylase, there is increased synthesis of the active hormone, 1,25(OH)₂D. Paradoxically, levels of this hormone are often normal in severe vitamin D deficiency. Therefore, measurements of 1,25(OH)₂D are not an accurate reflection of vitamin D stores and should not be used to diagnose vitamin D deficiency in patients with normal renal function.

Radiologic features of vitamin D deficiency in children include a widened, expanded growth plate, characteristic of rickets. These findings are not only apparent in the long bones but are also present at the costochondral junction, where the expansion of the growth plate leads to swellings

FIGURE 346-6 Radiograph of the scapula of a 58-year-old woman with phosphaturia as a cause of osteomalacia. The presence of a pseudofracture, or Looser's zone, is indicated by an arrow.

known as the "rachitic rosary." Impairment of intramembranous bone mineralization leads to delayed fusion of the calvarial sutures and a decrease in the radio-opacity of cortical bone in the long bones. If vitamin D deficiency occurs after epiphyseal fusion, the main radiologic finding is a decrease in cortical thickness and relative radiolucency of the skeleton. A specific radiologic feature of osteomalacia, whether associated with phosphate wasting or vitamin D deficiency, is pseudofractures, or Looser's zones (Fig. 346-6). These are radiolucent lines that occur where large arteries are in contact with the underlying skeletal elements; it is thought that the arterial pulsations lead to the radiolucencies. As a result, these pseudofractures are usually a few millimeters wide, several centimeters long, and are seen particularly in the scapula, the pelvis, and the femoral neck.

℞ VITAMIN D DEFICIENCY

Daily intake of a multivitamin (400 IU) is often insufficient to prevent vitamin D deficiency. Based on the observation that 800 IU of vitamin D, with calcium supplementation, decreases the risk of hip fractures in elderly women, this higher dose is thought to be an appropriate daily intake for prevention of vitamin D deficiency in adults. The safety margin for vitamin D is large, and vitamin D toxicity is usually observed only in patients taking doses in the range of 40,000 IU daily. Treatment of vitamin D deficiency should be directed at the underlying disorder, if possible, and should also be tailored to the severity of the condition. Vitamin D should always be repleted in conjunction with calcium supplementation since most, if not all, of the consequences of vitamin D deficiency are a result of impaired mineral ion homeostasis. In patients in whom 1α-hydroxylation is impaired, metabolites not requiring this activation step are the treatment of choice. These include 1,25(OH)₂D₃ [calcitriol (Rocaltrol), 0.25–0.5 µg/d] and 1,25-dihydroxyvitamin D₂ (Hectorol, 2.5–5 µg/d). If the pathway required for activation of vitamin D is intact, severe vitamin D deficiency can be treated with pharmacologic repletion initially (50,000 IU weekly for 3–12 weeks), followed by maintenance therapy (800 IU daily). Pharmacologic doses may be required for maintenance therapy in patients who are taking medications, such as barbiturates or phenytoin, that accelerate metabolism of or cause resistance to 1,25(OH)₂D. If intestinal malabsorption is a contributing factor, repletion can be performed with IM vitamin D (250,000 IU biannually). Calcium supplementation should include 1.5–2.0 g/d of elemental calcium. Normocalcemia is usually observed within 1 week of institution of therapy, although increases in PTH and alkaline phosphatase levels may persist for 3–6 months. The most efficacious methods to monitor treatment and resolution of vitamin D deficiency are serum and urinary calcium measurements. In patients who are vitamin D replete and taking adequate calcium supplementation, the 24-h urinary calcium excretion should be in the range of 100–250 mg/24 h. Lower levels suggest problems with adherence to the treatment regimen or with absorption of calcium or vitamin D supplements. Levels >250 mg/24 h predispose to nephrolithiasis and should lead to a reduction in vitamin D dosage and/or calcium supplementation.

FURTHER READINGS

BOYDEN LM et al: High bone density due to a mutation in LDL-receptor-related protein 5. N Engl J Med 346:1513, 2002

DELUCA HF: Overview of general physiologic features and functions of vitamin D. Am J Clin Nutr 80:1689S, 2004

HEANEY RP: Bone health. Am J Clin Nutr 85(1):300S, 2007

HOLICK MF: Vitamin D deficiency. N Engl J Med 357(3):266, 2007

KARSENTY G: The complexities of skeletal biology. Nature 316, 2003

KOBAYASHI T et al: Minireview: Transcriptional regulation in development of bone. Endocrinology 146:1012, 2005

TEITELBAUM SL, ROSS SP: Genetic regulation of osteoclast development and function. Nat Rev Genet 4:638, 2003

YU X, WHITE KE: FGF23 and disorders of phosphate homeostasis. Cytokine Growth Factor Rev 16:221, 2005

347 Diseases of the Parathyroid Gland and Other Hyper- and Hypocalcemic Disorders
John T. Potts, Jr.

The four parathyroid glands are located posterior to the thyroid gland. They produce parathyroid hormone (PTH), which is the primary regulator of calcium physiology. PTH acts directly on bone, where it induces calcium resorption, and on the kidney, where it stimulates calcium reabsorption and synthesis of 1,25-dihydroxyvitamin D [$1,25(OH)_2D$], a hormone that stimulates gastrointestinal calcium absorption. Serum PTH levels are tightly regulated by a negative feedback loop. Calcium, acting through the calcium-sensing receptor, and vitamin D, acting through its nuclear receptor, inhibit PTH release and synthesis. Understanding the hormone pathways that regulate calcium levels and bone metabolism is essential for effective diagnosis and management of a wide array of hyper- and hypocalcemic disorders.

Hyperparathyroidism (HPT), characterized by excess production of PTH, is a common cause of hypercalcemia and is usually the result of autonomously functioning adenomas or hyperplasia. Surgery for this disorder is highly effective and has been shown to reverse some of the deleterious effects of long-standing PTH excess on bone density. Hypercalcemia of malignancy is also common and is usually due to the overproduction of parathyroid hormone–related peptide (PTHrP) by cancer cells. The similarities in the biochemical characteristics of hyperparathyroidism and hypercalcemia of malignancy, first noted by Albright in 1941, are now known to reflect the actions of PTH and PTHrP through the same G protein–coupled PTH/PTHrP receptor.

The genetic basis of multiple endocrine neoplasia (MEN) types 1 and 2, familial hypocalciuric hypercalcemia (FHH), the different forms of pseudohypoparathyroidism (PHP), Jansen's syndrome, disorders of vitamin D synthesis and action, and the molecular events associated with parathyroid gland neoplasia have provided new insights into calcium metabolism. The advent of new drugs, including bisphosphonates and selective estrogen receptor modulators (SERMs), offers new avenues for the treatment and prevention of metabolic bone disease. PTH analogues are promising therapeutic agents for the treatment of postmenopausal or senile osteoporosis, and calcimimetic agents, which act through the calcium-sensing receptor, may provide new approaches for PTH suppression.

PARATHYROID HORMONE
PHYSIOLOGY

The primary function of PTH is to maintain the extracellular fluid (ECF) calcium concentration within a narrow normal range. The hormone acts directly on bone and kidney and indirectly on intestine through its effects on synthesis of $1,25(OH)_2D$ to increase serum calcium concentrations; in turn, PTH production is closely regulated by the concentration of serum ionized calcium. This feedback system is the critical homeostatic mechanism for maintenance of ECF calcium. Any tendency toward hypocalcemia, as might be induced by calcium-deficient diets, is counteracted by an increased secretion of PTH. This in turn (1) increases the rate of dissolution of bone mineral, thereby increasing the flow of calcium from bone into blood; (2) reduces the renal clearance of calcium, returning more of the calcium filtered at the glomerulus into ECF; and (3) increases the efficiency of calcium absorption in the intestine by stimulating the production of $1,25(OH)_2D$. Immediate control of blood calcium is due to PTH effects on bone and, to a lesser extent, on renal calcium clearance. Maintenance of steady-state calcium balance, on the other hand, probably results from the effects of $1,25(OH)_2D$ on calcium absorption (Chap. 346). The renal actions of the hormone are exerted at multiple sites and include inhibition of phosphate transport (proximal tubule), increased reabsorption of calcium (distal tubule), and stimulation of the renal $25(OH)D$-1α-hydroxylase. As much as 12 mmol (500 mg) calcium is transferred between the ECF and bone each day (a large amount in relation to the total ECF calcium pool), and PTH has a major effect on this transfer. The homeostatic role of the hormone can preserve calcium concentration in blood at the cost of bone destruction.

PTH has multiple actions on bone, some direct and some indirect. PTH-mediated changes in bone calcium release can be seen within minutes. The chronic effects of PTH are to increase the number of bone cells, both osteoblasts and osteoclasts, and to increase the remodeling of bone; these effects are apparent within hours after the hormone is given and persist for hours after PTH is withdrawn. Continuous exposure to elevated PTH (as in hyperparathyroidism or long-term infusions in animals) leads to increased osteoclast-mediated bone resorption. However, the intermittent administration of PTH, elevating hormone levels for 1–2 h each day, leads to a net stimulation of bone formation rather than bone breakdown. Striking increases, especially in trabecular bone in the spine and hip, have been reported with the use of PTH in combination with estrogen. PTH as monotherapy caused a highly significant reduction in fracture incidence in a worldwide placebo-controlled trial.

Osteoblasts (or stromal cell precursors), which have PTH receptors, are crucial to this bone-forming effect of PTH; osteoclasts, which mediate bone breakdown, lack PTH receptors. PTH-mediated stimulation of osteoclasts is believed to be indirect, acting in part through cytokines released from osteoblasts to activate osteoclasts; in experimental studies of bone resorption in vitro, osteoblasts must be present for PTH to activate osteoclasts to resorb bone (Chap. 346).

STRUCTURE

PTH is an 84-amino-acid single-chain peptide. The amino acid portion, PTH(1–34), is highly conserved and is critical for the biologic actions of the molecule. Modified synthetic fragments of the amino-terminal sequence as small as PTH(1–11) are sufficient to activate the major receptor (see below). The carboxyl-terminal region of PTH binds to a separate receptor (cPTH-R), but it has not yet been cloned. Fragments shortened at the amino terminus bind to cPTH-R and inhibit the actions of the full-length PTH(1–84) or the PTH(1–34) active fragments.

BIOSYNTHESIS, SECRETION, AND METABOLISM

Synthesis Parathyroid cells have multiple methods of adapting to increased needs for PTH production. Most rapid (within minutes) is secretion of preformed hormone in response to hypocalcemia. Second, within hours, PTH mRNA expression is induced by sustained hypocalcemia. Finally, protracted challenge leads within days to cellular replication to increase gland mass.

PTH is initially synthesized as a larger molecule (preproparathyroid hormone, consisting of 115 amino acids), which is then reduced in size by a second cleavage (proparathyroid hormone, 90 amino acids) before secretion as the 84-amino-acid peptide. In one kindred with hypoparathyroidism, a mutation in the preprotein region of the gene interferes with hormone transport and secretion.

Transcriptional suppression of the PTH gene by calcium is nearly maximal at physiologic calcium concentrations. Hypocalcemia increases transcriptional activity within hours. $1,25(OH)_2D_3$ strongly suppresses PTH gene transcription. In patients with renal failure, IV administration of supraphysiologic levels of $1,25(OH)_2D_3$ or analogues of the active metabolite can dramatically suppress PTH overproduction, which is sometimes difficult to control due to severe secondary HPT. Regulation of proteolytic destruction of preformed hormone (posttranslational regulation of hormone production) is an important mechanism for mediating rapid (minutes) changes in hormone availability. High calcium increases and low calcium inhibits the proteolytic destruction of hormone stores.

Regulation of PTH Secretion   PTH secretion increases steeply to a maximum value of five times the basal rate of secretion as calcium concentration falls from normal to the range of 1.9–2.0 mmol/L (7.5–8.0 mg/dL) (measured as total calcium). The ionized fraction of blood calcium is the important determinant of hormone secretion. Severe intracellular magnesium deficiency impairs PTH secretion (see below).

ECF calcium controls PTH secretion by interaction with a calcium sensor, a G protein–coupled receptor (GPCR) for which Ca^{2+} ions act as the ligand (see below). This receptor is a member of a distinctive subfamily of the GPCR superfamily that is characterized by a large extracellular domain suitable for "clamping" the small-molecule ligand. Stimulation of the receptor by high calcium levels suppresses PTH secretion. The receptor is present in parathyroid glands and the calcitonin-secreting cells (C cells) of the thyroid, as well as in other sites such as brain and kidney. Genetic evidence has revealed a key biologic role for the calcium-sensing receptor in parathyroid gland responsiveness to calcium and in renal calcium clearance. Point mutations associated with loss of function cause a syndrome FHH resembling hyperparathyroidism but with hypocalciuria. On the other hand, gain-of-function mutations cause a form of hypocalcemia resembling hypoparathyroidism (see below).

Metabolism   The secreted form of PTH is indistinguishable by immunologic criteria and by molecular size from the 84-amino-acid peptide (PTH 1–84) extracted from glands. However, much of the immunoreactive material found in the circulation is smaller than the extracted or secreted hormone. The principal circulating fragments of immunoreactive hormone lack a portion of the critical amino-terminal sequence required for biologic activity and, hence, are biologically inactive fragments (so-called middle- and carboxyl-terminal fragments). Much of the proteoly-

sis of hormone occurs in the liver and kidney. Peripheral metabolism of PTH does not appear to be regulated by physiologic states (high versus low calcium, etc.); hence peripheral metabolism of hormone, although responsible for rapid clearance of secreted hormone, appears to be a high-capacity, metabolically invariant catabolic process.

The rate of clearance of the secreted 84-amino-acid peptide from blood is more rapid than the rate of clearance of the biologically inactive fragment(s) corresponding to the middle- and carboxyl-terminal regions of PTH. Consequently, the interpretation of PTH immunoassays is influenced by the nature of the peptide fragments detected by the antibodies.

Although the problems inherent in PTH measurements have been largely circumvented by use of double-antibody assays that detect only the intact molecule, more recent evidence revealed larger PTH fragments that may affect the interpretation of most currently available double-antibody assays. Large amino-terminally truncated forms of PTH are present in normal and uremic individuals in addition to PTH(1–84). The concentration of these fragments relative to that of intact PTH(1–84) is higher with induced hypercalcemia than in eucalcemic or hypocalcemic conditions and is higher in patients with renal failure. These fragments have limited portions of the amino-terminal portion of the hormone degraded; PTH(7–84) has been identified as a major component of these amino-terminally truncated fragments. Growing evidence suggests that the PTH(7–84)-related amino-terminally truncated fragments can act as an inhibitor of PTH action and may be of clinical significance, particularly in renal failure. Efforts to prevent secondary HPT by a variety of measures (vitamin D analogues, higher calcium intake, and phosphate-lowering strategies) may have led to oversuppression of biologically active intact PTH since the amino-terminally truncated PTH reacts in many first-generation double-antibody PTH assays. The role, if any, of excessive PTH suppression due to inaccurate measurement of PTH in adynamic bone disease in renal failure (see below) is unknown. Newer assays with extreme amino-terminal epitopes that detect only full-length PTH(1–84) are being studied intensively.

PARATHYROID HORMONE–RELATED PROTEIN

The paracrine factor termed *PTHrP* is responsible for most instances of hypercalcemia of malignancy (Chap. 96), a syndrome that resembles HPT. Many different cell types produce PTHrP, including brain, pancreas, heart, lung, mammary tissue, placenta, endothelial cells, and smooth muscle. In fetal animals, PTHrP directs transplacental calcium transfer, and high concentrations of PTHrP are produced in mammary tissue and secreted into milk. Human and bovine milk contain very high concentrations of the hormone, the biologic significance of which is unknown. PTHrP may also play a role in uterine contraction and other biologic functions.

PTH and PTHrP, although distinctive products of different genes, exhibit considerable functional and structural homology (Fig. 347-1) and

FIGURE 347-1 Schematic diagram to illustrate similarities and differences in structure of human parathyroid hormone (PTH) and human PTH-related peptide (PTHrP). Close structural (and functional) homology exists between the first 30 amino acids of hPTH and hPTHrP. The PTHrP sequence may be ≥144 amino acid residues in length. PTH is only 84 residues long; after residue 30, there is little structural homology between the two. Dashed lines in the PTHrP sequence indicate identity; underlined residues, although different from those of PTH, still represent conservative changes (charge or polarity preserved). Eleven amino acids are identical, and a total of 21 of 30 are homologues.

may have evolved from a shared ancestral gene. The structure of the gene for human PTHrP, however, is more complex than that of PTH, containing multiple exons and multiple sites for alternate splicing patterns during formation of the mature mRNA. Protein products of 141, 139, and 173 amino acids are produced, and other molecular forms may result from tissue-specific degradation at accessible internal cleavage sites. The biologic roles of these various molecular species and the nature of the circulating forms of PTHrP are unclear. It is uncertain whether PTHrP circulates at any significant level in adults; as a paracrine factor, PTHrP may be produced, act, and be destroyed locally within tissues. In adults PTHrP appears to have little influence on calcium homeostasis, except in disease states, when large tumors, especially of the squamous cell type, lead to massive overproduction of the hormone.

PTH AND PTHRP HORMONE ACTION

Both PTH and PTHrP bind to and activate the PTH/PTHrP receptor. The 500-amino-acid PTH/PTHrP receptor (also known as the PTH-1 receptor, PTH1R) belongs to a subfamily of GPCRs that includes those for glucagon, secretin, and vasoactive intestinal peptide. The extracellular regions are involved in hormone binding, and the intracellular domains, after hormone activation, bind G protein subunits to transduce hormone signaling into cellular responses through stimulation of second messengers. A second receptor that binds PTH, originally termed the *PTH-2 receptor* (PTH2R), is expressed in brain, pancreas, and several other tissues. PTH1R responds equivalently to PTH and PTHrP, whereas PTH2R responds only to PTH. The endogenous ligand of this receptor is now believed to be a peptide distinct from PTH, a 39-amino-acid hypothalamic peptide (*tubular infundibular peptide*, TIP-39). PTH1R and PTH2R can be traced backward in evolutionary time to fish. Zebrafish PTH1R and PTH2R exhibit the same selective responses to PTH and PTHrP as do human PTH1R and PTH2R. The evolutionary conservation of structure and function suggests important biologic roles for these receptors, even in fish (which lack discrete parathyroid glands).

Studies using cloned PTH1R confirm that it can be coupled to more than one G protein and second-messenger kinase pathway, apparently explaining the multiplicity of pathways stimulated by PTH. Stimulation of protein kinases (A and C) and calcium transport channels is associated with a variety of hormone-specific tissue responses. These responses include inhibition of phosphate and bicarbonate transport, stimulation of calcium transport, and activation of renal 1α-hydroxylase in the kidney. The responses in bone include effects on collagen synthesis; increased alkaline phosphatase, ornithine decarboxylase, citrate decarboxylase, and glucose-6-phosphate dehydrogenase activities; DNA, protein, and phospholipid synthesis; and calcium and phosphate transport. Ultimately, these biochemical events lead to an integrated hormonal response in bone turnover and calcium homeostasis. PTH also activates Na^+/Ca^{2+} exchanges in renal distal tubular sites and stimulates translocation of preformed calcium transport channels, moving them from the interior to the apical surface to mediate increased tubular uptake of calcium. PTH-dependent stimulation of phosphate excretion (blocking reabsorption—the opposite effect from actions on calcium in the kidney) involves the sodium-dependent phosphate cotransporter, NPT-2, lowering its apical membrane content (and therefore function). Similar shifts may be involved in other renal tubular transport effects of PTH.

PTHrP exerts important developmental influences on fetal bone development and in adult physiology. A homozygous knockout of the PTHrP gene (or the gene for the PTH receptor) in mice causes a lethal deformity in which animals are born with severe skeletal deformities resembling chondrodysplasia (Fig. 347-2). The heterozygous PTHrP gene knockout animals display reduced mineral density consistent with osteoporosis. Experiments with these mouse models point to a hitherto unappreciated role of PTHrP as a paracrine/autocrine factor that modulates bone metabolism in adults as well as during bone development.

CALCITONIN (See also Chap. 345)

Calcitonin is a hypocalcemic peptide hormone that in several mammalian species acts as an antagonist to PTH. Calcitonin seems to be of

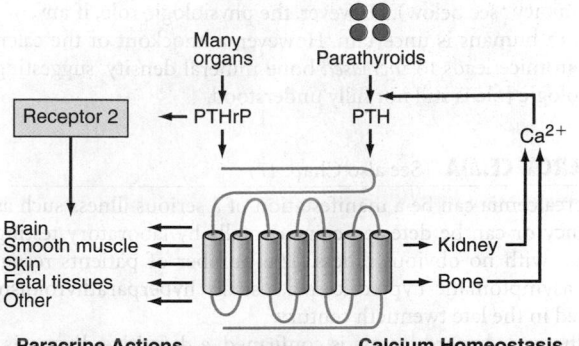

FIGURE 347-2 Dual role for the actions of the PTH/PTHrP receptor (PTH1R). Parathyroid hormone (PTH; endocrine-calcium homeostasis) and PTH-related peptide (PTHrP; paracrine–multiple tissue actions including growth plate cartilage in developing bone) use the single receptor for their disparate functions mediated by the amino-terminal 30 residues of either peptide. Other regions of both ligands interact with other receptors (not shown).

limited physiologic significance in humans, however, at least in calcium homeostasis. It is of medical significance because of its role as a tumor marker in sporadic and hereditary cases of medullary carcinoma and its medical use as an adjunctive treatment in severe hypercalcemia and in Paget's disease of bone.

The hypocalcemic activity of calcitonin is accounted for primarily by inhibition of osteoclast-mediated bone resorption and secondarily by stimulation of renal calcium clearance. These effects are mediated by receptors on osteoclasts and renal tubular cells. Calcitonin exerts additional effects through receptors present in brain, gastrointestinal tract, and the immune system. The hormone, for example, exerts analgesic effects directly on cells in the hypothalamus and related structures, possibly by interacting with receptors for related peptide hormones, such as calcitonin gene–related peptide (CGRP) or amylin. The latter ligands have specific high-affinity receptors and can also bind to and trigger calcitonin receptors. The calcitonin receptors are homologous in structure to PTH1R.

The thyroid is the major source of the hormone, and the cells involved in calcitonin synthesis arise from neural crest tissue. During embryogenesis, these cells migrate into the ultimobranchial body, derived from the last branchial pouch. In submammalian vertebrates, the ultimobranchial body constitutes a discrete organ, anatomically separate from the thyroid gland; in mammals, the ultimobranchial gland fuses with and is incorporated into the thyroid gland.

The naturally occurring calcitonins consist of a peptide chain of 32 amino acids. There is considerable sequence variability among species. Calcitonin from salmon, which is used therapeutically, is 10–100 times more potent than mammalian forms in lowering serum calcium.

There are two calcitonin genes, α and β; the transcriptional control of these genes is complex. Two different mRNA molecules are transcribed from the α gene; one is translated into the precursor for calcitonin, and the other message is translated into an alternative product, CGRP. CGRP is synthesized wherever the calcitonin mRNA is expressed, e.g., in medullary carcinoma of the thyroid. The β, or CGRP-2, gene is transcribed into the mRNA for CGRP in the central nervous system (CNS); this gene does not produce calcitonin, however. CGRP has cardiovascular actions and may serve as a neurotransmitter or play a developmental role in the CNS.

The circulating level of calcitonin in humans is lower than that in many other species. In humans, even extreme variations in calcitonin production do not change calcium and phosphate metabolism; no definite effects are attributable to calcitonin deficiency (totally thyroidectomized patients receiving only replacement thyroxine) or excess (patients with medullary carcinoma of the thyroid, a calcitonin-secreting tumor) (Chap. 345). Calcitonin has been a useful pharmacologic agent to suppress bone resorption in Paget's disease (Chap. 349) and osteoporosis (Chap. 348) and in the treatment of hypercalcemia of malignancy (see below). However, the physiologic role, if any, of calcitonin in humans is uncertain. However, a knockout of the calcitonin gene in mice leads to *increased* bone mineral density, suggesting that its biologic role is still not fully understood.

HYPERCALCEMIA (See also Chap. 47)

Hypercalcemia can be a manifestation of a serious illness such as malignancy or can be detected coincidentally by laboratory testing in a patient with no obvious illness. The number of patients recognized with asymptomatic hypercalcemia, usually hyperparathyroidism, increased in the late twentieth century.

Whenever hypercalcemia is confirmed, a definitive diagnosis must be established. Although hyperparathyroidism, a frequent cause of asymptomatic hypercalcemia, is a chronic disorder in which manifestations, if any, may be expressed only after months or years, hypercalcemia can also be the earliest manifestation of malignancy, the second most common cause of hypercalcemia in the adult. The causes of hypercalcemia are numerous (Table 347-1), but hyperparathyroidism and cancer account for 90% of cases.

Before undertaking a diagnostic workup, it is essential to be sure that true hypercalcemia, not a false-positive laboratory test, is present. A false-positive diagnosis of hypercalcemia is usually the result of inadvertent hemoconcentration during blood collection or elevation in serum proteins such as albumin. Hypercalcemia is a chronic problem, and it is cost-effective to obtain several serum calcium measurements; these tests need not be in the fasting state.

Clinical features are helpful in differential diagnosis. Hypercalcemia in an adult who is asymptomatic is usually due to primary hyperparathyroidism. In malignancy-associated hypercalcemia the disease is usually not occult; rather, symptoms of malignancy bring the patient to the physician, and hypercalcemia is discovered during the evaluation. In such patients the interval between detection of hypercalcemia and death, especially without vigorous treatment, is often <6 months. Accordingly, if an asymptomatic individual has had hypercalcemia or some manifestation of hypercalcemia, such as kidney stones, for >1 or 2 years, it is unlikely that malignancy is the cause. Nevertheless, differentiating primary hyperparathyroidism from *occult* malignancy can occasionally be difficult, and careful evaluation is required, particularly when the duration of the hypercalcemia is unknown. Hypercalcemia not due to hyperparathyroidism or malignancy can result from excessive vitamin D action, high bone turnover from any of several causes, or from renal failure (Table 347-1). Dietary history and a history of ingestion of vitamins or drugs are often helpful in diagnosing some of the less frequent causes.

TABLE 347-1 CLASSIFICATION OF CAUSES OF HYPERCALCEMIA

I. Parathyroid-related
   A. Primary hyperparathyroidism
      1. Solitary adenomas
      2. Multiple endocrine neoplasia
   B. Lithium therapy
   C. Familial hypocalciuric hypercalcemia
II. Malignancy-related
   A. Solid tumor with metastases (breast)
   B. Solid tumor with humoral mediation of hypercalcemia (lung, kidney)
   C. Hematologic malignancies (multiple myeloma, lymphoma, leukemia)
III. Vitamin D–related
   A. Vitamin D intoxication
   B. ↑ 1,25(OH)$_2$D; sarcoidosis and other granulomatous diseases
   C. Idiopathic hypercalcemia of infancy
IV. Associated with high bone turnover
   A. Hyperthyroidism
   B. Immobilization
   C. Thiazides
   D. Vitamin A intoxication
V. Associated with renal failure
   A. Severe secondary hyperparathyroidism
   B. Aluminum intoxication
   C. Milk-alkali syndrome

PTH immunoassays based on double-antibody methods serve as the principal laboratory test in differential diagnosis.

Hypercalcemia from any cause can result in fatigue, depression, mental confusion, anorexia, nausea, vomiting, constipation, reversible renal tubular defects, increased urination, a short QT interval in the electrocardiogram, and, in some patients, cardiac arrhythmias. There is a variable relation from one patient to the next between the severity of hypercalcemia and the symptoms. Generally, symptoms are more common at calcium levels >2.9–3 mmol/L (11.5–12.0 mg/dL), but some patients, even at this level, are asymptomatic. When the calcium level is >3.2 mmol/L (13 mg/dL), calcification in kidneys, skin, vessels, lungs, heart, and stomach occurs and renal insufficiency may develop, particularly if blood phosphate levels are normal or elevated due to impaired renal function. Severe hypercalcemia, usually defined as ≥3.7–4.5 mmol/L (15–18 mg/dL), can be a medical emergency; coma and cardiac arrest can occur.

Acute management of the hypercalcemia is usually successful. The type of treatment is based on the severity of the hypercalcemia and the nature of associated symptoms, as outlined below.

PRIMARY HYPERPARATHYROIDISM

Natural History and Incidence   Primary hyperparathyroidism is a generalized disorder of calcium, phosphate, and bone metabolism due to an increased secretion of PTH. The elevation of circulating hormone usually leads to hypercalcemia and hypophosphatemia. There is great variation in the manifestations. Patients may present with multiple signs and symptoms, including recurrent nephrolithiasis, peptic ulcers, mental changes, and, less frequently, extensive bone resorption. However, with greater awareness of the disease and wider use of multiphasic screening tests, including measurements of blood calcium, the diagnosis is frequently made in patients who have no symptoms and minimal, if any, signs of the disease other than hypercalcemia and elevated levels of PTH. The manifestations may be subtle, and the disease may have a benign course for many years or a lifetime. This milder form of the disease is usually termed *asymptomatic HPT*. Rarely, hyperparathyroidism develops or worsens abruptly and causes severe complications, such as marked dehydration and coma, so-called hypercalcemic parathyroid crisis.

The annual incidence of the disease is calculated to be as high as 0.2% in patients >60, with an estimated prevalence, including undiscovered asymptomatic patients, of ≥1%; some reports suggest the incidence may be declining. If confirmed, these changing estimates may reflect less frequent routine testing of serum calcium in recent years, earlier overestimates in incidence, or unknown factors. The disease has a peak incidence between the third and fifth decades but occurs in young children and in the elderly.

Etiology   Parathyroid tumors are most often encountered as an isolated adenomas without other endocrinopathy. They may also arise in hereditary syndromes, such as MEN syndromes. Parathyroid tumors may also arise as secondary to underlying disease (excessive stimulation in secondary hyperparathyroidism, especially chronic renal failure), or after other forms of excessive stimulation, such as lithium therapy. These etiologies are discussed below.

SOLITARY ADENOMAS   A single abnormal gland is the cause in ~80% of patients; the abnormality in the gland is usually a benign neoplasm or adenoma and rarely a parathyroid carcinoma. Some surgeons and pathologists report that the enlargement of multiple glands is common; double adenomas are reported. In ~15% of patients, all glands are hyperfunctioning; *chief cell parathyroid hyperplasia* is usually hereditary and frequently associated with other endocrine abnormalities.

HEREDITARY SYNDROMES AND MULTIPLE PARATHYROID TUMORS   Hereditary hyperparathyroidism can occur without other endocrine abnormalities but is usually part of a *multiple endocrine neoplasia* syndrome (Chap. 345). MEN 1 (Wermer's syndrome) consists of hyperparathyroidism and tumors of the pituitary and pancreas, often associated

FIGURE 347-3 A. Schematic diagram indicating molecular events in tumor susceptibility. The patient with the hereditary abnormality (multiple endocrine neoplasia, or MEN) is envisioned as having one defective gene inherited from the affected parent on chromosome 11, but one copy of the normal gene is present from the other parent. In the monoclonal tumor (benign tumor), a somatic event, here partial chromosomal deletion, removes the remaining normal gene from a cell. In nonhereditary tumors, two successive somatic mutations must occur, a process that takes a longer time. By either pathway, the cell, deprived of growth-regulating influence from this gene, has unregulated growth and becomes a tumor. A different genetic locus also involving loss of a tumor-suppressor gene termed HRPT2 is involved in the pathogenesis of parathyroid carcinoma. [*From A Arnold: J Clin Endocrine Metab 77(5):1108, 1993. Copyright 1993, The Endocrine Society.*] **B. Schematic illustration of the mechanism and consequences of gene rearrangement** and overexpression of the PRAD 1 protooncogene (pericentromeric inversion of chromosome 11) in parathyroid adenomas. The excessive expression of PRAD 1 (a cell cycle control protein, cyclin D_1) by the highly active PTH gene promoter in the parathyroid cell contributes to excess cellular proliferation. [*From J Habener et al, in L DeGroot, JL Jameson (eds): Endocrinology, 4th ed. Philadelphia, Saunders, 2001; with permission.*]

with gastric hypersecretion and peptic ulcer disease (Zollinger-Ellison syndrome). MEN 2A is characterized by pheochromocytoma and medullary carcinoma of the thyroid, as well as hyperparathyroidism; MEN 2B has additional associated features such as multiple neuromas but usually lacks hyperparathyroidism. Each of these MEN syndromes is transmitted in an apparent autosomal dominant manner, although, as noted below, the genetic basis of MEN 1 does not involve a dominant allele.

The *hyperparathyroidism jaw tumor* (HPT-JT) syndrome occurs in families with parathyroid tumors (sometimes carcinoma) in association with benign jaw tumors.

Some kindred exhibit hereditary hyperparathyroidism without other endocrinopathies. This disorder is often termed *nonsyndromic familial isolated hyperparathyroidism* (FIHP). There is speculation that these families may be examples of variable expression of the other syndromes, such as MEN 1, MEN 2, or the HPT-JT syndrome, but they may also have distinctive, still unidentified genetic causes.

Pathology Adenomas are most often located in the inferior parathyroid glands, but in 6–10% of patients, parathyroid adenomas may be located in the thymus, the thyroid, the pericardium, or behind the esophagus. Adenomas are usually 0.5–5 g in size but may be as large as 10–20 g (normal glands weigh 25 mg on average). Chief cells are predominant in both hyperplasia and adenoma. With chief cell hyperplasia, the enlargement may be so asymmetric that some involved glands appear grossly normal. If generalized hyperplasia is present, however, histologic examination reveals a uniform pattern of chief cells and disappearance of fat even in the absence of an increase in gland weight. Thus, microscopic examination of biopsy specimens of several glands is essential to interpret findings at surgery.

Parathyroid carcinoma is often not aggressive. Long-term survival without recurrence is common if at initial surgery the entire gland is removed without rupture of the capsule. Recurrent parathyroid carcinoma is usually slow-growing with local spread in the neck, and surgical

correction of recurrent disease may be feasible. Occasionally, however, parathyroid carcinoma is more aggressive, with distant metastases (lung, liver, and bone) found at the time of initial operation. It may be difficult to appreciate initially that a primary tumor is carcinoma; increased numbers of mitotic figures and increased fibrosis of the gland stroma may precede invasion. The diagnosis of carcinoma is often made in retrospect. Hyperparathyroidism from a parathyroid carcinoma may be indistinguishable from other forms of primary hyperparathyroidism but is usually more severe clinically. A potential clue to the diagnosis is offered by the degree of calcium elevation. Calcium values of 3.5–3.7 mmol/L (14–15 mg/dL) are frequent with carcinoma and may alert the surgeon to remove the abnormal gland with care to avoid capsular rupture. Recent findings concerning the genetic basis of parathyroid carcinoma (distinct from that of benign adenomas) indicate the need, in these kindreds, for family screening (see below).

GENETIC DEFECTS ASSOCIATED WITH HYPERPARATHYROIDISM As in many other types of neoplasia, two fundamental types of genetic defects have been identified in parathyroid gland tumors: (1) overactivity of protooncogenes, and (2) loss of function of tumor-suppressor genes. The former, by definition, can lead to uncontrolled cellular growth and function by activation (gain-of-function mutation) of a single allele of the responsible gene, whereas the latter requires loss of function of both allelic copies. Biallelic loss-of-function of a tumor-suppressor gene is usually characterized by a germ line defect (all cells) and an additional somatic deletion/mutation in the excised tumor (**Fig. 347-3**).

Mutations in the *MEN1* gene locus, encoding the protein MENIN, on chromosome 11q13 are responsible for causing MEN 1; the normal allele of this gene fits the definition of a tumor-suppressor gene. Inheritance of one mutated allele in this hereditary syndrome, followed by loss of the other allele via somatic cell mutation, leads to monoclonal expansion and tumor development. Also, in ~15–20% of sporadic parathyroid adenomas, both alleles of the *MEN1* locus on chromosome 11 are somatically deleted, implying that the same defect responsible for MEN 1 can also cause the sporadic disease (Fig. 347-3A). Consistent with the Knudson hypothesis for two-step neoplasia in certain inherited cancer syndromes (Chap. 79), the earlier onset of hyperparathyroidism in the hereditary syndromes reflects the need for only one mutational event to trigger the monoclonal outgrowth. In sporadic adenomas, typically occurring later in life, two different somatic events must occur before the MEN1 gene is silenced.

Other presumptive antioncogenes involved in hyperparathyroidism include a still unidentified gene mapped to chromosome 1p seen in 40% of sporadic parathyroid adenomas and a gene mapped to chromosome Xp11 in patients with secondary hyperparathyroidism and renal failure, who progressed to "tertiary" hyperparathyroidism, now known to reflect monoclonal outgrowths within previously hyperplastic glands.

A more complex pattern, still incompletely resolved, arises with genetic defects and carcinoma of the parathyroids seen in MEN 2. This appears to be due to biallelic loss of a functioning copy of a gene, HRPT2 (or CDC73), originally identified as the cause of the HPT-JT syndrome. Several inactivating mutations have been identified in HRPT2 (located on chromosome 1q25), which encodes a 531-amino acid protein called parafibromin. A protooncogene, RET, is mutated in all cases of MEN 2. With both types of genetically determined carcinoma syndromes (as with the loss of the MEN1 in parathyroid adenomas), the responsible genetic mutations in HRPT2 or RET appear to be necessary, but not sufficient, for the malignancies outlined below.

In general, the detection of additional genetic defects in these parathyroid tumor–related syndromes and the variations seen in phenotypic expression/penetrance indicate the multiplicity of the genetic factors responsible. Nonetheless, the ability to detect the presence of the major genetic contributors has greatly aided a more informed management of family members of patients identified in the hereditary syndromes such as MEN 1, MEN 2, and HPT-JT.

An important contribution from studies on the genetic origin of parathyroid carcinoma has been the realization that the mutations involve a different pathway than that involved with the benign gland enlargements. Unlike the pathogenesis of genetic alterations seen in colon cancer, where lesions evolve from benign adenomas to malignant disease by progressive genetic changes, the alterations commonly seen in most parathyroid cancers (HRPT2 mutations) are infrequently seen in sporadic parathyroid adenomas.

Abnormalities at the Rb gene were first noted in parathyroid cancer. The Rb gene, a tumor-suppressor gene located on chromosome 13q14, was initially associated with retinoblastoma but has since been implicated in other neoplasias, including parathyroid carcinoma. Early studies implicated allelic deletions of the Rb gene in many parathyroid carcinomas and decreased or absent expression of the Rb protein. However, because there are often large deletions in chromosome 13 that include many genes in addition to the Rb locus (with similar findings in some pituitary carcinomas), it remains possible that other tumor-suppressor genes on chromosome 13 may be playing a role in parathyroid carcinoma.

Study of the parathyroid cancers found in some patients with the HPT-JT syndrome has led to identification of a much larger role for mutations in the HRPT2 gene in most parathyroid carcinomas, including those that arise sporadically, without apparent association with the HPT-JT syndrome. Mutations in the coding region have been identified in 75–80% of all parathyroid cancers analyzed, leading to the conclusion that, with addition of presumed mutations in the noncoding regions, this genetic defect may be seen in essentially all parathyroid carcinomas. Of special importance was the discovery that, in some sporadic parathyroid cancers, germ-line mutations have been found; this, in turn, has led to careful investigation of the families of these patients and a new clinical indication for genetic testing in this setting.

Hypercalcemia occurring in family members (who are also found to have the germ-line mutations) can lead to the finding, at parathyroid surgery, of premalignant parathyroid tumors.

Overall, it seems there are multiple factors in parathyroid cancer, in addition to the HRPT2 gene, although the HRPT2 gene mutation is the most invariant abnormality. Deletions in the Rb gene locus may play an additional role in pathogenesis of parathyroid cancer, as well as other still uncharacterized genetic defects.

RET encodes a tyrosine kinase type receptor; specific inherited germ-line mutations lead to a constitutive activation of the receptor, thereby explaining the autosomal dominant mode of transmission and the relatively early onset of neoplasia. In the MEN 2 syndrome, the RET protooncogene may be responsible for the earliest disorder detected, the polyclonal disor-

der (C cell hyperplasia, which then is transformed into a clonal outgrowth—a medullary carcinoma with the participation of other, still uncharacterized genetic defects).

In some parathyroid adenomas, activation of a protooncogene has been identified (Fig. 347-3B). A reciprocal translocation involving chromosome 11 has been identified that juxtaposes the PTH gene promoter upstream of a gene product termed PRAD-1, encoding a cyclin D protein that plays a key role in normal cell division. This translocation plus other mechanisms that cause an equivalent overexpression of cyclin D1 are found in 20–40% of parathyroid adenomas

Mouse models have confirmed the role of several of the major identified genetic defects in parathyroid disease and the MEN syndromes. Loss of the MEN1 gene locus, or overexpression of the PRAD-1 protooncogene or the mutated RET protooncogene, have been analyzed by genetic manipulation in mice, with the expected onset of parathyroid tumors or medullary carcinoma, respectively.

Signs and Symptoms Half or more of patients with hyperparathyroidism are asymptomatic. In series in which patients are followed without operation, as many as 80% are classified as without symptoms. Manifestations of hyperparathyroidism involve primarily the kidneys and the skeletal system. Kidney involvement, due either to deposition of calcium in the renal parenchyma or to recurrent nephrolithiasis, was present in 60–70% of patients prior to 1970. With earlier detection, renal complications occur in <20% of patients in many large series. Renal stones are usually composed of either calcium oxalate or calcium phosphate. In occasional patients, repeated episodes of nephrolithiasis or the formation of large calculi may lead to urinary tract obstruction, infection, and loss of renal function. Nephrocalcinosis may also cause decreased renal function and phosphate retention.

The distinctive bone manifestation of hyperparathyroidism is *osteitis fibrosa cystica*, which occurred in 10–25% of patients in series reported 50 years ago. Histologically, the pathognomonic features are an increase in the giant multinucleated osteoclasts in scalloped areas on the surface of the bone (Howship's lacunae) and a replacement of the normal cellular and marrow elements by fibrous tissue. X-ray changes include resorption of the phalangeal tufts and replacement of the usually sharp cortical outline of the bone in the digits by an irregular outline (subperiosteal resorption). In recent years, osteitis fibrosa cystica is very rare in primary hyperparathyroidism, probably due to the earlier detection of the disease.

With the use of multiple markers of bone turnover, such as formation indices (bone-specific alkaline phosphatase, osteocalcin, and type I procollagen peptides) and bone resorption indices (including hydroxypyridinium collagen cross-links and telopeptides of type I collagen), increased skeletal turnover is detected in essentially all patients with established hyperparathyroidism.

Dual-energy x-ray absorptiometry (DEXA) of the spine provides reproducible quantitative estimates (within a few percent) of spinal bone density. Similarly, bone density in the extremities can be quantified by densitometry of the hip or of the distal radius at a site chosen to be primarily cortical. CT is a very sensitive technique for estimating spinal bone density, but reproducibility of standard CT is no better than 5%. Newer CT techniques (spiral, "extreme" CT) are more reproducible but are currently available in a limited number of medical centers. Cortical bone density is reduced while cancellous bone density, especially in the spine, is relatively preserved. Serial studies in patients who choose to be followed without surgery have indicated that in the majority of patients there is little further change over a number of years, consistent with laboratory data indicating relatively unchanged blood calcium and PTH levels. After an initial loss of bone mass in patients with mild asymptomatic hyperparathyroidism, a new equilibrium may be reached, with bone density and biochemical manifestations of the disease remaining relatively unchanged. However, some evidence suggests that there may be an increased fracture risk, including the spine, despite the relative preservation of spinal bone density; thus, some uncertainty about optimal management continues, even in asymptomatic patients (see below).

In symptomatic patients, dysfunctions of the CNS, peripheral nerve and muscle, gastrointestinal tract, and joints also occur. It has been reported that severe neuropsychiatric manifestations may be reversed by parathyroidectomy; it remains unclear, in the absence of controlled studies, whether this improvement has a defined cause-and-effect relationship. Generally, the fact that hyperparathyroidism is common in elderly patients, in whom there are often other problems, suggests the possibility that such coexisting problems as hypertension, renal deterioration, and depression may not be parathyroid-related and suggests caution in recommending parathyroid surgery as a cure for these manifestations.

When present, neuromuscular manifestations may include proximal muscle weakness, easy fatigability, and atrophy of muscles and may be so striking as to suggest a primary neuromuscular disorder. The distinguishing feature is the complete regression of neuromuscular disease after surgical correction of the hyperparathyroidism.

Gastrointestinal manifestations are sometimes subtle and include vague abdominal complaints and disorders of the stomach and pancreas. Again, cause and effect are unclear. In MEN 1 patients with hyperparathyroidism, duodenal ulcer may be the result of associated pancreatic tumors that secrete excessive quantities of gastrin (Zollinger-Ellison syndrome). Pancreatitis has been reported in association with hyperparathyroidism, but the incidence and the mechanism are not established.

In reports from European centers, the frequency of pathophysiologic deterioration, especially cardiovascular (as well as other systems), is more frequent than the U.S. experience with milder disease. The differences are not fully explained, but greater severity at initial diagnosis (fewer cases determined by routine screening) and vitamin D deficiency are possible explanations for the different manifestations of disease.

DIAGNOSIS

The diagnosis is typically made by detecting an elevated immunoreactive PTH level in a patient with asymptomatic hypercalcemia (see "Differential Diagnosis: Special Tests," below). Serum phosphate is usually low but may be normal, especially if renal failure has developed.

Many tests based on renal responses to excess PTH (renal calcium and phosphate clearance; blood phosphate, chloride, magnesium; urinary or nephrogenous cyclic AMP) were used in earlier decades. These tests have low specificity for hyperparathyroidism and are therefore not cost-effective; they have been replaced by PTH immunoassays combined with simultaneous blood calcium measurements (Fig. 347-4).

℞ HYPERPARATHYROIDISM

MEDICAL SURVEILLANCE VERSUS SURGICAL TREATMENT

The critical management question is whether the disease should be treated surgically. If severe hypercalcemia [3.7–4.5 mmol/L (15–18 mg/dL)] is present, surgery is mandatory as soon as the diagnosis can be confirmed by a PTH immunoassay. However, in most patients with hyperparathyroidism, hypercalcemia is mild and does not require urgent surgical or medical treatment.

The National Institutes of Health (NIH) held a Consensus Conference on Management of Asymptomatic Hyperparathyroidism in 1990. *Asymptomatic hyperparathyroidism* was defined as documented (presumptive) hyperparathyroidism without signs or symptoms attributable to the disease. The consensus was that patients <50 should undergo surgery, given the long surveillance that would be required. Other considerations that favored surgery included concern that consistent follow-up would be unlikely or that coexistent illness would complicate management. Patients >50 were deemed appropriate for medical monitoring if certain criteria were met, the patients wished to avoid surgery, or the guidelines for recommending surgery were not present (Table 347-2). Careful evaluation of patients over the subsequent 12 years provided reassurance that in some patients medical monitoring rather than surgery was still prudent yet promoted new questions about the natural history of the disease with or without surgery.

Data developed since the Consensus Conference indicated that a subgroup of patients had selective vertebral osteopenia out of proportion to bone loss at other sites and responded to surgery with striking restoration

FIGURE 347-4 Levels of immunoreactive parathyroid hormone (PTH) detected in patients with primary hyperparathyroidism, hypercalcemia of malignancy, and hypoparathyroidism. Boxed area represents the upper and normal limits of blood calcium and/or immunoreactive PTH. [*From SR Nussbaum, JT Potts, Jr, in L DeGroot, JL Jameson (eds): Endocrinology, 4th ed. Philadelphia, Saunders, 2001; with permission.*]

of bone mass (average >20%). Given reports of increased fracture risk by some centers, plus the advent of newer medical therapies and less invasive surgical procedures, the NIH convened a Workshop on Asymptomatic Hyperparathyroidism in 2002, and an independent (non-NIH) panel offered a revised set of recommendations. The changes reflect both practical considerations (such as the difficulty in creatinine clearance measurements and therefore substituting calculations based on serum creatinine) and concerns regarding potential deleterious skeletal effects in untreated patients (Tables 347-2 and 347-3). Accordingly, indications for surgical intervention were lowered (i.e., stricter serum calcium and bone density criteria). As before, it was emphasized that asymptomatic patients should be monitored regularly and that surgical correction of hyperparathyroidism can always be undertaken when indicated, if medically feasible, since the success rate is high (>90%), mortality is low, and morbidity is minimal. The goals of monitoring are early detection of worsening hypercalcemia, deteriorating bone or renal status, or other complications of hyperparathyroidism. No specific recommendations about medical therapy were made, but early data showed the promise of the newer agents, with the prediction that they would be used in future clinical practice to increase bone mass in patients not electing surgery as further experience is gained. Neither panel recommended estrogen use in patients for whom surgery was not elected because there was insufficient cumulative experience with such therapy to balance theoretical risks (breast and endometrial cancer)

TABLE 347-2	**GUIDELINES FOR PARATHYROID SURGERY IN ASYMPTOMATIC PRIMARY HYPERPARATHYROIDISM**[a]	
Measurement	**Guidelines, 1990**	**Guidelines, 2002**
Serum calcium (above upper limit of normal)	0.3–0.4 mmol/L (1–1.5 mg/dL) above normal	0.3 mmol/L (1.0 mg/dL) above normal
24-h urinary calcium	>400 mg	>400 mg
Creatinine clearance	Reduced by 30%	Reduced by 30%
Bone mineral density	Z-score <−2.0 (forearm)	T-score <−2.5 at any site
Age	<50	<50

[a]Surgery is also indicated in patients for whom medical surveillance is neither desired nor possible.

Source: From JP Bilezikian et al: J Clin Endocrinol Metab 87:5353, 2002.

TABLE 347-3 MANAGEMENT GUIDELINES FOR PATIENTS WITH ASYMPTOMATIC PRIMARY HYPERPARATHYROIDISM WHO DO NOT UNDERGO PARATHYROID SURGERY

Measurement	Older Guidelines	New Guidelines
Serum calcium	Biannually	Biannually
24-h urinary calcium	Annually	Not recommended[a]
Creatinine clearance	Annually	Not recommended[a]
Serum creatinine	Annually	Annually[b]
Bone density	Annually (forearm)	Annually (lumbar spine, hip, forearm)
Abdominal x-ray (+/− ultrasound)	Annually	Not recommended[a]

[a]Except at the time of initial evaluation.

[b]If the serum creatinine concentration suggests a change in the creatinine clearance when the Cockroft-Gault equation is applied, further, more direct assessments of the creatinine clearance are recommended.

Source: From JP Bilezikian et al: J Clin Endocrinol Metab 87:5353, 2002.

versus benefits. Raloxifene (Evista), the first of the SERMS, has been shown to have many of the bone-protective effects of estrogen in osteoporotic subjects yet at the same time lowers the incidence of breast cancer; preliminary use of this agent in a small series of hyperparathyroid patients led to increased bone density. As much as 5% increase in bone mineral density in the spine and hip was reported with alendronate use in asymptomatic patients. Experience with calcimimetics, drugs that selectively stimulate the calcium sensor and suppress PTH secretion, indicates that these agents decrease calcium levels to normal over 2 years of continuous use. Effects on PTH are less marked but significant.

SURGICAL TREATMENT Parathyroid exploration is challenging and should be undertaken by an experienced surgeon. Certain features help in predicting the pathology (e.g., multiple abnormal glands in familial cases). However, some critical decisions regarding management can be made only during the operation.

Increasingly, minimally invasive surgical procedures are being practiced. With conventional surgery, one approach is still based on the view that typically only one gland (the adenoma) is abnormal. If an enlarged gland is found, a normal gland should be sought. In this view, if a biopsy of a normal-sized second gland confirms its histologic (and presumed functional) normality, no further exploration, biopsy, or excision is needed. At the other extreme is the minority viewpoint that all four glands be sought and that most of the total parathyroid tissue mass should be removed. The concern with the former approach is that the recurrence rate of hyperparathyroidism may be high if a second abnormal gland is missed; the latter approach could involve unnecessary surgery and an unacceptable rate of hypoparathyroidism. When normal glands are found in association with one enlarged gland, excision of the single adenoma usually leads to cure or at least years free of symptoms. Long-term follow-up studies to establish true rates of recurrence are limited.

Recently, there has been growing experience with new surgical strategies that feature a minimally invasive approach guided by improved preoperative localization and intraoperative monitoring by PTH assays. Preoperative ^{99m}Tc sestamibi scans with single photon emission CT (SPECT) are used to predict the location of an abnormal gland and intraoperative sampling of PTH before and at 5-min intervals after removal of a suspected adenoma to confirm a rapid fall (>50%) to normal levels of PTH. In several centers, a combination of preoperative sestamibi imaging, cervical block anesthesia, minimal surgical incision, and intraoperative PTH measurements has allowed successful outpatient surgical management with a clear-cut cost benefit compared to general anesthesia and more extensive neck surgery. The use of these minimally invasive approaches requires clinical judgment to select patients unlikely to have multiple gland disease (e.g., MEN or secondary hyperparathyroidism). The growing acceptance of the technique and its relative ease for the patient has lowered the threshold for surgery.

Usually the severity of the hypercalcemia provides a preoperative clue to parathyroid carcinoma. In such cases, when neck exploration is undertaken, the tissue should be widely excised; care is taken to avoid rupture of the capsule to prevent local seeding of tumor cells.

Multiple gland hyperplasia, as predicted in familial cases, poses more difficult questions of surgical management. Once a diagnosis of hyperpla-

sia is established, all the glands must be identified. Two schemes have been proposed for surgical management. One is to totally remove three glands with partial excision of the fourth gland; care is taken to leave a good blood supply for the remaining gland. Other surgeons advocate total parathyroidectomy with immediate transplantation of a portion of a removed, minced parathyroid gland into the muscles of the forearm, with the view that surgical excision is easier from the ectopic site in the arm if there is recurrent hyperfunction.

In a minority of cases, if no abnormal parathyroid glands are found in the neck, the issue of further exploration must be decided. There are documented cases of five or six parathyroid glands and of unusual locations for adenomas, such as in the mediastinum.

When a second parathyroid exploration is indicated, the minimally invasive techniques for preoperative localization such as ultrasound, CT scan, and isotope scanning are combined with venous sampling and/or selective digital arteriography in one of the centers specializing in these procedures. Intraoperative monitoring of PTH levels by rapid PTH immunoassays may be useful in guiding the surgery. At one center, long-term cures have been achieved with selective embolization or injection of large amounts of contrast material into the end-arterial circulation feeding the parathyroid tumor.

A decline in serum calcium occurs within 24 h after successful surgery; usually blood calcium falls to low-normal values for 3–5 days until the remaining parathyroid tissue resumes full hormone secretion. Acute postoperative hypocalcemia is likely only if severe bone mineral deficits are present or if injury to all the normal parathyroid glands occurs during surgery. In general, there are few problems encountered in patients with uncomplicated disease such as a single adenoma (the clear majority), who do not have symptomatic bone disease nor a large deficit in bone mineral, who are vitamin D and magnesium sufficient, and who have good renal and gastrointestinal function. The extent of postoperative hypocalcemia varies with the surgical approach. If all glands are biopsied, hypocalcemia may be transiently symptomatic and more prolonged. Hypocalcemia is more likely to be symptomatic after second parathyroid explorations, particularly when normal parathyroid tissue was removed at the initial operation and when the manipulation and/or biopsy of the remaining normal glands is more extensive in the search for the missing adenoma.

Patients with hyperparathyroidism have efficient intestinal calcium absorption due to the increased levels of 1,25(OH)$_2$D stimulated by PTH excess. Once hypocalcemia signifies successful surgery, patients can be put on a high-calcium intake or be given oral calcium supplements. Despite mild hypocalcemia, most patients do not require parenteral therapy. If the serum calcium falls to <2 mmol/L (8 mg/dL), *and if the phosphate level rises simultaneously*, the possibility that surgery has caused hypoparathyroidism must be considered. With unexpected hypocalcemia, coexistent hypomagnesemia should be considered, as it interferes with PTH secretion and causes functional hypoparathyroidism (Chap. 346).

Signs of hypocalcemia include symptoms such as muscle twitching, a general sense of anxiety, and positive Chvostek and Trousseau signs coupled with serum calcium consistently <2 mmol/L (8 mg/dL). Parenteral calcium replacement at a low level should be instituted when hypocalcemia is symptomatic. The rate and duration of IV therapy are determined by the severity of the symptoms and the response of the serum calcium to treatment. An infusion of 0.5–2 (mg/kg)/h or 30–100 mL/h of a 1-mg/mL solution usually suffices to relieve symptoms. Usually, parenteral therapy is required for only a few days. If symptoms worsen or if parenteral calcium is needed for >2–3 days, therapy with a vitamin D analogue and/or oral calcium (2–4 g/d) should be started (see below). It is cost-effective to use calcitriol (doses of 0.5–1.0 μg/d) because of the rapidity of onset of effect and prompt cessation of action when stopped, in comparison to other forms of vitamin D. A rise in blood calcium after several months of vitamin D replacement may indicate restoration of parathyroid function to normal. It is also appropriate to monitor serum PTH serially to estimate gland function in such patients.

If magnesium deficiency was present, it can complicate the postoperative course. Magnesium deficiency impairs the secretion of PTH, and so hypomagnesemia should be corrected whenever detected. Magnesium replacement can be effective orally (e.g., MgCl$_2$, MgOH$_2$), but parenteral repletion is usual to ensure postoperative recovery, if magnesium deficiency is suspected due to low blood magnesium levels. Because the depressant effect of magnesium on central and peripheral nerve functions does not occur at levels <2 mmol/L (normal range 0.8–1.2 mmol/L), parenteral re-

FIGURE 347-5 Mutations in the calcium sensor receptor. The extracellular domain binds calcium, leading to conformational changes that stimulate Gq-coupled activation of the phospholipase C and suppression of PTH. The identified sequence alterations (X) cause loss of function and lead to inadequate suppression of parathyroid hormone release and, therefore, mild hypercalcemia (FHH). *, a gain-of-function mutation that causes hypocalcemia; •, conserved residues; ▲, acidic residues. (*From EM Brown et al: J Nutr 125:1965S, 1995; with permission.*)

placement can be given rapidly. A cumulative dose as great as 0.5–1 mmol/kg of body weight can be administered if severe hypomagnesemia is present; often, however, total doses of 20–40 mmol are sufficient.

OTHER PARATHYROID-RELATED CAUSES OF HYPERCALCEMIA

Lithium Therapy Lithium, used in the management of bipolar depression and other psychiatric disorders, causes hypercalcemia in ~10% of treated patients. The hypercalcemia is dependent on continued lithium treatment, remitting and recurring when lithium is stopped and restarted. The parathyroid adenomas reported in some hypercalcemic patients with lithium therapy may reflect the presence of an independently occurring parathyroid tumor; a permanent effect of lithium on parathyroid gland growth need not be implicated as most patients have complete reversal of hypercalcemia when lithium is stopped. However, long-standing stimulation of parathyroid cell replication by lithium may predispose to development of adenomas (as is documented in secondary hyperparathyroidism and renal failure).

At the levels achieved in blood in treated patients, lithium can be shown in vitro to shift the PTH secretion curve to the right in response to calcium; i.e., higher calcium levels are required to lower PTH secretion, probably acting at the calcium sensor (see below); this effect can cause elevated PTH levels and consequent hypercalcemia in otherwise normal individuals. Fortunately, there are usually alternative medications for the underlying psychiatric illness. Parathyroid surgery should not be recommended unless hypercalcemia and elevated PTH levels persist after lithium is discontinued.

GENETIC DISORDERS CAUSING HYPERPARATHYROID-LIKE SYNDROMES

Familial Hypocalciuric Hypercalcemia FHH (also called *familial benign hypercalcemia*) is inherited as an autosomal dominant trait. Affected individuals are discovered because of asymptomatic hypercalcemia. This disorder and Jansen's disease (discussed below) are variants of hyperparathyroidism. FHH involves excessive secretion of PTH, whereas Jans-

en's disease is caused by excessive biologic activity of the PTH receptor in target tissues. Neither disorder, however, involves a primary growth disorder of the parathyroids.

The pathophysiology of FHH is now understood. The primary defect is abnormal sensing of the blood calcium by the parathyroid gland and renal tubule, causing inappropriate secretion of PTH and excessive renal reabsorption of calcium. The calcium sensor is a member of the third family of GPCRs (type C, or III). The receptor responds to the ECF calcium concentration, suppressing PTH secretion through second messenger signaling, thereby providing negative-feedback regulation of PTH secretion. Many different mutations in the calcium-sensing receptor have been identified in patients with FHH (Fig. 347-5). These mutations lower the capacity of the sensor to bind calcium, and the mutant receptors function as though blood calcium levels were low; excessive secretion of PTH occurs from an otherwise normal gland. Approximately two-thirds of patients with FHH have mutations within the protein-coding region of the gene. The remaining one-third of kindreds may have mutations in the gene promoter or may involve still unknown mechanisms in other regions of the genome identified through mapping studies (e.g., chromosome 19).

Even before elucidation of the pathophysiology of FHH, abundant clinical evidence served to separate the disorder from primary hyperparathyroidism; these clinical features are still useful in differential diagnosis. Patients with primary hyperparathyroidism have <99% renal calcium reabsorption, whereas most patients with FHH have >99% reabsorption. The hypercalcemia in FHH is often detectable in affected members of the kindreds in the first decade of life, whereas hypercalcemia rarely occurs in patients with primary hyperparathyroidism or the MEN syndromes who are <10. PTH may be elevated in FHH, but the values are usually normal or lower for the same degree of calcium elevation than in patients with primary hyperparathyroidism. Parathyroid surgery performed in a few patients with FHH before the nature of the syndrome was understood led to permanent hypoparathyroidism; nevertheless, hypocalciuria persisted, establishing that hypocalciuria is not PTH-dependent (now known to be due to the abnormal calcium sensor in the kidney).

Few clinical signs or symptoms are present in patients with FHH, and other endocrine abnormalities are not present. Most patients are detected as a result of family screening after hypercalcemia is detected in a proband. In those patients inadvertently operated upon, the parathyroids appeared normal or moderately hyperplastic. Parathyroid surgery is not appropriate, nor, in view of the lack of symptoms, does medical treatment seem needed to lower the calcium. Calcimimetic agents that bind to the calcium sensor and elevate the set point are under investigation.

One striking exception to the rule against parathyroid surgery in this syndrome is the occurrence, usually in consanguineous marriages (due to the rarity of the gene mutation), of a homozygous or compound heterozygote state, resulting in complete loss of the calcium sensor function. In this condition, neonatal severe hypercalcemia, total parathyroidectomy is mandatory. Rare but well-documented cases of acquired hypocalciuric hypercalcemia are reported due to antibodies against the calcium sensor. They appear to be a complication of an underlying autoimmune disorder and respond to therapies directed against the underlying disorder.

Jansen's Disease Mutations in the PTH1R have been identified as responsible for this rare autosomal dominant syndrome. Because the mutations lead to constitutive receptor function, one abnormal copy of the mutant receptor is sufficient to cause the disease, thereby accounting for its dominant mode of transmission. The disorder leads to short-limbed dwarfism due to abnormal regulation of the bone growth plate. In adult life, there are numerous abnormalities in bone, including multiple cystic resorptive areas resembling those seen in severe hyperparathyroidism. Hypercalcemia and hypophosphatemia with undetectable or low PTH levels are typically seen. The pathogenesis of the disease has been confirmed by transgenic experiments in which targeted expression of the mutant receptor to the growth plate emulated several features of the disorder.

MALIGNANCY-RELATED HYPERCALCEMIA

Clinical Syndromes and Mechanisms of Hypercalcemia Hypercalcemia due to malignancy is common (occurring in as many as 20% of cancer patients, especially with certain types of tumor, such as lung carcinoma), often severe and difficult to manage, and on rare occasions, difficult to distinguish from primary hyperparathyroidism. Although malignancy is often clinically obvious or readily detectable by medical history, hypercalcemia can occasionally be due to an occult tumor. Previously, hypercalcemia associated with malignancy was thought to be due to local invasion and destruction of bone by tumor cells; many cases are now known to result from the elaboration by the malignant cells of humoral mediators of hypercalcemia. PTHrP is the responsible humoral agent in most solid tumors that cause hypercalcemia.

The histologic character of the tumor is more important than the extent of skeletal metastases in predicting hypercalcemia. Small-cell carcinoma (oat cell) and adenocarcinoma of the lung, although the most common lung tumors associated with skeletal metastases, rarely cause hypercalcemia. By contrast, many patients with squamous cell carcinoma of the lung develop hypercalcemia. Histologic studies of bone in patients with squamous cell or epidermoid carcinoma of the lung, in sites invaded by tumor as well as areas remote from tumor invasion, reveal increased bone resorption.

Two main mechanisms of hypercalcemia are operative in cancer hypercalcemia. Many solid tumors associated with hypercalcemia, particularly squamous cell and renal tumors, produce and secrete PTHrP that causes increased bone resorption and mediate the hypercalcemia through systemic actions on the skeleton. Alternatively, direct bone marrow invasion occurs with hematologic malignancies such as leukemia, lymphoma, and multiple myeloma. Lymphokines and cytokines (including PTHrP) produced by cells involved in the marrow response to the tumors promote resorption of bone through local destruction. Several hormones, hormone analogues, cytokines, and growth factors have been implicated as the result of clinical assays, in vitro tests, or chemical isolation. The etiologic factor produced by activated normal lymphocytes and by myeloma and lymphoma cells, originally termed *osteoclast activation factor*, now appears to represent the biologic action of several different cytokines, probably interleukin 1 and lymphotoxin or tumor necrosis factor. In some lymphomas, there is a third mechanism, caused by an increased blood level of $1,25(OH)_2D$, produced by the abnormal lymphocytes.

In the more common mechanism, usually termed *humoral hypercalcemia of malignancy*, solid tumors (cancers of the lung and kidney, in particular), in which bone metastases are absent, minimal, or not detectable clinically, secrete PTHrP measurable by immunoassay. Secretion by the tumors of the PTH-like factor, PTHrP, activates the PTH1R, resulting in a pathophysiology closely resembling hyperparathyroidism. The clinical picture resembles primary hyperparathyroidism (hypophosphatemia accompanies hypercalcemia), and elimination or regression of the primary tumor leads to disappearance of the hypercalcemia.

As in hyperparathyroidism, patients with the humoral hypercalcemia of malignancy have elevated urinary nephrogenous cyclic AMP excretion, hypophosphatemia, and increased urinary phosphate clearance. However, in humoral hypercalcemia of malignancy, immunoreactive PTH is undetectable or suppressed, making the differential diagnosis easier. Other features of the disorder differ from those of true hyperparathyroidism. The biologic actions of PTH and PTHrP are exerted through the same receptor, but subtle differences in responses must account for the discordance. Other cytokines elaborated by the malignancy may contribute to the variations from hyperparathyroidism in these patients. Patients may have low to normal levels of $1,25(OH)_2D$ instead of elevated levels as in true hyperparathyroidism. In some patients with the humoral hypercalcemia of malignancy, osteoclastic resorption is unaccompanied by an osteoblastic or bone-forming response, implying inhibition of the normal coupling of bone formation and resorption.

Several different assays (single- or double-antibody, different epitopes) have been developed to detect PTHrP. Most data indicate that circulating PTHrP levels are undetectable (or low) in normal individuals, elevated in most cancer patients with the humoral syndrome, and high in human milk. The etiologic mechanisms in cancer hypercalcemia may be multiple in the same patient. For example, in breast carcinoma (metastatic to bone) and in a distinctive type of T cell lymphoma/leukemia initiated by human T cell lymphotropic virus I, hypercalcemia is caused by direct local lysis of bone as well as by a humoral mechanism involving excess production of PTHrP. Hyperparathyroidism has been reported to coexist with the humoral cancer syndrome and, rarely, ectopic hyperparathyroidism due to tumor elaboration of true PTH is reported.

Diagnostic Issues Levels of PTH measured by the double-antibody technique are undetectable or extremely low in tumor hypercalcemia, as would be expected with the mediation of the hypercalcemia by a factor other than PTH (the hypercalcemia suppresses the normal parathyroid glands). In a patient with minimal symptoms referred for hypercalcemia, low or undetectable PTH levels would focus attention on a possible occult malignancy.

Ordinarily, the diagnosis of cancer hypercalcemia is not difficult because tumor symptoms are prominent when hypercalcemia is detected. Indeed, hypercalcemia may be noted incidentally during the workup of a patient with known or suspected malignancy. Clinical suspicion that malignancy is the cause of the hypercalcemia is heightened when there are other paraneoplastic signs or symptoms, such as weight loss, fatigue, muscle weakness, or unexplained skin rash, or when symptoms specific for a particular tumor are present. Squamous cell tumors are most frequently associated with hypercalcemia, particularly tumors of the lung, kidney, head and neck, and urogenital tract. Radiologic examinations can focus on these areas when clinical evidence is unclear. Bone scans with technetium-labeled bisphosphonate are useful for detection of osteolytic metastases; the sensitivity is high, but specificity is low; results must be confirmed by conventional x-rays to be certain that areas of increased uptake are due to osteolytic metastases per se. Bone marrow biopsies are helpful in patients with anemia or abnormal peripheral blood smears.

℞ MALIGNANCY-RELATED HYPERCALCEMIA

Treatment of the hypercalcemia of malignancy is first directed to control of tumor; reduction of tumor mass usually corrects hypercalcemia. If a patient has severe hypercalcemia yet has a good chance for effective tumor therapy, treatment of the hypercalcemia should be vigorous while awaiting the results of definitive therapy. If hypercalcemia occurs in the late stages of a tumor that is resistant to anti-tumor therapy, the treatment of the hypercalcemia should be judicious as high calcium levels can have a mild sedating effect. Standard therapies for hypercalcemia (discussed below) are applicable to patients with malignancy.

VITAMIN D–RELATED HYPERCALCEMIA

Hypercalcemia caused by vitamin D can be due to excessive ingestion or abnormal metabolism of the vitamin. Abnormal metabolism of the vitamin is usually acquired in association with a widespread granulomatous disorder. Vitamin D metabolism is carefully regulated, particularly the activity of renal 1α-hydroxylase, the enzyme responsible for the production of $1,25(OH)_2D$ (Chap. 346). The regulation of 1α-hydroxylase and the normal feedback suppression by $1,25(OH)_2D$ seem to work less well in infants than in adults and to operate poorly, if at all, in sites other than the renal tubule; these phenomena explain the occurrence of hypercalcemia secondary to excessive $1,25(OH)_2D_3$ production in infants with Williams' syndrome (see below) and in adults with sarcoidosis or lymphoma.

Vitamin D Intoxication Chronic ingestion of 40–100 times the normal physiologic requirement of vitamin D (amounts >40,000–100,000 U/d) is usually required to produce significant hypercalcemia in normal individuals. Nonetheless, an upper limit of dietary intake of 2000 U/d (50 μg/d) in adults is now recommended because of concerns about potential toxic effects of cumulative supraphysiologic doses. Vitamin D excess increases intestinal calcium absorption and, if severe, also increases bone resorption.

Hypercalcemia in vitamin D intoxication is due to an excessive biologic action of the vitamin, perhaps the consequence of increased levels of $25(OH)D$ rather than merely increased levels of the active metabolite $1,25(OH)_2D$ (the latter may not be elevated in vitamin D intoxication). $25(OH)D$ has definite, if low, biologic activity in intestine and bone. The production of $25(OH)D$ is less tightly regulated than is the production of $1,25(OH)_2D$. Hence concentrations of $25(OH)D$ are elevated severalfold in patients with excess vitamin D intake.

The diagnosis is substantiated by documenting elevated levels of $25(OH)D$. Hypercalcemia is usually controlled by restriction of dietary calcium intake and appropriate attention to hydration. These measures, plus discontinuation of vitamin D, usually lead to resolution of hypercalcemia. However, vitamin D stores in fat may be substantial, and vitamin D intoxication may persist for weeks after vitamin D ingestion is terminated. Such patients are responsive to glucocorticoids, which in doses of 100 mg/d of hydrocortisone or its equivalent, usually return serum calcium levels to normal over several days; severe intoxication may require intensive therapy.

Sarcoidosis and Other Granulomatous Diseases In patients with sarcoidosis and other granulomatous diseases, such as tuberculosis and fungal infections, excess $1,25(OH)_2D$ is synthesized in macrophages or other cells in the granulomas. Indeed, increased $1,25(OH)_2D$ levels have been reported in anephric patients with sarcoidosis and hypercalcemia. Macrophages obtained from granulomatous tissue convert $25(OH)D$ to $1,25(OH)_2D$ at an increased rate. There is a positive correlation in patients with sarcoidosis between $25(OH)D$ levels (reflecting vitamin D intake) and the circulating concentrations of $1,25(OH)_2D$, whereas normally there is no increase in $1,25(OH)_2D$ with increasing $25(OH)D$ levels due to multiple feedback controls on renal 1-hydroxylase (Chap. 346). The usual regulation of active metabolite production by calcium phosphate or PTH does not operate in these patients. Clearance of $1,25(OH)_2D$ from blood may be decreased in sarcoidosis as well. PTH levels are usually low and $1,25(OH)_2D$ levels are elevated, but primary hyperparathyroidism and sarcoidosis may coexist in some patients.

Management of the hypercalcemia can often be accomplished by avoiding excessive sunlight exposure and limiting vitamin D and calcium intake. Presumably, however, the abnormal sensitivity to vitamin D and abnormal regulation of $1,25(OH)_2D$ synthesis will persist as long as the disease is active. Alternatively, glucocorticoids in the equivalent of ≤100 mg/d of hydrocortisone control hypercalcemia. Glucocorticoids appear to act by blocking excessive production of $1,25(OH)_2D$ as well as the response to it in target organs.

Idiopathic Hypercalcemia of Infancy This rare disorder, usually referred to as *Williams syndrome*, is an autosomal dominant disorder characterized by multiple congenital development defects, including supravalvular aortic stenosis, mental retardation, and an elfin facies, in association with hypercalcemia due to abnormal sensitivity to vitamin D. The syndrome was first recognized in England after the fortification of milk with vitamin D. Levels of $1,25(OH)_2D$ are elevated, ranging from 46–120 nmol/L (150–500 pg/mL). The mechanism of the abnormal sensitivity to vitamin D and of the increased circulating levels of $1,25(OH)_2D$ is still unclear. Studies suggest that genetic mutations involving microdeletions at the elastin locus and perhaps other genes on chromosome 7 may play a role in the pathogenesis.

HYPERCALCEMIA ASSOCIATED WITH HIGH BONE TURNOVER

Hyperthyroidism As many as 20% of hyperthyroid patients have high-normal or mildly elevated serum calcium concentrations; hypercalciuria is even more common. The hypercalcemia is due to increased bone turnover, with bone resorption exceeding bone formation. Severe calcium elevations are not typical, and the presence of such suggests a concomitant disease such as hyperparathyroidism. Usually, the diagnosis is obvious, but signs of hyperthyroidism may occasionally be occult, particularly in the elderly (Chap. 335). Hypercalcemia is managed by treatment of the hyperthyroidism. Reports that thyroid-stimulating hormone (TSH) itself normally has a bone protective effect suggest that suppressed TSH levels also play a role in hypercalcemia.

Immobilization Immobilization is a rare cause of hypercalcemia in adults in the absence of an associated disease but may cause hypercalcemia in children and adolescents, particularly after spinal cord injury and paraplegia or quadriplegia. With resumption of ambulation, the hypercalcemia in children usually returns to normal.

The mechanism appears to involve a disproportion between bone formation and bone resorption. Hypercalciuria and increased mobilization of skeletal calcium can develop in normal volunteers subjected to extensive bed rest, although hypercalcemia is unusual. Immobilization of an adult with a disease associated with high bone turnover, however, such as Paget's disease, may cause hypercalcemia.

Thiazides Administration of benzothiadiazines (thiazides) can cause hypercalcemia in patients with high rates of bone turnover, such as patients with hypoparathyroidism treated with high doses of vitamin D. Traditionally, thiazides are associated with aggravation of hypercalcemia in primary hyperparathyroidism, but this effect can be seen in other high-bone-turnover states as well. The mechanism of thiazide action is complex. Chronic thiazide administration leads to reduction in urinary calcium; the hypocalciuric effect appears to reflect the enhancement of proximal tubular resorption of sodium and calcium in response to sodium depletion. Some of this renal effect is due to augmentation of PTH action and is more pronounced in individuals with intact PTH secretion. However, thiazides cause hypocalciuria in hypoparathyroid patients on high-dose vitamin D and oral calcium replacement if sodium intake is restricted. This finding is the rationale for the use of thiazides as an adjunct to therapy in hypoparathyroid patients, as discussed below. Thiazide administration to normal individuals causes a transient increase in blood calcium (usually within the high-normal range) that reverts to preexisting levels after a week or more of continued administration. If hormonal function and calcium and bone metabolism are normal, homeostatic controls are reset to counteract the calcium-elevating effect of the thiazides. In the presence of hyperparathyroidism or increased bone turnover from another cause, homeostatic mechanisms are ineffective. The abnormal effects of the thiazide on calcium metabolism disappear within days of cessation of the drug.

Vitamin A Intoxication Vitamin A intoxication is a rare cause of hypercalcemia and is most commonly a side effect of dietary faddism (Chap. 71). Calcium levels can be elevated into the 3–3.5 mmol/L (12–14 mg/dL) range after the ingestion of 50,000–100,000 units of vitamin A daily (10–20 times the minimum daily requirement). Typical features of severe hypercalcemia include fatigue, anorexia, and, in some, severe muscle and bone pain. Excess vitamin A intake is presumed to increase bone resorption.

The diagnosis can be established by history and by measurement of vitamin A levels in serum. Occasionally, skeletal x-rays reveal periosteal calcifications, particularly in the hands. Withdrawal of the vitamin is usually associated with prompt disappearance of the hypercalcemia and reversal of the skeletal changes. As in vitamin D intoxication, administration of 100 mg/d hydrocortisone or its equivalent leads to a rapid return of the serum calcium to normal.

HYPERCALCEMIA ASSOCIATED WITH RENAL FAILURE

Severe Secondary Hyperparathyroidism Secondary hyperparathyroidism occurs when partial resistance to the metabolic actions of PTH leads to excessive production of the hormone. Parathyroid gland hyperplasia occurs because resistance to the normal level of PTH leads to hypocalcemia, which, in turn, is a stimulus to parathyroid gland enlargement.

Secondary hyperparathyroidism occurs not only in patients with renal failure but also in those with osteomalacia due to multiple causes (Chap. 346), including deficiency of vitamin D action, and PHP (deficient response to PTH at the level of the receptor). Hypocalcemia seems to be the common denominator in initiating secondary hyperparathyroidism. Primary (1°) and secondary (2°) hyperparathyroidism can be distinguished conceptually by the autonomous growth of the parathyroid glands in primary hyperparathyroidism (presumably irreversible) and the adaptive response of the parathyroids in secondary hyperparathyroidism (typically reversible). In fact, reversal over weeks from an abnormal pattern of secretion, presumably accompanied by involution of parathyroid gland mass to normal, occurs in patients who have been treated effectively to reverse the resistance to PTH (such as with calcium and vitamin D in osteomalacia). However, it is now recognized that a true clonal outgrowth (irreversible) can arise in long-standing, inadequately treated chronic renal failure [e.g., tertiary (3°) hyperparathyroidism; see below].

Patients with secondary hyperparathyroidism may develop bone pain, ectopic calcification, and pruritus. The bone disease seen in patients with secondary hyperparathyroidism and renal failure is termed *renal osteodystrophy*. Osteomalacia (predominantly due to vitamin D and calcium deficiency) and/or osteitis fibrosa cystica (excessive PTH action on bone) may occur.

Two other skeletal disorders are associated with long-term dialysis in patients with renal failure. Aluminum deposition (see below) is associated with an osteomalacia-like picture. The other entity is a low-bone-turnover state termed "aplastic" or "adynamic" bone disease; PTH levels are lower than in typical secondary hyperparathyroidism. It is believed that the condition is caused, at least in part, by excessive PTH suppression, which may be even greater than previously appreciated in light of evidence that some of the immunoreactive PTH detected by most commercially available PTH assays is not the full-length biologically active molecule (as discussed above) but may consist of amino-terminally truncated fragments that do not activate the PTH1R.

℞ SECONDARY HYPERPARATHYROIDISM

Medical therapy to reverse secondary hyperparathyroidism includes reduction of excessive blood phosphate by restriction of dietary phosphate, the use of nonabsorbable antacids, and careful, selective addition of calcitriol (0.25–2.0 µg/d); calcium carbonate had been preferred over aluminum-containing antacids to prevent aluminum toxicity. However, synthetic gels that also bind phosphate (such as sevelamer; Chap. 274) are widely used, with the advantage of avoiding not only aluminum retention but excess calcium elevation. Intravenous calcitriol, administered as several pulses each week, helps control secondary hyperparathyroidism. Aggressive but carefully administered medical therapy can often, but not always, reverse hyperparathyroidism and its symptoms and manifestations.

Occasional patients develop severe manifestations of secondary hyperparathyroidism, including hypercalcemia, pruritus, extraskeletal calcifications, and painful bones, despite aggressive medical efforts to suppress the hyperparathyroidism. PTH hypersecretion no longer responsive to medical therapy, a state of severe hyperparathyroidism in patients with renal failure that requires surgery, has been referred to as *tertiary hyperparathyroidism*. Parathyroid surgery is necessary to control this condition. Based on genetic evidence from examination of tumor samples in these patients, the emergence of autonomous parathyroid function is due to a monoclonal outgrowth of one or more previously hyperplastic parathyroid glands. The adaptive response has become an independent contributor to disease; this finding seems to emphasize the importance of optimal medical management to reduce the proliferative response of the parathyroid cells that enables the irreversible genetic change.

Aluminum Intoxication Aluminum intoxication (and often hypercalcemia as a complication of medical treatment) may occur in patients on chronic dialysis; manifestations include acute dementia and unresponsive and severe osteomalacia. Bone pain, multiple nonhealing fractures, particularly of the ribs and pelvis, and a proximal myopathy may occur. Hypercalcemia develops when these patients are treated with vitamin D or calcitriol because of impaired skeletal responsiveness. Aluminum is present at the site of osteoid mineralization, osteoblastic activity is minimal, and calcium incorporation into the skeleton is impaired. Prevention is accomplished by avoidance of aluminum excess in the dialysis regimen; treatment of established disease involves mobilizing aluminum through the use of the chelating agent deferoxamine (Chap. 354).

Milk-Alkali Syndrome The milk-alkali syndrome is due to excessive ingestion of calcium and absorbable antacids such as milk or calcium carbonate. It is much less frequent since nonabsorbable antacids and other treatments became available for peptic ulcer disease. However, the increased use of calcium carbonate in the management of osteoporosis has led to reappearance of the syndrome. Several clinical presentations—acute, subacute, and chronic—have been described, all of which feature hypercalcemia, alkalosis, and renal failure. The chronic form of the disease, termed *Burnett's syndrome*, is associated with irreversible renal damage. The acute syndromes reverse if the excess calcium and absorbable alkali are stopped.

Individual susceptibility is important in the pathogenesis, as some patients are treated with calcium carbonate and alkali regimens without developing the syndrome. One variable is the fractional calcium absorption as a function of calcium intake. Some individuals absorb a high fraction of calcium, even with intakes ≥2 g of elemental calcium per day, instead of reducing calcium absorption with high intake, as occurs in most normal individuals. Resultant mild hypercalcemia after meals in such patients is postulated to contribute to the generation of alkalosis. Development of hypercalcemia causes increased sodium excretion and some depletion of total-body water. These phenomena and perhaps some suppression of endogenous PTH secretion due to mild hypercalcemia lead to increased bicarbonate resorption and to alkalosis in the face of continued calcium carbonate ingestion. Alkalosis per se selectively enhances calcium resorption in the distal nephron, thus aggravating the hypercalcemia. The cycle of mild hypercalcemia → bicarbonate retention → alkalosis → renal calcium retention → severe hypercalcemia perpetuates and aggravates hypercalcemia and alkalosis as long as calcium and absorbable alkali are ingested.

DIFFERENTIAL DIAGNOSIS: SPECIAL TESTS

Differential diagnosis of hypercalcemia is best achieved by using clinical criteria, but the immunoassay for PTH is especially useful in distinguishing among major causes (Fig. 347-6). The clinical features that deserve emphasis are the presence or absence of symptoms or signs of disease and evidence of chronicity. If one discounts fatigue or depression, >90% of patients with primary hyperparathyroidism have *asymptomatic hypercalcemia*; symptoms of malignancy are usually present in cancer-associated hypercalcemia. Disorders other than hyperparathyroidism and malignancy cause <10% of cases of hypercalcemia, and some of the nonparathyroid causes are associated with clear-cut manifestations such as renal failure.

Hyperparathyroidism is the likely diagnosis in patients with *chronic hypercalcemia*. If hypercalcemia has been manifest for >1 year, malignancy can usually be excluded as the cause. A striking feature of malignancy-associated hypercalcemia is the rapidity of the course, whereby signs and symptoms of the underlying malignancy are evident within months of the detection of hypercalcemia. Although clinical considerations are helpful in arriving at the correct diagnosis of the cause of hypercalcemia, appropriate laboratory testing is essential for definitive diagnosis. The immunoassay for PTH should separate hyperparathyroidism from all other causes of hypercalcemia. Patients with hyperparathyroidism have elevated PTH levels despite hypercalcemia, whereas patients with malignancy and the other causes of hypercalcemia (except for disorders mediated by PTH such as lithium-induced hypercalcemia) have levels of

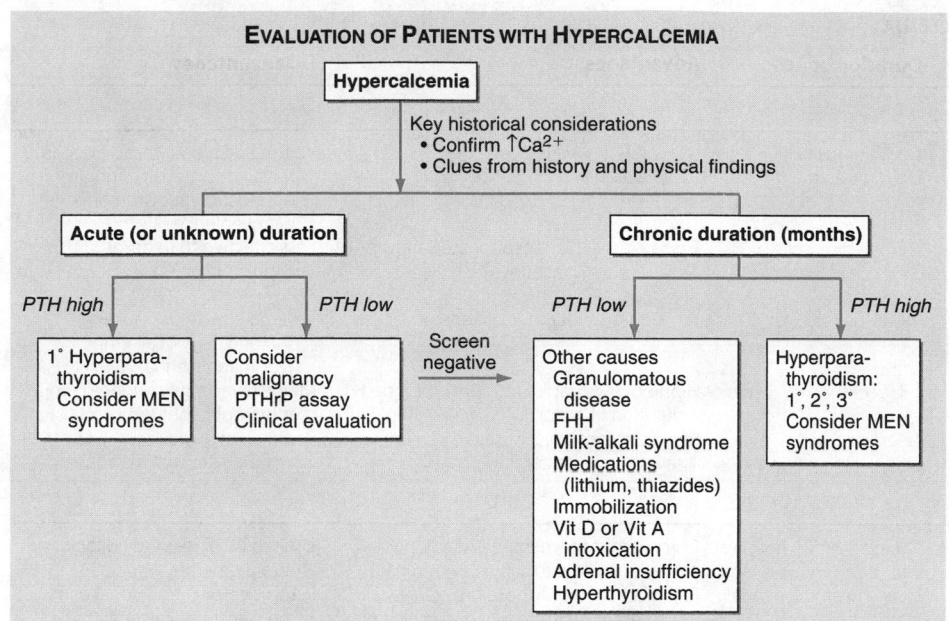

EVALUATION OF PATIENTS WITH HYPERCALCEMIA

FIGURE 347-6 Algorithm for the evaluation of patients with hypercalcemia. See text for details. FHH, familial hypocalciuric hypercalcemia; MEN, multiple endocrine neoplasia; PTH, parathyroid hormone; PTHrP, parathyroid hormone–related peptide.

hormone below normal or undetectable. Assays based on the double-antibody method for PTH exhibit very high sensitivity (especially if serum calcium is simultaneously evaluated) and specificity for the diagnosis of primary hyperparathyroidism (Fig. 347-4).

In summary, PTH values are elevated in >90% of parathyroid-related causes of hypercalcemia, undetectable or low in malignancy-related hypercalcemia, and undetectable or normal in vitamin D–related and high-bone-turnover causes of hypercalcemia. In view of the specificity of the PTH immunoassay and the high frequency of hyperparathyroidism in hypercalcemic patients, it is cost-effective to measure the PTH level in all hypercalcemic patients unless malignancy or a specific nonparathyroid disease is obvious. False-positive PTH assay results are rare. There are very rare reports of ectopic production of excess PTH by nonparathyroid tumors. Immunoassays for PTHrP are helpful in diagnosing certain types of malignancy-associated hypercalcemia. Although FHH is parathyroid-related, the disease should be managed distinctively from hyperparathyroidism. Clinical features and the low urinary calcium excretion can help make the distinction. Because the incidence of malignancy and hyperparathyroidism both increase with age, they can coexist as two independent causes of hypercalcemia.

$1,25(OH)_2D$ levels are elevated in many (but not all) patients with primary hyperparathyroidism. In other disorders associated with hypercalcemia, concentrations of $1,25(OH)_2D$ are low or, at the most, normal. However, this test is of low specificity and is not cost-effective, as not all patients with hyperparathyroidism have elevated $1,25(OH)_2D$ levels, and not all nonparathyroid hypercalcemic patients have suppressed $1,25(OH)_2D$. Measurement of $1,25(OH)_2D$ is, however, critically valuable in establishing the cause of hypercalcemia in sarcoidosis and certain lymphomas.

A useful general approach is outlined in Fig. 347-6. If the patient is *asymptomatic* and there is evidence of *chronicity* to the hypercalcemia, hyperparathyroidism is almost certainly the cause. If PTH levels (usually measured at least twice) are elevated, the clinical impression is confirmed and little additional evaluation is necessary. If there is only a short history or no data as to the duration of the hypercalcemia, *occult malignancy* must be considered; if the PTH levels are not elevated, then a thorough workup must be undertaken for malignancy, including chest x-ray, CT of chest and abdomen, and bone scan. Immunoassays for PTHrP may be especially useful in such situations. Attention should also be paid to clues for underlying hematologic disorders such as anemia, increased plasma globulin, and abnormal serum immunoelectrophoresis; bone scans can

be negative in some patients with metastases, such as in multiple myeloma. Finally, if a patient with chronic hypercalcemia is asymptomatic and malignancy therefore seems unlikely on clinical grounds, but PTH values are not elevated, it is useful to search for other chronic causes of hypercalcemia, such as occult sarcoidosis. A careful history of dietary supplements and drug use may suggest intoxication with vitamin D or vitamin A or the use of thiazides.

℞ HYPERCALCEMIC STATES

The approach to medical treatment of hypercalcemia varies with its severity (**Table 347-4**). Mild hypercalcemia, <3.0 mmol/L (12 mg/dL), can be managed by hydration. More severe hypercalcemia [levels of 3.2–3.7 mmol/L (13–15 mg/dL)] must be managed aggressively; above that level, hypercalcemia can be life-threatening and requires emergency measures. By using a combination of approaches in severe hypercalcemia, the serum calcium concentration can be decreased by 0.7–2.2 mmol/L (3–9 mg/dL) within 24–48 h in most patients, enough to relieve acute symptoms, prevent death from hypercalcemic crisis, and permit diagnostic evaluation. Therapy can then be directed at the underlying disorder—the second priority.

Hypercalcemia develops because of excessive skeletal calcium release, increased intestinal calcium absorption, or inadequate renal calcium excretion. Understanding the particular pathogenesis helps guide therapy. For example, hypercalcemia in patients with malignancy is primarily due to excessive skeletal calcium release and is, therefore, minimally improved by restriction of dietary calcium. On the other hand, patients with vitamin D hypersensitivity or vitamin D intoxication have excessive intestinal calcium absorption, and restriction of dietary calcium is beneficial. Decreased renal function or ECF depletion decreases urinary calcium excretion. In such situations, rehydration may rapidly reduce or reverse the hypercalcemia, even though increased bone resorption persists. As outlined below, the more severe the hypercalcemia, the greater the number of combined therapies that should be used. Rapid acting (hours) approaches—rehydration, forced diuresis, and calcitonin—can be used with the most effective antiresorptive agents, such as bisphosphonates (since severe hypercalcemia usually involves excessive bone resorption).

HYDRATION, INCREASED SALT INTAKE, MILD AND FORCED
DIURESIS The first principle of treatment is to restore normal hydration. Many hypercalcemic patients are dehydrated because of vomiting, inanition, and/or hypercalcemia-induced defects in urinary concentrating ability. The resultant drop in glomerular filtration rate is accompanied by an additional decrease in renal tubular sodium and calcium clearance. Restoring a normal ECF volume corrects these abnormalities and increases urine calcium excretion by 2.5–7.5 mmol/d (100–300 mg/d). Increasing urinary sodium excretion to 400–500 mmol/d increases urinary calcium excretion even further than simple rehydration. After rehydration has been achieved, saline can be administered or furosemide or ethacrynic acid can be given twice daily to depress the tubular reabsorptive mechanism for calcium (care must be taken to prevent dehydration). The combined use of these therapies can increase urinary calcium excretion to ≥12.5 mmol/d (500 mg/d) in most hypercalcemic patients. Since this is a substantial percentage of the exchangeable calcium pool, the serum calcium concentration usually falls 0.25–0.75 mmol/L (1–3 mg/dL) within 24 h. Precautions should be taken to prevent potassium and magnesium depletion; calcium-containing renal calculi are a potential complication.

Under life-threatening circumstances, the preceding approach can be pursued more aggressively, giving as much as 6 L isotonic saline (900 mmol sodium) daily plus furosemide or equivalent in doses up to 100 mg every 1–2 h or ethacrynic acid in doses to 40 mg every 1–2 h. Urinary calcium excretion may exceed 25 mmol/d (1000 mg/d), and the serum calcium may decrease

TABLE 347-4 THERAPIES FOR SEVERE HYPERCALCEMIA

Treatment	Onset of Action	Duration of Action	Advantages	Disadvantages
Most Useful Therapies				
Hydration with saline	Hours	During infusion	Rehydration invariably needed	Volume overload, cardiac decompensation, intensive monitoring, electrolyte disturbance, inconvenience
Forced diuresis; saline plus loop diuretic	Hours	During treatment	Rapid action	
Bisphosphonates 1st generation: etidronate	1–2 days	5–7 days in doses used	First available bisphosphonate; intermediate onset of action	Less effective than other bisphosphonates
2d generation: pamidronate	1–2 days	10–14 days to weeks	High potency; intermediate onset of action	Fever in 20% hypophosphatemia, hypocalcemia, hypomagnesemia
3d generation: zolendronate	1–2 days	>3 weeks	High potency; rapid infusion; prolonged duration of action	Minor; fever, rarely hypocalcemia or hypophosphatemia
Calcitonin	Hours	1–2 days	Rapid onset of action; useful as adjunct in severe hypercalcemia	Rapid tachyphylaxis
Special Use Therapies				
Phosphate Oral	24 h	During use	Chronic management (with hypophosphatemia); low toxicity if P < 4 mg/dL	Limited use except as adjuvant or chronic therapy
Intravenous	Hours	During use and 24–48 h afterward	Rapid action, highly potent but *rarely used* except with severe hypercalcemia and cardiac and renal decompensation present	Ectopic calcification; renal damage, fatal hypocalcemia
Glucocorticoids	Days	Days, weeks	Oral therapy, antitumor agent	Active only in certain malignancies; glucocorticoid side effects
Dialysis	Hours	During use and 24–48 h afterward	Useful in renal failure; onset of effect in hours; can immediately reverse life-threatening hypercalcemia	Complex procedure, reserved for extreme or special circumstances

by ≥1 mmol/L (4 mg/dL) within 24 h. Depletion of potassium and magnesium is inevitable unless replacements are given; pulmonary edema can be precipitated. The potential complications can be reduced by careful monitoring of central venous pressure and plasma or urine electrolytes; catheterization of the bladder may be necessary. This treatment approach should be supplemented with agents to block bone resorption. Though these agents do not become effective for several days, forced diuresis is difficult to sustain even in patients with good cardiopulmonary and renal function.

BISPHOSPHONATES The bisphosphonates are analogues of pyrophosphate, with high affinity for bone, especially in areas of increased bone turnover, where they are powerful inhibitors of bone resorption. These bone-seeking compounds are stable in vivo because phosphatase enzymes cannot hydrolyze the central carbon-phosphorus-carbon bond. The bisphosphonates are concentrated in areas of high bone turnover and are taken up by and inhibit osteoclast action; the mechanism of action is complex. Bisphosphonates alter osteoclast proton pump function or impair the release of acid hydrolases into the extracellular lysosomes contiguous with mineralized bone. They may also inhibit the differentiation of monocyte-macrophage precursors into osteoclasts and possibly have effects on osteoblasts as well. The bisphosphonate molecules that contain amino groups in the side chain structure (see below) interfere with prenylation of proteins and can lead to cellular apoptosis. The highly active non-amino group–containing bisphosphonates are also metabolized to cytotoxic products.

The initial bisphosphonate widely used in clinical practice, etidronate, was effective but had several disadvantages, including the capacity to inhibit bone formation as well as blocking resorption. Subsequently, a number of second-generation compounds have become the mainstays of antiresorptive therapy for treatment of hypercalcemia and osteoporosis. The newer bisphosphonates have a highly favorable ratio of blocking resorption versus inhibiting bone formation; they inhibit osteoclast-mediated skeletal resorption yet do not cause mineralization defects at ordinary doses. Though the bisphosphonates have similar structures, the routes of administration, efficacy, toxicity, and side effects vary. The potency of the compounds for inhibition of bone resorption varies over 10,000-fold, increasing in the order of etidronate, tiludronate, pamidronate, alendronate, risedronate, and zolendronate. Oral alendronate and risedronate are approved for the therapy of osteoporosis in the United States and elsewhere. The IV use of pamidronate and zolendronate is approved for the treatment of hypercalcemia in the United States; between 30 and 90 mg pamidronate, given as a single IV dose over a few hours, returns serum calcium to

normal within 24–48 h with an effect that lasts for weeks in 80–100% of patients. Zolendronate given in doses of 4 or 8 mg/5-min infusion has a more rapid and more sustained effort than pamidronate in direct comparison.

These drugs are used extensively in cancer patients. Absolute survival improvements are noted with pamidronate and zolendronate in multiple myeloma, for example. However, though still rare, there are increasing reports of jaw necrosis, especially after dental surgery, mainly in cancer patients treated with multiple doses of the more potent bisphosphonates.

CALCITONIN Calcitonin acts within a few hours of its administration, through receptors on osteoclasts, to block bone resorption and, in addition, to increase urinary calcium excretion by inhibition of renal tubular calcium reabsorption. If administered as a single agent, calcitonin, after 24 h of use, resulted in minimal lowering of calcium. Tachyphylaxis, a known phenomenon with this drug, seems to explain the results, since the drug is effective in the first hours of use. However, in life-threatening hypercalcemia, calcitonin can be used effectively within the first 24 h in combination with rehydration and saline diuresis while waiting for more sustained effects from a simultaneously administered bisphosphonate, such as pamidronate. Usual doses of calcitonin are 2–8 U/kg of body weight IV, SC, or IM every 6–12 h.

OTHER THERAPIES *Plicamycin* (formerly mithramycin), which inhibits bone resorption, has been a useful therapeutic agent but is now seldom used because of its toxicity and the effectiveness of bisphosphonates. Plicamycin must be given IV, either as a bolus or by slow infusion; the usual dose is 25 μg/kg body weight. *Gallium nitrate* exerts a hypocalcemic action by inhibiting bone resorption and altering the structure of bone crystals. It is not often used now because of superior alternatives.

Glucocorticoids have utility, especially in hypercalcemia complicating certain malignancies. They increase urinary calcium excretion and decrease intestinal calcium absorption when given in pharmacologic doses, but they also cause negative skeletal calcium balance. In normal individuals and in patients with primary hyperparathyroidism, glucocorticoids neither increase nor decrease the serum calcium concentration. In patients with hypercalcemia due to certain osteolytic malignancies, however, glucocorticoids may be effective as a result of antitumor effects. The malignancies in which hypercalcemia responds to glucocorticoids include multiple myeloma, leukemia, Hodgkin's disease, other lymphomas, and carcinoma of the breast, at least early in the course of the disease. Glucocorticoids are also effective in treating hypercalcemia due to vitamin D intoxication and sarcoidosis. Glucocorticoids are also useful in the rare form of hypercalcemia, now recognized in certain autoimmune disorders in which inactivating antibodies against the receptor imitate FHH. Elevated PTH and calcium levels are effectively lowered by the glucocorticoids. In all the preceding situations, the hypocalcemic effect develops over several days, and the usual glucocorticoid dosage is 40–100 mg prednisone (or its equivalent) daily in four divided doses. The side effects of chronic glucocorticoid therapy may be acceptable in some circumstances.

Dialysis is often the treatment of choice for severe hypercalcemia complicated by renal failure, which is difficult to manage medically. Peritoneal dialysis with calcium-free dialysis fluid can remove 5–12.5 mmol (200–500 mg) of calcium in 24–48 h and lower the serum calcium concentration by 0.7–3 mmol/L (3–12 mg/dL). Large quantities of phosphate are lost during dialysis, and serum inorganic phosphate concentrations usually fall, thus aggravating hypercalcemia. Therefore, the serum inorganic phosphate concentration should be measured after dialysis, and phosphate supplements should be added to the diet or to dialysis fluids if necessary.

Phosphate therapy, PO or IV, has a limited role in certain circumstances (Chap. 346). Correcting hypophosphatemia lowers the serum calcium concentration by several mechanisms, including bone/calcium exchange. The usual oral treatment is 1–1.5 g phosphorus per day for several days, given in divided doses. It is generally believed, but not established, that toxicity does not occur if therapy is limited to restoring serum inorganic phosphate concentrations to normal.

Raising the serum inorganic phosphate concentration above normal decreases serum calcium levels, sometimes strikingly. Intravenous phosphate is one of the most dramatically effective treatments available for severe hypercalcemia but is toxic and even dangerous (fatal hypocalcemia). For these reasons, it is used rarely and only in severely hypercalcemic patients with cardiac or renal failure where dialysis, the preferable alternative, is not feasible or is unavailable.

SUMMARY The various therapies for hypercalcemia are listed in Table 347-4. The choice depends on the underlying disease, the severity of the hypercalcemia, the serum inorganic phosphate level, and the renal, hepatic, and bone marrow function. Mild hypercalcemia [≤3 mmol/L (12 mg/dL)] can usually be managed by hydration. Severe hypercalcemia [≥3.7 mmol/L (15 mg/dL)] requires rapid correction. Calcitonin should be given for its rapid, albeit short-lived, blockade of bone resorption, and IV pamidronate or zolendronate should be administered, although its onset of action is delayed for 1–2 days. In addition, for the first 24–48 h, aggressive sodium-calcium diuresis with IV saline and, following rehydration, large doses of furosemide or ethacrynic acid, but only if appropriate monitoring is available and cardiac and renal function are adequate. Otherwise, dialysis may be necessary. Intermediate degrees of hypercalcemia between 3.0 and 3.7 mmol/L (12 and 15 mg/dL) should be approached with vigorous hydration and then the most appropriate selection for the patient of the combinations used with severe hypercalcemia.

HYPOCALCEMIA (See also Chap. 47)

PATHOPHYSIOLOGY OF HYPOCALCEMIA: CLASSIFICATION BASED ON MECHANISM

Chronic hypocalcemia is less common than hypercalcemia; causes include chronic renal failure, hereditary and acquired hypoparathyroidism, vitamin D deficiency, PHP, and hypomagnesemia.

Acute rather than chronic hypocalcemia is seen in critically ill patients or as a consequence of certain medications and often does not require specific treatment. Transient hypocalcemia is seen with severe sepsis, burns, acute renal failure, and extensive transfusions with citrated blood. Although as many as half of patients in an intensive care setting are reported to have calcium concentrations <2.1 mmol/L (8.5 mg/dL), most do not have a reduction in ionized calcium. Patients with severe sepsis may have a decrease in ionized calcium (true hypocalcemia), but in other severely ill individuals, hypoalbuminemia is the primary cause of the reduced total calcium concentration. Alkalosis increases calcium binding to proteins, and in this setting direct measurements of ionized calcium should be made.

Medications such as protamine, heparin, and glucagon may cause transient hypocalcemia. These forms of hypocalcemia are usually not associated with tetany and resolve with improvement in the overall medical condition. The hypocalcemia after repeated transfusions of citrated blood usually resolves quickly.

Patients with *acute pancreatitis* have hypocalcemia that persists during the acute inflammation and varies in degree with the severity of the pancreatitis. The cause of hypocalcemia remains unclear. PTH values are reported to be low, normal, or elevated, and both resistance to PTH and impaired PTH secretion have been postulated. Occasionally, a chronic low total calcium and low ionized calcium concentration are detected in an elderly patient without obvious cause and with a paucity of symptoms; the pathogenesis is unclear.

Chronic hypocalcemia, however, is usually symptomatic and requires treatment. Neuromuscular and neurologic manifestations of chronic hypocalcemia include muscle spasms, carpopedal spasm, facial grimacing, and, in extreme cases, laryngeal spasm and convulsions. Respiratory arrest may occur. Increased intracranial pressure occurs in some patients with long-standing hypocalcemia, often in association with papilledema. Mental changes include irritability, depression, and psychosis. The QT interval on the electrocardiogram is prolonged, in contrast to its shortening with hypercalcemia. Arrhythmias occur, and digitalis effectiveness may be reduced. Intestinal cramps and chronic malabsorption may occur. Chvostek's or Trousseau's sign can be used to confirm latent tetany.

The classification of hypocalcemia shown in Table 347-5 is based on an organizationally useful premise that PTH is responsible for minute-to-minute regulation of plasma calcium concentration and, therefore, that the occurrence of hypocalcemia must mean a failure of the homeostatic action of PTH. Failure of the PTH response can occur if there is hereditary or acquired parathyroid gland failure, if PTH is ineffective in target organs, or if the action of the hormone is overwhelmed by the loss of calcium from the ECF at a rate faster than it can be replaced.

PTH ABSENT

Whether hereditary or acquired, hypoparathyroidism has a number of common components. Symptoms of untreated hypocalcemia are shared by both types of hypoparathyroidism, although the onset of hereditary hypoparathyroidism is more gradual and is often associated with other developmental defects. Basal ganglia calcification and extrapyramidal syndromes are more common and earlier in onset in hereditary hypoparathyroidism. In earlier decades, acquired hypoparathyroidism secondary to surgery in the neck was more common than hereditary hypoparathyroidism, but the frequency of surgically induced parathyroid failure has diminished as a result of improved surgical techniques that spare the parathyroid glands and increased use of nonsurgical therapy for hyperthyroidism. PHP, an example of ineffective PTH action rather than a failure

TABLE 347-5	FUNCTIONAL CLASSIFICATION OF HYPOCALCEMIA (EXCLUDING NEONATAL CONDITIONS)
PTH Absent	
Hereditary hypoparathyroidism	Hypomagnesemia
Acquired hypoparathyroidism	
PTH Ineffective	
Chronic renal failure	Active vitamin D ineffective
Active vitamin D lacking	Intestinal malabsorption
↓ Dietary intake or sunlight	Vitamin D–dependent rickets type II
Defective metabolism:	Pseudohypoparathyroidism
Anticonvulsant therapy	
Vitamin D–dependent rickets type I	
PTH Overwhelmed	
Severe, acute hyperphosphatemia	Osteitis fibrosa after parathyroidectomy
Tumor lysis	
Acute renal failure	
Rhabdomyolysis	

Note: PTH, parathyroid hormone.

of parathyroid gland production, may share several features with hypoparathyroidism, including extraosseous calcification and extrapyramidal manifestations such as choreoathetotic movements and dystonia.

Papilledema and raised intracranial pressure may occur in both hereditary and acquired hypoparathyroidism, as do chronic changes in fingernails and hair and lenticular cataracts, the latter usually reversible with treatment of hypocalcemia. Certain skin manifestations, including alopecia and candidiasis, are characteristic of hereditary hypoparathyroidism associated with autoimmune polyglandular failure (Chap. 345).

Hypocalcemia associated with hypomagnesemia is associated with both deficient PTH release and impaired responsiveness to the hormone. Patients with hypocalcemia secondary to hypomagnesemia have absent or low levels of circulating PTH, indicative of diminished hormone release despite maximum physiologic stimulus by hypocalcemia. Plasma PTH levels return to normal with correction of the hypomagnesemia. Thus hypoparathyroidism with low levels of PTH in blood can be due to hereditary gland failure, acquired gland failure, or acute but reversible gland dysfunction (hypomagnesemia).

Genetic Abnormalities and Hereditary Hypoparathyroidism

Hereditary hypoparathyroidism can occur as an isolated entity without other endocrine or dermatologic manifestations (idiopathic hypoparathyroidism). More typically, it occurs in association with other abnormalities such as defective development of the thymus or failure of other endocrine organs such as the adrenal, thyroid, or ovary (Chap. 345). Idiopathic and hereditary hypoparathyroidism are often manifest within the first decade but may appear later.

Genetic defects associated with hypoparathyroidism are rare but serve to illuminate the complexity of organ development, hormonal biosynthesis and secretion, and tissue-specific patterns of endocrine effector function. Often, the hypoparathyroidism is isolated, signifying a highly specific functional disturbance. When the hypoparathyroidism is associated with other developmental or organ defects, treatment of the hypocalcemia can still be effective.

A rare form of hypoparathyroidism associated with defective development of both the thymus and the parathyroid glands is termed the DiGeorge syndrome, or the velocardiofacial syndrome. Congenital cardiovascular, facial, and other developmental defects are present, and most patients die in early childhood with severe infections, hypocalcemia and seizures, or cardiovascular complications. Some survive into adulthood, and milder, incomplete forms occur. Most cases are sporadic, but an autosomal dominant form involving microdeletions of chromosome 22q11.2 has been described. Smaller deletions in chromosome 22 are seen in incomplete forms of the DiGeorge syndrome, appearing in childhood or adolescence, that are manifest primarily by parathyroid gland failure. The chromosome 22 defect is now termed DSG1; more recently, a defect in chromosome 10p is also recognized—now called DSG2. The phenotypes seem similar. Studies on the chromosome 22 defect have pinpointed a transcription factor, TBX1. Deletions of the orthologous mouse gene shows a phenotype similar to the human syndrome.

Another autosomal dominant developmental defect, featuring hypoparathyroidism, deafness, and renal dysplasia (HDR) has been studied at a genetic level. Cytogenic abnormalities in some, but not all, kindred point to translocation defects on chromosome 10, as in DiGeorge syndrome. However, the lack of immunodeficiency and heart defects distinguishes the two syndromes. Mouse models, as well as deletional analysis in some HDR patients, has pointed to transcription factor GATA3, which is important in embryonic development and is expressed in developing kidney, ear structures, and the parathyroids.

Another pair of linked developmental disorders involving the parathyroids is recognized. Kenney-Caffey syndrome features hypoparathyroidism, short stature, osteosclerosis, and thick cortical bones. A defect seen in Middle Eastern patients, including Bedouin kindred, termed Sanjad-Sakati syndrome, also exhibits growth failure and other dysmorphic features. This syndrome, which is clearly autosomal recessive, involves a gene on chromosome 1q42-q43. Both syndromes apparently involve a chaperone protein, called TBCE, relevant to tubulin function.

Hypoparathyroidism can occur in association with a complex hereditary autoimmune syndrome involving failure of the adrenals, the ovaries, the immune system, and the parathyroids in association with recurrent mucocutaneous candidiasis, alopecia, vitiligo, and pernicious anemia (Chap. 345). The responsible gene on chromosome 21q22.3 has been identified. The protein product, which resembles a transcription factor, has been termed the autoimmune regulator, or AIRE. A stop codon mutation occurs in many Finnish families with the disorder, commonly referred to as polyglandular autoimmune type 1 deficiency.

Hypoparathyroidism is seen in two disorders associated with mitochondrial dysfunction and myopathy, one termed the Kearns-Sayre syndrome (KSS), with ophthalmoplegia and pigmentary retinopathy, and the other termed the MELAS syndrome, mitochondrial encephalopathy, lactic acidosis, and stroke-like episodes. Mutations or deletions in mitochondrial genes have been identified.

Several forms of hypoparathyroidism, each rare in frequency, are seen as isolated defects; the genetic mechanisms are varied. The inheritance includes autosomal dominant, autosomal recessive, and X-linked modes. Three separate autosomal defects involving the parathyroid gene have been recognized: one is dominant, the other two are recessive. The dominant form has a point mutation in the signal sequence, a critical region involved in intracellular transport of the hormone precursor. An Arg for Cys mutation interferes with processing of the precursor and seems to block the processing of the product of the normal allele. The other two forms are recessive. One point mutation also blocks cleavage of the PTH precursor but requires both alleles to cause hypoparathyroidism. The third involves a single nucleotide base change that results in an exon splicing defect; the lost exon contains the promoter—hence, the gene is silenced. An X-linked recessive form of hypoparathyroidism has been described in males and the defect has been localized to chromosome Xq26-q27, perhaps involving the SOX3 gene.

Abnormalities in the calcium-sensing receptor (CaSR) are detected in three distinctive hypocalcemic disorders. All are rare but at least 10 different gain-of-function mutations have been found in one form of hypocalcemia termed autosomal dominant hypocalcemic hypercalciuria (ADHH). The receptor senses the ambient calcium level as excessive and suppresses PTH secretion, leading to hypocalcemia. The hypocalcemia is aggravated by constitutive receptor activity in the renal tubule causing renal calcium wasting. Recognition of the syndrome is important because efforts to treat the hypocalcemia with vitamin D analogues and increased oral calcium exacerbate the already excessive urinary calcium secretion (several grams or more per 24 h), leading to irreversible renal damage from stones and ectopic calcification.

The Bartter syndrome is a group of disorders associated with disturbances in electrolyte and acid/base balance, sometimes with nephrocalcinosis and other features. Several types of ion channels or transporters are involved. Curiously, Bartter syndrome type V has the electrolyte and pH disturbances seen in the other syndromes but appears to be due to a gain-of-function in the CaSR. The defect may be more severe than in ADHH and explains the additional features seen beyond hypocalcemia and hypercalciuria.

As with autoimmune disorders that block the CaSR (discussed above under hypercalcemic conditions), there are autoantibodies that at least transiently activate the CaSR, leading to suppressed PTH secretion and hypocalcemia. This disorder, which may wax and wane, could be classified as an acquired form of hypoparathyroidism but is listed here with other disorders involving the CaSR.

Acquired Hypoparathyroidism

Acquired chronic hypoparathyroidism is usually the result of inadvertent surgical removal of all the parathyroid glands; in some instances, not all the tissue is removed, but the remainder undergoes vascular supply compromise secondary to fibrotic changes in the neck after surgery. In the past, the most frequent cause of acquired hypoparathyroidism was surgery for hyperthyroidism. Hypoparathyroidism now usually occurs after surgery for hyperparathyroidism when the surgeon, facing the dilemma of removing too little tissue and thus not curing the hyperparathyroidism, removes too much. Parathyroid function may not be totally absent in all patients with postoperative hypoparathyroidism.

Even rarer causes of acquired chronic hypoparathyroidism include radiation-induced damage subsequent to radioiodine therapy of hyperthyroidism and glandular damage in patients with hemochromatosis or hemosiderosis after repeated blood transfusions. Infection may involve one or more of the parathyroids but usually does not cause hypoparathyroidism because all four glands are rarely involved.

Transient hypoparathyroidism is frequent following surgery for hyperparathyroidism. After a variable period of hypoparathyroidism, normal parathyroid function may return due to hyperplasia or recovery of remaining tissue. Occasionally, recovery occurs months after surgery.

℞ ACQUIRED AND HEREDITARY HYPOPARATHYROIDISM

Treatment involves replacement with vitamin D or 1,25(OH)$_2$D$_3$ (calcitriol) combined with a high oral calcium intake. In most patients, blood calcium and phosphate levels are satisfactorily regulated, but some patients show resistance and a brittleness, with a tendency to alternate between hypocalcemia and hypercalcemia. For many patients, vitamin D in doses of 40,000–120,000 U/d (1–3 mg/d) combined with ≥1 g elemental calcium is satisfactory. The wide dosage range reflects the variation encountered from patient to patient; precise regulation of each patient is required. Compared to typical daily requirements in euparathyroid patients of 200 U/d (or in older patients as high as 800 U/d), the high dose of vitamin D (as much as 100-fold higher) reflects the reduced conversion of vitamin D to 1,25(OH)$_2$D. Many physicians now use 0.5–1.0 µg of calcitriol in management of such patients, especially if they are difficult to control. Because of its storage in fat, when vitamin D is withdrawn, weeks are required for the disappearance of the biologic effects, compared with a few days for calcitriol, which has a rapid turnover.

Oral calcium and vitamin D restore the overall calcium-phosphate balance but do not reverse the lowered urinary calcium reabsorption typical of hypoparathyroidism. Therefore, care must be taken to avoid excessive urinary calcium excretion after vitamin D and calcium replacement therapy; otherwise, kidney stones can develop. Thiazide diuretics lower urine calcium by as much as 100 mg/d in hypoparathyroid patients on vitamin D, provided they are maintained on a low-sodium diet. Use of thiazides seems to be of benefit in mitigating hypercalciuria and easing the daily management of these patients.

Hypomagnesemia Severe hypomagnesemia (<0.4 mmol/L; <0.8 meq/L) is associated with hypocalcemia (Chap. 346). Restoration of the total-body magnesium deficit leads to rapid reversal of hypocalcemia. There are at least two causes of the hypocalcemia—impaired PTH secretion and reduced responsiveness to PTH. For further discussion of causes and treatment of hypomagnesemia, see Chap. 46.

The effects of magnesium on PTH secretion are similar to those of calcium; hypermagnesemia suppresses and hypomagnesemia stimulates PTH secretion. The effects of magnesium on PTH secretion are normally of little significance, however, because the calcium effects dominate. Greater change in magnesium than in calcium is needed to influence hormone secretion. Nonetheless, hypomagnesemia might be expected to increase hormone secretion. It is therefore surprising to find that severe hypomagnesemia is associated with blunted secretion of PTH. The explanation for the paradox is that severe, chronic hypomagnesemia leads to intracellular magnesium deficiency, which interferes with secretion and peripheral responses to PTH. The mechanism of the cellular abnormalities caused by hypomagnesemia is unknown, although effects on adenylate cyclase (for which magnesium is a cofactor) have been proposed.

PTH levels are undetectable or inappropriately low in severe hypomagnesemia despite the stimulus of severe hypocalcemia, and acute repletion of magnesium leads to a rapid increase in PTH level. Serum phosphate levels are often not elevated, in contrast to the situation with acquired or idiopathic hypoparathyroidism, probably because phosphate deficiency is a frequent accompaniment of hypomagnesemia.

Diminished peripheral responsiveness to PTH also occurs in some patients, as documented by subnormal response in urinary phosphorus and urinary cyclic AMP excretion after administration of exogenous PTH to patients who are hypocalcemic and hypomagnesemic. Both blunted PTH secretion and lack of renal response to administered PTH can occur in the same patient. When acute magnesium repletion is undertaken, the restoration of PTH levels to normal or supranormal may precede restoration of normal serum calcium by several days.

℞ HYPOMAGNESEMIA

Repletion of magnesium cures the condition. Repletion should be parenteral. Attention must be given to restoring the intracellular deficit, which may be considerable. After IV magnesium administration, serum magnesium may return transiently to the normal range, but unless replacement therapy is adequate serum magnesium will again fall. If the cause of the hypomagnesemia is renal magnesium wasting, magnesium may have to be given chronically to prevent recurrence.

PTH INEFFECTIVE

PTH is ineffective when the hormone receptor–guanyl nucleotide–binding protein complex is defective (PHP, discussed below), when PTH action to promote calcium absorption from the diet is impaired because of vitamin D deficiency or because vitamin D is ineffective (receptor or synthesis defects), or in chronic renal failure in which the calcium-elevating action of PTH is impaired.

Typically, hypophosphatemia is more severe than hypocalcemia in vitamin D deficiency states because of the increased secretion of PTH, which, although only partly effective in elevating blood calcium, is capable of promoting phosphaturia.

PHP, on the other hand, has a pathophysiology different from the other disorders of ineffective PTH action. PHP resembles hypoparathyroidism (in which PTH synthesis is deficient) and is manifested by hypocalcemia and hyperphosphatemia, yet elevated PTH levels. The cause of the disorder is defective hormone activation of guanyl nucleotide–binding proteins, resulting in failure of PTH to increase intracellular cyclic AMP (see below).

Chronic Renal Failure Improved medical management of chronic renal failure now allows many patients to survive for years and hence time enough to develop features of renal osteodystrophy, which must be controlled to avoid its morbidity. Phosphate retention and impaired production of 1,25(OH)$_2$D are the principal factors that cause calcium deficiency, secondary hyperparathyroidism, and bone disease. Low levels of 1,25(OH)$_2$D due to hyperphosphatemia and destruction of renal tissue are critical in the development of hypocalcemia. The uremic state also causes impairment of intestinal absorption by mechanisms other than defects in vitamin D metabolism. Nonetheless, treatment with supraphysiologic amounts of vitamin D or calcitriol corrects the impaired calcium absorption.

Hyperphosphatemia in renal failure lowers blood calcium levels by several mechanisms, including extraosseous deposition of calcium and phosphate, impairment of the bone-resorbing action of PTH, and reduction in 1,25(OH)$_2$D production by remaining renal tissue.

℞ CHRONIC RENAL FAILURE

Therapy of chronic renal failure (Chap. 274) involves appropriate management of patients prior to dialysis and adjustment of regimens once dialysis is initiated. Attention should be paid to restriction of phosphate in the diet; avoidance of aluminum-containing phosphate-binding antacids to prevent the problem of aluminum intoxication; provision of an adequate calcium intake by mouth, usually 1–2 g/d; and supplementation with 0.25–1.0 µg/d calcitriol. Each patient must be monitored closely. The aim of therapy is to restore normal calcium balance to prevent osteomalacia and secondary hyperparathyroidism and, in light of evidence of genetic changes and monoclonal outgrowths of parathyroid glands in renal failure patients, to prevent secondary from becoming autonomous hyperparathyroidism. Reduction of hyperphosphatemia and restoration of normal intestinal calcium absorption by calcitriol can improve blood calcium levels and reduce the manifestations of secondary hyperparathyroidism. Since adynamic bone disease can occur in association with low PTH levels, it is important to avoid excessive suppression of the parathyroid glands while recognizing the beneficial effects of controlling the secondary hyperparathyroidism. These patients should probably be closely monitored with PTH assays that detect only the full-length PTH(1–84) to ensure that biologically active PTH and not inactive, inhibitory PTH fragments are measured.

Vitamin D Deficiency Due to Inadequate Diet and/or Sunlight
Vitamin D deficiency due to inadequate intake of dairy products enriched with vitamin D, lack of vitamin supplementation, and reduced sunlight exposure in the elderly, particularly during winter in northern latitudes, is more common in the United States than previously recognized. Biopsies of bone in elderly patients with hip fracture (documenting osteomalacia) and abnormal levels of vitamin D metabolites, PTH, calcium, and phosphate indicate that vitamin D deficiency may occur in as many as 25% of elderly patients, particularly in northern latitudes in the United States. Concentrations of 25(OH)D are low or low-normal in these patients. Quantitative histomorphometry of bone biopsy specimens reveals widened osteoid seams consistent with osteomalacia (Chap. 346). PTH hypersecretion compensates for the tendency for the blood calcium to fall but also induces renal phosphate wasting and results in osteomalacia.

Treatment involves adequate replacement with vitamin D and calcium until the deficiencies are corrected. Severe hypocalcemia rarely occurs in moderately severe vitamin D deficiency of the elderly, but vitamin D deficiency must be considered in the differential diagnosis of mild hypocalcemia.

Mild hypocalcemia, secondary hyperparathyroidism, severe hypophosphatemia, and a variety of nutritional deficiencies occur with gastrointestinal diseases. Hepatocellular dysfunction can lead to reduction in 25(OH)D levels, as in portal or biliary cirrhosis of the liver, and malabsorption of vitamin D and its metabolites, including $1,25(OH)_2D$, may occur in a variety of bowel diseases, hereditary or acquired. Hypocalcemia itself can lead to steatorrhea, due to deficient production of pancreatic enzymes and bile salts. Depending on the disorder, vitamin D or its metabolites can be given parenterally, guaranteeing adequate blood levels of active metabolites.

Defective Vitamin D Metabolism • ANTICONVULSANT THERAPY
Anticonvulsant therapy with any of several agents induces acquired vitamin D deficiency by increasing the conversion of vitamin D to inactive compounds and/or causing resistance to its action. The more marginal the vitamin D intake in the diet, the more likely that anticonvulsant therapy will lead to abnormal mineral and bone metabolism.

VITAMIN D–DEPENDENT RICKETS TYPE I
Rickets can be due to *resistance to the action* of vitamin D as well as to vitamin D deficiency. Vitamin D–dependent rickets type I, previously termed *pseudo-vitamin D–resistant rickets*, differs from true vitamin D–resistant rickets (vitamin D–dependent rickets type II, see below) in that it is less severe and the biochemical and radiographic abnormalities can be reversed with appropriate doses of the vitamin or the active metabolite, $1,25(OH)_2D_3$. Physiologic amounts of calcitriol cure the disease (Chap. 346). This finding fits with the pathophysiology of the disorder, which is autosomal recessive, and is now known to be caused by mutations in the gene encoding 25(OH)D-1α-hydroxylase. Both alleles are inactivated in all patients, and compound heterozygotes, harboring distinct mutations, are common.

Clinical features include hypocalcemia, often with tetany or convulsions, hypophosphatemia, secondary hyperparathyroidism, and osteomalacia, often associated with skeletal deformities and increased alkaline phosphatase. Treatment involves physiologic replacement doses of $1,25(OH)_2D_3$ (Chap. 346).

VITAMIN D–DEPENDENT RICKETS TYPE II
Vitamin D–dependent rickets type II results from end-organ resistance to the active metabolite $1,25(OH)_2D_3$. The clinical features resemble those of the type I disorder and include hypocalcemia, hypophosphatemia, secondary hyperparathyroidism, and rickets but also partial or total alopecia. Plasma levels of $1,25(OH)_2D$ are at least three times normal, in keeping with the refractoriness of the end organs. All of the genetically characterized phenotypes have mutations in the gene for the vitamin D receptor. Treatment is difficult, given the receptor defect (Chap. 346).

Pseudohypoparathyroidism
PHP is a hereditary disorder characterized by symptoms and signs of hypoparathyroidism, typically in association with distinctive skeletal and developmental defects. The hypoparathyroidism is due to a deficient end-organ response to PTH. Hyperplasia of the parathyroids, a response to hormone resistance, causes elevation of PTH levels. Studies, both clinical and basic, have clarified some aspects of this syndrome, including the variable clinical spectrum, the pathophysiology, the genetic defects, and the inheritance.

A working classification of the various forms of PHP is given in Table 347-6. The classification scheme is based on the signs of ineffective PTH action (low calcium and high phosphate), urinary cyclic AMP response to exogenous PTH, the presence or absence of *Albright's hereditary osteodystrophy* (AHO), and assays of the concentration of the $G_s\alpha$ subunit of the adenylate cyclase enzyme. Using these criteria, there are four types: PHP type I, subdivided into a and b categories; PHP-II; and pseudopseudohypoparathyroidism (PPHP).

PHP-IA AND PHP-IB
Individuals with PHP-I, the most common of the disorders, show a deficient urinary cyclic AMP response to administration of exogenous PTH. Patients with PHP-I are divided into type a, with AHO and reduced amounts of $G_s\alpha$ in in vitro assays with erythrocytes, and type b, lacking AHO and with normal amounts of $G_s\alpha$ in erythrocytes. There is a third type (PHP-Ic, reported in a few patients) that differs from PHP-Ia only in having normal erythrocyte levels of $G_s\alpha$ despite having AHO, hypocalcemia, and decreased urinary cyclic AMP responses to PTH (presumably with a post-$G_s\alpha$ defect in adenyl cyclase stimulation).

Most patients have PHP-Ia and reveal characteristic features of AHO, consisting of short stature, round face, skeletal anomalies (brachydactyly), and heterotopic calcification. Patients have low calcium and high phosphate levels, as with true hypoparathyroidism. PTH levels, however, are elevated, reflecting resistance to hormone action.

Amorphous deposits of calcium and phosphate are found in the basal ganglia in about half of patients. The defects in metacarpal and metatarsal bones are sometimes accompanied by short phalanges as well, possibly reflecting premature closing of the epiphyses. The typical findings are short fourth and fifth metacarpals and metatarsals. The defects are usually bilateral. Exostoses and radius curvus are frequent. Impairments in olfaction and taste and unusual dermatoglyphic abnormalities have been reported.

TABLE 347-6 CLASSIFICATION OF PSEUDOHYPOPARATHYROIDISM (PHP) AND PSEUDOPSEUDOHYPOPARATHYROIDISM (PPHP)

Type	Hypocalcemia, Hyperphosphatemia	Response of Urinary cAMP to PTH	Serum PTH	$G_s\alpha$ Subunit Deficiency	AHO	Resistance to Hormones in Addition to PTH
PHP-Ia	Yes	↓	↑	Yes	Yes	Yes
PHP-Ib	Yes	↓	↑	No	No	No
PHP-II	Yes	Normal	↑	No	No	No
PPHP	No	Normal	Normal	Yes	Yes	±

Note: ↓, decreased; ↑, increased; AHO, Albright's hereditary osteodystrophy; PTH, parathyroid hormone.

FIGURE 347-7 Paternal imprinting of renal parathyroid hormone (PTH) resistance (*GNAS-1* gene for $G_s\alpha$ subunit) in pseudohypoparathyroidism (PHPIa). An impaired excretion of urinary cyclic AMP and phosphate is observed in patients with PHP. In the renal cortex, there is selective silencing of the paternal $G_s\alpha$ gene mRNA. The disease becomes manifest only in patients who inherit the defective gene from an obligate female carrier (*left*). If the genetic defect is inherited from an obligate male gene carrier, there is no biochemical abnormality; administration of PTH causes an appropriate increase in the urinary cyclic AMP and phosphate concentration [pseudo-PHP (PPHP); *right*]. Both patterns of inheritance lead to Albright's hereditary osteodystrophy (AHO), perhaps because of haplotype insufficiency—i.e., both copies of $G_s\alpha$ must be active in the fetus for normal bone development.

Inheritance and Genetic Patterns

Multiple defects have now been identified in the *GNAS-1* gene in PHP-Ia and PPHP patients. This gene, which is located on chromosome 20q13, encodes the stimulatory G-protein subunit $G_s\alpha$, among other products (see below). Mutations include abnormalities in splice junctions associated with deficient mRNA production and point mutations that result in a protein with defective function; these mutations can be detected, as well as a 50% reduction in $G_s\alpha$ levels in erythrocytes, reflecting loss of the protein from the mutated allele.

Detailed analyses of disease transmission in affected kindreds have clarified many features of PHP-Ia, PPHP, and PHP-Ib (Fig. 347-7). The former two entities, traced through multiple kindreds, have an inheritance pattern consistent with gene imprinting—only females, not males, can transmit the full disease with hypocalcemia—and PHP and PPHP do not coexist in the same generation. The phenomenon of gene imprinting, independent of any mutation, involves selective inactivation of either the maternal or the paternal allele (Chap. 62). In the case of the $G_s\alpha$ transcript, it is paternally imprinted (silenced) in the renal cortex (where the disease manifestation is expressed), so that the disease PHP-Ia can never be inherited from the father carrying the defective allele but only from a mother whose allelic product is critical in the kidney. In the renal cortex, it is postulated that only the maternal allele is normally active (independent of any mutation), such that lack of activity from a defective paternal allele is not of consequence. This explains the occurrence in PHP-Ia of hypocalcemia, hyperphosphatemia, and other stigmata such as variable resistance to other hormones (since similar tissue-specific imprinting occurs in other endocrine organs). Strong evidence favoring this overall hypothesis comes from gene knockout studies in the mouse (ablating exon 2 of the gene responsible for $G_s\alpha$ synthesis). Mice inheriting the mutant allele from the female had undetectable $G_s\alpha$ protein in renal cortex and were hypocalcemic and resistant to renal actions of PTH. Offspring inheriting the mutant allele from the male showed no evidence of PTH resistance or hypercalcemia.

Imprinting is tissue selective. The defective *GNAS* allele is not imprinted or silenced in many tissues. It seems likely, therefore, that the AHO phenotype recognized in PPHP as well as PHP-Ia reflects haplotype insufficiency during embryonic development.

The complex mechanisms that control the *GNAS* gene contribute to challenges involved in unraveling the pathogenesis of these disorders, especially that of PHP-1b. Much intensive work with kindred having PHP-1b, as well as studies of the complex regulation of the *GNAS* gene locus, have now offered an explanation for the features of PHP-1b, particularly the absence of $G_s\alpha$ deficiency in erythrocytes used to determine $G_s\alpha$ subunit deficiency (Table 347-6), in the setting of defective urinary cyclic response to PTH, the absence of the AHO phenotype, and maternal inheritance of the disease.

The defect in PHP-Ib is not a mutation in the $G_s\alpha$ portion of the gene but rather upstream deletions on the maternal allele that interfere with the normal methylation patterns, such that in the renal cortex neither the paternal (normally imprinted) nor the usual maternally expressed allele is active in transcription of $G_s\alpha$. There is no $G_s\alpha$ in the renal cortex but normal expression in other tissues, hence the normal erythrocyte levels of $G_s\alpha$ and the normal development of bone (no AHO phenotype).

PHP-Ib, lacking the AHO phenotype, shares with PHP-Ia the resistance to PTH action, a blunted urinary cyclic AMP response to administered PTH, a standard test for hormone resistance (Table 347-6), and an inheritance pattern of disease transmission only from the mother. PHP-Ib patients, however, show normal levels of $G_s\alpha$ in erythrocytes. Bone responsiveness may be excessive rather than blunted in PHP-Ib compared to PHP-Ia patients, based on case reports that have emphasized an osteitis fibrosa–like pattern in some PHP patients who lack the AHO phenotype.

PHP-II refers to patients with hypocalcemia and hyperphosphatemia who have a normal urinary cyclic AMP response to PTH. These patients are assumed to have a defect in the response to PTH at a locus distal to cyclic AMP production, although at least some patients may instead have occult vitamin D deficiency.

The diagnosis of these hormone-resistant states can usually be made without difficulty when there is a positive family history for developmental defects and/or the presence of developmental anomalies, including brachydactyly, in association with the signs and symptoms of hypoparathyroidism. In both categories—PHP-Ia and -Ib—serum PTH levels are elevated, particularly when patients are hypocalcemic. However, patients with PHP-Ib or PHP-II do not have phenotypic abnormalities, only hypocalcemia with high PTH levels, confirming hormone resistance. In PHP-Ib, the response of urinary cyclic AMP to the administration of exogenous PTH is blunted. The diagnosis of PHP-II is more complex, in that cyclic AMP responses in urine are, by definition, normal. Since vitamin D deficiency itself can dissociate phosphaturic and urinary cyclic AMP responses to exogenous PTH, vitamin D deficiency must be excluded before the diagnosis of PHP-II can be entertained.

℞ PSEUDOHYPOPARATHYROIDISM

Treatment of PHP is similar to that of hypoparathyroidism, except that the doses of vitamin D and calcium are usually lower than those required in true hypoparathyroidism, presumably because the defect in PHP is only partial because of imprinting in specific tissues and tissue sites (renal cortex vs. renal medulla)—hence, urinary calcium clearance, a distal tubular function, is not affected. Variability in response makes it necessary to establish the optimal regimen for each patient, based on maintaining the appropriate blood calcium level and urinary calcium excretion.

PTH OVERWHELMED

Occasionally, loss of calcium from the ECF is so severe that PTH cannot compensate. Such situations include acute pancreatitis and severe, acute hyperphosphatemia, often in association with renal failure, conditions in which there is rapid efflux of calcium from the ECF. Severe hypocalcemia can occur quickly; PTH rises in response to hypocalcemia but does not return blood calcium to normal.

Severe, Acute Hyperphosphatemia Severe hyperphosphatemia is associated with extensive tissue damage or cell destruction (Chap. 346). The combination of increased release of phosphate from muscle and impaired ability to excrete phosphorus because of renal failure causes moderate to severe hyperphosphatemia, the latter causing calcium loss from the blood and mild to moderate hypocalcemia. Hypocalcemia is usually reversed with tissue repair and restoration of renal function as phosphorus and creatinine values return to normal. There may even be a mild hypercalcemic period in the oliguric phase of renal function recovery. This sequence, severe hypocalcemia followed by mild hypercalcemia, reflects widespread deposition of calcium in muscle and subsequent redistribution of some of the calcium to the ECF after phosphate levels return to normal.

Other causes of hyperphosphatemia include hypothermia, massive hepatic failure, and hematologic malignancies, either because of high cell turnover of malignancy or because of cell destruction by chemotherapy.

Rx SEVERE, ACUTE HYPERPHOSPHATEMIA

Treatment is directed toward lowering of blood phosphate by the administration of phosphate-binding antacids or dialysis, often needed for the management of renal failure. Although calcium replacement may be necessary if hypocalcemia is severe and symptomatic, calcium administration during the hyperphosphatemic period tends to increase extraosseous calcium deposition and aggravate tissue damage. The levels of $1,25(OH)_2D$ may be low during the hyperphosphatemic phase and return to normal during the oliguric phase of recovery.

Osteitis Fibrosis after Parathyroidectomy Severe hypocalcemia after parathyroid surgery is rare now that osteitis fibrosa cystica is an infrequent manifestation of hyperparathyroidism. When osteitis fibrosa cystica is severe, however, bone mineral deficits can be large. After parathyroidectomy, hypocalcemia can persist for days if calcium replacement is inadequate. Treatment may require parenteral administration of calcium; addition of calcitriol and oral calcium supplementation is sometimes needed for weeks to a month or two until bone defects are filled (which, of course, is of therapeutic benefit in the skeleton), making it possible to discontinue parenteral calcium and/or reduce the amount.

DIFFERENTIAL DIAGNOSIS OF HYPOCALCEMIA

Care must be taken to ensure that true hypocalcemia is present; in addition, acute transient hypocalcemia can be a manifestation of a variety of severe, acute illnesses, as discussed above. *Chronic hypocalcemia*, however, can usually be ascribed to a few disorders associated with absent or ineffective PTH. Important clinical criteria include the duration of the illness, signs or symptoms of associated disorders, and the presence of features that suggest a hereditary abnormality. A nutritional history can be helpful in recognizing a low intake of vitamin D and calcium in the elderly, and a history of excessive alcohol intake may suggest magnesium deficiency.

Hypoparathyroidism and PHP are typically lifelong illnesses, usually (but not always) appearing by adolescence; hence a recent onset of hypocalcemia in an adult is more likely due to nutritional deficiencies, renal failure, or intestinal disorders that result in deficient or ineffective vitamin D. Neck surgery, even long past, however, can be associated with a delayed onset of postoperative hypoparathyroidism. A history of seizure disorder raises the issue of anticonvulsive medication. Developmental defects may point to the diagnosis of PHP. Rickets and a variety of neuromuscular syndromes and deformities may indicate ineffective vitamin D action, either due to defects in vitamin D metabolism or to vitamin D deficiency.

A pattern of *low calcium with high phosphorus* in the absence of renal failure or massive tissue destruction almost invariably means hypoparathyroidism or PHP. A *low calcium and low phosphorus* points to absent or ineffective vitamin D, thereby impairing the action of PTH on calcium metabolism (but not phosphate clearance). The relative ineffectiveness of PTH in calcium homeostasis in vitamin D deficiency, anticonvulsant therapy, gastrointestinal disorders, and hereditary defects in vitamin D metabolism leads to secondary hyperparathyroidism as a compensation. The excess PTH on renal tubule phosphate transport accounts for renal phosphate wasting and hypophosphatemia.

Exceptions to these patterns may occur. Most forms of hypomagnesemia are due to long-standing nutritional deficiency as seen in chronic alcoholics. Despite the fact that the hypocalcemia is principally due to an acute absence of PTH, phosphate levels are usually low, rather than elevated as in hypoparathyroidism. Chronic renal failure is often associated with hypocalcemia and hyperphosphatemia, despite secondary hyperparathyroidism.

Diagnosis is usually established by application of the PTH immunoassay, tests for vitamin D metabolites, and measurements of the urinary cyclic AMP response to exogenous PTH. In hereditary and acquired hypoparathyroidism and in severe hypomagnesemia, PTH is either undetectable or in the normal range. This finding in a hypocalcemic patient is supportive of hypoparathyroidism, as distinct from ineffective PTH action, in which even mild hypocalcemia is associated with elevated PTH levels. Hence a failure to detect elevated PTH levels establishes the diagnosis of hypoparathyroidism; elevated levels suggest the presence of secondary hyperparathyroidism, as found in many of the situations in which the hormone is ineffective due to associated abnormalities in vitamin D action. Assays for 25(OH)D can be helpful. Low or low-normal 25(OH)D indicates vitamin D deficiency due to lack of sunlight, inadequate vitamin D intake, or intestinal malabsorption. Recognition that mild hypocalcemia, rickets, and hypophosphatemia are due to anticonvulsant therapy is made by history.

Rx HYPOCALCEMIC STATES

The management of hypoparathyroidism, PHP, chronic renal failure, and hereditary defects in vitamin D metabolism involves the use of vitamin D or vitamin D metabolites and calcium supplementation. Vitamin D itself is the least expensive form of vitamin D replacement and is frequently used in the management of uncomplicated hypoparathyroidism and some disorders associated with ineffective vitamin D action. When vitamin D is used prophylactically, as in the elderly or in those with chronic anticonvulsant therapy, there is a wider margin of safety than with the more potent metabolites. However, most of the conditions in which vitamin D is administered chronically for hypocalcemia require amounts 50–100 times the daily replacement dose because the formation of $1,25(OH)_2D$ is deficient. In such situations, vitamin D is no safer than the active metabolite because intoxication can occur with high-dose therapy (because of storage in fat). Calcitriol is more rapid in onset of action and also has a short biologic half-life.

Vitamin D [at least 2000 U/d (5 μg/d) (higher levels required in older persons)] or calcitriol (0.25–1.0 μg/d) is required to prevent rickets in normal individuals. In contrast, 40,000–120,000 U (1–3 mg) of vitamin D_2 or D_3 is typically required in hypoparathyroidism. The dose of calcitriol is unchanged in hypoparathyroidism, since the defect is in hydroxylation by the 25(OH)D-1α-hydroxylase. Calcitriol is also used in disorders of 25(OH)D-1α-hydroxylase; vitamin D receptor defects are much more difficult to treat.

Patients with hypoparathyroidism should be given 2–3 g elemental calcium PO each day. The two agents, vitamin D or calcitriol and oral calcium, can be varied independently. If hypocalcemia alternates with episodes of hypercalcemia in more brittle patients with hypoparathyroidism, administration of calcitriol and use of thiazides, as discussed above, may make management easier.

FURTHER READINGS

BASTEPE M, JÜPPNER H: *GNAS* locus and pseudohypoparathyroidism. Horm Res 63:65, 2005

BILEZIKIAN JP et al: Summary statement from a workshop on asymptomatic primary hyperparathyroidism: A perspective for the 21st century. J Bone Min Res 17(Suppl 2):N2, 2002

———, POTTS JT JR: Asymptomatic primary hyperparathyroidism: New issues and new questions—bridging the past with the future. J Bone Min Res 17(Suppl 2):N57, 2002

DEGROOT LJ, JAMESON JL (eds): *Endocrinology*, 5th ed. Philadelphia, Saunders, 2005

KREBS LJ et al: *HRPT2* mutational analysis of typical sporadic parathyroid adenomas. J Clin Endocrinol Metab 90:5015, 2005

PEACOCK M et al: Cinacalcet hydrochloride maintains long-term normocalcemia in patients with primary hyperparathyroidism. J Clin Endocrinol Metab 90:135, 2005

STEWART AF: Clinical practice: Hypercalcemia associated with cancer. N Engl J Med 352:373, 2005

WEINSTEIN LS et al: Minireview: GNAS: Normal and abnormal functions. Endocrinology 145:5459, 2004

348 Osteoporosis
Robert Lindsay, Felicia Cosman

Osteoporosis, a condition characterized by decreased bone strength, is prevalent among postmenopausal women but also occurs in men and women with underlying conditions or major risk factors associated with bone demineralization. Its chief clinical manifestations are vertebral and hip fractures, although fractures can occur at any skeletal site. Osteoporosis affects >10 million individuals in the United States, but only a small proportion are diagnosed and treated.

DEFINITION

Osteoporosis is defined as a reduction in the strength of bone leading to an increased risk of fractures. Loss of bone tissue is associated with deterioration in skeletal microarchitecture. The World Health Organization (WHO) operationally defines osteoporosis as a bone density that falls 2.5 standard deviations (SD) below the mean for young healthy adults of the same gender—also referred to as a *T-score* of –2.5. Postmenopausal women who fall at the lower end of the young normal range (a T-score of >1 SD below the mean) are defined as having low bone density and are also at increased risk of osteoporosis. More than 50% of the fractures, including hip fractures, among postmenopausal women occur in this group.

EPIDEMIOLOGY

In the United States, as many as 8 million women and 2 million men have osteoporosis (T-score < –2.5), and an additional 18 million individuals have bone mass levels that put them at increased risk of developing osteoporosis (e.g., bone mass T-score < –1.0). Osteoporosis occurs more frequently with increasing age as bone tissue is progressively lost. In women, the loss of ovarian function at menopause (typically about age 50) precipitates rapid bone loss such that most women meet the diagnostic criterion for osteoporosis by age 70–80.

The epidemiology of fractures follows the trend for bone density loss. Fractures of the distal radius increase in frequency before age 50 and plateau by age 60, with only a modest age-related increase thereafter. In contrast, incidence rates for hip fractures double every 5 years after age 70 (Fig. 348-1). This distinct epidemiology may be related to the way people fall as they age, with fewer falls on an outstretched hand and more falls directly on the hip. At least 1.5 million fractures

FIGURE 348-2 Lateral spine x-ray showing severe osteopenia and a severe wedge-type deformity (severe anterior compression).

occur each year in the United States as a consequence of osteoporosis. As the population continues to age, the total number of fractures will continue to escalate.

About 300,000 hip fractures occur each year in the United States, most of which require hospital admission and surgical intervention. The probability that a 50-year-old white individual will have a hip fracture during his or her lifetime is 14% for women and 5% for men; the risk for African Americans is lower (about half these rates). Hip fractures are associated with a high incidence of deep vein thrombosis and pulmonary embolism (20–50%) and a mortality rate between 5 and 20% during the year after surgery.

There are about 700,000 vertebral crush fractures per year in the United States. Only a fraction of these are recognized clinically, since many are relatively asymptomatic and are identified incidentally during radiography for other purposes (Fig. 348-2). Vertebral fractures rarely require hospitalization but are associated with long-term morbidity and a slight increase in mortality, primarily related to pulmonary disease. Multiple vertebral fractures lead to height loss (often of several inches), kyphosis, and secondary pain and discomfort related to altered biomechanics of the back. Thoracic fractures can be associated with restrictive lung disease, whereas lumbar fractures are associated with abdominal symptoms including distention, early satiety, and constipation.

Approximately 250,000 wrist fractures occur in the United States each year. Fractures of other bones (estimated to be ~300,000 per year) also occur with osteoporosis, which is not surprising given that bone loss is a systemic phenomenon. Fractures of the pelvis and proximal humerus are clearly associated with osteoporosis. Although some fractures are the result of major trauma, the threshold for fracture is reduced for an osteoporotic bone (Fig. 348-3). In addition to bone density there are a number of risk factors for fracture; the common ones are summarized in Table 348-1. Age, prior fractures, a family history of osteoporosis-re-

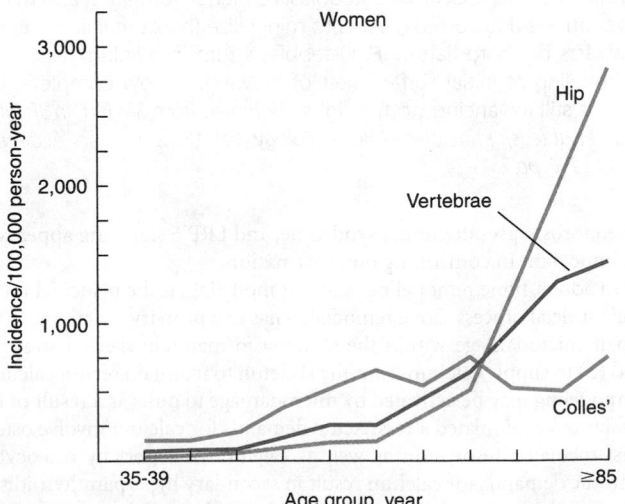

FIGURE 348-1 Epidemiology of vertebral, hip, and Colles' fractures with age. [Adapted from C Cooper, LJ Melton III: Trends Endocrinol Metab 3:224, 1992; with permission.]

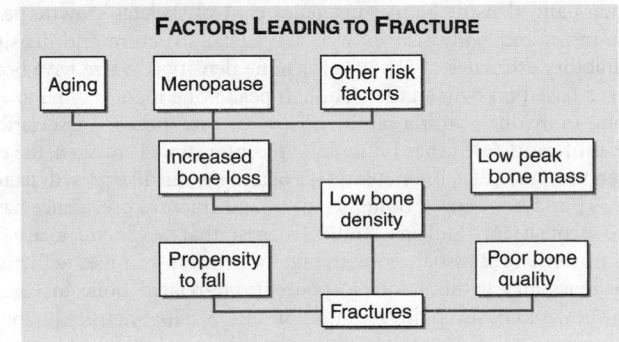

FIGURE 348-3 Factors leading to osteoporotic fractures.

TABLE 348-1	RISK FACTORS FOR OSTEOPOROSIS FRACTURE	
Nonmodifiable	Estrogen deficiency	
Personal history of fracture as an adult	Early menopause (<45 years) or bilateral ovariectomy	
History of fracture in first-degree relative	Prolonged premenstrual amenorrhea (>1 year)	
Female sex	Low calcium intake	
Advanced age	Alcoholism	
Caucasian race	Impaired eyesight despite adequate correction	
Dementia		
Potentially modifiable	Recurrent falls	
Current cigarette smoking	Inadequate physical activity	
Low body weight [<58 kg (127 lb)]	Poor health/frailty	

lated fractures, low body weight, cigarette consumption, and excessive alcohol use are each independent predictors of fracture. Chronic diseases with inflammatory components that increase skeletal remodeling, such as rheumatoid arthritis, increase the risk of osteoporosis, as do diseases associated with malabsorption. Chronic diseases that increase the risk of falling or frailty, including dementia, Parkinson's disease, and multiple sclerosis, also increase fracture risk.

In the United States and Europe, osteoporosis-related fractures are more common among women than men, presumably due to a lower peak bone mass as well as postmenopausal bone loss in women. However, this gender difference in bone density and age-related increase in hip fractures is not as apparent in some other cultures, possibly due to genetics, physical activity level, or diet.

Fractures are themselves risk factors for future fractures (Table 348-1). Vertebral fractures increase the risk of other vertebral fractures as well as fractures of the peripheral skeleton such as hip and wrist. Wrist fractures also increase the risk of vertebral and hip fractures. Consequently, among individuals over the age of 50, any fracture should be considered as potentially related to osteoporosis, irrespective of the circumstances of fracture. Osteoporotic bone is more likely to fracture than normal bone at any level of trauma, and a fracture in a person over 50 should trigger evaluation for osteoporosis.

PATHOPHYSIOLOGY

BONE REMODELING

Osteoporosis results from bone loss due to age-related changes in bone remodeling as well as extrinsic and intrinsic factors that exaggerate this process. These changes may be superimposed on a low peak bone mass. Consequently, understanding the bone remodeling process is fundamental to understanding the pathophysiology of osteoporosis (Chap. 346). During growth, the skeleton increases in size by linear growth and by apposition of new bone tissue on the outer surfaces of the cortex (Fig. 348-4). This latter process is called *modeling*, a process that also allows the long bones to adapt in shape to the stresses placed upon them. Increased sex hormone production at puberty is required for skeletal maturation, which reaches maximum mass and density in early adulthood. It is around puberty that the sexual dimorphism in skeletal size becomes obvious, although true bone density remains similar between sexes. Nutrition and lifestyle also play an important role in growth, though genetic factors primarily determine peak skeletal mass and density. Numerous genes control skeletal growth, peak bone mass, and body size, as well as skeletal structure and density. Heritability estimates of 50–80% for bone density and size have been derived based on twin studies. Though peak bone mass is often lower among individuals with a family history of osteoporosis, association studies of candidate genes [vitamin D receptor; type I collagen, the estrogen receptor (ER), interleukin (IL) 6; and insulin-like growth factor (IGF) I] and bone mass, bone turnover, and fracture prevalence have been inconsistent. Linkage studies suggest that a genetic locus on chromosome 11 is associated with high bone mass. Families with high bone mass and without much apparent age-related bone loss have been shown to have a point mutation in LRP 5, a low-density lipoprotein receptor–related protein. The role of this gene in the general population is not clear, although a nonfunctional mutation results in

FIGURE 348-4 Mechanism of bone remodeling. The basic molecular unit (BMU) moves along the trabecular surface at a rate of about 10 μm/d. The figure depicts remodeling over ~120 days. **A.** Origination of BMU-lining cells contract to expose collagen and attract preosteoclasts. **B.** Osteoclasts fuse into multinucleated cells that resorb a cavity. Mononuclear cells continue resorption and preosteoblasts are stimulated to proliferate. **C.** Osteoblasts align at bottom of cavity and start forming osteoid (black). **D.** Osteoblasts continue formation and mineralization. Previous osteoid starts to mineralize (horizontal lines). **E.** Osteoblasts begin to flatten. **F.** Osteoblasts turn into lining cells; bone remodeling at initial surface (left of drawing) is now complete, but BMU is still advancing (to the right). [*Adapted from SM Ott, in JP Bilezikian et al (eds): Principles of Bone Biology, vol. 18. San Diego, Academic Press, 1996, pp 231–241.*]

osteoporosis-pseudoglioma syndrome, and LRP 5 signaling appears to be important in controlling bone formation.

In adults, bone remodeling, and not modeling, is the principal metabolic skeletal process. Bone remodeling has two primary functions: (1) to repair microdamage within the skeleton to maintain skeletal strength, and (2) to supply calcium from the skeleton to maintain serum calcium. Remodeling may be activated by microdamage to bone as a result of excessive or accumulated stress. Acute demands for calcium involve osteoclast-mediated resorption as well as calcium transport by osteocytes. Chronic demands for calcium result in secondary hyperparathyroidism, increased bone remodeling, and overall loss of bone tissue.

Bone remodeling is also regulated by several circulating hormones, including estrogens, androgens, vitamin D, and parathyroid hormone (PTH), as well as locally produced growth factors such as IGF-I and -II,

A

B

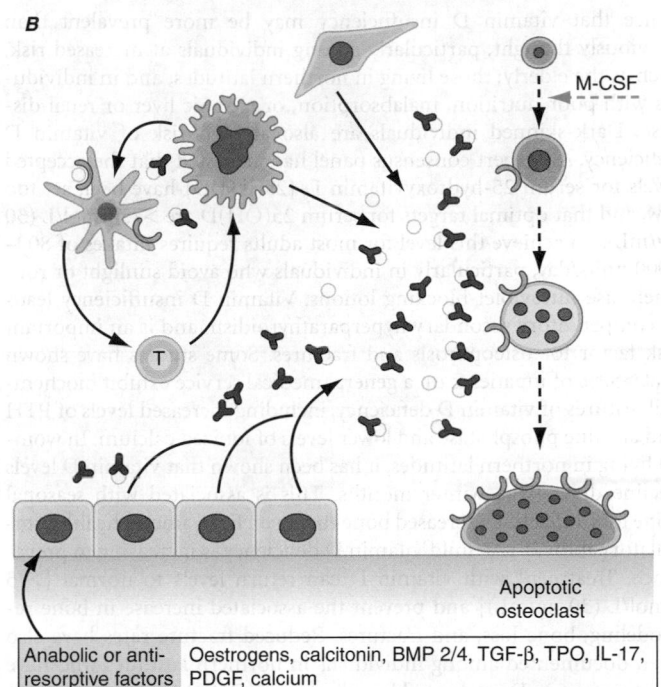

Pro-resorptive and calciotropic factors	1,25(OH)$_2$ vitamin D$_3$. PTH, PTHrP, PGE2, IL-1, IL-6, TNF, prolactin, corticosteroids, oncostatin M, LIF

Anabolic or anti-resorptive factors	Oestrogens, calcitonin, BMP 2/4, TGF-β, TPO, IL-17, PDGF, calcium

FIGURE 348-5 Hormonal control of bone resorption. A. Proresorptive and calcitropic factors; **B.** Anabolic and antiosteoclastic factors. RANKL expression is induced in osteoblasts, activated T cells, synovial fibroblasts, and bone marrow stromal cells. It binds to membrane-bound receptor RANK to promote osteoclast differentiation, activation, and survival. Conversely, osteoprotegerin (OPG) expression is induced by factors that block bone catabolism and promote anabolic effects. OPG binds and neutralizes RANKL, leading to a block in osteoclastogenesis and decreased survival of preexisting osteoclasts. RANKL, receptor activator of nuclear factor NFκB; PTH, parathyroid hormone; PGE2, prostaglandin E2; TNF, tumor necrosis factor; LIF, leukemia inhibitory factor; TPO, thrombospondin; PDGF, platelet-derived growth factor; OPG-L, osteoprotegerin-ligand; IL, interleukin; TGF-β, transforming growth factor β. *(From WJ Boyle et al: Nature 423: 337, 2003.)*

transforming growth factor (TGF) β, parathyroid hormone–related peptide (PTHrP), ILs, prostaglandins, and members of the tumor necrosis factor (TNF) superfamily. These factors primarily modulate the rate at which new remodeling sites are activated, a process that results initially in bone resorption by osteoclasts, followed by a period of repair during which new bone tissue is synthesized by osteoblasts. The cytokine responsible for communication between the osteoblasts, other marrow cells, and osteoclasts has been identified as RANK ligand (receptor activator of NF-kappa-B; RANKL). RANKL, a member of the TNF family, is secreted by osteoblasts and certain cells of the immune system (Chap. 346). The osteoclast receptor for this protein is referred to as *RANK*. Activation of RANK by RANKL is a final common path in osteoclast development and activation. A humoral decoy for RANKL, also secreted by osteoblasts, is referred to as *osteoprotegerin* (Fig. 348-5). Modulation of osteoclast recruitment and activity appears to be related to the interplay among these three factors. Additional influences include nutrition (particularly calcium intake) and physical activity level.

In young adults resorbed bone is replaced by an equal amount of new bone tissue. Thus, the mass of the skeleton remains constant after peak bone mass is achieved in adulthood. After age 30–45, however, the resorption and formation processes become imbalanced, and resorption exceeds formation. This imbalance may begin at different ages and varies at different skeletal sites; it becomes exaggerated in women after menopause. Excessive bone loss can be due to an increase in osteoclastic activity and/or a decrease in osteoblastic activity. In addition, an increase in remodeling activation frequency, and thus the number of remodeling sites, can magnify the small imbalance seen at each remodeling unit. Increased recruitment of bone remodeling sites produces a reversible reduction in bone tissue but can also result in permanent loss of tissue and disrupted skeletal architecture. In trabecular bone, if the osteoclasts penetrate trabeculae, they leave no template for new bone formation to occur and, consequently, rapid bone loss ensues and cancellous connectivity becomes impaired. A higher number of remodeling sites increases the likelihood of this event. In

cortical bone, increased activation of remodeling creates more porous bone. The effect of this increased porosity on cortical bone strength may be modest if the overall diameter of the bone is not changed. However, decreased apposition of new bone on the periosteal surface coupled with increased endocortical resorption of bone decreases the biomechanical strength of long bones. Even a slight exaggeration in normal bone loss increases the risk of osteoporosis-related fractures, due to the architectural changes that occur.

CALCIUM NUTRITION

Peak bone mass may be impaired by inadequate calcium intake during growth among other nutritional factors (calories, protein, and other minerals), thereby leading to increased risk of osteoporosis later in life. During the adult phase of life, insufficient calcium intake contributes to relative secondary hyperparathyroidism and an increase in the rate of bone remodeling to maintain normal serum calcium levels. PTH stimulates the hydroxylation of vitamin D in the kidney, leading to increased levels of 1,25-dihydroxyvitamin D [1,25(OH)$_2$D] and enhanced gastrointestinal calcium absorption. PTH also reduces renal calcium loss. Although these are all appropriate compensatory homeostatic responses for adjusting calcium economy, the long-term effects are detrimental to the skeleton because the increased remodeling rates and the ongoing imbalance between resorption and formation at remodeling sites combine to accelerate loss of bone tissue.

Total daily calcium intakes of <400 mg are detrimental to the skeleton, and intakes in the 600- to 800-mg range, which is about the average intake among adults in the United States, are also likely suboptimal. The recommended daily required intake of 1000–1200 mg for adults accommodates population heterogeneity in controlling calcium balance (Chap. 70).

VITAMIN D

(See also Chap. 346) Severe vitamin D deficiency causes rickets in children or osteomalacia in adults. However, there is accumulating evidence that vitamin D insufficiency may be more prevalent than previously thought, particularly among individuals at increased risk, such as the elderly; those living in northern latitudes; and in individuals with poor nutrition, malabsorption, or chronic liver or renal disease. Dark-skinned individuals are also at high risk of vitamin D deficiency. An expert consensus panel has suggested that the accepted levels for serum 25-hydroxyvitamin D [25(OH)D] have been set too low, and that optimal targets for serum 25(OH)D are >75 nmol/L (30 ng/mL). To achieve this level for most adults requires intakes of 800–1000 units/day, particularly in individuals who avoid sunlight or routinely use ultraviolet-blocking lotions. Vitamin D insufficiency leads to compensatory secondary hyperparathyroidism and is an important risk factor for osteoporosis and fractures. Some studies have shown that >50% of inpatients on a general medical service exhibit biochemical features of vitamin D deficiency, including increased levels of PTH and alkaline phosphatase and lower levels of ionized calcium. In women living in northern latitudes, it has been shown that vitamin D levels decline during the winter months. This is associated with seasonal bone loss, reflecting increased bone turnover. Even among healthy ambulatory individuals, mild vitamin D deficiency is increasing in prevalence. Treatment with vitamin D can return levels to normal [>75 μmol/L (30 ng/mL)] and prevent the associated increase in bone remodeling, bone loss, and fractures. Reduced fracture rates have also been documented among individuals in northern latitudes who have greater vitamin D intake and have higher 25(OH)D levels (see below). Vitamin D adequacy may also affect risk and/or severity of other diseases including cancers (colorectal, prostate, and breast), autoimmune diseases, and diabetes.

ESTROGEN STATUS

Estrogen deficiency probably causes bone loss by two distinct but interrelated mechanisms: (1) activation of new bone remodeling sites, and (2) exaggeration of the imbalance between bone formation and resorption. The change in activation frequency causes a transient bone loss until a new steady state between resorption and formation is achieved. The remodeling imbalance, however, results in a permanent decrement in mass. In addition, the very presence of more remodeling sites in the skeleton increases the probability that trabeculae will be penetrated, thereby eliminating the template upon which new bone can be formed and accelerating the loss of bony tissue.

The most frequent estrogen-deficient state is the cessation of ovarian function at the time of menopause, which occurs on average at the age of 51 (Chap. 342). Thus, with current life expectancy, an average woman will spend about 30 years without ovarian supply of estrogen. The mechanism by which estrogen deficiency causes bone loss is summarized in Fig. 348-5. Marrow cells (macrophages, monocytes, osteoclast precursors, mast cells) as well as bone cells (osteoblasts, osteocytes, osteoclasts) express ERs α and β. Loss of estrogen increases production of RANKL and may reduce production of osteoprogerin, increasing osteoclast recruitment. Estrogen may also play an important role in determining the life span of bone cells by controlling the rate of apoptosis. Thus, in situations of estrogen deprivation, the life span of osteoblasts may be decreased, whereas the longevity and activity of osteoclasts are increased.

Since remodeling is initiated at the surface of bone, it follows that trabecular bone—which has a considerably larger surface area (80% of the total) than cortical bone—will be preferentially affected by estrogen deficiency. Fractures occur earliest at sites where trabecular bone contributes most to bone strength; consequently, vertebral fractures are the most common early consequence of estrogen deficiency.

PHYSICAL ACTIVITY

Inactivity, such as prolonged bed rest or paralysis, results in significant bone loss. Concordantly, athletes have higher bone mass than the general population. These changes in skeletal mass are most marked when the stimulus begins during growth and before the age of puberty. Adults are less capable than children of increasing bone mass following restoration of physical activity. Epidemiologic data support the

TABLE 348-2	DISEASES ASSOCIATED WITH AN INCREASED RISK OF GENERALIZED OSTEOPOROSIS IN ADULTS
Hypogonadal states	Hematologic disorders/malignancy
Turner syndrome	Multiple myeloma
Klinefelter syndrome	Lymphoma and leukemia
Anorexia nervosa	Malignancy-associated parathyroid
Hypothalamic amenorrhea	hormone (PTHrP) production
Hyperprolactinemia	Mastocytosis
Other primary or secondary	Hemophilia
hypogonadal states	Thalassemia
Endocrine disorders	Selected inherited disorders
Cushing's syndrome	Osteogenesis imperfecta
Hyperparathyroidism	Marfan syndrome
Thyrotoxicosis	Hemochromatosis
Type 1 diabetes mellitus	Hypophosphatasia
Acromegaly	Glycogen storage diseases
Adrenal insufficiency	Homocystinuria
Nutritional and gastrointestinal	Ehlers-Danlos syndrome
disorders	Porphyria
Malnutrition	Menkes' syndrome
Parenteral nutrition	Epidermolysis bullosa
Malabsorption syndromes	Other disorders
Gastrectomy	Immobilization
Severe liver disease, especially	Chronic obstructive pulmonary
biliary cirrhosis	disease
Pernicious anemia	Pregnancy and lactation
Rheumatologic disorders	Scoliosis
Rheumatoid arthritis	Multiple sclerosis
Ankylosing spondylitis	Sarcoidosis
	Amyloidosis

beneficial effects on the skeleton of chronic high levels of physical activity. Fracture risk is lower in rural communities and in countries where physical activity is maintained into old age. However, when exercise is initiated during adult life, the effects of moderate exercise on the skeleton are modest, with a bone mass increase of 1–2% in short-term studies of <2 years' duration. It is argued that more active individuals are less likely to fall and are more capable of protecting themselves upon falling, thereby reducing fracture risk.

CHRONIC DISEASE

Various genetic and acquired diseases are associated with an increase in the risk of osteoporosis (Table 348-2). Mechanisms that contribute to bone loss are unique for each disease and typically result from multiple factors including nutrition, reduced physical activity levels, and factors that affect bone-remodeling rates. In most, but not all, circumstances the primary diagnosis is made before osteoporosis presents clinically.

MEDICATIONS

A large number of medications used in clinical practice have potentially detrimental effects on the skeleton (Table 348-3). *Glucocorticoids* are the most common cause of medication-induced osteoporosis. It is often not possible to determine the extent to which osteoporosis is related to the glucocorticoid or to other factors, as treatment is superimposed on the effects of the primary disease, which may in itself be associated with bone loss (e.g., rheumatoid arthritis). Excessive doses of thyroid hormone can accelerate bone remodeling and result in bone loss.

Other medications have less detrimental effects upon the skeleton than pharmacologic doses of glucocorticoids. *Anticonvulsants* are thought to increase the risk of osteoporosis, although many affected

TABLE 348-3	DRUGS ASSOCIATED WITH AN INCREASED RISK OF GENERALIZED OSTEOPOROSIS IN ADULTS
Glucocorticoids	Excessive thyroxine
Cyclosporine	Aluminum
Cytotoxic drugs	Gonadotropin-releasing hormone agonists
Anticonvulsants	Heparin
Excessive alcohol	Lithium
Aromatase inhibitors	

individuals have concomitant insufficiency of 1,25(OH)2D, as some anticonvulsants induce the cytochrome P450 system and vitamin D metabolism. Patients undergoing transplantation are at high risk for rapid bone loss and fracture, not only from glucocorticoids but also from treatment with other *immunosuppressants*, such as cyclosporine and tacrolimus (FK506). In addition, these patients often have underlying metabolic abnormalities, such as hepatic or renal failure, that predispose to bone loss.

Aromatase inhibitors, which potently block the aromatase enzyme that converts androgens and other adrenal precursors to estrogen, reduce circulating postmenopausal estrogen levels dramatically. These agents, used in various stages for breast cancer treatment, have also been shown to have a detrimental effect on bone density and risk of fracture.

CIGARETTE CONSUMPTION

The use of cigarettes over a long period has detrimental effects on bone mass. These effects may be mediated directly, by toxic effects on osteoblasts, or indirectly by modifying estrogen metabolism. On average, cigarette smokers reach menopause 1–2 years earlier than the general population. Cigarette smoking also produces secondary effects that can modulate skeletal status, including intercurrent respiratory and other illnesses, frailty, decreased exercise, poor nutrition, and the need for additional medications (e.g., glucocorticoids for lung disease).

MEASUREMENT OF BONE MASS

Several noninvasive techniques are now available for estimating skeletal mass or density. These include dual-energy x-ray absorptiometry (DXA), single-energy x-ray absorptiometry (SXA), quantitative CT, and ultrasound.

DXA is a highly accurate x-ray technique that has become the standard for measuring bone density in most centers. Though it can be used for measurements of any skeletal site, clinical determinations are usually made of the lumbar spine and hip. Portable DXA machines have been developed that measure the heel (calcaneus), forearm (radius and ulna), or finger (phalanges). DXA can also be used to measure body composition. In the DXA technique, two x-ray energies are used to estimate the area of mineralized tissue, and the mineral content is divided by the area, which partially corrects for body size. However, this correction is only partial since DXA is a two-dimensional scanning technique and cannot estimate the depths or posteroanterior length of the bone. Thus, small people tend to have lower-than-average bone mineral density (BMD). Bone spurs, which are frequent in osteoarthritis, tend to falsely increase bone density of the spine and are a particular problem in measuring the spine of older individuals. Because DXA instrumentation is provided by several different manufacturers, the output varies in absolute terms. Consequently, it has become standard practice to relate the results to "normal" values using T-scores, which compare individual results to those in a young population that is matched for race and gender. Z-scores compare individual results to those of an age-matched population that is also matched for race and gender. Thus, a 60-year-old woman with a Z-score of –1 (1 SD below mean for age) has a T-score of –2.5 (2.5 SD below mean for a young control group) (Fig. 348-6). A T-score below –2.5 in the lumbar spine, femoral neck, or total hip is taken as a diagnosis of osteoporosis.

CT is used primarily to measure the spine and more recently the hip. Peripheral CT is used to measure bone in the forearm or tibia. The results obtained from CT are different from all others currently available since this technique is three dimensional and can provide a true density (mass of bone tissue per unit volume). CT can also specifically analyze trabecular bone and cortical bone content and volume separately. However, CT remains expensive, involves greater radiation exposure, and is less reproducible than DXA. A new technique employing high-resolution CT scanning (called *Xtreme CT*) can also provide information on skeletal architecture, including cancellous connectivity.

Ultrasound is used to measure bone mass by calculating the attenuation of the signal as it passes through bone or the speed with which it

FIGURE 348-6 Relationship between Z-scores and T-scores in a 60-year-old woman (BMD, bone mineral density; SD, standard deviation).

traverses the bone. It is unclear whether ultrasound assesses properties of bone other than mass (e.g., quality), but this is a potential advantage of the technique. Because of its relatively low cost and mobility, ultrasound is amenable for use as a screening procedure.

All of these techniques for measuring BMD have been approved by the U.S. Food and Drug Administration (FDA) based upon their capacity to predict fracture risk. The hip is the preferred site of measurement in most individuals, since it predicts the risk of hip fracture, the most important consequence of osteoporosis, better than any other bone density measurement site. When hip measurements are performed by DXA, the spine can be measured at the same time. In younger individuals, such as perimenopausal or early postmenopausal women, spine measurements may be the most sensitive indicator of bone loss.

WHEN TO MEASURE BONE MASS

Clinical guidelines have been developed for use of bone densitometry in clinical practice. The original National Osteoporosis Foundation guidelines recommend bone mass measurements in postmenopausal women, assuming they have one or more risk factors for osteoporosis in addition to age, gender, and estrogen deficiency. The guidelines further recommend that bone mass measurement be considered in *all* women by age 65, a position ratified by the U.S. Preventive Health Services Task Force. Criteria approved for Medicare reimbursement of BMD are summarized in Table 348-4.

WHEN TO TREAT BASED UPON BONE MASS RESULTS

Most guidelines suggest that patients be considered for treatment when BMD is >2.5 SD below the mean value for young adults (T-score ≤ –2.5), a level consistent with the diagnosis of osteoporosis. Treatment should also be considered in postmenopausal women with risk factors, even if BMD is not in the osteoporosis range. It is important to consider the risk of fracture for individuals, including those whose BMD is within the premenopausal range. Risk factors (age, prior fracture, family history of hip fracture, low body weight, cigarette consumption, excessive alcohol, steroid use, and rheumatoid arthritis) can be combined with BMD to assess the likelihood of a fracture over a 5- or 10-year period. Treatment thresholds depend on cost-effectiveness analyses but will likely be ~1% per year of risk in the United States.

TABLE 348-4 FDA-APPROVED INDICATIONS FOR BMD TESTS[a]

Estrogen-deficient women at clinical risk of osteoporosis
Vertebral abnormalities on x-ray suggestive of osteoporosis (osteopenia, vertebral fracture)
Glucocorticoid treatment equivalent to ≥7.5 mg of prednisone, or duration of therapy >3 months
Primary hyperparathyroidism
Monitoring response to an FDA-approved medication for osteoporosis
Repeat BMD evaluations at >23-month intervals, or more frequently, if medically justified

[a]Criteria adapted from the 1998 Bone Mass Measurement Act.
Note: FDA, U.S. Food and Drug Administration; BMD, bone mineral density.

APPROACH TO THE PATIENT:
Osteoporosis

The perimenopausal transition is a good opportunity to initiate discussion about risk factors for osteoporosis and to consider indications for a BMD test. A careful history and physical examination should be performed to identify risk factors for osteoporosis. A low Z-score increases the suspicion of a secondary disease. Height loss > 2.5–3.8 cm (>1–1.5 in.) is an indication for radiography or vertebral fracture assessment by DXA to rule out asymptomatic vertebral fractures, as is the presence of significant kyphosis or back pain, particularly if it began after menopause. For patients who present with fractures, it is important to ensure that the fractures are not caused by an underlying malignancy. Usually this is clear on routine radiography, but on occasion, CT, MRI, or radionuclide scans may be necessary.

ROUTINE LABORATORY EVALUATION   There is no established algorithm for the evaluation of women presenting with osteoporosis. A general evaluation that includes complete blood count, serum and 24-h urine calcium, and renal and hepatic function tests is useful for identifying selected secondary causes of low bone mass, particularly for women with fractures or very low Z-scores. An elevated serum calcium level suggests hyperparathyroidism or malignancy, whereas a reduced serum calcium level may reflect malnutrition and osteomalacia. In the presence of hypercalcemia, a serum PTH level differentiates between hyperparathyroidism (PTH↑) and malignancy (PTH↓), and a high PTHrP level can help document the presence of humoral hypercalcemia of malignancy (Chap. 347). A low urine calcium (<50 mg/24 h) suggests osteomalacia, malnutrition, or malabsorption; a high urine calcium (>300 mg/24 h) is indicative of hypercalciuria and must be investigated further. Hypercalciuria occurs primarily in three situations: (1) a renal calcium leak, which is more frequent in males with osteoporosis; (2) absorptive hypercalciuria, which can be idiopathic or associated with increased 1,25(OH)$_2$D in granulomatous disease; or (3) hematologic malignancies or conditions associated with excessive bone turnover such as Paget's disease, hyperparathyroidism, and hyperthyroidism.

Individuals who have osteoporosis-related fractures or bone density in the osteoporotic range should have a measurement of serum 25(OH)D level, since the intake of vitamin D required to achieve a target level >32 ng/mL is very variable. Vitamin D levels should be optimized in all individuals being treated for osteoporosis. Hyperthyroidism should be evaluated by measuring thyroid-stimulating hormone (TSH).

When there is clinical suspicion of Cushing's syndrome, urinary free cortisol levels or a fasting serum cortisol should be measured after overnight dexamethasone. When bowel disease, malabsorption, or malnutrition is suspected, serum albumin, cholesterol, and a complete blood count should be checked. Asymptomatic malabsorption might be heralded by anemia (macrocytic–vitamin B$_{12}$ or folate deficiency; or microcytic-iron deficiency) or low serum cholesterol or urinary calcium levels. If these or other features suggest malabsorption, further evaluation is required. Asymptomatic celiac disease with selective malabsorption is being found with increasing frequency; the diagnosis can be made by testing for antigliadin, antiendomysial, or transglutaminase antibodies but may require endoscopic biopsy. A trial of a gluten-free diet can be confirmatory (Chap. 288). When osteoporosis is found associated with symptoms of rash, multiple allergies, diarrhea, or flushing, mastocytosis should be excluded using 24-h urine histamine collection or serum tryptase.

Myeloma can masquerade as generalized osteoporosis, although it more commonly presents with bone pain and characteristic "punched-out" lesions on radiography. Serum and urine electrophoresis and evaluation for light chains in urine are required to exclude this diagnosis. A bone marrow biopsy may be required to rule out myeloma (in patients with equivocal electrophoretic results) and can also be used to exclude mastocytosis, leukemia, and other marrow infiltrative disorders, such as Gaucher's disease.

TABLE 348-5   BIOCHEMICAL MARKERS OF BONE METABOLISM IN CLINICAL USE

Bone formation
  Serum bone-specific alkaline phosphatase
  Serum osteocalcin
  Serum propeptide of type I procollagen
Bone resorption
  Urine and serum cross-linked N-telopeptide
  Urine and serum cross-linked C-telopeptide
  Urine total free deoxypyridinoline

BONE BIOPSY   Tetracycline labeling of the skeleton allows determination of the rate of remodeling as well as evaluation for other metabolic bone diseases. The current use of BMD tests, in combination with hormonal evaluation and biochemical markers of bone remodeling, has largely replaced the clinical use of bone biopsy, although it remains an important tool in clinical research.

BIOCHEMICAL MARKERS   Several biochemical tests are now available that provide an index of the overall rate of bone remodeling (Table 348-5). Biochemical markers are usually characterized as those related primarily to *bone formation* or *bone resorption*. These tests measure the overall state of bone remodeling at a single point in time. Clinical use of these tests has been hampered by biologic variability (in part related to circadian rhythm) as well as to analytical variability, although the latter is improving.

For the most part, remodeling markers do not predict rates of bone loss well enough to use this information clinically. However, markers of bone resorption may help in the prediction of fracture risk, independently of bone density, particularly in older individuals. In women ≥65 years, when bone density results are greater than the usual treatment thresholds noted above, a high level of bone resorption should prompt consideration of treatment. The primary use of biochemical markers is for monitoring the response to treatment. With the introduction of antiresorptive therapeutic agents, bone remodeling declines rapidly, with the fall in resorption occurring earlier than the fall in formation. Inhibition of bone resorption is maximal within 3–6 months. Thus, measurement of bone resorption prior to initiating therapy and 4–6 months after starting therapy provides an earlier estimate of patient response than does bone densitometry. A decline in resorptive markers can be ascertained after treatment with bisphosphonates or estrogen; this effect is less marked after treatment with either raloxifene or intranasal calcitonin. A biochemical marker response to therapy is particularly useful for asymptomatic patients and might help to ensure long-term adherence to treatment. Bone turnover markers are also useful in monitoring the effects of 1-34hPTH, or teriparatide, which rapidly increases bone formation and later bone resorption.

℞ OSTEOPOROSIS

MANAGEMENT OF OSTEOPOROTIC FRACTURES   Treatment of the patient with osteoporosis frequently involves management of acute fractures as well as treatment of the underlying disease. Hip fractures almost always require surgical repair if the patient is to become ambulatory again. Depending on the location and severity of the fracture, condition of the neighboring joint, and general status of the patient, procedures may include open reduction and internal fixation with pins and plates, hemiarthroplasties, and total arthroplasties. These surgical procedures are followed by intense rehabilitation in an attempt to return patients to their prefracture functional level. Long bone fractures often require either external or internal fixation. Other fractures (e.g., vertebral, rib, and pelvic fractures) are usually managed with supportive care, requiring no specific orthopedic treatment.

Only ~25–30% of vertebral compression fractures present with sudden-onset back pain. For acutely symptomatic fractures, treatment with analgesics is required, including nonsteroidal anti-inflammatory agents and/or acetaminophen, sometimes with the addition of a narcotic agent (codeine or oxycodone). A few small, randomized clinical trials suggest that calcitonin may reduce pain related to acute vertebral compression fracture. A recently developed technique involves percutaneous injection of artificial cement (polymethylmethacrylate) into the vertebral body (vertebroplasty or kyphoplasty); this offers significant immediate pain relief in the majority of patients. Long-term effects are unknown, and conclusions are based on observational studies in patients with severe persistent back pain from acute or subacute vertebral fractures. There have been no long-term randomized controlled trials of either vertebroplasty or kyphoplasty to date. Short periods of bed rest may be helpful for pain management, but, in general, early mobilization is recommended as it helps prevent further bone loss associated with immobilization. Occasionally, use of a soft elastic-style brace may facilitate earlier mobilization. Muscle spasms often occur with acute compression fractures and can be treated with muscle relaxants and heat treatments.

Severe pain usually resolves within 6–10 weeks. Chronic pain is probably not bony in origin; instead, it is related to abnormal strain on muscles, ligaments, and tendons and to secondary facet-joint arthritis associated with alterations in thoracic and/or abdominal shape. Chronic pain is difficult to treat effectively and may require analgesics, sometimes including narcotic analgesics. Frequent intermittent rest in a supine or semireclining position is often required to allow the soft tissues, which are under tension, to relax. Back-strengthening exercises (paraspinal) may be beneficial. Heat treatments help relax muscles and reduce the muscular component of discomfort. Various physical modalities, such as ultrasound and transcutaneous nerve stimulation, may be beneficial in some patients. Pain also occurs in the neck region, not as a result of compression fractures (which almost never occur in the cervical spine as a result of osteoporosis) but because of chronic strain associated from trying to elevate the head in a person with a severe thoracic kyphosis.

Multiple vertebral fractures are often associated with psychological symptoms, not always commonly appreciated. The changes in body configuration and back pain can lead to marked loss of self-image and a secondary depression. Altered balance, precipitated by the kyphosis and the anterior movement of the body's center of gravity, leads to a fear of falling, a consequent tendency to remain indoors, and the onset of social isolation. These symptoms can sometimes be alleviated by family support and/or psychotherapy. Medication may be necessary when depressive features are present.

MANAGEMENT OF THE UNDERLYING DISEASE   **Risk Factor Reduction**   Patients should be thoroughly educated to reduce the impact of modifiable risk factors associated with bone loss and falling. Medications should be reviewed to ensure that all are necessary. Glucocorticoid medication, if present, should be evaluated to determine that it is truly indicated and is being given in doses as low as possible. For those on thyroid hormone replacement, TSH testing should be performed to determine that an excessive dose is not being used, as thyrotoxicosis can be associated with increased bone loss. In patients who smoke, efforts should be made to facilitate smoking cessation. Reducing risk factors for falling also includes alcohol abuse treatment and a review of the medical regimen for any drugs that might be associated with orthostatic hypotension and/or sedation, including hypnotics and anxiolytics. If nocturia occurs, the frequency should be reduced, if possible (e.g., by decreasing or modifying diuretic use), as arising in the middle of sleep is a common precipitant of a fall. Patients should be instructed about environmental safety with regard to eliminating exposed wires, curtain strings, slippery rugs, and mobile tables. Avoiding stocking feet on wood floors, checking carpet condition (particularly on stairs), and providing good light in paths to bathrooms and outside the home are important preventive measures. Treatment for impaired vision is recommended, particularly a problem with depth perception, which is specifically associated with increased falling risk. Elderly patients with neurologic impairment (e.g., stroke, Parkinson's disease, Alzheimer's disease) are particularly at risk of falling and require specialized supervision and care.

Nutritional Recommendations   *Calcium*   A large body of data indicates that optimal calcium intake reduces bone loss and suppresses bone turnover. Recommended intakes from an Institute of Medicine report are shown in **Table 348-6**. The National Health and Nutritional Evaluation Studies (NHANES) have consistently documented that average calcium intakes fall considerably short of these recommendations. The preferred source of calcium is from dairy products and other foods, but many patients require calcium supplementation. Food sources of calcium are dairy

TABLE 348-6   ADEQUATE CALCIUM INTAKE

Life Stage Group	Estimated Adequate Daily Calcium Intake, mg/d
Young children (1–3 years)	500
Older children (4–8 years)	800
Adolescents and young adults (9–18 years)	1300
Men and women (19–50 years)	1000
Men and women (51 and older)	1200

Note: Pregnancy and lactation needs are the same as for nonpregnant women (e.g., 1300 mg/d for adolescents/young adult and 1000 mg/d for ≥19 years).
Source: Adapted from the Standing Committee on the Scientific Evaluation of Dietary Reference Intakes. Food and Nutrition Board. Institute of Medicine. Washington, DC, 1997, National Academy Press.

products (milk, yogurt, and cheese) and fortified foods such as certain cereals, waffles, snacks, juices, and crackers. Some of these fortified foods contain as much calcium per serving as milk.

If a calcium supplement is required, it should be taken in doses ≤600 mg at a time, as the calcium absorption fraction decreases at higher doses. Calcium supplements should be calculated based on the elemental calcium content of the supplement, not the weight of the calcium salt **(Table 348-7)**. Calcium supplements containing carbonate are best taken with food since they require acid for solubility. Calcium citrate supplements can be taken at any time. To confirm bioavailability, calcium supplements can be placed in distilled vinegar. They should dissolve within 30 min.

Several controlled clinical trials of calcium plus vitamin D have confirmed reductions in clinical fractures, including fractures of the hip (~20–30% risk reduction). All recent studies of pharmacologic agents have been conducted in the context of calcium replacement (± vitamin D). Thus, it is standard practice to ensure an adequate calcium and vitamin D intake in patients with osteoporosis, whether they are receiving additional pharmacologic therapy or not. A systematic review confirmed a greater BMD response to anti-resorptive therapy when calcium intake was adequate.

Although side effects from supplemental calcium are minimal (eructation and constipation mostly with carbonate salts), individuals with a history of kidney stones should have a 24-h urine calcium determination before starting increased calcium to avoid significant hypercalciuria.

Vitamin D   Vitamin D is synthesized in skin under the influence of heat and ultraviolet light (Chap. 346). However, large segments of the population do not obtain sufficient vitamin D to maintain what is now considered an adequate supply [serum 25(OH)D consistently >75 μmol/L (30 ng/mL)]. Since vitamin D supplementation at doses that would achieve these serum levels is safe and inexpensive, the Institute of Medicine recommends daily intakes of 200 IU for adults <50 years of age, 400 IU for those from 50–70 years, and 600 IU for those >70 years. Multivitamin tablets usually contain 400 IU, and many calcium supplements also contain vitamin D. Some data suggest that higher doses (≥1000 IU) may be required in the elderly and chronically ill.

Other Nutrients   Other nutrients such as salt, high animal protein intakes, and caffeine may have modest effects on calcium excretion or absorption. Adequate vitamin K status is required for optimal carboxylation of osteocalcin. States in which vitamin K nutrition or metabolism is impaired, such as with long-term warfarin therapy, have been associated with reduced bone mass.

TABLE 348-7   ELEMENTAL CALCIUM CONTENT OF VARIOUS ORAL CALCIUM PREPARATIONS

Calcium Preparation	Elemental Calcium Content
Calcium citrate	60 mg/300 mg
Calcium lactate	80 mg/600 mg
Calcium gluconate	40 mg/500 mg
Calcium carbonate	400 mg/g
Calcium carbonate+ 5 μg vitamin D₂ (OsCal 250)	250 mg/tablet
Calcium carbonate (Tums 500)	500 mg/tablet

Source: Adapted from SM Krane and MF Holick, Chap. 355 in HPIM, 14 ed, 1998.

Research concerning cola intake is controversial but suggests a possible link to reduced bone mass through factors that are independent of caffeine.

Magnesium is abundant in foods, and magnesium deficiency is quite rare in the absence of a serious chronic disease. Magnesium supplementation may be warranted in patients with inflammatory bowel disease, celiac disease, chemotherapy, severe diarrhea, malnutrition, or alcoholism. Dietary phytoestrogens, which are derived primarily from soy products and legumes (e.g., garbanzo beans, chickpeas, and lentils), exert some estrogenic activity but are insufficiently potent to justify their use in place of a pharmacologic agent in the treatment of osteoporosis.

Patients with hip fracture are often frail and relatively malnourished. Some data suggest an improved outcome in such patients when they are provided calorie and protein supplementation. Excessive protein intake can increase renal calcium excretion, but this can be corrected by an adequate calcium intake.

PART 15
Endocrinology and Metabolism

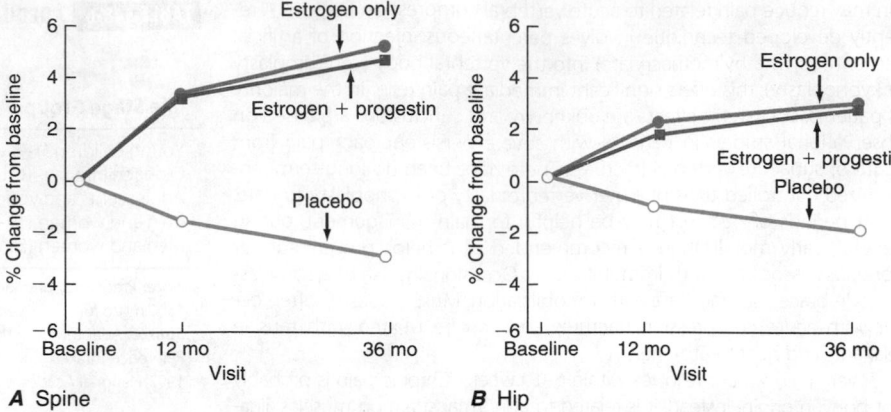

FIGURE 348-7 Results of hormone therapy regimens on bone mineral density (BMD) of the spine (**A**) and hip (**B**). Unadjusted mean percent change in BMD in the hip by treatment assignment and visit: adherent PEPI participants only. Results from the Postmenopausal Estrogen/Progestin Interventions (PEPI) Trial. Estrogen, conjugated equine estrogen 0.625 mg/d; progestin, medroxyprogesterone acetate 10 mg/d. (*Adapted from TL Bush et al: JAMA 276:1389, 1996.*)

Exercise   Exercise in young individuals increases the likelihood that they will attain the maximal genetically determined peak bone mass. Meta-analyses of studies performed in postmenopausal women indicate that weight-bearing exercise prevents bone loss but does not appear to result in substantial gain of bone mass. This beneficial effect wanes if exercise is discontinued. Most of the studies are short-term, and a more substantial effect on bone mass is likely if exercise is continued over a long period of time. Exercise also has beneficial effects on neuromuscular function, and it improves coordination, balance, and strength, thereby reducing the risk of falling. A walking program is a practical way to start. Other activities such as dancing, racquet sports, cross-country skiing, and use of gym equipment are also recommended, depending on the patient's personal preference and general condition. Even women who cannot walk benefit from swimming or water exercises, not so much for the effects on bone, which are quite minimal, but because of effects on muscle. Exercise habits should be consistent, optimally at least three times a week.

PHARMACOLOGIC THERAPIES   Until fairly recently, estrogen treatment, either by itself or in concert with a progestin, was the primary therapeutic agent for prevention or treatment of osteoporosis. However, a number of new drugs have appeared, and more are expected in the near future. Some are agents that specifically treat osteoporosis (bisphosphonates, calcitonin, PTH); others, such as selective estrogen response modulators (SERMs), have broader effects. The availability of these drugs allows therapy to be tailored to the needs of an individual patient.

Estrogens   A large body of clinical trial data indicates that various types of estrogens (conjugated equine estrogens, estradiol, estrone, esterified estrogens, ethinyl estradiol, and mestranol) reduce bone turnover, prevent bone loss, and induce small increases in bone mass of the spine, hip, and total body. The effects of estrogen are seen in women with natural or surgical menopause and in late postmenopausal women with or without established osteoporosis. Estrogens are efficacious when administered orally or transdermally. For both oral and transdermal routes of administration, combined estrogen/progestin preparations are now available in many countries, obviating the problem of taking two tablets or using a patch and oral progestin. One large study, referred to as PEPI (Postmenopausal Estrogen/Progestin Intervention Trial), indicated that C-21 progestins alone do not augment the effect of standard estrogen doses on bone mass (**Fig. 348-7**).

Dose of Estrogen   For oral estrogens, the standard recommended doses have been 0.3 mg/d for esterified estrogens, 0.625 mg/d for conjugated equine estrogens, and 5 μg/d for ethinyl estradiol. For transdermal estrogen, the commonly used dose supplies 50 μg estradiol per day, but a lower dose may be appropriate for some individuals. Dose response data for conjugated equine estrogens indicate that lower doses (0.3 and 0.45 mg/d) are effective. Doses even lower have been associated with bone mass protection.

Fracture Data   Epidemiologic databases indicate that women who take estrogen replacement have a 50% reduction, on average, of osteoporotic fractures, including hip fractures. The beneficial effect of estrogen is greatest among those who start replacement early and continue the treatment; the benefit declines after discontinuation such that there is no residual protective effect against fracture by 10 years after discontinuation. The first clinical trial evaluating fractures as secondary outcomes, the Heart and Estrogen-Progestin Replacement Study (HERS) trial, showed no effect of hormone therapy against hip or other clinical fractures in women with established coronary artery disease. These data made the results of the Women's Health Initiative (WHI) exceedingly important (Chap. 342). The estrogen-progestin arm of the WHI in >16,000 postmenopausal healthy women indicated that hormone therapy reduces the risk of hip and clinical spine fracture by 34% and all clinical fractures by 24%.

A few smaller clinical trials have evaluated spine fracture occurrence as an outcome with estrogen therapy. They have consistently shown that estrogen treatment reduces the incidence of vertebral compression fracture.

The WHI has now provided a vast amount of data on the multisystemic effects of hormone therapy. Although earlier observational studies suggested that estrogen replacement might reduce heart disease, the WHI showed that combined estrogen-progestin treatment increased risk of fatal and nonfatal myocardial infarction by ~29%, confirming data from the HERS study. Other important relative risks included a 40% increase in stroke, 100% increase in venous thromboembolic disease, and a 26% increase in risk of breast cancer. Subsequent analyses have confirmed the increased risk of stroke and shown a twofold increase in dementia. Benefits other than the fracture reductions noted above included a 37% reduction in risk of colon cancer. These relative risks have to be interpreted in light of absolute risk (**Fig. 348-8**). For example, out of 10,000 women treated with estrogen-progestin for 1 year, there will be 8 excess heart attacks, 8 excess breast cancers, 18 excess venous thromboembolic events, 5 fewer hip fractures, 44 fewer clinical fractures, and 6 fewer colorectal cancers. These numbers must be multiplied by years of hormone treatment. There was no effect of hormone treatment on risk of uterine cancer or total mortality.

It is important to note that these WHI findings apply specifically to hormone treatment in the form of conjugated equine estrogen plus medroxyprogesterone acetate. The relative benefits and risks of unopposed estrogen in women who had hysterectomy vary somewhat. They still show benefits against fracture occurrence and increased risk of venous thrombosis and stroke, similar in magnitude to the risks for combined hormone therapy. In contrast, though, the estrogen-only arm of WHI indicated no increased risk of heart attack or breast cancer. The data suggest that at least some of the detrimental effects of combined therapy are related to the progestin component.

Mode of Action   Two subtypes of ERs, α and β, have been identified in bone and other tissues. Cells of monocyte lineage express both ERα and -β, as do osteoblasts. Estrogen-mediated effects vary depending on the receptor type. Using ER knockout mouse models, elimination of ERα produces a modest reduction in bone mass, whereas mutation of ERβ has less effect on bone. A male patient with a homozygous mutation of ERα had markedly decreased bone density as well as abnormalities in epiphyseal

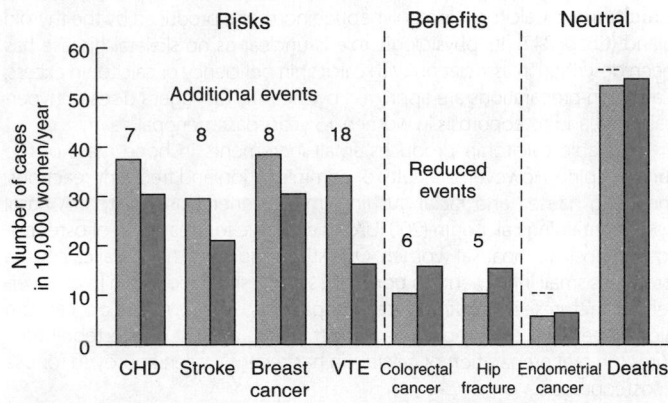

FIGURE 348-8 Effects of hormone therapy on event rates: green, placebo; purple, estrogen and progestin. (CHD, coronary heart disease; VTE, venous thromboembolic events.) *(Adapted from Women's Health Initiative. WHI HRT Update. Available at http://www.nhlbi.nih.gov/health/women/upd2002.htm.)*

closure, confirming the important role of ERα in bone biology. The mechanism of estrogen action in bone is an area of active investigation (Fig. 348-5). Although data are conflicting, estrogens may inhibit osteoclasts directly. However, the majority of estrogen (and androgen) effects on bone resorption are mediated indirectly through paracrine factors produced by osteoblasts. These actions include: (1) increasing IGF-I and TGF-β, and (2) suppressing IL-1 (α and β), IL-6, TNF-α, and osteocalcin synthesis. The indirect estrogen actions primarily decrease bone resorption.

Progestins In women with a uterus, daily progestin or cyclical progestins at least 12 days per month are prescribed in combination with estrogens to reduce the risk of uterine cancer. Medroxyprogesterone acetate and norethindrone acetate blunt the high-density lipoprotein response to estrogen, but micronized progesterone does not. Neither medroxyprogesterone acetate nor micronized progesterone appears to have an independent effect on bone; at lower doses of estrogen, norethindrone acetate might have an additive benefit. On breast tissue, progestins may increase the risk of breast cancer.

SERMs Two SERMs are currently being used in postmenopausal women: raloxifene, which is approved for prevention and treatment of osteoporosis, and tamoxifen, which is approved for the prevention and treatment of breast cancer.

Tamoxifen reduces bone turnover and bone loss in postmenopausal women compared to placebo groups. These findings support the concept that tamoxifen acts as an estrogenic agent in bone. There are limited data on the effect of tamoxifen on fracture risk, but the Breast Cancer Prevention study indicated a possible reduction in clinical vertebral, hip, and Colles' fractures. The major benefit of tamoxifen is on breast cancer occurrence. The breast cancer prevention trial indicated that tamoxifen administration over 4–5 years reduced the incidence of new invasive and noninvasive breast cancer by ~45% in women at increased risk of breast cancer. The incidence of ER-positive breast cancers was reduced by 65%. Tamoxifen increases the risk of uterine cancer in postmenopausal women, limiting its use for breast cancer prevention in women at low or moderate risk.

Raloxifene (60 mg/d) has effects on bone turnover and bone mass that are very similar to those of tamoxifen, indicating that this agent is also estrogenic on the skeleton. The effect of raloxifene on bone density (+1.4–2.8% versus placebo in the spine, hip, and total body) is somewhat less than that seen with standard doses of estrogens. Raloxifene reduces the occurrence of vertebral fracture by 30–50%, depending on the population; however, there are no data confirming that raloxifene can reduce the risk of nonvertebral fractures over 8 years of observation.

Raloxifene, like tamoxifen and estrogen, has effects in other organ systems. The most beneficial effect appears to be a reduction in invasive breast cancer (mainly decreased ER-positive) occurrence of ~65% in women who take raloxifene compared to placebo. In a head-to-head study, raloxifene was as effective as tamoxifen in preventing breast cancer in high-risk women, but in a separate study had no effect on heart disease in women with increased risk for this outcome. In contrast to tamoxifen, raloxifene is not associated with an increase in the risk of uterine cancer or benign uterine disease. Raloxifene increases the occurrence of hot flashes

but reduces serum total and low-density lipoprotein cholesterol, lipoprotein(a), and fibrinogen.

Mode of Action of SERMs All SERMs bind to the ER, but each agent produces a unique receptor-drug conformation. As a result, specific coactivator or co-repressor proteins are bound to the receptor (Chap. 332), resulting in differential effects on gene transcription that vary depending on other transcription factors present in the cell. Another aspect of selectivity is the affinity of each SERM for the different ERα and -β subtypes, which are expressed differentially in various tissues. These tissue-selective effects of SERMs offer the possibility of tailoring estrogen therapy to best meet the needs and risk factor profile of an individual patient.

Bisphosphonates Alendronate, risedronate, and ibandronate are approved for the prevention and treatment of postmenopausal osteoporosis. Risedronate and alendronate are approved for the treatment of steroid-induced osteoporosis, and risedronate is also approved for prevention of steroid-induced osteoporosis. Both alendronate and risedronate are approved for treatment of osteoporosis in men.

Alendronate has been shown to decrease bone turnover and increase bone mass in the spine by up to 8% versus placebo and by 6% versus placebo in the hip. Multiple trials have evaluated its effect on fracture occurrence. The Fracture Intervention Trial provided evidence in >2000 women with prevalent vertebral fractures that daily alendronate treatment (5 mg/d for 2 years and 10 mg/d for 9 months afterwards) reduces vertebral fracture risk by about 50%, multiple vertebral fractures by up to 90%, and hip fractures by up to 50% **(Fig. 348-9)**. Several subsequent trials have confirmed these findings. For example, in a study of >1900 women with low bone mass treated with alendronate (10 mg/d) versus placebo, the incidence of all nonvertebral fractures was reduced by ~47% after only 1 year.

Trials comparing once-weekly alendronate, 70 mg, with daily 10-mg dosing have shown equivalence with regard to bone mass and bone turnover responses. Consequently, once-weekly therapy is generally preferred

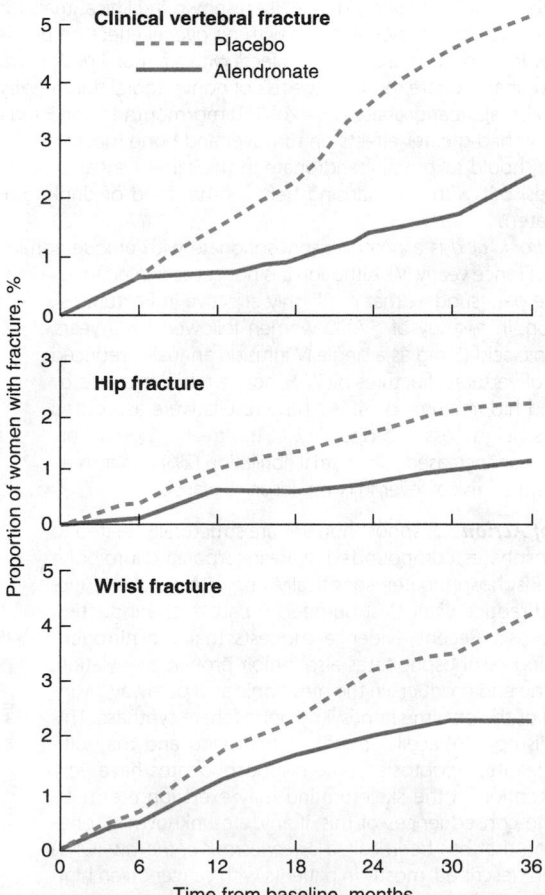

FIGURE 348-9 Cumulative proportions of women with osteoporosis who suffered clinical fracture (vertebral, hip, or wrist) during 3 years of treatment with alendronate or placebo (FIT 1). *(From DM Black et al: Lancet 348:1535, 1996.)*

because of the low incidence of gastrointestinal side effects and ease of administration. Alendronate should be given with a full glass of water before breakfast, as bisphosphonates are poorly absorbed. Because of the potential for esophageal irritation, alendronate is contraindicated in patients who have stricture or inadequate emptying of the esophagus. It is recommended that patients remain upright for at least 30 min after taking the medication to avoid esophageal irritation. Cases of esophagitis, esophageal ulcer, and esophageal stricture have been described, but the incidence appears to be low. In clinical trials, overall gastrointestinal symptomatology was no different with alendronate compared to placebo. Alendronate is also available in a preparation that contains vitamin D.

Risedronate also reduces bone turnover and increases bone mass. Controlled clinical trials have demonstrated 40–50% reduction in vertebral fracture risk over 3 years, accompanied by a 40% reduction in clinical nonspine fractures. The only clinical trial specifically designed to evaluate hip fracture outcome (HIP) indicated that risedronate reduced hip fracture risk in women in their seventies with confirmed osteoporosis by 40%. In contrast, risedronate was not effective at reducing hip fracture occurrence in older women (80+ years) without proven osteoporosis. Studies have shown that 35 mg of risedronate administered once weekly is therapeutically equivalent to 5 mg/d. Patients should take risedronate with a full glass of plain water, to facilitate delivery to the stomach, and should not lie down for 30 min after taking the drug. The incidence of gastrointestinal side effects in trials with risedronate was similar to that of placebo.

Etidronate was the first bisphosphonate to be approved, initially for use in Paget's disease and hypercalcemia. This agent has also been used in osteoporosis trials of smaller magnitude than those performed for alendronate and risedronate but is not approved by the FDA for treatment of osteoporosis. Etidronate probably has some efficacy against vertebral fracture when given as an intermittent cyclical regimen (2 weeks on, 2½ months off). There has not been any study of its effectiveness against nonvertebral fractures.

Ibandronate is the third amino-bisphosphonate approved in the United States. Ibandronate (2.5 mg/d) has been shown in clinical trials to reduce vertebral fracture risk by ~40% but with no overall effect on nonvertebral fractures. In a post hoc analysis of subjects with a femoral neck T-score of –3 or below, ibandronate reduced the risk of nonvertebral fractures by ~60%. In clinical trials, ibandronate doses of 150 mg/month PO or 3 mg every 3 months IV had greater effects on turnover and bone mass than 2.5 mg/d. Patients should take oral ibandronate in the same way as other bisphosphonates, but with 1 h elapsing before other food or drink (other than plain water).

Zoledronic acid is a potent bisphosphonate with unique administration regimens (once yearly IV). Although it is not yet approved for use in osteoporosis, the data suggest that it is highly effective in fracture risk reduction. In a study of >7000 women followed for 3 years, zoledronic acid (5 mg as a single IV infusion annually) reduced the risk of vertebral fractures by 70%, nonvertebral fractures by 25%, and hip fractures by 40%. These results were associated with less height loss and disability. In the treated population, there was an increased risk of atrial fibrillation (2%) and arthralgia and a 15% risk of fever, in comparison to placebo.

Mode of Action Bisphosphonates are structurally related to pyrophosphates, compounds that are incorporated into bone matrix. Bisphosphonates specifically impair osteoclast function and reduce osteoclast number, in part by the induction of apoptosis. Recent evidence suggests that the nitrogen-containing bisphosphonates also inhibit protein prenylation, one of the end products in the mevalonic acid pathway, by inhibition of the enzyme farnesyl pyrophosphate synthase. This effect disrupts intracellular protein trafficking and may ultimately lead to apoptosis. Some bisphosphonates have very long retention in the skeleton and may exert long-term effects. The consequences of this, if any, are unknown. A phenomenon that has been called *osteonecrosis of the jaw* (ONJ) has been described, mostly in patients with cancer given high doses of zoledronic acid or pamidronate. A few cases have been described in patients with osteoporosis treated with oral bisphosphonates. The background incidence of ONJ in this population is not known, and thus the attributable risk for bisphosphonates is not clear, but it appears to be relatively rare.

Calcitonin Calcitonin is a polypeptide hormone produced by the thyroid gland (Chap. 347). Its physiologic role is unclear as no skeletal disease has been described in association with calcitonin deficiency or calcitonin excess. Calcitonin preparations are approved by the FDA for Paget's disease, hypercalcemia, and osteoporosis in women >5 years past menopause.

Injectable calcitonin produces small increments in bone mass of the lumbar spine. However, difficulty of administration and frequent reactions, including nausea and facial flushing, make general use limited. A nasal spray containing calcitonin (200 IU/d) is available for treatment of osteoporosis in postmenopausal women. One study suggests that nasal calcitonin produces small increments in bone mass and a small reduction in new vertebral fractures in calcitonin-treated patients versus those on calcium alone. There has been no proven effectiveness against nonvertebral fractures. An oral preparation of calcitonin has recently been approved for use in osteoporosis.

Calcitonin is not indicated for prevention of osteoporosis and is not sufficiently potent to prevent bone loss in early postmenopausal women. Calcitonin might have an analgesic effect on bone pain, both in the SC and possibly the nasal form.

Mode of Action Calcitonin suppresses osteoclast activity by direct action on the osteoclast calcitonin receptor. Osteoclasts exposed to calcitonin cannot maintain their active ruffled border, which normally maintains close contact with underlying bone.

Parathyroid Hormone Endogenous PTH is an 84-amino-acid peptide that is largely responsible for calcium homeostasis (Chap. 347). Although chronic elevation of PTH, as occurs in hyperparathyroidism, is associated with bone loss (particularly cortical bone), PTH can also exert anabolic effects on bone. Consistent with this, some observational studies have indicated that mild elevations in PTH are associated with maintenance of trabecular bone mass. On the basis of these findings, several clinical trials have been performed using an exogenous PTH analogue (1-34hPTH; teriparatide) which is now approved for the treatment of established osteoporosis in both men and women. The first randomized controlled trial in postmenopausal women showed that PTH, when superimposed on ongoing estrogen therapy, produced substantial increments in bone mass (13% over a 3-year period compared to estrogen alone) and reduced the risk of vertebral compression deformity. In the pivotal study (median, 19 months' duration), 20 μg PTH(1-34) daily by SC injection reduced vertebral fractures by 65% and nonvertebral fractures by 45% **(Fig. 348-10)**. Treatment is administered as a single daily injection given for a maximum of 2 years. Teriparatide produces increases in bone mass and mediates architectural improvements in skeletal structure. These effects are lower when patients have been previously exposed to bisphosphonates, possibly in proportion

FIGURE 348-10 Number of incident vertebral deformities (15% and 20% reductions) in women with osteoporosis on hormone therapy (HT), compared to HT + PTH over 3 years. (HT, hormone therapy; PTH, parathyroid hormone.) *(From F Cosman et al: J Bone Miner Res 16:925, 2001.)*

to the potency of the antiresorptive effect. When 1-34hPTH is being considered for treatment-naïve patients, it is best administered as monotherapy and followed by an antiresorptive agent such as a bisphosphonate.

Side effects of teriparatide are generally mild and can include muscle pain, weakness, dizziness, headache, and nausea. Rodents given prolonged treatment with PTH in relatively high doses developed osteogenic sarcomas. One case of osteosarcoma has been described in a patient treated with teriparatide. At present this seems to equate to the background incidence of osteosarcoma in this population.

PTH use may be limited by its mode of administration; alternative modes of delivery are being investigated. The optimal frequency of administration also remains to be established, and it is possible that PTH might also be effective when used intermittently. Cost may also be a limiting factor.

Mode of Action Exogenously administered PTH appears to have direct actions on osteoblast activity, with biochemical and histomorphometric evidence of de novo bone formation early in response to PTH, prior to activation of bone resorption. Subsequently, PTH activates bone remodeling but still appears to favor bone formation over bone resorption. PTH stimulates IGF-I and collagen production and appears to increase osteoblast number by stimulating replication, enhancing osteoblast recruitment, and inhibiting apoptosis. Unlike all other treatments, PTH produces a true increase in bone tissue and an apparent restoration of bone microarchitecture (**Fig. 348-11**).

Fluoride Fluoride has been available for many years and is a potent stimulator of osteoprogenitor cells when studied in vitro. It has been used in multiple osteoporosis studies with conflicting results, in part related to use of varying doses and preparations. Despite increments in bone mass of up to 10%, there are no consistent effects of fluoride on vertebral or nonvertebral fracture; the latter might actually increase when high doses of fluoride are used. Fluoride remains an experimental agent, despite its long history and multiple studies.

Strontium ranelate is approved in several European countries for the treatment of osteoporosis. It increases bone mass throughout the skeleton; in clinical trials, the drug reduced the risk of vertebral fractures by 37% and nonvertebral fractures by 14%. It appears to be modestly antiresorptive, while at the same time not causing as much of a decrease in bone formation (measured biochemically). Strontium is incorporated into hydroxyapatite, replacing calcium, a feature that might explain some of its fracture benefits. Small increased risks of venous thrombosis, seizures, and abnormal cognition have been seen and require further study.

Other Potential Anabolic Agents Several small studies of growth hormone (GH), alone or in combination with other agents, have not shown consistent or substantial positive effects on skeletal mass. Many of these studies are relatively short-term, and the effects of GH, growth hormone–releasing hormone, and the IGFs are still under investigation. Anabolic steroids, mostly derivatives of testosterone, act primarily as antiresorptive agents to reduce bone turnover but may also stimulate osteoblastic activity. Effects on bone mass remain unclear but appear weak, in general, and use is limited by masculinizing side effects. Several recent observational studies suggest that the statin drugs, currently used to treat hypercholesterolemia, may be associated with increased bone mass and reduced fractures, but conclusions from clinical trials are mixed.

NONPHARMACOLOGIC APPROACHES Protective pads worn around the outer thigh, which cover the trochanteric region of the hip can prevent hip fractures in elderly residents in nursing homes. The use of hip protectors is limited largely by compliance and comfort, but new devices are being developed that may circumvent these problems and provide adjunctive treatments.

Kyphoplasty and *vertebroplasty* are also useful nonpharmacologic approaches for the treatment of painful vertebral fractures. However, no long-term data are available.

TREATMENT MONITORING There are currently no well-accepted guidelines for monitoring treatment of osteoporosis. Because most osteoporosis treatments produce small or moderate bone mass increments on average, it is reasonable to consider BMD as a monitoring tool. Changes must exceed ~4% in the spine and 6% in the hip to be considered significant in any individual. The hip is the preferred site due to larger surface area and greater reproducibility. Medication-induced increments may require several years to produce changes of this magnitude (if they do at all).

A   **B**

FIGURE 348-11 Effect of parathyroid hormone (PTH) treatment on bone microarchitecture. Paired biopsy specimens from a 64-year-old woman before (**A**) and after (**B**) treatment with PTH. *(From DW Dempster et al: J Bone Miner Res 16:1846, 2001.)*

Consequently, it can be argued that BMD should be repeated at intervals >2 years. Only significant BMD reductions should prompt a change in medical regimen, as it is expected that many individuals will not show responses greater than the detection limits of the current measurement techniques.

Biochemical markers of bone turnover may prove useful for treatment monitoring, but little hard evidence currently supports this concept; it remains unclear which endpoint is most useful. If bone turnover markers are used, a determination should be made before starting therapy and repeated ≥4 months after therapy is initiated. In general, a change in bone turnover markers must be 30–40% lower than the baseline to be significant because of the biologic and technical variability in these tests. A positive change in biochemical markers and/or bone density can be useful to help patients adhere to treatment regimens.

GLUCOCORTICOID-INDUCED OSTEOPOROSIS

Osteoporotic fractures are a well-characterized consequence of the hypercortisolism associated with Cushing's syndrome. However, the therapeutic use of glucocorticoids is by far the most common form of glucocorticoid-induced osteoporosis. Glucocorticoids are widely used in the treatment of a variety of disorders, including chronic lung disorders, rheumatoid arthritis and other connective tissue diseases, inflammatory bowel disease, and posttransplantation. Osteoporosis and related fractures are serious side effects of chronic glucocorticoid therapy. Because the effects of glucocorticoids on the skeleton are often superimposed upon the consequences of aging and menopause, it is not surprising that women and the elderly are most frequently affected. The skeletal response to steroids is remarkably heterogeneous, however, and even young, growing individuals treated with glucocorticoids can present with fractures.

The risk of fractures depends on the dose and duration of glucocorticoid therapy, although recent data suggest that there may be no completely safe dose. Bone loss is more rapid during the early months of treatment, and trabecular bone is more severely affected than cortical bone. As a result, fractures have been shown to increase within 3 months of steroid treatment. There is an increase in fracture risk in both the axial and appendicular skeleton, including risk of hip fracture. Bone loss can occur with any route of steroid administration including high-dose inhaled glucocorticoids and intraarticular injections. Alternate-day delivery does not appear to ameliorate the skeletal effects of glucocorticoids.

PATHOPHYSIOLOGY

Glucocorticoids increase bone loss by multiple mechanisms including: (1) inhibition of osteoblast function and an increase in osteoblast apoptosis, resulting in impaired synthesis of new bone; (2) stimulation of bone resorption, probably as a secondary effect; (3) impairment of the absorption of calcium across the intestine, probably by a vitamin D–independent effect; (4) increase of urinary calcium loss and perhaps induction of some degree of secondary hyperparathyroidism; (5) reduction of adrenal androgens and suppression of ovarian and testicular secretion of estrogens and androgens; and (6) induction of glucocorticoid myopathy, which may exacerbate effects on skeletal and calcium homeostasis as well as increase the risk of falls.

EVALUATION OF THE PATIENT

Because of the prevalence of glucocorticoid-induced bone loss, it is important to evaluate the status of the skeleton in all patients starting or already receiving long-term glucocorticoid therapy. Modifiable risk factors should be identified, including those for falls. Examination should include height and muscle strength testing. Laboratory evaluation should include an assessment of 24-h urinary calcium. All patients on long-term (>3 months) glucocorticoids should have measurement of bone mass at both the spine and hip using DXA. If only one skeletal site can be measured, it is best to assess the spine in individuals <60 years and the hip for those >60 years.

PREVENTION

Bone loss caused by glucocorticoids can be prevented, and the risk of fractures significantly reduced. Strategies must include using the lowest dose of glucocorticoid for disease management. Topical and inhaled routes of administration are preferred, where appropriate. Risk factor reduction is important, including smoking cessation, limitation of alcohol consumption, and participation in weight-bearing exercise, when appropriate. All patients should receive an adequate calcium and vitamin D intake from the diet or from supplements.

℞ GLUCOCORTICOID-INDUCED OSTEOPOROSIS

Only bisphosphonates have been demonstrated in large clinical trials to reduce the risk of fractures in patients being treated with glucocorticoids. Risedronate prevents bone loss and reduces vertebral fracture risk by ~70%. Similar beneficial effects are observed in studies of alendronate. Controlled trials of hormone therapy have shown bone-sparing effects, and calcitonin also has some protective effect in the spine. Thiazides reduce urine calcium loss, but their role in prevention of fractures is unclear. PTH has also been studied in a small group of women with glucocorticoid-induced osteoporosis, where bone mass increased substantially, and teriparatide is currently being investigated in a larger multicenter trial.

FURTHER READINGS

BARRETT-CONNOR E et al: Effects of raloxifene on cardiovascular events and breast cancer in postmenopausal women. N Engl J Med 355:125, 2006

COSMAN F: Anabolic therapy for osteoporosis: Parathyroid hormone. Curr Rheumatol Rep 8:63, 2006

DEROO BJ et al: Estrogen receptors and human disease. J Clin Invest 116:561, 2006

HEANEY RP: Bone health. Am J Clin Nutr 85:300S, 2007

LYLES KW et al: Zolendroic acid and clinical fractures and mortality after hip fracture. N Engl J Med 357:1799, 2007

MAUCK KF, CLARKE BL: Diagnosis, screening, prevention, and treatment of osteoporosis. Mayo Clin Proc 81:662, 2006

MULDER JE et al: Drug insight: Existing and emerging therapies for osteoporosis. Nat Clin Pract Endocrinol Metab 2:670, 2006

POOLE KE, COMPSTON JE: Osteoporosis and its management. BMJ 333:1251, 2006

VOGEL V et al: Effects of tamoxifen vs raloxifene on the risk of developing invasive breast cancer and other disease outcomes. JAMA 295:2727, 2006

349 Paget Disease and Other Dysplasias of Bone
Murray J. Favus, Tamara J. Vokes

PAGET DISEASE OF BONE

Paget disease is a localized bone disorder that affects widespread areas of the skeleton through increased bone remodeling. The pathologic process is initiated by overactive osteoclastic bone resorption followed by a compensatory increase in osteoblastic new bone formation. New pagetic bone is structurally disorganized and more susceptible to deformities and fractures. Although most patients are asymptomatic, a variety of symptoms and complications may result directly from bony involvement or secondarily from the expansion of bone and subsequent compression of surrounding neural tissue.

Epidemiology There is a marked geographic variation in the frequency of Paget disease, with high prevalence in Western Europe (Great Britain, France, and Germany but not Switzerland or Scandinavia) and among those who have immigrated to Australia, New Zealand, South Africa, and North and South America. The disease is rare in native populations of the Americas, Africa, Asia, and the Middle East. The prevalence is greater in males and increases with age. Autopsy series reveal Paget disease in about 3% of those over age 40. Prevalence of positive skeletal radiographs in patients over age 55 is 2.5% for men and 1.6% for women. Elevated alkaline phosphatase (ALP) levels in asymptomatic patients have an age-adjusted incidence of 12.7 and 7 per 100,000 person-years in men and women, respectively. The frequency of diagnosis by either radiographic or biochemical criteria has decreased during the past 20 years.

Etiology The etiology of Paget disease of bone remains unknown, but evidence supports both genetic and viral etiologies. A positive family history is found in 15–25% of patients and, when present, raises the prevalence of the disease seven- to tenfold among first-degree relatives.

A homozygous deletion of the *TNFRSF11B* gene, which encodes osteoprotegrin (Fig. 349-1), causes juvenile Paget disease, a disorder characterized by uncontrolled osteoclastic differentiation and resorption. Familial patterns of disease in several large kindred are consistent with an autosomal dominant pattern of inheritance with variable penetrance. A susceptibility locus for Paget disease has been mapped to chromosome 18q21–22, a region that contains a gene responsible for a rare Paget disease–like skeletal disorder known as *familial expansile osteolysis*. The gene encodes the receptor activator of nuclear factor-κB (RANK), a member of the tumor necrosis factor superfamily critical for osteoclast differentiation (Fig. 349-1). In other families, susceptibility loci have been mapped to loci on chromosomes 18q23, 6p21.3, 5q31, and 5q35. Mutations of the *SQSTM1* gene (sequestasome-1 or p62 protein) in the C-terminal ubiquitin-binding domain have been identified in familial and sporadic cases of Paget disease. The p62 protein is involved in NF–κB signaling and regulates osteoclastic differentiation. The phenotypic variability in patients with *SQSTM1* mutations suggests that additional factors, such as other genetic influences or viral infection, may influence clinical expression of the disease.

Several lines of evidence suggest that a viral infection may contribute to the clinical manifestations of Paget disease, including (1) the presence of cytoplasmic and nuclear inclusions resembling paramyxoviruses (measles and respiratory syncytial virus) in pagetic osteoclasts, and (2) viral mRNA in precursor and mature osteoclasts. The viral etiology is further supported by conversion of osteoclast precursors to pagetic-like osteoclasts by vectors containing the measles virus nucleocapsid or matrix genes. However, the viral etiology has been questioned by the inability to culture a live virus from pagetic bone and by failure to clone the full-length viral genes from material obtained from patients with Paget disease.

FIGURE 349-1 Diagram illustrating factors that promote differentiation and function of osteoclasts and osteoblasts and the role of the RANK pathway. Stromal bone marrow (mesenchymal) cells and differentiated osteoblasts produce multiple growth factors and cytokines, including macrophage colony-stimulating factor (M-CSF), to modulate osteoclastogenesis. RANKL (receptor activator of NFκB ligand) is produced by osteoblast progenitors and mature osteoblasts and can bind to a soluble decoy receptor known as OPG (osteoprotegrin) to inhibit RANKL action. Alternatively, a cell-cell interaction between osteoblast and osteoclast progenitors allows RANKL to bind to its membrane-bound receptor, RANK, thereby stimulating osteoclast differentiation and function. RANK binds intracellular proteins called TRAFS (tumor necrosis factor receptor–associated factors) that mediate receptor signaling through transcription factors such as NFκB. M-CSF binds to its receptor, c-fms, which is the cellular homologue of the *fms* oncogene. See text for the potential role of these pathways in disorders of osteoclast function such as Paget disease and osteopetrosis.

Pathophysiology The principal abnormality in Paget disease is the increased number and activity of osteoclasts. Pagetic osteoclasts are large, increased 10- to 100-fold in number, and have a greater number of nuclei (as many as 100 compared to 3–5 nuclei in the normal osteoclast). The overactive osteoclasts may create a sevenfold increase in resorptive surfaces and an erosion rate of 9 μg/d (normal is 1 μg/d). Several causes for the increased number and activity of pagetic osteoclasts have been identified: (1) osteoclastic precursors are hypersensitive to 1,25(OH)$_2$D$_3$; (2) osteoclasts are hyperresponsive to RANK ligand (RANKL), the osteoclast stimulatory factor that mediates the effects of most osteotropic factors on osteoclast formation; (3) marrow stromal cells from pagetic lesions have increased RANKL expression; (4) osteoclast precursor recruitment is increased by interleukin (IL) 6, which is increased in the blood of patients with active Paget disease and is overexpressed in pagetic osteoclasts; (5) expression of the proto-oncogene c-fos, which increases osteoclastic activity, is increased; and (6) the antiapoptotic oncogene Bcl-2 in pagetic bone is overexpressed. Numerous osteoblasts are recruited to active resorption sites and produce large amounts of new bone matrix. As a result, bone turnover is high and bone mass is normal or increased, not reduced.

The characteristic feature of Paget disease is increased bone resorption accompanied by accelerated bone formation. An initial osteolytic phase involves prominent bone resorption and marked hypervascularization. Radiographically, this manifests as an advancing lytic wedge, or "blade of grass" lesion. The second phase is a period of very active bone formation and resorption that replaces normal lamellar bone with haphazard (woven) bone. The mosaic pattern of woven bone is structurally inferior and can bow and fracture more readily. At the same time, fibrous connective tissue may replace normal bone marrow. In the final sclerotic phase, bone resorption declines progressively

and leads to a hard, dense, less vascular pagetic or mosaic bone, which represents the so-called burned-out phase of Paget disease. All three phases may be present at the same time at different skeletal sites.

Clinical Manifestations Asymptomatic patients are often diagnosed by discovery of an elevated ALP level on routine blood chemistry testing or from an abnormality on a skeletal radiograph obtained for another indication. The skeletal sites most commonly involved are the pelvis, vertebral bodies, skull, femur, and tibia. Numerous active sites of skeletal involvement are more common in familial cases with an early presentation.

Pain is the most common presenting symptom. It results from increased bony vascularity, expanding lytic lesions, fractures, bowing, or other deformities of the extremities. Bowing of the femur or tibia causes gait abnormalities and abnormal mechanical stresses with secondary osteoarthritis of the hip or knee joints. Long bone bowing also causes extremity pain by stretching the muscles attached to the bone softened by the pagetic process. Back pain results from enlarged pagetic vertebrae, vertebral compression fractures, spinal stenosis, degenerative changes of the joints, and altered body mechanics with kyphosis and forward tilt of the upper back. Rarely, spinal cord compression may result from bone enlargement or from the vascular steal syndrome. Skull involvement may cause headaches, symmetric or asymmetric enlargement of the parietal or frontal bones (frontal bossing), and increased head size. Cranial expansion may narrow cranial foramina and cause neurologic complications including hearing loss from cochlear nerve damage from temporal bone involvement, cranial nerve palsies, and softening of the base of the skull (*platybasia*) and the risk of brainstem compression. Pagetic involvement of the facial bones may cause facial deformity, loss of teeth and other dental conditions, and rarely, airway compression.

Fractures are serious complications of Paget disease and usually occur in long bones at areas of active or advancing lytic lesions. Common fracture sites are the femoral shaft and subtrochanteric regions. Neoplasms arising from pagetic bone are rare. The incidence of sarcoma appears to be decreasing, possibly because of earlier, more effective treatment with potent antiresorptive agents. The majority of tumors are osteosarcomas, which usually present with new pain in a long-standing pagetic lesion. Osteoclast-rich benign giant cell tumors may arise in areas adjacent to pagetic bone and respond to glucocorticoid therapy.

Cardiovascular complications may occur in patients with involvement of large (15–35%) portions of the skeleton and a high degree of disease activity (ALP four times above normal). The extensive arteriovenous shunting and marked increases in blood flow through the vascular pagetic bone lead to a high-output state and cardiac enlargement. However, high-output heart failure is relatively rare and usually develops in patients with concomitant cardiac pathology. In addition, calcific aortic stenosis and diffuse vascular calcifications have been associated with Paget disease.

Diagnosis The diagnosis may be suggested on clinical examination by the presence of an enlarged skull with frontal bossing, bowing of an extremity, or short stature with simian posturing. An extremity with an area of warmth and tenderness to palpation may suggest an underlying pagetic lesion. Other findings include bony deformity of the pelvis, skull, spine, and extremities; arthritic involvement of the joints adjacent to lesions; and leg length discrepancy resulting from deformities of the long bones.

Paget disease is usually diagnosed from radiologic and biochemical abnormalities. Radiographic findings typical of Paget disease include enlargement or expansion of an entire bone or area of a long bone, cortical thickening, coarsening of trabecular markings, and typical lytic and sclerotic changes. Skull radiographs (Fig. 349-2) reveal regions of "cotton wool," or osteoporosis circumscripta; thickening of diploic areas; and enlargement and sclerosis of a portion or all of one or more skull bones. Vertebral cortical thickening of the superior and inferior end plates creates a "picture frame" vertebra. Diffuse radiodense enlargement of a vertebra is referred to as "ivory vertebra." Pelvic radiographs may demonstrate disruption or fusion of the sacroiliac joints; porotic

FIGURE 349-2 A 48-year-old woman with Paget disease of the skull. *Left.* Lateral radiograph showing areas of both bone resorption and sclerosis. ***Right.*** ^{99m}Tc HDP bone scan with anterior, posterior, and lateral views of the skull showing diffuse isotope uptake by the frontal, parietal, occipital, and petrous bones.

and radiodense lesions of the ilium with whorls of coarse trabeculation; thickened and sclerotic ileopectinal line (Brim sign); and softening with protrusio acetabuli, with axial migration of the hips and functional flexion contracture. Radiographs of long bones reveal bowing deformity and typical pagetic changes of cortical thickening and expansion and areas of lucency and sclerosis (Fig. 349-3). Radionuclide ^{99m}Tc bone scans are less specific but are more sensitive than standard radiographs for identifying sites of active skeletal lesions. Suspected areas of malignant transformation are best distinguished from pagetic bone by CT or MRI. Definitive diagnosis of malignancy requires bone biopsy.

Biochemical evaluation is useful in the diagnosis and management of Paget disease. The marked increase in bone turnover can be monitored using biochemical markers of bone formation and resorption. The parallel rise in serum ALP and urinary hydroxyproline levels, markers of bone formation and resorption, respectively, confirm the coupling of bone formation and resorption in Paget disease. The degree of bone marker elevation reflects the extent and severity of the disease. Patients with the highest elevation of ALP (10 times the upper limit of normal) typically have involvement of the skull and at least one other skeletal site. Lower values suggest less extensive involvement

FIGURE 349-3 Radiograph of a 73-year-old man with Paget disease of the right proximal femur. Note the coarsening of the trabecular pattern with marked cortical thickening and narrowing of the joint space consistent with osteoarthritis secondary to pagetic deformity of the right femur.

or a quiescent phase of the disease. For most patients, serum total ALP remains the test of choice both for diagnosis and assessing response to therapy. Occasionally, a symptomatic patient with evidence of progression at a single site may have a normal total ALP level but increased bone-specific ALP. Serum osteocalcin, a marker of bone formation, is not always elevated in patients with active Paget disease and is not recommended for use in diagnosis or management.

Urinary and serum deoxypyridinoline, N-telopeptide, and C-telopeptide levels are products of type I collagen degradation and are more specific for bone resorption than hydroxyproline. These newer bone resorption markers have distinct advantages over measurement of 24-h or second-morning void hydroxyproline/creatinine ratio, which requires control of dietary gelatin intake and precise urine collection and analysis. The new resorption markers decrease more rapidly in response to therapy than does ALP.

Serum calcium and phosphate levels are normal in Paget disease. Immobilization of a patient with active Paget disease may rarely cause hypercalcemia and hypercalciuria and increase the risk for nephrolithiasis. However, the discovery of hypercalcemia, even in the presence of immobilization, should prompt a search for another cause of hypercalcemia. In contrast, hypocalcemia or mild secondary hyperparathyroidism may develop in Paget patients with very active bone formation and insufficient dietary calcium intake. Hypocalcemia can occur during bisphosphonate therapy when bone resorption is rapidly suppressed and active bone formation continues. Hypocalcemia may be prevented by adequate calcium and vitamin D intake.

Rx PAGET DISEASE OF BONE

The development of effective and potent pharmacologic agents (Table 349-1) has changed the treatment philosophy from treating only symptomatic patients to treating asymptomatic patients who are at risk for complications. Pharmacologic therapy is indicated in the following circumstances: to control symptoms caused by metabolically active Paget disease such as bone pain, fracture, headache, pain from pagetic radiculopathy or arthropathy, or neurologic complications; to decrease local blood flow and minimize operative blood loss in patients undergoing surgery at an active pagetic site; to reduce hypercalciuria that may occur during immobilization; and to decrease the risk of complications when disease activity is high (elevated ALP) and when the site of involvement involves weight-bearing bones, areas adjacent to major joints, vertebral bodies, and skull. Whether early therapy prevents late complications remains to be determined. However, the restoration of normal bone architecture following suppression of pagetic activity suggests that treatment may prevent further deformities and complications.

Agents approved for treatment of Paget disease suppress the very high rates of bone resorption and secondarily decrease the high rates of bone

TABLE 349-1 PHARMACOLOGIC AGENTS APPROVED FOR TREATMENT OF PAGET DISEASE

Name (Brand)	Potency[a]	Dose	Mode of Administration
Etidronate (Didronel)	1	400 mg/d for 6 mos	Fasting PO
Tiludronate (Skelid)	10	400 mg/d for 3 mos	Fasting PO
Pamidronate (Aredia)	100	30 mg/d for 3 doses *or* 60–90 mg once	IV
Alendronate (Fosamax)	700	30 mg/d for 2 mos	Fasting PO
Risedronate (Actonel)	1000	30 mg/d for 2 mos	Fasting PO
Zoledronate (Zometa)	NK	5 mg	IV
Calcitonin (Miacalcin)	NA	100 U daily	SC

[a]Potency is relative to etidronate. For each tablet, etidronate strength is 400 mg; tiludronate is 200 mg; alendronate is 40 mg; and risedronate is 30 mg. Miacalcin nasal spray is not approved for use in Paget disease.

Note: NK, not known; NA, does not apply.

formation (Table 349-1). As a result of decreasing bone turnover, pagetic structural patterns, including areas of poorly mineralized woven bone, are replaced by more normal cancellous or lamellar bone. The improvement in skeletal structure can be demonstrated on standard radiographs and ^{99m}Tc bone scans, which show decreased isotope accumulation in pagetic sites. Reduced bone turnover can be documented by a decline in urine or serum resorption markers (pyridinoline, deoxypyridinoline, N-telopeptide, C-telopeptide) and serum markers of bone formation (ALP, osteocalcin).

The potencies of various bisphosphonates are expressed relative to that of etidronate, the first clinically useful agent in this class. Etidronate use is now limited as the doses required to suppress bone resorption may impair mineralization. Thus, etidronate is administered in 6-month treatment cycles followed by a 6-month drug-free period. Failure to adhere to the cyclic regimen can produce osteomalacia manifested by bone pain and fractures. Etidronate should not be used in patients with advanced lytic lesions in weight-bearing bones. The major advantage of etidronate is that it is relatively well tolerated and only occasionally causes transient diarrhea or bone pain.

The second-generation oral bisphosphonates tiludronate, alendronate, and risedronate are more potent than etidronate in controlling bone turnover and thus induce a longer remission at a lower dose. The lower doses reduce the risks of impaired mineralization and osteomalacia. Oral bisphosphonates are poorly absorbed and have a potential to produce esophageal ulceration, reflux, and rarely, perforation. They should be taken first thing in the morning on an empty stomach, followed by maintenance of upright posture with no food or drink for 30–60 min. Other medications, liquids, and food should be delayed for at least 30–60 min after taking bisphosphonates to optimize absorption. Tiludronate daily for 3 months normalizes ALP in 24–35% of moderately affected patients. In patients with moderate to severe disease, alendronate for 6 months normalizes ALP in >67% of patients, with an overall fall in ALP of 79% compared to 44% with etidronate. In patients with moderately active disease, risedronate daily for 2–3 months reduces serum ALP by 80% and by 6 months after treatment normalizes indices of bone turnover in 73% of patients compared to 15% of those receiving etidronate.

Pamidronate is approved for IV use in Paget disease. The recommended dose is 30 mg dissolved in 500 mL of normal saline or dextrose IV over 4 h on three consecutive days. The dose can be adjusted to each patient's requirements. A single 60-mg IV dose of pamidronate may normalize bone turnover in patients with mild disease. In contrast, patients with moderate to severe disease (elevation of ALP of three to four times normal) may require two to four doses of pamidronate, 60–90 mg IV, every 1–2 weeks. Patients with very severe disease may require a total dose of pamidronate of 300–500 mg given weekly over several weeks. Although suppression of urinary bone markers occurs after a few days to weeks, normalization of serum ALP levels often requires at least 3 months. Consequently, the effects of pamidronate are best evaluated 3 months after the initial dose.

In 2006, IV zoledronate received approval by the U.S. Food and Drug Administration (FDA) for use in Paget disease. One 5-mg infusion of zoledronate normalizes ALP in about 90% of patients by 6 months, and the therapeutic effect persists for an additional 6 months in most patients.

Pamidronate and zoledronate are generally well tolerated; however, a small number of patients experience a flulike syndrome that may begin 24 h after the first infusion. In patients with high bone turnover, vitamin D (400–800 IU daily) and calcium (500 mg three times daily) should be provided to prevent hypocalcemia and secondary hyperparathyroidism. Indications for IV therapy include mild disease and normalization of bone turnover after a single infusion, previous prevention of disease progression, refractoriness to oral therapy, need for rapid response for those with neurologic symptoms or with severe bone pain due to a lytic lesion, or at risk of an impending fracture, and as pretreatment prior to elective surgery in an area of active disease. Remission following pamidronate and zoledronate therapy may persist for ≥ 1 year.

The subcutaneous injectable form of salmon calcitonin is approved for the treatment of Paget disease. Intranasal calcitonin spray is approved for osteoporosis at a dose of 200 U/d; however, the efficacy of this dose in Paget disease has not been thoroughly studied. The usual starting dose of injectable calcitonin (100 U/d) reduces ALP by 50% and may relieve skeletal symptoms. The dose may be reduced to 50 U/d three times weekly after an initial favorable response to 100 U daily; however, the lower dose may require long-term use to sustain efficacy. The common side effects of calcitonin therapy are nausea and facial flushing. Secondary resistance after prolonged use may be due to either the formation of anti-calcitonin antibodies or downregulation of osteoclastic cell–surface calcitonin receptors. The lower potency and injectable mode of delivery make this agent a less attractive treatment option that should be reserved for patients who either do not tolerate or do not respond to bisphosphonates.

SCLEROSING BONE DISORDERS

OSTEOPETROSIS

Osteopetrosis refers to a group of disorders caused by severe impairment of osteoclast-mediated bone resorption. Other terms that are often used include marble bone disease, which captures the solid x-ray appearance of the involved skeleton, and Albers-Schonberg disease, which refers to the milder, adult form of osteopetrosis also known as autosomal dominant osteopetrosis type II. The major types of osteopetrosis include malignant (severe, infantile, autosomal recessive) osteopetrosis and benign (adult, autosomal dominant) osteopetrosis types I and II. A rare autosomal recessive intermediate form has a more benign prognosis. Autosomal recessive carbonic anhydrase (CA) II deficiency produces osteopetrosis of intermediate severity associated with renal tubular acidosis and cerebral calcification.

Etiology and Genetics Naturally occurring and gene knockout animal models with phenotypes similar to those of the human disorders have been used to explore the genetic basis of osteopetrosis. The primary defect in osteopetrosis is the loss of osteoclastic bone resorption and preservation of normal osteoblastic bone formation. Osteoprotegerin (OPG) is a soluble decoy receptor that binds osteoblast-derived RANK ligand, which mediates osteoclast differentiation and activation (Fig. 349-1). Transgenic mice that overexpress OPG develop osteopetrosis, presumably by blocking RANK ligand. Mice deficient in RANK lack osteoclasts and develop severe osteopetrosis.

Recessive mutations of CA II prevent osteoclasts from generating an acid environment in the clear zone between its ruffled border and the adjacent mineral surface. Absence of CA II, therefore, impairs osteoclastic bone resorption. Other forms of human disease have less clear genetic defects. About one-half of the patients with malignant infantile osteopetrosis have a mutation in the *TCIRG1* gene encoding the osteoclast-specific subunit of the vacuolar proton pump, which mediates the acidification of the interface between bone mineral and the osteoclast ruffled border. Mutations in the *CICN7* chloride channel gene cause autosomal dominant osteopetrosis type II.

Clinical Presentation The incidence of autosomal recessive severe (malignant) osteopetrosis ranges from 1 in 200,000 to 1 in 500,000 live births. As bone and cartilage fail to undergo modeling, paralysis of one or more cranial nerves may occur due to narrowing of the cranial foramina. Failure of skeletal modeling also results in inadequate marrow space, leading to extramedullary hematopoiesis with hypersplenism and pancytopenia. Hypocalcemia due to lack of osteoclastic bone resorption may occur in infants and young children. The untreated infantile disease is fatal, often before age 5.

Adult (benign) osteopetrosis is an autosomal dominant disease that is usually diagnosed by the discovery of typical skeletal changes in young adults who undergo radiologic evaluation of a fracture. The prevalence is 1 in 100,000 to 1 in 500,000 adults. The course is not always benign, as fractures may be accompanied by loss of vision, deafness, psychomotor delay, mandibular osteomyelitis, and other complications usually associated with the juvenile form. In some kindred, nonpenetrance results in skip generations, while in other families severely affected children are born into families with benign disease. The milder form of the disease does not usually require treatment.

Radiography Typically, there are generalized symmetric increases in bone mass with thickening of both cortical and trabecular bone. Diaphyses and metaphyses are broadened, and alternating sclerotic and lucent bands may be seen in the iliac crests, at the ends of long bones, and in vertebral bodies. The cranium is usually thickened, particularly at the base of the skull, and the paranasal and mastoid sinuses are underpneumatized.

Laboratory Findings The only significant laboratory findings are elevated serum levels of osteoclast-derived tartrate-resistant acid phosphatase (TRAP) and the brain isoenzyme of creatine kinase. Serum calcium may be low in severe disease, and parathyroid hormone and 1,25-dihydroxyvitamin D levels may be elevated in response to hypocalcemia.

℞ OSTEOPETROSIS

Allogenic HLA-identical bone marrow transplantation has been successful in some children. Following transplantation, the marrow contains progenitor cells and normally functioning osteoclasts. A cure is most likely when children are transplanted before age 4. Marrow transplantation from nonidentical HLA-matched donors has a much higher failure rate. Limited studies in small numbers of patients have suggested variable benefits following treatment with interferon γ-1β, 1,25-dihydroxyvitamin D (which stimulates osteoclasts directly), methylprednisolone, and a low calcium/high-phosphate diet.

Surgical intervention is indicated to decompress optic or auditory nerve compression. Orthopedic management is required for the surgical treatment of fractures and their complications including mal-union and postfracture deformity.

PYKNODYSOSTOSIS

This is an autosomal recessive form of osteosclerosis that is believed to have affected the French impressionist painter Henri de Toulouse-Lautrec. The molecular basis involves mutations in the gene that encodes cathepsin K, a lysosomal metalloproteinase highly expressed in osteoclasts and important for bone matrix degradation. Osteoclasts are present but do not function normally. Pyknodysostosis is a form of short-limb dwarfism that presents with frequent fractures but usually normal life span. Clinical features include short stature; kyphoscoliosis and deformities of the chest; high arched palate; proptosis; blue sclerae; dysmorphic features including small face and chin, frontooccipital prominence, pointed beaked nose, large cranium, and obtuse mandibular angle; and small square hands with hypoplastic nails. Radiographs demonstrate a generalized increase in bone density, but in contrast to osteopetrosis, the long bones are normally shaped. Separated cranial sutures, including the persistent patency of the anterior fontanel, are characteristic of the disorder. There may also be hypoplasia of the sinuses, mandible, distal clavicles, and terminal phalanges. Persistence of deciduous teeth and sclerosis of the calvarium and base of the skull are also common. Histologic evaluation shows normal cor-

tical bone architecture with decreased osteoblastic and osteoclastic activities. Serum chemistries are normal, and unlike osteopetrosis, there is no anemia. There is no known treatment for this condition, and no reports of attempted bone marrow transplant.

PROGRESSIVE DIAPHYSEAL DYSPLASIA

Also known as *Camurati-Engelman disease*, progressive diaphyseal dysplasia is an autosomal dominant disorder that is characterized radiographically by diaphyseal hyperostosis and a symmetric thickening and increased diameter of the endosteal and periosteal surfaces of the diaphyses of the long bones, particularly the femur and tibia, and, less often, the fibula, radius, and ulna. The genetic defect responsible for the disease has been localized to the area of chromosome 19q13.2 encoding tumor growth factor (TGF)-β1. The mutation promotes activation of TGF-β1. The clinical severity is variable. The most common presenting symptoms are pain and tenderness of the involved areas, fatigue, muscle wasting, and gait disturbance. The weakness may be mistaken for muscular dystrophy. Characteristic body habitus includes thin limbs with little muscle mass yet prominent and palpable bones and, when the skull is involved, large head with prominent forehead and proptosis. Patients may also display signs of cranial nerve palsies, hydrocephalus, central hypogonadism, and Raynaud phenomenon. Radiographically, patchy progressive endosteal and periosteal new bone formation is observed along the diaphyses of the long bones. Bone scintigraphy shows increased radiotracer uptake in involved areas.

Treatment with low-dose glucocorticoids relieves bone pain and may reverse the abnormal bone formation. Intermittent bisphosphonate therapy has produced clinical improvement in a limited number of patients.

HYPEROSTOSIS CORTICALIS GENERALISATA

This is also known as *van Buchem disease*; it is an autosomal recessive disorder characterized by endosteal hyperostosis in which osteosclerosis involves the skull, mandible, clavicles, and ribs. The major manifestations are due to narrowed cranial foramina with neural compressions that may result in optic atrophy, facial paralysis, and deafness. Adults may have an enlarged mandible. Serum ALP levels may be elevated, which reflects the uncoupled bone remodeling with high osteoblastic formation rates and low osteoclastic resorption. As a result, there is increased accumulation of normal bone. Endosteal hyperostosis with syndactyly, known as *sclerosteosis*, is a more severe form. The genetic defects for both sclerosteosis and van Buchem disease have been assigned to the same region of the chromosome 17q12-q21. It is possible that both conditions may have deactivating mutations in the *BEER* (bone-expressed equilibrium regulator) gene.

MELORHEOSTOSIS

Melorheostosis (Greek, "flowing hyperostosis") may occur sporadically or follow a pattern consistent with an autosomal recessive disorder. The major manifestation is progressive linear hyperostosis in one or more bones of one limb, usually a lower extremity. The name comes from the radiographic appearance of the involved bone, which resembles melted wax that has dripped down a candle. Symptoms appear during childhood as pain or stiffness in the area of sclerotic bone. There may be associated ectopic soft tissue masses, composed of cartilage or osseous tissue, and skin changes overlying the involved bone, consisting of scleroderma-like areas and hypertrichosis. The disease does not progress in adults, but pain and stiffness may persist. Laboratory tests are unremarkable. No specific etiology is known. There is no specific treatment. Surgical interventions to correct contractures are often unsuccessful.

OSTEOPOIKILOSIS

The literal translation of osteopoikilosis is "spotted bones"; it is a benign autosomal dominant condition in which numerous small, variably shaped (usually round or oval) foci of bony sclerosis are seen in the epiphyses and adjacent metaphyses. The lesions may involve any bone except the skull, ribs, and vertebrae. They may be misidentified as metastatic lesions. The main differentiating points are that bony lesions of osteopoikilosis are stable over time and do not accumulate radionuclide on bone scanning. In some kindred, osteopoikilosis is associated with connective tissue nevi known as *dermatofibrosis lenticularis disseminata*, also known as *Buschke-Ollendorf syndrome*. Histologic inspection reveals thickened but otherwise normal trabeculae and islands of normal cortical bone. No treatment is indicated.

HEPATITS C–ASSOCIATED OSTEOSCLEROSIS

Hepatitis C–associated osteosclerosis (HCAO) is a rare acquired diffuse osteosclerosis in adults with prior hepatitis C infection. After a latent period of several years, patients develop diffuse appendicular bone pain and a generalized increase in bone mass with elevated serum ALP. Bone biopsy and histomorphometry reveal increased rates of bone formation, decreased bone resorption with a marked decrease in osteoclasts, and dense lamellar bone. One patient had increased serum OPG levels, and bone biopsy showed large numbers of osteoblasts positive for OPG and reduced osteoclast number. Empirical therapy includes pain control and there may be beneficial response to either calcitonin or bisphosphonate.

DISORDERS ASSOCIATED WITH DEFECTIVE MINERALIZATION

HYPOPHOSPHATASIA

This is a rare inherited disorder that presents as rickets in infants and children or osteomalacia in adults with paradoxically low serum levels of ALP. The frequency of the severe neonatal and infantile forms is about 1 in 100,000 live births in Canada, where the disease is most common because of its high prevalence among Mennonites and Hutterites. It is rare in African Americans. The severity of the disease is remarkably variable, ranging from intrauterine death associated with profound skeletal hypomineralization at one extreme, to premature tooth loss as the only manifestation in some adults. Severe cases are inherited in an autosomal recessive manner, but the genetic patterns are less clear for the milder forms. The disease is caused by a deficiency of tissue nonspecific (bone/liver/kidney) ALP (TNSALP), which, although ubiquitous, results only in bone abnormalities. Protein levels and functions of the other ALP isozymes (germ cell, intestinal, placental) are normal. Defective ALP permits accumulation of its major naturally occurring substrates including phosphoethanolamine (PEA), inorganic pyrophosphate (PPi), and pyridoxal 5'-phosphate (PLP). The accumulation of PPi interferes with mineralization through its action as a potent inhibitor of hydroxyapatite crystal growth.

Perinatal hypophosphatasia becomes manifest during pregnancy and is often complicated by polyhydroamnios and intrauterine death. The infantile form becomes clinically apparent before age 6 months with failure to thrive, rachitic deformities, functional craniosynostosis despite widely open fontanels (which are actually hypomineralized areas of the calvarium), raised intracranial pressure, and flail chest and predisposition to pneumonia. Hypercalcemia and hypercalciuria are common. This form has a mortality rate of about 50%. Prognosis seems to improve for the children who survive infancy. Childhood hypophosphatasia has variable clinical presentation. Premature loss of deciduous teeth (before age 5 years) is the hallmark of the disease. Rickets causes delayed walking with waddling gait, short stature, and dolichocephalic skull with frontal bossing. The disease often improves during puberty but may recur in adult life. Adult hypophosphatasia presents during middle age with painful, poorly healing metatarsal stress fractures or thigh pain due to femoral pseudofractures.

Laboratory investigation reveals low ALP levels and normal or elevated levels of serum calcium and phosphorus despite clinical and radiologic evidence of rickets or osteomalacia. Serum parathyroid hormone, 25-hydroxyvitamin D, and 1,25-dihydroxyvitamin D levels are normal. The elevation of PLP is specific for the disease and may even be present in asymptomatic parents of severely affected children. As vitamin B_6 increases PLP levels, vitamin B_6 supplements should be discontinued 1 week before testing.

There is no established medical therapy. In contrast to other forms of rickets and osteomalacia, calcium and vitamin D supplementation

should be avoided as they may aggravate hypercalcemia and hypercalciuria. A low-calcium diet, glucocorticoids, and calcitonin have been used in a small number of patients with variable responses. Because fracture healing is poor, placement of intramedullary rods is best for acute fracture repair and for prophylactic prevention of fractures.

AXIAL OSTEOMALACIA

This is a rare disorder characterized by defective skeletal mineralization despite normal serum calcium and phosphate levels. Clinically, the disorder presents in middle-aged or elderly men with chronic axial skeletal discomfort. Cervical spine pain may also be present. Radiographic findings are mainly osteosclerosis due to coarsened trabecular patterns typical of osteomalacia. Spine, pelvis, and ribs are most commonly affected. Histologic changes show defective mineralization and flat, inactive osteoblasts. The primary defect appears to be an acquired defect in osteoblast function. The course is benign and there is no established treatment. Calcium and vitamin D therapies are not effective.

FIBROGENESIS IMPERFECTA OSSIUM

This is a rare condition of unknown etiology. It presents in both sexes, in middle age or later, with progressive, intractable skeletal pain and fractures, worsening immobilization, and a debilitating course. Radiographic evaluation reveals generalized osteomalacia, osteopenia, and occasional pseudofractures. Histologic features include a tangled pattern of collagen fibrils with abundant osteoblasts and osteoclasts. There is no effective treatment. Spontaneous remission has been reported in a small number of patients. Calcium and vitamin D have not been beneficial.

FIBROUS DYSPLASIA AND McCUNE-ALBRIGHT SYNDROME

Fibrous dysplasia is a sporadic disorder characterized by the presence of one (monoostotic) or more (polyostotic) expanding fibrous skeletal lesions composed of bone-forming mesenchyme. The association of the polyostotic form with café-au-lait spots and hyperfunction of an endocrine system such as pseudo-precocious puberty of ovarian origin is known as *McCune-Albright syndrome* (MAS). A spectrum of the phenotypes is caused by activating mutations in the GNAS1 gene, which encodes the α subunit of the stimulatory G protein ($G_s\alpha$). As the postzygotic mutations occur at different stages of early development, the extent and type of tissue affected are variable and explain the mosaic pattern of skin and bone changes. GTP binding activates the $G_s\alpha$ regulatory protein and mutations in regions of $G_s\alpha$ that selectively inhibit GTPase activity, which results in constitutive stimulation of the cyclic AMP–protein kinase A signal transduction pathway. Such mutations of the $G_s\alpha$ protein–coupled receptor may cause autonomous function in bone (parathyroid hormone receptor); skin (melanocyte-stimulating hormone receptor); and various endocrine glands including ovary (follicle-stimulating hormone receptor), thyroid (thyroid-stimulating hormone receptor), adrenal (adrenocorticotropic hormone receptor), and pituitary (growth hormone–releasing hormone receptor). The skeletal lesions are composed largely of mesenchymal cells that do not differentiate into osteoblasts, resulting in the formation of imperfect bone. In some areas of bone, fibroblast-like cells develop features of osteoblasts in that they produce extracellular matrix that organizes into woven bone. Calcification may occur in some areas. In other areas, cells have features of chondrocytes and produce cartilage-like extracellular matrix.

Clinical Presentation   Fibrous dysplasia occurs with equal frequency in both sexes, whereas MAS with precocious puberty is more common (10:1) in girls. The monoostotic form is the most common and is usually diagnosed in patients between 20 and 30 years of age without associated skin lesions. The polyostotic form typically manifests in children <10 years of age and may progress with age. Early-onset disease is generally more severe. Lesions may become quiescent in puberty and progress during pregnancy or with estrogen therapy. In polyostotic fibrous dysplasia, the lesions most commonly involve the maxilla and other craniofacial bones, ribs, and metaphyseal or diaphyseal portions of the proximal femur or tibia. Expanding bone lesions may cause pain, deformity, fractures, and nerve entrapment. Sarcomatous degeneration involving the facial bones or femur is infrequent (<1%). The risk of malignant transformation is increased by radiation, which has proven to be ineffective treatment. In rare patients with widespread lesions, renal phosphate wasting and hypophosphatemia may cause rickets or osteomalacia. Hypophosphatemia may be due to production of a phosphaturic factor by the abnormal fibrous tissue.

MAS patients may have café-au-lait spots, which are flat, hyperpigmented skin lesions that have rough borders ("coast of Maine") in contrast to the café-au-lait lesions of neurofibromatosis that have smooth borders ("coast of California"). The most common endocrinopathy is isosexual pseudo-precocious puberty in girls. Other less common endocrine disorders include thyrotoxicosis, Cushing syndrome, acromegaly, hyperparathyroidism, hyperprolactinemia, and pseudo-precocious puberty in boys.

Radiographic Findings In long bones, the fibrous dysplastic lesions are typically well-defined, radiolucent areas with thin cortices and a ground-glass appearance. Lesions may be lobulated with trabeculated areas of radiolucency (**Fig. 349-4**). Involvement of facial bones usually presents as radiodense lesions, which may create a leonine appearance (leontiasis osea). Expansile cranial lesions may narrow foramina and cause optic lesions, reduce hearing, and create other manifestations of cranial nerve compression.

Laboratory Results Serum ALP is occasionally elevated but calcium, parathyroid hormone, 25-hydroxyvitamin D, and 1,25-dihydroxyvitamin D levels are normal. Patients with extensive polyostotic lesions may have hypophosphatemia, hyperphosphaturia, and osteomalacia. The hypophosphatemia and phosphaturia are directly related to the levels of fibroblast growth factor 23 (FGF-23). Biochemical markers of bone turnover may be elevated.

℞ FIBROUS DYSPLASIA AND McCUNE-ALBRIGHT SYNDROME

Spontaneous healing of the lesions does not occur, and there is no established effective treatment. Improvement in bone pain and partial or complete resolution of radiographic lesions have been reported after IV bisphosphonate therapy. Surgical stabilization is used to prevent pathologic fracture or destruction of a major joint space and to relieve nerve root or cranial nerve compression or sinus obstruction.

FIGURE 349-4 Radiograph of a 16-year-old male with fibrous dysplasia of the right proximal femur. Note the multiple cystic lesions, including the large lucent lesion in the proximal mid-shaft with scalloping of the interior surface. The femoral neck contains two lucent cystic lesions.

OTHER DYSPLASIAS OF BONE AND CARTILAGE

PACHYDERMOPERIOSTOSIS

Pachydermoperiostosis, or hypertrophic osteoarthropathy (primary or idiopathic), is an autosomal dominant disorder characterized by periosteal new bone formation that involves the distal extremities. The lesions present as clubbing of the digits and hyperhidrosis and thickening of the skin, primarily of the face and forehead. The changes usually appear during adolescence, progress over the next decade, and then become quiescent. During the active phase, progressive enlargement of the hands and feet produces a pawlike appearance, which may be mistaken for acromegaly. Arthralgias, pseudogout, and limited mobility may also occur. The disorder must be differentiated from secondary hypertrophic osteopathy that develops during the course of serious pulmonary disorders. The two conditions can be differentiated by standard radiography of the digits in which secondary pachydermoperiostosis has exuberant periosteal new bone formation and a smooth and undulating surface. In contrast, primary hypertrophic osteopathy has an irregular periosteal surface.

There are no diagnostic blood or urine tests. Synovial fluid does not have an inflammatory profile. There is no specific therapy, although a limited experience with colchicine suggests some benefit in controlling the arthralgias.

OSTEOCHONDRODYSPLASIAS

These include several hundred heritable disorders of connective tissue. These primary abnormalities of cartilage manifest as disturbances in cartilage and bone growth. Selected growth plate chondrodysplasias are described here. **For discussion of chondrodysplasias, see Chap. 357.**

Achondrodysplasia This is a relatively common form of short-limb dwarfism that occurs in 1 in 15,000 to 1 in 40,000 live births. The disease is caused by a mutation of the fibroblast growth factor receptor 3 (*FGFR3*) gene that results in a gain-of-function state. Most cases are sporadic mutations. However, when the disorder appears in families, the inheritance pattern is consistent with an autosomal dominant disorder. The primary defect is abnormal chondrocyte proliferation at the growth plate that causes development of short but proportionately thick long bones. Other regions of the long bones may be relatively unaffected. The disorder is manifest by the presence of short limbs (particularly the proximal portions), normal trunk, large head, saddle nose, and an exaggerated lumbar lordosis. Severe spinal deformity may lead to cord compression. The homozygous disorder is more serious than the sporadic form and may cause neonatal death. Pseudo-achondroplasia clinically resembles achondroplasia but has no skull abnormalities.

Enchondromatosis This is also called *dyschondroplasia*, or *Ollier disease*; it is also a disorder of the growth plate in which the primary cartilage is not resorbed. Cartilage ossification proceeds normally but it is not resorbed normally, leading to cartilage accumulation. The changes are most marked at the ends of long bones where the highest growth rates occur. Chondrosarcoma develops infrequently. The association of enchondromatosis and cavernous hemangiomas of the skin and soft tissues is known as *Maffucci syndrome*. Both Ollier disease and Maffucci syndrome are associated with various malignancies, including granulosa cell tumor of the ovary and cerebral glioma.

Multiple Exostoses This is also called *diaphyseal aclasis*, or *osteochondromatosis*; it is a genetic disorder that follows an autosomal dominant pattern of inheritance. In this condition, areas of growth plates become displaced, presumably by growing through a defect in the perichondrium. The lesion begins with vascular invasion of the growth plate cartilage, resulting in a characteristic radiographic finding of a mass that is in direct communication with the marrow cavity of the parent bone. The underlying cortex is resorbed. The disease is caused by inactivating mutations of the *EXT1* and *EXT2* genes, whose products normally regulate processing of chondrocyte cytoskeletal proteins. The products of the *EXT* gene likely function as tumor suppressors, with the loss-of-function mutation resulting in abnormal proliferation of growth plate cartilage. Solitary or multiple lesions are located in the metaphyses of long bones. Although usually asymptomatic, the lesions may interfere with joint or tendon function or compress peripheral nerves. The lesions stop growing when growth ceases but may recur during pregnancy. There is a small risk for malignant transformation into chondrosarcoma.

EXTRASKELETAL (ECTOPIC) CALCIFICATION AND OSSIFICATION

Deposition of calcium phosphate crystals (*calcification*) or formation of true bone (*ossification*) in nonosseous soft tissue may occur by one of three mechanisms: (1) metastatic calcification due to a supranormal calcium × phosphate concentration product in extracellular fluid; (2) dystrophic calcification due to mineral deposition into metabolically impaired or dead tissue despite normal serum levels of calcium and phosphate; and (3) ectopic ossification, or true bone formation. Disorders that may cause extraskeletal calcification or ossification are listed in Table 349-2.

METASTATIC CALCIFICATION

Soft tissue calcification may complicate diseases associated with significant hypercalcemia, hyperphosphatemia, or both. In addition, vitamin D and phosphate treatments or calcium administration in the presence of mild hyperphosphatemia, such as during hemodialysis, may induce ectopic calcification. Calcium phosphate precipitation may complicate any disorder when the serum calcium × phosphate concentration product > 75. The initial calcium phosphate deposition is in the form of small, poorly organized crystals, which subsequently organize into hydroxyapatite crystals. Calcifications that occur in hypercalcemic states with normal or low phosphate have a predilection for kidney, lungs, and gastric mucosa. Hyperphosphatemia with normal or low serum calcium may promote soft tissue calcification with predilection for the kidney and arteries. The disturbances of calcium and phosphate in renal failure and hemodialysis are common causes of soft tissue (metastatic) calcification.

TUMORAL CALCINOSIS

This is a rare genetic disorder characterized by masses of metastatic calcifications in soft tissues around major joints, most often shoulders, hips, and ankles. Tumoral calcinosis differs from other disorders in that the periarticular masses contain hydroxyapatite crystals or amorphous calcium phosphate complexes, while in fibrodysplasia ossificans progressiva (below), true bone is formed in soft tissues. About one-third of tumoral calcinosis cases are familial, with both autosomal recessive and autosomal dominant modes of inheritance reported. The disease is also associated with a variably expressed abnormality of dentition marked by short bulbous roots, pulp calcification, and radicular dentin deposited in swirls. The primary defect responsible for the metastatic calcification appears to be hyperphosphatemia resulting from the increased capacity of the renal tubule to reabsorb filtered phosphate. Spontaneous soft tissue calcification is related to the elevated serum phosphate, which along with normal serum calcium exceeds the concentration product of 75.

All of the North American patients reported have been African-American. The disease usually presents in childhood and continues lifelong. The calcific masses are typically painless and grow at variable rates, sometimes becoming large and bulky. The masses are often located near major joints but remain extracapsular. Joint range of motion is not usually restricted unless the tumors are very large. Complications include compression of neural structures and ulceration of the overlying skin with drainage of chalky fluid and risk of secondary infection. Small deposits not detected by standard radiographs may be detected by ^{99m}Tc bone scanning. The most common laboratory findings are hyperphosphatemia and elevated serum 1,25-dihydroxyvitamin D levels. Serum calcium, parathyroid hormone, and ALP levels are usually normal. Renal function is also usually normal. Urine calcium and phosphate excretions are low, and calcium and phosphate balances are positive.

An acquired form of the disease may occur with other causes of hyperphosphatemia, such as secondary hyperparathyroidism associated with hemodialysis, hypoparathyroidism, pseudohypoparathyroidism, and massive cell lysis following chemotherapy for leukemia. Tissue trauma from joint movement may contribute to the periarticular calcifications. Metastatic calcifications are also seen in conditions associated with hypercalcemia, such as in sarcoidosis, vitamin D intoxication, milk-alkali syndrome, and primary hyperparathyroidism. In these conditions, however, mineral deposits are more likely to occur in proton-transporting organs such as kidney, lungs, and gastric mucosa in which an alkaline milieu is generated by the proton pumps.

℞ TUMORAL CALCINOSIS

Therapeutic successes have been achieved with surgical removal of subcutaneous calcified masses, which tend not to recur if all calcification is removed from the site. Reduction of serum phosphate by chronic phosphorus restriction may be accomplished using low dietary phosphorus intake alone or in combination with oral phosphate binders. The addition of the phosphaturic agent acetazolamide may be useful. Limited experience using the phosphaturic action of calcitonin deserves further testing.

DYSTROPHIC CALCIFICATION

Posttraumatic calcification may occur with normal serum calcium and phosphate levels and normal ion solubility product. The deposited mineral is either in the form of amorphous calcium phosphate or hydroxyapatite crystals. Soft tissue calcification complicating connective tissue disorders such as scleroderma, dermatomyositis, and systemic lupus erythematosus may involve localized areas of the skin or deeper subcutaneous tissue and is referred to as *calcinosis circumscripta*. Mineral deposition at sites of deeper tissue injury including periarticular sites is called *calcinosis universalis*.

ECTOPIC OSSIFICATION

True extraskeletal bone formation that begins in areas of fasciitis following surgery, trauma, burns, or neurologic injury is referred to as *myositis ossificans*. The bone formed is organized as lamellar or trabecular, with normal osteoblasts and osteoclasts conducting active remodeling. Well-developed haversian systems and marrow elements may be present. A second cause of ectopic bone formation occurs in an inherited disorder, *fibrodysplasia ossificans progressiva*.

TABLE 349-2	DISEASES AND CONDITIONS ASSOCIATED WITH ECTOPIC CALCIFICATION AND OSSIFICATION
Metastatic calcification	Dystrophic calcification
Hypercalcemic states	Inflammatory disorders
Primary hyperparathyroidism	Scleroderma
Sarcoidosis	Dermatomyositis
Vitamin D intoxication	Systemic lupus erythematosus
Milk-alkali syndrome	Trauma-induced
Renal failure	Ectopic ossification
Hyperphosphatemia	Myositis ossificans
Tumoral calcinosis	Post surgery
Secondary hyperparathyroidism	Burns
Pseudohypoparathyroidism	Neurologic injury
Renal failure	Other trauma
Hemodialysis	Fibrodysplasia ossificans progressiva
Cell lysis following chemotherapy	
Therapy with vitamin D and phosphate	

FIBRODYSPLASIA OSSIFICANS PROGRESSIVA

This is also called *myositis ossificans progressiva*; it is a rare autosomal dominant disorder characterized by congenital deformities of the hands and feet and episodic soft tissue swellings that ossify. Ectopic bone formation occurs in fascia, tendons, ligaments, and connective tissue within voluntary muscles. Tender, rubbery induration, sometimes precipitated by trauma, develops in the soft tissue and gradually calcifies. Eventually, heterotopic bone forms at these sites of soft tissue trauma. Morbidity results from heterotopic bone interfering with normal movement and function of muscle and other soft tissues. Mortality is usually related to restrictive lung disease caused by an inability of the chest to expand. Laboratory tests are unremarkable.

There is no effective medical therapy. Bisphosphonates, glucocorticoids, and a low-calcium diet have largely been ineffective in halt-

ing progression of the ossification. Surgical removal of ectopic bone is not recommended, as the trauma of surgery may precipitate formation of new areas of heterotopic bone. Dental complications including frozen jaw may occur following injection of local anesthetics. Thus, CT imaging of the mandible should be undertaken to detect early sites of soft tissue ossification before they are appreciated by standard radiography.

FURTHER READINGS

HOCKING LJ et al: Domain-specific mutations in sequestosome 1 (SQSTM1) cause familial and sporadic Paget disease. Hum Mol Genet 11:2735, 2002

WHYTE MP: Paget's disease of bone. N Engl J Med 355:593, 2006

SECTION 3 | DISORDERS OF INTERMEDIARY METABOLISM

350 Disorders of Lipoprotein Metabolism

Daniel J. Rader, Helen H. Hobbs

Lipoproteins are complexes of lipids and proteins that are essential for the transport of cholesterol, triglycerides, and fat-soluble vitamins. Previously, lipoprotein disorders were the purview of specialized lipidologists, but the demonstration that lipid-lowering therapy significantly reduces the clinical complications of atherosclerotic cardiovascular disease (ASCVD) has brought the diagnosis and treatment of these disorders into the domain of the internist. The number of individuals who are candidates for lipid-lowering therapy has continued to increase. The development of safe, effective, and well-tolerated pharmacologic agents has greatly expanded the therapeutic armamentarium available to the physician to treat disorders of lipid metabolism. Therefore, the appropriate diagnosis and management of lipoprotein disorders is of critical importance in the practice of medicine. This chapter will review normal lipoprotein physiology, the pathophysiology of primary (inherited) disorders of lipoprotein metabolism, the diseases and environmental factors that cause secondary disorders of lipoprotein metabolism, and the practical approaches to their diagnosis and management.

LIPOPROTEIN METABOLISM

LIPOPROTEIN CLASSIFICATION AND COMPOSITION

Lipoproteins are large macromolecular complexes that transport hydrophobic lipids (primarily triglycerides, cholesterol, and fat-soluble vitamins) through body fluids (plasma, interstitial fluid, and lymph) to and from tissues. Lipoproteins play an essential role in the absorption of dietary cholesterol, long-chain fatty acids, and fat-soluble vitamins; the transport of triglycerides, cholesterol, and fat-soluble vitamins from the liver to peripheral tissues; and the transport of cholesterol from peripheral tissues to the liver.

Lipoproteins contain a core of hydrophobic lipids (triglycerides and cholesteryl esters) surrounded by hydrophilic lipids (phospholipids, unesterified cholesterol) and proteins that interact with body fluids. The plasma lipoproteins are divided into five major classes based on their relative density (**Fig. 350-1** and **Table 350-1**): chylomicrons, very low density lipoproteins (VLDLs), intermediate-density lipoproteins (IDLs), low-density lipoproteins (LDLs), and high-density lipoproteins (HDLs). Each lipoprotein class comprises a family of particles that vary slightly in density, size, migration during electrophoresis,

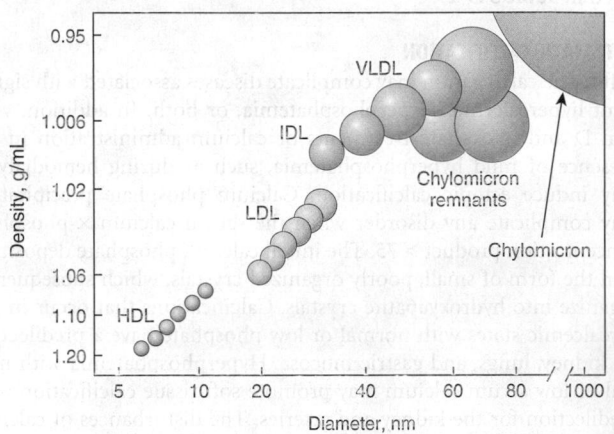

FIGURE 350-1 The density and size-distribution of the major classes of lipoprotein particles. Lipoproteins are classified by density and size, which are inversely related. VLDL, very low density lipoprotein; IDL, intermediate-density lipoprotein; LDL, low-density lipoprotein; HDL, high-density lipoprotein.

and protein composition. The density of a lipoprotein is determined by the amount of lipid per particle. HDL is the smallest and most dense lipoprotein, whereas chylomicrons and VLDLs are the largest and least dense lipoprotein particles. Most plasma triglyceride is transported in chylomicrons or VLDLs, and most plasma cholesterol is carried as cholesteryl esters in LDLs and HDLs.

The proteins associated with lipoproteins, called *apolipoproteins* (**Table 350-2**), are required for the assembly, structure, and function of lipoproteins. Apolipoproteins activate enzymes important in lipoprotein metabolism and act as ligands for cell surface receptors. ApoA-I, which is synthesized in the liver and intestine, is found on virtually all HDL particles. ApoA-II is the second most abundant HDL apolipoprotein and is on approximately two-thirds of all HDL particles. ApoB is the major structural protein of chylomicrons, VLDLs, IDLs, and LDLs; one molecule of apoB, either apoB-48 (chylomicron) or apoB-100 (VLDL, IDL or LDL), is present on each lipoprotein particle. The human liver synthesizes apoB-100, and the intestine makes apoB-48, which is derived from the same gene by mRNA editing. ApoE is present in multiple copies on chylomicrons, VLDL, and IDL, and it plays a critical role in the metabolism and clearance of triglyceride-rich particles. Three apolipoproteins of the C-series (apoC-I, apoC-II, and apoC-III) also participate in the metabolism of triglyceride-rich lipoproteins. The other apolipoproteins are listed in Table 350-2.

TABLE 350-1 MAJOR LIPOPROTEIN CLASSES

Lipoprotein	Density, g/mL[a]	Size, nm[b]	Electrophoretic Mobility[c]	Apolipoproteins Major	Other	Other Constituents
Chylomicrons	0.930	75–1200	Origin	ApoB-48	A-I, A-IV, C-I, C-II, C-III	Retinyl esters
Chylomicron remnants	0.930–1.006	30–80	Slow pre-β	ApoB-48	E, A-I, A-IV, C-I, C-II, C-III	Retinyl esters
VLDL	0.930–1.006	30–80	Pre-β	ApoB-100	E, A-I, A-II, A-V, C-I, C-II, C-III	Vitamin E
IDL	1.006–1.019	25–35	Slow pre-β	ApoB-100	E, C-I, C-II, C-III	Vitamin E
LDL	1.019–1.063	18–25	β	ApoB-100		Vitamin E
HDL	1.063–1.210	5–12	α	ApoA-I	A-II, A-IV, E, C-III	LCAT, CETP paroxonase
Lp(a)	1.050–1.120	25	Pre-β	ApoB-100	Apo(a)	

Note: All of the lipoprotein classes contain phospholipids, esterified and unesterified cholesterol, and triglycerides to varying degrees.
[a]The density of the particle is determined by ultracentrifugation.
[b]The size of the particle is measured using gel electrophoresis.
[c]The electrophoretic mobility of the particle on agarose gel electrophores reflects the size and surface charge of the particle, with β being the position of LDL and α being the position of HDL.

Abbreviations: VLDL, very low density lipoprotein; IDL, intermediate-density lipoprotein; LDL, low-density lipoprotein; HDL, high-density lipoprotein; Lp(a), lipoprotein A; LCAT, lecithin-cholesterol acyltransferase; CETP, cholesteryl ester transfer protein.

TRANSPORT OF DIETARY LIPIDS (EXOGENOUS PATHWAY)

The exogenous pathway of lipoprotein metabolism permits efficient transport of dietary lipids (Fig. 350-2). Dietary triglycerides are hydrolyzed by lipases within the intestinal lumen and emulsified with bile acids to form micelles. Dietary cholesterol, fatty acids, and fat-soluble vitamins are absorbed in the proximal small intestine. Cholesterol and retinol are esterified (by the addition of a fatty acid) in the enterocyte to form cholesteryl esters and retinyl esters, respectively. Longer-chain fatty acids (>12 carbons) are incorporated into triglycerides and packaged with apoB-48, cholesteryl esters, retinyl esters, phospholipids and cholesterol to form chylomicrons. Nascent chylomicrons are secreted into the intestinal lymph and delivered via the thoracic duct directly to the systemic circulation, where they are extensively processed by peripheral tissues before reaching the liver. The particles encounter lipoprotein lipase (LPL), which is anchored to proteoglycans that decorate the capillary endothelial surfaces of adipose tissue, heart and skeletal muscle (Fig. 350-2). The triglycerides of chylomicrons are hydrolyzed by LPL, and free fatty acids are released. ApoC-II, which is transferred to circulating chylomicrons from HDL, acts as a cofactor for LPL in this reaction. The released free fatty acids are taken up by adjacent myocytes or adipocytes and either oxidized to generate energy or reesterified and stored as triglyceride. Some of the released free fatty acids bind albumin before entering cells and are transported to other tissues, especially the liver. The chylomicron particle progressively shrinks in size as the hydrophobic core is hydrolyzed and the hydrophilic lipids (cholesterol and phospholipids) and apolipoproteins on the particle surface are transferred to HDL, creating chylomicron remnants. Chylomicron remnants are rapidly removed from the circulation by the liver through a process that requires apoE as a ligand for receptors in the liver. Consequently, few, if any, chylomicrons or chylomicron remnants are present in the blood after a 12-h fast, except in patients with disorders of chylomicron metabolism.

TRANSPORT OF HEPATIC LIPIDS (ENDOGENOUS PATHWAY)

The endogenous pathway of lipoprotein metabolism refers to the hepatic secretion of apoB-containing lipoproteins and their metabolism (Fig. 350-2). VLDL particles resemble chylomicrons in protein composition but contain apoB-100 rather than apoB-48 and have a higher ratio of cholesterol to triglyceride (~1 mg of cholesterol for every 5 mg of triglycer-

ide). The triglycerides of VLDL are derived predominantly from the esterification of long-chain fatty acids in the liver. The packaging of hepatic triglycerides with the other major components of the nascent VLDL particle (apoB-100, cholesteryl esters, phospholipids, and vitamin E) requires the action of the enzyme microsomal triglyceride transfer protein (MTP). After secretion into the plasma, VLDL acquires multiple copies of apoE and apolipoproteins of the C series by transfer from HDL. As with chylomicrons, the triglycerides of VLDL are hydrolyzed by LPL, especially in muscle and adipose tissue. After the VLDL remnants dissociate from LPL, they are referred to as IDLs, which contain roughly similar amounts of cholesterol and triglyceride. The liver removes approximately 40–60% of IDL by LDL receptor–mediated endocytosis via binding to apoE. The remainder of IDL is remodeled by hepatic lipase (HL) to form LDL. During this process, most of the triglyceride in the particle is hydrolyzed, and all apolipoproteins except apoB-100 are transferred to other lipoproteins. The cholesterol in LDL accounts for over half of the plasma cholesterol in most individuals. Approximately 70% of circulating LDL is cleared by LDL receptor–mediated endocytosis in the liver. *Lipoprotein(a)* [Lp(a)] is a lipoprotein similar to LDL in lipid and protein composition, but it contains an additional protein called *apolipoprotein(a)* [apo(a)]. Apo(a) is synthesized in the liver and attached to apoB-100 by a disulfide linkage. The major site of clearance of Lp(a) is the liver, but the uptake pathway is not known.

TABLE 350-2 MAJOR APOLIPOPROTEINS

Apolipo-protein	Primary Source	Lipoprotein Association	Function
ApoA-I	Intestine, liver	HDL, chylomicrons	Structural protein for HDL Activates LCAT
ApoA-II	Liver	HDL, chylomicrons	Structural protein for HDL
ApoA-IV	Intestine	HDL, chylomicrons	Unknown
ApoA-V	Liver	VLDL, chylomicrons	Promotes LPL-mediated triglyceride lipolysis
ApoB-48	Intestine	Chylomicrons	Structural protein for chylomicrons
ApoB-100	Liver	VLDL, IDL, LDL, Lp(a)	Structural protein for VLDL, LDL, IDL, Lp(a) Ligand for binding to LDL receptor
ApoC-I	Liver	Chylomicrons, VLDL, HDL	Unknown
ApoC-II	Liver	Chylomicrons, VLDL, HDL	Cofactor for LPL
ApoC-III	Liver	Chylomicrons, VLDL, HDL	Inhibits lipoprotein binding to receptors
ApoD	Spleen, brain, testes, adrenals	HDL	Unknown
ApoE	Liver	Chylomicron remnants, IDL, HDL	Ligand for binding to LDL receptor
ApoH	Liver	Chylomicrons, VLDL, LDL, HDL	B₂ glycoprotein I
ApoJ	Liver	HDL	Unknown
ApoL	Unknown	HDL	Unknown
ApoM	Liver	HDL	Unknown
Apo(a)	Liver	Lp(a)	Unknown

Note: HDL, high-density lipoprotein; LCAT, lecithin-cholesterol acyltransferase; VLDL, very low density lipoprotein; IDL, intermediate-density lipoprotein; LDL, low-density lipoprotein; Lp(a), lipoprotein A; LPL, lipoprotein lipase.

Exogenous

Dietary lipids

Bile acids + cholesterol

Small intestines

LDLR

Liver

ApoC's   ApoE

ApoB

Chylomicron   Chylomicron remnant

Capillaries

LPL

FFA

Muscle   Adipose

Endogenous

LDL

Peripheral tissues

VLDL   IDL

Capillaries

LPL

FFA

Muscle   Adipose

FIGURE 350-2 The exogenous and endogenous lipoprotein metabolic pathways. The exogenous pathway transports dietary lipids to the periphery and the liver. The endogenous pathway transports hepatic lipids to the periphery. LPL, lipoprotein lipase; FFA, free fatty acid; VLDL, very low density lipoprotein; IDL, intermediate-density lipoprotein; LDL, low-density lipoprotein; LDLR, low-density lipoprotein receptor.

HDL METABOLISM AND REVERSE CHOLESTEROL TRANSPORT

All nucleated cells synthesize cholesterol, but only hepatocytes and enterocytes can effectively excrete cholesterol from the body, into either the bile or the gut lumen. In the liver, cholesterol is excreted into the bile, either directly or after conversion to bile acids. Cholesterol in peripheral cells is transported from the plasma membranes of peripheral cells to the liver and intestine by a process termed "reverse cholesterol transport" that is facilitated by HDL (**Fig. 350-3**).

Nascent HDL particles are synthesized by the intestine and the liver. Newly secreted apoA-I rapidly acquires phospholipids and unesterified cholesterol from its site of synthesis (intestine or liver) via efflux promoted by the membrane protein ATP-binding cassette protein A1 (ABCA1). This process results in the formation of discoidal HDL particles, which then recruit additional unesterified cholesterol from the periphery. Within the HDL particle, the cholesterol is esterified by lecithin-cholesterol acyltransferase (LCAT), a plasma enzyme associated with HDL, and the more hydrophobic cholesteryl ester moves to the core of the HDL particle. As HDL acquires more cholesteryl ester it becomes spherical, and additional apolipoproteins and lipids are transferred to the particles from the surfaces of chylomicrons and VLDLs during lipolysis.

HDL cholesterol is transported to hepatocytes by both an indirect and a direct pathway. HDL cholesteryl esters can be transferred to apoB-containing lipoproteins in exchange for triglyceride by the cholesteryl ester transfer protein (CETP). The cholesteryl esters are then removed from the circulation by LDL receptor–

mediated endocytosis. HDL cholesterol can also be taken up directly by hepatocytes via the scavenger receptor class BI (SR-BI), a cell surface receptor that mediates the selective transfer of lipids to cells.

HDL particles undergo extensive remodeling within the plasma compartment by a variety of lipid transfer proteins and lipases. The phospholipid transfer protein has the net effect of transferring phospholipids from other lipoproteins to HDL. After CETP-mediated lipid exchange, the triglyceride-enriched HDL becomes a much better substrate for HL, which hydrolyzes the triglycerides and phospholipids to generate smaller HDL particles. A related enzyme called *endothelial lipase* hydrolyzes HDL phospholipids, generating smaller HDL particles that are catabolized faster. Remodeling of HDL influences the metabolism, function, and plasma concentrations of HDL.

DISORDERS OF LIPOPROTEIN METABOLISM

Frederickson and Levy classified hyperlipoproteinemias according to the type of lipoprotein particles that accumulate in the blood (Type I to Type V) (**Table 350-3**). A classification scheme based on the molecular etiology and pathophysiology of the lipoprotein disorders complements this system and forms the basis for this chapter. The identification and characterization of genes responsible for the genetic forms of hyperlipidemia have provided important molecular insights into the critical roles of structural apolipoproteins, enzymes, and receptors in lipid metabolism (**Table 350-4**).

PRIMARY DISORDERS OF ELEVATED APOB-CONTAINING LIPOPROTEINS

A variety of genetic conditions are associated with the accumulation in plasma of specific classes of lipoprotein particles. In general, these can divided into those causing elevated LDL-cholesterol (LDL-C) with normal triglycerides and those causing elevated triglycerides (Table 350-4).

Macrophage

Free cholesterol

Liver

Small intestines

ApoA-I

Nascent HDL

Peripheral cells

VLDL   IDL   LDL

CETP   ApoA-I

LCAT

CETP

Chylomicrons

Mature HDL

LDLR

SR-BI

FIGURE 350-3 HDL metabolism and reverse cholesterol transport. This pathway transports excess cholesterol from the periphery back to the liver for excretion in the bile. The liver and the intestine produce nascent HDLs. Free cholesterol is acquired from macrophages and other peripheral cells and esterified by LCAT, forming mature HDLs. HDL cholesterol can be selectively taken up by the liver via SR-BI (scavenger receptor class BI). Alternatively, HDL cholesteryl ester can be transferred by CETP from HDLs to VLDLs and chylomicrons, which can then be taken up by the liver. LCAT, lecithin-cholesterol acyltransferase; CETP, cholesteryl ester transfer protein; VLDL, very low density lipoprotein; IDL, intermediate-density lipoprotein; LDL, low-density lipoprotein; HDL, high-density lipoprotein; LDLR, low-density lipoprotein receptor; TG, triglyceride.

TABLE 350-3 FREDERICKSON CLASSIFICATION OF HYPERLIPOPROTEINEMIAS

Phenotype	I	IIa	IIb	III	IV	V
Lipoprotein, elevated	Chylomicrons	LDL	LDL and VLDL	Chylomicron and VLDL remnants	VLDL	Chylomicrons and VLDL
Triglycerides	++++	--	++	++ to +++	++	++++
Cholesterol	+ to ++	+++	++ to +++	++ to +++	-- to +	++ to +++
LDL-cholesterol	↓	↑	↑	↓	↓	↓
HDL-cholesterol	+++	+	++	++	++	+++
Plasma appearance	Lactescent	Clear	Clear	Turbid	Turbid	Lactescent
Xanthomas	Eruptive	Tendon, tuberous	None	Palmar, tuberoeruptive	None	Eruptive
Pancreatitis	+++	0	0	0	0	+++
Coronary atherosclerosis	0	+++	+++	+++	+/−	+/−
Peripheral atherosclerosis	0	+	+	++	+/−	+/−
Molecular defects	LPL and apoC-II	LDL receptor, ApoB-100, PCSK9, ARH, ABCG5 and ABCG8	Unknown	ApoE	ApoA-V and Unknown	ApoA-V and Unknown
Genetic nomenclature	FCS	FH, FDB, ADH, ARH, sitosterolemia	FCHL	FDBL	FHTG	FHTG

Note: LPL, lipoprotein lipase; apo, apolipoprotein; FCS, familial chylomicronemia syndrome; FH, familial hypercholesterolemia; FDB, familial defective apoB; ARH, autosomal recessive hypercholesterolemia; ADH, autosomal dominant hypercholesterolemia; FCHL, familial combined hyperlipidemia; FDBL, familial dysbetalipoproteinemia; FHTG, familial hypertriglyceridemia

Lipid Disorders Associated with Elevated LDL-C with Normal Triglycerides • *FAMILIAL HYPERCHOLESTEROLEMIA (FH)*

FH is an autosomal codominant disorder characterized by elevated plasma levels of LDL-C with normal triglycerides, tendon xanthomas, and premature coronary atherosclerosis. FH is caused by a large number (>900) of mutations in the LDL receptor gene. It has a higher incidence in certain founder populations, such as Afrikaners, Christian Lebanese, and French Canadians. The elevated levels of LDL-C in FH are due to an increase in the production of LDL from IDL and a delayed catabolism of LDL from the blood. There is a gene dose effect, in that individuals with two mutated LDL receptor alleles (FH homozygotes) are much more affected than those with one mutant allele (FH heterozygotes).

Homozygous FH occurs in approximately 1 in 1 million persons worldwide. Patients with homozygous FH can be classified into one of two groups based on the amount of LDL receptor activity measured in their skin fibroblasts: those patients with <2% of normal LDL receptor activity (receptor negative) and those patients with 2–25% of normal LDL receptor activity (receptor defective). Most patients with homozygous FH present in childhood with cutaneous xanthomas on the hands, wrists, elbows, knees, heels, or buttocks. Total cholesterol levels are usually >500 mg/dL and can be higher than 1000 mg/dL. The devastat-ing complication of homozygous FH is accelerated atherosclerosis, which can result in disability and death in childhood. Atherosclerosis often develops first in the aortic root, where it can cause aortic valvular or supravalvular stenosis, and typically extends into the coronary ostia, which become stenotic. Children with homozygous FH often develop symptomatic coronary atherosclerosis before puberty; symptoms can be atypical, and sudden death is common. Untreated, receptor-negative patients with homozygous FH rarely survive beyond the second decade; patients with receptor-defective LDL receptor defects have a better prognosis but almost invariably develop clinically apparent atherosclerotic vascular disease by age 30, and often much sooner. Carotid and femoral disease develops later in life and is usually not clinically significant.

A careful family history should be taken, and plasma lipid levels should be measured in the parents and other first-degree relatives of patients with homozygous FH. The diagnosis of homozygous FH can be confirmed by obtaining a skin biopsy and measuring LDL receptor activity in cultured skin fibroblasts, or by quantifying the number of LDL receptors on the surfaces of lymphocytes using cell sorting technology. Molecular assays are also available to define the mutations in the LDL receptor by DNA sequencing.

Combination therapy with an HMG-CoA reductase inhibitor and a cholesterol absorption inhibitor sometimes results in relatively modest

TABLE 350-4 PRIMARY HYPERLIPOPROTEINEMIAS CAUSED BY KNOWN SINGLE GENE MUTATIONS

Genetic Disorder	Gene Defect	Lipoproteins Elevated	Clinical Findings	Genetic Transmission	Estimated Incidence
Lipoprotein lipase deficiency	LPL (*LPL*)	Chylomicrons	Eruptive xanthomas, hepatosplenomegaly, pancreatitis	AR	1/1,000,000
Familial apolipoprotein C-II deficiency	ApoC-II (*APOC2*)	Chylomicrons	Eruptive xanthomas, hepatosplenomegaly, pancreatitis	AR	<1/1,000,000
ApoA-V deficiency	ApoA-V (*APOAV*)	Chylomicrons, VLDL	Eruptive xanthomas, hepatosplenomegaly, pancreatitis	AD	<1/1,000,000
Familial hepatic lipase deficiency	Hepatic lipase (*LIPC*)	VLDL remnants	Premature atherosclerosis, pancreatitis	AR	<1/1,000,000
Familial dysbetalipoproteinemia	apoE (*APOE*)	Chylomicron and VLDL remnants	Palmar and tuberoeruptive xanthomas, CHD, PVD	AR AD	1/10,000
Familial hypercholesterolemia	LDL receptor (*LDLR*)	LDL	Tendon xanthomas, CHD	AD	1/500
Familial defective apoB-100	apoB-100 (*APOB*) (Arg$_{3500}$ → Gln)	LDL	Tendon xanthomas, CHD	AD	<1/1000
Autosomal dominant hypercholesterolemia	PCSK9 (*PCSK9*)	LDL	Tendon xanthomas, CHD	AD	<1/1,000,000
Autosomal recessive hypercholesterolemia	ARH (*ARH*)	LDL	Tendon xanthomas, CHD	AR	<1/1,000,000
Sitosterolemia	*ABCG5* or *ABCG8*	LDL	Tendon xanthomas, CHD	AR	<1/1,000,000

Note: LPL, lipoprotein lipase; LDL, low-density lipoprotein; VLDL, very low density lipoprotein; ARH, autosomal recessive hypercholesterolemia; CHD, coronary heart disease; PVD, peripheral vascular disease; AR, autosomal recessive; AD, autosomal dominant.

reductions in plasma LDL-C in the FH homozygote. Patients with homozygous FH invariably require additional lipid-lowering therapy. Since the liver is quantitatively the most important tissue for removing circulating LDLs via the LDL receptor, liver transplantation is effective in decreasing plasma LDL-C levels in this disorder. Liver transplantation, however, is associated with substantial risks, including the requirement for long-term immunosuppression. The current treatment of choice for homozygous FH is LDL apheresis (a process by which the LDL particles are selectively removed from the circulation), which can promote regression of xanthomas and may slow the progression of atherosclerosis. Initiation of LDL apheresis should generally be delayed until approximately 5 years of age, except when evidence of atherosclerotic vascular disease is present.

Heterozygous FH is caused by the inheritance of one mutant LDL receptor allele and occurs in approximately 1 in 500 persons worldwide, making it one of the most common single-gene disorders. It is characterized by elevated plasma levels of LDL-C (usually 200–400 mg/dL) and normal levels of triglyceride. Patients with heterozygous FH have hypercholesterolemia from birth, although the disease is often not detected until adulthood, usually due to the detection of hypercholesterolemia on routine screening, the appearance of tendon xanthomas, or the development of symptomatic coronary atherosclerotic disease (CAD). Since the disease is codominant in inheritance and has a high penetrance (>90%), one parent and ~50% of the patient's siblings usually also have hypercholesterolemia. The family history is frequently positive for premature CAD on one side of the family. Corneal arcus is common, and tendon xanthomas involving the dorsum of the hands, elbows, knees, and especially the Achilles tendons are present in ~75% of patients. The age of onset of CAD is highly variable and depends in part on the molecular defect in the LDL receptor gene and also on coexisting cardiac risk factors. FH heterozygotes with elevated plasma levels of Lp(a) appear to be at greater risk for cardiovascular complications. Untreated men with heterozygous FH have a ~50% chance of having a myocardial infarction before age 60. Although the age of onset of atherosclerotic heart disease is later in women with FH, coronary heart disease (CHD) is significantly more common in women with FH than in the general female population.

No definitive diagnostic test for heterozygous FH is available. Although FH heterozygotes tend to have reduced levels of LDL receptor function in skin fibroblasts, significant overlap with the LDL receptor activity levels in normal fibroblasts exists. Molecular assays have recently become available to identify the mutation in the DNA sequence, but the clinical utility of pinpointing the mutation has not been demonstrated. The clinical diagnosis is usually not problematic, but it is critical that hypothyroidism, nephrotic syndrome, and obstructive liver disease be excluded before initiating therapy.

FH patients should be aggressively treated to lower plasma levels of LDL-C. Initiation of a low-cholesterol, low-fat diet is recommended, but almost all heterozygous FH patients require lipid-lowering drug therapy. Statins are effective in heterozygous FH, but combination drug therapy with the addition of a cholesterol absorption inhibitor is frequently required, and even a third drug, such as bile acid sequestrant or nicotinic acid, is sometimes needed. Heterozygous FH patients who cannot be adequately controlled on combination drug therapy are candidates for LDL apheresis.

Familial Defective ApoB-100 (FDB) This is a dominantly inherited disorder that clinically resembles heterozygous FH. FDB is a rare cause of hypercholesterolemia, except in populations with significant numbers of individuals of German descent where the frequency can be as high as 1 in 1000. The disease is characterized by elevated plasma LDL-C levels with normal triglycerides, tendon xanthomas, and an increased incidence of premature ASCVD. FDB is caused by mutations in the LDL receptor–binding domain of apoB-100. Most patients with FDB have a substitution of glutamine for arginine at position 3500 in apoB-100, although other rarer mutations have been reported to cause this disease. As a consequence of the mutation in

apoB-100, LDL binds the LDL receptor with reduced affinity, and LDL is removed from the circulation at a reduced rate. Patients with FDB cannot be clinically distinguished from patients with heterozygous FH, although patients with FDB tend to have lower plasma levels of LDL-C than FH heterozygotes. The apoB-100 gene mutation can be detected directly, but genetic diagnosis is not currently encouraged since the recommended management of FDB and heterozygous FH is identical.

AUTOSOMAL RECESSIVE HYPERCHOLESTEROLEMIA (ARH) ARH is a rare disorder (except on Sardinia, Italy) due to mutations in a protein (ARH, also called *LDLR adaptor protein*) involved in LDL receptor–mediated endocytosis in the liver. ARH clinically resembles homozygous FH and is characterized by hypercholesterolemia, tendon xanthomas, and premature coronary artery disease. The hypercholesterolemia tends to be intermediate between the levels seen in FH homozygotes and FH heterozygotes. LDL receptor function in cultured fibroblasts is normal or only modestly reduced in ARH, whereas LDL receptor function in lymphocytes and the liver is negligible. Unlike FH homozygotes, the hyperlipidemia responds partially to treatment with HMG-CoA reductase inhibitors, but these patients usually require LDL apheresis to lower plasma LDL-C to recommended levels.

AUTOSOMAL DOMINANT HYPERCHOLESTEROLEMIA (ADH) ADH is a rare disorder caused by gain-of-function mutations in proprotein convertase subtilisin/kexin type 9 (PCSK9). Increased activity of PCSK9 appears to cause dominant hypercholesterolemia by promoting the degradation of LDL receptors in the liver, thus reducing the clearance of circulating LDL. Interestingly, loss-of-function mutations in this gene cause low LDL-C levels (see below).

SITOSTEROLEMIA This is a rare autosomal recessive disease caused by mutations in one of two members of the ATP-binding cassette (ABC) transporter family, ABCG5 and ABCG8. These genes are expressed in the intestine and liver, where they form a functional complex and pump plant sterols, such as sitosterol and campesterol, and animal sterols, predominantly cholesterol, from enterocytes into the gut lumen and from hepatocytes into the bile. In normal individuals, <5% of dietary plant sterols are absorbed by the proximal small intestine and delivered to the liver. Plant sterols that are carried to the liver on chylomicrons are preferentially secreted into the bile such that the plant sterol levels in plasma and tissues are normally very low. In sitosterolemia, the intestinal absorption of plant sterols is increased and biliary excretion of the sterols is reduced, resulting in increased plasma and tissue levels of sitosterol and other plant sterols.

The trafficking of cholesterol is also impaired in sitosterolemia. Patients with sitosterolemia usually have elevated plasma levels of LDL cholesterol. Patients develop tendon xanthomas as well as premature atherosclerosis and can be mistaken for FH patients. Episodes of hemolysis, presumably secondary to the incorporation of plant sterols into the red blood cell membrane, are a distinctive clinical feature of this disease. The hypercholesterolemia in subjects with sitosterolemia is unusually responsive to reductions in dietary cholesterol content. Sitosterolemia should be suspected in patients in whom the plasma cholesterol level falls more than 40% on a low-cholesterol diet.

Sitosterolemia is confirmed by demonstrating an increase in the plasma level of sitosterol using gas chromatography. The hypercholesterolemia does not respond to HMG-CoA reductase inhibitors; however, bile acid sequestrants and cholesterol-absorption inhibitors, such as ezetimibe, are effective in reducing plasma sterol levels in these patients.

POLYGENIC HYPERCHOLESTEROLEMIA This condition is characterized by hypercholesterolemia due to elevated LDL-C with a normal plasma level of triglyceride in the absence of secondary causes of hypercholesterolemia. Plasma LDL-C levels are generally not as elevated as they are in FH and FDB. Family studies are useful to differentiate polygenic hypercholesterolemia from the single-gene disorders described above; half of the first-degree relatives of patients with FH and FDB are hypercholesterolemic, whereas <10% of first-degree relatives of patients with polygenic hypercholesterolemia have hypercholesterolemia. Treatment of polygenic hypercholesterolemia is identical to that of other forms of hypercholesterolemia.

Lipid Disorders Associated with Elevated Triglycerides • *FAMILIAL CHYLOMICRONEMIA SYNDROME (TYPE I HYPERLIPOPROTEINEMIA; LIPOPROTEIN LIPASE AND APOC-II DEFICIENCY)*
As noted above, LPL is required for the hydrolysis of triglycerides in chylomicrons and VLDLs, and apoC-II is a cofactor for LPL (Fig. 350-2). Genetic deficiency or inactivity of either protein results in impaired lipolysis and profound elevations in plasma chylomicrons. These patients can also have elevated plasma levels of VLDL, but chylomicronemia predominates. The fasting plasma is turbid, and if left at 4°C for a few hours, the chylomicrons float to the top and form a creamy supernatant. In these disorders, called *familial chylomicronemia syndromes*, fasting triglyceride levels are almost invariably >1000 mg/dL. Fasting cholesterol levels are also usually elevated but to a much lesser degree.

LPL deficiency has autosomal recessive inheritance and has a frequency of approximately 1 in 1 million in the population. *ApoC-II deficiency* is also recessive in inheritance pattern and is even less common than LPL deficiency. Multiple different mutations in the LPL and apoC-II genes cause these diseases. Obligate LPL heterozygotes have normal or mild-to-moderate elevations in plasma triglyceride levels, whereas individuals heterozygous for mutation in apoC-II do not have hypertriglyceridemia.

Both LPL and apoC-II deficiency usually present in childhood with recurrent episodes of severe abdominal pain due to acute pancreatitis. On fundoscopic examination the retinal blood vessels are opalescent (lipemia retinalis). Eruptive xanthomas, which are small, yellowish-white papules, often appear in clusters on the back, buttocks, and extensor surfaces of the arms and legs. These typically painless skin lesions may become puritic. Hepatosplenomegaly results from the uptake of circulating chylomicrons by reticuloendothelial cells in the liver and spleen. For unknown reasons, some patients with persistent and pronounced chylomicronemia never develop pancreatitis, eruptive xanthomas, or hepatosplenomegaly. Premature ASCVD is not a generally a feature of familial chylomicronemia syndromes.

The diagnoses of LPL and apoC-II deficiency are established enzymatically in specialized laboratories by assaying triglyceride lipolytic activity in postheparin plasma. Blood is sampled after an intravenous heparin injection to release the endothelial-bound LPL. LPL activity is profoundly reduced in both LPL and apoC-II deficiency; in patients with apoC-II deficiency, it normalizes after the addition of normal plasma (providing a source of apoC-II).

The major therapeutic intervention in familial chylomicronemia syndromes is dietary fat restriction (to as little as 15 g/d) with fat-soluble vitamin supplementation. Consultation with a registered dietician familiar with this disorder is essential. Caloric supplementation with medium-chain triglycerides, which are absorbed directly into the portal circulation, can be useful but may be associated with hepatic fibrosis if used for prolonged periods. If dietary fat restriction alone is not successful in resolving the chylomicronemia, fish oils have been effective in some patients. In patients with apoC-II deficiency, apoC-II can be provided by infusing fresh frozen plasma to resolve the chylomicronemia. Management of patients with familial chylomicronemia syndrome is particularly challenging during pregnancy when VLDL production is increased and may require plasmapheresis to remove the circulating chylomicrons.

APOA-V DEFICIENCY
A newly discovered apolipoprotein called *ApoA-V* circulates at much lower concentrations than most other apolipoproteins. Individuals who are compound heterozygotes for a mutation that causes premature truncation of ApoA-V and a sequence variant associated with increased triglyceride levels have late-onset chylomicronemia. The exact mechanism of action of ApoA-V is not known, but it appears to be required for the association of VLDL and chylomicrons with LPL.

HEPATIC LIPASE DEFICIENCY
HL is a member of the same gene family as LPL and hydrolyzes triglycerides and phospholipids in remnant lipoproteins and HDLs. HL deficiency is a very rare autosomal recessive disorder characterized by elevated plasma levels of cholesterol and triglycerides (mixed hyperlipidemia) due to the accumulation of circulating lipoprotein remnants and either a normal or elevated plasma level of HDL-C. The diagnosis is confirmed by measuring HL activity in postheparin plasma. Due to the small number of patients with HL deficiency, the association of this genetic defect with ASCVD is not clearly known, but lipid-lowering therapy is recommended.

FAMILIAL DYSBETALIPOPROTEINEMIA (TYPE III HYPERLIPOPROTEINEMIA)
Like HL deficiency, familial dysbetalipoproteinemia (FDBL) (also known as *type III hyperlipoproteinemia* or *familial broad β disease*) is characterized by a mixed hyperlipidemia due to the accumulation of remnant lipoprotein particles. ApoE is present in multiple copies on chylomicron and VLDL remnants and mediates their removal via hepatic lipoprotein receptors (Fig. 350-2). FDBL is due to genetic variations in apoE that interfere with its ability to bind lipoprotein receptors. The *APOE* gene is polymorphic in sequence, resulting in the expression of three common isoforms: apoE3, which is the most common; and apoE2 and apoE4, which both differ from apoE3 by a single amino acid. Although associated with slightly higher LDL-C levels and increased CHD risk, the apoE4 allele is not associated with FDBL. Patients with apoE4 have an increased incidence of late-onset Alzheimer's disease. ApoE2 has a lower affinity for the LDL receptor; therefore, chylomicron and VLDL remnants containing apoE2 are removed from plasma at a slower rate. Individuals who are homozygous for the E2 allele (the E2/E2 genotype) comprise the most common subset of patients with FDBL.

Approximately 0.5% of the general population are apoE2/E2 homozygotes, but only a small minority of these individuals develop FDBL. In most cases an additional, identifiable factor precipitates the development of hyperlipoproteinemia. The most common precipitating factors are a high-fat diet, diabetes mellitus, obesity, hypothyroidism, renal disease, estrogen deficiency, alcohol use, or certain drugs. Other mutations in apoE can cause a dominant form of FDBL where the hyperlipidemia is fully manifest in the heterozygous state, but these mutations are rare.

Patients with FDBL usually present in adulthood with xanthomas, premature coronary disease, and peripheral vascular disease. The disease seldom presents in women before menopause. Two distinctive types of xanthomas, tuberoeruptive and palmar, are seen in FCBL patients. Tuberoeruptive xanthomas begin as clusters of small papules on the elbows, knees, or buttocks and can grow to the size of small grapes. Palmar xanthomas (alternatively called *xanthomata striata palmaris*) are orange-yellow discolorations of the creases in the palms and wrists. In FDBL, the plasma levels of cholesterol and triglyceride are often elevated to a similar degree, the directly-measured LDL-C is low, and the HDL-C is usually normal (in contrast to the low HDL-C usually seen in patients with elevated triglyceride levels).

The traditional approaches to diagnosis of this disorder are lipoprotein electrophoresis (broad β band) or ultracentrifugation (ratio of VLDL-C to total plasma triglyceride >0.30). Protein methods (apoE phenotyping) or DNA-based methods (apoE genotyping) can be performed to confirm homozygosity for apoE2. However, absence of the apoE2/2 genotype does not rule out the diagnosis of FDBL, since other mutations in apoE can cause this condition.

Since FDBL is associated with increased risk of premature ASCVD, it should be treated aggressively. Subjects with FDBL have more peripheral vascular disease than is typically seen in FH. Other metabolic conditions that can worsen the hyperlipidemia (see above) should be actively treated. Patients with FDBL are typically very diet-responsive and can respond favorably to weight reduction and to low-cholesterol, low-fat diets. Alcohol intake should be curtailed. HMG-CoA reductase inhibitors, fibrates, and niacin are all generally effective in the treatment of FDBL, and sometimes combination drug therapy is required.

FAMILIAL HYPERTRIGLYCERIDEMIA (FHTG)
FHTG is a relatively common (~1 in 500) autosomal dominant disorder of unknown etiology

characterized by moderately elevated plasma triglycerides accompanied by more modest elevations in cholesterol. Since the major class of lipoproteins elevated in this disorder is VLDL, patients with this disorder are often referred to as having *Type IV hyperlipoproteinemia* (Frederickson classification, Table 350-3). The elevated plasma levels of VLDL are due to increased production of VLDL, impaired catabolism of VLDL, or a combination of these mechanisms. Some patients with FHTG have a more severe form of hyperlipidemia in which both VLDLs and chylomicrons are elevated (Type V hyperlipidemia), since these two classes of lipoproteins compete for the same lipolytic pathway. Increased intake of simple carbohydrates, obesity, insulin resistance, alcohol use, and estrogen treatment, all of which increase VLDL synthesis, can exacerbate this syndrome. FHTG appears not to be associated with increased risk of ASCVD in many families.

The diagnosis of FHTG is suggested by the triad of elevated levels of plasma triglycerides (250–1000 mg/dL), normal or only mildly increased cholesterol levels (<250 mg/dL), and reduced plasma levels of HDL-C. Plasma LDL-C levels are generally not increased and are often reduced due to defective metabolism of the triglyceride-rich particles. The identification of other first-degree relatives with hypertriglyceridemia is useful in making the diagnosis. FDBL and familial combined hyperlipidemia (FCHL) should also be ruled out since these two conditions are associated with a significantly increased risk of ASCVD. The plasma apoB levels are lower and the ratio of plasma TG to cholesterol is higher in FHTG than in either FDBL or FCHL.

It is important to consider and rule out secondary causes of the hypertriglyceridemia (Table 350-5) before making the diagnosis of FHTG. Lipid-lowering drug therapy can frequently be avoided with appropriate dietary and lifestyle changes. Patients with plasma triglyceride levels >500 mg/dL after a trial of diet and exercise should be considered for drug therapy to avoid the development of chylomicronemia and pancreatitis. Fibrate drugs or fish oils (omega 3 fatty acids) are reasonable first-line approaches for FHTG, and niacin can also be considered in this condition.

FAMILIAL COMBINED HYPERLIPIDEMIA FCHL is generally characterized by moderate elevations in plasma levels of triglycerides (VLDL) and cholesterol (LDL) and reduced plasma levels of HDL-C. It is the most common inherited lipid disorder, occurring in approximately 1 in 200 persons. Approximately 20% of patients who develop CHD under age 60 have FCHL. The disease is autosomal dominant in inheritance, and affected family members typically have one of three possible phenotypes: (1) elevated plasma levels of LDL-C, (2) elevated plasma levels of triglycerides due to elevation in VLDL-C, or (3) elevated plasma levels of both LDL-C and VLDL-C. A classic feature of FCHL is that the lipoprotein profile can switch among these three phenotypes over time and may depend on factors such as diet. FCHL can manifest in childhood but is usually not fully expressed until adulthood. A cluster of other metabolic risk factors are often found in association with this hyperlipidemia, including obesity, glucose intolerance, insulin resistance and hypertension (the so-called metabolic syndrome, Chap. 236). These patients do not develop xanthomas.

Patients with FCHL almost always have significantly elevated plasma levels of apoB. The levels of apoB are disproportionately high relative to the plasma LDL-C concentration, indicating the presence of small, dense LDL particles, which are characteristic of this syndrome. *Hyperapobetalipoproteinemia*, which has been used to describe the state of elevated plasma levels of apoB with normal plasma LDL-C levels, is probably a form of FCHL. Individuals with FCHL generally share the same metabolic defect, which is overproduction of VLDL by the liver. The molecular etiology of FCHL remains poorly understood, and it is likely that defects in several different genes can cause the phenotype of FCHL.

The presence of a mixed dyslipidemia (plasma triglyceride levels between 200–800 mg/dL and total cholesterol levels between 200–400 mg/dL, usually with HDL-C levels <40 mg/dL in men or <50 mg/dL in women) and a family history of hyperlipidemia and/or premature CHD strongly suggests the diagnosis of FCHL. The finding of an elevated plasma level of apoB level or the finding of an increased number of small, dense LDL particles in the plasma through advanced lipoprotein testing supports this diagnosis. FDBL should be considered and ruled out by beta quantification in suspected patients with a mixed hyperlipidemia.

Individuals with FCHL should be treated aggressively due to significantly increased risk of premature CHD. Decreased dietary intake of saturated fat and simple carbohydrates, aerobic exercise, and weight loss can all have beneficial effects on the lipid profile. Patients with diabetes should be aggressively treated to maintain good glucose control. Most patients with FCHL require lipid-lowering drug therapy to reduce lipoprotein levels to the recommended range and reduce the high risk of ASCVD. Statins are effective in this condition, but many patients will need a second drug (cholesterol absorption inhibitor, niacin, or fibrate) for optimal control of lipoprotein levels.

INHERITED CAUSES OF LOW LEVELS OF APOB-CONTAINING LIPOPROTEINS

Abetalipoproteinemia The synthesis and secretion of apoB-containing lipoproteins in the enterocytes of the proximal small bowel and in

TABLE 350-5 SECONDARY FORMS OF HYPERLIPIDEMIA

LDL		HDL		VLDL	IDL	Chylomicrons	Lp(a)
Elevated	**Reduced**	**Elevated**	**Reduced**	**Elevated**	**Elevated**	**Elevated**	**Elevated**
Hypothyroidism	Severe liver disease	Alcohol	Smoking	Obesity	Multiple myeloma	Autoimmune disease	Renal insufficiency
Nephrotic syndrome	Malabsorption	Exercise	DM type 2	DM type 2	Monoclonal gammopathy	DM type 2	Inflammation
Cholestasis	Malnutrition	Exposure to chlorinated hydrocarbons	Obesity	Glycogen storage disease	Autoimmune disease		Menopause
Acute intermittent porphyria	Gaucher's disease	Drugs: estrogen	Malnutrition	Hepatitis	Hypothyroidism		Orchidectomy
Anorexia nervosa	Chronic infectious disease		Gaucher's disease	Alcohol			Hypothyroidism
Hepatoma	Hyperthyroidism		Drugs: anabolic steroids, beta blockers	Renal failure			Acromegaly
Drugs: thiazides, cyclosporin, tegretol	Drugs: niacin toxicity			Sepsis			Nephrosis
				Stress			Drugs: growth hormone, isotretinoin
				Cushing's syndrome			
				Pregnancy			
				Acromegaly			
				Lipodystrophy			
				Drugs: estrogen, beta blockers, glucocorticoids, bile acid binding resins, retinoic acid			

Note: LDL, low-density lipoprotein; HDL, high-density lipoprotein; VLDL, very low density lipoprotein; IDL, intermediate-density lipoprotein; Lp(a), lipoprotein A; DM, diabetes mellitus.

the hepatocytes of the liver involve a complex series of events that coordinate the coupling of various lipids with apoB-48 and apoB-100, respectively. Abetalipoproteinemia is a rare autosomal recessive disease caused by loss-of-function mutations in the gene encoding MTP, a protein that transfers lipids to nascent chylomicrons and VLDLs in the intestine and liver, respectively. Plasma levels of cholesterol and triglyceride are extremely low in this disorder, and chylomicrons, VLDLs, LDLs, and apoB are undetectable in plasma. The parents of patients with abetalipoproteinemia (obligate heterozygotes) have normal plasma lipid and apoB levels. Abetalipoproteinemia usually presents in early childhood with diarrhea and failure to thrive and is characterized clinically by fat malabsorption, spinocerebellar degeneration, pigmented retinopathy, and acanthocytosis. The initial neurologic manifestations are loss of deep-tendon reflexes, followed by decreased distal lower extremity vibratory and proprioceptive sense, dysmetria, ataxia, and the development of a spastic gait, often by the third or fourth decade. Patients with abetalipoproteinemia also develop a progressive pigmented retinopathy presenting with decreased night and color vision, followed by reductions in daytime visual acuity and ultimately progressing to near-blindness. The presence of spinocerebellar degeneration and pigmented retinopathy in this disease has resulted in some patients with abetalipoproteinemia being misdiagnosed as having Friedreich's ataxia. Rarely, patients with abetalipoproteinemia develop a cardiomyopathy with associated life-threatening arrhythmias.

Most clinical manifestations of abetalipoproteinemia result from defects in the absorption and transport of fat-soluble vitamins. Vitamin E and retinyl esters are normally transported from enterocytes to the liver by chylomicrons, and vitamin E is dependent on VLDL for transport out of the liver and into the circulation. As a consequence of the inability of these patients to secrete apoB-containing particles, patients with abetalipoproteinemia are markedly deficient in vitamin E and are also mildly to moderately deficient in vitamin A and vitamin K. Patients with abetalipoproteinemia should be referred to specialized centers for confirmation of the diagnosis and appropriate therapy. Treatment consists of a low-fat, high-caloric, vitamin-enriched diet accompanied by large supplemental doses of vitamin E. It is imperative that treatment be initiated as soon as possible to help forestall the development of the neurologic sequelae, which generally eventually progress even with appropriate therapy. New therapies for this serious disease are needed.

Familial Hypobetalipoproteinemia Low plasma levels of LDL-C (the "beta lipoprotein") with a genetic or inherited basis are referred to generically as *familial hypobetalipoproteinemia*. Traditionally this term has been used to refer to the condition of low total cholesterol and LDL-C due to mutations in apoB. There is a range of mostly nonsense mutations in apoB that result in the translation of a truncated protein that has reduced secretion and/or accelerated catabolism. Individuals heterozygous for these mutations usually have LDL-C levels <80 mg/dL. They may be protected from the development of atherosclerotic vascular disease, though this has not been rigorously demonstrated. Some of these patients have evidence of increased hepatic fat. There are rare patients who have mutations in both apoB alleles and have plasma lipids similar to those in abetalipoproteinemia, but usually with a less severe neurologic phenotype. Patients with homozygous hypobetalipoproteinemia can be distinguished from individuals with abetalipoproteinemia by measuring the levels of LDL-C in the parents, which will also be low.

PCSK9 Deficiency A phenocopy of familial hypobetalipoproteinemia has recently been shown to result from loss-of-function mutations in PCSK9, a protein that circulates in the blood and regulates LDL receptor levels. This condition is more common in people of African descent. Individuals bearing these mutations have lower plasma levels of LDL-C and have a substantial reduction in lifetime risk of CHD with no apparent adverse consequences. The mechanism of the low LDL-C appears to involve upregulation of the hepatic LDL receptor and thus increased catabolism of LDL.

GENETIC DISORDERS OF HDL METABOLISM

Mutations in certain genes encoding critical proteins in HDL synthesis and catabolism cause marked variations in plasma levels of HDL-C. Unlike the genetic forms of hypercholesterolemia, which are invariably associated with premature coronary atherosclerosis, genetic forms of hypoalphalipoproteinemia (low HDL-C) are not always associated with accelerated atherosclerosis.

INHERITED CAUSES OF LOW LEVELS OF HDL-C

ApoA-I Deficiency and Structural Mutations Complete genetic deficiency of apoA-I due to deletion of the apoA-I gene results in the virtual absence of HDL from the plasma. The genes encoding apoA-I, apoC-III, apoA-IV, and apoA-V are clustered together on chromosome 11, and some of the patients with complete absence of apoA-I have deletions that include more than one of these genes in the complex. ApoA-I is required for LCAT function. Thus, plasma and tissue levels of free cholesterol are increased in this disease, resulting in the development of corneal opacities and planar xanthomas. Premature CHD is generally seen in the apoA-I deficient patients.

Missense and nonsense mutations in the apoA-I gene have been identified in selected patients with low plasma HDL levels (usually 15–30 mg/dL), but these are very rare causes of low HDL-C levels in the general population. Patients heterozygous for the apoA-I$_{Milano}$ Arg173Cys substitution have very low plasma levels of HDL due to the rapid catabolism of the mutant apolipoprotein, but they do not appear to have an increased risk of premature CHD. Most individuals with low plasma HDL-C levels due to missense mutations in apoA-I do not appear to have premature CHD or other clinical sequelae, though the disorder is too rare to study systematically. A few specific missense mutations in apoA-I cause systemic amyloidosis, and the mutant apoA-I has been found as the major component of the amyloid plaque.

Tangier Disease (ABCA1 Deficiency) Tangier disease is a very rare autosomal codominant form of low plasma HDL-C caused by mutations in the gene encoding ABCA1, a cellular transporter that facilitates efflux of unesterified cholesterol and phospholipids from cells to apoA-I (Fig. 350-3). ABCA1 plays a critical role in the generation and stabilization of the mature HDL particle. In its absence, HDL is rapidly cleared from the circulation. Patients with Tangier disease have plasma HDL-C levels <5 mg/dL and extremely low circulating levels of apoA-I. The disease is associated with cholesterol accumulation in the reticuloendothelial system, resulting in hepatosplenomegaly and pathognomonic enlarged, grayish yellow or orange tonsils. An intermittent peripheral neuropathy (mononeuritis multiplex) or a sphingomyelia-like neurologic disorder can also be seen. Tangier disease is associated with increased risk of premature atherosclerotic disease, although not as great as might be anticipated, given the markedly decreased plasma levels of HDL-C and apoA-I. Patients with Tangier disease have low plasma levels of LDL-C, which may attenuate the atherosclerotic risk. Obligate heterozygotes for ABCA1 mutations have moderately reduced plasma HDL-C levels (15–30 mg/dL) and are also at increased risk of premature CHD. ABCA1 mutations may be a cause of low HDL-C in a nontrivial minority of low HDL-C patients.

LCAT Deficiency This is a very rare autosomal recessive disorder caused by mutations in the gene encoding the plasma enzyme lecithin-cholesterol acyltransferase (Fig. 350-3). LCAT is synthesized in the liver and secreted into the plasma, where it circulates associated with lipoproteins. The enzyme mediates the esterification of cholesterol. Consequently, the proportion of free cholesterol in circulating lipoproteins is greatly increased (from ~25% to over 70% of total plasma cholesterol) in this disorder. Lack of normal cholesterol esterification impairs the formation of mature HDL particles and therefore results in rapid catabolism of circulating apoA-I. Two genetic forms of LCAT deficiency have been described in humans: complete deficiency (also called *classic LCAT deficiency*) and partial deficiency (also called *fish-eye disease*). Progressive corneal opacification due to the deposition of free cholesterol in the lens, very low plasma levels of HDL-C (usually <10 mg/dL), and variable hypertriglyceridemia are characteristic of both types. In partial LCAT deficiency, there are no other known clinical sequelae. In contrast, complete LCAT deficiency is characterized by a hemolytic anemia and progressive renal insufficiency that eventually leads to end-stage renal disease (ESRD). Remarkably, despite the extremely low plasma levels of HDL-C and apoA-I, premature ASCVD is not a consistent feature of either complete or partial LCAT deficiency, once again exemplifying the complex relationship between low plasma levels of HDL-C and the development of ASCVD. The diagnosis can be confirmed in a specialized laboratory by assaying plasma LCAT activity.

Primary Hypoalphalipoproteinemia   Low plasma levels of HDL-C (the "alpha lipoprotein") is referred to as *hypoalphalipoproteinemia*. Primary hypoalphalipoproteinemia is defined as a plasma HDL-C level below the tenth percentile in the setting of relatively normal cholesterol and triglyceride levels, no apparent secondary causes of low plasma HDL-C, and no clinical signs of LCAT deficiency or Tangier disease. This syndrome is often referred to as *isolated low HDL*. A family history of low HDL-C facilitates the diagnosis of an inherited condition, which usually follows an autosomal dominant pattern. The metabolic etiology of this disease appears to be primarily accelerated catabolism of HDL and its apolipoproteins. Some of these patients may have ABCA1 mutations and therefore technically have heterozygous Tangier disease. Several kindreds with primary hypoalphalipoproteinemia have been described in association with an increased incidence of premature CHD, although this is not an invariant association. Association of hypoalphalipoproteinemia with premature CHD may depend on the specific nature of the gene defect or the underlying metabolic defect responsible for the low plasma HDL-C level.

INHERITED CAUSES OF HIGH LEVELS OF HDL-C

CETP Deficiency   Loss-of-function mutations in both alleles of the gene encoding cholesteryl ester transfer protein (CETP) cause substantially elevated HDL-C levels (usually >150 mg/dL). As noted above, CETP facilitates the transfer of cholesteryl esters from HDL to apoB-containing lipoproteins (Fig. 350-3). The absence of this transfer results in reduced catabolism of HDL and increased plasma concentrations of large, cholesterol-rich HDL particles. CETP deficiency occurs almost exclusively in persons of Japanese descent. The relationship of CETP deficiency to risk of ASCVD has not been definitively resolved and remains a matter of substantial debate. Heterozygotes for CETP deficiency have only modestly elevated HDL-C levels. Based on the phenotype of high HDL in CETP deficiency, pharmacologic inhibition of CETP is under development as a new therapeutic approach to the treatment of low HDL-C and ASCVD.

Familial Hyperalphalipoproteinemia   The condition of high plasma levels of HDL-C is referred to as *hyperalphalipoproteinemia* and is defined as a plasma HDL-C level above the 90th percentile. This trait runs in families, and outside of Japan it is unlikely to be due to CETP deficiency. Most, but not all, persons with this condition appear to have a reduced risk of CHD and increased longevity. Other than CETP deficiency, the genetic basis of primary hyperalphalipoproteinemia is not known.

SECONDARY DISORDERS OF LIPOPROTEIN METABOLISM

Significant changes in plasma levels of lipoproteins are seen in a variety of diseases. It is critical that secondary causes of hyperlipidemias (Table 350-5) are considered prior to initiation of lipid-lowering therapy.

Obesity   (See also Chaps. 74 and 75) Obesity is frequently accompanied by hyperlipidemia. The increase in adipocyte mass and accompanying decreased insulin sensitivity associated with obesity has multiple effects on lipid metabolism. More free fatty acids are delivered from the expanded adipose tissue to the liver, where they are reesterified in hepatocytes to form triglycerides, which are packaged into VLDLs for secretion into the circulation. The increased insulin levels promote fatty acid synthesis in the liver. Increased dietary intake of simple carbohydrates

also drives hepatic production of VLDLs, resulting in elevations in VLDL and/or LDL in some obese subjects. Plasma levels of HDL-C tend to be low in obesity, due in part to reduced lipolysis. Weight loss is often associated with reductions in plasma levels of circulating apoB-containing lipoproteins and increases in the plasma levels of HDL-C.

Diabetes Mellitus   (See also Chap. 338) Patients with type I diabetes mellitus generally do not have hyperlipidemia if they remain under good glycemic control. Diabetic ketoacidosis is frequently accompanied by hypertriglyceridemia due to an increased hepatic influx of free fatty acids from adipose tissue. Patients with type II diabetes mellitus are usually dyslipidemic, even when under relatively good glycemic control. The high levels of insulin and insulin resistance associated with type II diabetes has multiple effects on fat metabolism: (1) a decrease in LPL activity resulting in reduced catabolism of chylomicrons and VLDLs, (2) an increase in the release of free fatty acid from the adipose tissue, (3) an increase in fatty acid synthesis in the liver, and (4) an increase in hepatic VLDL production. Patients with type II diabetes mellitus have several lipid abnormalities, including elevated plasma triglycerides (due to increased VLDL and lipoprotein remnants), elevated levels of dense LDL, and decreased plasma levels of HDL-C. In some diabetic patients, especially those with a genetic defect in lipid metabolism, the triglycerides can be extremely elevated, resulting in the development of pancreatitis. Elevated plasma LDL-C levels usually are not a feature of diabetes mellitus and suggest the presence of an underlying lipoprotein abnormality or may indicate the development of diabetic nephropathy. Patients with lipodystrophy, who have profound insulin resistance, have markedly elevated levels of VLDL and chylomicrons.

Thyroid Disease   (See also Chap. 335) Hypothyroidism is associated with elevated plasma LDL-C levels due primarily to a reduction in hepatic LDL receptor function and delayed clearance of LDL. Conversely, plasma levels of LDL-C are often reduced in the hyperthyroid patient. Hypothyroid patients also frequently have increased levels of circulating IDLs, and some patients with hypothyroidism also have mild hypertriglyceridemia. Because hypothyroidism is easily overlooked, all patients presenting with elevated plasma levels of LDL-C or IDL should be screened for hypothyroidism. Thyroid replacement therapy usually ameliorates the hypercholesterolemia; if not, the patient probably has a primary lipoprotein disorder and may require lipid-lowering drug therapy.

Renal Disorders   (See also Chap. 274) Nephrotic syndrome is often associated with pronounced hyperlipoproteinemia, which is usually mixed but can manifest as hypercholesterolemia or hypertriglyceridemia. The hyperlipidemia of nephrotic syndrome appears to be due to a combination of increased hepatic production and decreased clearance of VLDLs, with increased LDL production. Effective treatment of the underlying renal disease normalizes the lipid profile, but most patients with chronic nephrotic syndrome require lipid-lowering drug therapy.

ESRD is often associated with mild hypertriglyceridemia (<300 mg/dL) due to the accumulation of VLDLs and remnant lipoproteins in the circulation. Triglyceride lipolysis and remnant clearance are both reduced in patients with renal failure. Because the risk of ASCVD is increased in ESRD subjects with hyperlipidemia, they should be aggressively treated with lipid-lowering agents.

Patients with renal transplants usually have increased lipid levels due to the effect of the drugs required for immunosuppression (cyclosporine and glucocorticoids) and present a difficult management problem since HMG-CoA reductase inhibitors must be used cautiously in these patients.

Liver Disorders   (See also Chap. 295) Because the liver is the principal site of formation and clearance of lipoproteins, it is not surprising that liver diseases can profoundly affect plasma lipid levels in a variety of ways. Hepatitis due to infection, drugs, or alcohol is often associated with increased VLDL synthesis and mild to moderate hypertriglyceridemia. Severe hepatitis and liver failure are associated with dramatic reductions in plasma cholesterol and triglycerides due to reduced lipoprotein biosynthetic capacity. Cholestasis is associated with hypercholesterolemia, which can be very severe. A major pathway by which cholesterol is excreted from the body is via secretion into bile, either directly or after conversion to bile acids, and cholestasis blocks this critical excretory pathway. In cholestasis, free cholesterol, coupled with phospholipids, is secreted into the plasma as a constituent of a lamellar particle called *LP-X*. The particles can deposit in skin folds, producing lesions resembling those seen in patients with FDBL (xanthomata strata palmaris). Planar and eruptive xanthomas can also be seen in patients with cholestasis.

Alcohol   Regular alcohol consumption has a variable effect on plasma lipid levels. The most common effect of alcohol is to increase plasma triglyceride levels. Alcohol consumption stimulates hepatic secretion of VLDLs, possibly by inhibiting the hepatic oxidation of free fatty acids, which then promote hepatic triglyceride synthesis and VLDL secretion. The usual lipoprotein pattern seen with alcohol consumption is Type IV (increased VLDLs), but persons with an underlying primary lipid disorder may develop severe hypertriglyceridemia (Type V) if they drink alcohol. Regular alcohol use also raises plasma levels of HDL-C.

Estrogen   Estrogen administration is associated with increased VLDL and HDL synthesis, resulting in elevated plasma levels of both triglycerides and HDL-C. This lipoprotein pattern is distinctive since the levels of plasma triglyceride and HDL-C are typically inversely related. Plasma triglyceride levels should be monitored when birth control pills or postmenopausal estrogen therapy is initiated to ensure that the increase in VLDL production does not lead to severe hypertriglyceridemia. Use of low-dose preparations of estrogen or the estrogen patch can minimize the effect of exogenous estrogen on lipids.

Lysosomal Storage Diseases   (See also Chap. 355) Cholesteryl ester storage disease (due to deficiency in lysosomal acid lipase) and glycogen storage diseases such as von Gierke's disease (caused by mutations in glucose-6-phosphatase) are rare causes of secondary hyperlipidemias.

Cushing's Syndrome   (See also Chap. 336) Glucocorticoid excess is associated with increased VLDL synthesis and hypertriglyceridemia. Patients with Cushing's syndrome can also have mild elevations in plasma levels of LDL-C.

Drugs   Many drugs have an impact on lipid metabolism and can result in significant alterations in the lipoprotein profile (Table 350-5).

SCREENING

(See also Chaps. 218 and 236) Guidelines for the screening and management of lipid disorders have been provided by an expert Adult Treatment Panel (ATP) convened by the National Cholesterol Education Program (NCEP) of the National Heart Lung and Blood Institute. The NCEP ATPIII guidelines published in 2001 recommend that all adults over age 20 should have plasma levels of cholesterol, triglyceride, LDL-C, and HDL-C measured after a 12-hour overnight fast. In most clinical laboratories, the total cholesterol and triglycerides in the plasma are measured enzymatically, and then the cholesterol in the supernatant is measured after precipitation of apoB-containing lipoproteins to determine the HDL-C. The LDL-C is estimated using the following equation:

$$LDL\text{-}C = total\ cholesterol - (triglycerides/5) - HDL\text{-}C.$$

(The VLDL-C is estimated by dividing the plasma triglyceride by 5, reflecting the ratio of cholesterol to triglyceride in VLDL particles.) This formula is reasonably accurate if test results are obtained on fasting plasma and if the triglyceride level does not exceed ~300 mg/dL; by convention it cannot be used if the TGs are >400 mg/dL. The accurate determination of LDL-C levels in patients with triglyceride levels >300 mg/dL requires application of ultracentrifugation techniques or other direct assays for LDL-C. Further evaluation and treatment is based primarily on the plasma LDL-C level and the assessment of overall cardiovascular risk.

DIAGNOSIS

The critical first step in managing a lipid disorder is to determine the class or classes of lipoproteins that are increased or decreased in the patient. The Frederickson classification scheme for hyperlipoproteinemias (Table 350-3), though less commonly used now than in the past, can be helpful in this regard. Once the hyperlipidemia is accurately classified, efforts should be directed to rule out any possible secondary causes of the hyperlipidemia (Table 350-5). Although many patients with hyperlipidemia have a primary or genetic cause of their lipid disorder, secondary factors frequently contribute to the hyperlipidemia. A fasting glucose should be obtained in the initial work-up of all subjects with an elevated triglyceride level. Nephrotic syndrome and chronic renal insufficiency should be excluded by obtaining urine protein and serum creatinine. Liver function tests should be performed to rule out hepatitis and cholestasis. Hypothyroidism should be ruled out by measuring serum TSH. Patients with hyperlipidemia, especially hypertriglyceridemia, who drink alcohol or are obese should be encouraged to decrease their intake. Sedentary lifestyle, obesity, and smoking are all associated with low HDL-C levels, and patients should be counseled about these issues.

Once secondary causes for the elevated lipoprotein levels have been ruled out, attempts should be made to diagnose the primary lipid disorder since the underlying etiology has a significant effect on the risk of developing CHD, on the response to drug therapy, and on the management of other family members. Often, determining the correct diagnosis requires a detailed family medical history and, in some cases, lipid analyses in family members.

If the fasting plasma triglyceride level is >1000 mg/dL, the patient almost always has chylomicronemia and either has Type I or Type V hyperlipoproteinemia (Table 350-3). The plasma triglyceride to cholesterol ratio helps distinguish between these two possibilities and is higher in Type I than Type V hyperlipoproteinemia. If the patient has Type I hyperlipoproteinemia, a postheparin lipolytic assay should be performed to determine if the patient has LPL or apoC-II deficiency. Type V is a much more frequent form of chylomicronemia in the adult patient. Often treatment of secondary factors contributing to the hyperlipidemia (diet, obesity, glucose intolerance, alcohol ingestion, estrogen therapy) will change a Type V into a Type IV pattern, reducing the risk of developing acute pancreatitis.

If the levels of LDL-C are very high (>95th percentile), it is likely the patient has a genetic form of hyperlipidemia. The presence of severe hypercholesterolemia, tendon xanthomas, and an autosomal dominant pattern of inheritance are consistent with the diagnosis of either FH, FDB, or ADH due to mutations in PCSK9. At the present time there is no compelling reason to perform molecular studies to further refine the molecular diagnosis, since the treatment of FH and FDB is identical. Patients with more moderate hypercholesterolemia that does not segregate in families as a monogenic trait likely have polygenic hypercholesterolemia. Recessive forms of severe hypercholesterolemia are rare; a clue to the diagnosis of sitosterolemia is the response of the hypercholesterolemia to reductions in dietary cholesterol content and to bile acid resins.

The most common error in the diagnosis and treatment of lipid disorders is in patients with a mixed hyperlipidemia without chylomicronemia. Elevations in the plasma levels of both cholesterol and triglycerides are seen in patients with increased plasma levels of IDL (Type III) and of LDL and VLDL (Type IIB) and in patients with increased levels of VLDL (Type IV). The ratio of triglyceride to cholesterol is higher in Type IV than the other two disorders. A beta quantification to determine the VLDL-C to triglyceride ratio in plasma (see discussion of FDBL) or a direct measurement of the plasma LDL-C should be performed at least once prior to initiation of lipid-lowering therapy to determine if the hyperlipidemia is due to the accumulation of remnants or to an increase in both LDL and VLDL.

℞ LIPOPROTEIN DISORDERS

CLINICAL EVIDENCE THAT TREATMENT OF DYSLIPIDEMIA REDUCES RISK OF CHD Multiple epidemiologic studies have demonstrated a strong relationship between serum cholesterol and CHD. A direct connection between plasma cholesterol levels and the atherosclerotic process was made in humans when aortic fatty streaks in young persons were shown to be strongly correlated with serum cholesterol levels. The elucidation of homozygous familial hypercholesterolemia was proof that high cholesterol itself caused atherosclerotic vascular disease. Moreover, PCSK9 deficiency proves that very low LDL-C levels are associated with substantial lifetime reduction in cardiovascular risk.

LDL-C Reduction Early clinical trials of cholesterol (mostly LDL-C) reduction utilized niacin, bile acid sequestrants, and even the surgical approach of partial ileal bypass to reduce serum cholesterol levels. Although most of these studies found a small but significant reduction in cardiac events, no decrease in total mortality was seen, which tempered enthusiasm for aggressive, population-based treatment of hypercholesterolemia. The discovery of more potent and well-tolerated cholesterol-lowering agents, namely HMG-CoA reductase inhibitors (statins), ushered in a series of large cholesterol reduction trials that unequivocally established the benefit of cholesterol reduction. Some of these trials were performed in patients with preexisting stable CHD. The Scandinavian Simvastatin Survival Study in hypercholesterolemic men with CHD showed reduced major coronary events by 44% and total mortality by 30% with simvastatin. The Cholesterol and Recurrent Events (CARE) study and the Long-Term Intervention with Pravastatin in Ischemic Heart Disease (LIPID) study demonstrated reduced cardiac events and cardiovascular deaths in women and men with established CHD and normal to only mildly elevated LDL-C levels. Some of the early statin trials were in individuals without preexisting CHD. In the West of Scotland Coronary Prevention Study (WOSCOPS) with pravastatin, subjects had significantly elevated baseline LDL-C levels, whereas in the Air Force/Texas Coronary Atherosclerosis Study (AFCAPS/TexCAPS) with lovastatin, baseline LDL-C levels were only modestly elevated. Both trials demonstrated significant reductions in cardiovascular events and clearly established that drug therapy for hypercholesterolemia is an effective method of decreasing risk of cardiovascular events even in persons who do not have preexisting symptomatic CHD.

More recent studies have enrolled subjects with average or subaverage LDL-C levels and have involved targeting the on-treatment LDL-C to ever lower levels. The Heart Protection Study (HPS) included 20,536 men and women, ages 40–80 years, who had either established ASCVD or were at high risk for the development of CHD (primarily diabetes); the only lipid entry criterion was a total plasma cholesterol level of >135 mg/dL. Treatment with simvastatin for an average of 5 years resulted in a 24% reduction in major coronary events and a highly significant 13% reduction in all-cause mortality. Importantly, the relative benefit of statin therapy was similar across tertiles of baseline LDL-C, and even the large subgroup of individuals with an LDL-C <100 mg/dL at baseline experienced significant benefit from therapy. This study demonstrated that statin therapy is beneficial in high-risk subjects, even if the baseline LDL-C level is below the currently recommended targeted goal; it also helped to shift the emphasis from simply treating elevated cholesterol to treating patients at high risk of CHD.

The Anglo-Scandinavian Cardiac Outcomes Trial Lipid-Lowering Arm (ASCOT-LLA) involved 19,342 hypertensive patients with at least three other cardiovascular risk factors and with total cholesterol levels <242 mg/dL. The lipid-lowering arm involved the intervention of atorvastatin 10 mg vs. placebo, and was terminated after 3.3 years due to a highly significant 36% relative risk reduction in major cardiovascular events. In the Collaborative Atorvastatin Diabetes Study (CARDS), 2838 patients with type 2 diabetes were randomized to atorvastatin 10 mg or placebo and was also terminated early due to a significant 37% reduction in major cardiovascular events. Both of these studies involved on-treatment LDL-C levels well below recommended targets for the patients, but still involved comparison to placebo.

The most compelling data supporting the concept that "lower is better" come from studies in which different statin regimens were directly compared. In the Treat to New Targets (TNT) trial, 10,001 patients with CHD and LDL-C <130 mg/dL were randomized to atorvastatin 80 mg vs 10 mg daily. Atorvastatin 80 mg was associated with a significant 22% reduction in major cardio-

vascular events and a mean on-treatment LDL-C level of 77 mg/dL (compared with 101 mg/dL for the 10 mg dose). In the Pravastatin or Atorvastatin Evaluation and Infection Therapy (PROVE-IT) study, patients presenting with acute coronary syndromes were randomized to atorvastatin 80 mg (more intensive) or pravastatin 40 mg (less intensive). Atorvastatin 80 mg was associated with a significant 16% relative risk reduction in major cardiovascular events compared with the less-intensive pravastatin 40 mg regimen. The mean on-treatment LDL-C levels were 62 mg/dL in the atorvastatin 80 mg group and 95 mg/dL in the pravastatin 40 mg group. Based on several of these studies, a white paper was issued by the NCEP in 2004 establishing an "optional" LDL-C goal of <70 mg/dL in high-risk patients with CHD and of <100 mg/dL in very-high-risk patients without known CHD. These optional targets have been widely embraced, and clinical practice is clearly evolving to treating CHD and high-risk patients more aggressively for LDL reduction.

Treatment of the TG-HDL Axis Abnormalities of the TG-high-density lipoprotein (TG-HDL) axis are more common in patients with CHD or at risk for it than is elevated LDL-C. Yet the data supporting pharmacologic intervention in the TG-HDL axis is less abundant and compelling than the data supporting LDL-C reduction. Fibric acid derivatives (fibrates), nicotinic acid (niacin), and omega 3 fatty acids (fish oils) are the primary agents currently available for intervention regarding the TG-HDL axis. Fibrates have been used as lipid-lowering drugs for several decades and are more effective in reducing plasma TG levels and relatively less effective in increasing plasma HDL-C levels. The overall body of data with fibrates regarding cardiovascular outcomes trends is positive but mixed. The Helsinki Heart Study (HHS) compared gemfibrozil to placebo in hypercholesterolemic patients with no CHD and demonstrated a significant 36% reduction in coronary events. The Veteran Affairs High-Density Lipoprotein Cholesterol Intervention Trial (VA-HIT) examined the benefit of gemfibrozil in men with CHD, normal plasma levels of LDL-C levels, and low plasma levels of HDL-C levels and demonstrated a significant 22% reduction in nonfatal myocardial infarction and coronary death with gemfibrozil therapy. However, the Bezafibrate Infarction Prevention (BIP) trial of bezafibrate vs placebo in CHD patients with low HDL-C failed to demonstrate a statistically significant reduction in coronary events, though there was a positive trend. Similarly, the Fenofibrate Intervention and Event Lowering in Diabetes (FIELD) trial of fenofibrate in 9795 patients with type 2 diabetes also failed to show a significant reduction in its primary endpoint of nonfatal myocardial infarction and coronary death, though there was a positive trend (11% relative risk reduction) and significant reductions in total cardiovascular disease events. There was significantly greater "drop-in" of the placebo group into lipid-lowering therapy, mostly statins, making the interpretation complicated. Nevertheless, the overall body of data with fibrates and CVD risk reduction is mixed. Interestingly, despite the fact that fibrates are most effective in lowering triglycerides, no fibrate trial has ever been performed specifically in subjects with hypertriglyceridemia subjects; in addition, the benefit of the addition of a fibrate to baseline statin therapy has never been tested.

While niacin is the most effective HDL-raising drug currently available, it has never been tested for its ability to reduce cardiovascular risk in a trial in subjects with low HDL-C patients. The Coronary Drug Project showed that niacin modestly reduced cardiovascular events, but this was performed in hypercholesterolemic men with CHD. The AIM-HIGH trial is an ongoing study of the effect of niacin added to baseline statin therapy in patients with CHD and low HDL-C. Finally, while low-dose fish oils have been shown to reduce cardiovascular events, higher doses that reduce triglyceride levels have not been tested for their ability to reduce cardiovascular events. Definitive proof that treating the TG-HDL axis reduces cardiovascular events is likely to come from new therapies that are more effective in targeting these abnormalities.

LIPID-MODIFYING THERAPY The major goal of lipid-modifying therapy in most patients with disorders of lipid metabolism is to prevent ASCVD and its complications. Management of lipid disorders should be based on clinical trial data demonstrating that treatment reduces cardiovascular morbidity and mortality, although reasonable extrapolation of these data to specific subgroups is sometimes required. Clearly, elevated plasma levels of LDL-C are strongly associated with increased risk of ASCVD and treatment to lower the levels of plasma LDL-C decreases risk of clinical cardiovascular events in both secondary and primary prevention. Although the proportional benefit accrued from reducing plasma LDL-C appears to be similar over the entire range of LDL-C values, the absolute risk reduction depends on the baseline level of cardiovascular risk. The treatment guidelines developed by NCEP ATPIII incorporate these principles. As noted above, abnormalities in the TG-HDL axis (elevated TG, low HDL-C, or both) are commonly seen in patients with CHD or at high risk for developing it, but clinical trial data supporting the treatment of these abnormalities is much less compelling, and the pharmacologic tools for their management are more limited. Importantly, the NCEP ATPIII guidelines promote the use of the "non-HDL-C" as a secondary target of therapy in patients with TG levels >200 mg/dL. The goals for non-HDL-C are 30 mg/dL higher than the goals for LDL-C. Thus, many patients with abnormalities of the TG-HDL axis require additional therapy for reduction of non-HDL-C to recommended goals.

NONPHARMACOLOGIC TREATMENT

Diet Dietary modification is an important component in the management of dyslipidemia. The physician should assess the content of the patient's diet and provide suggestions for dietary modifications. In the patient with elevated LDL-C, dietary saturated fat and cholesterol should be restricted. For individuals with hypertriglyceridemia, the intake of simple carbohydrates should be curtailed. For severe hypertriglyceridemia (>1000 mg/dL), restriction of total fat intake is critical. The most widely used diet to lower the LDL-C level is the "Step I diet" developed by the American Heart Association. Most patients have a relatively modest (<10%) decrease in plasma levels of LDL-C on a step I diet in the absence of any associated weight loss. Almost all persons experience a decrease in plasma HDL-C levels with a reduction in the amount of total and saturated fat in their diet.

Foods and Additives Certain foods and dietary additives are associated with modest reductions in plasma cholesterol levels. Plant stanol and sterol esters are available in a variety of foods such as spreads, salad dressings, and snack bars. Plant sterol and sterol esters interfere with cholesterol absorption and reduce plasma LDL-C levels by ~10% when taken three times per day. The addition to the diet of psyllium, soy protein, or Chinese red yeast rice (which contains lovastatin) can have modest cholesterol-lowering effects. Other herbal approaches such as guggulipid have not been shown to reduce LDL-C. No controlled studies have been performed in which several of these nonpharmacologic options have been combined to address their additive or synergistic effects.

Weight Loss and Exercise The treatment of obesity, if present, can have a favorable impact on plasma lipid levels and should be actively encouraged. Plasma triglyceride levels tend to fall and HDL-C levels tend to increase in obese subjects after weight reduction. Regular aerobic exercise can also have a positive effect on lipids, in large measure due to the associated weight reduction. Aerobic exercise has a very modest elevating effect on plasma levels of HDL-C in most individuals but also has cardiovascular benefits that extend beyond the effects on plasma lipid levels.

PHARMACOLOGIC TREATMENT

The decision to use drug therapy depends on the level of cardiovascular risk. Drug therapy for hypercholesterolemia in patients with established CHD is well supported by clinical trial data, as reviewed above. Even patients with CHD or risk factors who have "average" LDL-C levels benefit from treatment. Drug treatment to lower LDL-C levels in patients with CHD is also highly cost-effective. Patients with diabetes mellitus without known CHD have similar cardiovascular risk to those without diabetes but with preexisting CHD. An effective way to estimate absolute risk of a cardiovascular event over 10 years is to use a scoring system based on the Framingham Heart Study database. Patients with a 10-year absolute CHD risk of >20% are considered "CHD risk equivalents." Current NCEP ATPIII guidelines call for drug therapy to reduce LDL-C to <100 mg/dL in patients with established CHD, other ASCVD (aortic aneurysm, peripheral vascular disease, or cerebrovascular disease), diabetes mellitus, or CHD risk equivalents; and "optionally" to reduce LDL-C to <70 mg/dL in high-risk CHD patients. Based on these guidelines, virtually all CHD and CHD risk-equivalent patients require cholesterol-lowering drug therapy. Moderate risk patients with two or more risk factors and a 10-year absolute risk of 10–20% should be treated to a goal LDL-C of <130 mg/dL or "optionally" to LDL-C <100 mg/dL.

Persons with markedly elevated plasma levels of LDL-C levels (>190 mg/dL) should be strongly considered for drug therapy even if their 10-year absolute CHD risk is not particularly elevated. The decision of whether to initiate drug treatment in individuals with plasma LDL-C levels between 130 and 190 mg/dL can be difficult. Although it is desirable to avoid drug treatment in patients who are unlikely to develop CHD, a very high proportion of patients who eventually develop CHD have plasma LDL-C levels that are in this range. Other clinical information can assist in the decision-making process. For example, a low plasma level of HDL-C (<40 mg/dL) supports a decision in favor of more aggressive therapy. Diagnosis of the metabolic syndrome also identifies a higher-risk individual who should be targeted for therapeutic lifestyle changes and might be a candidate for more aggressive drug therapy (Chap. 236). Other laboratory tests, such as an elevated plasma level of apoB, Lp(a) or high-sensitivity C-reactive protein, may help to identify additional high-risk individuals who should be considered for drug therapy when their LDL-C is in a "gray zone."

Drug treatment is also indicated in patients with triglycerides >1000 mg/dL who have been screened and treated for secondary causes of chylomicronemia. The goal is to reduce plasma triglycerides to below 500 mg/dL to prevent the risk of acute pancreatitis. When triglycerides are 500–1000 mg/dL, the decision to use drug therapy depends on the assessment of cardiovascular risk. Most major clinical endpoint trials with statins have excluded persons with triglyceride levels >350–450 mg/dL, and there are therefore few data regarding the effectiveness of statins in reducing cardiovascular risk in persons with triglycerides higher than this threshold. More data are needed regarding the relative effectiveness of statins, fibrates, niacin, and fish oils for reducing cardiovascular risk in this setting. Combination therapy is often required for optimal control of mixed dyslipidemia.

HMG-CoA Reductase Inhibitors (Statins) HMG-CoA reductase is the rate-limiting step in cholesterol biosynthesis, and inhibition of this enzyme decreases cholesterol synthesis. By inhibiting cholesterol biosynthesis, statins lead to increased hepatic LDL receptor activity and accelerated clearance of circulating LDL, resulting in a dose-dependent reduction in plasma levels of LDL-C. There is wide interindividual variation in the initial response to a statin, but once a patient is on a statin, the doubling of the statin dose produces a 6% further reduction in the level of plasma LDL-C. The statins currently available differ in their LDL-C reducing effects (**Table 350-6**). Statins also reduce plasma triglycerides in a dose-dependent fashion, which is proportional to their LDL-C lowering effects (if the triglycerides are <400 mg/dL). Statins have a modest HDL-raising effect (5–10%), and this effect is not dose-dependent.

Statins are well tolerated and can be taken in tablet form once a day. Potential side effects include dyspepsia, headaches, fatigue, and muscle or joint pains. Severe myopathy and even rhabdomyolysis occur rarely with statin treatment. The risk of statin-associated myopathy is increased by the presence of older age, frailty, renal insufficiency, and coadministration of drugs that interfere with the metabolism of statins, such as erythromycin and related antibiotics, antifungal agents, immunosuppressive drugs, and fibric acid derivatives (particularly gemfibrozil). Severe myopathy can usually be avoided by careful patient selection, avoidance of interacting drugs, and instructing the patient to contact the physician immediately in the event of unexplained muscle pain. In the event of muscle symptoms, the plasma creatine kinase (CK) level should be obtained to document the myopathy. Serum CK levels need not be monitored on a routine basis in patients taking statins, as an elevated CK in the absence of symptoms does not predict the development of myopathy and does not necessarily suggest the need for discontinuing the drug.

Another consequence of statin therapy can be elevation in liver transaminases (ALT and AST). They should be checked before starting therapy, at 2–3 months, and then annually. Substantial (greater than three times upper limit of normal) elevation in transaminases is relatively rare and mild to moderate (one to three times normal) elevation in transaminases in the absence of symptoms need not mandate discontinuing the medication. Severe clinical hepatitis associated with statins is exceedingly rare, and the trend is toward less frequent monitoring of transaminases in patients taking statins. The statin-associated elevation in liver enzymes resolves upon discontinuation of the medication.

Statins appear to be remarkably safe. Meta-analyses of large randomized controlled clinical trials with statins do not suggest an increase in any major noncardiac diseases. Statins are the drug class of choice for LDL-C reduction and are by far the most widely used class of lipid-lowering drugs.

Cholesterol Absorption Inhibitors Cholesterol within the lumen of the small intestine is derived from the diet (about one-third) and the bile (about two-thirds) and is actively absorbed by the enterocyte through a process that involves the protein NPC1L1. Ezetimibe (Table 350-6) is a cholesterol absorption inhibitor that binds directly to and inhibits NPC1L1 and blocks the intestinal absorption of cholesterol. In humans, ezetimibe at a dose of 10 mg was shown to inhibit cholesterol absorption by almost 60%. The result of inhibition of intestinal cholesterol absorption is likely to be reduction in hepatic cholesterol and an increase hepatic LDL receptor expression. The mean reduction in plasma LDL-C on ezetimibe (10 mg) is 18%, and the effect is additive when used in combination with a statin. Effects on TG and HDL-C levels are negligible, and no cardiovascular out-

TABLE 350-6 SUMMARY OF THE MAJOR DRUGS USED FOR THE TREATMENT OF HYPERLIPIDEMIA

Drug	Major Indications	Starting Dose	Maximal Dose	Mechanism	Common Side Effects
HMG-CoA reductase inhibitors (statins)	Elevated LDL-C			↓ Cholesterol synthesis, ↑ hepatic LDL receptors, ↓ VLDL production	Myalgias, arthralgias, elevated transaminases, dyspepsia
Lovastatin		20 mg daily	80 mg daily		
Pravastatin		40 mg qhs	80 mg qhs		
Simvastatin		20 mg qhs	80 mg qhs		
Fluvastatin		20 mg qhs	80 mg qhs		
Atorvastatin		10 mg qhs	80 mg qhs		
Rosuvastatin		10 mg qhs	40 mg qhs		
Cholesterol absorption inhibitors				↓ Intestinal cholesterol absorption	Elevated transaminases
Ezetimibe	Elevated LDL-C	10 mg daily	10 mg daily		
Bile acid sequestrants	Elevated LDL-C			↑ Bile acid excretion and ↑ LDL receptors	Bloating, constipation, elevated triglycerides
Cholestyramine		4 g daily	32 g daily		
Colestipol		5 g daily	40 g daily		
Colesevelam		3750 mg daily	4375 mg daily		
Nicotinic acid	Elevated LDL-C, low HDL-C, elevated TG			↓ VLDL hepatic synthesis	Cutaneous flushing, GI upset, elevated glucose, uric acid, and liver function tests
Immediate-release		100 mg tid	1 g tid		
Sustained-release		250 mg bid	1.5 g bid		
Extended-release		500 mg qhs	2 g qhs		
Fibric acid derivatives	Elevated TG, elevated remnants			↑ LPL, ↓ VLDL synthesis	Dyspepsia, myalgia, gallstones, elevated transaminases
Gemfibrozil		600 mg bid	600 mg bid		
Fenofibrate		145 mg qd	145 mg qd		
Omega 3 fatty acids	Elevated TG	3 g daily	6 g daily	↑ TG catabolism	Dyspepsia, diarrhea, fishy odor to breath

Note: LDL, low-density lipoprotein; VLDL, very low density lipoprotein; HDL, high-density lipoprotein; LDL-C, LDL-cholesterol; HDL-C, HDI-C, cholesterol; TG, triglyceride; LPL, lipoprotein lipase; GI, gastrointestinal.

come data have been reported. When used in combination with a statin, monitoring of liver transaminases is recommended. Ezetimibe has become the preferred drug to add to a statin in patients who require further LDL-C reduction and is also widely used in patients who are statin-intolerant.

Bile Acid Sequestrants (Resins) Bile acid sequestrants bind bile acids in the intestine and promote their excretion in the stool. To maintain the bile acid pool size, the liver diverts cholesterol to bile acid synthesis. The decreased hepatic intracellular cholesterol content results in upregulation of the LDL receptor and enhanced LDL clearance from the plasma. Bile acid sequestrants, including cholestyramine, colestipol, and colesevelam (Table 350-6), primarily reduce plasma LDL-C levels and can cause an increase in plasma triglycerides. Therefore, patients with hypertriglyceridemia should not be treated with bile acid binding resins. Cholestyramine and colestipol are insoluble resins that must be suspended in liquids. Colesevelam is available as tablets but generally requires up to six to seven tablets per day for effective LDL-C lowering. Most side effects of resins are limited to the gastrointestinal tract and include bloating and constipation. Since bile acid sequestrants are not systemically absorbed, they are very safe and the cholesterol-lowering drug of choice in children and in women of childbearing age who are lactating, pregnant, or could become pregnant. They are effective in combination with statins as well as in combination with ezetimibe and are particularly useful with one or both of these drugs for difficult-to-treat patients or those with statin intolerance.

Nicotinic Acid (Niacin) Nicotinic acid, or niacin, is a B-complex vitamin that has been used as a lipid-modifying agent for decades. It was previously shown to reduce the flux of nonesterified fatty acids (NEFAs) to the liver, resulting in reduced hepatic TG synthesis and VLDL secretion. Recently a receptor for nicotinic acid called GPR109A was discovered; it is expressed in adipocytes and, when activated, suppresses the release of NEFA by adipose. Niacin reduces plasma triglyceride and LDL-C levels and raises the plasma concentration of HDL-C (Table 350-6). Niacin is also the only currently available lipid-lowering drug that significantly reduces plasma levels of Lp(a). If properly prescribed and monitored, niacin is a safe and effective lipid-lowering agent.

The most frequent side effect of niacin is cutaneous flushing, which is mediated by activation of the same receptor GPR109A in the skin, leading to local generation of prostaglandin D2 production. Flushing can be reduced by formulations that slow the absorption and by taking aspirin prior to dosing. In addition, there is tachyphylaxis to the flushing. Niacin therapy is generally started at lower doses and titrated over time. Immediate-release crystalline niacin is generally administered three times per day, over-the-counter sustained-release niacin is taken twice a day, and a prescription form of extended release niacin is taken once a day. Mild elevations in transaminases occur in up

to 15% of patients treated with any form of niacin, but these elevations may require stopping the medication. Niacin potentiates the effect of warfarin, and these two drugs should be prescribed together with caution. Acanthosis nigricans, a dark-colored coarse skin lesion, and maculopathy are infrequent side effects of niacin. Niacin is contraindicated in patients with peptic ulcer disease and can exacerbate the symptoms of esophageal reflux. It can also raise plasma levels of uric acid and precipitate gouty attacks in susceptible patients.

Niacin can raise fasting plasma glucose levels. However, in one study in type 2 diabetics, niacin treatment was associated with only a slight increase in fasting glucose and no significant change from baseline in the HbA1c. In another, low-dose niacin was found to effectively reduce triglycerides and raise HDL-C without adversely impacting on glycemic control. Thus, niacin can be used in diabetic patients, but every effort should be made to optimize the diabetes management before initiating niacin, and glucose should be carefully monitored in nondiabetic patients with impaired fasting glucose after initiation of niacin therapy.

Successful therapy with niacin requires careful education and motivation on the part of the patient. Its advantages are its low cost and long-term safety. It is the most effective drug currently available for raising HDL-C levels. It is particularly useful in patients with combined hyperlipidemia and low plasma levels of HDL-C and is effective in combination with statins.

Fibric Acid Derivatives (Fibrates) Fibric acid derivatives are agonists of PPARα, a nuclear receptor involved in the regulation of carbohydrate and lipid metabolism. Fibrates stimulate LPL activity (enhancing triglyceride hydrolysis), reduce apoC-III synthesis (enhancing lipoprotein remnant clearance), and may reduce VLDL production. Fibrates are the most effective drugs available for reducing triglyceride levels and also raise HDL-C levels modestly (Table 350-6). They have variable effects on LDL-C and in hypertriglyceridemic patients can sometimes be associated with increases in plasma LDL-C levels.

Fibrates are generally very well tolerated. The most common side effect is dyspepsia. Myopathy and hepatitis occur rarely in the absence of other lipid-lowering agents. Fibrates promote cholesterol secretion into bile and are associated with an increased risk of gallstones. Importantly, fibrates can potentiate the effect of warfarin and certain oral hypoglycemic agents, so the anticoagulation status and plasma glucose levels should be closely monitored in patients on these agents.

Fibrates are the drug class of choice in patients with severe hypertriglyceridemia (> 1000 mg/dL) and are a reasonable consideration for first-line therapy in patients with moderate hypertriglyceridemia (500–1000 mg/dL) and FDBL. As noted above, the clinical trial data with fibrates overall suggests cardiovascular benefit, but the results are mixed. In patients with TG <500 mg/dL, the role of fibrates is primarily in combination with statins in selected patients with mixed dyslipidemia. In this setting, the risk of myopathy must be carefully weighed against the clinical benefit of the therapy.

Omega 3 Fatty Acids (Fish Oils)   N-3 polyunsaturated fatty acids (n-3 PUFAs) are present in high concentration in fish and in flax seeds. The most widely used n-3 PUFAs for the treatment of hyperlipidemias are the two active molecules in fish oil: eicosapentanoic acid (EPA) and decohexanoic acid (DHA). N-3 PUFAs have been concentrated into tablets and decrease fasting triglycerides in doses of 3–4 g/d. Fish oils can result in an increase in plasma LDL-C levels in some patients. Fish oil supplements can be used in combination with fibrates, niacin, or statins to treat hypertriglyceridemia. In general, fish oils are well tolerated and appear to be safe, at least at doses up to 3–4 g. Although fish oil administration is associated with a prolongation in the bleeding time, no increase in bleeding has been seen in clinical trials. A lower dose of omega 3 (about 1 g) has been associated with reduction in cardiovascular events in CHD patients and is used by some clinicians for this purpose.

Combination Drug Therapy   This type of therapy is often required in patients who do not reach lipid targets on monotherapy. Combination drug therapy is frequently used for (1) patients unable to reach LDL-C and non-HDL-C goals on statin monotherapy, (2) patients with combined elevated LDL-C and abnormalities of the TG-HDL axis, and (3) patients with severe hypertriglyceridemia who do not achieve non-HDL-C goal on a fibrate or fish oils alone. Inability to achieve LDL-C (and non-HDL-C) goals is not uncommon on statin monotherapy. In this setting, a cholesterol absorption inhibitor or bile acid sequestrant can be added. Combination of niacin with a statin is an attractive option for high-risk patients who do not attain their target LDL-C level on statin monotherapy and who have a low HDL-C as their primary lipid abnormality. Conversely, in high-risk patients on statin therapy who have elevated TG levels as their primary remaining lipid abnormality, addition of a fibrate or fish oils is a reasonable consideration. Hypertriglyceridemic patients treated with a fibrate often fail to reach LDL-C and non-HDL-C goals and are therefore candidates for the addition of a statin. Coadministration of statins and fibrates has obvious appeal in patients with combined hyperlipidemia, but no clinical trials have assessed the effectiveness of a statin-fibrate combination compared with either a statin or a fibrate alone in reducing cardiovascular events, and the long-term safety of this combination is not known. Statin-fibrate combinations are known to be associated with an increased incidence of severe myopathy (up to 2.5%) and rhabdomyolysis, and therefore patients treated with these two drugs must be carefully counseled and monitored. This combination of drugs should be used cautiously in patients with underlying renal or hepatic insufficiency; in the elderly, frail, and chronically ill; and in those on multiple medications.

OTHER APPROACHES   Occasionally, patients cannot tolerate any of the existing lipid-lowering drugs at doses required for adequate control of their lipid levels. A larger group of patients, most of whom have genetic lipid disorders, remain significantly hypercholesterolemic despite combination drug therapy. These patients are at high risk for development or progression of CHD and clinical CHD events. The preferred option for management of patients with severe refractory hypercholesterolemia is LDL apheresis. In this process, the patient's plasma is passed over a column that selectively removes the LDL, and the LDL-depleted plasma is returned to the patient. Patients on maximally tolerated combination drug therapy who have CHD and a plasma LDL-C level >200 mg/dL or no CHD and a plasma LDL-C level >300 mg/dL are candidates for every-other-week LDL apheresis and should be referred to a specialized lipid center.

MANAGEMENT OF LOW HDL-C   Severely reduced plasma levels of HDL-C (<20 mg/dL) accompanied by triglycerides <400 mg/dL usually indicate the presence of a genetic disorder, such as a mutation in apoA-I, LCAT deficiency, or Tangier disease. HDL-C levels <20 mg/dL are common

in the setting of severe hypertriglyceridemia, in which case the primary focus should be on the management of the triglycerides. HDL-C levels <20 mg/dL also occur in individuals using anabolic steroids. Secondary causes of more moderate reductions in plasma HDL (20–40 mg/dL) should be considered (Table 350-5). Smoking should be discontinued, obese persons should be encouraged to lose weight, sedentary persons should be encouraged to exercise, and diabetes should be optimally controlled. When possible, medications associated with reduced plasma levels of HDL-C should be discontinued. The presence of an isolated low plasma level of HDL-C in a patient with a borderline plasma level of LDL-C should prompt consideration of LDL-lowering drug therapy in high-risk individuals. Statins increase plasma levels of HDL-C only modestly (~5–10%). Fibrates also have only a modest effect on plasma HDL-C levels (increasing levels ~5–15%), except in patients with coexisting hypertriglyceridemia, where they can be more effective. Niacin is the most effective available HDL-C–raising therapeutic agent and can be associated with increases in plasma HDL-C by up to ~30%, although some patients do not respond to niacin therapy.

The issue of whether pharmacologic intervention should be used to specifically raise HDL-C levels has not been adequately addressed in clinical trials. In persons with established CHD and low HDL-C levels whose plasma LDL-C levels are at or below the goal, it may be reasonable to initiate therapy (with a fibrate or niacin) directed specifically at reducing plasma triglyceride levels and raising the level of plasma HDL-C. More data are required before broad recommendations are made to use drug therapy to specifically raise HDL-C levels to prevent cardiovascular events. New HDL-raising approaches are under development that may help to address this important issue.

FURTHER READINGS

BAIGENT C et al: Efficacy and safety of cholesterol-lowering treatment: Prospective meta-analysis of data from 90,056 participants in 14 randomised trials of statins. Lancet 366:1267, 2005

BRUNZELL JD: Clinical practice. Hypertriglyceridemia. N Engl J Med 357(10):1009, 2007

CANNON CP et al: Intensive versus moderate lipid lowering with statins after acute coronary syndromes. N Engl J Med 350:1495, 2004

CARLSON LA: Nicotinic acid: The broad-spectrum lipid drug. A 50th anniversary review. J Intern Med 258:94, 2005

DUFFY D, RADER DJ: Emerging therapies targeting high-density lipoprotein metabolism and reverse cholesterol transport. Circulation 113:1140, 2006

GRUNDY SM: The issue of statin safety: Where do we stand? Circulation 111:3016, 2005

——— et al: Implications of recent clinical trials for the National Cholesterol Education Program Adult Treatment Panel III guidelines. Circulation 110:227, 2004

LaROSA JC et al: Intensive lipid lowering with atorvastatin in patients with stable coronary disease. N Engl J Med 352:1425, 2005

NATIONAL CHOLESTEROL EDUCATION PROGRAM: Executive summary of the third report of the National Cholesterol Education Program (NCEP) Expert Panel on Detection, Evaluation, and Treatment of High Blood Cholesterol in Adults (Adult Treatment Panel III). JAMA 285:2486, 2001

RADER DJ et al: Monogenic hypercholesterolemia: New insights in pathogenesis and treatment. J Clin Invest 111:1795, 2003

SINGH IM et al: High-density lipoprotein as a therapeutic target: A systematic review. JAMA 298(7):786, 2007

351   Hemochromatosis
Lawrie W. Powell

DEFINITION

Hemochromatosis is a common inherited disorder of iron metabolism in which an inappropriate increase in intestinal iron absorption results in deposition of excessive amounts of iron in parenchymal cells with eventual tissue damage and impaired organ function. The iron-storage pigment in tissues was called *hemosiderin* because it was believed to be derived from the blood. The term *hemosiderosis* is used to describe the presence of stainable iron in tissues, but tissue iron must be quantified to assess body iron status accurately (see below and Chap. 98). *Hemochromatosis* refers to progressive iron overload, potentially leading to fibrosis and organ failure. Cirrhosis of the liver, diabetes mellitus, arthritis, cardiomyopathy, and hypogonadotropic hypogonadism are the major clinical manifestations.

TABLE 351-1 CLASSIFICATION OF IRON OVERLOAD STATES

Hereditary Hemochromatosis

Hemochromatosis, *HFE*-related (type 1)
  C282Y homozygosity
  C282Y/H63D compound heterozygosity
Hemochromatosis, non-*HFE*-related
  Juvenile hemochromatosis (type 2A) (hepcidin mutation)
  Juvenile hemochromatosis (type 2B) (hemojuvelin mutations)
  Mutated transferrin receptor 2 *TFR2* (type 3)
  Mutated ferroportin 1 gene, *SLC11A3* (type 4)

Acquired Iron Overload

Iron-loading anemias	Chronic liver disease
Thalassemia major	Hepatitis C
Sideroblastic anemia	Alcoholic cirrhosis, especially
Chronic hemolytic anemias	when advanced
Transfusional and parenteral iron	Nonalcoholic steatohepatitis
overload	Porphyria cutanea tarda
Dietary iron overload	Dysmetabolic iron overload
	syndrome
	Post–portacaval shunting

Miscellaneous

Iron overload in sub-Saharan Africa
Neonatal iron overload
Aceruloplasminemia
Congenital atransferrinemia

Although there is debate about definitions, the following terminology is widely accepted.

1. *Hereditary hemochromatosis* is most often caused by a mutant gene, termed *HFE*, which is tightly linked to the HLA-A locus on chromosome 6p (see "Genetic Basis," below). Rarer forms of non-*HFE* hemochromatosis caused by mutation in other genes involved in iron metabolism have recently been described (Table 351-1). The disease can be recognized during its early stages when iron overload and organ damage are minimal. At this stage the disease is best referred to as *early hemochromatosis* or *precirrhotic hemochromatosis*.
2. *Secondary iron overload* occurs as a result of an iron-loading anemia, such as thalassemia or sideroblastic anemia, in which erythropoiesis is increased but ineffective. In the acquired iron-loading disorders, massive iron deposits in parenchymal tissues can lead to the same clinical and pathologic features as in hemochromatosis.

PREVALENCE

HFE-associated hemochromatosis mutations are among the most common inherited disease alleles, although the prevalence varies in different ethnic groups. It is most common in populations of northern European extraction in whom approximately 1 in 10 persons are heterozygous carriers and 0.3–0.5% are homozygotes. However, expression of the disease is variable and modified by several factors, especially alcohol consumption and dietary iron intake, blood loss associated with menstruation and pregnancy, and blood donation. The clinical expression of the disease is 5–10 times more frequent in men than in women. Nearly 70% of affected patients develop the first symptoms between ages 40 and 60. The disease is rarely evident before age 20, although with family screening (see "Screening for Hemochromatosis," below) and periodic health examinations, asymptomatic subjects with iron overload can be identified, including young menstruating women. Recent studies in non–blood bank populations have revealed that 30–50% of homozygous individuals do not have overt clinical evidence of iron overload.

In contrast to *HFE*-associated hemochromatosis, the non-*HFE*-associated forms of hemochromatosis (Table 351-1) are rare.

GENETIC BASIS

The *HFE* gene was identified as the most common form of hemochromatosis in 1996. A homozygous G → A mutation resulting in a

cysteine to tyrosine substitution at position 282 (C282Y) is the most common mutation. It is identified in 85–90% of patients with hereditary hemochromatosis in populations of northern European descent but is found in only 60% of cases from Mediterranean populations (e.g., southern Italy). A second, relatively common *HFE* mutation (H63D) results in a substitution of histidine to aspartic acid at codon 63. Homozygosity for H63D is not associated with clinically significant iron overload. Some compound heterozygotes (e.g., one copy each of C282Y and H63D) have moderately increased body iron stores but develop clinical disease only with cofactors such as heavy alcohol intake or hepatic steatosis. Thus, *HFE*-associated hemochromatosis is inherited as an autosomal recessive trait; heterozygotes have no, or minimal, increase in iron stores. However, this slight increase in hepatic iron can act as a cofactor that modifies the expression of other diseases such as porphyria cutanea tarda (PCT) and nonalcoholic steatohepatitis.

Mutations in other genes involved in iron metabolism are responsible for non-*HFE*-associated hemochromatosis, including juvenile hemochromatosis, which affects persons in the second and third decade of life (Table 351-1). Mutations in the genes encoding hepcidin, transferrin receptor 2 (TfR2), and hemojuvelin (Fig. 351-1) result in clinicopathologic features indistinguishable from HFE-associated hemochromatosis. However, mutations in ferroportin, responsible for the efflux of iron from enterocytes and most other cell types, result in iron loading of reticuloendothelial cells and macrophages, as well as parenchymal cells.

PATHOPHYSIOLOGY

Normally, the body iron content of 3–4 g is maintained such that intestinal mucosal absorption of iron is equal to iron loss. This amount is approximately 1 mg/d in men and 1.5 mg/d in menstruating women. In hemochromatosis, mucosal absorption is greater than body requirements and amounts to 4 mg/d or more. The progressive accumulation of iron causes an early elevation in plasma iron, an increased saturation of transferrin, and progressive elevation of plasma ferritin level (Fig. 351-2). A liver-derived peptide, hepcidin, represses basolateral iron transport in the intestine and iron release from macrophages and other cells. Hepcidin, in turn, responds to signals in the liver mediated by HFE, TfR2, and hemojuvelin (Fig. 351-1). Hepcidin is thus a crucial molecule in iron metabolism, linking body stores with intestinal iron absorption.

The *HFE* gene encodes a 343-amino-acid protein that is structurally related to MHC class I proteins. The basic defect in *HFE*-associated hemochromatosis is a lack of cell surface expression of HFE (due to the C282Y mutation). The normal (wild-type) HFE protein forms a complex with β_2-microglobulin and transferrin receptor 1 (TfR1), and the C282Y mutation completely abrogates this interaction. As a result, the mutant HFE protein remains trapped intracellularly, reducing TfR1–mediated iron uptake by the intestinal crypt cell. This impaired TfR1-mediated iron uptake leads to upregulation of the divalent metal transporter (DMT1) on the brush border of the villus cells, causing inappropriately increased intestinal iron absorption (Fig. 351-1). In advanced disease, the body may contain 20 g or more of iron that is deposited mainly in parenchymal cells of the liver, pancreas, and heart. Iron may be increased 50- to 100-fold in the liver and pancreas and 5- to 25-fold in the heart. Iron deposition in the pituitary causes hypogonadotropic hypogonadism in both men and women. Tissue injury may result from disruption of iron-laden lysosomes, from lipid peroxidation of subcellular organelles by excess iron, or from stimulation of collagen synthesis by activated stellate cells.

Secondary iron overload with deposition in parenchymal cells occurs in chronic disorders of erythropoiesis, particularly in those due to defects in hemoglobin synthesis or ineffective erythropoiesis such as sideroblastic anemia and thalassemia (Chap. 99). In these disorders, iron absorption is increased. Moreover, these patients require blood transfusions and are frequently treated inappropriately with iron. PCT, a disorder characterized by a defect in porphyrin biosynthesis (Chap. 352), can also be associated with excessive parenchymal iron deposits. The magnitude of the iron load in PCT is usually insufficient to produce tissue damage. However, some patients with PCT also have mutations in the *HFE* gene, and some have associated hepatitis C virus (HCV) infection. Although the relationship among these disorders remains to be clarified, iron overload accentuates the inherited enzyme deficiency in PCT and

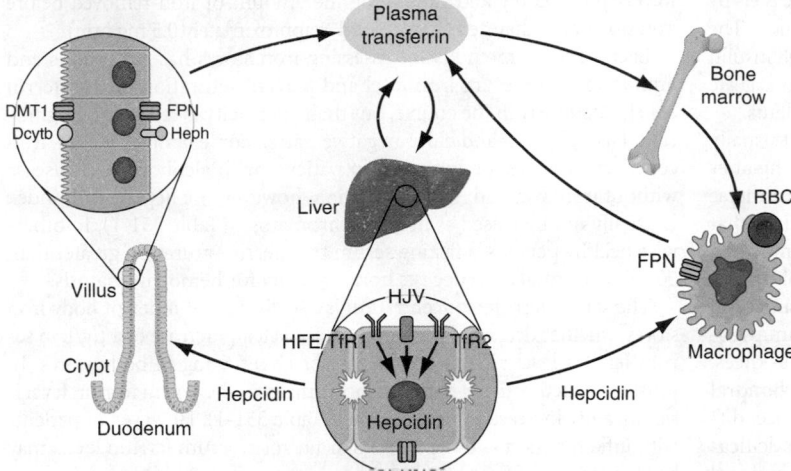

FIGURE 351-1 Pathways of normal iron homeostasis. Dietary inorganic iron traverses the brush border membrane of duodenal enterocytes via DMT1 after reduction of ferric (Fe^{3+}) iron to the ferrous (Fe^{2+}) state by duodenal cytochrome B (Dcytb). Iron then moves from the enterocyte into the circulation via a process requiring the basolateral iron exporter ferroportin (FPN) and the iron oxidase hephaestin (Heph). In the circulation, iron binds to plasma transferrin and is thereby distributed to sites of iron utilization and storage. Much of this diferric transferrin supplies iron to immature erythroid cells in the bone marrow for hemoglobin synthesis. At the end of their life, senescent red blood cells (RBC) are phagocytosed by macrophages and iron is returned to the circulation after export through ferroportin. The liver-derived peptide hepcidin represses basolateral iron transport in the gut as well as iron release from macrophages and other cells and serves as a central regulator of body iron traffic. Hepcidin responds to changes in body iron requirements by signals mediated by HFE, TfR2, and hemojuvelin (HJV). Heme is metabolized by heme oxygenase within the enterocytes, and the released iron then follows the same pathway.

Mutations in the genes encoding HFE, TfR2, hemojuvelin, and hepcidin all lead to decreased hepcidin release and increased iron absorption, resulting in hemochromatosis (Table 351-1).

should be avoided along with other agents (alcohol, estrogens, haloaromatic compounds) that may exacerbate PCT. Another cause of hepatic parenchymal iron overload is hereditary aceruloplasminemia. In this disorder, impairment of iron mobilization due to deficiency of ceruloplasmin (a ferroxidase) causes iron overload in hepatocytes.

Excessive iron ingestion over many years rarely results in hemochromatosis. An important exception has been reported in South Africa among groups who brew fermented beverages in vessels made of iron. Hemochromatosis has been described in apparently normal persons who have taken medicinal iron over many years, but such individuals probably had a genetic disorder.

The common denominator in all patients with hemochromatosis is *excessive amounts of iron in parenchymal tissues.* Parenteral administration of iron in the form of blood transfusions or iron preparations results predominantly in reticuloendothelial cell iron overload. This appears to lead to less tissue damage than iron loading of parenchymal cells.

In the liver, parenchymal iron is in the form of ferritin and hemosiderin. In the early stages these deposits are seen in the periportal parenchymal cells, especially within lysosomes in the pericanalicular cytoplasm of the hepatocytes. This stage progresses to perilobular fibrosis and eventually to deposition of iron in bile duct epithelium, Kupffer cells, and fibrous septa due to activation of stellate cells. In the advanced stage, a macronodular or mixed macro- and micronodular cirrhosis develops. Hepatic fibrosis and cirrhosis correlate significantly with hepatic iron concentration.

At autopsy, the enlarged nodular liver and pancreas are rusty in color. Histologically, iron is increased in many organs, particularly in the liver, heart, and pancreas, and to a lesser extent in the endocrine glands. The epidermis of the skin is thin, and melanin is increased in the cells of the basal layer and dermis. Deposits of iron are present around the synovial lining cells of the joints.

Many subjects with significant iron overload are asymptomatic. For example, in a study of 672 asymptomatic C282Y homozygous subjects—identified by either family screening or routine health examinations—there was hepatic iron overload (grades 2–4) in 56% and 34.5% of male and female subjects, respectively; hepatic fibrosis (stages 2–4) in 18.4% and 5.4%, respectively; and cirrhosis in 5.6% and 1.9%, respectively.

Initial symptoms are often nonspecific and include lethargy, arthralgia, change in skin color, loss of libido, and features of diabetes mellitus. Hepatomegaly, increased pigmentation, spider angiomas, splenomegaly, arthropathy, ascites, cardiac arrhythmias, congestive heart failure, loss of body hair, testicular atrophy, and jaundice are prominent in advanced disease.

The *liver* is usually the first organ to be affected, and hepatomegaly is present in more than 95% of symptomatic patients. Hepatic enlargement may exist in the absence of symptoms or of abnormal liver function tests. Manifestations of portal hypertension and esophageal varices occur less commonly than in cirrhosis from other causes. Hepatocellular carcinoma develops in about 30% of patients with cirrhosis, and it is the most common cause of death in treated patients—hence the importance of early diagnosis and therapy. Its incidence increases with age, it is more common in men, and it occurs almost exclusively in cirrhotic patients.

Excessive skin pigmentation is present in patients with advanced disease. The characteristic metallic or slate gray hue is sometimes referred to as *bronzing* and results from increased melanin and iron in the dermis. Pigmentation usually is diffuse and generalized, but it may be more pronounced on the face, neck, extensor aspects of the lower forearms, dorsa of the hands, lower legs, and genital regions, as well as in scars.

Diabetes mellitus occurs in about 65% of symptomatic patients and is more likely to develop in those with a family

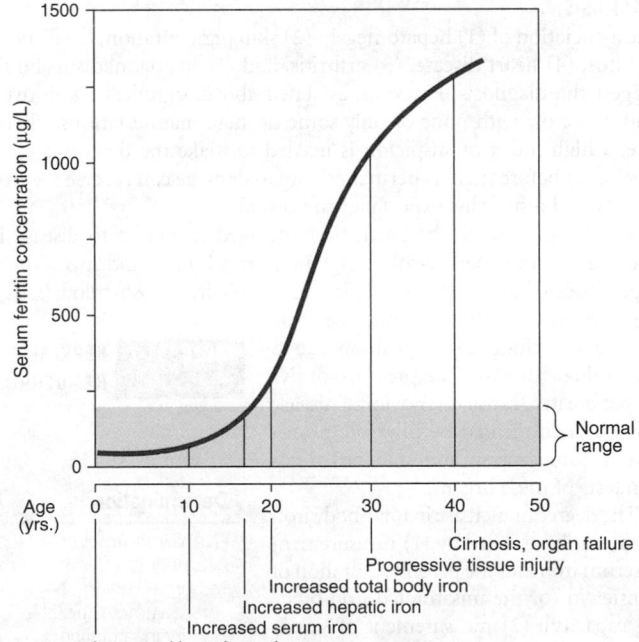

FIGURE 351-2 Sequence of events in genetic hemochromatosis and their correlation with the serum ferritin concentration. Increased iron absorption is present throughout life. Overt, symptomatic disease usually develops between ages 40 and 60, but latent disease can be detected long before this.

history of diabetes, suggesting that direct damage to the pancreatic islets by iron deposition occurs in combination with a genetic predisposition. The management is similar to that of other forms of diabetes, although insulin resistance is more common in association with hemochromatosis. Late complications are the same as seen in other causes of diabetes mellitus.

Arthropathy develops in 25–50% of symptomatic patients. It usually occurs after age 50 but may occur as a first manifestation, or long after therapy. The joints of the hands, especially the second and third metacarpophalangeal joints, are usually the first joints involved, a feature that helps to distinguish the chondrocalcinosis associated with hemochromatosis from the idiopathic form (Chap. 327). A progressive polyarthritis involving wrists, hips, ankles, and knees may also ensue. Acute brief attacks of synovitis may be associated with deposition of calcium pyrophosphate (chondrocalcinosis or pseudogout), mainly in the knees. Radiologic manifestations include cystic changes of the subchondral bones, loss of articular cartilage with narrowing of the joint space, diffuse demineralization, hypertrophic bone proliferation, and calcification of the synovium. The arthropathy tends to progress despite removal of iron by phlebotomy. Although the relation of these abnormalities to iron metabolism is not known, the fact that similar changes occur in other forms of iron overload suggests that iron is directly involved.

Cardiac involvement is the presenting manifestation in about 15% of symptomatic patients. The most common manifestation is congestive heart failure, which occurs in about 10% of young adults with the disease, especially those with juvenile hemochromatosis. Symptoms of congestive failure may develop suddenly, with rapid progression to death if untreated. The heart is diffusely enlarged; this may be misdiagnosed as idiopathic cardiomyopathy if other overt manifestations are absent. Cardiac arrhythmias include premature supraventricular beats, paroxysmal tachyarrhythmias, atrial flutter, atrial fibrillation, and varying degrees of atrioventricular block.

Hypogonadism occurs in both sexes and may antedate other clinical features. Manifestations include loss of libido, impotence, amenorrhea, testicular atrophy, gynecomastia, and sparse body hair. These changes are primarily the result of decreased production of gonadotropins due to impairment of hypothalamic-pituitary function by iron deposition. Adrenal insufficiency, hypothyroidism, and hypoparathyroidism are rare manifestations.

DIAGNOSIS

The association of (1) hepatomegaly, (2) skin pigmentation, (3) diabetes mellitus, (4) heart disease, (5) arthritis, and (6) hypogonadism should suggest the diagnosis. However, as stated above, significant iron overload may exist with none or only some of these manifestations. Therefore, a high index of suspicion is needed to make the diagnosis early. Treatment before there is permanent organ damage can reverse the iron toxicity and restore life expectancy to normal.

The history should be particularly detailed in regard to disease in other family members, alcohol ingestion, iron intake, and ingestion of large doses of ascorbic acid, which promotes iron absorption (Chap. 71). Appropriate tests should be performed to exclude iron deposition due to hematologic disease. The presence of liver, pancreatic, cardiac, and joint disease should be confirmed by physical examination, radiography, and standard function tests of these organs.

The degree of increase in total-body iron stores can be assessed by (1) measurement of serum iron and the percent saturation of transferrin (or the unsaturated iron-binding capacity); (2) measurement of serum ferritin concentration; (3) liver biopsy with measurement of the iron concentration and calculation of the hepatic iron index (**Table 351-2**); (4) MRI of the liver. In addition, a retrospective assessment of body iron storage is also provided by performing weekly phlebotomy and calculating the amount of iron removed before iron stores are exhausted (1 mL blood = approximately 0.5 mg iron).

Each of these methods for assessing iron stores has advantages and limitations. The serum iron level and percent saturation of transferrin are elevated early in the course, but their specificity is reduced by significant false-positive and false-negative rates. For example, serum iron concentration may be increased in patients with alcoholic liver disease without iron overload; in this situation, however, the hepatic iron index is usually not increased as in hemochromatosis (Table 351-1). In otherwise healthy persons, a fasting serum transferrin saturation greater than 50% is abnormal and suggests homozygosity for hemochromatosis.

The serum ferritin concentration is usually a good index of body iron stores, whether decreased or increased. In fact, an increase of 1 µg/L in serum ferritin level reflects an increase of about 5 mg in body stores. In most untreated patients with hemochromatosis, the serum ferritin level is significantly increased (Fig. 351-2 and Table 351-1). However, in patients with inflammation and hepatocellular necrosis, serum ferritin levels may be elevated out of proportion to body iron stores due to increased release from tissues. A repeat determination of serum ferritin should therefore be carried out after acute hepatocellular damage has subsided, e.g., in alcoholic liver disease. Ordinarily, the combined measurements of the percent transferrin saturation and serum ferritin level provide a simple and reliable screening test for hemochromatosis, including the precirrhotic phase of the disease. If either of these tests is abnormal, genetic testing for hemochromatosis should be performed (**Fig. 351-3**).

The role of liver biopsy in the diagnosis and management of hemochromatosis has been reassessed as a result of the widespread availability of genetic testing for the C282Y mutation. The absence of severe fibrosis can be accurately predicted in most patients using clinical and biochemical variables. Thus, there is virtually no risk of severe fibrosis in a C282Y homozygous subject with (1) serum ferritin level less than 1000 µg/L; (2) normal serum alanine amino transaminase values; (3) no hepatomegaly; and (4) no excess alcohol intake. However, it should be emphasized that liver biopsy is the only reliable method for establishing or excluding the presence of hepatic cirrhosis, which is the critical factor determining prognosis and the risk of developing hepatocellular carcinoma. Biopsy also permits histochemical estimation of tissue iron and measurement of hepatic iron concentration. Increased density of the liver due to iron deposition can be demonstrated by CT or MRI, and with improved technology, MRI is becoming more accurate in determining hepatic iron concentration.

SCREENING FOR HEMOCHROMATOSIS

When the diagnosis of hemochromatosis is established, it is important to counsel and screen other family members (Chap. 64). Asymptomatic as well as symptomatic family members with the disease usually have an increased saturation of transferrin and an increased serum ferritin concentration. These changes occur even before the iron stores are greatly increased (Fig. 351-2). All adult first-degree relatives of patients with hemochromatosis should be tested for the C282Y and H63D mutations and advised appropriately (Fig. 351-3). In affected individuals, it is im-

| TABLE 351-2 | REPRESENTATIVE IRON VALUES IN NORMAL SUBJECTS, PATIENTS WITH HEMOCHROMATOSIS, AND PATIENTS WITH ALCOHOLIC LIVER DISEASE |

Determination	Normal	Symptomatic Hemochromatosis	Homozygotes with Early, Asymptomatic Hemochromatosis	Heterozygotes	Alcoholic Liver Disease
Plasma iron, µmol/L (µg/dL)	9–27 (50–150)	32–54 (180–300)	Usually elevated	Elevated or normal	Often elevated
Total iron-binding capacity, µmol/L (µg/dL)	45–66 (250–370)	36–54 (200–300)	36–54 (200–300)	Elevated or normal	45–66 (250–370)
Transferrin saturation, percent	22–46	50–100	50–100	Normal or elevated	27–60
Serum ferritin, µg/L		900–6000	200–500	Usually <500	10–500
Men	20–250				
Women	15–150				
Liver iron, µg/g dry wt	300–1400	6000–18,000	2000–4000	300–3000	300–2000
Hepatic iron index	<1.0	>2	1.5–2.0	<2	<2

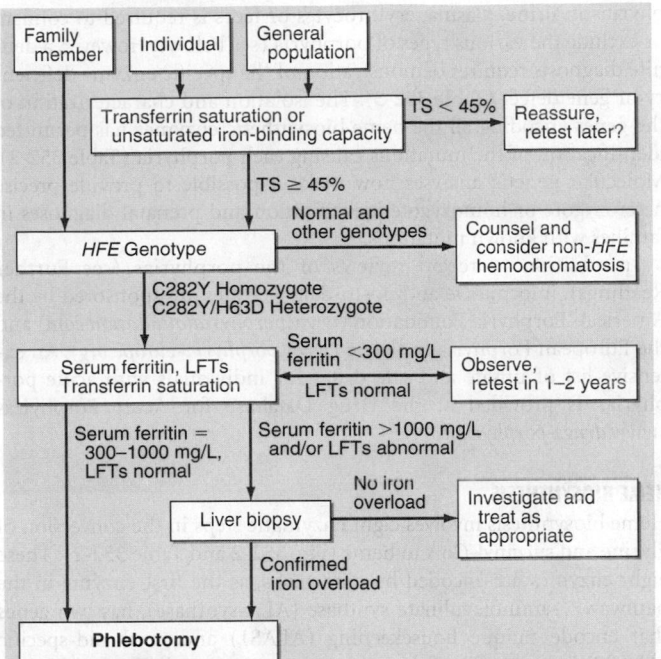

FIGURE 351-3 Algorithm for screening for *HFE*-associated hemochromatosis. LFT, liver function test; TS, transferrin saturation. (*From EJ Eijkelkamp et al: Can J Gastroenterol 14:121, 2000; with permission.*)

portant to confirm or exclude the presence of cirrhosis and begin therapy as early as possible. When children of a proband are affected, a homozygote-heterozygote mating is most likely. For practical purposes, children need not be checked before they are 18 years old.

The role of population screening for hemochromatosis is controversial. A recent study has shown that it is highly effective for primary care physicians to screen subjects using serum iron, transferrin saturation and serum ferritin levels. Such screening also detects iron deficiency. Genetic screening of the normal population is feasible, but its cost-effectiveness has not been established.

℞ HEMOCHROMATOSIS

The therapy of hemochromatosis involves removal of the excess body iron and supportive treatment of damaged organs. Iron removal is best accomplished by weekly or twice-weekly phlebotomy of 500 mL. Although there is an initial modest decline in the volume of packed red blood cells to about 35 mL/dL, the level stabilizes after several weeks. The plasma transferrin saturation remains increased until the available iron stores are depleted. In contrast, the plasma ferritin concentration falls progressively, reflecting the gradual decrease in body iron stores. One 500-mL unit of blood contains 200–250 mg iron, and up to 25 g iron or more may have to be removed. Therefore, weekly phlebotomy may be required for 1–2 years and it should be continued until the serum ferritin level is under 50 μg/L. Thereafter, phlebotomies are performed at appropriate intervals to maintain ferritin levels between 50 and 100 μg/L. Usually one phlebotomy every 3 months will suffice.

Chelating agents such as deferoxamine, when given parenterally, remove 10–20 mg iron per day, which is much less than that mobilized by once-weekly phlebotomy. Phlebotomy is also less expensive, more convenient, and safer for most patients. However, chelating agents are indicated when anemia or hypoproteinemia is severe enough to preclude phlebotomy. Subcutaneous infusion of deferoxamine using a portable pump is the most effective means of administration.

An effective oral iron chelating agent, deferasirox (Exjade), has recently become available. This agent is effective in thalassemia and secondary iron overload, but its role in primary iron overload has yet to be established.

Alcohol consumption should be severely curtailed or eliminated as it increases the risk of cirrhosis in hereditary hemochromatosis nearly tenfold. The management of hepatic failure, cardiac failure, and diabetes mellitus is similar to conventional therapy for these conditions. Loss of libido and change in secondary sex characteristics are managed with testosterone replacement or gonadotropin therapy (Chap. 340).

End-stage liver disease may be an indication for liver transplantation, although results are improved if the excess iron can be removed beforehand. The available evidence indicates that the fundamental metabolic abnormality in hemochromatosis is reversed by successful liver transplantation.

PROGNOSIS

The principal causes of death are cardiac failure, hepatocellular failure or portal hypertension, and hepatocellular carcinoma.

Life expectancy is improved by removal of the excessive stores of iron and maintenance of these stores at near-normal levels. The 5-year survival rate with therapy increases from 33 to 89%. With repeated phlebotomy, the liver decreases in size, liver function improves, pigmentation of skin decreases, and cardiac failure may be reversed. Diabetes improves in about 40%, but removal of excess iron has little effect on hypogonadism or arthropathy. Hepatic fibrosis may decrease, but established cirrhosis is irreversible. Hepatocellular carcinoma occurs as a late sequela in patients who are cirrhotic at presentation. The apparent increase in its incidence in treated patients is probably related to their increased life span. Hepatocellular carcinoma rarely develops if the disease is treated in the precirrhotic stage. Indeed, the life expectancy of homozygotes treated before the development of cirrhosis is normal.

The importance of family screening and early diagnosis and treatment cannot be overemphasized. Asymptomatic individuals detected by family studies should have phlebotomy therapy if iron stores are moderately to severely increased. Assessment of iron stores at appropriate intervals is also important. With this management approach, most manifestations of the disease can be prevented.

ROLE OF *HFE* MUTATIONS IN OTHER LIVER DISEASES

There is considerable interest in the role of *HFE* mutations and hepatic iron in several other liver diseases. Several studies have shown an increased prevalence of *HFE* mutations in PCT patients. Iron accentuates the inherited enzyme deficiency in PCT and clinical manifestations of PCT. The situation in non-alcoholic steatosis (NASH) is less clear, but some studies have shown an increased prevalence of one or two *HFE* mutations in NASH patients. The role of phlebotomy therapy, however, is unproven. In chronic HCV infection, *HFE* mutations are not more common but some subjects have increased hepatic iron. Before initiating antiviral therapy in these patients, it is reasonable to perform phlebotomy therapy to remove excess iron stores, as this reduces liver enzyme levels.

HFE mutations are not increased in frequency in alcoholic liver disease. Hemochromatosis in a heavy drinker can be distinguished from alcoholic liver disease by the presence of the C282Y mutation.

End-stage liver disease may also be associated with iron overload of the degree seen in hemochromatosis. The mechanism is uncertain, although hemolysis plays a role. *HFE* mutations are uncommon.

ACKNOWLEDGMENT

The author acknowledges the contribution of Dr. Kurt J. Isselbacher to this chapter in previous editions of Harrison's.

FURTHER READINGS

ALLEN KJ et al: A prospective study of mutations in the HFE gene and development of hereditary hemochromatosis disease. N Engl J Med, 2008 (in press)

ADAMS PC et al: Hemochromatosis and iron-overload screening in a racially diverse population. N Engl J Med 352:1769, 2005

PIETRANGELO A: Hemochromatosis: An endocrine liver disease. Hepatology. 46:1291, 2007

———: Non-HFE-linked hemochromatosis. Semin Liver Dis 25:450, 2005

———: Hereditary hemochromatosis—a new look at an old disease. N Engl J Med 350:2383, 2004

PIPERNO A et al: Blunted hepcidin response to oral iron challenge in HFE-hemochromatosis. Blood August 27 2007, epub ahead of print

POWELL LW et al: Screening for hemochromatosis in asymptomatic subjects with or without a family history. Arch Intern Med 166:294, 2006

ST. PIERRE TG et al: Noninvasive measurement and imaging of liver iron concentrations using proton magnetic resonance. Blood 105:855, 2005

CHAPTER 351 Hemochromatosis

352 The Porphyrias
Robert J. Desnick, Kenneth H. Astrin

The porphyrias are metabolic disorders, each resulting from the deficiency of a specific enzyme in the heme biosynthetic pathway (Fig. 352-1 and Table 352-1). These enzyme deficiencies are inherited as autosomal dominant or recessive traits, with the exception of porphyria cutanea tarda (PCT), which usually is sporadic (Table 352-1). The porphyrias are classified as either *hepatic* or *erythropoietic*, depending on the primary site of overproduction and accumulation of their respective porphyrin precursors or porphyrins (Tables 352-1 and 352-2), although some have overlapping features. For example, PCT, the most common porphyria, is hepatic and presents with blistering cutaneous photosensitivity. The major manifestations of the acute hepatic porphyrias are neurologic, including neuropathic abdominal pain, peripheral motor neuropathy, and mental disturbances, with attacks often precipitated by steroid hormones, certain drugs, and nutrition influences. While hepatic porphyrias are symptomatic primarily in adults, rare homozygous variants of the autosomal dominant hepatic porphyrias have been identified that usually manifest clinically prior to puberty.

In contrast, the erythropoietic porphyrias usually present with cutaneous photosensitivity at birth or in early childhood, or in the case of congenital erythropoietic porphyria (CEP), even in utero as nonimmune hydrops fetalis. Cutaneous sensitivity to sunlight results from excitation of excess porphyrins in the skin by long-wave ultraviolet light, leading to cell damage, scarring, and deformation. Thus, the porphyrias are metabolic disorders in which environmental, physiologic, and genetic factors interact to cause disease.

Because many symptoms of the porphyrias are nonspecific, diagnosis is often delayed. Laboratory measurement of porphyrin precursors [5′–aminolevulinic acid (ALA) and porphobilinogen (PBG)] or porphyrins in urine, plasma, erythrocytes or feces is required to confirm or exclude the various types of porphyria (see below). However, a definite diagnosis requires demonstration of the specific enzyme deficiency or gene defect (Table 352-3). The isolation and characterization of the genes encoding all the heme biosynthetic enzymes has permitted identification of the mutations causing each porphyria (Table 352-2). Molecular genetic analyses now make it possible to provide precise heterozygote or homozygote identification and prenatal diagnoses in families with known mutations.

In addition to recent reviews of the porphyrias (see Further Readings), informative and up-to-date websites are sponsored by the American Porphyria Foundation (*www.porphyriafoundation.com*) and the European Porphyria Initiative (*www.porphyria-europe.org*). An extensive list of unsafe and safe drugs for individuals with acute porphyrias is provided at the Drug Database for Acute Porphyrias (*www.drugs-porphyria.com*).

HEME BIOSYNTHESIS

Heme biosynthesis involves eight enzymatic steps in the conversion of glycine and succinyl-CoA to heme (Fig. 352-2 and Table 352-2). These eight enzymes are encoded by nine genes, as the first enzyme in the pathway, 5′-aminolevulinate synthase (ALA-synthase), has two genes that encode unique housekeeping (ALAS1) and erythroid-specific (ALAS2) isozymes. The first and last three enzymes in the pathway are located in the mitochondrion, whereas the other four are in the cytosol. Heme is required for a variety of hemoproteins such as hemoglobin, myoglobin, respiratory cytochromes, and the cytochrome P450 enzymes (CYPs). Hemoglobin synthesis in erythroid precursor cells accounts for approximately 85% of daily heme synthesis in humans. Hepatocytes account for most of the rest, primarily for synthesis of CYPs, which are especially abundant in the liver endoplasmic reticulum, and turn over more rapidly than many other hemoproteins, such as the mitochondrial respiratory cytochromes. As shown in Fig. 352-2, pathway intermediates are the porphyrin precursors, ALA and PBG, and porphyrins (mostly in their reduced forms, known as *porphyrinogens*). At least in humans, these intermediates do not accumulate in significant amounts under normal conditions or have important physiologic functions.

The first enzyme, ALA-synthase, catalyzes the condensation of glycine, activated by pyridoxal phosphate and succinyl coenzyme A, to form ALA. In the liver, this rate-limiting enzyme can be induced by a variety of drugs, steroids, and other chemicals. The distinct nonerythroid (e.g., housekeeping) and erythroid-specific forms of ALA-synthase are encoded by separate genes located on chromosome 3p21.1 (ALAS1) and Xp11.2 (ALAS2), respectively. Defects in the erythroid gene ALAS2 cause X-linked sideroblastic anemia (XLSA).

The second enzyme, 5′-aminolevulinate dehydratase (ALA-dehydratase), catalyzes the condensation of two molecules of ALA to form PBG. Hydroxymethylbilane synthase (HMB-synthase; also known as PBG-deaminase) catalyzes the head-to-tail condensation of four PBG molecules by a series of deaminations to form the linear tetrapyrrole, HMB. Uroporphyrinogen III synthase (URO-synthase) catalyzes the rearrangement and rapid cyclization of HMB to form the asymmetric, physiologic, octacarboxylate porphyrinogen uroporphyrinogen (URO) III.

The fifth enzyme in the pathway, uroporphyrinogen decarboxylase (URO-decarbox-

FIGURE 352-1 The human heme biosynthetic pathway indicating in linked boxes the enzyme that, when deficient, causes the respective porphyria. Hepatic porphyrias are shown in yellow boxes and erythropoietic porphyrias in pink boxes.

TABLE 352-1 HUMAN PORPHYRIAS: MAJOR CLINICAL AND LABORATORY FEATURES

Porphyria	Deficient Enzyme	Inheritance	Principal Symptoms NV or CP	Enzyme Activity % of Normal	Increased Porphyrin Precursors and/or Porphyrins Erythrocytes	Urine	Stool
Hepatic Porphyrias							
5-ALA dehydratase-deficient porphyria (ADP)	ALA-dehydratase	AR	NV	~5	Zn-protoporphyrin	ALA, Coproporphyrin III	—
Acute intermittent porphyria (AIP)	HMB-synthase	AD	NV	~50	—	ALA,[a] PBG, Uroporphyrin	
Porphyria cutanea tarda (PCT)	URO-decarboxylase	AD	CP	~20	—	Uroporphyrin, 7-carboxylate porphyrin	Isocoproporphyrin
Hereditary coproporphyria (HCP)	COPRO-oxidase	AD	NV & CP	~50	—	ALA, PBG, Coproporphyrin III	Coproporphyrin III
Variegate porphyria (VP)	PROTO-oxidase	AD	NV & CP	~50	—	ALA, PBG, Coproporphyrin III	Coproporphyrin III Protoporphyrin
Erythropoietic Porphyrias							
Congenital erythropoietic porphyria (CEP)	URO-synthase	AR	CP	1–5	Uroporphyrin I Coproporphyrin I	Uroporphyrin I Coproporphyrin I	Coproporphyrin I
Erythropoietic protoporphyria (EPP)	Ferrochelatase	AD[a]	CP	~20–30	Protoporphyrin	—	Protoporphyrin

[a]Polymorphism in intron 3 of wild-type allele affects level of enzyme activity and clinical expression.

Abbreviations: AD, autosomal dominant; ALA, 5′-aminolevulinic acid; AR, autosomal recessive; CP, cutaneous photosensitivity; COPRO, coproporphyrinogen; HMB, hydroxymethylbilane; ISOCOPRO, isocoproporphyrin; NV, neurovisceral; PBG, porphobilinogen; PROTO, protoporphyrinogen; URO, uroporphyrinogen.

ylase), catalyzes the sequential removal of the four carboxyl groups from the acetic acid side chains of URO III to form coproporphyrinogen (COPRO) III, a tetracarboxylate porphyrinogen. This compound then enters the mitochondrion, where COPRO-oxidase, the sixth enzyme, catalyzes the decarboxylation of two of the four propionic acid groups to form the two vinyl groups of protoporphyrinogen (PROTO) IX, a decarboxylate porphyrinogen. Next, PROTO-oxidase oxidizes PROTO IX to protoporphyrin IX by the removal of six hydrogen atoms. The product of the reaction is a porphyrin (oxidized form), in contrast to the preceding tetrapyrrole intermediates, which are porphyrinogens (reduced forms). Finally, ferrous iron is inserted into protoporphyrin IX to form heme, a reaction catalyzed by the eighth enzyme in the pathway, ferrochelatase (also known as heme synthetase or protoheme ferrolyase).

REGULATION OF HEME BIOSYNTHESIS

Regulation of heme synthesis differs in the two major heme-forming tissues, the liver and erythron. In the liver, "free" heme regulates the synthesis and mitochondrial translocation of the housekeeping form of ALA-synthase. Heme represses the synthesis of the ALA-synthase mRNA and interferes with the transport of the enzyme from the cytosol into mitochondria. Hepatic ALA-synthase is increased by many of the same chemicals that induce the cytochrome P450 enzymes in the endoplasmic reticulum of the liver. Because most of the heme in the liver is used for the synthesis of cytochrome P450 enzymes, hepatic ALA-synthase and the cytochrome P450s are regulated in a coordinated fashion, and many drugs that induce hepatic ALA-synthase also induce CYPs. The other hepatic heme biosynthetic enzymes are presumably expressed at constant levels, although their relative activities

TABLE 352-2 HUMAN HEME BIOSYNTHETIC ENZYMES AND GENES

Enzyme	Gene Symbol	Chromosomal Location	cDNA (bp)	Gene Size (kb)	Gene Exons[a]	Protein (aa)	Subcellular Location[b]	Known Mutations[c]	3D Structure[d]
ALA-synthase:									
Housekeeping	ALAS1	3p21.1	2199	17	11	640	M	—	
Erythroid-specific	ALAS2	Xp11.2	1937	22	11	587	M	26	—
ALA-dehydratase:									
Housekeeping	ALAD	9q32	1149	15.9	12 (1A + 2-12)	330	C	9	Y
Erythroid-specific	ALAD	9q32	1154	15.9	12 (1B + 2-12)	330	C	—	
HMB-synthase:									
Housekeeping	HMBS	11q23.3	1086	11	15 (1 + 3-15)	361	C	236	E
Erythroid-specific	HMBS	11q23.3	1035	11	15 (2-15)	344	C	10	
URO-synthase:									
Housekeeping	UROS	10q26.2	1296	34	10 (1 + 2B-10)	265	C	32	H
Erythroid-specific	UROS	10q26.2	1216	34	10 (2A+ 2B-10)	265	C	4	
URO-decarboxylase	UROD	1p34.1	1104	3	10	367	C	65	H
COPRO-oxidase	CPOX	3q12.1	1364	14	7	454	M	37	H
PROTO-oxidase	PPOX	1q23.3	1431	4.8	13	477	M	129	—
Ferrochelatase	FECH	18q21.31	1286	38.4	11	429	M	88	B

[a]Number of exons and those encoding separate housekeeping and erythroid-specific forms indicated in parentheses.

[b]M, mitochondria; C, cytoplasm.

[c]Number of known mutations from the Human Gene Mutation Database (www.hgmd.org), as of 2/1/2007.

[d]Crystallized from human (H), murine (M), E. coli (E), B. subtilis (B) or yeast (Y) purified enzyme; references in Protein Data Bank (www.rcsb.org).

Abbreviations: ALA, 5′-aminolevulinic acid; COPRO, coproporphyrin; HMB, hydroxymethylbilane; PROTO, protoporphyrin; URO, uroporphyrin.

Source: From KE Anderson et al., 2001.

TABLE 352-3 DIAGNOSIS OF ACUTE AND CUTANEOUS PORPHYRIAS

Symptoms	First Line Test	Possible Porphyria	Second Line Testing if First Line Testing Is Positive	Confirmatory Test
	Biochemical abnormality		To include: urine (U), plasma (P), and fecal (F) porphyrins; for acute porphyrias add red blood cell (RBC) HMB-synthase; for blistering skin lesions add P & RBC porphyrins	Enzyme assay and/or mutation analysis
Neurovisceral	**Spot U:** ↑↑ALA & normal PBG	ADP	**U porphyrins:** ↑↑, mostly coprophyrin III **P & F porphyrins:** normal or slightly ↑ **RBC HMB-synthase:** normal	Rule out other causes of elevated ALA; ↓↓ RBC ALA-dehydratase activity (<10%); ALAD mutation analysis
	Spot U: ↑↑ PBG	AIP	**U porphyrins:** ↑↑, mostly uroporphyrins & coproporphyrins **P & F porphyrins:** normal or slightly ↑ **RBC HMB-synthase:** usually ↓	HMBS mutation analysis
	Spot U: ↑↑ PBG	HCP	**U porphyrins:** ↑↑, mostly coproporphyrin III **P porphyrins:** normal or slightly ↑ (↑ if skin lesions present) **F porphyrins:** ↑↑, mostly coproporphyrin III	Measure RBC HMB-synthase: normal activity CPOX mutation analysis
	Spot U: ↑↑ PBG	VP	**U porphyrins:** ↑↑, mostly coproporphyrin III **P porphyrins:** ↑↑ (characteristic fluorescence peak at neutral pH) **F porphyrins:** ↑↑, mostly coproporphyrins & protoporphyrin	Measure RBC HMB-synthase: normal activity PPOX mutation analysis
Blistering Skin Lesions	**P:** ↑ porphyrins	PCT & HEP	**U porphyrins:** ↑↑, mostly uroporphyrins & heptacarboxylate porphyrin **P porphyrins:** ↑↑ **F porphyrins:** ↑↑, including increased isocoproporphyrin **RBC porphyrins:** ↑↑ zinc protoporphyrin in HEP[a]	RBC URO-decarboxylase activity: half-normal in familial PCT (~20% of all PCT cases); substantially deficient in HEP UROD mutation analysis: mutation(s) present in familial PCT (heterozygous) & HEP (homozygous)
	P: ↑ porphyrins	HCP & VP	See HCP & VP above. Also, U ALA & PBG: may be ↑	
	P: ↑ porphyrins	CEP	**RBC & U porphyrins:** ↑↑, mostly uroporphyrin I & coproporphyrin I **F porphyrins:** ↑↑; mostly coproporphyrin I	↓↓RBC URO-synthase activity (<15%) UROS mutation analysis
Nonblistering Photosensitivity	**P:** porphyrins usually ↑	EPP	**RBC porphyrins:** ↑↑, mostly free protoporphyrin **U porphyrins:** normal **F porphyrins:** normal or ↑, mostly protoporphyrin	FECH mutation analysis

[a]Nonspecific increases in zinc protoporphyrins are common in other porphyrias.

Abbreviations: ALA, 5-aminolevulinic acid; COPRO, coproporphyrinogen; HMB, hydroxy-methylbilane; PBG, porphobilinogen; PROTO, protoporphyrinogen; URO, uroporphyrinogen.

Source: KE Anderson et al, 2005.

and kinetic properties differ. For example, normal individuals have high activities of ALA-dehydratase but low activities of HMB-synthase, the latter being the second rate-limiting step in the pathway.

In the erythron, novel regulatory mechanisms allow for the production of the very large amounts of heme needed for hemoglobin synthesis. The response to stimuli for hemoglobin synthesis occurs during cell differentiation, leading to an increase in cell number. The erythroid-specific ALA-synthase is expressed at higher levels than the housekeeping enzyme, and erythroid-specific control mechanisms regulate other pathway enzymes as well as iron transport into erythroid cells. Separate erythroid-specific and nonerythroid or "house-keeping" transcripts are known for the first four enzymes in the pathway. As noted above, housekeeping and erythroid-specific ALA-synthases are encoded by genes on different chromosomes, but for each of the next three genes in the pathway, both erythroid and nonerythroid transcripts are transcribed by alternative promoters from their single respective genes.

CLASSIFICATION OF THE PORPHYRIAS

As mentioned above, the porphyrias can be classified as either *hepatic* or *erythropoietic*, depending on whether the heme biosynthetic intermediates that accumulate arise initially from the liver or developing erythrocytes, or as *acute* or *cutaneous*, based on their clinical manifestations. Table 352-1 lists the porphyrias, their principal symptoms and major biochemical abnormalities. Four of the five hepatic porphyrias—acute intermittent porphyria (AIP), hereditary coproporphyria (HCP), varie-

gate porphyria (VP) and ALA-dehydratase porphyria (ADP)—present during adult life with acute attacks of neurologic manifestations and elevated levels of one or both of the porphyrin precursors, ALA and PBG, and are thus classified as *acute porphyrias*. The fifth hepatic disorder, porphyria cutanea tarda (PCT), presents with blistering skin lesions. HCP and VP also may have cutaneous manifestations similar to PCT.

The erythropoietic porphyrias—congenital erythropoietic porphyria (CEP), and erythropoietic protoporphyria (EPP)—are characterized by elevations of porphyrins in bone marrow and erythrocytes and present with cutaneous photosensitivity. The skin lesions in CEP resemble PCT but are usually much more severe, whereas EPP causes a more immediate, painful, and nonblistering type of photosensitivity. EPP is the most common porphyria to cause symptoms before puberty. Around 20% of EPP patients develop minor abnormalities of liver function, with up to about 5% developing hepatic complications that can become life-threatening.

DIAGNOSIS OF PORPHYRIA

A few specific and sensitive first-line laboratory tests should be used whenever symptoms or signs suggest the diagnosis of porphyria (Table 352-3). If a first-line test is significantly abnormal, more comprehensive testing should follow to establish the type of porphyria.

Acute Porphyrias An acute porphyria should be suspected in patients with neurovisceral symptoms after puberty, such as abdominal

Mitochondria

Cytoplasm

FIGURE 352-2 The heme biosynthetic pathway showing the eight enzymes and their substrates and products. Four of the en-zymes are localized in the mitochondria and four in the cytosol.

pain, and when the initial clinical evaluation does not suggest another cause, the urinary porphyrin precursors (ALA and PBG) should be measured (Fig. 352-2). Urinary PBG is virtually always increased during acute attacks of AIP, HCP, and VP and is not substantially increased in any other medical condition. Therefore, this measurement is both sensitive and specific. A method for rapid, in-house testing for urinary PBG, such as the Trace PBG kit (Trace America/Trace Diagnostics, Louisville, Colorado), can be used. Results from spot (single void) urine specimens are highly informative because very substantial increases in PBG are expected during acute attacks of porphyria. A 24-h collection can unnecessarily delay diagnosis. The same spot urine specimen should be saved for quantitative determination of ALA and

PBG, in order to confirm the qualitative PBG result and also to detect patients with ALAD-deficient porphyria. Urinary porphyrins may remain increased longer than porphyrin precursors in HCP and VP. Therefore, it is useful to measure total urinary porphyrins in the same sample, keeping in mind that urinary porphyrin increases are often nonspecific. Measurement of urinary porphyrins alone should be avoided for screening, because these may be increased in disorders other than porphyrias, such as chronic liver disease, and misdiagnoses of porphyria can result from minimal increases in urinary porphyrins that have no diagnostic significance. Measurement of erythrocyte HMB-synthase is not useful as a first-line test in the acute setting because it does not differentiate latent from active AIP. Moreover, the enzyme activity is not decreased in all AIP patients, and is never deficient in other acute porphyrias.

Cutaneous Porphyrias   Blistering skin lesions due to porphyria are virtually always accompanied by increases in total plasma porphyrins. A fluorometric method is preferred, because the porphyrins in plasma in VP are mostly covalently linked to plasma proteins and may be less readily detected by HPLC. The normal range for plasma porphyrins is somewhat increased in patients with end-stage renal disease.

Although a total plasma porphyrin determination will usually detect EPP, an erythrocyte protoporphyrin determination is more sensitive. Increases in erythrocyte protoporphyrin occur in many other conditions. Therefore, the diagnosis of EPP must be confirmed by showing a predominant increase in free protoporphyrin rather than zinc protoporphyrin. Interpretation of laboratory reports can be difficult, because the term *free erythrocyte protoporphyrin* sometimes actually represents zinc protoporphyrin.

More extensive testing is justified when an initial test is positive. A substantial increase in PBG may be due to AIP, HCP, or VP. These acute porphyrias can be distinguished by measuring erythrocyte HMB-synthase, urinary porphyrins (using the same spot urine sample), fecal porphyrins, and plasma porphyrins. Assays for COPRO-oxidase or PROTO-oxidase are not widely available. The various porphyrias that cause blistering skin lesions are differentiated by measuring porphyrins in urine, feces, and plasma. Confirmation at the DNA level by the demonstration of the causative mutation(s) is important after the diagnosis is established by biochemical testing and also permits family studies. Further details are provided in the sections below on each type of porphyria.

Testing for Subclinical Porphyria   It is often difficult to diagnose or "rule out" porphyria in patients who have had suggestive symptoms months or years in the past, and in relatives of patients with acute porphyrias, because porphyrin precursors and porphyrins may be normal. More extensive testing and consultation with a specialist laboratory and physician may be needed. Before evaluating relatives, the diagnosis of porphyria should be firmly established in an index case, and the laboratory results reviewed to guide the choice of tests for the family members. The index case or another family member with confirmed porphyria should be retested if necessary. Identification of a disease-causing mutation in an index case greatly facilitates detection of additional carriers of mutations.

THE HEPATIC PORPHYRIAS

Markedly elevated plasma and urinary concentrations of the porphyrin precursors ALA or PBG, which originate from the liver, are especially evident during attacks of neurologic manifestations of the four acute porphyrias. In PCT, excess porphyrins also accumulate initially in the liver and cause chronic blistering of sun-exposed areas of the skin.

ALA-DEHYDRATASE DEFICIENT PORPHYRIA

ADP is a rare autosomal recessive acute hepatic porphyria caused by a severe deficiency of ALA-dehydratase activity. To date, there are only a few documented cases, some in children or young adults, in which specific gene mutations have been identified. These affected homozygotes had <10% of normal ALA-dehydratase activity in erythrocytes, but their clinically asymptomatic parents and heterozygous relatives had about half-normal levels of activity and did not excrete increased levels of ALA. The frequency of ADP is unknown, but the frequency of heterozygous individuals with <50% normal ALA-dehydratase activity was ~2% in a screening study in Sweden. Because there are multiple causes for deficient ALA-dehydratase activity, it is important to confirm the diagnosis of ADP by mutation analysis.

Clinical Features   The clinical presentation depends on the amount of residual ALA-dehydratase activity. Four of the six documented patients were male adolescents with symptoms resembling those of AIP, includ-

ing abdominal pain and neuropathy. One patient was an infant with more severe disease, including failure to thrive beginning at birth. The earlier age of onset and more severe manifestations in this patient reflect a more significant deficiency of ALA-dehydratase activity. Another patient developed an acute motor polyneuropathy at age 63 that was associated with a myeloproliferative disorder. He was heterozygous for an ALAD mutation that presumably was present in erythroblasts that underwent clonal expansion due to the bone marrow malignancy.

Diagnosis   All patients had significantly elevated levels of plasma and urinary ALA, urinary coproporphyrin III and ALAD activity in erythrocytes <10% of normal. Hereditary tyrosinemia type 1 (fumarylacetoacetase deficiency) and lead intoxication should be considered in the differential diagnosis since either succinylacetone (which accumulates in hereditary tyrosinemia and is structurally similar to ALA) or lead can inhibit ALA-dehydratase, increase urinary excretion of ALA and coproporphyrin, and cause manifestations that resemble those of the acute porphyrias. Heterozygotes are clinically asymptomatic and do not excrete increased levels of ALA but can be detected by demonstration of intermediate levels of erythrocyte ALA-dehydratase activity or a specific mutation in the ALAD gene. To date, molecular studies of ADP patients have identified eight point mutations, two splice-site mutations, and a two-base deletion in the ALAD gene (Human Gene Mutation Database; www.hgmd.org). The parents in each case were not consanguineous, and the index cases had inherited a different ALAD mutation from each parent. Prenatal diagnosis of this disorder is possible by determination of ALA-dehydratase activity and/or gene mutation in cultured chorionic villi or amniocytes.

℞ ALA-DEHYDRATASE DEFICIENT PORPHYRIA

The treatment of ADP acute attacks is similar to that of AIP (see below). The severely affected infant referred to above was supported by hyperalimentation and periodic blood transfusions, but did not respond to intravenous hemin and died after liver transplantation.

ACUTE INTERMITTENT PORPHYRIA

This hepatic porphyria is an autosomal dominant condition resulting from the half-normal level of HMB-synthase activity. The disease is widespread but is especially common in Scandinavia and Great Britain. Clinical expression is highly variable, and activation of the disease is often related to environmental or hormonal factors, such as drugs, diet, and steroid hormones. Attacks can be prevented by avoiding known precipitating factors. Rare homozygous dominant AIP also has been described in children (see below).

Clinical Features   Induction of the rate-limiting hepatic enzyme ALA-synthase in heterozygotes with half-normal HMB-synthase activity is thought to underlie the acute attacks in AIP. The disorder remains latent (or asymptomatic) in the great majority of those who are heterozygous for HMB-synthase mutations, and this is almost always the case prior to puberty. In those patients with no history of acute symptoms, porphyrin precursor excretion is usually normal, suggesting that half-normal hepatic HMB-synthase activity is sufficient and hepatic ALA-synthase activity is not increased. Under conditions where heme synthesis is increased in the liver, half-normal HMB-synthase activity may become limiting, and ALA, PBG, and other heme pathway intermediates may accumulate. Common precipitating factors include endogenous and exogenous steroids, porphyrinogenic drugs, alcohol ingestion, and low-calorie diets, usually instituted for weight loss.

The fact that AIP is almost always latent before puberty suggests that adult levels of steroid hormones are important for clinical expression. Symptoms are more common in women, suggesting a role for estrogens or progestins. Premenstrual attacks are probably due to endogenous progesterone. Acute porphyrias are sometimes exacerbated by exogenous steroids, including oral contraceptive preparations containing progestins. Surprisingly, pregnancy is usually well tolerat-

TABLE 352-4 UNSAFE DRUGS IN PORPHYRIA

Documented Porphyrinogenic	Probably Porphyrinogenic		Possibly Porphyrinogenic		
Carbamazepine	Altretamine	Lidocaine	Aceclofenac	Gramicidin	Pizotifen
Carisoprodol	Aminophylline	Lopinavir	Acitretin	Guaifenesin	Polidocanol
Chloramphenicol	Amiodarone	Lutropin alfa	Acrivastine	Hydrocortisone	Polyestradiol
Clindamycin	Amitriptyline	Lymecycline	Alfuzosin	Hydroxycarbamide	phosphate
Dextropropoxyphene	Amlodipine	Meclozine	Anastrozole	Hydroxychloroquine	Potassium
Dihydralazine	Amprenavir	Medroxyprogesterone	Auranofin	Ibutilide	canrenoate
Dihydroergotamine	Aprepitant	+ estrogen	Azelastine	Imatinib	Pravastatin
Drospirenone +	Atorvastatin	Metoclopramide	Benzatropine	Indomethacin	Prednisolone
estrogen	Azathioprine	Metronidazole	Benzydamine	Ketobemidone +	Prilocaine
Dydrogesterone	Bosentan	Metyrapone	Betaxolol	DDBA	Proguanil
Etonogestrel	Bromocriptine	Moxonidine	Bicalutamide	Ketorolac	Propafenone
Fosphenytoin sodium	Buspirone	Nandrolone	Biperiden	Lamotrigine	Pseudoephedrine
Hydralazine	Busulfan	Nefazodone	Bupropion	Letrozole	+ dexbromphe-
Hydroxyzine	Butylscopolamine	Nelfinavir	Carvedilol	Levodopa +	niramine
Indinavir	Cabergoline	Nevirapine	Chlorambucil	benserazide	Quillaia extract
Ketamine	Ceftriaxone + lidocaine	Nifedipine	Chlorcyclizine +	Levonorgestrel	Quinagolide
Ketoconazole	Cerivastatin	Nimodipine	guaifenesin	intrauterine	Quinine
Lidocaine	Cetirizine	Nitrazepam	Chloroquine	Levosimendan	Quinupristin +
Lynestrenol	Cholinetheophyllinate	Norethisterone	Chlorprothixene	Linezolid	dalfopristin
Lynestrenol +	Clarithromycin	Nortriptyline	Chlorzoxazone	Lofepramine	Reboxetine
estrogen	Clemastine	Oxcarbazepine	Chorionic	Lomustine	Repaglinide
Mecillinam	Clonidine	Oxytetracycline	gonadotrophin	Malathion	Rizatriptan
Medroxyprogesterone	Cyclizine	Paclitaxel	Ciclosporin	Maprotiline	Rofecoxib
Megestrol	Cyproterone	Paroxetine	Cisapride	Mebendazole	Ropinirole
Methylergometrine	Danazol	Phenazone + caffeine	Citalopram	Mefloquine	Ropivacaine
Methyldopa	Delavirdine	Pioglitazone	Clomethiazole	Melperone	Roxithromycin
Mifepristone	Desogestrel + estrogen	Probenecid	Clomiphene	Melphalan	Sertraline
Nicotinic acid/	Diazepam	Progesterone, vaginal	Clomipramine	Mepenzolate	Sevoflurane
meclozine/	Dienogest + estrogen	gel	Clopidogrel	Mepivacaine	Sibutramine
hydroxyzine	Diclofenac	Quinidine	Clotrimazole	Mercaptopurine	Sildenafil
Nitrofurantoin	Diltiazem	Rabeprazole	Cortisone	Methadone	Sirolimus
Norethisterone	Diphenhydramine	Raloxiphene	Cyclandelate	Methylprednisolone	Sodium aurothio-
Norgestimate +	Disopyramide	Rifabutin	Cyclophosphamide	Metixene	malate
estrogen	Disulfiram	Riluzole	Cyproheptadine	Metolazone	Sodium oleate +
Orphenadrine	Drospirenone + estrogen	Risperidone	Dacarbazine	Metronidazole	chlorocymol
Phenobarbital	Dydrogesterone	Rosiglitazone	Daunorubicin	Mexiletine	Stavudine
Phenytoin	Ergoloid mesylate	Saquinavir	Desogestrel	Mianserin	Sulindac
Pivampicillin	Erythromycin	Selegiline	Dichlorobenzyl alcohol	Midazolam	Sumatriptan
Pivmecillinam	Estramustine	Simvastatin	Dithranol	Minoxidil	Tacrolimus
Primidone	Ethosuximide	Sulfasalazine	Docetaxel	Mirtazapine	Tadalafil
Rifampicin	Etoposide	Telithromycin	Donepezil	Mitomycin	Tegafur + uracil
Ritonavir	Exemestane	Terbinafine	Doxycycline	Mitoxantrone	Telmisartan
Spironolactone	Felbamate	Terfenadine	Ebastine	Moclobemide	Thioridazine
Sulfadiazine +	Felodipine	Testosterone,	Econazole	Montelukast	Thioguanine
trimethoprim	Fluconazole	transdermal patch	Efavirenz	Morphine +	Tolphenamic acid
Tamoxifen	Flunitrazepam	Tetracycline	Escitalopram	scopolamine	Tolterodine
Testosterone, inj.	Fluvastatin	Theophylline	Esomeprazole	Multivitamins	Torsemide
Thiopental	Glibenclamide	Thiamazole	Estradiol/tablets	Mupirocin	Triamcinolone
Trimethoprim	Halothane	Tibolone	Estriol/tablets	Nabumetone	Trihexyphenidyl
Valproic acid	Hyoscyamine	Ticlopidine	Estrio/vainal crème,	Nafarelin	Trimipramine
	Ifosfamide	Tinidazole	tablet	Naltrexone	Valerian
	Imipramine	Thiotepa	Estrogen, conjug.	Nateglinide	Venlafaxine
	Irinotecan	Topiramate	Finasteride	Nilutamide	Vinblastine
	Isoniazid	Topotecan	Flecainide	Noscapine	Vincristine
	Isradipine	Toremifene	Flucloxacillin	Omeprazole	Vindesine
	Itraconazole	Tramadol	Fluoxetine	Oxybutynin	Vinorelbine
	Lamivudine +	Trimegestone +	Flupentixol	Oxycodone	Xylometazoline
	zidovudine	estrogen	Flutamide	Pantoprazole	Zaleplon
	Lansoprazole	Verapamil	Fluvoxamine	Papaverine	Ziprasidone
	Lercanidipine	Voriconazole	Follitropin alfa and beta	Parecoxib	Zolmitriptan
	Levonorgestrel	Zidovudine/AZT	Galantamine	Pentifylline	Zolpidem
			Glimepiride	Pentoxyverine	Zuclopenthixol
			Glipizide	Phenylpropanola-	
			Gonadorelin	mine + cinnarizine	

Note: Based on list in "Patient's and Doctor's Guide to Medication in Acute Porphyria," Swedish Porphyria Association and Porphyria Centre, Sweden. Also see the website Drug Database for Acute Porphyrias (*www.drugs-porphyria.com*) for a searchable list of safe and unsafe drugs.

ed, suggesting that beneficial metabolic changes may ameliorate the effects of high levels of progesterone. Table 352-4 provides a partial list of the major drugs that are harmful in AIP (and also in HCP and VP). Extensive lists of unsafe and safe drugs are available on websites sponsored by the American Porphyria Foundation (*www.porphyriafounda-tion.com*) and the European Porphyria Initiative (*www.porphyria-europe.org*), and at the Drug Database for Acute Porphyrias website (*www.drugs-porphyria.com*). Reduced intake of calories and carbohydrate, as may occur with illness or attempts to lose weight, can also increase porphyrin precursor excretion and induce attacks of porphyria.

Increased carbohydrate intake can ameliorate attacks. Studies in a knockout AIP mouse model indicate that hepatic ALAS1 gene is regulated by the peroxisome proliferator–activated receptor γ coactivator 1α (PGC-1α). Hepatic PGC-1α is induced by fasting, which in turn activates ALAS1 transcription, resulting in increased heme biosynthesis. This finding suggests an important link between nutritional status and the attacks in acute porphyrias. Attacks also can be provoked by infections, surgery, and ethanol.

Because the neurovisceral symptoms rarely occur before puberty and are often nonspecific, a high index of suspicion is required to make the diagnosis. The disease can be disabling but is rarely fatal. Abdominal pain, the most common symptom, is usually steady and poorly localized but may be cramping. Ileus, abdominal distention, and decreased bowel sounds are common. However, increased bowel sounds and diarrhea may occur. Abdominal tenderness, fever, and leukocytosis are usually absent or mild because the symptoms are neurologic rather than inflammatory. Nausea; vomiting; constipation; tachycardia; hypertension; mental symptoms; pain in the limbs, head, neck, or chest; muscle weakness; sensory loss; dysuria; and urinary retention are characteristic. Tachycardia, hypertension, restlessness, tremors, and excess sweating are due to sympathetic overactivity.

The peripheral neuropathy is due to axonal degeneration (rather than demyelination) and primarily affects motor neurons. Significant neuropathy does not occur with all acute attacks; abdominal symptoms are usually more prominent. Motor neuropathy affects the proximal muscles initially, more often in the shoulders and arms. The course and degree of involvement are variable and sometimes may be focal and involve cranial nerves. Deep tendon reflexes initially may be normal or hyperactive but become decreased or absent as the neuropathy advances. Sensory changes such as paresthesia and loss of sensation are less prominent. Progression to respiratory and bulbar paralysis and death occurs especially when diagnosis and treatment are delayed. Sudden death may result from sympathetic overactivity and cardiac arrhythmia.

Mental symptoms such as anxiety, insomnia, depression, disorientation, hallucinations, and paranoia can occur in acute attacks. Seizures can be due to neurologic effects or to hyponatremia. Treatment of seizures is difficult because most antiseizure drugs can exacerbate AIP (clonazepam may be safer than phenytoin or barbiturates). Hyponatremia results from hypothalamic involvement and inappropriate vasopressin secretion or from electrolyte depletion due to vomiting, diarrhea, poor intake, or excess renal sodium loss. Persistent hypertension and impaired renal function may occur. When an attack resolves, abdominal pain may disappear within hours, and paresis begins to improve within days and may continue to improve over several years.

Homozygous dominant AIP is a rare form of AIP in which patients inherit HMBS mutations from each of their heterozygous parents and, therefore, have very low (<2%) enzyme activity. The disease has been described in a Dutch girl, two young British siblings, and a Spanish boy. In these homozygous affected patients, the disease presented in infancy with failure to thrive, developmental delay, bilateral cataracts, and/or hepatosplenomegaly. Urinary ALA and PBG concentrations were markedly elevated. All of these patients' HMBS mutations (R167W, R167Q and R172Q) were in exon 10 within five bases of each other. Studies of the brain MRIs of children with homozygous AIP have suggested damage primarily in white matter that was myelinated postnatally, while tracks that myelinated prenatally were normal. Most children with homozygous AIP die at an early age.

Diagnosis ALA and PBG levels are substantially increased in plasma and urine, especially during acute attacks, and become normal only after prolonged latency. For example, urinary PBG excretion during an attack is usually 50–200 mg/24 h (220–880 μmol/24 h) [normal, 0–4 mg/24 h, (0–18 μmol/24 h)], and urinary ALA excretion is 20–100 mg/24 h (150–760 μmol/24 h) [normal, 1–7 mg/24 h (8–53 μmol/24 h)]. Because levels often remain high after symptoms resolve, the diagnosis of an acute attack in a patient with biochemically proven AIP is based primarily on clinical features. Excretion of ALA and PBG decrease dramatically after intravenous hemin. A normal urinary PBG level before hemin effectively excludes AIP as a cause for current symptoms. Fecal porphyrins are usually normal or minimally increased in AIP, in contrast to HCP and VP. Most heterozygotes with HMB-synthase deficiency with no history of symptoms have normal urinary excretion of ALA and PBG. Therefore, measurement of HMB-synthase in erythrocytes or, better, the detection of the family's HMBS mutation will diagnose asymptomatic family members.

The enzyme deficiency is detectable in erythrocytes from most AIP heterozygotes. Because the activity is higher in young erythrocytes, it may increase into the normal range if erythropoiesis is increased due to a concurrent condition. Furthermore, patients with HMBS mutations in the initiation of translation codon in exon 1 and in the intron 1 5′-splice donor site have normal enzyme levels in erythrocytes and deficient activity only in nonerythroid tissues. This occurs because the erythroid and housekeeping forms of HMB-synthase are encoded by a single gene, which has two promoters. More than 240 HMBS mutations have been identified in AIP, including missense, nonsense, and splicing mutations and insertions and deletions, with most mutations found in only one or a few families (Human Gene Mutation Database, www.hgmd.org). The prenatal diagnosis of a fetus at risk can be made with cultured amniotic cells or chorionic villi. However, this is seldom done, because the prognosis of individuals with HMBS mutations is generally favorable.

℞ ACUTE INTERMITTENT PORPHYRIA

During acute attacks, narcotic analgesics may be required for abdominal pain, and phenothiazines are useful for nausea, vomiting, anxiety, and restlessness. Chloral hydrate can be given for insomnia, and benzodiazepines are probably safe in low doses if a minor tranquilizer is required. Carbohydrate loading, usually with intravenous glucose (at least 300 g/dL daily) may be effective in milder acute attacks of porphyria (without paresis, hyponatremia, etc.). Because intravenous hemin is more effective and the response slower if treatment is delayed, it is no longer recommended that hemin therapy for a severe attack be started only after an unsuccessful trial of intravenous glucose for several days. Hemin should be used initially for severe attacks and for mild attacks that do not respond to carbohydrate loading within 1–2 days. The standard regimen is 3–4 mg/kg of heme, in the form of lyophilized hematin (Ovation Pharmaceuticals), heme albumin (hematin reconstituted with human albumin), or heme arginate (Orphan Europe), infused daily for 4 days. Heme arginate and heme albumin are chemically stable and are less likely than hematin to produce phlebitis or an anticoagulant effect. Recovery depends on the degree of neuronal damage and usually is rapid if therapy is started early. Recovery from severe motor neuropathy may require months or years. Identification and avoidance of inciting factors can hasten recovery from an attack and prevent future attacks. Inciting factors are usually multiple, and removal of one or more hastens recovery and helps prevent future attacks. Frequent attacks that occur during the luteal phase of the menstrual cycle may be prevented with a gonadotropin-releasing hormone analogue, which prevents ovulation and progesterone production.

The long-term risk of hypertension and chronic renal disease is increased in AIP; a number of patients have undergone successful renal transplantation. Chronic, low-grade abnormalities in liver function tests are common, and the risk of hepatocellular carcinoma is increased. Hepatic imaging is recommended at least yearly for early detection of these tumors.

An allogeneic liver transplant was performed on a 19-year-old female AIP heterozygote who had 37 acute attacks in the 29 months prior to transplantation. Posttransplantation, her elevated urinary ALA and BPG levels returned to normal in 24 h, and she did not experience acute neurologic attacks for more than 18 months posttransplant. Liver transplantation is a high-risk procedure and should not be considered as an established treatment for acute porphyrias.

PORPHYRIA CUTANEA TARDA

PCT, the most common of the porphyrias, can be either sporadic (type 1) or familial (types 2 and 3) and can also develop after exposure to halogenated aromatic hydrocarbons. Hepatic URO-decarboxylase is deficient in all types of PCT, and for clinical symptoms to manifest, this enzyme deficiency must be substantial (~20% of normal activity or less); it is currently attributed to generation of an URO-decarboxylase inhibitor specifically in the liver. Generation of a URO-decarboxylase inhibitor, specifically in the liver in the presence of iron and under conditions of oxidative stress, is suspected to cause this decrease, although it remains to be isolated and characterized.

The majority of PCT patients (~80%) have no UROD mutations and are said to have sporadic (type 1) disease, or type 3 if relatives are affected. PCT patients heterozygous for UROD mutations have familial (type 2) PCT. In these patients, inheritance of a UROD mutation from one parent results in half-normal enzyme activity in liver and all other tissues, which is a significant predisposing factor but is insufficient by itself to cause symptomatic PCT. As discussed below, other genetic and environmental factors contribute to susceptibility for all types of PCT. Because penetrance of the genetic trait is low, many patients with familial PCT have no family history of the disease. Hepatoerythropoietic porphyria (HEP) is an autosomal recessive form of porphyria that results from the marked systemic deficiency of URO-decarboxylase activity with clinical symptoms in childhood.

Clinical Features   Blistering skin lesions that appear most commonly on the backs of the hands are the major clinical feature (Fig. 352-3). These rupture and crust over, leaving areas of atrophy and scarring. Lesions may also occur on the forearms, face, legs, and feet. Skin friability and small white papules termed milia are common, especially on the backs of the hands and fingers. Hypertrichosis and hyperpigmentation, especially of the face, are especially troublesome in women. Occasionally, the skin over sun-exposed areas becomes severely thickened, with scarring and calcification that resembles systemic sclerosis. Neurologic features are absent.

A number of susceptibility factors, in addition to inherited UROD mutations in type 2 PCT, can be recognized clinically and can affect management. These include hepatitis C, HIV, excess alcohol, elevated iron levels, and estrogens. The importance of excess hepatic iron as a precipitating factor is underscored by the finding that the incidence of the common hemochromatosis-causing mutations, hemochromatosis gene (HFE) mutations C282Y and H63D, are increased in patients with types 1 and 2 PCT (Chap. 351). Excess alcohol is a long-recognized contributor, as is estrogen use in women. HIV is probably an independent but less common risk factor that, like hepatitis C, does not occur in isolation. Multiple susceptibility factors that appear to act synergistically can be identified in the individual patient with PCT. Patients with PCT characteristically have chronic liver disease and sometimes cirrhosis and are at risk for hepatocellular carcinoma. Various chemicals can also induce PCT; an epidemic of PCT occurred in east-

ern Turkey in the 1950s as a consequence of wheat contaminated with the fungicide hexachlorobenzene. PCT also occurs after exposure to other chemicals, including di- and trichlorophenols and 2,3,7,8-tetra-chlorodibenzo-(p)-dioxin (TCDD, dioxin).

Diagnosis   Porphyrins are increased in the liver, plasma, urine, and stool. The urinary ALA level may be slightly increased, but the PBG level is normal. Urinary porphyrins consist mostly of uroporphyrin and heptacarboxylate porphyrin, with lesser amounts of coproporphyrin and hexa- and pentacarboxylate porphyrins. Plasma porphyrins are also increased, and fluorometric scanning of diluted plasma at neutral pH can rapidly distinguish VP and PCT (Table 352-3). Isocoproporphyrins, which are increased in feces and sometimes in plasma and urine, are diagnostic for hepatic URO-decarboxylase deficiency.

Type 2 PCT and HEP can be distinguished from types 1 and 3 by finding decreased URO-decarboxylase in erythrocytes. URO-decarboxylase activity in liver, erythrocytes, and cultured skin fibroblasts in type 2 PCT is approximately 50% of normal in affected individuals and in family members with latent disease. In HEP, the UROD activity is markedly deficient, with typical levels of 3–10% of normal. Over 65 mutations have been identified in the UROD gene (Human Gene Mutation Database; *www.hgmd.org*). Of the mutations listed in the Human Gene Mutation Database, 57.4% are missense, 0.7% nonsense and 13.1% are splice-site mutations. Most UROD mutations have been identified in only one or two families.

Rx PORPHYRIA CUTANEA TARDA

Alcohol, estrogens, iron supplements, and, if possible, any drugs that may exacerbate the disease should be discontinued, but this step does not always lead to improvement. A complete response can almost always be achieved by the standard therapy, repeated phlebotomy, to reduce hepatic iron. A unit (450 mL) of blood can be removed every 1–2 weeks. The aim is to gradually reduce excess hepatic iron until the serum ferritin reaches the lower limits of normal. Because iron overload is not marked in most cases, remission may occur after only five or six phlebotomies; however, PCT patients with hemochromatosis may require more treatments to bring their iron levels down to the normal range. To document improvement in PCT, it is most convenient to follow the total plasma porphyrin concentration, which becomes normal some time after the target ferritin level is reached. Hemoglobin levels or hematocrits and serum ferritin should be followed closely to prevent development of iron deficiency and anemia. After remission, continued phlebotomy may not be needed. Plasma porphyrin levels are followed at 6–12 month intervals for early detection of recurrences, which are treated by additional phlebotomy.

An alternative when phlebotomy is contraindicated or poorly tolerated is a low-dose regimen of chloroquine or hydroxychloroquine, both of which complex with the excess porphyrins and promote their excretion. Small doses (e.g., 125 mg chloroquine phosphate twice weekly) should be given, because standard doses can induce transient, sometimes marked increases in photosensitivity and hepatocellular damage. Hepatic imaging can diagnose or exclude complicating hepatocellular carcinoma. Treatment of PCT in patients with end-stage renal disease is facilitated by administration of erythropoietin.

HEREDITARY COPROPORPHYRIA

HCP is an autosomal dominant hepatic porphyria that results from the half-normal activity of COPRO-oxidase. The disease presents with acute attacks, as in AIP. Cutaneous photosensitivity also may occur, but much less commonly than in VP. HCP patients may have acute attacks and cutaneous photosensitivity together or separately. HCP is less common than AIP and VP. Homozygous dominant HCP and harderoporphyria, a biochemically distinguishable variant of HCP, present with clinical symptoms in children (see below).

Clinical Features   HCP is influenced by the same factors that cause attacks in AIP. The disease is latent before puberty, and symptoms, which are virtually identical to those of AIP, are more common in women. HCP is generally less severe than AIP. Blistering skin lesions

FIGURE 352-3 Typical cutaneous lesions in a patient with porphyria cutanea tarda. Chronic, crusted lesions resulting from blistering due to photosensitivity are on the dorsum of the hand of a PCT patient. *(Courtesy of Dr. Karl E. Anderson; with permission.)*

are identical to PCT and VP and begin in childhood in rare homozygous cases.

Diagnosis COPRO III is markedly increased in the urine and feces in symptomatic disease and often persists, especially in feces, when there are no symptoms. Urinary ALA and PBG levels are increased (but less than in AIP) during acute attacks but may revert to normal more quickly than in AIP when symptoms resolve. Plasma porphyrins are usually normal or only slightly increased, but they may be higher in cases with skin lesions. The diagnosis of HCP is readily confirmed by increased fecal porphyrins consisting almost entirely of COPRO III, which distinguishes it from other porphyrias. An increase in the fecal COPRO III/COPRO I ratio is useful for detecting latent cases.

Although the diagnosis can be confirmed by measuring COPRO-oxidase activity, the assays for this mitochondrial enzyme are not widely available and require cells other than erythrocytes. The CPOX gene has been cloned and over 35 mutations, two-thirds of which are missense, have been identified in unrelated patients (Human Gene Mutation Database; *www.hgmd.org*).

℞ HEREDITARY COPROPORPHYRIA

Neurologic symptoms are treated as in AIP (see above). Phlebotomy and chloroquine are ineffective when cutaneous lesions are present.

VARIEGATE PORPHYRIA

VP is an autosomal dominant hepatic porphyria that results from the deficient activity of PROTO-oxidase, the seventh enzyme in the heme pathway, and can present with neurologic symptoms, photosensitivity, or both. VP is particularly common in South Africa, where 3 of every 1000 whites have the disorder. Most are descendants of a couple who emigrated from Holland to South Africa in 1688. In other countries, VP is less common than AIP. Rare cases of homozygous dominant VP, presenting in childhood with cutaneous symptoms, have also been reported.

Clinical Features VP can present with skin photosensitivity, acute neurovisceral crises, or both. In two large studies of VP patients, 59% had only skin lesions, 20% had only acute attacks, and 22% had both. Acute attacks are identical to those in AIP and are precipitated by the same factors as AIP (see above). Blistering skin manifestations are similar to those in PCT but are more difficult to treat and usually are of longer duration. Homozygous VP is associated with photosensitivity, neurologic symptoms, and developmental disturbances, including growth retardation, in infancy or childhood; all cases had increased erythrocyte levels of zinc protoporphyrin, a characteristic finding in all homozygous porphyrias so far described.

Diagnosis Urinary ALA and PBG levels are increased during acute attacks but may return to normal more quickly than in AIP. Increases in fecal protoporphyrin and COPRO III and in urinary COPRO III are more persistent. Plasma porphyrin levels also are increased, particularly when there are cutaneous lesions. VP can be distinguished rapidly from all other porphyrias by examining the fluorescence emission spectrum of porphyrins in plasma at neutral pH since VP has a unique fluorescence peak at neutral pH.

Assays of PROTO-oxidase activity in cultured fibroblasts or lymphocytes are not widely available. One hundred thirty mutations have been identified in PPOX gene from unrelated VP patients (Human Gene Mutation Database; *www.hgmd.org*). The missense mutation R59W is the common mutation in most South Africans with VP of Dutch descent. Five missense mutations were common in English and French VP patients; however, most mutations have been found in only one or two families.

℞ VARIEGATE PORPHYRIA

Acute attacks are treated as in AIP, and hemin should be started early in most cases. Other than avoiding sun exposure, there are few effective measures for treating the skin lesions. β-Carotene, phlebotomy, and chloroquine are not helpful.

THE ERYTHROPOIETIC PORPHYRIAS

In the erythropoietic porphyrias, excess porphyrins from bone marrow erythrocyte precursors are transported via the plasma to the skin and lead to cutaneous photosensitivity.

X-LINKED SIDEROBLASTIC ANEMIA

XLSA results from the deficient activity of the erythroid form of ALA-synthase and is associated with ineffective erythropoiesis, weakness, and pallor.

Clinical Features Typically, males with XLSA develop refractory hemolytic anemia, pallor, and weakness during infancy. They have secondary hypersplenism, become iron overloaded, and can develop hemosiderosis. The severity depends on the level of residual erythroid ALA-synthase activity and on the responsiveness of the specific mutation to pyridoxal 5′-phosphate supplementation (see below). Peripheral blood smears reveal a hypochromic, microcytic anemia with striking anisocytosis, poikilocytosis, and polychromasia; the leukocytes and platelets appear normal. Hemoglobin content is reduced, and the mean corpuscular volume and mean corpuscular hemoglobin concentration are decreased. Patients with milder, late-onset disease have been reported recently.

Diagnosis Bone marrow examination reveals hypercellularity with a left shift and megaloblastic erythropoiesis with an abnormal maturation. A variety of Prussian blue–staining sideroblasts are observed. Levels of urinary porphyrin precursors and of both urinary and fecal porphyrins are normal. The level of erythroid ALA-synthase is decreased in bone marrow, but this enzyme is difficult to measure in the presence of the normal ALA-synthase housekeeping enzyme. Definitive diagnosis requires the demonstration of mutations in the erythroid ALAS gene.

℞ X-LINKED SIDEROBLASTIC ANEMIA

The severe anemia may respond to pyridoxine supplementation. This cofactor is essential for ALA-synthase activity, and mutations in the pyridoxine binding site of the enzyme have been found in several responsive patients. Cofactor supplementation may make it possible to eliminate or reduce the frequency of transfusion. Unresponsive patients may be transfusion-dependent and require chelation therapy.

CONGENITAL ERYTHROPOIETIC PORPHYRIA

CEP, also known as Günther disease, is an autosomal recessive disorder. It is due to the markedly deficient, but not absent, activity of URO-synthase and the resultant accumulation of uroporphyrin I and coproporphyrin I isomers. CEP is associated with hemolytic anemia and cutaneous lesions.

Clinical Features Severe cutaneous photosensitivity begins in early infancy. The skin over light-exposed areas is friable, and bullae and vesicles are prone to rupture and infection. Skin thickening, focal hypo- and hyperpigmentation, and hypertrichosis of the face and extremities are characteristic. Secondary infection of the cutaneous lesions can lead to disfigurement of the face and hands. Porphyrins are deposited in teeth and in bones. As a result, the teeth are reddish-brown and fluoresce on exposure to long-wave ultraviolet light. Hemolysis is probably due to the marked increase in erythrocyte porphyrins and leads to splenomegaly. Adults with a milder form of the disease also have been described.

Diagnosis Uroporphyrin and coproporphyrin (mostly type I isomers) accumulate in the bone marrow, erythrocytes, plasma, urine, and feces.

The predominant porphyrin in feces is coproporphyrin I. The diagnosis of CEP can be confirmed by demonstration of markedly deficient URO-synthase activity and/or the identification of specific mutations in the UROS gene. The disease can be detected in utero by measuring porphyrins in amniotic fluid and URO-synthase activity in cultured amniotic cells or chorionic villi, or by the detection of the family's specific gene mutations. Molecular analyses of the mutant alleles from over 50 unrelated patients have revealed the presence of 35 mutations in the UROS gene, including four in the erythroid-specific promoter of the UROS gene. Genotype/phenotype correlations are seen in CEP.

℞ CONGENITAL ERYTHROPOIETIC PORPHYRIA

Severe cases often require transfusions for anemia. Chronic transfusions of sufficient blood to suppress erythropoiesis are effective in reducing porphyrin production but results in iron overload. Splenectomy may reduce hemolysis and decrease transfusion requirements. Protection from sunlight and from minor skin trauma is important. β-Carotene may be of some value. Complicating bacterial infections should be treated promptly. Recently, bone marrow and cord blood transplantation has proven effective in several transfusion-dependent children, providing the rationale for stem-cell gene therapy.

ERYTHROPOIETIC PROTOPORPHYRIA

EPP is an inherited disorder resulting from the partial deficiency of ferrochelatase activity, the last enzyme in the heme biosynthetic pathway. EPP is the most common erythropoietic porphyria in children and, after PCT, the second most common porphyria in adults. EPP patients have ferrochelatase activities as low as 15–25% in lymphocytes and cultured fibroblasts. Protoporphyrin accumulates in bone marrow reticulocytes and then appears in plasma, is taken up in the liver, and excreted in bile and feces. Protoporphyrins transported to the skin causes nonblistering photosensitivity. In most symptomatic patients (~90%), a disabling (i.e., causative) mutation in one FECH allele is combined with a relatively common (~10% normal Caucasians) intronic 3 (IVS3) single nucleotide alteration (IVS3-48T→C) in the normal allele, which results in decreased amounts of the normal enzyme. In a few families, two FECH mutations and a pattern of autosomal recessive inheritance has been found.

Clinical Features Skin photosensitivity, which differs from that in other porphyrias, usually begins in childhood and consists of pain, redness, and itching occurring within minutes of sunlight exposure (Fig. 352-4). Photosensitivity is associated with substantial elevations in erythrocyte protoporphyrin and occurs only in patients with genotypes that result in ferrochelatase activities below ~35% of normal. Vesicular lesions are uncommon. Redness, swelling, burning, and itching can develop shortly after sun exposure and resemble angioedema. Symptoms may seem out of proportion to the visible skin lesions. Sparse vesicles and bullae occur in 10% of cases. Chronic skin changes may include lichenification, leathery pseudovesicles, labial grooving, and nail changes. Severe scarring is rare, as are pigment changes, friability, and hirsutism. Unless hepatic or other complications develop, protoporphyrin levels and symptoms of photosensitivity remain remarkably stable over many years in most patients. Factors that exacerbate hepatic porphyrias play little or no role in EPP.

The primary source of excess protoporphyrin is the bone marrow reticulocytes. Erythrocyte protoporphyrin is free (not complexed with zinc) and is mostly bound to hemoglobin. In plasma, protoporphyrin is bound to albumin. Hemolysis and anemia are usually absent or mild.

Although EPP is an erythropoietic porphyria, up to 20% of EPP patients may have minor abnormalities of liver function, and in about 5% of these patients the accumulation of protoporphyrins causes chronic liver disease that can progress to liver failure and death. Protoporphyrin is insoluble, and excess amounts form crystalline structures in liver cells (Fig. 352-4) and can decrease hepatic bile flow. Studies in the mouse model of EPP have shown that the bile duct epithelium may be damaged by toxic bile, leading to biliary fibrosis. Thus, rapidly progressive liver

FIGURE 352-4 **Erythema and edema of the hands** due to acute photosensitivity in a 10-year-old boy with erythropoietic protoporphyria. *(From P Poblette-Gutierrez et al.)*

disease appears to be related to the cholestatic effects of protoporphyrins and is associated with increasing hepatic protoporphyrin levels due to impaired hepatobiliary excretion and increased photosensitivity. The hepatic complications are also often characterized by increasing levels of protoporphyrins in erythrocytes and plasma as well as severe abdominal and back pains, especially in the right upper quadrant. Gallstones composed at least in part of protoporphyrin occur in some patients.

Diagnosis A substantial increase in erythrocyte protoporphyrin, which is predominantly free and not complexed with zinc, is the hallmark of this disease. Protoporphyrin levels are also variably increased in bone marrow, plasma, bile, and feces. Erythrocyte protoporphyrin concentrations are increased in other conditions such as lead poisoning, iron deficiency, various hemolytic disorders, all homozygous forms of porphyria, and sometimes even in acute porphyrias. In all these conditions, however, in contrast to EPP, protoporphyrin is complexed with zinc. Therefore, after an increase in erythrocyte protoporphyrin is found in a suspected EPP patient, it is important to confirm the diagnosis by an assay that distinguishes free and zinc-complexed protoporphyrin. Erythrocytes in EPP also exhibit red fluorescence under a fluorescence microscopy at 620 nm. Urinary levels of porphyrins and porphyrin precursors are normal. Ferrochelatase activity in cultured lymphocytes or fibroblasts is decreased. DNA diagnosis by mutation analysis is recommended to detect the causative FECH mutation and the presence of the IVS3-48T→C alteration in the normal coding allele. To date, over 90 mutations have been identified in the FECH gene, many of which result in an unstable or absent enzyme protein (null alleles) (Human Gene Mutation Database; *www.hgmd.org*). Studies suggest that EPP patients with a null allele (and the IVS3-48T→C polymorphism) have a great risk for developing severe liver complications.

℞ ERYTHROPOIETIC PROTOPORPHYRIA

Avoiding sunlight exposure and wearing clothing designed to provide protection for conditions with chronic photosensitivity are essential. Oral β-carotene (120–180 mg/dL) improves tolerance to sunlight in many patients. The dosage may need to be adjusted to maintain serum carotene levels in the recommended range of 10–15 mmol/L (600–800 mg/dL). Mild skin discoloration due to carotenemia is the only significant side effect. The beneficial effects of β-carotene may involve quenching of singlet oxygen or free radicals.

Treatment of hepatic complications, which may be accompanied by motor neuropathy, is difficult. Cholestyramine and other porphyrin absorbents such as activated charcoal may interrupt the enterohepatic circulation of protoporphyrin and promote its fecal excretion, leading to some improvement. Splenectomy may be helpful when the disease is accompanied by hemolysis and significant splenomegaly. Plasmapheresis and intravenous hemin are sometimes beneficial.

Liver transplantation has been carried out in some EPP patients with severe liver complications and is often successful in the short term. However liver disease often recurs in the transplanted liver due to continued bone marrow production of excess protoporphyrin. In a retrospective study of 17 liver-transplanted EPP patients, 11 (65%) had recurrent EPP liver disease. Posttransplantation treatment with hematin and plasmapheresis should be considered to prevent the recurrence of liver disease. Bone marrow transplantation, which has been successful in human EPP and prevents liver disease in a mouse model, should be considered after the liver transplantation, if a suitable donor can be found.

ACKNOWLEDGMENT

The authors thank Dr. Karl E. Anderson for his review of the manuscript and helpful comments and suggestions.

FURTHER READINGS

ANDERSON KE et al: Recommendations for the diagnosis and treatment of the acute porphyrias. Ann Intern Med 142:439, 2005

ANDERSON KE et al: Disorders of heme biosynthesis: X-linked sideroblastic anemia and the porphyrias, in *The Metabolic and Molecular Bases of Inherited Diseases*, Scriver CR et al (eds). McGraw-Hill: New York, 2991–3062, 2001. *www.genetics.accessmedicine.com*

BISHOP DF et al: Uroporphyrinogen III synthase knock-in mice have the human congenital erythropoietic porphyria phenotype, including the characteristic light-induced cutaneous lesions. Am J Hum Genet 78:645, 2006

HANDSCHIN C et al: Nutritional regulation of hepatic heme biosynthesis and porphyria through PCG-1α. Cell 122:505, 2005

KAUPPINEN R: Porphyrias. Lancet 365:241, 2005

POBLETTE-GUTIERREZ P et al: The porphyrias: Clinical diagnosis and treatment. Eur J Dermatol 16:230, 2006

353 Disorders of Purine and Pyrimidine Metabolism
Robert L. Wortmann

Purines (adenine and guanine) and pyrimidines (cytosine, thymine, uracil) serve fundamental roles in the replication of genetic material, gene transcription, protein synthesis, and cellular metabolism. Disorders that involve abnormalities of nucleotide metabolism range from relatively common diseases such as hyperuricemia and gout, in which there is increased production or impaired excretion of a metabolic end product of purine metabolism (uric acid), to rare enzyme deficiencies that affect purine and pyrimidine synthesis or degradation. Understanding these biochemical pathways has led, in some instances, to the development of specific forms of treatment, such as the use of allopurinol to reduce uric acid production.

URIC ACID METABOLISM

Uric acid is the final breakdown product of purine degradation in humans. It is a weak acid with pK_as of 5.75 and 10.3. Urates, the ionized forms of uric acid, predominate in plasma extracellular fluid and synovial fluid, with ~98% existing as monosodium urate at pH 7.4.

Plasma is saturated with monosodium urate at a concentration of 415 μmol/L (6.8 mg/dL) at 37°C. At higher concentrations, plasma is therefore supersaturated, creating the potential for urate crystal precipitation. However, plasma urate concentrations can reach 4800 μmol/L (80 mg/dL) without precipitation, perhaps because of the presence of solubilizing substances.

The pH of urine greatly influences the solubility of uric acid. At pH 5.0, urine is saturated with uric acid at concentrations ranging from 360–900 μmol/L (6–15 mg/dL). At pH 7.0, saturation is reached at concentrations between 9480 and 12,000 μmol/L (158 and 200 mg/dL). Ionized forms of uric acid in urine include mono- and disodium, potassium, ammonium, and calcium urates.

Although purine nucleotides are synthesized and degraded in all tissues, urate is produced only in tissues that contain xanthine oxidase, primarily the liver and small intestine. Urate production varies with the purine content of the diet and the rates of purine biosynthesis, degradation, and salvage (Fig. 353-1). Normally, two-thirds to three-fourths of urate is excreted by the kidneys, and most of the remainder is eliminated through the intestines.

The kidneys clear urate from the plasma and maintain physiologic balance by utilizing specific organic anion transporters (OATs) including urate transporter 1 (URAT1) and human uric acid transporter (hUAT) (Fig. 353-2). URAT1 and other OATs carry urate into the tubular cells from the apical side of the lumen. Once inside the cell,

FIGURE 353-1 The total-body urate pool is the net result between urate production and excretion. Urate production is influenced by dietary intake of purines and the rates of de novo biosynthesis of purines from nonpurine precursors, nucleic acid turnover, and salvage by phosphoribosyltransferase activities. The formed urate is normally excreted by urinary and intestinal routes. Hyperuricemia can result from increased production, decreased excretion, or a combination of both mechanisms. When hyperuricemia exists, urate can precipitate and deposit in tissues as tophi.

urate must pass to the basolateral side of the lumen in a process controlled by the voltage-dependent carrier hUAT. Until recently, a four-component model has been used to describe the renal handling of urate/uric acid: (1) glomerular filtration, (2) tubular reabsorption, (3) secretion, and (4) postsecretory reabsorption. Although these processes have been considered sequential, it is now apparent that they are carried out in parallel by these transporters. URAT1 is a novel transporter expressed at the apical brush border of the proximal nephron. Uricosuric compounds (Table 353-1) directly inhibit URAT1 on the apical side of the tubular cell (so-called *cis*-inhibition). In contrast, antiuricosuric compounds (those that promote hyperuricemia), such as nicotinate, pyrazinoate, lactate, and other aromatic organic acids, serve as the exchange anion inside the cell, thereby stimulating anion exchange and urate reabsorption (*trans*-stimulation). The activities of URAT1, other OATs, and sodium anion transporter result in 8–12% of the filtered urate being executed as uric acid.

Most children have serum urate concentrations of 180–240 μmol/L (3.0–4.0 mg/dL). Levels begin to rise in males during puberty but remain low in females until menopause. Mean serum urate values of adult men and premenopausal women are 415 and 360 μmol/L (6.8 and 6.0 mg/dL), respectively. After menopause, values for women increase to approximate those of men. In adulthood, concentrations rise

FIGURE 353-2 Schematic for handling of uric acid by the kidney. Organic anion transporters (OATs) including urate transporter 1 (URAT1) carry uric acid into the tubular cell. Uricosuric compounds inhibit URAT1 on the apical side of the tubular cell.

steadily over time and vary with height, body weight, blood pressure, renal function, and alcohol intake.

HYPERURICEMIA

Hyperuricemia can result from increased production or decreased excretion of uric acid or from a combination of the two processes. Sustained hyperuricemia predisposes some individuals to develop clinical manifestations including gouty arthritis (Chap. 327), urolithiasis, and renal dysfunction (see below).

Hyperuricemia is defined as a plasma (or serum) urate concentration >408 μmol/L (6.8 mg/dL). The risk of developing gouty arthritis or urolithiasis increases with higher urate levels and escalates in proportion to the degree of elevation. Hyperuricemia is present in between 2.0 and 13.2% of ambulatory adults and is even more frequent in hospitalized individuals.

CAUSES OF HYPERURICEMIA
Hyperuricemia may be classified as primary or secondary depending on whether the cause is innate or is the result of an acquired disorder.

TABLE 353-1	MEDICATIONS WITH URICOSURIC ACTIVITY
Acetohexamide	Glyceryl guaiacolate
ACTH	Glycopyrrolate
Ascorbic acid	Halofenate
Azauridine	Losartan
Benzbromarone	Meclofenamate
Calcitonin	Phenolsulfonphthalein
Chlorprothixene	Phenylbutazone
Citrate	Probenecid
Dicumarol	Radiographic contrast agents
Diflunisal	Salicylates (>2 g/2d)
Estrogens	Sulfinpyrazone
Fenofibrate	Tetracycline that is outdated
Glucocorticoids	Zoxazolamine

TABLE 353-2	CLASSIFICATION OF HYPERURICEMIA BY PATHOPHYSIOLOGY

Urate Overproduction

Primary idiopathic	Myeloproliferative	Rhabdomyolysis
HPRT deficiency	diseases	Exercise
PRPP synthetase	Polycythemia vera	Alcohol
overactivity	Psoriasis	Obesity
Hemolytic processes	Paget's disease	Purine-rich diet
Lymphoproliferative	Glycogenosis III, V, and	
diseases	VII	

Decreased Uric Acid Excretion

Primary idiopathic	Starvation ketosis	Drug ingestion
Renal insufficiency	Berylliosis	Salicylates (>2 g/d)
Polycystic kidney	Sarcoidosis	Diuretics
disease	Lead intoxication	Alcohol
Diabetes insipidus	Hyperparathyroidism	Levodopa
Hypertension	Hypothyroidism	Ethambutol
Acidosis	Toxemia of pregnancy	Pyrazinamide
Lactic acidosis	Bartter's syndrome	Nicotinic acid
Diabetic ketoacidosis	Down syndrome	Cyclosporine

Combined Mechanism

Glucose-6-phosphatase	Fructose-1-phosphate	Alcohol
deficiency	aldolase deficiency	Shock

Note: HPRT, hypoxanthine phosphoribosyltransferase; PRPP, phosphoribosylpyrophosphate.

However, it is more useful to classify hyperuricemia in relation to the underlying pathophysiology, i.e., whether it results from increased production, decreased excretion, or a combination of the two (Fig. 353-1, Table 353-2).

Increased Urate Production Diet contributes to the serum urate in proportion to its purine content. Strict restriction of purine intake reduces the mean serum urate level by about 60 μmol/L (1.0 mg/dL) and urinary uric acid excretion by ~1.2 mmol/d (200 mg/d). Foods high in nucleic acid content include liver, "sweetbreads" (i.e., thymus and pancreas), kidney, and anchovy.

Endogenous sources of purine production also influence the serum urate level (Fig. 353-3). De novo purine biosynthesis is an 11-step process that forms inosine monophosphate (IMP). The rates of purine biosynthesis and urate production are determined, for the most part, by amidophosphoribosyltransferase (amidoPRT), which combines phosphoribosylpyrophosphate (PRPP) and glutamine. A secondary regulatory pathway is the salvage of purine bases by hypoxanthine phosphoribosyltransferase (HPRT). HPRT catalyzes the combination of the purine bases hypoxanthine and guanine with PRPP to form the respective ribonucleotides IMP and guanosine monophosphate (GMP).

Serum urate levels are closely coupled to the rates of de novo purine biosynthesis, which is driven in part by the level of PRPP, as evidenced by two X-linked inborn errors of purine metabolism. Both increased PRPP synthetase activity and HPRT deficiency are associated with overproduction of purines, hyperuricemia, and hyperuricaciduria (see below for clinical descriptions).

Accelerated purine nucleotide degradation can also cause hyperuricemia, i.e., with conditions of rapid cell turnover, proliferation, or cell death, as in leukemic blast crises, cytotoxic therapy for malignancy, hemolysis, or rhabdomyolysis. Hyperuricemia can result from excessive degradation of skeletal muscle ATP after strenuous physical exercise or status epilepticus and in glycogen storage diseases types III, V, and VII (Chap. 356). The hyperuricemia of myocardial infarction, smoke inhalation, and acute respiratory failure may also be related to accelerated breakdown of ATP.

Decreased Uric Acid Excretion Over 90% of individuals with sustained hyperuricemia have a defect in the renal handling of uric acid. Gouty individuals excrete ~40% less uric acid than nongouty individuals for

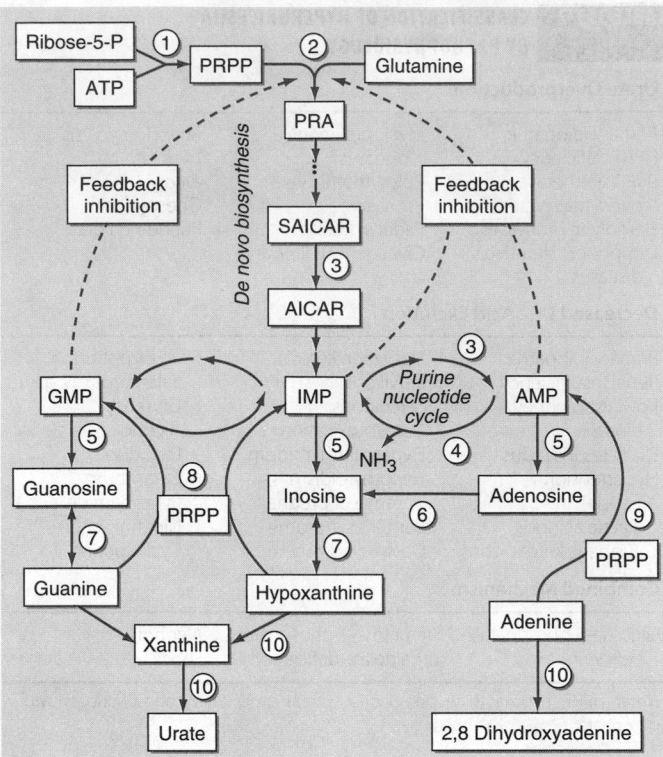

FIGURE 353-3 Abbreviated scheme of purine metabolism. (1) Phosphoribosylpyrophosphate (PRPP) synthetase, (2) amidophosphoribosyltransferase (amidoPRT), (3) adenylosuccinate lyase, (4) (myo-)adenylate (AMP) deaminase, (5) 5'-nucleotidase, (6) adenosine deaminase, (7) purine nucleoside phosphorylase, (8) hypoxanthine phosphoribosyltransferase (HPRT), (9) adenine phosphoribosyltransferase (APRT), and (10) xanthine oxidase. PRA, phosphoribosylamine; SAICAR, succinylaminoimidazole carboxamide ribotide; AICAR, aminoimidazole carboxamide ribotide; GMP, guanylate; IMP, inosine monophosphate.

any given plasma urate concentration. Uric acid excretion increases in gouty and nongouty individuals when plasma urate levels are raised by purine ingestion or infusion, but in those with gout, plasma urate concentrations must be 60–120 μmol/L (1–2 mg/dL) higher than normal to achieve equivalent uric acid excretion rates.

Altered uric acid excretion could theoretically result from decreased glomerular filtration, decreased tubular secretion, or enhanced tubular reabsorption. Decreased urate filtration does not appear to cause primary hyperuricemia but does contribute to the hyperuricemia of renal insufficiency. Although hyperuricemia is invariably present in chronic renal disease, the correlation between serum creatinine, urea nitrogen, and urate concentration is poor. Uric acid excretion per unit of glomerular filtration rate increases progressively with chronic renal insufficiency, but tubular secretory capacity tends to be preserved, tubular reabsorptive capacity is reduced, and extrarenal clearance of uric acid increases as renal damage becomes more severe.

Many agents that cause hyperuricemia exert their effects by stimulating reabsorption rather than inhibiting secretion. This appears to occur through a process of "priming" renal urate reabsorption through the sodium-dependent loading of proximal tubular epithelial cells with anions capable of *trans*-stimulating urate reabsorption. A transporter in the brush border of the proximal tubular cells mediates sodium-dependent resorption of components recognized to cause hyperuricemia by renal mechanisms. These include pyrazinoate (from pyrazinamide treatment), nicotinate (from niacin therapy), and the organic acids lactate, β-hydroxybutyrate, and acetoacetate. These monovalent anions are also substrates for URAT1. Thus, increased blood levels of these substances result in their increased glomerular filtration and greater reabsorption by proximal tubular cells. The increased intraepithelial cell concentrations lead to increased reabsorption of

urate by promoting URAT1-dependent anion exchange. Low doses of salicylates also promote hyperuricemia by this mechanism. In addition, sodium loading of proximal tubular cells stimulates brush border urate exchange, explaining urate retention provoked by reduced extracellular fluid volume and states of angiotensin II, insulin, and parathyroid hormone excess.

Alcohol promotes hyperuricemia because of increased urate production and decreased uric acid excretion. Excessive alcohol consumption accelerates hepatic breakdown of ATP to increase urate production. Alcohol consumption can also induce hyperlacticacidemia, which blocks uric acid secretion. The higher purine content in some alcoholic beverages such as beer may also be a factor.

EVALUATION

Hyperuricemia does not necessarily represent a disease, nor is it a specific indication for therapy. The decision to treat depends on the cause and the potential consequences of the hyperuricemia in each individual.

Quantification of uric acid excretion can be used to determine whether hyperuricemia is caused by overproduction or decreased excretion. On a purine-free diet, men with normal renal function excrete <3.6 mmol/d (600 mg/d). Thus, the hyperuricemia of individuals who excrete uric acid above this level while on a purine-free diet is due to purine overproduction; for those who excrete lower amounts on the purine-free diet, it is due to decreased excretion. If the assessment is performed while the patient is on a regular diet, the level of 4.2 mmol/d (800 mg/d) can be used as the discriminating value.

COMPLICATIONS

The most recognized complication of hyperuricemia is *gouty arthritis*. In the general population the prevalence of hyperuricemia ranges between 2.0 and 13.2%, and the prevalence of gout is between 1.3 and 3.7%. The higher the serum urate level, the more likely an individual is to develop gout. In one study, the incidence of gout was 4.9% for individuals with serum urate concentrations >540 μmol/L (9.0 mg/dL) compared with 0.5% for those with values between 415 and 535 μmol/L (7.0 and 8.9 mg/dL). The complications of gout correlate with both the duration and severity of hyperuricemia. **For further discussion of gout, see Chap. 327.**

Hyperuricemia also causes several renal problems: (1) nephrolithiasis; (2) urate nephropathy, a rare cause of renal insufficiency attributed to monosodium urate crystal deposition in the renal interstitium; and (3) uric acid nephropathy, a reversible cause of acute renal failure resulting from deposition of large amounts of uric acid crystals in the renal collecting ducts, pelvis, and ureters.

Nephrolithiasis Uric acid nephrolithiasis occurs most commonly, but not exclusively, in individuals with gout. In gout, the prevalence of nephrolithiasis correlates with the serum and urinary uric acid levels, reaching ~50% with serum urate levels of 770 μmol/L (13 mg/dL) or urinary uric acid excretion >6.5 mmol/d (1100 mg/d).

Uric acid stones can develop in individuals with no evidence of arthritis, only 20% of whom are hyperuricemic. Uric acid can also play a role in other types of kidney stones. Some nongouty individuals with calcium oxalate or calcium phosphate stones have hyperuricemia or hyperuricaciduria. Uric acid may act as a nidus on which calcium oxalate can precipitate or lower the formation product for calcium oxalate crystallization.

Urate Nephropathy Urate nephropathy, sometimes referred to as *urate nephrosis*, is a late manifestation of severe gout and is characterized histologically by deposits of monosodium urate crystals surrounded by a giant cell inflammatory reaction in the medullary interstitium and pyramids. The disorder is now rare and cannot be diagnosed in the absence of gouty arthritis. The lesions may be clinically silent or cause proteinuria, hypertension, and renal insufficiency.

Uric Acid Nephropathy This reversible cause of acute renal failure is due to precipitation of uric acid in renal tubules and collecting ducts that causes obstruction to urine flow. Uric acid nephropathy develops following sudden urate overproduction and marked hyperuricaciduria. Factors that favor uric acid crystal formation include dehydration and acidosis. This form of acute renal failure occurs most often during an aggressive "blastic" phase of leukemia or lymphoma prior to or coincident with cytolytic therapy but has also been observed in individuals with other neoplasms, following epileptic seizures, and after vigorous exercise with heat stress. Autopsy studies have demonstrated intraluminal precipitates of uric acid, dilated proximal tubules, and normal glomeruli. The initial pathogenic events are believed to include obstruction of collecting ducts with uric acid and obstruction of distal renal vasculature.

If recognized, uric acid nephropathy is potentially reversible. Appropriate therapy has reduced the mortality from about 50% to practically nil. Serum levels cannot be relied on for diagnosis because this condition has developed in the presence of urate concentrations varying from 720 to 4800 μmol/L (12 to 80 mg/dL). The distinctive feature is the urinary uric acid concentration. In most forms of acute renal failure with decreased urine output, urinary uric acid content is either normal or reduced, and the ratio of uric acid to creatinine is <1. In acute uric acid nephropathy the ratio of uric acid to creatinine in a random urine sample or 24-h specimen is >1, and a value that high is essentially diagnostic.

HYPERURICEMIA AND METABOLIC SYNDROME

Metabolic syndrome (Chap. 236) is characterized by abdominal obesity with visceral adiposity, impaired glucose tolerance due to insulin resistance with hyperinsulinemia, hypertriglyceridemia, increased low-density lipoprotein cholesterol, decreased high-density lipoprotein cholesterol, and hyperuricemia. Hyperinsulinemia reduces the renal excretion of uric acid and sodium. Not surprisingly, hyperuricemia resulting from euglycemic hyperinsulinemia may precede the onset of type 2 diabetes, hypertension, coronary artery disease, and gout in individuals with metabolic syndrome.

R_x HYPERURICEMIA

ASYMPTOMATIC HYPERURICEMIA Hyperuricemia is present in ~5% of the population and in up to 25% of hospitalized individuals. The vast majority are at no clinical risk. In the past, the association of hyperuricemia with cardiovascular disease and renal failure led to the use of urate-lowering agents for patients with asymptomatic hyperuricemia. This practice is no longer recommended except for individuals receiving cytolytic therapy for neoplastic disease, in which treatment is given in an effort to prevent uric acid nephropathy. Because hyperuricemia can be a component of the metabolic syndrome, its presence is an indication to screen for and aggressively treat any accompanying obesity, hyperlipidemia, diabetes mellitus, or hypertension.

Hyperuricemic individuals are at risk to develop gouty arthritis, especially those with higher serum urate levels. However, most hyperuricemic persons never develop gout and prophylactic treatment is not indicated. Furthermore, neither structural kidney damage nor tophi are identifiable before the first attack. Reduced renal function cannot be attributed to asymptomatic hyperuricemia, and treatment of asymptomatic hyperuricemia does not alter the progression of renal dysfunction in patients with renal disease. Increased risk of stone formation in those with asymptomatic hyperuricemia is not established.

Thus, because treatment with specific antihyperuricemic agents entails inconvenience, cost, and potential toxicity, routine treatment of asymptomatic hyperuricemia cannot be justified other than for prevention of acute uric acid nephropathy. In addition, routine screening for asymptomatic hyperuricemia is not recommended. If hyperuricemia is diagnosed, however, the cause should be determined. Causal factors should be corrected if the condition is secondary, and associated problems such as hypertension, hypercholesterolemia, diabetes mellitus, and obesity should be treated.

SYMPTOMATIC HYPERURICEMIA **Nephrolithiasis** (See Chap. 327 for treatment of gout.) Antihyperuricemic therapy is recommended for the individual who has both gouty arthritis and either uric acid– or calcium-containing stones, both of which may occur in association with hyperuric-

aciduria. Regardless of the nature of the calculi, fluid ingestion should be sufficient to produce a daily urine volume >2 L. Alkalinization of the urine with sodium bicarbonate or acetazolamide may be justified to increase the solubility of uric acid. Specific treatment of uric acid calculi requires reducing the urine uric acid concentration with a xanthine oxidase inhibitor, such as allopurinol or febuxostat. These agents decrease the serum urate concentration and the urinary excretion of uric acid in the first 24 h, with a maximum reduction occurring within 2 weeks. The average effective dose of allopurinol is 300–400 mg/d. Allopurinol can be given once a day because of the long half-life (18 h) of its active metabolite oxypurinol. The drug is effective in patients with renal insufficiency, but the dose should be reduced. Allopurinol is also useful in reducing the recurrence of calcium oxalate stones in gouty patients and in nongouty individuals with hyperuricemia or hyperuricaciduria. Febuxostat (80–240 mg/d) is also taken once daily, and doses do not need to be adjusted in the presence of mild to moderate renal dysfunction. Potassium citrate (30–80 mmol/d orally in divided doses) is an alternative therapy for patients with uric acid stones alone or mixed calcium/uric acid stones. A xanthine oxidase inhibitor is also indicated for the treatment of 2,8-dihydroxyadenine kidney stones.

Uric Acid Nephropathy Uric acid nephropathy is often preventable, and immediate, appropriate therapy has greatly reduced the mortality rate. Vigorous IV hydration and diuresis with furosemide dilute the uric acid in the tubules and promote urine flow to ≥100 mL/h. The administration of acetazolamide, 240–500 mg every 6–8 h, and sodium bicarbonate, 89 mmol/L, IV enhances urine alkalinity and thereby solubilizes more uric acid. It is important to ensure that the urine pH remains >7.0 and to watch for circulatory overload. In addition, antihyperuricemic therapy in the form of allopurinol in a single dose of 8 mg/kg is administered to reduce the amount of urate that reaches the kidney. If renal insufficiency persists, subsequent daily doses should be reduced to 100–200 mg because oxypurinol, the active metabolite of allopurinol, accumulates in renal failure. Despite these measures, hemodialysis may be required. Urate oxidase (Rasburicase) can also be administered IV to prevent or to treat tumor lysis syndrome.

HYPOURICEMIA

Hypouricemia, defined as a serum urate concentration <120 μmol/L (2.0 mg/dL) can result from decreased production of urate, increased excretion of uric acid, or a combination of both mechanisms. It occurs in <0.2% of the general population and <0.8% of hospitalized individuals. Hypouricemia causes no symptoms or pathology and therefore requires no therapy.

Most hypouricemia results from increased renal uric acid excretion. The finding of normal amounts of uric acid in a 24-h urine collection in an individual with hypouricemia is evidence for a renal cause. Medications with uricosuric properties (Table 353-1) include aspirin (at doses >2.0 g/d), losartan, fenofibrate, x-ray contrast materials, and glycerylguaiacholate. Total parenteral hyperalimentation can also cause hypouricemia, possibly a result of the high glycine content of the infusion formula. Other causes of increased urate clearance include conditions such as neoplastic disease, hepatic cirrhosis, diabetes mellitus, and inappropriate secretion of vasopressin; defects in renal tubular transport such as primary Fanconi syndrome and Fanconi syndromes caused by Wilson's disease, cystinosis, multiple myeloma, and heavy metal toxicity; and isolated congenital defects in the bidirectional transport of uric acid. Hypouricemia can be familial. Some of these cases result from a loss-of-function mutation in *SLC22A12*, the gene that encodes for URAT1.

SELECTED INBORN ERRORS OF PURINE METABOLISM (See also Table 353-3, Fig. 353-3.)

HPRT DEFICIENCY

The HPRT gene is located on the X chromosome. Affected males are hemizygous for the mutant gene; carrier females are asymptomatic. A complete deficiency of HPRT, the Lesch-Nyhan syndrome, is characterized by hyperuricemia, self-mutilative behavior, choreoathetosis, spasticity, and mental retardation. A partial deficiency

TABLE 353-3 INBORN ERRORS OF PURINE METABOLISM

Enzyme	Activity	Inheritance	Clinical Features	Laboratory Features
Hypoxanthine phosphoribo-syltransferase	Complete deficiency	X-linked	Self-mutilation, choreoathetosis, gout, and uric acid lithiasis	Hyperuricemia, hyperuricosuria
	Partial deficiency	X-linked	Gout, and uric acid lithiasis	Hyperuricemia, hyperuricosuria
Phosphoribosylpyrophos-phate synthetase	Overactivity	X-linked	Gout, uric acid lithiasis, and deafness	Hyperuricemia, hyperuricosuria
Adenine phosphoribosyl-transferase	Deficiency	Autosomal recessive	2,8-Dihydroxyadenine lithiasis	—
Xanthine oxidase	Deficiency	Autosomal recessive	Xanthinuria and xanthine lithiasis	Hypouricemia, hypouricosuria
Adenylosuccinate lyase	Deficiency	Autosomal recessive	Autism and psychomotor retardation	—
Myoadenylate deaminase	Deficiency	Autosomal recessive	Myopathy with exercise intolerance or asymptomatic	—
Adenosine deaminase	Deficiency	Autosomal recessive	Severe combined immunodefi-ciency disease and chrondro-osseous dysplasia	—
Purine nucleoside phosphorylase	Deficiency	Autosomal recessive	T cell–mediated immunodeficiency	—

of HPRT, the Kelley-Seegmiller syndrome, is associated with hyperuricemia but no central nervous system manifestations. In both disorders, the hyperuricemia results from urate overproduction and can cause uric acid crystalluria, nephrolithiasis, obstructive uropathy, and gouty arthritis. Early diagnosis and appropriate therapy with allopurinol can prevent or eliminate all the problems attributable to hyperuricemia but have no effect on the behavioral or neurologic abnormalities.

INCREASED PRPP SYNTHETASE ACTIVITY
Like the HPRT deficiency states, PRPP synthetase overactivity is X-linked and results in gouty arthritis and uric acid nephrolithiasis. Nerve deafness occurs in some families.

ADENINE PHOSPHORIBOSYLTRANSFERASE (APRT) DEFICIENCY
APRT deficiency is inherited as an autosomal recessive trait. Affected individuals develop kidney stones composed of 2,8-dihydroxyadenine. Caucasians with the disorder have a complete deficiency (type I), whereas Japanese subjects have some measurable enzyme activity (type II). Expression of the defect is similar in the two populations, as is the frequency of the heterozygous state (0.4–1.1 per 100). Allopurinol treatment prevents stone formation.

HEREDITARY XANTHINURIA
A deficiency of xanthine oxidase causes all purine in the urine to occur in the form of hypoxanthine and xanthine. About two-thirds of deficient individuals are asymptomatic. The remainder develop kidney stones composed of xanthine.

MYOADENYLATE DEAMINASE DEFICIENCY
Primary (inherited) and secondary (acquired) forms of myoadenylate deaminase deficiency have been described. The primary form is inherited as an autosomal recessive trait. Clinically, some may have relatively mild myopathic symptoms with exercise or other triggers, but most individuals with this defect are asymptomatic. Therefore, another explanation for the myopathy should be sought in symptomatic patients with this deficiency. The acquired deficiency occurs in association with a wide variety of neuromuscular disease, including muscular dystrophies, neuropathies, inflammatory myopathies, and collagen vascular diseases.

ADENYLOSUCCINATE LYASE DEFICIENCY
Deficiency of this enzyme is due to an autosomal recessive trait and causes profound psychomotor retardation,

seizures, and other movement disorders. All individuals with this deficiency are mentally retarded, and most are autistic.

ADENOSINE DEAMINASE DEFICIENCY AND PURINE NUCLEOSIDE PHOSPHORYLASE DEFICIENCY
See Chap. 310.

PYRIMIDINE DISORDERS

The pyrimidine, cytidine, is found in both DNA and RNA; it is a complementary base pair for guanine. Thymidine is found only in DNA where it is paired with adenine. Uridine is found only in RNA and can pair with either adenine or guanine in RNA secondary structures. Pyrimidines can be synthesized by a de novo pathway (Fig. 353-4) or reused in a salvage pathway. Although >25 different enzymes are involved in pyrimidine metabolism, disorders of these pathways are rare. Seven disorders of pyrimidine metabolism have been discovered (Table 353-4), three of which are discussed below.

FIGURE 353-4 Abbreviated scheme of pyrimidine metabolism. (1) thymidine kinase, (2) dihydropyrimidine dehydrogenase, (3) thymidylate synthase, (4) UMP synthase, (5) 5'-nucleotidase. CMP, cytidine-5'-monophosphate; UMP, uridine-5'-monophosphate; UDP, uridine-5'-diphosphate; dUMP, deoxyuridine-5'-monophosphate; dTMP, deoxythymidine-5'-monophosphate.

TABLE 353-4 INBORN ERRORS OF PYRIMIDINE METABOLISM

Enzyme	Activity	Inheritance	Clinical Features	Laboratory Features
Uridine-5′-monophosphate synthetase	Deficiency	Autosomal recessive	Orotic acid crystalluria; obstructive uropathy, hypochromic megaloblastic anemia	Orotic aciduria
Pyrimidine 5′-nucleotidase	Deficiency	Autosomal recessive	Hemolytic anemia	Basophilic stippling of erythrocytes; high levels of cytidine and uridine ribonucleotides
Pyrimidine 5′-nucleotidase	Superactivity	Uncertain	Developmental delay, seizures, ataxia, language deficit	Hypouricosuria
Thymidine phosphorylase	Deficiency	Autosomal recessive	Mitochondrial neurogastrointestinal encephalopathy	Hypouricosuria
Dihydropyrimidine dehydrogenase	Deficiency	Autosomal recessive	Seizures, motor and mental retardation	High levels of uracil, thymine, and 5-hydroxymethyluracil and low levels of dihydropyrimidines in urine
Dihydropyrimidinase	Deficiency	Uncertain	Seizures, mental retardation	Dihydropyrimidinuria
Ureidopropionase	Deficiency	Uncertain	Hypotonia, dystonia, developmental delay	High urinary excretion of N-carbamyl-β-alanine and N-carbamyl β-aminoisobutyric acid

OROTIC ACIDURIA

Hereditary orotic aciduria is caused by mutations in a bifunctional enzyme, uridine-5′-monophosphate (UMP) synthase, which converts orotic acid to UMP in the de novo synthesis pathway (Fig. 353-4). The disorder is characterized by hypochromic megaloblastic anemia that is unresponsive to vitamin B_{12} and folic acid, growth retardation, and neurologic abnormalities. Increased excretion of orotic acid causes crystalluria and obstructive uropathy. Replacement of uridine (100–200 mg/kg per day) corrects the anemia, reduces orotic acid excretion, and improves the other sequelae of the disorder.

PYRIMIDINE 5′-NUCLEOTIDASE DEFICIENCY

Pyrimidine 5′-nucleotidase catalyzes the removal of the phosphate group from pyrimidine ribonucleoside monophosphates (cytidine-5′-monophosphate or UMP) (Fig. 353-4). An inherited deficiency of this enzyme causes hemolytic anemia with prominent basophilic stippling of erythrocytes. The accumulation of pyrimidines or cytidine diphosphate choline (CDPC) is thought to induce hemolysis. There is no specific treatment. Acquired pyrimidine 5′-nucleotidase deficiency has been reported in lead poisoning and in thalassemia.

DIHYDROPYRIMIDINE DEHYDROGENASE DEFICIENCY

Dihydropyrimidine dehydrogenase (DPD) is the rate-limiting enzyme in the pathway of uracil and thymine degradation (Fig. 353-4). Deficiency of this enzyme causes excessive urinary excretion of uracil and thymine. DPD deficiency causes nonspecific cerebral dysfunction with convulsive disorders, motor retardation, and mental retardation. No specific treatment is available.

MEDICATION EFFECTS ON PYRIMIDINE METABOLISM

A variety of medications can influence pyrimidine metabolism. The anticancer agents fluorodeoxyuridine and 5-fluorouracil (5-FU) and the antimicrobial agent fluorocytosine cause cytotoxicity when converted to fluorodeoxyuridylate (FdUMP), a specific suicide inhibitor of thymidylate synthase. Fluorocytosine must be converted to 5-FU to be effective. This conversion is catalyzed by cytosine deaminase activity. Fluorocytosine's action is selective because cytosine deaminase is present in bacteria and fungi but not in human cells.

DPD is involved in the degradation of 5-FU. Consequently, deficiency of this enzyme is associated with 5-FU neurotoxicity.

Leflunomide, which is used to treat rheumatoid arthritis, inhibits de novo pyrimidine synthesis by inhibiting dihydroorotate dehydrogenase, resulting in an antiproliferative effect on T cells. Allopurinol, which is used to block xanthine oxidase and purine synthesis, also inhibits orotidine-5′-phosphate decarboxylase, a step in UMP synthesis. Consequently, allopurinol use is associated with increased excretion of orotidine and orotic acid; there are no known clinical effects of this inhibition.

FURTHER READINGS

BECKER MA et al: Febuxostat compared to allopurinol in patients with hyperuricemia and gout. N Engl J Med 353:2450, 2005

CHOI HK et al: Pathogenesis of gout. Ann Intern Med 143:499, 2005

LEE SJ, TERKELTAUB RA: New developments in clinically relevant mechanisms and treatment of gout. Curr Rheum Rep 8:224, 2006

SCRIVER CR et al (eds): Part 11. Purines and Pyrimidines, in The Metabolic and Molecular Bases of Inherited Disease, 8th ed. New York, McGraw-Hill, 2001, pp 2513–2702; OMMBID, 2006

WORTMANN RL, KELLEY WN: Gout and hyperuricemia, in Kelly's Textbook of Rheumatology, 7th ed, ED Harris, Jr et al (eds). Philadelphia, Saunders, 2005, pp 1402–1429

——— et al (eds): Crystal-Induced Arthropathies. New York, Informa Healthcare, 2006, pp 189–212, 255–276, 369–400

354 Wilson Disease
George J. Brewer

Wilson disease is an autosomal recessive disorder caused by mutations in the *ATP7B* gene, a membrane-bound copper-transporting ATPase. Clinical manifestations are caused by copper toxicity and primarily involve the liver and the brain. Because effective treatment is available, it is important to make this diagnosis early.

The frequency of Wilson disease in most populations is about 1 in 30,000–40,000, and the frequency of carriers of *ATP7B* mutations is thus ~1%. Siblings of a diagnosed patient have a 1 in 4 risk of Wilson disease, whereas children of an affected patient have about a 1 in 200 risk. Because a large number of inactivating mutations have been reported in the *ATP7B* gene, mutation screening for diagnosis is not yet practical, although this is likely in the near future. DNA haplotype analysis can be used to genotype siblings of an affected patient.

PATHOGENESIS

ATP7B protein deficiency impairs biliary copper excretion, resulting in positive copper balance, hepatic copper accumulation, and copper toxicity from oxidant damage. Excess hepatic copper is initially bound to metallothionein, but as this storage capacity is exceeded, liver damage begins as early as 3 years of age. Defective copper incorporation

TABLE 354-1 USEFUL TESTS FOR WILSON DISEASE

Test	Usefulness[a]	Normal Value	Heterozygous Carriers	Wilson Disease
Serum ceruloplasmin	+	180–350 mg/L (18–35 mg/dL)	Low in 20%	Low in 90%
KF rings	++	Absent	Absent	Present in 99% + if neurologic or psychiatric symptoms present Present in 30–50% in hepatic presentation and presymptomatic state
24-h urine Cu	+++	0.3–0.8 μmol (20–50 μg)	Normal to 1.3 μmol (80 μg)	>1.6 μmol (>100 μg) in symptomatic patients 0.9 to >1.6 μmol (60 to >100 μg) in presymptomatic patients
Liver Cu	++++	0.3–0.8 μmol/g (20–50 μg) tissue	Normal to 2.0 μmol (125 μg)	>3.1 μmol (>200 μg) (obstructive liver disease can cause false-positive results)
Haplotype analysis	++++ (Siblings only)	0 Matches	1 Match	2 Matches

[a]Usefulness: +, somewhat useful, to ++++, very useful.
Abbreviations: KF, Kayser-Fleischer; Cu, copper.

into apoceruloplasmin leads to excess catabolism and low blood levels of ceruloplasmin. Serum copper levels are usually lower than normal because of low blood ceruloplasmin, which normally binds >90% of serum copper. As the disease progresses, non-ceruloplasmin serum copper ("free" copper) levels increase, resulting in copper buildup in other parts of the body, such as the brain, leading to neurologic and psychiatric disease.

CLINICAL PRESENTATION

Hepatic Wilson disease may present as hepatitis, cirrhosis, or as hepatic decompensation, typically in the mid- to late-teenage years in western countries, although the age of presentation is quite broad and extends into the fifth decade of life.

An episode of hepatitis may occur, with elevated blood transaminase enzymes, with or without jaundice, and then spontaneously regress. Hepatitis often reoccurs, and most of these patients eventually develop cirrhosis.

Hepatic decompensation is associated with elevated serum bilirubin, reduced serum albumin and coagulation factors, ascites, peripheral edema, and hepatic encephalopathy. In severe hepatic failure, hemolytic anemia may occur because large amounts of copper derived from hepatocellular necrosis are released into the bloodstream. The association of hemolysis and liver disease makes Wilson disease a likely diagnosis.

Neurologic The neurologic manifestations of Wilson disease typically occur in patients in their early twenties, although the age of onset extends into the sixth decade of life. MRI and CT scans reveal damage in the basal ganglia and occasionally in the pons, medulla, thalamus, cerebellum, and subcortical areas. The three main movement disorders include: dystonia, incoordination, and tremor. Dysarthria and dysphagia are common. In some patients, the clinical picture closely resembles that of Parkinson disease. Dystonia can involve any part of the body and eventually leads to grotesque positions of the limbs, neck, and trunk. Autonomic disturbances may include orthostatic hypotension and sweating abnormalities as well as bowel, bladder, and sexual dysfunction. Memory loss, migraine-type headaches, and seizures may occur. Patients have difficulties focusing on tasks, but cognition is not usually grossly impaired. Sensory abnormalities and muscular weakness are not features of the disease.

Psychiatric A history of behavioral disturbances, with onset in the five years before diagnosis, is present in half of patients with neurologic disease. The features are diverse and may include loss of emotional control (temper tantrums, crying bouts), depression, hyperactivity, or loss of sexual inhibition.

Other Manifestations Some female patients have repeated spontaneous abortions, and most become amenorrheic prior to diagnosis. Cholelithiasis and nephrolithiasis occur with increased frequencies. Some patients may have osteoarthritis, particularly of the knee. Microscopic hematuria is common, and increased urinary excretion of phosphates, amino acids, glucose, or urates may occur; however, a full-blown Fanconi syndrome is rare. Sunflower cataracts and Kayser-Fleischer rings (copper deposits in the outer rim of the cornea) may be seen. Electrocardiographic and other cardiac abnormalities have been reported but are not common.

DIAGNOSIS

Diagnostic tests for Wilson disease are listed in Table 354-1. Serum ceruloplasmin levels should not be used for definitive diagnosis, because they are normal in up to 10% of affected patients and are reduced in 20% of carriers. Kayser-Fleischer rings (Fig. 354-1) can only be diagnosed definitively by an ophthalmologist using a slit lamp. They are present in >99% of patients with neurologic/psychiatric forms of the disease and have been described very rarely in the absence of Wilson disease. Kayser-Fleischer rings are present in only ~30–50% of patients diagnosed in the hepatic or presymptomatic state; thus, the absence of rings does not exclude the diagnosis.

Urine copper is an important diagnostic tool but must be collected carefully to avoid contamination. Symptomatic patients invariably have urine copper levels > 1.6 μmol (>100 μg) per 24 h. Heterozygotes have values <1.6 μmol (<100 μg) per 24 h. About half of presymptomatic patients who are ultimately affected have diagnostically elevated urine copper values, but the other half are in an intermediate range between 0.9 and 1.6 μmol (60 and 100 μg) per 24 h. Because heterozygotes may have values up to 1.3 μmol (80 μg) per 24 h, patients in this range may require a liver biopsy for definitive diagnosis.

The "gold standard" for diagnosis remains liver biopsy with quantitative copper assays. Affected patients have values >3.1 μmol/g (>200 μg/g) dry weight of liver. Copper stains are not reliable. False-positive results can occur with long-standing obstructive liver disease, which can elevate hepatic and urine copper and rarely causes Kayser-Fleischer rings.

FIGURE 354-1 A Kayser-Fleischer ring. Although in this case the brownish ring rimming the cornea is clearly visible to the naked eye, confirmation is usually by slit-lamp examination.

TABLE 354-2 RECOMMENDED ANTICOPPER DRUGS FOR WILSON DISEASE

Disease Status	First Choice	Second Choice
Initial hepatic		
Hepatitis or cirrhosis without decompensation	Zinc[a]	Trientine
Hepatic decompensation		
Mild	Trientine[b] and zinc	Penicillamine[b] and zinc
Moderate	Trientine and zinc	Hepatic transplantation
Severe	Hepatic transplantation	Trientine and zinc
Initial neurologic/psychiatric	Tetrathiomolybdate[c] and zinc	Zinc
Maintenance	Zinc	Trientine
Presymptomatic	Zinc	Trientine
Pediatric	Zinc	Trientine
Pregnant	Zinc	Trientine

[a]Zinc acetate is supplied as Galzin, manufactured by Gate Pharmaceutical. Recommended adult dose for all the above indications is 50 mg of elemental zinc three times daily, each dose separated from food and beverages other than water by at least 1 h, and separated from trientine or penicillamine doses by at least 1 h.
[b]Trientine is supplied as Syprine and penicillamine as Cuprimine, both manufactured by Merck. Recommended adult dosage for both drugs is 500 mg twice daily, each dose at least ½ h before or 2 h after meals.
[c]Tetrathiomolybdate is not yet commercially available but is expected to be marketed near the end of 2007.

℞ WILSON DISEASE

Recommended anticopper treatments are listed in **Table 354-2**. Penicillamine was previously the primary anticopper treatment but now plays a minor role because of its toxicity and because it often worsens existing neurologic disease if used as initial therapy. If penicillamine is given, it should always be accompanied by 25 mg/d of pyridoxine. Trientine is a less toxic chelator and is supplanting penicillamine when a chelator is indicated.

For patients with hepatitis or cirrhosis, but without evidence of hepatic decompensation or neurologic/psychiatric symptoms, zinc is the therapy of choice, although some advocate therapy with trientine. Zinc has proven efficacy in Wilson disease and is essentially nontoxic. It produces a negative copper balance by blocking intestinal absorption of copper, and it induces hepatic metallothionein synthesis, which sequesters additional toxic copper. All presymptomatic patients should be treated prophylactically, since the disease is close to 100% penetrant.

The first step in evaluating patients presenting with hepatic decompensation is to establish disease severity, which can be estimated using the Nazer prognostic index **(Table 354-3)**. Patients with scores <7 can usually be managed with medical therapy. Patients with scores >9 should be considered immediately for liver transplantation, and those with scores between 7 and 9 require clinical judgment as to whether to recommend transplantation or medical therapy. A combination of trientine and zinc has been used to treat patients with Nazer scores as high as 9, but such patients should be watched carefully for indications of hepatic deterioration, which mandates transplantation.

For initial medical therapy of patients with hepatic decompensation, a chelator (trientine is preferred) plus zinc is recommended (Table 354-2).

Zinc should not, however, be ingested simultaneously with trientine, as it will chelate zinc and form therapeutically ineffective complexes; the two drugs should be separated by at least 1 h.

For initial neurologic therapy, tetrathiomolybdate is emerging as the drug of choice because of its rapid action, preservation of neurologic function, and low toxicity. Penicillamine and trientine should be avoided because they each have a high risk of worsening the neurologic condition. Until tetrathiomolybdate is commercially available, zinc therapy is recommended. Although relatively slow-acting, zinc does not itself cause neurologic worsening. Although hepatic transplantation may improve neurologic symptoms, it does so only by removing copper, which can be done more safely and inexpensively with anticopper drugs. Pregnant patients should be treated with zinc or trientine throughout pregnancy, but without tight copper control, because copper deficiency can be teratogenic.

Anticopper therapy must be lifelong. With treatment, liver function usually recovers after about a year, although residual liver damage is usually present. Neurologic and psychiatric symptoms usually improve between 6 and 24 months of treatment.

MONITORING ANTICOPPER THERAPY When first using trientine or penicillamine, it is necessary to monitor for drug toxicity, particularly bone marrow suppression and proteinuria. Complete blood counts, standard biochemical profiles, and a urinalysis should be performed at weekly intervals for a month, then at 2-weekly intervals for 2–3 months, then at monthly intervals for 3 or 4 months, and at 4- to 6-monthly intervals thereafter.

The anticopper effects of trientine and penicillamine can be monitored by following 24-h "free" serum copper. Changes in urine copper are more difficult to interpret because excretion reflects the effect of the drug, as well as body loading with copper. Free serum copper is calculated by subtracting the ceruloplasmin copper from the total serum copper. Each 10 mg/L (mg/dL) of ceruloplasmin contributes 0.5 μmol/L (3.0 μg/dL) of serum copper. The normal free copper value is 1.6–2.4 μmol/L (10–15 μg/dL), and it often is as high as 7.9 μmol/L (50 μg/dL) in untreated Wilson disease. With treatment, free copper should be <3.9 μmol/L (<25 μg/dL).

Zinc treatment does not require blood or urine monitoring for toxicity. Its only significant side effect is gastric burning or nausea in ~10% of patients, usually with the first morning dose. This can be mitigated by taking the first dose an hour after breakfast or taking the zinc with a small amount of protein. Because zinc mainly affects stool copper, 24-h urine copper can be used to reflect body loading. The typical value in untreated symptomatic patients is >3.1 μmol (>200 μg) per 24 h. This level should decrease during the first 1–2 years of therapy to <2.0 μmol (<125 μg) per 24 h. A normal value [0.3 to 0.8 μmol (20 to 50 μg)] is rarely reached during the first decade of therapy and should raise concern about overtreatment (copper deficiency), the first sign of which is anemia and/or leukopenia.

GLOBAL CONSIDERATIONS

Age of onset of clinical disease may be considerably younger in India and far Eastern countries, often occurring in children only 5 or 6 years of age. The incidence of the disease may be increased in certain populations due to founder effects. For example, in Sardinia, the incidence may be 1 in 3000. In countries where penicillamine, trientine, and zinc acetate (as Galzin) are not available or cannot be afforded, zinc salts such as the gluconate or sulfate provide an alternative treatment option.

TABLE 354-3 PROGNOSTIC INDEX OF NAZER

Laboratory Measurement	Normal Value	Score (in Points)				
		0	1	2	3	4
Serum bilirubin[a]	0.2–1.2 mg/dL	<5.8	5.8–8.8	8.8–11.7	11.7–17.5	>17.5
Serum aspartate transferase (AST)	10–35 IU/L	<100	100–150	151–200	201–300	>300
Prolongation of prothrombin time (seconds)	—	<4	4–8	9–12	13–20	>20

[a]If hemolysis is present, the serum bilirubin cannot be used as a measure of liver function until the hemolysis subsides.
Source: Modified from H Nazer et al: Wilson's disease: Clinical presentation and use of prognostic index. Gut 27:1377, 1986; with permission from BMJ Publishing Group.

FURTHER READINGS

ALA A et al: Wilson's disease. Lancet 369(9559):397, 2007

ASKARI FK et al: Treatment of Wilson's disease with zinc XVIII. Initial treatment of the hepatic decompensation presentation with trientine and zinc. J Lab Clin Med 142:385, 2003

BREWER GJ: Recognition, diagnosis and management of Wilson's disease. Proc Soc Ex Biol Med 223:39, 2000

———, ASKARI FK: Wilson's disease: Clinical management and therapy. J Hepatol 42:S13, 2005

——— et al: Treatment of Wilson disease with ammonium tetrathiomolybdate: III. Initial therapy in 55 neurologically affected patients and follow-up with zinc therapy. Arch Neurol 60:379, 2003

——— et al: Treatment of Wilson's disease with ammonium tetrathiomolybdate: IV. Comparison of tetrathiomolybdate and trientine in a double blind study of treatment of the neurologic presentation of Wilson's disease. Arch Neurol 63:521, 2006

COX DW, ROBERTS EA: Wilson Disease. GeneClinics, University of Washington, Seattle. Online. Available at *http://www.geneclinics.org/profiles/wilson/details.html*

MERLE U et al: Clinical presentation, diagnosis, and long-term outcome of Wilson's disease: A cohort study. Gut 56:115, 2007

355 Lysosomal Storage Diseases
Robert J. Hopkin, Gregory A. Grabowski

Lysosomes are heterogeneous subcellular organelles containing specific hydrolyases that allow targeted processing or degradation of proteins, nucleic acids, carbohydrates, and lipids. There are >30 different lysosomal storage diseases, classified based on the nature of the stored material (Table 355-1). Several of the most prevalent disorders will be reviewed here, including Tay-Sachs disease, Fabry disease, Gaucher disease, Niemann-Pick disease, and mucopolysaccharidoses. Lysosomal storage diseases should be considered in the differential diagnosis of patients with neurologic, renal, or muscular degeneration and un-

TABLE 355-1 SELECTED LYSOSOMAL STORAGE DISEASES

Disorder[a]	Enzyme Deficiency (Specific Therapy)	Stored Material	Clinical Types (Onset)	Inheritance	Neurologic	Liver Spleen Enlargement	Skeletal Dysplasia
Mucopolysaccharidoses (MPS)							
MPS I H, Hurler (136)	α-L-Iduronidase (ET, BMT)	Dermatan sulfate Heparan sulfate	Infantile	AR	Mental retardation	+++	++++
MPS I H/S, Hurler/ Scheie			Intermediate				
MPS I S, Scheie			Adult		None		
MPS II, Hunter (136)	Iduronate sulfatase (ET)	Dermatan sulfate Heparan sulfate	Severe infantile Mild juvenile	X-linked	Mental retardation, less in mild form	+++	++++
MPS III A, Sanfilippo A (136)	Heparan-N-sulfatase	Heparan sulfate	Late infantile	AR	Severe mental retardation	+	+
MPS III B, Sanfilippo B	N-Acetyl-α-glucosaminidase	Heparan sulfate	Late infantile	AR	Severe mental retardation	+	+
MPS III C, Sanfilippo C	Acetyl-CoA: α-glucosaminide N-acetyltransferase	Heparan sulfate	Late infantile	AR	Severe mental retardation	+	+
MPS III D, Sanfilippo D	N-Acetylglucosamine-6-sulfate sulfatase	Heparan sulfate	Late infantile	AR	Severe mental retardation	+	+
MPS IV A, Morquio (136)	N-Acetylgalactosamine-6-sulfate sulfatase	Keratan sulfate Chondroitin-6 sulfate	Childhood	AR	None	+	++++
MPS VI B, Morquio (136)	β-Galactosidase		Childhood	AR	None	±	++++
MPS VI, Maroteaux-Lamy (136)	Arylsulfatase B (ET, BMT)	Dermatan sulfate	Late infantile	AR	None	++	++++
MPS VII (136)	β-Glucuronidase	Dermatan sulfate Heparan sulfate	Neonatal Infantile Adult	AR	Mental retardation, absent in some adults	+++	+++
GM₂ Gangliosidoses							
Tay-Sachs disease (153)	β-Hexosaminidase A	GM₂ gangliosides	Infantile Juvenile	AR	Mental retardation, seizures, later juvenile form	None	None
Sandhoff disease (153)	β-Hexosaminidases A and B	GM₂ gangliosides	Infantile	AR	Mental retardation, seizures	++	±
Neutral Glycosphingolipidoses							
Fabry disease (150)	α-Galactosidase A (ET)	Globotriaosylceramide	Childhood	X-linked	Painful acroparesthesias	None	None
Gaucher disease (146)	Acid β-glucosidase (ET, SRT)	Glucosylceramide	Type 1 Type 2 Type 3	AR	None ++++ ++	++++ +++ ++++	++++ + ++++
Niemann-Pick disease (144) A and B	Sphingomyelinase	Sphingomyelin	Neuronopathic, type A Nonneuronopathic, type B	AR	Mental retardation and seizures	++++	None Osteoporosis

explained hepatomegaly, splenomegaly, cardiomyopathy, or skeletal dysplasias and deformations. Physical findings are disease-specific, and definitive diagnosis is made by enzyme assays or genetic testing.

PATHOGENESIS OF LYSOSOMAL STORAGE DISEASES

Lysosomal biogenesis involves ongoing synthesis of lysosomal hydrolases, membrane constitutive proteins, and new membranes. Lysosomes originate from the fusion of *trans*-Golgi network (TGN) vesicles with late endosomes. Progressive vesicular acidification accompanies the maturation of TGN vesicles, and this gradient facilitates the pH-dependent dissociation of receptors and ligands, as well as activating lysosomal hydrolases.

Abnormalities at any biosynthetic step can impair enzyme activation and lead to a lysosomal storage disorder. Following leader sequence clipping, complex oligosaccharide modifications occur during transit through the Golgi, including the mannose-6-phosphate modification of high-mannose oligosaccharide chains of many soluble lysosomal hydrolases. Lysosomal integral or associated membrane proteins are sorted to the membrane or interior of the lysosome by several different signals. Phosphorylation, sulfation, additional proteolytic processing, and macromolecular assembly of heteromers occur concurrently. These are critical to enzyme function, and defects can result in multiple enzyme/protein deficiencies.

The final common pathway for lysosomal storage diseases is the accumulation of specific macromolecules within tissues and cells that normally have a high flux of these substrates. The majority of lysosomal enzyme deficiencies result from point mutations or genetic rearrangements at a locus that encodes a single lysosomal hydrolase. However, some mutations cause deficiencies of several different lysosomal hydrolases by altering the enzymes/proteins involved in targeting, active site modifications, or macromolecular association or trafficking. All are inherited as autosomal recessive disorders, except Hunter (mucopolysaccharidosis type II) and Fabry diseases, which are X-linked. Substrate accumulation leads to lysosomal distortion, which has significant pathologic consequences. In addition, abnormal amounts of metabolites may also have pharmacologic effects important to disease pathophysiology.

For many lysosomal diseases, the accumulated substrates are endogenously synthesized within particular tissue sites of pathology. Other diseases have greater exogenous substrate supplies, for example, they are delivered by low-density lipoprotein receptor–mediated uptake in Fabry and cholesteryl ester storage diseases or by phagocytosis in Gaucher disease type 1. The *threshold hypothesis* refers to a level of enzyme activity below which disease develops. Consequently, small changes in enzyme activity near the threshold can lead to or prevent disease. A critical element of this model is that enzymatic activity can be challenged by changes in substrate flux based on genetic background, cell turnover, recycling, or metabolic demands. Thus, a set level of residual enzyme may be adequate for substrate in some tissues or cells, but not in others. In addition, several variants of each lysosomal storage disease exist at a clinical level. These disorders therefore represent a continuum of manifestations that are not easily dissociated into discrete entities. The bases for such variations have not been elucidated in any detail.

SELECTED DISORDERS

TAY-SACHS DISEASE

About 1 in 30 Ashkenazi Jews is a carrier for Tay-Sachs disease, which is caused by total hexosaminidase A (Hex A) deficiency. The infantile form is a fatal neurodegenerative disease with macrocephaly, loss of motor skills, increased startle reaction, and a macular cherry red spot. The juvenile-onset form presents with ataxia and dementia, with death by age 10–15 years. The adult-onset disorder is characterized by clumsiness in childhood; progressive motor weakness in adolescence; and additional spinocerebellar, lower motor neuron symptoms, and dysarthria in adulthood. Intelligence declines slowly, and psychosis is common. Screening for Tay-Sachs disease carriers is recommended in the Ashkenazi Jewish population. *Sandhoff disease* is phenotypically similar to Tay-Sachs disease, but hepatosplenomegaly and bony dysplasias are also present.

FABRY DISEASE

Fabry disease is an X-linked disorder that results from mutations in the α-galactosidase gene. The estimated prevalence of hemizygous males is 1/40,000. Clinically, the disease manifests with angiokeratomas (telangiectatic skin lesions); hypohidrosis; corneal and lenticular opacities; acroparesthesia; and small-vessel disease of the kidney, heart, and brain.

The angiokeratomas and acroparesthesia may appear in childhood and lead to early diagnosis, if suspected. Angiokeratomas are punctate, dark red to blue-black, flat or slightly raised, and usually symmetric, and they do not blanch with pressure. They range from barely visible to several millimeters in diameter and have a tendency to increase in size and number with age. They usually are most dense between the umbili-

Clinical Features		
Ophthalmologic	**Hematologic**	**Unique Features**
Corneal clouding	Vacuolated lymphocytes	Coarse facies, cardiovascular involvement, joint stiffness
Retinal degeneration, no corneal clouding	Granulated lymphocytes	Coarse facies, cardiovascular, joint stiffness, distinctive pebbly skin lesions
None	Granulated lymphocytes	Mild coarse facies
None	Granulated lymphocytes	Mild coarse facies
None	Granulated lymphocytes	Mild coarse facies
None	Granulated lymphocytes	Mild coarse facies
Corneal clouding	Granulated neutrophils	Distinctive skeletal deformity, odontoid hypoplasia, aortic valve disease
Corneal clouding	Granulated neutrophils and lymphocytes	Coarse facies, valvular heart disease
Corneal clouding	Granulated neutrophils	Coarse facies, vascular involvement, hydrops fetalis in neonatal form
Cherry red spot in infantile form	None	Macrocephaly, hyperacusis in infantile form
Cherry red spot	None	Macrocephaly, hyperacusis
Corneal dystrophy, vascular lesions	None	Cutaneous angiokeratomas, hypohidrosis
None	Gaucher cells in bone marrow, cytopenias	Adult form highly variable
Eye movements		
Eye movements		
Macular degeneration	Foam cells in bone marrow	Pulmonary infiltrates Lung failure

(continued)

TABLE 355-1 SELECTED LYSOSOMAL STORAGE DISEASES (CONTINUED)

Disorder[a]	Enzyme Deficiency (Specific Therapy)	Stored Material	Clinical Types (Onset)	Inheritance	Neurologic	Liver Spleen Enlargement	Skeletal Dysplasia
Glycoproteinoses							
Fucosidosis (140)	α-Fucosidase	Glycopeptides, oligosaccharides	Infantile Juvenile	AR	Mental retardation	++	++
α-Mannosidosis (140)	α-Mannosidase	Oligosaccharides	Infantile Milder variant	AR	Mental retardation	+++	++
β-Mannosidosis (140)	β-Mannosidase	Oligosaccharides		AR	Seizures, mental retardation		++
Aspartylglucosaminuria (140)	Aspartylglucosaminidase	Aspartylglucosamine, glycopeptides	Young adult onset	AR	Mental retardation	±	++
Sialidosis (140)	Neuraminidase	Sialyloligosaccharides	Type I, congenital Type II, infantile and juvenile forms	AR	Myoclonus, mental retardation	++, less in type I	++, less in type I
Mucolipidoses (ML)							
ML-II, I-cell disease (138)	UDP-N-Acetylglucosamine-1-phosphotransferase	Glycoprotein, glycolipids	Infantile	AR	Mental retardation	±	++++
ML-III, pseudo-Hurler polydystrophy (138)	UDP-N-Acetylglucosamine-1-phosphotransferase	Glycoprotein, glycolipids	Late infantile	AR	Mild mental retardation	None	+++
Leukodystrophies							
Krabbe disease (147)	Galactosylceramidase (BMT)	Galactosylceramide, Galactosyl sphingosine	Infantile	AR	Mental retardation	None	None
Metachromatic leukodystrophy (148)	Arylsulfatase A	Cerebroside sulfate	Infantile Juvenile Adult	AR	Mental retardation, dementia, and psychosis in adult	None	None
Multiple sulfatase deficiency (149)	Active site cysteine to Cα-formylglycine-converting enzyme	Sulfatides, mucopolysaccharides	Late infantile	AR	Mental retardation	+	++
Disorders of Neutral Lipids							
Wolman disease (142)	Acid lysosomal lipase (BMT)	Cholesterol esters, triglycerides	Infantile	AR	Mild mental retardation	+++	None
Cholesteryl ester storage disease (142)	Acid lysosomal lipase	Cholesteryl esters	Childhood	AR	None	Hepatomegaly	None
Farber disease (142)	Acid ceramidase	Ceramide	Infantile Juvenile	AR	Occasional mental retardation	±	None
Pompe disease (135)	Acid α-glucosidase (ET)	Glycogen	Infantile late onset	AR	Neuromuscular	±	None

[a]Numbers in parentheses refer to the chapters in Scriver et al, 8th edition, for detailed reviews.
Note: AR, autosomal recessive; BMT, bone marrow (or stem cell) transplantation; ET, enzyme therapy; SRT, substrate reduction therapy.

cus and knees—"the bathing suit area"—but may occur anywhere, including the mucosal surfaces. Angiokeratomas also occur in Fordyce scrotal angiokeratoma and several other lysosomal storage diseases. Corneal and lenticular lesions, detectable on slit-lamp examination, may help in establishing a diagnosis of Fabry disease. Debilitating episodic burning pain of the hands, feet, and proximal extremities (acroparesthesia) can last from minutes to days and can be precipitated by changes in temperature, exercise, fatigue, or fever. Abdominal pain can resemble that from appendicitis or renal colic. Proteinuria, isosthenuria, and progressive renal dysfunction occur in the second to fourth decades. Hypertension, left ventricular hypertrophy, anginal chest pain with or without myocardial ischemia or infarction, and congestive heart failure can occur in the third to fourth decades. About 1–3% of patients with idiopathic hypertrophic myocardiopathy were found to

have Fabry disease. Leg lymphedema without hypoproteinemia and episodic diarrhea also occur. Death is due to renal failure or cardiovascular or cerebrovascular disease in untreated patients. Variants with residual α-galactosidase activity may have late-onset manifestations limited to the cardiovascular system that resemble hypertrophic cardiomyopathy. Variants with predominant cardiac, renal, or central nervous system (CNS) manifestations are becoming better defined. Up to 70% of heterozygous females may exhibit clinical manifestations, including acroparesthesia and CNS, cardiac, and renal disease.

Phenytoin and carbamazepine diminish the chronic and episodic acroparesthesia. Chronic hemodialysis or kidney transplantation can be life-saving in patients with renal failure. Enzyme therapy clears stored lipids from a variety of cells, particularly those of the renal, cardiac, and skin vascular endothelium. Renal insufficiency appears irre-

Clinical Features		
Ophthalmologic	**Hematologic**	**Unique Features**
None	Vacuolated lymphocytes, foam cells	Coarse facies, angiokeratomas in juvenile form
Cataracts, corneal clouding	Vacuolated lymphocytes, granulated neutrophils	Coarse facies, enlarged tongue
None	Vacuolated lymphocytes, foam cells	Angiokeratomas
None	Vacuolated lymphocytes, foam cells	Coarse facies
Cherry red spot	Vacuolated lymphocytes	MPS phenotype in type II
Corneal clouding	Vacuolated and granulated neutrophils	Coarse facies, absence of mucopolysacchariduria, gingival hypoplasia
Corneal clouding, mild retinopathy, hyperopic astigmatism		Coarse facies, stiffness of hands and shoulders
None	None	White matter globoid cells
Optic atrophy	None	Gait abnormalities in late infantile form
Retinal degeneration	Vacuolated and granulated cells	Absent activity of all known cellular sulfatases
None	None	Adrenal calcification
None	None	Cirrhosis
Macular degeneration	None	Arthropathy, subcutaneous nodules
None	None	Myocardiopathy

versible. Early institution of enzyme therapy may prevent or slow the progression of the life-threatening complications.

GAUCHER DISEASE

Gaucher disease is an autosomal recessive disorder that results from defective activity of acid β-glucosidase; >250 mutations have been described at the GBA locus of such patients. Disease variants are classified based on the absence or presence and progression of neuronopathic involvement.

Gaucher disease type 1 is a nonneuronopathic disease that can present in childhood to adulthood with slowly to rapidly progressive visceral disease. About 55–60% of such patients are diagnosed at <20 years in Caucasian populations and even younger in other groups. This pattern of presentation is distinctly bimodal, with peaks at <10 to 15 years and at ~25 years. Younger patients tend to have a greater degree of hepatosplenomegaly and accompanying blood cytopenias. In contrast, the older group has a greater tendency for chronic bone disease. Hepatosplenomegaly occurs in virtually all symptomatic patients and can be minor or massive. Accompanying anemia and thrombocytopenia are variable and are not directly related to liver or spleen volumes. Severe liver dysfunction is unusual. Splenic infarctions can resemble an acute abdomen. Pulmonary hypertension and alveolar Gaucher cell accumulation are uncommon, but life-threatening, and can occur at any age.

All patients with Gaucher disease have nonuniform infiltration of bone marrow by lipid-laden macrophages termed *Gaucher cells*. This can lead to marrow packing with subsequent infarction, ischemia, necrosis, and cortical bone destruction. Bone marrow involvement spreads from proximal to distal in the limbs and can involve the axial skeleton extensively, causing vertebral collapse. In addition to bone marrow involvement, bone remodeling is defective, with loss of total bone calcium leading to osteopenia, osteonecrosis, avascular infarction, and vertebral compression fractures and spinal cord involvement. Aseptic necrosis of the femoral head is common, as is fracture of the femoral neck. The mechanism by which diseased bone marrow macrophages interact with osteoclasts and/or osteoblasts to cause bone disease is not well understood. Chronic, ill-defined bone pain can be debilitating and poorly correlated with radiographic findings. "Bone crises" are associated with localized, excruciating pain, and, on occasion, local erythema, fever, and leukocytosis. Some patients have frequent crises, whereas other patients experience only one. These crises represent acute infarctions of bone, as evidenced in nuclear scans by localized absent uptake of pyrophosphate agents. Osteomyelitis should be excluded by appropriate cultures.

Decreased acid β-glucosidase activity (0–20% of normal) in nucleated cells makes the diagnosis. The enzyme is not present in bodily fluids. The sensitivity of enzyme testing is poor for heterozygote detection; molecular testing is preferred when the mutations are known. The disease frequency varies from about 1 in 1000 in Ashkenazi Jews to <1 in 100,000 in other populations. About 1 in 12–15 Ashkenazi Jews carries a Gaucher disease allele. Four common mutations account for ~85% of the mutations in that population of affected patients: N370S (1226G), 84GG (a G insertion at cDNA position 84), L444P (1448C), and IVS-2 (an intron 2 splice junction mutation).

Genotype/phenotype studies indicate a significant correlation, though not absolute, between disease type and severity and the acid β-glucosidase genotype. The most common mutation in the Ashkenazi Jewish population (N370S) shares a 100% association with nonneuronopathic or type 1 Gaucher disease. The N370S/N370S and N370S/other mutant allele genotypes are associated with later onset/less severe disease and with earlier onset/severe disease, respectively. As many as 50–60% of individuals with the N370S/N370S genotype have been calculated to be asymptomatic. Other alleles include L444P (very low activity), 84GG (null), or IVS-2 (null), and rare/private or uncharacterized alleles. The L444P/L444P patients almost always have life-threatening to very severe/early-onset disease, and many, though not all, develop CNS involvement in the first two decades of life.

Symptomatic management of the blood cytopenias and joint replacement surgeries continue to have important roles in management. However, enzyme therapy is currently the treatment of choice in significantly affected patients and is highly efficacious and safe in diminishing the hepatosplenomegaly and improving bone marrow involvement and hematologic findings. The bone disease is decreased but not eliminated by enzyme replacement therapy. Adult patients may benefit from adjunctive treatment with bisphosphonates to improve bone density. Patients who cannot be treated with enzyme replacement, either because it is not effective or because they have an allergy or other hypersensitivities, may be treated with medications that decrease the production of the complex lipid molecules that are broken down by acid β-glucosidase (substrate inhibition therapy). Other approaches to stabilize the abnormal enzyme produced by mutant alleles allowing improved enzyme function (referred to as *molecular chaperone therapy*) are under investigation as alternative treatments for Gaucher disease, Fabry disease, and other lysosomal diseases.

Gaucher disease type 2 is a rare, severe CNS disease that leads to death by 2 years of age. *Type 3 Gaucher disease* has highly variable manifestations in the CNS and viscera. It can present in early childhood with rapidly progressive, massive visceral disease and slowly progressive to static CNS involvement; in adolescence with dementia; or in early adulthood with rapidly progressive, uncontrollable myoclonic seizures and mild visceral disease. Visceral disease in type 3 is nearly identical to that in type 1 but is generally more severe. Early CNS findings may be limited to defects in lateral gaze tracking, which may remain static for decades. Mental retardation can be slowly progressive or static. This variant is most frequent among individuals of Swedish descent.

NIEMANN-PICK DISEASE

This is an autosomal recessive disorder that results from defects in acid sphingomyelinase. Types A and B are distinguished by an early age of onset and progressive CNS disease in type A. Type A typically has onset in the first 6 months, with rapidly progressive CNS deterioration, spasticity, failure to thrive, and massive hepatosplenomegaly. In contrast, type B has a later, more variable onset and progression of hepatosplenomegaly, with eventual development of cirrhosis and hepatic replacement by foam cells. Affected patients develop progressive pulmonary disease with dyspnea, hypoxemia, and a reticular infiltrative pattern on chest x-ray. Foam cells are present in alveoli, lymphatic vessels, and pulmonary arteries. Progressive hepatic or lung disease leads to demise in adolescence to early adulthood.

The diagnosis is established by markedly decreased (1–10% of normal) sphingomyelinase activity in nucleated cells. There is no specific treatment for Niemann-Pick disease. The efficacy of hepatic or bone marrow transplantation has not been proven. Clinical trials using enzyme therapy are anticipated in the near future.

MUCOPOLYSACCHARIDOSES

Mucopolysaccharidosis type I (MPS I) is an autosomal recessive disorder caused by deficiency of α-L-iduronidase. It has traditionally been divided into three categories: (1) Hurler disease for severe deficiency with neurodegeneration; (2) Scheie disease for later-onset disease without neurologic involvement and with relatively less severe disease in other organ systems; and (3) Hurler-Scheie disease for patients intermediate between these extremes. Hurler-Scheie disease is characterized by severe somatic disease without neurologic deterioration.

MPS I often presents in infancy or early childhood with chronic rhinitis, clouding of the corneas, and hepatosplenomegaly. As the disease progresses, nearly every organ system can be affected. For the more severe forms, cardiac and respiratory diseases become life-threatening in childhood. Skeletal disease can be quite severe, resulting in very limited mobility.

There are two current treatments for MPS I. Stem cell transplantation is the standard treatment for patients presenting in infancy who appear to have or are at risk for neurologic degeneration. Stem cell engraftment results in stabilization of the central nervous system disease and reverses the hepatosplenomegaly. It also improves the cardiac and respiratory disease. Stem cell transplantation does not eliminate the corneal disease or stop progression of the skeletal disease. The second currently available therapy is enzyme infusion therapy. Enzyme therapy effectively addresses the hepatosplenomegaly and improves cardiac and respiratory disease. It does not penetrate the CNS and is not a directly effective treatment for CNS disease. Enzyme therapy and stem cell transplant appear to have similar effects for signs and symptoms outside the CNS. Enzyme therapy has a lower risk for life-threatening complications and may therefore have advantages for patients without CNS degeneration. A combination of enzyme therapy and stem cell transplantation has been used with enzyme therapy started prior to transplantation in an attempt to decrease the disease burden prior to transplantation. However, there is little experience with this approach and its advantages over stem cell therapy alone are not clear.

Enzyme therapy has also recently received U.S. Food and Drug Administration (FDA) approval for treatment of Maroteaux-Lamy disease (MPS VI). This very rare autosomal recessive disorder is characterized by hepatosplenomegaly, bone disease, heart disease, and respiratory compromise similar to those seen in MPS I, but it is due to deficiency of arylsulfatase B and is not associated with neurologic degeneration.

Hunter disease (MPS II) is an X-linked disorder due to deficiency in iduronate sulfatase; it has manifestations very similar to MPS I, including neurologic degeneration, but there is no corneal clouding or other eye disease. Like MPS I, MPS II is clinically variable. Unfortunately, stem cell transplantation has not been successful in treating the CNS disease associated with MPS II. Enzyme replacement has been approved by the FDA and EMEA for treatment of patients with MPS II.

POMPE DISEASE

Acid maltase (acid α-glucosidase) deficiency, also called *Pompe disease*, is a glycogen and lysosomal storage disease with autosomal recessive inheritance. The classic severe infantile form presents with hypotonia, myocardiopathy, and hepatosplenomegaly. This variant is rapidly progressive and generally results in death in the first year of life. However, as with other lysosomal diseases, there are early- and late-onset forms of this disorder. The late-onset patients typically present with a slowly progressive myopathy that may resemble a limb-girdle muscular dystrophy. Respiratory insufficiency may develop with advancing disease. In late stages of the disease, patients may require mechanical ventilation, report swallowing difficulties, and experience loss of bowel and bladder control. Myocardiopathy is not usually seen in late-onset variants of Pompe disease.

The FDA has recently approved enzyme infusion therapy for Pompe disease. This is clearly beneficial in the infantile form, consistently resulting in improved cardiac function and prolonged survival. Improved respiratory function is seen in most treated infants. Some infants demonstrated marked improvement in motor functions while others had minor changes in muscle tone or strength. There are a few anecdotal reports of improvement with enzyme therapy in the late-onset forms, but studies are limited at this time. It is likely that there is benefit from early intervention with enzyme therapy in patients with late-onset acid α-glucosidase deficiency, but very advanced disease will have significant irreversible components.

FURTHER READINGS

CLARKE JT: Narrative review: Fabry disease. Ann Intern Med 146:425, 2007

GIUGLIANI R et al: Management guidelines for mucopolysaccharidosis VI. Pediatrics 120:405, 2007

MUENZER J et al: A phase I/II clinical trial of enzyme replacement therapy in mucopolysaccharidosis II (Hunter syndrome). Mol Genet Metab 90:329, 2007

RISCH N: Molecular epidemiology of Tay-Sachs disease. Adv Genet 44:233, 2001

SCHIFFMANN R, BRADY RO: New prospects for the treatment of lysosomal storage diseases. Drugs 62:733, 2002

SCRIVER CR et al (eds): *The Metabolic and Molecular Bases of Inherited Diseases*, 8th ed. New York, McGraw-Hill, 2001; *ommbid.com*, 2006

ZHAO H, GRABOWSKI GA: Gaucher disease: Perspectives on a prototype lysosomal disease. Cell Mol Life Sci 59:694, 2002

356 Glycogen Storage Diseases and Other Inherited Disorders of Carbohydrate Metabolism

Yuan-Tsong Chen

Carbohydrate metabolism plays a vital role in cellular function by providing the energy required for most metabolic processes. The relevant biochemical pathways involved in the metabolism of these carbohydrates are shown in Fig. 356-1. Glucose is the principle substrate of energy metabolism in humans. Metabolism of glucose generates ATP via glycolysis and mitochondrial oxidative phosphorylation. Dietary sources of glucose are obtained by ingesting polysaccharides, primarily starch, and disaccharides including lactose, maltose, and sucrose. Galactose and fructose are two other monosaccharides that provide fuel for cellular metabolism; however, their role as fuel sources is much less significant than that of glucose. Galactose is derived from lactose (galactose + glucose), which is found in milk products, and is an important component for certain glycolipids, glycoproteins, and glycosaminoglycans. The two dietary sources of fructose are sucrose (fructose + glucose), a commonly used sweetener, and fructose itself, which is found in fruits, vegetables, and honey.

Glycogen, the storage form of glucose in animal cells, is composed of glucose residues joined in straight chains by α1-4 linkages and branched at intervals of 4–10 residues by α1-6 linkages. Glycogen forms a treelike molecule and can have a molecular weight of many millions. Glycogen may aggregate to form structures recognizable by electron microscopy. Defects in glycogen metabolism typically cause an accumulation of glycogen in the tissues; hence the name *glycogen storage diseases*. The defects in gluconeogenesis or glycolytic pathways, including galactose and fructose metabolism, do not usually result in glycogen accumulation.

Clinical manifestations of the various disorders of carbohydrate metabolism differ markedly. The symptoms range from harmless to lethal. Unlike disorders of lipid metabolism, mucopolysaccharidoses, or other storage diseases, dietary therapy has been effective in many of the carbohydrate disorders. All of the genes responsible for the inherited defects of carbohydrate metabolism have been cloned, and mutations have been identified. Advances in our understanding of the molecular basis of these diseases are being used to improve diagnosis and management. Some of these disorders are candidates for enzyme replacement and early trials of gene therapy.

Historically, the glycogen storage diseases were categorized numerically in the order in which the enzymatic defects were identified. They are also classified by the organs involved and clinical manifestations. This is the system followed in this chapter (Table 356-1). The overall fre-

quency of all forms of glycogen storage disease is approximately 1 in 20,000 live births. Most are inherited as autosomal recessive traits; however, phosphoglycerate kinase deficiency and one form of phosphorylase kinase deficiency are X-linked disorders. The most common childhood disorders are glucose-6-phosphatase deficiency (type I), lysosomal acid α-glucosidase deficiency (type II), debrancher deficiency (type III), and liver phosphorylase kinase deficiency (type IX). The most common adult disorder is myophosphorylase deficiency (type V, or McArdle disease).

SELECTED LIVER GLYCOGENOSES

DISORDERS WITH HEPATOMEGALY AND HYPOGLYCEMIA

Type I Glycogen Storage Disease (Glucose-6-Phosphatase or Translocase Deficiency, von Gierke's Disease)   Type I glycogen storage disease is an autosomal recessive disorder caused by glucose-6-phosphatase deficiency in liver, kidney, and intestinal mucosa. It can be divided into two subtypes: type Ia, in which the glucose-6-phosphatase enzyme is defective, and type Ib, in which the translocase that transports glucose-6-phosphate across the microsomal membrane is defective. The

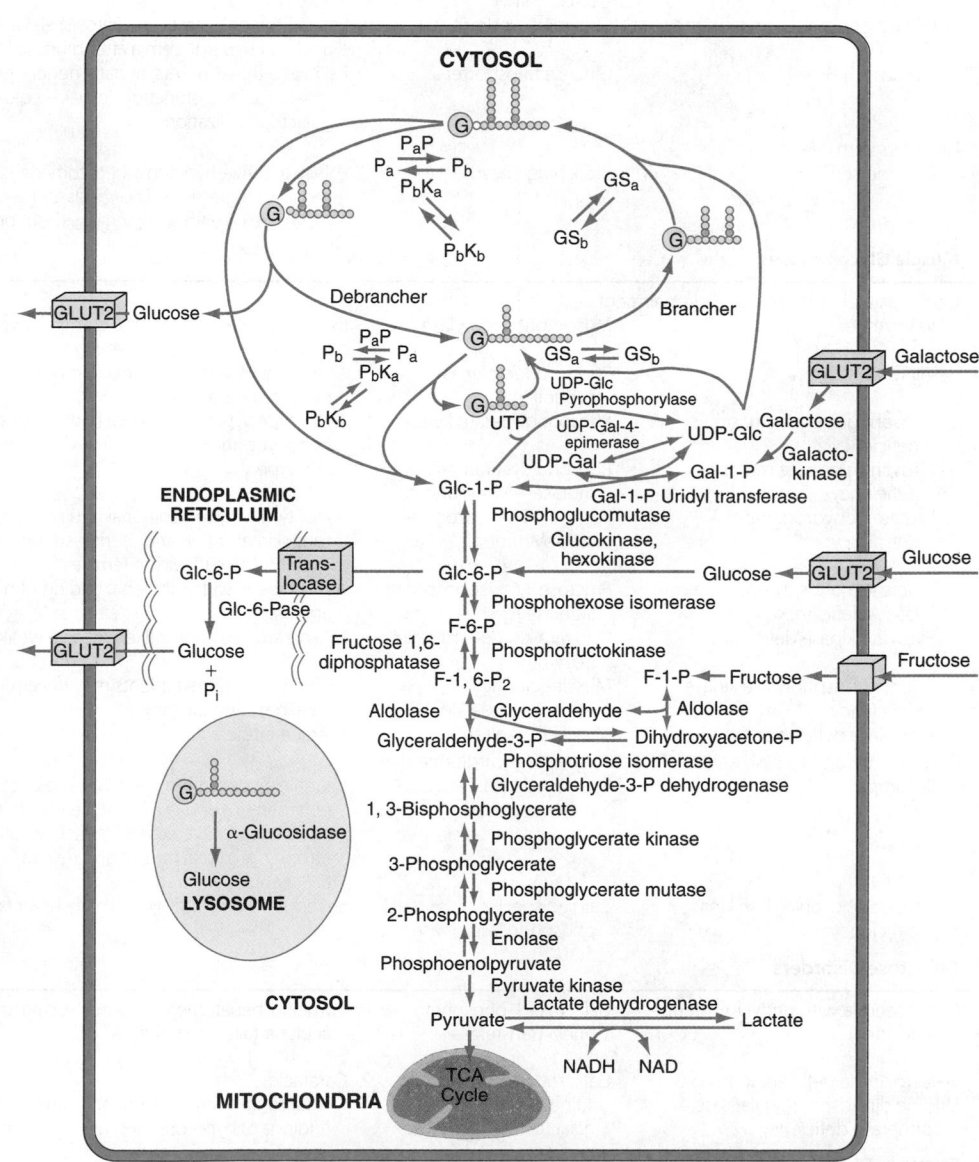

FIGURE 356-1 Metabolic pathways related to glycogen storage diseases and galactose and fructose disorders. Nonstandard abbreviations are as follows: GS$_a$, active glycogen synthase; GS$_b$, inactive glycogen synthase; P$_a$, active phosphorylase; P$_b$, inactive phosphorylase; P$_a$P, phosphorylase *a* phosphatase; P$_b$K$_a$, active phosphorylase *b* kinase; P$_b$K$_b$, inactive phosphorylase *b* kinase; G, glycogenin, the primer protein for glycogen synthesis. [*Modified from AR Beaudet, in KJ Isselbacher et al (eds): Harrison's Principles of Internal Medicine, 13th ed. New York: McGraw-Hill, 1994, p 1855.*]

TABLE 356-1 FEATURES OF GLYCOGEN STORAGE DISEASES AND GALACTOSE AND FRUCTOSE DISORDERS

Type/Common Name	Basic Defect	Clinical Features	Comments
Liver Glycogenoses			
Disorders with hepatomegaly and hypoglycemia			
Ia/von Gierke	Glucose-6-phosphatase	Growth retardation, enlarged liver and kidney, hypoglycemia, elevated blood lactate, cholesterol, triglycerides, and uric acid	Common, severe hypoglycemia Late complications in adulthood
Ib	Glucose-6-phosphate translocase	As for Ia, with additional findings of neutropenia and neutrophil dysfunction	~10% of type I
IIIa/Cori or Forbes	Liver and muscle debranching enzyme	Childhood: Hepatomegaly, growth retardation, muscle weakness, hypoglycemia, hyperlipidemia, elevated liver transaminases; liver symptoms improve with age	Common, intermediate severity of hypoglycemia Liver cirrhosis can occur
		Adulthood: muscle atrophy and weakness; onset: third to fourth decades; variable cardiomyopathy	
IIIb	Liver debranching enzyme (normal muscle debrancher activity)	Liver symptoms same as in type IIIa; no muscle symptoms	~15% of type III
VI/Hers	Liver phosphorylase	Hepatomegaly, mild hypoglycemia, hyperlipidemia and ketosis; symptoms improve with age	Rare, "benign" glycogenosis
IX/phosphorylase kinase deficiency	Liver phosphorylase kinase α subunit	As for VI	Common, "benign glycogenosis," X-linked
0/glycogen synthase deficiency	Glycogen synthase	Fasting hypoglycemia and ketosis, elevated lactic acid and hyperglycemia after glucose load	Decreased glycogen stores
XI/Fanconi-Bickel	Glucose transporter-2	Failure to thrive, rickets, hepatomegaly, proximal renal tubular dysfunction, impaired glucose and galactose utilization	Rare, consanguinity in 70%
Disorders with liver cirrhosis			
IV/Andersen	Branching enzyme	Failure to thrive, hypotonia, hepatomegaly, splenomegaly, progressive liver cirrhosis and failure (death usually before fifth year); some without progression	One of the rarer glycogenoses; other neuromuscular variants exist
Muscle Glycogenoses			
Disorders with muscle-energy impairment			
V/McArdle	Muscle phosphorylase	Exercise intolerance, muscle cramps, myoglobinuria on strenuous exercise, increased CK	Common, male predominance
VII/Tarui	Phosphofructokinase—M subunit	As for type V, with additional findings of a compensated hemolysis	Prevalent in Ashkenazi Jews and Japanese
Phosphoglycerate kinase deficiency	Phosphoglycerate kinase	As for type V, with additional findings of a hemolytic anemia and CNS dysfunction	Rare, X-linked
Phosphoglycerate mutase deficiency	Phosphoglycerate mutase—M subunit	As for type V	Rare; most patients are African American
Lactate dehydrogenase deficiency	Lactic acid dehydrogenase—M subunit	As for type V, with additional findings of erythematous skin eruption and uterine stiffness resulting in childbirth difficulty in female	Rare
Fructose 1,6-bisphosphate aldolase A deficiency	Fructose 1,6-bisphosphate aldolase A	As for type V, with additional finding of hemolytic anemia	Rare
Pyruvate kinase deficiency	Pyruvate kinase—muscle isozyme	Muscle cramps and/or fixed muscle weakness	Rare
Muscle phosphorylase kinase deficiency	Muscle-specific phosphorylase kinase	As for type V, some patients may have muscle weakness and atrophy	Rare, autosomal recessive
β-enolase deficiency	Muscle β-enolase	Exercise intolerance	Rare
Disorders with progressive skeletal myopathy and/or cardiomyopathy			
II/Pompe	Lysosomal acid α-glucosidase	Infantile: hypotonia, muscle weakness, cardiac enlargement and failure, fatal early; Juvenile and adult: progressive skeletal muscle weakness and atrophy, proximal muscle and respiratory muscle are seriously affected	Common, undetectable, or very low level of enzyme activity in infantile form; residual enzyme activity in late-onset
Cardiac phosphorylase kinase deficiency	Cardiac-specific phosphorylase kinase	Severe cardiomyopathy and early heart failure	Very rare
Galactose Disorders			
Galactosemia with uridyl transferase deficiency	Galactose 1-phosphate uridyl transferase	Vomiting, hepatomegaly, jaundice, cataracts, aminoaciduria, failure to thrive	Long-term complications exist despite early diagnosis and treatment
Galactokinase deficiency	Galactokinase	Cataracts	Benign
Uridine diphosphate galactose 4-epimerase deficiency	Uridine diphosphate galactose 4-epimerase	Similar to transferase deficiency with additional findings of hypotonia and nerve deafness	Benign variant exists
Fructose Disorders			
Essential fructosuria	Fructokinase	Asymptomatic, positive urine reducing substance	Benign
Hereditary fructose intolerance	Fructose 1-phosphate aldolase B	Vomiting, lethargy, failure to thrive, hepatic failure	Prognosis good with early diagnosis and fructose restriction
Fructose 1,6-diphosphatase deficiency	Fructose 1,6-diphosphatase	Episodic hypoglycemia and lactic acidosis	Avoid fasting, good prognosis

Note: CK, creatine kinase; M, muscle; CNS, central nervous system.

defects in both subtypes lead to inadequate conversion in the liver of glucose-6-phosphate to glucose and thus make affected individuals susceptible to fasting hypoglycemia.

CLINICAL AND LABORATORY FINDINGS Persons with type I disease may develop hypoglycemia and lactic acidosis during the neonatal period; however, more commonly, they present at 3–4 months of age with hepatomegaly. Hypoglycemia and lactic acidosis can develop after a short fast. These children often have doll-like faces with fat cheeks, relatively thin extremities, short stature, and a protuberant abdomen that is due to massive hepatomegaly. The kidneys are enlarged, but the spleen and heart are of normal size. The hepatocytes are distended by glycogen and fat with large and prominent lipid vacuoles. Despite hepatomegaly, liver enzymes are usually normal or near normal. Easy bruising and epistaxis are associated with a prolonged bleeding time as a result of impaired platelet aggregation/adhesion. Hyperuricemia is present. Hyperlipidemia includes elevation of triglycerides, cholesterol, and phospholipids. Type Ib patients have additional findings of neutropenia and impaired neutrophil function, resulting in recurrent bacterial infections and oral and intestinal mucosal ulceration.

LONG-TERM COMPLICATIONS Gout usually becomes symptomatic at puberty as a result of the long-term hyperuricemia. Puberty is often delayed. Virtually all females have ultrasound findings consistent with polycystic ovaries; however, the other clinical features of polycystic ovary syndrome, such as acne and hirsutism, are not seen. Secondary to the lipid abnormalities, there is an increased risk of pancreatitis. Frequent fractures and radiographic evidence of osteopenia are not uncommon in adult patients, and radial bone mineral content is significantly reduced in prepubertal patients. By the second or third decade, most patients with type I glycogen storage disease develop hepatic adenomas that can hemorrhage and, in some cases, become malignant. Renal disease is a serious late complication. Almost all patients older than 20 years have proteinuria, and many have hypertension, kidney stones, nephrocalcinosis, and altered creatinine clearance. In some patients, renal function deteriorates and progresses to complete failure, requiring dialysis or transplantation.

DIAGNOSIS The diagnosis of type I disease can be suspected on the basis of clinical presentation and abnormal plasma lactate and lipid values. Before the glucose-6-phosphatase and glucose-6-phosphate translocase genes were cloned, a definitive diagnosis required a liver biopsy to demonstrate a deficiency. Gene-based mutation analysis now provides a noninvasive way of diagnosis for most patients with types Ia and Ib disease.

℞ TYPE I GLYCOGEN STORAGE DISEASE

Treatment is designed to maintain normal blood glucose levels and is achieved by continuous nasogastric infusion of glucose or oral administration of uncooked cornstarch. Uncooked cornstarch acts as a slow-release form of glucose and can be given at a dose of 1.6 g/kg every 4 h for infants younger than 2 years. As the child grows older, the cornstarch regimen can be changed to every 6 h and given by mouth as a liquid (1:2, weight:volume) at a dose of 1.75–2.5 g/kg of body weight. Because fructose and galactose cannot be converted to free glucose, their dietary intake should be restricted. Dietary supplements of multivitamins and calcium are required. Allopurinol is given to lower uric acid levels. The hyperlipidemia can be reduced with lipid-lowering drugs such as HMG-CoA reductase inhibitors and fibric acids. Angiotensin-converting enzyme (ACE) inhibitors are beneficial for treating microalbuminuria, an early indicator of renal dysfunction in these patients. Citrate supplement may be beneficial in preventing or ameliorating nephrocalcinosis and development of urinary calculi.

Type III Glycogen Storage Disease (Debrancher Deficiency, Limit Dextrinosis) Type III glycogenoses are autosomal recessive disorders caused by a deficiency of glycogen debranching enzymes. Debranching enzyme and phosphorylase are responsible for complete degradation of glycogen. When the debranching enzyme is defective, glycogen breakdown is incomplete. Abnormal glycogen accumulates short outer chains and resembles dextrin.

CLINICAL AND LABORATORY FINDINGS Deficiency of glycogen debranching enzyme causes hepatomegaly, hypoglycemia, short stature, variable skeletal myopathy, and cardiomyopathy. The disorder usually involves both liver and muscle and is termed *type IIIa glycogen storage disease*. However, in about 15% of patients, the disease appears to involve only the liver and is classified as *type IIIb*. Hypoglycemia, hyperlipidemia, and elevated liver transaminases occur in children. In contrast to type I disease, fasting ketosis is prominent, and blood lactate and uric acid concentrations are usually normal. Serum creatine kinase (CK) levels can sometimes be used to identify patients with muscle involvement, but normal levels do not rule out muscle enzyme deficiency. In most patients with type III disease, hepatomegaly improves with age; however, liver cirrhosis and hepatocellular carcinoma may occur in late adulthood.

DIAGNOSIS In type IIIa glycogen storage disease, deficient debranching enzyme activity can be demonstrated in liver, skeletal muscle, and heart. In contrast, patients with type IIIb have debranching enzyme deficiency in the liver but not in muscle. In the past, definitive assignment of subtype required enzyme assays in both liver and muscle. DNA-based analyses now provide a noninvasive way of subtyping these disorders in most patients.

℞ TYPE III GLYCOGEN STORAGE DISEASE

Dietary management of type III disease is less demanding than that of type I. If hypoglycemia is present, frequent high-carbohydrate meals with cornstarch supplements or nocturnal gastric drip feedings are usually effective. A high-protein diet during the day plus overnight protein enteral infusion may be tried in patients with myopathy, but it is not established whether such a regimen is effective.

Type IX Glycogen Storage Disease (Liver Phosphorylase Kinase Deficiency) Defects of phosphorylase kinase cause a heterogeneous group of glycogenoses. The phosphorylase kinase enzyme complex consists of four subunits (α, β, γ, and δ). Each is encoded by different genes (X chromosome as well as autosomes) that are differentially expressed in various tissues. Phosphorylase kinase deficiency can be divided into several subtypes on the basis of the gene/subunit involved, the tissues primarily affected, and the mode of inheritance. The most common subtype is X-linked liver phosphorylase kinase deficiency, which is one of the most common liver glycogenoses. Phosphorylase kinase activity may also be deficient in erythrocytes and leukocytes but is normal in muscle. Typically, a child between the ages of 1 and 5 presents with growth retardation and hepatomegaly. Levels of cholesterol, triglycerides, and liver enzymes are mildly elevated. Ketosis may occur after fasting. Lactic and uric acid levels are normal. Hypoglycemia is mild, if present. Hepatomegaly and abnormal blood chemistries gradually return to normal with age. Most adults achieve a normal final height and are practically asymptomatic, despite a persistent phosphorylase kinase deficiency.

Treatment is symptomatic. A high-carbohydrate diet and frequent feedings are effective in preventing hypoglycemia. Some patients require no specific treatment. Prognosis is usually good, and adult patients have normal stature and minimal hepatomegaly.

Other subtypes of type IX include an autosomal recessive form of liver and muscle phosphorylase kinase deficiency, an autosomal recessive form of liver phosphorylase kinase deficiency that often develops into liver cirrhosis, a muscle-specific phosphorylase kinase deficiency that causes cramps and myoglobinuria with exercise, and a cardiac-specific phosphorylase kinase deficiency that is lethal during infancy because of massive glycogen deposition in the myocardium.

Other Liver Glycogenoses with Hepatomegaly and Hypoglycemia These disorders include glycogen synthase deficiency (type 0) and hepatic glycogenosis with renal Fanconi syndrome (type XI). The latter is caused by defects in the facilitative glucose transporter 2 (GLUT-2), which transports glucose in and out of hepatocytes, pancreatic cells, and the basolateral membranes of intestinal and renal epithelial cells. The disease is characterized by proximal renal tubular dysfunction, impaired glucose and galactose utilization, and accumulation of glycogen in liver and kidney.

SELECTED MUSCLE GLYCOGENOSES

DISORDERS WITH MUSCLE-ENERGY IMPAIRMENT

Type V Glycogen Storage Disease (Muscle Phosphorylase Deficiency, McArdle Disease) Type V glycogen storage disease is an autosomal recessive disorder caused by deficiency of muscle phosphorylase. McArdle disease is a prototypical muscle energy disorder as the enzyme deficiency limits ATP generation by glycogenolysis and results in glycogen accumulation.

CLINICAL AND LABORATORY FINDINGS Symptoms usually develop first in adulthood and are characterized by exercise intolerance with muscle cramps. Two types of activity tend to cause symptoms: (1) brief exercise of great intensity, such as sprinting or carrying heavy loads; and (2) less-intense but sustained activity, such as climbing stairs or walking uphill. Moderate exercise, such as walking on level ground, can be performed by most patients for long periods. About half of patients report burgundy-colored urine after exercise, the consequence of myoglobinuria secondary to rhabdomyolysis. Intense myoglobinuria after vigorous exercise may cause renal failure. In rare cases, electromyography (EMG) findings may suggest an inflammatory myopathy, a diagnosis that may be confused with polymyositis.

The level of serum CK is usually elevated at rest and increases after exercise. Exercise also increases the levels of blood ammonia, inosine, hypoxanthine, and uric acid. The latter abnormalities are attributed to accelerated recycling of muscle purine nucleotides in the face of insufficient ATP production.

DIAGNOSIS Lack of an increase in blood lactate and exaggerated blood ammonia elevations after an ischemic exercise test are indicative of muscle glycogenosis and suggest a defect in the conversion of glycogen or glucose to lactate. The abnormal exercise response, however, is not limited to type V disease and can occur with other defects in glycogenolysis or glycolysis, such as deficiencies of muscle phosphofructokinase or debranching enzyme (when the test is done after fasting). Definitive diagnosis is made by enzymatic assay in muscle tissue or by mutation analysis of the myophosphorylase gene.

℞ TYPE V GLYCOGEN STORAGE DISEASE

In general, avoidance of strenuous exercise can prevent major episodes of rhabdomyolysis; however, regular and moderate exercise is recommended to improve exercise capacity. Sucrose given before exercise can markedly improve tolerance in these patients. A high-protein diet may increase exercise endurance, and a creatine supplement has been shown to improve muscle function in some patients. In general, longevity does not appear to be affected.

DISORDERS WITH PROGRESSIVE SKELETAL MUSCLE MYOPATHY AND/OR CARDIOMYOPATHY

Type II Glycogen Storage Disease (Acid α-1,4 Glucosidase Deficiency, Pompe Disease) Type II disease is an autosomal recessive disorder caused by a deficiency of lysosomal acid α-1,4 glucosidase (acid maltase), an enzyme responsible for the degradation of glycogen in the lysosomes. It is characterized by the accumulation of glycogen in the lysosomes as opposed to accumulation in cytoplasm as in the other glycogenoses.

CLINICAL AND LABORATORY FINDINGS The disorder encompasses a range of phenotypes. Each includes myopathy but differs in the age of onset, organ involvement, and clinical severity. The most severe is the infantile-onset disease with cardiomegaly, hypotonia, and death before age 1. Infants appear normal at birth but soon develop generalized muscle weakness with feeding difficulties, macroglossia, hepatomegaly, and congestive heart failure due to a hypertrophic cardiomyopathy.

The juvenile, or late-childhood, form is characterized by skeletal muscle manifestations, usually without cardiac involvement, and a slowly progressive course. The juvenile form typically presents as delayed motor milestones (if age of onset is early enough) and difficulty in walking. These manifestations are followed by swallowing difficulties, proximal muscle weakness, and respiratory muscle involvement. Death may occur before the end of the second decade.

The adult form presents as a slowly progressive myopathy without cardiac involvement and has its onset between the second and seventh decades. The clinical picture is dominated by slowly progressive proximal muscle weakness with truncal involvement. The pelvic girdle, paraspinal muscles, and diaphragm are most seriously affected. The initial symptoms may be respiratory insufficiency manifested by somnolence, morning headache, orthopnea, and exertional dyspnea.

Laboratory findings include elevated levels of serum CK, aspartate transaminase, and lactate dehydrogenase, particularly in infants. Muscle biopsy shows the presence of vacuoles that stain positively for glycogen; muscle acid phosphatase is increased, presumably from a compensatory increase of lysosomal enzymes. EMG reveals myopathic features with irritability of muscle fibers and pseudomyotonic discharges. Serum CK is not always elevated in adults, and depending on the muscle biopsied or tested, muscle histology or EMG may not be abnormal. It is prudent to examine affected muscle.

DIAGNOSIS Diagnosis can be established by demonstrating the absence or reduced levels of acid α-glucosidase activity in muscle, cultured skin fibroblasts, or blood spots. Deficiency is usually more severe in the infantile form than in the juvenile and adult disorders.

℞ TYPE II GLYCOGEN STORAGE DISEASE

Nocturnal ventilatory support in late-onset patients improves the quality of life and is beneficial during a period of respiratory decompensation. A definitive therapy is now available using aglucosidase alfa (Myozyme), a recombinant human acid α-glucosidase at 20 mg/kg body weight every 2 weeks as an intravenous infusion. In the clinical trials, aglucosidase alfa has been shown to improve ventilator-free survival and motor function in patients with infantile-onset Pompe disease as compared to untreated controls.

GLYCOGEN STORAGE DISEASE MIMICKING HYPERTROPHIC CARDIOMYOPATHY

Deficiencies of lysosomal-associated membrane protein 2 (LAMP2, also called Danon's disease) and protein kinase, AMP-activated gamma 2 noncatalytic subunit (PRKAG2) result in the accumulation of glycogen in the heart and skeletal muscle. Clinically, these patients present primarily as hypertrophic cardiomyopathy, but this can be distinguished from the usual causes of hypertrophic cardiomyopathy due to defects in sarcomere-protein genes by their electrophysiologic abnormalities, particularly ventricular pre-excitation and conduction defects. The onset of cardiac symptoms, including chest pain, palpitation, syncope, and cardiac arrest, can occur between the ages of 8 and 15 years for LAMP2 deficiency, younger than the average age for patients with PRKAG2 deficiency, which is 33 years. The prognosis for LAMP2 deficiency is poor, with progressive end-stage heart failure early in adulthood. By contrast, cardiomyopathy due to PRKAG2 mutations is compatible with long-term survival, although some patients may necessitate the implantation of a pacemaker and aggressive control of arrhythmias.

SELECTED DISORDERS OF GALACTOSE METABOLISM

"Classic" *galactosemia* is due to galactose 1-phosphate uridyl transferase deficiency. It is a serious disease with an early onset of symptoms; the incidence is 1 in 60,000. The newborn infant normally receives up to 20% of caloric intake as lactose, which consists of glucose and galactose. Without the transferase, the infant is unable to metabolize galactose 1-phosphate (Fig. 356-1), the accumulation of which results in injury to parenchymal cells of the kidney, liver, and brain.

Widespread newborn screening for galactosemia has identified these infants early and allowed them to be placed on dietary restriction. Elimination of galactose from the diet reverses growth failure and renal and hepatic dysfunction, improving the prognosis. However, on long-term follow-up, these patients still have ovarian failure manifest as primary or secondary amenorrhea, as well as developmental delays and learning disabilities, which increase in severity with age. In addition, most patients have speech disorders, and a smaller number demonstrate poor growth and impaired motor function and balance (with or without overt ataxia). The treatment of galactosemia to prevent long-term complications remains a challenge.

Deficiency of *galactokinase* (Fig. 356-1) causes cataracts. Deficiency of *uridine diphosphate galactose 4-epimerase* can be benign when the enzyme deficiency is limited to blood cells but can be as severe as classic galactosemia when the enzyme deficiency is generalized.

SELECTED DISORDERS OF FRUCTOSE METABOLISM

Fructokinase deficiency (Fig. 356-1) causes a benign condition that is usually an incidental finding made through the detection of fructose as a reducing substance in the urine.

Deficiency of *fructose 1-phosphate aldolase* (aldolase B, hereditary fructose intolerance) is a serious disease in infants. These patients are healthy and asymptomatic until fructose or sucrose (table sugar) is ingested (usually from fruit, sweetened cereal, or sucrose-containing formula). Clinical manifestations may include jaundice, hepatomegaly, vomiting, lethargy, irritability, and convulsions. Laboratory findings include prolonged clotting time, hypoalbuminemia, elevation of bilirubin and transaminases, and proximal renal tubular dysfunction. If the disease is not diagnosed and intake of the noxious sugar persists, hypoglycemic episodes recur, and liver and kidney failure progresses, eventually leading to death. Treatment consists of the complete elimination of all sources of sucrose, fructose, and sorbitol from the diet. With this treatment, liver and kidney dysfunction improve, and catch-up growth is common. Intellectual development is usually unimpaired. As the patient matures, symptoms become milder, even after fructose ingestion, and the long-term prognosis is good.

Fructose 1,6-diphosphatase deficiency is characterized by childhood life-threatening episodes of acidosis, hypoglycemia, hyperventilation, convulsions, and coma. These episodes are triggered by febrile infections and gastroenteritis when oral food intake decreases. Laboratory findings include low blood glucose, high lactate and uric acid levels, and metabolic acidosis. In contrast to hereditary fructose intolerance, there is usually no aversion to sweets, and renal tubular and liver functions are normal. Treatment of acute attacks consists of correction of hypoglycemia and acidosis by intravenous infusion. Later, avoidance of fasting and elimination of fructose and sucrose from the diet prevent further episodes. For long-term prevention of hypoglycemia, a slowly released carbohydrate such as cornstarch is useful. Prognosis is good as patients who survive childhood develop normally.

FURTHER READINGS

ARAD M et al: Glycogen storage disease presenting as hypertrophic cardiomyopathy. N Engl J Med 352:362, 2005

BALI DS, CHEN YT: Glycogen storage disease, in *Encyclopedia of Diagnostic Genomics and Proteomics*, J Fuchs, M Podda (eds). New York, Dekker, 2004

KISHNANI PS et al: Chinese hamster ovary cell-derived recombinant human acid alpha-glucosidase in infantile-onset Pompe disease. J Pediatr 149:89, 2006

——— et al: Recombinant human acid ±-glucosidase: Major clinical benefits in patients with infantile-onset Pompe disease. Neurology 68:99, 2007

KOEBERL DD et al: Glycogen storage disease type I and II: Treatment updates. J Inherited Metab Dis 30:159, 2007

OZEN H: Glycogen storage diseases: New perspectives. World J Gastroenterol 13(18):2541, 2007

VESSING J, HALLER RG: The effect of oral sucrose on exercise tolerance in patients with McArdle's disease. N Engl J Med 349:2503, 2003

357 Heritable Disorders of Connective Tissue
Darwin J. Prockop, Malwina Czarny-Ratajczak

Heritable disorders that involve the major connective tissues of the body such as bone, skin, cartilage, blood vessels, and basement membranes are among the most common human genetic diseases. Here we focus primarily on those disorders that have severe manifestations, are relatively common, and are sufficiently understood at the molecular level to provide useful paradigms: osteogenesis imperfecta (OI), Ehlers-Danlos syndrome (EDS), chondrodysplasias (CDs), Marfan syndrome (MFS), epidermolysis bullosa (EB), and Alport syndrome (AS).

THE CHALLENGE OF CLASSIFYING THE DISEASES

The original classification of connective tissue diseases was based on the pattern of inheritance, the cluster of signs and symptoms, the histologic changes in tissues, and limited information about the molecular defects involved. This classification included about a dozen types and subtypes for OI, about the same number for the EDS, and over 200 for the CDs. However, identification of the genetic basis for these diseases has, in some instances, provided more accurate classifications. For example, the discovery that most patients with MFS have mutations in the gene for fibrillin-1 allowed more rigorous criteria to define the classical syndrome (type I). This discovery also identified a new subcategory of patients (type II) who do not meet the same criteria and have been shown to have mutations in other genes. In other diseases, the correlations between genotype and phenotype have been more difficult. For example,

most patients with OI have mutations in one of the two type I collagen genes, but only a few generalizations can be made about the nature of the mutation and the severity of the phenotype. Moreover, in a number of these diseases, the same mutation does not always produce the same phenotype in unrelated patients or in members of the same family. As a result, the current classifications tend to overemphasize the etiologic differences between severe genetic diseases that are apparent in infants and the more common diseases that appear much later in life. For example, a small subset of patients with postmenopausal osteoporosis have mutations in the procollagen I genes that are similar to the mutations that produce lethal variants of OI. Likewise, a subset of patients with familial aortic aneurysms have mutations in the procollagen III gene that are similar to the mutations that cause lethal variants of type IV EDS. Occasionally, patients with osteoarthritis have mutations in the procollagen II gene that are similar to the mutations that cause lethal CDs.

As noted above, molecular tests for mutations assist in the classification of the disorders (e.g., MFS). In several syndromes, the use of these tests has led to more rigorous clinical classification criteria, making the molecular tests less necessary for routine care, except to reassure the patients and families or to exclude mutations in family members with milder phenotypes. In other syndromes, the molecular tests have been less useful because correlations of genotype with phenotype have been difficult. Also, many of the tests are still costly because of the required reagents, instruments, and highly trained personnel. As a result, it is frequently difficult to maintain laboratories that provide the tests routinely, especially for the more rare disorders, or for those in which the same clinical phenotype can be produced by mutations in one of several genes.

DEFINITION AND COMPOSITION OF CONNECTIVE TISSUES

The distinguishing feature of connective tissues is that it consists of complex macromolecules that are assembled into an insoluble extracellular matrix (Table 357-1). The macromolecules include at least 28 different types of collagens along with many other matrix components. Differences in the connective tissues of bone, skin, and cartilage are partially explained by differences in the content of specific components (Table 357-1). For example, tendons and ligaments consist primarily of type I collagen fibrils and small amounts of other components that help organize the type I fibrils into thick fibers and fiber bundles. Cartilage consists primarily of fibrils of type II collagen in the form of arcades that are distended by highly charged proteoglycans and organized by a series other molecules that bind to collagen and proteoglycans. The extracellular matrix of the aorta contains collagens that provide tensile strength and elastin that provides elasticity. Differences among the connective tissues also depend on the three-dimensional organization of the molecular components. The type I collagen fibrils in tendon are packed into thick, parallel bundles of fibers, whereas type I collagen fibrils in skin are randomly oriented in the plane of the skin. In cortical bone, type I collagen fibrils form helical arrays around haversian canals. The forces that control three-dimensional organization of the components are still unknown.

BIOSYNTHESIS OF CONNECTIVE TISSUE

Connective tissues form in part by a process of self-assembly, in which a molecule of the correct size, shape, and surface property spontaneously binds to other molecules with the same or similar structure. The molecular mechanisms and driving forces are similar to those involved in crystal formation but are more complex because of the large number of components involved and the different rates at which they are secreted into the extracellular matrix.

Collagen Synthesis Collagens have a triple-helical conformation in which each of three polypeptide chains, referred to as an α chain, has a simple, repetitive amino acid sequence of about 1000 amino acids in which glycine (Gly) appears as every third amino acid. Therefore, the sequence of each chain can be designated as $(\text{-Gly-X-Y-})_{333}$, where X and Y represent amino acids other than glycine. To fold into a triple helix, every third amino acid in an chain must be glycine, the smallest amino acid, since this residue must fit in a sterically restricted space where the three chains of the triple helix come together. Many of the X- and Y-position amino acids are proline and hydroxyproline, which, because of their ring structures, provide rigidity to the triple helix.

Twenty-eight different collagens have been identified. Many are minor constituents that probably have highly specialized functions. The fibrillar collagens are abundant proteins that are found in tissues as long, highly ordered fibrils with a characteristic banding pattern revealed by electron microscopy. Type I collagen, the most abundant, is composed of two identical α1(I) chains and a third α2(I)chain that is the product of a different gene and differs slightly in its amino acid sequence. Type II collagen, the fibrillar collagen of cartilage, is composed of three identical α(II) chains. Type III collagen is composed of three identical α1(III) chains. It is found in small amounts in many tissues that contain type I collagen and in large amounts in major blood vessels. Type IV collagen is composed of three α chains synthesized from any of six different genes. It is found in basement membranes where it self-assembles with laminins and other macromolecules into a complex three-dimensional network to provide a diffusion barrier in the renal glomerulus, pulmonary alveolus, and other tissues.

Collagens are first synthesized as larger and more soluble precursors called *procollagens* that are composed of proα chains. As the proα chains of procollagen are synthesized on ribosomes, the free ends move into the cisternae of the rough endoplasmic reticulum (Fig. 357-1). Hydrophobic signal peptides at the N-termini are cleaved, and additional post-translational reactions begin. Proline residues in the Y position of the repeating -Gly-X-Y- sequences are converted to hydroxyproline by prolyl hydroxylase. The enzyme requires ascorbic acid as a cofactor, an observation that explains why wounds fail to heal in scurvy (Chap. 71). If sufficient proline residues are not converted to hydroxyproline, collagen cannot fold into a triple helix that is stable at body temperature. The abnormal protein accumulates in the cisternae of the rough endoplasmic reticulum and is slowly degraded. Lysine residues in the Y position are also hydroxylated to hydroxylysine by lysyl hydroxylase. Many of the hydroxylysine residues are glycosylated with galactose or with galactose and glucose. A large mannose-rich oligosaccharide is assembled on the C-terminal propeptide of each chain.

After secretion, procollagen is processed to collagen by cleavage of the N-propeptides by procollagen N-proteinase and of the C-propeptides by procollagen C-proteinase. The processing converts the precursor to type I collagen and thereby decreases the solubility of the protein about 1000-fold. The entropic energy that is released drives the spontaneous self-assembly of the collagen into fibrils. Self-assembled collagen fibers have considerable tensile strength, which is increased by cross-linking reactions that form covalent bonds between α chains in one molecule and α chains in adjacent molecules. The first step in cross-linking is oxidation by lysyl oxidase of amino groups on a few lysine or hydroxylysine residues to form aldehydes that interact to form stable covalent bonds.

During growth and development, the collagen fibrils in all tissues undergo repeated synthesis, degradation, and resynthesis. The degradation of collagen fibers in tissues is initiated by specific collagenases. In adults, collagen fibers in most tissues undergo very little metabolic turnover. One exception is bone where collagen fibrils are

TABLE 357-1	CONSTITUENTS OF CONNECTIVE TISSUES IN VARIOUS TISSUES		
Connective Tissue	**Major Constituents**	**Approximate Amounts, % dry wt**	**Characteristics or Functions**
Dermis, ligaments, tendons	Type I collagen	80	Bundles of fibrils
	Type III collagen	5–15	Thin fibrils
	Type IV collagen, laminin, nidogen	<5	In basal laminae under epithelium and endothelium
	Types V, VI, and VII collagens	<5	VII forms anchoring fibrils; others unknown
	Elastin, fibrillin	<5	Provides elasticity
	Fibronectin	<5	Associated with collagen fibers and cell surfaces
	Proteoglycans,[a] hyaluronate	0.5	Provide resiliency
Bone (demineralized)	Type I collagen	90	Complex fibril network
	Type VI collagen	1–2	Function unclear
	Proteoglycans[a]	1	Function unclear
	Osteonectin, osteopontin, osteocalcin, α2-glycoprotein, sialoproteins	1–5	May regulate mineralization
Aorta	Type I collagen	20–40	Fibril network
	Type III collagen	20–40	Thin fibrils
	Elastin, fibrillin	20–40	Provide elasticity
	Type IV collagen, laminin, nidogen	<5	Form basal lamina
	Types V and VI collagens	<2	Function unclear
	Proteoglycans[a]	<3	Provide resiliency
Cartilage	Type II collagen	40–50	Arcades of thin fibrils
	Type IX collagen	5–10	Links type II fibrils
	Type X collagen	5–10	Surrounds hypertrophic cells
	Type XI collagen	<10	Function unclear
	Proteoglycans,[a] hyaluronate	15–50	Provide resiliency

[a]As discussed in text, >30 proteoglycans have now been identified. They differ in the structures of their core proteins and their contents of glycosaminoglycan side chains of chondroitin-4-sulfate, chondroitin-6-sulfate, dermatan sulfate, and keratin sulfate. Basal lamina contain a proteoglycan with a side chain of heparan sulfate that resembles heparin.

FIGURE 357-1 Schematic representation of synthesis of a type I collagen fibril by a fibroblast. *A.* Intracellular steps in the assembly of the procollagen molecule. Hydroxylations and glycosylations of the proα chains begin soon after the amino termini pass into the cisternae of the rough endoplasmic reticulum and continue after the three chains associate through their carboxy-terminal propeptides and become disulfide linked. ***B.*** Cleavage of procollagen to collagen, self-assembly of the collagen molecule into quarter-staggered fibrils, and cross-linking of the molecules in the fibrils. Cleavage of the propeptides may occur within crypts of the fibroblast, as shown here, or some distance from the cell. Mutations (depicted by X) cause the synthesis of structurally abnormal proα1(I) or proα2(I) chains of type I procollagen by interfering either with protein assembly (procollagen suicide) (***A***) or with processing to normal collagen fibrils (***B***). *(From DJ Prockop et al: Am J Med Genet 34:60, 1989, with permission.)*

degraded and resynthesized as part of lifelong remodeling. Also, the rate of collagen turnover increases under some circumstances. In starvation, a large fraction of the collagen in skin and other connective tissues is degraded, thus providing amino acids for gluconeogenesis (Chap. 72). Large losses of collagen also occur in most connective tissues during immobilization or prolonged periods of low-gravitational stress. In rheumatoid arthritis, pannus invasion causes a rapid degradation of collagen in the articular cartilage. Glucocorticoids decrease the collagen content of most connective tissues, including bone, by decreasing the rate of collagen synthesis. Decreases in collagen weaken tissues. In many pathologic states, however, collagen is deposited in excess. With injury to tissue, inflammation is usually followed by increased deposition of collagen fibrils in the form of fibrotic tissue and scars. The deposition of collagen fibrils during the repair process is largely irreversible and is a major feature of the pathologic changes in hepatic cirrhosis, pulmonary fibrosis, atherosclerosis, and nephrosclerosis.

Elastin Synthesis Elastin assembly has some similarities to the assembly of collagen, since a few of the prolines in the protein are hydroxylated to hydroxyproline by prolyl hydroxylase. The elastin monomer, however, is a single polypeptide that does not fold into a defined three-dimensional structure and is not synthesized as a larger precursor molecule. Instead, it is slowly secreted from cells into extracellular compartments, where it forms amorphous deposits around previously deposited microfibrils. The elastin deposits then become covalently cross-linked through oxidation of lysine residues to aldehydes by the same lysyl oxidase

that initiates the cross-linking of collagen. The microfibrils in elastin deposits are largely composed of fibrillin, a large protein that forms beadlike strands.

Proteoglycan Synthesis The synthesis of proteoglycans begins in the cisternae of the rough endoplasmic reticulum with assembly of a core protein that undergoes sequential additions of sugars to generate large side chains of glycosaminoglycans. At least 30 proteoglycans have been identified by differences in the structures of their core proteins and their side chains. The major proteoglycan of cartilage, called *aggrecan*, has a core protein of about 2000 amino acids that is decorated with multiple side chains of chondroitin sulfate and keratin sulfate, polysaccharides consisting of highly charged and repetitive disaccharide sequences. The highly charged proteoglycan aggregate binds water and small ions that distend the collagen network and thereby make the tissue resilient to pressure.

SPECIFIC DISORDERS

OSTEOGENESIS IMPERFECTA

OI is predominantly characterized by a generalized decrease in bone mass (osteopenia) and by brittle bones. The disorder is frequently associated with blue sclerae, dental abnormalities (dentinogenesis imperfecta), progressive hearing loss, and a positive family history.

Classification The most common classification for OI was developed by Sillence (Table 357-2). Type I is the mildest form, and most patients have distinctly blue sclerae. Type II is lethal *in utero* or shortly after birth. Types III and IV are intermediate in severity between types I and II. They differ from type I because they are more severe and because sclerae are not blue or only slightly bluish in infancy and white in adulthood. Type III differs from type IV because it tends to become more severe with age, but the distinction between type IV and type III OI may not be clinically useful. Therefore, it may be sufficient to classify patients simply as mild (type I), lethal (type II), and moderately severe (type III). A few patients with many of the symptoms of OI were recently found not to have mutations in the genes for type I collagen. These patients have a characteristic lamellar patterning of bone, and distinctive clinical and radiological findings. They have been assigned the classifications of types V, VI, and VII OI.

The classification of mild and moderate forms of OI is not always prognostic because of variations in the clinical course. Some patients appear normal at birth and become progressively worse; others have multiple fractures in infancy and childhood, improve after puberty, and fracture more frequently later in life. Women are particularly

TABLE 357-2 EXPANDED CLASSIFICATION OF OSTEOGENESIS IMPERFECTA (OI)

Type	Bone Fragility	Blue Sclerae	Abnormal Dentition	Hearing Loss	Inheritance[a]
I	Mild	Present	Present in some	Present in most	AD
II	Extreme	Present	Present in some	Unknown	S, rarely AR
III	Severe	Bluish at birth	Present in some	High incidence	AD, rarely AR
IV	Variable	Absent	Absent in IVA, present in IVB	High incidence	AD
V	Moderate to severe	Absent	Absent		AD
VI	Moderate to severe	Absent	Absent		Unknown
VII	Moderate	Absent	Absent	Absent	AR

[a]AD, autosomal dominant; AR, autosomal recessive; S, sporadic.

prone to fracture during pregnancy and after menopause. A few women from families with mild variants of OI do not develop fractures until after menopause, and their disease may be difficult to distinguish from postmenopausal osteoporosis.

Incidence Type I OI has a frequency of about 1 in 30,000. Type II OI has a reported incidence at birth of about 1 in 60,000, but the combined incidence of the three severe forms that are recognizable at birth (types II, III, and IV) may be much higher. Only a few patients with types V, VI, and VII have been reported.

Skeletal Effects In type I OI, the fragility of bones may be severe enough to limit physical activity or be so mild that individuals are unaware of any disability. Radiographs of the skull in patients with mild disease may show a mottled appearance because of small islands of irregular ossification. In type II OI, bones and other connective tissues are so fragile that massive injuries can occur in utero or during delivery. Ossification of many bones is frequently incomplete. Continuously beaded or broken ribs and crumpled long bones (accordina femora) may be present. For reasons that are not apparent, the long bones may be either thick or thin. In types III and IV, multiple fractures from minor physical stress can produce severe deformities. Kyphoscoliosis can impair respiration, cause cor pulmonale, and predispose to pulmonary infections. The appearance of "popcorn-like" deposits of mineral in x-rays of the ends of long bones is an ominous sign. Progressive neurologic symptoms may result from basilar compression and communicating hydrocephalus. Type V OI is recognized by the presence of dislocated radial heads and hyperplastic callus formation. Rhizomelia and coxa vara are observed in patients with OI type VII.

In all forms of OI, bone mineral density is decreased. However, the degree of osteopenia may be difficult to evaluate because recurrent fractures limit exercise and thereby diminish bone mass. Surprisingly, fractures appear to heal normally.

Ocular Features The sclerae can be normal, slightly bluish, or bright blue. The color is probably caused by a thinness of the collagen layers of the sclerae that allows the choroid layers to be seen. Blue sclerae, however, are an inherited trait in some families who do not have increased bone fragility.

Dentinogenesis The teeth may be normal, moderately discolored, or grossly abnormal. The enamel generally appears normal, but the teeth may have a characteristic amber, yellowish brown, or translucent bluish gray color because of improper deposition or deficiency of dentin. The deciduous teeth are usually smaller than normal, whereas permanent teeth are frequently bell-shaped and restricted at the base. In some patients, the teeth readily fracture and need to be extracted. The defect in dentin is directly attributable to the fact that normal dentin is rich in type I collagen. Similar tooth defects, however, can be inherited without any evidence of OI.

Hearing Loss Hearing loss usually begins during the second decade of life and occurs in more than 50% of individuals over age 30. The loss can be conductive, sensorineural, or mixed, and it varies in severity. The middle ear usually exhibits maldevelopment, deficient ossification, persistence of cartilage in areas that are normally ossified, and abnormal calcium deposits.

Other Features Changes in other connective tissues can include thin skin that scars extensively, joint laxity with permanent dislocations indistinguishable from those of EDS, and, occasionally, cardiovascular manifestations such as aortic regurgitation, floppy mitral valves, mitral incompetence, and fragility of large blood vessels. For unknown reasons, some patients develop a hypermetabolic state with elevated serum thyroxine levels, hyperthermia, and excessive sweating.

Molecular Defects Most patients who meet the clinical criteria for OI are heterozygous for mutations in either the gene for the proα1(I)

chain or the gene for the proα2(I) chain of type I procollagen (the *COL1A1* and *COL1A2* genes). Surprisingly, null mutations that produce haploinsufficiency are found in patients with type I OI, the mildest forms of the disease. Over 90% of patients with type I OI and blue sclerae have mutations that reduce the synthesis of pro α1(I)chains to about one half. Mutations that reduce the synthesis of proα2(I) chains produce slightly more severe phenotypes that can overlap with EDS. The most severe variants (types II, III and IV) are caused by mutations that produce structurally abnormal, but partially functional, proα chains. These mutations include partial gene deletions, partial gene duplications, and splicing mutations. The most common mutations, however, are single base substitutions that introduce an amino acid with a bulky side chain for one of the glycine residues that appear as every third amino acid in the triple-helical domain of a proα chain. In effect, any of the 338 glycine residues in either the proα1(I) or proα2(I) chain is a potential site for a disease producing mutation. Mutations that cause structurally abnormal proα chains exert their effects through one of three mechanisms (Fig. 357-1). First, the presence of an abnormal proα chain in a procollagen molecule containing two normal proα chains can prevent folding of the protein into a triple-helical conformation and lead to degradation of the whole molecule in a process called *procollagen suicide*. Similar dominant negative mutations are seen with other multisubunit proteins. The net result of procollagen suicide is accumulation of the unfolded protein in the rough endoplasmic reticulum of cells and a reduction in the amount of collagen available for fibril assembly. Second, the presence of one abnormal proα chain in a procollagen molecule can interfere with cleavage of the N-propeptide from the protein. The persistence of the N-propeptide on a fraction of the molecules interferes with the self-assembly of normal collagen so that thin and irregular collagen fibrils are formed. Third, the substitution of a bulkier amino acid for glycine can produce a change in the conformation of the molecule and result in the assembly of collagen fibrils that are abnormally branched or abnormally thick and short. The data on the molecular consequences of mutations in the type I procollagen genes that cause OI have served as a paradigm for explaining the effects of mutations in other collagen genes.

Several generalizations can be made about mutations in collagen genes. One is that unrelated patients rarely have the same mutation in the same gene. Over 900 such "private" mutations have been identified with slightly more in the *COL1A1* gene than in the *COL1A2* gene. Another general trend is that similar mutations in different regions of the same gene can produce different disease syndromes, both in severity and in the major tissues involved. One reason for heterogeneity in clinical manifestations is that different regions of the large collagen molecule may be more important for its function in some connective tissues than in others. For example, some regions of the type I collagen molecule may be essential for the binding of mineralizing proteins in bone so that mutations in these regions cause fragile bones but do not impair function in skin and other nonmineralizing tissues. It is more difficult, however, to explain how the same mutation can produce a severe phenotype in some and a mild phenotype in other members of the same family. Such phenotypic variation appears to be characteristic of OI, where some family members are short and have multiple fractures from minor trauma, whereas others in the same family can be of normal stature and free of fractures. In the past, such phenotypic variation was explained by undefined variations in the genetic background of different family members. Studies in transgenic mice, however, demonstrate similar phenotypic variation with expression of a mutated collagen gene in an inbred strain of mice whose genetic background is uniform. Therefore, the phenotypic variation is probably caused by undefined stochastic or chance events during embryonic and fetal development. Although dramatic phenotypic variations are relatively rare in OI and related disorders, it is important to consider in counseling families about the consequences of inherited mutations. Recently, mutations in the gene for cartilage-associated protein (CASP or CRTAP) were detected in one family with the recessive form of type II OI and another family with type VII OI. CRTAP binds to prolyl 3-hydroxylase and appears to be essential for efficient hydroxylation of the 3-position carbon of a single prolyl residue in the X-position of collagen type I sequence. Prolyl 3-hydroxylase is encoded by the *LEPRE1* gene and null mutations in this gene were detected in five cases of a new recessive bone disorder resembling lethal/severe osteogenesis imperfecta.

Inheritance and Mosaicism in Germ-Line Cells and in Somatic Cells Type I OI is usually inherited as an autosomal dominant trait. However, some patients with type I OI appear to represent sporadic new mutations or the diagnosis may have been missed in earlier generations. Most lethal OI is the result of sporadic mutations that occur in the germ line in one of the parents. Because of the possibility for germ-line mosaicism for newly generated mutations, there is about a 7% probability that a second child could inherit a severe variant of OI.

Diagnosis OI is usually diagnosed on the basis of clinical criteria. The presence of fractures together with blue sclerae, dentinogenesis imperfecta, or family history of the disease is usually sufficient to make the diagnosis. Other causes of pathologic fractures must be excluded, including battered child syndrome, nutritional deficiencies, malignancies, and other inherited disorders such as CDs and hypophosphatasia. The absence of superficial bruises can be helpful in distinguishing OI from battered child syndrome. X-rays usually reveal a decrease in bone density that can be verified by photon or x-ray absorptiometry. Bone microscopy can be helpful in the diagnosis. A molecular defect in type I procollagen can be demonstrated in over two-thirds of patients by incubating skin fibroblasts with radioactive amino acids and then analyzing the proα chains by polyacrylamide gel electrophoresis. However, mutations in exons coding for the N-terminus of the helical region, where biochemical abnormalities do not result in overmodified collagen, are difficult to detect by gel electrophoresis. The mutations themselves can be defined in most patients by the sequencing of genomic DNA with tests that are available from specialized laboratories. Because each proband and each family usually has a private mutation, extensive analysis of about 10,000 bases in each of the two genes is required to identify the exact mutation. Analysis of collagen genes and most other large genes is usually performed by using about 100 polymerase chain reactions (PCRs) to amplify all the exons and exon/intron boundaries of the two large genes, followed by a screening of the PCR products for heteroduplexes of normal and mutated strands. If no mutation is detected with the screening technique, the PCR products are sequenced. After a mutation in a type I procollagen gene is identified, a simple PCR test can be used to screen family members at risk or for prenatal diagnosis. The DNA tests are useful for patients who do not meet all the criteria for OI, as an adjunct to prenatal diagnosis, to distinguish OI from battered child syndrome, and to reassure patients and family members.

℞ OSTEOGENESIS IMPERFECTA

Many patients with OI have successful careers despite severe deformities. Those with mild disorder may need little treatment when fractures decrease after puberty, but women require special attention during pregnancy and after menopause, when fractures again increase. More severely affected children require a comprehensive program of physical therapy, surgical management of fractures and skeletal deformities, and vocational education.

Many of the fractures are only slightly displaced and have little soft tissue swelling. Therefore, they can be treated with minimal support or traction for a week or two followed by a light cast. If fractures are relatively painless, physical therapy can be initiated early. A judicious amount of exercise prevents loss of bone mass secondary to physical inactivity. Some physicians advocate insertion of steel rods into long bones to correct limb deformities; the risk/benefits and cost/benefits of such procedures are difficult to evaluate. Aggressive conventional intervention is usually warranted for pneumonia and cor pulmonale. For severe hearing loss, stapedectomy or replacement of the stapes with a prosthesis may be successful. Moderately to severely affected patients should be evaluated periodically to anticipate possible neurologic problems. About half of children have a substantial increase in growth when

given growth hormone. Treatment with bisphosphonates to decrease bone loss has been introduced for moderate to severe forms of OI. Initial results are promising, but the long-term effects of decreasing bone resorption and bone turnover are still unknown. Also, a clinical trial has been performed in which patients were treated by intravenous infusion of cells from bone marrow referred to as mesenchymal stem cells, or multipotential stromal cells (MSCs), that home to sites of tissue injury and repair the tissues by a variety of mechanisms, including differentiating into osteoblasts (Chap. 67). In the first phase of the trial, four children with severe OI (type III) showed clinical improvement after marrow ablation and transplantation of whole bone marrow from an HLA-compatible sibling. The rationale of the trial was that the bone marrow from the donor might provide wild-type MSCs capable of differentiating into normal osteoblasts, thereby improving the quality of bone in the patients. In the second phase of the trial, the children showed further but temporary improvement after intravenous infusion of large numbers of wild-type MSCs from the same donors with whom the patients now shared an immune system. These results raise the possibility that it may be possible in the future to develop effective stem cell therapies for OI when effective and safe protocols are developed to correct the type I collagen mutation in a patient's own MSCs.

Counseling and emotional support are important for patients and their parents; lay organizations in some countries provide help in these areas. Prenatal ultrasonography will detect severely affected fetuses at about 16 weeks of pregnancy. Diagnosis by demonstrating synthesis of abnormal proα chains or by DNA sequencing can be carried out in chorionic villus biopsies at 8–12 weeks of pregnancy.

EHLERS-DANLOS SYNDROME

EDS is characterized by hyperelasticity of the skin and hypermobile joints.

Classification Several types of EDS have been defined, based on the extent to which the skin, joints, and other tissues are involved, mode of inheritance, and by molecular and biochemical analysis (Table 357-3). Classical EDS includes a severe form of the disease (type I) and a milder form (type II), both characterized by joint hypermobility and skin that is velvety in texture, hyperextensible, and easily scarred. In hypermobile EDS (type III), joint hypermobility is more prominent than skin changes. In vascular-type EDS (type IV), the skin changes are more prominent than joint changes, and the patients are predisposed to sudden death from rupture of large blood vessels or other hollow organs. EDS V is similar to EDS II but is inherited as an X-linked trait. The ocular-scoliotic type of EDS (type VI) is characterized by scoliosis, ocular fragility, and a cone-shaped deformity of the cornea (keratoconus). The arthrochalasic type of EDS (type VII A & B) is characterized by marked joint hypermobility that is difficult to distinguish from EDS III except by the specific molecular defects in the processing of type I procollagen to collagen. The periodontotic-type EDS (type VIII) is distinguished by prominent periodontal changes. EDS IX, X, and XI were defined on the basis of preliminary biochemical and clinical data. EDS due to tenascin X deficiency has not been assigned a type; it is an autosomal recessive form of the syndrome similar to EDS II. Because of overlapping signs and symptoms, many patients and families with some of the features of EDS cannot be assigned to any of the defined types.

Incidence The overall incidence of EDS is about 1 in 5,000 births, with a higher rate for blacks. Classical and hypermobile types of EDS are the most common. Patients with milder forms frequently do not seek medical attention.

Skin Skin changes vary from thin and velvety to skin that is either dramatically hyperextensible ("rubber man" syndrome) or easily torn or scarred. Patients with classical EDS develop characteristic "cigarette-paper" scars. In vascular-type EDS, extensive scars and hyperpigmentation develop over bony prominences, and the skin may be so thin that subcutaneous blood vessels are visible. In the periodontotic type of EDS, the skin is more fragile than hyperextensible, and it heals with atrophic, pigmented scars. Easy bruisability occurs in several types of EDS.

TABLE 357-3 DIFFERENT FORMS OF EHLERS-DANLOS SYNDROME

Type	Typical Features	Inheritance	Gene Defect	Protein Defect
Classic (EDS I - severe and EDS II – mild)	Skin hyperextensibility and fragility, joint hypermobility, tissue fragility manifested by widened atrophic scarring	AD	*COL5A1* *COL5A2*	Collagen V
		AD	*COL1A1*	Proα1 (I) and proα2 (I) chains of procollagen I
		AD, AR	*COL1A2*	
Hypermobile (EDS III)	Joint hypermobility, moderate skin involvement, absence of tissue fragility	AD	*TNX*	Tenascin X
Vascular (EDS IV)	Markedly reduced life span due to spontaneous rupture of internal organs such as arteries and intestines; skin is thin, translucent, and fragile, with extensive bruising; hypermobile minor joints; characteristic facial appearance	AD	*COL3A1*	Collagen III
X-linked EDS (EDS V)	Similar to classic type	X-linked recessive	Unknown	Unknown
Ocular-scoliotic EDS VI (EDS VIA and EDS VIB)	Features of classic EDS as well as severe muscular hypotonia after birth, progressive kyphoscoliosis, a Marfanoid habitus, osteopenia, occasionally rupture of the eye globe, and great arteries	AR	*PLOD1*	Deficiency of procollagen-lysine 5-dioxygenase activity (EDS VIA)
			Unknown for EDS VIB	Unknown for EDS VIB
Arthrochalasic EDS VII (EDS VIIA and EDS VIIB)	Congenital bilateral hip dislocation, hypermobile joints, moderate skin involvement, osteopenia	AD	*COL1A1* *COL1A2*	Mutations that prevent cleavage of the N-pro-peptides
Dermatosparactic EDS VII C	Redundant and fragile skin, prominent herniae, joint laxity, dysmorphic features	AR	*ADAMTS2*	Deficiency of procollagen I N-terminal proteinase
Periodontotic EDS VIII	Absorptive periodontosis with premature loss of permanent teeth, fragility of the skin, skin lesions	AD	Unknown	Unknown
EDS due to tenascin X deficiency	Similar to EDS II	AR	*TNX*	Tenascin X

Note: AD, autosomal dominant; AR, autosomal recessive.

Ligament and Joint Changes Laxity and hypermobility of joints vary from mild to unreducible dislocations of hips and other large joints. In mild forms, patients learn to reduce dislocations by limiting physical activity. In more severe forms, surgical repair may be required. Some patients have progressive difficulty with age.

Other Features Mitral valve prolapse and hernias occur, particularly with type I. Pes planus and mild to moderate scoliosis are common. Extreme joint laxity and repeated dislocations may lead to degenerative arthritis. In the ocular-scoliotic type of EDS, the eye may rupture with minimal trauma, and kyphoscoliosis can cause respiratory impairment. Also, sclerae may be blue.

Molecular Defects Many patients have mutations in structural genes for collagens or in the genes for the processing of procollagens (Table 357-3). However, a series of collagen and collagen-related genes have been excluded as loci for EDS, and mutations in other genes are probably involved. About 50% of patients with classical EDS (types I and II) have mutations in two of the three genes (*COL5A1* and *COL5A2*) for type V collagen, a minor collagen found in association with type I collagen in many tissues. In contrast to the mutations in collagen genes causing other syndromes, most of the mutations are null mutations causing haploinsufficiency; point mutations are rare. A few patients with the moderately severe classical EDS phenotype have mutations in the *COL1A2* gene. Some patients with the hypermobile EDS (type III) have mutations in the TNX gene that encodes tenascin X, another minor component of connective tissue that appears to regulate the assembly of collagen fibers. Most patients with the vascular EDS (type IV) have a defect in either the synthesis or the structure of type III procollagen, a precursor of a moderately abundant collagen found in many tissues in association with type I collagen. Most of the mutations in the type III procollagen gene are single base substitutions for glycine residues with consequences similar to those of glycine substitutions in other collagens (Fig. 357-1). The presence of mutations in the gene for type III collagen (*COL3A1*) is consistent with the fact that the patients are prone to spontaneous rupture of the aorta and intestines, tissues rich in type III collagen. The thinness and scarring of skin are more difficult to explain, since type III constitutes a small fraction of the collagen in skin (Table 357-1).

The ocular-scoliotic type of EDS (type VI) is caused by homozygous or compound heterozygous mutations in the *PLOD 1* gene that encodes procollagen-lysine 5-dioxygenase (lysyl hydroxylase 1). The decreased activity of the enzyme reduces the hydroxylysine content of collagen and produces weaker collagen because cross-links formed with lysine residues are less stable than those formed with hydroxylysine residues. Mutations in the *PLOD 1* gene were not detected in a small group of patients with EDS type VI that are classified as EDS type VIB.

Arthrochalasic type EDS occurs because of a defect in the conversion of procollagen to collagen caused either by mutations that make type I procollagen resistant to cleavage by procollagen N-proteinase or by mutations that decrease the activity of the enzyme. Mutations in EDS type VIIA alter the cleavage site in the proα1(I) chain, and mutations in EDS VIIB alter the cleavage site in the proα2(I) chain. Both types are dominantly inherited. Dermatosparactic-type EDS (type VIIC) is caused by mutations in the *ADAMTS2* gene that decrease the activity of procollagen N-proteinase, and it is inherited as an autosomal recessive trait. In all three forms of EDS type VII, the persistence of the N-propeptide causes the formation of collagen fibrils that are thin and irregular. Since most patients do not have clinical osteopenia, the thin and irregular fibrils apparently suffice for the structural integrity of bone but do not provide the necessary tensile strength for ligaments and joint capsules. However, some patients fracture easily, and their disorder is difficult to distinguish from variants of OI.

The cause of periodontotic-type EDS (type VIII) is unknown. Dominant mutations in tenacin X (*TNX*) are found in patients with EDS III (Table 357-3), but some patients with the symptoms of EDS II and recessive inheritance have mutations in both alleles of the gene associated with the fragmentation of the elastic fibers and reduction of collagen. A variant of EDS originally referred to as type IX is now more commonly classified as Menkes' syndrome and is caused by mutations in a gene coding for a copper-transporting ATPase (Chaps. 354 and 359). Initial observations suggested that EDS X may be caused by defects in fibronectin, but no specific mutations have been defined.

Diagnosis The diagnosis is based on clinical criteria. Biochemical assays and gene analyses for known molecular defects in EDS are difficult and time-consuming, but tests are sometimes available from specialized laboratories. Correlations between genotype and phenotype are challenging, but the tests are particularly useful for the diagnosis of vascular-type IV EDS with its dire prognosis.

As with other heritable diseases of connective tissue, there is a large degree of variability among members of the same family carrying the same mutation. Some patients have increased fractures and are difficult to distinguish from OI. A few families with heritable aortic aneurysms have mutations in the gene for type III collagen without any evidence of EDS or OI.

R℞ EHLERS-DANLOS SYNDROME

Surgical repair and tightening of joint ligaments require careful evaluation of individual patients, as the ligaments frequently do not hold sutures. Patients with easy bruisability should be evaluated for bleeding disorders. Patients with type IV EDS and members of their families should be evaluated at regular intervals for early detection of aneurysms, but surgical repair may be difficult because of friable tissues. Also, women with type IV EDS should be counseled about the increased risk of uterine rupture, bleeding, and other complications of pregnancy.

CHONDRODYSPLASIAS

(See also Chap. 349) Chondrodysplasias (CDs), also referred to as skeletal dysplasias, are heritable skeletal disorders that are characterized by dwarfism and abnormal body proportions. The category also includes some individuals with normal stature and body proportions who have features such as ocular changes or cleft palate that are common in more severe CDs. Many patients develop degenerative joint changes, and mild CD in adults may be difficult to differentiate from primary generalized osteoarthritis.

Classification   Over 200 distinct types and subtypes have been defined based on criteria such as "bringing death" (thanatophoric), causing "twisted" bones (diastrophic), affecting metaphyses (metaphyseal), affecting epiphyses (epiphyseal), affecting spine (spondylo-) and producing histologic changes such as an apparent increase in the fibrous material in the epiphyses (fibrochondrogenesis). Also, a number of eponyms are based on the first or most comprehensive case reports. Severe forms of the diseases produce gross distortions of most cartilaginous structures and of the eye. Mild forms are more difficult to classify. Among the features are cataracts, degeneration of the vitreous and retinal detachment, high forehead, hypoplastic facies, cleft palate, short extremities, and gross distortions of the epiphyses, metaphyses, and joint surfaces. Patients with Stickler syndrome (hereditary arthro-ophthalmopathy) have been classified into three types based on a combination of the ocular phenotype and mutated genes.

Incidence   Data on the frequency of most CDs are not available, but the incidence of the Stickler syndrome is 1 in 10,000. Therefore, the disease is probably among the most common heritable disorders of connective tissue.

Molecular Defects   A series of CDs are produced by mutations in the *COL2A1* gene for type II collagen. Patients with CDs can also have mutations in genes for the core protein of aggrecan, for four additional collagens (types VI, IX, X and XI), or for three structural macromolecules (cartilage oligomer matrix protein, matrilin-3 and perlecan) that modify the interactions between type II collagen and aggrecan. However, the mutated genes in a number of patients with CDs have not yet been identified.

The best correlation of mutations in the *COL2A1* gene with clinical findings is found in the Stickler syndrome. Mutations in the gene were initially found in some but not all patients with the syndrome. Subsequently, the patients were re-examined to develop more rigorous clinical criteria for what was defined as type I Stickler syndrome. The criteria are based on a numerical score for orofacial abnormalities, such as cleft palate and characteristic facies; auditory abnormalities,

such as high frequency sensorineural loss; skeletal changes, such as early osteoarthritis; and family history, with or without molecular data. Essentially, all patients who meet the clinical criteria have mutations in *COL2A1*. Most of the mutations are premature termination codons that produce haploinsufficiency. Many, but not all, patients who do not meet the criteria for type I Stickler syndrome, but who have several features of the syndrome, have mutations in two genes specific for type XI collagen, which is an unusual heterotrimer formed from α chains encoded by the gene for type II collagen (*COL2A1*) and two distinctive genes for type XI collagen (*COL11A1* and *COL11A2*). Mutations in the *COL11A1* gene are also found in patients with Marshall syndrome, which is similar to classic Stickler syndrome but with more severe hearing loss and dysmorphic features, such as a flat or retracted midface with flat nasal bridge, short nose, anteverted nostrils, long philtrum, and large-appearing eyes. Thick calvaria, abnormal frontal sinuses, and intracranial ossification are also typical radiological findings for Marshall syndrome.

Mutations in the *COL2A1* gene are also found in patients with CDs not classified as Stickler syndrome. Like mutations in the genes for other collagens, the phenotypes range from severe to mild, and a variety of mutations, including glycine substitutions, are found. The severe CDs are characterized by gross deformities of bones and cartilage, such as those found in spondyloepiphyseal dysplasia congenita, spondyloepimetaphyseal dysplasia congenita, hypochondrogenesis/achondrogenesis type II, and Kniest syndrome. However, mutations in the *COL2A1* gene are found in milder CDs and are also found in some families where few, if any, symptoms are present in childhood, but degenerative changes of osteoarthritis develop in midlife. As with mutations in other collagen genes, the correlation between genotype and the severity of the phenotype is variable.

Many individuals with Schmid metaphyseal CD have mutations in the gene for type X collagen, a short, network-forming collagen found primarily in the hypertrophic zone of endochondral cartilage. The syndrome is characterized by short stature, *coxa vara*, flaring metaphyses, and waddling gait.

Patients with achondroplasia have mutations in the gene for receptor for fibroblast growth factor (*FGFR3*). The syndrome is the most common cause of short-limbed dwarfism accompanied by macrocephaly and dysplasias of the metaphyses of long bones. The same single-base mutation in the gene that converts glycine to arginine at position 380 in the *FGFR3* gene is present in over 90% of patients. Most patients represent sporadic new mutations, and this nucleotide change must be one of the most common recurring mutations in the human genome. The mutation causes unregulated signal transduction through the receptor and inappropriate development of cartilage. Mutations that alter other domains of *FGFR3* have been found in patients with the more severe disorders of hypochondroplasia and thanatophoric dysplasia and in a few families with a variant of craniosynostosis. However, most patients with craniosynostosis appear to have mutations in the related *FGFR2* gene. The similarities between the phenotypes produced by mutations in genes for FGF receptors and mutations in structural proteins of cartilage is probably explained by the observation that the activity of FGFs is regulated in part by binding proteins sequestered in the extracellular matrix.

Patients with pseudoachondroplasia, or autosomal dominant multiple epiphyseal dysplasia, have mutations in the gene for the cartilage oligomeric matrix protein (*COMP*), a protein that interacts with both collagens and proteoglycans in cartilage. However, some families with multiple epiphyseal dysplasia have a defect in one of the three genes for type IX collagen (*COL9A1*, *COL9A2*, and *COL9A3*), or in matrilin-3, another extracellular protein found in cartilage. Patients with an autosomal recessive form of multiple epiphyseal dysplasia have mutations in a gene encoding a sulfate transporter protein (*DTDST*).

Diagnosis   The diagnosis of CDs is made on the basis of the physical appearance, slit-lamp eye examinations, x-ray findings, histologic changes, and clinical course. Evaluation of patients by specialists in the field is usually required for a diagnosis. DNA tests for mutations in some of the genes are available from specialized laboratories. For Stickler syndrome, more precise diagnostic criteria have made it possible to identify type I variants with mutations in the *COL2A1* gene with a high degree of accuracy. It has been suggested that the type II variant with mutations in the *COL11A1* gene can be identified on the basis of a "beaded" vitreous phenotype, and the type III variant with mutations in the *COL11A2* gene can be identified on the basis of the characteristic systemic features without the ocular involvement. Prenatal diagnosis based on analysis of DNA obtained from chorionic villus or amniotic fluid is possible.

℞ CHONDRODYSPLASIAS

The treatment is symptomatic and is directed to secondary features such as degenerative arthritis. Many patients require joint replacement surgery and corrective surgery for cleft palate. The eyes should be monitored carefully for the development of cataracts and the need for laser therapy to prevent retinal detachment. Patients should be advised to avoid obesity and contact sports. Counseling for the psychological problems of short stature is critical, and support groups have formed in many countries.

MARFAN SYNDROME

MFS includes features that primarily affect the skeleton, the cardiovascular system, and the eyes.

Classification   MFS was initially characterized by a triad of features: (a) skeletal changes that include long, thin extremities, frequently associated with loose joints; (b) reduced vision as the result of dislocations of the lenses (ectopia lentis); and (c) aortic aneurysms. Using the triad to define the disorder proved difficult because different patients displayed the features to varying degrees. The discovery that some, but not all, patients diagnosed with MFS had a mutation in the gene for fibrillin-1 (*FBN1*) prompted an international effort to develop more stringent "Ghent criteria" for diagnosis. With the more stringent criteria, more than 90% of the patients defined as type I MFS were found to have a mutation in the *FBN1* gene. Analyses of patients without mutations in the *FBN1* gene identified mutations in the gene that encodes transforming growth factor β receptor 2 (*TGFBR2*). These patients were classified as type II MFS. Patients with type II MFS were similar to patients with type I MFS but lacked the ocular changes. In subsequent studies, mutations in both *TGFB2* and the closely related *TGFB1* gene were found in patients with a new syndrome referred to as *Loeys-Dietz aneurysm syndrome* (LDAS). The patients with LDAS presented with aneurysms of the ascending aorta, tortuous arteries, cleft palate, and hypertelorism. In another series of analyses, mutations in fibrillin-2, a protein similar to fibrillin-1, were found in some patients originally classified as MFS. However, more careful evaluations indicated that these patients, including the original patient reported by Marfan, had some of the features of MFS and some of the features of OI, together with joint contractures. Therefore, they are classified as congenital contractual arachnodactyly (CCA).

Incidence and Inheritance   The incidence of MFS is about 1 in 3,000/ 5,000 in most racial and ethnic groups, with type I MFS being far more common than type II MFS, LDAS, or CCA. Most variants are inherited as autosomal dominant traits, but about one-fourth of patients have sporadic new mutations.

Skeletal Effects   Patients have long limbs and are usually tall compared to other members of the same family. The ratio of the upper segment (top of the head to the top of the pubic ramus) to the lower segment (top of the pubic ramus to the floor) is usually 2 SDs below mean for age, race, and sex. The fingers and hands are long and slender and have a spider-like appearance (arachnodactyly). Many patients have severe chest deformities, including depression (pectus excavatum), protrusion (pectus carinatum), or asymmetry. Scoliosis is frequent and usually accompanied by kyphosis. CT or MRI examinations of the lumbar sacral region frequently reveals enlargement of the neural canal, thinning of the pedicles and laminae, widening of the foraminae, or anterior meningocele (dural ectasia). High-arched palate and high pedal arches or pes planus are common. A few patients have severe joint hypermobility similar to EDS.

Cardiovascular Features   Cardiovascular abnormalities are the major source of morbidity and mortality (Chap. 242). Mitral valve prolapse develops early in life and progresses to mitral valve regurgitation of increasing severity in about one-quarter of patients. Dilatation of the root of the aorta and the sinuses of Valsalva are characteristic and ominous features of the disease that can develop at any age. The rate of dilatation is unpredictable, but it can lead to aortic regurgitation, dissection of the aorta, and rupture. Dilatation is probably accelerated by physical and emotional stress, as well as by pregnancy. Patients with familial aortic aneurysms tend to develop aneurysms at the base of the abdominal aorta. The location of the aneurysms, however, is somewhat variable, and the high incidence of aortic aneurysms in the general population (1 in 100) makes the differential diagnosis difficult unless other features of MFS are clearly present.

Ocular Features   Downward displacement of the lens is common. It is usually not progressive but may contribute to the formation of cataracts. The ocular globe is frequently elongated, most patients are myopic, and some develop retinal detachment. A few patients have lattice degeneration and retinal tears; most have adequate vision.

Other Features   Striae may occur over the shoulders and buttocks. A number of patients develop spontaneous pneumothorax. Inguinal and incisional hernias are common. Patients are typically thin with little subcutaneous fat, but adults may develop centripetal obesity.

Molecular Defects   Essentially all patients who meet the Ghent criteria for type I MFS are heterozygous for a mutation in the *FBN1* gene on chromosome 15. Over 550 different mutations that have been identified are scattered throughout the 65 coding exons of the gene. Most are private mutations, but about 10% are recurrent new mutations that are largely located in CpG sequences known to be "hot spots" for mutations. For reasons that are not apparent, mutations in nine central exons (24–32) account for most of the mutations in the rare, but most severe, form of MFS that is lethal in neonates. About a third of the mutations introduce premature termination codons that encode truncated forms of the protein. About two-thirds of the mutations are missense mutations that alter calcium-binding domains in the repetitive epidermal growth factor-like domains of the protein. The effects of the mutations are complex and include impaired trafficking of the protein, delayed secretion, or enhanced susceptibility to proteases because of alterations in the conformation of the protein. In general, the severity of the phenotype cannot be predicted from the nature of the mutation.

The glycoprotein fibrillin-1 is a major component of elastin-associated microfibrils that are abundant in large blood vessels and in other tissues, such as the suspensory ligaments of the lens. Therefore, it was initially reasoned that the symptoms of MFS are caused by a failure of the mechanical integrity of elastin fibers. The discovery that type II MFS is caused by mutations in *TGFB2* refocused attention on structural similarity between fibrillin-1 and TGF-β binding proteins that sequester TGF-β in the extracellular matrix. Therefore, some of the manifestations of type I MFS are probably produced by changes in binding sites that modulate the activity of TGF-β during early development of the skeleton and other tissues.

Diagnosis   All patients with a suspected diagnosis of MFS should have a slit-lamp examination and an echocardiogram. Also, homocystinuria should be ruled out by amino acid analysis of plasma (Chap. 358). The diagnosis of type I MFS according to the international Ghent standards places emphasis on major criteria that include presence of at least four skeletal abnormalities: ectopia lentis; dilation of the ascending aorta with or without dissection; dural ectasia; and a blood relative who meets the same criteria, with or without a DNA diagnosis. A final diagnosis is based on a balanced assessment of the major criteria together with several minor criteria. The absence of ocular changes suggests type II MFS, and the presence of contractures with some of the signs of OI suggests CCA.

Diagnostic tests based on detection of protein defects in fibrillin-1 in cultured skin fibroblasts or DNA analyses of the gene are now available from several laboratories. Because over 90% of patients who meet the Ghent criteria for type I MFS have mutations in the *FBN1* gene, analyses of the gene may not be helpful except to reassure the patients and families or to rapidly exclude the diagnosis in other family members. However, mutations in the *FBN1* gene can also cause isolated features of MFS. The same considerations apply to DNA analyses for type II MFS, LDAS, and CCA. DNA analyses of the genes are also available in several laboratories.

℞ MARFAN SYNDROME

Propranolol or other β-adrenergic blocking agents are effectively used to lower blood pressure and thereby delay or prevent aortic dilatation. Surgical correction of the aorta, aortic valve, and mitral valve has been successful in many patients, but tissues are frequently friable. Patients should be advised of the risks of severe physical and emotional stress and of pregnancy.

The scoliosis tends to be progressive and should be treated by mechanical bracing and physical therapy if >20° or by surgery if it progresses to >45°. Dislocated lenses rarely require surgical removal, but patients should be followed closely for retinal detachment.

ELASTIN-RELATED DISEASES

Because of the role of elastin in maintaining the elasticity of skin, mutations in the elastin gene (*ELN*) have been suspected to cause genetic forms of *cutis laxa*, a rare and heterogeneous group of disorders characterized by redundant, pendulous, and inelastic skin. Localized mutations in the *ELN* gene itself have been detected in only a small number of the patients with cutis laxa. In two families, the genetic mutations were associated with both cutis laxa and aortic aneurysms.

EPIDERMOLYSIS BULLOSA

EB is of a group of similar disorders in which the skin and related epithelial tissues break and blister as the result of minor trauma.

Classification and Incidence   Four types of EB are defined on the basis of the level at which blistering occurs: (1) EB simplex for blistering in the epidermis, (2) EB hemidesmosomal for fissures between kerotinocytes and the basal lamina, (3) EB junctional for blistering in the dermal-epidermal junction, and (4) EB dystrophica for blistering in the dermis.

The incidence of EB in the United States is about 1 in 50,000.

Molecular Defects   A series of patients with EB simplex were found to have mutations in either keratin 14 or keratin 5, two of the major keratins in basal epithelial cells. Patients with the related syndrome, epidermolytic icthyosis, have mutations in keratin 1 and keratin 10. The new disease phenotype of hemidesmosomal EB has three clinical variants caused by mutations in one of four genes: (1) a generalized atrophic and benign form of EB, caused by mutations in the *COL17A1* gene for type XVII collagen; (2) EB associated with pyloric atresia and other intestinal abnormalities, caused by mutations in either the gene for α6 integrin (*ITG A6*) or the gene for the β4 integrin (*ITGB4*); and (3) relatively mild blistering at birth, but associated with late-onset muscular dystrophy, caused by mutations in the gene for plectin (*PLEC-1*). Junctional EB is caused by mutations in any one of three genes for laminin (*LAMA-3, LAMB-3, LAMC-2*), a major component of the dermal-epidermal junction. The most severe dystrophic form of EB is caused by mutations in the gene for type VII collagen (*COL7A1*) that forms the anchoring fibers binding the epidermis to the dermis.

Diagnosis and Treatment   The diagnosis is based on skin that readily breaks and forms blisters. EB simplex and EB hemidesmosomal are generally milder than EB junctional or EB dystrophica. EB dystrophica variants usually cause large and prominent scars. Precise classification within subtypes usually requires electron microscopy. Also, DNA diagnostic tests are available. The treatment is symptomatic.

ALPORT SYNDROME

AS is an inherited disorder characterized by hematuria and several associated features. Four forms of the disease are now recognized: (1) classic AS, which is inherited as an X-linked disorder with hematuria, sensorineural deafness, and conical deformation of the anterior surface of the lens (lenticonus); (2) a subtype of the X-linked form associated with diffuse leiomyomatosis; (3) an autosomal recessive form; and (4) an autosomal dominant form. Both autosomal recessive and dominant forms can cause renal disease without deafness or lenticonus.

Incidence   The incidence of AS is about 1 in 10,000 in the general population and as high as 1 in 5,000 in some ethnic groups. About 80% of AS patients have the classical X-linked variant.

Molecular Defects   Most patients have mutations in four of the six genes for the chains of type IV collagen (*COL4A3, COL4A4, COL4A5,* and *COL4A6*). The genes for the proteins are arranged in tandem pairs on different chromosomes in an unusual head-to-head orientation and with overlapping promoters, i.e., the *COL4A1* and *COL4A2* genes are head-to-head on chromosome 13q34, the *COL4A3* and *COL4A4* genes are on chromosome 2q35-37, and the *COL4A5* and *COL4A6* genes are on chromosome Xq22. The X-linked variants are caused by either mutations in the COL4A5 gene or by partial deletions of both of the adjacent *COL4A4* and *COL4A5* genes. The autosomal recessive variants are caused by mutations in either the *COL4A3* or *COL4A4* genes. The mutations responsible for the autosomal dominant variants are still unknown, but they have been mapped to the same locus as the *COL4A3* and *COL4A4* genes.

Diagnosis   The diagnosis of classic AS is based on X-linked inheritance of hematuria, sensorineural deafness, and lenticonus. The lenticonus together with hematuria is pathognomonic of classic AS. The sensorineural deafness is primarily in the high-tone range. It can frequently be detected only by an audiogram and is usually not progressive. Because of the X-linked transmission, women are generally underdiagnosed and are usually less severely affected than men. The hematuria usually progresses to nephritis and may cause renal failure in late adolescence in affected males and at older ages in some women. Renal transplantation is usually successful.

ACKNOWLEDGMENTS

The authors acknowledge the contributions of Helena Kuivaniemi, Gerard Tromp, and Leena Ala-Kokko to this chapter in previous editions of Harrison's.

FURTHER READINGS

BOILEAU C et al: Molecular genetics of Marfan syndrome. Curr Opinions Cardiol 20:194, 2005

CABRAL WA et al: Prolyl 3-hydroxylase 1 deficiency causes a recessive metabolic bone disorder resembling lethal/severe osteogenesis imperfecta. Nat Genet 39(3):359, 2007

MORELLO R et al: CRTAP is required for prolyl 3-hydroxylation and mutations cause recessive osteogenesis imperfecta. Cell 127(2):291, 2006

RAMIREZ F, DIETZ HC: Marfan's syndrome: From molecular pathogenesis to clinical treatment. Curr Opin Genet Dev 17(3):252, 2007

RAUCH F, GLORIEUX FH: Osteogenesis imperfecta. Lancet 367:1377, 2004

ROSE PS et al: Stickler syndrome. Clinical characteristics and diagnostic criteria. Am J Med Genet 138A:199, 2005

ROYCE PM & STEINMANN B (eds): *Connective Tissue and Its Heritable Disorders*, 2d ed. New York, Wiley-Liss, 2002

ZWEERS MC et al: Elastic fiber abnormalities in hypermobility type Ehlers-Danlos syndrome patients with tenascin-X mutations. Clin Genet 67:330, 2005

358 Inherited Disorders of Amino Acid Metabolism in Adults
Nicola Longo

Amino acids are not only the building blocks of proteins but also serve as neurotransmitters (glycine, glutamate, γ-aminobutyric acid) or as precursors of hormones, coenzymes, pigments, purines, or pyrimidines. Eight amino acids, referred to as *essential*, cannot be synthesized by humans and must be obtained from dietary sources. The others are formed endogenously. Each amino acid has a unique degradative pathway by which its nitrogen and carbon components are used for the synthesis of other amino acids, carbohydrates, and lipids. Disorders of amino acid metabolism and transport (Chap. 359) are individually rare—the incidences range from 1 in 10,000 for cystinuria or phenylketonuria to 1 in 200,000 for homocystinuria or alkaptonuria—but collectively they affect perhaps 1 in 1000 newborns. Almost all are transmitted as autosomal recessive traits.

The features of inherited disorders of amino acid catabolism are summarized in Table 358-1. In general, these disorders are named for the compound that accumulates to highest concentration in blood (-*emias*) or urine (-*urias*). For many conditions (often called *aminoacidopathies*), the parent amino acid is found in excess; for others, generally referred to as *organic acidemias*, products in the catabolic pathway accumulate. Which compound(s) accumulates depends on the site of the enzymatic block, the reversibility of the reactions proximal to the lesion, and the availability of alternative pathways of metabolic "runoff." Biochemical and genetic heterogeneity are common. Five distinct forms of hyperphenylalaninemia, seven forms of homocystinuria, and seven types of methylmalonic acidemia are recognized. Such heterogeneity reflects the presence of an even larger array of molecular defects.

The manifestations of these conditions differ widely (Table 358-1). Some, such as sarcosinemia, produce no clinical consequences. At the other extreme, complete deficiency of ornithine transcarbamylase is lethal in the untreated neonate. Central nervous system (CNS) dysfunction, in the form of developmental retardation, seizures, alterations in sensorium, or behavioral disturbances, is present in more than half the disorders. Protein-induced vomiting, neurologic dysfunction, and hyperammonemia occur in many disorders of urea cycle intermediates. Metabolic ketoacidosis, often accompanied by hyperammonemia, is a frequent presenting finding in disorders of branched-chain amino acid metabolism. Some disorders produce focal tissue or organ involvement such as liver disease, renal failure, cutaneous abnormalities, or ocular lesions.

The analysis of plasma amino acids (by ion-exchange chromatography) and urine organic acids (by gas chromatography/mass spectrometry) is commonly used to diagnose and monitor most of these disorders. The diagnosis is confirmed by enzyme assay on cells or tissues from the patients or by DNA testing. The clinical manifestations in many of these conditions can be prevented or mitigated if a diagnosis is achieved early and appropriate treatment (e.g., dietary protein or amino acid restriction or vitamin supplementation) is instituted promptly. For this reason, newborn screening programs seek to identify several of these disorders. Infants with a positive screening test need additional metabolic testing (usually suggested by the newborn screening program) to confirm or exclude the diagnosis. Confirmed cases should be referred to a metabolic center for initiation of therapy. The parents need to be counseled about the recurrence risk of the disease in future pregnancies. In some cases, parents need testing to exclude metabolic alterations seen in carriers for some of these disorders (such as some forms of homocystinuria) or because they might have a disorder themselves (such as methylcrotonyl CoA carboxylase deficiency or fatty acid oxidation defects). Some metabolic disorders can remain asymptomatic until adult age, presenting only when fasting or severe stress require full activity of affected metabolic pathways to provide energy.

Selected disorders that illustrate the principles, properties, and problems presented by the disorders of amino acid metabolism are discussed in this chapter.

THE HYPERPHENYLALANINEMIAS

The hyperphenylalaninemias (Table 358-1) result from impaired conversion of phenylalanine to tyrosine. The most common and clinically important is *phenylketonuria* (frequency 1:10,000), which is an autosomal recessive disorder characterized by an increased concentration of phenylalanine and its by-products in body fluids and by severe mental retardation if untreated in infancy. It results from reduced activity of phenylalanine hydroxylase (phenylketonuria type I). The accumulation of phenylalanine inhibits the transport of other amino acids required for protein or neurotransmitter synthesis, reduces synthesis and increases degradation of myelin, and leads to inadequate formation of norepinephrine and serotonin. Phenylalanine is a competitive inhibitor of tyrosinase, a key enzyme in the pathway of melanin synthesis, and accounts for the hypopigmentation of hair and skin. Untreated children with classic phenylketonuria are normal at birth but fail to attain early developmental milestones, develop microcephaly, and demonstrate progressive impairment of cerebral function. Hyperactivity, seizures, and severe mental retardation are major clinical problems later in life. Electroencephalographic abnormalities; "mousy" odor of skin, hair, and urine (due to phenylacetate accumulation); and a tendency to hypopigmentation and eczema complete the devastating clinical picture. In contrast, affected children who are detected and treated at birth show none of these abnormalities.

℞ PHENYLKETONURIA

To prevent mental retardation, diagnosis and initiation of dietary treatment of classic phenylketonuria must occur before the child is 3 weeks of age. For this reason, most newborns in North America, Australia, and Europe are screened by determinations of blood phenylalanine levels. Abnormal values are confirmed using quantitative analysis of plasma amino acids. Dietary phenylalanine restriction is usually instituted if blood phenylalanine levels are >250 μmol/L (4 mg/dL). Treatment consists of a special diet low in phenylalanine and supplemented with tyrosine, since tyrosine becomes an essential amino acid in phenylalanine hydroxylase deficiency. With therapy, plasma phenylalanine concentrations should be maintained between 120 and 360 μmol/L (2 and 6 mg/dL). Dietary restriction should be continued and monitored indefinitely. Some patients with milder forms of phenylketonuria (phenylalanine <1200 μm at presentation) show increased tolerance to dietary proteins and improved metabolic control when treated with tetrahydrobiopterin (5–20 mg/kg per day), an essential cofactor of phenylalanine hydroxylase.

A number of women with phenylketonuria who have been treated since infancy will reach adulthood and become pregnant. If maternal phenylalanine levels are not strictly controlled before and during pregnancy, their offspring are at increased risk for congenital defects and microcephaly (*maternal phenylketonuria*). After birth, these children have severe mental and growth retardation. Pregnancy risks can be minimized by continuing lifelong phenylalanine-restricted diets and assuring strict phenylalanine restriction 2 months prior to conception and throughout gestation.

THE HOMOCYSTINURIAS (HYPERHOMOCYSTEINEMIAS)

The homocystinurias are seven biochemically and clinically distinct disorders (Table 358-1) characterized by increased concentration of the sulfur-containing amino acid homocystine in blood and urine.

Classic homocystinuria, the most common (frequency 1:200,000), results from reduced activity of cystathionine β-synthase (Fig. 358-1), the pyridoxal phosphate–dependent enzyme that condenses homocysteine with serine to form cystathionine. Most patients present between 3 and 5 years of age with dislocated optic lenses and mental retardation (in about half of cases). Some patients develop a marfanoid habitus and radiologic evidence of osteoporosis. Life-threatening vascular

TABLE 358-1 | **INHERITED DISORDERS OF AMINO ACID METABOLISM**

Aminoacid(s)	Condition	Enzyme Defect	Clinical Findings	Inheritance[a]
Phenylalanine	Phenylketonuria type I	Phenylalanine hydroxylase	Mental retardation, microcephaly, hypopigmented skin and hairs, eczema, "mousy" odor	AR
	Phenylketonuria type II	Dihydropteridine reductase	Mental retardation, hypotonia, spasticity, myoclonus	AR
	Phenylketonuria type III	6-Pyruvoyl-tetrahydropterin synthase	Dystonia, neurologic deterioration, seizures, mental retardation	AR
	GTP cyclohydrolase I deficiency	GTP cyclohydrolase I	Mental retardation, seizures, dystonia, temperature instability	AR
	Carbinolamine dehydratase deficiency	Pterin-4α-carbinolamine dehydratase	Transient hyperphenylalaninemia (benign)	AR
Tyrosine	Tyrosinemia type I (hepatorenal)	Fumarylacetoacetate hydrolase	Liver failure, cirrhosis, rickets, failure to thrive, peripheral neuropathy, "boiled cabbage" odor	AR
	Tyrosinemia type II (oculocutaneous)	Tyrosine transaminase	Palmoplantar keratosis, painful corneal erosions with photophobia, mental retardation (?)	AR
	Tyrosinemia type III	4-Hydroxyphenylpyruvate dioxygenase	Hypertyrosinemia with normal liver function, occasional mental delay	AR
	Hawkinsinuria	4-Hydroxyphenylpyruvate dioxygenase	Transient failure to thrive, metabolic acidosis in infancy	AD
	Alkaptonuria	Homogentisic acid oxidase	Ochronosis, arthritis, cardiac valve involvement, coronary artery calcification	AR
	Albinism (oculocutaneous)	Tyrosinase	Hypopigmentation of hair, skin, and optic fundus; visual loss; photophobia	AR
	Albinism (ocular)	Different enzymes or transporters	Hypopigmentation of optic fundus, visual loss	AR, XL
	DOPA-responsive dystonia	Tyrosine hydroxylase	Rigidity, truncal hypotonia, tremor, mental retardation	AR
GABA	4-Hydroxybutyric aciduria	Succinic semialdehyde dehydrogenase	Seizures, mental retardation, ataxia	AR
Tryptophan	Tryptophanuria	Unknown	Mental retardation, ataxia, skin photosensitivity	AR
	Hydroxykinureninuria	Kynureninase	Mental retardation, spasticity	AR
Histidine	Histidinemia	Histidine-ammonia lyase	Benign	AR
	Urocanic aciduria	Urocanase	Benign	AR
	Formiminoglutamic aciduria	Formiminotransferase	Occasional mental retardation	AR
Glycine	Glycine encephalopathy	Glycine cleavage (4 enzymes)	Infantile seizures, lethargy, apnea, profound mental retardation	AR
	Sarcosinemia	Sarcosine dehydrogenase	Benign	AR
	Hyperoxaluria type I	Alanine:glyoxylate aminotransferase	Calcium oxalate nephrolithiasis, renal failure	AR
	Hyperoxaluria type II	D-Glyceric acid dehydrogenase/ glyoxylate reductase	Calcium oxalate nephrolithiasis, renal failure	AR
Serine	Phosphoglycerate dehydrogenase deficiency	Phosphoglycerate dehydrogenase	Seizures, microcephaly, mental retardation	AR
Proline	Hyperprolinemia type I	Proline oxidase	Benign	AR
	Hyperprolinemia type II	Δ¹-Pyrroline-5-carboxylate dehydrogenase	Febrile seizures, mental retardation	AR
	Hyperhydroxyprolinemia	Hydroxyproline oxidase	Benign	AR
	Prolidase deficiency	Prolidase	Mild mental retardation, chronic dermatitis	AR
Methionine	Hypermethioninemia	Methionine adenosyltransferase	Usually benign	AR
	S-Adenosylhomocysteine hydrolase deficiency	S-Adenosylhomocysteine hydrolase	Hypotonia, mental retardation, absent tendon reflexes, delayed myelination	AR
	Glycine N-methyltransferase deficiency	Glycine N-methyltransferase	Elevated liver transaminases	AR
Homocystine	Homocystinuria	Cystathionine β-synthase	Lens dislocation, thrombotic vascular disease, mental retardation, osteoporosis	AR
	Homocystinuria	5,10-Methylenetetrahydrofolate reductase	Mental retardation, gait and psychiatric abnormalities, recurrent strokes	AR
	Homocystinuria	Methionine synthase (cblE, -G)	Mental retardation, hypotonia, seizures, megaloblastic anemia	AR
	Homocystinuria and methylmalonic acidemia	Vitamin B₁₂ lysosomal efflux and metabolism (cbl C, -D, -F)	Mental retardation, lethargy, failure to thrive, hypotonia, seizures, megaloblastic anemia	AR
Cystathionine	Cystathioninuria	β-Cystathioninase	Benign	AR
Cystine	Cystinosis	Cystinosin CTNS (lysosomal efflux)	Renal Fanconi syndrome, rickets, photophobia, hypotonia, renal failure	AR
S-Sulfo-L-cysteine	Sulfocysteinuria	Sulfate oxidase or molibdenum cofactor deficiency	Seizures, mental retardation, dislocated lenses	AR
Lysine	Hyperlysinemia, saccharopinuria	α-Aminoadipic semialdehyde synthase	Benign	AR
	Pyridoxine-dependent seizures	L-Δ¹-Piperideine-6-carboxilate dehydrogenase	Seizures	AR

(continued)

TABLE 358-1 **INHERITED DISORDERS OF AMINO ACID METABOLISM (CONTINUED)**

Aminoacid(s)	Condition	Enzyme Defect	Clinical Findings	Inheritance[a]
Lysine, tryptophan	α-Ketoadipic acidemia	α-Ketoadipic acid dehydrogenase	Benign	?
	Glutaric acidemia type I	Glutaryl-CoA dehydrogenase	Progressive severe dystonia and athetosis, mild mental retardation	AR
	Glutaric acidemia type II	Electron transfer flavoprotein or ETF:ubiquinone oxidoreductase	Hypoglycemia, metabolic acidosis, "sweaty feet" odor, hypotonia, cardiomyopathy	AR
Ornithine	Gyrate atrophy of the choroid and retina	Ornithine-δ-aminotransferase	Myopia, night blindness, loss of peripheral vision, cataracts, chorioretinal degeneration	AR
Urea cycle	Carbamylphosphate synthase-1 deficiency	Carbamylphosphate synthase-1	Lethargy progressing to coma, protein aversion, mental retardation, hyperammonemia	AR
	N-Acetylglutamate synthase deficiency	N-Acetylglutamate synthase	Lethargy progressing to coma, protein aversion, mental retardation, hyperammonemia	AR
	Ornithine transcarbamylase deficiency	Ornithine transcarbamylase	Lethargy progressing to coma, protein aversion, mental retardation, hyperammonemia	XL
	Citrullinemia type I	Argininosuccinate synthase	Lethargy progressing to coma, protein aversion, mental retardation, hyperammonemia	AR
	Argininosuccinic acidemia	Argininosuccinate lyase	Lethargy progressing to coma, protein aversion, mental retardation, hyperammonemia, trichorrhexis nodosa	AR
	Arginase deficiency	Arginase	Spastic tetraparesis, mental retardation, mild hyperammonemia	AR
	Hyperornithinemia, hyperammonemia, homocitrullinuria	Mitochondrial ornithine carrier ORNT1	Vomiting, lethargy, failure to thrive, mental retardation, episodic confusion, hyper-ammonemia, protein intolerance	AR
	Citrullinemia type 2	Mitochondrial aspartate/glutamate carrier CTLN2	Neonatal intrahepatic cholestasis, adult presentation with sudden behavioral changes and stupor, coma, hyperammonemia	AR
Proline, ornithine, arginine	Δ¹-pyrroline-5-carboxylate synthase deficiency	Δ¹-pyrroline-5-carboxylate synthase	Hypotonia, seizures, neurodegeneration, peripheral neuropathy, joint laxity, skin hyperelasticity, subcapsular cataracts, hyperammonemia	AR
Glutamine	Glutamine synthase deficiency	Glutamine synthase	Brain malformations, pachygyria, seizures, hypotonia, dysmorphic features	AR
Valine	Hypervalinemia	Valine aminotransferase	Vomiting, fever, failure to thrive, hypotonia	AR
	Isobutyryl-CoA dehydrogenase deficiency	Isobutyryl-CoA dehydrogenase	Failure to thrive, anemia, and dilated cardiomyopathy(?)	AR
Leucine, isoleucine	Hyperleucine-isoleucinemia	Leucine-isoleucine aminotransferase	Seizures, failure to thrive, mental retardation	?
Valine, leucine, isoleucine	Maple syrup urine disease (defective E1α, E1β, E2, E3)	Branched chain ketoacid dehydrogenase	Lethargy, vomiting, encephalopathy, seizures, mental retardation, "maple syrup" odor, protein intolerance	AR
Leucine	Isovaleric acidemia	Isovaleryl-CoA dehydrogenase	Acidosis, ketosis, vomiting, coma, hyper-ammonemia, "sweaty feet" odor, protein intolerance	AR
	3-Methylcrotonyl glycinuria	3-Methylcrotonyl-CoA carboxylase	Stress-induced metabolic acidosis, hypotonia, hypoglycemia, "cat's urine" odor	AR
	3-Methylglutaconic aciduria type I	3-Methylglutaconyl-CoA hydratase deficiency	Stress-induced acidosis, mental retardation, hypotonia, hepatomegaly	AR
	3-Hydroxy-3-methylglutaric aciduria	3-Hydroxy-3-methylglutaryl-CoA lyase	Stress-induced hypoketotic hypoglycemia and acidosis, encephalopathy, hyperammonemia	AR
Isoleucine	2-Methylbutyryl-glycinuria	2-Methylbutyryl-CoA dehydrogenase	Fasting-induced metabolic acidosis/hypoglycemia	AR
	2-Methyl-3-hydroxybutyryl-CoA dehydrogenase deficiency	2-Methyl-3-hydroxybutyryl-CoA dehydrogenase	Developmental regression, seizures, and rigidity sometimes triggered by illnesses	XL
	3-Oxothiolase deficiency	3-Oxothiolase	Fasting-induced acidosis and ketosis, vomiting, lethargy	AR
Valine, isoleucine, methionine, threonine	Propionic acidemia (pccA,-B,-C)	Propionyl-CoA carboxylase	Metabolic ketoacidosis, hyperammonemia, hypotonia, lethargy, coma, protein intolerance, mental retardation, hyperglycinemia	AR
	Multiple carboxylase/biotinidase deficiency	Holocarboxylase synthase or biotinidase	Metabolic ketoacidosis, diffuse rash, alopecia, seizures, mental retardation	AR
	Methylmalonic acidemia (mutase, cb1A, -B, racemase)	Methylmalonyl-CoA mutase/racemase or cobalamin reductase/adenosyltransferase	Metabolic ketoacidosis, hyperammonemia, hypertonia, lethargy, coma, protein intolerance, mental retardation, hyperglycinemia	AR

[a]AR, autosomal recessive; XL, X-linked, AD, autosomal dominant.

Note: GTP, guanosine 5'-triphosphate; DOPA, dihydroxyphenylalanine; GABA, γ-aminobutyric acid; Cbl, cobalamin.

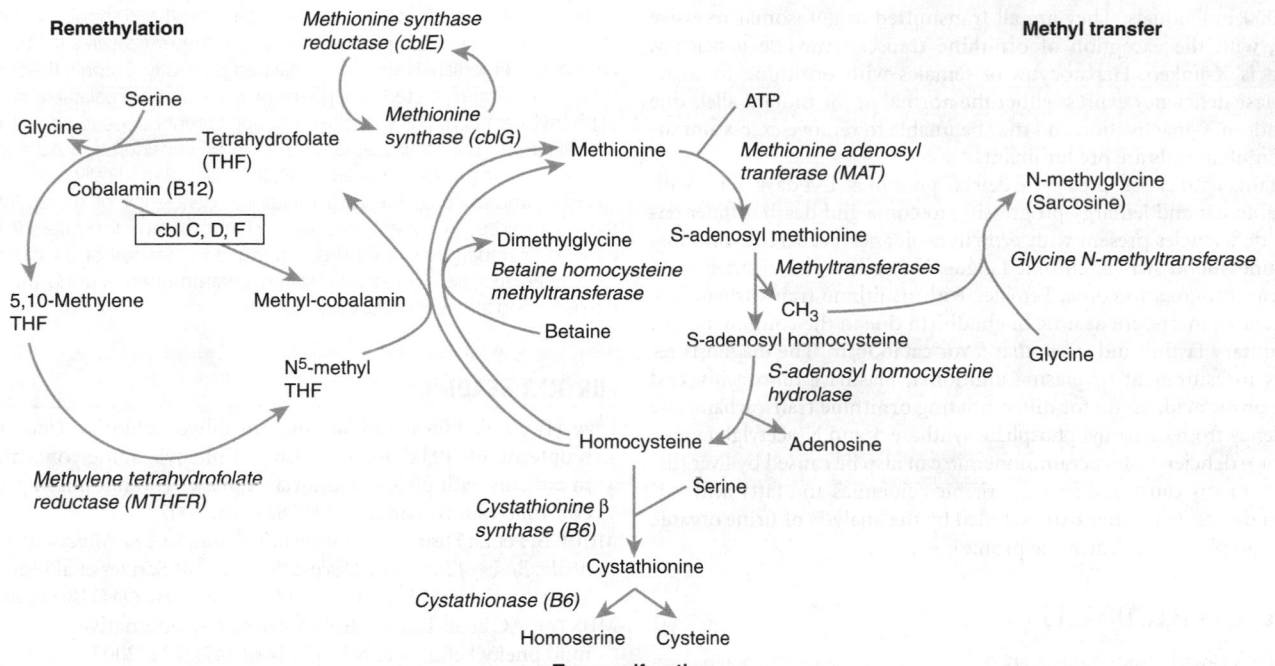

Remethylation / **Methyl transfer**

FIGURE 358-1 Pathways, enzymes, and coenzymes involved in the homocystinurias. Methionine transfers a methyl group during its conversion to homocysteine. Defects in methyl transfer or in the subsequent metabolism of homocysteine by the pyridoxal phosphate (vitamin B₆)-dependent cystathionine β-synthase increase plasma methionine levels. Homocysteine is transformed into methionine via re-methylation. This occurs through methionine synthase, a reaction requiring methylcobalamin and folic acid. Deficiencies in these enzymes or lack of cofactors is associated with decreased or normal methionine levels. In an alternative pathway, homocysteine can be remethylated by betaine:homocysteine methyl transferase.

complications (affecting coronary, renal, and cerebral arteries) can occur during the first decade of life and are the major cause of morbidity and mortality. Classic homocystinuria can be diagnosed with analysis of plasma amino acids, showing elevated methionine and presence of free homocystine. Total plasma homocysteine is also extremely elevated (usually >100 μM). Treatment consists of a special diet restricted in protein and methionine and supplemented with cystine. In approximately half of patients, oral pyridoxine (25–500 mg/d) produces a fall in plasma methionine and homocystine concentration in body fluids. Folate deficiency should be prevented by adequate supplementation. Betaine is also effective in reducing homocystine levels in pyridoxine-unresponsive patients.

The other forms of homocystinuria are the result of impaired remethylation of homocysteine to methionine. This can be caused by defective methionine synthase or reduced availability of two essential cofactors, 5-methyltetrahydrofolate and methylcobalamin (methyl-vitamin B₁₂).

Hyperhomocysteinemia refers to increased total plasma concentration of homocysteine with or without an increase in free homocystine (disulfide form). Hyperhomocysteinemia, in the absence of significant homocystinuria, is found in some heterozygotes for the genetic defects noted above or in homozygotes for milder variants. Changes of homocysteine levels are also observed with increasing age; with smoking; in postmenopausal women; in patients with renal failure, hypothyroidism, leukemias, inflammatory bowel disease, or psoriasis; and during therapy with drugs such as methotrexate, nitrous oxide, isoniazid, and some antiepileptic agents. Homocysteine acts as an atherogenic and thrombophilic agent. An increase in total plasma homocysteine represents an independent risk factor for coronary, cerebrovascular, and peripheral arterial disease as well as for deep-vein thrombosis (Chap. 235). Homocysteine is synergistic with hypertension and smoking, and it is additive with other risk factors that predispose to peripheral arterial disease. In addition, hyperhomocysteinemia and folate and vitamin B₁₂ deficiency have been associated with an increased risk of neural tube defects in pregnant women. Vitamin supplements are effective in reducing plasma homocysteine levels in these cases.

ALKAPTONURIA

Alkaptonuria is a rare (frequency 1:200,000) disorder of tyrosine catabolism in which deficiency of homogentisate 1,2-dioxygenase (also known as *homogentisic acid oxidase*) leads to excretion of large amounts of homogentisic acid in urine and accumulation of oxidized homogentisic acid pigment in connective tissues (*ochronosis*). Alkaptonuria may go unrecognized until middle life, when degenerative joint disease develops. Prior to this time, about half of patients might be diagnosed for the presence of dark urine. Foci of gray-brown scleral pigment and generalized darkening of the concha, anthelix, and, finally, helix of the ear usually develop after age 30. Low back pain usually starts between 30 and 40 years of age. *Ochronotic arthritis* is heralded by pain, stiffness, and some limitation of motion of the hips, knees, and shoulders. Acute arthritis may resemble rheumatoid arthritis, but small joints are usually spared. Pigmentation of heart valves, larynx, tympanic membranes, and skin occurs, and occasional patients develop pigmented renal or prostatic calculi. Degenerative cardiovascular disease is increased in older patients. The diagnosis should be suspected in a patient whose urine darkens to blackness. Homogentisic acid in urine is identified by urine organic acid analysis or by a specific colorimetric test. Ochronotic arthritis is treated symptomatically (Chap. 326). Ascorbic acid and protein restriction are not effective in reducing homogentisic acid production. By contrast, nitisone [2-(2-nitro-4-trifluoromethylbenzoyl)-1,3-cyclohexanedione], a drug used in tyrosinemia type I, reduces urinary excretion of homogentisic acid and, in conjunction with a low-protein diet, might prevent the long-term complications of alkaptonuria.

UREA CYCLE DEFECTS

Excess ammonia generated from protein nitrogen is removed by the urea cycle, a process mediated by several enzymes and transporters (Table 358-1). Complete absence of any of these enzymes usually causes severe hyperammonemia in newborns, while milder variants can be seen in adults. The accumulation of ammonia and glutamine leads to brain edema and direct neuronal toxicity. Deficiencies in urea cycle enzymes are individually rare, but as a group they affect about

1:25,000 individuals. They are all transmitted as autosomal recessive traits, with the exception of ornithine transcarbamylase deficiency, which is X-linked. Hepatocytes of females with ornithine transcarbamylase deficiency express either the normal or the mutant allele due to random X-inactivation and may be unable to remove excess ammonia if mutant cells are predominant.

Infants with classic urea cycle defects present at 1–4 days of life with refusal to eat and lethargy progressing to coma and death. Milder enzyme deficiencies present with protein avoidance, recurrent vomiting, migraine, mood swings, chronic fatigue, irritability, and disorientation that can progress to coma. Females with ornithine transcarbamylase deficiency can present at time of childbirth due to the combination of involuntary fasting and stress that favor catabolism. The diagnosis requires measurement of plasma ammonia, plasma amino acids, and urine orotic acid, useful for differentiating ornithine transcarbamylase deficiency from carbamyl phosphate synthase-1 and N-acetylglutamate synthase deficiency. Hyperammonemia can also be caused by liver disease from any cause and several organic acidemias and fatty acid oxidation defects (the latter two excluded by the analysis of urine organic acids and plasma acylcarnitine profile).

℞ UREA CYCLE DEFECTS

Therapy is aimed at stopping catabolism and ammonia production by providing adequate calories (as intravenous glucose and lipids in the comatose patient) and, if needed, insulin. Excess nitrogen is removed by intravenous phenylacetate and benzoate (0.25 g/kg for the priming dose and subsequently as an infusion over 24 h) that conjugate with glutamine and glycine, respectively, to form phenylacetylglutamine and hippuric acid, water-soluble molecules efficiently excreted in urine. Arginine (200 mg/kg/d) becomes an essential amino acid (except in arginase deficiency) and should be provided intravenously to resume protein synthesis. If these measures fail to reduce ammonia, hemodialysis should be initiated promptly. Chronic therapy consists of a protein-restricted diet, phenylbutyrate (a more palatable precursor of phenylacetate), arginine, or citrulline supplements, depending on the specific diagnosis. Liver transplantation should be considered in patients with severe urea cycle defects that are difficult to control medically.

Hyperammonemia due to a functional deficiency of glutamine synthase can occur in patients receiving chemotherapy for different malignancies or undergoing solid organ transplants. Several of these patients have been successfully rescued from hyperammonemia using the protocol described above for urea cycle defects.

FURTHER READINGS

Levy HL et al: Efficacy of sapropterin dihydrochloride (tetrahydrobiopterin, 6R-BH4) for reduction of phenylalanine concentration in patients with phenylketonuria: A phase III randomised placebo-controlled study. Lancet 370(9586):504, 2007

Mudd SH et al: Disorders of transulfuration, in *The Molecular & Metabolic Bases of Inherited Disease*, 8th ed., CR Scriver et al (eds). New York, McGraw-Hill, 2001, pp 2007–2056 www.OMMBID.com

Muntau AC et al: Tetrahydrobiopterin as an alternative treatment for mild phenylketonuria. N Engl J Med 347:2122, 2002

Nyhan WL et al: *Atlas of Metabolic Diseases*. London, Hodder Education, 2005

Phornphutkul C et al: Natural history of alkaptonuria. N Engl J Med 347:2111, 2002

Tuchman M et al: Hepatic glutamine synthetase deficiency in fatal hyperammonemia after lung transplantation. Ann Intern Med 127:446, 1997

359 Inherited Defects of Membrane Transport
Nicola Longo

Specific membrane transporters mediate the passage of a wide variety of substances across cellular membranes. Classes of substrates include amino acids, sugars, cations, anions, vitamins, and water. The number of inherited disorders of membrane transport continues to increase with the identification of new transporters and the clarification of the molecular basis of diseases with previously unknown pathophysiology. The first transport disorders identified affected the gut or the kidney, but transport processes are now proving essential for the normal function of every organ. Mutations in transporter molecules cause disorders of the heart, muscle, brain, and endocrine and sensory organs (Table 359-1). Inherited defects impairing the transport of selected amino acids that can present in adults are discussed here as examples of the abnormalities encountered; others are considered elsewhere in this text.

CYSTINURIA

Cystinuria (frequency of 1 in 10,000 to 1 in 15,000) is an autosomal recessive disorder caused by defective transporters in the apical brush border of proximal renal tubule and small intestinal cells. It is characterized by impaired reabsorption and excessive urinary excretion of the dibasic amino acids lysine, arginine, ornithine, and cystine. Because cystine is poorly soluble, its excess excretion predisposes to the formation of renal, ureteral, and bladder stones. Such stones are responsible for the signs and symptoms of the disorder.

There are two variants of cystinuria. Homozygotes for both variants have high urinary excretion of cystine, lysine, arginine, and ornithine. Type I heterozygotes usually have normal urinary amino, whereas most non-type I (formerly type II and type III) heterozygotes have moderately increased urinary excretion of each of the four amino acids. The gene for type I cystinuria (*SLC3A1*, chromosome 2p16.3) encodes a membrane glycoprotein. Non-type I cystinuria is caused by mutations in *SLC7A9* (chromosome 19q13) that encodes the b$^{0,+}$ amino acid transporter. The glycoprotein encoded by *SLC3A1* favors the correct processing of the b$^{0,+}$ membrane transporter, and explains why mutations in two different genes cause a similar disease.

Cystine stones account for 1–2% of all urinary tract calculi but are the most common cause of stones in children. Cystinuria homozygotes regularly excrete 2400–7200 μmol (600–1800 mg) of cystine daily. Since the maximum solubility of cystine in the physiologic urinary pH range of 4.5–7.0 is about 1200 μmol/L (300 mg/L), cystine needs to be diluted to 2.5–7 L of water to prevent crystalluria. Stone formation usually manifests in the second or third decade but may occur in the first year of life. Symptoms and signs are those typical of urolithiasis: hematuria, flank pain, renal colic, obstructive uropathy, and infection (Chap. 281). Recurrent urolithiasis may lead to progressive renal insufficiency.

Cystinuria is suspected after observing typical hexagonal crystals in the sediment of acidified, concentrated, chilled urine or after performing a urinary nitroprusside test. Quantitative urine amino acid analysis confirms the diagnosis of cystinuria by showing selective over excretion of cystine, lysine, arginine, and ornithine. Quantitative measurements are important for differentiating heterozygotes from homozygotes and for following free cystine excretion during therapy.

Management is aimed at preventing cystine crystal formation by increasing urinary volume and by maintaining an alkaline urine pH. Fluid ingestion in excess of 4 L/d is essential, and 5–7 L/d is optimal. Urinary cystine concentration should be <1000 μmol/L (250 mg/L). The daily fluid ingestion necessary to maintain this dilution of excreted cystine should be spaced over 24 h, with one-third of the total volume ingested between bedtime and 3 A.M. Cystine solubility rises sharply above pH 7.5, and urinary alkalinization (with bicarbonate or potassium citrate) can be therapeutic. Penicillamine (1–3 g/d) and tiopronin (α-mercaptopropionylglycine, 800–1200 mg/d in four divided doses) undergo sulfhydryl-disulfide exchange with cystine to form mixed disulfides. Since these disulfides are much more soluble than cystine, pharmacologic

TABLE 359-1 GENETIC DISORDERS OF MEMBRANE TRANSPORT (SELECTED EXAMPLES)

Class of Substance and Disorder	Individual Substrates	Tissues Manifesting Transport Defect	Molecular Defect	Major Clinical Manifestations	Inheritance
Amino Acids					
Cystinuria	Cystine, lysine, arginine, ornithine	Proximal renal tubule, jejunal mucosa	Shared dibasic-cystine transporter SLC3A1, SLC7A9	Cystine nephrolithiasis	AR
Dibasic aminoaciduria	Lysine, arginine, ornithine	Proximal renal tubule, jejunal mucosa	Dibasic transporter SLC7A7	Type I: Benign Type II: Protein intolerance, hyperammonemia, retardation	AR
Hartnup disease	Neutral amino acids	Proximal renal tubule, jejunal mucosa	Neutral amino acid transporter SLC6A19	Constant neutral aminoaciduria, intermittent symptoms of pellagra	AR
Methionine malabsorption	Methionine	Jejunal mucosa	Methionine transporter	White hair, mental retardation, convulsions, hyperpneic attacks, edema	Probable AR
Histidinuria	Histidine	Proximal renal tubule, jejunal mucosa	Histidine transporter	Mental retardation	AR
Iminoglycinuria	Glycine, proline, hydroxyproline	Proximal renal tubule, jejunal mucosa	Shared glycine–imino acid transporter	None	AR
Dicarboxylic aminoaciduria	Glutamic acid, aspartic acid	Proximal renal tubule, jejunal mucosa	Shared dicarboxylic amino acid transporter	None	Probable AR
Cystinosis	Cystine	Lysosomal membranes	Lysosomal cystine transporter	Renal failure, hypothyroidism, blindness	AR
Hexoses					
Glucose-galactose malabsorption	D-Glucose D-Galactose	Proximal renal tubule, jejunal mucosa	Sodium-dependent glucose/galactose transporter SGLT1	Watery diarrhea on feeding glucose, lactose, sucrose, or galactose	AR
Glucose-transport defect	D-Glucose	Ubiquitous blood brain barrier	Facilitative glucose transporter GLUT1	Seizures, mental retardation	AD
Fanconi-Bickel syndrome	D-Glucose	Liver, kidney, pancreas, intestine	Facilitative glucose transporter GLUT2	Growth retardation, rickets, hepatorenal glycogenosis, hypo- and hyperglycemia	AR
Urate					
Hypouricemia	Uric acid	Proximal renal tubule	Urate transporter SLC22A12	Hypouricemia, uric acid urolithiasis	AR
Anions					
Congenital chloridorrhea	Chloride, sulfate	Ileal and colonic mucosa	Cl⁻/HCO₃⁻ exchanger (DRA)	Hydramnios, watery diarrhea, elevated fecal chloride, metabolic alkalosis with volume depletion, hyperaldosteronism	AR
Dent disease, X-linked recessive hypophosphatemic rickets and nephrocalcinosis	Chloride, phosphate	Proximal renal tubule	Voltage-gated Cl⁻ channel CLCN5	Proteinuria, hypercalciuria, nephrocalcinosis, nephrolithiasis, rickets	XL
Cations					
Hyperinsulinemic hypoglycemia	Potassium	Pancreatic β cell	Sulfonylurea receptor SUR1, K⁺ channel KCNJ11	Neonatal hypoglycemia, hyperinsulinemia	AR
Benign familial neonatal epilepsy	Potassium	Brain	Voltage-gated K⁺ channels KCNQ2, KCNQ3	Neonatal seizures, normal development	AD
Water					
Nephrogenic diabetes insipidus type 2	Water	Renal collecting tubule	Aquaporin 2 (water channel)	Polyuria, dehydration, hypostenuria	AR
Vitamins					
Thiamine-responsive megaloblastic anemia	Thiamine	Ubiquitous	Thiamine transporter SLC19A2	Megaloblastic anemia, deafness, diabetes mellitus	AR
Other					
Carnitine deficiency	Carnitine	Kidney, muscle, heart	Carnitine transporter OCTN2	Hypoketotic hypoglycemia, cardiomyopathy, hypotonia	AR
Creatine deficiency	Creatine	Brain	Creatine transporter SLC6A8	Mental retardation, seizures, hypotonia	XL

Note: AR, autosomal recessive; AD, autosomal dominant; XL, X-linked recessive.

therapy can prevent and promote dissolution of calculi. Penicillamine can have significant side effects and should be reserved for patients who fail to respond to hydration alone or who are in a high-risk category (one remaining kidney, renal insufficiency). When medical management fails, shock wave lithotripsy, ureteroscopy, and percutaneous nephrolithotomy are effective for most stones. Open urologic surgery is considered for complex staghorn stones or when the patient has concomitant renal or ureteral abnormalities. Occasional patients progress to renal failure and require kidney transplantation.

DIBASIC AMINOACIDURIA

This disorder is characterized by a defect in renal tubular reabsorption of the three dibasic amino acids lysine, arginine, and ornithine but *not* cystine. There are two variants, transmitted as autosomal recessive traits. In the common form of dibasic aminoaciduria (type II), also known as *lysinuric protein intolerance*, homozygotes show defective intestinal transport of dibasic amino acids as well as exaggerated renal losses. It is most common in Finland (1 in 60,000), Southern Italy and Japan, but is rare elsewhere. The transport defect affects basolateral rather than luminal membrane transport and is associated with impairment of the urea cycle. The defective gene (*SLC7A7*, chromosome 14q11.2) encodes a unique membrane transporter, y+LAT, which associates with the cell-surface glycoprotein 4F2 heavy chain to form the complete sodium-independent transporter y+L.

Manifestations are related to the losses of ornithine, arginine, and lysine. Affected patients present in childhood with hepatosplenomegaly, protein intolerance, and episodic ammonia intoxication. Older patients may present with severe osteoporosis, impairment of kidney function, or interstitial changes in the lungs. Plasma concentrations of lysine, arginine, and ornithine are reduced, whereas urinary excretion of lysine and orotic acid are increased. Hyperammonemia may develop after the ingestion of protein loads or with infections, probably because of insufficient amounts of arginine and ornithine to maintain proper function of the urea cycle. The clinical features have been attributed to the hyperammonemia, to insufficient amounts of lysine to support protein synthesis during growth, and to decreased production of nitric oxide caused by arginine deficiency.

Therapy consists of dietary protein restriction and supplementation of citrulline (2–8 g/d), a neutral amino acid that fuels the urea cycle when metabolized to arginine and ornithine. Pulmonary disease responds to glycocorticoids or bronchoalveolar lavage in some patients. Women with lysinuric protein intolerance who become pregnant have an increased risk of anemia, toxemia, and bleeding complications during delivery. These can be minimized by aggressive nutritional therapy and control of blood pressure. Their infants can have intrauterine growth restriction but have normal neurologic function.

HARTNUP DISEASE

Hartnup disease (frequency 1 in 24,000) is an autosomal recessive disorder characterized by pellagra-like skin lesions, variable neurologic manifestations, and neutral and aromatic aminoaciduria. Alanine, serine, threonine, valine, leucine, isoleucine, phenylalanine, tyrosine, tryptophan, glutamine, asparagine, and histidine are excreted in urine in quantities 5–10 times greater than normal, and intestinal transport of these same amino acids is defective. The defective neutral amino acid transporter, B°AT1 encoded by the *SLC6A19* gene on chromosome 5p15, localizes to the apical membrane in renal tubular and intestinal cells.

The clinical manifestations result from nutritional deficiency of the essential amino acid tryptophan, caused by its intestinal and renal malabsorption, and of niacin, which derives in part from tryptophan metabolism. Only a small fraction of patients with the chemical findings of this disorder develop a pellagra-like syndrome, implying that manifestations depend on other factors in addition to the transport defect. The diagnosis of Hartnup disease should be suspected in any patient with clinical features of pellagra who does not have a history of dietary niacin deficiency (Chap. 71). The neurologic and psychiatric manifestations range from attacks of cerebellar ataxia to mild emotional lability to frank delirium, and they are usually accompanied by exacerbations of the erythematous, eczematoid skin rash. Fever, sunlight, stress, and sulfonamide therapy provoke clinical relapses. Diagnosis is made by detection of the neutral aminoaciduria, which does not occur in dietary niacin deficiency. Treatment is directed at niacin repletion and includes a high-protein diet and daily nicotinamide supplementation (50–250 mg).

FURTHER READINGS

Broer S, Wagner CA: *Membrane Transporter Diseases. Molecular Bases of Inherited Transport Defects.* New York, Kluver Academic/Plenum, 2003, 1–390

Kleta R et al: Mutations in SLC6A19, encoding B°AT1, cause Hartnup disorder. Nat Genet 36:999, 2004

Palacin M et al: The genetics of heteromeric amino acid transporters. Physiology (Bethesda) 20:112, 2005

Seow HF et al: Hartnup disorder is caused by mutations in the gene encoding the neutral amino acid transporter SLC6A19. Nat Genet 36:1003, 2004

360 Mechanisms of Neurologic Diseases
Stephen L. Hauser, M. Flint Beal

The human nervous system is the organ of consciousness, cognition, ethics, and behavior; as such, it is the most intricate structure known to exist. One-third of the 35,000 genes encoded in the human genome are expressed in the nervous system. Each mature brain is composed of 100 billion neurons, several million miles of axons and dendrites, and $>10^{15}$ synapses. Neurons exist within a dense parenchyma of multifunctional glial cells that synthesize myelin, preserve homeostasis, and regulate immune responses. Measured against this background of complexity, the achievements of molecular neuroscience have been extraordinary. This chapter reviews selected themes in neuroscience that provide a context for understanding fundamental mechanisms underlying neurologic disorders.

NEUROGENETICS

The landscape of neurology has been transformed by modern molecular genetics (Chap. 62). More than 350 different disease-causing genes have now been identified, and >1000 neurologic disorders have been genetically mapped to various chromosomal locations. The vast majority of these represent highly penetrant mutations that cause rare neurologic disorders; alternatively, they represent rare monogenic causes of common phenotypes. Examples of the latter include mutations of the amyloid precursor protein in familial Alzheimer's disease, the microtubule-associated protein tau (MAPT) in frontotemporal dementia, and α-synuclein in Parkinson's disease. These discoveries have been profoundly important because the mutated gene in the familial disorder often encodes a protein that is also pathogenetically involved (although not mutated) in the typical, sporadic form. The common mechanism involves disordered processing and, ultimately, aggregation of the protein, leading to cell death (see "Protein Aggregation and Neurodegeneration," below).

There is great optimism that complex genetic disorders, caused by combinations of both genetic and environmental factors, have now become tractable problems. The development of new genetic approaches, such as haplotype mapping for the efficient screening of variants genome-wide along with advances in high-throughput sequencing, are beginning to delineate incompletely penetrant genetic variants that influence susceptibility to, or modify the expression of, complex diseases including age-related macular degeneration, type 2 diabetes mellitus, and Alzheimer's disease.

Not all genetic diseases of the nervous system are caused by simple changes in the linear nucleotide sequence of genes. As the complex architecture of the human genome becomes better defined, many disorders that result from alterations in copy numbers of genes ("genedosage" effects) resulting from unequal crossing-over are likely to be identified. The first copy-number disorders to be recognized were Charcot-Marie-Tooth disease type 1A (CMT1A), caused by a duplication in the gene encoding the myelin protein PMP22, and the reciprocal deletion of the gene causing hereditary liability to pressure palsies (HNPP) (Chap. 379). Gene-dosage effects are causative in some cases of Parkinson's disease (α-synuclein), Alzheimer's disease (amyloid precursor protein), spinal muscular atrophy (survival motor neuron 2), the dysmyelinating disorder Pelizaeus-Merzbacher syndrome (pro-

teolipid protein 1), late-onset leukodystrophy (lamin B1), and a variety of developmental neurologic disorders. It is now evident that copy-number variations contribute substantially to normal human genomic variation for numerous genes involved in neurologic function, regulation of cell growth, and regulation of metabolism. It is also likely that gene-dosage effects will influence many behavioral phenotypes, learning disorders, and autism spectrum disorders.

The role of splicing variation as a contributor to neurologic disease is another area of active investigation. *Alternative splicing* refers to the inclusion of different combinations of exons in mature mRNA, resulting in the potential for many different protein products encoded by a single gene. Alternative splicing represents a powerful mechanism for generation of complexity and variation, and this mechanism appears to be highly prevalent in the nervous system, affecting key processes such as neurotransmitter receptors and ion channels. Numerous diseases are already known to result from abnormalities in alternative splicing. Increased inclusion of exon 10-containing transcripts of MAPT can cause frontotemporal dementia. Aberrant splicing also contributes to the pathogenesis of Duchenne, myotonic, and fascioscapulohumeral muscular dystrophies; ataxia telangiectasia; neurofibromatosis; some inherited ataxias; and fragile X syndrome; among other disorders. It is also likely that subtle variations of splicing will influence many genetically complex disorders. Recently a splicing variant of the interleukin 7 receptor α chain, resulting in production of more soluble and less membrane-bound receptor, was found to be associated with susceptibility to multiple sclerosis (MS) in multiple different populations.

Epigenetics refers to the mechanisms by which levels of gene expression can be exquisitely modulated, not by variations in the primary genetic sequence of DNA but rather by postgenomic alterations in DNA and chromatin structure, which influence how, when, and where genes are expressed. DNA methylation, as well as methylation and acetylation of histone proteins that interact with nuclear DNA to form chromatin, are key mediators of these events. Epigenetic processes appear to be dynamically active even in postmitotic neurons. *Imprinting* refers to an epigenetic feature, present for a subset of genes, in which the predominant expression of one allele is determined by its parent-of-origin. The distinctive neurodevelopmental disorders Prader-Willi syndrome (mild mental retardation and endocrine abnormalities) and Angelman syndrome (cortical atrophy, cerebellar dysmyelination, Purkinje cell loss) are classic examples of imprinting disorders whose distinctive features are determined by whether the paternal or maternal copy of chromosome of the critical genetic region 15q11-13 was responsible. Preferential allelic expression, whether due to imprinting, resistance to X-inactivation, or other mechanisms, is likely to play a major role in determining complex behaviors and susceptibility to many neurologic and psychiatric disorders.

ION CHANNELS AND CHANNELOPATHIES

The resting potential of neurons and the action potentials responsible for impulse conduction are generated by ion currents and ion channels. Most ion channels are gated, meaning that they can transition between conformations that are open or closed to ion conductance. Individual ion channels are distinguished by the specific ions they conduct; by their kinetics; and by whether they directly sense voltage, are linked to receptors for neurotransmitters or other ligands such as neurotrophins, or are activated by second messengers. The diverse characteristics of different ion channels provide a means by which neuronal excitability can be exquisitely modulated at both the cellular and the subcellular levels. Disor-

TABLE 360-1 EXAMPLES OF NEUROLOGIC CHANNELOPATHIES

Category	Disorder	Channel Type	Mutated Gene	Chap. Ref.
Genetic				
Ataxias	Episodic ataxia-1	K	KCNA1	368
	Episodic ataxia-2	Ca	CACNL1A	
	Spinocerebellar ataxia-6	Ca	CACNL1A	
Migraine	Familial hemiplegic migraine 1	Ca	CACNL1A	15
	Familial hemiplegic migraine 2	Na	SCN1A	
Epilepsy	Benign neonatal familial convulsions	K	KCNQ2, KCNQ3	363
	Generalized epilepsy with febrile convulsions plus	Na	SCN1B	
Periodic paralysis	Hyperkalemic periodic paralysis	Na	SCN4A	382
	Hypokalemic periodic paralysis	Ca	CACNL1A3	
Myotonia	Myotonia congenita	Cl	CLCN1	382
	Paramyotonia congenita	Na	SCN4A	
Deafness	Jorvell and Lange-Nielsen syndrome (deafness, prolonged QT interval, and arrythmia)	K	KCNQ1, KCNE1	30
	Autosomal dominant progressive deafness	K	KCNQ4	
Autoimmune				
Paraneoplastic	Limbic encephalitis	Kv1	—	97
	Acquired neuromyotonia	Kv1	—	97
	Cerebellar ataxia	Ca (P/Q type)	—	97
	Lambert-Eaton syndrome	Ca (P/Q type)	—	97

ders of ion channels—channelopathies—are responsible for a growing list of human neurologic diseases (Table 360-1). Most are caused by mutations in ion channel genes or by autoantibodies against ion channel proteins. One example is epilepsy, a syndrome of diverse causes characterized by repetitive, synchronous firing of neuronal action potentials. Action potentials are normally generated by the opening of sodium channels and the inward movement of sodium ions down the intracellular concentration gradient. Depolarization of the neuronal membrane opens potassium channels, resulting in outward movement of potassium ions, repolarization, closure of the sodium channel, and hyperpolarization. Sodium or potassium channel subunit genes have long been considered candidate disease genes in inherited epilepsy syndromes, and recently such mutations have been identified. These mutations appear to alter the normal gating function of these channels, increasing the inherent excitability of neuronal membranes in regions where the abnormal channels are expressed.

Whereas the specific clinical manifestations of channelopathies are quite variable, one common feature is that manifestations tend to be intermittent or paroxysmal, such as occurs in epilepsy, migraine, ataxia, myotonia, or periodic paralysis. Exceptions are clinically progressive channel disorders such as autosomal dominant hearing impairment. The genetic channelopathies identified to date are all uncommon disorders caused by obvious mutations in channel genes. As the full repertoire of human ion channels and related proteins is identified, it is likely that additional channelopathies will be discovered. In addition to rare disorders that result from obvious mutations, it is also likely that less penitrant allelic variations in channel genes or in their pattern of expression might underlie susceptibility to some common forms of epilepsy, migraine, or other disorders. For example, mutations in the T-type Ca channel gene *CACNA1H*, as well as a K channel (*KCND2*) and various GABA receptor genes, have been associated with an increased risk for epilepsy.

NEUROTRANSMITTERS AND NEUROTRANSMITTER RECEPTORS

Synaptic neurotransmission is the predominant means by which neurons communicate with each other. Classic neurotransmitters are synthesized in the presynaptic region of the nerve terminal; stored in vesicles; and released into the synaptic cleft, where they bind to receptors on the postsynaptic cell. Secreted neurotransmitters are eliminated by reuptake into the presynaptic neuron (or glia), by diffusion away from the synaptic cleft, and/or by specific inactivation. In addition to the classic neurotransmitters, many neuropeptides have been identified as definite or probable neurotransmitters; these include substance P, neurotensin, enkephalins, β-endorphin, histamine, vasoactive intestinal polypeptide, cholecystokinin, neuropeptide Y, and somatostatin. Peptide neurotransmitters are synthesized in the cell body rather than the nerve terminal and may colocalize with classic neurotransmitters in single neurons. Nitric oxide and carbon monoxide are gases that appear also to function as neurotransmitters, in part by signaling in a retrograde fashion from the postsynaptic to the presynaptic cell.

Neurotransmitters modulate the function of postsynaptic cells by binding to specific neurotransmitter receptors, of which there are two major types. *Ionotropic receptors* are direct ion channels that open after engagement by the neurotransmitter. *Metabotropic receptors* interact with G proteins, stimulating production of second messengers and activating protein kinases, which modulate a variety of cellular events. Ionotropic receptors are multiple subunit structures, whereas metabotropic receptors are composed of single subunits only. One important difference between ionotropic and metabotropic receptors is that the kinetics of ionotropic receptor effects are fast (generally <1 ms) because neurotransmitter binding directly alters the electrical properties of the postsynaptic cell, whereas metabotropic receptors function over longer time periods. These different properties contribute to the potential for selective and finely modulated signaling by neurotransmitters.

Neurotransmitter systems are perturbed in a large number of clinical disorders, examples of which are highlighted in Table 360-2. One example is the involvement of dopaminergic neurons originating in the substantia nigra of the midbrain and projecting to the striatum (nigrostriatal pathway) in Parkinson's disease and in heroin addicts after the ingestion of the toxin MPTP (1-methyl-4-phenyl-1,2,5,6-tetrahydropyridine).

A second important dopaminergic system arising in the midbrain is the mediocorticolimbic pathway, which is implicated in the pathogenesis of addictive behaviors including drug reward. Its key components include the midbrain ventral tegmental area (VTA), median forebrain bundle, and nucleus accumbens (Fig. 385-2). The cholinergic pathway originating in the nucleus basalis of Meynert plays a role in memory function in Alzheimer's disease.

Addictive drugs share the property of increasing dopamine release in the nucleus accumbens. Amphetamine increases intracellular release of dopamine from vesicles and reverses transport of dopamine through the dopamine transporters. Patients prone to addiction show increased activation of the nucleus accumbens following administration of amphetamine. Cocaine binds to dopamine transporters and inhibits its dopamine reuptake. Ethanol inhibits inhibitory neurons in the VTA, leading to increased dopamine release in the nucleus accumbens. Opioids also disinhibit these dopaminergic neurons by binding to μ receptors expressed by GABA-containing interneurons in the VTA. Nicotine increases dopamine release by activating nicotinic acetylcholine receptors on cell bodies and nerve terminals of dopaminergic VTA neurons. Tetrahydrocannabinol, the active ingredient of cannabis, also increases dopamine levels in the nucleus accumbens. Blockade of dopamine in the nucleus accumbens can terminate the rewarding effects of addictive drugs.

TABLE 360-2   **PRINCIPAL CLASSIC NEUROTRANSMITTERS**   2479

Neurotransmitter	Anatomy	Clinical Aspects
Acetylcholine (ACh) $CH_3\text{—}C(=O)\text{—}O\text{—}CH_2\text{—}N\text{—}(CH_3)_3$	Motor neurons in spinal cord → neuromuscular junction Basal forebrain → widespread cortex Interneurons in striatum Autonomic nervous system (preganglionic and postganglionic sympathetic)	Acetylcholinesterases (nerve gases) Myasthenia gravis (antibodies to ACh receptor) Congenital myasthenic syndromes (mutations in ACh receptor subunits) Lambert-Eaton syndrome (antibodies to Ca channels impair ACh release) Botulism (toxin disrupts ACh release by exocytosis) Alzheimer's disease (selective cell death) Autosomal dominant frontal lobe epilepsy (mutations in CNS ACh receptor) Parkinson's disease (tremor)
Dopamine HO, HO benzene ring $\text{—}CH_2\text{—}CH_2\text{—}NH_3$	Substantia nigra → striatum (nigrostriatal pathway) Substantia nigra → limbic system and widespread cortex Arcuate nucleus of hypothalamus → anterior pituitary (via portal veins)	Parkinson's disease (selective cell death) MPTP parkinsonism (toxin transported into neurons) Addiction, behavioral disorders Inhibits prolactin secretion
Norepinephrine (NE) HO, HO benzene ring $\text{—}CH(OH)\text{—}CH_2\text{—}NH_2$	Locus coeruleus (pons) → limbic system, hypothalamus, cortex Medulla → locus coeruleus, spinal cord Postganglionic neurons of sympathetic nervous system	Mood disorders (MAOA inhibitors and tricyclics increase NE and improve depression) Anxiety Orthostatic tachycardia syndrome (mutations in NE transporter)
Serotonin HO indole ring $\text{—}CH_2\text{—}CH_2\text{—}NH_2$	Pontine raphe nuclei → widespread projections Medulla/pons → dorsal horn of spinal cord	Mood disorders (SSRIs improve depression) Migraine pain pathway Pain pathway
γ-Aminobutyric acid (GABA) $H_2N\text{—}CH_2\text{—}CH_2\text{—}CH_2\text{—}COOH$	Major inhibitory neurotransmitter in brain; widespread cortical interneurons and long projection pathways	Stiff person syndrome (antibodies to glutamic acid decarboxylase, the biosynthetic enzyme for GABA) Epilepsy (gabapentin and valproic acid increase GABA)
Glycine $H_2N\text{—}CH_2\text{—}COOH$	Major inhibitory neurotransmitter in spinal cord	Spasticity Hyperekplexia (myoclonic startle syndrome) due to mutations in glycine receptor
Glutamate $H_2N\text{—}CH(COOH)\text{—}CH_2\text{—}CH_2\text{—}COOH$	Major excitatory neurotransmitter; located throughout CNS, including cortical pyramidal cells	Seizures due to ingestion of domoic acid (a glutamate analogue) Rasmussen's encephalitis (antibody against glutamate receptor 3) Excitotoxic cell death

Note: CNS, central nervous system; MPTP, 1-methyl-4-phenyl-1,2,3,6-tetrahydropyridine; MAOA, monoamine oxidase A; SSRI, selective serotonin reuptake inhibitor.

Not all cell-to-cell communication in the nervous system occurs via neurotransmission. Gap junctions provide for direct neuron-neuron electrical conduction and also create openings for the diffusion of ions and metabolites between cells. In addition to neurons, gap junctions are also widespread in glia, creating a syncytium that protects neurons by removing glutamate and potassium from the extracellular environment. Gap junctions consist of membrane-spanning proteins, termed *connexins*, that pair across adjacent cells. Mechanisms that involve gap junctions have been related to a variety of neurologic disorders. Mutations in connexin 32, a gap junction protein expressed by Schwann cells, are responsible for the X-linked form of CMT disease (Chap. 379). Mutations in either of two gap junction proteins expressed in the inner ear—connexin 26 and connexin 31—result in autosomal dominant progressive hearing loss (Chap. 30). Glial calcium waves mediated through gap junctions also appear to explain the phenomenon of spreading depression associated with migraine auras and the march of epileptic discharges. Spreading depression is a neural response that follows a variety of different stimuli and is characterized by a circumferentially expanding negative potential that propagates at a characteristic speed of 20 m/s and is associated with an increase in extracellular potassium.

SIGNALING PATHWAYS AND GENE TRANSCRIPTION

The fundamental issue of how memory, learning, and thinking are encoded in the nervous system is likely to be clarified by identifying the signaling pathways involved in neuronal differentiation, axon guidance, and synapse formation, and by understanding how these pathways are modulated by experience. Many families of transcription factors, each comprising multiple individual components, are expressed in the nervous system. Elucidation of these signaling pathways has already begun to provide insights into the cause of a variety of neurologic disorders, including inherited disorders of cognition such as X-linked mental retardation. This problem affects ~1 in 500 males, and linkage studies in different families suggest that as many as 60 different X-chromosome encoded genes may be responsible. Rett syndrome, a common cause of (dominant) X-linked progressive mental retardation in females, is due to a mutation in a gene (*MECP2*) encoding a DNA-binding protein involved in transcriptional repression. As the X chromosome comprises only ~3% of germline DNA, then by extrapolation the number of genes that potentially contribute to clinical disorders affecting intelligence in humans must be potentially very large. As discussed below, there is increasing evidence that abnormal gene transcription may play a role in neurodegenerative diseases, such as Huntington's disease, in which proteins with polyglutamine expansions bind to and sequester transcription factors. A critical transcription factor for neuronal survival is CREB (cyclic adenosine monophosphate responsive element-binding) protein, which also plays an important role in memory in the hippocampus.

MYELIN

Myelin is the multilayered insulating substance that surrounds axons and speeds impulse conduction by permitting action potentials to jump between naked regions of axons (nodes of Ranvier) and across myelinated segments. Molecular interactions between the myelin membrane and axon are required to maintain the stability, function, and normal lifespan of both structures. A single oligodendrocyte usually ensheaths multiple axons in the central nervous system (CNS), whereas in the peripheral nervous system (PNS) each Schwann cell typically myelinates a single axon. Myelin is a lipid-rich material formed by a spiraling process of the membrane of the myelinating cell around the axon, creating multiple membrane bilayers that are tightly apposed (compact myelin) by charged protein interactions. Several inhibitors of axon growth are expressed on the innermost (periaxonal) lamellae of the myelin membrane (see "Stem Cells and Transplantation," below). A number of clinically important neurologic disorders are caused by inherited mutations in myelin proteins of the CNS or PNS (Fig. 360-1). Constituents of myelin also have a propensity to be targeted as autoantigens in autoimmune demyelinating disorders (Fig. 360-2).

NEUROTROPHIC FACTORS

Neurotrophic factors (Table 360-3) are secreted proteins that modulate neuronal growth, differentiation, repair, and survival; some have additional functions, including roles in neurotransmission and in the synaptic reorganization involved in learning and memory. The neurotrophin (NT) family contains nerve growth factor (NGF), brain-derived neurotrophic factor (BDNF), NT3, and NT4/5. The neurotrophins act at TrK and p75 receptors to promote survival of neurons. Because of their survival-promoting and antiapoptotic effects, neurotrophic factors are in theory outstanding candidates for therapy of disorders characterized by premature death of neurons such as occurs in amyotrophic lateral sclerosis (ALS) and other degenerative motor neuron disorders. Knockout mice lacking receptors for ciliary neurotrophic factor (CNTF) or BDNF show loss of motor neurons, and experimental motor neuron death can be rescued by treatment with various neurotrophic factors including CNTF, BDNF, and vascular endothelial growth factor (VEGF). However, in phase 3 clinical trials, growth factors were ineffective in human ALS. The growth factor glial-derived neurotrophic factor (GDNF) is important for survival of dopaminergic neurons. It has shown promising neurorestorative effects in experimental models of Parkinson's disease and is being tested using gene therapy in early-stage human clinical trials.

STEM CELLS AND TRANSPLANTATION

The nervous system is traditionally considered to be a nonmitotic organ, in particular with respect to neurons. These concepts have been challenged by the finding that neural progenitor or stem cells exist in the adult CNS that are capable of differentiation, migration over long distances, and extensive axonal arborization and synapse formation with appropriate targets. These capabilities also indicate that the repertoire of factors required for growth, survival, differentiation, and migration of these cells exists in the mature nervous system. In rodents, neural stem cells, defined as progenitor cells capable of differentiating into mature cells of neural or glial lineage, have been experimentally propagated from fetal CNS and neuroectodermal tissues and also from adult germinal matrix and ependyma regions. Human fetal CNS tissue is also capable of differentiation into cells with neuronal, astrocyte, and

FIGURE 360-1 The molecular architecture of the myelin sheath illustrating the most important disease-related proteins. The illustration represents a composite of CNS and PNS myelin. Proteins restricted to CNS myelin are shown in green, proteins of PNS myelin are lavender, and proteins present in both CNS and PNS are red. In the CNS, the X-linked allelic disorders, Pelizaeus-Merzbacher disease and one variant of familial spastic paraplegia, are caused by mutations in the gene for proteolipid protein (PLP) that normally promotes extracellular compaction between adjacent myelin lamellae. The homologue of PLP in the PNS is the P_0 protein, mutations in which cause the neuropathy Charcot-Marie-Tooth disease (CMT) type 1B. The most common form of CMT is the 1A subtype caused by a duplication of the *PMP22* gene; deletions in *PMP22* are responsible for another inherited neuropathy termed *hereditary liability to pressure palsies* (Chap. 379).

In multiple sclerosis (MS), myelin basic protein (MBP) and the quantitatively minor CNS protein, myelin oligodendrocyte glycoprotein (MOG), are likely T cell and B cell antigens, respectively (Chap. 375). The location of MOG at the outermost lamella of the CNS myelin membrane may facilitate its targeting by autoantibodies. In the PNS, autoantibodies against myelin gangliosides are implicated in a variety of disorders, including GQ1b in the Fisher variant of Guillain-Barré syndrome, GM1 in multifocal motor neuropathy, and sulfatide constituents of myelin-associated glycoprotein (MAG) in peripheral neuropathies associated with monoclonal gammopathies (Chap. 380).

oligodendrocyte morphology when cultured in the presence of growth factors. Impressively, such cells could be stably engrafted into mouse CNS tissue, creating neural chimeras. Another approach is to use somatic cell nuclear transfer, in which cell nuclei are placed inside an enucleated oocyte and then differentiated into stem cells with an identical genetic background to the donor. This technique has been utilized successfully in animal models of Parkinson's disease. Once the repertoire of signals required for cell type specification is better understood, differentiation into specific neural or glial subpopulations can be directed in vitro; such cells could also be engineered to express therapeutic molecules. Another promising approach is to utilize growth factors, such as BDNF, to stimulate endogenous stem cells to proliferate and migrate to areas of neuronal damage. Administration of epidermal growth factor with fibroblast growth factor replenished up to 50% of hippocampal CA1 neurons a month after global ischemia in rats. The new neurons made connections and improved performance in a memory task.

Although stem cells hold tremendous promise for the treatment of debilitating neurologic diseases, such as Parkinson's disease and spinal cord injury, it should be emphasized that medical application is in its infancy. Major obstacles are the generation of position- and neurotransmitter-defined subtypes of neurons and their isolation as pure populations of the desired cells. This is crucial to avoid persistence of undifferentiated embryonic stem (ES) cells, which can generate tumors. The establishment of appropriate neural connections and afferent control is also critical. For instance, human ES motor neurons will need to be introduced at multiple segments in the neuraxis, and then their axons will need to regenerate from the spinal cord to distal musculature.

FIGURE 360-2 Involvement of mitochondria in cell death. A severe excitotoxic insult (**A**) results in cell death by necrosis, whereas a mild excitotoxic insult (**B**) results in apoptosis. After a severe insult (such as ischemia), there is a large increase in glutamate activation of NMDA receptors, an increase in intracellular Ca^{2+} concentrations, activation of nitric oxide synthase (NOS), and increased mitochondrial Ca^{2+} and superoxide generation followed by the formation of $ONOO^-$. This sequence results in damage to cellular macromolecules including DNA, leading to activation of poly-ADP-ribose polymerase (PARS). Both mitochondrial accumulation of Ca^{2+} and oxidative damage lead to activation of the permeability transition pore (PTP) that is linked to excitotoxic cell death. A mild excitotoxic insult can occur due either to an abnormality in an excitotoxicity amino acid receptor, allowing more Ca^{2+} flux, or to impaired functioning of other ionic channels or of energy production, which may allow the voltage-dependent NMDA receptor to be activated by ambient concentrations of glutamate. This event can then lead to increased mitochondrial Ca^{2+} and free radical production, yet relatively preserved ATP generation. The mitochondria may then release cytochrome c (Cytc), caspase 9, apoptosis-inducing factor (Aif), and perhaps other mediators that lead to apoptosis. The precise role of the PTP in this mode of cell death is still being clarified, but there does appear to be involvement of the adenine nucleotide transporter that is a key component of the PTP.

Experimental transplantation of human fetal dopaminergic neurons in patients with Parkinson's disease has shown that these transplanted cells can survive within the host striatum; however, some patients developed disabling dyskinesias and this approach is no longer in clinical development. Human ES cells can be differentiated into dopaminergic neurons, which reverse symptoms of Parkinson's disease in experimental animal models. Studies of transplantation for patients with Huntington's disease have also reported encouraging, although very preliminary, results. Oligodendrocyte precursor cells transplanted into mice with a dysmyelinating disorder effectively migrated in the new environment, interacted with axons, and mediated myelination; such experiments raise hope that similar transplantation strategies may be feasible in human disorders of myelin such as MS. The promise of stem cells for treatment of both neurodegenerative diseases and neural injury is great, but development has been slowed by unresolved concerns over safety (including the theoretical risk of malignant transformation of transplant-ed cells), ethics (particularly with respect to use of fetal tissue), and efficacy.

In developing brain, the extracellular matrix provides stimulatory and inhibitory signals that promote neuronal migration, neurite outgrowth, and axonal extension. After neuronal damage, reexpression of inhibitory molecules such as chondroitin sulfate proteoglycans may prevent tissue regeneration. Chondroitinase degraded these inhibitory molecules and enhanced axonal regeneration and motor recovery in a rat model of spinal cord injury. Several myelin proteins, specifically Nogo, oligodendrocyte myelin glycoprotein (OMGP), and myelin-associated glycoprotein (MAG), may also interfere with axon regeneration. Sialidase, which cleaves one class of receptors for MAG, enhances axonal outgrowth. Antibodies against Nogo promote regeneration after experimental focal ischemia or spinal cord injury. Nogo, OMGP, and MAG all bind to the same neural receptor, the Nogo receptor, which mediates its inhibitory function via the p75 neurotrophin receptor signaling.

CELL DEATH—EXCITOTOXICITY AND APOPTOSIS

Excitotoxicity refers to neuronal cell death caused by activation of excitatory amino acid receptors (Fig. 360-3). Compelling evidence for a role of excitotoxicity, especially in ischemic neuronal injury, is derived from experiments in animal models. Experimental models of stroke are associated with increased extracellular concentrations of the excitatory amino acid neurotransmitter glutamate, and neuronal damage is attenuated by denervation of glutamate-containing neurons or the administration of glutamate receptor antagonists. The distribution of cells sensitive to ischemia corresponds closely with that of *N*-methyl-D-aspartate (NMDA) receptors (except for cerebellar Purkinje cells, which are vulnerable to hypoxia-ischemia but lack NMDA receptors); and competitive and noncompetitive NMDA antagonists are effective in preventing focal ischemia. In global cerebral ischemia, non-NMDA receptors (kainic acid and AMPA) are activated, and antagonists to

TABLE 360-3 NEUROTROPHIC FACTORS

Neurotrophin family	Transforming growth factor β family
Nerve growth factor	Glial-derived neurotrophic family
Brain-derived neurotrophic factor	Neurturin
Neurotrophin-3	Persephin
Neurotrophin-4	Fibroblast growth factor family
Neurotrophin-6	Hepatocyte growth factor
Cytokine family	Insulin-like growth factor (IGF) family
Ciliary neurotrophic factor	IGF-1
Leukemia inhibitory factor	IGF-2
Interleukin-6	
Cardiotrophin-1	

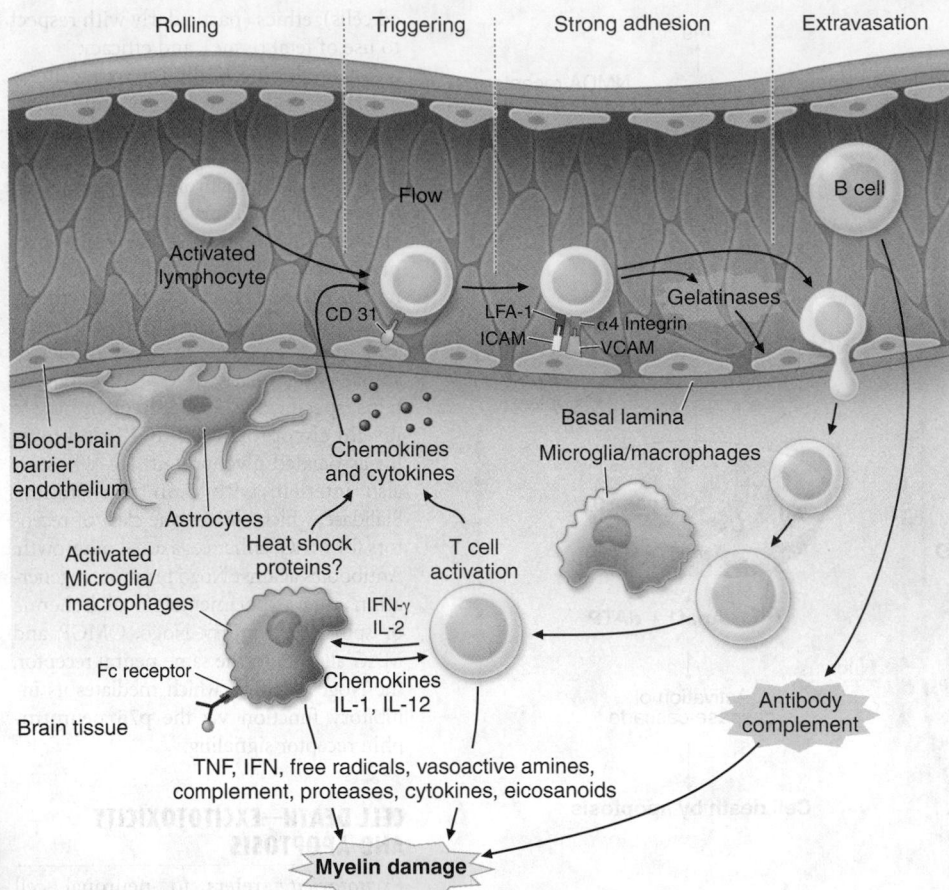

FIGURE 360-3 A model for experimental allergic encephalomyelitis (EAE). Crucial steps for disease initiation and progression include peripheral activation of preexisting autoreactive T cells; homing to the CNS and extravasation across the blood-brain barrier; reactivation of T cells by exposed autoantigens; secretion of cytokines; activation of microglia and astrocytes and recruitment of a secondary inflammatory wave; and immune-mediated myelin destruction. ICAM, intercellular adhesion molecule; LFA-1, leukocyte function-associated antigen-1; VCAM, vascular cell adhesion molecule; IFN, interferon; IL, interleukin; TNF, tumor necrosis factor.

these receptors are protective. Experimental brain damage induced by hypoglycemia is also attenuated by NMDA antagonists.

Excitotoxicity is not a single event but rather a cascade of cell injury. Excitotoxicity causes influx of calcium into cells, and much of the calcium is sequestered in mitochondria rather than in the cytoplasm. Increased cytoplasmic calcium causes metabolic dysfunction and free radical generation; activates protein kinases, phospholipases, nitric oxide synthase, proteases, and endonucleases; and inhibits protein synthesis. Activation of nitric oxide synthase generates nitric oxide (NO•), which can react with superoxide ($O^•_2$) to generate peroxynitrite (ONOO−), which may play a direct role in neuronal injury. Another critical pathway is activation of poly-ADP-ribose polymerase, which occurs in response to free radical–mediated DNA damage. Experimentally, mice with knockout mutations of neuronal nitric oxide synthase or poly-ADP-ribose polymerase, or those that overexpress superoxide dismutase, are resistant to focal ischemia.

Although excitotoxicity is clearly implicated in the pathogenesis of cell death in stroke, to date treatment with NMDA antagonists has not proven to be clinically useful. Transient receptor potentials (TRP) are calcium channels that are activated by oxidative stress in parallel with excitotoxic signal pathways. In addition, glutamate-independent pathways of calcium influx via acid-sensing ion channels have been identified. These channels transport calcium in the setting of acidosis and substrate depletion, and pharmacologic blockade of these channels markedly attenuates stroke injury. These channels offer a potential new therapeutic target for stroke.

Apoptosis, or programmed cell death, plays an important role in both physiologic and pathologic conditions. During embryogenesis, apoptot-

ic pathways operate to destroy neurons that fail to differentiate appropriately or reach their intended targets. There is mounting evidence for an increased rate of apoptotic cell death in a variety of acute and chronic neurologic diseases. Apoptosis is characterized by neuronal shrinkage, chromatin condensation, and DNA fragmentation, whereas necrotic cell death is associated with cytoplasmic and mitochondrial swelling followed by dissolution of the cell membrane. Apoptotic and necrotic cell death can coexist or be sequential events, depending on the severity of the initiating insult. Cellular energy reserves appear to have an important role in these two forms of cell death, with apoptosis favored under conditions in which ATP levels are preserved. Evidence of DNA fragmentation has been found in a number of degenerative neurologic disorders, including Alzheimer's disease, Huntington's disease, and ALS. The best characterized genetic neurologic disorder related to apoptosis is infantile spinal muscular atrophy (Werdnig-Hoffmann disease), in which two genes thought to be involved in the apoptosis pathways are causative.

Mitochondria are essential in controlling specific apoptosis pathways. The redistribution of cytochrome c, as well as apoptosis-inducing factor (AIF), from mitochondria during apoptosis leads to the activation of a cascade of intracellular proteases known as *caspases.* Caspase-independent apoptosis occurs after DNA damage, activation of poly-ADP-ribose polymerase, and translocation of AIF into the nucleus. Redistribution of cytochrome c is prevented by overproduction of the apoptotic protein BCL2 and is promoted by the proapoptotic protein BAX. These pathways may be triggered by activation of a large pore in the mitochondrial inner membrane known as the *permeability transition pore,* although in other circumstances they occur independently. Recent studies suggest that blocking the mitochondrial pore reduces both hypoglycemic and ischemic cell death. Mice deficient in cyclophilin D, a key protein involved in opening the permeability transition pore, are resistant to necrosis produced by focal cerebral ischemia.

PROTEIN AGGREGATION AND NEURODEGENERATION

The possibility that protein aggregation plays a role in the pathogenesis of neurodegenerative diseases is a major focus of current research. Protein aggregation is a major histopathologic hallmark of neurodegenerative diseases. Deposition of β-amyloid is strongly implicated in the pathogenesis of Alzheimer's disease. Genetic mutations in familial Alzheimer's disease cause increased production of β-amyloid with 42 amino acids, which has an increased propensity to aggregate, as compared to β-amyloid with 40 amino acids. Mutations in genes encoding the MAPT lead to altered splicing of tau and the production of neurofibrillary tangles in frontotemporal dementia and progressive supranuclear palsy. Familial Parkinson's disease is associated with mutations in α-synuclein, parkin, and the ubiquitin carboxy-terminal hydrolase. Parkin, which causes autosomal recessive early-onset Parkinson's disease, is a ubiquitin ligase. The characteristic histopathologic feature of Parkinson's disease is the Lewy body, an eosinophilic cytoplasmic inclusion that contains both neurofilaments and α-synuclein. Huntington's disease and cerebellar degenerations are associated with expansions of polyglutamine repeats in proteins, which aggregate to produce neuronal intranuclear inclusions. Familial ALS is associated with superoxide dismutase mutations and cytoplasmic inclusions containing superoxide dismutase. In autosomal dominant neurohypophyseal diabetes insipidus, mutations in vasopressin result in abnormal protein processing, accumulation in the endoplasmic reticulum, and cell death.

The current major scientific question is whether protein aggregates contribute to neuronal death or whether they are merely secondary bystanders. A major focus in all the neurodegenerative diseases is now on small protein aggregates termed *oligomers*. These may be the toxic species of β-amyloid, α-synuclein, and proteins with expanded polyglutamines such as are associated with Huntington's disease. Protein aggregates are usually ubiquinated, which targets them for degradation by the 26S component of the proteosome. An inability to degrade protein aggregates could lead to cellular dysfunction, impaired axonal transport, and cell death by apoptotic mechanisms.

In experimental models of Huntington's disease and cerebellar degeneration, protein aggregates are not well correlated with neuronal death and may be protective. A substantial body of evidence suggests that the mutant proteins with polyglutamine expansions in these diseases bind to transcription factors and that this contributes to disease pathogenesis. In Huntington's disease there is dysfunction of the transcriptional co-regulator, PGC-1α, a key regulator of mitochondrial biogenesis. Agents that upregulate gene transcription are neuroprotective in animal models of these diseases. A number of compounds have been developed to block β-amyloid production and/or aggregation, and these agents are being studied in early clinical trials in humans.

FIGURE 360-4 Mirror neuron systems are bilaterally activated during imitation. A. Bilateral activations (circled in yellow) in inferior frontal mirror neuron areas during imitation, as measured by BOLD fMRI signal changes. In red, activation during right hand imitation. In blue, activation during left hand imitation. **B.** In contrast, there is lateralized (contralateral) primary visual activation of the primary visual cortex for imitated actions presented to the right visual field (in red, left visual cortex) and to the left visual field (in blue, right visual cortex). **C.** Lateralized primary motor activation for hand actions imitated with the right hand (in red, left motor cortex) and with the left hand (in blue, right motor cortex). *(From L. Aziz-Zadeh et al: J Neurosci 26:2964, 2006.)*

SYSTEMS NEUROSCIENCE

Systems neuroscience refers to study of the functions of neurocircuits and how they relate to brain function, behavior, motor activity, and cognition. Brain imaging techniques, primarily functional MRI (fMRI) and position emission tomography (PET), have made it possible to investigate cognitive processes such as perception, making judgments, paying attention, and thinking. This has allowed insights into how networks of neurons operate to produce behavior. Many of these studies at present are based on determining the connectivity of neural circuits and how they operate, and how this can be then modeled to produce improved understanding of physiologic processes. fMRI uses contrast mechanisms related to physiologic changes in tissue, and brain perfusion can be studied by observing the time-course of changes in brain water signal as a bolus of injected paramagnetic gadolinium contrast moves through the brain. More recently, to study intrinsic contrast-related local changes in blood oxygenation with brain activity, blood-oxygen-level-dependent (BOLD) contrast has been used to provide a rapid noninvasive approach for functional assessment. These techniques have been reliably utilized in the field of both behavior and cognitive sciences. One example is the use of fMRI to demonstrate mirror neuron systems, imitative pathways activated when observing actions of others (Fig. 360-4). Mirror neurons are thought to be important for social conditioning and for many forms of learning, and abnormalities in mirror neurons may underlie some autism disorders. Data also suggest that enhancement of mirror neuron pathways might have potential for rehabilitation after stroke. Other examples of the use of fMRI include the study of memory. Recent studies have shown that not only is hippocampal activity correlated with declarative memory consolidation, but it also involves activation in the ventral medial prefrontal cortex. Consolidation of memory over time results in decreased activity of the hippocampus and progressively stronger activation in the ventral medial prefrontal region associated with retrieval of consolidated memories. An elegant study used MRI to identify the brain protein KIBRA as being significantly associated with human memory performance. This locus was initially identified in a genome-wide screen of three independent populations, which were studied in relation to the inability to perform verbal memory tasks. Several KIBRA alleles were associated with improved free recall performance. The authors then utilized fMRI to detect KIBRA allele–dependent differences in hippocampal activation during memory retrieval. These experiments provided strong evidence that KIBRA plays a direct role in human memory function. fMRI has also been utilized to identify sequences of brain activation involved in normal movements and alterations in their activation associated with both injury and recovery, and to plan neurosurgical operations. Diffusion tensor imaging is a recently developed MRI technique that can measure macroscopic axonal organization in nervous system tissues; it appears to be useful in assessing myelin and axonal injuries as well as brain development.

FURTHER READINGS

GOLDMAN S: Stem and progenitor cell-based therapy of the human central nervous system. Nat Biotechnol 23:862, 2005

IACOBONI M, MAZZIOTTA JC: Mirror neuron system: Basic findings and clinical applications. Ann Neurol 62:213, 2007

LEE JA, LUPSKI JR: Genomic rearrangements and gene copy-number alterations as a cause of nervous system disorders. Neuron 52:103, 2006

LICATALOSI DD, DARNELL RB: Splicing regulation in neurologic disease. Neuron 52:93, 2006

LIN MT, BEAL MF: Mitochondrial dysfunction and oxidative stress in neurodegenerative diseases. Nature 443:787, 2006

MATTHEWS PM et al: Applications of fMRI in translational medicine and clinical practice. Nat Rev Neurosci 7:732, 2006

PAPASSOTIROPOULOS A et al: Common Kibra alleles are associated with human memory performance. Science 314:475, 2006

PASINELLI P, BROWN RH: Molecular biology of amyotrophic lateral sclerosis: Insights from genetics. Nat Rev Neurosci 7:710, 2006

ROY NS et al: Functional engraftment of human ES cell–derived dopaminergic neurons enriched by coculture with telomerase-immortalized midbrain astrocytes. Nat Med 12:1259, 2006

SIMON R, XIONG S: Acidotoxicity in brain ischemia. Biochem Soc Trans 34:1356, 2006

STORKEBAUM E et al: Treatment of motoneuron degeneration by intracerebroventricular delivery of VEGF in a rat model of ALS. Nat Neurosci 8:85, 2005

TAKASHIMA A et al: Declarative memory consolidation in humans: A prospective functional magnetic resonance imaging study. Proc Natl Acad Sci USA 103:756, 2006

YANG LJS et al: Sialidase enhances spinal axon outgrowth in vivo. Proc Natl Acad Sci USA 103:11057, 2006

361 Approach to the Patient with Neurologic Disease

Daniel H. Lowenstein, Joseph B. Martin, Stephen L. Hauser

Neurologic diseases are common and costly. According to one estimate, 180 million Americans suffer from a nervous system disorder, resulting in an annual cost of over $700 billion. This aggregate cost is even greater than that for cardiovascular disease (Table 361-1). Globally, these disorders are responsible for 28% of all years lived with a disability. Most patients with neurologic symptoms seek care from internists and other generalists rather than from neurologists. Because therapies now exist for many neurologic disorders, a skillful approach to diagnosis is essential. Errors commonly result from an overreliance on costly neuroimaging procedures and laboratory tests, which, while useful, do not substitute for an adequate history and examination. The proper approach to the patient with a neurologic illness begins with the patient and focuses the clinical problem first in anatomic and then in pathophysiologic terms; only then should a specific diagnosis be entertained. This method ensures that technology is judiciously applied, a correct diagnosis is established in an efficient manner, and treatment is promptly initiated.

THE NEUROLOGIC METHOD

Locate the Lesion(s) The first priority is to identify the region of the nervous system that is likely to be responsible for the symptoms. Can the disorder be mapped to one specific location, is it multifocal, or is a diffuse process present? Are the symptoms restricted to the nervous system, or do they arise in the context of a systemic illness? Is the problem in the central nervous system (CNS), the peripheral nervous system (PNS), or both? If in the CNS, is the cerebral cortex, basal ganglia, brainstem, cerebellum, or spinal cord responsible? Are the pain-sensitive meninges involved? If in the PNS, could the disorder be located in peripheral nerves and, if so, are motor or sensory nerves primarily affected, or is a lesion in the neuromuscular junction or muscle more likely?

The first clues to defining the anatomic area of involvement appear in the history, and the examination is then directed to confirm or rule out these impressions and to clarify uncertainties. A more detailed examination of a particular region of the CNS or PNS is often indicated. For example, the examination of a patient who presents with a history of ascending paresthesias and weakness should be directed toward deciding, among other things, if the location of the lesion is in the spinal cord or peripheral nerves. Focal back pain, a spinal cord sensory level, and incontinence suggest a spinal cord origin, whereas a stocking-glove pattern of sensory loss suggests peripheral nerve disease; areflexia usually indicates peripheral neuropathy but may also be present with spinal shock in acute spinal cord disorders.

Deciding "where the lesion is" accomplishes the task of limiting the possible etiologies to a manageable, finite number. In addition, this strategy safeguards against making serious errors. Symptoms of recurrent vertigo, diplopia, and nystagmus should not trigger "multiple sclerosis" as an answer (etiology) but "brainstem" or "pons" (location); then a diagnosis of brainstem arteriovenous malformation will not be missed for lack of consideration. Similarly, the combination of optic neuritis and spastic ataxic paraparesis should initially suggest optic nerve and spinal cord disease; multiple sclerosis (MS), CNS syphilis, and vitamin B_{12} deficiency are treatable disorders that can produce this syndrome. Once the question, "Where is the lesion?" is answered, then the question, "What is the lesion?" can be addressed.

Define the Pathophysiology Clues to the pathophysiology of the disease process may also be present in the history. Primary neuronal (gray matter) disorders may present as early cognitive disturbances, movement disorders, or seizures, whereas white matter involvement produces predominantly "long tract" disorders of motor, sensory, visual, and cerebellar pathways. Progressive and symmetric symptoms often have a metabolic or degenerative origin; in such cases lesions are usually not sharply circumscribed. Thus, a patient with paraparesis and a clear spinal cord sensory level is unlikely to have vitamin B_{12} deficiency as the explanation. A Lhermitte symptom (electric shock–like sensations evoked by neck flexion) is due to ectopic impulse generation in white matter pathways and occurs with demyelination in the cervical spinal cord; among many possible causes, this symptom may indicate MS in a young adult or compressive cervical spondylosis in an older person. Symptoms that worsen after exposure to heat or exercise may indicate conduction block in demyelinated axons, as occurs in MS. A patient with recurrent episodes of diplopia and dysarthria associated with exercise or fatigue may have a disorder of neuromuscular transmission such as myasthenia gravis. Slowly advancing visual scotoma with luminous edges, termed *fortification spectra*, indicates spreading cortical depression, typically with migraine.

TABLE 361-1 PREVALENCE OF NEUROLOGIC AND PSYCHIATRIC DISEASES WORLDWIDE	
Disorder	**Patients, Millions**
Nutritional disorders and neuropathies	352
Migraine	326
Trauma	170
Depression	154
Alcoholism	91
Cerebrovascular diseases	61
Epilepsy	50
Schizophrenia	25
Dementia	24
Neurologic infections	18
Drug abuse	15

Source: World Health Organization estimates, 2002–2005.

THE NEUROLOGIC HISTORY

Attention to the description of the symptoms experienced by the patient and substantiated by family members and others often permits an accurate localization and determination of the probable cause of the complaints, even before the neurologic examination is performed. The history also helps to bring a focus to the neurologic examination that follows. Each complaint should be pursued as far as possible to elucidate the location of the lesion, the likely underlying pathophysiology, and potential etiologies. For example, a patient complains of weakness of the right arm. What are the associated features? Does the patient have difficulty with brushing hair or reaching upward (proximal) or buttoning buttons or opening a twist-top bottle (distal)? Negative associations may also be crucial. A patient with a right hemiparesis without a language deficit likely has a lesion (internal capsule, brainstem, or spinal cord) different from that of a patient with a right hemiparesis and aphasia (left hemisphere). Other pertinent features of the history include the following:

1. *Temporal course of the illness.* It is important to determine the precise time of appearance and rate of progression of the symptoms experienced by the patient. The rapid onset of a neurologic complaint, occurring within seconds or minutes, usually indicates a vascular event, a seizure, or migraine. The onset of sensory symptoms located in one extremity that spread over a few seconds to adjacent portions of that extremity and then to the other regions of the body suggests a seizure. A more gradual onset and less well localized symptoms point to the possibility of a transient ischemic attack (TIA). A similar but slower temporal march of symptoms accompanied by headache, nausea, or visual disturbance suggests migraine. The presence of "positive" sensory symptoms (e.g., tingling or sensations that are difficult to describe) or involuntary motor movements suggests a seizure; in contrast, transient loss of function (negative symptoms) suggests a TIA. A stuttering onset where symptoms appear, stabilize, and then progress over hours or days also suggests cerebrovascular disease; an additional history of transient remission or regression indicates that the process is more likely due to ischemia rather than hemorrhage. A gradual evolution of symptoms over hours or days suggests a toxic, metabolic, infectious, or inflammatory process. Progressing symptoms associated with the systemic manifestations of fever, stiff neck, and altered level of consciousness imply an infectious process. Relapsing and remitting symptoms involving different levels of the nervous system suggest MS or other inflammatory processes; these disorders can occasionally produce new symptoms that are rapidly progressive over hours. Slowly progressive symptoms without remissions are characteristic of neurodegenerative disorders, chronic infections, gradual intoxications, and neoplasms.

2. *Patients' descriptions of the complaint.* The same words often mean different things to different patients. "Dizziness" may imply impending syncope, a sense of disequilibrium, or true spinning vertigo. "Numbness" may mean a complete loss of feeling, a positive sensation such as tingling, or paralysis. "Blurred vision" may be used to describe unilateral visual loss, as in transient monocular blindness, or diplopia. The interpretation of the true meaning of the words used by patients to describe symptoms becomes even more complex when there are differences in primary languages and cultures.

3. *Corroboration of the history by others.* It is almost always helpful to obtain additional information from family, friends, or other observers to corroborate or expand the patient's description. Memory loss, aphasia, loss of insight, intoxication, and other factors may impair the patient's capacity to communicate normally with the examiner or prevent openness about factors that have contributed to the illness. Episodes of loss of consciousness necessitate that details be sought from observers to ascertain precisely what has happened during the event.

4. *Family history.* Many neurologic disorders have an underlying genetic component. The presence of a Mendelian disorder, such as Huntington's disease or Charcot-Marie-Tooth neuropathy, is often obvious if family data are available. More detailed questions about

family history are often necessary in polygenic disorders such as MS, migraine, and many types of epilepsy. It is important to elicit family history about all illnesses, in addition to neurologic and psychiatric disorders. A familial propensity to hypertension or heart disease is relevant in a patient who presents with a stroke. There are numerous inherited neurologic diseases that are associated with multisystem manifestations that may provide clues to the correct diagnosis (e.g., neurofibromatosis, Wilson's disease, neuro-ophthalmic syndromes).

5. *Medical illnesses.* Many neurologic diseases occur in the context of systemic disorders. Diabetes mellitus, hypertension, and abnormalities of blood lipids predispose to cerebrovascular disease. A solitary mass lesion in the brain may be an abscess in a patient with valvular heart disease, a primary hemorrhage in a patient with a coagulopathy, a lymphoma or toxoplasmosis in a patient with AIDS, or a metastasis in a patient with underlying cancer. Patients with malignancy may also present with a neurologic paraneoplastic syndrome (Chap. 97) or complications from chemotherapy or radiotherapy. Marfan's syndrome and related collagen disorders predispose to dissection of the cranial arteries and aneurysmal subarachnoid hemorrhage; the latter may also occur with polycystic kidney disease. Various neurologic disorders occur with dysthyroid states or other endocrinopathies. It is especially important to look for the presence of systemic diseases in patients with peripheral neuropathy. Most patients with coma in a hospital setting have a metabolic, toxic, or infectious cause.

6. *Drug use and abuse and toxin exposure.* It is essential to inquire about the history of drug use, both prescribed and illicit. Aminoglycoside antibiotics may exacerbate symptoms of weakness in patients with disorders of neuromuscular transmission, such as myasthenia gravis, and may cause dizziness secondary to ototoxicity. Vincristine and other antineoplastic drugs can cause peripheral neuropathy, and immunosuppressive agents such as cyclosporine can produce encephalopathy. Excessive vitamin ingestion can lead to disease; for example vitamin A and pseudotumor cerebri, or pyridoxine and peripheral neuropathy. Many patients are unaware that over-the-counter sleeping pills, cold preparations, and diet pills are actually drugs. Alcohol, the most prevalent neurotoxin, is often not recognized as such by patients, and other drugs of abuse such as cocaine and heroin can cause a wide range of neurologic abnormalities. A history of environmental or industrial exposure to neurotoxins may provide an essential clue; consultation with the patient's co-workers or employer may be required.

7. *Formulating an impression of the patient.* Use the opportunity while taking the history to form an impression of the patient. Is the information forthcoming, or does it take a circuitous course? Is there evidence of anxiety, depression, hypochondriasis? Are there any clues to defects in language, memory, insight, or inappropriate behavior? The neurologic assessment begins as soon as the patient comes into the room and the first introduction is made.

THE NEUROLOGIC EXAMINATION

The neurologic examination is challenging and complex; it has many components and includes a number of skills that can be mastered only through repeated use of the same techniques on a large number of individuals with and without neurologic disease. Mastery of the complete neurologic examination is usually important only for physicians in neurology and associated specialties. However, knowledge of the basics of the examination, especially those components that are effective in screening for neurologic dysfunction, is essential for all clinicians, especially generalists.

There is no single, universally accepted sequence of the examination that must be followed, but most clinicians begin with assessment of mental status followed by the cranial nerves, motor system, sensory system, coordination, and gait. Whether the examination is basic or comprehensive, it is essential that it be performed in an orderly and systematic fashion to avoid errors and serious omissions. Thus, the best way to learn and gain expertise in the examination is to choose one's own approach and practice it frequently and do it in the same exact sequence each time.

The detailed description of the neurologic examination that follows describes the more commonly used parts of the examination, with a particular emphasis on the components that are considered most helpful for the assessment of common neurologic problems. Each section also includes a brief description of the minimal examination necessary for adequate screening for abnormalities in a patient who has no symptoms suggesting neurologic dysfunction. A screening examination done in this way can be completed in 3–5 min.

Several additional points about the examination are worth noting. First, in recording observations, it is important to describe what is found rather than to apply a poorly defined medical term (e.g., "patient groans to sternal rub" rather than "obtunded"). Second, subtle CNS abnormalities are best detected by carefully comparing a patient's performance on tasks that require simultaneous activation of both cerebral hemispheres (e.g., eliciting a pronator drift of an outstretched arm with the eyes closed; extinction on one side of bilaterally applied light touch, also with eyes closed; or decreased arm swing or a slight asymmetry when walking). Third, if the patient's complaint is brought on by some activity, reproduce the activity in the office. If the complaint is of dizziness when the head is turned in one direction, have the patient do this and also look for associated signs on examination (e.g., nystagmus or dysmetria). If pain occurs after walking two blocks, have the patient leave the office and walk this distance and immediately return, and repeat the relevant parts of the examination. Finally, the use of tests that are individually tailored to the patient's problem can be of value in assessing changes over time. Tests of walking a 7.5-m (25-ft) distance (normal, 5–6 s; note assistance, if any), repetitive finger or toe tapping (normal, 20–25 taps in 5 s), or handwriting are examples.

Mental Status Examination

- *The bare minimum: During the interview, look for difficulties with communication and determine whether the patient has recall and insight into recent and past events.*

The mental status examination is underway as soon as the physician begins observing and talking with the patient. If the history raises any concern for abnormalities of higher cortical function or if cognitive problems are observed during the interview, then detailed testing of the mental status is indicated. The patient's ability to understand the language used for the examination, cultural background, educational experience, sensory or motor problems, or co-morbid conditions need to be factored into the applicability of the tests and interpretation of results.

The Folstein mini-mental status examination (MMSE) (Table 365-5) is a standardized screening examination of cognitive function that is extremely easy to administer and takes <10 min to complete. Using age-adjusted values for defining normal performance, the test is ~85% sensitive and 85% specific for making the diagnosis of dementia that is moderate or severe, especially in educated patients. When there is sufficient time available, the MMSE is one of the best methods for documenting the current mental status of the patient, and this is especially useful as a baseline assessment to which future scores of the MMSE can be compared.

Individual elements of the mental status examination can be subdivided into level of consciousness, orientation, speech and language, memory, fund of information, insight and judgment, abstract thought, and calculations.

Level of consciousness is the patient's relative state of awareness of the self and the environment, and ranges from fully awake to comatose. When the patient is not fully awake, the examiner should describe the responses to the minimum stimulus necessary to elicit a reaction, ranging from verbal commands to a brief, painful stimulus such as a squeeze of the trapezius muscle. Responses that are directed toward the stimulus and signify some degree of intact cerebral function (e.g., opening the eyes and looking at the examiner or reaching to push away a painful stimulus) must be distinguished from reflex responses of a spinal origin (e.g., triple flexion response—flexion at the ankle, knee, and hip in response to a painful stimulus to the foot).

Orientation is tested by asking the person to state his or her name, location, and time (day of the week and date); time is usually the first to be affected in a variety of conditions.

Speech is assessed by observing articulation, rate, rhythm, and prosody (i.e., the changes in pitch and accentuation of syllable and words).

Language is assessed by observing the content of the patient's verbal and written output, response to spoken commands, and ability to read. A typical testing sequence is to ask the patient to name successively more detailed components of clothing, a watch or a pen; repeat the phrase "No ifs, ands, or buts"; follow a three-step, verbal command; write a sentence; and read and respond to a written command.

Memory should be analyzed according to three main time scales: (1) immediate memory can be tested by saying a list of three items and having the patient repeat the list immediately, (2) short-term memory is assessed by asking the patient to recall the same three items 5 and 15 min later, and (3) long-term memory is evaluated by determining how well the patient is able to provide a coherent chronologic history of his or her illness or personal events.

Fund of information is assessed by asking questions about major historic or current events, with special attention to educational level and life experiences.

Abnormalities of *insight and judgment* are usually detected during the patient interview; a more detailed assessment can be elicited by asking the patient to describe how he or she would respond to situations having a variety of potential outcomes (e.g., "What would you do if you found a wallet on the sidewalk?").

Abstract thought can be tested by asking the patient to describe similarities between various objects or concepts (e.g., apple and orange, desk and chair, poetry and sculpture) or to list items having the same attributes (e.g., a list of four-legged animals).

Calculation ability is assessed by having the patient carry out a computation that is appropriate to the patient's age and education (e.g., serial subtraction of 7 from 100 or 3 from 20; or word problems involving simple arithmetic).

Cranial Nerve Examination

- *The bare minimum: Check the fundi, visual fields, pupil size and reactivity, extraocular movements, and facial movements.*

The cranial nerves (CN) are best examined in numerical order, except for grouping together CN III, IV, and VI because of their similar function.

CN I (OLFACTORY) Testing is usually omitted unless there is suspicion for inferior frontal lobe disease (e.g., meningioma). With eyes closed, ask the patient to sniff a mild stimulus such as toothpaste or coffee and identify the odorant.

CN II (OPTIC) Check visual acuity (with eyeglasses or contact lens correction) using a Snellen chart or similar tool. Test the visual fields by confrontation, i.e., by comparing the patient's visual fields to your own. As a screening test, it is usually sufficient to examine the visual fields of both eyes simultaneously; individual eye fields should be tested if there is any reason to suspect a problem of vision by the history or other elements of the examination, or if the screening test reveals an abnormality. Face the patient at a distance of approximately 0.6–1.0 m (2–3 ft) and place your hands at the periphery of your visual fields in the plane that is equidistant between you and the patient. Instruct the patient to look directly at the center of your face and to indicate when and where he or she sees one of your fingers moving. Beginning with the two inferior quadrants and then the two superior quadrants, move your index finger of the right hand, left hand, or both hands simultaneously and observe whether the patient detects the movements. A single small-amplitude movement of the finger is sufficient for a normal response. Focal perimetry and tangent screen examinations should be used to map out visual field defects fully or to search for subtle abnormalities. Optic fundi should be examined with an ophthalmoscope, and the color, size, and degree of swelling or elevation of the optic disc noted, as well as the color and texture of the retina. The retinal vessels should be checked for size, regularity, arterial-venous nicking at crossing points, hemorrhage, exudates, etc.

CN III, IV, VI (OCULOMOTOR, TROCHLEAR, ABDUCENS)   Describe the size and shape of pupils and reaction to light and accommodation (i.e., as the eyes converge while following your finger as it moves toward the bridge of the nose). To check extraocular movements, ask the patient to keep his or her head still while tracking the movement of the tip of your finger. Move the target slowly in the horizontal and vertical planes; observe any paresis, nystagmus, or abnormalities of smooth pursuit (saccades, oculomotor ataxia, etc.). If necessary, the relative position of the two eyes, both in primary and multidirectional gaze, can be assessed by comparing the reflections of a bright light off both pupils. However, in practice it is typically more useful to determine whether the patient describes diplopia in any direction of gaze; true diplopia should almost always resolve with one eye closed. Horizontal nystagmus is best assessed at 45° and not at extreme lateral gaze (which is uncomfortable for the patient); the target must often be held at the lateral position for at least a few seconds to detect an abnormality.

CN V (TRIGEMINAL)   Examine sensation within the three territories of the branches of the trigeminal nerve (ophthalmic, maxillary, and mandibular) on each side of the face. As with other parts of the sensory examination, testing of two sensory modalities derived from different anatomic pathways (e.g., light touch and temperature) is sufficient for a screening examination. Testing of other modalities, the corneal reflex, and the motor component of CN V (jaw clench—masseter muscle) is indicated when suggested by the history.

CN VII (FACIAL)   Look for facial asymmetry at rest and with spontaneous movements. Test eyebrow elevation, forehead wrinkling, eye closure, smiling, and cheek puff. Look in particular for differences in the lower versus upper facial muscles; weakness of the lower two-thirds of the face with preservation of the upper third suggests an upper motor neuron lesion, whereas weakness of an entire side suggests a lower motor neuron lesion.

CN VIII (VESTIBULOCOCHLEAR)   Check the patient's ability to hear a finger rub or whispered voice with each ear. Further testing for air versus mastoid bone conduction (Rinne) and lateralization of a 512-Hz tuning fork placed at the center of the forehead (Weber) should be done if an abnormality is detected by history or examination. Any suspected problem should be followed up with formal audiometry. **For further discussion of assessing vestibular nerve function in the setting of dizziness or coma, see Chaps. 22 and 268, respectively.**

CN IX, X (GLOSSOPHARYNGEAL, VAGUS)   Observe the position and symmetry of the palate and uvula at rest and with phonation ("aah"). The pharyngeal ("gag") reflex is evaluated by stimulating the posterior pharyngeal wall on each side with a sterile, blunt object (e.g., tongue blade), but the reflex is often absent in normal individuals.

CN XI (SPINAL ACCESSORY)   Check shoulder shrug (trapezius muscle) and head rotation to each side (sternocleidomastoid) against resistance.

CN XII (HYPOGLOSSAL)   Inspect the tongue for atrophy or fasciculations, position with protrusion, and strength when extended against the inner surface of the cheeks on each side.

Motor Examination

- *The bare minimum: Look for muscle atrophy and check extremity tone. Assess upper extremity strength by checking for pronator drift and strength of wrist or finger extensors. Tap the biceps, patellar, and Achilles reflexes. Test for lower extremity strength by having the patient walk normally and on heels and toes.*

The motor examination includes observations of muscle appearance, tone, strength, and reflexes. Although gait is in part a test of mo-

tor function, it is usually evaluated separately at the end of the examination.

APPEARANCE   Inspect and palpate muscle groups under good light and with the patient in a comfortable and symmetric position. Check for muscle fasciculations, tenderness, and atrophy or hypertrophy. Involuntary movements may be present at rest (e.g., tics, myoclonus, choreoathetosis), during maintained posture (pill-rolling tremor of Parkinson's disease), or with voluntary movements (intention tremor of cerebellar disease or familial tremor).

TONE   Muscle tone is tested by measuring the resistance to passive movement of a relaxed limb. Patients often have difficulty relaxing during this procedure, so it is useful to distract the patient to minimize active movements. In the upper limbs, tone is assessed by rapid pronation and supination of the forearm and flexion and extension at the wrist. In the lower limbs, while the patient is supine the examiner's hands are placed behind the knees and rapidly raised; with normal tone the ankles drag along the table surface for a variable distance before rising, whereas increased tone results in an immediate lift of the heel off the surface. Decreased tone is most commonly due to lower motor neuron or peripheral nerve disorders. Increased tone may be evident as spasticity (resistance determined by the angle and velocity of motion; corticospinal tract disease), rigidity (similar resistance in all angles of motion; extrapyramidal disease), or paratonia (fluctuating changes in resistance; frontal lobe pathways or normal difficulty in relaxing). Cogwheel rigidity, in which passive motion elicits jerky interruptions in resistance, is seen in parkinsonism.

STRENGTH   Testing for pronator drift is an extremely useful method for screening upper limb weakness. The patient is asked to hold both arms fully extended and parallel to the ground with eyes closed. This position should be maintained for ~10 s; any flexion at the elbow or fingers or pronation of the forearm, especially if asymmetric, is a sign of potential weakness. Muscle strength is further assessed by having the patient exert maximal effort for the particular muscle or muscle group being tested. It is important to isolate the muscles as much as possible, i.e., hold the limb so that only the muscles of interest are active. It is also helpful to palpate accessible muscles as they contract. Grading muscle strength and evaluating the patient's effort is an art that takes time and practice. Muscle strength is traditionally graded using the following scale:

  0 = no movement
  1 = flicker or trace of contraction but no
      associated movement at a joint
  2 = movement with gravity eliminated
  3 = movement against gravity but not against resistance
  4– = movement against a mild degree of resistance
  4 = movement against moderate resistance
  4+ = movement against strong resistance
  5 = full power

However, in many cases it is more practical to use the following terms:

  Paralysis = no movement
  Severe weakness = movement with gravity eliminated
  Moderate weakness = movement against gravity but not against
      mild resistance
  Mild weakness = movement against moderate resistance
  Full strength

Noting the pattern of weakness is as important as assessing the magnitude of weakness. Unilateral or bilateral weakness of the upper limb extensors and lower limb flexors ("pyramidal weakness") suggests a lesion of the pyramidal tract, bilateral proximal weakness suggests myopathy, and bilateral distal weakness suggests peripheral neuropathy.

REFLEXES *Muscle Stretch Reflexes* Those that are typically assessed include the biceps (**C5**, C6), brachioradialis (C5, **C6**), and triceps (**C7**, C8) reflexes in the upper limbs and the patellar or quadriceps (**L3**, L4) and Achilles (**S1**, S2) reflexes in the lower limbs. The patient should be relaxed and the muscle positioned midway between full contraction and extension. Reflexes may be enhanced by asking the patient to voluntarily contract other, distant muscle groups (Jendrassik maneuver). For example, upper limb reflexes may be reinforced by voluntary teeth-clenching, and the Achilles reflex by hooking the flexed fingers of the two hands together and attempting to pull them apart. For each reflex tested, the two sides should be tested sequentially, and it is important to determine the smallest stimulus required to elicit a reflex rather than the maximum response. Reflexes are graded according to the following scale:

0 = absent	3 = exaggerated
1 = present but diminished	4 = clonus
2 = normoactive	

Cutaneous Reflexes The plantar reflex is elicited by stroking, with a noxious stimulus such as a tongue blade, the lateral surface of the sole of the foot beginning near the heel and moving across the ball of the foot to the great toe. The normal reflex consists of plantar flexion of the toes. With upper motor neuron lesions above the S1 level of the spinal cord, a paradoxical extension of the toe is observed, associated with fanning and extension of the other toes (termed an *extensor plantar response*, or *Babinski sign*). Superficial abdominal reflexes are elicited by gently stroking the abdominal surface near the umbilicus in a diagonal fashion with a sharp object (e.g., the wooden end of a cotton-tipped swab) and observing the movement of the umbilicus. Normally, the umbilicus will pull toward the stimulated quadrant. With upper motor neuron lesions, these reflexes are absent. They are most helpful when there is preservation of the upper (spinal cord level T9) but not lower (T12) abdominal reflexes, indicating a spinal lesion between T9 and T12, or when the response is asymmetric. Other useful cutaneous reflexes include the cremasteric (ipsilateral elevation of the testicle following stroking of the medial thigh; mediated by L1 and L2) and anal (contraction of the anal sphincter when the perianal skin is scratched; mediated by S2, S3, S4) reflexes. It is particularly important to test for these reflexes in any patient with suspected injury to the spinal cord or lumbosacral roots.

Primitive Reflexes With disease of the frontal lobe pathways, several primitive reflexes not normally present in the adult may appear. The suck response is elicited by lightly touching the center of the lips, and the root response the corner of the lips, with a tongue blade; the patient will move the lips to suck or root in the direction of the stimulus. The grasp reflex is elicited by touching the palm between the thumb and index finger with the examiner's fingers; a positive response is a forced grasp of the examiner's hand. In many instances stroking the back of the hand will lead to its release. The palmomental response is contraction of the mentalis muscle (chin) ipsilateral to a scratch stimulus diagonally applied to the palm.

Sensory Examination

- *The bare minimum: Ask whether the patient can feel light touch and the temperature of a cool object in each distal extremity. Check double simultaneous stimulation using light touch on the hands.*

Evaluating sensation is usually the most unreliable part of the examination, because it is subjective and is difficult to quantify. In the compliant and discerning patient, the sensory examination can be extremely helpful for the precise localization of a lesion. With patients who are uncooperative or lack an understanding of the tests, it may be useless. The examination should be focused on the suspected lesion. For example, in spinal cord, spinal root, or peripheral nerve abnormalities, all major sensory modalities should be tested while looking for a pattern consistent with a spinal level and dermatomal or nerve distribution. In patients with lesions at or above the brainstem,

screening the primary sensory modalities in the distal extremities along with tests of "cortical" sensation is usually sufficient.

The five primary sensory modalities—light touch, pain, temperature, vibration, and joint position—are tested in each limb. Light touch is assessed by stimulating the skin with single, very gentle touches of the examiner's finger or a wisp of cotton. Pain is tested using a new pin, and temperature is assessed using a metal object (e.g., tuning fork) that has been immersed in cold and warm water. Vibration is tested using a 128-Hz tuning fork applied to the distal phalynx of the great toe or index finger just below the nailbed. By placing a finger on the opposite side of the joint being tested, the examiner compares the patient's threshold of vibration perception with his or her own. For joint position testing, the examiner grasps the digit or limb laterally and distal to the joint being assessed; small 1- to 2-mm excursions can usually be sensed. The Romberg maneuver is primarily a test of proprioception. The patient is asked to stand with the feet as close together as necessary to maintain balance while the eyes are open, and the eyes are then closed. A loss of balance with the eyes closed is an abnormal response.

"Cortical" sensation is mediated by the parietal lobes and represents an integration of the primary sensory modalities; testing cortical sensation is only meaningful when primary sensation is intact. Double simultaneous stimulation is especially useful as a screening test for cortical function; with the patient's eyes closed, the examiner lightly touches one or both hands and asks the patient to identify the stimuli. With a parietal lobe lesion, the patient may be unable to identify the stimulus on the contralateral side when both hands are touched. Other modalities relying on the parietal cortex include the discrimination of two closely placed stimuli as separate (two-point discrimination), identification of an object by touch and manipulation alone (stereognosis), and the identification of numbers or letters written on the skin surface (graphesthesia).

Coordination Examination

- *The bare minimum: Test rapid alternating movements of the hands and the finger-to-nose and heel-knee-shin maneuvers.*

Coordination refers to the orchestration and fluidity of movements. Even simple acts require cooperation of agonist and antagonist muscles, maintenance of posture, and complex servomechanisms to control the rate and range of movements. Part of this integration relies on normal function of the cerebellar and basal ganglia systems. However, coordination also requires intact muscle strength and kinesthetic and proprioceptive information. Thus, if the examination has disclosed abnormalities of the motor or sensory systems, the patient's coordination should be assessed with these limitations in mind.

Rapid alternating movements in the upper limbs are tested separately on each side by having the patient make a fist, partially extend the index finger, and then tap the index finger on the distal thumb as quickly as possible. In the lower limb, the patient rapidly taps the foot against the floor or the examiner's hand. Finger-to-nose testing is primarily a test of cerebellar function; the patient is asked to touch his or her index finger repetitively to the nose and then to the examiner's outstretched finger, which moves with each repetition. A similar test in the lower extremity is to have the patient raise the leg and touch the examiner's finger with the great toe. Another cerebellar test in the lower limbs is the heel-knee-shin maneuver; in the supine position the patient is asked to slide the heel of each foot from the knee down the shin of the other leg. For all these movements, the accuracy, speed, and rhythm are noted.

Gait Examination

- *The bare minimum: Observe the patient while walking normally, on the heels and toes, and along a straight line.*

Watching the patient walk is the most important part of the neurologic examination. Normal gait requires that multiple systems—including strength, sensation, and coordination—function in a highly integrated fashion. Unexpected abnormalities may be detected that prompt the examiner to return, in more detail, to other aspects of the examination. The patient should be observed while walking and turn-

TABLE 361-2	FINDINGS HELPFUL FOR LOCALIZATION WITHIN THE NERVOUS SYSTEM
	Signs
Cerebrum	Abnormal mental status or cognitive impairment
	Seizures
	Unilateral weakness[a] and sensory abnormalities including head and limbs
	Visual field abnormalities
	Movement abnormalities (e.g., diffuse incoordination, tremor, chorea)
Brainstem	Isolated cranial nerve abnormalities (single or multiple)
	"Crossed" weakness[a] and sensory abnormalities of head and limbs, e.g., weakness of right face and left arm and leg
Spinal cord	Back pain or tenderness
	Weakness[a] and sensory abnormalities sparing the head
	Mixed upper and lower motor neuron findings
	Sensory level
	Sphincter dysfunction
Spinal roots	Radiating limb pain
	Weakness[b] or sensory abnormalities following root distribution (see Figs. 25-2 and 25-3)
	Loss of reflexes
Peripheral nerve	Mid or distal limb pain
	Weakness[b] or sensory abnormalities following nerve distribution (see Figs. 25-2 and 25-3)
	"Stocking or glove" distribution of sensory loss
	Loss of reflexes
Neuromuscular junction	Bilateral weakness including face (ptosis, diplopia, dysphagia) and proximal limbs
	Increasing weakness with exertion
	Sparing of sensation
Muscle	Bilateral proximal or distal weakness
	Sparing of sensation

[a]Weakness along with other abnormalities having an "upper motor neuron" pattern, i.e., spasticity, weakness of extensors > flexors in the upper extremity and flexors > extensors in the lower extremity, hyperreflexia.

[b]Weakness along with other abnormalities having a "lower motor neuron" pattern, i.e., flaccidity and hyporeflexia.

ing normally, walking on the heels, walking on the toes, and walking heel-to-toe along a straight line. The examination may reveal decreased arm swing on one side (corticospinal tract disease), a stooped posture and short-stepped gait (parkinsonism), a broad-based unsta-ble gait (ataxia), scissoring (spasticity), or a high-stepped, slapping gait (posterior column or peripheral nerve disease), or the patient may appear to be stuck in place (apraxia with frontal lobe disease).

NEUROLOGIC DIAGNOSIS

The clinical data obtained from the history and examination are interpreted to arrive at an anatomic localization that best explains the clinical findings (Table 361-2), to narrow the list of diagnostic possibilities, and to select the laboratory tests most likely to be informative. The laboratory assessment may include (1) serum electrolytes; complete blood count; and renal, hepatic, endocrine, and immune studies; (2) cerebrospinal fluid examination; (3) focused neuroimaging studies (Chap. 362); or (4) electrophysiologic studies (**Chap. e31**). The anatomic localization, mode of onset and course of illness, other medical data, and laboratory findings are then integrated to establish an etiologic diagnosis.

The neurologic examination may be normal even in patients with a serious neurologic disease, such as seizures, chronic meningitis, or a TIA. A comatose patient may arrive with no available history, and in such cases the approach is as described in Chap. 268. In other patients, an inadequate history may be overcome by a succession of examinations from which the course of the illness can be inferred. In perplexing cases it is useful to remember that uncommon presentations of common diseases are more likely than rare etiologies. Thus, even in tertiary care settings, multiple strokes are usually due to emboli and not vasculitis, and dementia with myoclonus is usually Alzheimer's disease and not due to a prion disorder or a paraneoplastic cause. Finally, the most important task of a primary care physician faced with a patient who has a new neurologic complaint is to assess the urgency of referral to a specialist. Here, the imperative is to rapidly identify patients likely to have nervous system infections, acute strokes, and spinal cord compression or other treatable mass lesions and arrange for immediate care.

FURTHER READINGS

BLUMENTHAL H: *Neuroanatomy Through Clinical Cases.* Sunderland, Massachusetts, Sinauer Associates, 2002

CAMPBELL WW: *DeJong's The Neurological Examination,* 6th ed. Philadelphia, Lippincott Williams & Wilkins, 2005

ROPPER AH, BROWN RH: *Principles of Neurology,* 8th Ed. New York, McGraw-Hill, 2005

362 Neuroimaging in Neurologic Disorders
William P. Dillon

The clinician caring for patients with neurologic symptoms is faced with an expanding number of imaging options, including computed tomography (CT), CT angiography (CTA), perfusion CT (pCT), magnetic resonance imaging (MRI), MR angiography (MRA), functional MRI (fMRI), MR spectroscopy (MRS), MR neurography, diffusion and diffusion track imaging (DTI), and perfusion MRI (pMRI). In addition, an increasing number of interventional neuroradiologic techniques are available, including angiography; embolization, coiling, and stenting of vascular structures; and spine interventions such as discography, selective nerve root injection, and epidural injections. Recent developments, such as multidetector CTA and gadolinium-enhanced MRA, have narrowed the indications for conventional angiography, which is now reserved for patients in whom small-vessel detail is essential for diagnosis or for whom interventional therapies are planned (Table 362-1).

In general, MRI is more sensitive than CT for the detection of lesions affecting the central nervous system (CNS), particularly those of the spinal cord, cranial nerves, and posterior fossa structures. Diffusion MR, a sequence that detects reduction of microscopic motion of water, is the most sensitive technique for detecting acute ischemic stroke and is also useful in the detection of encephalitis, abscesses, and prion diseases. CT, however, can be quickly obtained and is widely available, making it a pragmatic choice for the initial evaluation of patients with acute changes in mental status, suspected acute stroke, hemorrhage, and intracranial or spinal trauma. CT is also more sensitive than MRI for visualizing fine osseous detail and is indicated in the initial evaluation of conductive hearing loss as well as lesions affecting the skull base and calvarium.

COMPUTED TOMOGRAPHY

TECHNIQUE

The CT image is a cross-sectional representation of anatomy created by a computer-generated analysis of the attenuation of x-ray beams passed through a section of the body. As the x-ray beam, collimated to the desired slice width, rotates around the patient, it passes through selected regions in the body. X-rays that are not attenuated by the body are detected by sensitive x-ray detectors aligned 180° from the x-ray tube. A computer calculates a "back projection" image from the 360° x-ray attenuation profile. Greater x-ray attenuation, e.g., as caused by bone, results in areas of high "density," while soft tissue

TABLE 362-1 GUIDELINES FOR THE USE OF CT, ULTRASOUND, AND MRI

Condition	Recommended Technique
Hemorrhage	
Acute parenchymal	CT, MR
Subacute/chronic	MRI
Subarachnoid hemorrhage	CT, CTA, lumbar puncture → angiography
Aneurysm	Angiography > CTA, MRA
Ischemic infarction	
Hemorrhagic infarction	CT or MRI
Bland infarction	MRI > CT, CTA, angiography
Carotid or vertebral dissection	MRI/MRA
Vertebral basilar insufficiency	CTA, MRI/MRA
Carotid stenosis	CTA > Doppler ultrasound, MRA
Suspected mass lesion	
Neoplasm, primary or metastatic	MRI + contrast
Infection/abscess	MRI + contrast
Immunosuppressed with focal findings	MRI + contrast
Vascular malformation	MRI +/− angiography
White matter disorders	MRI
Demyelinating disease	MRI +/− contrast
Dementia	MRI > CT
Trauma	
Acute trauma	CT (noncontrast)
Shear injury/chronic hemorrhage	MRI
Headache/migraine	CT (noncontrast) / MRI
Seizure	
First time, no focal neurologic deficits	?CT as screen +/− contrast
Partial complex/refractory	MRI with coronal T2W imaging
Cranial neuropathy	MRI with contrast
Meningeal disease	MRI with contrast
Spine	
Low back pain	
No neurologic deficits	MRI or CT after 4 weeks
With focal deficits	MRI > CT
Spinal stenosis	MRI or CT
Cervical spondylosis	MRI or CT myelography
Infection	MRI + contrast, CT
Myelopathy	MRI + contrast > myelography
Arteriovenous malformation	MRI, myelography/angiography

Note: CT, computed tomography; MRI, magnetic resonance imaging; MRA, MR angiography; CTA, CT angiography; T2W, T2-weighted.

structures, which have poor attenuation of x-rays, are lower in density. The resolution of an image depends on the radiation dose, the detector size or collimation (slice thickness), the field of view, and the matrix size of the display. A modern CT scanner is capable of obtaining sections as thin as 0.5–1 mm with submillimeter resolution at a speed of 0.5–1 s per rotation; complete studies of the brain can be completed in 2–10 s.

Helical or multidetector CT (MDCT) is now standard in most radiology departments. Continuous CT information is obtained while the patient moves through the x-ray beam. In the helical scan mode, the table moves continuously through the rotating x-ray beam, generating a "helix" of information that can be reformatted into various slice thicknesses. Single or multiple (from 4 to 256) detectors positioned 180 degrees to the x-ray source may result in multiple slices per revolution of the beam around the patient. Advantages of MDCT include shorter scan times, reduced patient and organ motion, and the ability to acquire images dynamically during the infusion of intravenous contrast that can be used to construct CT angiograms of vascular structures and CT perfusion images (Figs. 362-1*B*, 362-2*B*, and 362-3*B*). CTA images are post-processed for display in three dimensions to yield angiogram-like images (Fig. 362-1*C* and see Fig. 364-4). CTA has proved useful in assessing the cervical and intracranial arterial and venous anatomy.

Intravenous iodinated contrast is often administered prior to or during a CT study to identify vascular structures and to detect defects in the blood-brain barrier (BBB) that are associated with disorders such as tumors, infarcts, and infections. In the normal CNS, only ves-sels and structures lacking a BBB (e.g., the pituitary gland, choroid plexus, and dura) enhance after contrast administration. The use of iodinated contrast agents carries a risk of allergic reaction and adds additional expense and radiation dose. While helpful in characterizing mass lesions as well as essential for the acquisition of CTA studies, the decision to use contrast material should always be considered carefully.

INDICATIONS

CT is the primary study of choice in the evaluation of an acute change in mental status, focal neurologic findings, acute trauma to the brain and spine, suspected subarachnoid hemorrhage, and conductive hearing loss (Table 362-1). CT is complementary to MR in the evaluation of the skull base, orbit, and osseous structures of the spine. In the spine, CT is useful in evaluating patients with osseous spinal stenosis and spondylosis, but MRI is often preferred in those with neurologic deficits. CT can also be obtained following intrathecal contrast injection to evaluate the intracranial cisterns (*CT cisternography*) for cerebrospinal fluid (CSF) fistula, as well as the spinal subarachnoid space (*CT myelography*).

COMPLICATIONS

CT is safe, fast, and reliable. Radiation exposure depends on the dose used but is normally between 3 and 5 cGy for a routine brain CT study. Care must be taken to reduce exposure when imaging children. With the advent of MDCT, CTA, and CT perfusion, care must be taken to appropriately minimize radiation dose whenever possible. The most frequent complications are associated with use of intravenous contrast agents. Two broad categories of contrast media, ionic and nonionic, are in use. Although ionic agents are relatively safe and inexpensive, they are associated with a higher incidence of reactions and side effects. As a result, ionic agents have been largely replaced by safer nonionic compounds (Table 362-2).

Contrast nephropathy may result from hemodynamic changes, renal tubular obstruction and cell damage, or immunologic reactions to contrast agents. A rise in serum creatinine of at least 85 μmol/L (1 mg/dL) within 48 h of contrast administration is often used as a definition of contrast nephropathy, although other causes of acute renal failure must be excluded. The prognosis is usually favorable, with serum creatinine levels returning to baseline within 1–2 weeks. Risk factors for contrast nephropathy include advanced age (>80 years), preexisting renal disease (serum creatinine exceeding 2.0 mg/dL), solitary kidney, diabetes mellitus, dehydration, paraproteinemia, concurrent use of nephrotoxic medication or chemotherapeutic agents, and high contrast dose. Patients with diabetes and those with mild renal failure should be well hydrated prior to the administration of contrast agents, although careful consideration should be given to alternative imaging techniques, such as MR imaging or noncontrast examinations. Nonionic, low-osmolar media produce fewer abnormalities in renal blood flow and less endothelial cell damage but should still be used carefully in patients at risk for allergic reaction (Table 362-3).

Other side effects are rare but include a sensation of warmth throughout the body and a metallic taste during intravenous administration of iodinated contrast media. The most serious side effects are anaphylactic reactions, which range from mild hives to bronchospasm, acute anaphylaxis, and death. The pathogenesis of these allergic reactions is not fully understood but is thought to include the release of mediators such as histamine, antibody-antigen reactions, and complement activation. Severe allergic reactions occur in ~0.04% of patients receiving nonionic media, sixfold fewer than with ionic media. Risk factors include a history of prior contrast reaction, food allergies to shellfish, and atopy (asthma and hay fever). In such patients, a noncontrast CT or MRI procedure should be considered as an alternative to contrast administration. If iodinated contrast is absolutely required, a nonionic agent should be used in conjunction with pretreatment with glucocorticoids and antihistamines (Table 362-4). Patients with allergic reactions to iodinated contrast material do not usually react to gadolinium-based MR contrast material, although such reactions do

A **B**

C

**FIGURE 362-1 CT angiography (CTA) of ruptured anterior cerebral artery aneurysm in a patient presenting with acute headache. *A.* Noncontrast CT demonstrates subarachnoid hemorrhage and mild obstructive hydrocephalus. *B.* Axial maximum intensity projection from CT angiography demonstrates enlargement of the anterior cerebral artery (*arrow*). *C.* 3D surface reconstruction using a workstation confirms the anterior cerebral aneurysm and demonstrates its orientation and relationship to nearby vessels (*arrow*). CTA image is produced by 0.5–1 mm helical CT scans performed during a rapid bolus infusion of intravenous contrast medium.

gen proton in a tissue is influenced by local interactions with surrounding molecules and atomic neighbors. Two relaxation rates, T1 and T2, influence the signal intensity of the image. The T1 relaxation time is the time, measured in milliseconds, for 63% of the hydrogen protons to return to their normal equilibrium state, while the T2 relaxation is the time for 63% of the protons to become dephased owing to interactions among nearby protons. The intensity of the signal within various tissues and image contrast can be modulated by altering acquisition parameters, such as the interval between Rf pulses (TR) and the time between the Rf pulse and the signal reception (TE). So-called T1-weighted (T1W) images are produced by keeping the TR and TE relatively short. T2-weighted (T2W) images are produced by using longer TR and TE times. Fat and subacute hemorrhage have relatively shorter T1 relaxation rates and thus higher signal intensity than brain on T1W images. Structures containing more water, such as CSF and edema, have long T1 and T2 relaxation rates, resulting in relatively lower signal intensity on T1W images and a higher signal intensity on T2W images (Table 362-5). Gray matter contains 10–15% more water than white matter, which accounts for much of the intrinsic contrast between the two on MRI (Fig. 362-3). T2W images are more sensitive than T1W images to edema, demyelination, infarction, and chronic hemorrhage, while T1W imaging is more sensitive to subacute hemorrhage and fat-containing structures.

Many different MR pulse sequences exist, and each can be obtained in various planes (Figs. 362-3, 362-4, 362-5). The selection of a proper protocol that will best answer a clinical question depends on an accurate clinical history and indication for the examination. Fluid-attenuated inversion recovery (FLAIR) is a useful pulse sequence that produces T2W images in which the normally high signal intensity of CSF is suppressed (Fig. 362-5*A*). FLAIR images are more sensitive than standard spin echo images for any water-containing lesions or edema. Gradient echo imaging is most sensitive to magnetic susceptibility generated by blood, calcium, and air and is indicated in patients with traumatic brain injury to assess for subtle contusions and shear microhemorrhages. MR images can be generated in any plane without changing the patient's position. Each sequence, however, must be obtained separately and takes 1–5 min on average to complete. Three-dimensional volumetric imaging is also possible with MRI, resulting in a volume of data that can be reformatted in any orientation on a workstation to highlight certain disease processes.

MR Contrast Material The heavy-metal element gadolinium forms the basis of all currently approved intravenous MR contrast agents. Gadolinium is a paramagnetic substance, which means that it reduces the T1 and T2 relaxation times of nearby water protons, resulting in a high signal on T1W images and a low signal on T2W images (the latter requires a sufficient local concentration, usually in the form of an intravenous bolus). Unlike iodinated contrast agents, the effect of MR contrast agents depends on the presence of local hydrogen protons on which it must act to achieve the desired effect. Gadolinium is chelated to DTPA (diethylenetriaminepentaacetic acid), which allows safe renal excretion.

occur. It would be wise to pretreat patients with a prior allergic history to MR contrast administration in a similar fashion.

MAGNETIC RESONANCE IMAGING

TECHNIQUE

Magnetic resonance is a complex interaction between hydrogen protons in biologic tissues, a static magnetic field (the magnet), and energy in the form of radiofrequency (Rf) waves of a specific frequency introduced by coils placed next to the body part of interest. Field strength of the magnet is directly related to signal-to-noise ratio. While 1.5 Telsa magnets have become the standard high-field MRI units, 3T–8T magnets are now available and have distinct advantages in the brain and musculoskeletal systems. Spatial localization is achieved by magnetic gradients surrounding the main magnet, which impart slight changes in magnetic field throughout the imaging volume. The energy state of the hydrogen protons is transiently excited by Rf, which is administered at a frequency specific for the field strength of the magnet. The subsequent return to equilibrium energy state (*relaxation*) of the protons results in a release of Rf energy (the *echo*), which is detected by the coils that delivered the Rf pulses. The echo is transformed by Fourier analysis into the information used to form an MR image. The MR image thus consists of a map of the distribution of hydrogen protons, with signal intensity imparted by both density of hydrogen protons as well as differences in the relaxation times (see below) of hydrogen protons on different molecules. While clinical MRI currently makes use of the ubiquitous hydrogen proton, research into sodium and carbon imaging appears promising.

T1 and T2 Relaxation Times The rate of return to equilibrium of perturbed protons is called the *relaxation rate*. The relaxation rate varies among normal and pathologic tissues. The relaxation rate of a hydro-

A

B

C

D

E

FIGURE 362-2 Acute left hemiparesis due to middle cerebral artery occlusion. *A.* Axial noncontrast CT scan demonstrates high density within the right middle cerebral artery (*arrow*) associated with subtle low density involving the right putamen (*arrowheads*). *B.* Mean transit time map calculated from a CT perfusion study; prolongation of the mean transit time is visible throughout the right hemisphere (*arrows*). *C.* Axial maximum intensity projection from a CTA study through the Circle of Willis demonstrates an abrupt occlusion of the proximal right middle cerebral artery (*arrow*). Reconstitution of flow via collaterals is seen distal to the occlusion; however, the patient sustained a right basal ganglia infarction. *D.* Sagittal reformation through the right internal carotid artery demonstrates a low-density lipid laden plaque (*arrowheads*) narrowing the lumen (*black arrow*) *E.* 3D surface CTA images from a different patient demonstrate calcification and narrowing of the right internal carotid artery (*arrow*), consistent with atherosclerotic disease.

Approximately 0.2 mL/kg body weight is administered intravenously; the cost is ~$60 per dose. Gadolinium-DTPA does not normally cross the intact BBB immediately but will enhance lesions lacking a BBB (Fig. 362-4*A*) and areas of the brain that normally are devoid of the BBB (pituitary, choroid plexus). However, gadolinium contrast has been noted to slowly cross an intact BBB if given over time and especially in the setting of reduced renal clearance. The agents are generally well tolerated; severe allergic reactions are rare but have been reported. The adverse reaction rate in patients with a prior history of atopy or asthma is 3.7%;

TABLE 362-2	GUIDELINES FOR USE OF INTRAVENOUS CONTRAST IN PATIENTS WITH IMPAIRED RENAL FUNCTION
Serum Creatinine, μmol/L (mg/dL)[a]	**Recommendation**
<133 (<1.5)	Use either ionic or nonionic at 2 mL/kg to 150 mL total
133–177 (1.5–2.0)	Nonionic; hydrate diabetics 1 mL/kg per hour × 10h
>177 (>2.0)	Consider noncontrast CT or MRI; nonionic contrast if required
177–221 (2.0–2.5)	Nonionic only if required (as above); contraindicated in diabetics
>265 (>3.0)	Nonionic IV contrast given only to patients undergoing dialysis within 24 h

[a]Risk is greatest in patients with rising creatinine levels.
Note: CT, computed tomography; MRI, magnetic resonance imaging.

TABLE 362-3	INDICATIONS FOR USE OF NONIONIC CONTRAST MEDIA

- Prior adverse reaction to contrast media, with the exception of heat, flushing, or an episode of nausea or vomiting
- Asthma or other serious lung disease
- History of atopic allergies (pretreatment with steroid/antihistamines recommended)
- Children under the age of 2 years
- Renal failure or creatinine >177 μmol/L (>2.0 mg/dL)
- Cardiac dysfunction, including recent or imminent cardiac decompensation, severe arrhythmias, unstable angina pectoris, recent myocardial infarction, and pulmonary hypertension
- Diabetes
- Severe debilitation

TABLE 362-4	**GUIDELINES FOR PREMEDICATION OF PATIENTS WITH PRIOR CONTRAST ALLERGY**

12 h prior to examination:
 Prednisone, 50 mg PO *or* methylprednisolone, 32 mg PO
2 h prior to examination:
 Prednisone, 50 mg PO *or* methylprednisolone, 32 mg PO *and*
 Cimetidine, 300 mg PO *or* ranitidine, 150 mg PO
Immediately prior to examination:
 Benadryl, 50 mg IV (alternatively, can be given PO 2 h prior to exam)

however, the reaction rate increases to 6.3% in those patients with a prior history of unspecified allergic reaction to iodinated contrast agents. Gadolinium contrast material can be administered safely to children as well as adults, although these agents are generally avoided in those under 6 months of age. Renal failure does not occur.

A rare complication, nephrogenic systemic fibrosis (NSF), has recently been reported in patients with renal insufficiency who have been exposed to gadolinium contrast agents. The onset of NSF has been reported between 5 and 75 days following exposure; histologic features include thickened collagen bundles with surrounding clefts, mucin deposition, and increased numbers of fibrocytes and elastic fibers in skin.

TABLE 362-5	**SOME COMMON INTENSITIES ON T1- AND T2-WEIGHTED MRI SEQUENCES**

Image	TR	TE	Signal Intensity			
			CSF	Fat	Brain	Edema
T1W	Short	Short	Low	High	Low	Low
T2W	Long	Long	High	Low	High	High

Note: TR, interval between radiofrequency (Rf) pulses; TE, interval between Rf pulse and signal reception; CSF, cerebrospinal fluid; T1W and T2W, T1- and T2-weighted.

In addition to dermatologic symptoms, other manifestations include widespread fibrosis of the skeletal muscle, bone, lungs, pleura, pericardium, myocardium, kidney, muscle, bone, testes, and dura.

COMPLICATIONS AND CONTRAINDICATIONS

From the patient's perspective, an MRI examination can be intimidating, and a higher level of cooperation is required than with CT. The patient lies on a table that is moved into a long, narrow gap within the magnet. Approximately 5% of the population experiences severe claustrophobia in the MR environment. This can be reduced by mild sedation but re-

FIGURE 362-3 ***A.*** Axial noncontrast CT scan in a patient with left hemiparesis shows a subtle low density involving the right temporal and frontal lobes (*arrows*). The hyperdense middle cerebral artery (*arrowhead*) indicates an embolic occlusion of the middle cerebral artery. ***B.*** Mean transit time CT perfusion parametric map indicating prolonged mean transit time involving the right middle cerebral territory (*arrows*). ***C.*** Cerebral blood volume map shows reduced CBV involving an area within the defect shown in ***B***, indicating infarction (*arrows*). ***D.*** Coronal maximum intensity projection from MRA shows right middle cerebral artery (MCA) occlusion (*arrow*). ***E*** and ***F.*** Axial diffusion weighted image (***E***) and apparent diffusion coefficient image (***F***) documents the presence of a right middle cerebral artery infarction.

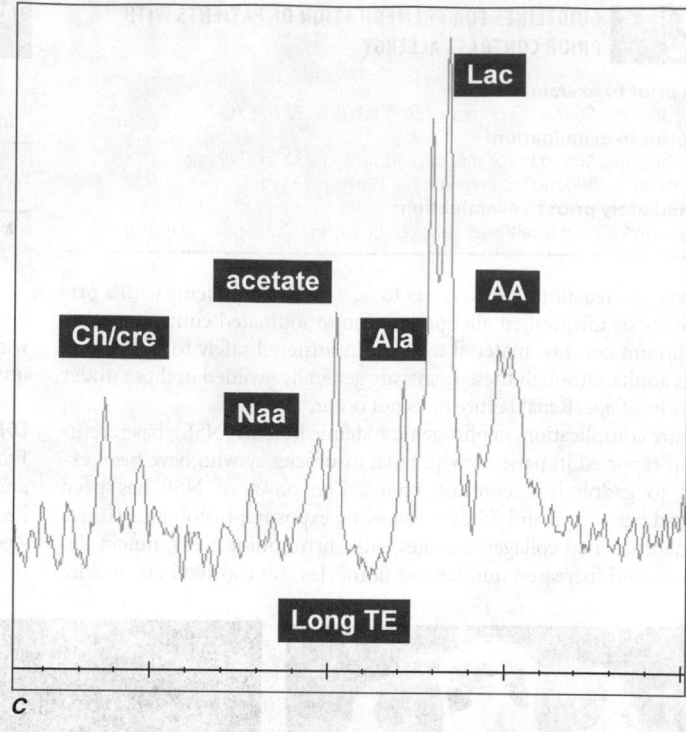

FIGURE 362-4 Cerebral abscess in a patient with fever and a right hemiparesis. A. Coronal postcontrast T1-weighted image demonstrates a ring enhancing mass in the left frontal lobe. **B.** Axial diffusion-weighted image demonstrates restricted diffusion (high signal intensity) within the lesion, which in this setting is highly suggestive of cerebral abscess. **C.** Single voxel proton spectroscopy (TE of 288 ms) reveals a reduced Naa peak and abnormal peaks for acetate, alanine (Ala), lactate (Lac), and amino acids (AA). These findings are highly suggestive of cerebral abscess; at biopsy a streptococcal abscess was identified.

mains a problem for some. Unlike CT, movement of the patient during an MR sequence distorts all the images; therefore, uncooperative patients should either be sedated for the MR study or scanned with CT. Generally, children under the age of 10 years usually require conscious sedation in order to complete the MR examination without motion degradation.

MRI is considered safe for patients, even at very high field strengths (>3–4 T). Serious injuries have been caused, however, by attraction of ferromagnetic objects into the magnet, which act as missiles if brought too close to the magnet. Likewise, ferromagnetic implants, such as aneurysm clips, may torque within the magnet, causing damage to vessels and even death. Metallic foreign bodies in the eye have moved and caused intraocular hemorrhage; screening for ocular metallic fragments is indicated in those with a history of metal work or ocular metallic foreign bodies. Implanted cardiac pacemakers are generally a contraindication to MRI owing to the risk of induced arrhythmias; however, some newer pacemakers have been shown to be safe. All health care personnel and patients must be screened and educated thoroughly to prevent such disasters as the magnet is always "on." Table 362-6 lists common contraindications for MRI.

MAGNETIC RESONANCE ANGIOGRAPHY

MR angiography (MRA) is a general term describing several MR techniques that result in vascular-weighted images. These provide a vascu-lar flow map rather than the anatomic map shown by conventional angiography. On routine spin echo MR sequences, moving protons (e.g., flowing blood, CSF) exhibit complex MR signals that range from high to low signal intensity relative to background stationary tissue. Fast-flowing blood returns no signal (flow void) on routine T1W or T2W spin echo MR images. Slower-flowing blood, as occurs in veins or distal to arterial stenosis, may appear high in signal. However, using special pulse sequences called *gradient echo sequences*, it is possible to increase the signal intensity of moving protons in contrast to the low signal background intensity of stationary tissue. This creates angiography-like images, which can be manipulated in three dimensions to highlight vascular anatomy and relationships.

Time-of-flight (TOF) imaging, currently the technique used most frequently, relies on the suppression of nonmoving tissue to provide a low-intensity background for the high signal intensity of flowing blood entering the section; arterial or venous structures may be highlighted. A typical TOF angiography sequence results in a series of contiguous, thin MR sections (0.6–0.9 mm thick), which can be viewed as a stack and manipulated to create an angiographic image data set that can be reformatted and viewed in various planes and angles, much like that seen with conventional angiography (Fig. 362-3D).

Phase-contrast MRA has a longer acquisition time than TOF MRA, but in addition to providing anatomic information similar to that of TOF im-

FIGURE 362-5 Herpes simplex encephalitis in a patient presenting with altered mental status and fever. A. Coronal T2-weighted FLAIR image demonstrates expansion and high signal intensity involving the left medial temporal lobe, insular cortex, and left cingulate gyrus. **B.** Diffusion-weighted image demonstrates high signal intensity indicating restricted diffusion involving the left medial temporal lobe and hippocampus (*arrows*). This is most consistent with neuronal death and can be seen in acute infarction as well as encephalitis and other inflammatory conditions. The suspected diagnosis of Herpes simplex encephalitis was confirmed by CSF PCR analysis. (*Courtesy of Howard Rowley, MD, University of Wisconsin; with permission.*)

aging, it can be used to reveal the velocity and direction of blood flow in a given vessel. Through the selection of different imaging parameters, differing blood velocities can be highlighted; selective venous and arterial MRA images can thus be obtained. One advantage of phase-contrast MRA is the excellent suppression of high signal intensity background structures.

MRA can also be acquired during infusion of contrast material. Advantages include faster imaging times (1–2 min vs. 10 min), fewer flow-related artifacts, and higher-resolution images. Recently, contrast-enhanced MRA has become the standard for extracranial vascular MRA. This technique entails rapid imaging using coronal three-dimensional TOF sequences during a bolus infusion of 15–20 mL of gadolinium-DTPA. Proper technique and timing of acquisition relative to bolus arrival are critical for success.

MRA has lower spatial resolution compared with conventional film-based angiography, and therefore the detection of small-vessel abnormalities, such as vasculitis and distal vasospasm, is problematic. MRA is also less sensitive to slowly flowing blood and thus may not reliably differentiate complete from near-complete occlusions. Motion, either by the patient or by anatomic structures, may distort the MRA images, creating artifacts. These limitations notwithstanding, MRA has proved useful in evaluation of the extracranial carotid and vertebral circulation as well as of larger-caliber intracranial arteries and dural sinuses. It has also proved useful in the noninvasive detection of intracranial aneurysms and vascular malformations.

TABLE 362-6 COMMON CONTRAINDICATIONS TO MR IMAGING

Cardiac pacemaker or permanent pacemaker leads
Internal defibrillatory device
Cochlear prostheses
Bone growth stimulators
Spinal cord stimulators
Electronic infusion devices
Intracranial aneurysm clips (some but not all)
Ocular implants (some) or ocular metallic foreign body
McGee stapedectomy piston prosthesis
Omniphase penile implant
Swan-Ganz catheter
Magnetic stoma plugs
Magnetic dental implants
Magnetic sphincters
Ferromagnetic IVC filters, coils, stents—safe 6 weeks after implantation
Tattooed eyeliner (contains ferromagnetic material and may irritate eyes)

ECHO-PLANAR MR IMAGING

Recent improvements in gradients, software, and high-speed computer processors now permit extremely rapid MRI of the brain. With echo-planar MRI (EPI), fast gradients are switched on and off at high speeds to create the information used to form an image. In routine spin echo imaging, images of the brain can be obtained in 5–10 min. With EPI, all of the information required for processing an image is accumulated in 50–150 ms, and the information for the entire brain is obtained in 1–2 min, depending on the degree of resolution required or desired. Fast MRI reduces patient and organ motion, permitting diffusion imaging and tractography (Figs. 362-3, 362-4, 362-5, 362-6; and see Fig. 364-16), perfusion imaging during contrast infusion, fMRI, and kinematic motion studies.

Perfusion and diffusion imaging are EPI techniques that are useful in early detection of ischemic injury of the brain and may be useful together to demonstrate infarcted tissue as well as ischemic but potentially viable tissue at risk of infarction (e.g., the ischemic penumbra). Diffusion-weighted imaging (DWI) assesses microscopic motion of water; restriction of motion appears as relative high signal intensity on diffusion-weighted images. DWI is the most sensitive technique for detection of acute cerebral infarction of <7 days' duration and is also sensitive to encephalitis and abscess formation, all of which have reduced diffusion and result in high signal on diffusion-weighted images.

Perfusion MRI involves the acquisition of EPI images during a rapid intravenous bolus of gadolinium contrast material. Relative perfusion abnormalities can be identified on images of the relative cerebral blood volume, mean transit time, and cerebral blood flow. Delay in mean transit time and reduction in cerebral blood volume and cerebral blood flow are typical of infarction. In the setting of reduced blood flow, a prolonged mean transit time of contrast but normal or elevated cerebral blood volume may indicate tissue supplied by collateral flow that is at risk of infarction. pMRI imaging can also be used in the assessment of brain tumors to differentiate intraaxial primary tumors from extraaxial tumors or metastasis.

Diffusion tract imaging (DTI) is derived from diffusion MRI techniques. Preferential microscopic motion of water along white matter tracts is detected by diffusion MR, which can also indicate the direction of white matter fiber tracts. This new technique has great potential in the assessment of brain maturation as well as disease entities that undermine the integrity of the white matter architecture (Fig. 362-7).

fMRI of the brain is an EPI technique that localizes regions of activity in the brain following task activation. Neuronal activity elicits a

FIGURE 362-6 Diffusion tractography in cerebral glioma. A. An axial fast spin echo T2-weighted image shows a high signal intensity glioma of the insular cortex lateral to the fibers of the internal capsule. **B** and **C.** Axial post-gadolinium images with diffusion tractography superimposed on the image. This shows the position of the internal capsule (*arrows*) relative to the enhancing tumor.

slight increase in the delivery of oxygenated blood flow to a specific region of activated brain. This results in an alteration in the balance of oxyhemoglobin and deoxyhemoglobin, which yields a 2–3% increase in signal intensity within veins and local capillaries. Further studies will determine whether these techniques are cost-effective or clinically useful, but currently preoperative somatosensory and auditory cortex localization is possible. This technique has proved useful to neuroscientists interested in interrogating the localization of certain brain functions.

FIGURE 362-7 Diffusion tractography in a healthy individual obtained at 3T demonstrates the normal subcortical fiber pathways. The direction of the tracts have been color-coded (red, left-right; green, anterior-posterior; blue, superior-inferior). (*Courtesy of Pratik Mukherjee, MD, PhD; with permission.*)

MAGNETIC RESONANCE NEUROGRAPHY

MR neurography is an MR technique that shows promise in detecting increased signal in irritated, inflamed, or infiltrated peripheral nerves. Images are obtained with fat-suppressed fast spin echo imaging or short inversion recovery sequences. Irritated or infiltrated nerves will demonstrate high signal on T2W imaging.

POSITRON EMISSION TOMOGRAPHY (PET)

PET relies on the detection of positrons emitted during the decay of a radionuclide that has been injected into a patient. The most frequently used moiety is 2-[^{18}F]fluoro-2-deoxy-D-glucose (FDG), which is an analogue of glucose and is taken up by cells competitively with 2-deoxyglucose. Multiple images of glucose uptake activity are formed after 45–60 min. Images reveal differences in regional glucose activity among normal and pathologic brain structures. A lower activity of FDG in the parietal lobes has been associated with Alzheimer's disease. FDG PET is used primarily for the detection of extracranial metastatic disease. Combination PET-CT scanners, in which both CT and PET are obtained at one sitting, are replacing PET scans alone for most clinical indications. Functional images superimposed on high-resolution CT scans result in more precise anatomic diagnoses.

MYELOGRAPHY

TECHNIQUE

Myelography involves the intrathecal instillation of specially formulated water-soluble iodinated contrast medium into the lumbar or cervical subarachnoid space. CT scanning is usually performed after myelography (*CT myelography*) to better demonstrate the spinal cord and roots, which appear as filling defects in the opacified subarachnoid space. *Low-dose CT myelography*, in which CT is performed after the subarachnoid injection of a small amount of relatively dilute contrast material, has replaced conventional myelography for many indications, thereby reducing exposure to radiation and contrast media. Newer multidetector scanners now obtain CT studies quickly so that reformations in sagittal and coronal planes, equivalent to traditional myelography projections, are now routine.

INDICATIONS

Myelography has been largely replaced by CT myelography and MRI for diagnosis of diseases of the spinal canal and cord (Table 362-1). Remaining indications for conventional plain-film myelography include the evaluation of suspected meningeal or arachnoid cysts and the localization of spinal dural arteriovenous or CSF fistulas. Conventional myelography and CT myelography provide the most precise information in patients with prior spinal fusion and spinal fixation hardware.

CONTRAINDICATIONS

Myelography is relatively safe; however, it should be performed with caution in any patient with elevated intracranial pressure, evidence of a spinal block, or a history of allergic reaction to intrathecal contrast media. In patients with a suspected spinal block, MR is the preferred technique. If myelography is necessary, only a small amount of contrast medium should be instilled below the lesion in order to minimize the risk of neurologic deterioration. Lumbar puncture is to be avoided in patients with bleeding disorders, including patients receiving anticoagulant therapy, as well as in those with infections of the soft tissues.

COMPLICATIONS

Headache, nausea, and vomiting are the most frequent complications of myelography and are reported to occur in up to 38% of patients. These symptoms result from either neurotoxic effects of the contrast agent, persistent leakage of CSF at the puncture site, or psychological reactions to the procedure. Vasovagal syncope may occur during lumbar puncture; it is accentuated by the upright position used during lumbar myelography. Adequate hydration before and after myelography will reduce the incidence of this complication. Postural headache (post–lumbar puncture headache) is generally due to leakage of CSF from the puncture site, resulting in CSF hypotension. Management of post-lumbar-puncture headache is discussed in Chap. 15.

If significant headache persists for longer than 48 hours, placement of an epidural blood patch should be considered. Hearing loss is a rare complication of myelography. It may result from a direct toxic effect of the contrast medium or from an alteration of the pressure equilibrium between CSF and perilymph in the inner ear. Puncture of the spinal cord is a rare but serious complication of cervical (C1–2) and high lumbar puncture. The risk of cord puncture is greatest in patients with spinal stenosis, Chiari malformations, or conditions that reduce CSF volume. In these settings, a low-dose lumbar injection followed by thin-section CT or MRI is a safer alternative to cervical puncture. Intrathecal contrast reactions are rare, but aseptic meningitis and encephalopathy may occur. The latter is usually dose-related and associated with contrast entering the intracranial subarachnoid space. Seizures occur following myelography in 0.1–0.3% of patients. Risk factors include a preexisting seizure disorder and the use of a total iodine dose of >4500 mg. Other reported complications include hyperthermia, hallucinations, depression, and anxiety states. These side effects have been reduced by the development of nonionic, water-soluble contrast agents, as well as by head elevation and generous hydration following myelography.

SPINE INTERVENTIONS

DISCOGRAPHY

The evaluation of back pain and radiculopathy may require diagnostic procedures that attempt either to reproduce the patient's pain or relieve it, indicating its correct source prior to lumbar fusion. Discography is performed by fluoroscopic placement of a 22- to 25-gauge needle into the intervertebral disc and subsequent injection of 1–3 mL of contrast media. The intradiscal pressure is recorded, as is an assessment of the patient's response to the injection of contrast material. Typically little or no pain is felt during injection of a normal disc, which does not accept much more than 1 mL of contrast material, even at pressures as high as 415–690 kPa (60–100 lbs/in^2). CT and plain films are obtained following the procedure.

SELECTIVE NERVE ROOT AND EPIDURAL SPINAL INJECTIONS

Percutaneous selective nerve root and epidural blocks with glucocorticoid and anesthetic mixtures may be both therapeutic as well as diagnostic, especially if a patient's pain is relieved. Typically, 1–2 mL of an equal mixture of a long-acting glucocorticoid such as betamethasone

and a long-acting anesthetic such as bupivicain 0.75% is instilled under CT or fluoroscopic guidance in the intraspinal epidural space or adjacent to an existing nerve root.

ANGIOGRAPHY

Catheter angiography is indicated for evaluating intracranial small-vessel pathology (such as vasculitis), for assessing vascular malformations and aneurysms, and in endovascular therapeutic procedures (Table 362-1). Angiography has been replaced for many indications by CT/CTA or MRI/MRA.

Angiography carries the greatest risk of morbidity of all diagnostic imaging procedures, owing to the necessity of inserting a catheter into a blood vessel, directing the catheter to the required location, injecting contrast material to visualize the vessel, and removing the catheter while maintaining hemostasis. Therapeutic transcatheter procedures (see below) have become important options for the treatment of some cerebrovascular diseases. The decision to undertake a diagnostic or therapeutic angiographic procedure requires careful assessment of the goals of the investigation and its attendant risks.

To improve tolerance to contrast agents, patients undergoing angiography should be well hydrated before and after the procedure. Since the femoral route is used most commonly, the femoral artery must be compressed after the procedure to prevent a hematoma from developing. The puncture site and distal pulses should be evaluated carefully after the procedure; complications can include thigh hematoma or lower extremity emboli.

COMPLICATIONS

A common femoral arterial puncture provides retrograde access via the aorta to the aortic arch and great vessels. The most feared complication of cerebral angiography is stroke. Thrombus can form on or inside the tip of the catheter, and atherosclerotic thrombus or plaque can be dislodged by the catheter or guide wire or by the force of injection and can embolize distally in the cerebral circulation. Risk factors for ischemic complications include limited experience on the part of the angiographer, atherosclerosis, vasospasm, low cardiac output, decreased oxygen-carrying capacity, advanced age, and prior history of migraine. The risk of a neurologic complication varies but is ~4% for transient ischemic attack and stroke, 1% for permanent deficit, and <0.1% for death.

Ionic contrast material injected into the cerebral vasculature can be neurotoxic if the BBB is breached, either by an underlying disease or by the injection of hyperosmolar contrast agent. Ionic contrast media are less well tolerated than nonionic media, probably because they can induce changes in cell membrane electrical potentials. Patients with dolichoectasia of the basilar artery can suffer reversible brainstem dysfunction and acute short-term memory loss during angiography, owing to the slow percolation of the contrast material and the consequent prolonged exposure of the brain. Rarely, an intracranial aneurysm ruptures during an angiographic contrast injection, causing subarachnoid hemorrhage, perhaps as a result of injection under high pressure.

SPINAL ANGIOGRAPHY

Spinal angiography may be indicated to evaluate vascular malformations and tumors and to identify the artery of Adamkiewicz (Chap. 372) prior to aortic aneurysm repair. The procedure is lengthy and requires the use of relatively large volumes of contrast; the incidence of serious complications, including paraparesis, subjective visual blurring, and altered speech, is ~2%. Gadolinium-enhanced MRA has been used successfully in this setting, as has iodinated contrast CTA, which has promise for replacing diagnostic spinal angiography for some indications.

INTERVENTIONAL NEURORADIOLOGY

This rapidly developing field is providing new therapeutic options for patients with challenging neurovascular problems. Available procedures include detachable coil therapy for aneurysms, particulate or liquid adhesive embolization of arteriovenous malformations, balloon angioplasty and stenting of arterial stenosis or vasospasm, transarterial or transvenous embolization of dural arteriovenous fistulas, balloon occlusion of carotid-cavernous and vertebral fistulas, endovascular treatment of vein-of-Galen malformations, preoperative embolization of tumors, and thrombolysis of acute arterial or venous thrombosis. Many of these disorders place the patient at high risk of cerebral hemorrhage, stroke, or death.

The highest complication rates are found with the therapies designed to treat the highest-risk diseases. The advent of electrolytically detachable coils has ushered in a new era in the treatment of cerebral aneurysms. One randomized trial found a 28% reduction of morbidity and mortality at 1 year among those treated for anterior circulation aneurysm with detachable coils compared with neurosurgical clip-

ping. It remains to be determined what the role of coils will be relative to surgical options, but in many centers, coiling has become standard therapy for many aneurysms.

FURTHER READINGS

BERMAN JI et al: Diffusion-tensor imaging-guided tracking of fibers of the pyramidal tract combined with intraoperative cortical stimulation mapping in patients with gliomas. J Neurosurg 101:66, 2004

GONZALEZ RG: Imaging-guided acute ischemic stroke therapy: From "time is brain" to "physiology is brain." AJNR 27:728, 2006

SCHAEFER PW: Diffusion-weighted imaging in acute stroke. Magn Reson Imaging Clin N Am 14:141, 2006

SECTION 2 — DISEASES OF THE CENTRAL NERVOUS SYSTEM

363 Seizures and Epilepsy
Daniel H. Lowenstein

A *seizure* (from the Latin *sacire*, "to take possession of") is a paroxysmal event due to abnormal, excessive, hypersynchronous discharges from an aggregate of central nervous system (CNS) neurons. Depending on the distribution of discharges, this abnormal CNS activity can have various manifestations, ranging from dramatic convulsive activity to experiential phenomena not readily discernible by an observer. Although a variety of factors influence the incidence and prevalence of seizures, ~5–10% of the population will have at least one seizure, with the highest incidence occurring in early childhood and late adulthood.

The meaning of the term *seizure* needs to be carefully distinguished from that of epilepsy. *Epilepsy* describes a condition in which a person has *recurrent* seizures due to a chronic, underlying process. This definition implies that a person with a single seizure, or recurrent seizures due to correctable or avoidable circumstances, does not necessarily have epilepsy. Epilepsy refers to a clinical phenomenon rather than a single disease entity, since there are many forms and causes of epilepsy. However, among the many causes of epilepsy there are various *epilepsy syndromes* in which the clinical and pathologic characteristics are distinctive and suggest a specific underlying etiology.

Using the definition of epilepsy as two or more unprovoked seizures, the incidence of epilepsy is ~0.3–0.5% in different populations throughout the world, and the prevalence of epilepsy has been estimated at 5–10 persons per 1000.

CLASSIFICATION OF SEIZURES

Determining the type of seizure that has occurred is essential for focusing the diagnostic approach on particular etiologies, selecting the appropriate therapy, and providing potentially vital information regarding prognosis. In 1981, the International League against Epilepsy (ILAE) published a modified version of the International Classification of Epileptic Seizures that has continued to be a useful classification system (Table 363-1). This system is based on the clinical features of seizures and associated electroencephalographic findings. Other potentially distinctive features such as etiology or cellular substrate are not considered in this classification system, although this will undoubtedly change in the future as more is learned about the pathophysiologic mechanisms that underlie specific seizure types.

A fundamental principle is that seizures may be either partial (synonymous with focal) or generalized. *Partial seizures* are those in which the seizure activity is restricted to discrete areas of the cerebral cortex.

Generalized seizures involve diffuse regions of the brain simultaneously. Partial seizures are usually associated with structural abnormalities of the brain. In contrast, generalized seizures may result from cellular, biochemical, or structural abnormalities that have a more widespread distribution.

PARTIAL SEIZURES

Partial seizures occur within discrete regions of the brain. If consciousness is fully preserved during the seizure, the clinical manifestations are considered relatively simple and the seizure is termed a *simple partial seizure*. If consciousness is impaired, the symptomatology is more complex and the seizure is termed a *complex partial seizure*. An important additional subgroup comprises those seizures that begin as partial seizures and then spread diffusely throughout the cortex, i.e., *partial seizures with secondary generalization*.

Simple Partial Seizures   Simple partial seizures cause motor, sensory, autonomic, or psychic symptoms without an obvious alteration in consciousness. For example, a patient having a partial motor seizure arising from the right primary motor cortex in the vicinity controlling hand movement will note the onset of involuntary movements of the contralateral, left hand. These movements are typically clonic (i.e., repetitive, flexion/extension movements) at a frequency of ~2–3 Hz; pure tonic posturing may be seen as well. Since the cortical region controlling hand movement is immediately adjacent to the region for facial expression, the seizure may also cause abnormal movements of the face synchronous with the movements of the hand. The electroencephalogram (EEG) recorded with scalp electrodes during the seizure (i.e., an ictal EEG) may show abnormal discharges in a very limited region over the appropriate area of cerebral cortex if the seizure focus involves the cerebral convexity. Seizure activity occurring within deeper

TABLE 363-1   **CLASSIFICATION OF SEIZURES**

1. Partial seizures
     a. Simple partial seizures (with motor, sensory, autonomic, or psychic signs)
     b. Complex partial seizures
     c. Partial seizures with secondary generalization
2. Primarily generalized seizures
     a. Absence (petit mal)
     b. Tonic-clonic (grand mal)
     c. Tonic
     d. Atonic
     e. Myoclonic
3. Unclassified seizures
     a. Neonatal seizures
     b. Infantile spasms

brain structures is often not recorded by the standard EEG, however, and may require intracranial electrodes for its detection.

Three additional features of partial motor seizures are worth noting. First, in some patients the abnormal motor movements may begin in a very restricted region such as the fingers and gradually progress (over seconds to minutes) to include a larger portion of the extremity. This phenomenon, described by Hughlings Jackson and known as a "Jacksonian march," represents the spread of seizure activity over a progressively larger region of motor cortex. Second, patients may experience a localized paresis (Todd's paralysis) for minutes to many hours in the involved region following the seizure. Third, in rare instances the seizure may continue for hours or days. This condition, termed *epilepsia partialis continua*, is often refractory to medical therapy.

Simple partial seizures may also manifest as changes in somatic sensation (e.g., paresthesias), vision (flashing lights or formed hallucinations), equilibrium (sensation of falling or vertigo), or autonomic function (flushing, sweating, piloerection). Simple partial seizures arising from the temporal or frontal cortex may also cause alterations in hearing, olfaction, or higher cortical function (psychic symptoms). This includes the sensation of unusual, intense odors (e.g., burning rubber or kerosene) or sounds (crude or highly complex sounds), or an epigastric sensation that rises from the stomach or chest to the head. Some patients describe odd, internal feelings such as fear, a sense of impending change, detachment, depersonalization, déjà vu, or illusions that objects are growing smaller (micropsia) or larger (macropsia). When such symptoms precede a complex partial or secondarily generalized seizure, these simple partial seizures serve as a warning, or *aura*.

Complex Partial Seizures Complex partial seizures are characterized by focal seizure activity accompanied by a transient impairment of the patient's ability to maintain normal contact with the environment. The patient is unable to respond appropriately to visual or verbal commands during the seizure and has impaired recollection or awareness of the ictal phase. The seizures frequently begin with an aura (i.e., a simple partial seizure) that is stereotypic for the patient. The start of the ictal phase is often a sudden behavioral arrest or motionless stare, which marks the onset of the period of amnesia. The behavioral arrest is usually accompanied by *automatisms*, which are involuntary, automatic behaviors that have a wide range of manifestations. Automatisms may consist of very basic behaviors such as chewing, lip smacking, swallowing, or "picking" movements of the hands, or more elaborate behaviors such as a display of emotion or running. The patient is typically confused following the seizure, and the transition to full recovery of consciousness may range from seconds up to an hour. Examination immediately following the seizure may show an anterograde amnesia or, in cases involving the dominant hemisphere, a postictal aphasia.

The routine interictal (i.e., between seizures) EEG in patients with complex partial seizures is often normal or may show brief discharges termed *epileptiform spikes*, or *sharp waves*. Since complex partial seizures can arise from the medial temporal lobe or inferior frontal lobe, i.e., regions distant from the scalp, the EEG recorded during the seizure may be nonlocalizing. However, the seizure focus is often detected using sphenoidal or surgically placed intracranial electrodes.

The range of potential clinical behaviors linked to complex partial seizures is so broad that extreme caution is advised before concluding that stereotypic episodes of bizarre or atypical behavior are not due to seizure activity. In such cases additional, detailed EEG studies may be helpful.

Partial Seizures with Secondary Generalization Partial seizures can spread to involve both cerebral hemispheres and produce a generalized seizure, usually of the tonic-clonic variety (discussed below). Secondary generalization is observed frequently following simple partial seizures, especially those with a focus in the frontal lobe, but may also be associated with partial seizures occurring elsewhere in the brain. A partial seizure with secondary generalization is often difficult to distinguish from a primary generalized tonic-clonic seizure, since bystanders tend to emphasize the more dramatic, generalized convulsive

phase of the seizure and overlook the more subtle, focal symptoms present at onset. In some cases, the focal onset of the seizure becomes apparent only when a careful history identifies a preceding aura (i.e., simple partial seizure). Often, however, the focal onset is not clinically evident and may be established only through careful EEG analysis. Nonetheless, distinguishing between these two entities is extremely important, as there may be substantial differences in the evaluation and treatment of partial versus generalized seizure disorders.

GENERALIZED SEIZURES

By definition, generalized seizures arise from both cerebral hemispheres simultaneously. However, it is currently impossible to exclude entirely the existence of a focal region of abnormal activity that initiates the seizure prior to rapid secondary generalization. For this reason, generalized seizures may be practically defined as bilateral clinical and electrographic events without any detectable focal onset. Fortunately, several types of generalized seizures have distinctive features that facilitate clinical diagnosis.

Absence Seizures (Petit Mal) Absence seizures are characterized by sudden, brief lapses of consciousness without loss of postural control. The seizure typically lasts for only seconds, consciousness returns as suddenly as it was lost, and there is no postictal confusion. Although the brief loss of consciousness may be clinically inapparent or the sole manifestation of the seizure discharge, absence seizures are usually accompanied by subtle, bilateral motor signs such as rapid blinking of the eyelids, chewing movements, or small-amplitude, clonic movements of the hands.

Absence seizures usually begin in childhood (ages 4–8) or early adolescence and are the main seizure type in 15–20% of children with epilepsy. The seizures can occur hundreds of times per day, but the child may be unaware of or unable to convey their existence. Since the clinical signs of the seizures are subtle, especially to new parents, it is not surprising that the first clue to absence epilepsy is often unexplained "daydreaming" and a decline in school performance recognized by a teacher.

The electrophysiologic hallmark of typical absence seizures is a generalized, symmetric, 3-Hz spike-and-wave discharge that begins and ends suddenly, superimposed on a normal EEG background. Periods of spike-and-wave discharges lasting more than a few seconds usually correlate with clinical signs, but the EEG often shows many more brief bursts of abnormal cortical activity than were suspected clinically. Hyperventilation tends to provoke these electrographic discharges and even the seizures themselves and is routinely used when recording the EEG.

Typical absence seizures are often associated with generalized, tonic-clonic seizures, but patients usually have no other neurologic problems and respond well to treatment with specific anticonvulsants. Although estimates vary, ~60–70% of such patients will have a spontaneous remission during adolescence.

Atypical Absence Seizures Atypical absence seizures have features that deviate both clinically and electrophysiologically from typical absence seizures. For example, the lapse of consciousness is usually of longer duration and less abrupt in onset and cessation, and the seizure is accompanied by more obvious motor signs that may include focal or lateralizing features. The EEG shows a generalized, slow spike-and-wave pattern with a frequency of ≤2.5/s, as well as other abnormal activity. Atypical absence seizures are usually associated with diffuse or multifocal structural abnormalities of the brain and therefore may accompany other signs of neurologic dysfunction such as mental retardation. Furthermore, the seizures are less responsive to anticonvulsants compared to typical absence seizures.

Generalized, Tonic-Clonic Seizures (Grand Mal) Primary generalized, tonic-clonic seizures are the main seizure type in ~10% of all persons with epilepsy. They are also the most common seizure type resulting from metabolic derangements and are therefore frequently encountered in many different clinical settings. The seizure usually begins abruptly without warning, although some patients describe vague premonitory symptoms in the hours leading up to the seizure. This prodrome is distinct from the stereotypic auras associated with focal seizures that secondarily generalize. The initial phase of the seizure is usually tonic contraction of muscles throughout the body, accounting for a number of the classic features of the event. Tonic contraction of the muscles of expiration and the larynx at the onset will produce a loud moan or "ictal cry." Respirations are impaired, secretions pool in the oropharynx, and cyanosis develops. Contraction of the jaw muscles may cause biting of the tongue. A marked enhancement of sympathetic tone leads to increases in heart rate, blood pressure, and pupillary size. After 10–20 s, the tonic phase of the seizure typically evolves into the clonic phase, produced by the superimposition of periods of muscle relaxation on the tonic muscle contraction. The periods of relaxation progressively increase until the end of the ictal phase, which usually lasts no more than 1 min. The postictal phase is characterized by unresponsiveness, muscular flaccidity, and excessive salivation that can cause stridorous breathing and partial airway obstruction. Bladder or bowel incontinence may occur at this point. Patients gradually regain consciousness over minutes to hours, and during this transition there is typically a period of postictal confusion. Patients subsequently complain of headache, fatigue, and muscle ache that can last for many hours. The duration of impaired consciousness in the postictal phase can be extremely long, i.e., many hours, in patients with prolonged seizures or underlying CNS diseases such as alcoholic cerebral atrophy.

The EEG during the tonic phase of the seizure shows a progressive increase in generalized low-voltage fast activity, followed by generalized high-amplitude, polyspike discharges. In the clonic phase, the high-amplitude activity is typically interrupted by slow waves to create a spike-and-wave pattern. The postictal EEG shows diffuse slowing that gradually recovers as the patient awakens.

There are many variants of the generalized tonic-clonic seizure, including pure tonic and pure clonic seizures. Brief tonic seizures lasting only a few seconds are especially noteworthy since they are usually associated with specific epileptic syndromes having mixed seizure phenotypes, such as the Lennox-Gastaut syndrome (discussed below).

Atonic Seizures Atonic seizures are characterized by sudden loss of postural muscle tone lasting 1–2 s. Consciousness is briefly impaired, but there is usually no postictal confusion. A very brief seizure may cause only a quick head drop or nodding movement, while a longer seizure will cause the patient to collapse. This can be extremely dangerous, since there is a substantial risk of direct head injury with the fall. The EEG shows brief, generalized spike-and-wave discharges followed immediately by diffuse slow waves that correlate with the loss of muscle tone. Similar to pure tonic seizures, atonic seizures are usually seen in association with known epileptic syndromes.

Myoclonic Seizures Myoclonus is a sudden and brief muscle contraction that may involve one part of the body or the entire body. A normal, common physiologic form of myoclonus is the sudden jerking movement observed while falling asleep. Pathologic myoclonus is most commonly seen in association with metabolic disorders, degenerative CNS diseases, or anoxic brain injury (Chap. 269). Although the distinction from other forms of myoclonus is imprecise, myoclonic seizures are considered to be true epileptic events since they are caused by cortical (versus subcortical or spinal) dysfunction. The EEG may show bilaterally synchronous spike-and-wave discharges synchronized with the myoclonus, although these can be obscured by movement artifact. Myoclonic seizures usually coexist with other forms of generalized seizure disorders but are the predominant feature of juvenile myoclonic epilepsy (discussed below).

UNCLASSIFIED SEIZURES

Not all seizure types can be classified as partial or generalized. This appears to be especially true of seizures that occur in neonates and infants. The distinctive phenotypes of seizures at these early ages likely result, in part, from differences in neuronal function and connectivity in the immature versus mature CNS.

EPILEPSY SYNDROMES

Epilepsy syndromes are disorders in which epilepsy is a predominant feature, and there is sufficient evidence (e.g., through clinical, EEG, radiologic, or genetic observations) to suggest a common underlying mechanism. Three important epilepsy syndromes are listed below; additional examples with a known genetic basis are shown in Table 363-2.

JUVENILE MYOCLONIC EPILEPSY

Juvenile myoclonic epilepsy (JME) is a generalized seizure disorder of unknown cause that appears in early adolescence and is usually characterized by bilateral myoclonic jerks that may be single or repetitive. The myoclonic seizures are most frequent in the morning after awakening and can be provoked by sleep deprivation. Consciousness is preserved unless the myoclonus is especially severe. Many patients also experience generalized tonic-clonic seizures, and up to one-third have absence seizures. The condition is otherwise benign, and although complete remission is uncommon, the seizures respond well to appropriate anticonvulsant medication. There is often a family history of epilepsy, and genetic linkage studies suggest a polygenic cause.

LENNOX-GASTAUT SYNDROME

Lennox-Gastaut syndrome occurs in children and is defined by the following triad: (1) multiple seizure types (usually including generalized tonic-clonic, atonic, and atypical absence seizures); (2) an EEG showing slow (<3 Hz) spike-and-wave discharges and a variety of other abnormalities; and (3) impaired cognitive function in most but not all cases. Lennox-Gastaut syndrome is associated with CNS disease or dysfunction from a variety of causes, including developmental abnormalities, perinatal hypoxia/ischemia, trauma, infection, and other acquired lesions. The multifactorial nature of this syndrome suggests that it is a nonspecific response of the brain to diffuse neural injury. Unfortunately, many patients have a poor prognosis due to the underlying CNS disease and the physical and psychosocial consequences of severe, poorly controlled epilepsy.

MESIAL TEMPORAL LOBE EPILEPSY SYNDROME

Mesial temporal lobe epilepsy (MTLE) is the most common syndrome associated with complex partial seizures and is an example of a symptomatic, partial epilepsy with distinctive clinical, electroencephalographic, and pathologic features (Table 363-3). High-resolution MRI can detect the characteristic hippocampal sclerosis that appears to be essential in the pathophysiology of MTLE for many patients (Fig. 363-1). Recognition of this syndrome is especially important because it tends to be refractory to treatment with anticonvulsants but responds extremely well to surgical intervention. Advances in the understanding of basic mechanisms of epilepsy have come through studies of experimental models of MTLE, discussed below.

THE CAUSES OF SEIZURES AND EPILEPSY

Seizures are a result of a shift in the normal balance of excitation and inhibition within the CNS. Given the numerous properties that control neuronal excitability, it is not surprising that there are many different ways to perturb this normal balance, and therefore many different causes of both seizures and epilepsy. Three clinical observations emphasize how a variety of factors determine why certain conditions may cause seizures or epilepsy in a given patient.

1. *The normal brain is capable of having a seizure under the appropriate circumstances, and there are differences between individuals in the susceptibility or threshold for seizures.* For example, seizures may be induced by high fevers in children who are otherwise normal and who never develop other neurologic problems, including epilepsy. However, febrile seizures occur only in a relatively small proportion of children. This implies there are various underlying *endoge-*

TABLE 363-2 EXAMPLES OF GENES ASSOCIATED WITH EPILEPSY SYNDROMES[a]

Gene (Locus)	Function of Gene	Clinical Syndrome	Comments
CHRNA4 (20q13.2)	Nicotinic acetylcholine receptor subunit; mutations cause alterations in Ca^{2+} flux through the receptor; this may reduce amount of GABA release in presynaptic terminals	Autosomal dominant nocturnal frontal lobe epilepsy (ADNFLE); childhood onset; brief, nighttime seizures with prominent motor movements; often misdiagnosed as primary sleep disorder	Rare; first identified in a large Australian family; other families found to have mutations in CHRNA2 or CHRNB2, and some families appear to have mutations at other loci
KCNQ2 (20q13.3)	Voltage-gated potassium channel subunits; mutation in pore regions may cause a 20–40% reduction of potassium currents, which will lead to impaired repolarization	Benign familial neonatal convulsions (BFNC); autosomal dominant inheritance; onset in 1st week of life in infants who are otherwise normal; remission usually within weeks to months; long-term epilepsy in 10–15%	Rare; other families found to have mutations in KCNQ3; sequence and functional homology to KCNQ1, mutations of which cause long QT syndrome and a cardiac-auditory syndrome
SCN1B (19q12.1)	β-subunit of a voltage-gated sodium channel; mutation disrupts disulfide bridge that is crucial for structure of extracellular domain; mutated β-subunit leads to slower sodium channel inactivation	Generalized epilepsy with febrile seizures plus (GEFS+); autosomal dominant inheritance; presents with febrile seizures at median 1 year, which may persist >6 years, then variable seizure types not associated with fever	Incidence uncertain; GEFS+ identified in other families with mutations in other sodium channel subunits (SCN1A and SCN2A) and GABA_A receptor subunit (GABRG2 and GABRA1); significant phenotypic heterogeneity within same family, including members with febrile seizures only
LGI1 (10q24)	Leucine-rich glioma-inactivated 1 gene; previous evidence for role in glial tumor progression; protein homology suggests a possible role in nervous system development	Autosomal dominant partial epilepsy with auditory features (ADPEAF); a form of idiopathic lateral temporal lobe epilepsy with auditory symptoms or aphasia as a major simple partial seizure manifestation; age of onset usually between 10 and 25 years	Mutations found in approximately 50% of families containing two or more subjects with idiopathic localization-related epilepsy with ictal auditory symptoms, suggesting that at least one other gene may underlie this syndrome. *LGI1* is the only gene identified so far in temporal lobe epilepsy
CSTB (21q22.3)	Cystatin B, a noncaspase cysteine protease inhibitor; normal protein may block neuronal apoptosis by inhibiting caspases directly or indirectly (via cathepsins), or controlling proteolysis	Progressive myoclonus epilepsy (PME) (Unverricht-Lundborg disease); autosomal recessive inheritance; age of onset between 6–15 years, myoclonic seizures, ataxia, and progressive cognitive decline; brain shows neuronal degeneration	Overall rare, but relatively common in Finland and Western Mediterranean (>1 in 20,000); precise role of cystatin B in human disease unknown, although mice with null mutations of cystatin B have similar syndrome
EPM2A (6q24)	Laforin, a protein tyrosine phosphatase (PTP); may influence glycogen metabolism, which is known to be regulated by phosphatases	Progressive myoclonus epilepsy (Lafora's disease); autosomal recessive inheritance; onset age 6–19 years, death within 10 years; brain degeneration associated with polyglucosan intracellular inclusion bodies in numerous organs	Most common PME in Southern Europe, Middle East, Northern Africa, and Indian subcontinent; genetic heterogeneity; unknown whether seizure phenotype due to degeneration or direct effects of abnormal laforin expression.
Doublecortin (Xq21-24)	Doublecortin, expressed primarily in frontal lobes; function unknown; potentially an intracellular signaling molecule	Classic lissencephaly associated with severe mental retardation and seizures in males; subcortical band heterotopia with more subtle findings in females (presumably due to random X-inactivation); X-linked dominant	Relatively rare but of uncertain incidence, recent increased ascertainment due to improved imaging techniques; relationship between migration defect and seizure phenotype unknown

[a]The first four syndromes listed in the table (ADNFLE, BFNC, GEFS+, and ADPEAF) are examples of idiopathic epilepsies associated with identified gene mutations. The last three syndromes are examples of the numerous Mendelian disorders in which seizures are one part of the phenotype.

Note: GABA, γ-aminobutyric acid; PME, progressive myoclonus epilepsy.

nous factors that influence the threshold for having a seizure. Some of these factors are clearly genetic, as it has been shown that a family history of epilepsy will influence the likelihood of seizures occurring in otherwise normal individuals. Normal development also plays an important role, since the brain appears to have different seizure thresholds at different maturational stages.

2. *There are a variety of conditions that have an extremely high likelihood of resulting in a chronic seizure disorder.* One of the best examples of this is severe, penetrating head trauma, which is associated with up to a 50% risk of subsequent epilepsy. The high propensity for severe traumatic brain injury to lead to epilepsy suggests that the injury results in a long-lasting pathologic change in the CNS that transforms a presumably normal neural network into one that is abnormally hyperexcitable. This process is known as *epileptogenesis*, and the specific changes that result in a lowered seizure threshold can be considered *epileptogenic factors*. Other processes associated with epileptogenesis include stroke, infections, and abnormalities of CNS development. Likewise, the genetic abnormalities associated with epilepsy likely involve processes that trigger the appearance of specific sets of epileptogenic factors.

3. *Seizures are episodic.* Patients with epilepsy have seizures intermittently and, depending on the underlying cause, many patients are completely normal for months or even years between seizures. This implies there are important provocative or *precipitating factors* that induce seizures in patients with epilepsy. Similarly, precipitating

TABLE 363-3 CHARACTERISTICS OF THE MESIAL TEMPORAL LOBE EPILEPSY SYNDROME

History

History of febrile seizures	Rare secondarily generalized seizures
Family history of epilepsy	Seizures may remit and reappear
Early onset	Seizures often intractable

Clinical observations

Aura common	Postictal disorientation, memory loss, dysphasia (with focus in dominant hemisphere)
Behavioral arrest/stare	
Complex automatisms	
Unilateral posturing	

Laboratory studies

Unilateral or bilateral anterior temporal spikes on EEG
Hypometabolism on interictal PET
Hypoperfusion on interictal SPECT
Material-specific memory deficits on intracranial amobarbital (Wada) test

MRI findings

Small hippocampus with increased signal on T2-weighted sequences
Small temporal lobe
Enlarged temporal horn

Pathologic findings

Highly selective loss of specific cell populations within hippocampus in most cases

Note: EEG, electroencephalogram; PET, positron emission tomography; SPECT, single photon emission computed tomography.

FIGURE 363-1 Mesial temporal lobe epilepsy. The EEG suggested a right temporal lobe focus. Coronal high-resolution T2-weighted fast spin echo magnetic resonance image obtained through the body of the hippocampus demonstrates abnormal high-signal intensity in the right hippocampus (*white arrows*; compare with the normal hippocampus on the left, *black arrows*) consistent with mesial temporal sclerosis.

factors are responsible for causing the single seizure in someone without epilepsy. Precipitants include those due to intrinsic physiologic processes, such as psychological or physical stress, sleep deprivation, or hormonal changes associated with the menstrual cycle. They also include exogenous factors such as exposure to toxic substances and certain medications.

These observations emphasize the concept that the many causes of seizures and epilepsy result from a dynamic interplay between endogenous factors, epileptogenic factors, and precipitating factors. The potential role of each needs to be carefully considered when determining the appropriate management of a patient with seizures. For example, the identification of predisposing factors (e.g., family history of epilepsy) in a patient with febrile seizures may increase the necessity for closer follow-up and a more aggressive diagnostic evaluation. Finding an epileptogenic lesion may help in the estimation of seizure recurrence and duration of therapy. Finally, removal or modification of a precipitating factor may be an effective and safer method for preventing further seizures than the prophylactic use of anticonvulsant drugs.

CAUSES ACCORDING TO AGE

In practice, it is useful to consider the etiologies of seizures based on the age of the patient, as age is one of the most important factors determining both the incidence and the likely causes of seizures or epilepsy (**Table 363-4**). During the *neonatal period and early infancy*, potential causes include hypoxic-ischemic encephalopathy, trauma, CNS infection, congenital CNS abnormalities, and metabolic disorders. Babies born to mothers using neurotoxic drugs such as cocaine, heroin, or ethanol are susceptible to drug-withdrawal seizures in the first few days after delivery. Hypoglycemia and hypocalcemia, which can occur as secondary complications of perinatal injury, are also causes of seizures early after delivery. Seizures due to inborn errors of metabolism usually present once regular feeding begins, typically 2–3 days after birth. Pyridoxine (vitamin B$_6$) deficiency, an important cause of neonatal seizures, can be effectively treated with pyridoxine replacement. The idiopathic or inherited forms of benign neonatal convulsions are also seen during this time period.

The most common seizures arising in *late infancy and early childhood* are febrile seizures, which are seizures associated with fevers but without evidence of CNS infection or other defined causes. The overall prevalence is 3–5% and even higher in some parts of the world, such as Asia. Patients often have a family history of febrile seizures or epilepsy. Febrile seizures usually occur between 3 months and 5 years of age and have a

TABLE 363-4	CAUSES OF SEIZURES
Neonates (<1 month)	Perinatal hypoxia and ischemia
	Intracranial hemorrhage and trauma
	Acute CNS infection
	Metabolic disturbances (hypoglycemia, hypocalcemia, hypomagnesemia, pyridoxine deficiency)
	Drug withdrawal
	Developmental disorders
	Genetic disorders
Infants and children (>1 mo and <12 years)	Febrile seizures
	Genetic disorders (metabolic, degenerative, primary epilepsy syndromes)
	CNS infection
	Developmental disorders
	Trauma
	Idiopathic
Adolescents (12–18 years)	Trauma
	Genetic disorders
	Infection
	Brain tumor
	Illicit drug use
	Idiopathic
Young adults (18–35 years)	Trauma
	Alcohol withdrawal
	Illicit drug use
	Brain tumor
	Idiopathic
Older adults (>35 years)	Cerebrovascular disease
	Brain tumor
	Alcohol withdrawal
	Metabolic disorders (uremia, hepatic failure, electrolyte abnormalities, hypoglycemia)
	Alzheimer's disease and other degenerative CNS diseases
	Idiopathic

Note: CNS, central nervous system.

peak incidence between 18 and 24 months. The typical scenario is a child who has a generalized, tonic-clonic seizure during a febrile illness in the setting of a common childhood infection such as otitis media, respiratory infection, or gastroenteritis. The seizure is likely to occur during the rising phase of the temperature curve (i.e., during the first day) rather than well into the course of the illness. A *simple* febrile seizure is a single, isolated event, brief, and symmetric in appearance. *Complex* febrile seizures are characterized by repeated seizure activity, duration >15 min, or by focal features. Approximately one-third of patients with febrile seizures will have a recurrence, but <10% have three or more episodes. Recurrences are much more likely when the febrile seizure occurs in the first year of life. Simple febrile seizures are not associated with an increase in the risk of developing epilepsy, while complex febrile seizures have a risk of 2–5%; other risk factors include the presence of preexisting neurologic deficits and a family history of nonfebrile seizures.

Childhood marks the age at which many of the well-defined epilepsy syndromes present. Some children who are otherwise normal develop idiopathic, generalized tonic-clonic seizures without other features that fit into specific syndromes. Temporal lobe epilepsy usually presents in childhood and may be related to mesial temporal lobe sclerosis (as part of the MTLE syndrome) or other focal abnormalities such as cortical dysgenesis. Other types of partial seizures, including those with secondary generalization, may be the relatively late manifestation of a developmental disorder, an acquired lesion such as head trauma, CNS infection (especially viral encephalitis), or very rarely a CNS tumor.

The period of *adolescence and early adulthood* is one of transition during which the idiopathic or genetically based epilepsy syndromes, including JME and juvenile absence epilepsy, become less common, while epilepsies secondary to acquired CNS lesions begin to predominate. Seizures that begin in patients in this age range may be associated with head trauma, CNS infections (including parasitic infections such as cysticercosis), brain tumors, congenital CNS abnormalities, illicit drug use, or alcohol withdrawal.

Head trauma is a common cause of epilepsy in adolescents and adults. The head injury can be caused by a variety of mechanisms, and

TABLE 363-5	DRUGS AND OTHER SUBSTANCES THAT CAN CAUSE SEIZURES

Alkylating agents (e.g., busulfan, chlorambucil)	Psychotropics
	Antidepressants
Antimalarials (chloroquine, mefloquine)	Antipsychotics
	Lithium
Antimicrobials/antivirals	Radiographic contrast agents
β-lactam and related compounds	Theophylline
Quinolones	Sedative-hypnotic drug withdrawal
Acyclovir	Alcohol
Isoniazid	Barbiturates (short-acting)
Ganciclovir	Benzodiazepines (short-acting)
Anesthetics and analgesics	Drugs of abuse
Meperidine	Amphetamine
Tramadol	Cocaine
Local anesthetics	Phencyclidine
Dietary supplements	Methylphenidate
Ephedra (ma huang)	Flumazenil[a]
Gingko	
Immunomodulatory drugs	
Cyclosporine	
OKT3 (monoclonal antibodies to T cells)	
Tacrolimus	
Interferons	

[a]In benzodiazepine-dependent patients.

the likelihood of developing epilepsy is strongly correlated with the severity of the injury. A patient with a penetrating head wound, depressed skull fracture, intracranial hemorrhage, or prolonged posttraumatic coma or amnesia has a 40–50% risk of developing epilepsy, while a patient with a closed head injury and cerebral contusion has a 5–25% risk. Recurrent seizures usually develop within 1 year after head trauma, although intervals of ≥10 years are well known. In controlled studies, mild head injury, defined as a concussion with amnesia or loss of consciousness of <30 min, was found to be associated with only a slightly increased likelihood of epilepsy. Nonetheless, most epileptologists know of patients who have partial seizures within hours or days of a mild head injury and subsequently develop chronic seizures of the same type; such cases may represent rare examples of chronic epilepsy resulting from mild head injury.

The causes of seizures in *older adults* include cerebrovascular disease, trauma (including subdural hematoma), CNS tumors, and degenerative diseases. Cerebrovascular disease may account for ~50% of new cases of epilepsy in patients older than 65. Acute seizures (i.e., occurring at the time of the stroke) are seen more often with embolic rather than hemorrhagic or thrombotic stroke. Chronic seizures typically appear months to years after the initial event and are associated with all forms of stroke.

Metabolic disturbances such as electrolyte imbalance, hypo- or hyperglycemia, renal failure, and hepatic failure may cause seizures at any age. Similarly, endocrine disorders, hematologic disorders, vasculitides, and many other systemic diseases may cause seizures over a broad age range. A wide variety of medications and abused substances are known to precipitate seizures as well (Table 363-5).

BASIC MECHANISMS

MECHANISMS OF SEIZURE INITIATION AND PROPAGATION

Partial seizure activity can begin in a very discrete region of cortex and then spread to neighboring regions, i.e., there is a *seizure initiation* phase and a *seizure propagation* phase. The initiation phase is characterized by two concurrent events in an aggregate of neurons: (1) high-frequency bursts of action potentials and (2) hypersynchronization. The bursting activity is caused by a relatively long-lasting depolarization of the neuronal membrane due to influx of extracellular calcium (Ca^{2+}), which leads to the opening of voltage-dependent sodium (Na^+) channels, influx of Na^+, and generation of repetitive action potentials. This is followed by a hyperpolarizing afterpotential mediated by γ-aminobutyric acid (GABA) receptors or potassium (K^+) channels, depending on

the cell type. The synchronized bursts from a sufficient number of neurons result in a so-called spike discharge on the EEG.

Normally, the spread of bursting activity is prevented by intact hyperpolarization and a region of surrounding inhibition created by inhibitory neurons. With sufficient activation there is a recruitment of surrounding neurons via a number of mechanisms. Repetitive discharges lead to the following: (1) an increase in extracellular K^+, which blunts hyperpolarization and depolarizes neighboring neurons; (2) accumulation of Ca^{2+} in presynaptic terminals, leading to enhanced neurotransmitter release; and (3) depolarization-induced activation of the *N*-methyl-D-aspartate (NMDA) subtype of the excitatory amino acid receptor, which causes Ca^{2+} influx and neuronal activation. The recruitment of a sufficient number of neurons leads to a loss of the surrounding inhibition and propagation of seizure activity into contiguous areas via local cortical connections, and to more distant areas via long commissural pathways such as the corpus callosum.

Many factors control neuronal excitability, and thus there are many potential mechanisms for altering a neuron's propensity to have bursting activity. Mechanisms *intrinsic* to the neuron include changes in the conductance of ion channels, response characteristics of membrane receptors, cytoplasmic buffering, second-messenger systems, and protein expression as determined by gene transcription, translation, and posttranslational modification. Mechanisms *extrinsic* to the neuron include changes in the amount or type of neurotransmitters present at the synapse, modulation of receptors by extracellular ions and other molecules, and temporal and spatial properties of synaptic and nonsynaptic input. Nonneural cells, such as astrocytes and oligodendrocytes, have an important role in many of these mechanisms as well.

Certain recognized causes of seizures are explained by these mechanisms. For example, accidental ingestion of domoic acid, which is an analogue of glutamate (the principal excitatory neurotransmitter in the brain), causes profound seizures via direct activation of excitatory amino acid receptors throughout the CNS. Penicillin, which can lower the seizure threshold in humans and is a potent convulsant in experimental models, reduces inhibition by antagonizing the effects of GABA at its receptor. The basic mechanisms of other precipitating factors of seizures, such as sleep deprivation, fever, alcohol withdrawal, hypoxia, and infection, are not as well understood but presumably involve analogous perturbations in neuronal excitability. Similarly, the endogenous factors that determine an individual's seizure threshold may relate to these properties as well.

Knowledge of the mechanisms responsible for initiation and propagation of most generalized seizures (including tonic-clonic, myoclonic, and atonic types) remains rudimentary and reflects the limited understanding of the connectivity of the brain at a systems level. Much more is understood about the origin of generalized spike-and-wave discharges in absence seizures. These appear to be related to oscillatory rhythms normally generated during sleep by circuits connecting the thalamus and cortex. This oscillatory behavior involves an interaction between $GABA_B$ receptors, T-type Ca^{2+} channels, and K^+ channels located within the thalamus. Pharmacologic studies indicate that modulation of these receptors and channels can induce absence seizures, and there is speculation that the genetic forms of absence epilepsy may be associated with mutations of components of this system.

MECHANISMS OF EPILEPTOGENESIS

Epileptogenesis refers to the transformation of a normal neuronal network into one that is chronically hyperexcitable. There is often a delay of months to years between an initial CNS injury such as trauma, stroke, or infection and the first seizure. The injury appears to initiate a process that gradually lowers the seizure threshold in the affected region until a spontaneous seizure occurs. In many genetic and idiopathic forms of epilepsy, epileptogenesis is presumably determined by developmentally regulated events.

Pathologic studies of the hippocampus from patients with temporal lobe epilepsy have led to the suggestion that some forms of epileptogenesis are related to *structural changes in neuronal networks*. For example, many patients with MTLE have a highly selective loss of neurons that may contribute to inhibition of the main excitatory neurons within the dentate gyrus. There is also evidence that, in response to the loss of neurons, there is reorganization or "sprouting" of surviving neurons in a way that affects the excitability of the network. Some of these changes can be seen in experimental models of prolonged electrical seizures or traumatic brain injury. Thus, an initial injury such as head injury may lead to a very focal, confined region of structural change that causes local hyperexcitability. The local hyperexcitability leads to further structural changes that evolve over time until the focal lesion produces clinically evident seizures. Similar models have also provided strong evidence for long-term alterations in *intrinsic, biochemical properties of cells* within the network, such as chronic changes in glutamate or GABA receptor function.

GENETIC CAUSES OF EPILEPSY

The most important recent progress in epilepsy research has been the identification of genetic mutations associated with a variety of epilepsy syndromes (Table 363-2). Although all of the mutations identified to date cause rare forms of epilepsy, their discovery has led to extremely important conceptual advances. For example, it appears that many of the inherited, idiopathic epilepsies (i.e., the relatively "pure" forms of epilepsy in which seizures are the phenotypic abnormality and brain structure and function are otherwise normal) are due to mutations affecting ion channel function. These syndromes are therefore part of the larger group of channelopathies causing paroxysmal disorders such as cardiac arrhythmias, episodic ataxia, periodic weakness, and familial hemiplegic migraine. In contrast, gene mutations observed in symptomatic epilepsies (i.e., disorders in which other neurologic abnormalities, such as cognitive impairment, coexist with seizures) are proving to be associated with pathways influencing CNS development or neuronal homeostasis. A current challenge is to identify the multiple susceptibility genes that underlie the more common forms of idiopathic epilepsies.

MECHANISMS OF ACTION OF ANTIEPILEPTIC DRUGS

Antiepileptic drugs appear to act primarily by blocking the initiation or spread of seizures. This occurs through a variety of mechanisms that modify the activity of ion channels or neurotransmitters, and in most cases the drugs have pleiotropic effects. The mechanisms include inhibition of Na^+-dependent action potentials in a frequency-dependent manner (e.g., phenytoin, carbamazepine, lamotrigine, topiramate, zonisamide), inhibition of voltage-gated Ca^{2+} channels (phenytoin), decrease of glutamate release (lamotrigine), potentiation of GABA receptor function (benzodiazepines and barbiturates), increase in the availability of GABA (valproic acid, gabapentin, tiagabine), and modulation of release of synaptic vesicles (levetiracetam). The two most effective drugs for absence seizures, ethosuximide and valproic acid, probably act by inhibiting T-type Ca^{2+} channels in thalamic neurons.

In contrast to the relatively large number of antiepileptic drugs that can attenuate seizure activity, there are currently no drugs known to prevent the formation of a seizure focus following CNS injury. The eventual development of such "antiepileptogenic" drugs will provide an important means of preventing the emergence of epilepsy following injuries such as head trauma, stroke, and CNS infection.

APPROACH TO THE PATIENT:
Seizure

When a patient presents shortly after a seizure, the first priorities are attention to vital signs, respiratory and cardiovascular support, and treatment of seizures if they resume (see "Rx: Seizures and Epilepsy"). Life-threatening conditions such as CNS infection, metabolic derangement, or drug toxicity must be recognized and managed appropriately.

When the patient is not acutely ill, the evaluation will initially focus on whether there is a history of earlier seizures (Fig. 363-2). If this is the first seizure, then the emphasis will be to (1) establish whether the reported episode was a seizure rather than another paroxysmal event, (2) determine the cause of the seizure by identifying risk factors and precipitating events, and (3) decide whether anticonvulsant therapy is required in addition to treatment for any underlying illness.

In the patient with prior seizures or a known history of epilepsy, the evaluation is directed toward (1) identification of the underlying cause and precipitating factors, and (2) determination of the adequacy of the patient's current therapy.

HISTORY AND EXAMINATION

The first goal is to determine whether the event was truly a seizure. An in-depth history is essential, for *in many cases the diagnosis of a seizure is based solely on clinical grounds—the examination and laboratory studies are often normal*. Questions should focus on the symptoms before, during, and after the episode in order to differentiate a seizure from other paroxysmal events (see "Differential Diagnosis of Seizures" below). Seizures frequently occur out-of-hospital, and the patient may be unaware of the ictal and immediate postictal phases; thus, witnesses to the event should be interviewed carefully.

The history should also focus on risk factors and predisposing events. Clues for a predisposition to seizures include a history of febrile seizures, earlier auras or brief seizures not recognized as such, and a family history of seizures. Epileptogenic factors such as prior head trauma, stroke, tumor, or infection of the nervous system should be identified. In children, a careful assessment of developmental milestones may provide evidence for underlying CNS disease. Precipitating factors such as sleep deprivation, systemic diseases, electrolyte or metabolic derangements, acute infection, drugs that lower the seizure threshold (Table 363-5), or alcohol or illicit drug use should also be identified.

The general physical examination includes a search for signs of infection or systemic illness. Careful examination of the skin may reveal signs of neurocutaneous disorders, such as tuberous sclerosis or neurofibromatosis, or chronic liver or renal disease. A finding of organomegaly may indicate a metabolic storage disease, and limb asymmetry may provide a clue to brain injury early in development. Signs of head trauma and use of alcohol or illicit drugs should be sought. Auscultation of the heart and carotid arteries may identify an abnormality that predisposes to cerebrovascular disease.

All patients require a complete neurologic examination, with particular emphasis on eliciting signs of cerebral hemispheric disease (Chap. 361). Careful assessment of mental status (including memory, language function, and abstract thinking) may suggest lesions in the anterior frontal, parietal, or temporal lobes. Testing of visual fields will help screen for lesions in the optic pathways and occipital lobes. Screening tests of motor function such as pronator drift, deep tendon reflexes, gait, and coordination may suggest lesions in motor (frontal) cortex, and cortical sensory testing (e.g., double simultaneous stimulation) may detect lesions in the parietal cortex.

LABORATORY STUDIES

Routine blood studies are indicated to identify the more common metabolic causes of seizures, such as abnormalities in electrolytes, glucose, calcium, or magnesium, and hepatic or renal disease. A screen for toxins in blood and urine should also be obtained from all patients in appropriate risk groups, especially when no clear precipitating factor has been identified. A lumbar puncture is indicated if there is any suspicion of meningitis or encephalitis, and it is mandatory in all patients infected with HIV, even in the absence of symptoms or signs suggesting infection.

ELECTROPHYSIOLOGIC STUDIES

All patients who have a possible seizure disorder should be evaluated with an EEG as soon as possible. Details about the EEG are covered in Chap. e31.

In the evaluation of a patient with suspected epilepsy, the presence of *electrographic seizure activity* during the clinically evident event—i.e., abnormal, repetitive, rhythmic activity having an abrupt onset and termination—clearly establishes the diagnosis. The absence of electrographic seizure activity does not exclude a seizure disorder, however, because simple or complex seizures may originate from a region of the cortex that is not within range of the scalp electrodes. The EEG is always abnormal during generalized tonic-clonic seizures. Since seizures are typically infrequent and unpredictable, it is often

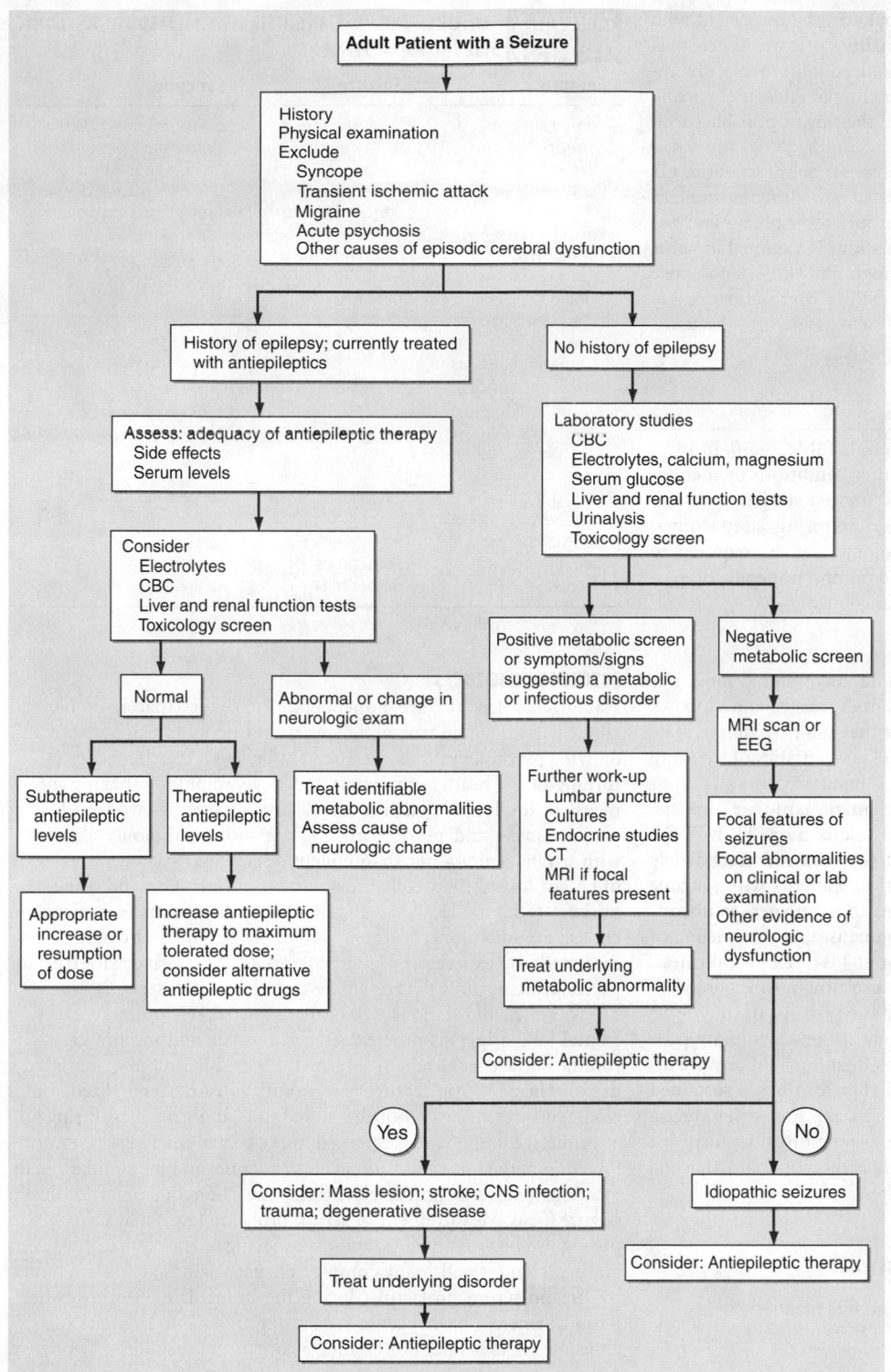

FIGURE 363-2 Evaluation of the adult patient with a seizure. CBC, complete blood count; CT, computed tomography; MRI, magnetic resonance imaging; EEG, electroencephalogram; CNS, central nervous system.

ity of the brain, it measures the small magnetic fields that are generated by this activity. Epileptiform activity seen on the MEG can be analyzed, and its source in the brain can be estimated using a variety of mathematical techniques. These source estimates can then be plotted on an anatomic image of the brain, such as an MRI (discussed below), to generate a magnetic source image (MSI). MSI can be useful to localize potential seizure foci.

The EEG may also be helpful in the interictal period by showing certain abnormalities that are highly supportive of the diagnosis of epilepsy. Such *epileptiform activity* consists of bursts of abnormal discharges containing spikes or sharp waves. The presence of epileptiform activity is not specific for epilepsy, but it has a much greater prevalence in patients with epilepsy than in normal individuals. However, even in an individual who is known to have epilepsy, the initial routine interictal EEG may be normal up to 60% of the time. Thus, the EEG cannot establish the diagnosis of epilepsy in many cases.

The EEG is also used for classifying seizure disorders and aiding in the selection of anticonvulsant medications. For example, episodic generalized spike-wave activity is usually seen in patients with typical absence epilepsy and may be seen with other generalized epilepsy syndromes. Focal interictal epileptiform discharges would support the diagnosis of a partial seizure disorder such as temporal lobe epilepsy or frontal lobe seizures, depending on the location of the discharges.

The routine scalp-recorded EEG may also be used to assess the prognosis of seizure disorders; in general, a normal EEG implies a better prognosis, whereas an abnormal background or profuse epileptiform activity suggests a poor outlook. Unfortunately, the EEG has not proved to be useful in predicting which patients with predisposing conditions, such as head injury or brain tumor, will go on to develop epilepsy, because in such circumstances epileptiform activity is commonly encountered regardless of whether seizures occur.

BRAIN IMAGING

Almost all patients with new-onset seizures should have a brain imaging study to determine whether there is an underlying structural abnormality that is responsible. The only potential exception to this rule is children who have an unambiguous history and examination suggestive of a benign, generalized seizure disorder such as absence epilepsy. MRI has been shown to be superior to CT for the detection of cerebral lesions associated with epilepsy. In some cases MRI will identify lesions such as tumors, vascular malformations, or other pathologies that need immediate therapy. The use of newer MRI methods, such as fluid-attenuated inversion recovery (FLAIR), has increased the sensitivity for detection of abnormalities of

not possible to obtain the EEG during a clinical event. Continuous monitoring for prolonged periods in video-EEG telemetry units for hospitalized patients or the use of portable equipment to record the EEG continuously on cassettes for ≥24 h in ambulatory patients has made it easier to capture the electrophysiologic accompaniments of clinical events. In particular, video-EEG telemetry is now a routine approach for the accurate diagnosis of epilepsy in patients with poorly characterized events or seizures that are difficult to control.

Magnetoencephalography (MEG) provides another way of looking noninvasively at cortical activity. Instead of measuring electrical activcortical architecture, including hippocampal atrophy associated with mesial temporal sclerosis, as well as abnormalities of cortical neuronal migration. In such cases the findings may not lead to immediate therapy, but they do provide an explanation for the patient's seizures and point to the need for chronic anticonvulsant therapy or possible surgical resection.

In the patient with a suspected CNS infection or mass lesion, CT scanning should be performed emergently when MRI is not immediately available. Otherwise, it is usually appropriate to obtain an MRI study within a few days of the initial evaluation. Functional imaging procedures such as positron emission tomography (PET) and single photon emission computed tomography (SPECT) are also used to evaluate certain patients with medically refractory seizures (discussed below).

DIFFERENTIAL DIAGNOSIS OF SEIZURES

Disorders that may mimic seizures are listed in Table 363-6. In most cases seizures can be distinguished from other conditions by meticulous attention to the history and relevant laboratory studies. On occasion, additional studies, such as video-EEG monitoring, sleep studies, tilt-table analysis, or cardiac electrophysiology, may be required to reach a correct diagnosis. Two of the more common nonepileptic syndromes in the differential diagnosis are detailed below.

SYNCOPE

(See also Chap. 21) The diagnostic dilemma encountered most frequently is the distinction between a generalized seizure and syncope. Observations by the patient and bystanders that can help differentiate between the two are listed in Table 363-7. Characteristics of a seizure include the presence of an aura, cyanosis, unconsciousness, motor manifestations lasting >30 s, postictal disorientation, muscle soreness, and sleepiness. In contrast, a syncopal episode is more likely if the event was provoked by acute pain or anxiety or occurred immediately after arising from the lying or sitting position. Patients with syncope often describe a stereotyped transition from consciousness to unconsciousness that includes tiredness, sweating, nausea, and tunneling of vision, and they experience a relatively brief loss of consciousness. Headache or incontinence usually suggests a seizure but may on occasion also occur with syncope. A brief period (i.e., 1–10 s) of convulsive motor activity is frequently seen immediately at the onset of a syncopal episode, especially if the patient remains in an upright posture after fainting (e.g., in a dentist's chair) and therefore has a sustained decrease in cerebral perfusion. Rarely, a syncopal episode can induce a full tonic-clonic seizure. In such cases the evaluation must focus on both the cause of the syncopal event as well as the possibility that the patient has a propensity for recurrent seizures.

TABLE 363-6   DIFFERENTIAL DIAGNOSIS OF SEIZURES

Syncope	Transient ischemic attack (TIA)
Vasovagal syncope	Basilar artery TIA
Cardiac arrhythmia	Sleep disorders
Valvular heart disease	Narcolepsy/cataplexy
Cardiac failure	Benign sleep myoclonus
Orthostatic hypotension	Movement disorders
Psychological disorders	Tics
Psychogenic seizure	Nonepileptic myoclonus
Hyperventilation	Paroxysmal choreoathetosis
Panic attack	Special considerations in children
Metabolic disturbances	Breath-holding spells
Alcoholic blackouts	Migraine with recurrent abdomi-
Delirium tremens	nal pain and cyclic vomiting
Hypoglycemia	Benign paroxysmal vertigo
Hypoxia	Apnea
Psychoactive drugs (e.g.,	Night terrors
hallucinogens)	Sleepwalking
Migraine	
Confusional migraine	
Basilar migraine	

TABLE 363-7   FEATURES THAT DISTINGUISH GENERALIZED TONIC-CLONIC SEIZURE FROM SYNCOPE

Features	Seizure	Syncope
Immediate precipitating factors	Usually none	Emotional stress, Valsalva, orthostatic hypotension, cardiac etiologies
Premonitory symptoms	None or aura (e.g., odd odor)	Tiredness, nausea, diaphoresis, tunneling of vision
Posture at onset	Variable	Usually erect
Transition to unconsciousness	Often immediate	Gradual over seconds[a]
Duration of unconsciousness	Minutes	Seconds
Duration of tonic or clonic movements	30–60 s	Never more than 15 s
Facial appearance during event	Cyanosis, frothing at mouth	Pallor
Disorientation and sleepiness after event	Many minutes to hours	<5 min
Aching of muscles after event	Often	Sometimes
Biting of tongue	Sometimes	Rarely
Incontinence	Sometimes	Sometimes
Headache	Sometimes	Rarely

[a]May be sudden with certain cardiac arrhythmias.

PSYCHOGENIC SEIZURES

Psychogenic seizures are nonepileptic behaviors that resemble seizures. They are often part of a conversion reaction precipitated by underlying psychological distress. Certain behaviors, such as side-to-side turning of the head, asymmetric and large-amplitude shaking movements of the limbs, twitching of all four extremities without loss of consciousness, and pelvic thrusting are more commonly associated with psychogenic rather than epileptic seizures. Psychogenic seizures often last longer than epileptic seizures and may wax and wane over minutes to hours. However, the distinction is sometimes difficult on clinical grounds alone, and there are many examples of diagnostic errors made by experienced epileptologists. This is especially true for psychogenic seizures that resemble complex partial seizures, since the behavioral manifestations of complex partial seizures (especially of frontal lobe origin) can be extremely unusual, and in both cases the routine surface EEG may be normal. Video-EEG monitoring is very useful when historic features are nondiagnostic. Generalized tonic-clonic seizures always produce marked EEG abnormalities during and after the seizure. For suspected complex partial seizures of temporal lobe origin, the use of additional electrodes beyond the standard scalp locations (e.g., sphenoidal electrodes) may be required to localize a seizure focus. Measurement of serum prolactin levels may also help to distinguish between organic and psychogenic seizures, since most generalized seizures and many complex partial seizures are accompanied by rises in serum prolactin (during the immediate 30-min postictal period), whereas psychogenic seizures are not. The diagnosis of psychogenic seizures does not exclude a concurrent diagnosis of epilepsy, since the two often coexist.

℞ SEIZURES AND EPILEPSY

Therapy for a patient with a seizure disorder is almost always multimodal and includes treatment of underlying conditions that cause or contribute to the seizures, avoidance of precipitating factors, suppression of recurrent seizures by prophylactic therapy with antiepileptic medications or surgery, and addressing a variety of psychological and social issues. Treatment plans must be individualized, given the many different types and causes of seizures as well as the differences in efficacy and toxicity of antiepileptic medications for each patient. In almost all cases a neurologist with experience in the treatment of epilepsy should design and oversee implementation of the treatment strategy. Furthermore, patients with refractory epilepsy or those who require polypharmacy with antiepileptic drugs should remain under the regular care of a neurologist.

TREATMENT OF UNDERLYING CONDITIONS If the sole cause of a seizure is a metabolic disturbance such as an abnormality of serum electrolytes or glucose, then treatment is aimed at reversing the metabolic problem and preventing its recurrence. Therapy with antiepileptic drugs is usually unnecessary unless the metabolic disorder cannot be corrected promptly and the patient is at risk of having further seizures. If the apparent cause of a seizure was a medication (e.g., theophylline) or illicit drug use (e.g., cocaine), then appropriate therapy is avoidance of the drug; there is usually no need for antiepileptic medications unless subsequent seizures occur in the absence of these precipitants.

Seizures caused by a structural CNS lesion such as a brain tumor, vascular malformation, or brain abscess may not recur after appropriate treatment of the underlying lesion. However, despite removal of the structural lesion, there is a risk that the seizure focus will remain in the surrounding tissue or develop de novo as a result of gliosis and other processes induced by surgery, radiation, or other therapies. Most patients are therefore maintained on an antiepileptic medication for at least 1 year, and an attempt is made to withdraw medications only if the patient has been completely seizure-free. If seizures are refractory to medication, the patient may benefit from surgical removal of the epileptic brain region (see below).

AVOIDANCE OF PRECIPITATING FACTORS Unfortunately, little is known about the specific factors that determine precisely when a seizure will occur in a patient with epilepsy. Some patients can identify particular situations that appear to lower their seizure threshold; these situations should be avoided. For example, a patient who has seizures in the setting of sleep deprivation should obviously be advised to maintain a normal sleep schedule. Many patients note an association between alcohol intake and seizures, and they should be encouraged to modify their drinking habits accordingly. There are also relatively rare cases of patients with seizures that are induced by highly specific stimuli such as a video game monitor, music, or an individual's voice ("reflex epilepsy"). If there is an association between stress and seizures, stress reduction techniques such as physical exercise, meditation, or counseling may be helpful.

ANTIEPILEPTIC DRUG THERAPY Antiepileptic drug therapy is the mainstay of treatment for most patients with epilepsy. The overall goal is to completely prevent seizures without causing any untoward side effects, preferably with a single medication and a dosing schedule that is easy for the patient to follow. Seizure classification is an important element in designing the treatment plan, since some antiepileptic drugs have different activities against various seizure types. However, there is considerable overlap between many antiepileptic drugs, such that the choice of therapy is often determined more by the patient's specific needs, especially his/her assessment of side effects.

When to Initiate Antiepileptic Drug Therapy Antiepileptic drug therapy should be started in any patient with recurrent seizures of unknown etiology or a known cause that cannot be reversed. Whether to initiate therapy in a patient with a single seizure is controversial. Patients with a single seizure due to an identified lesion such as a CNS tumor, infection, or trauma, in which there is strong evidence that the lesion is epileptogenic, should be treated. The risk of seizure recurrence in a patient with an apparently unprovoked or idiopathic seizure is uncertain, with estimates ranging from 31 to 71% in the first 12 months after the initial seizure. This uncertainty arises from differences in the underlying seizure types and etiologies in various published epidemiologic studies. Generally accepted risk factors associated with recurrent seizures include the following: (1) an abnormal neurologic examination, (2) seizures presenting as status epilepticus, (3) postictal Todd's paralysis, (4) a strong family history of seizures, or (5) an abnormal EEG. Most patients with one or more of these risk factors should be treated. Issues such as employment or driving may influence the decision whether to start medications as well. For example, a patient with a single, idiopathic seizure whose job depends on driving may prefer taking antiepileptic drugs rather than risk a seizure recurrence and the potential loss of driving privileges.

Selection of Antiepileptic Drugs Antiepileptic drugs available in the United States are shown in **Table 363-8**, and the main pharmacologic characteristics of commonly used drugs are listed in **Table 363-9**. Worldwide, older medications such as phenytoin, valproic acid, carbamazepine, and ethosuximide are generally used as first-line therapy for most seizure disorders since, overall, they are as effective as recently marketed drugs

TABLE 363-8 SELECTION OF ANTIEPILEPTIC DRUGS

Primary Generalized Tonic-Clonic	Partial[a]	Absence	Atypical Absence, Myoclonic, Atonic
First-Line			
Valproic acid Lamotrigine Topiramate	Carbamazepine Phenytoin Lamotrigine Oxcarbazepine Valproic acid	Valproic acid Ethosuximide	Valproic acid Lamotrigine Topiramate
Alternatives			
Zonisamide[b] Phenytoin Carbamazepine Oxcarbazepine Phenobarbital Primidone Felbamate	Levetiracetam[b] Topiramate Tiagabine[b] Zonisamide[b] Gabapentin[b] Phenobarbital Primidone Felbamate	Lamotrigine Clonazepam	Clonazepam Felbamate

[a]Includes simple partial, complex partial, and secondarily generalized seizures.
[b]As adjunctive therapy.

and significantly less expensive. Most of the new drugs that have become available in the past decade are used as add-on or alternative therapy, although some are now being used as first-line monotherapy.

In addition to efficacy, factors influencing the choice of an initial medication include the convenience of dosing (e.g., once daily versus three or four times daily) and potential side effects. In this regard, a number of the newer drugs have the advantage of a relative lack of drug-drug interactions and easier dosing. Almost all of the commonly used antiepileptic drugs can cause similar, dose-related side effects such as sedation, ataxia, and diplopia. Close follow-up is required to ensure these are promptly recognized and reversed. Most of the older drugs and some of the newer ones can also cause idiosyncratic toxicity such as rash, bone marrow suppression, or hepatotoxicity. Although rare, these side effects should be considered during drug selection, and patients must be instructed about symptoms or signs that should signal the need to alert their health care provider. For some drugs, laboratory tests (e.g., complete blood count and liver function tests) are recommended prior to the institution of therapy (to establish baseline values) and during initial dosing and titration of the agent.

Antiepileptic Drug Selection for Partial Seizures Carbamazepine (or a related drug, oxcarbazepine), phenytoin, lamotrigine and topiramate are currently the drugs of choice approved for the initial treatment of partial seizures, including those that secondarily generalize. Overall they have very similar efficacy, but differences in pharmacokinetics and toxicity are the main determinants for use in a given patient. For example, phenytoin has a relatively long half-life and offers the advantage of once or twice daily dosing compared to two or three times daily dosing for many of the other drugs. However, phenytoin shows properties of saturation kinetics, such that small increases in phenytoin doses above a standard maintenance dose can precipitate marked side effects. This is one of the main causes of acute phenytoin toxicity. Long-term use of phenytoin is associated with untoward cosmetic effects (e.g., hirsutism, coarsening of facial features, and gingival hypertrophy), and effects on bone metabolism, so it is often avoided in young patients who are likely to require the drug for many years. An advantage of carbamazepine (which is also available in an extended-release form) is that its metabolism follows first-order pharmacokinetics, and the relationship between drug dose, serum levels, and toxicity is linear. Carbamazepine can cause leukopenia, aplastic anemia, or hepatotoxicity and would therefore be contraindicated in patients with predispositions to these problems. Oxcarbazepine has the advantage of being metabolized in a way that avoids an intermediate metabolite associated with some of the side effects of carbamazepine. Oxcarbazepine also has fewer drug interactions than carbamazepine. Lamotrigine tends to be well-tolerated in terms of side effects. However, patients need to be particularly vigilant about the possibility of a skin rash during the initiation of therapy. This can be extremely severe and lead to Stevens-Johnson syndrome if unrecognized and if the medication is not discontinued immedi-

TABLE 363-9 DOSAGE AND ADVERSE EFFECTS OF COMMONLY USED ANTIEPILEPTIC DRUGS

Generic Name	Trade Name	Principal Uses	Typical Dose; Dose Interval	Half-Life	Therapeutic Range	Adverse Effects		Drug Interactions
						Neurologic	Systemic	
Phenytoin (diphenyl-hydantoin)	Dilantin	Tonic-clonic (grand mal) Focal-onset	300–400 mg/d (3–6 mg/kg, adult; 4–8 mg/kg, child); qd-bid	24 h (wide variation, dose-dependent)	10–20 μg/mL	Dizziness Diplopia Ataxia Incoordination Confusion	Gum hyperplasia Lymphade-nopathy Hirsutism Osteomalacia Facial coarsening Skin rash	Level increased by isoniazid, sulfonamides, fluoxetine Level decreased by enzyme-inducing drugs[a] Altered folate metabolism
Carbamaze-pine	Tegretol Carbatrol	Tonic-clonic Focal-onset	600–1800 mg/d (15–35 mg/kg, child); bid-qid	10–17 h	6–12 μg/mL	Ataxia Dizziness Diplopia Vertigo	Aplastic anemia Leukopenia Gastrointesti-nal irritation Hepatotoxicity Hyponatremia	Level decreased by enzyme-inducing drugs[a] Level increased by erythromycin, propoxyphene, isoniazid, cimeti-dine, fluoxetine
Valproic acid	Depakene Depakote Depakote ER	Tonic-clonic Absence Atypical absence Myoclonic Focal-onset	750–2000 mg/d (20–60 mg/kg); bid-qid	15 h	50–125 μg/mL	Ataxia Sedation Tremor	Hepatotoxicity Thrombocyto-penia Gastrointesti-nal irritation Weight gain Transient alopecia Hyperam-monemia	Level decreased by enzyme-inducing drugs[a]
Lamotrigine	Lamictal	Focal-onset Tonic-clonic Atypical absence Myoclonic Lennox-Gastaut syndrome	150–500 mg/d; bid	25 h 14 h (with enzyme-inducers) 59 h (with val-proic acid)	Not established	Dizziness Diplopia Sedation Ataxia Headache	Skin rash Stevens-Johnson syndrome	Level decreased by enzyme-inducing drugs[a] and oral contraceptives Level increased by valproic acid
Ethosuxi-mide	Zarontin	Absence (petit mal)	750–1250 mg/d (20–40 mg/kg); qd-bid	60 h, adult 30 h, child	40–100 μg/mL	Ataxia Lethargy Headache	Gastrointesti-nal irritation Skin rash Bone marrow suppression	
Gabapentin	Neurontin	Focal-onset	900–2400 mg/d; tid-qid	5–9 h	Not established	Sedation Dizziness Ataxia Fatigue	Gastrointesti-nal irritation Weight gain Edema	No known significant interactions
Topiramate	Topamax	Focal-onset Tonic-clonic Lennox-Gastaut syndrome	200–400 mg/d; bid	20–30 h	Not established	Psychomotor slowing Sedation Speech or language problems Fatigue Paresthesias	Renal stones (avoid use with other carbonic anhydrase inhibitors) Glaucoma Weight loss Hypohydrosis	Level decreased by enzyme-inducing drugs[a]
Tiagabine	Gabitril	Focal-onset Tonic-clonic	32–56 mg/d; bid-qid	7–9 h	Not established	Confusion Sedation Depression Dizziness Speech or language problems Paresthesias Psychosis	Gastrointesti-nal irritation	Level decreased by enzyme-inducing drugs[a]
Phenobar-bital	Luminol	Tonic-clonic Focal-onset	60–180 mg/d (1–4 mg/kg, adult); (3–6 mg/kg, child); qd	90 h (70 h in children)	10–40 μg/mL	Sedation Ataxia Confusion Dizziness Decreased libido Depression	Skin rash	Level increased by valproic acid, phenytoin
Primidone	Mysoline	Tonic-clonic Focal-onset	750–1000 mg/d (10–25 mg/kg); bid-tid	Primidone, 8–15 h Phenobarbital, 90 h	Primidone, 4–12 μg/mL Phenobarbital, 10–40 μg/mL	Same as pheno-barbital		

(continued)

Generic Name	Trade Name	Principal Uses	Typical Dose; Dose Interval	Half-Life	Therapeutic Range	Adverse Effects		Drug Interactions
						Neurologic	Systemic	
Clonazepam	Klonopin	Absence Atypical absence Myoclonic	1–12 mg/d (0.1–0.2 mg/kg); qd-tid	24–48 h	10–70 ng/mL	Ataxia Sedation Lethargy	Anorexia	Level decreased by enzyme-inducing drugs[a]
Felbamate	Felbatol	Focal-onset Lennox-Gastaut syndrome	2400–3600 mg/d, (45 mg/kg, child); tid-qid	16–22 h	Not established	Insomnia Dizziness Sedation Headache	Aplastic anemia Hepatic failure Weight loss Gastrointestinal irritation	Increases phenytoin, valproic acid, active carbamazepine metabolite
Levetirace-tam	Keppra	Focal-onset	1000–3000 mg/d; bid	6–8 h	Not established	Sedation Fatigue Incoordination Psychosis	Anemia Leukopenia	None known
Zonisamide	Zonegran	Focal-onset	200–400 mg/d; qd-bid	50–68 h	Not established	Sedation Dizziness Confusion Headache Psychosis	Anorexia Renal stones Hypohydrosis	Level decreased by enzyme-inducing drugs[a]
Oxcarbaz-epine	Trileptal	Focal-onset	900–2400 mg/d (30–45 mg/kg, child); bid	10–17 h (for active metabolite)	Not established	Fatigue Ataxia Dizziness Diplopia Vertigo Headache	See carbamaz-epine	Level decreased by enzyme-inducing drugs[a] May increase phenytoin

[a]Phenytoin, carbamazepine, phenobarbital.

ately. This risk can be reduced by slow introduction and titration. Lamotrigine must be started slowly when used as add-on therapy with valproic acid, since valproic acid inhibits lamotrigine metabolism, thereby substantially prolonging its half-life. Topiramate has recently been approved as monotherapy for partial and primary generalized seizures. Similar to some of the other antiepileptic drugs, topiramate can cause significant psychomotor slowing and other cognitive problems, and it should not be used in patients at risk for the development of glaucoma or renal stones.

Valproic acid is an effective alternative for some patients with partial seizures, especially when the seizures secondarily generalize. Gastrointestinal side effects are fewer when using the valproate semisodium formulation (Depakote). Valproic acid also rarely causes reversible bone marrow suppression and hepatotoxicity, and laboratory testing is required to monitor toxicity. This drug should generally be avoided in patients with preexisting bone marrow or liver disease. Irreversible, fatal hepatic failure appearing as an idiosyncratic rather than dose-related side effect is a relatively rare complication; its risk is highest in children <2 years old, especially those taking other antiepileptic drugs or with inborn errors of metabolism.

Levetiracetam, tiagabine, zonisamide, and gabapentin are additional drugs currently used for the treatment of partial seizures with or without secondary generalization. Phenobarbital and other barbiturate compounds were commonly used in the past as first-line therapy for many forms of epilepsy. However, the barbiturates frequently cause sedation in adults, hyperactivity in children, and other more subtle cognitive changes; thus, their use should be limited to situations in which no other suitable treatment alternatives exist.

Antiepileptic Drug Selection for Generalized Seizures   Valproic acid and lamotrigine are currently considered the best initial choice for the treatment of primary generalized, tonic-clonic seizures. Phenytoin, followed by topiramate, carbamazepine, and zonisamide are suitable alternatives. Valproic acid is also particularly effective in absence, myoclonic, and atonic seizures and is therefore the drug of choice in patients with generalized epilepsy syndromes having mixed seizure types. Importantly, both carbamazepine and phenytoin can worsen certain types of generalized seizures, including absence, myoclonic, tonic, and atonic seizures. Ethosuximide is a particularly effective drug for the treatment of uncomplicated absence seizures, but it is not useful for tonic-clonic or partial seizures.

Ethosuximide rarely causes bone marrow suppression, so that periodic monitoring of blood cell counts is required. Lamotrigine appears to be particularly effective in epilepsy syndromes with mixed, generalized seizure types such as JME and Lennox-Gastaut syndrome. Topiramate, zonisamide, and felbamate may have similar broad efficacy.

Initiation and Monitoring of Therapy   Because the response to any antiepileptic drug is unpredictable, patients should be carefully educated about the approach to therapy. The goal is to prevent seizures and minimize the side effects of therapy; determination of the optimal dose is often a matter of trial and error. This process may take months or longer if the baseline seizure frequency is low. Most anticonvulsant drugs need to be introduced relatively slowly to minimize side effects, and patients should expect that minor side effects such as mild sedation, slight changes in cognition, or imbalance will typically resolve within a few days. Starting doses are usually the lowest value listed under the dosage column in Table 363-9. Subsequent increases should be made only after achieving a steady state with the previous dose (i.e., after an interval of five or more half-lives).

Monitoring of serum antiepileptic drug levels can be very useful for establishing the initial dosing schedule. However, the published therapeutic ranges of serum drug concentrations are only an approximate guide for determining the proper dose for a given patient. The key determinants are the clinical measures of seizure frequency and presence of side effects, not the laboratory values. Conventional assays of serum drug levels measure the total drug (i.e., both free and protein-bound). However, it is the concentration of free drug that reflects extracellular levels in the brain and correlates best with efficacy. Thus, patients with decreased levels of serum proteins (e.g., decreased serum albumin due to impaired liver or renal function) may have an increased ratio of free to bound drug, yet the concentration of free drug may be adequate for seizure control. These patients may have a "subtherapeutic" drug level, but the dose should be changed only if seizures remain uncontrolled, not just to achieve a "therapeutic" level. It is also useful to monitor free drug levels in such patients. In practice, other than during the initiation or modification of therapy, monitoring of antiepileptic drug levels is most useful for documenting compliance.

If seizures continue despite gradual increases to the maximum tolerated dose and documented compliance, then it becomes necessary to switch to another antiepileptic drug. This is usually done by maintaining the patient on the first drug while a second drug is added. The dose of the

CHAPTER 363 Seizures and Epilepsy

second drug should be adjusted to decrease seizure frequency without causing toxicity. Once this is achieved, the first drug can be gradually withdrawn (usually over weeks unless there is significant toxicity). The dose of the second drug is then further optimized based on seizure response and side effects. Monotherapy should be the goal whenever possible.

When to Discontinue Therapy   Overall, about 70% of children and 60% of adults who have their seizures completely controlled with antiepileptic drugs can eventually discontinue therapy. The following patient profile yields the greatest chance of remaining seizure-free after drug withdrawal: (1) complete medical control of seizures for 1–5 years; (2) single seizure type, either partial or generalized; (3) normal neurologic examination, including intelligence; and (4) normal EEG. The appropriate seizure-free interval is unknown and undoubtedly varies for different forms of epilepsy. However, it seems reasonable to attempt withdrawal of therapy after 2 years in a patient who meets all of the above criteria, is motivated to discontinue the medication, and clearly understands the potential risks and benefits. In most cases it is preferable to reduce the dose of the drug gradually over 2–3 months. Most recurrences occur in the first 3 months after discontinuing therapy, and patients should be advised to avoid potentially dangerous situations such as driving or swimming during this period.

Treatment of Refractory Epilepsy   Approximately one-third of patients with epilepsy do not respond to treatment with a single antiepileptic drug, and it becomes necessary to try a combination of drugs to control seizures. Patients who have focal epilepsy related to an underlying structural lesion or those with multiple seizure types and developmental delay are particularly likely to require multiple drugs. There are currently no clear guidelines for rational polypharmacy, although in theory a combination of drugs with different mechanisms of action may be most useful. In most cases the initial combination therapy combines first-line drugs, i.e., carbamazepine, phenytoin, valproic acid, and lamotrigine. If these drugs are unsuccessful, then the addition of a newer drug such as levetiracetam or topiramate is indicated. Patients with myoclonic seizures resistant to valproic acid may benefit from the addition of clonazepam, and those with absence seizures may respond to a combination of valproic acid and ethosuximide. The same principles concerning the monitoring of therapeutic response, toxicity, and serum levels for monotherapy apply to polypharmacy, and potential drug interactions need to be recognized. If there is no improvement, a third drug can be added while the first two are maintained. If there is a response, the less effective or less well-tolerated of the first two drugs should be gradually withdrawn.

SURGICAL TREATMENT OF REFRACTORY EPILEPSY   Approximately 20–30% of patients with epilepsy are resistant to medical therapy despite efforts to find an effective combination of antiepileptic drugs. For some, surgery can be extremely effective in substantially reducing seizure frequency and even providing complete seizure control. Understanding the potential value of surgery is especially important when, at the time of diagnosis, a patient has an epilepsy syndrome that is considered likely to be drug-resistant. Rather than submitting the patient to years of unsuccessful medical therapy and the psychosocial trauma and increased mortality associated with ongoing seizures, the patient should have an efficient but relatively brief attempt at medical therapy and then be referred for surgical evaluation.

The most common surgical procedure for patients with temporal lobe epilepsy involves resection of the anteromedial temporal lobe (temporal lobectomy) or a more limited removal of the underlying hippocampus and amygdala (amygdalohippocampectomy). Focal seizures arising from extratemporal regions may be abolished by a focal neocortical resection with precise removal of an identified lesion (lesionectomy). When the cortical region cannot be removed, multiple subpial transection, which disrupts intracortical connections, is sometimes used to prevent seizure spread. Hemispherectomy or multilobar resection is useful for some patients with severe seizures due to hemispheric abnormalities such as hemimegalencephaly or other dysplastic abnormalities, and corpus callosotomy has been shown to be effective for disabling tonic or atonic seizures, usually when they are part of a mixed-seizure syndrome (e.g., Lennox-Gastaut syndrome).

Presurgical evaluation is designed to identify the functional and structural basis of the patient's seizure disorder. Inpatient video-EEG monitoring is used to define the anatomic location of the seizure focus and to correlate the abnormal electrophysiologic activity with behavioral manifestations of the seizure. Routine scalp or scalp-sphenoidal recordings are usually suffi-

cient for localization, and advances in neuroimaging have made the use of invasive electrophysiologic monitoring such as implanted depth electrodes or subdural electrodes less common. A high-resolution MRI scan is routinely used to identify structural lesions, and this is sometimes augmented with MEG. Functional imaging studies such as SPECT and PET are adjunctive tests that may help verify the localization of an apparent epileptogenic region. Once the presumed location of the seizure onset is identified, additional studies, including neuropsychological testing and the intracarotid amobarbital test (Wada test) may be used to assess language and memory localization and to determine the possible functional consequences of surgical removal of the epileptogenic region. In some cases, the exact extent of the resection to be undertaken is determined by performing cortical mapping at the time of the surgical procedure, allowing for a tailored resection. This involves electrocorticographic recordings made with electrodes on the surface of the brain to identify the extent of epileptiform disturbances. If the region to be resected is within or near brain regions suspected of having sensorimotor or language function, electrical cortical stimulation mapping is performed on the awake patient to determine the function of cortical regions in question in order to avoid resection of so-called eloquent cortex and thereby minimize postsurgical deficits.

Advances in presurgical evaluation and microsurgical techniques have led to a steady increase in the success of epilepsy surgery. Clinically significant complications of surgery are <5%, and the use of functional mapping procedures has markedly reduced the neurologic sequelae due to removal or sectioning of brain tissue. For example, about 70% of patients treated with temporal lobectomy will become seizure-free, and another 15–25% will have at least a 90% reduction in seizure frequency. Marked improvement is also usually seen in patients treated with hemispherectomy for catastrophic seizure disorders due to large hemispheric abnormalities. Postoperatively, patients generally need to remain on antiepileptic drug therapy, but the marked reduction of seizures following resective surgery can have a very beneficial effect on quality of life.

Not all medically refractory patients are suitable candidates for resective surgery. For example, some patients have seizures arising from more than one site, making the risk of ongoing seizures or potential harm from the surgery unacceptably high. Vagus nerve stimulation (VNS) may be useful in some of these cases, although the benefit for most patients seems to be very limited; i.e., the efficacy of VNS appears to be no greater than trying another drug, which rarely works if a patient has proved to be refractory to the first two to three drugs. The precise mechanism of action of VNS is unknown, although experimental studies have shown that stimulation of vagal nuclei leads to widespread activation of cortical and subcortical pathways and an associated increased seizure threshold. Adverse effects of the surgery are rare, and stimulation-induced side effects, including transient hoarseness, cough, and dyspnea, are usually mild.

Although still in development, there are some additional therapies that will likely be of benefit to patients with medically refractory epilepsy. Preliminary studies suggest that stereotactic radiosurgery may be effective in certain partial seizure disorders. There has also been great interest in the development of implantable devices that can detect the onset of a seizure (in some instances, before the seizure becomes clinically apparent) and deliver either an electrical stimulation or drug directly to the seizure focus to abort the event.

STATUS EPILEPTICUS

Status epilepticus refers to continuous seizures or repetitive, discrete seizures with impaired consciousness in the interictal period. Status epilepticus has numerous subtypes, including generalized convulsive status epilepticus (GCSE) (e.g., persistent, generalized electrographic seizures, coma, and tonic-clonic movements), and nonconvulsive status epilepticus (e.g., persistent absence seizures or partial seizures, confusion or partially impaired consciousness, and minimal motor abnormalities). The duration of seizure activity sufficient to meet the definition of status epilepticus has traditionally been specified as 15–30 min. However, a more practical definition is to consider status epilepticus as a situation in which the duration of seizures prompts the acute use of anticonvulsant therapy. For GCSE, this is typically when seizures last beyond 5 min.

GCSE is an emergency and must be treated immediately, since cardiorespiratory dysfunction, hyperthermia, and metabolic derangements can develop as a consequence of prolonged seizures, and these can lead to irreversible neuronal injury. Furthermore, CNS injury can occur even when the patient is paralyzed with neuromuscular blockade but continues to have electrographic seizures. The most common causes of GCSE are anticonvulsant withdrawal or noncompliance, metabolic disturbances, drug toxicity, CNS infection, CNS tumors, refractory epilepsy, and head trauma.

GCSE is obvious when the patient is having overt convulsions. However, after 30–45 min of uninterrupted seizures, the signs may become increasingly subtle. Patients may have mild clonic movements of only the fingers or fine, rapid movements of the eyes. There may be paroxysmal episodes of tachycardia, hypertension, and pupillary dilation. In such cases, the EEG may be the only method of establishing the diagnosis. Thus, if the patient stops having overt seizures, yet remains comatose, an EEG should be performed to rule out ongoing status epilepticus. This is obviously also essential when a patient with GCSE has been paralyzed with neuromuscular blockade in the process of protecting the airway.

The first step in the management of a patient in GCSE is to attend to any acute cardiorespiratory problems or hyperthermia, perform a brief medical and neurologic examination, establish venous access, and send samples for laboratory studies to identify metabolic abnormalities. Anticonvulsant therapy should then begin without delay; a treatment approach is shown in Fig. 363-3.

The treatment of nonconvulsive status epilepticus is somewhat less urgent than GCSE, since the ongoing seizures are not accompanied by the severe metabolic disturbances seen with GCSE. However, evidence suggests that nonconvulsive status epilepticus, especially that caused by ongoing, focal seizure activity, is associated with cellular injury in the region of the seizure focus, so that the condition should be treated as promptly as possible using the general approach described for GCSE.

BEYOND SEIZURES: OTHER MANAGEMENT ISSUES

INTERICTAL BEHAVIOR

The adverse effects of epilepsy often go beyond the occurrence of clinical seizures, and the extent of these effects largely depends on the etiology of the seizure disorder, the degree to which the seizures are controlled, and the presence of side effects from antiepileptic therapy. Many patients with epilepsy are completely normal between seizures and able to live highly successful and productive lives. In contrast, patients with seizures secondary to developmental abnormalities or acquired brain injury may have impaired cognitive function and other neurologic deficits. Frequent interictal EEG abnormalities have been shown to be associated with subtle dysfunction of memory and attention. Patients with many seizures, especially those emanating from the temporal lobe, often note an impairment of short-term memory that may progress over time.

Patients with epilepsy are at risk of developing a variety of psychiatric problems, including depression, anxiety, and psychosis. This risk varies considerably depending on many factors, including the etiology, frequency, and severity of seizures and the patient's age and previous history. Depression occurs in ~20% of patients, and the incidence of suicide is higher in epileptic patients than in the general population. Depression should be treated through counseling or medication. The selective serotonin reuptake inhibitors typically have no effect on seizures, while the tricyclic antidepressants may lower the seizure threshold. Anxiety can appear as a manifestation of a seizure, and anxious or psychotic behavior can sometimes be observed as part of a postictal delirium. Postictal psychosis is a rare phenomenon that typically occurs after a period of increased seizure frequency. There is usually a brief lucid interval lasting

FIGURE 363-3 Pharmacologic treatment of generalized tonic-clonic status epilepticus in adults. The horizontal bars indicate the approximate duration of drug infusions. IV, intravenous; PE, phenytoin equivalents.

up to a week, followed by days to weeks of agitated, psychotic behavior. The psychosis will usually resolve spontaneously but may require treatment with antipsychotic or anxiolytic medications.

There is ongoing controversy as to whether some patients with epilepsy (especially temporal lobe epilepsy) have a stereotypical "interictal personality." The predominant view is that the unusual or abnormal personality traits observed in such patients are, in most cases, not due to epilepsy but result from an underlying structural brain lesion, the effects of antiepileptic drugs, or psychosocial factors related to suffering from a chronic disease.

MORTALITY OF EPILEPSY

Patients with epilepsy have a risk of death that is roughly two to three times greater than expected in a matched population without epilepsy. Most of the increased mortality is due to the underlying etiology of epilepsy, e.g., tumors or strokes in older adults. However, a significant number of patients die from accidents, status epilepticus, and a syndrome known as *sudden unexpected death in epileptic patients* (SUDEP), which usually affects young people with convulsive seizures and tends to occur at night. The cause of SUDEP is unknown; it may result from brainstem-mediated effects of seizures on cardiac rhythms or pulmonary function.

PSYCHOSOCIAL ISSUES

There continues to be a cultural stigma about epilepsy, although it is slowly declining in societies with effective health education programs. Many patients with epilepsy harbor fears, such as the fear of becoming mentally retarded or dying during a seizure. These issues need to be carefully addressed by educating the patient about epilepsy and by ensuring that family members, teachers, fellow employees, and other associates are equally well informed. The Epilepsy Foundation of America (1-800-EFA-1000) is a patient advocacy organization and a useful source of educational material.

EMPLOYMENT, DRIVING, AND OTHER ACTIVITIES

Many patients with epilepsy face difficulty in obtaining or maintaining employment, even when their seizures are well controlled. Federal and state legislation is designed to prevent employers from discriminating against patients with epilepsy, and patients should be encouraged to

CHAPTER 363 Seizures and Epilepsy

understand and claim their legal rights. Patients in these circumstances also benefit greatly from the assistance of health providers who act as strong patient advocates.

Loss of driving privileges is one of the most disruptive social consequences of epilepsy. Physicians should be very clear about local regulations concerning driving and epilepsy, since the laws vary considerably among states and countries. In all cases, it is the physician's responsibility to warn patients of the danger imposed on themselves and others while driving if their seizures are uncontrolled (unless the seizures are not associated with impairment of consciousness or motor control). In general, most states allow patients to drive after a seizure-free interval (on or off medications) of between 3 months and 2 years.

Patients with incompletely controlled seizures must also contend with the risk of being in situations where an impairment of consciousness or loss of motor control could lead to major injury or death. Thus, depending on the type and frequency of seizures, many patients need to be instructed to avoid working at heights or with machinery, or to have someone close by for activities such as bathing and swimming.

SPECIAL ISSUES RELATED TO WOMEN AND EPILEPSY

CATAMENIAL EPILEPSY

Some women experience a marked increase in seizure frequency around the time of menses. This is thought to reflect either the effects of estrogen and progesterone on neuronal excitability or changes in antiepileptic drug levels due to altered protein binding. Acetazolamide (250–500 mg/d) may be effective as adjunctive therapy in some cases when started 7–10 days prior to the onset of menses and continued until bleeding stops. Some patients may benefit from increases in antiepileptic drug dosages during this time or from control of the menstrual cycle through the use of oral contraceptives. Natural progestins may be of benefit to a subset of women.

PREGNANCY

Most women with epilepsy who become pregnant will have an uncomplicated gestation and deliver a normal baby. However, epilepsy poses some important risks to a pregnancy. Seizure frequency during pregnancy will remain unchanged in ~50% of women, increase in 30%, and decrease in 20%. Changes in seizure frequency are attributed to endocrine effects on the CNS, variations in antiepileptic drug pharmacokinetics (such as acceleration of hepatic drug metabolism or effects on plasma protein binding), and changes in medication compliance. It is useful to see patients at frequent intervals during pregnancy and monitor serum antiepileptic drug levels. Measurement of the unbound drug concentrations may be useful if there is an increase in seizure frequency or worsening of side effects of antiepileptic drugs.

The overall incidence of fetal abnormalities in children born to mothers with epilepsy is 5–6%, compared to 2–3% in healthy women. Part of the higher incidence is due to teratogenic effects of antiepileptic drugs, and the risk increases with the number of medications used (e.g., 10% risk of malformations with three drugs). A syndrome comprising facial dysmorphism, cleft lip, cleft palate, cardiac defects, digital hypoplasia, and nail dysplasia was originally ascribed to phenytoin therapy, but it is now known to occur with other first-line antiepileptic drugs (i.e., valproic acid and carbamazepine) as well. Also, valproic acid and carbamazepine are associated with a 1–2% incidence of neural tube defects compared with a baseline of 0.5–1%. Little is currently known about the safety of newer drugs, although very recent reports suggest a higher than expected incidence of cleft lip with the use of lamotrigine during pregnancy.

Since the potential harm of uncontrolled seizures on the mother and fetus is considered greater than the teratogenic effects of antiepi-

leptic drugs, it is currently recommended that pregnant women be maintained on effective drug therapy. When possible, it seems prudent to have the patient on monotherapy at the lowest effective dose, especially during the first trimester. Patients should also take folate (1–4 mg/d), since the antifolate effects of anticonvulsants are thought to play a role in the development of neural tube defects, although the benefits of this treatment remain unproved in this setting.

Enzyme-inducing drugs such as phenytoin, phenobarbital, and primidone cause a transient and reversible deficiency of vitamin K–dependent clotting factors in ~50% of newborn infants. Although neonatal hemorrhage is uncommon, the mother should be treated with oral vitamin K (20 mg/d) in the last 2 weeks of pregnancy, and the infant should receive vitamin K (1 mg) at birth.

CONTRACEPTION

Special care should be taken when prescribing antiepileptic medications for women who are taking oral contraceptive agents. Drugs such as carbamazepine, phenytoin, phenobarbital, and topiramate can significantly antagonize the effects of oral contraceptives via enzyme induction and other mechanisms. Patients should be advised to consider alternative forms of contraception, or their contraceptive medications should be modified to offset the effects of the antiepileptic medications.

BREAST-FEEDING

Antiepileptic medications are excreted into breast milk to a variable degree. The ratio of drug concentration in breast milk relative to serum is ~80% for ethosuximide, 40–60% for phenobarbital, 40% for carbamazepine, 15% for phenytoin, and 5% for valproic acid. Given the overall benefits of breast-feeding and the lack of evidence for long-term harm to the infant by being exposed to antiepileptic drugs, mothers with epilepsy can be encouraged to breast-feed. This should be reconsidered, however, if there is any evidence of drug effects on the infant, such as lethargy or poor feeding.

FURTHER READINGS

CHANG B, LOWENSTEIN DH: Mechanisms of disease: Epilepsy. N Engl J Med 349:1257, 2003

DUNCAN JS et al: Adult epilepsy. Lancet 367:1087, 2006

FRENCH JA et al: Efficacy and tolerability of the new antiepileptic drugs I: Treatment of new onset epilepsy: Report of the Therapeutics and Technology Assessment Subcommittee and Quality Standards Subcommittee of the American Academy of Neurology and the American Epilepsy Society. Neurology 62:1252, 2004

———: Efficacy and tolerability of the new antiepileptic drugs II: Treatment of refractory epilepsy: Report of the Therapeutics and Technology Assessment Subcommittee and Quality Standards Subcommittee of the American Academy of Neurology and the American Epilepsy Society. Neurology 62:1261, 2004

KARCESKI S et al: Treatment of epilepsy in adults: Expert opinion, 2005. Epilepsy Behav 7(Suppl 1):S1, 2005

LOWENSTEIN DH, ALLDREDGE BK: Status epilepticus. N Engl J Med 338:970, 1998

LUCIANO AL, SHORVON SD: Results of treatment changes in patients with apparently drug-resistant chronic epilepsy. Ann Neurol 62:375, 2007

PACK AM, MORRELL MJ: Treatment of women with epilepsy. Semin Neurol 22:289, 2002

TAN NC et al: Genetic dissection of the common epilepsies. Curr Opin Neurol 19:157, 2006

WIEBE S et al: A randomized, controlled trial of surgery for temporal-lobe epilepsy. N Engl J Med 345:311, 2001

364 Cerebrovascular Diseases
Wade S. Smith, Joey D. English, S. Claiborne Johnston

Cerebrovascular diseases include some of the most common and devastating disorders: ischemic stroke, hemorrhagic stroke, and cerebrovascular anomalies such as intracranial aneurysms and arteriovenous malformations (AVMs). They cause ~200,000 deaths each year in the United States and are a major cause of disability. The incidence of cerebrovascular diseases increases with age, and the number of strokes is projected to increase as the elderly population grows, with a doubling in stroke deaths in the United States by 2030. Most cerebrovascular diseases are manifest by the abrupt onset of a focal neurologic deficit, as if the patient was "struck by the hand of God." A stroke, or cerebrovascular accident, is defined by this abrupt onset of a neurologic deficit that is attributable to a focal vascular cause. Thus, the definition of stroke is clinical, and laboratory studies including brain imaging are used to support the diagnosis. The clinical manifestations of stroke are highly variable because of the complex anatomy of the brain and its vasculature. *Cerebral ischemia* is caused by a reduction in blood flow that lasts longer than several seconds. Neurologic symptoms are manifest within seconds because neurons lack glycogen, so energy failure is rapid. If the cessation of flow lasts for more than a few minutes, *infarction* or death of brain tissue results. When blood flow is quickly restored, brain tissue can recover fully and the patient's symptoms are only transient: this is called a *transient ischemic attack* (TIA). The standard definition of TIA requires that all neurologic signs and symptoms resolve within 24 h regardless of whether there is imaging evidence of new permanent brain injury; stroke has occurred if the neurologic signs and symptoms last for >24 h. However, a newly proposed definition classifies those with new brain infarction as ischemic strokes regardless of whether symptoms persist. A generalized reduction in cerebral blood flow due to systemic hypotension (e.g., cardiac arrhythmia, myocardial infarction, or hemorrhagic shock) usually produces syncope (Chap. 21). If low cerebral blood flow persists for a longer duration, then infarction in the border zones between the major cerebral artery distributions may develop. In more severe instances, *global hypoxia-ischemia* causes widespread brain injury; the constellation of cognitive sequelae that ensues is called *hypoxic-ischemic encephalopathy* (Chap. 269). *Focal ischemia* or infarction, on the other hand, is usually caused by thrombosis of the cerebral vessels themselves or by emboli from a proximal arterial source or the heart. *Intracranial hemorrhage* is caused by bleeding directly into or around the brain; it produces neurologic symptoms by producing a mass effect on neural structures, from the toxic effects of blood itself, or by increasing intracranial pressure.

APPROACH TO THE PATIENT:
Cerebrovascular Disease

Rapid evaluation is essential for use of time-sensitive treatments such as thrombolysis. However, patients with acute stroke often do not seek medical assistance on their own, both because they are rarely in pain, as well as because they may lose the appreciation that something is wrong (anosagnosia); it is often a family member or a bystander who calls for help. Therefore, patients and their family members should be counseled to call emergency medical services immediately if they experience or witness the sudden onset of any of the following: loss of sensory and/or motor function on one side of the body (nearly 85% of ischemic stroke patients have hemiparesis); change in vision, gait, or ability to speak or understand; or if they experience a sudden, severe headache.

There are several common causes of sudden-onset neurologic symptoms that may mimic stroke, including seizure, intracranial tumor, migraine, and metabolic encephalopathy. An adequate history from an observer that no convulsive activity occurred at the onset reasonably excludes seizure. Tumors may present with acute neurologic symptoms due to hemorrhage, seizure, or hydrocephalus. Surprisingly, migraine can mimic stroke, even in patients without a significant migraine history. When it develops without head pain (*acephalgic migraine*), the diagnosis may remain elusive. Patients without any prior history of migraine may develop acephalgic migraine even after age 65. A sensory disturbance is often prominent, and the sensory deficit, as well as any motor deficits, tends to migrate slowly across a limb over minutes rather than seconds as with stroke. The diagnosis of migraine becomes more secure as the cortical disturbance begins to cross vascular boundaries or if typical visual symptoms are present, such as scintillating scotomata (Chap. 15). At times it may be difficult to make the diagnosis until multiple episodes have occurred leaving behind no residual symptoms and with a normal MRI study of the brain. Classically, metabolic encephalopathies produce fluctuating mental status without focal neurologic findings. However, in the setting of prior stroke or brain injury, a patient with fever or sepsis may manifest hemiparesis, which clears rapidly when the infection is remedied. The metabolic process serves to "unmask" a prior deficit.

Once the diagnosis of stroke is made, a brain imaging study is necessary to determine if the cause of stroke is ischemia or hemorrhage (Fig. 364-1). CT imaging of the brain is the standard imaging modality to detect the presence or absence of intracranial hemorrhage (see "Imaging Studies," below). If the stroke is ischemic, administration of recombinant tissue plasminogen activator (rtPA) or endovascular mechanical thrombectomy may be beneficial in restoring cerebral perfusion (see "Rx: Acute Ischemic Stroke"). Medical management to reduce the risk of complications becomes the next priority, followed by plans for secondary prevention. For ischemic stroke, several strategies can reduce the risk of subsequent stroke in all patients, while other strategies are effective for patients with specific causes of stroke such as cardiac embolus and carotid atherosclerosis. For hemorrhagic stroke, aneurysmal subarachnoid hemorrhage (SAH) and hypertensive intracranial hemorrhage are two important causes. The treatment and prevention of hypertensive intracranial hemorrhage are discussed later in this chapter. SAH is discussed in Chap. 269.

ISCHEMIC STROKE

PATHOPHYSIOLOGY OF ISCHEMIC STROKE

Acute occlusion of an intracranial vessel causes reduction in blood flow to the brain region it supplies. The magnitude of flow reduction is a function of collateral blood flow and this depends on individual vascular anatomy and the site of occlusion. A fall in cerebral blood flow to zero causes death of brain tissue within 4–10 min; values <16–18 mL/100 g tissue per min cause infarction within an hour; and values <20 mL/100 g tissue per min cause ischemia without infarction unless prolonged for several hours or days. If blood flow is restored prior to a significant amount of cell death, the patient may experience only transient symptoms, i.e., a TIA. Tissue surrounding the core region of infarction is ischemic but reversibly dysfunctional and is referred to as the *ischemic penumbra*. The penumbra may be imaged by using perfusion-diffusion imaging with MRI (see below and Fig. 364-16). The ischemic penumbra will eventually infarct if no change in flow occurs, and hence saving the ischemic penumbra is the goal of revascularization therapies.

Focal cerebral infarction occurs via two distinct pathways (Fig. 364-2): (1) a necrotic pathway in which cellular cytoskeletal breakdown is rapid, due principally to energy failure of the cell; and (2) an apoptotic pathway in which cells become programmed to die. Ischemia produces necrosis by starving neurons of glucose, which in turn results in failure of mitochondria to produce ATP. Without ATP, membrane ion pumps stop functioning and neurons depolarize, allowing intracellular calcium to rise. Cellular depolarization also causes glutamate release from synaptic terminals; excess extracellular glutamate produces neurotoxicity by activating postsynaptic glutamate receptors that increase neu-

ALGORITHM FOR STROKE AND TIA MANAGEMENT

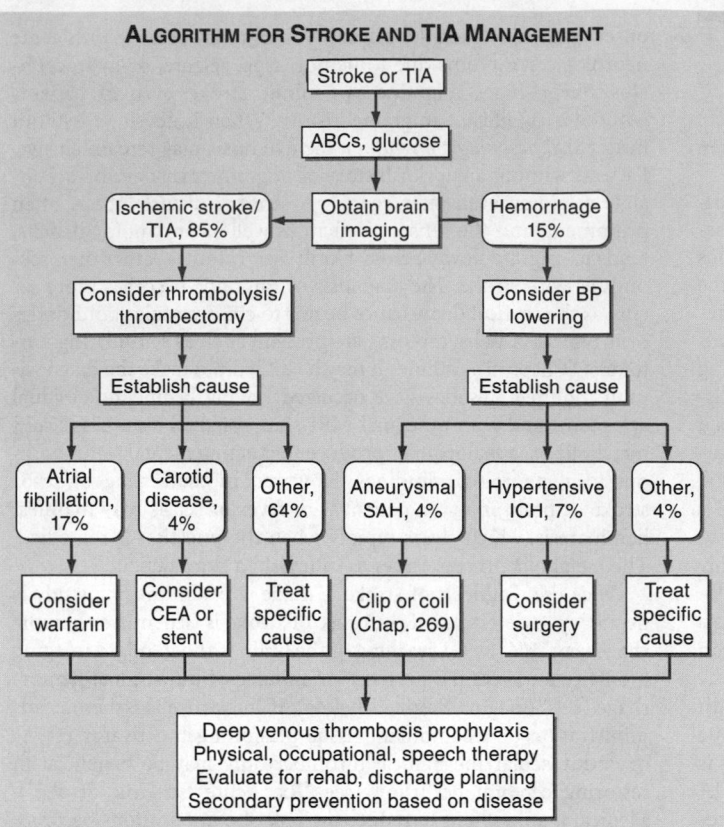

FIGURE 364-1 Medical management of stroke and TIA. Rounded boxes are diagnoses; rectangles are interventions. Numbers are percentages of stroke overall. Abbreviations: TIA, transient ischemic attack; ABCs, airway, breathing, circulation; BP, blood pressure; CEA, carotid endarterectomy, SAH, subarachnoid hemorrhage; ICH, intracerebral hemorrhage.

ronal calcium influx. Free radicals are produced by membrane lipid degradation and mitochondrial dysfunction. Free radicals cause catalytic destruction of membranes and likely damage other vital functions of cells. Lesser degrees of ischemia, as are seen within the ischemic penumbra, favor apoptotic cellular death causing cells to die days to weeks later. Fever dramatically worsens ischemia, as does hyperglycemia [glucose > 11.1 mmol/L (200 mg/dL)], so it is reasonable to suppress fever and prevent hyperglycemia as much as possible. Induced moderate hypothermia to mitigate stroke is the subject of continuing clinical research.

℞ ACUTE ISCHEMIC STROKE

After the clinical diagnosis of stroke is made, an orderly process of evaluation and treatment should follow (Fig. 364-1). The first goal is to prevent or reverse brain injury. Attend to the patient's airway, breathing, circulation, and treat hypoglycemia or hyperglycemia if identified. Perform an emergency noncontrast head CT scan in order to differentiate between ischemic stroke and hemorrhagic stroke; there are no reliable clinical findings that conclusively separate ischemia from hemorrhage, although a more depressed level of consciousness, higher initial blood pressure, or worsening of symptoms after onset favor hemorrhage, and a deficit that remits suggests ischemia. Treatments designed to reverse or lessen the amount of tissue infarction

and improve clinical outcome fall within six categories: (1) medical support (2) intravenous thrombolysis, (3) endovascular techniques, (4) antithrombotic treatment, (5) neuroprotection, and (6) stroke centers and rehabilitation.

MEDICAL SUPPORT When ischemic stroke occurs, the immediate goal is to optimize cerebral perfusion in the surrounding ischemic penumbra. Attention is also directed toward preventing the common complications of bedridden patients—infections (pneumonia, urinary tract, and skin) and deep venous thrombosis (DVT) with pulmonary embolism. Many physicians use pneumatic compression stockings to prevent DVT; subcutaneous heparin appears to be safe as well and can be used concomitantly.

Because collateral blood flow within the ischemic brain is blood pressure dependent, there is controversy about whether blood pressure should be lowered acutely. Blood pressure should be lowered if there is malignant hypertension (Chap. 241) or concomitant myocardial ischemia or if blood pressure is >185/110 mmHg and thrombolytic therapy is anticipated. When faced with the competing demands of myocardium and brain, lowering the heart rate with a β_1-adrenergic blocker (such as esmolol) can be a first step to decrease cardiac work and maintain blood pressure. Fever is detrimental and should be treated with antipyretics and surface cooling. Serum glucose should be monitored and kept at <6.1 mmol/L (110 mg/dL) using an insulin infusion.

Between 5 and 10% of patients develop enough cerebral edema to cause obtundation or brain herniation. Edema peaks on the second or third day but can cause mass effect for ~10 days. The larger the infarct, the greater the likelihood that clinically significant edema will develop. Water restriction and IV mannitol may be used to raise the serum osmolarity, but hypovolemia should be avoided as this may contribute to hypotension and worsening infarction. Combined analysis of three randomized European trials of hemicraniectomy (craniotomy and temporary removal of part of the skull) shows that this procedure markedly reduces mortality, and the clinical outcomes of survivors are acceptable.

Special vigilance is warranted for patients with cerebellar infarction. Such strokes may mimic labyrinthitis because of prominent vertigo and vomiting; the presence of head or neck pain should alert the physician to consider cerebellar stroke from vertebral artery dissection. Even small amounts of cerebellar edema can acutely increase intracranial pressure (ICP) or directly compress the brainstem. The resulting brainstem compression can result in coma and respiratory arrest and require emergen-

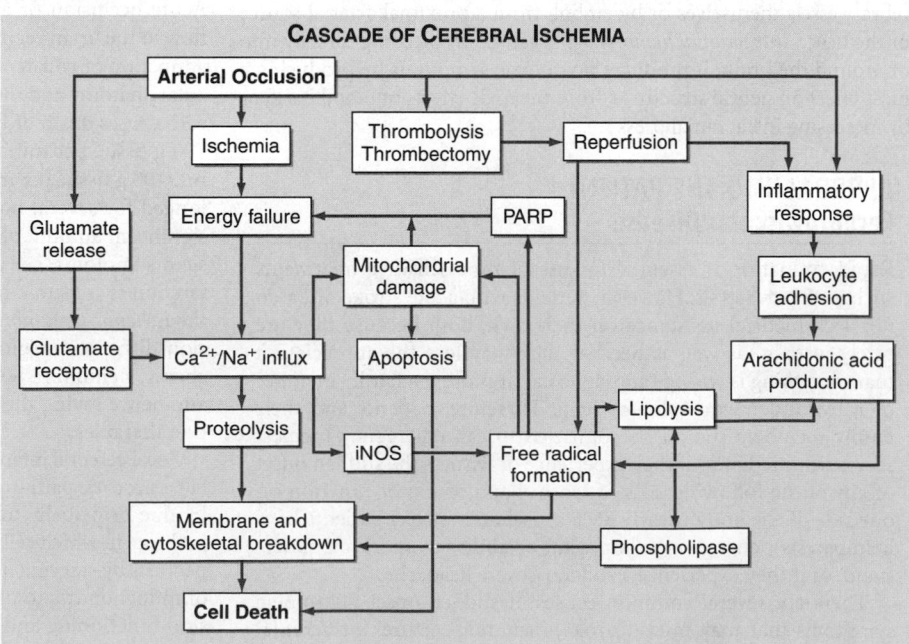

FIGURE 364-2 Major steps in the cascade of cerebral ischemia. See text for details. Abbreviations: PARP, poly-A ribose polymerase; iNOS, inducible nitric oxide synthase.

cy surgical decompression. Prophylactic suboccipital decompression of large cerebellar infarcts before brainstem compression, although not tested rigorously in a clinical trial, is practiced at most stroke centers.

INTRAVENOUS THROMBOLYSIS The National Institute of Neurological Disorders and Stroke (NINDS) recombinant tPA (rtPA) Stroke Study showed a clear benefit for IV rtPA in selected patients with acute stroke. The NINDS study used IV rtPA (0.9 mg/kg to a 90-mg max; 10% as a bolus, then the remainder over 60 min) vs. placebo in patients with ischemic stroke within 3 h of onset. Half of the patients were treated within 90 min. Symptomatic intracerebral hemorrhage occurred in 6.4% of patients on rtPA and 0.6% on placebo. There was a nonsignificant 4% reduction in mortality in patients on rtPA (21% on placebo and 17% on rtPA); there was a significant 12% absolute increase in the number of patients with only minimal disability (32% on placebo and 44% on rtPA.) Thus, despite an increased incidence of symptomatic intracerebral hemorrhage, treatment with IV rtPA within 3 h of the onset of ischemic stroke improved clinical outcome.

Results of other trials of rtPA have been negative, perhaps because of the dose of rtPA and timing of its delivery. The European Cooperative Acute Stroke Study (ECASS) I used a higher dose of rtPA (1.2 mg/kg), and ECASS-II tested the NINDS dose of rtPA (0.9 mg/kg; maximum dose, 90 mg) but allowed patients to receive drug up to the sixth hour. No significant benefit was found, but improvement was found in post hoc analyses. ATLANTIS tested the NINDS dosing of rtPA between 3 and 5 h and found no benefit. Because of the marked differences in trial design, including drug and dose used, time to thrombolysis, and severity of stroke, the precise efficacy of IV thrombolytics for acute ischemic stroke remains unclear. The risk of intracranial hemorrhage appears to rise with larger strokes, longer times from onset of symptoms, and higher doses of rtPA administered. The established dose of 0.9 mg/kg administered IV within 3 h of stroke onset appears safe. When data from all randomized IV rtPA trials are combined, efficacy is confirmed in the <3-h time window, and efficacy likely extends to 4.5 h. One may be able to select patients beyond the 3-h window who will benefit from thrombolysis using advanced neuroimaging (see neuroimaging section below), but this is currently investigational. The drug is now approved in the United States, Canada, and Europe for acute stroke when given within 3 h from the time the stroke symptoms began, and efforts should be made to give it as early in this 3-h window as possible. The time of stroke onset is defined as the time the patient's symptoms began or the time the patient was last seen as normal. Patients who awaken with stroke have the onset defined as when they went to bed. **Table 364-1** summarizes eligibility criteria and instructions for administration of IV rtPA.

ENDOVASCULAR TECHNIQUES Ischemic stroke from large-vessel intracranial occlusion results in high rates of mortality and morbidity. Occlusions in such large vessels [middle cerebral artery (MCA), internal carotid artery, and the basilar artery] generally involve a large clot volume and often fail to open with IV rtPA alone. Therefore, there is growing interest in using thrombolytics via an intraarterial route to increase the concentration of drug at the clot and minimize systemic bleeding complications. The Prolyse in Acute Cerebral Thromboembolism (PROACT) II trial found benefit for intraarterial pro-urokinase for acute MCA occlusions up to the sixth hour following onset of stroke. Intraarterial treatment of basilar artery occlusions may also be beneficial for selected patients. Intraarterial administration of a thrombolytic agent for acute ischemic stroke is not approved by the U.S. Food and Drug Administration (FDA); however, many stroke centers offer this treatment based on these data.

Endovascular mechanical thrombectomy has recently shown promise as an alternative treatment of acute stroke in patients who are ineligible for, or have contraindications to, thrombolytics or in those who have failed to have vascular recanalization with IV thrombolytics (see Fig. 364-15). The MERCI (Mechanical Embolus Removal in Cerebral Ischemia) single-arm trial investigated the ability of a novel endovascular thrombectomy device to restore patency of occluded intracranial vessels within 8 h of ischemic stroke symptoms. Recanalization of the target vessel occurred in 48% of treated patients and in 60% following use of adjuvant endovascular methods, and successful recanalization at 90 days correlated well with favorable outcome. Based upon these nonrandomized data, the FDA approved this device for revascularization of occluded vessels in acute ischemic stroke within 8 h of symptom onset. Recent trials have shown that it is safe to use this technique even in patients who have been given IV rtPA yet have failed to recanalize. Such a strategy allows primary stroke centers to admin-

TABLE 364-1	ADMINISTRATION OF INTRAVENOUS RECOMBINANT TISSUE PLASMINOGEN ACTIVATOR (RTPA) FOR ACUTE ISCHEMIC STROKE[a]

Indication
- Clinical diagnosis of stroke
- Onset of symptoms to time of drug administration ≤3 h
- CT scan showing no hemorrhage or edema of >$^1/_3$ of the MCA territory
- Age ≥18 years
- Consent by patient or surrogate

Contraindication
- Sustained BP >185/110 despite treatment
- Platelets <100,000; HCT <25%; glucose <50 or >400 mg/dL
- Use of heparin within 48 h and prolonged PTT, or elevated INR
- Rapidly improving symptoms
- Prior stroke or head injury within 3 months; prior intracranial hemorrhage
- Major surgery in preceding 14 days
- Minor stroke symptoms
- Gastrointestinal bleeding in preceding 21 days
- Recent myocardial infarction
- Coma or stupor

Administration of rtPA
- Intravenous access with two peripheral IV lines (avoid arterial or central line placement)
- Review eligibility for rtPA
- Administer 0.9 mg/kg intravenously (maximum 90 mg) IV as 10% of total dose by bolus, followed by remainder of total dose over 1 h
- Frequent cuff blood pressure monitoring
- No other antithrombotic treatment for 24 h
- For decline in neurologic status or uncontrolled blood pressure, stop infusion, give cryoprecipitate, and reimage brain emergently
- Avoid urethral catheterization for ≥2 h

[a]See Activase (tissue plasminogen activator) package insert for complete list of contraindications and dosing.
Note: BP, blood pressure; HCT, hematocrit; INR, international normalized ratio; MCA, middle cerebral artery; PTT, partial thromboplastin time.

ister rtPA to eligible patients, then rapidly refer such patients to comprehensive stroke centers that have endovascular capability.

ANTITHROMBOTIC TREATMENT **Platelet Inhibition** Aspirin is the only antiplatelet agent that has been proven effective for the acute treatment of ischemic stroke; there are several antiplatelet agents proven for the secondary prevention of stroke (see below). Two large trials, the International Stroke Trial (IST) and the Chinese Acute Stroke Trial (CAST), found that the use of aspirin within 48 h of stroke onset reduced both stroke recurrence risk and mortality minimally. Among 19,435 patients in IST, those allocated to aspirin, 300 mg/d, had slightly fewer deaths within 14 days (9.0 vs. 9.4%), significantly fewer recurrent ischemic strokes (2.8 vs. 3.9%), no excess of hemorrhagic strokes (0.9 vs. 0.8%), and a trend towards a reduction in death or dependence at 6 months (61.2 vs. 63.5%). In CAST, 21,106 patients with ischemic stroke received 160 mg/d of aspirin or a placebo for up to 4 weeks. There were very small reductions in the aspirin group in early mortality (3.3 vs. 3.9%), recurrent ischemic strokes (1.6 vs. 2.1%), and dependency at discharge or death (30.5 vs. 31.6%). These trials demonstrate that the use of aspirin in the treatment of acute ischemic stroke is safe and produces a small net benefit. For every 1000 acute strokes treated with aspirin, about 9 deaths or nonfatal stroke recurrences will be prevented in the first few weeks and ~13 fewer patients will be dead or dependent at 6 months.

The glycoprotein IIb/IIIa receptor inhibitor abciximab held promise as an acute treatment, but a recent clinical trial was stopped because of excess intracranial hemorrhage.

Anticoagulation Numerous clinical trials have failed to demonstrate any benefit of anticoagulation in the primary treatment of atherothrombotic cerebral ischemia. Several trials have investigated antiplatelet versus anticoagulant medications given within 12–24 h of the initial event. The U.S. Trial of Organon 10172 in Acute Stroke Treatment (TOAST), an investigational low-molecular-weight heparin, failed to show any benefit over aspirin. Use of SC unfractionated heparin versus aspirin was tested in IST. Heparin given SC afforded no additional benefit over aspirin and increased bleeding rates. Several trials of low-molecular-weight heparins have also shown no consistent benefit in acute ischemic stroke. Furthermore, trials generally have shown an excess risk of brain and systemic hemorrhage with acute anticoagulation. Therefore, trials do not support the use of heparin or other anticoagulants for patients with atherothrombotic stroke.

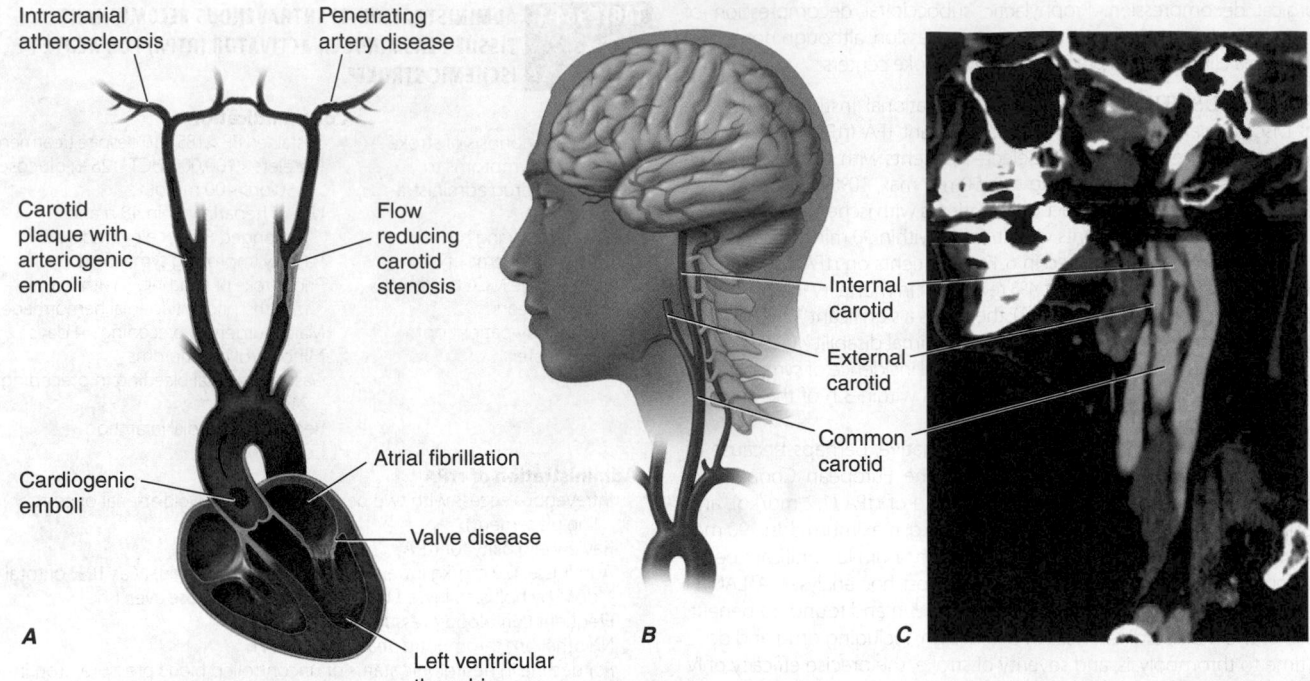

FIGURE 364-3 **Pathophysiology of ischemic stroke. A.** Diagram illustrating the three major mechanisms that underlie ischemic stroke: (1) occlusion of an intracranial vessel by an embolus that arises at a distant site (e.g., cardiogenic sources such as atrial fibrillation or artery-to-artery emboli from carotid atherosclerotic plaque), often affecting the large intracranial vessels; (2) in situ thrombosis of an intracranial vessel, typically affecting the small penetrating arteries that arise from the major intracranial arteries; (3) hypoperfusion caused by flow-limiting stenosis of a major extracranial (e.g., internal carotid) or intracranial vessel, often producing "watershed" ischemia. **B** and **C.** Diagram and reformatted CT angiogram of the common, internal, and external carotid arteries. High-grade stenosis of the internal carotid artery, which may be associated with either cerebral emboli or flow-limiting ischemia, was identified in this patient.

NEUROPROTECTION Neuroprotection is the concept of providing a treatment that prolongs the brain's tolerance to ischemia. Drugs that block the excitatory amino acid pathways have been shown to protect neurons and glia in animals, but despite multiple clinical trials, they have not yet been proven to be beneficial in humans. Hypothermia is a powerful neuroprotective treatment in patients with cardiac arrest (Chap. 269) and is neuroprotective in animal models of stroke, but it has not been adequately studied in patients with ischemic stroke.

STROKE CENTERS AND REHABILITATION Patient care in comprehensive stroke units followed by rehabilitation services improves neurologic outcomes and reduces mortality. Use of clinical pathways and staff dedicated to the stroke patient can improve care. Stroke teams that provide emergency 24-h evaluation of acute stroke patients for acute medical management and consideration of thrombolysis or endovascular treatments are important.

Proper rehabilitation of the stroke patient includes early physical, occupational, and speech therapy. It is directed toward educating the patient and family about the patient's neurologic deficit, preventing the complications of immobility (e.g., pneumonia, DVT and pulmonary embolism, pressure sores of the skin, and muscle contractures), and providing encouragement and instruction in overcoming the deficit. The goal of rehabilitation is to return the patient to home and to maximize recovery by providing a safe, progressive regimen suited to the individual patient. Additionally, the use of restraint therapy (immobilizing the unaffected side) has been shown to improve hemiparesis following stroke, even years following the stroke, suggesting that physical therapy can recruit unused neural pathways. This finding suggests that the human nervous system is more adaptable than originally thought and has stimulated active research into physical and pharmacologic strategies that can enhance long-term neural recovery.

ETIOLOGY OF ISCHEMIC STROKE

(Figs. 364-1 and 364-3 and Table 364-2) Although the initial management of acute ischemic stroke often does not depend on the etiology, establishing a cause is essential in reducing the risk of recurrence. Particular focus should be on atrial fibrillation and carotid atherosclerosis, as these etiologies have proved secondary prevention strategies. The clinical presentation and examination findings often establish the cause of stroke or narrow the possibilities to a few. Judicious use of laboratory testing and imaging studies completes the initial evaluation. Nevertheless, nearly 30% of strokes remain unexplained despite extensive evaluation.

Clinical examination should focus on the peripheral and cervical vascular system (carotid auscultation for bruits, blood pressure, and pressure comparison between arms), the heart (dysrhythmia, murmurs), extremities (peripheral emboli), and retina [effects of hypertension and cholesterol emboli (Hollenhorst plaques)]. A complete neurologic examination is performed to localize the site of stroke. An imaging study of the brain is nearly always indicated and is required for patients being considered for thrombolysis; it may be combined with CT- or MRI-based angiography to interrogate the neck and intracranial vessels (see "Imaging Studies," below). A chest x-ray, electrocardiogram (ECG), urinalysis, complete blood count, erythrocyte sedimentation rate, serum electrolytes, blood urea nitrogen, creatinine, blood sugar, serologic test for syphilis, serum lipid profile, prothrombin time, and partial thromboplastin time (PTT) are often useful and should be considered in all patients. An ECG may demonstrate arrhythmias or reveal evidence of recent myocardial infarction (MI).

Cardioembolic Stroke Cardioembolism is responsible for ~20% of all ischemic strokes. Stroke caused by heart disease is primarily due to embolism of thrombotic material forming on the atrial or ventricular wall or the left heart valves. These thrombi then detach and embolize into the arterial circulation. The thrombus may fragment or lyse quickly, producing only a TIA. Alternatively, the arterial occlusion may last longer, producing stroke. Embolic strokes tend to be sudden in onset, with maximum neurologic deficit at once. With reperfusion following more prolonged ischemia, petechial hemorrhage can occur within the ischemic territory. This is usually of no clinical significance

TABLE 364-2	CAUSES OF ISCHEMIC STROKE
Common Causes	**Uncommon Causes**
Thrombosis	Hypercoagulable disorders
Lacunar stroke (small vessel)	Protein C deficiency
Large vessel thrombosis	Protein S deficiency
Dehydration	Antithrombin III deficiency
Embolic occlusion	Antiphospholipid syndrome
Artery-to-artery	Factor V Leiden mutation[a]
Carotid bifurcation	Prothrombin G20210 mutation[a]
Aortic arch	Systemic malignancy
Arterial dissection	Sickle cell anemia
Cardioembolic	β-Thalassemia
Atrial fibrillation	Polycythemia vera
Mural thrombus	Systemic lupus erythematosus
Myocardial infarction	Homocysteinemia
Dilated cardiomyopathy	Thrombotic thrombocytopenic
Valvular lesions	purpura
Mitral stenosis	Disseminated intravascular
Mechanical valve	coagulation
Bacterial endocarditis	Dysproteinemias
Paradoxical embolus	Nephrotic syndrome
Atrial septal defect	Inflammatory bowel disease
Patent foramen ovale	Oral contraceptives
Atrial septal aneurysm	Venous sinus thrombosis[b]
Spontaneous echo contrast	Fibromuscular dysplasia
	Vasculitis
	Systemic vasculitis (PAN, Wegener's,
	Takayasu's, giant cell arteritis)
	Primary CNS vasculitis
	Meningitis (syphilis, tuberculosis,
	fungal, bacterial, zoster)
	Cardiogenic
	Mitral valve calcification
	Atrial myxoma
	Intracardiac tumor
	Marantic endocarditis
	Libman-Sacks endocarditis
	Subarachnoid hemorrhage vasospasm
	Drugs: cocaine, amphetamine
	Moyamoya disease
	Eclampsia

[a]Chiefly cause venous sinus thrombosis.
[b]May be associated with any hypercoagulable disorder.
Note: CNS, central nervous system; PAN, polyarteritis nodosa.

and should be distinguished from frank intracranial hemorrhage into a region of ischemic stroke where the mass effect from the hemorrhage can cause a decline in neurologic function.

Emboli from the heart most often lodge in the MCA, the posterior cerebral artery (PCA), or one of their branches; infrequently, the anterior cerebral artery (ACA) territory is involved. Emboli large enough to occlude the stem of the MCA (3–4 mm) lead to large infarcts that involve both deep gray and white matter and some portions of the cortical surface and its underlying white matter. A smaller embolus may occlude a small cortical or penetrating arterial branch. The location and size of an infarct within a vascular territory depend on the extent of the collateral circulation.

The most significant causes of cardioembolic stroke in most of the world are nonrheumatic (often called nonvalvular) atrial fibrillation, MI, prosthetic valves, rheumatic heart disease, and ischemic cardiomyopathy (Table 364-2). Cardiac disorders causing brain embolism are discussed in the respective chapters on heart diseases. A few pertinent aspects are highlighted here.

Nonrheumatic atrial fibrillation is the most common cause of cerebral embolism overall. The presumed stroke mechanism is thrombus formation in the fibrillating atrium or atrial appendage, with subsequent embolization. Patients with atrial fibrillation have an average annual risk of stroke of ~5%. The risk varies according to the presence of certain risk factors, including older age, hypertension, poor left ventricular function, prior cardioembolism, mitral stenosis, prosthetic heart valve, or diabetes. Patients <65 years with none of these risk factors have an annual risk for stroke of ~0.5%, while those with most of

TABLE 364-3	CONSENSUS RECOMMENDATION FOR ANTITHROMBOTIC PROPHYLAXIS IN ATRIAL FIBRILLATION

Age	Risk Factors[a]	Recommendation
Age ≤65	≥1	Warfarin INR 2–3
	0	Aspirin
Age 65–75	≥1	Warfarin INR 2–3
	0	Warfarin INR 2–3 or aspirin
Age >75		Warfarin INR 2–3

[a]Risk factors include previous transient ischemic attack or stroke, hypertension, heart failure, diabetes, systemic embolism, mitral stenosis, or prosthetic heart valve.
Source: Modified from DE Singer et al: Antithrombotic therapy in atrial fibrillation. Chest 126:429S, 2004; with permission.

the factors have a rate of ~15% per year. Left atrial enlargement and congestive heart failure are additional risk factors for formation of atrial thrombi. Rheumatic heart disease usually causes ischemic stroke when there is prominent mitral stenosis or atrial fibrillation. Guidelines for the use of warfarin and aspirin for secondary prevention are based on risk factors (Table 364-3).

Recent MI may be a source of emboli, especially when transmural and involving the anteroapical ventricular wall, and prophylactic anticoagulation following MI has been shown to reduce stroke risk. Mitral valve prolapse is not usually a source of emboli unless the prolapse is severe.

Paradoxical embolization occurs when venous thrombi migrate to the arterial circulation, usually via a patent foramen ovale or atrial septal defect. Bubble-contrast echocardiography (IV injection of agitated saline coupled with either transthoracic or transesophageal echocardiography) can demonstrate a right-to-left cardiac shunt, revealing the conduit for paradoxical embolization. Alternatively, a right-to-left shunt is implied if immediately following IV injection of agitated saline, the ultrasound signature of bubbles is observed during transcranial Doppler insonation of the MCA; pulmonary AVMs should be considered if this test is positive yet an echocardiogram fails to reveal an intracardiac shunt. Both techniques are highly sensitive for detection of right-to-left shunts. Besides venous clot, fat and tumor emboli, bacterial endocarditis, IV air, and amniotic fluid emboli at childbirth may occasionally be responsible for paradoxical embolization. The importance of right-to-left shunt as a cause of stroke is debated, particularly because such shunts are present in ~15% of the general population. Some studies have suggested that the risk is only elevated in the presence of a coexisting atrial septal aneurysm. The presence of a venous source of embolus, most commonly a deep venous thrombus, may provide confirmation of the importance of a right-to-left shunt in a particular case.

Bacterial endocarditis can cause valvular vegetations that can give rise to septic emboli. The appearance of multifocal symptoms and signs in a patient with stroke makes bacterial endocarditis more likely. Infarcts of microscopic size occur, and large septic infarcts may evolve into brain abscesses or cause hemorrhage into the infarct, which generally precludes use of anticoagulation or thrombolytics. Mycotic aneurysms caused by septic emboli give rise to SAH or intracerebral hemorrhage.

Artery-to-Artery Embolic Stroke Thrombus formation on atherosclerotic plaques may embolize to intracranial arteries producing an artery-to-artery embolic stroke. Alternatively, a diseased vessel may acutely thrombose; the resulting blockage causes stroke by producing ischemia within the region of brain it supplied. Unlike the myocardial vessels, artery-to-artery embolism, rather than local thrombosis, appears to be the dominant vascular mechanism causing ischemia. Any diseased vessel may be a source, including the aortic arch, common carotid, internal carotid, vertebral, and basilar arteries. Carotid bifurcation atherosclerosis is the most common source of artery-to-artery embolus, and specific treatments have proven efficacy in reducing risk.

CAROTID ATHEROSCLEROSIS Atherosclerosis within the carotid artery occurs most frequently within the common carotid bifurcation and proximal internal carotid artery. Additionally, the carotid siphon (por-

TABLE 364-4 **RISK FACTORS FOR STROKE**

Risk Factor	Relative Risk	Relative Risk Reduction with Treatment	Number Needed to Treat[a]	
			Primary Prevention	Secondary Prevention
Hypertension	2–5	38%	100–300	50–100
Atrial fibrillation	1.8–2.9	68% warfarin, 21% aspirin	20–83	13
Diabetes	1.8–6	No proven effect		
Smoking	1.8	50% at 1 year, baseline risk at 5 years post cessation		
Hyperlipidemia	1.8–2.6	16–30%	560	230
Asymptomatic carotid stenosis	2.0	53%	85	N/A
Symptomatic carotid stenosis (70–99%)		65% at 2 years	N/A	12
Symptomatic carotid stenosis (50–69%)		29% at 5 years	N/A	77

[a]Number needed to treat to prevent one stroke annually. Prevention of other cardiovascular outcomes is not considered here.

Note: N/A, not applicable.

tion within the cavernous sinus) is also vulnerable to atherosclerosis. Male gender, older age, smoking, hypertension, diabetes, and hypercholesterolemia are risk factors for carotid disease, as they are for stroke in general (Table 364-4). Carotid atherosclerosis produces an estimated 10% of ischemic stroke. **For further discussion of the pathogenesis of atherosclerosis, see Chap. 235.**

Carotid disease can be classified by whether the stenosis is symptomatic or asymptomatic and by the degree of stenosis (percent narrowing of the narrowest segment compared to a more distal internal carotid segment). Symptomatic carotid disease implies that the patient has experienced a stroke or TIA within the vascular distribution of the artery, and it is associated with a greater risk of subsequent stroke than asymptomatic stenosis, in which the patient is symptom free and the stenosis is detected through screening. Greater degrees of arterial narrowing are generally associated with a greater risk of stroke, except that those with near occlusions are at lower risk of stroke.

Rx CAROTID ATHEROSCLEROSIS

Carotid atherosclerosis can be removed surgically (endarterectomy) or mitigated with endovascular stenting with or without balloon angioplasty.

SURGICAL THERAPY *Symptomatic carotid stenosis* was studied in the North American Symptomatic Carotid Endarterectomy Trial (NASCET) and the European Carotid Surgery Trial (ECST). Both showed a substantial benefit for surgery in patients with a stenosis of ≥70%. In NASCET, the average cumulative ipsilateral stroke risk at 2 years was 26% for patients treated medically and 9% for those receiving the same medical treatment plus a carotid endarterectomy. This 17% *absolute* reduction in the surgical group is a 65% *relative* risk reduction favoring surgery (Table 364-4). NASCET also showed a significant, although less robust, benefit for patients with 50–70% stenosis. ECST found harm for patients with stenosis <30% treated surgically.

A patient's risk of stroke and possible benefit from surgery are related to the presence of retinal versus hemispheric symptoms, degree of arterial stenosis, extent of associated medical conditions (of note, NASCET and ECST excluded "high-risk" patients with significant cardiac, pulmonary, or renal disease), institutional surgical morbidity and mortality, timing of surgery relative to symptoms, and other factors. A recent meta-analysis of the NASCET and ECST trials demonstrated that endarterectomy is most beneficial when performed within 2 weeks of symptom onset. In addition, benefit is more pronounced in patients >75 years, and men appear to benefit more than women.

In summary, a patient with recent symptomatic hemispheric ischemia, high-grade stenosis in the appropriate internal carotid artery, and an institutional perioperative morbidity and mortality rate of ≤6% generally should undergo carotid endarterectomy. If the perioperative stroke rate is >6% for any particular surgeon, however, the benefits of carotid endarterectomy are questionable.

The indications for surgical treatment of *asymptomatic carotid disease* have been clarified by the results of the Asymptomatic Carotid Athero-

sclerosis Study (ACAS) and the Asymptomatic Carotid Surgery Trial (ACST). ACAS randomized asymptomatic patients with ≥60% stenosis to medical treatment with aspirin or the same medical treatment plus carotid endarterectomy. The surgical group had a risk over 5 years for ipsilateral stroke (and any perioperative stroke or death) of 5.1%, compared to a risk in the medical group of 11%. While this demonstrates a 53% *relative* risk reduction, the *absolute* risk reduction is only 5.9% over 5 years, or 1.2% annually (Table 364-4). Nearly half of the strokes in the surgery group were caused by preoperative angiograms. The recently published ACST randomized 3120 asymptomatic patients with >60% carotid stenosis to endarterectomy or medical therapy. The 5-year risk of stroke in the surgical group (including perioperative stroke or death) was 6.4%, compared to 11.8% in the medically treated group (46% relative risk reduction and 5.4% absolute risk reduction).

In both ACAS and ACST, the perioperative complication rate was higher in women, perhaps negating any benefit in the reduction of stroke risk within 5 years. It is possible that with longer follow-up, a clear benefit in women will emerge. At present, carotid endarterectomy in asymptomatic women remains particularly controversial.

In summary, the natural history of asymptomatic stenosis is a ~2% per year stroke rate, while symptomatic patients experience a 13% per year risk of stroke. Whether to recommend carotid revascularization for an asymptomatic patient is somewhat controversial and depends on many factors, including patient preference, degree of stenosis, age, gender, and comorbidities. Medical therapy for reduction of atherosclerosis risk factors, including cholesterol-lowering agents and antiplatelet medications, is generally recommended for patients with asymptomatic carotid stenosis. As with atrial fibrillation, it is imperative to counsel the patient about TIAs so that therapy can be revised if symptoms develop.

ENDOVASCULAR THERAPY Balloon angioplasty coupled with stenting is being used with increasing frequency to open stenotic carotid arteries and maintain their patency. These techniques can treat carotid stenosis not only at the bifurcation but also near the skull base and in the intracranial segments. The SAPPHIRE trial (Stenting and Angioplasty with Protection in Patients at High Risk for Endarterectomy) randomized high-risk patients (defined as patients with clinically significant coronary or pulmonary disease, contralateral carotid occlusion, restenosis after endarterectomy, contralateral laryngeal-nerve palsy, prior radical neck surgery or radiation, or age >80) with symptomatic carotid stenosis >50% or asymptomatic stenosis >80% to either stenting combined with a distal emboli-protection device or endarterectomy. The risk of death, stroke, or MI within 30 days and ipsilateral stroke or death within 1 year was 12.2% in the stenting group and 20.1% in the endarterectomy group ($p = .055$), suggesting that stenting is at the very least comparable to endarterectomy as a treatment option for this patient group at high risk of surgery. However, the outcomes with both interventions may not have been better than leaving the carotid stenoses untreated, particularly for the asymptomatic patients, and much of the benefit seen in the stenting group was due to a reduction in peri-procedure MI. Multicenter trials are currently underway comparing stenting with endarterectomy in lower-risk patients, the population previously studied in the NASCET, ECST, ACAS, and ACST trials (see above).

BYPASS SURGERY Extracranial-to-intracranial (EC-IC) bypass surgery has been proven ineffective for atherosclerotic stenoses that are inaccessible to conventional carotid endarterectomy. However, a trial is underway to evaluate whether patients with decreased brain perfusion based on positron emission tomography (PET) imaging will benefit from EC-IC bypass.

OTHER CAUSES OF ARTERY-TO-ARTERY EMBOLIC STROKE Intracranial atherosclerosis produces stroke either by an embolic mechanism or by in situ thrombosis of a diseased vessel. It is more common in patients of

Asian and African-American descent. The WASID (Warfarin-Aspirin Symptomatic Intracranial Disease) trial randomized patients with symptomatic stenosis (50–99%) of a major intracranial vessel to either high-dose aspirin (1300 mg/d) or warfarin (target INR, 2.0–3.0), with a combined primary endpoint of ischemic stroke, brain hemorrhage, or death from vascular cause other than stroke. The trial was terminated early because of an increased risk of adverse events related to warfarin anticoagulation. With a mean follow-up of 1.8 years, the primary endpoint was seen in 22.1% in the aspirin group and 21.8% of the warfarin group. Death from any cause was seen in 4.3% of the aspirin group and 9.7% of the warfarin group; 3.2% of patients on aspirin experienced major hemorrhage, compared to 8.3% of patients taking warfarin.

Given the worrisome natural history of symptomatic intracranial atherosclerosis (in the aspirin arm of the WASID trial, 15% of patients experienced a stroke within the first year, despite current standard aggressive medical therapy), some centers treat symptomatic lesions with intracranial angioplasty and stenting. This intervention has not been compared with medical therapy for stroke prevention in this patient population, but such clinical trials will likely be conducted in the near future. Likewise, it is unclear whether EC-IC bypass, or other grafting procedures of extracranial blood supply to the pial arteries, is of value in such patients.

Dissection of the internal carotid or vertebral arteries or even vessels beyond the circle of Willis is a common source of embolic stroke in young (age <60 years) patients. The dissection is usually painful and precedes the stroke by several hours or days. Extracranial dissections do not cause hemorrhage because of the tough adventitia of these vessels. Intracranial dissections, on the other hand, may produce SAH because the adventitia of intracranial vessels is thin and pseudoaneurysms may form, requiring treatment to prevent rerupture. Treating asymptomatic pseudoaneurysms following dissection is controversial. The cause of dissection is usually unknown and recurrence is rare. Ehlers-Danlos type IV, Marfan's disease, cystic medial necrosis, and fibromuscular dysplasia are associated with dissections. Trauma (usually a motor vehicle accident or a sports injury) can cause carotid and vertebral artery dissections. Spinal manipulative therapy is independently associated with vertebral artery dissection and stroke. Most dissections heal spontaneously, and stroke or TIA is uncommon beyond 2 weeks. Although there are no trials comparing anticoagulation to antiplatelet agents, many physicians treat acutely with anticoagulants for 3–6 months then convert to 6–9 months of antiplatelet therapy after demonstration of vascular recanalization.

Small-Vessel Stroke The term *lacunar infarction* refers to infarction following atherothrombotic or lipohyalinotic occlusion of a small artery (30–300 μm) in the brain. The term *small-vessel stroke* denotes occlusion of such a small penetrating artery and is now the preferred term. Small-vessel strokes account for ~20% of all strokes.

PATHOPHYSIOLOGY The MCA stem, the arteries comprising the circle of Willis (A1 segment, anterior and posterior communicating arteries, and P1 segment), and the

basilar and vertebral arteries all give rise to 30- to 300-μm branches that penetrate the deep gray and white matter of the cerebrum or brainstem (**Fig. 364-4**). Each of these small branches can occlude either by atherothrombotic disease at its origin or by the development of lipohyalinotic thickening. Thrombosis of these vessels causes small infarcts that are referred to as *lacunes* (Latin for "lake" of fluid noted at autopsy). These infarcts range in size from 3 mm to 2 cm in diameter. Hypertension and age are the principal risk factors.

CLINICAL MANIFESTATIONS The most common *lacunar syndromes* are the following: (1) *Pure motor hemiparesis* from an infarct in the posterior limb of the internal capsule or basis pontis; the face, arm, and leg are almost always involved; (2) *pure sensory stroke* from an infarct in the ventral thalamus; (3) *ataxic hemiparesis* from an infarct in the ventral pons or internal capsule; (4) and *dysarthria and a clumsy hand* or arm due to infarction in the ventral pons or in the genu of the internal capsule.

Transient symptoms (small vessel TIAs) may herald a small-vessel infarct; they may occur several times a day and last only a few minutes. Recovery from small-vessel strokes tends to be more rapid and complete than recovery from large-vessel strokes; in some cases, however,

FIGURE 364-4 Diagrams and reformatted CT angiograms in the coronal section illustrating the deep penetrating arteries involved in small-vessel strokes. In the anterior circulation, small penetrating arteries called lenticulostriates arise from the proximal portion of the anterior and middle cerebral arteries and supply deep subcortical structures (**upper panels**). In the posterior circulation, similar arteries arise directly from the vertebral and basilar arteries to supply the brainstem (**lower panels**). Occlusion of a single penetrating artery gives rise to a discrete area of infarct (pathologically termed a "lacune," or lake). Note that these vessels are too small to be visualized on CT angiography.

there is severe permanent disability. Often, institution of combined antithrombotic treatments does not prevent eventual stroke in "stuttering lacunes."

A large-vessel source (either thrombosis or embolism) may manifest initially as a lacunar syndrome with small-vessel infarction. Therefore, the search for embolic sources (carotid and heart) should not be completely abandoned in the evaluation of these patients. Secondary prevention of lacunar stroke involves risk factor modification, specifically reduction in blood pressure (see "Primary and Secondary Prevention," below).

LESS COMMON CAUSES OF STROKE

(Table 364-2) *Hypercoagulable disorders* (Chap. 59) primarily cause increased risk of venous thrombosis and therefore may cause venous sinus thrombosis. Protein S deficiency and homocysteinemia may cause arterial thromboses as well. Systemic lupus erythematosus with Libman-Sacks endocarditis can be a cause of embolic stroke. These conditions overlap with the antiphospholipid syndrome, which probably requires long-term anticoagulation to prevent further stroke.

Venous sinus thrombosis of the lateral or sagittal sinus or of small cortical veins (cortical vein thrombosis) occurs as a complication of oral contraceptive use, pregnancy and the postpartum period, inflammatory bowel disease, intracranial infections (meningitis), and dehydration. It is also seen with increased incidence in patients with laboratory-confirmed thrombophilia (Table 364-2) including polycythemia, sickle cell anemia, deficiencies of proteins C and S, factor V Leiden mutation (resistance to activated protein C), antithrombin III deficiency, homocysteinemia, and the prothrombin G20210 mutation. Women who take oral contraceptives and have the prothrombin G20210 mutation may be at particularly high risk for sinus thrombosis. Patients present with headache and may also have focal neurologic signs (especially paraparesis) and seizures. Often, CT imaging is normal unless an intracranial venous hemorrhage has occurred, but the venous sinus occlusion is readily visualized using magnetic resonance (MR) venography or conventional x-ray angiography. With greater degrees of sinus thrombosis, the patient may develop signs of increased ICP and coma. Intravenous heparin, regardless of the presence of intracranial hemorrhage, has been shown to reduce morbidity and mortality, and the long-term outcome is generally good. Heparin prevents further thrombosis and reduces venous hypertension and ischemia. If an underlying hypercoagulable state is not found, many physicians treat with warfarin sodium for 3–6 months then convert to aspirin, depending on the degree of resolution of the venous sinus thrombus. Anticoagulation is often continued indefinitely if thrombophilia is diagnosed.

Sickle cell anemia (SS disease) is a common cause of stroke in children. A subset of homozygous carriers of this hemoglobin mutation develop stroke in childhood and this may be predicted by documenting high-velocity blood flow within the MCAs using transcranial Doppler ultrasonography. In children who are identified to have high velocities, treatment with aggressive exchange transfusion dramatically reduces risk of stroke, and if exchange transfusion is ceased, their stroke rate increases again along with MCA velocities.

Fibromuscular dysplasia affects the cervical arteries and occurs mainly in women. The carotid or vertebral arteries show multiple rings of segmental narrowing alternating with dilatation. Occlusion is usually incomplete. The process is often asymptomatic but occasionally is associated with an audible bruit, TIAs, or stroke. Involvement of the renal arteries is common and may result in hypertension. The cause and natural history of fibromuscular dysplasia are unknown (Chap. 243). TIA or stroke generally occurs only when the artery is severely narrowed or dissects. Anticoagulation or antiplatelet therapy may be helpful.

Temporal (giant cell) arteritis (Chap. 319) is a relatively common affliction of elderly persons in which the external carotid system, particularly the temporal arteries, becomes the site of a subacute granulomatous inflammation with giant cells. Occlusion of posterior ciliary arteries derived from the ophthalmic artery results in blindness in one or both eyes and can be prevented with glucocorticoids. It rarely caus-

FIGURE 364-5 Cerebral angiogram from a 32-year-old male with central nervous system vasculitis. Dramatic beading (*arrow*) typical of vasculitis is seen.

es stroke as the internal carotid artery is usually not inflamed. Idiopathic giant cell arteritis involving the great vessels arising from the aortic arch (*Takayasu's arteritis*) may cause carotid or vertebral thrombosis; it is rare in the western hemisphere.

Necrotizing (or granulomatous) arteritis, occurring alone or in association with generalized polyarteritis nodosa or Wegener's granulomatosis, involves the distal small branches (<2 mm diameter) of the main intracranial arteries and produces small ischemic infarcts in the brain, optic nerve, and spinal cord. The cerebrospinal fluid (CSF) often shows pleocytosis, and the protein level is elevated. *Primary central nervous system vasculitis* is rare; small or medium-sized vessels are usually affected, without apparent systemic vasculitis. Brain biopsy or high-resolution conventional x-ray angiography is usually required to make the diagnosis (Fig. 364-5). The differential diagnosis includes infection (tubercular, fungal), atherosclerosis, emboli, connective tissue disease, sarcoidosis, angiocentric lymphoma, carcinomatous meningitis, vasospasm, and drug-associated causes. Some cases follow the postpartum period and are self-limited. Patients with any form of vasculitis may present with insidious progression of combined white and gray matter infarctions, prominent headache, and cognitive decline. Aggressive immunosuppression with glucocorticoids, and often cyclophosphamide, is usually necessary to prevent progression; a diligent investigation for infectious causes such as tuberculosis is essential prior to immunosuppression. Depending upon the duration of the disease, many patients can make an excellent recovery.

Drugs, in particular amphetamines and perhaps cocaine, may cause stroke on the basis of acute hypertension or drug-induced vasculitis. Abstinence appears to be the best treatment, as no data exist on use of any treatment. Phenylpropanolamine has been linked with intracranial hemorrhage, as has cocaine, perhaps related to a drug-induced vasculitis. Arteritis can also occur as a consequence of bacterial, tuberculous, and syphilitic meningitis.

Moyamoya disease is a poorly understood occlusive disease involving large intracranial arteries, especially the distal internal carotid artery and the stem of the MCA and ACA. Vascular inflammation is absent. The lenticulostriate arteries develop a rich collateral circulation around the occlusive lesion, which gives the impression of a "puff of smoke" (*moyamoya* in Japanese) on conventional x-ray angiography. Other collaterals include transdural anastomoses between the cortical surface branches of the meningeal and scalp arteries. The disease occurs mainly in Asian children or young adults, but the appearance may be identical in adults who have atherosclerosis, particularly in association with diabetes. The etiology of the childhood form is unknown. Because of the occurrence of intracranial hemorrhage from rupture of the transdural and pial anastomotic channels, anticoagulation is risky. Breakdown of dilated lenticulostriate arteries may produce parenchymal hemorrhage, and progressive occlusion of large surface arteries can occur, producing large-artery distribution strokes. Bypass of extracranial carotid arteries to the dura or MCAs may prevent stroke and hemorrhage.

Reversible posterior leukoencephalopathy can occur in head injury, migraine, sympathomimetic drug use, eclampsia, and the postpartum period. The etiology is unclear but likely involves widespread cerebral segmental vasoconstriction and cerebral edema. Patients complain of headache and manifest fluctuating neurologic symptoms and signs, especially visual symptoms. Sometimes cerebral infarction ensues, but typically the clinical and imaging findings suggest that ischemia reverses completely. Conventional x-ray angiography is the only means of establishing the diagnosis, but MRI findings are characteristic.

Leukoariosis, or *periventricular white matter disease*, is the result of multiple small-vessel infarcts within the subcortical white matter. It is readily seen on CT or MRI scans as areas of white matter injury surrounding the ventricles and within the corona radiata. Areas of lacunar infarction are often seen also. The pathophysiologic basis of the disease is lipohyalinosis of small penetrating arteries within the white matter, likely produced by chronic hypertension. Patients with periventricular white matter disease may develop a subcortical dementia syndrome, depending on the amount of white matter infarction.

CADASIL (cerebral autosomal dominant arteriopathy with subcortical infarcts and leukoencephalopathy) is an inherited disorder that presents as small-vessel strokes, progressive dementia, and extensive symmetric white matter changes visualized by MRI. Approximately 40% of patients have migraine with aura, often manifest as transient motor or sensory deficits. Onset is usually in the fourth or fifth decade of life. This autosomal dominant condition is caused by one of several mutations in Notch-3, a member of a highly conserved gene family characterized by epidermal growth factor repeats in its extracellular domain. Other monogenic ischemic stroke syndromes include cerebral autosomal recessive arteriopathy with subcortical infarcts and leukoencephalopathy (CARASIL) and hereditary endotheliopathy, retinopathy, nephropathy, and stroke (HERNS). Fabry's disease also produces both large-vessel arteriopathy and small-vessel infarcts by an unknown mechanism.

TRANSIENT ISCHEMIC ATTACKS

TIAs are episodes of stroke symptoms that last only briefly; the standard definition of duration is <24 h, but most TIAs last <1 h. The causes of TIA are similar to the causes of ischemic stroke, but because TIAs may herald stroke they are an important risk factor that should be considered separately. TIAs may arise from emboli to the brain or from in situ thrombosis of an intracranial vessel. With a TIA, the occluded blood vessel reopens and neurologic function is restored. However, infarcts of the brain do occur in 15–50% of TIAs even though neurologic signs and symptoms are absent. Newer definitions of TIA categorize those with new infarct as having ischemic stroke rather than TIA regardless of symptom duration, but the vast majority of studies have used the standard, time-based definition.

In addition to the stroke syndromes discussed below, one specific TIA symptom should receive special notice. *Amaurosis fugax*, or transient monocular blindness, occurs from emboli to the central retinal artery of one eye. This may indicate carotid stenosis as the cause or local ophthalmic artery disease.

The risk of stroke after a TIA is ~10–15% in the first 3 months, with most events occurring in the first 2 days. Therefore, urgent evaluation and treatment are justified. Since etiologies for stroke and TIA are identical, evaluation for TIA should parallel that of stroke (Figs. 364-1 and 364-3). The improvement characteristic of TIA is a contraindication to thrombolysis. However, since the risk of subsequent stroke in the first few days after a TIA is high, the opportunity to give rtPA more frequently and rapidly if a stroke occurs probably justifies hospital admis-

sion for most patients. Acute antiplatelet therapy has not been tested specifically after TIA but is likely to be effective and is recommended. No large-scale trial has evaluated acute anticoagulation after TIA, a setting in which the risk of hemorrhage may be lower than for other categories of stroke.

RISK FACTORS FOR ISCHEMIC STROKE AND TIA

Identification and control of modifiable risk factors is the best strategy to reduce the burden of stroke, and the total number of strokes could be reduced substantially by these means (Table 364-4).

PRIMARY AND SECONDARY PREVENTION OF STROKE AND TIA

General Principles   A number of medical and surgical interventions, as well as lifestyle modifications, are available for preventing stroke. Some of these can be widely applied because of their low cost and minimal risk; others are expensive and carry substantial risk but may be valuable for selected high-risk patients.

Evaluation of a patient's *clinical risk profile* can help determine which preventive treatments to offer. In addition to known risk factors for ischemic stroke (above), certain clinical characteristics also contribute to an increased risk of stroke (Table 364-4).

Atherosclerosis Risk Factors   The relationship of various factors to the risk of atherosclerosis is described in Chap. 235. Older age, family history of thrombotic stroke, diabetes mellitus, hypertension, tobacco smoking, abnormal blood cholesterol [particularly, low high-density lipoprotein (HDL) and/or high low-density lipoprotein (LDL)], and other factors are either proven or probable risk factors for ischemic stroke, largely by their link to atherosclerosis. Risk of stroke is much greater in those with prior stroke or TIA. Many cardiac conditions predispose to stroke, including atrial fibrillation and recent MI. Oral contraceptives and hormone replacement therapy increase stroke risk, and certain inherited and acquired hypercoagulable states predispose to stroke. Hypertension is the most significant of the risk factors; in general, all hypertension should be treated. The presence of known cerebrovascular disease is not a contraindication to treatment aimed at achieving normotension. Also, the value of treating systolic hypertension in older patients has been clearly established. Lowering blood pressure to levels below those traditionally defining hypertension appears to reduce the risk of stroke even further. Data are particularly strong in support of thiazide diuretics, angiotensin-converting enzyme inhibitors, and angiotensin receptor blockers.

Several trials have confirmed that statin drugs reduce the risk of stroke even in patients without elevated LDL or low HDL. The recently reported SPARCL (Stroke Prevention by Aggressive Reduction in Cholesterol Levels) trial showed benefit in secondary stroke reduction for patients with recent stroke or TIA who were prescribed atorvastatin, 80 mg/d. Although studies specifically targeting primary prevention of stroke are still underway, results for patients with cardiovascular risk factors or dyslipidemia have been compelling, with a 16–30% relative risk reduction for stroke. Therefore, a statin should be considered in all patients with prior ischemic stroke. Tobacco smoking should be discouraged in all patients (Chap. 390). Whether tight control of blood sugar in patients with diabetes lowers stroke risk is uncertain, but statins, more aggressive blood pressure control, and pioglitazone (an agonist of peroxisome proliferator-activated receptor gamma) are effective.

Antiplatelet Agents   *Platelet antiaggregation agents* can prevent atherothrombotic events, including TIA and stroke, by inhibiting the formation of intraarterial platelet aggregates. These can form on diseased arteries, induce thrombus formation, and occlude the artery or embolize into the distal circulation. Aspirin, clopidogrel, and the combination of aspirin plus extended-release dipyridamole are the antiplatelet agents most commonly used for this purpose. Ticlopidine has been largely abandoned because of its adverse effects.

Aspirin is the most widely studied antiplatelet agent. Aspirin acetylates platelet cyclooxygenase, which irreversibly inhibits the formation in platelets of thromboxane A_2, a platelet aggregating and vasoconstricting prostaglandin. This effect is permanent and lasts for the usual 8-day life of the platelet. Paradoxically, aspirin also inhibits the formation in endothelial cells of prostacyclin, an antiaggregating and vasodilating prostaglandin. This effect is transient. As soon as aspirin is cleared from the blood, the nucleated endothelial cells again produce prostacyclin. Aspirin in low doses given once daily inhibits the production of thromboxane A_2 in platelets without substantially inhibiting prostacyclin formation. Higher doses of aspirin have not been proven to be more effective than lower doses, and 50–325 mg/d of aspirin is generally recommended for stroke prevention.

Ticlopidine and clopidogrel block the ADP receptor on platelets and thus prevent the cascade resulting in activation of the glycoprotein IIb/IIIa receptor that leads to fibrinogen binding to the platelet and consequent platelet aggregation. Ticlopidine is more effective than aspirin; however, it has the disadvantage of causing diarrhea, skin rash, and, in rare instances, neutropenia and thrombotic thrombocytopenic purpura. Clopidogrel is not associated with these important side effects. However, the CAPRIE (Clopidogrel versus Aspirin in Patients at Risk of Ischemic Events) trial, which led to FDA approval, found that it was only marginally more effective than aspirin in reducing risk of stroke. The MATCH (Management of Atherothrombosis with Clopidogrel in High-Risk Patients) trial was a large multicenter, randomized double-blind study that compared clopidogrel in combination with aspirin to clopidogrel alone in the secondary prevention of TIA or stroke. The MATCH trial found no difference in TIA or stroke prevention with this combination, but did show a small but significant increase in major bleeding complications (3% vs. 1%). In the CHARISMA (Clopidogrel for High Atherothrombotic Risk and Ischemic Stabilization, Management, and Avoidance) trial, which included a subgroup of patients with prior stroke or TIA along with other groups at high risk of cardiovascular events, there was no benefit of clopidogrel combined with aspirin compared to aspirin alone. Thus, the use of clopidogrel in combination with aspirin is not generally recommended for stroke prevention. However, these trials did not enroll patients immediately after the stroke or TIA, and the benefits of combination therapy were greater among those treated earlier, so it is possible that clopidogrel combined with aspirin may be beneficial in this acute period. Ongoing studies are currently addressing this question.

Dipyridamole is an antiplatelet agent that inhibits the uptake of adenosine by a variety of cells, including those of the vascular endothelium. The accumulated adenosine is an inhibitor of aggregation. At least in part through its effects on platelet and vessel wall phosphodiesterases, dipyridamole also potentiates the antiaggregatory effects of prostacyclin and nitric oxide produced by the endothelium and acts by inhibiting platelet phosphodiesterase, which is responsible for the breakdown of cyclic AMP. The resulting elevation in cyclic AMP inhibits aggregation of platelets. Dipyridamole is erratically absorbed depending on stomach pH, but a newer formulation combines timed-release dipyridamole, 200 mg, with aspirin, 25 mg, and has better oral bioavailability. This combination drug was studied in two trials. The European Stroke Prevention Study (ESPS) II showed efficacy of both 50 mg/d of aspirin and extended-release dipyridamole in preventing stroke, and a significantly better risk reduction when the two agents were combined. The ESPRIT (European/Australasian Stroke Prevention in Reversible Ischaemia Trial) trial confirmed the ESPS-II results. This was an open-label, academic trial in which 2739 patients with stroke or TIA treated with aspirin were randomized to dipyridamole, 200 mg twice daily, or no dipyridamole. Primary outcome was the composite of death from all vascular causes, non-fatal stroke, non-fatal MI, or major bleeding complication. After 3.5 years of follow-up, 13% patients on aspirin and dipyridamole and 16% on aspirin alone (hazard ratio 0.80, 95% CI 0.66–0.98) met the primary outcome. A meta-analysis of all dypridamole data on secondary stroke prevention found an overall risk ratio for the composite of vascular death, stroke, or MI of 0.82 (95% CI 0.74–0.91). The principal side effect of the drug is headache. A combination capsule of extended-release dipyridamole and aspirin is approved for prevention of stroke.

Many large clinical trials have demonstrated clearly that most antiplatelet agents reduce the risk of all important vascular atherothrombotic events (i.e., ischemic stroke, MI, and death due to all vascular causes) in patients at risk for these events. The overall *relative* reduction in risk of nonfatal stroke is about 25–30% and of all vascular events is about 25%. The *absolute* reduction varies considerably, depending on the particular patient's risk. Individuals at very low risk for stroke seem to experience the same relative reduction, but their risk may be so low that the "benefit" is meaningless. On the other hand, individuals with a 10–15% risk of vascular events per year experience a reduction to about 7.5–11%.

Aspirin is inexpensive, can be given in low doses, and could be recommended for all adults to prevent both stroke and MI. However, it causes epigastric discomfort, gastric ulceration, and gastrointestinal hemorrhage, which may be asymptomatic or life-threatening. Consequently, not every 40- or 50-year-old should be advised to take aspirin regularly because the risk of atherothrombotic stroke is extremely low and is outweighed by the risk of adverse side effects. Conversely, every patient who has experienced an atherothrombotic stroke or TIA and has no contraindication should be taking an antiplatelet agent regularly because the average annual risk of another stroke is 8–10%; another few percent will experience a MI or vascular death. Clearly, the likelihood of benefit far outweighs the risks of treatment.

The choice of antiplatelet agent and dose must balance the risk of stroke, the expected benefit, and the risk and cost of treatment. However, there are no definitive data, and opinions vary. Many authorities believe low-dose (30–75 mg/d) and high-dose (650–1300 mg/d) aspirin are about equally effective. Some advocate very low doses to avoid adverse effects, and still others advocate very high doses to be sure the benefit is maximal. Most physicians in North America recommend 81–325 mg/d, while most Europeans recommend 50–100 mg. Similarly, the choice of aspirin, clopidogrel, or dipyridamole plus aspirin must balance the fact that the latter are more effective than aspirin but the cost is higher, and this is likely to affect long-term patient adherence.

Anticoagulation Therapy and Embolic Stroke Several trials have shown that anticoagulation (INR range, 2–3) in patients with chronic nonvalvular (nonrheumatic) atrial fibrillation prevents cerebral embolism and is safe. For primary prevention and for patients who have experienced stroke or TIA, anticoagulation with warfarin reduces the risk by about 67%, which clearly outweighs the 1% risk per year of a major bleeding complication.

The decision to use anticoagulation for primary prevention is based primarily on risk factors (Table 364-3). The presence of any risk factor tips the balance in favor of anticoagulation.

Because of the high annual stroke risk in untreated rheumatic heart disease, primary prophylaxis against stroke has not been studied in a double-blind fashion. These patients generally should receive long-term anticoagulation.

Anticoagulation also reduces the risk of embolism in acute MI. Most clinicians recommend a 3-month course of anticoagulation when there is anterior Q-wave infarction, substantial left ventricular dysfunction, congestive heart failure, mural thrombosis, or atrial fibrillation. Warfarin is recommended long-term if atrial fibrillation persists. Warfarin is currently being studied in patients with congestive heart failure.

Stroke secondary to thromboembolism is one of the most serious complications of prosthetic heart valve implantation. The intensity of anticoagulation and/or antiplatelet therapy is dictated by the type of prosthetic valve and its location. The Seventh American College of Chest Physicians Conference on Antithrombotic Therapy for Valvular Heart Disease published the following guidelines in 2004: (1) for St. Jude Medical bileaflet valves in the aortic position, long-term warfarin with a target INR of 2.5 (range 2.0–3.0), (2) for tilting disk valves and bileaflet mechanical valves in the mitral position, long-term warfarin with a target INR of 3.0; (range 2.5–3.5); (3) for caged ball or caged disk valves, long-term warfarin with target INR of 3.0 (range 2.5–3.5) in combination with aspirin (75–100 mg/d); (4) for bioprosthetic valves, warfarin anticoagulation with target INR 2.5 for 3 months, followed by long-term aspirin alone (75–100 mg/d), assuming there is no history of atrial fibrillation.

If the embolic source cannot be eliminated, anticoagulation should in most cases be continued indefinitely. Many neurologists recommend combining antiplatelet agents with anticoagulants for patients who "fail" anticoagulation (i.e., have another stroke or TIA).

Anticoagulation Therapy and Noncardiogenic Stroke Data do not support the use of long-term warfarin for preventing atherothrombotic stroke, for either intracranial or extracranial cerebrovascular disease. The WARSS (Warfarin-Aspirin Reinfarction Stroke Study) study found no benefit of warfarin sodium (INR, 1.4–2.8) over aspirin, 325 mg, for secondary prevention of stroke but did find a slightly higher bleeding rate in the warfarin group. A recent European study confirmed this finding. The WASID study (see above) demonstrated no benefit of warfarin (INR, 2–3) over aspirin in patients with symptomatic intracranial atherosclerosis, and also found higher bleeding complications.

Other Causes of Stroke · *CAROTID DISEASE* Surgical or endovascular repair of carotid atherosclerosis is preferred over medical therapy for symptomatic carotid artery disease (see section above). Anticoagulation has not been directly compared with antiplatelet therapy for carotid disease.

DURAL SINUS THROMBOSIS Limited evidence exists to support short-term usage of anticoagulants, regardless of the presence of intracranial hemorrhage for venous infarction following sinus thrombosis.

STROKE SYNDROMES

A careful history and neurologic examination can often localize the region of brain dysfunction; if this region corresponds to a particular arterial distribution, the possible causes responsible for the syndrome can be narrowed. This is of particular importance when the patient presents with a TIA and a normal examination. For example, if a patient develops language loss and a right homonymous hemianopia, a search for causes of left middle cerebral emboli should be performed. A finding of an isolated stenosis of the right internal carotid artery in that patient, for example, suggests an asymptomatic carotid stenosis, and the search for other causes of stroke should continue. The following sections describe the clinical findings of cerebral ischemia associated with cerebral vascular territories depicted in Figs. 364-4, and 364-6 through 364-14. Stroke syndromes are divided into: (1) large-vessel stroke within the anterior circulation, (2) large-vessel stroke within the posterior circulation, and (3) small-vessel disease of either vascular bed.

Stroke within the Anterior Circulation The internal carotid artery and its branches comprise the anterior circulation of the brain. These vessels can be occluded by intrinsic disease of the vessel (e.g., atherosclerosis or dissection) or by embolic occlusion from a proximal source as discussed above. Occlusion of each major intracranial vessel has distinct clinical manifestations.

MIDDLE CEREBRAL ARTERY Occlusion of the proximal MCA or one of its major branches is most often due to an embolus (artery-to-artery, cardiac, or of unknown source) rather than intracranial atherothrombosis. Atherosclerosis of the proximal MCA may cause distal emboli to the middle cerebral territory or, less commonly, may produce low-flow TIAs. Collateral formation via leptomeningeal vessels often prevents MCA stenosis from becoming symptomatic.

The cortical branches of the MCA supply the lateral surface of the hemisphere except for (1) the frontal pole and a strip along the superomedial border of the frontal and parietal lobes supplied by the ACA, and (2) the lower temporal and occipital pole convolutions supplied by the PCA (Figs. 364-6, 364-7, 364-8, and 364-9).

The proximal MCA (M1 segment) gives rise to penetrating branches (termed *lenticulostriate arteries*) that supply the putamen, outer globus pallidus, posterior limb of the internal capsule, the adjacent corona radiata, and most of the caudate nucleus (Fig. 364-6). In the sylvian fissure, the MCA in most patients divides into *superior* and *in-*

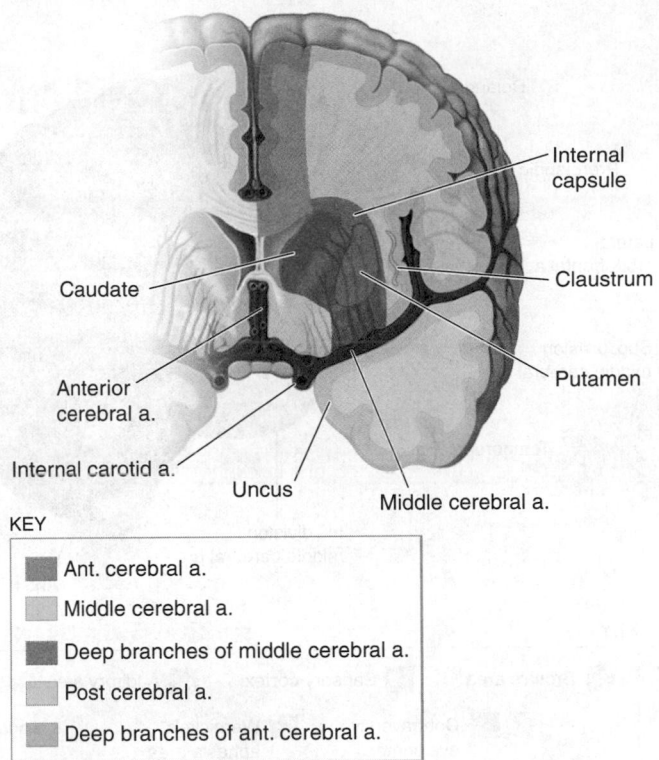

CHAPTER 364

Cerebrovascular Diseases

FIGURE 364-6 Diagram of a cerebral hemisphere in coronal section showing the territories of the major cerebral vessels that branch from the internal carotid arteries.

ferior divisions (M2 branches). Branches of the inferior division supply the inferior parietal and temporal cortex, and those from the superior division supply the frontal and superior parietal cortex (Fig. 364-7).

If the entire MCA is occluded at its origin (blocking both its penetrating and cortical branches) and the distal collaterals are limited, the clinical findings are contralateral hemiplegia, hemianesthesia, homonymous hemianopia, and a day or two of gaze preference to the ipsilateral side. Dysarthria is common because of facial weakness. When the dominant hemisphere is involved, global aphasia is present also, and when the nondominant hemisphere is affected, anosognosia, constructional apraxia, and neglect are found (Chap. 27).

Complete MCA syndromes occur most often when an embolus occludes the stem of the artery. Cortical collateral blood flow and differing arterial configurations are probably responsible for the development of many partial syndromes. Partial syndromes may also be due to emboli that enter the proximal MCA without complete occlusion, occlude distal MCA branches, or fragment and move distally.

Partial syndromes due to embolic occlusion of a single branch include hand, or arm and hand, weakness alone (brachial syndrome) or facial weakness with nonfluent (Broca) aphasia (Chap. 27), with or without arm weakness (frontal opercular syndrome). A combination of sensory disturbance, motor weakness, and nonfluent aphasia suggests that an embolus has occluded the proximal superior division and infarcted large portions of the frontal and parietal cortices (Fig. 364-7). If a fluent (Wernicke's) aphasia occurs without weakness, the inferior division of the MCA supplying the posterior part (temporal cortex) of the dominant hemisphere is probably involved. Jargon speech and an inability to comprehend written and spoken language are prominent features, often accompanied by a contralateral, homonymous superior quadrantanopia. Hemineglect or spatial agnosia without weakness indicates that the inferior division of the MCA in the nondominant hemisphere is involved.

Occlusion of a lenticulostriate vessel produces small-vessel (lacunar) stroke within the internal capsule (Fig. 364-6). This produces pure motor stroke or sensory-motor stroke contralateral to the lesion.

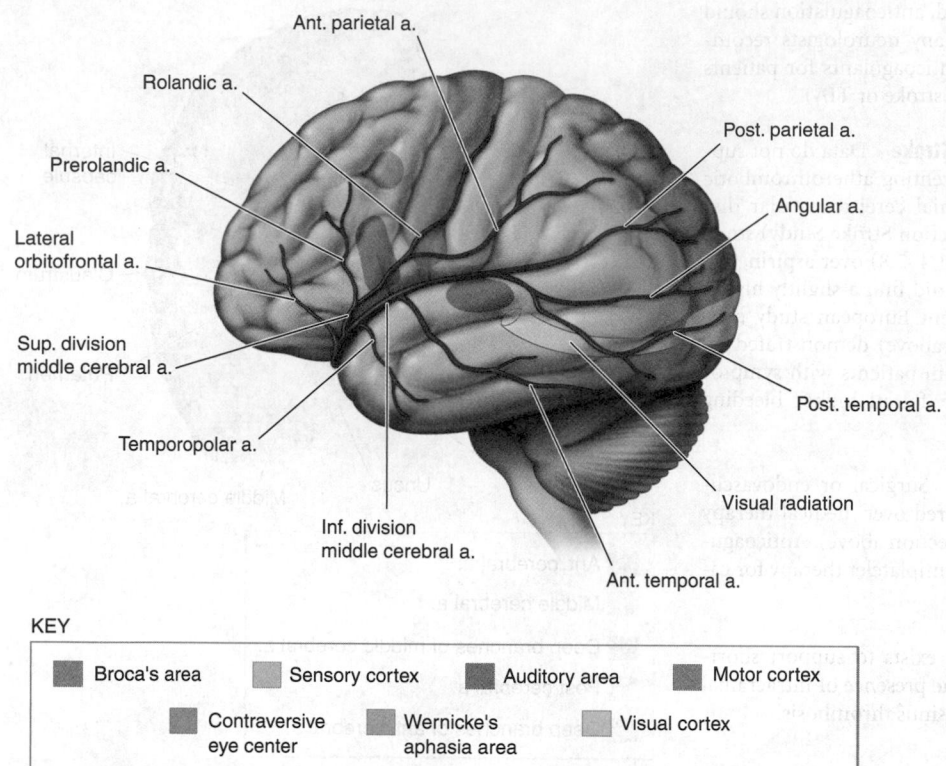

KEY

| ■ Broca's area | ■ Sensory cortex | ■ Auditory area | ■ Motor cortex |
| ■ Contraversive eye center | ■ Wernicke's aphasia area | ■ Visual cortex | |

FIGURE 364-7 Diagram of a cerebral hemisphere, lateral aspect, showing the branches and distribution of the middle cerebral artery and the principal regions of cerebral localization. Note the bifurcation of the middle cerebral artery into a superior and inferior division.

Signs and symptoms: *Structures involved*

Paralysis of the contralateral face, arm, and leg; sensory impairment over the same area (pinprick, cotton touch, vibration, position, two-point discrimination, stereognosis, tactile localization, barognosis, cutaneographia): *Somatic motor area for face and arm and the fibers descending from the leg area to enter the corona radiata and corresponding somatic sensory system*

Motor aphasia: *Motor speech area of the dominant hemisphere*

Central aphasia, word deafness, anomia, jargon speech, sensory agraphia, acalculia, alexia, finger agnosia, right-left confusion (the last four comprise the Gerstmann syndrome): *Central, suprasylvian speech area and parietooccipital cortex of the dominant hemisphere*

Conduction aphasia: *Central speech area (parietal operculum)*

Apractognosia of the nondominant hemisphere, anosognosia, hemiasomatognosia, unilateral neglect, agnosia for the left half of external space, dressing "apraxia," constructional "apraxia," distortion of visual coordinates, inaccurate localization in the half field, impaired ability to judge distance, upside-down reading, visual illusions (e.g., it may appear that another person walks through a table): *Nondominant parietal lobe (area corresponding to speech area in dominant hemisphere); loss of topographic memory is usually due to a nondominant lesion, occasionally to a dominant one*

Homonymous hemianopia (often homonymous inferior quadrantanopia): *Optic radiation deep to second temporal convolution*

Paralysis of conjugate gaze to the opposite side: *Frontal contraversive eye field or projecting fibers*

Ischemia within the genu of the internal capsule causes primarily facial weakness followed by arm then leg weakness as the ischemia moves posterior within the capsule. Alternatively, the contralateral hand may become ataxic and dysarthria will be prominent (clumsy hand, dysarthria lacunar syndrome). Lacunar infarction affecting the globus pallidus and putamen often has few clinical signs, but parkinsonism and hemiballismus have been reported.

ANTERIOR CEREBRAL ARTERY The ACA is divided into two segments: the precommunal (A1) circle of Willis, or stem, which connects the internal carotid artery to the anterior communicating artery, and the postcommunal (A2) segment distal to the anterior communicating artery (Figs. 364-4, 364-6, and 364-8). The A1 segment gives rise to several deep penetrating branches that supply the anterior limb of the internal capsule, the anterior perforate substance, amygdala, anterior hypothalamus, and the inferior part of the head of the caudate nucleus (Fig. 364-6).

Occlusion of the proximal ACA is usually well tolerated because of collateral flow through the anterior communicating artery and collaterals through the MCA and PCA. Occlusion of a single A2 segment results in the contralateral symptoms noted in Fig. 364-8. If both A2 segments arise from a single anterior cerebral stem (contralateral A1 segment atresia), the occlusion may affect both hemispheres. Profound abulia (a delay in verbal and motor response) and bilateral pyramidal signs with paraparesis and urinary incontinence result.

ANTERIOR CHOROIDAL ARTERY This artery arises from the internal carotid artery and supplies the posterior limb of the internal capsule and the white matter posterolateral to it, through which pass some of the geniculocalcarine fibers (Fig. 364-9). The complete syndrome of anterior choroidal artery occlusion consists of contralateral hemiplegia, hemianesthesia (hypesthesia), and homonymous hemianopia. However, because this territory is also supplied by penetrating vessels of the proximal MCA and the posterior communicating and posterior choroidal arteries, minimal deficits may occur, and patients frequently recover substantially. Anterior choroidal strokes are usually the result of in situ thrombosis of the vessel, and the vessel is particularly vulnerable to iatrogenic occlusion during surgical clipping of aneurysms arising from the internal carotid artery.

INTERNAL CAROTID ARTERY The clinical picture of internal carotid occlusion varies depending on whether the cause of ischemia is propagated thrombus, embolism, or low flow. The cortex supplied by the MCA territory is affected most often. With a competent circle of Willis, occlusion may go unnoticed. If the thrombus propagates up the internal carotid artery into the MCA or embolizes it, symptoms are identical to proximal MCA occlusion (see above). Sometimes there is massive infarction of the entire deep white matter and cortical surface. When the origins of both the ACA and MCA are occluded at the top of the carotid artery, abulia or stupor occurs with hemiplegia, hemianesthesia, and aphasia or anosognosia. When the PCA arises from the internal carotid artery (a configuration called a *fetal posterior cerebral artery*), it may also become occluded and give rise to symptoms referable to its peripheral territory (Figs. 364-8 and 364-9).

In addition to supplying the ipsilateral brain, the internal carotid artery perfuses the optic nerve and retina via the ophthalmic artery. In ~25% of symptomatic internal carotid disease, recurrent transient monocular blindness (amaurosis fugax) warns of the lesion. Patients typically describe a horizontal shade that sweeps down or up across the field of vision. They may also complain that their vision was blurred in that eye or that the upper or lower half of vision disappeared. In most cases, these symptoms last only a few minutes. Rarely, ischemia or infarction of the ophthalmic artery or central retinal arteries occurs at the time of cerebral TIA or infarction.

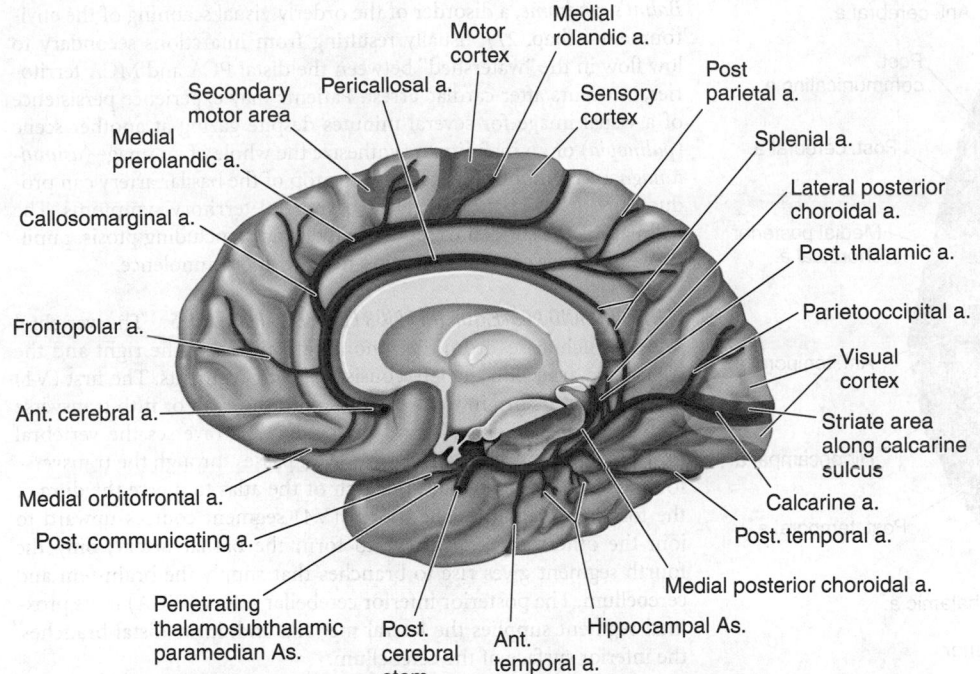

FIGURE 364-8 Diagram of a cerebral hemisphere, medial aspect, showing the branches and distribution of the anterior cerebral artery and the principal regions of cerebral localization.

Signs and symptoms: *Structures involved*

Paralysis of opposite foot and leg: *Motor leg area*

A lesser degree of paresis of opposite arm: *Arm area of cortex or fibers descending to corona radiata*

Cortical sensory loss over toes, foot, and leg: *Sensory area for foot and leg*

Urinary incontinence: *Sensorimotor area in paracentral lobule*

Contralateral grasp reflex, sucking reflex, gegenhalten (paratonic rigidity): *Medial surface of the posterior frontal lobe; likely supplemental motor area*

Abulia (akinetic mutism), slowness, delay, intermittent interruption, lack of spontaneity, whispering, reflex distraction to sights and sounds: *Uncertain localization—probably cingulate gyrus and medial inferior portion of frontal, parietal, and temporal lobes*

Impairment of gait and stance (gait apraxia): *Frontal cortex near leg motor area*

Dyspraxia of left limbs, tactile aphasia in left limbs: *Corpus callosum*

A high-pitched prolonged carotid bruit fading into diastole is often associated with tightly stenotic lesions. As the stenosis grows tighter and flow distal to the stenosis becomes reduced, the bruit becomes fainter and may disappear when occlusion is imminent.

COMMON CAROTID ARTERY All symptoms and signs of internal carotid occlusion may also be present with occlusion of the common carotid artery. Bilateral common carotid artery occlusions at their origin may occur in Takayasu's arteritis (Chap. 319).

Stroke within the Posterior Circulation The posterior circulation is composed of the paired vertebral arteries, the basilar artery, and the paired posterior cerebral arteries. The vertebral arteries join to form the basilar artery at the pontomedullary junction. The basilar artery divides into two posterior cerebral arteries in the interpeduncular fossa (Figs. 364-4, 364-8, and 364-9). These major arteries give rise to long and short circumferential branches and to smaller deep penetrating branches that supply the cerebellum, medulla, pons, midbrain, subthalamus, thalamus, hippocampus, and medial temporal and occipital lobes. Occlusion of each vessel produces its own distinctive syndrome.

POSTERIOR CEREBRAL ARTERY In 75% of cases, both PCAs arise from the bifurcation of the basilar artery; in 20%, one has its origin from the ipsilateral internal carotid artery via the posterior communicating artery; in 5%, both originate from the respective ipsilateral internal carotid arteries (Figs. 364-8 and 364-9). The precommunal, or P1, segment of the true posterior cerebral artery is atretic in such cases.

PCA syndromes usually result from atheroma formation or emboli that lodge at the top of the basilar artery; posterior circulation disease may also be caused by dissection of either vertebral artery and fibromuscular dysplasia.

Two clinical syndromes are commonly observed with occlusion of the PCA: (1) *P1 syndrome*: midbrain, subthalamic, and thalamic signs, which are due to disease of the proximal P1 segment of the PCA or its penetrating branches (thalamogeniculate, Percheron, and posterior choroidal arteries); and (2) *P2 syndrome*: cortical temporal and occipital lobe signs, due to occlusion of the P2 segment distal to the junction of the PCA with the posterior communicating artery.

P1 Syndromes Infarction usually occurs in the ipsilateral subthalamus and medial thalamus and in the ipsilateral cerebral peduncle and midbrain (Figs. 364-9 and 364-14). A third nerve palsy with contralateral ataxia (Claude's syndrome) or with contralateral hemiplegia (Weber's syndrome) may result. The ataxia indicates involvement of the red nucleus or dentatorubrothalamic tract; the hemiplegia is localized to the cerebral peduncle (Fig. 364-14). If the subthalamic nucleus is involved, contralateral hemiballismus may occur. Occlusion of the artery of Percheron produces paresis of upward gaze and drowsiness, and often abulia. Extensive infarction in the midbrain and subthalamus occurring with bilateral proximal PCA occlusion presents as coma, unreactive pupils, bilateral pyramidal signs, and decerebrate rigidity.

Occlusion of the penetrating branches of thalamic and thalamogeniculate arteries produces less extensive thalamic and thalamocapsular lacunar syndromes. The *thalamic Déjerine-Roussy syndrome* consists of contralateral hemisensory loss followed later by an agonizing, searing or burning pain in the affected areas. It is persistent and responds poorly to analgesics. Anticonvulsants (carbamazepine or gabapentin) or tricyclic antidepressants may be beneficial.

P2 Syndromes (See also Fig. 364-8 and 364-9) Occlusion of the distal PCA causes infarction of the medial temporal and occipital lobes. Contralateral homonymous hemianopia with macula sparing is the usual manifestation. Occasionally, only the upper quadrant of visual field is involved. If the visual association areas are spared and only the calcarine cortex is involved, the patient may be aware of visual defects. Medial temporal lobe and hippocampal involvement may cause an acute disturbance in memory, particularly if it occurs in the dominant hemisphere. The defect usually clears because memory has bilateral representation. If the dominant hemisphere is affected and the infarct extends to involve the splenium of the corpus callosum, the patient may demonstrate alexia without agraphia. Visual agnosia for faces, objects, mathematical symbols, and colors and anomia with paraphasic errors (amnestic aphasia) may also occur in this setting, even without callosal involvement. Occlusion of the posterior cerebral artery can produce *peduncular hallucinosis* (visual hallucinations of brightly colored scenes and objects).

Bilateral infarction in the distal PCAs produces cortical blindness (blindness with preserved pupillary light reaction). The patient is often

Internal carotid a.
Ant. cerebral a.
Post. communicating a.
Post. cerebral a.
Ant. choroidal a.
Medial posterior choroidal a.
Mesencephalic paramedian As.
Ant. temporal a.
Splenial a.
Parietooccipital a.
Calcarine a.
Hippocampal a.
Post. temporal a.
Post. thalamic a.
Visual cortex
Lateral posterior choroidal a.

FIGURE 364-9 Inferior aspect of the brain with the branches and distribution of the posterior cerebral artery and the principal anatomic structures shown.

Signs and symptoms: *Structures involved*

Peripheral territory (see also Fig. 364-12). Homonymous hemianopia (often upper quadrantic): *Calcarine cortex or optic radiation nearby.* Bilateral homonymous hemianopia, cortical blindness, awareness or denial of blindness; tactile naming, achromatopia (color blindness), failure to see to-and-fro movements, inability to perceive objects not centrally located, apraxia of ocular movements, inability to count or enumerate objects, tendency to run into things that the patient sees and tries to avoid: *Bilateral occipital lobe with possibly the parietal lobe involved.* Verbal dyslexia without agraphia, color anomia: *Dominant calcarine lesion and posterior part of corpus callosum.* Memory defect: *Hippocampal lesion bilaterally or on the dominant side only.* Topographic disorientation and prosopagnosia: *Usually with lesions of nondominant, calcarine, and lingual gyrus.* Simultanagnosia, hemivisual neglect: *Dominant visual cortex, contralateral hemisphere.* Unformed visual hallucinations, peduncular hallucinosis, metamorphopsia, teleopsia, illusory visual spread, palinopsia, distortion of outlines, central photophobia: *Calcarine cortex.* Complex hallucinations: *Usually nondominant hemisphere.*

Central territory. Thalamic syndrome: sensory loss (all modalities), spontaneous pain and dysesthesias, choreoathetosis, intention tremor, spasms of hand, mild hemiparesis: *Posteroventral nucleus of thalamus; involvement of the adjacent subthalamus body or its afferent tracts.* Thalamoperforate syndrome: crossed cerebellar ataxia with ipsilateral third nerve palsy (Claude's syndrome): *Dentatothalamic tract and issuing third nerve.* Weber's syndrome: third nerve palsy and contralateral hemiplegia: *Third nerve and cerebral peduncle.* Contralateral hemiplegia: *Cerebral peduncle.* Paralysis or paresis of vertical eye movement, skew deviation, sluggish pupillary responses to light, slight miosis and ptosis (retraction nystagmus and "tucking" of the eyelids may be associated): *Supranuclear fibers to third nerve, interstitial nucleus of Cajal, nucleus of Darkschewitsch, and posterior commissure.* Contralateral rhythmic, ataxic action tremor; rhythmic postural or "holding" tremor (rubral tremor): *Dentatothalamic tract.*

unaware of the blindness or may even deny it (*Anton's syndrome*). Tiny islands of vision may persist, and the patient may report that vision fluctuates as images are captured in the preserved portions. Rarely, only peripheral vision is lost and central vision is spared, resulting in "gunbarrel" vision. Bilateral visual association area lesions may result in

Balint's syndrome, a disorder of the orderly visual scanning of the environment (Chap. 27), usually resulting from infarctions secondary to low flow in the "watershed" between the distal PCA and MCA territories, as occurs after cardiac arrest. Patients may experience persistence of a visual image for several minutes despite gazing at another scene (*palinopia*) or an inability to synthesize the whole of an image (*asimultanagnosia*). Embolic occlusion of the top of the basilar artery can produce any or all of the central or peripheral territory symptoms. The hallmark is the sudden onset of bilateral signs, including ptosis, pupillary asymmetry or lack of reaction to light, and somnolence.

VERTEBRAL AND POSTERIOR INFERIOR CEREBELLAR ARTERIES The vertebral artery, which arises from the innominate artery on the right and the subclavian artery on the left, consists of four segments. The first (V1) extends from its origin to its entrance into the sixth or fifth transverse vertebral foramen. The second segment (V2) traverses the vertebral foramina from C6 to C2. The third (V3) passes through the transverse foramen and circles around the arch of the atlas to pierce the dura at the foramen magnum. The fourth (V4) segment courses upward to join the other vertebral artery to form the basilar artery; only the fourth segment gives rise to branches that supply the brainstem and cerebellum. The posterior inferior cerebellar artery (PICA) in its proximal segment supplies the lateral medulla and, in its distal branches, the inferior surface of the cerebellum.

Atherothrombotic lesions have a predilection for V1 and V4 segments of the vertebral artery. The first segment may become diseased at the origin of the vessel and may produce posterior circulation emboli; collateral flow from the contralateral vertebral artery or the ascending cervical, thyrocervical, or occipital arteries is usually sufficient to prevent low-flow TIAs or stroke. When one vertebral artery is atretic and an atherothrombotic lesion threatens the origin of the other, the collateral circulation, which may also include retrograde flow down the basilar artery, is often insufficient (Figs. 364-4 and 364-9). In this setting, low-flow TIAs may occur, consisting of syncope, vertigo, and alternating hemiplegia; this state also sets the stage for thrombosis. Disease of the distal fourth segment of the vertebral artery can promote thrombus formation manifest as embolism or with propagation as basilar artery thrombosis. Stenosis proximal to the origin of the PICA can threaten the lateral medulla and posterior inferior surface of the cerebellum.

If the subclavian artery is occluded proximal to the origin of the vertebral artery, there is a reversal in the direction of blood flow in the ipsilateral vertebral artery. Exercise of the ipsilateral arm may increase demand on vertebral flow, producing posterior circulation TIAs, or "subclavian steal."

Although atheromatous disease rarely narrows the second and third segments of the vertebral artery, this region is subject to dissection, fibromuscular dysplasia, and, rarely, encroachment by osteophytic spurs within the vertebral foramina.

Embolic occlusion or thrombosis of a V4 segment causes ischemia of the lateral medulla. The constellation of vertigo, numbness of the ipsilateral face and contralateral limbs, diplopia, hoarseness, dysarthria, dysphagia, and ipsilateral Horner's syndrome is called the *lateral medullary (or Wallenberg's) syndrome* (Fig. 364-10). Most cases result from ipsilateral vertebral artery occlusion; in the remainder, PICA occlusion is responsible. Occlusion of the medullary penetrating branches of the vertebral artery or PICA results in partial syndromes. *Hemiparesis is not a feature of vertebral artery occlusion, however, quadriparesis may result from occlusion of the anterior spinal artery.*

Rarely, a *medial medullary syndrome* occurs with infarction of the pyramid and contralateral hemiparesis of the arm and leg, sparing the face. If the medial lemniscus and emerging hypoglossal nerve fibers are involved, contralateral loss of joint position sense and ipsilateral tongue weakness occur.

Cerebellar infarction with edema can lead to *sudden respiratory arrest* due to raised ICP in the posterior fossa. Drowsiness, Babinski signs, dysarthria, and bifacial weakness may be absent, or present only briefly, before respiratory arrest ensues. Gait unsteadiness, headache,

FIGURE 364-10 Axial section at the level of the medulla, depicted schematically on the left, with a corresponding MR image on the right. Note that in Figs. 364-10 through 364-14, all drawings are oriented with the dorsal surface at the bottom, matching the orientation of the brainstem that is commonly seen in all modern neuroimaging studies. Approximate regions involved in medial and lateral medullary stroke syndromes are shown.

Signs and symptoms: *Structures involved*
1. Medial medullary syndrome (occlusion of vertebral artery or of branch of vertebral or lower basilar artery)
   On side of lesion
      Paralysis with atrophy of half the tongue: *Ipsilateral twelfth nerve*
   On side opposite lesion
      Paralysis of arm and leg, sparing face; impaired tactile and proprioceptive sense over half the body: *Contralateral pyramidal tract and medial lemniscus*
2. Lateral medullary syndrome (occlusion of any of five vessels may be responsible—vertebral, posterior inferior cerebellar, superior, middle, or inferior lateral medullary arteries)
   On side of lesion
      Pain, numbness, impaired sensation over half the face: *Descending tract and nucleus fifth nerve*
      Ataxia of limbs, falling to side of lesion: *Uncertain—restiform body, cerebellar hemisphere, cerebellar fibers, spinocerebellar tract (?)*
      Nystagmus, diplopia, oscillopsia, vertigo, nausea, vomiting: *Vestibular nucleus*

   Horner's syndrome (miosis, ptosis, decreased sweating): *Descending sympathetic tract*
   Dysphagia, hoarseness, paralysis of palate, paralysis of vocal cord, diminished gag reflex: *Issuing fibers ninth and tenth nerves*
   Loss of taste: *Nucleus and tractus solitarius*
   Numbness of ipsilateral arm, trunk, or leg: *Cuneate and gracile nuclei*
   Weakness of lower face: *Genuflected upper motor neuron fibers to ipsilateral facial nucleus*
   On side opposite lesion
      Impaired pain and thermal sense over half the body, sometimes face: *Spinothalamic tract*
3. Total unilateral medullary syndrome (occlusion of vertebral artery): Combination of medial and lateral syndromes
4. Lateral pontomedullary syndrome (occlusion of vertebral artery): Combination of lateral medullary and lateral inferior pontine syndrome
5. Basilar artery syndrome (the syndrome of the lone vertebral artery is equivalent): A combination of the various brainstem syndromes plus those arising in the posterior cerebral artery distribution.
   Bilateral long tract signs (sensory and motor; cerebellar and peripheral cranial nerve abnormalities): *Bilateral long tract; cerebellar and peripheral cranial nerves*
   Paralysis or weakness of all extremities, plus all bulbar musculature: *Corticobulbar and corticospinal tracts bilaterally*

dizziness, nausea, and vomiting may be the only early symptoms and signs and should arouse suspicion of this impending complication, which may require neurosurgical decompression, often with an excellent outcome. Separating these symptoms from those of viral labyrinthitis can be a challenge, but headache, neck stiffness, and unilateral dysmetria favor stroke.

BASILAR ARTERY Branches of the basilar artery supply the base of the pons and superior cerebellum and fall into three groups: (1) paramedian, 7–10 in number, which supply a wedge of pons on either side of the midline; (2) short circumferential, 5–7 in number, which supply the lateral two-thirds of the pons and middle and superior cerebellar peduncles; and (3) bilateral long circumferential (superior cerebellar and anterior inferior cerebellar arteries), which course around the pons to supply the cerebellar hemispheres.

Atheromatous lesions can occur anywhere along the basilar trunk but are most frequent in the proximal basilar and distal vertebral segments. Typically, lesions occlude either the proximal basilar and one or both vertebral arteries. The clinical picture varies depending on the availability of retrograde collateral flow from the posterior communicating arteries. Rarely, dissection of a vertebral artery may involve the basilar artery and, depending on the location of true and false lumen, may produce multiple penetrating artery strokes.

Although atherothrombosis occasionally occludes the distal portion of the basilar artery, emboli from the heart or proximal vertebral or basilar segments are more commonly responsible for "top of the basilar" syndromes.

Because the brainstem contains many structures in close apposition, a diversity of clinical syndromes may emerge with ischemia, reflecting involvement of the corticospinal and corticobulbar tracts, ascending sensory tracts, and cranial nerve nuclei (**Figs. 364-11, 364-12, 364-13,** and **364-14**).

The symptoms of transient ischemia or infarction in the territory of the basilar artery often do not indicate whether the basilar artery itself or one of its branches is diseased, yet this distinction has important implications for therapy. *The picture of complete basilar occlusion, how-*

FIGURE 364-11 Axial section at the level of the inferior pons, depicted schematically on the left, with a corresponding MR image on the right. Approximate regions involved in medial and lateral inferior pontine stroke syndromes are shown.

Signs and symptoms: *Structures involved*

1. Medial inferior pontine syndrome (occlusion of paramedian branch of basilar artery)

    On side of lesion

    Paralysis of conjugate gaze to side of lesion (preservation of convergence): *Center for conjugate lateral gaze*

    Nystagmus: *Vestibular nucleus*

    Ataxia of limbs and gait: Likely *middle cerebellar peduncle*

    Diplopia on lateral gaze: *Abducens nerve*

    On side opposite lesion

    Paralysis of face, arm, and leg: *Corticobulbar and corticospinal tract in lower pons*

    Impaired tactile and proprioceptive sense over half of the body: *Medial lemniscus*

2. Lateral inferior pontine syndrome (occlusion of anterior inferior cerebellar artery)

    On side of lesion

    Horizontal and vertical nystagmus, vertigo, nausea, vomiting, oscillopia: *Vestibular nerve or nucleus*

    Facial paralysis: *Seventh nerve*

    Paralysis of conjugate gaze to side of lesion: *Center for conjugate lateral gaze*

    Deafness, tinnitus: *Auditory nerve or cochlear nucleus*

    Ataxia: *Middle cerebellar peduncle and cerebellar hemisphere*

    Impaired sensation over face: *Descending tract and nucleus fifth nerve*

    On side opposite lesion

    Impaired pain and thermal sense over half the body (may include face): *Spinothalamic tract*

ever, is easy to recognize as a constellation of bilateral long tract signs (sensory and motor) with signs of cranial nerve and cerebellar dysfunction. A "locked-in" state of preserved consciousness with quadriplegia and cranial nerve signs suggests complete pontine and lower midbrain infarction. The therapeutic goal is to identify *impending* basilar occlusion before devastating infarction occurs. A series of TIAs and a slowly progressive, fluctuating stroke are extremely significant, as they often herald an atherothrombotic occlusion of the distal vertebral or proximal basilar artery.

TIAs in the proximal basilar distribution may produce vertigo (often described by patients as "swimming," "swaying," "moving," "unsteadiness," or "light-headedness"). Other symptoms that warn of basilar thrombosis include diplopia, dysarthria, facial or circumoral numbness, and hemisensory symptoms. In general, symptoms of basilar branch TIAs affect one side of the brainstem, whereas symptoms of basilar artery TIAs usually affect both sides, though a "herald" hemiparesis has been emphasized as an initial symptom of basilar occlusion. Most often TIAs, whether due to impending occlusion of the basilar artery or a basilar branch, are short-lived (5–30 min) and repetitive, occurring several times a day. The pattern suggests intermittent reduction of flow. Many neurologists treat with heparin to prevent clot propagation.

Atherothrombotic occlusion of the basilar artery with infarction usually causes *bilateral* brainstem signs. A gaze paresis or internuclear ophthalmoplegia associated with ipsilateral hemiparesis may be the only manifestation of bilateral brainstem ischemia. More often, unequivocal signs of bilateral pontine disease are present. Complete basilar thrombosis carries a high mortality.

Occlusion of a branch of the basilar artery usually causes *unilateral* symptoms and signs involving motor, sensory, and cranial nerves. As long as symptoms remain unilateral, concern over pending basilar occlusion should be reduced.

Occlusion of the superior cerebellar artery results in severe ipsilateral cerebellar ataxia, nausea and vomiting, dysarthria, and contralateral loss of pain and temperature sensation over the extremities, body, and face (spino- and trigeminothalamic tract). Partial deafness, ataxic tremor of the ipsilateral upper extremity, Horner's syndrome, and palatal myoclonus may occur rarely. Partial syndromes occur frequently (Fig. 364-13). With large strokes, swelling and mass effects may compress the midbrain or produce hydrocephalus; these symptoms may evolve rapidly. Neurosurgical intervention may be lifesaving in such cases.

Occlusion of the anterior inferior cerebellar artery produces variable degrees of infarction because the size of this artery and the territory it supplies vary inversely with those of the PICA. The principal symptoms include: (1) ipsilateral deafness, facial weakness, vertigo, nausea and vomiting, nystagmus, tinnitus, cerebellar ataxia, Horner's syndrome, and paresis of conjugate lateral gaze; and (2) contralateral loss of pain and temperature sensation. An occlusion close to the origin of the artery may cause corticospinal tract signs (Fig. 364-11).

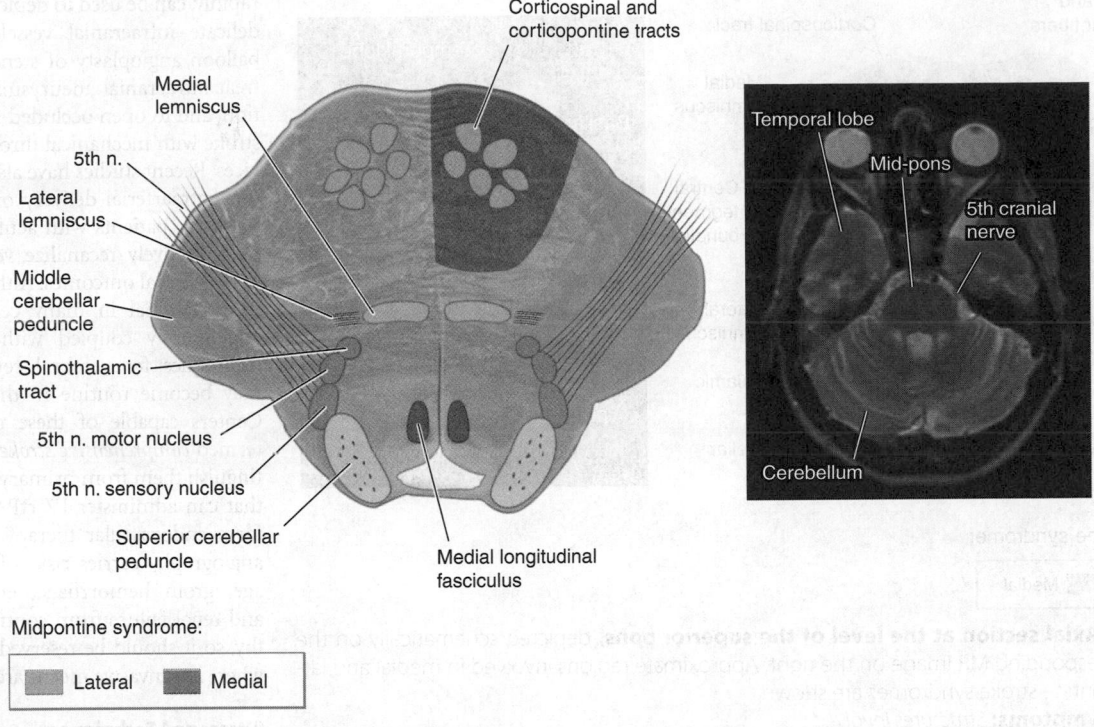

FIGURE 364-12 Axial section at the level of the mid pons, depicted schematically on the left, with a corresponding MR image on the right. Approximate regions involved in medial and lateral midpontine stroke syndromes are shown.

Signs and symptoms: *Structures involved*

1. Medial midpontine syndrome (paramedian branch of midbasilar artery)
   On side of lesion
     Ataxia of limbs and gait (more prominent in bilateral involvement): *Pontine nuclei*
   On side opposite lesion
     Paralysis of face, arm, and leg: *Corticobulbar and corticospinal tract*

Variable impaired touch and proprioception when lesion extends posteriorly: *Medial lemniscus*

2. Lateral midpontine syndrome (short circumferential artery)
   On side of lesion
     Ataxia of limbs: *Middle cerebellar peduncle*
     Paralysis of muscles of mastication: *Motor fibers or nucleus of fifth nerve*
     Impaired sensation over side of face: *Sensory fibers or nucleus of fifth nerve*
   On side opposite lesion
     Impaired pain and thermal sense on limbs and trunk: *Spinothalamic tract*

Occlusion of one of the short circumferential branches of the basilar artery affects the lateral two-thirds of the pons and middle or superior cerebellar peduncle, whereas occlusion of one of the paramedian branches affects a wedge-shaped area on either side of the medial pons (Figs. 364-11 through 364-13).

IMAGING STUDIES

See also Chap. 362.

CT Scans CT radiographic images identify or exclude hemorrhage as the cause of stroke, and they identify extraparenchymal hemorrhages, neoplasms, abscesses, and other conditions masquerading as stroke. Scans obtained in the first several hours after an infarction generally show no abnormality, and the infarct may not be seen reliably for 24–48 h. CT may fail to show small ischemic strokes in the posterior fossa because of bone artifact; small infarcts on the cortical surface may also be missed.

Contrast-enhanced CT scans add specificity by showing contrast enhancement of subacute infarcts and allow visualization of venous structures. Coupled with newer generation multi-detector scanners, CT angiography (CTA) can be performed with administration of IV iodinated contrast allowing visualization of the cervical and intracranial arteries, intracranial veins, aortic arch, and even the coronary arteries in one imaging session. Carotid disease and intracranial vascular occlusions are readily identified with this method (Fig. 364-3). After an IV bolus of contrast, deficits in brain perfusion produced by vascular occlusion can also be demonstrated (Fig. 364-15) and used to pre-

dict the region of infarcted brain and the brain at risk of further infarction (i.e., the ischemic penumbra). CT imaging is also sensitive for detecting SAH (though by itself does not rule it out), and CTA can readily identify intracranial aneurysms (Chap. 269). Because of its speed and wide availability, noncontrast head CT is the imaging modality of choice in patients with acute stroke (Fig. 364-1), and CTA and CT perfusion imaging may also be useful and convenient adjuncts.

MRI MRI reliably documents the extent and location of infarction in all areas of the brain, including the posterior fossa and cortical surface. It also identifies intracranial hemorrhage and other abnormalities but is less sensitive than CT for detecting acute blood. MRI scanners with magnets of higher field strength produce more reliable and precise images. Diffusion-weighted imaging is more sensitive for early brain infarction than standard MR sequences or CT (Fig. 364-16), as is FLAIR (fluid-attenuated inversion recovery) imaging (Chap. 362). Using IV administration of gadolinium contrast, MR perfusion studies can be performed. Brain regions showing poor perfusion but no abnormality on diffusion are considered equivalent to the ischemic penumbra (see "Pathophysiology of Ischemic Stroke," above and Fig. 364-16), and patients showing large regions of mismatch may be better candidates for acute revascularization. MR angiography is highly sensitive for stenosis of extracranial internal carotid arteries and of large intracranial vessels. With higher degrees of stenosis, MR angiography tends to overestimate the degree of stenosis when compared to conventional x-ray angiography. MRI with fat saturation is an imaging sequence used

Superior pontine syndrome:

▨ Lateral	■ Medial

FIGURE 364-13 Axial section at the level of the superior pons, depicted schematically on the left, with a corresponding MR image on the right. Approximate regions involved in medial and lateral superior pontine stroke syndromes are shown.

Signs and symptoms: *Structures involved*
1. Medial superior pontine syndrome (paramedian branches of upper basilar artery)
   On side of lesion
   Cerebellar ataxia (probably): *Superior and/or middle cerebellar peduncle*
   Internuclear ophthalmoplegia: *Medial longitudinal fasciculus*
   Myoclonic syndrome, palate, pharynx, vocal cords, respiratory apparatus, face, oculomotor apparatus, etc.: *Localization uncertain—central tegmental bundle, dentate projection, inferior olivary nucleus*
   On side opposite lesion
   Paralysis of face, arm, and leg: *Corticobulbar and corticospinal tract*
   Rarely touch, vibration, and position are affected: *Medial lemniscus*
2. Lateral superior pontine syndrome (syndrome of superior cerebellar artery)
   On side of lesion
   Ataxia of limbs and gait, falling to side of lesion: *Middle and superior cerebellar peduncles, superior surface of cerebellum, dentate nucleus*
   Dizziness, nausea, vomiting; horizontal nystagmus: *Vestibular nucleus*
   Paresis of conjugate gaze (ipsilateral): *Pontine contralateral gaze*
   Skew deviation: *Uncertain*
   Miosis, ptosis, decreased sweating over face (Horner's syndrome): *Descending sympathetic fibers*
   Tremor: Localization unclear—*Dentate nucleus, superior cerebellar peduncle*
   On side opposite lesion
   Impaired pain and thermal sense on face, limbs, and trunk: *Spinothalamic tract*
   Impaired touch, vibration, and position sense, more in leg than arm (there is a tendency to incongruity of pain and touch deficits): *Medial lemniscus (lateral portion)*

rapidly, can be used to deploy stents within delicate intracranial vessels, to perform balloon angioplasty of stenotic lesions, to treat intracranial aneurysms by embolization, and to open occluded vessels in acute stroke with mechanical thrombectomy devices. Recent studies have also documented that intraarterial delivery of thrombolytic agents to patients with acute MCA stroke can effectively recanalize vessels and improve clinical outcomes. Although its use is investigational in many centers, cerebral angiography coupled with endovascular techniques for cerebral revascularization may become routine in the near future. Centers capable of these techniques are termed *comprehensive stroke centers* to distinguish them from primary stroke centers that can administer IV rtPA but not perform endovascular therapy. Conventional angiography carries risks of arterial damage, groin hemorrhage, embolic stroke, and renal failure from contrast nephropathy, so it should be reserved for situations where less invasive means are inadequate.

Ultrasound Techniques Stenosis at the origin of the internal carotid artery can be identified and quantified reliably by ultrasonography that combines a B-mode ultrasound image with a Doppler ultrasound assessment of flow velocity ("duplex" ultrasound). Transcranial Doppler (TCD) assessment of MCA, ACA, and PCA flow and of vertebrobasilar flow is also useful. This latter technique can detect stenotic lesions in the large intracranial arteries because such lesions increase systolic flow velocity. In many cases, MR angiography combined with carotid and transcranial ultrasound studies eliminates the need for conventional x-ray angiography in evaluating vascular stenosis. Alternatively, CT angiography of the entire head and neck can be performed during the initial imaging of acute stroke. Because this images the entire arterial system relevant to stroke, with the exception of the heart, much of the clinician's stroke workup can be completed with one imaging study.

to visualize extra- or intracranial arterial dissection. This sensitive technique images clotted blood within the dissected vessel wall.

MRI is less sensitive for acute blood products than CT and is more expensive and time consuming and less readily available. Claustrophobia also limits its application. Most acute stroke protocols use CT because of these limitations. However, MRI may be useful outside the acute period by more clearly defining the extent of tissue injury and discriminating new from old regions of brain infarction. MRI may have particular utility in patients with TIA: it is also more likely to identify new infarction, which is a strong predictor of subsequent stroke.

Cerebral Angiography Conventional x-ray cerebral angiography is the "gold standard" for identifying and quantifying atherosclerotic stenoses of the cerebral arteries and for identifying and characterizing other pathologies, including aneurysms, vasospasm, intraluminal thrombi, fibromuscular dysplasia, arteriovenous fistula, vasculitis, and collateral channels of blood flow. Endovascular techniques, which are evolving

Perfusion Techniques Both xenon techniques (principally xenon-CT) and PET can quantify cerebral blood flow. These tools are generally used for research (Chap. 362) but can be useful for determining the significance of arterial stenosis and planning for revascularization surgery. Single photon emission tomography (SPECT) and MR perfusion techniques report relative cerebral blood flow. Since CT imaging is used as the initial imaging modality for acute stroke, some centers now combine both CT angiography and CT perfusion imaging together with the noncontrast CT scan. CT perfusion imaging increases the sensitivity for detecting ischemia, and can measure the ischemic penumbra (Fig. 364-15). Alternatively, MR perfusion can be combined with MR diffusion imaging to identify the ischemic penumbra as the mismatch between these two imaging sequences (Fig. 364-16). The ability to image the ischemic penumbra allows more judicious selection of patients who may or may not benefit from acute interventions such as thrombolysis, thrombectomy, or investigational neuroprotective strategies.

FIGURE 364-14 Axial section at the level of the midbrain, depicted schematically on the left, with a corresponding MR image on the right. Approximate regions involved in medial and lateral midbrain stroke syndromes are shown.

Signs and symptoms: *Structures involved*
1. Medial midbrain syndrome (paramedian branches of upper basilar and proximal posterior cerebral arteries)
   On side of lesion
   Eye "down and out" secondary to unopposed action of fourth and sixth cranial nerves, with dilated and unresponsive pupil: *Third nerve fibers*

On side opposite lesion
   Paralysis of face, arm, and leg: *Corticobulbar and corticospinal tract descending in crus cerebri*
2. Lateral midbrain syndrome (syndrome of small penetrating arteries arising from posterior cerebral artery)
   On side of lesion
   Eye "down and out" secondary to unopposed action of fourth and sixth cranial nerves, with dilated and unresponsive pupil: *Third nerve fibers and/or third nerve nucleus*
   On side opposite lesion
   Hemiataxia, hyperkinesias, tremor: *Red nucleus, dentatorubro-thalamic pathway*

INTRACRANIAL HEMORRHAGE

Hemorrhages are classified by their location and the underlying vascular pathology. Bleeding into subdural and epidural spaces is principally produced by trauma. SAHs are produced by trauma and rupture of intracranial aneurysms (Chap. 269). Intraparenchymal and intraventricular hemorrhage will be considered here.

DIAGNOSIS

Intracranial hemorrhage is often discovered on noncontrast CT imaging of the brain during the acute evaluation of stroke. Since CT is more sensitive than routine MRI for acute blood, CT imaging is the preferred method for acute stroke evaluation (Fig. 364-1). The location of the hemorrhage narrows the differential diagnosis to a few entities. Table 364-5 lists the causes and anatomic spaces involved in hemorrhages.

EMERGENCY MANAGEMENT

Close attention should be paid to airway management since a reduction in the level of consciousness is common and often progressive. The initial blood pressure should be maintained until the results of the CT scan are reviewed. There is growing evidence that intraparenchymal hemorrhage may be exacerbated by acutely elevated blood pressure, and current recommendations are to lower mean arterial blood pressure to <130 mmHg. Blood pressure should be lowered with nonvasodilating IV drugs such as nicardipine, labetalol, or esmolol. Patients with cerebellar hemorrhages or with depressed mental status and radiographic evidence of hydrocephalus should undergo urgent neurosurgical evaluation. Based on the clinical examination and CT findings, further imaging studies may be necessary, including MRI or conventional x-ray angiography. Stuporous or comatose patients generally are treated presumptively for elevated ICP, with tracheal intubation and hyperventila-

tion, mannitol administration, and elevation of the head of the bed while surgical consultation is obtained (Chap. 269).

INTRAPARENCHYMAL HEMORRHAGE

Intraparenchymal hemorrhage is the most common type of intracranial hemorrhage. It accounts for ~10% of all strokes and is associated with a 50% case fatality rate. Incidence rates are particularly high in Asians and African Americans. Hypertension, trauma, and cerebral amyloid angiopathy cause the majority of these hemorrhages. Advanced age and heavy alcohol consumption increase the risk, and cocaine use is one of the most important causes in the young.

Hypertensive Intraparenchymal Hemorrhage • *PATHOPHYSIOLOGY* Hypertensive intraparenchymal hemorrhage (hypertensive hemorrhage or hypertensive intracerebral hemorrhage) usually results from spontaneous rupture of a small penetrating artery deep in the brain. The most common sites are the basal ganglia (especially the putamen), thalamus, cerebellum, and pons. When hemorrhages occur in other brain areas or in nonhypertensive patients, greater consideration should be given to hemorrhagic disorders, neoplasms, vascular malformations, and other causes. The small arteries in these areas seem most prone to hypertension-induced vascular injury. The hemorrhage may be small or a large clot may form and compress adjacent tissue, causing herniation and death. Blood may dissect into the ventricular space, which substantially increases morbidity and may cause hydrocephalus.

Most hypertensive intraparenchymal hemorrhages develop over 30–90 min, whereas those associated with anticoagulant therapy may evolve for as long as 24–48 h. Within 48 h macrophages begin to phagocytize the hemorrhage at its outer surface. After 1–6 months, the hemorrhage is generally resolved to a slitlike orange cavity lined with glial scar and hemosiderin-laden macrophages.

FIGURE 364-15 Acute left middle cerebral artery (MCA) stroke with right hemiplegia but preserved language. A. CT perfusion mean-transit time map showing delayed perfusion of the left MCA distribution (blue). **B.** Predicted region of infarct (red) and penumbra (green) based on CT perfusion data. **C.** Conventional angiogram showing occlusion of the left internal carotid–MCA bifurcation (*left panel*), and revascularization of the vessels following successful thrombectomy 8 h after stroke symptom onset (*right panel*). **D.** The clot removed with a thrombectomy device (L5, Concentric Medical, Inc). **E.** CT scan of the brain 2 days later; note infarction in the region predicted in **B** but preservation of the penumbral region by successful revascularization.

CLINICAL MANIFESTATIONS   Although not particularly associated with exertion, intracerebral hemorrhages almost always occur while the patient is awake and sometimes when stressed. The hemorrhage generally presents as the abrupt onset of focal neurologic deficit. Seizures are uncommon. The focal deficit typically worsens steadily over 30–90 min and is associated with a diminishing level of consciousness and signs of increased ICP, such as headache and vomiting.

The putamen is the most common site for hypertensive hemorrhage, and the adjacent internal capsule is usually damaged (Fig. 364-17). Contralateral hemiparesis is therefore the sentinel sign. When mild, the face sags on one side over 5–30 min, speech becomes slurred, the arm and leg gradually weaken, and the eyes deviate away from the side of the hemiparesis. The paralysis may worsen until the affected limbs become flaccid or extend rigidly. When hemorrhages are large, drowsiness gives way to stupor as signs of upper brainstem compression appear. Coma ensues, accompanied by deep, irregular, or intermittent respiration, a dilated and fixed ipsilateral pupil, and decerebrate rigidity. In milder cases, edema in adjacent brain tissue may cause progressive deterioration over 12–72 h.

Thalamic hemorrhages also produce a contralateral hemiplegia or hemiparesis from pressure on, or dissection into, the adjacent internal capsule. A prominent sensory deficit involving all modalities is usually present. Aphasia, often with preserved verbal repetition, may occur after hemorrhage into the dominant thalamus, and constructional apraxia or

mutism occurs in some cases of nondominant hemorrhage. There may also be a homonymous visual field defect. Thalamic hemorrhages cause several typical ocular disturbances by virtue of extension inferiorly into the upper midbrain. These include deviation of the eyes downward and inward so that they appear to be looking at the nose, unequal pupils with absence of light reaction, skew deviation with the eye opposite the hemorrhage displaced downward and medially, ipsilateral Horner's syndrome, absence of convergence, paralysis of vertical gaze, and retraction nystagmus. Patients may later develop a chronic, contralateral pain syndrome (Déjerine-Roussy syndrome).

In pontine hemorrhages, deep coma with quadriplegia usually occurs over a few minutes. There is often prominent decerebrate rigidity and "pin-point" (1 mm) pupils that react to light. There is impairment of reflex horizontal eye movements evoked by head turning (doll's-head or oculocephalic maneuver) or by irrigation of the ears with ice water (Chap. 268). Hyperpnea, severe hypertension, and hyperhidrosis are common. Death often occurs within a few hours, but small hemorrhages are compatible with survival.

Cerebellar hemorrhages usually develop over several hours and are characterized by occipital headache, repeated vomiting, and ataxia of gait. In mild cases there may be no other neurologic signs other than gait ataxia. Dizziness or vertigo may be prominent. There is often paresis of conjugate lateral gaze toward the side of the hemorrhage, forced deviation of the eyes to the opposite side, or an ipsilateral sixth nerve palsy. Less frequent ocular signs include blepharospasm, involuntary closure of one eye, ocular bobbing, and skew deviation. Dysarthria and dysphagia may occur. As the hours pass, the patient often becomes stuporous and then comatose from brainstem compression or obstructive hydrocephalus; immediate surgical evacuation before brainstem compression occurs may be lifesaving. Hydrocephalus from fourth ventricle compression can be relieved by external ventricular drainage, but definitive hematoma evacuation is essential for survival. If the deep cerebellar nuclei are spared, full recovery is common.

Lobar Hemorrhage   Symptoms and signs appear over several minutes. Most lobar hemorrhages are small and cause a restricted clinical syndrome that simulates an embolus to an artery supplying one lobe. For example, the major neurologic deficit with an occipital hemorrhage is hemianopia; with a left temporal hemorrhage, aphasia and delirium; with a parietal hemorrhage, hemisensory loss; and with frontal hemorrhage, arm weakness. Large hemorrhages may be associated with stupor or coma if they compress the thalamus or midbrain. Most patients with lobar hemorrhages have focal headaches, and more than half vomit or are drowsy. Stiff neck and seizures are uncommon.

Other Causes of Intracerebral Hemorrhage   *Cerebral amyloid angiopathy* is a disease of the elderly in which arteriolar degeneration occurs and amyloid is deposited in the walls of the cerebral arteries. Amyloid angiopathy causes both single and recurrent lobar hemorrhages and is probably the most common cause of lobar hemorrhage in the elderly. It accounts for some intracranial hemorrhages associated with IV thrombolysis given for MI. This disorder can be suspected in patients who present with multiple hemorrhages (and infarcts) over several months or years, or in patients with "micro-bleeds" seen on brain MRI sequences sensitive for hemosiderin, but it is definitively diagnosed by pathologic demonstra-

FIGURE 364-17 Hypertensive hemorrhage. Transaxial noncontrast CT scan through the region of the basal ganglia reveals a hematoma involving the left putamen in a patient with rapidly progressive onset of right hemiparesis.

FIGURE 364-16 MRI of acute stroke. A. Perfusion defect within the right hemisphere (bright signal) imaged after administration of an IV bolus of gadolinium contrast. **B.** Cerebral blood flow measured at the same time as in **A**; darker signal reflects decreased blood flow. **C.** Diffusion-weighted image obtained 5 h after onset of a right middle cerebral artery stroke; bright signal indicates regions of restricted diffusion that will progress to infarction. The discrepancy between the region of poor perfusion shown in **A** and **B** and the diffusion deficit is called *diffusion-perfusion mismatch* and is a measure of the ischemic penumbra. Without specific therapy (as shown in Fig. 364-15) the region of infarction will expand to match the perfusion deficit, as shown in the diffusion weighted image in **D** obtained 5 days later. *(Courtesy of Gregory Albers and Vincent Thijs, MD, Stanford University; with permission.)*

tion of Congo red staining of amyloid in cerebral vessels. The ε2 and ε4 allelic variations of the apolipoprotein E gene are associated with increased risk of recurrent lobar hemorrhage and may therefore be markers of amyloid angiopathy. Currently, there is no specific therapy, though antiplatelet and anticoagulating agents are typically avoided.

Cocaine is a frequent cause of stroke in young (age < 45) patients. Intracerebral hemorrhage, ischemic stroke, and SAH are all associated with cocaine use. Angiographic findings vary from completely normal arteries to large-vessel occlusion or stenosis, vasospasm, or changes consistent with vasculitis. The mechanism of cocaine-related stroke is not known, but cocaine enhances sympathetic activity causing acute, sometimes severe, hypertension, and this may lead to hemorrhage. Slightly more than half of cocaine-related intracranial hemorrhages are intracerebral, and the rest are subarachnoid. In cases of SAH, a saccular aneurysm is usually identified. Presumably, acute hypertension causes aneurysmal rupture.

Head injury often causes intracranial bleeding. The common sites are intracerebral (especially temporal and inferior frontal lobes) and into the subarachnoid, subdural, and epidural spaces. Trauma must be considered in any patient with an unexplained acute neurologic deficit (hemiparesis, stupor, or confusion), particularly if the deficit occurred in the context of a fall (Chap. 373).

Intracranial hemorrhages associated with *anticoagulant therapy* can occur at any location; they are often lobar or subdural. Anticoagulant-related intracerebral hemorrhages may evolve slowly, over 24–48 h. Coagulopathy and thrombocytopenia should be reversed rapidly, as discussed below. Intracerebral hemorrhage associated with *hematologic disorders* (leukemia, aplastic anemia, thrombocytopenic purpura) can occur at any site and may present as multiple intracerebral hemorrhages. Skin and mucous membrane bleeding is usually evident and offers a diagnostic clue.

TABLE 364-5	**CAUSES OF INTRACRANIAL HEMORRHAGE**	
Cause	**Location**	**Comments**
Head trauma	Intraparenchymal: frontal lobes, anterior temporal lobes; subarachnoid	Coup and contracoup injury during brain deceleration
Hypertensive hemorrhage	Putamen, globus pallidus, thalamus, cerebellar hemisphere, pons	Chronic hypertension produces hemorrhage from small (~100 μm) vessels in these regions
Transformation of prior ischemic infarction	Basal ganglion, subcortical regions, lobar	Occurs in 1–6% of ischemic strokes with predilection for large hemispheric infarctions
Metastatic brain tumor	Lobar	Lung, choriocarcinoma, melanoma, renal cell carcinoma, thyroid, atrial myxoma
Coagulopathy	Any	Uncommon cause; often associated with prior stroke or underlying vascular anomaly
Drug	Lobar, subarachnoid	Cocaine, amphetamine, phenylpropranolamine
Arteriovenous malformation	Lobar, intraventricular, subarachnoid	Risk is ~2–4% per year for bleeding
Aneurysm	Subarachnoid, intraparenchymal, rarely subdural	Mycotic and nonmycotic forms of aneurysms
Amyloid angiopathy	Lobar	Degenerative disease of intracranial vessels; linkage to Alzheimer's disease, rare in patients <60
Cavernous angioma	Intraparenchymal	Multiple cavernous angiomas linked to mutations in KRIT1, CCM2, and PDCD10 genes
Dural arteriovenous fistula	Lobar, subarachnoid	Produces bleeding by venous hypertension
Capillary telangiectasias	Usually brainstem	Rare cause of hemorrhage

Hemorrhage into a *brain tumor* may be the first manifestation of neoplasm. Choriocarcinoma, malignant melanoma, renal cell carcinoma, and bronchogenic carcinoma are among the most common metastatic tumors associated with intracerebral hemorrhage. Glioblastoma multiforme in adults and medulloblastoma in children may also have areas of intracerebral hemorrhage.

Hypertensive encephalopathy is a complication of malignant hypertension. In this acute syndrome, severe hypertension is associated with headache, nausea, vomiting, convulsions, confusion, stupor, and coma. Focal or lateralizing neurologic signs, either transitory or permanent, may occur but are infrequent and therefore suggest some other vascular disease (hemorrhage, embolism, or atherosclerotic thrombosis). There are retinal hemorrhages, exudates, papilledema (hypertensive retinopathy), and evidence of renal and cardiac disease. In most cases ICP and CSF protein levels are elevated. The hypertension may be essential or due to chronic renal disease, acute glomerulonephritis, acute toxemia of pregnancy, pheochromocytoma, or other causes. Lowering the blood pressure reverses the process, but stroke can occur, especially if blood pressure is lowered too rapidly. Neuropathologic examination reveals multifocal to diffuse cerebral edema and hemorrhages of various sizes from petechial to massive. Microscopically, there are necrosis of arterioles, minute cerebral infarcts, and hemorrhages. The term *hypertensive encephalopathy* should be reserved for this syndrome and not for chronic recurrent headaches, dizziness, recurrent TIAs, or small strokes that often occur in association with high blood pressure.

Primary intraventricular hemorrhage is rare. It usually begins within the substance of the brain and dissects into the ventricular system without leaving signs of intraparenchymal hemorrhage. Alternatively, bleeding can arise from periependymal veins. Vasculitis, usually polyarteritis nodosa or lupus erythematosus, can produce hemorrhage into any region of the central nervous system; most hemorrhages are associated with hypertension, but the arteritis itself may cause bleeding by disrupting the vessel wall. *Sepsis* can cause small petechial hemorrhages throughout the cerebral white matter. *Moyamoya disease*, mainly an occlusive arterial disease that causes ischemic symptoms, may on occasion produce intraparenchymal hemorrhage, particularly in the young. Hemorrhages into the spinal cord are usually the result of an AVM or metastatic tumor. *Epidural spinal hemorrhage* produces a rapidly evolving syndrome of spinal cord or nerve root compression (Chap. 372). Spinal hemorrhages usually present with sudden back pain and some manifestation of myelopathy.

Laboratory and Imaging Evaluation Patients should have routine blood chemistries and hematologic studies. Specific attention to the platelet count and PT/PTT are important to identify coagulopathy. CT imaging reliably detects acute focal hemorrhages in the supratentorial space. Small pontine hemorrhages may not be identified because of motion and bone-induced artifact that obscure structures in the posterior fossa. After the first 2 weeks, x-ray attenuation values of clotted blood diminish until they become isodense with surrounding brain. Mass effect and edema may remain. In some cases, a surrounding rim of contrast enhancement appears after 2–4 weeks and may persist for months. MRI, though more sensitive for delineating posterior fossa lesions, is generally not necessary in most instances. Images of flowing blood on MRI scan may identify AVMs as the cause of the hemorrhage. MRI, CT angiography, and conventional x-ray angiography are used when the cause of intracranial hemorrhage is uncertain, particularly if the patient is young or not hypertensive and the hematoma is not in one of the four usual sites for hypertensive hemorrhage. For example, hemorrhage into the temporal lobe suggests rupture of a MCA saccular aneurysm.

Since patients typically have focal neurologic signs and obtundation, and often show signs of increased ICP, a lumbar puncture should be avoided as it may induce cerebral herniation.

℞ INTRACRANIAL HEMORRHAGE

ACUTE MANAGEMENT Nearly 50% of patients with a hypertensive intracerebral hemorrhage die, but others may have a good to complete recovery if they survive the initial hemorrhage. The volume and location of the hemato-

ma determine the prognosis. In general, supratentorial hematomas with volumes <30 mL have a good prognosis; 30–60 mL, an intermediate prognosis; and >60 mL, a poor prognosis during initial hospitalization. Extension into the ventricular system worsens the prognosis, as does advanced age, location within the posterior fossa, and depressed level of consciousness at initial presentation. Any identified coagulopathy should be reversed as soon as possible. For patients taking warfarin sodium, more rapid reversal of coagulopathy can be achieved by infusing prothrombin complex concentrates followed by fresh-frozen plasma and vitamin K. When intracerebral hemorrhage is associated with thrombocytopenia (platelet count < 50,000/μL), transfusion of fresh platelets is indicated. At present, little can be done about the hemorrhage itself. Hematomas may expand for several hours following the initial hemorrhage, so treating severe hypertension seems reasonable to prevent hematoma progression. Preliminary data suggest that treatment with recombinant factor VIIa, even in patients without coagulopathy, may decrease risk of hematoma expansion and improve clinical outcome; a multicenter randomized trial of this approach was recently completed.

Evacuation of supratentorial hematomas does not appear to improve outcome. The International Surgical Trial in Intracerebral Haemorrhage (STICH) randomized 1033 patients with supratentorial intracerebral hemorrhage to either early surgical evacuation or initial medical management. No benefit was found in the early surgery arm, though analysis was complicated by the fact that 26% of patients in the initial medical management group ultimately had surgery for neurologic deterioration. Overall, these data do not support routine surgical evacuation of supratentorial hemorrhages; however, many centers operate on patients with progressive neurologic deterioration. Surgical techniques continue to evolve, and minimally invasive endoscopic hematoma evacuation may prove beneficial in future trials.

For cerebellar hemorrhages, a neurosurgeon should be consulted immediately to assist with the evaluation; most cerebellar hematomas >3 cm in diameter will require surgical evacuation. If the patient is alert without focal brainstem signs and if the hematoma is <1 cm in diameter, surgical removal is usually unnecessary. Patients with hematomas between 1 and 3 cm require careful observation for signs of impaired consciousness and precipitous respiratory failure.

Tissue surrounding hematomas is displaced and compressed but not necessarily infarcted. Hence, in survivors, major improvement commonly occurs as the hematoma is reabsorbed and the adjacent tissue regains its function. Careful management of the patient during the acute phase of the hemorrhage can lead to considerable recovery.

Surprisingly, ICP is often normal even with large intraparenchymal hemorrhages. However, if the hematoma causes marked midline shift of structures with consequent obtundation, coma, or hydrocephalus, osmotic agents coupled with induced hyperventilation can be instituted to lower ICP (Chap. 269). These maneuvers will provide enough time to place a ventriculostomy or ICP monitor. Once ICP is recorded, further hyperventilation and osmotic therapy can be tailored to the individual patient. For example, if ICP is found to be high, CSF can be drained from the ventricular space and osmotic therapy continued; persistent or progressive elevation in ICP may prompt surgical evacuation of the clot or withdrawal of support. Alternately, if ICP is normal or only mildly elevated, induced hyperventilation can be reversed and osmotic therapy tapered. Since hyperventilation may actually produce ischemia by cerebral vasoconstriction, induced hyperventilation should be limited to acute resuscitation of the patient with presumptive high ICP and eliminated once other treatments (osmotic therapy or surgical treatments) have been instituted. Glucocorticoids are not helpful for the edema from intracerebral hematoma.

PREVENTION Hypertension is the leading cause of primary intracerebral hemorrhage. Prevention is aimed at reducing hypertension, excessive alcohol use, and use of illicit drugs such as cocaine and amphetamines.

VASCULAR ANOMALIES

Vascular anomalies can be divided into congenital vascular malformations and acquired vascular lesions.

CONGENITAL VASCULAR MALFORMATIONS

True *arteriovenous malformations* (AVMs), venous anomalies, and capillary telangiectasias are lesions that usually remain clinically silent through life. Although most AVMs are congenital, cases of acquired lesions have been reported.

True AVMs are congenital shunts between the arterial and venous systems that may present as headache, seizures, and intracranial hemorrhage. AVMs consist of a tangle of abnormal vessels across the cortical surface or deep within the brain substance. AVMs vary in size from a small blemish a few millimeters in diameter to a large mass of tortuous channels composing an arteriovenous shunt of sufficient magnitude to raise cardiac output. The blood vessels forming the tangle interposed between arteries and veins are usually abnormally thin and do not have a normal structure. AVMs occur in all parts of the cerebral hemispheres, brainstem, and spinal cord, but the largest ones are most frequently in the posterior half of the hemispheres, commonly forming a wedge-shaped lesion extending from the cortex to the ventricle.

Although the lesion is thought to be present from birth in most patients, bleeding or other symptoms are most common between the ages of 10 and 30, occasionally as late as the fifties. AVMs are more frequent in men, and rare familial cases have been described.

Headache (without bleeding) may be hemicranial and throbbing, like migraine, or diffuse. Focal seizures, with or without generalization, occur in ~30% of cases. Half of AVMs become evident as intracerebral hemorrhages. In most, the hemorrhage is mainly intraparenchymal with extension into the subarachnoid space in some cases. Blood is usually not deposited in the basal cisterns, and symptomatic cerebral vasospasm is rare. The risk of rerupture is ~2–4% per year and is particular high in the first few weeks. Hemorrhages may be massive, leading to death, or may be as small as 1 cm in diameter, leading to minor focal symptoms or no deficit. The AVM may be large enough to steal blood away from adjacent normal brain tissue or to increase venous pressure significantly to produce venous ischemia locally and in remote areas of the brain. This is seen most often with large AVMs in the territory of the MCA.

Large AVMs of the anterior circulation may be associated with a systolic and diastolic bruit (sometimes self-audible) over the eye, forehead, or neck and a bounding carotid pulse. Headache at the onset of AVM rupture is not generally as explosive as with aneurysmal rupture. MRI is better than CT for diagnosis, although noncontrast CT scanning sometimes detects calcification of the AVM and contrast may demonstrate the abnormal blood vessels. Once identified, conventional x-ray angiography is the gold standard for evaluating the precise anatomy of the AVM.

Surgical treatment of symptomatic AVMs, often with preoperative embolization to reduce operative bleeding, is usually indicated for accessible lesions. Stereotaxic radiation, an alternative to surgery, can produce a slow sclerosis of arterial channels over 2–3 years.

Patients with asymptomatic AVMs have about a ~2–4% per year risk for hemorrhage. Several angiographic features of the AVM can be used to help predict future bleeding risk. Paradoxically, smaller lesions seem to have a higher hemorrhage rate. The impact of recurrent hemorrhage on disability is relatively modest, so the indication for surgery in asymptomatic AVMs is debated. A large-scale randomized trial is currently addressing this question.

Venous anomalies are the result of development of anomalous cerebral, cerebellar, or brainstem drainage. These structures, unlike AVMs, are functional venous channels. They are of little clinical significance and should be ignored if found incidentally on brain imaging studies. Surgical resection of these anomalies may result in venous infarction and hemorrhage. Venous anomalies may be associated with cavernous malformations (see below), which do carry some bleeding risk. If resection of a cavernous malformation is attempted, the venous anomaly should not be disturbed.

Capillary telangiectasias are true capillary malformations that often form extensive vascular networks through an otherwise normal brain structure. The pons and deep cerebral white matter are typical locations, and these capillary malformations can be seen in patients with hereditary hemorrhagic telangiectasia (Osler-Rendu-Weber) syndrome. If bleeding does occur, it rarely produces mass effect or significant symptoms. No treatment options exist.

ACQUIRED VASCULAR LESIONS

Cavernous angiomas are tufts of capillary sinusoids that form within the deep hemispheric white matter and brainstem with no normal intervening neural structures. The pathogenesis is unclear. Familial cavernous angiomas have been mapped to several different chromosomal loci: KRIT1 (7q21-q22), CCM2 (7p13), and PDCD10 (3q26.1). Both KRIT1 and CCM2 are instrumental in blood vessel formation while PDCD10 is an apoptotic gene. Cavernous angiomas are typically <1 cm in diameter and are often associated with a venous anomaly. Bleeding is usually of small volume, causing slight mass effect only. The bleeding risk for single cavernous malformations is 0.7–1.5% per year and may be higher for patients with prior clinical hemorrhage or multiple malformations. Seizures may occur if the malformation is located near the cerebral cortex. Surgical resection eliminates bleeding risk and may reduce seizure risk, but it is reserved for those malformations that form near the brain surface. Radiation treatment has not been shown to be of benefit.

Dural arteriovenous fistulas are acquired connections usually from a dural artery to a dural sinus. Patients may complain of a pulse-synchronous cephalic bruit ("pulsatile tinnitus") and headache. Depending on the magnitude of the shunt, venous pressures may rise high enough to cause cortical ischemia or venous hypertension and hemorrhage, particularly subarachnoid hemorrhage. Surgical and endovascular techniques are usually curative. These fistulas may form because of trauma, but most are idiopathic. There is an association between fistulas and dural sinus thrombosis. Fistulas have been observed to appear months to years following venous sinus thrombosis, suggesting that angiogenesis factors elaborated from the thrombotic process may cause these anomalous connections to form. Alternatively, dural arteriovenous fistulas can produce venous sinus occlusion over time, perhaps from the high pressure and high flow through a venous structure.

FURTHER READINGS

ADAMS HP JR. et al: Guidelines for the Early Management of Adults with Ischemic Stroke. A Guideline from the American Heart Association/American Stroke Association Stroke Council, Clinical Cardiology Council, Cardiovascular Radiology and Intervention Council, and the Atherosclerotic Peripheral Vascular Disease and Quality of Care Outcomes in Research Interdisciplinary Working Groups. The American Academy of Neurology affirms the value of this guideline as an educational tool for neurologists. Stroke 38:1655, 2007

ALBERTS MJ et al: Recommendations for the establishment of primary stroke centers. Brain Attack Coalition. JAMA 238:3102, 2000

——— et al: Recommendations for comprehensive stroke centers: A consensus statement from the Brain Attack Coalition. Stroke 36:1597, 2005

CHOI JH, MOHR JP: Brain arteriovenous malformations in adults. Lancet Neurol 4:299, 2005

GOLDSTEIN LB et al: Primary prevention of ischemic stroke: A guideline from the American Heart Association/American Stroke Association Stroke Council: cosponsored by the Atherosclerotic Peripheral Vascular Disease Interdisciplinary Working Group; Cardiovascular Nursing Council; Clinical Cardiology Council; Nutrition, Physical Activity, and Metabolism Council; and the Quality of Care and Outcomes Research Interdisciplinary Working Group: The American Academy of Neurology affirms the value of this guideline. Stroke 37:1583, 2006

JOHNSTON SC et al: National Stroke Association guidelines for the management of transient ischemic attacks. Ann Neurol 60:301, 2006

LATCHAW RE et al: Guidelines and recommendations for perfusion imaging in cerebral ischemia: A scientific statement for healthcare professionals by the writing group on perfusion imaging, from the Council on Cardiovascular Radiology of the American Heart Association. Stroke 34:1084, 2003

MENDELOW AD et al: Early surgery versus initial conservative treatment in patients with spontaneous supratentorial intracerebral haematomas in the International Surgical Trial in Intracerebral Haemorrhage (STICH): A randomised trial. Lancet 365:387, 2005

MOHR JP et al: A comparison of warfarin and aspirin for the prevention of recurrent ischemic stroke. N Engl J Med. 345:1444, 2001

2536 ROTHWELL PM et al: Endarterectomy for symptomatic carotid stenosis in relation to clinical subgroups and timing of surgery. Lancet 363:915, 2004

SACCO RL et al: Guidelines for Prevention of Stroke in Patients with Ischemic Stroke and Transient Ischemic Attack: A Statement for Healthcare Professionals From the American Heart Association/American Stroke Association Council on Stroke. Stroke 37:577, 2006

SINGER DE et al: Antithrombotic therapy in atrial fibrillation: The Seventh ACCP Conference on Antithrombotic and Thrombolytic Therapy. Chest 126:429S, 2004

365 Dementia
Thomas D. Bird, Bruce L. Miller

Dementia, a syndrome with many causes, affects >4 million Americans and results in a total health care cost of >$100 billion annually. It is defined as an acquired deterioration in cognitive abilities that impairs the successful performance of activities of daily living. Memory is the most common cognitive ability lost with dementia; 10% of persons >70 and 20–40% of individuals >85 have clinically identifiable memory loss. In addition to memory, other mental faculties are also affected in dementia; these include language, visuospatial ability, calculation, judgment, and problem solving. Neuropsychiatric and social deficits also develop in many dementia syndromes, resulting in depression, withdrawal, hallucinations, delusions, agitation, insomnia, and disinhibition. The most common forms of dementia are progressive, but some dementing illnesses are static and unchanging or fluctuate dramatically from day to day. Most diagnoses of dementia require some sort of memory deficit, although there are many dementias, such as frontotemporal dementia, where memory loss is not a presenting feature. Memory and executive function are discussed in Chap. e6.

FUNCTIONAL ANATOMY OF THE DEMENTIAS

Dementia results from the disruption of cerebral neuronal circuits; the quantity of neuronal loss and the location of affected regions are factors that combine to cause the specific disorder (Chap. 27). Behavior and mood are modulated by noradrenergic, serotonergic, and dopaminergic pathways, while acetylcholine seems to be particularly important for memory. Therefore, the loss of cholinergic neurons in Alzheimer's disease (AD) may underlie the memory impairment, while in patients with non-AD dementias, the loss of serotonergic and glutaminergic neurons causes primarily behavioral symptoms, leaving memory relatively spared. Neurotrophins (Chap. 360) are also postulated to play a role in memory function, in part by preserving cholinergic neurons, and therefore represent a pharmacologic pathway toward slowing or reversing the effects of AD.

Dementias have anatomically specific patterns of neuronal degeneration that dictate the clinical symptomatology. AD begins in the entorhinal cortex, spreads to the hippocampus, and then moves to posterior temporal and parietal neocortex, eventually causing a relatively diffuse degeneration throughout the cerebral cortex. *Multi-infarct dementia* is associated with focal damage in a random patchwork of cortical regions. Diffuse white matter damage may disrupt intracerebral connections and cause dementia syndromes similar to those associated with leukodystrophies, multiple sclerosis, and Binswanger's disease (see below). Subcortical structures, including the caudate, putamen, thalamus, and substantia nigra, also modulate cognition and behavior in ways that are not yet well understood. The effect that these patterns of cortical degeneration have on disease symptomatology is clear: AD primarily presents as memory loss and is often associated with aphasia or other disturbances of language. In contrast, patients with frontal lobe or subcortical dementias such as *frontotemporal dementia* (FTD) or *Huntington's disease* (HD) are less likely to begin with memory problems and more likely to have difficulties with attention, judgment, awareness, and behavior.

Lesions of specific cortical-subcortical pathways have equally specific effects on behavior. The dorsolateral prefrontal cortex has connections with dorsolateral caudate, globus pallidus, and thalamus.

Lesions of these pathways result in poor organization and planning, decreased cognitive flexibility, and impaired judgment. The lateral orbital frontal cortex connects with the ventromedial caudate, globus pallidus, and thalamus. Lesions of these connections cause irritability, impulsiveness, and distractibility. The anterior cingulate cortex connects with the nucleus accumbens, globus pallidus, and thalamus. Interruption of these connections produces apathy and poverty of speech or even akinetic mutism.

The single strongest risk factor for dementia is increasing age. The prevalence of disabling memory loss increases with each decade over age 50 and is associated most often with the microscopic changes of AD at autopsy. Slow accumulation of mutations in neuronal mitochondria is also hypothesized to contribute to the increasing prevalence of dementia with age. Yet some centenarians have intact memory function and no evidence of clinically significant dementia. Whether dementia is an inevitable consequence of normal human aging remains controversial.

THE CAUSES OF DEMENTIA

The many causes of dementia are listed in Table 365-1. The frequency of each condition depends on the age group under study, the access of the group to medical care, the country of origin, and perhaps racial or ethnic background. AD is the most common cause of dementia in Western countries, representing more than half of demented patients. Vascular disease is the second most common cause of dementia in the United States, representing 10–20%. In populations with limited access to medical care, where vascular risk factors are undertreated, the prevalence of vascular dementia can be much higher. Dementia associated with Parkinson's disease (PD) is the next most common category, and in many instances these patients suffer from dementia with Lewy bodies (DLB). In patients under the age of 60, FTD rivals AD as the most common cause of dementia. Chronic intoxications, including those resulting from alcohol and prescription drugs, are an important and often treatable cause of dementia. Other disorders listed in the table are uncommon but important because many are reversible. The classification of dementing illnesses into two broad groups of reversible and irreversible disorders is a useful approach to the differential diagnosis of dementia.

In a study of 1000 persons attending a memory disorders clinic, 19% had a potentially reversible cause of the cognitive impairment and 23% had a potentially reversible concomitant condition. The three most common potentially reversible diagnoses were depression, hydrocephalus, and alcohol dependence (Table 365-1).

Subtle cumulative decline in episodic memory is a natural part of aging. This frustrating experience, often the source of jokes and humor, is referred to as *benign forgetfulness of the elderly*. *Benign* means that it is not so progressive or serious that it impairs reasonably successful and productive daily functioning, although the distinction between benign and more significant memory loss can be difficult to make. At age 85, the average person is able to learn and recall approximately one-half the number of items (e.g., words on a list) that he or she could at age 18. A cognitive problem that has begun to subtly interfere with daily activities is referred to as *mild cognitive impairment* (MCI). A sizeable proportion of persons with MCI will progress to frank dementia, usually caused by AD. The conversion rate from MCI to AD is ~12% per year. It remains unclear why some individuals show progression and others do not. Factors that predict progression from MCI to AD include a memory deficit >1.5 standard deviations from the norm, family history of dementia, the presence of an apolipoprotein ε4 (Apo ε4), and small hippocampal volumes. There is optimism

TABLE 365-1 DIFFERENTIAL DIAGNOSIS OF DEMENTIA

Most Common Causes of Dementia

Alzheimer's disease	Alcoholism[a]
Vascular dementia	Parkinson's disease
Multi-infarct	Drug/medication intoxication[a]
Diffuse white matter disease (Binswanger's)	

Less Common Causes of Dementia

Vitamin deficiencies
  Thiamine (B₁): Wernicke's encephalopathy[a]
  B₁₂ (pernicious anemia)[a]
  Nicotinic acid (pellagra)[a]
Endocrine and other organ failure
  Hypothyroidism[a]
  Adrenal insufficiency and Cushing's syndrome[a]
  Hypo- and hyperparathyroidism[a]
  Renal failure[a]
  Liver failure[a]
  Pulmonary failure[a]
Chronic infections
  HIV
  Neurosyphilis[a]
  Papovavirus (progressive multifocal
    leukoencephalopathy)
  Prion (Creutzfeldt-Jakob and Gerstmann-
    Sträussler-Scheinker diseases)
  Tuberculosis, fungal, and protozoal[a]
  Whipple's disease[a]
Head trauma and diffuse brain damage
  Dementia pugilistica
  Chronic subdural hematoma[a]
  Postanoxia
  Postencephalitis
  Normal-pressure hydrocephalus[a]
Neoplastic
  Primary brain tumor[a]
  Metastatic brain tumor[a]
  Paraneoplastic limbic encephalitis

Toxic disorders
  Drug, medication, and narcotic poisoning[a]
  Heavy metal intoxication[a]
  Dialysis dementia (aluminum)
  Organic toxins
Psychiatric
  Depression (pseudodementia)[a]
  Schizophrenia[a]
  Conversion reaction[a]
Degenerative disorders
  Huntington's disease
  Pick's disease
  Dementia with Lewy bodies
  Progressive supranuclear palsy (Steel-Richardson
    syndrome)
  Multisystem degeneration (Shy-Drager syndrome)
  Hereditary ataxias (some forms)
  Motor neuron disease [amyotrophic lateral sclerosis
    (ALS); some forms]
  Frontotemporal dementia
  Cortical basal degeneration
  Multiple sclerosis
  Adult Down's syndrome with Alzheimer's
  ALS–Parkinson's–Dementia complex of Guam
Miscellaneous
  Sarcoidosis[a]
  Vasculitis[a]
  CADASIL etc
  Acute intermittent porphyria[a]
  Recurrent nonconvulsive seizures[a]
Additional conditions in children or adolescents
  Hallervorden-Spatz disease
  Subacute sclerosing panencephalitis
  Metabolic disorders (e.g., Wilson's and Leigh's diseases,
    leukodystrophies, lipid storage diseases, mitochon-
    drial mutations)

[a]Potentially reversible dementia.

and neurologic findings; and neuroimaging features (Table 365-4).

HISTORY The history should concentrate on the onset, duration, and tempo of progression of the dementia. An acute or subacute onset of confusion may represent delirium and should trigger the search for intoxication, infection, or metabolic derangement. An elderly person with slowly progressive memory loss over several years is likely to suffer from AD. Nearly 75% of AD patients begin with memory symptoms, but other early symptoms include difficulty with managing money, driving, shopping, following instructions, finding words, or navigating. A change in personality, disinhibition, and gain of weight or food obsession suggests FTD, not AD. FTD is also suggested by the finding of apathy, loss of executive function, or progressive abnormalities in speech, or by a relative sparing of memory or spatial abilities. The diagnosis of DLB is suggested by the early presence of visual hallucinations; parkinsonism; delirium; REM sleep disorder (the merging of dream-states into wakefulness); or Capgras' syndrome, the delusion that a familiar person has been replaced by an impostor.

A history of sudden stroke with irregular stepwise progression suggests multi-infarct dementia. Multi-infarct dementia is also commonly seen in the setting of hypertension, atrial fibrillation, peripheral vascular disease, and diabetes. In patients suffering from cerebrovascular disease, it can be difficult to determine whether the dementia is due to AD, multi-infarct dementia, or a mixture of the two as many of the risk factors for vascular

that new positron emission tomography (PET) imaging techniques that label amyloid or tau in vivo might aid in early diagnosis of AD in the future.

The major degenerative dementias include AD, FTD and related disorders, DLB, HD, and prion disorders including Creutzfeldt-Jakob disease (CJD). These disorders are all associated with the abnormal aggregation of a specific protein: Aβ₄₂ in AD, tau or TDP-43 in FTD, α-synuclein in DLB, polyglutamine repeats in HD, and prions in CJD (Table 365-2).

APPROACH TO THE PATIENT:
Dementia

Three major issues should be kept in the forefront: (1) What is the most accurate diagnosis? (2) Is there a treatable or reversible component to the dementia? (3) Can the physician help to alleviate the burden on caregivers? A broad overview of the approach to dementia is shown in Table 365-3. The major degenerative dementias can usually be distinguished by the initial symptoms; neuropsychological, neuropsychiatric,

TABLE 365-2 THE MOLECULAR BASIS FOR DEGENERATIVE DEMENTIA

Dementia	Molecular Basis	Causal Genes and (Chromosome)	Susceptibility Genes	Pathology
AD	Aβ	<2% carry these mutations. *APP* (21), *PS-1* (14), *PS-2* (1) (most mutations are in *PS-1*)	*Apo ε4* (19)	Amyloid plaques, neurofibrillary tangles
FTD	Tau	Tau exon and intron mutations (17) (about 10% of familial cases) Progranulin (17) (10% of familial cases)	H1 tau haplotypes	Tau inclusions, Pick bodies, neurofibrillary tangles
DLB	α-synuclein	Very rare α-synuclein (4) (dominant)	Unknown	α-synuclein inclusions (Lewy bodies)
CJD	PrP^SC proteins	Prion (20) (up to 15% of cases carry these dominant mutations)	Codon 129 homozygosity for methionine or valine	Tau inclusions, spongiform changes, gliosis

Note: AD, Alzheimer's disease; FTD, frontotemporal dementia; DLB, dementia with Lewy bodies; CJD, Creutzfeldt-Jakob disease.

TABLE 365-3 EVALUATION OF THE PATIENT WITH DEMENTIA

Routine Evaluation	Optional Focused Tests	Occasionally Helpful Tests
History	Psychometric testing	EEG
Physical examination	Chest x-ray	Parathyroid function
Laboratory tests	Lumbar puncture	Adrenal function
Thyroid function (TSH)	Liver function	Urine heavy metals
Vitamin B$_{12}$	Renal function	RBC sedimentation rate
Complete blood count	Urine toxin screen	Angiogram
Electrolytes	HIV	Brain biopsy
CT/MRI	Apolipoprotein E	SPECT
	RPR or VDRL	PET

Diagnostic Categories

Reversible Causes	Irreversible/Degenerative Dementias	Psychiatric Disorders
Examples	Examples	Depression
Hypothyroidism	Alzheimer's	Schizophrenia
Thiamine deficiency	Frontotemporal dementia	Conversion reaction
Vitamin B$_{12}$ deficiency	Huntington's	
Normal-pressure hydrocephalus	Dementia with Lewy bodies	
Subdural hematoma	Vascular	
Chronic infection	Leukoencephalopathies	
Brain tumor	Parkinson's	
Drug intoxication		

Associated Treatable Conditions

Depression	Agitation
Seizures	Caregiver "burnout"
Insomnia	Drug side effects

Note: PET, positron emission tomography; RPR, rapid plasma reagin (test); SPECT, single photon emission CT; VDRL, Venereal Disease Research Laboratory (test for syphilis).

dementia, including diabetes, high cholesterol, elevated homocysteine and low exercise, are also risk factors for AD. Rapid progression of the dementia in association with motor rigidity and myoclonus suggests CJD. Seizures may indicate strokes or neoplasm. Gait disturbance is commonly seen with multi-infarct dementia, PD, or normal-pressure hydrocephalus (NPH). Multiple sex partners or intravenous drug use should trigger a search for central nervous system (CNS) infection, especially for HIV. A history of recurrent head trauma could indicate chronic subdural hematoma, dementia pugilistica, or NPH. Alcoholism may suggest malnutrition and thiamine deficiency. A remote history of gastric surgery resulting in loss of intrinsic factor can bring about vitamin B$_{12}$ deficiency. Certain occupations such as working in a battery or chemical factory might indicate heavy metal intoxication. Careful review of medication intake, especially of sedatives and tranquilizers, may raise the issue of chronic drug intoxication. A positive family of dementia is found in HD and in forms of familial Alzheimer's disease (FAD), FTD, or prion disorders. The recent death of a loved one, or depressive signs such as in-

somnia or weight loss, raises the possibility of pseudodementia due to depression.

PHYSICAL AND NEUROLOGIC EXAMINATION A thorough general and neurologic examination is essential to document dementia, look for other signs of nervous system involvement, and search for clues suggesting a systemic disease that might be responsible for the cognitive disorder. AD does not affect motor systems until later in the course. In contrast, FTD patients often develop axial rigidity, supranuclear gaze palsy, or features of amyotrophic lateral sclerosis (ALS). In DLB, initial symptoms may be the new onset of a parkinsonian syndrome (resting tremor, cogwheel rigidity, bradykinesia, festinating gait) with the dementia following later, or vice versa. Corticobasal degeneration (CBD) is associated with dystonia, alien hand, and asymmetric extrapyramidal, pyramidal, or sensory deficits or myoclonus. Progressive supranuclear palsy (PSP) is associated with unexplained falls, axial rigidity, dysphagia, and vertical gaze deficits. CJD is suggested by the presence of diffuse rigidity, an akinetic state, and myoclonus.

Hemiparesis or other focal neurologic deficits may occur in multi-infarct dementia or brain tumor. Dementia with a myelopathy and peripheral neuropathy suggests vita-

TABLE 365-4 CLINICAL DIFFERENTIATION OF THE MAJOR DEMENTIAS

Disease	First Symptom	Mental Status	Neuropsychiatry	Neurology	Imaging
AD	Memory loss	Episodic memory loss	Initially normal	Initially normal	Entorhinal cortex and hippocampal atrophy
FTD	Apathy; poor judgment/insight, speech/language; hyperorality	Frontal/executive, language; spares drawing	Apathy, disinhibition, hyperorality, euphoria, depression	Due to PSP/CBD overlap; vertical gaze palsy, axial rigidity, dystonia, alien hand	Frontal and/or temporal atrophy; spares posterior parietal lobe
DLB	Visual hallucinations, REM sleep disorder, delirium, Capgras' syndrome, parkinsonism	Drawing and frontal/executive; spares memory; delirium prone	Visual hallucinations, depression, sleep disorder, delusions	Parkinsonism	Posterior parietal atrophy; hippocampi larger than in AD
CJD	Dementia, mood, anxiety, movement disorders	Variable, frontal/executive, focal cortical, memory	Depression, anxiety	Myoclonus, rigidity, parkinsonism	Cortical ribboning and basal ganglia or thalamus hyperintensity on diffusion/flare MRI
Vascular	Often but not always sudden; variable; apathy, falls, focal weakness	Frontal/executive, cognitive slowing; can spare memory	Apathy, delusions, anxiety	Usually motor slowing, spasticity; can be normal	Cortical and/or subcortical infarctions, confluent white matter disease

Note: AD, Alzheimer's disease; FTD, frontotemporal dementia; PSP, progressive supranuclear palsy; CBD, cortical basal degeneration; DLB, dementia with Lewy bodies; CJD, Creutzfeldt-Jakob disease.

min B_{12} deficiency. A peripheral neuropathy could also indicate an underlying vitamin deficiency or heavy metal intoxication. Dry, cool skin, hair loss, and bradycardia suggest hypothyroidism. Confusion associated with repetitive stereotyped movements may indicate ongoing seizure activity. Hearing impairment or visual loss may produce confusion and disorientation misinterpreted as dementia. Such sensory deficits are common in the elderly but can be a manifestation of mitochondrial disorders.

COGNITIVE AND NEUROPSYCHIATRIC EXAMINATION Brief screening tools such as the mini-mental state examination (MMSE) help to confirm the presence of cognitive impairment and to follow the progression of dementia (Table 365-5). The MMSE, an easily administered 30-point test of cognitive function, contains tests of orientation, working memory (e.g., spell *world* backwards), episodic memory (orientation and recall), language comprehension, naming, and copying. In most patients with MCI and some with clinically apparent AD, the MMSE may be normal and a more rigorous set of neuropsychological tests will be required. Additionally, when the etiology for the dementia syndrome remains in doubt, a specially tailored evaluation should be performed that includes tasks of working and episodic memory, frontal executive function, language, and visuospatial and perceptual abilities. In AD the deficits involve episodic memory, category generation ("name as many animals as you can in one minute"), and visuoconstructive ability. Deficits in verbal or visual episodic memory are often the first neuropsychological abnormalities seen with AD, and tasks that require the patient to recall a long list of words or a series of pictures after a predetermined delay will demonstrate deficits in most AD patients. In FTD, the earliest deficits often involve frontal executive or language (speech or naming) function. DLB patients have more severe deficits in visuospatial function but do better on episodic memory tasks than patients with AD. Patients with vascular dementia often demonstrate a mixture of frontal executive and visuospatial deficits. In delirium, deficits tend to fall in the area of attention, working memory, and frontal function.

A functional assessment should also be performed. The physician should determine the day-to-day impact of the disorder on the patient's memory, community affairs, hobbies, judgment, dressing, and eating. Knowledge of the patient's day-to-day function will help the clinician and the family to organize a therapeutic approach.

Neuropsychiatric assessment is important for diagnosis, prognosis, and treatment. In the early stages of AD, mild depressive features, social withdrawal, and denial of illness are the most prominent psychiatric changes. However, patients often maintain their social skills into the middle stages of the illness, when delusions, agitation, and sleep disturbance become more common. In FTD, dramatic personality change, apathy, overeating, repetitive compulsions, disinhibition, euphoria, and loss of empathy are common. DLB shows visual hallucinations, delusions related to personal identity, and day-to-day fluctuation. Vascular dementia can present with psychiatric symptoms such as depression, delusions, disinhibition, or apathy.

LABORATORY TESTS The choice of laboratory tests in the evaluation of dementia is complex. The physician does not want to miss a reversible or treatable cause, yet no single etiology is common; thus, a screen must employ multiple tests, each of which has a low yield. Cost/benefit ratios are difficult to assess, and many laboratory screening algorithms for dementia discourage multiple tests. Nevertheless, even a test with only a 1–2% positive rate is probably worth undertaking if the alternative is missing a treatable cause of dementia. Table 365-3 lists most screening tests for dementia. Recently the American Academy of Neurology recommended the routine measurement of thyroid function, a vitamin B_{12} level test, and a neuroimaging study (CT or MRI).

Neuroimaging studies will identify primary and secondary neoplasms, locate areas of infarction, diagnose subdural hematomas, and suggest NPH or diffuse white matter disease. They also lend support to the diagnosis of AD, especially if there is hippocampal atrophy in addition to diffuse cortical atrophy. Focal frontal and/or anterior temporal atrophy suggests FTD. There is no specific pattern yet determined for DLB, although these patients tend to have less hippocampal atrophy than patients with AD. The use of diffusion-weighted imaging with MRI will detect abnormalities in the cortical ribbon and basal ganglia in the vast majority of patients with CJD. Large white-matter abnormalities correlate with a vascular etiology for dementia. The role of functional imaging in the diagnosis of dementia is still under study. Single photon emission computed tomography (SPECT) and PET scanning will show temporal-parietal hypoperfusion or hypometabolism in AD and frontotemporal hypoperfusion or hypometabolism in FTD, but most of these changes reflect atrophy. Recently, amyloid imaging has shown promise for the diagnosis of AD, and Pittsburgh Agent B appears to be a reliable agent for detecting brain amyloid due to the accumulation of $A\beta_{42}$ within plaques (Fig. 365-1). Similarly, MRI perfusion and brain activation studies using functional MRI are under active study as potential early diagnostic tools.

Lumbar puncture need not be done routinely in the evaluation of dementia, but it is indicated if CNS infection is a serious consideration. Cerebrospinal fluid (CSF) levels of tau protein and $A\beta_{42}$ amyloid show differing patterns with the various dementias; however, the sensitivity and specificity of these measures are not sufficiently high to warrant routine measurement. Formal psychometric testing, though not necessary in every patient with dementia, helps to document the severity of dementia, suggest psychogenic causes, and provide a semiquantitative method for following the disease course. EEG is rarely helpful except to suggest CJD (repetitive bursts of diffuse high voltage sharp waves) or an underlying nonconvulsive seizure disorder (epileptiform discharges). Brain biopsy (including meninges) is not advised except to diagnose vasculitis, potentially treatable neoplasms, unusual infections, or systemic disorders such as vasculitis or sarcoid, or in young persons where the diagnosis is uncertain. Angiography should be considered when cerebral vasculitis is a possible cause of the dementia.

SPECIFIC DEMENTIAS

ALZHEIMER'S DISEASE

Approximately 10% of all persons over the age of 70 have significant memory loss, and in more than half the cause is AD. It is estimated

TABLE 365-5 THE MINI-MENTAL STATUS EXAMINATION

	Points
Orientation	
Name: season/date/day/month/year	5 (1 for each name)
Name: hospital/floor/town/state/country	5 (1 for each name)
Registration	
Identify three objects by name and ask patient to repeat	3 (1 for each object)
Attention and calculation	
Serial 7s; subtract from 100 (e.g., 93–86–79–72–65)	5 (1 for each subtraction)
Recall	
Recall the three objects presented earlier	3 (1 for each object)
Language	
Name pencil and watch	2 (1 for each object)
Repeat "No ifs, ands, or buts"	1
Follow a 3-step command (e.g., "Take this paper, fold it in half, and place it on the table")	3 (1 for each command)
Write "close your eyes" and ask patient to obey written command	1
Ask patient to write a sentence	1
Ask patient to copy a design (e.g., intersecting pentagons)	1
Total	30

FIGURE 365-1 PET images obtained with the amyloid-imaging agent Pittsburgh Compound-B ([^{11}C]PIB) in a normal control (*left*); three different patients with mild cognitive impairment (MCI, *center*); and a mild AD patient (*right*). Some MCI patients have control-like levels of amyloid, some have AD-like levels of amyloid, and some have intermediate levels. PET, positron emission tomography; MCI, mild cognitive impairment; AD, Alzheimer's disease.

that the annual total cost of caring for a single AD patient in an advanced stage of the disease is >$50,000. The disease also exacts a heavy emotional toll on family members and caregivers. AD can occur in any decade of adulthood, but it is the most common cause of dementia in the elderly. AD most often presents with subtle onset of memory loss followed by a slowly progressive dementia that has a course of several years. Pathologically, there is diffuse atrophy of the cerebral cortex with secondary enlargement of the ventricular system. Microscopically, there are neuritic plaques containing Aβ amyloid, silver-staining neurofibrillary tangles (NFTs) in neuronal cytoplasm, and accumulation of Aβ$_{42}$ amyloid in arterial walls of cerebral blood vessels (see "Pathogenesis," below). The identification of four different susceptibility genes for AD has provided a foundation for rapid progress in understanding AD's biologic basis.

Clinical Manifestations The cognitive changes with AD tend to follow a characteristic pattern, beginning with memory impairment and spreading to language and visuospatial deficits. However, ~20% of AD patients present with nonmemory complaints such as word-finding, organizational, or navigational difficulty. In the early stages of the disease, the memory loss may go unrecognized or be ascribed to benign forgetfulness. Once the memory loss begins to affect day-to-day activities or falls below 1.5 standard deviations from normal on standardized memory tasks, the disease is defined as MCI. Approximately 50% of MCI individuals will progress to AD within 5 years. Slowly the cognitive problems begin to interfere with daily activities, such as keeping track of finances, following instructions on the job, driving, shopping, and housekeeping. Some patients are unaware of these difficulties (*anosognosia*), while others have considerable insight. Change of environment may be bewildering, and the patient may become lost on walks or while driving an automobile. In the middle stages of AD, the patient is unable to work, is easily lost and confused, and requires daily supervision. Social graces, routine behavior, and superficial conversation may be surprisingly intact. Language becomes impaired—first naming, then comprehension, and finally fluency. In some patients, *aphasia* is an early and prominent feature. Word-finding difficulties and circumlocution may be a problem even when formal testing demonstrates intact naming and fluency. *Apraxia* emerges, and patients have trouble performing sequential motor tasks. Visuospatial deficits begin to interfere with dressing, eating, solving simple puzzles, and copying geometric figures. Patients may be unable to do simple calculations or tell time.

In the late stages of the disease, some persons remain ambulatory but wander aimlessly. Loss of judgment, reason, and cognitive abilities is inevitable. Delusions are common and usually simple in quality, such as delusions of theft, infidelity, or misidentification. Approximately 10% of AD patients develop *Capgras' syndrome*, believing that a caregiver has been replaced by an impostor. In contrast to DLB, where

Capgras' syndrome is an early feature, in AD this syndrome emerges later in the course of the illness. Loss of inhibitions and aggression may occur and alternate with passivity and withdrawal. Sleep-wake patterns are prone to disruption, and nighttime wandering becomes disturbing to the household. Some patients develop a shuffling gait with generalized muscle rigidity associated with slowness and awkwardness of movement. Patients often look parkinsonian (Chap. 366) but rarely have a rapid, rhythmic, resting tremor. In end-stage AD, patients become rigid, mute, incontinent, and bedridden. Help may be needed with the simplest tasks, such as eating, dressing, and toilet function. They may show hyperactive tendon reflexes. Myoclonic jerks (sudden brief contractions of various muscles or the whole body) may occur spontaneously or in response to physical or auditory stimulation. Myoclonus raises the possibility of CJD (Chap. 378), but the course of AD is much more prolonged. Generalized seizures may also occur. Often death results from malnutrition, secondary infections, pulmonary emboli, or heart disease. The typical duration of AD is 8–10 years, but the course can range from 1 to 25 years. For unknown reasons, some AD patients show a steady downhill decline in function, while others have prolonged plateaus without major deterioration.

Differential Diagnosis Early in the disease course, other etiologies of dementia should be excluded. These include treatable entities such as thyroid disease, vitamin deficiencies, brain tumor, drug and medication intoxication, chronic infection, and severe depression (pseudodementia). Neuroimaging studies (CT and MRI) do not show a single specific pattern with AD and may be normal early in the course of the disease. As AD progresses, diffuse cortical atrophy becomes apparent, and MRI scans show atrophy of the hippocampus (Fig. 365-2A, B). Imaging helps to exclude other disorders, such as primary and secondary neoplasms, multi-infarct dementia, diffuse white matter disease, and NPH; it also helps to distinguish AD from other degenerative disorders with distinctive imaging patterns such as FTD or CJD. Functional imaging studies in AD reveal hypoperfusion or hypometabolism in the posterior temporal-parietal cortex (Fig. 365-2C, D). The EEG in AD is normal or shows nonspecific slowing. Routine spinal fluid examination is also normal. CSF Aβ amyloid levels are reduced, whereas levels of tau protein are increased, but the considerable overlap of these levels with those of the normal aged population limits the usefulness of these measurements in diagnosis. The use of blood Apo ε genotyping is discussed under "Pathogenesis," below. *Slowly progressive decline in memory and orientation, normal results on laboratory tests, and an MRI or CT scan showing only diffuse or posteriorly predominant cortical and hippocampal atrophy is highly suggestive of AD.* A clinical diagnosis of AD reached after careful evaluation is confirmed at autopsy about 90% of the time, with misdiagnosed cases usually representing one of the other dementing disorders described later in this chapter, a mixture of AD with vascular pathology, or DLB.

Relatively simple clinical clues are useful in the differential diagnosis. Early prominent gait disturbance with only mild memory loss suggests vascular dementia or, rarely, NPH (see below). Resting tremor with stooped posture, bradykinesia, and masked facies suggest PD (Chap. 366). The early appearance of parkinsonian features, visual hallucinations, delusional misidentification, or REM sleep disorder suggest DLB. Chronic alcoholism should prompt the search for vitamin deficiency. Loss of sensibility to position and vibration stimuli accompanied by Babinski responses suggests vitamin B$_{12}$ deficiency (Chap. 372). Early onset of a seizure suggests a metastatic or primary brain neoplasm (Chap. 374). A past history of depression suggests of AD, but this has not been confirmed in large prospective studies. Vascular disease, in particular stroke, seems to lower the threshold for the clinical expression of AD. Also, in many AD patients, amyloid angiopathy can lead to ischemic infarctions or hemorrhages. Diabetes increases the risk of AD threefold. Elevated homocysteine and cholesterol levels; hypertension; diminished serum levels of folic acid; low dietary intake of fruits, vegetables, and red wine; and low levels of exercise are all being explored as potential risk factors for AD.

Pathology At autopsy, the most severe pathology is usually found in the hippocampus, temporal cortex, and nucleus basalis of Meynert (lateral septum). The most important microscopic findings are neuritic "senile" plaques and NFTs. These lesions accumulate in small numbers during normal aging of the brain but occur in excess in AD. There is increasing evidence to suggest that soluble amyloid fibrils called *oligomers* lead to the dysfunction of the cell and may be the first biochemical injury in AD. Misfolded $A\beta_{42}$ molecules may be the most toxic form of this protein. Accumulation of oligomers eventually leads to formation of neuritic plaques (Fig. 365-3). The neuritic plaques contain a central core that includes $A\beta$ amyloid, proteoglycans, Apo $\epsilon 4$, α_1 antichymotrypsin, and other proteins. $A\beta$ amyloid is a protein of 39–42 amino acids that is derived proteolytically from a larger transmembrane protein named *amyloid precursor protein* (APP) when APP is cleaved by β and γ secretases. The normal function of $A\beta$ amyloid is unknown. APP has neurotrophic and neuroprotective activities. The plaque core is surrounded by the debris of degenerating neurons, microglia, and macrophages. The accumulation of $A\beta$ amyloid in cerebral arterioles is termed *amyloid angiopathy*. NFTs are silver-staining, twisted neurofilaments in neuronal cytoplasm that represent abnormally phosphorylated tau (τ) protein and appear as paired helical filaments by electron microscopy. Tau is a microtubule-associated protein that may function to assemble and stabilize the microtubules that convey cell organelles, glycoproteins, and other important materials throughout the neuron. The ability of tau protein to bind to microtubule segments is determined partly by the number of phosphate groups attached to it. Increased phosphorylation of tau protein disturbs this normal process. Finally, the co-association of AD with DLB and vascular pathology is extremely common.

Biochemically, AD is associated with a decrease in the cerebral cortical levels of several proteins and neurotransmitters, especially acetylcholine, its synthetic enzyme choline acetyltransferase, and nicotinic cholinergic receptors. Reduction of acetylcholine may be related in part to degeneration of cholinergic neurons in the nucleus basalis of Meynert that project to many areas of cortex. There is also reduction in norepinephrine levels in brainstem nuclei such as the locus coeruleus.

FIGURE 365-2 Alzheimer's disease. Axial T1-weighted MR images through the midbrain of a normal 86-year-old athlete (**A**) and a 77-year-old male (**B**) with AD. Note that both individuals have prominent sulci and slight dilatation of the lateral ventricles. However, there is a reduction in the volume of the hippocampus of the patient with AD (*arrows*) compared with that of the normal-for-age hippocampus (**A**). Fluorodeoxyglucose PET scans of a normal control (**C**) and a patient with AD (**D**). Note that the patient with AD has decreased activity in the parietal lobes bilaterally (*arrows*), a typical finding in this condition. AD, Alzheimer's disease; PET, positron emission tomography. *(Images courtesy of TF Budinger, University of California; with permission.)*

pseudodementia (see below). A history of treatment for insomnia, anxiety, psychiatric disturbance, or epilepsy suggests chronic drug intoxication. Rapid progression over a few weeks or months associated with rigidity and myoclonus suggests CJD (Chap. 378). Prominent behavioral changes with intact memory and lobar atrophy on brain imaging are typical of FTD. A positive family history of dementia suggests either one of the familial forms of AD or one of the other genetic disorders associated with dementia, such as HD (see below), FTD (see below), familial forms of prion diseases (Chap. 378), or rare forms of hereditary ataxias (Chap. 368).

Epidemiology The most important risk factors for AD are old age and a positive family history. The frequency of AD increases with each decade of adult life, reaching 20–40% of the population over the age of 85. A positive family history of dementia suggests a genetic cause of AD. Female gender may also be a risk factor independent of the greater longevity of women. Some AD patients have a past history of head trauma with concussion, but this appears to be a relatively minor risk factor. AD is more common in groups with very low educational attainment, but education influences test-taking ability, and it is clear that AD can affect persons of all intellectual levels. One study found that the capacity to express complex written language in early adulthood correlated with a decreased risk for AD. Numerous environmental factors, including aluminum, mercury, and viruses, have been proposed as causes of AD, but none has been demonstrated to play a significant role. Similarly, several studies suggest that the use of nonsteroidal anti-inflammatory agents is associated with a decreased risk

GENETIC CONSIDERATIONS Several genetic factors play important roles in the pathogenesis of at least some cases of AD. One is the *APP* gene on chromosome 21. Adults with trisomy 21 (Down's syn-

FIGURE 365-3 Mature neuritic plaque with a dense central amyloid core surrounded by dystrophic neurites (thioflavin S stain). *(Image courtesy of S DeArmond, University of California; with permission.)*

Step 1: Cleavage by either α- or β-secretase

APP

β ↓   ↓ α

Cell membrane

γ

β-Secretase product   α-Secretase product

Step 2: Cleavage by γ-secretase

$A\beta_{42}$ $A\beta_{40}$ P3
Toxic   Nontoxic   Nontoxic
Amyloidogenic

FIGURE 365-4 Amyloid precursor protein (APP) is catabolized by α-, β-, and γ-secretases. A key initial step is the digestion by either β-secretase (BASE) or α-secretase [ADAM10 or ADAM17 (TACE)], producing smaller nontoxic products. Cleavage of the β-secretase product by γ-secretase (step 2) results in either the toxic $A\beta_{42}$ or the nontoxic $A\beta_{40}$ peptide; cleavage of the α-secretase product by γ-secretase produces the nontoxic P3 peptide. Excess production of $A\beta_{42}$ is a key initiator of cellular damage in Alzheimer's disease. Current AD research is focused on developing therapies designed to reduce accumulation of $A\beta_{42}$ by antagonizing β- or γ-secretases, promoting α-secretase, or clearing $A\beta_{42}$ that has already formed by use of specific antibodies.

drome) consistently develop the typical neuropathologic hallmarks of AD if they survive beyond age 40. Many develop a progressive dementia superimposed on their baseline mental retardation. APP is a membrane-spanning protein that is subsequently processed into smaller units, including Aβ amyloid that is deposited in neuritic plaques. Aβ peptide results from cleavage of APP by β and γ secretases **(Fig. 365-4)**. Presumably the extra dose of the *APP* gene on chromosome 21 is the initiating cause of AD in adult Down's syndrome and results in an excess of cerebral amyloid. Furthermore, a few families with early-onset FAD have been discovered to have point mutations in the *APP* gene. Although very rare, these families were the first examples of a single-gene autosomal dominant genetic transmission of AD.

Investigation of large families with multigenerational FAD led to the discovery of two additional AD genes, termed the *presenilins*. Presenilin-1 (*PS-1*) is on chromosome 14 and encodes a protein called S182. Mutations in this gene cause an early-onset AD (onset before age 60 and often before age 50) transmitted in an autosomal dominant, highly penetrant fashion. More than 100 different mutations have been found in the *PS-1* gene in families from a wide range of ethnic backgrounds. Presenilin-2 (*PS-2*) is on chromosome 1 and encodes a protein called STM2. A mutation in the *PS-2* gene was first found in a group of American families with Volga German ethnic background. Mutations in *PS-1* are much more common than those in *PS-2*. The two genes (*PS-1* and *PS-2*) are highly homologous and encode similar proteins that at first appeared to have seven transmembrane domains (hence the designation *STM*), but subsequent studies have suggested eight such domains, with a ninth submembrane region. Both S182 and STM2 are cytoplasmic neuronal proteins that are widely expressed throughout the nervous system. They are homologous to a cell-trafficking protein, sel 12, found in the nematode *Coenorhabditis elegans*. Patients with mutations in these genes have elevated plasma levels of $A\beta_{42}$ amyloid, and *PS-1* mutations in cell cultures produce increased $A\beta_{42}$ amyloid in the media. There is evidence that *PS-1* is involved in the cleavage of APP at the gamma secretase site and mutations in either gene (*PS-1* or *APP*) may disturb this function. Mutations in *PS-1* have thus far proved to be the most common cause of early-onset FAD, representing perhaps 40–70% of this relatively rare syndrome. Mutations in *PS-1* tend to produce AD with an earlier age of onset (mean onset 45 years) and a shorter, more rapidly progressive course (mean duration 6–7 years) than the disease caused by mutations in *PS-2* (mean onset 53 years; duration 11 years). Some carriers of uncommon *PS-2* mutations have had onset of dementia after the age of 70. Mutations in the presenilins are rarely involved in the more common sporadic cases

of late-onset AD occurring in the general population. Molecular DNA blood testing for these uncommon mutations is now possible on a research basis, and mutation analysis of *PS-1* is commercially available. Such testing is likely to be positive only in early-onset familial cases of AD. Any testing of asymptomatic persons at risk must be done in the context of formal, thoughtful genetic counseling.

A discovery of great importance has implicated the *Apo ε* gene on chromosome 19 in the pathogenesis of late-onset familial and sporadic forms of AD. *Apo ε* is involved in cholesterol transport (Chap. 350) and has three alleles: 2, 3, and 4. The Apo ε4 allele has a strong association with AD in the general population, including sporadic and late-onset familial cases. Approximately 24–30% of the nondemented Caucasian population has at least one ε4 allele (12–15% allele frequency), and about 2% are ε4/4 homozygotes. Approximately 40–65% of AD patients have at least one ε4 allele, a highly significant difference compared with controls. On the other hand, many AD patients have no ε4 allele, and individuals with ε4 may never develop AD. Therefore, ε4 is neither necessary nor sufficient as a cause of AD. Nevertheless, it is clear that the Apo ε4 allele, especially in the homozygous 4/4 state, is an important risk factor for AD. It appears to act as a dose-dependent modifier of age of onset, with the earliest onset associated with the ε4/4 homozygous state. It is unknown how Apo ε functions as a risk factor modifying age of onset, but it may be involved with the clearance of amyloid, less efficiently in the case of Apo ε4. Apo ε is present in the neuritic amyloid plaques of AD, and it may also be involved in neurofibrillary tangle formation, because it binds to tau protein. Apo ε4 decreases neurite outgrowth in cultures of dorsal root ganglion neurons, perhaps indicating a deleterious role in the brain's response to injury. There is some evidence that the ε2 allele may be "protective," but that remains to be clarified. The use of Apo ε testing in the diagnosis of AD is controversial. It is not indicated as a predictive test in normal persons because its precise predictive value is unclear, and many individuals with the ε4 allele never develop dementia. However, some cognitively normal ε4 heterozygotes and homozygotes have been found by PET to have decreased cerebral cortical metabolic rates, suggesting possible presymptomatic abnormalities compatible with the earliest stage of AD. In demented persons who meet clinical criteria for AD, the finding of an ε4 allele increases the reliability of diagnosis. However, the absence of an ε4 allele does not eliminate the diagnosis of AD. Furthermore, all patients with dementia, including those with an ε4 allele, require a search for reversible causes of their cognitive impairment. Nevertheless, Apo ε4 remains the single most important biologic marker associated with risk for AD, and studies of its functional role and diagnostic usefulness are progressing rapidly. Its association (or lack thereof) with other dementing illnesses needs to be fully evaluated. The ε4 allele is not associated with FTD, DLB, or CJD. Additional genes are also likely to be involved in AD, but none have been reliably identified.

℞ ALZHEIMER'S DISEASE

The management of AD is challenging and gratifying, despite the absence of a cure or a robust pharmacologic treatment. The primary focus is on long-term amelioration of associated behavioral and neurologic problems.

Building rapport with the patient, family members, and other caregivers is essential to successful management. In the early stages of AD, memory aids such as notebooks and posted daily reminders can be helpful. Common sense and clinical studies show that family members should emphasize activities that are pleasant and deemphasize those that are unpleasant. Kitchens, bathrooms, and bedrooms need to be made safe, and eventually patients must stop driving. Loss of independence and change of environment may worsen confusion, agitation, and anger. Communication and repeated calm reassurance are necessary. Caregiver "burnout" is common, often resulting in nursing home placement of the patient, and respite breaks for the caregiver help to maintain successful long-term management of the patient. Use of adult day-care centers can be most helpful. Local and national support groups, such as the Alzheimer's Association, are valuable resources.

Donepezil, rivastigmine, galantamine, memantine, and tacrine are the drugs presently approved by the Food and Drug Administration (FDA) for treatment of AD. Due to hepatotoxicity, tacrine is no longer used. The pharmacologic action of donepezil, rivastigmine, and galantamine is inhibition of cholinesterase, with a resulting increase in cerebral levels of acetylcholine. Memantine appears to act by blocking overexcited N-methyl-D-aspartate (NMDA) channels. Double-blind, placebo-controlled, crossover studies with cholinesterase inhibitors and memantine have shown them to be associated with improved caregiver ratings of patients' functioning and with an apparent decreased rate of decline in cognitive test scores over periods of up to 3 years. The average patient on an anticholinesterase compound maintains his or her MMSE score for close to a year, whereas a placebo-treated patient declines 2–3 points over the same time period. Memantine, used in conjunction with cholinesterase inhibitors or by itself, seems to slow cognitive deterioration in patients with moderate to severe AD and is not approved for mild AD. These compounds have only modest efficacy for AD and offer even less benefit in the late stages. All the cholinesterase inhibitors are relatively easy to administer, and their major side effects are gastrointestinal symptoms (nausea, diarrhea, cramps), altered sleep with bad dreams, bradycardia (usually benign), and sometimes muscle cramps.

In a prospective observational study, the use of estrogen replacement therapy appeared to protect—by about 50%—against development of AD in women. This study seemed to confirm the results of two earlier case-controlled studies. Sadly, a prospective placebo-controlled study of a combined estrogen-progesterone therapy for asymptomatic postmenopausal women increased, rather than decreased, the prevalence of dementia. This study markedly dampened enthusiasm for hormone treatments for the prevention of dementia. Additionally, no benefit has been found in the treatment of AD with estrogen.

In patients with moderately advanced AD, a prospective trial of the antioxidants selegiline (Chap. 366), α-tocopherol (vitamin E), or both, slowed institutionalization and progression to death. Because vitamin E has less potential for toxicity than selegiline and is cheaper, the doses used in this study of 1000 IU twice daily are offered to many patients with AD. However, the beneficial effects of vitamin E remain controversial, and most investigators no longer give it in these high doses because of potential cardiovascular complications.

A randomized, double-blind, placebo-controlled trial of an extract of *Ginkgo biloba* found modest improvement in cognitive function in subjects with AD and vascular dementia. This study requires confirmation before *Ginkgo biloba* is used as a treatment for dementia because there was a high subject dropout rate and no improvement on a clinician's judgment scale. A comprehensive 6-year multicenter prevention study using *Ginkgo biloba* is underway.

Vaccination against Aβ42 has proved highly efficacious in mouse models of AD; it helped to clear amyloid from the brain and prevent further accumulation of amyloid. However, in human trials this approach led to life-threatening complications, including meningoencephalitis. Modifications of the vaccine approach using passive immunization with monoclonal antibodies are currently being evaluated in phase 3 trials. Another experimental approach to the treatment of AD has been the use of β and γ secretase inhibitors that diminish the production of Aβ42.

Several retrospective studies suggest that nonsteroidal anti-inflammatory agents and statins (HMG-CoA reductase inhibitors) may have a protective effect on dementia, and controlled prospective studies are being conducted. Similarly, prospective studies with the goal of lowering serum homocysteine levels are underway, suggesting an association of elevated homocysteine with dementia progression based on epidemiologic studies. Finally, there is now a strong interest in the relationship between diabetes and AD, and insulin-regulating studies are being conducted.

Mild to moderate depression is common in the early stages of AD and responds to antidepressants or cholinesterase inhibitors. Selective serotonin reuptake inhibitors (SSRIs) are commonly used due to their low anticholinergic side effects. Generalized seizures should be treated with an appropriate anticonvulsant, such as phenytoin or carbamazepine. Agitation, insomnia, hallucinations, and belligerence are especially troublesome characteristics of some AD patients, and these behaviors can lead to nursing home placement. The newer generation of atypical antipsychotics, such as risperidone, quetiapine, and olanzapine, are being used in low doses to treat these neuropsychiatric symptoms. The few controlled studies comparing drugs against behavioral intervention in the treatment of agitation suggest mild efficacy with significant side effects related to sleep, gait, and cardiovascular complications. All of the antipsychotics carry a black-box warning and should be used with caution. However, careful, daily, nonpharmacologic behavior management is often not available, rendering medications necessary.

VASCULAR DEMENTIA

Dementia associated with cerebral vascular disease can be divided into two general categories: multi-infarct dementia and diffuse white matter disease (also called *leukoaraiosis, subcortical arteriosclerotic encephalopathy* or *Binswanger's disease*). Cerebral vascular disease appears to be a more common cause of dementia in Asia than in Europe and North America. Individuals who have had several strokes may develop chronic cognitive deficits, commonly called *multi-infarct dementia*. The strokes may be large or small (sometimes lacunar) and usually involve several different brain regions. The occurrence of dementia depends partly on the total volume of damaged cortex, but it is also more common in individuals with left-hemisphere lesions, independent of any language disturbance. Patients typically report a history of discrete episodes of sudden neurologic deterioration. Many multi-infarct dementia patients have a history of hypertension, diabetes, coronary artery disease, or other manifestations of widespread atherosclerosis. Physical examination usually shows focal neurologic deficits such as hemiparesis, a unilateral Babinski reflex, a visual field defect, or pseudobulbar palsy. Recurrent strokes result in a stepwise progression of disease. Neuroimaging studies show multiple areas of infarction. Thus, the history and neuroimaging findings differentiate this condition from AD. However, both AD and multiple infarctions are common and sometimes occur together. With normal aging, there is also an accumulation of amyloid in cerebral blood vessels, leading to a condition called *cerebral amyloid angiopathy of aging* (not associated with dementia), which predisposes older persons to hemorrhagic lobar stroke. AD patients with amyloid angiopathy may be at increased risk for cerebral infarction.

Some individuals with dementia are discovered on MRI to have bilateral abnormalities of subcortical white matter, termed *diffuse white matter disease*, often occurring in association with lacunar infarctions (**Fig. 365-5**). The dementia may be insidious in onset and progress slowly, features that distinguish it from multi-infarct dementia, but other patients show a stepwise deterioration more typical of multi-infarct dementia. Early symptoms are mild confusion, apathy, changes in personality, depression, psychosis, memory, and spatial or executive deficits. Marked difficulties in judgment and orientation and dependence on others for daily activities develop later. Euphoria, elation, depression, or aggressive behaviors are common as the disease progresses.

FIGURE 365-5 Diffuse white matter disease (Binswanger's disease). Axial T2-weighted MR image through the lateral ventricles reveals multiple areas of abnormal high signal intensity involving the periventricular white matter as well as the corona radiata and lentiform nuclei (*arrows*). While seen in some individuals with normal cognition, this appearance is more pronounced in patients with dementia of a vascular etiology.

Both pyramidal and cerebellar signs may be present in the same patient. A gait disorder is present in at least half of these patients. With advanced disease, urinary incontinence and dysarthria with or without other pseudobulbar features (e.g., dysphagia, emotional lability) are frequent. Seizures and myoclonic jerks appear in a minority of patients. This disorder appears to result from chronic ischemia due to occlusive disease of small, penetrating cerebral arteries and arterioles (microangiopathy). Any disease-causing stenosis of small cerebral vessels may be the critical underlying factor, though most typically hypertension is the main cause. The term *Binswanger's disease* should be used with caution, because it does not really identify a single entity.

Other rare causes of white matter disease also present with dementia, such as adult metachromatic leukodystrophy (arylsulfatase A deficiency) and progressive multifocal leukoencephalopathy (papovavirus infection). A dominantly inherited form of diffuse white matter disease is known as *cerebral autosomal dominant arteriopathy with subcortical infarcts and leukoencephalopathy* (CADASIL). Clinically, there is a progressive dementia developing in the fifth to seventh decades in multiple family members who may also have a history of migraine and recurrent stroke without hypertension. Skin biopsy may show characteristic dense bodies in the media of arterioles. The disease is caused by mutations in the *notch 3* gene, and there is a commercially available genetic test. The frequency of this disorder is unknown, and there are no known treatments.

Mitochondrial disorders can present with strokelike episodes and can selectively injure basal ganglia or cortex. Many such patients show other findings suggestive of a neurologic or systemic disorder such as ophthalmoplegia, retinal degeneration, deafness, myopathy, neuropathy, or diabetes. Diagnosis is difficult but serum—especially CSF—levels of lactate and pyruvate may be abnormal, and biopsy of affected tissue is often diagnostic.

Treatment of vascular dementia must be focused on the underlying causes, such as hypertension, atherosclerosis, and diabetes. Recovery of lost cognitive function is not likely to occur, although fluctuations with periods of improvement are common. Anticholinesterase compounds are being studied as a treatment for vascular dementia.

FRONTOTEMPORAL DEMENTIA, PROGRESSIVE SUPRANUCLEAR PALSY, AND CORTICOBASAL DEGENERATION

Frontotemporal dementia (FTD) often begins when the patient is in the fifth to seventh decades, and in this age group it is nearly as common as AD. Most studies suggest that FTD is twice as common in men as it is in women. *Unlike AD, behavioral symptoms predominate in the early stages of FTD.* Genetics play a significant role in a sizable minority of cases. The clinical heterogeneity in familial and sporadic forms of FTD is remarkable, with patients demonstrating variable mixtures of disinhibition, dementia, PSP, CBD, and motor neuron disease. The most common genetic mutations that cause an autosomal dominant form of FTD involve the *tau* or *progranulin* genes, both on chromosome 17. *Tau* mutations lead to a change in the alternate splicing of tau or cause loss of function in the tau molecule. With *progranulin*, a missense mutation in the coding sequence of the gene is the underlying cause for the neurodegeneration. Progranulin appears to be a rare example of an autosomal dominant mutation leading to haploinsufficiency—too little of the progranulin protein. Both *tau* and *progranulin* mutations are associated with parkinsonian features, while ALS is rare in the setting of these mutations. In contrast, familial FTD with ALS has been linked to chromosome 9. Mutations in the valosin (chromosome 9) and ESCRTII molecules (chromosome 3) also lead to autosomal dominant forms of familial FTD.

In FTD, early symptoms are divided among cognitive, behavioral, and sometimes motor abnormalities, reflecting degeneration of the anterior frontal and temporal regions, basal ganglia, and motor neurons. Cognitive testing typically reveals spared memory but impaired planning, judgment, or language. Poor business decisions and difficulty organizing work tasks are common, and speech and language deficits often emerge. Patients with FTD often show an absence of insight into their condition. Common behavioral deficits include apathy, disinhibition, weight gain, food fetishes, compulsions, and euphoria.

Findings at the bedside are dictated by the anatomic localization of the disorder. Asymmetric left-frontal cases present with nonfluent aphasias, while left anterior temporal degeneration is characterized by loss of words and concepts related to language (semantic dementia). Nonfluent patients quickly progress to mutism, while those with semantic dementia develop features of multimodality agnosia, losing the ability to recognize faces, objects, words, and the emotions of others. Copying, calculating, and navigation often remain normal into later in the illness. Recently it has become apparent that many if not most patients with nonfluent aphasia progress to clinical syndromes that overlap with PSP and CBD and show these pathologies at autopsy. This left-hemisphere presentation of FTD has been called *primary progressive aphasia*. In contrast, right-frontal or temporal cases show profound alterations in social conduct, with loss of empathy, disinhibition, and antisocial behaviors predominating. Memory and visuospatial skills are relatively spared in most FTD patients. There is a striking overlap among FTD, PSP, CBD, and motor neuron disease; ophthalmoplegia, dystonia, swallowing symptoms, and fasciculations are common at presentation of FTD or emerge during the course of the illness.

The distinguishing anatomic hallmark of FTD is a marked lobar atrophy of temporal and/or frontal lobes, which can be visualized by neuroimaging studies and is readily apparent at autopsy (Figs. 365-6 and 365-7). The atrophy is sometimes asymmetric and may involve the basal ganglia. Two major pathologies have been linked to the clinical syndrome, one associated with tau inclusions, the other with inclusions that stain negatively for tau but positively for ubiquitin and TDP-43. Microscopic findings that are seen across all FTD cases include gliosis, neuronal loss, and spongiosis.

Approximately one-half of all cases show swollen or ballooned neurons containing cytoplasmic inclusions that stain positively for tau. These aggregates sometimes resemble those found in PSP and CBD, and tau plays a major role in the pathogenesis of all three conditions. A toxic gain of function related to tau underlies the pathogenesis of many familial cases and is presumed to be a factor in sporadic cases as well. Nearly 80% of FTD patients show involvement of the basal ganglia at autopsy, and 15% go on to develop motor neuron disease, underscoring the multisystem nature of this illness. Serotonergic losses

FIGURE 365-6 Frontotemporal dementia (FTD). Coronal MRI sections from one patient with frontally predominant FTD (*left*) and another with temporally predominant FTD (*right*). Prominent atrophy affecting the frontal gyri (*white arrows*) is present in frontally predominant FTD, particularly affecting the right frontal region; note also the thinning of the corpus callosum superior to the lateral ventricles. This patient presented with disinhibition and antisocial behavior. In the temporally predominant patient, severe atrophy in the left temporal lobe (*open arrows*) and amygdala (*white arrowheads*) is present; this patient presented with progressive aphasia. (*Images courtesy of H Rosen and G Schauer, University of California at San Francisco; with permission.*)

FIGURE 365-7 Voxel-based morphometry analysis showing differing patterns of brain atrophy in the frontal variant of frontotemporal dementia (red), temporal variant of frontotemporal dementia (green), and Alzheimer's disease (blue). This technique allows comparison of MRI gray matter volumes between groups of subjects. *(Image courtesy of M Gorno-Tempini, University of California at San Francisco; with permission.)*

are seen in many patients, and glutaminergic neurons are depleted. In contrast to AD, the cholinergic system is relatively spared in FTD, whereas serotonergic and glutaminergic neurons are depleted in many patients.

Historically, *Pick's disease* was described as a progressive degenerative disorder characterized clinically by selective involvement of the anterior frontal and temporal neocortex and pathologically by intracellular inclusions (*Pick bodies*). Classic Pick bodies stain positive with silver (argyrophilic) and tau, but many of the tau-positive inclusions in FTD cases are not labeled with silver stains (Fig. 365-8). Although the nomenclature for these patients has remained controversial, the term *FTD* is increasingly used to describe the clinical syndrome, while *Pick's disease* is used to classify patients in whom the pathology shows classic Pick bodies (only a minority of patients with the clinical features of FTD).

The burden on caregivers of FTD patients is extremely high. Treatment is symptomatic, and there are currently no therapies known to slow progression or improve cognitive symptoms. Many of the behaviors that accompany FTD, such as depression, hyperorality, compulsions, and irritability, can be ameliorated with serotonin-modifying antidepressants. The co-association with motor disorders necessitates the careful use of antipsychotics, which can exacerbate this problem.

Progressive supranuclear palsy (PSP) is a degenerative disease that involves the brainstem, basal ganglia, and neocortex. Clinically, this disorder begins with falls and vertical supranuclear gaze paresis and progresses to symmetrical rigidity and dementia. A stiff, unstable pos-

FIGURE 365-8 Classic intraneuronal Pick body (tau2 stain). These consist of loosely arranged paired and straight-helical filaments and stain positive for tau. Classic Pick bodies are seen in ~20% of all frontotemporal dementia cases.

ture with hyperextension of the neck and slow gait with frequent falls is characteristic of PSP. Early in the disease, patients have difficulty with downgaze and lose vertical opticokinetic nystagmus on downward movement of a target. Frequent unexplained and sometimes spectacular falls are common secondary to a combination of axial rigidity, inability to look down, and bad judgment. Although the patients have very limited voluntary eye movements, their eyes still retain oculocephalic reflexes (doll's head maneuver); thus, the eye-movement disorder is supranuclear. The dementia is similar to FTD with apathy, frontal/executive dysfunction, poor judgment, slowed thought processes, impaired verbal fluency, and difficulty with sequential actions and with shifting from one task to another all common at the time of presentation and often preceding the motor syndrome. Some patients begin with a nonfluent aphasia and progress to classical PSP. There is only a limited response to L-dopa; no other effective treatments exist. Death occurs within 5–10 years of onset. At autopsy, abnormal accumulation of tau is found within neurons and glia, often in the form of neurofibrillary tangles (NFTs). These tangles are found in multiple subcortical structures (including the subthalamus, globus pallidus, substantia nigra, locus coeruleus, periaqueductal gray, superior colliculi, and oculomotor nuclei) as well as in the neocortex. The NFTs have similar staining characteristics to those of AD, but on electron microscopy they are generally seen to consist of straight tubules rather than the paired helical filaments found in AD.

In addition to its overlap with FTD and CBD (see below), PSP is often confused with idiopathic *Parkinson's disease* (PD). Although elderly Parkinson's patients may have some difficulty with upgaze, they do not develop downgaze paresis or other abnormalities of voluntary eye movements typical of PSP. Dementia does occur in ~20% of PD patients, often secondary to DLB. Furthermore, the behavioral syndromes seen with DLB differ from PSP (see below). The occurrence of dementia in PD is more likely with increasing age, increasing severity of extrapyramidal signs, a long duration of disease, and the presence of depression. These patients also show cortical atrophy on brain imaging. Neuropathologically, there may be Alzheimer changes in the cortex (amyloid plaques and NFTs), neuronal Lewy body inclusions in both the substantia nigra and the cortex, or no specific microscopic changes other than gliosis and neuronal loss. Progressive supranuclear palsy and Parkinson's disease are discussed in detail in Chap. 366.

Cortical basal degeneration (CBD) is a slowly progressive dementing illness associated with severe gliosis and neuronal loss in both the neocortex and basal ganglia (substantia nigra and striatum). Occasionally there is a unilateral onset with rigidity, dystonia, and apraxia of one arm and hand, sometimes called the *alien hand*, while in other instances the disease presents as a progressive frontal syndrome or as progressive symmetrical parkinsonism. Some patients begin with a progressive nonfluent aphasia or a progressive motor disorder of speech. Eventually CBD becomes bilateral and leads to dysarthria, slow gait, action tremor, and dementia. The microscopic features include enlarged, achromatic neurons in the cortex with tau inclusions. Glial plaques with tau inclusions are pathognomonic of CBD. The condition is rarely familial, the cause is unknown, and there is no specific treatment.

DEMENTIA WITH LEWY BODIES

The parkinsonian dementia syndromes are under increasing study, with many cases unified by the presence of Lewy bodies in both the substantia nigra and the cortex at pathology. The clinical syndrome is characterized by visual hallucinations, parkinsonism, fluctuating alertness, falls, and often REM sleep behavior disorder. Dementia can precede or follow the appearance of parkinsonism. Hence, one pathway to DLB occurs in patients with longstanding PD without cognitive impairment who slowly develop a dementia that is associated with visual hallucinations, parkinsonism, and fluctuating alertness. In others, the dementia and neuropsychiatric syndrome precede the parkinsonism. DLB patients are highly susceptible to metabolic perturbations, and in some patients the first manifestation of illness is a delirium, often precipitated by an infection or other systemic disturbance. A delirium induced by L-dopa, prescribed for parkinsonian symptoms attributed to PD, may be the initial clue that the correct diagnosis is DLB. Even without an underlying precipitant, fluctuations can be marked in DLB patients, with the occurrence of episodic confusion admixed with lucid intervals. However, despite the fluctuating pattern, the clinical features persist over a long period of time, unlike delirium, which resolves following correction of the underlying precipitant. Cognitively, DLB patients tend to have relatively better memory but more severe visuospatial deficits than individuals with AD.

The key neuropathologic feature is the presence of Lewy bodies throughout the cortex, amygdala, cingulate cortex, and substantia nigra. Lewy bodies are intraneuronal cytoplasmic inclusions that stain with periodic acid–Schiff (PAS) and ubiquitin. They are composed of straight neurofilaments 7–20 nm long with surrounding amorphous material. They contain epitopes recognized by antibodies against phosphorylated and nonphosphorylated neurofilament proteins, ubiquitin, and a presynaptic protein called α-synuclein. Lewy bodies are traditionally found in the substantia nigra of patients with idiopathic PD. A profound cholinergic deficit is present in many patients with DLB and may be a factor responsible for the fluctuations and visual hallucinations present in these patients. In patients without other pathologic features, the condition is referred to as *diffuse Lewy body disease*. In patients whose brains also contain excessive amounts of amyloid plaques and NFTs, the condition is called the *Lewy body variant of Alzheimer's disease*. The quantity of Lewy bodies required to establish the diagnosis is controversial, but a definite diagnosis requires pathology. At autopsy, 10–30% of demented patients show cortical Lewy bodies.

Due to the overlap with AD and the cholinergic deficit in DLB, anticholinesterase compounds may be helpful. Exercise programs maximize the motor function of these patients. Similarly, antidepressants are often necessary to treat the depressive syndromes that accompany DLB. Atypical antipsychotics in low doses are sometimes needed to alleviate psychosis, although even low doses can increase extrapyramidal syndromes and may rarely lead to death. As noted above, patients with DLB are extremely sensitive to dopaminergic medications, which must be carefully titrated; tolerability may be improved by concomitant AD medications.

OTHER CAUSES OF DEMENTIA

Prion disorders such as *Creutzfeldt-Jakob disease* (CJD) are rare conditions (~1 per million population) that produce dementia. CJD is a rapidly progressive disorder associated with dementia, focal cortical signs, rigidity, and myoclonus, causing death in <1 year from the first symptoms. The rapidity of progression seen with CJD is uncommon in AD so that distinction between the two disorders is usually possible. However, CBD and DLB, more rapid degenerative dementias with prominent abnormalities in movement, are more likely to be mistaken for CJD. The differential diagnosis for CJD usually includes other rapidly progressive dementing conditions such as viral or bacterial encephalitides, Hashimoto's encephalitis, CNS vasculitis, lymphoma, or paraneoplastic syndromes. The markedly abnormal periodic EEG discharges and cortical and basal ganglia abnormalities on diffusion-weighted MRI are unique diagnostic features of CJD. Transmission from infected cattle to the human population in the United Kingdom has caused a small epidemic of atypical CJD in young adults. **Prion diseases are discussed in detail in Chap. 378.**

Huntington's disease (HD) (Chap. 367) is an autosomal dominant, degenerative brain disorder. A DNA repeat expansion (CAG repeat) of the mutant gene on chromosome 4 forms the basis of a diagnostic blood test for the disease gene. The clinical hallmarks of the disease are chorea, behavioral disturbance, and frontal executive disorder. Onset is usually in the fourth or fifth decade, but there is a wide range in age of onset, from childhood to >70 years. Memory is frequently not impaired until late in the disease, but attention, judgment, awareness, and executive functions may be seriously deficient at an early stage. Depression, apathy, social withdrawal, irritability, and intermittent disinhibition are common. Delusions and obsessive-compulsive behavior may occur. The disease duration is typically about 15 years but is quite variable. There is no specific treatment, but the adventitious movements may partially respond to first- and second-generation antipsychotics. Treatment of behavioral changes are discussed in "General Symptomatic Treatment of the Patient with Dementia," below. Asymptomatic adult children at risk for HD should receive careful genetic counseling prior to DNA testing, because a positive result may have serious emotional and social consequences.

Normal-pressure hydrocephalus (NPH) is a relatively uncommon syndrome with clinical, physiologic, and neuroimaging characteristics. Historically, many of the individuals who have been treated for NPH have suffered from other dementias, particularly AD, multi-infarct dementia, and DLB. For NPH the clinical triad includes an abnormal gait (ataxic or apractic), dementia (usually mild to moderate), and urinary incontinence. Neuroimaging studies reveal enlarged lateral ventricles (hydrocephalus) with little or no cortical atrophy. This syndrome is a communicating hydrocephalus with a patent aqueduct of Sylvius (Fig. 365-9), in contrast to congenital aqueductal stenosis, where the aqueduct is small. In many cases, periventricular edema is present. Lumbar puncture opening pressure is in the high normal range, and the CSF protein, sugar concentrations, and cell count are normal. NPH is presumed to be caused by obstruction to normal flow of CSF over the cerebral convexity and delayed absorption into the venous system. The indolent nature of the process results in enlarged lateral ventricles but relatively little increase in CSF pressure. There is presumed stretching and distortion of white matter tracts in the corona radiata, but the exact physiologic cause of the clinical syndrome is unclear. Some patients have a history of conditions producing scarring of the basilar meninges (blocking upward flow of CSF) such as previous meningitis, subarachnoid hemorrhage, or head trauma. Others with longstanding but asymptomatic congenital hydrocephalus may have adult-onset deterioration in gait or memory that is confused with NPH. In contrast to AD, the NPH patient has an early and prominent gait disturbance and no evidence of cortical atrophy on CT or MRI. A number of attempts have been made to use various special studies to improve the diagnosis of NPH and predict the success of ventricular shunting. These include radionuclide cisternography (showing a delay in CSF absorption over the convexity) and various attempts to monitor and alter CSF flow dynamics, including a constant-pressure infusion test. None has proven to be specific or consistently useful. There is sometimes a transient improvement in gait or cognition following lumbar puncture (or serial punctures) with removal of 30–50 mL of CSF, but this finding also has not proven to be consistently predictive of post-shunt improvement. AD often masquerades as NPH, because the gait may be abnormal in AD and cortical atrophy sometimes is difficult to determine by CT or MRI early in the disease. Hippocampal atrophy on MRI is a clue favoring AD. Approximately 30–50% of patients identified by careful diagnosis as having NPH will show improvement with a ventricular shunting procedure. Gait may improve more than memory. Transient, short-lasting improvement is common. Patients should be carefully selected for this operation, because subdural hematoma and infection are known complications.

Dementia can accompany *chronic alcoholism* (Chap. 387). This may be a result of associated malnutrition, especially of B vitamins and particularly thiamine. However, other poorly defined aspects of chronic alcohol ingestion may also produce cerebral damage. A rare idiopathic syndrome of dementia and seizures with degeneration of the corpus callosum has been reported primarily in male Italian drinkers of red wine (Marchiafava-Bignami disease).

Thiamine (vitamin B$_1$) deficiency causes Wernicke's encephalopathy (Chap. 269). The clinical presentation is a malnourished individual (frequently but not necessarily alcoholic) with confusion, ataxia, and diplopia from ophthalmoplegia. Thiamine deficiency damages the thalamus, mammillary bodies, midline cerebellum, periaqueductal grey matter of the midbrain, and peripheral nerves. Damage to the dorsomedial thalamic region correlates most closely with the memory loss. Prompt administration of parenteral thiamine (100 mg intravenously for 3 days followed by daily oral dosage) may reverse the dis-

A   **B**

FIGURE 365-9 Normal-pressure hydrocephalus. A. Sagittal T1-weighted MR image demonstrates dilatation of the lateral ventricle and stretching of the corpus callosum (*arrows*), depression of the floor of the third ventricle (*single arrowhead*), and enlargement of the aqueduct (*double arrowheads*). Note the diffuse dilatation of the lateral, third, and fourth ventricles with a patent aqueduct, typical of communicating hydrocephalus. **B.** Axial T2-weighted MR images demonstrate dilatation of the lateral ventricles. This patient underwent successful ventriculoperitoneal shunting.

ease if given in the first days of symptom onset. However, prolonged untreated thiamine deficiency can result in an irreversible dementia/ amnestic syndrome (Korsakoff's psychosis) or even death.

In *Korsakoff's syndrome*, the patient is unable to recall new information despite normal immediate memory, attention span, and level of consciousness. Memory for new events is seriously impaired, whereas memory of knowledge prior to the illness is relatively intact. Patients are easily confused, disoriented, and incapable of recalling new information for more than a brief interval. Superficially, they may be conversant, entertaining, and able to perform simple tasks and follow immediate commands. Confabulation is common, although not always present, and may result in obviously erroneous statements and elaborations. There is no specific treatment because the previous thiamine deficiency has produced irreversible damage to the medial thalamic nuclei and mammillary bodies. Mammillary body atrophy may be visible on high-resolution MRI (see Fig. 269-8).

Vitamin B_{12} deficiency, as can occur in pernicious anemia, causes a macrocytic anemia and may also damage the nervous system (Chaps. 100 and 372). Neurologically, it most commonly produces a spinal cord syndrome (myelopathy) affecting the posterior columns (loss of position and vibratory sense) and corticospinal tracts (hyperactive tendon reflexes with Babinski responses); it also damages peripheral nerves, resulting in sensory loss with depressed tendon reflexes. Damage to cerebral myelinated fibers may also cause dementia. The mechanism of neurologic damage is unclear but may be related to a deficiency of *S*-adenosylmethionine (required for methylation of myelin phospholipids) due to reduced methionine synthase activity or accumulation of methylmalonate, homocysteine, and propionate, providing abnormal substrates for fatty acids synthesis in myelin. The neurologic signs of vitamin B_{12} deficiency are usually associated with macrocytic anemia but on occasion may occur in its absence. Treatment with parenteral vitamin B_{12} (1000 μg intramuscularly daily for a week, weekly for a month, and monthly for life for pernicious anemia) stops progression of the disease if instituted promptly, but reversal of advanced nervous system damage will not occur.

Deficiency of nicotinic acid (*pellagra*) is associated with sun-exposed skin rash, glossitis, and angular stomatitis (Chap. 71). Severe dietary deficiency of nicotinic acid along with other B vitamins such as

pyridoxine may result in spastic paraparesis, peripheral neuropathy, fatigue, irritability, and dementia. This syndrome has been seen in prisoner-of-war and concentration camps. Low serum folate levels appear to be a rough index of malnutrition, but isolated folate deficiency has not been proven to be specific cause of dementia.

Infections of the CNS usually cause delirium and other acute neurologic syndromes (Chap. 269). However, some chronic CNS infections, particularly those associated with chronic meningitis (Chap. 377), may produce a dementing illness. The possibility of chronic infectious meningitis should be suspected in patients presenting with a dementia or behavioral syndrome who also have headache, meningismus, cranial neuropathy, and/or radiculopathy. Between 20 and 30% of patients in the advanced stages of infection with HIV become demented (Chap. 182). Cardinal features include psychomotor retardation, apathy, and impaired memory. This syndrome may result from secondary opportunistic infections but can also be caused by direct infection of CNS neurons with HIV. CNS syphilis (Chap. 162) was a common cause of dementia in the preantibiotic era; it is uncommon nowadays but can still be encountered in patients with multiple sex partners. Characteristic CSF changes consist of pleocytosis, increased protein, and a positive venereal disease research laboratory (VDRL) test.

Primary and metastatic *neoplasms of the CNS* (Chap. 374) usually produce focal neurologic findings and seizures rather than dementia. However, if tumor growth begins in the frontal or temporal lobes, the initial manifestations may be memory loss or behavioral changes. A paraneoplastic syndrome of dementia associated with occult carcinoma (often small cell lung cancer) is termed *limbic encephalitis* (Chap. 97). In this syndrome, confusion, agitation, seizures, poor memory, movement disorders, and frank dementia may occur in association with sensory neuropathy.

A *nonconvulsive seizure disorder* may underlie a syndrome of confusion, clouding of consciousness, and garbled speech. Psychiatric disease is often suspected, but an EEG demonstrates the seizure discharges. If recurrent or persistent, the condition may be termed *complex partial status epilepticus*. The cognitive disturbance often responds to anticonvulsant therapy. The etiology may be previous small strokes or head trauma; some cases are idiopathic.

It is important to recognize *systemic diseases* that indirectly affect the brain and produce chronic confusion or dementia. Such conditions include hypothyroidism; vasculitis; and hepatic, renal, or pulmonary disease. Hepatic encephalopathy may begin with irritability and confusion and slowly progress to agitation, lethargy, and coma (Chap. 268).

Isolated vasculitis of the CNS (CNS granulomatous vasculitis) (Chaps. 319 and 364) occasionally causes a chronic encephalopathy associated with confusion, disorientation, and cloudiness of consciousness. Headache is common, and strokes and cranial neuropathies may occur. Brain imaging studies may be normal or nonspecifically abnormal. CSF studies reveal a mild pleocytosis or elevation in the protein level. Cerebral angiography often shows multifocal stenosis and narrowing of vessels. A few patients have only small-vessel disease that is not revealed on angiography. The angiographic appearance is not specific and may be mimicked by atherosclerosis, infection, or other causes of vascular disease. Brain or meningeal biopsy demonstrates abnormal arteries with endothelial cell proliferation and infiltrates of mononuclear cells. The prognosis is often poor, although the disorder may remit spontaneously. Some patients respond to glucocorticoids or chemotherapy.

Chronic metal exposure may produce a dementing syndrome. The key to diagnosis is to elicit a history of exposure at work or home, or even as a consequence of a medical procedure such as dialysis. Chronic lead poisoning from inadequately fired glazed pottery has been reported. Fatigue, depression, and confusion may be associated with episodic abdominal pain and peripheral neuropathy. Gray lead lines appear in the gums. There is usually an anemia with basophilic stippling of red cells. The clinical presentation can resemble that of acute intermittent porphyria, including elevated levels of urine porphyrins as a result of the inhibition of δ-aminolevulinic acid dehydrase. The treatment is chelation therapy with agents such as ethylenediamine tetraacetic acid (EDTA). Chronic mercury poisoning produces dementia, peripheral neuropathy, ataxia, and tremulousness that may progress to a cerebellar intention tremor or choreoathetosis. The confusion and memory loss of chronic arsenic intoxication is also associated with nausea, weight loss, peripheral neuropathy, pigmentation and scaling of the skin, and transverse white lines of the fingernails (Mees' lines). Treatment is chelation therapy with dimercaprol (BAL). Aluminum poisoning has been best documented with the dialysis dementia syndrome, in which water used during renal dialysis was contaminated with excessive amounts of aluminum. This poisoning resulted in a progressive encephalopathy associated with confusion, nonfluent aphasia, memory loss, agitation, and, later, lethargy and stupor. Speech arrest and myoclonic jerks were common and associated with severe and generalized EEG changes. The condition has been eliminated by the use of deionized water for dialysis.

Recurrent head trauma in professional boxers may lead to a dementia sometimes called the "punch drunk" syndrome, or *dementia pugilistica*. The symptoms can be progressive, beginning late in a boxer's career or even long after retirement. The severity of the syndrome correlates with the length of the boxing career and number of bouts. Early in the condition, a personality change associated with social instability and sometimes paranoia and delusions occurs. Later, memory loss progresses to full dementia, often associated with parkinsonian signs and ataxia or intention tremor. At autopsy, the cerebral cortex may show changes similar to AD, although NFTs are usually more prominent than amyloid plaques (which are usually diffuse rather than neuritic). There may also be loss of neurons in the substantia nigra. Chronic subdural hematoma (Chap. 373) is also occasionally associated with dementia, often in the context of underlying cortical atrophy from conditions such as AD or HD. In these latter cases, evacuation of subdural hematoma will not alter the underlying degenerative process.

Transient global amnesia (TGA) is characterized by the sudden onset of a severe episodic memory deficit, usually occurring in persons >50. Often the memory loss occurs in the setting of an emotional stimulus or physical exertion. During the attack, the individual is alert and communicative, general cognition seems intact, and there are no other neurologic signs or symptoms. The patient may seem confused and repeatedly ask about present events. The ability to form new memories returns after a period of hours, and the individual returns to normal with no recall for the period of the attack. Frequently no cause is determined, but cerebrovascular disease, epilepsy (7% in one study), migraine, or cardiac arrhythmias have all been implicated. A Mayo Clinic review of 277 patients with TGA found a past history of migraine in 14% and cerebrovascular disease in 11%, but these conditions were not temporally related to the TGA episodes. Approximately one-quarter of the patients had recurrent attacks, but they were not at increased risk for subsequent stroke. Rare instances of permanent memory loss after sudden onset have been reported, usually representing ischemic infarction of the hippocampi or medial thalamic nuclei bilaterally.

The *ALS/parkinsonian/dementia complex of Guam* is a rare degenerative disease that has occurred in the Chamorro natives on the island of Guam. Individuals may have any combination of parkinsonian features, dementia, and motor neuron disease. The most characteristic pathologic features are the presence of NFTs in degenerating neurons

of the cortex and substantia nigra and loss of motor neurons in the spinal cord. Epidemiologic evidence supports a possible environmental cause, such as exposure to a neurotoxin with a long latency period. One interesting but unproven candidate neurotoxin occurs in the seed of the false palm tree, which Guamanians traditionally used to make flour. The ALS syndrome is decreasing in frequency in Guam, but a dementing illness with rigidity continues to be seen.

Rarely, adult-onset leukodystrophies, neuronal storage diseases, and other genetic disorders can present as dementia late in life. Metachromatic leukodystrophy can present as a dementia associated with large frontal white matter lesions. This syndrome is diagnosed by measuring arylsulfatase A enzyme activity in white blood cells. Adult presentations of adrenal leukodystrophy have been reported, and in these cases involvement of the spinal cord and posterior white matter is common. Adrenoleukodystrophy is diagnosed with measurement of plasma very long-chain fatty acids. CADASIL is another genetic syndrome associated with white matter disease, often frontally and temporally predominant. Diagnosis is made with biopsy of skin which shows osmophilic granules in arterioles; genetic testing for mutations in notch 3 is also possible (see above). The neuronal cerebrolipofuscinoses are a genetically heterogeneous group of disorders associated with myoclonus, seizures, and progressive dementia. Diagnosis is made by finding curvilinear inclusions within white blood cells or neuronal tissue.

Psychogenic amnesia for personally important memories is common, although whether this results from deliberate avoidance of unpleasant memories or from unconscious repression is currently unknown. The event-specific amnesia is more likely to occur after violent crimes such as homicide of a close relative or friend or sexual abuse. It may also develop in association with severe drug or alcohol intoxication and sometimes with schizophrenia. More prolonged psychogenic amnesia occurs in fugue states that also commonly follow severe emotional stress. The patient with a fugue state suffers from a sudden loss of personal identity and may be found wandering far from home. *In contrast to organic amnesia, fugue states are associated with amnesia for personal identity and events closely associated with the personal past.* At the same time, memory for other recent events and the ability to learn and use new information are preserved. The episodes usually last hours or days and occasionally weeks or months while the patient takes on a new identity. On recovery, there is a residual amnesia gap for the period of the fugue. Very rarely, selective loss of autobiographic information represents a focal injury in the brain areas involved with these functions.

Psychiatric diseases may mimic dementia. Severely depressed individuals may appear demented, a phenomenon called *pseudodementia*. Memory and language are usually intact when carefully tested in depressed persons, and a significant memory disturbance usually suggests an underlying dementia, even if the patient is depressed. The pseudodemented patient may feel confused and unable to accomplish routine tasks. Vegetative symptoms, such as insomnia, lack of energy, poor appetite, and concern with bowel function, are common. The onset is often abrupt, and the psychosocial milieu may suggest prominent reasons for depression. Such patients respond to treatment of the depression. Schizophrenia is usually not difficult to distinguish from dementia, but occasionally the distinction can be problematic. Schizophrenia generally has a much earlier age of onset (second and third decades) than most dementing illnesses, and is associated with intact memory. The delusions and hallucinations of schizophrenia are usually more complex and bizarre than those of dementia. Some chronic schizophrenics develop an unexplained progressive dementia late in life that is not related to AD. Conversely, FTD, HD, vascular dementia, DLB, AD, or leukoencephalopathy can begin with schizophrenia-like features, leading to the misdiagnosis of a psychiatric condition. The later age of onset, presence of significant deficits on cognitive testing, or the presence of abnormal neuroimaging findings point toward a degenerative condition. Memory loss may also be part of a conversion reaction. In this situation, patients commonly complain bitterly of memory loss, but careful cognitive testing either does not confirm the deficits or demonstrates inconsistent or unusual patterns of cognitive problems. The patient's behavior and "wrong" answers to questions often indicate that he or she understands the question and knows the correct answer.

Clouding of cognition by *chronic drug or medication use*, often prescribed by physicians, is an important cause of dementia. Sedatives, tranquilizers, and analgesics used to treat insomnia, pain, anxiety, or agitation may cause confusion, memory loss, and lethargy, especially in the elderly. Discontinuation of the offending medication often improves mentation.

R_x DEMENTIA

The major goals of management are to treat any correctable causes of the dementia and to provide comfort and support to the patient and caregivers. Treatment of underlying causes might include thyroid replacement for hypothyroidism; vitamin therapy for thiamine or B_{12} deficiency or for elevated serum homocysteine; antibiotics for opportunistic infections; ventricular shunting for NPH; and appropriate surgical, radiation, and/or chemotherapeutic treatment for CNS neoplasms. Removal of sedating or cognition-impairing drugs and medications is often beneficial. If the patient is depressed rather than demented (pseudodementia), the depression should be vigorously treated. Patients with degenerative diseases may also be depressed, and that portion of their condition may respond to antidepressant therapy. Antidepressants that are low in cognitive side effects, such as SSRIs (Chap. 386), are advisable when treatment is necessary. Anticonvulsants are used to control seizures.

Agitation, hallucinations, delusions, and confusion are difficult to treat. These behavioral problems represent major causes for nursing home placement and institutionalization. Before treating these behaviors with medications, a thorough search for potentially modifiable environmental or metabolic factors should be sought. Hunger, lack of exercise, toothache, constipation, urinary tract infection, or drug toxicity all represent easily correctable factors that can be treated without psychoactive drugs. Drugs such as phenothiazines and benzodiazepines may ameliorate the behavior problems but have untoward side effects such as sedation, rigidity, and dyskinesias. Despite their unfavorable side-effect profile, second-generation antipsychotics such as quetiapine (25 mg qd starting dose) are increasingly being used for patients with agitation, aggression, and psychosis. When patients do not respond to treatment, it is usually a mistake to advance to higher doses or to use anticholinergics or sedatives (such as barbiturates or benzodiazepines). It is important to recognize and treat depression; initial treatment can be with a low dose of an SSRI (e.g., escitalopram 10 mg/d) while monitoring for efficacy and toxicity. Sometimes apathy, visual hallucinations, depression, and other psychiatric symptoms respond to the cholinesterase inhibitors, obviating the need for other more toxic therapies.

Cholinesterase inhibitors are being used to treat AD, and other drugs, such as anti-inflammatory agents, are being investigated in the treatment or prevention of AD. Depression should be recognized and treated, initially with a low dose of an SSRI (Lexapro 10 mg), closely monitoring for efficacy and toxicity. These approaches are reviewed in the treatment section for AD, above.

A proactive strategy has been shown to reduce the occurrence of delirium in hospitalized patients. This strategy includes frequent orientation, cognitive activities, sleep-enhancement measures, vision and hearing aids, and correction of dehydration.

Nondrug behavior therapy has an important place in the management of dementia. The primary goal is to make the demented patient's life comfortable, uncomplicated, and safe. Preparing lists, schedules, calendars, and labels can be helpful. It is also useful to stress familiar routines, short-term tasks, walks, and simple physical exercises. For many demented patients, memory for facts is worse than that for routine activities, and they may still be able to take part in preserved physical activities such as walking, bowling, dancing, and golf. Demented patients usually object to losing control over familiar tasks such as driving, cooking, and handling finances. Attempts to help or take over may be greeted with complaints, depression, or anger. Hostile responses on the part of the caretaker are useless and sometimes harmful. Explanation, reassurance, distraction, and calm statements are more productive responses in this setting. Eventually, tasks such as finances and driving must be assumed by others, and the patient will conform and adjust. Safety is an important issue that includes not only driving but the environment of the kitchen, bathroom, and sleeping area. These areas need to be monitored, supervised, and made as safe as possible. A move to a retirement home, assisted-living center, or nursing home can initially increase confusion and agitation. Repeated reassurance, reorientation, and careful introduction to the new personnel will help to smooth the process. Provision of activities that are known to be enjoyable to the patient can be of considerable benefit. Attention should also be paid to frustration and depression in family members and caregivers. Caregiver guilt and burnout are common. Family members often feel overwhelmed and helpless and may vent their frustrations on the patient, each other, and health care providers. Caregivers should be encouraged to take advantage of day-care facilities and respite breaks. Education and counseling about dementia are important. Local and national support groups can be of considerable help, such as the Alzheimer's Association (*www.alz.org*).

FURTHER READINGS

KNOPMAN DS et al: Incidence and causes of nondegenerative nonvascular dementia: A population-based study. Arch Neurol 63:218, 2006

RAUSCHKA H: Late-onset metachromatic leukodystrophy: Genotype strongly influences phenotype. Neurology 67:859, 2006

ROBERSON ED, MUCKE L: 100 years and counting: Prospects for defeating Alzheimer's disease. Science 314:781, 2006

SEELEY WW et al: Early frontotemporal dementia targets neurons unique to apes and humans. Ann Neurol 60:660, 2006

SMALL GW et al: PET of brain amyloid and tau in mild cognitive impairment. N Engl J Med 355:2652, 2007

VAN OIJEN M et al: Atherosclerosis and risk for dementia. Ann Neurol 61:403, 2007

WILLIAMS DR et al: Characteristics of two distinct clinical phenotypes in pathologically proven progressive supranuclear palsy: Richardson's syndrome and PSP-parkinsonism. Brain 128:1247, 2005

ZUCCALA G et al: Correlate of cognitive impairment among patients with heart failure: Results of a multicenter survey. Am J Med 118:496, 2005

366 Parkinson's Disease and Other Extrapyramidal Movement Disorders

Mahlon R. DeLong, Jorge L. Juncos

PARKINSON'S DISEASE

Parkinson's disease (PD) is the most common form of a group of progressive neurodegenerative disorders characterized by the clinical features of parkinsonism, including bradykinesia (a paucity and slowness of movement), rest tremor, muscular rigidity, shuffling gait, and flexed posture. Although defined clinically as a movement disorder, it is now widely appreciated that PD can be accompanied by a variety of nonmotor symptoms, including autonomic, sensory, sleep, cognitive, and psychiatric disturbances. Nearly all forms of parkinsonism result from a reduction of dopaminergic transmission within the basal ganglia. The discovery of dopamine in the brain, the demonstration of its depletion in PD, and the success of dopamine replacement therapy by its precursor, levodopa, are all major landmarks in the field of neurology.

EPIDEMIOLOGY

PD afflicts ~1 million individuals in the United States (~1% of those over 55 years). Its peak age of onset is in the early 60s (range 35–85

TABLE 366-1 GENETICALLY BASED PARKINSON'S DISEASE

Locus	Gene	Protein	Function	Inheritance
PARK1	*SNCA*	α-Synuclein	Uncertain; ? vesicle trafficking	AD
PARK2	*PRKN*	Parkin	E3 ubiquitin ligase	AR
PARK4	*SNCA*	α-Synuclein (triplication or duplication)	Uncertain; ? vesicle trafficking	AD
PARK5	*UCH-L1*	UCH-L1 (Ubiquitin carboxy-terminal hydroxalase L1)	Proteosomal processing	AD
PARK6	*PINK1*	PINK1	Mitochondrial kinase	AR
PARK7	*DJ-1*	DJ-1	Oxidative stress response	AR
PARK8	*LRRK2*	Dardarin	Cytosolic kinase	AD

Note: See text for details. AD, autosomal dominant; AR, autosomal recessive.

years), and the course of the illness ranges between 10 and 25 years. PD accounts for ~75% of all cases of parkinsonism; the remaining cases result from other neurodegenerative disorders, cerebrovascular disease, and drugs. Familial forms of known autosomal dominant and recessive forms of PD (now numbering >10) comprise ~5% of cases (Table 366-1). These are generally characterized by an earlier age of onset (typically before age 45 years) and a longer course than cases of "sporadic" PD, although one genetic form, LLRK-2, causes PD in the same age range as sporadic PD. Although most patients with PD appear to have no strong genetic determinant, epidemiologic evidence points to a complex interaction between genetic vulnerability and environmental factors. Risk factors include a positive family history, male gender, head injury, exposure to pesticides, consumption of well water, and rural living. Factors associated with a reduced incidence of PD include coffee drinking, smoking, use of nonsteroidal anti-inflammatory drugs, and estrogen replacement in postmenopausal women.

CLINICAL FEATURES

A diagnosis of PD can be made with some confidence in patients who present with at least two of the three cardinal signs—rest tremor, rigidity, and bradykinesia. Tremor is particularly important, as it is present in 85% of patients with true PD; a diagnosis of PD is particularly difficult when tremor is absent. A unilateral and gradual onset of symptoms further supports the diagnosis. Masked facies, decreased eye blinking, stooped posture, and decreased arm swing complete the early picture. The onset may also be heralded by vague feelings of weakness, fatigue, aching, and discomfort.

MOTOR FEATURES

The most disabling motor feature of PD is bradykinesia, which interferes with all aspects of daily living including rising from a chair, walking, turning in bed, and dressing. Fine motor control is also impaired, as evidenced by decreased manual dexterity and micrographia. Soft speech (hypophonia) and sialorrhea are other troubling manifestations of (bulbar) bradykinesia. Rest tremor, at a frequency of 4–6 Hz, typically appears unilaterally, first distally, involving the digits and wrist, where it may have a "pill-rolling" character. Tremor usually spreads proximally and occasionally to the ipsilateral leg before appearing on the other side after a year or more. It may appear later in the lips, tongue, and jaw but spares the head and neck. Rigidity is felt as a uniform resistance to passive movement about a joint throughout the full range of motion, accompanied by a characteristic "plastic" quality to the movement. Brief, regular interruptions of resistance during passive movement, due to subclinical tremor, may give rise to a "cogwheeling" sensation. Dystonia involving the distal arm or leg may occur early in the disease, unrelated to treatment, especially in younger patients. It can also be provoked by antiparkinsonian drug therapy.

Gait disturbance with shuffling short steps and a tendency to turn en bloc is a prominent feature of PD. Festinating gait, a classic sign of parkinsonism, results from the combination of flexed posture and loss of postural reflexes, which cause the patient to accelerate in an effort to "catch up" with the body's center of gravity. Freezing of gait, a feature of more advanced PD, occurs commonly at the onset of locomotion (start hesitation), when attempting to change direction or turn around,

and upon entering a crowded room or narrow space such as a doorway.

Abnormalities of balance and posture tend to increase as the disease progresses. Flexion of the head, stooping and tilting of the upper trunk, and a tendency to hold the arm in a flexed posture while walking are common, as are changes in the posture of the fingers, hand, and arm. Postural instability is one of the most disabling features of advanced PD, contributing to falls and injuries and leading to major morbidity and mortality. It can be tested in the office with the "pull test" (Fig. 366-1). The development of postural instability and falls in the first years of the illness, however, strongly suggest a diagnosis of atypical PD. Patients are also at risk for hip fractures, which are associated with osteoporosis and vitamin D deficiency.

NON-MOTOR FEATURES

Non-motor aspects of PD include depression and anxiety, cognitive impairment, sleep disturbances, sensory abnormalities and pain, loss of smell (anosmia), and disturbances of autonomic function. Together these may contribute as much to the burden of the disease as the more obvious motor abnormalities. Some of these non-motor disturbances may be present long before the onset of motor signs. The physiologic basis of the non-motor signs and symptoms are explained in part by widespread involvement of brainstem, olfactory, thalamic, and cortical structures, as discussed below.

Sensory symptoms often manifest as a distressing sensation of inner restlessness presumed to be a form of akathisia. Aching pain and discomfort in the extremities can be a prominent presenting symptom or develop when antiparkinsonian medications are wearing off. Some patients may develop a subjective shortness of breath in the absence of any underlying cardiorespiratory pathology.

Sleep disorders and impaired daytime alertness are common in PD. Factors that disrupt sleep include nighttime reemergence of bradyki-

---

Testing for Postural Instability

I. Practice session

Explanation must be given that the patient will be pulled forcefully backward to test balance and that the patient must prevent himself or herself from falling, if necessary, by taking a step backward after he or she is pulled. At least one good practice session is carried out before the final test.

II. Patient stance

Patient must be upright and cannot lean forward in any way unless axial flexion prevents upright posture. Patient must not be pulled while off balance from a previous pull. Stance should be with feet comfortably apart.

III. Pull

Patient is pulled briskly and forcefully enough to trigger one step back.

IV. Examiner's response

Examiner is ready to catch the patient but allows enough space to move backward with the patient for at least three steps of recovery. The test is to be performed in a space long enough to differentiate between persistent but recovering retropulsion and no recovery.

FIGURE 366-1 Testing for postural instability. *(From: RP Munhox et al. Neurology 62:125, 2004; with permission.)*

nesia and rigidity, with difficulty turning in bed, as well as tremor and involuntary movements (e.g., myoclonic jerks or periodic leg movements). Restless legs and rapid eye movement behavioral disorder often precede the onset of motor signs of PD. Vivid dreams and hallucinations related to dopaminomimetic therapy may also contribute to sleep disruption. Finally, sleep apnea and other sleep disturbances can also occur. Correction of these sleep disorders may improve daytime functioning, but often alertness remains impaired, pointing to a separate disorder of arousal or to drug-induced sedation.

Autonomic dysfunction can produce diverse manifestations, including orthostatic hypotension, constipation, urinary urgency and frequency, excessive sweating, and seborrhea. Orthostatic hypotension is present in many patients resulting from impaired vasomotor reflexes, sympathetic denervation of the heart, or as a side effect of dopaminomimetic therapy. This rarely leads to syncope unless the patient has developed true autonomic failure or has an unrelated cardiac problem. Paroxysms of drenching sweats may occur in advanced PD, often related to the wearing off of antiparkinsonian medications.

NEUROPSYCHIATRIC SYMPTOMS

Changes in mood, cognition, and behavior are common accompaniments of PD, especially in its later stages, and may be the direct result of PD or its comorbid pathologies [e.g., Alzheimer's disease (AD), cortical dementia with Lewy bodies (DLB)] or may occur as a side effect of antiparkinsonian or concomitant therapy.

Depression affects approximately half of patients with PD and can occur at any phase of the illness. It is often difficult to diagnose due to the overlap between the somatic and vegetative symptoms of PD and depression. As a result, depression may go unrecognized and untreated. There is compelling evidence that depression in PD is an intrinsic part of the illness and not simply a reaction to disability. Recognizing even mild depression is particularly important since it can account for otherwise unexplained albeit reversible worsening of parkinsonian motor symptoms, new somatic symptoms, and sleep disruption. Depression can also be induced or aggravated iatrogenically by antiparkinsonian and psychotropic agents used to treat other symptoms. Finally, other causes for depressive symptoms and refractory depression should always be considered, including hypothyroidism, hypogonadism, and vitamin B_{12} deficiency.

Anxiety disorders in PD can appear in isolation or as an accompaniment of depression or progressive cognitive impairment. They can also be due to an akathisia equivalent provoked in part by undertreatment of motor symptoms. The development of drug-induced motor fluctuations can compound the problem by precipitating anxiety during the off periods that, in severe cases, may mimic panic attacks.

Mild or moderate cognitive abnormalities affect many patients with PD. These occur in the later stages of the illness and present as frontal lobe dysfunction. Difficulties with complex tasks, long-term planning, and memorizing or retrieving new information are common. Although some of these symptoms represent bradyphrenia (the cognitive equivalent of bradykinesia), it is now clear that the dysfunction also includes working memory, executive function, attention, mental flexibility, visuospatial function, and word fluency. In contrast, language and simple mathematical skills are relatively spared, unlike in patients with AD. Iatrogenic contributors to cognitive decline in vulnerable patients include the use of anticholinergics, amantadine, psychotropics, and even dopaminomimetic medications. Depression and intercurrent medical illnesses, especially infections (of the urinary tract or elsewhere) and dehydration, are important reversible causes of an acute change in cognitive function in PD.

The incidence of significant dementia in PD may be as high as six times that in age-matched controls and, in subspecialty clinics, can be as high as 70% or greater with long-term observation (≥ 8 years). In late stages the presence of substantial cognitive impairment may limit therapeutic options and contribute more to overall disability than the motor symptoms in PD. Predictors of dementia include late age of onset, akinetic-rigid phenotype, presence of severe depression, persistent hallucinations, and advanced stages of disease. In most instances, accumulating amyloid and α-synuclein pathologies in the frontal lobes,

basal forebrain, hippocampus, and amygdala account for the progression of these symptoms (see "Pathology," below).

Psychotic symptoms affect up to 40% of patients with PD, depending on the age, disease duration, and prevalence of dementia in the population surveyed. Early symptoms include visual illusions (e.g., shadows of the edge of the visual field) and formed visual hallucinations (usually people and animals), both with retained insight. Although depression and dementia are the most important risk factors for psychotic symptoms in PD, the symptoms are often triggered by drug therapy. Dopaminomimetics (especially dopamine agonists), anticholinergics, amantadine, and psychotropics are the chief drug offenders. Delusions are more disturbing than hallucinations because they place an even heavier burden on the family and caregivers. The prodrome to these psychotic symptoms includes sleep disturbances and subtle erratic behaviors with temperamental and sometimes unreasonable outbursts.

In recent years there has been increased recognition of insidious behavioral disturbances in a subset of patients with PD, referred to collectively as *impulse control disorders* (ICDs); these include pathologic gambling, hypersexuality, compulsive shopping, and compulsive eating and are associated primarily with the use of dopaminergic agents. A related disorder, termed *punding*, consists of stereotypical motor behavior in which there is an intense fascination with repetitive handling and examining of mechanical objects, such as picking at oneself, taking apart watches and radios, or sorting and arranging common objects. Current therapeutic approaches to these disorders include reduction or discontinuation of dopamine agonist therapy, psychosocial interventions, and in some cases consideration of deep brain stimulation with a goal of reducing the requirement for drugs.

PATHOLOGY

Gross examination of the brain in PD reveals mild frontal atrophy with loss of the normal dark melanin pigment of the midbrain. Microscopically there is degeneration of the dopaminergic cells with the presence of Lewy bodies (LBs) in the remaining neurons and processes of the substantia nigra pars compacta (SNpc); other brainstem nuclei; and regions such as the medial temporal, limbic, and frontal cortices. LBs have a high concentration of α-synuclein and are the pathologic hallmark of the disorder. Mutations in the α-synuclein gene can cause familial PD by promoting the formation of α-synuclein-positive filaments that aggregate into LBs and Lewy neurites (**Fig. 366-2**). It is now generally accepted that this pathology appears first in the anterior olfactory nuclei and lower brainstem (glosso-

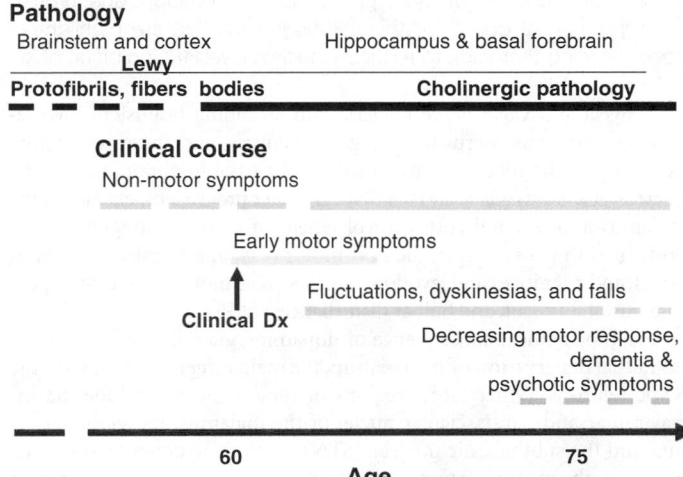

FIGURE 366-2 Proposed stages of Parkinson's disease (PD) based on extrapolations from pathologic, clinical and brain imaging studies. Broken black lines indicate that, by itself, Lewy (α-synuclein) protofibril or fiber pathology is not sufficient to make the pathologic diagnosis of PD. Broken blue lines represent non-motor signs that usually precede clinical recognition of PD, including impaired olfaction, sleep and mood disturbances, and constipation. Broken yellow lines indicate that fluctuations may be less apparent in the late stages of PD.

FIGURE 366-3 Pathogenesis of dopamine cell death in Parkinson's disease (PD) and possible sites for therapeutic intervention in PD. Studies on inherited forms of PD (see text) have led to the identification of genes that, when mutated, lead to dopaminergic cell loss. These genes are involved in cellular processes that include protein ubiquitination and degradation via the proteasomal system, response to oxidative stress, mitochondrial function, protein phosphorylation, and protein folding. Potential points for therapeutic intervention are highlighted: gene silencing therapies, to reduce synuclein levels (*i*); inhibition of sy- nuclein aggregation and/or processing (*ii*); interventions to down-regulate toxic substrates or up-regulate parkin or proteasomal function (*iii*); interventions to enhance mitochondrial function with factors such as CoQ_{10}, DJ-1, or PINK-1 (*iv*); free radical scavengers and antioxidants (*v*); kinase inhibitors to block LRRK2 activity or interventions to increase PINK-1 function (*vi*); and other therapies using tropic factors such as GDNF (see text), survival genes, or fetal/stem cell replacement that would protect or replace susceptible cells (*vii*). MPTP, 1-methyl-1,2,4,6 tetrahydropyridine. *(Reprinted from JM Savitt et al, with permission.)*

pharyngeal and vagal nerve nuclei), with ascending brainstem involvement of the locus coeruleus, n. gigantocellularis, and the raphe, before extending to the magnocellular nuclei of the basal forebrain, the central nucleus of the amygdala, and the SNpc. Further progression extends to the thalamus and cerebral cortex. Involvement of these extranigral areas is postulated to play a role in the non-motor (e.g., autonomic, sleep, emotional, and cognitive) and levodopa unresponsive motor aspects (e.g., postural instability, gait, and bulbar disturbances) of PD.

The biochemical consequence of dopaminergic cell loss in the SNpc is gradual denervation of the striatum, the main target projection for the SNpc neurons. Other target regions of these neurons include the intralaminar and parafascicular nuclei of the thalamus, the globus pallidus, and the subthalamic nucleus (STN). Dopamine denervation of the putamen, the motor portion of the striatum, leads to many of the motor symptoms of PD. Symptoms develop when striatal dopamine depletion reaches 50–70% of normal. Pharmacologic restoration of dopamine transmission is the basis for symptomatic drug treatment of PD.

GENETIC CONSIDERATIONS Although the vast majority of cases of PD appear to be sporadic, increasing evidence indicates that genetic factors play an important role in many forms of PD. Much of this evidence comes from studies of the concordance rates for PD among monozygotic and dizygotic twins. These studies suggest that heredity plays an important role in cases with age of onset <45 years and a less important role in older patients. Eight genes have been clearly linked to familial forms of PD (Table 366-1), and a number of other candidate genes or genetic loci have been identified as possibly causative of PD. Among the former, *PARK1*, *PARK4*, and *PARK5* lead to an autosomal dominant form of PD with atypical features such as early age of onset and rapid progression of symptoms. *PARK1* is due to a mutation in the gene for α-synuclein leading to abnormal aggregation of this protein (**Fig. 366-3**). *PARK2* and *PARK7* lead to autosomal recessive disorders also with atypical features, including juvenile forms of parkinsonism. *PARK2* encodes *parkin*, an E3 ubiquitin protein ligase. Mutations in parkin appear to be the major cause of autosomal recessive PD. Remarkably, *PARK5* codes for the ubiquitin carboxy-terminal hydroxylase L1 (UCH-L1), another component of the ubiquitin proteasomal system. Because ubiquitination of proteins targets them for degradation in the proteasome system, these findings suggest that abnormal proteasomal processing is important in the pathogenesis of at least some forms of PD. The most recently identified mutation is the gene for LRRK2. Most cases are slowly progressive and begin in late adulthood, closely resembling sporadic PD. The prevalence of causative LRRK2 mutations is highly dependent on the population under study, ranging from 1 to 2% of all PD cases, except in isolated pockets where the prevalence can be higher. Although the mechanism of action of the LRRK2 mutation is not certain, evidence suggests that abnormal kinase activity may mediate dopamine cell death;

a similar mechanism may be operative in *PARK6*, resulting from mutations in *PINK1* (Fig. 366-3). Other mutations with yet-to-be-identified genes include *PARK10*, a late-onset PD susceptibility gene. The identification of these and other mutations are proving invaluable in refining the correlation between genotypes and phenotypes, in generating animal models to study pathogenesis, and in identifying target pathways for possible therapeutic intervention.

PATHOGENESIS

In PD, nigral dopamine neurons and other cells die from a combination of factors, including: (1) genetic vulnerability (e.g., abnormal processing or folding of α-synuclein; Fig. 366-3, steps i, ii); (2) oxidative stress (steps iv, v); (3) proteasomal dysfunction (step iii); (4) abnormal kinase activity (step vi); and (5) environmental factors, most of which have yet to be identified.

Oxidative stress appears to play an important role in the sporadic forms of PD. Endogenous sources of oxidative stress include the free radicals produced by the metabolism of dopamine and melanin. Additional stress may come from defects in mitochondrial complex I of the oxidative phosphorylation chain. This defect has been detected in platelets and muscle and in postmortem tissue from the substantia nigra. Several agents have been shown to cause oxidative toxicity and dopamine cell death in animal models of PD, further strengthening the above hypothesis. The most important of these are MPTP, a meperidine derivative, and rotenone, a commonly used insecticide. Both cause oxidative damage by inhibiting complex I. In vitro, oxidative stress can lead to aggregation of α-synuclein and proteasomal dysfunction. Proteasomal system abnormalities have also been described in the substantia nigra from sporadic cases of PD. Other contributors to the selective dopamine neuron degeneration in PD are abnormal phosphorylation of proteins, microglial activation, low-grade inflammation, and apoptosis; each represents a potential target for therapeutic intervention.

DIFFERENTIAL DIAGNOSIS AND SCREENING EVALUATION

Primary and secondary causes must be considered in the differential diagnosis of parkinsonism (Table 366-2). Essential tremor (ET) is sometimes confused with rest tremor in PD, but the absence of other signs of parkinsonism, the bilaterality, higher frequency (8–10 Hz), and postural dependency of ET help differentiate this from the rest tremor of PD (Chap. 367). In individuals under 40, it is important to rule out Wilson disease (Chap. 354). In younger individuals, Huntington's disease (HD) sometimes presents with prominent parkinsonian features (Chap. 367). Although parkinsonian features are often present in AD, they occur late in the course and are greatly outweighed by cognitive and behavioral disturbances (Chap. 365). In DLB the parkinsonian features are compounded by the early appearance of hallucinations and disturbances in arousal and behavior (Chap. 365). Parkinsonism may also develop following exposure to certain neurotoxins such as carbon monoxide or manganese. MRI is useful in selected cases to rule out disorders such as normal pressure hydrocephalus, vascular disease, or mass lesions. Positron emission tomography (PET) is helpful in confirming the diagnosis but cannot reliably separate PD from the most common atypical forms. As yet, genetic screening has little place in general practice.

In evaluating individuals with PD, it is also important to rule out treatable conditions that may contribute to the disability, such as B₁₂ deficiency, hypothyroidism, testosterone deficiency, and vitamin D deficiency.

At present the frequency of misdiagnosis is still 10–25% even in the best of hands. The differentiation of sporadic (idiopathic) PD from atypical parkinsonism (see below) is often difficult, since early in their course these atypical forms may meet diagnostic criteria for PD (Table 366-3). Accordingly, it is important to watch for the development of early imbalance, falls, and characteristic abnormalities of vertical gaze that suggest progressive supranuclear palsy (PSP); and early urinary incontinence, orthostatic hypotension, and dysarthria suggestive of multiple system atrophy (MSA). The early appearance of drug-induced hallucinations strongly favors the diagnosis of DLB. As a rule, the different forms of atypical PD can be reliably differentiated from sporadic PD within the first 3–4 years of the illness.

TABLE 366-2 DIFFERENTIAL DIAGNOSIS OF PARKINSONISM

Primary Parkinsonism

Genetically based PD (see Table 366-1)
Idiopathic ("sporadic") PD (most common form)
  Phenotype may be influenced by "vulnerability" genes and environmental factors
Other neurodegenerative disorders
  Disorders associated with α-synuclein pathology
    Multiple system atrophies (glial and neuronal inclusions)
      Striatonigral degeneration
      Olivopontocerebellar atrophy
      Shy-Drager syndrome
      Motor neuron disease with PD features
    Dementia with Lewy bodies (cortical and brainstem neuronal inclusions)
  Disorders associated with primary tau pathology ("tauopathies")
    Progressive supranuclear palsy
    Corticobasal degeneration
    Frontotemporal dementia
  Disorders associated with primary amyloid pathology ("amyloidopathies")
    Alzheimer's disease with parkinsonism
Genetically mediated disorders with occasional parkinsonian features
  Wilson's disease
  Hallervorden-Spatz disease
  Chédiak-Hagashi syndrome
  SCA-3 spinocerebellar ataxia
  X-linked dystonia-parkinsonism (DYT3)
  Fragile X premutation associated ataxia-tremor-parkinsonism syndrome
  Huntington's disease (Westphalt variant)
  Prion disease
Miscellaneous acquired conditions
  Vascular parkinsonism
  Normal pressure hydrocephalus
  Catatonia
  Cerebral palsy

Secondary Parkinsonism

Repeated head trauma ("Dementia pugilistica" with parkinsonian features)
Infectious and postinfectious diseases
  Postencephalitic PD
  Neurosyphilis
Metabolic conditions
  Hypoparathyroidism or pseudohypoparathyroidism with basal ganglia calcifications
  Non-Wilsonian hepatolenticular degeneration
Drugs
  Neuroleptics (typical antipsychotics)
  Selected atypical antipsychotics (see text)
  Antiemetics (e.g., compazine, metoclopramide)
  Dopamine-depleting agents (reserpine, tetrabenazine)
  α-Methyldopa
  Lithium carbonate
  Valproic acid
  Fluoxetine
Toxins
  1-Methyl-1,2,4,6 tetrahydropyridine (MPTP)
  Manganese
  Cyanide
  Methanol
  Carbon monoxide
  Carbon disulfide
  Hexane

℞ PARKINSON'S DISEASE

GENERAL CONSIDERATIONS The goals of therapy in PD are to maintain function and quality of life and to avoid drug-induced complications. Bradykinesia, tremor, rigidity, and abnormal posture respond well to symptomatic therapy early in the course of the illness. In contrast, cognitive symptoms, hypophonia, autonomic dysfunction, and imbalance tend to respond poorly. Primary motor disability in PD is often aggravated by secondary disability resulting from physical deconditioning following a sedentary lifestyle. Prevention of secondary disability requires a consistent program of physical exercise. Multiple open-label studies of exercise in PD support the importance of regular activity; one controlled epidemiologic study revealed a hazard ratio of observed/expected deaths during the 4-

TABLE 366-3 HISTORY AND EXAMINATION FEATURES SUGGESTING DIAGNOSES OTHER THAN PARKINSON'S DISEASE

Symptoms/Signs	Alternative Diagnosis to Consider
History	
Falls as the first symptom	PSP
Exposure to neuroleptics	Drug-induced parkinsonism
Onset prior to age 40	If PD, think genetic causes
Associated unexplained liver disease	Wilson's disease
Early hallucinations	Lewy body dementia
Sudden onset of parkinsonian symptoms	Vascular parkinsonism
Physical Exam	
Dementia as first symptom	Dementia with Lewy bodies
Prominent orthostasis	MSA-p
Early dysarthria	MSA-c
Lack of tremor	Various Parkinson's-plus syndromes
High frequency (8–10 Hz) symmetric tremor	Essential tremor

year observation period of 1.8 in patients who did not exercise compared to those who did. Remaining mentally active is probably equally important for preservation of cognition in general.

As a general principle, patients should be treated as soon as symptoms begin to interfere with function in any way. Most specialists now have a low threshold for initiating symptomatic therapy. The concern that symptomatic therapy should be delayed as long as possible since the available compounds are effective for only a limited number of years is unfounded. Early initiation of therapy is often necessary to maintain an adequate level of physical and mental activity. Another common concern, that dyskinesias will develop sooner if levodopa is introduced "too early," is also unfounded. Recent studies (see below) have shown that the risk of "troublesome dyskinesias" in patients receiving levodopa therapy (up to 300 mg/d) appears to be considerably lower than previously reported.

A current priority is to move beyond symptom control to neuroprotective therapies. Unfortunately, no such therapy is yet available. High doses of coenzyme Q_{10}, oral creatine supplementation, intrastriatal infusion (or delivery via viral vectors) of neurotrophic factors, and possibly the use of newer monoamine oxidase B (MAO-B) inhibitors may hold promise in this regard and are under investigation. In animal models of PD, forced exercise (e.g., treadmill running) at moderate intensities appears to promote neuroprotection in dopamine neurons.

INITIATION OF THERAPY (**Fig. 366-4**) From a practical standpoint, dopaminomimetic therapy (**Table 366-4**) should be initiated as soon as the patient's symptoms begin to interfere with quality of life. The ideal first-line agent depends on the age and cognitive status of the patient and, to a lesser extent, the patient's clinical type and finances. The choices consist of either a dopamine agonist, a levodopa preparation, or one of the MAO-B inhibitors. Controlled studies support the view that, in early PD, monotherapy with any of the dopamine agonists is well tolerated and significantly improves motor function and disability. Using this approach, patients experience ~50% lower risk of dyskinesias and 25% lower risk of motor fluctuations compared to levodopa-treated patients. This difference lasts as long as the patient remains on monotherapy. Once a levodopa preparation is added, dyskinesias and motor fluctuations begin to emerge, suggesting that dopamine agonists delay the onset but do not prevent the development of these problems. In fact, about two-thirds of patients on agonist monotherapy require levodopa therapy by year 5 in order to maintain motor function.

Motor fluctuations, also known as "on-off" phenomena, are the exaggerated ebb and flow of parkinsonian signs experienced by many patients between doses of antiparkinsonian medications. *Dyskinesias* refer to choreiform and dystonic movements that can occur as a peak dose effect or at the beginning or end of the dose (diphasic dyskinesias). More than 50% of patients with PD treated over 5 years with levodopa will develop these complications.

Successful dopamine agonist monotherapy requires a higher dose of the agonist than is typically needed when the agonist is used to supplement levodopa (Table 366-4). In both cases, titration has to be slow and cautious to avoid unneces-

sary side effects. Patients benefit greatly from education and support during this titration. Most patients will require the addition of levodopa or another agent within 1–3 years of initiating dopamine agonist monotherapy. Preclinical studies suggest that the advantages of dopamine agonist monotherapy can be maintained with agonist-dominant therapy. In this case, dopamine agonists continue to provide the bulk of dopaminomimetic therapy, with levodopa playing a supplementary role.

Although dopamine agonist monotherapy is considered the initial treatment of choice for most patients with PD, the long-term benefits noted above must be balanced against a higher incidence of non-motor side effects and a slightly higher level of motor disability than with levodopa. These recommendations may need to be modified in patients with psychotic symptoms, behavioral disturbances, or severe daytime sleep disturbances. Older patients and those with akinetic rigid forms of PD have a lower risk of motor complications and dyskinesias compared to the average PD patient and may be satisfactorily treated with levodopa.

PHARMACOTHERAPY OF MOTOR SYMPTOMS The above practices in the initiation of therapy notwithstanding, levodopa remains the most effective treatment for PD. It significantly improves motor symptoms and increases quality of life and independence. The aim of all dopaminomimetic strategies is to restore dopamine transmission in the striatum. This is accomplished by stimulating postsynaptic receptors (directly with dopamine agonists), increasing dopamine precursor availability (levodopa), blocking the metabolism of levodopa in the periphery and in the brain, and blocking the catabolism of dopamine at the synapse.

Dopamine Agonists Dopamine agonists readily cross the blood-brain barrier and act directly on postsynaptic dopamine receptors (primarily D_2 type). Compared to levodopa, they are longer-acting and thus provide a more uniform stimulation of dopamine receptors. They are effective as monotherapeutic agents and as adjuncts to carbidopa/levodopa therapy. They can also be used in combination with anticholinergics and amantadine. Table 366-4 provides a guide to the doses and uses of these agents.

Available agents for PD include three non-ergot alkaloids—pramipexole, ropinirole, and, more recently, rotigotine—plus the ergot alkaloids bromocriptine, cabergoline, and lisuride (the latter two only in Europe). Pergolide is a dopamine agonist recently removed from the U.S. market

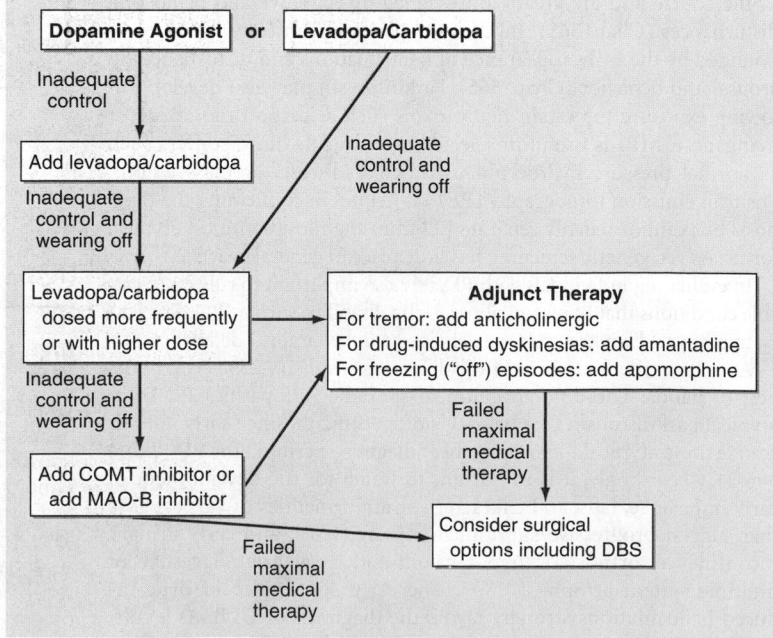

FIGURE 366-4 Treatment approaches to newly diagnosed idiopathic PD.

TABLE 366-4 LEVODOPA FORMULATIONS AND DOPAMINE AGONISTS USED IN PARKINSON'S DISEASE

Agents	LD Dose Equivalency	Available Strengths (mg)	Initial Dosing	Comments
Carbidopa/Levodopa (Typical Initial Strength)				
Carbidopa/levodopa IR 25/100	100 mg (levodopa anchor dose)	10/100 25/100 25/250	25/100; 0.5–1 tab tid	Usual range = 300–800 mg/d with typical schedules being q8h to q3h.
Carbidopa/levodopa CR 50/200	150 mg	25/100 50/200	50/200; 1 tab bid to tid	Increased bioavailability with food. Splitting the tablet negates the CR properties. Usual schedule is q8h to q4h.
Carbidopa/levodopa/entacapone 25/100/200	120 mg	12.5/50/200 25/100/200 37.5/150/200	25/100/200; 1 tab bid to tid	Do not split tablets. May combine with Sinemet IR. Usual schedule is q8h to q4h.
Parcopa 25/100	100 mg	25/100 25/250	25/100; 1 tab tid	Can be used as regular or supplemental rescue doses in cases of regular dose failure. Orally dissolved without water.

Dopamine Agonists				Approximate Target Doses		
	DA Equivalent to Above LD Anchor Dose	Available Strengths (mg)	Initial Dosing	Monotherapy	As Adjuncts to LD	Other Considerations
Non-ergot alkaloids						
Pramipexole	1 mg	0.125, 0.25, 1, 1.5	0.125 mg tid	1.5–4.5 mg/d	0.375–3.0 mg/d	Renal metabolism; dose adjustments needed in renal insufficiency. Occasionally associated with "sleep attacks."
Ropinirole	5 mg	0.25, 0.5, 1, 2, 3, 4, 5	0.25 mg tid	12–24 mg/d	6–16 mg/d	Hepatic metabolism; potential drug-drug interactions. Occasionally associated with "sleep attacks."
Ropinirole extended release	Availability pending.					
Rotigotine		2, 4, 6	2 mg/24 h	6 mg/d	2–6 mg/d	Available as transdermal patch.
Ergot alkaloids						
Bromocriptine	2 mg	2.5, 5.0	1.25 mg bid to tid	7.5–15 mg/d	3.75–7.5 mg/d	Rare reports of pulmonary and retroperitoneal fibrosis. Relative incidence of sleep attacks not well studied.
Pergolide	Removed from U.S. market in 2007. See text.					
Cabergoline	Used in select cases of PD in Europe. Not approved for the treatment of PD in the U.S.					

Note: Equivalency doses are approximations based on clinical experience, may not be accurate in individual patients, and are not intended to correlate with the in vitro binding affinities of these compounds.

Abbreviations: DA, dopamine agonist; IR, immediate release; CR, controlled release; LD, levodopa (with carbidopa).
Carbidopa/levodopa/entacapone = Stalevo.

due to its association with asymptomatic valvular heart disease in 28% of patients treated chronically. The incidence of symptomatic valvular disease is far lower, perhaps as low as <1%. Nonetheless, patients currently on pergolide need to be transferred to alternative therapy, perhaps equivalent doses of non-ergot dopamine agonists (Table 366-4). The dose equivalency of pergolide is ~1:1 with pramipexole.

Subcutaneous injectable apomorphine is approved in the United States as a "rescue therapy" for dose failure (usually due to erratic gastric emptying), motor fluctuations, and especially for the debilitating "off" spells that affect many patients with moderate to advanced disease. Finally, sumanirole is another potent experimental dopamine agonist that in a recent controlled study proved to be comparable in efficacy to ropinirole and better tolerated.

A long-acting formulation of ropinirole and a transdermal patch delivery system of rotigotine will soon be approved for use in PD. Based on pharmacokinetic data, these formulations can achieve levels of continuous dopaminergic stimulation that are closer to those achieved with subcutaneous infusions of apomorphine (not available in the United States). Compared with oral dopaminomimetics, infusion therapy has proved superior at controlling motor fluctuations and reducing dyskinesias over time. The convenience of these new formulations should overcome the major limitation of infusions: cost and site reactions. Experience with the patch delivery system thus far indicates that it is safe and well tolerated except for occasional skin reactions to the adhesive.

Dopamine agonists have been approved for the treatment of PD at every stage of disease and in combination with other antiparkinsonian agents;

however, the use of two dopamine agonists simultaneously cannot be recommended. Agonists are particularly effective in treating bradykinesia, loss of fine motor dexterity, tremor, and gait disturbances. When used as monotherapy, they are less effective than levodopa-based formulations. Accordingly, it is imperative to titrate the dose as needed to control motor function; the maximum dose provided in titration packs may be insufficient in some patients. As the dose is escalated it is equally important to remain vigilant to potential dose-dependent side effects, particularly when combining these drugs with carbidopa/levodopa and psychotropics.

Side effects of dopamine agonists include nausea, postural hypotension, psychiatric symptoms, daytime sedation, and occasional sleep attacks. These can be managed by decreasing the dose; by decreasing concomitant medication with similar side effects; or, in the case of nausea, by the introduction of peripheral dopamine blockers such as domperidone (not available in the United States) or a short course of trimethobenzamide or dronabinol until the patient develops tolerance to these symptoms. Patients should be cautioned about the potential for sleep attacks associated with dopamine agonists (and to a lesser extent with carbidopa/levodopa). These can occur without warning and have resulted in traffic accidents. When used as adjuncts to levodopa therapy, dopamine agonists can aggravate dyskinesias if the doses of carbidopa/levodopa are not adjusted accordingly. Furthermore, dopamine agonists are more expensive than carbidopa/levodopa, which is now available in generic form. Dopamine agonist–induced impulse control disorders (pathologic gambling, etc.) are discussed above under "Neuropsychiatric Symptoms."

Carbidopa/Levodopa Formulations Carbidopa/levodopa is available in regular, immediate release (IR) formulations (Sinemet, Atamet, and others; 10/100 mg, 25/100 mg, and 25/250 mg), controlled release (CR) formulations (Sinemet CR 25/100 mg, 50/200 mg), or more recently as Stalevo (Table 366-4). The latter combines variable doses of IR-carbidopa/levodopa (12.5/50, 25/100, 37.5/150) with 200 mg of entacapone (see below). In most individuals, at least 75 mg/d of carbidopa is necessary to block the peripheral decarboxylation of levodopa to dopamine, and to limit the symptoms of nausea and orthostasis associated with initiation of therapy. Initial target doses of these medications are summarized in Table 366-4. Individualized dosing and gradual dose escalation is recommended. Initiation of dosing at mealtimes will reduce the incidence and severity of nausea. As patients develop tolerance to nausea and other side effects, these medications can be administered on an empty stomach, which generally leads to a more brisk and predictable absorption.

Etilevodopa, the ethyl-ester pro-drug of levodopa, has greater solubility than levodopa in the stomach and a more rapid transit time to the duodenum, where it is quickly absorbed after being hydrolyzed to levodopa. In spite of these pharmacokinetic advantages, in a controlled study oral administration of etilevodopa (with carbidopa) proved no different from oral carbidopa/levodopa with respect to mean dose requirements, treatment failures, and hours of daily "off" time.

Levodopa Augmentation Strategies A number of drugs can augment dopamine transmission by blocking the breakdown of dopamine at the level of the synapse.

MAO-B Inhibitors These are selective and irreversible inhibitors of the catabolic breakdown of dopamine; they work by inhibiting MAO-B at the synapse. These compounds offer a modest symptomatic motor benefit when used as monotherapy and enhance the efficacy of carbidopa/levodopa formulations when used as adjuncts. Their potential additional role as neuroprotective agents remains unproven. Unlike patients taking unselective or MAO-A inhibitors who are subject to hypertensive crises from consumption of large doses of tyramine (the amino acid precursor of norepinephrine), patients taking MAO-B inhibitors do not require dietary tyramine restrictions. At the approved doses, rasagiline and oral zydis selegiline (i.e., orally disintegrating) carry little risk of a hypertensive complication.

Selegiline, a selective MAO-B inhibitor, was approved in 1989 for the treatment of PD. As monotherapy, it has a small symptomatic effect. As an adjunct to levodopa therapy, it increases "on" time while reducing motor fluctuations; the dose is 5 mg with breakfast and lunch. A significant side effect of selegiline is insomnia, probably due to an amphetamine-like metabolite.

In 2006, two additional, more potent MAO-B inhibitors with once-daily dosing were introduced for the treatment of PD. Rasagiline was approved for use as initial monotherapy and as adjunctive therapy. It is metabolized to an aminoindan metabolite that lacks the amphetamine-like properties of selegiline. As monotherapy in treatment-naïve patients it improves motor function compared to placebo, and as an adjunct it increases daily "on" time by about 1.8 h. The usual dose is 0.5–1 mg/d.

Zydis selegiline is an orally disintegrating, freeze-dried tablet that is absorbed through the oral mucosa; this results in higher levels of selegiline and lower levels of the plasma amphetamine-like metabolites compared with the usual oral route. Its usual dose is 1.25–2.5 mg/d in the morning. In a 2004 controlled study, Zydis selegiline in patients with PD and motor fluctuations increased dyskinesias-free "on" time by 1–1.5 h/d compared to placebo.

Although these compounds are generally well tolerated, side effects include dose-dependent nausea, dyspepsia, dizziness, insomnia, dyskinesias, orthostatic hypotension, confusion, and hallucinations. They should not be used with meperidine, tramadol, methadone, or propoxyphene. Rarely, a hyperserotonergic syndrome may result from use in combination with tricyclic antidepressants (TCAs) and selective serotonin reuptake inhibitors (SSRIs). This syndrome is characterized by anxiety, tremulousness, myoclonus, and alterations in mental status. Although the risk of this complication in PD appears to be small at the approved doses, it is judicious to remain vigilant to these possible side effects until more Phase IV safety information is available. In the interim, the lower dose of these compounds should be considered in older individuals with active cardiac disease, or in those who are prescribed concomitant antidepressant drugs.

COMT Inhibitors The catechol-*O*-methyltransferase (COMT) inhibitors entacapone and tolcapone offer yet another strategy to augment the effects of levodopa by blocking the enzymatic degradation of levodopa and dopamine. Entacapone is preferred to tolcapone because of the low but potentially serious incidence of hepatic and hematologic side effects of the latter. When used in conjunction with carbidopa/levodopa, these agents increase the plasma levodopa levels by >30% and alleviate wearing-off symptoms. Entacaprone (200 mg with each dose of carbidopa/levodopa) increases "on" time by <1 h/d, while tolcapone (100–200 mg tid) increases "on" time by about 1.8 h/d.

The more common side effects are gastrointestinal and hyperdopaminergic, including sleep disturbances and increased dyskinesias that may require reductions in the dose of carbidopa/levodopa. Hyperdopaminergic symptoms can be managed with appropriate decreases in the dose of other dopaminomimetics. Tolcapone can be associated with a dose-dependent increase in hepatic aminotransferase levels in 1–3% of cases and rare instances of acute fulminant liver failure. ALT/AST levels should be monitored every 2–4 weeks for the first 6 months and periodically thereafter. Tolcapone should not be used in patients with preexisting liver disease and should be discontinued if the ALT/AST levels exceed two times the upper limit of normal.

Other Well-Established Agents Anticholinergics and amantadine are appropriate adjuncts to dopaminomimetic therapy. Anticholinergics are particularly useful for controlling rest tremor and dystonia, and amantadine can reduce drug-induced dyskinesias by up to 70%. The mechanisms of action of amantadine are unknown, although there is evidence it has both anticholinergic and dopaminomimetic properties. Recently amantadine has been shown to have weak glutamate antagonist properties, a mechanism thought responsible for reducing drug-induced dyskinesias. The side effects of amantadine are nausea, headaches, edema, erythema, and livedo reticularis. In older patients, it may aggravate confusion and psychosis. Doses need to be decreased in patients with renal insufficiency.

THERAPY OF NON-MOTOR SYMPTOMS Patients with frequent nighttime awakenings due to nocturnal akinesia or tremor can be treated with supplemental doses of carbidopa/levodopa at night. A bedtime dose of a dopamine agonist helps restless leg symptoms and urinary urgency. Treatment of bladder symptoms will improve sleep in many elderly patients with PD. Depression typically responds to antidepressants (either TCAs or SSRIs). As discussed earlier, the combination of SSRIs and selegiline carries an exceedingly low risk of a hyperserotonergic syndrome (delirium with myoclonus and hyperpyrexia). Electroconvulsive therapy (ECT) is highly effective in drug-refractory cases or in patients intolerant of oral antidepressants. There are several reports indicating that ECT also has short-term benefit for parkinsonian motor symptoms.

In patients with psychotic symptoms or confusion, anticholinergics and amantadine should be eliminated first. Following this, MAO-B inhibitors and dopamine agonists should be reduced or discontinued as needed to control symptoms. This should be followed by gradual reductions as needed in nocturnal and then daytime doses of Sinemet CR, and finally carbidopa/levodopa. If the patient improves after only a modest reduction of antiparkinsonian therapy, the overall impact on the parkinsonian motor symptoms may be negligible. If in the process parkinsonian symptoms worsen, most specialists initiate treatment with an atypical antipsychotic that has a low incidence of extrapyramidal side effects rather than continuing to lower dopaminomimetic therapy. Clozapine (12.5–100 mg/d) is the best established agent for treatment of psychotic symptoms in PD. Quetiapine (12.5–100 mg) is sometimes used first because it lacks the small risk of agranulocytosis associated with clozapine. Both are dosed at night to promote sleep and minimize daytime sedation and orthostasis. Their use and that of all antipsychotics in PD are limited by dose-dependent sedation, orthostatic hypotension, dizziness, and confusion. Other atypical antipsychotics such as risperidone, olanzapine, and, more recently, aripiprazole are not well tolerated by most patients with PD due to a higher incidence of drug-induced parkinsonism (DIP) and akathisia.

Centrally acting acetylcholinesterase inhibitors can improve dementia symptoms in PD, providing the same stabilization of cognitive decline noted in AD. Rivastigmine is approved by the Food and Drug Administration for the treatment of dementia in PD, and donepezil also appears to be effective. Both appear to be well tolerated by most patients with PD and may also be useful for treatment of psychotic symptoms such as hallucinations and delusions.

Given the complexity of the above polypharmacy, the management of non-motor symptoms is best carried out in an interdisciplinary setting, coordinated by a neurologist who specializes in PD together with a psychiatrist and the patient's primary care physician.

NEUROPROTECTIVE THERAPY Slowing the progression of PD through neuroprotective or restorative therapy is a major focus of research. Epidemiologic studies suggest that the chronic use of nonsteroidal anti-inflammatory agents or the use of estrogen replacement in postmenopausal women may delay or prevent the onset of PD through yet-unclear mechanisms. Similarly, in large populations, the long-term use of nicotine and caffeine has been associated with a lower risk of PD.

From a pharmacologic standpoint, current strategies involve interrupting the cascade of biochemical events that leads to death of dopaminergic cells (Fig. 366-3). The first such clinical trial in PD was the large multicenter DATATOP study in which selegiline monotherapy delayed the need for levodopa therapy by 9–12 months in newly diagnosed patients. Most evidence indicates that this delay was due to a mild symptomatic effect of selegiline. The antioxidant vitamin E had no effect. Long-term follow-up of the DATATOP cohort revealed that patients who remained on selegiline for 7 years experienced slower motor decline compared to those who were changed to placebo after 5 years. The 7-year patient group was more likely to develop dyskinesias but less likely to develop freezing gait.

Coenzyme Q_{10}, an antioxidant and a cofactor of complex I of the mitochondrial oxidative chain, has been shown to have neuroprotective effects against multiple toxic agents in vitro and in animal models of PD. In a large controlled phase 2 trial, a dose of 1200 mg/d appeared to delay progression of disability in untreated patients with PD. Coenzyme Q_{10} was well tolerated and devoid of toxicity. A phase 3 trial will examine the disease-modifying effect of this compound in untreated patients receiving up to 2400 mg/d. Other potential neuroprotective agents under investigation are creatine monohydrate and acetyl-levo-carnitine. A phase 2 trial of creatine in early PD demonstrated promising results, and a phase 3 trial is now under way.

Dopamine agonists are also under investigation as putative agents to slow disease progression in PD, based on their possible antioxidant properties resulting in part from their in vitro ability to decrease dopamine turnover, scavenge free radicals, and interfere with proapoptotic cell signaling. Other promising agents include nitric oxide synthetase inhibitors and antiapoptotic agents such as Jun N-terminal kinase inhibitors and desmethylselegiline. The latter, a metabolite of selegiline, has been shown experimentally to have neuroprotective effects on dopamine neurons, possibly through modulation of cellular antiapoptotic mechanisms, including Bcl-2, glyceraldehyde-3-phosphate dehydrogenase (GAPDH); activation of the proteasome-ubiquitin complex; and the prevention of caspase 3 activation. Clinical trials to test the putative new effects of dopamine agonists are now under way.

SURGICAL TREATMENTS Over the past decade there has been a renaissance in the surgical treatment of PD and other movement disorders. Although both pallidotomy and thalamotomy were performed widely in the 1950s, the introduction of levodopa in the 1960s led to the virtual abandonment of surgery. The resurgence in the use of surgery has been motivated by the fact that after 5 or more years of treatment, many patients develop significant drug-induced motor fluctuations and dyskinesias. Advances in understanding the functional organization of the basal ganglia and the pathophysiologic basis of parkinsonism have provided a clearer rationale for the effectiveness of these procedures and guidance for targeting specific structures **(Fig. 366-5)**. The most common indications for surgery in PD are intractable tremor and drug-induced motor fluctuations or dyskinesias. The best candidates are patients with clear levodopa-responsive parkinsonism who are free of significant dementia or psychiatric comorbidities. In general, patients with atypical parkinsonism or dementia benefit little, or not at all. Currently the subthalamic nucleus is the preferred target, but controlled clinical trials comparing the pallidal and subthalamic targets are nearing completion. Deep brain stimulation (DBS) is most often performed bilaterally and simultaneously, but unilateral DBS can be highly effective for asymmetric cases. DBS in

these areas alleviates parkinsonian motor signs, particularly during "off" periods, and reduces troublesome dyskinesias, dystonia, and motor fluctuations that result from drug administration. Both procedures have been shown to strongly improve the patient's quality of life, and both are more effective than medical management in the target population of patients with advanced PD. Signs and symptoms not responding to levodopa, such as postural instability and falling, hypophonia, micrographia, drooling, and autonomic dysfunction, are unlikely to benefit from surgery. As a rule of thumb, the benefits from surgery are unlikely to exceed the best results from antiparkinsonian medications but provide relief from motor fluctuations, dyskinesias, and dystonia. In general, the decision for surgery should be made by a movement-disorder neurologist who is part of a team, including the neurosurgeon, neuropsychologist, and programmer.

The mechanism of action of DBS remains controversial. Since clinically it appears that ablation and stimulation of a given target have a similar effect, it has been assumed that stimulation causes a functional blockade. It is likely, however, that multiple factors are involved. The basis for improvement appears to be the replacement of abnormal neural activity by a more tolerable pattern of activity. Whatever the mechanism, it is clear that these approaches can offer impressive and enduring results in properly selected patients.

Neurotransplantation and Other Surgical Approaches Despite highly encouraging open-label pilot studies of fetal cell transplantation, this approach has produced considerable disappointment with the recent publication of the results from two large, well-controlled clinical trials. The first, using sham surgery, showed only modest benefit in patients under 60 and no benefit in those over 60. An unexpected complication in a number of patients was the development of symptomatic dyskinesias, occurring off medication. The second study has shown similar findings with regard to benefit and the development of dyskinesias. A puzzling feature of these studies is the apparent successful grafting observed by PET and at autopsy. Because of these disappointing results, the considerable obstacles to obtaining sufficient fetal tissue, and opposition to the use of fetal tissue on ethical grounds, this approach is now viewed as purely investigational. It is hoped that these issues can be addressed with the development of other strategies to enhance dopaminergic cell function (e.g., carotid body cells;

FIGURE 366-5 Schematic diagram of the basal ganglia–thalamocortical circuitry under normal conditions (A) and in Parkinson's disease (PD) (B). Inhibitory connections are shown as black arrows and excitatory connections as red arrows. Note that in PD, striatal dopamine denervation results in increased traffic in the indirect pathway and decreased traffic in the direct pathway. The downstream consequence of this is increased activity in striatal outflow stemming from the increased activity of STN and ultimately GPi/SNr neurons. Because striatal outflow is inhibitory to the thalamus (main neurotransmitter = γ-aminobutyric acid), there is a decrease in the ability of the thalamus to activate the frontal cortex leading to signs of parkinsonism. As discussed, changes in discharge pattern are also a major factor. D, direct pathway; I, indirect pathway; GPe, external segment of the globus pallidus; GPi, internal segment of the globus pallidus; SNr, substantia nigra, pars reticulata; SNc, substantia nigra, pars compacta; STN, subthalamic nucleus; VA/VL, ventral anterior/ventrolateral thalamus; CM, centromedian nucleus; PPN, pedunculopontine nucleus. *(Courtesy of T Wichmann, MD, Emory University School of Medicine; with permission.)*

stem cells; encapsulated and genetically engineered cells capable of producing levodopa, dopamine, and/or trophic factors). One approach uses genetically engineered retinal epithelial cells in gelatin capsules to ensure their survival following implantation, typically into the putamen. The cells produce levodopa, which then diffuses into the cerebral microenvironment, providing dopamine reinnervation to surrounding tissue. A controlled clinical trial is under way to examine the potential benefit of this approach in PD following positive results in a small open-label study.

The favorable response from direct infusion of glial cell–derived neurotrophic factor (GDNF) to the putamen in two small open-label trials in patients with PD raised hopes that this approach may offer neuroprotection. However, a well-controlled trial using bilateral GDNF infusion to the putamen failed to demonstrate significant improvement. There is currently a moratorium on further trials with GDNF due to the development of GDNF-neutralizing antibodies in four patients and to a toxicologic study revealing cerebellar degeneration in an exposed primate. However, trials are currently under way using alternative vehicles for these and other neurotrophins with actions similar to GDNF. These vehicles include recombinant adeno-associated virus, lentivirus, and pseudorabies virus. Stem cell transplantation in PD will need to await successful application of this technology in other areas of medicine.

DEMENTIA IN PARKINSON'S DISEASE

The incidence of dementia in PD may be as high as six times that in the general non-PD population. Approximately a quarter of patients will develop dementia of the Alzheimer type due to overlap of these two age-related pathologies. Pathologically, the incidence of AD-type findings in postmortem tissue from patients dying with PD is as high as 40%. Conversely, 25% of AD patients have at least mild clinical parkinsonian features such as rigidity and bradykinesia, and ≥ 60% have coexistent -synuclein pathology in the cortex. Patients with PD dementia (PDD) are more likely to have the akinetic/rigid PD phenotype rather than the tremor-predominant phenotype. In this population the presence of dementia makes management of the motor symptoms of PD more difficult due to the high incidence of cognitive side effects from antiparkinsonian therapy, particularly anticholinergics and amantadine. Central dopaminomimetic toxicity can present in many ways, ranging from sleep disruption with daytime sleepiness, personality changes, depression, and executive dysfunction (e.g., organization, planning, multitasking) to episodic confusion, hallucinations, and disruptive behaviors.

DLB is an increasingly recognized form of dementia with prominent parkinsonian features. The dementia may precede or follow the parkinsonian syndrome. In patients presenting with parkinsonian features, the dementia is often heralded by levodopa-induced sedation, myoclonus, and hallucinations. Early on, the phenotype can be indistinguishable from PD. Features that help differentiate this entity from PD include the presence of an action rather than a rest tremor; a rapidly fading response to levodopa; and rapidly fluctuating, spontaneous, and drug-induced problems with arousal. Another feature of DLB is the higher incidence of neuropsychiatric symptoms than in idiopathic PD. These symptoms include apathy, personality changes, depression, fixed delusions, and hallucinations. Finally, patients with DLB exhibit a heightened sensitivity to DIP when exposed to any dopamine blocker. The progression of symptoms in DLB is intermediate between the PD and PD/AD overlap. **DLB is discussed in detail in Chap. 365.**

OTHER PARKINSONIAN DISORDERS

PARKINSONIAN DISORDERS ASSOCIATED WITH ABNORMAL METABOLISM OF α-SYNUCLEIN (α-SYNUCLEINOPATHIES)

Multiple System Atrophy MSA comprises a group of sporadic disorders characterized by varying degrees of parkinsonism and cerebellar, corticospinal, and autonomic dysfunction. The average age of onset is 50 years (earlier than in PD) and the median survival 6–9 years. The clinical presentation is highly varied and may begin with any of the above clinical manifestations. The unifying pathologic hallmark is the presence of α-synuclein-positive inclusions located in various brain regions.

CLINICAL PHENOTYPES With disease progression, 90% of patients exhibit parkinsonian signs and 80% signs of autonomic failure; a similarly high percentage exhibit upper motor neuron signs. Tremor is common, but unlike in PD, this and other parkinsonian signs are more likely to present symmetrically. Parkinsonian symptoms are typically poorly responsive to dopaminergic therapy, although some patients may respond favorably for years. Drug-induced dyskinesias typically involve the face and neck rather than the trunk and limbs, as is the case in PD. Corticospinal signs consist of spasticity, involving the legs more than the arms, and pseudobulbar palsy. This aspect of the illness may mimic primary lateral sclerosis with lower motor neurons being occasionally involved. A few patients develop myoclonus.

Signs of autonomic failure include orthostatic hypotension, leg swelling not due to drug therapy, changes in sweating patterns, and autonomic storms with diaphoresis and flushing. Orthostatic hypotension can present with dizziness, faintness, or syncope. Once patients are successfully treated for syncope, they often develop fatigue and lassitude. This is due in part to chronic tissue hypoperfusion caused by marginal blood pressures while sitting or standing. More aggressive management of the blood pressure is warranted but not always successful. Urinary symptoms include urgency, retention, and incontinence. In men, impotence is one of the earliest and most prominent signs. The autonomic dysfunction can precede or follow the development of other neurologic signs by several years. Dementia may not be as frequent as in PD.

The clinical phenotype of MSA can fall into one of two broad categories, termed *MSA-p* (prominent parkinsonism at onset) and *MSA-c* (prominent cerebellar involvement at onset). Disorders that have now been reclassified as part of this new naming scheme include *striatonigral degeneration* (SND), *olivopontocerebellar atrophy* (OPCA), and *progressive autonomic failure* (PAF), either without parkinsonism or with parkinsonism (Shy-Drager syndrome). Patients presenting with a relatively pure form of akinetic rigid parkinsonism and a limited response to levodopa are designated as having MSA-p. Distinguishing these conditions from PD and each other can be difficult, particularly in the early stages of illness. Individuals with other signs such as ataxia, upper motor neuron and corticobulbar involvement, myoclonus, oculomotor abnormalities, peripheral neuropathy, and deafness fit into the category of MSA-c. This phenotype is notably heterogeneous, with both sporadic and hereditary forms. The sporadic forms tend to form part of the spectrum discussed in this section, while the hereditary forms usually represent one of the spinocerebellar ataxias (Chap. 368). Although MSA categories are clinically useful, as disease progresses there tends to be more clinical and pathologic overlap than separation between the different entities.

The spectrum of disease in MSA is determined by the location and density of the LB pathology. For instance, the LBs are confined to neurons in the brainstem in PD and to the brainstem, cortex, and hippocampus in DLB. In MSA these deposits take the form of glial α-synuclein-positive intracytoplasmic inclusions in the substantia nigra, putamen, inferior olives, pontine nuclei, pigmented nuclei of the brainstem, intermediolateral nucleus of the spinal cord, and the cerebellum. In addition, in MSA there is myelin degeneration and oligodendroglia containing argyrophilic glial cytoplasmic inclusions that are immunoreactive for ubiquitin and α-synuclein. Similar inclusions can be found in neuronal cell bodies and processes.

Several diagnostic tests help differentiate MSA from PD and other parkinsonian syndromes. In MSA-c, brain MRI reveals prominent atrophy of the cerebellum, pons, and olivary eminence of the medulla. In MSA-p, prominent volume loss and T2-weighted image hyperintensity in the putamen, globus pallidus, and white matter may be present. Electrodiagnostic studies may reveal rectal sphincter abnormalities with signs of degeneration with reinnervation due to anterior horn cell loss. Commercially available genetic tests are available for many of the spinocerebellar ataxias (Chap. 368) that present with features that overlap OPCA.

Rx # PARKINSONIAN DISORDERS OF α-SYNUCLEIN ABNORMAL METABOLISM

Early in the course of the illness, parkinsonian features may respond to dopaminomimetic agents. These have to be used with caution due to their tendency to provoke orthostatic hypotension. **Treatment of orthostatic hypotension and other autonomic symptoms is discussed in Chap. 370.**

PARKINSONIAN DISORDERS ASSOCIATED WITH ABNORMALITIES OF TAU METABOLISM (TAUOPATHIES)

As in the synucleopathies, the discovery of a group of familial and sporadic disorders with pathology involving the microtubule-associated protein tau has helped classify a group of disorders characterized by atypical parkinsonism and dementia. In the familial forms of these disorders, mutations in the *tau* gene have been linked to rare forms of parkinsonism and to frontotemporal dementia (Chap. 365). The two entities discussed below typically present as movement disorders. The first, progressive supranuclear palsy (PSP), has not been linked to mutations in the *tau* gene but is associated with overrepresentation of the H1 tau gene haplotype. These and other findings support the view that abnormal processing of tau may be directly linked to the pathogenesis of sporadic and familial tauopathies.

Progressive Supranuclear Palsy This is a sporadic neurodegenerative disorder of unknown etiology associated with tau pathology. It presents in the sixth to seventh decades and progresses more rapidly than PD, with death in 5–10 years. Risk factors include head trauma, vascular disease, dietary exposure to benzyl-tetrahydroisoquinolines (TIQ, reticuline), and beta-carbolines (reports from the West Indies).

PSP is characterized by akinetic rigid parkinsonism, dizziness, unsteadiness, slowness, falls, and pseudobulbar dysarthria. Tremor is distinctly uncommon. Supranuclear eye movement abnormalities affecting downgaze occur first, followed by variable limitations of upward and horizontal eye movement. Because the vestibular ocular reflex ("doll's eyes" maneuver) and the Bell's reflex (elevation and abduction of eyes on attempted lid closure) are intact, these abnormalities are termed *supranuclear*. Neurologic examination often reveals prominent stare and furrowed brow, axial (especially nuchal) and proximal limb rigidity and dystonia, as well as upper motor neuron and occasional cerebellar signs. Virtually all patients develop frontal-type cognitive dysfunction (Chap. 365), and a significant number may develop dementia with distinct subcortical features (e.g., abulia, mental inflexibility, and defects in memory retrieval). Brain MRI reveals midbrain atrophy (superior colliculus), and PET studies show symmetric frontal and striatal hypometabolism. The diagnosis is made on clinical grounds. Although some response may occur to levodopa and other antiparkinson medications, especially early in the course, treatment is generally not highly effective.

Pathologically, PSP is characterized by deposition of neurofibrillary tangles histochemically positive for tau (mostly 4-repeat tau) and negative for amyloid or α-synuclein. The deposits are associated with varying degrees of degeneration in the brainstem, basal ganglia, and cerebellum. There is loss of dopamine and dopamine receptors due to intrinsic striatal damage. This is thought to account for the poor response to therapy.

Corticobasal Degeneration (CBD) CBD, another sporadic tauopathy, is less common but has a broader range of clinical presentations than PSP. As with most atypical forms of parkinsonism, it begins insidiously in the sixth to seventh decades with varying degrees of asymmetric progressive apraxia, rigidity, dystonia, bradykinesia, and myoclonic jerks, with or without cortical sensory loss. The "alien limb" phenomenon, consisting of involuntary purposeful movements of a hand or limb, is a characteristic sign. The disorder progresses to become bilat-

eral over 2–5 years, leading to total incapacity with, ultimately, paraplegia in flexion. A significant number of cases present with frontotemporal dementia or progressive aphasia, followed by asymmetric cortical sensory signs, including abnormalities of graphesthesia and astereognosis (Chap. 365). Brain MRI reveals focal cortical loss in the contralateral superior frontal and parietal lobes with corresponding hypometabolic changes on PET scan as well as hyperintense signal abnormalities in white matter and sometimes atrophy of the corpus callosum. Treatment is largely ineffective.

Grossly, CBD is a focal cortical degenerative process with asymmetric pathology and volume loss in the parietal and frontal regions. Most of the damage is in the dorsal peri-Rolandic, superior frontal, and superior parietal cortices, whereas cases with aphasia show abnormalities in the peri-Sylvian regions. Histologically, gliosis and swollen (ballooned) achromatic neurons and neuronal loss are present in these cortical regions as well as in the nigra, caudate, putamen, and thalamus. Recent clinicopathologic evidence indicates that the syndrome can occur in the absence of basal ganglia or nigral degeneration.

SECONDARY PARKINSONISM

Drug-Induced Parkinsonism DIP typically presents bilaterally with bradykinesia or tremor. Asymmetry is far less prominent than in PD. It is commonly due to neuroleptics, some atypical antipsychotics, lithium carbonate, or antiemetic agents (especially metoclopramide). Less common causes include valproic acid and fluoxetine. DIP can also be induced by the chronic administration of antihypertensive agents such as reserpine and α-methyldopa. Exposure to manganese, carbon monoxide or disulfides, cyanide, and methanol can also lead to a parkinsonian state. The severity of the parkinsonian symptoms usually correlates with the dose or exposure to a medication or toxin. If due to medication, the symptoms tend to disappear within days to weeks after stopping the offending agent but may be permanent. Patients with permanent symptoms may have been in the process of developing parkinsonism. DIP may respond to anticholinergic agents, amantadine, and levodopa.

Vascular Parkinsonism The concept of vascular or atherosclerotic parkinsonism remains a topic of controversy. Generally, patients with vascular parkinsonism exhibit an akinetic-rigid syndrome with short mincing steps without tremor. Most have neurologic signs distinguishable from those associated with PD, including upper motor neuron signs, pseudobulbar palsy, or dementia. A poor response to levodopa therapy is characteristic. Imaging studies are heterogeneous and may reveal basal ganglia lacunes or multiple infarcts. The hypertensive and diabetic microangiopathy and diffuse white matter disease (Chap. 364) typically present with patchy, confluent, or diffuse white matter in the centrum semiovale. Other causes of microangiopathy can also rarely be responsible. The premortem diagnosis of these disorders is difficult to make with certainty, given the absence of disease markers.

FURTHER READINGS

DEUSCHL G et al: A randomized trial of deep-brain stimulation for Parkinson's disease. N Engl J Med 355:896, 2006

FACTOR S, WEINER W (eds): *Parkinson's Disease: Diagnosis and Clinical Management*, 2d ed. New York, Demos Medical Publishing, 2007

HARDY J et al: Genetics of Parkinson's disease and parkinsonism. Ann Neurol 60:389, 2006

LIPPA CF et al: DLB and PDD boundary issues: Diagnosis, treatment, molecular pathology, and biomarkers. Neurology 68:812, 2007

SAVITT JM et al: Diagnosis and management of Parkinson's disease: Molecules to medicine. J Clin Invest 116:1744, 2006

SCHADE R et al: Dopamine agonists and the risk of cardiac-valve regurgitation. N Engl J Med 356:29, 2007

TARNOPOLSKY MA, BEAL MF: Potential for creatine and other therapies targeting cellular energy dysfunction in neurologic disorders. Ann Neurol 49:561, 2001

WILLIAMS-GRAY CH et al: Evolution of cognitive dysfunction in an incident Parkinson's disease cohort. Brain 130:1787, 2007

367 Hyperkinetic Movement Disorders

C. Warren Olanow

HYPERKINETIC DISORDERS

Hyperkinetic movement disorders are characterized by the presence of a variety of different involuntary movements (Table 367-1). The major hyperkinetic movement disorders and the diseases with which they are associated are considered in this chapter.

ESSENTIAL TREMOR

Clinical Features Essential tremor (ET) is the most common involuntary movement disorder, affecting ~5–10 million individuals in the United States alone. It is a progressive disorder which can present in childhood but dramatically increases in prevalence over the age of 70. ET is characterized by a high-frequency tremor (up to 11Hz) that predominantly affects the upper extremities. The tremor is most prominent when trying to maintain a posture (postural tremor) or perform an action such as touching the finger to an object (kinetic tremor). It is typically bilateral and symmetric, but one side can be predominantly affected. Tremor may also affect the head (horizontal or vertical), and speech may be tremulous. The tremor characteristically improves with alcohol and may worsen with stress. Occasionally, subtle impairment of coordination or tandem walking may be present, but the neurologic examination is otherwise normal. ET can be differentiated from Parkinson's disease (PD) by the absence of resting tremor, bradykinesia, rigidity, micrographia, and other parkinsonian features. Tremor can also be observed with a variety of drugs, multiple sclerosis, degenerative disorders, and metabolic alterations.

Etiology and Pathophysiology The specific etiology and pathophysiology of ET are not known. Approximately 50% of cases have a positive family history with an autosomal dominant pattern of inheritance. Linkage studies have detected loci at chromosome 3q13 (*ETM-1*) and 2p22-25 (*ETM-2*), and it is likely that there are many other undiscovered loci. The cerebellum and inferior olives have been implicated as possible sites of a "tremor pacemaker" based on the presence of cerebellar signs in some patients and findings of increased metabolic activity and blood flow in these regions.

℞ ESSENTIAL TREMOR

Many cases are mild and require no treatment other than reassurance. Occasionally, tremor can be severe and interfere with eating, writing, and activities of daily living. Primidone (25–1000 mg/d) and propranolol (20–80 mg/d) are the standard drug therapies and can be administered alone or in combination. Primidone frequently causes sedation and should be started at low doses (12.5 mg) and gradually titrated to an effective dose. Propranolol and other beta blockers are contraindicated in patients with cardiac arrhythmias or asthma. Benefits with these drugs are attained in ~50% of patients but may not be sustained. Alprazolam, gabapentin, topiramate, clonazepam, clozapine, and nimodipine have been reported to improve tremor in some patients. Botulinum toxin injections may be helpful for limb or voice tremor, but treatment can be associated with muscle weakness. Surgical therapies targeting the VIM nucleus of the thalamus can be very effective in severe and drug-resistant cases.

DYSTONIA

Clinical Features Dystonia consists of sustained or repetitive involuntary muscle contractions, frequently causing twisting movements with abnormal postures. Dystonia can range from minor contractions in an individual muscle group to severe and disabling involvement of multiple muscle groups. The frequency is estimated at 300,000 cases in the United States but is likely greater since many cases are not recognized. Dystonia is often initially brought out by voluntary movements (action dystonia) and can later become sustained and extend to other body regions. It can be aggravated by stress and fatigue and attenuated by relaxation and sensory tricks such as touching the affected body part. Dystonia can be classified based on age of onset (childhood vs. adult), distribution (focal, multifocal, segmental, or generalized), or etiology (primary or secondary).

Primary Dystonias Idiopathic torsion dystonia (ITD), or Oppenheim's dystonia, is predominantly a childhood-onset form of dystonia with an autosomal dominant pattern of inheritance that primarily affects Ashkenazi Jewish families. The majority of patients have an age of onset younger than 26 years (mean 14 years). In young-onset patients, dystonia typically begins in a foot or arm and can progress to involve the other limbs as well as the head and neck. In severe cases, patients can suffer disabling postural deformities. Severity can vary even within a family, with some affected relatives having mild dystonia that may not even have been appreciated. Several gene mutations are associated with ITD. Most cases are linked to a mutation in the *DYT1* gene located on chromosome 9q34, which results in a trinucleotide GAG deletion with loss of one of a pair of glutamic acid residues in the protein torsin A. *DYT1* mutations are found in 90% of Ashkenazi Jewish patients with ITD and are probably related to a founder effect that occurred about 350 years ago. There is variable penetrance, with only about 30% of *DYT1* gene carriers expressing a clinical phenotype. The function of torsin A is not known, but it is a member of the AAA$^+$ (ATPase) family of proteins that resemble heat shock proteins and may thus be related to protein regulation. Indeed, postmortem studies have shown protein aggregates and inclusions in the region of the pedunculopontine nucleus (PPN). Transgenic mice that carry the DYT1 dystonia mutation express a hyperkinetic and dystonic phenotype and a similar pathology to human DYT1.

Dopa responsive dystonia (DRD) or the Segawa variant (DYT5) is a dominantly inherited form of childhood-onset dystonia due to a mutation in the gene that encodes for guanosine triphosphate (GTP) cyclohydrolase I, the rate-limiting enzyme for the synthesis of tetrahydrobiopterin. This mutation leads to a defect in the biochemical synthesis of tyrosine hydroxylase and dopamine. DRD typically presents in early childhood (1–12 years) and is characterized by foot dystonia that interferes with walking. Patients often experience diurnal fluctuations, with worsening of gait as the day progresses and improvement with sleep. DRD is typified by an excellent and sustained response to small doses of levodopa. Some patients may present with parkinsonian features but can be differentiated from juvenile PD by normal striatal fluorodopa uptake on positron emission tomography and the absence of levodopa-induced dyskinesias. DRD patients may occasionally present with spasticity, increased reflexes, and Babinski responses and be misdiagnosed as cerebral palsy. A mutation has also been identified in the epsilon-sarcoglycan gene on chromosome 7q21. These patients typically suffer from myoclonic dystonia frequently accompanied by psychiatric disturbances.

TABLE 367-1	HYPERKINETIC MOVEMENT DISORDERS
Disorders	**Movement Characteristics**
Athetosis	Slow, distal, writhing, involuntary movements with a propensity to affect the arms and hands.
Chorea	Rapid, semipurposeful, graceful, dancelike, nonpatterned involuntary movements involving distal or proximal muscle groups.
Dystonia	Involuntary patterned sustained or repeated muscle contractions, often leading to twisting movements and abnormal posture.
Myoclonus	Sudden, brief (<100 ms), shocklike, arrhythmic muscle twitches.
Tics	Brief, repeated, stereotyped muscle contractions that are often suppressible. Can be simple and involve a single muscle group or complex and affect a range of motor activities.
Tremor	Rhythmic oscillation of a body part due to intermittent muscle contractions.

Focal Dystonias These are the most common forms of dystonia. They typically present in the fourth to sixth decades and affect women more than men. The major types are:

1. *Blepharospasm*: dystonic contractions of the eyelids with increased blinking that can interfere with reading, watching TV, and driving.
2. *Oromandibular dystonia* (OMD): contractions of muscles of the lower face, lips, tongue, and jaw (opening or closing). Meige's syndrome is a combination of OMD and blepharospasm that predominantly affects women over the age of 60 years.
3. *Spasmodic dysphonia*: dystonic contractions of the vocal cords during phonation, causing impaired speech. Most cases affect the adductor muscles and cause speech to have a choking or strained quality. Less commonly, the abductors are affected, leading to speech with a breathy or whispering quality.
4. *Cervical dystonia*: dystonic contractions of neck muscles, causing the head to deviate to one side (*torticollis*), in a forward direction (*anterocollis*), or in a backward direction (*retrocollis*). Muscle contractions can be painful and associated with dystonic tremor and a secondary cervical radiculopathy.
5. *Limb dystonias*: these can be present in either arms or legs and are often brought out by task-specific activities such as handwriting (writer's cramp), playing a musical instrument (musician's cramp), or putting in golf (the yips).

Focal dystonias can extend to involve other body regions (~30% of cases) and are frequently misdiagnosed as psychiatric or orthopedic problems. Their cause is not known, but genetic factors, autoimmunity, and repeated trauma have been implicated.

Secondary Dystonias These occur as a consequence of drugs or other neurologic problems. Drug-induced dystonia is most commonly seen with neuroleptic drugs or after chronic levodopa treatment in PD patients (see below). Secondary dystonia can also be observed following discrete lesions in the striatum, pallidum, thalamus, cortex, and brainstem due to infarction, anoxia, trauma, tumor, infection, toxins such as manganese, or carbon monoxide. In these cases, dystonia often assumes a segmental distribution. More rarely, dystonia can develop following peripheral nerve injury.

Dystonia-Plus Syndromes Dystonia may occur as a part of neurodegenerative conditions such as Huntington's disease (HD), PD, Wilson's disease, corticobasal degeneration, progressive supranuclear palsy, the Lubag form of dystonia-parkinsonism (DYT3), and mitochondrial encephalopathies. In contrast to the primary dystonias, dystonia is usually not the dominant neurologic feature in these conditions.

Pathophysiology of Dystonia The pathophysiologic basis of dystonia is not known. The phenomenon is characterized by cocontracting bursts in agonist and antagonist muscle groups. This is associated with a loss of inhibition at multiple levels of the nervous system as well as increased cortical excitability and reorganization. Attention has focused on the basal ganglia as the site of origin of at least some types of dystonia as there are alterations in blood flow and metabolism in basal ganglia structures. Further, ablation or stimulation of the globus pallidus can both induce and ameliorate dystonia. The dopamine system has also been implicated in the pathogenesis of dystonia, as dopaminergic therapies can both induce and treat some forms of dystonia. Recent studies have demonstrated pathologic changes in the PPN, and electrical stimulation in this region induces dystonic muscle contractures, suggesting that the PPN might also be involved.

℞ DYSTONIA

Treatment is symptomatic for the most part, except in rare cases where treatment of a primary underlying condition is available. Wilson's disease should be ruled out in young patients with dystonia as well as in any young patient with a movement disorder. Levodopa should be tried in all cases of childhood-onset dystonia. High-dose anticholinergics (e.g., trihex-

yphenidyl 20–120 mg/d) may be beneficial in children but are less helpful in adults who can rarely tolerate such high doses because of cognitive impairment with hallucinations. Oral baclofen (25–120 mg) may be helpful, but benefits are usually modest, and side effects of sedation, weakness, and memory loss can be problematic. Intrathecal infusion of baclofen is more likely to be helpful, particularly with leg and trunk dystonia, but benefits are frequently not sustained and complications can be serious, including infection, seizures, and coma. Tetrabenazine (12.5–200 mg/d) may be helpful, but the drug is not readily available in the United States. Neuroleptics typically are not recommended because of the risk of extrapyramidal side effects. Clonazepam and diazepam are rarely effective. In general, dystonic patients are not satisfactorily controlled with drug therapies, particularly if they have a generalized dystonia.

On the other hand, botulinum toxin can be of great benefit for patients with focal dystonia, particularly if involvement is limited to small muscle groups such as in blepharospasm, torticollis, and spasmodic dysphonia. Botulinum toxin acts by blocking the release of acetylcholine at the neuromuscular junction, leading to muscle weakness and reduced dystonia. Two serotypes of botulinum toxin are available (A and B). Both are effective, and it is not clear if there are advantages of one over the other. No systemic side effects are encountered with the doses typically employed, but benefits are transient and repeat injections are required at 2- to 5-month intervals. Some patients fail to respond after having experienced an initial benefit. This has been attributed to induction of antibodies, but improper muscle selection, injection technique, and inadequate dose should be excluded.

Surgical therapy is an alternative for patients with severe dystonia who are not responsive to other treatments. Peripheral procedures such as rhizotomy and myotomy were used in the past to treat cervical dystonia but have been rarely employed since the introduction of botulinum toxin therapy. Bilateral deep brain stimulation (DBS) of the pallidum can provide dramatic benefits for patients with primary (DYT1) dystonia. This represents a major therapeutic advance as previously there was no consistently effective therapy for these patients. Patients with secondary dystonia are less likely to benefit from DBS. The value of DBS in patients with focal dystonia is currently being explored. Supportive treatments such as physical therapy and education are important and should be a part of the treatment regimen for all dystonia patients.

Physicians should be aware of dystonic storm, a potentially fatal condition that typically occurs in response to a stress situation such as surgery in patients with a preexisting history of dystonia. It consists of the acute onset of generalized and persistent dystonic contractions that can involve the vocal cords or laryngeal muscles, leading to airway obstruction. Patients may experience rhabdomyolysis with renal failure. Patients should be managed in an ICU and treated with one or a combination of anticholinergics, diphenhydramine, baclofen, benzodiazepines, or dopamine blockers. Spasms may be difficult to control, and anesthesia with muscle paralysis may be required.

CHOREAS

Huntington's Disease HD is a progressive, fatal, autosomal dominant disorder characterized by motor, behavioral, and cognitive dysfunction. The disease is named for George Huntington, a family physician who described cases on Long Island, New York, in the nineteenth century. Onset is typically between the ages of 25 and 45 years (range 3–70 years) with a prevalence of two to eight cases per 100,000. HD is characterized by rapid, nonpatterned, semipurposeful, involuntary choreiform movements. In the early stages the chorea tends to be focal or segmental, but it progresses over time to involve multiple body regions. Dysarthria, gait disturbance, and oculomotor abnormalities are common features. With advancing disease, there is a reduction in the chorea and emergence of dystonia, rigidity, bradykinesia, myoclonus, and spasticity. In younger patients (about 10% of cases), HD can present as an akinetic-rigid or parkinsonian syndrome (Westphall variant). HD patients eventually develop behavioral and cognitive disturbances which can be a major source of disability. Depression with suicidal tendencies, aggressive behavior, and psychosis can be prominent, and the majority of patients develop dementia. A clinical diagnosis of HD can be strongly suspected in cases of chorea with a positive family history. Neuropathologically, the disease predominant-

A

B

FIGURE 367-1 Huntington's disease. A. Coronal FLAIR MRI shows enlargement of the lateral ventricles reflecting typical caudate atrophy (*arrows*). **B.** Axial FLAIR image demonstrates abnormal high signal in the caudate and putamen (*arrows*).

ly strikes the striatum. Atrophy of the caudate nuclei, which form the lateral margins of the lateral ventricles, can be visualized on neuroimaging studies in the middle and late stages of the disease (Fig. 367-1). More diffuse cortical atrophy can be seen late in the disease. Genetic testing can be used to confirm the diagnosis and to detect affected individuals in the family, but this should be performed with caution and in conjunction with trained counselors, as positive results can lead to depressive and suicidal reactions.

ETIOLOGY HD is caused by an increase in the number of polyglutamine (CAG) repeats (>40) in the coding sequence of the Huntington gene located on the short arm of chromosome 4. The larger the number of repeats, the earlier the disease is manifest. Anticipation occurs, particularly in males, with subsequent generations having larger numbers of repeats and earlier age of disease onset. The gene encodes the highly conserved cytoplasmic protein huntingtin, which is widely distributed in neurons throughout the CNS, but whose function is not known. Models of HD with striatal pathology can be induced by excitotoxic agents such as kianic acid and 3-nitroproprionic acid, which promote calcium entry into the cell and cytotoxicity. Mitochondrial dysfunction has been observed in HD and has been theorized to promote "weak excitotoxicity" by reducing ATP formation necessary for maintaining the voltage-dependent magnesium blockade of calcium channels. Recent evidence indicates that fragments of the mutant huntingtin protein can be toxic, possibly by translocating into the nucleus and interfering with transcriptional regulatory proteins. Intraneuronal inclusions containing aggregates of ubiquitin and the mutant protein huntingtin are found in nuclei of neurons in the striatum and cerebral cortex. Neuronal inclusions found in affected regions in HD may represent a protective mechanism aimed at segregating and facilitating the clearance of these toxic proteins.

℞ HUNTINGTON'S DISEASE

Treatment involves a multidisciplinary approach with medical, neuropsychiatric, social, and genetic counseling for patients and their families. Dopamine-blocking agents may control the chorea but are generally not recommended because of their side-effect profile and potential to aggravate motor symptoms, and because the chorea tends to be self-limited and is usually not disabling. Depression and anxiety can be greater problems, and patients should be treated with appropriate antidepressant and anti-anxiety drugs and monitored for mania and suicidal ideations. Psychosis can be treated with atypical neuroleptics such as clozapine (50–600 mg/d), quetiapine (50–600 mg/d), and risperidone (2–8 mg/d). There is no ade-

quate treatment for the cognitive or motor decline. A neuroprotective therapy that slows or stops disease progression is the major unmet medical need in HD. Antiglutamate agents, bioenergetics, caspase inhibitors, inhibitors of protein aggregation, intracerebral delivery of neurotrophic factors, and transplantation of fetal striatal cells are all areas of active research, but none has as yet been demonstrated to have a disease-modifying effect.

Other Choreas Chorea can be seen in a number of disorders. Sydenham's chorea (originally called Saint Vitus' dance) is more common in females and is typically seen in childhood (5–15 years). It often develops in association with prior exposure to a group A streptococcal infection and is thought to be the result of an autoimmune-mediated inflammatory disorder. With the reduction in the incidence of rheumatic fever, the incidence of Sydenham's chorea has fallen, but it can still be seen in developing countries. It is characterized by the acute onset of choreiform movements, behavioral disturbances, and occasionally other motor dysfunctions. Chorea generally responds to dopamine-blocking agents, valproic acid, and carbamazepine but it tends to be self-limited, and treatment is generally restricted to those with severe chorea. Chorea may recur in later life, particularly in association with pregnancy (chorea gravidarum) or treatment with sex hormones. Neuroacanthocytosis is a progressive and typically fatal autosomal recessive disorder that is characterized by chorea coupled with red cell abnormalities on peripheral blood smear (acanthocytes). The chorea can be severe and associated with self-mutilating behavior, dystonia, tics, seizures, and a polyneuropathy. The cause is unknown, but linkage to chromosome 9q21 has been described. A phenotypically similar X-linked form of the disorder has been described in older individuals who have reactivity with Kell blood group antigens (McLeod syndrome).

Paroxysmal forms of chorea have been described in association with vascular diseases, hypo- and hyperglycemia, and a variety of infections and degenerative disorders. Paroxysmal kinesigenic dyskinesia is rare and characterized by brief episodes of chorea triggered by sudden voluntary movements. A benign senile chorea in older individuals and a benign inherited chorea of childhood have also been described. These conditions are somewhat controversial, and it is important to ensure that patients do not have HD.

Systemic lupus erythematosus (Chap. 313) is the most common systemic disorder that causes chorea; the chorea can last for days to years. Choreas can also be seen in patients with hyperthyroidism, various autoimmune disorders, infections including HIV, metabolic alterations, polycythemia rubra vera, following open heart surgery in the pediatric population, and in association with a wide variety of medications (especially anticonvulsants, cocaine, CNS stimulants, estrogens, and lithium).

℞ CHOREA

Diagnosis and treatment of the underlying condition, where possible, is the first priority. Tetrabenazine (not available in the United States), neuroleptics, dopamine-blocking agents, propranolol, clonazepam, and baclofen may be helpful. Treatment is not indicated if the condition is mild and self-limited.

Levodopa-Induced Dyskinesia Chronic levodopa treatment in PD patients is frequently associated with choreiform dyskinesias that affect the head, neck, torso, and extremities. They are usually associated

FIGURE 367-2 Schematic diagram of the basal ganglia–thalamo-cortical circuitry in normal (*left*) and hemiballismus (*right*) conditions. Inhibitory connections are shown as blue arrows and excitatory connections as green arrows. **A.** In the normal condition, the putamen connects to the GPi/SNr by direct and indirect pathways. Output neurons from the globus pallidus provide an inhibitory input to the VL thalamus and modulate its excitatory effect on cortical motor neurons. **B.** In hemiballismus, the lesion of the STN results in reduced excitatory input to the GPi/SNr and, in turn, reduced inhibition of thalamocortical neurons, leading to excessive activation of the cortex and the emergence of choreiform movements. Dopamine agonists may provide benefit in hemiballismus or chorea by blocking excitation of inhibitory neurons in the direct pathway (e.g., putamen → GPi/SNr) and preventing inhibition of remaining neurons in the excitatory indirect pathway (putamen → GPe → STN → GPi/SNr), thus increasing neuronal activity in GPi and inhibiting thalamic excitation of the cortex. Surgical lesions of the GPi are also beneficial, suggesting that abnormal neuronal discharge patterns in basal ganglia output neurons are an important contributing factor in the development of chorea. GPe, external segment of the globus pallidus; GPi, internal segment of the globus pallidus; SNr, substantia nigra, pars reticulata; SNc, substantia nigra, pars compacta; STN, subthalamic nucleus; VL, ventrolateral thalamus; PPN, pedunculopontine nucleus.

with the peak plasma levodopa level and maximal clinical effect (peak dose dyskinesia) but may occur at the onset and wearing off of the levodopa effect (diphasic dyskinesia). The dyskinesias can be disabling and can also limit the ability to fully utilize levodopa to control PD features. Levodopa-induced dyskinesias are thought to relate to plastic changes in basal ganglia neurons induced by intermittent nonphysiologic activation of striatal dopamine receptors due to the drug's short half-life. Medical management with levodopa dose manipulations, dopamine agonists, and amantadine may be helpful but frequently do not provide satisfactory control. Surgical therapies (ablation and stimulation) directed at the pallidum and subthalamic nucleus (STN) can be very effective in severe cases (Chap. 366). Recent studies suggest that dyskinesias can be prevented by more continuous delivery of levodopa or other dopaminergic agents. Levodopa does not cause dyskinesias in normal individuals.

Hemiballismus Hemiballismus is a violent form of chorea that comprises wild, flinging, large-amplitude movements on one side of the body. Proximal limb muscles tend to be predominantly affected. The movements may be so severe as to cause exhaustion, dehydration, local injury, and, in extreme cases, death. The most common cause is a partial lesion (infarct or hemorrhage) in the STN, but cases can also be seen with lesions in the putamen (Fig. 367-2). Fortunately, hemiballismus is usually self-limiting and tends to resolve spontaneously after weeks or months. The condition is difficult to treat pharmacologically.

The drugs most consistently beneficial are tetrabenazine (not available in the United States), haloperidol, propranolol, phenytoin, clonazepam, and baclofen. In extreme cases, pallidotomy can be very effective. Interestingly, surgically induced lesions of the STN in PD are usually not associated with hemiballismus.

TICS

Tourette Syndrome (TS)   TS is a neurobehavioral disorder named after the French neurologist Georges Gilles de la Tourette. It predominantly affects males, and prevalence is estimated to be 0.03–1.6%, but it is likely that many mild cases do not come to medical attention. TS is characterized by multiple motor tics and vocalizations. A *tic* is a brief, rapid, recurrent, and seemingly purposeless stereotyped motor contraction. Motor tics can be "simple," with movement only affecting an individual muscle group (e.g., blinking, twitching of the nose, jerking of the neck), or "complex," with coordinated involvement of multiple muscle groups [e.g., jumping, sniffing, head banging, and echopraxia (mimicking movements)]. Vocal tics can also be simple (e.g., grunting) or complex [e.g., echolalia (repeating other peoples words), palilalia (repeating your own words), and coprolalia (expression of obscene words)]. Patients may also experience sensory tics, consisting of unpleasant focal sensations in the face, head, or neck. Patients may experience an irresistible urge to express tics but characteristically can voluntarily suppress them for short periods of time. Tics vary in intensity and may be absent for days or weeks only to recur, occasionally in a different pattern. Tics tend to present between ages 2–15 years (mean 7 years) and often lessen or even disappear in adulthood. Associated behavioral disturbances include anxiety, depression, attention-deficit hyperactivity disorder and obsessive compulsive disorder. Patients may experience personality disorders, self-destructive behaviors, difficulties in school, and impaired interpersonal relationships. Tics may present in adulthood and can be seen in association with a variety of other disorders, including PD, HD, trauma, dystonia, drugs (e.g., levodopa, neuroleptics), and toxins.

ETIOLOGY AND PATHOPHYSIOLOGY   TS is thought to be a genetic disorder, but no specific gene has been identified as yet. Current evidence supports a complex inheritance pattern with one or more major genes, multiple loci, low penetrance, and environmental influences. The risk of a family with one affected child having a second is about 25%. The pathophysiology of TS is not known, but alterations in dopamine neurotransmission, opioids, and second messenger systems have been proposed.

℞ TOURETTE SYNDROME

Patients with mild disease often only require education and counseling (for themselves and family members). Drug treatment is indicated only when the tics are disabling and interfere with quality of life. Therapy is generally initiated with the α agonist clonidine, starting at low doses and gradually increasing the dose and frequency until satisfactory control is achieved. Guanfacine (0.5–2 mg/d) is a new α agonist that is preferred by many clinicians because it only requires once-a-day dosing. If these agents are not effective, antipsychotics can be employed. Atypical neuroleptics (risperidone 0.25–16 mg/d, olanzapine 2.5–15 mg/d, ziprasidone 20–200 mg/d) are preferred as they are associated with a reduced risk of extrapyramidal side effects. If they are not effective, classical neuroleptics such as haloperidol, fluphenazine, or pimozide can be tried. Botulinum toxin injections can be effective in controlling focal tics that involve small muscle groups. Behavioral features, and particularly anxiety and compulsions, can be a disabling feature of TS and should be treated. The potential value of DBS targeting the anterior portion of the internal capsule is currently being explored.

MYOCLONUS

Myoclonus is a brief, rapid (<100 ms), shocklike, jerky movement consisting of single or repetitive muscle discharges. Myoclonic jerks can be focal, multifocal, segmental, or generalized and can occur spontaneously, in association with voluntary movement (action myoclonus), or in response to an external stimulus (reflex or startle myoclonus). Negative myoclonus consists of a twitch due to a brief loss of muscle activity (e.g., asterixis in hepatic failure). Myoclonic jerks differ from tics in that they interfere with normal movement and are not suppressible. They can be seen in association with pathology in cortical, subcortical, or spinal cord regions, associated with hypoxic damage (especially following cardiac arrest), encephalopathy, and neurodegenerative disorders. Reversible myoclonus can be seen with metabolic disturbances (renal failure, electrolyte imbalance, hypocalcemia), toxins, and many medications. Essential myoclonus is a relatively benign familial condition characterized by multifocal lightning-like movements. Myoclonic jerks can be disabling when they interfere with normal movement. They can also be innocent and are commonly observed in normal people when waking up or falling asleep.

Rx MYOCLONUS

Treatment primarily consists of treating the underlying condition or removing an offending agent. Pharmacologic therapy involves one or a combination of GABAergic agents such as valproic acid (1200–3000 mg/d), piracetam (8–20 g/d), clonazepam (2–15 mg/d), or primidone (500–1000 mg/d). Recent studies suggest that levetiracetam may be particularly effective.

DRUG-INDUCED MOVEMENT DISORDERS

This important group of movement disorders is primarily associated with drugs that block dopamine receptors (neuroleptics) or central dopaminergic transmission. These drugs are mostly used in psychiatry but are also important in the treatment of nausea or vomiting (e.g., Compazine) or gastroesophageal disorders (e.g., metoclopramide). Hyperkinetic movement disorders secondary to neuroleptic drugs can be divided into those which present acutely, subacutely, or after prolonged exposure (tardive syndromes). Dopamine-blocking drugs can also be associated with a reversible parkinsonian syndrome for which anticholinergics are often concomitantly prescribed, but there is concern that this may increase the risk of developing a tardive syndrome.

Acute Dystonia is the most common acute hyperkinetic drug reaction. It is typically generalized in children and focal (e.g., blepharospasm, torticollis, or oromandibular dystonia) in adults. The reaction can develop within minutes of exposure and can be successfully treated in most cases with parenteral administration of anticholinergics (benztropine or diphenhydramine) or benzodiazepines (lorazepam or diazepam). Choreas, stereotypic behaviors, and tics may also be seen, particularly following acute exposure to CNS stimulants such as methylphenidate, cocaine, or amphetamines.

Subacute Akathisia is the commonest reaction in this category. It consists of motor restlessness with a need to move that is alleviated by movement. Therapy consists of removing the offending agent(s). When this is not possible, symptoms may be ameliorated with benzodiazepines, anticholinergics, beta blockers, or dopamine agonists.

Tardive Syndromes These disorders develop months to years after initiation of neuroleptic treatment. Tardive dyskinesia (TD) is the commonest and typically comprises choreiform movements involving the mouth, lips, and tongue. In severe cases the trunk, limbs, and respiratory muscles may be affected. Patients with affective disorders are more likely to develop TD than are patients with schizophrenia. In approximately one-third of patients, TD remits within 3 months of stopping the drug, and most patients gradually improve over the course of several years. The movements are often mild and more upsetting to the family than to the patient, but they can be severe and disabling, particularly in the context of an underlying psychiatric disorder. Atypical antipsychotics (e.g., clozapine, risperidone, olanzapine, quetiapine, ziprasidone, and aripiprazole) are associated with a significantly lower risk of TD in comparison to traditional antipsychotics. Younger patients have a lower risk of developing neuroleptic-induced TD, while the elderly, the edentulous, and those with underlying organic

cerebral dysfunction are at greater risk. Since TD can be permanent and resistant to treatment, antipsychotics should be used judiciously; atypical neuroleptics should be employed whenever possible, and the need for their continued use should be regularly monitored.

Treatment primarily consists of stopping the antipsychotic. If the patient is receiving a traditional antipsychotic and withdrawal is not possible, replacement with an atypical antipsychotic should be tried. Abrupt cessation of a neuroleptic should be avoided as acute withdrawal can induce transient worsening. TD can persist after withdrawal of antipsychotics and can be difficult to treat. Benefits may be achieved with valproic acid, anticholinergics, or botulinum toxin injections. In refractory cases, catecholamine depletors such as reserpine and tetrabenazine may be helpful. Tetrabenazine can be associated with dose-dependent sedation and orthostatic hypotension. Reserpine is an alternative, but it is frequently associated with depression and not often employed. Other approaches include baclofen (40–80 mg/d), clonazepam (1–8 mg/d), or valproic acid (750–3000 mg/d).

Chronic neuroleptic exposure can also be associated with tardive dystonia with preferential involvement of axial muscles and characteristic rocking movements of the trunk and pelvis. Tardive dystonia frequently persists despite stopping medication, and patients are often refractory to medical therapy. Valproic acid, anticholinergics, and botulinum toxin may occasionally be beneficial. Tardive akathisia and tardive Tourette syndromes are rare but may also occur after neuroleptic exposure.

Neuroleptic medications can also be associated with a neuroleptic malignant syndrome (NMS). NMS is characterized by muscle rigidity, elevated temperature, altered mental status, hyperthermia, tachycardia, labile blood pressure, and renal failure. Symptoms typically evolve within days or weeks after initiating the drug. NMS can also be precipitated by the abrupt withdrawal of antiparkinsonian medications in PD patients. Treatment involves immediate cessation of the offending antipsychotic drug and the introduction of a dopaminergic agent (e.g., dopamine agonists, levodopa), dantrolene, or benzodiazepines. Treatment also includes supportive measures such as control of body temperature (antipyretics and cooling blankets), hydration, electrolyte replacement, and control of renal function and blood pressure.

Drugs that have serotonin-like activity (tryptophan; MDMA, or "ecstasy"; meperidine) or that block serotonin reuptake can induce a rare, but potentially fatal, serotonin syndrome that is characterized by confusion, hyperthermia, tachycardia, and coma as well as rigidity, ataxia, and tremor. Myoclonus is often a prominent feature, in contrast to NMS, which it resembles. Patients can be managed with propranolol, diazepam, diphenhydramine, chlorpromazine, or cyproheptadine as well as supportive measures.

A variety of other drugs can also be associated with hyperkinetic movement disorders. Some examples include phenytoin (chorea, dystonia, tremor, myoclonus); carbamazepine (tics and dystonia); tricyclic antidepressants (dyskinesias, tremor, myoclonus); fluoxetine (myoclonus, chorea, dystonia); oral contraceptives (dyskinesia); adrenergics (tremor); buspirone (akathisia, dyskinesias, myoclonus); and digoxin, cimetidine, diazoxide, lithium, methadone, and fentanyl (dyskinesias).

PSYCHOGENIC DISORDERS

Virtually all movement disorders, including tremor, tics, dystonia, myoclonus, chorea, ballismus, and parkinsonism, can be psychogenic in origin. Tremor affecting the upper limbs is the most common psychogenic movement disorder. Psychogenic movements can result from a somatoform or conversion disorder, malingering (e.g., seeking financial gain), or a factitious disorder (e.g., seeking psychological gain). Psychogenic movement disorders are common (estimated 2–3% of patients in a movement disorder clinic), more prominent in women, disabling for the patient and family, and expensive for society (estimated $20 billion annually). Clinical features suggesting a psychogenic movement disorder include an acute onset and a pattern of abnormal movement that is inconsistent with a known movement disorder. Diagnosis is based on the nonorganic quality of the movement, the absence of findings of an organic disease process, and positive features that specifically point to a psychogenic illness such as variability and distractibility. For example, the magnitude of a psychogenic tremor is increased with attention and diminishes or even disappears when the patient is distracted by being asked to perform a different task or is unaware that he or she is being observed. This is the opposite of what occurs with organic movement disorders, which tend to worsen when the patient is distracted and abate with attention. Other positive features that suggest a psychogenic problem include a tremor frequency that is variable or entrains with the frequency of tapping in the contralateral limb and a positive response to placebo medication. Comorbid psychiatric problems such as anxiety, depression, and emotional trauma may be present but are not necessary for the diagnosis of a psychogenic movement disorder to be made. Psychogenic movement disorders can occur as an isolated entity or in association with an underlying organic problem. The diagnosis can often be made based on clinical features alone, and unnecessary tests or medications should be avoided. Underlying psychiatric problems should be identified and treated. Psychotherapy and hypnosis may be of value for patients with conversion reaction, and cognitive behavioral therapy may be helpful for patients with somatoform disorders. Patients with hypochondriasis, factitious disorders, and malingering have a poor prognosis.

FURTHER READINGS

DENG H et al: Genetics of essential tremor. Brain 130:1456, 2007

GUSELLA JF, MACDONALD ME: Huntington's disease: Seeing the pathogenic process through a genetic lens. Trends Biochem Sci 31:533, 2006

LOUIS ED: Essential tremor. Lancet Neurol 4:100, 2005

TARSY D, SIMON DK: Dystonia. N Engl J Med 355:818, 2006

VIDAILHET M et al: Bilateral deep-brain stimulation of the globus pallidus in primary generalized dystonia. N Engl J Med 352:459, 2005

WALKER FO: Huntington's disease. Lancet 369:218, 2007

368 Ataxic Disorders
Roger N. Rosenberg

APPROACH TO THE PATIENT:
Ataxic Disorders

Symptoms and signs of ataxia consist of gait impairment, unclear ("scanning") speech, visual blurring due to nystagmus, hand incoordination, and tremor with movement. These result from the involvement of the cerebellum and its afferent and efferent pathways, including the spinocerebellar pathways, and the frontopontocerebellar pathway originating in the rostral frontal lobe. True cerebellar ataxia must be distinguished from ataxia associated with vestibular nerve or labyrinthine disease, as the latter results in a disorder of gait associated with a significant degree of dizziness, light-headedness, or the perception of movement (Chap. 22). True cerebellar ataxia is devoid of these vertiginous complaints and is clearly an unsteady gait due to imbalance. Sensory disturbances can also on occasion simulate the imbalance of cerebellar disease; with sensory ataxia, imbalance dramatically worsens when visual input is removed (Romberg sign). Rarely, weakness of proximal leg muscles mimics cerebellar disease. In the patient who presents with ataxia, the rate and pattern of the development of cerebellar symptoms help to narrow the diagnostic possibilities (Table 368-1). A gradual and progressive increase in symptoms with bilateral and symmetric involvement suggests a biochemical, metabolic, immune, or toxic etiology. Conversely, focal, unilateral symptoms with headache and impaired level of consciousness accompanied by ipsilateral cranial nerve palsies and contralateral weakness imply a space-occupying cerebellar lesion.

SYMMETRIC ATAXIA Progressive and symmetric ataxia can be classified with respect to onset as acute (over hours or days), subacute (weeks or months), or chronic (months to years). Acute and reversible ataxias include those caused by intoxication with alcohol, phenytoin, lithium, barbiturates, and other drugs. Intoxication caused by toluene exposure, gasoline sniffing, glue sniffing, spray painting, or exposure to methyl mercury or bismuth are additional causes of acute or subacute ataxia, as is treatment with cytotoxic chemotherapeutic drugs such as fluorouracil and paclitaxel. Patients with a postinfectious syndrome (especially after varicella) may develop gait ataxia and mild dysarthria, both of which are reversible (Chap. 375). Rare infectious causes of acquired ataxia include poliovirus, coxsackievirus, echovirus, Epstein-Barr virus, toxoplasmosis, *Legionella*, and Lyme disease.

The subacute development of ataxia of gait over weeks to months (degeneration of the cerebellar vermis) may be due to the combined effects of alcoholism and malnutrition, particularly with deficiencies of vitamins B_1 and B_{12}. Hyponatremia has also been associated with ataxia. Paraneoplastic cerebellar ataxia is associated with a number of different tumors (and autoantibodies) such as breast and ovarian can-

TABLE 368-1 ETIOLOGY OF CEREBELLAR ATAXIA

Symmetric and Progressive Signs			Focal and Ipsilateral Cerebellar Signs		
Acute (Hours to Days)	**Subacute (Days to Weeks)**	**Chronic (Months to Years)**	**Acute (Hours to Days)**	**Subacute (Days to Weeks)**	**Chronic (Months to Years)**
Intoxication: alcohol, lithium, diphenylhydantoin, barbiturates (positive history and toxicology screen)	Intoxication: mercury, solvents, gasoline, glue; cytotoxic chemotherapeutic drugs	Paraneoplastic syndrome Anti-gliadin antibody syndrome Hypothyroidism	Vascular: cerebellar infarction, hemorrhage, or subdural hematoma Infectious: cerebellar abscess (mass lesion on MRI/CT, history in support of lesion)	Neoplastic: cerebellar glioma or metastatic tumor (positive for neoplasm on MRI/CT) Demyelinating: multiple sclerosis (history, CSF, and MRI are consistent)	Stable gliosis secondary to vascular lesion or demyelinating plaque (stable lesion on MRI/CT older than several months)
Acute viral cerebellitis (CSF supportive of acute viral infection) Postinfection syndrome	Alcoholic-nutritional (vitamin B_1 and B_{12} deficiency) Lyme disease	Inherited diseases Tabes dorsalis (tertiary syphilis) Phenytoin toxicity		AIDS-related multifocal leukoencephalopathy (positive HIV test and CD4+ cell count for AIDS)	Congenital lesion: Chiari or Dandy-Walker malformations (malformation noted on MRI/CT)

Abbreviations: CSF, cerebrospinal fluid; CT, computed tomography; MRI, magnetic resonance imaging.

cers (anti-Yo), small-cell lung cancer (anti-PQ type voltage-gated calcium channel), and Hodgkin's disease (anti-Tr) (Chap. 97). Another paraneoplastic syndrome associated with myoclonus and opsoclonus occurs with breast (anti-Ri) and lung cancers and neuroblastoma. Elevated serum anti-glutamic acid decarboxylase (GAD) antibodies have been associated with a progressive ataxic syndrome affecting speech and gait. For all of these paraneoplastic ataxias, the neurologic syndrome may be the presenting symptom of the cancer. Another immune-mediated progressive ataxia is associated with anti-gliadin (and anti-endomysium) antibodies and the HLA DQB1*0201 haplotype; in some affected patients, biopsy of the small intestine reveals villous atrophy consistent with gluten-sensitive enteropathy (Chap. 288). Finally, subacute progressive ataxia may be caused by a prion disorder, especially when an infectious etiology, such as transmission from contaminated human growth hormone, is responsible (Chap. 378).

Chronic symmetric gait ataxia suggests an inherited ataxia (discussed below), a metabolic disorder, or a chronic infection. Hypothyroidism must always be considered as a readily treatable and reversible form of gait ataxia. Infectious diseases that can present with ataxia are meningovascular syphilis and tabes dorsalis due to degeneration of the posterior columns and spinocerebellar pathways in the spinal cord.

FOCAL ATAXIA Acute focal ataxia commonly results from cerebrovascular disease, usually ischemic infarction, or cerebellar hemorrhage. These lesions typically produce cerebellar symptoms ipsilateral to the injured cerebellum and may be associated with an impaired level of consciousness due to brainstem compression and increased intracranial pressure; ipsilateral pontine signs, including sixth and seventh nerve palsies, may be present. Focal and worsening signs of acute ataxia should also prompt consideration of a posterior fossa subdural hematoma, bacterial abscess, or primary or metastatic cerebellar tumor. CT or MRI studies will reveal clinically significant processes of this type. Many of these lesions represent true neurologic emergencies, as sudden herniation, either rostrally through the tentorium or caudal herniation of cerebellar tonsils through the foramen magnum, can occur and is usually devastating. Acute surgical decompression may be required (Chap. 269). Lymphoma or progressive multifocal leukoencephalopathy (PML) in a patient with AIDS may present with an acute or subacute focal cerebellar syndrome. Chronic etiologies of progressive ataxia include multiple sclerosis (Chap. 375) and congenital lesions such as a Chiari malformation (Chap. 372) or a congenital cyst of the posterior fossa (Dandy-Walker syndrome).

THE INHERITED ATAXIAS

These may show autosomal dominant, autosomal recessive, or maternal (mitochondrial) modes of inheritance. A genomic classification (Table 368-2) has now largely superseded previous ones based on clinical expression alone.

Although the clinical manifestations and neuropathologic findings of cerebellar disease dominate the clinical picture, there may also be characteristic changes in the basal ganglia, brainstem, spinal cord, optic nerves, retina, and peripheral nerves. In large families with dominantly inherited ataxias, many gradations are observed from purely cerebellar manifestations to mixed cerebellar and brainstem disorders, cerebellar and basal ganglia syndromes, and spinal cord or peripheral nerve disease. Rarely, dementia is present as well. The clinical picture may be homogeneous within a family with dominantly inherited ataxia, but sometimes most affected family members show one characteristic syndrome, while one or several members have an entirely different phenotype.

AUTOSOMAL DOMINANT ATAXIAS

The autosomal spinocerebellar ataxias (SCAs) include SCA types 1 through SCA28, dentatorubropallidoluuysian atrophy (DRPLA), and episodic ataxia (EA) types 1 and 2 (Table 368-2). SCA1, SCA2, SCA3 [Machado-Joseph disease (MJD)], SCA6, SCA7, and SCA17 are caused by CAG triplet repeat expansions in different genes. SCA8 is due to an untranslated CTG repeat expansion, SCA12 is linked to an untranslated CAG repeat, and SCA10 is caused by an untranslated pentanucleotide repeat. The clinical phenotypes of these SCAs overlap. The genotype has become the "gold standard" for diagnosis and classification. CAG encodes glutamine, and these expanded CAG triplet repeat expansions result in expanded polyglutamine proteins, termed *ataxins*, that produce a toxic gain of function with autosomal dominant inheritance. Although the phenotype is variable for any given disease gene, a pattern of neuronal loss with gliosis is produced that is relatively unique for each ataxia. Immunohistochemical and biochemical studies have shown cytoplasmic (SCA2), neuronal (SCA1, MJD, SCA7), and nucleolar (SCA7) accumulation of the specific mutant polyglutamine-containing ataxin proteins. Expanded polyglutamine ataxins with more than ~40 glutamines are potentially toxic to neurons for a variety of reasons including the following: high levels of gene expression for the mutant polyglutamine ataxin in affected neurons; conformational change of the aggregated protein to a β-pleated structure; abnormal transport of the ataxin into the nucleus (SCA1, MJD, SCA7); binding to other polyglutamine proteins, including the TATA-binding transcription protein and the CREB-binding protein,

TABLE 368-2	CLASSIFICATION OF THE SPINOCEREBELLAR ATAXIAS	
Name	**Locus**	**Phenotype**
SCA1 (autosomal dominant type 1)	6p22-p23 with CAG repeats (exonic); leucine-rich acidic nuclear protein (LANP), region-specific interaction protein Ataxin-1	Ataxia with ophthalmoparesis, pyramidal and extrapyramidal findings
SCA2 (autosomal dominant type 2)	12q23-q24.1 with CAG repeats (exonic) Ataxin-2	Ataxia with slow saccades and minimal pyramidal and extrapyramidal findings
Machado-Joseph disease/SCA3 (autosomal dominant type 3)	14q24.3-q32 with CAG repeats (exonic); codes for ubiquitin protease (inactive with polyglutamine expansion); altered turnover of cellular proteins due to proteosome dysfunction MJD–ataxin-3	Ataxia with ophthalmoparesis and variable pyramidal, extrapyramidal, and amyotrophic signs
SCA4 (autosomal dominant type 4)	16q22.1-ter; pleckstrin homology domain-containing protein, family G, member 4; (PLEKHG4; puratrophin-1: Purkinje cell atrophy associated protein-1, including spectrin repeat and the guanine-nucleotide exchange factor, GEF for Rho GTPases)	Ataxia with normal eye movements, sensory axonal neuropathy, and pyramidal signs
SCA5 (autosomal dominant type 5)	11p12-q12; β-III spectrin mutations; (SPTBN2); stabilizes glutamate transporter EAAT4; descendants of President Abraham Lincoln	Ataxia and dysarthria

(continued)

Name	Locus	Phenotype
SCA6 (autosomal dominant type 6)	19p13.2 with CAG repeats in α_{1A}-voltage–dependent calcium channel gene (exonic); CACNA1A protein, P/Q type calcium channel subunit	Ataxia and dysarthria, nystagmus, mild proprioceptive sensory loss
SCA7 (autosomal dominant type 7)	3p14.1-p21.1 with CAG repeats (exonic); Ataxin-7; subunit of GCN5, histone acetyltransferase-containing complexes; ataxin 7 binding protein; Cbl-associated protein (CAP; SH3D5)	Ophthalmoparesis, visual loss, ataxia, dysarthria, extensor plantar response, pigmentary retinal degeneration
SCA8 (autosomal dominant type 8)	13q21 with CTG repeats; noncoding; 3′ untranslated region of transcribed RNA	Gait ataxia, dysarthria, nystagmus, leg spasticity, and reduced vibratory sensation
SCA10 (autosomal dominant type 10)	22q13; pentanucleotide repeat ATTCT repeat; noncoding, intron 9	Gait ataxia, dysarthria, nystagmus; partial complex and generalized motor seizures; polyneuropathy
SCA11 (autosomal dominant type 11)	15q14-q21.3 by linkage	Slowly progressive gait and extremity ataxia, dysarthria, vertical nystagmus, hyperreflexia
SCA12 (autosomal dominant type 12)	5q31-q33 by linkage; CAG repeat; protein phosphatase 2A, regulatory subunit B, (PPP2R2B); protein PP2A, serine/threonine phosphatase	Tremor, decreased movement, increased reflexes, dystonia, ataxia, dysautonomia, dementia, dysarthria
SCA13 (autosomal dominant type 13)	19q13.3-q14.4	Ataxia, legs>arms; dysarthria, horizontal nystagmus; delayed motor development; mental developmental delay; tendon reflexes increased; MRI: cerebellar and pontine atrophy
SCA14 (autosomal dominant type 14)	19q-13.4; protein kinase Cγ (PRKCG), missense mutations including in-frame deletion and a splice site mutation among others; serine/threonine kinase	Gait ataxia; leg>arm ataxia; dysarthria; pure ataxia with later onset; myoclonus; tremor of head and extremities; increased deep tendon reflexes at ankles; occasional dystonia and sensory neuropathy
SCA15 (autosomal dominant type 15)	3p24.2-3pter	Gait and extremity ataxia, dysarthria; nystagmus; MRI: superior vermis atrophy; sparing of hemispheres and tonsils
SCA16 (autosomal dominant type 16)	8q22.1-24.1	Pure cerebellar ataxia and head tremor, gait ataxia, and dysarthria; horizontal gaze–evoked nystagmus; MRI, cerebellar atrophy; no brainstem changes
SCA17 (autosomal dominant type 17)	6q27; CAG expansion in the TATA-binding protein (*TBP*) gene	Gait ataxia, dementia, parkinsonism, dystonia, chorea, seizures; hyperreflexia; dysarthria and dysphagia; MRI shows cerebral & cerebellar atrophy
SCA18 (autosomal dominant type 18)	7q22-q32	Ataxia; motor/sensory neuropathy; head tremor; dysarthria; extensor plantar responses in some patients; sensory axonal neuropathy; EMG denervation; MRI: cerebellar atrophy
SCA19 (autosomal dominant type 19)	1p21-q21	Ataxia, tremor, cognitive impairment, myoclonus; MRI: atrophy of cerebellum
SCA20 (assigned)	Chromosome 11	Dysarthria; gait ataxia; ocular gaze evoked saccades; palatal tremor; dentate calcification on CT; MRI: cerebral atrophy
SCA21 (autosomal dominant type 21)	7p21.3-p15.1	Ataxia, dysarthria, extrapyramidal features of akinesia, rigidity, tremor, cognitive defect; reduced deep tendon reflexes; MRI, cerebellar atrophy, normal basal ganglia and brainstem
SCA22 (autosomal dominant)	1p21-q23	Pure cerebellar ataxia; dysarthria; dysphagia; nystagmus; MRI: cerebellar atrophy
SCA23 (autosomal dominant)	20p13-12.3	Gait ataxia; dysarthria; extremity ataxia; ocular nystagmus, dysmetria; leg vibration loss; extensor plantar responses; MRI: cerebellar atrophy
SCA25 (autosomal dominant)	2p15-p21	Ataxia, nystagmus; vibratory loss in the feet; pain loss in some; abdominal pain; nausea and vomiting may be prominent; absent ankle reflexes; sensory nerve action potentials are absent; MRI: cerebellar atrophy, normal brainstem
SCA26 (autosomal dominant)	19p13.3	Gait ataxia; extremity ataxia; dysarthria; nystagmus; MRI: cerebellar atrophy
SCA27 (autosomal dominant)	13q34; fibroblast growth factor 14 protein; mutation F145S; produces reduced protein stability	Tremor extremities and head and orofacial dyskinesia; ataxia of arms>legs, gait ataxia; dysarthria; nystagmus; psychiatric symptoms; cognitive defect; MRI: cerebellar atrophy
SCA28 (autosomal dominant)	18p11.22-q11.2	Extremity and gait ataxia; dysarthria; nystagmus; ophthalmoparesis; leg hyperreflexia and extensor plantar responses; MRI: cerebellar atrophy
Dentatorubropallidoluysian atrophy (autosomal dominant)	12p13.31 with CAG repeats (exonic) Atrophin	Ataxia, choreoathetosis, dystonia, seizures, myoclonus, dementia
Friedreich's ataxia (autosomal recessive)	9q13-q21.1 with intronic GAA repeats, in intron at end of exon 1 Frataxin defective; abnormal regulation of mitochondrial iron metabolism; iron accumulates in mitochondria in yeast mutants	Ataxia, areflexia, extensor plantar responses, position sense deficits, cardiomyopathy, diabetes mellitus, scoliosis, foot deformities; optic atrophy; late onset form, as late as 50 years with preserved deep tendon reflexes, slower progression, reduced skeletal deformities, associated with an intermediate number of GAA repeats and missense mutations in one allele of frataxin
Friedreich's ataxia (autosomal recessive)	8q13.1-q13.3 (α-TTP deficiency)	Same as phenotype that maps to 9q but associated with vitamin E deficiency
Sensory ataxic neuropathy and ophthalmoparesis (SANDO) with dysarthria (autosomal recessive)	15q25; mutations in DNA polymerase-gamma (POLG) gene that leads to mtDNA deletions	Young-adult onset ataxia, sensory neuropathy, ophthalmoparesis, hearing loss, gastric symptoms; a variant of progressive external ophthalmoplegia; MRI: cerebellar and thalamic abnormalities; mildly increased lactate and creatine kinase
Von Hippel-Lindau syndrome (autosomal dominant)	3p26-p25	Cerebellar hemangioblastoma; pheochromocytoma

(continued)

CHAPTER 368

Ataxic Disorders

TABLE 368-2 **CLASSIFICATION OF THE SPINOCEREBELLAR ATAXIAS (CONTINUED)**

Name	Locus	Phenotype
Baltic myoclonus (Unverricht-Lundborg) (recessive)	21q22.3; cystatin B; extra repeats of 12 base pair tandem repeats	Myoclonus epilepsy; late onset ataxia; responds to valproic acid, Clonazepam; phenobarbital
Marinesco-Sjogren syndrome (recessive)	5q31; SIL 1 protein, nucleotide exchange factor for the heat-shock protein 70 (HSP70); chaperone HSPA5; homozygous 4-nucleotide duplication in exon 6; also compound heterozygote	Ataxia, dysarthria; nystagmus; retarded motor and mental maturation; rhabdomyolysis after viral illness; weakness; hypotonia; areflexia; cataracts in childhood; short stature; kyphoscoliosis; contractures; hypogonadism
Autosomal recessive spastic ataxia of Charlevoix-Saguenay (ARSACS)	Chromosome 13q12; SACS gene; loss of Sacsin peptide activity	Childhood onset of ataxia, spasticity, dysarthria, distal muscle wasting, foot deformity, retinal striations, mitral valve prolapse
Kearns-Sayre syndrome (sporadic)	mtDNA deletion and duplication mutations	Ptosis, ophthalmoplegia, pigmentary retinal degeneration, cardiomyopathy, diabetes mellitus, deafness, heart block, increased CSF protein, ataxia
Myoclonic epilepsy and ragged red fiber syndrome (MERRF) (maternal inheritance)	Mutation in mtDNA of the tRNA^{lys} at 8344; also mutation at 8356	Myoclonic epilepsy, ragged red fiber myopathy, ataxia
Mitochondrial encephalopathy, lactic acidosis, and stroke syndrome (MELAS) (maternal inheritance)	tRNA^{leu} mutation at 3243; also at 3271 and 3252	Headache, stroke, lactic acidosis, ataxia
Neuropathy; ataxia; retinitis pigmentosa (NARP)	ATPase6 (Complex 5); mtDNA point mutation at 8993	Neuropathy; ataxia; retinitis pigmentosa; dementia; seizures
Episodic ataxia, type 1 (EA-1) (autosomal dominant)	12p13; potassium voltage-gated channel gene, KCNA1; Phe249Leu mutation; variable syndrome	Episodic ataxia for minutes; provoked by startle or exercise; with facial and hand myokymia; cerebellar signs are not progressive; choreoathetotic movements; responds to phenytoin
Episodic ataxia, type 2 (EA-2) (autosomal dominant)	19p-13(CACNA1A) (allelic with SCA6) (α_{1A}-voltage–dependent calcium channel subunit); point mutations or small deletions; allelic with SCA6 and familial hemiplegic migraine	Episodic ataxia for days; provoked by stress, fatigue; with down-gaze nystagmus; nystagmus; vertigo; vomiting; headache; cerebellar atrophy results; progressive cerebellar signs; responds to acetazolamide
Episodic ataxia, type 3 (autosomal dominant)	1q42	Episodic ataxia; 1 min. to over 6 hrs.; induced by movement; vertigo and tinnitus; headache; responds to acetazolamide
Episodic ataxia, type 4 (autosomal dominant)	Not mapped	Episodic ataxia; vertigo; diplopia; ocular slow pursuit defect; no response to acetazolamide
Episodic ataxia, type 5 (autosomal dominant)	2q22-q23; CACNB4β4 protein	Episodic ataxia; hours to weeks; seizures
Episodic ataxia, type 6	5p13; SLC1A3; glutamate transporter in astrocytes	Episodic ataxia; seizures; cognitive impairment; under 24 h
Episodic ataxia, type 7 (autosomal dominant)	19q13	Episodic ataxia; vertigo, weakness; less than 24 h
Episodic ataxia with seizures, migraine, and alternating hemiplegia (autosomal dominant)	SLC1A3; 5p13; EAAT1 protein; missense mutations; glial glutamate transporter (GLAST); 1047 C to G; proline to arginine	Ataxia, duration 2–4 days; episodic hypotonia; delayed motor milestones; seizures; migraine; alternating hemiplegia; mild truncal ataxia; coma; febrile illness as a trigger; MRI: cerebellar atrophy
Fragile X tremor/ataxia syndrome (FXTAS) X-linked dominant	Xq27.3; CGG premutation expansion in FMR1 gene; expansions of 55–200 repeats in 5′ UTR of the FMR-1 mRNA; presumed dominant toxic RNA effect	Late onset ataxia with tremor, cognitive impairment, occasional parkinsonism; males typically affected, although affected females also reported; syndrome is of high concern if affected male has grandson with mental retardation; MRI shows increased T2 signal in middle cerebellar peduncles, cerebellar atrophy and occasional widespread brain atrophy
Ataxia telangiectasia (autosomal recessive)	11q22-23; ATM gene for regulation of cell cycle; mitogenic signal transduction and meiotic recombination	Telangiectasia, ataxia, dysarthria, pulmonary infections, neoplasms of lymphatic system; IgA and IgG deficiencies; diabetes mellitus, breast cancer
Early onset cerebellar ataxia with retained deep tendon reflexes (autosomal recessive)	13q11-12	Ataxia; neuropathy; preserved deep tendon reflexes; impaired cognitive and visuospatial functions; MRI, cerebellar atrophy
Ataxia with oculomotor apraxia (AOA1) (autosomal recessive)	9p13; protein is member of histidine triad superfamily, role in DNA repair	Ataxia; dysarthria; limb dysmetria; dystonia; oculomotor apraxia; optic atrophy; motor neuropathy; late sensory loss (vibration)
Ataxia with oculomotor apraxia 2 (AOA2) (autosomal recessive)	9q34; senataxin protein, involved in RNA maturation and termination; helicase superfamily 1	Gait ataxia; choreoathetosis; dystonia; oculomotor apraxia; neuropathy, vibration loss, position sense loss, and mild light touch loss; absent leg deep tendon reflexes; extensor plantar response
Cerebellar ataxia with muscle coenzyme Q10 deficiency (autosomal recessive)	9p13	Ataxia; hypotonia; seizures; mental retardation; increased deep tendon reflexes; extensor plantar responses; coenzyme Q10 levels reduced with about 25% of patients with a block in transfer of electrons to complex 3; may respond to coenzyme 10
Joubert syndrome (autosomal recessive)	9q34.3	Ataxia; ptosis; mental retardation; oculomotor apraxia; nystagmus; retinopathy; rhythmic tongue protrusion; episodic hyperpnea or apnea; dimples at wrists and elbows; telecanthus; micrognathia
Sideroblastic anemia and spinocerebellar ataxia (X-linked recessive)	Xq13; ATP-binding cassette 7 (ABCB7; ABC7) transporter; mitochondrial inner membrane; iron homeostasis; export from matrix to the intermembrane space	Ataxia; elevated free erythrocyte protoporphyrin levels; ring sideroblasts in bone marrow; heterozygous females may have mild anemia but not ataxia
Infantile-onset spinocerebellar ataxia of Nikali et al (autosomal recessive)	10q23.3-q24.1; twinkle protein(gene); homozygous for Tyr508Cys missense mutations	Infantile ataxia, sensory neuropathy; athetosis, hearing deficit, reduced deep tendon reflexes; ophthalmoplegia, optic atrophy; seizures; primary hypogonadism in females
Hypoceruloplasminemia with ataxia and dysarthria (autosomal recessive)	Ceruloplasmin gene; 3q23-q25 (trp 858 ter)	Gait ataxia and dysarthria; hyperreflexia; cerebellar atrophy by MRI; iron deposition in cerebellum, basal ganglia, thalamus, and liver; onset in the 4th decade
Spinocerebellar ataxia with neuropathy (SCAN1) (autosomal recessive)	Tryosyl-DNA phosphodiesterase-1 (TDP-1) 14q31-q32	Onset in 2nd decade; gait ataxia, dysarthria, seizures, cerebellar vermis atrophy on MRI, dysmetria

Abbreviations: MRI, magnetic resonance imaging; CSF, cerebrospinal fluid.

impairing their functions; altering the efficiency of the ubiquitin-proteosome system of protein turnover; and inducing neuronal apoptosis. An earlier age of onset (anticipation) and more aggressive disease in subsequent generations are due to further expansion of the CAG triplet repeat and increased polyglutamine number in the mutant ataxin. The most common disorders are discussed below.

SCA1 SCA1 was previously referred to as *olivopontocerebellar atrophy*, but genomic data have shown that that entity represents several different genotypes with overlapping clinical features.

SYMPTOMS AND SIGNS SCA1 is characterized by the development in early or middle adult life of progressive cerebellar ataxia of the trunk and limbs, impairment of equilibrium and gait, slowness of voluntary movements, scanning speech, nystagmoid eye movements, and oscillatory tremor of the head and trunk. Dysarthria, dysphagia, and oculomotor and facial palsies may also occur. Extrapyramidal symptoms include rigidity, an immobile face, and parkinsonian tremor. The reflexes are usually normal, but knee and ankle jerks may be lost, and extensor plantar responses may occur. Dementia may be noted but is usually mild. Impairment of sphincter function is common, with urinary and sometimes fecal incontinence. Cerebellar and brainstem atrophy are evident on MRI (Fig. 368-1).

Marked shrinkage of the ventral half of the pons, disappearance of the olivary eminence on the ventral surface of the medulla, and atrophy of the cerebellum are evident on gross postmortem inspection of the brain. Variable loss of Purkinje cells, reduced numbers of cells in the molecular and granular layer, demyelination of the middle cerebellar peduncle and the cerebellar hemispheres, and severe loss of cells in the pontine nuclei and olives are found on histologic examination. Degenerative changes in the striatum, especially the putamen, and loss of the pigmented cells of the substantia nigra may be found in cases with extrapyramidal features. More widespread degeneration in the central nervous system (CNS), including involvement of the posterior columns and the spinocerebellar fibers, is often present.

GENETIC CONSIDERATIONS SCA1 encodes a gene product, called ataxin-1, which is a novel protein of unknown function. The mutant allele has 40 CAG repeats located within the coding region, whereas alleles from unaffected individuals have ≤36 repeats. A few patients with 38–40 CAG repeats have been described. There is a direct correlation between a larger number of repeats and a younger age of onset for SCA1. Juvenile patients have higher numbers of repeats, and anticipation is present in subsequent generations. Transgenic mice carrying SCA1 developed ataxia and Purkinje cell pathology. Nuclear localization, but not aggregation, of ataxin-1 appears to be required for cell death initiated by the mutant protein.

SCA2 • ***SYMPTOMS AND SIGNS*** Another clinical phenotype, SCA2, has been described in patients from Cuba and India. Cuban patients probably are descendants of a common ancestor, and the population may be the largest homogeneous group of patients with ataxia yet described. The age of onset ranges from 2–65 years, and there is considerable clinical variability within families. Although neuropathologic and clinical findings are compatible with a diagnosis of SCA1, including slow saccadic eye movements, ataxia, dysarthria, parkinsonian rigidity, optic disk pallor, mild spasticity, and retinal degeneration, SCA2 is a unique form of cerebellar degenerative disease.

GENETIC CONSIDERATIONS The gene in SCA2 families also contains CAG repeat expansions coding for a polyglutamine-containing protein, ataxin-2. Normal alleles contain 15–32 repeats; mutant alleles have 35–77 repeats.

Machado-Joseph Disease/SCA3 MJD was first described among the Portuguese and their descendants in New England and California.

FIGURE 368-1 Sagittal MRI of the brain of a 60-year-old man with gait ataxia and dysarthria due to SCA1, illustrating cerebellar atrophy (*arrows*).

Subsequently, MJD has been found in families from Portugal, Australia, Brazil, Canada, China, England, France, India, Israel, Italy, Japan, Spain, Taiwan, and the United States. In most populations, it is the most common autosomal dominant ataxia.

SYMPTOMS AND SIGNS MJD has been classified into three clinical types. In type I MJD (amyotrophic lateral sclerosis–parkinsonism–dystonia type), neurologic deficits appear in the first two decades and involve weakness and spasticity of extremities, especially the legs, often with dystonia of the face, neck, trunk, and extremities. Patellar and ankle clonus are common, as are extensor plantar responses. The gait is slow and stiff, with a slightly broadened base and lurching from side to side; this gait results from spasticity, not true ataxia. There is no truncal titubation. Pharyngeal weakness and spasticity cause difficulty with speech and swallowing. Of note is the prominence of horizontal and vertical nystagmus, loss of fast saccadic eye movements, hypermetric and hypometric saccades, and impairment of upward vertical gaze. Facial fasciculations, facial myokymia, lingual fasciculations without atrophy, ophthalmoparesis, and ocular prominence are common early manifestations.

In type II MJD (ataxic type), true cerebellar deficits of dysarthria and gait and extremity ataxia begin in the second to fourth decades along with corticospinal and extrapyramidal deficits of spasticity, rigidity, and dystonia. Type II is the most common form of MJD. Ophthalmoparesis, upward vertical gaze deficits, and facial and lingual fasciculations are also present. Type II MJD can be distinguished from the clinically similar disorders SCA1 and SCA2.

Type III MJD (ataxic-amyotrophic type) presents in the fifth to the seventh decades with a pancerebellar disorder that includes dysarthria and gait and extremity ataxia. Distal sensory loss involving pain, touch, vibration, and position senses and distal atrophy are prominent, indicating the presence of peripheral neuropathy. The deep tendon reflexes are depressed to absent, and there are no corticospinal or extrapyramidal findings.

The mean age of onset of symptoms in MJD is 25 years. Neurologic deficits invariably progress and lead to death from debilitation within 15 years of onset, especially in patients with types I and II disease. Usually, patients retain full intellectual function.

The major pathologic findings are variable loss of neurons and glial replacement in the corpus striatum and severe loss of neurons in the pars compacta of the substantia nigra. A moderate loss of neurons occurs in the dentate nucleus of the cerebellum and in the red nucleus.

Purkinje cell loss and granule cell loss occur in the cerebellar cortex. Cell loss also occurs in the dentate nucleus and in the cranial nerve motor nuclei. Sparing of the inferior olives distinguishes MJD from other dominantly inherited ataxias.

GENETIC CONSIDERATIONS The gene for MJD maps to 14q24.3-q32. Unstable CAG repeat expansions are present in the MJD gene coding for a polyglutamine-containing protein named ataxin-3, or MJD-ataxin. An earlier age of onset is associated with longer repeats. Alleles from normal individuals have between 12 and 37 CAG repeats, while MJD alleles have 60–84 CAG repeats. Polyglutamine-containing aggregates of ataxin-3 (MJD-ataxin) have been described in neuronal nuclei undergoing degeneration. MJD ataxin codes for a ubiquitin protease, which is inactive due to expanded polyglutamines. Proteosome function is impaired, resulting in altered clearance of proteins and cerebellar neuronal loss.

SCA6 Genomic screening for CAG repeats in other families with autosomal dominant ataxia and vibratory and proprioceptive sensory loss have yielded another locus. Of interest is that different mutations in the same gene for the α_{1A} voltage-dependent calcium channel subunit (CACNLIA4; also referred to as the *CACNA1A* gene) at 19p13 result in different clinical disorders. CAG repeat expansions (21–27 in patients; 4–16 triplets in normal individuals) result in late-onset progressive ataxia with cerebellar degeneration. Missense mutations in this gene result in familial hemiplegic migraine. Nonsense mutations resulting in termination of protein synthesis of the gene product yield hereditary paroxysmal cerebellar ataxia or EA. Some patients with familial hemiplegic migraine develop progressive ataxia and also have cerebellar atrophy.

SCA7 This disorder is distinguished from all other SCAs by the presence of retinal pigmentary degeneration. The visual abnormalities first appear as blue-yellow color blindness and proceed to frank visual loss with macular degeneration. In almost all other respects, SCA7 resembles several other SCAs in which ataxia is accompanied by various noncerebellar findings, including ophthalmoparesis and extensor plantar responses. The genetic defect is an expanded CAG repeat in the SCA7 gene at 3p14-p21.1. The expanded repeat size in SCA7 is highly variable. Consistent with this, the severity of clinical findings varies from essentially asymptomatic to mild late-onset symptoms to severe, aggressive disease in childhood with rapid progression. Marked anticipation has been recorded, especially with paternal transmission. The disease protein, ataxin-7, forms aggregates in nuclei of affected neurons, as has also been described for SCA1 and SCA3/MJD.

SCA8 This form of ataxia is caused by a CTG repeat expansion in an untranslated region of a gene on chromosome 13q21. There is marked maternal bias in transmission, perhaps reflecting contractions of the repeat during spermatogenesis. The mutation is not fully penetrant. Symptoms include slowly progressive dysarthria and gait ataxia beginning at ~40 years of age with a range between 20 and 65 years. Other features include nystagmus, leg spasticity, and reduced vibratory sensation. Severely affected individuals are nonambulatory by the fourth to sixth decades. MRI shows cerebellar atrophy. The mechanism of disease may involve a dominant "toxic" effect occurring at the RNA level, as occurs in myotonic dystrophy.

Dentatorubropallidoluysian Atrophy DRPLA has a variable presentation that may include progressive ataxia, choreoathetosis, dystonia, seizures, myoclonus, and dementia. DRPLA is due to unstable CAG triplet repeats in the open reading frame of a gene named *atrophin* located on chromosome 12p12-ter. Larger expansions are found in patients with earlier onset. The number of repeats is 49 in patients with DRPLA and ≤26 in normal individuals. Anticipation occurs in successive generations, with earlier onset of disease in association with an increasing CAG repeat number in children who inherit the disease from their father. One well-characterized family in North Carolina has a

phenotypic variant known as the *Haw River syndrome*, now recognized to be due to the DRPLA mutation.

Episodic Ataxia EA types 1 and 2 are two rare dominantly inherited disorders that have been mapped to chromosomes 12p (a potassium channel gene) for type 1 and 19p for type 2. Patients with EA-1 have brief episodes of ataxia with myokymia and nystagmus that last only minutes. Startle, sudden change in posture, and exercise can induce episodes. Acetazolamide or anticonvulsants may be therapeutic. Patients with EA-2 have episodes of ataxia with nystagmus that can last for hours or days. Stress, exercise, or excessive fatigue may be precipitants. Acetazolamide may be therapeutic and can reverse the relative intracellular alkalosis detected by magnetic resonance spectroscopy. Stop codon, nonsense mutations causing EA-2 have been found in the *CACNA1A* gene, encoding the α_{1A} voltage-dependent calcium channel subunit (see "SCA6," above).

AUTOSOMAL RECESSIVE ATAXIAS

Friedreich's Ataxia This is the most common form of inherited ataxia, comprising one-half of all hereditary ataxias. It can occur in a classic form or in association with a genetically determined vitamin E deficiency syndrome; the two forms are clinically indistinguishable.

SYMPTOMS AND SIGNS Friedreich's ataxia presents before 25 years of age with progressive staggering gait, frequent falling, and titubation. The lower extremities are more severely involved than the upper ones. Dysarthria occasionally is the presenting symptom; rarely, progressive scoliosis, foot deformity, nystagmus, or cardiopathy is the initial sign.

The neurologic examination reveals nystagmus, loss of fast saccadic eye movements, truncal titubation, dysarthria, dysmetria, and ataxia of trunk and limb movements. Extensor plantar responses (with normal tone in trunk and extremities), absence of deep tendon reflexes, and weakness (greater distally than proximally) are usually found. Loss of vibratory and proprioceptive sensation occurs. The median age of death is 35 years. Women have a significantly better prognosis than men.

Cardiac involvement occurs in 90% of patients. Cardiomegaly, symmetric hypertrophy, murmurs, and conduction defects are reported. Moderate mental retardation or psychiatric syndromes are present in a small percentage of patients. A high incidence of diabetes mellitus (20%) is found and is associated with insulin resistance and pancreatic β-cell dysfunction. Musculoskeletal deformities are common and include pes cavus, pes equinovarus, and scoliosis. MRI of the spinal cord shows atrophy (**Fig. 368-2**).

The primary sites of pathology are the spinal cord, dorsal root ganglion cells, and the peripheral nerves. Slight atrophy of the cerebellum and cerebral gyri may occur. Sclerosis and degeneration occur predominantly in the spinocerebellar tracts, lateral corticospinal tracts, and posterior columns. Degeneration of the glossopharyngeal, vagus, hypoglossal, and deep cerebellar nuclei is described. The cerebral cortex is histologically normal except for loss of Betz cells in the precentral gyri. The peripheral nerves are extensively involved, with a loss of large myelinated fibers. Cardiac pathology consists of myocytic hypertrophy and fibrosis, focal vascular fibromuscular dysplasia with subintimal or medial deposition of periodic acid–Schiff (PAS)–positive material, myocytopathy with unusual pleomorphic nuclei, and focal degeneration of nerves and cardiac ganglia.

GENETIC CONSIDERATIONS The classic form of Friedreich's ataxia has been mapped to 9q13-q21.1, and the mutant gene, *frataxin*, contains expanded GAA triplet repeats in the first intron. There is homozygosity for expanded GAA repeats in >95% of patients. Normal persons have 7–22 GAA repeats, and patients have 200–900 GAA repeats. A more varied clinical syndrome has been described in compound heterozygotes who have one copy of the GAA expansion and the other copy a point mutation in the *frataxin* gene. When the point mutation is located in the region of the gene that encodes the amino-terminal half of frataxin, the phenotype is milder, often consisting of a spastic gait, retained or exaggerated reflexes, no dysarthria, and mild or absent ataxia.

FIGURE 368-2 Sagittal MRI of the brain and spinal cord of a patient with Friedreich's ataxia, demonstrating spinal cord atrophy.

Patients with Friedreich's ataxia have undetectable or extremely low levels of *frataxin* mRNA, as compared with carriers and unrelated individuals; thus, disease appears to be caused by a loss of expression of the frataxin protein. Frataxin is a mitochondrial protein involved in iron homeostasis. Mitochondrial iron accumulation due to loss of the iron transporter coded by the mutant *frataxin* gene results in oxidized intramitochondrial iron. Excess oxidized iron results in turn in the oxidation of cellular components and irreversible cell injury.

Two forms of hereditary ataxia associated with abnormalities in the interactions of vitamin E (α-tocopherol) with very low density lipoprotein (VLDL) have been delineated. These are abetalipoproteinemia (Bassen-Kornzweig syndrome) and ataxia with vitamin E deficiency (AVED). Abetalipoproteinemia is caused by mutations in the gene coding for the larger subunit of the microsomal triglyceride transfer protein (MTP). Defects in MTP result in impairment of formation and secretion of VLDL in liver. This defect results in a deficiency of delivery of vitamin E to tissues, including the central and peripheral nervous system, as VLDL is the transport molecule for vitamin E and other fat-soluble substitutes. AVED is due to mutations in the gene for α-tocopherol transfer protein (α-TTP). These patients have an impaired ability to bind vitamin E into the VLDL produced and secreted by the liver, resulting in a deficiency of vitamin E in peripheral tissues. Hence, either absence of VLDL (abetalipoproteinemia) or impaired binding of vitamin E to VLDL (AVED) causes an ataxic syndrome. Once again, a genotype classification has proved to be essential in sorting out the various forms of the Friedreich's disease syndrome, which may be clinically indistinguishable.

Ataxia Telangiectasia • *SYMPTOMS AND SIGNS* Patients with ataxia telangiectasia (AT) present in the first decade of life with progressive telangiectatic lesions associated with deficits in cerebellar function and nystagmus. The neurologic manifestations correspond to those in Friedreich's disease, which should be included in the differential diagnosis. Truncal and limb ataxia, dysarthria, extensor plantar responses, myoclonic jerks, areflexia, and distal sensory deficits may develop. There is a high incidence of recurrent pulmonary infections and neoplasms of the lymphatic and reticuloendothelial system in patients with AT. Thymic hypoplasia with cellular and humoral (IgA and IgG2) immunodeficiencies, premature aging, and endocrine disorders such as type 1 diabetes mellitus are described. There is an increased incidence of lymphomas, Hodgkin's disease, acute leukemias of the T cell type, and breast cancer.

The most striking neuropathologic changes include loss of Purkinje, granule, and basket cells in the cerebellar cortex as well as of neurons in the deep cerebellar nuclei. The inferior olives of the medulla may also

have neuronal loss. There is a loss of anterior horn neurons in the spinal cord and of dorsal root ganglion cells associated with posterior column spinal cord demyelination. A poorly developed or absent thymus gland is the most consistent defect of the lymphoid system.

GENETIC CONSIDERATIONS The gene for AT (the *ATM* gene) encodes a protein that is similar to several yeast and mammalian phosphatidylinositol-3′-kinases involved in mitogenic signal transduction, meiotic recombination, and cell cycle control. Defective DNA repair in AT fibroblasts exposed to ultraviolet light has been demonstrated. The discovery of *ATM* will make possible the identification of heterozygotes who are at risk for cancer (e.g., breast cancer) and permit early diagnosis.

Mitochondrial Ataxias Spinocerebellar syndromes have been identified with mutations in mitochondrial DNA (mtDNA). Thirty pathogenic mtDNA point mutations and 60 different types of mtDNA deletions are known, several of which cause or are associated with ataxia (Chap. 382).

℞ ATAXIC DISORDERS

The most important goal in management of patients with ataxia is to identify treatable disease entities. Mass lesions must be recognized promptly and treated appropriately. Paraneoplastic disorders can often be identified by the clinical patterns of disease that they produce, measurement of specific autoantibodies, and uncovering the primary cancer; these disorders are often refractory to therapy, but some patients improve following removal of the tumor or immunotherapy (Chap. 97). Ataxia with anti-gliadin antibodies and gluten-sensitive enteropathy may improve with a gluten-free diet. Malabsorption syndromes leading to vitamin E deficiency may lead to ataxia. The vitamin E deficiency form of Friedreich's ataxia must be considered, and serum vitamin E levels measured. Vitamin E therapy is indicated for these rare patients. Vitamin B_1 and B_{12} levels in serum should be measured, and the vitamins administered to patients having deficient levels. Hypothyroidism is easily treated. The cerebrospinal fluid should be tested for a syphilitic infection in patients with progressive ataxia and other features of tabes dorsalis. Similarly, antibody titers for Lyme disease and *Legionella* should be measured and appropriate antibiotic therapy should be instituted in antibody-positive patients. Aminoacidopathies, leukodystrophies, urea-cycle abnormalities, and mitochondrial encephalomyopathies may produce ataxia, and some dietary or metabolic therapies are available for these disorders. The deleterious effects of diphenylhydantoin and alcohol on the cerebellum are well known and these exposures should be avoided in patients with ataxia of any cause.

There is no proven therapy for any of the autosomal dominant ataxias (SCA1 to -28). There is preliminary evidence that idebenone, a free-radical scavenger, can improve myocardial hypertrophy in patients with classic Friedreich ataxia; there is no current evidence, however, that it improves neurologic function. Iron chelators and antioxidant drugs are potentially harmful in Friedreich's patients as they may increase heart muscle injury. Acetazolamide can reduce the duration of symptoms of episodic ataxia. At present, identification of an at-risk person's genotype, together with appropriate family and genetic counseling, can reduce the incidence of these cerebellar syndromes in future generations (Chap. 64).

FURTHER READINGS

BERKE SJ et al: Defining the role of ubiquitin-interacting motifs in the polyglutamine disease protein. J Biol Chem 280:32026, 2005

FOGEL BL, PERLMAN S: Clinical features and molecular genetics of autosomal recessive cerebellar ataxias. Lancet Neurol 6:245, 2007

HADJIVASSILIOU M et al: Gluten ataxia in perspective: Epidemiology, genetic susceptibility and clinical characteristics. Brain 136:685, 2003

ROSENBERG RN, PAULSON HL: The inherited ataxias, in *The Molecular and Genetic Basis of Neurologic and Psychiatric Disease*, 3d ed, RN Rosenberg et al (eds). Philadelphia, Elsevier Science, and Boston, Butterworth-Heinemann, 2003

http://www.neuro.wustl.edu/neuromuscular/ataxia, 2006

369 Amyotrophic Lateral Sclerosis and Other Motor Neuron Diseases

Robert H. Brown, Jr.

AMYOTROPHIC LATERAL SCLEROSIS

Amyotrophic lateral sclerosis (ALS) is the most common form of progressive motor neuron disease. It is a prime example of a neurodegenerative disease and is arguably the most devastating of the neurodegenerative disorders.

Pathology The pathologic hallmark of motor neuron degenerative disorders is death of lower motor neurons (consisting of anterior horn cells in the spinal cord and their brainstem homologues innervating bulbar muscles) and upper, or corticospinal, motor neurons (originating in layer five of the motor cortex and descending via the pyramidal tract to synapse with lower motor neurons, either directly or indirectly via interneurons) (Chap. 23). Although at its onset ALS may involve selective loss of function of only upper or lower motor neurons, it ultimately causes progressive loss of both categories of motor neurons. Indeed, in the absence of clear involvement of both motor neuron types, the diagnosis of ALS is questionable.

Other motor neuron diseases involve only particular subsets of motor neurons (Tables 369-1 and 369-2). Thus, in bulbar palsy and spinal muscular atrophy (SMA; also called progressive muscular atrophy), the lower motor neurons of brainstem and spinal cord, respectively, are most severely involved. By contrast, pseudobulbar palsy, primary lateral sclerosis (PLS), and familial spastic paraplegia (FSP) affect only upper motor neurons innervating the brainstem and spinal cord.

In each of these diseases, the affected motor neurons undergo shrinkage, often with accumulation of the pigmented lipid (lipofuscin) that normally develops in these cells with advancing age. In ALS, the motor neuron cytoskeleton is typically affected early in the illness. Focal enlargements are frequent in proximal motor axons; ultrastructurally, these "spheroids" are composed of accumulations of neurofilaments and other proteins. Also seen is proliferation of astroglia and microglia, the inevitable accompaniment of all degenerative processes in the central nervous system (CNS).

The death of the peripheral motor neurons in the brainstem and spinal cord leads to denervation and consequent atrophy of the corresponding muscle fibers. Histochemical and electrophysiologic evidence indicates that in the early phases of the illness denervated muscle can be reinnervated by sprouting of nearby distal motor nerve terminals, although reinnervation in this disease is considerably less extensive than in most other disorders affecting motor neurons (e.g., poliomyelitis, peripheral neuropathy). As denervation progresses, muscle atrophy is readily recognized in muscle biopsies and on clinical examination. This is the basis for the term *amyotrophy*. The loss of cortical motor neurons results in thinning of the corticospinal tracts that travel via the internal capsule (Fig. 369-1) and brainstem to the lateral and anterior white matter columns of the spinal cord. The loss of fibers in the lateral columns and resulting fibrillary gliosis impart a particular firmness (*lateral sclerosis*). A remarkable feature of the disease is the selectivity of neuronal cell death. By light microscopy, the entire sensory apparatus, the regulatory mechanisms for the control and coordination of movement, and the components of the brain that are needed for cognitive processes, remain intact. However, immunostaining indicates that neurons bearing ubiquitin, a marker for degeneration, are also detected in nonmotor systems. Moreover, studies of glucose metabolism in the illness also indicate that there is neuronal dysfunction outside of the motor system. Within the motor system, there is some selectivity of involvement. Thus, motor neurons required for ocular motility remain unaffected, as do the parasympathetic neurons in the sacral spinal cord (the nucleus of Onufrowicz, or Onuf) that innervate the sphincters of the bowel and bladder.

TABLE 369-1 ETIOLOGY AND INVESTIGATION OF MOTOR NEURON DISORDERS

Diagnostic Category	Investigations
Structural lesions	MRI scan of head (including foramen magnum), cervical spine[a]
Parasagittal or foramen magnum tumors	
Cervical spondylosis	
Chiari malformation or syrinx	
Spinal cord arteriovenous malformation	
Infections	CSF exam, culture[a]
Bacterial—tetanus, Lyme	Lyme antibody titer[a]
Viral—poliomyelitis, herpes zoster	Antiviral antibody titers
Retroviral myelopathy	HTLV-I titers
Intoxications, physical agents	
Toxins—lead, aluminum, others	24-h urine for heavy metals[a]
Drugs—strychnine, phenytoin	Serum for lead level[a]
Electric shock, x-irradiation	
Immunologic mechanisms	Complete blood count[a]
Plasma cell dyscrasias	Sedimentation rate[a]
Autoimmune polyradiculoneuropathy	Protein immunoelectrophoresis[a]
Motor neuropathy with conduction block	Anti-GM1 antibodies[a]
Paraneoplastic	Anti-Hu antibody
Paracarcinomatous/lymphoma	MRI scan, bone marrow biopsy
Metabolic	
Hypoglycemia	Fasting blood sugar (FBS), routine chemistries including calcium[a]
Hyperparathyroidism	PTH, calcium, phosphate
Hyperthyroidism	Thyroid function[a]
Deficiency of folate, vitamin B$_{12}$, vitamin E	Vitamin B$_{12}$, vitamin E, folate levels[a]
Malabsorption	24-h stool fat, carotene, prothrombin time
Mitochondrial dysfunction	Fasting lactate, pyruvate, ammonia Consider mtDNA analysis
Hereditary biochemical disorders	
Superoxide dismutase 1 gene mutation	White blood cell DNA analysis
Androgen receptor defect (Kennedy's disease)	Abnormal CAG insert in androgen receptor gene
Hexosaminidase deficiency	Lysosomal enzyme screen
Infantile (α-glucosidase deficiency/Pompe's disease)	α-glucosidase level
Hyperlipidemia	Lipid electrophoresis
Hyperglycinuria	Urine and serum amino acids
Methylcrotonylglycinuria	CSF amino acids

[a]Denotes studies that should be obtained in all cases.
Note: CSF, cerebrospinal fluid; HTLV, human T cell lymphotropic virus; PTH, parathyroid hormone.

Clinical Manifestations The manifestations of ALS are somewhat variable depending on whether corticospinal neurons or lower motor neurons in the brainstem and spinal cord are more prominently involved. With lower motor neuron dysfunction and early denervation, typically the first evidence of the disease is insidiously developing asymmetric weakness, usually first evident distally in one of the limbs. A detailed history often discloses recent development of cramping with volitional movements, typically in the early hours of the morning (e.g., while stretching in bed). Weakness caused by denervation is associated with progressive wasting and atrophy of muscles and, particularly early in the illness, spontaneous twitching of motor units, or fasciculations. In the hands, a preponderance of extensor over flexor weakness is common. When the initial denervation involves bulbar rather than limb muscles, the problem at onset is difficulty with chewing, swallowing, and movements of the face and tongue. Early involvement of the muscles of respiration may lead to death before the disease is far advanced elsewhere. With prominent corticospinal involvement, there is hyperactivity of the muscle-stretch reflexes (tendon jerks) and, often, spastic resistance to passive movements of the affected limbs. Patients with significant reflex hyperactivity complain of muscle stiffness often out of proportion to weakness. Degeneration of the corticobulbar projections innervating the

TABLE 369-2 SPORADIC MOTOR NEURON DISEASES

Chronic

Upper and lower motor neurons
    Amyotrophic lateral sclerosis
Predominantly upper motor neurons
    Primary lateral sclerosis
Predominantly lower motor neurons
    Multifocal motor neuropathy with conduction block
    Motor neuropathy with paraproteinemia or cancer
    Motor-predominant peripheral neuropathies
Other
    Associated with other degenerative disorders
    Secondary motor neuron disorders (see Table 369-1)

Acute

Poliomyelitis
Herpes zoster
Coxsackie virus

brainstem results in dysarthria and exaggeration of the motor expressions of emotion. The latter leads to involuntary excess in weeping or laughing (so-called pseudobulbar affect).

Virtually any muscle group may be the first to show signs of disease, but, as time passes, more and more muscles become involved until ultimately the disorder takes on a symmetric distribution in all regions. It is characteristic of ALS that, regardless of whether the initial disease involves upper or lower motor neurons, both will eventually be implicated. Even in the late stages of the illness, sensory, bowel and bladder, and cognitive functions are preserved. Even when there is severe brainstem disease, ocular motility is spared until the very late stages of the illness. Dementia is not a component of sporadic ALS. In some families, ALS is co-inherited with frontotemporal dementia, characterized by early behavioral abnormalities with prominent behavioral features indicative of frontal lobe dysfunction.

A committee of the World Federation of Neurology has established diagnostic guidelines for ALS. Essential for the diagnosis is simultaneous upper and lower motor neuron involvement with progressive weakness, and the exclusion of all alternative diagnoses. The disorder is ranked as "definite" ALS when three or four of the following are in-

FIGURE 369-1 Amyotrophic lateral sclerosis. Axial T2-weighted MRI scan through the lateral ventricles of the brain reveals abnormal high signal intensity within the corticospinal tracts (*arrows*). This MRI feature represents an increase in water content in myelin tracts undergoing Wallerian degeneration secondary to cortical motor neuronal loss. This finding is commonly present in ALS, but can also be seen in AIDS-related encephalopathy, infarction, or other disease processes that produce corticospinal neuronal loss in a symmetric fashion.

volved: bulbar, cervical, thoracic, and lumbosacral motor neurons. When two sites are involved, the diagnosis is "probable," and when only one site is implicated, the diagnosis is "possible." An exception is made for those who have progressive upper and lower motor neuron signs at only one site and a mutation in the gene encoding superoxide dismutase (SOD1; below).

Epidemiology The illness is relentlessly progressive, leading to death from respiratory paralysis; the median survival is from 3–5 years. There are very rare reports of stabilization or even regression of ALS. In most societies there is an incidence of 1–3 per 100,000 and a prevalence of 3–5 per 100,000. Several endemic foci of higher prevalence exist in the western Pacific (e.g., in specific regions of Guam or Papua New Guinea). In the United States and Europe, males are somewhat more frequently affected than females. Epidemiologic studies have incriminated risk factors for this disease including exposure to pesticides and insecticides, smoking and, in one report, service in the military. While ALS is overwhelmingly a sporadic disorder, some 5–10% of cases are inherited as an autosomal dominant trait.

Familial ALS Several forms of selective motor neuron disease are inheritable (Table 369-3). Two involve both corticospinal and lower motor neurons. The most common is familial ALS (FALS). Apart from its inheritance as an autosomal dominant trait, it is clinically indistinguishable from sporadic ALS. Genetic studies have identified mutations in the gene encoding the cytosolic, copper- and zinc-binding enzyme SOD1 as the cause of one form of FALS. However, this accounts for only 20% of inherited cases of ALS.

TABLE 369-3 GENETIC MOTOR NEURON DISEASES

Disease	Locus	Gene
I. Upper and lower motor neurons (familial ALS)		
A. Autosomal dominant	2p	Dynactin
	9q	Senataxin
	20q	Vesicle-associated protein B
	21q	Superoxide dismutase
	22q	Neurofilament heavy chain
B. Autosomal recessive	2q	Alsin
C. Mitochondrial	mtDNA	Cytochrome c oxidase
	mtDNA	tRNA-isoleucine
II. Lower motor neurons		
A. Spinal muscular atrophies	5q	Survival motor neuron protein
B. X-linked spinobulbar muscular atrophy	Xq	Androgen receptor
C. GM2 gangliosidosis		
1. Sandhoff disease	5q	Hexosaminidase B
2. AB variant	5q	GM2 activator protein
3. Adult Tay-Sach's disease	15q	Hexosaminidase A
III. Upper motor neuron (selected FSP's)		
A. Autosomal dominant	2p	Spastin
	11q	BSCL2
	12q	Kinesin heavy-chain KIF5A
	14q	Atlastin
	15q	NIPA1
B. Autosomal recessive	13q	Spartin
	15q	Maspardin
	16q	Paraplegin
C. X-linked	Xq	Proteolipid protein
	Xq	L1-CAM
D. Adrenomyeloneuropathy	Xq	Adrenoleukodystrophy protein
IV. ALS-plus syndromes		
Amyotrophy with behavioral disorder and Parkinsonism	17q	Tau protein

Note: ALS, amyotrophic lateral sclerosis; BSCL2, Bernadelli-Seip congenital lipodystrophy, 2B; FSP, familial spastic paraplegia

Rare mutations in other genes are also clearly implicated in ALS-like diseases. Thus, a familial, dominantly inherited motor disorder that in some individuals closely mimics the ALS phenotype arises from mutations in a gene that encodes a vesicle-binding protein. A predominantly lower motor neuron disease with early hoarseness due to laryngeal dysfunction has been ascribed to mutations in the gene encoding the cellular motor protein dynactin. Mutations in senataxin, a helicase, cause an early adult-onset, slowly evolving ALS variant. Kennedy's syndrome is an X-linked, adult-onset disorder that may mimic ALS, as described below.

Genetic analyses are also beginning to illuminate the pathogenesis of some childhood-onset motor neuron diseases. For example, a slowly disabling degenerative, predominantly upper motor neuron disease that starts in the first decade is caused by mutations in a gene that expresses a novel signaling molecule with properties of a guanine-exchange factor, termed *alsin*.

Differential Diagnosis Because ALS is currently untreatable, it is imperative that potentially remediable causes of motor neuron dysfunction be excluded (Table 369-1). This is particularly true in cases that are atypical by virtue of (1) restriction to either upper or lower motor neurons, (2) involvement of neurons other than motor neurons, and (3) evidence of motor neuronal conduction block on electrophysiologic testing. Compression of the cervical spinal cord or cervicomedullary junction from tumors in the cervical regions or at the foramen magnum or from cervical spondylosis with osteophytes projecting into the vertebral canal can produce weakness, wasting, and fasciculations in the upper limbs and spasticity in the legs, closely resembling ALS. The absence of cranial nerve involvement may be helpful in differentiation, although some foramen magnum lesions may compress the twelfth cranial (hypoglossal) nerve, with resulting paralysis of the tongue. Absence of pain or of sensory changes, normal bowel and bladder function, normal roentgenographic studies of the spine, and normal cerebrospinal fluid (CSF) all favor ALS. Where doubt exists, MRI scans and contrast myelography should be performed to visualize the cervical spinal cord.

Another important entity in the differential diagnosis of ALS is *multifocal motor neuropathy with conduction block* (MMCB), discussed below. A diffuse, lower motor axonal neuropathy mimicking ALS sometimes evolves in association with hematopoietic disorders such as lymphoma or multiple myeloma. In this clinical setting, the presence of an M-component in serum should prompt consideration of a bone marrow biopsy. Lyme disease (Chap. 166) may also cause an axonal, lower motor neuropathy, although typically with intense proximal limb pain and a CSF pleocytosis.

Other treatable disorders that occasionally mimic ALS are chronic lead poisoning and thyrotoxicosis. These disorders may be suggested by the patient's social or occupational history or by unusual clinical features. When the family history is positive, disorders involving the genes encoding cytosolic SOD1, hexosaminidase A, or α-glucosidase deficiency must be excluded (Chap. 355). These are readily identified by appropriate laboratory tests. Benign fasciculations are occasionally a source of concern because on inspection they resemble the fascicular twitchings that accompany motor neuron degeneration. The absence of weakness, atrophy, or denervation phenomena on electrophysiologic examination usually excludes ALS or other serious neurologic disease. Patients who have recovered from poliomyelitis may experience a delayed deterioration of motor neurons that presents clinically with progressive weakness, atrophy, and fasciculations. Its cause is unknown, but it is thought to reflect sublethal prior injury to motor neurons by poliovirus (Chap. 184).

Rarely, ALS develops concurrently with features indicative of more widespread neurodegeneration. Thus, one infrequently encounters otherwise typical ALS patients with a parkinsonian movement disorder or dementia. It remains unclear whether this reflects the unlikely simultaneous occurrence of two disorders or a primary defect triggering two forms of neurodegeneration. The latter is suggested by the observation that multisystem neurodegenerative diseases may be inherited. For example, prominent amyotrophy has been described as a dominantly inherited disorder in individuals with bizarre behavior and a movement disorder suggestive of parkinsonism; many such cases have now been ascribed to mutations that alter the expression of tau protein in brain (Chap. 365). In other cases, ALS develops simultaneously with a striking frontotemporal dementia. These disorders may be dominantly co-inherited; in some families, this trait is linked to a locus on chromosome 9p, although the underlying genetic defect is not established.

Pathogenesis The cause of sporadic ALS is not well defined. Several mechanisms that impair motor neuron viability have been elucidated in mice and rats induced to develop motor neuron disease by SOD1 transgenes with ALS-associated mutations. It is evident that excitotoxic neurotransmitters such as glutamate participate in the death of motor neurons in ALS. This may be a consequence of diminished uptake of synaptic glutamate by an astroglial glutamate transporter, EAAT2. It is striking that one cellular defense against such excitotoxicity is the enzyme SOD1, which detoxifies the free radical superoxide anion (Chap. 360). Precisely why the SOD1 mutations are toxic to motor nerves is not established, although it is clear the effect is not simply loss of normal scavenging of the superoxide anion. The mutant protein is conformationally unstable and prone to aberrant catalytic reactions. In turn, these features lead to aggregation of SOD1 protein, impairment of axonal transport, reduced production of ATP and other perturbations of mitochondrial function, activation of neuroinflammatory cascades within the ALS spinal cord, and ultimately induction of cell death via pathways that are at least partially dependent on caspases. Multiple recent studies have convincingly demonstrated that nonneuronal cells importantly influence the disease course, at least in ALS transgenic mice.

℞ AMYOTROPHIC LATERAL SCLEROSIS

No treatment arrests the underlying pathologic process in ALS. The drug riluzole (100 mg/d) was approved for ALS because it produces a modest lengthening of survival. In one trial, the survival rate at 18 months with riluzole was similar to placebo at 15 months. The mechanism of this effect is not known with certainty; riluzole may reduce excitotoxicity by diminishing glutamate release. Riluzole is generally well tolerated; nausea, dizziness, weight loss, and elevated liver enzymes occur occasionally. Pathophysiologic studies of mutant SOD1–related ALS in mice have disclosed diverse targets for therapy; consequently, multiple therapies are presently in clinical trails in ALS. These include studies of insulin-like growth factor I (IGF-I), which produced inconsistent results in ALS patients and is now undergoing further clinical trials and ceftriaxone, which may augment astroglial glutamate transport and thereby be anti-excitotoxic. Interventions such as antisense oligonucleotides (ASO) or inhibitory RNA that diminish expression of mutant SOD1 protein prolong survival in transgenic ALS mice and rats. Based on these data, a human trial of ASO is planned in SOD1-mediated ALS.

In the absence of a primary therapy for ALS, a variety of rehabilitative aids may substantially assist ALS patients. Foot-drop splints facilitate ambulation by obviating the need for excessive hip flexion and by preventing tripping on a floppy foot. Finger extension splints can potentiate grip. Respiratory support may be life-sustaining. For patients electing against long-term ventilation by tracheostomy, positive-pressure ventilation by mouth or nose provides transient (several weeks) relief from hypercarbia and hypoxia. Also extremely beneficial for some patients is a respiratory device (Cough Assist Device) that produces an artificial cough. This is highly effective in clearing airways and preventing aspiration pneumonia. When bulbar disease prevents normal chewing and swallowing, gastrostomy is uniformly helpful, restoring normal nutrition and hydration. Fortunately, an increasing variety of speech synthesizers are now available to augment speech when there is advanced bulbar palsy. These facilitate oral communication and may be effective for telephone use.

In contrast to ALS, several of the disorders (Tables 369-1 and 369-3) that bear some clinical resemblance to ALS are treatable. For this reason, a careful search for causes of secondary motor neuron disease is warranted.

OTHER MOTOR NEURON DISEASES

SELECTED LOWER MOTOR NEURON DISORDERS

In these motor neuron diseases, the peripheral motor neurons are affected without evidence of involvement of the corticospinal motor system (Tables 369-1 to 369-3).

X-Linked Spinobulbar Muscular Atrophy (Kennedy's Disease)   This is an X-linked lower motor neuron disorder in which progressive weakness and wasting of limb and bulbar muscles begins in males in mid-adult life and is conjoined with androgen insensitivity manifested by gynecomastia and reduced fertility (Chap. 340). In addition to gynecomastia, which may be subtle, two findings distinguishing this disorder from ALS are the absence of signs of pyramidal tract disease (spasticity) and the presence of a subtle sensory neuropathy in some patients. The underlying molecular defect is an expanded trinucleotide repeat (-CAG-) in the first exon of the androgen receptor gene on the X chromosome. DNA testing is available. An inverse correlation appears to exist between the number of -CAG- repeats and the age of onset of the disease.

Adult Tay-Sach's Disease   Several reports have described adult-onset, predominantly lower motor neuropathies arising from deficiency of the enzyme β-hexosaminidase (hex A). These tend to be distinguishable from ALS because they are very slowly progressive; dysarthria and radiographically evident cerebellar atrophy may be prominent. In rare cases, spasticity may also be present, although it is generally absent (Chap. 355).

Spinal Muscular Atrophy   The SMAs are a family of selective lower motor neuron diseases of early onset. Despite some phenotypic variability (largely in age of onset), the defect in the majority of families with SMA maps to a locus on chromosome 5 encoding a putative motor neuron survival protein (SMN, for survival motor neuron) that is important in the formation and trafficking of RNA complexes across the nuclear membrane. Neuropathologically these disorders are characterized by extensive loss of large motor neurons; muscle biopsy reveals evidence of denervation atrophy. Several clinical forms exist.

Infantile SMA (SMA I, Werdnig-Hoffmann disease) has the earliest onset and most rapidly fatal course. In some instances it is apparent even before birth, as indicated by decreased fetal movements late in the third trimester. Though alert, afflicted infants are weak and floppy (hypotonic) and lack muscle stretch reflexes. Death generally ensues within the first year of life. *Chronic childhood SMA* (SMA II) begins later in childhood and evolves with a more slowly progressive course. *Juvenile SMA* (SMA III, Kugelberg-Welander disease) manifests during late childhood and runs a slow, indolent course. Unlike most denervating diseases, in this chronic disorder weakness is greatest in the proximal muscles; indeed, the pattern of clinical weakness can suggest a primary myopathy such as limb-girdle dystrophy. Electrophysiologic and muscle biopsy evidence of denervation distinguish SMA III from the myopathic syndromes.

Multifocal Motor Neuropathy with Conduction Block   In this disorder lower motor neuron function is regionally and chronically disrupted by remarkably focal blocks in conduction. Many cases have elevated serum titers of mono- and polyclonal antibodies to ganglioside GM1; it is hypothesized that the antibodies produce selective, focal, paranodal demyelination of motor neurons. MMCB is not typically associated with corticospinal signs. In contrast with ALS, MMCB may respond dramatically to therapy such as IV immunoglobulin or chemotherapy; it is thus imperative that MMCB be excluded when considering a diagnosis of ALS.

Other Forms of Lower Motor Neuron Disease   In individual families, other syndromes characterized by selective lower motor neuron dysfunction in an SMA-like pattern have been described. There are rare X-linked and autosomal dominant forms of apparent SMA. There is an ALS variant of juvenile onset, the Fazio-Londe syndrome, that involves mainly the musculature innervated by the brainstem. A component of lower motor neuron dysfunction is also found in degenerative disorders such as Machado-Joseph disease and the related olivopontocerebellar degenerations (Chap. 368).

SELECTED DISORDERS OF THE UPPER MOTOR NEURON

Primary Lateral Sclerosis   This exceedingly rare disorder arises sporadically in adults in mid- to late life. Clinically PLS is characterized by progressive spastic weakness of the limbs, preceded or followed by spastic dysarthria and dysphagia, indicating combined involvement of the corticospinal and corticobulbar tracts. Fasciculations, amyotrophy, and sensory changes are absent; neither electromyography nor muscle biopsy shows denervation. On neuropathologic examination there is selective loss of the large pyramidal cells in the precentral gyrus and degeneration of the corticospinal and corticobulbar projections. The peripheral motor neurons and other neuronal systems are spared. The course of PLS is variable; while long-term survival is documented, the course may be as aggressive as in ALS, with ~3-year survival from onset to death. Early in its course, PLS raises the question of multiple sclerosis or other demyelinating diseases such as adrenoleukodystrophy as diagnostic considerations (Chap. 375). A myelopathy suggestive of PLS is infrequently seen with infection with the retrovirus human T cell lymphotropic virus (HTLV-I) (Chap. 372). The clinical course and laboratory testing will distinguish these possibilities.

Familial Spastic Paraplegia   In its pure form, FSP is usually transmitted as an autosomal trait; most adult-onset cases are dominantly inherited. Symptoms usually begin in the third or fourth decade, presenting as progressive spastic weakness beginning in the distal lower extremities; however, there are variants with onset so early that the differential diagnosis includes cerebral palsy. FSP typically has a long survival, presumably because respiratory function is spared. Late in the illness there may be urinary urgency and incontinence and sometimes fecal incontinence; sexual function tends to be preserved.

In pure forms of FSP, the spastic leg weakness is often accompanied by posterior column sensory loss and disturbance of bowel and bladder function. Some family members may have spasticity without clinical symptoms.

By contrast, particularly when recessively inherited, FSP may have complex or complicated forms in which altered corticospinal and dorsal column function is accompanied by significant involvement of other regions of the nervous system, including amyotrophy, mental retardation, optic atrophy, and sensory neuropathy.

Neuropathologically, in FSP there is degeneration of the corticospinal tracts, which appear nearly normal in the brainstem but show increasing atrophy at more caudal levels in the spinal cord; in effect, the pathologic picture is of a dying-back or distal axonopathy of long neuronal fibers within the CNS.

Defects at numerous loci underlie both dominantly and recessively inherited forms of FSP (Table 369-3). Eleven FSP genes have now been identified. The gene most commonly implicated in dominantly inherited FSP is *spastin,* which encodes a microtubule interacting protein. The most common childhood-onset dominant form arises from mutations in the *atlastin* gene. A kinesin heavy-chain protein implicated in microtubule motor function was found to be defective in a family with dominantly inherited FSP of variable onset age.

An infantile-onset form of X-linked, recessive FSP arises from mutations in the gene for myelin proteolipid protein (Chap. 360). This is an example of rather striking allelic variation, as most other mutations in the same gene cause not FSP but Pelizaeus-Merzbacher disease, a widespread disorder of CNS myelin. Another recessive variant is caused by defects in the *paraplegin* gene. Paraplegin has homology to metalloproteases that are important in mitochondrial function in yeast.

WEB SITES

Several web sites provide valuable information on ALS including those offered by the Muscular Dystrophy Association (*www.mdausa.org*), the Amyotrophic Lateral Sclerosis Association (*www.alsa.org*), and the World

Federation of Neurology and the Neuromuscular Unit at Washington University in St. Louis (*www.neuro.wustl.edu/neuromuscular*).

FURTHER READINGS

BOILLEE S et al: ALS: A disease of motor neurons and their nonneuronal neighbors. Neuron 52:39, 2006

BROWN RH et al: *Amyotrophic Lateral Sclerosis*, 2nd ed. London, Informa Healthcare, 2006

BRUIJN LI, CUDKOWICZ M: Therapeutic targets for amyotrophic lateral sclerosis: Current treatments and prospects for more effective therapies. Expert Rev Neurother 6:417, 2006

CLEMENT AM et al: Wild-type nonneuronal cells extend survival of SOD1 mutant motor neurons in ALS mice. Science, 302:113, 2003

DIGIORGIO et al: Non-cell autonomous effect of glia on motor neurons in an embryonic stem cell-based ALS model. Nat Neurosci 10:608, 2007

FINK JK: Hereditary spastic paraplegia. Curr Neurol Neurosci Rep 6:65, 2006

PASINELLI P, BROWN RH: Molecular biology of amyotrophic lateral sclerosis: Insights from genetics. Nat Rev Neurosci 7:710, 2006

RALPH GS et al: Silencing mutant SOD1 using RNAi protects against neurodegeneration and extends survival in an ALS model. Nat Med 11:429, 2005

SMITH RA et al: Antisense oligonucleotide therapy for neurodegenerative disease. J Clin Invest 116:2290, 2006

WEISSKOPF MG et al: Prospective study of military service and mortality from ALS. Neurology 64:32, 2005

370 Disorders of the Autonomic Nervous System

Phillip A. Low, John W. Engstrom

The autonomic nervous system (ANS) innervates the entire neuraxis and permeates all organ systems. It regulates blood pressure (BP), heart rate, sleep, and bladder and bowel function. It operates automatically; its full importance becomes recognized only when ANS function is compromised, resulting in dysautonomia. Hypothalamic disorders that cause disturbances in homeostasis are discussed in Chaps. 17 and 333.

ANATOMIC ORGANIZATION

The activity of the ANS is regulated by central neurons responsive to diverse afferent inputs. After central integration of afferent information, autonomic outflow is adjusted to permit the functioning of the major organ systems in accordance with the needs of the organism as a whole. Connections between the cerebral cortex and the autonomic centers in the brainstem coordinate autonomic outflow with higher mental functions.

The preganglionic neurons of the parasympathetic nervous system leave the central nervous system (CNS) in the third, seventh, ninth, and tenth cranial nerves as well as the second and third sacral nerves, while the preganglionic neurons of the sympathetic nervous system exit the spinal cord between the first thoracic and the second lumbar segments (Fig. 370-1). The postganglionic neurons, located in ganglia outside the CNS, give rise to the postganglionic autonomic nerves that innervate organs and tissues throughout the body. Responses to sympathetic and parasympathetic stimulation are frequently antagonistic (Table 370-1), reflecting highly coordinated interactions within the CNS; the resultant changes in parasympathetic and sympathetic activity provide more precise control of autonomic responses than could be achieved by the modulation of a single system.

Acetylcholine (ACh) is the preganglionic neurotransmitter for both divisions of the ANS as well as the postganglionic neurotransmitter of the parasympathetic neurons. Norepinephrine (NE) is the neurotransmitter of the postganglionic sympathetic neurons, except for cholinergic neurons innervating the eccrine sweat glands.

CLINICAL EVALUATION

CLASSIFICATION

Disorders of the ANS may result from pathology of either the CNS or the peripheral nervous system (PNS) (Table 370-2). Signs and symptoms may result from interruption of the afferent limb, CNS processing centers, or efferent limb of reflex arcs controlling autonomic responses.

For example, a lesion of the medulla produced by a posterior fossa tumor can impair BP responses to postural changes and result in orthostatic hypotension (OH). OH can also be caused by lesions of the spinal cord or peripheral vasomotor nerve fibers (e.g., diabetic autonomic neuropathy). The site of reflex interruption is usually established by the clinical context in which the dysautonomia arises, combined with judicious use of ANS testing and neuroimaging studies. The presence or absence of CNS signs (pathophysiology and prognosis differ), association with sensory or motor polyneuropathy, medical illnesses, medication use, and family history are often important considerations. Some syndromes do not fit easily into any classification scheme.

SYMPTOMS OF AUTONOMIC DYSFUNCTION

Clinical manifestations result from a loss of function (e.g., impaired baroreflexes leading to OH), overactivity (e.g., hyperhidrosis, hypertension, tachycardia), or loss of regulation (e.g., autonomic storms, autonomic dysreflexia) of autonomic circuits. Symptoms may be widespread or regional in distribution. An autonomic history focuses on systemic functions (BP, heart rate, sleep, thermoregulation) and involvement of individual organ systems (pupils, bowel, bladder, sexual function). More formal assessment is possible using a standardized instrument such as the autonomic symptom profile. It is also important to recognize the modulating effects of age and gender. For instance, OH commonly results in lightheadedness in the young, whereas cognitive slowing is more common in the elderly. Specific symptoms of orthostatic intolerance are diverse (Table 370-3). Autonomic symptoms may vary dramatically, reflecting the dynamic nature of autonomic control over homeostatic function. For example, OH might be manifest only in the early morning, following a meal, or with exercise, depending upon the regional vascular bed affected by dysautonomia.

Early symptoms may be overlooked. Impotence, although not specific for autonomic failure, often heralds autonomic failure in men and may precede other symptoms by years (Chap. 49). A decrease in the frequency of spontaneous early morning erections may occur months before loss of nocturnal penile tumescence and development of total impotence. Bladder dysfunction may appear early in men and

TABLE 370-1	FUNCTIONAL CONSEQUENCES OF NORMAL ANS ACTIVATION	
	Sympathetic	**Parasympathetic**
Heart rate	Increased	Decreased
Blood pressure	Increased	Mildly decreased
Bladder	Increased sphincter tone	Voiding (decreased tone)
Bowel motility	Decreased motility	Increased
Lung	Bronchodilation	Bronchoconstriction
Sweat glands	Sweating	—
Pupils	Dilation	Constriction
Adrenal glands	Catecholamine release	—
Sexual function	Ejaculation, orgasm	Erection
Lacrimal glands	—	Tearing
Parotid glands	—	Salivation

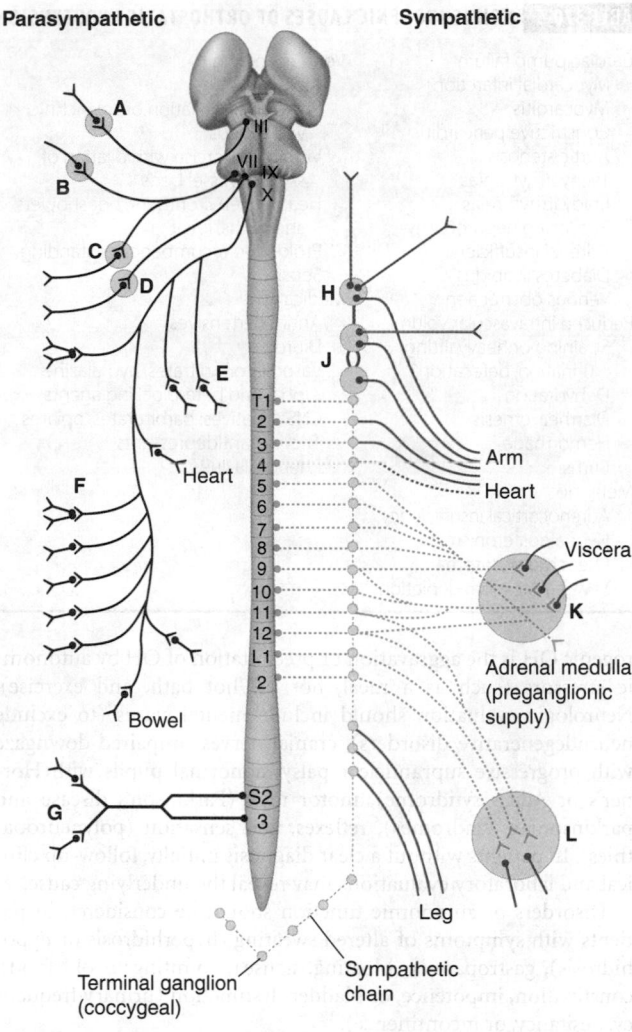

Parasympathetic   **Sympathetic**

Parasympathetic system
from cranial nerves III, VII, IX, X
and from sacral nerves 2 and 3

Sympathetic system
from T1-L2
Preganglionic fibers ··········
Postganglionic fibers ———

A Ciliary ganglion
B Sphenopalatine
(pterygopalatine) ganglion
C Submandibular ganglion
D Otic ganglion
E Vagal ganglion cells
in the heart wall
F Vagal ganglion cells in
bowel wall
G Pelvic ganglia

H Superior cervical ganglion
J Middle cervical ganglion and
inferior cervical (stellate)
ganglion including T1
ganglion
K Coeliac and other
abdominal ganglia
L Lower abdominal
sympathetic ganglia

FIGURE 370-1 Schematic representation of the autonomic nervous system. *(From M Moskowitz: Clin Endocrinol Metab 6:77, 1977.)*

women, particularly in those with CNS involvement. Brain and spinal cord disease above the level of the lumbar spine results first in urinary frequency and small bladder volumes and eventually in incontinence (upper motor neuron or spastic bladder). Disease of PNS autonomic nerve fibers results in large bladder volumes, urinary frequency, and overflow incontinence (lower motor neuron flaccid bladder). Measurement of bladder volume (post-void residual) is a useful bedside test for distinguishing between upper and lower motor neuron bladder dysfunction in the early stages of dysautonomia. Gastrointestinal autonomic dysfunction typically presents as severe constipation. Diarrhea occurs occasionally (as in diabetes mellitus) due to rapid transit of contents or uncoordinated small-bowel motor activity, or on an osmotic basis from bacterial overgrowth associated with small-bowel stasis. Impaired glandular secretory function may cause difficulty with

TABLE 370-2 CLASSIFICATION OF CLINICAL AUTONOMIC DISORDERS

I. Autonomic disorders with brain involvement
  A. Associated with multisystem degeneration
    1. Multisystem degeneration: autonomic failure clinically prominent
      a. Multiple system atrophy (MSA)
      b. Parkinson's disease with autonomic failure
      c. Diffuse Lewy body disease (some cases)
    2. Multisystem degeneration: autonomic failure clinically not usually prominent
      a. Parkinson's disease
      b. Other extrapyramidal disorders (inherited spinocerebellar atrophies, progressive supranuclear palsy, corticobasal degeneration, Machado-Joseph disease)
  B. Unassociated with multisystem degeneration
    1. Disorders mainly due to cerebral cortex involvement
      a. Frontal cortex lesions causing urinary/bowel incontinence
      b. Partial complex seizures
    2. Disorders of the limbic and paralimbic circuits
      a. Shapiro's syndrome (agenesis of corpus callosum, hyperhidrosis, hypothermia)
      b. Autonomic seizures
    3. Disorders of the hypothalamus
      a. Wernicke-Korsakoff syndrome
      b. Diencephalic syndrome
      c. Neuroleptic malignant syndrome
      d. Serotonin syndrome
      e. Fatal familial insomnia
      f. Antidiuretic hormone (ADH) syndromes (diabetes insipidus, inappropriate ADH)
      g. Disturbances of temperature regulation (hyperthermia, hypothermia)
      h. Disturbances of sexual function
      i. Disturbances of appetite
      j. Disturbances of BP/HR and gastric function
      k. Horner's syndrome
    4. Disorders of the brainstem and cerebellum
      a. Posterior fossa tumors
      b. Syringobulbia and Arnold-Chiari malformation
      c. Disorders of BP control (hypertension, hypotension)
      d. Cardiac arrhythmias
      e. Central sleep apnea
      f. Baroreflex failure
      g. Horner's syndrome
II. Autonomic disorders with spinal cord involvement
  A. Traumatic quadriplegia
  B. Syringomyelia
  C. Subacute combined degeneration
  D. Multiple sclerosis
  E. Amyotrophic lateral sclerosis
  F. Tetanus
  G. Stiff-man syndrome
  H. Spinal cord tumors
III. Autonomic neuropathies
  A. Acute/subacute autonomic neuropathies
    1. Subacute autoimmune autonomic neuropathy (panautonomic neuropathy, pandysautonomia)
      a. Subacute paraneoplastic autonomic neuropathy
      b. Guillain-Barré syndrome
      c. Botulism
      d. Porphyria
      e. Drug induced autonomic neuropathies
      f. Toxic autonomic neuropathies
  B. Chronic peripheral autonomic neuropathies
    1. Distal small fiber neuropathy
    2. Combined sympathetic and parasympathetic failure
      a. Amyloid
      b. Diabetic autonomic neuropathy
      c. Autoimmune autonomic neuropathy (paraneoplastic and idiopathic)
      d. Sensory neuronopathy with autonomic failure
      e. Familial dysautonomia (Riley-Day syndrome)

Note: BP, blood pressure; HR, heart rate.

food intake due to decreased salivation or eye irritation due to decreased lacrimation. Occasionally, temperature elevation and vasodilation can result from anhidrosis because sweating is normally important for heat dissipation (Chap. 17).

TABLE 370-3 SYMPTOMS OF ORTHOSTATIC INTOLERANCE

Lightheadedness (dizziness)	88%
Weakness or tiredness	72%
Cognitive difficulty (thinking/concentrating)	47%
Blurred vision	47%
Tremulousness	38%
Vertigo	37%
Pallor	31%
Anxiety	29%
Palpitations	26%
Clammy feeling	19%
Nausea	18%

Source: From PA Low et al: Mayo Clin Proc 70:617,1995.

OH (also called *postural hypotension*) is perhaps the most disabling feature of autonomic dysfunction. The prevalence of OH is relatively high, especially when OH associated with aging and diabetes mellitus is included (Table 370-4). OH can cause a variety of symptoms, including dimming or loss of vision, lightheadedness, diaphoresis, diminished hearing, pallor, and weakness. Syncope results when the drop in BP impairs cerebral perfusion. Other manifestations of impaired baroreflexes are supine hypertension, a heart rate that is fixed regardless of posture, postprandial hypotension, and an excessively high nocturnal BP. Many patients with OH have a preceding diagnosis of hypertension or have concomitant supine hypertension, reflecting the great importance of baroreflexes in maintaining postural and supine normotension. The appearance of OH in patients receiving antihypertensive treatment may indicate overtreatment or the onset of an autonomic disorder. The most common causes of OH are not neurologic in origin; these must be distinguished from the neurogenic causes (Table 370-5). **Neurocardiogenic and cardiac syncope are considered in Chap. 21.**

APPROACH TO THE PATIENT:
Orthostatic Hypotension and Other ANS Disorders

The first step in the evaluation of symptomatic OH is the exclusion of treatable causes. The history should include a review of medications that may affect the autonomic system (Table 370-6). The main classes of drugs that may cause OH are diuretics, antihypertensives, antidepressants, phenothiazines, ethanol, narcotics, insulin, dopamine agonists, barbiturates, and calcium channel blocking agents. However, the precipitation of OH by medications may also be the first sign of an underlying autonomic disorder. The history may reveal an underlying cause for symptoms (e.g., diabetes, Parkinson's disease) or specific underlying mechanisms (e.g., cardiac pump failure, reduced intravascular volume). The relationship of symptoms to meals (splanchnic pooling), standing on awakening in the morning (intravascular volume depletion), ambient warming (vasodilatation), or exercise (muscle arteriolar vasodilatation) should be sought.

Physical examination includes measurement of supine and standing pulse and BP. OH is defined as a sustained drop in systolic ($\geq$20 mmHg) or diastolic ($\geq$10 mmHg) BP within 3 min of standing. In nonneurogenic causes of OH (such as hypovolemia), the BP drop is accompanied by a compensatory increase in heart rate of >15 beats/min. An important clinical clue that the patient has neu-

TABLE 370-4 PREVALENCE OF ORTHOSTATIC HYPOTENSION IN DIFFERENT DISORDERS

Disorder	Prevalence
Aging	14–20%
Diabetic neuropathy	10%
Other autonomic neuropathies	10–50 per 100,000
Multiple system atrophy	5–15 per 100,000
Pure autonomic failure	10–30 per 100,000

TABLE 370-5 NONNEUROGENIC CAUSES OF ORTHOSTATIC HYPOTENSION

Cardiac pump failure	Venous pooling
Myocardial infarction	Alcohol
Myocarditis	Postprandial dilation of splanchnic
Constrictive pericarditis	vessel beds
Aortic stenosis	Vigorous exercise with dilation of
Tachyarrhythmias	skeletal vessel beds
Bradyarrhythmias	Heat: hot environment, hot showers
Salt-losing nephropathy	and baths, fever
Adrenal insufficiency	Prolonged recumbency or standing
Diabetes insipidus	Sepsis
Venous obstruction	Medications
Reduced intravascular volume	Antihypertensives
Straining or heavy lifting,	Diuretics
urination, defecation	Vasodilators: nitrates, hydralazine
Dehydration	Alpha- and beta-blocking agents
Diarrhea, emesis	CNS sedatives: barbiturates, opiates
Hemorrhage	Tricyclic antidepressants
Burns	Phenothiazines
Metabolic	
Adrenocortical insufficiency	
Hypoaldosteronism	
Pheochromocytoma	
Severe potassium depletion	

rogenic OH is the aggravation or precipitation of OH by autonomic stressors (such as a meal, hot tub/hot bath, and exercise). Neurologic evaluation should include mental status (to exclude neurodegenerative disorders), cranial nerves (impaired downgaze with progressive supranuclear palsy; abnormal pupils with Horner's or Adie's syndrome), motor tone (Parkinson's disease and parkinsonian syndromes), reflexes, and sensation (polyneuropathies). In patients without a clear diagnosis initially, follow-up clinical and laboratory evaluations may reveal the underlying cause.

Disorders of autonomic function should be considered in patients with symptoms of altered sweating (hyperhidrosis or hypohidrosis), gastroparesis (bloating, nausea, vomiting of old food), constipation, impotence, or bladder dysfunction (urinary frequency, hesitancy, or incontinence).

AUTONOMIC TESTING Autonomic function tests (Table 370-7) are helpful when the history and examination findings are inconclusive, to detect subclinical involvement, or to follow the course of an autonomic disorder.

Heart Rate Variation with Deep Breathing This is a test of parasympathetic function on cardiovascular reflexes, via the vagus nerve. Results are influenced by the subject's posture, rate and depth of respiration [6 breaths per minute and a forced vital capacity (FVC) >1.5 L are optimal], age, medications, and degree of

TABLE 370-6 SOME DRUGS THAT AFFECT AUTONOMIC FUNCTION

Symptom	Drug Class	Specific Examples
Impotence	Opioids	Tylenol #3
	Anabolic steroids	—
	Some antiarrhythmics	Prazosin
	Some antihypertensives	Clonidine
	Some diuretics	Benazepril
	Some SSRIs	Venlafaxine
Urinary retention	Opioids	Fentanyl
	Decongestants	Brompheniramine
		Diphenhydramine
Diaphoresis	Some antihypertensives	Amlodipine
	Some SSRIs	Citalopram
	Opioids	Morphine
Hypotension	Tricyclics	Amitriptyline
	Beta blockers	Propranolol
	Diuretics	HCTZ
	CCBs	Verapamil

Note: SSRIs, selective serotonin reuptake inhibitors; HCTZ, hydrochlorothiazide; CCBs, calcium channel blockers.

TABLE 370-7	NEURAL PATHWAYS UNDERLYING SOME STANDARDIZED AUTONOMIC TESTS	
Test Evaluated	**Procedure**	**Autonomic Function**
HRBD	6 deep breaths/min	Cardiovagal function
Valsalva ratio	Expiratory pressure, 40 mmHg for 10–15 s	Cardiovagal function
QSART	Axon-reflex test 4 limb sites	Postganglionic sudomotor function
BP$_{BB}$ to VM	BP$_{BB}$ response to VM	Adrenergic function: baroreflex adrenergic control of vagal and vasomotor function
HUT	BP$_{BB}$ and heart rate response to HUT	Adrenergic and cardiovagal responses to HUT

Note: HRDB, heart rate response to deep breathing; BP$_{BB}$, beat-to-beat blood pressure; QSART, quantitative sudomotor axon-reflex test; VM, Valsalva maneuver; HUT, head-up tilt.

hypocapnia. Interpretation of results requires comparison of test data with results from normal individuals collected under the same test conditions. For example, the lower limit of normal heart rate variation with deep breathing in persons <20 years is >15–20 beats/min, but for persons over age 60 it is 5–8 beats/min. Heart rate variation with deep breathing (respiratory sinus arrhythmia) is abolished by atropine but is unaffected by sympathetic blockade (e.g., propranolol).

Valsalva Response This response (Table 370-7) assesses the integrity of the baroreflex control of heart rate (parasympathetic) and BP (adrenergic). The response is obtained with the subject supine. A constant expiratory pressure of 40 mmHg is maintained for 15 s while measuring changes in heart rate and beat-to-beat BP. There are four phases of BP and heart rate response to the Valsalva maneuver. Phases I and III are mechanical and related to changes in intrathoracic and intraabdominal pressure. In early phase II, reduced venous return results in a fall in stroke volume and BP, counteracted by a combination of reflex tachycardia and increased total peripheral resistance. Increased total peripheral resistance arrests the BP drop ~5–8 s after the onset of the maneuver. Late phase II begins with a progressive rise in BP towards or above baseline. Venous return and cardiac output return to normal in phase IV. Persistent peripheral arteriolar vasoconstriction and increased cardiac adrenergic tone results in a temporary BP overshoot and phase IV bradycardia (mediated by the baroreceptor reflex).

Autonomic function during the Valsalva maneuver can be measured using beat-to-beat blood pressure or heart rate changes. The *Valsalva ratio* is defined as the maximum phase II tachycardia divided by the minimum phase IV bradycardia. The ratio reflects cardiovagal function.

Sudomotor Function Sweating is induced by release of ACh from sympathetic postganglionic fibers. The quantitative sudomotor axon reflex test (QSART) is a measure of regional autonomic function mediated by ACh-induced sweating. A reduced or absent response indicates a lesion of the postganglionic sudomotor axon. For example, sweating may be reduced in the legs as a result of peripheral neuropathy (e.g., diabetes) before other signs of autonomic dysfunction emerge. The thermoregulatory sweat test (TST) is a qualitative measure of regional sweat production in response to an elevation of body temperature. An indicator powder placed on the anterior surface of the body changes color with sweat production during temperature elevation. The pattern of color changes is a measure of regional sweat secretion. Combining TST and QSART results will determine the site of the lesion. A postganglionic lesion is present if both QSART and TST show absent sweating. In a preganglionic lesion, QSART is intact but TST shows anhidrosis. Measurement of galvanic skin responses in the limbs after an induced electrical potential is a simple qualitative test for detecting the presence or absence of sweating.

Orthostatic BP Recordings Beat-to-beat BP measurements determined in supine, 70° tilt, and tilt-back positions are useful to quantitate orthostatic failure of BP control. It is important to allow a 20-min period of supine rest before assessing changes in BP during tilting. The BP change combined with heart rate monitoring can be useful for the evaluation of patients with suspected OH, unexplained syncope, or to detect vagally mediated syncope.

Tilt Table Testing for Syncope The great majority of patients with syncope do not have autonomic failure. Tilt-table testing can be used to make the diagnosis of vasovagal syncope with sensitivity, specificity, and reproducibility. A standardized protocol is used that specifies the tilt apparatus, angle and duration of tilt, and procedure for provocation of vasodilation (e.g., sublingual or spray nitroglycerin). A positive nitroglycerin-stimulated test predicts recurrence of syncope. Recommendations for the performance of tilt study for syncope have been incorporated in consensus guidelines.

Pharmacologic Tests Pharmacologic assessments can help localize an autonomic defect to the CNS or the PNS. A useful method to evaluate the systemic adrenergic response is the measurement of plasma NE, first with the patient supine and then after standing for at least 5 min. Supine values are reduced in postganglionic disorders (such as autonomic neuropathy or pure autonomic failure) and may fail to increase in preganglionic or postganglionic disorders (e.g., multiple system atrophy).

Administration of tyramine (releases NE from postganglionic terminals) and phenylephrine (denervation supersensitivity—directly acting α_1 agonist) is used to evaluate postganglionic adrenergic function. In a postganglionic lesion, the response to tyramine is reduced and there is an excessive response to subthreshold doses of phenylephrine. Other strategies include ganglionic blockade with trimethaphan (greater fall in resulting BP with a preganglionic lesion) or administration of arginine vasopressin (to evaluate afferent central pathways).

SPECIFIC SYNDROMES OF ANS DYSFUNCTION

MULTIPLE SYSTEM ATROPHY

Multiple system atrophy (MSA) is an uncommon entity that comprises autonomic failure (OH and/or a neurogenic bladder are required for diagnosis) combined with either striatonigral degeneration (Shy-Drager syndrome) or sporadic olivopontocerebellar atrophy (Chap. 366). The Parkinsonism is usually unassociated with rest tremor and is not responsive to levodopa. Levodopa-induced dyskinesia is also uncommon. Autonomic function tests can usually differentiate MSA from Parkinson's disease; the severity and distribution of autonomic failure are more severe and generalized in MSA. Cardiac postganglionic adrenergic innervation, measured as labeled metaiodobenzylguanidine (MIBG) uptake on single photon emission computed tomography or fluorodopamine on positron emission tomography, is markedly impaired in the dysautonomia of Parkinson's disease but is normal in MSA.

MSA generally progresses relentlessly to death 7–10 years after onset. Neuropathologic changes include neuronal loss and gliosis in many CNS regions, including the brainstem, cerebellum, striatum, and intermediolateral cell column of the thoracolumbar spinal cord.

Autonomic dysfunction is a common feature in dementia with Lewy bodies (Chap. 365); the severity is usually less than that found in MSA or Parkinson's disease.

SPINAL CORD

Spinal cord lesions from any cause may result in focal autonomic deficits or autonomic hyperreflexia. Spinal cord transection or hemisection may be attended by autonomic hyperreflexia affecting bowel, bladder, sexual, temperature-regulation, or cardiovascular functions. Dangerous increases or decreases in body temperature may result from an inability to experience the sensory accompaniments of heat or cold exposure below the level of the injury. Quadriparetic patients exhibit both supine hypertension and OH after upward tilting. Markedly increased autonomic discharge can be elicited by stimulation of the bladder, skin, or muscles; suprapubic palpation of the bladder, a distended bladder, catheter insertion, catheter obstruction, or urinary infection are common and correctable precipitants. This phenomenon, termed *autonomic dysreflexia*, affects 85% of patients with a traumatic spinal cord lesion above the C6 level. In patients with supine hypertension, BP can be lowered by tilting the head upward. Vasodilator drugs may be used to treat acute elevations in BP. Clonidine is used prophylactically to reduce the hypertension resulting from bladder stimulation. Sudden, dramatic increases in BP can lead to intracranial hemorrhage and death.

PERIPHERAL NERVE AND NEUROMUSCULAR JUNCTION DISORDERS

Peripheral neuropathies (Chap. 379) are the most common cause of chronic autonomic insufficiency. Neuropathies that affect small myelinated and unmyelinated fibers of the sympathetic and parasympathetic nerves commonly occur in diabetes mellitus, amyloidosis, chronic alcoholism, porphyria, and Guillain-Barré syndrome. Neuromuscular junction disorders accompanied by autonomic involvement include botulism and Lambert-Eaton syndrome.

Diabetes Mellitus Autonomic neuropathy typically begins ~10 years after the onset of diabetes (Chap. 338) and slowly progresses. The earliest autonomic abnormalities, typically asymptomatic, consist of vagal disturbances, which can be detected as reduced heart rate variation with deep breathing, and loss of distal sudomotor function, detected by QSART. Loss of small myelinated and unmyelinated nerve fibers in the splanchnic distribution, carotid sinus, and vagus nerves is characteristic. In advanced disease, widespread enteric neuropathy can cause profound disturbances in gut motility (*gastroparesis*), nausea and vomiting, malnutrition, achlorhydria, and bowel incontinence. Other symptoms can include impotence, urinary incontinence, pupillary abnormalities, and OH. Typical symptoms and signs of hypoglycemia may fail to appear because damage to the sympathetic innervation of the adrenal gland can result in a lack of epinephrine release. Insulin increases flow through arteriovenous shunts and may also aggravate OH. Autonomic dysfunction may lengthen the QT interval, increasing the risk of sudden death due to cardiac arrhythmia. Hyperglycemia appears to be a direct risk factor for autonomic involvement in diabetes. Biochemical and pharmacologic studies in diabetic neuropathy are compatible with autonomic failure localized to the PNS.

Amyloidosis Autonomic neuropathy occurs in both sporadic and familial forms of amyloidosis (Chap. 324). The AL (immunoglobulin light chain) type is associated with primary amyloidosis or amyloidosis secondary to multiple myeloma. The ATTR type, with transthyretin as the primary protein component, is responsible for the most common form of inherited amyloidosis. Although patients usually present with a distal painful neuropathy accompanied by sensory loss, autonomic insufficiency can precede the development of the polyneuropathy or occur in isolation. Diagnosis can be made by protein electrophoresis of blood and urine, tissue biopsy (abdominal fat pad, rectal mucosa, or sural nerve) to search for amyloid deposits, and genetic testing for transthyretin in familial cases. Treatment of familial cases with liver transplantation can be successful. The response of primary amyloidosis to melphalan and stem cell transplantation has been mixed. Death is usually due to cardiac or renal involvement. Postmortem studies reveal amyloid deposition in many organs, including two sites that contribute to autonomic failure: intraneural blood vessels and autonomic ganglia. Pathologic examination reveals a loss of unmyelinated and myelinated nerve fibers.

Alcoholic Neuropathy Abnormalities in parasympathetic vagal and efferent sympathetic function are usually mild in individuals with alcoholic polyneuropathy. Pathologic changes can be demonstrated in the parasympathetic (vagus) and sympathetic fibers, and in ganglia. OH is usually due to brainstem involvement. Impotence is a major problem, but concurrent gonadal hormone abnormalities may ob-

scure the parasympathetic component. Clinical symptoms of autonomic failure generally appear when the polyneuropathy is severe, and there is usually coexisting Wernicke's encephalopathy (Chap. 269). Autonomic involvement may contribute to the high mortality rates associated with alcoholism (Chap. 387).

Porphyria Although each of the porphyrias can cause autonomic dysfunction, the condition is most extensively documented in the acute intermittent type (Chap. 352). Autonomic symptoms include tachycardia, sweating, urinary retention, hypertension, or (less commonly) hypotension. Other prominent symptoms include anxiety, abdominal pain, nausea, and vomiting. Abnormal autonomic function can occur both during acute attacks and during remissions. Elevated catecholamine levels during acute attacks correlate with the degree of tachycardia and hypertension that is present.

Guillain-Barré Syndrome (Chap. 380) BP fluctuations and arrhythmias can be severe. It is estimated that between 2 and 10% of patients with severe Guillain-Barré syndrome suffer fatal cardiovascular collapse. Gastrointestinal autonomic involvement, sphincter disturbances, abnormal sweating, and pupillary dysfunction also occur. Demyelination has been described in the vagus and glossopharyngeal nerves, the sympathetic chain, and the white rami communicantes. Interestingly, the degree of autonomic involvement appears to be independent of the severity of motor or sensory neuropathy.

Autoimmune Autonomic Neuropathy This disorder presents with the subacute development of autonomic failure with OH, enteric neuropathy (gastroparesis, ileus, constipation/diarrhea), and cholinergic failure; the latter consists of loss of sweating, sicca complex, and a tonic pupil. Autoantibodies against the ganglionic ACh receptor (A$_3$ AChR) are present in the serum of many patients and are now considered to be diagnostic of this syndrome. In general, the antibody titer correlates with the severity of autonomic failure. Symptoms of cholinergic failure are also associated with a high antibody titer. Onset of the neuropathy follows a viral infection in approximately half of cases. Some patients appear to respond to immunotherapy. The spectrum of autoimmune autonomic neuropathy (AAN) is now broader than originally thought; some antibody-positive cases have an insidious onset and slow progression with a pure autonomic failure (see below) phenotype. A recent report describes a dramatic clinical response to repeated plasma exchange combined with immunosuppression in a patient with longstanding AAN.

AAN can have a paraneoplastic basis (Chap. 97). The clinical features of the autonomic neuropathy may be indistinguishable from the nonparaneoplastic form, or a coexisting paraneoplastic syndrome, such as cerebellar involvement or dementia, may be present (see Tables 97-2 and 97-3). The neoplasm may be truly occult and possibly suppressed by the autoantibody.

Botulism Botulinum toxin binds presynaptically to cholinergic nerve terminals and, after uptake into the cytosol, blocks ACh release. Manifestations consist of motor paralysis and autonomic disturbances that include blurred vision, dry mouth, nausea, unreactive or sluggishly reactive pupils, constipation, and urinary retention (Chap. 134).

PURE AUTONOMIC FAILURE (PAF)

This sporadic syndrome consists of postural hypotension, impotence, bladder dysfunction, and defective sweating. The disorder begins in the middle decades and occurs in women more often than men. The symptoms can be disabling, but the disease does not shorten life span. The clinical and pharmacologic characteristics suggest primary involvement of postganglionic sympathetic neurons. There is a severe reduction in the density of neurons within sympathetic ganglia that results in low supine plasma NE levels and noradrenergic supersensitivity. Some studies have questioned the specificity of PAF as a distinct clinical entity. Some cases are ganglionic antibody–positive and thus represent a type of AAN. Between 10 and 15% of cases evolve into MSA.

POSTURAL ORTHOSTATIC TACHYCARDIA SYNDROME (POTS)

This syndrome is characterized by symptomatic orthostatic intolerance (not OH) and by either an increase in heart rate to >120 beats/min or an increase of 30 beats/min with standing that subsides on sitting or lying down. Women are affected approximately five times more often than men, and most develop the syndrome between the ages of 15 and 50. Approximately half of affected patients report an antecedent viral infection. Syncopal symptoms (lightheadedness, weakness, blurred vision) combined with symptoms of autonomic overactivity (palpitations, tremulousness, nausea) are common. Recurrent unexplained episodes of dysautonomia and fatigue also occur. The pathogenesis is unclear in most cases; hypovolemia, venous pooling, impaired brainstem regulation, or β-receptor supersensitivity may play a role. In one affected individual, a mutation in the NE transporter, which resulted in impaired NE clearance from synapses, was responsible. Some cases are due to an underlying limited autonomic neuropathy. Although ~80% of patients improve, only one-quarter eventually resume their usual daily activities (including exercise and sports). Expansion of fluid volume and postural training (see Rx: Autonomic Failure) are initial approaches to treatment. If these approaches are inadequate, then midodrine, fludrocortisone, phenobarbital, beta blockers, or clonidine may be used with some success.

INHERITED DISORDERS

There are five known hereditary sensory and autonomic neuropathies (HSAN I–V). The most important ones are HSAN I and HSAN III (Riley-Day syndrome; familial dysautonomia). HSAN I is dominantly inherited and often presents as a distal small-fiber neuropathy (burning feet syndrome). The responsible gene, on chromosome 9q, is designated *SPTLC1*. SPTLC is an important enzyme in the regulation of ceramide. Cells from HSAN I patients affected by mutation of *SPTLC1* produce higher-than-normal levels of glucosyl ceramide, perhaps triggering apoptosis.

HSAN III, an autosomal recessive disorder of infants and children that occurs among Ashkenazi Jews, is much less prevalent than HSAN I. Decreased tearing, hyperhidrosis, reduced sensitivity to pain, areflexia, absent fungiform papillae on the tongue, and labile BP may be present. Episodic abdominal crises and fever are common. Pathologic examination of nerves reveals a loss of small myelinated and unmyelinated nerve fibers. The defective gene, named *IKBKAP*, is also located on the long arm of chromosome 9. Pathogenic mutations may prevent normal transcription of important molecules in neural development.

PRIMARY HYPERHIDROSIS

This syndrome presents with excess sweating of the palms of the hands and soles of the feet. The disorder affects 0.6–1.0% of the population; the etiology is unclear, but there may be a genetic component. While not dangerous, the condition can be socially embarrassing (e.g., shaking hands) or disabling (e.g., inability to write without soiling the paper). Onset of symptoms is usually in adolescence; the condition tends to improve with age. Topical antiperspirants are occasionally helpful. More useful are potent anticholinergic drugs such as glycopyrrolate (1–2 mg po tid). T2 ganglionectomy or sympathectomy is successful in >90% of patients with palmar hyperhidrosis. The advent of endoscopic transaxillary T2 sympathectomy has lowered the complication rate of the procedure. The most common postoperative complication is compensatory hyperhidrosis, which improves spontaneously over months; other potential complications include recurrent hyperhidrosis (16%), Horner's syndrome (<2%), gustatory sweating, wound infection, hemothorax, and intercostal neuralgia. Local injection of botulinum toxin has also been used to block cholinergic, postganglionic sympathetic fibers to sweat glands in patients with palmar hyperhidrosis. This approach is limited by the need for repetitive injections (the effect usually lasts 4 months before waning), pain with injection, the high cost of botulinum toxin, and the possibility of temporary intrinsic hand muscle weakness.

ACUTE AUTONOMIC SYNDROMES

The physician may be confronted occasionally with an acute autonomic syndrome, either acute autonomic failure (acute AAN syndrome) or a state of sympathetic overactivity. An *autonomic storm* is an acute state of sustained sympathetic surge that results in variable combinations of alterations in blood pressure and heart rate, body temperature, respiration and sweating. Causes of autonomic storm are brain and spinal cord injury, toxins and drugs, autonomic neuropathy, and chemodectomas (e.g., pheochromocytoma).

Brain injury is most commonly a cause of autonomic storm following severe head trauma (with diffuse axonal injury) and in post-resuscitation encephalopathy following anoxic-ischemic brain insult. Autonomic storm can also occur with other acute intracranial lesions such as hemorrhage, cerebral infarction, rapidly expanding tumors, subarachnoid hemorrhage, hydrocephalus, or (less commonly) an acute spinal cord lesion. Lesions involving the diencephalon may be more prone to present with dysautonomia, but the most consistent setting is that of an acute intracranial catastrophe of sufficient size and rapidity to produce a massive catecholaminergic surge. The surge can cause seizures, neurogenic pulmonary edema, and myocardial injury. Manifestations include fever, tachycardia, hypertension, tachypnea, hyperhidrosis, pupillary dilatation, and flushing.

Drugs and toxins may also be responsible, including sympathomimetics such as phenylpropanolamine, cocaine, amphetamines, and tricyclic antidepressants; tetanus; and, less often, botulinum. Phenylpropanolamine, now off the market, was in the past a potent cause of this syndrome. Cocaine, including "crack," can cause a hypertensive state with CNS hyperstimulation. Tricyclic overdose, such as amitriptyline, can cause flushing, hypertension, tachycardia, fever, mydriasis, anhidrosis, and a toxic psychosis. *Neuroleptic malignant syndrome* refers to a syndrome of muscle rigidity, hyperthermia, and hypertension in psychotic patients treated with phenothiazines.

The hyperadrenergic state with Guillain-Barré syndrome can produce a moderate autonomic storm. Pheochromocytoma presents with a paroxysmal or sustained hyperadrenergic state, headache, hyperhidrosis, palpitations, anxiety, tremulousness, and hypertension.

Management of autonomic storm includes ruling out other causes of autonomic instability, including malignant hyperthermia, porphyria, and epilepsy. Sepsis and encephalitis need to be excluded with appropriate studies. EEG should be done to detect epileptiform activity; MRI of the brain and spine are often necessary. The patient should be managed in an intensive care unit. Management with morphine sulphate (10 mg every 4 h) and labetalol (100–200 mg twice daily) have worked relatively well. Treatment may need to be maintained for several weeks.

MISCELLANEOUS

Other conditions associated with autonomic failure include infections, poisoning (organophosphates), malignancy, and aging. Disorders of the hypothalamus can affect autonomic function and produce abnormalities in temperature control, satiety, sexual function, and circadian rhythms (Chap. 333).

REFLEX SYMPATHETIC DYSTROPHY AND CAUSALGIA

The failure to identify a primary role of the ANS in the pathogenesis of these disorders has resulted in a change of nomenclature. Complex regional pain syndrome (CRPS) types I and II are now used in place of reflex sympathetic dystrophy (RSD) and causalgia, respectively.

CRPS type I is a regional pain syndrome that usually develops after tissue trauma. Examples of associated trauma include myocardial infarction, minor shoulder or limb injury, and stroke. *Allodynia* (the perception of a nonpainful stimulus as painful), *hyperpathia* (an exaggerated pain response to a painful stimulus), and spontaneous pain occur. The symptoms are unrelated to the severity of the initial trauma and are not confined to the distribution of a single peripheral nerve. CRPS type II is a regional pain syndrome that develops after injury to a peripheral nerve, usually a major nerve trunk. Spontaneous pain initially develops within the territory of the affected nerve but eventually may spread outside the nerve distribution.

Pain is the primary clinical feature of CRPS. Vasomotor dysfunction, sudomotor abnormalities, or focal edema may occur alone or in combination but must be present for diagnosis. Limb pain syndromes that do not meet these criteria are best classified as "limb pain—not otherwise specified." In CRPS, localized sweating (increased resting sweat output) and changes in blood flow may produce temperature differences between affected and unaffected limbs.

CRPS type I (RSD) has classically been divided into three clinical phases but is now considered to be more variable. Phase I consists of pain and swelling in the distal extremity occurring within weeks to 3 months after the precipitating event. The pain is diffuse, spontaneous, and either burning, throbbing, or aching in quality. The involved extremity is warm and edematous, and the joints are tender. Increased sweating and hair growth develop. In phase II (3–6 months after onset), thin, shiny, cool skin appears. After an additional 3–6 months (phase III), atrophy of the skin and subcutaneous tissue plus flexion contractures complete the clinical picture.

The natural history of typical CRPS may be more benign than reflected in the literature. A variety of surgical and medical treatments have been developed, with conflicting reports of efficacy. Clinical trials suggest that early mobilization with physical therapy or a brief course of glucocorticoids may be helpful for CRPS type I. Other medical treatments include the use of adrenergic blockers, nonsteroidal anti-inflammatory drugs, calcium channel blockers, phenytoin, opioids, and calcitonin. Stellate ganglion blockade is a commonly used invasive therapeutic technique that often provides temporary pain relief, but the efficacy of repetitive blocks is uncertain.

℞ AUTONOMIC FAILURE

Management of autonomic failure is aimed at specific treatment of the cause and alleviation of symptoms. Of particular importance is the removal of drugs or amelioration of underlying conditions that cause or aggravate the autonomic symptoms, especially in the elderly. For instance, OH can be caused or aggravated by angiotensin-converting enzyme inhibitors, calcium channel blocking agents, tricyclic antidepressants, levodopa, alcohol, or insulin. A summary of drugs that can cause OH by class, putative mechanism, and magnitude of the BP drop, is shown in Table 370-6.

PATIENT EDUCATION OH can be asymptomatic or symptomatic. Neurogenic OH requires treatment, but only a minority of patients require pharmacologic treatment. All patients should be taught the mechanisms of postural normotension (volume status, resistance and capacitance bed, autoregulation) and the nature of orthostatic stressors (time of day and the influence of meals, heat, standing, and exercise). Patients should learn to recognize orthostatic symptoms early in their evolution (especially subtle cognitive symptoms, weakness, and fatigue) and to modify activities that provoke episodes. Other helpful measures may include keeping a BP log, dietary education (salt/fluids), and recognizing medications and situations to avoid. Learning physical countermaneuvers that reduce standing OH, practicing postural and resistance training, and learning to manage worsening OH in specific situations and at specific times are helpful measures.

SYMPTOMATIC TREATMENT Nonpharmacologic approaches are summarized in **Table 370-8**. Adequate intake of salt and fluids to produce a voiding volume between 1.5 and 2.5 L of urine (containing >170 meq of Na+) each 24 h is essential. Sleeping with the head of the bed elevated will minimize the effects of supine nocturnal hypertension. Prolonged recumbency should be avoided when possible. Patients are advised to sit with legs dangling over the edge of the bed for several minutes before attempting to stand in the morning; other postural stresses should be similarly approached in a gradual manner. Physical countermaneuvers that can reduce OH include leg-crossing, with maintained contraction of leg muscles for 30 s. Such maneuvers compress leg veins and increase systemic resistance. Compressive garments, such as compression stockings and

TABLE 370-8	INITIAL TREATMENT OF ORTHOSTATIC HYPOTENSION (OH)

Patient education: mechanisms and stressors of OH
High-salt diet (10–20 g/d)
High-fluid intake (2 L/D)
Elevate head of bed 10 cm (4 in.)
Maintain postural stimuli
Learn physical countermaneuvers
Compression garments
Correct anemia

abdominal binders, are helpful on occasion but uncomfortable for some patients. Anemia should be corrected with erythropoietin, administered subcutaneously at doses of 25–75 U/kg three times per week. The hematocrit increases after 2–6 weeks. A weekly maintenance dose is usually necessary. The increased intravascular volume that accompanies the rise in hematocrit can exacerbate supine hypertension.

If these measures are not sufficient, drug treatment may be necessary. Midodrine is effective, but at higher doses it can aggravate supine hypertension. The drug is a directly acting α_1-agonist that does not cross the blood-brain barrier. It has a duration of action of 2–4 h. The usual dose is 5–10 mg orally tid, but some patients respond best to a decremental dose (e.g., 15 mg on awakening, 10 mg at noon, and 5 mg in the afternoon). Midodrine should not be taken after 6 P.M. Side effects include pruritus, uncomfortable piloerection, and supine hypertension. Pyridostigmine appears to improve OH without aggravating supine hypertension by enhancing ganglionic transmission (maximal when orthostatic, minimal supine). Fludrocortisone will reduce OH, but it aggravates supine hypertension. At doses between 0.1 mg/d and 0.3 mg bid orally, it enhances renal sodium conservation and increases the sensitivity of arterioles to NE. Susceptible patients may develop fluid overload, congestive heart failure, supine hypertension, or hypokalemia. Potassium supplements are often necessary with chronic administration of fludrocortisone. Sustained elevations of supine BP >180/110 mmHg should be avoided.

Postprandial OH may respond to several measures. Frequent, small, low-carbohydrate meals may diminish splanchnic shunting of blood after meals and reduce postprandial OH. Prostaglandin inhibitors (ibuprofen or indomethacin) taken with meals or midodrine (10 mg with the meal) can be helpful. The somatostatin analogue octreotide can be useful in the treatment of postprandial syncope by inhibiting the release of gastrointestinal peptides that have vasodilator and hypotensive effects. The subcutaneous dose ranges from 25 μg bid to 100–200 μg tid.

The patient should be taught to self-treat transient worsening of OH. Drinking two 250-mL (8-oz) glasses of water can raise standing BP 20–30 mmHg for about 2 h, beginning ~20 min after the fluid load. The patient can increase intake of salt and fluids (bouillon treatment), increase use of physical countermaneuvers, temporarily resort to a full-body stocking (compression pressure 30–40 mmHg), or increase the dose of midodrine. Supine hypertension (>180/110 mmHg) can be self-treated by avoiding the supine position and reducing fludrocortisone. A daily glass of wine, if requested by the patient, can be taken shortly before bedtime. If these simple measures are not adequate, drugs to be considered include oral hydralazine (25 mg qhs), oral procardia (10 mg qhs), or a nitroglycerin patch.

FURTHER READINGS

SCHROEDER C et al: Plasma exchange for primary autoimmune autonomic failure. N Engl J Med 353:1585, 2005

THAISETTHAWATKUL P et al: Autonomic dysfunction in dementia with Lewy bodies. Neurology 62:1804, 2004

THIEBEN MJ et al: Postural orthostatic tachycardia syndrome: The Mayo clinic experience. Mayo Clin Proc 82:308, 2007

VINIK AI, ZIEGLER D: Diabetic cardiovascular autonomic neuropathy. Circulation 115:387, 2007

371 Trigeminal Neuralgia, Bell's Palsy, and Other Cranial Nerve Disorders

M. Flint Beal, Stephen L. Hauser

Symptoms and signs of cranial nerve pathology are common in internal medicine. They often develop in the context of a widespread neurologic disturbance, and in such situations cranial nerve involvement may represent the initial manifestation of the illness. In other disorders, involvement is largely restricted to one or several cranial nerves; these distinctive disorders are reviewed in this chapter. Disorders of ocular movement are discussed in Chap. 29, disorders of hearing in Chap. 30, and vertigo and disorders of vestibular function in Chap. 22.

FACIAL PAIN OR NUMBNESS

ANATOMIC CONSIDERATIONS

The trigeminal (fifth cranial) nerve supplies sensation to the skin of the face and anterior half of the head (Fig. 371-1). Its motor part innervates the masseter and pterygoid masticatory muscles.

TRIGEMINAL NEURALGIA (TIC DOULOUREUX)

Clinical Manifestations Trigeminal neuralgia is characterized by excruciating paroxysms of pain in the lips, gums, cheek, or chin and, very rarely, in the distribution of the ophthalmic division of the fifth nerve. The pain seldom lasts more than a few seconds or a minute or two but may be so intense that the patient winces, hence the term *tic*. The paroxysms, experienced as single jabs or clusters, tend to recur frequently, both day and night, for several weeks at a time. They may occur spontaneously or with movements of affected areas evoked by speaking, chewing, or smiling. Another characteristic feature is the presence of trigger zones, typically on the face, lips, or tongue, that provoke attacks; patients may report that tactile stimuli—e.g. washing the face, brushing the teeth, or exposure to a draft of air—generate excruciating pain. *An essential feature of trigeminal neuralgia is that objective signs of sensory loss cannot be demonstrated on examination.*

Trigeminal neuralgia is relatively common, with an estimated annual incidence of 4.5 per 100,000 individuals. Middle-aged and elderly persons are affected primarily, and ~60% of cases occur in women. Onset is typically sudden, and bouts tend to persist for weeks or months before remitting spontaneously. Remissions may be long-lasting, but in most patients the disorder ultimately recurs.

FIGURE 371-1 The three major sensory divisions of the trigeminal nerve consist of the ophthalmic, maxillary, and mandibular nerves.

Pathophysiology Symptoms result from ectopic generation of action potentials in pain-sensitive afferent fibers of the fifth cranial nerve root just before it enters the lateral surface of the pons. Compression or other pathology in the nerve leads to demyelination of large myelinated fibers that do not themselves carry pain sensation but become hyperexcitable and electrically coupled with smaller unmyelinated or poorly myelinated pain fibers in close proximity; this may explain why tactile stimuli, conveyed via the large myelinated fibers, can stimulate paroxysms of pain. Compression of the trigeminal nerve root by a blood vessel, most often the superior cerebellar artery or on occasion a tortuous vein, is the source of trigeminal neuralgia in a substantial proportion of patients. In cases of vascular compression, age-related brain sagging and increased vascular thickness and tortuosity may explain the prevalence of trigeminal neuralgia in later life.

Differential Diagnosis Trigeminal neuralgia must be distinguished from other causes of face and head pain (Chap. 15) and from pain arising from diseases of the jaw, teeth, or sinuses. Pain from migraine or cluster headache tends to be deep-seated and steady, unlike the superficial stabbing quality of trigeminal neuralgia; rarely, cluster headache is associated with trigeminal neuralgia, a syndrome known as *cluster-tic*. In temporal arteritis, superficial facial pain is present but is not typically shocklike, the patient frequently complains of myalgias and other systemic symptoms, and an elevated erythrocyte sedimentation rate (ESR) is usually present (Chap. 319). When trigeminal neuralgia develops in a young adult or is bilateral, multiple sclerosis is a key consideration, and in such cases the cause is a demyelinating plaque at the root entry zone of the fifth nerve in the pons; often, evidence of facial sensory loss can be found on careful examination. Cases that are secondary to mass lesions—such as aneurysms, neurofibromas, acoustic schwannomas, or meningiomas—usually produce objective signs of sensory loss in the trigeminal nerve distribution (trigeminal neuropathy, see below).

Laboratory Evaluation An ESR is indicated if temporal arteritis is suspected. In typical cases of trigeminal neuralgia, neuroimaging studies are usually unnecessary but may be valuable if multiple sclerosis is a consideration or in assessing overlying vascular lesions in order to plan for decompression surgery.

℞ TRIGEMINAL NEURALGIA

Drug therapy with carbamazepine is effective in ~50–75% of patients. Carbamazepine should be started as a single daily dose of 100 mg taken with food and increased gradually (by 100 mg daily every 1–2 days) until substantial (>50%) pain relief is achieved. Most patients require a maintenance dose of 200 mg qid. Doses >1200 mg daily provide no additional benefit. Dizziness, imbalance, sedation, and rare cases of agranulocytosis are the most important side effects of carbamazepine. If treatment is effective, it is usually continued for 1 month and then tapered as tolerated. If carbamazepine is not well tolerated or is ineffective, phenytoin, 300–400 mg daily, can be tried; other anticonvulsants may also be effective. Baclofen may also be administered, either alone or in combination with carbamazepine or phenytoin. The initial dose is 5–10 mg tid, gradually increasing as needed to 20 mg qid.

If drug treatment fails, surgical therapy should be offered. The most widely applied procedure creates a heat lesion of the trigeminal (gasserian) ganglion or nerve, a method termed *radiofrequency thermal rhizotomy*. This procedure produces short-term relief in >95% of patients; however, long-term studies indicate that pain recurs in up to one-third of treated patients. These procedures result in partial numbness of the face, sometimes with unpleasant dysesthesias. Masseter (jaw) weakness is another potential complication, especially following bilateral procedures. When used for first-division trigeminal neuralgia, there is also a risk of corneal denervation with secondary keratitis.

Gamma knife radiosurgery is also utilized for treatment and results in complete pain relief in more than two-thirds of patients; the response is often long-lasting. Compared with thermal rhizotomy, gamma knife surgery appears to be somewhat less effective but has a lower risk of serious complications.

A third surgical treatment, microvascular decompression to relieve pressure on the trigeminal nerve as it exits the pons, requires a suboccipital craniotomy. This procedure has a >70% efficacy rate and a low rate of pain recurrence in responders; in a small number of cases, there is perioperative damage to the eighth or seventh cranial nerves or to the cerebellum. High-resolution magnetic resonance angiography is useful preoperatively to visualize the relationships between the fifth cranial nerve root and nearby blood vessels.

TRIGEMINAL NEUROPATHY

A variety of diseases may affect the trigeminal nerve (Table 371-1). Most present with sensory loss on the face or with weakness of the jaw muscles. Deviation of the jaw on opening indicates weakness of the pterygoids on the side to which the jaw deviates. Some cases are due to Sjögren's syndrome or a collagen-vascular disease such as systemic lupus erythematosus, scleroderma, or mixed connective tissue disease. Among infectious causes, herpes zoster and leprosy should be considered. Tumors of the middle cranial fossa (meningiomas), of the trigeminal nerve (schwannomas), or of the base of the skull (metastatic tumors) may cause a combination of motor and sensory signs. Lesions in the cavernous sinus can affect the first and second divisions of the trigeminal nerve, and lesions of the superior orbital fissure can affect the first (ophthalmic) division; the accompanying corneal anesthesia increases the risk of ulceration (neurokeratitis).

Loss of sensation over the chin (mental neuropathy) can be the only manifestation of systemic malignancy. Rarely, an idiopathic form of trigeminal neuropathy is observed. It is characterized by numbness and paresthesias, sometimes bilaterally, with loss of sensation in the territory of the trigeminal nerve but without weakness of the jaw. Gradual recovery is the rule. Tonic spasm of the masticatory muscles, known as *trismus*, is symptomatic of tetanus (Chap. 133) or may occur in patients treated with phenothiazine drugs.

FACIAL WEAKNESS

ANATOMIC CONSIDERATIONS

(Fig. 371-2) The seventh cranial nerve supplies all the muscles concerned with facial expression. The sensory component is small (the nervus intermedius); it conveys taste sensation from the anterior two-thirds of the tongue and probably cutaneous impulses from the anterior wall of the external auditory canal. The motor nucleus of the seventh nerve lies anterior and lateral to the abducens nucleus. After leaving the pons, the seventh nerve enters the internal auditory meatus with the acoustic nerve. The nerve continues its course in its own bony channel, the facial canal, and exits from the skull via the stylomastoid foramen. It then passes through the parotid gland and subdivides to supply the facial muscles.

A complete interruption of the facial nerve at the stylomastoid foramen paralyzes all muscles of facial expression. The corner of the mouth droops, the creases and skinfolds are effaced, the forehead is unfurrowed, and the eyelids will not close. Upon attempted closure of the lids, the eye on the paralyzed side rolls upward (*Bell's phenomenon*). The lower lid sags and falls away from the conjunctiva, permitting tears to spill over the cheek. Food collects between the teeth and lips, and saliva may dribble from the corner of the mouth. The patient complains of a heaviness or numbness in the face, but sensory loss is rarely demonstrable and taste is intact.

If the lesion is in the middle-ear portion, taste is lost over the anterior two-thirds of the tongue on the same side. If the nerve to the stapedius is interrupted, there is hyperacusis (sensitivity to loud sounds). Lesions in the internal auditory meatus may affect the adjacent auditory and vestibular nerves, causing deafness, tinnitus, or dizziness. Intrapontine lesions that paralyze the face usually affect the abducens nucleus as well, and often the corticospinal and sensory tracts.

If the peripheral facial paralysis has existed for some time and recovery of motor function is incomplete, a continuous

diffuse contraction of facial muscles may appear. The palpebral fissure becomes narrowed, and the nasolabial fold deepens. Attempts to move one group of facial muscles may result in contraction of all (associated movements, or *synkinesis*). Facial spasms, initiated by movements of the face, may develop (*hemifacial spasm*). Anomalous regeneration of seventh nerve fibers may result in other troublesome phenomena. If fibers originally connected with the orbicularis oculi come to innervate the orbicularis oris, closure of the lids may cause a retraction of the mouth, or if fibers originally connected with muscles of the face later innervate the lacrimal gland, anomalous tearing ("crocodile tears") may occur with any activity of the facial muscles, such as eating. Another facial synkinesia is triggered by jaw opening, causing closure of the eyelids on the side of the facial palsy (jaw-winking).

BELL'S PALSY

The most common form of facial paralysis is *Bell's palsy*. The annual incidence of this idiopathic disorder is ~25 per 100,000 annually, or about 1 in 60 persons in a lifetime.

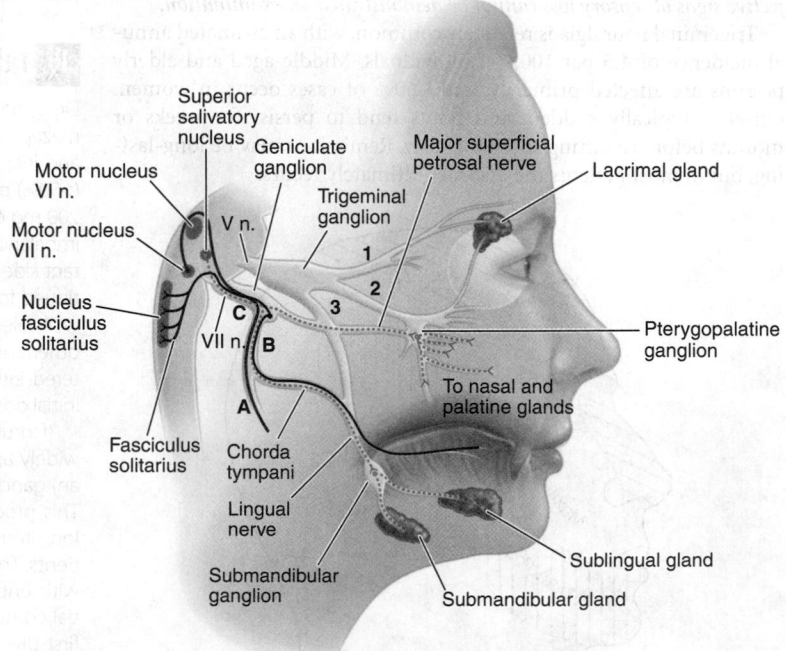

FIGURE 371-2 The facial nerve. A, B, and C denote lesions of the facial nerve at the stylomastoid foramen, distal and proximal to the geniculate ganglion, respectively. Green lines indicate the parasympathetic fibers, red line indicates motor fibers, and purple lines indicate visceral afferent fibers (taste). (*Adapted from Carpenter.*)

FIGURE 371-3 Axial and coronal T1 weighted images post-Gadolinium with fat suppression demonstrate diffuse smooth linear enhancement of the left facial nerve, involving the genu, tympanic, and mastoid segments within the temporal bone (*arrows*), without evidence of mass lesion. Although highly suggestive of Bell's palsy, similar findings may be seen with other etiologies such as Lyme disease, sarcoidosis, and perineural malignant spread.

Clinical Manifestations The onset of Bell's palsy is fairly abrupt, maximal weakness being attained by 48 h as a general rule. Pain behind the ear may precede the paralysis for a day or two. Taste sensation may be lost unilaterally, and hyperacusis may be present. In some cases there is mild cerebrospinal fluid lymphocytosis. MRI may reveal swelling and uniform enhancement of the geniculate ganglion and facial nerve and, in some cases, entrapment of the swollen nerve in the temporal bone. Approximately 80% of patients recover within a few weeks or months. Electromyography may be of some prognostic value; evidence of denervation after 10 days indicates there has been axonal degeneration, that there will be a long delay (3 months as a rule) before regeneration occurs, and that it may be incomplete. The presence of incomplete paralysis in the first week is the most favorable prognostic sign.

Pathophysiology Bell's palsy is associated with the presence of herpes simplex virus (HSV) type 1 DNA in endoneurial fluid and posterior auricular muscle, suggesting that a reactivation of this virus in the geniculate ganglion may be responsible. However, a causal role for HSV in Bell's palsy is unproven. An increased incidence of Bell's palsy was also reported among recipients of inactivated intranasal influenza vaccine, and it was hypothesized that this could have resulted from the *Escherichia coli* enterotoxin used as adjuvant or to reactivation of latent virus.

Differential Diagnosis There are many other causes of acute facial palsy that must be considered in the differential diagnosis of Bell's palsy. Lyme disease can cause unilateral or bilateral facial palsies; in endemic areas, 10% or more of cases of facial palsy are likely due to infection with *Borrelia burgdorferi* (Chap. 166). The *Ramsay Hunt syndrome*, caused by reactivation of herpes zoster in the geniculate ganglion, consists of a severe facial palsy associated with a vesicular eruption in the external auditory canal and sometimes in the pharynx and other parts of the cranial integument; often the eighth cranial nerve is affected as well. Facial palsy that is often bilateral occurs in sarcoidosis (Chap. 322) and in *Guillain-Barré syndrome* (Chap. 380). Leprosy frequently involves the facial nerve, and facial neuropathy may also occur in diabetes mellitus, connective tissue diseases including Sjögren's syndrome, and amyloidosis. The rare *Melkersson-Rosenthal syndrome* consists of recurrent facial paralysis; recurrent—and eventually permanent—facial (particularly labial) edema; and, less constantly, plication of the tongue. Its cause is unknown. *Acoustic neuromas* frequently involve the facial nerve by local compression. Infarcts, demyelinating lesions of multiple sclerosis, and tumors are the common pontine lesions that interrupt the facial nerve fibers; other signs of brainstem involvement are usually present. Tumors that invade the temporal bone (carotid body, cholesteatoma, dermoid) may produce a facial palsy, but the onset is insidious and the course progressive.

All these forms of nuclear or peripheral facial palsy must be distinguished from the supranuclear type. In the latter, the frontalis and orbicularis oculi muscles are involved less than those of the lower part of the face, since the upper facial muscles are innervated by corticobulbar pathways from both motor cortices, whereas the lower facial muscles are innervated only by the opposite hemisphere. In supranuclear lesions there may be a dissociation of emotional and voluntary facial movements and often some degree of paralysis of the arm and leg, or an aphasia (in dominant hemisphere lesions) is present.

Laboratory Evaluation The diagnosis of Bell's palsy can usually be made clinically in patients with (1) a typical presentation, (2) no risk factors or preexisting symptoms for other causes of facial paralysis, (3) absence of cutaneous lesions of herpes zoster in the external ear canal, and (4) a normal neurologic examination with the exception of the facial nerve. Particular attention to the eighth cranial nerve, which courses near to the facial nerve in the pontomedullary junction and in the temporal bone, and to other cranial nerves is essential. In atypical or uncertain cases, an ESR, testing for diabetes mellitus, a Lyme titer, angiotensin-converting enzyme and chest imaging studies for possible sarcoidosis, a lumbar puncture for possible Guillain-Barré syndrome, or MRI scanning may be indicated. MRI often shows swelling and enhancement of the facial nerve in idiopathic Bell's palsy (Fig. 371-3).

℞ BELL'S PALSY

Symptomatic measures include (1) the use of paper tape to depress the upper eyelid during sleep and prevent corneal drying, and (2) massage of the weakened muscles. A course of glucocorticoids, given as prednisone 60–80 mg daily during the first 5 days and then tapered over the next 5 days, appears to shorten the recovery period and modestly improve the functional outcome. A recently published randomized trial found no added benefit of acyclovir (400 mg five times daily for 10 days) compared to prednisolone alone for treatment of acute Bell's palsy; the value of valacyclovir (usual dose 1000 mg daily for 5–7 days) either alone or in combination with glucocorticoids is not known.

OTHER MOTOR DISORDERS OF THE FACE

Hemifacial spasm consists of painless irregular involuntary contractions on one side of the face. Symptoms may develop as a sequela to Bell's palsy but may also be due to an irritative lesion of the facial nerve (e.g., an acoustic neuroma, an aberrant artery that compresses the nerve, or a basilar artery aneurysm). However, in the most common form of hemifacial spasm, the cause and pathology are unknown. Mild cases can be treated with carbamazepine, gabapentin, or, if these drugs fail, with baclofen. Local injections of botulinum toxin into affected muscles can relieve spasms for 3–4 months, and the injections can be repeated. Refractory cases due to vascular compression usually respond to surgical decompression of the facial nerve. *Blepharospasm* is an involuntary recurrent spasm of both eyelids that usually occurs in elderly persons as an isolated phenomenon or with varying degrees of spasm of other facial muscles. Severe, persistent cases of blepharospasm can be treated by local injection of botulinum toxin into the orbicularis oculi. *Facial myokymia* refers to a fine rippling activity of the facial muscles; it may be caused by multiple sclerosis or follow Guillain-Barré syndrome (Chap. 380).

TABLE 371-2 CRANIAL NERVE SYNDROMES

Site	Cranial Nerves	Usual Cause
Sphenoid fissure (superior orbital)	III, IV, first division V, VI	Invasive tumors of sphenoid bone; aneurysms
Lateral wall of cavernous sinus	III, IV, first division V, VI, often with proptosis	Infection, thrombosis, aneurysm, or fistula of cavernous sinus; invasive tumors from sinuses and sella turcica; benign granuloma responsive to glucocorticoids
Retrosphenoid space	II, III, IV, V, VI	Large tumors of middle cranial fossa
Apex of petrous bone	V, VI	Petrositis; tumors of petrous bone
Internal auditory meatus	VII, VIII	Tumors of petrous bone (dermoids, etc.); infectious processes; acoustic neuroma
Pontocerebellar angle	V, VII, VIII, and sometimes IX	Acoustic neuroma; meningioma
Jugular foramen	IX, X, XI	Tumors and aneurysms
Posterior laterocondylar space	IX, X, XI, XII	Tumors of parotid gland and carotid body and metastatic tumors
Posterior retroparotid space	IX, X, XI, XII and Horner syndrome	Tumors of parotid gland, carotid body, lymph nodes; metastatic tumor; tuberculous adenitis

Facial hemiatrophy occurs mainly in women and is characterized by a disappearance of fat in the dermal and subcutaneous tissues on one side of the face. It usually begins in adolescence or early adult years and is slowly progressive. In its advanced form, the affected side of the face is gaunt, and the skin is thin, wrinkled, and brown. The facial hair may turn white and fall out, and the sebaceous glands become atrophic. Bilateral involvement may occur. A limited form of systemic sclerosis (scleroderma) may be the cause of some cases. Treatment is cosmetic, consisting of transplantation of skin and subcutaneous fat.

OTHER CRANIAL NERVE DISORDERS

GLOSSOPHARYNGEAL NEURALGIA

This form of neuralgia involves the ninth (glossopharyngeal) and sometimes portions of the tenth (vagus) cranial nerves. It resembles trigeminal neuralgia in many respects but is much less common. The pain is intense and paroxysmal; it originates on one side of the throat, approximately in the tonsillar fossa. In some cases the pain is localized in the ear or may radiate from the throat to the ear because of involvement of the tympanic branch of the glossopharyngeal nerve. Spasms of pain may be initiated by swallowing or coughing. There is no demonstrable motor or sensory deficit; the glossopharyngeal nerve supplies taste sensation to the posterior third of the tongue and, together with the vagus nerve, sensation to the posterior pharynx. Cardiac symptoms—bradycardia or asystole, hypotension, and fainting—have been reported. Medical therapy is similar to that for trigeminal neuralgia, and carbamazepine is generally the first choice. If drug therapy is unsuccessful, surgical procedures—including microvascular decompression if vascular compression is evident—or rhizotomy of glossopharyngeal and vagal fibers in the jugular bulb is frequently successful.

Very rarely, herpes zoster involves the glossopharyngeal nerve. Glossopharyngeal neuropathy in conjunction with vagus and accessory nerve palsies may also occur with a tumor or aneurysm in the posterior fossa or in the jugular foramen. Hoarseness due to vocal cord paralysis, some difficulty in swallowing, deviation of the soft palate to the intact side, anesthesia of the posterior wall of the pharynx, and weakness of the upper part of the trapezius and sternocleidomastoid muscles make up the jugular foramen syndrome (Table 371-2).

DYSPHAGIA AND DYSPHONIA

When the intracranial portion of one vagus (tenth cranial) nerve is interrupted, the soft palate droops ipsilaterally and does not rise in phonation. There is loss of the gag reflex on the affected side, as well as of the "curtain movement" of the lateral wall of the pharynx, whereby the faucial pillars move medially as the palate rises in saying "ah." The voice is hoarse and slightly nasal, and the vocal cord lies immobile

midway between abduction and adduction. Loss of sensation at the external auditory meatus and the posterior pinna may also be present.

The pharyngeal branches of both vagal nerves may be affected in diphtheria; the voice has a nasal quality, and regurgitation of liquids through the nose occurs during the act of swallowing.

The vagus nerve may be involved at the meningeal level by neoplastic and infectious processes and within the medulla by tumors, vascular lesions (e.g., the lateral medullary syndrome), and motor neuron disease. This nerve may be involved by infection with herpes zoster virus. Polymyositis and dermatomyositis, which cause hoarseness and dysphagia by direct involvement of laryngeal and pharyngeal muscles, may be confused with diseases of the vagus nerves. Dysphagia is also a symptom in some patients with myotonic dystrophy. **Nonneurologic causes of dysphagia are discussed in Chap. 38.**

The recurrent laryngeal nerves, especially the left, are most often damaged as a result of intrathoracic disease. Aneurysm of the aortic arch, an enlarged left atrium, and tumors of the mediastinum and bronchi are much more frequent causes of an isolated vocal cord palsy than are intracranial disorders. However, a substantial number of cases of recurrent laryngeal palsy remain idiopathic.

When confronted with a case of laryngeal palsy, the physician must attempt to determine the site of the lesion. If it is intramedullary, there are usually other signs, such as ipsilateral cerebellar dysfunction, loss of pain and temperature sensation over the ipsilateral face and contralateral arm and leg, and an ipsilateral Horner syndrome. If the lesion is extramedullary, the glossopharyngeal and spinal accessory nerves are frequently involved (jugular foramen syndrome). If it is extracranial in the posterior laterocondylar or retroparotid space, there may be a combination of ninth, tenth, eleventh, and twelfth cranial nerve palsies and a Horner syndrome (Table 371-2). If there is no sensory loss over the palate and pharynx and no palatal weakness or dysphagia, the lesion is below the origin of the pharyngeal branches, which leave the vagus nerve high in the cervical region; the usual site of disease is then the mediastinum.

NECK WEAKNESS

Isolated involvement of the accessory (eleventh cranial) nerve can occur anywhere along its route, resulting in partial or complete paralysis of the sternocleidomastoid and trapezius muscles. More commonly, involvement occurs in combination with deficits of the ninth and tenth cranial nerves in the jugular foramen or after exit from the skull (Table 371-2). An idiopathic form of accessory neuropathy, akin to Bell's palsy, has been described, and it may be recurrent in some cases. Most but not all patients recover.

TONGUE PARALYSIS

The hypoglossal (twelfth cranial) nerve supplies the ipsilateral muscles of the tongue. The nucleus of the nerve or its fibers of exit may be involved by intramedullary lesions such as tumor, poliomyelitis, or most often motor neuron disease. Lesions of the basal meninges and the occipital bones (platybasia, invagination of occipital condyles, Paget's disease) may compress the nerve in its extramedullary course or in the hypoglossal canal. Isolated lesions of unknown cause can occur. Atrophy and fasciculation of the tongue develop weeks to months after interruption of the nerve.

MULTIPLE CRANIAL NERVE PALSIES

Several cranial nerves may be affected by the same disease process. In this situation, the main clinical problem is to determine whether the lesion lies within the brainstem or outside it. Lesions that lie on the surface of the brainstem are characterized by involvement of adjacent cranial nerves (often occurring in succession) and late and rather slight involvement of the long sensory and motor pathways and segmental structures lying within the brainstem. The opposite is true of primary lesions within the brainstem. The extramedullary lesion is more likely to cause bone erosion or enlargement of the foramens of exit of cranial nerves. The intramedullary lesion involving cranial nerves often produces a crossed sensory or motor paralysis (cranial nerve signs on one side of the body and tract signs on the opposite side).

Involvement of multiple cranial nerves outside the brainstem is frequently the result of diabetes or trauma, localized infections such as herpes zoster, infectious and noninfectious (especially carcinomatous) causes of meningitis (Chaps. 376 and 377), granulomatous diseases such as Wegener's granulomatosis, Behçet's disease, enlarging saccular aneurysms, or tumors. Among the tumors, nasopharyngeal cancers, lymphomas, neurofibromas, meningiomas, chordomas, cholesteatomas, carcinomas, and sarcomas have all been observed to involve a succession of lower cranial nerves. Owing to their anatomic relationships, the multiple cranial nerve palsies form a number of distinctive syndromes, listed in Table 371-2. Sarcoidosis is the cause of some cases of multiple cranial neuropathy, and chronic glandular tuberculosis the cause of a few others. Platybasia, basilar invagination of the skull, and the adult Chiari malformation are additional causes. A purely motor disorder without atrophy always raises the question of myasthenia gravis (Chap. 381). As noted above, Guillain-Barré syndrome commonly affects the facial nerves bilaterally. In the Fisher variant of the Guillain-Barré syndrome, oculomotor paresis occurs with ataxia and areflexia in the limbs (Chap. 380). Wernicke encephalopathy can cause a severe ophthalmoplegia combined with other brainstem signs.

The *cavernous sinus syndrome* (Fig. 371-4) is a distinctive and frequently life-threatening disorder. It often presents as orbital or facial pain; orbital swelling and chemosis due to occlusion of the ophthalmic veins; fever; oculomotor neuropathy affecting the third, fourth, and sixth cranial nerves; and trigeminal neuropathy affecting the ophthalmic (V_1) and occasionally the maxillary (V_2) divisions of the trigeminal nerve. Cavernous sinus thrombosis, often secondary to infection from orbital cellulitis (frequently *Staphylococcus aureus*), a cutaneous source on the face, or sinusitis (especially with mucormycosis in diabetic patients), is the most frequent cause; other etiologies include aneurysm of the carotid artery, a carotid-cavernous fistula (orbital bruit may be present), meningioma, nasopharyngeal carcinoma, other tumors, or an idiopathic granulomatous disorder (Tolosa-Hunt syndrome). The two cavernous sinuses directly communicate via intercavernous channels; thus, involvement on one side may extend to become bilateral. Early diagnosis is essential, especially when due to infection, and treatment depends on the underlying etiology. In infectious cases, prompt administration of broad-spectrum antibiotics, drainage of any abscess cavities, and identification of the offending organism are essential. Anticoagulant

FIGURE 371-4 Anatomy of the cavernous sinus in coronal section, illustrating the location of the cranial nerves in relation to the vascular sinus, internal carotid artery (which loops anteriorly to the section), and surrounding structures.

therapy may benefit cases of primary thrombosis. Repair or occlusion of the carotid artery may be required for treatment of fistulas or aneurysms. The Tolosa-Hunt syndrome generally responds to glucocorticoids. A dramatic improvement in pain is usually evident within a few days; oral prednisone (60 mg daily) is usually continued for several weeks and then gradually tapered.

An idiopathic form of multiple cranial nerve involvement on one or both sides of the face is occasionally seen. The syndrome consists of a subacute onset of boring facial pain, followed by paralysis of motor cranial nerves. The clinical features overlap those of the Tolosa-Hunt syndrome and appear to be due to idiopathic inflammation of the dura mater, which may be visualized by MRI. The syndrome is frequently responsive to glucocorticoids.

ACKNOWLEDGMENT
The authors acknowledge the contributions of Dr. Joseph B. Martin to this chapter in previous editions.

FURTHER READINGS

ALBERTON DL, ZED PJ: Bell's palsy: A review of treatment using antiviral agents. Ann Pharmacother 40:1838, 2006

GILDEN DH: Clinical practice. Bell's Palsy. N Engl J Med 351:13, 2004

GROGAN PM, GRONSETH GS: Practice parameter: Steroids, acyclovir, and surgery for Bell's palsy (an evidence-based review). Report of the Quality Standards Subcommittee of the American Academy of Neurology. Neurology 56:830, 2001

HATO N et al: Valacyclovir and prednisolone treatment for Bell's palsy: A randomized, placebo-controlled study. Otol Neurotol 28:408, 2007

LOVE S, COAKHAM HB: Trigeminal neuralgia: Pathology and pathogenesis. Brain 124:2347, 2002

PEARCE JMS: Glossopharyngeal neuralgia. Eur Neurol 55:49, 2006

SULLIVAN FM et al: Early treatment with prednisolone or acyclovir in Bell's palsy. N Engl J Med 357:1598, 2007

SWEENEY CJ, GILDEN DH: Ramsay Hunt syndrome. J Neurol Neurosurg Psychiatry 71:149, 2001

372 Diseases of the Spinal Cord
Stephen L. Hauser, Allan H. Ropper

Diseases of the spinal cord are frequently devastating. They produce quadriplegia, paraplegia, and sensory deficits far beyond the damage they would inflict elsewhere in the nervous system because the spinal cord contains, in a small cross-sectional area, almost the entire motor output and sensory input of the trunk and limbs. Many spinal cord diseases are reversible if recognized and treated at an early stage (Table 372-1); thus, they are among the most critical of neurologic emergencies. The efficient use of diagnostic procedures, guided by knowledge of the anatomy and the clinical features of spinal cord diseases, is required for a successful outcome.

APPROACH TO THE PATIENT:
Spinal Cord Disease

SPINAL CORD ANATOMY RELEVANT TO CLINICAL SIGNS The spinal cord is a thin, tubular extension of the central nervous system contained within the bony spinal canal. It originates at the medulla and continues caudally to the conus medullaris at the lumbar level; its fibrous extension, the filum terminale, terminates at the coccyx. The adult spinal cord is ~46 cm (18 in.) long, oval in shape, and enlarged in the cervical and lumbar regions, where neurons that innervate the upper and lower extremities, respectively, are located. The white matter tracts containing ascending sensory and descending motor pathways are located peripherally, whereas nerve cell bodies are clustered in an inner region shaped like a four-leaf clover that surrounds the central canal (anatomically an extension of the fourth ventricle). The membranes that cover the spinal cord—the pia, arachnoid, and dura—are continuous with those of the brain.

The spinal cord has 31 segments, each defined by an exiting ventral motor root and entering dorsal sensory root. During embryologic development, growth of the cord lags behind that of the vertebral column, and the mature spinal cord ends at approximately the first lumbar vertebral body. The lower spinal nerves take an increasingly downward course to exit via intervertebral foramina. The first seven pairs of cervical spinal nerves exit above the same-numbered vertebral bodies, whereas all the subsequent nerves exit below the same-numbered vertebral bodies because of the presence of eight cervical spinal cord segments but only seven cervical vertebrae. The relationship between spinal cord segments and the corresponding vertebral bodies is shown in Table 372-2. These relationships assume particular importance for localization of lesions that cause spinal cord compression. A T10 spinal cord sensory level, for example, indicates involvement of the cord adjacent to the seventh or eighth thoracic vertebral body (Figs. 25-2 and 25-3). In addition, at every level the main ascending and descending tracts are somatotopically organized with a laminated distribution that reflects the origin or destination of nerve fibers.

Determining the Level of the Lesion The presence of a horizontally defined level below which sensory, motor, and autonomic function is impaired is a hallmark of spinal cord disease. This *sensory level* is sought by asking the patient to identify a pinprick or cold stimulus (e.g., a dry tuning fork after immersion in cold water) applied to the proximal legs and lower trunk and sequentially moved up toward the neck on each side. The sensory level indicates damage to the spinothalamic tract one to two segments above the perceived level of a unilateral spinal cord lesion and at the level of a bilateral lesion. That is the result of the ascent of second-order sensory fibers, which originate in the dorsal horn, proceed to cross anterior to the central canal while ascending to join the opposite spinothalamic tract. Lesions that transect the descending corticospinal and other motor tracts cause paraplegia or quadriplegia, with the evolution over time of increased muscle tone, heightened

TABLE 372-1 TREATABLE SPINAL CORD DISORDERS

Compressive
  Epidural, intradural, or intramedullary neoplasm
  Epidural abscess
  Epidural hemorrhage
  Cervical spondylosis
  Herniated disc
  Posttraumatic compression by fractured or displaced vertebra or
    hemorrhage
Vascular
  Arteriovenous malformation
  Antiphospholipid syndrome and other hypercoagulable states
Inflammatory
  Multiple sclerosis
  Neuromyelitis optica
  Transverse myelitis
  Sarcoidosis
  Vasculitis
Infectious
  Viral: VZV, HSV-1 and -2, CMV, HIV, HTLV-I, others
  Bacterial and mycobacterial: *Borrelia*, *Listeria*, syphilis, others
  Mycoplasma pneumoniae
  Parasitic: schistosomiasis, toxoplasmosis
Developmental
  Syringomyelia
  Meningomyelocoele
  Tethered cord syndrome
Metabolic
  Vitamin B_{12} deficiency (subacute combined degeneration)
  Copper deficiency

Note: VZV, varicella-zoster virus; HSV, herpes simplex virus; CMV, cytomegalovirus; HTLV, human T cell lymphotropic virus.

deep tendon reflexes, and Babinski signs (the upper motor neuron syndrome). Such lesions also typically produce autonomic disturbances consisting of absent sweating below the implicated cord level and bladder, bowel, and sexual dysfunction.

The uppermost level of a spinal cord lesion can also be localized by attention to the *segmental signs* corresponding to disturbed motor or sensory innervation by an individual cord segment. A band of altered sensation (hyperalgesia or hyperpathia) at the upper end of the sensory disturbance, fasciculations or atrophy in muscles innervated by one or several segments, or a muted or absent deep tendon reflex may be noted at this level. These signs also occur with focal root or peripheral nerve disorders; thus, segmental signs are most useful when they occur together with signs of long tract damage. With severe and acute transverse lesions, the limbs initially may be flaccid rather than spastic. This state of "spinal shock" lasts for several days, rarely for weeks, and should not be mistaken for extensive damage to many segments of the cord or for an acute polyneuropathy.

The main features of transverse damage at each level of the spinal cord are summarized below.

Cervical Cord Upper cervical cord lesions produce quadriplegia and weakness of the diaphragm. Lesions at C4-C5 produce quadriplegia; at C5-C6, there is loss of power and reflexes in the biceps; at C7 weakness is found only in finger and wrist extensors and triceps; and at C8, finger and wrist flexion are impaired. Horner's syndrome (miosis, ptosis, and facial hypohidrosis) may accompany a cervical cord lesion at any level.

TABLE 372-2 SPINAL CORD LEVELS RELATIVE TO THE VERTEBRAL BODIES

Spinal Cord Level	Corresponding Vertebral Body
Upper cervical	Same as cord level
Lower cervical	1 level higher
Upper thoracic	2 levels higher
Lower thoracic	2 to 3 levels higher
Lumbar	T10-T12
Sacral	T12-L1

Thoracic Cord Lesions here are localized by the sensory level on the trunk and by the site of midline back pain if it accompanies the syndrome. Useful markers for localization are the nipples (T4) and umbilicus (T10). Leg weakness and disturbances of bladder and bowel function accompany the paralysis. Lesions at T9-T10 paralyze the lower—but not the upper—abdominal muscles, resulting in upward movement of the umbilicus when the abdominal wall contracts (*Beevor's sign*).

Lumbar Cord Lesions at the L2-L4 spinal cord levels paralyze flexion and adduction of the thigh, weaken leg extension at the knee, and abolish the patellar reflex. Lesions at L5-S1 paralyze only movements of the foot and ankle, flexion at the knee, and extension of the thigh, and abolish the ankle jerks (S1).

Sacral Cord/Conus Medullaris The conus medullaris is the tapered caudal termination of the spinal cord, comprising the lower sacral and single coccygeal segments. The conus syndrome is distinctive, consisting of bilateral saddle anesthesia (S3-S5), prominent bladder and bowel dysfunction (urinary retention and incontinence with lax anal tone), and impotence. The bulbocavernosus (S2-S4) and anal (S4-S5) reflexes are absent (Chap. 361). Muscle strength is largely preserved. By contrast, lesions of the cauda equina, the cluster of nerve roots derived from the lower cord, are characterized by low back and radicular pain, asymmetric leg weakness and sensory loss, variable areflexia in the lower extremities, and relative sparing of bowel and bladder function. Mass lesions in the lower spinal canal often produce a mixed clinical picture in which elements of both cauda equina and conus medullaris syndromes coexist. Cauda equina syndromes are also discussed in Chap. 16.

Special Patterns of Spinal Cord Disease The location of the major ascending and descending pathways of the spinal cord are shown in Fig. 372-1. Most fiber tracts—including the posterior columns and the spinocerebellar and pyramidal tracts—are situated on the side of the body they innervate. However, afferent fibers mediating pain and temperature sensation ascend in the spinothalamic tract contralateral to the side they supply. The anatomic configurations of these tracts produce characteristic syndromes that provide clues to the underlying disease process.

Brown-Sequard Hemicord Syndrome This consists of ipsilateral weakness (corticospinal tract) and loss of joint position and vibratory sense (posterior column), with contralateral loss of pain and temperature sense (spinothalamic tract) one or two levels below the lesion. Segmental signs, such as radicular pain, muscle atrophy, or loss of a deep tendon reflex, are unilateral. This classical pattern is rare, and partial forms are more commonly encountered.

Central Cord Syndrome The central cord syndrome results from damage to the gray matter nerve cells and crossing spinothalamic tracts near the central canal. In the cervical cord, the central cord syndrome produces arm weakness out of proportion to leg weakness and a "dissociated" sensory loss, signify-ing a loss of pain and temperature sense in a cape distribution over the shoulders, lower neck, and upper trunk in contrast to preservation of light touch, joint position, and vibration sense in these regions. Trauma, syringomyelia, tumors, and anterior spinal artery ischemia (including from aortic dissection) are the main causes.

Anterior Spinal Artery Syndrome Infarction of the cord is generally the result of occlusion or diminished flow in this artery. The result is extensive bilateral tissue destruction that spares the posterior columns. All spinal cord functions—motor, sensory, and autonomic—are lost below the level of the lesion, with the striking exception of retained vibration and position sensation.

Foramen Magnum Syndrome Lesions in this area interrupt decussating pyramidal tract fibers destined for the legs, which cross caudal to those of the arms, resulting in weakness of the legs (*crural paresis*). Compressive lesions near the foramen magnum may produce weakness of the ipsilateral shoulder and arm followed by weakness of the ipsilateral leg, then the contralateral leg, and finally the contralateral arm, an "around the clock" pattern that may begin in any of the four limbs. There is typically suboccipital pain spreading to the neck and shoulders.

Intramedullary and Extramedullary Syndromes It is useful to differentiate *intramedullary* processes, arising within the substance of the cord, from *extramedullary* ones that compress the spinal cord or its vascular supply. The differentiating features are only relative and serve as clinical guides. With extramedullary lesions, radicular pain is often prominent, and there is early sacral sensory loss (lateral spinothalamic tract) and spastic weakness in the legs (corticospinal tract) due to the superficial location of leg fibers in the corticospinal tract. Intramedullary lesions tend to produce poorly localized burning pain rather than radicular pain and spare sensation in the perine-

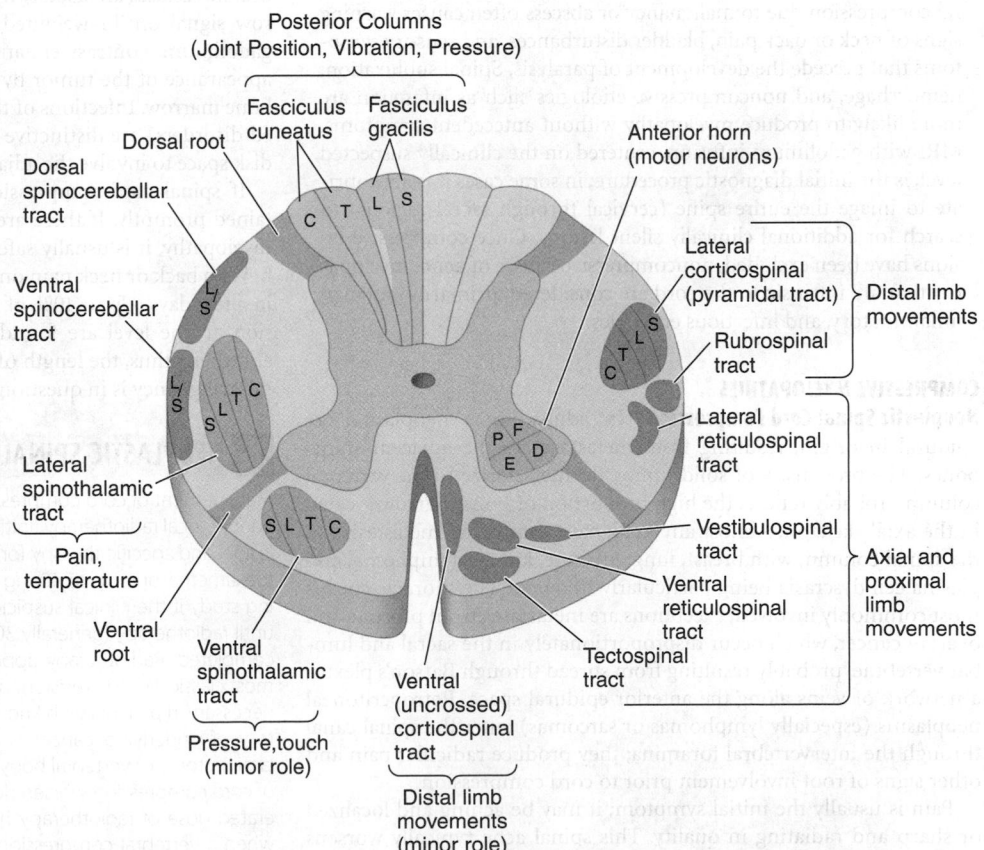

Posterior Columns
(Joint Position, Vibration, Pressure)

Fasciculus cuneatus   Fasciculus gracilis
Dorsal root
Dorsal spinocerebellar tract
Ventral spinocerebellar tract
Lateral spinothalamic tract
Pain, temperature
Ventral root
Ventral spinothalamic tract
Pressure, touch (minor role)
Ventral (uncrossed) corticospinal tract
Distal limb movements (minor role)

Anterior horn (motor neurons)
Lateral corticospinal (pyramidal tract) — Distal limb movements
Rubrospinal tract
Lateral reticulospinal tract
Vestibulospinal tract — Axial and proximal limb movements
Ventral reticulospinal tract
Tectospinal tract

FIGURE 372-1 Transverse section through the spinal cord, composite representation, illustrating the principal ascending (**left**) and descending (**right**) pathways. The lateral and ventral spinothalamic tracts ascend contralateral to the side of the body that is innervated. C, cervical; T, thoracic; L, lumbar; S, sacral; P, proximal; D, distal; F, flexors; E, extensors.

CHAPTER 372 Diseases of the Spinal Cord

al and sacral areas ("sacral sparing"), reflecting the laminated configuration of the spinothalamic tract with sacral fibers outermost; corticospinal tract signs appear later. Regarding extramedullary lesions, a further distinction is made between extradural and intradural masses, as the former are generally malignant and the latter benign (neurofibroma being a common cause). Consequently, a long duration of symptoms favors an intradural origin.

ACUTE AND SUBACUTE SPINAL CORD DISEASES

The initial symptoms of disease that evolve over days or weeks are focal neck or back pain, followed by various combinations of paresthesias, sensory loss, motor weakness, and sphincter disturbance evolving over hours to several days. There may be only mild sensory symptoms or a devastating functional transection of the cord. Partial lesions selectively involve the posterior columns or anterior spinothalamic tracts or are limited to one side of the cord. Paresthesias or numbness typically begins in the feet and ascends symmetrically or asymmetrically. These symptoms initially simulate Guillain-Barré syndrome, but involvement of the trunk with a sharply demarcated spinal cord level indicates the myelopathic nature of the process. In severe and abrupt cases, areflexia reflecting spinal shock may be present, but hyperreflexia supervenes over days or weeks; persistent areflexic paralysis with a sensory level indicates necrosis over multiple segments of the spinal cord.

APPROACH TO THE PATIENT:
Compressive and Noncompressive Myelopathy

DISTINGUISHING COMPRESSIVE FROM NONCOMPRESSIVE MYELOPATHY The first priority is to exclude a treatable compression of the cord by a mass. The common causes are tumor, epidural abscess or hematoma, herniated disc, or vertebral pathology. Epidural compression due to malignancy or abscess often causes warning signs of neck or back pain, bladder disturbances, and sensory symptoms that precede the development of paralysis. Spinal subluxation, hemorrhage, and noncompressive etiologies such as infarction are more likely to produce myelopathy without antecedent symptoms. MRI with gadolinium infusion, centered on the clinically suspected level, is the initial diagnostic procedure; in some cases it is appropriate to image the entire spine (cervical through sacral regions) to search for additional clinically silent lesions. Once compressive lesions have been excluded, noncompressive causes of acute myelopathy that are intrinsic to the cord are considered, primarily vascular, inflammatory, and infectious etiologies.

COMPRESSIVE MYELOPATHIES
Neoplastic Spinal Cord Compression In adults, most neoplasms are epidural in origin, resulting from metastases to the adjacent spinal bones. The propensity of solid tumors to metastasize to the vertebral column probably reflects the high proportion of bone marrow located in the axial skeleton. Almost any malignant tumor can metastasize to the spinal column, with breast, lung, prostate, kidney, lymphoma, and plasma cell dyscrasia being particularly frequent. The thoracic cord is most commonly involved; exceptions are metastases from prostate and ovarian cancer, which occur disproportionately in the sacral and lumbar vertebrae, probably resulting from spread through Batson's plexus, a network of veins along the anterior epidural space. Retroperitoneal neoplasms (especially lymphomas or sarcomas) enter the spinal canal through the intervertebral foramina; they produce radicular pain and other signs of root involvement prior to cord compression.

Pain is usually the initial symptom; it may be aching and localized or sharp and radiating in quality. This spinal ache typically worsens with movement, coughing, or sneezing and characteristically awakens patients at night. A recent onset of persistent back pain, particularly if in the thoracic spine (which is uncommonly involved by spondylosis), should prompt consideration of vertebral metastasis. Rarely, pain is

FIGURE 372-2 Epidural spinal cord compression due to breast carcinoma. Sagittal T1-weighted (**A**) and T2-weighted (**B**) MRI scans through the cervicothoracic junction reveal an infiltrated and collapsed second thoracic vertebral body with posterior displacement and compression of the upper thoracic spinal cord. The low-intensity bone marrow signal in *A* signifies replacement by tumor.

mild or absent. Plain radiographs of the spine and radionuclide bone scans have only a limited role in diagnosis because they do not identify 15–20% of metastatic vertebral lesions and fail to detect paravertebral masses that reach the epidural space through the intervertebral foramina. MRI provides excellent anatomic resolution of the extent of spinal tumors (Fig. 372-2) and is able to distinguish between malignant lesions and other masses—epidural abscess, tuberculoma, or epidural hemorrhage, among others—that present in a similar fashion. Vertebral metastases are usually hypointense relative to a normal bone marrow signal on T1-weighted MRI scans; after the administration of gadolinium, contrast enhancement may deceptively "normalize" the appearance of the tumor by increasing its intensity to that of normal bone marrow. Infections of the spinal column (osteomyelitis and related disorders) are distinctive in that, unlike tumor, they may cross the disk space to involve the adjacent vertebral body.

If spinal cord compression is suspected, imaging should be obtained promptly. If there are radicular symptoms but no evidence of myelopathy, it is usually safe, if necessary, to defer imaging for 24–48 h. With back or neck pain only, imaging studies may be obtained within a few days. Up to 40% of patients who present with cord compression at one level are found to have asymptomatic epidural disease elsewhere; thus, the length of the spine should be imaged when epidural malignancy is in question.

℞ NEOPLASTIC SPINAL CORD COMPRESSION

Management of cord compression includes glucocorticoids to reduce cord edema, local radiotherapy (initiated as early as possible) to the symptomatic lesion, and specific therapy for the underlying tumor type. Glucocorticoids (dexamethasone, up to 40 mg daily) can be administered before the imaging study if the clinical suspicion is strong and continued at a lower dose until radiotherapy (generally 3000 cGy administered in 15 daily fractions) is completed. Radiotherapy appears to be as effective as surgery, even for most classically radioresistant metastases. Biopsy of the epidural mass is unnecessary in patients with known preexisting cancer but is indicated if a history of underlying cancer is lacking. Surgery, either decompression by laminectomy or vertebral body resection, should be considered when signs of cord compression worsen despite radiotherapy, when the maximum tolerated dose of radiotherapy has been delivered previously to the site, or when a vertebral compression fracture or spinal instability contributes to cord compression. A good response to radiotherapy can be expected in individuals who are ambulatory at presentation; new weakness is prevented, and some recovery of motor function occurs in approximately half of treated patients. Fixed motor deficits (paraplegia or quadriplegia), once estab-

FIGURE 372-3 MRI of a thoracic meningioma. Coronal T1-weighted post-contrast image through the thoracic spinal cord demonstrates intense and uniform enhancement of a well-circumscribed extramedullary mass (*arrows*) which displaces the spinal cord to the left.

lished for >12 h, do not usually improve, and beyond 48 h the prognosis for substantial motor recovery is poor.

In contrast to tumors of the epidural space, most intradural mass lesions are slow-growing and benign. Meningiomas and neurofibromas account for most of these, with occasional cases caused by chordoma, lipoma, dermoid, or sarcoma. Meningiomas (Fig. 372-3) are often located posterior to the thoracic cord or near the foramen magnum, although they can arise from the meninges anywhere along the spinal canal. Neurofibromas are benign tumors of the nerve sheath that typically arise near the posterior root; when multiple, neurofibromatosis is the likely etiology. Symptoms usually begin with radicular sensory symptoms followed by an asymmetric, progressive spinal cord syndrome. Therapy is by surgical resection.

Primary intramedullary tumors of the spinal cord are uncommon. They present as central cord or hemicord syndromes, often in the cervical region; there may be poorly localized burning pain in the extremities and sparing of sacral sensation. In adults, these lesions are ependymomas, hemangioblastomas, or low-grade astrocytomas (Fig. 372-4). Complete resection of an intramedullary ependymoma is often possible with microsurgical techniques. Debulking of an intramedullary astrocytoma can also be helpful, as these are often slowly growing lesions; the value of adjunctive radiotherapy and chemotherapy is uncertain. Secondary (metastatic) intramedullary tumors are also common, especially in patients with advanced metastatic disease (Chap. 374).

Spinal Epidural Abscess Spinal epidural abscess presents as a clinical triad of midline dorsal pain, fever, and progressive limb weakness. Prompt recognition of this distinctive process will in most cases prevent permanent sequelae. Aching pain is almost always present, either over the spine or in a radicular pattern. The duration of pain prior to presentation is generally ≤2 weeks but may on occasion be several months or longer. Fever is usual, accompanied by elevated white blood cell count and sedimentation rate. As the abscess expands, further spinal cord damage results from venous congestion and thrombosis. Once weakness and other signs of myelopathy appear, progression may be rapid. A more chronic sterile granulomatous form of abscess is also known, usually after treatment of an acute epidural infection.

Risk factors include an impaired immune status (diabetes mellitus, renal failure, alcoholism, malignancy), intravenous drug abuse, and in-

FIGURE 372-4 MRI of an intramedullary astrocytoma. Sagittal T1-weighted post-contrast image through the cervical spine demonstrates expansion of the upper cervical spine by a mass lesion emanating from within the spinal cord at the cervicomedullary junction. Irregular peripheral enhancement occurs within the mass (*arrows*).

fections of the skin or other tissues. Two-thirds of epidural infections result from hematogenous spread of bacteria from the skin (furunculosis), soft tissue (pharyngeal or dental abscesses), or deep viscera (bacterial endocarditis). The remainder arise from direct extension of a local infection to the subdural space; examples of local predisposing conditions are vertebral osteomyelitis, decubitus ulcers, lumbar puncture, epidural anesthesia, or spinal surgery. Most cases are due to *Staphylococcus aureus*; gram-negative bacilli, *Streptococcus*, anaerobes, and fungi can also cause epidural abscesses. Tuberculosis from an adjacent vertebral source, Pott's disease, remains an important cause in the underdeveloped world.

MRI scans (Fig. 372-5) localize the abscess and exclude other causes of myelopathy. Lumbar puncture is only required if encephalopathy or other clinical signs raise the question of associated meningitis, a feature that is found in <25% of cases. The level of the puncture should be planned to minimize the risk of meningitis due to passage of the needle through infected tissue or herniation due to decompression below an area of obstruction to the flow of cerebrospinal fluid (CSF). A high cervical tap is often the safest approach. CSF abnormalities in subdural abscess consist of pleocytosis with a preponderance of polymorphonuclear cells, an elevated protein level, and a reduced glucose

FIGURE 372-5 MRI of a spinal epidural abscess due to tuberculosis. ***A.*** Sagittal T2-weighted free spin-echo MR sequence. A hypointense mass replaces the posterior elements of C3 and extends epidurally to compress the spinal cord (*arrows*). ***B.*** Sagittal T1-weighted image after contrast administration reveals a diffuse enhancement of the epidural process (*arrows*) with extension into the epidural space.

level, but the responsible organism is not cultured unless there is associated meningitis. Blood cultures are positive in <25% of cases.

Rx SPINAL EPIDURAL ABSCESS

Treatment is by decompressive laminectomy with debridement combined with long-term antibiotic treatment. Surgical evacuation prevents development of paralysis and may improve or reverse paralysis in evolution, but it is unlikely to improve deficits of more than several days duration. Antibiotics should be started empirically before surgery and then modified on the basis of culture results; medication is continued for at least 4 weeks. If surgery is contraindicated or if there is a fixed paraplegia or quadriplegia that is unlikely to improve following surgery, long-term administration of systemic and oral antibiotics can be used; in such cases, the choice of antibiotics may be guided by results of blood cultures. However, paralysis may develop or progress during antibiotic therapy; thus, initial surgical management remains the treatment of choice unless the abscess is limited in size and causes few or no neurologic signs.

Spinal Epidural Hematoma Hemorrhage into the epidural (or subdural) space causes acute focal or radicular pain followed by variable signs of a spinal cord or conus medullaris disorder. Therapeutic anticoagulation, trauma, tumor, or blood dyscrasia are predisposing conditions. Rare cases complicate lumbar puncture or epidural anesthesia, sometimes in association with use of low-molecular-weight heparin. MRI and CT confirm the clinical suspicion and can delineate the extent of the bleeding. Treatment consists of prompt reversal of any underlying clotting disorder and surgical decompression. Surgery may be followed by substantial recovery, especially in patients with some preservation of motor function preoperatively. Because of the risk of hemorrhage, lumbar puncture should be avoided whenever possible in patients with severe thrombocytopenia or other coagulopathies.

Hematomyelia Hemorrhage into the substance of the spinal cord is a rare result of trauma, intraparenchymal vascular malformation (see below), vasculitis due to polyarteritis nodosa or systemic lupus erythematosus (SLE), bleeding disorders, or a spinal cord neoplasm. Hematomyelia presents as an acute painful transverse myelopathy. With large lesions, extension into the subarachnoid space may occur, resulting in subarachnoid hemorrhage (Chap. 269). Diagnosis is by MRI or CT. Therapy is supportive, and surgical intervention is generally not useful. An exception is hematomyelia due to an underlying vascular malformation, for which selective spinal angiography may be indicated, followed by surgery to evacuate the clot and remove the underlying vascular lesion.

NONCOMPRESSIVE MYELOPATHIES

The most frequent causes of noncompressive acute transverse myelopathy (ATM) are spinal cord infarction; systemic inflammatory disorders, including SLE and sarcoidosis; demyelinating diseases, including multiple sclerosis (MS) and neuromyelitis optica; postinfectious or idiopathic transverse myelitis, which is presumed to be an immune condition related to acute disseminated encephalomyelitis (Chap. 375); and infectious (primarily viral) causes. After spinal cord compression is excluded, the evaluation generally requires a lumbar puncture and a search for underlying systemic disease (Table 372-3).

Spinal Cord Infarction The cord is supplied by three arteries that course vertically over its surface: a single anterior spinal artery and paired posterior spinal arteries. In addition to the vertebral arteries, the anterior spinal artery is fed by radicular vessels that arise at C6, at an upper thoracic level, and, most consistently, at T11-L2 (artery of Adamkiewicz). At each segment, paired penetrating vessels branch from the anterior spinal artery to supply the anterior two-thirds of the spinal cord; the posterior spinal arteries, which often become less distinct below the midthoracic level, supply the posterior columns.

Spinal cord ischemia can occur at any level; however, the presence of the artery of Adamkiewicz creates a watershed of marginal blood flow in

TABLE 372-3	EVALUATION OF ACUTE TRANSVERSE MYELOPATHY

1. MRI of spinal cord with and without contrast (exclude compressive causes).
2. CSF studies: Cell count, protein, glucose, IgG index/synthesis rate, oligoclonal bands, VDRL; Gram's stain, acid-fast bacilli, and India ink stains; PCR for VZV, HSV-2, HSV-1, EBV, CMV, HHV-6, enteroviruses, HIV; antibody for HTLV-I, *B. burgdorferi*, *M. pneumoniae*, and *Chlamydia pneumoniae*; viral, bacterial, mycobacterial, and fungal cultures.
3. Blood studies for infection: HIV; RPR; IgG and IgM enterovirus antibody; IgM mumps, measles, rubella, group B arbovirus, *Brucella melitensis*, *Chlamydia psittaci*, *Bartonella henselae*, schistosomal antibody; cultures for *B. melitensis*. Also consider nasal/pharyngeal/anal cultures for enteroviruses; stool O&P for *Schistosoma* ova.
4. Immune-mediated disorders: ESR; ANA; ENA; dsDNA; rheumatoid factor; anti-SSA; anti-SSB, complement levels; antiphospholipid and anticardiolipin antibodies; p-ANCA; antimicrosomal and antithyroglobulin antibodies; if Sjögren syndrome suspected, Schirmer test, salivary gland scintography, and salivary/lacrimal gland biopsy.
5. Sarcoidosis: Serum angiotensin-converting enzyme; serum Ca; 24 hour urine Ca; chest x-ray; chest CT; total body gallium scan; lymph node biopsy.
6. Demyelinating disease: Brain MRI scan, evoked potentials, CSF oligoclonal bands, neuromyelitis optica antibody (aquaporin-4).
7. Vascular causes: CT myelogram; spinal angiogram.

Note: VDRL, Venereal Disease Research Laboratory; PCR, polymerase chain reaction; VZV, varicella-zoster virus; HHV, human herpes virus; RPR, rapid plasma reagin (test); O&P, ova and parasites; ESR, erythrocyte sedimentation rate; ANA, antinuclear antibodies; ENA, epithelial neutrophil-activating peptide.

the upper thoracic segments. With systemic hypotension, cord infarction occurs at the level of greatest ischemic risk, usually T3-T4, and also at boundary zones between the anterior and posterior spinal artery territories. The latter may result in a rapidly progressive syndrome over hours of weakness and spasticity with little sensory change.

Acute infarction in the territory of the *anterior spinal artery* produces paraplegia or quadriplegia, dissociated sensory loss affecting pain and temperature sense but sparing vibration and position sense, and loss of sphincter control ("anterior cord syndrome"). Onset may be sudden and dramatic but more typically is progressive over minutes or a few hours, quite unlike stroke in the cerebral hemispheres. Sharp midline or radiating back pain localized to the area of ischemia is frequent. Areflexia due to spinal shock is often present initially; with time, hyperreflexia and spasticity appear. Less common is infarction in the territory of the *posterior spinal arteries*, resulting in loss of posterior column function.

Spinal cord infarction results from aortic atherosclerosis, dissecting aortic aneurysm (manifest as chest or back pain with diminished pulses in legs), vertebral artery occlusion or dissection in the neck, or profound hypotension from any cause. Cardiogenic emboli, vasculitis related to collagen vascular disease [particularly SLE and the antiphospholipid antibody syndrome (see below)], and surgical interruption of aortic aneurysms are other causative conditions. Occasional cases develop from *embolism of nucleus pulposus* material into spinal vessels, usually from local spine trauma. In a substantial number of cases no cause can be found, and thromboembolism in arterial feeders is suspected. The MRI may fail to demonstrate limited infarctions of the cord, especially in the first day, but as often it is abnormal at the affected level.

In cord infarction due to presumed thromboembolism, acute anticoagulation is probably not indicated, with the exception of the unusual transient ischemic attack or incomplete infarction with a stuttering or progressive course. The antiphospholipid antibody syndrome is treated with anticoagulation. Drainage of spinal fluid has reportedly been successful in some cases of cord infarction but has not been studied systematically.

Inflammatory and Immune Myelopathies (Myelitis) This broad category includes MS and postinfectious myelitis, both of which are demyelinating in nature (see below), as well as connective tissue disease. In approximately one-quarter of cases of myelitis, no underlying cause can be identified. Some will later manifest additional symptoms of a systemic immune-mediated disease such as SLE or, more often, MS. *Recurrent episodes of myelitis* are usually due to an immune-mediated disease such as a demyelinating disease, SLE, or sarcoid; or to infection with herpes simplex virus (HSV) type 2 (below).

SYSTEMIC INFLAMMATORY DISORDERS Myelitis occurs in a small number of patients with SLE (Chap. 313), many cases of which are associated with antiphospholipid antibodies. The CSF is usually normal or shows a mild lymphocytic pleocytosis; oligoclonal bands are a variable finding. Responses to glucocorticoids and/or cyclophosphamide have been reported, but there is no systematic evidence of their benefit. Other immune-mediated myelitides include cases associated with Sjögren's syndrome (Chap. 317), mixed connective tissue disease (Chap. 316), Behçet's syndrome (Chap. 320), and vasculitis with perinuclear antineutrophilic cytoplasmic (p-ANCA) antibodies (Chap. 319).

Another important consideration in this group is sarcoid myelopathy (Chap. 322), in which an edematous swelling of the spinal cord may mimic tumor; there is almost always gadolinium enhancement of the lesion and of the adjacent surface of the cord. The CSF profile consists of variable lymphocytic pleocytosis; oligoclonal bands are present in one-third of cases. The diagnosis is particularly difficult when systemic manifestations of sarcoid are minor or absent (nearly 50% of cases) or when other classic neurologic manifestations of the disease—such as cranial neuropathy, hypothalamic involvement, or meningeal enhancement visualized by MRI—are lacking. A slit-lamp examination of the eye to search for uveitis, chest x-ray and CT to assess pulmonary involvement and mediastinal lymphadenopathy, serum angiotensin-converting enzyme (ACE; positive in only one-quarter of cases), serum calcium, and a gallium scan may assist in the diagnosis. The usefulness of spinal fluid ACE is uncertain. Initial treatment is with oral glucocorticoids; immunosuppressant drugs are used for resistant cases.

DEMYELINATING MYELOPATHIES Multiple sclerosis (Chap. 375) may present with myelitis, particularly in individuals of Asian or African ancestry. In Caucasians, MS rarely causes a complete transverse myelopathy (i.e., acute bilateral signs), but it is among the most common causes of a partial syndrome. Neuromyelitis optica (NMO) is a demyelinating syndrome consisting of a severe myelopathy associated with optic neuritis; the optic neuritis is often bilateral and may precede or follow myelitis by weeks or months (Chap. 375). A specific serum antibody test is available. NMO is also associated with SLE and antiphospholipid antibodies (see above) as well as with other connective tissue diseases.

MRI findings in MS-associated myelitis typically consist of mild swelling and edema of the cord and diffuse or multifocal areas of abnormal signal on T2-weighted sequences. Contrast enhancement, indicating disruption in the blood-brain barrier associated with inflammation, is present in many acute cases. A brain MRI is most helpful in gauging the likelihood that a case of myelitis represents an initial attack of MS. A normal scan indicates that the risk of evolution to MS is low, ~10–15% over 5 years; in contrast, the finding of multiple periventricular T2-bright lesions indicates a much higher risk, >50% over 5 years and >90% by 14 years. The CSF may be normal, but more often there is a mild pleocytosis, occasionally up to several hundred mononuclear cells per microliter, with normal or mildly elevated CSF protein levels; oligoclonal bands are variable, but when bands are present, a diagnosis of MS is more likely. These bands are generally absent in neuromyelitis optica.

There are no adequate trials of therapy for MS-associated transverse myelitis. Intravenous methylprednisolone (500 mg qd for 3 days) followed by oral prednisone (1 mg/kg per day for several weeks, then gradual taper) has been used as initial treatment. A course of plasma exchange is indicated for severe cases if glucocorticoids are ineffective. Preliminary data suggest that treatment with anti-CD20 (anti-B cell) monoclonal antibody may protect against relapses in patients with NMO.

POSTINFECTIOUS MYELITIS Many cases of myelitis, termed *postinfectious* or *postvaccinal*, follow an infection or vaccination. Numerous organisms have been implicated, including Epstein-Barr virus (EBV),

cytomegalovirus (CMV), mycoplasma, influenza, measles, varicella, rubeola, and mumps. As in the related disorder acute disseminated encephalomyelitis (Chap. 375), postinfectious myelitis often begins as the patient appears to be recovering from an acute febrile infection, or in the subsequent days or weeks, but an infectious agent cannot be isolated from the nervous system or spinal fluid. The presumption is that the myelitis represents an autoimmune disorder triggered by infection and is not due to direct infection of the spinal cord. Treatment is usually with glucocorticoids or, in fulminant cases, plasma exchange. There are no trials by which to adequately judge these therapies.

ACUTE INFECTIOUS MYELITIS Many viruses have been associated with an acute myelitis that is infectious in nature rather than postinfectious. Nonetheless, the two processes are often difficult to distinguish. Herpes zoster is the best characterized viral myelitis, but HSV types 1 and 2, EBV, CMV, and rabies virus are other well-described causes. HSV-2 (and less commonly HSV-1) produces a distinctive syndrome of recurrent sacral myelitis in association with outbreaks of genital herpes mimicking MS. Poliomyelitis is the prototypic viral myelitis, but it is more or less restricted to the gray matter of the cord. Chronic viral myelitic infections, such as that due to HIV, are discussed below.

Bacterial and mycobacterial myelitis (most are essentially abscesses) are far less common than viral causes. Almost any pathogenic species may be responsible, including *Listeria monocytogenes*, *Borrelia burgdorferi* (Lyme disease), and *Treponema pallidum* (syphilis). *Mycoplasma pneumoniae* may be a cause of myelitis, but its status is uncertain since many cases are more properly classified as postinfectious.

Schistosomiasis (Chap. 212) is an important cause of parasitic myelitis in endemic areas. The process is intensely inflammatory and granulomatous, caused by a local response to tissue-digesting enzymes from the ova of the parasite. Toxoplasmosis (Chap. 207) can occasionally cause a focal myelopathy, and this diagnosis should be considered, particularly in patients with AIDS.

In cases of suspected viral myelitis, it may be appropriate to begin specific therapy pending laboratory confirmation. Herpes zoster, HSV, and EBV myelitis are treated with intravenous acyclovir (10 mg/kg q8h) or oral valacyclovir (2 gm tid) for 10–14 days; CMV with ganciclovir (5 mg/kg IV bid) plus foscarnet (60 mg/kg IV tid), or cidofovir (5 mg/kg per week for 2 weeks).

CHRONIC MYELOPATHIES

SPONDYLITIC MYELOPATHY

Spondylitic myelopathy is one of the most common causes of gait difficulty in the elderly. Neck and shoulder pain with stiffness are early symptoms; impingement of bone and soft tissue overgrowth on nerve roots results in radicular arm pain, most often in a C5 or C6 distribution. Compression of the cervical cord, which occurs in fewer than one-third of cases, produces a slowly progressive spastic paraparesis, at times asymmetric and often accompanied by paresthesias in the feet and hands. Vibratory sense is diminished in the legs, there is a Romberg sign, and occasionally there is a sensory level for vibration on the upper thorax. In some cases, coughing or straining produces leg weakness or radiating arm or shoulder pain. Dermatomal sensory loss in the arms, atrophy of intrinsic hand muscles, increased deep-tendon reflexes in the legs, and extensor plantar responses are common. Urinary urgency or incontinence occurs in advanced cases, but there are many alternative causes of these problems in older individuals. A tendon reflex in the arms is often diminished at some level; the biceps is most often affected (C5-C6). In individual cases, radicular, myelopathic, or combined signs may predominate. The diagnosis should be considered in cases of progressive cervical myelopathy, paresthesias of the feet and hands, or wasting of the hands.

Diagnosis is made by MRI or myelography. Extrinsic cord compression and deformation is appreciated on axial MRI views, and T2-weighted sequences may reveal areas of high signal intensity within the cord adjacent to the site of compression. A cervical collar may be helpful in milder cases, but definitive therapy consists of surgical decompression. Posterior laminectomy or an anterior approach with resection of the protruded disc and bony material may be required. Cervical spondylosis and related degenerative diseases of the spine are discussed in Chap. 16.

VASCULAR MALFORMATIONS OF THE CORD AND DURA

Although uncommon, vascular malformations of the cord and overlying dura are treatable causes of progressive myelopathy. True arteriovenous malformations (AVMs) are located posteriorly along the surface of the cord or within the dura, where they are more properly classified as fistulas. Most are at or below the midthoracic level. The typical presentation is a middle-aged man with a progressive myelopathy that worsens slowly or intermittently and may have periods of apparent remission resembling MS. Acute deterioration due to hemorrhage into the spinal cord or subarachnoid space may also occur but is rare. A saltatory progression is most common and is the result of local ischemia and edema from venous congestion. Most patients have incomplete sensory, motor, and bladder disturbances. The motor disorder may predominate and produce a mixture of upper and restricted lower motor neuron signs, simulating amyotrophic lateral sclerosis (ALS). Pain over the dorsal spine, dysesthesias, or radicular pain may be present. Other symptoms suggestive of AVM include intermittent claudication, symptoms that change with posture, exertion such as singing, menses, or fever. A rare AVM process presents as a progressive thoracic myelopathy with paraparesis developing over weeks or several months, characterized pathologically by abnormally thick, hyalinized vessels within the cord (Foix-Alajouanine syndrome).

Spinal bruits are infrequent but should be sought at rest and after exercise in suspected cases. High-resolution MRI with contrast administration detects many but not all AVMs (Fig. 372-6). A small number not detected by MRI may be visualized by CT myelography as enlarged vessels along the surface of the cord. Definitive diagnosis requires selective spinal angiography, which defines the feeding vessels and the extent of the malformation. Endovascular embolization of the major feeding vessels may stabilize a progressive neurologic deficit or allow for gradual recovery.

RETROVIRUS-ASSOCIATED MYELOPATHIES

The myelopathy associated with the human T cell lymphotropic virus type I (HTLV-I), formerly called tropical spastic paraparesis, is a slowly progressive spastic syndrome with variable sensory and bladder disturbance (Chap. 181). Approximately half of patients have mild back or leg pain. The neurologic signs may be asymmetric, often lacking a well-defined sensory level; the only sign in the arms may be hyperreflexia after several years of illness. The onset is insidious, and the illness is slowly progressive at a variable rate; most patients are unable to walk within 10 years of onset. This presentation may resemble primary progressive MS or a thoracic AVM. Diagnosis is made by demonstration of HTLV-I–specific antibody in serum by enzyme-linked immunosorbent assay (ELISA), confirmed by radioimmunoprecipitation or western blot analysis. There is no effective treatment, but symptomatic therapy for spasticity and bladder symptoms may be helpful.

A progressive myelopathy may also result from HIV infection (Chap. 182). It is characterized by vacuolar degeneration of the posterior and lateral tracts, resembling subacute combined degeneration (see below).

SYRINGOMYELIA

Syringomyelia is a developmental cavitary expansion of the cervical cord that is prone to enlarge and produce progressive myelopathy. Symptoms begin insidiously in adolescence or early adulthood, progress irregularly, and may undergo spontaneous arrest for several years. Many young patients acquire a cervical-thoracic scoliosis. More than half of all cases are associated with Chiari type 1 malformations in which the cerebellar tonsils protrude through the foramen magnum and into the cervical spinal canal. The pathophysiology of syrinx expansion is controversial, but some interference with the normal flow of CSF seems likely, perhaps by the Chiari malformation. Acquired cavitations of the cord in areas of necrosis are also termed *syrinx cavities*; these follow trauma, myelitis, necrotic spinal cord tumors, and chronic arachnoiditis due to tuberculosis and other etiologies.

The classic presentation is a central cord syndrome consisting of a dissociated sensory loss and areflexic weakness in the upper limbs. The sensory deficit is recognizable by loss of pain and temperature sensation with sparing of touch and vibration in a distribution that is "suspended" over the nape of the neck, shoulders, and upper arms (cape distribution) or in the hands. Most cases begin asymmetrically with unilateral sensory loss in the hands that leads to injuries and burns that are not appreciated by the patient. Muscle wasting in the lower neck, shoulders, arms, and hands with asymmetric or absent reflexes in the arms reflects expansion of the cavity into the gray matter of the cord. As the cavity enlarges and further compresses the long tracts, spasticity and weakness of the legs, bladder and bowel dysfunction, and a Horner's syndrome appear. Some patients develop facial numbness and sensory loss from damage to the descending tract of the trigeminal nerve (C2 level or above). In cases with Chiari malformations, cough-induced headache and neck, arm, or facial pain are reported. Extension of the syrinx into the medulla, syringobulbia, causes palatal or vocal cord paralysis, dysarthria, horizontal or vertical nystagmus, episodic dizziness, and tongue weakness.

MRI scans accurately identify developmental and acquired syrinx cavities and their associated spinal cord enlargement (Fig. 372-7). MRI scans of the brain and the entire spinal cord should be obtained to delineate the full longitudinal extent of the syrinx, assess posterior fossa structures for the Chiari malformation, and determine whether hydrocephalus is present.

FIGURE 372-6 Arteriovenous malformation. Sagittal MR scans of the thoracic spinal cord: T2 fast spin-echo technique (*left*) and T1 post-contrast image (*right*). On the T2-weighted image (*left*), abnormally high signal intensity is noted in the central aspect of the spinal cord (*arrowheads*). Numerous punctate flow voids indent the dorsal and ventral spinal cord (*arrow*). These represent the abnormally dilated venous plexus supplied by a dural arteriovenous fistula. After contrast administration (*right*), multiple, serpentine, enhancing veins (*arrows*) on the ventral and dorsal aspect of the thoracic spinal cord are visualized, diagnostic of arteriovenous malformation. This patient was a 54-year-old man with a 4-year history of progressive paraparesis.

℞ SYRINGOMYELIA

Treatment of syringomyelia is generally unsatisfactory. The Chiari tonsillar herniation is usually decompressed, generally by suboccipital craniectomy, upper cervical laminectomy, and placement of a dural graft. Obstruction of fourth ventricular outflow is reestablished by this procedure. If the syrinx cavity is large, some surgeons recommend direct decompression or drainage by one of a number of methods, but the added benefit of this procedure is uncertain, and morbidity is common. With Chiari malformations, shunting of hydrocephalus should generally precede any attempt to correct the syrinx. Surgery may stabilize the neurologic deficit, and some patients improve.

FIGURE 372-7 MRI of syringomyelia associated with a Chiari malformation. Sagittal T1-weighted image through the cervical and upper thoracic spine demonstrates descent of the cerebellar tonsils and vermis below the level of the foramen magnum (*black arrows*). Within the substance of the cervical and thoracic spinal cord, a CSF collection dilates the central canal (*white arrows*).

Syringomyelia secondary to trauma or infection is treated with a decompression and drainage procedure in which a small shunt is inserted between the syrinx cavity and the subarachnoid space; alternatively, the cavity can be fenestrated. Cases due to intramedullary spinal cord tumor are generally managed by resection of the tumor.

CHRONIC MYELOPATHY OF MULTIPLE SCLEROSIS

A chronic progressive myelopathy is the most frequent cause of disability in both primary progressive and secondary progressive forms of MS. Involvement is typically bilateral but asymmetric and produces motor, sensory, and bladder/bowel disturbances. Fixed motor disability appears to result from extensive loss of axons in the corticospinal tracts; thus, the symptoms are not simply due to demyelination. Diagnosis is facilitated by identification of earlier attacks such as optic neuritis. MRI, CSF, and evoked response testing are confirmatory. Therapy with interferon β, glatiramer acetate, or natalizumab is indicated for patients with progressive myelopathy who also have coexisting MS relapses. These therapies are sometimes also offered to patients without relapses, despite the lack of evidence supporting their value in this setting. MS is discussed in Chap. 375.

SUBACUTE COMBINED DEGENERATION (VITAMIN B₁₂ DEFICIENCY)

This treatable myelopathy presents with subacute paresthesias in the hands and feet, loss of vibration and position sensation, and a progressive spastic and ataxic weakness. Loss of reflexes due to an associated peripheral neuropathy in a patient who also has Babinski signs, is an important diagnostic clue. Optic atrophy and irritability or other mental changes may be prominent in advanced cases and are rarely the presenting symptoms. The myelopathy of subacute combined degeneration tends to be diffuse rather than focal; signs are generally symmetric and reflect predominant involvement of the posterior and lateral tracts, including Romberg's sign. The diagnosis is confirmed by the finding of macrocytic red blood cells, a low serum B_{12} concentration, elevated serum levels of homocysteine and methylmalonic acid, and in uncertain cases a positive Schilling test (Chap. 288). Treatment is by replacement therapy, beginning with 1000 μg of intramuscular vitamin B_{12} repeated at regular intervals or by subsequent oral treatment.

HYPOCUPRIC MYELOPATHY

This recently described myelopathy is virtually identical to subacute combined degeneration (described above) and probably explains many cases previously described with normal serum levels of B_{12}. Low levels of serum copper are found and often there is also a low level of serum ceruloplasmin. Some cases follow gastrointestinal procedures that result in impaired copper absorption, but many others are idiopathic. Improvement or at least stabilization may be expected with reconstitution of copper stores by oral supplementation. The pathophysiology and pathology are not known.

TABES DORSALIS

The classic syndromes of tabes dorsalis and meningovascular syphilis of the spinal cord are now less frequent than in the past but must be considered in the differential diagnosis of spinal cord disorders. The characteristic symptoms of tabes are fleeting and repetitive lancinating pains, primarily in the legs or less often in the back, thorax, abdomen, arms, and face. Ataxia of the legs and gait due to loss of position sense occurs in half of patients. Paresthesias, bladder disturbances, and acute abdominal pain with vomiting (visceral crisis) occur in 15–30% of patients. The cardinal signs of tabes are loss of reflexes in the legs; impaired position and vibratory sense; Romberg's sign; and, in almost all cases, bilateral Argyll Robertson pupils, which fail to constrict to light but accommodate. Diabetic polyradiculopathy may simulate tabes.

FAMILIAL SPASTIC PARAPLEGIA

Many cases of slowly progressive myelopathy are genetic in origin (Chap. 369). More than 20 different causative loci have been identified, including autosomal dominant, autosomal recessive, and X-linked forms. Most patients present with almost imperceptibly progressive spasticity and weakness in the legs, usually but not always symmetrical. Sensory symptoms and signs are absent or mild, but sphincter disturbances may be present. In some families additional neurologic signs are prominent, including nystagmus, ataxia, or optic atrophy. The onset may be as early as the first year of life or as late as middle adulthood. Only symptomatic therapies for the spasticity are currently available.

ADRENOMYELONEUROPATHY

This X-linked disorder is a variant of adrenoleukodystrophy. Affected males usually have a history of adrenal insufficiency beginning in childhood and then develop a progressive spastic (or ataxic) paraparesis beginning in early adulthood; some patients also have a mild peripheral neuropathy. Female heterozygotes may develop a slower, insidiously progressive spastic myelopathy beginning later in adulthood and without adrenal insufficiency. Diagnosis is usually made by demonstration of elevated levels of very long chain fatty acids in plasma and in cultured fibroblasts. The responsible gene encodes ADLP, a peroxisomal membrane transporter that is a member of the ATP-binding cassette (ABC) family. Steroid replacement is indicated if hypoadrenalism is present, and bone marrow transplantation and nutritional supplements have been attempted for this condition without clear evidence of efficacy.

OTHER CHRONIC MYELOPATHIES

Primary lateral sclerosis (Chap. 369) is a degenerative disorder characterized by progressive spasticity with weakness, eventually accompanied by dysarthria and dysphonia; bladder symptoms occur in approximately half of patients. Sensory function is spared. The disorder resembles ALS and is considered a variant of the motor neuron degenerations, but without the characteristic lower motor neuron disturbance. Some cases may represent familial spastic paraplegia, particularly autosomal recessive or X-linked varieties in which a family history may be absent.

There are a number of rare toxic causes of spastic myelopathy, including lathyrism due to ingestion of chick peas containing the excitotoxin β-N-oxalylaminoalanine (BOAA), seen primarily in the developing world, and nitrous oxide inhalation producing a myelopathy identical to subacute combined degeneration. SLE (Chap. 313), Sjögren's syndrome (Chap. 317), and sarcoidosis (Chap. 322) may each cause a myelopathy without overt evidence of systemic disease. Cancer-related causes of chronic myelopathy, besides the common neoplastic compressive myelopathy discussed earlier, include a rare paraneoplastic myelopathy (Chap. 97) or radiation injury (Chap. 374). It is notable that metastases to the cord are probably more common than

TABLE 372-4 EXPECTED NEUROLOGIC FUNCTION FOLLOWING COMPLETE CORD LESIONS

Level	Self-Care	Transfers	Maximum Mobility
High quadriplegia (C1-C4)	Dependent on others; requires respiratory support	Dependent on others	Motorized wheelchair
Low quadriplegia (C5-C8)	Partially independent with adaptive equipment	May be dependent or independent	May use manual wheelchair, drive an automobile with adaptive equipment
Paraplegia (below T1)	Independent	Independent	Ambulates short distances with aids

Source: Adapted from JF Ditunno, CS Formal: Chronic spinal cord injury. N Engl J Med 330:550, 1994; with permission.

either of these. In obscure cases, a cause can often be identified through periodic reassessment.

REHABILITATION OF SPINAL CORD DISORDERS

The prospects for recovery from an acute destructive spinal cord lesion fade after ~6 months. There are currently no effective means to promote repair of injured spinal cord tissue; promising experimental approaches include the use of factors that influence reinnervation by axons of the corticospinal tract, nerve and neural sheath graft bridges, and the local introduction of stem cells. The disability associated with irreversible spinal cord damage is determined primarily by the level of the lesion and by whether the disturbance in function is complete or incomplete (Table 372-4). Even a complete high cervical cord lesion may be compatible with a productive life. The primary goals are development of a rehabilitation plan framed by realistic expectations and attention to the neurologic, medical, and psychological complications that commonly arise.

Many of the usual symptoms associated with medical illnesses, especially somatic and visceral pain, may be lacking because of the destruction of afferent pain pathways. Unexplained fever, worsening of spasticity, or deterioration in neurologic function should prompt a search for infection, thrombophlebitis, or an intraabdominal pathology. The loss of normal thermoregulation and inability to maintain normal body temperature can produce recurrent fever (*quadriplegic fever*), although most episodes of fever are due to infection of the urinary tract, lung, skin, or bone.

Bladder dysfunction generally results from loss of supraspinal innervation of the detrusor muscle of the bladder wall and the sphincter musculature. Detrusor spasticity is treated with anticholinergic drugs (oxybutinin, 2.5–5 mg qid) or tricyclic antidepressants with anticholinergic properties (imipramine, 25–200 mg/d). Failure of the sphincter muscle to relax during bladder emptying (urinary dyssynergia) may be managed with the α-adrenergic blocking agent terazosin hydrochloride (1–2 mg tid or qid), with intermittent catheterization, or, if that is not feasible, by use of a condom catheter in men or a permanent indwelling catheter. Surgical options include the creation of an artificial bladder by isolating a segment of intestine that can be catheterized intermittently (enterocystoplasty) or can drain continuously to an external appliance (urinary conduit). Bladder areflexia due to acute spinal shock or conus lesions is best treated by catheterization. Bowel regimens and disimpaction are necessary in most patients to ensure at least biweekly evacuation and avoid colonic distention or obstruction.

Patients with acute cord injury are at risk for venous thrombosis and pulmonary embolism. During the first 2 weeks, use of calf-compression devices and anticoagulation with heparin (5000 U subcutaneously every 12 h) or warfarin (INR, 2–3) are recommended. In cases of persistent paralysis, anticoagulation should probably be continued for 3 months.

Prophylaxis against decubitus ulcers should involve frequent changes in position in a chair or bed, the use of special mattresses, and cushioning of areas where pressure sores often develop, such as the sacral prominence and heels. Early treatment of ulcers with careful cleansing, surgical or enzyme debridement of necrotic tissue, and appropriate dressing and drainage may prevent infection of adjacent soft tissue or bone.

Spasticity is aided by stretching exercises to maintain mobility of joints. Drug treatment is effective but may result in reduced function, as some patients depend upon spasticity as an aid to stand, transfer, or walk. Baclofen (15–240 mg/d in divided doses) is effective; it acts by facilitating GABA-mediated inhibition of motor reflex arcs. Diazepam acts by a similar mechanism and is useful for leg spasms that interrupt sleep (2–4 mg at bedtime). Tizanidine (2–8 mg tid), an α₂ adrenergic agonist that increases presynaptic inhibition of motor neurons, is another option. For nonambulatory patients, the direct muscle inhibitor dantrolene (25–100 mg qid) may be used, but it is potentially hepatotoxic. In refractory cases, intrathecal baclofen administered via an implanted pump, botulinum toxin injections, or dorsal rhizotomy may be required to control spasticity.

A paroxysmal autonomic hyperreflexia may occur following lesions above the major splanchnic sympathetic outflow at T6. Headache, flushing, and diaphoresis above the level of the lesion, as well as hypertension with bradycardia or tachycardia, are the major symptoms. The trigger is typically a noxious stimulus—for example, bladder or bowel distention, a urinary tract infection, or a decubitus ulcer—below the level of the cord lesion. Treatment consists of removal of offending stimuli; ganglionic blocking agents (mecamylamine, 2.5–5 mg) or other short-acting antihypertensive drugs are useful in some patients.

Attention to these details allows longevity and a productive life for patients with complete transverse myelopathies.

FURTHER READINGS

DE SEZE J et al: Acute myelopathies: Clinical, laboratory and outcome profiles in 79 cases. Brain 124:1509, 2001

KALB RG: Getting the spinal cord to think for itself. Arch Neurol 60:805, 2003

KAPLIN AI et al: Diagnosis and management of acute myelopathies. Neurologist 11:2, 2005

KUMAR N: Copper deficiency myelopathy (human swayback). Mayo Clin Proc 81:1371, 2006

PRASAD D, SCHIFF D: Malignant spinal-cord compression Lancet Oncol 6:15, 2005

TRANSVERSE MYELITIS CONSORTIUM WORKING GROUP: Proposed diagnostic criteria and nosology of acute transverse myelitis. Neurology 59:499, 2002

TRAUL DE et al: Part I: Spinal-cord neoplasms—intradural neoplasms. Lancet Oncol 8:35, 2007

373 Concussion and Other Head Injuries
Allan H. Ropper

Almost 10 million head injuries occur annually in the United States, about 20% of which are serious enough to cause brain damage.

Among men <35 years, accidents, usually motor vehicle collisions, are the chief cause of death, and >70% of these involve head injury. Furthermore, minor head injuries are so common that almost all physicians will be called upon to provide immediate care or to see patients who are suffering from various sequelae.

Medical personnel caring for head injury patients should be aware that (1) spinal injury often accompanies head injury and care must be taken to prevent compression of the spinal cord due to instability of the spinal column; (2) intoxication is an important accompaniment of traumatic brain injury and, when appropriate, testing should be carried out for drugs and alcohol; and (3) accompanying systemic injuries, including rupture of abdominal organs, may produce vascular collapse or respiratory compromise requiring immediate attention.

TYPES OF HEAD INJURIES

CONCUSSION

This classically refers to an immediate but transient loss of consciousness that is associated with a short period of amnesia. Some patients do not lose consciousness after a minor head injury and instead may appear dazed, confused or report feeling "star struck." The mechanics of concussion involve a blunt forward impact that creates sudden deceleration of the head and an anterior-posterior movement of the brain within the skull. Severe concussion may precipitate a brief convulsion or autonomic signs such as facial pallor, bradycardia, faintness with mild hypotension, or sluggish pupillary reaction, but most patients are soon neurologically normal. The loss of consciousness in concussion is believed to be a transient electrophysiologic dysfunction of the reticular activating system in the upper midbrain caused by rotation of the cerebral hemispheres on the relatively fixed brainstem (Chap. 268).

Gross and light-microscopic changes in the brain are usually absent following concussion, but biochemical and ultrastructural changes, such as mitochondrial ATP depletion and local disruption of the blood-brain barrier, suggest that transient abnormalities occur. CT and MRI scans are usually normal; however, a small number of patients will be found to have an intracranial hemorrhage or brain contusion.

A brief period of both retrograde and anterograde amnesia is typical of concussion and disappears rapidly in alert patients. The memory loss spans the moments before impact but with severe injuries loss of memory may encompass the previous days or weeks (rarely months). The extent of retrograde amnesia roughly correlates with the severity of injury. Memory is regained in an orderly way from the most distant to recent memories, with islands of amnesia occasionally remaining. The mechanism of amnesia is not known. Hysterical posttraumatic amnesia is not uncommon after head injury and should be suspected when inexplicable abnormalities of behavior occur, such as recounting events that cannot be recalled on later testing, a bizarre affect, forgetting one's own name, or a persistent anterograde deficit that is excessive in comparison with the degree of injury. A further discussion of amnesia is provided in Chap. 27.

A single, uncomplicated concussion only infrequently produces permanent neurobehavioral changes in patients who are free of preexisting psychiatric problems and substance abuse. Nonetheless, residual minor problems in memory and concentration may have an anatomic correlate in microscopic cerebral lesions (see below).

CONTUSION, BRAIN HEMORRHAGE, AND AXONAL SHEARING LESIONS

A surface bruise of the brain, or *contusion*, consists of varying degrees of petechial hemorrhage, edema, and tissue destruction. Contusions and deeper hemorrhages result from mechanical forces that displace and compress the hemispheres forcefully and by deceleration of the brain against the inner skull, either under a point of impact (coup lesion) or, as the brain swings back, in the antipolar area (contrecoup lesion). Trauma sufficient to cause prolonged unconsciousness usually produces some degree of contusion. Blunt deceleration impact, as from an automobile dashboard or from falling forward while drunk, causes contusions on the orbital surfaces of the frontal lobes and the anterior and basal portions of the temporal lobes. With lateral forces, as from impact on an automobile door frame, the contusions are situated on the lateral convexity of the hemisphere. The clinical signs are determined by the location and size of the contusion; often, there are no focal neurologic abnormalities. A hemiparesis or gaze preference is fairly typical of moderately sized contusions. Large bilateral contusions produce coma with extensor posturing, while those limited to the frontal lobes cause a taciturn state. Contusions in the temporal lobe may cause delirium or an aggressive, combative syndrome.

Contusions are easily visible on CT and MRI scans, appearing as inhomogeneous hyperdensities on CT and as hyperintensities on MRI;

FIGURE 373-1 Traumatic cerebral contusion. Noncontrast CT scan demonstrating a hyperdense hemorrhagic region in the anterior temporal lobe.

the signal changes reflect small scattered areas of cortical and subcortical blood and localized brain edema (Fig. 373-1); there is usually some subarachnoid bleeding detected by scans or lumbar puncture. Blood in the cerebrospinal fluid (CSF) resulting from trauma may provoke a mild inflammatory reaction. Over a few days, contusions acquire a surrounding contrast enhancement and edema that may be mistaken for tumor or abscess. Glial and macrophage reactions result in scarred, hemosiderin-stained depressions on the cortex (*plaques jaunes*) that are the main source of posttraumatic epilepsy.

Torsion or shearing forces within the brain cause hemorrhages of the basal ganglia and other deep regions. Large hemorrhages after minor trauma suggest that there is a bleeding diathesis or cerebrovascular amyloidosis. For unexplained reasons, deep cerebral hemorrhages may not develop until several days after injury. Sudden neurologic deterioration in a comatose patient or a sudden rise in intracranial pressure (ICP) should therefore prompt investigation with a CT scan.

Another type of deep white matter lesion consists of widespread acute disruption, or shearing, of axons at the time of impact. Most characteristic are small areas of tissue injury in the corpus callosum and dorsolateral pons. The presence of widespread axonal damage in both hemispheres, a state called *diffuse axonal injury*, is proposed to explain persistent coma and the vegetative state after closed head injury (Chap. 268), but small ischemic-hemorrhagic lesions in the midbrain and thalamus are as often the cause of this clinical state. Only severe shearing lesions that contain blood are visualized by CT, usually in the corpus callosum and centrum semiovale (Fig. 373-2); however, special imaging sequences of the MRI can demonstrate such lesions throughout the white matter.

SKULL FRACTURES

A blow to the skull causes fracture if the elastic tolerance of the bone is exceeded. Intracranial lesions accompany roughly two-thirds of skull fractures, and the presence of a skull fracture increases manyfold the chances of an underlying subdural or epidural hematoma. Consequently, fractures are primarily markers of the site and severity of injury. They also provide potential pathways for entry of bacteria (meningitis) or air (pneumocephalus) to the CSF and for leakage of CSF out through the dura.

Most fractures are linear and extend from the point of impact toward the base of the skull. Basilar skull fractures are often extensions of adjacent linear fractures over the convexity of the skull but may occur independently owing to stresses on the floor of the middle cranial fossa or occiput. Basilar fractures are usually parallel to the petrous bone or along the sphenoid bone and directed toward the sella turcica and ethmoidal groove. Although most basilar fractures are uncomplicated, they can cause CSF leakage, pneumocephalus, and cavernous-

FIGURE 373-2 Multiple small areas of hemorrhage and tissue disruption in the white matter of the frontal lobes on noncontrast CT scan. These appear to reflect an extreme type of the diffuse axonal shearing lesions that occur with closed head injury.

carotid fistulas. Hemotympanum (blood behind the tympanic membrane), delayed ecchymosis over the mastoid process (Battle sign), or periorbital ecchymosis ("raccoon sign") are associated signs. Because routine x-ray examination may fail to disclose basilar fractures, they should be suspected if these clinical signs are present.

CSF may leak through the cribriform plate or the adjacent sinus and allow a watery discharge from the nose (CSF rhinorrhea). Persistent rhinorrhea and recurrent meningitis are indications for surgical repair of torn dura underlying the fracture. The site of the leak is often difficult to determine, but useful diagnostic tests include the instillation of water-soluble contrast into the CSF followed by CT with the patient in various positions, or injection of radionuclide compounds or fluorescein into the CSF and the insertion of absorptive nasal pledgets. The site of an intermittent leak is rarely delineated, and many resolve spontaneously.

Sellar fractures, even those associated with serious neuroendocrine dysfunction, may be radiologically occult or are evident by an air-fluid level in the sphenoid sinus. Fractures of the dorsum sella cause sixth or seventh nerve palsies or optic nerve damage.

Petrous bone fractures, especially those oriented along the long axis of the bone, may be associated with facial palsy, disruption of ear ossicles, and CSF otorrhea. Transverse petrous fractures are less common; they almost always damage the cochlea or labyrinths and often the facial nerve as well. External bleeding from the ear is usually from local abrasion of the external canal but can also result from petrous fracture.

Fractures of the frontal bone are usually depressed, involving the frontal and paranasal sinuses and the orbits; permanent anosmia results if the olfactory filaments in the cribriform plate are disrupted. Depressed skull fractures are typically compound, but they are often asymptomatic because the impact energy is dissipated in breaking the bone; however, a few have underlying brain contusions. Debridement and exploration of compound fractures are required in order to avoid infection; simple fractures do not require surgery.

CRANIAL NERVE INJURIES

The cranial nerves most often injured with head trauma are the olfactory, optic, oculomotor, and trochlear; the first and second branches of the trigeminal nerve; and the facial and auditory nerves. Anosmia and an apparent loss of taste (actually a loss of perception of aromatic flavors, with elementary taste perception retained) occur in ~10% of persons with serious head injuries, particularly after falls on the back of the head. This is the result of displacement of the brain and shearing of the olfactory nerve filaments and may occur in the absence of a fracture. At least partial recovery of olfactory and gustatory function is the rule, but if bilateral anosmia persists for several months, the prognosis

is poor. Partial optic nerve injuries from closed trauma result in blurring of vision, central or paracentral scotomas, or sector defects. Direct orbital injury may cause short-lived blurred vision for close objects due to reversible iridoplegia. Diplopia limited to downward gaze and corrected when the head is tilted away from the side of the affected eye indicates trochlear nerve damage. It occurs frequently as an isolated problem after minor head injury or may develop after a delay of several days without pathophysiologic explanation. Direct facial nerve injury caused by a basilar fracture is present immediately in up to 3% of severe injuries; it may also be delayed 5–7 days. Fractures through the petrous bone, particularly the less common transverse type, are liable to produce facial palsy. Delayed palsy, the mechanism of which is unknown, has a good prognosis. Injury to the eighth cranial nerve from a fracture of the petrous bone causes loss of hearing, vertigo, and nystagmus immediately after injury. Deafness from eighth nerve injury must be distinguished from that due to rupture of the eardrum, blood in the middle ear, or disruption of the ossicles from fracture through the middle ear. Dizziness and high-tone hearing loss occur with direct cochlear concussion.

SEIZURES

Convulsions are surprisingly uncommon immediately after a head injury, but a brief period of tonic extensor posturing or a few clonic movements of the limbs just after the moment of impact can occur. However, the cortical scars that evolve from contusions are highly epileptogenic and may later manifest as seizures, even after many years (Chap. 363). The severity of injury roughly determines the risk of future seizures. It has been estimated that 17% of individuals with brain contusion, subdural hematoma, or prolonged loss of consciousness will develop a seizure disorder and that this risk extends for an indefinite period of time, whereas the risk is ≤2% after mild injury. The majority of convulsions in the latter group occurs within 5 years of injury but may be delayed for decades. Penetrating injuries have a much higher rate of subsequent epilepsy.

SUBDURAL AND EPIDURAL HEMATOMAS

Hemorrhages beneath the dura (subdural) or between the dura and skull (epidural) each have characteristic clinical and radiologic features. They are associated with underlying contusions and other injuries, often making it difficult to determine the relative contribution of each component to the clinical state. The mass effect and raised ICP caused by these hematomas may be life threatening, making it imperative to identify them rapidly by CT or MRI scan and to remove them when appropriate.

Acute Subdural Hematoma   (Fig. 373-3) Up to one-third of patients have a lucid interval lasting minutes to hours before coma supervenes, but most are drowsy or comatose from the moment of injury. Direct cranial trauma may be minor and is not required for acute subdural hemorrhage to occur, especially in the elderly and those taking anticoagulant medications. Acceleration forces alone, as from whiplash, are sometimes sufficient to produce subdural hemorrhage. A unilateral headache and slightly enlarged pupil on the same side are frequently but not invariably present. Stupor or coma, hemiparesis, and unilateral pupillary enlargement are signs of larger hematomas. In an acutely deteriorating patient, burr (drainage) holes or an emergency craniotomy are required. Small subdural hematomas may be asymptomatic and usually do not require evacuation.

A subacutely evolving syndrome due to subdural hematoma occurs days or weeks after injury with drowsiness, headache, confusion, or mild hemiparesis; it usually arises in alcoholics and in the elderly, often after only minor trauma.

On imaging studies subdural hematomas appear as crescentic collections over the convexity of one or both hemispheres, most commonly in the frontotemporal region, and less often in the inferior middle fossa or over the occipital poles (Fig. 373-3). Interhemispheric, posterior fossa, or bilateral convexity hematomas are less frequent and are difficult to diagnose clinically, although drowsiness and the signs

FIGURE 373-3 Acute subdural hematoma. Noncontrast CT scan reveals a hyperdense clot which has an irregular border with the brain and causes more horizontal displacement (mass effect) than might be expected from its thickness. The disproportionate mass effect is the result of the large rostral-caudal extent of these hematomas. Compare to Fig. 373-4.

expected for damage in each region can usually be detected. The bleeding that causes larger hematomas is primarily venous in origin, although additional arterial bleeding sites are sometimes found at operation and a few large hematomas have a purely arterial origin.

Epidural Hematoma (Fig. 373-4) These evolve more rapidly than subdural hematomas and are correspondingly more treacherous. They occur in up to 10% of cases of severe head injury but are associated with underlying cortical damage less often than are subdural hematomas. Most patients are unconscious when first seen. A "lucid interval" of several minutes to hours before coma supervenes is most characteristic of epidural hemorrhage, but it is still uncommon, and epidural hemorrhage is by no means the only cause of this temporal sequence. Rapid surgical evacuation and ligation or cautery of the damaged vessel that is the source of bleeding, usually the middle meningeal artery that has been lacerated by an overlying skull fracture, is indicated.

Chronic Subdural Hematoma A history of trauma may or may not be elicited in relation to chronic subdural hematoma. The causative injury may have been trivial and forgotten; 20–30% of patients recall no head

FIGURE 373-4 Acute epidural hematoma. The tightly attached dura is stripped from the inner table of the skull, producing a characteristic lenticular-shaped hemorrhage on noncontrast CT scan. Epidural hematomas are usually caused by tearing of the middle meningeal artery following fracture of the temporal bone.

FIGURE 373-5 CT scan of chronic bilateral subdural hematomas of different ages. The collections began as acute hematomas and have become hypodense in comparison to the adjacent brain after a period during which they were isodense and difficult to appreciate. Some areas of resolving blood are contained on the more recently formed collection on the left (*arrows*).

injury, particularly the elderly and those with clotting disorders. Headache is common but not invariable. Additional features may include slowed thinking, vague change in personality, seizure, or a mild hemiparesis. The headache may fluctuate in severity, sometimes with changes in head position. Bilateral chronic subdural hematomas produce perplexing clinical syndromes. Focal signs such as hemiparesis may be lacking, and the initial clinical impression may be of a stroke, brain tumor, drug intoxication, depression, or a dementing illness because drowsiness, inattentiveness, and incoherence of thought are more prominent than focal signs such as hemiparesis. Patients with undetected bilateral subdural hematomas have a low tolerance for surgery, anesthesia, and drugs that depress the nervous system, remaining drowsy or confused for long periods. Chronic hematomas rarely cause brief episodes of hemiparesis or aphasia that are indistinguishable from transient ischemic attacks; on occasion a chronic collection can expand over a period of days or weeks and clinically resemble a brain tumor.

Skull x-rays are usually normal except for a shift of the calcified pineal body to one side or an occasional unexpected fracture. In long-standing cases an irregular calcification of membranes that surround the hematoma may be appreciated. CT without contrast infusion shows a low-density mass over the convexity of the hemisphere (Fig. 373-5), but between 2 and 6 weeks after the initial bleeding the hemorrhage becomes isodense compared to adjacent brain and is then inapparent. Many subdural hematomas that are a week or more in age contain areas of blood adjacent to intermixed serous fluid. Bilateral chronic hematomas may fail to be detected because of the absence of lateral tissue shifts; this circumstance is suggested by a "hypernormal" CT scan with fullness of the cortical sulci and small ventricles in an older patient. The infusion of contrast material demonstrates enhancement of the vascular fibrous capsule surrounding the collection. MRI reliably identifies subacute and chronic hematomas.

Clinical observation coupled with serial imaging is a reasonable approach to patients with few symptoms and small chronic subdural collections. Treatment with glucocorticoids alone is sufficient for some hematomas, but surgical evacuation is more often successful. The fibrous membranes that grow from the dura and encapsulate the collection require removal to prevent recurrent fluid accumulation. Small hematomas are resorbed, leaving only the organizing membranes. On imaging studies very chronic subdural hematomas may be difficult to distinguish from hygromas, which are collections of CSF from a rent in the arachnoid membrane. As noted, cortical damage underlying a chronic hematoma may serve as the origin of seizures.

MINOR INJURY

The patient who is fully alert and attentive minutes after head injury but who has one or more symptoms of headache, dizziness, faintness, nausea, a single episode of emesis, difficulty with concentration, or slight blurring of vision has a good prognosis with little risk of subsequent deterioration. Such patients have usually sustained a concussion and are expected to have a brief amnestic period. Children are particularly prone to drowsiness, vomiting, and irritability, which are sometimes delayed for several hours after apparently minor injuries. Vasovagal syncope that follows injury may cause undue concern. Constant generalized or frontal headache is common in the following days. It may be migrainous (throbbing and hemicranial) in nature or aching and bilateral. After several hours of observation, patients with minor injury may be accompanied home and observed for a day by a family member or friend; written instructions to return if symptoms worsen should be provided.

Persistent severe headache and repeated vomiting in the context of normal alertness and no focal neurologic signs are usually benign, but radiologic studies should be obtained and a period of observation in the hospital is justified. The decision to perform imaging tests depends largely on clinical signs that indicate the impact was severe (e.g., prolonged concussion, periorbital or mastoid hematoma, repeated vomiting, palpable skull fracture), on the seriousness of other bodily injuries, and on the degree of surveillance that can be anticipated after discharge. Two prospective studies have suggested that older age, two or more episodes of vomiting, >30 min of retrograde or persistent anterograde amnesia, seizure, and concurrent drug or alcohol intoxication are sensitive (but not specific) indicators of intracranial hemorrhage that justify CT scanning. It is appropriate to be more liberal in obtaining CT scans in children since a small number, even without loss of consciousness, will display intracranial lesions.

Concussion in Sports   In the current absence of adequate data, a common sense approach has been taken to returning an athlete who has suffered a concussion to physical activities. It is generally advisable to avoid contact sports for several days at least, and for weeks after a severe concussion or after more than one minor concussion or if there are protracted neurologic symptoms (Table 373-1). These guidelines are designed to avoid cognitive decline and an extremely rare complication of recurrent head injury, termed the *second impact syndrome*, in which cerebral swelling follows a minor head injury. There is some evidence that repeated concussions in football and soccer players are associated with mild but cumulative cognitive deficits, but this topic is controversial.

INJURY OF INTERMEDIATE SEVERITY

Patients who have persistent confusion, behavioral changes, subnormal alertness, extreme dizziness, or focal neurologic signs such as hemiparesis should be admitted to the hospital and soon thereafter have a CT scan. Usually a cerebral contusion or hematoma is found. The common clinical syndromes in this group include (1) delirium with a disinclination to be examined or moved, expletive speech, and resistance if disturbed (anterior temporal lobe contusions); (2) a quiet, disinterested, slowed mental state (abulia) with dull facial expression alternating with irascibility (inferior frontal and frontopolar contusions); (3) a focal deficit such as aphasia or mild hemiparesis (due to subdural hematoma or convexity contusion, or, less often but frequently missed, carotid artery dissection); (4) confusion and inattention, poor performance on simple mental tasks, and fluctuating or slightly erroneous orientation (associated with several types of injuries, including those described above as well as medial frontal contusions and interhemispheric subdural hematoma); (5) repetitive vomiting, nystagmus, drowsiness, and unsteadiness (usually from labyrinthine concussion, but occasionally due to a posterior fossa subdural hematoma or vertebral artery dissection); and (6) diabetes insipidus (damage to the median eminence or pituitary stalk). *Injuries of this degree are often complicated by drug or alcohol intoxication, and clinically inapparent cervical spine injury may be present.*

TABLE 373-1   GUIDELINES FOR MANAGEMENT OF CONCUSSION IN SPORTS

Severity of Concussion

Grade 1: Transient confusion, no loss of consciousness (LOC), all symptoms resolve within 15 min.
Grade 2: Transient confusion, no LOC, but concussive symptoms or mental status abnormalities persist longer than 15 min.
Grade 3: Any LOC, either brief (seconds) or prolonged (minutes).

On-site Evaluation

1. Mental status testing
   a. Orientation—time, place, person, circumstances of injury
   b. Concentration—digits backward, months of year in reverse order
   c. Memory—names of teams, details of contest, recent events, recall of three words and objects at 0 and 5 min
2. Finger-to-nose with eyes open and closed
3. Pupillary symmetry and reaction
4. Romberg and tandem gait
5. Provocative testing—40-yard sprint, 5 push ups, 5 sit ups, 5 knee bends (development of dizziness, headaches, or other symptoms is abnormal)

Management Guidelines

Grade 1: Remove from contest. Examine immediately and at 5 min intervals. May return to contest if exam clears within 15 min. A second grade 1 concussion eliminates player for 1 week, with return contingent upon normal neurologic assessment at rest and with exertion.
Grade 2: Remove from contest, cannot return for at least 1 week. Examine at frequent intervals on sideline. Formal neurologic exam the next day. If headache or other symptoms persist for 1 week or longer, CT or MRI scan is indicated. After 1 full asymptomatic week, repeat neurologic assessment at rest and with exercise before cleared to resume play. A second grade 2 concussion eliminates player for at least 2 weeks following complete resolution of symptoms at rest or with exertion. If imaging shows abnormality, player is removed from play for the season.
Grade 3: Transport by ambulance to emergency department if still unconscious or worrisome signs are present; cervical spine stabilization may be indicated. Neurologic exam and, when indicated, CT or MRI scan will guide subsequent management. Hospital admission indicated when signs of pathology are present or if mental status remains abnormal. If findings are normal at the time of the initial medical evaluation, the athlete may be sent home, but daily exams as an outpatient are indicated. A brief (LOC for seconds) grade 3 concussion eliminates player for 1 week, and a prolonged (LOC for minutes) grade 3 concussion for 2 weeks, following complete resolution of symptoms. A second grade 3 concussion should eliminate player from sports for at least 1 month following resolution of symptoms. Any abnormality on CT or MRI scans should result in termination of the season for the athlete, and return to play at any future time should be discouraged.

Source: Modified from Quality Standards Subcommittee of the American Academy of Neurology: *The American Academy of Neurology Practice Handbook.* The American Academy of Neurology, St. Paul, MN, 1997.

Most patients in this category, after appropriate surgical removal of hematomas, improve over several days or weeks. During the first week the state of alertness, memory, and other cognitive functions often fluctuates, and irascibility or agitation is common. Behavioral changes are worse at night, as with many other encephalopathies, and may be treated with small doses of antipsychotic medications. Subtle abnormalities of attention, intellect, spontaneity, and memory tend to return to normal weeks or months after the injury, sometimes surprisingly abruptly. Persistent problems in cognition are discussed below.

SEVERE INJURY

Patients who are comatose from the onset require immediate neurologic attention and resuscitation. After intubation, with care taken to immobilize the cervical spine, the depth of coma, pupillary size and reactivity, limb movements, and Babinski responses are assessed. As soon as vital functions permit and cervical spine x-rays and a CT scan have been obtained, the patient should be transported to a critical care unit where systemic complications that follow severe brain injury can be treated. Hypoxia should be reversed and normal saline used as the preferred resuscitation fluid. The finding of an epidural or subdural hematoma or large intracerebral hemorrhage is an indication for

TABLE 373-2 GLASGOW COMA SCALE FOR HEAD INJURY

Eye opening (E)		Verbal response (V)	
Spontaneous	4	Oriented	5
To loud voice	3	Confused, disoriented	4
To pain	2	Inappropriate words	3
Nil	1	Incomprehensible sounds	2
Best motor response (M)		Nil	1
Obeys	6		
Localizes	5		
Withdraws (flexion)	4		
Abnormal flexion posturing	3		
Extension posturing	2		
Nil	1		

Note: Coma score = E + M + V. Patients scoring 3 or 4 have an 85% chance of dying or remaining vegetative, while scores >11 indicate only a 5–10% likelihood of death or vegetative state and 85% chance of moderate disability or good recovery. Intermediate scores correlate with proportional chances of recovery.

prompt surgery and intracranial decompression in an otherwise salvageable patient. The use of prophylactic anticonvulsants has been recommended by some neurosurgeons but there is little supportive data. **Management of raised ICP, a frequent feature of severe head injury, is discussed in Chap. 269.**

GRADING AND PROGNOSIS

In severe head injury, the clinical features of eye opening, motor responses of the limbs, and verbal output have been found to be generally predictive of outcome. These three features are summarized in the Glasgow Coma Scale; a score between 3 and 15 is assigned based on responses (Table 373-2). Over 85% of patients with aggregate scores of <5 die within 24 h. However, a number of patients with slightly higher scores and a poor initial prognosis, including a few without pupillary light responses, survive, suggesting that an initially aggressive approach is justified in most patients. Patients <20 years, particularly children, may make remarkable recoveries after having grave early neurologic signs. In one large study of severe head injury, 55% of children had a good outcome at 1 year, compared with 21% of adults. Older age, increased ICP, early hypoxia or hypotension, and evidence on imaging of compression of the cisterns surrounding the brainstem and shift of midline structures are all poor prognostic signs. A delay in the evacuation of large intracerebral hemorrhages is also associated with a poorer prognosis.

374 Primary and Metastatic Tumors of the Nervous System
Stephen M. Sagar, Mark A. Israel

Malignant primary tumors of the central nervous system (CNS) occur in ~16,500 individuals and account for an estimated 13,000 deaths in the United States annually, a mortality rate of 6 per 100,000. The age-adjusted incidence appears to be about the same worldwide. An approximately equal number of benign tumors of the CNS are diagnosed, with a much lower mortality rate. Glial tumors account for 50–60% of primary brain tumors, meningiomas for 25%, schwannomas for 10%, and other CNS tumors for the remainder.

Brain and vertebral metastases from systemic cancer are far more prevalent than primary CNS tumors. About 15% of patients who die of cancer (80,000 individuals each year in the United States) have symptomatic brain metastases; an additional 5% suffer spinal cord involvement. Brain and spinal metastases therefore pose a major problem in the management of systemic cancer.

POSTCONCUSSION SYNDROME

The *postconcussion syndrome* refers to a state of nervous instability following mild or moderate head injury. The main features are fatigue, dizziness, headache, and difficulty in concentration. The syndrome is at times difficult to distinguish from asthenia and depression. Based largely on experimental models, it has been proposed that subtle axonal shearing lesions or as yet undefined biochemical alterations account for the cognitive symptoms. In moderate and severe trauma, neuropsychological changes such as difficulty with attention, memory, and other cognitive deficits are undoubtedly present, sometimes severe, but many deficits identified by formal testing do not impact daily functioning. Test scores tend to improve rapidly during the first 6 months after injury, then more slowly for years.

℞ CONCUSSION

Management of the various symptoms of the postconcussive syndrome requires the identification and treatment of depression, sleeplessness, anxiety, persistent headache, and dizziness. A clear explanation of the problems that may follow concussion has been shown to reduce subsequent complaints. Care is taken to avoid prolonged use of drugs that produce dependence. Vestibular exercises (Chap. 30) and small doses of vestibular suppressants such as phenergan may be helpful when dizziness is the main problem. Patients who after minor or moderate injury report difficulty with memory or with complex cognitive tasks at work may also be reassured that these problems usually improve over 6–12 months. It is helpful to obtain serial and quantified neuropsychological testing in order to adjust the work environment to the patient's current abilities and to document improvement over time. Whether cognitive exercises are useful is uncertain, but patients certainly report them to be so. Previously energetic individuals usually have the best recoveries. In patients with persistent symptoms, the possibility exists of malingering or prolongation as a result of litigation.

FURTHER READINGS

LOVELL MR et al: Recovery from concussion in high school athletes. J Neurosurg 98:296, 2003

ROPPER AH (ed): *Neurological and Neurosurgical Intensive Care*, 4th ed. Philadelphia, Lippincott Williams & Wilkins, 2004

——, GORSON KC: Concussion. N Engl J Med 356:166, 2007

SAVOLA O, HILBLOM M: Early predictors of post-concussion symptoms in patients with mild head injury. Eur J Neurol 10:175, 2003

APPROACH TO THE PATIENT:
Brain Tumors

CLINICAL FEATURES Brain tumors usually present with one of three syndromes: (1) subacute progression of a focal neurologic deficit; (2) seizure; or (3) nonfocal neurologic disorder such as headache, dementia, personality change, or gait disorder. The presence of systemic symptoms such as malaise, weight loss, anorexia, or fever suggests a metastatic rather than a primary brain tumor.

Progressive focal neurologic deficits result from compression of neurons and white matter tracts by expanding tumor and surrounding edema. Less commonly, a brain tumor presents with a sudden stroke-like onset of a focal neurologic deficit. Although this presentation may be caused by hemorrhage into the tumor, often no hemorrhage can be demonstrated and the mechanism is obscure. Tumors frequently associated with hemorrhage include high-grade gliomas, metastatic melanoma, and choriocarcinoma.

Seizures may result from disruption of cortical circuits. Tumors that invade or compress the cerebral cortex, even small meningiomas, are more likely to be associated with seizures than subcortical neoplasms. Nonfocal neurologic dysfunction usually reflects increased intracranial pressure (ICP), hydrocephalus, or diffuse tumor spread. Tumors in some areas of the brain may produce behavioral disorders; for example, frontal lobe tumors may present with personality change, dementia, or depression.

Headache may result from focal irritation or displacement of pain-sensitive structures (Chap. 15) or from a generalized increase in ICP. A headache that worsens rather than abates with recumbency is suggestive of a mass lesion. Headaches from increased ICP are usually holocephalic and episodic, occurring more than once a day. They typically develop rapidly over several minutes, persist for 20–40 min, and subside quickly. They may awaken the patient from a sound sleep, generally 60–90 min after retiring. Vomiting may occur with severe headaches. As elevated ICP becomes sustained, the headache becomes continuous but varying in intensity. Elevated ICP may cause papilledema (Chap. 29), although it is often not present in infants or patients >55 years.

The Karnofsky performance scale is useful in assessing patients with brain tumors (Chap. 77). A score ≥70 indicates that the patient is ambulatory and independent in self-care activities; it is often taken as a level of function justifying aggressive therapy.

NEUROIMAGING CT and MRI can reveal mass effect and contrast enhancement. Mass effect reflects the volume of neoplastic tissue as well as surrounding edema. Brain tumors typically produce a vasogenic pattern of edema, with accumulation of excess water in surrounding white matter. Contrast enhancement reflects a breakdown of the blood-brain barrier within the tumor, permitting leakage of contrast agent. Low-grade gliomas typically do not exhibit contrast enhancement.

Positron emission tomography (PET) and single-photon emission tomography (SPECT) have ancillary roles in the imaging of brain tumors, primarily in distinguishing tumor recurrence from tissue necrosis that can occur after irradiation (see below). Functional imaging with PET, MRI, or magnetoencephalography may be of use in surgical or radiosurgical planning to define the anatomic relationship of the tumor to critical brain regions such as the primary motor or language cortex.

LABORATORY EXAMINATION Primary brain tumors typically do not produce serologic abnormalities such as an elevated sedimentation rate or tumor-specific antigens. In contrast, metastases to the nervous system, depending on the type and extent of the primary tumor, may be associated with systemic signs of malignancy (Chap. 77). Lumbar puncture is generally not useful in the diagnosis of brain tumors. The cerebrospinal fluid (CSF) rarely contains malignant cells, with the important exceptions of leptomeningeal metastases; primary CNS lymphoma; and primitive neuroectodermal tumors, including medulloblastoma. The primary use of lumbar puncture in the evaluation of a brain tumor is to exclude other diagnoses, such as infection or demyelinating disease. Moreover, lumbar puncture may precipitate brain herniation in patients with mass lesions and should be performed only in patients in whom imaging studies have demonstrated the basilar cisterns to be patent.

Rx BRAIN TUMORS

SYMPTOMATIC Glucocorticoids decrease the volume of edema surrounding brain tumors and improve neurologic function; dexamethasone (initially 12–20 mg/d in divided doses PO or IV) is used because it has relatively little mineralocorticoid activity. Because of the toxicities of long-term glucocorticoid administration, the dexamethasone dose is rapidly tapered to the lowest dose that relieves symptoms.

The treatment of epilepsy associated with brain tumors is identical to the treatment of other forms of partial epilepsy. The first-line agents phenytoin, carbamazepine, and valproic acid are equally effective; leviractam and oxcarbazepine are also coming into wide use (Chap. 363). It is common practice to administer anti-epileptic drugs prophylactically to all patients with supratentorial brain tumors, although there are no good data supporting this practice.

Gliomas and primary CNS lymphomas are associated with an increased risk for deep vein thrombosis and pulmonary embolism, probably because these tumors secrete procoagulant factors into the systemic circulation. Even though hemorrhage within gliomas is a frequent histopathologic finding, patients are at no increased risk for symptomatic intracranial bleeding following treatment with an anticoagulant. Prophylaxis with low-dose SC heparin should be employed for patients with brain tumors who have lower limb immobility, which places them at risk for deep venous thrombosis.

PRIMARY BRAIN TUMORS

ETIOLOGY

Exposure to ionizing radiation is the only well-documented environmental risk factor for the development of gliomas. A number of hereditary syndromes are associated with an increased risk of brain tumors (Table 374-1). Genes that contribute to the development of brain tumors, as well as other malignancies, fall into two general classes, *tumor-suppressor genes* and *oncogenes* (Chap. 79). Whereas germ-line mutations of such genes do occur in patients with hereditary predisposition syndromes (Table 374-1), most brain tumors do not occur in patients with such recognizable syndromes. As is the case in all other tumor types, somatic mutations are almost invariably present in malignant brain tumor tissue. Amplification of the *EGFR* gene occurs in approximately one-third of cases of glioblastoma multiforme (GBM), the highest grade astrocytoma. Moreover, cytogenetic analysis often reveals characteristic changes that can signal the alteration in cancer-related genes within these chromosomal regions. In astrocytic tumors, DNA is commonly lost on chromosomes 10p, 17p, 13q, and 9. Oligodendrogliomas frequently have deletions of 1p and 19q, resulting from a centromeric translocation and loss of one of the translocated chromosomes. In meningiomas portions of 22q, which contains the gene for neurofibromatosis (NF) type 2, are often lost.

The particular constellation of genetic alterations varies among individual gliomas, even those that are histologically indistinguishable. Moreover, gliomas are genetically unstable. Genetic abnormalities tend to accumulate with time, and these changes correspond with an increasingly malignant phenotype. There are at least two genetic routes for the development of GBM (Fig. 374-1). One route involves the progression, generally over years, from a low-grade astrocytoma with deletions of chromosome 17 and inactivation of the *p53* gene to a highly malignant glioma with additional chromosomal alterations. The second route is characterized by the de novo appearance of a malignant glioma with amplification of the *EGFR* gene and an intact *p53* gene in association with other genetic abnormalities.

ASTROCYTOMAS

Tumors with astrocytic cytologic features are the most common primary intracranial neoplasms (Fig. 374-2). The most widely used histologic grading system is the World Health Organization four-tiered grading system. Grade I is reserved for special histologic variants of astrocytoma that occur mainly in childhood and can have an excellent prognosis after surgical excision. These include *juvenile pilocytic astrocytoma*, *subependymal giant cell astrocytoma* (which most often occurs in patients with tuberous sclerosis), and *pleiomorphic xanthoastrocytoma*. At the other extreme is grade IV GBM, a clinically aggressive tumor. *Astrocytoma* (grade II) and *anaplastic astrocytoma* (grade III) are intermediate in their histologic and clinical manifestations. The histologic features associated with higher grade are hypercellularity, nuclear and cytoplasmic atypia, endothelial proliferation, mitotic activity, and necrosis. Endothelial proliferation and necrosis are strong predictors of aggressive behavior.

Quantitative measures of mitotic activity also correlate with prognosis. The proliferation index can be determined by immunohistochemical staining with antibodies to the proliferating cell nuclear antigen (PCNA) or with a monoclonal antibody termed *Ki-67*, which recognizes a histone protein expressed in proliferating but not quiescent cells.

The prognosis of brain tumor patients is closely associated with the histologic grade of the tumor. In a representative Finnish population, the

TABLE 374-1 HEREDITARY SYNDROMES ASSOCIATED WITH BRAIN TUMORS

Syndrome	Gene (Locus)	Gene Product (Function)	Nervous System Neoplasms
Neurofibromatosis type 1 (von Recklinghausen's Disease)[a]	NF1 (17q)	Neurofibromin (GTPase activating protein)	Neuroma, schwannoma, meningioma, optic glioma
Neurofibromatosis type 2[a]	NF2 (22q)	Merlin (cytoskeletal protein)	Schwannoma, glioma, ependymoma, meningioma
Tuberous sclerosis	TSC1 (9q) TSC2 (16p)	Hamartin (unknown function) Tuberin (GTPase activating protein)	Astrocytoma
von Hippel-Lindau[a]	VHL (3p)	pVHL (modulator of cellular hypoxic response)	Hemangioblastoma of retina, cerebellum and spinal cord; pheochromocytoma
Li-Fraumeni[a]	p53 (17p)	TP53 (cell cycle and transcriptional regulator)	Malignant glioma
Retinoblastoma[a]	RB1 (13q)	RB (cell cycle regulator)	Retinoblastoma, pineoblastoma, malignant glioma
Turcot	APC (5q) (adenomatous polyposis coli)	APC (cell adhesion)	Medulloblastoma, malignant glioma
Gorlin (basal cell nevus syndrome)	PTCH (9q) (patched)	PTH (developmental regulator)	Medulloblastoma
Multiple endocrine neoplasia 1 (Werner syndrome)[a]	MEN1 (11q13)	Menin (cofactor for transcription)	Pituitary adenoma, malignant schwannoma

[a]Genetic testing possible.

median survival was 93.5 months for patients with grade I or II astrocytomas, 12.4 months for patients with grade III (anaplastic astrocytoma), and 5.1 months for patients with grade IV (GBM) tumors. Although these survival rates are somewhat lower than are generally reported, they represent a population-based experience and are not influenced by selection bias. Clinical features correlating with poor prognosis include age >65 and a poor functional status, as defined by the Karnofsky performance scale.

Low-Grade Astrocytoma Low-grade astrocytomas are more common in children than adults. Pilocytic astrocytoma, named for its characteristic spindle-shaped cells, is the most common childhood brain tumor and is typically benign. It frequently occurs in the cerebellum and is well demarcated from adjacent brain. Complete surgical excision usually produces long-term, disease-free survival.

The median overall survival of grade II astrocytoma is 5–6 years. The optimum timing of surgery and radiation therapy for these patients is unknown. Since astrocytomas infiltrate surrounding brain, total surgical excision is impossible. Moreover, they are genetically unstable and accumulate mutations over time, leading to more aggressive behavior. For patients who are symptomatic from mass effect or poorly controlled epilepsy, surgical excision can relieve symptoms. For patients who are asymptomatic or minimally symptomatic at presentation, a diagnostic biopsy should be performed and, when surgically feasible, the tumor may be resected. Whether radiation therapy is administered immediately postoperatively or at the time of tumor progression is not thought to affect overall survival, but immediate radiation therapy does delay tumor progression. No role for chemotherapy in the management of low-grade astrocytoma has been defined.

High-Grade Astrocytoma The large majority of astrocytomas arising in adults are high grade, supratentorial, and do not have a clearly defined margin between normal and malignant tissue. Neoplastic cells

FIGURE 374-1 Model for the pathogenesis of human astrocytoma. Glioblastoma multiforme (GBM) typically presents without evidence of a precursor lesion, referred to as de novo GBM, frequently associated with amplification of the epidermal growth factor receptor (EGFR) gene. Less commonly, GBM arises in association with progressive genetic alterations after the diagnosis of a lower grade astrocytoma. These tumors are referred to as secondary GBM. The most widely described alterations are mutations of p53 and INK4a. Other genes implicated in the development of these primary brain tumors include CDK4, MDM2, DDC, and PDGFR. LOH, loss of heterozygosity.

FIGURE 374-2 Malignant astrocytoma (glioblastoma). Coronal proton density–weighted MR scan through the temporal lobes demonstrates a heterogeneous right temporal lobe mass (*arrows*) compressing the third and lateral ventricles. The area of hypointense signal (*double arrows*) indicates either hemorrhage or calcification. Heterogeneous MR signal intensity is typical of glioblastoma.

migrate away from the main tumor mass and infiltrate adjacent brain, often tracking along white matter pathways. Imaging studies do not indicate the full extent of the tumor. These tumors are almost all eventually fatal. Median survival of patients with grade III astrocytoma is <3 years and for those with a grade IV tumor, <1 year. Longer survival correlates with younger age, better performance status, and greater extent of surgical resection. Late in their course, astrocytomas, especially those located in the posterior fossa, can metastasize along CSF pathways to the spine. Metastases outside the CNS are rare.

High-grade astrocytomas are managed with glucocorticoids, surgery, radiation therapy, and chemotherapy. Dexamethasone is generally administered at the time of diagnosis and continued for the duration of radiation therapy. After completion of radiation therapy, dexamethasone is tapered to the lowest possible dose.

Because astrocytomas infiltrate adjacent normal brain, total surgical excision is not possible. Nevertheless, retrospective studies indicate that the extent of tumor resection correlates with survival in younger patients. Therefore, accessible astrocytomas are generally resected aggressively. Surgery is indicated to obtain tissue for pathologic diagnosis and to control mass effect.

Postoperative radiation therapy prolongs survival and improves quality of life. Treated with dexamethasone alone following surgery, the mean survival of patients <65 years with glioblastoma is 7–9 months. Survival is prolonged to 11–13 months with radiation therapy. For primary glial tumors, radiation is generally administered to the tumor mass, as defined by contrast enhancement on a CT or MRI scan, plus a 2-cm margin. A total dose of 5000–7000 cGy is administered in 25–35 equal fractions, 5 days per week.

The roles of stereotaxic radiosurgery and interstitial brachytherapy in glioma treatment are uncertain. *Stereotaxic radiosurgery* is the administration of a focused high dose of radiation to a precisely defined volume of tissue in a single treatment. Stereotaxic radiosurgery can potentially achieve tumor ablation within the treated volume. A major limitation of stereotaxic radiosurgery is that it can be used for only relatively small tumors, generally <4 cm in maximum diameter. *Interstitial brachytherapy*, the implantation of radioactive material into the tumor mass, is generally reserved for tumor recurrence because of its associated toxicity, necrosis of adjacent brain tissue.

Chemotherapy is marginally effective and is often used as an adjuvant therapy following surgery and radiation therapy. Temozolomide, an orally administered alkylating agent, has replaced nitrosureas, including carmustine (BCNU) and lomustine (CCNU), as the most widely used chemotherapeutic agent for high-grade gliomas. Temozolomide is generally better tolerated than nitrosoureas, notably producing less fatigue and pulmonary toxicity, and has the advantage of oral administration. Moreover, a randomized trial of radiation therapy plus temozolomide for the adjuvant treatment of GBM compared to radiation therapy alone was the first clinical trial to demonstrate a clear-cut advantage of adjuvant chemotherapy for that disease. The patients who received radiation therapy plus temozolomide had a median survival $2^{1}/_{2}$ months longer than those who received radiation therapy alone. The modest survival benefit appears to be restricted to a subgroup of patients with methylation and silencing of the promoter for the *MGMT* gene coding for O^{6}-methylguanine-DNA methyltransferase.

An alternative approach to the chemotherapy of high-grade gliomas that has shown survival benefit in controlled trials is the surgical implantation directly into

the tumor resection cavity of polymer wafers that release BCNU locally into surrounding brain. The efficacy of this approach is similar to but probably slightly less than that of temozolomide, although without the attendant systemic toxicity of chemotherapy.

Experimental approaches to brain tumor chemotherapy include efforts to bypass the blood-brain barrier using local injection of chemotherapeutic agents into the tumor mass or the intraarterial injection of chemotherapy following osmotic disruption of the blood-brain barrier. Molecularly targeted therapies are also being tested in patients with GBM. In particular, since mutation or overexpression of EGFR is common in GBM, EGFR antagonists or inhibitors of its signaling pathways are being evaluated in patients with GBM in clinical trials.

Gliomatosis cerebri is a rare form of astrocytoma in which there is diffuse infiltration of the brain by malignant astrocytes without a focal enhancing mass. It generally presents as a multifocal CNS syndrome or a more generalized disorder including dementia, personality change, or seizures. Neuroimaging studies are often nonspecific, and biopsy is required to establish the diagnosis. Gliomatosis cerebri is treated with whole-brain radiation therapy or temozolomide; in selected patients, radiation to the entire neuroaxis is employed.

OLIGODENDROGLIOMAS

Oligodendrogliomas, which comprise about 15% of gliomas in adults, have a more benign course and are more responsive to cytotoxic treatment than astrocytomas. For grade II oligodendrogliomas, the median survival is 7–8 years, and there are a substantial number of patients with prolonged survival (>10 years). For grade III or anaplastic oligodendrogliomas, median survival is ~5 years. Oligodendrogliomas occur chiefly in supratentorial locations; in adults, ~30% contain areas of calcification (Fig. 374-3).

As a rule, oligodendrogliomas are less infiltrative than astrocytomas, permitting more complete surgical excision. Histologic features of mitoses, necrosis, and nuclear atypia are associated with a more aggressive clinical course. If these features are prominent, the tumor is termed an *anaplastic oligodendroglioma*. Some gliomas contain mixtures of cells with astrocytic and oligodendroglial features. If this mixed histology is prominent, the tumor is termed a *mixed glioma*, or an *oligoastrocytoma*. The greater the oligodendroglial component, the more benign the clinical course.

Surgery, at minimum a stereotaxic biopsy, is necessary to establish a diagnosis. Many oligodendrogliomas are amenable to gross total surgical

FIGURE 374-3 Oligodendroglioma. *A.* Noncontrast CT scan reveals a calcified mass involving the left temporal lobe (*arrows*) associated with mild mass effect but little edema. ***B.*** An MR T2-weighted image demonstrates a heterogeneous mass with hypointense signal (*black arrows*) surrounded by a zone of higher signal intensity (*white arrows*), consistent with a calcified temporal lobe mass. The tumor extends into the left medial temporal lobe and compresses the midbrain.

resection. In addition, oligodendrogliomas may respond dramatically to systemic combination chemotherapy with procarbazine, lomustine, and vincristine (PCV), or to temozolomide, which, although not approved by the U.S. Food and Drug Administration (FDA) for this indication, is currently much more widely used than PCV. Oligodendrogliomas with deletions of chromosome 1p always respond to chemotherapy, but only ~25% of oligodendrogliomas lacking the 1p deletion respond. The simultaneous deletion of 1p and 19q, which results from a centromeric translocation of chromosomes 1 and 19, predicts a durable response to chemotherapy (>31 months on average) and a much longer survival. It appears that the chromosomal translocation identifies a subgroup of anaplastic oligodendrogliomas with a less aggressive natural course, and response to chemotherapy is another marker of that favorable phenotype.

EPENDYMOMAS

In adults, the most frequent histologic type is myxopapillary ependymoma, which typically arises from the filum terminale of the spinal cord and appears in the lumbosacral region. The term *myxopapillary* refers to the papillary arrangement of tumor cells, which produce mucin. Ependymomas in adults may also occur intracranially or at higher levels of the spinal cord. On CT or MRI, ependymomas typically appear as diffusely enhancing masses relatively well demarcated from adjacent neural tissue. Following gross total resection, the prognosis is good, with >80% 5-year disease-free survival. Ependymomas that cannot be totally resected are treated with stereotaxic radiosurgery or with a course of external beam radiation therapy.

MEDULLOBLASTOMAS AND PRIMITIVE NEUROECTODERMAL TUMORS (PNET)

These highly cellular malignant tumors are thought to arise from neural precursor cells. Medulloblastomas occur in the posterior fossa and, along with astrocytomas, are the most frequent malignant brain tumors of children. PNET is a term applied to tumors histologically indistinguishable from medulloblastoma but occurring either in adults or supratentorially in children. In adults, >50% present in the posterior fossa. These tumors frequently disseminate along CSF pathways.

If possible, these tumors should be surgically excised; the less residual tumor left behind, the better the prognosis. In adults, surgical excision of a PNET should be followed by irradiation of the entire neuraxis, with a boost in radiation dose to the primary tumor. If the tumor is not disseminated at presentation, the prognosis is generally favorable. Aggressive treatment can result in prolonged survival, although half of adult patients relapse within 5 years of treatment. Whereas chemotherapy is widely used in medulloblastoma and PNET in children, its role in adults is not yet defined.

CNS LYMPHOMA

Primary CNS Lymphoma Primary CNS lymphoma is typically a high-grade B cell malignancy that presents within the neuraxis without evidence of systemic lymphoma. These occur most frequently in immunocompromised individuals, specifically organ transplant recipients and patients with AIDS (Chap. 182). In immunocompromised patients, CNS lymphomas are invariably associated with Epstein-Barr virus infection of the tumor cells.

In immunocompetent patients, neuroimaging studies most often reveal a uniformly enhancing mass lesion. Stereotaxic needle biopsy can be used to establish the diagnosis. There is no benefit of surgical resection unless there is a need for immediate decompression of a life-threatening mass effect. Leptomeningeal involvement is present in ~15% of patients at presentation and in 50% at some time during the course of the illness. Moreover, the disease extends to the eyes in up to 15% of patients. Therefore, a slit-lamp examination and, if indicated, anterior chamber paracentesis or vitreous biopsy is necessary to define radiation ports.

The prognosis of primary CNS lymphoma is poor compared to histologically similar lymphoma occurring outside the CNS. Many patients experience a dramatic clinical and radiographic response to glucocorticoids; however, relapse almost invariably occurs within weeks. The mainstay of definitive therapy is chemotherapy. A single dose of rituximab is generally administered prior to cytotoxic chemotherapy as long as an enhancing mass lacking a blood-tumor barrier is present. Chemotherapy includes high-dose methotrexate, but multiagent chemotherapy, usually adding vincristine and procarbazine, appears to be more effective than methotrexate alone. Chemotherapy is followed in patients <60 years with whole-brain radiation therapy (WBRT). WBRT is postponed as long as possible or administered at reduced doses in patients >60 years because of the risk of dementia, gait disorder, and incontinence as manifestations of late-delayed radiation toxicity. Consolidation therapy is typically with high-dose cytarabine. Intraarterial chemotherapy with or without blood-brain barrier disruption is an alternative. Intrathecal chemotherapy with methotrexate can be added if leptomeningeal disease is present, but it has not proven to offer added benefit if high-dose methotrexate is used. Despite aggressive therapy, >90% of patients develop recurrent CNS disease. The median survival of patients who tolerate treatment with high-dose methotrexate is >3 years.

In immunodeficient patients, primary CNS lymphoma may be ring-enhancing rather than diffusely enhancing on CT or MRI (Fig. 374-4). It may therefore be impossible by imaging criteria to distinguish primary CNS lymphoma from metastatic malignancies or infections, particularly toxoplasmosis. The standard approach to this dilemma in a neurologically stable patient is to administer antibiotics to treat toxoplasmosis for 2–3 weeks and then repeat neuroimaging. If the imaging shows clear improvement, antibiotic treatment is continued. If not, a stereotaxic brain biopsy, which has substantially more risk in an immunodeficient than an immunocompetent patient, is performed. Alternatively, when the clinical situation permits a safe lumbar puncture, a CSF examination demonstrating Epstein-Barr virus DNA in CSF in an immunodeficient patient with neuroimaging findings consistent with lymphoma is diagnostic of primary CNS lymphoma. In organ transplant recipients, reversal of the immunosuppressed state can improve outcome. Survival with AIDS-related primary CNS lymphoma is very poor, generally ≤3 months; pretreatment performance status, the degree of immunosuppression, and the extent of CNS dissemination at diagnosis all appear to influence outcome.

Secondary CNS Lymphoma Secondary CNS lymphoma is a manifestation of systemic disease and almost always occurs in adults with progressive B cell lymphoma or B cell leukemia who have tumor involvement of bone, bone marrow, testes, or the cranial sinuses. The leptomeninges are the most common site of CNS metastasis. Leptomeningeal lymphoma is usually detectable with contrast-enhanced CT or gadolinium-enhanced MRI of the brain and spine or by CSF examination. Treatment consists of systemic chemotherapy, intrathecal chemotherapy, and CNS irradiation. It is usually possible to suppress the leptomeningeal disease effectively, although the overall prognosis is determined by the course of the systemic lymphoma. Intraparenchymal lymphoma metastases may be treated with radiation therapy or systemic chemotherapy.

MENINGIOMAS

Meningiomas are derived from mesoderm, probably from cells giving rise to the arachnoid granulations. These tumors are usually benign and attached to the dura. They may invade the skull but only infrequently invade the brain. Meningiomas most often occur along the sagittal sinus, over the cerebral convexities, in the cerebellar-pontine angle, and along the dorsum of the spinal cord. They are more frequent in women than men, with a peak incidence in middle age.

Meningiomas may be found incidentally on a CT or MRI scan or may present with a focal seizure, a slowly progressive neurologic deficit, or symptoms of raised ICP. The radiologic image of a dural-based, extraaxial mass with dense, uniform contrast enhancement is essentially diagnostic, although a dural metastasis must also be considered (Fig. 374-5). A meningioma may have a "dural tail," a streak of dural enhancement flanking the main tumor mass; however, this finding may also be present with other dural tumors.

Total surgical resection of benign meningiomas is curative. If a total resection cannot be achieved, local external beam radiotherapy or ster-

FIGURE 374-4 CNS lymphoma. A. Proton density–weighted MR image through the temporal lobe demonstrates a low signal intensity nodule (*small arrows*) surrounded by a ring of high signal intensity edema (*larger arrows*). **B.** T1-weighted contrast-enhanced axial MRI demonstrates ring enhancement surrounded by a nonenhanced rim of edema. In this patient with AIDS, a solitary lesion of this type is consistent with either lymphoma or toxoplasmosis; the presence of multiple lesions favors toxoplasmosis. **C.** In a different patient with lymphomatous meningitis, an axial postcontrast T1-weighted MRI through the midbrain demonstrates multiple areas of abnormal enhancement in periventricular and subependymal regions (*arrows*). Lymphoma tends to spread subependymally at interfaces of CSF and brain parenchyma.

eotaxic radiosurgery reduces the recurrence rate to <10%. For meningiomas that are not surgically accessible, radiosurgery is the treatment of choice. Small asymptomatic meningiomas incidentally discovered in older patients can safely be followed radiologically; these tumors grow at an average rate of a few millimeters in diameter per year and only rarely become symptomatic.

Rare meningiomas invade the brain or have histologic evidence of malignancy such as nuclear pleomorphism and cellular atypia. A high mitotic index is also predictive of aggressive behavior. *Hemangiopericytoma*, although not strictly a meningioma, is a meningeal tumor with an especially aggressive behavior. Meningiomas with features of aggressiveness and hemangiopericytomas, even if totally excised by gross inspection, frequently recur and should receive postoperative radiotherapy. Chemotherapy has no proven benefit.

FIGURE 374-5 Meningioma. Coronal postcontrast T1-weighted MR image demonstrates an enhancing extraaxial mass arising from the falx cerebri (*arrows*). There is a "dural tail" of contrast enhancement extending superiorly along the intrahemispheric septum.

SCHWANNOMAS

These tumors are also called *neuromas*, *neurinomas*, or *neurolemmomas*. They arise from Schwann cells of nerve roots, most frequently in the eighth cranial nerve (*vestibular schwannoma*, formerly termed *acoustic schwannoma* or *acoustic neuroma*). The fifth cranial nerve is the second most frequent site; however, schwannomas may arise from any cranial or spinal root except the optic and olfactory nerves, which are myelinated by oligodendroglia rather than Schwann cells. Neurofibromatosis (NF) type 2 (see below) strongly predisposes to vestibular schwannoma. Schwannomas of spinal nerve roots also occur in patients with NF type 2 as well as patients with NF type 1.

Eighth cranial nerve schwannomas typically arise from the vestibular division of the nerve. On MRI they are densely and uniformly enhancing neoplasms (**Fig. 374-6**). Vestibular schwannomas enlarge the internal auditory canal, an imaging feature that helps distinguish them from other cerebellopontine angle masses. Because the vestibular system adapts to slow destruction of the eighth nerve, patients with vestibular schwannomas characteristically present with progressive unilateral hearing loss rather than with dizziness or other vestibular symptoms. Unexplained unilateral hearing loss merits evaluation with audiometry and an MRI scan (Chap. 30). As a vestibular schwannoma grows, it can compress the cerebellum, pons, or facial nerve. With rare exceptions schwannomas are histologically and clinically benign.

Whenever possible, schwannomas should be surgically excised. When the tumors are small, it is usually possible to preserve hearing in the involved ear. In the case of large tumors, the patient is usually deaf at presentation; nonetheless, surgery is indicated to prevent further compression of posterior fossa structures. Stereotaxic radiosurgery is also effective treatment for schwannoma and has a complication rate equivalent to that of surgery.

OTHER BENIGN BRAIN TUMORS

Epidermoid tumors are cystic tumors with proliferative epidermal cells at the periphery and more mature epidermal cells towards the center of the cyst. The mature cells desquamate into the liquid center of the cyst. Epidermoid tumors are thought to arise from embryonic epidermal rests within the cranium. They occur extraaxially near the midline, in the middle cranial fossa, the suprasellar region, or the cerebellopontine angle. These well-demarcated lesions are amenable to complete surgical excision. Postoperative radiation therapy is unnecessary.

FIGURE 374-6 Vestibular schwannoma. A. Axial noncontrast MR scan through the cerebellopontine angle demonstrates an extraaxial mass that extends into a widened internal auditory canal, displacing the pons (*arrows*). **B.** Postcontrast T1-weighted image demonstrates intense enhancement of the vestibular schwannoma (*white arrow*). Abnormal enhancement of the left fifth nerve (*black arrow*) most likely represents another schwannoma in this patient with neurofibromatosis type 2.

Dermoid cysts are thought to arise from embryonic rests of skin tissue trapped within the CNS during closure of the neural tube. The most frequent locations are in the midline supratentorially or at the cerebellopontine angle. Histologically, they are composed of multiple elements of the dermis including epidermis, hair follicles, and sweat glands; they frequently calcify. Treatment is surgical excision.

Craniopharyngiomas are thought to arise from remnants of Rathke's pouch, the mesodermal structure from which the anterior pituitary gland is derived (Chap. 333). Craniopharyngiomas typically present as suprasellar masses. Because of their location, they may present as growth failure in children, endocrine dysfunction in adults, or visual loss in either age group. Histologically, craniopharyngiomas resemble epidermoid tumors; they are usually cystic, and in adults 80% are calcified. Treatment is surgical excision; postoperative external beam radiation or stereotaxic radiosurgery is added if total surgical removal cannot be achieved.

Colloid cysts are benign tumors of unknown cellular origin that occur within the third ventricle and can obstruct CSF flow. Other *rare benign primary brain tumors* include neurocytomas, subependymomas, and pleomorphic xanthoastrocytomas. Surgical excision of these neoplasms is the primary treatment and can be curative.

Pituitary tumors are discussed in Chap. 333.

NEUROCUTANEOUS SYNDROMES

This group of genetic disorders, also known as the *phakomatoses*, produces a variety of developmental abnormalities of skin along with an increased risk of nervous system tumors (Table 374-1). These disorders are inherited as autosomal dominant conditions with variable penetrance.

NEUROFIBROMATOSIS TYPE 1 (VON RECKLINGHAUSEN'S DISEASE)

NF1 is characterized by cutaneous *neurofibromas*, pigmented lesions of the skin called *café au lait spots*, freckling in non-sun-exposed areas such as the axilla, hamartomas of the iris termed *Lisch nodules*, and pseudoarthrosis of the tibia. Neurofibromas are benign peripheral nerve tumors composed of proliferating Schwann cells and fibroblasts. They present as multiple, palpable, rubbery, cutaneous tumors. They are generally asymptomatic; however, if they grow in an enclosed space, e.g., the intervertebral foramen, they may produce a compressive radiculopathy or neuropathy. Aqueductal stenosis with hydrocephalus, scoliosis, short stature, hypertension, epilepsy, and mental retardation may also occur.

Patients with NF1 are at increased risk of developing nervous system neoplasms, including plexiform neurofibromas, optic pathway gliomas, ependymomas, meningiomas, astrocytomas, and pheochro-

mocytomas. Neurofibromas may undergo secondary malignant degeneration and become sarcomatous.

Mutation of the *NF1* gene on chromosome 17 causes von Recklinghausen's disease. The *NF1* gene is a tumor-suppressor gene; it encodes a protein, *neurofibromin*, which modulates signal transduction through the *ras* GTPase pathway.

NEUROFIBROMATOSIS TYPE 2

NF2 is characterized by the development of bilateral vestibular schwannomas in >90% of individuals who inherit the gene. Patients with NF2 also have a predisposition for the development of meningiomas, gliomas, and schwannomas of cranial and spinal nerves. In addition, a characteristic type of cataract, juvenile posterior subcapsular lenticular opacity, occurs in NF2. Multiple café au lait spots and peripheral neurofibromas occur rarely.

In patients with NF2, vestibular schwannomas are usually associated with progressive unilateral deafness early in the third decade of life. Bilateral vestibular schwannomas are generally detectable by MRI at that time (Fig. 374-6). Surgical management is designed to treat the underlying tumor and preserve hearing as long as possible.

This syndrome is caused by mutation of the *NF2* gene on chromosome 22q. *NF2* encodes a protein called *neurofibromin 2, schwannomin*, or *merlin*, with homology to a family of cytoskeletal proteins that includes moesin, ezrin, and radixin.

TUBEROUS SCLEROSIS (BOURNEVILLE'S DISEASE)

Tuberous sclerosis is characterized by cutaneous lesions, seizures, and mental retardation. The cutaneous lesions include adenoma sebaceum (facial angiofibromas), ash leaf–shaped hypopigmented macules (best seen under ultraviolet illumination with a Wood's lamp), shagreen patches (yellowish thickenings of the skin over the lumbosacral region of the back), and depigmented nevi. Recognizable by neuroimaging studies, the presence of subependymal nodules, which may be calcified, is characteristic. Tuberous sclerosis patients are at increased risk of developing ependymomas and childhood astrocytomas, of which >90% are *subependymal giant cell astrocytomas*. These are benign neoplasms that may develop in the retina or along the border of the lateral ventricles. They may obstruct the foramen of Monro and produce hydrocephalus. Rhabdomyomas of the myocardium and angiomyomas of the kidney, liver, adrenals, and pancreas may also occur.

Treatment is symptomatic. Anticonvulsants for seizures, shunting for hydrocephalus, and behavioral and educational strategies for mental retardation are the mainstays of management. Severely affected individuals generally die before age 30.

Mutations in either the *TSC-1* gene at 9q or the *TSC-2* gene at 16p are associated with tuberous sclerosis. These genes encode *tuberins*, proteins that modulate the GTPase activity of other cellular signaling proteins.

VON HIPPEL–LINDAU SYNDROME

This syndrome consists of retinal, cerebellar, and spinal hemangioblastomas, which are slowly growing cystic tumors. Hypernephroma, renal cell carcinoma, pheochromocytoma, and benign cysts of the kidneys, pancreas, epididymis, or liver may also occur. Erythropoietin produced by hemangioblastomas may result in polycythemia. Mutation of the von Hippel–Lindau (*VHL*) gene on chromosome 3p, a tumor-suppressor gene, causes this disorder. *VHL* encodes a protein with multiple functions, including modulation of signal transduction in response to cellular hypoxia.

TUMORS METASTATIC TO BRAIN

MECHANISMS OF BRAIN METASTASES

Brain metastases arise from hematogenous spread. The anatomic distribution of brain metastases generally parallels regional cerebral blood flow, with a predilection for the gray matter–white matter junction and

TABLE 374-2 FREQUENCY OF NERVOUS SYSTEM METASTASES BY COMMON PRIMARY TUMORS

Site of Primary Tumor	Brain Metastases, %	Leptomeningeal Metastases, %	Spinal Cord Compression, %
Lung	40	24	18
Breast	19	41	24
Melanoma	10	12	4
Gastrointestinal tract	7	13	6
Genitourinary tract	7		18
Other	17	10	30

for the border zone between middle cerebral and posterior cerebral artery distributions. The lung is the most common origin of brain metastases; both primary lung cancer and cancers metastatic to the lung frequently metastasize to the brain. Breast cancer (especially ductal carcinoma) has a propensity to metastasize to the cerebellum and the posterior pituitary gland. Other common origins of brain metastases are gastrointestinal malignancies and melanoma (Table 374-2). Certain less common tumors have a special propensity to metastasize to brain, including germ cell tumors and thyroid cancer. By contrast, prostate cancer, ovarian cancer, and Hodgkin's disease rarely metastasize to the brain.

EVALUATION OF METASTASES FROM KNOWN CANCER

On MRI scans brain metastases typically appear as well-demarcated, approximately spherical lesions that are hypointense or isointense relative to brain on T1-weighted images and bright on T2-weighted images. They invariably enhance with gadolinium, reflecting extravasation of gadolinium through tumor vessels that lack a blood-tumor barrier (Fig. 374-7). Small metastases often enhance uniformly. Larger metastases typically produce ring enhancement surrounding a central mass of nonenhancing necrotic tissue that develops as the metastasis outgrows its blood supply. Metastases are surrounded by variable amounts of edema. Blood products may also be seen, reflecting hemorrhage of abnormal tumor vessels.

The radiologic appearance of a brain metastasis is not specific. The differential diagnosis of ring-enhancing lesions includes brain abscess, radiation necrosis, toxoplasmosis, granulomas, tuberculosis, sarcoidosis, demyelinating lesions, primary brain tumors, primary CNS lymphoma, stroke, hemorrhage, and trauma. Contrast-enhanced CT scanning is less sensitive than MRI for the detection of brain metastases. Cytologic

examination of the CSF is not indicated, since intraparenchymal brain metastases almost never shed cells into the CSF.

BRAIN METASTASES WITHOUT A KNOWN PRIMARY TUMOR

In general hospital populations, up to one-third of patients presenting with brain metastases do not have a previously known underlying cancer. These patients generally present with either a seizure or a progressive neurologic deficit. Neuroimaging studies typically demonstrate one or multiple ring-enhancing lesions. In individuals who are not immunocompromised and not at risk for brain abscesses, this radiologic pattern is most likely due to brain metastasis.

Diagnostic evaluation begins with a search for the primary tumor. Blood tests should include carcinoembryonic antigen and liver function tests. Examination of the skin for melanoma and the thyroid gland for masses should be carried out. The search for a primary cancer most often discloses lung cancer (particularly small cell lung cancer) or melanoma. In 30% of patients no primary tumor can be identified, even after extensive evaluation. A CT scan of the chest, abdomen, and pelvis should be obtained. If these are all negative, further imaging studies, including bone scan, other radionuclide scans, mammography, and upper and lower gastrointestinal barium studies, are unlikely to be productive.

A tissue diagnosis is essential. If a primary tumor is found, it will usually be more accessible to biopsy than a brain lesion. If a single brain lesion is found in a surgically accessible location, if a primary tumor is not found, or if the primary tumor is in a location difficult to biopsy, the brain metastasis should be biopsied or resected.

Rx TUMORS METASTATIC TO BRAIN

Once a systemic cancer metastasizes to the brain it is, with rare exception, incurable. Therapy is therefore palliative, designed to prevent disability and suffering and, if possible, to prolong life. Published outcome studies have focused on survival as the primary endpoint, leaving questions regarding quality of life unanswered. There is, however, widespread agreement that glucocorticoids, anticonvulsants, radiation therapy, and surgery (see below) can contribute to the management of these patients.

GENERAL MEASURES   Glucocorticoids frequently ameliorate symptoms of brain metastases. Improvement is often dramatic, occurring within 24 h, and is sustained with continued administration, although the toxicity of glucocorticoids is cumulative. Therefore, if possible, a more definitive therapy for metastases should be instituted to permit withdrawal of glucocorticoid therapy. One-third of patients with brain metastases have one or more seizures; anticonvulsants are used empirically for seizure prophylaxis.

SPECIFIC MEASURES   Radiation Therapy
Radiation therapy is the primary treatment for brain metastases. Since multiple microscopic deposits of tumor cells throughout the brain are likely to be present in addition to metastases visualized by neuroimaging studies, WBRT is usually used. Its benefit has been established in controlled studies, but no clear dose response has been shown. Usually, 30–37.5 Gy is administered in 10–15 fractions; an additional dose ("boost") of focal irradiation to a single or large metastasis may also be administered. Stereotaxic radiosurgery is of benefit in patients with four or fewer metastases demonstrable by MRI. The addition of WBRT to stereotaxic radiosurgery delays tumor recurrence in the brain but does not prolong survival.

Surgery   Up to 40% of patients with brain metastases have only a single tumor mass identified by CT. Accessible single metastases may be surgically excised as a palliative measure. If the systemic disease is under control, total resection of a single brain lesion has been demonstrated to improve survival and minimize disability. Survival is further improved if surgery is followed by WBRT.

FIGURE 374-7 Brain metastasis. A. Axial T2-weighted MRI through the lateral ventricles reveals two isodense masses, one in the subependymal region and one near the cortex (*arrows*). **B.** T1-weighted postcontrast image at the same level as **A** reveals enhancement of the two masses seen on the T2-weighted image as well as a third mass in the left frontal lobe (*arrows*).

Chemotherapy Brain metastases of certain tumors, including breast cancer, small cell lung cancer, and germ cell tumors, are often responsive to systemic chemotherapy. Although metastases frequently do not respond as well as the primary tumor, dramatic responses to systemic chemotherapy or hormonal therapy may occur in some cases. In patients who are neurologically asymptomatic, two to four cycles of systemic chemotherapy may be administered initially to reduce tumor mass and render the residual tumor more amenable to radiation therapy. Even if a complete radiologic remission is achieved from chemotherapy, WBRT should then be administered. Gene therapy, immunotherapy, intraarterial chemotherapy, and chemotherapy administered following osmotic disruption of the blood-brain barrier are currently under investigation.

LEPTOMENINGEAL METASTASES

Leptomeningeal metastases are also called *carcinomatous meningitis, meningeal carcinomatosis*, and, in the case of specific tumors, *leukemic meningitis* or *lymphomatous meningitis*. Clinical evidence of leptomeningeal metastases is present in 8% of patients with metastatic solid tumors; at necropsy, the prevalence is as high as 19%. Among solid tumors, adenocarcinomas of the breast, lung, and gastrointestinal tract and melanoma are the most common cause of leptomeningeal metastases (Table 374-2). In one-quarter of patients the systemic cancer is under control, and especially in these patients the effective control of leptomeningeal disease can improve the quality and duration of life.

Cancer usually metastasizes to the meninges via the bloodstream. Alternatively, cells may invade the subarachnoid space directly from a superficially located parenchymal brain metastasis. Some tumors, including squamous cell carcinoma of the skin and some non-Hodgkin's lymphomas, have a propensity to grow along peripheral nerves and may seed the meninges by that route.

CLINICAL FEATURES

Leptomeningeal metastases present with signs and symptoms at multiple levels of the nervous system, most often in a setting of known systemic malignancy. Encephalopathy is frequent, and cranial neuropathy or spinal radiculopathy from nodular nerve root compression is characteristic. Hydrocephalus can result from obstruction of CSF outflow. Focal neurologic deficits reflect coexisting intraparenchymal metastases.

LABORATORY AND IMAGING EVALUATION

Leptomeningeal metastases are diagnosed by cytologic demonstration of malignant cells in the CSF, by MRI demonstration of nodular tumor deposits or diffuse enhancement in the meninges (Fig. 374-8), and by meningeal biopsy. CSF findings are usually those of an inflammatory meningitis consisting of lymphocytic pleocytosis, elevated protein levels, and normal or low CSF glucose. A positive CSF cytology is unequivocal evidence of tumor spread to the subarachnoid space. CSF examination is more likely to be informative when larger volumes of CSF are submitted for cytology and when up to three CSF examinations are performed. A complete MRI examination of the neuraxis is indicated in all cases of suspected leptomeningeal metastases; in addition to nodular meningeal lesions, hydrocephalus due to obstruction of CSF pathways may be found.

℞ LEPTOMENINGEAL METASTASES

Although the prognosis of patients with leptomeningeal metastases is poor, ~20% of patients treated aggressively can expect a response of ≥6 months. Intrathecal therapy exposes meningeal tumor implants to high concentrations of chemotherapy with minimal systemic toxicity. Methotrexate can be safely administered intrathecally and is effective against leptomeningeal metastases from a variety of solid tumors including lymphoma; cytarabine and thiotepa are alternative agents. Liposomal cytarabine provides prolonged cytotoxic levels of cytarabine in the CSF, requiring administration only every 2 weeks, in contrast to weekly or twice weekly administration of other agents. Intrathecal chemotherapy may be administered either by repeated lumbar puncture or through an indwelling Ommaya reservoir, which consists of a catheter in one lateral ventricle attached to a reservoir implanted

FIGURE 374-8 Carcinomatous meningitis. Sagittal postcontrast MRI through the lower thoracic region demonstrates diffuse pial enhancement along the surface of the spinal cord (*arrows*), typical of CSF spread of neoplasm.

under the scalp. If there is a question of patency of CSF pathways, a radionuclide flow study through the reservoir may be performed.

Large, nodular deposits of tumor on the meninges or along nerve roots are unlikely to respond to intrathecal chemotherapy, as the barrier to diffusion is too great. Therefore, external beam radiation is employed, and these patients may also benefit from systemic chemotherapy. Hydrocephalus is treated with a ventriculoperitoneal shunt, although seeding of the peritoneum by tumor is a risk.

MALIGNANT SPINAL CORD COMPRESSION

Spinal cord compression from solid tumor metastases usually results from growth of a vertebral metastasis into the epidural space. Primary tumors that frequently metastasize to bone include lung, breast, and prostate cancer. Back pain is usually the first symptom and is prominent at presentation in 90% of patients. The pain is typically dull, aching, and may be associated with localized tenderness. If a nerve root is compressed, radicular pain is also present. The thoracic cord is most often affected. Weakness, sensory loss, and autonomic dysfunction (urinary urgency and incontinence, fecal incontinence, and sexual impotence in men) are hallmarks of spinal cord compression. Once signs of spinal cord compression appear, they tend to progress rapidly. It is thus essential to recognize and treat this serious complication of malignancy promptly to prevent irreversible neurologic deficits. Diagnosis and management are discussed in Chap. 372.

METASTASES TO THE PERIPHERAL NERVOUS SYSTEM

Systemic cancer may compress or invade peripheral nerves. Compression of the brachial plexus may occur by direct extension of Pancoast's tumors (cancer of the apex of the lung), by lymphoma, or by extension of local lymph node metastases in breast or lung cancer. The lumbosacral plexus may be compressed by retroperitoneal tumor invasion such as occurs in cases of prostate or ovarian cancer or lymphoma. Skull metastases may compress cranial nerve branches as they pass through the skull, and pituitary metastases may extend into the cavernous sinus.

The epineurium generally provides an effective barrier to invasion of the peripheral nerves by solid tumors, but certain tumors characteristically invade and spread along peripheral nerves. Squamous cell carcinoma of the skin may spread along the trigeminal nerve and extend intracranially. Non-Hodgkin's lymphoma may be neurotrophic and cause polyradiculopathy or a syndrome resembling mononeuropathy multiplex (Chap. 379). Focal external beam radiation may reduce

FIGURE 374-9 Radiation injury. A. Late delayed radiation injury 1 year after whole-brain radiation (5500 cGy). T2-weighted MR image at the level of the temporal lobes reveals high signal intensity abnormality in periventricular white matter (*arrows*). **B** and **C.** Focal radiation necrosis 3 years after radiotherapy (7000 cGy) for carcinoma of the nasopharynx. Axial T2-weighted MRI (**B**) demonstrates a mass in the right frontal lobe with surrounding vasogenic edema. Abnormal signal changes are also present on the left. T1-weighted postcontrast MRI (**C**) reveals a heterogeneously enhancing mass in the right cingulate gyrus.

pain, prevent irreversible loss of peripheral nerve function, and possibly restore function.

In patients with cancer who have brachial or lumbosacral plexopathy, it may be difficult to distinguish tumor invasion from radiation injury. High radiation dose or the presence of myokymia (rippling contractions of muscle) suggests radiation injury, whereas pain suggests tumor. Radiographic imaging studies may be equivocal, and surgical exploration is sometimes required.

COMPLICATIONS OF THERAPY

RADIATION TOXICITY

The nervous system is vulnerable to injury by therapeutic radiation. Histologically, there is demyelination, degeneration of small arterioles, and eventually brain infarction and necrosis.

Acute radiation injury to the brain occurs during or immediately after therapy. It is rarely seen with current protocols of external beam radiation but may occur after stereotaxic radiosurgery. Manifestations include headache, sleepiness, and worsening of preexisting neurologic deficits.

Early delayed radiation injury occurs within 4 months of therapy. It is associated with an increased white matter T2 signal on MRI scans. In children, the *somnolence syndrome* is a common form of early delayed radiation injury in which somnolence and ataxia develop after WBRT. Irradiation of the cervical spine may cause Lhermitte's phenomenon, an electricity-like sensation evoked by neck flexion. Symptoms resulting from acute and early delayed radiation injury often respond to glucocorticoid administration, are self-limited, and usually resolve without residual deficits. These injuries do not increase the risk of late radiation injury.

Late delayed radiation injury produces permanent damage to the nervous system. It occurs >4 months (generally 8–24 months) after completion of therapy; onset as late as 15 years after therapy has been described. Following focal brain irradiation, radiation necrosis can occur within the radiation field, producing a contrast-enhancing (frequently ring-enhancing) mass with surrounding white matter signal abnormalities (Fig. 374-9). MRI or CT scans are often unable to distinguish radiation necrosis from recurrent tumor, but PET or SPECT scans may demonstrate the increased glucose metabolism typical of tumor tissue or the decreased metabolism of necrotic tissue. Magnetic resonance spectroscopy may demonstrate a high lactate concentration with relatively low choline concentration in areas of necrosis. Biopsy is frequently required to establish the correct diagnosis. Peripheral nerves, including the brachial and lumbosacral plexuses, may also develop late delayed radiation injury.

If untreated, radiation necrosis of the CNS may act as an expanding mass lesion. Symptoms may resolve spontaneously or respond to treatment with glucocorticoids. Progressive radiation necrosis is best treated with surgical resection if the patient has a life expectancy of at least 6 months and a Karnofsky performance score >70. There are anecdotal reports that anticoagulation with heparin or warfarin may be beneficial. After WBRT, progressive dementia can occur, often accompanied by gait apraxia and urinary incontinence. Radiation injury of large arteries also accelerates the development of atherosclerosis, but an increase in the risk of stroke becomes significant only years after radiation treatment.

Endocrine dysfunction resulting in hypopituitarism frequently follows exposure of the hypothalamus or pituitary gland to therapeutic radiation. Growth hormone is the pituitary hormone most sensitive to radiation therapy, and thyroid-stimulating hormone is the least sensitive; ACTH, prolactin, and the gonadotropins have an intermediate sensitivity.

Development of a second neoplasm is another risk of therapeutic radiation that generally occurs many years after radiation exposure. Depending on the irradiated field, the risk of gliomas, meningiomas, sarcomas, and thyroid cancer is increased.

TOXICITIES OF CHEMOTHERAPY

Chemotherapy regimens used to treat primary brain tumors generally include alkylating agents, either temozolomide or nitrosoureas, and are relatively well tolerated. Infrequently, drugs used to treat CNS neoplasms are associated with the development of altered mental states (e.g., confusion, depression), ataxia, and seizures. Chemotherapy for systemic malignancy is a more frequent cause of nervous system toxicity and is more often toxic to the peripheral than the central nervous system. Cisplatin commonly produces tinnitus and high-frequency bilateral hearing loss, especially in younger patients. At cumulative doses > 450 mg/m², cisplatin can produce a symmetric, large-fiber axonal neuropathy that is predominantly sensory; paclitaxel (Taxol) produces a similar picture. Fluorouracil and high-dose cytarabine can cause cerebellar dysfunction that resolves after discontinuation of therapy. Vincristine, which is commonly used to treat lymphoma, may cause an acute ileus and is frequently associated with development of a progressive distal, symmetric sensory motor neuropathy with foot drop and paresthesias.

FURTHER READINGS

BATCHELOR T, LOEFFLER JS: Primary CNS lymphoma. J Clin Oncol 24:1281, 2006

DEANGELIS L: Chemotherapy for brain tumors—a new beginning. N Engl J Med 352:1036, 2005

FRIEDMAN HS, BIGNER DD: Glioblastoma multiforme and the epidermal growth factor receptor. N Engl J Med 353:1997, 2005

KEIME-GUIBERT F et al: Radiotherapy for glioblastoma in the elderly. N Engl J Med 356:1527, 2007

MCKUSICK VA (ed): *Online Mendelian Inheritance in Man.* URL: *www.ncbi.nlm.nih.gov/Omim/.* Washington, DC, National Library of Medicine, 2007

375 Multiple Sclerosis and Other Demyelinating Diseases

Stephen L. Hauser, Douglas S. Goodin

Demyelinating disorders are characterized by inflammation and selective destruction of central nervous system (CNS) myelin. The peripheral nervous system (PNS) is spared, and most patients have no evidence of an associated systemic illness.

MULTIPLE SCLEROSIS

Multiple sclerosis (MS) is characterized by a triad of inflammation, demyelination, and gliosis (scarring); the course can be relapsing-remitting or progressive. Lesions of MS typically occur at different times and in different CNS locations (i.e., disseminated in time and space). MS affects ~350,000 individuals in the United States and 2.5 million individuals worldwide. In Western societies, MS is second only to trauma as a cause of neurologic disability beginning in early to middle adulthood. Manifestations of MS vary from a benign illness to a rapidly evolving and incapacitating disease requiring profound lifestyle adjustments.

PATHOGENESIS

Anatomy   The lesions of MS (plaques) vary in size from 1 or 2 mm to several centimeters. Acute MS lesions are characterized by perivenular cuffing with inflammatory mononuclear cells, predominantly T cells and macrophages, which also infiltrate the surrounding white matter. At sites of inflammation, the blood-brain barrier (BBB) is disrupted, but unlike vasculitis, the vessel wall is preserved. In many lesions, myelin-specific autoantibodies are present, presumably promoting demyelination directly as well as stimulating macrophages and microglial cells (bone marrow–derived CNS phagocytes) that scavenge the myelin debris. As lesions evolve, there is prominent astrocytic proliferation (gliosis). Surviving oligodendrocytes or those that differentiate from precursor cells may partially remyelinate the surviving naked axons, producing so-called shadow plaques. In many lesions, oligodendrocyte precursors are present in large numbers but fail to remyelinate. Ultrastructural studies of MS lesions suggest that fundamentally different underlying pathologies may exist in different patients. Heterogeneity has been observed in terms of (1) whether the inflammatory cell infiltrate is associated with antibody deposition and activation of complement, and (2) whether the target of the immunopathologic process is the myelin sheath itself or the cell body of the oligodendrocyte. Although relative sparing of axons is typical of MS, partial or total axonal destruction can also occur, especially within highly inflammatory lesions. Evidence also suggests that axonal loss is a major contributor to irreversible neurologic disability in MS (see "Neurodegeneration," below).

Physiology   Nerve conduction in myelinated axons occurs in a saltatory manner, with the nerve impulse jumping from one node of Ranvier to the next without depolarization of the axonal membrane underlying the myelin sheath between nodes (**Fig. 375-1**). This produces considerably faster conduction velocities (~70 m/s) than the slow velocities (~1 m/s) produced by continuous propagation in unmyelinated nerves. Conduction block occurs when the nerve impulse is unable to traverse the demyelinated segment. This can happen when the resting axon membrane becomes hyperpolarized due to the exposure of voltage-dependent potassium channels that are normally buried underneath the myelin sheath. A temporary conduction block often follows a demyelinating event before sodium channels (originally concentrated at the nodes) redistribute along the naked axon (Fig. 375-1). This redistribution ultimately allows continuous propagation of nerve action potentials through the demyelinated segment. On occasion, conduction block is incomplete, affecting, for example, high- but not low-frequency volleys of impulses. Variable conduction block can occur with raised body temperature or metabolic alterations and may explain clinical fluctuations that vary from hour to hour or appear with fever or exercise. Conduction slowing occurs when the demyelinated segments support only (slow) continuous nerve impulse propagation.

Epidemiology   MS is approximately threefold more common in women than men. The age of onset is typically between 20 and 40 years (slightly later in men than in women), but the disease can present across the lifespan. Approximately 10% of cases begin before age 18 years of age, and extremes with onset as early as 1–2 years of age or as late as the eighth decade have been described.

Geographical gradients have been repeatedly observed in MS, with prevalence rates increasing at higher latitudes. The highest known prevalence for MS (250 per 100,000) occurs in the Orkney Islands, located north of Scotland, and similarly high rates are found throughout northern Europe, the northern United States, and Canada. By contrast, the prevalence is low in Japan (6 per 100,000), in other parts of Asia, in equatorial Africa, and in the Middle East.

One proposed explanation for the latitude effect on MS is that there is a protective effect of sun exposure. Ultraviolet radiation from sun is the most important source of vitamin D in most individuals, and low levels of vitamin D are common at high latitudes where sun exposure

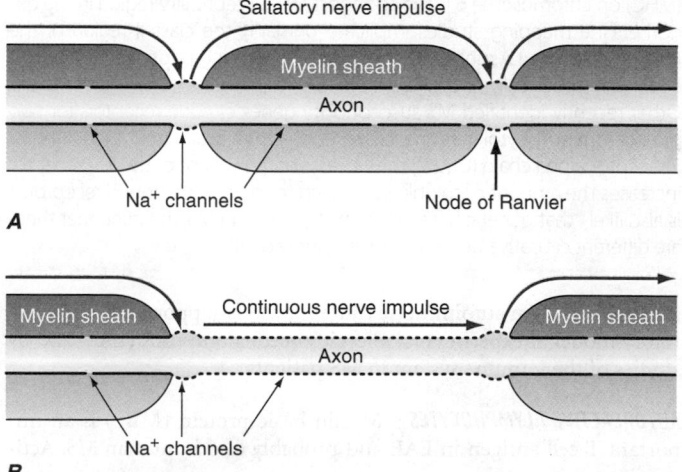

FIGURE 375-1 Nerve conduction in myelinated and demyelinated axons. *A.* Saltatory nerve conduction in myelinated axons occurs with the nerve impulse jumping from one node of Ranvier to the next. Sodium channels (shown as breaks in the solid black line) are concentrated at the nodes where axonal depolarization occurs. ***B.*** Following demyelination, additional sodium channels are redistributed along the axon itself, thereby allowing continuous propagation of the nerve action potential despite the absence of myelin.

may be low, particularly during winter months. Prospective studies have confirmed that vitamin D deficiency is associated with an increase in MS risk. Immunoregulatory effects of vitamin D could explain this possible relationship.

Migration studies and identification of possible point epidemics provide additional support for an environmental effect on MS risk. Migration studies suggest that some MS-related exposure occurs in childhood and years before MS is clinically evident. In some studies, migration early in life from a low- to high-risk area was found to increase MS risk, and conversely, migration from a high- to a low-risk area decreased risk. With respect to possible point epidemics, the most convincing example occurred in the Faeroe Islands north of Denmark after the British occupation during World War II.

The prevalence of MS appears to have steadily increased over the past century; furthermore, this increase has occurred primarily in women. Interestingly, recent epidemiologic data suggests that the latitude effect on MS may currently be decreasing, for unknown reasons.

MS risk also correlates with high socioeconomic status, which may reflect improved sanitation and delayed initial exposures to infectious agents. By analogy, some viral infections (e.g., poliomyelitis and measles viruses) produce neurologic sequelae more frequently when the age of initial infection is delayed. Occasional reports seem to implicate a specific infectious agent such as human herpes virus type 6 (HHV-6) or *Chlamydia pneumoniae*, although, in general, the available reports have been inconsistent.

Most intriguingly, the evidence of a remote Epstein-Barr virus (EBV) infection playing some role in MS is supported by a number of epidemiologic and laboratory studies. A higher risk of infectious mononucleosis (associated with relatively late EBV infection) and higher-antibody titers to latency-associated EBV nuclear antigen are associated with MS; conversely, individuals never infected with EBV are at low MS risk. At this time, however, a causal role for EBV or for any specific infectious agent in MS remains uncertain.

GENETIC CONSIDERATIONS Evidence also supports an important genetic influence on MS. Caucasians are inherently at higher risk for MS than Africans or Asians, even when residing in a similar environment. MS also aggregates within some families, and adoption, half-sibling, twin, and spousal studies indicate that familial aggregation is due to genetic, and not environmental, factors **(Table 375-1)**.

Susceptibility to MS is polygenic, with each gene contributing a relatively small amount to the overall risk. The major histocompatibility complex (MHC) on chromosome 6 is the strongest MS susceptibility region in the genome. Fine mapping studies implicate primarily the class II region of the MHC (encoding HLA molecules involved in presenting peptide antigens to T cells) and specifically the DR2 (molecular designation DRB1*1501) allele. Other recently identified MS susceptibility genes encode receptors for two proinflammatory cytokines, the IL-7 receptor alpha chain (CD127) and the IL-2 receptor alpha chain (CD25); the MS associated variant of the IL-7 receptor increases the amount of soluble compared to membrane bound receptor. It is also likely that genetic heterogeneity is present in MS, meaning that there are different causative genes in different individuals.

Immunology An autoimmune cause for MS is supported by the laboratory model of experimental allergic encephalomyelitis (EAE) and by studies of the immune system in MS patients.

AUTOREACTIVE T LYMPHOCYTES Myelin basic protein (MBP) is an important T cell antigen in EAE and probably also in human MS. Activated MBP-reactive T cells have been identified in the blood, in cerebrospinal fluid (CSF), and within MS lesions. Moreover, DR2 may influence the autoimmune response because it binds with high affinity to a fragment of MBP (spanning amino acids 89–96), stimulating T cell responses to this self-protein.

HUMORAL AUTOIMMUNITY B cell activation and antibody responses also appear to be necessary for the full development of demyelinating lesions to occur, both in experimental models and in human MS. Increased numbers of clonally expanded B cells with properties of postgerminal center memory or antibody-producing lymphocytes are present in MS lesions and in CSF. Myelin-specific autoantibodies, some directed against myelin oligodendrocyte glycoprotein (MOG), have been detected bound to vesiculated myelin debris in MS plaques. In the CSF, elevated levels of locally synthesized immunoglobulins and oligoclonal antibodies derived from expansion of clonally restricted plasma cells are also characteristic of MS. The pattern of oligoclonal banding is unique to each individual, and attempts to identify the targets of these antibodies have been largely unsuccessful, although one recent report indicated that some bands recognized EBV antigens.

CYTOKINES Cytokines and chemokines appear to regulate many of the cellular interactions that operate in MS. Proinflammatory T_H1 cytokines including interleukin (IL) 2, tumor necrosis factor (TNF) α, and interferon (IFN) γ play key roles in activating and maintaining autoimmune responses, and TNF-α and IFN-γ may directly injure oligodendrocytes or the myelin membrane.

TRIGGERS Studies reveal that in patients with early relapsing remitting MS, serial MRI has demonstrated bursts of focal inflammatory disease activity occurring far more frequently than would have been predicted by the frequency of relapses. Thus, early in MS, most disease activity is clinically silent. The triggers causing these bursts are unknown, although the fact that patients may experience relapses after nonspecific upper respiratory infections suggests that either molecular mimicry between viruses and myelin antigens or viral superantigens activating pathogenic T cells may play a role in MS pathogenesis (Chap. 312).

Neurodegeneration Axonal damage occurs in every newly formed MS lesion, and cumulative axonal loss is considered to be the major cause of progressive and irreversible neurological disability in MS. As many as 70% of axons are lost from the lateral corticospinal tracts in patients with advanced paraparesis from MS, and longitudinal MRI studies suggest there is progressive axonal loss over time within established, inactive, lesions. Knowledge of the mechanisms responsible for axonal injury is incomplete, and it is even unclear whether demyelination is a prerequisite for axonal injury in MS. Demyelination can result in reduced trophic support for axons, redistribution of ion channels, and destabilization of action potential membrane potentials. Axons can initially adapt, but eventually distal and retrograde degeneration occurs. Therefore the early promotion of remyelination and preservation of oligodendrocytes remain important therapeutic goals in MS. Some evidence suggests that axonal damage is mediated directly by resident and invading inflammatory cells and their toxic products, in particular by microglia, macrophages, and CD8 T lymphocytes. Activated microglia are particularly likely to cause axonal injury through the release of NO and oxygen radicals and via glutamate, which is toxic to oligodendrocytes and neurons.

CLINICAL MANIFESTATIONS

The onset of MS may be abrupt or insidious. Symptoms may be severe or seem so trivial that a patient may not seek medical attention for months or years. Indeed, at autopsy some individuals who were asymptomatic during life will be found, unexpectedly, to have MS. In others, an MRI scan obtained for an unrelated reason may show evidence of asymptomatic MS. Symptoms of MS are extremely varied and depend on the location and severity of lesions within the CNS

TABLE 375-1	RISK OF DEVELOPING MS
1 in 3	If an identical twin has MS
1 in 15	If a fraternal twin has MS
1 in 25	If a sibling has MS
1 in 50	If a parent or half-sibling has MS
1 in 100	If a first cousin has MS
1 in 1000	If a spouse has MS
1 in 1000	If no one in the family has MS

Symptom	Percent of Cases	Symptom	Percent of Cases
TABLE 375-2	**INITIAL SYMPTOMS OF MS**		
Sensory loss	37	Lhermitte	3
Optic neuritis	36	Pain	3
Weakness	35	Dementia	2
Paresthesias	24	Visual loss	2
Diplopia	15	Facial palsy	1
Ataxia	11	Impotence	1
Vertigo	6	Myokymia	1
Paroxysmal attacks	4	Epilepsy	1
Bladder	4	Falling	1

Source: After WB Matthews et al, *McAlpine's Multiple Sclerosis,* New York, Churchill Livingstone, 1991.

(Table 375-2). Examination generally reveals evidence of neurologic dysfunction, often in asymptomatic locations. For example, a patient may present with symptoms in one leg but signs in both.

Weakness of the limbs may manifest as loss of strength or dexterity, fatigue, or a disturbance of gait. Exercise-induced weakness is a characteristic symptom of MS. The weakness is of the upper motor neuron type (Chap. 23) and is usually accompanied by other pyramidal signs such as spasticity, hyperreflexia and Babinski signs. Occasionally a tendon reflex may be lost (simulating a lower motor neuron lesion) if an MS lesion disrupts the afferent reflex fibers in the spinal cord.

Spasticity (Chap. 23) is often associated with spontaneous and movement-induced muscle spasms. More than 30% of MS patients have moderate to severe spasticity, especially in the legs. This is often accompanied by painful spasms, interfering with ambulation, work, or self-care. Occasionally spasticity provides support for the body weight during ambulation, and in these cases treatment of spasticity may actually do more harm than good.

Optic neuritis (ON) presents as diminished visual acuity, dimness, or decreased color perception (desaturation) in the central field of vision. These symptoms may be mild or may progress to severe visual loss. Rarely, there is complete loss of light perception. Visual symptoms are generally monocular but may be bilateral. Periorbital pain (aggravated by eye movement) often precedes or accompanies the visual loss. An afferent pupillary defect (Chap. 29) is usually present. Funduscopic examination may be normal or reveal optic disc swelling (papillitis). Pallor of the optic disc (optic atrophy) commonly follows ON. Uveitis is rare and should raise the possibility of alternative diagnoses.

Visual blurring in MS may result from ON or diplopia; if the symptom resolves when either eye is covered, the cause is diplopia.

Diplopia may result from internuclear ophthalmoplegia (INO) or from palsy of the sixth cranial nerve (rarely the third or fourth). An INO consists of impaired adduction of one eye due to a lesion in the ipsilateral medial longitudinal fasciculus (Chap. 29). Prominent nystagmus is often observed in the abducting eye, along with a small skew deviation. A bilateral INO is particularly suggestive of MS. Other common gaze disturbances in MS include (1) a horizontal gaze palsy, (2) a "one and a half" syndrome (horizontal gaze palsy plus an INO), and (3) acquired pendular nystagmus.

Sensory symptoms are varied and include both paresthesias (e.g., tingling, prickling sensations, formications, "pins and needles," or painful burning) and hypesthesia (e.g., reduced sensation, numbness, or a "dead" feeling). Unpleasant sensations (e.g., feelings that body parts are swollen, wet, raw, or tightly wrapped) are also common. Sensory impairment of the trunk and legs below a horizontal line on the torso (a sensory level) indicates that the spinal cord is the origin of the sensory disturbance. It is often accompanied by a bandlike sensation of tightness around the torso. Pain is a common symptom of MS, experienced by >50% of patients. Pain can occur anywhere on the body and can change locations over time.

Ataxia usually manifests as cerebellar tremors (Chap. 368). Ataxia may also involve the head and trunk or the voice, producing a characteristic cerebellar dysarthria (scanning speech).

Bladder dysfunction is present in >90% of MS patients, and in a third of patients, dysfunction results in weekly or more frequent episodes of incontinence. During normal reflex voiding, relaxation of the bladder sphincter (α-adrenergic innervation) is coordinated with contraction of the detrusor muscle in the bladder wall (muscarinic cholinergic innervation). *Detrusor hyperreflexia*, due to impairment of suprasegmental inhibition, causes urinary frequency, urgency, nocturia, and uncontrolled bladder emptying. *Detrusor sphincter dyssynergia*, due to loss of synchronization between detrusor and sphincter muscles, causes difficulty in initiating and/or stopping the urinary stream, producing hesitancy, urinary retention, overflow incontinence, and recurrent infection.

Constipation occurs in >30% of patients. Fecal urgency or *bowel incontinence* is less common (15%) but can be socially debilitating.

Cognitive dysfunction can include memory loss, impaired attention, difficulties in problem solving, slowed information processing, and problems shifting between cognitive tasks. Euphoria (elevated mood) was once thought to be characteristic of MS but is actually uncommon, occurring in <20% of patients. Cognitive dysfunction sufficient to impair activities of daily living is rare.

Depression, experienced by approximately half of patients, can be reactive, endogenous, or part of the illness itself and can contribute to fatigue. Suicide in MS patients is 7.5-fold more common than in age-matched controls.

Fatigue is experienced by 90% of patients; this symptom is the most common reason for work-related disability in MS. Fatigue can be exacerbated by elevated temperatures, by depression, by expending exceptional effort to accomplish basic activities of daily living, or by sleep disturbances (e.g., from frequent nocturnal awakenings to urinate).

Sexual dysfunction may manifest as decreased libido, impaired genital sensation, impotence in men, and diminished vaginal lubrication or adductor spasms in women.

Facial weakness due to a lesion in the pons may resemble idiopathic Bell's palsy (Chap. 371). Unlike Bell's palsy, facial weakness in MS is usually not associated with ipsilateral loss of taste sensation or retroauricular pain.

Vertigo may appear suddenly from a brainstem lesion, superficially resembling acute labyrinthitis (Chap. 22). *Hearing loss* may also occur in MS but is uncommon.

Ancillary Symptoms *Heat sensitivity* refers to neurologic symptoms produced by an elevation of the body's core temperature. For example, unilateral visual blurring may occur during a hot shower or with physical exercise (*Uhthoff's symptom*). It is also common for MS symptoms to worsen transiently, sometimes dramatically, during febrile illnesses (see "Acute Attacks or Initial Demyelinating Episodes," below). Such heat-related symptoms probably result from transient conduction block (see above).

Lhermitte's symptom is an electric shocklike sensation (typically induced by flexion or other movements of the neck) that radiates down the back into the legs. Rarely, it radiates into the arms. It is generally self-limited but may persist for years. Lhermitte's symptom can also occur with other disorders of the cervical spinal cord (e.g., cervical spondylosis).

Paroxysmal symptoms are distinguished by their brief duration (10 s to 2 min), high frequency (5–40 episodes per day), lack of any alteration of consciousness or change in background electroencephalogram during episodes, and a self-limited course (generally lasting weeks to months). They may be precipitated by hyperventilation or movement. These syndromes may include Lhermitte's symptom; tonic contractions of a limb, face, or trunk (tonic seizures); paroxysmal dysarthria and ataxia; paroxysmal sensory disturbances; and several other less well-characterized syndromes. Paroxysmal symptoms probably result from spontaneous discharges, arising at the edges of demyelinated plaques and spreading to adjacent white matter tracts.

Trigeminal neuralgia, hemifacial spasm, and *glossopharyngeal neuralgia* (Chap. 371) can occur when the demyelinating lesion involves the root entry (or exit) zone of the fifth, seventh, and ninth cranial

FIGURE 375-2 Clinical course of multiple sclerosis (MS). *A.* Relapsing/remitting MS. ***B.*** Secondary progressive MS. ***C.*** Primary progressive MS. ***D.*** Progressive/relapsing MS.

nerve, respectively. Trigeminal neuralgia (tic douloureux) is a very brief lancinating facial pain often triggered by an afferent input from the face or teeth. Most cases of trigeminal neuralgia are not MS-related; however, atypical features such as onset before age 50 years, bilateral symptoms, objective sensory loss, or nonparoxysmal pain should raise concerns that MS could be responsible.

Facial myokymia consists of either persistent rapid flickering contractions of the facial musculature (especially the lower portion of the orbicularis oculus) or a contraction that slowly spreads across the face. It results from lesions of the corticobulbar tracts or brainstem course of the facial nerve.

DISEASE COURSE

Four clinical types of MS have been described (Fig. 375-2):

1. *Relapsing/remitting MS* (RRMS) accounts for 85% of MS cases at onset and is characterized by discrete attacks that generally evolve over days to weeks (rarely over hours). There is often complete recovery over the ensuing weeks to months (Fig. 375-2*A*). However, when ambulation is severely impaired during an attack, approximately half will fail to improve. Between attacks, patients are neurologically stable.

2. *Secondary progressive MS* (SPMS) always begins as RRMS (Fig. 375-2*B*). At some point, however, the clinical course changes so that the patient experiences a steady deterioration in function unassociated with acute attacks (which may continue or cease during the progressive phase). SPMS produces a greater amount of fixed neurologic disability than RRMS. For a patient with RRMS, the risk of developing SPMS is ~2.5% each year, meaning that the great majority of RRMS ultimately evolves into SPMS. SPMS appears to represent a late stage of the same underlying illness as RRMS.

3. *Primary progressive MS* (PPMS) accounts for ~15% of cases. These patients do not experience attacks but only a steady functional decline from disease onset (Fig. 375-2*C*). Compared to RRMS, the sex distribution is more even, the disease begins later in life (mean age ~40 years), and disability develops faster (at least relative to the onset of the first clinical symptom). Whether PPMS is an uncommon form of the same underlying illness as RRMS or whether these are distinct illnesses is uncertain.

4. *Progressive/relapsing MS* (PRMS) overlaps PPMS and SPMS and accounts for ~5% of MS patients. Like patients with PPMS, these patients experience a steady deterioration in their condition from disease onset. However, like SPMS patients, they experience occasional attacks superimposed upon their progressive course (Fig. 375-2*D*).

TABLE 375-3 DIAGNOSTIC CRITERIA FOR MS

1. Examination must reveal *objective* abnormalities of the CNS.
2. Involvement must reflect predominantly disease of white matter long tracts, usually including (a) pyramidal pathways, (b) cerebellar pathways, (c) medial longitudinal fasciculus, (d) optic nerve, and (e) posterior columns.
3. Examination or history must implicate involvement of two or more areas of the CNS.
   a. MRI may be used to document a second lesion when only one site of abnormality has been demonstrable on examination. A confirmatory MRI must have either four lesions involving the white matter or three lesions if one is periventricular in location. Acceptable lesions must be >3 mm in diameter. For patients older than 50 years, two of the following criteria must also be met: (a) lesion size >5 mm, (b) lesions adjacent to the bodies of the lateral ventricles, and (c) lesion(s) present in the posterior fossa.
   b. Evoked response testing may be used to document a second lesion not evident on clinical examination.
4. The clinical pattern must consist of (a) two or more separate episodes of worsening involving different sites of the CNS, each lasting at least 24 h and occurring at least 1 month apart, or (b) gradual or stepwise progression over at least 6 months if accompanied by increased IgG synthesis or two or more oligoclonal bands. MRI may be used to document dissemination in time if a new T2 lesion or a Gd-enhancing lesion is seen 3 or more months after a clinically isolated syndrome.
5. The patient's neurologic condition could not better be attributed to another disease.

Diagnostic Categories

1. *Definite MS:* All five criteria fulfilled.
2. *Probable MS: All* five criteria fulfilled except (a) only one objective abnormality despite two symptomatic episodes or (b) only one symptomatic episode despite two or more objective abnormalities.
3. *At risk for MS:* Criteria 1, 2, 3, and 5 fulfilled; patient has only one symptomatic episode and one objective abnormality.

Note: CNS, central nervous system; MRI, magnetic resonance imaging; Gd, gadolinium.

DIAGNOSIS

There is no definitive diagnostic test for MS. Diagnostic criteria for clinically definite MS require documentation of two or more episodes of symptoms and two or more signs that reflect pathology in anatomically noncontiguous white matter tracts of the CNS (Table 375-3). Symptoms must last for >24 h and occur as distinct episodes that are separated by a month or more. At least one of the two required signs must be present on neurologic examination. The second may be documented by abnormal paraclinical tests such as MRI or evoked potentials (EPs). Similarly, in the most recent diagnostic scheme, the second clinical event (in time) may be supported solely by paraclinical information, usually the development of new focal white matter lesions on MRI. In patients who experience gradual progression of disability for ≥6 months without superimposed relapses, documentation of intrathecal IgG may be used to support the diagnosis.

DIAGNOSTIC TESTS

Magnetic Resonance Imaging MRI has revolutionized the diagnosis and management of MS (Fig. 375-3); characteristic abnormalities are found in >95% of patients. An increase in vascular permeability from a breakdown of the BBB is detected by leakage of intravenous gadolinium (Gd) into the parenchyma. Such leakage occurs early in the development of an MS lesion and serves as a useful marker of inflammation. Gd enhancement persists for approximately 1 month, and the residual MS plaque remains visible indefinitely as a focal area of hyperintensity (a lesion) on spin-echo (T2-weighted) and proton-density images. Lesions are frequently oriented perpendicular to the ventricular surface, corresponding to the pathologic pattern of perivenous demyelination (Dawson's fingers). Lesions are multifocal within the brain, brainstem, and spinal cord. Lesions larger than 6 mm located in the corpus callosum, periventricular white matter, brainstem, cerebellum, or spinal cord are particularly helpful diagnostically. Different criteria for the use of MRI in the diagnosis of MS have been proposed (Table 375-3).

The total volume of T2-weighted signal abnormality (the "burden of disease") shows a significant (albeit weak) correlation with clinical

FIGURE 375-3 MRI findings in MS. A. Axial first-echo image from T2-weighted sequence demonstrates multiple bright signal abnormalities in white matter, typical for MS. **B.** Sagittal T2-weighted FLAIR (fluid attenuated inversion recovery) image in which the high signal of CSF has been suppressed. CSF appears dark, while areas of brain edema or demyelination appear high in signal as shown here in the corpus callosum (*arrows*). Lesions in the anterior corpus callosum are frequent in MS and rare in vascular disease. **C.** Sagittal T2-weighted fast spin echo image of the thoracic spine demonstrates a fusiform high-signal-intensity lesion in the mid thoracic spinal cord. **D.** Sagittal T1-weighted image obtained after the intravenous administration of gadolinium DTPA reveals focal areas of blood-brain barrier disruption, identified as high-signal-intensity regions (*arrows*).

ically uninvolved. For example, in a patient with a remitting and relapsing spinal cord syndrome with sensory deficits in the legs, an abnormal somatosensory EP following posterior tibial nerve stimulation provides little new information. By contrast, an abnormal visual EP in this circumstance would permit a diagnosis of clinically definite MS (Table 375-3). Abnormalities on one or more EP modalities occur in 80–90% of MS patients. EP abnormalities are not specific to MS, although a marked delay in the latency of a specific EP component (as opposed to a reduced amplitude or distorted waveshape) is suggestive of demyelination.

Cerebrospinal Fluid CSF abnormalities found in MS include a mononuclear cell pleocytosis and an increased level of intrathecally synthesized IgG. The total CSF protein is usually normal or slightly elevated. Various formulas distinguish intrathecally synthesized IgG from IgG that may have entered the CNS passively from the serum. One formula, the CSF IgG index, expresses the ratio of IgG to albumin in the CSF divided by the same ratio in the serum. The IgG synthesis rate uses serum and CSF IgG and albumin measurements to calculate the rate of CNS IgG synthesis. The measurement of oligoclonal banding (OCB) in the CSF also assesses intrathecal production of IgG. OCBs are detected by agarose gel electrophoresis. Two or more OCBs are found in 75–90% of patients with MS. OCBs may be absent at the onset of MS, and in individual patients the number of bands may increase with time. It is important that paired serum samples be studied to exclude a peripheral (i.e., non-CNS) origin of any OCBs detected in the CSF.

A mild CSF pleocytosis (>5 cells/μL) is present in ~25% of cases, usually in young patients with RRMS. A pleocytosis of >75 cells/μL, the presence of polymorphonuclear leukocytes, or a protein concentration of >1.0 g/L (>100 mg/dL) in CSF should raise concern that the patient may not have MS.

disability, as do measures of brain atrophy. Approximately one-third of T2-weighted lesions appear as hypointense lesions (black holes) on T1-weighted imaging. Black holes may be a marker of irreversible demyelination and axonal loss, although even this measure depends on the timing of the image acquisition (e.g., most acute Gd-enhancing T2 lesions are T1 dark).

Newer MRI measures such as magnetization transfer ratio (MTR) imaging and proton magnetic resonance spectroscopic imaging (MRSI) may ultimately serve as surrogate markers of clinical disability. For example, MRSI can quantitate molecules such as *N*-acetyl aspartate, which is a marker of axonal integrity, and MTR may be able to distinguish demyelination from edema.

Evoked Potentials EP testing assesses function in afferent (visual, auditory, and somatosensory) or efferent (motor) CNS pathways. EPs use computer averaging to measure CNS electric potentials evoked by repetitive stimulation of selected peripheral nerves or of the brain. These tests provide the most information when the pathways studied are clin-

DIFFERENTIAL DIAGNOSIS

No single clinical sign or test is diagnostic of MS. The diagnosis is readily made in a young adult with relapsing and remitting symptoms involving different areas of CNS white matter. The possibility of an alternative diagnosis should always be considered (Table 375-4), particularly when (1) symptoms are localized exclusively to the posterior fossa, craniocervical junction, or spinal cord; (2) the patient is <15 or >60 years of age; (3) the clinical course is progressive from onset; (4) the patient has never experienced visual, sensory, or bladder symptoms; or (5) laboratory findings (e.g., MRI, CSF, or EPs) are atypical. Similarly, uncommon or rare symptoms in MS (e.g., aphasia, parkinsonism, chorea, isolated dementia, severe muscular atrophy, peripheral neuropathy, episodic loss of consciousness, fever, headache, seizures, or coma) should increase concern about an alternative diagnosis. Diagnosis is also difficult in patients with a rapid or explosive (strokelike) onset or with mild symptoms and a normal neurologic examination. Rarely, intense inflammation and swelling may produce a mass lesion that mimics a primary or metastatic

TABLE 375-4 DISORDERS THAT CAN MIMIC MS

Acute disseminated encephalomyelitis (ADEM)
Antiphospholipid antibody syndrome
Behçet's disease
Cerebral autosomal dominant arteriopathy, subcortical infarcts, and
  leukoencephalopathy (CADASIL)
Congenital leukodystrophies (e.g., adrenoleukodystrophy, metachromatic
  leukodystrophy)
Human immunodeficiency virus (HIV) infection
Ischemic optic neuropathy (arteritic and nonarteritic)
Lyme disease
Mitochondrial encephalopathy with lactic acidosis and stroke (MELAS)
Neoplasms (e.g., lymphoma, glioma, meningioma)
Sarcoid
Sjögren's syndrome
Stroke and ischemic cerebrovascular disease
Syphilis
Systemic lupus erythematosus and related collagen vascular disorders
Tropical spastic paraparesis (HTLV I/II infection)
Vascular malformations (especially spinal dural AV fistulas)
Vasculitis (primary CNS or other)
Vitamin B_{12} deficiency

Note: HTLV, human T cell lymphotropic virus; AV, arteriovenous; CNS, central nervous system.

tumor. The specific tests required to exclude alternative diagnoses will vary with each clinical situation; however, an erythrocyte sedimentation rate, serum B_{12} level, ANA, and treponemal antibody should probably be obtained in all patients with suspected MS.

PROGNOSIS

Most patients with MS ultimately experience progressive neurologic disability. Fifteen years after onset, only 20% of patients have no functional limitation; between one-third and one-half will have progressed to SPMS and will require assistance with ambulation. Twenty-five years after onset, ~80% of MS patients will have reached this level of disability. In 1998, it was estimated that the total annual economic burden of MS in the United States exceeded $6.8 billion.

However, even if the prognosis for disability is grave for the average patient, the prognosis in an individual is difficult to establish. Certain clinical features suggest a more favorable prognosis, including ON or sensory symptoms at onset; fewer than two relapses in the first year of illness; and minimal impairment after 5 years. By contrast, patients with truncal ataxia, action tremor, pyramidal symptoms, or a progressive disease course are more likely to become disabled.

Importantly, some MS patients have a benign variant of MS and never develop neurologic disability. The likelihood of having benign MS is thought to be <20%. Patients with benign MS 15 years after onset who have entirely normal neurologic examinations are likely to maintain their benign course.

In patients with their first demyelinating event (i.e., a clinically isolated syndrome), the brain MRI provides prognostic information. With three or more typical T2-weighted lesions, the risk of developing MS after 10 years is 70–80%. Conversely, with a normal brain MRI, the likelihood of developing MS is <20%. Similarly, two or more Gd-enhancing lesions at baseline is highly predictive of future MS, as is the appearance of either new T2-weighted lesions or new Gd enhancement ≥3 months after the initial episode.

Mortality as a direct consequence of MS is uncommon, although it has been estimated that the 25-year survival is only 85% of expected. Death can occur during an acute MS attack, although this is distinctly rare. More commonly, death occurs as a complication of MS (e.g., pneumonia in a debilitated individual). Death also results from suicide.

Effect of Pregnancy Pregnant MS patients experience fewer attacks than expected during gestation (especially in the last trimester), but more attacks than expected in the first 3 months postpartum. When considering the pregnancy year as a whole (i.e., 9 months pregnancy plus 3 months postpartum), the overall disease course is unaffected. Decisions about childbearing should thus be made based on (1) the

mother's physical state, (2) her ability to care for the child, and (3) the availability of social support. Disease-modifying therapy is generally discontinued during pregnancy, although the actual risk from the interferons and glatiramer acetate (see below) appears to be low.

℞ MULTIPLE SCLEROSIS

Therapy for MS can be divided into several categories: (1) treatment of acute attacks as they occur, (2) treatment with disease-modifying agents that reduce the biological activity of MS, and (3) symptomatic therapy. Treatments that promote remyelination or neural repair do not currently exist but would be highly desirable.

The Kurtzke Expanded Disability Status Score (EDSS) is a useful measure of neurologic impairment in MS **(Table 375-5)**. Most patients with EDSS scores <3.5 have RRMS, walk normally, and are generally not disabled; by contrast, patients with EDSS scores >5.5 have progressive MS (SPMS or PPMS), are gait-impaired and, typically, are occupationally disabled.

ACUTE ATTACKS OR INITIAL DEMYELINATING EPISODES

When patients experience acute deterioration, it is important to consider whether this change reflects new disease activity or a "pseudoexacerbation" resulting from an increase in ambient temperature, fever, or an infection. In such instances, glucocorticoid treatment is inappropriate. Glucocorticoids are used to manage either first attacks or acute exacerbations. They provide short-term clinical benefit by reducing the severity and shortening the duration of attacks. Whether treatment provides any long-term benefit on the course of the illness is less clear. Therefore, mild attacks are often not treated. Physical and occupational therapy can help with mobility and manual dexterity.

Glucocorticoid treatment is usually administered as intravenous methylprednisolone, 500–1000 mg/d for 3–5 days, either without a taper or followed by a course of oral prednisone beginning at a dose of 60–80 mg/d and gradually tapered over 2 weeks. Outpatient treatment is usually possible. If intravenous therapy is unavailable or inconvenient, oral glucocorticoids can be substituted.

Side effects of short-term glucocorticoid therapy include fluid retention, potassium loss, weight gain, gastric disturbances, acne, and emotional lability. Concurrent use of a low-salt, potassium-rich diet and avoidance of potassium-wasting diuretics is advisable. Lithium carbonate (300 mg orally bid) may help to manage emotional lability and insomnia associated with glucocorticoid therapy. Patients with a history of peptic ulcer disease may require cimetidine (400 mg bid) or ranitidine (150 mg bid).

Plasma exchange (seven exchanges: 40–60 mL/kg per exchange, every other day for 14 days) may benefit patients with fulminant attacks of demyelination (not only MS) that are unresponsive to glucocorticoids. However, the cost is high, and the evidence of efficacy is only preliminary.

DISEASE-MODIFYING THERAPIES FOR RELAPSING FORMS OF MS (RRMS, SPMS WITH EXACERBATIONS) Five such agents are approved in the United States: (1) IFN-β-1a (Avonex), (2) IFN-β-1a (Rebif), (3) IFN-β-1b (Betaseron), (4) glatiramer acetate (Copaxone), and (5) natalizumab (Tysabri). Each of these treatments is also used in SPMS patients who continue to experience attacks, because SPMS can be difficult to distinguish from RRMS, and because clinical trials suggest that such patients also derive therapeutic benefit. In Phase III clinical trials, recipients of IFN-β-1b, IFN-β-1a, glatiramer acetate, and natalizumab experienced fewer clinical exacerbations and fewer new MRI lesions compared to placebo recipients **(Table 375-6)**. Mitoxantrone (Novantrone), an immune suppressant, has also been approved in the United States, although it is generally reserved for patients with progressive disability who have failed other treatments because of its potential toxicity.

Interferon β, Glatiramer Acetate, and Natalizumab IFN-β is a class I interferon originally identified by its antiviral properties. Efficacy in MS probably results from immunomodulatory properties including (1) downregulating expression of MHC molecules on antigen-presenting cells, (2) inhibiting proinflammatory and increasing regulatory cytokine levels, (3) inhibition of T cell proliferation, and (4) limiting the trafficking of inflammatory cells in the CNS. Glatiramer acetate is a synthetic, random polypeptide composed of four amino acids (L-glutamic acid, L-lysine, L-alanine, and L-tyrosine). Its mechanism of action may include (1) induction of antigen-specific suppressor T cells; (2) binding to MHC molecules, thereby displacing bound MBP; or (3) altering the balance between proinflammatory and regulatory cytokines.

TABLE 375-5 SCORING SYSTEMS FOR MS

Kurtzke Expanded Disability Status Score (EDSS)

0.0 = Normal neurologic exam [all grade 0 in functional status (FS)]
1.0 = No disability, minimal signs in one FS (i.e., grade 1)
1.5 = No disability, minimal signs in more than one FS (more than one grade 1)
2.0 = Minimal disability in one FS (one FS grade 2, others 0 or 1)
2.5 = Minimal disability in two FS (two FS grade 2, others 0 or 1)
3.0 = Moderate disability in one FS (one FS grade 3, others 0 or 1) or mild disability in three or four FS (three/four FS grade 2, others 0 or 1) though fully ambulatory
3.5 = Fully ambulatory but with moderate disability in one FS (one grade 3) and one or two FS grade 2; or two FS grade 3; or five FS grade 2 (others 0 or 1)
4.0 = Ambulatory without aid or rest for ≥ 500 m
4.5 = Ambulatory without aid or rest for ≥ 300 m
5.0 = Ambulatory without aid or rest for ≥ 200 m
5.5 = Ambulatory without aid or rest for ≥ 100 m

6.0 = Unilateral assistance required to walk about 100 m with or without resting
6.5 = Constant bilateral assistance required to walk about 20 m without resting
7.0 = Unable to walk beyond about 5 m even with aid; essentially restricted to wheelchair; wheels self and transfers alone
7.5 = Unable to take more than a few steps; restricted to wheelchair; may need aid to transfer
8.0 = Essentially restricted to bed or chair or perambulated in wheelchair, but out of bed most of day; retains many self-care functions; generally has effective use of arms
8.5 = Essentially restricted to bed much of the day; has some effective use of arm(s); retains some self-care functions
9.0 = Helpless bed patient; can communicate and eat
9.5 = Totally helpless bed patient; unable to communicate or eat
10.0 = Death due to MS

Functional Status (FS) Score

A. Pyramidal functions
  0 = Normal
  1 = Abnormal signs without disability
  2 = Minimal disability
  3 = Mild or moderate paraparesis or hemiparesis, or severe monoparesis
  4 = Marked paraparesis or hemiparesis, moderate quadriparesis, or monoplegia
  5 = Paraplegia, hemiplegia, or marked quadriparesis
  6 = Quadriplegia
B. Cerebellar functions
  0 = Normal
  1 = Abnormal signs without disability
  2 = Mild ataxia
  3 = Moderate truncal or limb ataxia
  4 = Severe ataxia all limbs
  5 = Unable to perform coordinated movements due to ataxia
C. Brainstem functions
  0 = Normal
  1 = Signs only
  2 = Moderate nystagmus or other mild disability
  3 = Severe nystagmus, marked extraocular weakness, or moderate disability of other cranial nerves
  4 = Marked dysarthria or other marked disability
  5 = Inability to swallow or speak
D. Sensory functions
  0 = Normal
  1 = Vibration or figure-writing decrease only, in 1 or 2 limbs
  2 = Mild decrease in touch or pain or position sense, and/or moderate decrease in vibration in 1 or 2 limbs, or vibratory decrease alone in 3 or 4 limbs
  3 = Moderate decrease in touch or pain or position sense, and/or essentially lost vibration in 1 or 2 limbs, or mild decrease in touch or pain, and/or moderate decrease in all proprioceptive tests in 3 or 4 limbs
  4 = Marked decrease in touch or pain or loss of proprioception, alone or combined, in 1 or 2 limbs or moderate decrease in touch or pain and/or severe proprioceptive decrease in more than 2 limbs

  5 = Loss (essentially) of sensation in 1 or 2 limbs or moderate decrease in touch or pain and/or loss of proprioception for most of the body below the head
  6 = Sensation essentially lost below the head
E. Bowel and bladder functions
  0 = Normal
  1 = Mild urinary hesitancy, urgency, or retention
  2 = Moderate hesitancy, urgency, retention of bowel or bladder, or rare urinary incontinence
  3 = Frequent urinary incontinence
  4 = In need of almost constant catheterization
  5 = Loss of bladder function
  6 = Loss of bowel and bladder function
F. Visual (or optic) functions
  0 = Normal
  1 = Scotoma with visual acuity (corrected) better than 20/30
  2 = Worse eye with scotoma with maximal visual acuity (corrected) of 20/30 to 20/59
  3 = Worse eye with large scotoma, or moderate decrease in fields, but with maximal visual acuity (corrected) of 20/60 to 20/99
  4 = Worse eye with marked decrease of fields and maximal acuity (corrected) of 20/100 to 20/200; grade 3 plus maximal acuity of better eye of 20/60 or less
  5 = Worse eye with maximal visual acuity (corrected) less than 20/200; grade 4 plus maximal acuity of better eye of 20/60 or less
  6 = Grade 5 plus maximal visual acuity of better eye of 20/60 or less
G. Cerebral (or mental) functions
  0 = Normal
  1 = Mood alteration only (does not affect EDSS score)
  2 = Mild decrease in mentation
  3 = Moderate decrease in mentation
  4 = Marked decrease in mentation
  5 = Chronic brain syndrome—severe or incompetent

Source: After JF Kurtzke: Rating neurologic impairment in multiple sclerosis: An expanded disability status scale (EDSS). Neurology 33:1444, 1983.

Natalizumab is a humanized monoclonal antibody directed against the α_4 subunit of $\alpha_4\beta_1$ integrin, a cellular adhesion molecule expressed on the surface of lymphocytes. It prevents lymphocytes from binding to endothelial cells, thereby preventing lymphocytes from penetrating the BBB and entering the CNS.

IFN-β reduces the attack rate and improves disease severity measures such as EDSS progression and MRI-documented disease burden. IFN-β should be considered in patients with either RRMS or SPMS with superimposed relapses. In patients with SPMS but without relapses, efficacy has not been established. Higher IFN-β doses appear to have slightly greater efficacy but are also more likely to induce neutralizing antibodies, which may reduce the clinical benefit (see below).

Glatiramer acetate also reduces the attack rate (whether measured clinically or by MRI) in RRMS. Glatiramer acetate may also benefit disease severity measures, although this is less well-established than for the relapse rate. Therefore, glatiramer acetate should be considered in RRMS patients. Its usefulness in progressive disease is entirely unknown.

Natalizumab dramatically reduces the attack rate and significantly improves all measures of disease severity in MS. However, because of the development of progressive multifocal leukoencephalopathy (PML) in two patients treated with natalizumab in combination with IFN-β-1a (Avonex), and a third case in a patient treated (in combination with other immunosuppressant drugs) for Crohn's disease, natalizumab is currently recommended only for patients who have failed other therapies or who have particularly aggressive presentations. Its usefulness in the treatment of progressive disease has not been studied.

The long-term efficacy of these treatments remains uncertain, although several recent studies suggest that these agents can improve the long-term outcome of MS when administered in the RRMS stage of the illness. Beneficial effects seen in early MS include a reduction in the relapse rate and a reduction in CNS inflammation as measured by MRI. Unfortunately, already established progressive symptoms do not respond to treatment with these disease-modifying therapies. Because progressive symptoms are likely to result from delayed effects of earlier focal demyelinating epi-

TABLE 375-6 TWO-YEAR OUTCOMES FOR FDA-APPROVED THERAPIES FOR MULTIPLE SCLEROSIS[a]

Dose, Route, and Schedule	Clinical Outcomes[b]		MRI Outcomes[c]	
	Attack Rate, Mean	Change in Disease Severity	New T2 Lesions[d]	Total Burden of Disease
IFN-β-1b, 250 μg SC qod	-34%[e]	-29% (ns)	-83%[f]	-17%[e]
IFN-β-1a, 30 μg IM qw	-18%[g]	-37%[g]	-36%[f]	-4% (ns)
IFN-β-1a, 44 μg SC tiw	-32%[e]	-30%[g]	-78%[e]	-15%[e]
GA, 20 mg SC qd	-29%[f]	-12% (ns)	-38%[f]	-8%[f]
MTX, 12 mg/m² IV q3mo	-66%[e]	-75%[g]	-79%[g]	nr
NTZ, 300 mg IV qmo	-68%[e]	-42%[e]	-83%[e]	-18%[e]

[a]Percentage reductions (or increases) have been calculated by dividing the reported rates in the treated group by the comparable rates in the placebo group, except for MRI disease burden, which was calculated as the difference in the median % change between the treated and placebo groups.

[b]Severity = 1 point EDSS progression, sustained for 3 months (in the IFN-β-1a 30 μg qw trial, this change was sustained for 6 months; in the IFN-β-1b trial, this was over 3 years).

[c]Different studies measured these MRI measures differently, making comparisons difficult (numbers for new T2 represent the best case scenario for each trial).

[d]New lesions seen on T₂-weighted MRI.

[e]p = .001.

[f]p = .01.

[g]p = .05.

Abbreviations: IFN-β, interferon β; GA, glatiramer acetate; MTX, mitoxantrone; NTZ, natalizumab; IM, intramuscular; SC, subcutaneous; IV, intravenous; qod, every other day; qw, once per week; tiw, three times per week; qd, daily; q3mo, once every 3 months; qmo, once per month; ns, not significant; nr, not reported.

sodes, many experts now believe that very early treatment with a disease-modifying drug is appropriate for most MS patients. It is reasonable to delay initiating treatment in patients with (1) normal neurologic exams, (2) a single attack or a low attack frequency, and (3) a low burden of disease as assessed by brain MRI. Untreated patients should be followed closely with periodic brain MRI scans; the need for therapy is reassessed if scans reveal evidence of ongoing, subclinical disease.

Most treated patients with relapsing forms of MS receive IFN-β or glatiramer acetate as first-line therapy. Regardless of which agent is chosen

first, treatment should probably be changed in patents who continue to have frequent attacks or progressive disability (Fig. 375-4). The value of combination therapy is unknown.

IFN-β-1a (Avonex), 30 μg, is administered by intramuscular injection once every week. IFN-β-1a (Rebif), 44 μg, is administered by subcutaneous injection three times per week. IFN-β-1b (Betaseron), 250 μg, is administered by subcutaneous injection every other day. Glatiramer acetate, 20 mg, is administered by subcutaneous injection every day. Natalizumab, 300 μg, is administered by IV infusion each month. Common side effects of IFN-β therapy include flulike symptoms (e.g., fevers, chills, and myalgias) and mild abnormalities on routine laboratory evaluation (e.g., elevated liver function tests or lymphopenia). Rarely, more severe hepatotoxicity may occur. Subcutaneous IFN-β also causes reactions at the injection site (e.g., pain, redness, induration, or, rarely, skin necrosis). Side effects can usually be managed with concomitant nonsteroidal anti-inflammatory medications and with the use of an autoinjector. Depression, increased spasticity, and cognitive changes have been reported, although these symptoms can also be due to the underlying disease. In any event, side effects to IFN-β therapy usually subside with time.

Approximately 2–10% of IFN-β-1a (Avonex) recipients, 15–25% of IFN-β-1a (Rebif) recipients, and 30–40% of IFN-β-1b (Betaseron) recipients develop neutralizing antibodies to IFN-β, which may disappear over time. Some evidence suggests that neutralizing antibodies reduce efficacy, especially for MRI outcomes. The current clinical data, however, are quite conflicted.

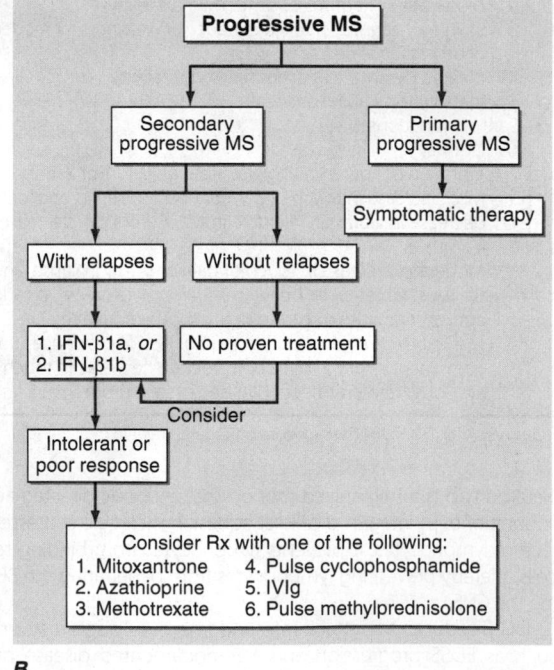

FIGURE 375-4 Therapeutic decision-making for MS.

Moreover, there are few situations where measurement of antibodies is necessary. Thus, for a patient doing well on therapy, the presence of antibodies should not affect treatment. Conversely, for a patient doing poorly on therapy, alternative treatment should be considered, even if there are no detectable antibodies.

Injection-site reactions also occur with glatiramer acetate but are less severe than with IFN-β-1b. Approximately 15% of patients experience one or more episodes of flushing, chest tightness, dyspnea, palpitations, and anxiety after injection. This systemic reaction is unpredictable, brief (duration <1 h), and tends not to recur.

Treatment with natalizumab is, in general, well tolerated. A small percentage (<10%) of patients experience hypersensitivity reactions (including anaphylaxis) and ~6% develop neutralizing antibodies to the molecule. As noted above, of greater potential concern was the occurrence of PML in three patients.

Mitoxantrone Hydrochloride Mitoxantrone (Novantrone), an anthracenedione, exerts its antineoplastic action by (1) intercalating into DNA and producing both strand breaks and interstrand cross-links, (2) interfering with RNA synthesis, and (3) inhibiting topoisomerase II (involved in DNA repair). The U.S. Food and Drug Administration (FDA) approved mitoxantrone on the basis of a single (relatively small) phase III clinical trial in Europe, in addition to an even smaller phase II study completed earlier. Mitoxantrone received (from the FDA) the broadest indication of any current treatment for MS. Thus, mitoxantrone is indicated for use in SPMS, in PRMS, and in patients with worsening RRMS (defined as patients whose neurologic status remains significantly abnormal between MS attacks). Despite this broad indication, however, the data supporting its efficacy are weaker than for other approved therapies.

Mitoxantrone can be cardiotoxic (e.g., cardiomyopathy, reduced left ventricular ejection fraction, and irreversible congestive heart failure). As a result, a cumulative dose >140 mg/m^2 is not recommended. At currently approved doses (12 mg/m^2 every 3 months), the maximum duration of therapy can be only 2–3 years. Furthermore, >40% of women will experience amenorrhea, which may be permanent. Finally, there is risk of acute leukemia, and this complication has already been reported in several mitoxantrone-treated MS patients.

Given these risks, mitoxantrone should not be used as a first-line agent in either RRMS or relapsing SPMS. It is reasonable to consider mitoxantrone in selected patients with a progressive course who have failed other approved therapies.

DISEASE-MODIFYING THERAPIES FOR SPMS High-dose IFN-β probably has a beneficial effect in patients with SPMS who are still experiencing acute relapses. IFN-β is probably ineffective in patients with SPMS who are not having acute attacks. Glatiramer acetate and natalizumab have not been studied in this patient population.

Although mitoxantrone has been approved for patients with progressive MS, this is not the population studied in the pivotal trial. Therefore no evidence-based recommendation can be made with regard to its use in this setting.

PPMS No currently available therapies have shown any promise for treating PPMS at this time. A phase III clinical trial of glatiramer acetate in PPMS was recently stopped because of lack of efficacy. Trials of mitoxantrone and rituximab in PPMS are currently underway.

OFF-LABEL TREATMENT OPTIONS FOR RRMS AND SPMS *Azathioprine* (2–3 mg/kg/per day) has been used primarily in SPMS. Meta-analysis of published trials suggests that azathioprine is marginally effective at lowering relapse rates, although a benefit on disability progression has not been demonstrated.

Methotrexate (7.5–20 mg/wk) was shown in one study to slow the progression of upper-extremity dysfunction in SPMS. Because of the possibility of developing irreversible liver damage, some experts recommend a blind liver biopsy after 2 years of therapy.

Cyclophosphamide (700 mg/m^2, every other month) may be helpful for treatment-refractory patients who are (1) otherwise in good health, (2) ambulatory, and (3) <40 years of age. Because cyclophosphamide can be used for periods in excess of 3 years, it may be preferable to mitoxantrone in these circumstances.

Intravenous immunoglobulin (IVIg), administered in monthly pulses (up to 1 g/kg) for up to 2 years, appears to reduce annual exacerbation rates. However, its use is limited because of its high cost, questions about optimal dose, and uncertainty about its effect on long-term disability outcome.

Methylprednisolone administered in one study as monthly high-dose intravenous pulses, reduced disability progression (see above).

OTHER THERAPEUTIC CLAIMS Many purported treatments for MS have never been subjected to scientific scrutiny. These include dietary therapies (e.g., the Swank diet in addition to others), megadose vitamins, low-dose naltrexone, calcium orotate, bee stings, cow colostrum, hyperbaric oxygen, procarin (a combination of histamine and caffeine), chelation, acupuncture, acupressure, various Chinese herbal remedies, and removal of mercury-amalgam tooth fillings, among many others. Patients should avoid costly or potentially hazardous unproven treatments. Many such treatments lack biologic plausibility. For example, no reliable case of mercury poisoning resembling typical MS has ever been described.

Although potential roles for EBV, HHV-6, or chlamydia have been suggested for MS, these reports are unconfirmed, and treatment with antiviral agents or antibiotics is not currently appropriate.

SYMPTOMATIC THERAPY Potassium channel blockers (e.g., 4-aminopyridine, 10–40 mg/d; and 3,4-di-aminopyridine, 40–80 mg/d) may be helpful for *weakness*, especially for heat-sensitive symptoms. At high doses they may cause seizures. These agents are not FDA-approved but can be obtained from compounding pharmacies around the United States.

Ataxia/tremor is often intractable. Clonazepam, 1.5–20 mg/d; mysoline, 50–250 mg/d; propranolol, 40–200 mg/d; or ondansetron, 8–16 mg/d may help. Wrist weights occasionally reduce tremor in the arm or hand. Thalamotomy or deep-brain stimulation has been tried with mixed success.

Spasticity and *spasms* may improve with physical therapy, regular exercise, and stretching. Avoidance of triggers (e.g., infections, fecal impactions, bed sores) is extremely important. Effective medications include lioresal (20–120 mg/d), diazepam (2–40 mg/d), tizanidine (8–32 mg/d), dantrolene (25–400 mg/d), and cyclobenzaprine hydrochloride (10–60 mg/d). For severe spasticity, a lioresal pump (delivering medication directly into the CSF) can provide substantial relief.

Pain is treated with anticonvulsants (carbamazepine, 100–1000 mg/d; phenytoin, 300–600 mg/d; gabapentin, 300–3600 mg/d; or pregabalin, 50–300 mg/d), antidepressants (amitriptyline, 25–150 mg/d; nortriptyline, 25–150 mg/d; desipramine, 100–300 mg/d; or venlafaxine, 75–225 mg/d), or antiarrhythmics (mexiletine, 300–900 mg/d). If these approaches fail, patients should be referred to a comprehensive pain management program.

Bladder dysfunction management is best guided by urodynamic testing. Evening fluid restriction or frequent voluntary voiding may help *detrusor hyperreflexia*. If these methods fail, propantheline bromide (10–15 mg/d), oxybutynin (5–15 mg/d), hyoscyamine sulfate (0.5–0.75 mg/d), tolterodine tartrate (2–4 mg/d), or solifenacin (5–10 mg/d) may help. Coadministration of pseudoephedrine (30–60 mg) is sometimes beneficial.

Detrusor/sphincter dyssynergia may respond to phenoxybenzamine (10–20 mg/d) or terazosin hydrochloride (1–20 mg/d). Loss of reflex bladder wall contraction may respond to bethanechol (30–150 mg/d). However, both conditions often require catheterization.

Urinary tract infections should be treated promptly. Patients with large post-void residual urine volumes are predisposed to infections. Prevention by urine acidification (with cranberry juice or vitamin C) inhibits some bacteria. Prophylactic administration of antibiotics is sometimes necessary but may lead to colonization by resistant organisms. Intermittent catheterization may help to prevent recurrent infections.

Treatment of *constipation* includes high-fiber diets and fluids. Natural or other laxatives may help. *Fecal incontinence* may respond to a reduction in dietary fiber.

Depression should be treated. Useful drugs include the selective serotonin reuptake inhibitors (fluoxetine, 20–80 mg/d, or sertraline, 50–200 mg/d); the tricyclic antidepressants (amitriptyline, 25–150 mg/d, nortriptyline, 25–150 mg/d, or desipramine, 100–300 mg/d); and the nontricyclic antidepressants (venlafaxine, 75–225 mg/d).

Fatigue may improve with assistive devices, help in the home, or successful management of spasticity. Patients with frequent nocturia may benefit from anticholinergic medication at bedtime. Primary MS fatigue may respond to amantadine (200 mg/d), methylphenidate (5–25 mg/d), or modafinil (100–400 mg/d).

Cognitive problems may respond to the cholinesterase inhibitor donepezil hydrochloride (10 mg/d).

Paroxysmal symptoms respond dramatically to low-dose anticonvulsants (acetazolamide, 200–600 mg/d; carbamazepine, 50–400 mg/d; phenytoin, 50–300 mg/d; or gabapentin, 600–1800 mg/d).

Heat sensitivity may respond to heat avoidance, air-conditioning, or cooling garments.

Sexual dysfunction may be helped by lubricants to aid in genital stimulation and sexual arousal. Management of pain, spasticity, fatigue, and bladder/bowel dysfunction may also help. Sildenafil (50–100 mg) taken 1–2 h before sex, is now the standard treatment for maintaining erections.

PROMISING EXPERIMENTAL THERAPIES Numerous clinical trials are currently underway. These include: (1) combination therapies; (2) higher-dose IFN-β than currently prescribed; (3) monoclonal antibodies against CD20 to deplete B cells, against the IL-2 receptor, or against CD52 to induce global lymphocyte depletion; (4) an oral sphingosine-1-phosphate receptor antagonist to sequester lymphocytes in the secondary lymphoid organs; (5) use of MBP, or an altered peptide ligand resembling MBP, to induce antigen-specific tolerance; (6) an oral inhibitor of the enzyme dihydroorotate dehydrogenase involved in pyrimidine synthesis; (7) use of statins as immunomodulators; (8) estriol to induce a pregnancy-like state; and (9) bone marrow transplantation.

CLINICAL VARIANTS OF MS

Neuromyelitis optica (NMO), or Devic's syndrome, consists of separate attacks of acute ON and myelitis. ON may be unilateral or bilateral and precede or follow an attack of myelitis by days, months, or years. In contrast to MS, patients with NMO do not experience brainstem, cerebellar, and cognitive involvement, and the brain MRI is typically normal. A focal enhancing region of swelling and cavitation, extending over three or more spinal cord segments, is typically seen on MRI. Histopathology of these lesions may reveal thickening of blood-vessel walls and deposition of antibody and complement. Occasional patients with apparent NMO also have brain MRI changes indicating involvement of the cerebral hemispheres.

NMO, which is uncommon in Caucasians compared with Asians and Africans, is best understood as a syndrome with diverse causes. Some patients have a systemic autoimmune disorder, often systemic lupus erythematosus, Sjögren's syndrome, p-ANCA (perinuclear antineutrophil cytoplasmic antibody) associated vasculitis, or mixed connective tissue disease. In others, onset may be associated with acute infection with varicella-zoster virus, EBV, HIV, or tuberculosis. More frequently, however, NMO is idiopathic and probably represents an MS variant; in such cases the course can be monophasic but is more often recurrent.

A highly specific autoantibody directed against the water channel protein aquaporin-4 is present in the sera of more than half of patients who have a clinical diagnosis of NMO. Aquaporin-4 is localized to the foot processes of astrocytes in close apposition to endothelial surfaces. The role of aquaporin-4 antibodies in the pathogenesis of NMO, however, is unknown.

Disease-modifying therapies for MS have not been rigorously studied in NMO. Acute attacks are usually treated with high-dose glucocorticoids as for MS exacerbations (see above). Because of the possibility that NMO is antibody-mediated, plasma exchange has also been used empirically for acute episodes that fail to respond to glucocorticoids. Immunosuppressants (cyclophosphamide or azathioprine with glucocorticoids) are sometimes used in the hope that further relapses will be prevented. More recently, in a small open-case series, B cell depletion with anti-CD20 monoclonal antibody (rituxan) appeared to show promise in preventing relapses of NMO.

Acute MS (Marburg's variant) is a fulminant demyelinating process that in some cases progresses inexorably to death within 1–2 years. Typically, there are no remissions. When acute MS presents as a solitary, usually cavitary, lesion, a brain tumor is often suspected. In such cases a brain biopsy is usually required to establish the diagnosis. An antibody-mediated process appears to be responsible for most cases. Marburg's variant does not seem to follow infection or vaccination, and it is unclear whether this syndrome represents an extreme form of MS or another disease altogether. No controlled trials of therapy exist;

high-dose glucocorticoids, plasma exchange, and cyclophosphamide have been tried, with uncertain benefit.

ACUTE DISSEMINATED ENCEPHALOMYELITIS (ADEM)

ADEM has a monophasic course and is frequently associated with antecedent immunization (postvaccinal encephalomyelitis) or infection (postinfectious encephalomyelitis). The hallmark of ADEM is the presence of widely scattered small foci of perivenular inflammation and demyelination. In its most explosive form, acute hemorrhagic leukoencephalitis, the lesions are vasculitic and hemorrhagic, and the clinical course is devastating.

Postvaccinal encephalomyelitis may follow the administration of smallpox and certain rabies vaccines. Postinfectious encephalomyelitis is most frequently associated with the viral exanthems of childhood. Infection with measles virus is the most common antecedent (1 in 1000 cases). Worldwide, measles encephalomyelitis is still common, although use of the live measles vaccine has dramatically reduced its incidence in developed countries. An ADEM-like illness rarely follows vaccination with live measles vaccine (1–2 in 10^6 immunizations). ADEM is now most frequently associated with varicella (chickenpox) infections (1 in 4000–10,000 cases). It may also follow infection with rubella, mumps, influenza, parainfluenza, infectious mononucleosis viruses, and *Mycoplasma*. Some patients may have a nonspecific upper respiratory infection or no known antecedent illness.

All forms of ADEM presumably result from a cross-reactive immune response to the infectious agent or vaccine that then triggers an inflammatory demyelinating response. Autoantibodies to MBP and to other myelin antigens have been detected in the CSF from many patients with ADEM. Attempts to demonstrate direct viral invasion of the CNS have been unsuccessful.

CLINICAL MANIFESTATIONS

In severe cases, onset is abrupt and progression rapid (hours to days). In postinfectious ADEM, the neurologic syndrome generally begins late in the course of the viral illness as the exanthem is fading. Fever reappears, and headache, meningismus, and lethargy progressing to coma may develop. Seizures are common. Signs of disseminated neurologic disease are consistently present (e.g., hemiparesis or quadriparesis, extensor plantar responses, lost or hyperactive tendon reflexes, sensory loss and brainstem involvement). In ADEM due to chickenpox, cerebellar involvement is often conspicuous. CSF protein is modestly elevated [0.5–1.5 g/L (50–150 mg/dL)]. Lymphocytic pleocytosis, generally 200 cells/μl, occurs in 80% of patients. Occasional patients have higher counts or a mixed polymorphonuclear-lymphocytic pattern during the initial days of the illness. Transient CSF oligoclonal banding has been reported. MRI may reveal extensive gadolinium enhancement of white matter in brain and spinal cord.

DIAGNOSIS

The diagnosis is easily established when there is a history of recent vaccination or exanthematous illness. In severe cases with predominantly cerebral involvement, acute encephalitis due to infection with herpes simplex or other viruses may be difficult to exclude. The simultaneous onset of disseminated symptoms and signs is common in ADEM and rare in MS. Similarly, meningismus, drowsiness, coma, or seizures suggest ADEM rather than MS. Unlike in MS, in ADEM optic nerve involvement is generally bilateral and transverse myelopathy complete. MRI findings that may support a diagnosis of ADEM include extensive and relatively symmetric white matter abnormalities and Gd enhancement of all abnormal areas, indicating active disease and a monophasic course.

℞ ACUTE DISSEMINATED ENCEPHALOMYELITIS

Initial treatment is with high-dose glucocorticoids as for exacerbations of MS (see above); depending on the response, treatment may need to be continued for 4–8 weeks. Patients who fail to respond within a few days may benefit from a course of plasma exchange or intravenous immunoglobulin. The prognosis reflects the severity of the underlying acute illness. Measles encephalomyelitis is associated with a mortality rate of 5–20%, and most survivors have permanent neurologic sequelae. Children who recover may have persistent seizures and behavioral and learning disorders.

FURTHER READINGS

CREE BA et al: An open label study of the effects of rituximab in neuromyelitis optica. Neurology 64:1270, 2005

GOODIN DS et al: Disease modifying therapies in multiple sclerosis: Report of the Therapeutics and Technology Assessment Subcommittee of the American Academy of Neurology. Neurology 58:169, 2002

HAUSER SL, OKSENBERG JR: The neurobiology of multiple sclerosis: genes, inflammation, and neurodegeneration. Neuron 52:61, 2006

KAPPOS L et al: Effect of early vs delayed interferon beta-1b treatment on disability after a first clinical event suggestive of multiple sclerosis: A 3-year follow-up analysis of the BENEFIT study. Lancet 370:389, 2007

LENNON VA et al: A serum autoantibody marker of neuromyelitis optica: Distinction from multiple sclerosis. Lancet 364:2106, 2004

MILLER DH, LEARY SM: Primary-progressive multiple sclerosis. Lancet Neurol 6:903, 2007

THE INTERNATIONAL MULTIPLE SCLEROSIS GENETICS CONSORTIUM: Risk alleles for multiple sclerosis identified by a genomewide study. N Engl J Med July 29 2007, epub ahead of print

RANSOHOFF RM: Natalizumab for multiple sclerosis. N Engl J Med 356:2622, 2007

TROJANO M et al: New natural history of interferon-beta-treated relapsing multiple sclerosis. Ann Neurol 61:300, 2007

376 Meningitis, Encephalitis, Brain Abscess, and Empyema
Karen L. Roos, Kenneth L. Tyler

Acute infections of the nervous system are among the most important problems in medicine because early recognition, efficient decision-making, and rapid institution of therapy can be lifesaving. These distinct clinical syndromes include acute bacterial meningitis, viral meningitis, encephalitis, focal infections such as brain abscess and subdural empyema, and infectious thrombophlebitis. Each may present with a nonspecific prodrome of fever and headache, which in a previously healthy individual may initially be thought to be benign, until (with the exception of viral meningitis) altered consciousness, focal neurologic signs, or seizures appear. Key goals of early management are to emergently distinguish between these conditions, identify the responsible pathogen, and initiate appropriate antimicrobial therapy.

APPROACH TO THE PATIENT

(Fig. 376-1) The first task is to identify whether an infection predominantly involves the subarachnoid space (*meningitis*) or whether there is evidence of either generalized or focal involvement of brain tissue in the cerebral hemispheres, cerebellum, or brainstem. When brain tissue is directly injured by a viral infection the disease is referred to as *encephalitis*, whereas focal bacterial, fungal, or parasitic infections involving brain tissue are classified as either *cerebritis* or *abscess*, depending on the presence or absence of a capsule.

Nuchal rigidity ("stiff neck") is the pathognomonic sign of meningeal irritation and is present when the neck resists passive flexion. Kernig's and Brudzinski's signs are also classic signs of meningeal irritation. *Kernig's sign* is elicited with the patient in the supine position. The thigh is flexed on the abdomen, with the knee flexed; attempts to passively extend the knee elicit pain when meningeal irritation is present. *Brudzinski's sign* is elicited with the patient in the supine position and is positive when passive flexion of the neck results in spontaneous flexion of the hips and knees. Although commonly tested on physical examinations, the sensitivity and specificity of Kernig's and Brudzinski's signs are uncertain. Both may be absent or reduced in very young or elderly patients, immunocompromised individuals, or patients with a severely depressed mental status. The high prevalence of cervical spine disease in older individuals may result in false-positive tests for nuchal rigidity.

Initial management can be guided by several considerations: (1) Empirical therapy should be initiated promptly whenever bacterial meningitis is a significant diagnostic consideration. (2) All patients who have had recent head trauma, are immunocompromised, have known malignant lesions or central nervous system (CNS) neoplasms, or have focal neurologic findings that include papilledema or a depressed level of consciousness should undergo CT or MRI of the brain prior to lumbar puncture (LP). In these cases empirical antibiotic therapy should not be delayed pending test results but should be administered prior to neuroimaging and LP. (3) A significantly depressed level of consciousness (e.g., somnolence, coma), seizures, or focal neurologic deficits do not occur in viral (*aseptic*) meningitis; patients with these symptoms should be hospitalized for further evaluation and treated empirically for bacterial and viral meningoencephalitis. (4) Immunocompetent patients with a normal level of consciousness, no prior antimicrobial treatment, and a cerebrospinal fluid (CSF) profile consistent with viral meningitis (lymphocytic pleocytosis and a normal glucose concentration) can often be treated as outpatients if appropriate contact and monitoring can be ensured. Failure of a patient with suspected viral meningitis to improve within 48 h should prompt a reevaluation including follow-up neurologic and general medical examination and repeat imaging and laboratory studies, often including a second LP.

ACUTE BACTERIAL MENINGITIS

DEFINITION

Bacterial meningitis is an acute purulent infection within the subarachnoid space. It is associated with a CNS inflammatory reaction that may result in decreased consciousness, seizures, raised intracranial pressure (ICP), and stroke. The meninges, the subarachnoid space, and the brain parenchyma are all frequently involved in the inflammatory reaction (*meningoencephalitis*).

EPIDEMIOLOGY

Bacterial meningitis is the most common form of suppurative CNS infection, with an annual incidence in the United States of >2.5 cases/100,000 population. The epidemiology of bacterial meningitis has changed significantly in recent years, reflecting a dramatic decline in the incidence of meningitis due to *Haemophilus influenzae*, and a smaller decline in that due to *Neisseria meningitidis*, following the introduction and increasingly widespread use of vaccines for both these organisms. Currently, the organisms most commonly responsible for community-acquired bacterial meningitis are *Streptococcus pneumoniae* (~50%), *N. meningitidis* (~25%), group B streptococci (~15%), and *Listeria monocytogenes* (~10%). *H. influenzae* now accounts for <10% of cases of bacterial meningitis in most series.

ETIOLOGY

S. pneumoniae (Chap. 130) is the most common cause of meningitis in adults >20 years of age, accounting for nearly half the reported cases (1.1

2622

per 100,000 persons per year). There are a number of predisposing conditions that increase the risk of pneumococcal meningitis, the most important of which is pneumococcal pneumonia. Additional risk factors include coexisting acute or chronic pneumococcal sinusitis or otitis media, alcoholism, diabetes, splenectomy, hypogammaglobulinemia, complement deficiency, and head trauma with basilar skull fracture and CSF rhinorrhea. Mortality remains ~20% despite antibiotic therapy.

N. meningitidis (Chap. 136) accounts for 25% of all cases of bacterial meningitis (0.6 cases per 100,000 persons per year) and for up to 60% of cases in children and young adults between the ages of 2 and 20. The presence of petechial or purpuric skin lesions can provide an important clue to the diagnosis of meningococcal infection. In some patients the disease is fulminant, progressing to death within hours of symptom onset. Infection may be initiated by nasopharyngeal colonization, which can result in either an asymptomatic carrier state or invasive meningococcal disease. The risk of invasive disease following nasopharyngeal colonization depends on both bacterial virulence factors and host immune defense mechanisms, including the host's capacity to produce antimeningococcal antibodies and to lyse meningococci by both classic and alternative complement pathways. Individuals with deficiencies of any of the complement components, including properdin, are highly susceptible to meningococcal infections.

Enteric gram-negative bacilli are an increasingly common cause of meningitis in individuals with chronic and debilitating diseases such as diabetes, cirrhosis, or alcoholism and in those with chronic urinary tract infections. Gram-negative meningitis can also complicate neurosurgical procedures, particularly craniotomy.

Group B streptococcus, or *S. agalactiae*, was previously responsible for meningitis predominantly in neonates, but it has been reported with increasing frequency in individuals >50 years of age, particularly those with underlying diseases.

L. monocytogenes (Chap. 132) has become an increasingly important cause of meningitis in neonates (<1 month of age), pregnant women, individuals >60 years, and immunocompromised individuals of all ages. Infection is acquired by ingesting foods contaminated by *Listeria*. Foodborne human listerial infection has been reported from contaminated coleslaw, milk, soft cheeses, and several types of "ready-to-eat" foods, including delicatessen meat and uncooked hotdogs.

The frequency of *H. influenzae* type b meningitis in children has declined dramatically since the introduction of the Hib conjugate vaccine, although rare cases of Hib meningitis in vaccinated children have been reported. More frequently, *H. influenzae* causes meningitis in unvaccinated children and adults.

Staphylococcus aureus and coagulase-negative staphylococci (Chap. 129) are important causes of meningitis that occurs following invasive neurosurgical procedures, particularly shunting procedures for hydrocephalus, or as a complication of the use of subcutaneous Ommaya reservoirs for administration of intrathecal chemotherapy.

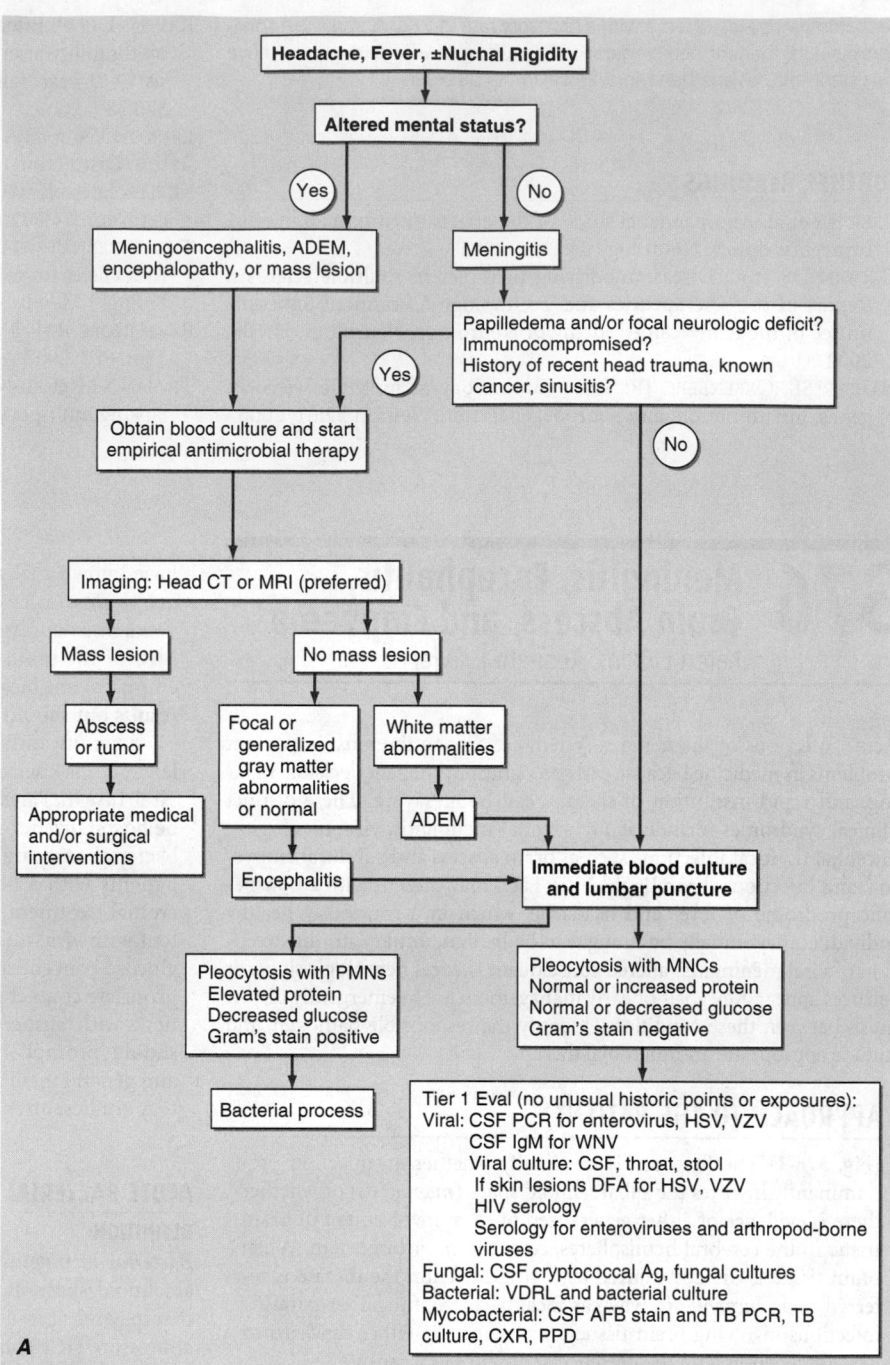

FIGURE 376-1 The management of patients with suspected CNS infection. ADEM, acute disseminated encephalomyelitis; CT, computed tomography; MRI, magnetic resonance imaging; PMNs, polymorphonuclear leukocytes; MNCs, mononuclear cells; CSF, cerebrospinal fluid; PCR, polymerase chain reaction; HSV, herpes simplex virus; VZV, varicella-zoster virus; WNV, West Nile virus; DFA, direct fluorescent antibody; Ag, antigen; VDRL, Venereal Disease Research Laboratory; AFB, acid-fast bacillus; TB, tuberculosis; CXR, chest x-ray; PPD, purified protein derivative; EBV, Epstein-Barr virus; CTFV, Colorado tick fever virus; HHV, human herpesvirus; LCMV, lymphocytic choriomeningitis virus.

PATHOPHYSIOLOGY

The most common bacteria that cause meningitis, *S. pneumoniae* and *N. meningitidis*, initially colonize the nasopharynx by attaching to nasopharyngeal epithelial cells. Bacteria are transported across epithelial cells in membrane-bound vacuoles to the intravascular space or invade the intravascular space by creating separations in the apical tight junctions of columnar epithelial cells. Once in the bloodstream, bacteria are able to avoid phagocytosis by neutrophils and classic complement–mediated bactericidal activity because of the presence of a polysaccharide

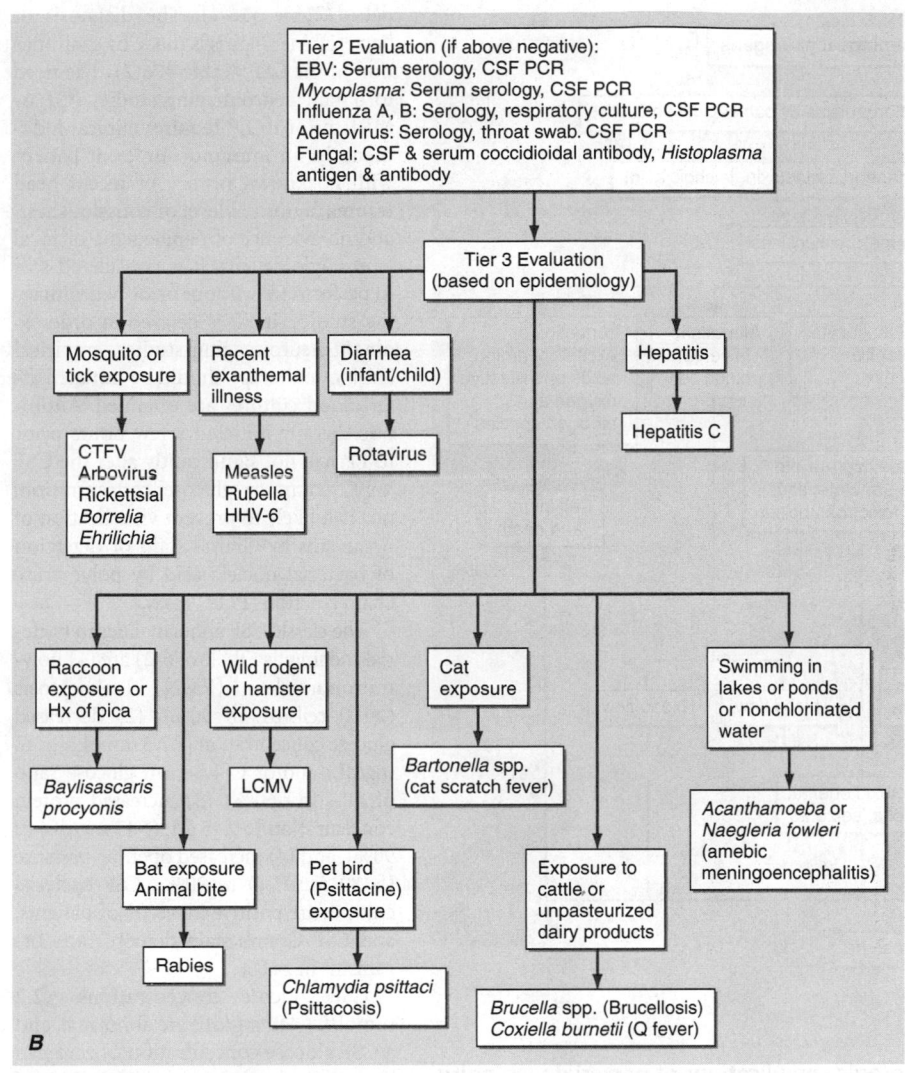

Tier 2 Evaluation (if above negative):
EBV: Serum serology, CSF PCR
Mycoplasma: Serum serology, CSF PCR
Influenza A, B: Serology, respiratory culture, CSF PCR
Adenovirus: Serology, throat swab. CSF PCR
Fungal: CSF & serum coccidioidal antibody, *Histoplasma* antigen & antibody

Tier 3 Evaluation
(based on epidemiology)

Mosquito or tick exposure

Recent exanthemal illness

Diarrhea (infant/child)

Hepatitis

Hepatitis C

CTFV
Arbovirus
Rickettsial
Borrelia
Ehrilichia

Measles
Rubella
HHV-6

Rotavirus

Raccoon exposure or Hx of pica

Wild rodent or hamster exposure

Cat exposure

Swimming in lakes or ponds or nonchlorinated water

Baylisascaris procyonis

LCMV

Bartonella spp. (cat scratch fever)

Acanthamoeba or *Naegleria fowleri* (amebic meningoencephalitis)

Bat exposure
Animal bite

Pet bird (Psittacine) exposure

Exposure to cattle or unpasteurized dairy products

Rabies

Chlamydia psittaci (Psittacosis)

Brucella spp. (Brucellosis)
Coxiella burnetii (Q fever)

B

FIGURE 376-1 *(Continued.)*

capsule. Bloodborne bacteria can reach the intraventricular choroid plexus, directly infect choroid plexus epithelial cells, and gain access to the CSF. Some bacteria, such as *S. pneumoniae*, can adhere to cerebral capillary endothelial cells and subsequently migrate through or between these cells to reach the CSF. Bacteria are able to multiply rapidly within CSF because of the absence of effective host immune defenses. Normal CSF contains few white blood cells (WBCs) and relatively small amounts of complement proteins and immunoglobulins. The paucity of the latter two prevents effective opsonization of bacteria, an essential prerequisite for bacterial phagocytosis by neutrophils. Phagocytosis of bacteria is further impaired by the fluid nature of CSF, which is less conducive to phagocytosis than a solid tissue substrate.

A critical event in the pathogenesis of bacterial meningitis is the inflammatory reaction induced by the invading bacteria. Many of the neurologic manifestations and complications of bacterial meningitis result from the immune response to the invading pathogen rather than from direct bacteria-induced tissue injury. As a result, neurologic injury can progress even after the CSF has been sterilized by antibiotic therapy.

The lysis of bacteria with the subsequent release of cell-wall components into the subarachnoid space is the initial step in the induction of the inflammatory response and the formation of a purulent exudate in the subarachnoid space (Fig. 376-2). Bacterial cell-wall components, such as the lipopolysaccharide (LPS) molecules of gram-negative bacteria and teichoic acid and peptidoglycans of *S. pneumoniae*, induce meningeal inflammation by stimulating the production of inflammatory cytokines and chemokines by microglia, astrocytes, monocytes, microvascular endothelial cells, and CSF leukocytes. In experimental models of meningitis, cytokines including tumor necrosis factor (TNF) and interleukin 1 (IL-1) are present in CSF within 1–2 h of intracisternal inoculation of LPS. This cytokine response is quickly followed by an increase in CSF protein concentration and leukocytosis. Chemokines (cytokines that induce chemotactic migration in leukocytes) and a variety of other proinflammatory cytokines are also produced and secreted by leukocytes and tissue cells that are stimulated by IL-1 and TNF. In addition, bacteremia and the inflammatory cytokines induce the production of excitatory amino acids, reactive oxygen and nitrogen species (free oxygen radicals, nitric oxide, and peroxynitrite), and other mediators that can induce death of brain cells.

Much of the pathophysiology of bacterial meningitis is a direct consequence of elevated levels of CSF cytokines and chemokines. TNF and IL-1 act synergistically to increase the permeability of the blood-brain barrier, resulting in induction of vasogenic edema and the leakage of serum proteins into the subarachnoid space (Fig. 376-2). The subarachnoid exudate of proteinaceous material and leukocytes obstructs the flow of CSF through the ventricular system and diminishes the resorptive capacity of the arachnoid granulations in the dural sinuses, leading to obstructive and communicating hydrocephalus and concomitant interstitial edema.

Inflammatory cytokines upregulate the expression of selectins on cerebral capillary endothelial cells and leukocytes, promoting leukocyte adherence to vascular endothelial cells and subsequent migration into the CSF. The adherence of leukocytes to capillary endothelial cells increases the permeability of blood vessels, allowing for the leakage of plasma proteins into the CSF, which adds to the inflammatory exudate. Neutrophil degranulation results in the release of toxic metabolites that contribute to cytotoxic edema, cell injury, and death. Contrary to previous beliefs, CSF leukocytes probably do little to contribute to the clearance of CSF bacterial infection.

During the very early stages of meningitis, there is an increase in cerebral blood flow, soon followed by a decrease in cerebral blood flow and a loss of cerebrovascular autoregulation (Chap. 269). Narrowing of the large arteries at the base of the brain due to encroachment by the purulent exudate in the subarachnoid space and infiltration of the arterial wall by inflammatory cells with intimal thickening (*vasculitis*) also occur and may result in ischemia and infarction, obstruction of branches of the middle cerebral artery by thrombosis, thrombosis of the major cerebral venous sinuses, and thrombophlebitis of the cerebral cortical veins. The combination of interstitial, vasogenic, and cytotoxic edema leads to raised ICP and coma. Cerebral herniation usually results from the effects of cerebral edema, either focal or generalized; hydrocephalus and dural sinus or cortical vein thrombosis may also play a role.

CLINICAL PRESENTATION

Meningitis can present as either an acute fulminant illness that progresses rapidly in a few hours or as a subacute infection that progressively worsens over several days. The classic clinical triad of meningitis is fever, headache, and nuchal rigidity. A decreased level of consciousness occurs in >75% of patients and can vary from lethargy to coma. Nausea, vomiting, and photophobia are also common complaints.

Seizures occur as part of the initial presentation of bacterial meningitis or during the course of the illness in 20–40% of patients. Focal

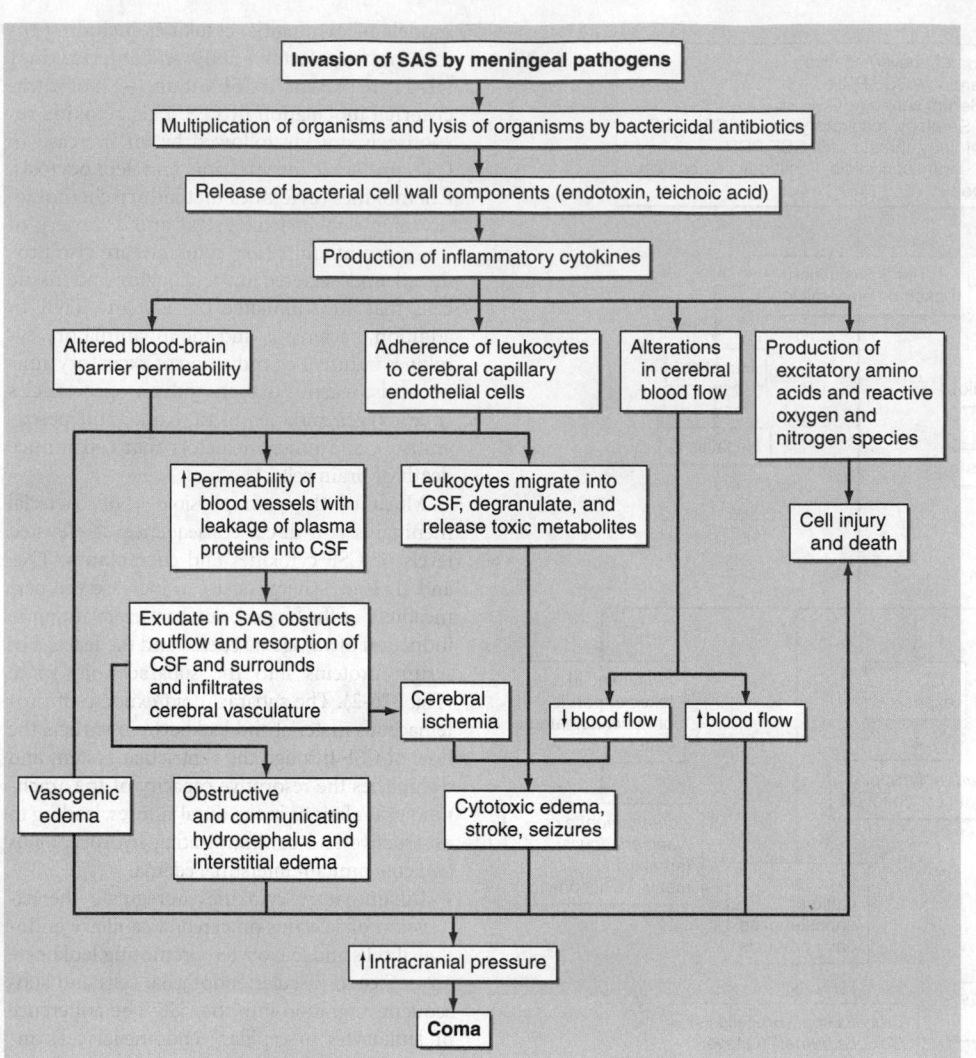

FIGURE 376-2 The pathophysiology of the neurologic complications of bacterial meningitis. SAS, subarachnoid space; CSF, cerebrospinal fluid.

seizures are usually due to focal arterial ischemia or infarction, cortical venous thrombosis with hemorrhage, or focal edema. Generalized seizure activity and status epilepticus may be due to hyponatremia, cerebral anoxia, or, less commonly, the toxic effects of antimicrobial agents such as high-dose penicillin.

Raised ICP is an expected complication of bacterial meningitis and the major cause of obtundation and coma in this disease. More than 90% of patients will have a CSF opening pressure >180 mmH₂O, and 20% have opening pressures >400 mmH₂O. Signs of increased ICP include a deteriorating or reduced level of consciousness, papilledema, dilated poorly reactive pupils, sixth nerve palsies, decerebrate posturing, and the Cushing reflex (bradycardia, hypertension, and irregular respirations). The most disastrous complication of increased ICP is cerebral herniation. The incidence of herniation in patients with bacterial meningitis has been reported to occur in as few as 1% to as many as 8% of cases.

Specific clinical features may provide clues to the diagnosis of individual organisms and are discussed in more detail in specific chapters devoted to individual pathogens. The most important of these clues is the rash of meningococcemia, which begins as a diffuse erythematous maculopapular rash resembling a viral exanthem; however, the skin lesions of meningococcemia rapidly become petechial. Petechiae are found on the trunk and lower extremities, in the mucous membranes and conjunctiva, and occasionally on the palms and soles.

DIAGNOSIS

When bacterial meningitis is suspected, blood cultures should be immediately obtained and empirical antimicrobial therapy initiated without

delay (Table 376-1). The diagnosis of bacterial meningitis is made by examination of the CSF (Table 376-2). The need to obtain neuroimaging studies (CT or MRI) prior to LP requires clinical judgment. In an immunocompetent patient with no known history of recent head trauma, a normal level of consciousness, and no evidence of papilledema or focal neurologic deficits, it is considered safe to perform LP without prior neuroimaging studies. If LP is delayed in order to obtain neuroimaging studies, empirical antibiotic therapy should be initiated after blood cultures are obtained. Antibiotic therapy initiated a few hours prior to LP will not significantly alter the CSF WBC count or glucose concentration, nor is it likely to prevent visualization of organisms by Gram's stain or detection of bacterial nucleic acid by polymerase chain reaction (PCR) assay.

The classic CSF abnormalities in bacterial meningitis (Table 376-2) are (1) polymorphonuclear (PMN) leukocytosis (>100 cells/μL in 90%), (2) decreased glucose concentration [<2.2 mmol/L (<40 mg/dL) and/or CSF/serum glucose ratio of <0.4 in ~60%], (3) increased protein concentration [>0.45 g/L (>45 mg/dL) in 90%], and (4) increased opening pressure (>180 mmH₂O in 90%). CSF bacterial cultures are positive in >80% of patients, and CSF Gram's stain demonstrates organisms in >60%.

CSF glucose concentrations <2.2 mmol/L (<40 mg/dL) are abnormal, and a CSF glucose concentration of zero can be seen in bacterial meningitis. Use of the CSF/serum glucose ratio corrects for hyperglycemia that may mask a relative decrease in the CSF glucose concentration. The CSF glucose concentration is low when the CSF/serum glucose ratio is <0.6. A CSF/serum glucose ratio <0.4 is highly suggestive of bacterial meningitis but may also be seen in other conditions, including fungal, tuberculous, and carcinomatous meningitis. It takes from 30 min to several hours for the concentration of CSF glucose to reach equilibrium with blood glucose levels; therefore, administration of 50 mL of 50% glucose (D50) prior to LP, as commonly occurs in emergency room settings, is unlikely to alter CSF glucose concentration significantly unless more than a few hours have elapsed between glucose administration and LP.

A broad-range PCR can detect small numbers of viable and nonviable organisms in CSF and is expected to be useful for making a diagnosis of bacterial meningitis in patients who have been pretreated with oral or parenteral antibiotics and in whom Gram's stain and CSF culture are negative. When the broad-range PCR is positive, a PCR that uses specific bacterial primers to detect the nucleic acid of *S. pneumoniae*, *N. meningitidis*, *Escherichia coli*, *L. monocytogenes*, *H. influenzae*, and *S. agalactiae* can be obtained based on the clinical suspicion of the meningeal pathogen. The latex agglutination (LA) test for the detection of bacterial antigens of *S. pneumoniae*, *N. meningitidis*, *H. influenzae* type b, group B streptococcus, and *E. coli* K1 strains in the CSF has been useful for making a diagnosis of bacterial meningitis but is being replaced by the CSF bacterial PCR assay. The CSF LA test has a *specificity* of 95–100% for *S. pneumoniae* and *N. meningitidis*, so a positive test is virtually diagnostic of bacterial meningitis caused by these organisms. However, the *sensitivity* of the CSF LA test is only 70–100% for detection of *S. pneumoniae* and 33–70% for detection of *N. menin-*

TABLE 376-1 ANTIBIOTICS USED IN EMPIRICAL THERAPY OF BACTERIAL MENINGITIS AND FOCAL CNS INFECTIONS[a]

Indication	Antibiotic
Preterm infants to infants <1 month	Ampicillin + cefotaxime
Infants 1–3 mos	Ampicillin + cefotaxime or ceftriaxone
Immunocompetent children >3 mos and adults <55	Cefotaxime or ceftriaxone + vancomycin
Adults >55 and adults of any age with alcoholism or other debilitating illnesses	Ampicillin + cefotaxime or ceftriaxone + vancomycin
Hospital-acquired meningitis, posttraumatic or postneurosurgery meningitis, neutropenic patients, or patients with impaired cell-mediated immunity	Ampicillin + ceftazidime + vancomycin

Antimicrobial Agent	Total Daily Dose and Dosing Interval	
	Child (>1 month)	Adult
Ampicillin	200 (mg/kg)/d, q4h	12 g/d, q4h
Cefepime	150 (mg/kg)/d, q8h	6 g/d, q8h
Cefotaxime	200 (mg/kg)/d, q6h	12 g/d, q4h
Ceftriaxone	100 (mg/kg)/d, q12h	4 g/d, q12h
Ceftazidime	150 (mg/kg)/d, q8h	6 g/d, q8h
Gentamicin	7.5 (mg/kg)/d, q8h[b]	7.5 (mg/kg)/d, q8h
Meropenem	120 (mg/kg)/d, q8h	3 g/d, q8h
Metronidazole	30 (mg/kg)/d, q6h	1500–2000 mg/d, q6h
Nafcillin	100–200 (mg/kg)/d, q6h	9–12 g/d, q4h
Penicillin G	400,000 (U/kg)/d, q4h	20–24 million U/d, q4h
Vancomycin	60 (mg/kg)/d, q6h	2 g/d, q12h[b]

[a]All antibiotics are administered intravenously; doses indicated assume normal renal and hepatic function.

[b]Doses should be adjusted based on serum peak and trough levels: gentamicin therapeutic level: peak: 5–8 μg/mL; trough: <2 μg/mL; vancomycin therapeutic level: peak: 25–40 μg/mL; trough: 5–15 μg/mL.

gitidis antigens, so a negative test does not exclude infection by these organisms. The Limulus amebocyte lysate assay is a rapid diagnostic test for the detection of gram-negative endotoxin in CSF and thus for making a diagnosis of gram-negative bacterial meningitis. The test has a specificity of 85–100% and a sensitivity approaching 100%. Thus, a positive Limulus amebocyte lysate assay occurs in virtually all patients with gram-negative bacterial meningitis, but false positives may occur.

Almost all patients with bacterial meningitis will have neuroimaging studies performed during the course of their illness. MRI is preferred over CT because of its superiority in demonstrating areas of cerebral edema and ischemia. In patients with bacterial meningitis, diffuse meningeal enhancement is often seen after the administration of gadolinium. Meningeal enhancement is not diagnostic of meningitis but occurs in any CNS disease associated with increased blood-brain barrier permeability.

Petechial skin lesions, if present, should be biopsied. The rash of meningococcemia results from the dermal seeding of organisms with vascular endothelial damage, and biopsy may reveal the organism on Gram's stain.

TABLE 376-2 CEREBROSPINAL FLUID (CSF) ABNORMALITIES IN BACTERIAL MENINGITIS

Opening pressure	>180 mmH$_2$O
White blood cells	10/μL to 10,000/μL; neutrophils predominate
Red blood cells	Absent in nontraumatic tap
Glucose	<2.2 mmol/L (<40 mg/dL)
CSF/serum glucose	<0.4
Protein	>0.45 g/L (>45 mg/dL)
Gram's stain	Positive in >60%
Culture	Positive in >80%
Latex agglutination	May be positive in patients with meningitis due to S. pneumoniae, N. meningitidis, H. influenzae type b, E. coli, group B streptococci
Limulus lysate	Positive in cases of gram-negative meningitis
PCR	Detects bacterial DNA

Note: PCR, polymerase chain reaction.

DIFFERENTIAL DIAGNOSIS

Viral meningoencephalitis, and particularly herpes simplex virus (HSV) encephalitis, can mimic the clinical presentation of bacterial meningitis (see "Encephalitis," below). HSV encephalitis typically presents with headache, fever, altered consciousness, focal neurologic deficits (e.g., dysphasia, hemiparesis), and focal or generalized seizures. The findings on CSF studies, neuroimaging, and electroencephalogram (EEG) distinguish HSV encephalitis from bacterial meningitis. The typical CSF profile with viral CNS infections is a lymphocytic pleocytosis with a normal glucose concentration, in contrast to PMN pleocytosis and hypoglycorrhachia characteristic of bacterial meningitis. MRI abnormalities (other than meningeal enhancement) are not seen in uncomplicated bacterial meningitis. By contrast, in HSV encephalitis, on T2-weighted and fluid-attenuated inversion recovery (FLAIR) MRI images, high signal intensity lesions are seen in the orbitofrontal, anterior, and medial temporal lobes in the majority of patients within 48 h of symptom onset. Some patients with HSV encephalitis have a distinctive periodic pattern on EEG (see below).

Rickettsial disease can resemble bacterial meningitis (Chap. 167). Rocky Mountain spotted fever (RMSF) is transmitted by a tick bite and caused by the bacteria *Rickettsia rickettsii*. The disease may present acutely with high fever, prostration, myalgia, headache, nausea, and vomiting. Most patients develop a characteristic rash within 96 h of the onset of symptoms. The rash is initially a diffuse erythematous maculopapular rash that may be difficult to distinguish from that of meningococcemia. It progresses to a petechial rash, then to a purpuric rash and, if untreated, to skin necrosis or gangrene. The color of the lesions changes from bright red to very dark red, then yellowish-green to black. The rash typically begins in the wrist and ankles and then spreads distally and proximally within a matter of a few hours, involving the palms and soles. Diagnosis is made by immunofluorescent staining of skin biopsy specimens. Ehrlichioses are also transmitted by a tick bite. These are small gram-negative coccobacilli of which two species cause human disease. *Anaplasma phagocytophilum* causes human granulocytic ehrlichiosis (anaplasmosis), and *Ehrlichia chaffeensis* causes human monocytic ehrlichiosis. The clinical and laboratory manifestations of the infections are similar. Patients present with fever, headache, nausea, and vomiting. Twenty percent of patients have a maculopapular or petechial rash. There is laboratory evidence of leukopenia, thrombocytopenia and anemia, and mild to moderate elevations in alanine aminotransferases, alkaline phosphatase, and lactate dehydrogenase. Patients with RMSF and those with ehrlichial infections may have an altered level of consciousness ranging from mild lethargy to coma, confusion, focal neurologic signs, cranial nerve palsies, hyperreflexia, and seizures.

Focal suppurative CNS infections (see below), including subdural and epidural empyema and brain abscess, should also be considered, especially when focal neurologic findings are present. MRI should be performed promptly in all patients with suspected meningitis who have focal features, both to detect the intracranial infection and to search for associated areas of infection in the sinuses or mastoid bones.

A number of noninfectious CNS disorders can mimic bacterial meningitis. Subarachnoid hemorrhage (SAH; Chap. 269) is generally the major consideration. Other possibilities include chemical meningitis due to rupture of tumor contents into the CSF (e.g., from a cystic glioma or craniopharyngioma epidermoid or dermoid cyst); drug-induced hypersensitivity meningitis; carcinomatous or lymphomatous meningitis; meningitis associated with inflammatory disorders such as sarcoid, systemic lupus erythematosus (SLE), and Behçet's syndrome; pituitary apoplexy; and uveomeningitic syndromes (Vogt-Koyanagi-Harada syndrome).

On occasion, subacutely evolving meningitis (Chap. 377) may be considered in the differential diagnosis of acute meningitis. The principal causes include *Mycobacterium tuberculosis* (Chap. 158), *Cryptococcus neoformans* (Chap. 195), *Histoplasma capsulatum* (Chap. 192), *Coccidioides immitis* (Chap. 193), and *Treponema pallidum* (Chap. 162).

℞ ACUTE BACTERIAL MENINGITIS

EMPIRICAL ANTIMICROBIAL THERAPY (Table 376-1) Bacterial meningitis is a medical emergency. The goal is to begin antibiotic therapy within 60 min of a patient's arrival in the emergency room. Empirical antimicrobial therapy is initiated in patients with suspected bacterial meningitis before the results of CSF Gram's stain and culture are known. *S. pneumoniae* (Chap. 128) and *N. meningitidis* (Chap. 136) are the most common etiologic organisms of community-acquired bacterial meningitis. Due to the emergence of penicillin- and cephalosporin-resistant *S. pneumoniae*, empirical therapy of community-acquired suspected bacterial meningitis in children and adults should include a combination of dexamethasone, a third-generation cephalosporin (e.g., ceftriaxone or cefotaxime) and vancomycin, plus acyclovir, as HSV encephalitis is the leading disease in the differential diagnosis, and doxycycline during tick season to treat tick-borne bacterial infections. Ceftriaxone or cefotaxime provide good coverage for susceptible *S. pneumoniae*, group B streptococci, and *H. influenzae* and adequate coverage for *N. meningitidis*. Cefepime is a broad-spectrum fourth-generation cephalosporin with in vitro activity similar to that of cefotaxime or ceftriaxone against *S. pneumoniae* and *N. meningitidis* and greater activity against *Enterobacter* species and *Pseudomonas aeruginosa*. In clinical trials, cefepime has been demonstrated to be equivalent to cefotaxime in the treatment of penicillin-sensitive pneumococcal and meningococcal meningitis, and it has been used successfully in some patients with meningitis due to *Enterobacter* species and *P. aeruginosa*. Ampicillin should be added to the empirical regimen for coverage of *L. monocytogenes* in individuals <3 months of age, those >55, or those with suspected impaired cell-mediated immunity because of chronic illness, organ transplantation, pregnancy, malignancy, or immunosuppressive therapy. In hospital-acquired meningitis, and particularly meningitis following neurosurgical procedures, staphylococci and gram-negative organisms including *P. aeruginosa* are the most common etiologic organisms. In these patients, empirical therapy should include a combination of vancomycin and ceftazidime, cefepime, or meropenem. Ceftazidime, cefepime, or meropenem should be substituted for ceftriaxone or cefotaxime in neurosurgical patients and in neutropenic patients, as ceftriaxone and cefotaxime do not provide adequate activity against CNS infection with *P. aeruginosa*. Meropenem is a carbapenem antibiotic that is highly active in vitro against *L. monocytogenes*, has been demonstrated to be effective in cases of meningitis caused by *P. aeruginosa*, and shows good activity against penicillin-resistant pneumococci. In experimental pneumococcal meningitis, meropenem was comparable to ceftriaxone and inferior to vancomycin in sterilizing CSF cultures. The number of patients with bacterial meningitis enrolled in clinical trials of meropenem has not been sufficient to definitively assess the efficacy of this antibiotic.

SPECIFIC ANTIMICROBIAL THERAPY   Meningococcal Meningitis

(Table 376-3) Although ceftriaxone and cefotaxime provide adequate empirical coverage for *N. meningitidis*, penicillin G remains the antibiotic of choice for meningococcal meningitis caused by susceptible strains. Isolates of *N. meningitidis* with moderate resistance to penicillin have been identified, but patients infected with these strains have still been successfully treated with penicillin. CSF isolates of *N. meningitidis* should be tested for penicillin and ampicillin susceptibility, and if resistance is found, cefotaxime or ceftriaxone should be substituted for penicillin. A 7-day course of intravenous antibiotic therapy is adequate for uncomplicated meningococcal meningitis. The index case and all close contacts should receive chemoprophylaxis with a 2-day regimen of rifampin (600 mg every 12 h for 2 days in adults and 10 mg/kg every 12 h for 2 days in children >1 year). Rifampin is not recommended in pregnant women. Alternatively, adults can be treated with one dose of ciprofloxacin (750 mg), one dose of azithromycin (500 mg), or one intramuscular dose of ceftriaxone (250 mg). Close contacts are defined as those individuals who have had contact with oropharyngeal secretions, either through kissing or by sharing toys, beverages, or cigarettes.

Pneumococcal Meningitis   Antimicrobial therapy of pneumococcal meningitis is initiated with a cephalosporin (ceftriaxone, cefotaxime, or cefepime) and vancomycin. All CSF isolates of *S. pneumoniae* should be tested for sensitivity to penicillin and the cephalosporins. Once the results of antimicrobial susceptibility tests are known, therapy can be modified accordingly (Table 376-3). For *S. pneumoniae* meningitis, an isolate of *S. pneumoniae* is considered to be susceptible to penicillin with a minimal inhibitory concentration (MIC) <0.06 μg/mL, to have intermediate resistance when the MIC is 0.1–1.0 μg/mL, and to be highly resistant when the MIC >1.0 μg/mL. Isolates of *S. pneumoniae* that have cephalosporin MICs ≤0.5 μg/mL are considered sensitive to the cephalosporins (cefotaxime, ceftriaxone, cefepime). Those with MICs of 1 μg/mL are considered to have intermediate resistance, and those with MICs ≥2 μg/mL are considered resistant. For meningitis due to pneumococci with cefotaxime or ceftriaxone MICs ≤0.5 μg/mL, treatment with cefotaxime or ceftriaxone is usually adequate. If the MIC >1 μg/mL, vancomycin is the antibiotic of choice. Rifampin can be added to vancomycin for its synergistic effect but is inadequate as monotherapy because resistance develops rapidly when it is used alone. A 2-week course of intravenous antimicrobial therapy is recommended for pneumococcal meningitis.

Patients with *S. pneumoniae* meningitis should have a repeat LP performed 24–36 h after the initiation of antimicrobial therapy to document sterilization of the CSF. Failure to sterilize the CSF after 24–36 h of antibiotic therapy should be considered presumptive evidence of antibiotic resistance. Patients with penicillin- and cephalosporin-resistant strains of *S. pneumoniae* who do not respond to intravenous vancomycin alone may benefit from the addition of intraventricular vancomycin. The intraventricular route of administration is preferred over the intrathecal route because adequate concentrations of vancomycin in the cerebral ventricles are not always achieved with intrathecal administration.

***Listeria* Meningitis**   Meningitis due to *L. monocytogenes* is treated with ampicillin for at least 3 weeks (Table 376-3). Gentamicin is often added (2 mg/kg loading dose, then 7.5 mg/kg per day given every 8 h and adjusted for serum levels and renal function). The combination of trimethoprim [10–20 (mg/kg)/d] and sulfamethoxazole [50–100 (mg/kg)/d] given every 6 h may provide an alternative in penicillin-allergic patients.

Staphylococcal Meningitis   Meningitis due to susceptible strains of *S. aureus* or coagulase-negative staphylococci is treated with nafcillin (Table 376-3). Vancomycin is the drug of choice for methicillin-resistant staphylococci and for patients allergic to penicillin. In these patients, the CSF should be monitored during therapy. If the CSF is not sterilized after 48 h of intravenous vancomycin therapy, then either intraventricular or intrathecal vancomycin, 20 mg once daily, can be added.

Gram-Negative Bacillary Meningitis   The third-generation cephalosporins—cefotaxime, ceftriaxone, and ceftazidime—are equally efficacious for the treatment of gram-negative bacillary meningitis, with the exception of meningitis due to *P. aeruginosa*, which should be treated with ceftazidime, cefepime, or meropenem (Table 376-3). A 3-week course of intravenous antibiotic therapy is recommended for meningitis due to gram-negative bacilli.

ADJUNCTIVE THERAPY   The release of bacterial cell-wall components by bactericidal antibiotics leads to the production of the inflammatory cytokines IL-1 and TNF in the subarachnoid space. Dexamethasone exerts its beneficial effect by inhibiting the synthesis of IL-1 and TNF at the level of mRNA, decreasing CSF outflow resistance, and stabilizing the

TABLE 376-3	ANTIMICROBIAL THERAPY OF CNS BACTERIAL INFECTIONS BASED ON PATHOGEN[a]

Organism	Antibiotic
Neisseria meningitides	
Penicillin-sensitive	Penicillin G or ampicillin
Penicillin-resistant	Ceftriaxone or cefotaxime
Streptococcus pneumoniae	
Penicillin-sensitive	Penicillin G
Penicillin-intermediate	Ceftriaxone or cefotaxime
Penicillin-resistant	(Ceftriaxone or cefotaxime) + vancomycin
Gram-negative bacilli (except *Pseudomonas* spp.)	Ceftriaxone or cefotaxime
Pseudomonas aeruginosa	Ceftazidime or cefepime or meropenem
Staphylococci spp.	
Methicillin-sensitive	Nafcillin
Methicillin-resistant	Vancomycin
Listeria monocytogenes	Ampicillin + gentamicin
Haemophilus influenzae	Ceftriaxone or cefotaxime
Streptococcus agalactiae	Penicillin G or ampicillin
Bacteroides fragilis	Metronidazole
Fusobacterium spp.	Metronidazole

[a]Doses are as indicated in Table 376-1.

blood-brain barrier. The rationale for giving dexamethasone 20 min before antibiotic therapy is that dexamethasone inhibits the production of TNF by macrophages and microglia only if it is administered before these cells are activated by endotoxin. Dexamethasone does not alter TNF production once it has been induced. The results of clinical trials of dexamethasone therapy in children, predominantly with meningitis due to *H. influenzae* and *S. pneumoniae*, have demonstrated its efficacy in decreasing meningeal inflammation and neurologic sequelae such as the incidence of sensorineural hearing loss.

A prospective European trial of adjunctive therapy for acute bacterial meningitis in 301 adults found that dexamethasone reduced the number of unfavorable outcomes (15% vs. 25%, *p* = .03) including death (7% vs. 15%, *p* = .04). The benefits were most striking in patients with pneumococcal meningitis. Dexamethasone (10 mg intravenously) was administered 15–20 min before the first dose of an antimicrobial agent, and the same dose was repeated every 6 h for 4 days. These results were confirmed in a second trial of dexamethasone in adults with pneumococcal meningitis. Therapy with dexamethasone should ideally be started 20 min before, or not later than concurrent with, the first dose of antibiotics. It is unlikely to be of significant benefit if started >6 h after antimicrobial therapy has been initiated. Dexamethasone may decrease the penetration of vancomycin into CSF, and it delays the sterilization of CSF in experimental models of *S. pneumoniae* meningitis. As a result, its potential benefit should be carefully weighed when vancomycin is the antibiotic of choice. Alternatively, vancomycin can be administered by the intraventricular route.

INCREASED INTRACRANIAL PRESSURE   Emergency treatment of increased ICP includes elevation of the patient's head to 30–45°, intubation and hyperventilation (Pa$_{CO_2}$ 25–30 mmHg), and mannitol. Patients with increased ICP should be managed in an intensive care unit; accurate ICP measurements are best obtained with an ICP monitoring device. **Treatment of increased intracranial pressure is discussed in detail in Chap. 269.**

PROGNOSIS

Mortality is 3–7% for meningitis caused by *H. influenzae*, *N. meningitidis*, or group B streptococci; 15% for that due to *L. monocytogenes*; and 20% for *S. pneumoniae*. In general, the risk of death from bacterial meningitis increases with (1) decreased level of consciousness on admission, (2) onset of seizures within 24 h of admission, (3) signs of increased ICP, (4) young age (infancy) and age >50, (5) the presence of comorbid conditions including shock and/or the need for mechanical ventilation, and (6) delay in the initiation of treatment. Decreased CSF glucose concentration [<2.2 mmol/L (<40 mg/dL)] and markedly increased CSF protein concentration [>3 g/L (>300 mg/dL)] have been predictive of increased mortality and poorer outcomes in some series. Moderate or severe sequelae occur in ~25% of survivors, although the exact incidence varies with the infecting organism. Common sequelae include decreased intellectual function, memory impairment, seizures, hearing loss and dizziness, and gait disturbances.

ACUTE VIRAL MENINGITIS

CLINICAL MANIFESTATIONS

Patients with viral meningitis usually present with headache, fever, and signs of meningeal irritation coupled with an inflammatory CSF profile (see below). The headache of viral meningitis is usually frontal or retroorbital and is often associated with photophobia and pain on moving the eyes. Nuchal rigidity is present in most cases but may be mild and present only near the limit of neck anteflexion. Constitutional signs can include malaise, myalgia, anorexia, nausea and vomiting, abdominal pain, and/or diarrhea. Patients often have mild lethargy or drowsiness; however, profound alterations in consciousness, such as stupor, coma, or marked confusion, are unusual in viral meningitis and suggest the presence of encephalitis or other alternative diagnoses. Similarly, seizures or focal neurologic signs or symptoms or neuroimaging abnormalities indicative of brain parenchymal involvement are not typical of viral meningitis and suggest the presence of encephalitis or another CNS infectious or inflammatory process.

TABLE 376-4   VIRUSES CAUSING ACUTE MENINGITIS AND ENCEPHALITIS IN NORTH AMERICA

Acute Meningitis

Common	Less Common
Enteroviruses (coxsackieviruses, echoviruses, and human enteroviruses 68–71)	Varicella zoster virus
	Epstein-Barr virus
	Lymphocytic choriomeningitis virus
Herpes simplex virus 2	
Arthropod-borne viruses	
HIV	

Acute Encephalitis

Common	Less Common
Herpesviruses	Rabies
Herpes simplex virus 1	Eastern equine encephalitis virus
Varicella zoster virus	Western equine encephalitis virus
Epstein-Barr virus	Powassan virus
Arthropod-borne viruses	Cytomegalovirus*a*
La Crosse virus	Enteroviruses*a*
West Nile virus	Colorado tick fever
St. Louis encephalitis virus	Mumps

*a*Immunocompromised host.

ETIOLOGY

Using a variety of diagnostic techniques, including CSF PCR, culture, and serology, a specific viral cause can be found in 75–90% of cases of viral meningitis. The most important agents are enteroviruses, HSV type 2 (HSV-2), and arboviruses (Table 376-4). CSF cultures are positive in 30–70% of patients, the frequency of isolation depending on the specific viral agent. Approximately two-thirds of culture-negative cases of aseptic meningitis have a specific viral etiology identified by CSF PCR testing (see below).

EPIDEMIOLOGY

Viral meningitis is not a nationally reportable disease; however, it has been estimated that the incidence is ~75,000 cases per year. In temperate climates, there is a substantial increase in cases during the summer and early fall months, reflecting the seasonal predominance of enterovirus and arthropod-borne virus (arbovirus) infections, with a peak monthly incidence of about 1 reported case per 100,000 population.

LABORATORY DIAGNOSIS

CSF Examination   The most important laboratory test in the diagnosis of viral meningitis is examination of the CSF. The typical profile is a lymphocytic pleocytosis (25–500 cells/μL), a normal or slightly elevated protein concentration [0.2–0.8 g/L (20–80 mg/dL)], a normal glucose concentration, and a normal or mildly elevated opening pressure (100–350 mmH$_2$O). Organisms are *not* seen on Gram's or acid-fast stained smears or India ink preparations of CSF. Rarely, PMNs may predominate in the first 48 h of illness, especially with infections due to echovirus 9, eastern equine encephalitis (EEE) virus, or mumps. A pleocytosis of polymorphonuclear neutrophils also occurs in 45% of patients with West Nile virus (WNV) meningitis and can persist for a week or longer before shifting to a lymphocytic pleocytosis. Despite these exceptions, the presence of a CSF PMN pleocytosis in a patient with suspected viral meningitis should always prompt consideration of alternative diagnoses, including bacterial meningitis or parameningeal infections. The total CSF cell count in viral meningitis is typically 25–500/μL, although cell counts of several thousand/μL are occasionally seen, especially with infections due to lymphocytic choriomeningitis virus (LCMV) and mumps virus. The CSF glucose concentration is typically normal in viral infections, although it may be decreased in 10–30% of cases due to mumps or LCMV. Rare instances of decreased CSF glucose concentration occur in cases of meningitis due to echoviruses and other enteroviruses, HSV-2, and varicella-zoster virus (VZV). As a rule, a lymphocytic pleocytosis with a low glucose concentration should suggest fungal or tuberculous meningitis, *Listeria* meningoencephalitis, or noninfectious disorders (e.g., sarcoid, neoplastic meningitis).

A number of tests measuring levels of various CSF proteins, enzymes, and mediators—including C-reactive protein, lactic acid, lactate dehydrogenase, neopterin, quinolinate, IL-1β, IL-6, soluble IL-2 receptor, β$_2$-microglobulin, and TNF—have been proposed as potential discriminators between viral and bacterial meningitis or as markers of specific types of viral infection (e.g., infection with HIV), but they remain of uncertain sensitivity and specificity and are not widely used for diagnostic purposes.

Polymerase Chain Reaction Amplification of Viral Nucleic Acid Amplification of viral-specific DNA or RNA from CSF using PCR amplification has become the single most important method for diagnosing CNS viral infections. In both enteroviral and HSV infections of the CNS, PCR has become the diagnostic procedure of choice and is substantially more sensitive than viral cultures. HSV PCR is also an important diagnostic test in patients with recurrent episodes of "aseptic" meningitis, many of whom have amplifiable HSV DNA in CSF despite negative viral cultures. CSF PCR is also used routinely to diagnose CNS viral infections caused by cytomegalovirus (CMV), Epstein-Barr virus (EBV), VZV, and human herpesvirus 6 (HHV-6). CSF PCR tests are available for WNV but are not as sensitive as CSF IgM. PCR is also useful in the diagnosis of CNS infection caused by *Mycoplasma pneumoniae*, which can mimic viral meningitis and encephalitis.

Viral Culture The sensitivity of CSF cultures for the diagnosis of viral meningitis and encephalitis, in contrast to its utility in bacterial infections, is generally poor. In addition to CSF, specific viruses may also be isolated from throat swabs, stool, blood, and urine. Enteroviruses and adenoviruses may be found in feces; arboviruses, some enteroviruses, and LCMV in blood; mumps and CMV in urine; and enteroviruses, mumps, and adenoviruses in throat washings. During enteroviral infections, viral shedding in stool may persist for several weeks. The presence of enterovirus in stool is not diagnostic and may result from residual shedding from a previous enteroviral infection; it also occurs in some asymptomatic individuals during enteroviral epidemics.

Serologic Studies For some viruses, including many arboviruses such as WNV, serologic studies remain a crucial diagnostic tool. Serum antibody determination is less useful for viruses with high seroprevalence rates in the general population such as HSV, VZV, CMV, and EBV. For viruses with low seroprevalence rates, diagnosis of acute viral infection can be made by documenting seroconversion between acute-phase and convalescent sera (typically obtained after 2–4 weeks) or by demonstrating the presence of virus-specific IgM antibodies. Documentation of synthesis of virus-specific antibodies in CSF, as shown by an increased IgG index or the presence of CSF IgM antibodies, is more useful than serum serology alone and can provide presumptive evidence of CNS infection. Although serum and CSF IgM antibodies generally persist for only a few months after acute infection, there are exceptions to this rule. For example, WNV IgM has been shown to persist in some patients for >1 year following acute infection. Unfortunately, the delay between onset of infection and the host's generation of a virus-specific antibody response often means that serologic data are useful mainly for the retrospective establishment of a specific diagnosis, rather than in aiding acute diagnosis or management.

CSF oligoclonal gamma globulin bands occur in association with a number of viral infections. The associated antibodies are often directed against viral proteins. Oligoclonal bands occur commonly in certain noninfectious neurologic diseases (e.g., multiple sclerosis) and may be found in nonviral infections (e.g., neurosyphilis, Lyme neuroborreliosis).

Other Laboratory Studies All patients with suspected viral meningitis should have a complete blood count and differential, liver and renal function tests, erythrocyte sedimentation rate (ESR) and C-reactive protein, electrolytes, glucose, creatine kinase, aldolase, amylase, and lipase. Neuroimaging studies (MRI, CT) are not necessary in patients with uncomplicated viral meningitis but should be performed in pa-

tients with altered consciousness, seizures, focal neurologic signs or symptoms, or atypical CSF profiles.

DIFFERENTIAL DIAGNOSIS
The most important issue in the differential diagnosis of viral meningitis is to consider diseases that can mimic viral meningitis, including (1) untreated or partially treated bacterial meningitis; (2) early stages of meningitis caused by fungi, mycobacteria, or *Treponema pallidum* (neurosyphilis), in which a lymphocytic pleocytosis is common, cultures may be slow growing or negative, and hypoglycorrhachia may not be present early; (3) meningitis caused by agents such as *Mycoplasma*, *Listeria* spp., *Brucella* spp., *Coxiella* spp., *Leptospira* spp., and *Rickettsia* spp.; (4) parameningeal infections; (5) neoplastic meningitis; and (6) meningitis secondary to noninfectious inflammatory diseases, including hypersensitivity meningitis, SLE and other rheumatologic diseases, sarcoidosis, Behçet's syndrome, and the uveomeningitic syndromes.

SPECIFIC VIRAL ETIOLOGIES
Enteroviruses (Chap. 184) are the most common cause of viral meningitis, accounting for >75% of cases in which a specific etiology can be identified. CSF reverse transcriptase PCR (RT-PCR) is the diagnostic procedure of choice and is both sensitive (>95%) and specific (>100%). Enteroviruses are the most likely cause of viral meningitis in the summer months, especially in children (<15 years), although cases occur at reduced frequency year round. Although the incidence of enteroviral meningitis declines with increasing age, some outbreaks have preferentially affected older children and adults. Meningitis outside the neonatal period is usually benign. Patients present with sudden onset of fever; headache; nuchal rigidity; and often constitutional signs, including vomiting, anorexia, diarrhea, cough, pharyngitis, and myalgias. The physical examination should include a careful search for stigmata of enterovirus infection, including exanthemata, hand-foot-mouth disease, herpangina, pleurodynia, myopericarditis, and hemorrhagic conjunctivitis. The CSF profile is typically a lymphocytic pleocytosis (100–1000 cells/µL) with normal glucose and normal or mildly elevated protein concentration. In rare cases, PMNs may predominate during the first 48 h of illness. Treatment is supportive, and patients usually recover without sequelae. Chronic and severe infections can occur in neonates and in individuals with hypo- or agammaglobulinemia.

Arbovirus infections (Chap. 189) occur predominantly in the summer and early fall. Arboviral meningitis should be considered when clusters of meningitis and encephalitis cases occur in a restricted geographic region during the summer or early fall. In WNV epidemics, avian deaths may serve as sentinel infections for subsequent human disease. A history of tick exposure or travel or residence in the appropriate geographic area should suggest the possibility of Colorado tick fever virus or Powassan virus infection, although nonviral tick-borne diseases, including RMSF and Lyme neuroborreliosis, may present similarly. Arbovirus meningoencephalitis is typically associated with a CSF lymphocytic pleocytosis, normal glucose concentration, and normal or mildly elevated protein concentration. However, 40–45% of patients with WNV meningoencephalitis have CSF neutrophilia, which can persist for a week or more. The rarity of hypoglycorrhachia in WNV infection as well as the absence of positive Gram's stains and the negative cultures helps distinguish these patients from those with bacterial meningitis. The presence of increased numbers of plasmacytoid cells or Mollaret-like large mononuclear cells in the CSF may be a clue to the diagnosis of WNV infection. Definitive diagnosis of arboviral meningoencephalitis is based on demonstration of viral-specific IgM in CSF or seroconversion. CSF PCR tests are available for some viruses in selected diagnostic laboratories and at the Centers for Disease Control and Prevention (CDC), but in the case of WNV, sensitivity (~70%) of CSF PCR is less than that of CSF serology.

HSV-2 meningitis (Chap. 172) occurs in ~25% of women and 11% of men at the time of an initial (primary) episode of genital herpes. Of these patients, 20% go on to have recurrent attacks of meningitis. HSV-2 has been increasingly recognized as a major cause of viral meningitis in adults, and overall it is probably second in importance to enteroviruses as a cause of viral meningitis. Diagnosis of HSV meningitis is usually by HSV CSF PCR as cultures may be negative, especially in patients with recurrent meningitis. Demonstration of intrathecal synthesis of HSV-specific antibody may also be useful in diagnosis, although antibody tests are less sensitive and less specific than PCR and may not become positive until after the first week of infection. In contrast to HSV encephalitis in adults in which >90% of cases are due to HSV-1, the overwhelming majority of HSV meningitis is due to HSV-2. Although a history of or the presence of HSV genital lesions is an important diagnostic clue, many patients with HSV meningitis give no history and have no evidence of active genital herpes at the time of presentation. Most cases of recurrent viral or "aseptic" meningitis, including cases previously diagnosed as Mollaret's meningitis, are likely due to HSV.

VZV meningitis should be suspected in the presence of concurrent chickenpox or shingles. However, it is important to recognize that in some series, up to 40% of VZV meningitis cases have been reported to occur in the absence of rash. The frequency of VZV as a cause of meningitis is extremely variable, ranging from as low as 3% to as high as 20% in different series. Diagnosis is usually based on CSF PCR, although the sensitivity of this test may not be as high as for the other herpesviruses. In patients with negative CSF PCR results, the diagnosis of VZV CNS infection can be made by the demonstration of VZV-specific intrathecal antibody synthesis and/or the presence of VZV CSF IgM antibodies, or by positive CSF cultures.

EBV infections may also produce aseptic meningitis, with or without associated infectious mononucleosis. The presence of atypical lymphocytes in the CSF or peripheral blood is suggestive of EBV infection but may occasionally be seen with other viral infections. EBV is almost never cultured from CSF. Serum and CSF serology can help establish the presence of acute infection, which is characterized by IgM viral capsid antibodies (VCAs), antibodies to early antigens (EA), and the absence of antibodies to EBV-associated nuclear antigen (EBNA). CSF PCR is another important diagnostic test, although positive results may reflect viral reactivation associated with other infectious or inflammatory processes.

HIV meningitis should be suspected in any patient presenting with a viral meningitis with known or suspected risk factors for HIV infection. Meningitis may occur following primary infection with HIV in 5–10% of cases and less commonly at later stages of illness. Cranial nerve palsies, most commonly involving cranial nerves V, VII, or VIII, are more common in HIV meningitis than in other viral infections. Diagnosis can be confirmed by detection of HIV genome in blood or CSF. Seroconversion may be delayed, and patients with negative HIV serologies who are suspected of having HIV meningitis should be monitored for delayed seroconversion. For further discussion of HIV infection, see Chap. 182.

Mumps (Chap. 187) should be considered when meningitis occurs in the late winter or early spring, especially in males (male/female ratio 3:1). With the widespread use of the live attenuated mumps vaccine in the United States since 1967, the incidence of mumps meningitis has fallen by >95%. The presence of parotitis, orchitis, oophoritis, pancreatitis, or elevations in serum lipase and amylase are suggestive of mumps meningitis; however, their absence does not exclude the diagnosis. Clinical meningitis occurs in up to 30% of patients with mumps parotitis, and CSF pleocytosis occurs in >50%. Mumps infection confers lifelong immunity, so a documented history of previous infection excludes this diagnosis. Patients with meningitis have a CSF pleocytosis that can exceed 1000 cells/μL in 25%. Lymphocytes predominate in 75%, although CSF neutrophilia occurs in 25%. Hypoglycorrhachia, occurs in 10–30% of patients and may be a clue to the diagnosis when present. Diagnosis is typically made by culture of virus from CSF or by detecting IgM antibodies or seroconversion. CSF PCR is available in some diagnostic and research laboratories. The frequency of mumps meningitis has declined dramatically with the widespread use of the live-attenuated mumps vaccine. Rare cases of vaccine-associated meningitis occur, with a frequency of 10–100/100,000 doses typically 2–4 weeks after vaccination.

LCMV infection (Chap. 189) should be considered when aseptic meningitis occurs in the late fall or winter and in individuals with a history of

exposure to house mice (*Mus musculus*), pet or laboratory rodents (e.g., hamsters, rats, mice), or their excreta. Some patients have an associated rash, pulmonary infiltrates, alopecia, parotitis, orchitis, or myopericarditis. Laboratory clues to the diagnosis of LCMV, in addition to the clinical findings noted above, may include the presence of leukopenia, thrombocytopenia, or abnormal liver function tests. Some cases present with a marked CSF pleocytosis (>1000 cells/μL) and hypoglycorrhachia (<30%). Diagnosis is based on serology and/or culture of virus from CSF.

℞ ACUTE VIRAL MENINGITIS

Treatment of almost all cases of viral meningitis is primarily symptomatic and includes use of analgesics, antipyretics, and antiemetics. Fluid and electrolyte status should be monitored. Patients with suspected bacterial meningitis should receive appropriate empirical therapy pending culture results (see above). Hospitalization may not be required in immunocompetent patients with presumed viral meningitis and no focal signs or symptoms, no significant alteration in consciousness, and a classic CSF profile (lymphocytic pleocytosis, normal glucose, negative Gram's stain) if adequate provision for monitoring at home and medical follow-up can be ensured. Immunocompromised patients; patients with significant alteration in consciousness, seizures, or the presence of focal signs and symptoms suggesting the possibility of encephalitis or parenchymal brain involvement; and those patients who have an atypical CSF profile should be hospitalized. Oral or intravenous acyclovir may be of benefit in patients with meningitis caused by HSV-1 or -2 and in cases of severe EBV or VZV infection. Data concerning treatment of HSV, EBV, and VZV meningitis are extremely limited. Seriously ill patients should probably receive intravenous acyclovir (15–30 mg/kg per day in three divided doses), which can be followed by an oral drug such as acyclovir (800 mg, five times daily), famciclovir (500 mg tid), or valacyclovir (1000 mg tid) for a total course of 7–14 days. Patients who are less ill can be treated with oral drugs alone. Patients with HIV meningitis should receive highly active antiretroviral therapy (Chap. 182).

Patients with viral meningitis who are known to have deficient humoral immunity (e.g., X-linked agammaglobulinemia) and who are not already receiving either intramuscular gamma globulin or intravenous immunoglobulin (IVIg), should be treated with these agents. Intraventricular administration of immunoglobulin through an Ommaya reservoir has been tried in some patients with chronic enteroviral meningitis who have not responded to intramuscular or intravenous immunoglobulin.

An investigational drug, pleconaril, has shown efficacy against a variety of enteroviral infections and has good oral bioavailability and excellent CNS penetration. Clinical trials in patients with enteroviral meningitis indicated that pleconaril decreased the duration of symptoms compared to placebo. Most cases of enteroviral CNS infection are benign and self-limited and do not require specific antiviral therapy. However, pleconaril treatment might benefit patients with chronic CNS enteroviral infections in the setting of agammaglobulinemia or those who develop poliomyelitis as a complication of polio vaccine administration. Unfortunately, the availability of pleconaril for compassionate-use purposes is currently uncertain.

Vaccination is an effective method of preventing the development of meningitis and other neurologic complications associated with poliovirus, mumps, and measles infection. A live attenuated VZV vaccine (Varivax) is available in the United States. Clinical studies indicate an effectiveness rate of 70–90% for this vaccine, but a booster may be required to maintain immunity. An inactivated varicella vaccine is available for transplant recipients.

PROGNOSIS

In adults, the prognosis for full recovery from viral meningitis is excellent. Rare patients complain of persisting headache, mild mental impairment, incoordination, or generalized asthenia for weeks to months. The outcome in infants and neonates (<1 year) is less certain; intellectual impairment, learning disabilities, hearing loss, and other lasting sequelae have been reported in some studies.

VIRAL ENCEPHALITIS

DEFINITION

In contrast to viral meningitis, where the infectious process and associated inflammatory response are limited largely to the meninges, in encephalitis the brain parenchyma is also involved. Many patients with encephalitis also have evidence of associated meningitis (meningoencephalitis) and, in some cases, involvement of the spinal cord or nerve roots (encephalomyelitis, encephalomyeloradiculitis).

CLINICAL MANIFESTATIONS

In addition to the acute febrile illness with evidence of meningeal involvement characteristic of meningitis, the patient with encephalitis commonly has an altered level of consciousness (confusion, behavioral abnormalities), or a depressed level of consciousness, ranging from mild lethargy to coma, and evidence of either focal or diffuse neurologic signs and symptoms. Patients with encephalitis may have hallucinations, agitation, personality change, behavioral disorders, and, at times, a frankly psychotic state. Focal or generalized seizures occur in many patients with encephalitis. Virtually every possible type of focal neurologic disturbance has been reported in viral encephalitis; the signs and symptoms reflect the sites of infection and inflammation. The most commonly encountered focal findings are aphasia, ataxia, upper or lower motor neuron patterns of weakness, involuntary movements (e.g., myoclonic jerks, tremor), and cranial nerve deficits (e.g., ocular palsies, facial weakness). Involvement of the hypothalamic-pituitary axis may result in temperature dysregulation, diabetes insipidus, or the development of the syndrome of inappropriate secretion of antidiuretic hormone (SIADH). Despite the clear neuropathologic evidence that viruses differ in the regions of the CNS they injure, it is often impossible to distinguish reliably on clinical grounds alone one type of viral encephalitis (e.g., that caused by HSV) from others (see "Differential Diagnosis," below).

ETIOLOGY

In the United States, there are ~20,000 reported cases of encephalitis per year, although the actual number of cases is likely to be significantly larger. Hundreds of viruses are capable of causing encephalitis, although only a limited subset is responsible for most cases in which a specific cause is identified (Table 376-4). The same organisms responsible for aseptic meningitis are also responsible for encephalitis, although the relative frequencies with which specific organisms cause these two patterns of infection often differ. The most important viruses causing sporadic cases of encephalitis in immunocompetent adults are herpesviruses (HSV, VZV, EBV). Epidemics of encephalitis are caused by arboviruses, which belong to several different viral taxonomic groups including *Alphaviruses* (e.g., EEE virus, western equine encephalitis virus), *Flaviviruses* (e.g., WNV, St. Louis encephalitis virus, Japanese encephalitis virus, Powassan virus), and *Bunyaviruses* (e.g., California encephalitis virus serogroup, LaCrosse virus). Historically, the largest number of cases of arbovirus encephalitis in the United States has been due to St. Louis encephalitis virus and the California encephalitis virus serogroup. However, since 2002, WNV has been responsible for the majority of arbovirus meningitis and encephalitis cases in the United States. The 2003 epidemic was the largest epidemic of arboviral neuroinvasive disease (encephalitis + meningitis) ever recorded in the United States, with 2860 cases and 264 deaths. Since 2003, WNV has accounted for ~1100–1300 cases of neuroinvasive disease per year and 100–120 deaths in the United States. New causes of viral CNS infections are constantly appearing, as evidenced by the recent outbreak of cases of encephalitis in Southeast Asia caused by Nipah virus, a newly identified member of the Paramyxovirus family, and of meningitis in Europe caused by Toscana virus, an arbovirus belonging to the Bunyavirus family.

LABORATORY DIAGNOSIS

CSF Examination CSF examination should be performed in all patients with suspected viral encephalitis unless contraindicated by the presence of severely increased ICP. The characteristic CSF profile is indistinguishable from that of viral meningitis and typically consists of a lymphocytic pleocytosis, a mildly elevated protein concentration, and a normal glucose concentration. A CSF pleocytosis (>5 cells/μL) occurs in >95% of patients with documented viral encephalitis. In rare cases, a pleocytosis may be absent on the initial LP but present on subsequent LPs. Patients who are severely immunocompromised by HIV infection, glucocorticoid or other immunosuppressant drugs, chemotherapy, or lymphoreticular malignancies may fail to mount a CSF inflammatory response. CSF cell counts exceed 500/μL in only about 10% of patients with encephalitis. Infections with certain arboviruses (e.g., EEE virus or California encephalitis virus), mumps, and LCMV may occasionally result in cell counts >1000/μL, but this degree of pleocytosis should suggest the possibility of nonviral infections or other inflammatory processes. Atypical lymphocytes in the CSF may be seen in EBV infection and less commonly with other viruses, including CMV, HSV, and enteroviruses. Increased numbers of plasmacytoid or Mollaret-like large mononuclear cells have been reported in WNV encephalitis. Polymorphonuclear pleocytosis occurs in ~40% of patients with WNV encephalitis. Large numbers of CSF PMNs may be present in patients with encephalitis due to EEE virus, echovirus 9, and, more rarely, other enteroviruses. However, persisting CSF neutrophilia should prompt consideration of bacterial infection, leptospirosis, amebic infection, and noninfectious processes such as acute hemorrhagic leukoencephalitis. About 20% of patients with encephalitis will have a significant number of red blood cells (>500/μL) in the CSF in a nontraumatic tap. The pathologic correlate of this finding may be a hemorrhagic encephalitis of the type seen with HSV; however, CSF red blood cells occur with similar frequency and in similar numbers in patients with nonherpetic focal encephalitides. A decreased CSF glucose concentration is distinctly unusual in viral encephalitis and should suggest the possibility of bacterial, fungal, tuberculous, parasitic, leptospiral, syphilitic, sarcoid, or neoplastic meningitis. Rare patients with mumps, LCMV, or advanced HSV encephalitis may have low CSF glucose concentrations.

CSF PCR CSF PCR has become the primary diagnostic test for CNS infections caused by CMV, EBV, VZV, HHV-6, and enteroviruses (see "Viral Meningitis," above). The sensitivity and specificity of CSF PCRs varies with the virus being tested. The sensitivity (~96%) and specificity (~99%) of HSV CSF PCR is equivalent to or exceeds that of brain biopsy. It is important to recognize that HSV CSF PCR results need to be interpreted after considering the likelihood of disease in the patient being tested, the timing of the test in relationship to onset of symptoms, and the prior use of antiviral therapy. A negative HSV CSF PCR test performed by a qualified laboratory at the appropriate time during illness in a patient with a high likelihood of HSV encephalitis based on clinical and laboratory abnormalities significantly reduces the likelihood of HSV encephalitis but does not exclude it. For example, in a patient with a pretest probability of 35% of having HSV encephalitis, a negative HSV CSF PCR reduces the posttest probability to ~2%, and for a patient with a pretest probability of 60%, a negative test reduces the posttest probability to ~6%. In both situations a positive test makes the diagnosis almost certain (98–99%). There have been several recent reports of initially negative HSV CSF PCR tests that were obtained early (≤72 h) following symptom onset, and that became positive when repeated 1–3 days later. The frequency of positive HSV CSF PCRs in patients with herpes encephalitis also decreases as a function of the duration of illness, with only ~20% of cases remaining positive after ≥14 days. PCR results are generally not affected by ≤1 week of antiviral therapy. In one study, 98% of CSF specimens remained PCR-positive during the first week of initiation of antiviral therapy, but the numbers fell to ~50% by 8–14 days and to ~21% by >15 days after initiation of antiviral therapy.

The sensitivity and specificity of CSF PCR tests for viruses other than herpes simplex have not been definitively characterized. Enteroviral CSF PCR appears to have a sensitivity and specificity of >95%. The specificity of EBV CSF PCR has not been established. Positive EBV CSF PCRs associated with positive tests for other pathogens have been reported and may reflect reactivation of EBV latent in lymphocytes that enter the CNS as a result of an unrelated infectious or inflammatory process. In patients with CNS infection due to VZV, CSF antibody and PCR studies should be considered complementary, as patients may have evidence of intrathecal synthesis of VZV-specific antibodies and negative CSF PCRs. In the case of WNV infection, CSF PCR appears to be less sensitive (~70% sensitivity) than detection of WNV-specific CSF IgM, although PCR testing remains useful in immunocompromised patients who may not mount an effective anti-WNV antibody response.

CSF Culture Attempts to culture viruses from the CSF in cases of encephalitis are often disappointing. Cultures are negative in >95% of cases of HSV-1 encephalitis.

Serologic Studies and Antigen Detection The basic approach to the serodiagnosis of viral encephalitis is identical to that discussed earlier for viral meningitis. In patients with HSV encephalitis, both antibodies to HSV-1 glycoproteins and glycoprotein antigens have been detected in the CSF. Optimal detection of both HSV antibodies and antigen typically occurs after the first week of illness, limiting the utility of these tests in acute diagnosis. Nonetheless, HSV CSF antibody testing is of value in selected patients whose illness is >1 week in duration and who are CSF PCR–negative for HSV. Demonstration of WNV IgM antibodies is diagnostic of WNV encephalitis as IgM antibodies do not cross the blood-brain barrier, and their presence in CSF is therefore indicative of intrathecal synthesis. Timing of antibody collection may be important as the rate of CSF WNV IgM seropositivity increases by ~10% per day during the first week after illness onset.

MRI, CT, EEG Patients with suspected encephalitis almost invariably undergo neuroimaging studies and often EEG. These tests help identify or exclude alternative diagnoses and assist in the differentiation between a focal, as opposed to a diffuse, encephalitic process. Focal findings in a patient with encephalitis should always raise the possibility of HSV encephalitis. Examples of focal findings include: (1) areas of increased signal intensity in the frontotemporal, cingulate, or insular regions of the brain on T2-weighted, FLAIR, or diffusion-weighted MRI images (Fig. 376-3); (2) focal areas of low absorption, mass effect, and contrast enhancement on CT; or (3) periodic focal temporal lobe spikes on a background of slow or low-amplitude ("flattened") activity on EEG. Approximately 10% of patients with PCR-documented HSV encephalitis will have a normal MRI, although nearly 80% will have abnormalities in the temporal lobe, and an additional 10% in ex-

tratemporal regions. The lesions are typically hyperintense on T2-weighted images. CT is less sensitive than MRI and is normal in up to 33% of patients. The addition of FLAIR and diffusion-weighted images to the standard MRI sequences enhances sensitivity. EEG abnormalities occur in >90% of PCR-documented cases of HSV encephalitis; they typically involve the temporal lobes but are often nonspecific. Some patients with HSV encephalitis have a distinctive EEG pattern consisting of periodic, stereotyped, sharp-and-slow complexes originating in one or both temporal lobes and repeating at regular intervals of 2–3 s. The periodic complexes are typically noted between the 2nd and 15th day of the illness and are present in two-thirds of pathologically proven cases of HSV encephalitis.

Significant MRI abnormalities are found in only ~50% of patients with WNV encephalitis, a frequency less than that with HSV encephalitis. When present, abnormalities often involve deep brain structures, including the thalamus, basal ganglia, and brainstem, rather than the cortex and may only be apparent on FLAIR images. EEGs typically show generalized slowing that may be more anteriorly prominent rather than the temporally predominant pattern of sharp or periodic discharges more characteristic of HSV encephalitis. Patients with VZV encephalitis may show multifocal areas of hemorrhagic and ischemic infarction reflecting the tendency of this virus to produce a CNS vasculopathy rather than a true encephalitis. Immunocompromised adult patients with CMV often have enlarged ventricles with areas of increased T2 signal on MRI outlining the ventricles and sub-ependymal enhancement on T1-weighted post-contrast images. Table 376-5 highlights specific diagnostic test results in encephalitis that can be useful in clinical decision-making.

Brain Biopsy Brain biopsy is now generally reserved for patients in whom CSF PCR studies fail to lead to a specific diagnosis, who have focal abnormalities on MRI, and who continue to show progressive

FIGURE 376-3 Coronal FLAIR magnetic resonance image from a patient with herpes simplex encephalitis. Note the area of increased signal in the right temporal lobe (left side of image) confined predominantly to the gray matter. This patient had predominantly unilateral disease; bilateral lesions are more common but may be quite asymmetric in their intensity.

TABLE 376-5 USE OF DIAGNOSTIC TESTS IN ENCEPHALITIS

The best test for WNV encephalitis is the *CSF IgM antibody test*. The prevalence of positive CSF IgM tests increases by about 10%/day after illness onset and reaches 70–80% by the end of the first week. Serum WNV IgM can provide evidence for recent WNV infection, but in the absence of other findings does not establish the diagnosis of neuroinvasive disease (meningitis, encephalitis, acute flaccid paralysis).

Approximately 80% of patients with proven HSV encephalitis have *MRI* abnormalities involving the temporal lobes. This percentage likely increases to >90% when FLAIR and DWI MR sequences are also utilized. The absence of temporal lobe lesions on MR reduces the likelihood of HSV encephalitis and should prompt consideration of other diagnostic possibilities.

The *CSF HSV PCR* test may be negative in the first 72 h of symptoms of HSV encephalitis. A repeat study should be considered in patients with an initial early negative PCR in whom diagnostic suspicion of HSV encephalitis remains high and no alternative diagnosis has yet been established.

Detection of *intrathecal synthesis* (increased CSF/serum HSV antibody ratio corrected for breakdown of the blood-brain barrier) of *HSV-specific antibody* may be useful in diagnosis of HSV encephalitis in patients in whom only late (>1 week post-onset) CSF specimens are available and PCR studies are negative. Serum serology alone is of no value in diagnosis of HSV encephalitis due to the high seroprevalence rate in the general population.

Negative *CSF viral cultures* are of no value in excluding the diagnosis of HSV or EBV encephalitis.

VZV CSF IgM antibodies may be present in patients with a negative VZV CSF PCR. Both tests should be performed in patients with suspected VZV CNS disease.

The specificity of *EBV CSF PCR* for diagnosis of CNS infection is unknown. Positive tests may occur in patients with a CSF pleocytosis due to other causes. Detection of EBV CSF IgM or intrathecal synthesis of antibody to VCA supports the diagnosis of EBV encephalitis. Serological studies consistent with acute EBV infection (e.g., IgM VCA, presence of antibodies against EA but not against EBNA) can help support the diagnosis.

Note: CSF, cerebrospinal fluid; IgM, immunoglobulin M; WNV, West Nile virus; HSV, herpes simplex virus; MRI, magnetic resonance imaging; FLAIR, fluid attenuated inversion recovery; DWI, diffusion-weighted imaging; PCR, polymerase chain reaction; EBV, Epstein-Barr virus; VZV, varicella-zoster virus; CNS, central nervous system; VCA, viral capsid antibody; EA, early antigen; EBNA, EBV-associated nuclear antigen.

clinical deterioration despite treatment with acyclovir and supportive therapy.

DIFFERENTIAL DIAGNOSIS

Infection by a variety of other organisms can mimic viral encephalitis. In studies of biopsy-proven HSV encephalitis, common infectious mimics of focal viral encephalitis included mycobacteria, fungi, rickettsia, *Listeria* and other bacteria (including *Bartonella* sp.), and *Mycoplasma*.

Infection caused by the ameba *Naegleria fowleri* can also cause acute meningoencephalitis (primary amebic meningoencephalitis), whereas that caused by *Acanthamoeba* and *Balamuthia* more typically produces subacute or chronic granulomatous amebic meningoencephalitis. *Naegleria* thrive in warm, iron-rich pools of water, including those found in drains, canals, and both natural and human-made outdoor pools. Infection has typically occurred in immunocompetent children with a history of swimming in potentially infected water. The CSF, in contrast to the typical profile seen in viral encephalitis, often resembles that of bacterial meningitis with a neutrophilic pleocytosis and hypoglycorrhachia. Motile trophozoites can be seen in a wet mount of warm, fresh CSF. No effective treatment has been identified, and mortality approaches 100%.

Encephalitis can be caused by the raccoon pinworm *Baylisascaris procyonis*. Clues to the diagnosis include a history of raccoon exposure, and especially of playing in or eating dirt potentially contaminated with raccoon feces. Most patients are children, and many have an associated eosinophilia.

Once nonviral causes of encephalitis have been excluded, the major diagnostic challenge is to distinguish HSV from other viruses that cause encephalitis. This distinction is particularly important because in virtually every other instance the therapy is supportive, whereas specific and effective antiviral therapy is available for HSV, and its efficacy is enhanced when it is instituted early in the course of infection. HSV encephalitis should be considered when clinical features suggesting involvement of the inferomedial frontotemporal regions of the brain are present, including prominent olfactory or gustatory hallucinations, anosmia, unusual or bizarre behavior or personality alterations, or memory disturbance. HSV encephalitis should always be suspected in patients with focal findings on clinical examination, neuroimaging studies, or EEG. The diagnostic procedure of choice in these patients is CSF PCR analysis for HSV. A positive CSF PCR establishes the diagnosis, and a negative test dramatically reduces the likelihood of HSV encephalitis (see above).

The anatomic distribution of lesions may provide an additional clue to diagnosis. Patients with rapidly progressive encephalitis and prominent brainstem signs, symptoms, or neuroimaging abnormalities may be infected by flaviviruses (WNV, St. Louis encephalitis virus, Japanese encephalitis virus), HSV, rabies, or *L. monocytogenes*. Significant involvement of deep gray matter structures, including the basal ganglia and thalamus, should also suggest possible flavivirus infection. These patients may present clinically with prominent movement disorders (tremor, myoclonus) or parkinsonian features. Patients with WNV infection can also present with a poliomyelitis-like acute flaccid paralysis, as can patients infected with enterovirus 71 and, less commonly, other enteroviruses. Acute flaccid paralysis is characterized by the acute onset of a lower motor neuron type of weakness with flaccid tone, reduced or absent reflexes, and relatively preserved sensation. Despite an aggressive World Health Organization poliovirus eradication initiative, >1200 cases of wild-type poliovirus-induced poliomyelitis have been reported worldwide in 2006, with 88% occurring in Nigeria and India and >20 cases each from Somalia, Afghanistan, and Namibia. There have been recent small outbreaks of poliomyelitis associated with vaccine strains of virus that have reverted to virulence through mutation or recombination with circulating wild-type enteroviruses in Hispaniola, China, the Philippines, and Madagascar.

Epidemiologic factors may provide important clues to the diagnosis of viral meningitis or encephalitis. Particular attention should be paid to the season of the year; the geographic location and travel history; and

possible exposure to animal bites or scratches, rodents, and ticks. Although transmission from the bite of an infected dog remains the most common cause of rabies worldwide, in the United States very few cases of dog rabies occur, and the most common risk factor is exposure to bats—although a clear history of a bite or scratch is often lacking. The classic clinical presentation of encephalitic (furious) rabies is of fever, fluctuating consciousness, and autonomic hyperactivity. Phobic spasms of the larynx, pharynx, neck muscles, and diaphragm can be triggered by attempts to swallow water (*hydrophobia*) or by inspiration (*aerophobia*). Patients may also present with paralytic (dumb) rabies characterized by acute ascending paralysis. Rabies due to the bite of a bat has a different clinical presentation than classic rabies. Patients present with focal neurologic deficits, myoclonus, seizures, and hallucinations; phobic spasms are not a typical feature. Patients with rabies have a CSF lymphocytic pleocytosis and may show areas of increased T2 signal abnormality in the brainstem, hippocampus, and hypothalamus. Diagnosis can be made by finding rabies virus antigen in brain tissue or in the neural innervation of hair follicles at the nape of the neck. PCR amplification of viral nucleic acid from CSF and saliva or tears may also enable diagnosis. Serology is frequently negative in both serum and CSF in the first week after onset of infection, which limits its acute diagnostic utility. No specific therapy is available, and cases are almost invariably fatal, with isolated survivors having devastating neurologic sequelae.

State public health authorities provide a valuable resource concerning isolation of particular agents in individual regions. Regular updates concerning the number, type and distribution of cases of arboviral encephalitis can be found on the CDC and U.S. Geological Survey (USGS) websites (*http://www.cdc.gov* and *http://diseasemaps.usgs.gov*).

The major noninfectious etiologies that should be included in the differential diagnosis of acute encephalitis are nonvasculitic autoimmune meningoencephalitis, which may or may not be associated with serum antithyroid microsomal and antithyroglobulin antibodies; limbic encephalitis associated with antineuronal antibodies; limbic encephalopathy not associated with cancer; acute disseminated encephalomyelitis and related fulminant demyelinating disorders (Chap. 375); and lymphoma. Finally, Creutzfeldt-Jakob disease (Chap. 378) can rarely present in an explosive fashion mimicking viral encephalitis.

℞ VIRAL ENCEPHALITIS

Specific antiviral therapy should be initiated when appropriate. Vital functions, including respiration and blood pressure, should be monitored continuously and supported as required. In the initial stages of encephalitis, many patients will require care in an intensive care unit. Basic management and supportive therapy should include careful monitoring of ICP, fluid restriction, avoidance of hypotonic intravenous solutions, and suppression of fever. Seizures should be treated with standard anticonvulsant regimens, and prophylactic therapy should be considered in view of the high frequency of seizures in severe cases of encephalitis. As with all seriously ill, immobilized patients with altered levels of consciousness, encephalitis patients are at risk for aspiration pneumonia, stasis ulcers and decubiti, contractures, deep venous thrombosis and its complications, and infections of indwelling lines and catheters.

Acyclovir is of benefit in the treatment of HSV and should be started empirically in patients with suspected viral encephalitis, especially if focal features are present, while awaiting viral diagnostic studies. Treatment should be discontinued in patients found not to have HSV encephalitis, with the possible exception of patients with severe encephalitis due to VZV or EBV. HSV, VZV, and EBV all encode an enzyme, deoxypyrimidine (thymidine) kinase, that phosphorylates acyclovir to produce acyclovir-5′-monophosphate. Host cell enzymes then phosphorylate this compound to form a triphosphate derivative. It is the triphosphate that acts as an antiviral agent by inhibiting viral DNA polymerase and by causing premature termination of nascent viral DNA chains. The specificity of action depends on the fact that uninfected cells do not phosphorylate significant amounts of acyclovir to acyclovir-5′-monophosphate. A second level of specificity is provided by the fact that the acyclovir triphosphate is a more potent inhibitor of viral DNA polymerase than of the analogous host cell enzymes.

Adults should receive a dose of 10 mg/kg of acyclovir intravenously every 8 h (30 mg/kg per day total dose) for a minimum of 14 days. CSF PCR can be repeated at the completion of the 14-day course, with PCR-positive patients receiving an additional 7 days of treatment, followed by a repeat CSF PCR test. Neonatal HSV CNS infection is less responsive to acyclovir therapy than HSV encephalitis in adults; it is recommended that neonates with HSV encephalitis receive 20 mg/kg of acyclovir every 8 h (60 mg/kg per day total dose) for a minimum of 21 days.

Prior to intravenous administration, acyclovir should be diluted to a concentration ≤7 mg/mL. (A 70-kg person would receive a dose of 700 mg, which would be diluted in a volume of 100 mL.) Each dose should be infused slowly over 1 h rather than by rapid or bolus infusion, to minimize the risk of renal dysfunction. Care should be taken to avoid extravasation or intramuscular or subcutaneous administration. The alkaline pH of acyclovir can cause local inflammation and phlebitis (9%). Dose adjustment is required in patients with impaired renal glomerular filtration. Penetration into CSF is excellent, with average drug levels ~50% of serum levels. Complications of therapy include elevations in blood urea nitrogen and creatinine levels (5%), thrombocytopenia (6%), gastrointestinal toxicity (nausea, vomiting, diarrhea) (7%), and neurotoxicity (lethargy or obtundation, disorientation, confusion, agitation, hallucinations, tremors, seizures) (1%). Acyclovir resistance may be mediated by changes in either the viral deoxypyrimidine kinase or DNA polymerase. To date, acyclovir-resistant isolates have not been a significant clinical problem in immunocompetent individuals. However, there have been reports of clinically virulent acyclovir-resistant HSV isolates from sites outside the CNS in immunocompromised individuals, including those with AIDS.

Oral antiviral drugs with efficacy against HSV, VZV, and EBV, including acyclovir, famciclovir, and valacyclovir, have not been evaluated in the treatment of encephalitis either as primary therapy or as supplemental therapy following completion of a course of parenteral acyclovir. A National Institute of Allergy and Infectious Disease (NIAID)/National Institute of Neurological Disorders and Stroke–sponsored phase III trial of supplemental oral valacyclovir therapy (2 g tid for 3 months) following the initial 14- to 21-day course of therapy with parenteral acyclovir is ongoing in patients with HSV encephalitis; this may help clarify the role of extended oral antiviral therapy.

Ganciclovir and foscarnet, either alone or in combination, are often utilized in the treatment of CMV-related CNS infections, although their efficacy remains unproven. Cidofovir (see below) may provide an alternative in patients who fail to respond to ganciclovir and foscarnet, although data concerning its use in CMV CNS infections is extremely limited.

Ganciclovir is a synthetic nucleoside analogue of 2'-deoxyguanosine. The drug is preferentially phosphorylated by virus-induced cellular kinases. Ganciclovir triphosphate acts as a competitive inhibitor of the CMV DNA polymerase, and its incorporation into nascent viral DNA results in premature chain termination. Following intravenous administration, CSF concentrations of ganciclovir are 25–70% of coincident plasma levels. The usual dose for treatment of severe neurologic illnesses is 5 mg/kg every 12 h given intravenously at a constant rate over 1 h. Induction therapy is followed by maintenance therapy of 5 mg/kg every day for an indefinite period. Induction therapy should be continued until patients show a decline in CSF pleocytosis and a reduction in CSF CMV DNA copy number on quantitative PCR testing (where available). Doses should be adjusted in patients with renal insufficiency. Treatment is often limited by the development of granulocytopenia and thrombocytopenia (20–25%), which may require reduction in or discontinuation of therapy. Gastrointestinal side effects, including nausea, vomiting, diarrhea, and abdominal pain, occur in ~20% of patients. Some patients treated with ganciclovir for CMV retinitis have developed retinal detachment, but the causal relationship to ganciclovir treatment is unclear. Valganciclovir is an orally bioavailable prodrug that can generate high serum levels of ganciclovir, although studies of its efficacy in treating CMV CNS infections are limited.

Foscarnet is a pyrophosphate analogue that inhibits viral DNA polymerases by binding to the pyrophosphate-binding site. Following intravenous infusion, CSF concentrations range from 15 to 100% of coincident plasma levels. The usual dose for serious CMV-related neurologic illness is 60 mg/kg every 8 h administered by constant infusion over 1 h. Induction therapy for 14–21 days is followed by maintenance therapy (60–120 mg/kg per day). Induction therapy may need to be extended in patients who fail to show a decline in CSF pleocytosis and a reduction in CSF CMV DNA copy number on quantitative PCR tests (where available). Approximately one-third of patients develop renal impairment during treatment, which is reversible following discontinuation of therapy in most, but not all, cases. This is often associated with elevations in serum creatinine and proteinuria and is less frequent in patients who are adequately hydrated. Many pa-

tients experience fatigue and nausea. Reduction in serum calcium, magnesium, and potassium occur in ~15% of patients and may be associated with tetany, cardiac rhythm disturbances, or seizures.

Cidofovir is a nucleotide analogue that is effective in treating CMV retinitis and equivalent or better than ganciclovir in some experimental models of murine CMV encephalitis, although data concerning its efficacy in human CMV CNS disease are limited. The usual dose is 5 mg/kg intravenously once weekly for 2 weeks, then biweekly for two or more additional doses, depending on clinical response. Patients must be prehydrated with normal saline (e.g., 1 L over 1–2 h) prior to each dose and treated with probenecid (e.g., 1 g 3 h before cidofovir and 1 g 2 and 8 h after cidofovir). Nephrotoxicity is common; the dose should be reduced if renal function deteriorates.

Intravenous ribavirin (15–25 mg/kg per day in divided doses given every 8 h) has been reported to be of benefit in isolated cases of severe encephalitis due to California encephalitis (LaCrosse) virus. Ribavirin might be of benefit for the rare patients, typically infants or young children, with severe adenovirus or rotavirus encephalitis and in patients with encephalitis due to LCMV or other arenaviruses. However, clinical trials are lacking. Hemolysis, with resulting anemia, has been the major side effect limiting therapy.

No specific antiviral therapy of proven efficacy is currently available for treatment of WNV encephalitis. Patients have been treated with α-interferon, ribavirin, WNV-specific antisense oligonucleotides, and an Israeli IVIg preparation that contains high-titer anti-WNV antibody (Omr-IgG-am). WNV chimeric vaccines, in which WNV envelope and premembrane proteins are inserted into the background of another flavivirus, are already undergoing human clinical testing for safety and immunogenicity. Both chimeric and killed inactivated WNV vaccines have been found to be safe and effective in preventing equine WNV infection, and several effective flavivirus vaccines are already in human use, creating optimism that a safe and effective human WNV vaccine can also be developed.

SEQUELAE

There is considerable variation in the incidence and severity of sequelae in patients surviving viral encephalitis. In the case of EEE virus infection, nearly 80% of survivors have severe neurologic sequelae. At the other extreme are infections due to EBV, California encephalitis virus, and Venezuelan equine encephalitis virus, where severe sequelae are unusual. For example, approximately 5–15% of children infected with LaCrosse virus have a residual seizure disorder, and 1% have persistent hemiparesis. Detailed information about sequelae in patients with HSV encephalitis treated with acyclovir is available from the NIAID-CASG trials. Of 32 acyclovir-treated patients, 26 survived (81%). Of the 26 survivors, 12 (46%) had no or only minor sequelae, 3 (12%) were moderately impaired (gainfully employed but not functioning at their previous level), and 11 (42%) were severely impaired (requiring continuous supportive care). The incidence and severity of sequelae were directly related to the age of the patient and the level of consciousness at the time of initiation of therapy. Patients with severe neurologic impairment (Glasgow coma score 6) at initiation of therapy either died or survived with severe sequelae. Young patients (<30 years) with good neurologic function at initiation of therapy did substantially better (100% survival, 62% with no or mild sequelae) compared with their older counterparts (>30 years; 64% survival, 57% no or mild sequelae). Some recent studies using quantitative HSV CSF PCR tests indicate that clinical outcome following treatment also correlates with the amount of HSV DNA present in CSF at the time of presentation. Many patients with WNV infection have acute sequelae, including cognitive impairment; weakness; and hyper- or hypokinetic movement disorders, including tremor, myoclonus, and parkinsonism. Improvement in these symptoms may occur over the subsequent 6–12 months, although detailed clinical studies of the duration and severity of WNV sequelae are not yet available.

SUBACUTE MENINGITIS

CLINICAL MANIFESTATIONS

Patients with subacute meningitis typically have an unrelenting headache, stiff neck, low-grade fever, and lethargy for days to several weeks before they present for evaluation. Cranial nerve abnormalities and night sweats may be present. This syndrome overlaps that of chronic meningitis, discussed in detail in Chap. 377.

ETIOLOGY

Common causative organisms include *M. tuberculosis, C. neoformans, H. capsulatum, C. immitis,* and *T. pallidum.* Initial infection with *M. tuberculosis* is acquired by inhalation of aerosolized droplet nuclei. Tuberculous meningitis in adults does not develop acutely from hematogenous spread of tubercle bacilli to the meninges. Rather, millet seed–size (miliary) tubercles form in the parenchyma of the brain during hematogenous dissemination of tubercle bacilli in the course of primary infection. These tubercles enlarge and are usually caseating. The propensity for a caseous lesion to produce meningitis is determined by its proximity to the subarachnoid space (SAS) and the rate at which fibrous encapsulation develops. Subependymal caseous foci cause meningitis via discharge of bacilli and tuberculous antigens into the SAS. Mycobacterial antigens produce an intense inflammatory reaction that leads to the production of a thick exudate that fills the basilar cisterns and surrounds the cranial nerves and major blood vessels at the base of the brain.

Fungal infections are typically acquired by the inhalation of airborne fungal spores. The initial pulmonary infection may be asymptomatic or present with fever, cough, sputum production, and chest pain. The pulmonary infection is often self-limited. A localized pulmonary fungal infection can then remain dormant in the lungs until there is an abnormality in cell-mediated immunity that allows the fungus to reactivate and disseminate to the CNS. The most common pathogen causing fungal meningitis is *C. neoformans.* This fungus is found worldwide in soil and bird excreta. *H. capsulatum* is endemic to the Ohio and Mississippi River valleys of the central United States and to parts of Central and South America. *C. immitis* is endemic to the desert areas of the southwest United States, northern Mexico, and Argentina.

Syphilis is a sexually transmitted disease that is manifest by the appearance of a painless chancre at the site of inoculation. *T. pallidum* invades the CNS early in the course of syphilis. Cranial nerves VII and VIII are most frequently involved.

LABORATORY DIAGNOSIS

The classic CSF abnormalities in tuberculous meningitis are as follows: (1) elevated opening pressure, (2) lymphocytic pleocytosis (10–500 cells/μL), (3) elevated protein concentration in the range of 1–5 g/L (10–500 mg/dL), and (4) decreased glucose concentration in the range of 1.1–2.2 mmol/L (20–40 mg/dL). *The combination of unrelenting headache, stiff neck, fatigue, night sweats, and fever with a CSF lymphocytic pleocytosis and a mildly decreased glucose concentration is highly suspicious for tuberculous meningitis.* The last tube of fluid collected at LP is the best tube to send for a smear for acid-fast bacilli (AFB). If there is a pellicle in the CSF or a cobweb-like clot on the surface of the fluid, AFB can best be demonstrated in a smear of the clot or pellicle. Positive smears are typically reported in only 10–40% of cases of tuberculous meningitis in adults. Cultures of CSF take 4–8 weeks to identify the organism and are positive in ~50% of adults. Culture remains the "gold standard" to make the diagnosis of tuberculous meningitis. PCR for the detection of *M. tuberculosis* DNA has a sensitivity of 70–80% but is limited at the present time by a high rate of false-positive results.

The characteristic CSF abnormalities in fungal meningitis are a mononuclear or lymphocytic pleocytosis, an increased protein concentration, and a decreased glucose concentration. There may be eosinophils in the CSF in *C. immitis* meningitis. Large volumes of CSF are often required to demonstrate the organism on India ink smear or grow the organism in culture. If spinal fluid examined by LP on two separate occasions fails to yield an organism, CSF should be obtained by high-cervical or cisternal puncture.

The cryptococcal polysaccharide antigen test is a highly sensitive and specific test for cryptococcal meningitis. A reactive CSF cryptococcal antigen test establishes the diagnosis. The detection of the histoplasma polysaccharide antigen in CSF establishes the diagnosis of a fungal meningitis but is not specific for meningitis due to *H. capsulatum.* It may be falsely positive in coccidioidal meningitis. The CSF complement fixation antibody test is reported to have a specificity of 100% and a sensitivity of 75% for coccidioidal meningitis.

The diagnosis of syphilitic meningitis is made when a reactive serum treponemal test [fluorescent treponemal antibody absorption test (FTA-ABS) or microhemagglutination-*T. pallidum* (MHA-TP)] is associated with a CSF lymphocytic or mononuclear pleocytosis and an elevated protein concentration, or when the CSF VDRL (Venereal Disease Research Laboratory) is positive. A reactive CSF FTA-ABS is not definitive evidence of neurosyphilis. The CSF FTA-ABS can be falsely positive from blood contamination. A negative CSF VDRL does not rule out neurosyphilis. A negative CSF FTA-ABS or MHA-TP rules out neurosyphilis.

℞ SUBACUTE MENINGITIS

Empirical therapy of tuberculous meningitis is often initiated on the basis of a high index of suspicion without adequate laboratory support. Initial therapy is a combination of isoniazid (300 mg/d), rifampin (10 mg/kg per day), pyrazinamide (30 mg/kg per day in divided doses), ethambutol (15–25 mg/kg per day in divided doses), and pyridoxine (50 mg/d). If the clinical response is good, pyrazinamide and ethambutol can be discontinued after 8 weeks and isoniazid and rifampin continued alone for the next 6–12 months. A 6-month course of therapy is acceptable, but therapy should be prolonged for 9–12 months in patients who have an inadequate resolution of symptoms of meningitis or who have positive mycobacterial cultures of CSF during the course of therapy. Dexamethasone therapy is recommended for patients who develop hydrocephalus.

Meningitis due to *C. neoformans* is treated with amphotericin B (0.7 mg/kg IV per day) or AmBisome (5 mg/kg per day), plus flucytosine (100 mg/kg per day in four divided doses) for 2 weeks or until CSF culture is sterile. This treatment is followed by an 8–10-week course of fluconazole (400–800 mg/d PO). If the CSF culture is sterile after 10 weeks of acute therapy, the dose of fluconazole is decreased to 200 mg/d for 6 months to a year. Patients with HIV infection may require indefinite maintenance therapy. Meningitis due to *H. capsulatum* is treated with amphotericin B (0.7–1.0 mg/kg per day) for 4–12 weeks. A total dose of 30 mg/kg is recommended. Therapy with amphotericin B is not discontinued until fungal cultures are sterile. After completing a course of amphotericin B, maintenance therapy with itraconazole 200 mg twice daily is initiated and continued for at least 6 months to a year. *C. immitis* meningitis is treated with either high-dose fluconazole (1000 mg daily) as monotherapy or intravenous amphotericin B (0.5–0.7 mg/kg per day) for >4 weeks. Intrathecal amphotericin B (0.25–0.75 mg/d three times weekly) may be required to eradicate the infection. Lifelong therapy with fluconazole (200–400 mg daily) is recommended to prevent relapse. AmBisome (5 mg/kg per day) or amphotericin B lipid complex (5 mg/kg per day) can be substituted for amphotericin B in patients who have or who develop significant renal dysfunction. The most common complication of fungal meningitis is hydrocephalus. Patients who develop hydrocephalus should receive a CSF diversion device. A ventriculostomy can be used until CSF fungal cultures are sterile, at which time the ventriculostomy is replaced by a ventriculoperitoneal shunt.

Syphilitic meningitis is treated with aqueous penicillin G in a dose of 3–4 million units intravenously every 4 h for 10–14 days. An alternative regimen is 2.4 million units of procaine penicillin G intramuscularly daily with 500 mg of oral probenecid four times daily for 10–14 days. Either regimen is followed with 2.4 million units of benzathine penicillin G intramuscularly once a week for 3 weeks. The standard criterion for treatment success is reexamination of the CSF. The CSF should be reexamined at 6-month intervals for 2 years. The cell count is expected to normalize within 12 months, and the VDRL titer to decrease by two dilutions or revert to nonreactive within 2 years of completion of therapy. Failure of the CSF pleocytosis to resolve or an increase in the CSF VDRL titer by two or more dilutions requires retreatment.

CHRONIC ENCEPHALITIS

PROGRESSIVE MULTIFOCAL LEUKOENCEPHALOPATHY

Clinical Features and Pathology Progressive multifocal leukoencephalopathy (PML) is a progressive disorder characterized pathologically by multifocal areas of demyelination of varying size distributed throughout the brain but sparing the spinal cord and optic nerves. In addition to demyelination, there are characteristic cytologic alterations in both astrocytes and oligodendrocytes. Astrocytes are enlarged and contain hyperchromatic, deformed, and bizarre nuclei and frequent mitotic figures. Oligodendrocytes have enlarged, densely staining nuclei that contain viral inclusions formed by crystalline arrays of JC virus (JCV) particles. Patients often present with visual deficits (45%), typically a homonymous hemianopia; mental impairment (38%) (dementia, confusion, personality change); weakness, including hemi- or monoparesis; and ataxia. Seizures occur in ~20% of patients, predominantly in those with lesions abutting the cortex.

Almost all patients have an underlying immunosuppressive disorder. In recent series, the most common associated conditions were AIDS (80%), hematologic malignancies (13%), transplant recipients (5%), and chronic inflammatory diseases (2%). It has been estimated that up to 5% of AIDS patients will develop PML. There have been three cases of PML occurring in patients being treated for multiple sclerosis and inflammatory bowel disease with natalizumab, a humanized monoclonal antibody that inhibits lymphocyte trafficking into CNS and bowel mucosa by binding to α_4 integrins. Risk in these patients has been estimated at 1 PML case per 1000 treated patients after a mean of 18 months of therapy. The basic clinical and diagnostic features are similar in AIDS and non-AIDS–associated PML.

Diagnostic Studies The diagnosis of PML is frequently suggested by MRI. MRI reveals multifocal asymmetric, coalescing white matter lesions located periventricularly, in the centrum semiovale, in the parietal-occipital region, and in the cerebellum. These lesions have increased signal on T2 and FLAIR images and decreased signal on T1-weighted images. PML lesions are classically nonenhancing (90%) but may rarely show ring enhancement, especially in more immunocompetent patients. PML lesions are not typically associated with edema or mass effect. CT scans, which are less sensitive than MRI for the diagnosis of PML, often show hypodense nonenhancing white matter lesions.

The CSF is typically normal, although mild elevation in protein and/or IgG may be found. Pleocytosis occurs in <25% of cases, is predominantly mononuclear, and rarely exceeds 25 cells/μL. PCR amplification of JCV DNA from CSF has become an important diagnostic tool. The presence of a positive CSF PCR for JCV DNA in association with typical MRI lesions in the appropriate clinical setting is diagnostic of PML, reflecting the assay's relatively high specificity (92–100%); however, sensitivity is variable. In HIV-negative patients and HIV-positive patients not receiving highly active antiviral therapy (HAART), sensitivity is likely 70–90%. In HAART-treated patients, sensitivity may be closer to 60%, reflecting the lower JCV CSF viral load in this relatively more immunocompetent group. Studies with quantitative JCV CSF PCR indicate that patients with low JCV loads (<100 copies/μL) have a generally better prognosis than those with higher viral loads. Patients with negative CSF PCR studies may require brain biopsy for definitive diagnosis. In biopsy or necropsy specimens of brain, JCV antigen and nucleic acid can be detected by immunocytochemistry, in situ hybridization, or PCR amplification. Detection of JCV antigen or genomic material should only be considered diagnostic of PML if accompanied by characteristic pathologic changes, since both antigen and genomic material have been found in the brains of normal patients.

Serologic studies are of no utility in diagnosis due to high basal seroprevalence level (>80%).

℞ PROGRESSIVE MULTIFOCAL LEUKOENCEPHALOPATHY

No effective therapy for PML is available. Intravenous and/or intrathecal cytarabine were not shown to be of benefit in a randomized controlled trial in HIV-associated PML. Another randomized controlled trial of cidofovir in HIV-associated PML also failed to show significant benefit. Some patients with HIV-associated PML have shown disease stabilization and, in rare cases, improvement associated with improvement in their immune status following institution of HAART. In HIV-positive patients treated with HAART, 1-year survival is ~50%, although up to 80% of survivors may have significant neurologic sequelae. HIV-positive patients with higher CD4 counts (>300

mm³) and low or nondetectable HIV viral loads have a better prognosis than those with lower CD4 counts and higher viral loads.

SUBACUTE SCLEROSING PANENCEPHALITIS (SSPE)

SSPE is a rare chronic, progressive demyelinating disease of the CNS associated with a chronic nonpermissive infection of brain tissue with measles virus. The frequency has been estimated at 1 in 100,000–500,000 measles cases. An average of five cases per year are reported in the United States. The incidence has declined dramatically since the introduction of a measles vaccine. Most patients give a history of primary measles infection at an early age (2 years), which is followed after a latent interval of 6–8 years by the development of progressive neurologic disorder. Some 85% of patients are between 5 and 15 years old at diagnosis. Initial manifestations include poor school performance and mood and personality changes. Typical signs of a CNS viral infection, including fever and headache, do not occur. As the disease progresses, patients develop progressive intellectual deterioration, focal and/or generalized seizures, myoclonus, ataxia, and visual disturbances. In the late stage of the illness, patients are unresponsive, quadriparetic, and spastic, with hyperactive tendon reflexes and extensor plantar responses.

Diagnostic Studies MRI is often normal early, although areas of increased T2 signal develop in the white matter of the brain and brainstem as disease progresses. The EEG may initially show only nonspecific slowing, but with disease progression, patients develop a characteristic periodic pattern with bursts of high-voltage, sharp, slow waves every 3–8 s, followed by periods of attenuated ("flat") background. The CSF is acellular with a normal or mildly elevated protein concentration and a markedly elevated gamma globulin level (>20% of total CSF protein). CSF antimeasles antibody levels are invariably elevated, and oligoclonal antimeasles antibodies are often present. Measles virus can be cultured from brain tissue using special cocultivation techniques. Viral antigen can be identified immunocytochemically, and viral genome can be detected by in situ hybridization or PCR amplification.

℞ SUBACUTE SCLEROSING PANENCEPHALITIS

No definitive therapy for SSPE is available. Treatment with isoprinosine (Inosiplex, 100 mg/kg per day), alone or in combination with intrathecal or intraventricular alpha interferon, has been reported to prolong survival and produce clinical improvement in some patients but has never been subjected to a controlled clinical trial.

PROGRESSIVE RUBELLA PANENCEPHALITIS

This is an extremely rare disorder that primarily affects males with congenital rubella syndrome, although isolated cases have been reported following childhood rubella. After a latent period of 8–19 years, patients develop progressive neurologic deterioration. The manifestations are similar to those seen in SSPE. CSF shows a mild lymphocytic pleocytosis, slightly elevated protein concentration, markedly increased gamma globulin, and rubella virus–specific oligoclonal bands. No therapy is available. Universal prevention of both congenital and childhood rubella through the use of the available live attenuated rubella vaccine would be expected to eliminate the disease.

BRAIN ABSCESS

DEFINITION

A brain abscess is a focal, suppurative infection within the brain parenchyma, typically surrounded by a vascularized capsule. The term *cerebritis* is often employed to describe a nonencapsulated brain abscess.

EPIDEMIOLOGY

A bacterial brain abscess is a relatively uncommon intracranial infection, with an incidence of ~0.3–1.3/100,000 persons per year. Predisposing conditions include otitis media and mastoiditis, paranasal sinusitis, pyogenic infections in the chest or other body sites, penetrating head trauma or neurosurgical procedures, and dental infections. In immunocompetent individuals the most important pathogens are *Streptococcus* spp. [anaerobic, aerobic, and viridans (40%)], Enterobacteriaceae [*Proteus* spp., *E. coli* sp., *Klebsiella* spp. (25%)], anaerobes [e.g., *Bacteroides* spp., *Fusobacterium* spp. (30%)], and staphylococci (10%). In immunocompromised hosts with underlying HIV infection, organ transplantation, cancer, or immunosuppressive therapy, most brain abscesses are caused by *Nocardia* spp., *Toxoplasma gondii*, *Aspergillus* spp., *Candida* spp., and *C. neoformans*. In Latin America and in immigrants from Latin America, the most common cause of brain abscess is *Taenia solium* (neurocysticercosis). In India and the Far East, mycobacterial infection (tuberculoma) remains a major cause of focal CNS mass lesions.

ETIOLOGY

A brain abscess may develop (1) by direct spread from a contiguous cranial site of infection, such as paranasal sinusitis, otitis media, mastoiditis, or dental infection; (2) following head trauma or a neurosurgical procedure; or (3) as a result of hematogenous spread from a remote site of infection. In up to 25% of cases, no obvious primary source of infection is apparent (cryptogenic brain abscess).

Approximately one-third of brain abscesses are associated with otitis media and mastoiditis, often with an associated cholesteatoma. Otogenic abscesses occur predominantly in the temporal lobe (55–75%) and cerebellum (20–30%). In some series, up to 90% of cerebellar abscesses are otogenic. Common organisms include streptococci, *Bacteroides* spp., *Pseudomonas* spp., *Haemophilus* spp., and Enterobacteriaceae. Abscesses that develop as a result of direct spread of infection from the frontal, ethmoidal, or sphenoidal sinuses and those that occur due to dental infections are usually located in the frontal lobes. Approximately 10% of brain abscesses are associated with paranasal sinusitis, and this association is particularly strong in young males in their second and third decades of life. The most common pathogens in brain abscesses associated with paranasal sinusitis are streptococci (especially *S. milleri*), *Haemophilus* spp., *Bacteroides* spp., *Pseudomonas* spp., and *S. aureus*. Dental infections are associated with ~2% of brain abscesses, although it is often suggested that many "cryptogenic" abscesses are in fact due to dental infections. The most common pathogens in this setting are streptococci, staphylococci, *Bacteroides* spp., and *Fusobacterium* spp.

Hematogenous abscesses account for ~25% of brain abscesses. Hematogenous abscesses are often multiple, and multiple abscesses often (50%) have a hematogenous origin. These abscesses show a predilection for the territory of the middle cerebral artery (i.e., posterior frontal or parietal lobes). Hematogenous abscesses are often located at the junction of the gray and white matter and are often poorly encapsulated. The microbiology of hematogenous abscesses is dependent on the primary source of infection. For example, brain abscesses that develop as a complication of infective endocarditis are often due to viridans streptococci or *S. aureus*. Abscesses associated with pyogenic lung infections such as lung abscess or bronchiectasis are often due to streptococci, staphylococci, *Bacteroides* spp., *Fusobacterium* spp., or Enterobacteriaceae. Abscesses that follow penetrating head trauma or neurosurgical procedures are frequently due to methicillin-resistant *S. aureus* (MRSA), *S. epidermidis*, Enterobacteriaceae, *Pseudomonas* spp., and *Clostridium* spp. Enterobacteriaceae and *P. aeruginosa* are important causes of abscesses associated with urinary sepsis. Congenital cardiac malformations that produce a right-to-left shunt, such as tetralogy of Fallot, patent ductus arteriosus, and atrial and ventricular septal defects, allow bloodborne bacteria to bypass the pulmonary capillary bed and reach the brain. Similar phenomena can occur with pulmonary arteriovenous malformations. The decreased arterial oxygenation and saturation from the right-to-left shunt and polycythemia may cause focal areas of cerebral ischemia, thus providing a nidus for microorganisms that bypassed the pulmonary circulation to multiply and form an abscess. Streptococci are the most common pathogens in this setting.

PATHOGENESIS AND HISTOPATHOLOGY

Results of experimental models of brain abscess formation suggest that for bacterial invasion of brain parenchyma to occur, there must be preexisting or concomitant areas of ischemia, necrosis, or hypoxia in brain tissue. The intact brain parenchyma is relatively resistant to infection. Once bacteria have established infection, brain abscess frequently evolves through a series of stages, influenced by the nature of the infecting organism and by the immunocompetence of the host. The early cerebritis stage (days 1–3) is characterized by a perivascular infiltration of inflammatory cells, which surround a central core of coagulative necrosis. Marked edema surrounds the lesion at this stage. In the late cerebritis stage (days 4–9), pus formation leads to enlargement of the necrotic center, which is surrounded at its border by an inflammatory infiltrate of macrophages and fibroblasts. A thin capsule of fibroblasts and reticular fibers gradually develops, and the surrounding area of cerebral edema becomes more distinct than in the previous stage. The third stage, early capsule formation (days 10–13), is characterized by the formation of a capsule that is better developed on the cortical than on the ventricular side of the lesion. This stage correlates with the appearance of a ring-enhancing capsule on neuroimaging studies. The final stage, late capsule formation (day 14 and beyond), is defined by a well-formed necrotic center surrounded by a dense collagenous capsule. The surrounding area of cerebral edema has regressed, but marked gliosis with large numbers of reactive astrocytes has developed outside the capsule. This gliotic process may contribute to the development of seizures as a sequelae of brain abscess.

CLINICAL PRESENTATION

A brain abscess typically presents as an expanding intracranial mass lesion rather than as an infectious process. Although the evolution of signs and symptoms is extremely variable, ranging from hours to weeks or even months, most patients present to the hospital 11–12 days following onset of symptoms. The classic clinical triad of headache, fever, and a focal neurologic deficit is present in <50% of cases. The most common symptom in patients with a brain abscess is headache, occurring in >75% of patients. The headache is often characterized as a constant, dull, aching sensation, either hemicranial or generalized, and it becomes progressively more severe and refractory to therapy. Fever is present in only 50% of patients at the time of diagnosis, and its absence should not exclude the diagnosis. The new onset of focal or generalized seizure activity is a presenting sign in 15–35% of patients. Focal neurologic deficits including hemiparesis, aphasia, or visual field defects are part of the initial presentation in >60% of patients.

The clinical presentation of a brain abscess depends on its location, the nature of the primary infection if present, and the level of the ICP. Hemiparesis is the most common localizing sign of a frontal lobe abscess. A temporal lobe abscess may present with a disturbance of language (dysphasia) or an upper homonymous quadrantanopia. Nystagmus and ataxia are signs of a cerebellar abscess. Signs of raised ICP—papilledema, nausea and vomiting, and drowsiness or confusion—can be the dominant presentation of some abscesses, particularly those in the cerebellum. Meningismus is not present unless the abscess has ruptured into the ventricle or the infection has spread to the subarachnoid space.

DIAGNOSIS

Diagnosis is made by neuroimaging studies. MRI (Fig. 376-4) is better than CT for demonstrating abscesses in the early (cerebritis) stages and is superior to CT for identifying abscesses in the posterior fossa. Cerebritis appears on MRI as an area of low-signal intensity on T1-weighted images with irregular postgadolinium enhancement and as an area of increased signal intensity on T2-weighted images. Cerebritis is often not visualized by CT scan but, when present, appears as an area of hypodensity. On a contrast-enhanced CT scan, a mature brain abscess appears as a focal area of hypodensity surrounded by ring enhancement with surrounding edema (hypodensity). On contrast-enhanced T1-weighted MRI, a mature brain abscess has a capsule that enhances surrounding a hypodense center and surrounded by a hypodense area of edema. On T2-weighted MRI, there is a hyperintense central area of pus surrounded by a well-defined hypointense capsule and a hyperintense surrounding area of edema. It is important to recognize that the CT and MR appearance, particularly of the capsule, may be altered by treatment with glucocorticoids. The distinction between a brain abscess and other focal CNS lesions such as primary or metastatic tumors may be facilitated by the use of diffusion-weighted imaging sequences on which brain abscesses typically show increased signal and low apparent diffusion coefficient.

Microbiologic diagnosis of the etiologic agent is most accurately determined by Gram's stain and culture of abscess material obtained by stereotactic needle aspiration. Aerobic and anaerobic bacterial cultures and mycobacterial and fungal cultures should be obtained. Up to 10% of patients will also have positive blood cultures. LP should not be performed in patients with known or suspected focal intracranial infections such as abscess or empyema; CSF analysis contributes nothing to diagnosis or therapy, and LP increases the risk of herniation.

Additional laboratory studies may provide clues to the diagnosis of brain abscess in patients with a CNS mass lesion. About 50% of patients have a peripheral leukocytosis, 60% an elevated ESR, and 80% an elevated C-reactive protein. Blood cultures are positive in ~10% of cases overall but may be positive in >85% of patients with abscesses due to *Listeria*.

DIFFERENTIAL DIAGNOSIS

Conditions that can cause headache, fever, focal neurologic signs, and seizure activity include brain abscess, subdural empyema, bacterial meningitis, viral meningoencephalitis, superior sagittal sinus thrombosis, and acute disseminated encephalomyelitis. When fever is absent, primary and metastatic brain tumors become the major differential diagnosis. Less commonly, cerebral infarction or hematoma can have an MRI or CT appearance resembling brain abscess.

Rx BRAIN ABSCESS

Optimal therapy of brain abscesses involves a combination of high-dose parenteral antibiotics and neurosurgical drainage. Empirical therapy of community-acquired brain abscess in an immunocompetent patient typically includes a third-generation cephalosporin (e.g., cefotaxime or ceftriaxone) and metronidazole (see Table 376-1 for antibiotic dosages). In patients with penetrating head trauma or recent neurosurgical procedures, treatment should include ceftazidime as the third-generation cephalosporin to enhance coverage of *Pseudomonas* spp. and vancomycin for coverage of staphylococci. Meropenem plus vancomycin also provides good coverage in this setting.

Aspiration and drainage of the abscess under stereotactic guidance are beneficial for both diagnosis and therapy. Empirical antibiotic coverage should be modified based on the results of Gram's stain and culture of the abscess contents. Complete excision of a bacterial abscess via craniotomy or craniectomy is generally reserved for multiloculated abscesses or those in which stereotactic aspiration is unsuccessful.

Medical therapy alone is not optimal for treatment of brain abscess and should be reserved for patients whose abscesses are neurosurgically inaccessible, for patients with small (<2–3 cm) or nonencapsulated abscesses (cerebritis), and patients whose condition is too tenuous to allow performance of a neurosurgical procedure. All patients should receive a minimum of 6–8 weeks of parenteral antibiotic therapy. The role, if any, of supplemental oral antibiotic therapy following completion of a standard course of parenteral therapy has never been adequately studied.

FIGURE 376-4 Pneumococcal brain abscess. Note that the abscess wall has hyperintense signal on the axial T1-weighted MRI (**A**, *black arrow*), hypointense signal on the axial proton density images (**B**, *black arrow*), and enhances prominently after gadolinium administration on the coronal T1-weighted image (**C**). The abscess is surrounded by a large amount of vasogenic edema and has a small "daughter" abscess (**C**, *white arrow*). (*Courtesy of Joseph Lurito, MD; with permission.*)

In addition to surgical drainage and antibiotic therapy, patients should receive prophylactic anticonvulsant therapy because of the high risk (~35%) of focal or generalized seizures. Anticonvulsant therapy is continued for at least 3 months after resolution of the abscess, and decisions regarding withdrawal are then based on the EEG. If the EEG is abnormal, anticonvulsant therapy should be continued. If the EEG is normal, anticonvulsant therapy can be slowly withdrawn, with close follow-up and repeat EEG after the medication has been discontinued.

Glucocorticoids should not be given routinely to patients with brain abscesses. Intravenous dexamethasone therapy (10 mg every 6 h) is usually reserved for patients with substantial periabscess edema and associated mass effect and increased ICP. Dexamethasone should be tapered as rapidly as possible to avoid delaying the natural process of encapsulation of the abscess.

Serial MRI or CT scans should be obtained on a monthly or twice-monthly basis to document resolution of the abscess. More frequent studies (e.g., weekly) are probably warranted in the subset of patients who are receiving antibiotic therapy alone. A small amount of enhancement may remain for months after the abscess has been successfully treated.

PROGNOSIS

The mortality of brain abscess has declined in parallel with the development of enhanced neuroimaging techniques, improved neurosurgical procedures for stereotactic aspiration, and improved antibiotics. In modern series, the mortality is typically <15%. Significant sequelae, including seizures, persisting weakness, aphasia, or mental impairment, occur in ≥20% of survivors.

NONBACTERIAL CAUSES OF INFECTIOUS FOCAL CNS LESIONS

ETIOLOGY

Neurocysticercosis is the most common parasitic disease of the CNS worldwide. Humans acquire cysticercosis by the ingestion of food contaminated with the eggs of the parasite *T. solium*. Toxoplasmosis is a parasitic disease caused by *T. gondii* and acquired from the ingestion of undercooked meat and from handling cat feces.

CLINICAL PRESENTATION

The most common manifestation of neurocysticercosis is new-onset partial seizures with or without secondary generalization. Cysticerci may develop in the brain parenchyma and cause seizures or focal neurologic deficits. When present in the subarachnoid or ventricular spaces, cysticerci can produce increased ICP by interference with CSF flow. Spinal cysticerci can mimic the presentation of intraspinal tumors. When the cysticerci first lodge in the brain, they frequently cause little in the way of an inflammatory response. As the cysticercal cyst degenerates, it elicits an inflammatory response that may present clinically as a seizure. Eventually the cyst dies, a process that may take several years and is typically associated with resolution of the inflammatory response and, often, abatement of seizures.

Primary *toxoplasma* infection is often asymptomatic. However, during this phase parasites may spread to the CNS, where they become latent. Reactivation of CNS infection is almost exclusively associated with immunocompromised hosts, particularly those with HIV infection. During this phase patients present with headache, fever, seizures, and focal neurologic deficits.

DIAGNOSIS

The lesions of neurocysticercosis are readily visualized by MRI or CT scans. Lesions with viable parasites appear as cystic lesions. The scolex can often be visualized on MRI. Lesions may appear as contrast-enhancing lesions surrounded by edema. A very early sign of cyst death is hypointensity of the vesicular fluid on T2-weighted images when compared with CSF. Parenchymal brain calcifications are the most common finding and evidence that the parasite is no longer viable. MRI findings of toxoplasmosis consist of multiple lesions in the deep white matter, the thalamus, and basal ganglia and at the gray-white junction in the cerebral hemispheres. With contrast administration, the majority of the lesions enhance in a ringed, nodular, or homogeneous pattern and are surrounded by edema. In the presence of the characteristic neuroimaging abnormalities of *T. gondii* infection, serum IgG antibody to *T. gondii* should be obtained and, when positive, the patient should be treated.

℞ INFECTIOUS FOCAL CNS LESIONS

Anticonvulsant therapy is initiated when the patient with neurocysticercosis presents with a seizure. There is controversy about whether or not antihelminthic therapy should be given to all patients. Such therapy does not necessarily reduce the risk of seizure recurrence. Cysticerci appearing as cystic lesions or as enhancing lesions in the brain parenchyma or in the subarachnoid space at the convexity of the cerebral hemispheres should be treated with anticysticidal therapy. Cysticidal drugs accelerate the destruction of the parasites, resulting in a faster resolution of the infection. Albendazole and praziquantel are used in the treatment of neurocysticercosis. Approximately 85% of parenchymal cysts are destroyed by a single course of albendazole, and ~75% are destroyed by a single course of praziquantel. The dose of albendazole is 15 mg/kg per day in two doses for 8 days. The dose of praziquantel is 50 mg/kg per day for 15 days, although a number of other dosage regimens are also frequently cited. Antiepileptic therapy can be stopped once the follow-up CT scan shows resolution of the lesion. Long-term antiepileptic therapy is recommended when seizures occur after resolution of edema and resorption or calcification of the degenerating cyst.

CNS toxoplasmosis is treated with a combination of sulfadiazine, 1.5–2.0 g orally qid, plus pyrimethamine, 100 mg orally to load then 75–100 mg orally qd, plus folinic acid, 10–15 mg orally qd. Folinic acid is added to the regimen to prevent megaloblastic anemia. Therapy is continued until there is no evidence of active disease on neuroimaging studies, which typically takes at least 6 weeks, and then the dose of sulfadiazine is reduced to 2–4 g/d and pyrimethamine to 50 mg/d. Clindamycin plus pyrimethamine is an alternative therapy for patients who cannot tolerate sulfadiazine, but the combination of pyrimethamine and sulfadiazine is more effective.

SUBDURAL EMPYEMA

A subdural empyema (SDE) is a collection of pus between the dura and arachnoid membranes (Fig. 376-5).

EPIDEMIOLOGY

SDE is a rare disorder that accounts for 15–25% of focal suppurative CNS infections. Sinusitis is the most common predisposing condition and typically involves the frontal sinuses, either alone or in combination with the ethmoid and maxillary sinuses. Sinusitis-associated empyema has a striking predilection for young males, possibly reflecting sex-related differences in sinus anatomy and development. It has been suggested that SDE may complicate 1–2% of cases of frontal sinusitis severe enough to require hospitalization. As a consequence of this epi-

FIGURE 376-5 Subdural empyema.

demiology, SDE shows an ~3:1 male:female predominance, with 70% of cases occurring in the second and third decades of life. SDE may also develop as a complication of head trauma or neurosurgery. Secondary infection of a subdural effusion may also result in empyema, although secondary infection of hematomas, in the absence of a prior neurosurgical procedure, is rare.

ETIOLOGY

Aerobic and anaerobic streptococci, staphylococci, Enterobacteriaceae, and anaerobic bacteria are the most common causative organisms of sinusitis-associated SDE. Staphylococci and gram-negative bacilli are often the etiologic organisms when SDE follows neurosurgical procedures or head trauma. Up to one-third of cases are culture-negative, possibly reflecting difficulty in obtaining adequate anaerobic cultures.

PATHOPHYSIOLOGY

Sinusitis-associated SDE develops as a result of either retrograde spread of infection from septic thrombophlebitis of the mucosal veins draining the sinuses or contiguous spread of infection to the brain from osteomyelitis in the posterior wall of the frontal or other sinuses. SDE may also develop from direct introduction of bacteria into the subdural space as a complication of a neurosurgical procedure. The evolution of SDE can be extremely rapid because the subdural space is a large compartment that offers few mechanical barriers to the spread of infection. In patients with sinusitis-associated SDE, suppuration typically begins in the upper and anterior portions of one cerebral hemisphere and then extends posteriorly. SDE is often associated with other intracranial infections, including epidural empyema (40%), cortical thrombophlebitis (35%), and intracranial abscess or cerebritis (>25%). Cortical venous infarction produces necrosis of underlying cerebral cortex and subcortical white matter, with focal neurologic deficits and seizures (see below).

CLINICAL PRESENTATION

A patient with SDE typically presents with fever and a progressively worsening headache. The diagnosis of SDE should always be suspected in a patient with known sinusitis who presents with new CNS signs or symptoms. Patients with underlying sinusitis frequently have symptoms related to this infection. As the infection progresses, focal neurologic deficits, seizures, nuchal rigidity, and signs of increased ICP commonly occur. Headache is the most common complaint at the time of presentation; initially it is localized to the side of the subdural infection, but then it becomes more severe and generalized. Contralat-

FIGURE 376-6 Subdural empyema. There is marked enhancement of the dura and leptomeninges (**A**, **B**, *straight arrows*) along the left medial hemisphere. The pus is hypointense on T1-weighted images (**A**, **B**) but markedly hyperintense on the proton density–weighted (**C**, *curved arrow*) image. *(Courtesy of Joseph Lurito, MD; with permission.)*

eral hemiparesis or hemiplegia is the most common focal neurologic deficit and can occur from the direct effects of the SDE on the cortex or as a consequence of venous infarction. Seizures begin as partial motor seizures that then become secondarily generalized. Seizures may be due to the direct irritative effect of the SDE on the underlying cortex or result from cortical venous infarction (see above). In untreated SDE, the increasing mass effect and increase in ICP cause progressive deterioration in consciousness, leading ultimately to coma.

DIAGNOSIS

MRI (Fig. 376-6) is superior to CT in identifying SDE and any associated intracranial infections. The administration of gadolinium greatly improves diagnosis by enhancing the rim of the empyema and allowing the empyema to be clearly delineated from the underlying brain parenchyma. Cranial MRI is also extremely valuable in identifying sinusitis, other focal CNS infections, cortical venous infarction, cerebral edema, and cerebritis. CT may show a crescent-shaped hypodense lesion over one or both hemispheres or in the interhemispheric fissure. Frequently the degree of mass effect, exemplified by midline shift, ventricular compression, and sulcal effacement, is far out of proportion to the mass of the SDE.

CSF examination should be avoided in patients with known or suspected SDE as it adds no useful information and is associated with the risk of cerebral herniation.

DIFFERENTIAL DIAGNOSIS

The differential diagnosis of the combination of headache, fever, focal neurologic signs, and seizure activity that progresses rapidly to an altered level of consciousness includes subdural hematoma, bacterial meningitis, viral encephalitis, brain abscess, superior sagittal sinus thrombosis, and acute disseminated encephalomyelitis. The presence of nuchal rigidity is unusual with brain abscess or epidural empyema and should suggest the possibility of SDE when associated with significant focal neurologic signs and fever. Patients with bacterial meningitis also have nuchal rigidity but do not typically have focal deficits of the severity seen with SDE.

℞ SUBDURAL EMPYEMA

SDE is a medical emergency. Emergent neurosurgical evacuation of the empyema, either through burr-hole drainage or craniotomy, is the definitive step in the management of this infection. Empirical antimicrobial therapy should include a combination of a third-generation cephalosporin (e.g., cefotaxime or ceftriaxone), vancomycin, and metronidazole (see Table 376-1 for dosages). Parenteral antibiotic therapy should be continued for a minimum of 4 weeks. Specific diagnosis of the etiologic organisms is made based on Gram's stain and culture of fluid obtained via either burr holes or craniotomy; the initial empirical antibiotic coverage can be modified accordingly.

PROGNOSIS

Prognosis is influenced by the level of consciousness of the patient at the time of hospital presentation, the size of the empyema, and the speed with which therapy is instituted. Long-term neurologic sequelae, which include seizures and hemiparesis, occur in up to 50% of cases.

EPIDURAL ABSCESS

Cranial epidural abscess is a suppurative infection occurring in the potential space between the inner skull table and dura (Fig. 376-7).

ETIOLOGY AND PATHOPHYSIOLOGY

Epidural abscess is less common than either brain abscess or SDE and accounts for <2% of focal suppurative CNS infections. A cranial epidural abscess develops as a complication of a craniotomy or compound skull fracture or as a result of spread of infection from the frontal sinuses, middle ear, mastoid, or orbit. An epidural abscess may develop contiguous to an area of osteomyelitis, when craniotomy is complicated by infection of the wound or bone flap, or as a result of direct infection of the epidural space. Infection in the frontal sinus, middle ear, mastoid, or orbit can reach the epidural space through retrograde spread of infection from septic thrombophlebitis in the emissary veins that drain these areas or by way of direct spread of infection through areas of osteomyelitis. Unlike the subdural space, the epidural space is really a potential rather than an actual compartment. The dura is normally tightly adherent to the inner skull table, and infection must dissect the dura away from the skull table as it spreads. As a result, epidural abscesses are often smaller than SDEs. Cranial epidural abscesses, unlike brain abscesses, only rarely result from hematogenous spread of infection from extracranial primary sites. The bacteriology of a cranial epidural abscess is similar to that of SDE (see above). The etiologic organisms of an epidural abscess that arises from frontal sinusitis, middle ear infections, or mastoiditis are usually streptococci or anaerobic organisms. Staphylococci or gram-negative organisms are the usual cause of an epidural abscess that develops as a complication of craniotomy or compound skull fracture.

CLINICAL PRESENTATION

Patients present with fever (60%), headache (40%), nuchal rigidity (35%), seizures (10%), and focal deficits (5%). Periorbital edema and Potts puffy tumor, reflecting underlying associated frontal bone osteomyelitis, are present in ~40%. In patients with a recent neurosurgical procedure, wound infection is invariably present, but other symptoms may be subtle and can include altered mental status (45%), fever

Epidural abscess

FIGURE 376-7 Cranial epidural abscess is a collection of pus between the dura and the inner table of the skull.

(35%), and headache (20%). The diagnosis should also be considered when fever and headache follow recent head trauma or occur in the setting of frontal sinusitis, mastoiditis, or otitis media.

DIAGNOSIS

Cranial MRI is the procedure of choice to demonstrate a cranial epidural abscess. The sensitivity of CT is limited by the presence of signal artifacts arising from the bone of the inner skull table. The CT appearance of an epidural empyema is that of a lens or crescent-shaped hypodense extraaxial lesion. On MRI, an epidural empyema appears as a lentiform or crescent-shaped fluid collection that is hyperintense compared to CSF on T2-weighted images. On T1-weighted images, the fluid collection has a signal intensity that is intermediate between that of brain tissue and CSF. Following the administration of gadolinium, a significant enhancement of the dura is seen on T1-weighted images. In distinction to subdural empyema, signs of mass effect or other parenchymal abnormalities are uncommon.

℞ EPIDURAL ABSCESS

Immediate neurosurgical drainage is indicated. Empirical antimicrobial therapy, pending the results of Gram's stain and culture of the purulent material obtained at surgery, should include a combination of a third-generation cephalosporin, vancomycin, and metronidazole (Table 376-1). Ceftazidime or meropenem should be substituted for ceftriaxone or cefotaxime in neurosurgical patients. When the organism has been identified, antimicrobial therapy can be modified accordingly. Antibiotics should be continued for at least 3 weeks after surgical drainage.

PROGNOSIS

Mortality is <5% in modern series, and full recovery is the rule in most survivors.

SUPPURATIVE THROMBOPHLEBITIS

DEFINITION

Suppurative intracranial thrombophlebitis is septic venous thrombosis of cortical veins and sinuses. This may occur as a complication of bacterial meningitis; SDE; epidural abscess; or infection in the skin of the face, paranasal sinuses, middle ear, or mastoid.

ANATOMY AND PATHOPHYSIOLOGY

The cerebral veins and venous sinuses have no valves; therefore, blood within them can flow in either direction. The superior sagittal sinus is the largest of the venous sinuses (Fig. 376-8). It receives blood from the frontal, parietal, and occipital superior cerebral veins and the diploic veins, which communicate with the meningeal veins. Bacterial meningi-

tis is a common predisposing condition for septic thrombosis of the superior sagittal sinus. The diploic veins, which drain into the superior sagittal sinus, provide a route for the spread of infection from the meninges, especially in cases where there is purulent exudate near areas of the superior sagittal sinus. Infection can also spread to the superior sagittal sinus from nearby SDE or epidural abscess. Dehydration from vomiting, hypercoagulable states, and immunologic abnormalities, including the presence of circulating antiphospholipid antibodies, also contribute to cerebral venous sinus thrombosis. Thrombosis may extend from one sinus to another, and at autopsy thrombi of different histologic ages can often be detected in several sinuses. Thrombosis of the superior sagittal sinus is often associated with thrombosis of superior cortical veins and small parenchymal hemorrhages.

The superior sagittal sinus drains into the transverse sinuses (Fig. 376-8). The transverse sinuses also receive venous drainage from small veins from both the middle ear and mastoid cells. The transverse sinus becomes the sigmoid sinus before draining into the internal jugular vein. Septic transverse/sigmoid sinus thrombosis can be a complication of acute and chronic otitis media or mastoiditis. Infection spreads from the mastoid air cells to the transverse sinus via the emissary veins or by direct invasion. The cavernous sinuses are inferior to the superior sagittal sinus at the base of the skull. The cavernous sinuses receive blood from the facial veins via the superior and inferior ophthalmic veins. Bacteria in the facial veins enter the cavernous sinus via these veins. Bacteria in the sphenoid and ethmoid sinuses can spread to the cavernous sinuses via the small emissary veins. The sphenoid and ethmoid sinuses are the most common sites of primary infection resulting in septic cavernous sinus thrombosis.

CLINICAL MANIFESTATIONS

Septic thrombosis of the superior sagittal sinus presents with headache, fever, nausea and vomiting, confusion, and focal or generalized seizures. There may be a rapid development of stupor and coma. Weakness of the lower extremities with bilateral Babinski signs or hemiparesis is often present. When superior sagittal sinus thrombosis occurs as a complication of bacterial meningitis, nuchal rigidity and Kernig's and Brudzinski's signs may be present.

The oculomotor nerve, the trochlear nerve, the abducens nerve, the ophthalmic and maxillary branches of the trigeminal nerve, and the internal carotid artery all pass through the cavernous sinus (see Fig. 371-4). The symptoms of *septic cavernous sinus thrombosis* are fever, headache, frontal and retroorbital pain, and diplopia. The classic signs are ptosis, proptosis, chemosis, and extraocular dysmotility due to deficits of cranial nerves III, IV, and VI; hyperesthesia of the ophthalmic and maxillary divisions of the fifth cranial nerve and a decreased corneal reflex may be detected. There may be evidence of dilated, tortuous retinal veins and papilledema.

Headache and earache are the most frequent symptoms of *transverse sinus thrombosis*. A transverse sinus thrombosis may also present with otitis media, sixth nerve palsy, and retroorbital or facial pain (*Gradinego's syndrome*). Sigmoid sinus and internal jugular vein thrombosis may present with neck pain.

DIAGNOSIS

The diagnosis of septic venous sinus thrombosis is suggested by an absent flow void within the affected venous sinus on MRI and confirmed by magnetic resonance venography, CT angiogram, or the venous phase of cerebral angiography. The diagnosis of thrombophlebitis of intracerebral and meningeal veins is suggested by the presence of intracerebral hemorrhage but requires cerebral angiography for definitive diagnosis.

℞ SUPPURATIVE THROMBOPHLEBITIS

Septic venous sinus thrombosis is treated with antibiotics, hydration, and removal of infected tissue and thrombus in septic lateral or cavernous sinus thrombosis. The choice of antimicrobial therapy is based on the bacteria responsible for the predisposing or associated condition. Optimal duration of therapy is unknown, but antibiotics are usually continued for 6 weeks or until there is radiographic evidence of resolution of thrombosis. Anticoagulation with dose-adjusted heparin has been reported to be beneficial in patients with aseptic venous sinus thrombosis; it is also used in the treatment of sep-

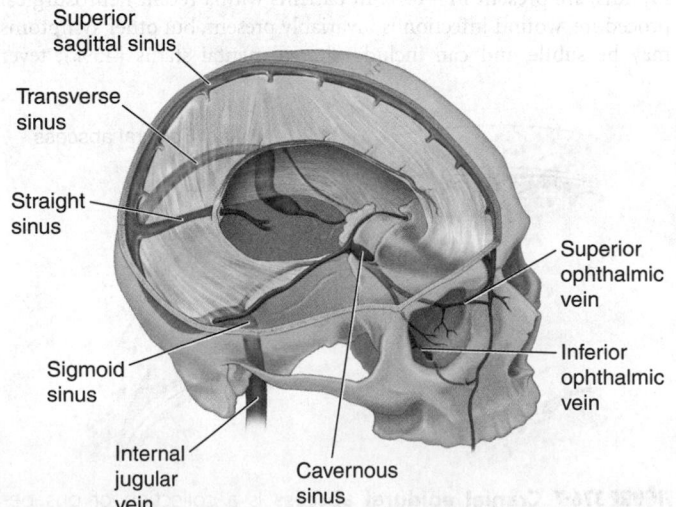

FIGURE 376-8 Anatomy of the cerebral venous sinuses.

Superior sagittal sinus

Transverse sinus

Straight sinus

Sigmoid sinus

Internal jugular vein

Cavernous sinus

Superior ophthalmic vein

Inferior ophthalmic vein

tic venous sinus thrombosis complicating bacterial meningitis in patients who are worsening despite antimicrobial therapy and intravenous fluids. The presence of a small intracerebral hemorrhage from septic thrombophlebitis is not an absolute contraindication to heparin therapy. Successful management of aseptic venous sinus thrombosis has been reported with catheter-directed urokinase therapy and with a combination of intrathrombus recombinant tissue plasminogen activator (rtPA) and intravenous heparin, but there has not been enough experience with these therapies in septic venous sinus thrombosis to make recommendations regarding their use.

FURTHER READINGS

DE GANS J, VAN DE BEEK D: Dexamethasone in adults with bacterial meningitis. N Engl J Med 347:1549, 2002

BARTT RE: Multiple sclerosis, natalizumab therapy, and progressive multifocal leukoencephalopathy. Curr Opin Neurol 19:341, 2006

GLASER CA et al: In search of encephalitis etiologies: Diagnostic challenges from the California Encephalitis project, 1998–2000. Clin Infect Dis 36:731, 2003

LU CH et al: Bacterial brain abscess: Microbiological features, epidemiological trends and therapeutic outcomes. QJM 95:501, 2002

ROSENSTEIN NE et al: Meningococcal disease. N Engl J Med 344:1378, 2001

SOLOMON T et al: West Nile encephalitis. BMJ 326:865, 2003

STEPHENS DS et al: Epidemic meningitis, meningococcaemia, and Neisseria meningitidis. Lancet 369:2196, 2007

TUNKEL AR et al: Practice guidelines for the management of bacterial meningitis. Clin Infect Dis 39:1267, 2004

377 Chronic and Recurrent Meningitis

Walter J. Koroshetz, Morton N. Swartz

Chronic inflammation of the meninges (pia, arachnoid, and dura) can produce profound neurologic disability and may be fatal if not successfully treated. The condition is most commonly diagnosed when a characteristic neurologic syndrome exists for > 4 weeks and is associated with a persistent inflammatory response in the cerebrospinal fluid (CSF) (white blood cell count >5/µL). The causes are varied, and appropriate treatment depends on identification of the etiology. Five categories of disease account for most cases of chronic meningitis: (1) meningeal infections, (2) malignancy, (3) noninfectious inflammatory disorders, (4) chemical meningitis, and (5) parameningeal infections.

CLINICAL PATHOPHYSIOLOGY

Neurologic manifestations of chronic meningitis (Table 377-1) are determined by the anatomic location of the inflammation and its consequences. Persistent headache with or without stiff neck, hydrocephalus, cranial neuropathies, radiculopathies, and cognitive or personality changes are the cardinal features. These can occur alone or in combination. When they appear in combination, widespread dissemination of the inflammatory process along CSF pathways has occurred. In some cases, the presence of an underlying systemic illness points to a specific agent or class of agents as the probable cause. The diagnosis of chronic meningitis is usually made when the clinical presentation prompts the astute physician to examine the CSF for signs of inflammation. CSF is produced by the choroid plexus of the cerebral ventricles, exits through nar-

row foramina into the subarachnoid space surrounding the brain and spinal cord, circulates around the base of the brain and over the cerebral hemispheres, and is resorbed by arachnoid villi projecting into the superior sagittal sinus. CSF flow provides a pathway for rapid spread of infectious and other infiltrative processes over the brain, spinal cord, and cranial and spinal nerve roots. Spread from the subarachnoid space into brain parenchyma may occur via the arachnoid cuffs that surround blood vessels that penetrate brain tissue (Virchow-Robin spaces).

Intracranial Meningitis Nociceptive fibers of the meninges are stimulated by the inflammatory process, resulting in headache or neck or back pain. Obstruction of CSF pathways at the foramina or arachnoid villi may produce *hydrocephalus* and symptoms of raised intracranial pressure (ICP), including headache, vomiting, apathy or drowsiness, gait instability, papilledema, visual loss, impaired upgaze, or palsy of the sixth cranial nerve (CN) (Chap. 371). Cognitive and behavioral changes during the course of chronic meningitis may also result from vascular damage, which may similarly produce seizures, stroke, or myelopathy. Inflammatory deposits seeded via the CSF circulation are often prominent around the brainstem and cranial nerves and along the undersurface of the frontal and temporal lobes. Such cases, termed *basal meningitis*, often present as multiple cranial neuropathies, with visual loss (CN II), facial weakness (CN VII), hearing loss (CN VIII), diplopia (CNs III, IV, and VI), sensory or motor abnormalities of the oropharynx (CNs IX, X, and XII), decreased olfaction (CN I), or facial sensory loss and masseter weakness (CN V).

Spinal Meningitis Injury may occur to motor and sensory roots as they traverse the subarachnoid space and penetrate the meninges. These cases present as multiple radiculopathies with combinations of radicular pain, sensory loss, motor weakness, and sphincter dysfunction. Meningeal inflammation can encircle the cord, resulting in myelopathy. Patients with slowly progressive involvement of multiple cranial nerves and/or spinal nerve roots are likely to have chronic meningitis. Electrophysiologic testing (electromyography, nerve conduction studies, and evoked response testing) may be helpful in determining whether there is involvement of cranial and spinal nerve roots.

Systemic Manifestations In some patients, evidence of systemic disease provides clues to the underlying cause of chronic meningitis. A careful history and physical examination are essential before embarking on a diagnostic workup, which may be costly, prolonged, and associated with risk from invasive procedures. A complete history of travel, sexual practice, and exposure to infectious agents should be sought. Infectious causes are often associated with fever, malaise, anorexia, and signs of localized or disseminated infection outside the nervous system. Infectious causes are of major concern in the immunosuppressed patient, especially in patients with AIDS, in whom chronic meningitis may present without headache or fever. Noninfectious inflammatory disorders often produce systemic manifestations, but meningitis may be the initial manifestation. Carcinomatous meningitis may or may not be accompanied by clinical evidence of the primary neoplasm.

TABLE 377-1	SYMPTOMS AND SIGNS OF CHRONIC MENINGITIS
Symptom	**Sign**
Chronic headache	+/– Papilledema
Neck or back pain	Brudzinski's or Kernig's sign of meningeal irritation
Change in personality	Altered mental status—drowsiness, inattention, disorientation, memory loss, frontal release signs (grasp, suck, snout), perseveration
Facial weakness	Peripheral seventh CN palsy
Double vision	Palsy of CNs III, IV, VI
Visual loss	Papilledema, optic atrophy
Hearing loss	Eighth CN palsy
Arm or leg weakness	Myelopathy or radiculopathy
Numbness in arms or legs	Myelopathy or radiculopathy
Sphincter dysfunction	Myelopathy or radiculopathy Frontal lobe dysfunction (hydrocephalus)
Clumsiness	Ataxia

Note: CN, cranial nerve.

APPROACH TO THE PATIENT:
Chronic Meningitis

The occurrence of chronic headache, hydrocephalus, cranial neuropathy, radiculopathy, and/or cognitive decline in a patient should prompt consideration of a lumbar puncture for evidence of meningeal inflammation. On occasion the diagnosis is made when an imaging study (CT or MRI) shows contrast enhancement of the meninges, which is always abnormal with the exception of dural enhancement after lumbar puncture, neurosurgical procedures, or spontaneous CSF leakage. Once chronic meningitis is confirmed by CSF examination, effort is focused on identifying the cause (Tables 377-2 and 377-3) by (1) further analysis of the CSF, (2) diagnosis of an underlying systemic infection or noninfectious inflammatory condition, or (3) pathologic examination of meningeal biopsy specimens.

TABLE 377-2   INFECTIOUS CAUSES OF CHRONIC MENINGITIS

Causative Agent	CSF Formula	Helpful Diagnostic Tests	Risk Factors and Systemic Manifestations
Common Bacterial Causes			
Partially treated suppurative meningitis	Mononuclear or mixed mononuclear-polymorphonuclear cells	CSF culture and Gram stain	History consistent with acute bacterial meningitis and incomplete treatment
Parameningeal infection	Mononuclear or mixed polymorphonuclear-mononuclear cells	Contrast-enhanced CT or MRI to detect parenchymal, subdural, epidural, or sinus infection	Otitis media, pleuropulmonary infection, right-to-left cardiopulmonary shunt for brain abscess; focal neurologic signs; neck, back, ear, or sinus tenderness
Mycobacterium tuberculosis	Mononuclear cells except polymorphonuclear cells in early infection (commonly <500 WBC/μL); low CSF glucose, high protein	Tuberculin skin test may be negative; AFB culture of CSF (sputum, urine, gastric contents if indicated); tuberculostearic acid detection in CSF; identify tubercle bacillus on acid-fast stain of CSF or protein pellicle; PCR	Exposure history; previous tuberculous illness; immunosuppressed or AIDS; young children; fever, meningismus, night sweats, miliary TB on X-ray or liver biopsy; stroke due to arteritis
Lyme disease (Bannwarth's syndrome) *Borrelia burgdorferi*	Mononuclear cells; elevated protein	Serum Lyme antibody titer; Western blot confirmation; (patients with syphilis may have false-positive Lyme titer)	History of tick bite or appropriate exposure history; erythema chronicum migrans skin rash; arthritis, radiculopathy, Bell's palsy, meningoencephalitis–multiple sclerosis-like syndrome
Syphilis (secondary, tertiary) *Treponema pallidum*	Mononuclear cells; elevated protein	CSF VDRL; serum VDRL (or RPR); fluorescent treponemal antibody-absorbed (FTA) or MHA-TP; serum VDRL may be negative in tertiary syphilis	Appropriate exposure history; HIV seropositive individuals at increased risk of aggressive infection; "dementia"; cerebral infarction due to endarteritis
Uncommon Bacterial Causes			
Actinomyces	Polymorphonuclear cells	Anaerobic culture	Parameningeal abscess or sinus tract (oral or dental focus); pneumonitis
Nocardia	Polymorphonuclear; occasionally mononuclear cells; often low glucose	Isolation may require weeks; weakly acid fast	Associated brain abscess may be present
Brucella	Mononuclear cells (rarely polymorphonuclear); elevated protein; often low glucose	CSF antibody detection; serum antibody detection	Intake of unpasteurized dairy products; exposure to goats, sheep, cows; fever, arthralgia, myalgia, vertebral osteomyelitis
Whipple's disease *Tropheryma whippelii*	Mononuclear cells	Biopsy of small bowel or lymph node; CSF PCR for *T. whippelii*; brain and meningeal biopsy (with PAS stain and EM examination)	Diarrhea, weight loss, arthralgias, fever; dementia, ataxia, paresis, ophthalmoplegia, oculomasticatory myoclonus
Rare Bacterial Causes			
Leptospirosis (occasionally if left untreated may last 3–4 weeks)			
Fungal Causes			
Cryptococcus neoformans	Mononuclear cells; count not elevated in some patients with AIDS	India ink or fungal wet mount of CSF (budding yeast); blood and urine cultures; antigen detection in CSF	AIDS and immune suppression; pigeon exposure; skin and other organ involvement due to disseminated infection
Coccidioides immitis	Mononuclear cells (sometimes 10–20% eosinophils); often low glucose	Antibody detection in CSF and serum	Exposure history—southwestern US; increased virulence in dark-skinned races
Candida sp.	Polymorphonuclear or mononuclear	Fungal stain and culture of CSF	IV drug abuse; post surgery; prolonged intravenous therapy; disseminated candidiasis
Histoplasma capsulatum	Mononuclear cells; low glucose	Fungal stain and culture of large volumes of CSF; antigen detection in CSF, serum, and urine; antibody detection in serum, CSF	Exposure history—Ohio and central Mississippi River Valley; AIDS; mucosal lesions
Blastomyces dermatitidis	Mononuclear cells	Fungal stain and culture of CSF; biopsy and culture of skin, lung lesions; antibody detection in serum	Midwestern and southeastern USA; usually systemic infection; abscesses, draining sinus, ulcers
Aspergillus sp.	Mononuclear or polymorphonuclear	CSF culture	Sinusitis; granulocytopenia or immunosuppression
Sporothrix schenckii	Mononuclear cells	Antibody detection in CSF and serum; CSF culture	Traumatic inoculation; IV drug use; ulcerated skin lesion

(continued)

TABLE 377-2 INFECTIOUS CAUSES OF CHRONIC MENINGITIS (CONTINUED) 2643

Causative Agent	CSF Formula	Helpful Diagnostic Tests	Risk Factors and Systemic Manifestations
Rare Fungal Causes			
Xylohypha (formerly *Cladosporium*) *trichoides* and other dark-walled (demateaceous) fungi such as *Curvularia, Drechslera; Mucor, Pseudoallescheria boydii*			
Protozoal Causes			
Toxoplasma gondii	Mononuclear cells	Biopsy or response to empirical therapy in clinically appropriate context (including presence of antibody in serum)	Usually with intracerebral abscesses; common in HIV seropositive patients
Trypanosomiasis *Trypanosoma gambiense, T. rhodesiense*	Mononuclear cells, elevated protein	Elevated CSF IgM; identification of trypanosomes in CSF and blood smear	Endemic in Africa; chancre, lymphadenopathy; prominent sleep disorder
Rare Protozoal Causes			
Acanthamoeba sp. causing granulomatous amebic encephalitis and meningoencephalitis in immunocompromised and debilitated individuals			
Helminthic Causes			
Cysticercosis (infection with cysts of *Taenia solium*)	Mononuclear cells; may have eosinophils; glucose level may be low	Indirect hemagglutination assay in CSF; ELISA immunoblotting in serum	Usually with multiple cysts in basal meninges and hydrocephalus; cerebral cysts, muscle calcification
Gnathostoma spinigerum	Eosinophils, mononuclear cells	Peripheral eosinophilia	History of eating raw fish; common in Thailand and Japan; subarachnoid hemorrhage; painful radiculopathy
Angiostrongylus cantonensis	Eosinophils, mononuclear cells	Recovery of worms from CSF	History of eating raw shellfish; common in tropical Pacific regions; often benign
Baylisascaris procyonis (raccoon ascarid)	Eosinophils, mononuclear cells		Infection follows accidental ingestion of *B. procyonis* eggs from raccoon feces; fatal meningoencephalitis
Rare Helminthic Causes			
Trichinella spiralis (trichinosis); *Echinococcus* cysts; *Schistosoma* sp. The former may produce a lymphocytic pleocytosis whereas the latter two may produce an eosinophilic response in CSF associated with cerebral cysts (*Echinococcus*) or granulomatous lesions of brain or spinal cord			
Viral Causes			
Mumps	Mononuclear cells	Antibody in serum	No prior mumps or immunization; may produce meningoencephalitis; may persist for 3–4 weeks
Lymphocytic choriomeningitis	Mononuclear cells	Antibody in serum	Contact with rodents or their excreta; may persist for 3–4 weeks
Echovirus	Mononuclear cells; may have low glucose	Virus isolation from CSF	Congenital hypogammaglobulinemia; history of recurrent meningitis
HIV (acute retroviral syndrome)	Mononuclear cells	p24 antigen in serum and CSF; high level of HIV viremia	HIV risk factors; rash, fever, lymphadenopathy; lymphopenia in peripheral blood; syndrome may persist long enough to be considered as "chronic meningitis"; or chronic meningitis may develop in later stages (AIDS) due to HIV
Herpes simplex (HSV)	Mononuclear cells	PCR for HSV, CMV DNA; CSF antibody for HSV, EBV	Recurrent meningitis due to HSV-2 (rarely HSV-1) often associated with genital recurrences; EBV associated with myeloradiculopathy, CMV with polyradiculopathy

Abbreviations: AFB, acid-fast bacillus; CMV, cytomegalovirus; CSF, cerebrospinal fluid; CT, computed tomography; EBV, Epstein-Barr virus; ELISA, enzyme-linked immunosorbent assay; EM, electron microscopy; FTA, fluorescent treponemal antibody absorption test; HSV, herpes simplex virus; MHA-TP, microhemagglutination assay–*T. pallidum*; MRI, magnetic resonance imaging; PAS, periodic acid–Schiff; PCR, polymerase chain reaction; RPR, rapid plasma reagin test; TB, tuberculosis; VDRL, Venereal Disease Research Laboratories test.

CHAPTER 377

Chronic and Recurrent Meningitis

Two clinical forms of chronic meningitis exist. In the first, the symptoms are chronic and persistent, whereas in the second there are recurrent, discrete episodes of illness. In the latter group, all symptoms, signs, and CSF parameters of meningeal inflammation resolve completely between episodes without specific therapy. In such patients, the likely etiologies include herpes simplex virus (HSV) type 2; chemical meningitis due to leakage into CSF of contents from an epidermoid tumor, craniopharyngioma, or cholesteatoma; primary inflammatory conditions, including Vogt-Koyanagi-Harada syndrome, Behçet's syndrome (Chap. 320), systemic lupus erythematosus (SLE; Chap. 313); and drug hypersensitivity with repeated administration of the offending agent.

The epidemiologic history is of considerable importance and may provide direction for selection of laboratory studies. Pertinent features include a history of tuberculosis or exposure to a likely case; past travel to areas endemic for fungal infections (the San Joaquin Valley in California and southwestern states for coccidioidomycosis, midwestern states for histoplasmosis, southeastern states for blastomycosis); travel to the Mediterranean region or ingestion of imported unpasteurized dairy products (*Brucella*); time spent in wooded areas endemic for Lyme disease; exposure to sexually transmitted disease (syphilis); exposure of an immunocompromised host to pigeons and their droppings (*Cryptococcus*); gardening (*Sporothrix schenkii*); ingestion of poorly cooked

TABLE 377-3 NONINFECTIOUS CAUSES OF CHRONIC MENINGITIS

Causative Agents	CSF Formula	Helpful Diagnostic Tests	Risk Factors and Systemic Manifestations
Malignancy	Mononuclear cells, elevated protein, low glucose	Repeated cytologic examination of large volumes of CSF; CSF exam by polarizing microscopy; clonal lymphocyte markers; deposits on nerve roots or meninges seen on myelogram or contrast-enhanced MRI; meningeal biopsy	Metastatic cancer of breast, lung, stomach, or pancreas; melanoma, lymphoma, leukemia; meningeal gliomatosis; meningeal sarcoma; cerebral dysgerminoma; meningeal melanoma or B cell lymphoma
Chemical compounds (may cause recurrent meningitis)	Mononuclear or PMNs, low glucose, elevated protein; xanthochromia from subarachnoid hemorrhage in week prior to presentation with "meningitis"	Contrast-enhanced CT scan or MRI Cerebral angiogram to detect aneurysm	History of recent injection into the subarachnoid space; history of sudden onset of headache; recent resection of acoustic neuroma or craniopharyngioma; epidermoid tumor of brain or spine, sometimes with dermoid sinus tract; pituitary apoplexy
Primary inflammation			
CNS sarcoidosis	Mononuclear cells; elevated protein; often low glucose	Serum and CSF angiotensin-converting enzyme levels; biopsy of extraneural affected tissues or brain lesion/meningeal biopsy	CN palsy, especially of CN VII; hypothalamic dysfunction, especially diabetes insipidus; abnormal chest radiograph; peripheral neuropathy or myopathy
Vogt-Koyanagi-Harada syndrome (recurrent meningitis)	Mononuclear cells		Recurrent meningoencephalitis with uveitis, retinal detachment, alopecia, lightening of eyebrows and lashes, dysacousia, cataracts, glaucoma
Isolated granulomatous angiitis of the nervous system	Mononuclear cells, elevated protein	Angiography or meningeal biopsy	Subacute dementia; multiple cerebral infarctions; recent zoster ophthalmicus
Systemic lupus erythematosus	Mononuclear or PMNs	Anti-DNA antibody, antinuclear antibodies	Encephalopathy; seizures; stroke; transverse myelopathy; rash; arthritis
Behçet's syndrome (recurrent meningitis)	Mononuclear or PMNs, elevated protein		Oral and genital aphthous ulcers; iridocyclitis; retinal hemorrhages; pathergic lesions at site of skin puncture
Chronic benign lymphocytic meningitis	Mononuclear cells		Recovery in 2–6 months, diagnosis by exclusion
Mollaret's meningitis (recurrent meningitis)	Large endothelial cells and PMNs in first hours, followed by mononuclear cells	PCR for herpes; MRI/CT to rule out epidermoid tumor or dural cyst	Recurrent meningitis; exclude HSV-2; rare cases due to HSV-1; occasional case associated with dural cyst
Drug hypersensitivity	PMNs; occasionally mononuclear cells or eosinophils		Exposure to ibuprofen, sulfonamides, isoniazid, tolmetin, ciprofloxacin, phenazopyridine; improvement after discontinuation of drug; recurrent episodes with recurrent exposure
Wegener's granulomatosis	Mononuclear cells	Chest and sinus radiographs; urinalysis; ANCA antibodies in serum	Associated sinus, pulmonary, or renal lesions; CN palsies; skin lesions; peripheral neuropathy
Other: multiple sclerosis, Sjögren's syndrome, neonatal onset multisystemic inflammatory disease (NOMID), and rarer forms of vasculitis (e.g., Cogan's syndrome)			

Abbreviations: ANCA, anti-neutrophil cytoplasmic antibodies; CN, cranial nerve; CSF, cerebrospinal fluid; CT, computed tomography; HSV, herpes simplex virus; MRI, magnetic resonance imaging; PCR, polymerase chain reaction; PMNs, polymorphonuclear cells.

meat or contact with a household cat (*Toxoplasma gondii*); residence in Thailand or Japan (*Gnathostoma spinigerum*), Latin America (*Paracoccidioides brasiliiensis*), or the South Pacific (*Angiostrongylus cantonensis*); rural residence and raccoon exposure (*Baylisascaris procyonis*); and residence in Latin America, the Philippines, or Southeast Asia when eosinophilic meningitis is present (*Taenia solium*).

The presence of focal cerebral signs in a patient with chronic meningitis suggests the possibility of a brain abscess or other parameningeal infection; identification of a potential source of infection (chronic draining ear, sinusitis, right-to-left cardiac or pulmonary shunt, chronic pleuropulmonary infection) supports this diagnosis. In some cases, diagnosis may be established by recognition and biopsy of unusual skin lesions (Behçet's syndrome, cryptococcosis, blastomycosis, SLE, Lyme disease, IV drug use, sporotrichosis, trypanosomiasis) or enlarged lymph nodes (lymphoma, tuberculosis, sarcoid, infection with HIV, secondary syphilis, or Whipple's disease). A careful ophthalmologic examination may reveal uveitis [Vogt-Koyanagi-Harada syndrome, sarcoid, or central nervous system (CNS) lymphoma], keratoconjunctivitis sicca (Sjögren's syndrome), or iridocyclitis (Behçet's syndrome) and is essential to assess visual loss from papilledema. Aphthous oral lesions, genital

ulcers, and hypopyon suggest Behçet's syndrome. Hepatosplenomegaly suggests lymphoma, sarcoid, tuberculosis, or brucellosis. Herpetic lesions in the genital area or on the thighs suggests HSV-2 infection. A breast nodule, a suspicious pigmented skin lesion, focal bone pain, or an abdominal mass directs attention to possible carcinomatous meningitis.

IMAGING Once the clinical syndrome is recognized as a potential manifestation of chronic meningitis, proper analysis of the CSF is essential. However, if the possibility of raised ICP exists, a brain imaging study should be performed before lumbar puncture. If ICP is elevated because of a mass lesion, brain swelling, or a block in ventricular CSF outflow (obstructive hydrocephalus), then lumbar puncture carries the potential risk of brain herniation. Obstructive hydrocephalus usually requires direct ventricular drainage of CSF. In patients with open CSF flow pathways, elevated ICP can still occur due to impaired resorption of CSF by arachnoid villi. In such patients, lumbar puncture is usually safe, but repetitive or continuous lumbar drainage may be necessary to prevent relatively sudden death from raised ICP. In some patients, especially with cryptococcal meningitis, fatal levels of raised ICP can occur without enlarged ventricles.

FIGURE 377-1 Primary central nervous system lymphoma. A 24-year-old man, immunosuppressed due to intestinal lymphangiectasia, developed multiple cranial neuropathies. CSF findings consisted of 100 lymphocytes/μL and a protein of 2.5 g/L (250 mg/dL); cytology and cultures were negative. Gadolinium-enhanced T1 MRI revealed diffuse, multifocal meningeal enhancement surrounding the brainstem (**A**), spinal cord and cauda equina (**B**).

Contrast-enhanced MRI or CT studies of the brain and spinal cord can identify meningeal enhancement, parameningeal infections (including brain abscess), encasement of the spinal cord (malignancy or inflammation and infection), or nodular deposits on the meninges or nerve roots (malignancy or sarcoidosis) (Fig. 377-1). Imaging studies are also useful to localize areas of meningeal disease prior to meningeal biopsy.

Cerebral angiography may be indicated in patients with chronic meningitis and stroke to identify cerebral arteritis (granulomatous angiitis, other inflammatory arteritides, or infectious arteritis).

CEREBROSPINAL FLUID ANALYSIS The CSF pressure should be measured and samples sent for bacterial, fungal, and tuberculous culture; Venereal Disease Research Laboratories (VDRL) test; cell count and differential; Gram's stain; and measurement of glucose and protein. Wet mount for fungus and parasites, India ink preparation and culture, culture for fastidious bacteria and fungi, assays for cryptococcal antigen and oligoclonal immunoglobulin bands, and cytology should be performed. Other specific CSF tests (Tables 377-2 and 377-3) or blood tests and cultures should be ordered as indicated on the basis of the history, physical examination, or preliminary CSF results (i.e., eosinophilic, mononuclear, or polymorphonuclear meningitis). Rapid diagnosis may be facilitated by serologic tests and polymerase chain reaction (PCR) testing to identify DNA sequences in the CSF that are specific for the suspected pathogen.

In most categories of chronic (not recurrent) meningitis, mononuclear cells predominate in the CSF. When neutrophils predominate after 3 weeks of illness, the principal etiologic considerations are *Nocardia asteroides*, *Actinomyces israelii*, *Brucella*, *Mycobacterium tuberculosis* (5–10% of early cases only), various fungi (*Blastomyces dermatitidis*, *Candida albicans*, *Histoplasma capsulatum*, *Aspergillus* spp., *Pseudallescheria boydii*, *Cladophialophora bantiana*), and noninfectious causes (SLE, exogenous chemical meningitis). When eosinophils predominate or are present in limited numbers in a primarily mononuclear cell response in the CSF, the differential diagnosis includes parasitic diseases (*A. cantonensis*, *G. spinigerum*, *B. procyonis*, or *Toxocara canis* infection, cysticercosis, schistosomiasis, echinococcal disease, *T. gondii* infection), fungal infections (6–20% eosinophils along with a predominantly lymphocyte pleocytosis, particularly with coccidioidal meningitis), neoplastic disease (lymphoma, leukemia, metastatic carcinoma), or other inflammatory processes (sarcoidosis, hypereosinophilic syndrome).

It is often necessary to broaden the number of diagnostic tests if the initial workup does not reveal the cause. In addition, repeated samples of large volumes of CSF may be required to diagnose certain infectious and malignant causes of chronic meningitis. For instance, lymphomatous or carcinomatous meningitis may be diagnosed by examination of sections cut from a cell block formed by spinning down the sediment from a large volume of CSF. The diagnosis of fungal meningitis may require large volumes of CSF for culture of sediment. If standard lumbar puncture is unrewarding, a cervical cisternal tap to sample CSF near to the basal meninges may be fruitful.

LABORATORY INVESTIGATION In addition to the CSF examination, an attempt should be made to uncover pertinent underlying illnesses. Tuberculin skin test, chest radiograph, urine analysis and culture, blood count and differential, renal and liver function tests, alkaline phosphatase, sedimentation rate, antinuclear antibody, anti-Ro, anti-La antibody and serum angiotensin-converting enzyme level are often indicated. Liver or bone marrow biopsy may be diagnostic in some cases of miliary tuberculosis, disseminated fungal infection, sarcoidosis, or metastatic malignancy. Abnormalities discovered on chest radiograph or chest CT can be pursued by bronchoscopy or transthoracic needle biopsy.

MENINGEAL BIOPSY A meningeal biopsy should be strongly considered in patients who are severely disabled, who need chronic ventricular decompression, or whose illness is progressing rapidly. The activities of the surgeon, pathologist, microbiologist, and cytologist should be coordinated so that a large enough sample is obtained and the appropriate cultures and histologic and molecular studies, including electron-microscopic and PCR studies, are performed. The diagnostic yield of meningeal biopsy can be increased by targeting regions that enhance with contrast on MRI or CT. With current microsurgical techniques, most areas of the basal meninges can be accessed for biopsy via a limited craniotomy. In a series from the Mayo Clinic reported by Cheng et al., MRI demonstrated meningeal enhancement in 47% of patients undergoing meningeal biopsy. Biopsy of an enhancing region was diagnostic in 80% of cases; biopsy of nonenhancing regions was diagnostic in only 9%; sarcoid (31%) and metastatic adenocarcinoma (25%) were the most common conditions identified. Tuberculosis is the most common condition identified in many reports from outside the United States.

APPROACH TO THE ENIGMATIC CASE In approximately one-third of cases, the diagnosis is not known despite careful evaluation of CSF and potential extraneural sites of disease. A number of the organisms that cause chronic meningitis may take weeks to be identified by cultures. In enigmatic cases several options are available, determined by the extent of the clinical deficits and rate of progression. It is prudent to wait until cultures are finalized if the patient is asymptomatic or symptoms are mild and not progressive. Unfortunately, in many cases progressive neurologic deterioration occurs, and rapid treatment is required. Ventricular-peritoneal shunts may be placed to relieve hydrocephalus, but the risk of disseminating the undiagnosed inflammatory process into the abdomen must be considered.

Empirical Treatment Diagnosis of the causative agent is essential because effective therapies exist for many etiologies of chronic meningitis, but if the condition is left untreated, progressive damage to the CNS and cranial nerves and roots is likely to occur. Occasionally, empirical therapy must be initiated when all attempts at diagnosis fail. In general, empirical therapy in the United States consists of antimycobacterial agents, amphotericin for fungal infection, or glucocorticoids for noninfectious inflammatory causes. It is important to direct empirical therapy of lymphocytic meningitis at tuberculosis, particularly if the condition is associated with hypoglycorrhachia and sixth and other CN palsies, since untreated disease is fatal in 4–8 weeks. In the Mayo Clinic series, the most useful empirical therapy was administration of glucocorticoids rather than antituberculous therapy. Carcinomatous or lymphomatous meningitis may be difficult to diagnose initially, but the diagnosis becomes evident with time.

Chronic meningitis is not uncommon in the course of HIV infection. Pleocytosis and mild meningeal signs often occur at the onset of HIV infection, and occasionally low-grade meningitis persists. Toxoplasmosis commonly presents as intracranial abscesses and may also be associated with meningitis. Other important causes of chronic meningitis in AIDS include infection with *Cryptococcus, Nocardia, Candida,* or other fungi; syphilis; and lymphoma (Fig. 377-1). Toxoplasmosis, cryptococcosis, nocardiosis, and other fungal infections are important etiologic considerations in individuals with immunodeficiency states other than AIDS, including those due to immunosuppressive medications. Because of the increased risk of chronic meningitis and the attenuation of clinical signs of meningeal irritation in immunosuppressed individuals, CSF examination should be performed for any persistent headache or unexplained change in mental state.

FURTHER READINGS

CAWS M et al: Role of IS6110-targeted PCR, culture, biochemical, clinical, and immunological criteria for diagnosis of tuberculous meningitis. J Clin Microbiol 38(9):3150, 2000

GILDEN DH et al: Herpesvirus infections of the nervous system. Nat Clin Pract Neurol 3:82, 2007

GLEISSNER B, CHAMBERLAIN MC: Neoplastic meningitis. Lancet Neurol 5:443, 2006

HALPERIN JJ et al: Practice parameter: Treatment of nervous system Lyme disease (an evidence-based review): Report of the Quality Standards Subcommittee of the American Academy of Neurology. Neurology 69:91, 2007

LAN SH et al: Cerebral infarction in chronic meningitis: A comparison of tuberculous meningitis and cryptococcal meningitis. Q J Med 94(5):247, 2001

LILIANG PC et al: Use of ventriculoperitoneal shunts to treat uncontrollable intracranial hypertension in patients who have cryptococcal meningitis without hydrocephalus. Clin Infect Dis 34(12):E64, 2002

THURTELL MJ et al: Tuberculous cranial pachymeningitis. Neurology 68:298, 2007

378 Prion Diseases
Stanley B. Prusiner, Bruce Miller

Prions are infectious proteins that cause degeneration of the central nervous system (CNS). Prion diseases are disorders of protein conformation, the most common of which in humans is called Creutzfeldt-Jakob disease (CJD). CJD typically presents with dementia and myoclonus, is relentlessly progressive, and generally causes death within a year of onset. Most CJD patients are between 50 and 75 years of age; however, patients as young as 17 and as old as 83 have been recorded.

In mammals, prions reproduce by binding to the normal, cellular isoform of the *prion* protein (PrP^C) and stimulating conversion of PrP^C into the disease-causing isoform (PrP^Sc). PrP^C is rich in α-helix and has little β-structure, while PrP^Sc has less α-helix and a high amount of β-structure (Fig. 378-1). This α-to-β structural transition in the prion protein (PrP) is the fundamental event underlying prion diseases (Table 378-1).

Four new concepts have emerged from studies of prions: (1) Prions are the only known infectious pathogens that are devoid of nucleic acid; all other infectious agents possess genomes composed of either RNA or DNA that direct the synthesis of their progeny. (2) Prion diseases may be manifest as infectious, genetic, and sporadic disorders; no other group of illnesses with a single etiology presents with such a wide spectrum of clinical manifestations. (3) Prion diseases result from the accumulation of PrP^Sc, the conformation of which differs substantially from that of its precursor, PrP^C. (4) PrP^Sc can exist in a variety of different conformations, each of which seems to specify a particular disease phenotype. How a specific conformation of a PrP^Sc molecule is imparted to PrP^C during prion replication to produce nascent PrP^Sc with the same conformation is unknown. Additionally, it is unclear what factors determine where in the CNS a particular PrP^Sc molecule will be deposited.

SPECTRUM OF PRION DISEASES

The sporadic form of CJD is the most common prion disorder in humans. Sporadic CJD (sCJD) accounts for ~85% of all cases of human prion disease, while inherited prion diseases account for 10–15% of all cases (Table 378-2). Familial CJD (fCJD), Gerstmann-Sträussler-Scheinker (GSS) disease, and fatal familial insomnia (FFI) are all dominantly inherited prion diseases that are caused by mutations in the PrP gene.

Although infectious prion diseases account for <1% of all cases and infection does not seem to play an important role in the natural history of these illnesses, the transmissibility of prions is an important biologic feature. *Kuru* of the Fore people of New Guinea is thought to have resulted from the consumption of brains from dead relatives during ritualistic cannibalism. With the cessation of ritualistic cannibalism in the late 1950s, kuru has nearly disappeared, with the ex-

FIGURE 378-1 Structures of prion proteins. A. NMR structure of Syrian hamster recombinant (rec) PrP(90–231). Presumably, the structure of the α-helical form of recPrP(90–231) resembles that of PrP^C. recPrP(90–231) is viewed from the interface where PrP^Sc is thought to bind to PrP^C. Shown are: α-helices A (residues 144–157), B (172–193), and C (200–227). Flat ribbons depict β-strands S1 (129–131) and S2 (161–163). (**A,** *from SB Prusiner: N Engl J Med 344:1516, 2006; with permission.*) **B.** Structural model of PrP^Sc. The 90–160 region has been modeled onto a β-helical architecture while the COOH terminal helices B and C are preserved as in PrP^C. (*Image prepared by C. Govaerts.*)

TABLE 378-1	GLOSSARY OF PRION TERMINOLOGY
Prion	*Pro*teinaceous *in*fectious particle that lacks nucleic acid. Prions are composed largely, if not entirely, of PrP^Sc molecules. They can cause scrapie in sheep and goats, and related neurodegenerative diseases of humans such as Creutzfeldt-Jakob disease (CJD).
PrP^Sc	Disease-causing isoform of the prion protein. This protein is the only identifiable macromolecule in purified preparations of scrapie prions.
PrP^C	Cellular isoform of the prion protein. PrP^C is the precursor of PrP^Sc.
PrP 27-30	A fragment of PrP^Sc, generated by truncation of the NH2-terminus by limited digestion with proteinase K. PrP 27-30 retains prion infectivity and polymerizes into amyloid.
PRNP	PrP gene located on human chromosome 20.
Prion rod	An aggregate of prions composed largely of PrP 27-30 molecules. Created by detergent extraction and limited proteolysis of PrP^Sc. Morphologically and histochemically indistinguishable from many amyloids.
PrP amyloid	Amyloid containing PrP in the brains of animals or humans with prion disease; often accumulates as plaques.

TABLE 378-2 THE PRION DISEASES

Disease	Host	Mechanism of Pathogenesis
Human		
Kuru	Fore people	Infection through ritualistic cannibalism
iCJD	Humans	Infection from prion-contaminated hGH, dura mater grafts, etc.
vCJD	Humans	Infection from bovine prions
fCJD	Humans	Germ-line mutations in *PRNP*
GSS	Humans	Germ-line mutations in *PRNP*
FFI	Humans	Germ-line mutation in *PRNP* (D178N, M129)
sCJD	Humans	Somatic mutation or spontaneous conversion of PrP^C into PrP^Sc?
sFI	Humans	Somatic mutation or spontaneous conversion of PrP^C into PrP^Sc?
Animal		
Scrapie	Sheep, goats	Infection in genetically susceptible sheep
BSE	Cattle	Infection with prion-contaminated MBM
TME	Mink	Infection with prions from sheep or cattle
CWD	Mule deer, elk	Unknown
FSE	Cats	Infection with prion-contaminated beef
Exotic ungulate encephalopathy	Greater kudu, nyala, or oryx	Infection with prion-contaminated MBM

Abbreviations: BSE, bovine spongiform encephalopathy; CJD, Creutzfeldt-Jakob disease; fCJD, familial Creutzfeldt-Jakob disease; iCJD, iatrogenic Creutzfeldt-Jakob disease; sCJD, sporadic Creutzfeldt-Jakob disease; vCJD, variant Creutzfeldt-Jakob disease; CWD, chronic wasting disease; FFI, fatal familial insomnia; sFI, sporadic fatal insomnia; FSE, feline spongiform encephalopathy; GSS, Gerstmann-Sträussler-Scheinker disease; hGH, human growth hormone; MBM, meat and bone meal; TME, transmissible mink encephalopathy.

ception of a few recent patients exhibiting incubation periods of >40 years. Iatrogenic CJD (iCJD) seems to be the result of the accidental inoculation of patients with prions. Variant CJD (vCJD) in teenagers and young adults in Europe is the result of exposure to tainted beef from cattle with bovine spongiform encephalopathy (BSE).

Six diseases of animals are caused by prions (Table 378-2). Scrapie of sheep and goats is the prototypic prion disease. Mink encephalopathy, BSE, feline spongiform encephalopathy, and exotic ungulate encephalopathy are all thought to occur after the consumption of prion-infected foodstuffs. The BSE epidemic emerged in Britain in the late 1980s and was shown to be due to industrial cannibalism. Whether BSE began as a sporadic case of BSE in a cow or started with scrapie in sheep is unknown. The origin of chronic wasting disease (CWD), a prion disease endemic in deer and elk in regions of North America, is uncertain.

EPIDEMIOLOGY

CJD is found throughout the world. The incidence of sCJD is approximately one case per million population, and thus it accounts for about one in every 10,000 deaths. Because sCJD is an age-dependent neurodegenerative disease, its incidence is expected to increase steadily as older segments of populations in developed and developing countries continue to expand. Although many geographic clusters of CJD have been reported, each has been shown to segregate with a PrP gene mutation. Attempts to identify common exposure to some etiologic agent have been unsuccessful for both the sporadic and familial cases. Ingestion of scrapie-infected sheep or goat meat as a cause of CJD in humans has not been demonstrated by epidemiologic studies, although speculation about this potential route of inoculation continues. Of particular interest are deer hunters who develop CJD, because up to 90% of culled deer in some game herds have been shown to harbor CWD prions. Whether prion disease in deer or elk can be passed to cows, sheep, or directly to humans remains unknown. Studies with Syrian hamsters demonstrate that oral infection with prions can occur, but the process is inefficient compared to intracerebral inoculation.

PATHOGENESIS

The human prion diseases were initially classified as neurodegenerative disorders of unknown etiology on the basis of pathologic changes being confined to the CNS. With the transmission of kuru and CJD to apes, investigators began to view these diseases as infectious CNS illnesses caused by slow viruses. Even though the familial nature of a subset of CJD cases was well described, the significance of this observation became more obscure with the transmission of CJD to animals. Eventually the meaning of heritable CJD became clear with the discovery of

mutations in the PRNP gene of these patients. The prion concept explains how a disease can manifest as a heritable as well as an infectious illness. Moreover, the hallmark of all prion diseases, whether sporadic, dominantly inherited, or acquired by infection, is that they involve the aberrant metabolism of PrP.

A major feature that distinguishes prions from viruses is the finding that both PrP isoforms are encoded by a chromosomal gene. In humans, the PrP gene is designated *PRNP* and is located on the short arm of chromosome 20. Limited proteolysis of PrP^Sc produces a smaller, protease-resistant molecule of ~142 amino acids designated PrP 27 30; PrP^C is completely hydrolyzed under the same conditions (Fig. 378-2). In the presence of detergent, PrP 27-30 polymerizes into amyloid. Prion rods formed by limited proteolysis and detergent extraction are indistinguishable from the filaments that aggregate to form PrP amyloid plaques in the CNS. Both the rods and the PrP amyloid filaments found in brain tissue exhibit similar ultrastructural morphology and green-gold birefringence after staining with Congo red dye.

Prion Strains The existence of prion strains raised the question of how heritable biologic information can be enciphered in a molecule other than nucleic acid. Various strains of prions have been defined by incubation times and the distribution of neuronal vacuolation. Subsequently, the patterns of PrP^Sc deposition were found to correlate with vacuolation profiles, and these patterns were also used to characterize prion strains.

Persuasive evidence that strain-specific information is enciphered in the tertiary structure of PrP^Sc comes from transmission of two different inherited human prion diseases to mice expressing a chimeric human-mouse PrP transgene. In FFI, the protease-resistant fragment of PrP^Sc after deglycosylation has a molecular mass of 19 kDa, whereas in fCJD and most sporadic prion diseases, it is 21 kDa (Table 378-3). This difference in molecular mass was shown to be due to different sites of proteolytic cleavage at the NH$_2$ termini of the two human PrP^Sc molecules, reflecting different tertiary structures. These distinct conformations were not unexpected because the amino acid sequences of the PrPs differ.

Extracts from the brains of patients with FFI transmitted disease into mice expressing a chimeric human-mouse PrP transgene and in-

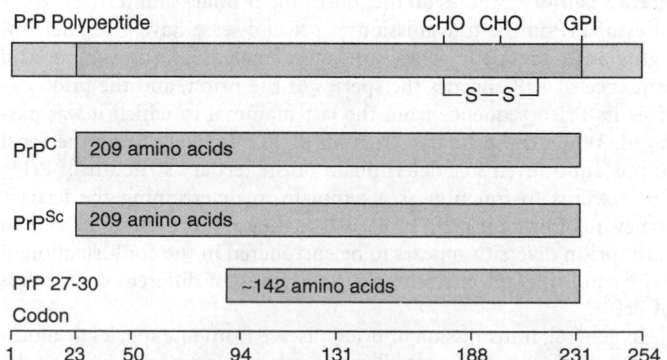

FIGURE 378-2 Prion protein isoforms. Bar diagram of Syrian hamster PrP, which consists of 254 amino acids. After processing of the NH$_2$ and COOH termini, both PrP^C and PrP^Sc consist of 209 residues. After limited proteolysis, the NH$_2$ terminus of PrP^Sc is truncated to form PrP 27–30 composed of ~142 amino acids.

TABLE 378-3 DISTINCT PRION STRAINS GENERATED IN HUMANS WITH INHERITED PRION DISEASES AND TRANSMITTED TO TRANSGENIC MICE[a]

Inoculum	Host Species	Host PrP Genotype	Incubation Time [days ± SEM] (n/n_0)	PrP^{Sc} (kDa)
None	Human	FFI(D178N, M129)		19
FFI	Mouse	Tg(MHu2M)	206 ± 7 (7/7)	19
FFI → Tg(MHu2M)	Mouse	Tg(MHu2M)	136 ± 1 (6/6)	19
None	Human	fCJD(E200K)		21
fCJD	Mouse	Tg(MHu2M)	170 ± 2 (10/10)	21
fCJD → Tg(MHu2M)	Mouse	Tg(MHu2M)	167 ± 3 (15/15)	21

[a]Tg(MHu2M) mice express a chimeric mouse-human PrP gene.

Note: Clinicopathologic phenotype is determined by the conformation of PrP^{Sc} in accord with the results of the transmission of human prions from patients with FFI to transgenic mice. FFI, fatal familial insomnia; fCJD, familial Creutzfeldt-Jakob disease.

duced formation of the 19-kDa PrP^{Sc}, whereas brain extracts from fCJD and sCJD patients produced the 21-kDa PrP^{Sc} in mice expressing the same transgene. On second passage, these differences were maintained, demonstrating that chimeric PrP^{Sc} can exist in two different conformations based on the sizes of the protease-resistant fragments, even though the amino acid sequence of PrP^{Sc} is invariant.

This analysis was extended when patients with sporadic fatal insomnia (sFI) were identified. Although they did not carry a *PRNP* gene mutation, the patients demonstrated a clinical and pathologic phenotype that was indistinguishable from that of patients with FFI. Furthermore, 19-kDa PrP^{Sc} was found in their brains, and on passage of prion disease to mice expressing a chimeric human-mouse PrP transgene, 19-kDa PrP^{Sc} was also found. These findings indicate that the disease phenotype is dictated by the conformation of PrP^{Sc} and not the amino acid sequence. PrP^{Sc} acts as a template for the conversion of PrP^C into nascent PrP^{Sc}. On the passage of prions into mice expressing a chimeric hamster-mouse PrP transgene, a change in the conformation of PrP^{Sc} was accompanied by the emergence of a new strain of prions.

New strains of prions were also generated from recombinant (rec) PrP produced in bacteria. In these studies, recPrP was polymerized into amyloid fibrils and inoculated into transgenic mice expressing very high levels of truncated mouse PrP^C; about 500 days later, the mice died of prion disease. These "synthetic prions" were found to be much more stable than any prions previously isolated from animals or humans with naturally occurring prion diseases. Surprisingly, studies of synthetic and naturally occurring prions indicate that the incubation time is directly proportional to the stability of the prion. As the stability increases, the incubation time lengthens; thus, less-stable prions replicate more rapidly. These studies also showed that PrP^{Sc} can adopt a continuum of conformational states, each of which enciphers a distinct incubation-time phenotype.

Species Barrier Studies on the role of the primary and tertiary structures of PrP in the transmission of prion disease have given new insights into the pathogenesis of these maladies. The amino acid sequence of PrP encodes the species of the prion, and the prion derives its PrP^{Sc} sequence from the last mammal in which it was passaged. While the primary structure of PrP is likely to be the most important or even sole determinant of the tertiary structure of PrP^C, PrP^{Sc} seems to function as a template in determining the tertiary structure of nascent PrP^{Sc} molecules as they are formed from PrP^C. In turn, prion diversity appears to be enciphered in the conformation of PrP^{Sc}, and thus prion strains seem to represent different conformers of PrP^{Sc}.

In general, transmission of prion disease from one species to another is inefficient, in that not all intracerebrally inoculated animals develop disease, and those that fall ill do so only after long incubation times that can approach the natural life span of the animal. This "species barrier" to transmission is correlated with the degree of similarity between the amino acid sequences of PrP^C in the inoculated host and of PrP^{Sc} in the prion inoculum. The importance of sequence similarity

between the host and donor PrP argues that PrP^C directly interacts with PrP^{Sc} in the prion conversion process.

SPORADIC AND INHERITED PRION DISEASES

Several different scenarios might explain the initiation of sporadic prion disease: (1) A somatic mutation may be the cause and thus follow a path similar to that for germ-line mutations in inherited disease. In this situation, the mutant PrP^{Sc} must be capable of targeting wild-type PrP^C, a process known to be possible for some mutations but less likely for others. (2) The activation barrier separating wild-type PrP^C from PrP^{Sc} could be crossed on rare occasions when viewed in the context of a population. Most individuals would be spared while presentations in the elderly with an incidence of ~1 per million would be seen. (3) PrP^{Sc} may be present at very low levels in some normal cells, where it performs some important, as yet unknown, function. The level of PrP^{Sc} in such cells is hypothesized to be sufficiently low as to be not detected by bioassay. In some altered metabolic states, the cellular mechanisms for clearing PrP^{Sc} might become compromised and the rate of PrP^{Sc} formation would then begin to exceed the capacity of the cell to clear it. The third possible mechanism is attractive since it suggests PrP^{Sc} is not simply a misfolded protein, as proposed for the first and second mechanisms, but that it is an alternatively folded molecule with a function. Moreover, the multitude of conformational states that PrP^{Sc} can adopt, as described above, raises the possibility that PrP^{Sc} or another prion-like protein might function in a process like short-term memory where information storage occurs in the absence of new protein synthesis.

More than 30 different mutations resulting in nonconservative substitutions in the human *PRNP* gene have been found to segregate with inherited human prion diseases. Missense mutations and expansions in the octapeptide repeat region of the gene are responsible for familial forms of prion disease. Five different mutations of the *PRNP* gene have been linked genetically to heritable prion disease.

Although phenotypes may vary dramatically within families, specific phenotypes tend to be observed with certain mutations. A clinical phenotype indistinguishable from typical sCJD is usually seen with substitutions at codons 180, 183, 200, 208, 210, and 232. Substitutions at codons 102, 105, 117, 198, and 217 are associated with the GSS variant of prion disease. The normal human PrP sequence contains five repeats of an eight-amino-acid sequence. Insertions from two to nine extra octarepeats frequently cause variable phenotypes ranging from a condition indistinguishable from sCJD to a slowly progressive dementing illness of many years' duration to an early-age-of-onset disorder that is similar to Alzheimer's disease. A mutation at codon 178 resulting in substitution of asparagine for aspartic acid produces FFI if a methionine is encoded at the polymorphic 129 residue on the same allele. Typical CJD is seen if a valine is encoded at position 129 of the same allele.

HUMAN PRNP GENE POLYMORPHISMS

Polymorphisms influence the susceptibility to sporadic, inherited, and infectious forms of prion disease. The methionine/valine polymorphism at position 129 not only modulates the age of onset of some inherited prion diseases but can also determine the clinical phenotype. The finding that homozygosity at codon 129 predisposes to sCJD supports a model of prion production that favors PrP interactions between homologous proteins.

Substitution of the basic residue lysine at position 218 in mouse PrP produced dominant-negative inhibition of prion replication in transgenic mice. This same lysine at position 219 in human PrP has been found in 12% of the Japanese population, and this group appears to be resistant to prion disease. Dominant-negative inhibition of prion replication was also found with substitution of the basic residue arginine at position 171; sheep with arginine are resistant to scrapie prions but are susceptible to BSE prions that were inoculated intracerebrally.

INFECTIOUS PRION DISEASES

IATROGENIC CJD

Accidental transmission of CJD to humans appears to have occurred with corneal transplantation, contaminated electroencephalogram (EEG) electrode implantation, and surgical procedures. Corneas from donors with inapparent CJD have been transplanted to apparently healthy recipients who developed CJD after prolonged incubation periods. The same improperly decontaminated EEG electrodes that caused CJD in two young patients with intractable epilepsy caused CJD in a chimpanzee 18 months after their experimental implantation.

Surgical procedures may have resulted in accidental inoculation of patients with prions, presumably because some instrument or apparatus in the operating theater became contaminated when a CJD patient underwent surgery. Although the epidemiology of these studies is highly suggestive, no proof for such episodes exists.

Dura Mater Grafts More than 160 cases of CJD after implantation of dura mater grafts have been recorded. All of the grafts were thought to have been acquired from a single manufacturer whose preparative procedures were inadequate to inactivate human prions. One case of CJD occurred after repair of an eardrum perforation with a pericardium graft.

Human Growth Hormone and Pituitary Gonadotropin Therapy The possibility of transmission of CJD from contaminated human growth hormone (hGH) preparations derived from human pituitaries has been raised by the occurrence of fatal cerebellar disorders with dementia in >180 patients ranging in age from 10 to 41 years. These patients received injections of hGH every 2–4 days for 4–12 years. If it is assumed that these patients developed CJD from injections of prion-contaminated hGH preparations, the possible incubation periods range from 4 to 30 years. Even though several investigations argue for the efficacy of inactivating prions in hGH fractions prepared from human pituitaries with 6 *M* urea, it seems doubtful that such protocols will be used for purifying hGH because recombinant hGH is available. Four cases of CJD have occurred in women receiving human pituitary gonadotropin.

VARIANT CJD

The restricted geographic occurrence and chronology of vCJD raised the possibility that BSE prions have been transmitted to humans through the consumption of tainted beef. More than 190 cases of vCJD have occurred, with >90% of these in Britain. vCJD has also been reported in people either living in or originating from France, Ireland, Italy, Netherlands, Portugal, Spain, Saudi Arabia, United States, Canada, and Japan.

Because the number of vCJD cases is still small, it not possible to decide if we are at the beginning of a prion disease epidemic in Europe, similar to those seen for BSE and kuru, or if the number of vCJD cases will remain small. What is certain is that prion-tainted meat should be prevented from entering the human food supply.

The most compelling evidence that vCJD is caused by BSE prions was obtained from experiments in mice expressing the bovine PrP transgene. Both BSE and vCJD prions were efficiently transmitted to these transgenic mice and with similar incubation periods. In contrast to sCJD prions, vCJD prions did not transmit disease efficiently to mice expressing a chimeric human-mouse PrP transgene. Earlier studies with nontransgenic mice suggested that vCJD and BSE might be derived from the same source because both inocula transmitted disease with similar but very long incubation periods.

Attempts to determine the origin of BSE and vCJD prions have relied on passaging studies in mice, some of which are described above, as well as studies of the conformation and glycosylation of PrP^{Sc}. One scenario suggests that a particular conformation of bovine PrP^{Sc} was selected for heat resistance during the rendering process and was then reselected multiple times as cattle infected by ingesting prion-contam-

inated meat and bone meal (MBM) were slaughtered and their offal rendered into more MBM.

NEUROPATHOLOGY

Frequently the brains of patients with CJD have no recognizable abnormalities on gross examination. Patients who survive for several years have variable degrees of cerebral atrophy.

On light microscopy, the pathologic hallmarks of CJD are spongiform degeneration and astrocytic gliosis. The lack of an inflammatory response in CJD and other prion diseases is an important pathologic feature of these degenerative disorders. Spongiform degeneration is characterized by many 1- to 5-μm vacuoles in the neuropil between nerve cell bodies. Generally the spongiform changes occur in the cerebral cortex, putamen, caudate nucleus, thalamus, and molecular layer of the cerebellum. Astrocytic gliosis is a constant but nonspecific feature of prion diseases. Widespread proliferation of fibrous astrocytes is found throughout the gray matter of brains infected with CJD prions. Astrocytic processes filled with glial filaments form extensive networks.

Amyloid plaques have been found in ~10% of CJD cases. Purified CJD prions from humans and animals exhibit the ultrastructural and histochemical characteristics of amyloid when treated with detergents during limited proteolysis. In first passage from some human Japanese CJD cases, amyloid plaques have been found in mouse brains. These plaques stain with antibodies raised against PrP.

The amyloid plaques of GSS disease are morphologically distinct from those seen in kuru or scrapie. GSS plaques consist of a central dense core of amyloid surrounded by smaller globules of amyloid. Ultrastructurally, they consist of a radiating fibrillar network of amyloid fibrils, with scant or no neuritic degeneration. The plaques can be distributed throughout the brain but are most frequently found in the cerebellum. They are often located adjacent to blood vessels. Congophilic angiopathy has been noted in some cases of GSS disease.

In vCJD, a characteristic feature is the presence of "florid plaques." These are composed of a central core of PrP amyloid, surrounded by vacuoles in a pattern suggesting petals on a flower.

CLINICAL FEATURES

Nonspecific prodromal symptoms occur in about a third of patients with CJD and may include fatigue, sleep disturbance, weight loss, headache, malaise, and ill-defined pain. Most patients with CJD present with deficits in higher cortical function. These deficits almost always progress over weeks or months to a state of profound dementia characterized by memory loss, impaired judgment, and a decline in virtually all aspects of intellectual function. A few patients present with either visual impairment or cerebellar gait and coordination deficits. Frequently the cerebellar deficits are rapidly followed by progressive dementia. Visual problems often begin with blurred vision and diminished acuity, rapidly followed by dementia.

Other symptoms and signs include extrapyramidal dysfunction manifested as rigidity, masklike facies, or choreoathetoid movements; pyramidal signs (usually mild); seizures (usually major motor) and, less commonly, hypoesthesia; supranuclear gaze palsy; optic atrophy; and vegetative signs such as changes in weight, temperature, sweating, or menstruation.

Myoclonus Most patients (~90%) with CJD exhibit myoclonus that appears at various times throughout the illness. Unlike other involuntary movements, myoclonus persists during sleep. Startle myoclonus elicited by loud sounds or bright lights is frequent. It is important to stress that myoclonus is neither specific nor confined to CJD. Dementia with myoclonus can also be due to Alzheimer's disease (AD) (Chap. 365), dementia with Lewy bodies (Chap. 365), cryptococcal encephalitis (Chap. 195), or the myoclonic epilepsy disorder Unverricht-Lundborg disease (Chap. 363).

Clinical Course In documented cases of accidental transmission of CJD to humans, an incubation period of 1.5–2.0 years preceded the development of clinical disease. In other cases, incubation periods of up to 30 years have been suggested. Most patients with CJD live 6–12 months after the onset of clinical signs and symptoms, whereas some live for up to 5 years.

The constellation of dementia, myoclonus, and periodic electrical bursts in an afebrile 60-year-old patient generally indicates CJD. Clinical abnormalities in CJD are confined to the CNS. Fever, elevated sedimentation rate, leukocytosis in blood, or a pleocytosis in cerebrospinal fluid (CSF) should alert the physician to another etiology to explain the patient's CNS dysfunction.

Variations in the typical course appear in inherited and transmitted forms of the disease. fCJD has an earlier mean age of onset than sCJD. In GSS disease, ataxia is usually a prominent and presenting feature, with dementia occurring late in the disease course. GSS disease typically presents earlier than CJD (mean age 43 years) and is typically more slowly progressive than CJD; death usually occurs within 5 years of onset. FFI is characterized by insomnia and dysautonomia; dementia occurs only in the terminal phase of the illness. Rare sporadic cases have been identified. vCJD has an unusual clinical course, with a prominent psychiatric prodrome that may include visual hallucinations and early ataxia, while frank dementia is usually a late sign of vCJD.

DIFFERENTIAL DIAGNOSIS

Many conditions may mimic CJD superficially. Dementia with Lewy bodies (Chap. 365) is the most common disorder to be mistaken for CJD. It can present in a subacute fashion with delirium, myoclonus, and extrapyramidal features. Other neurodegenerative disorders to consider include AD, frontotemporal dementia, progressive supranuclear palsy, ceroid lipofuscinosis (Chap. 365), and myoclonic epilepsy with Lafora bodies (Chap. 363). The absence of abnormalities on diffusion-weighted and FLAIR MRI will usually distinguish these dementing conditions from CJD.

Hashimoto's encephalopathy, which presents as a subacute progressive encephalopathy with myoclonus and periodic triphasic complexes on the EEG, should be excluded in every case of suspected CJD. It is diagnosed by the finding of high titers of antithyroglobulin or antithyroid peroxidase (antimicrosomal) antibodies in the blood and improves with glucocorticoid therapy. Unlike CJD, fluctuations in severity typically occur in Hashimoto's encephalopathy.

Intracranial vasculitides (Chap. 319) may produce nearly all of the symptoms and signs associated with CJD, sometimes without systemic abnormalities. Myoclonus is exceptional with cerebral vasculitis, but focal seizures may confuse the picture. Prominent headache, absence of myoclonus, stepwise change in deficits, abnormal CSF, and focal white matter changes on MRI or angiographic abnormalities all favor vasculitis.

Paraneoplastic conditions, particularly limbic encephalitis and cortical encephalitis, can also mimic CJD. In many of these patients, dementia appears prior to the diagnosis of a tumor, and in some, no tumor is ever found. Detection of the paraneoplastic antibodies is often the only way to distinguish these cases from CJD.

Other diseases that can simulate CJD include neurosyphilis (Chap. 162), AIDS dementia complex (Chap. 182), progressive multifocal leukoencephalopathy (Chap. 376), subacute sclerosing panencephalitis, progressive rubella panencephalitis, herpes simplex encephalitis, diffuse intracranial tumor (gliomatosis cerebri; Chap. 374), anoxic encephalopathy, dialysis dementia, uremia, hepatic encephalopathy, and lithium or bismuth intoxication.

LABORATORY TESTS

The only specific diagnostic tests for CJD and other human prion diseases measure PrP^{Sc}. The most widely used method involves limited proteolysis that generates PrP 27-30, which is detected by immunoassay after denaturation. The conformation-dependent immunoassay (CDI) is based on immunoreactive epitopes that are exposed in PrP^C but buried in PrP^{Sc}. The CDI is extremely sensitive and quantitative and is likely to find wide application in both the post- and antemortem detection of prions. In humans, the diagnosis of CJD can be established by brain biopsy if PrP^{Sc} is detected. If no attempt is made to measure PrP^{Sc}, but the constellation of pathologic changes frequently found in CJD is seen in a brain biopsy, then the diagnosis is reasonably secure (see "Neuropathology," above). Because PrP^{Sc} is not uniformly distributed throughout the CNS, the apparent absence of PrP^{Sc} in a limited sample such as a biopsy

FIGURE 378-3 T2-weighted (FLAIR) MRI showing hyperintensity in the cortex in a patient with sporadic CJD. This so-called "cortical ribboning" along with increased intensity in the basal ganglia on T2 or diffusion-weighted imaging can aid in the diagnosis of CJD.

does not rule out prion disease. At autopsy, sufficient brain samples should be taken for both PrP^{Sc} immunoassay, preferably by CDI, and immunohistochemistry of tissue sections.

To establish the diagnosis of either sCJD or familial prion disease, sequencing the *PRNP* gene must be performed. Finding the wild-type *PRNP* gene sequence permits the diagnosis of sCJD if there is no history to suggest infection from an exogenous source of prions. The identification of a mutation in the *PRNP* gene sequence that encodes a nonconservative amino acid substitution argues for familial prion disease.

CT may be normal or show cortical atrophy. MRI is valuable for distinguishing sCJD from most other conditions. On FLAIR sequences and diffusion-weighted imaging, ~90% of patients show increased intensity in the basal ganglia and cortical ribboning (Fig. 378-3). This pattern is not seen with other neurodegenerative disorders but has been seen infrequently with viral encephalitis, paraneoplastic syndromes, or seizures. When the typical MRI pattern is present, in the proper clinical setting, diagnosis is facilitated. However, some cases of sCJD do not show this typical pattern, and other early diagnostic approaches are still needed.

CSF is nearly always normal but may show protein elevation and, rarely, mild pleocytosis. Although the stress protein 14-3-3 is elevated in the CSF of some patients with CJD, similar elevations of 14-3-3 are found in patients with other disorders; thus this elevation is not specific.

The EEG is often useful in the diagnosis of CJD, although only about 60% of individuals show the typical pattern. During the early phase of CJD, the EEG is usually normal or shows only scattered theta activity. In most advanced cases, repetitive, high-voltage, triphasic, and polyphasic sharp discharges are seen, but in many cases their presence is transient. The presence of these stereotyped periodic bursts of <200 ms duration, occurring every 1–2 s, makes the diagnosis of CJD very likely. These discharges are frequently but not always symmetric; there may be a one-sided predominance in amplitude. As CJD progresses, normal background rhythms become fragmentary and slower.

CARE OF CJD PATIENTS

Although CJD should not be considered either contagious or communicable, it is transmissible. The risk of accidental inoculation by aerosols is very small; nonetheless, procedures producing aerosols should be performed in certified biosafety cabinets. Biosafety level 2 practices, containment equipment, and facilities are recommended by the Centers for Disease Control and Prevention and the National Institutes of Health. The primary problem in caring for patients with CJD is the inadvertent infection of health care workers by needle and stab wounds. The transmission of prions through the air has never been documented. Electroencephalographic and electromyographic needles should not be reused after studies on patients with CJD have been performed.

There is no reason for pathologists or other morgue employees to resist performing autopsies on patients whose clinical diagnosis was CJD. Standard microbiologic practices outlined here, along with specific recommendations for decontamination, seem to be adequate precautions for the care of patients with CJD and the handling of infected specimens.

DECONTAMINATION OF CJD PRIONS

Prions are extremely resistant to common inactivation procedures, and there is some disagreement about the optimal conditions for sterilization. Some investigators recommend treating CJD-contaminated materials once with 1 N NaOH at room temperature, but we believe this procedure may be inadequate for sterilization. Autoclaving at 134°C for 5 h or treatment with 2 N NaOH for several hours is recommended for sterilization of prions. The term *sterilization* implies complete destruction of prions; any residual infectivity can be hazardous. Recent studies show that sCJD prions bound to stainless steel surfaces are resistant to inactivation by autoclaving at 134°C for 2 h; exposure of bound prions to an acidic detergent solution prior to autoclaving rendered prions susceptible to inactivation.

PREVENTION AND THERAPEUTICS

There is no known effective therapy for preventing or treating CJD. The finding that phenothiazines and acridines inhibit PrP^{Sc} formation in cultured cells led to clinical studies of quinacrine in CJD patients. Although quinacrine seems to slow the rate of decline in some CJD patients, no cure of the disease has been observed. In wild-type mice, quinacrine treatment has been ineffective. Recent studies indicate that inhibition of the P-glycoprotein (Pgp) transport system results in sub-stantially increased quinacrine levels in the brains of mice. Whether such an approach can be used to treat CJD remains to be established.

Like the acridines, anti-PrP antibodies have been shown to eliminate PrP^{Sc} from cultured cells. Additionally, such antibodies in mice, either administered by injection or produced from a transgene, have been shown to prevent prion disease when prions are introduced by a peripheral route, such as intraperitoneal inoculation. Unfortunately, the antibodies were ineffective in mice inoculated intracerebrally with prions. Several drugs, including pentosan polysulfate and porphyrin derivatives, delay the onset of disease in animals inoculated intracerebrally with prions if the drugs are given intracerebrally beginning soon after inoculation.

Structure-based drug design predicated on dominant-negative inhibition of prion formation has produced several promising compounds. Modified quinacrine compounds that are more potent than the parent drug have been found. Whether improving the efficacy of such small molecules will provide general methods for developing novel therapeutics for other neurodegenerative disorders, including AD and Parkinson's disease as well as amyotrophic lateral sclerosis (ALS), remains to be established.

Disclosure: SBP has a financial interest in InPro Biotechnology, Inc.

FURTHER READINGS

PRUSINER SB: Prions, in *Fields Virology*, 5th ed., DM Knipe, PM Howley (eds.), Philadelphia, Pennsylvania, Lippincott Williams & Wilkins, 2007, pp 3059–3092

SAFAR JG et al: Diagnosis of human prion disease. Proc Natl Acad Sci USA 102:3501, 2005

WILL RG et al: Diagnosis of new variant Creutzfeldt-Jakob disease. Ann Neurol 47:575, 2000

SECTION 3   NERVE AND MUSCLE DISORDERS

379   Peripheral Neuropathy
Vinay Chaudhry

Peripheral neuropathy describes disorders of peripheral nerves, including the dorsal or ventral nerve roots; dorsal root ganglia; brachial or lumbosacral plexus; cranial nerves (except I and II); and other sensory, motor, autonomic, or mixed nerves; the term *peripheral* indicates that the disorder is outside the central nervous system (brain and spinal cord). Peripheral neuropathy affects ~2–8% of adults; the incidence increases with age. Evaluation begins with a history focusing on the time course of the illness, symptoms, medical conditions that predispose to neuropathy (e.g., diabetes mellitus, connective tissue disease, nutritional deficiency), toxic exposures (drug or environmental), and family history. Physical examination assesses the function of small sensory fibers (pain and temperature), large sensory fibers (vibration, proprioception, reflex changes), and/or motor nerves (weakness). The distribution of sensory, motor, and reflex changes determines whether the neuropathy is asymmetric or symmetric. Electrodiagnostic studies (EDx) help to classify the neuropathy into one of three major categories: axonal, demyelinating, or neuronal. Focused laboratory tests are then performed based on the history, examination, and EDx. An underlying cause can be identified in ~75% of neuropathies.

APPROACH TO THE PATIENT:
Peripheral Neuropathy

A stepwise approach to diagnosis is presented in Fig. 379-1. The following questions should be addressed initially:

1. *Is this a peripheral neuropathy?* The initial symptoms of peripheral neuropathy are often intermittent, and examination can be normal. Patients may present with positive and/or negative symptoms (Table 379-1). In most situations, sensory symptoms precede motor symptoms. Small-fiber neuropathies often present with dysesthesias and paresthesias, terms used interchangeably to describe unpleasant, unusual, or abnormal sensations such as burning or cutting pain, electric shock–like sensations, tingling, pins and needles, formication, prickly feelings such as a limb falling asleep, or cramp-like sensations (Chap. 25). Large-fiber neuropathies can present as numbness, tingling, or a gait disturbance (sensory ataxia). In most cases, the abnormal sensation originates in the toes and feet and ascends proximally to the legs in a stocking distribution. Only when the sensation reaches the level of the knee or thigh do symptoms appear in the hands, producing a length-dependent, or stocking-glove, pattern. Paresthesias that begin in one hand suggest an entrapment neuropathy such as carpal tunnel syndrome.

Motor symptoms usually have a later onset than sensory symptoms. In long-standing inherited neuropathies, patients may present with isolated weakness of the feet without sensory symptoms; the ankle jerk, the most distal deep tendon reflex, is invariably absent. When confronted with a length-dependent pattern of sensory symptoms, the diagnosis of a peripheral neuropathy is not difficult. However, in cases with pure motor weakness or wasting, localization may be difficult, and in such cases the presence of distal weakness is helpful in differentiating a peripheral neuropathy from muscle or neuromuscular junction disorders, which typical-

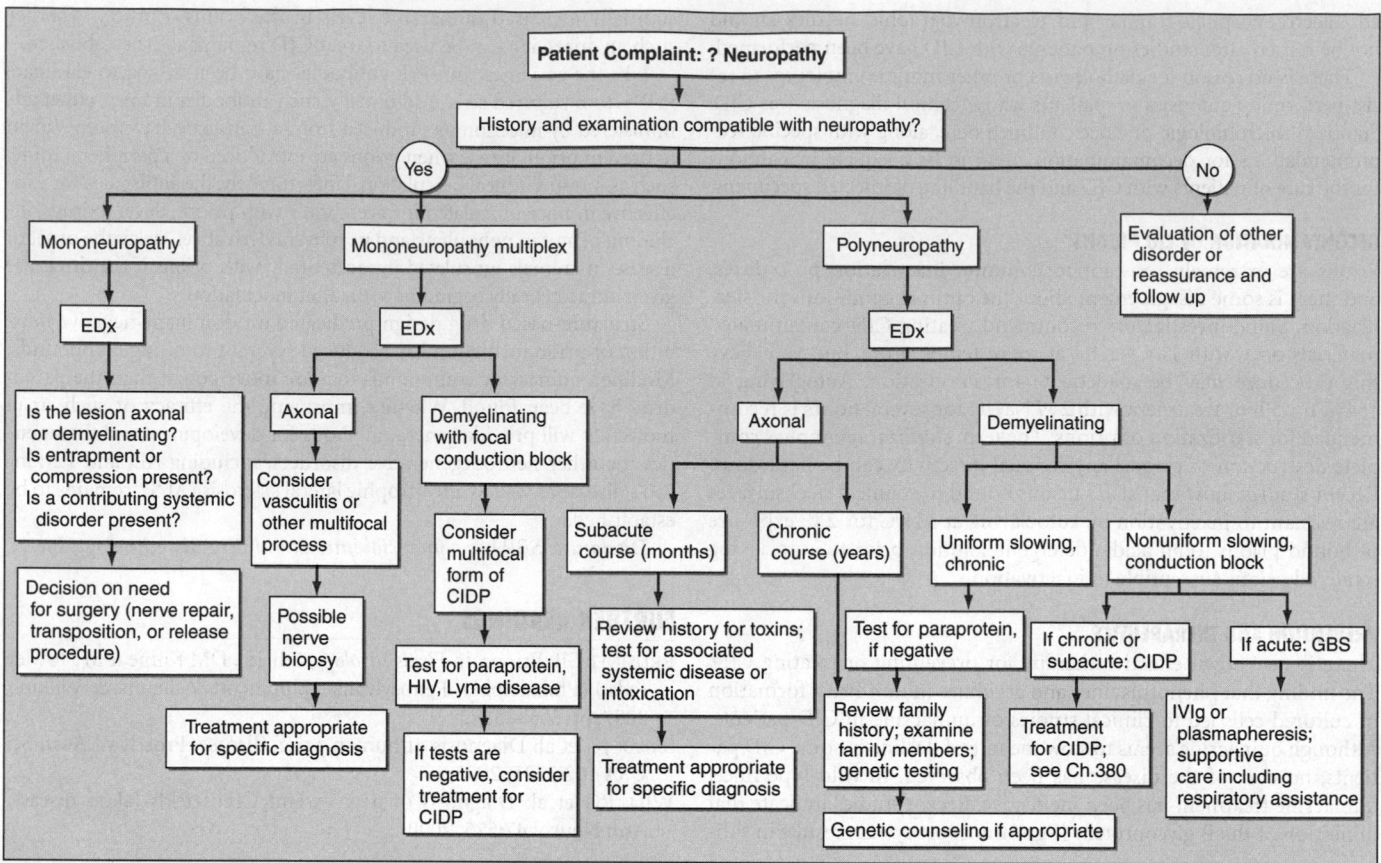

FIGURE 379-1 Approach to the evaluation of peripheral neuropathies. CIDP, chronic inflammatory demyelinating polyradiculoneuropathy; GBS, Guillain-Barré syndrome.

ly present with proximal weakness. Motor neuron disease can also present with distal weakness and wasting; however, the findings are not in the distribution of an individual nerve.

2. *What is its distribution?* Polyneuropathy involves widespread and symmetric dysfunction of the peripheral nerves; mononeuropathy involves a single peripheral nerve; multiple mononeuropathy involves multiple individual peripheral nerves (Table 379-2 and Fig. 379-1). Mononeuropathies are usually due to compression, trauma, or vascular causes. Multiple mononeuropathies (also referred to as mononeuropathy multiplex) can be a result of multiple entrapments, infiltration, or vasculitis. Plexopathies (brachial or lumbosacral) also involve multiple peripheral nerves, in an asymmetric fashion.

3. *Which fibers are affected?* In a polyneuropathy, manifestations can be classified as small-fiber sensory, large-fiber sensory, motor, and/or autonomic (Table 379-3). Often there is overlap, but if there is predominant involvement of one fiber group, the differential diagnosis and evaluation can be narrowed. For example, if a patient has burning pain in the feet, a small-fiber neuropathy is likely and diabetes mellitus is a possible etiology. If a patient has sensory ataxia, large fibers are likely affected and Sjögren's syndrome or a paraneoplastic process should be considered.

4. *What is the anatomic pattern?* Clinical evaluation is often helpful in categorizing a neuropathy as axonal, demyelinating, or neuronal [dorsal root ganglion (DRG)] (Table 379-4). Most axonal neuropathies follow a length-dependent (stocking-glove)

pattern with sensory (small fiber more than large fiber) symptoms and signs predominating over motor manifestations; distal reflexes are absent. In contrast, most demyelinating neuropathies affect motor fibers and sensory fibers (large fiber more than small fiber) equally, and areflexia or hyporeflexia is more generalized. DRG lesions involve purely sensory fibers in a non-length-dependent fashion; sensory ataxia and generalized loss of reflexes are usually found. EDx studies are also important in defining the anatomy of a neuropathy.

TABLE 379-1 SYMPTOMS, SIGNS, AND TESTS IN PERIPHERAL NEUROPATHY

Large Fiber	Small Fiber	Motor	Autonomic
Symptoms			
Numbness "Pins and needles" Tingling Poor balance	Pain: burning, shock-like, stabbing, prickling, shooting, lancinating Allodynia	Cramps Weak grip Footdrop Twitching	Decreased or increased sweating Dry eyes, mouth, Erectile dysfunction Gastroparesis/diarrhea Faintness, light-headedness
Signs			

Decreased
  Vibration
  Joint-position sense
  Reflexes
	Decreased
	  Pin prick
	  Temperature sensation
		Reduced
		  Strength
		  Reflexes
			Orthostasis
			Unequal pupil size

Tests			
NCS-EMG Nerve biopsy LP	Skin biopsy QST Nerve biopsy	NCS-EMG	QSART Tilt table R-R interval Valsalva

Note: NCS-EMG, nerve conduction studies/electromyography; QSART, quantitative sudomotor axon reflex testing; QST, quantitative sensory test; LP, lumbar puncture.

TABLE 379-2 CLASSIFICATION OF NEUROPATHY BY LOCATION

Polyneuropathy
Fairly symmetric
Distal stocking-glove
May or may not be painful
Sensorimotor
Symmetrically decreased
reflexes

Plexopathy
Asymmetric
Painful onset
Multiple nerves in a single limb
Rapid onset of weakness,
atrophy
Isolated reflex loss

Multiple Mononeuropathy
In distribution of single nerve(s)
Setting: diabetes, pressure, vasculitis
May or may not be painful
Isolated reflex loss

Not a Neuropathy
Upper motor neuron signs (brisk
reflexes)
Prominent bladder and bowel
involvement
Unilateral (arm, leg, face) symptoms
Sensory level
Hyperventilation

TABLE 379-3 CLASSIFICATION OF NEUROPATHY BY FIBER TYPE

Small-fiber sensory (painful neuropathies and dissociated sensory loss)
Hereditary sensory neuropathies (early)
Lepromatous leprosy
Diabetic (includes glucose intolerance) small-fiber neuropathy
Amyloidosis
Analphalipoproteinemia (Tangier disease)
Fabry's disease (pain predominates)
Dysautonomia (Riley-Day syndrome)
HIV and antiretroviral therapy neuropathy
Large-fiber sensory (ataxic-neuropathies)
Sjögren's syndrome
Vitamin B_{12} neuropathy (from dorsal column involvement)
Cisplatin neuropathy
Pyridoxine toxicity
Friedreich's ataxia
Small- and large-fiber: Global sensory loss
Carcinomatous sensory neuropathy
Hereditary sensory neuropathies (recessive and dominant)
Diabetic sensory neuropathy
Vacor intoxication
Xanthomatous neuropathy of primary biliary cirrhosis (tabes dorsalis)
Motor-predominant neuropathies
Immune neuropathies: acute (Guillain-Barré syndrome); relapsing
Heritable motor-sensory neuropathies
Acute intermittent porphyria
Diphtheritic neuropathy
Lead neuropathy
Brachial neuritis
Diabetic lumbosacralplexus neuropathy (diabetic amyotrophy)
Autonomic
Acute: Acute pandysautonomic neuropathy, botulism, porphyria, GBS,
vacore, amiodarone, vincristine
Chronic: Amyloid, diabetes, Sjögren's, HSAN I and III (Riley-Day), Chagas,
paraneoplastic

Note: GBS, Guillain-Barré syndrome; HSAN, hereditary sensory and autonomic neuropathy.

5. *What is the time course?* Rapidly evolving peripheral neuropathies are usually inflammatory [Guillain-Barré syndrome (GBS)] or toxic in origin. Subacute evolution suggests an inflammatory, toxic, or nutritional cause (Table 379-5). Chronic neuropathies, especially those that are long-standing over many years, are usually hereditary, such as Charcot-Marie-Tooth (CMT) disease.

6. *What is the likely etiology?* It is helpful to consider potential etiologies by category: metabolic (diabetes mellitus, renal failure, amyloid, porphyria); infectious [HIV, Lyme disease, cytomegalovirus (CMV), syphilis, leprosy, diphtheria]; immune-mediated [GBS, chronic inflammatory demyelinating neuropathy (CIDP), multifocal motor neuropathy, anti-myelin-associated glycoprotein (MAG) neuropathy]; hereditary (CMT); toxic (HIV drugs, anticancer drugs, alcohol, heavy metals, tick bite); vasculitic (polyarteritis nodosa, Churg-Strauss syndrome, cryoglobulinemia, isolated vasculitis of the peripheral nervous system); paraneoplastic (especially lung); nutritional (vitamin B_{12}, B_1, B_6 deficiencies); and miscellaneous causes (celiac disease, Fabry disease, hypothyroidism).

7. *What tests are indicated?* These may include fasting blood glucose and hemoglobin A_{1C} (HbA_{1C}); serum vitamin B_{12}; tests for systemic vasculitis or collagen vascular disease; measurement of neuropathy-associated autoantibodies; urine screen for heavy metals; spinal fluid analysis; autonomic function testing (Chap. 370); and genetic tests for hereditary neuropathies. An impaired glucose tolerance test is found in more than half of patients with idiopathic sensory neuropathy and is more sensitive than tests of fasting glucose or HbA_{1C}. Diagnostic tests to further characterize the neuropathy include quantitative sensory testing, EDx studies, sural nerve biopsy, and muscle biopsy. Diagnostic tests and procedures are more likely to be informative in patients with asymmetric, motor-predominant, rapid-onset or demyelinating neuropathies than in patients with slowly evolving length-dependent sensory > motor types.

8. *What treatment is appropriate?* Treatment of the underlying disorder, pain management, and supportive care to protect and rehabilitate damaged tissue all need to be considered. Examples of therapies directed at the underlying etiology include glycemic control for diabetic neuropathy, vitamin replacement for B_{12} deficiency, immunosuppression for vasculitis, surgery for entrapment neuropathy, enzyme replacement for Fabry disease, liver or bone marrow transplant for amyloid neuropathy, and treatment for immune-mediated neuropathies (Chap. 380).

Pain management usually begins with tricyclic antidepressants (TCAs) such as amitriptyline, imipramine, and desipramine, which can reduce burning, aching, sharp, throbbing, and stinging (Table 379-6; see also Table 12-1). Duloxetine hydrochloride, a dual reuptake inhibitor of serotonin and norepinephrine, is approved for the management of neuropathic pain from diabetes. Tramadol is also effective for painful diabetic neuropathy. Anticonvulsants such as phenytoin, carbamazepine, clonazepam, gabapentin, topiramate, lamotrigine, and pregabalin are effective for lancinating pains. Topical anesthetic agents including lidocaine, mexiletine, and capsaicin creams provide transient relief for focal neuropathic pain. Narcot-

TABLE 379-4 CLASSIFICATION OF NEUROPATHY BY HISTOPATHOLOGY

	Demyelinating	**Axonal**	**Neuronal**
Pattern	Proximal = distal	Distal > proximal; length-dependent	Non-length-dependent; UE, LE, face
Onset	Acute/subacute	Slow evolution	Rapid
Symptoms	Paresthesia and weakness	Dysesthesias and distal weakness	Paresthesias, gait ataxia
Sensory signs	Vibration and proprioception > pain and temperature	Pain and temperature affected > vibration and proprioception	Vibration and proprioception > pain and temperature
Motor	Distal and proximal weakness	Distal weakness	Proprioceptive weakness
DTRs	Areflexia	Distal areflexia	Areflexia
NCS	Velocity affected > amplitude	Amplitudes affected > velocity	Sensory amplitudes affected; radial > sural
Nerve biopsy	Demyelination and remyelination	Axonal degeneration and regeneration	Axonal degeneration but no regeneration
Prognosis	Rapid recovery	Slow recovery	Poor recovery
Causes	GBS, diphtheria, CIDP, DM, MMN	Toxic, metabolic, HIV, CMT2, DM	Sjögren's, cisplatin, pyridoxine

Note: UE, LE, upper, lower extremities; DTRs, deep tendon reflexes; NCS, nerve conduction studies; GBS, Guillain-Barré syndrome; CIDP, chronic inflammatory demyelinating neuropathy; DM, diabetes mellitus; MMN, multifocal motor neuropathy; CMT, Charcot-Marie-Tooth.

TABLE 379-5   CLASSIFICATION OF NEUROPATHY BY TIME COURSE

Acute
  GBS, porphyria, toxic (triorthocresyl phosphate, vacor, thallium), diphtheria, brachial neuritis
Subacute
  Toxic (hexacarbon, acrylamid), angiopathic, nutritional, alcoholic
Chronic
  Diabetic, CIDP, paraneoplastic, paraprotein
Longstanding heritable
  CMT, Friedreich's ataxia
Recurrent
  Relapsing CIDP, porphyria, Refsum's disease, HNPP

Note: GBS, Guillain-Barré syndrome; CIDP, chronic inflammatory demyelinating neuropathy; CMT, Charcot-Marie-Tooth (disease); HNPP, hereditary neuropathy with pressure palsies.

ics may be required for severe cases of refractory neuropathic pain. Treatment of pain is discussed in detail in Chap. 12.

The role of physical therapy, occupational therapy, and assistive devices (such as a foot brace) should not be overlooked. Trophic changes in a denervated/immobile extremity, combined with recurrent, unnoticed, painless trauma, predisposes to skin ulceration, poor healing, tissue resorption, neurogenic arthropathy, and mutilation; amputation may be required. This unfortunate sequence of events is avoidable with proper care of the denervated areas.

ELECTROPHYSIOLOGIC STUDIES (See Chap. e31)

Electrophysiologic studies serve as an extension of the neurologic examination and thus play an important role in the evaluation of pe-

TABLE 379-6   TREATMENT OF PAINFUL NEUROPATHY

First-Line Therapy

Antidepressants
  Tricyclic
    Amitriptyline, nortriptyline, imipramine, desimipramine, doxepin (10–150 mg qd)
  Serotonin-noradrenaline reuptake inhibitors (SNRI)
    Duloxetine (60–120 mg qd)
    Venlafaxine (150–225 mg qd)
Antiepileptics
  Carbamazepine 100–800 mg qd
  Oxcarabazepine 1200–2400 mg qd
  Lamotrigine 200–400 mg qd
  Topiramate 300–400 mg qd
  Gabapentin 900–3600 mg qd
  Pregabalin 150–600 mg qd
  Valproic acid 1000–1200 mg qd

Second-Line Therapy

Opioids
  Oxycodone 40–160 mg qd
  Morphine 90–360 mg qd PO
  Tramadol 50–400 mg qd
  Fentanyl patch 25–75 µg/h q 3 days
Antiarrhythmics
  Mexilitine 600–1200 mg qd
Topical
  Capsaicin 0.075% topical tid or qid
  Lidocaine 5% patch bid
  Isosorbide dinitrate spray 30 mg qhs
Others
  Clonidine 0.1–2.4 mg qd
  Memantine 55 mg qd
  Dextromethorphan 400 mg
  Levodopa 100 mg tid
  Alpha-lipoic acid (thioctic acid) 600 mg
  Spinal cord stimulator
  Transcutaneous electrical nerve stimulation (TENS)
Alternative
  Acupuncture
  Pain psychologist/counselor

ripheral neuropathies (**Chap. e31**). The following information should be obtained from nerve conduction studies and electromyography (NCS-EMG):

1. Is the process axonal or demyelinating? This determination is one of the main goals of an NCS-EMG study since approaches to management and prognosis hinge largely on this distinction. In general, axonal processes affect sensory fibers more than motor fibers, whereas equal involvement is characteristic of most demyelinating processes.
2. Are the findings focal or generalized and are they symmetric or asymmetric?
3. Is this a length-dependent neuropathy? A distal axonopathy generally gives rise to length-dependent findings. The order of nerves affected, as measured by sensory NCS, for example, is sural, followed by ulnar, median, and radial. By contrast, a neuronopathy (or ganglionopathy) may affect the radial nerve before the sural or ulnar nerve.
4. How severe is the lesion? The complete absence of a response may reflect complete loss of fibers or complete conduction block.
5. What is the approximate age of the lesion? In axonal processes, the compound muscle action potential amplitudes are lost early (7 days) compared with sensory amplitudes (10 days). In demyelinating lesions it is often useful to follow progression of findings with serial studies (Chap. 380).
6. Is this a hereditary or acquired neuropathy? A uniform slowing of NCS suggests a hereditary neuropathy, although exceptions exist, such as x-linked CMT and hereditary neuropathy with liability to pressure palsies (HNPP).
7. Is there a subclinical neuropathy? In patients receiving chemotherapy or other potentially neurotoxic drugs, directed examination and limited NCS may help the physician adjust therapy before a significant neuropathy develops.
8. What is the prognosis? For both demyelinating and axonal neuropathies, the degree of axonal loss serves as a guide to prognosis.

It is important to recognize that EDx studies have limitations, and that not all patients with neuropathic symptoms will have informative findings.

MONONEUROPATHIES (Table 379-7)

Mononeuropathy refers to disease or damage of a single nerve. The most common causes are compression, entrapment, and trauma. Extrinsic compression usually occurs when a limb is maintained in a fixed position that produces sustained pressure on the nerve. The neuropathy is often reversible if the position is changed. However, if the patient is unable to move (e.g., during anesthesia or with intoxication), permanent injury can result. Intrinsic factors such as arthritis, fluid retention (pregnancy), amyloid, tumors, and diabetes mellitus may make nerves at entrapment sites more susceptible to injury. Often both extrinsic and intrinsic factors contribute to neuropathy, e.g., an anatomically narrowed region coupled with repetitive activity, poor posture or position. Common entrapment neuropathies include the median nerve at the wrist (carpal tunnel), ulnar nerve at the cubital tunnel or in the ulnar groove, lower trunk of the brachial plexus at the thoracic outlet, common peroneal nerve at the fibular head, posterior tibial nerve at the tarsal tunnel, and lateral femoral cutaneous nerve at the inguinal ligament. Symptoms and signs of various entrapment neuropathies are listed in Table 379-7. Histologic changes of subacute compression consist of a mixture of segmental demyelination and Wallerian degeneration reflecting retrograde axonal injury.

Since most entrapped nerves contain both motor and sensory fibers, both types of symptoms occur, usually in the distribution of the affected nerve. Sensory symptoms may include numbness, pins and needles, tingling, prickling, burning, or electric shock sensations. Light touch is often more affected than pinprick, and subtle sensory abnormalities may be revealed by measuring two-point discrimination. Aching and nondescript pain can also occur proximal to the site of nerve compression. In mild cases, no motor symptoms are evident,

TABLE 379-7 **MONONEUROPATHIES** 2655

	Symptoms	Precipitating Activities	Examination	Electro-Diagnosis	Differential Diagnosis	Treatment
Carpal tunnel syndrome	Numbness, pain or paresthesias in fingers	Sleep or repetitive hand activity	Sensory loss in thumb, second, and third fingers Weakness in thenar muscles; inability to make a circle with thumb and index finger Tinel and Phalen signs	Slowing of sensory and motor conduction across carpal tunnel	C6 radiculopathy	Splint Surgery definitive treatment
Ulnar nerve entrapment at the elbow (UNE)	Numbness or paresthesias in ulnar aspect of hand	Elbow flexion during sleep; elbow resting on desk	Sensory loss in the little finger and ulnar half of ring finger Weakness of the interossei and thumb adductor; claw-hand	Focal slowing of nerve conduction velocity at the elbow	Thoracic outlet syndrome C8-T1 radiculopathy	Elbow pads Avoid further injury Surgery when conservative treatment fails
Ulnar nerve entrapment at the wrist	Numbness or weakness in the ulnar distribution in the hand	Unusual hand activities with tools, bicycling	Like UNE but sensory examination spares dorsum of the hand, and selected hand muscles affected	Prolongation of distal motor latency in the hand	UNE	Avoid precipitating activities
Radial neuropathy at the spiral groove	Wrist drop	Sleeping on arm after inebriation with alcohol—"Saturday night palsy"	Wrist drop with sparing of elbow extension (triceps sparing); finger and thumb extensors paralyzed; sensory loss in radial region of wrist	Early—conduction block along the spiral groove Late—denervation in radial muscles; reduced radial SNAP	Posterior cord lesion; deltoid also weak Posterior interosseous nerve (PIN); isolated finger drop C7 radiculopathy	Splint Spontaneous recovery provided no ongoing injury
Thoracic outlet syndrome	Numbness, paresthesias in medial arm, forearm, hand, and fingers	Lifting heavy objects with the hand	Sensory loss resembles ulnar nerve and motor loss resembles median nerve	Absent ulnar sensory response and reduced median motor response	UNE	Surgery if correctable lesion present
Femoral neuropathy	Buckling of knee, numbness or tingling in thigh/medial leg	Abdominal hysterectomy; lithotomy position; hematoma, diabetes	Wasting and weakness of quadriceps; absent knee jerk; sensory loss in medial thigh and lower leg	EMG of quadriceps, iliopsoas, paraspinal muscles, adductor muscles	L2-4 radiculopathy Lumbar plexopathy	Physiotherapy to strengthen quadriceps and mobilize hip joint Surgery if needed
Obturator neuropathy	Weakness of the leg, thigh numbness	Stretch during hip surgery; pelvic fracture; childbirth	Weakness of hip adductors; sensory loss in upper medial thigh	EMG—denervation limited to hip adductors sparing the quadriceps	L3-4 radiculopathy Lumbar plexopathy	Conservative management Surgery if needed
Meralgia paresthetica	Pain or numbness in the anterior lateral thigh	Standing or walking Recent weight gain	Sensory loss in the pocket of the pant distribution	Sometimes slowing of sensory response can be demonstrated across the inguinal ligament	L2 radiculopathy	Usually resolves spontaneously
Peroneal nerve entrapment at the fibular head	Footdrop	Usually an acute compressive episode identifiable; weight loss	Weak dorsiflexion, eversion of the foot Sensory loss in the anterolateral leg and dorsum of the foot	Focal slowing of nerve conduction across fibular head Denervation in tibialis anterior and peroneus longus muscles	L5 radiculopathy	Foot brace; remove external source of compression
Sciatic neuropathy	Flail foot and numbness in foot	Injection injury; fracture/dislocation of hip; prolonged pressure on hip (comatose patient)	Weakness of hamstring, plantar and dorsiflexion of foot; sensory loss in tibial and peroneal nerve distribution	NCS—abnormal sural, peroneal, and tibial amplitudes EMG—denervation in sciatic nerve distribution sparing glutei and paraspinal	L5-S1 radiculopathies Common peroneal neuropathy (partial sciatic nerve injury) LS plexopathies	Conservative follow up for partial sciatic nerve injuries Brace and physiotherapy Surgical exploration if needed
Tarsal tunnel syndrome	Pain and paresthesias in the sole of the foot but not in the heel	At the end of the day after standing or walking; nocturnal	Sensory loss in the sole of the foot Tinel's sign at tarsal tunnel	Reduced amplitude in sensory or motor components of medial and planter nerves	Polyneuropathy, foot deformity, poor circulation	Surgery if no external cause identified

but in more affected patients, weakness, wasting, or fasciculations may occur. Knowledge of the anatomy of individual nerves is important to be able to localize the site of the lesion to the root, plexus, or nerves or their branches. Sensory testing may occasionally provoke paresthesias. Reflexes are generally unaffected since most entrapped nerves are distal to the deep tendon reflexes typically examined. Percussion of the nerve at the affected site may induce paresthesias (Tinel's sign); however, this may also occur in normal individuals and is not a reliable sign. Placing the limb in a posture known to aggravate the compression may accentuate symptoms (e.g., Phalen's sign evoked by flexing the wrist for carpal tunnel syndrome).

EDx studies confirm the clinical diagnosis and provide information about location, severity, and prognosis. Focal demyelination is detected as a focally reduced nerve conduction velocity along the length of the sensory and/or motor fibers. Wallerian degeneration is reflected in a reduction of distal amplitudes and as denervation potentials. The latter is associated with a relatively poor prognosis for recovery. Bone or joint abnormalities and soft tissue masses can be revealed by appropriate imaging techniques. MR neurography and ultrasonography are useful in identifying thickening of nerves at sites of compression; these studies are useful for proximal entrapments (brachial plexus, lumbosacral plexus, or sciatic or gluteal nerve lesions).

℞ MONONEUROPATHIES

Treatment for acute and subacute compressive neuropathies consists of identifying and removing extrinsic contributors and the use of splints to avoid further compression. In patients with chronic compressive neuropathies, exacerbating factors should be identified and treated before surgical correction is considered. The use of splints, a change of work habits to avoid activities or movements that precipitate the neuropathy, or anti-inflammatory medication for tenosynovitis may be helpful (see below).

Surgical treatment may be required for management of chronic compressive neuropathies when conservative measures have failed and the site of entrapment is clearly delineated.

MONONEUROPATHY MULTIPLEX

Mononeuropathy multiplex refers to the multifocal involvement of individual peripheral nerves. Although multiple compressive neuropathies can present in this manner, more often an inflammatory cause is responsible, and in such cases the disorder is referred to as *mononeuritis multiplex*. Both systemic (67%) and nonsystemic (33%) vasculitis may present as mononeuritis multiplex; less commonly, vasculitic neuropathy can present as an asymmetric or distal symmetric neuropathy. Among the systemic vasculitides, polyarteritis nodosa, rheumatoid arthritis, systemic lupus erythematosus (SLE), Churg-Strauss syndrome, Wegener's granulomatosis, and hypersensitivity vasculitis should be considered; these are often associated with constitutional symptoms such as fever and weight loss (Chap. 319). The common fibular nerve (previously called the common peroneal nerve) is affected in ~75% of patients with vasculitic neuropathy; symptoms consist of a painful foot drop. The ulnar, median, and radial nerves may also be involved.

℞ MONONEURITIS MULTIPLEX

Therapy of the necrotizing systemic vasculitides can stabilize and in some cases improve the neuropathy. Glucocorticoids [prednisone (1.5 mg/kg per day)] plus a cytotoxic agent (usually oral cyclophosphamide at 2 mg/kg per day) is the treatment of choice (Chap. 319). Aggressive therapy is warranted since the prognosis for survival of untreated patients is poor. Prednisone can be changed to an alternate-day regimen after 1 month to minimize side effects. Once a clinical response is documented, prednisone may be tapered by 5 mg every 2–4 weeks. The cytotoxic agent is usually continued for 1 year. Therapy of hypersensitivity vasculitis is focused primarily upon removal of the offending antigen trigger. Treatment of localized vasculitis restricted to the peripheral nervous system can be less aggressive than for systemic vasculitis because the risk of death from untreated disease is very low. Monotherapy with either oral glucocorticoids or a brief course of cyclophosphamide (3–6 months) may be sufficient. A tissue diagnosis of vasculitis should be obtained before initiating therapy; a positive nerve biopsy helps to justify long-term immunosuppressive treatment, and pathologic confirmation of the diagnosis is often difficult after treatment has commenced.

POLYNEUROPATHIES

DIABETIC NEUROPATHY

Diabetes mellitus is associated with various neuropathy syndromes that differ in their etiology, natural history, and treatment. The overall prevalence of neuropathy is 66% for type 1 and 59% for type 2 diabetes. Neuropathy can be broadly divided into symmetric and asymmetric types, although a great deal of overlap exists between these categories. Symmetric neuropathies may present as small-fiber in-

volvement (e.g., dysesthesias in the feet) or autonomic dysfunction (e.g., sexual impotence), but often both occur together; examination usually reveals additional evidence of large-fiber involvement and of an underlying generalized neuropathy.

The asymmetric neuropathies are divided into those with acute onset and those with gradual onset. Asymmetric abrupt-onset neuropathies include diabetic truncal radiculoneuropathy (DTRN), diabetic lumbosacral radiculoplexus neuropathy (DLSRPN), and oculomotor (third or sixth nerve) neuropathy. These monophasic conditions are thought to be due to vascular causes such as infarction. Neuropathies of more gradual onset are usually caused by entrapment or compression and include median neuropathy at the wrist, ulnar neuropathy at the elbow, peroneal neuropathy at the fibular head, and lateral cutaneous neuropathy at the thigh at the inguinal ligament (meralgia paresthetica).

Symmetric Diabetic Neuropathy   By far the most common form of diabetic neuropathy is a length-dependent diabetic sensorimotor polyneuropathy (DSPN). The lifetime prevalence is ~55% for type 1 and 45% for type 2 diabetes. DSPN is a mixed neuropathy with small- and large-fiber sensory, autonomic, and motor nerve involvement in various combinations, although sensory and autonomic symptoms are more prominent than motor ones (Table 379-1). Proposed criteria for the diagnosis of DSPN are two or more of the following: symptoms or signs of neuropathy, abnormal EDx studies, quantitative sensation test abnormalities, heart rate decrease with deep breathing or Valsalva maneuver.

DSPN has an insidious, progressive course. Initial symptoms may consist of numbness, tingling, buzzing, burning, or prickling sensation affecting the toes and feet. Paresthesias ascend up to the legs and then hands in a stocking-glove distribution. Over time, gait disturbance and distal weakness may occur. Painful or insensitive extremities predispose to foot ulcers; amputation is sometimes required. Examination shows a distal sensory loss to pin, temperature, touch, and vibration sense. Ankle reflexes are invariably reduced or absent. Weakness, if present, is mild and involves toe flexors and extensors. The length-dependent pattern of neuropathy is evident in the stocking-glove sensory loss, and some patients also show sensory loss in the anterior abdominal region in a wedge-shaped distribution. Autonomic symptoms including impotence, nocturnal diarrhea, difficulty voiding, abnormalities of sweating, and abnormal fullness after eating and orthostatic hypotension may be present.

The diagnosis of DSPN is usually straightforward, although other contributors to the neuropathy should be excluded, including nutritional (vitamins B_1 and B_{12} and folate deficiencies), toxic (alcohol, vitamin B_6 toxicity), immune-mediated (paraprotein), and inherited causes. An alternative diagnosis should be sought in patients with rapidly progressive or asymmetric weakness, a family history of neuropathy, exposure to toxins, or prior malignancy. A glucose tolerance test is indicated in all patients presenting with neuropathy. EDx studies show mixed findings of axonal loss and demyelination in a length-dependent pattern. Nerve biopsy and lumbar puncture are not necessary unless alternative diagnoses are being considered.

Various hypotheses have been invoked to account for DSPN. Increased neuronal concentrations of glucose induce the conversion of glucose to sorbitol by aldose reductase using NADPH as a coenzyme. Sorbitol decreases levels of *myo*-inositol and phosphoinositides, leading to a decrease in diacylglycerol, protein kinase C, and Na^+, K^+, ATPase activity. This sequence of events leads to axonal loss and demyelination and is the basis of trials using aldose reductase inhibitors and high *myo*-inositol diets. A second hypothesis proposes insufficient blood flow: increased aldose reductase activity results in competitive inhibition of nitric oxide synthetase for NADPH, resulting in decreased nitric oxide and reduced blood flow in the vasa nervorum. Altered metabolism of fatty acids, reduced concentrations of nerve growth factor, and oxidative stress are possible additional contributing factors.

℞ DIABETIC SENSORIMOTOR POLYNEUROPATHY

Treatment consists of strict glucose control, which prevents the neuropathy from worsening; established neuropathy does not usually reverse. Aldose reductase inhibitors to treat and prevent diabetic neuropathy have been studied in >30 trials. Although controlled trials of the aldose reductase inhibitors sorbinol and tolrestat were found to improve electrophysiologic or morphometric markers of DSPN, any clinically meaningful improvement in pain or sensation has been inconsistent. Treatment with recombinant nerve growth factor was ineffective. Alpha lipoic acid (thioctic acid), an antioxidant, has been shown to improve experimental diabetic neuropathy, and a meta-analysis of clinical trials suggested that the treatment (600 mg/d IV for 3 weeks) is safe and improves symptoms and signs of neuropathy. Pancreatic transplantation can halt progression of DSPN but is a realistic therapy only for patients who have renal failure and are undergoing combined kidney and pancreas transplantation.

Glycemic control is essential for the prevention of diabetic autonomic neuropathy. Once neuropathy is established, few effective treatments exist.

Asymmetric Diabetic Neuropathy · *CRANIAL NEUROPATHIES* The
oculomotor nerves (in decreasing order of frequency the sixth, third, and rarely fourth nerves) are most often affected. In general, cranial neuropathy occurs in patients over the age of 50 who already have evidence of DSPN. Abducens (sixth) nerve palsy manifests as the sudden onset of painless double vision, and examination shows paralysis of abduction on the affected side (Chap. 29). In a patient with diabetes who has no other clinical findings the diagnosis is straightforward. Spontaneous recovery typically occurs within 3–5 months and no treatment except an eye patch or prism is necessary. Diabetic third nerve palsy is also abrupt in onset but is often heralded by intense retroorbital pain that may be present for several days. Symptoms include double vision, unilateral ptosis, and restriction of medial gaze and upgaze. Unlike compressive etiologies (e.g., aneurysms of the superior cerebellar or posterior communicating arteries), which present with an enlarged ("blown") pupil, the pupil is nearly always spared in diabetic third nerve palsy. This is due to the fact that pupillomotor fibers are present on the outer layers of the third nerve fascicle, and an ischemic lesion tends to involve the center of the fascicle. In atypical cases, such as those with pupillary involvement or without pain, a neuroimaging study, usually MRI or MR angiography (MRA), is indicated to exclude an aneurysm. Most patients improve spontaneously in 3–6 months without any treatment. Symptomatic treatment with eye prisms is often helpful. Idiopathic neuropathy of the facial nerve (seventh; Bell's palsy) is also more common in older diabetics than in nondiabetics. The clinical features and prognosis are similar to the nondiabetic form (Chap. 371).

LIMB MONONEUROPATHIES Diabetics are also susceptible to entrapment neuropathies, including median neuropathy at the wrist (carpal tunnel syndrome), ulnar neuropathy at the elbow, fibular (peroneal) neuropathy at the fibular head, and lateral cutaneous neuropathy at the inguinal ligament (meralgia paresthetica). The special susceptibility of diabetic nerves may be related to endoneurial edema and vascular factors. Patients typically present with several weeks or months of pain, numbness, or weakness in the distribution of the affected nerve. The approach to these entrapments is similar to that in individuals without diabetes. Decompressive surgery may be needed if there is associated weakness, numbness, or pain in the distribution of the affected nerves and if no reversible extrinsic source of compression (position/habits) can be identified.

RADICULOPATHIES AND PLEXOPATHIES *Diabetic truncal radiculoneuropathy* occurs in diabetics in middle or later life, usually in association with underlying DSPN. Patients present with an abrupt onset, typically over days to weeks, of severe pain in the thoracic spine, flank, rib cage, or upper abdomen. The pain is described as burning, stabbing, or belt-like. Contact hyperesthesia is present in the area of pain. Associated, sometimes profound, weight loss is often described; this can also be seen in diabetic amyotrophy (see below). Examination may be normal or may reveal variable sensory loss in the distribution of one or several intercostal nerves and their branches. Anterior abdominal wall weakness may be noted as focal bulging of the weakened region when the patient attempts to sit up. A needle EMG of the affected muscles may

confirm denervation in the abdominal or intercostal muscles; the paraspinal muscles may be spared. This finding, and a reduced fiber density measured by skin biopsy from symptomatic regions, suggests that the injury in diabetic truncal radiculoneuropathy is at, or distal to, the sensory ganglion. The differential diagnosis in this elderly population should include herpes zoster infection (without rash) and an abdominal malignancy. Most patients improve spontaneously, although the pain may persist for weeks to months. Pain management may be difficult and includes topical capsaicin and narcotics. The abrupt onset and spontaneous recovery suggest a vascular cause to this syndrome, although an inflammatory etiology can not be excluded.

Diabetic amyotrophy (femoral neuropathy; proximal diabetic neuropathy) occurs in older patients, usually with type 2 diabetes. Patients present with the abrupt onset of severe pain affecting the anterior thigh. Buttock and lower back pain may also be present. The pain is worse at night and is described as burning. Weakness and wasting in the thigh muscles leads to difficulty climbing stairs and walking. Males are more likely to be affected, and weight loss, at times dramatic, is invariably present. Although symptoms may be bilateral, one side is more severely affected than the other. Examination shows prominent wasting of the quadriceps muscle unilaterally with weakness of the knee extensor and hip flexor and, variably, ankle dorsiflexor, accompanied by sensory loss in the thigh and leg in the distribution of the femoral nerve, and a reduced knee jerk on the affected side. The syndrome progresses over weeks to months, then stabilizes and gradually improves. EDx studies show findings of radiculopathy (L2-4), lumbar plexopathy, or femoral neuropathy along with a distal sensorimotor neuropathy. An MRI of the lumbosacral spine and plexus is indicated to exclude a compressive cause. Cerebrospinal fluid (CSF) examination and nerve biopsy should be considered whenever the diagnosis is uncertain. The level of CSF protein is often elevated, and biopsy of the intermediate femoral cutaneous nerve may show microvasculitis. The condition may be quite painful and require opiates for pain control. Treatment with high-dose glucocorticoids or intravenous immunoglobulin (IVIg) has been effective in case reports, although controlled trials have not shown clear benefit. Physiotherapy and orthotic devices are helpful. The prognosis is generally favorable; improvement occurs over several months in most patients treated with symptomatic measures only. A similar condition may also occur in nondiabetic patients.

Uncommon Diabetic Neuropathies *Diabetic neuropathic cachexia* (acute painful neuropathy of diabetes) is an uncommon painful sensory neuropathy occurring in type 1 diabetics in the setting of poor glucose control and weight loss. Manifestations include severe pain in the feet ascending up to the legs and trunk with associated allodynia. Examination may reveal distal sensory loss to pinprick and vibration and reduced or absent ankle jerks. Strength is preserved. EDx studies may show a distal neuropathy. Unlike DSPN, the prognosis is favorable with glucose control. The painful symptoms reverse over months to a year.

Insulin neuritis describes a painful neuropathy seen with initiation of insulin treatment for diabetes. The clinical presentation is similar to the acute painful neuropathy of diabetes, and most patients improve.

A reversible sensory and motor polyneuropathy has been reported in association with diabetic ketoacidosis. Most patients also have upper and lower motor neuron signs, as well as a preexisting neuropathy. The etiology is not clear; critical illness neuropathy may be the underlying cause. Finally, chronic inflammatory demyelinating neuropathy (CIDP) occurs in diabetics; the disease resembles that seen in nondiabetics.

TOXIC INCLUDING CHEMOTHERAPY-INDUCED NEUROPATHIES
Most toxic neuropathies are distal axonal degenerations that develop gradually over time. The causes are varied, including drugs, heavy metals, and industrial and environmental substances (Table 379-8). Novel anticancer drugs and antiretroviral agents are the most common drugs implicated, although over-the-counter medications (especially pyridoxine) can also cause neuropathy. A temporal relationship between introduction of the toxic substance and the onset of neuropathy is usually noted, as is a dose-response relationship. In general, a

TABLE 379-8 TOXIC NEUROPATHIES

	Circumstances of Toxicity	Neuropathy	Comments
Axonopathy			
Nonpharmaceutical toxins			
Acrylamide monomer	Flocculators, grouting agents	Sensory ataxia; large fiber	Numbness, excessive sweating, exfoliative dermatitis
Allyl chloride	Epoxy resin, glycerin	Dysesthesia and distal weakness	
Arsenic (inorganic)	Copper/lead smelting, contaminant in recreational drugs, suicide/homicide (herbicide/insecticide)	S > M; painful; usually subacute or chronic; may be acute following large doses	Skin: hyperkeratosis, "rain-drop" pigmentation of skin, Mees' line in nails
Carbon disulphide	Viscose rayon, cellophane; airborne industrial exposure	SM	Slow NCS
Dimethylaminopropio-nitrile (DMAPN)	Polyurethane foam	SM	Small-fiber neuropathy with prominent bladder symptoms and impotence
Ethylene oxide	Sterilization of biomedicals		
Hexacarbons (paranodal giant axonal)	Solvents, adhesives Substance abuse (glues and thinners)	SM	Neurofilament swelling of axons; CNS
Lead	Batteries, smelting metal ores, paints	M > S; wrist drop	Burton's line, anemia, basophilic stippling
Mercury (inorganic)	Environmental/workplace	CNS > PNS; neuropathy uncommon	Tremor, insomnia, behavioral change
Methyl bromide	Fumigant, insecticide, refrigerant, fire extinguisher	Variable recovery	Encephalitis, ataxia
Organophosphorus esters	Insecticide, petroleum, plastics	SM	Acute toxicity presents as cholinergic crisis
Thallium (rat poison)	Rodenticides, insecticides	Painful SM	Thallium (alopecia, Mees' line, hyperkeratosis)
Vacor	Rodenticide, suicide	Rapid onset of severe axonopathy and autonomic dysfunction	Diabetic ketoacidosis a feature of acute toxicity
Pharmaceutical agents			
Chloramphenicol	Mean cumulative dose 255 g, duration	S > M	Also optic neuropathy
Colchicine	Chronic dosing at 1.2 mg/d especially in the presence of renal dysfunction	Distal paresthesias and proximal weakness	Also myopathy with elevated serum CK
Dapsone	200–400 mg/d over many months	Pure motor, especially upper limbs	May look like motor neuron disease
Disulfiram	250–500 mg/d after several months used for alcoholism	SM	Difficult to distinguish from alcohol neuropathy
Ethambutol	>20 mg/kg per day over many months	Sensory neuropathy	Also optic neuropathy
Ethionamide	>15 mg/kg	Sensory neuropathy	Limited by GI, dermatologic and CNS side effects
Gold	Controversial, as rheumatoid arthritis can cause neuropathy Not dose dependent	S > M with myokymia	Rash, pruritus
Isoniazid	>5 mg/kg over weeks or about 6 months, depending on acetylator status	Dose-dependent SM neuropathy	Add pyridoxine 50 mg/d when using INH
Metronidazole	Cumulative dose > 30 g	Sensory (small and large fiber)	
Misonidazole	Cumulative dose > 18 g/m²	Sensory axonopathy	Dose-limiting side effect
Nitrofurantoin	Standard dose of 200 mg/day over a few weeks	Mild SM neuropathy	
Nitrous oxide	Dental surgery, anesthesia, substance abuse	S >> M	Toxic myeloneuropathy resembles cobalamin deficiency
Nucleoside analogues (ddC, ddI, 4dT)	>12.5 mg/kg per day for ddI, 0.02 mg/kg per day for ddC, and 0.5 mg/kg per day for 4dT	Painful sensory neuropathy	Difficult to distinguish from HIV neuropathy
Pyridoxine	>200 mg a day over several months	Length-dependent axonopathy	Neuronopathy at higher doses
Suramin	Peak serum concentration of 350 μg/mL	S > M; may be demyelinating	
Taxol	Cumulative dose of >1500 mg/m²	S > M	Higher single doses may cause neuronopathy
Thalidomide	100 mg/d for 6 months.	S > M	Thalidomide (brittle nails, palmar erythema)
Vincristine and other vinca alkaloids	Almost all patients	S > M but autonomic fibers also affected	Vacuolar myopathy
Myelinopathy			
Amiodarone	400 mg/day for 6–36 months, serum concentration of 2.4 mg/L	SM; dose-dependent	Tremor
Perhexiline	Not dose-related	S (large fiber) and M, facial, autonomic	Hepatic toxicity
Polychlorinated biphenyls	Plasticizers, electrical insulators	SM	Acne, brown nails
Suramin	Not dose-related	?Demyelinating like subacute GBS	
Trichloroethylene	Dry-cleaning, rubber, degreasing agent	Mainly cranial nerves: trigeminal, facial, oculomotor, optic	Limbs rarely affected
Sensory Neuronopathy			
Platinum compounds, e.g., cisplatin	Cumulative dose more than 900 mg/m²	Large-fiber sensory	Irreversible
High-dose pyridoxine	Massive parenteral doses in grams over days	Sensory neuronopathy; gait ataxia, pseudoathetosis	May be irreversible
Taxol	Single dose of ≥250 mg/m²	Sensory ataxia	May be irreversible

Note: S, sensory; M, motor; SM, sensorimotor; NCS, nerve conduction studies; CNS/PNS, central/peripheral nervous system; CK, creatine kinase; GI, gastrointestinal; GBS, Guillain- Barré syndrome; EDx, electrodiagnosis; CSF, cerebrospinal fluid; CMV, cytomegalovirus; DSPN, diabetic sensory polyneuropathy.

lower dose over a longer period of time is less toxic than a higher dose for a short period, even if the eventual cumulative doses are similar. Onset following introduction of the agent and reversal or at least arrest following its removal provide the best evidence of a toxic neuropathy, along with the symptoms and signs typically caused by the suspected agent. The neuropathy may first manifest or may continue to progress after discontinuing the substance; this phenomenon, known as *coasting*, is seen with the platinum cancer drugs, hexacarbons, nucleoside analogue reverse transcriptase inhibitors, and pyridoxine.

Clinical evaluation includes a history focusing on the temporal relationship between exposure and onset of sensory or motor symptoms, comorbid diseases that may cause neuropathy, and symptoms of systemic toxicity. Nerve biopsy occasionally demonstrates pathognomonic features such as osmiophillic Schwann cell inclusions in amiodarone, perhexiline and chloroquine neuropathies, and paranodal giant axonal swellings in hexacarbon neuropathies. Levels of some toxins can be measured in certain tissues: heavy metals such as lead, arsenic, and thallium can be measured in urine; arsenic can be measured in hair or nails. Blood levels of drugs are also useful.

Table 379-8 lists some of the better-documented neurotoxic substances. Awareness of the types of industries in which toxic exposure can occur is important in identifying occupational exposure. Lower dosages and shorter durations of exposure may produce neuropathy in susceptible individuals such as those with underlying inherited neuropathy. An acute onset of neuropathy occurs with drugs such as paclitaxel, suramin, and vacor, and with biologic agents such as ciguatera, puffer fish (tetrodotoxin), and buckthorn. Some toxic agents that otherwise require long-term exposure to produce chronic neuropathy may do so acutely when used at higher doses; examples include arsenic, thallium, and pyridoxine. The combination of two toxic drugs, commonly seen with anticancer therapy (e.g., paclitaxel and cisplatin), may produce greater nerve toxicity than either one alone. Patients with underlying conditions may be predisposed to neuropathy when exposed to some compounds, e.g., vitamin B_{12}–deficient patients who receive nitrous oxide anesthesia, or patients with porphyria who receive barbiturates. Usually, however, toxic neuropathy is subacute in onset, developing over a period of months. Vincristine, amiodarone, nitrofurantoin, isoniazid, dimethylaminopropionitrile (DMAPN), inorganic mercury, and thallium all cause a subacute neuropathy. The insidious onset of a chronic neuropathy occurs with exposure to industrial toxins at low dosages over a prolonged period of time. Examples include acrylamide, allyl chloride, hexacarbons, carbon disulfide, ethylene oxide, lead, and arsenic. In addition to preexisting neuropathy, other host factors, including diabetes, hepatic or renal impairment, and alcohol abuse, may reduce the threshold for neurotoxicity. The neuropathy may be predominantly motor with lead, inorganic mercury, organophosphates, buckthorn, dapsone, and vincristine; small-fiber sensory with DMAPN, thallium, nucleoside analogue reverse transcriptase inhibitors (dideoxycytidine ddC, dideoxyinosine ddI, stavudine d4T), ethionamide, metronidazole, and taxane; or large-fiber sensory with cisplatin, high doses of taxol, pyridoxine, or acrylamide. Autonomic dysfunction can occur with vincristine, vacor, perhexiline, high dose-pyridoxine, and platinum. Other toxins that may involve autonomic nerves include acrylamide (acral and pedal hyperhidrosis), DMAPN (urologic and sexual dysfunction), and hexacarbons (hyperhidrosis and impotence). Some toxic neuropathies also involve the cranial nerves. These include trichloroethylene, which causes acute dysfunction of the cranial nerves V, VII, III, and II; thallium and acute fulminant vacor poisonings, which cause facial diplegia with generalized neuropathy resembling Guillain-Barré syndrome; perhexiline, which causes facial diplegia and perioral numbness; vincristine and paclitaxel, which may be associated with numbness in the trigeminal nerve distribution; and chloramphenicol, ethambutol, and nitrous oxide, all of which may cause optic neuropathy. Asymmetric neuropathy or mononeuritis multiplex is rare but may be seen with lead, which may cause unilateral wrist drop; or with DMAPN, which causes sacral dermatomal sensory loss. Signs of toxicity to kidney, liver, or other organs can in some cases alert the clinician to the possibility that a neuropathy could be toxic in origin.

Cisplatin Cisplatin (*cis*-diaminodichloroplatinum) is a heavy metal used to treat a variety of solid tumors. Cisplatin is toxic to dorsal root ganglia neurons, producing a dose-related large-fiber sensory neuropathy (*neuronopathy*). It also injures hair cells of the cochlea, causing hearing loss. Peripheral neuropathy is the dose-limiting toxicity of cisplatin. A cumulative cisplatin dose of at least 300 mg/m^2 may lead to paresthesias in the extremities and numbness. Lhermitte's sign, an electric shock–like sensation evoked by flexion of the neck, may occur due to retrograde degeneration of axons in the posterior columns of the spinal cord. Patients with preexisting neuropathy and those who receive combination chemotherapy may develop symptoms after lower cumulative doses. Sensory ataxia may be disabling in patients who have severe neuropathy. Small-fiber sensation (e.g., pain and temperature) and strength are generally spared.

Oxaliplatin Oxaliplatin can cause an early acute and a late chronic neuropathy. The acute neuropathy begins during the infusion, within minutes to hours, or within 1–2 days of administration. Patients complain of paresthesias in the hands or feet, mouth, or throat along with myalgias, cramps, or stiffness. Shortness of breath or difficulty swallowing may occur. Symptoms are often triggered by exposure to cold. Neuromyotonia may be seen on EMG. Although this acute toxicity occurs in >90% of patients, it is often self-limited and resolves within days. A channelopathy is thought to be the underlying mechanism. A chronic large-fiber ataxic neuropathy, similar to that caused by cisplatin, occurs with cumulative doses ≥ 780 mg/m^2, generally after eight or nine treatment cycles. Even though the signs and symptoms (paresthesias, distal sensory loss, and loss of reflexes) are similar to those caused by cisplatin, oxaliplatin neuropathy is more likely to be reversible.

Paclitaxel Paclitaxel, a diterpene alkaloid drug, is widely used as a chemotherapeutic agent. Peripheral neuropathy, which can be severe, is the dose-limiting toxicity. A symmetric, length-dependent neuropathy with prominent sensory (large more than small fiber) and minor motor manifestations, is typically present. Preexisting neuropathy is a risk factor. The neuropathy is dose-dependent, and both single and cumulative doses are important. The drug affects microtubule assembly, causing disruption of axonal transport and a "dying back" axonal neuropathy.

Vincristine Vincristine, an alkaloid derived from the perinwinkle plant, vinca rosea, causes a dose-dependent sensorimotor neuropathy. Lower cumulative doses (4–19 mg) cause only reflex changes, while higher doses progressively cause paresthesias, sensory loss (upper extremity more than lower), weakness with footdrop, and hand weakness and clumsiness. Autonomic neuropathy can manifest as cardiac arrhythmias, orthostasis, urinary bladder dysfunction, constipation, or paralytic ileus. Cranial neuropathies have also been described.

Suramin Suramin is a polysulfonated naphthylurea that has been used as an antineoplastic agent and as a treatment for certain parasitic diseases. Suramin causes a length-dependent distal axonal neuropathy in over half of patients and a subacute inflammatory demyelinating neuropathy in ~15% of patients. Neuropathy occurs with peak plasma concentrations > 300 μg/mL.

Thalidomide Peripheral neuropathy remains the dose-limiting toxicity of thalidomide, which causes a length-dependent painful sensory axonal neuropathy; a sensory neuronopathy has also been reported. Peripheral neuropathy occurs in up to 75% of patients and is dose-dependent, rarely occurring with cumulative doses < 20 g, but invariably noted at cumulative doses > 100 g. The risk of neuropathy is minimized at doses ≤ 150 mg/d. Serial sensory action potential measurements are important in the early detection of the neuropathy. Symptoms often, though not always, improve with cessation or dose reduction. The neuropathy develops at a lower dose and is typically more severe in patients with a preexisting diabetic neuropathy.

Bortezomib Bortezomib (Velcade), a novel proteosome inhibitor used in the treatment of multiple myeloma, induces a length-dependent, sensory more than motor, axonal polyneuropathy that is dose-dependent, increasing with increasing cycles of treatment. Both small- and large-fiber sensory symptoms occur. In a few patients the symptoms stabilize or improve after stopping treatment. A toxic acquired demyelinating neuropathy has also been reported.

Rx TOXIC NEUROPATHIES

Removal of the toxic substance is the most important step. Specific treatments are available for some toxic neuropathies. Treatment for heavy metal toxicity includes chelation therapy: penicillamine or calcium-EDTA for lead toxicity; penicillamine or British anti-Lewisite (BAL) for arsenic toxicity; and potassium chloride or Prussian blue for thallium toxicity. Pyridoxine (10–50 mg/d) can be used to prevent and treat isoniazid neurotoxicity. Niacin and pyridoxine are recommended for ethionamide neurotoxicity. There may be some benefit from the use of neuroprotective agents. Vitamin E (tocopherol) was reported to be neuroprotective in one small, unblinded study, but these results have not been confirmed. Org 2766, glutathione, diethyldithiocarbamate, and amifostine have also been tried without conclusive outcomes. Studies are under way to evaluate the possible efficacy of nerve growth factor.

Prognosis for recovery depends on both the site of pathology and the severity of the neuropathy. Involvement of the dorsal root ganglion is associated with a poor prognosis. Severe axonopathy requires years for recovery. Demyelinating disorders, if detected early, generally are associated with a relatively rapid recovery. Most toxic neuropathies, even if advanced, will at least stabilize, and some will improve, when exposure to the toxic agent is stopped.

NUTRITIONAL NEUROPATHIES
(See also Chap. 71)

Thiamine (Vitamin B₁) (Dry Beriberi) Thiamine deficiency can be a result of inadequate intake, as may occur in alcoholism, anorexia, intentional dieting, starvation, or bulimia. Protracted vomiting, e.g., in patients receiving chemotherapy or in pregnant women with hyperemesis gravidarum, may also cause thiamine deficiency. Neuropathy from thiamine deficiency presents as the acute or subacute onset of paresthesias, dysesthesias, and mild weakness in the legs. On examination a stocking-glove sensory loss, distal weakness in the legs, and loss of ankle jerks is typical. Nerve conduction tests and sural nerve biopsies show axonal degeneration. Erythrocyte transketolase activity is reduced in the blood. Treatment consists of oral thiamine replacement, 100 mg/d. Alcohol-induced neuropathy develops in some patients without any identifiable nutritional deficiencies, suggesting that alcohol itself may cause sensory neuropathy. It predominantly affects small fibers and is painful, but there is considerable overlap with thiamine deficiency neuropathy.

Pyridoxine (Vitamin B₆) A subacute length-dependent axonal neuropathy occurs as a result of pyridoxine deficiency. Causes include dietary deficiency and drugs such as isoniazid, cycloserine, and penicillamine, which act as pyridoxine antagonists by combining to the aldehyde moiety of the vitamin. Dietary deficiency of pyridoxine is uncommon, although the requirement is increased in pregnancy. Measurement of xanthurenic acid after tryptophan loading can help confirm the diagnosis. Treatment consists of oral pyridoxine, 30 mg/d. Pyridoxine supplements are recommended for prophylaxis during pregnancy and for patients taking isoniazid. Overzealous treatment with pyridoxine should be avoided, as high doses of pyridoxine cause a toxic sensory neuronopathy.

Vitamin B₁₂ (Cobalamin) Peripheral neuropathy is a minor part of the vitamin B₁₂ deficiency syndrome; subacute combined degeneration of the spinal cord is more prominent. Distal sensory loss predominantly involving large-fiber modalities, dysequilibrium, Lhermitte's sign, and the combination of an absent ankle jerk and upgoing toe may be present. Pancytopenia, megaloblastic anemia, and glossitis are other signs. The principal dietary sources of vitamin B₁₂ are meat and dairy products; enteric processing and absorption typically occur in the terminal ileum. Common causes of vitamin B₁₂ deficiency include inadequate intake, malabsorption (including post-gastrectomy), and pernicious anemia. Borderline vitamin B₁₂ deficiency may develop after exposure to nitrous oxide during anesthesia or with chronic recreational use. Diagnosis of vitamin B₁₂ deficiency is made by low serum cobalamin levels and raised levels of methylmalonic acid and homocysteine. Autoantibodies to intrinsic factor and gastric parietal cells are present in pernicious anemia. Treatment is with parenteral administration of cobalamin (vitamin B₁₂) (see Chap. 100).

Riboflavin, Nicotinic Acid and Other B-Group Vitamins Riboflavin and nicotinic acid deficiencies have been incriminated in neuropathies, usually in association with deficiencies of other water-soluble vitamins. Peripheral neuropathy may be accompanied by dermatitis, diarrhea, and dementia (pellagra). The diagnosis is made on clinical grounds, and treatment consists of administration of 40–250 mg niacin daily. *Strachan's syndrome* is characterized by a painful sensory neuropathy associated with orogenital dermatitis, amblyopia, and deafness. This syndrome was first reported in Jamaica and later in malnourished field workers and prisoners of war. Distal sensory loss with hyporeflexia at the ankles (peripheral nerve lesion), combined with hyperreflexia at the knees and an ataxic gait (spinal cord involvement), indicate the combined peripheral and central axonal loss that is characteristic of this deficiency state. Treatment with vitamin B complex frequently improves the symptoms.

Vitamin E Deficiency Vitamin E deficiency can occur from fat malabsorption or from abetalipoproteinemia. The clinical features of vitamin E deficiency resemble those of Friedreich's ataxia (Chap. 368), with severe large-fiber loss and a non-length-dependent reduction of sensory nerve action potentials suggestive of dorsal root ganglionopathy. The diagnosis is confirmed by measurement of serum α tocopherol and the ratio of vitamin E to total serum lipids. Treatment consists of administration of α tocopherol (400 mg bid), which may reverse or prevent progression of the sensory neuronopathy.

INFECTIONS AND PERIPHERAL NEUROPATHY

HIV Infection (See also Chap. 182) HIV infection is associated with polyradiculopathies, distal symmetric polyneuropathies, inflammatory demyelinating polyneuropathies, multifocal mononeuropathies, cranial neuropathies, and neuropathies induced by antiretroviral drugs (Table 379-9).

Lumbosacral polyradiculopathies are usually due to CMV infection and occur with advanced HIV/AIDS. These present with pain, incontinence, and rapidly progressive asymmetric lower extremity weakness leading to paraplegia. Saddle anesthesia is always present. Deep tendon reflexes are often preserved. EMG reveals findings of both peripheral neuropathy and lumbosacral radiculopathy. CSF analysis shows pleocytosis with polymorphonuclear cells; polymerase chain reaction for CMV is positive. The differential diagnosis includes GBS; other infections including herpes viruses, treponema, or tuberculosis; and carcinomatous meningoradiculitis from lymphoma. Aggressive and rapid treatment with ganciclovir, foscarnet, or cidofovir should be considered.

DISTAL SYMMETRIC POLYNEUROPATHY ASSOCIATED WITH HIV HIV distal sensory symmetric polyneuropathy presents as a painful, predominantly small-fiber neuropathy. This syndrome cannot be distinguished reliably from neuropathy caused by antiretroviral drugs (nucleoside reverse transcriptase inhibitors); its onset with respect to exposure to the offending drugs may be the only clue. It is estimated that ~30% of hospitalized patients with AIDS and 100% of individuals dying with AIDS have evidence of neuropathy. The prevalence is lower in less advanced HIV infection, occurring in only 3% of those with CD4 cell counts > 200/μL. Older age, associated nutritional deficiencies, and toxic exposures are additional risk factors for AIDS-related neuropathy. Most patients present with painful burning, tingling, and numbness in the feet. Symp-

TABLE 379-9 **NEUROPATHIES ASSOCIATED WITH HIV INFECTION** 2661

HIV Neuropathy	Symptoms and Signs	Typical CD4 Counts, cells/µL	Diagnostic Tests
Distal symmetric polyneuropathy	Painful paresthesias, distal sensory loss, absent ankle jerk	<200	EDx studies Skin biopsy
GBS, CIDP	Progressive weakness, areflexia, numbness	<500; >50	EDx studies CSF studies: elevated protein, variable pleocytosis
Mononeuropathy multiplex (cryoglobulinemia, hepatitis C)	Footdrop, wrist drop, facial weakness	<500; >50	EDx studies, nerve biopsy
CMV polyradiculopathy	Flaccid paraparesis, saddle anesthesia, urinary retention	<50	EDx, CSF studies
Herpes zoster, tuberculosis, lymphoma	Depends on specific etiology	<50	EDx, CSF studies Nerve biopsy
Toxic neuropathy	Similar to DSPN	<500	Eliminate drug: stavudine (d4T), didanosine (ddI), zalcidabine (ddC)

Note: GBS, Guillain-Barré syndrome; CIDP, chronic inflammatory demyelinating polyneuropathy; EDx, electrodiagnosis; CSF, cerebrospinal fluid; CMV, cytomegalovirus; DSPN, diabetic sensory polyneuropathy.

toms are typically bilateral, gradual in onset, and worse at night (features common to all painful neuropathies). Examination usually shows distal loss to pin and temperature sensation and absent or decreased ankle jerk. Weakness is either not detected or is confined to the intrinsic foot muscles. Asymmetric presentations suggest the possibility of vasculitis (nerve biopsy indicated) or an entrapment neuropathy. The possibility of a confounding neuropathy from diabetes, alcohol, nutritional causes, or toxin exposure should always be considered.

Nerve biopsy shows a length-dependent axonal degeneration of sensory fibers, with little evidence of nerve-fiber regeneration. Both large myelinated and unmyelinated nerve fibers are lost. Inflammatory infiltrates of lymphocytes and activated macrophages and reduced numbers of DRG neurons may be seen.

TOXIC NEUROPATHY FROM ANTIRETROVIRAL DRUGS A toxic neuropathy follows exposure to specific dideoxynucleosides (d4T, ddI, and especially ddC), particularly in advanced HIV disease. Sural nerve biopsy shows severe axonal destruction, most prominently in unmyelinated fibers, along with mitochondrial abnormalities. Serum lactate concentrations are elevated and acetylcarnitine levels are reduced as a result of mitochondrial dysfunction. Dideoxynucleosides have also been shown in vitro to inhibit gamma DNA polymerase, whereas zidovudine, lamivudine, and abacavir (drugs that are not associated with neuropathy) have only limited effects on this enzyme.

℞ **TOXIC NEUROPATHY FROM ANTIRETROVIRAL DRUGS**

Treatment consists of discontinuing the offending dideoxynucleoside and changing the highly active antiretroviral therapy (HAART) regimen, provided that there is another regimen to offer. Failing this, a patient may need to continue the regimen with the addition of pain-modifying drugs. Prescribing patterns have changed in the developed world to limit the use of specific dideoxynucleosides. However, in resource-limited countries, generic antiretroviral combinations typically contain d4T. After discontinuation of a toxic dideoxynucleoside, symptomatic improvement can be expected in most individuals within ~3 months.

Various pain-modifying drugs have been tried without success, including tricyclic antidepressants and anticonvulsants. Lamotrigine was reported to be efficacious in a subgroup of patients in one class I trial, but results of a smaller class II trial were contradictory. Some positive results have been achieved with topical capsaicin or topical lidocaine, especially in patients with symptoms confined to the feet. Patients with severe neuropathies may require narcotic analgesics for pain relief, and long-acting narcotics such as transdermal fentanyl, morphine, or oxycodone preparations are particularly useful. Specific prescribing guidelines should be used, par-

ticularly if there is any history of substance abuse. Regenerative strategies, including trials of recombinant human nerve growth factor, have been attempted.

Neuropathies with Lyme Disease (See also Chap. 166) A focal or multifocal radiculoneuropathy may occur with *Borrelia burgdorferi* infection. Subacute cranial neuropathy (especially VII) or painful radiculopathy may occur in the acute phase of Lyme disease, with or without associated meningitis. The radiculitis is dysesthetic or painful and is variable in distribution. CSF pleocytosis with intrathecal production of *B. burgdorferi* antibodies is typical. The radiculitis is dysesthetic or painful and is variable in distribution. Most patients improve either spontaneously or after IV ceftriaxone treatment. In the chronic phase, a mild, chronic distal polyneuropathy (sensory more than motor) has been described; however, the CSF is normal and the association may be coincidental.

Herpes Zoster (See also Chap. 173) Reactivation of varicella zoster virus (VZV) in dorsal root ganglia produces lancinating pain and hyperalgesia in a dermatomal distribution. The pain is followed 3–4 days later by the appearance of a blistering skin rash. The inflammation may at times involve the adjacent motor nerve roots, causing weakness and wasting. Ophthalmoplegic zoster causes weakness in the division of one or more oculomotor nerves; facial zoster causes facial palsy (Ramsay Hunt syndrome); thoracolumbar zoster causes rash and sensory loss in a thoracic or lumbar nerve root. Although pain usually subsides after a few days to a week, it sometimes persists (postherpetic neuralgia). Herpes zoster and postherpetic neuralgia both occur more commonly in the elderly and in immunosuppressed individuals. In the acute setting acyclovir, famciclovir, or valacyclovir are equally effective, although acyclovir must be given five times a day as opposed to three times a day for the other two drugs. Glucocorticoids are of unproven benefit. Treatment of postherpetic neuralgia includes tricyclic antidepressants, duloxetin, gabapentin, pregabalin, oxycodone, morphine sulfate, tramodol, lidocaine patch, and topical capsaicin. A zoster vaccine (Zostavax) has been approved to prevent VZV in elderly patients; the incidence of shingles is reduced by 50% and postherpetic neuralgia by 67%.

Leprous Neuritis (See also Chap. 159) *Mycobacterium leprae* causes mononeuropathy multiplex affecting peripheral nerves in cooler regions of the body, reflecting the predilection for this bacterium to thrive at cooler temperatures. The deformities caused by untreated leprous neuritis have led to the fear and stigma attached to this disease. Although the incidence of leprous neuritis has declined, it remains a leading cause of neuropathy worldwide. Leprosy is classified into tuberculoid, lepromatous, and borderline types; peripheral nerves may be affected in all three types, and involved nerves are often palpably thickened. In tuberculoid leprosy, a single patch of hypesthetic or anesthetic skin may occur in any location. The area is generally hypopigmented, thickened, or red. A mononeuropathy involving a nearby superficial nerve may occur. Lepromatous leprosy produces more widespread skin thickening, hypesthesia, and anhidrosis affecting the pinnae of ears, dorsum of hands or feet, dorsomedial surfaces of the forearm, and anteromedial aspects of the legs. The sensory loss spares the midline of the trunk anteriorly, the groin, axilla, and scalp; these are the warmer regions of the body. The fifth and seventh cranial nerves, greater auricular nerve in the neck, median and ulnar nerves, and peroneal nerves can all be involved. Over the long term, untreated leprosy leads to claw hand deformity (from ulnar and median nerve weakness), footdrop, and inability to close the eyelids due to orbicularis oculi weakness.

CHAPTER 379 Peripheral Neuropathy

CHARCOT-MARIE-TOOTH DISEASE

Clinical Features CMT neuropathy is the most common heritable neuromuscular disorder with an estimated incidence of 17–40 cases per 100,000 (Table 379-10). It is a chronic distal sensory and motor neuropathy presenting as longstanding gait difficulty with frequent tripping, followed by difficulty with buttoning, handling keys, turning door knobs, and opening jars. There is often a history of clumsiness, frequent ankle injuries, inability to jump well or to keep up with other children in races, and being unathletic. In some patients the history suggests a more recent onset. If carefully sought, a family history can often be obtained. Wasting and weakness of the distal muscles of the legs (inverted champagne bottle appearance) with hammer toes and high arched feet (pes cavus) are commonly present, along with steppage gait, distal sensory loss, and distal loss of reflexes. Pes cavus and hammer toes indicate that the neuropathy dates from early life. An inability to walk on the heels or perform tandem gait is often present. The differential diagnosis is limited if there is an early age of onset, a positive family history, and longstanding symptoms. If

TABLE 379-10 FORMS OF CHARCOT-MARIE-TOOTH DISEASE (HEREDITARY MOTOR AND SENSORY NEUROPATHY) AND RELATED DISORDERS

Disorder	Locus	Gene	Inheritance
Charcot-Marie-Tooth Type 1			
(HMSNI)			
CMT1A	17p11.2-p12	PMP22	AD
CMT1B	1q22-q23	P₀	AD
CMT1C	16p12-p13	SIMPLE	AD
CMT1D	10q21-q22	EGR2	AD/AR
CMT1X	Xq13.1	GJB1	X-linked
CMT5X	Xq21.32-24	PRPS1	X-linked
CMT4A	8q13-q21	GDAP1	AR
CMT4B1	11q22	MTMR2	AR
CMT4B2	11p15	SBF2	AR
CMT4D (HMSN-Lom)	8q24	NDRG1	AR
CMT4E	10q21.1-q22.1	EGR2	AR
CMT4F	19q13	PRX	AR
CMT4J	6q21	FIG4	AR
Charcot-Marie-Tooth Type 2			
(HMSNII)			
CMT2A	1p35-p36	KIF1B	AD
CMT2B	3q13-q22	RAB7	AD
CMT2C	12q23-q24	Unknown	AD
CMT2D	7p14	GARS	AD
CMT2E	8p21	NEF-L	AD
CMT2B1	11q21	LMNA	AR
Déjerine-Sottas			
(HMSNIII)			
DSS	17p11.2-p12	PMP22	AD
	1q22-p23	P₀	AD
	10q21-q22	EGR2	AD/AR
	19q13	PRX	AD
Congenital Hypomyelination			
CHN	1q22-23	P₀	AD
	10q21-q22	EGR2	AR/AD
Hereditary Neuropathy with Pressure Palsies			
HNPP	17p11.2-p12	PMP22	AD

Abbreviations: HMSN, hereditary motor and sensory neuropathies; PMP22, peripheral myelin protein 22; P₀, myelin protein zero; SIMPLE, small integral membrane protein of late endosome; Cx32, connexin32; EGR2 (Krox-20) early growth response 2 gene; GDAP1, ganglioside-induced differentiation-associated protein-1; MTMR2, myotubularin-related protein-2; SBF2, SET binding factor 2; NDRG1, N-myc downstream regulated gene1; PRX, periaxin; KIF1B, kinesin family member 1B; RAB7, ras-associated protein 7; GARS, Glycyl-tRNA synthetase; NEFL, neurofilament, light polypeptide; LMNA, lamin A.

the EDx findings indicate a demyelinating process, the diagnosis of CMT can be made with confidence, although genetic testing may be needed to confirm the precise genotype. If the EDx findings are axonal, or if the family history is uncertain or negative, CMT becomes a diagnosis of exclusion. Diabetes, as well as nutritional, toxic, endocrine, inflammatory, paraprotein-associated, and infectious causes, may all need to be excluded. Physical examination and EDx studies of at-risk family members can be more useful diagnostically than additional laboratory testing of the patient. Treatment is supportive; patients often need foot braces but rarely, if ever, become wheelchair dependent. CMT does not reduce the life span and only rarely involves respiratory muscles.

Classification Demyelinating forms of CMT are classified as CMT1, and axonal forms as CMT2. Patients with nerve conduction velocities (NCVs) intermediate between CMT1 and CMT2 are classified as having "intermediate CMT," and most of these cases are X-linked. CMT is usually transmitted as an autosomal dominant trait, but X-linked-dominant CMT is responsible for ~10% of CMT cases. Rare autosomal recessive forms, designated CMT4, tend to have an early onset and are more severe than the dominant types. In total, ~35 different loci and >24 genes have been identified in CMT.

Charcot-Marie-Tooth 1 (CMT1) Demyelinating Neuropathies CMT1 is the most common of the heritable neuropathies; inheritance is autosomal dominant. Distal weakness, wasting, and sensory loss with distal reduction of tendon reflexes and foot deformities occur as with other forms of CMT. The onset is in the first or second decade of life, although patients may not come to attention until much later in life. EDx studies show a pattern of generalized demyelination with NCVs that are uniformly and proportionally slowed in distal, intermediate, and proximal segments of the same nerve on the opposite side, and in adjacent nerves. Findings suggestive of heterogeneous demyelination, such as conduction block or dispersion, are not seen. Electrophysiologic evidence of demyelination may be prominent even in patients who are clinically asymptomatic. Nerve biopsies show evidence of repeated bouts of demyelination and remyelination. Proliferation of Schwann cells occurs in an attempt to remyelinate; the supernumerary Schwann cells are concentrically arranged around demyelinated and remyelinated axons, giving a characteristic "onion bulb" appearance. There is also increased collagen between the layers of Schwann cells leading to palpably thickened nerves.

CMT1 is classified into several genetically distinct subtypes (Table 379-10), all of which are clinically similar. In addition, distinct phenotypes with overlapping genotypes are identified. These include HNPP; infantile-onset or severe childhood forms, which include Déjerine-Sottas syndrome (DSS) and congenital hypomyelinating neuropathies (CHN); and Roussy-Lévy syndrome.

CMT1A This is the most common form; it is associated with the 17p11.2-p12 duplication in the *PMP22* gene expressed by Schwann cells. The duplication involves a large segment of DNA (~1.4 Mb) encoding a 160-amino-acid protein localized to compact myelin in peripheral nerves. CMT1A accounts for up to 90% of CMT1 and 50% of all CMT. Deletion of the *PMP22* gene produces a different phenotype—HNPP (see below). Commercial testing for *PMP22* duplication/deletion is widely available. *PMP22* appears to be important in the initiation of myelin spirals; regulation and growth of Schwann cells; and control of thickness, stability, and maintenance of myelin sheaths.

CMT1B CMT1B accounts for <5% of CMT1 cases. It is due to a mutation in the myelin protein zero (*MPZ*, or P₀) gene. Different mutations in the same gene can produce a wide spectrum of phenotypes including DSS, CHN, or CMT2. P₀ is quantitatively the major structural protein of peripheral nerve myelin and is important in myelin compaction. CMT1B is clinically indistinguishable from CMT1A; a late adult-onset form with footdrop can occur. Genetic testing is available.

CMT1X This is an X-linked dominant form of CMT that can also affect heterozygote females. It is responsible for up to 10% of CMT.

Males are more often affected, and female carriers are usually mildly affected or asymptomatic. Male-to-male transmission does not occur. Onset in males is between the ages of 5 and 20; symptoms include difficulty running, sprained ankles, footdrop, distal wasting, weakness, sensory loss, and reduced reflexes. These features do not distinguish CMT1X from other forms of CMT1. Signs of central nervous system (CNS) involvement, including ataxia, dysarthria, weakness, aphasia, disorientation, and hearing loss, may be present, especially in males. Spontaneously resolving confluent white matter changes may be seen on MRI. NCVs are in an intermediate range, although males have slower conduction velocities (25–45 m/s), which may be nonuniform with conduction block and dispersion. This nonuniform pattern may mimic findings of an acquired disorder such as CIDP. The mutated gene, *GJB1*, encodes the gap junction protein connexin-32, which is expressed at the paranodal regions and at the Schmidt-Lanterman incisures of noncompact myelin.

HEREDITARY NEUROPATHY WITH LIABILITY TO PRESSURE PALSIES
This is also called *tomaculous neuropathy*. It is an autosomal dominant disorder that presents as recurrent episodes of focal entrapment neuropathy with attacks of numbness and weakness in peroneal, ulnar, radial, and median nerves (in descending order) or in a brachial plexus distribution. Malposition of a limb or trauma may provoke episodes of neuropathy. Some patients present with a progressive length-dependent polyneuropathy rather than with recurrent mononeuropathies, and others remain entirely asymptomatic. Increased distal latencies in median and peroneal nerves and reduced velocities across the elbow of the ulnar and fibular head segment of the peroneal nerves may be found. Tomaculae are sausage-shaped bodies that indicate segmental demyelination. CMT1A and HNPP are both associated with copy number changes in the *PMP22* gene—a duplication causing CMT1A and deletion causing HNPP. Hence, CMT1A and HNPP are the reciprocal products of unequal crossing-over during meiosis. When HNPP presents as a painless brachial plexus neuropathy, it should be distinguished from brachial plexus neuritis and from hereditary neuralgic amyotrophy, a familial disorder with painful weakness and sensory loss in the brachial plexus distribution. Treatment for HNPP is supportive. Avoiding further compression or trauma to the entrapment sites is preferred over surgical release or transposition.

DÉJERINE-SOTTAS SYNDROME AND CONGENITAL HYPOMYELINATING NEUROPATHY
These are severe childhood forms of CMT1. DSS and CHN both present with muscle weakness at birth or infancy, with absent or very slow NCVs. Delayed motor milestones are noted in early childhood. Patients either never ambulate or lose their ability to ambulate in infancy or childhood. NCVs are markedly slow (typically 10 m/s); CSF protein is elevated. Clinically DSS and CHN are indistinguishable. DSS can be either autosomal dominant or recessive; CHN is autosomal recessive. Nerve biopsy can distinguish the two, with DSS showing a thin myelin sheath surrounded by onion bulbs composed of concentric layers of basal lamina (Schwann cells are degenerated leaving the basal lamina), while CHN shows lack of onion bulbs and absent myelin sheaths. DSS may be caused by mutations of *PMP22*, myelin protein zero (*MPZ*), or early growth response gene (*ERG2*); *EGR2* or *MPZ* mutations underlie CHN.

ROUSSY-LÉVY SYNDROME
This describes a combination of demyelinating CMT with postural and action tremor. The original family members had the *MPZ* mutation, but mutations in *PMP22* (CMT1A), *MPZ* (CMT1B), or *GJB1* (CMT1X) genes may also cause this syndrome.

Charcot-Marie-Tooth 2 (CMT2) Axonal Neuropathies
CMT2, an autosomal dominant neuropathy, is responsible for one-third of CMT disease, although the number of patients is increasing as more genetic abnormalities are being identified. CMT2 has a later age of onset than CMT1; family members may be affected subclinically. Although typical length-dependent sensory and motor loss develops over the years, intrinsic hand weakness and atrophy, present in CMT1, do not develop.

CMT2A (classic CMT2) is caused by mutations in *MFN2* and represents 10% of dominant CMT2; CMT2B is caused by mutations in *RAB7*, a member of the Rab family of *ras*-related GTPases that function in intracellular membrane trafficking; it presents with severe sensory involvement and limb ulcerations. CMT2B overlaps with hereditary sensory neuropathy (HSN) type I with prominent sensory loss and severe sensory loss to touch and pain (see below). CMT2C is associated with vocal cord and respiratory (diaphragm) involvement; the genetic defects have not been identified. CMT2D is an axonal CMT with upper limb predominance associated with mutations in the glycyl-tRNA synthetase gene; predominant hand involvement with atrophy of distal hand muscles in a patient with a positive family history suggests CMT2D.

Autosomal Recessive Forms of CMT Autosomal recessive CMTs account for <10% of inherited neuropathy cases in the Western world but may be more common in regions of the world where consanguinity is common. Several genes have been identified, especially in inbred families. Demyelinating autosomal recessive forms, designated CMT4, are usually characterized by early onset and more severe involvement, with congenital or delayed motor milestones, facial weakness, bulbar weakness, sensorineural deafness, diaphragm weakness, and vocal cord paralysis.

Molecular Testing The phenotype, the inheritance pattern, and electrophysiologic data guide the approach to the diagnosis of an inherited neuropathy. **Figure 379-2** summarizes an approach to genetic testing for CMT. If the proband has CMT1, a single nerve study (median motor forearm conduction velocity) in family members is a quick screening tool. However, if the proband has axonal CMT (CMT2), more detailed evaluation of family members may be required. Evaluation for HNPP employs the same molecular test as for the CMT1A duplication. Most CMT1 and CMT2 pedigrees are autosomal dominant. X-linked inheritance should be suspected if males are more often affected, there is no male-to-male transmission, and EDx studies show heterogeneous findings. Sporadic cases are difficult to evaluate since family members may not be available. Testing for the CMT1A duplication/deletion and for *GJB1* mutation can diagnose ~80% of all cases of CMT.

OTHER INHERITED NEUROPATHIES
Hereditary Motor Neuropathies (HMN)
The distal HMNs present with distal motor weakness with sparing of sensory fibers. Seven subtypes have been described based on the age of onset and mode of inheritance, which is usually autosomal dominant or recessive. The common HMNs present as footdrop with severe wasting and weakness distally. Some variants may manifest with predominantly upper limb involvement, vocal cord paralysis, or with upper motor neuron signs mimicking amyotrophic lateral sclerosis (Chap. 369); the prognosis is relatively good.

Hereditary Sensory Neuropathies (HSN)
HSNs, also called *hereditary sensory and autonomic neuropathies* (HSANs), are a heterogeneous group of disorders affecting the sensory and/or autonomic neurons. The predominant clinical presentation is of progressive distal sensory loss, although some weakness and wasting is also observed. The classification of HSN and HSAN is based on the age of onset and mode of inheritance. Five subtypes are described. The most common is HSN 1 (also called HSAN 1), an autosomal dominant neuropathy presenting with predominant small-fiber sensory involvement with lancinating pain, loss of pain and temperature sensation, and foot ulceration. Of note, CMT2B (see above) also presents with predominantly sensory loss to all modalities and foot ulcerations. HSN 2–5 are all autosomal recessive. HSN 2 presents in the first two decades of life with prominent sensory loss and mutilation in hands and feet. HSN 3 (HSAN 3), also called *Riley-Day syndrome*, has prominent dysautonomia. HSN 4 (HSAN 4) presents with episodic fever, anhidrosis, and reduced response to painful stimuli. HSAN 5 presents with congenital insensitivity to pain; mutations in a sodium channel (SCN1.7) are causative.

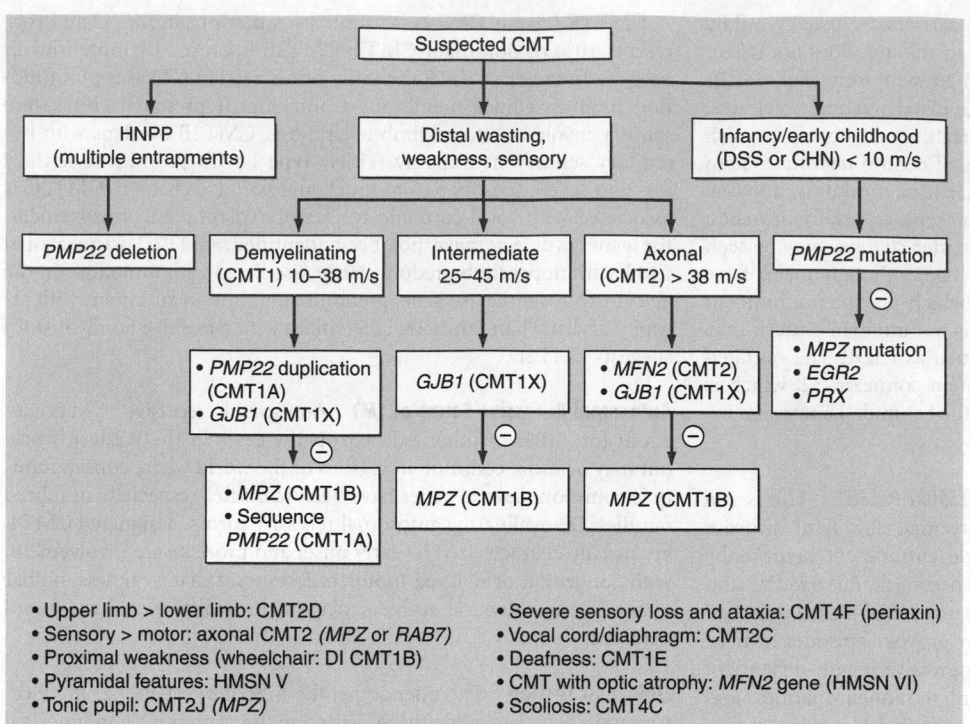

• Upper limb > lower limb: CMT2D
• Sensory > motor: axonal CMT2 (*MPZ* or *RAB7*)
• Proximal weakness (wheelchair): DI CMT1B
• Pyramidal features: HMSN V
• Tonic pupil: CMT2J (*MPZ*)

• Severe sensory loss and ataxia: CMT4F (periaxin)
• Vocal cord/diaphragm: CMT2C
• Deafness: CMT1E
• CMT with optic atrophy: *MFN2* gene (HMSN VI)
• Scoliosis: CMT4C

FIGURE 379-2 Diagnostic approach to Charcot-Marie-Tooth disease (CMT). HNPP, hereditary neuropathy with pressure palsies; DSS, Déjerine-Sottas syndrome; CHN, congenital hypomyelinating neuropathy; HMSN, hereditary motor and sensory neuropathy.

Refsum Disease This is an autosomal recessive hypertrophic neuropathy caused by defective oxidation of phytanic acid, a branched-chain fatty acid found in dairy products, beef, lamb, and fish. The onset is in late childhood or adolescence, with a slowly progressive course of a sensorimotor demyelinating neuropathy with sensorineural deafness, cerebellar ataxia, and anosmia. Retinitis pigmentosa presenting as night blindness often precedes the onset of neuropathy. Thickened skin (ichthyosis), syndactyly and shortening of the fourth toe, cardiomyopathy, and cataracts are other features. CSF protein is typically elevated. Abnormally high plasma and urinary levels of phytanic acid are diagnostic. Although a diet low in phytanic acid may prevent the onset of some of the complications, compliance with this diet is usually poor. Plasma exchange and dialysis may be helpful for episodes of worsening.

Familial Amyloid Neuropathy This is an autosomal dominant disorder in which there is extracellular deposition of amyloid in peripheral nerves and other organs (Chap. 324). A painful sensory neuropathy with early involvement of autonomic nerves and cardiomyopathy is typically present. Age of onset can vary from 18–83 years. Small fibers (pain and temperature) are more affected than large fibers (vibration and proprioception); anhidrosis, gastrointestinal disturbances (diarrhea alternating with constipation), impotence, orthostatic intolerance, visual changes, and arrhythmias are additional features. Mutations in transthyretin (FAP 1 and 2), apolipoprotein A1 (FAP 3) or gelosin (FAP 4) are responsible. Transthyretin is most often implicated in peripheral neuropathy. Nearly 100 different mutations have been identified in the *TTR* gene, the most common being the *Val30Met* mutation. Liver transplantation halts disease progression.

Tangier Disease (TD) This is a rare syndrome caused by a severe deficiency of high-density lipoproteins (HDL) in plasma (Chap. 350). Peripheral neuropathy is the most disabling feature of TD and affects ~50% of patients. Three patterns are recognized: a transient or relapsing, often asymmetric neuropathy (including isolated cranial nerve deficits); a slowly progressive symmetric neuropathy most marked in the distal upper limbs (syringomyelia-like); and a slowly progressive symmetric sensory motor neuropathy most marked in the lower limbs. Mononeuropathies involving the oculomotor nerve, long thoracic nerve, or any of the limb nerves may occur. The syringomyelic presentation includes wasting of hand muscles, loss of pain and temperature sensation, and facial diplegia. The length-dependent sensorimotor neuropathy pattern is the least common variant. Deposits of cholesterol esters in tonsils, liver, spleen, rectal mucosa, and cornea lead to the other non-neurologic manifestations of TD. There is no treatment available; a low-cholesterol diet or other dietary changes do not modify the natural history. Gene therapy may be possible in the future.

Porphyric Neuropathy Peripheral neuropathy accompanies the inherited hepatic porphyrias (Chap. 352). The triad of acute neuropathy, psychiatric symptoms, and abdominal involvement are similar in all hepatic porphyrias. Variegate porphyria and hereditary coproporphyria are characterized by additional skin lesions (blisters and bullae) in ~50% of patients. Most patients with porphyria are asymptomatic between attacks. Attacks can occur spontaneously or be precipitated by certain drugs, stress, hormonal factors, and reduced caloric intake. Abdominal pain, constipation, vomiting, and mental changes frequently herald the attacks. Peripheral neuropathy has an acute onset and may be preceded or accompanied by autonomic manifestations such as tachycardia, hypertension, and postural hypotension. The neuropathy is usually subacutely progressive (over 2–4 weeks) with diffuse weakness (often proximal more than distal) and areflexia. Sensory loss is generally mild and may be more prominent proximally in a "bathing trunk" distribution. Porphyric neuropathy should be considered in the differential diagnosis of GBS, the most common cause of rapidly progressive ascending paralysis.

CSF is acellular but the protein level is elevated, similar to that in GBS. Acute attacks are invariably associated with increased urinary excretion of aminolevulinic acid and/or porphobilinogen. Measuring 24-h urinary excretion of porphobilinogen and aminolevulinic acid and 24-h fecal excretion of protoporphyrin and coproporphyrin during a symptomatic period is the most helpful method of determining whether symptoms are due to acute porphyria. Since porphyrins are light sensitive, specimens must be stored in the dark and tested as soon as possible.

Treatment is largely supportive during the acute crisis and includes fluid management, ventilatory support, management of heart rate and blood pressure (autonomic dysfunction), and avoidance of medications that are known to precipitate an acute attack. Oral and IV glucose and heme arginate are the mainstays of treatment (Chap. 352). Recovery from an acute attack may take several months.

Critical Illness Neuropathy See Chap. 269.

SPECIAL PERIPHERAL NEUROPATHY PRESENTATIONS
AUTONOMIC NEUROPATHY

Symptoms may include orthostatic hypotension (syncope, light headedness, dizziness, fatigue, and lethargy), heat intolerance, abnormal (reduced or increased) sweating, constipation, diarrhea, incontinence, sexual dysfunction, dry eyes, dry mouth, or visual blurriness. Autonomic neuropathy is usually a manifestation of a more generalized polyneuropathy, as in diabetes, GBS, and alcoholic poly-neuropathy, but occasionally syndromes of pure pandysautonomia are encountered. Other causes include amyloidosis and multiple drugs and tox-ins. Autonomic neuropathies are discussed in detail in Chap. 370.

PURE MOTOR NEUROPATHY

Examples of predominantly motor neuropathies include acute inflammatory neuropathies such as GBS; chronic neuropathies such as CIDP and mul-tifocal motor neuropathy (MMN) (Chap. 380); some inherited neuropathies; brachial neuropathy; diabetic lumbosacral radiculoplexus neuropathy (diabetic amyotrophy); and neuropathy due to spinal muscular atrophy, acute intermittent por-phyria, diphtheria, lead, and dapsone. Motor neu-ronopathies include the lower-motor form of amyotrophic lateral sclerosis, poliomyelitis, heredi-tary spinal muscular atrophies, and an adult vari-ant of hexosaminidase A deficiency (Chap. 369). Neuromuscular junction disorders (e.g., Lambert-Eaton myasthenic syndrome, tick bite paralysis, and other types of toxic neuromuscular blockade) are purely motor and can be recognized and local-ized electrodiagnostically (Chap. 381).

PURE SENSORY NEUROPATHY

Causes include Friedreich's ataxia, idiopathic sensory neuropathy, sen-sory neuropathy associated with Sjögren syndrome, vitamin B_{12} neu-ropathy (dorsal column involvement is the major factor), pyridoxine toxicity, and cisplatin neuropathy. The most severe and widespread of these pure sensory syndromes exhibit poor or no recovery, suggesting irreversible lesions of nerve cell bodies in dorsal root and trigeminal ganglia (neuronopathy). A painful sensory neuropathy is an early fea-ture of hereditary sensory neuropathies, lepromatous leprosy, diabetic small-fiber neuropathy, amyloidosis, TD, Fabry's disease, and dysauto-nomia. Global sensory loss can occur with carcinomatous sensory neuropathy, hereditary sensory neuropathies, diabetic sensory neu-ropathy, vacor intoxication, and xanthoma-tous neuropathy of primary biliary cirrhosis.

PLEXOPATHY

This refers to disorders of either the brachial or the lumbosacral plexus. *Brachial plexopa-thy* is a broad term used to define any injury, traumatic or otherwise, to the brachial plexus. Causes include birth injury, trauma, neo-plasm, radiation, and familial and immune-mediated processes (Fig. 379-3; Table 379-11). Trauma to the plexus is responsible for up to 70% of brachial plexus lesions; the upper plex-us is the most vulnerable. Brachial neuritis (neuralgic amyotrophy; Chap. 16), character-ized by sudden onset of pain in the shoulder region followed by weakness and atrophy, is the second most common cause. In this dis-order, the shoulder girdle muscles are most frequently affected, and individual peripheral nerves tend to be more commonly involved. Other causes include a cervical rib or band, in-filtration by malignant tumor, or prior radia-tion therapy.

Brachial plexus lesions demonstrate charac-teristic motor and sensory signs. When the up-per parts of the brachial plexus (cervical roots 5–7) are affected, weakness and atrophy of shoulder girdle and upper arm muscles occurs.

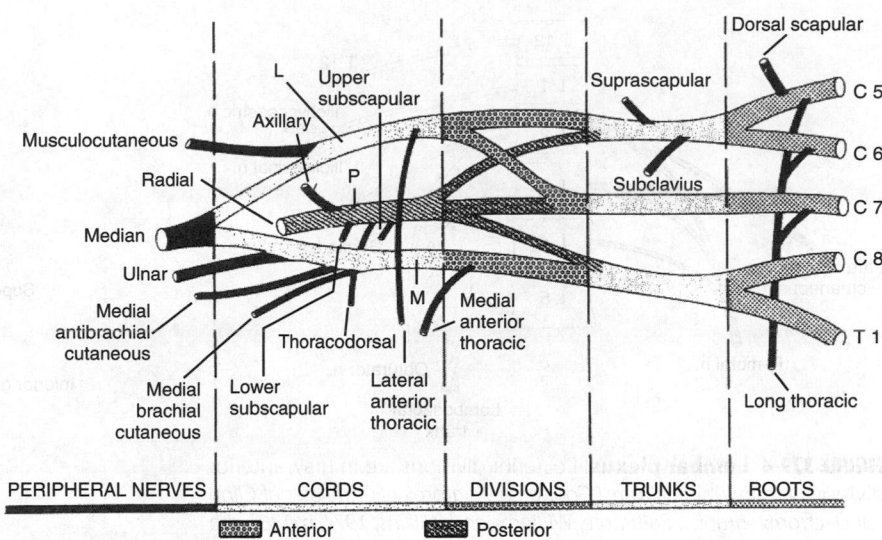

FIGURE 379-3 Brachial plexus anatomy. L, lateral; M, medial; P, posterior. *(From J Goodgold: Anatomical Correlates of Clinical Electromyography. Baltimore, Williams and Wilkins, 1974, p. 126, with permission.)*

Injuries to the lower brachial plexus (C8-T1 roots) produce distal arm weakness, atrophy, and focal sensory deficits in the forearm and hand. In general, idiopathic brachial neuritis, irradiation with >60 Gy (6000 rad), and specific types of trauma (arm jerked downward) result in damage to the upper portions of the brachial plexus. In contrast, infil-tration by malignant tumor, a cervical rib or band, and specific types of trauma (arm jerked upward) cause damage to the lower brachial plexus.

The *lumbosacral plexus* is formed by the ventral primary rami of L1-S4. Although often considered as a single entity, it can be divided into a lumbar plexus (ventral rami of L1–L4) and a sacral plexus (lumbosa-cral trunk L4 and L5 and ventral rami of S1–S4) (Figs. 379-4 and 379-5). The femoral and obturator nerves are the main nerves formed from the lumbar plexus, and the sciatic, gluteal, and pudendal nerves

TABLE 379-11 BRACHIAL PLEXUS LESIONS

Site of Injury	Nerves/Nerve Roots	Muscles Affected	Sensory Loss	Common Causes
Upper trunk	C-5 and C-6	Weakness of shoulder abduction (supra-spinatus & deltoid), external rotation (infraspinatus) and el-bow flexion (biceps)	Small patch of skin overlying the deltoid	Birth injury during difficult delivery (Erb-Duchenne palsy); brachial neuritis, also called neuralgica my-otrophy (Parsonage-Turner syndrome)
Lower trunk	C-8 and T-1	Weakness and wast-ing of small muscles of the hand (claw-hand deformity)	Ulnar border of the hand and inner forearm	Birth injury, especially breech delivery (Déjerine-Klumpke paralysis), compres-sion by cervical rib or band (thoracic outlet syndrome), tumor infiltration
Lateral cord	Musculocuta-neous nerve and lateral part of me-dian nerve	Weakness of flexion and pronation of forearm	Radial border of forearm and hand	Trauma, stretch
Medial cord	Medial part of median nerve and ulnar nerve	Weakness and wast-ing of small muscles of the hand (claw hand deformity)	Ulnar border of the hand and inner forearm	Trauma
Posterior cord	Axillary and radial nerves	Deltoid, extensors of el-bow, wrist, and fingers	Outer aspect of upper arm	Trauma, shoulder dislocation

FIGURE 379-4 Lumbar plexus. Posterior divisions are in gray, anterior divisions are in white. *(From J Goodgold: Anatomical Correlates of Clinical Electromyography. Baltimore, Williams and Wilkins, 1974, p. 126, with permission.)*

PART 16 Neurologic Disorders

are the main nerves formed by the sacral plexus. The lumbosacral plexus courses near the paravertebral psoas muscle and the sacroiliac notch and sacral ala, where it is relatively well protected from injury, unlike its upper extremity counterpart. Disorders affecting the lumbosacral plexus include: trauma, intraoperative damage, retroperitoneal hemorrhage, radiotherapy, neoplastic invasion, diabetes mellitus, pregnancy and labor, retroperitoneal abscess or hemorrhage, abdominal aortic aneurysm, and idiopathic lumbosacral plexopathy (**Table 379-12**). Most patients present with varying degrees of pain, sensory deficits, and weakness in the lower limbs, generally in an asymmetric distribution. The onset may be acute, subacute, or insidious depending on the etiology; the course may vary from being monophasic, stepwise, or progressive. EDx studies are invaluable aids for diagnosis and localization.

PERIPHERAL NERVE INJURY

Physical damage to peripheral nerves may result from sudden compression, crush, transection, or stretching of a nerve. The mildest form of nerve injury results when a stretch or pressure injury distorts the myelin overlying the nodes of Ranvier and produces focal conduction block. This type of injury, with conduction block but without Wallerian degeneration, is referred to as *neurapraxia*, or *class 1 injury*. This results in a transient sensation of numbness in an extremity, as occurs after lying or sitting in a certain position. Nerve injury that interrupts the axon's continuity and results in Wallerian degeneration of the nerve distal to the lesion is considered moderate or severe. If the endoneurium is preserved, the lesion is considered moderate and is called *axonotmesis*, or *class 2 injury*. If the endoneurium is destroyed, the lesion is considered severe and is called *neurotmesis*. Peripheral nerve lesions are often mixed; neurapraxia and axonotmesis may coexist. Similarly, one fascicle may be completely disrupted while another is only partially affected. If the clinical and electrophysiologic examinations show that the lesion is complete, and if the mechanism of injury is known to be a clean laceration, then surgical repair should be considered within 24 h of the injury. If the mechanism of injury is contusion, stretch, traction, or compression, nerve conduction studies to determine whether the lesion is neurapraxic or axonotmesic should be delayed for 3 weeks. If neurapraxic, a return of function can be expected, provided care is taken to ensure that there is no ongoing compressive injury. If clinical and electrophysiologic examinations (no motor units seen by EMG) fail to reveal evidence of return of function after 3 months, the lesion was most likely neurotmesic, and exploration and surgical repair may need to be un-

FIGURE 379-5 Lumbosacral plexus. Posterior divisions are in black, anterior divisions are in white. *(From J Goodgold: Anatomical Correlates of Clinical Electromyography. Baltimore, Williams and Wilkins, 1974, p. 126, with permission.)*

dertaken. If the lesion is incomplete, follow-up evaluations should be performed monthly; if no improvement is seen, then surgery may be required. Approximately 80% of closed injuries resolve spontaneously, because these lesions are in continuity. The appearance of an advancing Tinel's sign in the distribution of the injured nerve indicates that the nerve is in continuity and justifies postponement of surgery. The growth rate of regenerating axons is about 2.5 cm/month. The time required for regeneration is dependent on the distance from the site of injury to the first muscle innervated below the lesion. Since this distance is greater for proximal nerve lesions, severe proximal injuries are associated with poor recovery. Brachial plexus injuries during birth carry a better prognosis for spontaneous recovery than do those in adults.

PERIPHERAL NERVE TUMORS

Peripheral nerve tumors, which can present as peripheral neuropathy, are mostly benign and can arise in any nerve trunk or nerve twig. Although peripheral nerve tumors can occur anywhere in the body, including the spinal roots and cauda equina, many are subcutaneous in location and present as a soft swelling, sometimes with a purplish discoloration of the skin. Symptoms can include tingling or pain when the lesion is touched. Diagnostic studies may include imaging (CT/MRI),

TABLE 379-12	LUMBOSACRAL PLEXUS LESIONS			
Site	Nerve Roots	Muscles	Sensory Loss	Common Causes
Upper plexus	L-2, L-3, L4	Weakness of thigh flexion (psoas), thigh adduction, and knee extension (quadriceps)	Anterior thigh and medial leg; absent knee jerk	Diabetic amyotrophy; abdominal surgery—either directly/retraction, or due to positioning; lumbosacral plexitis
Lower plexus	L-4, L-5, S-1, and S-2	Weakness of thigh extension (glutei), knee flexion (hamstrings), foot dorsiflexion and plantar flexion	Posterior thigh, lateral leg, and entire foot; absent ankle jerk	Lumbosacral plexitis, perioperative, cancer infiltration, radiation

EMG and nerve conduction studies, and tumor biopsy. Two major categories of peripheral nerve tumors are recognized: neurilemmoma (schwannoma) and neurofibroma. Neurilemmomas are usually solitary and grow in the nerve sheath, rendering the tumor relatively easy to dissect free. In contrast, neurofibromas tend to be multiple and grow in the endoneurial substance, which renders them difficult to dissect. They may undergo malignant changes. Neurofibromas are the hallmark of von Recklinghausen's neurofibromatosis (NF1) (Chap. 374).

FURTHER READINGS

BROMBERG MB, SMITH AG (eds): *Handbook of Peripheral Neuropathy.* Taylor & Francis Group, FL, 2005

DYCK PJ et al (eds): *Peripheral Neuropathy.* Saunders, Philadelphia, 2005

HARATI Y (ed): *Neurologic Clinics. Peripheral Neuropathies.* Elsevier Saunders, Philadelphia, 2007, pp 1–330

MENDELL JR et al: *Diagnosis and Management of Peripheral Nerve Disorders.* Oxford University Press, NY, 2001

MYGLAND A: Approach to the patient with chronic polyneuropathy. Acta Neurol Scand Suppl 187:15, 2007

PAREYSON E et al: Clinical and electrophysiological aspects of Charcot-Marie-Tooth disease. Neuromol Med 8:559, 2006

PRESTON DC, SHAPIRO BE (eds): *Electromyography and Neuromuscular Disorders, Clinical Electrophysiological Correlations,* 2d ed. Elsevier, Butterworth Heinemann, Philadelphia, 2005

SAID G: Diabetic neuropathy—a review. Nat Clin Pract Neurol 3:331, 2007

STEWART JD: *Focal Peripheral Neuropathies,* 3d ed. Lippincott Williams & Wilkins, Philadelphia, 2000

380 Guillain-Barré Syndrome and Other Immune-Mediated Neuropathies
Stephen L. Hauser, Arthur K. Asbury

GUILLAIN-BARRÉ SYNDROME

Guillain-Barré syndrome (GBS) is an acute, frequently severe, and fulminant polyradiculoneuropathy that is autoimmune in nature. It occurs year-round at a rate of about one case per million per month, or ~3500 cases per year in the United States and Canada. Males are at 1.5-fold higher risk for GBS than females, and in western countries adults are more frequently affected than children.

Clinical Manifestations GBS manifests as rapidly evolving areflexic motor paralysis with or without sensory disturbance. The usual pattern is an ascending paralysis that may be first noticed as rubbery legs. Weakness typically evolves over hours to a few days and is frequently accompanied by tingling dysesthesias in the extremities. The legs are usually more affected than the arms, and facial diparesis is present in 50% of affected individuals. The lower cranial nerves are also frequently involved, causing bulbar weakness with difficulty handling secretions and maintaining an airway; the diagnosis in these patients may initially be mistaken for brainstem ischemia. Pain in the neck, shoulder, back, or diffusely over the spine is also common in the early stages of GBS, occurring in ~50% of patients. Most patients require hospitalization, and almost 30% require ventilatory assistance at some time during the illness. Fever and constitutional symptoms are absent at the onset and, if present, cast doubt on the diagnosis. Deep tendon reflexes attenuate or disappear within the first few days of onset. Cutaneous sensory deficits (e.g., loss of pain and temperature sensation) are usually relatively mild, but functions subserved by large sensory fibers, such as deep tendon reflexes and proprioception, are more severely affected. Bladder dysfunction may occur in severe cases but is usually transient. If bladder dysfunction is a prominent feature and comes early in the course, diagnostic possibilities other than GBS should be considered, particularly spinal cord disease. Once clinical worsening stops and the patient reaches a plateau (almost always within 4 weeks of onset), further progression is unlikely.

Autonomic involvement is common and may occur even in patients whose GBS is otherwise mild. The usual manifestations are loss of vasomotor control with wide fluctuation in blood pressure, postural hypotension, and cardiac dysrhythmias. These features require close monitoring and management and can be fatal. Pain is another common feature of GBS; in addition to the acute pain described above, a deep aching pain may be present in weakened muscles that patients liken to having overexercised the previous day. Other pains in GBS include dysesthetic pain in the extremities as a manifestation of sensory nerve fiber involvement. These pains are self-limited and often respond to standard analgesics (Chap. 12).

Several subtypes of GBS are recognized, as determined primarily by electrodiagnostic and pathologic distinctions (Table 380-1). These include the axonal variants, which are often clinically severe—either acute motor axonal neuropathy (AMAN) or acute motor sensory axonal neuropathy (AMSAN). In addition, a range of limited or regional GBS syndromes are also encountered. Notable among these is the Miller Fisher syndrome (MFS; Table 380-1), which presents as rapidly evolving ataxia and areflexia of limbs without weakness, and ophthalmoplegia, often with pupillary paralysis. The MFS variant accounts for ~5% of all GBS cases and is strongly associated with antibodies to the ganglioside GQ1b (see "Immunopathogenesis," below). Other regional variants of GBS include (1) pure sensory forms; (2) ophthalmoplegia with anti-GQ1b antibodies as part of severe motor-sensory GBS; (3) GBS with severe bulbar and facial paralysis, sometimes associated with antecedent cytomegalovirus (CMV) infection and anti-GM2 antibodies; and (4) acute pandysautonomia (Chap. 370).

Antecedent Events Approximately 70% of cases of GBS occur 1–3 weeks after an acute infectious process, usually respiratory or gastrointestinal. Culture and seroepidemiologic techniques show that 20–30% of all cases occurring in North America, Europe, and Australia are preceded by infection or reinfection with *Campylobacter jejuni*. A similar proportion is preceded by a human herpes virus infection, often CMV or Epstein-Barr virus. Other viruses and also *Mycoplasma pneumoniae* have been identified as agents involved in antecedent infections, as have recent immunizations. The swine influenza vaccine, administered widely in the United States in 1976, is the most notable example; influenza vaccines in use from 1992–1994, however, resulted in only one additional case of GBS per million persons vaccinated. Older-type rabies vaccine, prepared in nervous system tissue, is implicated as a trigger of GBS in developing countries where it is still used; the mechanism is presumably immunization against neural antigens. GBS also occurs more frequently than can be attributed to chance alone in patients with lymphoma (including Hodgkin's disease), in HIV-seropositive individuals, and in patients with systemic lupus erythematosus (SLE). *C. jejuni* has also been implicated in summer outbreaks of AMAN among children and young adults exposed to chickens in rural China.

Immunopathogenesis Several lines of evidence support an autoimmune basis for acute inflammatory demyelinating polyneuropathy (AIDP), the most common and best-studied type of GBS; the concept extends to all of the subtypes of GBS (Table 380-1).

It is likely that both cellular and humoral immune mechanisms contribute to tissue damage in AIDP. T cell activation is suggested by

TABLE 380-1 SUBTYPES OF GUILLAIN-BARRÉ SYNDROME (GBS)

Subtype	Features	Electrodiagnosis	Pathology
Acute inflammatory demyelinating poly-neuropathy (AIDP)	Adults affected more than children; 90% of cases in western world; recovery rapid; anti-GM1 antibodies (<50%)	Demyelinating	First attack on Schwann cell surface; widespread myelin damage, macrophage activation, and lymphocytic infiltration; variable secondary axonal damage
Acute motor axonal neuropathy (AMAN)	Children and young adults; prevalent in China and Mexico; may be seasonal; recovery rapid; anti-GD1a antibodies	Axonal	First attack at motor nodes of Ranvier; macrophage activation, few lymphocytes, frequent periaxonal macrophages; extent of axonal damage highly variable
Acute motor sensory axonal neuropathy (AMSAN)	Mostly adults; uncommon; recovery slow, often incomplete; closely related to AMAN	Axonal	Same as AMAN, but also affects sensory nerves and roots; axonal damage usually severe
M. Fisher syndrome (MFS)	Adults and children; uncommon; ophthalmoplegia, ataxia, and areflexia; anti-GQ1b antibodies (90%)	Demyelinating	Few cases examined; resembles AIDP

the finding that elevated levels of cytokines and cytokine receptors are present in serum [interleukin (IL) 2, soluble IL-2 receptor] and in cerebrospinal fluid (CSF) (IL-6, tumor necrosis factor α, interferon-γ). AIDP is also closely analogous to an experimental T cell–mediated immunopathy designated *experimental allergic neuritis* (EAN); EAN is induced in laboratory animals by immune sensitization against protein fragments derived from peripheral nerve proteins, and in particular against the P2 protein. Based on analogy to EAN, it was initially thought that AIDP was likely to be primarily a T cell–mediated disorder; however, abundant data now suggest that autoantibodies directed against nonprotein determinants may be central to many cases.

Circumstantial evidence suggests that all GBS results from immune responses to nonself antigens (infectious agents, vaccines) that misdirect to host nerve tissue through a resemblance-of-epitope (molecular mimicry) mechanism (Fig. 380-1). The neural targets are likely to be glycoconjugates, specifically gangliosides (Table 380-2; Fig. 380-2). Gangliosides are complex glycosphingolipids that contain one or more sialic acid residues; various gangliosides participate in cell-cell interactions (including those between axons and glia), modulation of receptors, and regulation of growth. They are typically exposed on the plasma membrane of cells, rendering them susceptible to an antibody-mediated attack. Gangliosides and other glycoconjugates are present in large quantity in human nervous tissues and in key sites, such as nodes of Ranvier. Antiganglioside antibodies, most frequently to GM1, are common in GBS (20–50% of cases), particularly in those preceded by *C. jejuni* infection. Furthermore, isolates of *C. jejuni* from stool cultures of patients with GBS have surface glycolipid structures that antigenically cross react with gangli-

osides, including GM1, concentrated in human nerves. Another line of evidence is derived from experience in Europe with parenteral use of purified bovine brain gangliosides for treatment of various neuropathic disorders. Between 5 and 15 days after injection some recipients developed acute motor axonal GBS with high titers of anti-GM1 antibodies that recognized epitopes at nodes of Ranvier and motor endplates. Experimentally, anti-GM1 antibodies can trigger complement-mediated injury at paranodal axon-glial junctions, disrupting the clustering of sodium channels and likely contributing to conduction block (see "Pathophysiology," below).

Anti-GQ1b IgG antibodies are found in >90% of patients with MFS (Table 380-2; Fig. 380-2), and titers of IgG are highest early in the course. Anti-GQ1b antibodies are not found in other forms of GBS unless there is extraocular motor nerve involvement. A possible explanation for this association is that extraocular motor nerves are enriched in GQ1b gangliosides in comparison to limb nerves. In addition, a monoclonal anti-GQ1b antibody raised against *C. jejuni* isolated from a patient with MFS blocked neuromuscular transmission experimentally.

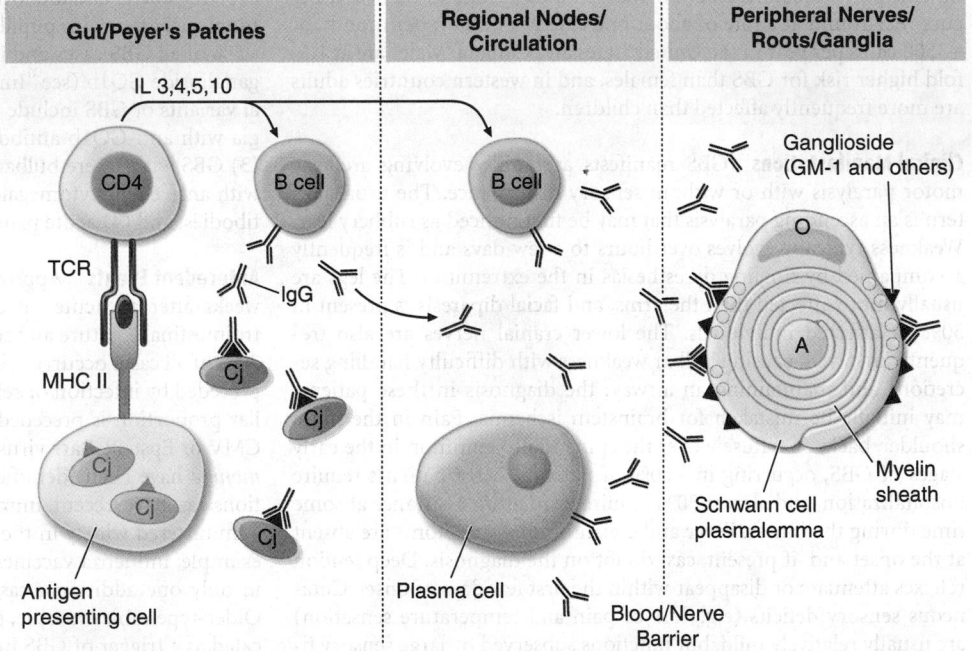

FIGURE 380-1 Postulated immunopathogenesis of GBS associated with *C. jejuni* infection. B cells recognize glycoconjugates on *C. jejuni* (Cj) (triangles) that cross-react with ganglioside present on Schwann cell surface and subjacent peripheral nerve myelin. Some B cells, activated via a T cell–independent mechanism, secrete primarily IgM (not shown). Other B cells (upper left side) are activated via a partially T cell–dependent route and secrete primarily IgG; T cell help is provided by CD4 cells activated locally by fragments of Cj proteins that are presented on the surface of antigen-presenting cells (APC). A critical event in the development of GBS is the escape of activated B cells from Peyer's patches into regional lymph nodes. Activated T cells probably also function to assist in opening of the blood-nerve barrier, facilitating penetration of pathogenic autoantibodies. The earliest changes in myelin (right) consist of edema between myelin lamellae and vesicular disruption (shown as circular blebs) of the outermost myelin layers. These effects are associated with activation of the C5b-C9 membrane attack complex and probably mediated by calcium entry; it is possible that the macrophage cytokine tumor necrosis factor (TNF) also participates in myelin damage. B, B cell; MHC II, class II major histocompatibility complex molecule; TCR, T cell receptor; A, axon; O, oligodendrocyte.

TABLE 380-2	PRINCIPAL ANTI-GLYCOLIPID ANTIBODIES IMPLICATED IN IMMUNE NEUROPATHIES		
Clinical Presentation		**Antibody Target**	**Usual Isotype**
Acute Immune Neuropathies (Guillain-Barré Syndrome)			
Acute inflammatory demyelinating polyneuropathy (AIDP)		No clear patterns GM1 most common	IgG (polyclonal)
Acute motor axonal neuropathy (AMAN)		GD1a, GM1, GM1b, GalNAc–GD1a (<50% for any)	IgG (polyclonal)
Miller Fisher syndrome (MFS)		GQ1b (>90%)	IgG (polyclonal)
Acute pharyngeal cervico-brachial neuropathy (APCBN)		GT1a (? Most)	IgG (polyclonal)
Chronic Immune Neuropathies			
Chronic inflammatory demyelinating polyneuropathy (CIDP) (75%)		Po in some	No clear pattern
CIDPa (MGUS associated) (25%)		Neural binding sites	IgG, IgA (monoclonal)
Chronic sensory > motor neuropathy		SPGP, SGLPG (on MAG) (50%)	IgM (monoclonal)
		Uncertain (50%)	IgM (monoclonal)
Multifocal motor neuropathy (MMN)		GM1, GalNAc–GD1a, others (25–50%)	IgM (polyclonal, monoclonal)
Chronic sensory ataxic neuropathy		GD1b, GQ1b, and other b-series gangliosides	IgM (monoclonal)

Note: MGUS, monoclonal gammopathy of undetermined significance; MAG, myelin-associated glycoprotein.
Source: Modified from HJ Willison, N Yuki: Brain 125:2591, 2002.

Taken together, these observations provide strong but still inconclusive evidence that autoantibodies play an important pathogenic role in GBS. Although anti-ganglioside antibodies have been studied most intensively, other antigenic targets may also be important. One report identified IgG antibodies against Schwann cells and neurons

FIGURE 380-2 Glycolipids implicated as antigens in immune-mediated neuropathies. (*Modified from HJ Willison, N Yuki: Brain 125:2591, 2002.*)

(nerve growth cone region) in some GBS cases. Proof that these antibodies are pathogenic requires that they be capable of mediating disease following direct passive transfer to naïve hosts; this has not yet been demonstrated, although one case of apparent maternal-fetal transplacental transfer of GBS has been described.

In ADEM, an early step in the induction of tissue damage appears to be complement deposition along the outer surface of the Schwann cell. Activation of complement initiates a characteristic vesicular disintegration of the myelin sheath, and also leads to recruitment of activated macrophages, which participate in damage to myelin and axons. In AMAN, the pattern is different in that complement is deposited along with IgG at the nodes of Ranvier along large motor axons.

Pathophysiology In the demyelinating forms of GBS, the basis for flaccid paralysis and sensory disturbance is conduction block. This finding, demonstrable electrophysiologically, implies that the axonal connections remain intact. Hence, recovery can take place rapidly as remyelination occurs. In severe cases of demyelinating GBS, secondary axonal degeneration usually occurs; its extent can be estimated electrophysiologically. More secondary axonal degeneration correlates with a slower rate of recovery and a greater degree of residual disability. When a severe primary axonal pattern is encountered electrophysiologically, the implication is that axons have degenerated and become disconnected from their targets, specifically the neuromuscular junctions, and must therefore regenerate for recovery to take place. In motor axonal cases in which recovery is rapid, the lesion is thought to be localized to preterminal motor branches, allowing regeneration and reinnervation to take place quickly. Alternatively, in mild cases, collateral sprouting and reinnervation from surviving motor axons near the neuromuscular junction may begin to reestablish physiologic continuity with muscle cells over a period of several months.

Laboratory Features CSF findings are distinctive, consisting of an elevated CSF protein level [1–10 g/L (100–1000 mg/dL)] without accompanying pleocytosis. The CSF is often normal when symptoms have been present for ≤48 h; by the end of the first week the level of protein is usually elevated. A transient increase in the CSF white cell count (10–100/μL) occurs on occasion in otherwise typical GBS; however, a sustained CSF pleocytosis suggests an alternative diagnosis (viral myelitis) or a concurrent diagnosis such as unrecognized HIV infection. Electrodiagnostic features are mild or absent in the early stages of GBS and lag behind the clinical evolution. In cases with demyelination (Table 380-1), prolonged distal latencies, conduction velocity slowing, evidence of conduction block, and temporal dispersion of compound action potential are the usual features. In cases with primary axonal pathology, the principal electrodiagnostic finding is reduced amplitude of compound action potentials without conduction slowing or prolongation of distal latencies.

Diagnosis GBS is a descriptive entity. The diagnosis is made by recognizing the pattern of rapidly evolving paralysis with areflexia, absence of fever or other systemic symptoms, and characteristic antecedent events (Table 380-3). Other disorders that may enter into the differential diagnosis include acute myelopathies (especially with prolonged back pain and sphincter disturbances); botulism (pupillary reactivity lost early); diphtheria (early oropharyngeal disturbances); Lyme polyradiculitis and other tick-borne paralyses; porphyria (abdominal pain, seizures, psychosis); vasculitic neuropathy (check erythrocyte sedimentation rate, described below); poliomyelitis (fever and meningismus common); CMV polyradiculitis (in immunocompromised patients); critical illness neuropathy; neuromuscular disorders such as myasthenia gravis; poisonings with organophosphates, thallium, or arsenic; tick paralysis; paralytic shellfish poisoning; or severe hypophosphatemia (rare). Laboratory tests are helpful primarily to exclude mimics of GBS. Electrodiagnostic features may be minimal, and the CSF protein level may not rise until the end of the first week. If the diagnosis is strongly suspected, treatment should be initiated without waiting for evolution of the characteristic electrodiagnostic and CSF

CHAPTER 380 Guillain-Barré Syndrome and Other Immune-Mediated Neuropathies

TABLE 380-3 DIAGNOSTIC CRITERIA FOR GUILLAIN-BARRÉ SYNDROME

Required

1. Progressive weakness of 2 or more limbs due to neuropathy[a]
2. Areflexia
3. Disease course <4 weeks
4. Exclusion of other causes [e.g., vasculitis (polyarteritis nodosa, systemic lupus erythematosus, Churg-Strauss syndrome), toxins (organophosphates, lead), botulism, diphtheria, porphyria, localized spinal cord or cauda equina syndrome]

Supportive

1. Relatively symmetric weakness
2. Mild sensory involvement
3. Facial nerve or other cranial nerve involvement
4. Absence of fever
5. Typical CSF profile (acellular, increase in protein level)
6. Electrophysiologic evidence of demyelination

[a]Excluding M. Fisher and other variant syndromes.
Source: Modified from AK Asbury, DR Cornblath: Ann Neurol 27:S21, 1990.

findings to occur. Both tau and 14-3-3 protein levels are reported to be elevated early (during the first few days of symptoms) in some cases of GBS. Tau increases in CSF may reflect axonal damage and predict a residual deficit. GBS patients with risk factors for HIV or with CSF pleocytosis should have a serologic test for HIV.

℞ GUILLAIN-BARRÉ SYNDROME

In the vast majority of patients with GBS, treatment should be initiated as soon after diagnosis as possible. Each day counts; ~2 weeks after the first motor symptoms, immunotherapy is no longer effective. Either high-dose intravenous immune globulin (IVIg) or plasmapheresis can be initiated, as they are equally effective. A combination of the two therapies is not significantly better than either alone. IVIg is often the initial therapy chosen because of its ease of administration and good safety record. IVIg is administered as five daily infusions for a total dose of 2 g/kg body weight. There is some evidence that GBS autoantibodies are neutralized by anti-idiotypic antibodies present in IVIg preparations, perhaps accounting for the therapeutic effect. A course of plasmapheresis usually consists of ~40–50 mL/kg plasma exchange (PE) four times over a week. Meta-analysis of randomized clinical trials indicates that treatment reduces the need for mechanical ventilation by nearly half (from 27% to 14% with PE), and increases the likelihood of full recovery at 1 year (from 55% to 68%). In patients who are treated early in the course of GBS and improve, relapse may occur in the second or third week. Brief retreatment with the original therapy is usually effective. Glucocorticoids have not been found to be effective in GBS. Occasional patients with very mild forms of GBS, especially those who appear to have already reached a plateau when initially seen, may be managed conservatively without IVIg or PE.

In the worsening phase of GBS, most patients require monitoring in a critical care setting, with particular attention to vital capacity, heart rhythm, blood pressure, nutrition, deep vein thrombosis prophylaxis, cardiovascular status, early consideration (after 2 weeks of intubation) of tracheotomy, and chest physiotherapy. As noted, ~30% of patients with GBS require ventilatory assistance, sometimes for prolonged periods of time (several weeks or longer). Frequent turning and assiduous skin care are important, as are daily range-of-motion exercises to avoid joint contractures and daily reassurance as to the generally good outlook for recovery.

Prognosis and Recovery Approximately 85% of patients with GBS achieve a full functional recovery within several months to a year, although minor findings on examination (such as areflexia) may persist. The mortality rate is <5% in optimal settings; death usually results from secondary pulmonary complications. The outlook is worst in patients with severe proximal motor and sensory axonal damage. Such axonal damage may be either primary or secondary in nature (see "Pathophysiology," above), but in either case successful regeneration cannot occur. Other factors that worsen the outlook for recovery are

advanced age, a fulminant or severe attack, and a delay in the onset of treatment. Between 5 and 10% of patients with typical GBS have one or more late relapses; such cases are then classified as chronic inflammatory demyelinating polyneuropathy (CIDP).

CHRONIC INFLAMMATORY DEMYELINATING POLYNEUROPATHY

CIDP is distinguished from GBS by its chronic course. In other respects, this neuropathy shares many features with the common demyelinating form of GBS, including elevated CSF protein levels and the electrodiagnostic findings of acquired demyelination. Most cases occur in adults, and males are affected slightly more often than females. The incidence of CIDP is lower than that of GBS, but due to the protracted course the prevalence is greater.

Clinical Manifestations Onset is usually gradual, sometimes subacute; in a few, the initial attack is indistinguishable from that of GBS. An acute-onset form of CIDP should be considered when GBS deteriorates >9 weeks after onset or relapses at least three times. Symptoms are both motor and sensory in most cases. Weakness of the limbs is usually symmetric but can be strikingly asymmetric. There is considerable variability from case to case. Some patients experience a chronic progressive course, whereas others, usually younger patients, have a relapsing and remitting course. Some have only motor findings, and a small proportion present with a relatively pure syndrome of sensory ataxia. Tremor occurs in ~10% and may become more prominent during periods of subacute worsening or improvement. A small proportion have cranial nerve findings, including external ophthalmoplegia. CIDP tends to ameliorate over time with treatment; the result is that many years after onset nearly 75% of patients have reasonable functional status. Death from CIDP is uncommon.

Diagnosis The diagnosis rests on characteristic clinical, CSF, and electrophysiologic findings. The CSF is usually acellular with an elevated protein level, sometimes several times normal. Electrodiagnostically, variable degrees of conduction slowing, prolonged distal latencies, temporal dispersion of compound action potentials, and conduction block are the principal features. In particular, the presence of conduction block is a certain sign of an acquired demyelinating process. Evidence of axonal loss, presumably secondary to demyelination, is present in >50% of patients. Serum protein electrophoresis with immunofixation is indicated to search for monoclonal gammopathy and associated conditions (see "Monoclonal Gammopathy of Undetermined Significance," below). In all patients with presumptive CIDP, it is also reasonable to exclude vasculitis, collagen vascular disease (especially SLE), chronic hepatitis, HIV infection, and diabetes mellitus. Other associated conditions include inflammatory bowel disease and Hodgkin's lymphoma.

Pathogenesis Although there is evidence of immune activation in CIDP, the precise mechanisms of pathogenesis are unknown. Biopsy typically reveals little inflammation and onion-bulb changes (imbricated layers of attenuated Schwann cell processes surrounding an axon) that result from recurrent demyelination and remyelination (Fig. 380-1). The response to therapy suggests that CIDP is immune-mediated; CIDP responds to glucocorticoids, whereas GBS does not. Passive transfer of demyelination into experimental animals has been accomplished using IgG purified from the serum of some patients with CIDP, lending support for a humoral autoimmune pathogenesis. Although the target antigen or antigens in CIDP have not yet been identified, the myelin protein Po has been implicated as a potential autoantigen in some patients. It is also of interest that a CIDP-like illness developed spontaneously in the nonobese diabetic (NOD) mouse when the immune co-stimulatory molecule B7-2 (CD86) was genetically deleted; this suggests that CIDP can result from altered triggering of T cells by antigen-presenting cells.

Approximately 25% of patients with clinical features of CIDP also have a monoclonal gammopathy of undetermined significance (MGUS).

Cases associated with monoclonal IgA or IgG usually respond to treatment as favorably as cases without a monoclonal gammopathy. Patients with IgM monoclonal gammopathy tend to have more sensory findings, a more protracted course, and may have a less satisfactory response to treatment, although this is an area of controversy.

Rx CHRONIC INFLAMMATORY DEMYELINATING POLYNEUROPATHY

Most authorities initiate treatment for CIDP when progression is rapid or walking is compromised. If the disorder is mild, management can be expectant, awaiting spontaneous remission. Controlled studies have shown that high-dose IVIg, PE, and glucocorticoids are all more effective than placebo. Initial therapy is usually with IVIg, administered as 0.4 g/kg body weight daily for 5 days; most patients require periodic re-treatment at ~6-week intervals. PE, which appears to be as effective as IVIg, is initiated at two to three treatments per week for 6 weeks; periodic re-treatment may also be required. Treatment with glucocorticoids is another option (60–80 mg prednisone PO daily for 1–2 months, followed by a gradual dose reduction of 10 mg per month as tolerated), but long-term adverse effects including bone demineralization, gastrointestinal bleeding, and cushingoid changes are problematic. Anecdotal experience suggested that glucocorticoids might be harmful to some patients with a purely motor form of CIDP, thus glucocorticoids should probably be avoided when sensory findings are absent. Approximately one-half of patients with CIDP fail to respond adequately to the initial therapy chosen; a different treatment should then be tried. Patients who fail therapy with IVIg, PE, and glucocorticoids may benefit from treatment with immunosuppressive agents such as azathioprine, methotrexate, cyclosporine, and cyclophosphamide, either alone or as adjunctive therapy. Early experience with anti-CD20 (rituximab) has also shown promise. Use of these therapies requires periodic reassessment of their risks and benefits.

MULTIFOCAL MOTOR NEUROPATHY

Multifocal motor neuropathy (MMN) is a distinctive but uncommon neuropathy that presents as slowly progressive motor weakness and atrophy evolving over years in the distribution of selected nerve trunks, associated with sites of persistent focal motor conduction block in the same nerve trunks. Sensory fibers are relatively spared. The arms are affected more frequently than the legs, and >75% of all patients are male. Some cases have been confused with lower motor neuron forms of amyotrophic lateral sclerosis (Chap. 369). Approximately 50% of patients present with high titers of polyclonal IgM antibody to the ganglioside GM1. It is uncertain how this finding relates to the discrete foci of persistent motor conduction block, but high concentrations of GM1 gangliosides are normal constituents of nodes of Ranvier in peripheral nerve fibers. Pathology reveals demyelination and mild inflammatory changes at the sites of conduction block.

Most patients with MMN respond to high-dose IVIg (dosages as for CIDP, above); periodic re-treatment is required in more than half of responders to maintain the benefit. Some refractory patients have responded to cyclophosphamide. Glucocorticoids and PE are not effective.

NEUROPATHIES WITH MONOCLONAL GAMMOPATHY

MULTIPLE MYELOMA

Clinically overt polyneuropathy occurs in ~5% of patients with the commonly encountered type of multiple myeloma, which exhibits either lytic or diffuse osteoporotic bone lesions. These neuropathies are sensorimotor, are usually mild and slowly progressive but may be severe, and generally do not reverse with successful suppression of the myeloma. In most cases, electrodiagnostic and pathologic features are consistent with a process of axonal degeneration.

In contrast, myeloma with osteosclerotic features, although representing only 3% of all myelomas, is associated with polyneuropathy in one-half of cases. These neuropathies, which may also occur with solitary plasmacytoma, are distinct because they (1) are usually demyelinating in nature; (2) often respond to radiation therapy or removal of the primary lesion; (3) are associated with different monoclonal proteins and light chains (almost always lambda as opposed to primarily kappa in the lytic type of multiple myeloma); and (4) may occur in association with other systemic findings including thickening of the skin, hyperpigmentation, hypertrichosis, organomegaly, endocrinopathy, anasarca, and clubbing of fingers. These are features of the POEMS syndrome (polyneuropathy, organomegaly, endocrinopathy, M protein, and skin changes). The pathogenesis of this uncommon syndrome and the explanation for its association with lambda light chains are unknown. Treatment of the neuropathy is best directed at the osteosclerotic myeloma using surgery, radiotherapy, or chemotherapy, as indicated.

Neuropathies are also encountered in other systemic conditions with gammopathy including Waldenström's macroglobulinemia, primary systemic amyloidosis, and cryoglobulinemic states (mixed essential cryoglobulinemia, some cases of hepatitis C).

MONOCLONAL GAMMOPATHY OF UNDETERMINED SIGNIFICANCE

Chronic polyneuropathies occurring in association with MGUS are usually associated with the immunoglobulin isotypes IgG, IgA, and IgM. From a clinical standpoint, many of these patients are indistinguishable from patients with CIDP without monoclonal gammopathy (see "Chronic Inflammatory Demyelinating Polyneuropathy," above), and their response to immunosuppressive agents is also similar. An exception is the syndrome of IgM kappa monoclonal gammopathy associated with an indolent, longstanding, sometimes static sensory neuropathy, frequently with tremor and sensory ataxia. Most patients are male and over age 50. In the majority, the monoclonal IgM immunoglobulin binds to a normal peripheral nerve constituent, myelin-associated glycoprotein (MAG), found in the paranodal regions of Schwann cells. Binding appears to be specific for a polysaccharide epitope that is also found in other normal peripheral nerve myelin glycoproteins, P0 and PMP22, and also in other normal nerve-related glycosphingolipids (Fig. 380-1). In the MAG-positive cases, IgM paraprotein is incorporated into the myelin sheaths of affected patients and widens the spacing of the myelin lamellae, thus producing a distinctive ultrastructural pattern. Demyelination and remyelination are the hallmarks of the lesions. The chronic demyelinating neuropathy appears to result from a destabilization of myelin metabolism rather than activation of an immune response. Therapy with chlorambucil, or cyclophosphamide combined with glucocorticoids or PE, often results in improvement of the neuropathy associated with a prolonged reduction in the levels in the circulating paraprotein; chronic use of these alkylating agents is associated with significant risks. Recent preliminary data also suggest that anti-CD20 (rituximab) therapy may be effective. In a small proportion of patients (30% at 10 years), MGUS will in time evolve into frankly malignant conditions such as multiple myeloma or lymphoma.

VASCULITIC NEUROPATHY

Peripheral nerve involvement is common in polyarteritis nodosa (PAN), appearing in half of all cases clinically and in 100% of cases at postmortem studies (Chap. 319). The most common pattern is multifocal (asymmetric) motor-sensory neuropathy (mononeuropathy multiplex) due to ischemic lesions of nerve trunks and roots; however, some cases of vasculitic neuropathy present as a distal, symmetric sensorimotor polyneuropathy. Symptoms of neuropathy are a common presenting complaint in patients with PAN. The electrodiagnostic findings are those of an axonal process. Small- to medium-sized arteries of the vasa nervorum, particularly the epineural vessels, are affected in PAN, resulting in a widespread ischemic neuropathy. A high frequency of neuropathy occurs in allergic angiitis and granulomatosis (Churg-Strauss syndrome).

Systemic vasculitis should always be considered when a subacute or chronically evolving mononeuropathy multiplex occurs in conjunction with constitutional symptoms (fever, anorexia, weight loss, loss of energy, malaise, and nonspecific pains). Diagnosis of suspected vasculitic neuropathy is made by a combined nerve and muscle biopsy, with serial section or skip-serial techniques (Chap. 379).

Approximately one-third of biopsy-proven cases of vasculitic neuropathy are "nonsystemic" in that the vasculitis appears to affect only peripheral nerves. Constitutional symptoms are absent, and the course is more indolent than that of PAN. The erythrocyte sedimentation rate may be elevated, but other tests for systemic disease are negative. Nevertheless, clinically silent involvement of other organs is likely, and vasculitis is frequently found in muscle biopsied at the same time as nerve.

Vasculitic neuropathy may also be seen as part of the vasculitis syndrome occurring in the course of other connective tissue disorders (Chap. 319). The most frequent is rheumatoid arthritis, but ischemic neuropathy due to involvement of vasa nervorum may also occur in mixed cryoglobulinemia, Sjögren's syndrome, Wegener's granulomatosis, hypersensitivity angiitis, and progressive systemic sclerosis. Management of these neuropathies, including the "nonsystemic" vasculitic neuropathy, consists of treatment of the underlying condition as well as the aggressive use of glucocorticoids and other immunosuppressant drugs. One reasonable starting regimen is daily prednisone (initial dose 1 mg/kg per day PO with a gradual taper after 1 month) plus IV pulse (or daily oral) cyclophosphamide for 3–6 months.

ANTI-HU PARANEOPLASTIC NEUROPATHY

This uncommon immune-mediated disorder manifests as a sensory neuronopathy (i.e., selective damage to sensory nerve bodies in dorsal root ganglia). The onset is often asymmetric with dysesthesias and sensory loss in the limbs that soon progress to affect all limbs, the torso, and face. Marked sensory ataxia, pseudoathetosis, and inability to walk, stand, or even sit unsupported are frequent features and are secondary to the extensive deafferentation. Subacute sensory neuronopathy may be idiopathic, but more than half of cases are paraneoplastic, primarily related to lung cancer, and most of those are small cell lung cancer (SCLC). Diagnosis of the underlying SCLC requires awareness of the association, paraneoplastic testing, and often PET scanning for the tumor. The target antigens are a family of RNA binding proteins (HuD, HuC, and Hel-N1) that in normal tissues are only expressed by neurons. The same proteins are usually expressed by SCLC, triggering in some patients an immune response characterized by antibodies and cytotoxic T cells that cross-react with the Hu proteins of the dorsal root ganglion neurons, resulting in immune-mediated neuronal destruction. An encephalomyelitis may accompany the sensory neuronopathy and presumably has the same pathogenesis. Neurologic symptoms usually precede, by ≤ 6 months, the identification of SCLC. The sensory neuronopathy runs its course in a few weeks or months and stabilizes, leaving the patient disabled. Most cases are unresponsive to treatment with glucocorticoids, IVIg, PE, or immunosuppressant drugs.

FURTHER READINGS

GORSON KC: Vasculitic neuropathies. An update. The Neurologist 13:12, 2007

HADDEN RDM et al: European Federation of Neurological Societies/Peripheral Nerve Society guideline on management of paraproteinemic demyelinating neuropathies: Report of a joint task force of the European Federation of Neurological Societies and the Peripheral Nerve Society. Eur J Neurol 13:809, 2006

HUGHES RAC et al: European Federation of Neurological Societies/Peripheral Nerve Society guideline on management of chronic inflammatory demyelinating polyradiculoneuropathy: Report of a joint task force of the European Federation of Neurological Societies and the Peripheral Nerve Society. Eur J Neurol 13:326, 2006

—— et al: Immunotherapy for Guillain-Barré syndrome: A systematic review. Brain. March 2, 2007, epub ahead of print

MATHEW L et al: Treatment of vasculitic peripheral neuropathy: A retrospective analysis of outcome. QJ Med 100:41, 2007

RUTS L et al: Distinguishing acute-onset CIDP from Guillain-Barré syndrome with treatment-related fluctuations. Neurology 65(1):138, 2005

SUSUKI K et al: Anti-GM1 antibodies cause complement-mediated disruption of sodium channel clusters in peripheral motor nerve fibers. J Neurosci 27:3956, 2007

VAN SCHAIK IN et al: European Federation of Neurological Societies/Peripheral Nerve Society guideline on management of multifocal motor neuropathy. Eur J Neurol 13:802, 2006

381 Myasthenia Gravis and Other Diseases of the Neuromuscular Junction
Daniel B. Drachman

Myasthenia gravis (MG) is a neuromuscular disorder characterized by weakness and fatigability of skeletal muscles. The underlying defect is a decrease in the number of available acetylcholine receptors (AChRs) at neuromuscular junctions due to an antibody-mediated autoimmune attack. Treatment now available for MG is highly effective, although a specific cure has remained elusive.

PATHOPHYSIOLOGY

In the neuromuscular junction (Fig. 381-1), acetylcholine (ACh) is synthesized in the motor nerve terminal and stored in vesicles (quanta). When an action potential travels down a motor nerve and reaches the nerve terminal, ACh from 150–200 vesicles is released and combines with AChRs that are densely packed at the peaks of postsynaptic folds. The structure of the AChR has been fully elucidated; it consists of five subunits (2α, 1β, 1δ, and 1γ or ϵ) arranged around a central pore. When ACh combines with the binding sites on the α subunits of the AChR, the channel in the AChR opens, permitting the rapid entry of cations, chiefly sodium, which produces depolarization at the end-plate region of the muscle fiber. If the depolarization is sufficiently large, it initiates an ac-

tion potential that is propagated along the muscle fiber, triggering muscle contraction. This process is rapidly terminated by hydrolysis of ACh by acetylcholinesterase (AChE), which is present within the synaptic folds, and by diffusion of ACh away from the receptor.

In MG, the fundamental defect is a decrease in the number of available AChRs at the postsynaptic muscle membrane. In addition, the postsynaptic folds are flattened, or "simplified." These changes result in decreased efficiency of neuromuscular transmission. Therefore, although ACh is released normally, it produces small end-plate potentials that may fail to trigger muscle action potentials. Failure of transmission at many neuromuscular junctions results in weakness of muscle contraction.

The amount of ACh released per impulse normally declines on repeated activity (termed *presynaptic rundown*). In the myasthenic patient, the decreased efficiency of neuromuscular transmission combined with the normal rundown results in the activation of fewer and fewer muscle fibers by successive nerve impulses and hence increasing weakness, or *myasthenic fatigue*. This mechanism also accounts for the decremental response to repetitive nerve stimulation seen on electrodiagnostic testing.

The neuromuscular abnormalities in MG are brought about by an autoimmune response mediated by specific anti-AChR antibodies. The anti-AChR antibodies reduce the number of available AChRs at neuromuscular junctions by three distinct mechanisms: (1) accelerated turnover of AChRs by a mechanism involving cross-linking and rapid endocytosis of the receptors; (2) blockade of the active site of the AChR, i.e., the site that normally binds ACh; and (3) damage to the postsynaptic muscle membrane by the antibody in collaboration with complement. An immune response to muscle-specific kinase (MuSK) can also result in myasthenia gravis, possibly by interfering with AChR

FIGURE 381-1 Diagrams of (A) normal and (B) myasthenic neuromuscular junctions. AChE, acetylcholinesterase. See text for description of normal neuromuscular transmission. The MG junction demonstrates a normal nerve terminal; a reduced number of AChRs (stippling); flattened, simplified postsynaptic folds; and a widened synaptic space. *(Modified from DB Drachman: N Engl J Med 330:1797, 1994; with permission.)*

clustering. The pathogenic antibodies are IgG and are T cell dependent. Thus, immunotherapeutic strategies directed against T cells are effective in this antibody-mediated disease.

How the autoimmune response is initiated and maintained in MG is not completely understood. However, the thymus appears to play a role in this process. The thymus is abnormal in ~75% of patients with MG; in ~65% the thymus is "hyperplastic," with the presence of active germinal centers detected histologically, though the hyperplastic thymus is not necessarily enlarged. An additional 10% of patients have thymic tumors (thymomas). Muscle-like cells within the thymus (myoid cells), which bear AChRs on their surface, may serve as a source of autoantigen and trigger the autoimmune reaction within the thymus gland.

CLINICAL FEATURES

MG is not rare, having a prevalence of 1–7 in 10,000. It affects individuals in all age groups, but peaks of incidence occur in women in their twenties and thirties and in men in their fifties and sixties. Overall, women are affected more frequently than men, in a ratio of ~3:2. The cardinal features are *weakness* and *fatigability* of muscles. The weakness increases during repeated use (fatigue) and may improve following rest or sleep. The course of MG is often variable. Exacerbations and remissions may occur, particularly during the first few years after the onset of the disease. Remissions are rarely complete or permanent. Unrelated infections or systemic disorders often lead to increased myasthenic weakness and may precipitate "crisis" (see below).

The distribution of muscle weakness often has a characteristic pattern. The cranial muscles, particularly the lids and extraocular muscles, are often involved early in the course of MG, and diplopia and ptosis are common initial complaints. Facial weakness produces a "snarling" expression when the patient attempts to smile. Weakness in chewing is most noticeable after prolonged effort, as in chewing meat. Speech may have a nasal timbre caused by weakness of the palate or a dysarthric "mushy" quality due to tongue weakness. Difficulty in swallowing may occur as a result of weakness of the palate, tongue, or pharynx, giving rise to nasal regurgitation or aspiration of liquids or food. Bulbar weakness is especially prominent in MuSK antibody–positive MG. In ~85% of patients, the weakness becomes generalized, affecting the limb muscles as well. If weakness remains restricted to the extraocular muscles for 3 years, it is likely that it will not become generalized, and these patients are said to have *ocular MG*. The limb weakness in MG is often proximal and may be asymmetric. Despite the muscle weakness, deep tendon reflexes are preserved. If weakness of respiration becomes so severe as to require respiratory assistance, the patient is said to be in *crisis*.

DIAGNOSIS AND EVALUATION

(Table 381-1) The diagnosis is suspected on the basis of weakness and fatigability in the typical distribution described above, without loss of reflexes or impairment of sensation or other neurologic function. The suspected diagnosis should always be confirmed definitively before treatment is undertaken; this is essential because (1) other treatable conditions may closely resemble MG, and (2) the treatment of MG may involve surgery and the prolonged use of drugs with adverse side effects.

Antibodies to AChR or MuSK As noted above, anti-AChR antibodies are detectable in the serum of ~85% of all myasthenic patients but in only about 50% of patients with weakness confined to the ocular muscles. The presence of anti-AChR antibodies is virtually diagnostic of MG, but a negative test does not exclude the disease. The measured level of anti-AChR antibody does not correspond well with the severity of MG in different patients. However, in an individual patient, a treatment-induced fall in the antibody level often correlates with clinical improvement. Antibodies to MuSK have been found to be present in ~40% of AChR antibody-negative patients with generalized MG, and their presence is a useful diagnostic test in these patients. MuSK antibodies are rarely present in AChR antibody-positive patients or in patients with MG limited to ocular muscles. These antibodies may interfere with clustering of AChRs at neuromuscular junctions, as MuSK is known to do during early development. There is also evidence that MG patients without demonstrable antibodies to either AChR or MuSK have other—as yet undefined—antibodies that impair neuromuscular transmission.

Electrodiagnostic Testing Repetitive nerve stimulation often provides helpful diagnostic evidence of MG. Anti-AChE medication is stopped 6–24 h before testing. It is best to test weak muscles or proximal muscle groups. Electric shocks are delivered at a rate of two or three per second to the appropriate nerves, and action potentials are recorded from the muscles. In normal individuals, the amplitude of the evoked muscle action potentials does not change at these rates of stimulation.

TABLE 381-1	DIAGNOSIS OF MYASTHENIA GRAVIS (MG)

History
    Diplopia, ptosis, weakness
    Weakness in characteristic distribution
    Fluctuation and fatigue: worse with repeated activity, improved by rest
    Effects of previous treatments
Physical examination
    Ptosis, diplopia
    Motor power survey: quantitative testing of muscle strength
    Forward arm abduction time (5 min)
    Vital capacity
    Absence of other neurologic signs
Laboratory testing
    Anti-AChR radioimmunoassay: ~85% positive in generalized MG; 50% in ocular MG; definite diagnosis if positive; negative result does not exclude MG. ~40% of AChR antibody-negative patients with generalized MG have anti-MuSK antibodies.
    Repetitive nerve stimulation; decrement of >15% at 3 Hz: highly probable
    Single-fiber electromyography: blocking and jitter, with normal fiber density; confirmatory, but not specific
    Edrophonium chloride (Tensilon) 2 mg + 8 mg IV; highly probable diagnosis if unequivocally positive
    For ocular or cranial MG: exclude intracranial lesions by CT or MRI

Note: AChR, acetylcholine receptor; MuSK, muscle-specific tyrosine kinase.
Source: From RT Johnson, JW Griffin (eds): *Current Therapy in Neurologic Disease*, 4th ed. St. Louis, Mosby Year Book, 1994; with permission.

TABLE 381-2 THE CONGENITAL MYASTHENIC SYNDROMES

Type	Clinical Features	Electrophysiology	Genetics	End-Plate Effects	Treatment
Slow channel	Most common; weak forearm extensors; onset 2d to 3d decade; variable severity	Repetitive muscle response on nerve stimulation; prolonged channel opening and MEPP duration	Autosomal dominant; α, β, ε AChR mutations	Excitotoxic end-plate myopathy; decreased AChRs; postsynaptic damage	Quinidine: decreases end-plate damage; made worse by anti-AChE
Low-affinity fast channel	Onset early; moderately severe; ptosis, EOM involvement; weakness and fatigue	Brief and infrequent channel openings; opposite of slow channel syndrome	Autosomal recessive; may be heteroallelic	Normal end-plate structure	3,4-DAP; anti-AChE
Severe AChR deficiencies	Early onset; variable severity; fatigue; typical MG features	Decremental response to repetitive nerve stimulation; decreased MEPP amplitudes	Autosomal recessive; ε mutations most common; many different mutations	Increased length of end plates; variable synaptic folds	Anti-AChE; ?3,4-DAP
AChE deficiency	Early onset; variable severity; scoliosis; may have normal EOM, absent pupillary responses	Decremental response to repetitive nerve stimulation	Mutant gene for AChE's collagen anchor	Small nerve terminals; degenerated junctional folds	Worse with anti-AChE drugs

Abbreviations: AChR, acetylcholine receptor; AChE, acetylcholinesterase; EOM, extraocular muscles; MEPP, miniature end-plate potentials; 3,4-DAP, 3-4-diaminopyridine.

However, in myasthenic patients there is a rapid reduction of >10–15% in the amplitude of the evoked responses. As a further test, a single dose of edrophonium may be given to prevent or diminish this decremental response.

Anticholinesterase Test Drugs that inhibit the enzyme AChE allow ACh to interact repeatedly with the limited number of AChRs, producing improvement in the strength of myasthenic muscles. Edrophonium is used most commonly for diagnostic testing because of the rapid onset (30 s) and short duration (~5 min) of its effect. An objective end-point must be selected to evaluate the effect of edrophonium, such as weakness of extraocular muscles, impairment of speech, or the length of time that the patient can maintain the arms in forward abduction. An initial IV dose of 2 mg of edrophonium is given. If definite improvement occurs, the test is considered positive and is terminated. If there is no change, the patient is given an additional 8 mg IV. The dose is administered in two parts because some patients react to edrophonium with side effects such as nausea, diarrhea, salivation, fasciculations, and rarely with severe symptoms of syncope or bradycardia. Atropine (0.6 mg) should be drawn up in a syringe, ready for IV administration if these symptoms become troublesome.

False-positive tests occur in occasional patients with other neurologic disorders, such as amyotrophic lateral sclerosis, and in placebo-reactors. False-negative or equivocal tests may also occur. In some cases it is helpful to use a longer-acting drug such as neostigmine (15 mg PO), since this permits more time for detailed evaluation of strength. The edrophonium test is now reserved for patients with clinical findings that are suggestive of MG but who have negative antibody and electrodiagnostic test results.

Inherited Myasthenic Syndromes The congenital myasthenic syndromes (CMS) comprise a heterogeneous group of disorders of the neuromuscular junction that are not autoimmune but rather are due to genetic mutations in which virtually any component of the neuromuscular junction may be affected. Alterations in function of the presynaptic nerve terminal or in the various subunits of the AChR or AChE have been identified in the various forms of CMS. These disorders share many of the clinical features of autoimmune MG, including weakness and fatigability of skeletal muscles, in some cases involving extraocular muscles (EOMs), lids, and proximal muscles, similar to the distribution in autoimmune MG. CMS should be suspected when symptoms of myasthenia have begun in infancy or childhood and AChR antibody tests are consistently negative. Features of four of the most common forms of CMS are summarized in Table 381-2. Although clinical features and electrodiagnostic and pharmacologic tests may suggest the correct diagnosis, molecular analysis is required for precise elucidation of the defect; this may lead to helpful treatment as well as genetic counseling. In the forms that involve the AChR, a wide variety of mutations have been identified in each of the subunits, but the ε subunit is affected in ~75% of these cases. In most of the recessively inherited forms of CMS, the mutations are heteroallelic; that is, different mutations affecting each of the two alleles are present.

Differential Diagnosis Other conditions that cause weakness of the cranial and/or somatic musculature include the nonautoimmune CMS discussed above, drug-induced myasthenia, Lambert-Eaton myasthenic syndrome (LEMS), neurasthenia, hyperthyroidism, botulism, intracranial mass lesions, and progressive external ophthalmoplegia. Treatment with penicillamine (used for scleroderma or rheumatoid arthritis) may result in true autoimmune MG, but the weakness is usually mild, and recovery occurs within weeks or months after discontinuing its use. Aminoglycoside antibiotics or procainamide can cause exacerbation of weakness in myasthenic patients; very large doses can cause neuromuscular weakness in normal individuals.

LEMS is a presynaptic disorder of the neuromuscular junction that can cause weakness similar to that of MG. The proximal muscles of the lower limbs are most commonly affected, but other muscles may be involved as well. Cranial nerve findings, including ptosis of the eyelids and diplopia, occur in up to 70% of patients and resemble features of MG. However, the two conditions are readily distinguished, since patients with LEMS have depressed or absent reflexes, experience autonomic changes such as dry mouth and impotence, and have incremental rather than decremental responses on repetitive nerve stimulation. LEMS is caused by autoantibodies directed against P/Q type calcium channels at the motor nerve terminals, which can be detected in ~85% of LEMS patients by radioimmunoassay. These autoantibodies result in impaired release of ACh from nerve terminals. Most patients with LEMS have an associated malignancy, most commonly small cell carcinoma of the lung, which may express calcium channels that stimulate the autoimmune response. The diagnosis may signal the presence of a tumor long before it would otherwise be detected, permitting early removal. Treatment of LEMS involves plasmapheresis and immunosuppression, as for MG. 3,4-Diaminopyridine (3,4-DAP) and pyridostigmine may also be symptomatically helpful. 3,4-DAP acts by blocking potassium channels, which results in prolonged depolarization of the motor nerve terminals and thus enhances ACh release. Pyridostigmine prolongs the action of ACh, allowing repeated interactions with AChRs.

Botulism is due to a potent bacterial toxin produced by *Clostridium botulinum*. The toxin interferes with the release of acetylcholine from the presynaptic neuromuscular junction, thereby interfering with neuromuscular transmission. The most common form is food-borne botulism from ingestion of food containing toxin; in wound and intestinal botulism spores germinate and give rise to organisms that produce toxin. Patients present with bulbar weakness (e.g., diplopia, dysarthria, dysphagia), but lack sensory symptoms and signs; deep tendon reflexes are preserved early in the disease course. Weakness generalizes to the limbs and may result in respiratory failure; reflexes may be diminished as the disease progresses. Mentation is normal. Autonomic findings include paralytic ileus, constipation, urinary retention, dilated or poorly reactive pupils, and dry mouth. The demonstration of toxin in serum by bioassay is definitive, but may be negative. Nerve conduction studies reveal findings of presynaptic neuromuscular blockade with reduced compound muscle action potentials (CMAPs) that increase in amplitude following high frequency repetitive stimulation. Treatment may include intubation for airway protection, ventilatory support, or aggressive inpatient supportive care (e.g., nutrition, DVT prophylaxis). Equine antitoxin is given rapidly before the results of laboratory studies are available. The prognosis is better among patients with type B infection who are under the age of 60 years. A vaccine is available for highly exposed individuals.

Neurasthenia is the historic term for a myasthenia-like fatigue syndrome without an organic basis. These patients may present with subjective symptoms of weakness and fatigue, but muscle testing usually reveals the "jerky release" or "give-away weakness" characteristic of nonorganic disorders; the complaint of fatigue in these patients means tiredness or apathy rather than decreasing muscle power on repeated effort. Hyperthyroidism is readily diagnosed or excluded by tests of thyroid function, which should be carried out routinely in patients with suspected MG. Abnormalities of thyroid function (hyper- or hypothyroidism) may increase myasthenic weakness. Botulism can cause myasthenic-like weakness, but the pupils are often dilated, and repetitive nerve stimulation gives an incremental response. Diplopia resembling that in MG may occasionally be due to an intracranial mass lesion that compresses nerves to the EOMs (e.g., sphenoid ridge meningioma), but MRI of the head and orbits usually reveals the lesion.

Progressive external ophthalmoplegia is a rare condition resulting in weakness of the EOMs, which may be accompanied by weakness of the proximal muscles of the limbs and other systemic features. Most patients with this condition have mitochondrial disorders that can be detected on muscle biopsy (Chap. 382).

Search for Associated Conditions

(Table 381-3) Myasthenic patients have an increased incidence of several associated disorders. Thymic abnormalities occur in ~75% of patients, as noted above. Neoplastic change (thymoma) may produce enlargement of the thymus, which is detected by CT or MRI scanning of the anterior mediastinum. A thymic shadow on CT scan may normally be present through young adulthood, but enlargement of the thymus in a patient >40 years old is highly suspicious of thymoma. Hyperthyroidism occurs in 3–8% of patients and may aggravate the myasthenic weakness. Thyroid function tests should be obtained in all patients with suspected MG. Because of the association of MG with other autoimmune disorders, blood tests for rheumatoid factor and antinuclear antibodies should also be carried out. Chronic infection of any kind can exacerbate MG and should be sought carefully. Finally, measurements of ventilatory function are valuable because of the frequency and seriousness of respiratory impairment in myasthenic patients.

Because of the side effects of glucocorticoids and other immunosuppressive agents used in the treatment of MG, a thorough medical investigation should be undertaken, searching specifically for evidence of chronic or latent infection (such as tuberculosis or hepatitis), hypertension, diabetes, renal disease, and glaucoma.

℞ MYASTHENIA GRAVIS

The prognosis has improved strikingly as a result of advances in treatment; virtually all myasthenic patients can be returned to full productive lives

TABLE 381-3 DISORDERS ASSOCIATED WITH MYASTHENIA GRAVIS AND RECOMMENDED LABORATORY TESTS

Associated disorders
  Disorders of the thymus: thymoma, hyperplasia
  Other autoimmune disorders: Hashimoto's thyroiditis, Graves' disease, rheumatoid arthritis, lupus erythematosus, skin disorders, family history of autoimmune disorder
  Disorders or circumstances that may exacerbate myasthenia gravis: hyperthyroidism or hypothyroidism, occult infection, medical treatment for other conditions (see Table 381-4)
  Disorders that may interfere with therapy: tuberculosis, diabetes, peptic ulcer, gastrointestinal bleeding, renal disease, hypertension, asthma, osteoporosis, obesity
Recommended laboratory tests or procedures
  CT or MRI of mediastinum
  Tests for lupus erythematosus, antinuclear antibody, rheumatoid factor, antithyroid antibodies
  Thyroid-function tests
  PPD skin test
  Chest radiography
  Fasting blood glucose measurement, hemoglobin A1c
  Pulmonary-function tests
  Bone densitometry in older patients

Note: PPD, purified protein derivative.
Source: From RT Johnson, JW Griffin (eds): *Current Therapy in Neurologic Disease*, 4th ed. St. Louis, Mosby Year Book, 1993, p 379; with permission.

with proper therapy. The most useful treatments for MG include anticholinesterase medications, immunosuppressive agents, thymectomy, and plasmapheresis or intravenous immunoglobulin (IVIg) **(Fig. 381-2)**.

ANTICHOLINESTERASE MEDICATIONS Anticholinesterase medication produces at least partial improvement in most myasthenic patients, although improvement is complete in only a few. Pyridostigmine is the most widely used anticholinesterase drug. As a rule, the beneficial action of oral pyridostigmine begins within 15–30 min and lasts for 3–4 h, but individual responses vary. Treatment is begun with a moderate dose, e.g., 30–60 mg three to four times daily. The frequency and amount of the dose should be tailored to the patient's individual requirements throughout the day. For example, patients with weakness in chewing and swallowing may benefit by taking the medication before meals so that peak strength coincides with mealtimes. Long-acting pyridostigmine may occasionally be useful to get the patient through the night but should never be used for daytime medication because of variable absorption. The maximum useful dose of pyridostigmine rarely exceeds 120 mg every 3–6 h during daytime. Overdosage with anticholinesterase medication may cause increased weakness and other side effects. In some patients, muscarinic side effects of the anticholinesterase medication (diarrhea, abdominal cramps, salivation, nausea) may limit the dose tolerated. Atropine/diphenoxylate or loperamide is useful for the treatment of gastrointestinal symptoms.

THYMECTOMY Two separate issues should be distinguished: (1) surgical removal of thymoma, and (2) thymectomy as a treatment for MG. Surgical removal of a thymoma is necessary because of the possibility of local tumor spread, although most thymomas are histologically benign. In the absence of a tumor, the available evidence suggests that up to 85% of patients experience improvement after thymectomy; of these, ~35% achieve drug-free remission. However, the improvement is typically delayed for months to years. The advantage of thymectomy is that it offers the possibility of long-term benefit, in some cases diminishing or eliminating the need for continuing medical treatment. In view of these potential benefits and of the negligible risk in skilled hands, thymectomy has gained widespread acceptance in the treatment of MG. It is the consensus that thymectomy should be carried out in all patients with generalized MG who are between the ages of puberty and at least 55 years. Whether thymectomy should be recommended in children, in adults >55 years of age, and in patients with weakness limited to the ocular muscles is still a matter of debate. There is also evidence that patients with MuSK antibody–positive MG may not respond to thymectomy. Thymectomy must be carried out in a hospital where it is performed regularly and where the staff is experienced in the pre- and postoperative management, anesthesia, and surgical techniques of total thymectomy.

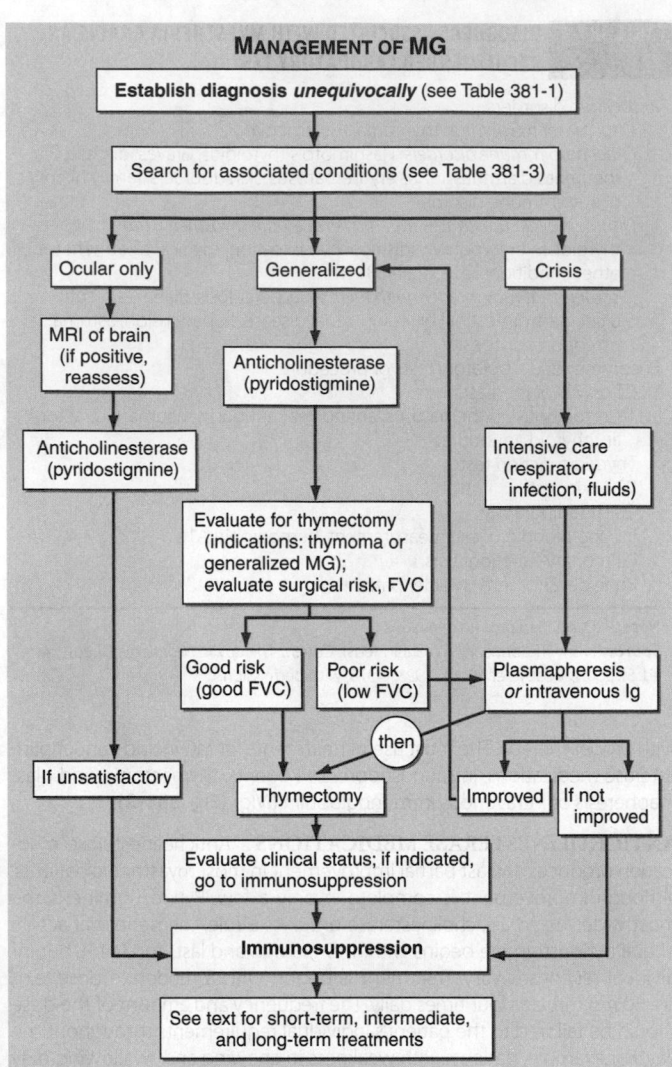

MANAGEMENT OF MG

Establish diagnosis *unequivocally* (see Table 381-1)

Search for associated conditions (see Table 381-3)

Ocular only → MRI of brain (if positive, reassess) → Anticholinesterase (pyridostigmine) → If unsatisfactory

Generalized → Anticholinesterase (pyridostigmine) → Evaluate for thymectomy (indications: thymoma or generalized MG); evaluate surgical risk, FVC → Good risk (good FVC) / Poor risk (low FVC) → Plasmapheresis *or* intravenous Ig

then → Thymectomy → Improved / If not improved

Crisis → Intensive care (respiratory infection, fluids) → Plasmapheresis *or* intravenous Ig

Evaluate clinical status; if indicated, go to immunosuppression

Immunosuppression

See text for short-term, intermediate, and long-term treatments

FIGURE 381-2 Algorithm for the management of myasthenia gravis. FVC, forced vital capacity.

IMMUNOSUPPRESSION

Immunosuppression using glucocorticoids, azathioprine, and other drugs is effective in nearly all patients with MG. The choice of drugs or other immunomodulatory treatments should be guided by the relative benefits and risks for the individual patient and the urgency of treatment. It is helpful to develop a treatment plan based on short-term, intermediate-term, and long-term objectives. For example, if immediate improvement is essential either because of the severity of weakness or because of the patient's need to return to activity as soon as possible, IVIg should be administered or plasmapheresis should be undertaken. For the intermediate term, glucocorticoids and cyclosporine or tacrolimus generally produce clinical improvement within a period of 1–3 months. The beneficial effects of azathioprine and mycophenolate mofetil usually begin after many months (up to a year), but these drugs have advantages for the long-term treatment of patients with MG. For the occasional patient with MG that is genuinely refractory to optimal treatment with conventional immunosuppressive agents, a course of high-dose cyclophosphamide may induce long-lasting (possibly permanent) benefit by "rebooting" the immune system. At high doses, cyclophosphamide eliminates mature lymphocytes, but hematopoietic precursors (stem cells) are spared, because they express the enzyme aldehyde dehydrogenase, which hydrolyzes cyclophosphamide. At present, this procedure is reserved for refractory patients and should be administered only in a facility fully familiar with this approach.

Glucocorticoid Therapy Glucocorticoids, when used properly, produce improvement in myasthenic weakness in the great majority of patients. To minimize adverse side effects, prednisone should be given in a single dose rather than in divided doses throughout the day. The initial dose should be relatively low (15–25 mg/d) to avoid the early weakening that occurs in about one-third of patients treated initially with a high-dose regimen. The dose is increased stepwise, as tolerated by the patient (usually by 5 mg/d at 2- to 3-day intervals), until there is marked clinical improvement or a dose of 50–60 mg/d is reached. This dose is maintained for 1–3 months and then is gradually modified to an alternate-day regimen over the course of an additional 1–3 months; the goal is to reduce the dose on the "off day" to zero or to a minimal level. Generally, patients begin to improve within a few weeks after reaching the maximum dose, and improvement continues to progress for months or years. The prednisone dosage may gradually be reduced, but usually months or years may be needed to determine the minimum effective dose, and close monitoring is required. Few patients are able to do without immunosuppressive agents entirely. Patients on long-term glucocorticoid therapy must be followed carefully to prevent or treat adverse side effects. The most common errors in glucocorticoid treatment of myasthenic patients include (1) insufficient persistence—improvement may be delayed and gradual; (2) too early, too rapid, or excessive tapering of dosage; and (3) lack of attention to prevention and treatment of side effects. **The management of patients treated with glucocorticoids is discussed in Chap. 336.**

Other Immunosuppressive Drugs Mycophenolate mofetil, azathioprine, cyclosporine, tacrolimus, and occasionally cyclophosphamide are effective in many patients, either alone or in various combinations.

Mycophenolate mofetil has become one of the most widely used drugs in the treatment of MG because of its effectiveness and relative lack of side effects. A dose of 1–1.5 g bid is recommended. Its mechanism of action involves inhibition of purine synthesis by the de novo pathway. Since lymphocytes lack the alternative salvage pathway that is present in all other cells, mycophenolate inhibits proliferation of lymphocytes but not proliferation of other cells. It does not kill or eliminate preexisting autoreactive lymphocytes, and therefore clinical improvement may be delayed for many months to a year, until the preexisting autoreactive lymphocytes die spontaneously. The advantage of mycophenolate lies in its relative lack of adverse side effects, with only occasional production of diarrhea and rare development of leukopenia. This drug has become the choice for long-term treatment of myasthenic patients. Unfortunately, the cost of mycophenolate is still very high (~$6400 U.S. annually for 1g bid).

Until recently, azathioprine has been the most widely used of these drugs because of its relative safety in most patients and long track record. Its therapeutic effect may add to that of glucocorticoids and/or allow the glucocorticoid dose to be reduced. However, up to 10% of patients are unable to tolerate azathioprine because of idiosyncratic reactions consisting of flulike symptoms of fever and malaise, bone marrow depression, or abnormalities of liver function. An initial dose of 50 mg/d should be used to test for adverse side effects. If this dose is tolerated, it is increased gradually until the white blood count falls to ~3000–4000/μL. In patients who are receiving glucocorticoids concurrently, leukocytosis precludes the use of this measure. A reduction of the lymphocyte count to <1000/μL and/or an increase of the mean corpuscular volume of red blood cells may be used as indications of adequacy of azathioprine dosage. The typical dosage range is 2–3 mg/kg total body weight. The beneficial effect of azathioprine takes at least 3–6 months to begin and even longer to peak. In patients taking azathioprine, allopurinol should never be used to treat hyperuricemia, because the two drugs share a common degradation pathway; the result may be severe bone marrow depression due to increased effects of the azathioprine.

The calcineurin inhibitors cyclosporine and tacrolimus (FK506) are approximately as effective as azathioprine and are being used increasingly in the management of MG. Their beneficial effect appears more rapidly than that of azathioprine. Either drug may be used alone, but they are usually used as an adjunct to glucocorticoids to permit reduction of the glucocorticoid dose. The usual dose of cyclosporine is 4–5 mg/kg per day, and the average dose of tacrolimus is 0.1 mg/kg per day, given in two equally divided doses (to minimize side effects). Side effects of these drugs include hypertension and nephrotoxicity, which must be closely monitored. "Trough" blood levels are measured 12 h after the evening dose. The therapeutic range for cyclosporine is 150–200 ng/L, and for tacrolimus it is 5–15 ng/L.

Cyclophosphamide is reserved for occasional patients refractory to the other drugs (see above for discussion of high-dose cyclophosphamide treatment).

PLASMAPHERESIS AND INTRAVENOUS IMMUNOGLOBULIN

Plasmapheresis has been used therapeutically in MG. Plasma, which contains the pathogenic antibodies, is mechanically separated from the blood cells, which are returned to the patient. A course of five exchanges (3–4 L per exchange) is generally administered over a 10- to 14-day period. Plasmapheresis produces a short-term reduction in anti-AChR antibodies, with clinical improvement in many patients. It is useful as a temporary expedient in seriously affected patients or to improve the patient's condition prior to surgery (e.g., thymectomy).

The indications for the use of IVIg are the same as those for plasma exchange: to produce rapid improvement to help the patient through a difficult period of myasthenic weakness or prior to surgery. This treatment has the advantages of not requiring special equipment or large-bore venous access. The usual dose is 2 g/kg, which is typically administered over 5 days (400 mg/kg per day). If tolerated, the course of IVIg can be shortened to administer the entire dose over a 3-day period. Improvement occurs in ~70% of patients, beginning during treatment, or within a week, and continuing for weeks to months. The mechanism of action of IVIg is not known; the treatment has no consistent effect on the measurable amount of circulating AChR antibody. Adverse reactions are generally not serious but include headache, fluid overload, and rarely aseptic meningitis or renal failure. IVIg should rarely be used as a long-term treatment in place of rationally managed immunosuppressive therapy. Unfortunately, there is a tendency for physicians unfamiliar with immunosuppressive treatments to rely on repeated IVIg infusions, which are inconvenient, usually produce only intermittent benefit, and are costly. The intermediate and long-term treatment of myasthenic patients requires other methods of therapy outlined earlier in this chapter.

MANAGEMENT OF MYASTHENIC CRISIS Myasthenic crisis is defined as an exacerbation of weakness sufficient to endanger life; it usually consists of respiratory failure caused by diaphragmatic and intercostal muscle weakness. Crisis rarely occurs in properly managed patients. Treatment should be carried out in intensive care units staffed with teams experienced in the management of MG, respiratory insufficiency, infectious disease, and fluid and electrolyte therapy. The possibility that deterioration could be due to excessive anticholinesterase medication ("cholinergic crisis") is best excluded by temporarily stopping anticholinesterase drugs. The most common cause of crisis is intercurrent infection. This should be treated immediately, because the mechanical and immunologic defenses of the patient can be assumed to be compromised. The myasthenic patient with fever and early infection should be treated like other immunocompromised patients. Early and effective antibiotic therapy, respiratory assistance, and pulmonary physiotherapy are essentials of the treatment program. As discussed above, plasmapheresis or IVIg is frequently helpful in hastening recovery.

DRUGS TO AVOID IN MYASTHENIC PATIENTS Many drugs have been reported to have adverse effects in patients with MG (**Table 381-4**). However, not all patients react adversely to all these drugs. Conversely, not

TABLE 381-4 DRUGS WITH INTERACTIONS IN MYASTHENIA GRAVIS (MG)

Drugs That May Exacerbate MG

Antibiotics
  Aminoglycosides: e.g., streptomycin, tobramycin, kanamycin
  Quinolones: e.g., ciprofloxacin, levofloxacin, ofloxacin, gatifloxacin
  Macrolides: e.g., erythromycin, azithromycin, telithromycin
Nondepolarizing muscle relaxants for surgery
  D-Tubocurarine (curare), pancuronium, vecuronium, atracurium
Beta-blocking agents
  Propranolol, atenolol, metoprolol
Local anesthetics and related agents
  Procaine, xylocaine in large amounts
  Procainamide (for arrhythmias)
Botulinum toxin
  Botox exacerbates weakness
Quinine derivatives
  Quinine, quinidine, chloroquine, mefloquine (Lariam)
Magnesium
  Decreases ACh release
Penicillamine
  May cause MG

Drugs with Important Interactions in MG

Cyclosporine
  Broad range of drug interactions, which may raise or lower cyclosporine levels.
Azathioprine
  Avoid allopurinol—combination may result in myelosuppression.

History	Myasthenia Gravis Worksheet			
General	Normal	Good	Fair	Poor
Diplopia	None	Rare	Occasional	Constant
Ptosis	None	Rare	Occasional	Constant
Arms	Normal	Slightly limited	Some ADL impairment	Definitely limited
Legs	Normal	Walks/runs fatigues	Can walk limited distances	Minimal walking
Speech	Normal	Dysarthric	Severely dysarthric	Unintelligible
Voice	Normal	Fades	Impaired	Severely impaired
Chew	Normal	Fatigue on normal foods	Fatigue on soft foods	Feeding tube
Swallow	Normal	Normal foods	Soft foods only	Feeding tube
Respiration	Normal	Dyspnea on unusual effort	Dyspnea on any effort	Dyspnea at rest

Examination

BP _____ Pulse _____ Wt _____   Arm abduction time R_____ L_____
Edema _____   Deltoids R_____ L_____
Vital capacity_____   Biceps R_____ L_____
Cataracts? R _____ L _____   Triceps R_____ L_____
EOMS _____   Grip R_____ L_____
Ptosis time _____   Iliopsoas R_____ L_____
Face _____   Quadriceps R_____ L_____
   Hamstrings R_____ L_____
   Other R_____ L_____

FIGURE 381-3 Abbreviated interval assessment form for use in evaluating treatment for myasthenia gravis.

all "safe" drugs can be used with impunity in patients with MG. As a rule, the listed drugs should be avoided *whenever possible*, and myasthenic patients should be followed closely when *any new drug* is introduced.

PATIENT ASSESSMENT
In order to evaluate the effectiveness of treatment as well as drug-induced side effects, it is important to assess the patient's clinical status systematically at baseline and on repeated interval examinations. Because of the variability of symptoms of MG, the interval history and physical findings on examination must be taken into account. The most useful clinical tests include forward arm abduction time (up to a full 5 min), forced vital capacity, range of eye movements, and time to development of ptosis on upward gaze. Manual muscle testing or, preferably, quantitative dynamometry of limb muscles, especially proximal muscles, is also important. An interval form can provide a succinct summary of the patient's status and a guide to treatment results; an abbreviated form is shown in Fig. 381-3. A progressive reduction in the patient's AChR antibody level also provides clinically valuable confirmation of the effectiveness of treatment; conversely, a rise in AChR antibody levels during tapering of immunosuppressive medication may predict clinical exacerbation. For reliable quantitative measurement of AChR antibody levels, it is best to compare antibody levels from prior frozen serum aliquots with current serum samples in simultaneously run assays.

FURTHER READINGS

DRACHMAN DB et al: Treatment of refractory myasthenia gravis: "Rebooting" with high dose cyclophosphamide. Ann Neurol 53:29, 2003

LINDSTROM JM: Acetylcholine receptors and myasthenia. Muscle Nerve 23:453, 2000

SCHNEIDER-GOLD C et al: Mycophenolate mofetil and tacrolimus: New therapeutic options in neuroimmunological diseases. Muscle Nerve 34:284, 2006

ZINMAN L et al: IV immunoglobulin in patients with myasthenia gravis: A randomized controlled trial. Neurology 68:837, 2007

CHAPTER 381

Myasthenia Gravis and Other Diseases of the Neuromuscular Junction

382 Muscular Dystrophies and Other Muscle Diseases

Robert H. Brown, Jr., Anthony A. Amato, Jerry R. Mendell

Skeletal muscle diseases, or myopathies, are disorders with structural changes or functional impairment of muscle. These conditions can be differentiated from other diseases of the motor unit (e.g., lower motor neuron or neuromuscular junction pathologies) by characteristic clinical and laboratory findings. Myasthenia gravis and related disorders are discussed in Chap. 381; dermatomyositis, polymyositis, and inclusion body myositis are discussed in Chap. 383.

CLINICAL FEATURES

The most common clinical findings of a myopathy are proximal, symmetric limb weakness (arms or legs) with preserved reflexes and sensation. An associated sensory loss suggests injury to peripheral nerve or the central nervous system (CNS) rather than myopathy. On occasion, disorders affecting the motor nerve cell bodies in the spinal cord (anterior horn cell disease), the neuromuscular junction, or peripheral nerves can mimic findings of myopathy.

Muscle Weakness Symptoms of muscle weakness can be either intermittent or persistent. Disorders causing *intermittent weakness* (Fig. 382-1) include myasthenia gravis, periodic paralyses (hypokalemic, hyperkalemic, and paramyotonia congenita), and metabolic energy deficiencies of glycolysis (especially myophosphorylase deficiency) and fatty acid utilization (carnitine palmitoyltransferase deficiency and some mitochondrial myopathies). The states of energy deficiency cause activity-related muscle breakdown accompanied by myoglobinuria, appearing as light-brown- to dark-brown-colored urine.

Most muscle disorders cause *persistent weakness* (Fig. 382-2). In the majority of these, including most types of muscular dystrophy, polymyositis, and dermatomyositis, the proximal muscles are weaker than the distal and are symmetrically affected, and the facial muscles are spared, a pattern referred to as *limb-girdle*. The differential diagnosis is more restricted for other patterns of weakness. Facial weakness (difficulty with eye closure and impaired smile) and scapular winging (Fig. 382-3) are characteristic of facioscapulohumeral dystrophy. Facial and distal limb weakness associated with hand grip myotonia is virtually diagnostic of myotonic dystrophy. When other cranial nerve muscles are weak, causing ptosis or extraocular muscle weakness, the most important disorders to consider include neuromuscular junction disorders, oculopharyngeal muscular dystrophy, mitochondrial myopathies, or some of the congenital myopathies (Table 382-1). A pathognomonic pattern characteristic of inclusion body myositis is atrophy and weakness of the flexor forearm (e.g., wrist and finger flexors) and quadriceps muscles that is often asymmetric. Less frequently, but important diagnostically, is the presence of a dropped head syndrome indicative of selective neck extensor muscle weakness. The most important neuromuscular diseases associated with this pattern of weakness include myasthenia gravis, amyotrophic lateral sclerosis, late-onset nemaline myopathy, hyperparathyroidism, focal myositis, and some forms of inclusion body myopathy. A final pattern, recognized because of preferential distal extremity weakness, is typical of a unique category of muscular dystrophy, the distal myopathies.

It is important to examine functional capabilities to help disclose certain patterns of weakness (Table 382-2). The Gowers' sign (Fig. 382-4) is particularly useful. Observing the gait of an individual may disclose a lordotic posture caused by combined trunk and hip weakness, frequently exaggerated by toe walking (Fig. 382-5). A waddling gait is caused by the inability of weak hip muscles to prevent hip drop or hip dip. Hyperextension of the knee (genu recurvatum or back-kneeing) is characteristic of quadriceps muscle weakness; and a steppage gait, due to footdrop, accompanies distal weakness.

Any disorder causing muscle weakness may be accompanied by *fatigue*, referring to an inability to maintain or sustain a force (pathologic fatigability). This condition must be differentiated from asthenia, a type of fatigue caused by excess tiredness or lack of energy. Associated symptoms may help differentiate asthenia and pathologic fatigability. Asthenia is often accompanied by a tendency to avoid physical activities, complaints of daytime sleepiness, necessity for frequent naps, and difficulty concentrating on activities such as reading. There may be feelings of overwhelming stress and depression. Thus, asthenia is not a myopathy. In contrast, pathologic fatigability occurs in disorders of neuromuscular transmission and in disorders altering energy production, including defects in glycolysis, lipid metabolism, or mitochondrial energy production. Pathologic fatigability also occurs in chronic myopathies because of difficulty accomplishing a task with less muscle. Pathologic fatigability is accompanied by abnormal clinical or lab-

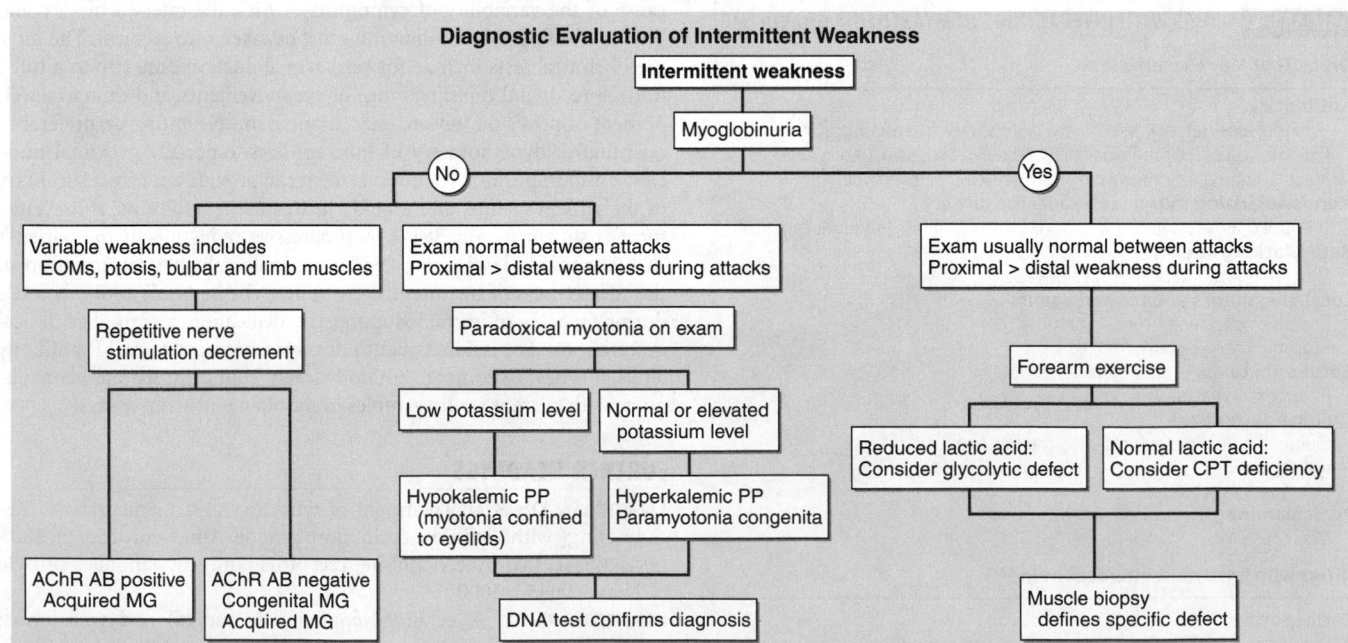

FIGURE 382-1 Diagnostic evaluation of intermittent weakness. EOMs, extraocular muscles; AChR AB, acetylcholine receptor antibody; PP, periodic paralysis; CPT, carnitine palmitoyltransferase; MG, myasthenia gravis.

Diagnostic Evaluation of Persistent Weakness

Persistent Weakness

↓

Patterns of Weakness on Neurologic Exam

| Proximal > distal PM; DM; muscular dystrophies | Ptosis, EOMs OPMD; mitochondrial myopathy; myotubular myopathy | Facial and scapular winging FSHD | Facial, distal, quadriceps; handgrip myotonia Myotonic muscular dystrophy | Proximal & distal (hand grip), & quadriceps IBM | Distal Distal myopathy | Dropped head MG; PM; ALS |

↓

Myopathic EMG confirms muscle disease and excludes ALS
Repetitive nerve stimulation indicates MG
CK elevation supports myopathy

↓

May need DNA testing for further distinction of inherited myopathies

↓

Muscle biopsy will help distinguish many disorders

FIGURE 382-2 Diagnostic evaluation of persistent weakness. Examination reveals one of seven patterns of weakness. The pattern of weakness in combination with the laboratory evaluation leads to a diagnosis. EOM, extraocular muscles; OPMD, oculopharyngeal muscular dystrophy; FSHD, facioscapulohumeral dystrophy; IBM, inclusion body myositis; DM, dermatomyositis; PM, polymyositis; MG, myasthenia gravis; ALS, amyotrophic lateral sclerosis; CK, creatine kinase.

oratory findings. Fatigue without those supportive features almost never indicates a primary muscle disease.

Muscle Pain (Myalgias), Cramps, and Stiffness Muscle pain can be associated with cramps, spasms, contractures, and stiff or rigid muscles. In distinction, true myalgia (muscle aching), which can be localized or generalized, may be accompanied by weakness, tenderness to palpation, or swelling. Certain drugs cause true myalgia (Table 382-3).

There are two painful muscle conditions of particular importance, neither of which is associated with muscle weakness. *Fibromyalgia* is a common, yet poorly understood type of myofascial pain syndrome. Patients complain of severe muscle pain and tenderness and have specific painful trigger points, sleep disturbances, and easy fatigability. Serum creatine kinase (CK), erythrocyte sedimentation rate (ESR), electromyography (EMG), and muscle biopsy are normal (Chap. 329). *Polymyalgia rheumatica* occurs mainly in patients >50 years and is characterized by stiffness and pain in the shoulders, lower back, hips, and thighs (Chap. 319). The ESR is elevated, while serum CK, EMG, and muscle biopsy are normal. Temporal arteritis, an inflammatory disorder of medium- and large-sized arteries, usually involving one or more branches of the carotid artery, may accompany polymyalgia rheumatica. Vision is threatened by ischemic optic neuritis. Glucocorticoids can relieve the myalgias and protect against visual loss.

Localized muscle pain is most often traumatic. A common cause of sudden abrupt-onset pain is a ruptured tendon, which leaves the muscle belly appearing rounded and shorter in appearance compared to the normal side. The biceps brachii and Achilles tendons are particularly vulnerable to rupture. Infection or neoplastic infiltration of the muscle is a rare cause of localized muscle pain.

A *muscle cramp* or *spasm* is a painful, involuntary, localized, muscle contraction with a visible or palpable hardening of the muscle. Cramps are abrupt in onset, short in duration, and may cause abnormal posturing of the joint. The EMG shows firing of motor units, reflecting an origin from spontaneous neural discharge. Muscle cramps often occur in neurogenic disorders, especially motor neuron disease (Chap. 369), radiculopathies, and polyneuropathies (Chap. 379), but are not a feature of most primary muscle diseases. Duchenne muscular dystrophy is an exception since calf muscle complaints are a common complaint. Muscle cramps are also common during pregnancy.

FIGURE 382-3 Facioscapulohumeral dystrophy with prominent scapular winging.

TABLE 382-1 NEUROMUSCULAR CAUSES OF PTOSIS OR OPHTHALMOPLEGIA

Peripheral neuropathy
 Guillain-Barré syndrome
 Miller-Fisher syndrome
Neuromuscular junction
 Botulism
 Lambert-Eaton syndrome
 Myasthenia gravis
 Congenital myasthenia
Myopathy
 Mitochondrial myopathies
  Kearns-Sayre syndrome
  Progressive external ophthalmoplegia
 Oculopharyngeal and oculopharyngodistal muscular dystrophy
 Myotonic dystrophy (ptosis only)
 Congenital myopathy
  Myotubular
  Nemaline (ptosis only)
 Hyperthyroidism/Graves disease (ophthalmoplegia without ptosis)

TABLE 382-2 OBSERVATIONS ON EXAMINATION THAT DISCLOSE MUSCLE WEAKNESS

Functional Impairment	Muscle Weakness
Inability to forcibly close eyes	Upper facial muscles
Impaired pucker	Lower facial muscles
Inability to raise head from prone position	Neck extensor muscles
Inability to raise head from supine position	Neck flexor muscles
Inability to raise arms above head	Proximal arm muscles (may be only scapular stabilizing muscles)
Inability to walk without hyperextending knee (backkneeing or genu recurvatum)	Knee extensor muscles
Inability to walk with heels touching the floor (toe walking)	Shortening of the Achilles tendon
Inability to lift foot while walking (steppage gait or footdrop)	Anterior compartment of leg
Inability to walk without a waddling gait	Hip muscles
Inability to get up from the floor without climbing up the extremities (Gowers' sign)	Hip muscles
Inability to get up from a chair without using arms	Hip muscles

FIGURE 382-5 Lordotic posture, exaggerated by standing on toes, associated with trunk and hip weakness.

A *muscle contracture* is different from a muscle cramp. In both conditions, the muscle becomes hard, but a contracture is associated with energy failure in glycolytic disorders. The muscle is unable to relax after an active muscle contraction. The EMG shows electrical silence. Confusion is created because contracture also refers to a muscle that cannot be passively stretched to its proper length (fixed contracture) because of fibrosis. In some muscle disorders, especially in Emery-Dreifuss muscular dystrophy and Bethlem myopathy, fixed contractures occur early and represent distinctive features of the disease.

Muscle stiffness can refer to different phenomena. Some patients with inflammation of joints and periarticular surfaces feel stiff. This condition is different from the disorders of hyperexcitable motor nerves causing stiff or rigid muscles. In *stiff-person syndrome* spontaneous discharges of the motor neurons of the spinal cord cause involuntary muscle contractions mainly involving the axial (trunk) and proximal lower extremity muscles. The gait becomes stiff and labored, with hyperlordosis of the lumbar spine. Superimposed episodic muscle spasms are precipitated by sudden movements, unexpected noises, and emotional upset. The muscles relax during sleep. Serum antibodies against glutamic acid decarboxylase are present in approximately two-thirds of cases. In *neuromyotonia* (Isaacs' syndrome) there is hyperexcitability of the peripheral nerves manifesting as continuous muscle fiber activity. *Myokymia* (groups of fasciculations associated with continuous undulations of muscle) and impaired muscle relax-

FIGURE 382-4 Gowers' sign showing a patient using arms to climb up the legs in attempting to get up from the floor.

TABLE 382-3 DRUGS THAT CAUSE TRUE MYALGIA

Cimetidine
Cocaine
Cyclosporine
Danazol
Emetine
Epsilon aminocaproic acid
Gold
Heroin
Labetalol
Methadone
D-Penicillamine
Statins and other cholesterol-lowering agents
L-Tryptophan
Zidovudine

ation are the result. Muscles of the leg are stiff, and the constant contractions of the muscle cause increased sweating of the extremities. This peripheral nerve hyperexcitability is antibody-mediated, targeted against voltage-gated potassium channels. The site of origin of the spontaneous nerve discharges is principally in the distal portion of the motor nerves.

Myotonia is a condition of prolonged muscle contraction followed by slow muscle relaxation. It always follows muscle activation (action myotonia), usually voluntary, but may be elicited by mechanical stimulation (percussion myotonia) of the muscle. Myotonia typically causes difficulty in releasing objects after a firm grasp. In myotonic muscular dystrophy type 1 (DM1), distal weakness usually accompanies myotonia, whereas in DM2 proximal muscles are more affected; thus the related term *proximal myotonic myopathy* (PROMM) is used to describe this condition. Myotonia also occurs with *myotonia congenita* (a chloride channel disorder), but in this condition muscle weakness is not prominent. Myotonia may also be seen in individuals with sodium channel mutations (*hyperkalemic periodic paralysis* or *potassium-sensitive myotonia*). Another sodium channelopathy, *paramyotonia congenita*, also is associated with muscle stiffness. In contrast to other disorders associated with myotonia in which the myotonia is eased by repetitive activity, paramyotonia congenita is named for a paradoxical phenomenon whereby the myotonia worsens with repetitive activity.

Muscle Enlargement and Atrophy

In most myopathies muscle tissue is replaced by fat and connective tissue, but the size of the muscle is usually not affected. However, in many limb-girdle muscular dystrophies (and particularly the dystrophinopathies) enlarged calf muscles are typical. The enlargement represents true muscle hypertrophy, thus the term "pseudohypertrophy" should be avoided when referring to these patients. The calf muscles remain very strong even late in the course of these disorders. Muscle enlargement can also result from infiltration by sarcoid granulomas, amyloid deposits, bacterial and parasitic infections, and focal myositis. In contrast, muscle atrophy is characteristic of other myopathies. In dysferlinopathies (LGMD2B) there is a predilection for early atrophy of the gastrocnemius muscles. Atrophy of the humeral muscles is characteristic of facioscapulohumeral muscular dystrophy.

LABORATORY EVALUATION

A limited battery of tests can be used to evaluate a suspected myopathy. Nearly all patients require serum enzyme level measurements and electrodiagnostic studies as screening tools to differentiate muscle disorders from other motor unit diseases. The other tests described—DNA studies, the forearm exercise test, and muscle biopsy—are used to diagnose specific types of myopathies.

Serum Enzymes

CK is the preferred muscle enzyme to measure in the evaluation of myopathies. Damage to muscle causes the CK to leak from the muscle fiber to the serum. The MM isoenzyme predominates in skeletal muscle, while CK-MB is the marker for cardiac muscle. Serum CK can be elevated in normal individuals without provocation, presumably on a genetic basis or after strenuous activity, minor trauma (including the EMG needle), a prolonged muscle cramp, or a generalized seizure. Aspartate aminotransferase (AST), alanine aminotransferase (ALT), aldolase, and lactic dehydrogenase (LDH) are enzymes sharing an origin in both muscle and liver. Problems arise when the levels of these enzymes are found to be elevated in a routine screening battery, leading to the erroneous assumption that liver disease is present when in fact muscle could be the cause. An elevated γ-glutamyl transferase (GGT) helps to establish a liver origin since this enzyme is not found in muscle.

Electrodiagnostic Studies

EMG, repetitive nerve stimulation, and nerve conduction studies (**Chap. e31**) are essential methods for evaluation of the patient with suspected muscle disease. In combination they provide the information necessary to differentiate myopathies from neuropathies and neuromuscular junction diseases. Routine nerve conduction studies are typically normal in myopathies but reduced amplitudes of com-

TABLE 382-4 **MYOTONIC DISORDERS**
Myotonic dystrophy type 1
Myotonic dystrophy type 2/Proximal myotonic myopathy
Myotonia congenita
Paramyotonia congenita
Hyperkalemic periodic paralysis
Chondrodystrophic myotonia (Schwartz-Jampel syndrome)
Centronuclear/myotubular myopathy[a]
Drug-induced
Cholesterol-lowering agents (statin medications, fibrates)
Cyclosporine
Chloroquine
Glycogen storage disorders[a] (Pompe disease, debrancher deficiency, branching enzyme deficiency)
Myofibrillar myopathies[a]

[a]Associated with myotonic discharges on EMG but no clinical myotonia.

pound muscle action potentials may be seen in atrophied muscles. The needle EMG may reveal irritability on needle placement suggestive of a necrotizing myopathy (inflammatory myopathies, dystrophies, toxic myopathies, myotonic myopathies), whereas a lack of irritability is characteristic of long-standing myopathic disorders (muscular dystrophies, endocrine myopathies, disuse atrophy, and many of the metabolic myopathies). In addition, the EMG may demonstrate myotonic discharges that will narrow the differential diagnosis (Table 382-4). Another important EMG finding is the presence of short-duration, small-amplitude, polyphasic motor unit action potentials (MUAPs). Such MUAPs can be seen in both myopathic and neuropathic disorders; however, the recruitment or firing pattern is different. In myopathies, the MUAPs fire early but at a normal rate to compensate for the loss of individual muscle fibers, whereas in neurogenic disorders the MUAPs fire faster. The EMG is usually normal in steroid or disuse myopathy, both of which are associated with type 2 fiber atrophy; this is because the EMG preferentially assesses the physiologic function of type 1 fibers. The EMG can also be invaluable in helping to choose an appropriately affected muscle to sample for biopsy.

DNA Analysis

This now serves as an important tool for the definitive diagnosis of many muscle disorders. Nevertheless, there are a number of limitations in currently available molecular diagnostics. For example, in Duchenne and Becker dystrophies, two-thirds of patients have deletion or duplication mutations that are easy to detect, while the remainder have point mutations that are much more difficult to find. For patients without identifiable gene defects, the muscle biopsy remains the main diagnostic tool.

Forearm Exercise Test

In myopathies with intermittent symptoms, and especially those associated with myoglobinuria, there may be a defect in glycolysis. Many variations of the forearm exercise test exist. For safety, the test should not be performed under ischemic conditions to avoid an unnecessary insult to the muscle, causing rhabdomyolysis. The test is performed by placing a small indwelling catheter into an antecubital vein. A baseline blood sample is obtained for lactic acid and ammonia. The forearm muscles are exercised by asking the patient to vigorously open and close the hand for 1 min. Blood is then obtained at intervals of 1, 2, 4, 6, and 10 min for comparison with the baseline sample. A three- to fourfold rise of lactic acid is typical. The simultaneous measurement of ammonia serves as a control, since it should also rise with exercise. In patients with myophosphorylase deficiency or other glycolytic defects, the lactic acid rise will be absent or below normal, while the rise in ammonia will reach control values. If there is lack of effort, neither lactic acid nor ammonia will rise. Patients with selective failure to increase ammonia may have myoadenylate deaminase deficiency. This condition has been reported to be a cause of myoglobinuria, but deficiency of this enzyme in asymptomatic individuals makes interpretation controversial.

Muscle Biopsy

Muscle biopsy is an important step in establishing the diagnosis of a suspected myopathy. The biopsy is usually obtained from a

TABLE 382-5 PROGRESSIVE MUSCULAR DYSTROPHIES

Type	Inheritance	Defective Gene/Protein	Onset Age	Clinical Features	Other Organ Systems Involved
Duchenne	XR	Dystrophin	Before 5 years	Progressive weakness of girdle muscles Unable to walk after age 12 Progressive kyphoscoliosis Respiratory failure in 2d or 3d decade	Cardiomyopathy Mental impairment
Becker	XR	Dystrophin	Early childhood to adult	Progressive weakness of girdle muscles Able to walk after age 15 Respiratory failure may develop by 4th decade	Cardiomyopathy
Limb-girdle	AD/AR	Several (Tables 382-6, 382-7)	Early childhood to early adult	Slow progressive weakness of shoulder and hip girdle muscles	± Cardiomyopathy
Emery-Dreifuss	XR/AD	Emerin/Lamins A/C	Childhood to adult	Elbow contractures, humeral and peroneal weakness	Cardiomyopathy
Congenital	AR	Several	At birth or within first few months	Hypotonia, contractures, delayed milestones Progression to respiratory failure in some; static course in others	CNS abnormalities (hypomyelination, malformation) Eye abnormalities
Myotonic[a] (DM1, DM2)	AD	DM1: Expansion CTG repeat DM2: Expansion CCTG repeat	Usually 2d decade May be infancy if mother affected (DM1 only)	Slowly progressive weakness of face, shoulder girdle, and foot dorsiflexion Preferential proximal weakness in DM2	Cardiac conduction defects Mental impairment Cataracts Frontal baldness Gonadal atrophy
Facioscapulo-humeral	AD	Deletion, distal 4q	Before age 20	Slowly progressive weakness of face, shoulder girdle, and foot dorsiflexion	Deafness Coats' (eye) disease
Oculopharyn-geal	AD	Expansion, poly-A RNA binding protein	5th to 6th decade	Slowly progressive weakness of extraocular, pharyngeal, and limb muscles	—

[a] Two forms of myotonic dystrophy, DM1 and DM2, have been identified. Many features overlap (see text).

Abbreviations: XR, X-linked recessive; AD, autosomal dominant; AR, autosomal recessive; CNS, central nervous system.

quadriceps or biceps brachii muscle, less commonly from a deltoid muscle. Evaluation includes a combination of techniques—light microscopy, histochemistry, immunocytochemistry with a battery of antibodies, and electron microscopy. Not all techniques are needed for every case. A specific diagnosis can be established in many disorders. A combination of stains to identify mononuclear cells (polymyositis), complement (dermatomyositis), and amyloid (inclusion body myositis) helps to distinguish the inflammatory myopathies. In addition, the congenital myopathies have distinctive light and electron microscopy features essential for diagnosis. Mitochondrial and metabolic (e.g., myophosphorylase and acid maltase deficiencies) myopathies also demonstrate distinctive histochemical and electron-microscopic profiles. Biopsied muscle tissue can be sent for metabolic enzyme or mitochondrial DNA analyses. A battery of antibodies is available for the identification of missing components of the dystrophin-glycoprotein complex and related proteins to help diagnose specific types of muscular dystrophies. Western blot analysis on muscle specimens can be performed to determine whether specific muscle proteins are reduced in quantity or are of abnormal size.

HEREDITARY MYOPATHIES

Muscular dystrophy refers to a group of hereditary progressive diseases each with unique phenotypic and genetic features (**Tables 382-5, 382-6,** and **382-7**).

DUCHENNE MUSCULAR DYSTROPHY

This X-linked recessive disorder, sometimes also called *pseudohypertrophic muscular dystrophy,* has an incidence of ~30 per 100,000 live-born males.

Clinical Features Duchenne dystrophy is present at birth, but the disorder usu-

ally becomes apparent between ages 3 and 5. The boys fall frequently and have difficulty keeping up with friends when playing. Running, jumping, and hopping are invariably abnormal. By age 5, muscle weakness is obvious by muscle testing. On getting up from the floor, the patient uses his hands to climb up himself [Gowers' maneuver (Fig. 382-4)]. Contractures of the heel cords and iliotibial bands become apparent by age 6, when toe walking is associated with a lordotic posture. Loss of muscle strength is progressive, with predilection for proximal limb muscles and the neck flexors; leg involvement is more severe than arm involvement. Between ages 8 and 10 walking may require the use of braces; joint contractures and limitations of hip flexion, knee, elbow, and wrist extension are made worse by prolonged sitting. By age 12, most patients are wheelchair dependent. Contrac-

TABLE 382-6 AUTOSOMAL DOMINANT LIMB-GIRDLE MUSCULAR DYSTROPHIES (LGMDS)

Disease	Clinical Features	Laboratory Features	Locus or Gene
LGMD1A	Onset 3d to 4th decade Muscle weakness affects distal limb muscles, vocal cords, and pharyngeal muscles	Serum CK 2 × normal EMG mixed myopathy/neuropathy NCS normal	Myotilin
LGMD1B	Onset 1st or 2d decade Proximal lower limb weakness and cardiomyopathy with conduction defects Some cases indistinguishable from Emery-Dreifuss muscular dystrophy with joint contractures	Serum CK 3–5 × normal NCS normal EMG myopathic	Lamin A/C
LGMD1C	Onset in early childhood Proximal weakness Gowers' sign, calf hypertrophy Exercise-related muscle cramps	Serum CK 4–25 × normal NCS normal EMG myopathic	Caveolin-3
LGMD1D	Onset 3d to 5th decade Proximal muscle weakness Cardiomyopathy and arrhythmias	Serum CK 2–4 × normal NCS normal EMG myopathic	Linked to chromosome 7q Gene unidentified
LGMD1E	Childhood onset Proximal muscle weakness	Serum CK usually normal NCS normal EMG myopathic	Linked to chromosome 6q23 Gene unidentified

Abbreviations: CK, creatine kinase; NCS, nerve conduction studies; EMG, electromyography.

Disease	Clinical Features	Laboratory Features	Locus or Gene
LGMD2A	Onset 1st or 2d decade Tight heel cords Contractures at elbows, wrists, and fingers; rigid spine in some Proximal and distal weakness	Serum CK 3–15 × normal NCS normal EMG myopathic	Calpain-3
LGMD2B	Onset 2d or 3d decade Proximal muscle weakness at onset, later distal (calf) muscles affected Miyoshi myopathy is variant of LGMD2B with calf muscles affected at onset	Serum CK 3–100 × normal NCS normal EMG myopathic Inflammation on muscle biopsy may simulate polymyositis	Dysferlin
LGMD2C–F	Onset in childhood to teenage yrs Clinical condition similar to Duchenne and Becker muscular dystrophies Cardiomyopathy uncommon Cognitive function normal	Serum CK 5–100 × normal NCS normal EMG myopathic	γ, α, β, δ sarcoglycans
LGMD2G	Onset age 10 to 15 Proximal and distal muscle weakness	Serum CK 3–17 × normal NCS normal EMG myopathic	Telethonin
LGMD2H	Onset 1st to 3d decade Proximal muscle weakness	Serum CK 2–25 × normal NCS normal EMG myopathic	TRIM32 gene
LGMD2I	Onset 1st to 3d decade Clinical condition similar to Duchenne or Becker dystrophies Cardiomyopathy (some not all) Cognitive function normal	Serum CK 10–30 × normal NCS normal EMG myopathic	Fukutin-related protein
LGMD2J[a]	Onset 1st to 3d decade Proximal lower limb weakness Mild distal weakness Progressive weakness causes loss of ambulation	Serum CK 1.5–2 × normal NCS normal EMG myopathic	Titin

[a]Tibial muscular dystrophy is a form of titin deficiency with only distal muscle weakness (see Table 382-8).
Abbreviations: CK, creatine kinase; NCS, nerve conduction studies; EMG, electromyography.

tures become fixed, and a progressive scoliosis often develops that may be associated with pain. The chest deformity with scoliosis impairs pulmonary function, which is already diminished by muscle weakness. By age 16 to 18, patients are predisposed to serious, sometimes fatal pulmonary infections. Other causes of death include aspiration of food and acute gastric dilation.

A cardiac cause of death is uncommon despite the presence of a cardiomyopathy in almost all patients. Congestive heart failure seldom occurs except with severe stress such as pneumonia. Cardiac arrhythmias are rare. The typical electrocardiogram (ECG) shows an increase net RS in lead V_1; deep, narrow Q waves in the precordial leads; and tall right precordial R waves in V_1. Intellectual impairment in Duchenne dystrophy is common; the average intelligence quotient (IQ) is ~1 SD below the mean. Impairment of intellectual function appears to be nonprogressive and affects verbal ability more than performance.

Laboratory Features Serum CK levels are invariably elevated to between 20 and 100 times normal. The levels are abnormal at birth but decline late in the disease because of inactivity and loss of muscle mass. EMG demonstrates features typical of myopathy. The muscle biopsy shows muscle fibers of varying size as well as small groups of necrotic and regenerating fibers. Connective tissue and fat replace lost muscle fibers. A definitive diagnosis of Duchenne dystrophy can be established on the basis of dystrophin deficiency in a biopsy of muscle tissue or mutation analysis on peripheral blood leukocytes, as discussed below.

Duchenne dystrophy is caused by a mutation of the gene that encodes dystrophin, a 427-kDa protein localized to the inner surface of the sarcolemma of the muscle fiber. The dystrophin gene is >2000 kb in size and thus is one of the largest identified human genes. It is localized to the short arm of the X chromosome at Xp21. The most common gene mutation is a deletion. The size varies but does not correlate with disease severity. Deletions are not uniformly distributed over the

gene but rather are most common near the beginning (5′ end) and middle of the gene. Less often, Duchenne dystrophy is caused by a gene duplication or point mutation. Identification of a specific mutation allows for an unequivocal diagnosis, makes possible accurate testing of potential carriers, and is useful for prenatal diagnosis.

A diagnosis of Duchenne dystrophy can also be made by Western blot analysis of muscle biopsy specimens, revealing abnormalities on the quantity and molecular weight of dystrophin protein. In addition, immunocytochemical staining of muscle with dystrophin antibodies can be used to demonstrate absence or deficiency of dystrophin localizing to the sarcolemmal membrane. Carriers of the disease may demonstrate a mosaic pattern, but dystrophin analysis of muscle biopsy specimens for carrier detection is not reliable.

Pathogenesis Dystrophin is part of a large complex of sarcolemmal proteins and glycoproteins (Fig. 382-6). Dystrophin binds to F-actin at its amino terminus and to β-dystroglycan at the carboxyl terminus. β-Dystroglycan complexes to α-dystroglycan, which binds to laminin in the extracellular matrix (ECM). Laminin has a heterotrimeric molecular structure arranged in the shape of a cross with one heavy chain and two light chains, β1 and γ1. The laminin heavy chain of skeletal muscle is designated laminin α2. Collagen proteins IV and VI are also found in the ECM. Like β-dystroglycan, the transmembrane sarcoglycan proteins also bind to dystrophin; these five proteins (designated α- through ε-sarcoglycan) complex tightly with each other. More recently, other membrane proteins implicated in muscular dystrophy have been found to be loosely affiliated with constituents of the dystrophin complex. These include caveolin-3, α7 integrin, and collagen VI.

The dystrophin-glycoprotein complex appears to confer stability to the sarcolemma, although the function of each individual component of the complex is incompletely understood. Deficiency of one member of the complex may cause abnormalities in other components. For example, a primary deficiency of dystrophin (Duchenne dystrophy) may lead to secondary loss of the sarcoglycans and dystroglycan. The primary loss of a single sarcoglycan (see "Limb-Girdle Muscular Dystrophy," below) results in a secondary loss of other sarcoglycans in the membrane without uniformly affecting dystrophin. In either instance, disruption of the dystrophin-glycoprotein complexes weakens the sarcolemma, causing membrane tears and a cascade of events leading to muscle fiber necrosis. This sequence of events occurs repeatedly during the life of a patient with muscular dystrophy.

℞ DUCHENNE MUSCULAR DYSTROPHY

Glucocorticoids, administered as prednisone in a dose of 0.75 mg/kg per day, significantly slow progression of Duchenne dystrophy for up to 3 years. Some patients cannot tolerate glucocorticoid therapy; weight gain and increased risk of fractures in particular represent a significant deterrent for some boys. As in other recessively inherited dystrophies presumed to arise from loss of function of a critical muscle gene, there is optimism that Duchenne disease may benefit from novel therapies that either replace the defective gene or missing protein or implement downstream corrections (e.g., skipping mutated exons or reading through mutations that introduce stop codons).

FIGURE 382-6 Selected muscular dystrophy–associated proteins in the cell membrane and Golgi complex. Dystrophin localizes to the cytoplasmic face of the muscle cell membrane. It complexes with two transmembrane protein complexes, the dystroglycans and the sarcoglycans. The dystroglycans bind to the extracellular matrix protein merosin, which is also complexed with β_1 and α_7 integrins (Tables 382-5, 382-6, 382-7). Dysferlin complexes with caveolin-3 (which binds to neuronal nitric oxide synthase, or nNOS) but not with the dystrophin-associated proteins or the integrins. In each of four congenital dystrophies, there is loss of function of different Golgi-associated proteins: POMT1, POMGnT1, Fukutin, and Fukutin-related protein.

BECKER MUSCULAR DYSTROPHY

This less severe form of X-linked recessive muscular dystrophy results from allelic defects of the same gene responsible for Duchenne dystrophy. Becker muscular dystrophy is ~10 times less frequent than Duchenne, with an incidence of about 3 per 100,000 live-born males.

Clinical Features The pattern of muscle wasting in Becker muscular dystrophy closely resembles that seen in Duchenne. Proximal muscles, especially of the lower extremities, are prominently involved. As the disease progresses, weakness becomes more generalized. Significant facial muscle weakness is not a feature. Hypertrophy of muscles, particularly in the calves, is an early and prominent finding.

Most patients with Becker dystrophy first experience difficulties between ages 5 and 15 years, although onset in the third or fourth decade or even later can occur. By definition, patients with Becker dystrophy walk beyond age 15, while patients with Duchenne dystrophy are typically in a wheelchair by the age of 12. Patients with Becker dystrophy have a reduced life expectancy, but most survive into the fourth or fifth decade.

Mental retardation may occur in Becker dystrophy, but it is not as common as in Duchenne. Cardiac involvement occurs in Becker dystrophy and may result in heart failure; some patients manifest with only heart failure. Other less common presentations are asymptomatic hyper-CK-emia, myalgias without weakness, and myoglobinuria.

Laboratory Features Serum CK levels, results of EMG, and muscle biopsy findings closely resemble those in Duchenne dystrophy. The diagnosis of Becker muscular dystrophy requires Western blot analysis of muscle biopsy samples demonstrating a reduced amount or abnormal size of dystrophin or mutation analysis of DNA from peripheral blood leukocytes. Genetic testing reveals deletions or duplications of the dystrophin gene in 65% of patients with Becker dystrophy, approximately the same percentage as in Duchenne dystrophy. In both Becker and

Duchenne dystrophies, the size of the DNA deletion does not predict clinical severity; however, in ~95% of patients with Becker dystrophy, the DNA deletion does not alter the translational reading frame of messenger RNA. These "in-frame" mutations allow for production of some dystrophin, which accounts for the presence of altered rather than absent dystrophin on western blot analysis.

℞ BECKER MUSCULAR DYSTROPHY

The use of glucocorticoids has not been adequately studied in Becker dystrophy.

LIMB-GIRDLE MUSCULAR DYSTROPHY

The syndrome of limb-girdle muscular dystrophy (LGMD) represents more than one disorder. Both males and females are affected, with onset ranging from late in the first decade to the fourth decade. The LGMDs typically manifest with progressive weakness of pelvic and shoulder girdle musculature. Respiratory insufficiency from weakness of the diaphragm may occur, as may cardiomyopathy.

A systematic classification of LGMD is based on autosomal dominant (LGMD1) and autosomal recessive (LGMD2) inheritance. Superimposed on the backbone of LGMD1 and LGMD2, the classification employs a sequential alphabetical lettering system (LGMD1A, LGMD2A, etc.). Disorders receive letters in the order in which they are found to have chromosomal linkage. This results in an ever-expanding list of conditions. Presently there are 5 autosomal dominant and 10 autosomal recessive disorders, summarized in Tables 382-6 and 382-7. None of the conditions is as common as the dystrophinopathies; however, prevalence data for the LGMDs have not been systematically gathered for any large heterogeneous population. In referral-based clinical populations, Fukutin-related protein (FKRP) deficiency (LGMD2I), calpainopathies (LGMD2A), and to a lesser extent dysferlinopathies (LGMD2B) have emerged as the most common disorders.

EMERY-DREIFUSS MUSCULAR DYSTROPHY

There are two genetically distinct forms of Emery-Dreifuss muscular dystrophy (EDMD). One is inherited as an X-linked disorder, while the other is autosomal dominant. The latter is classified under the rubric of LGMD1B, but clinically the conditions are closely related.

Clinical Features Prominent contractures can be recognized in early childhood and teenage years, often preceding muscle weakness. The contractures persist throughout the course of the disease and are present at the elbows, ankles, and neck. Muscle weakness affects humeral and peroneal muscles at first and later spreads to a limb-girdle distribution. The cardiomyopathy is potentially life threatening and may result in sudden death. A spectrum of atrial rhythm and conduction defects includes atrial fibrillation and paralysis and atrioventricular heart block. Some patients have a dilated cardiomyopathy. Female carriers of the X-linked variant may have cardiac manifestations that become clinically significant.

Laboratory Features Serum CK may be elevated two- to tenfold. EMG is myopathic. Muscle biopsy shows nonspecific dystrophic features. Immunohistochemistry reveals absent emerin staining of myonuclei in X-lined EDMD. ECGs demonstrate atrial and atrioventricular rhythm disturbances.

X-linked EDMD arises from defects in the emerin gene encoding a nuclear envelope protein. The autosomal dominant disease is caused by mutations of the *LMNA* gene on chromosome 1q21.2 encoding the lamin proteins A and C. These proteins are alternatively spliced products of the *LMNA* gene that are essential components of the filamentous network underlying the inner nuclear membrane. Loss of structural integrity of the nuclear envelope from defects in emerin or lamin A/C accounts for overlapping phenotypes (**Fig. 382-7**).

℞ EMERY-DREIFUSS MUSCULAR DYSTROPHY

Supportive care should be offered for neuromuscular disability, including ambulatory aids, if necessary. Stretching of contractures is difficult. Man-

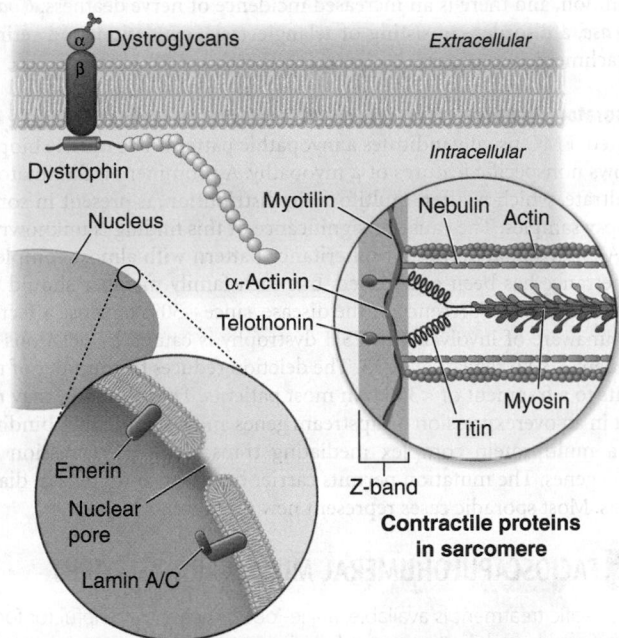

FIGURE 382-7 Selected muscular dystrophy–associated proteins in the nuclear membrane and sarcomere. As shown in the exploded view, emerin and lamin A/C are constituents of the inner nuclear membrane. Several dystrophy-associated proteins are represented in the sarcomere including titin, nebulin, calpain, telothonin, actinin, and myotilin. The position of the dystrophin-dystroglycan complex is also illustrated.

agement of cardiomyopathy and arrhythmias (e.g., early use of a cardiac pacemaker) may be life saving.

CONGENITAL MUSCULAR DYSTROPHY (CMD)

This is not one entity but rather a group of disorders with varying degrees of muscle weakness, central nervous system impairment, and eye abnormalities.

Clinical Features   As a group, CMDs present at birth or in the first few months of life with hypotonia and proximal or generalized muscle weakness. Calf muscle hypertrophy is seen in some patients. Facial muscles may be weak, but other cranial nerve–innervated muscles are spared (e.g., extraocular muscles are normal). Most patients have joint contractures of varying degrees at elbows, hips, knees, and ankles. Contractures present at birth are referred to as *arthrogryposis*. Respiratory failure may be seen in some cases.

The CNS is affected in some forms of CMD. In merosin and FKRP deficiency, cerebral hypomyelination may be seen by MRI, though only a small number of patients have mental retardation and seizures. Three forms of congenital muscular dystrophy have severe brain impairment. These include Fukuyama congenital muscular dystrophy (FCMD), muscle-eye-brain (MEB) disease, and Walker-Warburg syndrome (WWS). Patients are severely disabled in all three of these conditions. In MEB disease and WWS, but not in FCMD, ocular abnormalities impair vision. WWS is the most severe congenital muscular dystrophy, causing death by 1 year of age.

Laboratory Features   Serum CK is markedly elevated in all of these conditions. The EMG is myopathic and muscle biopsies show nonspecific dystrophic features. Merosin, or laminin α2 chain (a basal lamina protein), is deficient surrounding muscle fibers in merosin deficiency. Skin biopsies can also demonstrate defects in laminin α2 chain. In the other disorders (FKRP deficiency, FCMD, MEB disease, WWS) there is abnormal alpha-dystroglycan staining in muscle. In merosin deficiency, cerebral hypomyelination is common, and a host of brain malformations are seen in FCMD, MEB disease, and WWS.

All forms of CMD are inherited as autosomal recessive disorders. Chromosomal linkage and specific gene defects are presented in Table 382-11 online. With the exception of merosin, the other gene defects affect posttranslational glycosylation of alpha-dystroglycan. This abnormality is thought to impair binding with merosin and leads to weakening of the dystrophin-glycoprotein complex, instability of the muscle membrane, and/or abnormalities in muscle contraction. CMDs with brain and eye phenotypes probably involve defective glycosylation of additional proteins, accounting for the more extensive phenotypes.

CONGENITAL MUSCULAR DYSTROPHY

There is no specific treatment for CMD. Proper wheelchair seating is important. Management of epilepsy and cardiac manifestations is necessary for some patients.

MYOTONIC DYSTROPHY

Myotonic dystrophy is also known as *dystrophia myotonica* (DM). The condition is composed of at least two clinical disorders with overlapping phenotypes and distinct molecular genetic defects: myotonic dystrophy type 1 (DM1), the classic disease originally described by Steinert, and myotonic dystrophy type 2 (DM2), also called *proximal myotonic myopathy* (PROMM).

Clinical Features   The clinical expression of myotonic dystrophy varies widely and involves many systems other than muscle. Affected patients have a typical "hatchet-faced" appearance due to temporalis, masseter, and facial muscle atrophy and weakness. Frontal baldness is also characteristic of the disease. Neck muscles, including flexors and sternocleidomastoids, and distal limb muscles are involved early. Weakness of wrist extensors, finger extensors, and intrinsic hand muscles impairs function. Ankle dorsiflexor weakness may cause footdrop. Proximal muscles remain stronger throughout the course, although preferential atrophy and weakness of quadriceps muscles occur in many patients. Palatal, pharyngeal, and tongue involvement produce a dysarthric speech, nasal voice, and swallowing problems. Some patients have diaphragm and intercostal muscle weakness, resulting in respiratory insufficiency.

Myotonia, which usually appears by age 5 years, is demonstrable by percussion of the thenar eminence, the tongue, and wrist extensor muscles. Myotonia causes a slow relaxation of hand grip after a forced voluntary closure. Advanced muscle wasting makes myotonia more difficult to detect.

Cardiac disturbances occur commonly in patients with DM1. ECG abnormalities include first-degree heart block and more extensive conduction system involvement. Complete heart block and sudden death can occur. Congestive heart failure occurs infrequently but may result from cor pulmonale secondary to respiratory failure. Mitral valve prolapse also occurs commonly. Other associated features include intellectual impairment, hypersomnia, posterior subcapsular cataracts, gonadal atrophy, insulin resistance, and decreased esophageal and colonic motility.

Congenital myotonic dystrophy is a more severe form of DM1 and occurs in ~25% of infants of affected mothers. It is characterized by severe facial and bulbar weakness, transient neonatal respiratory insufficiency, and mental retardation.

DM2, or PROMM, has a distinct pattern of muscle weakness affecting mainly proximal muscles. Other features of the disease overlap with DM1, including cataracts, testicular atrophy, insulin resistance, constipation, hypersomnia, and cognitive defects. Cardiac conduction defects occur but are less common, and the hatchet face and frontal baldness are less consistent features. A very striking difference is the failure to clearly identify a congenital form of DM2.

Laboratory Features   The diagnosis of myotonic dystrophy can usually be made on the basis of clinical findings. Serum CK levels may be normal or mildly elevated. EMG evidence of myotonia is present in most cases of DM1 but may be more patchy in DM2. Muscle biopsy shows muscle atrophy, which selectively involves type 1 fibers in 50% of cases, and ringed fibers in DM1 but not in DM2. Typically, numerous internalized nuclei can be seen in individual muscle fibers as well as atrophic fibers with pyknotic nuclear clumps in both DM1 and DM2. Necrosis of muscle fibers and increased connective tissue, common in other muscular dystrophies, are less apparent in myotonic dystrophy.

DM1 and DM2 are both autosomal dominant disorders. New mutations do not appear to contribute to the pool of affected individuals. DM1 is transmitted by an intronic mutation consisting of an unstable expansion of a CTG trinucleotide repeat in a serine-threonine protein kinase gene (named *DMPK*) on chromosome 19q13.3. An increase in the severity of the disease phenotype in successive generations (genetic anticipation) is accompanied by an increase in the number of trinucleotide repeats. A similar type of mutation has been identified in fragile X syndrome (Chap. 62). The unstable triplet repeat in myotonic dystrophy can be used for prenatal diagnosis. Congenital disease occurs almost exclusively in infants born to affected mothers; it is possible that sperm with greatly expanded triplet repeats do not function well.

DM2 is caused by a DNA expansion mutation consisting of a CCTG repeat in intron 1 of the *ZNF9* gene located at chromosome 3q13.3-q24. The gene is believed to encode an RNA binding protein expressed in many different tissues, including skeletal and cardiac muscle.

The DNA expansions in DM1 and DM2 almost certainly impair muscle function by a toxic gain of function of the mutant mRNA. In both DM1 and DM2, the mutant RNA appears to form intranuclear inclusions composed of aberrant RNA. These RNA inclusions sequester RNA binding proteins essential for proper splicing of a variety of other mRNAs. This leads to abnormal transcription of multiple proteins in a variety of tissues/organ systems, in turn causing the systemic manifestations of DM1 and DM2.

℞ MYOTONIC DYSTROPHY

The myotonia in DM1 rarely warrants treatment, though some patients with DM2 are significantly bothered by the discomfort related to the associated muscle stiffness. Phenytoin and mexiletine are the preferred agents for the occasional patient who requires an antimyotonia drug; other agents, particularly quinine and procainamide, may worsen cardiac conduction. A cardiac pacemaker should be considered for patients with unexplained syncope, advanced conduction system abnormalities with evidence of second-degree heart block, or trifascicular conduction disturbances with marked prolongation of the PR interval. Molded ankle-foot orthoses help prevent footdrop in patients with distal lower extremity weakness. Excessive daytime somnolence with or without sleep apnea is not uncommon. Sleep studies, noninvasive respiratory support (BiPAP), and treatment with modafinil may be beneficial.

FACIOSCAPULOHUMERAL (FSH) MUSCULAR DYSTROPHY

This form of muscular dystrophy has a prevalence of ~1 in 20,000. It is distinct from a similar disorder known as scapuloperoneal dystrophy.

Clinical Features   The condition typically has an onset in childhood or young adulthood. In most cases, facial weakness is the initial manifestation, appearing as an inability to smile, whistle, or fully close the eyes. Weakness of the shoulder girdles, rather than the facial muscles, usually brings the patient to medical attention. Loss of scapular stabilizer muscles makes arm elevation difficult. Scapular winging (Fig. 382-3) becomes apparent with attempts at abduction and forward movement of the arms. Biceps and triceps muscles may be severely affected, with relative sparing of the deltoid muscles. Weakness is invariably worse for wrist extension than for wrist flexion, and weakness of the anterior compartment muscles of the legs may lead to footdrop.

In most patients, the weakness remains restricted to facial, upper extremity, and distal lower extremity muscles. In 20% of patients, weakness progresses to involve the pelvic girdle muscles, and severe functional impairment and possible wheelchair dependency result.

Characteristically, patients with FSH dystrophy do not have involvement of other organ systems, although labile hypertension is common, and there is an increased incidence of nerve deafness. *Coats' disease*, a disorder consisting of telangiectasia, exudation, and retinal detachment, also occurs.

Laboratory Features   The serum CK level may be normal or mildly elevated. EMG usually indicates a myopathic pattern. The muscle biopsy shows nonspecific features of a myopathy. A prominent inflammatory infiltrate, which is often multifocal in distribution, is present in some biopsy samples. The cause or significance of this finding is unknown.

An autosomal dominant inheritance pattern with almost complete penetrance has been established, but each family member should be examined for the presence of the disease, since ~30% of those affected are unaware of involvement. FSH dystrophy is caused by deletions of tandem 3.3-kb repeats at 4q35. The deletion reduces the number of repeats to a fragment of <35 kb in most patients. This mutation may result in an overexpression of upstream genes and a loss of DNA binding of a multiprotein complex mediating transcriptional repression of 4q35 genes. The mutation permits carrier detection and prenatal diagnosis. Most sporadic cases represent new mutations.

℞ FACIOSCAPULOHUMERAL MUSCULAR DYSTROPHY

No specific treatment is available; ankle-foot orthoses are helpful for footdrop. Scapular stabilization procedures improve scapular winging but may not improve function.

OCULOPHARYNGEAL DYSTROPHY

This form of muscular dystrophy represents one of several disorders characterized by progressive external ophthalmoplegia, which consists of slowly progressive ptosis and limitation of eye movements with sparing of pupillary reactions for light and accommodation. Patients usually do not complain of diplopia, in contrast to patients having conditions with a more acute onset of ocular muscle weakness (e.g., myasthenia gravis).

Clinical Features   Oculopharyngeal muscular dystrophy has a late onset; it usually presents in the fourth to sixth decade with ptosis and/or dysphagia. The extraocular muscle impairment is less prominent in the early phase but may be severe later. The swallowing problem may become debilitating and result in pooling of secretions and repeated episodes of aspiration. Mild weakness of the neck and extremities also occurs.

Laboratory Features   The serum CK level may be two to three times normal. Myopathic EMG findings are typical. On biopsy, muscle fibers are found to contain rimmed vacuoles, which by electron microscopy are shown to contain membranous whorls, accumulation of glycogen, and other nonspecific debris related to lysosomes. A distinct feature of oculopharyngeal dystrophy is the presence of tubular filaments, 8.5 nm in diameter, in muscle cell nuclei.

Oculopharyngeal dystrophy has an autosomal dominant inheritance pattern with complete penetrance. The incidence is high in French-Canadians and in Spanish-American families of the southwestern United States. Large kindreds of Italian and of eastern European Jewish descent have been reported. The molecular defect in oculopharyngeal muscular dystrophy is a subtle expansion of a modest polyalanine repeat tract in a poly-RNA binding protein (PABP2) in muscle.

℞ OCULOPHARYNGEAL DYSTROPHY

Dysphagia can cause inanition, making oculopharyngeal muscular dystrophy a potentially life-threatening disease. Cricopharyngeal myotomy may improve swallowing, although it does not prevent aspiration. Eyelid crutches can improve vision when ptosis obstructs vision; candidates for ptosis surgery must be carefully selected—those with severe facial weakness are not suitable.

DISTAL MYOPATHIES

A group of muscle diseases, the distal myopathies, are notable for their preferential distal distribution of muscle weakness in contrast to most

TABLE 382-8 DISTAL MYOPATHIES

2687

Disease	Clinical Features	Laboratory Features	Inheritance/Locus or Gene
Welander distal myopathy	Onset in fifth decade Weakness begins in hands Slow progression with spread to distal lower extremities Lifespan normal	Serum CK 2–3 × normal EMG myopathic NCS normal Muscle biopsy shows dystrophic features	AD Chromosome 2p13
Tibial muscular dystrophy (Udd)	Onset 4th to 8th decade Distal lower extremity weakness (tibial distribution) Upper extremities usually normal Lifespan normal	Serum CK 2–4 × normal EMG myopathic NCS normal Muscle biopsy shows dystrophic features Titin absent in M-line of muscle	AD Titin
Markesbery-Griggs distal myopathy	Onset 4th to 8th decade Distal lower extremity weakness (tibial distribution) with progression to distal arms and proximal muscles	Serum CK is usually mildly elevated EMG reveals irritative myopathy Muscle biopsies demonstrate rimmed vacuoles and features of myofibrillar myopathy	AD Z-band alternatively spliced PDX motif-containing protein (ZASP)
Laing distal myopathy	Onset childhood to 3d decade Distal lower extremity weakness (tibial distribution) and neck flexors affected early	Serum CK is normal or slightly elevated Muscle biopsies do not show rimmed vacuoles Large deposits of myosin heavy chain are seen in type 1 muscle fibers	AD Myosin heavy chain 7
Nonaka distal myopathy (autosomal recessive hereditary inclusion body myopathy)	Onset 2d to 3d decade Lower extremity distal weakness Mild distal upper limb weakness may be present early Progression to other muscles sparing quadriceps Ambulation may be lost in 10–15 years	Serum CK 3–10 × normal EMG myopathic NCS normal Dystrophic features on muscle biopsy plus rimmed vacuoles and 15- to 19-nm filaments within vacuoles	AR*GNE* gene: UDP-*N*-acetylglucosamine 2-epimerase/*N*-acetylmannosamine kinase Allelic to hereditary inclusion body myopathy
Miyoshi myopathy	Onset 2d to 3d decade Lower extremity weakness in posterior compartment muscles Progression leads to weakness in other muscle groups Ambulation lost after 10–15 years in about one-third of cases	Serum CK 20–100 × normal EMG myopathic NCS normal Muscle biopsy shows nonspecific dystrophic features often with prominent inflammatory cell infiltration; no rimmed vacuoles	AR Allelic to LGMD2B (see Table 382-7) Dysferlin
Myofibrillar myopathies	Onset from early childhood to late adult life Weakness may be distal, proximal, or generalized Cardiomyopathy and respiratory involvement is not uncommon	Serum CKs can be normal or moderately elevated EMG is myopathic and often associated with myopathic discharges Muscle biopsy demonstrates abnormal accumulation of desmin and other proteins, rimmed vacuoles, and myofibrillar degeneration	Genetically heterogeneous AD: Myotilin (also known as LGMD 1A) ZASP (see Markesbery-Griggs distal myopathy) Filamin-C Desmin Alpha B crystallin AR: Desmin Selenoprotein N1

Abbreviations: CK, creatine kinase; AD, autosomal dominant; AR, autosomal recessive; EMG, electromyography; NCS, nerve conduction studies.

muscle conditions associated with proximal weakness. The major distal myopathies are summarized in Table 382-8.

Clinical Features *Welander, Udd,* and *Markesbery-Griggs distal myopathies* are all late-onset, dominantly inherited disorders of distal limb muscles, usually beginning after age 40 years. Welander distal myopathy preferentially involves the wrist and finger extensors, whereas the others are associated with anterior tibial weakness leading to progressive footdrop. *Laing distal myopathy* is also a dominantly inherited disorder heralded by tibial weakness; however, it is distinguished by onset in childhood or early adult life. *Nonaka distal myopathy* and *Miyoshi myopathy* are distinguished by autosomal recessive inheritance and onset in the late teens or twenties. Nonaka myopathy entails anterior tibial weakness, whereas Miyoshi myopathy is unique in that gastrocnemius muscles are preferentially affected at onset. Finally, the *myofibrillar myopathies* (MFM) are a clinically and genetically heterogeneous group of disorders that can be associated with prominent distal weakness; they can be inherited in an autosomal dominant or recessive pattern.

Confounding these clinical features is the observation that proximal muscles can be affected as each of these disorders progresses (less so for Welander disease than the others). In contrast to many other inherited muscle diseases, the distal myopathies are for the most part limited to skeletal muscle.

Laboratory Features Serum CK level is particularly helpful in diagnosing Miyoshi myopathy since it is very elevated. In the other conditions serum CK is only slightly increased. EMGs are myopathic. In the myofibrillar myopathies (MFM), myotonic or pseudomyotonic discharges are common. Muscle biopsy shows nonspecific dystrophic features and, with the exception of Laing and Nonaka distal myopathies, often shows rimmed vacuoles. MFM is associated with the accumulation of dense inclusions, as well as amorphous material best seen on Gomori trichrome and myofibrillar disruption on electron microscopy. Immune staining sometimes demonstrates accumulation of desmin and other proteins in MFM, large deposits of myosin heavy chain in the subsarcolemmal region of type 1 muscle fibers in Laing myopathy, and reduced or absent dysferlin in Miyoshi myopathy.

The affected genes and their gene products are listed in Table 382-8. The gene for Welander disease awaits identification.

Rx DISTAL MYOPATHIES

Occupational therapy is offered for loss of hand function; ankle-foot orthoses can support distal lower limb muscles. The MFMs can be associated with cardiomyopathy (congestive heart failure or arrhythmias) and respiratory failure that may require medical management.

CONGENITAL MYOPATHIES

These rare disorders are distinguished from muscular dystrophies by the presence of specific histochemical and structural abnormalities in muscle. Although primarily disorders of infancy or childhood, three forms that may present in adulthood are described here: central core disease, nemaline (rod) myopathy, and centronuclear (myotubular) myopathy. Other types, such as minicore myopathy (multi-minicore disease), fingerprint body myopathy, and sarcotubular myopathy, are not discussed.

CENTRAL CORE DISEASE

Patients with central core disease may have decreased fetal movements and breech presentation. Hypotonia and delay in motor milestones, particularly in walking, are common. Later in childhood, patients develop problems with stair climbing, running, and getting up from the floor. On examination, there is mild facial, neck-flexor, and proximal-extremity muscle weakness. Legs are more affected than arms. Skeletal abnormalities include congenital hip dislocation, scoliosis, and pes cavus; clubbed feet also occur. Most cases are nonprogressive, but exceptions are well documented. Susceptibility to malignant hyperthermia must be considered as a potential risk factor for patients with central core disease.

The serum CK level is usually normal. Needle EMG demonstrates a myopathic pattern. Muscle biopsy shows fibers with single or multiple central or eccentric discrete zones (cores) devoid of oxidative enzymes. Cores occur preferentially in type 1 fibers and represent poorly aligned sarcomeres associated with Z disk streaming.

Autosomal dominant inheritance is characteristic; sporadic cases also occur. The disease is caused by point mutations of the ryanodine receptor gene on chromosome 19q, encoding the calcium-release channel of the sarcoplasmic reticulum of skeletal muscle; mutations of this gene also account for some cases of inherited malignant hyperthermia (Chap. 17). Malignant hyperthermia is an allelic condition; C-terminal mutations of the *RYR1* gene predispose to this complication.

Specific treatment is not required, but establishing a diagnosis of central core disease is extremely important because these patients have a known predisposition to malignant hyperthermia during anesthesia.

NEMALINE MYOPATHY

The term *nemaline* refers to the distinctive presence in muscle fibers of rods or threadlike structures (Greek *nema*, "thread"). Nemaline myopathy is clinically heterogeneous. A severe neonatal form presents with hypotonia and feeding and respiratory difficulties, leading to early death. Nemaline myopathy usually presents in infancy or childhood with delayed motor milestones. The course is nonprogressive or slowly progressive. The physical appearance is striking because of the long, narrow facies, high-arched palate, and open-mouthed appearance due to a prognathous jaw. Other skeletal abnormalities include pectus excavatum, kyphoscoliosis, pes cavus, and clubfoot deformities. Facial and generalized muscle weakness, including respiratory muscle weakness, is common. An adult-onset disorder with progressive proximal weakness may be seen. Myocardial involvement is occasionally present in both the childhood and adult-onset forms. The serum CK level is usually normal or slightly elevated. The EMG demonstrates a myopathic pattern. Muscle biopsy shows clusters of small rods (nemaline bodies), which occur preferentially, but not exclusively, in the sarcoplasm of type 1 muscle fibers. Occasionally, the rods are also apparent in myonuclei. The muscle often shows type 1 muscle fiber predominance. Rods originate from the Z disk material of the muscle fiber.

Five genes have been associated with nemaline myopathy. All code for thin filament–associated proteins, suggesting disturbed assembly or interplay of these structures as a pivotal mechanism. Mutations of the nebulin (*NEB*) gene account for most cases, including both severe neonatal and early childhood forms, inherited as autosomal recessive disorders. Neonatal and childhood cases, inherited as predominantly autosomal dominant disorders, are caused by mutations of the skeletal muscle α-actinin (*ACTA1*) gene. In milder forms of the disease with autosomal dominant inheritance, mutations have been identified in both the slow α-tropomyosin (*TPM3*) and β-tropomyosin (*TPM2*) genes accounting for <3% of cases. Muscle troponin T (*TNNT1*) gene mutations appear to be limited to the Amish population in North America. No specific treatment is available.

CENTRONUCLEAR (MYOTUBULAR) MYOPATHY

Three distinct variants of centronuclear myopathy occur. A neonatal form, also known as *myotubular myopathy*, presents with severe hypotonia and weakness at birth. The late infancy–early childhood form presents with delayed motor milestones. Later, difficulty with running and stair climbing becomes apparent. A marfanoid, slender body habitus, long narrow face, and high-arched palate are typical. Scoliosis and clubbed feet may be present. Most patients exhibit progressive weakness, some requiring wheelchairs. Progressive external ophthalmoplegia with ptosis and varying degrees of extraocular muscle impairment are characteristic of both the neonatal and the late-infantile forms. A third variant, the late childhood–adult form, has an onset in the second or third decade. Patients have full extraocular muscle movements and rarely exhibit ptosis. There is mild, slowly progressive limb weakness that may be distally predominant [some of these patients have been classified as having Charcot-Marie-Tooth disease type 2 (CMT2; Chap. 379)].

Normal or slightly elevated CK levels occur in each of the forms. Nerve conduction studies may reveal reduced amplitudes of distal compound muscle action potentials, in particular in adult-onset cases that resemble CMT2. EMG studies often give distinctive results, showing positive sharp waves and fibrillation potentials, complex and repetitive discharges, and rarely myotonic discharges. Muscle biopsy specimens in longitudinal section demonstrate rows of central nuclei, often surrounded by a halo. In transverse sections, central nuclei are found in 25–80% of muscle fibers.

A gene for the neonatal form of centronuclear myopathy has been localized to Xq28; this gene encodes myotubularin, a protein tyrosine phosphatase. Missense, frameshift, and splice-site mutations predict loss of myotubularin function in affected individuals. Carrier identification and prenatal diagnosis are possible. The inheritance pattern for the late infancy–early childhood disorder is probably autosomal recessive, and for the late childhood–adult form is probably autosomal dominant. No specific treatment is available. Some of the autosomal dominant late-onset cases, which are allelic to a form of CMT2, are associated with mutations in the gene that encodes dynamin-2.

DISORDERS OF MUSCLE ENERGY METABOLISM

There are two principal sources of energy for skeletal muscle—fatty acids and glucose. Abnormalities in either glucose or lipid utilization can be associated with distinct clinical presentations that can range from an acute, painful syndrome with rhabdomyolysis and myoglobinuria to a chronic, progressive muscle weakness simulating muscular dystrophy.

GLYCOGEN STORAGE AND GLYCOLYTIC DEFECTS
Disorders of Glycogen Storage Causing Progressive Weakness • *α-GLU-COSIDASE, OR ACID MALTASE, DEFICIENCY (POMPE'S DISEASE)*   Three clinical forms of α-glucosidase, or acid maltase, deficiency (*type II glycogenosis*) can be distinguished. The infantile form is the most common, with onset of symptoms in the first 3 months of life. Infants develop severe muscle weakness, cardiomegaly, hepatomegaly, and respiratory insufficiency. Glycogen accumulation in motor neurons of the spinal cord and brainstem contributes to muscle weakness. Death usually occurs

by 1 year of age. In the childhood form, the picture resembles muscular dystrophy. Delayed motor milestones result from proximal limb muscle weakness and involvement of respiratory muscles. The heart may be involved, but the liver and brain are unaffected. The adult form usually begins in the third or fourth decade but can present as late as the seventh decade. Respiratory failure and diaphragmatic weakness are often initial manifestations, heralding progressive proximal muscle weakness. The heart and liver are not involved.

The serum CK level is 2 to 10 times normal in infantile or childhood-onset Pompe disease but can be normal in adult-onset cases. EMG examination demonstrates a myopathic pattern, but other features are especially distinctive, including myotonic discharges, trains of fibrillation and positive waves, and complex repetitive discharges. EMG discharges are very prominent in the lumbosacral paraspinal muscles. The muscle biopsy in infants typically reveals vacuoles containing glycogen and the lysosomal enzyme acid phosphatase. Electron microscopy reveals membrane-bound and free tissue glycogen. However, muscle biopsies in late-onset Pompe's disease may demonstrate only nonspecific abnormalities. Enzyme analysis of dried blood spots is a new and sensitive technique to screen for Pompe's disease. A definitive diagnosis is established by enzyme assay in muscle or cultured fibroblasts or by genetic testing.

Acid maltase deficiency is inherited as an autosomal recessive disorder caused by mutations of the α-glucosidase gene. Recently, replacement therapy with IV recombinant human α-glucosidase has been shown to be beneficial in infantile-onset Pompe disease and was approved by the U.S. Food and Drug Administration (FDA). The efficacy in later-onset cases is under study. Clinical benefits in the infantile disease include reduced heart size, improved muscle function, reduced need for ventilatory support, and longer life.

OTHER GLYCOGEN STORAGE DISEASES WITH PROGRESSIVE WEAKNESS In *debranching enzyme deficiency* (*type III glycogenosis*), a slowly progressive form of muscle weakness can develop after puberty. Rarely, myoglobinuria may be seen. Patients are usually diagnosed in infancy, however, because of hypotonia and delayed motor milestones, hepatomegaly, growth retardation, and hypoglycemia. *Branching enzyme deficiency* (*type IV glycogenosis*) is a rare and fatal glycogen storage disease characterized by failure to thrive and hepatomegaly. Hypotonia and muscle wasting may be present, but the skeletal muscle manifestations are minor compared to liver failure.

Disorders of Glycolysis Causing Exercise Intolerance Several glycolytic defects are associated with recurrent myoglobinuria: *myophosphorylase deficiency* (*type V glycogenosis*), *phosphofructokinase deficiency* (*type VII glycogenosis*), *phosphoglycerate kinase deficiency* (*type IX glycogenosis*), *phosphoglycerate mutase deficiency* (*type X glycogenosis*), *lactate dehydrogenase deficiency* (*glycogenosis type XI*), and *beta-enolase deficiency*. Myophosphorylase deficiency, also known as *McArdle's disease*, is by far the most common of the glycolytic defects associated with exercise intolerance. These glycolytic defects result in a common failure to support energy production at the initiation of exercise, although the exact site of energy failure remains controversial.

Clinical muscle manifestations in these conditions usually begin in adolescence. Symptoms are precipitated by brief bursts of high-intensity exercise, such as running or lifting heavy objects. A history of myalgia and muscle stiffness usually precedes the intensely painful muscle contractures, which may be followed by myoglobinuria. Acute renal failure accompanies significant pigmenturia.

Certain features help distinguish some enzyme defects. In McArdle's disease exercise tolerance can be enhanced by a slow induction phase (warm-up) or brief periods of rest, allowing for the start of the "second-wind" phenomenon (switching to utilization of fatty acids). Varying degrees of hemolytic anemia accompany deficiencies of both phosphofructokinase (mild) and phosphoglycerate kinase (severe). In phosphoglycerate kinase deficiency, the usual clinical presentation is a seizure disorder associated with mental retardation; exercise intolerance is an infrequent manifestation.

In all of these conditions, the serum CK levels fluctuate widely and may be elevated even during symptom-free periods. CK levels >100 times normal are expected, accompanying myoglobinuria. All patients with suspected glycolytic defects leading to exercise intolerance should undergo a forearm exercise test. An impaired rise in venous lactate is highly indicative of a glycolytic defect. In lactate dehydrogenase deficiency, venous levels of lactate do not increase, but pyruvate rises to normal. A definitive diagnosis of glycolytic disease is made by muscle biopsy and subsequent enzyme analysis or by genetic testing.

Myophosphorylase deficiency, phosphofructokinase deficiency, and phosphoglycerate mutase deficiency are inherited as autosomal recessive disorders. Phosphoglycerate kinase deficiency is X-linked recessive. Mutations can be found in the respective genes encoding the abnormal proteins in each of these disorders.

Training may enhance exercise tolerance, perhaps by increasing perfusion to muscle. Dietary intake of free glucose or fructose prior to activity may improve function but care must be taken to avoid obesity from ingesting too many calories.

LIPID AS AN ENERGY SOURCE AND ASSOCIATED DEFECTS

Lipid is an important muscle energy source during rest and during prolonged, submaximal exercise. Fatty acids are derived from circulating very low density lipoprotein (VLDL) in the blood or from triglycerides stored in muscle fibers. Oxidation of fatty acids occurs in the mitochondria. To enter the mitochondria, a fatty acid must first be converted to an "activated fatty acid," acyl-CoA. The acyl-CoA must be linked with carnitine by the enzyme carnitine palmitoyltransferase (CPT) I for transport into the mitochondria. CPT I is present on the inner side of the outer mitochondrial membrane. Carnitine is removed by CPT II, an enzyme attached to the inside of the inner mitochondrial membrane, allowing transport of acyl-CoA into the mitochondrial matrix for β-oxidation.

Carnitine Palmitoyltransferase Deficiency CPT II deficiency is the most common recognizable cause of recurrent myoglobinuria, more common than the glycolytic defects. Onset is usually in the teenage years or early twenties. Muscle pain and myoglobinuria typically occur after prolonged exercise but can also be precipitated by fasting or infections; up to 20% of patients do not exhibit myoglobinuria, however. Strength is normal between attacks. In contrast to disorders caused by defects in glycolysis, in which muscle cramps follow short, intense bursts of exercise, the muscle pain in CPT II deficiency does not occur until the limits of utilization have been exceeded and muscle breakdown has already begun. Episodes of rhabdomyolysis may produce severe weakness. In young children and newborns, CPT II deficiency can present with a very severe clinical picture including hypoketotic hypoglycemia, cardiomyopathy, liver failure, and sudden death.

Serum CK levels and EMG findings are both usually normal between episodes. A normal rise of venous lactate during forearm exercise distinguishes this condition from glycolytic defects, especially myophosphorylase deficiency. Muscle biopsy does not show lipid accumulation and is usually normal between attacks. The diagnosis requires direct measurement of muscle CPT or genetic testing.

CPT II deficiency is much more common in men than women (5:1); nevertheless, all evidence indicates autosomal recessive inheritance. A mutation in the gene for CPT II (chromosome 1p36) causes the disease in some individuals. Attempts to improve exercise tolerance with frequent meals and a low-fat, high-carbohydrate diet, or by substituting medium-chain triglycerides in the diet, have not proven to be beneficial.

Myoadenylate Deaminase Deficiency The muscle enzyme myoadenylate deaminase converts adenosine 5′-monophosphate (5′-AMP) to inosine monophosphate (IMP) with liberation of ammonia. Myoadenylate deaminase may play a role in regulating adenosine triphosphate (ATP) levels in muscles. Most individuals with myoadenylate deaminase deficiency have no symptoms. There have been a few reports of patients with this disorder who have exercise-exacerbated myalgia and myoglobinuria. Many questions have been raised about the clinical effects of myoadenylate deaminase deficiency, and, specifically, its relationship to exertional myalgia and fatigability, but there is no consensus.

MITOCHONDRIAL MYOPATHIES

In 1972, Olson and colleagues recognized that muscle fibers with significant numbers of abnormal mitochondria could be highlighted with the modified trichrome stain; the term *ragged red fibers* was coined. By electron microscopy, the mitochondria in ragged red fibers are enlarged and often bizarrely shaped and have crystalline inclusions. Since that seminal observation, the understanding of these disorders of muscle and other tissues has expanded (Chap. 62).

Mitochondria play a key role in energy production. Oxidation of the major nutrients derived from carbohydrate, fat, and protein leads to the generation of reducing equivalents. The latter are transported through the respiratory chain in the process known as *oxidative phosphorylation*. The energy generated by the oxidation-reduction reactions of the respiratory chain is stored in an electrochemical gradient coupled to ATP synthesis.

A novel feature of mitochondria is their genetic composition. Each mitochondrion possesses a DNA genome that is distinct from that of the nuclear DNA. Human mitochondrial DNA (mtDNA) consists of a double-strand, circular molecule comprising 16,569 base pairs. It codes for 22 transfer RNAs, 2 ribosomal RNAs, and 13 polypeptides of the respiratory chain enzymes. The genetics of mitochondrial diseases differ from the genetics of chromosomal disorders. The DNA of mitochondria is directly inherited from the cytoplasm of the gametes, mainly from the oocyte. The sperm contributes very little of its mitochondria to the offspring at the time of fertilization. Thus, mitochondrial genes are derived almost exclusively from the mother, accounting for maternal inheritance of some mitochondrial disorders.

Patients with mitochondrial disorders have clinical manifestations that fall into three groups: chronic progressive external ophthalmoplegia (CPEO), skeletal muscle–CNS syndromes, and pure myopathy simulating muscular dystrophy or metabolic myopathy.

PROGRESSIVE EXTERNAL OPHTHALMOPLEGIA SYNDROMES WITH RAGGED RED FIBERS

The single most common sign of a mitochondrial myopathy is CPEO, occurring in >50% of all mitochondrial myopathies. Varying degrees of ptosis and weakness of extraocular muscles are seen, usually in the absence of diplopia, a point of distinction from disorders with fluctuating eye weakness (e.g., myasthenia gravis).

KEARNS-SAYRE SYNDROME (KSS)

KSS is a widespread multiorgan system disorder with a defined triad of clinical findings: onset before age 20, CPEO, and pigmentary retinopathy plus one or more of the following features: complete heart block, cerebrospinal fluid (CSF) protein > 1.0 g/L (100 mg/dL), or cerebellar ataxia. Some patients with CPEO and ragged red fibers may not fulfill all of the criteria for KSS. The cardiac disease includes syncopal attacks and cardiac arrest related to the abnormalities in the cardiac conduction system: prolonged intraventricular conduction time, bundle branch block, and complete atrioventricular block. Death attributed to heart block occurs in ~20% of the patients. Varying degrees of progressive limb muscle weakness and easy fatigability affect activities of daily living. Endocrine abnormalities are common, including gonadal dysfunction in both sexes with delayed puberty, short stature, and infertility. Diabetes mellitus is a cardinal sign of mitochondrial disorders and is estimated to occur in 13% of KSS patients. Other less common endocrine disorders include thyroid disease, hyperaldosteronism, Addison's disease, and hypoparathyroidism. Both mental retardation and dementia are common accompaniments to this disorder. Serum CK levels are normal or slightly elevated. Serum lactate and pyruvate levels may be elevated. EMG is myopathic. Nerve conduction studies may be abnormal related to an associated neuropathy. Muscle biopsies reveal ragged red fibers, highlighted in oxidative enzyme stains, many showing defects in cytochrome oxidase. By electron microscopy there are increased numbers of mitochondria that often appear enlarged and contain paracrystalline inclusions.

KSS is a sporadic disorder. The disease is caused by single mtDNA deletions presumed to arise spontaneously in the ovum or zygote. The most common deletion, occurring in about one-third of patients, removes 4977 bp of contiguous mtDNA. Monitoring for cardiac conduction defects is critical. Prophylactic pacemaker implantation is indicated when ECGs demonstrate a bifascicular block. In KSS no benefit has been shown for supplementary therapies, including multivitamins or coenzyme Q10. Of all the proposed options, exercise might be the most applicable but must be approached cautiously because of defects in the cardiac conduction system.

PROGRESSIVE EXTERNAL OPHTHALMOPLEGIA (PEO)

This condition is caused by nuclear DNA mutations affecting mtDNA copy number and integrity and is thus inherited in a Mendelian fashion. Onset is usually after puberty. Fatigue, exercise intolerance, and complaints of muscle weakness are typical. Some patients notice swallowing problems. The neurologic examination confirms the ptosis and ophthalmoplegia, usually asymmetric in distribution. A sensorineural hearing loss may be encountered. Mild facial, neck flexor, and proximal weakness are typical. Rarely, respiratory muscles may be progressively affected and may be the direct cause of death. Serum CK is normal or mildly elevated. The resting lactate level is normal or slightly elevated but may rise excessively after exercise. CSF protein is normal. The EMG is myopathic, and nerve conduction studies are usually normal. Ragged red fibers are prominently displayed in the muscle biopsy. Southern blots of muscle reveal a normal mtDNA band at 16.6 kb and several additional mtDNA deletion bands with genomes varying from 0.5 to 10 kb.

This autosomal dominant form of CPEO has been linked to loci on three chromosomes: 4q35, 10q24, and 15q22-26. In the chromosome 4q–related form of disease, mutations of the gene encoding the heart and skeletal muscle–specific isoform of the adenine nucleotide translocator 1 (*ANT1*) gene are found. This highly abundant mitochondrial protein forms a homodimeric inner mitochondrial channel through which ADP enters and ATP leaves the mitochondrial matrix. In the chromosome 10q–related disorder, mutations of the gene *C10orf2* are found. Its gene product, *twinkle*, co-localizes with the mtDNA and is named for its punctate, starlike staining properties. The function of twinkle is presumed to be critical for lifetime maintenance of mitochondrial integrity. In the cases mapped to chromosome 15q, a mutation affects the gene encoding mtDNA polymerase (*POLG*), an enzyme important in mtDNA replication. Autosomal recessive PEO has also been described with mutations in the *POLG* gene. Point mutations have been identified within various mitochondrial tRNA (Leu, Ile, Asn, Trp) genes in families with maternal inheritance of PEO.

Exercise may improve function but will depend on the patients' ability to participate.

AUTOSOMAL RECESSIVE CARDIOMYOPATHY AND OPHTHALMOPLEGIA (ARCO)

ARCO is a rare mitochondrial disorder clinically important because of an associated life-threatening cardiomyopathy. CPEO is the initial manifestation, occurring between ages 8 and 10. Exercise intolerance and fatigue follow the early symptoms, accompanied by palpitations and chest pain. Examination reveals extraocular muscle weakness, ptosis, facial weakness, reduced muscle bulk, and limb weakness, greater in proximal muscles. A dilated cardiomyopathy is typical, and some patients have conduction system involvement. Death from congestive heart failure occurs as early as age 13. Serum lactate is normal at rest but increases with mild exercise. Serum CK is increased two- to fourfold. EMG is normal or myopathic. Muscle biopsy demonstrates typical ragged red fibers. Multiple mtDNA deletions are seen on Southern blots of muscle. Echocardiograms show reduced ejection fraction. Conduction block is seen on ECGs. The disease is inherited as an autosomal recessive disorder. The gene has not been identified. Heart failure may require orthotopic cardiac transplantation. Cardiac pacemakers are appropriate for patients with heart block.

Feature	Calcium Channel	Sodium Channel		Potassium Channel
	Hypokalemic PP	**Hyperkalemic PP**	**Paramyotonia Congenita**	**Anderson's Syndrome**[b]
Mode of inheritance	AD	AD	AD	AD
Age of onset	Adolescence	Early childhood	Early childhood	Early childhood
Myotonia[a]	No	Yes	Yes	No
Episodic weakness	Yes	Yes	Yes	Yes
Frequency of attacks of weakness	Daily to yearly	May be 2–3/d	With cold, usually rare	Daily to yearly
Duration of attacks of weakness	2–12 h	From 1–2 h to >1 day	2–24 h	2–24 h
Serum K+ level during attacks of weakness	Decreased	Increased or normal	Usually normal	Variable
Effect of K+ loading	No change	Increased myotonia, then weakness	Increased myotonia	No change
Effect of muscle cooling	No change	Increased myotonia	Increased myotonia, then weakness	No change
Fixed weakness	Yes	Yes	Yes	Yes

[a]May be paradoxical in paramyotonia congenita.
[b]Dysmorphic features and cardiac arrhythmias are distinguishing features (see text).

Abbreviations: AD, autosomal dominant; PP, periodic paralysis.

mtDNA SKELETAL MUSCLE–CENTRAL NERVOUS SYSTEM SYNDROMES

Myoclonic Epilepsy with Ragged Red Fibers (MERRF) The onset of MERRF is variable, ranging from late childhood to middle adult life. Characteristic features include myoclonic epilepsy, cerebellar ataxia, and progressive muscle weakness. The seizure disorder is an integral part of the disease and may be the initial symptom. Cerebellar ataxia precedes or accompanies epilepsy. It is slowly progressive and generalized. The third major feature of the disease is muscle weakness in a limb-girdle distribution. Other more variable features include dementia, peripheral neuropathy, optic atrophy, hearing loss, and diabetes mellitus.

Serum CK levels are normal or slightly increased. The serum lactate may be elevated. EMG is myopathic, and in some patients nerve conduction studies show a neuropathy. The electroencephalogram is abnormal, corroborating clinical findings of epilepsy. Typical ragged red fibers are seen on muscle biopsy. MERRF is caused by maternally inherited point mutations of mitochondrial tRNA genes. The most common mutation found in 80% of MERRF patients is an A to G substitution at nucleotide 8344 of tRNA lysine (A8344G tRNA^{lys}). Other tRNA^{lys} mutations include base-pair substitutions T8356C and G8363A. Only supportive treatment is possible, with special attention to epilepsy.

Mitochondrial Myopathy, Encephalopathy, Lactic Acidosis, and Stroke-Like Episodes (MELAS)

MELAS is the most common mitochondrial encephalomyopathy. The term *stroke-like* is appropriate because the cerebral lesions do not conform to a strictly vascular distribution. The onset in the majority of patients is before age 20. Seizures, usually partial motor or generalized, are common and may represent the first clearly recognizable sign of disease. The cerebral insults that resemble strokes cause hemiparesis, hemianopia, and cortical blindness. A presumptive stroke occurring before age 40 should place this mitochondrial encephalomyopathy high in the differential diagnosis. Associated conditions include hearing loss, diabetes mellitus, hypothalamic pituitary dysfunction causing growth hormone deficiency, hypothyroidism, and absence of secondary sexual characteristics. In its full expression MELAS leads to dementia, a bedridden state, and a fatal outcome. Serum lactic acid is typically elevated. The CSF protein is also increased but is usually ≤1.0 g/L (100 mg/dL). Muscle biopsies show ragged red fibers. Neuroimaging demonstrates basal ganglia calcification in a high percentage of cases. Focal lesions that mimic infarction are present predominantly in the occipital and parietal lobes. Strict vascular territories are not respected, and cerebral angiography fails to demonstrate lesions of the major cerebral blood vessels.

MELAS is caused by maternally inherited point mutations of mitochondrial tRNA genes. Most of the tRNA mutations are lethal, accounting for the paucity of multigeneration families with this syndrome. The A3243G point mutation in tRNA$^{Leu(UUR)}$ is the most common, occurring in ~80% of MELAS cases. About 10% of MELAS

patients have other mutations of the tRNA$^{Leu(UUR)}$ gene including 3252G, 3256T, 3271C, and 3291C. Other tRNA gene mutations have also been reported in MELAS including G583A tRNA^{Phe}, G1642A tRNA^{Val}, G4332A tRNA^{Glu}, and T8316C tRNA^{Lys}. Mutations have also been reported in mtDNA polypeptide-coding genes. Two mutations were found in the ND5 subunit of complex I of the respiratory chain. A missense mutation has been reported at mtDNA position 9957 in the gene for subunit III of cytochrome C oxidase. No specific treatment is available. Supportive treatment is essential for the stroke-like episodes, seizures, and endocrinopathies.

PURE MYOPATHY SYNDROMES

Muscle weakness and fatigue can be the predominant manifestations of mtDNA mutations. When the condition affects exclusively muscle (pure myopathy), the disorder becomes difficult to recognize. Occasionally, mitochondrial myopathies can present with recurrent myoglobinuria without fixed weakness and thus resemble a glycogen storage disorder or CPT deficiency.

Mitochondrial DNA Depletion Myopathy This disorder, clinically indistinguishable from muscular dystrophy, usually presents in the neonatal period with weakness, hypotonia, and delayed motor milestones. Some cases are rapidly fatal, with death before age 2. A milder form affects patients at a slightly later age. These patients have slowly evolving proximal muscle weakness simulating Duchenne muscular dystrophy. In some, seizures and cardiomyopathy may be present. Serum CK can reach levels of 20 to 30 times normal. Resting lactate varies from normal to mildly elevated. The EMG is myopathic, and ragged red fibers are seen on muscle biopsy. The mtDNA depletion syndrome is inherited as an autosomal recessive condition. Mutations have been identified in the *TK2* gene on chromosome 16q22 encoding thymidine kinase-2. The affected gene controls the supply of deoxyribonucleotides used for the synthesis of mtDNA. No specific treatment is available. Supportive care follows the approaches outlined for muscular dystrophy.

DISORDERS OF MUSCLE MEMBRANE EXCITABILITY

Muscle membrane excitability is affected in a group of disorders referred to as *channelopathies*. The heart may also be involved, resulting in life-threatening complications (Table 382-9).

CALCIUM CHANNEL DISORDERS OF MUSCLE

Hypokalemic Periodic Paralysis (HypoKPP) Onset occurs at adolescence. Men are more often affected because of decreased penetrance in women. Episodic weakness with onset after age 25 is almost never due to periodic paralyses with the exception of thyrotoxic periodic paralysis (see below). Attacks are often provoked by meals high in carbohydrates or sodium and may accompany rest following prolonged exercise.

Weakness usually affects proximal limb muscles more than distal. Ocular and bulbar muscles are less likely to be affected. Respiratory muscles are usually spared but when they are involved, the condition may prove fatal. Weakness may take as long as 24 h to resolve. Life-threatening cardiac arrhythmias related to hypokalemia may occur during attacks. As a late complication, patients commonly develop severe, disabling proximal lower extremity weakness.

Attacks of thyrotoxic periodic paralysis resemble those of primary HypoKPP. Despite a higher incidence of thyrotoxicosis in women, men, particularly those of Asian descent, are more likely to manifest this complication. Attacks abate with treatment of the underlying thyroid condition.

A low serum potassium level during an attack, excluding secondary causes, establishes the diagnosis. Interattack muscle biopsies show the presence of single or multiple centrally placed vacuoles or tubular aggregates. Provocative tests with glucose and insulin to establish a diagnosis are usually not necessary and are potentially hazardous.

In the midst of an attack of weakness, motor conduction studies may demonstrate reduced amplitudes, whereas EMG may show electrical silence in severely weak muscles. In between attacks, the EMG and nerve conduction studies are normal, with the exception that myopathic motor unit action potentials may be seen in patients with fixed weakness.

HypoKPP is caused by mutations in either of two genes. HypoKPP type 1, the most common form, is inherited as an autosomal dominant disorder with incomplete penetrance. These patients have mutations in the voltage-sensitive, skeletal muscle calcium channel gene, *CALCL1A3* (Fig. 382-8). Approximately 10% of cases are HypoKPP type 2, arising from mutations in the voltage-sensitive sodium channel gene (*SCN4A*).

℞ HYPOKALEMIC PERIODIC PARALYSIS

The acute paralysis improves after the administration of potassium. Muscle strength and ECG should be monitored. Oral KCl (0.2–0.4 mmol/kg) should be given every 30 min. Only rarely is IV therapy necessary (e.g., when swallowing problems or vomiting is present). Administration of potassium in a glucose solution should be avoided because it may further reduce serum potassium levels. Mannitol is the preferred vehicle for administration of IV potassium. The long-term goal of therapy is to avoid attacks. This may reduce late-onset, fixed weakness. Patients should be made aware of the importance of a low-carbohydrate, low-sodium diet and consequences of intense exercise. Prophylactic administration of acetazolamide (125–1000 mg/d in divided doses) reduces or may abolish attacks in HypoKPP type 1. Paradoxically the potassium is lowered, but this is offset by the beneficial effect of metabolic acidosis. If attacks persist on acetazolamide, oral KCl should be added. Some patients require treatment with triamterine (25–100 mg/d) or spironolactone (25–100 mg/d). However, in patients with HypoKPP type 2, attacks of weakness can be exacerbated with acetazolamide.

SODIUM CHANNEL DISORDERS OF MUSCLE
Hyperkalemic Periodic Paralysis (HyperKPP) The term *hyperkalemic* is misleading since patients are often normokalemic during attacks. The fact that attacks are precipitated by potassium administration best defines the disease. The onset is in the first decade. Attacks are brief and mild, usually lasting 30 min to 4 h. Weakness affects proximal muscles, sparing bulbar muscles. Attacks are precipitated by rest following exercise and fasting. In a variant of this disorder, the predominant symptom is myotonia without weakness (*potassium-aggravated myotonia*). The symptoms are aggravated by cold, and myotonia makes the muscles stiff and painful. This disorder can be confused with paramyotonia congenita, myotonia congenita, and proximal myotonic myopathy (DM2).

Potassium may be slightly elevated but may also be normal during an attack. As in HypoKPP, nerve conduction studies in HyperKPP muscle may demonstrate reduced motor amplitudes and the EMG may be silent in very weak muscles. In between attacks of weakness, the conduction studies are normal. The EMG will often demonstrate myotonic discharges during and between attacks.

FIGURE 382-8 The sodium and calcium channels are depicted here as containing four homologous domains, each with six membrane-spanning segments. The fourth segment of each domain bears positive charges and acts as the "voltage sensor" for the channel. The association of the four domains is thought to form a pore through which ions pass. Sodium channel mutations are shown along with the phenotype that they confer. HyperKPP, hyperkalemic periodic paralysis; PC, paramyotonia congenita; PAM, potassium-aggravated myotonia. See text for details.

The chloride channel is envisioned to have ten membrane-spanning domains. The positions of mutations causing dominantly and recessively inherited myotonia congenita are indicated, along with mutations that cause this disease in mice and goats.

The muscle biopsy shows vacuoles that are smaller, less numerous, and more peripheral compared to the hypokalemic form or tubular aggregates. Provocative tests by administration of potassium can induce weakness but are usually not necessary to establish the diagnosis. HyperKPP and potassium-aggravated myotonia are inherited as autosomal dominant disorders. Mutations of the voltage-gated sodium channel *SCN4A* gene (Fig. 382-8) cause these conditions. For patients with frequent attacks, acetazolamide (125–1000 mg/d) is helpful. We have found mexiletine to be helpful in patients with significant myotonia.

Paramyotonia Congenita In paramyotonia congenita (PC) the attacks of weakness are cold-induced or occur spontaneously and are mild. Myotonia is a prominent feature but worsens with muscle activity (paradoxical myotonia). This is in contrast to classic myotonia in which exercise alleviates the condition. Attacks of weakness are seldom severe enough to require emergency room treatment. Over time patients develop interattack weakness as they do in other forms of periodic paralysis. PC is usually associated with normokalemia or hyperkalemia.

Serum CK is usually mildly elevated. Routine sensory and motor nerve conduction studies are normal. Cooling of the muscle often dramatically reduces the amplitude of the compound muscle action potentials. EMG reveals diffuse myotonic potentials in PC. Upon local cooling of the muscle the myotonic discharges disappear as the patient becomes unable to activate motor unit action potentials.

PC is inherited as an autosomal dominant condition; voltage-gated sodium channel mutations (Fig. 382-8) are responsible and thus this disorder is allelic with HyperKPP and potassium-aggravated myotonia. Patients with PC seldom seek treatment during attacks. Oral administration of glucose or other carbohydrates hastens recovery. Since interattack weakness may develop after repeated episodes, prophylactic treatment is usually indicated. Thiazide diuretics (e.g., chlorothiazide, 250–1000 mg/d) and mexiletine (slowly increase dose from 450 mg/d) are reported to be helpful. Patients should be advised to increase carbohydrates in their diet.

POTASSIUM CHANNEL DISORDERS

Andersen-Tawil Syndrome   This rare disease is characterized by episodic weakness, cardiac arrhythmias, and dysmorphic features (short stature, scoliosis, clinodactyly, hypertelorism, small or prominent low set ears, micrognathia, and broad forehead). The cardiac arrhythmias are potentially serious and life threatening. They include long QT, ventricular ectopy, bidirectional ventricular arrhythmias, and tachycardia. For many years the classification of this disorder was uncertain because episodes of weakness are associated with elevated, normal, or reduced levels of potassium during an attack. In addition, the potassium levels differ among kindreds but are consistent within a family. Inheritance is autosomal dominant, with incomplete penetrance and variable expressivity. The disease is caused by mutations of the inwardly rectifying potassium channel (*Kir 2.1*) gene. The treatment is similar to that for other forms of periodic paralysis and must include cardiac monitoring. The episodes of weakness may differ between patients because of potassium variability. Acetazolamide decreases the attack frequency and severity.

CHLORIDE CHANNEL DISORDERS

Two forms of this disorder, autosomal dominant (*Thomsen's disease*) and autosomal recessive (*Becker's disease*) are related to the same gene abnormality. Symptoms are noted in infancy and early childhood. The severity lessens in the third to fourth decade. Myotonia is worsened by cold and improved by activity. The gait may appear slow and labored at first but improves with walking. In Thomsen's disease muscle strength is normal, but in Becker's, which is usually more severe, there may be muscle weakness. Muscle hypertrophy is usually present. Myotonic discharges are prominently displayed by EMG recordings.

Serum CK is normal or mildly elevated. The muscle biopsy shows hypertrophied fibers. The disease is inherited as dominant or recessive and is caused by mutations of the chloride channel gene (Fig. 382-8). Many patients will not require treatment and learn that the symptoms improve with activity. Medications that can be used to decrease myotonia include quinine, phenytoin, and mexiletine.

ENDOCRINE AND METABOLIC MYOPATHIES

Many endocrine disorders cause weakness. Muscle fatigue is more common than true weakness. The cause of weakness in these disorders is not well defined. It is not even clear that weakness results from disease of muscle as opposed to another part of the motor unit, since the serum CK level is often normal (except in hypothyroidism) and the muscle histology is characterized by atrophy rather than destruction of muscle fibers. Nearly all endocrine myopathies respond to treatment.

THYROID DISORDERS

(See also Chap. 335) Abnormalities of thyroid function can cause a wide array of muscle disorders. These conditions relate to the important role of thyroid hormones in regulating the metabolism of carbohydrates and lipids as well as the rate of protein synthesis and enzyme production. Thyroid hormones also stimulate calorigenesis in muscle, increase muscle demand for vitamins, and enhance muscle sensitivity to circulating catecholamines.

Hypothyroidism   Patients with hypothyroidism have frequent muscle complaints, and proximal muscle weakness occurs in about one-third of them. Muscle cramps, pain, and stiffness are common. Some patients have enlarged muscles. Features of slow muscle contraction and relaxation occur in 25% of patients; the relaxation phase of muscle stretch reflexes is characteristically prolonged and best observed at the ankle or biceps brachii reflexes. The serum CK level is often elevated (up to 10 times normal), even when there is minimal clinical evidence of muscle disease. EMG is typically normal. The cause of muscle enlargement has not been determined, and muscle biopsy shows no distinctive morphologic abnormalities.

Hyperthyroidism   Patients who are thyrotoxic commonly have proximal muscle weakness and atrophy on examination, but they rarely complain of myopathic symptoms. Activity of deep tendon reflexes may be enhanced. Bulbar, respiratory, and even esophageal muscles may occasionally be affected, causing dysphagia, dysphonia, and aspiration. When bulbar involvement occurs, it is usually accompanied by chronic proximal limb weakness, but occasionally it presents in the absence of generalized thyrotoxic myopathy. Fasciculations may be apparent and, when coupled with increased muscle stretch reflexes, may lead to an erroneous diagnosis of amyotrophic lateral sclerosis. Other neuromuscular disorders occur in association with hyperthyroidism, including acquired hypokalemic periodic paralysis, myasthenia gravis, and a progressive ocular myopathy associated with proptosis (*Graves' ophthalmopathy*). Serum CK levels are not elevated in thyrotoxic myopathy, the EMG is normal, and muscle histology usually shows only atrophy of muscle fibers.

PARATHYROID DISORDERS

(See also Chap. 347)

Hyperparathyroidism   Muscle weakness is an integral part of primary and secondary hyperparathyroidism. Proximal muscle weakness, muscle wasting, and brisk muscle stretch reflexes are the main features of this endocrinopathy. Some patients develop neck extensor weakness (part of the dropped head syndrome). Serum CK levels are usually normal or slightly elevated. Serum parathyroid hormone levels are elevated. Serum calcium and phosphorus levels show no correlation with the clinical neuromuscular manifestations. Muscle biopsies show only varying degrees of atrophy without muscle fiber degeneration.

Hypoparathyroidism   An overt myopathy due to hypocalcemia rarely occurs. Neuromuscular symptoms are usually related to localized or generalized tetany. Serum CK levels may be increased secondary to muscle damage from sustained tetany. Hyporeflexia or areflexia is usually present and contrasts with the hyperreflexia in hyperparathyroidism.

ADRENAL DISORDERS

(See also Chap. 336) Conditions associated with glucocorticoid excess cause a myopathy; in fact, steroid myopathy is the most commonly diagnosed endocrine muscle disease. Glucocorticoid excess, either endogenous or exogenous (see "Drug-Induced Myopathies," below), produces various degrees of proximal limb weakness. Muscle wasting may be striking. A cushingoid appearance usually accompanies clinical signs of myopathy. Histologic sections demonstrate muscle fiber atrophy, preferentially affecting type 2b fibers, rather than degeneration or necrosis of muscle fibers. Adrenal insufficiency commonly causes muscle fatigue. The degree of weakness may be difficult to assess but is typically mild. In primary hyperaldosteronism (*Conn's syndrome*), neuromuscular complications are due to potassium depletion. The clinical picture is one of persistent muscle weakness. Long-standing hyperaldosteronism may lead to proximal limb weakness and wasting. Serum CK levels may be elevated, and a muscle biopsy may demonstrate degenerating fibers, some with vacuoles. These changes relate to hypokalemia and are not a direct effect of aldosterone on skeletal muscle.

PITUITARY DISORDERS

(See also Chap. 333) Patients with acromegaly usually have mild proximal weakness without muscle atrophy. Muscles often appear enlarged but exhibit decreased force generation. The duration of acromegaly, rather than the serum growth hormone levels, correlates with the degree of myopathy.

DIABETES MELLITUS

(See also Chap. 338) Neuromuscular complications of diabetes mellitus are most often related to neuropathy, with cranial and peripheral nerve palsies or distal sensorimotor polyneuropathy. *Diabetic amyotrophy* is a clumsy term since the condition represents a neuropathy affecting the proximal major nerve trunks and lumbosacral plexus. More appropriate terms for this disorder include *diabetic proximal neuropathy* and *lumbosacral radiculoplexus neuropathy*.

The only notable myopathy of diabetes mellitus is ischemic infarction of leg muscles, usually involving one of the thigh muscles but on occasion affecting the distal leg. This condition occurs in patients with poorly controlled diabetes and presents with abrupt onset of pain, tenderness, and edema of one thigh. The area of muscle infarction is hard and indurated. The muscles most often affected include the vastus lateralis, thigh adductors, and biceps femoris. CT or MRI can demonstrate focal abnormalities in the affected muscle. Diagnosis by imaging is preferable to muscle biopsy, if possible, as hemorrhage into the biopsy site can occur.

VITAMIN DEFICIENCY

Vitamin D deficiency (Chap. 71) due to either decreased intake, decreased absorption, or impaired vitamin D metabolism (as occurs in renal disease) may lead to chronic muscle weakness. Pain reflects the underlying bone disease (*osteomalacia*). Vitamin E deficiency may result from malabsorption. Clinical manifestations include ataxic neuropathy due to loss of proprioception and myopathy with proximal weakness. Progressive external ophthalmoplegia is a distinctive finding. It has not been established that deficiency of other vitamins causes a myopathy.

MYOPATHIES OF SYSTEMIC ILLNESS

Systemic illnesses such as chronic respiratory, cardiac, or hepatic failure are frequently associated with severe muscle wasting and complaints of weakness. Fatigue is usually a more significant problem than weakness, which is typically mild.

Myopathy may be a manifestation of chronic renal failure, independent of the better known uremic polyneuropathy. Abnormalities of calcium and phosphorus homeostasis and bone metabolism in chronic renal failure result from a reduction in 1,25-dihydroxyvitamin D, leading to decreased intestinal absorption of calcium. Hypocalcemia, further accentuated by hyperphosphatemia due to decreased renal phosphate clearance, leads to secondary hyperparathyroidism. Renal osteodystrophy results from the compensatory hyperparathyroidism, which leads to osteomalacia from reduced calcium availability and to osteitis fibrosa from the parathyroid hormone excess. The clinical picture of the myopathy of chronic renal failure is identical to that of primary hyperparathyroidism and osteomalacia. There is proximal limb weakness with bone pain.

Gangrenous calcification represents a separate, rare, and sometimes fatal complication of chronic renal failure. In this condition, widespread arterial calcification occurs and results in ischemia. Extensive skin necrosis may occur, along with painful myopathy and even myoglobinuria.

DRUG-INDUCED MYOPATHIES

Drug-induced myopathies are relatively uncommon in clinical practice with the exception of those caused by the cholesterol-lowering agents and glucocorticoids. Others impact practice to a lesser degree but are important to consider in specific situations. Table 382-10 provides a comprehensive list of drug-induced myopathies with their distinguishing features.

MYOPATHY FROM LIPID-LOWERING AGENTS

All classes of lipid-lowering agents have been implicated in muscle toxicity including fibrates (clofibrate, gemfibrozil), HMG-CoA reductase inhibitors (referred to as *statins*), niacin (nicotinic acid), and ezetimibe.

TABLE 382-10 DRUG-INDUCED MYOPATHIES

Drugs	Major Toxic Reaction

Lipid-lowering agents
  Fibric acid derivatives
  HMG-CoA reductase inhibitors
  Niacin (nicotinic acid)
	Drugs belonging to all three of the major classes of lipid-lowering agents can produce a spectrum of toxicity: asymptomatic serum creatine kinase elevation, myalgias, exercised-induced pain, rhabdomyolysis, and myoglobinuria.

Glucocorticoids	Acute, high-dose glucocorticoid treatment can cause acute quadriplegic myopathy. These high doses of steroids are often combined with nondepolarizing neuromuscular blocking agents but the weakness can occur without their use. Chronic steroid administration produces predominantly proximal weakness.
Nondepolarizing neuromuscular blocking agents	Acute quadriplegic myopathy can occur with or without concomitant glucocorticoids.
Zidovudine	Mitochondrial myopathy with ragged red fibers.

Drugs of abuse
  Alcohol
  Amphetamines
  Cocaine
  Heroin
  Phencyclidine
  Meperidine
	All drugs in this group can lead to widespread muscle breakdown, rhabdomyolysis, and myoglobinuria. Local injections cause muscle necrosis, skin induration, and limb contractures.

Autoimmune toxic myopathy D-Penicillamine	Use of this drug may cause polymyositis and myasthenia gravis.

Amphophilic cationic drugs
  Amiodarone
  Chloroquine
  Hydroxychloroquine
	All amphophilic drugs have the potential to produce painless, proximal weakness associated with autophagic vacuoles in the muscle biopsy.

Antimicrotubular drugs Colchicine	This drug produces painless, proximal weakness especially in the setting of renal failure. Muscle biopsy shows autophagic vacuoles.

Myalgia, malaise, and muscle tenderness are the most common manifestations. Muscle pain may be related to exercise. Patients may exhibit proximal weakness. Varying degrees of muscle necrosis are seen, and in severe reactions rhabdomyolysis and myoglobinuria occur. Concomitant use of statins with fibrates and cyclosporine is more likely to cause adverse reactions than use of one agent alone. Elevated serum CK is an important indication of toxicity. Muscle weakness is accompanied by a myopathic EMG, and muscle necrosis is observed by muscle biopsy. Severe myalgias, muscle weakness, significant elevations in serum CK (> three times baseline), and myoglobinuria are indications for stopping the drug. Patients usually improve with drug cessation, although this may take several weeks. Rare cases continue to progress after the offending agent is discontinued. It is possible that in such cases the statin may have triggered an immune-mediated necrotizing myopathy, as these individuals may respond to glucocorticoid therapy.

GLUCOCORTICOID-RELATED MYOPATHIES

Glucocorticoid myopathy occurs with chronic treatment or as "acute quadriplegic" myopathy secondary to high-dose, IV glucocorticoids. Chronic administration produces proximal weakness accompanied by cushingoid manifestations, which can be quite debilitating; the chronic use of prednisone at a daily dose of ≥30 mg/d is most often associated with toxicity. Patients taking fluorinated glucocorticoids (triamcinolone, betamethasone, dexamethasone) appear to be at especially high risk for myopathy. Patients receiving high-dose, IV glucocorticoids for status asthmaticus, chronic obstructive pulmonary disease, or other indications may develop severe generalized weakness. Involvement of the diaphragm and intercostal muscles causes respiratory failure and requires ventilatory support. In this setting, the use of glucocorticoids in combination with nondepolarizing neuromuscular blocking agents to further decrease airway resistance is particularly likely to lead to this complication. In chronic steroid myopathy the serum CK is usually normal. Serum potassium may be low. The muscle biopsy in chronic cases shows preferential type 2 muscle fiber atrophy; this is not reflected in the EMG, which is usually normal. In acute cases with quadriplegic myopathy the muscle biopsy is abnormal, showing a distinctive loss of thick filaments (myosin) by electron microscopy. By light microscopy there is focal loss of ATPase staining in central or paracentral areas of the muscle fiber. Calpain stains show diffusely reactive atrophic fibers. Withdrawal of glucocorticoids will improve the chronic myopathy. In acute quadriplegic myopathy, recovery is slow. Patients require supportive care and rehabilitation.

MYOPATHY OF NONDEPOLARIZING NEUROMUSCULAR BLOCKING AGENTS

Patients may receive nondepolarizing neuromuscular blocking agents because of life-threatening airway resistance. Acute quadriplegic myopathy may result, with or without glucocorticoid use. The clinical features are identical to acute quadriplegic myopathy secondary to glucocorticoids.

DRUG-INDUCED MITOCHONDRIAL MYOPATHY

Zidovudine, used in the treatment of HIV infection, is a thymidine analogue that inhibits viral replication by interrupting reverse transcriptase. Myopathy is a well-established complication of this agent. Patients present with myalgias, muscle weakness, and atrophy affecting the thigh and calf muscles. The complication occurs in about 17% of patients treated with doses of 1200 mg/d for 6 months. The introduction of protease inhibitors for treatment of HIV infection has led to lower doses of zidovudine therapy and a decreased incidence of myopathy. Serum CK is elevated and EMG is myopathic. Muscle biopsy shows ragged red fibers with minimal inflammation; the lack of inflammation serves to distinguish zidovudine toxicity from HIV-related myopathy. If the myopathy is thought to be drug-related, the medication should be stopped or the dosage reduced.

DRUGS OF ABUSE AND RELATED MYOPATHIES

Myotoxicity is a potential consequence of addiction to alcohol and illicit drugs. Ethanol is one of the most commonly abused substances with potential to damage muscle. Other potential toxins include cocaine, heroin, and amphetamines. The most deleterious reactions occur from overdosing leading to coma and seizures, causing rhabdomyolysis, myoglobinuria, and renal failure. Direct toxicity can occur from cocaine, heroin, and amphetamines causing muscle breakdown and varying degrees of weakness. The effects of alcohol are more controversial. Direct muscle damage is less certain, since toxicity usually occurs in the setting of poor nutrition and possible contributing factors such as hypokalemia and hypophosphatemia. Alcoholics are also prone to neuropathy and a variety of CNS disorders (Chap. 387).

Focal myopathies from self-administration of meperidine, heroin, and pentazocine can cause pain, swelling, muscle necrosis, and hemorrhage. The cause is multifactorial; needle trauma, direct toxicity of the drug or vehicle, and infection may all play a role. When severe, there may be overlying skin induration and contractures with replacement of muscle by connective tissue. Elevated serum CK and myopathic EMG are characteristic of these reactions. The muscle biopsy shows widespread or focal areas of necrosis. In conditions leading to rhabdomyolysis, patients need adequate hydration to reduce serum myoglobin and protect renal function. In all of these conditions, counseling is essential to limit drug abuse.

DRUG-INDUCED AUTOIMMUNE MYOPATHIES

The most consistent drug-related inflammatory or antibody-mediated myopathy is caused by D-penicillamine. This drug chelates copper and is used in the treatment of Wilson's disease. It is also used to treat other disorders including scleroderma, rheumatoid arthritis, and primary biliary cirrhosis. Adverse events include drug-induced polymyositis, indistinguishable from the spontaneous disease. The incidence of this inflammatory muscle disease is about 1%. Myasthenia gravis is also induced by D-penicillamine, with a higher incidence estimated at 7%. These disorders resolve with drug withdrawal, although immunosuppressive therapy may be warranted in severe cases.

Scattered reports of other drugs causing an inflammatory myopathy are rare and include a heterogeneous group of agents: cimetidine, phenytoin, procainamide, and propylthiouracil. In most cases, a cause-and-effect relationship is uncertain. A complication of interest was related to L-tryptophan. In 1989 an epidemic of eosinophilia-myalgia syndrome (EMS) in the United States was caused by a contaminant in the product from one manufacturer. The product was withdrawn, and incidence of EMS diminished abruptly following this action.

OTHER DRUG-INDUCED MYOPATHIES

Certain drugs produce painless, largely proximal, muscle weakness. These drugs include the amphophilic cationic drugs (amiodarone, chloroquine, hydroxychloroquine) and antimicrotubular drugs (colchicine) (Table 382-10). Muscle biopsy can be useful in the identification of toxicity since autophagic vacuoles are prominent pathologic features of these toxins.

FURTHER READINGS

ABU-BAKER A, ROULEAU GA: Oculopharyngeal muscular dystrophy: Recent advances in the understanding of the molecular pathogenic mechanisms and treatment strategies. Biochim Biophys Acta 772:173, 2007

CANNON SC: Pathomechanisms in channelopathies of skeletal muscle and brain. Ann Rev Neurosci 29:387, 2006

DAVIES KE, NOWAK KJ: Molecular mechanisms of muscular dystrophies: Old and new players. Nat Rev Mol Cell Biol 7:762, 2006

DIMAURO S, DAVIDZON G: Mitochondrial DNA and disease. Ann Med 37:222, 2005

GLOVER L, BROWN RH Jr: Dysferlin in membrane trafficking and patch repair. Traffic 8:785, 2007

GODFREY C et al: Fukutin mutations in steroid-responsive limb girdle muscular dystrophy. Ann Neurol 60:603, 2006

LUECK JD et al: Chloride channelopathy in myotonic dystrophy resulting from loss of post-transcriptional regulation for CLCN1. Am J Physiol Cell Physiol 292:C1291, 2007

MENDELL JR et al: The congenital muscular dystrophies: Recent advances and molecular insights. Pediatr Devel Path 9:427, 2006

MOORE SA et al: Limb girdle dystrophy in the United States. J Neuropath Exp Neurol 65:995, 2006

RANUM LPW, COOPER TA: RNA-mediated neuromuscular disorders. Ann Rev Neurosci 29:259, 2006

RODINO-KLAPAC LR et al: Gene therapy for Duchenne muscular dystrophy: Expectations and challenges. Arch Neurol 64:1236, 2007

SAMPAOLESI M et al: Mesangioblast stem cells ameliorate muscle function in dystrophic dogs. Nature 444:574, 2006

VAN DE MAAREL SM et al: Facioscapuloperoneal muscular dystrophy. Biochim Biophys Acta 189:697, 2007

WELCH E et al: PTC124 targets genetic disorders caused by nonsense mutations. Nature 447:87, 2007

383 Polymyositis, Dermatomyositis, and Inclusion Body Myositis

Marinos C. Dalakas

The inflammatory myopathies represent the largest group of acquired and potentially treatable causes of skeletal muscle weakness. They are classified into three major groups: polymyositis (PM), dermatomyositis (DM), and inclusion body myositis (IBM).

CLINICAL FEATURES

The prevalence of the inflammatory myopathies is estimated at 1 in 100,000. PM as a stand-alone entity is a rare disease affecting adults. DM affects both children and adults and women more often than men. IBM is three times more frequent in men than in women, more common in Caucasians than blacks, and is most likely to affect persons >50 years of age.

These disorders present as progressive and symmetric muscle weakness except for IBM, which can have an asymmetric pattern. Patients usually report increasing difficulty with everyday tasks requiring the use of proximal muscles, such as getting up from a chair, climbing steps, stepping onto a curb, lifting objects, or combing hair. Fine-motor movements that depend on the strength of distal muscles, such as buttoning a shirt, sewing, knitting, or writing, are affected only late in the course of PM and DM, but fairly early in IBM. Falling is common in IBM because of early involvement of the quadriceps muscle with buckling of the knees. Ocular muscles are spared, even in advanced, untreated cases; if these muscles are affected, the diagnosis of inflammatory myopathy should be questioned. Facial muscles are unaffected in PM and DM, but mild facial muscle weakness is common in patients with IBM. In all forms of inflammatory myopathy, pharyngeal and neck-flexor muscles are often involved, causing dysphagia or difficulty in holding up the head (*head drop*). In advanced and rarely in acute cases, respiratory muscles may also be affected. Severe weakness, if untreated, is almost always associated with muscle wasting. Sensation remains normal. The tendon reflexes are preserved but may be absent in severely weakened or atrophied muscles, especially in IBM where atrophy of the quadriceps and the distal muscles is common. Myalgia and muscle tenderness may occur in a small number of patients, usually early in the disease, and particularly in DM associated with connective tissue disorders. Weakness in PM and DM progresses subacutely over a period of weeks or months and rarely acutely; by contrast, IBM progresses very slowly, over years, simulating a late-life muscular dystrophy (Chap. 382) or slowly progressive motor neuron disorder (Chap. 369).

SPECIFIC FEATURES

(Table 383-1)

Polymyositis The actual onset of PM is often not easily determined, and patients typically delay seeking medical advice for several months. This is in contrast to DM, in which the rash facilitates early recognition (see below). PM mimics many other myopathies and is a diagnosis of exclusion. It is a subacute inflammatory myopathy affecting adults, and rarely children, who *do not have* any of the following: rash, involvement of the extraocular and facial muscles, family history of a neuromuscular disease, history of exposure to myotoxic drugs or toxins, endocrinopathy, neurogenic disease, muscular dystrophy, biochemical muscle disorder (deficiency of a muscle enzyme), or IBM as excluded by muscle biopsy analysis (see below). As an isolated entity, PM is a rare (and overdiagnosed) disorder; more commonly, PM occurs in association with a systemic autoimmune or connective tissue disease, or with a known viral or bacterial infection. Drugs, especially D-penicillamine or zidovudine (AZT), may also produce an inflammatory myopathy similar to PM.

Dermatomyositis DM is a distinctive entity identified by a characteristic rash accompanying, or more often preceding, muscle weakness.

The rash may consist of a blue-purple discoloration on the upper eyelids with edema (heliotrope rash; see Fig. 55-3), a flat red rash on the face and upper trunk, and erythema of the knuckles with a raised violaceous scaly eruption (*Gottron's sign*; see Fig. 55-4). The erythematous rash can also occur on other body surfaces, including the knees, elbows, malleoli, neck and anterior chest (often in a *V sign*), or back and shoulders (*shawl sign*), and may worsen after sun exposure. In some patients the rash is pruritic, especially on the scalp, chest, and back. Dilated capillary loops at the base of the fingernails are also characteristic. The cuticles may be irregular, thickened, and distorted, and the lateral and palmar areas of the fingers may become rough and cracked, with irregular, "dirty" horizontal lines, resembling *mechanic's hands*. The weakness can be mild, moderate, or severe enough to lead to quadriparesis. At times, the muscle strength appears normal, hence the term *dermatomyositis sine myositis*. When muscle biopsy is performed in such cases, however, significant perivascular and perimysial inflammation is often seen.

DM usually occurs alone but may overlap with scleroderma and mixed connective tissue disease. Fasciitis and thickening of the skin, similar to that seen in chronic cases of DM, have occurred in patients with the *eosinophilia-myalgia syndrome* associated with the ingestion of contaminated L-tryptophan.

Inclusion Body Myositis In patients ≥50 years of age, IBM is the most common of the inflammatory myopathies. It is often misdiagnosed as PM and is suspected only later when a patient with presumed PM does not respond to therapy. Weakness and atrophy of the distal muscles, especially foot extensors and deep finger flexors, occur in almost all cases of IBM and may be a clue to early diagnosis. Some patients present with falls because their knees collapse due to early quadriceps weakness. Others present with weakness in the small muscles of the

TABLE 383-1 FEATURES ASSOCIATED WITH INFLAMMATORY MYOPATHIES

Characteristic	Polymyositis	Dermatomyositis	Inclusion Body Myositis
Age at onset	>18 yr	Adulthood and childhood	>50 yr
Familial association	No	No	Yes, in some cases
Extramuscular manifestations	Yes	Yes	Yes
Associated conditions			
Connective tissue diseases	Yes[a]	Scleroderma and mixed connective tissue disease (overlap syndromes)	Yes, in up to 20% of cases[a]
Systemic autoimmune diseases[b]	Frequent	Infrequent	Infrequent
Malignancy	No	Yes, in up to 15% of cases	No
Viruses	Yes[c]	Unproven	Yes[c]
Drugs[d]	Yes	Yes, rarely	No
Parasites and bacteria[e]	Yes	No	No

[a]Systemic lupus erythematosus, rheumatoid arthritis, Sjögren's syndrome, systemic sclerosis, mixed connective tissue disease.

[b]Crohn's disease, vasculitis, sarcoidosis, primary biliary cirrhosis, adult celiac disease, chronic graft-versus-host disease, discoid lupus, ankylosing spondylitis, Behçet's syndrome, myasthenia gravis, acne fulminans, dermatitis herpetiformis, psoriasis, Hashimoto's disease, granulomatous diseases, agammaglobulinemia, monoclonal gammopathy, hypereosinophilic syndrome, Lyme disease, Kawasaki disease, autoimmune thrombocytopenia, hypergammaglobulinemic purpura, hereditary complement deficiency, IgA deficiency.

[c]HIV (human immunodeficiency virus) and HTLV-I (human T cell lymphotropic virus type I).

[d]Drugs include penicillamine (dermatomyositis and polymyositis), zidovudine (polymyositis), and contaminated tryptophan (dermatomyositis-like illness). Other myotoxic drugs may cause myopathy but not an inflammatory myopathy (see text for details).

[e]Parasites (protozoa, cestodes, nematodes), tropical and bacterial myositis (pyomyositis).

hands, especially finger flexors, and complain of inability to hold objects such as golf clubs or perform tasks such as turning keys or tying knots. On occasion, the weakness and accompanying atrophy can be asymmetric and selectively involve the quadriceps, iliopsoas, triceps, biceps, and finger flexors, resembling a lower motor neuron disease. Dysphagia is common, occurring in up to 60% of IBM patients, and may lead to episodes of choking. Sensory examination is generally normal; some patients have mildly diminished vibratory sensation at the ankles that presumably is age-related. The pattern of distal weakness, which superficially resembles motor neuron or peripheral nerve disease, results from the myopathic process affecting distal muscles selectively. Disease progression is slow but steady, and most patients require an assistive device such as cane, walker, or wheelchair within several years of onset.

In at least 20% of cases, IBM is associated with systemic autoimmune or connective tissue diseases. Familial aggregation of typical IBM may occur; such cases have been designated as *familial inflammatory IBM*. This disorder is distinct from *hereditary inclusion body myopathy* (h-IBM), which describes a heterogeneous group of recessive, and less frequently dominant, inherited syndromes; the h-IBMs are noninflammatory myopathies. A subset of h-IBM that spares the quadriceps muscles has emerged as a distinct entity. This disorder, originally described in Iranian Jews and now seen in many ethnic groups, is linked to chromosome 9p1 and results from mutations in the UDP-*N*-acetylglucosamine 2-epimerase/*N*-acetylmannosamine kinase (*GNE*) gene.

ASSOCIATED CLINICAL FINDINGS

Extramuscular Manifestations   These may be present to a varying degree in patients with PM or DM, and include:

1. *Systemic symptoms*, such as fever, malaise, weight loss, arthralgia, and Raynaud's phenomenon, especially when inflammatory myopathy is associated with a connective tissue disorder.
2. *Joint contractures*, mostly in DM and especially in children.
3. *Dysphagia and gastrointestinal symptoms*, due to involvement of oropharyngeal striated muscles and upper esophagus, especially in DM and IBM.
4. *Cardiac disturbances*, including atrioventricular conduction defects, tachyarrhythmias, dilated cardiomyopathy, a low ejection fraction, and congestive heart failure, may rarely occur, either from the disease itself or from hypertension associated with long-term use of glucocorticoids.
5. *Pulmonary dysfunction*, due to weakness of the thoracic muscles, interstitial lung disease, or drug-induced pneumonitis (e.g., from methotrexate), which may cause dyspnea, nonproductive cough, and aspiration pneumonia. Interstitial lung disease may precede myopathy or occur early in the disease and develops in up to 10% of patients with PM or DM, most of whom have antibodies to t-RNA synthetases, as described below.
6. *Subcutaneous calcifications*, in DM, sometimes extruding on the skin and causing ulcerations and infections.
7. *Arthralgias*, synovitis, or deforming arthropathy with subluxation in the interphalangeal joints can occur in some patients with DM and PM who have Jo-1 antibodies (see below).

Association with Malignancies   Although all the inflammatory myopathies can have a chance association with malignant lesions, especially in older age groups, the incidence of malignant conditions appears to be specifically increased only in patients with DM and not in those with PM or IBM. The most common tumors associated with DM are ovarian cancer, breast cancer, melanoma, colon cancer, and non-Hodgkin lymphoma. The extent of the search that should be conducted for an occult neoplasm in adults with DM depends on the clinical circumstances. Tumors in these patients are usually uncovered by abnormal findings in the medical history and physical examination and not through an extensive blind search. The weight of evidence argues against performing expensive, invasive, and nondirected tumor searches. A complete annual physi-

cal examination with pelvic, breast (mammogram, if indicated), and rectal examinations (with colonoscopy according to age and family history); urinalysis; complete blood count; blood chemistry tests; and a chest film should suffice in most cases. In Asians, nasopharyngeal cancer is common, and a careful examination of ears, nose, and throat is indicated.

Overlap Syndromes   These describe the association of inflammatory myopathies with connective tissue diseases. A well-characterized overlap syndrome occurs in patients with DM who also have manifestations of systemic sclerosis or mixed connective tissue disease, such as sclerotic thickening of the dermis, contractures, esophageal hypomotility, microangiopathy, and calcium deposits (Table 383-1). By contrast, signs of rheumatoid arthritis, systemic lupus erythematosus, or Sjögren's syndrome are very rare in patients with DM. Patients with the overlap syndrome of DM and systemic sclerosis may have a specific antinuclear antibody, the anti-PM/Scl, directed against a nucleolar-protein complex.

PATHOGENESIS

An autoimmune etiology of the inflammatory myopathies is indirectly supported by an association with other autoimmune or connective tissue diseases; the presence of various autoantibodies; an association with specific major histocompatibility complex (MHC) genes; demonstration of T cell–mediated myocytotoxicity or complement-mediated microangiopathy; and a response to immunotherapy.

Autoantibodies and Immunogenetics   Various autoantibodies against nuclear antigens (antinuclear antibodies) and cytoplasmic antigens are found in up to 20% of patients with inflammatory myopathies. The antibodies to cytoplasmic antigens are directed against ribonucleoproteins involved in protein synthesis (anti-synthetases) or translational transport (anti-signal-recognition particles). The antibody directed against the histidyl-transfer RNA synthetase, called *anti-Jo-1*, accounts for 75% of all the anti-synthetases and is clinically useful because up to 80% of patients with anti-Jo-1 antibodies have interstitial lung disease. Some patients with the anti-Jo-1 antibody also have Raynaud's phenomenon, nonerosive arthritis, and the MHC molecules DR3 and DRw52. DR3 haplotypes (molecular designation DRB1*0301, DQB1*0201) occur in up to 75% of patients with PM and IBM, whereas in juvenile DM there is an increased frequency of DQA1*0501 (Chap. 309).

Immunopathologic Mechanisms   In DM, humoral immune mechanisms are implicated, resulting in a microangiopathy and muscle ischemia (Fig. 383-1). Endomysial inflammatory infiltrates are composed of B cells located in proximity to CD4 T cells, dendritic cells, and macrophages; there is a relative absence of lymphocytic invasion of nonnecrotic muscle fibers. Activation of the complement C5b-9 membranolytic attack complex is thought to be a critical early event that triggers release of proinflammatory cytokines and chemokines, induces expression of vascular cell adhesion molecule (VCAM) 1 and intracellular adhesion molecule (ICAM) 1 on endothelial cells, and facilitates migration of activated lymphoid cells to the perimysial and endomysial spaces. Necrosis of the endothelial cells, reduced numbers of endomysial capillaries, ischemia, and muscle-fiber destruction resembling microinfarcts occur. The remaining capillaries often have dilated lumens in response to the ischemic process. Larger intramuscular blood vessels may also be affected in the same pattern. Residual perifascicular atrophy reflects the endofascicular hypoperfusion that is prominent in the periphery of the muscle fascicles.

By contrast, in PM and IBM a mechanism of T cell–mediated cytotoxicity is likely. CD8 T cells, along with macrophages, initially surround and eventually invade and destroy healthy, nonnecrotic muscle fibers that aberrantly express class I MHC molecules. MHC-I expression, absent from the sarcolemma of normal muscle fibers, is probably induced by cytokines secreted by activated T cells and macrophages. The CD8/MHC-I complex is characteristic of PM and IBM; its detection can aid in confirming the histologic diagnosis of PM, as discussed below. The cytotoxic CD8 T cells contain perforin and granzyme gran-

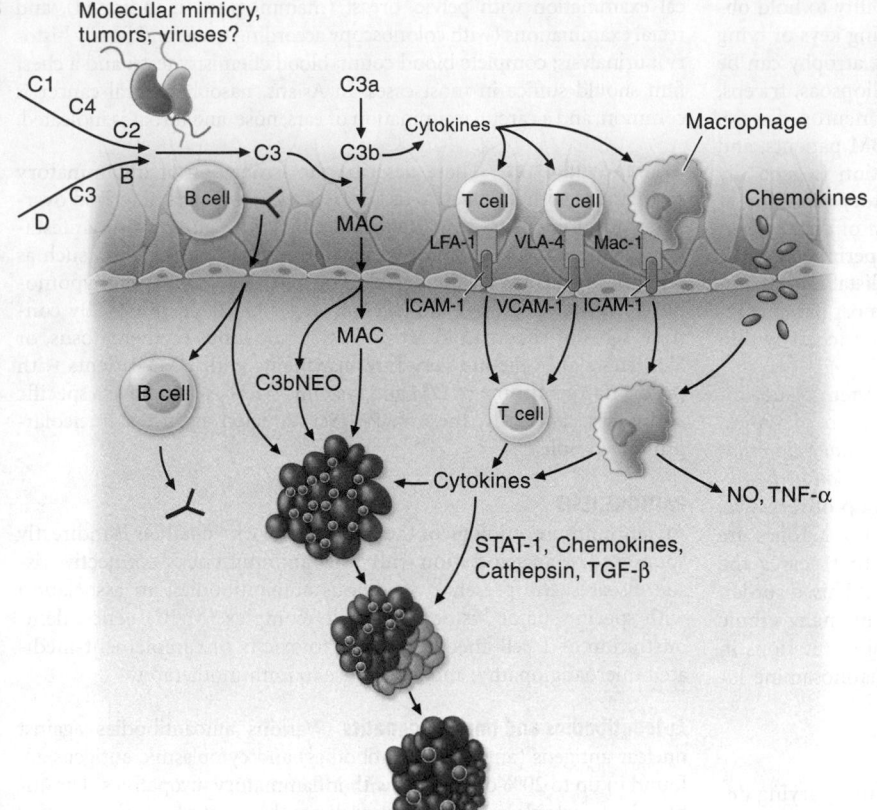

FIGURE 383-1 Immunopathogenesis of dermatomyositis. Activation of complement, possibly by autoantibodies (Y), against endothelial cells and formation of C3 via the classic or alternative pathway. Activated C3 leads to formation of C3b, C3bNEO, and membrane attack complexes (MAC), which are deposited in and around the endothelial cell wall of the endomysial capillaries. Deposition of MAC leads to destruction of capillaries, ischemia, or microinfarcts most prominent in the periphery of the fascicles, and perifascicular atrophy. B cells, CD4 T cells, and macrophages traffic from the circulation to the muscle. Endothelial expression of vascular cell adhesion molecule (VCAM) and intercellular adhesion molecule (ICAM) is induced by cytokines released by the mononuclear cells. Integrins, specifically very late activation antigen (VLA)-4 and leukocyte function-associated antigen (LFA)-1, bind VCAM and ICAM and promote T cell and macrophage infiltration of muscle through the endothelial cell wall.

ules directed towards the surface of the muscle fibers and capable of inducing myonecrosis. Analysis of T cell receptor molecules expressed by the infiltrating CD8 cells have revealed clonal expansion and conserved sequences in the antigen-binding region, both suggesting an antigen-driven T cell response. Whether the putative antigens are endogenous (e.g., muscle) or exogenous (e.g., viral) sequences is unknown. Viruses have not been identified within the muscle fibers. Co-stimulatory molecules and their counterreceptors, which are fundamental for T cell activation and antigen recognition, are strongly upregulated in PM and IBM. Key molecules involved in T cell–mediated cytotoxicity are depicted in Fig. 383-2.

The Role of Nonimmune Factors in IBM In IBM, the presence of β-amyloid deposits within vacuolated muscle fibers and abnormal mitochondria with cytochrome oxidase–negative fibers suggest that, in addition to the autoimmune component, there is also a degenerative process. Similar to Alzheimer's disease, the amyloid deposits in IBM are immunoreactive against amyloid precursor protein (APP), chymotrypsin, apolipoprotein E, and phosphorylated tau, but it is unclear whether these deposits are directly pathogenic or represent secondary phenomena. The same is true for the mitochondrial abnormalities, which may also be secondary to the effects of aging or a bystander effect of upregulated cytokines. Expression of cytokines and upregula-

tion of MHC class I by the muscle fibers may cause an endoplasmic reticulum stress response resulting in intracellular accumulation of misfolded glycoproteins and activation of nuclear factor κB (NFκB), leading to further cytokine activation.

Association with Viral Infections and the Role of Retroviruses Several viruses, including coxsackieviruses, influenza, paramyxoviruses, mumps, cytomegalovirus, and Epstein-Barr virus, have been indirectly associated with myositis. For the coxsackieviruses, an autoimmune myositis triggered by molecular mimicry has been proposed because of structural homology between histidyl-transfer RNA synthetase that is the target of the Jo-1 antibody (see above) and genomic RNA of an animal picornavirus, the encephalomyocarditis virus. Sensitive polymerase chain reaction (PCR) studies, however, have repeatedly failed to confirm the presence of such viruses in muscle biopsies.

The best evidence of a viral connection in PM and IBM is with the retroviruses. Some individuals infected with HIV or with human T cell lymphotropic virus I (HTLV-I) develop PM or IBM; a similar disorder has been described in nonhuman primates infected with the simian immunodeficiency virus. The inflammatory myopathy may occur as the initial manifestation of a retroviral infection, or myositis may develop later in the disease course. Retroviral antigens have been detected only in occasional endomysial macrophages and not within the muscle fibers themselves, suggesting that persistent infection and viral replication within the muscle do not occur. Histologic findings are identical to retroviral-negative PM or IBM. The infiltrating T cells in the muscle are clonally driven and a number of them are retroviral-specific. This disorder should be distinguished from a toxic myopathy related to long-term therapy with AZT, characterized by fatigue, myalgia, mild muscle weakness, and mild elevation of creatine kinase (CK). AZT-induced myopathy, which generally improves when the drug is discontinued, is a mitochondrial disorder characterized histologically by "ragged-red" fibers. AZT inhibits γ-DNA polymerase, an enzyme found solely in the mitochondrial matrix.

DIFFERENTIAL DIAGNOSIS
The clinical picture of the typical skin rash and proximal or diffuse muscle weakness has few causes other than DM. However, proximal muscle weakness without skin involvement can be due to many conditions other than PM or IBM.

Subacute or Chronic Progressive Muscle Weakness This may be due to denervating conditions such as the spinal muscular atrophies or amyotrophic lateral sclerosis (Chap. 369). In addition to the muscle weakness, upper motor neuron signs in the latter and signs of denervation detected by electromyography (EMG) aid in the diagnosis. The muscular dystrophies (Chap. 382) may be additional considerations; however, these disorders usually develop over years rather than weeks or months and rarely present after the age of 30. It may be difficult, even with a muscle biopsy, to distinguish chronic PM from a rapidly advancing muscular dystrophy. This is particularly true of facioscapulohumeral muscular dystrophy, dysferlin myopathy, and the dystrophinopathies where inflammatory cell infiltration is often found early in the disease. Such doubtful cases should always be given an adequate trial of glucocorticoid therapy and undergo genetic testing to exclude muscular dystrophy. Identification of the MHC/CD8 lesion by muscle biopsy is helpful to

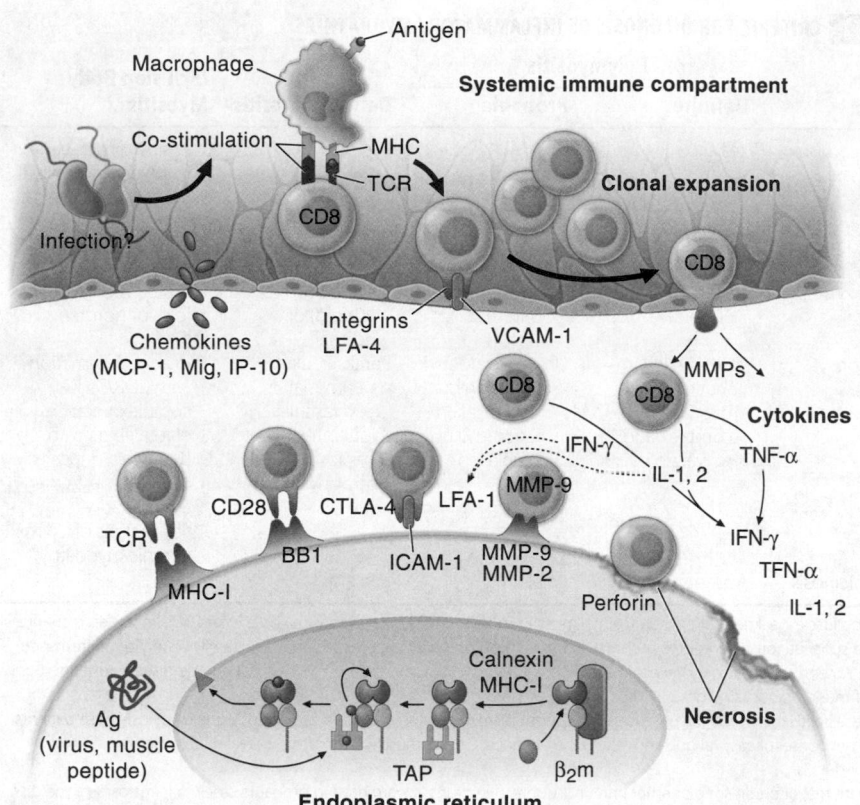

FIGURE 383-2 Cell-mediated mechanisms of muscle damage in polymyositis (PM) and inclusion body myositis (IBM). Antigen-specific CD8 cells are expanded in the periphery, cross the endothelial barrier, and bind directly to muscle fibers via T cell receptor (TCR) molecules that recognize aberrantly expressed MHC-I. Engagement of co-stimulatory molecules (BB1 and ICOSL) with their ligands (CD28, CTLA-4, and ICOS) along with ICAM-1/LFA-1, stabilize the CD8–muscle fiber interaction. Metalloproteinases (MMP) facilitate the migration of T cells and their attachment to the muscle surface. Muscle fiber necrosis occurs via perforin granules released by the autoaggressive T cells. A direct myocytotoxic effect exerted by the cytokines interferon (IFN) γ, interleukin (IL) 1, or tumor necrosis factor (TNF) α may also play a role. Death of the muscle fiber is mediated by necrosis. MHC class I molecules consist of a heavy chain and a light chain [β_2 microglobulin (β_2m)] complexed with an antigenic peptide that is transported into the endoplasmic reticulum by TAP proteins (Chap. 309).

identify cases of PM. Some metabolic myopathies, including glycogen storage disease due to myophosphorylase or acid maltase deficiency, lipid storage myopathies due to carnitine deficiency, and mitochondrial diseases produce weakness that is often associated with other characteristic clinical signs; diagnosis rests upon histochemical and biochemical studies of the muscle biopsy. The endocrine myopathies such as those due to hypercorticosteroidism, hyper- and hypothyroidism, and hyper- and hypoparathyroidism require the appropriate laboratory investigations for diagnosis. Muscle wasting in patients with an underlying neoplasm may be due to disuse, cachexia, or rarely to a paraneoplastic neuromyopathy (Chap. 97).

Diseases of the neuromuscular junction, including myasthenia gravis or the Lambert-Eaton myasthenic syndrome, cause fatiguing weakness that also affects ocular and other cranial muscles (Chap. 381). Repetitive nerve stimulation and single-fiber EMG studies aid in diagnosis.

Acute Muscle Weakness This may be caused by an acute neuropathy such as Guillain-Barré syndrome (Chap. 380), transverse myelitis (Chap. 372), a neurotoxin (Chap. 382), or a neurotropic viral infection such as poliomyelitis or West Nile virus (Chap. 376). When acute weakness is associated with painful muscle cramps, rhabdomyolysis, and myoglobinuria, it may be due to a viral infection or a metabolic disorder such as myophosphorylase deficiency or carnitine palmitoyl-

transferase deficiency (Chap. 382). Several animal parasites, including protozoa (*toxoplasma, trypanosoma*), cestodes (cysticerci), and nematodes (trichinae), may produce a focal or diffuse inflammatory myopathy known as *parasitic polymyositis. Staphylococcus aureus, Yersinia, Streptococcus*, or anaerobic bacteria may produce a suppurative myositis, known as *tropical polymyositis*, or *pyomyositis*. Pyomyositis, previously rare in the west, is now occasionally seen in AIDS patients. Other bacteria, such as *Borrelia burgdorferi* (Lyme disease) and *Legionella pneumophila* (Legionnaire's disease) may infrequently cause myositis.

Patients with periodic paralysis experience recurrent episodes of acute muscle weakness without pain, always beginning in childhood. Chronic alcoholics may develop painful myopathy with myoglobinuria after a bout of heavy drinking. Acute painless muscle weakness with myoglobinuria may occur with prolonged hypokalemia, or hypophosphatemia and hypomagnesemia, usually in chronic alcoholics or in patients on nasogastric suction receiving parenteral hyperalimentation.

Myofasciitis This distinctive inflammatory disorder affecting muscle and fascia presents as diffuse myalgias, skin induration, fatigue, and mild muscle weakness; mild elevations of serum CK are usually present. The most common form is eosinophilic myofasciitis characterized by peripheral blood eosinophilia and eosinophilic infiltrates in the endomysial tissue. In some patients, the eosinophilic myositis/fasciitis occurs in the context of parasitic infections, vasculitis, mixed connective tissue disease, hypereosinophilic syndrome, or toxic exposures (e.g., toxic oil syndrome, contaminated L-tryptophan) or with mutations in the calpain gene. A distinct subset of myofasciitis is characterized by pronounced infiltration of the connective tissue around the muscle by sheets of periodic acid–Schiff-positive macrophages and occasional CD8 T cells (macrophagic myofasciitis). Such histologic involvement is focal and limited to sites of previous vaccinations, which may have been administered months or years earlier. This disorder, which to date has not been observed outside of France, has been linked to an aluminum-containing substrate in vaccines. Most patients respond to glucocorticoid therapy, and the overall prognosis seems favorable.

Necrotizing Myositis This is an increasingly recognized entity that has distinct features, even though it is often labeled as PM. It presents often in the fall or winter as an acute or subacute onset of symmetric muscle weakness; CK is typically extremely high. The weakness can be severe. Coexisting interstitial lung disease and cardiomyopathy may be present. The disorder may develop after a viral infection or in association with cancer. Some patients have antibodies against signal recognition particle (SRP). The muscle biopsy demonstrates necrotic fibers infiltrated by macrophages but only rare, if any, T cell infiltrates. Muscle MHC-I expression is only slightly and focally upregulated. The capillaries may be swollen with hyalinization, thickening of the capillary wall, and deposition of complement. Some patients respond to immunotherapy, but others are resistant.

Drug-Induced Myopathies D-Penicillamine and procainamide may produce a true myositis resembling PM, and a DM-like illness had been associated with the contaminated preparations of L-tryptophan. As noted above, AZT causes a mitochondrial myopathy. Other drugs may elicit a toxic noninflammatory myopathy that is histologically different from

DM, PM, or IBM. These include cholesterol-lowering agents such as clofibrate, lovastatin, simvastatin, or provastatin, especially when combined with cyclosporine or gemfibrozil. Rhabdomyolysis and myoglobinuria have been rarely associated with amphotericin B, ε-aminocaproic acid, fenfluramine, heroin, and phencyclidine. The use of amiodarone, chloroquine, colchicine, carbimazole, emetine, etretinate, ipecac syrup, chronic laxative or licorice use resulting in hypokalemia, and glucocorticoids or growth hormone administration have also been associated with myopathic muscle weakness. Some neuromuscular blocking agents such as pancuronium, in combination with glucocorticoids, may cause an acute critical illness myopathy. A careful drug history is essential for diagnosis of these drug-induced myopathies, which do not require immunosuppressive therapy.

"Weakness" Due to Muscle Pain and Muscle Tenderness

A number of conditions including *polymyalgia rheumatica* (Chap. 319) and arthritic disorders of adjacent joints may enter into the differential diagnosis of inflammatory myopathy, even though they do not cause myositis. The muscle biopsy is either normal or discloses type II muscle fiber atrophy. Patients with *fibrositis* and *fibromyalgia* (Chap. 329) complain of focal or diffuse muscle tenderness, fatigue, and aching, which is sometimes poorly differentiated from joint pain. Some patients, however, have muscle tenderness, painful muscles on movement, and signs suggestive of a collagen vascular disorder, such as an increased erythrocyte sedimentation rate, C-reactive protein, antinuclear antibody, or rheumatoid factor, along with modest elevation of the serum CK and aldolase. They demonstrate a "give-way" pattern of weakness with difficulty sustaining effort but not true muscle weakness. The muscle biopsy is usually normal or nonspecific. Many such patients show some response to nonsteroidal anti-inflammatory agents or glucocorticoids, though most continue to have indolent complaints. An indolent fasciitis in the setting of an ill-defined connective tissue disorder may be present, and these patients should not be labeled as having a psychosomatic disorder. *Chronic fatigue syndrome*, which may follow a viral infection, can present with debilitating fatigue, fever, sore throat, painful lymphadenopathy, myalgia, arthralgia, sleep disorder, and headache (Chap. 384). These patients do not have muscle weakness, and the muscle biopsy is normal.

DIAGNOSIS

The clinically suspected diagnosis of PM, DM, or IBM is confirmed by examining the serum muscle enzymes, EMG findings, and muscle biopsy (Table 383-2).

The most sensitive enzyme is CK, which in active disease can be elevated as much as 50-fold. Although the CK level usually parallels disease activity, it can be normal in some patients with active IBM or DM, especially when associated with a connective tissue disease. The CK is always elevated in patients with active PM. Along with the CK, the serum glutamic-oxaloacetic and glutamate pyruvate transaminases, lactate dehydrogenase, and aldolase may be elevated.

Needle EMG shows myopathic potentials characterized by short-duration, low-amplitude polyphasic units on voluntary activation and increased spontaneous activity with fibrillations, complex repetitive discharges, and positive sharp waves. Mixed potentials (polyphasic units

of short and long duration) indicating a chronic process and muscle fiber regeneration are often present in IBM. These EMG findings are not diagnostic of an inflammatory myopathy but are useful to identify the presence of active or chronic myopathy and to exclude neurogenic disorders.

MRI is not routinely used for the diagnosis of PM, DM, or IBM. However, it may guide the location of the muscle biopsy in certain clinical settings.

Muscle biopsy is the definitive test for establishing the diagnosis of inflammatory myopathy and for excluding other neuromuscular diseases. Inflammation is the histologic hallmark for these diseases; however, additional features are characteristic of each subtype (Figs. 383-3, 383-4, and 383-5).

In PM the inflammation is *primary*, a term used to indicate that T cell infiltrates, located primarily within the muscle fascicles (endomysially), surround individual, healthy muscle fibers and result in phagocytosis and necrosis (Fig. 383-3). The MHC-I molecule is ubiquitously expressed on the sarcolemma, even in fibers not invaded by CD8+ cells. The CD8/MHC-I lesion is now fundamental for confirming or establishing the diagnosis and to exclude disorders with secondary, nonspecific, inflammation. When the disease is chronic, connective tissue is increased and may react positively with alkaline phosphatase.

In DM the endomysial inflammation is predominantly perivascular or in the interfascicular septae and around, rather than within, the muscle fascicles (Fig. 383-4). The intramuscular blood vessels show endothelial hyperplasia with tuboluloreticular profiles, fibrin thrombi, and obliteration of capillaries. The muscle fibers undergo necrosis, degeneration, and phagocytosis, often in groups involving a portion of a muscle fasciculus in a wedgelike shape or at the periphery of the fascicle, due to microinfarcts within the muscle. This results in perifascicular atrophy, characterized by 2–10 layers of atrophic fibers at the periphery of the fascicles. The presence of perifascicular atrophy is diagnostic of DM, *even in the absence of inflammation*.

TABLE 383-2 CRITERIA FOR DIAGNOSIS OF INFLAMMATORY MYOPATHIES

Criterion	Polymyositis Definite	Polymyositis Probable	Dermatomyositis	Inclusion Body Myositis
Myopathic muscle weakness[a]	Yes	Yes	Yes[b]	Yes; slow onset, early involvement of distal muscles, frequent falls
Electromyographic findings	Myopathic	Myopathic	Myopathic	Myopathic with mixed potentials
Muscle enzymes	Elevated (up to 50-fold)	Elevated (up to 50-fold)	Elevated (up to 50-fold) or normal	Elevated (up to 10-fold) or normal
Muscle biopsy findings[c]	"Primary" inflammation with the CD8/MHC-I complex and no vacuoles	Ubiquitous MCH-I expression but minimal inflammation and no vacuoles[d]	Perifascicular, perimysial, or perivascular infiltrates, perifascicular atrophy	Primary inflammation with CD8/MHC-I complex; vacuolated fibers with β-amyloid deposits; cytochrome oxygenase–negative fibers; signs of chronic myopathy[e]
Rash or calcinosis	Absent	Absent	Present[f]	Absent

[a]Myopathic muscle weakness, affecting proximal muscles more than distal ones and sparing eye and facial muscles, is characterized by a subacute onset (weeks to months) and rapid progression in patients who have no family history of neuromuscular disease, no endocrinopathy, no exposure to myotoxic drugs or toxins, and no biochemical muscle disease (excluded on the basis of muscle-biopsy findings).

[b]In some cases with the typical rash, the muscle strength is seemingly normal (dermatomyositis sine myositis); these patients often have new onset of easy fatigue and reduced endurance. Careful muscle testing may reveal mild muscle weakness.

[c]See text for details.

[d]An adequate trial of prednisone or other immunosuppressive drugs is warranted in probable cases. If, in retrospect, the disease is unresponsive to therapy, another muscle biopsy should be considered to exclude other diseases or possible evolution in inclusion body myositis.

[e]If the muscle biopsy does not contain vacuolated fibers but shows chronic myopathy with hypertrophic fibers, primary inflammation with the CD8/MHC-I complex and cytochrome oxygenase–negative fibers, the diagnosis is probable inclusion body myositis.

[f]If rash is absent but muscle biopsy findings are characteristic of dermatomyositis, the diagnosis is probable DM.

FIGURE 383-3 Cross section of a muscle biopsy from a patient with polymyositis demonstrates scattered inflammatory foci with lymphocytes invading or surrounding muscle fibers. Note lack of chronic myopathic features (increased connective tissue, atrophic or hypertrophic fibers) as seen in inclusion body myositis.

In IBM (Fig. 383-5), there is endomysial inflammation with T cells invading MHC-I-expressing nonvacuolated muscle fibers; basophilic granular deposits distributed around the edge of slitlike vacuoles (rimmed vacuoles); loss of fibers, replaced by fat and connective tissue, hypertrophic fibers, and angulated or round fibers; eosinophilic cytoplasmic inclusions; abnormal mitochondria characterized by the presence of ragged-red fibers or cytochrome oxidase–negative fibers; amyloid deposits within or next to the vacuoles; and filamentous inclusions seen by electron microscopy in the vicinity of the rimmed vacuoles.

℞ INFLAMMATORY MYOPATHIES

The goal of therapy is to improve muscle strength, thereby improving function in activities of daily living, and ameliorate the extramuscular manifestations (rash, dysphagia, dyspnea, fever). When strength improves, the serum CK falls concurrently; however, the reverse is not always true. Unfortunately, there is a common tendency to "chase" or treat the CK level instead of the muscle weakness, a practice that has led to prolonged and unnecessary use of immunosuppressive drugs and erroneous assessment of their efficacy. It is prudent to discontinue these drugs if, after an adequate trial, there is no objective improvement in muscle strength whether or not CK levels are reduced. Agents used in the treatment of PM and DM include:

1. *Glucocorticoids*. Oral prednisone is the initial treatment of choice; the effectiveness and side effects of this therapy determine the future need for stronger immunosuppressive drugs. High-dose prednisone, at least 1 mg/kg per day, is initiated as early in the disease as possible. After 3–4 weeks, prednisone is tapered slowly over a period of 10 weeks to 1 mg/kg every other day. If there is evidence of efficacy and no serious side effects, the dosage is then further reduced by 5 or 10 mg every 3–4 weeks until the lowest possible dose that controls the disease is reached. The efficacy of prednisone is determined by an objective increase in muscle strength and activities of daily living, which almost always occurs by the third month of therapy. A feeling of increased energy or a reduction of the CK level without a concomitant increase in muscle strength is not a reliable sign of improvement. If prednisone provides no objective benefit after ~3 months of high-dose therapy, the disease is probably unresponsive to the drug and tapering should be accelerated while the next-in-line immunosuppressive drug is started. Although controlled trials have not been performed, almost all patients with true PM or DM respond to glucocorticoids to *some degree and for some period of time*; in general, DM responds better than PM.

   The long-term use of prednisone may cause increased weakness associated with a normal or unchanged CK level; this effect is referred to as *steroid myopathy*. In a patient who previously responded to high doses of prednisone, the development of new weakness may be related to

steroid myopathy or to disease activity that either will respond to a higher dose of glucocorticoids or has become glucocorticoid-resistant. In uncertain cases, the prednisone dosage can be steadily increased or decreased as desired: the cause of the weakness is usually evident in 2–8 weeks.

2. *Other immunosuppressive* drugs. Approximately 75% of patients ultimately require additional treatment. This occurs when a patient fails to respond adequately to glucocorticoids after a 3-month trial, the patient becomes glucocorticoid-resistant, glucocorticoid-related side effects appear, attempts to lower the prednisone dose repeatedly result in a new relapse, or rapidly progressive disease with evolving severe weakness and respiratory failure develops.

   The following drugs are commonly used but have never been tested in controlled studies: (1) *Azathioprine* is well tolerated, has few side effects, and appears to be as effective for long-term therapy as other drugs. The dose is up to 3 mg/kg daily. (2) *Methotrexate* has a faster onset of action than azathioprine. It is given orally starting at 7.5 mg weekly for the first 3 weeks (2.5 mg every 12 h for 3 doses), with gradual dose escalation by 2.5 mg per week to a total of 25 mg weekly. A rare side effect is methotrexate pneumonitis, which can be difficult to distinguish from the interstitial lung disease of the primary myopathy associated with Jo-1 antibodies (described above). (3) *Mycophenolate mofetil* also has a faster onset of action than azathioprine. At doses up to 2.5 mg/d, it is well tolerated and appears promising for long-term use. (4) Monoclonal anti-CD20 (rituximab) has been shown in a small uncontrolled series to benefit patients with DM. (5) *Cyclosporine* has inconsistent and mild benefit. (6) *Cyclophosphamide* (0.5–1 g IV monthly for 6 months) has limited success and significant toxicity. (7) Tacrolimus (formerly known as Fk506) has been effective in some difficult cases of PM.

3. *Immunomodulation*. In a controlled trial of patients with refractory DM, intravenous immunoglobulin (IVIg) improved not only strength and rash but also the underlying immunopathology. The benefit is often short-lived (≤8 weeks); repeated infusions every 6–8 weeks are generally required to maintain improvement. A dose of 2 g/kg divided over 2–5 days per course is recommended. Uncontrolled observations suggest that IVIg may also be beneficial for patients with PM. Neither plasmapheresis nor leukapheresis appears to be effective in PM and DM.

The following sequential empirical approach to the treatment of PM and DM is suggested: *Step 1*: high-dose prednisone; *Step 2*: azathioprine, mycophenolate, or methotrexate for steroid-sparing effect; *Step 3*: IVIg; *Step 4*: a trial, with guarded optimism, of one of the following agents, chosen according to the patient's age, degree of disability, tolerance, experience with the drug, and general health: rituximab, cyclosporine, cyclophosphamide, or tacrolimus. Patients with interstitial lung disease may benefit from aggressive treatment with cyclophosphamide or tacrolimus.

A patient with presumed PM who has not responded to any form of immunotherapy most likely has IBM or another disease, usually a metabolic myopathy, a muscular dystrophy, a drug-induced myopathy, or an endo-

FIGURE 383-4 Cross section of a muscle biopsy from a patient with dermatomyositis demonstrates atrophy of the fibers at the periphery of the fascicle (perifascicular atrophy).

FIGURE 383-5 Cross sections of a muscle biopsy from a patient with inclusion body myositis demonstrate the typical features of vacuoles with lymphocytic infiltrates surrounding nonvacuolated or necrotic fibers (**A**), tiny endomysial deposits of amyloid visualized with crystal violet (**B**), cytochrome oxidase-negative fibers, indicative of mitochondrial dysfunction (**C**), and ubiquitous MHC-I expression at the periphery of all fibers (**D**).

crinopathy. In these cases, a repeat muscle biopsy and a renewed search for another cause of the myopathyis indicated.

Calcinosis, a manifestation of DM, is difficult to treat; however, new calcium deposits may be prevented if the primary disease responds to the available therapies. Bisphosphonates, aluminum hydroxide, probenecid, colchicine, low doses of warfarin, calcium blockers, and surgical excision have all been tried without success.

IBM is generally resistant to immunosuppressive therapies. Prednisone together with azathioprine or methotrexate is often tried for a few months in newly diagnosed patients, although results are generally disappointing. Because occasional patients may feel subjectively weaker after these drugs are discontinued, some clinicians prefer to maintain some patients on low-dose, every-other-day prednisone or weekly methotrexate in an effort to slow disease progression, even though there is no objective evidence or controlled study to support this practice. In two controlled studies of IVIg in IBM, minimal benefit in up to 30% of patients was found; the strength gains, however, were not of sufficient magnitude to justify its routine use. Another trial of IVIg combined with prednisone was ineffective. Nonetheless, many experts believe that a 2- to 3-month trial with IVIg may be reasonable for selected patients with IBM who experience rapid progression of muscle weakness or choking episodes due to worsening dysphagia.

PROGNOSIS

The 5-year survival rate for treated patients with PM and DM is ~95% and the 10-year survival 84%; death is usually due to pulmo-nary, cardiac, or other systemic complications. Patients severely affected at presentation or treated after long delays, those with severe dysphagia or respiratory difficulties, older patients, and those with associated cancer have a worse prognosis. DM responds more favorably to therapy than PM and thus has a better prognosis. Most patients improve with therapy, and many make a full functional recovery, which is often sustained with maintenance therapy. Up to 30% may be left with some residual muscle weakness. Relapses may occur at any time.

IBM has the least favorable prognosis of the inflammatory myopathies. Most patients will require the use of an assistive device such as a cane, walker, or wheelchair within 5–10 years of onset. In general, the older the age of onset in IBM, the more rapidly progressive is the course.

FURTHER READINGS

ASKANAS V et al: Inclusion-body myositis: Clinical and pathologic aspects, and basic research potentially relevant to treatment. Neurology 24:66(Suppl 1), 2006

DALAKAS MC: Signaling pathways and immunobiology of inflammatory myopathies. Nat Clin Pract Rheumatol 2:219, 2006

——— et al: Inclusion body myositis with human immunodeficiency virus infection: Four cases with clonal expansion of viral-specific T cells. Ann Neurol 61:466, 2007

———: Sporadic inclusion body myositis: Diagnosis, pathogenesis and therapeutic strategies. Nat Clin Pract Neurol 2:437, 2006

———, HOHLFELD R: Polymyositis and dermatomyositis. Lancet 362:971, 2003

ENGEL AG, HOHLFELD R: The polymyositis and dermatomyositis syndromes, in *Myology*, 3d ed, AG Engel, C Franzini-Armstrong (eds). New York, McGraw-Hill, 2004, pp 1321–1366

HILTON-JONES D: Inflammatory myopathies. Curr Opin Neurol 14:591, 2001

MARIE I et al: Polymyositis and dermatomyositis: Short term and long term outcome and predictive factors of prognosis. J Rheumatol 28:2230, 2001

MASTAGLIA FL: Inflammatory myopathies: Clinical, diagnostic and therapeutic aspects. Muscle Nerve 27:407, 2003

MIKOL J, ENGEL AG: Inclusion body myositis, in: *Myology*, 3d ed, AG Engel, C Franzini-Armstrong (eds). New York, McGraw-Hill, 2004, pp 1367–1388

SONTHEIMER RD: Dermatomyositis: An overview of recent progress with emphasis on dermatologic aspects. Dermatol Clin 20:387, 2002

SECTION 4 CHRONIC FATIGUE SYNDROME

384 Chronic Fatigue Syndrome
Stephen E. Straus†

DEFINITION

Chronic fatigue syndrome (CFS) is the current name for a disorder characterized by debilitating fatigue and several associated physical, constitutional, and neuropsychological complaints (Table 384-1). This syndrome is not new; in the past, patients diagnosed with conditions such as the vapors, neurasthenia, effort syndrome, chronic brucellosis, epidemic neuromyasthenia, myalgic encephalomyelitis, hypoglycemia, multiple chemical sensitivity syndrome, chronic candidiasis, chronic mononucleosis, chronic Epstein-Barr virus (EBV) infection, and postviral fatigue syndrome may have had what is now called CFS. A subset of ill veterans of military campaigns suffer from CFS. The U.S. Centers for Disease Control and Prevention (CDC) has developed diagnostic criteria for CFS based upon symptoms and the exclusion of other illnesses (Table 384-2).

EPIDEMIOLOGY

Patients with CFS are twice as likely to be women as men and are generally 25–45 years old, although cases in childhood and in later life have been described.

Cases are recognized in many developed countries. Most arise sporadically, but many clusters have also been reported. Famous outbreaks of CFS occurred in Los Angeles County Hospital in 1934; in Akureyri, Iceland, in 1948; in the Royal Free Hospital, London, in 1955; and in Incline Village, Nevada, in 1985. While these clustered cases suggest a common environmental or infectious cause, none has been identified.

Estimates of the prevalence of CFS have depended on the case definition used and the method of study. Chronic fatigue itself is a common symptom, occurring in as many as 20% of patients attending general medical clinics; CFS is far less common. Community-based studies find that 100–300 individuals per 100,000 population in the United States meet the current CDC case definition.

PATHOGENESIS

The diverse names for the syndrome reflect the many and controversial hypotheses about its etiology. Several common themes underlie attempts to understand the disorder: (1) it is often postinfectious; (2) it is associated with mild immunologic disturbances and sedentary behavior during childhood; and (3) it is commonly accompanied by neuropsychological complaints, somatic preoccupation, and/or depression.

Many studies over the past quarter century sought to link CFS to acute and/or persisting infections with EBV, cytomegalovirus, human herpesvirus type 6, retroviruses, enteroviruses, *Candida albicans*, *Mycoplasma* spp., or *Coxiella burnetii*, among other microbial pathogens.

TABLE 384-1 SPECIFIC SYMPTOMS REPORTED BY PATIENTS WITH CHRONIC FATIGUE SYNDROME

Symptom	Percentage
Fatigue	100
Difficulty concentrating	90
Headache	90
Sore throat	85
Tender lymph nodes	80
Muscle aches	80
Joint aches	75
Feverishness	75
Difficulty sleeping	70
Psychiatric problems	65
Allergies	55
Abdominal cramps	40
Weight loss	20
Rash	10
Rapid pulse	10
Weight gain	5
Chest pain	5
Night sweats	5

Source: From SE Straus: J Infect Diseases 157:405, 1988; with permission.

Compared to findings in age-matched control subjects, the titers of antibodies to some microorganisms are elevated in CFS patients. Reports that viral antigens and nucleic acids could be specifically identified in patients with CFS, however, have not been confirmed. One study from the United Kingdom failed to detect any association between acute infections and subsequent prolonged fatigue. Another study found that chronic fatigue did not develop after typical upper

TABLE 384-2 CDC CRITERIA FOR DIAGNOSIS OF CHRONIC FATIGUE SYNDROME

A case of chronic fatigue syndrome is defined by the presence of:
1. Clinically evaluated, unexplained, persistent or relapsing fatigue that is of new or definite onset; is not the result of ongoing exertion; is not alleviated by rest; and results in substantial reduction of previous levels of occupational, educational, social, or personal activities; and
2. Four or more of the following symptoms that persist or recur during six or more consecutive months of illness and that do not predate the fatigue:
   - Self-reported impairment in short-term memory or concentration
   - Sore throat
   - Tender cervical or axillary nodes
   - Muscle pain
   - Multijoint pain without redness or swelling
   - Headaches of a new pattern or severity
   - Unrefreshing sleep
   - Postexertional malaise lasting ≥24 h

Note: CDC, U.S. Centers for Disease Control and Prevention.
Source: Adapted from K Fukuda et al: Ann Intern Med 121:953, 1994; with permission.

†Deceased.

respiratory infections but did in some individuals after infectious mononucleosis. Thus, while antecedent infections are associated with CFS, a direct microbial causality is unproven and unlikely.

Changes in numerous immune parameters of uncertain functional significance have been reported in CFS. Modest elevations in titers of antinuclear antibodies, reductions in immunoglobulin subclasses, deficiencies in mitogen-driven lymphocyte proliferation, reductions in natural killer cell activity, disturbances in cytokine production, and shifts in lymphocyte subsets have been described. None of these immune findings appears in most patients, nor do any correlate with the severity of CFS. Comparison of monozygotic twin pairs discordant for CFS showed no substantive immunologic differences between affected and unaffected individuals. In theory, symptoms of CFS could result from excessive production of a cytokine, such as interleukin 1, that induces asthenia and other flulike symptoms; however, compelling data in support of this hypothesis are lacking. A recently published population-based study from Wichita, Kansas, reported differences in gene expression patterns and in candidate gene polymorphisms between CFS patients and controls; these results are controversial and await confirmation.

In some but not the more recent studies, patients with CFS commonly manifested sensitivity to sustained upright posture or tilting, resulting in hypotension and syncope, so as to suggest a form of dysautonomia.

Disturbances in hypothalamic-pituitary-adrenal function have been identified in several controlled studies of CFS, with some evidence for normalization in patients whose fatigue abates. These neuroendocrine abnormalities could contribute to the impaired energy and depressed mood of patients.

Mild to moderate depression is present in half to two-thirds of patients. Much of this depression may be reactive, but its prevalence exceeds that seen in other chronic medical illnesses. Some propose that CFS is fundamentally a psychiatric disorder and that the various neuroendocrine and immune disturbances arise secondarily.

MANIFESTATIONS

Typically, CFS arises suddenly in a previously active individual. An otherwise unremarkable flulike illness or some other acute stress leaves unbearable exhaustion in its wake. Other symptoms, such as headache, sore throat, tender lymph nodes, muscle and joint aches, and frequent feverishness, lead to the belief that an infection persists, and medical attention is sought. Over weeks to months, despite reassurances that "nothing serious is wrong," the symptoms persist and other features of the syndrome become evident—disturbed sleep, difficulty in concentration, and depression (Table 384-1).

Depending on the dominant symptoms and the beliefs of the patient, additional consultations may be sought from allergists, rheumatologists, infectious disease specialists, psychiatrists, ecologic therapists, homeopaths, or other professionals, frequently with unsatisfactory results. Once the pattern of illness is established, the symptoms may fluctuate somewhat. Many patients report that CFS symptoms, including cognitive problems, are exacerbated by intensive physical or other stressors, yet recent prospective studies have not confirmed this impression.

Most patients remain capable of meeting family, work, or community obligations despite their symptoms; discretionary activities are abandoned first. Some feel unable to engage in any gainful employment. A minority of individuals requires help with the activities of daily living. Econometric analyses conducted by the CDC have confirmed that CFS exacts a significant toll on household and workforce productivity.

Ultimately, isolation, frustration, and pathetic resignation can mark the protracted course of illness. Patients may become angry at physicians for failing to acknowledge or resolve their plight. Fortunately, CFS does not appear to progress. On the contrary, many patients experience gradual improvement, and a minority recover fully.

DIAGNOSIS

A thorough history, physical examination, and judicious use of laboratory tests are required to exclude other causes of the patient's symptoms.

Prominent abnormalities argue strongly in favor of alternative diagnoses. No laboratory test, however, can diagnose this condition or measure its severity. In most cases, elaborate, expensive workups are not helpful. Early claims that MRI or single photon emission CT can identify abnormalities in the brain of CFS patients have not withstood further study. The dilemma for patient and clinician alike is that CFS has no pathognomonic features and remains a constellation of symptoms and a diagnosis of exclusion. Often the patient presents with features that also meet criteria for other subjective disorders such as fibromyalgia and irritable bowel syndrome. Questions have been raised as to the relative merits of rendering a diagnosis of CFS. Being diagnosed can provide validation of a patient's perceived symptoms but may also perpetuate or exacerbate them. Refusal to label a patient as having CFS, however, can deny the patient the opportunity to undertake treatments that are of proven merit.

℞ CHRONIC FATIGUE SYNDROME

After other illnesses have been excluded, there are several points to address in the long-term care of a patient with chronic fatigue.

The patient should be educated about the illness and what is known of its pathogenesis; potential impact on the physical, psychological, and social dimensions of life; and prognosis. Periodic reassessment is appropriate to identify a possible underlying process that is late in declaring itself and to address intercurrent symptoms that should not be simply dismissed as additional subjective complaints.

Many symptoms of CFS respond to treatment. Nonsteroidal anti-inflammatory drugs alleviate headache, diffuse pain, and feverishness. Allergic rhinitis and sinusitis are common; when present, antihistamines or decongestants may be helpful. Although the patient may be averse to psychiatric diagnoses, depression and anxiety are often prominent and should be treated. Expert psychiatric assessment is sometimes advisable. Nonsedating antidepressants improve mood and disordered sleep and may attenuate the fatigue. Even modest improvements in symptoms can make an important difference in the patient's degree of self-sufficiency and ability to appreciate life's pleasures.

Practical advice should be given regarding life-style. Sleep disturbances are common; consumption of heavy meals, alcohol, and caffeine at night can make sleep even more elusive, compounding fatigue. Total rest leads to further deconditioning and the self-image of being an invalid, whereas overexertion may worsen exhaustion and lead to total avoidance of exercise. A carefully graded exercise regimen should be encouraged and has been proven to relieve symptoms and enhance exercise tolerance.

Controlled therapeutic trials have established that acyclovir, fludrocortisone, galantamine, modafinil, and IV immunoglobulin, among other agents, offer no significant benefit in CFS. Low doses of hydrocortisone provide modest benefit but may lead to adrenal suppression. Countless anecdotes circulate regarding other traditional and nontraditional therapies. It is important to guide patients away from those therapeutic modalities that are toxic, expensive, or unreasonable.

The physician should promote the patient's efforts to recover. Several controlled trials conducted in the United Kingdom, in Australia, and in the Netherlands showed cognitive-behavioral therapy to be helpful in adolescents and adults with CFS. This approach aims to dispel misguided beliefs and fears about CFS that can contribute to inactivity and despair. For CFS, as for many other conditions, a comprehensive approach to physical, psychological, and social aspects of well-being is in order.

FURTHER READINGS

BAKER R, SHAW EJ: Diagnosis and management of chronic fatigue syndrome or myalgic encephalitis (or encephalopathy): Summary of NICE guidance. BMJ 335:446, 2007

PRINS JB et al: Chronic fatigue syndrome. Lancet 367:346, 2006

VERNON SD, REEVES WC: The challenge of integrating high-content data: Epidemiological, clinical and laboratory data collected during an in-hospital study of chronic fatigue syndrome. Pharmacogenomics 7:341, 2006

385 Biology of Psychiatric Disorders
Steven E. Hyman, Eric Kandel

Psychiatric disorders are a diverse group of brain disorders with symptoms that primarily involve emotion, higher cognitive function, and the ability to control complex behaviors. A compendium of psychiatric disorders can be found in the *Diagnostic and Statistical Manual of Mental Disorders* of the American Psychiatric Association 4th edition (DSM-IV). This compendium illustrates that the boundary between psychiatric and neurologic disorders, another heterogeneous group of brain disorders, is arbitrary and shifting. In areas of overlap such as autism, Tourette's disorder, and Alzheimer's disease, the disorder is often treated by either a psychiatrist or a neurologist. The term *mental disorders*, while still widely used, fails to acknowledge the neural substrates of these disturbances and their effects on physiology and behavior.

The major psychiatric disorders are common and often run a chronic course. The chronic disorders include anxiety disorders, attention deficit hyperactivity disorder, autism, obsessive-compulsive disorder, and schizophrenia. Other psychiatric disorders such as depressive disorders recur across the life span, but even bipolar disorder, classically characterized as episodic, can run a chronic course.

The symptoms of psychiatric disorders often begin early, impairing the ability of children and adolescents to learn and compromising the functioning of adults at work and in other life roles. As a result of their high prevalence, early onset, and persistence, psychiatric disorders contribute substantially to the burden of illness in all countries in which they have been studied. In the United States they are not only a leading cause of disability but also a significant cause of premature death, because mood disorders, schizophrenia, and to some extent other psychiatric disorders constitute the most potent risk factors for suicide, a leading cause of death worldwide.

ANATOMY

Progress in understanding the pathophysiology of psychiatric disorders has been slow, despite its fundamental importance. Perhaps the most significant challenge is posed by the difficulties inherent in understanding the high-level cognitive and affective functions of the brain that are disrupted in psychiatric disorders. As a result, unlike many neurologic disorders, the common psychiatric disorders appear to involve widely distributed neural networks and lack an obvious, localized neuropathology, which, if present, would help to narrow the hunt for cellular pathology and for underlying biochemical and molecular causes. Thus, the motor disturbances in Parkinson's disease, Huntington's disease, and amyotrophic lateral sclerosis result from discrete macroscopic lesions in different parts of the motor system. By contrast, in psychiatric disorders, when candidate regions have been identified, as in schizophrenia, depression, and autism, it has proven difficult to differentiate convincingly, these abnormalities from normal variation partly because these target regions form only one component of a disorder involving a much larger neural circuit (Chap. 27).

GENETIC CONSIDERATIONS Given the challenges of identifying relatively subtle neuropathology, it has long been hoped that the identification of genetic variants conferring risk for psychiatric disorders would provide effective clues to those underlying neural abnormalities that contribute to the psychiatric disorder in question. This hope is based on the significant body of data derived from family, twin, and adoption studies demonstrating that heredity plays a significant role in the risk of major psychiatric disorders, including schizophrenia, bipolar disorder, depressive disorders, and many others. For example, the rate of schizophrenia in the general population is ~1%. However, when one member of a monozygotic twin pair is diagnosed with schizophrenia, the other twin, who is genetically identical, has nearly a 50% chance of also manifesting the disease. A first-degree relative of an affected proband (who shares on average 50% of DNA sequences) has a 9% risk of schizophrenia. Adoption-at-birth studies provide additional strong support for a genetic contribution to schizophrenia spectrum disorders; in one study from Finland, a schizophrenia-related illness was present in nearly one-quarter of adoptees whose biologic mother carried a similar diagnosis.

While there continue to be promising leads in the search for risk-conferring alleles, research over the past two decades has not succeeded in identifying with certainty risk genes for psychiatric disorders. There have been large efforts using a variety of strategies, including linkage studies and candidate gene studies, in attempts to identify genes responsible for schizophrenia, and more recently several groups have begun to undertake whole-genome association studies. The strongest candidates include: disrupted in schizophrenia (*DISC1*), a gene that was disrupted by a balanced chromosomal translocation in a Scottish family with schizophrenia-like symptoms; distrobrevin-binding protein 1 (*DTNBP1*); and neuroregulin 1 (*NRG1*), which encodes a protein involved in neuronal migration and in expression of *N*-methyl-*D*-aspartate (NMDA) glutamate receptors. Other potential candidates include *DAOA*, *RGS4*, and *AKT1*, but the evidence supporting them is weaker **(Table 385-1)**.

One problem in identifying risk genes for psychiatric diseases has been the failure to replicate convincingly the discovery of putative risk genes. The failure stems in large part from the complex nature of risk for psychiatric disorders, which appears to involve multiple genes of small effect interacting with nongenetic factors. In addition, there appear to be different risk genes in different population groups, perhaps reflecting new or recent mutations.

It is now relatively straightforward to identify genes that exert large causal effects on disease. Several less common neurologic disorders result from deleterious mutations within single genes. Thus, genes have been identified that contribute to the muscular dystrophies, triplet repeat disorders such as Huntington's disease and fragile X, and Down's syndrome. The discovery of the Huntington gene was followed by the development of powerful tools to investigate the neural basis of the disease by putting the mutated gene into worms, flies, or mice in order to study the mechanisms of pathogenesis. While such tools are only a beginning, and indeed have not yet led to development of therapies, gene identification and the study of its function have already created a strong platform for investigation. It permits, for example, the spatiotemporal characterization in the brain of the expression of disease-related genes, the generation of antibodies against the normal and altered proteins, and the production by genetic engineering of worm, fly, and mouse models that could serve as assays for testing possible therapies. Moreover, the identification of rare, Mendelian forms of Parkinson's disease, Alzheimer's disease, amyotrophic lateral sclerosis, and epilepsy has provided significant insights into the more common forms of these disorders. Thus far, however, no Mendelian form of any of the common early-onset psychiatric disorders of the brain has been identified convincingly. A small number of Mendelian disorders have symptoms that overlap with those of common psychiatric disorders. For example, Rett syndrome, which results from mutations in the methyl DNA binding protein MECP2, includes autistic-like symptoms but also many severe symptoms that are not characteristic of autism.

In psychiatric disorders such as schizophrenia, genes are not, by themselves, causative; other factors, a "second hit," must contribute. Unfortunately, these potential environmental factors, the "second hits," have been difficult to identify. One interesting finding, documented in the Netherlands following World War II and in China, is that maternal famine during gestation is correlated with an increased incidence of schizophrenia, perhaps by contributing to de novo germ-line mutations. Other potential risk factors include urban birth, migration, increasing paternal age, and intrauterine exposure to viral infection.

New genetic technologies are now available for the investigation of genetically complex disorders; these include more complete maps of human

TABLE 385-1 **SCHIZOPHRENIA CANDIDATE GENES**

Protein	Gene	CH Location	Evidence	Function
Disrupted in schizophrenia	DISC1	1q42	Initially identified through a balanced translocation in a single family with schizophrenia and affective disorder; confirmed by linkage and association in different populations.	Roles in microtubular transport and neuronal migration (via interactions with Lis1 and NudEL); influences postsynaptic responses (interactions with Citron); activates phosphodiesterase 4B, increasing cAMP (target of antidepressant rolipram).
Dysbindin (dystrobrevin-binding protein 1)	DTNBP1	6p22	Linkage and association; no coding region mutations; no consistent allele or haplotype implicated in different studies; negative symptoms of schizophrenia may associate with a specific haplotype of DTNBP1; expression decreased in schizophrenia brain.	Wide distribution in CNS; expression in synaptic terminals of hippocampus; in vitro, reduced levels decrease glutamate in neurons.
Neuregulin 1	NRG1	8p12-21	Linkage and association; no coding region mutations; no consistent allele or haplotype implicated in different studies; expression increased in schizophrenia brain.	Suppresses function of NMDA receptors; role in neuronal differentiation and migration.
D-Amino oxidase activator	DAOA	13q32-34	Linkage and association; no consistent allele or haplotype implicated in different studies.	Activates D-amino oxidase which oxidies D-serine, an agonist at NMDA receptors; reduced D-serine levels reported in blood and CSF in schizophrenia.
Regulator of G-protein signaling 4	RGS4	1q21-22	Linkage and association; susceptibility allele may impair working memory and regionally reduce brain volumes	Modulates postsynaptic signal transduction, including downregulation of 5HT1a (serotonin) receptors.
V-akt murine thymoma viral oncogene homologue 1	AKT1	14q22-32	Inconsistent linkage, association, and brain expression studies.	Phosphorylates and inactivates glycogen synthase kinase (GSK) 3 beta.

Note: CH, chromosome; CNS, central nervous system; CSF, cerebrospinal fluid; NMDA, N-methyl-D-aspartate.

genetic variability, high-density whole-genome association methods, and efficient high-throughput sequencing technologies using single nucleotide polymorphism (SNP) arrays. The use of these tools has already begun to yield significant results for several common complex disorders, such as inflammatory bowel disease, age-related macular degeneration, and type 2 diabetes mellitus. Psychiatric disorders are well positioned to benefit from these new approaches. In addition, it is expected that additional emerging technologies, including cost-efficient methods for whole-genome sequencing, will soon be available, further increasing the likelihood that risk-conferring alleles for psychiatric disorders will be identified within the next few years. To take full advantage of these new methods, the psychiatric research community will need to collect very large populations for sufficiently powered genetic studies, and identify (by high-resolution imaging, gene expression patterns, or other markers) biologically meaningful phenotypes for stratification of the genetic data.

CHALLENGES WITH PHENOTYPING

Psychiatric disorders have an additional obstacle to the identification of risk genes or pathophysiologic processes that cannot be addressed simply by improving genetic technologies. There are at the moment no objective diagnostic measures for any of the common psychiatric disorders. There is not, as yet, a well-defined neuropathology for psychiatric disorders nor are there biologic markers. The diagnostic classification scheme (e.g., DSM-IV) upon which both research and clinical practice rely is derived from expert consensus based on clusters of symptoms and signs and disease course. As a result, failure to delineate well-defined disease entities and to reliably assign individuals to affected versus nonaffected status have bedeviled psychiatric research.

The lack of objective tests for phenotyping presents enormous difficulties for genetic and other forms of investigation. While type 2 diabetes mellitus and hypertension, for example, are both highly heterogeneous disorders, the measurement of glucose tolerance or of systolic and diastolic blood pressure creates a strong framework within which subtyping can occur, generally based on additional objective measures. In contrast, it is not at all certain that the boundaries currently drawn around disorders in the DSM-IV lead to an underlying and distinguishable set of neurobiologic factors. For example, there is much debate about the boundaries of schizophrenia. The DSM-IV lists three psychotic disorders as being independent—schizophrenia, schizoaffective disorder, and schizophreniform disorder (American Psychiatric Association, 2000). Yet there is little agreement on whether the latter two are sufficiently homogeneous clinical entities to warrant independent recognition.

Despite the problems with current disease classification in psychiatry, there is agreement on the core symptoms and strong cross-cultural similarity of disease manifestation. In addition, there is a strong familial nature to major psychiatric disorders and also a potent role for heredity, which can be inferred from twin and adoption studies. These findings suggest that the central criteria for diagnosing schizophrenia, bipolar disorder, autism, and other major psychiatric disorders identify, however imperfectly, distinctive, naturally occurring brain diseases.

NEUROIMAGING

In parallel with improved classification and genetic studies, attempts are being made using neuroimaging to define anatomic abnormalities as objective, measurable phenotypes of the disease. For example, new quantitative methods combined with structural MRI have suggested that, in schizophrenia, there may be disease-specific patterns of gray matter loss in frontal and temporal cerebral cortex. Longitudinal studies of individuals with childhood-onset schizophrenia have documented an accelerated loss of gray matter. More recently, attempts have been made to associate specific DISC1 haplotypes with reduced frontal gray matter. While these approaches are in their early stages, the effort to define objective brain-based phenotypes for genetic and clinical studies appears very promising.

Functional imaging of individuals with depression similarly has pinpointed abnormal activity in Brodman area 25, the subgenual prefrontal cortex, a brain region that connects to the amygdala and is thought to play a critical role in the processing of emotion-related information (Fig. 385-1). Area 25 exhibits excessive metabolic activity in major depression, which reverses with successful antidepressant treatment. This region is also activated in normal subjects in whom sadness is induced by means of emotion laden stimuli. This information serves as the basis for an experimental approach to severe depression involving the use of deep-brain stimulation of the subgenual prefrontal cortex using implanted electrodes. In an initial series, four of six patients with severe depression unresponsive to all currently proven treatments, including electroconvulsive therapy, had immediate and sustained responses; however, due to the invasiveness, risk, and cost, this approach may not become a widespread treatment. Its significance lies in the putative iden-

Subgenual
PFC

$x = -3$

$y = 31$

CC

t value

0

−2.8

−5.5

FIGURE 385-1 Some patients with unipolar and bipolar disease show a functional abnormality in the prefrontal cortex ventral to the genu of the corpus callosum. *(From ER Kandel et al: Principles of Neural Science, 4th ed. New York, McGraw-Hill, 2000; with permission.)*

tification of a circuit involved in mood regulation that can be manipulated to produce therapeutic benefit.

℞ PSYCHIATRIC DISORDERS

The high prevalence and serious consequences of psychiatric disorders make the availability of effective treatments a matter of great importance for public health. Since the middle of the twentieth century, several classes of pharmacologic treatments (antipsychotic drugs, antidepressant drugs, lithium, benzodiazepines, and anticonvulsants) and several standardized short-term psychotherapies have been developed and found to be efficacious in clinical trials. The result is an armamentarium of useful treatments for many of the common disorders; however, as is the case for many common, chronic medical disorders, there are no cures for psychiatric disorders. Residual symptoms and recurrences are common, and many pharmacologic treatments have significant side effects.

This state of affairs is typified by schizophrenia, where a large number of drugs have been developed. Initially these drugs were thought to be useful only in the treatment of schizophrenia; however, they are now commonly used to treat any psychosis, irrespective of origin. In schizophrenia, in addition to the psychotic symptoms of hallucinations and delusions, referred to as *positive symptoms*, there are also *negative symptoms* (social withdrawal, impoverished speech, lack of motivation) and *cognitive symptoms* (poor executive function). Both positive and negative symptoms are thought to be related to dopaminergic systems in the brain **(Fig. 385-2)**. The primary clinical benefit of antipsychotic drugs is the amelioration of the positive psychotic symptoms. With the exception of clozapine, often described as an atypical antipsychotic drug, which produces improvement in some patients who do not respond to other drugs, all the existing antipsychotic drugs have similar efficacy and differ primarily in their pattern of side effects. Clozapine and some other atypical drugs are thought to exert at least a modest therapeutic effect on the negative symptoms of schizophrenia. None of the drugs, however, is effective against the cognitive symptoms

A Midsagittal section

Nucleus accumbens (ventral striatum)

Frontal cortex

Mesolimbic and mesocortical system

Hippocampal formation

Ventral tegmental area

B Coronal section

Neocortex

Mesocortical system: ? involved in the negative symptoms of schizophrenia

Limbic forebrain

Hippocampal formation

Ventral tegmental area

Midbrain

Mesolimbic system: ? involved in the positive symptoms of schizophrenia

FIGURE 385-2 The major dopaminergic tracts of the brain. *(From ER Kandel et al: Principles of Neural Science, 4th ed. New York, McGraw-Hill, 2000.)*

FIGURE 385-3 The key steps in the synthesis and degradation of dopamine and the sites of action of various psychoactive substances at the dopaminergic synapse. *(From ER Kandel et al: Principles of Neural Science, 4th ed. New York, McGraw-Hill, 2000.)*

are central to the illness. Furthermore, their residual presence throughout the course of the illness contributes substantially to the persistence of disability over the patient's lifetime. The search for new drugs to treat schizophrenia now focuses extensively on the ability to modify its cognitive symptoms. All antipsychotic drugs in current use block or diminish the action of dopamine at its D_2 receptors **(Fig. 385-3)**; they differ in their relative affinity at D_2 receptors and by their actions at other neurotransmitter receptors. These drugs represent important progress, but safer and more effective treatments are very much needed.

Drugs useful in depression act by increasing synaptic levels of serotonin, norepinephrine, or less commonly dopamine **(Fig. 385-4)**. The term *antidepressant* is a misnomer for this diverse class of drugs, however, because their spectrum of action is much broader than depression. These drugs are also effective in treating fear-based anxiety disorders such as panic disorder and generalized anxiety disorder. In high doses, the selective serotonin uptake inhibitors are effective for obsessive-compulsive disorder. The antidepressants are effective in the treatment of depression, but only moderately so. Many patients require sequential trials with a number of different drugs alone or in combination to achieve clinically meaningful benefit, and ~30% of patients derive no benefit at all. When pharmacologic modalities fail in depression, electroconvulsive therapy continues to be an effective treatment option. Lithium and several anticonvulsants dampen mood swings in bipolar disorder and also treat acute manic episodes; however, residual depressive symptoms, recurrences, and significant side effects are the rule. The exact mechanism of action of lithium is not known. At therapeutic levels, lithium interacts with two important signaling pathways: (1) it blocks inositol monophosphatase, thus influencing signaling via inositol phosphates, such as IP_3; and (2) it also blocks glycogen synthase kinase 3 beta (GSK3beta).

Unfortunately, there are currently very few promising drug targets that can be exploited to produce medications with truly novel mechanisms of action. Indeed, all of the major classes of drugs used to treat psychiatric disorders were identified through empirical observations of drug effects in patient populations rather than as a result of understanding pathophysiology. The molecular targets of these drugs were identified by the study of efficacious drugs and then exploited to produce improved compounds within the same class.

Cognitive-behavioral psychotherapy designed to focus on the management of specific symptoms has shown benefit in mild to moderately severe depression, fear-based anxiety disorders, and obsessive-compulsive disorder. A significant improvement in the treatment of depression in the past decade has been the standardization of psychotherapy and its evaluation in clinical trials. Instruments such as the Depression Inventory and Sui-

cide Intent Scale are now available for measuring mental illness; these have helped to objectify research in psychopathology.

New insights into the etiology of depression have also helped to guide therapy. Depressed patients have a systematic negative bias in their cognitive styles—in the way they think about themselves and their future. These distorted patterns of thinking reflect not simply an unconscious conflict within the psyche but a disorder in cognitive style and behavior that is a key etiologic agent in maintaining the disorder.

An approach that focuses on distorted thinking, cognitive therapy has been shown in randomized trials to be an effective psychological treatment for depression. This approach is based on increasing the patients' objectivity regarding their misinterpretations of everyday situations (their cognitive distortions), their misevaluation of their internal processes (body sensations, intrusive thoughts and images), and their negative expectancies. A wide range of professionals can use the methods with highly positive results.

Cognitive therapy has also proved beneficial in individuals at risk for suicide. Validated instruments exist to classify and assess suicidal behaviors, making it possible to identify high-risk individuals prospectively. Of particular importance has been the identification of clinical and psychological variables that predict future suicide. Hopelessness and consequent suicidal ideation, which are better predictors of suicide than clinical depression per se, can be quantified and substantially reduced by cognitive interventions. Several studies with individuals who had recently attempted suicide have demonstrated that a short-term cognitive intervention can significantly reduce subsequent suicide attempts when compared to a control group.

This therapy has been extended to the treatment of other disorders including anxiety states and obsessive-compulsive disorder. With respect to obsessive-compulsive disorders, cognitive therapy has been shown to reverse a metabolic abnormality, identified by neuroimaging, in parallel with the clinical improvement **(Fig. 385-5)**.

Cognitive therapy has replaced psychoanalytically based dynamic psychotherapy as the principal psychological treatment provided by specialists in certain countries. Its success has stimulated the development of other forms of short-term psychotherapy, including Interpersonal Psychiatry and Psychoanalytic-Oriented Insight Therapy. These therapies are now also being tested in controlled clinical trials and have been found to be effective in a variety of clinical situations.

Thus, paradoxically, one of the significant advances in the era of the new brain-based biologic psychiatry has been the development of evidence-based psychotherapy, a development based on the evidence that insofar as psychotherapy and other psychiatric treatments work, they do so by altering the functioning and perhaps even the structure of the brain.

A Serotonergic neurons

☐ Depressant
☐ Antidepressant

1 **Inhibition of synthesis** (p-chlorophenylalanine, p-propyldopacetamide)

Tryptophan

↓

5-OH-Tryptophan

↓

5-HT

→ 5-HIAA

2 **Interference with vesicular storage** (reserpine, tetrabenazine)

5-HT

5-HT

5-HT

3a **Stimulation of autoreceptor agonist** 8-Hydroxy-dipropylamino-tetraline (8-OH-DPAT)

MAO

5 **Inhibition of enzyme that oxidizes 5-HT** (iproniazid, clorgyline)   MAO inhibitors

3b **Stimulation of 5-HT receptors as partial agonist** (lysergic acid diethylamide)

4 **Inhibition of reuptake** (Imipramine, amitryptyline, fluoxetine, sertraline)   Tricyclics and selective serotonin reuptake inhibitors

5-HT

5-HT receptor

B Noradrenergic neurons

Tyrosine hydroxylase

1a **Inhibition of synthesis** (α-methyltyrosine)

Deaminated products

↓

DOPA

1b **Inhibition of synthesis** (FLA 63)

↓

Dopamine

2 **Interference with vesicular storage** (reserpine, tetrabenazine)

NE

7 **Inhibition of enzyme that oxidizes NE** (pargyline)   MAO inhibitors

3 **Stimulation of release of NE at nerve terminals** (amphetamine)

NE

MAO

4a **Stimulation of receptors** (clonidine)

Receptor

6 **Inhibition of reuptake** (desipramine)   Tricyclics

→ NM

4b **Blocking of receptors** (phenoxybenzamine and phentolamine)

COMT

5 **Inhibition of enzyme that inactivates NE** (tropolone)   Inactivation inhibitor

FIGURE 385-4 Actions of antidepressant and other drugs at serotonergic and noradrenergic synapses. (From ER Kandel et al: Principles of Neural Science, 4th ed. New York, McGraw-Hill, 2000.)

Medication therapy
Pre

Post

Psychotherapy
Pre

Post

FIGURE 385-5 Patients with obsessive-compulsive disorder tend to show hyperactivity in the head of the caudate. (From ER Kandel et al: Principles of Neural Science, 4th ed. New York, McGraw-Hill, 2000.)

FURTHER READINGS

CANNON T et al: Association of DISC1/TRAX haplotypes with schizophrenia, reduced prefrontal gray matter, and impaired short- and long-term memory. Arch Gen Psychiatry 62:1205, 2005

DORPH-PETERSEN KA et al: Primary visual cortex volume and total neuron number are reduced in schizophrenia. J Comp Neurol 501:290, 2007

FREITAG CM: The genetics of autistic disorders and its clinical relevance: A review of the literature. Mol Psychiat 12:2, 2007

HAHN CG et al: Altered neuregulin 1-erbB4 signaling contributes to NMDA receptor hypofunction in schizophrenia. Nature Med 12: 824, 2006

2710 HYMAN SE: Can neuroscience be integrated into the DSM-V? Nat Rev Neurosci 9:725, 2007

KANDEL ER et al: *Principles of Neural Science*, 4th ed. New York, McGraw-Hill, 2000

KENDLER KS et al: A Swedish national twin study of lifetime major depression. Am J Psychiatry 163:107, 2006

MACDONALD AW 3d et al: Specificity of prefrontal dysfunction and context processing deficits to schizophrenia in never-medicated patients with first-episode psychosis. Am J Psychiatry 162:475, 2005

MAYBERG HS et al: Deep brain stimulation for treatment-resistant depression. Neuron 45:651, 2005

MCCLELLAN JM et al: Maternal famine, de novo mutations, and schizophrenia. JAMA 296: 582, 2006

ROSS CA et al: Neurobiology of schizophrenia. Neuron 52:139, 2006

TIENARI P et al: Genetic boundaries of the schizophrenia spectrum: Evidence from the Finnish adoptive family study of schizophrenia. Am J Psychiatry 160:1587, 2003

386 Mental Disorders
Victor I. Reus

Mental disorders are common in medical practice and may present either as a primary disorder or as a comorbid condition. The prevalence of mental or substance use disorders in the United States is approximately 30%. Only one-third of these individuals are currently receiving treatment. Global burden of disease statistics indicate that 4 out of the 10 most important causes of disease worldwide are psychiatric in origin.

The revised 4th edition for use by primary care physicians of the *Diagnostic and Statistical Manual* (DSM-IV-PC) provides a useful synopsis of mental disorders most likely to be seen in primary care practice. The current system of classification is multiaxial and includes the presence or absence of a major mental disorder (axis I), any underlying personality disorder (axis II), general medical condition (axis III), psychosocial and environmental problems (axis IV), and overall rating of general psychosocial functioning (axis V).

Changes in health care delivery underscore the need for primary care physicians to assume responsibility for the initial diagnosis and treatment of the most common mental disorders. Prompt diagnosis is essential to ensure that patients have access to appropriate medical services and to maximize the clinical outcome. Validated patient-based questionnaires have been developed that systematically probe for signs and symptoms associated with the most prevalent psychiatric diagnoses and guide the clinician into targeted assessment. Prime MD (and a self-report form, the PHQ) and the Symptom-Driven Diagnostic System for Primary Care (SDDS-PC) are inventories that require only 10 min to complete and link patient responses to the formal diagnostic criteria of anxiety, mood, somatoform, and eating disorders and to alcohol abuse or dependence.

A physician who refers patients to a psychiatrist should know not only when doing so is appropriate but also how to refer, since societal misconceptions and the stigma of mental illness impede the process. Primary care physicians should base referrals to a psychiatrist on the presence of signs and symptoms of a mental disorder and not simply on the absence of a physical explanation for a patient's complaint. The physician should discuss with the patient the reasons for requesting the referral or consultation and provide reassurance that he or she will continue to provide medical care and work collaboratively with the mental health professional. Consultation with a psychiatrist or transfer of care is appropriate when physicians encounter evidence of psychotic symptoms, mania, severe depression, or anxiety; symptoms of posttraumatic stress disorder (PTSD); suicidal or homicidal preoccupation; or a failure to respond to first-order treatment. Eating disorders are discussed in Chap. 76, and the pathogenesis of psychiatric and addictive disorders in Chap. 385.

ANXIETY DISORDERS

Anxiety disorders, the most prevalent psychiatric illnesses in the general community, are present in 15–20% of medical clinic patients. Anxiety, defined as a subjective sense of unease, dread, or foreboding, can indicate a primary psychiatric condition or can be a component of, or reaction to, a primary medical disease. The primary anxiety disorders are classified according to their duration and course and the existence and nature of precipitants.

When evaluating the anxious patient, the clinician must first determine whether the anxiety antedates or postdates a medical illness or is due to a medication side effect. Approximately one-third of patients presenting with anxiety have a medical etiology for their psychiatric symptoms, but an anxiety disorder can also present with somatic symptoms in the absence of a diagnosable medical condition.

PANIC DISORDER

Clinical Manifestations Panic disorder is defined by the presence of recurrent and unpredictable panic attacks, which are distinct episodes of intense fear and discomfort associated with a variety of physical symptoms, including palpitations, sweating, trembling, shortness of breath, chest pain, dizziness, and a fear of impending doom or death (Table 386-1). Paresthesias, gastrointestinal distress, and feelings of unreality are also common. Diagnostic criteria require at least 1 month of concern or worry about the attacks or a change in behavior related to them. The lifetime prevalence of panic disorder is 1–3%. Panic attacks have a sudden onset, developing within 10 min and usually resolving over the course of an hour, and they occur in an unexpected fashion. The frequency and severity of panic attacks vary, ranging from once a week to clusters of attacks separated by months of well-being. The first attack is usually outside the home, and onset is typically in late adolescence to early adulthood. In some individuals, anticipatory anxiety develops over time and results in a generalized fear and a progressive avoidance of places or situations in which a panic attack might recur. *Agoraphobia*, which occurs commonly in patients with panic disorder, is an acquired irrational fear of being in places where one might feel trapped or unable to escape (Table 386-2). Typically, it leads the patient into a progressive restriction in lifestyle and, in a literal sense, in geography. Frequently, patients are embarrassed that they are housebound and dependent on the company of others to go out into the world and do not volunteer this information;

TABLE 386-1 DIAGNOSTIC CRITERIA FOR PANIC ATTACK

A discrete period of intense fear or discomfort, in which four or more of the following symptoms developed abruptly and reached a peak within 10 min:

1. Palpitations, pounding heart, or accelerated heart rate
2. Sweating
3. Trembling or shaking
4. Sensations of shortness of breath or smothering
5. Feeling of choking
6. Chest pain or discomfort
7. Nausea or abdominal distress
8. Feeling dizzy, unsteady, lightheaded, or faint
9. Derealization (feelings of unreality) or depersonalization (being detached from oneself)
10. Fear of losing control or going crazy
11. Fear of dying
12. Paresthesias (numbness or tingling sensations)
13. Chills or hot flushes

Source: *Diagnostic and Statistical Manual of Mental Disorders*, 4th ed. Washington, DC, American Psychiatric Association, 2000.

TABLE 386-2 DIAGNOSTIC CRITERIA FOR AGORAPHOBIA

1. Anxiety about being in places or situations from which escape might be difficult (or embarrassing) or in which help may not be available in the event of having an unexpected or situationally predisposed panic attack or panic-like symptoms. Agoraphobic fears typically involve characteristic clusters of situations that include being outside the home alone; being in a crowd or standing in a line; being on a bridge; and traveling in a bus, train, or automobile.

2. The situations are avoided (e.g., travel is restricted) or else are endured with marked distress or with anxiety about having a panic attack or panic-like symptoms, or require the presence of a companion.

3. The anxiety or phobic avoidance is not better accounted for by another mental disorder, such as social phobia (e.g., avoidance limited to social situations because of fear of embarrassment), specific phobia (e.g., avoidance limited to a single situation like elevators), obsessive-compulsive disorder (e.g., avoidance of dirt in someone with an obsession about contamination), posttraumatic stress disorder (e.g., avoidance of stimuli associated with a severe stressor), or separation anxiety disorder (e.g., avoidance of leaving home or relatives).

Source: *Diagnostic and Statistical Manual of Mental Disorders*, 4th ed. Washington, DC, American Psychiatric Association, 2000.

thus physicians will fail to recognize the syndrome if direct questioning is not pursued.

Differential Diagnosis A diagnosis of panic disorder is made after a medical etiology for the panic attacks has been ruled out. A variety of cardiovascular, respiratory, endocrine, and neurologic conditions can present with anxiety as the chief complaint. Patients with true panic disorder will often focus on one specific feature to the exclusion of others. For example, 20% of patients who present with syncope as a primary medical complaint have a primary diagnosis of a mood, anxiety, or substance-abuse disorder, the most common being panic disorder. The differential diagnosis of panic disorder is complicated by a high rate of comorbidity with other psychiatric conditions, especially alcohol and benzodiazepine abuse, which patients initially use in an attempt at self-medication. Some 75% of panic disorder patients will also satisfy criteria for major depression at some point in their illness.

When the history is nonspecific, physical examination and focused laboratory testing must be used to rule out anxiety states resulting from medical disorders such as pheochromocytoma, thyrotoxicosis, or hypoglycemia. Electrocardiogram (ECG) and echocardiogram may detect some cardiovascular conditions associated with panic, such as paroxysmal atrial tachycardia and mitral valve prolapse. In two studies, panic disorder was the primary diagnosis in 43% of patients with chest pain who had normal coronary angiograms and was present in 9% of all outpatients referred for cardiac evaluation. Panic disorder has also been diagnosed in many patients referred for pulmonary function testing or with symptoms of irritable bowel syndrome.

Etiology and Pathophysiology The etiology of panic disorder is unknown but appears to involve a genetic predisposition, altered autonomic responsivity, and social learning. Panic disorder shows familial aggregation; the disorder is concordant in 30–45% of monozygotic twins, and genome-wide screens have identified suggestive risk loci. Acute panic attacks appear to be associated with increased noradrenergic discharges in the locus coeruleus. Intravenous infusion of sodium lactate evokes an attack in two-thirds of panic disorder patients, as do the α_2-adrenergic antagonist yohimbine, cholecystokinin tetrapeptide (CCK-4), and carbon dioxide inhalation. It is hypothesized that each of these stimuli activates a pathway involving noradrenergic neurons in the locus coeruleus and serotonergic neurons in the dorsal raphe. Agents that block serotonin reuptake can prevent attacks. Panic-disorder patients have a heightened sensitivity to somatic symptoms, which triggers increasing arousal, setting off the panic attack; accordingly, therapeutic intervention involves altering the patient's cognitive interpretation of anxiety-producing experiences as well as preventing the attack itself.

℞ PANIC DISORDER

Achievable goals of treatment are to decrease the frequency of panic attacks and to reduce their intensity. The cornerstone of drug therapy is antidepressant medication (Tables 386-3, 386-4, and 386-5). Selective serotonin reuptake inhibitors (SSRIs) benefit the majority of panic disorder patients and do not have the adverse effects of tricyclic antidepressants (TCAs). Fluoxetine, paroxetine, and sertraline have received approval from the U.S. Food and Drug Administration (FDA) for this indication. SSRIs should be started at one-third to one-half of their usual antidepressant dose (e.g., 5–10 mg fluoxetine, 25–50 mg sertraline, 10 mg paroxetine). Monoamine oxidase inhibitors (MAOIs) are also effective and may specifically benefit patients who have comorbid features of atypical depression (i.e., hypersomnia and weight gain). Insomnia, orthostatic hypotension, and the need to maintain a low-tyramine diet (avoidance of cheese and wine) have limited their use, however. Antidepressants typically take 2–6 weeks to become effective, and doses may need to be adjusted based upon the clinical response.

Because of anticipatory anxiety and the need for immediate relief of panic symptoms, benzodiazepines are useful early in the course of treatment and sporadically thereafter (Table 386-6). For example, alprazolam, starting at 0.5 mg qid and increasing to 4 mg/d in divided doses, is effective, but patients must be monitored closely, as some develop dependence and begin to escalate the dose of this medication. Clonazepam, at a final maintenance dose of 2–4 mg/d, is also helpful; its longer half-life permits twice-daily dosing, and patients appear less likely to develop dependence on this agent.

Early psychotherapeutic intervention and education aimed at symptom control enhances the effectiveness of drug treatment. Patients can be taught breathing techniques, educated about physiologic changes that occur with panic, and learn to expose themselves voluntarily to precipitating events in a treatment program spanning 12–15 sessions. Homework assignments and monitored compliance are important components of successful treatment. Once patients have achieved a satisfactory response, drug treatment should be maintained for 1–2 years to prevent relapse. Controlled trials indicate a success rate of 75–85%, although the likelihood of complete remission is somewhat lower.

GENERALIZED ANXIETY DISORDER

Clinical Manifestations Patients with generalized anxiety disorder (GAD) have persistent, excessive, and/or unrealistic worry associated with muscle tension, impaired concentration, autonomic arousal, feeling "on edge" or restless, and insomnia (Table 386-7). Onset is usually before age 20, and a history of childhood fears and social inhibition may be present. The lifetime prevalence of GAD is 5–6%; the risk is higher in first-degree relatives of patients with the diagnosis. Interestingly, family studies indicate that GAD and panic disorder segregate independently. Over 80% of patients with GAD also suffer from major depression, dysthymia, or social phobia. Comorbid substance abuse is common in these patients, particularly alcohol and/or sedative/hypnotic abuse. Patients with GAD worry excessively over minor matters, with life-disrupting effects; unlike in panic disorder, complaints of shortness of breath, palpitations, and tachycardia are relatively rare.

Etiology and Pathophysiology Anxiogenic agents share in common the property of altering the binding of benzodiazepines to the γ-aminobutyric acid (GABA)$_A$ receptor/chloride ion channel complex, implicating this neurotransmitter system in the pathogenesis of anxiety and panic attacks. Benzodiazepines are thought to bind two separate GABA$_A$ receptor sites: type I, which has a broad neuroanatomic distribution, and type II, which is concentrated in the hippocampus, striatum, and neocortex. The antianxiety effects of the various benzodiazepines and side effects such as sedation and memory impairment are influenced by their relative binding to type I and type II receptor sites. Serotonin [5-hydroxytryptamine (5HT)] and 3α-reduced neuractive steroids (allosteric modulators of GABA$_A$) also appear to have a role in anxiety, and buspirone, a partial 5HT$_{1A}$ receptor agonist, and certain 5HT$_{2A}$ and 5HT$_{2C}$ receptor antagonists (e.g., nefazodone) may have beneficial effects.

TABLE 386-3 ANTIDEPRESSANTS

Name	Usual Daily Dose, mg	Side Effects	Comments
SSRIs			
Fluoxetine (Prozac)	10–80	Headache; nausea and other GI effects; jitteriness; insomnia; sexual dysfunction; can affect plasma levels of other meds (except sertraline); akathisia rare	Once daily dosing, usually in A.M.; fluoxetine has very long half-life; must not be combined with MAOIs
Sertraline (Zoloft)	50–200		
Paroxetine (Paxil)	20–60		
Fluvoxamine (Luvox)	100–300		
Citalopram (Celexa)	20–60		
Escitalopram (Lexapro)	10–30		
TCAs			
Amitriptyline (Elavil)	150–300	Anticholinergic (dry mouth, tachycardia, constipation, urinary retention, blurred vision); sweating; tremor; postural hypotension; cardiac conduction delay; sedation; weight gain	Once daily dosing, usually qhs; blood levels of most TCAs available; can be lethal in O.D. (lethal dose = 2 g); nortriptyline best tolerated, especially by elderly
Nortriptyline (Pamelor)	50–200		
Imipramine (Tofranil)	150–300		
Desipramine (Norpramin)	150–300		
Doxepin (Sinequan)	150–300		
Clomipramine (Anafranil)	150–300		
Mixed norepinephrine/serotonin reuptake inhibitors			
Venlafaxine (Effexor)	75–375	Nausea; dizziness; dry mouth; headaches; increased blood pressure; anxiety and insomnia	Bid-tid dosing (extended release available); lower potential for drug interactions than SSRIs; contraindicated with MAOI
Duloxetine (Cymbalta)	40–60	Nausea, dizziness, headache, insomnia, constipation	May have utility in treatment of neuropathic pain and stress incontinence
Mirtazapine (Remeron)	15–45	Somnolence; weight gain; neutropenia rare	Once daily dosing
Mixed-action drugs			
Bupropion (Wellbutrin)	250–450	Jitteriness; flushing; seizures in at-risk patients; anorexia; tachycardia; psychosis	Tid dosing, but sustained release also available; fewer sexual side effects than SSRIs or TCAs; may be useful for adult ADD
Trazodone (Desyrel)	200–600	Sedation; dry mouth; ventricular irritability; postural hypotension; priapism rare	Useful in low doses for sleep because of sedating effects with no anticholinergic side effects
Nefazodone (Serzone)	300–600	Sedation; headache; dry mouth; nausea; constipation	Discontinued sale in United States and several other countries due to risk of liver failure
Amoxapine (Asendin)	200–600	Sexual dysfunction	Lethality in overdose; EPS possible
MAOIs			
Phenelzine (Nardil)	45–90	Insomnia; hypotension; anorgasmia; weight gain; hypertensive crisis; toxic reactions with SSRIs	May be more effective in patients with atypical features or treatment-refractory depression
Tranylcypromine (Parnate)	20–50		
Isocarboxazid (Marplan)	20–60		
Transdermal selegiline (Emsam)	6–12	Local skin reaction; hypertension	No dietary restrictions with 6-mg dose

Note: ADD, attention deficit disorder; MAOI, monoamine oxidase inhibitor; SSRI, selective serotonin reuptake inhibitor; TCA, tricyclic antidepressant; EPS, extrapyramidal symptoms.

tency, half-life, lipid solubility, metabolic pathways, and presence of active metabolites. Agents that are absorbed rapidly and are lipid soluble, such as diazepam, have a rapid onset of action and a higher abuse potential. Benzodiazepines should generally not be prescribed for >4–6 weeks because of the development of tolerance and the risk of abuse and dependence. Withdrawal must be closely monitored as relapses can occur. It is important to warn patients that concomitant use of alcohol or other sedating drugs may be neurotoxic and impair their ability to function. An optimistic approach that encourages the patient to clarify environmental precipitants, anticipate his or her reactions, and plan effective response strategies is an essential element of therapy.

Adverse effects of benzodiazepines generally parallel their relative half-lives. Longer-acting agents, such as diazepam, chlordiazepoxide, flurazepam, and clonazepam, tend to accumulate active metabolites, with resultant sedation, impairment of cognition, and poor psychomotor performance. Shorter-acting compounds, such as alprazolam and oxazepam, can produce daytime anxiety, early morning insomnia, and, with discontinuation, rebound anxiety and insomnia. Although patients develop tolerance to the sedative effects of benzodiazepines, they are less likely to habituate to the adverse psychomotor effects. Withdrawal from the longer half-life benzodiazepines can be accomplished through gradual, stepwise dose reduction (by 10% every 1–2 weeks) over 6–12 weeks. It is usually more difficult to taper patients off shorter-acting benzodiazepines. Physicians may need to switch the patient to a benzodiazepine with a longer half-life or use an adjunctive medication, such as a beta blocker or carbamazepine, before attempting to discontinue the benzodiazepine. Withdrawal reactions vary in severity and duration; they can include depression, anxiety, lethargy, diaphoresis, autonomic arousal, and, rarely, seizures.

Buspirone is a nonbenzodiazepine anxiolytic agent. It is nonsedating, does not produce tolerance or dependence, does not interact with benzodiazepine receptors or alcohol, and has no abuse or disinhibition potential. However, it requires several weeks to take effect and requires thrice-daily dosing. Patients who were previously responsive to a benzodiazepine are unlikely to rate buspirone as equally effective, but patients with head injury or dementia who have symptoms of anxiety and/or agitation may do well with this agent. Escitalopram, paroxetine, and venlafaxine are FDA approved for the treatment of GAD, usually at doses that are comparable to their efficacy in major depression. Benzodiazepines are contraindicated during pregnancy and breast-feeding.

Anticonvulsants with GABAergic properties may also be effective against anxiety. Gabapentin, oxcarbazepine, tiagabine, pregabalin, and divalproex have all shown some degree of benefit in a variety of anxiety-related syndromes. Agents that selectively target $GABA_A$ receptor subtypes are cur-

℞ GENERALIZED ANXIETY DISORDER

A combination of pharmacologic and psychotherapeutic interventions is most effective in GAD, but complete symptomatic relief is rare. A short course of a benzodiazepine is usually indicated, preferably lorazepam, oxazepam, or temazepam. (The first two of these agents are metabolized via conjugation rather than oxidation and thus do not accumulate if hepatic function is altered.) Administration should be initiated at the lowest dose possible and prescribed on an as-needed basis as symptoms warrant. Benzodiazepines differ in their milligram per kilogram po-

TABLE 386-4 MANAGEMENT OF ANTIDEPRESSANT SIDE EFFECTS

Symptoms	Comments and Management Strategies
Gastrointestinal	
Nausea, loss of appetite	Usually short-lived and dose-related; consider temporary dose reduction or administration with food and antacids
Diarrhea	Famotidine, 20–40 mg/d
Constipation	Wait for tolerance; try diet change, stool softener, exercise; avoid laxatives
Sexual dysfunction	Consider dose reduction; drug holiday
Anorgasmia/ impotence; impaired ejaculation	Bethanechol, 10–20 mg, 2 h before activity, or cyproheptadine, 4–8 mg 2 h before activity, or bupropion, 100 mg bid or amantadine, 100 mg bid/tid
Orthostasis	Tolerance unlikely; increase fluid intake, use calf exercises/support hose; fludrocortisone, 0.025 mg/d
Anticholinergic	Wait for tolerance
Dry mouth, eyes	Maintain good oral hygiene; use artificial tears, sugar-free gum
Tremor/jitteriness	Antiparkinsonian drugs not effective; use dose reduction/slow increase; lorazepam, 0.5 mg bid, or propranolol, 10–20 mg bid
Insomnia	Schedule all doses for the morning; trazodone, 50–100 mg qhs
Sedation	Caffeine; schedule all dosing for bedtime; bupropion, 75–100 mg in afternoon
Headache	Evaluate diet, stress, other drugs; try dose reduction; amitriptyline, 50 mg/d
Weight gain	Decrease carbohydrates; exercise; consider fluoxetine
Loss of therapeutic benefit over time	Related to tolerance? Increase dose or drug holiday; add amantadine, 100 mg bid, buspirone, 10 mg tid, or pindolol, 2.5 mg bid

TABLE 386-5 POSSIBLE DRUG INTERACTIONS WITH SELECTIVE SEROTONIN REUPTAKE INHIBITORS

Agent	Effect
Monoamine oxidase inhibitors	Serotonin syndrome[a]—absolute contraindication
Serotonergic agonists, e.g., tryptophan, fenfluramine	Potential serotonin syndrome
Drugs that are metabolized by P450 isoenzymes: tricyclics, other SSRIs, antipsychotics, beta blockers, codeine, triazolobenzodiazepines, calcium channel blockers	Delayed metabolism resulting in increased blood levels and potential toxicity—possible fatality secondary to QT prolongation with terfenadine or astemizole
Drugs that are bound tightly to plasma proteins, e.g., warfarin	Increased bleeding secondary to displacement
Drugs that inhibit the metabolism of SSRIs by P450 isoenzymes, e.g., quinidine	Increased SSRI side effects

[a]See Rx Depressive Disorders, below.
Note: SSRI, selective serotonin reuptake inhibitor.

mal phobia were found to be 23% for monozygotic twins and 15% for dizygotic twins. A twin study of fear conditioning, a model for the acquisition of phobias, demonstrated a heritability of 35–45%, and a genome-wide linkage scan identified a risk locus on chromosome 14 in a region previously implicated in a mouse model of fear. Animal studies of fear conditioning have indicated that processing of the fear stimulus occurs through the lateral nucleus of the amygdala, extending through the central nucleus and projecting to the periaqueductal gray region, lateral hypothalamus, and paraventricular hypothalamus.

Rx PHOBIC DISORDERS

Beta blockers (e.g., propranolol, 20–40 mg orally 2 h before the event) are particularly effective in the treatment of "performance anxiety" (but not

rently under development, and it is hoped that these will lack the sedating, memory-impairing, and addicting properties of benzodiazepines.

PHOBIC DISORDERS

Clinical Manifestations The cardinal feature of phobic disorders is a marked and persistent fear of objects or situations, exposure to which results in an immediate anxiety reaction. The patient avoids the phobic stimulus, and this avoidance usually impairs occupational or social functioning. Panic attacks may be triggered by the phobic stimulus or may occur spontaneously. Unlike patients with other anxiety disorders, individuals with phobias usually experience anxiety only in specific situations. Common phobias include fear of closed spaces (claustrophobia), fear of blood, and fear of flying. Social phobia is distinguished by a specific fear of social or performance situations in which the individual is exposed to unfamiliar individuals or to possible examination and evaluation by others. Examples include having to converse at a party, use public restrooms, and meet strangers. In each case, the affected individual is aware that the experienced fear is excessive and unreasonable given the circumstance. The specific content of a phobia may vary across gender, ethnic, and cultural boundaries.

Phobic disorders are common, affecting ~10% of the population. Full criteria for diagnosis are usually satisfied first in early adulthood, but behavioral avoidance of unfamiliar people, situations, or objects dating from early childhood is common.

In one study of female twins, concordance rates for agoraphobia, social phobia, and ani-

TABLE 386-6 ANXIOLYTICS

Name	Equivalent PO dose, mg	Onset of Action	Half-life, h	Comments
Benzodiazepines				
Diazepam (Valium)	5	Fast	20–70	Active metabolites; quite sedating
Flurazepam (Dalmane)	15	Fast	30–100	Flurazepam is a pro-drug; metabolites are active; quite sedating
Triazolam (Halcion)	0.25	Intermediate	1.5–5	No active metabolites; can induce confusion and delirium, especially in elderly
Lorazepam (Ativan)	1	Intermediate	10–20	No active metabolites; direct hepatic glucuronide conjugation; quite sedating
Alprazolam (Xanax)	0.5	Intermediate	12–15	Active metabolites; not too sedating; may have specific antidepressant and antipanic activity; tolerance and dependence develop easily
Chlordiazepoxide (Librium)	10	Intermediate	5–30	Active metabolites; moderately sedating
Oxazepam (Serax)	15	Slow	5–15	No active metabolites; direct glucuronide conjugation; not too sedating
Temazepam (Restoril)	15	Slow	9–12	No active metabolites; moderately sedating
Clonazepam (Klonopin)	0.5	Slow	18–50	No active metabolites; moderately sedating
Non-benzodiazepines				
Buspirone (BuSpar)	7.5	2 weeks	2–3	Active metabolites; tid dosing— usual daily dose 10–20 mg tid; nonsedating; no additive effects with alcohol; useful for agitation in demented or brain-injured patients

TABLE 386-7 DIAGNOSTIC CRITERIA FOR GENERALIZED ANXIETY DISORDER

A. Excessive anxiety and worry (apprehensive expectation), occurring more days than not for at least 6 months, about a number of events or activities (such as work or school performance).
B. The person finds it difficult to control the worry.
C. The anxiety and worry are associated with three (or more) of the following six symptoms (with at least some symptoms present for more days than not for the past 6 months): (1) restlessness or feeling keyed up or on edge; (2) being easily fatigued; (3) difficulty concentrating or mind going blank; (4) irritability; (5) muscle tension; (6) sleep disturbance (difficulty falling or staying asleep, or restless unsatisfying sleep).
D. The focus of the anxiety and worry is not confined to features of an Axis I disorder, e.g., the anxiety or worry is not about having a panic attack (as in panic disorder), being embarrassed in public (as in social phobia), being contaminated (as in obsessive-compulsive disorder), being away from home or close relatives (as in separation anxiety disorder), gaining weight (as in anorexia nervosa), having multiple physical complaints (as in somatization disorder), or having a serious illness (as in hypochondriasis), and the anxiety and worry do not occur exclusively during posttraumatic stress disorder.
E. The anxiety, worry, or physical symptoms cause clinically significant distress or impairment in social, occupational, or other important areas of functioning.
F. The disturbance is not due to the direct physiologic effects of a substance (e.g., a drug of abuse, a medication) or a general medical condition (e.g., hyperthyroidism) and does not occur exclusively during a mood disorder, a psychotic disorder, or a pervasive developmental disorder.

Source: Diagnostic and Statistical Manual of Mental Disorders, 4th ed. Washington, DC, American Psychiatric Association, 2000.

general social phobia) and appear to work by blocking the peripheral manifestations of anxiety, such as perspiration, tachycardia, palpitations, and tremor. MAOIs alleviate social phobia independently of their antidepressant activity, and paroxetine, sertraline, and venlafaxine have received FDA approval for treatment of social anxiety. Benzodiazepines can be helpful in reducing fearful avoidance, but the chronic nature of phobic disorders limits their usefulness.

Behaviorally focused psychotherapy is an important component of treatment, as relapse rates are high when medication is used as the sole treatment. Cognitive-behavioral strategies are based upon the finding that distorted perceptions and interpretations of fear-producing stimuli play a major role in perpetuation of phobias. Individual and group therapy sessions teach the patient to identify specific negative thoughts associated with the anxiety-producing situation and help to reduce the patient's fear of loss of control. In desensitization therapy, hierarchies of feared situations are constructed and the patient is encouraged to pursue and master gradual exposure to the anxiety-producing stimuli.

Patients with social phobia, in particular, have a high rate of comorbid alcohol abuse, as well as of other psychiatric conditions (e.g., eating disorders), necessitating the need for parallel management of each disorder if anxiety reduction is to be achieved.

STRESS DISORDERS

Clinical Manifestations   Patients may develop anxiety after exposure to extreme traumatic events such as the threat of personal death or injury or the death of a loved one. The reaction may occur shortly after the trauma (*acute stress disorder*) or be delayed and subject to recurrence (PTSD) (Table 386-8). In both syndromes, individuals experience associated symptoms of detachment and loss of emotional responsivity. The patient may feel depersonalized and unable to recall specific aspects of the trauma, though typically it is reexperienced through intrusions in thought, dreams, or flashbacks, particularly when cues of the original event are present. Patients often actively avoid stimuli that precipitate recollections of the trauma and demonstrate a resulting increase in vigilance, arousal, and startle response. Patients with stress disorders are at risk for the development of other disorders related to anxiety, mood, and substance abuse (especially alcohol). Between 5 and 10% of Americans will at some time in their life satisfy criteria for PTSD, with women more likely to be affected than men.

TABLE 386-8 DIAGNOSTIC CRITERIA FOR POSTTRAUMATIC STRESS DISORDER

A. The person has been exposed to a traumatic event in which both of the following were present:
  1. The person experienced, witnessed, or was confronted with an event or events that involved actual or threatened death or serious injury, or a threat to the physical integrity of self or others.
  2. The person's response involved intense fear, helplessness, or horror.
B. The traumatic event is persistently reexperienced in one (or more) of the following ways:
  1. Recurrent and intrusive distressing recollections of the event, including images, thoughts, or perceptions.
  2. Recurrent distressing dreams of the event.
  3. Acting or feeling as if the traumatic event were recurring (includes a sense of reliving the experience, illusions, hallucinations, and dissociative flashback episodes, including those that occur on awakening or when intoxicated).
  3. Intense psychological distress at exposure to internal or external cues that symbolize or resemble an aspect of the traumatic event.
  4. Physiologic reactivity on exposure to internal or external cues that symbolize or resemble an aspect of the traumatic event.
C. Persistent avoidance of stimuli associated with the trauma and numbing of general responsiveness (not present before the trauma), as indicated by three or more of the following:
  1. Efforts to avoid thoughts, feelings, or conversations associated with the trauma
  2. Efforts to avoid activities, places, or people that arouse recollections of the trauma
  3. Inability to recall an important aspect of the trauma
  4. Markedly diminished interest or participation in significant activities
  5. Feeling of detachment or estrangement from others
  6. Restricted range of affect (e.g., unable to have loving feelings)
  7. Sense of a foreshortened future (e.g., does not expect to have a career, marriage, children, or a normal life span)
D. Persistent symptoms of increased arousal (not present before the trauma), as indicated by two (or more) of the following:
  1. Difficulty falling or staying asleep
  2. Irritability or outbursts of anger
  3. Difficulty concentrating
  4. Hypervigilance
  5. Exaggerated startle response
E. Duration of the disturbance (symptoms in criteria B, C, and D) is more than 1 month.
F. The disturbance causes clinically significant distress or impairment in social, occupational, or other important areas of functioning.

Source: Diagnostic and Statistical Manual of Mental Disorders, 4th ed. Washington, DC, American Psychiatric Association, 2000.

Risk factors for the development of PTSD include a past psychiatric history and personality characteristics of high neuroticism and extroversion. Twin studies show a substantial genetic influence on all symptoms associated with PTSD, with less evidence for an environmental effect.

Etiology and Pathophysiology   It is hypothesized that in PTSD there is excessive release of norepinephrine from the locus coeruleus in response to stress and increased noradrenergic activity at projection sites in the hippocampus and amygdala. These changes theoretically facilitate the encoding of fear-based memories. Greater sympathetic responses to cues associated with the traumatic event occur in PTSD, although pituitary adrenal responses are blunted.

℞ STRESS DISORDERS

Acute stress reactions are usually self-limited, and treatment typically involves the short-term use of benzodiazepines and supportive/expressive psychotherapy. The chronic and recurrent nature of PTSD, however, requires a more complex approach employing drug and behavioral treatments. PTSD is highly correlated with peritraumatic dissociative symptoms and the development of an acute stress disorder at the time of the trauma. TCAs such as imipramine and amitriptyline, the MAOI phenelzine, and the SSRIs can all reduce anxiety, symptoms of intrusion, and avoidance behaviors, as can prazosin, an α_1 antagonist. Propranolol given during the acute stress period may have beneficial effects in preventing the development of PTSD. Trazodone, a sedating antidepressant, is frequently used at night to help with insomnia (50–150 mg qhs). Carbamazepine, valproic acid, or alprazolam have also independently produced improvement in uncontrolled trials. Psychotherapeutic strategies for PTSD help the patient overcome avoidance behaviors and demoralization and master fear of recurrence of the trauma; therapies that encourage the patient to dismantle avoidance behaviors through stepwise focusing on the experience of the traumatic event are the most effective.

OBSESSIVE-COMPULSIVE DISORDER

Clinical Manifestations Obsessive-compulsive disorder (OCD) is characterized by obsessive thoughts and compulsive behaviors that impair everyday functioning. Fears of contamination and germs are common, as are handwashing, counting behaviors, and having to check and recheck such actions as whether a door is locked. The degree to which the disorder is disruptive for the individual varies, but in all cases obsessive-compulsive activities take up >1 h/d and are undertaken to relieve the anxiety triggered by the core fear. Patients often conceal their symptoms, usually because they are embarrassed by the content of their thoughts or the nature of their actions. Physicians must ask specific questions regarding recurrent thoughts and behaviors, particularly if physical clues such as chafed and reddened hands or patchy hair loss (from repetitive hair pulling, or trichotillomania) are present. Comorbid conditions are common, the most frequent being depression, other anxiety disorders, eating disorders, and tics. OCD has a lifetime prevalence of 2–3% worldwide. Onset is usually gradual, beginning in early adulthood, but childhood onset is not rare. The disorder usually has a waxing and waning course, but some cases may show a steady deterioration in psychosocial functioning.

Etiology and Pathophysiology A genetic contribution to OCD is suggested by twin studies. Family studies show an aggregation with Tourette's disorder. OCD is also more common in males and in first-born children.

The anatomy of obsessive-compulsive behavior is thought to include the orbital frontal cortex, caudate nucleus, and globus pallidus. The caudate nucleus appears to be involved in the acquisition and maintenance of habit and skill learning, and interventions that are successful in reducing obsessive-compulsive behaviors also decrease metabolic activity measured in the caudate.

℞ OBSESSIVE-COMPULSIVE DISORDER

Clomipramine, fluoxetine, fluvoxamine, and sertraline are approved for the treatment of OCD. Clomipramine is a TCA that is often tolerated poorly owing to anticholinergic and sedative side effects at the doses required to treat the illness (25–250 mg/d). Its efficacy in OCD is unrelated to its antidepressant activity. Fluoxetine (5–60 mg/d), fluvoxamine (25–300 mg/d), and sertraline (50–150 mg/d) are as effective as clomipramine and have a more benign side-effect profile. Only 50–60% of patients with OCD show adequate improvement with pharmacotherapy alone. In treatment-resistant cases, augmentation with other serotonergic agents, such as buspirone, or with a neuroleptic or benzodiazepine may be beneficial. When a therapeutic response is achieved, long-duration maintenance therapy is usually indicated.

For many individuals, particularly those with time-consuming compulsions, behavior therapy will result in as much improvement as that afforded by medication. Effective techniques include the gradual increase in exposure to stressful situations, maintenance of a diary to clarify stressors, and homework assignments that substitute new activities for compulsive behaviors.

MOOD DISORDERS

Mood disorders are characterized by a disturbance in the regulation of mood, behavior, and affect. Mood disorders are subdivided into (1) depressive disorders, (2) bipolar disorders, and (3) depression in association with medical illness or alcohol and substance abuse (Chaps. 387, 388, and 389). Depressive disorders are differentiated from bipolar disorders by the absence of a manic or hypomanic episode. The relationship between pure depressive syndromes and bipolar disorders is not well understood; depression is more frequent in families of bipolar individuals, but the reverse is not true. In the Global Burden of Disease Study conducted by the World Health Organization, unipolar major depression ranked fourth among all diseases in terms of disability-adjusted life-years and was projected to rank second by the year 2020. In the United States, lost productivity directly related to mood disorders has been estimated at $55.1 billion per year.

DEPRESSION IN ASSOCIATION WITH MEDICAL ILLNESS

Depression occurring in the context of medical illness is difficult to evaluate. Depressive symptomatology may reflect the psychological stress of coping with the disease, may be caused by the disease process itself or by the medications used to treat it, or may simply coexist in time with the medical diagnosis.

Virtually every class of *medication* includes some agent that can induce depression. Antihypertensive drugs, anticholesterolemic agents, and antiarrhythmic agents are common triggers of depressive symptoms. Among the antihypertensive agents, β-adrenergic blockers and, to a lesser extent, calcium channel blockers are the most likely to cause depressed mood. Iatrogenic depression should also be considered in patients receiving glucocorticoids, antimicrobials, systemic analgesics, antiparkinsonian medications, and anticonvulsants. To decide whether a causal relationship exists between pharmacologic therapy and a patient's change in mood, it may sometimes be necessary to undertake an empirical trial of an alternative medication.

Between 20 and 30% of *cardiac* patients manifest a depressive disorder; an even higher percentage experience depressive symptomatology when self-reporting scales are used. Depressive symptoms following unstable angina, myocardial infarction, cardiac bypass surgery, or heart transplant impair rehabilitation and are associated with higher rates of mortality and medical morbidity. Depressed patients often show decreased variability in heart rate (an index of reduced parasympathetic nervous system activity); this has been proposed as one mechanism by which depression may predispose individuals to ventricular arrhythmia and increased morbidity. Depression also appears to increase the risk of developing coronary heart disease; increased serotonin-induced platelet aggregation has been implicated as a possible cause. TCAs are contraindicated in patients with bundle branch block, and TCA-induced tachycardia is an additional concern in patients with congestive heart failure. SSRIs appear not to induce ECG changes or adverse cardiac events and thus are reasonable first-line drugs for patients at risk for TCA-related complications. SSRIs may interfere with hepatic metabolism of anticoagulants, however, causing increased anticoagulation.

In patients with *cancer*, the mean prevalence of depression is 25%, but depression occurs in 40–50% of patients with cancers of the pancreas or oropharynx. This association is not due to the effect of cachexia alone, as the higher prevalence of depression in patients with pancreatic cancer persists when compared to those with advanced gastric cancer. Initiation of antidepressant medication in cancer patients has been shown to improve quality of life as well as mood. Psychotherapeutic approaches, particularly group therapy, may have some effect on short-term depression, anxiety, and pain symptoms.

Depression occurs frequently in patients with *neurologic disorders*, particularly cerebrovascular disorders, Parkinson's disease, dementia, multiple sclerosis, and traumatic brain injury. One in five patients with left-hemisphere stroke involving the dorsolateral frontal cortex experiences major depression. Late-onset depression in otherwise cognitively normal individuals increases the risk of a subsequent diagnosis of Alzheimer's disease. Both TCA and SSRI agents are effective against these depressions, as are stimulant compounds and, in some patients, MAOIs.

The reported prevalence of depression in patients with *diabetes mellitus* varies from 8–27%, with the severity of the mood state correlating with the level of hyperglycemia and the presence of diabetic complications. Treatment of depression may be complicated by effects of antidepressive agents on glycemic control. MAOIs can induce hypoglycemia and weight gain. TCAs can produce hyperglycemia and carbohydrate craving. SSRIs, like MAOIs, may reduce fasting plasma glucose, but they are easier to use and may also improve dietary and medication compliance.

Hypothyroidism is frequently associated with features of depression, most commonly depressed mood and memory impairment. Hyperthyroid states may also present in a similar fashion, usually in geriatric populations. Improvement in mood usually follows normalization of thyroid function, but adjunctive antidepressant medication is sometimes required. Patients with subclinical hypothyroidism can also experience symptoms of depression and cognitive difficulty that respond to thyroid replacement.

The lifetime prevalence of depression in *HIV-positive* individuals has been estimated at 22–45%. The relationship between depression and disease progression is multifactorial and likely to involve psychological and social factors, alterations in immune function, and central nervous system disease. Chronic hepatitis C infection is also associated with depression, which may worsen with interferon-α treatment.

Some chronic disorders of uncertain etiology, such as chronic fatigue syndrome (Chap. 384) and fibromyalgia (Chap. 329), are strongly associated with depression and anxiety; patients may benefit from antidepressant treatment, usually at lower than normal dosing.

DEPRESSIVE DISORDERS
Clinical Manifestations *Major depression* is defined as depressed mood on a daily basis for a minimum duration of 2 weeks (Table 386-9). An episode may be characterized by sadness, indifference, apathy, or irritability and is usually associated with: changes in sleep patterns, appetite, and weight; motor agitation or retardation; fatigue; impaired concentration and decision-making; feelings of shame or guilt; and thoughts of death or dying. Patients with depression have a profound loss of plea-

TABLE 386-9 CRITERIA FOR MAJOR DEPRESSIVE EPISODE

A. Five (or more) of the following symptoms have been present during the same 2-week period and represent a change from previous functioning; at least one of the symptoms is either (1) depressed mood or (2) loss of interest or pleasure. **Note:** Do not include symptoms that are clearly due to a general medical condition, or mood-incongruent delusions or hallucinations.

1. Depressed mood most of the day, nearly every day, as indicated by either subjective report (e.g., feels sad or empty) or observation made by others (e.g., appears tearful)
2. Markedly diminished interest or pleasure in all, or almost all, activities most of the day, nearly every day (as indicated by either subjective account or observation made by others)
3. Significant weight loss when not dieting or weight gain (e.g., a change of >5% of body weight in a month), or decrease or increase in appetite nearly every day
4. Insomnia or hypersomnia nearly every day
5. Psychomotor agitation or retardation nearly every day (observable by others, not merely subjective feelings of restlessness or being slowed down)
6. Fatigue or loss of energy nearly every day
7. Feelings of worthlessness or excessive or inappropriate guilt (which may be delusional) nearly every day (not merely self-reproach or guilt about being sick)
8. Diminished ability to think or concentrate, or indecisiveness, nearly every day (either by subjective account or as observed by others)
9. Recurrent thoughts of death (not just fear of dying), recurrent suicidal ideation without a specific plan, or a suicide attempt or a specific plan for committing suicide

B. The symptoms do not meet criteria for a mixed episode
C. The symptoms cause clinically significant distress or impairment in social, occupational, or other important areas of functioning
D. The symptoms are not due to the direct physiologic effects of a substance (e.g., a drug of abuse, a medication) or a general medical condition (e.g., hypothyroidism)
E. The symptoms are not better accounted for by bereavement; i.e., after the loss of a loved one, the symptoms persist for >2 months or are characterized by marked functional impairment, morbid preoccupation with worthlessness, suicidal ideation, psychotic symptoms, or psychomotor retardation

Source: *Diagnostic and Statistical Manual of Mental Disorders,* 4th ed. Washington, DC, American Psychiatric Association, 2000.

sure in all enjoyable activities, exhibit early morning awakening, feel that the dysphoric mood state is qualitatively different from sadness, and often notice a diurnal variation in mood (worse in morning hours).

Approximately 15% of the population experiences a major depressive episode at some point in life, and 6–8% of all outpatients in primary care settings satisfy diagnostic criteria for the disorder. Depression is often undiagnosed, and, even more frequently, it is treated inadequately. If a physician suspects the presence of a major depressive episode, the initial task is to determine whether it represents unipolar or bipolar depression or is one of the 10–15% of cases that are secondary to general medical illness or substance abuse. Physicians should also assess the risk of suicide by direct questioning, as patients are often reluctant to verbalize such thoughts without prompting. If specific plans are uncovered or if significant risk factors exist (e.g., a past history of suicide attempts, profound hopelessness, concurrent medical illness, substance abuse, or social isolation), the patient must be referred to a mental health specialist for immediate care. The physician should specifically probe each of these areas in an empathic and hopeful manner, being sensitive to denial and possible minimization of distress. The presence of anxiety, panic, or agitation significantly increases near-term suicidal risk. Approximately 4–5% of all depressed patients will commit suicide; most will have sought help from a physician within 1 month of their death.

In some depressed patients, the mood disorder does not appear to be episodic and is not clearly associated with either psychosocial dysfunction or change from the individual's usual experience in life. *Dysthymic disorder* consists of a pattern of chronic (at least 2 years), ongoing, mild depressive symptoms that are less severe and less disabling than those found in major depression; the two conditions are sometimes difficult to separate, however, and can occur together ("double depression"). Many patients who exhibit a profile of pessimism, disinterest, and low self-esteem respond to antidepressant treatment. Dysthymic disorder exists in ~5% of primary care patients. The term *minor depression* is used for individuals who experience at least two depressive symptoms for 2 weeks but who do not meet the full criteria for major depression. Despite its name, minor depression is associated with significant morbidity and disability and also responds to pharmacologic treatment.

Depression is approximately twice as common in women as in men, and the incidence increases with age in both sexes. Twin studies indicate that the liability to major depression in adult women is largely genetic in origin. Negative life events can precipitate and contribute to depression, but genetic factors influence the sensitivity of individuals to these stressful events. In most cases, both biologic and psychosocial factors are involved in the precipitation and unfolding of depressive episodes. The most potent stressors appear to involve death of a relative, assault, or severe marital or relationship problems.

Unipolar depressive disorders usually begin in early adulthood and recur episodically over the course of a lifetime. The best predictor of future risk is the number of past episodes; 50–60% of patients who have a first episode have at least one or two recurrences. Some patients experience multiple episodes that become more severe and frequent over time. The duration of an untreated episode varies greatly, ranging from a few months to ≥1 year. The pattern of recurrence and clinical progression in a developing episode are also variable. Within an individual, the nature of episodes (e.g., specific presenting symptoms, frequency and duration) may be similar over time. In a minority of patients, a severe depressive episode may progress to a psychotic state; in elderly patients, depressive symptoms may be associated with cognitive deficits mimicking dementia ("pseudodementia"). A seasonal pattern of depression, called *seasonal affective disorder*, may manifest with onset and remission of episodes at predictable times of the year. This disorder is more common in women, whose symptoms are anergy, fatigue, weight gain, hypersomnia, and episodic carbohydrate craving. The prevalence increases with distance from the equator, and improvement may occur by altering light exposure.

Etiology and Pathophysiology Although evidence for genetic transmission of unipolar depression is not as strong as in bipolar disorder, monozygotic twins have a higher concordance rate (46%) than dizygotic siblings (20%), with little support for any effect of a shared family environment. There is some evidence that a functional polymorphism in the serotonin transporter (*5-HTT*) gene may interact with stressful life events to markedly increase risk of depression and suicide. Positron emission tomography (PET) studies show decreased metabolic activity in the caudate nuclei and frontal lobes in depressed patients that returns to normal with recovery. Single-photon emission computed tomography (SPECT) studies show comparable changes in blood flow.

Postmortem examination of brains of suicide victims indicate altered noradrenergic activity, including increased binding to α_1-, α_2-, and β-adrenergic receptors in the cerebral cortex and decreased numbers of noradrenergic neurons in the locus coeruleus. Involvement of the serotonin system is suggested by findings of reduced plasma tryptophan levels, a decreased cerebrospinal fluid level of 5-hydroxyindolacetic acid (the principal metabolite of serotonin in brain), and decreased platelet serotonergic transporter binding. An increase in brain serotonin receptors in suicide victims and decreased expression of the cyclic AMP response element-binding (CREB) protein are also reported. Depletion of blood tryptophan, the amino acid precursor of serotonin, rapidly reverses the antidepressant benefit in depressed patients who have been successfully treated. However, a decrement in mood after tryptophan reduction is considerably less robust in untreated patients, indicating that, if presynaptic serotonergic dysfunction occurs in depression, it likely plays a contributing rather than a causal role.

Neuroendocrine abnormalities that reflect the neurovegetative signs and symptoms of depression include (1) increased cortisol and corticotropin-releasing hormone (CRH) secretion, (2) an increase in adrenal size, (3) a decreased inhibitory response of glucocorticoids to dexamethasone, and (4) a blunted response of thyroid-stimulating hormone (TSH) level to infusion of thyroid-releasing hormone (TRH). Antidepressant treatment leads to normalization of these pituitary-adrenal abnormalities. Major depression is also associated with an upregulation of proinflammatory cytokines, which normalizes with antidepressant treatment.

Diurnal variations in symptom severity and alterations in circadian rhythmicity of a number of neurochemical and neurohumoral factors suggest that biologic differences may be secondary to a primary defect in regulation of biologic rhythms. Patients with major depression show consistent findings of a decrease in rapid eye movement (REM) sleep onset (REM latency), an increase in REM density, and, in some subjects, a decrease in stage IV delta slow-wave sleep.

Although antidepressant drugs inhibit neurotransmitter uptake within hours, their therapeutic effects typically emerge over several weeks, implicating adaptive changes in second messenger systems and transcription factors as possible mechanisms of action. Antidepressant drugs have been shown to regulate neural plasticity and cell survival by increasing the expression of brain-derived neurotrophic factor (BDNF) through upregulation of the CREB protein and to alter stress responsivity through an increase in glucocorticoid receptor transcription. Secondary effects on activation of the mitogen-activated protein (MAP) kinase and phosphoinositol-3 kinase/AKT pathways and increased expression of the antiapoptotic protein, Bcl-2, are also thought to be critical to antidepressant actions.

R̶x̶ DEPRESSIVE DISORDERS

Treatment planning requires coordination of short-term strategies to induce remission combined with longer term maintenance designed to prevent recurrence. The most effective intervention for achieving remission and preventing relapse is medication, but combined treatment, incorporating psychotherapy to help the patient cope with decreased self-esteem and demoralization, improves outcome **(Fig. 386-1)**. Approximately 40% of primary care patients with depression drop out of treatment and discontinue medication if symptomatic improvement is not noted within a month, unless additional support is provided. Outcome improves with (1) increased intensity and frequency of visits during the first 4–6 weeks of treatment, (2) supplemental educational materials, and (3) psychiatric consultation as indicated. Despite the widespread use of SSRIs and other second-generation antidepressant drugs, there is no convincing evidence

FIGURE 386-1 A guideline for the medical management of major depressive disorder. SSRI, selective serotonin reuptake inhibitor; TCA, tricyclic antidepressant.

that this class of antidepressant is more efficacious than TCAs. Between 60 and 70% of all depressed patients respond to any drug chosen, if it is given in a sufficient dose for 6–8 weeks. There is no ideal antidepressant; no current compound combines rapid onset of action, moderate half-life, a meaningful relationship between dose and blood level, a low side-effect profile, minimal interaction with other drugs, and safety in overdose.

A rational approach to selecting which antidepressant to use involves matching the patient's preference and medical history with the metabolic and side effect profile of the drug (Tables 386-4 and 386-5). A previous response, or a family history of a positive response, to a specific antidepressant often suggests that that drug be tried first. Before initiating antidepressant therapy, the physician should evaluate the possible contribution of comorbid illnesses and consider their specific treatment. In individuals with suicidal ideation, particular attention should be paid to choosing a drug with low toxicity if taken in overdose. The SSRIs and other newer antidepressant drugs are distinctly safer in this regard; nevertheless, the advantages of TCAs have not been completely superseded. The existence of generic equivalents make TCAs relatively cheap, and for several tricyclics, particularly nortriptyline, imipramine, and desipramine, well-defined relationships among dose, plasma level, and therapeutic response exist. The steady-state plasma level achieved for a given drug dose can vary more than tenfold between individuals. Plasma levels may help in interpreting apparent resistance to treatment and/or unexpected drug toxicity. The principal side effects of TCAs are antihistamine (sedation) and anticholinergic (constipation, dry mouth, urinary hesitancy, blurred vision). Cardiac toxicity due to conduction block or arrhythmias can also occur but is uncommon at therapeutic levels. TCAs are contraindicated in patients with serious cardiovascular risk factors. Overdoses of tricyclic agents can be lethal, with desipramine carrying the greatest risk. It is judicious to prescribe only a 10-day supply when suicide is a risk. Most patients require a daily dose of 150–200 mg of imipramine or amitriptyline or its equivalent to achieve a therapeutic blood level of 150–300 ng/mL and a satisfactory remission; some patients show a partial effect at lower doses. Geriatric patients may require a low starting dose and slow escalation. Ethnic differences in drug metabolism are significant; Hispanic, Asian, and African-American patients generally require lower doses than Caucasians to achieve a comparable blood level. P450 profiling using genetic chip technology may be clinically useful in predicting individual sensitivity.

Second-generation antidepressants include amoxapine, maprotiline, trazodone, and bupropion. Amoxapine is a dibenzoxazepine derivative that blocks norepinephrine and serotonin reuptake and has a metabolite that shows a degree of dopamine blockade. Long-term use of this drug carries a risk of tardive dyskinesia. Maprotiline is a potent noradrenergic reuptake blocker that has little anticholinergic effect but may produce seizures. Bupropion is a novel antidepressant whose mechanism of action is thought to involve enhancement of noradrenergic function. It has no anticholinergic, sedating, or orthostatic side effects and has a low incidence of sexual side effects. It may, however, be associated with stimulant-like side effects, may lower seizure threshold, and has an exceptionally short half-life, requiring frequent dosing. An extended-release preparation is available.

SSRIs such as fluoxetine, sertraline, paroxetine, citalopram, and escitalopram cause a lower frequency of anticholinergic, sedating, and cardiovascular side effects but a possibly greater incidence of gastrointestinal complaints, sleep impairment, and sexual dysfunction than do TCAs. Akathisia, involving an inner sense of restlessness and anxiety in addition to increased motor activity, may also be more common, particularly during the first week of treatment. One concern is the risk of "serotonin syndrome," thought to result from hyperstimulation of brainstem $5HT_{1A}$ receptors and characterized by myoclonus, agitation, abdominal cramping, hyperpyrexia, hypertension, and potentially death. Serotonergic agonists taken in combination should be monitored closely for this reason. Considerations such as half-life, compliance, toxicity, and drug-drug interactions may guide the choice of a particular SSRI. Fluoxetine and its principal active metabolite, norfluoxetine, for example, have a combined half-life of almost 7 days, resulting in a delay of 5 weeks before steady-state levels are achieved and a similar delay for complete drug excretion once its use is discontinued. All the SSRIs may impair sexual function, resulting in diminished libido, impotence, or difficulty in achieving orgasm. Sexual dysfunction frequently results in noncompliance and should be asked about specifically. Sexual dysfunction can sometimes be ameliorated by lowering the dose, by instituting weekend drug holidays (two or three times a month), or by treatment with amantadine (100 mg tid), bethanechol (25 mg tid), buspirone (10 mg tid), or bupropion (100–150 mg/d). Paroxetine appears to be more anticholinergic than either fluoxetine or sertraline, and sertraline carries a lower risk of producing an adverse drug interaction than the other two. Rare side effects of SSRIs include angina due to vasospasm and prolongation of the prothrombin time. Escitalopram is the most specific of currently available SSRIs and appears to have no specific inhibitory effects on the P450 system.

Venlafaxine and duloxetine block the reuptake of both norepinephrine and serotonin but produce relatively little in the way of traditional tricyclic side effects. Unlike the SSRIs, venlafaxine has a relatively linear dose-response curve. Patients should be monitored for a possible increase in diastolic blood pressure, and multiple daily dosing is required because of the drug's short half-life. An extended-release form is available and has a somewhat lower incidence of gastrointestinal side effects. Mirtazapine is a tetracyclic antidepressant that has a unique spectrum of activity. It increases noradrenergic and serotonergic neurotransmission through a blockade of central α_2-adrenergic receptors and postsynaptic $5HT_2$ and $5HT_3$ receptors. It is also strongly antihistaminic and, as such, may produce sedation.

With the exception of citalopram and escitalopram, each of the SSRIs may inhibit one or more cytochrome P450 enzymes. Depending on the specific isoenzyme involved, the metabolism of a number of concomitantly administered medications can be dramatically affected. Fluoxetine and paroxetine, for example, by inhibiting 2D6, can cause dramatic increases in the blood level of type 1C antiarrhythmics, while sertraline, by acting on 3A4, may alter blood levels of carbamazepine, or digoxin.

The MAOIs are highly effective, particularly in atypical depression, but the risk of hypertensive crisis following intake of tyramine-containing food or sympathomimetic drugs makes them inappropriate as first-line agents. Transdermal selegiline may avert this risk at low dose. Common side effects include orthostatic hypotension, weight gain, insomnia, and sexual dysfunction. MAOIs should not be used concomitantly with SSRIs, because of the risk of serotonin syndrome, or with TCAs, because of possible hyperadrenergic effects.

Electroconvulsive therapy is at least as effective as medication, but its use is reserved for treatment-resistant cases and delusional depressions. Transcranial magnetic stimulation (TMS) is an investigational treatment of depression that has been shown to have efficacy in several controlled trials; it is uncertain whether the observed benefits were clinically meaningful, however. Vagus nerve stimulation (VNS) has recently been approved for treatment-resistant depression, but its degree of efficacy is controversial.

Regardless of the treatment undertaken, the response should be evaluated after ~2 months. Three-quarters of patients show improvement by this time, but if remission is inadequate the patient should be questioned about compliance and an increase in medication dose should be considered if side effects are not troublesome. If this approach is unsuccessful, referral to a mental health specialist is advised. Strategies for treatment then include selection of an alternative drug, combinations of antidepressants, and/or adjunctive treatment with other classes of drugs, including lithium, thyroid hormone, and dopamine agonists. A large randomized trial (STAR-D) was unable to show preferential efficacy. Patients whose response to an SSRI wanes over time may benefit from the addition of buspirone (10 mg tid) or pindolol (2–5 mg tid) or small amounts of a TCA such as desipramine (25 mg bid or tid). Most patients will show some degree of response but aggressive treatment should be pursued until remission is achieved, and drug treatment should be continued for at least 6–9 more months to prevent relapse. In patients who have had two or more episodes of depression, indefinite maintenance treatment should be considered.

It is essential to educate patients both about depression and the benefits and side effects of medications they are receiving. Advice about stress reduction and cautions that alcohol may exacerbate depressive symptoms and impair drug response are helpful. Patients should be given time to describe their experience, their outlook, and the impact of the depression on them and their families. Occasional empathic silence may be as helpful for the treatment alliance as verbal reassurance. Controlled trials have shown that cognitive-behavioral and interpersonal therapies are effective in improving psychological and social adjustment and that a combined treatment approach is more successful than medication alone for many patients.

BIPOLAR DISORDER

Clinical Manifestations Bipolar disorder is characterized by unpredictable swings in mood from mania (or hypomania) to depression. Some patients suffer only from recurrent attacks of *mania*, which in its pure form is associated with increased psychomotor activity; excessive social extroversion; decreased need for sleep; impulsivity and impairment in judgment; and expansive, grandiose, and sometimes irritable mood (Table 386-10). In severe mania, patients may experience delusions and paranoid thinking indistinguishable from schizophrenia. Half of patients with bipolar disorder present with a mixture of psychomotor agitation and activation with dysphoria, anxiety, and irritability. It may be difficult to distinguish *mixed mania* from *agitated depression*. In some bipolar patients (*bipolar II disorder*), the full criteria for mania are lacking, and the requisite recurrent depressions are separated by periods of mild activation and increased energy (hypomania). In *cyclothymic disorder*, there are numerous hypomanic periods, usually of relatively short duration, alternating with clusters of depressive symptoms that fail, either in severity or duration, to meet the criteria of major depression. The mood fluctuations are chronic and should be present for at least 2 years before the diagnosis is made.

Manic episodes typically emerge over a period of days to weeks, but onset within hours is possible, usually in the early morning hours. An untreated episode of either depression or mania can be as short as several weeks or last as long as 8–12 months, and rare patients have an unremitting chronic course. The term *rapid cycling* is used for patients who have four or more episodes of either depression or mania in a given year. This pattern occurs in 15% of all patients, almost all of whom are women. In some cases, rapid cycling is linked to an underlying thyroid dysfunction and, in others, it is iatrogenically triggered by prolonged antidepressant treatment. Approximately half of patients have sustained difficulties in work performance and psychosocial functioning.

Bipolar disorder is common, affecting ~1.5% of the population in the United States. Onset is typically between 20 and 30 years of age, but many individuals report premorbid symptoms in late childhood or early adolescence. The prevalence is similar for men and women; women are likely to have more depressive and men more manic episodes over a lifetime.

TABLE 386-10 CRITERIA FOR A MANIC EPISODE

A. A distinct period of abnormally and persistently elevated, expansive, or irritable mood, lasting at least 1 week (or any duration if hospitalization is necessary)

B. During the period of mood disturbance, three (or more) of the following symptoms have persisted (four if the mood is only irritable) and have been present to a significant degree:
1. Inflated self-esteem or grandiosity
2. Decreased need for sleep (e.g., feels rested after only 3 hours of sleep)
3. More talkative than usual or pressure to keep talking
4. Flight of ideas or subjective experience that thoughts are racing
5. Distractibility (i.e., attention too easily drawn to unimportant or irrelevant external stimuli)
6. Increase in goal-directed activity (either socially, at work or school, or sexually) or psychomotor agitation
7. Excessive involvement in pleasurable activities that have a high potential for painful consequences (e.g., engaging in unrestrained buying sprees, sexual indiscretions, or foolish business investments)

C. The symptoms do not meet criteria for a mixed episode.

D. The mood disturbance is sufficiently severe to cause marked impairment in occupational functioning or in usual social activities or relationships with others, or to necessitate hospitalization to prevent harm to self or others, or there are psychotic features.

E. The symptoms are not due to the direct physiologic effects of a substance (e.g., a drug of abuse, a medication, or other treatment) or a general medical condition (e.g., hyperthyroidism).

Note: Manic-like episodes that are clearly caused by somatic antidepressant treatment (e.g., medication, electroconvulsive therapy, light therapy) should not count toward a diagnosis of bipolar I disorder.

Source: *Diagnostic and Statistical Manual of Mental Disorders*, 4th ed. Washington, DC, American Psychiatric Association, 2000.

Differential Diagnosis The differential diagnosis of mania includes toxic effects of stimulant or sympathomimetic drugs as well as secondary mania induced by hyperthyroidism, AIDS, or neurologic disorders, such as Huntington's or Wilson's disease, or cerebrovascular accidents. Comorbidity with alcohol and substance abuse is common, either because of poor judgment and increased impulsivity or because of an attempt to self-treat the underlying mood symptoms and sleep disturbances.

Etiology and Pathophysiology Genetic predisposition to bipolar disorder is evident from family studies; the concordance rate for monozygotic twins approaches 80%. Multiple genes are likely to be involved.

The pathophysiologic mechanisms underlying the profound and recurrent mood swings of bipolar disorder remain unknown. Neuroimaging studies have reported anatomic changes in amygdala volume as well as increases in white matter hyperintensities. Molecular studies have implicated changes in membrane Na^+- and K^+-activated ATPase and disordered signal transduction involving the phosphoinositol system and GTP-binding proteins as possible contributing mechanisms. Patients with bipolar disorder also appear to have altered circadian rhythmicity, and lithium may exert its therapeutic benefit through a resynchronization of intrinsic rhythms keyed to the light/dark cycle.

℞ BIPOLAR DISORDER

(Table 386-11) Lithium carbonate is the mainstay of treatment in bipolar disorder, although sodium valproate and olanzapine are equally effective in acute mania, as is lamotrigine in the depressed phase. The response rate to lithium carbonate is 70–80% in acute mania, with beneficial effects appearing in 1–2 weeks. Lithium also has a prophylactic effect in prevention of recurrent mania and, to a lesser extent, in the prevention of recurrent depression. A simple cation, lithium is rapidly absorbed from the gastrointestinal tract and remains unbound to plasma or tissue proteins. Some 95% of a given dose is excreted unchanged through the kidneys within 24 h.

Serious side effects from lithium are rare, but minor complaints such as gastrointestinal discomfort, nausea, diarrhea, polyuria, weight gain, skin eruptions, alopecia, and edema are common. Over time, urine-concentrating ability may be decreased, but significant nephrotoxicity does not usually occur. Lithium exerts an antithyroid effect by interfering with the

TABLE 386-11 CLINICAL PHARMACOLOGY OF MOOD STABILIZERS

Agent and Dosing	Side Effects and Other Effects

Lithium
  Starting dose: 300 mg bid or tid
  Therapeutic blood level: 0.8–1.2 meq/L
	Common side effects: Nausea/anorexia/diarrhea, fine tremor, thirst, polyuria, fatigue, weight gain, acne, folliculitis, neutrophilia, hypothyroidism
	Blood level is increased by thiazides, tetracyclines, and NSAIDs
	Blood level is decreased by bronchodilators, verapamil, and carbonic anhydrase inhibitors
	Rare side effects: Neurotoxicity, renal toxicity, hypercalcemia, ECG changes

Valproic acid
  Starting dose: 250 mg tid
  Therapeutic blood level: 50–125 µg/mL
	Common side effects: Nausea/anorexia, weight gain, sedation, tremor, rash, alopecia
	Inhibits hepatic metabolism of other medications
	Rare side effects: Pancreatitis, hepatotoxicity, Stevens-Johnson syndrome

Carbamazepine/oxcarbazepine Starting dose: 200 mg bid for carbamazepine, 150 bid for oxcarbazepine Therapeutic blood level: 4–12 µg/mL for carbamazepine	*Common side effects:* Nausea/anorexia, sedation, rash, dizziness/ataxia Carbamazepine, but not oxcarbazepine, induces hepatic metabolism of other medications *Rare side effects:* Hyponatremia, agranulocytosis, Stevens-Johnson syndrome
Lamotrigine Starting dose: 25 mg/d	*Common side effects:* Rash, dizziness, headache, tremor, sedation, nausea *Rare side effect:* Stevens-Johnson syndrome

Note: NSAID, nonsteroidal anti-inflammatory drug; ECG, electrocardiogram.

synthesis and release of thyroid hormones. More serious side effects include tremor, poor concentration and memory, ataxia, dysarthria, and incoordination. There is suggestive, but not conclusive, evidence that lithium is teratogenic, inducing cardiac malformations in the first trimester.

In the treatment of acute mania, lithium is initiated at 300 mg bid or tid, and the dose is then increased by 300 mg every 2–3 days to achieve blood levels of 0.8–1.2 meq/L. Because the therapeutic effect of lithium may not appear until after 7–10 days of treatment, adjunctive usage of lorazepam (1–2 mg every 4 h) or clonazepam (0.5–1 mg every 4 h) may be beneficial to control agitation. Antipsychotics are indicated in patients with severe agitation who respond only partially to benzodiazepines. Patients using lithium should be monitored closely, since the blood levels required to achieve a therapeutic benefit are close to those associated with toxicity.

Valproic acid may be better than lithium for patients who experience rapid cycling (i.e., more than four episodes a year) or who present with a mixed or dysphoric mania. Tremor and weight gain are the most common side effects; hepatotoxicity and pancreatitis are rare toxicities.

Carbamazepine and oxcarbazepine, although not formally approved by the FDA for bipolar disorder, have clinical efficacy in the treatment of acute mania. Second-generation antipsychotic drugs (olanzapine, quetiapine, risperidone, ziprasidone, and aripiprazole) have also been shown to be effective, either alone or in combination with a mood stabilizer. An increased risk of weight gain and other metabolic abnormalities is a concern with these agents.

The recurrent nature of bipolar mood disorder necessitates maintenance treatment. A sustained blood lithium level of at least 0.8 mEq/L is important for optimal prophylaxis and has been shown to reduce risk of suicide, a finding not yet apparent for other mood stabilizers. Compliance is frequently an issue and often requires enlistment and education of concerned family members. Efforts to identify and modify psychosocial factors that may trigger episodes are important, as is an emphasis on lifestyle regularity. Antidepressant medications are sometimes required for the treatment of severe breakthrough depressions, but their use should generally be avoided during maintenance treatment because of the risk of precipitating mania or accelerating the cycle frequency. Loss of efficacy over time may be observed with any of the mood-stabilizing agents. In such situations, an alternative agent or combination therapy is usually helpful.

Consensus guidelines for the treatment of acute mania and bipolar depression are described in **Table 386-12**.

TABLE 386-12 CONSENSUS GUIDELINES FOR DRUG TREATMENT OF ACUTE MANIA AND BIPOLAR DEPRESSION

Condition	Preferred Agents
Euphoric mania	Lithium
Mixed/dysphoric mania	Valproic acid
Mania with psychosis	Valproic acid with olanzapine, conventional antipsychotic, or risperidone
Hypomania	Lithium, lamotrigine, or valproic acid alone
Severe depression with psychosis	Venlafaxine, bupropion, or paroxetine *plus* lithium *plus* olanzapine, *or* risperidone; consider ECT
Severe depression without psychosis	Bupropion, paroxetine, sertraline, venlafaxine, *or* citalopram *plus* lithium
Mild to moderate depression	Lithium *or* lamotrigine alone; add bupropion if needed

Note: ECT, electroconvulsive therapy.
Source: From GS Sachs et al: Postgrad Med, April, 2000.

SOMATOFORM DISORDERS

Clinical Manifestations Patients with multiple somatic complaints that cannot be explained by a known medical condition or by the effects of alcohol or of recreational or prescription drugs are commonly seen in primary care practice; one survey indicated a prevalence of such complaints of 5%. In *somatization disorder*, the patient presents with multiple physical complaints referable to different organ systems (Table 386-13). Onset is usually before age 30, and the disorder is persistent. Formal diagnostic criteria require the recording of at least four pain, two gastrointestinal, one sexual, and one pseudoneurologic symptom. Patients with somatization disorder often present with dramatic complaints, but the complaints are inconsistent. Symptoms of comorbid anxiety and mood disorder are common and may be the result of drug interactions due to regimens initiated independently by different physicians. Patients with somatization disorder may be impulsive and demanding and frequently qualify for a

TABLE 386-13 DIAGNOSTIC CRITERIA FOR SOMATIZATION DISORDER

A. A history of many physical complaints beginning before age 30 that occur over a period of several years and result in treatment being sought or significant impairment in social, occupational, or other important areas of functioning.

B. Each of the following criteria must have been met, with individual symptoms occurring at any time during the course of the disturbance:
  1. *Four pain symptoms:* a history of pain related to at least four different sites or functions (e.g., head, abdomen, back, joints, extremities, chest, rectum, during menstruation, during sexual intercourse, or during urination)
  2. *Two gastrointestinal symptoms:* a history of at least two gastrointestinal symptoms other than pain (e.g., nausea, bloating, vomiting other than during pregnancy, diarrhea, or intolerance of several different foods)
  3. *One sexual symptom:* a history of at least one sexual or reproductive symptom other than pain (e.g., sexual indifference, erectile or ejaculatory dysfunction, irregular menses, excessive menstrual bleeding, vomiting throughout pregnancy)
  4. *One pseudoneurologic symptom:* a history of at least one symptom or deficit suggesting a neurologic condition not limited to pain (conversion symptoms such as impaired coordination or balance, paralysis or localized weakness, difficulty swallowing or lump in throat, aphonia, urinary retention, hallucinations, loss of touch or pain sensation, double vision, blindness, deafness, seizures; dissociative symptoms such as amnesia; or loss of consciousness other than fainting)

C. Either of the following:
  1. After appropriate investigation, each of the symptoms in criterion B cannot be fully explained by a known general medical condition or the direct effects of a substance (e.g., a drug of abuse, a medication)
  2. When there is a related general medical condition, the physical complaints or resulting social or occupational impairment are in excess of what would be expected from the history, physical examination, or laboratory findings

D. The symptoms are not intentionally produced or feigned (as in factitious disorder or malingering).

Source: *Diagnostic and Statistical Manual of Mental Disorders*, 4th ed. Washington, DC, American Psychiatric Association, 2000.

formal comorbid psychiatric diagnosis. In *conversion disorder*, the symptoms focus on deficits that involve motor or sensory function and on psychological factors that initiate or exacerbate the medical presentation. Like somatization disorder, the deficit is not intentionally produced or simulated, as is the case in factitious disorder (malingering). In *hypochondriasis*, the essential feature is a belief of serious medical illness that persists despite reassurance and appropriate medical evaluation. As with somatization disorder, patients with hypochondriasis have a history of poor relationships with physicians stemming from their sense that they have been evaluated and treated inappropriately or inadequately. Hypochondriasis can be disabling in intensity and is persistent, with waxing and waning symptomatology.

In *factitious illnesses*, the patient consciously and voluntarily produces physical symptoms of illness. The term *Munchausen's syndrome* is reserved for individuals with particularly dramatic, chronic, or severe factitious illness. In true factitious illness, the sick role itself is gratifying. A variety of signs, symptoms, and diseases have been either simulated or caused by factitious behavior, the most common including chronic diarrhea, fever of unknown origin, intestinal bleeding or hematuria, seizures, and hypoglycemia. Factitious disorder is usually not diagnosed until 5–10 years after its onset, and it can produce significant social and medical costs. In *malingering*, the fabrication derives from a desire for some external reward, such as a narcotic medication or disability reimbursement.

℞ SOMATOFORM DISORDERS

Patients with somatization disorders are frequently subjected to many diagnostic tests and exploratory surgeries in an attempt to find their "real" illness. Such an approach is doomed to failure and does not address the core issue. Successful treatment is best achieved through behavior modification, in which access to the physician is tightly regulated and adjusted to provide a sustained and predictable level of support that is less clearly contingent on the patient's level of presenting distress. Visits can be brief and should not be associated with a need for a diagnostic or treatment action. Although the literature is limited, some patients with somatization disorder may benefit from antidepressant treatment.

Any attempt to confront the patient usually creates a sense of humiliation and causes the patient to abandon treatment from that caregiver. A better strategy is to introduce psychological causation as one of a number of possible explanations and to include factitious illness as an option in the differential diagnoses that are discussed. Without directly linking psychotherapeutic intervention to the diagnosis, the patient can be offered a face-saving means by which the pathologic relationship with the health care system can be examined and alternative approaches to life stressors developed.

PERSONALITY DISORDERS

Clinical Manifestations Personality disorders are characteristic patterns of thinking, feeling, and interpersonal behavior that are relatively inflexible and cause significant functional impairment or subjective distress for the individual. The observed behaviors are not secondary to another mental disorder, nor are they precipitated by substance abuse or a general medical condition. This distinction is often difficult to make in clinical practice, as personality change may be the first sign of serious neurologic, endocrine, or other medical illness. Patients with frontal lobe tumors, for example, can present with changes in motivation and personality while the results of the neurologic examination remain within normal limits. Individuals with personality disorders are often regarded as "difficult patients" in clinical medical practice because they are seen as excessively demanding and/or unwilling to follow recommended treatment plans. Although DSM-IV portrays personality disorders as qualitatively distinct categories, there is an alternative perspective that personality characteristics vary as a continuum between normal functioning and formal mental disorder.

Personality disorders have been grouped into three overlapping clusters. *Cluster A* includes paranoid, schizoid, and schizotypal personality disorders. It includes individuals who are odd and eccentric and who maintain an emotional distance from others. Individuals have a restricted emotional range and remain socially isolated. Patients with schizotypal personality disorder frequently have unusual perceptual experiences and express magical beliefs about the external world. The essential feature of paranoid personality disorder is a pervasive mistrust and suspiciousness of others to an extent that is unjustified by available evidence. *Cluster B* disorders include antisocial, borderline, histrionic, and narcissistic types and describe individuals whose behavior is impulsive, excessively emotional, and erratic. *Cluster C* incorporates avoidant, dependent, and obsessive-compulsive personality types; enduring traits are anxiety and fear. The boundaries between cluster types are to some extent artificial, and many patients who meet criteria for one personality disorder also meet criteria for aspects of another. The risk of a comorbid major mental disorder is increased in patients who qualify for a diagnosis of personality disorder.

℞ PERSONALITY DISORDERS

Dialectical behavior therapy (DBT) is a cognitive-behavioral approach that focuses on behavioral change while providing acceptance, compassion, and validation of the patient. Several randomized trials have demonstrated the efficacy of DBT in the treatment of personality disorders. Antidepressant medications and low-dose antipsychotic drugs have some efficacy in cluster A personality disorders, while anticonvulsant mood-stabilizing agents and MAOIs may be considered for patients with cluster B diagnoses who show marked mood reactivity, behavioral dyscontrol, and/or rejection hypersensitivity. Anxious or fearful cluster C patients often respond to medications used for axis I anxiety disorders (see above). It is important that the physician and the patient have reasonable expectations vis-à-vis the possible benefit of any medication used and its side effects. Improvement may be subtle and observable only over time.

SCHIZOPHRENIA

Clinical Manifestations Schizophrenia is a heterogeneous syndrome characterized by perturbations of language, perception, thinking, social activity, affect, and volition. There are no pathognomonic features. The syndrome commonly begins in late adolescence, has an insidious (and less commonly acute) onset, and, often, a poor outcome, progressing from social withdrawal and perceptual distortions to recurrent delusions and hallucinations. Patients may present with positive symptoms (such as conceptual disorganization, delusions, or hallucinations) or negative symptoms (loss of function, anhedonia, decreased emotional expression, impaired concentration, and diminished social engagement) and must have at least two of these for a 1-month period and continuous signs for at least 6 months to meet formal diagnostic criteria. As individuals age, positive psychotic symptoms tend to attenuate and some measure of social and occupational function may be regained. "Negative" symptoms predominate in one-third of the schizophrenic population and are associated with a poor long-term outcome and a poor response to drug treatment. However, marked variability in the course and individual character of symptoms is typical.

The four main subtypes of schizophrenia are catatonic, paranoid, disorganized, and residual. Many individuals have symptoms of more than one type. *Catatonic-type* describes patients whose clinical presentation is dominated by profound changes in motor activity, negativism, and echolalia or echopraxia. *Paranoid-type* describes patients who have a prominent preoccupation with a specific delusional system and who otherwise do not qualify as having *disorganized-type* disease, in which disorganized speech and behavior are accompanied by a superficial or silly affect. In *residual-type* disease, negative symptomatology exists in the absence of delusions, hallucinations, or motor disturbance. The term *schizophreniform disorder* describes patients who meet the symptom requirements but not the duration requirements for schizophrenia, and *schizoaffective disorder* is used for those who manifest symptoms of schizophrenia and independent periods of mood disturbance. Prognosis depends not on symptom severity but on the response to antipsychotic medication. A permanent remission

without recurrence does occasionally occur. About 10% of schizophrenic patients commit suicide.

Schizophrenia is present in 0.85% of individuals worldwide, with a lifetime prevalence of ~1–1.5%. An estimated 300,000 episodes of acute schizophrenia occur annually in the United States, resulting in direct and indirect costs of $62.7 billion.

Differential Diagnosis The diagnosis is principally one of exclusion, requiring the absence of significant associated mood symptoms, any relevant medical condition, and substance abuse. Drug reactions that cause hallucinations, paranoia, confusion, or bizarre behavior may be dose-related or idiosyncratic; parkinsonian medications, clonidine, quinacrine, and procaine derivatives are the most common prescription medications associated with these symptoms. Drug causes should be ruled out in any case of newly emergent psychosis. The general neurologic examination in patients with schizophrenia is usually normal, but motor rigidity, tremor, and dyskinesias are noted in one-quarter of untreated patients.

Epidemiology and Pathophysiology Epidemiologic surveys identify several risk factors for schizophrenia including genetic susceptibility, early developmental insults, winter birth, and increasing parental age. Genetic factors are involved in at least a subset of individuals who develop schizophrenia. Schizophrenia is observed in ~6.6% of all first-degree relatives of an affected proband. If both parents are affected, the risk for offspring is 40%. The concordance rate for monozygotic twins is 50%, compared to 10% for dizygotic twins. Schizophrenia-prone families are also at risk for other psychiatric disorders, including schizoaffective disorder and *schizotypal* and *schizoid personality disorders*, the latter terms designating individuals who show a lifetime pattern of social and interpersonal deficits characterized by an inability to form close interpersonal relationships, eccentric behavior, and mild perceptual distortions.

Despite evidence for a genetic causation, the results of molecular genetic linkage studies in schizophrenia are inconclusive. Major gene effects appear unlikely. Possible susceptibility genes include: neuregulin-1 (chromosome 8p21); dysbindin (6p22.3); proline dehydrogenase (22q11); D-amino-acid oxidase activator (13q34); disrupted in schizophrenia 1, (DISC1), (1q42); and catechol-O-methyl transferase (COMT). Neuregulin-1, dysbindin, and D-amino-acid oxidase activator appear to be involved in glutamatergic function, increasing interest in *N*-methyl-D-aspartate (NMDA)–mediated glutamate signaling as a possible therapeutic target for treatment. COMT is involved in the removal of dopamine from synapses, and DISC1 is a scaffolding protein that participates in a variety of protein-protein interactions important in neuronal development. One group has reported risk variants in the α7 nicotinic acetylcholine receptor subunit gene and linked it to a specific auditory processing deficit.

Schizophrenia is also associated with gestational and perinatal complications, including Rh factor incompatibility, fetal hypoxia, prenatal exposure to influenza during the second trimester, and prenatal nutritional deficiency. Studies of monozygotic twins discordant for schizophrenia have reported neuroanatomic differences between affected and unaffected siblings, supporting a "two-strike" etiology involving both genetic susceptibility and an environmental insult. The latter might involve localized hypoxia during critical stages of brain development.

A number of structural and functional abnormalities have been identified in schizophrenia, including (1) cortical atrophy and ventricular enlargement; (2) specific volume losses in the amygdala, hippocampus, right prefrontal cortex, fusiform gyrus, and thalamus; (3) progressive reduction in cortical volume over time; (4) reduced metabolism in the thalamus and prefrontal cortex; (5) abnormalities of the planum temporale; and (6) changes in the size, orientation, and density of cells in the hippocampus and prefrontal cortex, and decreased numbers of cortical interneurons. These observations have suggested that schizophrenia may result from a disturbance in a cortical striatal–thalamic circuit resulting in abnormalities in sensory filtering and attention.

Schizophrenic individuals are highly distractible and demonstrate deficits in perceptual-motor speed, ability to shift attention, and filtering out of background stimuli. Event-related evoked potential studies of schizophrenia have defined a reduction in P300 amplitude to a novel stimulus,

TABLE 386-14 ANTIPSYCHOTIC AGENTS

Name	Usual PO Daily Dose, mg	Side Effects	Sedation	Comments
First-Generation Antipsychotics				
Low-potency				
Chlorpromazine (Thorazine)	100–1000	Anticholinergic effects; orthostasis; photosensitivity; cholestasis; QT prolongation	+ + +	EPSEs usually not prominent; can cause anticholinergic delirium in elderly patients
Thioridazine (Mellaril)	100–600			
Clozapine (Clozaril)	150–600	Agranulocytosis (1%); weight gain; seizures; drooling; hyperthermia	+ +	Requires weekly WBC for first 6 months, then biweekly if stable
Mid-potency				
Trifluoperazine (Stelazine)	2–50	Fewer anticholinergic side effects; fewer EPSEs than with higher potency agents.	+ +	Well tolerated by most patients
Perphenazine (Trilafon)	4–64		++	
Loxapine (Loxitane)	30–100	Frequent EPSEs	+ +	
Molindone (Moban)	30–100	Frequent EPSEs	0	Little weight gain
High-potency				
Haloperidol (Haldol)	.5–20	No anticholinergic side effects; EPSEs often prominent	0/+	Often prescribed in doses that are too high; long-acting injectable forms of haloperidol and fluphenazine available
Fluphenazine (Prolixin)	1–20	Frequent EPSEs	0/+	
Thiothixene (Navane)	2–50	Frequent EPSEs	0/+	
Second-Generation Antipsychotics				
Risperidone (Risperdal)	2–8	Orthostasis	+	Requires slow titration; EPSEs observed with doses >6 mg qd
Olanzapine (Zyprexa)	10–30	Weight gain	+ +	Mild prolactin elevation
Quetiapine (Seroquel)	350–800	Sedation; weight gain; anxiety	+ + +	Bid dosing
Ziprasidone (Geodon)	120–200	Orthostatic hypotension	+/++	Minimal weight gain; increases QT interval
Aripiprazole (Abilify)	10–30	Nausea, anxiety, insomnia	0/+	Mixed agonist/antagonist

Note: EPSEs, extrapyramidal side effects; WBC, white blood count.

which implicates an impairment in cognitive processing. Impaired information processing is also found in unaffected family members.

The *dopamine hypothesis* of schizophrenia is based on the discovery that agents that diminish dopaminergic activity also reduce the acute symptoms and signs of psychosis, specifically agitation, anxiety, and hallucinations. Amelioration of delusions and social withdrawal is less dramatic. Thus far, however, evidence for increased dopaminergic activity in schizophrenia is indirect, although decreased D_2 receptor occupancy by dopamine has been shown in drug-naïve patients. An increase in the activity of nigrostriatal and mesolimbic systems and a decrease in mesocortical tracts innervating the prefrontal cortex is hypothesized, although it is likely that other neurotransmitters, including serotonin, acetylcholine, glutamate, and GABA, also contribute to the pathophysiology of the illness. Possible involvement of excitatory amino acids is supported by the genetic data cited above and findings that NMDA receptor antagonists and channel blockers, such as phencyclidine (PCP) and ketamine, produce characteristic signs of schizophrenia in normal individuals; cycloserine, an NMDA receptor agonist, can decrease the negative symptoms of psychosis.

℞ SCHIZOPHRENIA

Antipsychotic agents (Table 386-14) are the cornerstone of acute and maintenance treatment of schizophrenia and are effective in the treatment of hallucinations, delusions and thought disorders, regardless of etiology. The mechanism of action involves, at least in part, binding to dopamine D_2/D_3 receptors in the ventral striatum; the clinical potencies of traditional antipsychotic drugs parallel their affinities for the D_2 receptor, and even the newer "atypical" agents exert some degree of D_2 receptor blockade. All neuroleptics induce expression of the immediate-early gene c-*fos* in the nucleus accumbens, a dopaminergic site connecting prefrontal and limbic cortices. The clinical efficacy of newer atypical neuroleptics, however, may involve NMDA receptor blockade, α_1- and α_2-noradrenergic activity, altering the relationship between $5HT_2$ and D_2 receptor activity, as well as faster dissociation of D_2 binding and effects on neuroplasticity.

Conventional neuroleptics differ in their potency and side-effect profile. Older agents, such as chlorpromazine and thioridazine, are more sedating and anticholinergic and more likely to cause orthostatic hypotension, while higher potency antipsychotics, such as haloperidol, perphenazine, and thiothixene, are more likely to induce extrapyramidal side effects. The model first-generation antipsychotic agent is *clozapine*, a dibenzodiazepine that has a greater potency in blocking the $5HT_2$ than the D_2 receptor and a much higher affinity for the D_4 than the D_2 receptor. Its principal disadvantage is a risk of blood dyscrasias. Unlike other antipsychotics, clozapine does not cause a rise in prolactin level. Approximately 30% of patients who do not benefit from conventional antipsychotic agents will have a better response to this drug, which also has a demonstrated superiority to other antipsychotic agents in preventing suicide; however, its side-effect profile makes it most appropriate for treatment-resistant cases. *Risperidone*, a benzisoxazole derivative, is more potent at $5HT_2$ than D_2 receptor sites, like clozapine, but it also exerts significant α_2 antagonism, a property that may contribute to its perceived ability to improve mood and increase motor activity. Risperidone is not as effective as clozapine in treatment-resistant cases but does not carry a risk of blood dyscrasias. *Olanzapine* is similar neurochemically to clozapine but has a significant risk of inducing weight gain. *Quetiapine* is distinct in having a weak D_2 effect but potent α_1 and histamine blockade. *Ziprasidone* causes minimal weight gain and is unlikely to increase prolactin but may increase QT prolongation. *Aripiprazole* also has little risk of weight gain or prolactin increase but may increase anxiety, nausea, and insomnia as a result of its partial agonist properties.

Antipsychotic agents are effective in 70% of patients presenting with a first episode. Improvement may be observed within hours or days, but full remission usually requires 6–8 weeks. The choice of agent depends principally on the side-effect profile and cost of treatment or on a past personal or family history of a favorable response to the drug in question. Atypical agents appear to be more effective in treating negative symptoms and improving cognitive function. An equivalent treatment response can usually be achieved with relatively low doses of any drug selected, i.e., 4–6 mg/d of haloperidol, 10–15 mg of olanzapine, or 4–6 mg/d of risperidone. Doses in this range result in >80% D_2 receptor blockade, and there is little evidence that higher doses increase either the rapidity or degree of response. Maintenance treatment requires careful attention to the possibility of relapse and monitoring for the development of a movement disorder. Intermittent drug treatment is less effective than regular dosing, but gradual dose reduction is likely to improve social functioning in many schizophrenic patients who have been maintained at high doses. If medications are completely discontinued, however, the relapse rate is 60% within 6 months. Long-acting injectable preparations (risperidone) are considered when noncompliance with oral therapy leads to relapses. In treatment-resistant patients, a transition to clozapine usually results in rapid improvement, but a prolonged delay in response in some cases necessitates a 6- to 9-month trial for maximal benefit to occur.

Antipsychotic medications can cause a broad range of side effects, including lethargy, weight gain, postural hypotension, constipation, and dry mouth. Extrapyramidal symptoms such as dystonia, akathisia, and akinesia are also frequent with first-generation agents and may contribute to poor adherence if not specifically addressed. Anticholinergic and parkinsonian symptoms respond well to trihexyphenidyl, 2 mg bid, or benztropine mesylate, 1–2 mg bid. Akathisia may respond to beta blockers. In rare cases, more serious and occasionally life-threatening side effects may emerge, including ventricular arrhythmias, gastrointestinal obstruction, retinal pigmentation, obstructive jaundice, and neuroleptic malignant syndrome (characterized by hyperthermia, autonomic dysfunction, muscular rigidity, and elevated creatine phosphokinase levels). The most serious adverse effects of clozapine are agranulocytosis, which has an incidence of 1%, and induction of seizures, which has an incidence of 10%. Weekly white blood cell counts are required, particularly during the first 3 months of treatment.

The risk of type 2 diabetes mellitus appears to be increased in schizophrenia, and second-generation agents as a group produce greater adverse effects on glucose regulation, independent of effects on obesity, than traditional agents. Clozapine, olanzapine, and quetiapine seem more likely to cause hyperglycemia, weight gain, and hypertriglyceridemia than other atypical antipsychotic drugs. Close monitoring of plasma glucose and lipid levels are indicated with the use of these agents.

A serious side effect of long-term use of first generation antipsychotic agents is *tardive dyskinesia*, characterized by repetitive, involuntary, and potentially irreversible movements of the tongue and lips (bucco-linguo-masticatory triad), and, in approximately half of cases, choreoathetosis. Tardive dyskinesia has an incidence of 2–4% per year of exposure, and a prevalence of 20% in chronically treated patients. The prevalence increases with age, total dose, and duration of drug administration. The risk associated with second-generation agents appears to be much lower. The cause may involve formation of free radicals and perhaps mitochondrial energy failure. Vitamin E may reduce abnormal involuntary movements if given early in the syndrome.

The CATIE study, a large scale investigation of the effectiveness of antipsychotic agents in "real world" patients, revealed a high rate of discontinuation of treatment over 18 months. Olanzapine showed greater effectiveness than quetiapine, risperidone, perphenazine, or ziprasidone but also a higher discontinuation rate due to weight gain and metabolic effects. Surprisingly, perphenazine, a first-generation agent, showed little evidence of inferiority to newer drugs.

Drug treatment of schizophrenia is by itself insufficient. Educational efforts directed toward families and relevant community resources have proved to be necessary to maintain stability and optimize outcome. A treatment model involving a multidisciplinary case-management team that seeks out and closely follows the patient in the community has proved particularly effective.

ASSESSMENT AND EVALUATION OF VIOLENCE

Primary care physicians may encounter situations in which family, domestic, or societal violence is discovered or suspected. Such an awareness can carry legal and moral obligations; many state laws mandate reporting of child, spousal, and elder abuse. Physicians are frequently the first point of contact for both victim and abuser. Approximately 2 million older Americans and 1.5 million U.S. children are thought to experience some form of physical maltreatment each year. Spousal abuse is thought to be even more prevalent. An interview study of 24,000 women in ten countries found a lifetime prevalence of physical or sexual violence that ranged from 15–71%; these individuals are more likely to suffer from depression, anxiety, somatization disorder, and substance abuse and to have attempted suicide.

In addition, abused individuals frequently express low self-esteem, vague somatic symptomatology, social isolation, and a passive feeling of loss of control. Although it is essential to treat these elements in the victim, the first obligation is to ensure that the perpetrator has taken responsibility for preventing any further violence. Substance abuse and/or dependence and serious mental illness in the abuser may contribute to the risk of harm and require direct intervention. Depending on the situation, law enforcement agencies, community resources such as support groups and shelters, and individual and family counseling can be appropriate components of a treatment plan. A safety plan should be formulated with the victim, in addition to providing information about abuse, its likelihood of recurrence, and its tendency to increase in severity and frequency. Antianxiety and antidepressant medications may sometimes be useful in treating the acute symptoms, but only if independent evidence for an appropriate psychiatric diagnosis exists.

MENTAL HEALTH PROBLEMS IN THE HOMELESS

There is a high prevalence of mental disorders and substance abuse among homeless and impoverished individuals. Depending on the definition used, estimates of the total number of homeless individuals in the United States range from 800,000 to 2 million, one-third of whom qualify as having a serious mental disorder. Poor hygiene and nutrition, substance abuse, psychiatric illness, physical trauma, and exposure to the elements combine to make the provision of medical care challenging. Only a minority of these individuals receive formal mental health care; the main points of contact are outpatient medical clinics and emergency departments. Primary care settings represent a critical site in which housing needs, treatment of substance dependence, and evaluation and treatment of psychiatric illness can most efficiently take place. Successful intervention is dependent on breaking down traditional administrative barriers to health care and recognizing the physical constraints and emotional costs imposed by homelessness. Simplifying health care instructions and follow-up, allowing frequent visits, and dispensing medications in limited amounts that require ongoing contact are possible techniques for establishing a successful therapeutic relationship.

FURTHER READINGS

AMERICAN PSYCHIATRIC ASSOCIATION: *American Psychiatric Association Practice Guidelines for the Treatment of Psychiatric Disorders*: Compendium 2006. Washington, DC, APA Press, 2006

GALE C, DAVIDSON O: Generalised anxiety disorder. BMJ 334:579, 2007

KARLIN BE, FULLER JD: Meeting the mental health needs of older adults. Geriatrics 62:26, 2007

LESPERANCE F et al: Effects of citalopram and interpersonal psychotherapy on depression in patients with coronary artery disease: The Canadian Cardiac Randomized Evaluation of Antidepressant and Psychotherapy Efficacy (CREATE) trial. JAMA 297:367, 2007

LIEBERMAN JA: Effectiveness of antipsychotic drugs in patients with chronic schizophrenia: Efficacy, safety and cost outcomes of CATIE and other trials. J Clin Psychiatry 68:e04, 2007

MAURER D, COLT R: An evidence-based approach to the management of depression. Prim Care 33:923, 2007

SACHS GS et al: Effectiveness of adjunctive antidepressant treatment for bipolar depression. N Engl J Med 356:1711, 2007

SCHANZER B et al: Homelessness, health status, and health care use. Am J Public Health 97:464, 2007

STEIN DJ et al: Post-traumatic stress disorder: Medicine and politics. Lancet 369:139, 2007

STEPHENSON DT, PRICE JR: Medically unexplained physical symptoms in emergency medicine. Emerg Med J 23:595, 2006

TYLEE A, WALTERS P: Underrecognition of anxiety and mood disorders in primary care: Why does the problem exist and what can be done? J Clin Pyschiatry 68(Suppl 2):27, 2007

387 Alcohol and Alcoholism

Marc A. Schuckit

Alcohol, a drug, is consumed at some time by up to 80% of the population. At low doses alcohol can have some beneficial effects such as decreased rates of myocardial infarction, stroke, gallstones, and possibly vascular and Alzheimer's dementias. However, the consumption of more than two standard drinks per day increases the risk for health problems in many organ systems. Heavy repetitive drinking, as is seen in alcohol abuse and dependence, cuts short the life span by an estimated decade in both genders, all cultural groups, and all socioeconomic strata. Unless an individual stops drinking, a diagnosis of alcohol dependence carries a ≥80% risk for continued severe problems over the next 5 years. In addition, even relatively low doses of alcohol can adversely affect many preexisting disease states and alter the effectiveness or blood levels of most over-the-counter and prescribed medications.

PHARMACOLOGY AND NUTRITIONAL IMPACT OF ETHANOL

Ethanol is a weakly charged molecule that moves easily through cell membranes, rapidly equilibrating between blood and tissues. The level of alcohol in the blood is expressed as milligrams or grams of ethanol per deciliter (e.g., 100 mg/dL or 0.10 g/dL), with blood values of about 0.02 g/dL resulting from the ingestion of one typical drink. In round figures, 340 mL (12 oz) of beer, 115 mL (4 oz) of nonfortified wine, and 43 mL (1.5 oz) (a shot) of 80-proof beverage such as whisky, gin, or vodka each contain ~10–15 g of ethanol; 0.5 L (1 pint) of 80-proof beverage contains ~160 g (about 16 standard drinks), and 1 L of wine contains ~80 g of ethanol. These beverages also have additional components, called *congeners*, that affect the taste and effects; congeners include low-molecular-weight alcohols (e.g., methanol and butanol), aldehydes, esters, histamine, phenols, tannins, iron, lead, and cobalt. Such congeners might also contribute to the adverse health consequences associated with heavy drinking.

Ethanol is a central nervous system (CNS) depressant that decreases neuronal activity, although some behavioral stimulation is observed at low blood levels. This drug has cross-tolerance with other depressants, including benzodiazepines and barbiturates, and all produce similar behavioral alterations. Alcohol is absorbed from mucous membranes of the mouth and esophagus (in small amounts), from the stomach and large bowel (in modest amounts), and from the proximal portion of the small intestine (the major site). The rate of absorption is increased by

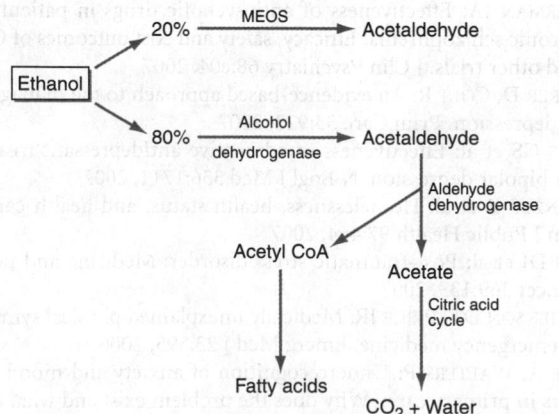

FIGURE 387-1 The metabolism of alcohol. MEOS, microsomal ethanol-oxidizing system.

rapid gastric emptying (as can be induced by carbonated beverages); by the absence of proteins, fats, or carbohydrates (which interfere with absorption); by the absence of congeners; and by dilution to a modest percentage of ethanol (maximum at ~20% by volume).

Between 2% (at low blood alcohol concentrations) and 10% (at high blood alcohol concentrations) of ethanol is excreted directly through the lungs, urine, or sweat, but the greater part is metabolized to acetaldehyde, primarily in the liver. The most important pathway occurs in the cell cytosol where alcohol dehydrogenase (ADH) produces acetaldehyde, which is then rapidly destroyed by aldehyde dehydrogenase (ALDH) in the cytosol and mitochondria (Fig. 387-1). A second pathway in the microsomes of the smooth endoplasmic reticulum (the microsomal ethanol-oxidizing system, or MEOS), is responsible for ≥10% of ethanol oxidation at high blood alcohol concentrations.

While alcohol supplies calories (a drink contains ~300 kJ, or 70–100 kcal), these are devoid of nutrients such as minerals, proteins, and vitamins. Alcohol can also interfere with absorption of vitamins in the small intestine and decreases their storage in the liver with modest effects on folate (folacin or folic acid), pyridoxine (B_6), thiamine (B_1), nicotinic acid (niacin, B_3), and vitamin A.

An ethanol load in a fasting, healthy individual is likely to produce transient hypoglycemia within 6–36 h, secondary to the acute actions of ethanol on gluconeogenesis. This can temporarily result in abnormal glucose tolerance tests (with a resulting erroneous diagnosis of diabetes mellitus) until the alcoholic has abstained for 2–4 weeks. Alcohol ketoacidosis, probably reflecting a decrease in fatty acid oxidation coupled with poor diet or recurrent vomiting, can be misdiagnosed as diabetic ketosis. With the former, patients show an increase in serum ketones along with a mild increase in glucose but a large anion gap, a mild to moderate increase in serum lactate, and a β-hydroxybutyrate/lactate ratio of between 2:1 and 9:1 (with normal being 1:1).

BEHAVIORAL EFFECTS, TOLERANCE, AND DEPENDENCE

The acute effects of a drug depend on many factors. These include the dose, the rate of increase in plasma, the concomitant presence of other drugs, and the past experience with the agent. With alcohol, an additional factor is whether blood alcohol levels are rising or falling; the effects are more intense during the former period.

"Legal intoxication" in the United States requires a blood alcohol concentration of at least 0.08–0.10 g/dL, while levels of 0.04 or even lower are cited in some other countries. However, behavioral, psychomotor, and cognitive changes are seen at levels as low as 0.02–0.03 g/dL (i.e., after one to two drinks) (Table 387-1). Deep but disturbed sleep can be seen at twice the legal intoxication level, and death can occur with levels between 0.30 and 0.40 g/dL. Beverage alcohol is probably responsible for more overdose deaths than any other drug.

The intoxicating effects of alcohol reflect the actions of this drug on a wide range of neurotransmitters, receptors, and transporters. Most prominently, alcohol acutely enhances actions at γ-aminobutyric acid

TABLE 387-1	EFFECTS OF BLOOD ALCOHOL LEVELS IN THE ABSENCE OF TOLERANCE
Blood Level, g/dL	**Usual Effect**
0.02	Decreased inhibitions, a slight feeling of intoxication
0.08	Decrease in complex cognitive functions and motor performance
0.20	Obvious slurred speech, motor incoordination, irritability, and poor judgment
0.30	Light coma and depressed vital signs
0.40	Death

A (GABA$_A$) receptors and inhibits N-methyl-D-aspartate (NMDA) receptors. There are also effects on adenosine, with an inhibition of uptake of this transmitter, and a translocation of the cyclic AMP–dependent protein kinase catalytic subunit from the cytoplasm to the nucleus. Alcohol also affects opioid systems and cannabinol receptors, enhances activity of the dopamine-rich reward system, increases serotonin actions, and directly or indirectly affects most other neurochemical systems. As with most depressants, neurons adapt quickly to these actions, and tolerance to many effects develops; after repeated exposure, abrupt decreases in blood alcohol levels are likely to produce physiologic changes that are opposite to the acute effects of this drug (i.e., withdrawal). The presence of tolerance and/or withdrawal characterizes physical dependence.

Tolerance is a complex phenomenon involving at least three types of compensatory mechanisms. (1) After 1–2 weeks of daily drinking, *metabolic or pharmacokinetic tolerance* can be seen, with up to a 30% increase in the rate of hepatic ethanol metabolism. This alteration disappears almost as rapidly as it develops. (2) *Cellular or pharmacodynamic tolerance* develops through neurochemical changes that maintain relatively normal physiologic functioning despite the presence of alcohol. Subsequent decreases in blood levels contribute to symptoms of withdrawal. (3) Individuals learn to adapt their behavior so that they can function better than expected under influence of the drug (*behavioral tolerance*).

The cellular changes caused by chronic ethanol exposure may not resolve for several weeks or longer following cessation of drinking. The resulting withdrawal syndrome is most intense during the first 5 days, but some symptoms (e.g., disturbed sleep and anxiety) can take up to 4–6 months to resolve.

THE EFFECTS OF ETHANOL ON ORGAN SYSTEMS

Although one to two drinks per day in an otherwise healthy and nonpregnant individual can have some beneficial cardiovascular effects, at higher doses alcohol is toxic to most organ systems. Knowledge about the deleterious effects of alcohol helps the physician to identify alcoholic patients and provides information that can be used to help motivate patients to abstain. The information offered here generally applies to all, regardless of age or gender, although some differences apply. It is important to remember that the typical white- or blue-collar alcoholic often functions at a fairly high level for years, holding a job and maintaining ties with friends and relatives who may be unaware of the severity of the drinking problem. Not everyone develops each of the problems described below.

NERVOUS SYSTEM

Approximately 35% of drinkers (and a much higher proportion of alcoholics) experience a *blackout*, an episode of temporary anterograde amnesia, in which the person forgets all or part of what occurred during a drinking evening. Another common problem, one seen after as few as several drinks, is disturbed sleep. Although alcohol might initially help a person to fall asleep, it disrupts sleep throughout the rest of the night. The stages of sleep are also altered, and time spent in rapid eye movement (REM) and deep sleep is reduced. Patients may experience prominent and sometimes disturbing dreams. Alcohol relaxes muscles in the pharynx, which can cause snoring and exacerbate sleep apnea; symptoms of the latter occur in 75% of alcoholic men over age 60. Another common consequence of alcohol use is impaired judgment and coordination, increasing the risk of accidents and injury; 40% of drinkers in the United States have at some time driven while intoxicated. Heavy drinking can also be associated with headache, thirst, nausea, vomiting, and fatigue the following day, a hangover syndrome that is responsible for significant financial losses in most work environments.

The effect of alcohol on the nervous system is even more pronounced among alcohol-dependent individuals. Chronic high doses cause *peripheral neuropathy* in 5–15% of alcoholics: similar to diabetes, patients experience bilateral limb numbness, tingling, and paresthesias, all of which are more pronounced distally. Approximately 1%

of alcoholics develop cerebellar degeneration or atrophy. This is a syndrome of progressive unsteady stance and gait often accompanied by mild nystagmus; neuroimaging studies reveal atrophy of the cerebellar vermis. Fortunately, very few alcoholics (perhaps as few as 1 in 500) develop *Wernicke's* (ophthalmoparesis, ataxia, and encephalopathy) and *Korsakoff's* (retrograde and anterograde amnesia) *syndromes*. These occur as the result of thiamine deficiency, especially in predisposed individuals, e.g., those with transketolase deficiency. Alcoholics can manifest *cognitive problems* lasting for weeks to months after an alcoholic binge. Brain atrophy, evident as ventricular enlargement and widened cortical sulci on MRI and CT scans, occurs in ~50% of chronic alcoholics; these changes are often reversible if abstinence is maintained. There is no single alcoholic dementia syndrome; rather, this label is used to describe patients who have apparently irreversible cognitive changes (possibly from diverse causes) in the context of chronic alcoholism.

As many as two-thirds of alcohol-dependent individuals meet the criteria for a psychiatric syndrome in the *Fourth Diagnostic and Statistical Manual* (DSM-IV) of the American Psychiatric Association (Chap. 386). Half of these relate to a preexisting antisocial personality manifesting as impulsivity and disinhibition. The lifetime risk is 3% in males, and ≥80% of such individuals demonstrate alcohol and/or drug dependence. Another common co-morbidity occurs with dependence on illicit substances. The remaining third of alcoholics with psychiatric syndromes have preexisting conditions such as schizophrenia or manic depressive disease and anxiety disorders such as panic disorder. The reasons for the co-morbidities of alcoholism with independent psychiatric disorders are not known, but they might represent an overlap in genetic vulnerabilities, impaired judgment resulting from the independent psychiatric condition, or an attempt to use alcohol to alleviate some of the symptoms of the disorder or side effects of medications.

Many psychiatric syndromes can be seen temporarily during heavy drinking and subsequent withdrawal. These include an intense *sadness* lasting for days to weeks in the midst of heavy drinking seen in 40% of alcoholics (alcohol-induced mood disorder); temporary severe *anxiety* in 10–30% of alcoholics, often beginning during alcohol withdrawal, and which can persist for a month or more after cessation of drinking (alcohol-induced anxiety disorder); and auditory *hallucinations* and/or paranoid delusions in a person who is alert and oriented, seen in 3–5% of alcoholics (*alcohol-induced psychotic disorder*).

Treatment of all forms of alcohol-induced psychopathology includes helping patients achieve abstinence and offering supportive care, as well as reassurance and "talk therapy" such as cognitive-behavioral approaches. However, with the exception of short-term antipsychotics for substance-induced psychosis, substance-induced psychiatric conditions only rarely require medications. Recovery is likely within several days to 4 weeks of abstinence. A history of alcohol intake is an important consideration in any patient with one of these psychiatric symptoms.

The distinction between long term, independent psychiatric conditions and temporary alcohol-induced syndromes is important because their prognoses and optimal treatments are quite different. Independent syndromes can be recognized because they often began before the alcohol dependence and/or remain after a period of a month or more of abstinence.

THE GASTROINTESTINAL SYSTEM

Esophagus and Stomach Alcohol intake can result in inflammation of the esophagus and stomach causing epigastric distress and gastrointestinal bleeding. Alcohol is one of the most common causes of hemorrhagic gastritis. Violent vomiting can produce severe bleeding through a Mallory-Weiss lesion, a longitudinal tear in the mucosa at the gastroesophageal junction.

Pancreas and Liver The incidence of acute pancreatitis (~25 per 1000 per year) is almost threefold higher in alcoholics than in the general population, accounting for an estimated 10% or more of the total cases. Alcohol impairs gluconeogenesis in the liver, resulting in a fall in the amount of glucose produced from glycogen, increased lactate production, and decreased oxidation of fatty acids. This contributes to an increase in fat accumulation in liver cells. In healthy individuals these changes are reversible, but with repeated exposure to ethanol, more severe changes in the liver occur, including alcohol-induced hepatitis, perivenular sclerosis, and cirrhosis, with the latter observed in an estimated 15% of alcoholics (Chap. 301).

CANCER

Drinking as few as 1.5 drinks per day increases a woman's risk of breast cancer 1.4-fold. For both genders, four drinks per day increases the risk for oral and esophageal cancers approximately threefold and rectal cancers by a factor of 1.5; seven to eight or more drinks per day enhances approximately fivefold the risks for many cancers.

HEMATOPOIETIC SYSTEM

Ethanol causes an increase in red blood cell size [mean corpuscular volume, (MCV)], which reflects its effects on stem cells. If heavy drinking is accompanied by folic acid deficiency, there can also be hypersegmented neutrophils, reticulocytopenia, and a hyperplastic bone marrow; if malnutrition is present, sideroblastic changes can be observed. Chronic heavy drinking can decrease production of white blood cells, decrease granulocyte mobility and adherence, and impair delayed-hypersensitivity responses to novel antigens (with a possible false-negative tuberculin skin test). Finally, many alcoholics have mild thrombocytopenia, which usually resolves within a week of abstinence unless there is hepatic cirrhosis or congestive splenomegaly.

CARDIOVASCULAR SYSTEM

Acutely, ethanol decreases myocardial contractility and causes peripheral vasodilation, with a resulting mild decrease in blood pressure and a compensatory increase in cardiac output. Exercise-induced increases in cardiac oxygen consumption are higher after alcohol intake. These acute effects have little clinical significance for the average healthy drinker but can be problematic in men and women with persisting cardiac disease.

The consumption of three or more drinks per day results in a dose-dependent increase in blood pressure, which returns to normal within weeks of abstinence. Thus, heavy drinking is an important factor in mild to moderate hypertension. Chronic heavy drinkers have a sixfold increased risk for coronary artery disease as well as an increased risk for cardiomyopathy. Symptoms range from unexplained arrhythmias in the presence of left ventricular impairment to heart failure with dilation of all four heart chambers and hypocontractility of heart muscle. Perhaps one-third of cases of cardiomyopathy are alcohol-induced. Mural thrombi can form in the left atrium or ventricle, while heart enlargement >25% can cause mitral regurgitation. Atrial or ventricular arrhythmias, especially paroxysmal tachycardia, can also occur after a drinking binge in individuals showing no other evidence of heart disease—a syndrome known as the "holiday heart." This condition is observed transiently in the majority of alcoholics entering treatment.

Chronic intake of modest doses of alcohol can have some beneficial effects. A maximum of one to two drinks per day may decrease the risk for cardiovascular death, perhaps through an increase in high-density lipoprotein (HDL) cholesterol or changes in clotting mechanisms. In one large national study, cardiovascular mortality was reduced by 30–40% among individuals reporting one or more drinks daily compared to nondrinkers, with overall mortality lowest among those consuming approximately one drink per day. Recent data have also corroborated that regular light drinking decreases the risk for ischemic, but not hemorrhagic, stroke.

GENITOURINARY SYSTEM CHANGES, SEXUAL FUNCTIONING, AND FETAL DEVELOPMENT

Acutely, modest ethanol doses (e.g., blood alcohol concentrations of 0.06 gm/dL) can increase sexual drive but also decrease erectile capacity in men. Even in the absence of liver impairment, a significant minority of chronic alcoholic men show irreversible testicular atrophy with shrinkage of the seminiferous tubules, decreases in ejaculate volume, and a lower sperm count (Chap. 340).

The repeated ingestion of high doses of ethanol by women can result in amenorrhea, a decrease in ovarian size, absence of corpora lutea with associated infertility, and an increased risk of spontaneous abortion. Heavy drinking during pregnancy results in the rapid placental transfer of both ethanol and acetaldehyde, which may have serious consequences for fetal development. The *fetal alcohol syndrome* can include any of the following: facial changes with epicanthal eye folds; poorly formed ear concha; small teeth with faulty enamel; cardiac atrial or ventricular septal defects; an aberrant palmar crease and limitation in joint movement; and microcephaly with mental retardation. The amount of ethanol required and the time of vulnerability during pregnancy have not been defined, making it advisable for pregnant women to abstain completely.

OTHER EFFECTS OF ETHANOL

Between one-half and two-thirds of alcoholics have skeletal muscle weakness caused by acute *alcoholic myopathy*, a condition that improves but which might not fully remit with abstinence. Effects of repeated heavy drinking on the *skeletal system* include changes in calcium metabolism, lower bone density, and decreased growth in the epiphyses, leading to an increased risk for fractures and osteonecrosis of the femoral head. *Hormonal changes* include an increase in cortisol levels, which can remain elevated during heavy drinking; inhibition of vasopressin secretion at rising blood alcohol concentrations and enhanced secretion at falling blood alcohol concentrations (with the final result that most alcoholics are likely to be slightly overhydrated); a modest and reversible decrease in serum thyroxine (T_4); and a more marked decrease in serum triiodothyronine (T_3). Hormone irregularities should be reevaluated after a month of abstinence.

ALCOHOLISM (ALCOHOL ABUSE OR DEPENDENCE)

Because many drinkers occasionally imbibe to excess, temporary alcohol-related pathology is common in nonalcoholics, especially those in the late teens to the late twenties. When repeated problems in multiple life areas develop, the individual is likely to meet criteria for alcohol abuse or dependence.

DEFINITIONS AND EPIDEMIOLOGY

Alcohol dependence is defined in DSM-IV as repeated alcohol-related difficulties in at least three of seven areas of functioning that cluster together over a 12-month period. Two of these seven items, tolerance and withdrawal, may have special importance as they are associated with a more severe clinical course. Alcohol dependence is seen in all countries where alcohol is available and occurs in men and women from all socioeconomic strata and all racial backgrounds. The diagnosis of alcohol dependence predicts a course of recurrent problems with the use of alcohol and the consequent shortening of the life span by a decade on average.

Alcohol abuse is defined as repetitive problems with alcohol in any one of four life areas—social, interpersonal, legal, and occupational—or repeated use in hazardous situations such as driving while intoxicated. If an individual is not alcohol dependent, he or she still may be given a diagnosis of alcohol abuse.

The lifetime risk for alcohol dependence in most western countries is about 10–15% for men and 5–8% for women. Rates are generally similar in the United States, Canada, Germany, Australia, and England; rates tend to be lower in most Mediterranean countries, such as Italy, Greece, and Israel, and may be higher in Ireland, France, and Scandinavia. Even higher rates have been reported for several native cultures including American Indians, Eskimos, Maori groups, and aboriginal tribes of Australia. These differences reflect both cultural and genetic influences, as described below. When alcohol abuse is also considered, the rates of alcohol use disorders increase. In western countries, the typical alcoholic does not fulfill the common stereotype of a "skid-row" denizen but is more often a blue- or white-collar worker or homemaker. The lifetime risk for alcoholism among physicians is similar to that of the general population.

GENETICS OF ALCOHOLISM

Several separate and distinct characteristics appear to contribute to the risk. For example, some families carry a risk for both alcoholism and drug dependence associated with the characteristic of high levels of impulsivity, as can be seen in the antisocial personality disorder. In other families, the risk for both alcohol and drug dependence may relate to a genetic vulnerability to schizophrenia, panic disorder, or manic depressive disease. A third and different mechanism increases only the alcoholism risk (e.g., in some offspring of alcoholics and Native Americans) through a low response to alcohol and subsequent drinking higher doses to achieve the desired effects. The relatively low response to alcohol contributes to attitudes and drinking patterns that increase the risk for alcohol-related problems and alcoholism. By contrast, a decreased risk for heavy drinking can result from a more intense response to alcohol, as seen in approximately half of Asian men and women. This is due primarily to a mutation that causes the production of an inactive form of the enzyme ALDH, which results in higher levels of acetaldehyde following alcohol ingestion.

NATURAL HISTORY

Although the age of the first drink is similar in alcoholics and nonalcoholics, earlier onset of regular drinking and drunkenness is associated with a higher risk for later problems. By the early to mid-twenties, most nonalcoholic men and women moderate their drinking (perhaps learning from minor problems), whereas alcoholics are likely to escalate their patterns of drinking despite difficulties. The first major life problem from alcohol often appears in the early to mid-twenties. Once established, the course of alcoholism is likely to be one of exacerbations and remissions. As a rule, there is little difficulty in stopping alcohol use when problems develop, and this step is often followed by days to months of abstinence and then a period of carefully controlled drinking. Unless abstinence is maintained, however, these phases almost inevitably give way to escalations in alcohol intake and subsequent problems. The course is not hopeless; following treatment, between half and two-thirds of alcoholics maintain abstinence for years, and often permanently. Even without formal treatment or self-help groups there is at least a 20% chance of spontaneous remission with long-term abstinence. However, should the alcoholic continue to drink, the life span is shortened by 10–15 years on average, with the leading causes of death, in decreasing order, the result of heart disease, cancer, accidents, and suicide.

IDENTIFICATION OF THE ALCOHOLIC AND INTERVENTION

Even in affluent areas ~20% of patients have an alcohol use disorder. It is important to pay attention to the alcohol-related symptoms and signs as well as laboratory tests that are likely to be abnormal in the context of regular consumption of six to eight or more drinks per day. The two blood tests with ≥70% sensitivity and specificity for heavy alcohol consumption are γ-glutamyl transferase (GGT) (>35 U) and carbohydrate-deficient transferrin (CDT) (>20 U/L); the combination of the two is likely to be more accurate than either alone. Physicians should consider using these tests to screen all patients as indicators of possible alcoholism. These serologic markers of heavy drinking can also be useful in monitoring abstinence, as they are likely to return toward normal within several weeks of the cessation of drinking; thus, increases in values of as little as 10% are likely to indicate a resumption of heavy alcohol intake. Other blood tests that can be useful in identifying individuals consuming six or more standard drinks per day include high-normal MCVs (≥91 μm^3) and serum uric acid (>416 mol/L, or 7 mg/dL). Physical signs and symptoms that can be useful in identifying alcoholism include mild and fluctuating hypertension, repeated infections such as pneumonia, and otherwise unexplained cardiac arrhythmias. Other disorders suggestive of dependence include cancer of the head and neck, esophagus, or stomach as well as cirrhosis, unexplained hepatitis, pancreatitis, bilateral parotid gland swelling, and peripheral neuropathy.

The clinical diagnosis of alcohol abuse or dependence ultimately rests on the documentation of a pattern of repeated difficulties associated with alcohol use; the definition is not based on the quantity and frequency of alcohol consumption. Thus, in screening it is important to probe for life problems and then attempt to tie in use of alcohol or another substance. Information regarding marital or job problems, legal difficulties, histories of accidents, medical problems, evidence of tolerance, etc., are important. While all physicians should be able to take the time needed to gather such information, some standardized questionnaires can be helpful, including the 10-item Alcohol Use Disorder Screening Test (AUDIT) (Table 387-2). However, these are only screening tools, and a careful face-to-face interview is still required for a meaningful diagnosis.

After alcoholism is identified, the diagnosis must be shared with the patient as part of an intervention. The presenting complaint can be used as an entrée to the alcohol problem. For instance, the patient with insomnia or hypertension can be told that these are clinically important problems which, in conjunction with other physical findings and laboratory tests, indicate that alcohol is increasing the risk for further medical and psychological problems. The physician should share information about the course of alcoholism and explore possible avenues of addressing the problem. This process can be carried out by any physician or other health care provider. Several protocols, categorized as *brief interventions* and *motivational interviewing,* are available for health care workers to follow. The technique of brief interventions has been shown to be effective in decreasing alcohol use and problems when instituted as two 15-min sessions 1 month apart, along with a telephone follow-up reminder. Motivational interviewing uses the clinician's level of concern and understanding of the need for patients to progress through their own stages of enhanced understanding of their problems to optimize their ability to alter their drinking behaviors.

The process of intervention is rarely accomplished in one session. Multiple sessions to explain the problem, the optimal treatments, and the benefits of making certain lifestyle changes are often required. For the person who refuses to stop drinking at the first intervention, a logical step is to "keep the door open," establishing future meetings so that help is available as problems escalate. In the meantime the family may benefit from counseling or referral to self-help groups such as Al-

TABLE 387-2	THE ALCOHOL USE DISORDERS IDENTIFICATION TEST (AUDIT)^a

Item	5-Point Scale (Least to Most)
1. How often do you have a drink containing alcohol?	Never (0) to 4+ per week (4)
2. How many drinks containing alcohol do you have on a typical day?	1 or 2 (0) to 10+ (4)
3. How often do you have six or more drinks on one occasion?	Never (0) to daily or almost daily (4)
4. How often during the last year have you found that you were not able to stop drinking once you had started?	Never (0) to daily or almost daily (4)
5. How often during the last year have you failed to do what was normally expected from you because of drinking?	Never (0) to daily or almost daily (4)
6. How often during the last year have you needed a first drink in the morning to get yourself going after a heavy drinking session?	Never (0) to daily or almost daily (4)
7. How often during the last year have you had a feeling of guilt or remorse after drinking?	Never (0) to daily or almost daily (4)
8. How often during the last year have you been unable to remember what happened the night before because you had been drinking?	Never (0) to daily or almost daily (4)
9. Have you or someone else been injured as a result of your drinking?	No (0) to yes, during the last year (4)
10. Has a relative, friend, doctor or other health worker been concerned about your drinking or suggested that you should cut down?	No (0) to yes, during the last year (4)

^{a}The AUDIT is scored by simply summing the values associated with the endorsed response.

Source: Adapted from DF Reinert, GP Allen: *Alcoholism: Clinical & Experimental Research* 26:272, 2002, and from MA Schuckit, 2006.

Anon (the Alcoholics Anonymous group for family members) and Alateen (for teenage children of alcoholics).

THE ALCOHOL WITHDRAWAL SYNDROME

Once the brain has been repeatedly exposed to high doses of alcohol, any sudden decrease in intake can produce withdrawal symptoms, many of which are the opposite of those produced by intoxication. Features include tremor of the hands (shakes or jitters); agitation and anxiety; autonomic nervous system overactivity including an increase in pulse, respiratory rate, and body temperature; and insomnia, sometimes accompanied by frightening dreams. Because alcohol has a short half-life, these withdrawal symptoms generally begin within 5–10 h of decreasing ethanol intake, peak in intensity on day 2 or 3, and improve by day 4 or 5. Anxiety, insomnia, and mild levels of autonomic dysfunction may persist to some degree for 4–6 months as a protracted abstinence syndrome, which may contribute to the tendency to return to drinking.

At some point in their lives, between 2 and 5% of alcoholics experience withdrawal seizures, often within 48 h of stopping drinking. These rare events usually involve a single generalized seizure, and electroencephalographic abnormalities generally return to normal within several days.

The term *delirium tremens* (DTs) refers to an uncommon state of intense acute withdrawal that includes delirium (mental confusion, agitation, and fluctuating levels of consciousness) associated with a tremor and autonomic overactivity (e.g., marked increases in pulse, blood pressure, and respirations). Fortunately, this serious and potentially life-threatening complication of alcohol withdrawal is seen in <5% of alcohol-dependent individuals; the chance of DTs during any single withdrawal is <1%. DTs are most likely to develop in patients with concomitant severe medical disorders and can usually be avoided by identifying and treating the underlying medical conditions.

℞ ALCOHOL-RELATED CONDITIONS

ACUTE INTOXICATION The first priority is to assess vital signs and manage respiratory depression, cardiac arrhythmia, or blood pressure instability, if present. The possibility of intoxication with other drugs should be considered, and blood and urine samples are obtained to screen for opioids or other CNS depressants such as benzodiazepines or barbiturates. Other medical conditions that must be considered include hypoglycemia, hepatic failure, or diabetic ketoacidosis.

Patients who are medically stable should be placed in a quiet environment. If recumbent, patients should lie on their side to minimize the risk of aspiration. When the intoxicated person is aggressive or violent, hospital procedures should be followed, including planning for the possibility of a show of force with an intervention team. In the context of aggressiveness, patients should be reminded in a clear and nonthreatening way that the staff wants to help them to feel better and to avoid problems. If the aggressive behavior continues, relatively low doses of a short-acting benzodiazepine such as lorazepam (e.g., 1–2 mg PO or IV) may be used and can be repeated as needed, but care must be taken so that the addition of this second CNS depressant does not destabilize vital signs or worsen confusion. An alternative approach is to use an antipsychotic medication (e.g., 0.5–5 mg of haloperidol PO or IM every 48 h if needed), but this has the potential danger of lowering the seizure threshold. Two other medications useful for agitation are ziprasidone (10 mg IM every 2h as needed, up to 40 mg) and olanzapine (2.5–10 mg IM repeated at 2 h and 6 h, if needed). If aggression escalates, the patient might require a short-term admission to a locked ward, where medications can be used more safely and vital signs more closely monitored.

WITHDRAWAL The first step is to perform a thorough physical examination in all alcoholics who are considering stopping drinking, including a search for evidence of liver failure, gastrointestinal bleeding, cardiac arrhythmia, infection, and glucose or electrolyte imbalance.

The second step is to offer reassurance that the acute withdrawal is short lived and to offer adequate nutrition and rest. All patients should be given oral multiple B vitamins, including 50–100 mg of thiamine daily for a week or more. Because most alcoholics who enter withdrawal are either normally hydrated or mildly overhydrated, IV fluids should be avoided unless there is evidence of significant recent bleeding, vomiting, or diarrhea. Medications can usually be administered orally.

The third step in treatment is to recognize that most withdrawal symptoms are caused by the rapid removal of a CNS depressant, in this case, alcohol. The symptoms can be controlled by administering any drug of this class in doses that decrease the agitation, and gradually taper the dose over 3–5 days. While most CNS depressants are effective, benzodiazepines (Chap. 386) have the highest margin of safety and lowest cost and are, therefore, the preferred class of drugs. Benzodiazepines with short half-lives are especially useful for patients with serious liver impairment or evidence of preexisting encephalopathy or brain damage. However, short-acting benzodiazepines such as lorazepam can produce rapidly changing drug blood levels and must be given every 4 h to avoid abrupt fluctuations that may increase the risk for seizures. Therefore, most clinicians use drugs with longer half-lives, such as diazepam or chlordiazepoxide, administering enough drug on day 1 to alleviate most of the symptoms of withdrawal (e.g., the tremor and elevated pulse) and then gradually decreasing the dose over a period of 3–5 days. The approach is flexible; the dose is increased if signs of withdrawal escalate, and the medication is withheld if the patient is sleeping or shows signs of increasing orthostatic hypotension. The average patient requires 25–50 mg of chlordiazepoxide or 10 mg of diazepam given PO every 4–6 h on the first day.

Treatment of the patient with DTs can be challenging, and the condition is likely to run a course of 3–5 days regardless of the therapy employed. The focus of care is to identify and correct medical problems and to control behavior and prevent injuries. Many clinicians recommend the use of high doses of a benzodiazepine (as much as 800 mg/d of chlordiazepoxide has been reported), a treatment that will decrease agitation and raise the seizure threshold but probably does little to improve the confusion. Other clinicians recommend the use of antipsychotic medications, such as haloperidol, ziprasidone, or olanzapine as discussed above, although these drugs have not been directly evaluated for DTs. Antipsychotics are less likely to exacerbate confusion but may increase the risk of seizures; they have no place in the treatment of mild withdrawal symptoms.

Generalized withdrawal seizures rarely require aggressive pharmacologic intervention beyond that given to the usual patient undergoing withdrawal, i.e., adequate doses of benzodiazepines. There is little evidence that anticonvulsants such as phenytoin or gabapentin are effective in drug-withdrawal seizures, and the risk of seizures has usually passed by the time effective drug levels are reached. The rare patient with status epilepticus must be treated aggressively (Chap. 363).

While alcohol withdrawal is often treated in a hospital, efforts at reducing costs have resulted in the development of outpatient detoxification for relatively mild abstinence syndromes. This is appropriate for patients in good physical condition who demonstrate mild signs of withdrawal despite low blood alcohol concentrations and for those without prior history of DTs or withdrawal seizures. Such individuals still require a careful physical examination, appropriate blood tests, and vitamin supplementation. Benzodiazepines can be given in a 1- to 2-day supply to be administered to the patient by a spouse or other family member four times a day. Patients are asked to return daily for evaluation of vital signs and to come to the emergency room if signs and symptoms of withdrawal escalate.

REHABILITATION OF ALCOHOLICS After completing alcoholic rehabilitation, ≥60% of alcoholics, especially middle class patients, maintain abstinence for at least a year, and many achieve lifetime sobriety.

The core of treatment begins with helping patients recognize the need to change, while working with them to alter their behaviors to enhance compliance. Therapeutic maneuvers fall into several general categories, which are applied to all patients regardless of age or ethnic group. The manner in which the treatments are used should be sensitive to the practices and needs of specific populations. The first step is to help the alcoholic achieve and maintain a high level of motivation toward abstinence. This includes education about alcoholism and instructions to family and/or friends to stop protecting the patient from problems caused by alcohol. The second step is to help the patient readjust to life without alcohol and to reestablish a functional lifestyle through counseling, vocational rehabilitation, and self-help groups such as Alcoholics Anonymous (AA). The third component, called *relapse prevention*, helps the patient to identify situations in which a return to drinking is likely, formulate ways of managing these risks, and develop coping strategies that increase the chances of a return to abstinence if a slip occurs.

For many patients, especially those who are highly motivated and have supportive social systems, treatment can be on an outpatient basis. However, more intense interventions work better than less intensive measures, and some alcoholics do not respond to outpatient approaches. The decision to hospitalize or utilize residential care can be made if (1) the patient has medical problems that are difficult to treat outside a hospital; (2) depression, confusion, or psychosis interferes with outpatient care; (3) there is a severe life crisis that makes it difficult to work in an outpatient setting; (4) outpatient treatment has failed; or (5) the patient lives too far from the treatment center to participate in an outpatient program. The best predictors of continued abstinence include evidence of higher levels of life stability (e.g., supportive family and friends) and higher levels of functioning (e.g., job skills, higher levels of education, and absence of crimes unrelated to alcohol).

Whether the treatment begins in an inpatient or an outpatient setting, subsequent outpatient contact should be maintained for a minimum of 6 months and preferably a full year after abstinence is achieved. Counseling with an individual physician or through groups focuses on day-to-day living, emphasizing areas of improved functioning in the absence of alcohol (i.e., why it is a good idea to continue to abstain) and helping the patient to manage free time without alcohol, develop a nondrinking peer group, and handle stresses on the job.

The physician serves an important role in identifying the alcoholic, diagnosing and treating associated medical or psychiatric syndromes, overseeing detoxification, referring the patient to rehabilitation programs, and providing counseling. Physicians are also responsible for selecting which (if any) medication might be appropriate during alcoholism rehabilitation. Patients often complain of continuing sleep problems or anxiety when acute withdrawal treatment is over, problems that may be a component of protracted withdrawal. In general, hypnotics or antianxiety drugs should be avoided in this situation. Patients should be reassured that the trouble sleeping is normal after alcohol withdrawal and will improve over the subsequent weeks and months. Patients should follow a rigid bedtime and awakening schedule and avoid naps or the use of caffeine in the evenings. The sleep pattern will improve with time, and the patient can avoid the rebound insomnia associated with most hypnotics and the risk for developing dependence on another depressant. Anxiety can be addressed by helping the person to gain insight into the temporary nature of the symptoms and to develop strategies to achieve relaxation as well as by using forms of cognitive therapy.

While the mainstay of alcoholic rehabilitation involves counseling, education, and cognitive approaches, several medications might be useful. The optimal length of time to continue these drugs in the context of a positive response is unclear, but most clinicians would recommend 6–12 months. The first is the opioid-antagonist drug naltrexone, 50–150 mg/d, which has been reported to decrease the probability of a return to drinking and to shorten periods of relapse. Recently a once-per-month injection of this drug (380 mg) has been developed to help improve compliance. By blocking opioid receptors, naltrexone may decrease activity in the dopamine-rich ventral tegmental reward system, or decrease the feeling of pleasure or reward if alcohol is imbibed. The improved rate of functioning and abstinence with this drug is modest. The side effects are relatively few at the recommended doses and include gastrointestinal distress. A second medication, acamprosate (Campral), 2 g/d, has been widely tested in patients in the United States and Europe; results are generally similar to those reported for naltrexone. This drug inhibits the actions of NMDA receptors and has been hypothesized to act by decreasing mild symptoms of protracted withdrawal. There are few side effects, aside from mild gastrointestinal distress. Several long-term trials of combined naltrexone and acamprosate using doses similar to those noted above have reported that the combination may be superior to either drug alone, although not all studies agree.

Disulfiram, an ALDH inhibitor, has been used extensively in the past for treatment of alcoholism. In doses of 250 mg/d this drug produces an unpleasant (and potentially dangerous) reaction in the presence of alcohol, a phenomenon related to rapidly rising blood levels of the first metabolite of alcohol, acetaldehyde. Few adequate controlled trials have demonstrated a clear superiority of disulfiram over placebo. Drinking alcohol while taking disulfiram produces a reaction involving an increased pulse, changes in blood pressure, and vomiting and diarrhea. This can be dangerous, especially for patients with heart disease, stroke, diabetes mellitus, or hypertension. The drug itself has also been reported to carry potential risks of depression, psychotic symptoms, peripheral neuropathy, and liver damage. Thus, most clinicians reserve this medication for patients who have a clear history of longer-term abstinence associated with prior use of disulfiram, and for those who might take the drug under the supervision of another individual (such as a spouse), especially during discrete periods identified as representing high-risk drinking situations for them (such as the Christmas holiday). Other drugs under investigation for possible use in alcoholism rehabilitation include the serotonin antagonist ondansetron; topiramate, an anticonvulsant with possible effects on dopamine; and the cannabinol receptor antagonist ramonibant; at present, there are insufficient data to support their use in clinical settings.

Additional support for alcoholics and their relatives and friends is available through self-help programs such as AA. These groups, which typically consist of recovering alcoholics, offer an effective model of abstinence, provide a sober peer group, and make crisis intervention freely available when the urge to drink escalates. This can help patients optimize their chances for recovery, especially when incorporated into a more structured treatment milieu.

FURTHER READINGS

BABOR TF et al: Brief interventions for at-risk drinking: Patient outcomes and cost-effectiveness in managed care organizations. Alcohol 41:624, 2006

GELERNTER J et al: Opioid receptor gene (*OPRM1*, *OPRK1*, and *OPRD1*) variants and response to naltrexone treatment for alcohol dependence: Results from the VA Cooperative Study. Alcohol Clin Exp Res 31:555, 2007

LAWRENCE AJ: Therapeutics for alcoholism: What's the future? Drug Alcohol Rev 26:3, 2007

388 Opioid Drug Abuse and Dependence
Marc A. Schuckit

It is difficult to imagine modern medical practice without the use of opioid analgesics. These drugs have been part of health care since 300 B.C. Opium and codeine were isolated in the early nineteenth century, opioid-like substances produced by the body were recognized in the 1970s, and the first endogenous opioid was isolated in 1995. As important as these substances are to modern medicine, opioid drugs have many disadvantages, including overdosage and dependency; close to 1 million individuals in the United States are opioid-dependent. All opioid drugs are capable of producing a heroin-like intoxication, as well as tolerance and withdrawal.

PHARMACOLOGY

The prototypic opiates, morphine and codeine (3-methoxymorphine), are derived from the juice of the poppy *Papaver somniferum*. The semisynthetic drugs produced from morphine or thebane molecules include hydromorphone, diacetylmorphine (heroin), and oxycodone. The purely synthetic opioids and their cousins include meperidine, propoxyphene, diphenoxylate, fentanyl, buprenorphine, tramadol, methadone, and pentazocine.

The body's own endogenous opioid peptides (e.g., enkephalins, endorphins, dynorphins, and others) have distinct distributions in the central nervous system (CNS) and appear to be natural ligands for

TABLE 388-1	ACTIONS OF OPIOID RECEPTORS
Receptor Type	**Actions**
Mu (μ) (e.g., morphine)	Analgesia, reinforcement euphoria, cough and appetite suppression, decreased respirations, decreased GI motility, sedation, hormone changes, dopamine and acetylcholine release
Kappa (κ) (e.g., butorphanol)	Decreased dysphoria, decreased GI motility, decreased appetite, decreased respiration, psychotic symptoms, sedation, diuresis, analgesia
Delta (δ) (e.g., etorphine)	Hormone changes, appetite suppression, dopamine release

Note: GI, gastrointestinal.

opioid receptors. As summarized in Table 388-1, the receptors with which opioid peptides interact differentially produce analgesia, respiratory depression, constipation, euphoria, and other actions. Substances capable of antagonizing one or more of these actions include nalorphine, levallorphan, cyclazocine, butorphanol, buprenorphine, and pentazocine, each of which has mixed agonist and antagonist properties, as well as naloxone, nalmefene, and naltrexone, which are pure opiate antagonists.

The availability of relatively specific antagonists has helped identify at least three receptor subtypes. These include μ receptors, which influence some of the more classic opioid actions such as pain control, reinforcement, constipation, hormone levels, and respiration; κ receptors, with possible similar functions along with sedation and effects on hormones; and δ receptors, thought to relate mostly to analgesia, mood, reinforcement, and breathing. A fourth possible receptor subtype, sensitive to another endogenous peptide, is sometimes called *nociceptin* or *orphanin* and may influence pain. The major features of tolerance, dependence, and withdrawal are thought to be mediated primarily by μ receptors, and these are affected by all prescription opioids.

The most rapid and pronounced effects of opioids occur through IV administration, with only slightly less efficient absorption after smoking or inhaling the vapor ("chasing the dragon"). The slowest onset and least intense effects occur after oral consumption. Most of the metabolism of opioids occurs in the liver, primarily through conjugation with glucuronic acid, and only small amounts are excreted directly in the urine or feces. The plasma half-lives of these drugs range from 2.5–3 h for morphine to >22 h for methadone.

Street heroin is typically only 5–10% pure and is usually mixed with sugars, quinine, powdered milk, phenacetin, caffeine, antipyrine, and strychnine. Unexpected increases in the purity of street drugs can cause unintentional lethal overdoses.

ACUTE AND CHRONIC EFFECTS OF OPIOIDS

With the exception of overdose and physical dependence, most opioid effects are rapidly reversible. A major danger, however, comes through the use of contaminated needles by IV users, which increases the risk of hepatitis B and C, bacterial endocarditis, and infection with HIV (Chap. 182).

Effects on Organ Systems   Euphoria and rewarding effects of opioids are due, at least in part, to stimulation of dopaminergic pathways originating in the midbrain and terminating in the nucleus accumbens. Effects on other neurotransmitter systems also occur. CNS effects of opioid drugs include nausea and vomiting (medulla), decreased pain perception (spinal cord, thalamus, and periaqueductal gray region), and sedation (reticular activating system). The adulterants added to street drugs may contribute to nervous system damage, including peripheral neuropathy, amblyopia, myelopathy, and leukoencephalopathy. Acute opioid administration inhibits release of some hormones from the hypothalamus, including corticotropin-releasing factor (CRF) and luteinizing hormone, with a subsequent reduction in some sex hormones, actions that might contribute to a decreased sex drive and problems in handling stress. Other hormonal changes include a decrease in the release of thyrotropin and increases in prolactin and possibly growth hormone (Chap. 333).

Acute changes in the respiratory system include a CNS-mediated decrease in the cough reflex (which can be useful as an antitussive) and respiratory depression, which result from a decreased response of the brainstem to carbon dioxide tension, a component of the drug overdose syndrome described below. At even low drug doses, this effect can be clinically significant for individuals with pulmonary disease. Aspiration pneumonia is an additional risk. The gastrointestinal effects of opioids can include decreased gut motility (useful in treating diarrhea), nausea, constipation, and anorexia with weight loss. Cardiovascular changes following modest doses tend to be relatively mild, with no direct opioid effect on heart rhythm or myocardial contractility, but orthostatic hypotension can occur, probably secondary to histamine release and dilation of peripheral vessels. Bacterial endocarditis with septic emboli and stroke can occur from contaminated needles.

Opioid Toxicity and Overdosage   High doses of opioids can result in a potentially lethal overdose. This occurs at some point in over half of opioid-dependent persons, especially with the more potent drugs such as fentanyl (80–100 times more powerful than morphine). The typical syndrome, which occurs immediately with IV overdose, includes shallow and slow respirations, pupillary miosis (with mydriasis once brain anoxia develops), bradycardia, hypothermia, and stupor or coma (Chap. 268). If not treated rapidly, respiratory depression, cardiorespiratory arrest, and death can ensue. Postmortem examination reveals few specific changes except for diffuse cerebral edema. An "allergic-like" reaction to IV heroin, perhaps in part related to adulterants, can also occur and is characterized by decreased alertness, frothy pulmonary edema, and an elevation in the blood eosinophil count.

℞ OPIOID OVERDOSE

The first step in managing overdose is to support vital signs, using intubation if needed. Definitive treatment is the administration of a narcotic antagonist such as naloxone, 0.4–2 mg IV or IM. A response should occur in 1–2 min, but if needed, the dose can be repeated every 2–3 min up to 10 mg. With the exception of buprenorphene overdoses, a lack of response after 10 mg makes a toxic reaction due solely to opioids unlikely. It is important to titrate the dose relative to the patient's symptoms to ameliorate the respiratory depression but not provoke a severe withdrawal state; the latter cannot be aggressively treated until overdose-related vital signs are relatively stable. Because the effects of naloxone diminish within several hours, the individual must be monitored for at least 24 h after a heroin overdose and 72 h after an overdose of a longer-acting drug such as methadone. If there is little response to an opioid antagonist, the possibility of a concomitant overdose with a benzodiazepine should be considered and a challenge with IV flumazenil, 0.2 mg/min up to a maximum of 3 mg in an hour, might be used. This drug should be administered with caution as it can precipitate seizures and increase intracranial pressure.

Treatment of either the typical or the "allergic" type of opioid toxic reaction requires continued respiratory support (often with oxygen supplementation and positive-pressure breathing for the "allergic" type of overdose), IV fluids, and pressor agents when needed to support blood pressure. Activated charcoal (e.g., 1 g/kg suspended in water) should be considered if ingestion of large doses of oral opioids is suspected; alternatively, gastric lavage can be used to remove any remaining drug. Intubation is often required to prevent aspiration in the stuporous or comatose patient. Cardiac arrhythmias and/or seizures may also be part of the opioid toxic reaction, especially with codeine, propoxyphene, or meperidine.

OPIOID ABUSE AND DEPENDENCE

Definition and Epidemiology   The *Fourth Diagnostic and Statistical Manual* (DSM-IV) of the American Psychiatric Association defines dependence as repeated use of a drug to the point of causing repetitive problems in multiple life areas. The definition requires evidence of three or more such problems clustered together within the same 12-month period of time, including tolerance, withdrawal, use of greater amounts of opiates than intended, and use despite consequences. Patients who do not have dependence but demonstrate repeated opioid-related difficulties with the law, impaired ability to meet obligations, use in hazardous situations, or continued use despite problems can be labeled as having abuse.

The use of opioids for intoxication is less prevalent than the use of alcohol, marijuana, and stimulants such as cocaine or amphetamines. A national survey of adolescents and young adults published in 2005 reported that 13.5% of 12th graders (high school seniors) had tried an opioid outside of a doctor's prescription, including 1.5% who had used heroin. Figures for young adults and college students were almost 17.6% and 1.9%, respectively. In all studies, prevalence rates were only slightly higher in males than females. The prevalence of opioid dependence is estimated as a lifetime risk of about 1%.

Genetics Genetic factors appear to influence an individual's specific risk for opioid dependence as well as a more general vulnerability toward substance-related problems. The proportion of the total risk explained by genes is estimated at ~50%. Specific genes potentially include variations in the α_2 subunit of the γ-aminobutyric acid (GABA)-A receptor; this might affect the risk of abuse or dependence on a wide range of substances through effects on impulsivity and sensation-seeking. All genetic influences operate in the context of environmental factors as well.

Natural History While an opioid use disorder can develop in anyone, at least three groups are at increased risk for dependence or misuse. First, a minority of persons with chronic pain syndromes (e.g., back, joint, and muscle disorders) misuse their prescribed drugs. If physical dependence is established, any drop in opioid blood levels can intensify the pain and promote continued drug intake. Physicians can avoid contributing to physical dependence by helping the patient to accept the goal of moderation rather than disappearance of the pain, and to recognize that discomfort may not be completely eliminated (Chap. 12). Analgesic medication should be only one component of treatment and should be limited to the oral administration of the least potent analgesic that is able to "take the edge off" the pain (e.g., naproxen or ibuprofen). Behavior-modification techniques, such as muscle relaxation and meditation, and carefully selected exercises should be used as appropriate to help increase function and decrease pain. Finally, nonmedicinal approaches, including electrical transcutaneous neurostimulation for muscle and joint disease, may be useful.

The second group at high risk consists of physicians, nurses, and pharmacists, primarily because of easy access to opioids. Physicians may begin use to help with sleep or to reduce stress or physical aches and pains, and then escalate doses as tolerance develops. Because of the growing awareness of these problems, programs have been developed to identify and aid substance-impaired physicians, providing peer support and education before problems escalate to the point of licensure revocation. All physicians are advised never to prescribe opioids for themselves or family members

The third group are those who buy illicit drugs to get high. While some of these individuals have severe antisocial problems, many had a relatively high level of premorbid functioning. The typical person begins using opioids occasionally, often after experimenting with tobacco, then alcohol, then marijuana, and then brain depressants or stimulants. Occasional opioid use, or "chipping," might continue for some time, and some individuals never escalate their intake to the point of developing dependence. For others, the frequency of use and quantity needed increase, tolerance develops, excuses are made for associated problems, and a full dependence syndrome appears.

Opioid-dependent individuals are not likely to give up their intake of other drugs. Alcohol may be used to moderate withdrawal problems, to enhance the opioid high, and to serve as a substitute when the opioid is not available, including during methadone or other maintenance or antagonist treatments. Problematic drinking, including alcohol dependence, is seen in about half of opioid-dependent persons. Cocaine appears to be taken for many of the same reasons, and is often administered IV with the opioid in a mixture known as a "speedball." Another relevant class of drugs is the benzodiazepines, taken for a high

or alleviation of withdrawal symptoms, especially among people in methadone maintenance.

Once persistent opioid use is established, severe problems are likely to develop. At least 25% of opioid-dependent individuals die within 10–20 years (a mortality rate 15-fold higher than the general population) from suicide, homicide, accidents, or infectious diseases such as tuberculosis, hepatitis, or AIDS. The latter has become an epidemic among injection drug users, with as many as 60% of these men and women in some locales carrying the HIV virus (Chap. 182). Although the majority of opioid-dependent persons experience frequent exacerbations and remissions, it is important to remember that even without treatment ~35% achieve long-term, often permanent, abstinence, especially after the age of 40. As is true with most drugs of abuse, a favorable prognosis is associated with a prior history of marital and employment stability and fewer prior criminal activities unrelated to drugs.

℞ **OPIOID ABUSE AND DEPENDENCE**

The first step in treatment is to identify the problem. It is important to discard the erroneous stereotype that opioid-dependent individuals are unemployed and homeless. Abuse or dependence is possible in any patient who demonstrates symptoms of what might be opioid withdrawal; anyone who has a chronic pain syndrome; physicians, nurses, and pharmacists or others with easy access to opioids; and patients who repeatedly seek out prescription analgesics. Before prescribing an opioid analgesic, it is important to gather a complete history that elucidates patterns of life problems and any history of opioid use. If a problem with opioids is suspected, gathering further data from a relative or close friend can be helpful. Additionally, clinicians should search for physical stigmata of misuse (e.g., needle marks) and, when appropriate, screen blood or urine for opioids.

After identifying opioid dependence, the next step is intervention as described for alcoholism in Chap. 387. Motivational interviewing techniques of empathy, careful listening, presenting options, and gauging the patient's motivational readiness to change are important, as are efforts to enlist the help of relatives and friends. Ongoing treatment even after the patient achieves abstinence is important; this includes offering help in establishing a drug-free lifestyle.

SYMPTOMS OF WITHDRAWAL Withdrawal symptoms (which are generally the opposite of the acute effects of the drug) include nausea, diarrhea, coughing, lacrimation, mydriasis, rhinorrhea, profuse sweating, twitching of muscles, and piloerection (or "goose bumps") as well as mild elevations in body temperature, respiratory rate, and blood pressure. In addition, diffuse body pain, insomnia, and yawning occur, along with intense drug craving. Withdrawal from opioids with shorter half-lives, such as morphine or heroin, usually causes symptoms within 8–16 h of the last dose; intensity peaks within 36–72 h after discontinuation of the drug; and the acute syndrome disappears within 5–8 days. A protracted abstinence phase of mild moodiness, autonomic dysfunction, and changes in pain threshold and sleep patterns may persist for ≥6 months and probably contributes to relapse. For longer-acting opioids such as methadone or continuous-release morphine, symptoms may not appear for several days, and may not peak until 7–10 days later.

TREATMENT OF THE WITHDRAWAL SYNDROME A thorough physical examination, including an assessment of neurologic function and a search for focal and systemic infections, especially abscesses, is essential. Laboratory testing includes assessment of liver function and, in IV users, HIV and hepatitis B and C status.

One treatment approach to withdrawal is to administer an opioid (e.g., 10–25 mg of methadone bid) on day 1 to decrease symptoms. After several days of a stabilized drug dose, the opioid is then decreased by 10–20% of the original day's dose each day. However, the use of opioids for detoxification is proscribed or limited in most states. Thus, pharmacologic treatments often center on relief of symptoms of diarrhea with loperamide, of "sniffles" with decongestants, and pain with nonopioid analgesics (e.g., ibuprofen). Comfort can be enhanced with administration of the α_2-adrenergic agonist clonidine in doses up to 0.3 mg given two to four times a day to decrease sympathetic nervous system overactivity. Blood pressure must be closely monitored. Some clinicians augment this regimen with low to moderate doses of benzodiazepines for 2–5 days to decrease agitation and promote sleep. An ultra-rapid detoxification procedure using deep sedation and withdrawal precipitated by naltrexone has been proposed but has many inherent dangers and few, if any, advantages.

REHABILITATION   The basic strategy, similar to that for alcoholics, includes detoxification and the establishment of realistic goals for abstinence and improvement of life functioning, along with counseling and education to increase motivation toward abstinence. A long-term commitment by the patient to maintain a lifestyle without illicit substances is essential for preventing relapse.

In most programs, patients are educated about their responsibility for improving their lives, and motivation for abstinence is increased by providing information about the medical and psychological problems that can be expected if dependence continues. Patients and families are encouraged to establish an opioid-free lifestyle by learning to cope with chronic pain and develop realistic vocational planning. The dependent person is also advised to establish a drug-free peer group and to participate in self-help groups such as Narcotics or Alcoholics Anonymous; the latter is appropriate for substance-dependent persons regardless of their usual drug of abuse. Another important treatment component is relapse prevention aimed at identifying triggers for a return to drugs and developing appropriate coping strategies.

Much of this advice and counseling can be given by the physician or by referring patients to formal drug programs, including methadone maintenance clinics, programs using narcotic antagonists, and therapeutic communities. Long-term follow-up of treated patients indicates that approximately one-third are completely drug free, and 60% no longer use opioids.

Opioid Maintenance   Maintenance programs with methadone or buprenorphene should be used only in combination with education and counseling. The goal is to provide a substitute drug that is legally accessible, safer, can be taken orally, and has a relatively long half-life so that it can be taken once a day. This can help persons who have repeatedly failed in drug-free programs to improve functioning within the family and job, to decrease legal problems, and to improve health. Individuals who stay in methadone maintenance are likely to show less antisocial behavior and improvement in employment status.

Methadone is a long-acting opioid optimally dosed at 80–120 mg/d (a goal met through slow, careful increases over time). This dose is effective in blocking heroin-induced euphoria while decreasing craving, thereby helping patients to maintain abstinence from illegal opioids. Over three-quarters of patients in well-supervised methadone clinics are likely to remain heroin-free for ≥6 months. Methadone is usually administered as an oral liquid given once a day at the program, with weekend doses taken at home. After a period of maintenance (usually 6 months to ≥1 year), the clinician can work to slowly decrease the dose by ~5% per week. Some individuals however, are unable to taper off the drug and require long-term maintenance.

An alternative medication that has been used for maintenance treatment is buprenorphine, a μ opioid agonist and antagonist. A dose of 6–12 mg buprenorphine is roughly equivalent to 35–60 mg of methadone. Administered either as a sublingual liquid or tablet, doses can be gradually increased to 8–16 mg/d over the first 2 months. Doses of 16–32 mg per treatment day may be needed if the drug is given three times per week. Buprenorphine is available as monotherapy or in combination with the antagonist naltrexone (2–8 mg buprenorphine with 0.5–2 mg naltrexone), which precipitates withdrawal if the patient dissolves the pills and injects them IV. Buprenorphine has several advantages including low overdose danger, potentially easier detoxification than is seen with methadone, and a probable ceiling effect in which higher doses do not increase euphoria. It can also be given in the doctor's office by physicians who have completed a required training program. While some studies report equal effectiveness of buprenorphine and methadone, others suggest higher dropout rates or more concomitant illicit drug use with buprenorphine compared to methadone. As with all opioids, there is a danger of misuse of this drug.

In the past, the British have used heroin maintenance with goals and guidelines similar to those of current methadone programs. There is no evidence that heroin maintenance has any advantages over methadone maintenance, but the heroin approach increases the risk that the drug will be sold on the streets.

Opioid Antagonists   The opioid antagonists (e.g., naltrexone) compete with heroin and other opioids at receptors, reducing the effects of the opioid agonists. Administered over long periods with the intention of blocking the opioid "high," these drugs can be useful as part of an overall treatment approach that includes counseling and support. Naltrexone doses of 50 mg/d antagonize 15 mg of heroin for 24 h, and the possibly more effective higher doses (125–150 mg) block the effects of 25 mg of IV heroin for up to 3 days. To avoid precipitating a withdrawal syndrome, patients must be free of opioids for a minimum of 5 days before beginning treatment with naltrexone and should first be challenged with 0.4 or 0.8 mg of the shorter-acting agent naloxone to be certain they can tolerate the long-acting antagonist. A test dose of 10 mg of naltrexone is then given, which can produce withdrawal symptoms in 0.5–2 h. If none appear, the patient can begin with the usual dose of 40–150 mg three times per week.

Drug-Free Programs   Most opioid-dependent individuals enter treatment programs that are based primarily on the cognitive behavioral approaches of enhancing commitment to abstinence, helping individuals to rebuild their lives without substances, and preventing relapse. Whether carried out in inpatient, residential, or outpatient settings, patients usually do not receive maintenance medications.

A variation of this approach can be used for persons who are having problems maintaining a drug-free state. Here, the basic elements of treatment are incorporated into long-term (often a year or more) residence in a therapeutic community. The person begins with almost full immersion in the environment in which other individuals at various stages of recovery become the primary support group, offering advice and a drug-free atmosphere in which the opioid-dependent person progresses through ever-increasing levels of independence, including assuming a job outside the therapeutic atmosphere.

As is true for treatments of all substance-use disorders, it is likely that counseling, behavioral treatments, and relatively simple approaches to psychotherapy add significantly to a positive outcome. Most programs focus on teaching participants to cope with stress, enhancing their understanding of personality attributes, teaching better cognitive styles, and, through the process of relapse prevention, addressing issues that might contribute to increased craving, easy access to drugs, or periods of decreased motivation. A combination of these therapies with the approaches described above appears to give the best results.

Finally, it is important to discuss prevention. Except for the terminally ill, physicians should carefully monitor opioid drug use in their patients, keeping doses as low as is practical while still controlling pain, and administering opioids over as short a period as the level of pain would warrant in the average person. Physicians must be vigilant regarding their own risk for opioid abuse and dependence, never prescribing these drugs for themselves. For the nonmedical IV drug–dependent person, all possible efforts must be made to prevent AIDS, hepatitis, bacterial endocarditis, and other consequences of contaminated needles both through methadone maintenance and by considering needle-exchange programs.

FURTHER READINGS

JOHNSTON LD et al: *Monitoring the Future: National Results on Adolescent Drug Use: Overview of Key Findings*, 2005. Bethesda, MD, National Institute on Drug Abuse

SCHUCKIT MA: *Drug and Alcohol Abuse: A Clinical Guide to Diagnosis and Treatment*, 6th ed. New York, Springer, 2006

STRANG J et al: Does prescribing for opiate addiction change after national guidelines? Methadone and buprenorphine prescribing to opiate addicts by general practitioners and hospital doctors in England, 1995–2005. Addiction 102(5):761, 2007

389 Cocaine and Other Commonly Abused Drugs

Jack H. Mendelson, Nancy K. Mello

Initiation and perpetuation of the abuse of cocaine and other psychostimulants are determined by a complex interaction between the pharmacologic properties and relative availability of each drug, the personality and expectations of the user, and the environmental context in which the drug is used. Polydrug abuse, the concurrent use of several drugs with different pharmacologic effects, is increasingly common. Some forms of polydrug abuse, such as the combined use of heroin and cocaine intravenously, are especially dangerous and remain a major problem in hospital emergency rooms. Sometimes one drug is used to enhance the effects of another, as with the combined use of benzodiazepines and methadone, or cocaine and heroin in methadone-maintained patients.

Chronic cocaine and psychostimulant abuse may cause a number of adverse health consequences, ranging from pulmonary disease to reproductive dysfunction. Preexisting disorders such as hypertension and cardiac disease may be exacerbated by drug abuse, and the combined use of two or more drugs may accentuate medical complications associated with abuse of one of them. The adverse health consequences of drug abuse are further complicated by increased vulnerability to infections.

Drug abuse increases the risk of exposure to HIV. Cocaine and psychostimulant abuse contribute to the risk for HIV infection in part by suppression of immune function. In addition, concurrent use of cocaine and opiates (the "speedball") is frequently associated with needle-sharing by IV drug users. Intravenous drug abusers continue to represent the largest single group of persons with HIV infection in several major metropolitan areas in the United States as well as in urban areas in Scotland, Italy, Spain, Thailand, and China.

COCAINE

Cocaine is a stimulant and local anesthetic with potent vasoconstrictor properties. The leaves of the *coca* plant (*Erythroxylon coca*) contain ~0.5–1% cocaine. The drug produces physiologic and behavioral effects when administered PO, intranasally, IV, or via inhalation following pyrolysis (smoking). The reinforcing effects of cocaine appear to be related to activation of dopaminergic neurons in the mesolimbic system. Cocaine increases synaptic concentrations of the monamine neurotransmitters dopamine, norepinephrine, and serotonin by binding to transporter proteins in presynaptic neurons and blocking reuptake.

Prevalence of Cocaine Use   Cocaine is widely available throughout the United States, and cocaine abuse occurs in virtually all social and economic strata of society. The prevalence of cocaine abuse in the general population has been accompanied by an increase in cocaine abuse by heroin-dependent persons, including those in methadone maintenance programs. Intravenous cocaine is often used concurrently with IV heroin. This combination purportedly attenuates the postcocaine "crash" and substitutes a cocaine "high" for the heroin "high" blocked by methadone.

Acute and Chronic Intoxication   There has been an increase in both IV administration and inhalation of pyrolyzed cocaine via smoking. Following intranasal administration, changes in mood and sensation are perceived within 3–5 min, and peak effects occur at 10–20 min. The effects rarely last more than 1 h. Inhalation of pyrolyzed materials includes inhaling crack/cocaine or smoking coca paste, a product made by extracting cocaine preparations with flammable solvents, and cocaine free-base smoking. Free-base cocaine, including the free base prepared with sodium bicarbonate (crack), has become increasingly popular because of the relative high potency of the compound and its rapid onset of action (8–10 s following smoking).

Cocaine produces a brief, dose-related stimulation and enhancement of mood and an increase in cardiac rate and blood pressure. Body temperature usually increases following cocaine administration, and high doses of cocaine may induce lethal pyrexia or hypertension. Because cocaine inhibits reuptake of catecholamines at adrenergic nerve endings, the drug potentiates sympathetic nervous system activity. Cocaine has a short plasma half-life of approximately 45–60 min. Cocaine is metabolized by plasma esterases, and cocaine metabolites are excreted in urine. The very short duration of the euphorigenic effects of cocaine observed in chronic abusers is probably due to both acute and chronic tolerance. Frequent self-administration of the drug (two to three times per hour) is often reported by chronic cocaine abusers. Alcohol is used to modulate both the cocaine high and the dysphoria associated with the abrupt disappearance of cocaine's effects. A metabolite of cocaine, cocaethylene, has been detected in blood and urine of persons who concurrently abuse alcohol and cocaine. Cocaethylene induces changes in cardiovascular function similar to those of cocaine alone, and the pathophysiologic consequences of alcohol abuse plus cocaine abuse may be additive when both are used together.

The prevalent assumption that cocaine inhalation or IV administration is relatively safe is contradicted by reports of death from respiratory depression, cardiac arrhythmias, and convulsions associated with cocaine use. In addition to generalized seizures, neurologic complications may include headache, ischemic or hemorrhagic stroke, or subarachnoid hemorrhage. Disorders of cerebral blood flow and perfusion in cocaine-dependent persons have been detected with magnetic resonance spectroscopy (MRS) studies. Severe pulmonary disease may develop in individuals who inhale crack cocaine; this effect is attributed both to the direct effects of cocaine and to residual contaminants in the smoked material. Hepatic necrosis has been reported to occur following crack/cocaine use.

Although men and women who abuse cocaine may report that the drug enhances libidinal drive, chronic cocaine use causes significant loss of libido and adversely affects reproductive function. Impotence and gynecomastia have been observed in male cocaine abusers, and these abnormalities often persist for long periods following cessation of drug use. Women who abuse cocaine may experience major derangements in menstrual cycle function including galactorrhea, amenorrhea, and infertility. Chronic cocaine abuse may cause persistent hyperprolactinemia as a consequence of disordered dopaminergic inhibition of prolactin secretion by the anterior pituitary. Cocaine abuse by pregnant women, particularly the smoking of crack, has been associated with both an increased risk of congenital malformations in the fetus and perinatal cardiovascular and cerebrovascular disease in the mother. However, cocaine abuse per se is probably not the sole cause of these perinatal disorders, since many problems associated with maternal cocaine abuse, including poor nutrition and health care status as well as polydrug abuse, also contribute to the risk for perinatal disease.

Protracted cocaine abuse may cause paranoid ideation and visual and auditory hallucinations, a state that resembles alcoholic hallucinosis. Psychological dependence on cocaine, indicated by inability to abstain from frequent compulsive use, has also been reported. Although the occurrence of withdrawal syndromes involving psychomotor agitation and autonomic hyperactivity remains controversial, severe depression ("crashing") following cocaine intoxication may accompany drug withdrawal.

℞ COCAINE OVERDOSE AND CHRONIC ABUSE

Treatment of cocaine overdose is a medical emergency that is usually best managed in an intensive care unit. Cocaine toxicity produces a hyperadrenergic state characterized by hypertension, tachycardia, tonic-clonic seizures, dyspnea, and ventricular arrhythmias. Intravenous diazepam in doses up to 0.5 mg/kg administered over an 8-h period has been shown to be effective for control of seizures. Ventricular arrhythmias have been managed successfully by administration of 0.5–1.0 mg of propranolol IV. Since many instances of cocaine-related mortality have been associated with concurrent use of other illicit drugs (particularly heroin), the physician must be prepared to institute effective emergency treatment for multiple drug toxicities.

Treatment of chronic cocaine abuse requires the combined efforts of primary care physicians, psychiatrists, and psychosocial care providers. Early abstinence from cocaine use is often complicated by symptoms of depression and guilt, insomnia, and anorexia, which may be as severe as those observed in major affective disorders. Individual and group psychotherapy, family therapy, and peer group assistance programs are often useful for inducing prolonged remission from drug use. A number of medications used for the treatment of various medical and psychiatric disorders have been administered to reduce the duration and severity of cocaine abuse and dependence. However, no available medication is both safe and highly effective for either cocaine detoxification or maintenance of abstinence. Some psychotherapeutic interventions may be effective; however, no specific form of psychotherapy or behavioral modification is uniquely beneficial.

MARIJUANA AND CANNABIS COMPOUNDS

Cannabis sativa contains >400 compounds in addition to the psychoactive substance, delta-9-tetrahydrocannabinol (THC). Marijuana cigarettes are prepared from the leaves and flowering tops of the plant, and a typical marijuana cigarette contains 0.5–1 g of plant material. Although the usual THC concentration varies between 10 and 40 mg, concentrations >100 mg per cigarette have been detected. Hashish is prepared from concentrated resin of *C. sativa* and contains a THC concentration of between 8 and 12% percent by weight. "Hash oil," a lipid-soluble plant extract, may contain a THC concentration of 25–60% and may be added to marijuana or hashish to enhance its THC concentration. Smoking is the most common mode of marijuana or hashish use. During pyrolysis, >150 compounds in addition to THC are released in the smoke. Although most of these compounds do not have psychoactive properties, they do have potential physiologic effects.

THC is quickly absorbed from the lungs into blood and is then rapidly sequestered in tissues. It is metabolized primarily in the liver, where it is converted to 11-hydroxy-THC, a psychoactive compound, and >20 other metabolites. Many THC metabolites are excreted through the feces at a rate of clearance that is relatively slow in comparison to that of most other psychoactive drugs.

Specific cannabinoid receptors (CB_1 and CB_2) have been identified in the central nervous system, including the spinal cord, and in the peripheral nervous system. High densities of these receptors have been found in the cerebral cortex, basal ganglia, and hippocampus. T and B lymphocytes also have cannabinoid receptors, and these appear to mediate anti-inflammatory and immunoregulatory properties of cannabinoids. A naturally occurring THC-like ligand has been identified in the nervous system, where it is widely distributed.

Prevalence of Use Marijuana is the most commonly used illegal drug in the United States. Use is particularly prevalent among adolescents; studies suggest that ~37% of high school students in the United States have used marijuana. Marijuana is relatively inexpensive and is often considered to be less hazardous than other controlled drugs and substances. Very potent forms of marijuana (sinsemilla) are now available in many communities, and concurrent use of marijuana with crack/cocaine and phencyclidine is increasing.

Acute and Chronic Intoxication Acute intoxication from marijuana and cannabis compounds is related to both the dose of THC and the route of administration. THC is absorbed more rapidly from marijuana smoking than from orally ingested cannabis compounds. Acute marijuana intoxication usually consists of a subjective perception of relaxation and mild euphoria resembling mild to moderate alcohol intoxication. This condition is usually accompanied by some impairment in thinking, concentration, and perceptual and psychomotor function. Higher doses of cannabis may produce behavioral effects analogous to severe alcohol intoxication. Although the effects of acute

marijuana intoxication are relatively benign in normal users, the drug can precipitate severe emotional disorders in individuals who have antecedent psychotic or neurotic problems. As with other psychoactive compounds, both set (user's expectations) and setting (environmental context) are important determinants of the type and severity of behavioral intoxication.

As with abuse of cocaine, opioids, and alcohol, chronic marijuana abusers may lose interest in common socially desirable goals and steadily devote more time to drug acquisition and use. However, THC does not cause a specific and unique "amotivational syndrome." The range of symptoms sometimes attributed to marijuana use is difficult to distinguish from mild to moderate depression and the maturational dysfunctions often associated with protracted adolescence. Chronic marijuana use has also been reported to increase the risk of psychotic symptoms in individuals with a past history of schizophrenia. Persons who initiate marijuana smoking before the age of 17 may subsequently develop severe cognitive and neuropsychological disorders, and they may also be at higher risk for polydrug and alcohol abuse problems in later life.

Physical Effects Conjunctival injection and tachycardia are the most frequent immediate physical concomitants of smoking marijuana. Tolerance for marijuana-induced tachycardia develops rapidly among regular users. However, marijuana smoking may precipitate angina in persons with a history of coronary insufficiency. Exercise-induced angina may be increased after marijuana use to a greater extent than after tobacco cigarette smoking. Patients with cardiac disease should be strongly advised not to smoke marijuana or use cannabis compounds.

Significant decrements in pulmonary vital capacity have been found in regular daily marijuana smokers. Because marijuana smoking typically involves deep inhalation and prolonged retention of marijuana smoke, marijuana smokers may develop chronic bronchial irritation. Impairment of single-breath carbon monoxide diffusion capacity (DL_{CO}) is greater in persons who smoke both marijuana and tobacco than in tobacco smokers.

Although marijuana has also been associated with a number of other adverse effects, many of these studies await replication and confirmation. A reported correlation between chronic marijuana use and decreased testosterone levels in males has not been confirmed. Decreased sperm count and sperm motility and morphologic abnormalities of spermatozoa following marijuana use have been reported. Prospective studies demonstrated a correlation between impaired fetal growth and development and heavy marijuana use during pregnancy. Marijuana has also been implicated in derangements of the immune system; in chromosomal abnormalities; and in inhibition of DNA, RNA, and protein synthesis; however, these findings have not been confirmed or related to any specific physiologic effect in humans.

Tolerance and Physical Dependence Habitual marijuana users rapidly develop tolerance to the psychoactive effects of marijuana and often smoke more frequently and try to secure more potent cannabis compounds. Tolerance for the physiologic effects of marijuana develops at different rates; e.g., tolerance develops rapidly for marijuana-induced tachycardia but more slowly for marijuana-induced conjunctival injection. Tolerance for both behavioral and physiologic effects of marijuana decreases rapidly upon cessation of marijuana use.

Withdrawal signs and symptoms have been reported in chronic cannabis users, with the severity of symptoms related to dosage and duration of use. These include tremor, nystagmus, sweating, nausea, vomiting, diarrhea, irritability, anorexia, and sleep disturbances. Withdrawal signs and symptoms observed in chronic marijuana users are usually relatively mild in comparison to those observed in heavy opiate or alcohol users and rarely require medical or pharmacologic intervention. More severe and protracted abstinence syndromes may occur after sustained use of high-potency cannabis compounds.

Therapeutic Use of Marijuana Marijuana, administered as cigarettes or as a synthetic oral cannabinoid (dronabinol), has been proposed to have a number of medicinal properties that may be clinically useful in some situations. These include antiemetic effects in chemotherapy recipients, appetite-promoting effects in AIDS patients, reduction of intraocular pressure in glaucoma, and reduction of spasticity in multiple sclerosis and other neurologic disorders. With the possible exception of AIDS-related cachexia, none of these attributes of marijuana compounds is clearly superior to other readily available therapies.

METHAMPHETAMINE

Methamphetamine is also referred to as "meth," "speed," "crank," "chalk," "ice," "glass," or "crystal." In the United States, hospital admissions for treatment of methamphetamine abuse increased substantially (from 3–8%) between 1994 and 2004. This increase occurred despite drug seizures, closures of clandestine laboratories that produce methamphetamine illegally, and an increase in methamphetamine abuse prevention programs.

Methamphetamine can be self-administered PO or by smoking, snorting, and IV injection. Individuals who abuse or become dependent upon methamphetamine report that use of this drug induces feelings of euphoria and decreases fatigue associated with difficult life situations. Adverse consequences of methamphetamine abuse include headache, difficulty concentrating, diminished appetite, abdominal pain, vomiting or diarrhea, disordered sleep, paranoid or aggressive behavior, and psychosis. Chronic methamphetamine abuse can result in severe dental caries, described as blackened, rotting, crumbling teeth. Severe, life-threatening methamphetamine toxicity may present as hypertension, cardiac arrhythmia or failure, subarachnoid hemorrhage, ischemic stroke, intracerebral hemorrhage, convulsions, or coma. Methamphetamines increase the release of monoamine neurotransmitters (dopamine, norepinephrine, and serotonin) from presynaptic neurons. It is thought that the euphoric and reinforcing effects of this class of drugs are mediated through dopamine and the mesolimbic system, whereas the cardiovascular effects are related to norepinephrine. MRS studies of the brain suggest that chronic abusers have neuronal damage in the frontal areas and basal ganglia.

Therapy of acute methamphetamine overdose is largely symptomatic. Ammonium chloride may be useful to acidify the urine and enhance clearance of the drug. Hypertension may respond to sodium nitroprusside or α-adrenergic antagonists. Sedatives may reduce agitation and other signs of central nervous system hyperactivity. Treatment of chronic methamphetamine dependence may be accomplished in either an inpatient or outpatient setting using strategies similar to those described above for cocaine abuse.

MDMA (3,4-methylenedioxymethamphetamine), or *Ecstasy*, is a derivative of methamphetamine. Ecstasy is usually taken PO but may be injected or inhaled; its effects last for 3–6 h. In addition to amphetamine-like effects, MDMA can induce hyperthermia and vivid hallucinations and other perceptual distortions.

During the past decade, an eighteenfold increase in MDMA-related emergency room incidents has been reported in the United States. Recent studies have revealed that MDMA use is associated with cognitive and memory impairment and a mild withdrawal syndrome after cessation of use. The long-term consequences of recreational use of MDMA by young persons are poorly understood.

LYSERGIC ACID DIETHYLAMIDE (LSD)

The discovery of the psychedelic effects of LSD in 1947 led to an epidemic of LSD abuse during the 1960s. Imposition of stringent constraints on the manufacture and distribution of LSD (classified as a Schedule I substance by the U.S. Food and Drug Administration), as well as public recognition that psychedelic experiences induced by LSD were a health hazard, have resulted in a reduction in LSD abuse. LSD still remains popular among adolescents and young adults, and there are indications that LSD use among young persons has been increasing in some communities in the United States.

LSD is a very potent drug; oral doses as low as 20 μg may induce profound psychological and physiologic effects. Tachycardia, hypertension, pupillary dilation, tremor, and hyperpyrexia occur within

minutes following oral administration of 0.5–2 μg/kg. A variety of bizarre and often conflicting perceptual and mood changes, including visual illusions, synesthesias, and extreme lability of mood, usually occur within 30 min after LSD intake. These effects of LSD may persist for 12–18 h, even though the half-life of the drug is only 3 h.

Tolerance develops rapidly for LSD-induced changes in psychological function when the drug is used one or more times per day for >4 days. Abrupt abstinence following continued use does not produce withdrawal signs or symptoms. There have been no clinical reports of death caused by the direct effects of LSD.

The most frequent acute medical emergency associated with LSD use is a panic episode (the "bad trip"), which may persist up to 24 h. Management of this problem is best accomplished by supportive reassurance ("talking down") and, if necessary, administration of small doses of anxiolytic drugs. Adverse consequences of chronic LSD use include enhanced risk for schizophreniform psychosis and derangements in memory function, problem solving, and abstract thinking. Treatment of these disorders is best carried out in specialized psychiatric facilities.

PHENCYCLIDINE

Phencyclidine (PCP), a cyclohexylamine derivative, is widely used in veterinary medicine to briefly immobilize large animals and is sometimes described as a dissociative anesthetic. PCP binds to ionotropic *n*-methyl-*d*-aspartate (NMDA) receptors in the nervous system, blocking ion current through these channels. PCP is easily synthesized; its abusers are primarily young people and polydrug users. It is used PO, by smoking, or by IV injection. It is also used as an adulterant in THC, LSD, amphetamine, or cocaine. The most common street preparation, *angel dust*, is a white granular powder that contains 50–100% percent of the drug. Low doses (5 mg) produce agitation, excitement, impaired motor coordination, dysarthria, and analgesia. Users may have horizontal or vertical nystagmus, flushing, diaphoresis, and hyperacusis. Behavioral changes include distortions of body image, disorganization of thinking, and feelings of estrangement. Higher doses of PCP (5–10 mg) may produce profuse salivation, vomiting, myoclonus, fever, stupor, or coma. PCP doses of ≥10 mg cause convulsions, opisthotonus, and decerebrate posturing, which may be followed by prolonged coma.

The diagnosis of PCP overdose is difficult because the patient's initial symptoms may suggest an acute schizophrenic reaction. Confirmation of PCP use is possible by determination of PCP levels in serum or urine. PCP assays are available at most toxicologic centers. PCP remains in urine for 1–5 days following high-dose intake.

PCP overdose requires life-support measures, including treatment of coma, convulsions, and respiratory depression in an intensive care unit. There is no specific antidote or antagonist for PCP. PCP excretion from the body can be enhanced by gastric lavage and acidification of urine. Death from PCP overdose may occur as a consequence of some combination of pharyngeal hypersecretion, hyperthermia, respiratory depression, severe hypertension, seizures, hypertensive encephalopathy, and intracerebral hemorrhage.

Acute psychosis associated with PCP use should be considered a psychiatric emergency since patients may be at high risk for suicide or extreme violence toward others. Phenothiazines should not be used for treatment because these drugs potentiate PCP's anticholinergic effects. Haloperidol (5 mg IM) has been administered on an hourly basis to induce suppression of psychotic behavior. PCP, like LSD and mescaline, produces vasospasm of cerebral arteries at relatively low doses. Chronic PCP use has been shown to induce insomnia, anorexia, severe social and behavioral changes, and, in some cases, chronic schizophrenia.

POLYDRUG ABUSE

Although drug abusers often report a preference for a particular drug, such as alcohol or opiates, the concurrent use of other drugs is common. Polydrug abuse often involves substances that may have different pharmacologic effects from the preferred drug. For example, concurrent use of such dissimilar compounds as stimulants and opiates or stimulants and alcohol is not unusual. The diversity of reported drug use combinations suggests that achieving some perceptible change in state, rather than any particular direction of change (stimulation or sedation), may be the primary reinforcer in polydrug use and abuse. There is also evidence that intoxication with alcohol or opiates is associated with increased tobacco smoking. There is relatively little systematic information available about multiple drug abuse interactions. However, the combined use of cocaine, heroin, and alcohol increases the risk for toxic effects and adverse medical consequences over risks associated with use of a single drug. One determinant of polydrug use patterns is the relative availability and cost of the drugs. There are many examples of situationally determined drug use patterns. For example, alcohol abuse, with its attendant medical complications, is one of the most serious problems encountered in former heroin addicts participating in methadone maintenance programs.

The physician must recognize that perpetuation of polydrug abuse and drug dependence is not necessarily a symptom of an underlying emotional disorder. Neither alleviation of anxiety nor reduction of depression accounts for initiation and perpetuation of polydrug abuse. Severe depression and anxiety are as frequently the consequences of polydrug abuse as they are the antecedents. There is also evidence that some of the most adverse consequences of drug use may be reinforcing and contribute to the continuation of polydrug abuse.

℞ POLYDRUG ABUSE

Adequate treatment of polydrug abuse, as well as other forms of drug abuse, requires innovative programs of intervention. The first step in successful treatment is detoxification, a process that may be difficult because of the abuse of several drugs with different pharmacologic actions (e.g., alcohol, opiates, and cocaine). Since patients may not recall or may deny simultaneous multiple drug use, diagnostic evaluation should always include urinalysis for qualitative detection of psychoactive substances and their metabolites. Treatment of polydrug abuse often requires hospitalization or inpatient residential care during detoxification and the initial phase of drug abstinence. When possible, specialized facilities for the care and treatment of chemically dependent persons should be used. Outpatient detoxification of polydrug abuse patients is likely to be ineffective and may be dangerous.

Drug abuse disorders often respond to effective treatment, but episodes of relapse may occur unpredictably. The physician should continue to assist patients during relapse and recognize that occasional recurrent drug use is not unusual in this complex behavioral disorder.

FURTHER READINGS

CAMI J, FARRE M: Mechanisms of disease: Drug addiction. N Engl J Med 349:975, 2003

HALPERN JH et al: Diminished interleukin-6 response to pro-inflammatory challenge in men and women after intravenous cocaine administration. J Clin Endocrinol Metabol 88:1188, 2003

TOUMBOUROU JW et al: Interventions to reduce harm associated with adolescent substance use. Lancet 369:1391, 2007

VOCCI FJ et al: Medication development for addictive disorders: The state of the science. Am J Psychiatry 162:1432, 2005

VOLKOW ND et al: Cocaine cues and dopamine in dorsal striatum: Mechanism of craving in cocaine addiction. J Neurosci 26:6583, 2006

390 Nicotine Addiction
David M. Burns

The use of tobacco leaf to create and satisfy nicotine addiction was introduced to Columbus by Native Americans and spread rapidly to Europe. The use of tobacco as cigarettes, however, became popular in the twentieth century and so is a modern phenomenon, as is the epidemic of disease caused by this form of tobacco.

Nicotine is the principal constituent of tobacco responsible for its addictive character. Addicted smokers regulate their nicotine intake and blood levels by adjusting the frequency and intensity of their tobacco use both to obtain the desired psychoactive effects and avoid withdrawal.

Unburned cured tobacco contains nicotine, carcinogens, and other toxins capable of causing gum disease, oral cancer, and possibly a slight increase in the risk of heart disease. When tobacco is burned, the resultant smoke contains, in addition to nicotine, 4000 other compounds that result from volatilization, pyrolysis, and pyrosynthesis of tobacco and various chemical additives used in making different tobacco products. The smoke is composed of a fine aerosol and a vapor phase; aerosolized particles are of a size range that results in deposition in the airways and alveolar surfaces of the lungs. The bulk of the toxicity and carcinogenicity of the smoke resides in the aerosolized particulate phase, which contains a large number of toxic constituents and carcinogenic compounds. The aggregate of particulate matter, after subtracting nicotine and moisture, is referred to as tar. The vapor phase contains carbon monoxide, respiratory irritants, and ciliotoxins as well as many of the volatile compounds responsible for the distinctive smell of cigarette smoke.

The alkaline pH of smoke from blends of tobacco utilized for pipes and cigars allows sufficient absorption of nicotine across the oral mucosa to satisfy the smoker's need for this drug. Therefore, smokers of pipes and cigars tend not to inhale the smoke into the lung, confining the toxic and carcinogenic exposure (and the increased rates of disease) largely to the upper airway for most users of these products. The acidic pH of smoke generated by the tobacco used in cigarettes dramatically reduces absorption of nicotine in the mouth, necessitating inhalation of the smoke into the larger surface of the lungs in order to absorb quantities of nicotine sufficient to satisfy the smoker's addiction. The shift to using tobacco as cigarettes, with resultant increased deposition of smoke in the lung, has created the epidemic of heart disease, lung disease, and lung cancer that dominates the current disease manifestations of tobacco use.

Several genes have been associated with nicotine addiction. Some reduce the clearance of nicotine, and others have been associated with an increased likelihood of becoming dependent on tobacco and other drugs as well as a higher incidence of depression. It is unlikely that genetic factors are the principal determinants of addiction. Rates of smoking cessation have increased, and rates of nicotine addiction have decreased dramatically, since the mid-1950s, suggesting that factors other than genetics are important. It is more likely that genetic susceptibility can influence the probability that adolescent experimentation with tobacco will lead to addiction as an adult.

Adult cigarette smoking prevalence has declined to about 20% in the United States, with similar declines in Canada and most European countries. Male smoking prevalence is falling but remains high in most Asian countries, with increasing smoking prevalence among women in those countries. The highest rates of smoking and least cessation are observed in the former Soviet block countries. Of particular concern is the rapidly rising smoking rate observed in the developing world; it is hoped that the recently ratified World Health Organization Framework Convention on Tobacco Control will encourage effective tobacco control approaches in these countries in order to prevent a future epidemic of tobacco-related illness.

DISEASE MANIFESTATIONS OF CIGARETTE SMOKING

Over 400,000 individuals die prematurely each year in the United States from cigarette use; this represents approximately one out of every five deaths in the United States. Approximately 40% of cigarette smokers will die prematurely due to cigarette smoking unless they are able to quit.

TABLE 390-1 RELATIVE RISKS FOR CURRENT SMOKERS OF CIGARETTES		
	Current Smokers	
Disease or Condition	Males	Females
Coronary heart disease		
Age 35–64	2.8	3.1
Age ≥65	1.5	1.6
Cerebrovascular disease		
Age 35–64	3.3	4
Age ≥65	1.6	1.5
Aortic aneurysm	6.2	7.1
Chronic airway obstruction	10.6	13.1
Cancer		
Lung	23.3	12.7
Larynx	14.6	13
Lip, oral cavity, pharynx	10.9	5.1
Esophagus	6.8	7.8
Bladder, other urinary organs	3.3	2.2
Kidney	2.7	1.3
Pancreas	2.3	2.3
Stomach	2	1.4
Cervix		1.6
Acute myeloid leukemia	1.4	1.4
Sudden infant death syndrome		2.3
Infant respiratory distress syndrome		1.3
Low birth weight at delivery		1.8

The major diseases caused by cigarette smoking are listed in Table 390-1. The ratio of smoking-related disease rates in smokers compared to never smokers (relative risk) is greater at younger ages, particularly for coronary artery disease and stroke. At older ages, the background rate of disease in nonsmokers increases, diminishing the fractional contribution of smoking and the relative risk; however, absolute excess rates of disease mortality found in smokers compared to nonsmokers increase with increasing age. The organ damage caused by smoking and the number of smokers who die from smoking are both greater among the elderly, as one would expect from a process of cumulative injury.

CARDIOVASCULAR DISEASES

Cigarette smokers are more likely than nonsmokers to develop large-vessel atherosclerosis as well as small-vessel disease. Approximately 90% of peripheral vascular disease in the nondiabetic population can be attributed to cigarette smoking, as can ~50% of aortic aneurysms. In contrast, 20–30% of coronary artery disease and ~10% of occlusive cerebrovascular disease are caused by cigarette smoking. There is a multiplicative interaction between cigarette smoking and other cardiac risk factors such that the increment in risk produced by smoking among individuals with hypertension or elevated serum lipids is substantially greater than the increment in risk produced by smoking for individuals without these risk factors.

In addition to its role in promoting atherosclerosis, cigarette smoking also increases the likelihood of myocardial infarction and sudden cardiac death by promoting platelet aggregation and vascular occlusion. Reversal of these effects may explain the rapid benefit of smoking cessation for a new coronary event demonstrable among those who have survived a first myocardial infarction. This effect may also explain the substantially higher rates of graft occlusion among continuing smokers following vascular bypass surgery for cardiac or peripheral vascular disease.

Cessation of cigarette smoking reduces the risk of a second coronary event within 6–12 months; rates of first myocardial infarction or death from coronary heart disease also decline within the first few years following cessation. After 15 years of cessation, the risk of a new myocardial infarction or death from coronary heart disease in former smokers is similar to that for those who have never smoked.

CANCER

Tobacco smoking causes cancer of the lung, oral cavity, naso-, oro-, and hypopharynx, nasal cavity and paranasal sinuses, larynx, esophagus, stomach, pancreas, liver, kidney (body and pelvis), ureter, urinary bladder, and uterine cervix and also causes myeloid leukemia. There is evi-

dence suggesting that cigarette smoking may play a role in increasing the risk of colorectal and possibly premenopausal breast cancer, but there is no association with postmenopausal breast cancer. There does not appear to be a causal link between cigarette smoking and cancer of the endometrium, and there is a lower risk of uterine cancer among postmenopausal women who smoke. The risks of cancer increase with the increasing number of cigarettes smoked per day and with increasing duration of smoking. Additionally, there are synergistic interactions between cigarette smoking and alcohol use for cancer of the oral cavity, esophagus, and possibly lung. Several occupational exposures also synergistically increase lung cancer risk among cigarette smokers, most notably occupational asbestos and radon exposure.

Cessation of cigarette smoking reduces the risk of developing cancer relative to continuing smoking, but even 20 years after cessation there is a modest persistent increased risk of developing lung cancer.

RESPIRATORY DISEASE

Cigarette smoking is responsible for 90% of chronic obstructive pulmonary disease. Within 1–2 years of beginning to smoke regularly, many young smokers will develop inflammatory changes in their small airways, although lung function measures of these changes do not predict development of chronic airflow obstruction. After 20 years of smoking, pathophysiologic changes in the lungs develop and progress proportional to smoking intensity and duration. Chronic mucous hyperplasia of the larger airways results in a chronic productive cough in as many as 80% of smokers >60 years. Chronic inflammation and narrowing of the small airways and/or enzymatic digestion of alveolar walls resulting in pulmonary emphysema can result in reduced expiratory airflow sufficient to produce clinical symptoms of respiratory limitation in ~15% of smokers.

Changes in the small airways of young smokers will reverse after 1–2 years of cessation. There may also be a small increase in measures of expiratory airflow among individuals who have developed chronic airflow obstruction, but the major change following cessation is a slowing of the rate of decline in lung function with advancing age rather than a return of lung function toward normal.

PREGNANCY

Cigarette smoking is associated with several maternal complications of pregnancy: premature rupture of membranes, abruptio placentae, and placenta previa; there is also a small increase in the risk of spontaneous abortion among smokers. Infants of smoking mothers are more likely to experience preterm delivery, have a higher perinatal mortality, be small for their gestational age, and have higher rates of infant respiratory distress syndrome; they are more likely to die of sudden infant death syndrome, and appear to have a developmental lag for at least the first several years of life.

OTHER CONDITIONS

Smoking delays healing of peptic ulcers; increases the risk of osteoporosis, senile cataracts, and macular degeneration; and results in premature menopause, wrinkling of the skin, gallstones and cholecystitis in women, and male impotence.

ENVIRONMENTAL TOBACCO SMOKE

Long-term exposure to environmental tobacco smoke increases the risk of lung cancer and coronary artery disease among nonsmokers. It also increases the incidence of respiratory infections, chronic otitis media, and asthma in children as well as causing exacerbation of asthma in children.

PHARMACOLOGIC INTERACTIONS

Cigarette smoking may interact with a variety of other drugs (Table 390-2). Cigarette smoking induces the cytochrome P450 system, which may alter the metabolic clearance of drugs such as theophylline. This may result in inadequate serum levels in smokers as outpatients when the dosage is established in the hospital under nonsmoking conditions.

TABLE 390-2 INTERACTIONS OF SMOKING AND PRESCRIPTION DRUGS

Drug	Interaction
Benzodiazepines	Less sedation
Beta-blockers	Reduced lowering of heart rate and blood pressure
Caffeine	Faster metabolic clearance
Chlorpromazine	Decreased serum concentrations[a]
Clomipramine	Decreased serum concentrations[a]
Clozapine	Decreased serum concentrations[a]
Dextropropoxyphene	Less analgesia
Oral estrogens	Increased hepatic clearance
Flecainide	Increased first-pass clearance
Fluphenazine	Decreased serum concentrations[a]
Fluvoxamine	Decreased serum concentrations[a]
Haloperidol	Decreased serum concentrations[a]
Heparin	Faster clearance
Imipramine	Decreased serum concentrations[a]
Insulin	Delayed absorption due to skin vasoconstriction
Lidocaine	Increased first-pass clearance
Mexiletine	Increased first-pass clearance
Olanzapine	Faster clearance
Pentazocine	Less analgesia, possible increased clearance
Propanolol	Increased first-pass clearance
Tacrine	Faster metabolic clearance
Theophylline	Faster metabolic clearance
Thiothixene	Faster metabolic clearance
Trazodone	Decreased serum concentrations[a]

[a]Clinical implications uncertain.

Correspondingly, serum levels may rise when smokers are hospitalized and not allowed to smoke. Smokers may also have higher first-pass clearance for drugs such as lidocaine, and the stimulant effects of nicotine may reduce the effect of benzodiazepines or beta blockers.

OTHER FORMS OF TOBACCO USE

Other major forms of tobacco use are moist snuff deposited between the cheek and gum, chewing tobacco, pipes and cigars, and recently bidi (tobacco wrapped in tendu or temburni leaf; commonly used in India), clove cigarettes, and water pipes. Oral tobacco use leads to gum disease and can result in oral cancer. All forms of burned tobacco generate toxic and carcinogenic smoke similar to that of cigarette smoke. The differences in disease consequences of use relate to frequency of use and depth of inhalation. The risk of upper airway cancers is similar among cigarette and cigar smokers, while those who have smoked only cigars have a much lower risk of lung cancer, heart disease, and chronic obstructive pulmonary disease. However, cigarette smokers who switch to pipes or cigars do tend to inhale the smoke, increasing their risk; and it is likely that comparable inhalation and frequency of exposure to tobacco smoke from any of these forms of tobacco use will lead to comparable disease outcomes.

A resurgence of cigar, bidi, and water pipe use among adolescents of both genders has raised concerns that these older forms of tobacco use are once again causing a public health problem.

LOWER TAR AND NICOTINE CIGARETTES

Filtered cigarettes with lower machine-measured yields of tar and nicotine have been recommended as offering lower disease risks. However, these cigarettes commonly use ventilation holes in the filters and other engineering designs to artificially lower the machine measurements. Smokers, however, can compensate and preserve their intake of nicotine (and tar) by changing the manner in which they puff on the cigarette or the number of cigarettes smoked per day. There is no meaningful disease-reduction benefit for smokers who switch to lower-yield cigarettes, and smokers should be discouraged from thinking of low-yield cigarettes as an alternative to cessation.

CESSATION

The process of stopping smoking is often a cyclical one, with the smoker sometimes making multiple attempts to quit and failing before finally being successful. Approximately 70–80% of smokers would like to quit smoking, approximately one-third of current smokers attempt to quit each year, and 90% of these unassisted attempts fail. Clinician-based smoking interventions should encourage smokers to try to quit and to use different forms of cessation assistance with each new cessation attempt rather than focusing exclusively on immediate cessation at the time of the first visit.

Advice from a physician to quit smoking, particularly around an acute illness, is a powerful trigger for cessation attempts, with up to half of patients who are advised to quit making a cessation effort. Other triggers include the cost of cigarettes, media campaigns, and changes in rules to restrict smoking in the workplace.

PHYSICIAN INTERVENTION (Table 390-3)

All patients should be asked whether they smoke, their past experience with quitting, and whether they are currently interested in quitting. Those who are not interested in quitting should be encouraged and motivated to quit; provided a clear, strong, and personalized physician message that smoking is an important health concern; and offered assistance if they become interested in quitting in the future. There is a relationship between the amount of assistance a patient is willing to accept and the success of the cessation attempt. A quit date should be negotiated, usually not the day of the visit but within the next few weeks, and a follow-up contact by office staff around the time of the quit date should be provided.

There are a variety of nicotine-replacement products, including over-the-counter nicotine patches, gum, and lozenges, as well as nicotine nasal and oral inhalers available by prescription. These products can be used for up to 3–6 months, and some products are formulated to allow a gradual step-down in dosage with increasing duration of abstinence. Antidepressants such as bupropion (300 mg in divided doses for up to 6 months) have also been shown to be effective, as has varenicline, a partial agonist for the nicotinic acetylcholine receptor (initial dose 0.5 mg daily increasing to 1 mg twice daily at day 8; treatment duration up to 6 months). Some evidence supports the combined use of nicotine-replacement therapy and antidepressants as well as the use of gum or lozenges for acute cravings in patients using patches. Nicotine-replacement therapy is provided in different dosages with higher doses being recommended for more intense smokers. Clonidine or nortriptyline may be useful for patients who have failed on first-line pharmacologic treat-

TABLE 390-3 CLINICAL PRACTICE GUIDELINES

Physician actions
  Ask: Systematically identify all tobacco users at every visit
  Advise: Strongly urge all smokers to quit
  Identify smokers willing to quit
  Assist the patient in quitting
  Arrange follow-up contact
Effective pharmacologic interventions[a]
  First-line therapies
    Nicotine gum (1.5)
    Nicotine patch (1.9)
    Nicotine nasal inhaler (2.7)
    Nicotine oral inhaler (2.5)
    Nicotine lozenge (2.0)
    Bupropion (2.1)
    Varenicline (2.7)
  Second-line therapies
    Clonidine (2.1)
    Nortriptyline (3.2)
Other Effective Interventions[a]
  Physician or other medical personnel counseling (10 min) (1.3)
  Intensive smoking cessation programs (at least 4–7 sessions of 20–30
    min duration lasting at least 2 and preferably 8 weeks) (2.3)
  Clinic-based smoking status identification system (3.1)
  Counseling by nonclinicians and social support by family and friends
  Telephone counseling (1.2)

[a]Numerical value following the intervention is the multiple for cessation success compared to no intervention.

ment or who are unable to use other therapies. Antidepressants are more effective in those with a history of depression symptoms.

Current recommendations are to offer pharmacologic treatment, usually with nicotine replacement therapy (NRT) and bupropion, to all who will accept it and to provide counseling and other support as a part of the cessation attempt. Currently, indications approved by the U.S. Food and Drug Administration for NRT products limit their use to short-term use in conjunction with a cessation attempt. Nevertheless, it is not uncommon for individual smokers to use these products, particularly the products available over the counter, for longer durations and sometimes with no intent to stop. There are some data to suggest that longer-term use of NRT may enable cessation in some smokers who are unable to quit with shorter duration use and that some individuals are able to achieve abstinence from tobacco through use of NRT chronically. It is useful for the practicing physician to recognize that these patterns of use exist among smokers trying to quit and that they may contribute to successful abstinence in some smokers. Cessation advice alone by a physician or his or her staff is likely to increase success compared with no intervention; a more comprehensive approach with advice, pharmacologic assistance, and counseling can increase cessation success by almost threefold.

Incorporation of cessation assistance into a practice requires a change of the care delivery infrastructure. Simple changes include: (1) adding questions about smoking and interest in cessation on patient-intake questionnaires, (2) asking patients whether they smoke as part of the initial vital sign measurements made by office staff, (3) listing smoking as a problem in the medical record, and (4) automating follow-up contact with the patient on the quit date. These changes are essential to institutionalizing smoking intervention within the practice setting; without this institutionalization, the best intentions of physicians to intervene with their patients who smoke are often lost in the time crush of a busy practice.

PREVENTION

Approximately 90% of individuals who will become cigarette smokers initiate the behavior during adolescence. Factors that promote adolescent initiation are parental or older generation cigarette smoking, tobacco advertising and promotional activities, the availability of cigarettes, and the social acceptability of smoking. The need for an enhanced self-image and to imitate adult behavior is greatest for those adolescents who have the least external validation of their self-worth, which may explain in part the enormous differences in adolescent smoking prevalence by socioeconomic and school performance strata.

Prevention of smoking initiation must begin early, preferably in the elementary school years. Physicians who treat adolescents should be sensitive to the prevalence of this problem. Physicians should ask all adolescents whether they have experimented with tobacco or currently use tobacco, reinforce the facts that most adolescents and adults do not smoke, and explain that all forms of tobacco are both addictive and harmful.

FURTHER READINGS

FRIEDEN TR, BLOOMBERG MR: How to prevent 100 million deaths from tobacco. Lancet 369:1758, 2007

INTERNATIONAL AGENCY FOR RESEARCH ON CANCER: *Reversal of Risk After Quitting Smoking.* IARC Handbooks of Cancer Prevention, Tobacco Control, Volume 11. Lyon, France, IARC, 2006

US DEPARTMENT OF HEALTH AND HUMAN SERVICES: *The Health Consequences of Tobacco Use: A Report of the Surgeon General.* National Center for Chronic Disease Prevention and Health Promotion, Office on Smoking and Health, 2004

———: *Treating Tobacco Use and Dependence.* Clinical Practice Guideline, Public Health Service, DHHS, 2000

391 Disorders Caused by Reptile Bites and Marine Animal Exposures

Paul S. Auerbach, Robert L. Norris

This chapter outlines general principles for evaluation and management of victims of envenomation by venomous snakes and marine creatures. Because the incidence of serious bites and stings is relatively low in developed nations, there remains a paucity of relevant clinical research, and therapeutic decision-making is often based on anecdotal information.

VENOMOUS SNAKEBITE

EPIDEMIOLOGY

Venomous snakes of the world belong to the families Viperidae (subfamily Viperinae: Old World vipers; subfamily Crotalinae: New World and Asian pit vipers), Elapidae (including cobras, kraits, coral snakes, and all Australian venomous snakes), Hydrophiidae (sea snakes), Atractaspididae (burrowing asps), and Colubridae (a large family, of which most species are nonvenomous and only a few are dangerously toxic to humans). Bite rates are highest in temperate and tropical regions where the population subsists by manual agriculture. Estimates indicate >5 million bites annually by venomous snakes worldwide, with >125,000 deaths.

SNAKE ANATOMY/IDENTIFICATION

The typical snake-venom apparatus consists of bilateral venom glands located below and behind the eye and connected by ducts to hollow, anterior maxillary teeth. In viperids (vipers and pit vipers), these teeth are long mobile fangs that retract against the roof of the mouth when the animal is at rest. In elapids and sea snakes, the fangs are smaller and are relatively fixed in an erect position. In ~20% of pit viper bites and higher percentages of other snakebites (e.g., up to 75% for sea snakes), no venom is released ("dry" bites). Significant envenomation probably occurs in ~50% of all venomous snakebites.

Differentiation of venomous from nonvenomous snake species can be difficult. Viperids are characterized by somewhat triangular heads (a feature shared with many harmless snakes); elliptical pupils (also seen in some nonvenomous snakes, such as boas and pythons); enlarged maxillary fangs; and, in pit vipers, paired heat-sensing pits (foveal organs) on each side of the head. The New World rattlesnakes generally have a series of interlocking keratin plates (the rattle) on the tip of the tail; the rattle is used to warn potentially threatening intruders. Color pattern is notoriously misleading in identifying most venomous snakes. Many harmless snakes have color patterns that closely mimic venomous snakes found in the same region.

VENOMS AND CLINICAL MANIFESTATIONS

Snake venoms are complex mixtures of enzymes, low-molecular-weight polypeptides, glycoproteins, and metal ions. Among the deleterious components are hemorrhagins that promote vascular leakage and cause both local and systemic bleeding. Proteolytic enzymes cause local tissue necrosis, affect the coagulation pathway at various steps, and impair organ function. Myocardial depressant factors reduce cardiac output, and neurotoxins act either pre- or postsynaptically to inhibit peripheral nerve impulses. Most snake venoms have multisystem effects in their victims.

Envenomations by most viperids and some elapids with necrotizing venoms typically cause progressive local swelling, pain, ecchymosis (Fig. 391-1), and (over a period of hours or days) hemorrhagic bullae and serum-filled vesicles. In serious bites, tissue loss can be significant (Fig. 391-2). Systemic findings can include changes in taste, mouth numbness, muscle fasciculations, tachycardia or bradycardia, hypotension, pulmonary edema, hemorrhage (from essentially any anatomic site), and renal dysfunction. Envenomations by neurotoxic elapids such as kraits (*Bungarus* spp.), many Australian elapids [e.g., death adders (*Atractaspis* spp.) and tiger snakes (*Notechis* spp.)], some cobras (*Naja* spp.), and some viperids [e.g., the South American rattlesnake (*Crotalus durissus*) and some Indian Russell's vipers (*Daboia russelii*)] cause neurologic dysfunction. Early findings may consist of cranial nerve weakness (e.g., manifested by ptosis) and altered mental status. Severe poisoning may result in paralysis, including the muscles of respiration, and lead to death due to respiratory failure and aspiration. After elapid bites, the time of onset of venom intoxication varies from minutes to hours depending on the species involved, the anatomic location of the bite, and the amount of venom injected. Sea snake envenomation usually causes local pain (variable), myalgias, rhabdomyolysis, and neurotoxicity; these manifestations are occasionally delayed for hours.

℞ VENOMOUS SNAKEBITE

Field Management The most important aspect of prehospital care of a victim bitten by a venomous snake is rapid delivery to a medical facility equipped to provide supportive care (airway, breathing, and circulation) and antivenom administration. Most first aid recommendations made in

FIGURE 391-1 Northern Pacific rattlesnake (*Crotalus oreganus oreganus*) envenomations. *Left:* Moderately severe envenomation. Note edema and early ecchymosis 2 h after a bite to the finger. *Right:* Severe envenomation. Note extensive ecchymosis 5 days after a bite to the ankle.

FIGURE 391-2 Early stages of severe, full-thickness necrosis 5 days after a **Russell's viper (*Daboia russelii*) bite** in southwestern India.

the past are of little benefit, and some can actually worsen outcome. It is reasonable to apply a splint to the bitten extremity in order to lessen bleeding and discomfort and, if possible, to keep the extremity at approximately heart level. In developing regions, indigenous people should be encouraged to seek care quickly at health care facilities equipped with antivenoms as opposed to consulting traditional healers.

Although mechanical suction has been recommended in the field management of venomous snakebite for many years, there is now evidence that this intervention is of no benefit and can actually be deleterious in terms of local tissue damage.

Techniques or devices used for centuries in an effort to limit venom spread remain controversial. Lympho-occlusive bandages or tourniquets may limit spread only at the cost of greater local tissue damage, particularly with necrotic venoms. Because tourniquets lead to higher rates of amputation and loss of function, they absolutely should not be used. Elapid venoms that are primarily neurotoxic and have no significant local tissue effects may be localized by pressure-immobilization, in which the entire limb is immediately wrapped with a bandage (e.g., crepe or elastic) and then splinted. The wrap pressure must reach ~40–70 mmHg to be effective. Furthermore, if more than a few minutes from medical care, the victim must be carried out from the scene of the bite. Otherwise, muscular pumping will promote venom dispersal, even in bites to the upper extremities. In short, pressure-immobilization should be used only in cases where the offending snake is reliably identified and has a primarily neurotoxic venom, the rescuer is skilled in pressure-wrap application, and the victim can be carried to medical care—an uncommon combination of conditions. Besides tourniquets, other forbidden measures include incising or cooling the bite site, giving the victim alcoholic beverages, and applying electric shocks. The best first aid advice, as coined by Dr. Ian Simpson of the World Health Organization's Snakebite Treatment Group, is to "do it 'RIGHT'": *r*eassure the victim, *i*mmobilize the extremity, *g*et to the *h*ospital, and inform the physician of *t*elltale symptoms and signs.

Hospital Management In the hospital, the victim should be closely monitored (vital signs, cardiac rhythm, oxygen saturation, urine output) while a history is quickly obtained and a rapid, thorough physical examination is performed. Victims of neurotoxic envenomation should be watched carefully for evidence of difficulty swallowing or respiratory insufficiency, which should prompt definitive securing of the airway by endotracheal intubation. To provide objective evidence of the progression of envenomation,

the level of swelling in a bitten extremity should be marked and limb circumferences measured in several locations every 15 min until swelling has stabilized. Large-bore IV access in unaffected extremities should be established. Early hypotension is due to pooling of blood in the pulmonary and splanchnic vascular beds. Later, hemolysis and loss of intravascular volume into soft tissues may play important roles. Fluid resuscitation with isotonic saline should be initiated for clinical shock. If the blood pressure response to administration of crystalloid (20–40 mL/kg) is inadequate, a trial of 5% albumin (10–20 mL/kg) is prudent. If tissue perfusion fails to respond to volume resuscitation and antivenom infusion (see below), vasopressors (e.g., dopamine) can be added. Invasive hemodynamic monitoring (central venous and/or pulmonary arterial pressures) can be helpful in such cases, although obtaining access is risky if coagulopathy has developed.

Blood should be drawn for typing and cross-matching and for laboratory evaluation as soon as possible. Important studies include a complete blood count (to evaluate degree of hemorrhage or hemolysis and effects on platelet count), studies of renal and hepatic function, coagulation studies (to identify consumptive coagulopathy), and testing of urine for blood or myoglobin. In developing regions, the 20-min whole-blood clotting test (WBCT) can be used to diagnose coagulopathy reliably. A few milliliters of fresh blood are placed in a new, plain glass receptacle (e.g., test tube) and left undisturbed for 20 min. The tube is then tipped once to 45° to determine whether a clot has formed. If not, coagulopathy is diagnosed. In severe envenomations or with significant comorbidity, arterial blood gas studies, electrocardiography, and chest radiography may be helpful. Any arterial puncture in the setting of coagulopathy, however, requires great caution and must be performed at an anatomic site amenable to direct-pressure tamponade. After antivenom therapy (see below), laboratory values should be rechecked every 6 h until clinical stability is achieved.

The key to management of venomous snakebite is the administration of specific antivenom. Circulating venom components bind quickly with heterologous antibodies produced in animals immunized with the venom in question (or a very closely related venom). Antivenoms may be monospecific (for a particular snake species) or polyspecific (covering several medically important species in the region) but rarely offer cross-protection against snake species other than those used in their production unless the species are known to have homologous venoms. In the United States, assistance in finding antivenom can be obtained 24 h a day from regional poison control centers.

Indications for antivenom administration in victims of viperid bites include any evidence of systemic envenomation (systemic symptoms or signs; laboratory abnormalities) and (possibly) significant, progressive local findings (e.g., soft tissue swelling crossing a joint or involving more than half the bitten limb in the absence of a tourniquet). Care must be used in determining the significance of isolated soft-tissue swelling as, in many countries, the saliva of some relatively harmless snakes causes mild edema at the bite site. In such bites, antivenoms are unhelpful and unnecessary.

In the developing world (e.g., much of Asia and Africa), elapid bites are generally treated similarly to viperid bites. Systemic symptoms such as ptosis, other manifestations of cranial nerve impairment, or respiratory compromise constitute grounds for antivenom administration. Decisions about antivenom administration to victims with isolated local signs or symptoms are based on the criteria listed above for viperid bites.

Production of the only antivenom currently available in the United States for coral snake bites has been discontinued, and remaining stocks will be exhausted or will expire shortly. Until a suitable substitute is produced or imported, physicians caring for victims of *Micrurus* bites may have to rely on sound supportive care, especially airway management and respiratory support.

The package insert for the selected antivenom can be consulted regarding species covered, method of administration, starting dose, and need (if any) for re-dosing. The information in antivenom package inserts, however, is not always accurate and reliable. Whenever possible, it is advisable for treating physicians to seek advice from experts in snakebite management regarding indications for and dosing of antivenom. For viperid bites, antivenom administration should generally be continued as needed until the victim shows definite improvement (e.g., stabilized vital signs, reduced pain, restored coagulation). Neurotoxicity from elapid bites may be harder to reverse with antivenom. Once neurotoxicity is established and endotracheal intubation is required, further doses of antivenom are unlikely to be beneficial. In such cases, the victim must be maintained on mechanical ventilation until recovery occurs, which may take days to weeks.

TABLE 391-1 COMPARISON OF ANTIVENOMS RECENTLY AVAILABLE FOR TREATMENT OF PIT VIPER BITES IN THE UNITED STATES

	Antivenin (Crotalidae) Polyvalent[a]	CroFab[b]
Available since	1954	2000
Origin	Equine	Ovine
Snakes used in manufacture	*Crotalus adamanteus*	*C. adamanteus*
	C. atrox	*C. atrox*
	C. durissus terrificus	*C. scutulatus*
	Bothrops atrox	*Agkistrodon piscivorus*
Snakes covered	All North, Central, and South American and some Asian pit vipers	All North American pit vipers (and possibly other Latin American pit vipers)
Contains	IgG, equine albumin	Fab fragments
Skin testing recommended by manufacturer	Yes	No
Pretreatment with antihistamines recommended	Yes	No
Dosing (for North American pit viper bites only)[c]		
Dry bite	None	None
Mild	0 or 5 vials	4 vials
Moderate	10 vials	4–6 vials
Severe	15–20 vials	6 vials
Repeat dosing	As needed	Repeat starting dose if patient fails to stabilize. After stabilization, give 2 vials q6h for 3 more doses. (Alternatively, re-dose on an as-needed basis with close observation for recurrence of abnormalities.)
Volume of diluent	1000 mL[d]	250 mL
Administer over	2 h	1 h
Incidence of anaphylactic/-oid reaction	23–56%[e]	14%[f]
Incidence of delayed serum sickness	18–86%[g]	3%

[a]Wyeth-Ayerst Laboratories, Philadelphia, PA.
[b]Fougera, Melville, NY.
[c]Degrees of envenomation: mild = progressive local findings (no systemic findings and normal laboratory tests); moderate = local findings plus either mild systemic findings or mild laboratory abnormalities; and severe = local findings plus either severe systemic findings or severe laboratory abnormalities.
[d]Reduce for children and for patients with congestive heart failure.
[e]Some reactions have been severe, and some have been fatal.
[f]To date, all reactions have been relatively mild.
[g]Incidence is higher with larger doses.

The newest available antivenom in the United States (CroFab; Fougera, Melville, NY) is an ovine, Fab fragment antivenom that covers systemic venom effects of all North American pit viper species and carries a low risk of allergic sequelae. **Table 391-1** compares the two antivenoms recently available for the treatment of pit viper bites in the United States. The manufacturer of Antivenin (Crotalidae) Polyvalent has recently discontinued its production, leaving CroFab as the current drug of choice for the management of indigenous pit viper envenomations in the United States. Use of any heterologous serum product carries a risk of anaphylactoid reactions and delayed-hypersensitivity reactions (serum sickness). Skin testing for potential allergy is insensitive and nonspecific and should be omitted. Worldwide, the quality and availability of antivenoms are highly variable. In many developing countries, antivenom resources are scarce, contributing to high morbidity and mortality rates in these regions. The rates of acute anaphylactoid reactions to some of these products exceed 50%. If the risk of allergic reaction is significant, pretreatment with appropriate loading doses of IV antihistamines (e.g., diphenhydramine, 1 mg/kg to a maximum of 100 mg; and cimetidine, 5–10 mg/kg to a maximum of 300 mg) may be considered. In some regions, a prophylactic SC or IM dose of epinephrine is given in an effort to reduce the risk of reaction. Further research is necessary to determine whether any pretreatment measures are truly beneficial. Modest expansion of the patient's intravascular volume with crystalloids could blunt an acute adverse reaction.

Pretreatment is not recommended by the manufacturer of CroFab. Epinephrine should, however, always be immediately available, and the antivenom dose to be administered should be diluted in an appropriate volume of crystalloid according to the package insert. Antivenom should be given only by the IV route, and the infusion should be started slowly, with the physician at the bedside during the initial period to intervene immediately at the first signs of any acute reaction. The rate of infusion can be increased gradually in the absence of a reaction until the full starting dose has been administered (over a total period of ~1 h). Further antivenom may be necessary if the patient's clinical condition fails to stabilize or worsens. After stabilization, additional doses of CroFab are often recommended as the small-molecular-weight Fab fragments are rapidly cleared from the circulation. Larger, whole IgG or F(ab)$_2$ antivenoms have longer half-lives that eliminate the need for re-dosing after initial stabilization unless definitive symptoms of envenomation reappear.

If the patient develops an acute reaction to antivenom, the infusion should be temporarily stopped and the reaction immediately treated with IM epinephrine and IV antihistamine and steroids (Chap. 311). If the severity of envenomation warrants additional antivenom, the dose should be further diluted in isotonic saline and restarted as soon as possible. Rarely, in recalcitrant cases, a concomitant IV infusion of epinephrine may be required to hold allergic sequelae at bay while further antivenom is administered. The patient must be very closely monitored, preferably in an intensive care setting, during such therapy.

Blood products are rarely necessary in the management of the envenomated patient. The venoms of many snake species can cause a drop in platelet count or hematocrit and depletion of coagulation factors. Nevertheless, these components usually rebound within hours after administration of adequate antivenom. If the need for blood products is thought to be great (e.g., for a dangerously low platelet count in a hemorrhaging patient), these products still should be given only after adequate antivenom administration to avoid adding fuel to ongoing consumptive coagulopathy.

Rhabdomyolysis and hemolysis should be managed in standard fashion. Victims who develop acute renal failure should be evaluated by a nephrologist and referred for dialysis (peritoneal or hemodialysis) as needed. Such renal failure, usually due to acute tubular necrosis, is frequently reversible. If bilateral cortical necrosis occurs, however, the prognosis for renal recovery is more grim, and long-term dialysis with possible renal transplantation may be necessary.

Acetylcholinesterase inhibitors (e.g., edrophonium and neostigmine) may promote neurologic improvement in patients bitten by snakes with postsynaptic neurotoxins. Victims with objective evidence of neurologic dysfunction after snakebite should receive a trial of acetylcholinesterase inhibitors as outlined in **Table 391-2**. If they respond, additional doses of long-acting neostigmine can be continued as needed. Special vigilance is required to prevent aspiration if repetitive dosing of neostigmine is used in an attempt to obviate endotracheal intubation.

Care of the bite wound includes application of a dry sterile dressing and splinting of the extremity with padding between the digits. Once the administration of an indicated antivenom has been initiated, the extremity should be elevated above heart level to relieve edema. Tetanus immunization should be updated as appropriate. Prophylactic antibiotics are generally unnecessary after bites by North American snakes, as the incidence of secondary infection is low. Antibiotics can be considered, however, if misguided first-aid efforts have included incisions or mouth suction. In some regions of the world, secondary bacterial infection is more common and the consequences are dire. In these regions, prophylactic antibiotics (e.g., cephalosporins) are commonly used.

Most snake envenomations involve subcutaneous deposition of venom. On occasion, however, venom can be injected more deeply into muscle

CHAPTER 391

Disorders Caused by Reptile Bites and Marine Animal Exposures

TABLE 391-2 USE OF ACETYLCHOLINESTERASE INHIBITORS IN NEUROTOXIC SNAKE ENVENOMATION

1. Patients with clear, objective evidence of neurotoxicity after snakebite (e.g., ptosis or inability to maintain upward gaze) should receive a trial of edrophonium (if available) or neostigmine.
   a. Pretreat with atropine: 0.6 mg IV (children, 0.02 mg/kg; minimum of 0.1 mg)
   b. Follow with:
      Edrophonium: 10 mg IV (children, 0.25 mg/kg)
      or
      Neostigmine: 1.5–2.0 mg IM (children, 0.025–0.08 mg/kg)
2. If objective improvement is evident at 5 min, continue neostigmine at a dose of 0.5 mg (children, 0.01 mg/kg) every 30 min as needed, with continued administration of atropine by continuous infusion of 0.6 mg over 8 h (children, 0.02 mg/kg over 8 h).
3. Maintain vigilance regarding aspiration risk, and secure the airway with endotracheal intubation as needed.

compartments. If swelling in the bitten extremity raises concern that subfascial muscle edema may be impeding tissue perfusion (muscle-compartment syndrome), intracompartmental pressures (ICPs) should be checked by any minimally invasive technique—e.g., wick catheter or ICP monitor (Stryker Instruments, Kalamazoo, MI). If any ICP is high (>30–40 mmHg), the extremity should be kept elevated while further antivenom is given. A dose of IV mannitol (1 g/kg) can be given in an effort to reduce muscle edema if the patient's hemodynamic status is stable. If, after 1 h of such therapy, the ICP remains elevated, a surgical consultation for possible fasciotomy should be obtained. While evidence from studies of animals suggests that fasciotomy may actually worsen myonecrosis, compartmental decompression is still required to preserve nerve function. Fortunately, the incidence of muscle-compartment syndrome is very low following snakebite.

Wound care in the days after the bite may require careful aseptic debridement of clearly necrotic tissue once coagulation has been restored. Intact serum-filled vesicles or hemorrhagic blebs should be left undisturbed. If ruptured, they should be debrided with sterile technique.

Physical therapy should be started when pain allows in order to return the victim to a functional state. The incidence of long-term loss of function (e.g., reduced range of motion, impaired sensory function) is unclear but is probably quite high (>30%), particularly after viperid bites.

Any patient with signs of venom poisoning should be observed in the hospital for at least 24 h. In North America, a patient with an apparently "dry" viperid bite should be watched for at least 8 h before discharge, as significant toxicity occasionally develops after a delay of several hours. The onset of systemic symptoms is commonly delayed for a number of hours after bites by several of the elapids (including coral snakes), some non–North American viperids [e.g., the hump-nosed pit viper (*Hypnale hypnale*)], and sea snakes. Patients bitten by these reptiles should be observed in the hospital for at least 24 h. Unstable patients should be admitted to a monitored setting.

At discharge, victims of venomous snakebite should be warned about signs and symptoms of wound infection and serum sickness as well as other potential long-term sequelae, such as pituitary insufficiency in Russell's viper (*D. russelii*) bites. If the victim had evidence of coagulopathy early on, this abnormality can recur during the first 2–3 weeks after the bite. Such victims should be warned to avoid elective surgery or activities posing a high risk of trauma during this period. Outpatient analgesic treatment and physical therapy should be continued.

In the event of serum sickness (fever, chills, urticaria, myalgias, arthralgias, and possibly renal or neurologic dysfunction developing 1–2 weeks after antivenom administration), the victim should be treated with systemic glucocorticoids (e.g., oral prednisone, 1–2 mg/kg daily) until all findings resolve, at which point the dose is tapered over 1–2 weeks. Oral antihistamines (e.g., diphenhydramine in standard doses) provide additional relief of symptoms.

MORBIDITY AND MORTALITY

The overall mortality rates for venomous snakebite are low in areas with rapid access to medical care and appropriate antivenoms. In the United States, for example, the mortality rate is <1% for victims who receive antivenom. Eastern and western diamondback rattlesnakes (*Crotalus adamanteus* and *C. atrox*, respectively) are responsible for the few snakebite deaths occurring in the United States. Snakes responsible for large numbers of deaths in other regions include cobras (*Naja* spp.), carpet and saw-scaled vipers (*Echis* spp.), Russell's vipers (*D. russelii*), large African vipers (*Bitis* spp.), lancehead pit vipers (*Bothrops* spp.), and tropical rattlesnakes (*C. durissus*).

The incidence of morbidity—defined as permanent functional loss in a bitten extremity—is difficult to estimate but is substantial. Morbidity may be due to muscle, nerve, or vascular injury or to scar contracture. In the United States, such loss tends to be more common and severe after rattlesnake bites than after bites by copperheads (*Agkistrodon contortrix*) or water moccasins (*A. piscivorus*).

MARINE ENVENOMATIONS

Management of venom poisoning by marine creatures is similar to that of venomous snakebite in that much of the treatment administered is supportive in nature. A specific marine antivenom can be used when appropriate.

INVERTEBRATES

Hydroids, fire coral, jellyfish, Portuguese man-of-war, and *sea anemones* possess specialized living stinging cells called *cnidocytes*, which encapsulate intracytoplasmic stinging organelles called *cnidae* (including nematocysts). The venoms from these organisms are mixtures of proteins, carbohydrates, and other components. Victims usually report immediate prickling or burning, pruritus, paresthesias, and painful throbbing with radiation. The skin becomes reddened, darkened, edematous, and/or blistered. A legion of neurologic, cardiovascular, respiratory, rheumatologic, gastrointestinal, renal, and ocular symptoms have been described. Anaphylaxis sometimes develops. During stabilization, the skin should immediately be decontaminated with a generous application of vinegar (5% acetic acid), which is the all-purpose agent most useful in inactivating the nematocysts. Rubbing alcohol (40–70% isopropyl alcohol), baking soda (sodium bicarbonate), papain (unseasoned meat tenderizer), fresh lemon or lime juice, household ammonia, olive oil, or sugar may be effective, depending on the species of stinging creature. For the sting of the venomous box-jellyfish (*Chironex fleckeri*), vinegar should be used. Perfume, aftershave lotion, and high-proof ethanol are not efficacious and may be detrimental; formalin, ether, gasoline, and other organic solvents should not be used. Shaving the skin helps remove remaining nematocysts. Freshwater irrigation and rubbing lead to further stinging by adherent nematocysts and should be avoided. Commercial (chemical) cold packs or real ice packs applied over a thin dry cloth or plastic membrane have been shown to be effective in alleviating mild or moderate *Physalia utriculus* (bluebottle jellyfish) stings. Recent observations suggest that local application of heat [up to 45°C (113°F)] may be as effective as or more effective than application of cold. After decontamination, application of anesthetic ointment (lidocaine, benzocaine), antihistamine (diphenhydramine), or steroid (hydrocortisone) topical preparations may be helpful. Persistent severe pain after decontamination may be treated with morphine, meperidine, fentanyl, or another narcotic analgesic. Muscle spasms may respond to 10% calcium gluconate (5–10 mL) or diazepam (2–5 mg, titrated upward as necessary) given IV. An ovine-derived antivenom is available from Commonwealth Serum Laboratories (see section on antivenom sources, below) for stings from the box-jellyfish found in Australian and Indo-Pacific waters. As of this writing, this antivenom has not yet been used to treat envenomation by the box-shaped jellyfish (possibly of the genus *Chiropsalmus*) that has been found in Florida waters. The pressure-immobilization technique is no longer recommended for venom containment in the setting of a jellyfish sting. Safe Sea, a "jellyfish-safe" sunblock (*www.nidaria.com*) applied to the skin before an individual enters the water, inactivates the recognition and discharge mechanisms of nematocysts, has been tested successfully against a number of marine stingers, and may prevent or diminish the effects of coelenterate stings.

Touching a *sea sponge* may result in dermatitis. The afflicted skin should be gently dried and adhesive tape used to remove embedded spicules. Vinegar should be applied immediately and then for 10–30 min three or four times a day. Rubbing alcohol may be used if vinegar is unavailable. After spicule removal and skin decontamination, steroid or antihistamine cream may be applied to the skin. Severe vesiculation should be treated with a 2-week course of systemic glucocorticoids.

Annelid worms (bristleworms) possess rows of soft, cactus-like spines capable of inflicting painful stings. Contact results in symptoms similar to those of nematocyst envenomation. Without treatment, pain usually subsides over several hours, but inflammation may persist for up to a week. Victims should resist the urge to scratch, since scratching may fracture retrievable spines. Visible bristles should be removed with forceps and adhesive tape or a commercial facial peel; alternatively, a thin layer of rubber cement can be used to entrap the spines. Use of vinegar, rubbing alcohol, or dilute ammonia or a brief application of unseasoned meat tenderizer (papain) may provide additional relief. Local inflammation should be treated with topical or systemic glucocorticoids.

Sea urchins possess either hollow, venom-filled, calcified spines or triple-jawed, globiferous pedicellariae with venom glands. The venom contains toxic components, including steroid glycosides, hemolysins, proteases, serotonin, and cholinergic substances. Contact with either venom apparatus produces immediate and intensely painful stings. The affected part should be immersed immediately in hot water (see below). Accessible embedded spines should be removed but may break off and remain lodged in the victim. Residual dye from the surface of a spine remaining after the spine's removal may mimic a retained spine but is otherwise of no consequence. Soft tissue radiography or MRI can confirm the presence of retained spines, which may warrant referral for attempted surgical removal if the spines are located near vital structures (e.g., joints, neurovascular bundles). Retained spines may cause the formation of granulomas that are amenable to excision or to intralesional injection with triamcinolone hexacetonide (5 mg/mL). Local and diffuse neuropathies have been observed after penetration by multiple spines of the black sea urchin (*Diadema* spp.). The pathophysiology of this phenomenon has not yet been determined.

Serious envenomations and deaths have followed bites of the *Australian blue-ringed octopuses* (*Octopus maculosus* and *O. lunulata*). Although these animals rarely exceed 20 cm in length, their venom contains a potent neurotoxin (maculotoxin) that inhibits peripheral nerve transmission by blocking sodium conductance. Oral and facial numbness develop within several minutes of a serious envenomation and rapidly progress to total flaccid paralysis, including failure of respiratory muscles. Immediately after envenomation, a circumferential pressure-immobilization dressing 15 cm wide should be applied over a gauze pad (~$7 \times 7 \times 2$ cm) that has been placed directly over the sting. The dressing should be applied at venous-lymphatic pressure, with the preservation of distal arterial pulses. Once the victim has been transported to the nearest medical facility, the bandage can be released. Since there is no antidote, treatment is supportive. If respirations are assisted, the victim may remain awake although completely paralyzed. Even with serious envenomations, significant recovery often takes place within 4–10 h. Sequelae are uncommon unless related to hypoxia.

VERTEBRATES

A *stingray* injury is both an envenomation and a traumatic wound. The venom, which contains serotonin, 5′-nucleotidase, and phosphodiesterase, causes immediate, intense pain that may last up to 48 h. The wound often becomes ischemic in appearance and heals poorly, with adjacent soft tissue swelling and prolonged disability. Systemic effects include weakness, diaphoresis, nausea, vomiting, diarrhea, dysrhythmias, syncope, hypotension, muscle cramps, fasciculations, paralysis, and (in rare cases) death.

The designation *scorpionfish* encompasses members of the family Scorpaenidae and includes not only scorpionfish but also lionfish and stonefish. A complex venom with neuromuscular toxicity is delivered through 12 or 13 dorsal, 2 pelvic, and 3 anal spines. In general, the sting of a stonefish is regarded as the most serious (severe to life-threatening); that of the scorpionfish is of intermediate seriousness; and that of the lionfish is the least serious. Like that of a stingray, the sting of a scorpionfish is immediately and intensely painful. Pain from a stonefish envenomation may last for days. Systemic manifestations of scorpionfish stings are similar to those of stingray envenomations but may be more pronounced, particularly in the case of a stonefish sting. The rare deaths following stonefish envenomation usually occur within 6–8 h.

Two species of marine catfish—*Plotosus lineatus* (the oriental catfish) and *Galeichthys felis* (the common sea catfish)—as well as several species of freshwater catfish are capable of stinging humans. Venom is delivered through a single dorsal spine and two pectoral spines. Clinically, a catfish sting is comparable to that of a stingray, although marine catfish envenomations are generally more severe than those of their freshwater counterparts. Surgeonfish (doctorfish, tang), weeverfish, ratfish, and horned venomous sharks have also envenomated humans.

℞ MARINE VERTEBRATE STINGS

The stings of all marine vertebrates are treated in a similar fashion. Except for stonefish and serious scorpionfish envenomations (see below), no antivenom is available. The affected part should be immersed immediately in nonscalding hot water (45°C/113°F) for 30–90 min or until there is significant relief of pain. Recurrent pain may respond to repeated hot-water treatment. Cryotherapy is contraindicated. Opiates will help alleviate the pain, as will local wound infiltration or regional nerve block with 1% lidocaine, 0.5% bupivacaine, and sodium bicarbonate mixed in a 5:5:1 ratio. After soaking and anesthetic administration, the wound must be explored and debrided. Radiography (in particular, MRI) may be helpful in identification of foreign bodies. After exploration and debridement, the wound should be vigorously irrigated with warm sterile water, saline, or 1% povidone-iodine in solution. Bleeding can usually be controlled by sustained local pressure for 10–15 min. In general, wounds should be left open to heal by secondary intention or treated by delayed primary closure. Tetanus immunization should be updated. Antibiotic treatment should be considered for serious wounds and for envenomation in immunocompromised hosts. The initial antibiotics should cover *Staphylococcus* and *Streptococcus* spp. If the victim is immunocompromised, if a wound is primarily repaired and is more than minor, or if an infection develops, antibiotic coverage should be broadened to include *Vibrio* spp.

APPROACH TO THE PATIENT:
Marine Envenomations

It is useful to be familiar with the local marine fauna and to recognize patterns of injury.

A large puncture wound or jagged laceration (particularly on the lower extremity) that is more painful than one would expect from the size and configuration of the wound is likely to be a stingray envenomation. Smaller punctures, as described above, represent the activity of a sea urchin or starfish. Stony corals cause rough abrasions and, in rare instances, lacerations or puncture wounds.

Coelenterate (marine invertebrate) stings sometimes create diagnostic skin patterns. A diffuse urticarial rash on exposed skin is often indicative of exposure to fragmented hydroids or larval anemones. A linear, whiplike print pattern appears where a jellyfish tentacle has contacted the skin. In the case of the dreaded box-jellyfish (Fig. 391-3), a cross-hatched, sometimes frosted appearance, followed by development of dark purple coloration within a few hours of the sting, heralds skin necrosis. The frosted appearance may be augmented by aluminum salt–based remedies applied to the wound. An encounter with fire coral causes immediate pain and swollen red skin irritation in the pattern of contact, similar to but more severe than the imprint left by exposure to an intact feather hydroid. Seabather's eruption, caused by thimble jellyfishes and larval anemones, may produce a diffuse rash that consists of clusters of erythematous macules or raised papules, accompanied by intense itching (Fig. 391-4). Toxic sponges create a burning and painful red rash on exposed skin, which may blister and later desquamate. Virtually all marine stingers invoke the sequelae of inflammation, so that local erythema, swelling, and adenopathy are fairly nonspecific.

FIGURE 391-3 Skin lesions caused by *Chironex fleckeri* sting. *(Courtesy of Dr. V. Pranava Murthy; with permission.)*

SOURCES OF ANTIVENOMS AND OTHER ASSISTANCE

The best way to locate a specific antivenom in the United States is to call a regional poison control center and ask for assistance. Divers Alert Network, a nonprofit organization designed to assist in the care of injured divers, may also help with the treatment of marine injuries. The network can be reached on the Internet at www.diversalertnetwork.org or by telephone 24 hours a day at (919) 684-8111. An antivenom for stonefish (and severe scorpionfish) envenomation is made in Australia by the Commonwealth Serum Laboratories (CSL; 45 Poplar Road, Parkville, Victoria, Australia 3052; *www.csl.com.au*; 61-3-389-1911). Polyvalent sea snake antivenom is also available from CSL. It is no longer recommended that tiger snake antivenom be used if sea snake antivenom is unavailable.

MARINE POISONINGS

CIGUATERA

Ciguatera poisoning is the most common nonbacterial food poisoning associated with fish in the United States; most U.S. cases occur in Florida and Hawaii. The poisoning almost exclusively involves tropical and semitropical marine coral reef fish common in the Indian Ocean, the South Pacific, and the Caribbean Sea. Of reported cases, 75% (except in Hawaii) involve the barracuda, snapper, jack, or grouper. The ciguatera syndrome is associated with at least five polyether sodium channel activator toxins that originate in photosynthetic dinoflagel-

FIGURE 391-4 Erythematous, papular rash typical of seabather's eruption caused by thimble jellyfish and larval anemones.

lates (such as *Gambierdiscus toxicus*) and accumulate in the food chain. Three major ciguatoxins are found in the flesh and viscera of ciguateric fishes: CTX-1, -2, and -3. Most, if not all, ciguatoxins are unaffected by freeze-drying, heat, cold, and gastric acid. None of the toxins affects the odor, color, or taste of fish. Cooking methods may alter the relative concentrations of the various toxins.

The onset of symptoms may come within 15–30 min of ingestion and typically takes place within 2–6 h. Symptoms increase in severity over the ensuing 4–6 h. Most victims develop symptoms within 12 h of ingestion, and virtually all are afflicted within 24 h. The >150 symptoms reported include abdominal pain, nausea, vomiting, diarrhea, chills, paresthesias, pruritus, tongue and throat numbness or burning, sensation of "carbonation" during swallowing, odontalgia or dental dysesthesias, dysphagia, dysuria, dyspnea, weakness, fatigue, tremor, fasciculations, athetosis, meningismus, aphonia, ataxia, vertigo, pain and weakness in the lower extremities, visual blurring, transient blindness, hyporeflexia, seizures, nasal congestion and dryness, conjunctivitis, maculopapular rash, skin vesiculations, dermatographism, sialorrhea, diaphoresis, headache, arthralgias, myalgias, insomnia, bradycardia, hypotension, central respiratory failure, and coma. Death is rare.

Diarrhea, vomiting, and abdominal pain usually develop 3–6 h after ingestion of a ciguatoxic fish. Symptoms may persist for 48 h and then generally resolve (even without treatment). A pathognomonic symptom is the reversal of hot and cold tactile perception, which develops in some persons after 3–5 days and may last for months. Tachycardia and hypertension have been described, in some cases after potentially severe transient bradycardia and hypotension. More severe reactions tend to occur in persons previously stricken with the disease. Persons who have ingested parrotfish (scaritoxin) may develop classic ciguatera poisoning as well as a "second-phase" syndrome (after 5–10 days' delay) of disequilibrium with locomotor ataxia, dysmetria, and resting or kinetic tremor. This syndrome may persist for 2–6 weeks.

The differential diagnosis of ciguatera includes paralytic shellfish poisoning, eosinophilic meningitis, type E botulism, organophosphate insecticide poisoning, tetrodotoxin poisoning, and psychogenic hyperventilation. At present, the diagnosis of ciguatera poisoning is made on clinical grounds because no routinely used laboratory test detects ciguatoxin in human blood. High-performance liquid chromatography (HPLC) is available for ciguatoxins and okadaic acid but is of limited clinical value because most health care institutions do not have the equipment needed to perform the test. A ciguatoxin enzyme immunoassay or radioimmunoassay may be used to test small portions of the suspected fish, but even these tests may not detect the very small amount of toxin (0.1 ppb) necessary to render fish flesh toxic.

℞ CIGUATERA POISONING

Therapy is supportive and based on symptoms. Nausea and vomiting may be controlled with an antiemetic, such as prochlorperazine (2.5–5 mg IV). Hypotension may require the administration of IV crystalloid and, in rare cases, a pressor drug. Bradyarrhythmias that lead to cardiac insufficiency and hypotension generally respond well to atropine (0.5 mg IV, up to 2 mg). Cool showers or the administration of hydroxyzine (25 mg PO every 6–8 h) may relieve pruritus. Amitriptyline (25 mg PO twice a day) reportedly ameliorates pruritus and dysesthesias. In three cases unresponsive to amitriptyline, tocainide appeared to be efficacious. Nifedipine has been used to treat headache. IV infusion of mannitol may be beneficial in moderate or severe cases, particularly for the relief of distressing neurologic or cardiovascular symptoms, although the efficacy of this therapy has been challenged and has not been definitively proven. The infusion is rendered initially as 1 g/kg per day over 45–60 min during the acute phase (days 1–5). If symptoms improve, a second dose may be given within 3–4 h and repeated on the following day. Care must be taken to avoid dehydration in the treated patient. The mechanism of the benefit against ciguatera intoxication is perhaps hyperosmotic water-drawing action, which reverses ciguatoxin-induced Schwann cell edema. Mannitol may also act in some fashion as a "hydroxyl scavenger" or may competitively inhibit ciguatoxin at the cell membrane.

During recovery from ciguatera poisoning, the victim should exclude the following from the diet: fish (fresh or preserved), fish sauces, shellfish, shellfish sauces, alcoholic beverages, nuts, and nut oils. Consumption of fish in ciguatera-endemic regions should be avoided. All oversized fish of any predacious reef species should be suspected of harboring ciguatoxin. Neither moray eels nor the viscera of tropical marine fish should ever be eaten.

PARALYTIC SHELLFISH POISONING

Paralytic shellfish poisoning is induced by ingestion of any of a variety of feral or aquacultured filter-feeding organisms, including clams, oysters, scallops, mussels, chitons, limpets, starfish, and sand crabs. The origin of their toxicity is the chemical toxin they accumulate and concentrate by feeding on various planktonic dinoflagellates (e.g., *Protogonyaulax*, *Ptychodiscus*, and *Gymnodinium*) and protozoan organisms. The unicellular phytoplanktonic organisms form the foundation of the food chain, and in warm summer months these organisms "bloom" in nutrient-rich coastal temperate and semitropical waters. These planktonic species can release massive amounts of toxic metabolites into the water and cause mortality in bird and marine populations. The paralytic shellfish toxins are water-soluble as well as heat- and acid-stable; they cannot be destroyed by ordinary cooking. The best-characterized and most frequently identified paralytic shellfish toxin is saxitoxin, which takes its name from the Alaska butter clam *Saxidomus giganteus*. A toxin concentration of >75 μg/100 g of foodstuff is considered hazardous to humans. In the 1972 New England "red tide," the concentration of saxitoxin in blue mussels exceeded 9000 μg/100 g of foodstuff. Saxitoxin appears to block sodium conductance, inhibiting neuromuscular transmission at the axonal and muscle membrane levels.

The onset of intraoral and perioral paresthesias (notably of the lips, tongue, and gums) comes within minutes to a few hours after ingestion of contaminated shellfish, and these paresthesias progress rapidly to involve the neck and distal extremities. The tingling or burning sensation later changes to numbness. Other symptoms rapidly develop and include lightheadedness, disequilibrium, incoordination, weakness, hyperreflexia, incoherence, dysarthria, sialorrhea, dysphagia, thirst, diarrhea, abdominal pain, nausea, vomiting, nystagmus, dysmetria, headache, diaphoresis, loss of vision, chest pain, and tachycardia. Flaccid paralysis and respiratory insufficiency may follow 2–12 h after ingestion. In the absence of hypoxia, the victim often remains alert but paralyzed.

℞ PARALYTIC SHELLFISH POISONING

Treatment is supportive and based on symptoms. If the victim comes to medical attention within the first few hours after poison ingestion, the stomach should be emptied by gastric lavage and then irrigated with 2 L (in 200-mL aliquots) of a solution of 2% sodium bicarbonate; this intervention has not been proved to be of benefit but is based on the notion that gastric acidity may enhance the potency of saxitoxin. Because breathing difficulty can be rapid in onset, induction of emesis is not advised. The administration of activated charcoal (50–100 g) and a cathartic (sorbitol, 20–50 g) makes empirical sense since these shellfish toxins are believed to bind well to charcoal. Some authors advise against administration of magnesium-based solutions (e.g., certain cathartics), cautioning that hypermagnesemia may contribute to suppression of nerve conduction.

The most serious problem is respiratory paralysis. The victim should be closely observed in a hospital for at least 24 h for respiratory distress. With prompt recognition of ventilatory failure, endotracheal intubation and assisted ventilation prevent anoxic myocardial and brain injury.

A direct human serum assay to identify the toxin responsible for paralytic shellfish poisoning is not yet clinically available; the mouse bioassay in widespread use may be replaced by an automated tissue culture bioassay. Polyclonal enzyme-linked immunosorbent assay (ELISA) to measure specific toxins is under development, as is fluorimetric HPLC.

DOMOIC ACID INTOXICATION (AMNESTIC SHELLFISH POISONING)

In late 1987 in eastern Canada, an outbreak of gastrointestinal and neurologic symptoms (amnestic shellfish poisoning) was documented in persons who had consumed mussels found to be contaminated with domoic acid. In this outbreak, the source of the toxin was *Nitzschia pungens*, a diatom ingested by the mussels. In 1991, an epidemic of domoic acid poisoning in the state of Washington was attributed to the consumption of razor clams. A heat-stable neuroexcitatory amino acid whose biochemical analogues are kainic acid and glutamic acid, domoic acid binds to the kainate type of glutamate receptor with three times the affinity of kainic acid and is 20 times as powerful a toxin. Shellfish can be tested for domoic acid by mouse bioassay and HPLC. The regulatory limit for domoic acid in shellfish is 20 parts per million.

The abnormalities noted within 24 h of ingesting contaminated mussels (*Mytilus edulis*) include arousal, confusion, disorientation, and memory loss. The median time of onset is 5.5 h. Other prominent symptoms include severe headache, nausea, vomiting, diarrhea, abdominal cramps, hiccoughs, arrhythmias, hypotension, seizures, ophthalmoplegia, pupillary dilation, piloerection, hemiparesis, mutism, grimacing, agitation, emotional lability, coma, copious bronchial secretions, and pulmonary edema. Histologic study of brain tissue taken at autopsy has shown neuronal necrosis or cell loss and astrocytosis, most prominently in the hippocampus and the amygdaloid nucleus—findings similar to those in animals poisoned with kainic acid. Several months after the primary intoxication, victims still display chronic residual memory deficits and motor neuronopathy or axonopathy. Nonneurologic illness does not persist.

℞ DOMOIC ACID INTOXICATION

Therapy is supportive and based on symptoms. Since kainic acid neuropathology seems to be nearly entirely seizure-mediated, an emphasis should be placed on anticonvulsive therapy, for which diazepam appears to be as effective as any other drug.

SCOMBROID POISONING

Scombroid (mackerel-like) fish include the albacore, bluefin, and yellowfin tuna; mackerel; saury; needlefish; wahoo; skipjack; and bonito. Nonscombroid fish that produce scombroid poisoning include the dolphinfish (Hawaiian mahimahi, *Coryphaena hippurus*), kahawai, sardine, black marlin, pilchard, anchovy, herring, amberjack, and Australian ocean salmon. In the northeastern and mid-Atlantic United States, bluefish (*Pomatomus saltatrix*) has been linked to scombroid poisoning. Because greater numbers of nonscombroid fish are being recognized as scombrotoxic, the syndrome may more appropriately be called *pseudoallergic fish poisoning*.

Under conditions of inadequate preservation or refrigeration, the musculature of these dark- or red-fleshed fish undergoes bacterial decomposition, which includes decarboxylation of the amino acid L-histidine to histamine, histamine phosphate, and histamine hydrochloride. Histamine levels of 20–50 mg/100 g are noted in toxic fish, with levels >400 mg/100 g on occasion. However, it is possible that some other compound may be responsible for this intoxication, since large doses of oral histamine do not reproduce the affliction. Whatever toxin(s) are involved are heat-stable and are not destroyed by domestic or commercial cooking. Affected fish typically have a sharply metallic or peppery taste; however, they may be normal in appearance, color, and flavor. Not all persons who eat a contaminated fish necessarily become ill, perhaps because of uneven distribution of decay within the fish.

Symptoms develop within 15–90 min of ingestion and include flushing (sharply demarcated; exacerbated by ultraviolet exposure; particularly pronounced on the face, neck, and upper trunk), a sensation of warmth without elevated core temperature, conjunctival hyperemia, pruritus, urticaria, angioneurotic edema, bronchospasm, nausea, vomiting, diarrhea, epigastric pain, abdominal cramps, dysphagia, headache, thirst, pharyngitis, gingival burning, palpitations, tachycardia, dizziness, and hypotension. Without treatment, the symptoms generally resolve within 8–12 h. Because of blockade of gastrointestinal tract histaminase, the reaction may be more severe in a person who is concurrently ingesting isoniazid.

Rx SCOMBROID POISONING

Therapy is directed at reversing the histamine effect with antihistamines, either H-1 or H-2. If bronchospasm is severe, an inhaled bronchodilator—or in rare, extremely severe circumstances, injected epinephrine—may be used. Glucocorticoids are of no proven benefit. Protracted nausea and vomiting, which may empty the stomach of toxin, may be controlled with a specific antiemetic, such as prochlorperazine. The persistent headache of scombroid poisoning may respond to cimetidine or a similar antihistamine if standard analgesics are not effective.

FURTHER READINGS

AUERBACH PS (ed): *Wilderness Medicine*, 5th ed. St. Louis, Mosby, 2007

BUSH SP, HARDY DL: Immediate removal of Extractor is recommended. Ann Emerg Med 38:607, 2001

———— et al: Effects of a negative pressure venom extraction device (Extractor) on local tissue injury after artificial rattlesnake envenomation in a porcine model. Acad Emerg Med 7:495, 2000

DART RC et al: A randomized multicenter trial of Crotalinae polyvalent immune Fab (ovine) antivenom for the treatment for crotaline snakebite in the United States. Arch Intern Med 161:2030, 2001

GOLD BS et al: Bites of venomous snakes. N Engl J Med 347:347, 2002

MEBS D: *Venomous and Poisonous Animals*. Boca Raton, FL, CRC Press, 2002

MEIER J, WHITE J (eds): *Handbook of Clinical Toxicology of Animal Venoms and Poisons*. Boca Raton, FL, CRC Press, 1996, pp 89–176

MEYER WP et al: First clinical experiences with a new ovine Fab *Echis ocellatus* snake bite antivenom in Nigeria: Randomized comparative trial with Institute Pasteur Serum (Ipser) Africa antivenom. Am J Trop Med Hyg 56:291, 1997

PEARN J: Neurology of ciguatera. J Neurol Neurosurg Psychiatry 70:4, 2001

SIMPSON ID, NORRIS RL: Snakes of medical importance in India: Is the "big 4" still relevant and useful? Wilderness Environ Med 18:2, 2007

392 Ectoparasite Infestations and Arthropod Bites and Stings
Richard J. Pollack, James H. Maguire

Ectoparasites are arthropods or helminths that infest the skin or hair of other animals, from which they derive sustenance and shelter. They may penetrate beneath the surface of the host or attach superficially by their mouthparts. These organisms damage their hosts by inflicting direct injury, by eliciting a hypersensitivity reaction, or by inoculating toxins or pathogens. The main medically important ectoparasites are arachnids (including mites and ticks), insects (including lice, fleas, bedbugs, and flies), pentastomes (tongue worms), and leeches. Arthropods may also harm humans through brief encounters during which they take a blood meal or attempt to defend themselves by biting, stinging, or exuding venoms. Various arachnids (spiders, scorpions), insects (bees, hornets, wasps, ants, flies, bugs, caterpillars, and beetles), millipedes, and centipedes produce ill effects in this manner, as do certain ectoparasites of animals, including ticks, biting mites, and fleas. In the United States, more people die each year as a consequence of arthropod stings than from the bites of poisonous snakes.

SCABIES

The human itch mite, *Sarcoptes scabiei*, is a common cause of itching dermatosis infesting ~300 million persons worldwide. Gravid female mites, measuring ~0.3 mm in length, burrow superficially beneath the stratum corneum, depositing three or fewer eggs per day. Nymphs mature in ~2 weeks and then emerge as adults to the surface of the skin, where they mate and (re)invade the skin of the same or another host. Transfer of newly fertilized female mites from person to person occurs mainly by intimate contact and is facilitated by crowding, poor hygiene, and multiple sexual partners. Generally, these mites die within a day or so in the absence of host contact. Transmission via sharing of contaminated bedding or clothing is therefore infrequent. In the United States, scabies may account for up to 5% of visits to dermatologists. Outbreaks occur in nursing homes, mental institutions, and hospitals.

The itching and rash associated with scabies derive from a sensitization reaction directed against the excreta that the mite deposits in its burrow. An initial infestation remains asymptomatic for up to 6 weeks, and a reinfestation produces a hypersensitivity reaction without delay. Burrows become surrounded by infiltrates of eosinophils, lymphocytes, and histiocytes, and a generalized hypersensitivity rash later develops in remote sites. Immunity and associated scratching limit most infestations to <15 mites per person. Hyperinfestation with thousands of mites, a condition known as *crusted scabies* or *Norwegian scabies*, may result from glucocorticoid use, immunodeficiency, and neurologic and psychiatric illnesses that limit itching and scratching.

Intense itching worsens at night and after a hot shower. Typical burrows may be difficult to find because they are few in number and may be obscured by excoriations. Burrows appear as dark wavy lines in the epidermis and measure up to 15 mm. Lesions occur most frequently on the volar wrists, between the fingers, on the elbows, and on the penis. Small papules and vesicles, often accompanied by eczematous plaques, pustules, or nodules, are symmetrically distributed in these sites and in skin folds under the breasts and around the navel, axillae, belt line, buttocks, upper thighs, and scrotum. Except in infants, the face, scalp, neck, palms, and soles are spared. Crusted scabies resembles psoriasis in its typical widespread erythema, thick keratotic crusts, scaling, and dystrophic nails. Characteristic burrows are not seen in crusted scabies, and patients usually do not itch, although their infestations are highly contagious and have been responsible for outbreaks of classic scabies in hospitals.

Scabies should be considered in patients with pruritus and symmetric polymorphic skin lesions in characteristic locations, particularly if there is a history of household contact with a case. Burrows should be sought and unroofed with a sterile needle or scalpel blade, and the scrapings should be examined microscopically for the mite, its eggs, and its fecal pellets. Biopsies, scrapings of papulovesicular lesions, and microscopic inspection of clear adhesive tape lifted from lesions may also be diagnostic. In the absence of identifiable mites or mite products, the diagnosis is based on clinical presentation and history. Diverse kinds of dermatitis due to other causes are frequently misdiagnosed as scabies.

Rx SCABIES

Permethrin cream (5%) is less toxic than 1% lindane preparations and is effective against lindane-tolerant infestations. Scabicides are applied thinly but thoroughly behind the ears and from the neck down after bathing and are removed 8 h later with soap and water. Successful treatment of crusted scabies requires pre-application of a keratolytic agent such as 6% salicylic acid and then of scabicides to the scalp, face, and ears. Repeated treatments or the sequential use of several agents may be necessary. Although ivermectin has not yet been approved by the U.S. Food and Drug Administration (FDA) for use against any form of scabies, a single oral dose (200 μg/kg) effectively treats scabies in otherwise-healthy persons; patients with crusted scabies may require two doses separated by an interval of 1–2 weeks.

Although effectively treated scabies infestations become noninfectious within a day, itching and rash due to hypersensitivity to the dead mites and their excreted and secreted products frequently persist for weeks or months. Unnecessary re-treatment with topical agents may provoke contact dermatitis. Antihistamines, salicylates, and calamine lotion relieve itching during treatment, and topical glucocorticoids are useful for pruritus that lingers after effective treatment. To prevent reinfestations, bedding and clothing should be washed and/or dried on high heat or heat-pressed, and close contacts, even if asymptomatic, should be treated simultaneously.

CHIGGERS AND OTHER BITING MITES

Chiggers are the larvae of trombiculid (harvest) mites that normally feed on mice in grassy or brush-covered sites in the tropics and subtropics and less frequently in temperate areas during warm months. They wait for hosts on low vegetation and attach themselves to passing animals or to humans. The larva pierces the skin of its host and produces a secreted tube-like structure (*stylostome*) in the dermis through which it imbibes tissue fluids. The stylostome is highly antigenic and causes an exceptionally pruritic papular, papulovesicular, or papulourticarial lesion (≤2 cm in diameter) that develops within hours of attachment in persons previously sensitized to mite antigen. Feeding mites appear as tiny red vesicles adjacent to hair follicles. Scratching invariably destroys the body of a mite. Generally, lesions vesiculate and develop a hemorrhagic base. Itching and burning persist for weeks. The rash is common on the ankles and where clothing obstructs the further wanderings of the mites. Repellents are useful for preventing chigger bites.

Diverse mites associated with birds and rodents can be particularly bothersome when they invade homes and bite human inhabitants. In North America, the northern fowl mite, the chicken mite, the tropical rat mite, and the house mouse mite normally feed on poultry, various songbirds, or small mammals and are abundant in and near their hosts' nests. These mites invade homes after their natural hosts die or leave their nests. Although the mites often are not seen because of their small size, their bites can be painful and pruritic. Painful bite-like sensations associated only with certain rooms of a home may be due to biting mites. Rodent- and bird-associated mites are best eliminated by excluding hosts, removing nests, and cleaning and treating the nesting area with appropriate acaricides. *Pyemotes* and other mites that infest grain, straw, cheese, or other animal products occasionally produce similar episodes of rash and discomfort.

Diagnosis of mite-induced dermatitides (including those caused by chiggers) relies on a history of exposure to the source of the mite. Antihistamines or topical steroids effectively reduce mite-induced pruritus.

TICK BITES AND TICK PARALYSIS

Ticks attach and feed painlessly; blood is their only food. Their secretions produce local reactions, a febrile illness, or paralysis and transmit diverse pathogens. Generally, soft ticks attach for <1 h and may produce erythematous macular lesions ≤3 cm in diameter. Some species in Africa, the western United States, and Mexico produce painful hemorrhagic lesions. In contrast, hard ticks attach and feed for several days or sometimes for >1 week. At the site of hard-tick bites, small areas of induration with surrounding erythema and occasionally necrotic ulcers develop. Chronic nodules (tick granulomas) reach several centimeters in diameter and may require surgical excision. Tick-induced fever, associated with headache, nausea, and malaise, usually resolves ≤36 h after the tick is removed.

Tick paralysis, an ascending flaccid paralysis, is believed to be caused by a toxin in tick saliva that produces neuromuscular block and decreases nerve conduction. Throughout the world, this rare complication has followed the bites of >40 kinds of ticks; in the United States, dog and wood ticks are most commonly involved. Weakness begins in the lower extremities ≤6 days after the tick's attachment and ascends symmetrically over several days to result in complete paralysis of the extremities and cranial nerves. Deep tendon reflexes are diminished or lacking altogether, but sensory examination and findings on lumbar puncture are typically normal. Removal of the tick generally results in improvement within a few hours and complete recovery after several days. Failure to remove the tick may lead to dysarthria, dysphagia, and ultimately death from aspiration or respiratory paralysis. Diagnosis

FIGURE 392-1 Deer ticks (*Ixodes scapularis*, black-legged ticks) on a U.S. penny: larva (*below ear*), nymph (*right*), adult male (*above*), and adult female (*left*).

depends on finding the tick, which is often hidden beneath hair. An antiserum to the saliva of *Ixodes holocyclus*, the usual cause of tick paralysis in Australia, effectively reverses paralysis caused by these ticks.

Ticks should be removed by firm traction with a forceps placed near the point of attachment. Use of occlusive dressings, heat, or other substances merely delays tick removal. The site of attachment should be disinfected. Tick mouthparts remaining in the skin generally are shed within days without excision. Removal of ticks during the first 48 h of attachment nearly always prevents transmission of the agents of Lyme disease, babesiosis, anaplasmosis, and ehrlichiosis. Gentle handling (to avoid rupture of ticks) and use of gloves may avert accidental contamination with tick fluids containing pathogens. Rather than awaiting results of tick testing or seroconversion to Lyme disease, patients with bites thought to be associated with deer ticks (Fig. 392-1) may be treated presumptively with a short course of oral doxycycline.

PEDICULIASIS (LOUSE INFESTATION)

Nymphs and adults of all three kinds of human lice feed at least once a day, ingesting human blood exclusively. Head lice (*Pediculus capitis*) infest mainly the hair of the scalp, body lice (*Pediculus humanus*) the clothing, and crab or pubic lice (*Phthirus pubis*) mainly the hair of the pubis. The saliva of lice produces an intensely irritating maculopapular or urticarial rash in sensitized persons. Female head and pubic lice cement their eggs firmly to hair and female body lice to clothing. A nymph hatches after ~10 days of development. The empty egg (nit) may remain affixed for months thereafter.

In North America, head lice infest ~1% of elementary school–aged children. Head lice are transmitted mainly by direct head-to-head contact rather than by fomites (shared headgear, grooming implements, bedding). Infestations by head lice tend to be asymptomatic. Pruritus, due mainly to hypersensitivity to the louse's saliva, generally is transient and mild. Head lice removed from a person succumb to desiccation and starvation within ~1 day. Head lice are unimportant as vectors of pathogenic agents.

Body lice remain on clothing except when feeding and generally succumb in ≤2 days if separated from their host. These lice mainly infest disaster victims or indigent people who are in close contact with other infested individuals. Body lice are acquired by direct contact or by sharing of clothing and bedding. These lice are vectors for the agents of louse-borne typhus (Chap. 167), louse-borne relapsing fever (Chap. 165), and trench fever (Chap. 153). Pruritic lesions are particularly common around the neckline. Chronic infestations result in a postinflammatory hyperpigmentation and thickening of skin known as *vagabonds' disease*.

The crab or pubic louse is transmitted mainly by sexual contact. These lice occur mainly on pubic hair and less frequently on hair of the axillae and the face, including the eyelashes. Children and adults may acquire pubic lice by sexual or close nonsexual contact. Intensely

FIGURE 392-2 Adult female human head louse (*Pediculus capitis*) on a nit (louse-egg) comb.

pruritic lesions and blue macules ~3 mm in diameter (*maculae ceruleae*) develop at the site of bites. Blepharitis commonly accompanies infestations of the eyelashes.

Pediculiasis may be suspected upon the detection of nits on hairs or in clothing, but confirmation should be based upon discovery of a live louse.

℞ PEDICULIASIS

Generally, treatment is warranted only if live lice are discovered. The presence of nits alone is evidence of former—but not current—infestation. Mechanical removal of lice and their eggs by means of a fine-toothed louse or nit comb (**Fig. 392-2**) often fails to eliminate infestations. Treatment of newly identified active infestations generally relies upon a 10-min application of ~1% permethrin or pyrethrins, with a second application 10 days later. Lice persisting after this treatment may be resistant to pyrethroids (see below). Chronic infestations may be treated for ≤12 h with 0.5% malathion. Lindane is applied for just 4 min but seems less effective and may pose a greater risk of adverse reaction, particularly when misused. Resistance of head lice to permethrin, malathion, and lindane has been reported. Ivermectin may be useful in cases of resistance to malathion and permethrin but has not been approved for this purpose by the FDA. Although children infested by head lice are frequently isolated or excluded from school, this practice is increasingly seen as unjustified.

Body lice are usually eliminated by bathing and by changing to laundered clothes. Application of topical pediculicides from head to foot may be necessary for hirsute patients. Clothes and bedding are effectively deloused by heating in a clothes dryer at ≥55°C for 30 min or by heat-pressing. Emergency mass delousing of persons and clothing may be warranted during periods of civil strife and after natural disasters to reduce the risk of pathogen transmission by body lice.

Pubic lice infestations are treated with topical pediculicides except for eyelid infestations (*phthiriasis palpebrum*), which generally respond to a coating of petrolatum applied for 3–4 days.

MYIASIS (FLY INFESTATION)

Myiasis refers to infestations by fly larvae (maggots) that invade living or necrotic tissue or body cavities and produce different clinical syndromes, depending on the species of fly.

In forested parts of Central and South America, larvae of the human botfly *Dermatobia hominis* produce boil-like subcutaneous nodules ≤3 cm in diameter. The adult female captures a mosquito or another bloodsucking insect and deposits her eggs on its abdomen. When the carrier insect attacks a human or bovine host several days later, the warmth and moisture of the host's surface stimulate the larvae to hatch. The larvae promptly penetrate intact skin. After 6–12 weeks of development, mature larvae emerge from the skin and drop to the ground. The African tumbu fly *Cordylobia anthropophaga* deposits its eggs on sand or drying laundry contaminated with urine or sweat. Larvae hatch on contact with the body, penetrate the skin, and produce boils from which they emerge ~9 days later. Furuncular myiasis is suggested by uncomfortable lesions with a central breathing pore that emits bubbles when submerged in water. A sensation of movement under the patient's skin may lead to severe emotional distress. Botfly larvae may be induced to emerge if the air pore is coated with petrolatum or another occlusive substance. Removal may be facilitated by injection of a local anesthetic into the surrounding tissue, but sur-

gical excision is often necessary because upward-pointing spines of some species hold the larva firmly in place.

Larvae of the horse botfly *Gasterophilus intestinalis* do not mature after penetrating human skin but migrate for weeks in the epidermis. The resulting pruritic and serpiginous eruption resembles cutaneous larva migrans caused by hookworms (Chap. 209). Horseback riders become infested when eggs deposited on the flank of the horse hatch against their bare legs. Larvae are removed with a needle. The larvae of the cattle botfly invade more deeply and produce boil-like swellings.

Certain flies are attracted to blood and pus, and their newly hatched larvae enter wounds or diseased skin. Larvae of the green bottle fly usually remain superficial and confined to necrotic tissue. Larvae of screwworm flies and the flesh fly invade viable tissue more deeply and produce large suppurating lesions. Larvae that infest wounds may also infest body cavities such as the mouth, nose, ears, sinuses, anus, vagina, and lower urinary tract, particularly in unconscious or otherwise debilitated patients. The consequences range from harmless colonization to destruction of the nose, meningitis, and deafness. Treatment involves removal of maggots and debridement of tissue.

The maggots responsible for furuncular and wound myiasis may also cause ophthalmomyiasis. Sequelae include nodules in the eyelid, retinal detachment, and destruction of the globe. Most instances in which maggots are found in human feces are the result of larviposition by flesh flies on recently passed stools.

PENTASTOMIASIS

Pentastomids (tongue worms) inhabit the respiratory passages of reptiles and carnivorous mammals. Human infestation by *Linguatula serrata* is common in the Middle East and results from the ingestion of encysted larval stages in raw liver or lymph nodes of sheep and goats—the intermediate hosts. Larvae migrate to the nasopharynx and produce an acute self-limiting syndrome known as *Halzoun* or *Marrara*, which is characterized by pain and itching of the throat and ears, coughing, hoarseness, dysphagia, and dyspnea. Severe edema may cause obstruction that necessitates tracheostomy; ocular invasion has been described. Diagnostic larvae measuring ≤10 mm in length appear in copious nasal discharge or vomitus. Individuals become infected with *Armillifer armillatus* by ingesting eggs in contaminated food or drink or after handling the definitive host, the African python. Larvae encyst in various organs but rarely cause symptoms. Cysts occasionally require surgical removal as they enlarge during molting, but they are usually encountered as an incidental finding at autopsy. Cutaneous larva migrans syndromes due to other pentastomes have been reported from Southeast Asia and Central America.

LEECH INFESTATIONS

Medically important leeches are annelid worms that attach to their hosts with chitinous cutting jaws and draw blood through muscular suckers. The medicinal leech *Hirudo medicinalis* is still used occasionally to reduce venous congestion in surgical flaps or replanted body parts. This practice has been complicated by wound infections, myonecrosis, and sepsis due to *Aeromonas hydrophila*, which colonizes the gullets of commercially available leeches.

Ubiquitous aquatic leeches that parasitize fish, frogs, and turtles readily attach to the skin of humans and avidly suck blood. More notorious are the land leeches that live among moist vegetation of tropical rain forests. Attachment is usually painless. Hirudinin, a powerful anticoagulant secreted by the leech, causes continued bleeding after the leech has detached. Healing of the wound is slow, and bacterial infections are not uncommon. Several kinds of aquatic leeches in Africa, Asia, and southern Europe can enter through the mouth, nose, and genitourinary tract and attach to mucosal surfaces at sites as deep as the esophagus and trachea. Externally attached leeches generally drop off after they have engorged, but removal is hastened by gentle scraping aside of the anterior and posterior suckers and traction or by application of alcohol, salt, vinegar, insect repellent, or a flame or heated instrument to the leech. Internally attached leeches may detach on exposure to gargled saline or may be removed by forceps.

SPIDER BITES

Of the >30,000 recognized species of spiders, only ~100 defend themselves aggressively and have fangs sufficiently long to penetrate human skin. The venom that spiders use to immobilize and digest their prey can cause necrosis of skin and systemic toxicity. Whereas the bites of most spiders are painful but not harmful, envenomations of the brown or fiddle spiders (*Loxosceles* species) and widow spiders (*Latrodectus* species) may be life-threatening. Identification of the offending spider should be attempted, both because specific treatments exist for bites of widow and brown recluse spiders and because injuries attributed to spiders are frequently due to other causes. Except in cases where the patient actually observes a spider immediately associated with the bite or fleeing from the site, lesions reported to be due to spider bites are most often due to other injuries or bacterial infections.

Recluse Spider Bites and Necrotic Arachnidism Severe necrosis of skin and subcutaneous tissue follows envenomation by the brown recluse spider, which is found mainly in the southern and midwestern United States, and by its close relatives in the Americas, Africa, and the Middle East. Necrotic ulcerations also result from bites of the hobo spider in the Pacific Northwest and sac spiders throughout the United States and abroad. These spiders are not aggressive toward human beings and bite only if threatened or pressed against the skin. They hide under rocks and logs or in caves and animal burrows. They invade homes and seek dark and undisturbed hiding spots in closets, in folds of clothing, or under furniture and rubbish in storage rooms, garages, and attics. Despite their impressive abundance in some homes, these spiders only infrequently bite humans. Bites tend to occur while the victim is dressing and are sustained primarily on the arms, neck, and lower abdomen.

The venoms of these spiders contain an esterase, alkaline phosphatase, proteases, and other enzymes that produce tissue necrosis and hemolysis. Sphingomyelinase B, the most important dermonecrotic factor, binds cell membranes and promotes chemotaxis of neutrophils, leading to vascular thrombosis and an Arthus-like reaction. Initially, the bite is painless or produces a stinging sensation. Within the next few hours, the site becomes painful and pruritic, with central induration surrounded by a pale zone of ischemia and a zone of erythema. In most cases, the lesion resolves without treatment in just a few days. In severe cases, the erythema spreads, and the center of the lesion becomes hemorrhagic and necrotic with an overlying bulla. A black eschar forms and sloughs several weeks later, leaving an ulcer that may eventually result in a depressed scar. Healing usually takes place in ≤6 months but may take as long as 3 years if adipose tissue is involved. Local complications include injury to nerves and secondary infection. Fever, chills, weakness, headache, nausea, vomiting, myalgia, arthralgia, maculopapular rash, and leukocytosis may develop ≤72 h after the bite. In rare instances, acute complications such as hemolytic anemia, hemoglobinuria, and renal failure are fatal.

Rx RECLUSE SPIDER BITES

Initial management includes local cleansing, application of sterile dressings and cold compresses, and elevation and loose immobilization of the affected limb. Analgesics, antihistamines, antibiotics, and tetanus prophylaxis should be administered if indicated. Within the first 48–72 h, the oral administration of dapsone (50–100 mg twice daily after glucose-6-phosphate dehydrogenase deficiency has been ruled out) may halt the progression of necrosis. Debridement and later skin grafting may be necessary after signs of acute inflammation have subsided, but immediate surgical excision of the wound is detrimental. Patients should be monitored closely for signs of hemolysis, renal failure, and other systemic complications.

Widow Spider Bites The bites of the female widow spiders are notorious for their potent neurotoxins. The black widow, which is best known and most abundant in the southeastern United States, measures ≤1 cm in body length and 5 cm in leg span and is shiny black with a red hourglass marking on the ventral abdomen. Other dangerous *Latrodectus* species occur elsewhere in temperate and subtropical parts of the world.

Widow spiders spin their webs under stones, logs, plants, or rock piles or in dark spaces in barns, garages, and outhouses. Bites are most common in the summer and early autumn and occur when the web is disturbed or when the spider is trapped or provoked. The initial bite goes unnoticed or is perceived as a sharp pinprick. Two small red marks, mild erythema, and edema develop at the fang entrance site. The venom that is injected does not produce local necrosis, and some persons experience no other symptoms. α-Latrotoxin, the most active component of the venom, binds irreversibly to nerves and causes release and eventual depletion of acetylcholine, norepinephrine, and other neurotransmitters from presynaptic terminals. Painful cramps may spread within 60 min from the bite site to large muscles of the extremities and trunk. Extreme rigidity of the abdominal muscles and excruciating pain may suggest peritonitis, but the abdomen is not tender on palpation. The pain begins to subside during the first 12 h but may recur during several days or weeks before resolving spontaneously. Other features include salivation, diaphoresis, vomiting, hypertension, tachycardia, labored breathing, anxiety, headache, weakness, fasciculations, paresthesia, hyperreflexia, urinary retention, uterine contractions, and premature labor. Rhabdomyolysis and renal failure have been reported, and respiratory arrest, cerebral hemorrhage, or cardiac failure may end fatally, especially in very young, elderly, or debilitated persons.

Rx WIDOW SPIDER BITES

Treatment consists of local cleansing, application of ice packs, and tetanus prophylaxis. Hypertension that does not respond to analgesics and antispasmodics (e.g., benzodiazepines or methocarbamol) requires specific antihypertensive medication. IV administration of a widely available equine antivenom rapidly relieves pain and can be life-saving. Because of the risk of anaphylaxis and serum sickness, antivenom should be reserved for severe cases involving respiratory arrest, uncontrollable hypertension, seizures, or pregnancy.

Tarantulas and Other Spiders Tarantulas are hairy spiders of which 30 species are found in the United States, mainly in the Southwest. The tarantulas that have become popular household pets are usually imported species. Tarantulas bite only when threatened and cause no more harm than a bee sting, but the venom occasionally provokes deep pain and swelling. Tarantulas of several species are covered with urticating hairs that are brushed off in the thousands when a threatened spider rubs its hind legs across its dorsal abdomen. These hairs penetrate human skin and produce pruritic papules that may persist for weeks. Failure to wear gloves or to wash the hands after handling the Chilean Rose tarantula, a popular pet spider, has resulted in transfer of hairs to the eye and devastating ocular inflammation. Treatment of bites includes local washing and elevation of the bitten area, tetanus prophylaxis, and analgesic administration. Antihistamines and topical or systemic glucocorticoids are given for exposure to urticating hairs.

Atrax robustus, a funnel-web spider of Australia, and *Phoneutria* species, the South American banana spiders, are among the most dangerous spiders in the world because of their aggressive behavior and potent neurotoxins. Envenomation by *A. robustus* causes a rapidly progressive neuromotor syndrome that can be fatal within 2 h. The bite of a banana spider causes severe local pain followed by profound systemic symptoms and respiratory paralysis that can lead to death within 2–6 h. Specific antivenoms for envenomation by each of these spiders are available.

SCORPION STINGS

Scorpions are arachnids that feed on ground-dwelling arthropods and small lizards, which they paralyze by injecting venom from a stinger on the tip of the tail. Painful but relatively harmless scorpion stings need to be distinguished from the potentially lethal envenomations that are produced by ~30 of the ~1000 known species and that cause >5000 deaths worldwide each year. Scorpions feed at night and remain hidden during the day in crevices or burrows or under wood, loose bark, or rocks on the ground. They seek cool spots under buildings and often enter houses, where they hide in shoes, clothing, or bedding or enter bathtubs and sinks in search of water. Scorpions sting human beings only when disturbed.

Of the 40 or so scorpion species in the United States, only the bark scorpion (*Centruroides sculpturatus* or *C. exilicauda*) produces venom that can be lethal. Its venom contains neurotoxins that cause sodium channels to remain open and neurons to fire repetitively. Such envenomations are usually associated with little swelling, but prominent pain, paresthesia, and hyperesthesia can be accentuated by tapping on the affected area (the tap test). These symptoms soon spread to other locations; dysfunction of cranial nerves and hyperexcitability of skeletal muscles develop within hours. Patients present with restlessness, blurred vision, abnormal eye movements, profuse salivation, lacrimation, rhinorrhea, slurred speech, difficulty in handling secretions, diaphoresis, nausea, and vomiting. Muscle twitching, jerking, and shaking may be mistaken for a seizure. Complications include tachycardia, arrhythmias, hypertension, hyperthermia, rhabdomyolysis, and acidosis. Symptoms progress to maximal severity in ~5 h and subside within a day or two, although pain and paresthesia can last for weeks. Fatal respiratory arrest is most common among young children and the elderly.

Envenomations by *Leiurus quinquestriatus* in the Middle East and North Africa, by *Mesobuthus tamulus* in India, by *Androctonus* species along the Mediterranean littoral and in North Africa and the Middle East, and by *Tityus serrulatus* in Brazil cause massive release of endogenous catecholamines with hypertensive crises, arrhythmias, pulmonary edema, and myocardial damage. Acute pancreatitis occurs with stings of *Tityus trinitatis* in Trinidad, and central nervous toxicity complicates stings of *Parabuthus* and *Buthotus* scorpions of South Africa. Tissue necrosis and hemolysis may follow stings of the Iranian *Hemiscorpius lepturus*.

Stings of most other species cause immediate sharp local pain followed by edema, ecchymosis, and a burning sensation. Symptoms typically resolve within a few hours, and skin does not slough. Allergic reactions to the venom sometimes develop.

Rx SCORPION STINGS

Identification of the offending scorpion aids in planning therapy. Stings of nonlethal species require at most ice packs, analgesics, or antihistamines. Because most victims experience only local discomfort, they can be managed at home with instructions to return to the emergency department if signs of cranial-nerve or neuromuscular dysfunction develop. Aggressive supportive care and judicious use of antivenom can reduce or eliminate deaths from more severe envenomations. Keeping the patient calm and applying pressure dressings and cold packs to the sting site are measures that decrease the absorption of venom. A continuous IV infusion of midazolam controls the agitation, flailing, and involuntary muscle movements produced by scorpion stings. Close monitoring during treatment with this drug and other sedatives or narcotics is necessary for persons with neuromuscular symptoms because of the risk of respiratory arrest. Hypertension and pulmonary edema respond to nifedipine, nitroprusside, hydralazine, or prazosin, and bradyarrhythmias can be controlled with atropine.

Commercially prepared antivenoms are available in several countries for some of the most dangerous species. A *C. sculpturatus* antivenom (not yet approved by the FDA) is available as an investigational drug only in Arizona. IV administration of antivenom rapidly reverses cranial-nerve dysfunction and muscular symptoms but does not affect pain and paresthesia. The benefit of scorpion antivenom has not been established in controlled trials.

HYMENOPTERA STINGS

Insects that sting to defend their colonies or subdue their prey belong to the order Hymenoptera, which includes apids (bees and bumble-bees), vespids (wasps, hornets, and yellow jackets), and formicids (ants). Their venoms contain a wide array of amines, peptides, and enzymes that cause local and systemic reactions. Although the toxic effect of multiple stings can be fatal, nearly all of the ≥100 deaths due to hymenopteran stings in the United States each year are the result of allergic reactions.

Bee and Wasp Stings Honeybees often lose their stinging apparatus and the attached venom sac in the act of stinging and subsequently die, while other bees, ants, and vespids can sting numerous times in succession. The familiar honeybees (*Apis mellifera*) and bumblebees (*Bombus* and other genera) generally attack only when a colony is disturbed. Africanized honeybees, however, respond to minimal intrusions more aggressively. Since their introduction into Brazil in 1957, these "killer bees" have spread through South and Central America to the southern and western United States.

In bees and wasps, venom is produced in glands at the posterior end of the abdomen and is expelled rapidly by contraction of muscles of the venom sac, which has a capacity of up to 0.1 mL. The venoms of different species of hymenopterans are biochemically and immunologically distinct. Direct toxic effects are mediated by mixtures of low-molecular-weight compounds such as serotonin, histamine, and acetylcholine and several kinins. Polypeptide toxins in honeybee venom include mellitin, which damages cell membranes; mast cell–degranulating protein, which causes histamine release; apamin, a neurotoxin; and adolapin, which has anti-inflammatory activity. Enzymes in venom include hyaluronidase, which allows the spread of other venom components, and phospholipases, which may be among the major venom allergens. There appears to be little cross-sensitization between honeybee and wasp venoms.

Uncomplicated stings cause immediate pain, a wheal-and-flare reaction, and local edema and swelling that subside in a few hours. Stings from accidentally swallowed insects may induce life-threatening edema of the upper airways. Multiple stings can lead to vomiting, diarrhea, generalized edema, dyspnea, hypotension, and collapse. Rhabdomyolysis and intravascular hemolysis may cause renal failure. Death from the direct effects of venom has followed 300–500 honeybee stings.

Large local reactions that spread ≥10 cm around the sting site over 24–48 h are not uncommon. These reactions may resemble cellulitis but are caused by hypersensitivity rather than secondary infection. Such reactions tend to recur on subsequent exposure but are seldom accompanied by anaphylaxis and are not prevented by venom immunotherapy.

An estimated 0.4–4.0% of the U.S. population exhibits clinical immediate-type hypersensitivity to insect stings, and 15% may have asymptomatic sensitization manifested by positive skin tests. Persons who experience severe allergic reactions are likely to have similar reactions after subsequent stings; occasionally, adults who have had mild reactions later experience serious reactions. Mild anaphylactic reactions from insect stings, as from other causes, consist of nausea, abdominal cramping, generalized urticaria, flushing, and angioedema. Serious reactions, including upper airway edema, bronchospasm, hypotension, and shock, may be rapidly fatal. Severe reactions usually begin within 10 min of the sting and only rarely develop after 5 h.

Rx BEE AND WASP STINGS

Stingers from honeybees embedded in the skin should be removed as promptly as possible, using any method available, to limit the quantity of venom delivered. The previously suggested approach of scraping or brushing off the stinger with a blade or a fingernail but not removing it with forceps simply delays removal and exacerbates the consequences. The site should be cleansed and disinfected and ice packs applied to slow the spread of venom. Elevation of the affected site and administration of analgesics, oral antihistamines, and topical calamine lotion relieve symptoms. Large local reactions may require a short course of oral therapy with glucocorticoids. Patients with numerous stings should be monitored for 24 h for evidence of renal failure or coagulopathy.

Anaphylaxis is treated with SC injection of 0.3–0.5 mL of epinephrine hydrochloride in a 1:1000 dilution; treatment is repeated every 20–30 min as necessary. IV epinephrine (2–5 mL of a 1:10,000 solution administered by slow push) is indicated for profound shock. A tourniquet may slow the spread of venom. Parenteral antihistamines, fluid resuscitation, bronchodilators, oxygen, intubation, and vasopressors may be required. Patients should be observed for 24 h for recurrent anaphylaxis.

Persons with a history of allergy to insect stings should carry a sting kit with a preloaded syringe containing epinephrine for self-administration. These patients should seek medical attention immediately after using the kit.

Repeated injections of purified venom produce a blocking IgG antibody response to venom and reduce the incidence of recurrent anaphylaxis. Honeybee, wasp, yellow jacket, and mixed vespid venoms are commercially available for desensitization and for skin testing. Results of skin tests and venom-specific radioallergosorbent tests aid in the selection of patients for immunotherapy and guide the design of such treatment.

Stinging Ants Stinging fire ants are an important medical problem in the United States. Imported fire ants infest southern states from Texas to North Carolina, with colonies in California, New Mexico, Arizona, and Virginia. Slight disturbances of their mound nests have provoked massive outpourings of ants and as many as 10,000 stings on a single person. Elderly and immobile persons are at high risk for attacks when fire ants invade dwellings.

Fire ants attach to skin with powerful mandibles and rotate their bodies while repeatedly injecting venom with posteriorly situated stingers. The alkaloid venom consists of cytotoxic and hemolytic piperidines and several proteins with enzymatic activity. The initial wheal-and-flare reaction, burning, and itching resolve in ~30 min, and a sterile pustule develops within 24 h. The pustule ulcerates over the next 48 h and then heals in ≥1 week. Large areas of erythema and edema lasting several days are not uncommon and in extreme cases may compress nerves and blood vessels. Anaphylaxis occurs in ≤2% of persons, and seizures and mononeuritis have been reported. Stings are treated with ice packs, topical glucocorticoids, and oral antihistamines. Covering pustules with bandages and antibiotic ointment may prevent bacterial infection. Epinephrine and supportive measures are indicated for anaphylactic reactions. Whole-body extracts are available for skin testing and immunotherapy, which appears to lower the rate of anaphylactic reactions.

The western United States is home to harvester ants. The painful local reaction following harvester ant stings often extends to lymph nodes and may be accompanied by anaphylaxis.

Dipteran (Fly and Mosquito) Bites In the process of feeding on vertebrate blood, adults of certain fly species inflict painful bites, produce local allergic reactions, or transmit pathogenic agents. Bites of mosquitoes, tiny "no-see-um" midges, and phlebotomine sand flies typically produce a wheal and a pruritic papule. Nodular lesions at the site of midge bites may last for months. Bites of small humpbacked black flies or simuliids leave a bleeding laceration and a painful and pruritic sore that are slow to heal; regional lymphadenopathy, fever, or anaphylaxis occasionally ensues. The widely distributed deer and horse flies as well as the tsetse flies of Africa are stout flies measuring ≤25 mm in length that attack during the day and produce large and painful bleeding punctures.

Rx FLY AND MOSQUITO BITES

Treatment of fly bites is symptom-based. Topical application of antipruritic agents, glucocorticoids, or antiseptic lotions may relieve itching and pain. Allergic reactions may require oral antihistamines. Antibiotics may be necessary for the treatment of large bite wounds that become secondarily infected.

Flea Bites Common human-biting fleas include the dog and cat fleas (*Ctenocephalides* species) and the rat flea (*Xenopsylla cheopis*), which inhabit the nests and resting sites of their hosts. Sensitized persons develop erythematous pruritic papules, urticaria, and occasionally vesi-

cles and bacterial superinfection at the site of the bite. Treatment consists of antihistamines and antipruritics.

Flea infestations are eliminated by frequent cleaning of nesting sites and of the host's bedding and by application of contact insecticides. Flea infestations in the home may abate if pets are treated with veterinary antiparasitic agents and insect growth regulators.

Tunga penetrans, like other fleas, is a wingless, laterally flattened insect that feeds on blood. Also known as the chigoe flea, sand flea, or jigger, it occurs in tropical regions of Africa and the Americas. Adults live in sandy soil and burrow under the skin between toes, under nails, or on the soles of bare feet. Chigoes engorge on blood and grow from pinpoint to pea size during a 2-week period. The lesions they produce resemble a white pustule with a central black depression and may be pruritic or painful. Occasional complications include tetanus, bacterial infections, and autoamputation of toes. Tungiasis is treated by removal of the intact flea with a sterile needle or scalpel, tetanus vaccination, and topical application of antibiotics.

Hemipteran (True Bug) Bites Several true bugs of the family Reduviidae inflict bites that produce allergic reactions and are sometimes painful. The cone-nose bugs, so called because of their elongated heads, include the assassin and wheel bugs, which feed on other insects and bite vertebrates only in self-defense, and the kissing bugs, which routinely feed on vertebrate blood. The bites of the nocturnally feeding kissing bugs are painless. Reactions to such bites depend on prior sensitization and include tender and pruritic papules, vesicular or bullous lesions, giant urticaria, fever, lymphadenopathy, and anaphylaxis. Bug bites are treated with topical antipruritics or oral antihistamines. Persons with anaphylactic reactions to reduviid bites should keep an epinephrine kit available. The cosmopolitan bedbugs (*Cimex* species) hide in crevices of mattresses, bed frames and other furniture, walls, and picture frames and under loose wallpaper. Bedbugs have become resurgent, recently attaining populations and spreading to an extent not encountered since the mid-twentieth century. These bugs are now a fairly common nuisance in homes, dormitories, and hotels and on cruise ships. The bugs hide during the day and take their blood meal at night. Their bite is painless, but sensitized persons develop erythema, itching, and wheals around a central hemorrhagic punctum. Bedbugs are not known to transmit pathogens.

Centipede Bites and Millipede Dermatitis The fangs of centipedes of the genus *Scolopendra* can penetrate human skin and deliver a venom that produces intense burning pain, swelling, erythema, and lymphangitis. Dizziness, nausea, and anxiety are occasionally described, and rhabdomyolysis and renal failure have been reported. Treatment includes washing of the site, application of cold dressings, oral analgesic administration or local lidocaine infiltration, and tetanus prophylaxis.

Millipedes, unlike centipedes, do not bite, but some secrete defensive fluids that burn and discolor human skin. Affected skin turns brown overnight and may blister and exfoliate. Secretions in the eye cause intense pain and inflammation that may lead to corneal ulceration and blindness. Management includes irrigation with copious amounts of water or saline, use of analgesics, and local care of denuded skin.

Caterpillar Stings and Dermatitis The surface of caterpillars of several moth species is covered with hairs or spines that produce mechanical irritation and may contain or be coated with venom. Contact with these caterpillars causes an immediate burning sensation followed by local swelling and erythema and occasionally by regional lymphadenopathy, nausea, vomiting, and headache; shock, seizures, and coagulopathy are rare complications. In the United States, dermatitis is most often associated with io, puss, saddleback, and brown-tail moths. Contact with even detached hairs of other caterpillars, such as gypsy moth larvae, can later produce a pruritic urticarial or papular rash. Spines may be deposited on tree trunks and drying laundry or may be airborne and cause irritation of the eyes and upper airways. Treatment of caterpillar stings consists of repeated application of adhesive or cellophane tape to remove the hairs, which can then be identified microscopically. Local ice packs, topical steroids, and oral antihistamines relieve symptoms.

 Beetle Vesication When disturbed, blister beetles extrude cantharidin, a low-molecular-weight toxin that produces thin-walled blisters measuring ≤5 cm in diameter 2–5 h after contact. The blisters are not painful or pruritic unless broken and resolve without treatment in ≤10 days. Nephritis may follow unusually heavy cantharidin exposure. Contact occurs when individuals sit on the ground, work in the garden, or deliberately handle the beetles. The hemolymph of certain rove beetles contains paederin, a potent vesicant. When these beetles are crushed or brushed against the skin, the released fluid may provoke erythematous and bullous lesions. These beetles occur worldwide but are most numerous and problematic in parts of Africa and Asia. Ocular lesions are common from impacts with the flying beetles at night or transfer of the vesicant on the fingers. Treatment is rarely necessary, although ruptured blisters should be kept clean and bandaged.

DELUSIONAL INFESTATIONS

The groundless conviction that one is infested with arthropods or other parasites is an extremely difficult disorder to treat and unfortunately is not rare. Patients report infestations of their skin, clothing, or homes and describe sensations of something moving in or on their skin. Excoriations often accompany reports of pruritus or insect bites. Frequently, patients submit as evidence of infestation specimens that consist of plant-feeding and nonbiting peridomestic arthropods, pieces of skin, vegetable matter, or inanimate objects. It is imperative to rule out true infestations and bites by arthropods, endocrinopathies, neuropathies, drug use, environmental irritants (e.g., fragments or threads of glass insulation), and other causes of tingling or prickling sensations. Frequently, such patients repeatedly seek medical consultations, resist alternative explanations for their symptoms, and exacerbate their discomfort by self-treatment. Pharmacotherapy with pimozide has been more helpful than psychotherapy in treating this disorder.

FURTHER READINGS

ARLIAN LG: Arthropod allergens and human health. Annu Rev Entomol 47:395, 2002

BURGESS IF: Human lice and their control. Annu Rev Entomol 49:457, 2004

CORAPI KM et al: Strategies for primary and secondary prevention of Lyme disease. Nat Clin Pract Rheumatol 3:20, 2007

FRADIN MS: Mosquitoes and mosquito repellents: A clinician's guide. Ann Intern Med 128:931, 1998

GODDARD J: *Physician's Guide to Arthropods of Medical Importance*, 4th ed. Boca Raton, FL, CRC Press, 2002

HALL M, WALL R: Myiasis of humans and domestic animals. Adv Parasitol 35:257, 1995

HAYES EB, PIESMAN J: How can we prevent Lyme disease? N Engl J Med 348:2424, 2003

LEONE PA: Scabies and pediculosis pubis: An update of treatment regimens and general review. Clin Infect Dis 44:S153, 2007

MULLEN G, DURDEN L: *Medical and Veterinary Entomology*. Amsterdam, Academic Press, 2002

PETERS W: *A Colour Atlas of Arthropods in Clinical Medicine*. London, Wolfe, 1992

POLLACK RJ, MARCUS L: A travel medicine guide to arthropods of medical importance. Infect Dis Clin North Am 19:169, 2005

SAUCIER JR: Arachnid envenomation. Emerg Med Clin North Am 22:405, 2004

STEEN CJ et al: Insect sting reactions to bees, wasps, and ants. Int J Dermatol 44:91, 2005

SWANSON DL, VETTER RS: Bites of brown recluse spiders and suspected necrotic arachnidism. N Engl J Med 352:700, 2005

VETTER RS, BUSH SP: Reports of presumptive brown recluse spider bites reinforce improbable diagnosis in regions of North America where the spider is not endemic. Clin Infect Dis 35:442, 2002

VISSCHER PK et al: Removing bee stings: Speed matters, method doesn't. Lancet 348:301, 1996

WONG HC: Importance of proper identification of stinging insects. Ann Intern Med 132:418, 2000

Appendix: Laboratory Values of Clinical Importance

Alexander Kratz, Michael A. Pesce, Daniel J. Fink

INTRODUCTORY COMMENTS

The following are tables of reference values for laboratory tests, special analytes, and special function tests. A variety of factors can influence reference values. Such variables include the population studied, the duration and means of specimen transport, laboratory methods and instrumentation, and even the type of container used for the collection of the specimen. The reference or "normal" ranges given in this appendix may therefore not be appropriate for all laboratories, and these values should only be used as general guidelines. Whenever possible, reference values provided by the laboratory performing the testing should be utilized in the interpretation of laboratory data. Values supplied in this Appendix reflect typical reference ranges in adults. Pediatric reference ranges may vary significantly from adult values.

In preparing the Appendix, the authors have taken into account the fact that the system of international units (SI, système international d'unités) is used in most countries and in some medical journals. However, clinical laboratories may continue to report values in "conventional" units. Therefore, both systems are provided in the Appendix. The dual system is also used in the text except for (1) those instances in which the numbers remain the same but only the terminology is changed (mmol/L for meq/L or IU/L for mIU/mL), when only the SI units are given; and (2) most pressure measurements (e.g., blood and cerebrospinal fluid pressures), when the conventional units (mmHg, mmH$_2$O) are used. In all other instances in the text the SI unit is followed by the traditional unit in parentheses.

REFERENCE VALUES FOR LABORATORY TESTS

TABLE 1 HEMATOLOGY AND COAGULATION

Analyte	Specimen[a]	SI Units	Conventional Units
Activated clotting time	WB	70–180 s	70–180 seconds
Activated protein C resistance (Factor V Leiden)	P	Not applicable	Ratio > 2.1
Alpha$_2$ antiplasmin	P	0.87–1.55	87–155%
Antiphospholipid antibody panel			
PTT-LA (Lupus anticoagulant screen)	P	Negative	Negative
Platelet neutralization procedure	P	Negative	Negative
Dilute viper venom screen	P	Negative	Negative
Anticardiolipin antibody	S		
IgG		0–15 arbitrary units	0–15 GPL
IgM		0–15 arbitrary units	0–15 MPL
Antithrombin III	P		
Antigenic		220–390 mg/L	22–39 mg/dL
Functional		0.7–1.30 U/L	70–130%
Anti-Xa assay (heparin assay)	P		
Unfractionated heparin		0.3–0.7 kIU/L	0.3–0.7 IU/mL
Low-molecular-weight heparin		0.5–1.0 kIU/L	0.5–1.0 IU/mL
Danaparoid (Orgaran)		0.5–0.8 kIU/L	0.5–0.8 IU/mL
Autohemolysis test	WB	0.004–0.045	0.4%–4.50%
Autohemolysis test with glucose	WB	0.003–0.007	0.3%–0.7%
Bleeding time (adult)		<7.1 min	<7.1 min
Bone marrow: see Table 8			
Clot retraction	WB	0.50–1.00/2 h	50–100%/2 h
Cryofibrinogen	P	Negative	Negative
D-Dimer	P	0.22–0.74 µg/mL	0.22–0.74 µg/mL
Differential blood count	WB		
Neutrophils		0.40–0.70	40–70%
Bands		0.0–0.05	0–5%
Lymphocytes		0.20–0.50	20–50%
Monocytes		0.04–0.08	4–8%
Eosinophils		0.0–0.6	0–6%
Basophils		0.0–0.02	0–2%
Eosinophil count	WB	150–300/µL	150–300/mm^3
Erythrocyte count	WB		
Adult males		4.30–5.60 × 10^{12}/L	4.30–5.60 × 10^6/mm^3
Adult females		4.00–5.20 × 10^{12}/L	4.00–5.20 × 10^6/mm^3
Erythrocyte life span	WB		
Normal survival		120 days	120 days
Chromium labeled, half life ($t_{1/2}$)		25–35 days	25–35 days
Erythrocyte sedimentation rate	WB		
Females		0–20 mm/h	0–20 mm/h
Males		0–15 mm/h	0–15 mm/h
Euglobulin lysis time	P	7200–14400 s	120–240 min
Factor II, prothrombin	P	0.50–1.50	50–150%
Factor V	P	0.50–1.50	50–150%
Factor VII	P	0.50–1.50	50–150%
Factor VIII	P	0.50–1.50	50–150%
Factor IX	P	0.50–1.50	50–150%
Factor X	P	0.50–1.50	50–150%
Factor XI	P	0.50–1.50	50–150%
Factor XII	P	0.50–1.50	50–150%
Factor XIII screen	P	Not applicable	Present
Factor inhibitor assay	P	< 0.5 Bethesda Units	< 0.5 Bethesda Units

(continued)

TABLE 1   **HEMATOLOGY AND COAGULATION (CONTINUED)**

Analyte	Specimen[a]	SI Units	Conventional Units
Fibrin(ogen) degradation products	P	0–1 mg/L	0–1 µg/mL
Fibrinogen	P	2.33–4.96 g/L	233–496 mg/dL
Glucose-6-phosphate dehydrogenase (erythrocyte)	WB	< 2400 s	<40 min
Ham's test (acid serum)	WB	Negative	Negative
Hematocrit	WB		
Adult males		0.388–0.464	38.8–46.4
Adult females		0.354–0.444	35.4–44.4
Hemoglobin			
Plasma	P	6–50 mg/L	0.6–5.0 mg/dL
Whole blood	WB		
Adult males		133–162 g/L	13.3–16.2 g/dL
Adult females		120–158 g/L	12.0–15.8 g/dL
Hemoglobin electrophoresis	WB		
Hemoglobin A		0.95–0.98	95–98%
Hemoglobin A$_2$		0.015–0.031	1.5–3.1%
Hemoglobin F		0–0.02	0–2.0%
Hemoglobins other than A, A$_2$, or F		Absent	Absent
Heparin-induced thrombocytopenia antibody	P	Negative	Negative
Joint fluid crystal	JF	Not applicable	No crystals seen
Joint fluid mucin	JF	Not applicable	Only type I mucin present
Leukocytes			
Alkaline phosphatase (LAP)	WB	0.2–1.6 µkat/L	13–100 µ/L
Count (WBC)	WB	3.54–9.06 × 10^9/L	3.54–9.06 × 10^3/mm^3
Mean corpuscular hemoglobin (MCH)	WB	26.7–31.9 pg/cell	26.7–31.9 pg/cell
Mean corpuscular hemoglobin concentration (MCHC)	WB	323–359 g/L	32.3–35.9 g/dL
Mean corpuscular hemoglobin of reticulocytes (CH)	WB	24–36 pg	24–36 pg
Mean corpuscular volume (MCV)	WB	79–93.3 fL	79–93.3 µm^3
Mean platelet volume (MPV)	WB	9.00–12.95 fL	9.00–12.95 µm^3
Osmotic fragility of erythrocytes	WB		
Direct		0.0035–0.0045	0.35–0.45%
Index		0.0030–0.0065	0.30–0.65%
Partial thromboplastin time, activated	P	26.3–39.4 s	26.3–39.4 s
Plasminogen	P		
Antigen		84–140 mg/L	8.4–14.0 mg/dL
Functional		0.70–1.30	70–130%
Plasminogen activator inhibitor 1	P	4–43 µg/L	4–43 ng/mL
Platelet aggregation	PRP	Not applicable	> 65% aggregation in response to adenosine diphosphate, epinephrine, collagen, ristocetin, and arachidonic acid
Platelet count	WB	165–415 × 10^9/L	165–415 × 10^3/mm^3
Platelet, mean volume	WB	6.4–11 fL	6.4–11.0 µm^3
Prekallikrein assay	P	0.50–1.5	50–150%
Prekallikrein screen	P		No deficiency detected
Protein C	P		
Total antigen		0.70–1.40	70–140%
Functional		0.70–1.30	70–130%
Protein S	P		
Total antigen		0.70–1.40	70–140%
Functional		0.65–1.40	65–140%
Free antigen		0.70–1.40	70–140%
Prothrombin gene mutation G20210A	WB	Not applicable	Not present
Prothrombin time	P	12.7–15.4 s	12.7–15.4 s
Protoporphyrin, free erythrocyte	WB	0.28–0.64 µmol/L of red blood cells	16–36 µg/dL of red blood cells
Red cell distribution width	WB	< 0.145	< 14.5%
Reptilase time	P	16–23.6 s	16–23.6 s
Reticulocyte count	WB		
Adult males		0.008–0.023 red cells	0.8–2.3% red cells
Adult females		0.008–0.020 red cells	0.8–2.0% red cells
Reticulocyte hemoglobin content	WB	>26 pg/cell	>26 pg/cell
Ristocetin cofactor (functional von Willebrand factor)	P		
Blood group O		0.75 mean of normal	75% mean of normal
Blood group A		1.05 mean of normal	105% mean of normal
Blood group B		1.15 mean of normal	115% mean of normal
Blood group AB		1.25 mean of normal	125% mean of normal
Sickle cell test	WB	Negative	Negative
Sucrose hemolysis	WB	<0.1	<10% hemolysis
Thrombin time	P	15.3–18.5 s	15.3–18.5 s
Total eosinophils	WB	150–300 × 10^6/L	150–300/mm^3
Transferrin receptor	S, P	9.6–29.6 nmol/L	9.6–29.6 nmol/L
Viscosity			
Plasma	P	1.7–2.1	1.7–2.1
Serum	S	1.4–1.8	1.4–1.8

(continued)

TABLE 1 HEMATOLOGY AND COAGULATION (CONTINUED)

Analyte	Specimen[a]	SI Units	Conventional Units
Von Willebrand factor (vWF) antigen (factor VIII:R antigen)	P		
Blood group O		0.75 mean of normal	75% mean of normal
Blood group A		1.05 mean of normal	105% mean of normal
Blood group B		1.15 mean of normal	115% mean of normal
Blood group AB		1.25 mean of normal	125% mean of normal
Von Willebrand factor multimers	P	Normal distribution	Normal distribution
White blood cells: see "leukocytes"			

[a]P, plasma; JF, joint fluid; PRP, platelet-rich plasma; S, serum; WB, whole blood.

TABLE 2 CLINICAL CHEMISTRY AND IMMUNOLOGY

Analyte	Specimen[a]	SI Units	Conventional Units
Acetoacetate	P	20–99 μmol/L	0.2–1.0 mg/dL
Adrenocorticotropin (ACTH)	P	1.3–16.7 pmol/L	6.0–76.0 pg/mL
Alanine aminotransferase (AST, SGPT)	S	0.12–0.70 μkat/L	7–41 U/L
Albumin	S		
Female		41–53 g/L	4.1–5.3 g/dL
Male		40–50 g/L	4.0–5.0 g/L
Aldolase	S	26–138 nkat/L	1.5–8.1 U/L
Aldosterone (adult)			
Supine, normal sodium diet	S, P	55–250 pmol/L	2–9 ng/dL
Upright, normal sodium diet	S, P		2–5-fold increase over supine value
Supine, low-sodium diet	S, P		2–5-fold increase over normal sodium diet level
	U	6.38–58.25 nmol/d	2.3–21.0 μg/24 h
Alpha fetoprotein (adult)	S	0–8.5 μg/L	0–8.5 ng/mL
Alpha₁ antitrypsin	S	1.0–2.0 g/L	100–200 mg/dL
Ammonia, as NH₃	P	11–35 μmol/L	19–60 μg/dL
Amylase (method dependent)	S	0.34–1.6 μkat/L	20–96 U/L
Androstenedione (adult)	S	1.75–8.73 nmol/L	50–250 ng/dL
Angiotensin-converting enzyme (ACE)	S	0.15–1.1 μkat/L	9–67 U/L
Anion gap	S	7–16 mmol/L	7–16 mmol/L
Apo B/Apo A-1 ratio		0.35–0.98	0.35–0.98
Apolipoprotein A-1	S	1.19–2.40 g/L	119–240 mg/dL
Apolipoprotein B	S	0.52–1.63 g/L	52–163 mg/dL
Arterial blood gases			
[HCO₃⁻]		22–30 mmol/L	22–30 meq/L
P_CO₂		4.3–6.0 kPa	32–45 mmHg
pH		7.35–7.45	7.35–7.45
P_O₂		9.6–13.8 kPa	72–104 mmHg
Aspartate aminotransferase (AST, SGOT)	S	0.20–0.65 μkat/L	12–38 U/L
Autoantibodies			
Anti-adrenal antibody	S	Not applicable	Negative at 1:10 dilution
Anti-double-strand (native) DNA	S	Not applicable	Negative at 1:10 dilution
Anti–glomerular basement membrane antibodies	S		
Qualitative		Negative	Negative
Quantitative		<5 kU/L	<5 U/mL
Anti-granulocyte antibody	S	Not applicable	Negative
Anti-Jo-1 antibody	S	Not applicable	Negative
Anti-La antibody	S	Not applicable	Negative
Anti-mitochondrial antibody	S	Not applicable	Negative
Antineutrophil cytoplasmic autoantibodies, cytoplasmic (C-ANCA)	S		
Qualitative		Negative	Negative
Quantitative (antibodies to proteinase 3)		< 2.8 kU/L	< 2.8 U/mL
Antineutrophil cytoplasmic autoantibodies, perinuclear (P-ANCA)	S		
Qualitative		Negative	Negative
Quantitative (antibodies to myeloperoxidase)		< 1.4 kU/L	< 1.4 U/mL
Antinuclear antibody	S	Not applicable	Negative at 1:40
Anti–parietal cell antibody	S	Not applicable	Negative at 1:20
Anti-Ro antibody	S	Not applicable	Negative
Anti-platelet antibody	S	Not applicable	Negative
Anti-RNP antibody	S	Not applicable	Negative
Anti-Scl 70 antibody	S	Not applicable	Negative
Anti-Smith antibody	S	Not applicable	Negative
Anti-smooth-muscle antibody	S	Not applicable	Negative at 1:20
Anti-thyroglobulin	S	Not applicable	Negative
Anti-thyroid antibody	S	< 0.3 kIU/L	<0.3 IU/mL

(continued)

Analyte	Specimen[a]	SI Units	Conventional Units
B type natriuretic peptide (BNP)	P	Age and gender specific: < 167 ng/L	Age and gender specific: < 167 pg/mL
Bence Jones protein, serum	S	Not applicable	None detected
Bence Jones protein, urine, qualitative	U	Not applicable	None detected in 50× concentrated urine
Bence Jones Protein, urine, quantitative	U		
Kappa		<25 mg/L	<2.5 mg/dL
Lambda		<50 mg/L	<5.0 mg/dL
β_2-Microglobulin			
	S	<2.7 mg/L	<0.27 mg/dL
	U	<120 µg/d	<120 µg/day
Bilirubin	S		
Total		5.1–22 µmol/L	0.3–1.3 mg/dL
Direct		1.7–6.8 µmol/L	0.1–0.4 mg/dL
Indirect		3.4–15.2 µmol/L	0.2–0.9 mg/dL
C peptide (adult)	S, P	0.17–0.66 nmol/L	0.5–2.0 ng/mL
C1-esterase-inhibitor protein	S		
Antigenic		124–250 mg/L	12.4–24.5 mg/dL
Functional		Present	Present
CA 125	S	0–35 kU/L	0–35 U/mL
CA 19-9	S	0–37 kU/L	0–37 U/mL
CA-15-3	S	0–34 kU/L	0–34 U/mL
CA27-29	S	0–40 kU/L	0–40 U/mL
Calcitonin	S		
Male		3–26 ng/L	3–26 pg/mL
Female		2–17 ng/L	2–17 pg/mL
Calcium	S	2.2–2.6 mmol/L	8.7–10.2 mg/dL
Calcium, ionized	WB	1.12–1.32 mmol/L	4.5–5.3 mg/dL
Carbon dioxide content (TCO₂)	P (sea level)	22–30 mmol/L	22–30 meq/L
Carboxyhemoglobin (carbon monoxide content)	WB		
Nonsmokers		0–0.04	0–4%
Smokers		0.04–0.09	4–9%
Onset of symptoms		0.15–0.20	15–20%
Loss of consciousness and death		>0.50	>50%
Carcinoembryonic antigen (CEA)	S		
Nonsmokers		0.0–3.0 µg/L	0.0–3.0 ng/mL
Smokers	S	0.0–5.0 µg/L	0.0–5.0 ng/mL
Ceruloplasmin	S	250–630 mg/L	25–63 mg/dL
Chloride	S	102–109 mmol/L	102–109 meq/L
Cholesterol: see Table 5			
Cholinesterase	S	5–12 kU/L	5–12 U/mL
Complement			
C3	S	0.83–1.77 g/L	83–177 mg/dL
C4	S	0.16–0.47 g/L	16–47 mg/dL
Total hemolytic complement (CH50)	S	50–150%	50–150%
Factor B	S	0.17–0.42 g/L	17–42 mg/dL
Coproporphyrins (types I and III)	U	150–470 µmol/d	100–300 µg/d
Cortisol			
Fasting, 8 A.M.–12 noon	S	138–690 nmol/L	5–25 µg/dL
12 noon–8 P.M.		138–414 nmol/L	5–15 µg/dL
8 P.M.–8 A.M.		0–276 nmol/L	0–10 µg/dL
Cortisol, free	U	55–193 nmol/24 h	20–70 µg/24 h
C-reactive protein	S	0.2–3.0 mg/L	0.2–3.0 mg/L
Creatine kinase (total)	S		
Females		0.66–4.0 µkat/L	39–238 U/L
Males		0.87–5.0 µkat/L	51–294 U/L
Creatine kinase-MB	S		
Mass		0.0–5.5 µg/L	0.0–5.5 ng/mL
Fraction of total activity (by electrophoresis)		0–0.04	0–4.0%
Creatinine	S		
Female		44–80 µmol/L	0.5–0.9 ng/mL
Male		53–106 µmol/L	0.6–1.2 ng/mL
Cryoproteins	S	Not applicable	None detected
Dehydroepiandrosterone (DHEA) (adult)			
Male	S	6.2–43.4 nmol/L	180–1250 ng/dL
Female		4.5–34.0 nmol/L	130–980 ng/dL
Dehydroepiandrosterone (DHEA) sulfate	S		
Male (adult)		100–6190 µg/L	10–619 µg/dL
Female (adult, premenopausal)		120–5350 µg/L	12–535 µg/dL
Female (adult, postmenopausal)		300–2600 µg/L	30–260 µg/dL
Deoxycorticosterone (DOC) (adult)	S	61–576 nmol/L	2–19 ng/dL
11-Deoxycortisol (adult) (compound S) (8:00 A.M.)	S	0.34–4.56 nmol/L	12–158 ng/dL
Dihydrotestosterone			
Male	S, P	1.03–2.92 nmol/L	30–85 ng/dL
Female		0.14–0.76 nmol/L	4–22 ng/dL

(continued)

| TABLE 2 | CLINICAL CHEMISTRY AND IMMUNOLOGY (CONTINUED) | | |

Analyte	Specimen[a]	SI Units	Conventional Units
Dopamine	P	< 475 pmol/L	< 87 pg/mL
Dopamine	U	425–2610 nmol/d	65–400 µg/d
Epinephrine	P		
Supine (30 min)		< 273 pmol/L	< 50 pg/mL
Sitting		< 328 pmol/L	< 60 pg/mL
Standing (30 min)		< 491pmol/L	< 90 pg/mL
Epinephrine	U	0–109 nmol/d	0–20 µg/d
Erythropoietin	S	4–27 U/L	4–27 U/L
Estradiol	S, P		
Female			
Menstruating:			
Follicular phase		74–532 pmol/L	<20–145 pg/mL
Mid-cycle peak		411–1626 pmol/L	112–443 pg/mL
Luteal phase		74–885 pmol/L	<20–241 pg/mL
Postmenopausal		217 pmol/L	<59 pg/mL
Male		74 pmol/L	< 20 pg/mL
Estrone	S, P		
Female			
Menstruating:			
Follicular phase		55–555 pmol/L	15–150 pg/mL
Luteal phase		55–740 pmol/L	15–200 pg/mL
Postmenopausal		55–204 pmol/L	15–55 pg/mL
Male		55–240 pmol/L	15–65 pg/mL
Fatty acids, free (nonesterified)	P	<0.28–0.89 mmol/L	<8–25 mg/dL
Ferritin	S		
Female		10–150 µg/L	10–150 ng/mL
Male		29–248 µg/L	29–248 ng/mL
Follicle stimulating hormone (FSH)	S, P		
Female			
Menstruating:			
Follicular phase		3.0–20.0 IU/L	3.0–20.0 mIU/mL
Ovulatory phase		9.0–26.0 IU/L	9.0–26.0 mIU/mL
Luteal phase		1.0–12.0 IU/L	1.0–12.0 mIU/mL
Postmenopausal		18.0–153.0 IU/L	18.0–153.0 mIU/mL
Male		1.0–12.0 IU/L	1.0–12.0 mIU/mL
Free testosterone, adult			
Female	S	2.1–23.6 pmol/L	0.6–6.8 pg/mL
Male		163–847 pmol/L	47–244 pg/mL
Fructosamine	S	<285 µmol/L	<285 µmol/L
Gamma glutamyltransferase	S	0.15–0.99 µkat/L	9–58 U/L
Gastrin	S	<100 ng/L	<100 pg/mL
Glucagon	P	20–100 ng/L	20–100 pg/mL
Glucose (fasting)	P		
Normal		4.2–6.1 mmol/L	75–110 mg/dL
Impaired glucose tolerance		6.2–6.9 mmol/L	111–125 mg/dL
Diabetes mellitus		>7.0 mmol/L	>125 mg/dL
Glucose, 2 h postprandial	P	3.9–6.7 mmol/L	70–120 mg/dL
Growth hormone (resting)	S	0.5–17.0 µg/L	0.5–17.0 ng/mL
Hemoglobin A$_{1c}$	WB	0.04–0.06 Hb fraction	4.0–6.0%
High-density lipoprotein (HDL) (see Table 5)			
Homocysteine	P	4.4–10.8 µmol/L	4.4–10.8 µmol/L
Human chorionic gonadotropin (hCG)	S		
Non-pregnant female		< 5 IU/L	< 5 mIU/mL
1–2 weeks postconception		9–130 IU/L	9–130 mIU/mL
2–3 weeks postconception		75–2600 IU/L	75–2600 mIU/mL
3–4 weeks postconception		850–20,800 IU/L	850–20,800 mIU/mL
4–5 weeks postconception		4000–100,200 IU/L	4000–100,200 mIU/mL
5–10 weeks postconception		11,500–289,000 IU/L	11,500–289,000 mIU/mL
10–14 weeks postconception		18,300–137,000 IU/L	18,300–137,000 mIU/mL
Second trimester		1400–53,000 IU/L	1400–53,000 mIU/mL
Third trimester		940–60,000 IU/L	940–60,000 mIU/mL
β-Hydroxybutyrate	P	0–290 µmol/L	0–3 mg/dL
5-Hydroindoleacetic acid [5-HIAA]	U	10.5–36.6 µmol/d	2–7 mg/d
17-Hydroxyprogesterone (adult)	S		
Male		0.15–7.5 nmol/L	5–250 ng/dL
Female			
Follicular phase		0.6–3.0 nmol/L	20–100 ng/dL
Midcycle peak		3–7.5 nmol/L	100–250 ng/dL
Luteal phase		3–15 nmol/L	100–500 ng/dL
Postmenopausal		≤ 2.1 nmol/L	≤ 70 ng/dL
Hydroxyproline	U, 24 hour	38–500 µmol/d	38–500 µmol/d
Immunofixation	S	Not applicable	No bands detected

(continued)

Analyte	Specimen[a]	SI Units	Conventional Units
Immunoglobulin, quantitation (adult)			
IgA	S	0.70–3.50 g/L	70–350 mg/dL
IgD	S	0–140 mg/L	0–14 mg/dL
IgE	S	24–430 μg/L	10–179 IU/mL
IgG	S	7.0–17.0 g/L	700–1700 mg/dL
IgG$_1$	S	2.7–17.4 g/L	270–1740 mg/dL
IgG$_2$	S	0.3–6.3 g/L	30–630 mg/dL
IgG$_3$	S	0.13–3.2 g/L	13–320 mg/dL
IgG$_4$	S	0.11–6.2 g/L	11–620 mg/dL
IgM	S	0.50–3.0 g/L	50–300 mg/dL
Insulin	S, P	14.35–143.5 pmol/L	2–20 μU/mL
Iron	S	7–25 μmol/L	41–141 μg/dL
Iron-binding capacity	S	45–73 μmol/L	251–406 μg/dL
Iron-binding capacity saturation	S	0.16–0.35	16–35%
Joint fluid crystal	JF	Not applicable	No crystals seen
Joint fluid mucin	JF	Not applicable	Only type I mucin present
Ketone (acetone)	S, U	Negative	Negative
17 Ketosteroids	U	0.003–0.012 g/d	3–12 mg/d
Lactate	P, arterial	0.5–1.6 mmol/L	4.5–14.4 mg/dL
	P, venous	0.5–2.2 mmol/L	4.5–19.8 mg/dL
Lactate dehydrogenase	S	2.0–3.8 μkat/L	115–221 U/L
Lactate dehydrogenase isoenzymes	S		
Fraction 1 (of total)		0.14–0.26	14–26%
Fraction 2		0.29–0.39	29–39%
Fraction 3		0.20–0.25	20–26%
Fraction 4		0.08–0.16	8–16%
Fraction 5		0.06–0.16	6–16%
Lipase (method dependent)	S	0.51–0.73 μkat/L	3–43 U/L
Lipids: see Table 5			
Lipoprotein (a)	S	0–300 mg/L	0–30 mg/dL
Low-density lipoprotein (LDL) (see Table 5)			
Luteinizing hormone (LH)	S, P		
Female			
Menstruating			
Follicular phase		2.0–15.0 U/L	2.0–15.0 U/L
Ovulatory phase		22.0–105.0 U/L	22.0–105.0 U/L
Luteal phase		0.6–19.0 U/L	0.6–19.0 U/L
Postmenopausal		16.0–64.0 U/L	16.0–64.0 U/L
Male		2.0–12.0 U/L	2.0–12.0 U/L
Magnesium	S	0.62–0.95 mmol/L	1.5–2.3 mg/dL
Metanephrine	P	<0.5 nmol/L	<100 pg/mL
Metanephrine	U	30–211 mmol/mol creatinine	53–367 μg/g creatinine
Methemoglobin	WB	0.0–0.01	0–1%
Microalbumin urine	U		
24-h urine		0.0–0.03 g/d	0–30 mg/24 h
Spot urine		0.0–0.03 g/g creatinine	0–30 μg/mg creatinine
Myoglobin	S		
Male		19–92 μg/L	19–92 μg/L
Female		12–76 μg/L	12–76 μg/L
Norepinephrine	U	89–473 nmol/d	15–80 μg/d
Norepinephrine	P		
Supine (30 min)		650–2423 pmol/L	110–410 pg/mL
Sitting		709–4019 pmol/L	120–680 pg/mL
Standing (30 min)		739–4137 pmol/L	125–700 pg/mL
N-telopeptide (cross linked), NTx	S		
Female, premenopausal		6.2–19.0 nmol BCE	6.2–19.0 nmol BCE
Male		5.4–24.2 nmol BCE	5.4–24.2 nmol BCE
Bone collagen equivalent (BCE)			
N-telopeptide (cross linked), NTx	U		
Female, premenopausal		17–94 nmol BCE/mmol creatinine	17–94 nmol BCE/mmol creatinine
Female, postmenopausal		26–124 nmol BCE/mmol creatinine	26–124 nmol BCE/mmol creatinine
Male		21–83 nmol BCE/mmol creatinine	21–83 nmol BCE/mmol creatinine
Bone collagen equivalent (BCE)			
5' Nucleotidase	S	0.02–0.19 μkat/L	0–11 U/L
Osmolality	P	275–295 mOsmol/kg serum water	275–295 mOsmol/kg serum water
	U	500–800 mOsmol/kg water	500–800 mOsmol/kg water
Osteocalcin	S	11–50 μg/L	11–50 ng/mL
Oxygen content	WB		
Arterial (sea level)		17–21	17–21 vol%
Venous (sea level)		10–16	10–16 vol%
Oxygen percent saturation (sea level)	WB		
Arterial		0.97	94–100%
Venous, arm		0.60–0.85	60–85%

(continued)

TABLE 2 **CLINICAL CHEMISTRY AND IMMUNOLOGY (CONTINUED)**

Analyte	Specimen[a]	SI Units	Conventional Units
Parathyroid hormone (intact)	S	8–51 ng/L	8–51 pg/mL
Phosphatase, alkaline	S	0.56–1.63 µkat/L	33–96 U/L
Phosphorus, inorganic	S	0.81–1.4 mmol/L	2.5–4.3 mg/dL
Porphobilinogen	U	None	None
Potassium	S	3.5–5.0 mmol/L	3.5–5.0 meq/L
Prealbumin	S	170–340 mg/L	17–34 mg/dL
Progesterone	S, P		
Female			
Follicular		<3.18 nmol/L	<1.0 ng/mL
Midluteal		9.54–63.6 nmol/L	3–20 ng/mL
Male		<3.18 nmol/L	< 1.0 ng/mL
Prolactin	S	0–20 µg/L	0–20 ng/mL
Prostate-specific antigen (PSA)	S		
Male			
<40 years		0.0–2.0 µg/L	0.0–2.0 ng/mL
>40 years		0.0–4.0 µg/L	0.0–4.0 ng/mL
PSA, free; in males 45–75 years, with PSA values between 4 and 20 µg/mL	S	>0.25 associated with benign prostatic hyperplasia	>25% associated with benign prostatic hyperplasia
Protein fractions	S		
Albumin		35–55 g/L	3.5–5.5 g/dL (50–60%)
Globulin		20–35 g/L	2.0–3.5 g/dL (40–50%)
Alpha$_1$		2–4 g/L	0.2–0.4 g/dL (4.2–7.2%)
Alpha$_2$		5–9 g/L	0.5–0.9 g/dL (6.8–12%)
Beta		6–11 g/L	0.6–1.1 g/dL (9.3–15%)
Gamma		7–17 g/L	0.7–1.7 g/dL (13–23%)
Protein, total	S	67–86 g/L	6.7–8.6 g/dL
Pyruvate	P, arterial	40–130 µmol/L	0.35–1.14 mg/dL
	P, venous	40–130 µmol/L	0.35–1.14 mg/dL
Rheumatoid factor	S, JF	<30 kIU/L	<30 IU/mL
Serotonin	WB	0.28–1.14 µmol/L	50–200 ng/mL
Serum protein electrophoresis	S	Not applicable	Normal pattern
Sex hormone binding globulin (adult)	S		
Male		13–71 nmol/L	13–71 nmol/L
Female		18–114 nmol/L	18–114 nmol/L
Sodium	S	136–146 mmol/L	136–146 meq/L
Somatomedin-C (IGF-1) (adult)	S		
16–24 years		182–780 µg/L	182–780 ng/mL
25–39 years		114–492 µg/L	114–492 ng/mL
40–54 years		90–360 µg/L	90–360 ng/mL
>54 years		71–290 µg/L	71–290 ng/mL
Somatostatin	P	<25 ng/L	<25 pg/mL
Testosterone, total, morning sample	S		
Female		0.21–2.98 nmol/L	6–86 ng/dL
Male		9.36–37.10 nmol/L	270–1070 ng/dL
Thyroglobulin	S	0.5–53 µg/L	0.5–53 ng/mL
Thyroid-binding globulin	S	13–30 mg/L	1.3–3.0 mg/dL
Thyroid-stimulating hormone	S	0.34–4.25 mIU/L	0.34–4.25 µIU/mL
Thyroxine, free (fT$_4$)	S	10.3–21.9 pmol/L	0.8–1.7 ng/dL
Thyroxine, total (T$_4$)	S	70–151 nmol/L	5.4–11.7 µg/dL
(Free) thyroxine index	S	6.7–10.9	6.7–10.9
Transferrin	S	2.0–4.0 g/L	200–400 mg/dL
Triglycerides (see Table 5)	S	0.34–2.26 mmol/L	30–200 mg/dL
Triiodothyronine, free (fT$_3$)	S	3.7–6.5 pmol/L	2.4–4.2 pg/mL
Triiodothyronine, total (T$_3$)	S	1.2–2.1 nmol/L	77–135 ng/dL
Troponin I	S		
Normal population, 99 %tile		0–0.08 µg/L	0–0.08 ng/mL
Cut-off for MI		>0.4 µg/L	>0.4 ng/mL
Troponin T	S		
Normal population, 99 %tile		0–0.1 µg/L	0–0.01 ng/mL
Cut-off for MI		0–0.1 µg/L	0–0.1 ng/mL
Urea nitrogen	S	2.5–7.1 mmol/L	7–20 mg/dL
Uric acid	S		
Females		0.15–0.33 µmol/L	2.5–5.6 mg/dL
Males		0.18–0.41 µmol/L	3.1–7.0 mg/dL
Urobilinogen	U	0.09–4.2 µmol/d	0.05–25 mg/24 h
Vanillylmandelic acid (VMA)	U, 24h	<30 µmol/d	<6 mg/d
Vasoactive intestinal polypeptide	P	0–60 ng/L	0–60 pg/mL

[a]P, plasma; S, serum; U, urine; WB, whole blood; JF, joint fluid.

Drug	Therapeutic Range		Toxic Level	
	SI Units	Conventional Units	SI Units	Conventional Units
Acetaminophen	66–199 µmol/L	10–30 µg/mL	>1320 µmol/L	>200 µg/mL
Amikacin				
Peak	34–51 µmol/L	20–30 µg/mL	>60 µmol/L	>35 µg/mL
Trough	0–17 µmol/L	0–10 µg/mL	>17 µmol/L	>10 µg/mL
Amitriptyline/nortriptyline (total drug)	430–900 nmol/L	120–250 ng/mL	>1800 nmol/L	>500 ng/mL
Amphetamine	150–220 nmol/L	20–30 ng/mL	>1500 nmol/L	>200 ng/mL
Bromide				
Sedation	1.3–6.3 mmol/L	10–50 mg/dL		
Epilepsy	9.4–18.8 mmol/L	75–150 mg/dL		
Mild toxicity			6.4–18.8 mmol/L	51–150 mg/dL
Severe toxicity			>18.8 mmol/L	>150 mg/dL
Lethal			>37.5 mmol/L	>300 mg/dL
Carbamazepine	17–42 µmol/L	4–10 µg/mL	85 µmol/L	>20 µg/mL
Chloramphenicol				
Peak	31–62 µmol/L	10–20 µg/mL	>77 µmol/L	>25 µg/mL
Trough	15–31 µmol/L	5–10 µg/mL	>46 µmol/L	>15 µg/mL
Chlordiazepoxide	1.7–10 µmol/L	0.5–3.0 µg/mL	>17 µmol/L	>5.0 µg/mL
Clonazepam	32–240 nmol/L	10–75 ng/mL	>320 nmol/L	>100 ng/mL
Clozapine	0.6–2.1 µmol/L	200–700 ng/mL	>3.7 µmol/L	>1200 ng/mL
Cocaine			>3.3 µmol/L	>1.0 µg/mL
Codeine	43–110 nmol/mL	13–33 ng/mL	>3700 nmol/mL	>1100 ng/mL, lethal
Cyclosporine				
Renal transplant				
0–6 months	208–312 nmol/L	250–375 ng/mL	>312 nmol/L	>375 ng/mL
6–12 months after transplant	166–250 nmol/L	200–300 ng/mL	>250 nmol/L	>300 ng/mL
>12 months	83–125 nmol/L	100–150 ng/mL	>125 nmol/L	>150 ng/mL
Cardiac transplant				
0–6 months	208–291 nmol/L	250–350 ng/mL	>291 nmol/L	>350 ng/mL
6–12 months after transplant	125–208 nmol/L	150–250 ng/mL	>208 nmol/L	>250 ng/mL
>12 months	83–125 nmol/L	100–150 ng/mL	>125 nmol/L	>150 ng/mL
Lung transplant				
0–6 months	250–374 nmol/L	300–450 ng/mL	>374 nmol/L	>450 ng/mL
Liver transplant				
0–7 days	249–333 nmol/L	300–400 ng/mL	>333 nmol/L	>400 ng/mL
2–4 weeks	208–291 nmol/L	250–350 ng/mL	>291 nmol/L	>350 ng/mL
5–8 weeks	166–249 nmol/L	200–300 ng/mL	>249 nmol/L	>300 ng/mL
9–52 weeks	125–208 nmol/L	150–250 ng/mL	>208 nmol/L	>250 ng/mL
>1 year	83–166 nmol/L	100–200 ng/mL	>166 nmol/L	>200 ng/mL
Desipramine	375–1130 nmol/L	100–300 ng/mL	>1880 nmol/L	>500 ng/mL
Diazepam (and metabolite)				
Diazepam	0.7–3.5 µmol/L	0.2–1.0 µg/mL	>7.0 µmol/L	>2.0 µg/mL
Nordiazepam	0.4–6.6 µmol/L	0.1–1.8 µg/mL	>9.2 µmol/L	>2.5 µg/mL
Digoxin	0.64–2.6 nmol/L	0.5–2.0 ng/mL	>3.1 nmol/L	>2.4 ng/mL
Disopyramide	>7.4 µmol/L	2.5 µg/mL	20.6 µmol/L	>7 µg/mL
Doxepin and nordoxepin				
Doxepin	0.36–0.98 µmol/L	101–274 ng/mL	>1.8 µmol/L	>503 ng/mL
Nordoxepin	0.38–1.04 µmol/L	106–291 ng/mL	>1.9 µmol/L	>531 ng/mL
Ethanol				
Behavioral changes			>4.3 mmol/L	>20 mg/dL
Legal limit			≥17 mmol/L	≥80 mg/dL
Critical with acute exposure			>54 mmol/L	>250 mg/dL
Ethylene glycol				
Toxic			>2 mmol/L	>12 mg/dL
Lethal			>20 mmol/L	>120 mg/dL
Ethosuximide	280–700 µmol/L	40–100 µg/mL	>700 µmol/L	>100 µg/mL
Flecainide	0.5–2.4 µmol/L	0.2–1.0 µg/mL	>3.6 µmol/L	>1.5 µg/mL
Gentamicin				
Peak	10–21 µmol/mL	5–10 µg/mL	>25 µmol/mL	>12 µg/mL
Trough	0–4.2 µmol/mL	0–2 µg/mL	>4.2 µmol/mL	>2 µg/mL
Heroin (diacetyl morphine)			>700 µmol/L	>200 ng/mL (as morphine)
Ibuprofen	49–243 µmol/L	10–50 µg/mL	>97 µmol/L	>200 µg/mL
Imipramine (and metabolite)				
Desimipramine	375–1130 nmol/L	100–300 ng/mL	>1880 nmol/L	>500 ng/mL
Total imipramine + desimipramine	563–1130 nmol/L	150–300 ng/mL	>1880 nmol/L	>500 ng/mL
Lidocaine	5.1–21.3 µmol/L	1.2–5.0 µg/mL	>38.4 µmol/L	>9.0 µg/mL
Lithium	0.5–1.3 mmol/L	0.5–1.3 meq/L	>2 mmol/L	>2 meq/L
Methadone	1.3–3.2 µmol/L	0.4–1.0 µg/mL	>6.5 µmol/L	>2 µg/mL
Methamphetamine	1.3–4.0 µmol/L	2–6 µg/dL	4.0–33.5 µmol/L 67.0–268.0 µmol/L	60–500-1.0 µg/dL, toxic 1000–4000 µg/dL, lethal

(continued)

| TABLE 3 | TOXICOLOGY AND THERAPEUTIC DRUG MONITORING (CONTINUED) |

| Drug | Therapeutic Range | | Toxic Level | |
	SI Units	Conventional Units	SI Units	Conventional Units
Methanol			>6 mmol/L	>20 mg/dL, toxic
			>16 mmol/L	>50 mg/dL, severe toxicity
			>28 mmol/L	>89 mg/dL, lethal
Methotrexate				
Low-dose	0.01–0.1 µmol/L	0.01–0.1 µmol/L	>0.1 mmol/L	>0.1 mmol/L
High-dose (24 h)	<5.0 µmol/L	<5.0 µmol/L	>5.0 µmol/L	>5.0 µmol/L
High-dose (48 h)	<0.50 µmol/L	<0.50 µmol/L	>0.5 µmol/L	>0.5 µmol/L
High-dose (72 h)	<0.10 µmol/L	<0.10 µmol/L	>0.1 µmol/L	>0.1 µmol/L
Morphine	35–250 µmol/L	10–70 ng/mL	180–14000 µmol/L	50–4000 ng/mL
Nitroprusside (as thiocyanate)	103–499 µmol/L	6–29 µg/mL	860 µmol/L	>50 µg/mL
Nortriptyline	190–569 nmol/L	50–150 ng/mL	>1900 nmol/L	>500 ng/mL
Phenobarbital	65–172 µmol/L	15–40 µg/mL	>215 µmol/L	>50 µg/mL
Phenytoin	40–79 µmol/L	10–20 µg/mL	>118 µmol/L	>30 µg/mL
Phenytoin, free	4.0–7.9 µmol/L	1–2 µg/mL	>13.9 µmol/L	>3.5 µg/ml
% Free	0.08–0.14	8–14%		
Primidone and metabolite				
Primidone	23–55 µmol/L	5–12 µg/mL	>69 µmol/L	>15 µg/mL
Phenobarbital	65–172 µmol/L	15–40 µg/mL	>215 µmol/L	>50 µg/mL
Procainamide				
Procainamide	17–42 µmol/L	4–10 µg/mL	>51 µmol/L	>12 µg/mL
NAPA (N-acetylprocainamide)	22–72 µmol/L	6–20 µg/mL	>126 µmol/L	>35 µg/mL
Quinidine	6.2–15.4 µmol/L	2.0–5.0 µg/mL	>31 µmol/L	>10 µg/mL
Salicylates	145–2100 µmol/L	2–29 mg/dL	>2172 µmol/L	>30 mg/dL
Sirolimus (trough level)				
Kidney transplant	4.4–13.1 nmol/L	4–12 ng/mL	>16 nmol/L	>15 ng/mL
Tacrolimus (FK506) (trough)				
Kidney and liver				
0–2 months posttransplant	12–19 nmol/L	10–15 ng/mL	>25 nmol/L	>20 ng/mL
> 2 months posttransplant	6–12 nmol/L	5–10 ng/mL		
Heart				
0–2 months posttransplant	19–25 nmol/L	15–20 ng/mL	>25 nmol/L	>20 ng/mL
3–6 months posttransplant	12–19 nmol/L	10–15 ng/mL		
>6 months posttransplant	10–12 nmol/L	8–10 ng/mL		
Theophylline	56–111 µmol/L	10–20 µg/mL	>140 µmol/L	>25 µg/mL
Thiocyanate				
After nitroprusside infusion	103–499 µmol/L	6–29 µg/mL	860 µmol/L	>50 µg/mL
Nonsmoker	17–69 µmol/L	1–4 µg/mL		
Smoker	52–206 µmol/L	3–12 µg/mL		
Tobramycin				
Peak	11–22 µmol/L	5–10 µg/mL	>26 µmol/L	>12 µg/mL
Trough	0–4.3 µmol/L	0–2 µg/mL	>4.3 µmol/L	>2 µg/mL
Valproic acid	350–700 µmol/L	50–100 µg/mL	>1000 µmol/L	>150 µg/mL
Vancomycin				
Peak	14–28 µmol/L	20–40 µg/mL	>55 µmol/L	>80 µg/mL
Trough	3.5–10.4 µmol/L	5–15 µg/mL	>14 µmol/L	>20 µg/mL

TABLE 4 **VITAMINS AND SELECTED TRACE MINERALS**

		Reference Range	
Specimen	**Analyte**[a]	**SI Units**	**Conventional Units**
Aluminum	S	<0.2 μmol/L	<5.41 μg/L
	U, random	0.19–1.11 μmol/L	5–30 μg/L
Arsenic	WB	0.03–0.31 μmol/L	2–23 μg/L
	U, 24 h	0.07–0.67 μmol/d	5–50 μg/d
Cadmium	WB	<44.5 nmol/L	<5.0 μg/L
Coenzyme Q10 (ubiquinone)	P	433–1532 μg/L	433–1532 μg/L
B carotene	S	0.07–1.43 μmol/L	4–77 μg/dL
Copper			
	S	11–22 μmol/L	70–140 μg/dL
	U, 24 h	<0.95 μmol/d	<60 μg/d
Folic acid	RC	340–1020 nmol/L cells	150–450 ng/mL cells
Folic acid	S	12.2–40.8 nmol/L	5.4–18.0 ng/mL
Lead (adult)	S	<0.5 μmol/L	<10 μg/dL
Mercury			
	WB	3.0–294 nmol/L	0.6–59 μg/L
	U, 24 h	<99.8 nmol/L	<20 μg/L
Selenium	S	0.8–2.0 μmol/L	63–160 μg/L
Vitamin A	S	0.7–3.5 μmol/L	20–100 μg/dL
Vitamin B$_1$ (thiamine)	S	0–75 nmol/L	0–2 μg/dL
Vitamin B$_2$ (riboflavin)	S	106–638 nmol/L	4–24 μg/dL
Vitamin B$_6$	P	20–121 nmol/L	5–30 ng/mL
Vitamin B$_{12}$	S	206–735 pmol/L	279–996 pg/mL
Vitamin C (ascorbic acid)	S	23–57 μmol/L	0.4–1.0 mg/dL
Vitamin D$_3$, 1,25-dihydroxy	S	60–108 pmol/L	25–45 pg/mL
Vitamin D$_3$, 25-hydroxy	P		
Summer		37.4–200 nmol/L	15–80 ng/mL
Winter		34.9–105 nmol/L	14–42 ng/mL
Vitamin E	S	12–42 μmol/L	5–18 μg/mL
Vitamin K	S	0.29–2.64 nmol/L	0.13–1.19 ng/mL
Zinc	S	11.5–18.4 μmol/L	75–120 μg/dL

[a]P, plasma; RC, red cells; S, serum; WB, whole blood; U, urine.

TABLE 5 **CLASSIFICATION OF LDL, TOTAL, AND HDL CHOLESTEROL**

LDL cholesterol, mg/dL (mmol/L)

<70 (<1.81)	Therapeutic option for very high risk patients
<100 (<2.59)	Optimal
100–129 (2.59–3.34)	Near optimal/above optimal
130–159 (3.36–4.11)	Borderline high
160–189 (4.14–4.89)	High
≥190 (≥4.91)	Very high

Total cholesterol, mg/dL (mmol/L)

<200 (<5.17)	Desirable
200–239 (5.17–6.18)	Borderline high
≥240 (≥6.21)	High

HDL cholesterol, mg/dL (mmol/L)

<40 (<1.03)	Low
≥60 (≥1.55)	High

Note: LDL, low-density lipoprotein; HDL, high-density lipoprotein
Source: Executive summary of the third report of the National Cholesterol Education Program (NCEP) expert panel on detection, evaluation, and treatment of high blood cholesterol in adults (adult treatment panel III). JAMA 285:2486, 2001; and Implications of recent clinical trials for the National Cholesterol Education Program Adult Treatment Panel III Guidelines: SM Grundy et al for the Coordinating Committee of the National Cholesterol Education Program. Circulation 110:227, 2004.

TABLE 6 CEREBROSPINAL FLUID (CSF)[a]

Constituent	Reference Range SI Units	Reference Range Conventional Units
Osmolarity	292–297 mmol/kg water	292–297 mosmol/L
Electrolytes		
Sodium	137–145 mmol/L	137–145 meq/L
Potassium	2.7–3.9 mmol/L	2.7–3.9 meq/L
Calcium	1.0–1.5 mmol/L	2.1–3.0 meq/L
Magnesium	1.0–1.2 mmol/L	2.0–2.5 meq/L
Chloride	116–122 mmol/L	116–122 meq/L
CO_2 content	20–24 mmol/L	20–24 meq/L
P_{CO_2}	6–7 kPa	45–49 mmHg
pH	7.31–7.34	
Glucose	2.22–3.89 mmol/L	40–70 mg/dL
Lactate	1–2 mmol/L	10–20 mg/dL
Total protein		
Lumbar	0.15–0.5 g/L	15–50 mg/dL
Cisternal	0.15–0.25 g/L	15–25 mg/dL
Ventricular	0.06–0.15 g/L	6–15 mg/dL
Albumin	0.066–0.442 g/L	6.6–44.2 mg/dL
IgG	0.009–0.057 g/L	0.9–5.7 mg/dL
IgG index[b]	0.29–0.59	
Oligoclonal bands	<2 bands not present in matched serum sample	
Ammonia	15–47 µmol/L	25–80 µg/dL
Creatinine	44–168 µmol/L	0.5–1.9 mg/dL
Myelin basic protein	<4 µg/L	
CSF pressure		50–180 mmH₂O
CSF volume (adult)	~150 mL	
Red blood cells	0	0
Leukocytes		
Total	0–5 mononuclear cells per µL	0–5 mononuclear cells per mm³
Differential		
Lymphocytes	60–70%	
Monocytes	30–50%	
Neutrophils	None	

[a]Since cerebrospinal fluid concentrations are equilibrium values, measurements of the same parameters in blood plasma obtained at the same time are recommended. However, there is a time lag in attainment of equilibrium, and cerebrospinal levels of plasma constituents that can fluctuate rapidly (such as plasma glucose) may not achieve stable values until after a significant lag phase.

[b]IgG index = CSF IgG(mg/dL) × serum albumin(g/dL)/Serum IgG(g/dL) × CSF albumin(mg/dL).

TABLE 7   URINE ANALYSIS   A-11

TABLE 7 URINE ANALYSIS

	Reference Range SI Units	Reference Range Conventional Units
Acidity, titratable	20–40 mmol/d	20–40 meq/d
Ammonia	30–50 mmol/d	30–50 meq/d
Amylase		4–400 U/L
Amylase/creatinine clearance ratio [(Cl_am/Cl_cr) × 100]	1–5	1–5
Calcium (10 meq/d or 200 mg/d dietary calcium)	<7.5 mmol/d	<300 mg/d
Creatine, as creatinine		
Female	<760 µmol/d	<100 mg/d
Male	<380 µmol/d	<50 mg/d
Creatinine	8.8–14 mmol/d	1.0–1.6 g/d
Eosinophils	<100,000 eosinophils/L	<100 eosinophils/mL
Glucose (glucose oxidase method)	0.3–1.7 mmol/d	50–300 mg/d
5-Hydroxyindoleacetic acid (5-HIAA)	10–47 µmol/d	2–9 mg/d
Iodine, spot urine		
WHO classification of iodine deficiency		
Not iodine deficient	>100 µg/L	>100 µg/L
Mild iodine deficiency	50–100 µg/L	50–100 µg/L
Moderate iodine deficiency	20–49 µg/L	20–49 µg/L
Severe iodine deficiency	<20 µg/L	<20 µg/L
Microalbumin		
Normal	0.0–0.03 g/d	0–30 mg/d
Microalbuminuria	0.03–0.30 g/d	30–300 mg/d
Clinical albuminuria	>0.3 g/d	>300 mg/d
Microalbumin/creatinine ratio		
Normal	0–3.4 g/mol creatinine	0–30 µg/mg creatinine
Microalbuminuria	3.4–34 g/mol creatinine	30–300 µg/mg creatinine
Clinical albuminuria	>34 g/mol creatinine	>300 µg/mg creatinine
Oxalate		
Male	80–500 µmol/d	7–44 mg/d
Female	45–350 µmol/d	4–31 mg/d
pH	5.0–9.0	5.0–9.0
Phosphate (phosphorus) (varies with intake)	12.9–42.0 mmol/d	400–1300 mg/d
Potassium (varies with intake)	25–100 mmol/d	25–100 meq/d
Protein	<0.15 g/d	<150 mg/d
Sediment		
Red blood cells	0–2/high power field	
White blood cells	0–2/high power field	
Bacteria	None	
Crystals	None	
Bladder cells	None	
Squamous cells	None	
Tubular cells	None	
Broad casts	None	
Epithelial cell casts	None	
Granular casts	None	
Hyaline casts	0–5/low power field	
Red blood cell casts	None	
Waxy casts	None	
White cell casts	None	
Sodium (varies with intake)	100–260 mmol/d	100–260 meq/d
Specific gravity	1.001–1.035	1.001–1.035
Urea nitrogen	214–607 mmol/d	6–17 g/d
Uric acid (normal diet)	1.49–4.76 mmol/d	250–800 mg/d

Note: WHO, World Health Organization.

TABLE 8 DIFFERENTIAL NUCLEATED CELL COUNTS OF BONE MARROW ASPIRATES[a]

	Observed Range, %	95% Confidence Intervals, %	Mean, %
Blast cells	0–3.2	0–3.0	1.4
Promyelocytes	3.6–13.2	3.2–12.4	7.8
Neutrophil myelocytes	4–21.4	3.7–10.0	7.6
Eosinophil myelocytes	0–5.0	0–2.8	1.3
Metamyelocytes	1–7.0	2.3–5.9	4.1
Neutrophils			
Males	21.0–45.6	21.9–42.3	32.1
Females	29.6–46.6	28.8–45.9	37.4
Eosinophils	0.4–4.2	0.3–4.2	2.2
Eosinophils plus eosinophil myelocytes	0.9–7.4	0.7–6.3	3.5
Basophils	0–0.8	0–0.4	0.1
Erythroblasts			
Male	18.0–39.4	16.2–40.1	28.1
Females	14.0–31.8	13.0–32.0	22.5
Lymphocytes	4.6–22.6	6.0–20.0	13.1
Plasma cells	0–1.4	0–1.2	0.6
Monocytes	0–3.2	0–2.6	1.3
Macrophages	0–1.8	0–1.3	0.4
M:E ratio			
Males	1.1–4.0	1.1–4.1	2.1
Females	1.6–5.4	1.6–5.2	2.8

[a]Based on bone marrow aspirate from 50 healthy volunteers (30 men, 20 women).
Source: From BJ Bain: The bone marrow aspirate of healthy subjects. Br J Haematol 94(1):206, 1996.

TABLE 9 STOOL ANALYSIS

	Reference Range	
	SI Units	Conventional Units
Amount	0.1–0.2 kg/d	100–200 g/24 h
Coproporphyrin	611–1832 nmol/d	400–1200 µg/24 h
Fat		
Adult		<7 g/d
Adult on fat-free diet		<4 g/d
Fatty acids	0–21 mmol/d	0–6 g/24 h
Leukocytes	None	None
Nitrogen	<178 mmol/d	<2.5 g/24 h
pH	7.0–7.5	
Occult blood	Negative	Negative
Trypsin		20–95 U/g
Urobilinogen	85–510 µmol/d	50–300 mg/24 h
Uroporphyrins	12–48 nmol/d	10–40 µg/24 h
Water	<0.75	<75%

Source: Modified from FT Fishbach, MB Dunning III: *A Manual of Laboratory and Diagnostic Tests,* 7th ed., Lippincott Williams & Wilkins, Philadelphia, 2004.

TABLE 10	RENAL FUNCTION TESTS	
	Reference Range	
	SI Units	**Conventional Units**
Clearances (corrected to 1.72 m² body surface area)		
Measures of glomerular filtration rate		
Inulin clearance (CI)		
Males (mean ± 1 SD)	2.1 ± 0.4 mL/s	124 ± 25.8 mL/min
Females (mean ± 1 SD)	2.0 ± 0.2 mL/s	119 ± 12.8 mL/min
Endogenous creatinine clearance	1.5–2.2 mL/s	91–130 mL/min
Measures of effective renal plasma flow and tubular function		
p-Aminohippuric acid clearance (CI$_{PAH}$)		
Males (mean ± 1 SD)	10.9 ± 2.7 mL/s	654 ± 163 mL/min
Females (mean ± 1 SD)	9.9 ± 1.7 mL/s	594 ± 102 mL/min
Concentration and dilution test		
Specific gravity of urine		
After 12-h fluid restriction	>1.025	>1.025
After 12-h deliberate water intake	≤1.003	≤1.003
Protein excretion, urine	<0.15 g/d	<150 mg/d
Specific gravity, maximal range	1.002–1.028	1.002–1.028
Tubular reabsorption, phosphorus	0.79–0.94 of filtered load	79–94% of filtered load

TABLE 11	CIRCULATORY FUNCTION TESTS	
	Results: Reference Range	
Test	**SI Units (Range)**	**Conventional Units (Range)**
Arteriovenous oxygen difference	30–50 mL/L	30–50 mL/L
Cardiac output (Fick)	2.5–3.6 L/m² of body surface area per min	2.5–3.6 L/m² of body surface area per min
Contractility indexes		
Max. left ventricular $dp/dt(dp/dt)$/DP when DP = 5.3 kPa (40 mmHg) (DP, diastolic pressure)	220 kPa/s (176–250 kPa/s) (37.6 ± 12.2)/s	1650 mmHg/s (1320–1880 mmHg/s) (37.6 ± 12.2)/s
Mean normalized systolic ejection rate (angiography)	3.32 ± 0.84 end-diastolic volumes per second	3.32 ± 0.84 end-diastolic volumes per second
Mean velocity of circumferential fiber shortening (angiography)	1.83 ± 0.56 circumferences per second	1.83 ± 0.56 circumferences per second
Ejection fraction: stroke volume/end-diastolic volume (SV/EDV)	0.67 ± 0.08 (0.55–0.78)	0.67 ± 0.08 (0.55–0.78)
End-diastolic volume	70 ± 20.0 mL/m² (60–88 mL/m²)	70 ± 20.0 mL/m² (60–88 mL/m²)
End-systolic volume	25 ± 5.0 mL/m² (20–33 mL/m²)	25 ± 5.0 mL/m² (20–33 mL/m²)
Left ventricular work		
Stroke work index	50 ± 20.0 (g•m)/m² (30–110)	50 ± 20.0 (g•m)/m² (30–110)
Left ventricular minute work index	1.8–6.6 [(kg•m)/m²]/min	1.8–6.6 [(kg•m)/m²]/min
Oxygen consumption index	110–150 mL	110–150 mL
Maximum oxygen uptake	35 mL/min (20–60 mL/min)	35 mL/min (20–60 mL/min)
Pulmonary vascular resistance	2–12 (kPa•s)/L	20–130 (dyn•s)/cm⁵
Systemic vascular resistance	77–150 (kPa•s)/L	770–1600 (dyn•s)/cm⁵

Source: E Braunwald et al: *Heart Disease*, 6th ed, Philadelphia, Saunders, 2001.

TABLE 12 **GASTROINTESTINAL TESTS**

Test	Results SI Units	Results Conventional Units
Absorption tests		
D-Xylose: after overnight fast, 25 g xylose given in oral aqueous solution		
Urine, collected for following 5 h	25% of ingested dose	25% of ingested dose
Serum, 2 h after dose	2.0–3.5 mmol/L	30–52 mg/dL
Vitamin A: a fasting blood specimen is obtained and 200,000 units of vitamin A in oil is given orally	Serum level should rise to twice fasting level in 3–5 h	Serum level should rise to twice fasting level in 3–5 h
Bentiromide test (pancreatic function): 500 mg bentiromide (chymex) orally; *p*-aminobenzoic acid (PABA) measured		
Plasma		>3.6 (±1.1) µg/mL at 90 min
Urine	>50% recovered in 6 h	>50% recovered in 6 h
Gastric juice		
Volume		
24 h	2–3 L	2–3 L
Nocturnal	600–700 mL	600–700 mL
Basal, fasting	30–70 mL/h	30–70 mL/h
Reaction		
pH	1.6–1.8	1.6–1.8
Titratable acidity of fasting juice	4–9 µmol/s	15–35 meq/h
Acid output		
Basal		
Females (mean ± 1 SD)	0.6 ± 0.5 µmol/s	2.0 ± 1.8 meq/h
Males (mean ± 1 SD)	0.8 ± 0.6 µmol/s	3.0 ± 2.0 meq/h
Maximal (after SC histamine acid phosphate, 0.004 mg/kg body weight, and preceded by 50 mg promethazine, or after betazole, 1.7 mg/kg body weight, or pentagastrin, 6 µg/kg body weight)		
Females (mean ± 1 SD)	4.4 ± 1.4 µmol/s	16 ± 5 meq/h
Males (mean ± 1 SD)	6.4 ± 1.4 µmol/s	23 ± 5 meq/h
Basal acid output/maximal acid output ratio	≤0.6	≤0.6
Gastrin, serum	0–200 µg/L	0–200 pg/mL
Secretin test (pancreatic exocrine function): 1 unit/kg body weight, IV		
Volume (pancreatic juice) in 80 min	>2.0 mL/kg	>2.0 mL/kg
Bicarbonate concentration	>80 mmol/L	>80 meq/L
Bicarbonate output in 30 min	>10 mmol	>10 meq

TABLE 13 **NORMAL VALUES OF DOPPLER ECHOCARDIOGRAPHIC MEASUREMENTS IN ADULTS**

	Range	Mean
RVD (cm), measured at the base in apical 4-chamber view	2.6–4.3	3.5 ± 0.4
LVID (cm), measured in the parasternal long axis view	3.6–5.4	4.7 ± 0.4
Posterior LV wall thickness (cm)	0.6–1.1	0.9 ± 0.4
IVS wall thickness (cm)	0.6–1.1	0.9 ± 0.4
Left atrial dimension (cm), antero-posterior dimension	2.3–3.8	3.0 ± 0.3
Aortic root dimension (cm)	2.0–3.5	2.4 ± 0.4
Aortic cusps separation (cm)	1.5–2.6	1.9 ± 0.4
Percentage of fractional shortening	34–44%	36%
Mitral flow (m/s)	0.6–1.3	0.9
Tricuspid flow (m/s)	0.3–0.7	0.5
Pulmonary artery (m/s)	0.6–0.9	0.75
Aorta (m/s)	1.0–1.7	1.35

Note: RVD, right ventricular dimension; LVID, left ventricular internal dimension; LV, left ventricle; IVS, interventricular septum.

Source: From A Weyman: *Principles and Practice of Echocardiography*, 2d ed., Philadelphia, Lea & Febiger, 1994.

| TABLE 14 | SUMMARY OF VALUES USEFUL IN PULMONARY PHYSIOLOGY |

| | | Typical Values | |
	Symbol	Man, Age 40, 75 kg, 175 cm Tall	Woman, Age 40, 60 kg, 160 cm Tall
Pulmonary Mechanics			
Spirometry—volume-time curves			
Forced vital capacity	FVC	4.8 L	3.3 L
Forced expiratory volume in 1 s	FEV_1	3.8 L	2.8 L
FEV_1/FVC	$FEV_1\%$	76%	77%
Maximal midexpiratory flow	MMF (FEF 25–27)	4.8 L/s	3.6 L/s
Maximal expiratory flow rate	MEFR (FEF 200–1200)	9.4 L/s	6.1 L/s
Spirometry—flow-volume curves			
Maximal expiratory flow at 50% of expired vital capacity	V_{max} 50 (FEF 50%)	6.1 L/s	4.6 L/s
Maximal expiratory flow at 75% of expired vital capacity	V_{max} 75 (FEF 75%)	3.1 L/s	2.5 L/s
Resistance to airflow			
Pulmonary resistance	RL (R_L)	<3.0 (cmH_2O/s)/L	
Airway resistance	Raw	<2.5 (cmH_2O/s)/L	
Specific conductance	SGaw	>0.13 cmH_2O/s	
Pulmonary compliance			
Static recoil pressure at total lung capacity	Pst TLC	25 ± 5 cmH_2O	
Compliance of lungs (static)	CL	0.2 L cmH_2O	
Compliance of lungs and thorax	C(L + T)	0.1 L cmH_2O	
Dynamic compliance of 20 breaths per minute	C dyn 20	0.25 ± 0.05 L/cmH_2O	
Maximal static respiratory pressures			
Maximal inspiratory pressure	MIP	>90 cmH_2O	>50 cmH_2O
Maximal expiratory pressure	MEP	>150 cmH_2O	>120 cmH_2O
Lung Volumes			
Total lung capacity	TLC	6.4 L	4.9 L
Functional residual capacity	FRC	2.2 L	2.6 L
Residual volume	RV	1.5 L	1.2 L
Inspiratory capacity	IC	4.8 L	3.7 L
Expiratory reserve volume	ERV	3.2 L	2.3 L
Vital capacity	VC	1.7 L	1.4 L
Gas Exchange (Sea Level)			
Arterial O_2 tension	Pa_{O_2}	12.7 ± 0.7 kPa (95 ± 5 mmHg)	
Arterial CO_2 tension	Pa_{CO_2}	5.3 ± 0.3 kPa (40 ± 2 mmHg)	
Arterial O_2 saturation	Sa_{O_2}	0.97 ± 0.02 (97 ± 2%)	
Arterial blood pH	pH	7.40 ± 0.02	
Arterial bicarbonate	HCO_3^-	24 + 2 meq/L	
Base excess	BE	0 ± 2 meq/L	
Diffusing capacity for carbon monoxide (single breath)	DL_{CO}	0.42 mL CO/s/mmHg (25 mL CO/min/mmHg)	
Dead space volume	V_D	2 mL/kg body wt	
Physiologic dead space; dead space-tidal volume ratio	V_D/V_T		
Rest		≤35% V_T	
Exercise		≤20% V_T	
Alveolar-arterial difference for O_2	$P(A - a)_{O_2}$	≤2.7 kPa ≤20 kPa (≤20 mmHg)	

TABLE 15 — BODY FLUIDS AND OTHER MASS DATA

	Reference Range	
	SI Units	Conventional Units
Ascitic fluid: See Table 44-1		
Body fluid,		
Total volume (lean) of body weight	50% (in obese) to 70%	
Intracellular	0.3–0.4 of body weight	
Extracellular	0.2–0.3 of body weight	
Blood		
Total volume		
Males	69 mL per kg body weight	
Females	65 mL per kg body weight	
Plasma volume		
Males	39 mL per kg body weight	
Females	40 mL per kg body weight	
Red blood cell volume		
Males	30 mL per kg body weight	1.15–1.21 L/m² of body surface area
Females	25 mL per kg body weight	0.95–1.00 L/m² of body surface area
Body mass index	18.5–24.9 kg/m²	18.5–24.9 kg/m²

TABLE 16 — RADIATION-DERIVED UNITS

Quantity	Old Unit	SI Unit	Name for SI Unit (and Abbreviation)	Conversion
Activity	curie (Ci)	Disintegrations per second (dps)	becquerel (Bq)	1 Ci = 3.7 × 10¹⁰ Bq 1 mCi = 37 mBq 1 μCi = 0.037 MBq or 37 GBq 1 Bq = 2.703 × 10⁻¹¹ Ci
Absorbed dose	rad	joule per kilogram (J/kg)	gray (Gy)	1 Gy = 100 rad 1 rad = 0.01 Gy 1 mrad = 10⁻³ cGy
Exposure	roentgen (R)	coulomb per kilogram (C/kg)	—	1 C/kg = 3876 R 1 R = 2.58 × 10⁻⁴ C/kg 1 mR = 258 pC/kg
Dose equivalent	rem	joule per kilogram (J/kg)	sievert (Sv)	1 Sv = 100 rem 1 rem = 0.01 Sv 1 mrem = 10 μSv

ACKNOWLEDGMENT

The authors acknowledge the contributions of Dr. Patrick M. Sluss, Dr. James L. Januzzi, and Dr. Kent B. Lewandrowski to this chapter in previous editions.

FURTHER READINGS

KRATZ A et al: Case records of the Massachusetts General Hospital. Weekly clinicopathological exercises. Laboratory reference values. N Engl J Med 351(15):1548, 2004

LEHMAN HP, HENRY JB: SI units, in *Henry's Clinical Diagnosis and Management by Laboratory Methods*, 21st ed, RC McPherson, MR Pincus (eds). Philadelphia, Elsevier Saunders, 2007, pp 1404–1418

PESCE MA: Reference ranges for laboratory tests and procedures, in *Nelson's Textbook of Pediatrics*, 18th ed, RM Klegman et al (eds). Philadelphia, Elsevier Saunders, 2007, pp 2943–2949

SOLBERG HE: Establishment and use of reference values, in *Tietz Textbook of Clinical Chemistry and Molecular Diagnostics*, 4th ed, CA Burtis et al (eds). Philadelphia, Elsevier Saunders, 2006, pp 425–448

Bold number indicates the start of the main discussion of the topic; numbers followed by "f" or "t" refer to pages of figures and tables; numbers preceded by "e" refer to the e-chapter pages on the DVD; "V" refers to the videos on the DVD; numbers preceded by "A" refer to the Appendix.

INDEX

INDEX